Williams Textbook of
ENDOCRINOLOGY

EDITION 11

Williams Textbook of ENDOCRINOLOGY

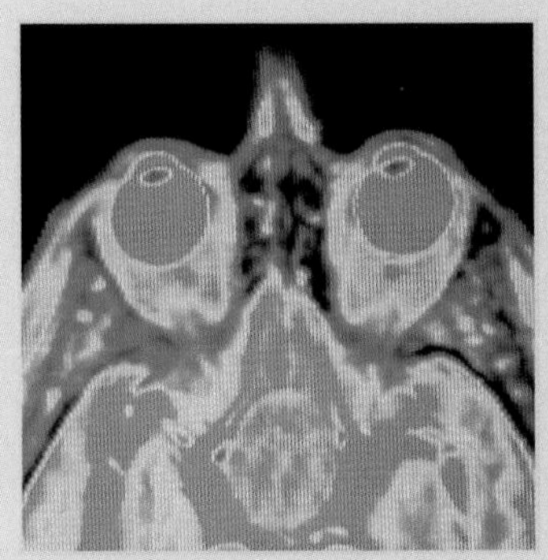
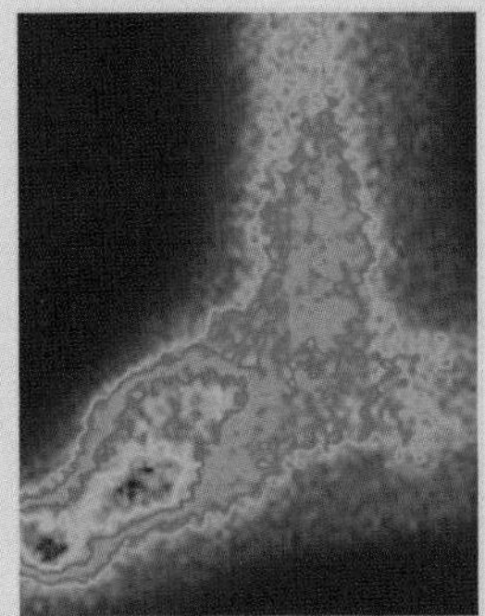
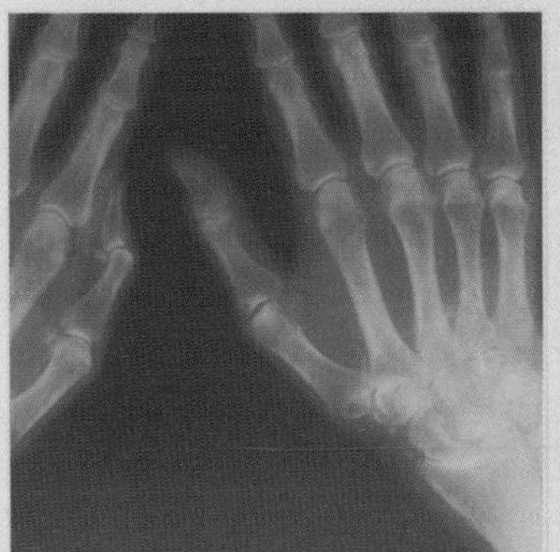
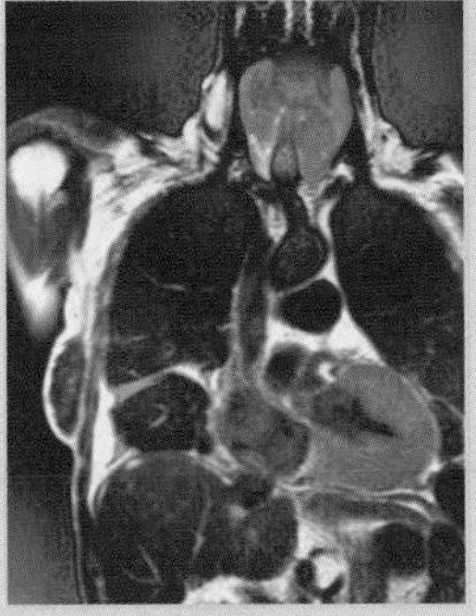

Henry M. Kronenberg, MD
Professor of Medicine
Harvard Medical School
Chief, Endocrine Unit
Massachusetts General Hospital
Boston, Massachusetts

Shlomo Melmed, MD, FRCP
Helene and Philip Hixon Chair in Investigative Medicine
Senior Vice President for Academic Affairs
Cedars Sinai Medical Center
Los Angeles, California

Kenneth S. Polonsky, MD
Adolphus Busch Professor and Chairman
Department of Medicine
Washington University School of Medicine
St. Louis, Missouri

P. Reed Larsen, MD, FACP, FRCP
Professor of Medicine
Harvard Medical School
Chief, Division of Endocrinology, Diabetes, and Hypertension
Brigham and Women's Hospital
Boston, Massachusetts

SAUNDERS

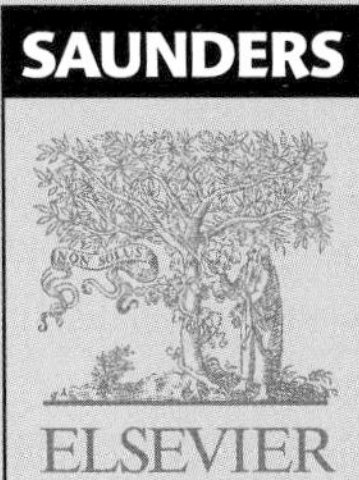

ELSEVIER

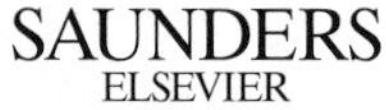

SAUNDERS
ELSEVIER

1600 John F. Kennedy Blvd.
Suite 1800
Philadelphia, PA 19103-2899

WILLIAMS TEXTBOOK OF ENDOCRINOLOGY ISBN: 9781416029113

Notice

Knowledge and best practice in this field are constantly changing. As new research and experience broaden our knowledge, changes in practice, treatment, and drug therapy may become necessary or appropriate. Readers are advised to check the most current information provided (i) on procedures featured or (ii) by the manufacturer of each product to be administered, to verify the recommended dose or formula, the method and duration of administration, and contraindications. It is the responsibility of the practitioner, relying on his or her experience and knowledge of the patient, to make diagnoses, to determine dosages and the best treatment for each individual patient, and to take all appropriate safety precautions. To the fullest extent of the law, neither the Publisher nor the Editors assume any liability for any injury and/or damage to persons or property arising out of or related to any use of the material contained in this book.

The Publisher

Library of Congress Cataloging-in-Publication Data (in PHL)

Williams textbook of endocrinology.—11th ed. / Henry M. Kronenberg . . . [et al.].
p. ; cm
Includes bibliographical references and index.
ISBN 978-1-4160-2911-3
1. Endocrinology. 2. Endocrine glands–Diseases. I. Kronenberg, Henry. II. Williams, Robert Hardin. III. Title: Textbook of endocrinology.
[DNLM: 1. Endocrine Glands. 2. Endocrine System Diseases. WK 100 W721 2008]
RC648.T46 2008
616.4—dc22 2007026873

Acquisitions Editor: Dolores Meloni
Developmental Editor: Anne Snyder
Publishing Services Manager: Frank Polizzano
Senior Project Manager: Peter Faber
Design Direction: Ellen Zanolle

Printed in Canada

Last digit is the print number: 9 8 7 6 5 4 3 2 1

CONTRIBUTORS

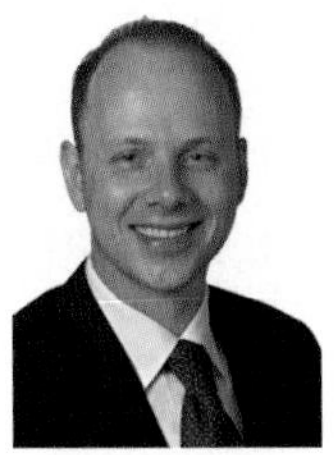

JOHN C. ACHERMANN, MD
Wellcome Trust Senior Research Fellow in Clinical Science, Developmental Endocrinology Research Group, UCL Institute of Child Health; Honorary Consultant in Paediatric Endocrinology, Great Ormond Street Hospital for Children NHS Trust, London, United Kingdom
DISORDERS OF SEX DEVELOPMENT

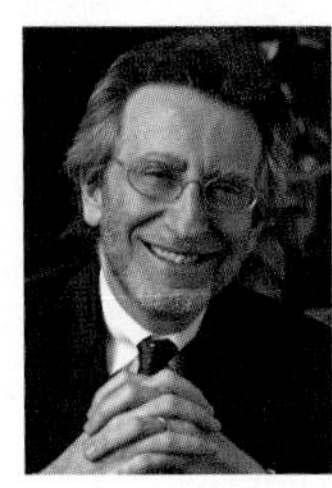

ELI Y. ADASHI, MD
Dean of Medicine and Biological Sciences, Division of Biology and Medicine, Brown University Medical School, Providence, Rhode Island
THE PHYSIOLOGY AND PATHOLOGY OF THE FEMALE REPRODUCTIVE AXIS

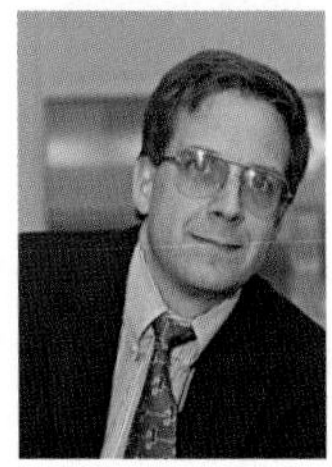

LLOYD P. AIELLO, MD, PHD
Head, Section of Eye Research, Director, Beetham Eye Institute, Joslin Diabetes Center; Associate Professor of Ophthalmology, Harvard Medical School, Boston, Massachusetts
COMPLICATIONS OF DIABETES MELLITUS

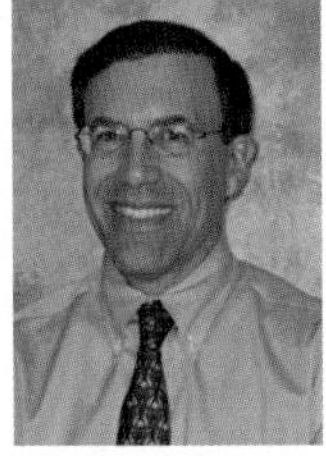

ANDREW ARNOLD, MD
Murray-Heilig Chair in Molecular Medicine and Professor of Medicine and Genetics, University of Connecticut School of Medicine; Chief, Division of Endocrinology and Metabolism, and Director, Center for Molecular Medicine, University of Connecticut Health Center, Farmington, Connecticut
PATHOGENESIS OF ENDOCRINE TUMORS

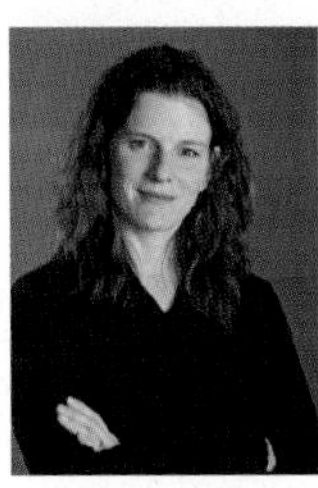

JENNIFER M. BARKER, MD
Assistant Professor of Pediatrics, University of Colorado School of Medicine; Endocrinologist, Barbara Davis Center for Childhood Diabetes, Aurora, Colorado
THE IMMUNOENDOCRINOPATHY SYNDROMES

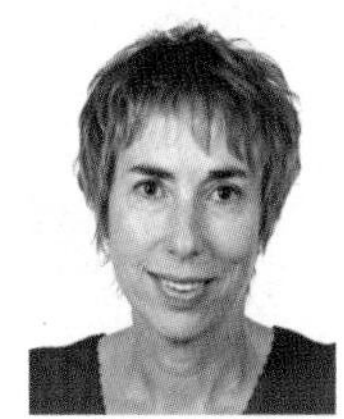

ROSEMARY BASSON, MD, FRCP(UK)
Clinical Professor, University of British Colombia Faculty of Medicine; Director, UBC Sexual Medicine Program, University of British Columbia; Director, Sexual Medicine Program, Vancouver Hospital, Vancouver, British Columbia, Canada
SEXUAL DYSFUNCTION IN MEN AND WOMEN

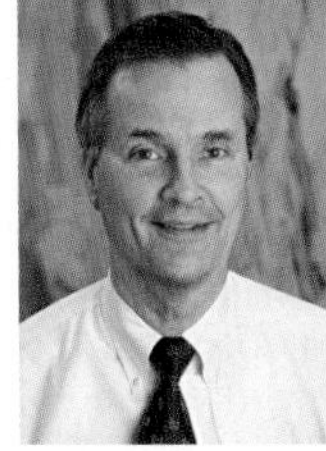

THOMAS P. BERSOT, MD, PHD
Associate Investigator, Gladstone Institute of Cardiovascular Disease, Professor of Medicine, University of California, San Francisco
DISORDERS OF LIPID METABOLISIM

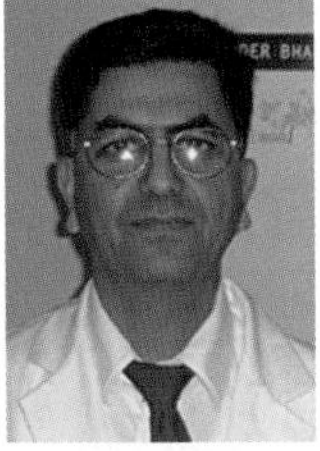

SHALENDER BHASIN, MD
Professor of Medicine, Section of Endocrinology, Diabetes, and Nutrition, Boston University School of Medicine; Chief, Section of Endocrinology, Diabetes, and Nutrition, Boston Medical Center, Boston, Massachusetts
TESTICULAR DISORDERS
SEXUAL DYSFUNCTION IN MEN AND WOMEN

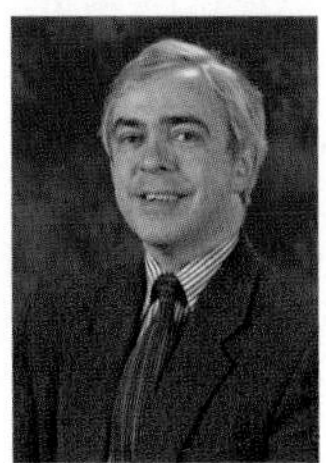

ANDREW J. M. BOULTON, MD, FRCP
Professor of Medicine, University of Manchester, Consultant Physician, Manchester Royal Infirmary, Manchester, United Kingdom; Division of Endocrinology, Metabolism, and Diabetes, University of Miami School of Medicine, Miami, Florida
COMPLICATIONS OF DIABETES MELLITUS

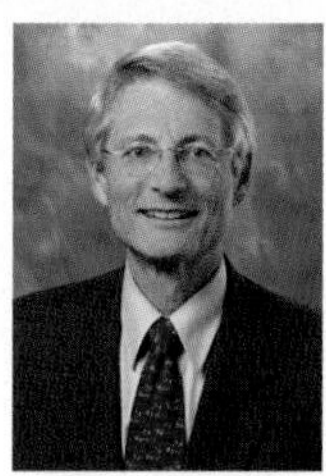

GLENN D. BRAUNSTEIN, MD
Professor of Medicine, David Geffen School of Medicine at UCLA; Chairman, Department of Medicine, and James R. Klinenberg Chair in Medicine, Cedars-Sinai Medical Center, Los Angeles, California
ENDOCRINE CHANGES IN PREGNANCY

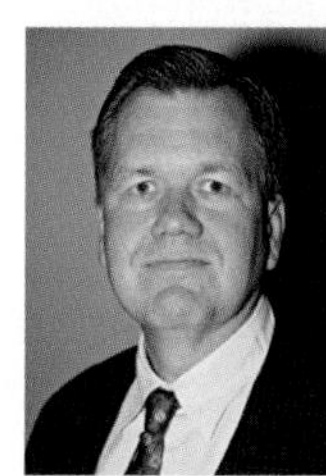

GREGORY A. BRENT, MD
Professor of Medicine and Physiology, David Geffen School of Medicine at UCLA; Chief, Endocrinology and Diabetes Division, VA Greater Los Angeles Healthcare System, Los Angeles, California
HYPOTHYROIDISM AND THYROIDITIS

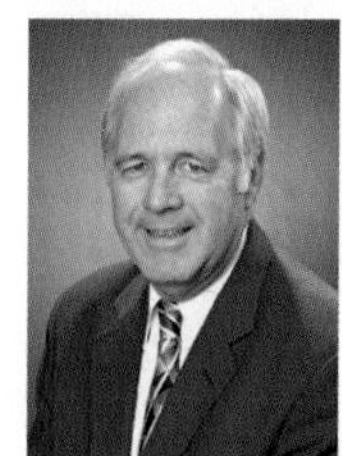

F. RICHARD BRINGHURST, MD
Associate Professor of Medicine Harvard Medical School, Physician, Endocrine Division, Massachusetts General Hospital, Boston, Massachusetts
HORMONES AND DISORDERS OF MINERAL METABOLISM

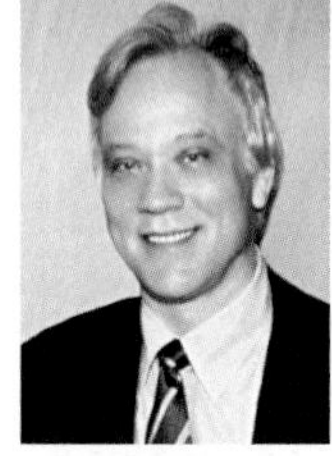

MICHAEL BROWNLEE, MD
Anita and Jack Saltz Professor of Diabetes Research, Director, JDRF International Center for Diabetic Complications Research, Department of Medicine and Pathology, Albert Einstein College of Medicine, Bronx, New York
COMPLICATIONS OF DIABETES MELLITUS

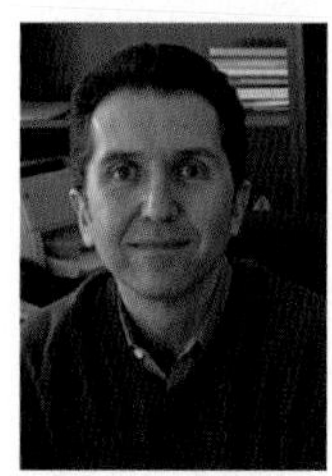

SERDAR E. BULUN, MD
George H. Gardner Professor of Clinical Gynecology and Chief, Division of Reproductive Biology Research, Department of Obstetrics and Gynecology, Northwestern University Feinberg School of Medicine, Chicago, Illinois
THE PHYSIOLOGY AND PATHOLOGY OF THE FEMALE REPRODUCTIVE AXIS

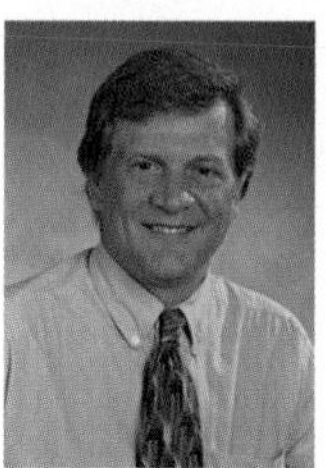

CHARLES F. BURANT, MD, PHD
Professor of Internal Medicine University of Michigan Health System Ann Arbor, Michigan
TYPE 2 DIABETES MELLITUS

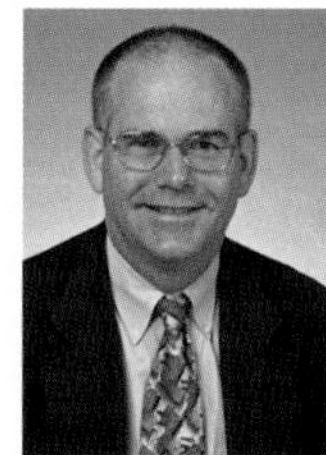

JOHN B. BUSE, MD, PHD
Professor of Medicine, University of North Carolina at Chapel Hill School of Medicine, Chapel Hill, North Carolina
TYPE 2 DIABETES MELLITUS
TYPE 1 DIABETES MELLITUS

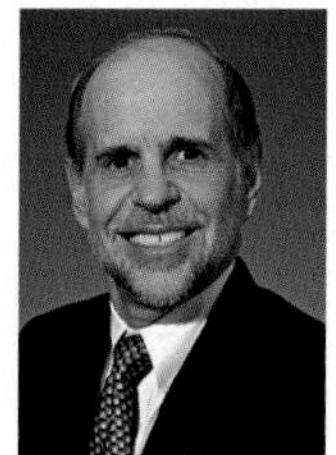

DAVID A. BUSHINSKY, MD
Professor of Medicine, Pharmacology and Physiology, University of Rochester School of Medicine and Dentistry; Chief, Division of Nephrology, University of Rochester Medical Center, Rochester, New York
KIDNEY STONES

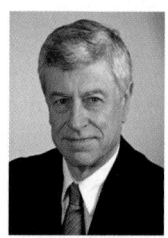

ERNESTO CANALIS, MD
Professor of Medicine, University of Connecticut School of Medicine, Farmington; Director of Research, St. Francis Hospital Medical Center, Hartford, Connecticut
METABOLIC BONE DISEASE

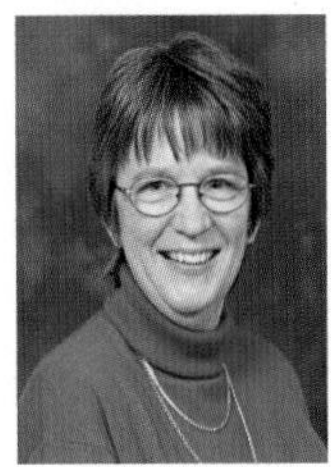

CHRISTIN CARTER-SU, PhD
Professor of Molecular and Integrative Physiology, Associate Director and Head of the Michigan Diabetes Research and Training Center, University of Michigan Medical School, Ann Arbor, Michigan
MECHANISM OF ACTION OF HORMONES THAT ACT AT THE CELL SURFACE

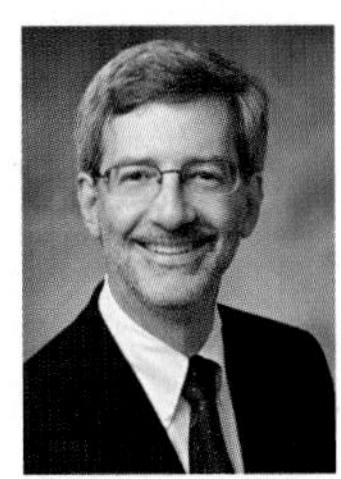

ROGER D. CONE, PhD
Director, Center for the Study of Weight Regulation and Associated Disorders, Oregon Health and Science University, Portland;
Senior Scientist, Vollum Institute, Oregon Health and Science University, Portland, Oregon
NEUROENDOCRINE CONTROL OF ENERGY STORES

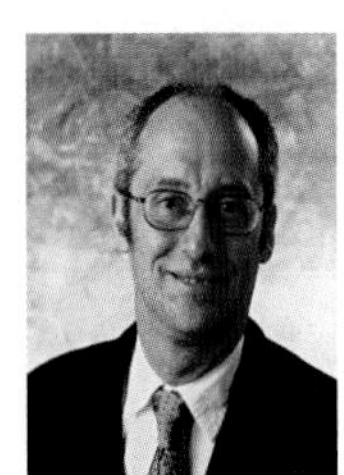

MARK E. COOPER, MBBS, PhD, FRACP
Professor of Medicine and Immunology, Eastern Clinical School, Monash University; Professor of Medicine and Physiology, University of Melbourne, Senior Endocrinologist, Alfred Hospital, Melbourne; Head, JDRF Danielle Alberti Memorial Centre for Diabetic Complications, Diabetes and Metabolism Division, Baker Heart Research Institute, Melbourne, Victoria, Australia
COMPLICATIONS OF DIABETES MELLITUS

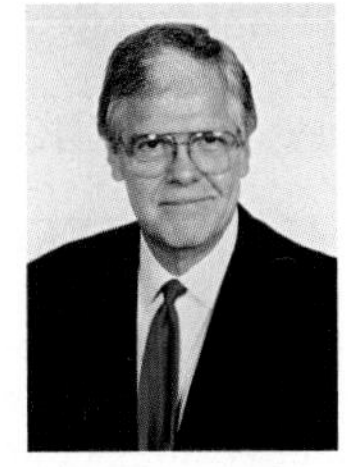

PHILIP E. CRYER, MD
Irene E. and Michael M. Karl Professor of Endocrinology and Metabolism in Medicine, Washington University in St. Louis School of Medicine; Physician, Barnes-Jewish Hospital, St. Louis, Missouri
GLUCOSE HOMEOSTASIS AND HYPOGLYCEMIA

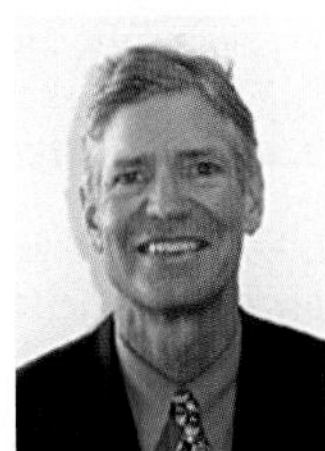

PHILIP D. DARNEY, MD, MSc
Professor of Obstetrics, Gynecology, and Reproductive Sciences, University of California, San Francisco, School of Medicine; Chief, Obstetrics and Gynecology, San Francisco General Hospital, San Francisco, California
HORMONAL CONTRACEPTION

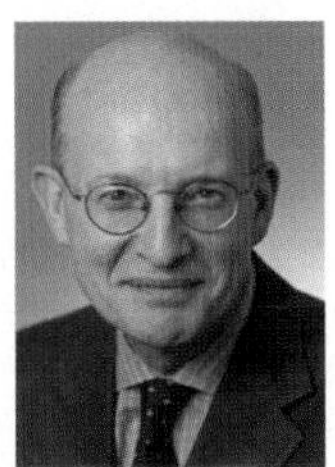

TERRY F. DAVIES, MBBS, MD, FRCP, FACE
Florence and Theodore Baumritter Professor of Medicine, Mount Sinai School of Medicine; Attending Physician, Mount Sinai Hospital; Director, Division of Endocrinology and Metabolism, James J. Peters VA Medical Center, New York, New York
THYROID PHYSIOLOGY AND DIAGNOSTIC EVALUATION OF PATIENTS WITH THYROID DISORDERS
THYROTOXICOSIS
HYPOTHYROIDISM AND THYROIDITIS

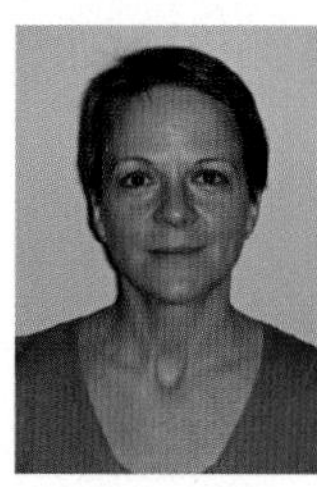

MARIE B. DEMAY, MD
Associate Professor of Medicine, Harvard Medical School, Massachusetts General Hospital; Boston, Massachusetts
HORMONES AND DISORDERS OF MINERAL METABOLISM

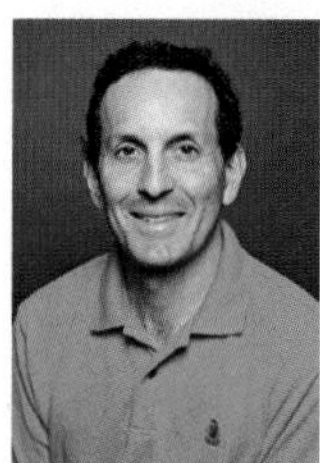

DANIEL J. DRUCKER, MD
Director, Banting and Best Diabetes Centre, University of Toronto, Toronto General Hospital, Toronto, Ontario, Canada
GASTROINTESTINAL HORMONES AND GUT ENDOCRINE TUMORS

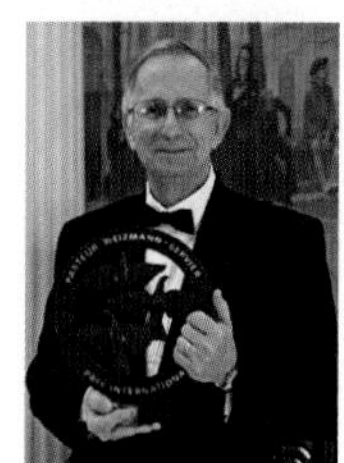

GEORGE S. EISENBARTH, MD, PHD
Professor, Departments of Pediatrics, Medicine, and Immunology, University of Colorado School of Medicine, Denver; Executive Director, Barbara Davis Center for Childhood Diabetes, Aurora; Physician, University Hospital and The Children's Hospital, Denver, Colorado
TYPE 1 DIABETES MELLITUS
THE IMMUNOENDOCRINOPATHY SYNDROMES

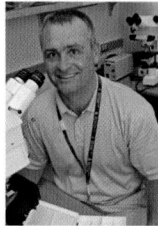

JOEL K. ELMQUIST, DVM, PHD
Maclin Family Professor in Medical Science, in Honor of Dr. Roy A. Brinkley, Departments of Medicine and Pharmacology; Director, Division of Hypothalamic Research, University of Texas Southwestern Medical Center, Dallas, Texas
NEUROENDOCRINE CONTROL OF ENERGY STORES

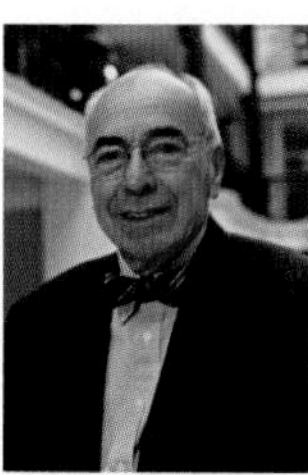

DANIEL D. FEDERMAN, MD
Carl W. Walter Distinguished Professor of Medicine, Harvard Medical School, Boston, Massachusetts
THE ENDOCRINE PATIENT

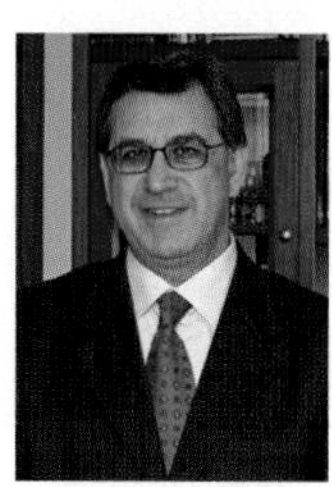

SEBASTIANO FILETTI, MD
Professor of Internal Medicine, Department of Clinical Sciences, University of Rome La Sapienza School of Medicine; Head, Department of Internal Medicine, Policlinico Umberto I, Rome, Italy
NONTOXIC DIFFUSE AND NODULAR GOITER AND THYROID NEOPLASIA

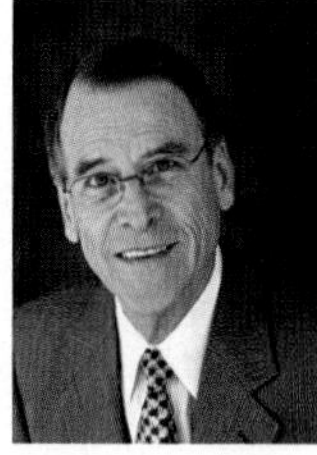

DELBERT A. FISHER, MD
Professor of Pediatrics and Medicine Emeritus, David Geffen School of Medicine at UCLA, Los Angeles; Chairman Emeritus, Department of Pediatrics, and Serous Scientist, Walter Martin Research Center, Harbor-UCLA Medical Center, Torrance, California
ENDOCRINOLOGY OF FETAL DEVELOPMENT

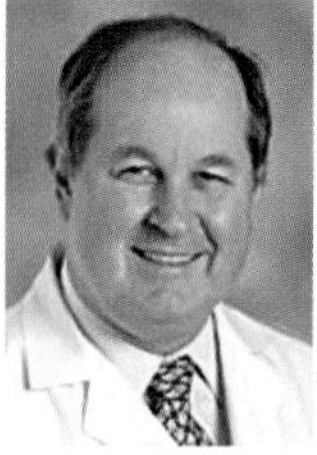

ROBERT F. GAGEL, MD
Professor and Head, Division of Internal Medicine, The University of Texas MD Anderson Cancer Center; Professor of Cell Biology, Baylor College of Medicine, Houston, Texas
MULTIPLE ENDOCRINE NEOPLASIA

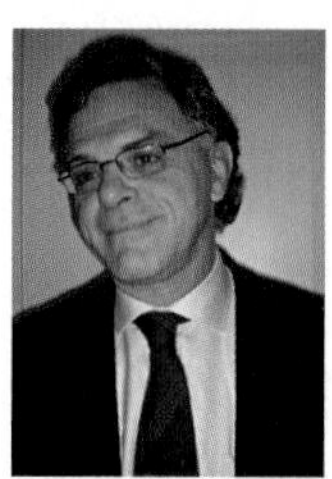

EZIO GHIGO, MD
Professor of Endocrinology, Department of Internal Medicine, University of Turin Faculty of Medicine; Chief, Division of Endocrinology and Metabolism, University Hospital, Turin, Italy
HORMONES AND ATHLETIC PERFORMANCE

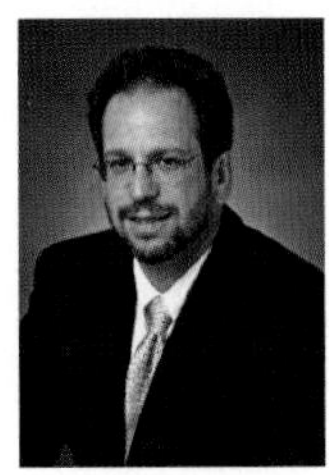

PETER A. GOTTLIEB, MD
Associate Professor of Pediatrics and Medicine, University of Colorado School of Medicine, Aurora; Physician, University of Colorado Hospital and the Children's Hospital, Denver, Colorado
The Immunoendocrinopathy Syndromes

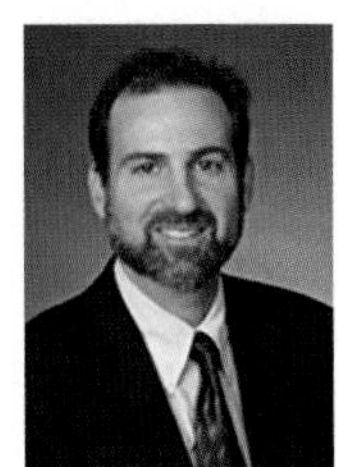

STEVEN K. GRINSPOON, MD
Associate Professor of Medicine, Harvard Medical School; Director, MGH Program in Nutritional Metabolism, and Clinical Director, Neuroendocrine Clinical Center, Massachusetts General Hospital, Boston, Massachusetts
Endocrinology of HIV/AIDS

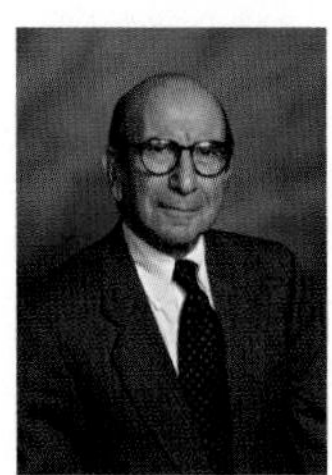

MELVIN M. GRUMBACH, MD
Edward B. Shaw Emeritus Professor of Pediatrics and Emeritus Chairman, Department of Pediatrics, University of California, San Francisco, California
Puberty: Ontogeny, Neuroendocrinology, Physiology, and Disorders

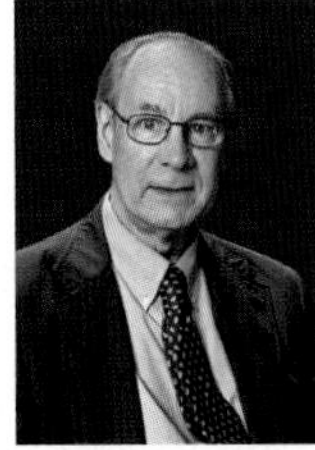

JOEL F. HABENER, MD
Professor of Medicine, Harvard Medical School; Associate Physician, Massachusetts General Hospital, Boston, Massachusetts
Genetic Control of Peptide Hormone Formation

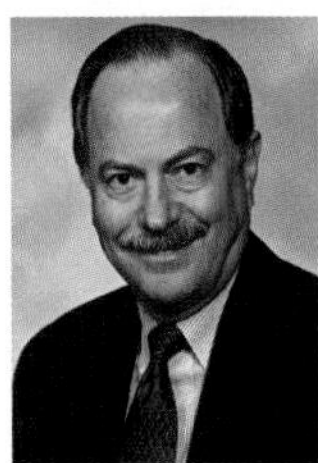

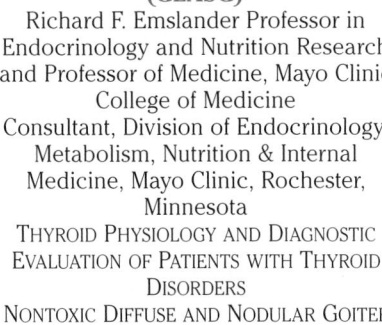

IAN D. HAY, BSc, MBChB, PhD, MRCP(UK), FACE, FACP, FRCP (EDIN & LOND), FRCPI (HON), FRCPS (GLASG)
Richard F. Emslander Professor in Endocrinology and Nutrition Research and Professor of Medicine, Mayo Clinic College of Medicine
Consultant, Division of Endocrinology, Metabolism, Nutrition & Internal Medicine, Mayo Clinic, Rochester, Minnesota
Thyroid Physiology and Diagnostic Evaluation of Patients with Thyroid Disorders
Nontoxic Diffuse and Nodular Goiter and Thyroid Neoplasia

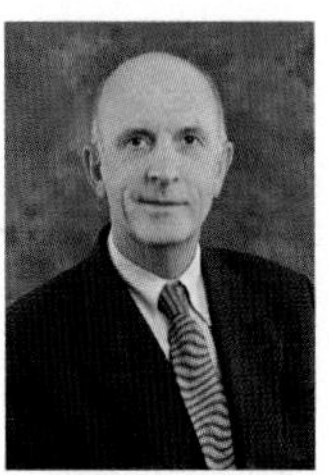

IEUAN A. HUGHES, MD, FRCP, FRCPCh, FMedSci
Professor of Paediatrics and Head, Department of Paediatrics, University of Cambridge; Addenbrooke's Hospital, Cambridge, United Kingdom
Disorders of Sex Development

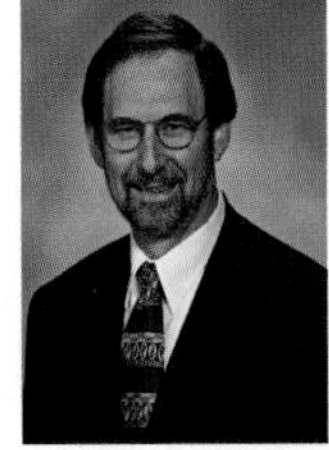

GEORGE G. KLEE, MD, PhD
Professor of Laboratory Medicine, Mayo Medical School; Consultant, Mayo Clinic, Rochester, Minnesota
Laboratory Techniques for Recognition of Endocrine Disorders

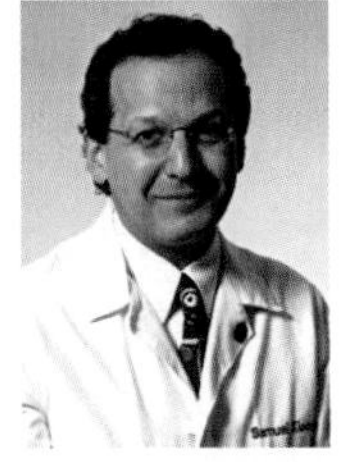

SAMUEL KLEIN, MD
William H. Danforth Professor of Medicine and Nutritional Science, Washington University in St. Louis, School of Medicine; Attending Physician, Barnes-Jewish Hospital, St. Louis, Missouri
Obesity

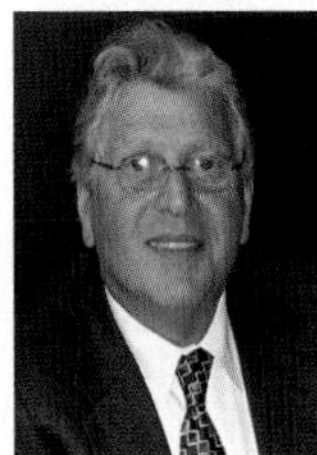

DAVID KLEINBERG, MD
Professor of Medicine, Director, Neuroendocrine Unit, New York University School of Medicine; Chief of Endocrinology, Veterans Administration Medical Center, New York, New York
Anterior Pituitary

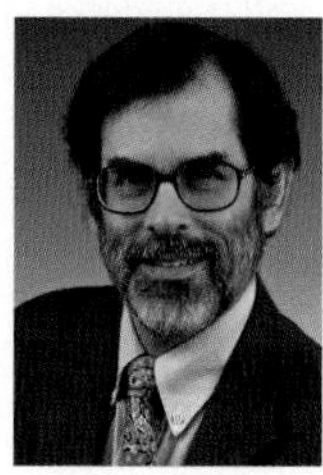

HENRY M. KRONENBERG, MD
Professor of Medicine, Harvard Medical School; Chief, Endocrine Unit, Massachusetts General Hospital, Boston, Massachusetts
PRINCIPLES OF ENDOCRINOLOGY
HORMONES AND DISORDERS OF MINERAL METABOLISM

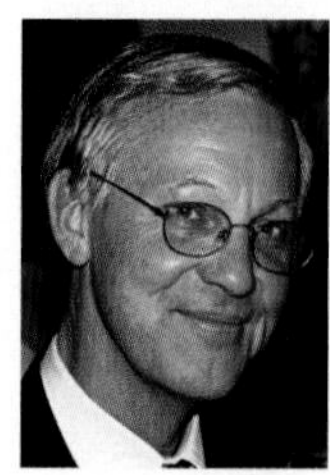

STEVEN W.J. LAMBERTS, MD, PhD
Professor of Medicine, Erasmus University Faculty of Medicine; Endocrinologist, Erasmus Medical Center, Rotterdam, The Netherlands
ENDOCRINOLOGY AND AGING

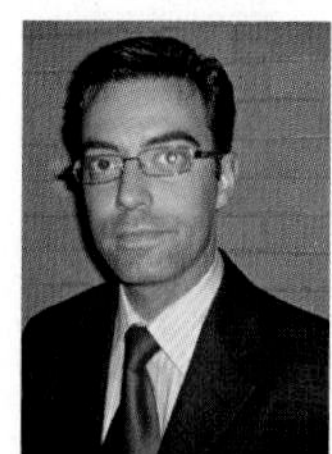

FABIO LANFRANCO, MD
Assistant Professor of Endocrinology, Department of Internal Medicine, University of Turin Faculty of Medicine; Clinical Practice in Endocrinology, University Hospital, Turin, Italy
HORMONES AND ATHLETIC PERFORMANCE

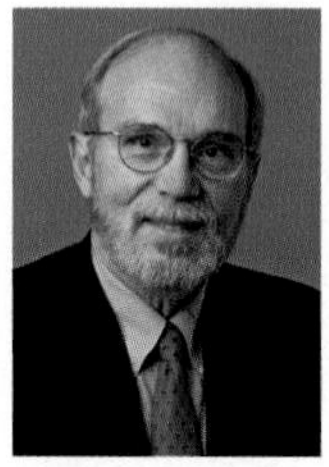

P. REED LARSEN, MD, FACP, FRCP
Professor of Medicine, Harvard Medical School; Chief, Division of Endocrinology, Diabetes, and Hypertension, Brigham and Women's Hospital, Boston, Massachusetts
PRINCIPLES OF ENDOCRINOLOGY
THYROID PHYSIOLOGY AND DIAGNOSTIC EVALUATION OF PATIENTS WITH THYROID DISORDERS
THYROTOXICOSIS
HYPOTHYROIDISM AND THYROIDITIS

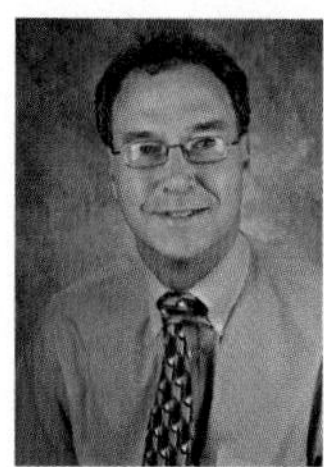

MITCHELL A. LAZAR, MD, PhD
Sylvan H. Eisman Professor of Medicine and Professor of Genetics; Chief, Division of Endocrinology, Diabetes, and Metabolism; and Director, Institute for Diabetes, Obesity, and Metabolism, University of Pennsylvania School of Medicine, Philadelphia, Pennsylvania
MECHANISM OF ACTION OF HORMONES THAT ACT ON NUCLEAR RECEPTORS

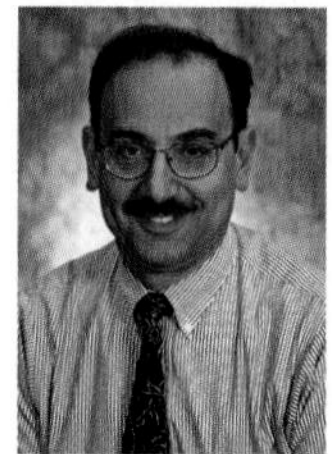

JOSEPH A. LORENZO, MD
Professor of Medicine, University of Connecticut School of Medicine; Director, Bone Biology Research, University of Connecticut Health Center; Attending Physician, John Dempsey Hospital, Farmington, Connecticut
METABOLIC BONE DISEASE

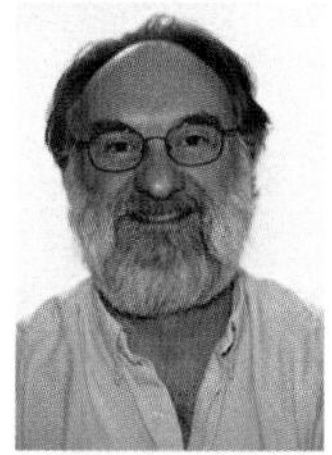

MALCOLM J. LOW, MD, PhD
Senior Scientist and Associate Director, Center for the Study of Weight Regulation; Professor of Behavioral Neuroscience, School of Medicine; Affiliate Scientist, Vollum Institute, Oregon Health & Science University, Portland, Oregon
NEUROENDOCRINOLOGY

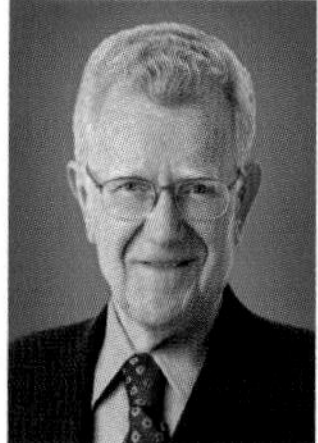

ROBERT W. MAHLEY, MD, PhD
President, The J. David Gladstone Institutes, Senior Investigator, Gladstone Institute of Cardiovascular Disease; Professor of Pathology and Medicine, University of California, San Francisco, California
DISORDERS OF LIPID METABOLISM

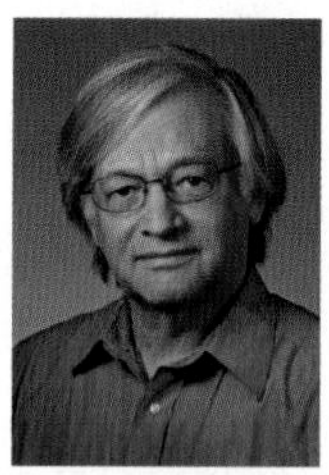

STEPHEN J. MARX, MD
Chief, Metabolic Diseases Branch, Genetics and Endocrinology Section, National Institute of Diabetes and Digestive and Kidney Diseases, National Institutes of Health, Bethesda, Maryland
MULTIPLE ENDOCRINE NEOPLASIA

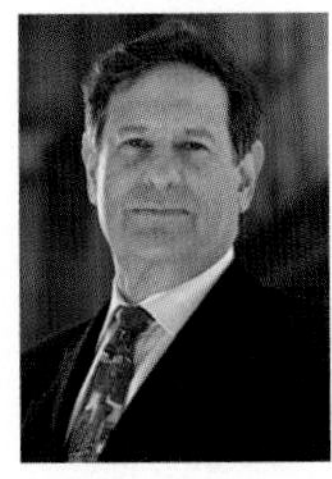

SHLOMO MELMED, MD, FRCP
Helene and Philip Hixon Chair in Investigative Medicine,
Senior Vice President for Academic Affairs, Cedars Sinai Medical Center, Los Angeles, California
PRINCIPLES OF ENDOCRINOLOGY
ANTERIOR PITUITARY

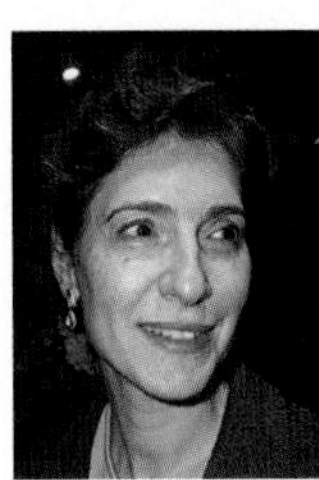

REBECA D. MONK, MD
Associate Professor of Medicine, University of Rochester School of Medicine and Dentistry, Rochester, New York
KIDNEY STONES

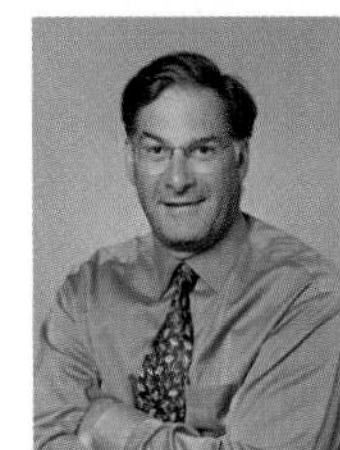

RICHARD W. NESTO, MD
Associate Professor of Medicine, Harvard Medical School, Boston; Chair, Department of Cardiovascular Medicine, Lahey Clinic Medical Center, Burlington, Massachusetts
COMPLICATIONS OF DIABETES MELLITUS

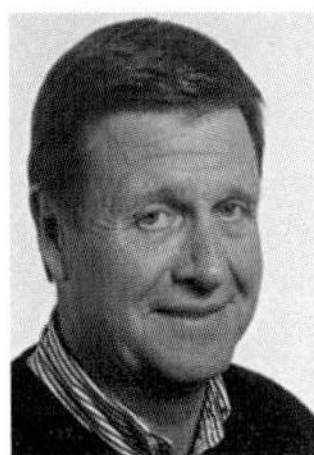

KJELL E. ÖBERG, MD, PHD
Professor, Department of Medical Sciences, and Dean, Medical Faculty, Uppsala University; Attending, Department of Endocrine Oncology, University Hospital, Uppsala, Sweden
CARCINOID TUMORS, CARCINOID SYNDROME, AND RELATED DISORDERS

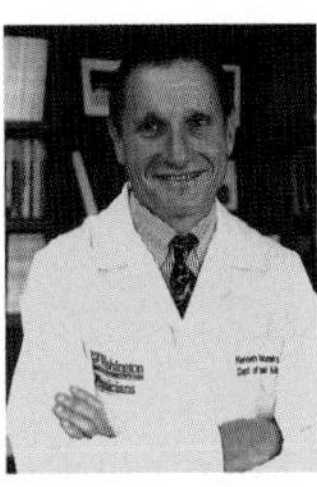

KENNETH S. POLONSKY, MD
Adolphus Busch Professor and Chairman, Department of Medicine, Washington University in St. Louis, School of Medicine, St. Louis, Missouri
PRINCIPLES OF ENDOCRINOLOGY
TYPE 2 DIABETES MELLITUS
TYPE 1 DIABETES MELLITUS

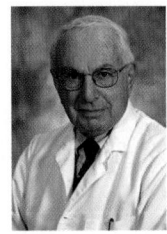

LAWRENCE G. RAISZ, MD
Board of Trustees Distinguished Professor of Medicine, University of Connecticut School of Medicine; Physician, John Dempsey Hospital, Farmington, Connecticut
METABOLIC BONE DISEASE

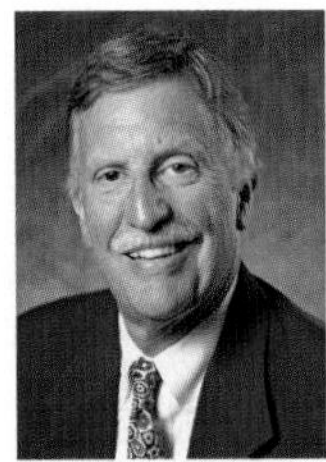

EDWARD O. REITER, MD
Professor of Pediatrics, Tufts University School of Medicine, Boston; Chair, Department of Pediatrics, Baystate Children's Hospital, Springfield, Massachusetts
NORMAL AND ABERRANT GROWTH

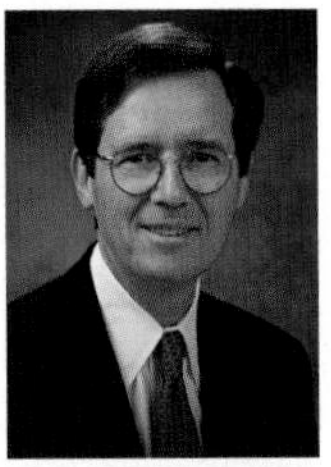

ALAN G. ROBINSON, MD
Professor of Medicine and Executive Associate Dean, David Geffen School of Medicine at UCLA; Associate Vice Chancellor, Medical Sciences, University of California at Los Angeles, Los Angeles, California
POSTERIOR PITUITARY

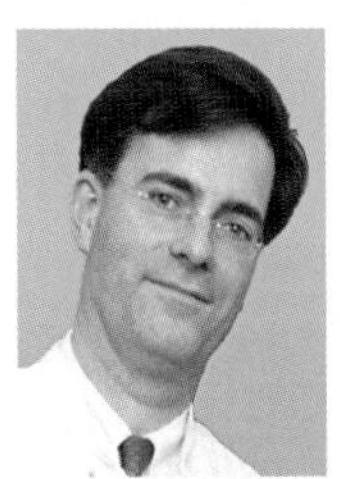

JOHANNES A. ROMIJN, MD, PHD
Professor, Department of Endocrinology, Leiden University Medical School; Physician, Department of Endocrinology, Leiden University Medical Center, Leiden, The Netherlands
OBESITY

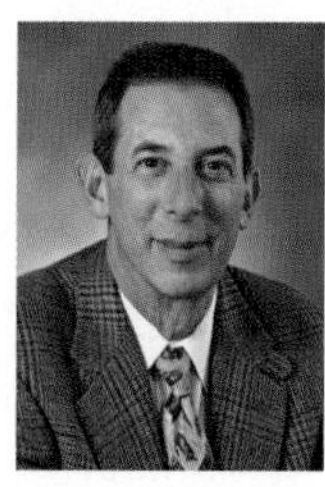

RON G. ROSENFELD, MD
Professor of Pediatrics, Oregon Health & Science University School of Medicine, Portland, Oregon, and Stanford University School of Medicine, Stanford, California; Senior Vice-President for Medical Affairs, Lucile Packard Foundation for Children's Health, Palo Alto, California
NORMAL AND ABERRANT GROWTH

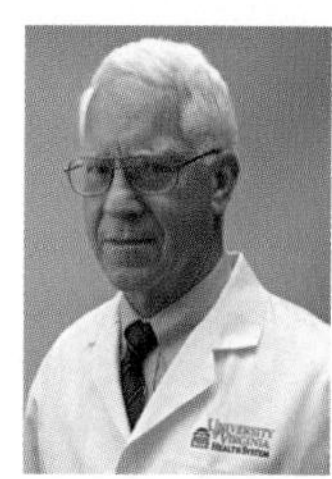

RICHARD SANTEN, MD
Professor of Medicine, University of Virginia School of Medicine; Associate Director, Clinical Research, Division of Endocrinology and Metabolism, University of Virginia Health System, Charlottesville, Virginia
ENDOCRINE-RESPONSIVE CANCER

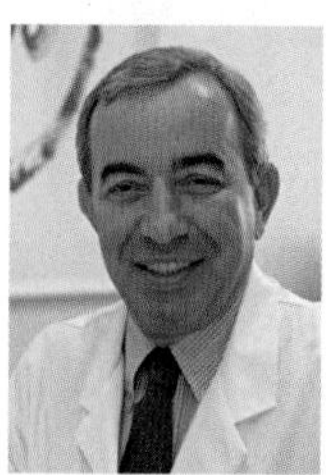

MARTIN-JEAN SCHLUMBERGER, MD
Professor of Oncology, University of Paris, Paris SWD; Chairman, Department of Nuclear Medicine and Endocrine Oncology, Institute Gustave Roussy, Villejuif, France
THYROID PHYSIOLOGY AND DIAGNOSTIC EVALUATION OF PATIENTS WITH THYROID DISORDERS
NONTOXIC DIFFUSE AND NODULAR GOITER AND THYROID NEOPLASIA

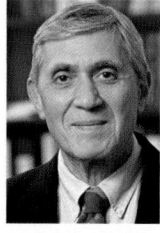

ALLEN SPIEGEL, MD
Marilyn and Stanley M. Katz Dean, Albert Einstein College of Medicine, Bronx, New York
MECHANISM OF ACTION OF HORMONES THAT ACT AT THE CELL SURFACE

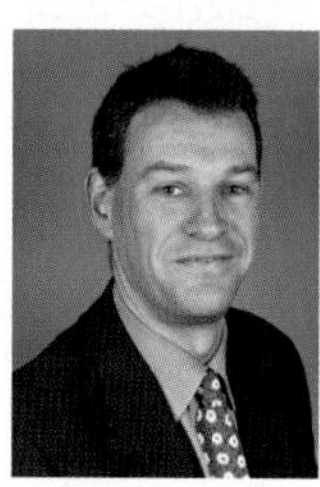

PAUL M. STEWART, MD, FRCP, FMEDSCI
Professor of Medicine, The University of Birmingham Institute of Biomedical Research; Honorary Consultant Physician, Department of Medicine, University Hospital Birmingham Foundation, NHS Trust, Birmingham, United Kingdom
THE ADRENAL CORTEX

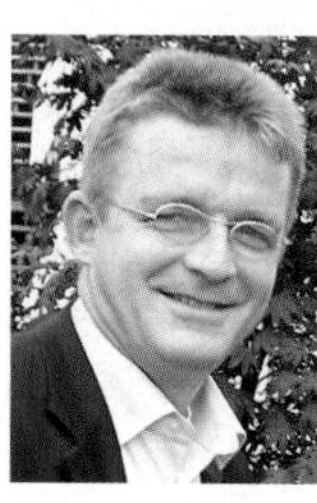

CHRISTIAN J. STRASBURGER, MD
Professor of Clinical Endocrinology and Division Chief, Department of Medicine, Charité Universitätsmedizin Berlin, Berlin, Germany
HORMONES AND ATHLETIC PERFORMANCE

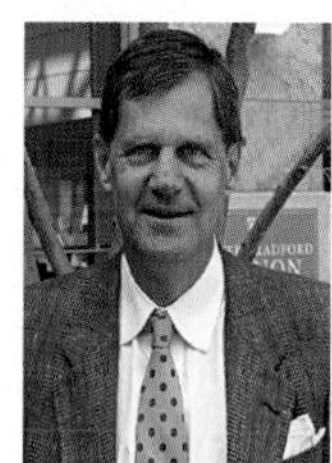

GORDON J. STREWLER, MD
Vice-Chairman, Department of Medicine, Beth Israel Deaconess Medical Center; Professor of Medicine; Master, Walter Bradford Cannon Society, Harvard Medical School, Boston, Massachusetts
HUMORAL MANIFESTATIONS OF MALIGNANCY

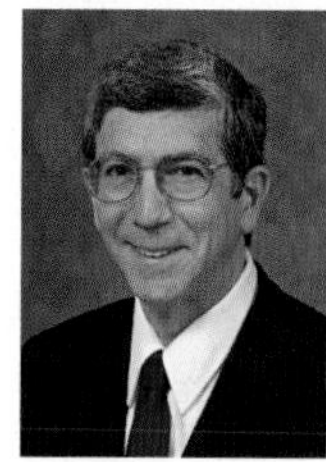

DENNIS M. STYNE, MD
Rumsey Chair of Pediatric Endocrinology, Professor of Pediatrics, University of California, Davis School of Medicine, Sacramento, California
PUBERTY: ONTOGENY, NEUROENDOCRINOLOGY, PHYSIOLOGY, AND DISORDERS

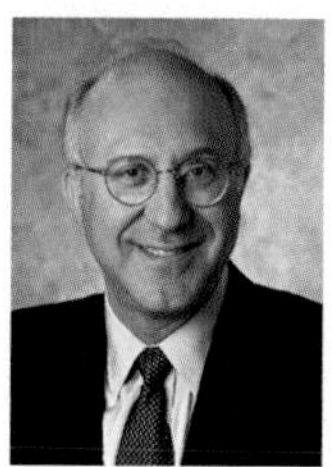

SIMEON I. TAYLOR, MD, PHD
Vice President, Discovery Biology, Pharmaceutical Research Institute, Bristol-Myers Squibb, Hopewell, New Jersey
MECHANISM OF ACTION OF HORMONES THAT ACT AT THE CELL SURFACE

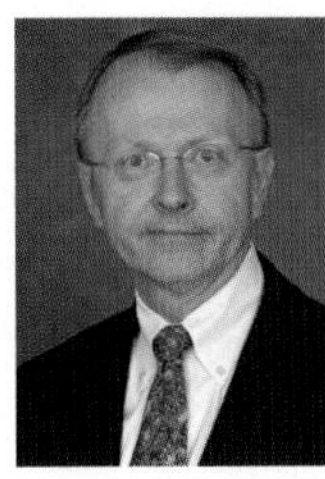

JOSEPH G. VERBALIS, MD
Professor of Medicine and Physiology and Interim Chair, Department of Medicine, Georgetown University School of Medicine; Physician-in-Chief of Medicine, Georgetown University Hospital, Washington, DC
POSTERIOR PITUITARY

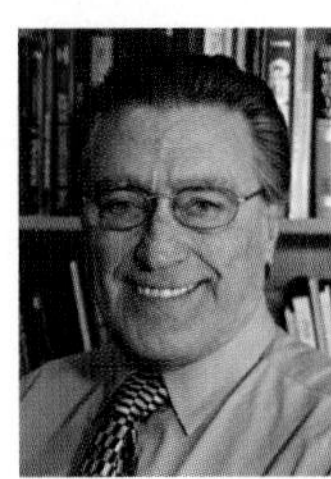

AARON I. VINIK, MD, PHD
Professor, Internal Medicine, Pathology, Neurobiology, Eastern Virginia Medical School; Director, Strelitz Diabetes Research Institutes, Norfolk, Virginia
COMPLICATIONS OF DIABETES MELLITUS

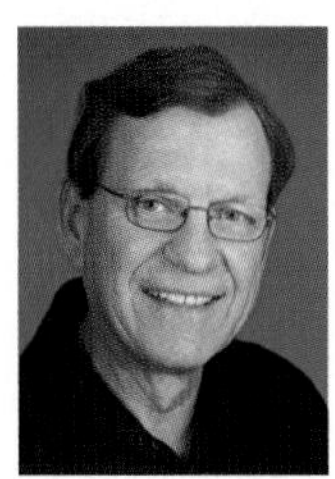

KARL H. WEISGRABER, PHD
Professor of Pathology, University of California, San Francisco, School of Medicine; Senior Investigator, Gladstone Institute of Neurological Disease, San Francisco, California
DISORDERS OF LIPID METABOLISM

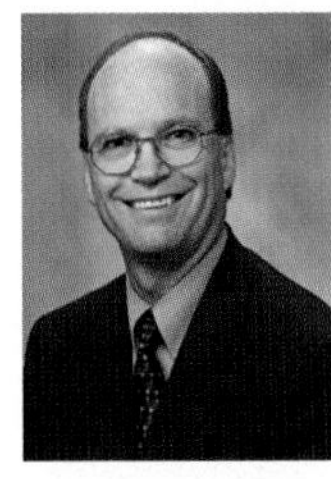

WILLIAM F. YOUNG, JR., MD, MSC
Professor of Medicine, Mayo Clinic College of Medicine; Consultant, Division of Endocrinology, Diabetes, Metabolism, and Nutrition, Mayo Clinic, Rochester, Minnesota
ENDOCRINE HYPERTENSION

PREFACE

Welcome to the eleventh edition of *Willams Textbook of Endocrinology*. Although Robert Williams inaugurated this book more than 50 years ago, the goals of the text have not changed. Williams stated his goal as "a condensed and authoritative discussion of the management of clinical endocrinopathies based upon the application of fundamental information obtained from chemical and physiological investigation." Of course, today we would add "genetic and epidemiologic investigation, as well as the wealth of clinical trial data" as sources of information that aids clinical management. The immense and ongoing new information from multiple disciplines, in fact, makes a synthetic exercise like this textbook more relevant than ever to help guide endocrinologists in the care of their patients. To encourage the goal of synthesis, we continue to ask a small number of distinguished authors to work together to present entire areas of endocrine science. The mandate for concise presentations acknowledges both the time pressures on today's physicians and the desire to make the text affordable and easily navigated.

This edition displays many important innovations. Three entirely new chapters focus on "Hormones and Athletic Performance," "Neuroendocrine Control of Appetite and Body Weight," and the "Endocrinology of HIV/AIDS." The latter two chapters join the revised chapters on "Obesity," "Disorders of Lipid Metabolism," and "Gastrointestinal Hormones and Gut Endocrine Tumors" to form a new Section entitled "Body Fat and Lipid Metabolism." All chapters have been extensively revised, and 12 new authors have joined the book's faculty.

For the first time, full color figures are placed throughout the text to enable effective communication. A uniform style has been used to facilitate identification and use of clinical algorithms.

We express our deep gratitude to the co-workers in our offices, Irma Sabbag, Lynn Moulton, Grace Labrado, Louise Ishibashi, and Sherri Turner, whose great and continuing efforts have made this work possible. We also thank our colleagues at Elsevier, Dolores Meloni and Anne Snyder, who navigated the ever-changing world of medical publishing without deviating from our goals, while keeping us on deadline. Their efforts have been essential in ensuring the successful publication of this high quality textbook.

Henry M. Kronenberg

Shlomo Melmed

Kenneth S. Polonsky

P. Reed Larsen

CONTENTS

SECTION I

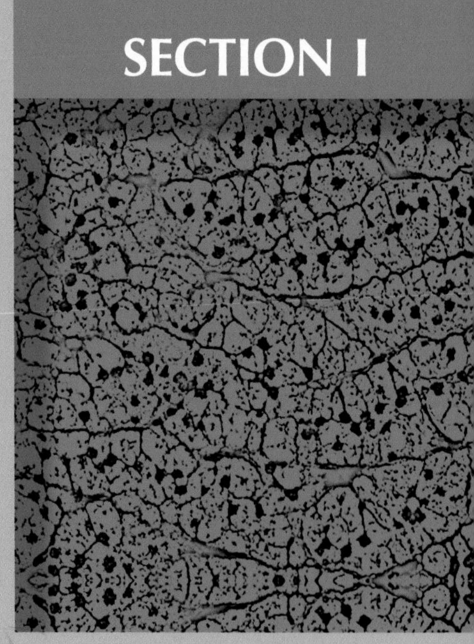

Hormones and Hormone Action

CHAPTER 1

PRINCIPLES OF ENDOCRINOLOGY

Henry M. Kronenberg, Shlomo Melmed, P. Reed Larsen, and Kenneth S. Polonsky

Introduction

Roughly a hundred years ago, Starling coined the term "hormone" to describe secretin, a substance secreted by the small intestine into the bloodstream to stimulate pancreatic secretion. In his Croonian Lectures, Starling considered the endocrine and nervous systems as two distinct mechanisms for coordination and control of organ function. Thus, endocrinology found its first home in the discipline of mammalian physiology.

Work over the next several decades by biochemists, physiologists, and clinical investigators led to the characterization of many hormones secreted into the bloodstream from discrete glands or other organs. These investigators showed that diseases such as hypothyroidism and diabetes could be treated successfully for the first time by replacing specific hormones. These initial triumphs formed the foundation of the clinical specialty of endocrinology.

Advances in cell biology, molecular biology, and genetics over the ensuing years began to explain the mechanisms of endocrine diseases and of hormone secretion and action. Even though these advances have embedded endocrinology in the framework of molecular cell biology, they have not changed the essential subject of endocrinology—the signaling that coordinates and controls the functions of multiple organs and processes. Herein we survey the general themes and principles that underpin the diverse approaches used by clinicians, physiologists, biochemists, cell biologists, and geneticists to understand the endocrine system.

The Evolutionary Perspective

Hormones can be defined as chemical signals secreted into the bloodstream that act on distant tissues, usually in a regulatory fashion. Hormonal signaling represents a special case of the more general process of signaling between cells. Even unicellular organisms, such as baker's yeast, *Saccharomyces cerevisiae*, secrete short peptide mating factors that act on receptors of other yeast cells to trigger mating between the two cells. These receptors resemble the ubiquitous family of mammalian 7-transmembrane spanning receptors that respond to ligands as diverse as photons and glycoprotein hormones. Because these yeast receptors trigger activation of heterotrimeric G proteins just as mammalian receptors do, this conserved signaling pathway must have been present in the common ancestor of yeast and humans.

Signals from one cell to adjacent cells, so-called paracrine signals, often trigger cellular responses that use the same molecular pathways used by hormonal signals. For example, the sevenless receptor controls the differentiation of retinal cells in the Drosophila eye by responding to a membrane-anchored signal from an adjacent cell. Sevenless is a membrane-spanning receptor with an intracellular tyrosine kinase domain that signals in a way that closely resembles the signaling by hormone receptors such as the insulin receptor tyrosine kinase. Because paracrine factors and hormones can share signaling machinery, it is not surprising that hormones can, in some settings, act as paracrine factors. Testosterone, for example, is secreted into the bloodstream but also acts locally in the testes to control spermatogenesis. Insulin-like growth factor I (IGF-I) is a hormone secreted into the bloodstream from the liver and other tissues, but is also a paracrine factor made locally in most tissues to control cell proliferation. Furthermore, one receptor can mediate actions of a hormone, such as parathyroid hormone, and of a paracrine factor, such as parathyroid hormone–related protein. In some cases, the paracrine actions of "hormones" have functions quite unrelated to the hormonal functions. For example, macrophages synthesize the active form of vitamin D (1,25(OH)$_2$vitaminD$_3$), which can then bind to vitamin D receptors in the same cells and stimulate production of antimicrobial peptides.[1] The vitamin D 1α-hydroxylase responsible for activating 25(OH)-vitamin D is synthesized in multiple tissues in which it has functions not apparently related to the calcium homeostatic actions of the 1,25(OH)$_2$vitaminD$_3$ hormone. One can speculate that the hormonal actions of vitamin D might have evolved well after the paracrine vitamin D system provided the raw materials for the hormonal system.

Target cells respond similarly to signals that reach them from the bloodstream (hormones) or from the cell next door (paracrine factors); the cellular response machinery does not distinguish the sites of origin of signals. The shared final common pathways used by hormonal and paracrine signals should not, however, obscure important differences between hormonal and paracrine signaling systems (Fig. 1–1). Paracrine signals do not travel very far; consequently, the specific site of origin of a paracrine factor determines where it will act and provides specificity to that action. When the paracrine factor BMP4 is secreted by cells in the developing kidney, BMP4 regulates the differentiation of renal cells; when the same factor is secreted by cells in bone, it regulates bone formation. Thus, the site of origin of BMP4 determines its physiologic role. In contrast, because hormones are secreted into the bloodstream, their sites of origin are often divorced from their functions. We know nothing about thyroid hormone function, for example, that requires that the thyroid gland be in the neck.

Because the specificity of paracrine factor action is so dependent on its precise site of origin, elaborate mechanisms have evolved to regulate and constrain the diffusion of paracrine factors. Paracrine factors of the hedgehog family, for example, are covalently bound to cholesterol to constrain the diffusion of these molecules in the extracellular milieu. Most paracrine factors interact with binding proteins that block their action and control their diffusion. Chordin, noggin, and many other distinct proteins all bind to various members of the BMP family to regulate their action, for example. Proteases such as tolloid then destroy the binding proteins at specific sites to liberate BMPs so that they can act on appropriate target cells.

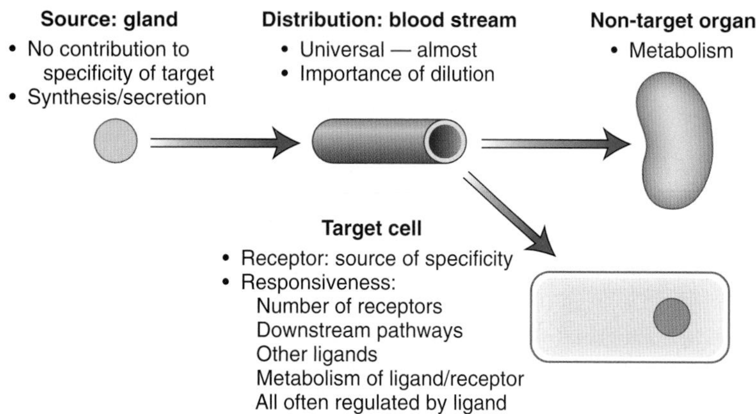

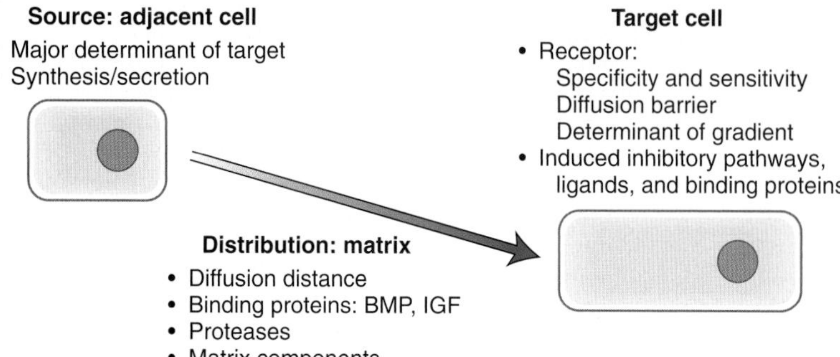

Figure 1–1 ▪ Comparison of determinants of endocrine and paracrine signaling.

Hormones have rather different constraints. Because they diffuse throughout the body, they must be synthesized in enormous amounts relative to the amounts of paracrine factors needed at specific locations. This synthesis usually occurs in specialized cells designed for that specific purpose. Hormones must then be able to travel in the bloodstream and diffuse in effective concentrations into tissues. Therefore, for example, lipophilic hormones bind to soluble proteins that allow them to travel in the aqueous media of blood at relatively high concentrations. The ability of hormones to diffuse through the extracellular space means that the local concentration of hormone at target sites will rapidly decrease when glandular secretion of the hormone stops. Because hormones diffuse throughout extracellular fluid quickly, hormonal metabolism can occur in specialized organs such as the liver and kidney in a way that determines the effective concentration of the hormones in other tissues.

Thus, paracrine factors and hormones use several distinct strategies to control their biosynthesis, sites of action, transport, and metabolism. These differing strategies probably explain partly why a hormone such as IGF-I, unlike its close relative, insulin, has multiple binding proteins that control its action in tissues. As noted earlier, IGF-I has a double life as both a hormone and a paracrine factor. Presumably, the local actions of IGF-I mandate an elaborate binding protein apparatus.

All the major hormonal signaling programs—G protein–coupled receptors, tyrosine kinase receptors, serine/threonine kinase receptors, ion channels, cytokine receptors, nuclear receptors—are also used by paracrine factors. In contrast, several paracrine signaling programs are used only by paracrine factors and are probably not used by hormones. For example, Notch receptors respond to membrane-based ligands to control cell fate, but no blood-borne ligands use Notch-type signaling (at least, none is currently known). Perhaps the intracellular strategy used by Notch, which involves cleavage of the receptor and subsequent nuclear actions of the receptor's cytoplasmic portion, is too inflexible to serve the purposes of hormones.

The analyses of the complete genomes of multiple bacterial species, the yeast *S. cerevisiae,* the fruit fly *Drosophila melanogaster,* the worm *Caenorhabitis elegans,* the plant *Aradopsis thaliana,* humans, and many other species have allowed a comprehensive view of the signaling machinery used by various forms of life. As noted already, *S. cerevisiae* uses G protein–linked receptors; this organism, however, lacks tyrosine kinase receptors and nuclear receptors that resemble the estrogen/thyroid receptor family. In contrast, the worm and fly share with humans the use of each of these signaling pathways, although with substantial variation in numbers of genes committed to each pathway. For example, the *Drosophila* genome encodes 20 nuclear receptors, the *C. elegans* genome encodes 270, and the human genome encodes (tentatively) more than 50. These patterns suggest that ancient multicellular animals must have already established the signaling systems that are the foundation of the endocrine system as we know it in mammals.

Even before the sequencing of the human genome, sequence analyses had made clear that many receptor genes are found in mammalian genomes for which no clear ligand or function was known. The analyses of these "orphan" receptors have succeeded in broadening the current understanding of hormonal signaling. For example, the LXR receptor was one such orphan receptor found when searching for unknown nuclear receptors. Subsequent experiments showed that oxygenated derivatives of cholesterol are the ligands for LXR, which regulates genes involved in cholesterol and fatty acid metabolism.[2] The examples of LXR and many others raise the question of what constitutes a hormone. The classic view of hormones is that they are synthesized in discrete glands and have no function other than activating receptors on cell membranes or in the nucleus. Cholesterol, which is converted in cells to oxygenated derivatives that activate the LXR receptor, in contrast, uses a hormonal strategy to regulate its own metabolism. Other orphan nuclear receptors similarly respond to ligands such as bile acids and fatty acids. These "hormones" have important metabolic roles quite separate from their signaling properties, although the hormone-like signaling serves to allow regulation of the metabolic function. The calcium-sensing receptor is an example from the G protein–linked receptor family of receptors that responds to a nonclassic ligand, ionic calcium. Calcium is released into the bloodstream from bone, kidney, and intestine and acts on the calcium-sensing receptor on parathyroid cells, renal tubular cells, and other cells to coordinate cellular responses to calcium. Thus, many important metabolic factors have taken on hormonal properties as part of a regulatory strategy.

Endocrine Glands

Hormone formation may occur either in localized collections of specific cells, the endocrine glands, or in cells that have additional roles. Many protein hormones, such as growth hormone, parathyroid hormone, prolactin, insulin, and glucagon, are produced in dedicated cells by standard protein synthetic mechanisms common to all cells. These secretory cells usually contain specialized secretory granules designed to store large amounts of hormone and to release the hormones in response to specific signals. Formation of small hormone molecules initiates with commonly found precursors, usually in specific glands such as the adrenals, gonads, or thyroid. In the case of the steroid hormones, the precursor is cholesterol, which is modified by various hydroxylations, methylations, and demethylations to form the glucocorticoids, androgens, estrogens, and their biologically active derivatives. In contrast, the precursor of vitamin D, 7-dehydrocholesterol, is produced in skin keratinocytes, again from cholesterol, by a photochemical reaction. Leptin, which regulates appetite and energy expenditure, is formed in adipocytes, thus providing a specific signal reflecting the nutritional state to the central nervous system.

Thyroid hormone synthesis occurs via a unique pathway. The thyroid cell synthesizes a 660,000-kd homodimer, thyroglobulin, which is then iodinated at specific iodotyrosines. Certain of these "couple" to form the iodothyronine molecule within thyroglobulin, which is then stored in the lumen of the thyroid follicle. In order for this to occur, the thyroid cell must concentrate the trace quantities of iodide from the blood and oxidize it via a specific peroxidase. Release of thyroxine (T_4) from the thyroglobulin requires its phagocytosis and cathepsin-catalyzed digestion by the same cells.

Hormones are synthesized in response to biochemical signals generated by various modulating systems. Many of these systems are specific to the effects of the hormone product, for example, parathyroid hormone synthesis is regulated by the concentration of ionized calcium. For others, such as gonadal, adrenal, and thyroid hormones, control of hormone synthesis is achieved by the hormonostatic function of the hypothalamic-pituitary axis. Cells in the hypothalamus and pituitary monitor the circulating hormone concentration and secrete tropic hormones, which activate specific pathways for hormone synthesis and release. Typical examples are luteinizing hormone, follicle-stimulating hormone, thyroid-stimulating hormone, and adrenocorticotropic hormone (LH, FSH, TSH, and ACTH, respectively).

These trophic hormones increase rates of hormone synthesis and secretion, and they may induce target cell division, thus causing enlargement of the various target glands. For example, in hypothyroid individuals living in iodine-deficient areas of the world, TSH secretion causes a marked hyperplasia of thyroid cells. In such regions, the thyroid gland may be 20- to 50-fold times its normal size. Adrenal hyperplasia occurs in patients with genetic deficiencies in cortisol formation. Hypertrophy and hyperplasia of parathyroid cells, in this case initiated by an intrinsic response to the stress of hypocalcemia, occurs in patients with renal insufficiency or calcium malabsorption.

Hormones may be fully active when released into the bloodstream (e.g., growth hormone or insulin), or they may require activation in specific cells to produce their biologic effects. These activation steps are often highly regulated. For example, the T_4 released from the thyroid cell is a prohormone that must undergo a specific deiodination to form the active 3,5,3′ triiodothyronine (T_3). This deiodination reaction can occur in target tissues, such as in the central nervous system, in the thyrotrophs, where T_3 provides feedback regulation of TSH production, or in hepatic and renal cells from which it is released into the circulation for uptake by all tissues. A similar post-secretory activation step catalyzed by a 5α-reductase causes tissue-specific activation of testosterone to dihydrotestosterone in target tissues including the male urogenital tract and genital skin, as well as in liver. Vitamin D undergoes hydroxylation at the 25 position in the liver, and in the 1 position in the kidney. Both hydroxylations must occur to produce the active hormone $1,25(OH)_2$ vitamin D. The activity of the 1α-hydroxylase, but not the 25-hydroxylase, is stimulated by parathyroid hormone and reduced plasma phosphate but is inhibited by calcium, $1,25(OH)_2$ vitamin D, and FGF23.

Hormones are synthesized as required on a daily, hourly, or minute-to-minute basis with minimal storage, but there are significant exceptions. One is the thyroid gland, which contains enough stored hormone to last for about 2 months. This permits a constant supply of this hormone despite significant variations in the availability of iodine. However, if iodine deficiency is prolonged, the normal reservoirs of thyroxine can be depleted.

The various feedback signaling systems exemplified above provide the hormonal *homeostasis* characteristic of virtually all endocrine systems. Regulation may include the central nervous system or local signal recognition mechanisms in the glandular cells, such as the calcium-sensing receptor of the parathyroid cell. Superimposed, centrally programmed increases and decreases in hormone secretion or activation through neuroendocrine pathways also occur. Examples include the circadian variation in the secretion of ACTH directing the synthesis and release of cortisol. The monthly menstrual cycle exemplifies a system with much longer periodicity that requires a complex synergism between central and peripheral axes of the endocrine glands. Disruption of hormonal homeostasis due to glandular or central regulatory system dysfunction has both clinical and laboratory consequences. Recognition and correction of these are the essence of clinical endocrinology.

Transport of Hormones in Blood

Protein hormones and some small molecules, such as the catecholamines, are water-soluble and are readily transported via the circulatory system. Others are nearly insoluble in water (e.g., the steroid and thyroid hormones) and their distribution presents special problems. Such molecules are bound to 50- to 60-kd carrier plasma glycoproteins such as thyroxine-binding globulin (TBG), sex hormone-binding globulin (SHBG), and corticosteroid-binding globulin (CBG), as well as to albumin. These ligand-protein complexes serve as reservoirs of these hormones, ensure ubiquitous distribution of their water-insoluble ligands, and protect the small molecules from rapid inactivation or excretion in the urine or bile. Without these proteins, it is unlikely that hydrophobic molecules would be transported much beyond the veins draining the glands in which they are formed. The protein-bound hormones exist in rapid equilibrium with the often minute quantities of hormone in the aqueous plasma. It is this "free" fraction of the circulating hormone that is taken up by the cell. It has been shown, for example, that if tracer thyroid hormone is injected into the portal vein in a protein-free solution, it is bound to hepatocytes at the periphery of the hepatic sinusoid. When the same experiment is repeated with a protein-containing solution, there is a uniform distribution of the tracer hormone throughout the hepatic lobule.[3] Despite the very high affinity of some of the binding proteins for their ligands, one specific protein may not be essential for hormone distribution. For example, in humans with a congenital deficiency of TBG, other proteins, transthyretin (TTR) and albumin, subsume its role. Because the affinity of these secondary thyroid hormone transport proteins is several orders of magnitude lower than that of TBG, it is possible for the hypothalamic-pituitary feedback system to maintain free thyroid hormone in the normal range at a much lower total hormone concentration. The fact that the "free" hormone concentration is normal in subjects with TBG deficiency indicates that it is this free moiety that is defended by the hypothalamic-pituitary axis and is the active hormone.[4]

The availability of gene targeting techniques has allowed specific tests of the physiologic role of several hormone-binding proteins. For example, mice with targeted inactivation of the vitamin D–binding protein (DBP) have been generated.[5] While the absence of DBP markedly reduces the circulating concentration of vitamin D, the mice are otherwise normal. However, they do show enhanced susceptibility to a vitamin D–deficient diet because of the reduced reservoir of this sterol. In addition, the absence of DBP markedly reduces the half-life of $25(OH)D_2$ by accelerating its hepatic uptake, making the mice less susceptible to vitamin D intoxication.

In rodents, transthyretin (TTR) carries retinol-binding protein and is also the principal thyroid hormone–binding protein. This protein is synthesized in the liver and in choroid plexus. It is the major thyroid hormone–binding protein in the cerebrospinal fluid of both rodents and humans and was thought to perhaps serve an important role in thyroid hormone transport into the central nervous system. This hypothesis has been disproved by the fact that mice without TTR have normal concentrations of T_4 in the brain as well as of free T_4 in the plasma.[6,7] To be sure, the serum concentrations of vitamin A and total T_4 are decreased, but the knockout mice have no signs of vitamin A deficiency or hypothyroidism. Such studies suggest that these proteins primarily serve distributive and reservoir functions.

Protein hormones and some small ligands (e.g., catecholamines) produce their effects by interacting with cell-surface receptors. Others, such as the steroid and thyroid hormones, must enter the cell to bind to cytosolic or nuclear receptors. In the past, it has been thought that much of the transmembrane transport of hormones was passive. Evidence is now in-hand that there are specific transporters involved in cellular uptake of thyroid hormone.[8] This may be found to be the case for other small ligands as well, revealing yet another mechanism for ensuring the distribution of a hormone to its site of action. Studies in mice missing megalin, a large, cell-surface protein in the LDL receptor family, suggest that estrogen and testosterone, bound to SHBG, uses megalin to enter certain tissues while still bound to SHBG.[9] In this case, therefore, the hormone bound to SHBG, rather than "free" hormone, is the active moiety that enters cells. It is unclear how generally this apparent exception to the "free hormone" hypothesis occurs.

Target Cells as Active Participants

Hormones determine cellular target actions by binding with high specificity to receptor proteins. Whether or not a peripheral cell is hormonally responsive, depends to a large extent on the presence and function of specific and selective hormone receptors. Receptor expression thus determines which cells will respond, as well as the nature of the intracellular effector pathways activated by the hormone signal. Receptor proteins may be localized to the cell membrane, cytoplasm, and nucleus. Broadly, polypeptide hormone receptors are cell membrane–associated, while soluble intracellular proteins selectively bind to steroid hormones (Fig. 1–2). This idea of selective localization has, however, recently been challenged, because related sequences can be found in multiple cellular compartments.

Membrane-associated receptor proteins usually consist of extracellular sequences that recognize and bind ligand, transmembrane anchoring hydrophobic sequences, and intracellular sequences, which initiate intracellular signaling. Intracellular signaling is mediated by soluble second messengers (e.g., cyclic adenosine monophosphate) or by activation of intracellular signaling molecules (e.g., STAT proteins). Receptor-dependent activation of heterotrimeric G proteins, comprising α, β, and γ subunits, may either induce or suppress effector enzymes or ion channels.

Several growth factors and hormone receptors (e.g., for insulin) behave as intrinsic tyrosine kinases or activate intracellular protein tyrosine kinases. Ligand activation may cause receptor dimerization (e.g., GH) or heterodimerization (e.g., interleukin-6), followed by activation of intracellular phosphorylation cascades. These activated proteins ultimately determine specific nuclear gene expression.

Both the number of receptors expressed per cell, as well as their responses, are also regulated, thus providing a further level of control for hormone action. Several mechanisms account for altered receptor function. Receptor endocytosis causes internalization of cell-surface receptors; the hormone-receptor complex is subsequently dissociated, resulting in abrogation of the hormone signal. Receptor trafficking may then result in recycling back to the cell-surface (e.g., as for insulin), or the internalized receptor may undergo lysosomal degradation. Both these mechanisms triggered by activation of receptors effectively lead to impaired hormone signaling by down-regulation of these receptors. The hormone signaling pathway may also be down-regulated by receptor desensitization (e.g., as for epinephrine); ligand-mediated receptor phosphorylation leads to a reversible deactivation of the receptor. Desensitization mechanisms can be activated by a receptor's ligand (homologous desensitization) or by another signal (heterologous desensitization), thereby attenuating receptor signaling in the continued presence of ligand. Receptor function may also be limited by action of specific phosphatases (e.g., SHP) or by intracellular negative regulation of the signaling cascade (e.g., SOCS proteins inhibiting JAK-STAT signaling).

Mutational changes in receptor structure can also determine hormone action. Constitutive receptor activation may be induced by activating mutations (e.g., TSH receptor) leading to endocrine organ hyperfunction, even in the absence of hormone. Conversely, inactivating receptor mutations may lead to endocrine hypofunction (e.g., testosterone or vasopressin receptors). These syndromes are well-characterized and are well-described in this volume (Fig. 1–3).

The functional diversity of receptor signaling also results in overlapping or redundant intracellular pathways. For example,

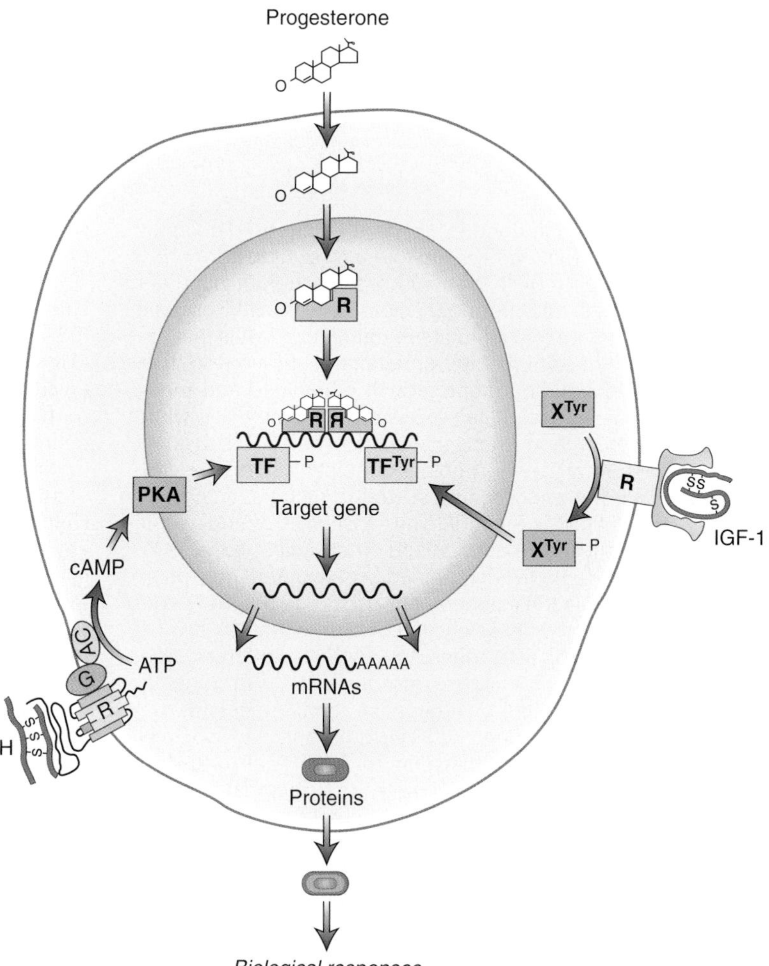

Figure 1–2 ■ Hormonal signaling by cell-surface and intracellular receptors. The receptors for the water-soluble polypeptide hormones, LH, and IGF-I are integral membrane proteins located at the cell surface. They bind the hormone-utilizing extracellular sequences and transduce a signal by the generation of second messengers: cyclic adenosine monophosphate for the LH receptor and tyrosine-phosphorylated substrates for the insulin-like growth factor I receptor. Although effects on gene expression are indicated, direct effects on cellular proteins (e.g., ion channels) are also observed. In contrast, the receptor for the lipophilic steroid hormone progesterone resides in the cell nucleus. It binds the hormone and becomes activated and capable of directly modulating target gene transcription.) *R,* Receptor molecule; *TF,* transcription factor. (Reproduced from Mayo K. In Conn PM, Melmed S, eds. Endocrinology: Basic and Clinical Principles. Totowa, NJ: Humana Press, 1997:11.)

Diseases caused by mutations in G protein-coupled receptors			
Condition	**Receptor**	**Inheritance**	**Δ Function**
Retinitis pigmentosa	Rhodopsin	AD/AR	Loss
Nephrogenic diabetes insipidus	Vasopressin V2	X-linked	Loss
Isolated glucocorticoid deficiency	ACTH	AR	Loss
Color blindness	Red/green opsins	X-linked	Loss
Familial precocious puberty	LH	AD (male)	Gain
Familial hypercalcemia	Ca^{2+} sensing	AD	Loss
Neonatal severe parathyroidism	Ca^{2+} sensing	AR	Loss
Dominant form hypocalcemia	Ca^{2+} sensing	AD	Gain
Congenital hyperthyroidism	TSH	AD	Gain
Resistance to thyroid hormone	TSH	AR (comp het)	Loss
Hyperfunctioning thyroid adenoma	TSH	Somatic	Gain
Metaphyseal chondrodysplasia	PTH-PTHrP	Somatic	Gain
Hirschsprung's disease	Endothelin-B	Multigenic	Loss
Coat color alteration (*E* locus, mice)	MSH	AD/AR	Loss and gain
Dwarfism (*little* locus, mice)	GHRH	AR	Loss

Figure 1–3 ▪ Diseases caused by mutations in G-protein–coupled receptors. All are human conditions with the exception of the final two entries, which refer to the mouse. *AD,* Autosomal dominant; *AR,* autosomal recessive inheritance. Loss of function refers to inactivating mutations of the receptor, and gain of function to activating mutations. Abbreviations for G-protein–coupled receptors: *ACTH,* Adrenocorticotropic hormone; *LH,* luteinizing hormone; *TSH,* thyroid-stimulating hormone; *PTH-PTHrP,* parathyroid hormone and parathyroid hormone–related peptide; *MSH,* melanocyte-stimulating hormone; *GHRH,* growth hormone–releasing hormone; *FSH,* follicle-stimulating hormone. (Reproduced from Mayo K. In Conn PM, Melmed S, eds. Endocrinology: Basic and Clinical Principles. Totowa, NJ: Humana Press, 1997:27.)

both GH and cytokines activate JAK-STAT signaling, whereas the distal effects of these stimuli clearly differ. Thus, despite common signaling pathways, hormones elicit highly specific cellular effects. Tissue or cell-type genetic programs or receptor-receptor interactions at the cell surface (e.g., dopamine D2 with SRIF receptor hetero-oligonization) may also confer specific cellular response to a hormone and provide an additive cellular effect.[10]

Control of Hormone Secretion

Anatomically distinct endocrine glands are composed of highly differentiated cells that synthesize, store, and secrete hormones. Circulating hormone concentrations are a function of glandular secretory patterns and hormone clearance rates. Hormone secretion is tightly regulated to attain circulating levels that are most conducive to elicit the appropriate target tissue response. For example, longitudinal bone growth is initiated and maintained by exquisitely regulated levels of circulating GH, while mild GH hypersecretion results in gigantism and GH deficiency causes growth retardation. Ambient circulating hormone concentrations are not uniform, and secretion patterns determine appropriate physiologic function. Thus, insulin secretion occurs in short pulses elicited by nutrient and other signals, gonadotrophin secretion is episodic, determined by a hypothalamic pulse generator, and prolactin secretion appears to be relatively continuous with secretory peaks elicited during suckling.

Hormone secretion also adheres to rhythmic patterns. Circadian rhythms serve as adaptive responses to environmental signals and are controlled by a circadian timing mechanism.[11] Light is the major environmental cue adjusting the endogenous clock. The retinohypothalamic tract entrains circadian pulse generators situated within hypothalamic suprachiasmatic nuclei. These signals subserve timing mechanisms for the sleep-wake cycle and determine patterns of hormone secretion and action. Disturbed circadian timing results in hormonal dysfunction, and may also be reflective of entrainment or pulse generator lesions. For example, adult GH deficiency due to a damaged hypothalamus or pituitary is associated with elevations in integrated 24-hour leptin concentrations, decreased leptin pulsatility, and yet preserved circadian rhythm of leptin. GH replacement restores leptin pulsatility, followed by loss of body fat mass.[12] Sleep is also an important cue regulating hormone pulsatility. About 70% of overall GH secretion occurs during slow-wave sleep, and increasing age is associated with declining slow-wave sleep and concomitant decline in GH and elevation of cortisol secretion.[13] Most pituitary hormones are secreted in a circadian (day-night) rhythm, best exemplified by ACTH peaks before 9 AM, whereas ovarian steroids follow a 28-day menstrual rhythm. Disrupted episodic rhythms are often a hallmark of endocrine dysfunction. Thus, loss of circadian ACTH secretion with high midnight cortisol levels is a feature of Cushing's disease.

Hormone secretion is induced by multiple specific biochemical and neural signals. Integration of these stimuli results in the net temporal and quantitative secretion of the hormone (Fig. 1–4). Thus, signals elicited by hypothalamic hormones (GHRH, SRIF), peripheral hormones (IGF-I, sex steroids, thyroid hormone), nutrients, adrenergic pathways, stress, and other neuropeptides, all converge on the somatotroph cell, resulting in the ultimate pattern and quantity of GH secretion. Networks of reciprocal interactions allow for dynamic adaptation and shifts in environmental signals. These regulatory systems embrace the hypothalamic pituitary and target endocrine glands, as well as the adipocyte and lymphocyte. Peripheral inflammation and stress elicit cytokine signals that interface with the neuroendocrine system, resulting in hypothalamic-pituitary axis activation. The parathyroid and pancreatic secreting cells are less tightly controlled by the hypothalamus, but their functions are tightly regulated by the effects they elicit. Thus, parathyroid hormone (PTH) secretion is induced when serum calcium levels fall, and the signal for sustained PTH secretion is abrogated by rising calcium levels.

Several tiers of control subserve the ultimate net glandular secretion. First, central nervous system signals including stress, afferent stimuli, and neuropeptides signal the synthesis and secretion of hypothalamic hormones and neuropeptides (Fig. 1–5). Four hypothalamic-releasing hormones (GHRH, CRH, TRH, and GnRH) traverse the hypothalamic portal vessels and

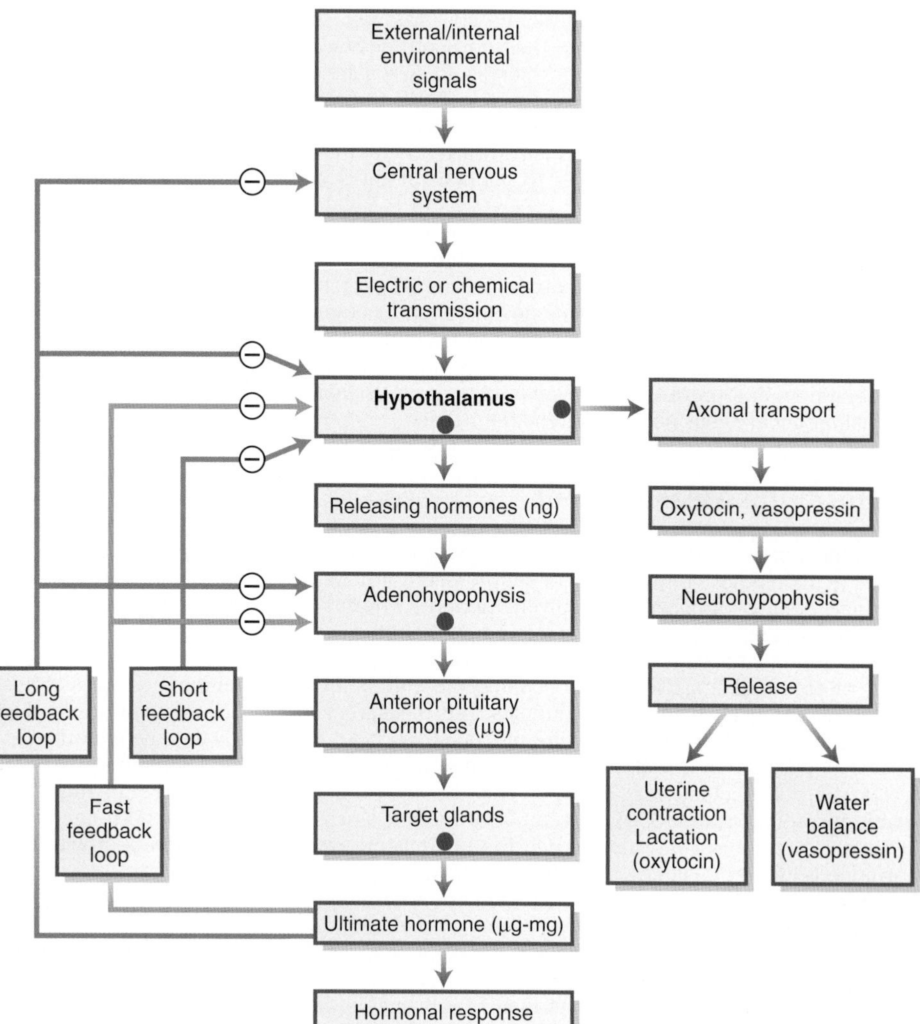

Figure 1–4 ▪ Peripheral feedback mechanism and a million-fold amplifying cascade of hormonal signals. Environmental signals are transmitted to the central nervous system, which innervates the hypothalamus, which responds by secreting nanogram amounts of a specific hormone. Releasing hormones are transported down a closed portal system, pass the blood-brain barrier at either end through fenestrations, and bind to specific anterior pituitary cell membrane receptors to elicit secretion of micrograms of specific anterior pituitary hormones. These enter the venous circulation through fenestrated local capillaries, bind to specific target gland receptors, trigger release of micrograms to milligrams of daily hormone amounts, and elicit responses by binding to receptors in distal target tissues. Peripheral hormone receptors enable widespread cell signaling by a single initiating environmental signal, thus facilitating intimate homeostatic association with the external environment. *Arrows* with a black dot at their origin indicate a secretory process. (Reproduced from Normal AW, Litwack G. Hormones, ed 2. New York: Academic Press, 1997:14.)

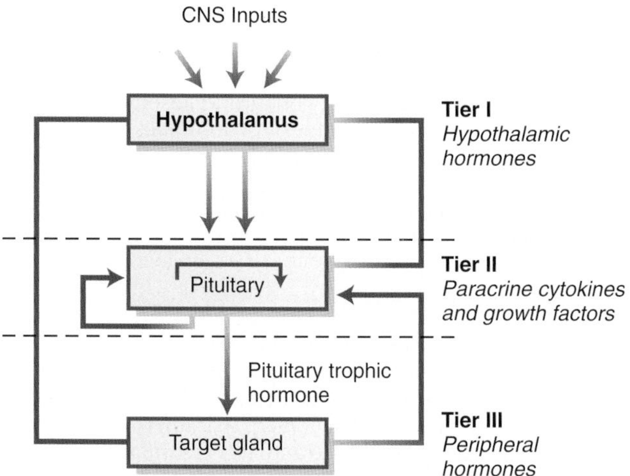

Figure 1–5 ▪ Model for regulation of anterior pituitary hormone secretion by three tiers of control. Hypothalamic hormones impinge directly on their respective target cells. Intrapituitary cytokines and growth factors regulate tropic cell function by paracrine (and autocrine) control. Peripheral hormones exert negative feedback inhibition of respective pituitary trophic hormone synthesis and secretion. (Reproduced from Ray D, Melmed S. Pituitary cytokine and growth factor expression and action. Endocrin Rev 1997;18:206-228.)

impinge upon their respective transmembrane trophic hormone-secreting cell receptors. These distinct cells express GH, ACTH, TSH, and gonadotrophins. In contrast, hypothalamic somatostatin and dopamine suppress GH, PRL, or TSH secretion. Trophic hormones also maintain the structural-functional integrity of endocrine organs, including the thyroid and adrenal glands, and the gonads. Target hormones, in turn, serve as powerful negative feedback regulators of their respective trophic hormone; they often also suppress secretion of hypothalamic-releasing hormones. In certain circumstances (e.g., during puberty), peripheral sex steroids may positively induce the hypothalamic-pituitary-target gland axis. Thus, LH induces ovarian estrogen secretion, which feeds back positively to induce further LH release. Pituitary hormones themselves, in a short feedback loop, may also regulate their own respective hypothalamic-controlling hormone. Hypothalamic-releasing hormones are secreted in nanogram amounts, and have short half-lives of a few minutes. Anterior pituitary hormones are produced in microgram amounts and have longer half-lives, while peripheral hormones can be produced in up to milligram amounts daily, with much longer half-lives.

A further level of secretion control occurs within the gland itself. Thus, intraglandular paracrine or autocrine growth peptides serve to autoregulate pituitary hormone secretion, as exemplified by EGF control of prolactin or IGF-I control of GH secretion. Molecules within the endocrine cell may also subserve an intracellular feedback loop. Thus, corticotrope SOCS-3 induction by gp130-linked cytokines serves to abrogate the ligand-induced JAK-STAT cascade and block POMC transcription and ACTH secretion. This rapid on-off regulation of ACTH secretion provides a plastic endocrine response to changes in environmental signaling and serves to maintain homeostatic integrity.[14]

In addition to the central-neuroendocrine interface mediated by hypothalamic chemical signal transduction, the central nervous system directly controls several hormonal secretory processes. Posterior pituitary hormone secretion occurs as direct efferent neural extensions. Postganglionic sympathetic nerves also regulate rapid changes in renin, insulin, and glucagon secretion, and preganglionic sympathetic nerves signal to adrenal medullary cells eliciting adrenaline release.

Hormone Measurement

Endocrine function can be assessed by measuring levels of basal circulating hormone, evoked or suppressed hormone, or hormone binding proteins. Alternatively, peripheral hormone receptor function can be assessed. Meaningful strategies for timing hormonal measurements vary from system to system. In some cases, circulating hormone concentrations can be measured in randomly collected serum samples. This measurement, when standardized for fasting, environmental stress, age, and gender is reflective of true hormone concentrations only when levels do not fluctuate appreciably. For example, thyroid hormone, prolactin, and IGF-I levels can be accurately assessed in fasting morning serum samples. On the other hand, when hormone secretion is clearly episodic, timed samples may be required over a defined time course to reflect hormone bioavailability. Thus, early morning and late evening cortisol measurements are most appropriate. Twenty-four–hour sampling for GH measurements, with samples collected every 2, 10, or 20 minutes, are expensive and cumbersome, yet may yield valuable diagnostic information. Random sampling may also reflect secretion peaks or nadirs, thus confounding adequate interpretation of results.

In general, confirmation of failed glandular function is made by attempting to evoke hormone secretion by recognized stimuli. Thus, testing of pituitary hormone reserve may be accomplished by injecting appropriate hypothalamic releasing hormones. Injection of trophic hormones, including TSH and ACTH, evokes specific target gland hormone secretion. Pharmacologic stimuli (e.g., metoclopramide for induction of PRL secretion) may also be useful tests of hormone reserve. In contrast, hormone hypersecretion can be diagnosed by suppressing glandular function. Thus, failure to appropriately suppress GH levels after a standardized glucose load implies inappropriate GH hypersecretion.

Radioimmunoassays utilize highly specific antibodies unique to the hormone, or a hormone fragment, to quantify hormone levels. Enzyme-linked immunosorbent assays (ELISAs) employ enzymes instead of radioactive hormone markers, and enzyme activity is reflective of hormone concentration. This sensitive technique has allowed ultrasensitive measurements of physiologic hormone concentrations. Hormone-specific receptors may be employed in place of the antibody in a radioreceptor assay.

Endocrine Diseases

Endocrine diseases fall into four broad categories: (1) hormone overproduction, (2) hormone underproduction, (3) altered tissue responses to hormones, and (4) tumors of endocrine glands.

Hormone Overproduction

Occasionally, hormones are secreted in increased amounts because of genetic abnormalities that cause abnormal regulation of hormone synthesis or release. For example, in glucocorticoid-remediable hyperaldosteronism, an abnormal chromosomal crossing over event puts the aldosterone synthetase gene under the control of the ACTH-regulated 11β-hydroxylase gene. More often, diseases of hormone overproduction are associated with an increase in the total number of hormone-producing cells. For example, the hyperthyroidism of Graves' disease, in which antibodies mimic TSH and activate the TSH receptors on thyroid cells, is associated with dramatic increase in thyroid cell proliferation, as well as with increased synthesis and release of thyroid hormone from each thyroid cell. In this example, the increase in thyroid cell number represents a polyclonal expansion of thyroid cells, in which large numbers of thyroid cells proliferate in response to an abnormal stimulus. However, most endocrine tumors are not polyclonal expansions, but instead represent monoclonal expansions of one mutated cell. Pituitary and parathyroid tumors, for example, are usually monoclonal expansions in which somatic mutations in multiple tumor suppressor genes and proto-oncogenes occur. These mutations lead to an increase in proliferation and/or survival of the mutant cells. Sometimes, this proliferation is associated with abnormal secretion of hormone from each tumor cell as well. For example, mutant G_s α proteins in somatotrophs can lead to both increased cellular proliferation and increased secretion of growth hormone from each tumor cell.

Hormone Underproduction

Underproduction of hormone can result from a wide variety of processes, ranging from surgical removal of parathyroid glands during neck surgery, to tuberculous destruction of adrenal glands, or to iron deposition in β cells in hemochromatosis. A frequent cause of destruction of hormone-producing cells is autoimmunity. Autoimmune destruction of β cells in type 1 diabetes mellitus or of thyroid cells in Hashimoto's thyroiditis are two of the most common disorders treated by endocrinologists. More uncommonly, a host of genetic abnormalities can also lead to decreased hormone production. These disorders can result from abnormal development of hormone-producing cells (e.g., hypogonadotrophic hypogonadism caused by KAL gene mutations), from abnormal synthesis of hormones (e.g., deletion of the growth hormone gene), or from abnormal regulation of hormone secretion (e.g., the hypoparathyroidism associated with activating mutations of the parathyroid cell's calcium-sensing receptor).

Altered Tissue Responses

Resistance to hormones can be caused by a variety of genetic disorders. Examples include mutations in the growth hormone receptor in Laron dwarfism and mutations in the G_s α gene in the hypoparathyroidism of pseudohypoparathyroidism type 1a. The insulin resistance in muscle and liver central to the etiology of type 2 diabetes mellitus appears to be polygenic in origin. Type 2 diabetes is also an example of a disease in which end organ insensitivity is worsened by signals from other organs, in this case by signals originating in fat cells. In other cases, the target organ of hormone action is more directly abnormal, as in the PTH resistance of renal failure.

Increased end organ function can be caused by mutations in signal reception and propagation. For example, activating mutations in TSH, LH, and PTH receptors can cause increased activity of thyroid cells, Leydig cells, and osteoblasts, even in the absence of ligand. Similarly, activating mutations in the G_s α protein can cause precocious puberty, hyperthyroidism, and acromegaly in McCune-Albright syndrome.

Tumors of Endocrine Glands

Tumors of endocrine glands, as noted above, often result in hormone overproduction. Some tumors of endocrine glands produce little if any hormone, but cause disease by causing local compressive symptoms or by metastatic spread. Examples include so-called nonfunctioning pituitary tumors, which are usually benign but can cause a variety of symptoms due to compression on adjacent structures, and thyroid cancer, which can spread throughout the body without causing hyperthyroidism.

Therapeutic Strategies

In general, hormones are employed pharmacologically for both their replacement or suppressive effects. Hormones may also be utilized for diagnostic stimulatory effects (e.g., hypothalamic hormones) to evoke target organ responses, or to diagnose endocrine hyperfunction by suppressing hormone hypersecretion (e.g., T_3). Ablation of endocrine gland function due to genetic or acquired causes can be restored by hormone replacement therapy. In general, steroid and thyroid hormones are replaced orally, whereas peptide hormones (e.g., insulin, growth hormone) require injection. Gastrointestinal absorption and first pass kinetics determine oral hormone dosage and availability. Physiologic replacement can achieve both appropriate hormone levels (e.g., thyroid) as well as approximate hormone secretory patterns (e.g., GnRH delivered intermittently via a pump). Hormones can also be used to treat diseases associated with glandular hyperfunction. Long-acting depot preparations of somatostatin analogues suppress GH hypersecretion in acromegaly or 5-HIAA hypersecretion in carcinoid syndrome. Estrogen receptor antagonists (e.g., tamoxifen) are useful for some patients with breast cancer, and GnRH analogues may down-regulate the gonadotrophin axis and benefit patients with prostate cancer.

Novel formulations of receptor-specific hormone ligands are now being clinically developed (e.g., estrogen agonists/antagonists, somatostatin receptor subtype ligands), resulting in more selective therapeutic targeting. Modes of hormone injection (e.g., for PTH) may also determine therapeutic specificity and efficacy. Improved hormone delivery systems, including computerized minipumps, intranasal sprays (e.g., for DDAVP), pulmonary inhalations, and depot intramuscular injections, will also allow added patient compliance and ease of administration. Insulin delivered by inhalation has already been approved for use, and inhaled growth hormone is under investigation, for example.

Despite this tremendous progress, some therapies, such as insulin delivery to rigorously control blood sugar, still require tremendous patient involvement and await innovative approaches. Hormones are biologically powerful molecules that exert therapeutic benefit and effectively replace pathologic deficits. They should not be prescribed without clear-cut indications and should not be administered without careful evaluation by an appropriately qualified medical practitioner.

REFERENCES

1. Liu PT, Stenger S, Li H, et al. Toll-like receptor triggering of a vitamin D-mediated human antimicrobial response. Science, 2006;311:1770-1773.
2. Chawla A, Repa JJ, Evans RM, et al. Nuclear receptors and lipid physiology: opening the X-files. Science 2001;294:1866-1870.
3. Mendel CM, Weisiger RA, Jones AL, et al. Thyroid hormone-binding proteins in plasma facilitate uniform distribution of thyroxine within tissues: a perfused rat liver study. Endocrinology 1987;120:1742-1749.
4. Mendel CM. The free hormone hypothesis: physiologically based mathematical model. Endocr Rev 1989;10(3):232-274.
5. Safadi FF, Thornton P, Magiera H, et al. Osteopathy and resistance to vitamin D toxicity in mice null for vitamin D binding protein. J Clin Invest 1999;103:239-251.
6. Palha JA, Fernandes R, de Escobar GM, et al. Transthyretin regulates thyroid hormone levels in the choroid plexus, but not in the brain parenchyma: study in a transthyretin-null mouse model. Endocrinology 2000;141:3267-3272.
7. Palha JA, Episkopou V, Maeda S, et al. Thyroid hormone metabolism in a transthyretin-null mouse strain. J Biol Chem 1994;269: 32767.
8. Friesema EC, Jansen J, Heuer H, et al. Mechanisms of disease: Psychomotor retardation and high T_3 levels caused by mutations in monocarboxylate transporter 8. Nat Clin Pract Endocrinol Metab 2006;2:512-523.
9. Hammes A, Andreassen TK, Spoelgen R, et al. Role of endocytosis in cellular uptake of sex steroids. Cell 2005;122:751-762.
10. Rocheville M, Lange DC, Kumar U, et al. Receptors for dopamine and somatostatin: formation of hetero-oligomers with enhanced functional activity. Science 2000;288:154-157.
11. Moore RY. Circadian rhythms: basic neurobiology and clinical applications. Ann Rev Med 1997;48:253-266.
12. Aftab MA, Guzder R, Wallace AM, et al. Circadian and ultradian rhythm and leptin pulsatility in adult GH deficiency: effects of GH replacement. J Clin Endocrinol Metab 2001;86:3499-3506.
13. Cauter EV, Leproult R, Plat L. Age-related changes in slow wave sleep and REM sleep and relationship with growth hormone and cortisol levels in healthy men. JAMA 2000;284:861-868.
14. Melmed S. The immuno-neuroendocrine interface. J Clin Invest 2001;108:1563-1566.

CHAPTER 2

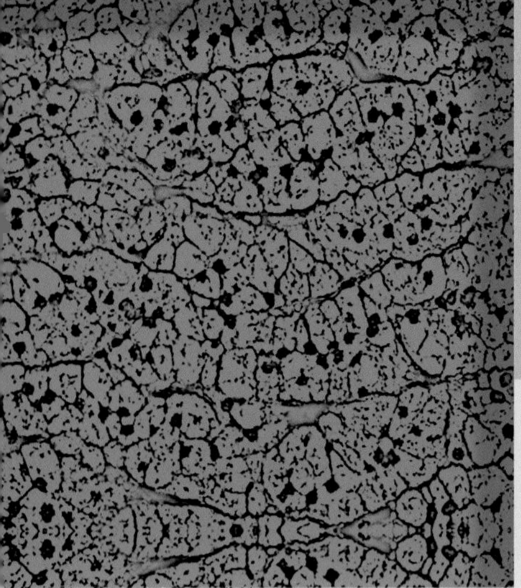

THE ENDOCRINE PATIENT

Daniel D. Federman

A textbook of medicine is inevitably about disease, but the practice of medicine deals with illness, that is, a person experiencing a disease. This is why the present chapter has been entitled "The Endocrine Patient." This chapter lays out the general issues and approaches applicable to caring for patients with endocrine disorders. The topics to be discussed include initial evaluation and the nature of referral, the fact-finding required in clinical evaluation, the use of the laboratory and imaging, the formulation of a differential diagnosis, decision making, and management. In each case, the steps are portrayed from the patient's point of view. Except for acute adrenal insufficiency, endocrine disorders are seldom life-threatening. They have enormous effect on the quality of life, however, and successful intervention can be extremely important to both patient and family.

General Considerations

Many features of being an endocrine patient are common to all experiences of illness. Most often, a perceived change in bodily function, a symptom, gets one to the doctor. Although generations of medical students have described new patients as being "in no acute distress," most patients are, in fact, worried and anxious when they see a physician, the more so when the physician is not known to them. A few minutes spent in getting to know the patient pays enormous dividends in the accuracy of the history obtained and in setting the stage for further cooperation with testing and treatment.

Inasmuch as most endocrine consultation is elective rather than emergent, I favor asking a few simple questions, such as "Where are you from?" "What do you do?" "How did you come to us?" "Were you referred?" and so on. Almost always, some common experience or acquaintance is discovered that provides the basis for a rapport that does not emerge from formal medical questioning. This approach also immediately conveys that you are interested in the patient as a person and not just the patient's disease. It also provides reassurance that you have the time to listen to the person, a simple luxury often omitted in the current maelstrom of medicine.

Special Features of Endocrine Illness

Traditionally a consultation begins with either a telephone call or letter from the referring physician. But this invaluable step is today honored more in the breach than the fact.

Discovery through Screening

Numerous special features of endocrine disease make patient presentation quite different from that seen in general medicine. One feature is the discovery of abnormality through screening of asymptomatic individuals, for example, a high serum calcium level discovered through multiphasic screening or a high blood glucose level discovered in a shopping mall kiosk. The very absence of symptoms lends an unreality to the moment and should become an explicit topic of the patient-doctor interaction. In this circumstance, it is worth emphasizing the value of early discovery and prevention of greater morbidity.

Quantitative Rather than Qualitative Abnormalities

A second special feature of endocrine disorders is that they are quantitative, rather than qualitative, departures from normal. No endocrine disorder is due to a novel hormone. Everyone has cortisol circulating as a determining feature of his or her life. Hypercorticism and adrenal insufficiency represent just more or less of the natural hormone. Similarly, all hormones found in excess or in deficiency in disease are physiologic determinants of stature, weight, complexion, hairiness, temperament, and behavior. In contrast, no one has a little pneumonia or a little inflammatory bowel disease as a constitutive status. In addition, most endocrine glands have both a basal and a stimulable or reserve function. It is common to have partial diminution of capacity in which the basal function is adequate but a reserve called upon during part of each day—or, more dramatically, in emergencies—is not available.

Overlap with Other Diseases

The symptoms of endocrine disorders overlap a great range of normal characteristics, including body contour, facial configurations, weight distributions, skin and hair coloring, and muscular capacity. They also overlap with other conditions that are far more common, including depression, obesity, and normal aging. The added adipose tissue of hyperadrenocorticism is more difficult to recognize in a person who is already obese. The nervousness associated with hyperthyroidism is less apparent in a thin, hyperkinetic man than in a person of moderate body weight. The effects of an androgen-producing adrenal tumor are less likely to be noticed in a family of swarthy, hirsute individuals.

Finally, most endocrine disorders evolve gradually over months to years instead of appearing suddenly, such as a heart attack or an acute infection. This combination of varied host background and slow evolution of disease leads to considerable delay in diagnosis: both the patient and primary care physician adapt to the changes as part of the person, and definitive evaluation, now relatively easy for most disorders, is not undertaken. Hypothyroidism and acromegaly are good examples of this phenomenon. Published series for both diseases show a remarkable delay in diagnosis despite sometimes disabling symptoms.

Hormones have more distant effects than local effects. This, of course, reflects their messenger status. Unlike an abscess, a myocardial infarction, or an esophageal cancer, endocrine disorders seldom produce symptoms near the gland of origin. (Subacute thyroiditis and large pituitary tumors, of course, are exceptions.) But because in most endocrinopathies the excess or missing hormone works on several or many systems, the resulting syndrome can be enigmatic.

Several endocrine disorders are important not because of their incidence but because of their curability: Cushing's disease, acromegaly, and pheochromocytoma are cases in point. Although these disorders enter the differential diagnosis of common problems such as diabetes, their occurrence is so rare that the primary care physician does not easily think of them, thus the maxim: "What you don't see often you don't see."

Unique Features of Reproductive Disorders

Reproductive disorders have symptoms and signs that have no parallel in other areas. This is the one system in which sexual dimorphism is inherent rather than epiphenomenal; it is also the one with the greatest span of developmental change. Once the heart starts beating in the embryo, it goes on doing so until the last moment of life; but puberty, adult sexual functioning, and menopause establish time lines against which all symptoms are to be assessed. Thus, vaginal bleeding has entirely different meanings when it occurs on the first day of life, as a natural appearance at age 12, during pregnancy, as a harbinger of menopause at age 46 years, or as a highly probable symptom of cancer at age 66 years.

Physical appearance and function are important features of self-image. Thus, hirsutism, thinness, obesity, sexual arousal, and erectile capacity bear considerable psychological import to the endocrine patient. The clinician should be constantly aware of both spoken and unspoken thoughts that may be troubling the patient.

The Couple as a Clinical Unit

The ultimate goal of reproductive capacity is, of course, a fertile union. This means that the couple, rather than the individual, is the unit of clinical concern. It is thus the principal area in medicine wherein two people and their interaction, rather than a single person and her capacities, are studied and treated. In addition, there are dimensions of successful sexual function that are important at other times than when fertility is sought. Sex drive, erotic responsiveness, affection, and tenderness are all important aspects of life whether or not fertility is a current issue.

Evaluation of Patients with Endocrine Disorders

I have emphasized previously the belief that establishing an interested and warm relationship is the beginning of excellence in any elective medical interaction. In addition to its affective power, the relationship elicits a more informative history, establishes better cooperation in both testing and treatment, and provides a platform for informed decision making by the patient.

History

As in most areas of medicine, precision of diagnosis and economy of investigation begin with a carefully wrought history. An open-ended question, combined with an attentive silence, allows the patient to provide the background for the clinical moment. After the patient has spoken spontaneously, the physician elicits a guided expansion of the information. Details of timing, sequence, changes of diet or activity, relationship to the menstrual cycle, changes in weight or size, and alterations in mood or sleep pattern—all of these may provide clues to underlying endocrine abnormality.

A good example of the power of the history is the interpretation of irregular periods in a woman of reproductive age. The simple statement, "I've never been regular," points to a presumptive diagnosis of polycystic ovary syndrome in a way that a very convoluted sequence of questions might actually fail to do. That statement is to be contrasted with this one: "I used to be regular, but in the last year or so, I never know when my period is going to come." If the presenting symptom is irregular periods, the simple invitation, "Tell me about your periods," is likely to be the key to the diagnosis.

Careful questioning about use of complementary and alternative medicines is an important and, occasionally, a very revealing step.

A thorough family history has become increasingly important as the genetic basis for more and more endocrine diseases becomes established. For practical purposes, I favor diagramming a pedigree of the first-order relatives—parents, siblings, children—of all patients, not just those for whom a genetic disorder is already suspected. Known disorders are readily revealed this way, and unknown conjunctions of clinical and genetic factors may also be disclosed (Fig. 2–1).

Physical Examination

General Examination

It is said that the history is 80% or more of clinical diagnosis, and that is no less true in endocrine disorders than in general medicine. Yet the physical examination is a critical element in arriving at a diagnosis, and here I call particular attention to the first impression.

Cushing's syndrome, Addison's disease, hyperthyroidism, hypothyroidism, acromegaly, polycystic ovary syndrome, hypogonadism, and Turner's syndrome—these and other endocrine disorders should be considered from the first moment one encounters a new patient. Otherwise, one risks accepting that the appearance of the patient is just that and no more. In other words, as soon as one accepts that the initial impression is what the person looks like naturally, the quantitative departure from normal that is the essence of endocrine disease fails to be impressive. This, incidentally, is why both families and primary care physicians often miss a diagnosis that seems obvious to the consultant endocrinologist.

A quantification of this last point may be helpful. If the signs of hypothyroidism or acromegaly, for example, take 3 years to become striking, the person living with the patient is exposed to 1/1095th of fractional change per day—well below the threshold of just noticeable difference. Similarly, a primary care physician seeing the patient perhaps four times a year for a general checkup and management of hypertension is exposed to 91/1095th fractional change. This can sometimes lead to a diagnosis but often does not. When one sees the patient for the first time, however, the imprint of the disease catches attention and the constitutional appearance is in the background.

Although a consultant participates because of a special area of interest and expertise, he or she is a general physician first and should be alert to all dimensions of the physical examination: What is the height-to-weight ratio? What is the basic degree of muscularity? Is there evidence of heart disease to explain the chest pain and dyspnea one has heard about in the history? What is the degree of hirsutism? Are there signs of liver disease, malnutrition, or poor or excellent physical training? What is the blood pressure with the patient standing as well as lying or sitting? These and many other points of a general examination begin to modify the thinking one has undertaken on the basis of history.

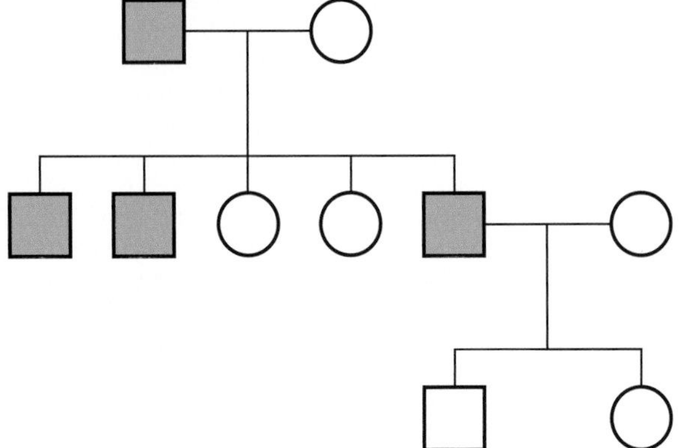

Figure 2–1 ▪ Simple pedigree of the propositus *(arrow)* and first-order relatives should be the standard family history in a new patient workup. If the patient has children, their health status should be included as well.

Targeted Examination

The targeted physical examination of any consultant is a dynamic interplay of general and specific goals. Theoretically, any experienced clinician should undertake a general examination and come to all the findings pertinent to an underlying endocrine disorder. In fact, however, the physical examination is greatly influenced by the hypotheses generated in the history. Let us look at a few examples.

If a patient reports weight loss despite a good appetite, there is only a very restricted differential diagnosis, principally malabsorption or hypermetabolism. In doing a physical examination, therefore, I would pay particular attention to signs of malabsorption (muscular wasting, vitamin deficiencies, purpura) and to signs of thyroid disease with its generalized hypermetabolism and localized autoimmune phenomena, including ophthalmopathy.

Similarly, if a patient complains of hirsutism or other signs of androgen excess, one is immediately thrust into a consideration of ethnic hair distribution and quality. Is there temporal recession of the hairline? Does the hair on the abdomen come up over the umbilicus? Is hair present on the back (rare without marked hyperandrogenism)? How much acne is there? Is acanthosis nigricans present? At the extreme, is there evidence of clitoral enlargement?

Finally, and most important, does the patient look like or unlike the other women in her family?

Direct Assessment of Endocrine Glands

Three endocrine glands are palpable—the thyroid, the testis, and the ovary. Specific attention should be given to each of these.

The thyroid gland should be approached first by inspection—while the patient swallows—for size, symmetry, or localized enlargement. Many thyroid nodules are visible, and inspection often calls attention to lesions that would be missed on palpation. The thyroid should then be felt while the patient swallows, from the front with your thumbs or from behind the patient with the index and third fingers. It is crucial to keep your own fingers from moving while the patient is swallowing. The principal observation is whether there is diffuse enlargement of the thyroid gland (most often Graves' hyperplasia or Hashimoto's thyroiditis) or one or more nodules. Although the consistency of the gland is to be noted, in fact it is often not concordant with the pathology.

Functioning tumors of the testis may be too small to be felt with the fingers, and most internists and general physicians are not skilled in palpation of the ovaries. For this reason, ultrasound and other forms of imaging have become key features of gonadal evaluation and are discussed later.

The size of one other endocrine gland, the pituitary, can be inferred from physical examination for what Cushing called "neighborhood signs." As a pituitary tumor or diffuse enlargement proceeds, it pushes up on the optic chiasm from below, producing a bitemporal hemianopsia first manifested in the upper quadrants, often to a blinking or flashing red light. This finding is too subtle for confidence, however, and pituitary assessment depends on formal visual fields and imaging.

Indirect Assessment of Endocrine Status

Many consequences of hormone action can be detected on physical examination; the results combine with the history to produce a highly reliable differential diagnosis and thus an informed basis for laboratory evaluation and imaging. Among the things to be looked for are the eye signs and dermopathy of Graves' disease, acanthosis nigricans as a clue to insulin resistance, muscular wasting and tremor, changes in the voice due to hypothyroidism or acromegaly, and a general impression of nutrition and its adequacy or excess. Each of these findings is described in more detail with the specific disorder in subsequent chapters.

Laboratory Testing of Endocrine Function

Modern endocrine laboratory evaluation began with the introduction of radioimmunoassay by Berson and Yalow. The precise measurement of hormone concentrations, determined by competitive displacement of specific antibodies, was soon succeeded by competitive binding assays and, more recently, by immunofluorescent and radioluminescent determinations of even greater sensitivity and specificity. It should theoretically be possible to enter the name of a hormone on a laboratory slip and expect to get back a definitive reflection of the status of the patient for that gland. For practical purposes, that has become true of thyroid-stimulating hormone (TSH). Reliable determinations of elevated, normal, and suppressed levels of this hormone by radiochemiluminescent determination have made it the standard of care for thyroid disease and a model for all endocrine laboratory tests. However, it is an exception rather than the rule, and it is worthwhile reviewing why other testing is not as easy and why considerable judgment is required. The following examples illustrate this point.

Pulsatile Hormone Secretion

Many hormones are secreted in pulses rather than steadily. The peaks or valleys of hormones secreted in pulsatile fashion, such as luteinizing hormone or growth hormone, may fall above or below the ostensibly normal range. If such a value is obtained by chance, it can erroneously suggest hypofunction or hyperfunction. Repeating the test with three samples drawn at 30-minute intervals and pooled can clarify this type of problem.

Diurnal Variation

The hypothalamic-pituitary-adrenal axis of cortisol secretion is typically maximal during the day and lower in the evening and night. A plasma cortisol level of 12 μg/dL is normal at 8 AM, but the same value at 8 PM reflects a loss of diurnal rhythm resulting from either stress or hypercorticism. A plasma cortisol sample drawn at midnight is an excellent test for evaluation of overactive adrenal function.

Cyclic Variation

The menstrual cycle provides the most extreme "normal variation" of any hormone level. From the first day of a menstrual period, when estrogen levels may be indistinguishable from those of a normal man, the level rises extraordinarily rapidly and at the 14th day can be as high as in early pregnancy. As a consequence, an estrogen level must be evaluated in the light of the stage of the cycle at which it is drawn.

Age

All clinicians are aware that gonadal hormones show marked differences reflective of the individual's stage of life. It is not as widely known that the adrenal hormone dehydroepiandrosterone (DHEA) is barely secreted during childhood, is actively put out by the adrenal glands from age 8 or so to age 55, and then disappears as mysteriously as it came. At present, there is no clear understanding of the physiologic role of its presence or absence, nor of its control.

Sleep Entrainment

Both prolactin and growth hormone have a sleep-entrained secretory pulse shortly after sleep begins. In people who work at night and sleep during the day, this secretion is clearly related to sleep and not to clock time.

Hormone Antagonism

Certain hormones antagonize the effects of other hormones; it is thus necessary to know the value of each hormone to interpret the clinical phenomenon. The opposite effects of estrogen and androgen on the male breast are a good example. A normal testosterone level combined with an elevated estrogen level, or a normal estrogen level but a decreased androgen level, easily accounts for gynecomastia.

Dynamic Testing

Many endocrine glands have a basal secretory level and a reserve secretion elicited by either a tropic hormone or a change in metabolic or physiologic state. Cortisol secretion can increase 5- to 10-fold in response to stress or adrenocorticotropic hormone (ACTH). Insulin release is stimulated by both glucose and amino acids and by distinct pathways.

Baseline hormone levels can be misleading. The test results in Table 2–1 were obtained from a 30-year-old woman who complained of fatigue and amenorrhea 6 months after a pregnancy during which she had been markedly anemic (hemoglobin, 9 g/dL); she had never been in shock and had received no transfusions.

TABLE 2–1 BASELINE HORMONAL VALUES

	INSULIN IV		TRH IV		GnRH IV	
Time 0	**Glucose 80 mg/dL**	**Cortisol 7.7 μg/dL**	**TSH 3.2 mU/L**	**Prolactin 6.6 ng/mL**	**FSH 8.9 mIU/mL**	**LH 6.7 mIU/mL**
15	47	8.2	5.6	7.6	5.9	9.3
30	23	8.6				
45	30	7.7				
60	38	13.0				
90	50	9.7				
120	63	9.6				

FSH, Follicle-stimulating hormone; *GnRH,* gonadotropin-releasing hormone; *IV,* intravenous; *LH,* luteinizing hormone; *TRH,* thyrotropin-releasing hormone; *TSH,* thyroid-stimulating hormone.

In this study, all basal values are within normal limits. Note, however, that intravenous insulin lowers the blood glucose levels but does not elicit an adequate release of cortisol. Thyrotropin-releasing hormone (TRH) does not induce a normal rise in thyrotropin (TSH) or prolactin. Gonadotropin-releasing hormone (GnRH) evokes a submaximal increase in follicle-stimulating hormone (FSH) and luteinizing hormone (LH).

Hormone and Metabolite Interaction

Insulin is a good example of a hormone whose absolute level is less meaningful than its relationship to the blood glucose level. A plasma insulin of 70 is a normal response to a meal, when the blood glucose level is rising. In contrast, an insulin value of 10 or 12 is abnormal (is not appropriately suppressed) if the glucose level is 40 mg/dL. Indeed, the lower insulin level in a fasting hypoglycemic patient is distinct evidence of spontaneous hyperinsulinism, such as in an islet cell tumor.

Growth hormone represents another instance in which a single random sample cannot be given much meaning. During a day, plasma growth hormone levels vary from values that, if sustained, would be diagnostic of acromegaly to values that, again if sustained, would point to hypopituitarism. In normal people, growth hormone secretion is suppressed by glucose intake. A plasma growth hormone of 8 within an hour of a standard meal containing glucose would be pathologically elevated; it should be less than 2. Similarly, however, a growth hormone value of 2 in a fasting person who had run up a flight of stairs suggests deficient pituitary function.

Most hormones are part of a feedback loop in which an artificial increase, especially by ingestion of the hormone in a medication, decreases endogenous secretion. If a normal person takes 0.1 to 0.3 mg of thyroxine (T_4), hypothalamic secretion of TRH and pituitary secretion of thyrotropin (TSH) are suppressed. Plasma levels of T_4 and triiodothyronine (T_3) may not change, but TSH levels would be decreased and reflections of TSH effect, such as radioactive iodine uptake, would similarly be suppressed. Although ultrasensitive TSH testing has replaced tests of suppressibility for the diagnosis of thyroid disease, tests of suppressibility are the standard approach to evaluating growth hormone and ACTH/cortisol regulation.

Protein Binding

Hormones such as T_4 and cortisol are compartmentalized into a fraction attached to a transport protein (and thus physiologically unavailable) and a free portion able to diffuse into cells and initiate a hormone effect. It is the free or unbound portion that is physiologically regulated; the level of the binding protein may be increased or decreased without physiologic consequence if the free portion is unchanged. The measurement of free T_4 or a free T_4 index (FT_4I) (see Chapter 10) has become the standard second step if a screening TSH value is abnormally high or low.

Testosterone is even more complicated because it is trebly partitioned among sex hormone–binding globulin, albumin, and a free portion. Measurement of the free hormone level is often necessary, particularly when the binding protein level has been artifactually raised or lowered (see Chapter 6).

Laboratory Error

Laboratory error may seem too obvious a source of confusion to mention, but it provides a reminder for an important caution about laboratory testing. It is easy to be seduced by numbers and to consider the laboratory report the final arbiter. In fact, it is the history and physical examination, plus the clinician's judgment, that establish the prior probability of a given diagnosis. Both in choosing and in interpreting laboratory tests, the endocrinologist should establish his or her own expectations before testing. If the physician feels strongly that a particular condition is present, discordant initial laboratory results should not be dissuasive. More detailed testing, as discussed in subsequent chapters, is then appropriate. The clinician's judgment is still a key component of the process.

Imaging

The extraordinary power of modern imaging, particularly ultrasound, computed tomography (CT), and magnetic resonance imaging (MRI), has enriched endocrinology as it has all of medicine. However, the role of imaging in endocrinology is, to my mind, different from its contribution elsewhere.

For one thing, several endocrine glands (the thyroid, the pituitary, and the adrenals in particular) frequently contain clinically insignificant, nonfunctioning adenomas and cysts. Second, functioning and nonfunctioning lesions other than in the thyroid gland can be difficult to distinguish from each other. Thus, except in an emergency (e.g., suspected pituitary apoplexy), the clinician should define the functional state of the gland before requesting imaging. In other words, one should be clear from hormone measurements, including dynamic testing, whether the gland is overactive, underactive, or normal.

In addition, one should have a clear idea of how the radiologist can be expected to help. Such clarity reduces costs by targeting the selection of imaging and making the radiologic findings a truly complementary element of evaluation. The best imaging modalities for the various glands are discussed in their respective chapters. The approach suggested here, however, is broadly applicable.

Conveying Results

Both sophisticated imaging and thorough laboratory testing produce results after the actual office visit. Patients are understandably anxious about the findings and deserve a prompt response. The best approach depends on the circumstance. A new patient with Cushing's syndrome or acromegaly should be given an early in-person visit. A patient with hypothyroidism who understands the disease well and just needs a slight change in T_4 dose can easily be informed with a telephone call. Someone with negative results can be left a message of reassurance and can be encouraged to call back, both to confirm receipt of the information and to get questions answered.

Some New Features of Clinical Endocrinology

Genetics

The decoding of the human genome promises to change the face of medical practice. Ironically, the first human disease in which cancer was prevented by application of genetic testing in susceptible families was the screening for medullary thyroid carcinoma in pedigrees of multiple endocrine neoplasia type 2 (MEN-2). The screening at that time was done by pentagastrin or calcium provocation of calcitonin release. Now the screening for endocrine manifestations of MEN-2 is secondary to screening families for the *RET* proto-oncogene defect that is the basis of the disease. Endocrine testing, such as measurement of calcitonin or plasma catecholamines, is restricted to patients who have the genetic abnormality. In the dangerous variant of the MEN-2 syndrome in which medullary thyroid carcinomas appear in the first year of life, aggressive genetic screening is done during that year, and endocrine testing in patients at risk can justify surgical thyroidectomy before the first birthday.

Hereditary predispositions will certainly emerge for other endocrine disorders and will make it crucial for the clinician to take a revealing family history and follow up even minor clues.

The Internet

Never in history has so much medical information been available to patients. I now routinely ask patients what they already know about their condition or their symptoms. A bit sheepishly in some cases, many patients admit to looking up topics on the World Wide Web and are about to compare what I tell them with what they have already read. Much of that information is accurate, but some is nonsense, and it requires patience and clear explanation before such patients go away satisfied.

Electronic Mail

Although opinions differ widely, I find e-mail an extremely useful advance in communicating with patients who have computers, provided there is a doctor-patient relationship already established personally. Patients have access to you between appointments and on a time frame of mutual convenience. The computer thus reduces anxiety on the patient's part, particularly regarding questions or findings for which they might otherwise hesitate to make an appointment. Reporting laboratory test results is expedited, and accompanying the report with a few sentences of interpretation can be as useful as a telephone call.

It is wise to keep copies of e-mails so that a clear record of the exchange is available. There are, however, several important caveats. Never let an e-mail exchange substitute for a true evaluation, including history and physical examination. I believe that one should not prescribe for a patient whom one has not seen, and one should not provide much interpretation of history or laboratory tests without very fundamental disclaimers. But in an established patient-doctor relationship, e-mail as the patient's choice can be very helpful.

Managed Care

The effort to control health care costs by limiting reimbursement for physician services, laboratory testing, and imaging has had a profound impact throughout medicine. Without taking on the whole issue, I want to comment on several practical consequences.

"Curbsiding"—the request by a physician for patient guidance without being asked to see the patient—has increased strikingly. Consultants can provide some general help to primary care physicians without seeing the patient; however, effectiveness hinges on the history and physical examination done by the primary care physician. The failure to realize that hyperthyroidism is due to a hot nodule, for example, totally distorts the picture and will lead to an erroneous recommendation for treatment. The failure to distinguish a recent onset of amenorrhea and virilization from a polycystic ovary-like syndrome may hide the presence of a readily curable virilizing tumor. The failure to recognize hypoglycemic unresponsiveness may perpetuate a dangerous degree of overinsulinization and elicit inappropriate advice from the consultant. Thus, the consultant must set boundaries and at some point indicate that it is important for a formal consultation to take place.

Costs

Some endocrine workups can be expensive and invite challenge from third-party insurers. The best approach to this concern is a careful history and physical examination, clear establishment of the prior probabilities of certain diagnoses, and then effective use of screening tests before embarking on an unnecessarily extensive evaluation. For example, in a patient with suspected Cushing's syndrome, it is mandatory to establish the presence of hypercorticism before embarking on a search for its cause. Once this lethal but curable disorder has been properly diagnosed, however, no cost should deter one from finding the cause and correcting it. One argument I make is that expensive tests and imaging should be amortized rather than considered an extravagant or unnecessary one-time expense. If a young woman age 30, with a life expectancy of 80 years or more, has a husband and two children to whom her life matters, the $3000 evaluation breaks down to $20 per loved one per year of life expectancy. Any plan manager has to see that this is an appropriate cost.

Management

There are few more gratifying experiences in medicine than recognizing and correcting an endocrine disorder. Patients feel that they have been rescued from a mysterious overtaking of their identity. Body contour, facial appearance, temperament, and well-being are restored to the patient's constitutive status. Deterioration previously attributed to aging or depression or chronic disease is reversed. In brief, something almost miraculous takes place. Even when these goals cannot be achieved, as in diabetes, a major impact on mortality and morbidity can be. Of course, these optimal outcomes require accuracy of diagnosis—but that is only the beginning. A true sharing by patient and physician, based on a sound knowledge of normal physiology, provides the best foundation for choice of therapy and maintenance of a continuing program. The result can be, simply put, wonderful.

CHAPTER 3

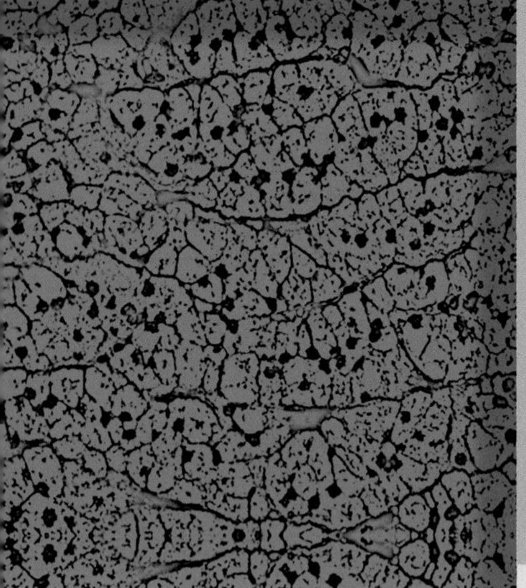

GENETIC CONTROL OF PEPTIDE HORMONE FORMATION

Joel F. Habener

Advances in the fields of molecular and cellular biology have provided new insights into the mechanistic workings of cells. Recombinant deoxyribonucleic acid (DNA) technology and the sequencing (decoding) of the entire human and mouse genomes now make it possible to analyze the precise structure and function of DNA, the genetic substance that is the basis for life. The discovery of the unique biochemical and structural properties of DNA provided the conceptual framework with which to begin a systematic investigation of the origins, development, and organization of life forms.[1]

The completion of the entire sequences of the human and mouse genomes was accomplished in the years 2003 and 2004, and the annotation of the encoded information is nearing completion. The availability of a complete blueprint of the structure and organization of all expressed genes now provides profound insights into the basis of genetically determined diseases. Within the next decade, genotyping of individuals shortly after birth likely will be possible. Therapeutic approaches for the correction of genetic defects by techniques of gene replacement are likely to become a reality, thereby providing insights into relative risks for developing diseases.

The polypeptide hormones constitute a critically important and diverse set of regulatory molecules encoded by the genome whose functions are to convey specific information among cells and organs. This type of molecular communication arose early in the development of life and evolved into a complex system for the control of growth, development, and reproduction and for the maintenance of metabolic homeostasis. These hormones, including the many chemokines and cytokines primarily involved in the regulation of the immune system, consist of approximately 400 or more small proteins ranging from as few as three amino acids (thyrotropin-releasing hormone, or TRH) to 192 amino acids (growth hormone). In a broader sense, these polypeptides function both as hormones, whose actions on distant organs are mediated by way of their transport through the bloodstream, and as local cell-to-cell communicators (Fig. 3–1). The latter function of the polypeptide hormones is exemplified by their elaboration and secretion within neurons of the central, autonomic, and peripheral nervous systems, where they act as neurotransmitters, and in leukocytes where they modulate immune responses. These multiple modes of expression of the polypeptide hormone genes have aroused great interest in the specific functions of these peptides and the mechanisms of their synthesis and release.

This chapter reviews the diverse structures of genes encoding peptide hormones and the multiple mechanisms that govern their expression. The synthesis of nonpeptide hormones (e.g., catecholamines, thyroid hormones, and steroid hormones)

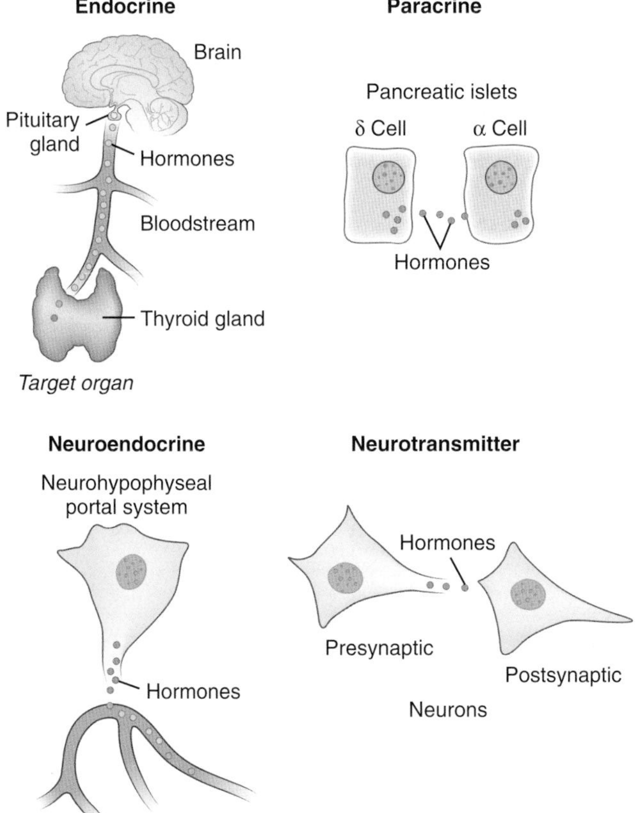

Figure 3–1 ▪ Different modes of utilization of polypeptide hormones in expression of their biologic actions. The peptide hormones are expressed in at least four ways in fulfilling their functions as cellular messenger molecules: (1) endocrine mode, for purposes of communication among organs (e.g., pituitary-thyroid axis); (2) paracrine mode, for communication among adjacent cells, often located within endocrine organs; (3) neuroendocrine mode, for synthesis and release of peptides from specialized peptidergic neurons for action on distant organs through the bloodstream (e.g., neuroendocrine peptides of hypothalamus); and (4) neurotransmitter mode, for action of peptides in concert with classic amino acid–derived aminergic transmitters in the neuronal communication network. Identical polypeptides are often utilized in the nervous system both as neuroendocrine hormones and as neurotransmitters. In some instances, the same gene product is used in all four modes of expression.

involves the action of multiple enzymes and hence the expression of multiple genes; these are discussed in the individual chapters devoted to such hormones.

Evolution of Peptide Hormones and Their Functions

Peptide hormones arose early in the evolution of life. Indeed, polypeptides that are structurally similar to mammalian peptides are present in lower vertebrates, insects, yeasts, and bacteria.[2] An example of the early evolution of regulatory peptides is the α-factor (mating pheromone) of yeast, which is similar in structure to gonadotropin-releasing hormone (GnRH).[3] The oldest member of the cholecystokinin-gastrin family of peptides appeared at least 500 million years ago in the protochordate *Ciona intestinalis*.[4]

Thus, the genes encoding polypeptide hormones, and particularly regulatory peptides, evolved early in the development of life and initially fulfilled the function of cell-to-cell communication to cope with problems concerning nourishment, growth, development, and reproduction. As specialized organs connected by a circulatory system developed during evolution, similar, if not identical, gene products became hormones for purposes of organ-to-organ communication.

Steps in Expression of a Protein-Encoding Gene

The steps involved in transfer of information encoded in the polynucleotide language of DNA to the poly–amino acid language of biologically active proteins involve gene transcription, posttranscriptional processing of ribonucleic acids (RNAs), translation, and posttranslational processing of the proteins. The expression of genes and protein synthesis can be considered in terms of several major processes, any one or more of which may serve as specific control points in the regulation of gene expression (Fig. 3–2).

Rearrangements and Transpositions of DNA Segments. These processes occur over many years (eons) in evolution, with the exception of uncommon mechanisms of somatic gene rearrangements such as the rearrangements in the immunoglobulin genes during the lifetime of an individual.

Transcription. Synthesis of RNA results in the formation of RNA copies of the two gene alleles and is catalyzed by the basal RNA polymerase II–associated transcription factors.

Posttranscriptional Processing. Specific modifications of the RNA include the formation of messenger RNA (mRNA) from the precursor RNA by way of excision and rejoining of RNA segments (introns and exons) and modifications of the 3′ end of the RNA by polyadenylation and of the 5′ end by addition of 7-methylguanine “caps.”

Translation. Amino acids are assembled by base pairing of the nucleotide triplets (anticodons) of the specific “carrier” aminoacylated transfer RNAs to the corresponding codons of the mRNA bound to polyribosomes and are polymerized into the polypeptide chains.

Posttranslational Processing and Modification. Final steps in protein synthesis may involve one or more cleavages of peptide bonds, which result in the conversion of biosynthetic precursors (prohormones), to intermediate or final forms of the protein; derivatization of amino acids (e.g., glycosylation, phosphorylation, acetylation, myristoylation); and the folding of the processed polypeptide chain into its native conformation.

Each of the specific steps of gene expression requires the integration of precise enzymatic and other biochemical reactions. These processes have developed to provide high fidelity in the reproduction of the encoded information and to provide control points for the expression of the specific phenotype of cells.

The posttranslational processing of proteins creates diversity in gene expression through modifications of the protein. Although the functional information contained in a protein is ultimately encoded in the primary amino acid sequence, the specific biologic activities are a consequence of the higher order secondary, tertiary, and quaternary structures of the polypeptide. Given the wide range of possible specific modifications of the amino acids, such as glycosylation, phosphorylation, acetylation, amidation, lipidation, and sulfation,[5] any one of which may affect the conformation or function of the protein, a single gene may ultimately encode a wide variety of specific proteins as a result of posttranslational processes.

Polypeptide hormones are synthesized in the form of larger precursors that appear to fulfill several functions in biologic systems (Fig. 3–3), including (1) intracellular trafficking, by which the cell distinguishes among specific classes of proteins

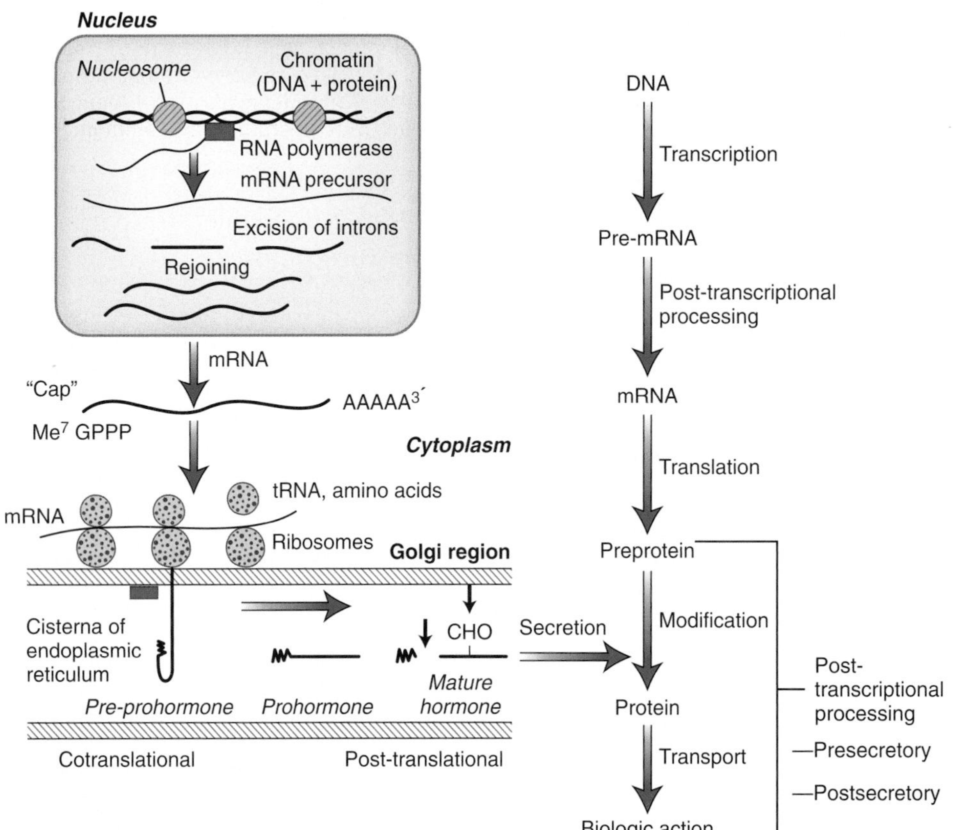

Figure 3–2 ▪ Steps in the cellular synthesis of polypeptide hormones. Steps that take place within the nucleus include transcription of genetic information into a messenger ribonucleic acid (mRNA) precursor (pre-mRNA) followed by posttranscriptional processing, which includes RNA cleavage, excision of introns, and rejoining of exons, resulting in formation of mRNA. Ends of mRNA are modified by addition of methylguanosine caps at the 5′ end and addition of poly(A) tracts at the 3′ ends. The cytoplasmic mRNA is assembled with ribosomes. Amino acids, carried by aminoacylated transfer RNAs (tRNAs), are then polymerized into a polypeptide chain. The final step in protein synthesis is that of posttranslational processing. These processes take place both during growth of the nascent polypeptide chain (cotranslational) and after release of the completed chain (posttranslational), and they include proteolytic cleavages of polypeptide chain (conversion of pre-prohormones or prohormones to hormones), derivatizations of amino acids (e.g., glycosylation, phosphorylation), and cross-linking and assembly of the polypeptide chain into its conformed structure. The diagram depicts posttranslational synthesis and processing of a typical secreted polypeptide, which requires vectorial or unidirectional transport of the polypeptide chain across the membrane bilayer of the endoplasmic reticulum, thus resulting in sequestration of the polypeptide in the cisterna of the endoplasmic reticulum, a first step in the export of proteins destined for secretion from the cell (see Fig. 3–6). Most translational processing occurs within the cell as depicted (presecretory) and in some instances outside the cell, when further proteolytic cleavages or modifications of the protein may take place (postsecretory). *CHO,* carbohydrate.

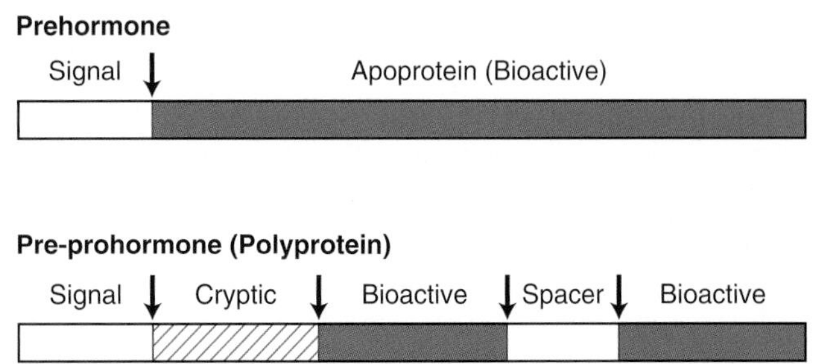

Figure 3–3 ▪ Diagrammatic depiction of two configurations of precursors of polypeptide hormones. Diagrams represent polypeptide backbones of protein sequences encoded in mRNA. One form of precursor consists of the NH_2-terminal signal, or presequence, followed by the apoprotein portion of the polypeptide that needs no further proteolytic processing for activity. A second form of precursor is a pre-prohormone that consists of the NH_2-terminal signal sequence followed by a polyprotein, or prohormone, sequence consisting of two or more peptide domains linked together that are subsequently liberated by cleavages during posttranslational processing of the prohormone. The reason for synthesis of polypeptide hormones in the form of precursors is only partly understood. Clearly, NH_2-terminal signal sequences function in the early stages of transport of polypeptide into the secretory pathway. Prohormones, or polyproteins, often serve to provide a source of multiple bioactive peptides (see Fig. 3–4). However, many prohormones contain peptide sequences that are removed by cleavage and have no known biologic activity, and they are referred to as *cryptic peptides,* perhaps awaiting the discovery of unique biologic activities. Other peptides may serve as spacer sequences between two bioactive peptides (e.g., the C peptide of proinsulin). In instances in which a bioactive peptide is located at the COOH terminus of the prohormone, the NH_2-terminal prohormone sequence may simply facilitate the cotranslational translocation of polypeptide in endoplasmic reticulum (see Fig. 3–6).

and directs them to their sites of action, and (2) the generation of multiple biologic activities from a common genetically encoded protein by regulated or cell-specific variations in the posttranslational modifications (Fig. 3–4).

All the peptide hormones and regulatory peptides studied thus far contain signal or leader sequences at the amino termini; these hydrophobic helical sequences recognize specific sites on the membranes of the rough endoplasmic reticulum, which results in the transport of nascent polypeptides into the secretory pathway of the cell (see Figs. 3–2 and 3–3).[6] The consequence of the specialized signal sequences of the precursor proteins is that proteins destined for secretion are selected from a great many other cellular proteins for sequestration and subsequent packaging into secretory granules and export from the cell. In addition, most, if not all, of the smaller hormones and regulatory peptides are produced as a consequence of posttranslational cleavages of the precursors within the Golgi complex of secretory cells.

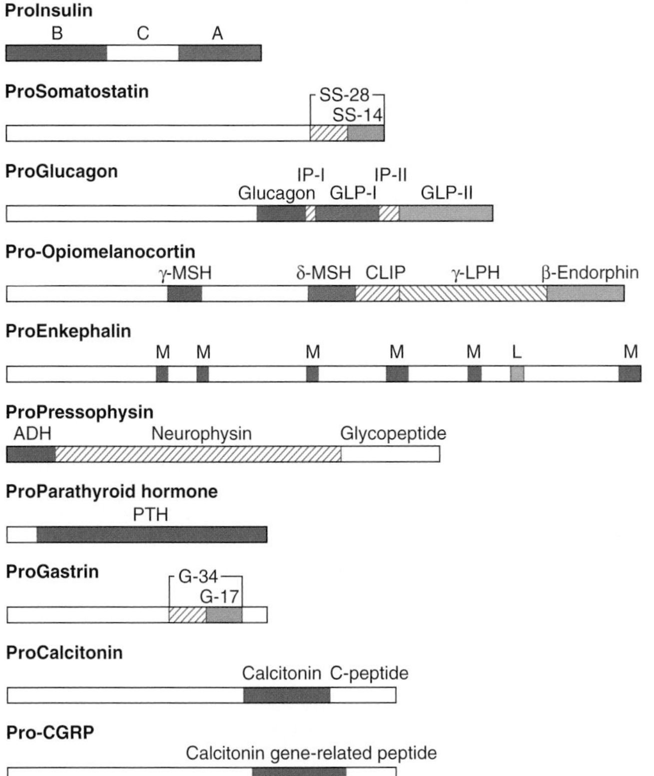

Figure 3–4 ▪ Diagrammatic illustration of primary structures of several prohormones. The *darkly shaded areas* of prohormones denote regions of sequence that constitute known biologically active peptides after their posttranslational cleavage from prohormones. Sequences indicated by *hatching* denote regions of precursor that alter the biologic specificity of that region of precursor. For example, the precursor contains the sequence of γ-melanocyte-stimulating hormone (γ-MSH), but when the latter is covalently attached to the CLIP peptide, it constitutes adrenocorticotropic hormone (corticotropin, ACTH). Somatostatin-28 (SS-28) is an NH_2-terminally extended form of somatostatin-14 (SS-14) that has higher potency than SS-14 on certain receptors. The neurophysin sequence linked to the COOH terminus of vasopressin (ADH) functions as a carrier protein for the ADH hormone during its transport down the axon of neurons in which it is synthesized. The precursor proenkephalin represents a polyprotein that contains multiple similar peptides within its sequence, either met-enkephalin (M) or leu-enkephalin (L). Procalcitonin and procalcitonin gene–related product (CGRP) share identical NH_2-terminal sequences but differ in their COOH-terminal regions as a result of alternative splicing during the posttranscriptional processing of the RNA precursor. *γ-LPH,* γ-Lipotropin; *GLP,* glucagon-like peptide; *IP,* intervening peptide.

Subcellular Structure of Cells that Secrete Protein Hormones

Cells whose principal functions are the synthesis and export of proteins contain highly developed, specialized subcellular organelles for the translocation of secreted proteins and their packaging into secretory granules. The subcellular pathways utilized in protein secretion have been elucidated largely through the early efforts of Palade[7] (reviewed by Jamieson[8]). Secretory cells contain an abundance of endoplasmic reticulum, Golgi complexes, and secretory granules (Fig. 3–5). The proteins that are to be secreted from the cells are transferred during their synthesis into these subcellular organelles, which transport the proteins to the plasma membrane.

Protein secretion begins with translation of the mRNA encoding the precursor of the protein on the rough endoplasmic reticulum, which consists of polyribosomes attached to elaborate membranous saccules that contain cavities (cisternae). The newly synthesized, nascent proteins are discharged into the cisternae by transport across the lipid bilayer of the membrane. Within the cisternae of the endoplasmic reticulum, proteins are carried to the Golgi complex by mechanisms that are incompletely understood. The proteins gain access to the Golgi complex either by direct transfer from the cisternae, which are in continuity with the membranous channels of the Golgi complex, or by way of shuttling vesicles known as transition elements (see Fig. 3–5).

Within the Golgi complex, the proteins are packaged into secretory vesicles or secretory granules by their budding from the Golgi stacks in the form of immature granules. Immature granules undergo maturation through condensation of the proteinaceous material and application of a specific coat around the initial Golgi membrane. On receiving the appropriate extracellular stimuli (regulated pathway of secretion), the granules migrate to the cell surface and fuse to become continuous with the plasma membrane, which results in the release of proteins into the extracellular space, a process known as *exocytosis.*

The second pathway of intracellular transport and secretion involves the transport of proteins contained within secretory vesicles and immature secretory granules (see Fig. 3–5). Although the use of this alternative vesicle-mediated transport pathway remains to be demonstrated conclusively (it is generally considered to be a constitutive, or unregulated, pathway), different extracellular stimuli may modulate hormone secretion differently, depending on the pathway of secretion. For example, in the parathyroid gland and in the pituitary cell line derived from corticotropic cells (AtT-20), newly synthesized hormone is released more rapidly than hormone synthesized earlier. These findings suggest that the newly synthesized hormone may be transported by way of a vesicle-mediated pathway without incorporation into mature storage granules.

Intracellular Segregation and Transport of Polypeptide Hormones

Specific amino acid sequences encoded in the proteins serve as directional signals in the sorting of proteins within subcellular organelles.[6,9,10] A typical eukaryotic cell synthesizes an estimated 5000 different proteins during its lifespan. These different proteins are synthesized by a common pool of polyribosomes. However, each of the different proteins is directed to a specific location within the cell, where its biologic function is expressed. For example, specific groups of proteins are transported into mitochondria, into membranes, into the nucleus, or into other subcellular organelles, where they serve as regulatory proteins, enzymes, or structural proteins. A subset of proteins is specifi-

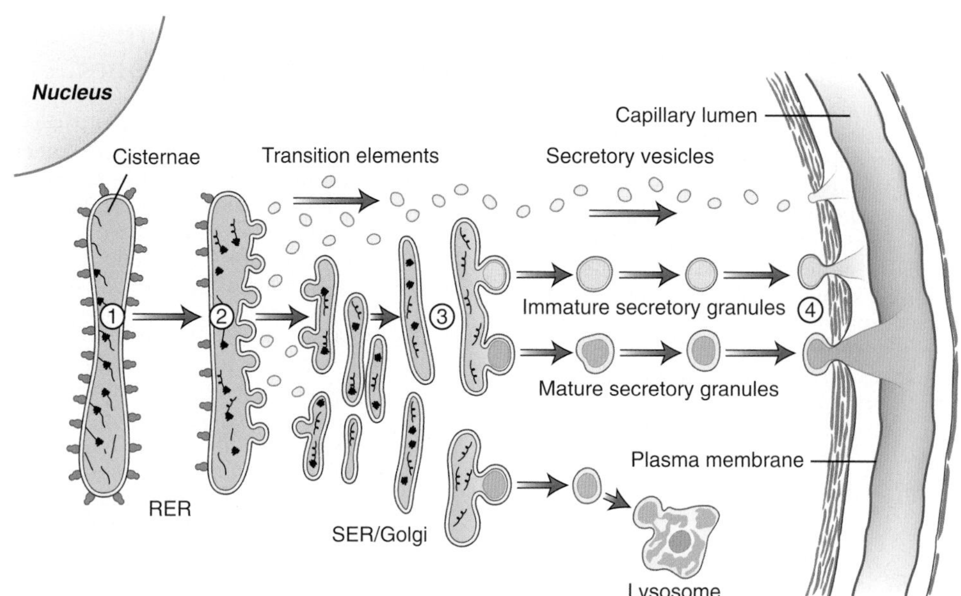

Figure 3–5 ▪ Schematic representation of subcellular organelles involved in transport and secretion of polypeptide hormones or other secreted proteins within a protein-secreting cell. (1) Synthesis of proteins on polyribosomes attached to endoplasmic reticulum (RER) and vectorial discharge of proteins through the membrane into the cisterna. (2) Formation of shuttling vesicles (transition elements) from endoplasmic reticulum followed by their transport to and incorporation by the Golgi complex. (3) Formation of secretory granules in the Golgi complex. (4) Transport of secretory granules to the plasma membrane, fusion with the plasma membrane, and exocytosis resulting in the release of granule contents into the extracellular space. Note that secretion may occur by transport of secretory vesicles and immature granules as well as mature granules. Some granules are taken up and hydrolyzed by lysosomes (crinophagy). *Golgi,* Golgi complex; *RER,* rough endoplasmic reticulum; *SER,* smooth endoplasmic reticulum. (From Habener JF. Hormone biosynthesis and secretion. In Felig P, Baxter JD, Broadus AE, et al, eds. Endocrinology and Metabolism. New York: McGraw-Hill, 1981: 29-59.)

cally designed for export from the cell (e.g., immunoglobulins, serum albumin, blood coagulation factors, and protein and polypeptide hormones).

This process of directional transport of proteins involves sophisticated informational signals. Because the information for these translocation processes must reside either wholly or in part within the primary structure or in the conformational properties of the protein, sequential posttranslational modifications may be crucial for determining the specificity of protein function. Continued investigations of protein sorting and trafficking in cells have revealed increased complexities beyond the simple paradigm illustrated in Figure 3–5.[11] The sequential sorting of proteins to their final destinations, be they export from the cells (secretion) or targeting to a subcellular compartment or organelle, takes place not only in the Golgi apparatus but also pre-Golgi in the endoplasmic reticulum and post-Golgi in endosomes and tubulosaccules.[12] It is interesting to contemplate that each and every one of the 5000 or so proteins expressed in a given cell contains a specific targeting signal responsible for directing the protein to its final destination. These targeting signals consist of short stretches of amino acids in the proteins that serve as "ZIP codes" to ensure their accurate delivery. Modern approaches using proteomics and bioinformatics are able to predict localization in cells based on the characteristics of these targeting signals.[13]

Signal Sequences in Peptide Prohormone Processing and Secretion

The early processes of protein secretion that result in the specific transport of exported proteins into the secretory pathway are now becoming better understood.[6,10-15] Initial clues to this process came from determinations of the amino acid sequences of the proteins programmed by the cell-free translation of mRNAs encoding secreted polypeptides.[16] Secreted proteins are synthesized as precursors that are extended at their NH_2 termini by sequences of 15 to 30 amino acids, called *signal* or *leader sequences.* Signal sequence extensions, or their functional equivalents, are required for targeting the ribosomal or nascent protein to specific membranes and for the vectorial transport of the protein across the membrane of the endoplasmic reticulum. On emergence of the signal sequence from the large ribosomal subunit, the ribosomal complex specifically makes contact with the membrane, which results in translocation of the nascent polypeptide across the endoplasmic reticulum membrane into the cisterna as the first step in the transport of the polypeptide within the secretory pathway. These observations initially left unanswered the question of how specific polyribosomes that translate mRNAs encoding secretory proteins recognize and attach to the endoplasmic reticulum (Fig. 3–6).

Because microsomal membranes in vitro reproduce the processing activity of intact cells, it was possible to identify macromolecules responsible for processing of the precursor and for translocation activities.[17] The endoplasmic reticulum and the cytoplasm contain an aggregate of molecules, called a *signal recognition particle complex,* that consists of at least 16 different proteins, including three guanosine triphosphatases to generate energy[18] and a 7S RNA.[6,10,19] (Most recently reviewed in reference 20). This complex, or particle, binds to the polyribosomes involved in the translation of mRNAs encoding secretory polypeptides when the NH_2-terminal signal sequence first emerges from the large subunit of the ribosome.

The specific interaction of the signal recognition particle with the nascent signal sequence and the polyribosome arrests further translation of mRNA. The nascent protein remains in a

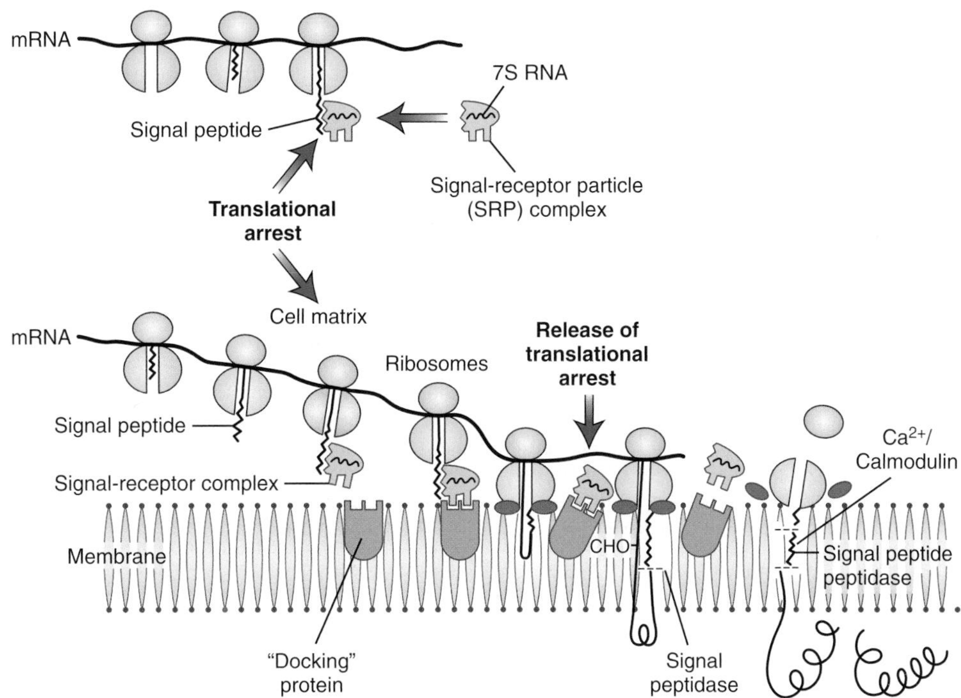

Figure 3–6 ▪ Diagram depicting cellular events in initial stages of synthesis of a polypeptide hormone according to the signal hypothesis. In this schema, a signal recognition particle, consisting of a complex of six proteins and an RNA (7S RNA), interacts with the NH_2-terminal signal peptide of the nascent polypeptide chain after approximately 70 amino acids are polymerized, which results in the arrest of further growth of the polypeptide chain. The complex of the signal recognition particle and the polyribosome nascent chain remains in a state of translational arrest until it recognizes and binds to a docking protein, which is a receptor protein located on the cytoplasmic face of the endoplasmic reticular membrane. This interaction of the signal recognition particle complex with docking protein releases the translational block, and protein synthesis resumes. The nascent polypeptide chain is discharged across the membrane bilayer into the cisterna of the endoplasmic reticulum and is released from the signal peptide by cleavage with a signal peptidase located in the cisternal face of the membrane. In this model, the signal peptide is cleaved from the polypeptide chain by signal peptidase before the chain is completed (cotranslational cleavage). The configuration of the polypeptide during transport across the membrane and the forces and mechanisms responsible for its translocation are unknown. The loop, or hairpin, configuration of the chain that is shown is an arbitrary model; other models are equally possible.

state of arrested translation until it finds a high-affinity binding protein on the endoplasmic reticulum, the signal recognition particle receptor, or docking protein.[6] On interaction with the specific docking protein, the translational block is released and protein synthesis resumes. The protein is then transferred across the membrane of the endoplasmic reticulum through a proteinaceous tunnel called the *translocon*.[20]

At some point, near the termination of synthesis of the polypeptide chain, the NH_2-terminal signal sequence is cleaved from the polypeptide by a specific signal peptidase located on the cisternal surface of the endoplasmic reticulum membrane. The removal of the hydrophobic signal sequence frees the protein (prohormone or hormone) so that it may assume its characteristic secondary structure during transport through the endoplasmic reticulum and the Golgi apparatus. Interestingly, after its cleavage from the protein by signal peptidase, the signal peptide may sometimes be further cleaved in the endoplasmic reticulum membrane to produce a biologically active peptide. The signal sequence of preprolactin of 30 amino acids, for example, is cleaved by a signal peptide peptidase to give a charged peptide of 20 amino acids that is released into the cytosol, where it binds to calmodulin and inhibits Ca^{2+}-calmodulin-dependent phosphodiesterase.[21]

This sequence in the directional transport of specific polypeptides ensures optimal cotranslational processing of secretory proteins, even when synthesis commences on free ribosomes. The presence of a cytoplasmic form of the signal recognition particle complex that blocks translation guarantees that the synthesis of the presecretory proteins is not completed in the cytoplasm; the efficient transfer of proteins occurs only after contact has been made with the specific receptor or docking protein on the membrane. Although the identification of the signal recognition particle and the docking protein explains the specificity of the binding of ribosomes containing mRNAs encoding the secretory proteins, it does not explain the mode of translocation of the nascent polypeptide chain across the membrane bilayer. Further dissection and analysis of the membrane have identified other macromolecules that are responsible for the transport process.[6]

Cellular Processing of Prohormones

The signal sequences of prehormones and pre-prohormones are involved in the transport of these molecules, but the function of the intermediate hormone precursors (prohormones) is not fully understood. The conversion of prohormones to their final products begins in the Golgi apparatus. For example, the time that elapses between the synthesis of pre-proparathyroid hormone and the first appearance of parathyroid hormone correlates closely with the time required for radioautographic grains to reach the Golgi apparatus.[22] Similarly, the conversion of proinsulin to insulin takes place about an hour after the synthesis of proinsulin is complete, and processing of proinsulin to insulin and C peptide takes place during the transport within the secretory granule.[23] The conversion of prohormones to hormones can also be blocked by inhibitors of cellular energy production such as antimycin A and dinitrophenol[24] and by drugs that interfere with the functions of microtubules (vinblastine, colchicine).[25] Thus, the translocation of the prohormone from the rough endoplasmic reticulum to the Golgi complex depends on metabolic energy and probably involves microtubules.

There is no evidence that sequences that are specific to the prohormone contribute to or are chemically involved in transport of the newly synthesized protein from the rough endoplasmic reticulum to the Golgi apparatus or that they are involved in the packaging of the hormone in the vesicles or granules. Analyses of the structures of the primary products of translation of mRNAs encoding secretory proteins indicate that many of these are not synthesized in the form of prohormone intermediates (see Fig. 3–3). It remains puzzling that some secretory proteins (e.g., parathyroid hormone, insulin, serum albumin) are formed by way of intermediate precursors, whereas others (e.g., growth hormone, prolactin, albumin) are not.

Size constraints may be placed on the length of a secretory polypeptide. When the bioactivity of peptides resides at the COOH termini of the precursors (e.g., somatostatin, calcitonin, gastrin), NH_2-terminal extensions may be required to provide a sufficient "spacer" sequence to allow the signal sequence on the growing nascent polypeptide chain to emerge from the large ribosome subunit for interaction with the signal recognition particle and to provide adequate polypeptide length to span the large ribosomal subunit and the membrane of the endoplasmic reticulum during vectorial transport of the nascent polypeptide across the membrane (see Fig. 3–6). When the final hormonal product is 100 amino acids long or longer (e.g., growth hormone, prolactin, or the α and β subunits of the glycoprotein hormones), there may be no requirement for a prohormone intermediate.

Although the exact functions of prohormones remain unknown, certain details of their cleavages have been established. Unlike the situation with prehormones, in which the amino acids at the cleavage site between the signal sequence and the remainder of the molecule (hormone or prohormone) vary from one hormone to the next, the cleavage sites of the prohormone intermediates consist of the basic amino acid lysine or arginine, or both, usually two to three in tandem. This sequence is preferentially cleaved by endopeptidases with trypsin-like activities.

Specific *prohormone-converting enzymes* (PCs) consist of a family of at least eight such enzymes.[26-28] The most studied of the isozymes are PC2 and PC1/3, which are responsible for the cleavages of proinsulin between the A chain/C peptide and B chain/C peptide, respectively. A rare patient missing PC1 presented with childhood obesity, hypogonadotropic hypogonadism, and hypercortisolism and was found to have elevated proinsulin levels and presumably widespread abnormalities in neuropeptide modification.[29] Targeted disruption of the PC2 gene in mice resulted in incomplete processing of proinsulin, leaving the A chain and C peptide intact.[30] Notably, proglucagon in the pancreas remains completely unprocessed, indicating that PC2 is required for the formation of glucagon. As a consequence of defective PC2 activity and low levels of glucagon, the mice have severe chronic hypoglycemia.

After endopeptidase cleavage, the remaining basic residues are selectively removed by exopeptidases with activity resembling that of carboxypeptidase B. In the instances in which the COOH terminal residue of the peptide hormone is amidated, a process that appears to enhance the stability of a peptide by conferring resistance to carboxypeptidase, specific amidation enzymes (peptide amidating monooxygenases) in the Golgi complex work in concert with the cleavage enzymes for modification of the COOH terminal of the bioactive peptides.[31,32]

All proproteins and prohormones are cleaved by PC enzymatic processes within the Golgi complex of cells of diverse origins. The significance of specific cleavages of specific prohormones remains incompletely understood, as does the reason for the existence of prohormone intermediates in some but not all secretory proteins. As indicated earlier, precursor peptides removed from the prohormones may have intrinsic biologic activities that are as yet unrecognized.

Processes of Hormone Secretion

Specific extracellular stimuli control the secretion of polypeptide hormones. The stimuli consist of changes in homeostatic balance; the hormonal products released in response to the stimuli act on the respective target organs to reestablish homeostasis (Fig. 3–7). Endocrine systems typically consist of closed-loop feedback mechanisms such that, if hormones from organ A stimulate organ B, organ B in turn secretes hormones that

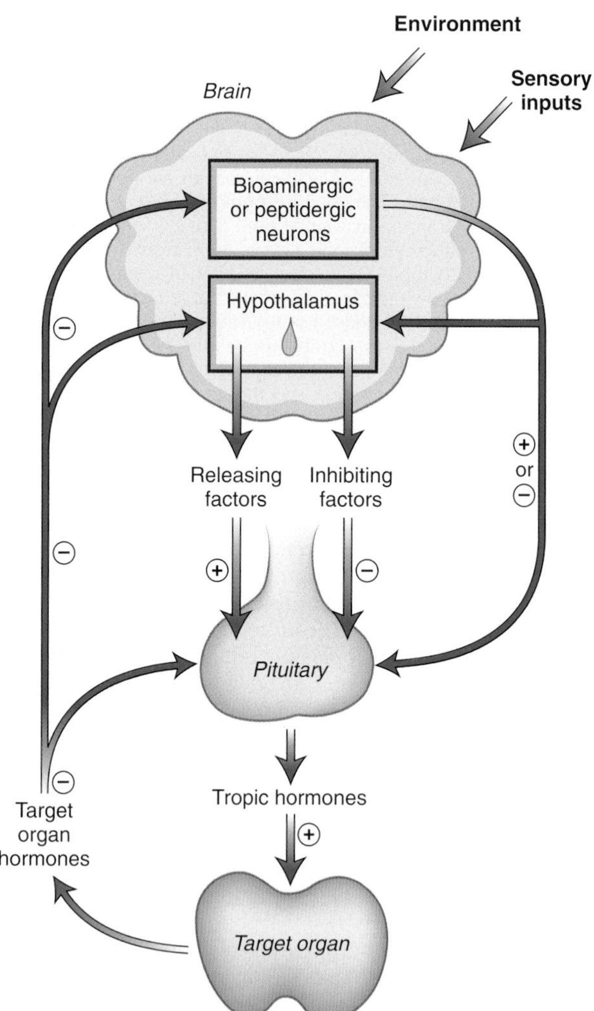

Figure 3–7 ▪ Regulatory feedback loops of the hypothalamic-pituitary-target organ axis. Being a combination of both stimulatory and inhibitory factors, hormones often act in concert to maintain homeostatic balance in the presence of physiologic or pathophysiologic perturbations. The concerted actions of hormones typically establish closed feedback loops by stimulatory and inhibitory effects coupled to maintain homeostasis.

inhibit the secretion of hormones from organ A. The concerted actions of both positive and negative hormonal influences thereby maintain homeostasis. An example of such negative feedback regulation is the control of the secretion of adrenocorticotropic hormone (ACTH) by the anterior pituitary gland. Increased ACTH stimulates the adrenal cortex to produce and secrete cortisol, which in turn feeds back to suppress further pituitary secretion of ACTH. These regulatory processes may also include feedback loops in which nonhormonal substances controlled by the target organs regulate hormone secretion. For example, an increase in the concentration of plasma electrolytes as a consequence of dehydration stimulates the release of arginine vasopressin (also called antidiuretic hormone [ADH]) in the neural lobe of the pituitary gland, and vasopressin in turn acts on the kidney to increase the reabsorption of water from the renal tubule, thereby readjusting serum electrolyte concentrations toward normal levels.

In many instances, endocrine regulation is complex and involves the responses of several endocrine glands and their respective target organs. After a meal, the release of a dozen or more hormones is triggered as a result of gastric distention, variations in the pH of the contents of the stomach and duodenum, and increased concentrations of glucose, fatty acids, and amino acids in the blood. The rise in plasma glucose and amino acid levels stimulates the release of insulin and the incretin hormones glucagon-like peptide 1 and glucose-dependent insulinotropic peptide and suppresses the release of glucagon from the pancreas. Both effects promote the net uptake of glucose by the liver; insulin increases cellular transport and uptake of glucose, and the lower blood levels of glucagon decrease the outflow of glucose because of diminished rates of glycogenolysis and gluconeogenesis.

Structure of a Gene Encoding a Polypeptide Hormone

Structural analyses of gene sequences have resulted in at least three major discoveries that are important for understanding the expression of peptide-encoding genes. First, sequences of almost all the known biologically active hormonal peptides are contained within larger precursors that often encode other peptides, many of which are of unknown biologic activity. Second, the transcribed regions of genes (exons) are interrupted by sequences (introns) that are transcribed but subsequently cleaved from the initial RNA transcripts during their nuclear processing and assembly into specific mRNAs. Third, specific regulatory sequences reside in the regions of DNA flanking the structural genes as well as within introns, and these DNA sequences constitute specific targets for the interactions of DNA-binding proteins that determine the level of expression of the gene.

The DNA of higher organisms is wound around proteins forming tightly and regularly packed chromosomal structures called *nucleosomes*.[33,34] Nucleosomes are composed of four or five different histone subunits that form a core structure about which approximately 140 base pairs of genomic DNA are wound. The nucleosomes are arranged similarly to beads on a string, and coils of nucleosomes form the fundamental organizational units of the eukaryotic chromosome.

The nucleosomal structure serves several purposes. For example, nucleosomes enable the large amount of DNA ($\sim 2 \times 10^9$ pairs) of the genome to be compacted into a small volume. Nucleosomes are involved in the replication of DNA and gene transcription. In addition to histones, other proteins are associated with DNA, and the complex nucleoprotein structure provides specific recognition sites for regulatory proteins and enzymes involved in DNA replication, rearrangements of DNA segments, and gene expression. The acetylation and deacetylation of histone-rich chromatin is involved in the regulation of gene transcription.

The topography of a typical protein-encoding gene consists of two functional units (Fig. 3–8): (1) A transcriptional region and (2) A promoter or regulatory region.

Transcriptional Regions

The transcriptional unit is the segment of the gene that is transcribed into an mRNA precursor. The sequences corresponding to the mature mRNA consist of the exon sequences that are spliced from the primary transcript during the cotranscriptional and posttranscriptional processing of the precursor RNA; these exons contain the code for the mRNA sequence that is translated into protein and for untranslated sequences at the 5′- and 3′-flanking regions. The 5′ sequence typically begins with a methylated guanine residue known as the *cap site.* The 3′-untranslated region contains within it a short sequence, AATAAA, that signals the site of cleavage of the 3′ end of the RNA and the addition of a poly(A) tract of 100 to 200 nucleotides located approximately 20 bases from the AATAAA sequence. Although the functions of these modifications of the ends of mRNAs are not completely understood, they appear to provide signals for leaving the nucleus; enhance stability, perhaps through providing resistance to degradation by exonucleases; and stimulate initiation of mRNA translation. The protein-coding sequence of the mRNA begins with the codon AUG for methionine and ends with the codon immediately preceding one of the three nonsense, or stop, codons (UGA, UAA, and UAG).

The nature of the enzymatic splicing mechanisms that result in the excision of intron-coded sequences and the rejoining of exon-coded sequences is incompletely understood. Helpful interpretations of the splicing processes are provided in recent reviews.[35,36] Short "consensus" sequences of nucleotides reside at the splice junctions—for example, the bases GT and AG at the 5′ and 3′ ends of the introns, respectively, are invariant—and a polypyrimidine stretch is found near the AG.[37] Splicing involves a series of cleavage and ligation steps that remove the introns as a lariat structure with its 5′ end ligated near the 3′ end of the introns and ligate the two adjacent exons together. An elaborate machinery (the spliceosome) consisting of five *small nuclear RNAs* (snRNAs) and roughly 50 proteins direct these steps, guided by base pairing between three of the snRNAs and the mRNA precursor.

Regulatory Regions

The molecular mechanisms involved in the regulation of the expression of genes that encode polypeptides are becoming understood in some detail. As a result of experiments involving the deletions of 5′ sequence segments that reside upstream from structural genes, followed by analyses of the expression of the genes after introduction into cell lines, several insights have been obtained. These regulatory sequences, termed *promoters* and *enhancers,* consist of short polynucleotide sequences (see Fig. 3–8). They can be divided into at least four groups with respect to their functions and distances from the transcriptional initiation site.

First, the sequence *TATAA* (TATA, or Goldberg-Hogness, box) is usually present in the more proximal promoter within 25 to 30 nucleotides upstream from the point of transcriptional initiation. The TATA sequence is required to ensure the accuracy of initiation of transcription at a particular site. The TATA box directs the binding of a complex of several proteins, including RNA polymerase II. The proteins, referred to as *TATA box transcription factors* (TFs), number six or more basal factors (IIA,

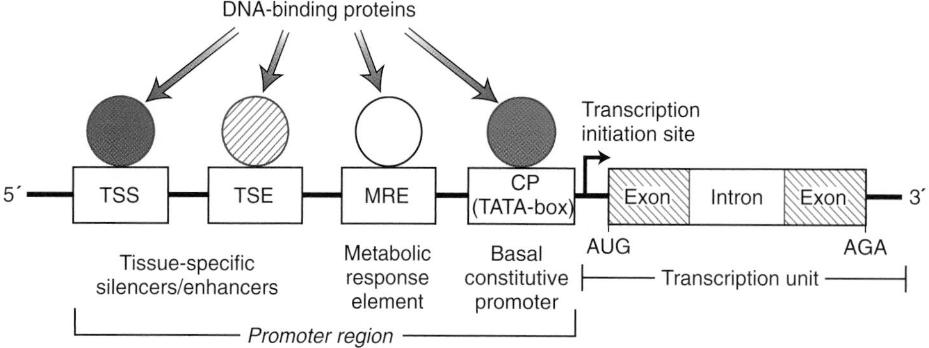

Figure 3–8 ▪ Diagrammatic structure of a "consensus" gene encoding a prototypical polypeptide hormone. Such a gene typically consists of a promoter region and a transcription unit. The transcription unit is the region of deoxyribonucleic acid (DNA) composed of exons and introns that is transcribed into a messenger ribonucleic acid (mRNA) precursor. Transcription begins at the cap site sequence in DNA and extends several hundred bases beyond the poly(A) addition site in the 3′ region. During posttranscriptional processing of the RNA precursor, the 5′ end of mRNA is capped by addition of methylguanosine residues. The transcript is then cleaved at the poly(A) addition site approximately 20 bases 3′ to the AATAAA signal sequence, and the poly(A) tract is added to the 3′ end of the RNA. Introns are cleaved from the RNA precursor, and exons are joined together. Dinucleotides GT and AG are invariably found at the 5′ and 3′ ends of introns. Translation of mRNA starts with the codon ATG for methionine. Translation is terminated when the polyribosome reaches the stop codon TGA, TAA, or TAG. The promoter region of the gene located 5′ to the cap site contains numerous short regulatory DNA sequences that are targets for interactions with specific DNA-binding proteins. These sequences consist of the basal constitutive promoter (TATA box), metabolic response elements that modulate transcription (e.g., in response to cAMP, steroid hormone receptors, and thyroid hormone receptors), and tissue-specific enhancers and silencers that permit or prevent transcription of the gene, respectively. The enhancer and silencer elements direct expression of specific subsets of genes to cells of a given phenotype. Whether a gene is or is not expressed in a particular cellular phenotype depends on complex interactions of the various DNA-binding proteins among themselves and, most important, with the TATA box proteins of the basal constitutive promoter.

IIB, IID, IIE, IIF, IIH) and, along with RNA polymerase II, form the general or basal transcriptional machinery required for the initiation of RNA synthesis.[38-40]

The other three groups of regulatory sequences consist of *tissue-specific silencers* (TSSs), which function by binding repressor proteins; *tissue-specific enhancers* (TSEs), which are activated by the binding of transcriptional activator proteins; and *metabolic response elements* (MREs), which are regulated by the binding of specialized proteins whose transcriptional activities (repressor or activator) are regulated by metabolic signaling, often involving changes in their phosphorylation.

Introns and Exons

Genes encoding proteins and ribosomal RNAs in eukaryotes are interrupted by intervening DNA sequences (introns) that separate them into coding blocks (exons).[35,36,41] In bacterial genes, the nucleotide sequences of the chromosomal genes match precisely the corresponding sequences in the mRNAs. Interruption of the continuity of genetic information appears to be unique to nucleated cells. The reasons for such interruption are not completely understood, but introns appear to separate exons into functional domains with respect to the proteins that they encode. An example is the gene for proglucagon, a precursor of glucagon in which five introns separate six exons, three of which encode glucagon and the two glucagon-related peptides contained within the precursor (Fig. 3–9).[42] A second example is the growth hormone gene, which is divided into five exons by four introns that separate the promoter region of the gene from the protein-coding region and the latter into three partly homologous repeated segments, two coding for the growth-promoting activity of the hormone and the third for its carbohydrate metabolic functions.[43] As a rule, the genes for the precursors of hormones and regulatory peptides contain introns at or about the region where the signal peptides join the apoproteins or prohormones, thus separating the signal sequences from the components of the precursor that are exported from the cell as hormones or peptides.

There are exceptions to the *one exon, one function theory* in mammalian cells. The genes of several precursors of peptide hormones are not interrupted by introns in a manner that corresponds to the separation of the functional components of the precursor. Notable in this regard is the precursor pro-opiomelanocortin, from which the peptides ACTH, α-melanocyte-stimulating hormone, and β-endorphin are cleaved during the posttranslational processing of the precursor. The protein-coding region of the pro-opiomelanocortin gene is devoid of introns. Likewise, no introns interrupt the protein-coding region of the gene for the proenkephalin precursor, which contains seven copies of the enkephalin sequences. It is possible that, in the past, introns separated each of these coding domains and were lost during the course of evolution.

A precedent for the selective loss of introns appears to be exemplified by the rat insulin genes. The rat genome harbors two nonallelic insulin genes: one containing two introns and the other containing a single intron. The most likely explanation is that an ancestral gene containing two introns was transcribed into RNA and spliced; then that RNA was copied back into DNA by a cellular reverse transcriptase and inserted back into the genome at a new site.

Regulation of Gene Expression

The regulation of expression of genes encoding polypeptide hormones can take place at one or more levels in the pathway of hormone biosynthesis (Fig. 3–10)[44-46]:

- DNA synthesis (cell growth and division)
- Transcription
- Posttranscriptional processing of mRNA
- Translation
- Posttranslational processing

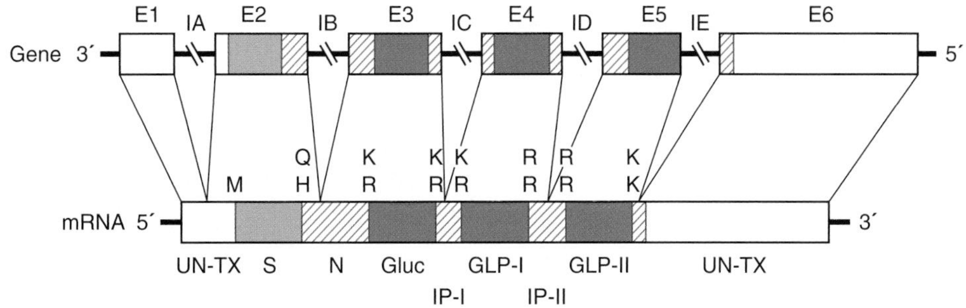

Figure 3–9 ▪ Diagram of the pancreatic glucagon gene and its encoded messenger RNA (mRNA) (complementary DNA). The glucagon gene is an example of a gene in which exons precisely encode separate functional domains. The gene consists of six exons (E1 to E6) and five introns (1A to 1E). The mRNA encoding pre-proglucagon, the protein precursor of glucagon, consists of 10 specific regions: from left to right, a 5′-untranslated sequence (UN-TX, *unshaded*), a signal sequence (S, *stippled*), an NH_2-terminal extension sequence (N, *hatched*), glucagon (Gluc, *shaded*), a first intervening peptide (IP-I, *hatched*), a first glucagon-like peptide (GLP-I, *shaded*), a second intervening peptide (IP-II, *hatched*), a second glucagon-like peptide (GLP-II, *shaded*), a dilysyl dipeptide *(hatched)* after the glucagon-like peptide II sequence, and an untranslated region (UN-TX, *unshaded*). Exons from left to right encode the 5′-untranslated region, signal sequence, glucagon, glucagon-like peptide I, glucagon-like peptide II, and 3′-untranslated sequence. Letters shown above the mRNA denote amino acids located at positions in pre-proglucagon that are cleaved during cellular processing of precursor. The amino acid methionine (M) marks the initiation of translation of mRNA into pre-proglucagon. *H,* Histidine; *K,* lysine; *Q,* glutamine; *R,* arginine.

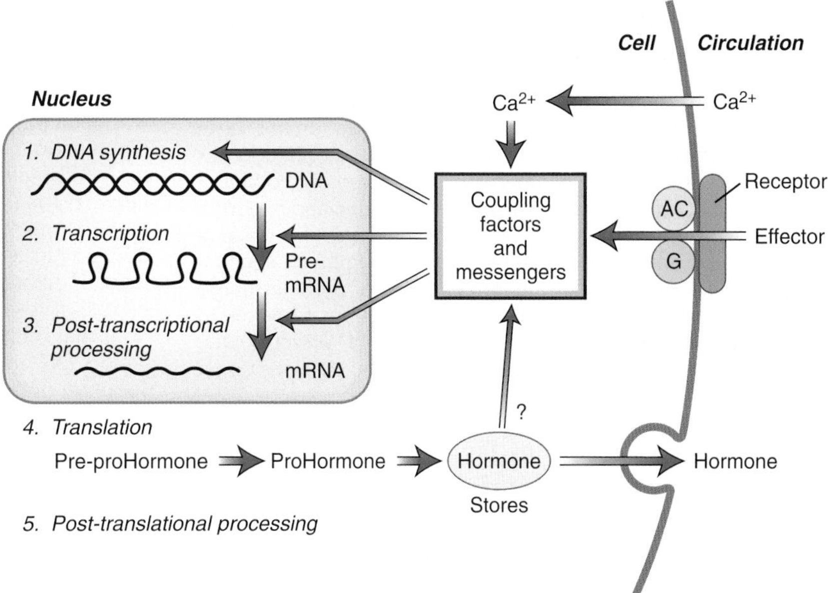

Figure 3–10 ▪ Diagram of an endocrine cell showing potential control points for regulation of gene expression in hormone production. Specific effector substances bind either to plasma membrane receptors (peptide effectors) or to cytosolic or nuclear receptors (steroids), which leads to initiation of a series of events that couple the effector signal with gene expression. In the illustration shown, peptide effector-receptor complex interactions act initially through activation of adenylate cyclase (AC) coupled with a guanosine triphosphate-binding protein (G). Coupling factors and substances such as glucose, cyclic adenosine monophosphate, and cations activate protein kinases, resulting in a series of phosphorylations of macromolecules. As discussed in the text, specific effectors for various endocrine cells appear to act at one or more of the indicated five levels of gene expression, with the possible exception of posttranslational processing of prohormones, for which no definite examples of metabolic regulation have yet been found.

In different endocrine cells, one or more levels may serve as specific control points for regulation of production of a hormone (see Generation of Biologic Diversification).

Levels of Gene Control

Newly synthesized prolactin transcripts are formed within minutes after exposure of a prolactin-secreting cell line to TRH.[47] Cortisol stimulates growth hormone synthesis in both somatotropic cell lines and pituitary slices through increases in rates of gene transcription and enhancement of the stability of mRNA.[48,49] The time required for cortisol to enhance transcription of the growth hormone gene is 1 to 2 hours, which is considerably longer than the time required for the action of TRH on prolactin gene transcription. Regulation of proinsulin biosynthesis appears to take place primarily at the level of translation.[50,51] Within minutes after raising the plasma glucose level, the rate of proinsulin biosynthesis increases 5- to 10-fold. Glucose acts either directly or indirectly to enhance the efficiency of initiation of translation of proinsulin mRNA.[52]

Rapid metabolic regulation at the level of posttranscriptional processing of mRNA precursors is not yet clearly established. However, alternative exon splicing plays a major role in the regulation of the formation of mRNAs during development (see Generation of Biologic Diversification). For example, the primary RNA transcripts derived from the calcitonin gene are alternatively spliced to provide two or more tissue-specific mRNAs that encode chimeric protein precursors with both common and different amino acid sequences, indicating that regulation takes place at the level of processing of the calcitonin gene transcripts.

In many instances, the level of gene expression under regulatory control is optimal for meeting the secretory and biosynthetic demands of the endocrine organ. For example, after a meal there is an immediate requirement for the release of large amounts of insulin. This release depletes insulin stores of the pancreatic β cells within a few minutes, and increasing the translational efficiency of preformed proinsulin mRNA provides additional hormone rapidly.

Tissue-Specific Gene Expression

Differentiated cells have a remarkable capacity for selective expression of specific genes. In one cell type, a single gene may account for a large fraction of the total gene expression, and in another cell type the same gene may be expressed at undetectable levels.

When a gene can be expressed in a particular cell type, the associated chromatin is loosely arranged; when the same gene is never expressed in a particular cell type, the chromatin organization is more compact. Thus, the DNA within the chromatin of expressed genes is more susceptible to cleavage by deoxyribonuclease than is the DNA in tissues in which the genes are quiescent.[53-55] This looseness may facilitate access of RNA polymerase to the gene for purposes of transcription. In addition, inactive genes appear to have a higher content of methylated cytosine residues than the same genes in tissues in which they are expressed.[56,57]

Determinants for the tissue-specific transcriptional expression of genes exist in control sequences usually residing within 1000 base pairs of the 5′-flanking region of the transcriptional sequence. Enhancer sequences in animal cell genes were first described for immunoglobulin genes, a finding that extended the earlier observations of enhancer control elements in viral genomes.[58] Historically, the first clear demonstrations of these elements directing transcription to cells of distinct phenotypes came from studies of the comparative expression of two model genes, insulin and chymotrypsin, in the endocrine and exocrine pancreas, respectively.[59] The restricted expression of genes in a cell-specific manner is determined by the assembly of specific combinations of DNA-binding proteins on a predetermined array of control elements of the promoter regions of genes to create a transcriptionally active complex of proteins that includes the components of the general or basal transcriptional apparatus.

Transcription Factors in Developmental Organogenesis of Endocrine Systems

Certain families of transcription factors are critical for organogenesis and the development of the body plan. Among these factors are the homeodomain proteins[60] and the nuclear receptor proteins.[61-63] The family of homeotic selector, or homeodomain, proteins are highly conserved throughout the animal kingdom from flies to humans. The orchestrated spatial and temporal expression of these proteins and the target genes that they activate determine the orderly development of the body plan of specific tissues, limbs, and organs. Similarly, the actions of families of nuclear receptors (steroid and thyroid hormones, retinoic acid, and others) are critical for normal development to occur. Inactivating mutations in the genes encoding these essential transcription factors predictably result in loss or impairment of the development of the specific organ whose development they direct.

Three examples are described of impaired organogenesis attributable to mutations in essential transcription factors:

- Partial anterior pituitary agenesis (Pit-1)
- Adrenal and gonadal agenesis (SF-1, DAX-1)
- Pancreatic agenesis (IPF-1)

Partial Pituitary Agenesis

The transcription factor Pit-1 is a member of a family of pou-homeodomain proteins, which is a specialized subfamily of the larger family of homeodomain proteins.[64] Pit-1 is a key transcriptional activator of the promoters of the growth hormone, prolactin, and thyroid-stimulating hormone β genes, produced in the anterior pituitary somatotrophs, lactotrophs, and thyrotrophs, respectively. Pit-1 is also the major enhancer activating factor for the promoter of the growth hormone-releasing factor receptor gene.[65] Mutations in Pit-1 that impair its DNA-binding and transcriptional activation functions are responsible for the phenotype of the Jackson and Snell dwarf mice.[64]

Mutations in the gene encoding Pit-1 have been found in patients with combined pituitary hormone deficiency in which there is no production of growth hormone, prolactin, or thyroid-stimulating hormone, resulting in growth impairment and mental deficiency.[66] Notably, the production of the other two of the five hormones secreted by the anterior pituitary gland, adrenocorticotropin and the gonadotropin luteinizing hormone (LH) and follicle-stimulating hormone (FSH), is unaffected.[66] In these human Pit-1 mutations, Pit-1 can bind to its cognate DNA control elements but is defective in *trans*-activating gene transcription. Furthermore, the mutated Pit-1 acts as a dominant negative inhibitor of Pit-1 actions on the unaffected allele.

Pancreatic Agenesis

The homeodomain protein pancreas duodenum homeobox 1 or PDX-1 (somatostatin transcription factor 1 [STF-1], islet duodenum homeobox 1 [IDX-1], insulin promoter factor 1 [IPF-1]) appears to be responsible for the development and growth of the pancreas. Targeted disruption of the PDX-1 gene in mice resulted in a phenotype of pancreatic agenesis.[67] A child born without a pancreas was shown to be homozygous for inactivating mutations in the IPF-1 gene (IPF-1 in the human nomenclature).[68] Notably, the parents and their ancestors who are heterozygous for the affected allele have a high incidence of maturity-onset (type 2) diabetes mellitus, suggesting that a decrease in gene dosage of IPF-1 may predispose to the development of diabetes. The possibility that a mutated IPF-1 allele may be one of several "diabetes genes" is supported by the observation that PDX-1/IPF-1 and the helix-loop-helix transcription factors E47 and β-2 appear to be key up-regulators of the transcription of the insulin gene.[69]

Agenesis of the Adrenal Gland and Gonads

Two nuclear receptor transcription factors have been identified as critical for the development of the adrenal gland, gonads, pituitary gonadotrophs, and the ventral medial hypothalamus. These nuclear receptors are SF-1 (steroidogenic factor 1)[70] and DAX-1 (dosage-sensitive sex reversal, adrenal hypoplasia congenita, X chromosome).[71] SF-1 binds to half-sites of estrogen response elements that bind estrogen receptors in the promoters of genes. DAX-1 binds to retinoic acid receptor (RAR) binding sites in promoters and inhibits RAR actions. Targeted disruption of SF-1 in mice results in a phenotype of adrenal and gonadal agenesis. In addition, pituitary gonadotrophs are absent and the ventral medial hypothalamus is severely underdeveloped.[72,73]

X-linked adrenal hypoplasia congenita is an X-linked, developmental disorder of the human adrenal gland that is lethal if untreated. The gene responsible for adrenal hypoplasia congenita has been identified by positional cloning and encodes DAX-1, a member of the nuclear receptor proteins related to RAR.[71] Several inactivating mutations identified in the DAX-1 gene result in the syndrome of adrenal hypoplasia congenita and hypogonadotropic hypogonadism. Thus, genetically defined and transmitted defects in the genes encoding the transcription factors SF-1 and DAX-1 result in profound arrest in the development of the target organs regulated by the hypothalamic-pituitary-adrenal axis involved in steroidogenesis—the adrenal gland (glucocorticoids, mineralocorticoids) and the gonads (estrogens and androgens).

Coupling of Effector Action to Cellular Response

Another mode of gene control consists of the induction and suppression of genes that are normally expressed in a specific tissue. These processes are at work in the minute-to-minute and day-to-day regulation of rates of production of the specific proteins produced by the cells (e.g., production of polypeptide hormones in response to extracellular stimuli).

At least two classes of signaling pathways—protein phosphorylation and activation of steroid hormone receptors by hormone binding—appear to be involved in the physiologic regulation of hormone gene expression. These two pathways mediate the actions of peptide and steroid hormones, respectively. Peptide ligands bind to receptor complexes on the plasma membrane, which results in enzyme activation, mobilization of calcium, formation of phosphorylated nucleotide intermediates, activation of protein kinases, and phosphorylation of specific regulatory proteins such as transcription factors (see Chapter 5).[74,75]

Steroidal compounds, because of their hydrophobic composition, readily diffuse through the plasma membrane, bind to specific receptor proteins, and interact with other macromolecules in the nucleus, including specific domains on the chromatin located in and around the gene that is activated (see Chapter 4).[61-63] Phosphorylated nucleotides such as cyclic adenosine monophosphate (cAMP), adenosine triphosphate, and guanosine triphosphate, as well as calcium, appear to have important functions in secretory processes. In particular, fluxes of calcium from the extracellular fluid into the cell and from intracellular organelles (e.g., endoplasmic reticulum) into the cytosol are closely coupled to secretion.[76,77]

The cellular signaling pathways that involve protein phosphorylations are multiple and complex. They typically consist of sequential phosphorylations and dephosphorylations of molecules referred to as *protein kinase* or *phosphatase cascades.*[78] These cascades are initiated by hormones, sensor molecules known as ligands, that bind to and activate receptors located on the surface of cells, resulting in the generation of small second messenger molecules such as cAMP, diacylglycerol, or calcium ions. These second messengers then activate protein kinases that phosphorylate and thereby activate key target proteins (Fig. 3–11). The final step in the signaling pathways is the phosphorylation and activation of important transcription factors, resulting in gene expression (or repression).

Insight has been gained into the identities of some of the phosphoproteins. As discussed earlier, a specific group of transcription factors, DNA-binding proteins, interacts with cAMP-responsive and phorbol ester-responsive DNA elements to stimulate gene transcription mediated by the cAMP-protein kinase A, diacylglycerol-protein kinase C, and calcium-calmodulin signal transduction pathways (see Fig. 3–11). These proteins are encoded by a complex family of genes and bind to the DNA elements in the form of heterodimers or homodimers through a coiled-coil helical structure known as a leucine zipper motif.[79] There is evidence that phosphorylation of these proteins modulates dimerization, DNA recognition and binding, and transcriptional *trans*-activation activities. Phosphorylation of the protein substrates might change their conformations and activate the proteins, which, in turn, interact with coactivator proteins such as the cAMP response element-binding (CREB) protein and the protein components of the basal transcriptional machinery, thereby allowing RNA polymerase to initiate gene transcription.[80]

Generally, the second messengers activate serine/threonine kinases, which phosphorylate serine or threonine residues, or both, on proteins, whereas the receptor kinases are tyrosine-specific kinases that phosphorylate tyrosine residues.[78,81] Examples of receptor tyrosine kinases are growth factor receptors such as those for insulin, insulin-like growth factor (IGF), epidermal growth factor, and platelet-derived growth factor. Receptors in the cytokine receptor family, which include leptin, growth hormone, and prolactin, activate associated tyrosine kinases in a variation on the theme.

The different types of signal transduction pathways are described as more or less distinct pathways for semantic

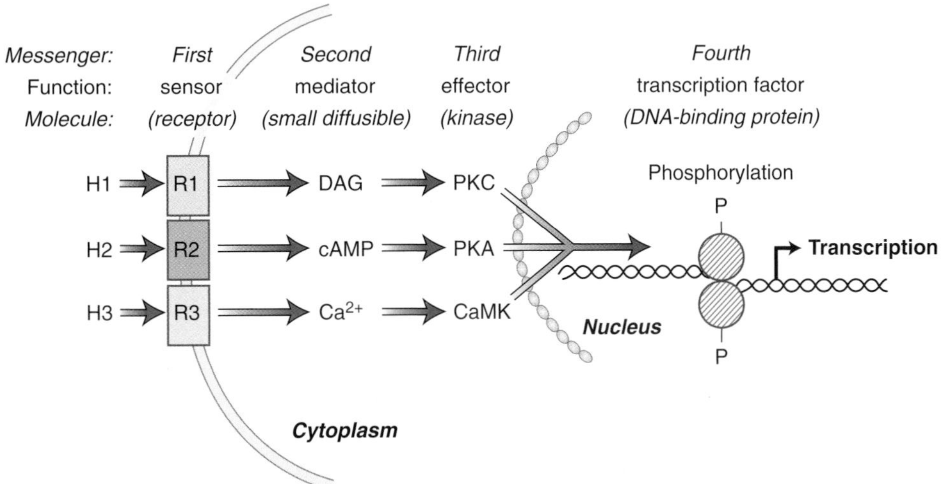

Figure 3–11 ▪ Diagram showing three cell-surface receptor-coupled signal transduction pathways involved in the activation of a superfamily of nuclear transcription factors. Peptide hormone molecules (H1, H2, and H3) interact with sensor receptors (R1, R2, and R3) coupled to the diacylglycerol (DAG)-protein kinase C (PKC), the cyclic adenosine monophosphate (cAMP)-protein kinase A (PKA), and the calcium-calmodulin pathways in which small diffusible second messenger molecules are generated (DAG, cAMP, Ca^{2+}). The third messengers or effector protein kinases are generated and phosphorylate transcription factors such as members of the CREB/ATF and jun/AP-1 families of DNA-binding proteins to modulate DNA-binding affinities or transcriptional activation, or both. The various proteins bind as dimers determined by a poorly understood code that is not promiscuous in as much as only certain homodimer or heterodimer combinations are permissible. *AP-1,* Activator protein 1; *ATF,* activating transcription factor; *CaMK,* calcium/calmodulin-dependent protein kinase; *CREB,* cAMP response element-binding protein.

purposes. In reality, there is considerable cross-talk among the different pathways that occur developmentally and in cell type-specific settings. An active area of research in endocrine systems is attempting to understand these complex interactions among different signal transduction pathways. Although the growth factor and cytokine receptors are similar in some respects, they differ in other respects. For example, growth factor receptor tyrosine kinases activate transcription factors through cascades that involve both tyrosine phosphorylation and serine/threonine kinases such as mitogen-activated protein kinases, whereas the Janus kinases (JAKs) activated by cytokine receptors directly tyrosine phosphorylate the signal transducer and activator of transcription (STAT) factors.[81,82]

Generation of Biologic Diversification

In addition to providing control points for the regulation of gene expression, the various steps involved in transfer of information encoded in the DNA of the gene to the final bioactive protein are a means for diversification of information stored in the gene (Fig. 3–12). Five steps in gene expression can be arbitrarily described: (1) gene duplication and copy number, (2) transcription, (3) posttranscriptional RNA processing, (4) translation, and (5) posttranslational processing.

Gene Duplications

At the level of DNA, diversification of genetic information comes about by way of gene duplication and amplification. Many of the polypeptide hormones are derived from families of multiple, structurally related genes. Examples include the growth hormone family, consisting of growth hormone, prolactin, and placental lactogen; the glucagon family, consisting of glucagon, vasoactive intestinal peptide, secretin, gastric inhibitory peptide, and growth hormone-releasing hormone; and the glycoprotein hormone family, thyrotropin, luteinizing hormone, follicle-stimulating hormone, and chorionic gonadotropin.

A remarkable example of diversification at the level of gene amplifications is the extraordinarily large number of genes encoding the pheromone and odorant receptors.[83] It is estimated that as many as 1000 such receptor genes may exist in mouse and rat genomes, each receptive to a particular odorant ligand. Over the course of evolution, an ancestral gene encoding a prototypic polypeptide representative of each of these families was duplicated one or more times and, through mutation and selection, the progeny proteins of the ancestral gene assumed different biologic functions. The exonic-intronic structural organization of the genomes of higher animals lends itself to gene recombination and RNA copying of genetic sequences with subsequent reintegration of DNA reverse-transcribed sequences back into the genome, resulting in rearrangement of transcriptional units and regulatory sequences.[84,85]

Transcription

In addition to duplication of genes and their promoters, another way to create diversity in expression is at the level of gene transcription by providing genes with alternative promoters[86] and by utilizing a large array of *cis*-regulatory elements in the promoters regulated by complex combinations of transcription factors.

Alternative Promoters

Many of the genes encoding hormones and their receptors utilize more than one promoter during development or when

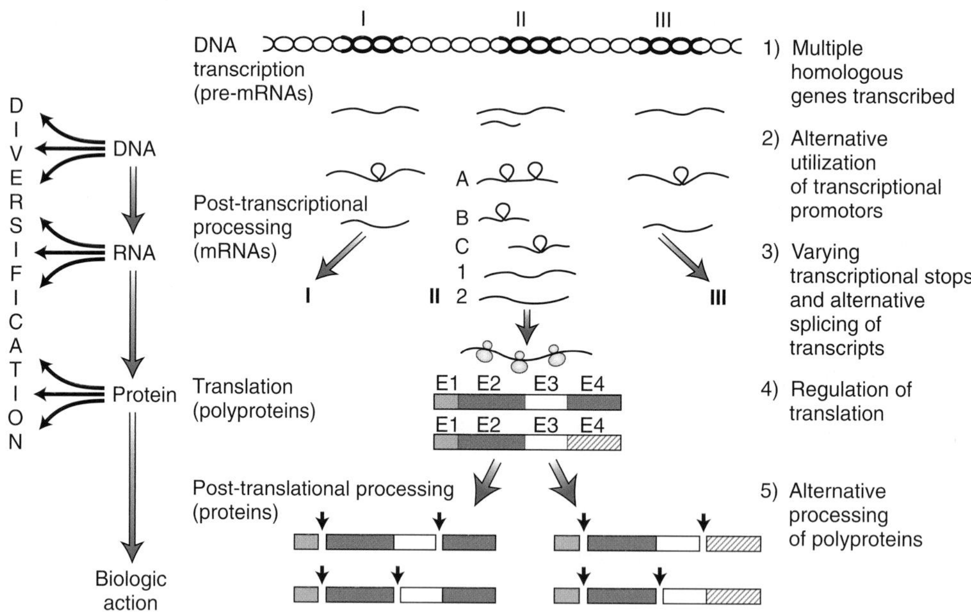

Figure 3–12 ▪ Schema indicating levels in expression of genetic information at which diversification of information encoded in a gene may take place. The three major levels of genetic diversification are (1) gene duplication, a process that occurs in terms of evolutionary time; (2) variation in the processing of ribonucleic acid (RNA) precursors, which results in formation of two or more messenger RNAs (mRNAs) by way of alternative pathways of splicing of transcript (see Figs. 3–13 and 3–14); and (3) use of alternative patterns in processing of protein biosynthetic precursors (polyproteins, or prohormones). These three levels in gene expression provide a means for diversification of gene expression at levels of deoxyribonucleic acid (DNA), RNA, or protein. One or a combination of these processes leads to formation of the final biologically active peptide or hormone. In the diagram, loops depicted in transcripts denote introns; in diagrammatic structures of proteins, the *stippled, shaded,* and *unshaded* areas denote exons. See text for details.

expressed in different tissue types. The employment of alternative promoters results in the formation of multiple transcripts that differ at their 5′ ends (Fig. 3–13). It is presumed that some genes have multiple promoters because they provide flexibility in the control of expression of the genes. For example, in some cases, expression of genes in more than one tissue or developmental stage may require distinct combinations of tissue-specific transcription factors. This flexibility enables genes in different cell types to respond to the same signal transduction pathways or genes in the same cell type to respond to different signal transduction pathways. A single promoter may not be adequate to respond to a complex array of transcription factors and a changing environment of cellular signals.

The organization of alternative promoters in genes is manifested in several patterns within exons or introns in the 5′ noncoding sequence or the coding sequence (see Fig. 3–13). The most common occurrence of alternative promoters is within the 5′ noncoding or leader exons. The utilization of different promoters in the 5′ untranslated region of a gene, often accompanied by alternative exon splicing, results in the formation of mRNAs with different 5′ sequences. The alternative usage of promoters in 5′ leader exons can affect gene expression and generate diversity in several different ways. These include the developmental stage-specific and temporal expression of genes, the tissue-type specificity of expression, the levels of expression, the responsivity of gene expression to specific metabolic signals conveyed through signal transduction pathways, the stability of the mRNAs, the efficiencies of translation, and the structures of the amino termini of proteins encoded by the genes.[86]

Examples of genes that use alternative 5′ leader promoters during development are those encoding IGF-I, IGF-II, the retinoic acid receptors, and glucokinase, all of which are regulated by multiple promoters that are active in a variety of embryonic and adult tissues and are subject to developmental and tissue-specific regulation.[86] During fetal development, promoters P2, P3, and P4 of the IGF-II gene are active in the liver. These promoters are shut off after birth, at which time the P1 promoter is activated. The P1 and P2 promoters of the IGF-I gene are differentially responsive to growth hormone: P2 expressed in liver is responsive to growth hormone, whereas P1 expressed in muscle is not.

The retinoic acid receptor exists in three isoforms (RARα, RARβ, and RARγ) encoded by separate genes that give rise to at least 17 different mRNAs generated by a combination of multiple promoters and alternative splicing.[87] The RAR isoforms appear to differ in their specificity for retinoic acid-responsive promoters, in their affinities for ligand isoforms, and in *trans*-activating capabilities. The different RAR isoforms are expressed at different times in different tissues during development. It has been proposed that the different RAR isoforms provide a means of achieving a diverse set of cellular responses to a single, simple ligand, retinoic acid.[87]

Glucokinase is an example of the alternative use of 5′ leader promoters that have different metabolic responsiveness.[88] Expression of glucokinase in pancreatic beta cells and some other neuroendocrine cells utilizes an upstream promoter (1 β), whereas in liver a promoter (IL) 26 kb downstream of the 1 β promoter is used exclusively. In β cells, expression of the glucokinase gene is apparently not responsive to hormones. In contrast, in liver expression mediated by the IL promoter it is intensely up-regulated by insulin and down-regulated by glucagon.

The α-amylase gene provides an example in which two alternative promoters in the 5′ noncoding exons expressed in two different tissues have dramatically different strengths of expression.[86] A strong upstream promoter directs expression within the parotid gland, contrasting with weak expression directed by an alternative downstream promoter in liver.

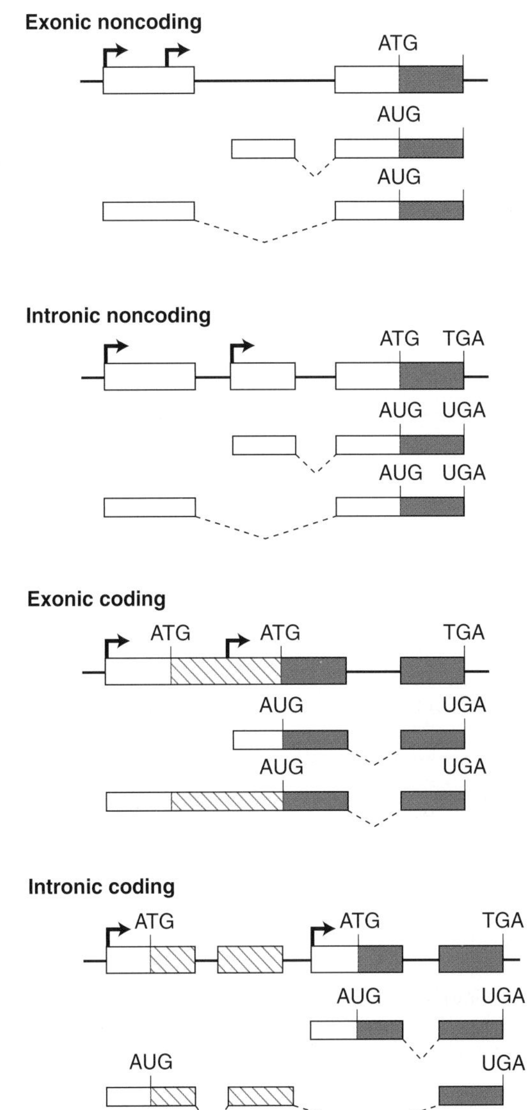

Figure 3–13 ▪ Utilization of alternative promoters in the expression of genes as a means to generate biologic diversification of gene expression. The use of alternative promoters allows a gene to be expressed in a variety of unique contexts that alter the properties of the messenger ribonucleic acid (mRNA) that is expressed. Such alternative promoter usage may render the mRNA more or less stable, affect translational efficiencies, or switch the translation of one protein isoform to another. The use of alternative promoters in genes characteristically occurs during development, or after development is completed, to designate tissue-specific patterns of expression of the gene. Exons are shown as boxes whose protein-coding regions are *shaded*. Introns are designated by *horizontal lines*. *Dashed lines* indicate introns that are spliced out. (Adapted from Ayoubi TAY, Van De Ven WJM. Regulation of gene expression by alternative promoters. FASEB J 1996;10:453-460.)

Examples of the alternative usage of promoters in the coding regions of genes are the progesterone receptor (PR) and the transcription factor cAMP response element modulator (CREM). In both of these examples, different protein isoforms are produced that have markedly different functional activities. The genes encoding the chicken and human progesterone receptors express two isoforms of the receptor (isoforms A and B).[89] Isoform A initiates translation at a methionine residue located 164 amino acids downstream from the methionine that initiates the translation of the longer form B. Analyses of the mechanisms responsible for the synthesis of two different isoforms revealed that two promoters exist in the human PR gene: one upstream of the 5′ leader exon and the other in the first protein coding exon. The two isoforms of the human PR differ markedly in their capabilities to *trans*-activate transcription from different progesterone responsive elements (PRE). Both human PR isoforms equivalently activate a canonical PRE. Isoform B is much more efficient than A at activating the PRE in the mouse mammary tumor virus promoter, whereas isoform A, but not B, activates transcription from the ovalbumin promoter.[89]

The utilization of an alternative intronic promoter within the protein coding sequence of a gene is exemplified by the CREM gene.[90] The CREM gene employs a constitutively active, unregulated promoter (P1) that encodes predominantly activator forms of CREM and an internal promoter (P2) located in the fourth intron that is regulated by cAMP signaling and encodes a repressor isoform, ICER (inducible cAMP early response). The remarkable complexity of the alternative mechanisms of expression of the CREM and CREB genes is discussed subsequently.

Diversity of Transcription Factors

Another mechanism to create diversity at the level of gene transcription is that of the interplay of multiple transcription factors on multiple *cis*-regulatory sequences. The promoters of typical genes may contain 20 or 30 or more *cis*-acting control elements, either enhancers or silencers. These control elements may respond to ubiquitous transcription factors found in all cell types and to cell type-specific factors.

Unique patterns of control of gene expression can be affected by several different mechanisms acting in concert. The spacing, relative locations, and juxtapositioning of control elements with respect to each other and to the basal transcriptional machinery influences levels of expression. Transcription factors often act in the form of dimers or higher oligomers among factors of the same or different classes. A given transcription factor may act as either an activator or a repressor as a consequence of the existing circumstances. The ambient concentrations of transcription factors within the nucleus in conjunction with their relative DNA-binding affinities and *trans*-activation potencies may determine the levels of expression of genes.

Posttranscriptional Processing (Alternative Exon Splicing)

Identification of the mosaic structure of transcriptional units encoding polypeptide hormones and other proteins that consist of exons and introns raised the possibility that the use of alternative pathways in RNA splicing could provide informationally distinct molecules. Different proteins could arise either by inclusion or exclusion of specific exonic segments or by utilization of parts of introns in one mRNA as exons in another mRNA. In addition, differences in the splice sites would result in expression of new translational reading frames. Alternative splicing utilizes two distinct mechanisms (Fig. 3–14). One is that of exon skipping or switching in or out of exons. The other mechanism, known as intron slippage, is to include part of an intron in an exon, to splice out part of an exon along with the intron, or to include a "coding" intron.

There are many examples of both mechanisms used to generate diversity in endocrine systems. Included among the genes encoding prohormones in which the pre-mRNAs are alternatively spliced by exon skipping or switching are those for procalcitonin/calcitonin gene-related peptide, prosubstance P/K, and the prokininogens. Alternative processing of the RNA transcribed from the calcitonin gene results in production of an mRNA in neural tissues that is distinct from that formed in the C cells of the thyroid gland.[91] The thyroid mRNA encodes a precursor to calcitonin, whereas the mRNA in the neural tissues generates a neuropeptide known as calcitonin gene-related peptide. Immunocytochemical analyses of the distribution of the peptide in brain and other tissues suggest functions for the peptide in perception of pain, ingestive behavior, and modulation of the autonomic and endocrine systems.

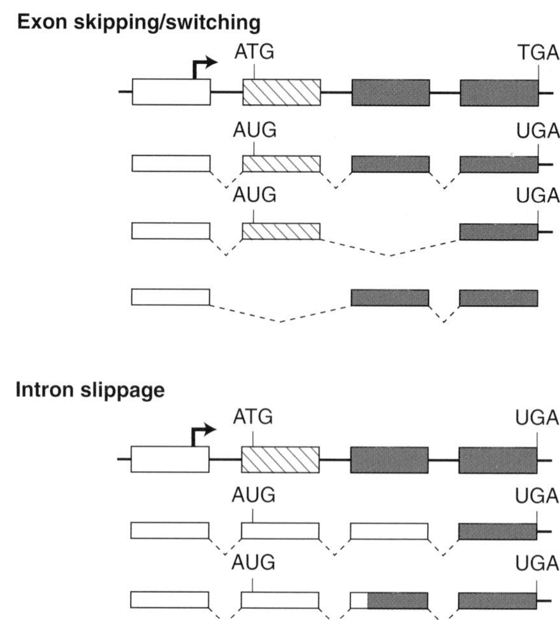

Figure 3–14 ▪ Alternative exon splicing provides a means to generate biologic diversification of gene expression. Mechanisms of exon skipping or switching and intron slippage are frequently utilized in the alternative processing of pre–messenger ribonucleic acids (mRNAs) to provide unique mRNAs and encoded proteins during development and in a tissue-specific pattern of expression in the fully differentiated tissues or organs. Exons are shown as boxes with protein-coding regions *shaded* to designate origin of protein isoforms. Introns are depicted as *horizontal lines*. *Dashed lines* denote spliced-out introns.

The splicing of the RNA precursor that encodes substance P can take place in at least two ways.[92] One splicing pattern results in the mRNA that encodes substance P and another peptide, called *substance K*, in a common protein precursor. Other mRNAs are apparently spliced so as to exclude the coding sequence for substance K. An alternative RNA splicing pattern also occurs in the processing of transcripts arising from the gene encoding bradykinin.[93] The high-molecular-weight and low-molecular-weight kininogens are translated from mRNAs that differ by the alternative use of 3′-end exons encoding the COOH termini of the prohormones, a situation similar to that found in the transcription of the calcitonin gene.

Other examples of genetic diversification arise from the programmed flexibility in the choice of splice acceptor sites within coding regions (intron slippage), which allows an array of coding sequences (exons) to be put together in a number of useful combinations. For example, the coding sequences of the growth hormone, lutropin-choriogonadotropin,[94] and leptin receptors[95] can be brought together in two different ways, one to include, the other to exclude, an exonic coding sequence specifying the transmembrane spanning domains of the polypeptide chains that anchor the receptors to the surface of cells. If mRNA splicing excludes the anchor's peptide sequence, a secreted rather than a surface protein is produced.

Translation

The process of translation provides a fourth level for the creation of diversity of gene expression. As discussed earlier under

Regulation of Gene Expression, the rate of translational initiation can be regulated as typified by the proinsulin and prohormone convertase mRNAs, in which translation is augmented by glucose and cAMP. Molecular diversity of translation, however, is generated by the developmentally regulated utilization of alternative translation initiation (start) codons (methionine codons, AUGs). The mechanism of translation initiation involves the assembly of the 40S ribosome subunit on the 5′ methyl guanosine cap of the mRNA.[96] The ribosome subunit then scans 5′ to 3′ along the mRNA until it encounters an AUG sequence in a context of surrounding nucleotides favorable for the initiation of protein synthesis. Upon encountering such a favorable AUG, the subunit pauses and recruits the 60S subunit plus a number of other essential translation initiation factors, allowing the polymerization of amino acids.

The use of an alternative downstream start codon for translation can occur by mechanisms of loose scanning and reinitiation (Fig. 3–15).[97] Loose scanning is believed to occur when the most 5′ AUG codon is not in a strongly favorable context and allows the 40S ribosomal subunit to continue scanning until it encounters a more favorable AUG downstream. Thus, in the loose scanning mechanism, both translational start codons are used. In contrast, the mechanism of translational reinitiation involves the termination of translation followed by the reinitiation of translation at a downstream start codon. Thus, two proteins are encoded from the same mRNA by a start and stop mechanism.

This process of translational reinitiation can occur either by continued scanning of the 40S ribosomal subunit after termination of translation followed by reinitiation, as in loose scanning, or by complete dissociation of the ribosomal subunits at the time of termination followed by complete reassembly at a downstream start codon, referred to as an *internal ribosomal entry site* (IRES). Such utilization of alternative translation start codons occurs in mRNAs encoding certain classes of transcription factors illustrated by the basic leucine zipper (bZIP) proteins CREB, CREM, and certain of the CCAAT/enhancer binding proteins (C/EBPs), the C/EBPα and C/EBPβ isoforms. In all four of these DNA-binding proteins, the alternative use of internal start codons results in a switch from activators to repressors.

The CREB gene uses translational reinitiation by the somewhat novel mechanism of alternative exon switching that occurs during spermatogenesis.[98] At developmental stages IV and V of the seminiferous tubule of the rat, an exon (exon W) is spliced into the CREB mRNA. Exon W introduces an in-frame stop codon, thereby terminating translation approximately 40 amino acids upstream of the DNA-binding domain.[99,100] The termination of translation then permits reinitiation of translation at each of two downstream start codons, resulting in the synthesis of two repressor or inhibitor isoforms of CREB known as I-CREBs that are powerful dominant negative inhibitors of activator forms of CREB and CREM because they consist of the DNA-binding domain devoid of any *trans*-activation domains.[98-100] The function, if any, of the amino-terminal truncated protein consisting of the activation domains devoid of the DNA-binding domain is unknown. It has been postulated that the role of the alternative splicing of exon W in the CREB pre-mRNA is to interrupt a forward positive feedback loop during spermatogenesis.

CREM, C/EBPα, and C/EBPβ mRNAs utilize alternative downstream start codons to synthesize repressors during development. Like the I-CREBs, these repressors consist of the DNA-binding domains and lack *trans*-activation domains. The CREM repressor (S-CREM) is expressed during brain development.[90] The C/EBPα-30 and C/EBPα-20 isoforms are expressed during the differentiation of adipoblasts to adipocytes, and the C/EBP repressor liver inhibitory protein (LIP) is expressed during the development of the liver.[90]

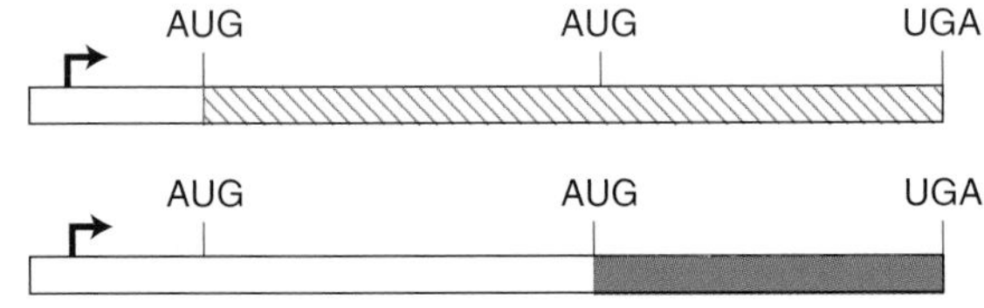

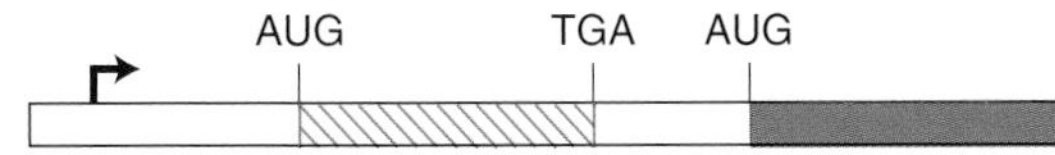

Figure 3–15 ▪ Alternative translational initiation sites are used to change the coding sequences of messenger ribonucleic acids to encode different protein isoforms. The two mechanisms illustrated involve loose scanning and reinitiation of translation. See text.

Posttranslational Processing

A fifth level of gene expression at which diversification of biologic information can take place is that of posttranslational processing. Many precursors of polypeptide hormones, particularly those encoding small peptides, contain multiple peptides that are cleaved during posttranslational processing of the prohormones.[101] Certain polyprotein precursors, however, contain several copies of the peptide. Examples of prohormones that contain multiple identical peptides are the precursors encoding TRH[102] and the α mating factor of yeast,[103] each of which contains four copies of the respective peptide. Polyproteins that contain several distinct peptides include proenkephalins,[104] pro-opiomelanocortin,[105] and proglucagon.[106]

In many instances, biologic diversification at the level of posttranslational processing occurs in a tissue-specific manner. The processing of pro-opiomelanocortin differs markedly in the anterior compared with the intermediate lobe of the pituitary gland. In the anterior pituitary the primary peptide products are ACTH and β-endorphin, whereas in the intermediate lobe of the pituitary one of the primary products is α-melanocyte-stimulating hormone. The smaller peptides produced are extensively modified by acetylation and phosphorylation of amino acid residues.

The processing of proglucagon in the pancreatic A cells and that in the intestinal L cells are also different (see Fig. 3–15).[42] In the pancreatic A cells, the predominant bioactive product of the processing of proglucagon is glucagon itself; the two glucagon-like peptides are not processed efficiently from proglucagon in the A cells and are biologically inactive by virtue of having NH_2-terminal and COOH-terminal extensions. On the other hand, in the intestinal L cell, the glucagon immunoreactive product is a molecule, called *glicentin,* that consists of the NH_2-terminal extension of the proglucagon plus glucagon and the small COOH-terminal peptide known as intervening peptide I.

Glicentin has no glucagon-like biologic activity, and therefore the bioactive peptide (or peptides) in the intestinal L cells must be one or both of the glucagon-like peptides. In fact, glucagon-like peptide I in its shortened form of 31 amino acids, GLP-I (7-37), is a potent insulinotropic hormone in its actions of stimulating insulin release from pancreatic beta cells.[107] This peptide is released from the intestines into the bloodstream in response to oral nutrients and appears to be a potent intestinal incretin factor implicated in the augmented release of insulin in response to oral compared with systemic (intravenous) nutrients. This potential for diversification of biologic information provided by the alternative pathways of gene expression is impressive when one considers that these pathways can occur in multiple combinations.

Unexpectedly Low Numbers of Expressed Genes in Genomes of Mammals (Humans and Mice)

A somewhat surprising initial conclusion, heralded in the lay press when the results of the sequencing of the human and mouse genomes were revealed, was that the number of genes in the human and mouse was approximately 30,000. This number was viewed as remarkably low because the number of genes in yeast *(Saccharomyces cerevisiae)*, worm (*Caenorhabditis elegans*), and fly *(Drosophila melanogaster)* is about 20,000. However, it seems quite clear from the complexities of the mRNAs expressed in humans and mice, as exemplified by the growing database of expressed sequence tags, that tissue-specific alternative exon splicing and alternative promoter usage occur much more frequently in humans and mice than in yeast, worms, and flies. Considering the as yet incomplete database of expressed genes at the mRNA level, it seems reasonable to extrapolate that the human genome may actually express as many as 100,000 to 200,000 mRNAs that encode proteins with distinct, specific functions. This extrapolation is based on the observation that alternative exon splicing and promoter usage appear to be on the order of 5 to 10 times more frequent in higher vertebrate mammals than in yeasts and flies.

ACKNOWLEDGMENTS

I am indebted to the members of the laboratory whose forbearance and helpful discussions of this chapter were invaluable. I thank Apolo Ndyabahika for help in the preparation of the manuscript.

REFERENCES

1. Watson JD, Crick FHC. Molecular structure of nucleic acids. Nature 1953;171:737-738.
2. Roth J, LeRoith D, Shiloach J, et al. The evolutionary origins of hormones, neurotransmitters, and other extracellular chemical messengers. N Engl J Med 1982;306:523-527.
3. Loumaye E, Thorner J, Catt KJ. Yeast mating pheromone activates mammalian gonadotrophs: evolutionary conservation of a reproductive hormone? Science 1982;218:1323-1325.
4. Johnsen AH. Phylogeny of the cholecystokinin/gastrin family. Front Neuroendocrinol 1998;19:73-99.
5. Uy R, Wold F. Post-translational covalent modification of proteins. Science 1977;198:890-896.
6. Martoglio B, Dobberstein B. Signal sequences: more than just greasy peptides. Trends Cell Biol 1998;8:410-415.
7. Palade G. Intracellular aspects of the process of protein synthesis. Science 1975;189:347-358.
8. Jamieson JD. The Golgi complex: perspectives and prospectives. Biochim Biophys Acta 1998;1404:3-7.
9. Blobel G. Intracellular protein topogenesis. Proc Natl Acad Sci U S A 1980;77:1496-1500.
10. Hegde RS, Lingappa VR. Regulation of protein biogenesis at the endoplasmic reticulum membrane. Trends Cell Biol 1999;9:132-137.
11. van Vliet C, Thomas EC, Merino-Trigo A, et al. Intracellular sorting and transport of proteins. Prog Biophys Mol Biol 2003;83:1-45.
12. Rodriguez-Boulan E, Musch A. Protein sorting in the Golgi complex: shifting paradigms. Biochim Biophys Acta 2005;1744: 455-464.
13. Schneider G, Fechner U. Advances in the prediction of protein targeting signals. Proteomics 2004;4:1571-1580.
14. Nelson DL, Cox MM. Lehninger's Principles of Biochemistry, 3rd ed. New York: Worth, 2000.
15. Agarraberes FA, Dice JF. Protein translocation across membranes. Biochim Biophys Acta 2001;1513:1-24.
16. Blobel G, Dobberstein B. Transfer to proteins across membranes. II. Reconstitution of functional rough microsomes from heterologous components. J Cell Biol 1975;67:852-862.
17. Walter P, Blobel F. Signal recognition particle contains a 7S RNA essential for protein translocation across the endoplasmic reticulum. Nature 1982;299:691-698.
18. Bacher G, Pool M, Dobberstein B. The ribosome regulates the GTPase of the beta-subunit of the signal recognition particle receptor. J Cell Biol 1999;146:723-730.
19. Wang L, Dobberstein B. Oligomeric complexes involved in translocation of proteins across the membrane of the endoplasmic reticulum. FEBS Lett 1999;457:316-322.
20. Nagai K, Oubridge C, Kuglstatter A, et al. Structure, function and evolution of the signal recognition particle. EMBO J 2003;22:3479-3485.
21. Martoglio B, Graf R, Dobberstein B. Signal peptide fragments of preprolactin and NIV-1 p-gp160 interact with calmodulin. EMBO J 1997;16:6636-6645.
22. Habener JF, Amgerdt M, Ravazzola M, et al. Parathyroid hormone biosynthesis. J Cell Biol 1979;80:715-731.
23. Steiner DF, Docherty K, Carroll R. Golgi/granule processing of peptide hormone and neuropeptide precursors: a minireview. J Cell Biochem 1984;24:121-130.
24. Chu LLH, MacGregor RR, Cohn DV. Energy-dependent intracellular translocation of proparathormone. J Cell Biol 1977;72:1-10.
25. Kemper B, Habener JF, Rich A, et al. Microtubules and the intracellular conversion of proparathyroid hormone to parathyroid hormone. Endocrinology 1975;96:902-912.
26. Steiner DF. The proprotein convertases. Curr Opin Chem Biol 1998;2:31-39.
27. Muller L, Lindberg I. The cell biology of the prohormone convertases PC1 and PC2. Prog Nucleic Acid Res Mol Biol 1999;63: 69-108.
28. Seidah NG, Chretien M. Proprotein and prohormone convertases: a family of subtilases generating diverse bioactive polypeptides. Brain Res 1999;848:45-62.
29. Jackson RS, Creemers JW, Ohagi S, et al. Obesity and impaired prohormone processing associated with mutations in the human prohormone convertase 1 gene. Nat Genet 1997;16:303-306.
30. Furuta M, Yano H, Zhou A, et al. Defective prohormone processing and altered pancreatic islet morphology in mice lacking active SPC2. Proc Natl Acad Sci U S A 1997;94:6646-6651.
31. Bradbury AF, Smyth DG. Peptide amidation. Trends Biochem Sci 1991;16:112-115.
32. Prigge ST, Mains RE, Eipper BA, et al. New insights into copper monooxygenases and peptide amidation: structure, mechanism and function. Cell Mol Life Sci 2000;57:1236-1259.
33. Kornberg RD. Eukaryotic transcriptional control. Trends Cell Biol 1999;9:M46-M49.
34. Wolffe AP, Kurumizaka H. The nucleosome: a powerful regulator of transcription. Prog Nucleic Acid Res Mol Biol 1998;61: 379-422.
35. Blencowe BJ. Alternative splicing: new insights from global analyses. Cell 2006;126:37-47.
36. Roy SW, Gilbert W. The evolution of spliceosomal introns: patterns, puzzles and progress. Nat Rev Genet 2006;7:211-221.
37. Sharp PA. Split genes and RNA splicing. Cell 1994;77:805-815.
38. Albright SR, Tjian R. TAFs revisited: more data reveal new twists and confirm old ideas. Gene 2000;242:1-13.
39. Levine M, Tjian R. Transcription regulation and animal diversity. Nature 2003;424:147-151.
40. Taatjes DJ, Marr MT, Tjian R. Regulatory diversity among metazoan co-activator complexes. Nat Rev Mol Cell Biol 2004;5:403-410.
41. Crick F. Split genes and RNA splicing. Science 1979;204:264-271.
42. Mojsov S, Heinrich G, Wilson IB, et al. Preproglucagon gene expression in pancreas and intestine diversifies at the level of post-translational processing. J Biol Chem 1986;261:11880-11889.
43. Miller W, Eberhardt NL. Structure and evolution of the growth hormone gene family. Endocr Rev 1983;4:97-130.
44. Brown DD. Gene expression in eukaryotes. Science 1981;211:667-674.
45. Darnell JE. Variety in the level of gene control in eukaryotic cells. Nature 1982;297:365-371.
46. Brivanlou AH, Darnell JE Jr. Signal transduction and the control of gene expression. Science 2002;295:813-818.

47. Murdoch GH, Franco R, Evans RM, et al. Polypeptide hormone regulation of gene expression. J Biol Chem 1983;258:15329-15335.
48. Baxter JD, Ivarie RD. Regulation of gene expression by glucocorticoid hormones: studies of receptors and responses in cultured cells. Receptors Horm Action 1978;2:251-284.
49. Wegnez M, Schachter BS, Baxter JD, et al. Hormonal regulation of growth hormone mRNA. DNA 1982;1:145-153.
50. Itoh N, Okamoto H. Translational control of proinsulin synthesis by glucose. Nature 1980;283:100-102.
51. Skelly RH, Schuppin GT, Ishihara H, et al. Glucose-regulated translational control of proinsulin biosynthesis with that of the proinsulin endopeptidases PC2 and PC3 in the insulin-producing MIN6 cell line. Diabetes 1996;45:37-43.
52. Itoh, N. and H. Okamoto. "Translational control of proinsulin synthesis by glucose." Nature 1980;283:100-102.
53. Wu C, Gilbert W. Tissue-specific exposure of chromatin structure at the 5′ terminus of the preproinsulin II gene. Proc Natl Acad Sci U S A 1981;78:1577-1580.
54. Barton MC, Crowe AJ. Chromatin alteration, transcription and replication: what's the opening line to the story? Oncogene 2001;20: 3094-3099.
55. Feil R, Khosla S. Genomic imprinting in mammals: an interplay between chromatin and DNA methylation? Trends Genet 1999;15: 431-435.
56. Stallcup MR. Role of protein methylation in chromatin remodeling and transcriptional regulation. Oncogene 2001;20:3014-3020.
57. Wade PA. Methyl CpG binding proteins: coupling chromatin architecture to gene regulation. Oncogene 2001;20:3166-3173.
58. Marx JL. Immunoglobulin genes have enhancers. Science 1983; 221:735-757.
59. Walker MD, Edlund T, Boulet AM, et al. Cell-specific expression controlled by the 5′-flanking region of insulin and chymotrypsin genes. Nature 1983;306:557-561.
60. Krumlauf R. Hox genes in vertebrate development. Cell 1994;78: 191-201.
61. Beato M, Klug J. Steroid hormone receptors: an update. Hum Reprod Update 2000;6:225-236.
62. McKenna NJ, Lanz RB, O'Malley BW. Nuclear receptor coregulators: cellular and molecular biology. Endocr Rev 1999;20:321-344.
63. Rosenfeld MG, Glass CK. Coregulator codes of transcriptional regulation by nuclear receptors. J Biol Chem 2001;276:36865-36868.
64. Rosenfeld MG. POU-domain transcription factors: pou-er-ful developmental regulators. Genes Dev 1991;5:897-907.
65. Lin C, Lin S-C, Chang C-P, et al. Pit-1-dependent expression of the receptor for growth hormone releasing factor mediates pituitary cell growth. Nature 1992;360:765-768.
66. Latchman DS. Transcription-factor mutations and disease. N Engl J Med 1996;334:28-33.
67. Jonsson J, Carlsson L, Edlund T, et al. Insulin-promoter-factor 1 is required for pancreas development in mice. Nature 1994;371: 606-609.
68. Stoffers DA, Zinkin NT, Stonojevic V, et al. Pancreatic agenesis attributable to a single nucleotide deletion in the human *IPF1* gene coding sequence. Nat Genet 1996;15:106-110.
69. Peers B, Leonard J, Sharma S, et al. Insulin expression in pancreatic islet cells relies on cooperative interactions between the helix-loop-helix factor E47 and the homeobox factor STF-1. Mol Endocrinol 1994;8:1798-1806.
70. Luo X, Ikeda Y, Parker KL. A cell-specific nuclear receptor is essential for adrenal and gonadal development and sexual differentiation. Cell 1994;77:481-490.
71. Zanaria E, Muscatelli F, Bardoni B, et al. An unusual member of the nuclear hormone receptor superfamily responsible for X-linked adrenal hypoplasia congenita. Nature 1994;372:635-641.
72. Hammer GD, Parker KL, Schimmer BP. Minireview: transcriptional regulation of adrenocortical development. Endocrinology 2005; 146:1018-1024.
73. Niakan KK, McCabe ER. DAX1 origin, function, and novel role. Mol Genet Metab 2005;86:70-83.
74. Cohen P. Signal integration at the level of protein kinases, protein phosphatases and their substrates. Trends Biochem Sci 1992;17: 408-413.
75. Krebs EG, Graves JD. Interactions between protein kinases and proteases in cellular signaling and regulation. Adv Enzyme Regul 2000;40:441-470.
76. Berridge MJ. Elementary and global aspects of calcium signalling. J Physiol (Lond) 1997;499:291-306.
77. Bootman MD, Collins TJ, Peppiatt CM, et al. Calcium signalling: an overview. Semin Cell Dev Biol 2001;12:3-10.
78. Hill CS, Treisman R. Transcriptional regulation by extracellular signals: mechanisms and specificity. Cell 1995;80:199-211.
79. Habener JF, Miller CP, Vallejo M. Cyclic AMP-dependent regulation of gene transcription by CREB and CREM. Vitam Horm 1995;51: 1-57.
80. Janknecht R, Hunter T. A growing coactivator network. Nature 1996;383:22-23.
81. Cobb MH, Goldsmith EJ. How MAP kinases are regulated. J Biol Chem 1995;270:14843-14846.
82. Schindler C, Darnell JE Jr. Transcriptional responses to polypeptide ligands: the JAK-STAT pathway. Annu Rev Biochem 1995;64: 621-651.
83. Axel R. The molecular logic of smell. Sci Am 1995;273(4): 154-159.
84. Dover G. Molecular drive: a cohesive mode of species evolution. Nature 1982;299:111-117.
85. Reanney D. Genetic noise in evolution. Nature 1984;307:318-319.
86. Ayoubi TAY, Van De Ven WJM. Regulation of gene expression by alternative promoters. FASEB J 1996;10:453-460.
87. Leid M, Kastner P, Chambon P. Multiplicity generates diversity in the retinoic acid signaling pathways. Trends Biochem Sci 1992;117: 427-433.
88. Davidson EH, Jacobs HT, Britten RJ. Very short repeats and coordinate induction of genes. Nature 1983;301:468-470.
89. Kastner P, Krust A, Turcotte B, et al. Two distinct estrogen-regulated promoters generate transcripts encoding the two functionally different human progesterone receptor forms A and B. EMBO J 1990;9:1603-1614.
90. Foulkes NS, Sassone-Corsi P. More is better: activators and repressors from the same gene. Cell 1992;68:411-414.
91. Rosenfeld MG, Mermod JJ, Amara SG, et al. Production of a novel neuropeptide encoded by the calcitonin gene via tissue-specific RNA processing. Nature 1983;304:129-135.
92. Nawa H, Hirose T, Takashima H, et al. Nucleotide sequences of cloned cDNAs for two types of bovine brain substance P precursor. Nature 1983;306:32-36.
93. Kitamura N, Takagaki Y, Furuto S, et al. A single gene for bovine high molecular weight and low molecular weight kininogens. Nature 1983;305:545-549.
94. Segaloff DL, Ascoli M. The lutropin/choriogonadotropin receptor . . . 4 years later. Endocr Rev 1993;14:324-347.
95. Lee G-H, Proenca R, Montez JM, et al. Abnormal splicing of the leptin receptor in diabetic mice. Nature 1996;379:632-635.
96. Dreyfuss G, Hentze M, Lamond AI, et al. From transcript to protein. Cell 1996;85:963-972.
97. Kozak M. The scanning model for translation: an update. J Cell Biol 1989;108:229-241.
98. Walker WH, Sanborn BM, Habener JF. An isoform of transcription factor CREM expressed during spermatogenesis lacks the phosphorylation domain and represses cAMP-induced transcription. Proc Natl Acad Sci U S A 1994;91:12423-12427.
99. Walker WH, Girardet C, Habener JF. An alternatively spliced, polycistronic mRNA controls a switch from activator to repressor isoforms of transcription factor CREB during spermatogenesis. J Biol Chem 1996;271:20145-20158.
100. Walker WH, Habener JF. Role of transcription factors CREB and CREM in cAMP-induced regulation of transcription during spermatogenesis. Trends Endocrinol Metab 1996;4:133-138.
101. Neurath H. Proteolytic processing and regulation. Enzyme 1991;45: 239-243.
102. Lechan RM, Wu P, Jackson IME, et al. Thyrotropin-releasing hormone precursor: characterization in rat brain. Science 1986;231: 159-161.
103. Kurjan J, Herskowitz I. Structure of a yeast pheromone gene (MF): a putative factor precursor contains four tandem copies of mature factor. Cell 1982;30:933-943.
104. Noda M, Teranishi Y, Yakahashi T, et al. Isolation and structural organization of the human preproenkephalin gene. Nature 1982;297:431-434.

105. Nakanishi S, Inoue A, Kita T, et al. Nucleotide sequence of cloned cDNA for bovine corticotropin-β-lipotropin precursor. Nature 1979;278:423-427.
106. Heinrich G, Gros P, Lund PK, et al. Pre-proglucagon messenger RNA: nucleotide and encoded amino acid sequences of the rat pancreatic cDNA. Endocrinology 1984;115:2176-2181.
107. Mojsov S, Weir GC, Habener JF. Insulinotropin: glucagon-like peptide I (7-37) coencoded in the glucagon gene is a potent stimulator of insulin release in perfused rat pancreas. J Clin Invest 1987;79:616-619.

CHAPTER 4

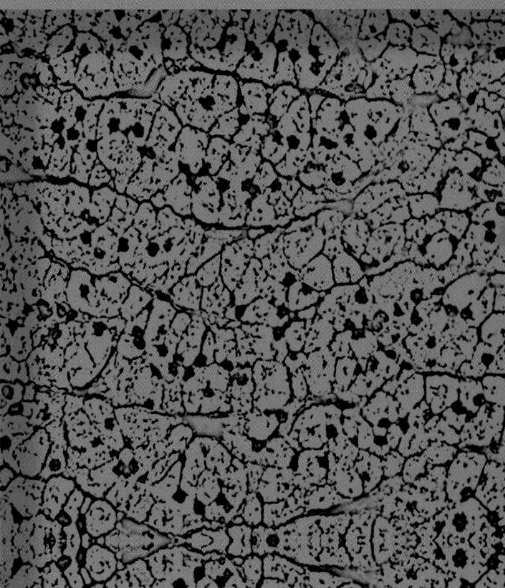

MECHANISM OF ACTION OF HORMONES THAT ACT ON NUCLEAR RECEPTORS

Mitchell A. Lazar

Hormones can be divided into two groups on the basis of where they function in a target cell. The first group includes hormones that do not enter cells; instead, they signal via second messengers generated by interacting with receptors at the cell surface. All polypeptide hormones, as well as monoamines and prostaglandins, utilize cell surface receptors (see Chapter 5, "Mechanism of Action of Hormones That Act at the Cell Surface"). The second group, the focus of this chapter, includes hormones that can enter cells. These hormones bind to intracellular receptors that function in the nucleus of the target cell to regulate gene expression. Classical hormones that utilize intracellular receptors include thyroid and steroid hormones.

Hormones serve as a major form of communication between different organs and tissues, allowing specialized cells in complex organisms to respond in a coordinated manner to changes in the internal and external environments. Classical endocrine hormones, such as thyroid and steroid hormones, are secreted by ductless glands and are distributed throughout the body via the bloodstream. These hormones were discovered by purifying the biologically active substances from clearly definable glands.

It is recognized that numerous other signaling molecules share with thyroid and steroid hormones the ability to function in the nucleus to convey intercellular and environmental signals. Not all of these molecules are produced in glandular tissues. Furthermore, whereas some of these signaling molecules arrive at target tissues via the bloodstream like classical endocrine hormones, others have paracrine functions (i.e., they act on adjacent cells) or autocrine functions (i.e., they act on the cell of origin).

In addition to the classical steroid and thyroid hormones, lipophilic signaling molecules that utilize nuclear receptors include the following: derivatives of vitamins A and D; endogenous metabolites such as oxysterols and bile acids; and non-natural chemicals encountered in the environment (xenobiotics). These molecules are referred to generically as *ligands for nuclear receptors*. The nuclear receptors for all of these signaling molecules are structurally related and collectively referred to as the *nuclear receptor superfamily.*[1-3] The study of these receptors is a fast moving and evolving field, and readers interested in updates and more detailed information are encouraged to visit The Nuclear Receptor Signaling Atlas (http://www.nursa.org/index.cfm).

Ligands that Act Via Nuclear Receptors

General Features of Nuclear Receptor Ligands

Unlike polypeptide hormones that function via cell surface receptors, no ligands for nuclear receptors are directly encoded in the genome. To the contrary, all nuclear receptor ligands are small (molecular weight <1000 daltons [d]) and lipophilic, enabling them to enter cells. Cellular uptake of nuclear receptor ligands may be a passive process, but in some cases a membrane transport protein is involved. For example, the oatp3 organic anion transporter mediates thyroid hormone entry into cells.[4] The lipophilicity of nuclear receptor ligands also allows them to be absorbed from the gastrointestinal tract, thus facilitating their use in replacement of pharmacologic therapies of disease states.

Another common feature of naturally occurring nuclear receptor ligands is that all are derived from dietary, environmental, and metabolic precursors. In this sense, the function of these ligands and their receptors is to translate cues from the external and internal environments into changes in gene expression. Their critical role in maintaining homeostasis in multicellular organisms is highlighted by the fact that nuclear receptors are found in all vertebrates as well as insects but not in single-cell organisms such as yeast.[5]

Because nuclear receptor ligands are lipophilic, most are readily absorbed from the gastrointestinal tract. This makes nuclear receptors excellent targets for pharmaceutical interventions. Hence, in addition to natural ligands, many drugs in clinical use target nuclear receptors. These range from those used to treat specific hormone deficiencies to those used to treat common multigenic diseases such as inflammation, cancer, and type 2 diabetes.

Subclasses of Nuclear Receptor Ligands

One classification of nuclear receptor ligands is outlined in Table 4–1 and is described next.

TABLE 4–1 NUCLEAR RECEPTOR LIGANDS AND THEIR RECEPTORS

Classical Hormones
Thyroid Hormone: Thyroid hormone receptor (TR), subtypes α, β
Estrogen: Estrogen receptor (ER), subtypes α, β
Testosterone: Androgen receptor (AR)
Progesterone: Progesterone receptor (PR)
Aldosterone: Mineralocorticoid receptor (MR)
Cortisol: Glucocorticoid receptor (GR)

Vitamins
1, 25-$(OH)_2$-Vitamin D_3: Vitamin D receptor (VDR)
All-*trans*-retinoic acid: Retinoic acid receptor, subtypes α, β, γ)
9-*cis*-retinoic acid: Retinoid X receptor (RXR), subtypes α, β, γ)

Metabolic Intermediates and Products
Fatty acids: Peroxisome proliferator activated receptor (PPAR), subtypes α, δ, γ)
Oxysterols: Liver X receptor (LXR), subtypes α, β)
Bile acids: Bile acid receptor (BAR)

Xenobiotics
Pregnane X receptor (PXR), Constitutive androstane receptor (CAR)

Classical Hormones

The classical hormones that utilize nuclear receptors for signaling are thyroid hormone and steroid hormones. Steroid hormones include cortisol, aldosterone, estradiol, progesterone, and testosterone. In some cases (e.g., thyroid hormone receptor [TR] α and β genes, estrogen receptor [ER] α and β), there are multiple receptor genes encoding multiple receptors. Multiple receptors for the same hormone can also derive from a single gene either by alternative promoter usage or alternative splicing (e.g., TR β1 and β2).

Finally, some receptors can mediate the signal of multiple hormones. For example, the mineralocorticoid (aldosterone) receptor (MR) has equal affinity for cortisol[6] and probably functions as a glucocorticoid receptor in some tissues, such as the brain, and the androgen receptor (AR) binds and responds to both testosterone and dihydrotestosterone (DHT).[7]

Vitamins

Vitamins were discovered as essential constituents of a healthful diet. Two fat-soluble vitamins, A and D, are precursors of important signaling molecules that function as ligands for nuclear receptors.

Precursors of vitamin D are synthesized and stored in skin and activated by ultraviolet light; vitamin D can also be derived from dietary sources. Vitamin D is then converted in the liver to 25(OH) vitamin D and in the kidney to 1,25-$(OH)_2$-vitamin D_3, the most potent natural ligand of the vitamin D receptor (VDR). The 1-hydroxylation of 25(OH) vitamin D is tightly regulated, and 1,25-$(OH)_2$-vitamin D_3 acts as a circulating hormone.

Vitamin A is stored in the liver and is activated by metabolism to all-*trans*-retinoic acid, which is a high-affinity ligand for retinoic acid receptors (RARs). Retinoic acid is likely to function as a signaling molecule in paracrine as well as endocrine pathways. Retinoic acid is also converted to its 9-*cis*-isomer, which is a ligand for another nuclear receptor called the retinoid X receptor (RXR).[8] These retinoids and their receptors are essential for normal life and development of multiple organs and tissues.[9] They also have pharmaceutical utility for conditions ranging from skin diseases to leukemia.

Metabolic Intermediates and Products

Certain nuclear receptors have been discovered to respond to naturally occurring, endogenous metabolic products. The peroxisome proliferator-activated receptors (PPARs) constitute the best defined subfamily of metabolite-sensing nuclear receptors.[10] There are three subtypes, and all are activated by polyunsaturated fatty acids. No single fatty acid has particularly high affinity for any PPAR, and it is possible that these receptors may function as integrators of the concentration of a number of fatty acids.

PPARα is expressed primarily in liver; to date, the natural ligand with highest affinity for PPARα is an eicosanoid, 8(S)-hydroxyeicosatetraenoic acid,[11,12] although recent evidence suggests that the natural ligand may be a fatty acid derived from lipolysis of circulating triglyceride-rich lipoproteins.[13] The fibrate class of lipid-lowering pharmaceuticals are potent ligands for PPARα, and the name of PPARα is derived from the ability of these compounds to induce the proliferation of peroxisomes in the liver.[14] Indeed, stimulation of fatty acid oxidation is one of the main physiologic roles of PPARα.

The other PPARs (δ and γ) are structurally related but are not activated by peroxisome proliferators. PPAR-δ (also known as PPAR-β) is ubiquitous, and its ligands—other than fatty acids—are not well characterized. Activation of PPARδ appears to increase oxidative metabolism in fat and skeletal muscle. PPARγ is expressed primarily in fat cells (adipocytes) and is necessary for differentiation along the adipocyte lineage.[15] PPARγ is also expressed in other cell types, including colonocytes, macrophages, and vascular endothelial cells, where it may play physiologic as well as pathologic roles. The natural ligand for PPARγ is not known, although prostaglandin J derivatives have the highest affinity (in the micromolar range).[16-18] It is exciting that PPARγ appears to be the target of thiazolidinedione antidiabetic drugs that improve insulin sensitivity.[15,19] These pharmaceutical agents bind to PPARγ with nanomolar affinities, and non-thiazolidinedione PPARγ ligands are also insulin sensitizers, further implicating PPARγ in this physiologic role.

Another metabolite-responsive nuclear receptor, called liver X receptor (LXR), is activated by oxysterol intermediates in cholesterol biosynthesis. Mice lacking LXR-α have dramatically impaired ability to metabolize cholesterol.[20] Another "orphan receptor," bile acid receptor (BAR), also known as FXR, or "Farnesyl X receptor," is likely to play a role in regulation of bile synthesis and circulation in normal as well as disease states.[8]

Xenobiotics

Other nuclear receptors appear to function as integrators of exogenous environmental signals, including natural endobiotics (e.g., medicinals and toxins found in plants) and xenobiotics (compounds that are not naturally occurring).[14] In these cases, the role of the activated nuclear receptor is to induce cytochrome P450 enzymes that facilitate detoxification of potentially dangerous compounds in the liver. Receptors in this class include SXR, or sterol and xenobiotic receptor (also known as pregnane X receptor, or PXR),[15] and CAR, or constitutive androstane receptor.[16] Intriguingly, PPARα is also activated by certain environmental chemicals.

Unlike other nuclear receptors that have high affinity for very specific ligands, xenobiotic receptors have low affinity for a large number of ligands, reflecting their function in defense from a varied and challenging environment. Although these xenobiotic compounds are clearly not "hormones" in the classical sense, the function of these nuclear receptors is consistent with the general theme of helping the organism to cope with environmental challenges.

Orphan Receptors

The nuclear receptor superfamily is one of the largest families of transcription factors. The hormones and vitamins just described account for the functions of only a fraction of the total number of nuclear receptors. The remainder have been designated as orphan receptors because their putative ligands are not known.[21]

From analyses of mice and humans with mutations in various orphan receptors, it is clear that many of these receptors are required for life or development of specific organs ranging from brain nuclei to endocrine glands. Some orphan receptors appear to be active in the absence of any ligand ("constitutively active") and may not respond to a natural ligand. Nevertheless, all of the receptors known to respond to metabolites and environmental compounds were originally discovered as orphans. Thus, it is likely that future research will find that additional orphan receptors function as receptors for physiologic, pharmacologic, or environmental ligands.

Variant Receptors

As discussed, the carboxyl (C-) terminus of the nuclear receptors is responsible for hormone binding. In the case of a few nuclear receptors, including TRα and the glucocorticoid receptor, alternative splicing leads to the production of variant receptors with unique C-termini that do not bind to ligand.[22,23] These variant receptors are normally expressed, but their biologic relevance is uncertain. It has been speculated that they modulate the action of the classical receptor to which they are related by inhibiting its function.

Other types of normally occurring variant nuclear receptors lack a classic deoxyribonucleic acid (DNA) binding domain (see "Target Gene Recognition by Receptors"). These include DAX-1, which is mutated in human disease,[24] and SHP-1.[25] Their ligands, if any, are not known, and it is likely that DAX-1 and SHP-1 bind to and repress the actions of other receptors.

Rare, naturally occurring mutations of hormone receptors can cause hormone resistance in affected patients.[26] Inheritance of the hormone resistance phenotype can be dominant if the mutant receptor inhibits the action of the normal receptor, as with resistance to thyroid hormone or PPARγ ligands.[26] Inheritance is recessive if the mutation results in a complete loss of receptor function, as with the syndrome of hereditary 1,25-dihydroxyvitamin D–resistant rickets.[27] Inheritance can also be X-linked, as with the mutated androgen receptor in androgen insensitivity syndromes, including testicular feminization.[28]

Regulation of Ligand Levels

Ligand levels can be regulated in a number of ways (Table 4–2). A dietary precursor may not be available in required amounts, as occurs in hypothyroidism due to iodine deficiency. Pituitary hormones (e.g., thyroid-stimulating hormone) regulate the synthesis and secretion of classical thyroid and steroid hormones. When the glands that synthesize these hormones fail, hormone deficiency can occur.

Many of the nuclear receptor ligands are enzymatically converted from inactive prohormones to the biologically active hormone (e.g., 5′ deiodination of thyroxine [T_4] to triiodothyronine [T_3]; see Chapter 10). In other cases, one hormone is precursor for another (e.g., aromatization of testosterone to estradiol). Biotransformation may occur in a specific tissue that is not the main target of the hormone (e.g., renal 1-hydroxylation of vitamin D; see Chapter 27) or it may occur primarily in target tissues (e.g., 5α-reduction of testosterone to DHT; see Chapter

TABLE 4–2 MECHANISMS REGULATING LIGAND LEVELS
Precursor availability
Synthesis
Secretion
Activation (prohormone → active hormone)
Deactivation (active hormone → inactive hormone)
Elimination (hepatic, renal clearance)

18). Deficiency or pharmacologic inhibition of such an enzyme can also reduce hormone levels.[29]

Hormones can be inactivated by standard hepatic or renal clearance mechanisms or by more specific enzymatic processes. In the latter case, reduction in enzyme activity due to gene mutations or pharmacologic agents can result in hormone excess syndromes, for example, the renal deactivation of cortisol by 11-β-hydroxysteroid dehydrogenase (11β-OHSD). Because, as noted earlier, cortisol can activate the mineralocorticoid receptor, insufficient 11β-OHSD activity due to licorice ingestion, gene mutation, or extremely high cortisol levels causes syndromes of apparent mineralocorticoid excess.[30]

Nuclear Receptor Signaling Mechanisms

Nuclear receptors are multifunctional proteins that transduce the signals of their cognate ligands. General features of nuclear receptor signaling are illustrated in Fig. 4–1.

First and foremost, the ligand and the nuclear receptor must get to the nucleus. The nuclear receptor must also bind to its ligand with high affinity. Because a major function of the receptor is to selectively regulate target gene transcription, it must recognize and bind to promoter elements in appropriate target genes. One discriminatory mechanism is dimerization of a receptor with a second copy of itself or with another nuclear receptor. The DNA-bound receptor must also work in the context of chromatin to signal the basal transcription machinery to increase or decrease transcription of the target gene.

Throughout the following discussion on the mechanisms and regulation of signaling by nuclear receptors, it should be kept in mind that some basic mechanisms are generally used by many or all members of the nuclear receptor superfamily, whereas other mechanisms impart the specificity that is crucial to the vastly different biologic effects of the many hormones and ligands that utilize these related receptors.

Domain Structure of Nuclear Receptors

The nuclear receptors are proteins whose molecular weights are generally between 50,000 and 100,000 d. They all share a common series of domains, referred to as A to F (Fig. 4–2). This linear depiction of the receptors is useful for describing and comparing the receptors, but it does not capture the role of

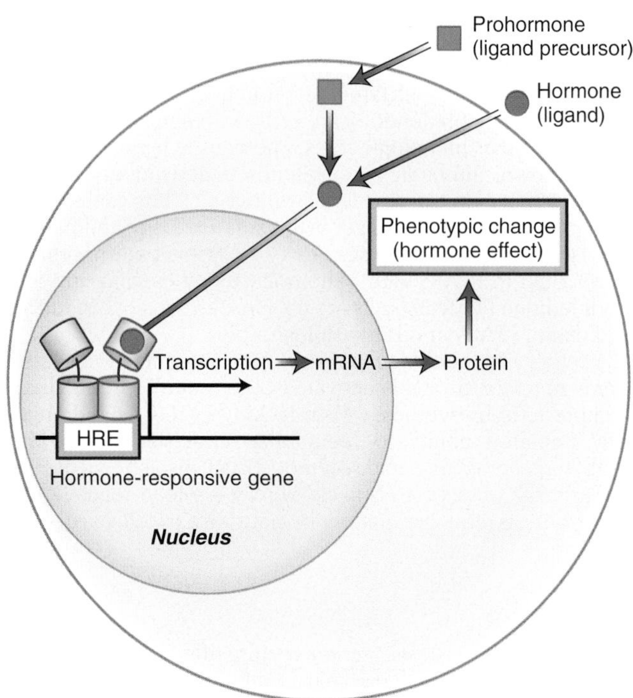

Figure 4–1 ▪ Signal transduction by hormones and other ligands that act via nuclear receptors. *HRE,* Hormone response element; *mRNA,* messenger ribonucleic acid.

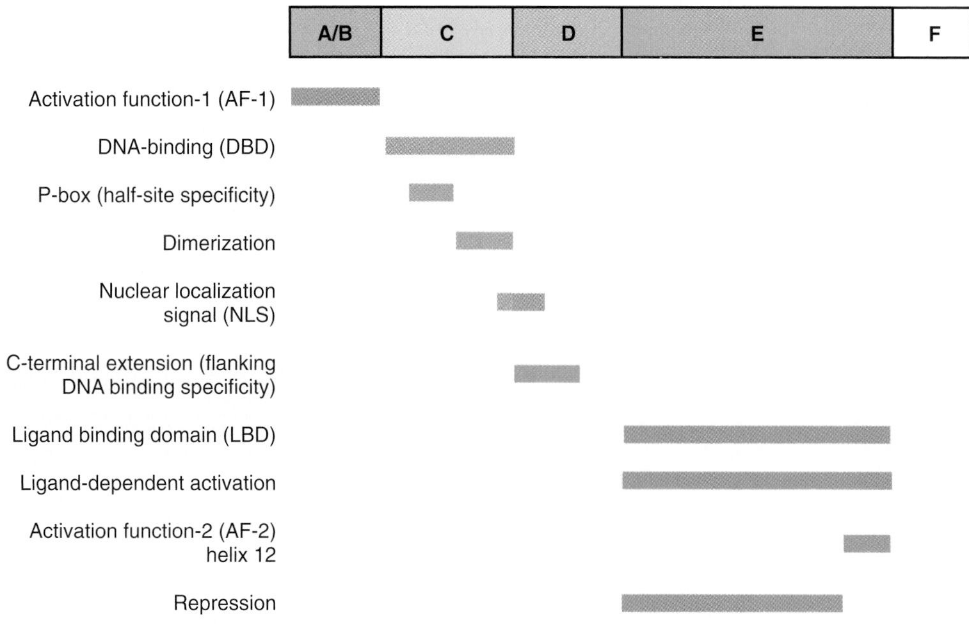

Figure 4–2 ▪ Domain structure of nuclear receptors.

protein folding and tertiary structure in mediating the various receptor functions. As of this writing, no full-length nuclear hormone receptor has been crystallized, but structures of individual domains have been extremely revealing, as becomes clear in the discussions of specific receptor functions that follow.

Nuclear Localization

The nuclear receptors, like all cellular proteins, are synthesized on ribosomes that reside outside the nucleus. Import of the nuclear receptors into the nucleus requires the nuclear localization signal (NLS), located near the border of the C and D domains (see Fig. 4–2). As a result of their nuclear localization signals, most of the nuclear receptors reside in the nucleus in the absence, as well as in presence, of ligand. A major exception is the glucocorticoid receptor (GR), which, in the absence of hormone, is tethered in the cytoplasm to a complex of chaperone molecules, including heat shock proteins (hsps). Hormone binding to GR induces a conformational change that results in dissociation of the chaperone complex, thereby allowing the hormone-activated GR to translocate to the nucleus via its nuclear localization signal.

Hormone Binding

High-affinity binding of a lipophilic ligand is a shared characteristic of many nuclear receptors. This defining function of the receptor is mediated by the C-terminal ligand-binding domains (LBDs), domains D and E in Fig. 4–2. This region of the receptor also has many other functions, including induction of dimerization and transcriptional regulation (see "Receptor Dimerization" and "Receptor Regulation of Gene Transcription" below).

The structure of the LBD has been solved for a number of receptors. All share a similar overall structure consisting of 12 α-helical segments in a highly folded tertiary structure (Fig. 4–3A). The ligand binds within a hydrophobic pocket composed of amino acids in helix 3 (H3), H4, and H5. The major structural

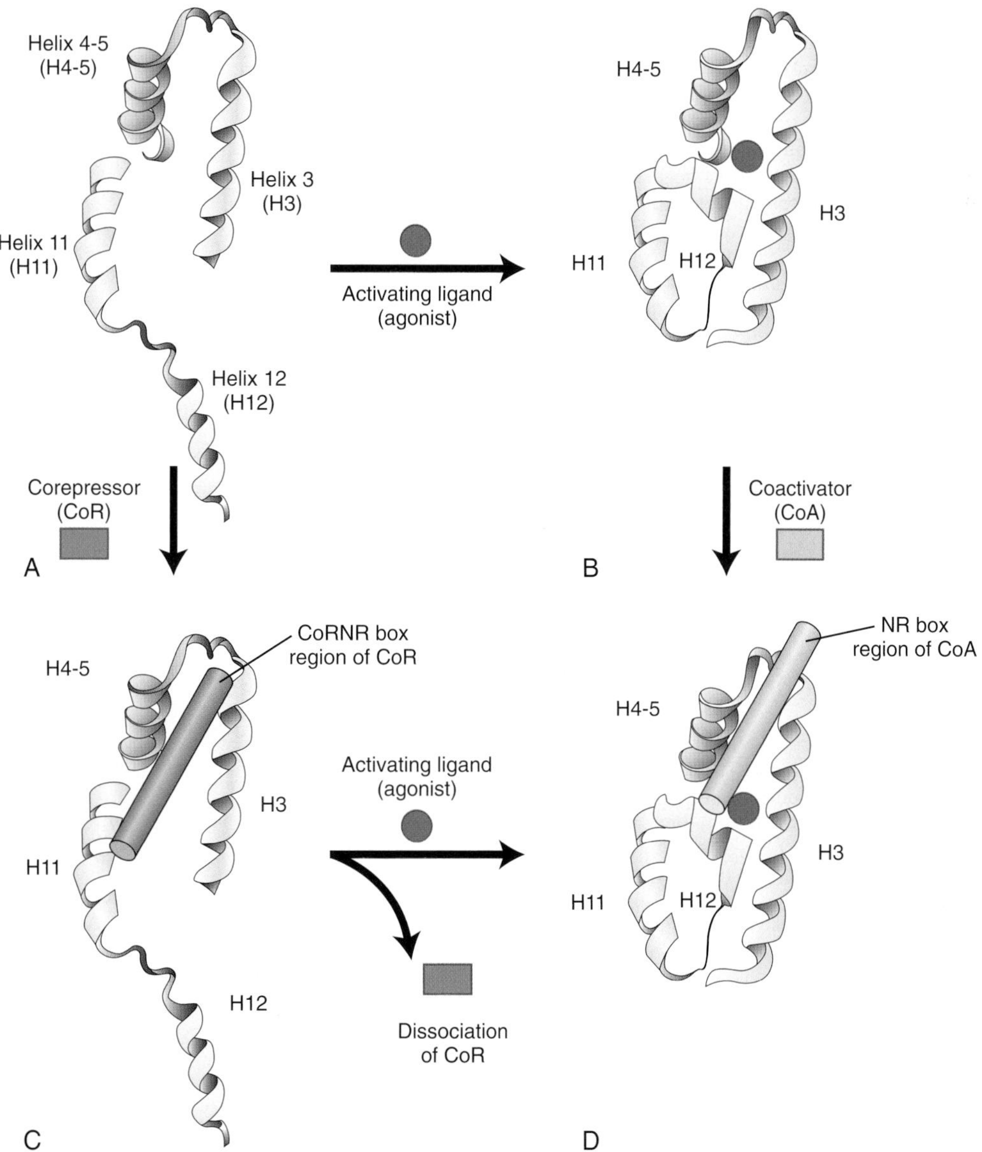

Figure 4–3 ▪ Structural basis of nuclear receptor ligand binding and cofactor recruitment. **A** and **B**, Apo-receptor (no ligand bound); **B** and **D**, ligand-bound receptor. **C** and **D**, Structures showing the positional binding of corepressor **(C)** or coactivator **(D)**.

change induced by ligand binding is an internal folding of the most C-terminal helix (H12), which forms a cap on the ligand-binding pocket (see Fig. 4–3B). Although the overall mechanism of ligand binding is similar for all receptors, the details are crucial in determining ligand specificity.[31,32] Although the molecular details of ligand binding are beyond the scope of this chapter, this is the most critical determinant of receptor specificity.

Target Gene Recognition by Receptors

Another crucial specificity factor for nuclear receptors is their ability to recognize and bind to the subset of genes that is to be regulated by their cognate ligand. Target genes contain specific DNA sequences that are called hormone response elements (HREs). Binding to the HRE is mediated by the central C domain of the nuclear receptors (see Fig. 4–2). This region is typically composed of 66 to 68 amino acids, including two subdomains called *zinc fingers* because the structure of each subdomain is maintained by four cysteine residues that coordinate with a zinc atom.

The first of these zinc-ordered modules contains basic amino acids that contact DNA; as with the LBD, the overall structure of the DNA-binding domain (DBD) is very similar for all members of the nuclear receptor superfamily. The specificity of DNA binding is determined by multiple factors (Table 4–3). All steroid hormone receptors, except for the estrogen receptor (ER), bind to the double-stranded DNA sequence AGAACA (Fig. 4–4).

By convention, the double-stranded sequence is described by the sequence of one of the complementary strands, with the bases ordered from the 5′ to the 3′ end. Other nuclear receptors recognize the sequence AGGTCA. The primary determinant of this specificity is a group of amino acid residues in the so-called P-box of the DBD (see Fig. 4–4). These hexamer DNA sequences are referred to as *half-sites*. The only two differences between these hexameric half-sites are the central two base pairs (underlined). For some nuclear receptors, the C-terminal extension of the DBD contributes specificity for extended half-sites containing additional, highly specific DNA sequences 5′ to the hexamer (see Fig. 4–2). Another source of specificity for target genes is the spacing and orientation of these half-sites, which in most cases are bound by receptor dimers.

Receptor Dimerization

As noted earlier, the nuclear receptor DBD has affinity for the hexameric half-site, or extended half-sites; many HREs, however, are composed of repeats of the half-site sequence, and most nuclear receptors bind such HREs as dimers. Steroid receptors, including ER, function primarily as homodimers, which preferentially bind to two half-sites oriented toward each other (inverted repeats) with three base pairs in between (IR3) (see Fig. 4–4A). The major dimerization domain in steroid receptors is within the C-domain, although the LBD contributes. Ligand-binding facilitates dimerization and DNA binding of steroid hormone receptors. Most other receptors, including TR, RAR, VDR, PPAR, LXR, and VDR, bind to DNA as heterodimers with RXR (see Fig. 4–4B).

Heterodimerization with RXR is mediated by two distinct interactions, one involving LBDs and the other involving DBDs. The receptor LBD mediates the strongest interaction, which occurs even in the absence of DNA. These receptor heterodimers bind to two half-sites arranged as direct repeats (DRs) with variable numbers of base pairs in between.

TABLE 4–3 DETERMINANTS OF TARGET GENE SPECIFICITY OF NUCLEAR RECEPTORS

Specificity Factor	Region of Receptor
Binding to DNA	DNA-binding domain (DBD, C domain)
Binding to specific hexamer (AGGTCA vs. AGAACA)	P-Box in C-domain
Binding to sequences 5′ to hexamer	C-terminal extension of DBD
Binding to hexamer repeats	Dimerization domain (C domain for steroid receptors, D-E-F for others)
Recognition of hexamer spacing	Heterodimerization with RXR (nonsteroid receptors, C domain)

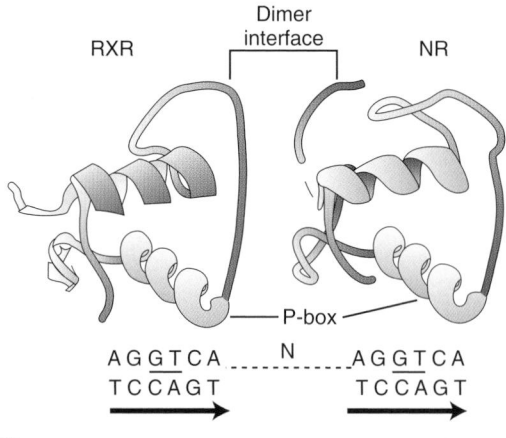

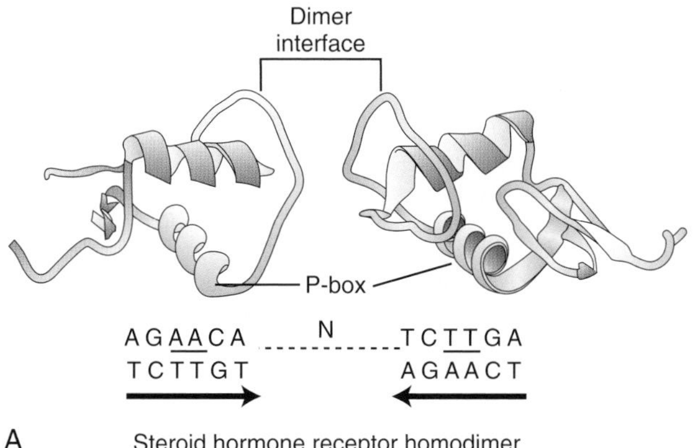

Figure 4–4 ▪ Structural basis of nuclear receptor (NR) DNA-binding specificity. Ribbon diagrams of receptor DNA-binding domains (DBDs) are shown. **A,** Steroid hormone receptor binding as homodimer to inverted repeat (*arrows*) of AGAACA half-site. **B,** RXR-NR heterodimer binding to direct repeat of AGGTCA. The position of the P-box, the region of the DBD that makes direct contact with DNA, is shown. *N,* Number of base pairs between the two half-sites; *RXR,* retinoid X receptor.

The spacing of the half-sites is a major determinant of target gene specificity. This is due to the second receptor-receptor interaction, which involves the DBDs and is highly sensitive to the spacing of the half-sites. For example, VDR/RXR heterodimers bind preferentially to direct repeats separated by three bases (DR3 sites), TR/RXR binds DR4, and RAR/RXR binds DR5 with highest affinity.[33]

The structural basis of this restriction on DNA binding is related to the fact that the RXR binds to the upstream half-site (farthest from the start of transcription). As a result of the periodicity of the DNA helix, each base pair separating the half-sites leads to a rotation of about 36 degrees of one half-site relative to the other. Subtle differences in the structure of the receptor LBDs make the DBD interactions more or less favorable at the different degrees of rotation.[34]

Receptor Regulation of Gene Transcription

Nuclear receptors mediate a variety of effects on gene transcription. The most common modes of regulation are ligand-dependent gene activation, ligand-independent repression of transcription, and ligand-dependent negative regulation of transcription (Table 4–4). The remainder of this chapter describes these mechanisms.

Ligand-Dependent Activation

Ligand-dependent activation is the most well understood function of nuclear receptors and their ligands. In this case, the ligand-bound receptor increases transcription of a target gene to which it is bound. The DBD serves to bring the receptor domains that mediate transcriptional activation to a specific gene. Transcriptional activation itself is mediated primarily by the LBD, which can function in the same way even when it is transferred to a DNA-binding protein that is not related to nuclear receptors. The activation function (AF) of the LBD is referred to as *AF-2* (see Fig. 4–2).

Gene transcription is mediated by a large complex of factors that ultimately regulate the activity of ribonucleic acid (RNA) polymerase, the enzyme that uses the chromosomal DNA template to direct the synthesis of messenger RNA. Most mammalian genes are transcribed by RNA polymerase II, utilizing a large set of cofactor proteins, including basal transcription factors, and associated factors collectively referred to here as general transcription factors (GTFs). Details about GTFs are of fundamental importance and are available elsewhere.[35]

The ligand-bound nuclear receptor communicates stimulatory signals to GTFs on the gene to which it is bound. Ligands specifically recruit a set of proteins to the nuclear receptor LBD.[36] Positively acting cofactors, called coactivators, specifically recognize the ligand-bound conformation of the LBD and bind to the nuclear receptor on DNA only when an activating ("agonist") hormone or ligand is bound.[37] A number of coactivator proteins that bind to liganded nuclear receptors have been described (Table 4–5).[37]

The most important determinant of coactivator binding is the position of H12, which changes dramatically when activating ligands bind receptors (see Fig. 4–3D). Along with H3, H4, and H5, H12 forms a hydrophobic cleft that is bound by short polypeptide regions of the coactivator molecules.[38-40] These polypeptides, called NR boxes, have characteristic sequences of LxxLL, where L is leucine and xx can be any two amino acids.[41]

Coactivators increase the rate of gene transcription. This is accomplished by enzymatic functions, including DNA unwinding activity as well as histone acetyltransferase (HAT) activity.[42] HAT activity is critically important for activation because chromosomal DNA is tightly wrapped around nucleosomal units composed of core histone proteins. Acetylation of lysine tails on histones "opens up" this chromatin structure.

The best understood class of coactivator proteins is the so-called p160 family, whose name is based on their size (~160 kd). There are at least three such molecules, each with numerous names (see Table 4–5).[43] These factors possess HAT activity and also recruit other coactivators (CBP and p300), which are also HATs. A third HAT, called p300/CBP-associated factor (pCAF), is also recruited by liganded receptors. Together these HATs, along with a complex of molecules called Swi/Snf, which directs adenosine triphosphate (ATP)-dependent DNA unwinding, create a chromatin structure that favors transcription (Fig. 4–5).[44]

It is possible that the recruitment of multiple HATs reflects different specificities for core histones and potentially other, nonhistone proteins. Some HATs also interact directly with GTFs and further enhance their activities. An important complex that also links nuclear receptors to GTFs is the TRAP (TR-associated protein) or DRIP (D receptor–associated protein) complex.[45,46] The HATs and TRAP factors are both recruited to the liganded, target-gene bound receptor in an ordered manner that also involves cycling on and off receptor gene targets by a mechanism that is not yet understood.[47]

Repression of Gene Expression by Unliganded Receptor

Although DNA binding is ligand-dependent for steroid hormone receptors, other nuclear receptors are bound to DNA even in the

TABLE 4–4 REGULATION OF GENE TRANSCRIPTION BY NUCLEAR RECEPTORS

1. Ligand-dependent gene activation: DNA binding and recruitment of coactivators
2. Ligand-independent gene repression: DNA binding and recruitment of corepressors
3. Ligand-dependent negative regulation of gene expression: DNA binding and recruitment of corepressors *or* recruitment of coactivators off DNA

TABLE 4–5 NUCLEAR RECEPTOR COACTIVATORS AND COREPRESSORS

COACTIVATORS
1. Chromatin Remodeling Swi/Snf complex 2. Histone Acetyl Transferase p160 family (SRC-1, GRIP-1, pCIP) p300/CBP pCAF (p300/CBP-associated factor) 3. Activation TRAP/DRIP (thyroid receptor associated proteins/D-receptor interacting proteins)
COREPRESSORS
N-CoR (Nuclear receptor corepressor) SMRT (Silencing mediator for retinoid and thyroid hormone receptors)

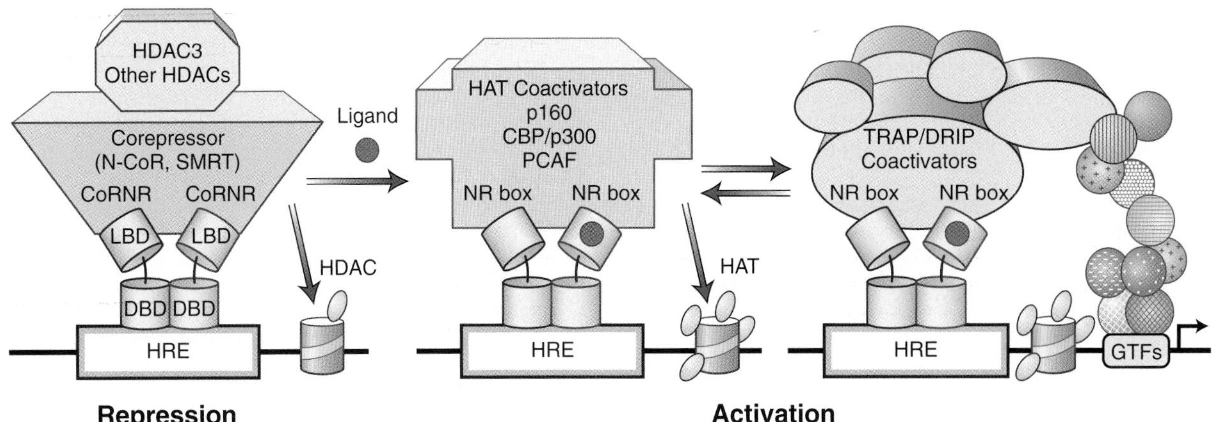

Figure 4–5 ▪ Coactivators and corepressors in transcriptional regulation by nuclear receptors. *CBP,* Calcium-binding protein; *DRIP,* D receptor-interacting protein; *HRE,* hormone response element; *HAT,* histone acetyltransferase; *HDAC,* histone deacetylase; *N-CoR,* nuclear receptor corepressor; *NR,* nuclear receptor; *PCAF,* CBP/p300-associated factor; *SMRT,* silencing mediator of retinoid and thyroid receptors; *TRAP,* thyroid hormone receptor-associated protein.

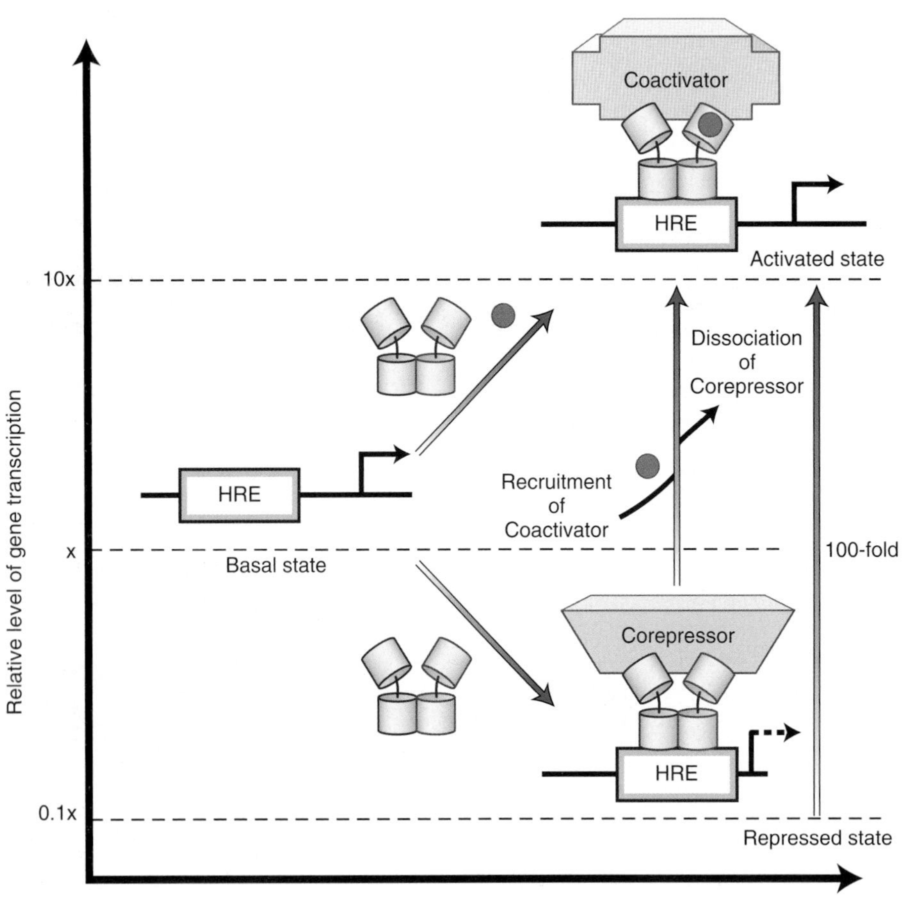

Figure 4–6 ▪ Repression and activation functions augmenting the dynamic range of transcriptional regulation by nuclear receptors. *HRE,* Hormone response element. The magnitude of activation and repression were arbitrarily set at 10-fold for this theoretical example. In cells these magnitudes vary as a function of coactivator and corpressor concentration, as well as in a target-gene-specific manner.

absence of their cognate ligand. The unliganded DNA-bound receptor is not passively waiting for hormone; instead, it actively represses transcription of the target gene. This repression both "turns off" the target gene and amplifies the magnitude of the subsequent activation by hormone or ligand. For instance, if the level of gene transcription in the repressed state is 10% of the basal level in the absence of receptor, a hormone-activation to 10-fold above that basal level represents a 100-fold difference of transcription rate between hormone-deficient (repressed) genes and hormone-activated genes (Fig. 4–6).[48]

In many ways, the molecular mechanism of repression is the mirror image of ligand-dependent activation. The unliganded nuclear receptor recruits negatively acting factors (corepressors) to the target gene (see Fig. 4–3C). The two major corepressors are large (~270 kd) proteins, called nuclear receptor corepressor (N-CoR) and silencing mediator for retinoid and thyroid receptors (SMRT).[49] N-CoR and SMRT specifically recognize the unliganded conformation of nuclear receptors and use an amphipathic helical sequence similar to the NR box of coactivators to bind to a hydrophobic pocket in the receptor.

For corepressors, the peptide responsible for receptor binding is called the CoRNR box and contains the sequence (I or L) xx (I or V)I (where I is isoleucine, L is leucine, V is valine, and xx represents any two amino acids).[50] The receptor utilizes helices 3 to 5 to form the hydrophobic pocket, as in coactivator binding, but H12 does not promote and even hinders corepressor binding. This negative role of H12 highlights the role of the ligand-dependent change in the position of H12 as the switch that determines repression and activation by nuclear receptors (see Fig. 4–5).[51]

The transcriptional functions of N-CoR and SMRT are the opposite of those of the coactivators. The corepressors themselves do not possess enzyme activity but do recruit histone deacetylases (HDACs) to the target gene, thereby reversing the effects of histone acetylation described earlier and leading to a compact, repressed state of chromatin. Although the mammalian genome contains multiple HDACs, several of which may play a role in nuclear receptor function, the main one involved in repression is HDAC3, whose enzyme activity actually depends on interaction with N-CoR or SMRT.[52] The corepressors also interact directly with GTFs to inhibit their transcriptional activities, and they exist in large multiprotein complexes whose range of functions is not yet fully understood.

Ligand-Dependent Negative Regulation of Gene Expression (Transrepression)

The ligand-dependent switch between the repressed and activated receptor conformations explains how hormones activate gene expression. However, many important gene targets of hormones are turned off in the presence of the ligand. This is referred to as ligand-dependent negative regulation of transcription, or transrepression, to distinguish it from the repression of basal transcription by unliganded receptors.

The mechanism of negative regulation is less well understood than ligand-dependent activation, and, indeed, there may be more than one mechanism.[53] One mechanism involves nuclear receptor binding to DNA binding sites that reverse the paradigm of ligand-dependent activation (negative response elements). Ligand-bound receptors recruit corepressors and HDAC activity to such binding sites. For example, when the unliganded TR binds to the negative response element of the gene for the β subunit of thyroid-stimulating hormone (TSH), transcription is activated. Ligand binding recruits corepressors and HDAC to the TR and leads to suppression of transcription. In other cases, it has been postulated that negative regulation may result from ligand binding to nuclear receptors that bind to other transcription factors without binding DNA. This interaction leads to removal of coactivators such as p300 and CBP from the other transcription factors that positively regulate the gene. In this model, inhibition of the activity of the positively acting factors results in the observed negative regulation.

Role of Other Nuclear Receptor Domains

The N-terminal A/B domain of the nuclear receptors is the most variable region among all members of the superfamily in terms of length and amino acid sequence. Even subtypes of the same receptor often have completely different A/B domains. The function of this domain is least well defined. It is not required for unliganded repression or ligand-dependent activation. In many receptors, the A/B domain contains a positive transcriptional activity, often referred to as *AF-1* (see Fig. 4–2), that is ligand-independent but probably interacts with coactivators and may influence the magnitude of activation by agonists or partial agonists. This activation function is tissue-specific and tends to be more important for steroid hormone receptors, whose A/B domains are notably longer than those of other members of the superfamily.[54] The F domain of the nuclear receptors is hypervariable in length and sequence, and its function is not known.

TABLE 4–6 FACTORS MODULATING RECEPTOR ACTIVITY IN DIFFERENT TISSUES

Receptor concentration
Ligand concentration
Ligand function (agonist, partial agonist, antagonist)
Concentrations and types of coactivators and corepressors
Phosphorylation state of nuclear receptor

Cross-talk with Other Signaling Pathways

Hormones and cytokines that signal via cell surface receptors also regulate gene transcription, often by activating protein kinases that phosphorylate transcription factors such as cAMP-response element-binding protein (CREB). Such signals can also lead to phosphorylation of nuclear receptors. Multiple signal-dependent kinases can phosphorylate nuclear receptors, leading to conformational changes that regulate function.[55] Phosphorylation can lead to changes in DNA binding, ligand binding, or coactivator binding; these variable consequences depend on the specific kinase, receptor, and domain of the receptor that is phosphorylated. The properties of coactivators and corepressor molecules are also regulated by phosphorylation.

Receptor Antagonists

Certain ligands function as receptor antagonists by competing with agonists for the ligand-binding site. In the case of steroid hormone receptors, the position of H12 in the antagonist-bound receptor is not identical to that in the unliganded receptor or the agonist-bound receptor. H12, which itself has a sequence that resembles the NR box, binds to the coactivator-binding pocket of the receptor and thereby prevents coactivator binding.[56] This antagonist-bound conformation of the receptor also favors corepressor binding to steroid hormone receptors.

Tissue-Selective Ligands

Some ligands function as antagonists in some tissues but as full or partial agonists in others. These selective receptor modulators include compounds such as tamoxifen, a selective estrogen receptor modulator (SERM). SERMs are estrogen receptor antagonists with respect to the functions of AF-2, including coactivator binding, and require the AF-1 function for their agonist activity.[57] Such agonism, like AF-1 activity, tends to be tissue-specific and therefore has great therapeutic utility.[58]

In addition to drugs, certain endogenous ligands (e.g., testosterone, DHT) also mediate tissue-specific effects. The molecular basis of tissue-specific activity is not well understood but is probably due to the expression or activity of transcriptional cofactors that differentiate between receptors bound to different ligands. Table 4–6 summarizes factors contributing to tissue-specificity of receptor activity.

REFERENCES

1. Chambon P. The nuclear receptor superfamily: a personal retrospect on the first two decades. Mol Endocrinol 2005;19:1418-1428.
2. Evans RM. The nuclear receptor superfamily: a Rosetta Stone for physiology. Mol Endocrinol 2005;19:1429-1438.
3. O'Malley BW. A life-long search for the molecular pathways of steroid hormone action. Mol Endocrinol 2005;19:1402-1411.
4. Abe T, et al. Molecular characterization and tissue distribution of a new organic anion transporter subtype (oatp3) that transports

thyroid hormones and taurocholate and comparison with oatp2. J Biol Chem 1998;273:22395-22401.
5. Escriva H, Delaunay F, Laudet V. Ligand binding and nuclear receptor evolution. Bioassays 2000;22:717-727.
6. Arriza JL, et al. Cloning of human mineralocorticoid receptor complementary cDNA: structure and functional kinship with the glucocorticoid receptor. Science 1987;237:268-275.
7. Roy AK, et al. Androgen receptor: structural domains and functional dynamics after ligand-receptor interaction. Ann N Y Acad Sci 2001;949:44-57.
8. Mangelsdorf DJ, Evans RM. The RXR heterodimers and orphan receptors. Cell 1995;83:841-850.
9. Chambon P. A decade of molecular biology of retinoic acid receptors. FASEB J 1996;10:940-954.
10. Desvergne B, Michalik L, Wahli W. Be fit or be sick: peroxisome proliferator-activated receptors are down the road. Mol Endocrinol 2004;18:1321-1332.
11. Forman BM, Chen J, Evans RM. Hypolipidemic drugs, polyunsaturated fatty acids, and eicosanoids are ligands for peroxisome proliferator-activated receptors α and δ. Proc Natl Acad Sci U S A. 1997;94:4312-4317.
12. Yu K, et al. Differential activation of peroxisome proliferator-activated receptors by eicosanoids. J Biol Chem 1995;270:23975-23983.
13. Ziouzenkova O, et al. Lipolysis of triglyceride-rich lipoproteins generates PPAR ligands: evidence for an antiinflammatory role for lipoprotein lipase. Proc Natl Acad Sci U S A 2003;100:2730-2735.
14. Issemann I, Green S. Activation of a member of the steroid hormone receptor superfamily by peroxisome proliferators. Nature 1990;347:645-650.
15. Rangwala SM, Lazar MA. Peroxisome proliferator-activated receptor gamma in diabetes and metabolism. Trends Pharmacol Sci 2004;25:331-336.
16. Forman BM, et al. 15-deoxy, delta 12, 14-prostaglandin J2 is a ligand for the adipocyte determination factor PPARγ. Cell 1995;83:803-812.
17. Kliewer SA, et al. A prostaglandin J2 metabolite binds peroxisome proliferator-activated receptor γ and promotes adipocyte differentiation. Cell 1995;83:813-819.
18. Yu C, et al. Mechanism by which fatty acids inhibit insulin activation of IRS-1 associated phosphatidylinositol 3-kinase activity in muscle. J Biol Chem 2002;277:50230-50236.
19. Lehmann JM, et al. An antidiabetic thiazolidinedione is a high affinity ligand for the nuclear peroxisome proliferator-activated receptor γ (PPARγ). J Biol Chem 1995;270:12953-12956.
20. Tontonoz P, Mangelsdorf DJ. Liver X receptor signaling pathways in cardiovascular disease. Mol Endocrinol 2003;17:985-993.
21. Giguere V. Orphan nuclear receptors: from gene to function. Endocr Rev 1999;20:689-725.
22. Lu NZ, Cidlowski JA. The origin and functions of multiple human glucocorticoid receptor isoforms. Ann N Y Acad Sci 2004;1024:102-123.
23. Zhang J, Lazar MA. The mechanism of action of thyroid hormone receptors. Ann Rev Physiol 2000;62:439-466.
24. Achermann JC, Jameson JL. Fertility and infertility: genetic contributions from the hypothalamic-pituitary-gonadal axis. Mol Endocrinol 1999;13:812-818.
25. Seol W, Choi HS, Moore DD. An orphan nuclear hormone receptor that lacks a DNA binding domain and heterodimerizes with other receptors. Science 1996;272:1336-1339.
26. Gurnell M, Chatterjee VK. Nuclear receptors in disease: thyroid receptor beta, peroxisome-proliferator-activated receptor gamma and orphan receptors. Essays Biochem 2004;40:169-189.
27. Niu DM, et al. Contributions of bone maturation measurements to the differential diagnosis of neonatal transient hypothyroidism versus dyshormonogenetic congenital hypothyroidism. Acta Paediatr 2004;93:1301-1306.
28. McPhaul MJ. Molecular defects of the androgen receptor. Recent Prog Horm Res 2002;57:181-194.
29. Palermo M, Quinkler M, Stewart PM. Apparent mineralocorticoid excess syndrome: an overview. Arq Bras Endocrinol Metabol 2004;48:687-696.
30. Stewart PM, Krozowski ZS. 11 beta-hydroxysteroid dehydrogenase. Vitam Horm 1999;57:249-324.
31. Moras D, Gronemeyer H. The nuclear receptor ligand-binding domain: structure and function. Curr Opin Cell Biol 1998;10:384-391.
32. Weatherman RV, Fletterick RJ, Scanlan TS. Nuclear receptor ligands and ligand-binding domains. Ann Rev Biochem 1999;68:559-581.
33. Umesono K, Murakami KK, Thompson CC, et al. Direct repeats as selective response elements for the thyroid hormone, retinoic acid, and vitamin D3 receptors. Cell 1991;65:1255-1266.
34. Rastinejad F, Perlmann T, Evans RM, et al. Structural determinants of nuclear receptor assembly on DNA direct repeats. Nature 1995;375:203-211.
35. Roeder RG. Role of general and gene-specific cofactors in the regulation of eukaryotic transcription. Cold Spring Harb Symp Quant Biol 1998;63:201-218.
36. Halachmi S, et al. Estrogen receptor-associated proteins: possible mediators of hormone-induced transcription. Science 1994;264:1455-1458.
37. Smith CL, O'Malley BW. Coregulator function: a key to understanding tissue specificity of selective receptor modulators. Endocr Rev 2004;25:45-71.
38. Feng W, et al. Hormone-dependent coactivator binding to a hydrophobic cleft on nuclear receptors. Science 1998;280:1747-1749.
39. Nolte RT, et al. Ligand binding and co-activator assembly of the peroxisome proliferator-activated receptor-γ. Nature 1998;395:137-143.
40. Shiau AK, et al. The structural basis of estrogen receptor/coactivator recognition and the antagonism of this interaction by tamoxifen. Cell 1998;95:927-937.
41. Heery DM, Kalkhoven E, Hoare S, Parker MG. A signature motif in transcriptional co-activators mediates binding to nuclear receptors. Nature 1997;387:733-736.
42. Fischle W, Wang Y, Allis CD. Histone and chromatin cross-talk. Curr Opin Cell Biol 2003;15:172-183.
43. Glass CK, Rose DW, Rosenfeld MG. Nuclear receptor coactivators. Curr Opin Cell Biol 1997;9:222-232.
44. Aoyagi S, Trotter KW, Archer TK. ATP-dependent chromatin remodeling complexes and their role in nuclear receptor-dependent transcription in vivo. Vitam Horm 2005;70:281-307.
45. Ito M, et al. Identity between TRAP and SMCC complexes indicates novel pathways for the function of nuclear receptors and diverse mammalian activators. Mol Cell 1999;3:361-370.
46. Rachez C, et al. A novel protein complex that interacts with the vitamin D3 receptor in a ligand-dependent manner and enhances VDR transactivation in a cell-free system. Genes Dev 1998;12:1787-1800.
47. Shang Y, Hu X, DiRenzo J, et al. Cofactor dynamics and sufficiency in estrogen receptor-regulated transcription. Cell 2000;103:843-852.
48. Hu X, Lazar MA. Transcriptional repression by nuclear hormone receptors. Trends Endocrinol Metab 2000;11:6-10.
49. Privalsky ML. The role of corepressors in transcriptional regulation by nuclear hormone receptors. Annu Rev Physiol 2004;66:315-360.
50. Hu X, Lazar MA. The CoRNR motif controls the recruitment of corepressors to nuclear hormone receptors. Nature 1999;402:93-96.
51. Glass CK, Rosenfeld MG. The coregulator exchange in transcriptional functions of nuclear receptors. Genes Dev 2000;14:121-141.
52. Ishizuka T, Lazar MA. The nuclear receptor corepressor deacetylase activating domain is essential for repression by thyroid hormone receptor. Mol Endocrinol 2005;19:1443-1451.
53. Lazar MA. Thyroid hormone action: a binding contract. J Clin Invest 2003;112:497-499.
54. Kumar R, Thompson EB. Transactivation functions of the N-terminal domains of nuclear hormone receptors: protein folding and coactivator interactions. Mol Endocrinol 2003;17:1-10.
55. Shao D, Lazar MA. Modulating nuclear receptor function: may the phos be with you. J Clin Invest 1999;103:1617-1618.
56. Gronemeyer H, Gustafsson JA, Laudet V. Principles for modulation of the nuclear receptor superfamily. Nat Rev Drug Discov 2004;3:950-964.
57. Osborne CK, Zaho H, Fuqua SA. Selective estrogen receptor modulators: structure, function, and clinical use. J Clin Oncol 2000;18:3172-3186.
58. Shang Y, Brown M. Molecular determinants for the tissue specificity of SERMs. Science 2002;295:2465-2468.

CHAPTER 5

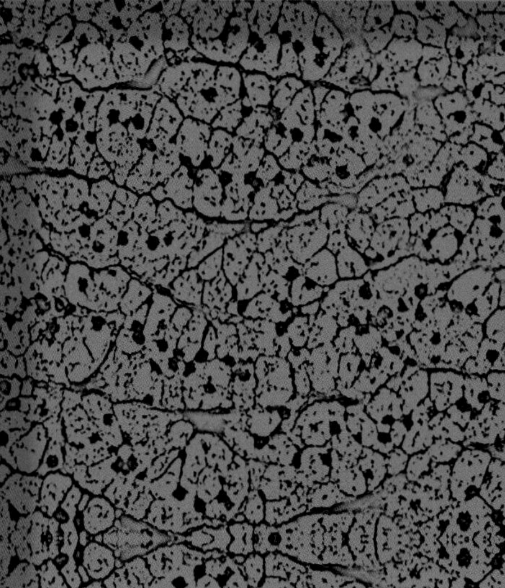

MECHANISM OF ACTION OF HORMONES THAT ACT AT THE CELL SURFACE

Allen Spiegel, Christin Carter-Su, and Simeon I. Taylor

Hormones are secreted into the blood and act upon target cells at a distance from the secretory gland. In order to respond to a hormone, a target cell must contain the essential components of a signaling pathway. First, there must be a receptor to bind the hormone. Second, there must be an effector—or example, an enzymatic activity that is regulated when the hormone binds to its receptor. Finally, there must be appropriate downstream signaling pathways to mediate the physiologic responses to the hormone. In fact, this type of mechanism involving receptors, effectors, and downstream signaling pathways is quite general and also functions in nonendocrine systems such as those regulated by neurotransmitters, cytokines, and paracrine and autocrine factors. This chapter reviews several examples of endocrine signaling pathways that begin with activation of receptors located on the surface of target cells, with particular attention to the molecular mechanisms that function in normal physiology and to the molecular pathology causing disease.

Receptors

Definition and Classification

There are two essential functions that define hormone receptors: (1) the ability to bind the hormone and (2) the ability to couple hormone binding to hormone action. Both components of the definition are essential; for example, many hormones bind to binding proteins that are distinct from receptors because the binding proteins do not trigger the signaling pathways that mediate hormone action.

Many classes of receptors are of interest in endocrinology. Some receptors are located within the cell and function as transcription factors (e.g., receptors for steroid and thyroid hormones). Other receptors are located on the cell surface and function primarily to transport their ligands into the cell by a process referred to as *receptor-mediated endocytosis* (e.g., low-density lipoprotein receptors). In this chapter, we focus upon cell-surface receptors that trigger intracellular signaling pathways. These cell-surface receptors can be classified according to the molecular mechanisms by which they accomplish their signaling function:

1. Ligand-gated ion channels (e.g., nicotinic acetylcholine receptors)
2. Receptor tyrosine kinases (e.g., receptors for insulin and insulin-like growth factor I [IGF-I])
3. Receptor serine/threonine kinases (e.g., receptors for activins and inhibins)
4. Receptor guanylate cyclase (e.g., atrial natriuretic factor receptor)
5. G protein–coupled receptors (e.g., receptors for adrenergic agents, muscarinic cholinergic agents, glycoprotein hormones, glucagon, and parathyroid hormone)
6. Cytokine receptors (e.g., receptors for growth hormone, prolactin, and leptin)

The receptors belonging to classes 1 to 4 are bifunctional molecules that can bind hormone as well as serve as effectors by functioning either as ion channels or as enzymes. In contrast, the receptors belonging to classes 5 and 6 have the ability to bind the hormone but must recruit a separate molecule to catalyze the effector function. For example, as the name implies, G protein–coupled receptors utilize G proteins to regulate downstream effector molecules. Similarly, cytokine receptors recruit cytosolic tyrosine kinases (e.g., Janus family tyrosine kinases, or JAKs) as effectors to trigger downstream signaling pathways.

Hormone Binding

As predicted by the fact that hormones circulate in relatively low concentrations in the plasma, the binding interaction between a hormone and its receptor is characterized by high binding affinity. Furthermore, hormone binding has a high degree of specificity. Generally, the receptor binds its cognate hormone more tightly than it binds other hormones. However, some receptors may bind structurally related hormones with lower affinity. For example, the insulin receptor binds insulin-like growth factors (IGFs) with approximately 100-fold lower affinity than it binds insulin. Similarly, the thyrotropin receptor binds human chorionic gonadotropin with lower affinity than it binds thyrotropin. This phenomenon has been referred to as *specificity spillover* and provides an explanation of several pathologic conditions, such as hypoglycemia caused by tumors secreting IGF-II and hyperthyroidism associated with choriocarcinoma.[1]

Binding of a hormone (H) to its receptor (R) can be described mathematically as an equilibrium reaction:

$$H + R \leftrightharpoons HR$$

At equilibrium, $K_a = (HR)/(H)(R)$, where K_a is the association constant for the formation of the hormone receptor complex (HR). As originally shown by Scatchard, it is possible to rearrange this equation in terms of the total concentration of receptor binding sites, $R_0 = (R) + (RH)$, as follows:

$$K_a = (HR)/\{[R_0 - (HR)](H)\}$$

$$(HR) = K_a[R_0 - (HR)](H)$$

$$(HR)/(H) = K_aR_0 - K_a(HR)$$

A straight line is obtained when (HR)/(H) (i.e., the ratio of bound to free hormone) is plotted as a function of (HR) (the concentration of bound hormone). The slope of the line is $-K_a$, and the line intercepts the horizontal axis at the point where $(HR) = R_0$ = the total number of binding sites. This type of plot is referred to as a *Scatchard plot* and has been used as a graphic method to estimate the affinity with which a receptor binds its hormone. Although the binding properties of some receptors are described more or less accurately by these simple equations, other receptors exhibit more complex properties. This simple algebraic derivation of the Scatchard equation implicitly assumes that there is only one class of receptors and that the binding sites on the receptors do not interact with one another. If these assumptions do not apply to the interaction of a particular hormone with its receptor, the Scatchard plot may not be linear.

Several molecular mechanisms may contribute to nonlinearity of the Scatchard plot. For example, there may be more than one type of receptor that binds the hormone (e.g., a high-affinity, low-capacity site and a low-affinity, high-capacity site). Alternatively, some receptors have more than one binding site, and there may be cooperative interactions among the binding sites (e.g., the insulin receptor). In addition, the interaction between a G protein and a G protein–coupled receptor may affect the affinity with which the receptor binds its ligand; moreover, the effect on binding affinity depends on whether guanosine diphosphate (GDP) or guanosine triphosphate (GTP) is bound to the G protein. However, a detailed discussion of these complexities is beyond the scope of this chapter.

Regulation of Hormone Sensitivity

Early in the history of endocrinology, attention was focused on the regulation of hormone secretion as the most important mechanism for regulating physiology. However, it has become apparent that the target cell is not passive. Rather, there are many influences that can alter the sensitivity of the target cell's response to a given concentration of hormone. For example, the number of receptors can be regulated. All things being equal, hormone sensitivity is directly related to the number of hormone receptors expressed on the cell surface. In addition, posttranslational modifications of the receptor can modify either the affinity of hormone binding or the efficiency of coupling to downstream signaling pathways. Moreover, all of the downstream components in the hormone action pathway are subject to similar types of regulatory influences, which can have a significant impact on the ability of the target cell to respond to hormone.

Just as hormone sensitivity is subject to normal physiologic regulation, pathologic influences can cause disease by targeting components of the hormone action pathway. Multiple etiologic factors can impair the hormone action pathway, such as genetic influences, autoimmune processes, and exogenous toxins. For example, disease mechanisms can alter the functions of cell-surface receptors, effectors such as G proteins, and other components of the downstream signaling pathways. This chapter describes several examples illustrating these principles.

Receptor Tyrosine Kinases

Receptor tyrosine kinases have several structural features in common: an extracellular domain containing the ligand-binding site, a single transmembrane domain, and an intracellular portion that includes the tyrosine kinase catalytic domain (Fig. 5–1). Analysis of the sequence of the human genome suggests that there are approximately 100 receptor tyrosine kinases. The tyrosine kinase domain is the most highly conserved sequence among all the receptors in this family. In contrast, there is considerable variation among the sequences of the extracellular domains. Indeed, the family of receptor tyrosine kinases can be

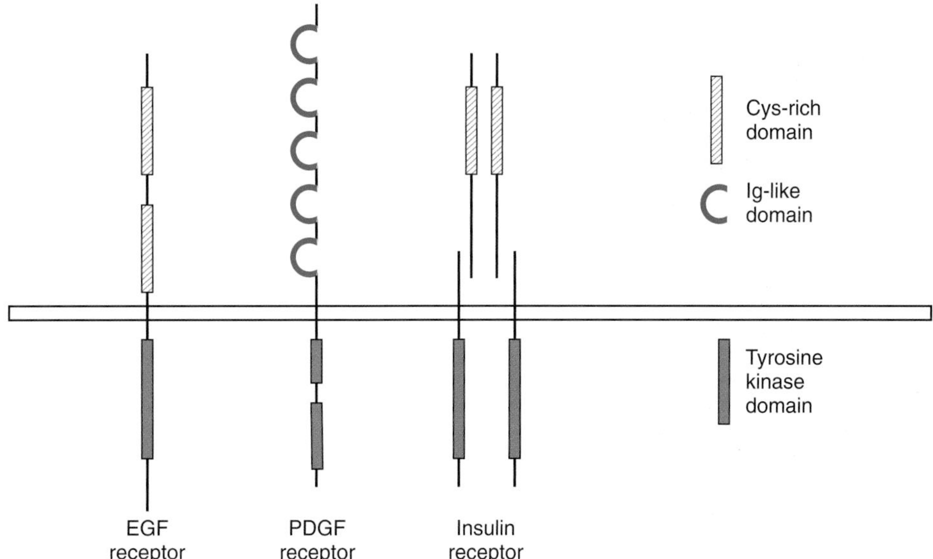

Figure 5–1 ▪ Receptor tyrosine kinases. This diagram illustrates 3 of the 16 families of receptor tyrosine kinases.[2,3] All receptor tyrosine kinases possess an extracellular domain containing the ligand-binding site, a single transmembrane domain, and an intracellular domain containing the tyrosine kinase domain. Several structural motifs (i.e., cysteine-rich domain, immunoglobulin-like domain, tyrosine kinase domain) in these receptor tyrosine kinases are indicated on the right side of the figure. *Cys,* Cysteine; *EGF,* epidermal growth factor; *Ig,* immunoglobulin; *PDGF,* platelet-derived growth factor.

classified into 16 subfamilies, primarily on the basis of the differences in the structure of the extracellular domain.[2] Furthermore, receptor tyrosine kinases mediate the biologic actions of a wide variety of ligands, including insulin, epidermal growth factor (EGF), platelet-derived growth factor (PDGF), and vascular endothelial cell–derived growth factor. The variation in the sequences of the extracellular domains enables the receptors to bind this structurally diverse collection of ligands.

The EGF receptor was the first cell-surface receptor demonstrated to possess tyrosine kinase activity[4] and it was the first receptor tyrosine kinase to be cloned.[5] Like most receptor tyrosine kinases, the EGF receptor exists primarily as a monomer in the absence of ligand. However, binding of ligand induces receptor dimerization. As discussed later in this chapter, ligand-induced dimerization is central to the mechanism whereby the receptor mediates the biologic activity of EGF. In addition to the ability to form homodimers, the EGF receptor can form heterodimers with other members of the same subfamily of receptor tyrosine kinases. Because a small number of receptors can combine in a large number of pairings, heterodimer formation has the potential to fine-tune the specificity of receptors with respect to both ligand binding and downstream signaling.

The insulin receptor is of special interest to endocrinologists because diabetes is among the most common diseases of the endocrine system. Furthermore, the insulin receptor closely resembles the type 1 receptor for IGFs.[6] This is the receptor that mediates the biologic actions of IGF-I and therefore also plays an important role in the physiology of growth hormone (GH) in vivo. Although the kinase domains of receptors for insulin and IGF-I closely resemble other receptor tyrosine kinases, at least two distinctive features set them apart. First, the receptors are synthesized as proreceptors that undergo proteolytic cleavage into two subunits (α and β). The α subunit contains the ligand-binding site; the β subunit includes the transmembrane and tyrosine kinase domains. Second, both receptors exist as $\alpha_2\beta_2$ heterotetramers that are stabilized by intersubunit disulfide bonds. In contrast to other receptor tyrosine kinases, which are thought to dimerize in response to ligand binding, the insulin receptor exists as a dimer of αβ monomers even in the absence of ligand. The remainder of this section reviews the molecular mechanisms whereby receptor tyrosine kinases mediate biologic action, with special emphasis on the insulin receptor as an illustrative example.

Receptor Activation: Role of Receptor Dimerization

Dimerization plays a central role in the mechanism whereby most receptor tyrosine kinases are activated by their cognate ligands.[2,7] Although receptor dimerization is a common theme, the detailed molecular mechanisms differ from receptor to receptor. The following are three examples of the mechanisms of receptor dimerization (Fig. 5–2).[8-12]

Dimeric Ligand

PDGF and vascular endothelial cell-derived growth factor are examples of dimeric ligands (see Fig. 5–2).[8,9,13] Because each subunit of ligand can bind one receptor molecule, simultaneous binding of two receptor molecules drives receptor dimerization. Direct support for this type of mechanism is provided by the crystal structure of vascular endothelial cell–derived growth factor bound to its receptor (Flt-1).[13]

Two Receptor Binding Sites on a Monomeric Ligand

Although this mechanism is important for many receptor tyrosine kinases, it was first shown rigorously for the GH receptor, which is not a member of the receptor tyrosine kinase family (see Fig. 5–2).[10-12] As illustrated by the crystal structure of GH bound to its receptor, one molecule of ligand can bind two molecules of receptor. In fact, there are two distinct receptor-binding sites on each GH molecule, and this enables the ligand to promote receptor dimerization. This observation has an important implication for pharmacology. By abolishing one of the two receptor-binding sites, it is possible to design mutant ligands that lack the ability to promote receptor dimerization and therefore lack the ability to trigger hormone action. Nevertheless, by binding to receptors, the mutant ligand acquires the ability to inhibit the action of the endogenous hormone. Such mutant GH molecules have been developed as therapeutic agents, for example, in conditions such as acromegaly.

Preexisting Receptor Dimers

The insulin receptor represents a paradox. The insulin receptor exists as a dimer even in the absence of ligand. (Actually, it is

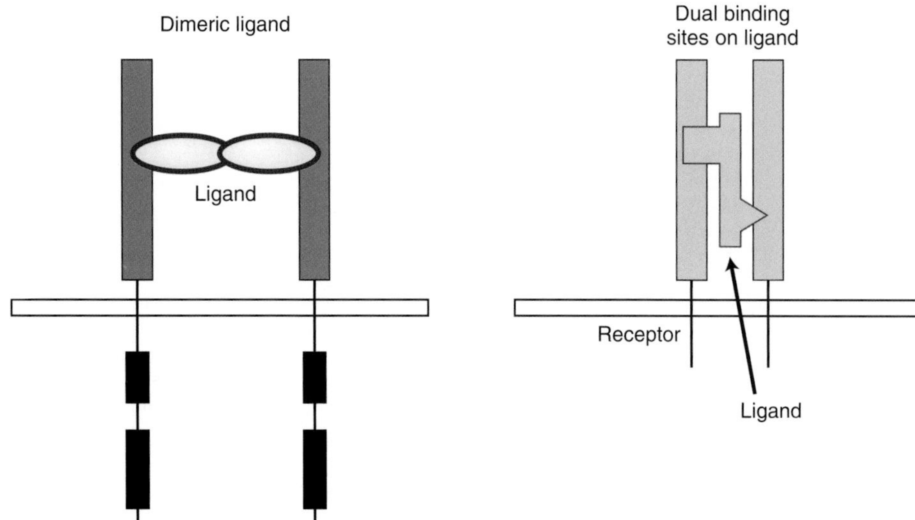

Figure 5–2 ▪ Ligand-induced dimerization of receptors. Two molecular mechanisms of ligand-induced receptor dimerization are illustrated. In the case of the platelet-derived growth factor, the ligand is dimeric and therefore contains two receptor binding sites.[8,9] In the case of growth hormone, a single ligand molecule contains two binding sites so that it can bind simultaneously to two receptor molecules.[10-12]

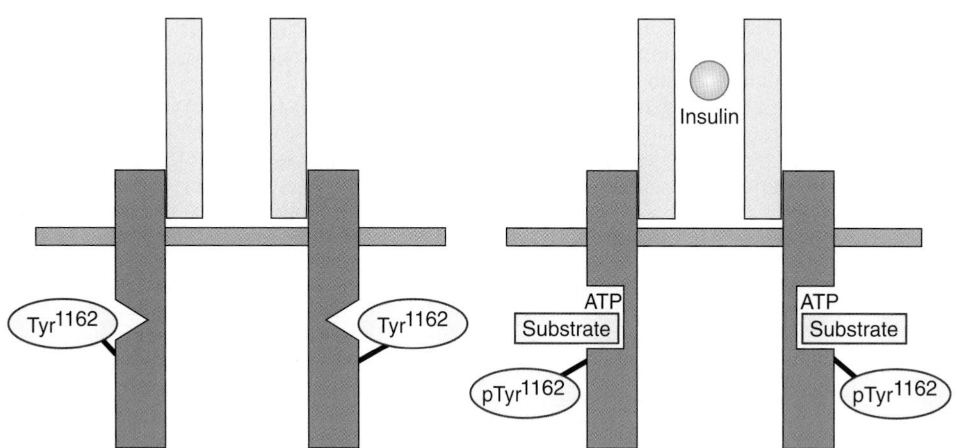

Figure 5–3 ▪ Phosphorylation of tyrosine residues in the activation loop leads to activation of the insulin receptor tyrosine kinase. A hypothetical mechanism for ligand-stimulated activation of the insulin receptor tyrosine kinase is illustrated. The model is based on the three-dimensional structure of the isolated insulin receptor tyrosine kinase as determined by x-ray crystallography.[19,20,23] In the inactive insulin receptor kinase (*left*), Tyr1162 blocks the active site so that substrates cannot bind. In contrast, when the tyrosine residues in the activation loop (including Tyr1162) become phosphorylated (*right*), Tyr1162 moves out of the way, and there is a conformational change that allows binding of adenosine triphosphate (ATP) and protein substrate so that the kinase reaction can proceed.

an $\alpha_2\beta_2$ heterotetramer, which is a *dimer* of $\alpha\beta$ monomers.) If the receptor is already dimerized, why is it not active? Although the molecular details remain to be elucidated, it seems likely that the two halves of the insulin receptor are not oriented in an optimal way to permit receptor activation in the absence of ligand. Perhaps, insulin binding triggers a conformational change that somehow mimics the effects of dimerization in other receptor tyrosine kinases. In any case, several studies have demonstrated that receptor dimerization is necessary for the ability of insulin to activate its receptor. For example, $\alpha\beta$ monomers retain the ability to bind insulin but are not activated in response to insulin binding.[14,15] Furthermore, indirect evidence suggests that a single insulin molecule binds simultaneously to both α subunits of the insulin receptor[16,17]; the ability to bind simultaneously to both halves of the dimeric receptor appears to be essential to the ability of insulin to activate its receptor.

Receptor Activation: Conformational Changes in the Kinase Domain

When ligand binds to the extracellular domain, it stimulates the tyrosine kinase activity of the intracellular domain. Although the detailed mechanisms of transmembrane signaling are not completely understood, considerable progress has been made in elucidating the molecular mechanisms of receptor activation. Investigations of the three-dimensional structure of the insulin receptor tyrosine kinase domain help explain why the receptor is maintained in a low-activity state in the absence of insulin (Fig. 5–3).[18-20] In the inactive form of the insulin receptor kinase, Tyr1162 is located in a position so that it blocks protein substrates from binding to the active site. Furthermore, in the inactive state of the tyrosine kinase domain, the active site assumes a conformation that does not accommodate magnesium adenosine triphosphate (ATP). Thus, the tyrosine kinase is inactive because the active site cannot bind either of its substrates. How does insulin activate the receptor? Insulin binding triggers autophosphorylation of three tyrosine residues (Tyr1158, Tyr1162, and Tyr1163) in the "activation loop." When the three tyrosine residues in the activation loop become phosphorylated, an important conformational change occurs. As a result of the movement of the activation loop, the active site acquires the ability to bind both ATP and protein substrates. Thus, the conformational change induced by autophosphorylation activates the receptor to phosphorylate other substrates.[21,22]

It remains unclear how this process is initiated. Because the inactive state of the tyrosine kinase cannot bind ATP, it seems unlikely that phosphorylation of Tyr1162 proceeds by a true *auto*phosphorylation mechanism. Rather, it is likely that Tyr1162 in one β subunit is transphosphorylated by the second β subunit in the $\alpha_2\beta_2$ heterotetramer molecule.[2,23] However, this proposed mechanism poses a "chicken and egg" problem. It requires that at least one of the β subunits is active before the Tyr residues in the activation loop become phosphorylated. Perhaps the activation loop is somewhat mobile so that some molecules of unphosphorylated tyrosine kinase can assume an active conformation and initiate a chain reaction of transphosphorylation and receptor activation.

Receptor Tyrosine Kinases Phosphorylate Other Intracellular Proteins

Once activated, tyrosine kinases are capable of phosphorylating other protein substrates. Several factors determine which proteins are phosphorylated under physiologic conditions within the cell.

Amino Acid Sequence Context of Tyr Residue

Tyrosine kinases do not exhibit strict specificity with respect to the amino acid sequence of the phosphorylation site. Nevertheless, most tyrosine phosphorylation sites are located in the vicinity of acidic amino acid residues (i.e., Glu or Asp).[2]

Binding to the Tyrosine Kinase

Some protein substrates bind directly to the intracellular domain of the receptor. The binding interaction brings the substrate into close proximity to the kinase, thereby promoting phosphorylation of the substrate. For example, the insulin receptor substrate (IRS) proteins are characterized by a highly conserved phosphotyrosine-binding (PTB) domain that binds to a conserved motif (Asn-Pro-Xaa-pTyr) in the juxtamembrane domain of the insulin receptor.[24-26] Binding of the PTB domain to the insulin receptor requires phosphorylation of the Tyr residue in the Asn-Pro-Xaa-pTyr motif. This provides another mechanism (in addition to activation of the intrinsic receptor tyrosine kinase) whereby autophosphorylation of the receptor enhances phosphorylation of IRS proteins. Similarly, substrates for some tyrosine kinases contain Src homology 2 (SH2) domains, highly conserved domains that bind phosphotyrosine residues (see Functional Significance of Tyrosine Phosphorylation). For example, the activated PDGF receptor contains a phosphotyrosine residue near its C-terminus that binds the SH2 domain of phospholipase Cγ. This enables the PDGF receptor to phosphorylate and activate phospholipase Cγ.[2,27]

Subcellular Localization

Because receptor tyrosine kinases are located in the plasma membrane, they are in close proximity to other plasma membrane proteins. This colocalization has the potential to promote phosphorylation. For example, the insulin receptor has been reported to phosphorylate pp120/hepatocyte antigen-4 (HA4).[28,29] Like the insulin receptor, pp120/HA4 is an integral membrane glycoprotein associated with the plasma membrane of hepatocytes. Similarly, FGF receptor substrate-2 (FRS2), a substrate of the fibroblast-derived growth factor receptor, is targeted to the plasma membrane by an N-terminal myristoylation site.[30]

Functional Significance of Tyrosine Phosphorylation

There are at least two distinct mechanisms whereby tyrosine phosphorylation regulates protein function. First, tyrosine phosphorylation can induce a conformational change in a protein, thereby altering its function. For example, as discussed earlier, phosphorylation of the three Tyr residues in the activation loop of the insulin receptor changes the conformation of the active site, thereby facilitating binding of substrates and activating the receptor tyrosine kinase.[18-20] However, most of the effects of tyrosine phosphorylation on protein function are mediated indirectly by regulating protein-protein interactions. In order to understand how tyrosine phosphorylation regulates protein-protein interactions, it is useful to review the biochemistry of c-src, the prototype of a nonreceptor tyrosine kinase. When the amino acid sequence of c-src is analyzed, it is apparent that there are three highly conserved domains in the molecule: the kinase catalytic domain and two noncatalytic domains that are referred to as src homology domains 2 and 3 (SH2 and SH3, respectively).

SH2 Domains

SH2 domains consist of conserved sequences (approximately 100 amino acid residues) that are present in many proteins that function in signaling pathways. From a functional point of view, SH2 domains share the ability to bind pTyr residues. However, individual SH2 domains vary with respect to their binding specificity. The binding affinity of an SH2 is determined by the three amino acid residues downstream from the pTyr residue. For example, the SH2 domains of phosphatidylinositol (PI) 3-kinase exhibit a preference for pTyr-(Met/Xaa)-Xaa-Met, whereas the SH2 domain of growth factor receptor binding protein 2 (Grb-2) prefers to bind pTyr-Xaa-Asn-Xaa. Thus, a given SH2 domain binds to a tyrosine-phosphorylated protein if and only if the pTyr residue is located in a context that corresponds to the binding specificity of the SH2 domain.

SH3 Domains

SH3 domains consist of conserved sequences (approximately 50 amino acid residues) that bind to proline-rich sequences. Like SH2 domains, SH3 domains are found in many proteins that function in signaling pathways.

Downstream Signaling Pathways

Receptor tyrosine kinases mediate the action of a wide variety of ligands in a wide variety of cell types. The bewildering complexity of the downstream signaling pathways corresponds to the huge number of physiologic processes that are regulated by receptor tyrosine kinases. Although it is beyond the scope of this chapter to attempt an encyclopedic review of all the downstream signaling pathways, we have selected examples to illustrate general principles.

As discussed earlier, the activated insulin receptor phosphorylates multiple substrates including IRS-1, IRS-2, IRS-3, and IRS-4.[31] Each of these substrates contains multiple tyrosine phosphorylation sites, many of which correspond to consensus sequences for SH2 domains in important signaling molecules. Thus, IRS proteins serve as docking proteins that bind SH2 domain-containing proteins. Among these, two of the most important are PI 3-kinase and Grb-2. Binding of SH2 domains triggers multiple downstream signaling pathways.

Phosphatidylinositol 3-Kinase

The catalytic subunit of PI 3-kinase (p110; molecular mass approximately 110,000) is bound to a regulatory subunit. The classical isoforms of the regulatory subunit (p85; molecular mass approximately 85,000) contain two SH2 domains, both of which bind to pTyr in the context of pTyr-(Met/Xaa)-Xaa-Met motifs. Binding of pTyr residues to both SH2 domains of p85 leads to maximal activation of PI 3-kinase catalytic activity. (Submaximal activation can be achieved with occupancy of a single SH2 domain in p85.) Because all four IRS molecules (IRS-1, IRS-2, IRS-3, and IRS-4) contain multiple tyrosine phosphorylation sites that conform to the Tyr-(Met/Xaa)-Xaa-Met consensus sequence, insulin-stimulated phosphorylation promotes binding of IRS proteins to the SH2 domains in the regulatory subunit PI 3-kinase, thereby increasing the enzymatic activity of the catalytic subunit.[32-35] Activation of PI 3-kinase triggers activation of a cascade of downstream kinases, beginning with phosphoinositide-dependent kinases 1 and 2. These phosphoinositide-dependent kinases phosphorylate and activate multiple downstream protein kinases including protein kinase B and atypical isoforms of protein kinase C.[36-42]

A large body of evidence demonstrates that the pathways downstream from PI 3-kinase mediate the metabolic activities of insulin (e.g., activation of glucose transport into skeletal muscle, activation of glycogen synthesis, and inhibition of transcription of the phosphoenolpyruvate carboxykinase gene). Among other lines of evidence, PI 3-kinase inhibitors (e.g., LY294002 and wortmannin) block the metabolic actions of insulin.[43] Similarly, overexpression of dominant negative mutants of the p85 regulatory subunit of PI 3-kinase also inhibits the metabolic actions of insulin.[36] Although it is generally agreed that activation of PI 3-kinase is necessary, it is controversial whether it is sufficient to trigger the metabolic actions of insulin. For example, a second parallel pathway may also be required. The latter pathway involves tyrosine phosphorylation of Cbl, another protein that can be phosphorylated by the insulin receptor in some cell types.[44-46]

Grb-2 and the Activation of Ras

Grb-2 is a short adaptor molecule that contains an SH2 domain[47] capable of binding to pTyr residues in several signaling molecules, for example, IRS-1 and Shc, another PTB domain-containing protein that is phosphorylated by several receptor tyrosine kinases including the insulin receptor.[48,49] The SH2 domain of Grb-2 is flanked by two SH3 domains,[47] which bind to proline-containing sequences in mSos (the mammalian homologue of *Drosophila* son-of-sevenless).[50] mSos is capable of activating Ras, a small G protein that plays an important role in intracellular signaling pathways. mSos activates Ras by catalyzing the exchange of GTP for GDP in the guanine nucleotide-binding site of Ras. This, in turn, triggers the activation of a cascade of serine/threonine-specific protein kinases including Raf, mitogen-activated protein/extracellular signal-regulated kinase (MEK), and mitogen-activated protein (MAP) kinase. These pathways downstream from Ras contribute to the ability of tyrosine kinases to promote cell growth and regulate the expression of various genes.

We have focused on the signaling pathways downstream from the insulin receptor because of the importance of insulin and IGF-I in endocrinology (Fig. 5–4). In many ways, the molecular mechanisms closely resemble those downstream from other receptor tyrosine kinases. However, the insulin signaling pathway is atypical in at least one respect. The insulin receptor phosphorylates docking proteins (e.g., IRS-1), which bind SH2

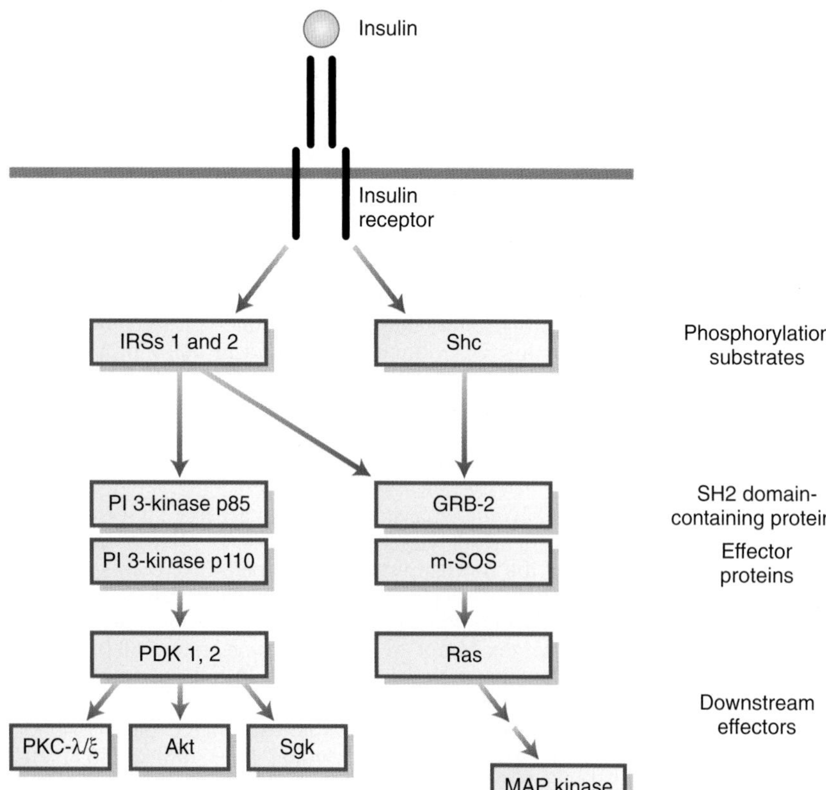

Figure 5–4 ▪ Simplified model of signaling pathways downstream from the insulin receptor. Insulin binds to the insulin receptor, thereby activating the receptor tyrosine kinase to phosphorylate tyrosine residues on insulin receptor substrates (IRSs) including IRS-1 and IRS-2.[31] Consequently, phosphotyrosine residues in IRS molecules bind to Src homology 2 (SH2) domains in molecules such as growth factor receptor-binding protein 2 (GRB-2) and the p85 regulatory subunit of phosphatidylinositol (PI) 3-kinase. These SH2 domain-containing proteins initiate two distinct branches of the signaling pathway. Activation of PI 3-kinase leads to activation of phosphoinositide-dependent kinases (PDKs) 1 and 2, which activates multiple protein kinases including Akt/protein kinase B, atypical protein kinase C (PKC) isoforms, and serum/glucocorticoid-activated protein kinases (Sgk).[53] Grb-2 interacts with m-SOS, a guanine nucleotide exchange factor that activates Ras.[54] Activation of Ras triggers a cascade of protein kinases leading to the activation of mitogen-activated protein (MAP) kinase.

domain-containing proteins (e.g., PI 3-kinase and Grb-2). In contrast, the intracellular domains of most receptor tyrosine kinases contain binding sites for SH2 domains. For example, the SH2 domain of Grb-2 binds to pTyr716 in the activated PDGF receptor.[2] Similarly, the PDGF receptor contains two Tyr-(Met/Xaa)-Xaa-Met motifs in the kinase insert domain that bind to the two SH2 domains in the p85 subunit of PI 3-kinase.[2,51] It is not clear why some tyrosine kinases (e.g., the PDGF receptor) activate PI 3-kinase through a direct binding interaction, whereas others (e.g., the insulin receptor) utilize an indirect mechanism involving docking proteins. However, in contrast to PDGF receptors, which are associated with the plasma membrane, IRS proteins appear to be associated with the cytoskeleton.[52] Perhaps this differential subcellular localization contributes to signaling specificity. In other words, if insulin and PDGF receptors trigger translocation of PI 3-kinase to different locations within the cell, this compartmentation may permit two different receptors to elicit different biologic responses even though both responses are mediated by the same signaling molecule (i.e., PI 3-kinase).

Off Signals: Termination of Hormone Action

Just as there are complex biochemical pathways that mediate hormone action, there are also mechanisms to terminate the biologic response. The necessity for these mechanisms is illustrated by the following example. After we eat a meal, the concentration of plasma glucose increases. This elicits an increase in insulin secretion, which in turn leads to a decrease in plasma glucose levels. If these processes went on unchecked, the level of glucose in the plasma would eventually fall so low that it would lead to symptomatic hypoglycemia. How is insulin action terminated? The answers to this question are not yet entirely clear, but several mechanisms contribute to turning off the insulin signaling pathway.

Receptor-Mediated Endocytosis

Insulin binding to its receptor triggers endocytosis of the receptor. Although most of the internalized receptors are recycled to the plasma membrane, some receptors are transported to lysosomes, where they are degraded.[55,56] As a result, insulin binding accelerates the rate of receptor degradation, thereby down-regulating the number of receptors on the cell surface. Furthermore, endosomes contain proton pumps, which acidify the lumen; the acidic pH within the endosome promotes dissociation of insulin from its receptor. Ultimately, insulin is transported to the lysosome for degradation. In fact, receptor-mediated endocytosis is the principal mechanism whereby insulin is cleared from the plasma.[57] Binding of ligands to other receptor tyrosine kinases also triggers receptor-mediated endocytosis by similar mechanisms.

Protein Tyrosine Phosphatases

Protein phosphorylation is a dynamic process. Tyrosine kinases catalyze the phosphorylation of tyrosine residues, but there are also protein tyrosine phosphatases (PTPases) to remove the phosphates.[2] Thus, PTPases antagonize the action of tyrosine kinases. Studies with knockout mice have demonstrated that the absence of PTPase-1B is associated with increased insulin sensitivity and also protects against weight gain.[58,59] Nevertheless, the human genome encodes a large number of PTPases, and it is an important goal of research to elucidate their physiologic functions. If one could develop selective inhibitors of the PTPases that oppose the effects of the insulin receptor tyrosine kinase, it is possible that these inhibitors would provide novel therapies for diabetes.

Serine/Threonine Kinases

Most receptor tyrosine kinases, including the insulin receptor, are substrates for phosphorylation by Ser/Thr-specific protein kinases. Interestingly, the Ser/Thr phosphorylation appears to inhibit the action of the tyrosine kinase. Similarly, other phosphotyrosine-containing proteins are subject to inhibitory influences of Ser/Thr phosphorylation resistance. For example, it has been reported that Ser/Thr phosphorylation of IRS-1 may inhibit insulin action, thereby causing insulin resistance.[60-64]

Mechanisms of Disease

The simplest forms of endocrine disease are caused by either a deficiency or an excess of a hormone. However, hormone resistance syndromes resulting from defects in the signaling pathways can masquerade as hormone deficiency states. Similarly, diseases associated with constitutively activated receptors can mimic states of hormone excess. In some cases, the abnormality in hormone action is genetic in origin, resulting from a mutation in a gene encoding one of the proteins in the signaling pathway. Similar syndromes can also be caused by other mechanisms; for example, there are autoimmune syndromes caused by autoantibodies directed against cell-surface receptors. These clinical syndromes illustrate the principle that understanding the biochemical pathways of hormone action can provide important insights into the pathophysiology of human disease.

Genetic Defects in Receptor Function

At least two distinct major types of genetic defects can cause hormone resistance.[65] First, mutations can lead to a decrease in the number of receptors. For example, in the case of the insulin receptor, mutations have been identified that decrease receptor number by at least three mechanisms: (1) impairing receptor biosynthesis, (2) inhibiting the transport of receptors to their normal location in the plasma membrane, and (3) accelerating the rate of receptor degradation. Second, mutations can impair the intrinsic activities of the receptor. In the case of the insulin receptor, mutations have been reported that decrease the affinity of insulin binding or inhibit receptor tyrosine kinase activity.

Receptor dimerization is known to play a central role in the mechanisms whereby ligands activate many cell-surface receptors. This role has been shown most convincingly in the case of the GH receptor (a member of the family of cytokine receptors) but has also been postulated for receptor tyrosine kinases. The syndromes of multiple endocrine neoplasia types 2A and 2B and familial medullary carcinoma of the thyroid are caused by mutations in the gene encoding the Ret tyrosine kinase (a subunit of the receptor for glial cell–derived growth factor).[66] Ordinarily, cysteine residues in the extracellular domain of Ret participate in the formation of intramolecular disulfide bonds. Mutation of one of the cysteine residues leaves an unpaired cysteine residue that promotes dimerization of Ret molecules, thereby activating the Ret receptor tyrosine kinase (Fig. 5–5). Activation of the Ret tyrosine kinase through this germ line mutation converts Ret into an oncogene.

Autoantibodies Directed against Cell-Surface Receptors

Inhibitory antireceptor autoantibodies were first identified in myasthenia gravis.[69] In this neurologic disease, antibodies to the

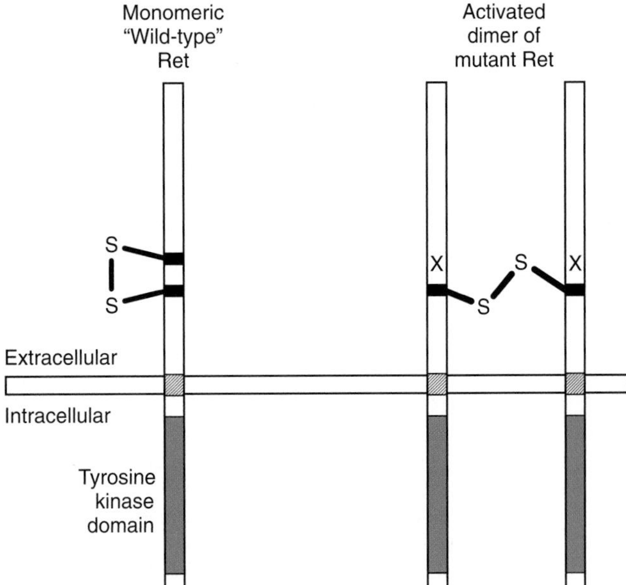

Figure 5–5 ▪ Mutations leading to constitutive activation of Ret. "Wild-type" Ret has intramolecular disulfide bonds formed by two cysteine residues in the same receptor molecule (*left*). When one of the two cysteine residues is mutated, the unpaired cysteine residue is available to form an intermolecular disulfide bond with a cysteine residue on another receptor molecule. This leads to receptor dimerization (*right*), which in turn leads to constitutive activation of the receptor tyrosine kinase.[66-68] This type of mutation has been identified in patients with multiple endocrine neoplasia type 2.

nicotinic acetylcholine receptor impair neuromuscular transmission, apparently by accelerating receptor degradation. Subsequently, autoantibodies to the insulin receptor were demonstrated to block insulin action in the syndrome of type B extreme insulin resistance.[70] Insulin resistance is caused by at least two mechanisms: (1) the antireceptor antibodies inhibit insulin binding to the receptor[71] and (2) the antibodies accelerate receptor degradation.[72]

Graves' disease provided the first example of stimulatory antireceptor autoantibodies.[73] In Graves' disease, there are autoantibodies directed against the thyroid-stimulating hormone (TSH) receptor. These antireceptor antibodies activate the TSH receptor, thereby stimulating growth of the thyroid gland as well as hypersecretion of thyroid hormone. This "experiment of nature" demonstrates that the receptor can be activated by ligands other than the physiologic ligand and that the normal spectrum of biologic actions can be triggered by this unphysiologic ligand (i.e., the antireceptor antibody). Similarly, antibodies to the insulin receptor have been demonstrated to activate the insulin receptor by mimicking insulin action. Although it is more common for a patient with anti–insulin receptor autoantibodies to present with insulin resistance, patients with anti–insulin receptor autoantibodies have also been reported to experience fasting hypoglycemia.[74,75]

Receptor Serine Kinases

Receptor serine kinases[76] have several features in common with receptor tyrosine kinases. For example, both classes of receptors possess (1) N-terminal extracellular domains, which bind ligand, (2) a single transmembrane domain, and (3) C-terminal intracellular domains, which possess protein kinase activity. However, the two classes of receptors differ with respect to enzymatic specificity. Whereas receptor tyrosine kinases phosphorylate tyrosine residues, receptor serine kinases phosphorylate serine and threonine residues in their protein substrates. There are two types of receptor serine kinases: type I and type II. The human genome contains 12 genes encoding receptor serine kinases—seven type I and five type II receptors—each of which is approximately 500 amino acids in length.

Receptor Activation: Role of Receptor Dimerization

Receptor serine kinases mediate the biologic actions (Fig. 5–6) of a single, large family of ligands: the transforming growth factor (TGF)-β family of ligands, which are characterized by the presence of six conserved cysteine residues.[76] The human genome contains 42 genes encoding cytokines in the TGF-β family, which are divided into two classes: (1) the activin/TGF-β family and (2) the müllerian inhibitory substance (MIS)/bone morphogenic protein (BMP) family. Activin and the related inhibin, as well as MIS, are of particular interest within the field of reproductive endocrinology (see Chapters 8 and 16).

When ligands bind to the receptors, this promotes a physical interaction between the type I receptor (RI) and the type II receptor (RII) (see Fig. 5–6). As a consequence of this physical interaction, the RII receptor activates the RI receptor by phosphorylating one or more serine residues in the GS domain (TTSGSGSG sequence) of the RI receptor.[76] How does the ligand trigger receptor activation? In the case of the MIS/BMP family of cytokines, the ligand binds to the isolated RI receptor with high affinity and the RII receptor with relatively low affinity. Because the ligand can bind simultaneously to both RI and RII, this provides a ready explanation for the ability to promote a physical interaction between RI with RII. The mechanism is different in the case of the activin/TGF-β family of cytokines. For example, TGF-β binds with high affinity to RII but does not interact directly with RI. However, TGF-β binding appears to induce a conformational change in RII, thereby promoting a direct binding interaction between the intracellular domains of RII and RI. Furthermore, cytokines such as TGF-β exist as dimers, which permits them to bind simultaneously to two RII molecules so that the activated receptor complex probably exists as a heterotetramer: $(RI)_2(RII)_2$.

There is an additional level of complexity that contributes to the regulation of receptor serine kinases.[76] The biology related to activin provides several examples. Follistatin is a "ligand trap," a soluble protein that binds activin, thereby blocking access to RI and RII. Inhibin is a peptide that inhibits activin signaling by binding to the receptor without activating the phosphorylation of RI. Betaglycan is a membrane-anchored protein, which functions as a coreceptor for inhibin by promoting inhibin binding to the activin receptor. Interestingly, betaglycan does not bind activin.

Receptor Serine Kinases Phosphorylate Other Intracellular Proteins

Once activated, receptor serine kinases are capable of phosphorylating other protein substrates. Receptor-regulated Smad proteins (R-Smad) function as the immediate downstream effectors of receptor serine kinases (see Fig. 5–6).[76] Smad proteins are the mammalian homologs of the proteins encoded by the drosophila Mad (Mothers against decapentaplegic) gene and the *C. elegans* Sma genes. There are five human R-Smad proteins. Smad2 and Smad3 mediate the actions of the activin/TGF-β family of cytokines; Smad1, Smad5, and Smad8 mediate the actions of the MIS/BMP family of cytokines.

The mechanism of action of TGF-β has been studied in considerable detail[71] and provides a prototype for the mechanism

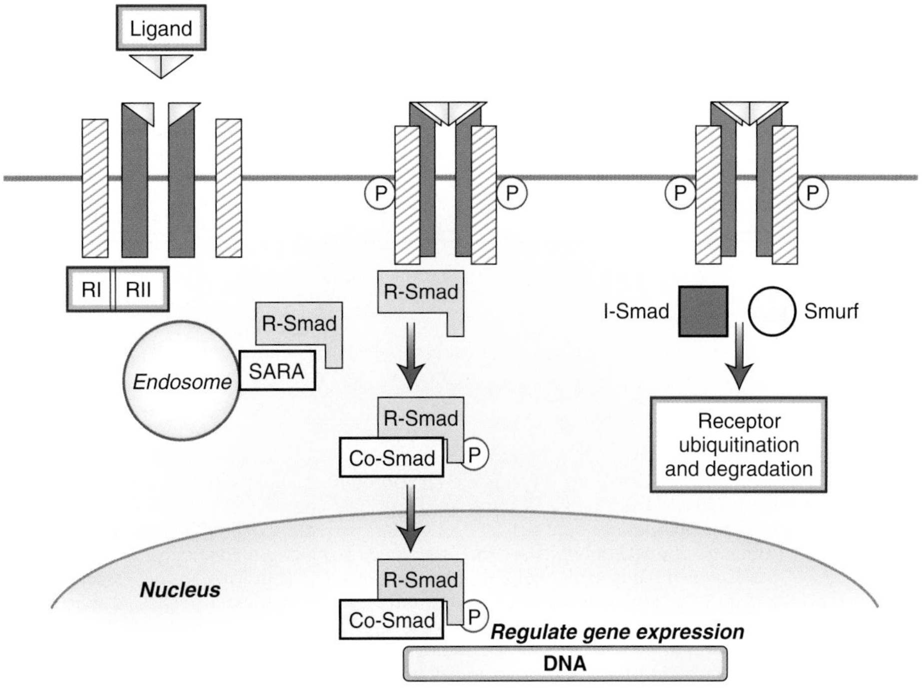

Figure 5–6 ▪ Mechanism of action of receptor serine kinases. Binding of dimeric ligand to the RII subunit triggers assembly of the receptor into the heterotetrameric $[(RI)_2(RII)_2]$ state. RII transphosphorylates RI, thereby activating phosphorylation of the R-Smad (bound to SARA in endosomes). The phosphorylated R-Smad associates with a Co-Smad. Eventually, the R-Smad is translocated into the nucleus, where it binds to DNA, enabling it to regulate gene transcription. The I-Smad can also bind to the activated receptor, thereby promoting ubiquitination and degradation of the receptor.

of action of receptor serine kinases.[76] When RI becomes phosphorylated in its GS domain in response to TGF-β, this increases the binding affinity for R-Smad proteins such as Smad2 (see Fig. 5–6). This, in turn, leads to phosphorylation of the two C-terminal serine residues in the SSXS sequence at the C-terminus of Smad2. Receptor-mediated phosphorylation of the R-Smad, Smad2, takes place when Smad 2 is bound to the Smad anchor for receptor activation (SARA), which is located in early endosomes. When the two C-terminal serine residues in Smad2 become phosphorylated, this promotes dissociation of Smad2 from SARA and also promotes binding of Smad2 to the co-mediator (Co-Smad), Smad4. Thus, phosphorylation of the R-Smad promotes the assembly of heteromeric complexes of R-Smad molecules with the Co-Smad.

Smads also contain sites for phosphorylation by other protein kinases, which provides an opportunity for regulatory cross-talk from other cellular signaling systems.

Smad7 is an inhibitory Smad (I-Smad), which binds to activated receptors in competition with R-Smads. Binding of Smad7 promotes receptor ubiquitination and degradation mediated by E3 ubiquitin ligases and Smad ubiquitination regulatory factors (Smurfs). These processes represent a negative feedback system, which contributes to the termination of TGF-β signaling (see Fig. 5–6).

Smad Proteins Regulate Gene Expression

Some R-Smads contain lysine-rich nuclear localization signals (KKLKK), which bind to importin, thereby mediating translocation into the nucleus.[76] It is possible that direct binding to components of the nuclear pore complex also contribute to the mechanism whereby Smads are translocated into the nucleus. Most R-Smads (with the exception of Smad2) bind to DNA in a sequence-specific fashion. The minimum Smad binding element is a 4 base pair (bp) sequence: 5′-AGAC-3′. This sequence is quite short, and would not be expected to provide a high degree of specificity. Therefore, it seems likely that other factors also contribute to the specificity of gene regulation.

Receptors that Signal through Associated Tyrosine Kinases

Overview

Members of the cytokine family of receptors resemble receptor tyrosine kinases in their mechanism of action, with one important difference. Instead of the tyrosine kinase being intrinsic to the receptor, enzymatic activity resides in a protein that associates with the cytokine receptor. As with receptor tyrosine kinases, ligand binding to the cytokine receptor activates the associated kinase. The more than 25 known ligands that bind to members of the cytokine receptor family have diverse functions. Three of the ligands are hormones: (1) GH, which is vital for normal body height; (2) prolactin (PRL), which is required for reproduction and lactation; and (3) leptin, which suppresses appetite and stimulates energy expenditure. Other ligands of cytokine receptors, for example, erythropoietin, most interleukins, and interferons α, β, and γ, regulate hematopoiesis or the immune response. A number of genetic diseases can be traced to defects in cytokine receptors. For example, Laron dwarfism is caused by autosomal recessive mutations of the GH receptor[77] and autosomal recessive mutations of the leptin receptor can cause morbid obesity.[78]

Cytokine Receptors Are Composed of Multiple Subunits

Members of the cytokine family of receptors share homology in both the extracellular and cytoplasmic domains. Some cytokine receptors, including the receptors for GH, PRL, and leptin, are thought to be composed of dimers of a single receptor subunit (Fig. 5–7). One ligand is thought to bind to both receptor subunits as discussed earlier for the GH receptor. However, most cytokine receptors are composed of two or more different subunits, with as many as six subunits constituting a single receptor.[79,80] Some of these receptors are thought to bind ligand dimers. One or more of these receptor subunits is shared by

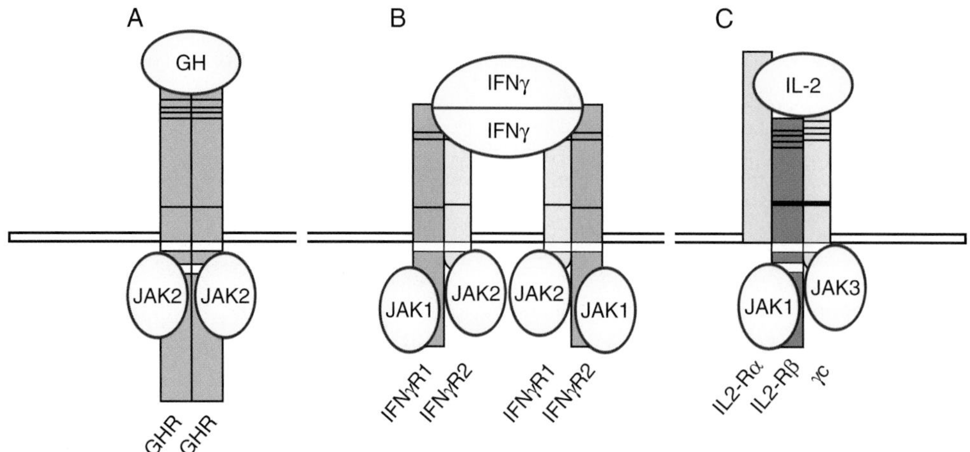

Figure 5–7 ■ Cytokine receptors are composed of multiple subunits and bind to one or more members of the Janus kinase (JAK) family of tyrosine kinases. **A,** Growth hormone (GH), like prolactin and leptin, binds to receptor homodimers and activates JAK2. **B,** Interferon-γ (IFN-γ) homodimers bind to their ligand-binding γR1 subunits. The γR2 subunits are then recruited, leading to activation of JAK1, which binds to γR1 subunit, and JAK2, which binds to γR2 subunit. Both subunits and both JAKs are necessary for responses to IFN-γ. **C,** Interleukin-2 (IL-2) binds to receptors composed of three subunits: a γc subunit shared with receptors for ILs 4, 7, 9 and 15; an IL-2Rβ subunit shared with the IL-15 receptor; and a noncytokine receptor subunit, IL-2Rα subunit. IL-2 activates both JAK3, bound to the γc subunit, and JAK1, bound to IL2-Rβ. Extracellular regions of homology are indicated by the *black lines* and *patterns.* Intracellular regions of homology are indicated by the *white boxes.* Identical subunits are indicated by *identical colors.*

receptors for other cytokines. This phenomenon of "mixing and matching" receptor subunits is an efficient way for the cell to fine-tune its cellular responses and increase the number of ligands a group of receptor subunits can bind. For example, a receptor composed of gp130 and leukemia inhibitory factor receptor β subunit binds leukemia inhibitory factor, a pleiotropic cytokine with multiple functions that appears to serve as a molecular interface between the neuroimmune and endocrine systems.[81] The same receptor subunits, when combined with a ciliary neurotrophic factor receptor subunit, show a preference for ciliary neurotrophic factor, a trophic factor for motor neurons in the ciliary ganglion and spinal cord and a potent appetite suppressor.[82] Combine two gp130 subunits with an interleukin-6 (IL-6) receptor subunit and the new receptor shows a preference for IL-6, an inducer of the acute phase response with additional antiinflammatory properties.[83]

Cytokine Receptors Activate Members of the Janus Family of Tyrosine Kinases

Members of the cytokine family of receptors do not themselves exhibit enzymatic activity. Rather, they bind members of the Janus family of tyrosine kinases (JAKs) via a proline-rich region (see Fig. 5–7). There are four known JAKs, designated JAK1, JAK2, JAK3, and TYK2. As do the cytokine receptors themselves, the JAKs mix and match in that some receptors show a strong preference for a single JAK, some require two different JAKs, and others appear to activate multiple JAK family members. For example, GH, PRL, and leptin preferentially activate JAK2. Interferon-γ activates JAK1 and JAK2, and IL-2 activates JAK1 and JAK3.[79,84]

Binding of ligand to a cytokine receptor activates the appropriate JAK family member or members. In some cases (e.g., PRL), the JAKs appear to be constitutively associated with the cytokine receptor and ligand binding increases their activity.[85] In other cases (e.g., the GH receptor), ligand binding increases both the affinity of JAKs for the cytokine receptor and the activity of the associated JAKs.[86] Activation of JAKs requires receptor oligomerization, presumably to bring two or more JAKs into sufficiently close proximity to transphosphorylate each other on the activating tyrosine in the kinase domain, as described earlier in the chapter for the receptor tyrosine kinases. Both receptor dimerization and ligand-induced changes in receptor conformation appear to be required for receptor activation.[87] Transphosphorylation is believed to cause a conformational change that exposes the ATP- or substrate-binding site, or both. Once the JAKs are activated, they phosphorylate themselves and their associated receptor subunits on multiple tyrosines. JAKs appear to be vital for normal human function. Mutations in the JAK3 gene have been linked to an autosomal recessive form of severe combined immunodeficiency disease.[88] Targeted disruption of the JAK2 gene in mice is embryonic lethal.[89]

Signaling Pathways Initiated by Cytokine Receptor–JAK Complexes

Phosphorylated tyrosines within the cytokine receptor subunits and their associated JAKs form binding sites for various signaling proteins containing phosphotyrosine binding domains, such as SH2 and PTB domains. Each cytokine receptor–JAK complex would be expected to have some tyrosine-containing motifs shared with many other cytokine receptor–JAK complexes (e.g., tyrosines within JAKs) and some ligand-specific tyrosine-containing motifs (e.g., tyrosines within a specific combination of receptor subunits). Thus, ligand binding to cytokine receptors would be expected to initiate some signaling pathways that are shared by many cytokines and some that are more specialized to a particular cytokine receptor. The signaling proteins known to be recruited to subsets of cytokine receptor–JAK complexes are generally the same as those recruited to receptor tyrosine kinases. Examples include the IRS proteins, the adaptor proteins Shc and Grb-2 that lead to activation of the Ras-MAP kinase pathway, phospholipase Cγ, and PI 3-kinase. However, there is one family of signaling proteins that appears to be particularly important for the function of cytokines—signal transducers and activators of transcription (STATs) (Fig. 5–8). STAT proteins are latent cytoplasmic transcription factors. STATs bind, through their SH2 domains, to one or more phosphorylated tyrosines in

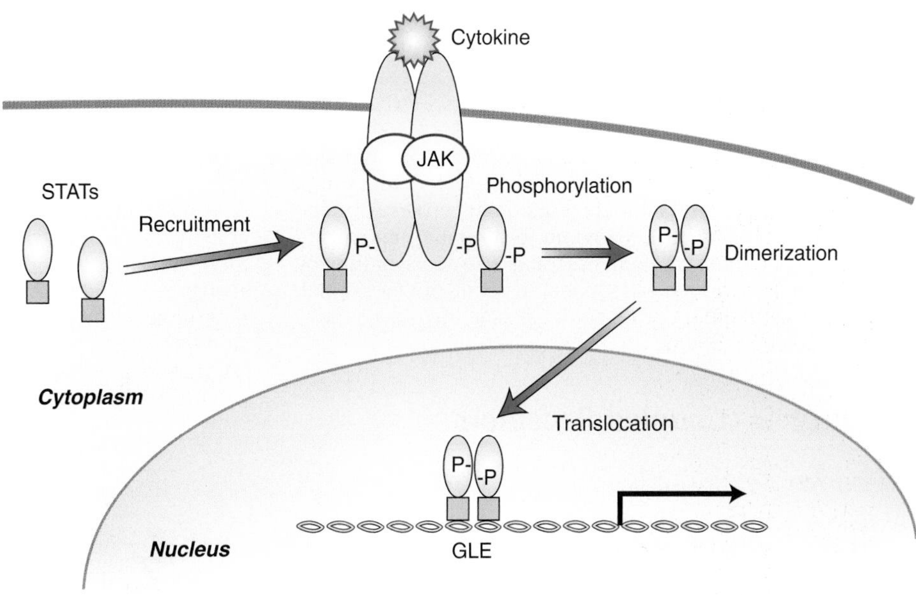

Figure 5–8 ▪ Cytokines activate signal transducers and activators of transcription (STATs). STAT proteins are latent cytoplasmic transcription factors. STATs bind, through Src homology 2 (SH2) domains, to one or more phosphorylated tyrosines in activated receptor-JAK complexes. Once bound, they themselves are tyrosyl phosphorylated, presumably by the receptor-associated JAKs. STATs then dissociate from the receptor-JAK complexes, homodimerize or heterodimerize with other STAT proteins, move to the nucleus, and bind to gamma-activated sequence–like elements (GLEs) in the promoters of cytokine-responsive genes. (Adapted from figure by J. Herrington, with permission.)

activated receptor-JAK complexes. Once bound, they themselves are tyrosyl phosphorylated, presumably by the receptor-associated JAKs. STATs then dissociate from the receptor-JAK complexes, homodimerize or heterodimerize with other STAT proteins, move to the nucleus, and bind to gamma-activated sequence–like elements in the promoters of cytokine-responsive genes.[90] The transcriptional response depends on how many STAT binding sites exist in the receptor-JAK complex, with which of the seven known STATs a particular STAT heterodimerizes, to what other proteins a particular STAT binds, the degree of serine or threonine phosphorylation of the STAT, and what other transcription factors are also activated. For example, leukemia inhibitory factor, whose receptor contains seven STAT3 binding motifs (YXXQ, where Y = tyrosine, X = any amino acid, and Q = glutamine) is a particularly potent activator of STAT-STAT3.[91] The transcriptional activity of STAT5 is enhanced by its forming a complex with the glucocorticoid, mineralocorticoid, and progesterone receptors but is diminished by its forming a complex with the estrogen receptor.[92] The importance of STAT5b for GH signaling is illustrated by the finding that severe growth failure is associated with point mutations in the STAT5b gene that result in a defective SH2 domain or an unstable, truncated form of STAT5b.[93,94]

Precise Regulation of the Cytokine Receptors is Required for Normal Function

Ligand binding to cytokine receptors normally activates JAKs rapidly and transiently. Conversely, constitutively activated JAKs and STATs are associated with cellular transformation. For example, a single acquired activating point mutation in *JAK2* is present in the majority of patients with a myeloproliferative disorder.[95] Constitutively active JAKs and STATs are also a common characteristic of leukemias,[96] and both JAK2 and STAT5b have been identified as fusion partners in translocations in leukemias. The Tel-JAK2 fusion protein is constitutively active, leading to constitutively active STAT proteins. Thus, an understanding of what turns off cytokine receptor signaling is of utmost importance in understanding normal signaling via cytokine receptors.

As with the receptor tyrosine kinases, several steps have been hypothesized to serve as points of signal termination for cytokine signaling. These include receptor degradation (e.g., through a ubiquination/proteosome pathway) and dephosphorylation of tyrosines within JAK or receptor (e.g., by a tyrosine phosphatase that binds to receptor-JAK complexes). The suppressors of cytokine-signaling (SOCSs) are thought to be particularly important players in the termination or suppression of cytokine signaling pathways. SOCS proteins are an excellent example of an effective negative feedback loop. They are generally synthesized in response to cytokines. The newly synthesized SOCS proteins in turn bind, through their SH2 domain, to phosphorylated tyrosines within the cytokine receptor–JAK complex and inhibit further cytokine signaling. In some cases (i.e., SOCS1), SOCS proteins are thought to bind to phosphotyrosines in the kinase domain of JAK and inhibit kinase activity.[97] In other cases (i.e., SOCS3), SOCS proteins bind to phosphorylated tyrosines in the receptor and inhibit JAK activity.[98] Finally, in some cases (i.e., cytokine-inducible SH2 protein [CIS]), SOCS proteins bind to phosphorylated tyrosines in the receptor and block STAT binding and activation.[99] SOCS proteins can also be synthesized in response to noncytokine receptors, suggesting a mechanism whereby prior exposure to one ligand suppresses subsequent responses to another. For example, SOCS proteins have been implicated in the well-known ability of endotoxin to cause resistance to GH.[100]

Summary

Hormones, growth factors, and cytokines that bind to members of the cytokine family of receptors activate JAK family tyrosine kinases. The activated kinases in turn phosphorylate tyrosines in themselves and associated receptors. The phosphorylated tyrosines form binding sites for other signaling proteins, including STAT proteins and a variety of other phosphotyrosine-binding proteins. STAT proteins promote the regulation of cytokine-sensitive genes, including SOCS proteins that serve a negative feedback function of terminating ligand activation of JAKs or STATs, or both.

Although this gives the general picture, it should be recognized that the picture is becoming much more complex every day. For example, there are reports that members of the Src family of tyrosine kinases can also be activated by some cytokine receptors (e.g., PRL receptor),[101] that some JAK-binding proteins (e.g., SH2-B) are potent activators of JAK2,[102] and that other proteins contribute to the down-regulation of cytokine-signaling pathways, including protein inhibitors of activated STAT (PIAS) proteins that bind to specific STATs and negatively regulate their activity.[103] Cytokine receptors, JAKs, STATs, and/or SOCS proteins have also been shown to interact with or be components of signaling downstream of some receptor tyrosine kinases (e.g., receptors for insulin, IGF-I, epidermal growth factor) as well as several G protein–coupled receptors (e.g., the receptors for angiotensin II, serotonin, α-thrombin, luteinizing hormone). In contrast to their essential role in signaling by cytokine receptors, JAKs do not appear to be the primary signaling mediator with either the receptor tyrosine kinases or the G protein–coupled receptors.

G Protein–Coupled Receptors

Overview

G protein–coupled receptors (GPCRs) are an evolutionarily conserved gene superfamily with members in all eukaryotes from yeast to mammals. They transduce a wide variety of extracellular signals including photons of light; chemical odorants; divalent cations; monoamine, amino acid, and nucleoside neurotransmitters; lipids; and peptide and protein hormones.[104] All members of the GPCR superfamily share a common structural feature, seven membrane-spanning helices, but various subfamilies diverge in primary amino acid sequence and in the domains that serve in ligand binding, G protein coupling, and interaction with other effector proteins (Fig. 5–9).

All GPCRs act as guanine nucleotide exchange factors. In their activated (agonist-bound) conformation, they catalyze exchange of GDP tightly bound to the α subunit of heterotrimeric G proteins for GTP (Fig. 5–10). This in turn leads to activation of the α subunit and its dissociation from the G protein βγ dimer. Both G protein subunits are capable of regulating effector activity.[105] Identified G protein–regulated effectors include enzymes of second messenger metabolism such as adenylyl cyclase and phospholipase C-β and a variety of ion channels. Agonist binding to GPCRs thus alters intracellular second messenger and ion concentrations with resultant rapid effects on hormone secretion, muscle contraction, and a variety of other physiologic functions. Long-term changes in gene expression are also seen as a result of second messenger-stimulated phosphorylation of transcription factors.

The G protein subunits are encoded by three distinct genes. The α subunit binds guanine nucleotides with high affinity and specificity and has intrinsic guanosine triphosphatase (GTPase) activity. The β and γ polypeptides are tightly but noncovalently associated in a functional dimer subunit. The three-dimensional structures of the individual and associated subunits have been determined.[105,106] There is considerable diversity in G protein subunits, with multiple genes encoding all three subunits and alternative gene splicing resulting in additional polypeptide products. There are at least 16 distinct α subunit genes in

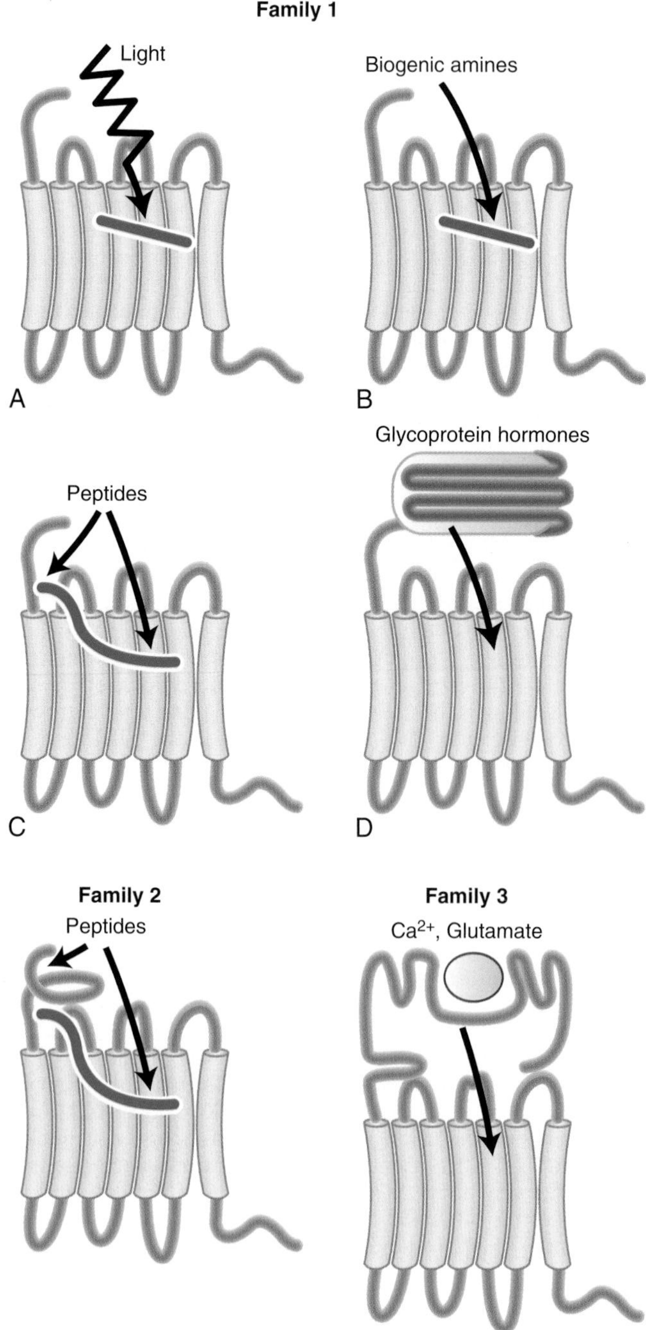

Figure 5–9 ▪ The G protein–coupled receptor (GPCR) superfamily: diversity in ligand binding and structure. Each panel depicts various members of the GPCR superfamily in cartoon form. The seven membrane-spanning α helices are shown as cylinders with the extracellular amino terminus and three extracellular loops above and the intracellular carboxyl terminus and three intracellular loops below. The superfamily can be divided into three subfamilies on the basis of amino acid sequence conservation within the transmembrane helices. Family 1 includes **(A)** the opsins, in which light (*jagged arrow*) causes isomerization of retinal covalently bound within the pocket created by the transmembrane helices (*bar*); **(B)** monoamine receptors, in which agonists (*arrow*) bind noncovalently within the pocket created by the transmembrane helices (*bar*); **(C)** receptors for peptides such as vasopressin, in which agonist binding (*arrow*) may involve parts of the extracellular amino terminus and loops as well as the transmembrane helices (*bar*); and **(D)** glycoprotein hormone receptors, in which agonists (*oval*) bind to the large extracellular amino terminus, thereby activating the receptor through as yet undefined interactions with the extracellular loops or transmembrane helices (*arrow*). Family 2 includes receptors for peptide hormones such as parathyroid hormone (PTH) and secretin. Agonists (*arrow*) may bind to residues in the extracellular amino terminus and loops as well as transmembrane helices (*bar*). Family 3 includes the extracellular Ca^{2+} sensing receptor and metabotropic glutamate receptors. Agonists (*sphere*) bind in a cleft of the Venus flytrap–like domain in the large extracellular amino terminus, thereby activating the receptor through as yet undefined interactions with the extracellular loops or transmembrane helices (*arrow*).

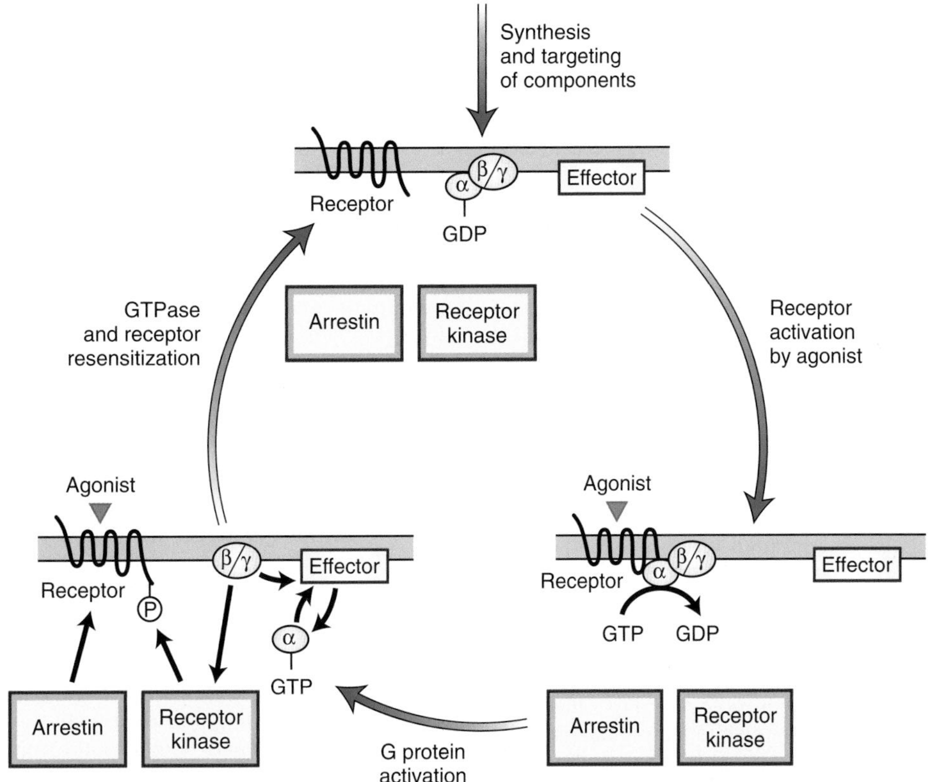

Figure 5–10 ▪ The G protein guanosine triphosphatase (GTPase) and G protein–coupled receptor (GPCR) desensitization-resensitization cycle. In each panel, the *stippled region* denotes the plasma membrane with extracellular above and intracellular below. In the basal state, the G protein is a heterotrimer with guanosine diphosphate (GDP) tightly bound to the α subunit. The agonist-activated GPCR catalyzes release of GDP, which permits guanosine triphosphate (GTP) to bind. The GTP-bound α subunit dissociates from the βγ dimer. *Arrows* from α subunit to effector and from βγ dimer to effector indicate regulation of effector activity by the respective subunits. *Arrow* from effector to α subunit indicates regulation of its GTPase activity by effector interaction. Under physiologic conditions, effector regulation by G protein subunits is transient and is terminated by the GTPase activity of the α subunit. The latter converts bound GTP to GDP, thus returning the α subunit to its inactivated state with high affinity for the βγ dimer, which reassociates to form the heterotrimer in the basal state. In the basal state, the receptor kinase and arrestin are shown as cytosolic proteins. Dissociation of the GTP-bound α subunit from the βγ dimer permits the latter to facilitate binding of receptor kinase to the plasma membrane (*arrow* from βγ dimer to receptor kinase). Plasma membrane binding permits the receptor kinase to phosphorylate the agonist-bound GPCR (depicted here as "P" occurring on the carboxyl-terminal tail of the GPCR, but sites on intracellular loops are also possible). GPCR phosphorylation in turn facilitates arrestin binding to GPCR, resulting in desensitization. Endocytic trafficking of arrestin-bound GPCR and recycling to the plasma membrane during resensitization are not depicted here.

mammals. These vary widely in range of expression. Some, such as Gs-α, which couples many GPCRs to stimulation of adenylyl cyclase, are ubiquitous; others, such as Gtl-α, which couples the GPCR rhodopsin to cyclic guanosine monophosphate phos-phodiesterase in retinal rod photoreceptor cells, are highly localized.

Because multiple distinct GPCRs, G proteins, and effectors are expressed within any given cell, the degree and basis for specificity in G protein coupling to GPCRs and to effectors are major subjects of investigation with implications for drug action and disease mechanisms.[106] Since the pioneering work of Rodbell[107] in discovering G proteins and showing that G protein–mediated signal transduction involves three separable components (receptor, G protein, and effector), additional complexity has emerged.

A large new gene family termed RGS (for regulators of G protein signaling) has been identified. RGS proteins bind to a transition state of the GTP-activated G protein α subunit and accelerate its GTPase activity, thus helping deactivate the α subunit. RGS domains have also been found in modular proteins with additional functions, in certain cases linking heterotrimeric G protein signaling with the function of low-molecular-weight GTP-binding proteins in the ras superfamily.[106] Lefkowitz[108] has shown that a family of GPCR kinases and of arrestin proteins is involved in GPCR desensitization after agonist binding. In addition, it is now clear that GPCRs interact directly with a number of other proteins in addition to G proteins. Not only are GPCRs important targets for treatment of many diseases, but also mutations in genes encoding GPCRs have been identified as the cause of a number of endocrine as well as nonendocrine disorders.

G Protein–Coupled Receptor Structure and Function

Structure

Hydropathy analysis of the primary sequence of all GPCRs predicts seven membrane-spanning α helices connected by three intracellular loops and three extracellular loops with an extracellular amino terminus and an intracellular carboxyl terminus (see Fig. 5–9). This basic structure has now been verified by x-ray crystallography for rhodopsin.[109] Although there was already evidence that visual transduction in the retina and hormone activation of adenylyl cyclase shared common features, the discovery that the β-adrenergic receptor has the same topographic structure as rhodopsin came as a surprise.[108] Cloning of the complementary deoxyribonucleic acids (cDNAs) for a vast number of GPCRs followed elucidation of the primary sequence of the β-adrenergic receptor, and in every case the same core structure was predicted by hydropathy analysis.

In addition to the predicted core structure, certain other common features (with exceptions in some subsets of the GPCR superfamily) were noted[104]: (1) a disulfide bridge connecting the first and second extracellular loops; (2) one or more N-linked glycosylation sites, usually in the amino terminus but occasionally in extracellular loops; (3) palmitoylation of one or more cysteines in the carboxyl terminus, effectively creating a fourth intracellular loop; (4) potential phosphorylation sites in the carboxyl terminus and occasionally the third intracellular loop. Glycosylation appears to be important for proper folding and trafficking to the plasma membrane rather than for ligand binding. The disulfide bridge may help in proper arrangement of the transmembrane helices.

Superimposed on the basic structure of GPCRs are a number of variations relevant to differences in ligand binding, G protein coupling, and interaction with other proteins.[104] First, there are major differences in amino acid sequence among members of the GPCR superfamily. Sequence alignment, especially of the transmembrane helices, allows one to divide the superfamily into subfamilies (see Fig. 5–9). Of these, family 1 is the largest and itself can be subdivided. The largest subset includes opsins; odorant receptors; and monoamine, purinergic, and opiate receptors. These are characterized by a short amino terminus. The next subset includes chemokine, protease-activated, and certain peptide hormone receptors characterized by a slightly longer amino terminus. The last subset comprises receptors for the large glycoprotein hormones, TSH, luteinizing hormone, and follicle-stimulating hormone. These have an approximately 400-residue extracellular amino terminus.

Family 2 shows essentially no sequence homology to family 1 even within the transmembrane helices and is characterized by an approximately 100-residue amino terminus. Members include receptors for a number of peptide hormones such as parathyroid hormone (PTH), calcitonin, vasoactive intestinal peptide, and corticotropin-releasing hormone.

Family 3, in addition to a unique primary sequence, has other unique features such as an approximately 200-residue carboxyl terminus and an approximately 600-residue amino terminus. The latter consists of a putative "Venus flytrap–like" domain and a cysteine-rich domain. Members include the metabotropic glutamate receptors, an extracellular Ca^{2+}-sensing receptor, and putative taste and pheromone receptors.[110] The determination of the three-dimensional crystal structure of part of the extracellular amino terminus of one of the metabotropic glutamate receptors verifies the Venus flytrap structure.[110]

Ligand Binding

Given the diversity of ligands (>1000) that bind to GPCRs, it is not surprising that considerable diversity is evident in both the sequence and structure of presumptive GPCR ligand-binding domains. The opsins are unique among GPCRs in that the ligand, retinal, is covalently bound to a lysine in the seventh transmembrane helix.[109] Ligand binding for other members of family 1 with a short extracellular amino terminus, for example, adrenergic and other monoamine receptors, probably involves a pocket within the transmembrane helices as demonstrated for rhodopsin (see Fig. 5–9). For other family 1 GPCRs, the extracellular amino terminus, perhaps together with extracellular loops and portions of the transmembrane helices, is involved in ligand binding. In the case of the glycoprotein hormone receptors, the large extracellular amino terminus plays the principal role in hormone binding. In a model for peptide binding to family 2 receptors, the extracellular amino terminus is responsible for initial binding to the peptide carboxy-terminus followed by peptide amino-terminus binding to the seven-transmembrane domain.[111] For family 3 GPCRs, the three-dimensional structure of the type 1 metabotropic glutamate receptor shows that agonist binding occurs within a cleft between the lobes of the Venus flytrap.[110]

G Protein Coupling

Because the number of potential G proteins to which GPCRs couple is much more limited than the number of ligands that bind GPCRs, more conservation of the domains involved in G protein coupling would be expected. Although GPCRs can be broadly divided into those that couple to Gs, those that couple to the Gq subfamily, and those that couple to the Gi-Go subfamily, the situation is probably more complicated.[106] Specificity of coupling to the most recently identified G proteins, Gl2 and G13, is still uncertain. Also, some GPCRs evidently can couple to both Gs and Gq.

A vast number of studies have been performed to define the sites of ligand binding and G protein coupling of GPCRs.[106,112] Considerable evidence points to the third intracellular loop (particularly its membrane-proximal portions) and to the membrane-proximal portion of the carboxyl terminus as key determinants of G protein coupling specificity. For example, exchanging only the third intracellular loop between different GPCRs confers the G protein coupling specificity of the exchanged loop upon the recipient GPCR.[113] In contrast, the second intracellular loop, although important for G protein coupling, appears to play a role in the activation mechanism rather than in determining specificity of coupling.[113] A tripeptide motif (D/E, R, Y/W) at the start of the second intracellular loop that is highly conserved in family 1 GPCRs is critical for G protein activation.[112]

Mechanism of Activation

The precise mechanism of activation after agonist binding remains to be defined for most GPCRs, but studies of rhodopsin provide the clearest picture available. In the ground state, retinal covalently bound to the seventh transmembrane helix in rhodopsin holds the transmembrane helices in an inactive conformation. Isomerization of retinal upon absorption of light of the appropriate wavelength converts an antagonist ligand into an agonist. The rhodopsin crystal structure identifies the residues in the transmembrane helices that interact with retinal and suggests a mechanism for movement of the helices upon photoactivation of retinal.[109] Movement of the transmembrane helices in turn leads to changes in conformation of cytoplasmic loops that promote G protein activation.

For family 1 receptors related to rhodopsin, the determination of its three-dimensional structure validates the idea that a change in conformation of transmembrane helices is the direct result of agonist versus antagonist binding to residues within the helices. Further refinements in understanding the mechanism of activation for opsin-related GPCRs should come as additional three-dimensional structures are determined. Until then, molecular modeling by computer on the basis of the rhodopsin structure and then experimental testing offer a useful approach.[114] For other GPCRs whose presumptive site of agonist binding does not involve direct contact with transmembrane helices (families 2 and 3 and the glycoprotein hormone receptors in family 1), much remains to be learned about how agonist binding to the extracellular domain of such GPCRs leads to presumptive changes in conformation of transmembrane helices and receptor activation. Determination of the structure of the extracellular domain of the FSH receptor bound to FSH provides important insights into the general mechanism of glycoprotein hormone binding to their cognate GPCRs, and resultant interactions with the seven-transmembrane domain leading to activation.[115] A general hypothesis of GPCR activation postulates that GPCRs are in equilibrium between an activated state and an inactive state. These states presumably differ in the disposition of the transmembrane helices and, in turn, the cytoplasmic domains that determine G protein coupling. Agonists, according to this ternary complex model, are viewed as stabilizing the activated state. Antagonists may be neutral; that is, they simply compete with agonists for receptor binding but their binding does not influence this equilibrium. Alternatively, they may be "inverse" agonists; that is, their binding stabilizes the inactive state of the receptor.[116] Refinements of the ternary complex model based on kinetic and biophysical studies suggest added complexity.[117]

Dimerization

Members of the tyrosine kinase receptor family have long been known to require dimerization as part of their activation mechanism. It is now apparent that many GPCRs likewise form homodimers and heterodimers.[104] Residues within transmembrane helix 6 may foster dimerization of small family 1 GPCRs,[118] and intermolecular disulfide bonds in the extracellular amino-terminal domain are involved in homodimerization of most family 3 GPCRs.[110,119,120] A coiled-coil interaction in the carboxyl terminus of γ-aminobutyric acid B receptor subtypes is responsible for heterodimerization, and this is critical for proper receptor function.[121] Modifications of ligand binding, signaling, and receptor sequestration have been demonstrated upon heterodimerization of angiotensin with bradykinin receptors, of κ with δ opioid receptors, and of opioid with β-adrenergic receptors.[122] Further studies are needed to elucidate the physiologic relevance of GPCR homodimerization and heterodimerization.

G Protein–Coupled Receptor Desensitization

Pharmacologists long ago appreciated that continued exposure to agonist leads to a diminished response, so-called desensitization. This phenomenon has been extensively studied in GPCRs. Two forms are defined: heterologous, in which binding of agonist to one GPCR leads to a diminished response of a different GPCR to its agonist, and homologous, in which desensitization occurs only for the GPCR to which agonist is bound. Both forms of desensitization involve GPCR phosphorylation but by different kinases and at different sites. Stimulation of cyclic adenosine monophosphate formation by agonist binding to a Gs-coupled GPCR leads to activation of protein kinase A, which in turn can phosphorylate and desensitize the GPCR. Such phosphorylation may also alter G protein–coupling specificity.[104] Similarly, protein kinase C activation resulting from GPCR coupling to Gq family members may cause protein kinase C–catalyzed phosphorylation of GPCRs with desensitization.

In retinal photoreceptors, a specific rhodopsin kinase and a protein termed arrestin were implicated in attenuation of the light response. Just as parallels were identified between rhodopsin and GPCR structure, so were parallels identified in this desensitization mechanism. Rhodopsin kinase is but one member of a family of GPCR kinases and arrestin only one of a family of related proteins that function in desensitization of many members of the GPCR superfamily.[108] GPCR kinases preferentially phosphorylate the agonist-bound form of a GPCR, thus ensuring homologous desensitization. Upon GPCR phosphorylation by GPCR kinase, arrestins bind to the third intracellular loop and carboxyl-terminal tail of the GPCR, thereby blocking G protein binding (see Fig. 5–10). GPCR kinases and arrestins not only act to desensitize GPCRs but also mediate other functions including receptor internalization and interaction with other effectors (see next section).

G Protein–Coupled Receptor Interactions with Other Proteins

The initial paradigm of GPCR function postulated that G protein activation is the sole outcome of agonist binding to GPCRs. With the identification of GPCR interactions with GPCR kinases and arrestins, this concept was modified to include these proteins involved in GPCR desensitization. Later evidence, however, suggests that GPCR interaction with arrestins may also permit recruitment of other proteins to the GPCR. For example, the src tyrosine kinase may interact with the β-adrenergic receptor, with β-arrestin serving as an adaptor.[123] Arrestins may also recruit proteins involved in endocytosis. GPCR kinases may also serve to recruit additional signaling proteins to the GPCR.[123]

Other classes of proteins may interact with specific GPCRs without recruitment by GPCR kinases and arrestins. These include SH2 domain-containing proteins, small GTP-binding proteins, and PDZ (for *p*ostsynaptic density protein-95/*d*iscs large/*z*ona occluden-1) domain-containing proteins. Examples of the latter include binding of the Na^+/H^+ exchanger regulatory factor to the carboxyl terminus of the β-adrenergic receptor.[123] The long carboxyl terminus of family 3 GPCRs such as metabotropic glutamate receptors contains polyproline motifs involved in binding members of the Homer family. The latter can facilitate functional interactions with yet other proteins such as the inositol triphosphate receptor.[124] Receptor activity-modifying proteins (RAMPs), a new family of single-transmembrane-domain proteins, appear to heterodimerize with certain GPCRs, assisting them in proper folding and membrane trafficking.[125] Interestingly, when the calcitonin receptor-like GPCR associates with RAMP1, it forms a calcitonin gene-related peptide receptor, whereas when it associates with RAMP2, it becomes an adrenomedullin receptor. Clearly, this rapidly evolving aspect of GPCR function holds many further interesting developments in store.

G Protein–Coupled Receptors in Disease Pathogenesis and Treatment

Because of their diverse and critical roles in normal physiology, their accessibility on the cell surface, and the ability to synthesize selective agonists and antagonists, GPCRs have long been a major target for drug development. One estimate is that about 65% of prescription drugs are targeted against GPCRs. Drugs targeting GPCRs may act not only as agonists or antagonists, but also as allosteric modulators. So-called calcimimetic drugs inhibit parathyroid hormone release, for example, by binding to the seven-transmembrane domain and acting as positive allosteric modulators of the Ca^{2+}-sensing receptor.[120] With the cloning of GPCR cDNAs, much greater diversity of receptor subclasses became evident than had been anticipated on the basis of pharmacologic studies. For example, five muscarinic receptor subtypes and an even greater number of serotoninergic GPCRs were identified.[112] This has allowed the development of highly specific, subtype-selective drugs that have fewer side effects than those produced by previously available agents.

Another result of the cloning of GPCR cDNAs by homology screening and polymerase chain reaction-based approaches is the identification of "orphan" GPCRs, that is, receptors with the canonical, predicted seven-transmembrane-domain structure of GPCRs but without knowledge of their physiologic agonist. There have been substantial efforts to identify the relevant ligands for such orphan receptors. Krebs cycle intermediates, succinate and α-ketoglutarate, for example, were shown to be the physiologically relevant activators of orphan GPCRs, GPR91 and GPR99, respectively, and thereby to regulate renin release and blood pressure.[126] GPR40, another orphan receptor selectively expressed in β cells, is activated by free fatty acids and may play a role in linking obesity to type 2 diabetes.[127] In addition to revealing new physiologic and pathophysiologic mechanisms, GPCR "deorphanization" provides novel targets for drug development.

Beyond drug development, defects in GPCRs are an important cause of a wide variety of human diseases.[128] GPCR mutations can cause loss of function by impairing any of several steps in the normal GPCR-GTPase cycle (see Fig. 5–10). These include failure to synthesize GPCR protein altogether, failure of synthesized GPCR to reach the plasma membrane, failure of GPCR to bind or be activated by agonist, and failure of GPCR to couple to or activate G protein. Because in most cases clinically significant impairment of signal transduction requires loss of both alleles of the GPCR gene, most such diseases are inherited in autosomal recessive fashion (Table 5–1).

Most of these diseases are manifested as resistance to the action of the normal agonist and thus mimic deficiency of the agonist. For example, TSH receptor loss-of-function mutations cause a form of hypothyroidism mimicking TSH deficiency, but serum TSH is actually elevated in such cases, reflecting resistance to the hormone's action caused by defective receptor function. Interestingly, hypogonadotropic hypogonadism may be caused by loss of function mutations of either the GnRH receptor or of the orphan GPCR, GPR54. In the former, there is resistance to the action of GnRH. The latter may be due to failure to release GnRH, but the precise mechanism has not been defined.[129] Nephrogenic diabetes insipidus (renal vasopressin resistance) is caused by loss-of-function mutations in the V2 vasopressin receptor gene located on the X chromosome. Thus, males with a single copy of the gene experience the disease when they inherit a mutant gene, whereas most females do not show overt disease because random X inactivation leaves them with an average 50% of normal gene function. Most V2 vasopressin receptor mutations associated with nephrogenic diabetes insipidus cause loss of function by impairing normal synthesis or folding of the receptor, or both. A novel mechanism for receptor loss of function elucidated for a V2 vasopressin receptor missense mutation associated with nephrogenic diabetes insipidus involves constitutive arrestin-mediated desensitization.[130]

The extracellular Ca^{2+}-sensing receptor appears to be an interesting exception to the association between GPCR loss-of-function mutations and hormone resistance. Loss-of-function mutations of the Ca^{2+}-sensing receptor mimic a hormone hypersecretion state, primary hyperparathyroidism. In fact, Ca^{2+}-sensing receptor loss-of-function mutations do cause hormone resistance, but in this case extracellular Ca^{2+} is the hormonal agonist that acts through this receptor to inhibit PTH secretion. A loss-of-function mutation of one copy of the receptor gene typically causes mild resistance to extracellular Ca^{2+} manifested as familial hypocalciuric hypercalcemia. If two defective copies are inherited, extreme Ca^{2+} resistance causing neonatal severe primary hyperparathyroidism results (see Table 5–1). In some cases, a heterozygous receptor loss-of-function mutation may be associated with neonatal severe primary hyperparathyroidism, perhaps reflecting a dominant negative effect caused by dimerization of wild-type and mutant receptors.[131]

GPCR gain-of-function mutations (Table 5–2) are also an important cause of disease.[128] Given the dominant nature of activating mutations, most such diseases are inherited in an autosomal dominant manner. Activating TSH receptor mutations may be inherited in autosomal dominant fashion and cause diffuse thyroid enlargement in familial nonautoimmune hyperthyroidism, or they may occur as somatic mutations causing focal, sporadic hyperfunctional thyroid nodules.[132] Likewise, activating, germline LH receptor mutations cause familial male precocious puberty due to LH-independent Leydig cell

TABLE 5–1 DISEASES CAUSED BY G PROTEIN–COUPLED RECEPTOR LOSS-OF-FUNCTION MUTATIONS

Receptor	Disease	Inheritance
V2 vasopressin	Nephrogenic diabetes insipidus	X-linked
ACTH	Familial ACTH resistance	Autosomal recessive
GHRH	Familial GH deficiency	Autosomal recessive
GnRH	Hypogonadotropic hypogonadism	Autosomal recessive
GPR54	Hypogonadotropic hypogonadism	Autosomal recessive
FSH	Hypergonadotropic ovarian dysgenesis	Autosomal recessive
LH	Male pseudohermaphroditism	Autosomal recessive
TSH	Familial hypothyroidism	Autosomal recessive
Ca^{2+} sensing	Familial hypocalciuric hypercalcemia, neonatal severe primary hyperparathyroidism	Autosomal dominant autosomal recessive
Melanocortin 4	Obesity	Autosomal recessive
PTH/PTHrP	Blomstrand chondrodysplasia	Autosomal recessive

ACTH, Adrenocorticotropic hormone; *FSH,* follicle-stimulating hormone; *GH,* growth hormone; *GHRH,* growth hormone–releasing hormone; *GnRH,* gonadotropin-releasing hormone; *LH,* luteinizing hormone; *PTH,* parathyroid hormone; *PTHrP,* parathyroid hormone–related protein; *TSH,* thyroid-stimulating hormone.

TABLE 5–2 DISEASES CAUSED BY G PROTEIN–COUPLED RECEPTOR GAIN-OF-FUNCTION MUTATIONS

Receptor	Disease	Inheritance
LH	Familial male precocious puberty	Autosomal dominant
TSH	Sporadic hyperfunctional thyroid nodules	Noninherited (somatic)
TSH	Familial nonautoimmune hyperthyroidism	Autosomal dominant
Ca^{2+} sensing	Familial hypocalcemic hypercalciuria	Autosomal dominant
PTH/PTHrP	Jansen's metaphyseal chondrodysplasia	Autosomal dominant
V2 vasopressin	Nephrogenic inappropriate antidiuresis	Autosomal dominant

LH, Luteinizing hormone; *PTH,* parathyroid hormone; *PTHrP,* parathyroid hormone–related protein; *TSH,* thyroid-stimulating hormone.

hyperfunction, while somatic LH receptor mutations may cause focal Leydig cell tumors.[132]

Unlike loss-of-function mutations, which may be missense as well as nonsense or frameshift mutations that truncate the normal receptor protein, GPCR gain-of-function mutations are almost always missense mutations. The location and nature of naturally occurring, disease-causing mutations offer important insights into GPCR structure and function. The basis for defective receptor function is clear with mutations that truncate receptor synthesis prematurely. More subtle missense mutations may impair function if they involve highly conserved residues in transmembrane helices critical for normal protein folding. Activating missense mutations often involve residues within or bordering transmembrane helices and are thought to disrupt normal inhibitory constraints that maintain the receptor in its inactive conformation.[133] Mutations disrupting these constraints mimic the effects of agonist binding and shift the equilibrium toward the activated state of the receptor. A striking example is the activating, missense mutations in the V2 vasopressin receptor of arginine 137, part of the "DRY" motif at the intracellular border of transmembrane helix 3 conserved in most family 1 GPCRs, leading to the syndrome of nephrogenic inappropriate antidiuresis.[134]

Clinically, diseases caused by activating GPCR mutations therefore mimic states of agonist excess, but direct measurement shows that agonist concentrations are actually low, reflecting normal negative feedback mechanisms. Again, the Ca^{2+}-sensing receptor is an apparent exception, with activating mutations causing functional hypoparathyroidism. For most GPCRs, disease-associated gain-of-function mutations cause constitutive, agonist-independent, activation but with rare exceptions, the Ca^{2+}-sensing receptor gain-of-function mutations cause increased sensitivity to extracellular Ca^{2+} rather than to Ca^{2+}-independent activation.[131]

Naturally occurring animal models of human disease have revealed additional examples of etiologic GPCR mutations. For example, a loss-of-function mutation in the hypocretin (orexin) type 2 receptor gene was identified in canine narcolepsy.[135] Dozens of mouse GPCR gene knockout models have been created, many revealing interesting and in some cases unexpected phenotypes. Characterization of the phenotype resulting from disruption of a mouse GPCR gene may accurately predict the clinical picture resulting from the corresponding mutation in humans, such as with disruption of the melanocortin-4 receptor gene resulting in obesity in mouse[136] and human[137] and disruption of the PTH/PTH-related protein receptor gene impairing normal bone growth and development in mouse[138] and in the human disease Blomstrand chondrodysplasia.[139] Further knockout models and further detailed studies of these models can be expected to increase substantially our understanding of GPCR function and to address questions such as the unique roles of multiple subtypes of various GPCR subclasses, for example, the β3-adrenergic receptor subtype.[140] Availability of mouse knockout models of human diseases should also facilitate testing of novel therapies including gene transfer. For example, aminoglycosides, which are known to suppress premature termination codons, were shown to rescue expression and function in mice with nephrogenic diabetes insipidus caused by a nonsense mutant in the V2 vasopressin receptor.[141] Many disease-causing loss of function mutations in GPCRs lead to defective protein folding and/or protein routing. Novel therapeutic approaches such as use of molecular "chaperones" and modulation of the cell's "quality control" mechanisms have shown promise in in vitro studies.[142]

Screening of GPCR genes for mutations as the potential cause of additional human disorders may continue to turn up new examples, but it is also becoming clear that variations in GPCR gene sequence can have profound consequences beyond simply causing resistance to, or activation independent of, the cognate hormone agonist. Familial spontaneous ovarian hyperstimulation syndrome occurring in early pregnancy, for example, was shown to be caused by missense mutations in the transmembrane helix domain of the FSH receptor.[143,144] Such mutations increase receptor basal activity, and permit low affinity binding of hCG to the ectodomain to activate the FSH receptor. Studies are needed to determine whether variable susceptibility to iatrogenic ovarian hyperstimulation occurring in the context of in vitro fertilization might be due to such variations in FSH receptor sequence.[144]

As more polymorphisms are discovered in the human genome, many examples of variations in GPCR gene sequence will be found and the challenge will be to elucidate their possible functional significance. In vitro studies may reveal functional differences, such as differences in G protein coupling seen with a four-amino-acid polymorphism in the third intracellular loop of the α_{2C}-adrenergic receptor,[145] but further studies are required to determine whether such differences are important in individual variation in response to various drugs (pharmacogenomics) or in other subtle physiologic differences that could confer susceptibility to disease (complex disease genes). Given the high proportion of the human genome devoted to GPCR genes, it is clear that studies of this gene superfamily will play a prominent role in the post-human genome sequence era.

REFERENCES

1. Fradkin JE, Eastman RC, Lesniak MA, et al. Specificity spillover at the hormone receptor—exploring its role in human disease. N Engl J Med 1989;320:640-645.
2. Hunter T. The Croonian Lecture 1997. The phosphorylation of proteins on tyrosine: its role in cell growth and disease. Philos Trans R Soc Lond B Biol Sci 1998;353:583-605.
3. Hanks SK, Hunter T. Protein kinases 6. The eukaryotic protein kinase superfamily: kinase (catalytic) domain structure and classification. FASEB J 1995;9:576-596.
4. Ushiro H, Cohen S. Identification of phosphotyrosine as a product of epidermal growth factor-activated protein kinase in A-431 cell membranes. J Biol Chem 1980;255:8363-8365.
5. Ullrich A, Coussens L, Hayflick JS, et al. Human epidermal growth factor receptor cDNA sequence and aberrant expression of the amplified gene in A431 epidermoid carcinoma cells. Nature 1984;309:418-425.
6. Ullrich A, Gray A, Tam AW, et al. Insulin-like growth factor I receptor primary structure: comparison with insulin receptor suggests structural determinants that define functional specificity. EMBO J 1986;5:2503-2512.
7. Weiss A, Schlessinger J. Switching signals on or off by receptor dimerization. Cell 1998;94:277-280.
8. Westermark B, Claesson-Welsh L, Heldin CH. Structural and functional aspects of the receptors for platelet-derived growth factor. Prog Growth Factor Res 1989;1:253-266.
9. Heldin CH, Ostman A, Ronnstrand L. Signal transduction via platelet-derived growth factor receptors. Biochim Biophys Acta 1998;1378:F79-F113.
10. Cunningham BC, Ultsch M, De Vos AM, et al. Dimerization of the extracellular domain of the human growth hormone receptor by a single hormone molecule. Science 1991;254:821-825.
11. de Vos AM, Ultsch M, Kossiakoff AA. Human growth hormone and extracellular domain of its receptor: crystal structure of the complex. Science 1992;255:306-312.
12. Wells JA. Binding in the growth hormone receptor complex. Proc Natl Acad Sci U S A 1996;93:1-6.
13. Wiesmann C, Fuh G, Christinger HW, et al. Crystal structure at 1.7 Å resolution of VEGF in complex with domain 2 of the Flt-1 receptor. Cell 1997;91:695-704.
14. Boni-Schnetzler M, Rubin JB, Pilch PF. Structural requirements for the transmembrane activation of the insulin receptor kinase. J Biol Chem 1986;261:15281-15287.

15. Boni-Schnetzler M, Scott W, Waugh SM, et al. The insulin receptor: structural basis for high affinity ligand binding. J Biol Chem 1987;262:8395-8401.
16. Taouis M, Levy-Toledano R, Roach P, et al. Structural basis by which a recessive mutation in the alpha-subunit of the insulin receptor affects insulin binding. J Biol Chem 1994;269: 14912-14918.
17. De Meyts P. The structural basis of insulin and insulin-like growth factor-I receptor binding and negative co-operativity, and its relevance to mitogenic versus metabolic signalling. Diabetologia 1994;37:S135-S148.
18. Hubbard SR, Wei L, Ellis L, et al. Crystal structure of the tyrosine kinase domain of the human insulin receptor. Nature 1994;372: 746-754.
19. Hubbard SR. Crystal structure of the activated insulin receptor tyrosine kinase in complex with peptide substrate and ATP analog. EMBO J 1997;16:5572-5581.
20. Hubbard SR, Mohammadi M, Schlessinger J. Autoregulatory mechanisms in protein-tyrosine kinases. J Biol Chem 1998;273:11987-11990.
21. Herrera R, Rosen OM. Regulation of the protein kinase activity of the human insulin receptor. J Recept Res 1987;7:405-415.
22. Tornqvist HE, Avruch J. Relationship of site-specific beta subunit tyrosine autophosphorylation to insulin activation of the insulin receptor (tyrosine) protein kinase activity. J Biol Chem 1988;263: 4593-4601.
23. Ullrich A, Schlessinger J. Signal transduction by receptors with tyrosine kinase activity. Cell 1990;61:202-203.
24. Kavanaugh WM, Williams LT. An alternative to SH2 domains for binding tyrosine-phosphorylated proteins. Science 1994;266:1862-1865.
25. Blaikie P, Immanuel D, Wu J, et al. A region in Shc distinct from the SH2 domain can bind tyrosine-phosphorylated growth factor receptors. J Biol Chem 1994;269:32031-32034.
26. Gustafson TA, He W, Craparo A, et al. Phosphotyrosine-dependent interaction of Shc and insulin receptor substrate 1 with the NPEY motif of the insulin receptor via a novel non-SH2 domain. Mol Cell Biol 1995;15:2500-2508.
27. Anderson D, Koch CA, Grey L, et al. Binding of SH2 domains of phospholipase Cg 1, GAP, and Src to activated growth factor receptors. Science 1990;250:979-982.
28. Perrotti N, Accili D, Marcus-Samuels B, et al. Insulin stimulates phosphorylation of a 120-kDa glycoprotein substrate (pp120) for the receptor-associated protein kinase in intact H-35 hepatoma cells. Proc Natl Acad Sci U S A 1987;84:3137-3140.
29. Najjar SM, Philippe N, Suzuki Y, et al. Insulin-stimulated phosphorylation of recombinant pp120/HA4, an endogenous substrate of the insulin receptor tyrosine kinase. Biochemistry 1995;34: 9341-9349.
30. Kouhara H, Hadari YR, Spivak-Kroizman T, et al. A lipid-anchored Grb2-binding protein that links FGF-receptor activation to the Ras/ MAPK signaling pathway. Cell 1997;89:692-693.
31. White MF, Yenush L. The IRS-signaling system: a network of docking proteins that mediate insulin and cytokine action. Curr Top Microbiol Immunol 1998;228:178-179.
32. Sun XJ, Rothenberg P, Kahn CR, et al. Structure of the insulin receptor substrate IRS-1 defines a unique signal transduction protein. Nature 1991;352:73-77.
33. Sun XJ, Wang LM, Zhang Y, et al. Role of IRS-2 in insulin and cytokine signaling. Nature 1995;377:173-177.
34. Lavan BE, Lane WS, Lienhard GE. The 60-kDa phosphotyrosine protein in insulin-treated adipocytes is a new member of the insulin receptor substrate family. J Biol Chem 1997;272:11439-11443.
35. Sciacchitano S, Taylor SI. Cloning, tissue expression, and chromosomal localization of the mouse IRS-3 gene. Endocrinology 1997;138:4931-4940.
36. Quon MJ, Chen H, Ing BL, et al. Roles of 1-phosphatidylinositol 3-kinase and ras in regulating translocation of GLUT4 in transfected rat adipose cells. Mol Cell Biol 1995;15:5403-5411.
37. Kohn AD, Summers SA, Birnbaum MJ, et al. Expression of a constitutively active Akt Ser/Thr kinase in 3T3-L1 adipocytes stimulates glucose uptake and glucose transporter 4 translocation. J Biol Chem 1996;271:31372-31378.
38. Cong LN, Chen H, Li Y, et al. Physiological role of Akt in insulin-stimulated translocation of GLUT4 in transfected rat adipose cells. Mol Endocrinol 1997;11:1881-1890.
39. Standaert ML, Galloway L, Karnam P, et al. Protein kinase C-zeta as a downstream effector of phosphatidylinositol 3-kinase during insulin stimulation in rat adipocytes. Potential role in glucose transport. J Biol Chem 1997;272:30075-30082.
40. Kitamura T, Ogawa W, Sakaue H, et al. Requirement for activation of the serine-threonine kinase Akt (protein kinase B) in insulin stimulation of protein synthesis but not of glucose transport. Mol Cell Biol 1998;18:3708-3717.
41. Alessi DR, Deak M, Casamayor A, et al. 3-Phosphoinositide-dependent protein kinase-1 (PDK1): structural and functional homology with the *Drosophila* DSTPK61 kinase. Curr Biol 1997;7:776-779.
42. Alessi DR, Downes CP. The role of PI 3-kinase in insulin action. Biochim Biophys Acta 1998;1436:151-154.
43. Cheatham B, Vlahos CJ, Cheatham L, et al. Phosphatidylinositol 3-kinase activation is required for insulin stimulation of pp70 S6 kinase, DNA synthesis, and glucose transporter translocation. Mol Cell Biol 1994;14:4902-4911.
44. Watson R, Shigematsu S, Chiang S, et al. Lipid raft microdomain compartmentalization of TC10 is required for insulin signaling and GLUT4 translocation. J Cell Biol 2001;154:829-840.
45. Baumann CA, Ribon V, Kanzaki M, et al. CAP defines a second signalling pathway required for insulin-stimulated glucose transport. Nature 2000;407:202-207.
46. Chiang SH, Baumann CA, Kanzaki M, et al. Insulin-stimulated GLUT4 translocation requires the CAP-dependent activation of TC10. Nature 2001;410:944-948.
47. Lowenstein EJ, Daly RJ, Batzer AG, et al. The SH2 and SH3 domain-containing protein GRB2 links receptor tyrosine kinases to ras signaling. Cell 1992;70:431-432.
48. Pronk GJ, McGlade J, Pelicci G, et al. Insulin-induced phosphorylation of the 46- and 52-kDa Shc proteins. J Biol Chem 1993;268: 5748-5753.
49. Skolnik EY, Lee CH, Batzer A, et al. The SH2/SH3 domain-containing protein GRB2 interacts with tyrosine-phosphorylated IRS1 and Shc: implications for insulin control of ras signalling. EMBO J 1993;12:1929-1936.
50. Li N, Batzer A, Daly R, et al. Guanine-nucleotide-releasing factor hSos1 binds to Grb2 and links receptor tyrosine kinases to Ras signalling. Nature 1993;363:85-88.
51. Yarden Y, Escobedo JA, Kuang WJ, et al. Structure of the receptor for platelet-derived growth factor helps define a family of closely related growth factor receptors. Nature 1986;323:226-232.
52. Clark SF, Martin S, Carozzi AJ, et al. Intracellular localization of phosphatidylinositide 3-kinase and insulin receptor substrate-1 in adipocytes: potential involvement of a membrane skeleton. J Cell Biol 1998;140:1211-1225.
53. Belham C, Wu S, Avruch J. Intracellular signalling: PDK1-a kinase at the hub of things. Curr Biol 1999;9:R93-R96.
54. Avruch J, Khokhlatchev A, Kyriakis JM, et al. Ras activation of the Raf kinase: tyrosine kinase recruitment of the MAP kinase cascade. Recent Prog Horm Res 2001;56:127-155.
55. Carpentier JL. Insulin receptor internalization: molecular mechanisms and physiopathological implications. Diabetologia 1994;37: S117-S124.
56. Carpentier JL, Hamer I, Gilbert A, et al. Molecular and cellular mechanisms governing the ligand-specific and non-specific steps of insulin receptor internalization. Z Gastroenterol 1996;34: 73-75.
57. Flier JS, Minaker KL, Landsberg L, et al. Impaired in vivo insulin clearance in patients with severe target-cell resistance to insulin. Diabetes 1982;31:132-135.
58. Elchebly M, Payette P, Michaliszyn E, et al. Increased insulin sensitivity and obesity resistance in mice lacking the protein tyrosine phosphatase-1B gene. Science 1999;283:1544-1548.
59. Klaman LD, Boss O, Peroni OD, et al. Increased energy expenditure, decreased adiposity, and tissue-specific insulin sensitivity in protein-tyrosine phosphatase 1B-deficient mice. Mol Cell Biol 2000;20:5479-5489.
60. Hotamisligil GS, Peraldi P, Budavari A, et al. IRS-1-mediated inhibition of insulin receptor tyrosine kinase activity in TNF-alpha-and obesity-induced insulin resistance. Science 1996;271:665-668.

61. De Fea K, Roth RA. Modulation of insulin receptor substrate-1 tyrosine phosphorylation and function by mitogen-activated protein kinase. J Biol Chem 1997;272:31400-31406.
62. Li J, DeFea K, Roth RA. Modulation of insulin receptor substrate-1 tyrosine phosphorylation by an Akt/phosphatidylinositol 3-kinase pathway. J Biol Chem 1999;274:9351-9356.
63. Aguirre V, Uchida T, Yenush L, et al. The c-Jun NH_2 terminal kinase promotes insulin resistance during association with insulin receptor substrate-1 and phosphorylation of Ser(307). J Biol Chem 2000;275:9047-9054.
64. Rui L, Aguirre V, Kim JK, et al. Insulin/IGF-1 and TNF-alpha stimulate phosphorylation of IRS-1 at inhibitory Ser307 via distinct pathways. J Clin Invest 2001;107:181-189.
65. Taylor SI. Lilly lecture: molecular mechanisms of insulin resistance. Lessons from patients with mutations in the insulin-receptor gene. Diabetes 1992;41:1473-1490.
66. Carlomagno F, Salvatore G, Cirafici AM, et al. The different RET-activating capability of mutations of cysteine 620 or cysteine 634 correlates with the multiple endocrine neoplasia type 2 disease phenotype. Cancer Res 1997;57:391-395.
67. Mulligan LM, Kwok JB, Healey CS, et al. Germ-line mutations of the *RET* proto-oncogene in multiple endocrine neoplasia type 2A. Nature 1993;363:458-460.
68. Santoro M, Carlomagno F, Romano A, et al. Activation of *RET* as a dominant transforming gene by germline mutations of *MEN2A* and *MEN2B*. Science 1995;267:381-383.
69. Drachman DB. Myasthenia gravis. N Engl J Med 1994;330: 1797-1810.
70. Kahn CR, Flier JS, Bar RS, et al. The syndromes of insulin resistance and acanthosis nigricans: insulin-receptor disorders in man. N Engl J Med 1976;294:739-745.
71. Flier JS, Kahn CR, Roth J, et al. Antibodies that impair insulin receptor binding in an unusual diabetic syndrome with severe insulin resistance. Science 1975;190:63-65.
72. Taylor SI, Marcus-Samuels B. Anti-receptor antibodies mimic the effect of insulin to down-regulate insulin receptors in cultured human lymphoblastoid (IM-9) cells. J Clin Endocrinol Metab 1984;58:182-186.
73. Weetman AP. Graves' disease. N Engl J Med 2000;343:1236-1248.
74. Flier JS, Bar RS, Muggeo M, et al. The evolving clinical course of patients with insulin receptor autoantibodies: spontaneous remission or receptor proliferation with hypoglycemia. J Clin Endocrinol Metab 1978;47:985-995.
75. Taylor SI, Grunberger G, Marcus-Samuels B, et al. Hypoglycemia associated with antibodies to the insulin receptor. N Engl J Med 1982;307:1422-1426.
76. Shi Y, Massague J. Mechanisms of TGF-β signaling from cell membrane to the nucleus. Cell 2003;113:685-700.
77. Amselem S, Duquesnoy P, Attree O, et al. Laron dwarfism and mutations of the growth hormone-receptor gene. N Engl J Med 1989;321:989-995.
78. Clement K, Vaisse C, Lahlou N, et al. A mutation in the human leptin receptor gene causes obesity and pituitary dysfunction. Nature 1998;392:398-401.
79. Smit LS, Meyer DJ, Argetsinger LS, et al. Molecular events in growth hormone-receptor interaction and signaling. In Kostyo JS, Goodman HM, eds. Handbook of Physiology. New York: Oxford University Press, 1999:445-480.
80. Bravo J, Heath JK. Receptor recognition by gp130 cytokines. EMBO J 2000; 19:2399-2411.
81. Auernhammer CJ, Melmed S. Leukemia-inhibitory factor-neuroimmune modulator of endocrine function. Endocr Rev 2000;21:313-345.
82. Lambert PD, Anderson KD, Sleeman MW, et al. Ciliary neurotrophic factor activates leptin-like pathways and reduces body fat, without cachexia or rebound weight gain, even in leptin-resistant obesity. Proc Natl Acad Sci U S A 2001;98:4652-4657.
83. Opal SM, DePalo VA. Anti-inflammatory cytokines. Chest 2000;117: 1162-1172.
84. Heim MH. The JAK-STAT pathway: cytokine signalling from the receptor to the nucleus. J Recept Signal Transduct Res 1999;19: 75-120.
85. Campbell GS, Argetsinger LS, Ihle JN, et al. Activation of JAK2 tyrosine kinase by prolactin receptors in Nb2 cells and mouse mammary gland explants. Proc Natl Acad Sci U S A 1994;91:5232-5236.
86. Argetsinger LS, Campbell GS, Yang X, et al. Identification of JAK2 as a growth hormone receptor-associated tyrosine kinase. Cell 1993;74:237-244.
87. Brown RJ, Adams JJ, Pelekanos RA, et al. Model for growth hormone receptor activation based on subunit rotation within a receptor dimer. Nat Struct Mol Biol 2005;12:814-821.
88. Noguchi M, Yi H, Rosenblatt HM, et al. Interleukin-2 receptor gamma chain mutation results in X-linked severe combined immunodeficiency in humans. Cell 1993;73:147-157.
89. Parganas E, Wang D, Stravopodis D, et al. JAK2 is essential for signaling through a variety of cytokine receptors. Cell 1998;93:385-395.
90. Ihle JN, Thierfelder W, Teglund S, et al. Signaling by the cytokine receptor superfamily. Ann N Y Acad Sci 1998;865:1-9.
91. Stahl N, Boulton TG, Farruggella T, et al. Association and activation of JAK-Tyk kinases by CNTF-LIF-OSM-IL-6 beta receptor components. Science 1994;263:92-95.
92. Stoecklin E, Wissler M, Schaetzle D, et al. Interactions in the transcriptional regulation exerted by STAT5 and by members of the steroid hormone receptor family. J Steroid Biochem Mol Biol 1999;69:195-204.
93. Kofoed EM, Hwa V, Little B, et al. Growth hormone insensitivity associated with a STAT5b mutation. N Engl J Med 2003;349:1139-1147.
94. Hwa V, Little B, Adiyaman P, et al. Severe growth hormone insensitivity resulting from total absence of signal transducer and activator of transcription 5b. J Clin Endocrinol Metab 2005;90:4260-4266.
95. Baxter EJ, Scott LM, Campbell PJ, et al. Acquired mutation of the tyrosine kinase JAK2 in human myeloproliferative disorders. Lancet 2005;365:1054-1061.
96. Lin TS, Mahajan S, Frank DA. STAT signaling in the pathogenesis and treatment of leukemias. Oncogene 2000;19:2496-2504.
97. Yasukawa H, Misawa H, Sakamoto H, et al. The JAK-binding protein JAB inhibits Janus tyrosine kinase activity through binding in the activation loop. EMBO J 1999;18:1309-1320.
98. Hansen JA, Lindberg K, Hilton DJ, et al. Mechanism of inhibition of growth hormone receptor signaling by suppressor of cytokine signaling proteins. Mol Endocrinol 1999;13:1832-1843.
99. Ram PA, Waxman DJ. SOCS/CIS protein inhibition of growth hormone-stimulated STAT5 signaling by multiple mechanisms. J Biol Chem 1999;274:35553-35561.
100. Mao Y, Ling PR, Fitzgibbons TP, et al. Endotoxin-induced inhibition of growth hormone receptor signaling in rat liver in vivo. Endocrinology 1999;140:5505-5515.
101. Clevenger CV, Medaglia MV. The protein tyrosine kinase P59fyn is associated with prolactin (PRL) receptor and is activated by PRL stimulation of T-lymphocytes. Mol Endocrinol 1994;8:674-681.
102. Rui L, Carter-Su C. Identification of SH2-Bb as a potent cytoplasmic activator of the tyrosine kinase Janus kinase 2. Proc Natl Acad Sci U S A 1999;96:7172-7177.
103. Shuai K, Liu B. Regulation of gene-activation pathways by PIAS proteins in the immune system. Nat Rev Immunol 2005;5: 593-605.
104. Bockaert J, Pin JP. Molecular tinkering of G protein-coupled receptors: an evolutionary success. EMBO J 1999;18:1723-1729.
105. Neer EJ. Heterotrimeric G proteins: organizers of transmembrane signals. Cell 1995;80:249-257.
106. Cabrera-Vera TM, Vanhauwe J, Thomas TO, et al. Insights into G protein structure, function and regulation. Endocr Rev 2003;24: 765-781.
107. Rodbell M. The role of GTP-binding proteins in signal transduction: from the sublimely simple to the conceptually complex. Curr Top Cell Regul 1992;32:1-47.
108. Lefkowitz RJ. Historical review: a brief history and personal retrospective of seven-transmembrane receptors. Trends Pharmacol Sci 2004;25:413-422.
109. Palczewski K, Kumasaka T, Hori T, et al. Crystal structure of rhodopsin: a G protein-coupled receptor. Science 2000;289:739-745.
110. Kunishima N, Shimada Y, Tsuji Y, et al. Structural basis of glutamate recognition by a dimeric metabotropic glutamate receptor. Nature 2000;407:971-977.

111. Hoare SRJ. Mechanisms of peptide and nonpeptide ligand binding to class B G protein-coupled receptors. Drug Discovery Today 2005;10:417-427.
112. Wess J, ed. Structure-Function Analysis of G Protein-Coupled Receptors. New York: Wiley-Liss, 1999.
113. Yamashita T, Terakita A, Shichida Y. Distinct roles of the second and third cytoplasmic loops of bovine rhodopsin in G protein activation. J Biol Chem 2000;275:34272-34279.
114. Gershengorn M, Osman R. Insights into G protein-coupled receptor function using molecular models. Endocrinology 2001;142:2-10.
115. Fan QR, Hendrickson WA. Structure of the human follicle-stimulating hormone in complex with its receptor. Nature 2005;433:269-277.
116. Soudijn W, Wijngaarden IV, Ijzerman AP. Structure-activity relationships of inverse agonists for G protein-coupled receptors. Medicinal Res Rev 2005;25:398-426.
117. Perez D, Karnik S. Multiple signaling states of G protein-coupled receptors. Pharm Rev 2005;57:147-161.
118. Herbert TE, Moffett S, Morello JP, et al. A peptide derived from a β2-adrenergic receptor transmembrane domain inhibits both receptor dimerization and activation. J Biol Chem 1996;271: 16384-16392.
119. Ray K, Hauschild BC, Steinbach PJ, et al. Identification of the cysteine residues in the amino-terminal extracellular domain of the human Ca^{2+} receptor critical for dimerization. J Biol Chem 1999;274:27642-27650.
120. Pin J-P, Kniazeff J, Liu J, et al. Allosteric functioning of dimeric class C G protein-coupled receptors. FEBS J 2005;272:2947-2955.
121. Kaupmann K, Malitschek B, Schuler V, et al. GABA-B receptor subtypes assemble into functional heteromeric complexes. Nature 1998;396:683-687.
122. Maggio R, Novi F, Scarselli M, et al. The impact of G protein-coupled receptor hetero-oligomerization on function and pharmacology. FEBS J 2005;272:2939-2946.
123. Lefkowitz RJ, Shenoy SK. Transduction of receptor signals by β-arrestins. Science 2005;308:512-517.
124. Tu JC, Xiao B, Yuan JP, et al. Homer binds a novel proline-rich motif and links group 1 metabotropic glutamate receptors with IP3 receptors. Neuron 1998;21:717-726.
125. McLatchie L, Fraser N, Main M, et al. RAMPs regulate the transport and ligand specificity of the calcitonin-like receptor. Nature 1998;393:333-339.
126. Hebert SC. Orphan detectors of metabolism. Nature 2004;429: 143-145.
127. Steneberg P, Rubins N, Bartoov-Shifman R, et al. The FFA receptor GPR40 links hyperinsulinemia, hepatic steatosis, and impaired glucose homeostasis in mouse. Cell Metabolism 2005;1:245-258.
128. Spiegel AM, Weinstein LS. Inherited diseases involving G proteins and G protein-coupled receptors. Ann Rev Med 2004;55:27-39.
129. Seminara SB, Messager S, Chatzidaki EE, et al. The GPR54 gene as a regulator of puberty. N Engl J Med 2003;349:1614-1627.
130. Barak LS, Oakley RH, Laporte SA, et al. Constitutive arrestin-mediated desensitization of a human vasopressin receptor mutant associated with nephrogenic diabetes insipidus. Proc Natl Acad Sci U S A 2001;98:93-98.
131. Hu J, Spiegel AM. Naturally occurring mutations of the extracellular Ca-sensing receptor: implications for its structure and function. Trends Endocrinol Metab 2003;14:282-288.
132. Van Sande J, Parma J, Tonacchera M, et al. Somatic and germline mutations of the TSH receptor gene in thyroid diseases. J Clin Endocrinol Metab 1995;80:2577-2585.
133. Javitch JA, Fu D, Liapakis G, Chen J. Constitutive activation of the β2-adrenergic receptor alters the orientation of its sixth membrane-spanning segment. J Biol Chem 1997;272:18546-18549.
134. Feldman BJ, Rosenthal SM, Vargas GA, et al. Nephrogenic syndrome of inappropriate antidiuresis. N Engl J Med 2005;352: 1884-1890.
135. Lin L, Faraco J, Li R, et al. The sleep disorder canine narcolepsy is caused by a mutation in the hypocretin (orexin) receptor 2 gene. Cell 1999;98:365-376.
136. Huszar D, Lynch CA, Fairchild-Huntress V, et al. Targeted disruption of the melanocortin-4 receptor results in obesity in mice. Cell 1997;88:131-141.
137. Farooqi IS, Keough JM, Yeo GS, et al. Clinical spectrum of obesity and mutations in the melanocortin 4 receptor gene. N Engl J Med 2003;348:1085-1095.
138. Lanske B, Karaplis AC, Lee K, et al. PTH/PTHrP receptor in early development and Indian hedgehog-regulated bone growth. Science 1996;273:663-666.
139. Jobert AS, Zhang P, Couvineau A, et al. Absence of functional receptors for parathyroid hormone and parathyroid hormone-related peptide in Blomstrand chondrodysplasia. J Clin Invest 1998;102:34-40.
140. Susulic VS, Frederich RC, Lawitts J, et al. Targeted disruption of the β3-adrenergic receptor gene. J Biol Chem 1995;270:29483-29492.
141. Sangkuhl K, Schulz A, Rompler H, et al. Aminoglycoside-mediated rescue of a disease-causing nonsense mutation in the V2 vasopressin receptor gene *in vitro* and *in vivo*. Hum Mol Gen 2004;13: 893-903.
142. Castro-Fernandez C, Maya-Nunez G, Conn PM. Beyond the signal sequence: protein routing in health and disease. Endocr Rev 2005;26:479-503.
143. Kaiser UB. The pathogenesis of the ovarian hyperstimulation syndrome. N Engl J Med 2003;349:729-732.
144. Monanelli L, Delbaere A, Di Carlo C, et al. A mutation in the follicle-stimulating hormone receptor as a cause of familial spontaneous ovarian hyperstimulation syndrome. J Clin Endocrinol Metab 2004;89:1255-1258.
145. Small KM, Forbes SL, Rahman FF, et al. A four amino acid deletion polymorphism in the third intracellular loop of the human α_{2C}-adrenergic receptor confers impaired coupling to multiple effectors. J Biol Chem 2000;275:23059-23064.

CHAPTER 6

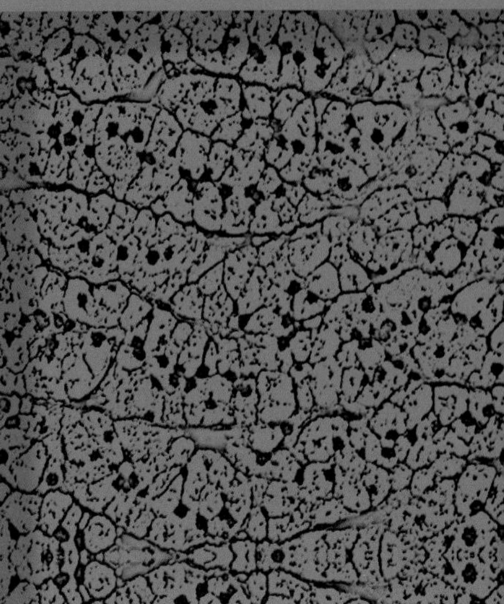

LABORATORY TECHNIQUES FOR RECOGNITION OF ENDOCRINE DISORDERS

George G. Klee

Endocrinology is a practice of medicine that is highly dependent on accurate laboratory measurements because small changes in hormone levels often may be more specific and more sensitive for early disease than the classic physical signs and symptoms. Because most endocrinologists currently do not have facilities to develop and validate laboratory assays, they rely on commercial analytic assays or send a patient's specimen to specialized laboratories. Even most hospital and commercial laboratories have minimal expertise for developing analytic assays. This critical dependence on quality laboratory measurements, combined with minimal information about the performance of these tests, places endocrinologists in a potentially vulnerable position.

This chapter provides an overview of the strengths and weaknesses of the analytic techniques typically used for endocrine measurements in blood and urine. Concentrations of most hormones are much lower than those of general chemistry analytes, and specialized techniques are necessary to measure these low concentrations.

Four major types of assays for measuring hormones are described: immunoassays (both competitive and sandwich), chromatography, mass spectrometry, and nucleic acid–based assays for evaluation of genetic alterations.

The analytic performance validation required by the Federal Government for laboratories testing specimens of Medicare patients is outlined, along with explanations of these performance parameters. This information should help endocrinologists better assess the performance of the analytic systems that they are using. Techniques to investigate discordant laboratory test values also are presented to help clinicians work with their laboratories to reconcile test values that do not match clinical presentations.

Hormone concentrations are reported in molar units, mass units, or standardized units, such as World Health Organization (WHO) International Units (IU). When these measurements are expressed in molar units, most hormones in blood and urine are present in concentrations of 10^{-6} to 10^{-12} M/L (Fig. 6–1). The terms used to describe these concentrations are micromolar (10^{-6} M/L), nanomolar (10^{-9} M/L), and picomolar (10^{-12} M/L). The range—from the lowest to the highest concentrations—is more than a million-fold difference. Therefore, laboratory techniques must be targeted to the levels of each given hormone.

The major techniques for measuring the lower picomolar concentrations are immunoassay and mass spectrometry, whereas the higher nanomolar and micromolar concentrations can be measured by these methods as well as chromatography and chemical detection systems. Some hormones, such as thyrotropin (TSH), have very low concentrations in the femtomolar (10^{-15} M/L) range in patients with diseases such as thyrotoxicosis. Exquisitely sensitive immunometric assays are usually used to measure these very low concentrations.[1,2]

Types of Assays

The four major techniques used for endocrine measurements are as follows: (1) antibody-based immunologic assays, of which there are two subcategories: competitive immunoassays and immunometric (sandwich) assays, (2) chromatographic assays, (3) mass spectrometry, and (4) nucleic acid–based assays.

Competitive Immunoassays

The term *competitive radioimmunoassay* refers to a measurement method in which an antigen (e.g., a hormone) in a

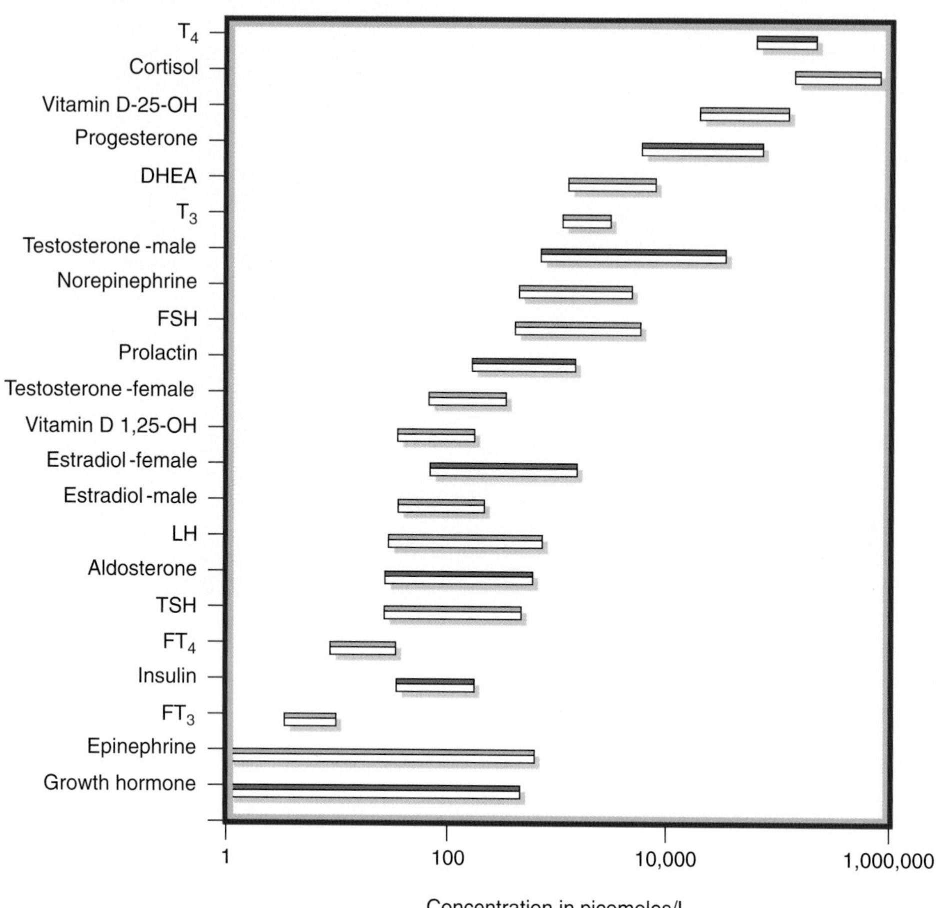

Figure 6–1 ▪ Six-logarithm range of normal concentrations for the plasma concentrations of endocrine tests. *DHEA,* Dehydroepiandrosterone; *FSH,* follicle-stimulating hormone; *FT_4,* free thyroxine; *FT_3,* free triiodothyronine; *LH,* luteinizing hormone; *T_3,* triiodothyronine; *T_4,* thyroxine; *TSH,* thyrotropin.

specimen competes with radiolabeled reagent antigen for a limited number of binding sites on a reagent antibody. The three basic components of a competitive immunoassay are (1) antiserum specific for a unique epitope on a hormone or antigen, (2) labeled antigen that binds to this antiserum, (3) unlabeled antigen in the specimen or standard that is to be measured.[3,4]

The antiserum is diluted to a concentration in which the number of binding sites available on the antibodies is fewer than the number of antigen molecules (labeled and unlabeled) in the reaction mixture. The labeled and unlabeled antigens compete for this limited number of binding sites on the antiserum. The competition is not always equal because the labeled antigen *(tracer)* may react differently with the antibody compared with the native antigen. This disparity in reactivity may be caused by alteration of the antigen due to the chemical attachment of the label or by differences in the endogenous antigen versus the form of the antigen used in the reagents. As long as the reactions are reproducible, these differences in reactivity are not important because the reaction can be *calibrated* with standard reference materials having known concentrations.

Figure 6–2 illustrates the concepts of a competitive immunoassay. In the schematic diagram, 8 units of antibody react with 16 units of labeled antigen and 4 units of native antigen. At equilibrium (assuming equal reactivity), 6 units of label and 2 units of native antigen are bound to the limited supply of antibody. The antigen bound to the antibody is separated from the liquid antigen by any of several methods, and the amount of labeled antigen in the bound portion is quantitated. The assay is calibrated by measuring standards with known concentrations and cross-plotting the signal (i.e., counts of the gamma rays emitted from the radioactive label) versus the concentration of the standards to generate a dose-response curve. As the concentration increases, the signal decreases exponentially.

Generally, the antiserum used in a competitive assay is diluted to a titer that binds between 40% and 50% of the labeled antigen when no unlabeled antigen is present. Further dilution of the antiserum increases the analytic sensitivity but decreases both the signal and the range of the assay.

The precision of competitive immunoassays is related to the rate of change of the signal compared with the rate of change of concentration (i.e., the slope of the dose-response curve).[5] In Figure 6–2B, the slope is much lower at higher concentrations, causing the assay precision to be less at higher concentrations. Most competitive immunoassays also have a relatively flat dose-response curve at very low concentrations, causing poor precision at the low end of the assay. Consequently, the precision profile for most immunoassays is U-shaped, having the best coefficients of variation in the center of the dose-response curve.

As shown in Figure 6–2, the higher the concentration of the unlabeled antigen, the lower the amount of radiolabeled antigen that binds to the limited amount of antiserum. The signal decreases exponentially from the approximately half-maximum at zero concentration to a minimum value at high concentrations. This minimal binding, or *nonspecific binding* (NSB), is a valuable control parameter. Elevations in NSB usually signify impurities in the label that bind to the sides of the tubes and are not competitively displaced. Most assays add surfactants and proteins to minimize the NSB. Monitoring of changes in the NSB provides an early warning of potential assay problems.

Statistical data processing techniques are needed to translate the assay signals into concentrations. As illustrated, these dose-response curves generally are not linear, and numerous

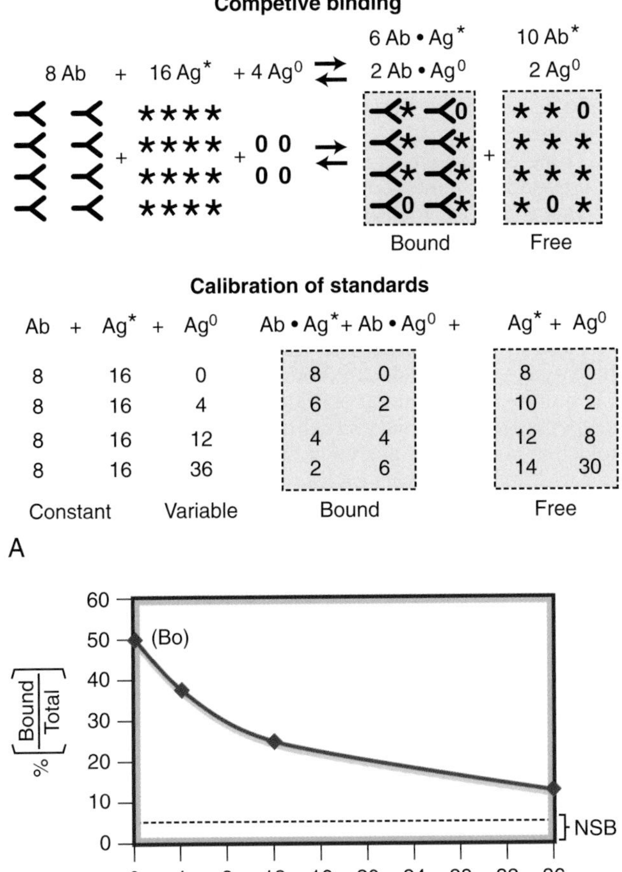

Ab	Ag*	Ag0	Ab • Ag*	Ab • Ag0	Ag*	Ag0
8	16	0	8	0	8	0
8	16	4	6	2	10	2
8	16	12	4	4	12	8
8	16	36	2	6	14	30

Figure 6–2 ▪ **A,** Principles of competitive binding assays. **B,** Typical dose-response curve.

curve-fitting algorithms have been developed. Before the introduction of microprocessors, tedious error-prone, manual calculations were required to mathematically transform the data into linear models. A commonly used model was to cross-plot the logit of the normalized signal versus the logarithm of the concentration and to use linear regression lines to establish the dose-response curve.[5] Fortunately, today this procedure of curve fitting usually is accomplished electronically by using programs that automatically test the robustness of fit of multiparameter curves after statistically eliminating discordant data points.[6] However, users of these systems must understand the limitations and should pay attention to any warnings presented by the programs during processing of the data.

In radioimmunoassays, radioactive iodine (^{125}I) is usually used to label the antigen. The immune complexes are separated from the unbound molecules by precipitation with centrifugation after reaction with secondary antisera and precipitating reagents (e.g., polyethylene glycol).[7] These radioimmunoassays are labor intensive and may require special handling and licensure to ensure safety of the radioisotopes. The statistical counting errors associated with the relatively low radioactive counts and the poor reproducibility associated with the multiple manual steps generally necessitate that most laboratories perform the measurements in duplicate.[8] Even when the averages of duplicate measurements are used, many manual radioimmunoassays have coefficients of variation between 10% and 15%.

It is important that key quality control parameters for radioimmunoassays be carefully monitored. In addition to NSB, another key quality control parameter is the percentage binding of the radiolabel when zero antigen (Bo) is present. As the label deteriorates, because of aging, the binding often decreases, resulting in a less reliable assay.

Another important quality control parameter is the slope of the dose-response curve. This parameter can be tracked by monitoring the concentration corresponding to half-maximum binding (50% of B/Bo). If this concentration increases significantly, the slope of the response curve decreases and the assay may not be capable of reliably measuring patient specimens at clinically important concentrations.

Many commercial kits and automated immunoassays use nonisotopic signal systems to measure hormone concentrations. These assays often use colorimetric, fluorometric, or chemiluminescent signals rather than radioactivity to quantitate the response. The advantages of these alternate signals are biosafety, longer reagent shelf-life, and ease of automation. On the other hand, these signals are more subject to matrix interferences than radioactive iodine.

Radioactivity is not affected by changes in protein concentration, hemolysis, color, or drugs (except for other radioactive compounds), whereas many of the current signal systems may yield spurious results when such interferences are present. In addition, many automated immunoassays are read kinetically before the reactions reach equilibrium. This step accentuates the effects of matrix differences between the reference standards and patient specimens. Later in this chapter potential troubleshooting steps are outlined to help clinicians evaluate the integrity of test measurements when spurious results are suspected.

Solid-phase reactions often are used in current immunoassays to facilitate the separation of the bound antibody-antigen complexes from the free reactants.[9] Three frequently used solid-phase materials are (1) microtiter plates, (2) polystyrene beads, and (3) paramagnetic particles.[10] Typically, the antibody is attached to the solid phase, and the separation of the immune complexes from the unbound moieties is accomplished by plate washers, bead washers, or magnetic wash stations, eliminating the need for centrifugation. Another novel way of accomplishing this separation is to attach high-affinity linkers to antiserum, which then can be coupled to a complementary linker on the solid phase.

An excellent pair of linkers are biotin and streptavidin. These compounds bind with affinity constants of approximately 10^{15} L/M.[11] Biotin is a relatively small molecule that can be easily covalently attached to antiserum and used with streptavidin (a 70-kd tetrameric nonglycosylated protein) conjugated to microtiter plates, beads, or paramagnetic particles to facilitate separation. This technique allows the antibody-antigen reaction to proceed faster with less stearic hindrance than when the antibody is directly coupled to the solid phase.

The antiserum used in these assays is a crucial component. Most earlier immunoassays used *polyclonal* antiserum produced in animals. The process of generating these antisera is a combination of art, science, and luck. Generally, a relatively pure form of the antigen is conjugated to a carrier protein (especially if the antigen is less than 10,000 d), mixed with adjuvant (e.g., Freud's complete adjuvant), and injected intradermally into the host animal. After several boosts with conjugated protein plus Freud's incomplete adjuvant, the host animal recognizes the material as foreign and develops immune responses. The antiserum then is harvested from the animal's blood. Under optimal conditions, moderate quantities of high-affinity antisera, which react only with the specific target antigen, are developed. The analytic sensitivity of a competitive immunoassay is approximately inversely related to the affinity of the antiserum, such that an antiserum with an affinity constant of 10^9 L/M can be used to measure analytes in the nanomolar concentration range.

The polyclonal antiserum developed by immunizing animals represents a composite of many immunologic clones, with each clone having a different affinity and different immunologic specificity. Most clones have affinities in the 10^7 to 10^8 L/M range, with only rare clones having affinities above 10^{12} L/M. Various techniques are used to develop a specific antiserum, including (1) altering the form of the antigen by blocking cross-reacting epitopes and (2) purifying the antiserum using affinity chromatography to select antibodies directed toward the epitope of interest. Affinity-column purification also can be used for immunoextraction of higher affinity antisera by selectively eluting antiserum from the column by means of a series of buffers with increasing acidity.[12]

The major disadvantage of a polyclonal antiserum is the limited quantity. The large quantities needed by commercial suppliers of immunoassay reagents often require them to use multiple sources of antisera. These changes in antisera can cause significant changes in assay performance. In many instances, laboratories and clinicians are not informed about these changes, which may cause problems in medical decisions.

Monoclonal antisera are used in many current immunoassays. These antisera are made by immunizing animals (usually mice) using techniques similar to those used for polyclonal antisera; instead of harvesting the antisera from the blood, however, the animal is killed and the spleen is removed.[13] The lymphocytes in the spleen are fused with myeloma cells to make cells that will grow in culture and produce antisera.

These fused cells are separated into clones by means of serial plating techniques similar to those used in subculturing bacteria. The supernatant of these monoclonal cell lines (or ascites fluid if the cells are transplanted into carrier mice) contains monoclonal antisera. The selection processes used to separate the initial clones can be targeted to identify specific clones producing antisera with high affinities and low cross-reactivity to related compounds.

The high specificity of monoclonal antisera can cause problems for some endocrine assays. Many hormones circulate in the blood as heterogeneous mixtures of multiple forms. Some of these forms are caused by genetic differences in patients, whereas other forms are related to metabolic precursors and degradation products of the hormone. Genetic differences cause some patients to produce variant forms of a hormone such as luteinizing hormone (LH). These genetic differences can cause marked variations in measurements made using assays with specific monoclonal antisera compared with more uniform measurements made using assays with polyclonal antisera that cross-react with the multiple forms.[14] Well-characterized monoclonal antisera can be mixed together to make an "engineered polyclonal antiserum" with improved sensitivity and specificity.[15] Cross-reactivity with precursor forms of the analytes and with metabolic degradation products can cause major differences in assays. For example, cross-reactivity with six molecular forms of human chorionic gonadotropin (hCG) causes differences in hCG assays, and cross-reactivity with metabolic fragments causes differences in parathyroid hormone (PTH) assays.[16,17] Cortisol is another analyte wherein major cross-reactivity with other steroids such as corticosterone, 11-deoxycortisol, cortisone, and numerous synthetic steroids causes significant immunoassay interferences.[18]

Extraction of hormones from serum and urine specimens before measurement is a technique that can enhance both sensitivity and specificity of immunoassays. Numerous extraction systems have been developed, including (1) organic-aqueous partitioning to remove water-soluble interferences seen with steroids, (2) solid-phase extraction with absorption and selective elution from resins such as silica gels, and (3) immunoaffinity chromatography.[19,20] Unfortunately, extraction and purification before immunoassay are seldom used in clinical assays. These techniques are difficult to automate and require skills and equipment not available in many clinical laboratories. Although commercial assays generally use reagents having adequate sensitivity and specificity to measure *most* patient specimens, some patient specimens may give spurious results and some disease states may require more analytic sensitivity to ensure sound clinical decisions. In these cases, extraction of specimens before measurement may provide more reliable information.

Immunoassays measure concentrations rather than biologic activity. For most hormones, there is a strong correlation between the concentration of the protein or steroid being measured and the biologic activity, but this is not universally true. The reactive site for most antibodies is relatively small, about 5 to 10 amino acids for linear peptides. Some antiserum reactions are specific for the tertiary structure that corresponds to unique molecular configurations, but immunoassays seldom react with the exact antigenic structure that confers biologic activity.

Figure 6–3 presents a schematic illustration of the difference between immunologic binding site and biologic receptor binding site on a hormone. Indirect immunoassays have been developed using cultured cells that synthesize second messengers such as cyclic adenosine monophosphate (cAMP) at rates proportional to the concentration of hormone in the specimen. An example of this technique is the immunoassay measurement of cAMP produced by osteosarcoma cells to quantitate PTH bioactivity in serum.[21] Unfortunately, these assays are tedious and generally are not reproducible. Techniques using recombinant receptors as immunoassay binders may provide improved specificity with good reliability.[22-24]

Immunometric (Sandwich) Assays

A second immunologic technique used to measure hormones is the immunometric (sandwich) assay. The three basic components of a sandwich assay are (1) an antigen large enough to allow two antibodies to bind concurrently on different binding sites, (2) a *capture* antiserum directed to one of the antigenic sites on the antigen—this antiserum is attached to a solid phase to permit immunologic extraction of the immune complexes, and (3) a *signal* antiserum directed to a second antigenic site on the antigen—this antiserum is attached to an assay signal system.

In contrast to competitive immunoassays, these assays use a large excess of antiserum-binding sites compared with the concentration of antigen. The capture antibody immunoextracts the antigen from the sample and the signal antibody binds

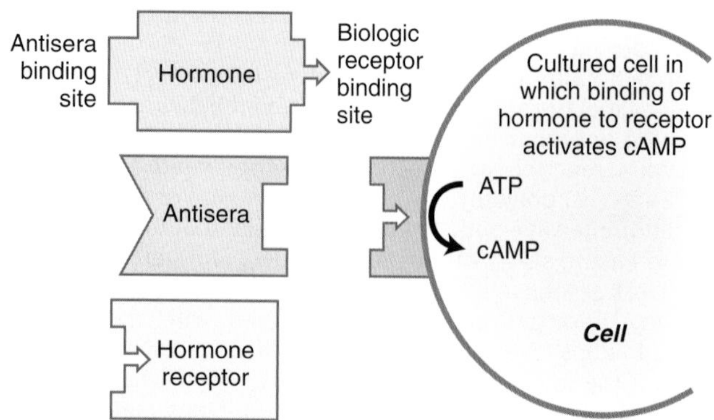

Figure 6–3 ▪ Comparison of an immunologic technique for measuring hormone concentration versus a receptor technique for measuring hormone activity. *ATP,* Adenosine triphosphate; *cAMP,* cyclic adenosine monophosphate.

to the capture-antibody-antigen complex to form a tertiary complex. As the antigen concentration increases, the signal increases progressively.

Figure 6–4 schematically illustrates these concepts. The capture antiserum (ATB1) is attached to biotin *(see solid circles)*. The signal antiserum (ATB2) is labeled with a detection system *(see asterisks)*. The ATB1-antigen-ATB2 complexes are immunologically extracted using a streptavidin solid phase *(see horizontal cups)*. After the complex is bound to the solid phase, most of the unbound signal antibody is washed away.

As shown in Figure 6–4, the signal increases progressively with the concentration. For lower concentrations, the signal generally increases proportionally to the assay concentrations (after the offset caused by the NSB). At higher concentrations, the signal generally is less than proportional, so that nonlinear curve-fitting techniques are used to generate the dose-response curves. Again, the relative imprecision, expressed as a coefficient of variation, depends on the slope of the dose-response curve; consequently, the relative precision is less at higher concentrations.

In immunometric assays, the background level of signal is associated with very low concentrations. This background signal is caused by the NSB. The analytic sensitivity of immunometric assays is related to the ratio of the true signal to the NSB signal. Therefore, assays can be made more sensitive either by increasing the response signal or by decreasing NSB. Inadvertent increases in NSB caused by specimen interference or reagent deterioration can significantly alter the assay performance.

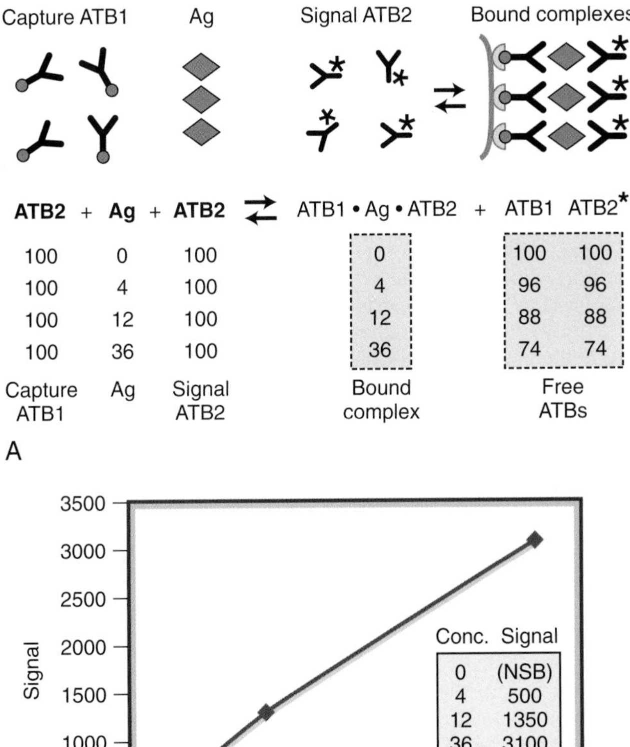

Figure 6–4 ▪ **A,** Principles of immunometric assays. *Ag,* Antigen; *ATB1,* capture antiserum; *ATB2,* signal antiserum. **B,** Typical dose-response curve. *NSB,* Nonspecific binding.

In immunometric assays, it is also important that a large excess of capture antibody be used. When the antigen concentration approaches the effective binding capacity of the capture antibody system, the signal no longer increases. If the antigen concentration exceeds the binding capacity of the capture antibody, the signal may actually decrease.

Figure 6–5 illustrates this *high-dose hook effect* for immunometric assays caused by insufficient amounts of capture or signal antiserum.[25] The signal increases progressively until the hormone concentration exceeds the binding capacity; the signal then decreases, apparently as a result of the removal of some of the weaker binding antigen-antibody complexes during the wash cycle on the assay.[26-28] This is a potentially dangerous phenomenon because very high concentrations can give the same "answer" as lower concentrations. If this artifact is suspected, the specimen can be diluted and reanalyzed. If the answer for the diluted specimen is higher than the original answer, a high-dose hook effect probably is present.

Most manufacturers are aware of this potential problem and configure assays with relatively large amounts of capture antibody; however, some patients produce high concentrations of hormones or antigens that may exceed assay limits. Laboratories are able to detect this phenomenon by analyzing specimens at two dilutions, but this practice generally is not cost-effective. Therefore, feedback to the laboratory about results that are inconsistent with clinical findings is essential.

Another potential problem for immunometric assays consists of endogenous heterophile antibodies that cross-react with reagent antiserum.[29] Normally, the signal antibody does not form a "sandwich" with the capture antibody unless the specific antigen is present; however, divalent heterophile antibodies may mimic the antigen by simultaneously binding to the signal and capture reagent antibodies, thereby causing "falsely" elevated results.[30,31]

Figure 6–6 schematically illustrates this situation. The problem is most common with monoclonal antibodies but may also occur with polyclonal antibodies. Immunoglobulins contain both a *constant* (Fc) region and a *variable* (Fab) region. As implied in the name, the Fc region is constant, or similar, for all immunoglobulins from that species. Therefore, if a patient receives immunotherapy or imaging reagents containing mouse immunoglobulin, he or she is likely to develop human anti-mouse antibodies (HAMAs) directed to the Fc fragment.[32] Some patients may develop heterophile antibodies after exposure to foreign proteins from domestic pets or food contaminants. When these endogenous antibodies are present in a patient's specimen, they may bridge across the reagent antibodies used in immunometric assays and may cause falsely high values. These antibodies also may bind to sites on the reagent

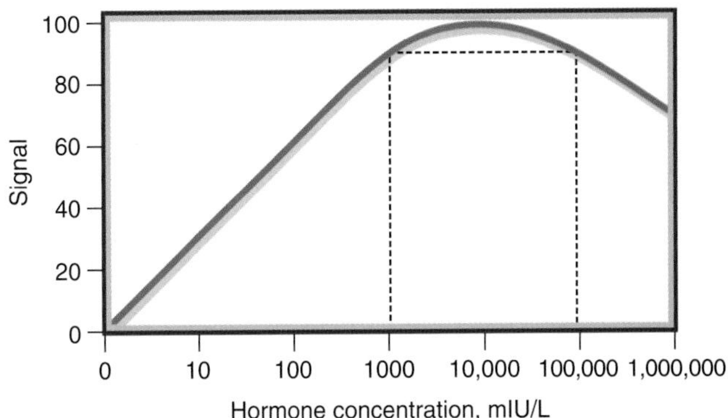

Figure 6–5 ▪ Immunometric "high-dose hook effect." The response signal reaches a maximum and then decreases when the antigen concentration exceeds the limit of the assay.

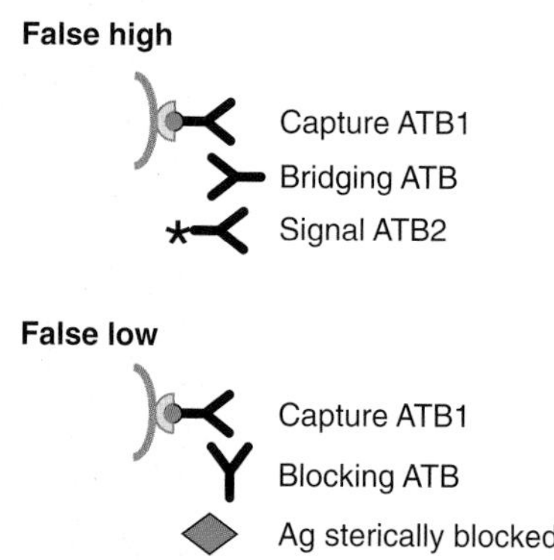

Figure 6–6 ▪ Assay interferences caused by heterophile antibodies, which result in either false high or false low results. *Ag,* Antigen; *ATB1,* capture antiserum; *ATB2,* signal antiserum.

TABLE 6–1 EFFECT OF IMMUNOASSAY SPECIFICITY ON CALIBRATION OF HUMAN CHORIONIC GONADOTROPIN (hCG) ASSAY

	Assay 1	Assay 2	Assay 3
Specificity for intact hCG standard	100%	100%	100%
Cross-reactivity with free β-hCG	0%	100%	200%
Value of specimen with no free β-hCG, IU/L	10.0	10.0	10.0
Value of specimen with 10% free β-hCG, IU/L	9.0	10.0	11.0
Value specimen with 50% free β-hCG, IU/L	5.0	10.0	15.0

antibodies, which sterically block the binding of the specific antigen and give falsely low test values. Most manufacturers include nonimmune immunoglobulin in the assays to help block these interferences; as with the high-dose hook effect, however, the amounts added are not always adequate and some patients with high titer antibodies thus may still show in vitro assay interference.[33]

The combined specificity of the two antibodies used in an immunometric assay can produce exquisitely sensitive and specific immunoassays. In the past, a common problem with early competitive immunoassays was cross-reactivity among the structurally similar gonadotropins: LH, follicle-stimulating hormone (FSH), TSH, and hCG. The α subunits of each of these hormones are almost identical, and the β subunits have considerable structural homology. Many individual antisera (especially polyclonal antisera) used for measuring one of these hormones may have cross-reactivity for the other gonadotropins. The cross-reactivity of a pair of antibodies is less than the cross-reactivity of each of the individual antibodies because any cross-reacting substance must contain both of the binding epitopes in order to simultaneously bind to both antibodies.

For example, consider two antibodies for LH, each having 1% cross-reactivity with hCG. The cross-reactivity of the pair is less than the product of the two cross-reactivities or, in this case, less than 0.01%. Most current immunoassays for LH have a cross-reactivity of less than 0.01%. This low cross reactivity is important because pregnant patients and patients with choriocarcinoma may have very high hCG concentrations that could interfere with measurements of the other gonadotropin hormones.

Multiple forms of most hormones circulate in the blood. Some hormones (e.g., prolactin, growth hormone) circulate with macro forms, which can cause difficulty in their analysis if specimens are not pretreated.[7] For hormones composed of subunits (e.g., the gonadotropins), both the intact and the free subunits circulate in blood. Immunometric assays can be made specific for intact molecules by pairing an antibody specific for the α-β bridge site of the subunits with a second antibody specific for the β subunit. Assays using these antibody pairs retain the two-antibody, low cross-reactivity needed for measuring gonadotropins and do not react with the free subunit forms of the hormones.

The heterogeneous forms of circulating hormones and differences in specificity characteristics of immunoassays for these forms make calibration and harmonization difficult. Two immunoassays calibrated with the same reference preparation can give widely varying measurements on patient specimens. Consider the example of hCG in Table 6–1. The three assays are calibrated with a pure preparation of intact hCG, such as the WHO Third International Reference Preparation.[33] The three assays differ in their cross-reactivity with free β-hCG (0, 100%, and 200%, respectively). These assays give identical measurements for a specimen containing only intact hCG but progressively disparate values as the percentage of free β-hCG in the specimen increases. In reality, the standardization issue is much more complex because multiple forms of hormones (i.e., intact, free subunits, nicked forms, glycosylated forms, degradation products) circulate in patients and each assay has different cross-reactivities for these forms.[16,34]

Free (Unbound) Hormone Assays

Many hormones are tightly bound to specific plasma-binding proteins and loosely bound to albumin. The unbound (free) forms as well as some of the loosely bound forms are biologically active.

Multiple methods are available to measure these free, unbound forms of a hormone. Theoretically, the best procedure is direct measurement of the free hormone concentration after physical separation of free-form bound hormone by equilibrium dialysis, ultrafiltration, or gel filtration. Unfortunately, this method is difficult to perform, is thus not readily available, and is subject to technical errors.

The two major clinical applications for free hormone measurements are for thyroid hormones (thyroxine [FT_4] and triiodothyronine [FT_3]) and steroids (testosterone and estradiol). Four techniques are commonly used to estimate free thyroid hormone concentrations: indirect index methods, two-step labeled hormone methods, one-step labeled hormone analogue methods, and labeled antibody methods.

Indirect Index Methods

The *indirect indices* involve two measurements: one for total hormone concentration and another for the thyroxine-binding globulin (TBG), followed by calculation of the ratio or a normalized index (FT4I or FT3I). The availability of test results for both the total T_4 and the T_4 binding capacity has the advantage of assessing these two different quantities, but has the disadvantage that ratios and indices are subject to the combined error of both measurements. These methods correct for routine changes in TBG associated with estrogen levels, but they may produce inappropriately abnormal values in patients with extreme variations in TBG levels found in patients with congenital disorders of the TBG gene, familial dysalbuminemic hyperthyroxinemia, thyroid hormone autoantibodies, and nonthyroidal illnesses. Because of the necessity for two measurements and the sensitivity of these methods to interference with drugs, these indirect methods are being used less frequently.

Two-Step Labeled Hormone Methods

These methods immunologically bind the free and loosely bound thyroid hormone to a solid phase. The other serum components are washed away, and the residual binding sites are back-titrated with labeled hormone. When calibrated with appropriate serum standards, these methods are thought to pose fewer problems with binding protein abnormalities.

One-Step Labeled Hormone Analogue Methods

These methods use synthetic analogues of T_4 and T_3 that bind to the measurement antibody but do not bind to normal TBG. These methods are seldom used because performance has been poor in patients with abnormal albumin concentrations, abnormal free fatty acid concentrations, and all conditions that interfere with the indirect indices.[35]

Labeled Antibody Methods

These methods use kinetic reactions of antibodies with selected affinities that bind preferentially with the free form of the hormone. These methods work best for automated testing instruments and have become popular.

Complexities in Testing

Each of these methods works well for correcting for minor changes in TBG levels, but each has problems with some patient sera, especially those containing interfering substances such as inhibitors and heterophilic antibodies. Unfortunately, most manufacturers have not fully validated their methods in patients with these abnormalities.[36]

Multiple methods are also available for measuring both the free and the biologically active forms of steroid hormones. The preferred method for measurement of free hormones consists of direct physical separation and high-sensitivity assays similar to those recommended for the thyroid hormones. One-step labeled hormone-analogue methods also have been developed, but these are associated with interference problems similar to the problems with free thyroid hormone assays. The measurement of free testosterone has been problematic. Most immunoassays are unreliable at low concentrations and the concentration of free testosterone is much lower than total testosterone.

Another complexity in regard to steroid hormones is that in addition to the free hormones, testosterone and estrogen bound to albumin also are biologically active. The concentration of the biologically active forms can be estimated using indirect indices calculated from measurements of the total hormones and sex hormone–binding globulin (SHBG) or by measurement of the residual free and albumin-bound steroids after separation of the SHBG-bound forms after differential precipitation with ammonium sulfate. Recent work with tandem mass spectrometry shows promise as a more reliable test method (see later sections of this chapter).[37]

Chromatographic Assays

Another major method of measuring hormone concentrations involves chromatographically separating the various biochemical forms and quantitating specific characteristics of the molecules. High-performance liquid chromatography (HPLC) systems utilize multiple forms of detection, including light absorption, fluorescence, electrochemical properties, and mass spectrometry.[38,39]

There are two major advantages of these techniques: (1) they can be used to simultaneously measure multiple forms of an analyte, and (2) they are not dependent on unique immunologic reagents. Therefore, harmonization of measurements made with different assays is more feasible. The major disadvantages of these methods are their complexity and their limited availability.

Many chemical separation techniques are based on chromatography, but the two most commonly used for liquid chromatography are (1) *normal-phase* HPLC and (2) *reverse-phase* HPLC.[26] In both systems, a bonded solid-phase column is made that interacts with the analytes as they flow past in a liquid solvent. In normal-phase HPLC, the functional groups of the stationary phase are polar (e.g., amino or nitrile ions) relative to the nonpolar stationary phase (e.g., hexane); in reverse-phase HPLC, a nonpolar stationary phase (e.g., C-18 octadecylsilane molecules bonded to silica) is used.

More recently, polymeric packings made of mixed copolymers have been made with C4, C8, and C18 functional groups directly incorporated so that they are more stable over a wide pH range. The mobile and stationary phases are selected to optimize adherence of the analytes to the stationary phase. The adhered molecules can be eluted differentially from the solid phase after washing to separate specific forms of the analyte from interfering substances as follows: When the composition of the mobile phase remains constant throughout the run, the process is called an *isocratic elution*. If the mobile-phase composition is abruptly changed, a *step elution* occurs. If the composition is gradually changed throughout the run, a *gradient elution* occurs.

The efficiency of separation in a chromatography system is a function of the flow rates of the different substances.[40] The resolution of the system is a measure of the separation of the two solute bands in terms of their relative retention volumes (V_r) and their bandwidths (ω). Resolution (R_s) of solutes A and B is shown as:

$$R_s = \frac{2[V_r(B) - V_r(A)]}{\omega(A) + \omega(B)}$$

Values of R_s less than 0.8 result in inadequate separation, and values greater than 1.25 correspond to baseline separation. The resolution of a chromatography column is a function of flow rates and thermodynamic factors.

The simultaneous measurement of the three catecholamines (epinephrine, norepinephrine, and dopamine) can be performed with reverse-phase HPLC with a C-18 column and electrochemical detection system[41] or fluorometric detection.[42] Prior extraction by absorption on activated alumina and acid elution helps improve specificity. Dihydroxybenzylamine, a molecule similar to endogenous catecholamines, can be used as an internal standard.

Mass Spectrometry

The technique of mass spectrometry involves fragmentation of target molecules, followed by separation and measurement of the mass to charge ratio of the components.[40] When coupled with liquid chromatography, a mass spectrometer can function as a unique detector to provide structural information about the composition of individual solutes.[43] Inclusion of internal standards in the specimens, which are molecularly similar to the measured compounds, allows precise quantitation of the concentration of the eluting analytes. The measurement of specific mass fragments makes possible the quantitation of multiple specific analytes in complex mixtures.

The basic components of a quadrupole mass spectrometer are an ionizer, an ion analyzer, and a detector (Fig. 6–7). The initial step in mass spectrometry is the fragmentation of the target compound into charged ions. Multiple techniques are used to generate these charged ions, including *chemical ionization* and *electron-impact ionization*.

Chemical ionization uses reagent gas molecules, such as methane, ammonia, water, and isobutane, to transfer protons.

This process produces less fragmentation than other techniques because the process is not highly excited.

The electron impact bombards gas molecules from the sample, with electrons emitted from a heated filament. The process occurs in a vacuum to prevent the filament from burning out. *Electron-spray ionization* is a process in which a solution containing the analyte is introduced into a gas phase and is sprayed across an ionizing potential.[44] The charged droplets are desolvinated and analyzed in a mass spectrometer.

The ion analyzer uses four charged rods to systematically set up a charged field that selects only certain ions with particular mass-to-charge ratios and facilitates their movement along a path to the detector. Regular calibration is necessary to ensure accuracy of the instrument.

A *mass spectrum* is a bar graph in which the heights of the bars correspond to the relative abundance of a particular ion plotted as a function of the mass-to-charge ratio. Modern mass spectrometers can measure molecular masses so accurately and precisely that the elemental composition of a compound can be predicted by comparison with stored spectral libraries.

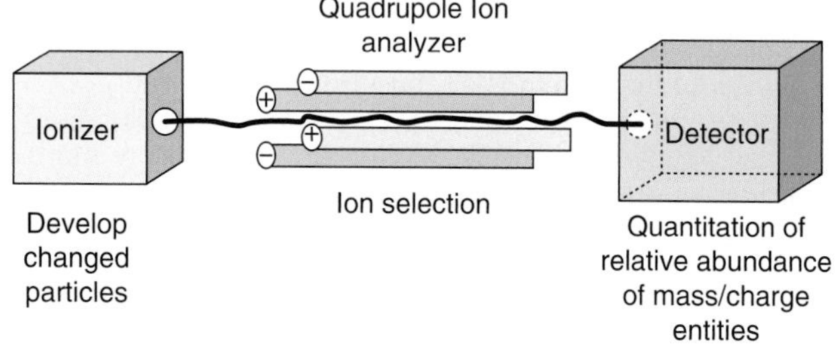

Figure 6–7 ▪ Basic components of quadrupole mass spectrometer.

When these systems are used to measure only a few select compounds having known spectrums, the mass spectrometer can be programmed to focus only on these selected ions.

Stable isotopes of the compounds of interest can be used as internal standards through a technique called *isotope dilution mass spectrometry.* Stable isotopes generally perform the same as the native compounds in terms of extraction, chromatography, and mass spectrometry and are thus ideal internal standards. However, they must have a sufficient number of isotopic atoms to ensure that their mass is different from naturally occurring substances that may be in the specimen.

Tandem mass spectrometry (MS/MS) is a powerful new tool consisting of two mass analyzers separated by an ion-activation device.[45,46] The first analyzer is used to isolate and dissociate the ion of interest by activation, and the second mass analyzer is used to analyze its dissociation products. This technique can be used to provide rapid, definitive measurements of multiple endocrine analytes.[43] For example, liquid chromatography and tandem mass spectrometry can be used to simultaneously quantitate multiple steroid compounds.[47-51] In Figure 6–8, the chromatograph shows peaks for nine steroids in a standard solution.[49] The nine steroids investigated in positive-ion mode and their respective deuterated internal standards were separated well in 18 minutes. These chromatograms were run on a SCIEX (Applied Biosystems/MDS SCIEX, Foster City, CA/Concord, Ontario, Canada) API-3000 triple quadrupole tandem MS equipped with an APPI (Applied Biosystems/MDS SCIEX) source. The column eluate was fed directly into an electro-spray ionization device in a triple-quadrupole mass spectrometer (API 3000, Perkin-Elmer SCIEX, Foster City, CA). The stable isotopes were from Cambridge Isotope Laboratories (Andover, MA). A 10-minute analysis provided quantitation of the 10 compounds: cortisone, cortisol, 21-deoxycortisol, corticosterone, 11-deoxycortisol, androstenedione, deoxycorticosterone (DOC), 17-hydroxyprogesterone, progesterone, and pregnenolone. The sensitivity for cortisol using d_4 cortisol calibration was 0.1 cg/dL.

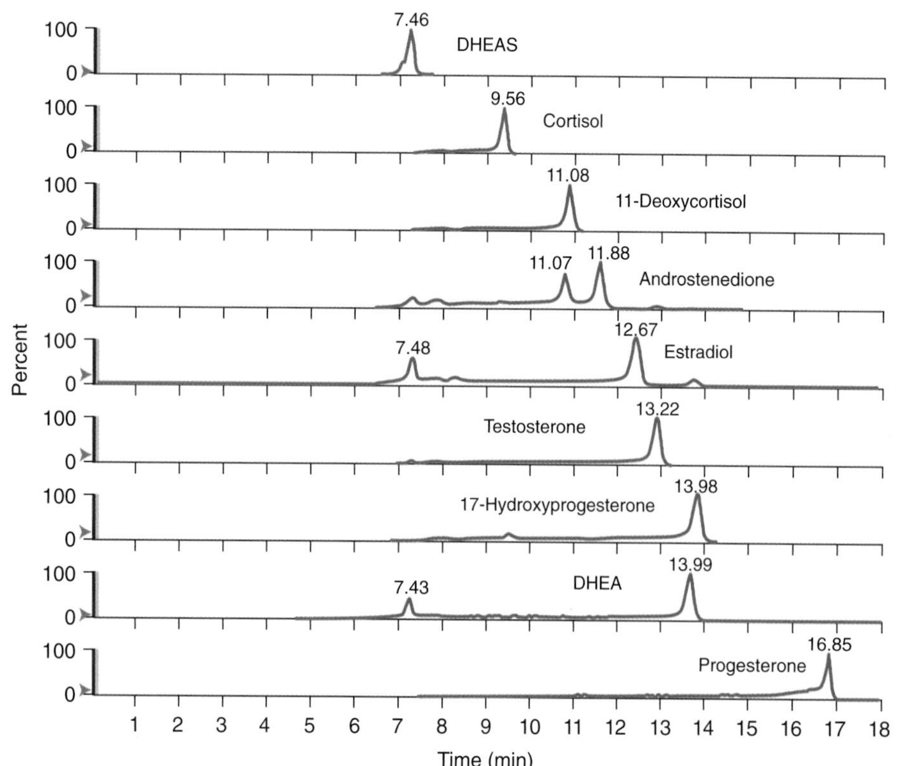

Figure 6–8 ▪ Liquid chromatography-tandem mass spectroscopy profiles of nine steroids.[49] *DHEAS,* Dehydroepiandrosterone 3-sulfate; *DHEA,* dehydroepiandrosterone. (Reproduced with permission from Archives of Pathology of Laboratory Medicine).

Nucleic Acid–Based Assays

The decoding of the human genome has set the stage for an enormous increase in nucleic acid–based gene assays. The basic principles of nucleic acid–based assays have been known for several decades, but the identification of specific genes and the mapping of gene defects to clinical disease states have now made these measurements clinically useful.[52,53] Four concepts important for nucleic acid measurements are (1) hybridization, (2) amplification, (3) restriction fragment length polymorphisms (RFLPs), and (4) electrophoretic separation.[54]

Hybridization

Nucleic acid molecules have a unique ability to fuse with complementary base-pair sequences. When a fragment of a known sequence (probe) is mixed under specific conditions with a specimen containing a complementary sequence, hybridization occurs. This feature is analogous to the antibody-antigen binding used in immunoassays. Many of the formats used for immunoassay have been adopted to nucleic acid assays, including some of the same signal systems (e.g., radioactivity, fluorescence, chemiluminescence) and the same solid-phase capture systems (e.g., magnetic beads, biotin-streptavidin binding). In situ hybridization, which involves the binding of probes to intact tissue and cells, provides information about morphologic localization analogous to immunohistochemistry.

Amplification

Nucleic acid assays have an advantage that low concentrations can be amplified in vitro before quantitation. The best known amplification procedure is the polymerase chain reaction (PCR), first reported by Mullis and Faloona.[55] The three steps in the process (denaturation, annealing, and elongation) occur rapidly at different temperatures. Each "cycle" of amplification can occur in less than 90 seconds by cycling the temperature. The target double-stranded DNA is denatured at high temperature to make two single-stranded DNA fragments. Oligonucleotide primers, which are specific for target region, are annealed to the DNA when the temperature is lowered. Addition of DNA polymerase allows the primer DNA to extend across the amplification region, thus doubling the number of DNA copies.

At 85% to 90% efficiency, this process can amplify the DNA by about 250,000-fold in 20 cycles. This huge amplification is subject to major problems with contamination if special precautions are not taken. In one control technique, a psoralen derivative is used to prevent subsequent copying by polymerase during exposure to ultraviolet light.

Restriction Fragment Length Polymorphisms

Some diseases (e.g., sickle cell anemia) are associated with a specific gene mutation; generally, however, a series of deletions and additions of DNA are involved with the disease. A number of restriction enzymes that cleave DNA at specific locations have been identified. Changes in the sequence of DNA result in different fragment lengths. This technique, or RFLP, is particularly helpful in family studies for disorders that have a unique *genetic fingerprint.*

Electrophoretic Separation

E. M. Southern invented an electrophoretic separation technique known as *Southern blotting.*[56] Restriction enzymes are used to digest a sample of DNA into fragments, and the product is subjected to electrophoresis. The separated bands of DNA are then transferred to a solid support and hybridized. *Northern blotting* is a similar technique, in which RNA is used as the starting material. *Western blotting* refers to electrophoresis and transfer of proteins.

Analytic Validation

Clinicians generally assume that laboratory methods have been validated and that they function correctly. Although this assumption is generally true, it is helpful to understand the level of assay validation performed and the appropriateness of the validation criteria for each clinical application of a test.[57,58]

In the United States, the Federal Government regulates all laboratories performing complex tests for patients receiving Medicare.[59] These regulations, published in the Federal Register, outline the validation requirements for both Food and Drug Administration (FDA)-approved instruments, kits, and test systems as well as methods developed in-house. Laboratories must document analytic accuracy, precision, reportable ranges, and reference ranges for all procedures. The regulations for in-house procedures and modifications of approved commercial procedures are more extensive and require laboratories to further document (1) analytic sensitivity; (2) analytic specificity, including interfering substances; and (3) other performance characteristics required for testing patient specimens.

Although the details of method validation may be unique to a specific procedure, the following analytic validation studies have proved valuable for most procedures: (1) method comparison, (2) precision, (3) linearity, (4) recovery, (5) detection limit, (6) reportable range, (7) analytic interference, (8) carryover, (9) reference interval, (10) specimen stability, and (11) specimen type. Laboratories should have documentation for each of these performance characteristics, either from the diagnostics manufacturer or from direct studies.

Method Comparison

Ideally, the system should be compared with an established reference method; however, many endocrine tests do not have reference methods and many laboratories do not have the facilities to perform reference methods when they exist. As a minimum, the assay should be compared with an analytic system that has been clinically validated with specimens from healthy subjects and specimens from patients with the diseases being investigated.[60] The system should be traceable to established reference standards, such as those from the WHO and the National Institute of Standards and Technology (NIST).[61-63] Between 100 and 200 different specimens distributed over the assay range are recommended for method comparisons.[64]

A cross-plot displaying the new method on the vertical axis versus the established method on the horizontal axis, along with the identity line, reference value lines, and regression statistics, is a useful way of displaying these comparisons. An alternative display method is the Bland-Altman difference plot, in which the difference between the test method and the reference method is plotted against the reference method values.

Although acceptable performance criteria for method comparisons are not well established, some important characteristics to examine are as follows:

- Any grossly discordant test values.
- The degree of scatter about the regression curve
- The size of the regression offset on the vertical axis
- The number of points crossing between the low, normal, and high reference intervals for the two methods.

The European Union (EU) has enacted the In Vitro Diagnostics Directive, which requires manufacturers marketing in the European Union after the year 2003 to establish that their products are "traceable to reference standards and reference procedures of a higher order" when these references exist. Hopefully, medically relevant performance characteristics that define the allowable ranges for differences between a specific assay's test values and the traceable standards will be linked with this traceability requirement.[65] This combination of traceability and allowable error requirements could serve to harmonize many test methods worldwide because most diagnostic companies market internationally.[66]

Precision

Precision is a measure of the replication of repeated measurements of the same specimen; it is a function of the time between repeats and the concentration of the analyte. Both short-term precision (within a run or within a day) and long-term precision (across calibrations and across batches of reagents) should be documented at clinically appropriate concentration levels.[67]

In general, normal range, abnormally low range, and abnormally high range targets are chosen for precision studies; however, targets focused on critical medical decision limits may be more appropriate for some analytes. Twenty measurements are recommended at each level for both short-term and long-term precision validations. Precision generally is expressed as the coefficient of variation, calculated as 100 times the standard deviation divided by the average of the replicate measurements.[68]

There is no universal agreement on the performance criteria for analytic precision, although numerous recommendations have been put forth. Two major approaches to defining these criteria have been (1) comparison with biologic variation and (2) expert opinion of clinicians based on their perceived impact of laboratory variation on clinical decisions.

The total variation clinically observed in test measurements is a combination of the analytic and biologic variations, for instance: If the analytic standard deviation (SD) is less than one fourth of the biologic SD, the analytic component increases the SD of the total error by less than 3%. If the analytic precision is less than one half of the biologic SD, the total error increases by only 12%.

These observations have led to recommendations for maintaining precision of less than one fourth or one-half of the biologic variation. The expert opinion precision recommendations are based on estimates of the magnitude of change of a test value that would cause clinicians to alter their clinical decisions. Table 6–2 lists some precision recommendations for selected endocrine tests.[69-71]

TABLE 6–2 RECOMMENDED ANALYTIC PERFORMANCE LIMITS*

Analyte	Biologic CVi (%)	Precision (%)	Accuracy (%)
Calcium	1.8	0.9†	0.7
Glucose	4.4	2.2†	1.9
Thyroxine	7.6	3.4†	4.1
Potassium	4.4	2.4†	1.6
Triiodothyronine	8.7†	4.0‡	5.5‡
Thyrotropin	20.2†	8.1‡	8.9‡
Cortisol	15.2†	(7.6)*	
Estradiol	21.7†	(10.9)*	
Follicle-stimulating hormone	30.8†	(15.4)*	
Luteinizing hormone	14.5†	(7.2)*	
Prolactin	40.5†	(20.2)*	
Testosterone	8.3†	(4.1)*	
Insulin	15.2†	(7.6)*	
Dehydroepiandrosterone	5.6†	(2.8)*	
11-deoxycortisol	21.3†	(10.6)*	

*Data from Stockl D, et al. Eur J Clin Chem Clin Biochem 1995;33:157-169[69]. Numbers in parentheses correspond to one-half of within individual coefficient of variation.
†Data from Fraser CG. Arch Pathol Lab Med 1992;116:916-923.
‡Data from Fraser CG, et al. Eur J Clin Chem Clin Biochem 1992;30:311-317.

Linearity

Patient specimens commonly contain several different forms of the hormones to be measured compared with the pure form contained in the reference standards and calibrators used to establish the assay dose-response curve.[72] When a patient specimen is diluted, the measured value for these dilutions should parallel the dose-response curve and give results proportional to the dilution. Linearity can be evaluated by measuring serial dilutions of patient specimens with high concentrations diluted in the appropriate assay diluent.[73,74] The product of the measured value multiplied by the dilution factor should be approximately constant. There are no performance standards for linearity, but a reasonable expectation for most hormones is that dilutions are comparable within 10% of the undiluted value.

Recovery

Two methods of assessing the recovery of assays are (1) measuring the increase in test values after the reference analyte is added and (2) measuring the proportional changes caused by mixing high-concentration and low-concentration specimens. Some analytes circulate in the blood in multiple forms, and some of these forms may be bound to carrier proteins. The recovery rate of pure substances added to a specimen may be low if the assay does not measure some of the bound forms. Mixtures of patient specimens may not be measured correctly if one of the specimens contains cross-reacting substances such as autoantibodies. A thorough understanding of the chemical forms of the analyte and their cross-reactivities in the assay is important during assessment of recovery data.

Detection Limit

The minimal analytic detection limit is the smallest concentration that can be statistically differentiated from zero. This concentration is mathematically determined as the upper 95% limit of replicate measurements of the *zero standard,* calculated from the average signal plus 2.0 SD. This minimal detection limit is valid *only* for the average of multiple replicate measurements. When individual determinations are performed on a specimen having a true concentration exactly at the minimal detection limit, the probability that the measurement is above the noise level of the assay is only about 50%.

A second term for the lowest level of reliable measurement for an assay is the *functional detection limit,* or the *limit of quantitation.* For this parameter to be measured, multiple pools with low concentrations are made and analyzed in the replicate. A cross-plot of the coefficient of variation of the measurements versus the concentration allows one to generate a precision profile. The concentration corresponding to a coefficient of variation of 20% is the functional detection limit.[1] This term generally applies to across-assay variation, but it also can be calculated using within-assay variation if one uses the tests to evaluate results measured within one run (e.g., provocative and suppression tests).

Reportable Range

The reportable range of an assay generally spans from the functional detection limit to the concentration of the highest standard. Values above the highest standard may be reported if they are diluted and the measured value is multiplied by the dilution factor. The validity of the analytic range is documented by the linearity and recovery studies. Some laboratories erroneously report the exact values displayed by the test systems even if they are outside of the analytic range. Therefore, it is important for clinicians to understand the limitations of valid measurements and not inappropriately use meaningless numbers that may be reported.

Another potential source of error is failure of the technologist to multiply the measured value of diluted specimens by the dilution factor to correct for the dilution. In addition, care should be taken to define the number of significant figures used for reporting test values and to establish an appropriate algorithm for rounding test values to the significant number of digits.

Analytic Interference

The cross-reactivity and potential interference of other analytes that may react in a test system should be documented.[71] The choice of potential interfering substances that must be evaluated requires an understanding of both the analytic system and the pathophysiology of the analyte being evaluated. In immunoassays, for example, compounds with similar structures as well as precursor forms and degradation products should be tested.[75-78] Drugs commonly prescribed for the diseases under evaluation should be assessed for interference both by addition of the drug to a specimen and by analysis of specimens from patients before and after receiving the drug.[79,81] Most assays also are evaluated for the effects of hemolysis, lipemia, and icterus.

Carryover Studies

Many diagnostic systems use automated sample-handling devices. If a specimen to be tested is preceded by a specimen with a very high concentration, a trace amount of the first specimen may significantly increase the reported concentration of the second specimen. The choice of the concentration that should be tested for carryover depends on the pathophysiology of the disease, but high values may need to be tested because some endocrine disorders may produce these high values. A prudent procedure would be to retest all specimens following a specimen with an extraordinarily high value. One also should document that carryover from the sampling probe has not inadvertently contaminated subsequent specimen vials, thereby invalidating subsequently repeated measurements.

Reference Intervals

The development and validation of reference intervals for endocrine tests can be a very complex task.[82,83] The normal reference interval for most laboratory tests is based on estimates of the central 95 percentile limits of measurements in healthy subjects.[84] A minimum of 120 subjects is needed to reliably define the 2.5 and 97.5 percentiles. The reference intervals for many endocrine tests depend on gender, age, developmental status, and other test values. Formal statistical consultation is recommended to determine the appropriate number of subjects to test and to develop statistical models for defining multivariate reference ranges.

Full evaluation of the adrenal, gonadal, and thyroid axes requires simultaneous measurement of the trophic and target hormones. Bivariate displays of these hormone concentrations along with their multivariate reference intervals facilitate the interpretation.[85] Preanalytic conditions should be well defined and controlled during evaluation of both healthy reference subjects and patients.

Specimen Stability

Analyte stability is a function of storage conditions and specimen type.[86] Although most hormones are relatively stable in serum or urine if they are rapidly frozen and stored in hermetically sealed vials at –70°C, multiple freeze/thaw cycles may damage analytes, and storage in frost-free freezers that repeatedly cycle through thawing temperatures can adversely affect stability. Blood specimens collected in edetate (EDTA) often are more stable than serum or heparinized specimens because edetate chelates calcium and magnesium ions, which function as coenzymes for some proteases. The addition of protease inhibitors (e.g., aprotinin) to blood specimens may also improve specimen stability.[87]

Types of Specimens

Most hormones are measured in blood or urine, but alternative testing sources, such as saliva and transdermal membrane monitors, are also used.

Urine Specimens

The 24-hour urine specimen is used for many endocrine tests. Urine specimens represent a time average that integrates over the multiple pulsatile spikes of hormone secretion occurring throughout the day. The 24-hour urine specimen also has the advantage of better analytic sensitivity for some hormones.[88,89] Urine often contains not only the original hormone but also key metabolites that may or may not have biologic activity.

Drawbacks include the inconvenience of and delays in collecting the 24-hour specimen. Another limitation of urine specimens is the uncertainty of the completeness of the collection. Measurement of urinary creatinine concentrations helps in monitoring collection completeness, especially when it is compared with the patient's muscle mass. Many urinary hormones are conjugated to carrier proteins before excretion. Therefore, both hepatic function and, to a lesser degree, renal function may alter urinary hormone values.

Blood Specimens

Blood specimens have both the advantage and the limitation of time dependency. The ability to direct rapid changes to a provocative stimulus is a strong advantage, whereas the unsuspected changes due to pulsatile secretions may be a major limitation. Most hormones undergo significant biologic variations, including ultradian, diurnal, menstrual, and seasonal changes.[90-92] Many hormones have short half-lives and are thus rapidly cleared from the blood. The half-life is particularly important when one is attempting to measure the response to a provocative drug, such as the effect of gonadotropin-releasing hormone (GnRH).[93] The development of rapid intraoperative methods for measuring PTH and growth hormone has highlighted the importance of plasma specimens, which do not require extra waiting time for the blood to clot to make serum.[94,95]

Saliva Specimens

Saliva is becoming an alternative specimen for measuring non–protein-bound hormones and small molecules.[96-100] Small analytes in blood pass into oral fluid by crossing capillary walls and basement membranes and by passage through lipophilic membranes of epithelial cells.[100] This transport involves passive diffusion, ultrafiltration, and/or active transport. The concentration in saliva depends on the concentration of the non–protein-bound analyte in blood as well as salivary pH, the pKa of the analyte, and the size of the analyte. Analytes entering saliva by passive diffusion generally are less than 500 d, non–protein-bound, and nonionized. Saliva measurements correlate with blood measurements in some hormones like cortisol, progesterone, estradiol, and testosterone, but they do not correlate well for others (e.g., thyroid and pituitary hormones).[101-103]

Multiple preanalytic variables can affect the salivary measurement. Stimulation of oral fluid production by chewing or the use of candy or drops containing stimulants like citric acid can increase oral fluid volume and stabilize pH, but this stimulation may alter some analyte concentrations. Several commercial devices are available for collection of oral fluid; however, these devices need to be validated for each analyte and each assay system to ensure they adequately recover each of the analytes.

Blood Drops

Blood drops collected on filter paper from punctures of a finger or heel are a convenient system for collecting, transporting, and measuring hormones.[104,105] If standardized collection conditions and extraction techniques are used, these measurements correlate well with serum measurements. Integration of immunochemistry with computer chip technology has also led to immunochips that can measure multiple analytes using a single drop of blood.[106]

Noninvasive Measurements

Noninvasive transcutaneous measurements also have been developed for some endocrine tests.[107] Transcutaneous glucose measurements using near-infrared spectroscopy correlate well with blood measurements.[108] The GlucoWatch device is also being marketed for noninvasive monitoring of glucose.[109]

Quality Assurance

Quality Control Systems

Laboratory quality control programs are intended to ensure that the test procedures are being performed within defined limits. A critical component of control systems is the definition of acceptable performance criteria.[110,111] Unfortunately, these criteria often are not well defined and many laboratories use floating criteria that change when assays change.[112] Control limits are often set at the mean ± *2 or 3 Standard Deviations (SDs),* where the mean and SD are arbitrarily assigned based on measurements made in that laboratory. When reagents or equipment change, new limits are assigned. These types of control systems provide some assurance that the laboratory is functioning at a level of performance similar to that of the recent past, but they provide little assurance that measurements are adequate for clinical decisions.

Statistically, there are two major forms of analytic errors: random and systematic. *Random error* relates to reproducibility; *systematic error* relates to the offset or bias of the test values from the target or reference value. Performance criteria can be defined for each of these parameters, and quality control systems can be programmed to monitor compliance with these criteria. Control systems must have low false-positive rates as well as high statistical power to detect assay deviations. The multirule algorithms developed by Westgard and colleagues[113] use combinations of control rules, such as two consecutive controls outside of *warning limits,* one control outside of *action limits,* or moving average trend analyzers outside of limits to achieve good statistical error detection characteristics.[114]

Traditionally, quality control programs have focused primarily on precision; however, analytic bias also can cause major clinical problems. When fixed decision levels are used to trigger clinical actions, such as therapy and additional investigations, changes in the analytic set-point of an assay can cause major changes in the number of follow-up cases.[114] This concept is illustrated in Figure 6–9 for TSH measurements.

Under stable laboratory testing conditions, approximately 122 per 1000 patients tested have TSH values above 5.0 mIU/L.

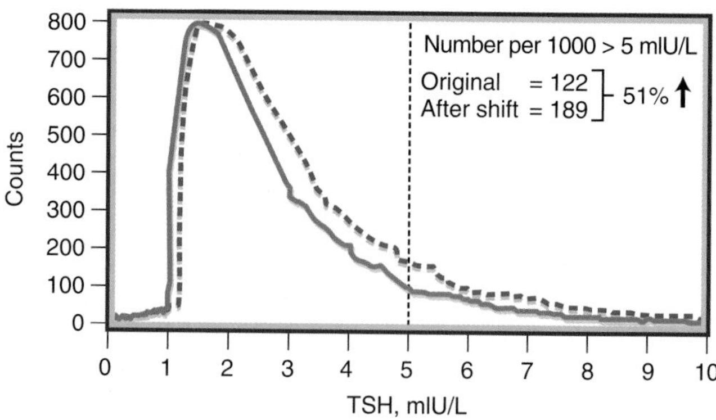

Figure 6–9 ▪ Effect of analytic bias, or shift, on the number of patients with elevated levels of thyrotropin (TSH).

If the test shifts upward by 20%, the number of patients with TSH values above 5.0 mIU/L increases to 189, which equates to more than a 50% increase in the number of patients flagged as abnormal. These changes in test value distributions often can be sensed by clinicians who encounter multiple patients with unexpected elevated test values, causing them to call the laboratory and inquire whether the "test is running high today." Some modern quality control systems use moving averages of patient test values to help monitor changes in analytic bias.[115]

Some medical facilities are linking together into networks to provide more integrated patient care. This crossover of both physicians and patients is increasing the importance of *harmonized* testing systems. For endocrine tests, harmonization is best achieved when all the laboratories in the network use the same test systems. Differences in analytic specificity may cause across-method differences in patient test distributions even when the methods use the same reference standard. Full harmonization of testing requires not only standardization of equipment but also standardization of reagents (including using the same lot numbers) and standardization of laboratory protocols. Real-time quality control monitors with peer group comparisons across the laboratories in the health care network are necessary to ensure uniformity of testing.

Investigation of Discordant Test Values

The practice of modern endocrinology depends extensively on reliable and accurate test values; even in the best laboratories, however, erroneous results sometimes are reported. Careful correlation of pathophysiology with test values can help to identify values that are "discordant."[85] Some of these discordant test values may be analytically correct, but others may be erroneous. Clinicians can help investigate these suspicious test values by requesting laboratories to perform a few simple validation procedures.

Repeated testing of the same specimen is a valuable first step. If the specimen has been stored under stable conditions, the absolute value of the difference between the initial and the repeated measurements should be less than *3 analytic SDs* 95% of the time. Normally, the 95% confidence range is associated with the mean ±2 *SDs;* with repeated laboratory tests, however, errors are associated with the first as well as the second measurement. The confidence interval for the uncertainty of the difference between two measurements can be calculated using the statistical rules for propagation of errors.

To better understand this propagation of error, consider:

$$D = X_1 - X_2$$

where X_1 is the first measurement, X_2 is the repeated measurement, and D is the difference.

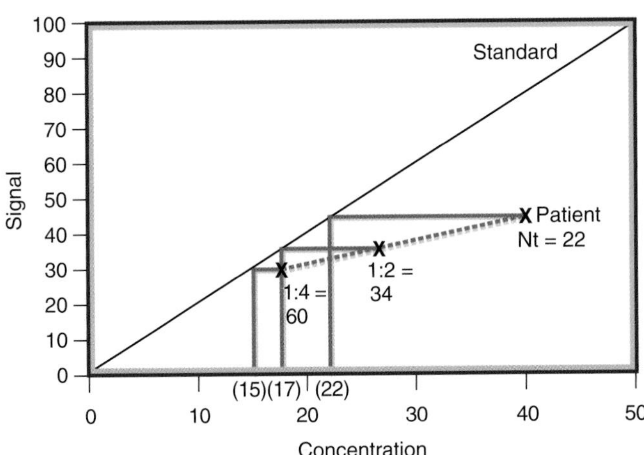

Figure 6–10 ▪ Nonproportional dilutions. Discordant values are produced when samples do not dilute linearly. (Nt = undiluted [neat])

$$\text{Variance(D)} = \text{Variance}(X_1) + \text{Variance}(X_2)$$
$$\text{Variance(D)} = 2\ \text{Variance(X)}$$
$$\text{SD(D)} = \sqrt{2\ \text{Variance(X)}}$$
$$\text{SD(D)} = \sqrt{2}\text{SD(X)}$$

The variance of D is the *sum* of the variance of X_1 and the variance of X_2. The SD of D is the square root of the variance of D, or the square root of twice the variance of X_1. The SD of D equates to square root of 2 multiplied by the SD of S. Therefore, 95% of the absolute values for D should be within 2 times $\sqrt{2}$ SD(X), or approximately 3 SD(X). If a repeat measurement exceeds this 3 SD(X) limit, the initial (or reagent) measurement is probably in error.

Linearity and recovery are valuable techniques for evaluating test validity. If the initial test value is elevated, serially diluting the specimen in the assay diluent and reassaying should be considered. If the specimen dilutes nonproportionately (Fig. 6–10), no meaningful value can be reported with that assay.

In the example, the undiluted specimen reads 22, the twofold dilution multiplies back to 34 (2 × 17), and the fourfold dilution multiplies back to 60 (4 × 15). Therefore, the result depends on the dilution factor, so that no reliable answer can be reported.

If the initial value is low, one may consider adding known quantities of the analyte to part of the specimen. Analyzing these spiked or diluted specimens with the original specimen allows one to evaluate both reproducibility and recovery. It may be helpful to analyze the linearity or recovery of the assay standards at the same time to provide internal controls of the dilution or spiking procedures and the appropriateness of the diluent and spiking material.

If the replication, dilution, or recovery experiment appears successful, further analytic troubleshooting will vary according to the method used. Immunoassays may be affected by interference caused by heterophile antibodies. Addition of nonimmune mouse serum or heterophile antibody-blocking solutions may neutralize these effects.[116,117] Chromatographic assays are usually more robust than immunoassays. Specimens with suspected interference on one type of assay can be reanalyzed by means of an alternative methodology.

Water-soluble interferences have been reported for some direct assays for steroid measurements.[19,20,118] Extraction of the hormones into organic solvents, followed by drying down and reconstitution in the assay zero standard, removes these interferences. Similarly, interferences with cross-reacting drugs and metabolic products can be minimized with selective extraction.

The analytic methods of assessing endocrine problems in patients are continually expanding. The newer systems are often based on analytic techniques similar to those outlined in this chapter, but the configurations are generally more user-friendly. These advances make the systems more convenient, but they also become more of a "black box" that conceals most of the details of the system. The performance validation steps outlined in this chapter become important procedures for ensuring that these systems continue to provide the reliable measurements needed for quality medical care.

REFERENCES

1. Spencer CA, LoPresti JS, Patel A, et al. Applications of a new chemiluminometric thyrotropin assay to subnormal measurement. J Clin Endocrinol Metab 1990;70:453.
2. Klee GG, Hay ID. Biochemical testing of thyroid function. Endocrinol Metab Clin North Am 1997;26:763-775.
3. Thorell JI, Larson SM. Radioimmunoassay and related techniques. St Louis: CV Mosby, 1978.
4. Price CP, Newman DJ, eds. Principles and Practice of Immunoassay, 2nd ed. New York: Stockton Press, 1996.
5. Rodbard D. Data processing for radioimmunoassays: an overview. In Natelson S, Pesce AJ, Dietz AA, eds. Clinical Chemistry and Immunochemistry (AACC): Chemical and Cellular Bases and Applications in Disease. Washington, DC: AACC, 1978:477-494.
6. Gosling JP. A decade of development in immunoassay methodology. Clin Chem 1990;36:1408-1427.
7. Vieira JG, Tachibana TT, Obara LH, et al. Extensive experience and validation of polyethylene glycol precipitation as a screening method for macroprolactinemia. Clin Chem 1998;44(8 Pt 1): 1758-1759.
8. Klee GG, Post G. Effect of counting errors on immunoassay precision. Clin Chem 1989;35:1362-1366.
9. Butler JE, ed. Immunochemistry of Solid-Phase Immunoassay. Boston: CRC Press, 1991.
10. Hersh LS, Yaverbaum S. Magnetic solid-phase radioimmunoassay. Clin Chem Acta 1975;63:69.
11. Suter M. Streptavidin: production, purification, and use in antibody immobilization. In Butler JE, ed. Immunochemistry of Solid-Phase Immunoassay. Boston: CRC Press, 1991:269-276.
12. Hage DS. Survey of recent advances in analytical applications of immunoaffinity chromatography. J Chromatogr B Biomed Sci Appl 1998;715:3-28.
13. Vetterlein D. Monoclonal antibodies: production, purification, and technology. Adv Clin Chem 1989;27:303-354.
14. Pettersson KS, Soderholm JRM. Individual differences in lutropin immunoreactivity revealed by monoclonal antibodies. Clin Chem 1991;37:333-340.
15. Ehrlich PH, Moyle WR. Cooperative immunoassays: ultrasensitive assays with mixed monoclonal antibodies. Science 1983;221: 279-281.
16. Bristow A, Berger P, Bidart JM, et al. Establishment, value assignment, and characterization of new WHO reference reagents for six molecular forms of human chorionic gonadotropin. Clin Chem 2005;51(1):177-182.
17. Gao P, D'Amour P. Evolution of the parathyroid hormone (PTH) assay—importance of circulating PTH immunoheterogeneity and of its regulation. Clin Lab 2005;51(1-2):21-29.
18. Roberts RF, Roberts WL. Performance characteristics of five automated serum cortisol immunoassays. Clin Biochem 2004;37: 489-493.
19. Fitzgerald RL, Herold DA. Serum total testosterone: immunoassay compared with negative chemical ionization gas chromatography-mass spectrometry. Clin Chem 1996;42:749-755.
20. Leung Y, Dees K, Cyr R, et al. Falsely increased serum estradiol results in direct estradiol assays. Clin Chem 1997;43:1250-1251.
21. Klee GG, Preissner CM, Schloegel IW, et al. Bioassay of parathyrin: analytical characteristics and clinical performance in patients with hypercalcemia. Clin Chem 1988;34:482-488.
22. Di Lorenzo D, Ruggeri G, Iacobello C, et al. Evaluation of a radioreceptor assay to assess exogenous estrogen activity in serum of patients with breast cancer. Int J Biol Markers 1991;6: 151-158.

23. Strasburger CJ, Wu Z, Pflaum CD, et al. Immunofunctional assay of human growth hormone (hGH) in serum: a possible consensus for quantitative hGH measurement. J Clin Endocrinol Metab 1996;81:2613-2620.
24. Hoare SR, de Vries G, Usdin TB. Measurement of agonist and antagonist ligand-binding parameters at the human parathyroid hormone type 1 receptor: evaluation of receptor states and modulation by guanine nucleotide. J Pharm Exp Ther 1999;289: 1323-1333.
25. Zweig MH, Csako G. High-dose hook effect in a two-site IRMA for measuring thyrotropin. Ann Clin Biochem 1990;27(Pt 5):494-495.
26. Pesce MA. "High-dose hook effect" with the Centocor CA 125 assay. Clin Chem 1993;39:1347.
27. Ooi DS, Escares EA. "High-dose hook effect" in IRMA-Count PSA assay of prostate-specific antigen. Clin Chem 1991;37:771-772.
28. Wolf E, Brem G. "High-dose hook effect" as a pitfall in quantifying transgene expression in metallothionein-human growth hormone (MT-hGH) transgenic mice. Clin Chem 1991;37:763-765.
29. Ellis MJ, Livesey JH. Techniques for identifying heterophile antibody interference are assay specific: study of seven analytes on two automated immunoassay analyzers. Clin Chem 2005;51(3): 639-641.
30. Klee GG. Human anti-mouse antibodies. Arch Pathol Lab Med 2000;124:921-923.
31. Reinsberg J. Interference by human antibodies with tumor marker assays. Hybridoma 1995;14:205-208.
32. Baum RP, Nielsen A, Hertel A, et al. Activating anti-idiotypic human anti-mouse antibodies for immunotherapy of ovarian carcinoma. Cancer 1994;73:1121-1125.
33. Preissner M, Dodge LA, O'Kane DJ, et al. Prevalence of heterophilic antibody interference in eight automated tumor marker immunoassays. Technical Brief. Clin Chem 2005;51(1):208-210.
34. Cole LA. Immunoassay of human chorionic gonadotropin: its free subunits and metabolites. Clin Chem 1997;43:2233-2243.
35. Ekins R. Analytic measurements of free thyroxine. Clin Lab Med 1993;13:599-630.
36. Demers LM, Spencer CA, eds. In Laboratory Medicine Practice Guidelines. Laboratory Support for the Diagnosis and Monitoring of Thyroid Disease. National Academy of Clinical Biochemistry, Thyroid Standards Of Laboratory Practice thyroid 2003;13(1):1-126, 2000.
37. Klee GG, Heser DW. Techniques to measure testosterone in the elderly. Mayo Clin Proc 2000;75(suppl):S19-S25.
38. Anderson DJ. High-performance liquid chromatography in clinical analysis. Anal Chem 1999;71(12):314R-327R.
39. Volin P. High-performance liquid chromatographic analysis of corticosteroids. J Chromatogr B Biomed Appl 1995;671(1-2):319-340.
40. Ullman MD, Bowers LD, Burtis CA. Chromatography/mass spectrometry. In Burtis CA, Ashwood ER, eds. Tietz Textbook of Clinical Chemistry, 3rd ed. Philadelphia: WB Saunders, 1999:164-204.
41. Clauson RC. High performance liquid chromatographic separation and determination of catecholamines. In Mark and Rodnight, eds. Research Methods in Neurochemistry, Vol 6. New York: Plenum, 1985.
42. Willemsen JJ, Ross HA, Jacobs MC, et al. Highly sensitive and specific HPLC with fluorometric detection for determination of plasma epinephrine and norepinephrine applied to kinetic studies in humans. Clin Chem 1995;41:1455-1460.
43. Niessen WM. Advances in instrumentation in liquid chromatography-mass spectrometry and related liquid-introduction techniques. J Chromatogr A 1998;794(1-2):407-435.
44. Strege MA. High-performance liquid chromatographic-electrospray ionization mass spectrometry analyses for the integration of natural products with modern high-throughput screening. J Chromatogr B 1999;725:67-78.
45. Dongre AR, Eng JK, Yates JR 3rd. Emerging tandem mass spectrometry techniques for the rapid identification of proteins. Trends Biotechnol 1997;15:418-425.
46. Magera MJ, Lacey JM, Casetta B, et al. Method for the determination of total homocysteine in plasma and urine by stable isotope dilution and electrospray tandem mass spectrometry. Clin Chem 1999;45:1517-1522.
47. Park S, Magera MJ, Lacey JM, et al. Profiling of the conjugated forms of steroid hormones and their metabolites using HPLC-tandem mass spectrometry. Clin Chem 2000;46(suppl 6):A127.
48. Machacek DA, Magera JM, Park S, et al. Diagnosis of adrenal dysfunction using liquid chromatography with tandem spectrometry. Clin Chem 2000;46(suppl 6):A127.
49. Guo T, Chan M, Soldin SJ. Steroid profiles using liquid chromatography-tandem mass spectrometry with atmospheric pressure photoionization source. Arch Pathol Lab Med 2004;128:469-475.
50. Shou WZ, Jiang X, Naidong W. Development and validation of a high-sensitivity liquid chromatography/tandem mass spectrometry (LC/MS/MS) method with chemical derivatization for the determination of ethinyl estradiol in human plasma. Biomed Chromatogr 2004;18:414-421.
51. Tai AA, Welch MJ. Development and evaluation of a candidate reference method for the determination of total cortisol in human serum using isotope dilution liquid chromatography/tandem mass spectrometry. Anal Chem 2004;76:1008-1014.
52. Coleman WD, Tsongalis GJ. Molecular Diagnostics for the Clinical Laboratory. Totowa, NJ: Humana Press, 1997.
53. Stowasser M, Bachmann AW, Jonsson JR, et al. Clinical, biochemical and genetic approaches to the detection of familial hyperaldosteronism type 1. J Hypertens 1995;13(12 Pt 2):1610-1613.
54. Unger ER, Piper MA. Nucleic acid biochemistry and diagnostic applications. In Burtis CA, Ashwood ER, eds. Tietz Textbook of Clinical Chemistry, 3rd ed. Philadelphia: WB Saunders, 1999:421-443.
55. Mullis KB, Faloona FA. Specific synthesis of DNA in vitro via a polymerase-catalyzed chain reaction. Methods Enzymol 1987; 155:335-350.
56. Southern EM. Detection of specific sequences among DNA fragments separated by gel electrophoresis. J Mol Biol 1975;98: 503-517.
57. National Committee for Clinical Laboratory Standards (NCCLS). Preliminary Evaluation of Quantitative Clinical Laboratory Methods: Approved Guideline EP10-A. Wayne, PA: NCCLS, 1998.
58. Carey RN, Garber CC. Evaluation of methods. In Kaplan LA, Pesce AJ, eds. Clinical Chemistry: Theory, Practice and Correlation, 2nd ed. St Louis: CV Mosby, 1989:290-310.
59. Department of Health and Human Services, Health Care Financing Administration. Clinical Laboratory Improvement Amendments of 1988: Final Rule. Federal Register, No. 7165[42CFR493. 1217], February 28, 1992.
60. National Committee for Clinical Laboratory Standards (NCCLS). Method Comparison and Bias Estimation Using Patient Samples: Approved Guideline EP9-A. Wayne, PA: NCCLS, 1995.
61. Taylor BN (U.S. ed). The International System of Units (SI). Special Publication 330. Gaithersburg, MD: National Institute of Standards and Technology (NIST), 1991:62. Periodically revised; available from Superintendent of Documents, Code No. NSPUE2, U.S. Government Printing Office, Washington, DC 20402-9325.
62. Hilleman MR. International biological standardization in historic and contemporary perspective. Dev Biol Stand 1999;100:19-30.
63. Rose MP. Follicle-stimulating hormone international standards and reference preparations for the calibration of immunoassays and bioassays. Clin Chim Acta 1998;273:103-117.
64. Linnet K. Necessary sample size for method comparison studies based on regression analysis. Clin Chem 1999;45:882-894.
65. The European Parliament and the Council of the European Union Directive 98/79/EC of the European Parliament and of the Council of October 27, 1998, on in vitro diagnostic medical devices. OJ L 220, 30.8.1993:23.
66. Powers DM. Regulations and Standards: Traceability of assay calibrators: The EU's IVD Directive raises the bar. IVD Technol 2000:26-33.
67. Fraser CG, Petersen PH. Analytical performance characteristics should be judged against objective quality specifications. Clin Chem 1999;45:321-333.
68. National Committee for Clinical Laboratory Standards (NCCLS). Evaluation of Precision Performance of Clinical Chemistry Devices: Approved Guideline EP5-A. Wayne, PA: NCCLS, 1999.
69. Stockl D, Baadenhuijsen H, Fraser CG, et al. Desirable routine analytical goals for quantities assayed in serum. Eur J Clin Chem Clin Biochem 1995;33:157-169.
70. Fraser CG: Biological variation in clinical chemistry: an update-collated data, 1988-1991. Arch Pathol Lab Med 1992;116: 916-923.

71. Fraser CG, Petersen PH, Ricos C, et al. Proposed quality specifications for the imprecision and inaccuracy of analytical systems for clinical chemistry. Eur J Clin Chem Clin Biochem 1992;30: 311-317.
72. Kroll MH, Emancipator K. A theoretical evaluation of linearity. Clin Chem 1993;39:405-413.
73. National Committee for Clinical Laboratory Standards (NCCLS). Evaluation of Matrix Effects: Proposed Guideline EP14-P. Wayne, PA: NCCLS, 1998.
74. National Committee for Clinical Laboratory Standards (NCCLS). Evaluation of the Linearity of Quantitative Analytical Methods: Proposed Guideline EP6-P. Wayne, PA: NCCLS, 1986.
75. National Committee for Clinical Laboratory Standards (NCCLS). Interference Testing in Clinical Chemistry: Proposed Guideline EP7-P. Wayne, PA: NCCLS, 1986.
76. Levine S, Noth R, Loo A, et al. Anomalous serum thyroxin measurements with the Abbott TDx procedure. Clin Chem 1990;36: 1838-1840.
77. Mbuyi-Kalala A, Ehrenstein G. Anomalous effects of hormone fragments on the measurement of parathyroid hormone by radioimmunoassay. Methods Find Exp Clin Pharmacol 1996;18:87-99.
78. Micallef JV, Hayes MM, Latif A, et al. Serum binding of steroid tracers and its possible effects on direct steroid immunoassay. Ann Clin Biochem 1995;32:566-574.
79. Cook NJ, Read GF. Oestradiol measurement in women on oral hormone replacement therapy: the validity of commercial test kits. Br J Biomed Sci 1995;52:97-101.
80. Cummings EA, Salisbury SR, Givner ML, et al. Testolactone-associated high androgen levels: a pharmacologic effect or a laboratory artifact? J Clin Endocrinol Metab 1998;83:784-787.
81. Thomas CM, van den Berg RJ, Segers MF, et al. Inaccurate measurement of 17 beta-estradiol in serum of female volunteers after oral administration of milligram amounts of micronized 17 beta-estradiol. Clin Chem 1993;39(11 Pt 1):2341-2342.
82. O'Brien PC, Dyck PJ. Procedures for setting normal values. Neurology 1995;45:17-23.
83. Solberg HE. Establishment and use of reference values. In Burtis CA, Ashwood ER, eds. Tietz Textbook of Clinical Chemistry, 2nd ed. Philadelphia: WB Saunders, 1994:454-484.
84. National Committee for Clinical Laboratory Standards (NCCLS). How to Define and Determine Reference Intervals in the Clinical Laboratory: Approved Guideline C28-A2, 2nd ed. Wayne, PA: NCCLS, 2000.
85. Klee GG. Maximizing efficacy of endocrine tests: importance of decision-focused testing strategies and appropriate patient preparation. Clin Chem 1999;45(8B):1323-1330.
86. Heins M, Heil W, Withold W. Storage of serum or whole blood samples? Effects of time and temperature on 22 serum analytes. Eur J Clin Chem Clin Biochem 1995;33:231-238.
87. Tateishi K, Klee GG, Cunningham JM, Lennon VA. Stability of bombesin in serum, plasma, urine, and culture media. Clin Chem 1985;31:276-278.
88. Demir A, Alfthan H, Stenman UH, et al. A clinically useful method for detecting gonadotropins in children: assessment of luteinizing hormone and follicle-stimulating hormone from urine as an alternative to serum by ultrasensitive time-resolved immunofluorometric assays. Pediatr Res 1994;36:221-226.
89. Hourd P, Edwards R. Current methods for the measurement of growth hormone in urine. Clin Endocrinol 1994;40:155-170.
90. Maes M, Mommen K, Hendrickx D, et al. Components of biological variation, including seasonality, in blood concentrations of TSH, TT_3, FT_4, PRL, cortisol, and testosterone in healthy volunteers. Clin Endocrinol 1997;46:587-598.
91. Sebastian-Gambaro MA, Liron-Hernandez FJ, Fuentes-Arderiu X. Intra- and interindividual biological variability bank. J Clin Chem Clin Biochem 1997;35:845-852.
92. Leppaluoto J, Ruskoaho H. Atrial natriuretic peptide, renin activity, aldosterone, urine volume and electrolytes during a 24-hour sleep-wake cycle in man. Acta Physiol Scand 1990;139:47-53.
93. Demers LM. Pituitary function. In Burtis CA, Ashwood ER, eds. Tietz Textbook of Clinical Chemistry, 3rd ed. Philadelphia: WB Saunders, 1999:1470-1495.
94. Bergenfelz A, Isaksson A, Lindblom P, et al. Measurement of parathyroid hormone in patients with primary hyperparathyroidism undergoing first and reoperative surgery. Br J Surg 1998;85:1129-1132.
95. Abe T, Ludecke DK. Recent primary transnasal surgical outcomes associated with intraoperative growth hormone measurement in acromegaly. Clin Endocrinol 1999; 50:27-35.
96. Hansen AM, Garde AH, Christensen JM, Eller NH, Netterstrom B. Evaluation of a radioimmunoassay and establishment of a reference interval for salivary cortisol in healthy subjects in Denmark. Scand J Clin Lab Invest 2003;63:303-310.
97. Chiu SK, Collier CP, Clark AF, Wynn-Edwards KE. Salivary cortisol on ROCHE Elecsys immunoassay system: pilot biological variation studies. Clin Biochem 2003;36:211-214.
98. Horvat-Gordon M, Granger DA, Schwartz EB, et al. Oxytocin is not a valid biomarker when measured in saliva by immunoassay. Physiol Behav 2005;84:445-448.
99. Lawrence HP. Salivary markers of systemic disease: noninvasive diagnosis of disease and monitoring of general health. J Can Dental Assoc 2002;68(3):170-174.
100. Choo RE, Huestis MA. Oral fluid as a diagnostic tool. Clin Chem Lab Med 2004;42(11):1273-1287.
101. Vining RF, McGinley RA. The measurement of hormones in saliva: possibilities and pitfalls. Steroid Biochem 1987;27:81-94.
102. Granger DA, Schwartz EB, Booth A, et al. Assessing dehydroepiandrosterone in saliva: a simple radioimmunoassay for use in studies of children, adolescents and adults. Psychoneuroendocrinology 1999;24:567-579.
103. O'Rorke A, Kane MM, Gosling JP, et al. Development and validation of a monoclonal antibody enzyme immunoassay for measuring progesterone in saliva. Clin Chem 1994;403:454-458.
104. Worthman CM, Stallings JF. Hormone measures in finger-prick blood spot samples: new field methods for reproductive endocrinology. Am J Phys Anthropol 1997;104:1-21.
105. Howe CJ, Handelsman DJ. Use of filter paper for sample collection and transport in steroid pharmacology. Clin Chem 1997;43: 1408-1415.
106. Kricka LJ. Miniaturization of analytical systems. Clin Chem 1998; 44:2008-2014.
107. Gabriely I, Kaplan J, Wozniak R. Transcutaneous glucose measurement using near-infrared spectroscopy during hypoglycemia. Diabetes Care 1999;22:2026-2032.
108. Tamada JA, Garg S, Jovanovic L, et al. Noninvasive glucose monitoring: comprehensive clinical results. JAMA 1999;282:1839-1844.
109. Garg SK, Potts RO, Ackerman NR, et al. Correlation of fingerstick blood glucose measurements with GlucoWatch biographer glucose results in young subjects with type 1 diabetes. Diabetes Care 1999;22:1708-1714.
110. Westgard JO, Klee GG. Quality management. In Burtis CA, Ashwood ER, eds. Tietz Textbook of Clinical Chemistry, 4th ed. Philadelphia: WB Saunders, 2006:485-531.
111. Browning MCK. Analytical goals for quantities used to assess thyrometabolic status. Ann Clin Biochem 1989;26:1-2.
112. Tietz NW. Accuracy in clinical chemistry: does anybody care? Clin Chem 1994;40:859-861.
113. Westgard JO, Barry PL, Hunt MR, et al. A multi-rule Shewhart chart for quality control on clinical chemistry. Clin Chem 1981;27: 493-501.
114. Klee GG, Schryver PG, Kisabeth RM. Analytic bias specifications based on the analysis of effects on performance of medical guidelines. Scand J Clin Lab Invest 1999;59:509-512.
115. Smith FA, Kroft SH. Optimal procedures for detecting analytic bias using patient samples. Am J Clin Pathol 1997;108:254-268.
116. Reinsberg J. Different efficacy of various blocking reagents to eliminate interferences by human antimouse antibodies with a two-site immunoassay. Clin Biochem 1996;29:145-148.
117. Nicholson S, Fox M, Epenetos A, et al. Immunoglobulin inhibiting reagent: evaluation of a new method for eliminating spurious elevations in CA 125 caused by HAMA. Int J Biol Markers 1996;11: 46-49.
118. Wheeler MJ, D'Souza A, Matadeen J, et al. Ciba Corning ACS: 180 testosterone assays evaluated. Clin Chem 1996;42:1445-1449.

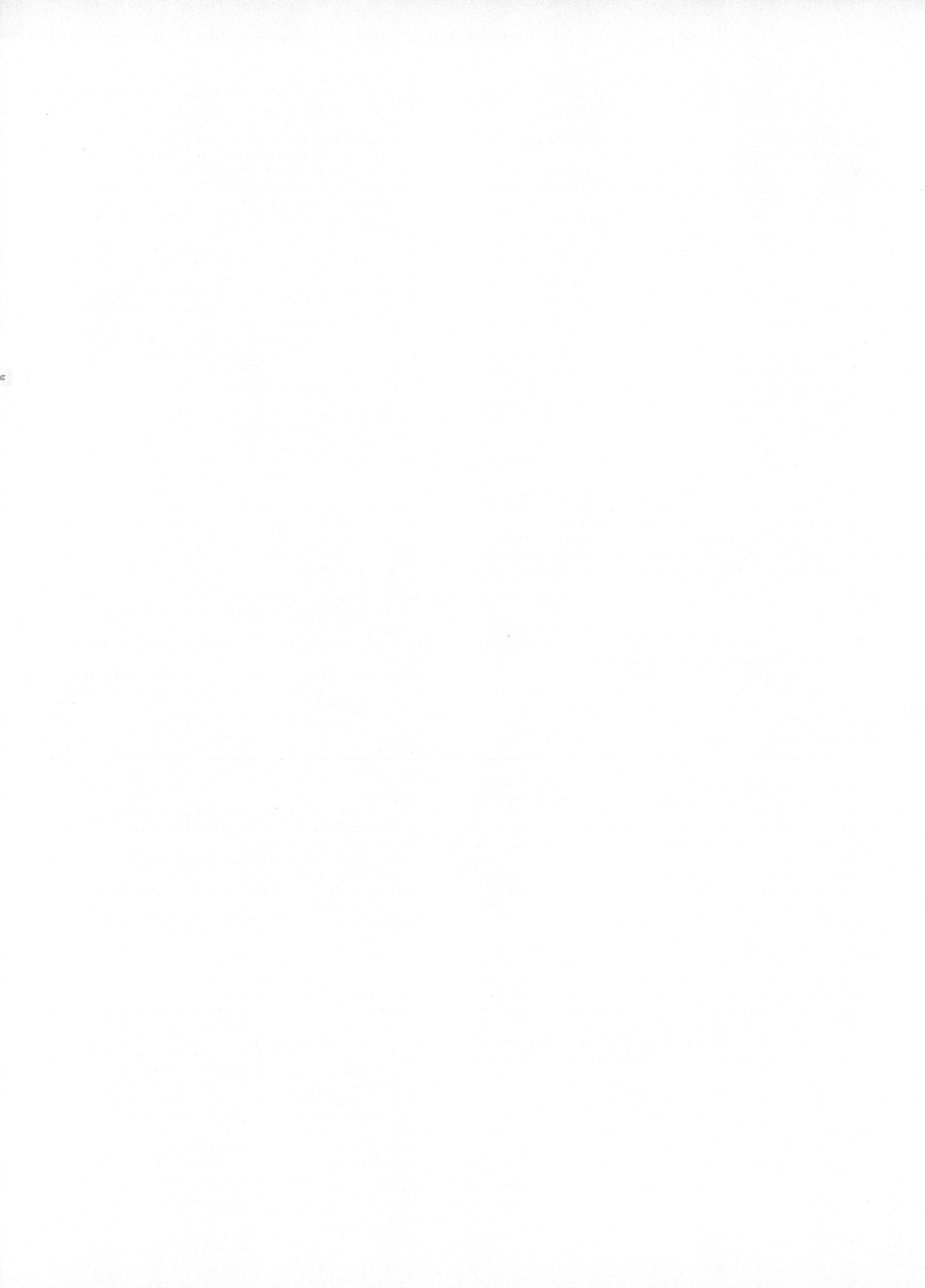

SECTION II

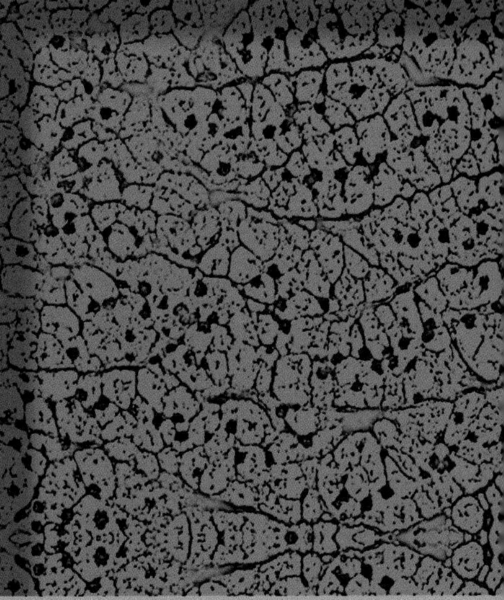

Hypothalamus and Pituitary

CHAPTER 7

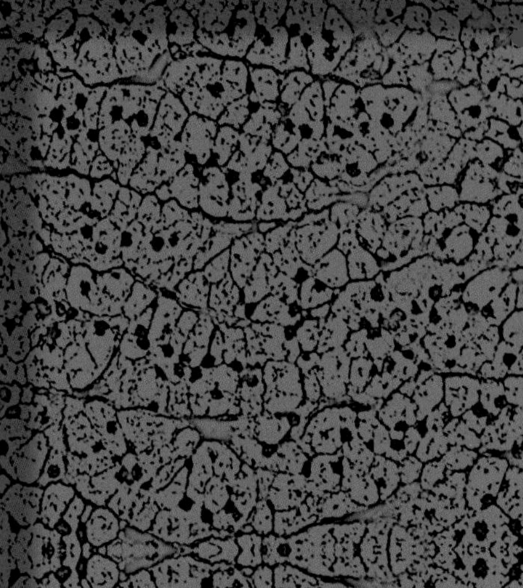

NEUROENDOCRINOLOGY

Malcolm J. Low

HISTORICAL PERSPECTIVE

The field of neuroendocrinology has expanded from its original focus on the control of pituitary hormone secretion by the hypothalamus to encompass multiple reciprocal interactions between the central nervous system (CNS) and endocrine systems in the control of homeostasis and physiologic responses to environmental stimuli. Although many of these concepts are relatively recent, the intimate interaction of the hypothalamus and the pituitary gland was recognized more than a century ago. For example, at the end of the nineteenth century, clinicians including Alfred Fröhlich described an obesity and infertility condition referred to as *adiposogenital dystrophy* in patients with sellar tumors.[1] This condition subsequently became known as Fröhlich's syndrome and was most often associated with the accumulation of excessive subcutaneous fat, hypogonadotrophic hypogonadism, and growth retardation.

Whether this syndrome was due to injury to the pituitary gland itself or to the overlying hypothalamus was extremely controversial. Several leaders in the field of endocrinology, including Cushing and his colleagues, argued that the syndrome was due to disruption of the pituitary gland.[2] However, experimental evidence began to accumulate that the hypothalamus was somehow involved in the control of the pituitary gland. For example, Aschner demonstrated in dogs that the precise removal of the pituitary gland without damage to the overlying hypothalamus did not result in obesity.[3] Later, seminal studies by Hetherington and Ranson demonstrated that stereotaxic destruction of the medial basal hypothalamus with electrolytic lesions, which spared the pituitary gland, resulted in morbid obesity and neuroendocrine derangements similar to those of the patients described by Fröhlich.[4] This and subsequent studies clearly established that an intact hypothalamus is required for normal endocrine function. However, the mechanisms by which the hypothalamus was involved in endocrine regulation remained unsettled for years to come. We now know that the phenotypes of Fröhlich's syndrome and the ventromedial hypothalamic lesion syndrome are probably due to dysfunction or destruction of key hypothalamic neurons that regulate pituitary hormone secretion and energy homeostasis.

The field of neuroendocrinology took a major step forward when several groups, especially Ernst and Berta Scharrer, recognized that neurons in the hypothalamus were the source of the axons that constitute the neural lobe (see Neurosecretion). The hypothalamic control of the anterior pituitary gland remained unclear, however. For example, Popa and Fielding identified the pituitary portal vessels linking the median eminence of the hypothalamus and the anterior pituitary gland.[5] Although they appreciated the fact that this vasculature provided a link between hypothalamus and pituitary gland, they hypothesized at the time that blood flowed from the pituitary up to the brain. Anatomic studies by Wislocki and King supported the concept that blood flow was from the hypothalamus to the pituitary.[6] Later studies, including the seminal work of Geoffrey Harris, established the flow of blood from the hypothalamus at the median eminence to the anterior pituitary gland.[7] This supported the concept that the hypothalamus controlled anterior pituitary gland function indirectly and led to the now accepted hypophyseal-portal chemotransmitter hypothesis.

Subsequently, several important studies, especially those from Schally and colleagues and the Guillemin group, established that the anterior pituitary is tightly controlled by the hypothalamus.[8,9] Both groups identified several putative peptide hormone-releasing factors (see later sections). These fundamental studies resulted in the awarding of the Nobel Prize in Medicine in 1977 to Andrew Schally and Roger Guillemin.[10,11] Of course, we now know that these releasing factors are the fundamental link between the central nervous system (CNS) and the control of endocrine function. Furthermore, these neuropeptides are highly conserved across species and are essential for reproduction, growth, and metabolism. The anatomy, physiology, and genetics of these factors constitute a major portion of this chapter.

Over the past 2 decades, work in the field of neuroendocrinology has continued to advance across several fronts. Cloning and characterization of the specific G protein–coupled receptors used by the hypothalamic-releasing factors have helped define signaling mechanisms utilized by the releasing factors. Characterization of the distribution of these receptors has universally demonstrated receptor expression in the brain and in peripheral tissues other than the pituitary, arguing for multiple physiologic roles for the neuropeptide releasing factors. Finally, the last 2 decades have also seen tremendous advances in our understanding of both regulatory neuronal and humoral inputs to the hypophyseotropic neurons.

The adipostatic hormone leptin, discovered in 1994,[12] is an example of a humoral factor that has profound effects on multiple neuroendocrine circuits. Reduction in circulating leptin is responsible for suppression of the thyroid and reproductive axes during the starvation response. The subsequent discovery of ghrelin,[13] a stomach peptide that regulates appetite and also acts on multiple neuroendocrine axes, demonstrates that much remains to be learned regarding the regulation of the hypothalamic-releasing hormones. Traditionally, it has been extremely difficult to study releasing factor gene expression or the specific regulation of the releasing factor neurons because of their small numbers and, in some cases, diffuse distribution. Transgenic experiments have produced mice in which expression of fluorescent marker proteins has been specifically targeted to gonadotropin-releasing hormone (GnRH) neurons[14] and arcuate pro-opiomelanocortin (POMC) neurons[15] among others. This technology will allow detailed study of the electrophysiologic properties of hypothalamic neurons in the more native context of slice preparations or organotypic cultures.

As just described, much of the field of neuroendocrinology has focused on hypothalamic-releasing factors and their control of reproduction, growth, development, fluid balance, and the stress response through their control of pituitary hormone production. More broadly, however, neuroendocrinology has become a rubric to define the study of interaction of the endocrine and nervous systems in the regulation of homeostasis. The field of neuroendocrinology has been further expanded, however, because diverse areas of basic research have often been fundamental to understanding the neuroendocrine system and thus championed by its investigators. These areas include studies of neuropeptide structure, function, and mechanism of action; neural secretion; hypothalamic neuroanatomy; G protein–coupled receptor structure, function, and signaling; transport of substances into the brain; and the action of hormones on the brain. Many homeostatic systems involve integrated endocrine, autonomic, and behavioral responses. Thus, many homeostatic systems exist in which the classic neuroendocrine axes are important but not autonomous pathways, such as energy homeostasis and immune function, and these subjects also are studied often in the context of neuroendocrinology.

This chapter first presents the concepts of neural secretion, the neuroanatomy of the hypothalamic-pituitary unit, and the CNS structures most relevant to the control of the neurohypophysis and adenohypophysis. It then covers each classical hypothalamic-pituitary axis, including a consideration of the immune system and its integration with neuroendocrine function. Finally, the chapter reviews the pathophysiology of disorders of neural regulation of endocrine function. The neuroendocrinology of energy homeostasis is fully considered in Chapter 34.

NEURAL CONTROL OF GLANDULAR SECRETION

A fundamental principle of neuroendocrinology encompasses the regulated secretion of hormones, neurotransmitters, or neuromodulators by specialized cells.[16] Endocrine cells and neurons are prototypical secretory cells. Both have electrically excitable plasma membranes and specific ion conductances that regulate exocytosis of their signaling molecules from storage vesicles. In addition, secretory cells are broadly classified by their topographic mechanisms of secretion. For example, endocrine cells secrete their contents directly into the bloodstream, allowing these substances to act globally as hormones. Cells classified as paracrine secrete their contents into the extracellular space and predominantly affect the function of closely neighboring cells. Similarly, autocrine secretory cells affect their own function by the local actions of their secretions. In contrast, secretory cells within exocrine glands secrete proteinaceous substances including enzymes into the lumen of ductal systems.

Neurosecretion

Neurons are secretory cells that send their axons throughout the nervous system to release their neurotransmitters and neuromodulators predominantly at specialized chemical synapses. Neurohumoral or neurosecretory cells constitute a unique subset of neurons whose axon terminals are not associated with synapses. Two examples of neurosecretory cells are neurohypophyseal and hypophyseotropic cells. The prototypical neurohypophyseal cells are the magnicellular neurons of the paraventricular and supraoptic nuclei in the hypothalamus. Hypophyseotropic cells are neurons that secrete their products into the pituitary portal vessels at the median eminence (Fig. 7–1).

In the most basic sense, neurosecretory cells are neurons that secrete substances directly into the bloodstream to act as hormones. The theory of neurosecretion evolved from the seminal work of Scharrer and Scharrer,[16,17] who used morphologic techniques to identify stained secretory granules in the supraoptic and paraventricular hypothalamic neurons. They found that cutting the pituitary stalk led to an accumulation of these granules in the hypothalamus. These findings led them to hypothesize that the source of substances secreted by the neural lobe (posterior pituitary) was hypothalamic neurons. Although the Scharrers' concept initially raised great skepticism among contemporary researchers, we now know that the axon terminals in the neural lobe arise from the supraoptic and paraventricular magnicellular neurons that contain oxytocin and arginine vasopressin (AVP).

The modern definition of neurosecretion has evolved to include the release of any neuronal secretory product from a neuron. Indeed, a fundamental tenet of neuroscience is that all neurons in the CNS, including neurons that secrete AVP and oxytocin in the neural lobe, receive multiple synaptic inputs largely onto their dendrites and cell bodies. In addition, neurons have the basic ability to detect and integrate input from multiple neurons through specific receptors. They in turn fire action potentials that result in the release of neurotransmitters and neuromodulators into synapses formed with postsynaptic

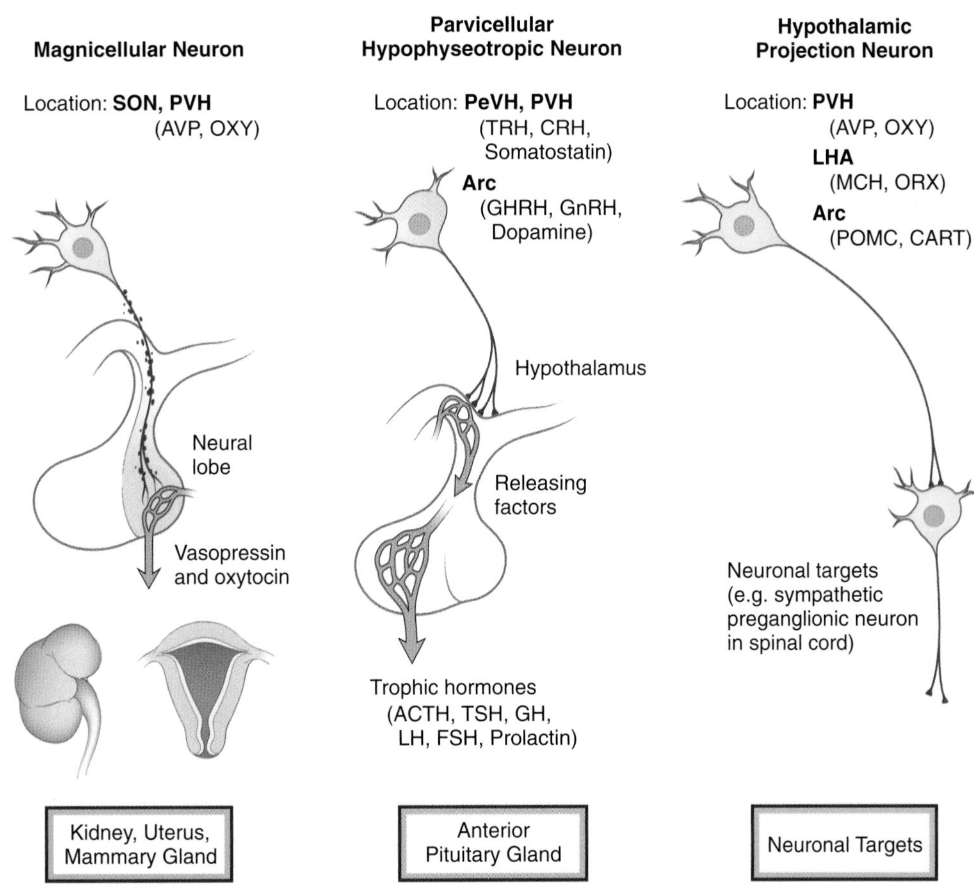

Figure 7–1 ▪ Three types of hypothalamic neurosecretory cells. **Left,** A magnicellular neuron that secretes arginine vasopressin (AVP) or oxytocin (OXY). The cell body, which is located in the supraoptic (SON) or paraventricular hypothalamic nucleus (PVH), projects its neuronal process into the neural lobe, and neurohormone is released from nerve endings. **Center,** Similar peptidergic neurons are located in the medial basal hypothalamus in nuclear groups including the periventricular hypothalamic nucleus (PeVH), PVH, and arcuate nucleus of the hypothalamus (Arc). The neuropeptides in this case are released into the specialized blood supply to the pituitary to regulate its secretion. **Right,** A third category of hypothalamic peptidergic neurons terminates at chemical synapses on other neurons. These projection neurons are found in sites including the PVH, Arc, and lateral hypothalamic area (LHA) that innervate multiple central nervous system nuclei, including autonomic preganglionic neurons in the brain stem and spinal cord. Such substances act as neurotransmitters or neuromodulators. *ACTH,* Corticotropin; *CART,* cocaine- and amphetamine-regulated transcript; *CRH,* corticotropin-releasing hormone; *FSH,* follicle-stimulating hormone; *GH,* growth hormone; *GHRH,* growth hormone–releasing hormone; *GnRH,* gonadotropin-releasing hormone; *LH,* luteinizing hormone; *MCH,* melanin-concentrating hormone; *ORX,* orexin/hypocretin; *POMC,* pro-opiomelanocortin; *TRH,* thyrotropin-releasing hormone; *TSH,* thyrotropin.

neurons. The vast majority of communications between neurons is accomplished by "classical" fast-acting neurotransmitters (e.g., glutamate, γ-aminobutyric acid [GABA], acetylcholine) and neuromodulators (e.g., neuropeptides) acting at chemical synapses.[11,18] Thus, neurosecretion represents a fundamental concept in understanding the mechanisms used by the nervous system to control behavior and maintain homeostasis.

In the era of the elucidation of the human genome, the importance of these early observations often is not fully appreciated. However, accounts of these early studies are illuminating. Moreover, it is not an overstatement that the confirmation of the neurosecretion hypothesis represented one of the major advances in the field of neuroscience and neuroendocrinology. Indeed, this and other early experiments, including the pioneering work of Geoffrey Harris,[7,19] led to the fundamental concept that the hypothalamus releases hormones directly into the bloodstream (neurohypophyseal cells). These observations provided the principles on which the modern discipline of neuroendocrinology is built.

The Autonomic Nervous System's Contribution to Endocrine Control

Another major precept of neuroendocrinology is that the nervous system controls or modifies the function of both endocrine and exocrine glands. The exquisite control of the anterior pituitary gland is accomplished by the action of releasing factor hormones (see Hypophyseotropic Hormone, and Neuroendocrine Axes). Other endocrine and exocrine organs (e.g., pancreas, adrenal, pineal, salivary glands) are also regulated through direct innervation from the cholinergic and noradrenergic inputs from the autonomic nervous system. Although it is beyond the scope of this chapter, an appreciation of the functional anatomy and pharmacology of the parasympathetic and sympathetic nervous systems is fundamental in understanding the neural control of endocrine function.

The efferent arms of the autonomic nervous system comprise the sympathetic and parasympathetic systems. Each system has a similar wiring diagram characterized by a preganglionic neuron that innervates a postganglionic neuron that in turn targets an end organ.[20] Preganglionic and postganglionic parasympathetic neurons are cholinergic. In contrast, preganglionic sympathetic neurons are cholinergic and postganglionic neurons are noradrenergic (except for those innervating sweat glands, which are cholinergic). Another basic concept is that autonomic neurons coexpress several neuropeptides. This coexpression is a common feature of neurons in the central and peripheral nervous systems.[11,18,21] For example, postganglionic noradrenergic neurons coexpress somatostatin and neuropeptide Y (NPY). Postganglionic cholinergic neurons coexpress neuropeptides including vasoactive intestinal polypeptide (VIP) and calcitonin gene-related peptide (CGRP).

The majority of sympathetic preganglionic neurons lie in the intermediolateral cell column in the thoracolumbar regions of the spinal cord.[20] Most postganglionic neurons are located in sympathetic ganglia lying near the vertebral column (e.g., sympathetic chain and superior cervical ganglia). Postganglionic fibers, in turn, innervate target organs. Thus, as a rule, sympathetic preganglionic fibers are relatively short and the postganglionic fibers are long. In contrast, the parasympathetic preganglionic neurons lie in the midbrain (Edinger-Westphal nucleus of the third cranial nerve), the medulla oblongata (e.g., dorsal motor nucleus of the vagus and nucleus ambiguus), and the sacral spinal cord. Postganglionic neurons that innervate the eye and salivary glands arise from the ciliary, pterygopalatine, submandibular, and otic ganglia. Postganglionic parasympathetic neurons in the thorax and abdomen typically lie within the target organs including the gut wall and pancreas.[20] Consequently, parasympathetic preganglionic fibers are relatively long and the postganglionic fibers are short.

A dual autonomic innervation of the pancreas illustrates the importance of coordinated neural control of endocrine organs. The endocrine pancreas receives sympathetic (noradrenergic) and parasympathetic (cholinergic) innervation.[20,22] The latter activity is provided by the vagus nerve (dorsal motor nucleus of the vagus) and is an excellent example of neural modulation because cholinergic tone of β cells affects their secretion of insulin. For example, vagal input is thought to modulate insulin secretion before (cephalic phase), during, and after ingestion of food.[23] In addition, noradrenergic stimulation of the endocrine pancreas can alter the secretion of glucagon and inhibits insulin release.[22] It should be noted, of course, that a major regulator of insulin secretion is the extracellular concentration of glucose.[24] In fact, glucose can induce insulin secretion in the absence of neural input. However, the exquisite control by the nervous system is illustrated by the fact that populations of neurons in the brain stem and hypothalamus, like the β cell, have the ability to sense glucose levels in the bloodstream.[25] This information is integrated by the hypothalamus and ultimately results in alterations in the activity of the autonomic nervous system innervating the pancreas. Thus, neural control of the endocrine pancreas probably contributes to the physiologic control of insulin secretion and may contribute to the pathophysiology of disorders such as diabetes mellitus. Certainly, an increased understanding of this complex interplay between the CNS and endocrine function is necessary to diagnose and clinically manage endocrine disorders.

HYPOTHALAMIC-PITUITARY UNIT

The hypothalamus is one of the most evolutionarily conserved and essential regions of the mammalian brain. Indeed, the hypothalamus is the ultimate brain structure that allows mammals to maintain homeostasis, and destruction of the hypothalamus is not compatible with life. Hypothalamic control of homeostasis stems from the ability of this collection of neurons to orchestrate coordinated endocrine, autonomic, and behavioral responses. A key principle is that the hypothalamus receives sensory inputs from the external environment (e.g., light, pain, temperature, odorants) and information regarding the internal environment (e.g., blood pressure, blood osmolality, blood glucose levels). In addition, of particular relevance to neuroendocrine control, hormones (e.g., glucocorticoids, estrogen, testosterone, thyroid hormone) exert both negative and positive feedback directly on the hypothalamus.

The hypothalamus integrates diverse sensory and hormonal inputs and provides coordinated responses through motor outputs to key regulatory sites. These include the anterior pituitary gland, posterior pituitary gland, cerebral cortex, premotor and motor neurons in the brain stem and spinal cord, and parasympathetic and sympathetic preganglionic neurons. The patterned hypothalamic outputs to these effector sites ultimately result in coordinated endocrine, behavioral, and autonomic responses that maintain homeostasis. The focus of this section, the hypothalamic–pituitary unit, is an exquisitely controlled system and underlies the ability of mammals to coordinate endocrine functions that are necessary for survival.

Development and Differentiation of Hypothalamic Nuclei

Tremendous advances in our knowledge of the molecular and genetic basis for embryonic development of the hypothalamic-pituitary unit have occurred in the past 2 decades as a result of the genome sequencing projects and use of transgenic model systems.[26] Pituitary development is discussed in detail in Chapter 8. Therefore, only a few key points most relevant to the physiology and pathophysiology of the neuroendocrine hypothalamus are presented in this section.

There has been considerable debate concerning the extent to which developmental studies in the rodent hypothalamic-pituitary system are applicable to the human. However, accumulating data suggest that the similarities outweigh the differences. Ontogenic analyses of the organization of the human hypothalamus utilizing a battery of neurochemical markers have reinforced its homologies to the better studied rat brain.[27] The cytoarchitectonic boundaries of hypothalamic nuclei are much more easily discerned in fetal human brain than in the adult's, and for the most part correspond to homologous structures in the rat hypothalamus. This finding has important implications for the validity of interspecies comparative analyses. Two examples further illustrate this point. First, the ventromedial nucleus (VMH) of the hypothalamic core, which plays a role in energy balance and in female sexual behavior, differentiates from neuroblasts at a time-point intermediate to the earlier differentiation of lateral hypothalamic nuclei and later differentiation of the midline nuclei (including the suprachiasmatic [SCN], arcuate, and paraventricular nuclei [PVH]) in both humans and rodents.[27,28] Expression of the transcription factor SF1 has been shown to be restricted both temporally and spatially to cells in the VMH and knockout of the SF1 gene in mice alters VMH development by influencing the migration of cells and hence their ultimate location.[28] A second example of interspecies homologies in hypothalamic development is the migration of gonadotropin-releasing hormone neurons from their origins in rostral neuroepithelium to the anterior hypothalamus.[29] As discussed in later sections of this chapter, spontaneous and inherited mutations in genes that affect the migration of these neurons are an important cause of Kallman's syndrome or hypogonadotropic hypogonadism associated with anosmia.

A growing list of genes in addition to SF1 and those associated with Kallman's syndrome, primarily encoding transcription factors, have been implicated in human neuroendocrine disorders and characterized experimentally in rodent models.[30] This list includes the homeobox transcription factor OTP and the heterodimeric complex formed by the helix-loop-helix (bHLH) factors SIM1 and ARNT2. These factors are required for the proper development of the PVH and supraoptic nucleus (SON) and expression of many key hypophyseotropic neuropeptide genes. The physiologic importance of SIM1 is illustrated by the development of an obesity phenotype in both mice and humans with a haploinsufficiency of SIM1 expression.[30]

Two key concepts involved in CNS development, which also apply to the hypothalamus, are the balance between neurogenesis and cell death in the establishment of nuclei and the role of circulating hormones in providing organizational signals that regulate cell number and synaptic remodeling. The most thoroughly characterized examples are the effects of sex steroid hormones on the developing brain that result in key sexual dimorphisms of functional importance in later reproductive behaviors.[31] This principle has been extended recently to include organizational effects of other classes of hormones. Notably, leptin plays an important role in the development of medial-basal hypothalamic circuits important for energy homeostasis by mediating axonal projections between hypothalamic nuclei.[32]

Anatomy of the Hypothalamic-Pituitary Unit

The pituitary gland is regulated by three interacting elements: hypothalamic inputs (releasing factors or hypophyseotropic hormones), feedback effects of circulating hormones, and paracrine and autocrine secretions of the pituitary itself. In humans, the pituitary gland (hypophysis) can be divided into two major parts, the adenohypophysis and the neurohypophysis, which are easily distinguishable from each other by T1-weighted magnetic resonance imaging (MR T1WI) (Fig. 7–2).[33] The adenohypophysis in turn can be subdivided into three distinct lobes, the pars distalis (anterior lobe), pars intermedia (intermediate lobe), and pars tuberalis. Whereas a well-developed intermediate lobe is found in most mammals, only rudimentary vestiges of the intermediate lobe are detectable in adult humans with the bulk of intermediate lobe cells being dispersed in the anterior and posterior lobes.

The neurohypophysis is composed of the pars nervosa (also known as the neural or posterior lobe), the infundibular stalk, and the median eminence. The infundibular stalk is surrounded by the pars tuberalis, and together they constitute the hypophyseal stalk. The pituitary gland lies in the sella turcica (the Turkish saddle) of the sphenoid bone and underlies the base of the hypothalamus. This anatomic location explains the hypotha-

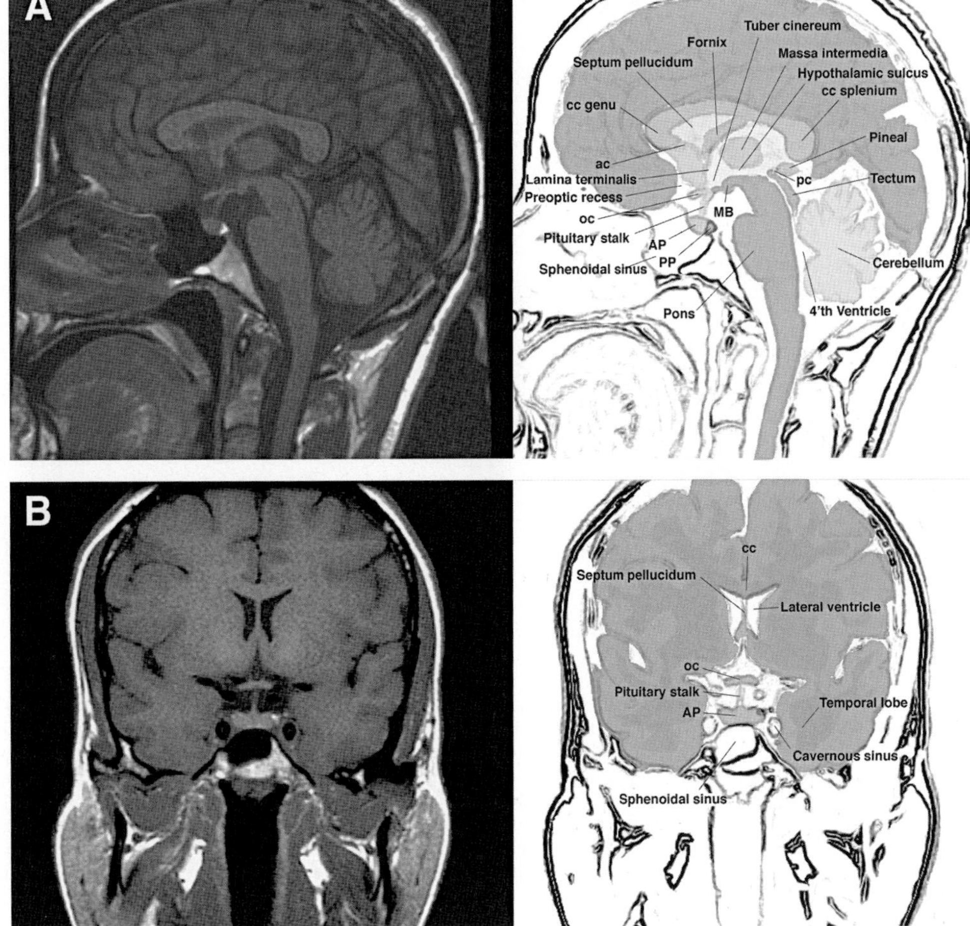

Figure 7–2 ■ Normal anatomy of the human hypothalamic-pituitary unit in sagittal **(A)** and coronal planes **(B)**. Structures that are visible in the T1-weighted magnetic resonance images (*left panels*) are identified in the corresponding diagrams (*right panels*). The hypothalamus is bounded anteriorly by the optic chiasm, laterally by the sulci formed with the temporal lobes, and posteriorly by the mammillary bodies (in which the mammillary nuclei are located). Dorsally, the hypothalamus is delineated from the thalamus by the hypothalamic sulcus. The smooth, rounded base of the hypothalamus is the tuber cinereum; the pituitary stalk descends from its central region, which is termed the median eminence. The median eminence stands out from the rest of the tuber cinereum because of its dense vascularity, which is formed by the primary plexus of the hypophyseal-portal system. The long portal veins run along the ventral surface of the pituitary stalk. Note the location of the pituitary stalk, the hyperintense signal (*white*) from the posterior pituitary (panel A, left), and the anatomic relationships of the pituitary gland to the optic chiasm, the optic nerves, and the cavernous sinuses. (MRI images courtesy of Dr. David M. Cook, Oregon Health & Science University.)

lamic damage described by Fröhlich.[1] In humans, the base of the hypothalamus forms a mound called the tuber cinereum, the central region of which gives rise to the median eminence (see Fig. 7–2).[34]

The anterior and intermediate lobes of the pituitary derive from a dorsal invagination of the pharyngeal epithelium, called *Rathke's pouch,* in response to inductive signals from the overlying neuroepithelium of the ventral diencephalon. Precursor cells within the pouch undergo steps of organ determination and cell fate commitment to a pituitary phenotype, proliferation, and migration during development.[26] The intermediate lobe is in direct contact with the neural lobe and is the least prominent of the three lobes. With age, the human intermediate lobe decreases in size to leave a small, residual collection of POMC cells. In nonprimate species, these cells are responsible for secreting the POMC-derived product α-melanocyte–stimulating hormone (α-MSH).[35]

The major component of the neural lobe is a collection of axon terminals arising from magnicellular secretory neurons located in the PVH and SON of the hypothalamus (see Fig. 7–1; Fig. 7–3). These axon terminals are in close association with a capillary plexus, and they secrete substances including AVP and oxytocin into the hypophyseal veins and into the general circulation (Table 7–1). The blood supply to the neurohypophysis arises from the inferior hypophyseal artery (a branch of the internal carotid artery). Glial-like cells called pituicytes are scattered among the nerve terminals. As the source of AVP to the general circulation, the PVH and SON and their axon terminals in the neural lobe are the effector arms of the central regulation of blood osmolality, fluid balance, and blood pressure (see Chapter 9).

The secretion of oxytocin by magnicellular neurons is critical at parturition, resulting in uterine myometrial contraction. In addition, the secretion of oxytocin is regulated by the classic milk let-down reflex.[36] Although the exact neuroanatomic substrate underlying this response is still unclear, apparently mechanosensory information from the nipple reaches the magnicellular neurons, directly or indirectly, from the dorsal horn of the spinal cord, resulting in release of oxytocin into the general circulation.[37] Oxytocin acts on receptors on myoepithelial cells in the mammary gland acini, leading to release of milk into the ductal system and ultimately the release of milk from the mammary gland.

The Median Eminence and Hypophyseotropic Neuronal System

The median eminence is the functional link between the hypothalamus and the anterior pituitary gland, lies in the center of the tuber cinereum, and is composed of an extensive array of blood vessels and nerve endings (see Fig. 7–2; Fig. 7–4).[17,34,38] Its extremely rich blood supply arises from the superior hypophyseal artery (a branch of the internal carotid artery), which sends off

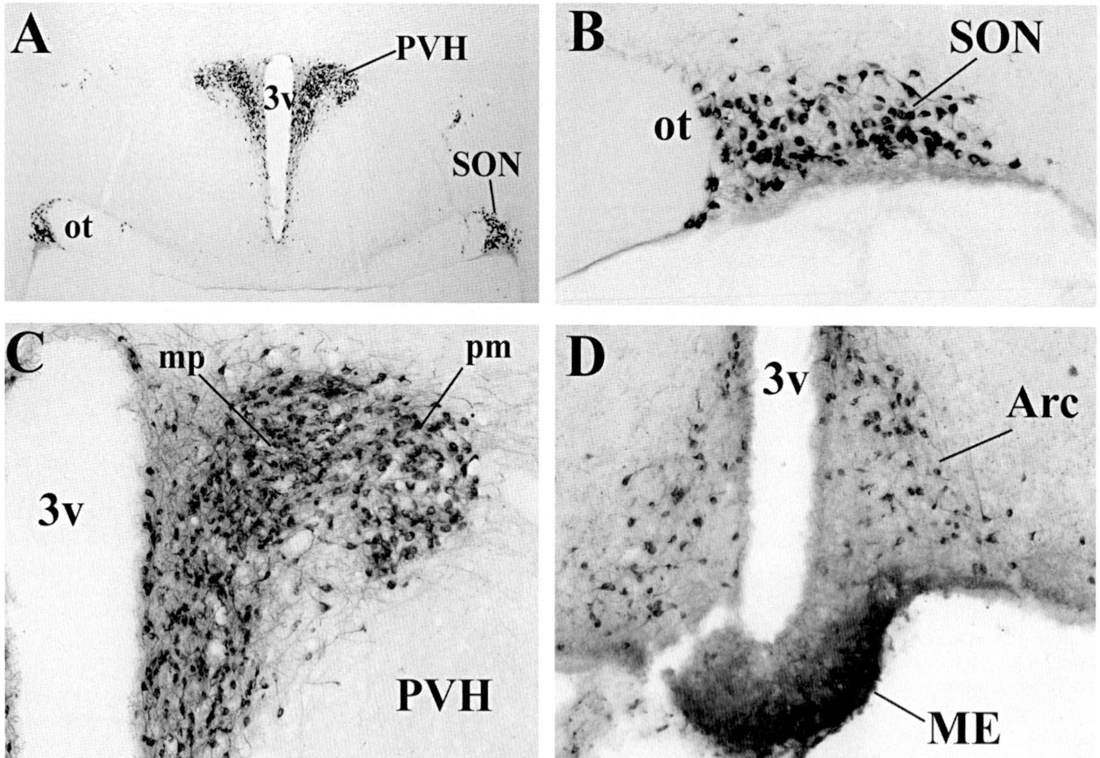

Figure 7–3 ■ The tuberoinfundibular system is revealed by retrograde transport of cholera toxin subunit B (CtB). The location of hypothalamic cell bodies of neurons projecting to the median eminence (ME) and the posterior pituitary can be identified by microinjecting a small volume of the retrograde tracer CtB into the median eminence of the rat. **A,** Retrogradely labeled cells can be seen in the paraventricular (PVH) and supraoptic nuclei of the hypothalamus (SON). **B,** Magnicellular neurons are observed in the SON. **C,** Labeled neurons are found in the posterior magnicellular group (pm) as well as the medial parvicellular subdivision (mp). The labeled cells in the PVH include those that contain corticotropin-releasing hormone (CRH) and thyrotropin-releasing hormone (TRH). **D,** Retrogradely labeled cells are also found in the arcuate nucleus of the hypothalamus (Arc). These include neurons that release growth hormone-releasing hormone (GHRH) and dopamine. *3v,* Third ventricle; *ot,* optic tract. (Photomicrographs courtesy of Dr. R. M. Lechan.)

TABLE 7–1 NEUROTRANSMITTERS AND NEUROMODULATORS IN THE PARAVENTRICULAR NUCLEUS AND THE ARCUATE NUCLEUS OF THE HYPOTHALAMUS

Paraventricular Nucleus	Arcuate Nucleus
Magnicellular Division	Acetylcholine
Angiotensin II	γ-Aminobutyric acid (GABA)
Cholecystokinin (CCK)	Agouti-related peptide (AGRP)
Dynorphins	Cocaine- and amphetamine-regulated transcript (CART)
Nitric oxide (NO)	
Oxytocin	Dopamine
Vasopressin	Endocannabinoids
	Enkephalins
Parvicellular Divisions	Galanin
γ-Aminobutyric acid (GABA)	Galanin-like peptide (GALP)
Angiotensin II	Glutamate
Atrial natriuretic factor (ANF)	Gonadotropin-releasing hormone (GnRH)
Bombesin-like peptides	
	Growth hormone–releasing hormone (GHRH)
Cholecystokinin (CCK)	
	Kisspeptins
Corticotropin-releasing hormone (CRH)	Neuromedin U
Dopamine	Neuropeptide Y (NPY)
Endocannabinoids	Neurotensin
Enkephalins	Nociceptin/orphanin FQ (OFQ)
Galanin	Pancreatic polypeptide
Glutamate	Prolactin
Interleukin-1 (IL-1)	Pro-opiomelanocortin
Neuropeptide Y (NPY)	Melanocortins (ACTH, α-MSH, β-MSH, γ-MSH)
Neurotensin	
Nitric Oxide (NO)	Opioids (β-endorphin)
RFRP (RF amide-related peptides)	QRFP (pyro-glutamyl-RFamide peptide)
Somatostatin	Somatostatin
Thyrotropin-releasing hormone (TRH)	Substance P
Vasopressin	
Vasoactive intestinal peptide (VIP)	

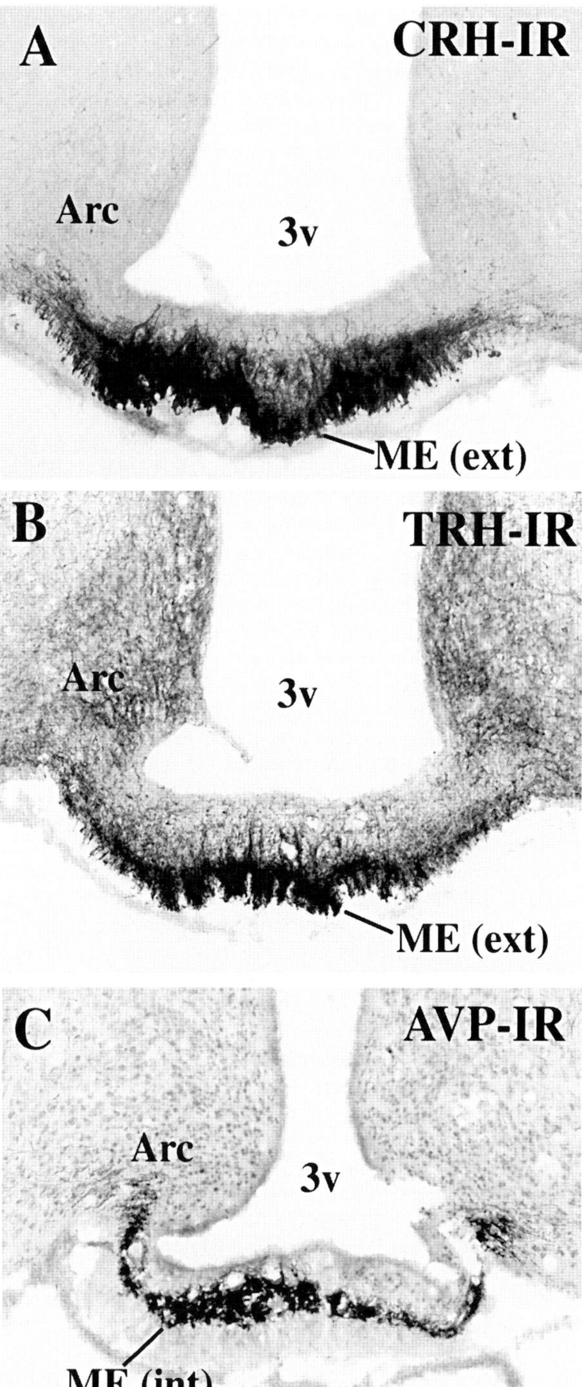

Figure 7–4 ▪ The median eminence is the functional connection of the hypothalamus and the pituitary gland. **A** and **B,** Distribution of corticotropin-releasing hormone and thyrotropin-releasing hormone (CRH-IR and TRH-IR) immunoreactivity in the external layer of the median eminence (ME ext) of the rat. CRH and TRH cell bodies reside in the medial division of the paraventricular hypothalamic nucleus. **C,** Arginine vasopressin (AVP) immunoreactivity in nerve endings in the internal layer of the median eminence (ME int). *Arc,* Arcuate nucleus; *3v,* third ventricle. (Photomicrographs courtesy of Dr. R. M. Lechan.)

many small branches that form capillary loops. The small capillary loops extend into the internal and external zones (see next paragraph), form anastomoses, and drain into sinusoids that become the pituitary portal veins that enter the vascular pool of the pituitary gland.[38-40] The flow of blood in these short loops is thought to be predominantly (if not exclusively) in a hypothalamic-to-pituitary direction.[40] This well-developed plexus results in a tremendous increase in the vascular surface area. In addition, the vessels are fenestrated, allowing diffusion of the peptide-releasing factors to their site of action in the anterior pituitary gland. This vascular complex in the base of the hypothalamus and its "arteriolized" venous drainage to the pituitary compose a circulatory system analogous to the portal vein system of the liver, hence the term *hypophyseal-portal circulation.*

Three distinct compartments of the median eminence are recognized: the innermost ependymal layer, the internal zone, and the external zone (see Fig. 7–4).[38] Ependymal cells form the floor of the third ventricle and are unique in that they have microvilli rather than cilia. Tight junctions at the ventricular pole of the ependymal cells prevent the diffusion of large-molecular-weight substances between the cerebrospinal fluid (CSF) and the extracellular space within the median eminence. The ependymal layer also contains specialized cells called tanycytes that send processes into the other layers of the median eminence.[41] Tight junctions between tanycytes at the lateral edges of the median eminence likely prevent the diffusion of releasing factors back into the medial basal hypothalamus.

The internal zone of the median eminence is composed of axons of passage of the supraoptic and paraventricular magnicellular neurons en route to the posterior pituitary (see Fig. 7–4C) and the axons of the hypophyseotropic neurons destined for the external layer of the median eminence (see Fig. 7–4A and B). In addition, supportive cells populate this layer.

Finally, the external zone of the median eminence represents the exchange point of the hypothalamic-releasing factors and the pituitary portal vessels.[38] Two general types of tuberohypophyseal neurons project to the external zone: (1) peptide-secreting (peptidergic) neurons including thyrotropin-releasing hormone (TRH), corticotropin-releasing hormone (CRH), and gonadotropin-releasing hormone (GnRH) (see Fig. 7–1) and (2) neurons containing monoamines (e.g., dopamine and serotonin). Although the secretion of these substances into the portal circulation is an important control mechanism, some peptides and neurotransmitters in nerve endings are not released into the hypophyseal-portal circulation but instead function to regulate the secretion of other nerve terminals.[42] The anatomic relationships of nerve endings, basement membranes, interstitial spaces, fenestrated (windowed) capillary endothelia, and glia in the median eminence are similar to those in the neural lobe. As in the case of neurohormone secretion from the neurohypophysis, depolarization of hypothalamic cells leads to the release of neuropeptides and monoamines at the median eminence.

Nonneuronal supporting cells in the hypothalamus also play a dynamic role in hypophyseotropic regulation. For example, nerve terminals in the neurohypophysis are enveloped by pituicytes; when the gland is inactive they surround the nerve endings, whereas they retract to expose the terminals when AVP secretion is enhanced as in states of dehydration. Within the median eminence, GnRH nerve endings are enveloped by the tanycytes, which also cover or uncover neurons with changes in functional status.[41,43] Thus, supporting elements, with their own sets of receptors, can change the neuroregulatory milieu within the hypothalamus, median eminence, and pituitary.

The site of production, the genetics, and the regulation of synthesis and release of individual peptide-releasing factors are discussed in detail in later sections. Briefly, the cell groups in the hypothalamus that contain releasing factors that are secreted into the pituitary portal circulation are located in several cell groups of the medial hypothalamus (Table 7–2).[34,44] These cell groups include the arcuate (infundibular) nucleus (see Fig. 7–3D), the PVH (see Fig. 7–3A and C), the periventricular nucleus, and a group of cells in the medial preoptic area near the organum vasculosum of the lamina terminalis (OVLT) (Fig. 7–5). As discussed earlier, magnicellular neurons in the SON and PVH send axons that predominantly traverse the median eminence to terminate in the neural lobe of the pituitary. In addition, a smaller number of magnicellular axons project directly to the external zone of the median eminence, but their functional significance is unknown.

The third structure often grouped as a component of the median eminence is the pars tuberalis. The pars tuberalis is a subdivision of the adenohypophysis and is a thin sheet of glandular tissue that lies around the infundibulum and pituitary stalk. In some animals, the epithelial component may make up as much as 10% of the total glandular tissue of the anterior pituitary. The pars tuberalis contains cells making pituitary tropic hormones including luteinizing hormone (LH) and thyrotropin (thyroid stimulating hormone [TSH]). A definitive physiologic function of the pars tuberalis is not established, but melatonin receptors are expressed in the pars tuberalis.

TABLE 7–2 STRUCTURAL FORMULAS OF PRINCIPAL HUMAN HYPOTHALAMIC PEPTIDES DIRECTLY RELATED TO PITUITARY SECRETION

Vasopressin
Cys-Tyr-Phe-Gln-Asn-Cys-Pro-Arg-Gly-NH_2 (MW = 1084.38)

Oxytocin
Cys-Tyr-Ile-Gln-Asn-Cys-Pro-Leu-Gly-NH_2 (MW = 1007.35)

Thyrotropin-Releasing Hormone
pGlu-His-Pro-NH_2 (MW = 362.42)

Gonadotropin-Releasing Hormone
pGlu-His-Trp-Ser-Tyr-Gly-Leu-Arg-Pro-Gly-NH_2 (MW = 1182.39)

Corticotropin-Releasing Hormone
Ser-Glu-Glu-Pro-Pro-Ile-Ser-Leu-Asp-Leu-Thr-Phe-His-Leu-Leu-Arg-Glu-Val-Leu-Glu-Met-Ala-Arg-Ala-Glu-Gln-Leu-Ala-Gln-Gln-Ala-His-Ser-Asn-Arg-Lys-Leu-Met-Glu-Ile-Ile-NH_2 (MW = 4758.14)

Growth Hormone–Releasing Hormone (GHRH 1-40; 1-44-NH_2, Human)
Tyr-Ala-Asp-Ala-Ile-Phe-Thr-Asn-Ser-Tyr-Arg-Lys-Val-Leu-Gly-Gln-Leu-Ser-Ala-Arg-Lys-Leu-Leu-Gln-Asp-Ile-Met-Ser-Arg-Gln-Gln-Gly-Glu-Ser-Asn-Gln-Glu-Arg-Gly-Ala (MW = 4544.73); [-Arg-Ala-Arg-Leu-NH_2] (MW = 5040.4)

Somatostatin
Ala-Gly-Cys-Lys-Asn-Phe-Phe-Trp-Lys-Thr-Phe-Thr-Ser-Cys (MW = 1638.12)

Somatostatin-28
Ser-Ala-Asn-Ser-Asn-Pro-Ala-Met-Ala-Pro-Arg-Glu-Arg-Lys-Ala-Gly-Cys-Lys-Asn-Phe-Phe-Trp-Lys-Thr-Phe-Thr-Ser-Cys (MW = 3149.0)

Somatostatin-28 (1-12)
Ser-Ala-Asn-Ser-Asn-Pro-Ala-Met-Ala-Pro-Arg-Glu (MW = 1244.49)

Vasoactive Intestinal Peptide
His-Ser-Asp-Ala-Val-Phe-Thr-Asp-Asn-Tyr-Thr-Arg-Leu-Arg-Lys-Gln-Met-Ala-Val-Lys-Lys-Tyr-Leu-Asn-Ser-Ile-Leu-Asn-NH_2 (MW = 3326.26)

Prolactin-Releasing-Peptide (PrRP31; PrRP20)
[Ser-Arg-Thr-His-Arg-His-Ser-Met-Glu-Ile-Arg]-Thr-Pro-Asp-Ile-Asn-Pro-Ala-Trp-Tyr-Ala-Ser-Arg-Gly-Ile-Arg-Pro-Val-Gly-Arg-Phe-NH_2 (MW = 3665.16; 2273.58)

Ghrelin
Gly-Ser-Ser-Phe-Leu-Ser-Pro-Glu-His-Gln-Arg-Val-Gln-Gln-Arg-Lys-Glu-Ser-Lys-Lys-Pro-Pro-Ala-Lys-Leu-Gln-Pro-Arg (MW = 3314.9) [Ser 3 is *n*-octanoylated]

Disulfide bonds between pairs of cystines that produce cyclization of the peptides are indicated by brackets above the sequences.
MW, Molecular weight; *pGlu*, pyro-glutamyl.

CIRCUMVENTRICULAR ORGANS

A fundamental principle of physiology and neuropharmacology is that the brain, including the hypothalamus, resides in an environment that is protected from humoral signals.[41,45,46] The exclusion of macromolecules is due to the structural vascular specializations that make up the blood-brain barrier. These specializations include tight junctions of brain vascular endothelial cells that preclude the free passage of polarized macromolecules including peptides and hormones. In addition, astrocytic foot processes and perivascular microglial cells contribute to the integrity of the blood-brain barrier.[46] However, to exert

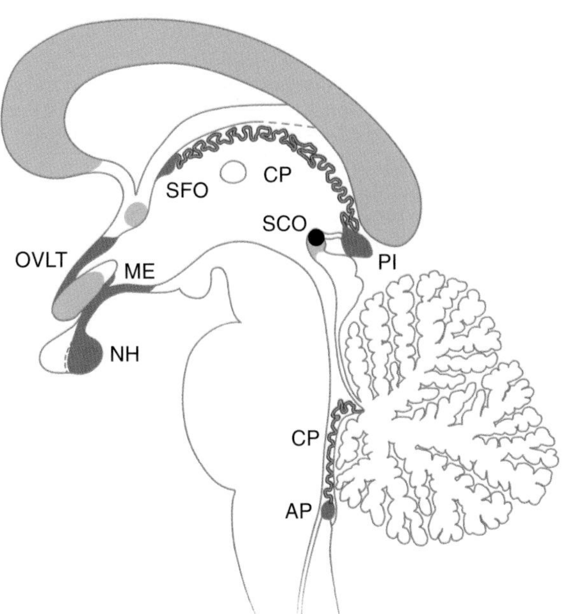

Figure 7–5 ■ Median sagittal section through the human brain to show the circumventricular organs (*black*). Cross-hatched areas are the optic chiasm, corpus callosum, anterior and posterior commisures. *AP,* Area postrema; *ME,* median eminence; *NH,* neurohypophysis; *OVLT,* organum vasculosum of the lamina terminalis; *PI,* pineal body; *SFO,* subfornical organ; *SCO,* subcommissural organ; *CP,* choroid plexus. (From Weindl A. Neuroendocrine aspects of circumventricular organs. In Ganong WF, Martini L, eds. Frontiers in Neuroendocrinology, Vol 3. New York: Oxford University Press, 1973:3-32.)

homeostatic control, the brain must assess key sensory information from the bloodstream including hormone levels, metabolites, and potential toxins. For example, to monitor key signals, the brain has "windows on the circulation" or circumventricular organs (CVOs) that serve as a conduit of peripheral cues into key neuronal cell groups that maintain homeostasis.[45,46]

As the name implies, CVOs are specialized structures that lie on the midline of the brain along the third and fourth ventricles. These structures include the OVLT, subfornical organ (SFO), median eminence, neurohypophysis (posterior pituitary), subcommissural organ, and the area postrema (see Fig. 7–5). Unlike the vasculature in the rest of the brain, the blood vessels in CVOs have fenestrated capillaries that allow relatively free passage of molecules such as proteins and peptide hormones. Thus, neurons and glial cells that reside within the CVOs have access to these macromolecules. In addition to the distinct nature of the vessels themselves, the CVOs have an unusually rich blood supply, allowing them to act as integrators at the interface of the blood-brain barrier. As discussed in more detail in the following subsections, several of the CVOs have major projections to hypothalamic nuclear groups that regulate homeostasis. Thus, the CVOs serve as a critical link between peripheral metabolic cues, hormones, and potential toxins and cell groups within the brain that regulate coordinated endocrine, autonomic, and behavioral responses. Detailed discussion of the physiologic roles of individual CVOs is beyond the scope of this chapter, but several in-depth reviews have assessed the function of each.[45-48]

Median Eminence

The median eminence and neurohypophysis contain the neurosecretory axons that control pituitary function. The role of the median eminence as a link between the hypothalamus and the pituitary gland is detailed in other sections of this chapter (see Figs. 7–2 and 7–4 and see Hypothalamic-Pituitary Unit). However, it is important to understand that the anatomic location of the median eminence places it in a position to serve as an afferent sensory organ as well. Specifically, the median eminence is located adjacent to several neuroendocrine and autonomic regulatory nuclei at the tuberal level of the hypothalamus (see Fig. 7–3). These nuclear groups include the arcuate, ventromedial, dorsomedial, and paraventricular nuclei.[34]

A role of hypothalamic nuclei surrounding the median eminence as afferent sensory centers is supported by several observations. For example, toxins such as monosodium glutamate and gold thioglucose damage neurons in cell groups overlying the median eminence, resulting in obesity and hyperphagia. Experimental evidence suggests that the median eminence is a portal of entry for hormones such as leptin. Indeed, administration of radiolabeled peptides or hormones, such as α-MSH or leptin, led to their accumulation around the median eminence.[49,50] Moreover, leptin receptor messenger ribonucleic acid (mRNA) and leptin-induced gene expression are densely localized in the arcuate, ventromedial, dorsomedial, and ventral premammillary hypothalamic nuclei.[51] Leptin is an established mediator of body weight and neuroendocrine function that acts on several cells in the hypothalamus including POMC neurons that reside in the arcuate nucleus.[15,51,52] Notably, POMC neurons are also found embedded within the median eminence. Thus, it is likely that the median eminence is involved in conveying information from humoral factors such as leptin to key hypothalamic regulatory neurons in the medial basal hypothalamus.[41]

Organum Vasculosum of the Lamina Terminalis and the Subfornical Organ

The OVLT and the SFO are located at the front wall of the third ventricle, the lamina terminalis. The OVLT and SFO lie at the ventral and dorsal boundaries of the third ventricle, respectively (see Fig. 7–5).[45] Because it lies at the rostral and ventral tip of the third ventricle, the OVLT is surrounded by cell groups of the preoptic region of the hypothalamus. Like other CVOs, the OVLT is composed of neurons, glial cells, and tanycytes. It is also noteworthy that axon terminals containing several neuropeptides and neurotransmitters including GnRH, somatostatin, angiotensin, dopamine, norepinephrine, serotonin, acetylcholine, oxytocin, AVP, and TRH innervate the OVLT. In the rodent, neurons that contain GnRH surround the OVLT. In addition, the OVLT in the rat brain contains estrogen receptors and the application of estrogen or electric stimulation at this site is capable of stimulating ovulation through GnRH-containing neurons that project to the median eminence, suggesting that the region regulates sexual behavior in the rat.[43]

The region of the hypothalamus that immediately surrounds the OVLT regulates a diverse array of autonomic processes. However, as the OVLT is potentially involved in the maintenance of so many processes, definitive studies ascribing specific functions to the OVLT are inherently difficult. For example, lesions of the OVLT and surrounding preoptic area led to altered febrile responses after immunologic stimulation and disruptions in fluid and electrolyte balance, blood pressure, reproduction, and thermoregulation. Indeed, large lesions of the OVLT attenuated lipopolysaccharide (LPS)-induced fever.[53] Consistent with this finding, it has been demonstrated that receptors for prostaglandin E_2 (PGE_2) are located within and immediately surrounding the OVLT.[54] Because PGE_2 is thought to be an obligate endogenous pyrogen, the OVLT may be a critical regulator of febrile responses.

The OVLT is also likely to be involved in sensing serum osmolality because lesions of the OVLT attenuate vasopressin and oxytocin secretion in response to osmotic stimuli. In addition, hypertonic saline administration to rats induced c-Fos (a marker of neuronal activation) in OVLT neurons.[55] The efferent projections of the OVLT are not well defined because of the inherent difficulty of injecting this small structure with specific neuroanatomic tracers without contaminating surrounding preoptic nuclei. However, the neurons in the OVLT apparently have a remarkably restricted range of projections that include the paraventricular and supraoptic nuclei, the dorsomedial hypothalamic nucleus, and the lateral hypothalamic area (Elmquist JK, Sherin JE, and Saper CB, unpublished observations.)

The SFO is located in the roof of the third ventricle below the fornix. This CVO critically regulates fluid homeostasis and contributes to blood pressure regulation.[45] Consistent with these functions, the SFO has receptors for angiotensin II and atrial natriuretic peptide.[47,56] In addition to expressing these key receptors, the SFO is thought to regulate fluid homeostasis because of its specific and massive projections to key hypothalamic regulatory sites. Notable among these are the inputs to oxytocin and AVP magnicellular neurons in the supraoptic and paraventricular nuclei. Parvicellular neurons in the PVH concerned with neuroendocrine and autonomic control also receive innervation from the SFO. In addition, the SFO densely innervates the paramedian preoptic region of the hypothalamus (often known as the anteroventral third ventricular region) and other hypothalamic sites including the perifornical area of the lateral hypothalamus. A major cell group within the anteroventral third ventricular region is the median preoptic nucleus, which receives dense innervation from the SFO.[57] Several neuroanatomic studies have demonstrated that the median preoptic nucleus is a major source of afferents to the magnicellular neuroendocrine neurons in the paraventricular and supraoptic hypothalamic nuclei.

In addition to the preceding neuroanatomic findings, physiologic evidence suggests that the SFO is critical in maintaining fluid balance. For example, Simpson and Routtenberg demonstrated that substances such as angiotensin II induced drinking behavior only when the SFO was intact. Specifically, they found that low doses of angiotensin II when injected into the SFO elicited drinking.[58] Later studies demonstrated that SFO neurons have electrophysiologic responses to angiotensin II.[47] In addition, stimulation of the SFO elicited vasopressin secretion. Like the OVLT, the SFO expressed c-Fos after stimulation by hypertonic saline administration.[55] Thus, the SFO provides dense direct and indirect innervation to the magnicellular neuroendocrine neurons in the paraventricular and supraoptic nuclei that are critical in the maintenance of fluid balance and blood pressure.

Area Postrema

The area postrema lies at the caudal end of the fourth ventricle adjacent to the nucleus of the solitary tract (see Fig. 7–5). In experimental animals such as the rat and mouse, it is a midline structure lying above the nucleus of the solitary tract.[46,59] However, in humans the area postrema is a bilateral structure. As the area postrema overlies the nucleus of the solitary tract, it also receives direct visceral afferent input from the glossopharyngeal nerve (including the carotid sinus nerve) and the vagus nerve. In addition, the area postrema receives direct input from several hypothalamic nuclei. The efferent projections of the area postrema include projections to the nucleus of the solitary tract, ventral lateral medulla, and the parabrachial nucleus. Consistent with its role as a sensory organ, the area postrema is enriched with receptors for several neuropeptides including glucagon-like peptide-I and cholecystokinin (CCK).[60,61] It also contains chemosensory neurons that include osmoreceptors.[45] Notably, the area postrema is thought to be critical in the detection of potential toxins and can induce vomiting in response to foreign substances. In fact, the area postrema is often referred to as the chemoreceptor trigger zone.[59]

The best-described physiologic role of the area postrema is the coordinated control of blood pressure.[45,46] For example, the area postrema contains binding sites for angiotensin II, AVP, and atrial natriuretic peptide. Moreover, lesions of the area postrema in rats blunt the rise in blood pressure induced by angiotensin II.[62] Finally, administration of angiotensin II induces the expression of c-Fos in neurons of the area postrema. The area postrema has also been hypothesized to play a role in responding to inflammatory cytokines during the acute febrile response.

Subcommissural Organ

The subcommissural organ (SCO) is located near the junction of the third ventricle and cerebral aqueduct below the posterior commissure and the pineal gland (see Fig. 7–5).[45] It is composed of specialized ependymal cells that secrete a highly glycosylated protein of unknown function. The secretion of this protein leads to aggregation and formation of the so-called Reissner's fibers.[48] The glycoproteins are extruded through the aqueduct, the fourth ventricle, and the spinal cord lumen to terminate in the caudal spinal canal. In humans, intracellular secretory granules are identifiable in the SCO but Reissner's fibers are absent. The SCO secretion in humans is therefore presumed to be more soluble and to be absorbed directly from the CSF. Compared with other CVOs, the physiologic role of the SCO is largely unknown. Hypothesized roles for the SCO include clearance of substances from the CSF.[48]

PINEAL GLAND

Historically, the functional significance of the pineal gland has been obscure. For example, Descartes called the pineal gland the "seat of the soul." The pineal gland is both an endocrine and a circumventricular organ; it is derived from cells from the roof of the third ventricle and lies above the posterior commissure near the level of the habenular complex and the sylvian aqueduct. The pineal gland is composed of two cell types, pinealocytes and interstitial (glial-like) cells. Histologic studies suggest that the pineal gland cells are secretory in nature, and indeed the pineal is the principal source of melatonin in mammals. As discussed subsequently, the pineal gland integrates information encoded by light into coordinated secretions that underlie biologic rhythmicity.[63,64]

The pineal is an epithalamic structure and consists of primordial photoreceptive cells. The pineal retains its light sensitivity in lower vertebrates such as fish and amphibians but lacks photosensitivity in mammals and has evolved as a strictly secretory organ in higher vertebrates. However, neuroanatomic studies have established that light-encoded information is relayed to the pineal by a polysynaptic pathway. This series of synapses ultimately results in innervation of the gland by noradrenergic sympathetic nerve terminals that are critical regulators of melatonin production and release. Specifically, the retina provides direct innervation to the SCN of the hypothalamus through the retinohypothalamic tract.[65] The SCN in turn provides input to the dorsal parvicellular PVH, a key cell group in neuroendocrine and autonomic control. This input is provided through direct and indirect pathways by intrahypothalamic projections.[66,67]

The PVH in turn provides direct innervation to sympathetic preganglionic neurons in the intermediolateral cell column of the thoracic regions of the spinal cord.[68] Sympathetic preganglionic neurons innervate postganglionic neurons in the superior cervical ganglion,[69] which in turn provide the noradrenergic innervation to the pineal (see Hypothalamic-Pituitary Unit). This rather circuitous pathway represents the anatomic substrate for light to regulate the secretion of melatonin. It is important to note that in the absence of light input, the pineal gland rhythms persist but are not entrained to the external light-dark cycle.

The Pineal Is the Source of Melatonin

The predominant hormone secreted by the pineal gland is melatonin. However, the pineal contains other biogenic amines, peptides, and GABA. Pineal-derived melatonin is synthesized from tryptophan, through serotonin, with the rate-limiting step catalyzed by the enzyme arylalkylamine *N*-acetyltransferase (AANAT) (Fig. 7–6).[70,71] Hydroxyindole-*O*-methyltransferase (HIOMT) catalyzes the final step of melatonin synthesis. These enzymes are expressed in a pineal specific manner; however, HIOMT is also expressed in the retina and red blood cells. Melatonin plays a key role in regulating a myriad of circadian rhythms, and a fundamental principle of circadian biology is that the synthesis of melatonin is exquisitely controlled.[63] This control is exerted at several levels. AANAT mRNA levels, AANAT activity, and melatonin synthesis and release are regulated in a circadian fashion and are entrained by the light-dark cycle, with darkness thought to be the most important signal.[64,70,71] For example, melatonin and AANAT levels are highest during the dark and decrease sharply with the onset of light. Melatonin is not stored to any significant degree and thus is released into blood or CSF directly after its biosynthesis in proportion to AANAT activity.

The CNS control of melatonin secretion during the dark is mediated by the neuroanatomic pathway outlined above. Lack of light ultimately results in the release of norepinephrine from postganglionic sympathetic nerve terminals that act on β-adrenergic receptors in pinealocytes, resulting in an increase in adenylyl cyclase activity and synthesis of cyclic adenosine monophosphate (cAMP) from ATP.[70] Increased levels of intracellular cAMP activate downstream signal transduction cascades, including the catalytic subunits of protein kinase A and phosphorylation of cAMP response element-binding protein. Notably, cAMP response elements have been identified in the promoter of AANAT.[70,72] Thus, light (or lack of it) acting through the sympathetic nervous system induces an increase in cAMP, representing a fundamental regulator of AANAT transcription and melatonin synthesis that ultimately results in a dramatic change of melatonin levels across the day.

Physiologic Roles of Melatonin

One of the best characterized roles of melatonin is the regulation of the reproductive axis, including gonadotropin secretion[73] and the timing and onset of puberty (see Gonadotropin-Releasing Hormone and Control of the Reproductive Axis). The potent regulation of the reproductive axis by melatonin is established in rodents and domestic animals such as the sheep. It was observed experimentally with the demonstration that removal of the pineal leads to precocious puberty and ameliorates the effects of constant darkness to induce gonadal involution. In addition, male rats exposed to constant darkness or blinded by enucleation display testicular atrophy and decreased levels of testosterone. These profound effects are normalized by removal of the pineal gland.[74] The physiologic significance of melatonin is probably most important in species referred to as seasonal breeders. Indeed, the role of melatonin in regulating reproductive capacity in species such as the sheep and the horse is now established. This type of reproductive strategy probably evolved to synchronize the length of day with the gestational period of the species to ensure that the offspring are born at favorable times of the year and maximize the viability of the young. Interestingly, although there is a strong and consistent correlation between altered melatonin secretion, day length, and seasonal breeding in diverse species, the valence of the signal can be either positive or negative dependent on the ecologic niche for each species.

Despite the potent effects of day length on reproduction in these species, exact mechanisms of melatonin regulation of GnRH release are unsettled. However, melatonin inhibits LH release from the rat pars tuberalis.[73] The role of the pineal in human reproduction is even less understood.[75] Earlier onset of menarche in blind women has been reported. In addition, a decline in melatonin at puberty has been described in some, but not other studies.

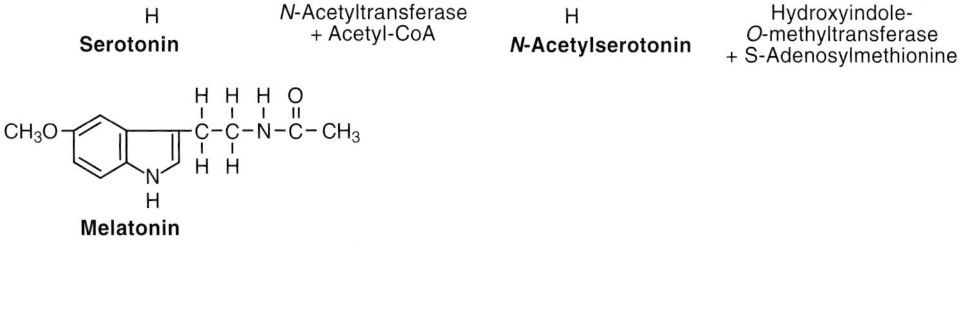

Tryptophan → (Tryptophan hydroxylase) → 5-Hydroxytryptophan → (5-Hydroxytryptophan decarboxylase) → Serotonin → (*N*-Acetyltransferase + Acetyl-CoA) → *N*-Acetylserotonin → (Hydroxyindole-*O*-methyltransferase + S-Adenosylmethionine) → Melatonin

Figure 7–6 ▪ Biosynthesis of melatonin from tryptophan in the pineal gland. Step 1 is catalyzed by tryptophan hydroxylase, step 2 by aromatic-l-amino acid decarboxylase, step 3 by arylalkylamine *N*-acetyltransferase, and step 4 by hydroxyindole-*O*-methyltransferase. (From Wurtman RJ, Axelrod J, Kelly DE, eds. Biochemistry of the pineal gland. In The Pineal. New York: Academic Press, 1968:47-75.)

Interspecies comparative studies of melatonin's physiologic function must be tempered by knowledge of key differences between rodent and human melatonin regulation. Significantly more light, as much as 4 log units, is required in humans to produce an equivalent nocturnal suppression of melatonin[76] and the control of AANAT is largely posttranscriptional in humans rather than transcriptional.[71]

Melatonin Receptors

Melatonin mediates its effects by acting on a family of G protein–coupled receptors, which have been characterized by pharmacologic, neuroanatomic, and molecular approaches.[63,64,71] The first member of the family, MT1 (Mel_{1a}), is a high-affinity receptor that was isolated originally from *Xenopus* melanophores. The second, MT2 (Mel_{1b}), has approximately 60% homology with MT1. A third receptor in mammals, *MT3,* is not a GPCR but instead a high-affinity binding site on the cytosolic enzyme quinone reductase 2 that is involved in cellular detoxification and might account for some of melatonin's effects as an antioxidant.[64,71]

The mechanisms for melatonin's effects on regulating and entraining circadian rhythms are becoming increasingly understood. For example, melatonin inhibits the activity of neurons in the SCN of the hypothalamus, the master circadian pacemaker in the mammalian brain.[63,77,78] Melatonin can entrain several mammalian circadian rhythms, probably by the inhibition of neurons in the SCN. Neuroanatomic evidence suggests that many of the effects of melatonin on circadian rhythms involve actions on MT1 receptors in that the distribution of MT1 mRNA overlaps with radiolabeled melatonin-binding sites in the relevant brain regions. These sites include the SCN, the retina, and the pars tuberalis of the adenohypophysis. The MT2 receptor is also expressed in retina and brain, particularly the SCN, but evidently at much lower levels.[63,71,77]

Genetic studies in mice have also helped illuminate the relative roles of each melatonin receptor in mediating the effects of this hormone. Targeted deletion (knockout) of the MT1 but not the MT2 receptor abolished the ability of melatonin to inhibit the activity of SCN neurons.[78,79] Several studies have suggested that the inhibition of SCN neurons by melatonin is of great physiologic significance. For example, Reppert and colleagues have suggested that elevations of melatonin at night could decrease the responsiveness of the SCN to activity-related stimuli that could result in phase shifts. As noted, light potently inhibits melatonin synthesis and release. Thus, melatonin may underlie the mechanism by which light induces phase shifts. However, it should be noted that lack of the MT1 gene does not block the ability of melatonin to induce phase shifts. These unexpected and somewhat confusing results have resulted in the hypothesis that MT2 is involved in melatonin-induced phase shifts, because this receptor may be expressed in the SCN in human brain.[71]

Melatonin Therapy in Humans

Melatonin is purported to exert multiple beneficial functions that include slowing or reversing the progression of aging, protecting against ischemic damage after vascular reperfusion, and enhancing immune function.[64,71] However, the most studied and established role of melatonin in humans is that of phase shifting and resetting circadian rhythms. In this context, melatonin has been used to treat jet lag and may be effective in treating circadian-based sleep disorders.[80] In addition, melatonin administration has been shown to regulate sleep in humans. Specifically, melatonin has a hypnotic effect at relatively low doses. Melatonin therapy has also been suggested as a way to treat seasonal affective disorders. However, two recent metaanalyses of the published reports on melatonin for the treatment of either primary or secondary sleep disorders concluded that there is limited evidence for significant clinical efficacy, but melatonin is safe with short-term use (≤3 months).[81,82] Because melatonin is now available over the counter and without a prescription throughout the United States, it is important that further controlled clinical studies be conducted to assess fully the therapeutic potential and safety of long-term melatonin use in humans.

HYPOPHYSEOTROPIC HORMONES AND NEUROENDOCRINE AXES

With the demonstration by the first half of the 1900s that pituitary secretion was controlled by hypothalamic hormones released into the portal circulation, the search was on for the hypothalamic-releasing factors. The search for hypothalamic neurohormones with anterior pituitary regulating properties focused on extracts of stalk median eminence, neural lobe, and hypothalamus from sheep and pigs. To give some idea of the Herculean nature of this effort, approximately 250,000 hypothalamic fragments were required to purify and characterize the first such factor, TRH.[9] Such hypophyseotropic substances were initially called *releasing factors* but are now more commonly called *releasing hormones.*

All of the hypothalamic-pituitary regulating hormones are peptides with the notable exception of dopamine, which is a biogenic amine and the principal prolactin-inhibiting factor (PIF) (see Table 7–2). All are available for clinical investigations or diagnostic tests, and therapeutic analogues for dopamine, GnRH, and somatostatin are widely prescribed.

In addition to regulating hormone release, some hypophyseotropic factors control pituitary cell differentiation and proliferation and hormone synthesis. Somatostatin and dopamine are inhibitory, and some act on more than one pituitary hormone. For example, TRH is a potent releaser of prolactin (PRL) and of TSH, and under some circumstances releases corticotropin (adrenocorticotropic hormone [ACTH]) and growth hormone (GH). GnRH releases both LH and follicle-stimulating hormone (FSH). Somatostatin inhibits the secretion of GH, TSH, and a wide variety of nonpituitary hormones. The principal inhibitor of PRL secretion, dopamine, also inhibits secretion of TSH, gonadotropins and, under certain conditions, GH. Dual control is exerted by the interaction of inhibitory and stimulatory hypothalamic hormones. For example, somatostatin interacts with growth hormone–releasing hormone (GHRH) and TRH to control secretion of GH and TSH, respectively, and dopamine interacts with prolactin-releasing factors (PRFs) to regulate PRL secretion. Some hypothalamic hormones act synergistically; for example, CRH and vasopressin act together to regulate the release of pituitary ACTH.

Secretion of the releasing hormones in turn is regulated by neurotransmitters and neuropeptides released by a complex array of neurons synapsing with hypophyseotropic neurons. Control of secretion is also exerted through feedback control by hormones such as glucocorticoids, gonadal steroids, thyroid hormone, anterior pituitary hormones (short-loop feedback control), and hypophyseotropic factors themselves (ultrashort-loop feedback control).

The distribution of the hypophyseotropic hormones is not limited to the hypothalamus. Most are produced in nonhypophyseotropic hypothalamic neurons, in extrahypothalamic regions of the brain, and in peripheral organs where they mediate functions unrelated to pituitary regulation (e.g., effects on behavior or homeostasis). A majority of the peptides, hormones, and neurotransmitters involved in the regulation of hypothalamic-pituitary control transduce their signals through members of the extensive G protein–coupled receptor family (Table 7–3).

Feedback Concepts in Neuroendocrinology

In order to understand the regulation of each hypothalamic-pituitary-target organ axis, it is important to understand some basic concepts of homeostatic systems. A simplified account of feedback control in relation to neuroendocrine regulation is presented in this section.[83-85] Hormonal systems form part of a feedback loop in which the controlled variable (generally the blood hormone level or some biochemical surrogate of the hormone) determines the rate of secretion of the hormone. In negative feedback systems, the controlled variable inhibits hormone output, and in positive feedback control systems, the controlled variable increases hormone secretion. Both negative and positive endocrine feedback control systems can be part of a closed loop, in which regulation is entirely restricted to the interacting regulatory glands, or an open loop, in which the nervous system influences the feedback loop. All pituitary feedback systems have nervous system inputs that either alter the set-point of the feedback control system or introduce open-loop elements that can influence or override the closed-loop control elements.

In engineering formulations of feedback, three controlled variables can be identified: a sensing element that detects the concentration of the controlled variable, a reference input that defines the proper control levels, and an error signal that determines the output of the system. The reference input is the set-point of the system.

Hormonal feedback control systems resemble engineering systems in that the concentration of the hormone in the blood (or some function of the hormone) regulates the output of the controlling gland. Hormonal feedback differs from engineering systems in that the sensor element and the reference input element are not readily distinguishable. The set-point of the controlled variable is determined by a complex cascade beginning with the kinetics of binding to a receptor and the activities of successive intermediate messengers. Sophisticated models incorporating control elements, compartmental analysis, and hormone production and clearance rates exist for many systems.

Endocrine Rhythms

Virtually all functions of living animals (regardless of their position on the evolutionary scale) are subject to periodic or cyclic changes, many of which are influenced mainly by the nervous system (see Table 7–4 for definitions).[86-89] Most periodic changes are free-running; that is, they are intrinsic to the organism, independent of the environment, and driven by a biologic "clock."

Most free-running rhythms are coordinated (entrained) by external signals (cues), such as light-dark changes, meal patterns, cycles of the lunar periods, or the ratio of the length of day to the length of night. External signals of this type (zeitgeber or "time givers") do not bring about the rhythm but provide the synchronizing time cue. Many endogenous rhythms have a period of approximately 24 hours (circadian [around a day] or diurnal rhythms). Circadian changes follow an intrinsic program that is about 24 hours long, whereas diurnal rhythms can be either circadian or dependent on shifts in light and dark. Rhythms that occur more frequently than once a day are ultradian. Infradian rhythms have a period longer than 1 day, as in the approximately 27-day human menstrual cycle and the yearly breeding patterns of some animals.

Most endocrine rhythms are circadian (Fig. 7–7). The secretion of GH and PRL in humans is maximal shortly after the onset of sleep, and that of cortisol is maximal between 2 and 4 AM. TSH secretion is lowest in the morning between 9 AM and 12 noon and maximal between 8 PM and midnight. Gonadotropin secretion in adolescents is increased at night. Superimposed on the circadian cycle are ultradian bursts of hormone secretion. LH secretion during adolescence is characterized by rapid, high-amplitude pulsations at night, whereas in sexually mature individuals secretory episodes are lower in amplitude and occur throughout the 24 hours. GH, ACTH, and PRL are also secreted in brief, fairly regular pulses. The short-term fluctuations in hormonal secretion have important functional significance. In the case of LH, the normal endogenous rhythm of pituitary secretion reflects the pulsatile release of GnRH. The period of approximately 90 minutes between the peak of pulses corresponds to the optimal timing to induce maximal pituitary stimulation. Episodic secretion of GH also enhances its biopotency, but for many rhythms, the function is not clear. Most homeostatic activities are also rhythmic, including body temperature, water balance, blood volume, sleep, and activity.[90,91]

Assessment of endocrine function must take into account the variability of hormone levels in the blood, and appropriately obtained samples at different times of day or night may provide useful dynamic indicators of hypothalamic-pituitary function. For example, the loss of diurnal rhythm of GH and ACTH secretion may be an early sign of hypothalamic dysfunction. Furthermore, the optimal timing for the administration of glucocorticoids to suppress ACTH secretion (as in therapy for congenital adrenal hyperplasia) must take into account the varying suppressibility of the axis at different times of day.

The best understood neural structures responsible for circadian rhythms are the SCN, paired structures in the anterior hypothalamus above the optic chiasm.[87,91] In addition to the retinohypothalamic projection from the retina described earlier, the SCN receives neuronal input from many nuclei. Individual cells of the SCN have an intrinsic capacity to oscillate in a circadian pattern,[92] and the nucleus is organized to permit many reciprocal neuron-neuron interactions through direct synaptic contacts. It is especially rich in neuropeptides, including somatostatin, VIP, NPY, and neurotensin, and microinjections of pancreatic polypeptide into the SCN reset the timing cycle of some circadian rhythms in hamsters. The SCN also responds to the pineal hormone melatonin through melatonin receptors.[64,71] Interestingly, recent studies have indicated that intrinsic pacemaker function is not unique to neurons of the SCN. Circadian oscillators are also found in multiple peripheral tissues.[91]

Metabolic changes in the SCN, such as increased uptake of 2-deoxyglucose and an increased level of VIP, accompany circadian rhythms. This nucleus projects to the pineal gland indirectly via the PVH and the autonomic nervous system (see earlier section on the pineal gland) and regulates its activity.[87] However, the bulk of SCN outflow occurs in a trunk coursing dorsal-laterally through the ventral subparaventricular zone and terminating in the dorsal medial nucleus of the hypothalamus. Polysynaptic pathways involving these latter structures are responsible for the actions of the SCN to produce the circadian rhythms in thermoregulation, glucocorticoid secretion, sleep, arousal, and feeding.[87]

Circadian rhythms during fetal life are regulated by maternal circadian rhythms.[93] Circadian changes can be detected 2 to 3 days before birth, and SCN from fetuses of this age display spontaneous rhythmicity in vitro. Maternal regulation of fetal circadian rhythms may be mediated by circulating melatonin or

TABLE 7–3 RECEPTORS FOR NEUROTRANSMITTERS AND NEUROPEPTIDES INVOLVED IN HYPOTHALAMIC-PITUITARY CONTROL AND NEUROENDOCRINE HOMEOSTASIS

Group and Ligand	Receptor Family	Receptor Protein*	Receptor Gene	Mode of Action⁺
Classic Neurotransmitters				
Catecholamines (NE, E)	α1-Adrenoreceptors	ADA1A (α1A)	ADRA1A	7-TM, $G_{q/11}$
		ADA1B (α1B)	ADRA1B	7-TM, $G_{q/11}$
		ADA1D (α1D)	ADRA1D	7-TM, $G_{q/11}$
	α2-Adrenoreceptors	ADA2A (α2A)	ADRA2A	7-TM, $G_{i/o}$
		ADA2B (α2B)	ADRA2B	7-TM, $G_{i/o}$
		ADA2C (α2C)	ADRA2C	7-TM, $G_{i/o}$
	β-Adrenoreceptors	ADRB1 (β1)	ADRB1	7-TM, G_S
		ADRB3 (β2)	ADRB2	7-TM, G_S
		ADRB3 (β3)	ADRB3	7-TM, G_S
Serotonin (5-OH-tryptamine)	5-HT1 receptors	5HT1A (5HT1A-α)	HTR1A	7-TM, $G_{i/o}$
		5HT1B (5HT1D-β)	HTR1B	7-TM, $G_{i/o}$
		5HT1D (5HT1D-α)	HTR1D	7-TM, $G_{i/o}$
		5HT1E	HTR1E	7-TM, $G_{i/o}$
	5-HT2 receptors	5HT2A	HTR2A	7-TM, $G_{q/11}$
		5HT2B	HTR2B	7-TM, $G_{q/11}$
		5HT2C (5HT1C)	HTR2C	7-TM, $G_{q/11}$
	5-HT3 receptors	5HT3	Pentamer	Cation flux
		Subunit genes:	HTR3A, HTR3B	
	5-HT4 receptors	5HT4R	HTR4	7-TM, G_S
Dopamine	Dopamine receptors	DRD1 (D1-R, D1A)	DRD1	7-TM, G_S
		DRD2 (D2-R)	DRD2	7-TM, $G_{i/o}$
		DRD3 (D3-R)	DRD3	7-TM, $G_{i/o}$
		DRD4 (D4-R, D2C)	DRD4	7-TM, $G_{i/o}$
		DRD5 (D5-R, D1B)	DRD5	7-TM, G_S
Histamine	Histamine receptors	HRH1 (H1-R)	HRH1	7-TM, $G_{q/11}$
		HRH2 (H2-R)	HRH2	7-TM, G_S
		HRH3 (H3-R)	HRH3	7-TM, $G_{i/o}$
Melatonin	Melatonin receptors	MT1RA (Mel1AR, MT1)	MTNR1A	7-TM, $G_{i/o}$, PLC-β
		MT1RB (Mel1BR, MT2)	MTNR1B	7-TM, $G_{i/o}$, $G_{q/11}$
		MT3 (quinone reductase 2)	NQO2	cytosolic enzyme
Trace amines	Trace amine receptor	TAAR1 (TaR-1)	TAAR1	7-TM, ••
Acetylcholine	Muscarinic receptors	ACM1 (M1)	CHRM1	7-TM, $G_{q/11}$
		ACM2 (M2)	CHRM2	7-TM, $G_{q/11}$
		ACM3 (M3)	CHRM3	7-TM, $G_{q/11}$
		ACM4 (M4)	CHRM4	7-TM, $G_{i/o}$
		ACM5 (M5)	CHRM5	7-TM, $G_{q/11}$
	Nicotinic receptors	ACHA-P, ACH1-7	Pentamer	Cation flux
		Subunit genes:	CHRNA, CHRNB	
Glutamate	Ionotropic receptors	NMDA (NR1, NR2A-D)	Oligomer	Cation flux
		NMZ1 subunit gene:	GRIN1 (NMDAR1)	
		AMPA (GluR1-4)	Oligomer	Cation flux
		GRIA1 subunit gene:	GRIA1 (GLUR1)	
		Kainate (GluR5-7, KA-1/2)	Oligomer	Cation flux
		LK1 subunit gene:	GRIK1 (GLUR5)	
	Metabotropic receptors	MGR1 (mGluR1)	GRM1	7-TM, $G_{q/11}$
		MGR2 (mGluR2)	GRM2	7-TM, $G_{i/o}$
		MGR3 (mGluR3)	GRM3	7-TM, $G_{i/o}$
		MGR4 (mGluR4)	GRM4	7-TM, $G_{i/o}$
		MGR5 (mGluR5)	GRM5	7-TM, $G_{q/11}$
		MGR6 (mGluR6)	GRM6	7-TM, $G_{i/o}$
		MGR7 (mGluR7)	GRM7	7-TM, $G_{i/o}$
γ-aminobutyric acid (GABA)	Ionotropic	GAA-E (GABA-A-R)	Pentamer	[Cl^-] ion flux
		GAA1 (α1) subunit gene	GABRA1	
	Heterodimeric	GABR1 (GABA-B-R1)	GABBR1	7-TM, $G_{i/o}$
		GABR2 (GABA-B-R2)	GABBR2	7-TM, $G_{i/o}$
Neuropeptides				
Neurohypophyseal hormones				
Vasopressin	Vasopressin receptors	V1AR (V1a)	AVPR1A	7-TM, $G_{q/11}$
		V1BR (V1b, V3)	AVPR1B	7-TM, $G_{q/11}$
		V2R (ADH-R)	AVPR2	7-TM, G_S
Oxytocin	Oxytocin receptor	OXYR (OT-R)	OXTR	7-TM, $G_{q/11}$
Hypophyseotropic hormones				
TRH	TRH receptor	TRFR (TRH-R)	TRHR	7-TM, $G_{q/11}$
GHRH	GHRH receptor	GHRHR (GRFR)	GHRHR	7-TM, G_S
GHRP/Ghrelin	GHS receptor	GHSR (GHRP-R)	GHSR	7-TM, $G_{q/11}$
GnRH	GnRH receptor	GNRHR (GnRH-R)	GNRHR	7-TM, $G_{q/11}$
GRH/Urocortin	CRH receptors	CRFR1 (CRH-R1)	CRHR1	7-TM, G_S
		CRFR2 (CRH-R2)	CRHR2	7-TM, G_S

Table continued on following page 99

TABLE 7–3 RECEPTORS FOR NEUROTRANSMITTERS AND NEUROPEPTIDES INVOLVED IN HYPOTHALAMIC-PITUITARY CONTROL AND NEUROENDOCRINE HOMEOSTASIS (Continued)

Group and Ligand	Receptor Family	Receptor Protein*	Receptor Gene	Mode of Action⁺
Somatostatin/Cortistatin	Somatostatin receptors	SSR1 (SS1R, SRIF-2)	SSTR1	7-TM, $G_{i/o}$
		SSR2 (SS2R, SRIF-1)	SSTR2	7-TM, $G_{i/o}$
		SSR3 (SS3R, SSR-28)	SSTR3	7-TM, $G_{i/o}$
		SSR4 (SS4R)	SSTR4	7-TM, $G_{i/o}$
		SSR5 (SS5R)	SSTR5	7-TM, $G_{i/o}$
Endogenous opioid peptides				
β-endorphin	Mu opioid receptor	OPRM (μ, MOR-1)	OPRM1	7-TM, $G_{i/o}$
Enkephalin	Delta opioid receptor	OPRD (δ, DOR-1)	OPRD1	7-TM, $G_{i/o}$
Dynorphin	Kappa opioid receptor	OPRK (κ, KOR-1)	OPRK1	7-TM, $G_{i/o}$
Nociceptin/OFQ	OFQ opioid receptor	OPRX (KOR-3)	OPRL1	7-TM, $G_{i/o}$
Melanocortin peptides				
MSH	MSH receptor	MSHR (MC1-R)	MC1R	7-TM, G_S
ACTH	ACTH receptor	ACTHR (MC2-R)	MC2R	7-TM, G_S
γMSH, MSH	Melanocortin receptor 3	MC3R (MC3-R)	MC3R	7-TM, G_S
MSH, βMSH	Melanocortin receptor 4	MC4R (MC4-R)	MC4R	7-TM, G_S
MSH	Melanocortin receptor 5	MC5R (MC5-R)	MC5R	7-TM, G_S
Tachykinins (neurokinins)				
Substance P	Neurokinin receptors	NK1R (SPR)	TACR1	7-TM, $G_{i/o}$
Substance K		NK2R (SKR)	TACR2	7-TM, $G_{i/o}$
Neurokinin B		NKR3 (NKR)	TACR3	7-TM, $G_{i/o}$
Vasoactive peptides				
Angiotensin II	Angiotensin receptors	AGTR1 (AT1)	AGTR1	7-TM, $G_{q/11}$
		AGTR2 (AT2)	AGTR2	7-TM, $G_{i/o}$
Atrial natriuretic peptide	ANP receptors	ANPRA (NPR-A)	NPR1	cGMP, 1-TM
		ANPRB (NPR-B)	NPR2	cGMP, 1-TM
Endothelin	Endothelin receptors	ENDRA (ETA-R)	EDNRA	7-TM, $G_{q/11}$
		ENDRB (ETB-R)	EDNRB	7-TM, $G_{q/11}$
Miscellaneous neuropeptides				
CART	No receptor identified			•• 7-TM, $G_{i/o}$
Orexin/hypocretin	Orexin receptors	OX1R (HCRTR-1)	HCRTR1	7-TM, many
		OX2R (HCRTR-2)	HCRTR2	7-TM, many
Melanin-concentrating hormone	MCH receptor	MCHR1 (GPCR24)	MCHR1	7-TM, $G_{i/q}$
Prolactin-releasing peptide	PRP receptor	PRLHR (GPCR10)	PRLHR	7-TM, $G_{i/o/q}$
Kisspeptins/Metastin	Kisspeptin receptor	KISSR (GPCR54)	KISS1R	7-TM, $G_{q/11}$
Neuromedin U	Neuromedin receptors	NMUR1 (GPCR66)	NMUR1	7-TM, $G_{q/11}$
		NUMR2	NMUR2	7-TM, $G_{q/11}$
Neurotensin	Neurotensin receptor	NTR1 (NTRH)	NTSR1	7-TM, $G_{q/11}$
PACAP	PACAP receptor	PACR (PACAP-R-1)	ADCYAR1R1	7-TM, G_S
Vasoactive intestinal peptide	VIP receptors	VIPR1 (PACAP-R-2)	VIPR1	7-TM, G_S
		VIPR2 (PACAP-R-3)	VIPR3	7-TM, G_S
Galanin/GALP	Galanin receptors	GALR1 (GAL1-R)	GALR1	7-TM, $G_{i/o}$
		GALR2 (GAL2-R)	GALR2	7-TM, $G_{i/o}$
		GALR3 (GAL3-R)	GALR3	7-TM, $G_{i/o}$
Glucagon-like peptide	GLP receptor	GLP1R	GLP1R	7-TM, G_S
CCK/Gastrin	CCK receptors	CCKAR (CCK1-R)	CCKAR	7-TM, $G_{q/11}$
		GASR (CCK2-R)	CCKBR	7-TM, $G_{q/11}$
Neuropeptide Y	NPY/PYY/PP receptors	NPY1R (NPY-Y1)	NPY1R	7-TM, $G_{i/o}$
PYY (3-32)		NPY2R (NPY-Y2)	NPY2R	7-TM, $G_{i/o}$
Pancreatic polypeptide		NPY4R (PP1)	PPYR1	7-TM, $G_{i/o}$
Neuropeptide Y		NPY5R (NPY-Y5)	NPY5R	7-TM, $G_{i/o}$
Other				
Cannabinoid	Cannabinoid receptor	CNR1 (CB1)	CNR1	7-TM, $G_{i/o}$

*Receptors cited are human. Swiss-Prot identifiers and alternative names (in parentheses) are provided for each receptor and were obtained with the use of the GPCRDB information system (http://www.gpcr.org/7tm/) described in: Horn F, Bettler E, Oliveira L, Campagne F, Cohen FE, Vriend G (2003) GPCRDB information system for G protein-coupled receptors. *Nucleic Acids Res.* 31:294-297.

⁺The mode of action designation is oversimplified. It is common for seven transmembrane (7-TM) G-protein coupled receptors (GPCR) to interact with multiple different G-protein complexes depending on the specific cell. $G_{i/o}$, GPCR coupled to the $G_{i/o}$ family, inhibits adenylyl cyclase and decreases intracellular cAMP, opens K^+ channels and closes $Ca2^+$ channels; $G_{q/11}$, GPCR coupled to the $G_{q/11}$ family, stimulates phosphoinositol cascade; G_S, GPCR coupled to the G_S family, stimulates adenylyl cyclase and increases intracellular cAMP; PLC-ß, GPCR coupled to G protein that activates phospholipase Cß (PLC-ß); cGMP, Guanylate cyclase activity intrinsic to these 1 trans-membrane pass receptors.

AMPA, α-amino-3-hydroxy-5-methyl-4-isoxazdeproprionic acid; *CART,* cocaine and amphetamine responsive transcript; *CCK,* cholecystokinin; *CRH,* corticotropin-releasing hormone; *E,* epinephrine; *GALP,* galanin-like peptide; *GHRH,* growth hormone-releasing hormone; *GnRH,* gonadotropin-releasing hormone; *NE,* norepinephrine; *NMDA,* N-methyl-d-aspartate; *OFQ,* orphanin FQ; *PACAP,* pituitary adenylyl cyclase activating peptide; *PYY,* peptide YY; *TRH,* thyrotropin-releasing hormone.

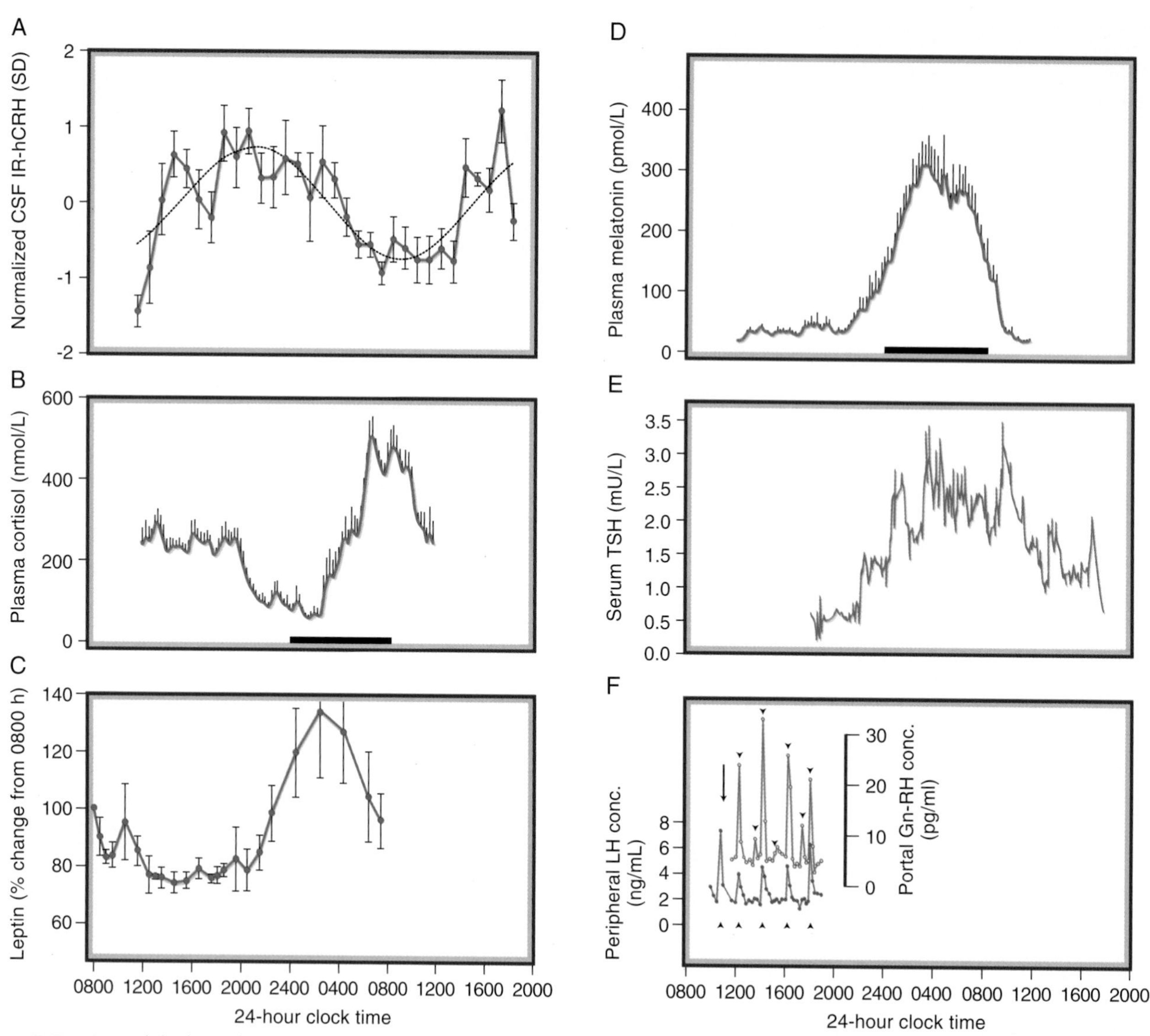

Figure 7–7 ▪ Diurnal rhythms of corticotropin-releasing hormone (CRH) (A), cortisol (B), leptin (C), melatonin (D), and thyrotropin (TSH) in humans (E), and the relationship between gonadotropin-releasing hormone (GnRH) and luteinizing hormone (LH) secretion in sheep (F). *CSF,* Cerebrospinal fluid; *IR,* immunoreactive. (From Kling MA, DeBellis MD, O'Rourke DK, et al. Diurnal variation of cerebrospinal fluid immunoreactive corticotropin-releasing hormone levels in healthy volunteers. J Clin Endocrinol Metab 1994;79:233-239, Fig 3; van Coevorden A, Mockel J, Laurent E, et al. Neuroendocrine rhythms and sleep in aging men. Am J Physiol 1991;260:E651-E661, Fig 1A and C; Sinha MK, Ohannesian JP, Heiman ML, et al. Nocturnal rise of leptin in lean, obese,and non-insulin-dependent diabetes mellitus subjects. J Clin Invest 1996;97:1344-1347, Fig 2; Brabant G, Prank K, Ranft U, et al. Physiological regulation of circadian and pulsatile thyrotropin secretion in normal man and woman. J Clin Endocrinol Metab 1990;70:403-409, Fig 2B; and Clarke IJ, Cummins JT. The temporal relationship between gonadotropin releasing hormone [GnRH] and luteinizing hormone [LH] secretion in ovariectomized ewes. Endocrinology 1982;111:1737-1739, Fig 2A.)

by cyclic changes in the food intake of the mother. The timing of the circadian pacemaker can be shifted in humans by the administration of triazolam, a short-acting benzodiazepine, or melatonin, as described earlier, or by altered patterns of intense illumination.[76]

Thyrotropin-Releasing Hormone

Chemistry and Evolution

TRH, the smallest known peptide-releasing hormone, is the tripeptide pyroGlu-His-Pro-NH_2. Six copies of the TRH peptide sequence are encoded within the human TRH pre-prohormone gene (Fig. 7–8).[94] The rat pro-TRH precursor contains five TRH peptide repeats flanked by dibasic residues (Lys-Arg or Arg-Arg), along with seven or more non-TRH peptides.[95] Two prohormone convertases, PC1 and PC2, cleave the TRH tripeptides at the dibasic residues within the regulated secretory pathway. Carboxypeptidase E then removes the dibasic residues, leaving the sequence Gln-His-Pro-Gly. This peptide is then amidated at the C-terminus by peptidylglycine α-amidating monooxygenase (PAM), with Gly acting as the amide donor. The amino-terminal pyro-Glu residue results from cyclization of the Gln.

Although the TRH tripeptide is the only established hormone encoded within its large prohormone, rat pro-TRH yields seven additional peptides that have unique tissue distributions.[96] Several biologic activities of these peptides have been observed: pro-TRH(160-169) may be a hypophyseotropic factor because it is released from hypothalamic slices and potentiates the TSH-releasing effects of TRH. Pro-TRH(178-199) is also released from the median eminence and appears to inhibit ACTH release. TRH is a phylogenetically ancient peptide, which has been isolated

TABLE 7–4 TERMS USED TO DESCRIBE CYCLIC ENDOCRINE PHENOMENA

Period	Length of the cycle
Circadian	Around a day (24 h)
Diurnal	Exactly a day
Ultradian	Less than a day, i.e., minutes or hours
Infradian	Longer than a day, i.e., month or year
Mean	Arithmetic mean of all values within a cycle
Range	Difference between the highest and lowest values
Nadir	Minimal level (inferred from mathematical curve fitting calculations)
Acrophase	Time of maximal levels (inferred from curve fitting)
Zeitgeber	"Time-giver" (German), the external cue, usually the light-dark cycle that synchronizes endogenous rhythms
Entrainment	The process by which an endogenous rhythm is regulated by a zeitgeber
Phase shift	Induced change in an endogenous rhythm
Intrinsic clock	Neural structures that possess intrinsic capacity for spontaneous rhythms; for circadian rhythms these are located in the suprachiasmatic nucleus

Adapted from Van Cauter E, Turek FW. Endocrine and other biological rhythms. In DeGroot LJ, ed. Endocrinology, 3rd ed. Philadelphia: WB Saunders, 1995:2497-2548.

from primitive vertebrates such as the lamprey, and even invertebrates such as the snail. TRH is widely expressed in both the CNS and periphery in amphibians, reptiles, and fishes but does not stimulate TSH release in these poikilothermic vertebrates. Thus, TRH has multiple peripheral and central activities and was co-opted as a hypophyseotropic factor midway during the evolution of vertebrates, perhaps specifically as a factor needed for coordinated regulation of temperature homeostasis.

Effects on the Pituitary Gland and Mechanism of Action

After intravenous injection of TRH in humans, serum TSH levels rise within a few minutes,[97] followed by a rise in serum triiodothyronine (T_3) levels; there is an increase in thyroxine (T_4) release as well, but a change in blood levels of T_4 is usually not demonstrable because the pool of circulating T_4 (most of which is bound to carrier proteins) is so large. The clinical applications of TRH testing are discussed later in this chapter and in Chapter 10. TRH action on the pituitary is blocked by previous treatment with thyroid hormone, which is a crucial element in feedback control of pituitary TSH secretion.

TRH is also a potent PRF.[97] The time course of response of blood PRL levels to TRH, the dose-response characteristics, and the suppression by thyroid hormone pretreatment (all of which parallel changes in TSH secretion) suggest that TRH may be involved in the regulation of PRL secretion. Moreover, TRH is present in the hypophyseal-portal blood of lactating rats. However, it is unlikely to be a physiologic regulator of PRL secretion because the PRL response to nursing in humans is unaccompanied by changes in plasma TSH levels[98] and mice lacking TRH have normal lactotrophs and basal prolactin secretion.[99] Nevertheless, TRH may occasionally cause hyperprolactin-emia (with or without galactorrhea) in patients with hypothyroidism.

In normal individuals, TRH has no influence on the secretion of pituitary hormones other than TSH and PRL, but it enhances the release of GH in acromegaly and of ACTH in some patients

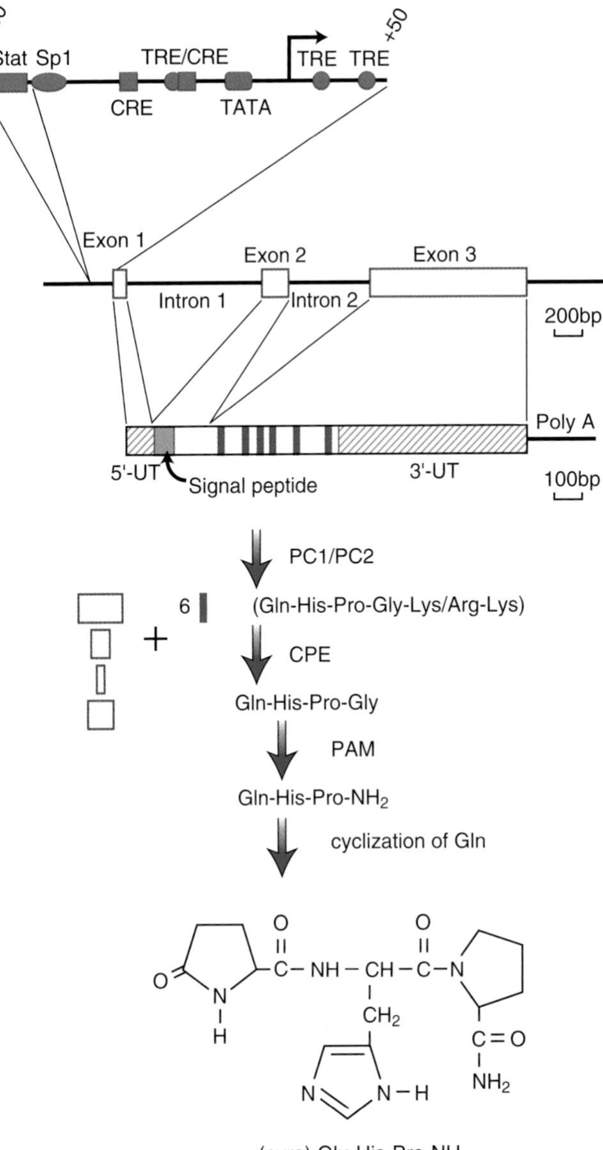

Figure 7–8 ▪ Structure of the human thyrotropin-releasing hormone (TRH) gene, cDNA, and prohormone, showing six repeating codons for the TRH peptide sequence. *CPE,* Carboxypeptidase E; *PAM,* peptidylglycine alpha-amidating monooxygenase; *PC1/PC2,* prohormone convertases 1 and 2. (Adapted from data in Yamada M, Radovick S, Wondisford FE, et al. Cloning and structure of human genomic DNA and hypothalamic cDNA encoding human preprothyrotropin-releasing hormone. Mol Endocrinol 1990;4:551-556.)

with Cushing's disease. Furthermore, prolonged stimulation of the normal pituitary with GHRH can sensitize it to the GH-releasing effects of TRH. TRH also causes the release of GH in some patients with uremia, hepatic disease, anorexia nervosa, and psychotic depression and in children with hypothyroidism.[97] TRH inhibits sleep-induced GH release through its actions in the CNS (see later in the section on extrapituitary actions of TRH).

Stimulatory effects of TRH are initiated by binding of the peptide to specific receptors on the plasma membrane of the thyrotroph.[100] Neither thyroid hormone nor somatostatin, both of which antagonize the effects of TRH, interfere with its binding. TRH action is mediated mainly through hydrolysis of phosphatidylinositol, with phosphorylation of key protein kinases and an increase in intracellular free Ca^{2+} as the crucial step in postreceptor activation (see Chapter 5).[101] TRH effects can be mimicked by exposure to a Ca^{2+} ionophore and are partially abolished by a Ca^{2+}-free medium. TRH stimulates the formation of mRNAs coding for TSH and PRL in addition to regulating their secretion and stimulates the mitogenesis of thyrotrophs.

TRH is degraded to acid TRH and to the dipeptide histidylprolineamide, which cyclizes nonenzymatically to histidylproline diketopiperazine (cyclic His-Pro). Acid TRH has some behavioral effects in rats that are similar to those of TRH but no other proven actions. Cyclic His-Pro is reported to act as a PRF and to have other neural effects, including reversal of ethanol-induced sleep (TRH is also effective in this system), elevation of brain cyclic guanosine monophosphate levels, an increase in stereotypical behavior, modification of body temperature, and inhibition of eating behavior. Some of the effects of TRH may be mediated through cyclic His-Pro, but the fact that cyclic His-Pro is abundant in some areas and is not proportional to the amount of TRH suggests that the peptide may not be derived solely from TRH. This latter assertion appears to be confirmed by the detection of substantial amounts of the dipeptide in brains of TRH knockout mice.[99]

Extrapituitary Function

TRH is present in virtually all parts of the brain: cerebral cortex, circumventricular structures, neurohypophysis, pineal gland, and spinal cord.[102] TRH is also found in pancreatic islet cells and in the gastrointestinal tract. Although it exists in low concentration, the total amount in extrahypothalamic tissues exceeds the amount in the hypothalamus.

The extensive extrahypothalamic distribution of TRH, its localization in nerve endings, and the presence of TRH receptors in brain tissue suggest that TRH serves as a neurotransmitter or neuromodulator outside the hypothalamus. TRH is a general stimulant and induces hyperthermia on intracerebroventricular injection, suggesting a role in central thermoregulation.[102] Studies in TRH knockout mice are expected to further clarify the nonhypophyseotropic actions of TRH.[99]

Clinical Applications

The use of TRH for the diagnosis of hyperthyroidism is less common since the development of ultrasensitive assays for thyroid-stimulating hormone (TSH)[97] (see Chapter 10); its use to discriminate between hypothalamic and pituitary causes of TSH deficiency has also declined because of the test's poor specificity,[97] but the application of ultrasensitive assays in conjunction with the TRH test has not been fully evaluated. TRH testing also is not of value in the differential diagnosis of causes of hyperprolactinemia but is useful for the demonstration of residual abnormal somatotropin-secreting cells in acromegalic patients who release hGH in response to TRH before treatment.

Studies of the effect of TRH on depression have shown inconsistent results, possibly because of poor blood-brain barrier penetration.[102] Intrathecal administration of TRH may improve responses in depressed patients, but its clinical utility is unknown.[103] Although a role for TRH in depression is not established, many depressed patients have a blunted TSH response to TRH and changes in TRH responsiveness correlate with the clinical course. The mechanism by which blunting occurs is unknown.

TRH has been evaluated for the treatment of diverse neurobiologic disorders (for review, see reference 102) including spinal muscle atrophy and amyotrophic lateral sclerosis; transient improvement in strength was reported in both disorders, but the combined experience at many centers using a variety of treatment protocols including long-term intrathecal administration failed to confirm efficacy. TRH administration also reduces the severity of experimentally induced spinal and ischemic shock; preliminary studies in humans suggest that TRH treatment may improve recovery after spinal cord injury and head trauma. TRH has been used to treat children with neurologic disorders including West's syndrome, Lennox-Gastaut syndrome, early infantile epileptic encephalopathy, and intractable epilepsy.[104] TRH has been proposed to be an analeptic agent. Sleeping or drug-sedated animals were awakened by the administration of TRH, TRH reportedly reversed sedative effects of ethanol in humans, and TRH is said to have awakened a patient with a profound sleep disorder caused by a hypothalamic and midbrain eosinophilic granuloma.[102]

Regulation of TSH Release

The secretion of TSH is regulated by two interacting elements: negative feedback by thyroid hormone and open-loop neural control by hypothalamic hypophyseotropic factors (Fig. 7–9). TSH secretion is also modified by other hormones, including estrogens, glucocorticoids, and possibly GH, and is inhibited by cytokines in the pituitary and hypothalamus.[97,105] Aspects of the pituitary-thyroid axis are also considered in Chapter 10.

Feedback Control: Pituitary-Thyroid Axis

In the context of a feedback system, the level of thyroid hormone in blood or of its unbound fraction is the controlled variable and the set-point is the normal resting level of plasma thyroid hormone. Secretion of TSH is inversely regulated by the level of thyroid hormone so that deviations from the set-point of control lead to appropriate changes in the rate of TSH secretion (Fig. 7–10). Factors that determine the rate of TSH secretion required to maintain a given level of thyroid hormone include the rate at which TSH and thyroid hormone disappear from the blood (turnover rate) and the rate at which T_4 is converted to its more active form, T_3.

Thyroid hormones act on both the pituitary and the hypothalamus. Feedback control of the pituitary by thyroid hormone is remarkably precise. Administration of small doses of T_3 and T_4 inhibited the TSH response to TRH, and barely detectable decreases in plasma thyroid hormone levels were sufficient to sensitize the pituitary to TRH. TRH stimulates TSH secretion within a few minutes through its action on a membrane receptor, whereas thyroid hormone actions, mediated by intranuclear receptors, require several hours to take effect (see Chapter 10).

The secretion of hypothalamic TRH is also regulated by thyroid hormone feedback. Systemic injections of T_3 or implantations of tiny T_3 pellets in the PVH of hypothyroid rats[106] (Fig. 7–11A and B) reduced the concentration of TRH mRNA and TRH prohormone in TRH-secreting cells. Thyroid hormone also suppressed TRH secretion into hypophyseal-portal blood in sheep.

T_4 in the blood gains access to TRH-secreting neurons in the hypothalamus by way of the CSF. The hormone is taken up by epithelial cells of the choroid plexus of the lateral ventricle of the brain, bound within the cell to locally produced transthyretin (T_4-binding prealbumin), and then secreted across the blood-brain barrier.[107] Within the brain, T_4 is converted to T_3 by type II deiodinase, and T_3 interacts with subtypes of the thyroid hormone receptor, $TR\alpha_1$, $TR\beta_1$, and $TR\beta_2$, in the PVH and other brain cells (see Chapter 10). Thereby the set-point of the pituitary-thyroid axis is determined by thyroid hormone levels within the brain.[108] T_3 in the circulation is not transported into brain in this manner but presumably gains access to the paraventricular TRH neurons across the blood-brain barrier. The

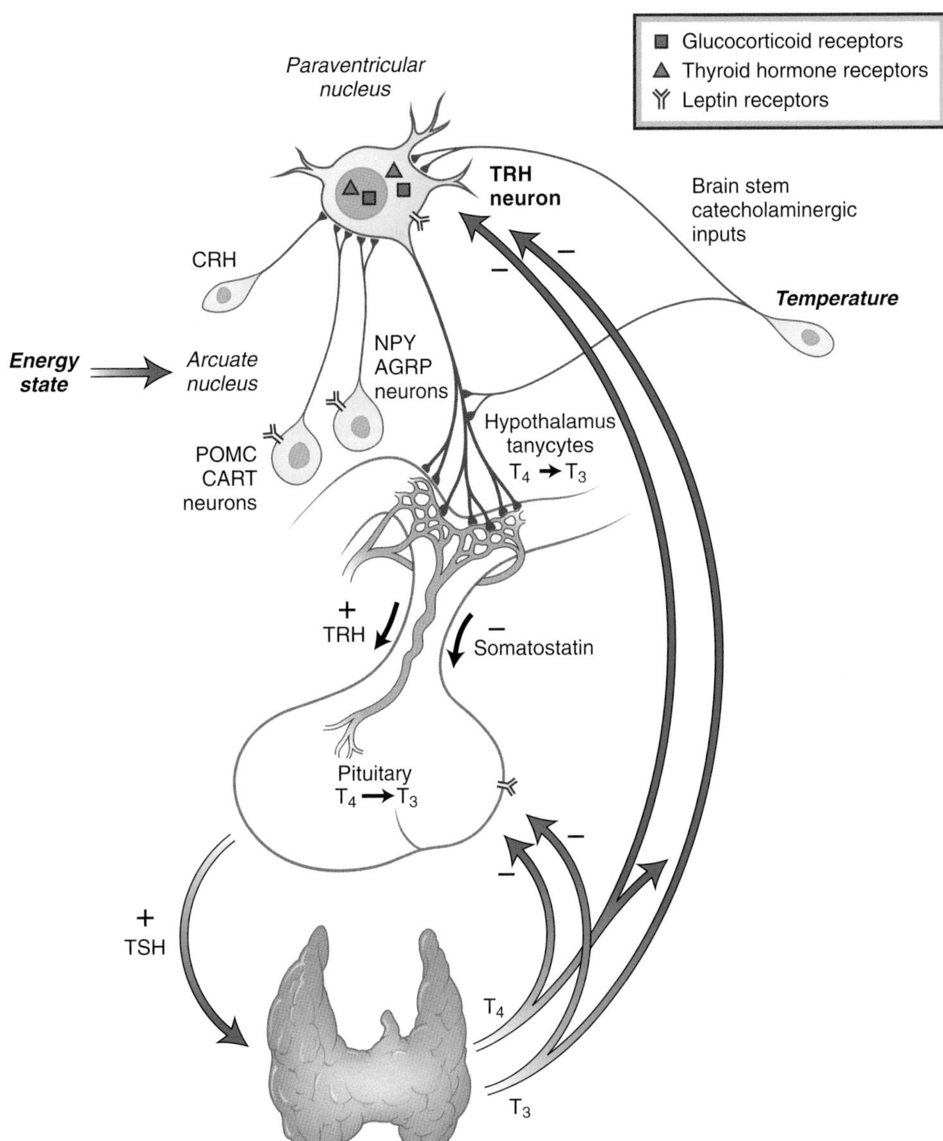

Figure 7–9 ▪ Regulation of the hypothalamic-pituitary-thyroid axis. *AGRP,* Agouti-related protein; *CART,* cocaine- and amphetamine-regulated transcript; *CRH,* corticotropin-releasing hormone; *NPY,* neuropeptide Y; *POMC,* proopiomelanocortin; *T_3,* triiodothyronine; *T_4,* thyroxine; *TRH,* thyrotropin-releasing hormone; *TSH,* thyrotropin.

brain T_4 transport and deiodinase system account for the fact that higher blood levels of T_3 are required to suppress pituitary-thyroid function after administration of T_3 than after administration of T_4.[108,109]

Transthyretin is present in the brain of early reptiles and in addition is synthesized by the liver in warm-blooded animals.[107] During embryogenesis in mammals, transthyretin is first detected when the blood-brain barrier appears, ensuring thyroid hormone access to the developing nervous system.

Neural Control

The hypothalamus determines the set-point of feedback control around which the usual feedback regulatory responses are elicited. Lesions of the thyrotropic area lower basal thyroid hormone levels and make the pituitary more sensitive to inhibition by thyroid hormone, and high doses of TRH raise TSH and thyroid hormone levels. Synthesis of TRH in the paraventricular nuclei is regulated by feedback actions of thyroid hormones.[108] The hypothalamus can override normal feedback control through an open-loop mechanism involving neuronal inputs to the hypophyseotropic TRH neurons (see Fig. 7–9). For example, cold exposure causes a sharp increase in TSH release in animals and in human newborns. Circadian changes in TSH secretion are another example of brain-directed changes in the set-point of feedback control, but if thyroid hormone levels are sufficiently elevated, as in hyperthyroidism, TRH cannot overcome the inhibition.

Hypothalamic regulation of TSH secretion is also influenced by two inhibitory factors, somatostatin and dopamine. Antisomatostatin antibodies increase basal TSH levels and potentiate the response to stimuli that normally induce TSH release in the rat, such as cold exposure and TRH administration.[110] Thyroid hormone in turn inhibits the release of somatostatin, implying coordinated, reciprocal regulation of TRH and somatostatin by thyroid hormone. GH stimulates hypothalamic somatostatin synthesis and can inhibit TSH secretion. The role of somatostatin in the regulation of TSH secretion in humans is uncertain.

Dopamine has modest effects on TSH secretion, and blockade of dopamine receptors (in the human) stimulates TSH secretion slightly. Changes in the metabolism of thyroid hormone also influence T_3 homeostasis within the brain. In states of thyroid hormone deficiency, brain T_3 levels are maintained by an increase in the deiodinase that converts T_4 to T_3.[41]

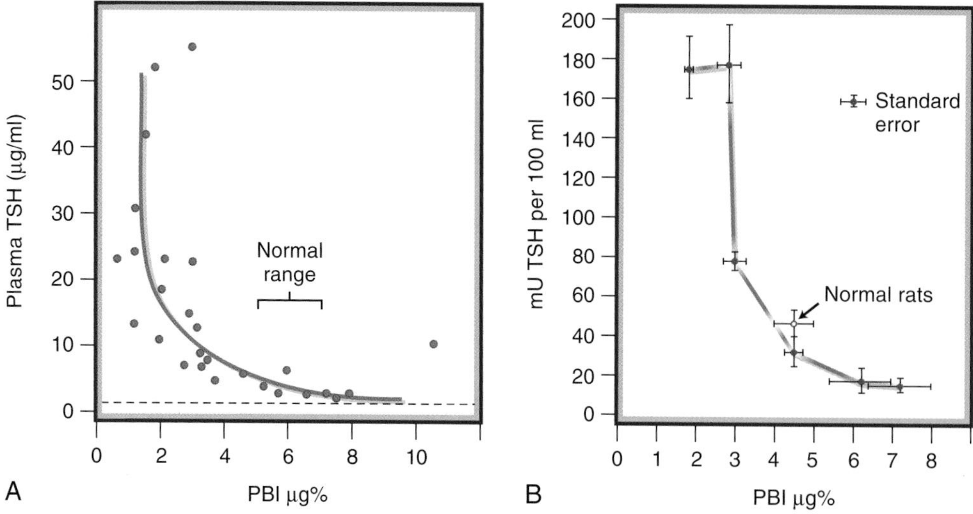

Figure 7–10 ▪ Relationship between plasma thyrotropin levels and thyroid hormone as determined by plasma protein-bound iodine (PBI) measurements in humans and rats. These curves illustrate, in the human **(A)** and the rat **(B)**, that plasma thyrotropin levels are a curvilinear function of plasma thyroid hormone level. Human studies were carried out by giving myxedematous patients successive increments of thyrotropin T_4 at approximately 10-day intervals. Each point represents simultaneous measurements of plasma PBI and plasma thyrotropin at various times in the six patients studied. The rat studies were performed by treating thyroidectomized animals with various doses of T_4 for 2 weeks before assay of plasma thyrotropin and plasma PBI. These curves illustrate that the secretion of thyrotropin is regulated over the entire range of thyroid hormone levels. At the normal set-point for T_4, the small changes above and below the control level are followed by appropriate increases or decreases in plasma thyrotropin. *T_4*, Thyroxine, *TSH*, thyrotropin. (*A* from Reichlin S, Utiger RD. Regulation of the pituitary thyroid axis in man: relationship of TSH concentration to concentration of free and total thyroxine in plasma. J Clin Endocrinol Metab 1967;27:251-255, copyright by The Endocrine Society. *B* from Reichlin S, Martin JB, Boshans RL, et al. Measurement of TSH in plasma and pituitary of the rat by a radioimmunoassay utilizing bovine TSH: effect of thyroidectomy or thyroxine administration on plasma TSH levels. Endocrinology 1970;87:1022-1031, copyright by The Endocrine Society.)

The pineal gland has been reported to inhibit thyroid function in some but not all studies. The pineal gland contains TRH, and in the frog its content changes with the season and with light and dark cycles independently of hypothalamic TRH.

Circadian Rhythm

Plasma TSH in humans is characterized by a circadian periodicity, with a maximum between 9 PM and 5 AM and a minimum between 4 PM and 7 PM.[111] Smaller ultradian TSH peaks occur every 90 to 180 minutes, probably because of bursts of TRH release from the hypothalamus, and are physiologically important in controlling the synthesis and glycosylation of TSH. Glycosylation is a determinant of TSH potency.[112]

Temperature

External cold exposure activates and high ambient temperature inhibits the pituitary-thyroid axis in animals, and analogous changes occur in humans under certain conditions.[113] Exposure of infants to cold at the time of delivery causes an increase in blood TSH levels, possibly because of alterations in the turnover and degradation of the thyroid hormones. Blood thyroid hormone levels are higher in the winter than in the summer in individuals in cold climates but not in other climates. However, it is difficult to show that changes in environmental or body temperature in adults influence TSH secretion. For example, exposure to cold ambient temperature or central hypothalamic cooling does not modify TSH levels in young men. Behavioral changes, activation of the sympathetic nervous system, and shivering appear to be more important in temperature regulation in adults than the thyroid response.

The autonomic nervous system and the thyroid axis work together to maintain temperature homeostasis in mammals, and TRH plays a role in both pathways.[113] Hypothalamic TRH release is rapidly (30 to 45 minutes) increased in rats exposed to cold. Rapid inhibition of somatostatin release in the median eminence also has been documented, and both changes appear to play important roles in the rise in plasma TSH induced by cold exposure. TRH mRNA is elevated within an hour of cold exposure (see Fig. 7–11C and D).[114] The regulation of hypophyseotropic TRH release and expression by cold is largely mediated by catecholamines. Noradrenergic and adrenergic fibers, originating in the brain stem, are found in close proximity to TRH nerve endings in the median eminence, and a rapid rise in TRH release was seen after norepinephrine treatment of hypothalamic fragments containing mainly median eminence. Brain stem adrenergic and noradrenergic fibers also make synaptic contacts with TRH neurons in the PVH (see Fig. 7–9), and thus catecholamines are likely to be involved in the regulation of TRH gene expression by cold. TRH neurons in the PVH are densely innervated by NPY terminals,[115] and a portion of the NPY terminals arising from the C1, C2, C3, and A1 cell groups of the brain stem and projecting to the PVH are known to be catecholaminergic. Somatostatin, dopamine, and serotonin also play a variety of roles in the regulation of TRH.

Stress

Stress is another determinant of TSH secretion.[105] In humans, physical stress inhibits TSH release, as indicated by the finding that in the euthyroid sick syndrome low levels of T_3 and T_4 do not cause compensatory increases in TSH secretion as would occur in normal individuals.[116]

A number of observations demonstrate interactions between the thyroid and adrenal axes. Physiologically, the bulk of evidence suggests that glucocorticoids in humans and rodents act

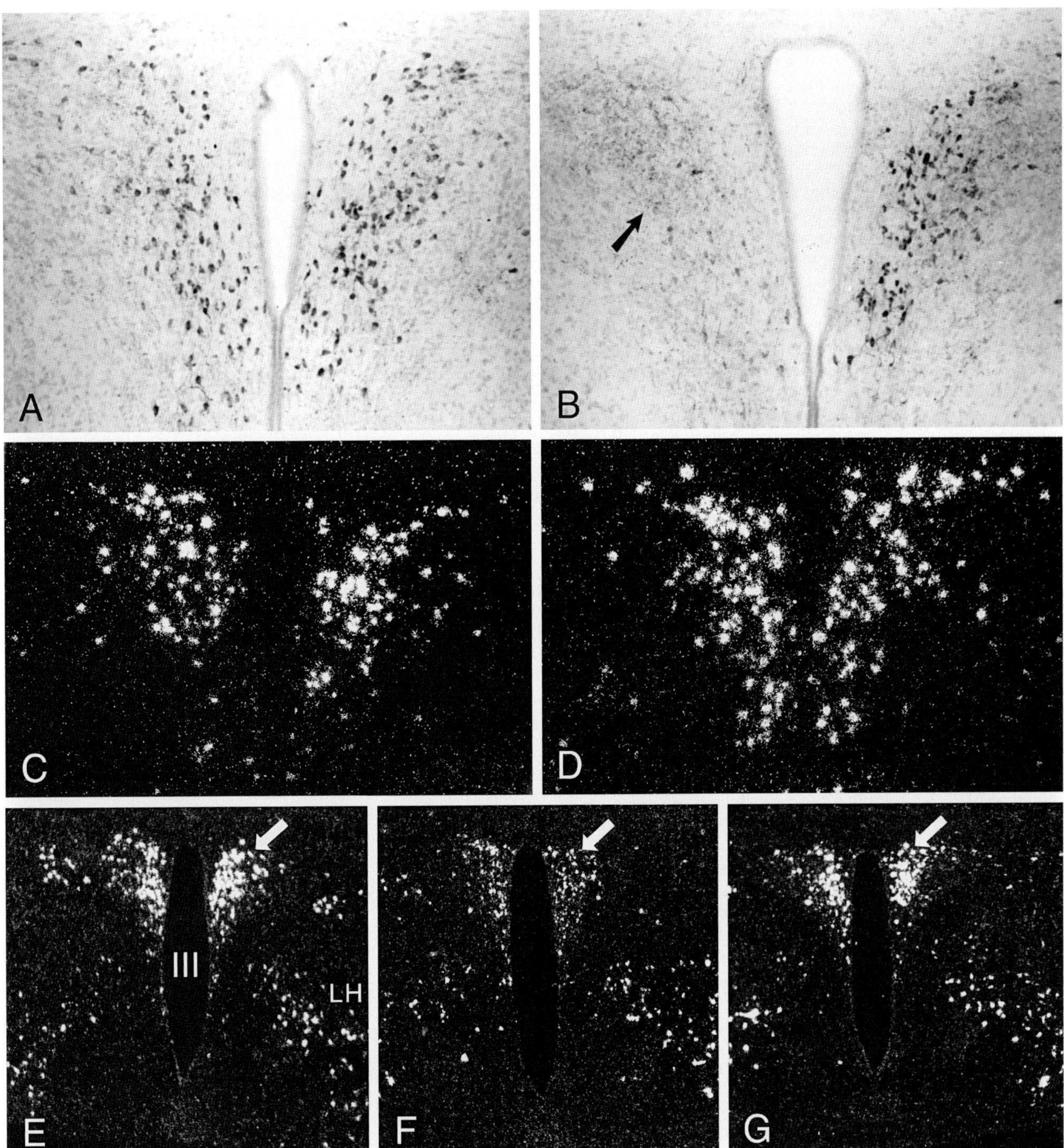

Figure 7–11 ▪ **A** and **B,** Direct effects of triiodothyronine (T_3) on thyrotropin-releasing hormone (TRH) synthesis in the rat hypothalamic paraventricular nucleus (parvicellular division) were shown in this experiment by immunohistochemical detection of pre-proTRH(25-50) after implantation of a pellet of either T_3 **(B)** or inactive diiodotyrosine (T_2) as a control **(A).** The T_2 pellet had no effect on the concentration of pre-proTRH **(A).** In contrast, the TRH prohormone **(B)** concentrations were markedly reduced (the black arrow indicates the unilateral pellet implantation). These studies indicate that thyroid hormone regulates the hypothalamic component of the pituitary-thyroid axis as well as the pituitary thyrotrope itself. **C** and **D,** Effects of 1 hour at 4°C on TRH messenger ribonucleic acid (mRNA). **E** to **G,** Effects on TRH mRNA levels of starvation **(F)** and leptin replacement during starvation **(G)** (the white arrows show the location of the paraventricular nucleus; III, 3rd ventricle; LH, lateral Lypothalamus). (Photomicrographs in panels A, B, E–G courtesy of Dr. R. M. Lechan. From Dyess EM, Segerson TP, Liposits Z, et al. Triiodothyronine exerts direct cell-specific regulation of thyrotropin-releasing hormone gene expression in the hypothalamic paraventricular nucleus. Endocrinology 1988;123:2291-2297, copyright by The Endocrine Society; Photomicrographs in panels C and D courtesy of Dr. Patricia Joseph-Bravo.)

to blunt the thyroid axis through actions in the CNS.[117] Some actions may be direct because the TRH gene (see Fig. 7–8) contains the glucocorticoid response element consensus sequence[95] and hypophyseotropic TRH neurons appear to contain glucocorticoid receptors.[118] The diurnal rhythm of cortisol is opposite that of TSH (see Fig. 7–7) and acute administration of glucocorticoids can block the nocturnal rise in TSH, but disruption of cortisol synthesis with metyrapone only modestly affects the TSH circadian rhythm.

Several lines of evidence, however, identify conditions in which elevated glucocorticoids are associated with stimulation of the thyroid axis. Human depression is often associated with hypercortisolism and hyperthyroxinemia, and TRH mRNA levels are elevated by glucocorticoids in a number of cell lines as well as in cultured fetal hypothalamic TRH neurons from the rat. Thus, although glucocorticoids probably stimulate TRH production in TRH neurons, their overall inhibitory effect on the thyroid axis results from indirect glucocorticoid negative feedback on structures such as the hippocampus. Disruption of hippocampal suppression of the hypothalamic-pituitary-adrenal (HPA) axis is proposed to be involved in the hypercortisolemia commonly seen in affective illness, and disruption of hippocampal inputs to the hypothalamus have been shown to produce a rise in hypophyseotropic TRH in the rat.[119]

Starvation

The thyroid axis is depressed during starvation, presumably to help conserve energy by depressing metabolism (see Fig. 7–11E to G). In humans, reduced T_3, T_4, and TSH are seen during starvation or fasting.[120] There are also changes in the thyroid axis in anorexia nervosa, such as low blood levels of T_3 and low normal levels of T_4 (see Chapter 10). Inappropriately low levels of TSH are found, suggesting defective activation of TRH production by low thyroid hormone levels. During starvation in rodents, reduced TRH release into hypophyseal portal blood and reduced pro-TRH mRNA levels are seen, despite lowered thyroid hormone levels.[121] Reduced basal TSH levels are also usually present.

The hypothyroidism seen in fasting or in the leptin-deficient *ob/ob* mouse can be reversed by administration of leptin,[122] and the evidence suggests that the mechanism involves leptin's ability to up-regulate TRH gene expression in the PVH (see Fig. 7–11E to G).[123] Leptin appears to act both directly through leptin receptors on hypophyseotropic TRH neurons and indirectly through its actions on other hypothalamic cell groups, such as arcuate nucleus POMC and NPY-agouti-related peptide (AgRP) neurons.[124,125] TRH neurons in the PVH receive dense NPY-AgRP and POMC projections from the arcuate and express NPY and melanocortin-4 receptors (MC4R),[126] and α-MSH administration partially prevents the fasting-induced drop in thyroid hormone levels.[124,125] Indeed, the TRH promoter contains a signal transducer and activator of transcription (STAT) response element and a cAMP response element that have been demonstrated to mediate induction of TRH gene expression by leptin and α-MSH, respectively, in a heterologous cell system (see Fig. 7–8).[126] The regulation of TRH by metabolic state is likely to be under redundant control, however, because, unlike rodents, leptin-deficient children are euthyroid,[127] and both MC4R-deficient rodents and humans are euthyroid.[128]

Infection and Inflammation

The molecular basis of infection- or inflammation-induced TSH suppression is partially established. Sterile abscesses or the injection of interleukin-1β (IL-1β; endogenous pyrogen, a secretory peptide of activated lymphocytes)[129] or of tumor necrosis factor α (TNF-α) inhibits TSH secretion, and IL-1β stimulates the secretion of somatostatin.[130] TNF-α inhibits TSH secretion directly and induces functional changes in the rat characteristic of the "sick euthyroid" state.[131] It is likely that the TSH inhibition in animal models of the sick euthyroid syndrome is due to cytokine-induced changes in hypothalamic and pituitary function.[132] IL-6, IL-1, and TNF-α contribute to the suppression of TSH in the sick euthyroid syndrome.[133]

Corticotropin-Releasing Hormone

Chemistry and Evolution

The HPA axis is the humoral component of an integrated neural and endocrine system that functions to respond to internal and external challenges to homeostasis (stressors). The system comprises the neuronal pathways linked to release of catecholamines from the adrenal medulla (fight-or-flight response) and the hypothalamic-pituitary control of ACTH release in the control of glucocorticoid production by the adrenal cortex. Pituitary ACTH release is stimulated primarily by CRH and to a lesser extent by AVP (see Chapter 8). The hypophyseotropic CRH neurons are located in the parvicellular division of the PVH and project to the median eminence (see Figs. 7–3 and 7–4).

In a broader context, the CRH system in the CNS is also vitally important in the behavioral response to stress. This complex system includes not only nonhypophyseotropic CRH neurons but also three CRH-like peptides (urocortin I, urocortin II or stresscopin-like peptide, and urocortin III or stresscopin), at least two cognate receptors (CRH-R1 and CRH-R2), and a high-affinity CRH-binding protein, each with distinct and complex distributions in the CNS.

The Schally and Guillemin laboratories demonstrated in 1955 that extracts from the hypothalamus stimulated ACTH release from the pituitary. The principal bioactive peptide, CRH, was purified and characterized from the sheep in 1981 by Vale and colleagues. Human CRH is an amidated 41-amino-acid peptide that is cleaved from the carboxyl terminus of a 196-amino-acid pre-prohormone precursor by PC1 and PC2 (Fig. 7–12).[134] In general, the peptide is highly conserved; the human peptide is identical in sequence to the mouse and rat peptides but differs at seven residues from the ovine sequence. Mammalian CRH and urocortin I, II, and III, fish urotensin, anuran sauvagine, and the insect diuretic peptides are members of an ancient family of peptides that evolved from an ancestral precursor early in the evolution of metazoans, approximately 500 million years ago.[135] Comparison of peptide sequences in vertebrates suggests a grouping of the peptides into two families, CRH-urotensin-urocortin-sauvagine and urocortin II-urocortin III (Fig. 7–13).[136] Urocortin and sauvagine appear to represent tetrapod orthologues of fish urotensin. Sauvagine, isolated originally from *Phyllomedusa sauvagei,* is an osmoregulatory peptide produced in the skin of certain frogs; urotensin is an osmoregulatory peptide produced in the caudal neurosecretory system of the fish. Whereas isolation of CRH required 250,000 ovine hypothalami, the cloning of urocortin II and III was accomplished by computer search of the human genome database.[136]

The CRH peptides signal by binding to CRH-R1[137,138] and CRH-R2 [139] receptors that couple to G_s and activation of adenylyl cyclase. Two splice variants of the latter that differ in the extracellular amino-terminal domain, CRH-R2α and CRH-R2β, have been found in both rodents and humans,[140] and a third N-terminal splice variant, CRH-R2γ, has been reported in the human.[141]

CRH, urotensin, and sauvagine are all potent agonists of CRH-R1, urocortin is a potent agonist of both receptors, and urocortins II and III are specific agonists of CRH-R2. CRH-activation of the HPA axis is mediated exclusively through CRH-R1 expressed in the corticotroph. The PVH is the site of the majority of CRH neurons projecting to the median eminence,

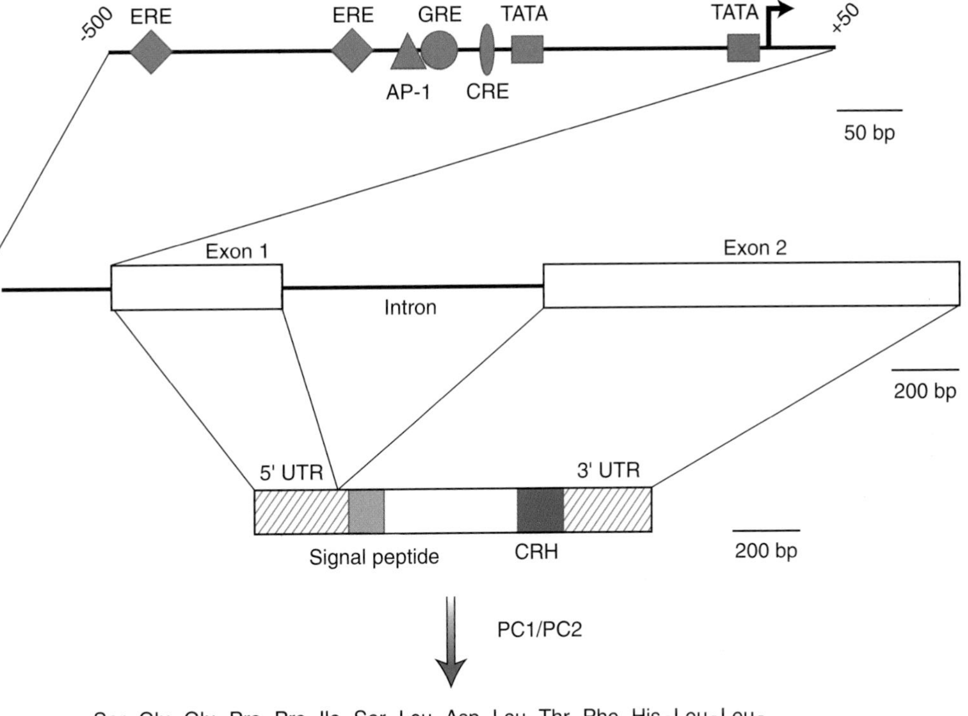

Ser - Glu - Glu - Pro - Pro - Ile - Ser - Leu - Asp - Leu - Thr - Phe - His - Leu - Leu -
Arg - Glu - Val - Leu - Glu - Met - Ala - Arg - Ala - Glu - Gln - Leu - Ala - Gln - Gln -
Ala - His - Ser - Asn - Arg - Lys - Leu - Met - Glu - Ile - Ile - Gly - Lys

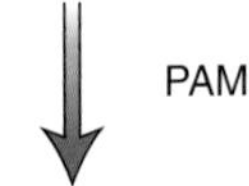

Ser - Glu - Glu - Pro - Pro - Ile - Ser - Leu - Asp - Leu - Thr - Phe - His - Leu - Leu -
Arg - Glu - Val - Leu - Glu - Met - Ala - Arg - Ala - Glu - Gln - Leu - Ala - Gln - Gln -
Ala - His - Ser - Asn - Arg - Lys - Leu - Met - Glu - Ile - Ile - NH_2

Figure 7–12 ▪ Structure of the human corticotropin-releasing hormone (CRH) gene, cDNA, and protein. The sequence coding for CRH occurs at the carboxyl-terminus of the prohormone. Cleavage sites and the terminal Gly position are shown. *CRE,* Cyclic AMP-responsive element; *ERE,* estrogen response element; *GRE,* glucocorticoid response element; *PAM,* peptidylglycine alpha-amidating monooxygenase; *PC1/PC2,* prohormone convertases 1 and 2; TATA, Goldstein-Hogness box involued in binding RNA polymerase; *UTR,* untranslated. (Redrawn from data of Shibahara S, Morimoto Y, Furutani Y, et al. Isolation and sequence analysis of the human corticotropin-releasing factor precursor gene. EMBO J 1983;2:775-779.)

Frog sauvagine	QG**PPISIDLS**LE**LL**RKM**IE**IE**K**QEKE**K**Q**QA**AN**NR**L**L**L**D**T**I**
Carp urotensin-I	NDD**PPISIDLTF**H**LL**RNM**IE**M**AR**NENQ**R**E**QA**GL**NR**KYL**D**E**V**
Human urocortin	DN**P**S**LSIDLTF**H**LL**RTL**LE**L**AR**TQSQ**R**ER**A**EQ**NR**I**I**F**D**S**V**
Human CRH	SEE**PPISLDLTF**H**LL**REV**LE**M**AR**AEQLAQ**QA**HS**NR**K**L**M**E**I**I**
Human SRP	HPGSRIV**LSLDV**PIG**LL**QIL**LE**Q**AR**ARAA**R**E**QA**TT**N**AR**I**LAR**V**GHC
Human SCP	TKFT**LSLDV**PTN**I**MNLLFNI**AK**AKNL**R**A**QA**AA**N**AH**L**MAQ**I**GRRK

Figure 7–13 ▪ Sequence comparison of members of the corticotropin-releasing hormone (CRH) peptide family. Identical or highly conserved amino acids are indicated in bold letters. *SCP,* Stresscopin; *SRP,* stresscopin-related peptide.

although some CRH neurons projecting to the median eminence are found in most hypothalamic nuclei (Fig. 7–14A). Some CRH fibers in the PVH also project to the brain stem, and nonhypophyseotropic CRH neurons are abundant elsewhere, primarily in limbic structures involved in processing sensory information and in regulating the autonomic nervous system. Sites include the prefrontal, insular, and cingulate cortices; amygdala; substantia nigra; periaqueductal gray; locus coeruleus; nucleus of the solitary tract; and parabrachial nucleus. In the periphery, CRH is found in human placenta, where it is up-regulated 6- to 40-fold during the third trimester; lymphocytes; autonomic nerves; and gastrointestinal tract. Urocortin is expressed at highest levels in the Edinger-Westphal nucleus, lateral superior olive, and SON of the rodent brain, with additional sites including the substantia nigra, ventral tegmental area, and dorsal raphe (see Fig. 7–14B). In the human, urocortin is widely distributed with highest levels in the frontal cortex, temporal cortex, and hypothalamus[142] and has also been reported in the Edinger-Westphal and olivary nuclei.[143] In the periphery, urocortin is seen in placenta, mucosal inflammatory cells in the gastrointestinal tract, lymphocytes, and cardiomyocytes. There is limited information concerning the tissue distribution of urocortins II and III, particularly in the brain.

In addition to its expression in pituitary corticotrophs, CRH-R1 is found in the neocortex and cerebellar cortex, subcortical limbic structures, and amygdala, with little to no expression in the hypothalamus (Fig. 7–14C). CRH-R1 also is found in a variety of peripheral sites in humans, including ovary, endometrium,

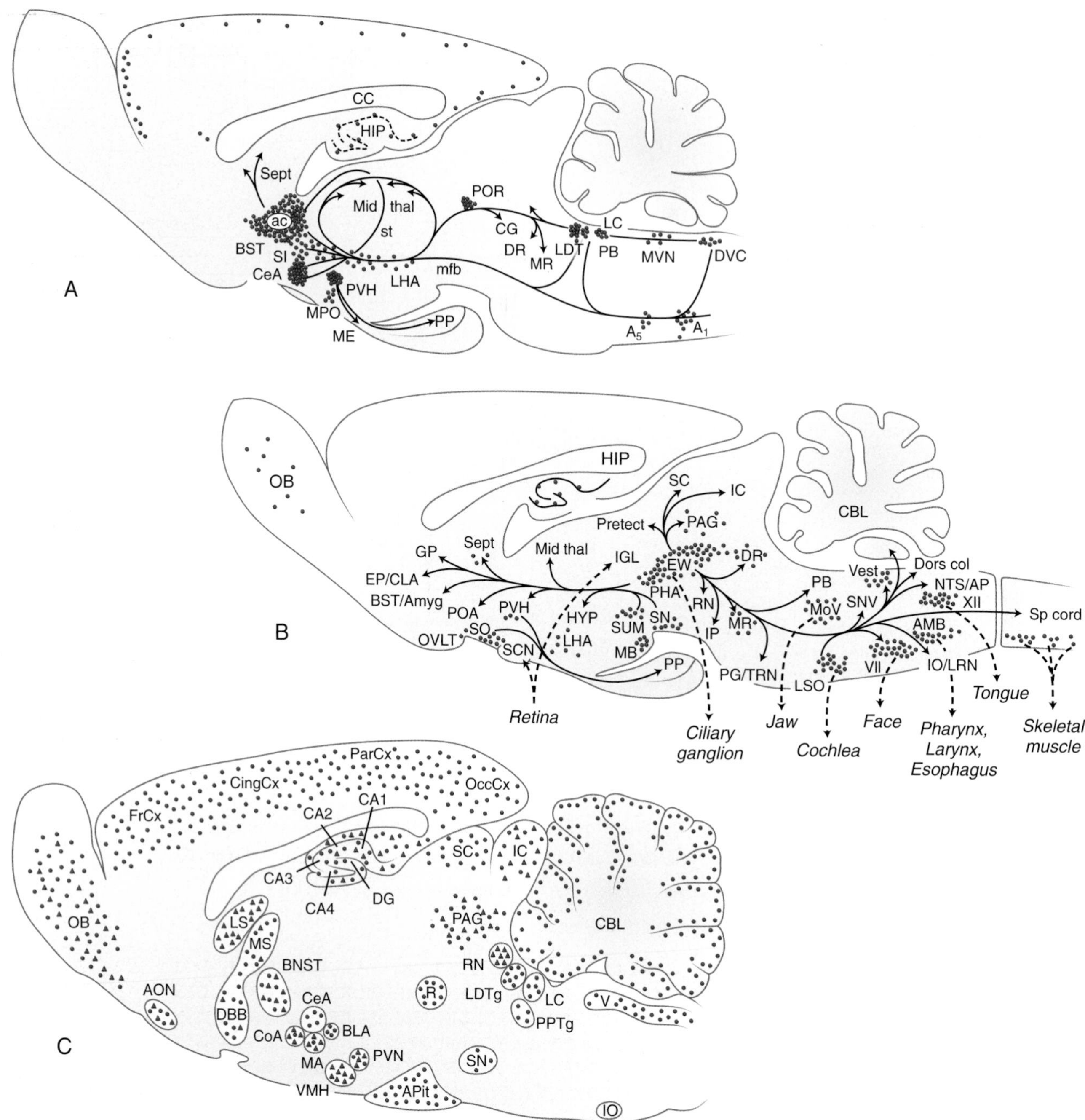

Figure 7–14 ▪ Distribution of corticotropin-releasing hormone (CRH) **(A),** urocortin **(B),** and the CRH receptor 1 (CRH-R1) (**C,** circles) and CRH-R2 (**C,** triangles) mRNA sequences in the rat brain. *A_1,* Noradrenergic cell group 1; *A_5,* noradrenergic cell group 5; *ac,* anterior commissure; *BST/BNST,* bed nucleus of the stria terminalis; *cc,* corpus callosum; *CeA,* central nucleus amygdala; CBL, cerebellum; *CG,* central gray; *DR,* dorsal raphe; *DVC,* dorsal vagal complex; *HIP,* hippocampus; *LC,* locus coeruleus; *LDT,* laterodorsal tegmental nucleus; *LHA,* lateral hypothalamic area; *ME,* median eminence; *MID THAL,* midline thalamic nuclei; *mfb,* medial forebrain bundle; *MPO,* medial preoptic area; *MR,* medial raphe; *MVN,* medial vestibular nucleus; OB, olfactory bulb; *PB,* parabrachial nucleus; *POR,* perioculomotor nucleus; *PP,* posterior pituitary; *PVH,* paraventricular nucleus; SiEPT, septal region; *SI,* substantia innominata; *st,* stria. (From Swanson LW, Sawchenko PE, Rivier J, et al. Organization of ovine corticotropin-releasing factor immunoreactive cells and fibers in the rat brain: an immunohistochemical study. Neuroendocrinology 1983;36:165-186; Bittencourt JC, Vaughan J, Arias C, et al. Urocortin expression in rat brain: evidence against a pervasive relationship of urocortin-containing projections with targets bearing type 2 CRF receptors. J Comp Neurol 1999;415:285-312, Fig. 17; Steckler T, Holsboer F. Corticotropin-releasing hormone receptor subtypes and emotion. Biol Psychol 1999;46:1480-1508, Fig. 1.)

and skin. CRH-R2α is found mainly in the brain in rodents, with high levels of expression seen in the ventromedial hypothalamic nucleus and lateral septum (see Fig. 7–14C).[144] CRH-R2β is seen centrally in cerebral arterioles and peripherally in gastrointestinal tract, heart, and muscle.[139,145] In contrast, in humans CRH-R2α is seen in brain and periphery, and the β and γ subtypes are primarily central.[140,141] Little CRH-R2 message is seen in pituitary. Although CRH-R1 appears to be exclusively involved in regulation of pituitary ACTH synthesis and release, both receptors are expressed in the rodent adrenal cortex. Data suggest that this intraadrenal CRH-ACTH system may be involved in fine-tuning of adrenocortical corticosterone release.

The CRH system is also regulated in both brain and periphery by a 37-kd high-affinity CRH-binding protein.[146-148] This factor was initially postulated from the observation that CRH levels rise dramatically during the second and third trimesters of pregnancy without activating the pituitary-adrenal axis. Among hypophyseotropic factors, CRH is the only one for which a specific binding protein (in addition to the receptor) exists in tissue or blood. The placenta is the principal source of pregnancy-related CRH-binding protein. Human and rat CRH-binding proteins are homologous (85% amino acid identity), but in the rat the protein is expressed only in brain. The binding protein is species specific; bovine CRH, which is almost identical in sequence to rat-human CRH, has a lower affinity of binding to the human binding protein.

The functional significance of the CRH-binding protein is not fully understood. CRH-binding protein does not bind to the CRH receptor but does inhibit CRH action. For this reason CRH-binding protein probably acts to modulate CRH actions at the cellular level. Corticotroph cells in the anterior pituitary have membrane CRH receptors and intracellular CRH-binding protein; conceivably, the binding protein acts to sequester or terminate the action of membrane-bound CRH. CRH-binding protein is present in many regions of the CNS, including cells that synthesize CRH and cells that receive innervation from CRH-containing neurons. The anatomic distribution of the protein, the variability of its location in relation to the presence of CRH, and its relative sparseness in the CRH tuberohypophyseal neuronal system suggest a control system that is as yet poorly understood. Transgenic mouse models with both overexpression and gene deletion of the CRH-binding protein have been produced with little effect on basal or stress-activation of the HPA axis (reviewed in reference 149).

Structure-activity relationship studies have demonstrated that C-terminal amidation and an α-helical secondary structure are both important for biologic activity of CRH. The first CRH antagonist described was termed α-helical CRH_{9-41}.[150] A second, more potent antagonist, termed *astressin*, has the structure cyclo(30-33)(d-Phe^{12}, Nle^{12}, Glu^{12}, Lys^{12})$hCRH_{12-41}$.[151] Both peptides are somewhat nonspecific, antagonizing both CRH-R1 and CRH-R2. Because of the anxiogenic activity of CRH and urocortin, a number of pharmaceutical companies have developed small-molecule CRH antagonists; several of the molecules are currently in clinical trials for anxiety and depression (discussed in more detail later). Thus far, this structurally diverse group of small molecule compounds, such as antalarmin, CP-154,526, and NBI27914, are potent antagonists of CRH-R1, with little activity at CRH-R2. The efficacy of these compounds across the entire behavioral, neuroendocrine, and autonomic repertoire of response to stress has been demonstrated in a number of laboratory animal studies. For example, oral administration of antalarmin in a social stress model in the primate (introduction of strange males) reduced behavioral measures of anxiety such as lack of exploratory behavior, decreased plasma ACTH and cortisol, and reduced plasma epinephrine and norepinephrine.[152] Other preclinical studies in rhesus monkeys have compared the pharmacologic profiles of astressin B and antalarmin.[153] A peptide antagonist with 100-fold selectivity for the CRH 2β receptor, (d-Phe,[11] His[12])sauvagine 11-40 or anti-sauvagine-30, has also been described.[154]

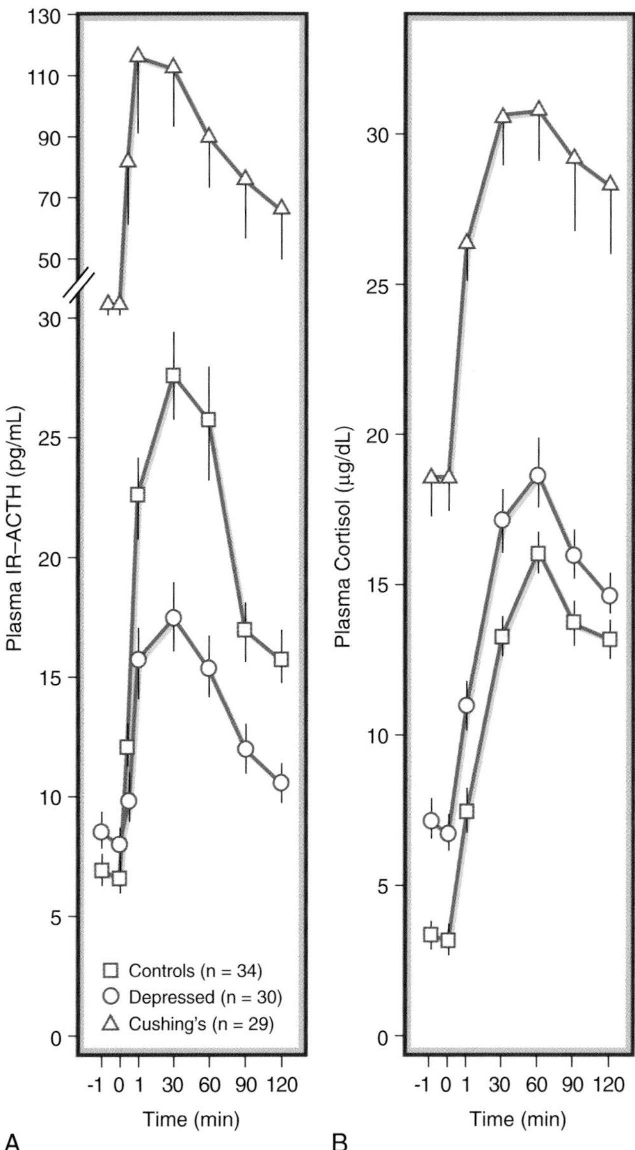

Figure 7–15 ▪ Comparison of plasma immunoreactive adrenocorticotropic hormone (IR-ACTH) **(A)** and plasma cortisol **(B)** responses to ovine corticotropin-releasing hormone in control subjects, patients with depression, and patients with Cushing's disease. (From Gold PW, Loriaux DL, Roy A, et al. Responses to corticotropin-releasing hormone in the hypercortisolism of depression and Cushing's disease. Pathophysiologic and diagnostic implications. N Engl J Med 1986;314:1329-1335.)

Effects on the Pituitary and Mechanism of Action

Administration of CRH to humans causes prompt release of ACTH into the blood, followed by secretion of cortisol (Fig. 7–15) and other adrenal steroids including aldosterone. Most studies have used ovine CRH, which is more potent and longer acting than human CRH, but human and porcine CRHs appear to have equal diagnostic value. The effect of CRH is specific to ACTH release and is inhibited by glucocorticoids.

As mentioned earlier, CRH acts on the pituitary corticotroph primarily by binding to CRH-R1 and activating adenylyl cyclase. The concentration of cAMP in the tissue is increased in parallel with the biologic effects and is reduced by glucocorticoids. The rate of transcription of the mRNA that encodes the ACTH prohormone POMC is also enhanced by CRH.

Extrapituitary Functions

CRH and the urocortin peptides have a wide range of biologic activities in addition to the hypophyseotropic role of CRH in regulating ACTH synthesis and release. Centrally, these peptides have behavioral activities in anxiety, mood, arousal, locomotion, reward, and feeding[155,156] and increase sympathetic activation. Many of the nonhypophyseotropic behavioral and autonomic functions of these peptides can be viewed as complementary to activation of the HPA axis in the maintenance of homeostasis under exposure to stress. In the periphery, activities have been reported in immunity, cardiac function, gastrointestinal function, and reproduction.[157]

The CRH and urocortin peptides have a repertoire of behavioral and autonomic actions after central administration that suggests a role for these pathways in mediating the behavioral-autonomic components of the stress response. Hyperactivity of the HPA axis is a common neuroendocrine finding in affective disorders (see Fig. 7–15).[155,158] Furthermore, normalization of HPA regulation is highly predictive of successful treatment. Defective dexamethasone suppression of CRH release, implying defective corticosteroid receptor signaling, is seen not only in depressed patients but also in healthy subjects with a family history of depression.[159] Depressed patients also show elevated levels of CRH in the CSF.[160] Extensive behavioral testing in a variety of mutant mouse models with genetically altered expression of either the CRH ligands or receptors generally supports the hypothesis that activation of central CRH pathways is a critical neurobiologic substrate of anxiety and depressive states.[149,156]

Central administration of CRH or urocortin activates neuronal cell groups involved in cardiovascular control and increases blood pressure, heart rate, and cardiac output.[161] However, urocortin is expressed in cardiac myocytes, and intravenous administration of CRH or urocortin decreases blood pressure and increases heart rate in most species, including humans.[161] This hypotensive effect is probably mediated peripherally because ganglion blockade did not disrupt the hypotensive effects of intravenous urocortin. Furthermore, high levels of CRH-R2β have been seen in the cardiac atria and ventricles,[139,145] and knockout of the CRH-R2 gene in the mouse eliminated the hypotensive effects of intravenous urocortin administration.[162,163]

Cytokines have an important role in extinguishing inflammatory responses through activation of CRH and AVP neurons in the PVH and subsequent elevation of anti-inflammatory glucocorticoids. Interestingly, CRH is generally proinflammatory in the periphery, where it is found in sympathetic efferents, sensory afferent nerves, leukocytes, and in macrophages in some species.[157,164] CRH also functions as a paracrine factor in the endometrium, where it may play a role in decidualization and implantation and act as a uterine vasodilator.[157]

The relative contributions of each of the CRH-urocortin peptides and receptors to the different biologic functions reported has been the topic of considerable analysis, given the receptor-specific antagonists already described as well as the CRH, CRH-R1, and CRH-R2 knockout mice available for study (reviewed in references 149 and 156). Examination of three potent stressors—restraint, ether, and fasting—demonstrated that other ACTH secretagogues, such as AVP, oxytocin, and catecholamines, could not replace CRH in its role in mounting the stress response. In contrast, augmentation of glucocorticoid secretion by a stressor after prolonged stress was not defective in the CRH knockout mouse, implicating CRH-independent mechanisms.

Although CRH is a potent anxiogenic peptide, the CRH knockout mouse exhibits normal anxiety behaviors in, for example, conditioned fear paradigms. The nonpeptide CRH-R1 specific antagonist CP-154,526 was anxiolytic in a shock-induced freezing paradigm in both wild-type and CRH knockout mice, suggesting that the anxiogenic activity is a CRH-like peptide acting at the CRH-R1 receptor.

CRH and urocortin peptides also have potent anorexigenic activity, implicating the CRH system in stress-induced inhibition of feeding. Stress-induced inhibition of feeding remained intact, however, in the CRH knockout mouse. Likewise, suppression of the proestrous LH surge by restraint was intact in the CRH knockout mouse. Both CRH-R1 and CRH-R2 knockout strains had normal weight and feeding behavior but were distinctly different from wild-type mice in the anorexigenic response to centrally administered urocortin or CRH. The CRH-R1-deficient mice lacked the acute anorexigenic response (0 to 1.5 hours) to urocortin seen in wild-type mice. Both wild-type and CRH-R1 knockout mice exhibited comparable reduction in feeding 3 to 11 hours after administration. In contrast, the late phase of urocortin responsiveness appeared to depend on the presence of CRH-R2. Thus, signaling through CRH-R1 and CRH-R2 appears to play a complex role in the acute effects of stress on feeding behavior.

Clinical Applications

No approved therapeutic application of CRH or CRH-like peptides exists, although the peptide has been demonstrated to have a number of activities in human and primate studies. For example, intravenous administration of CRH was found to stimulate energy expenditure and has been proposed for use in weight loss. CRH is used diagnostically, often in combination with dexamethasone suppression or inferior petrosal venous sampling, in the evaluation of Cushing's syndrome to differentiate between pituitary and ectopic sources of ACTH (reviewed in reference 165; see Chapters 8 and 14).

The development of small molecule, orally available, CRH-R1 antagonists has, however, produced considerable interest in their potential for treatment of anxiety and depression.[166,167] In particular the compound R121919 was studied in phase I and IIa clinical trials before its discontinuance. These studies of 20 patients demonstrated significant reductions in scores of anxiety and depression, using ratings determined by either patient or clinician, and also demonstrated the compound's safety and favorable side-effect profile including a lack of effect on endocrine function or body weight gain.[168-170]

Feedback Control

The administration of glucocorticoids inhibits ACTH secretion; removal of the adrenals (or administration of drugs that impair secretion of glucocorticoids) leads to increased ACTH release. The set-point of pituitary feedback is determined by the hypothalamus acting through hypothalamic-releasing hormones CRH and AVP (see Chapter 8).[171-174] Glucocorticoids act on both the pituitary corticotrophs and the hypothalamic neurons that secrete CRH and AVP. These regulatory actions are analogous to the control of the pituitary-thyroid axis. However, whereas TSH becomes completely unresponsive to TRH when thyroid hormone levels are sufficiently high, severe neurogenic stress and large amounts of CRH can break through the feedback inhibition by glucocorticoids. A still higher level of feedback control is exerted by glucocorticoid-responsive neurons in the hippocampus that project to the hypothalamus; these neurons affect the activity of CRH hypophyseotropic neurons and determine the set-point of pituitary responsiveness to glucocorticoids.[174] A recent comprehensive review of glucocorticoid effects on CRH and AVP and regulation of the HPA axis has emphasized the complexity of this control beyond that of a simple closed-loop feedback.[175]

Glucocorticoids are lipid soluble and freely enter the brain through the blood-brain barrier.[173] In brain and pituitary they can bind to two receptors, type I (the mineralocorticoid receptor, so named because it binds aldosterone and glucocorticoids with high affinity) and type II (glucocorticoid receptor, which has low affinity for mineralocorticoids).[172-174] Classic glucocorticoid action involves binding of the steroid-receptor complex to regulator sequences in the genome. Type I receptors are saturated by basal levels of glucocorticoids, whereas type II receptors are not saturated under basal conditions but approach saturation during peak phases of the circadian rhythm and during stress. These differences and differences in regional distribution within the brain suggest that type I receptors determine basal activity of the hypothalamic-pituitary axis and that type II receptors mediate stress responses.

In the pituitary, glucocorticoids inhibit secretion of ACTH and the synthesis of POMC mRNA; in the hypothalamus, the secretion of CRH and AVP and the synthesis of their respective mRNAs are inhibited, although with distinct temporal patterns.[173-175] Neuron membrane excitability and ion transport properties are suppressed by changes in glucocorticoid-directed synthesis of intracellular protein. Recent studies indicate that glucocorticoids can exert additional rapid signaling events in neurons including an endocannabinoid-mediated suppression of synaptic excitation.[176] These rapid events involve membrane-associated complexes and are independent of changes in gene transcription or acute protein translation, but the exact mechanisms and nature of the receptors are still under investigation.[177]

Glucocorticoids block stress-induced ACTH release. The latency of the inhibitory effect is so short (less than 30 minutes) that it is likely that gene regulation is not the sole basis of the response.[177] Long-term suppression (more than 1 hour) clearly acts through genomic mechanisms.

Glucocorticoid receptors are also found outside the hypothalamus in the septum and amygdala,[173,174] structures that are involved in the psychobehavioral changes in hypercortisolism and hypocortisolism. It is worth noting that in all these areas, apart from CRH neurons of the PVH, glucocorticoids have either a stimulatory or a neutral effect on CRH gene expression.[175] Hippocampal neurons are reduced in number by prolonged elevation of glucocorticoids during chronic stress.[174]

Neural Control

Significant physiologic or psychological stressors evoke an adaptive response that commonly includes activation of both the HPA axis and the sympathoadrenal axis. The end products of these pathways then help to mobilize resources to cope with the physiologic demands in emergency situations, acutely through the fight-or-flight response and over the long term through systemic effects of glucocorticoids on functions such as gluconeogenesis and energy mobilization (see Chapter 33). The HPA axis also has unique stress-specific homeostatic roles, the best example being the role of glucocorticoids in down-regulating immune responses after infection and other events that stimulate cytokine production by the immune system.

The PVH is the primary hypothalamic nucleus responsible for providing the integrated whole-animal response to stress.[175,178,179] This nucleus contains three major types of effector neurons that are spatially distinct from one another within it: (1) magnicellular oxytocin and AVP neurons that project to the posterior pituitary and participate in the regulation of blood pressure, fluid homeostasis, lactation, and parturition; (2) neurons projecting to the brain stem and spinal cord that regulate a variety of autonomic responses including sympathoadrenal activation; and (3) parvicellular CRH neurons that project to the median eminence and regulate ACTH synthesis and release. Many CRH neurons coexpress AVP, which acts as an auxiliary ACTH secretagogue, synergistic with CRH. AVP is regulated quite differently in parvicellular versus magnicellular neurons but is also regulated somewhat differently from CRH by stressors in parvicellular cells expressing both peptides.[175] Different stressors result in different patterns of activation of the three major visceromotor cell groups within the PVH, as measured by the general neuronal activation marker c-Fos (Fig. 7–16). For example, salt loading down-regulates CRH mRNA in parvicellular CRH cells, up-regulates CRH in a small number of magnicellular CRH cells, but only activates magnicellular cells. Hemorrhage activates every division of the PVH, whereas cytokine administration primarily activates parvicellular CRH cells with some minor activation of magnicellular and autonomic divisions.

The synthesis and release of AVP, which regulates renal water absorption and vascular smooth muscle, are controlled mainly by the volume and tonicity of the blood. This information is relayed to the magnicellular AVP cell through the nucleus of the solitary tract and A1 noradrenergic cell group of the ventrolateral medulla and projections from a triad of CVOs lining the third ventricle, the SFO, medial preoptic nucleus (MePO), and OVLT. Oxytocin is primarily involved in reproductive functions, such as parturition, lactation, and milk ejection, although it is cosecreted with AVP in response to osmotic and volume challenges, and oxytocin cells receive direct projections from the nucleus of the solitary tract as well as from the SFO, MePO, and OVLT. In contrast to the neurosecretory neurons functionally defined by the three peptides, CRH, oxytocin, and AVP, PVH neurons projecting to brain stem and spinal cord include neurons expressing each of these peptides.

In the rodent, a wide variety of stressors have been determined to activate parvicellular CRH neurons, including cytokine injection, salt loading, hemorrhage, adrenalectomy, restraint, foot shock, hypoglycemia, fasting, and ether exposure. Thus, in contrast to the simplicity of inputs to magnicellular cells (Fig. 7–17A), it is not surprising that parvicellular CRH neurons receive a diverse and complex assortment of inputs (Fig. 7–18; see Fig. 7–17B). These inputs are divided into three major categories: brain stem, limbic forebrain, and hypothalamus. Because the PVH is not known to receive any direct projections from the cerebral cortex or thalamus, stressors involving emotional or cognitive processing must involve indirect relay to the PVH.

Visceral sensory input to the PVH involves primarily two pathways. The nucleus of the solitary tract, the primary recipient of sensory information from the thoracic and abdominal viscera, sends dense catecholaminergic projections to the PVH, both directly and through relays in the ventrolateral medulla. These brain stem projections account for about half of the NPY fibers present in the PVH. A second major input responsible for transducing signals from blood-borne substances derives from three CVOs adjacent to the third ventricle, the SFO, OVLT, and MePO. These pathways account for activation of CRH neurons by what are referred to as *systemic* or *physiologic stressors.*[179]

By contrast, what are termed *neurogenic, emotional,* or *psychological* stressors involve, in addition, nociceptive or somatosensory pathways as well as cognitive and affective brain centers. Using elevation of c-Fos as an indicator of neuronal activation, detailed studies have compared PVH-projecting neurons activated by IL-1 treatment (systemic stressor) versus foot shock (neurogenic stressor).[179] Only catecholaminergic solitary tract nucleus and ventrolateral medulla neurons were activated by moderate doses of IL-1. In contrast, foot–shock mediated activation of neurons of the solitary tract nucleus and ventrolateral medulla but also cell groups in the limbic forebrain and hypothalamus. Notably, pharmacologic or mechanical disruption of the ascending catecholaminergic fibers blocked IL-1–mediated activation but not foot–shock–mediated activation of the HPA axis. Data suggest that pathways activated by other neurogenic and systemic stressors may overlap significantly with those activated by foot–shock and IL-1 treatment, respectively.[178,179]

Except for the catecholaminergic neurons of the nucleus of the solitary tract and ventrolateral medulla, parts of the bed nucleus of the stria terminalis, and the dorsomedial nucleus of the hypothalamus, many inputs to the PVH, such as those deriving from the prefrontal cortex and lateral septum, are thought to act indirectly through local hypothalamic glutamatergic[180] and GABAergic neurons[181] with direct synapses to the CRH neurons. The bed nucleus of the stria terminalis is the only

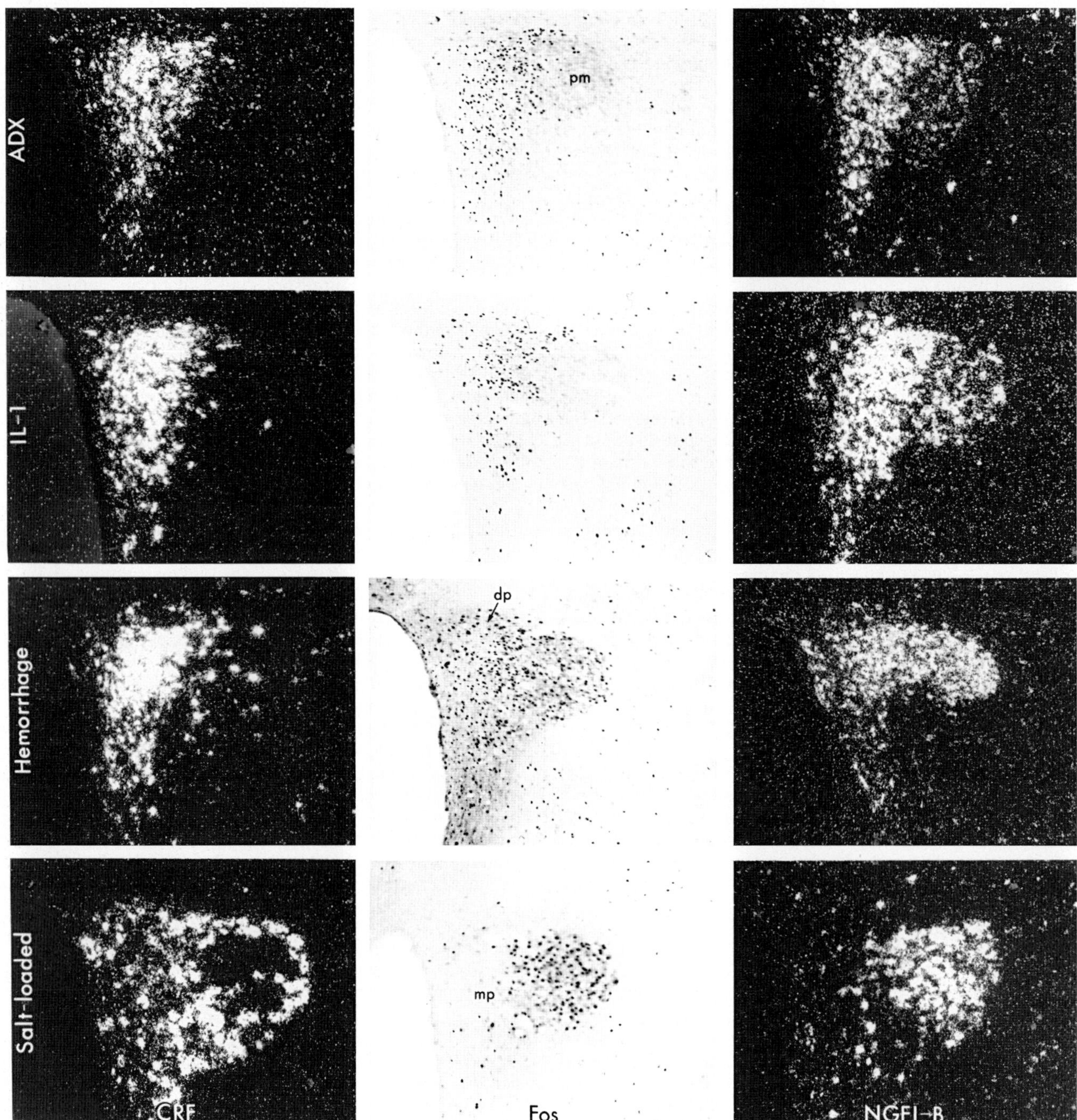

Figure 7–16 ▪ Regulation of neurons of the paraventricular nucleus (PVH) by diverse stressors. *ADX,* Adrenalectomy; CRF, corticotropin-releasing factor in situ hybridization (dark-field); *dp,* dorsal PVH; Fos, c-Fos immunoreactivity (bright-field); *IL-1,* interleukin-1; *pm,* magnicellular PVH; *NGFI-B,* nerve growth factor I-B in situ hybridization (dark field); *mp,* medial PVH. (From Sawchenko PE, Brown ER, Chan RK, et al. The paraventricular nucleus of the hypothalamus and the functional neuroanatomy of visceromotor responses to stress. Prog Brain Res 1996; 107:201-222.)

limbic region with prominent direct projections to the PVH. With substantial projections from the amygdala, hippocampus, and septal nuclei, it may thus serve as a key integrative center for transmission of limbic information to the PVH.[178]

Inflammation and Cytokines

Stimulation of the immune system by foreign pathogens leads to a stereotyped set of responses orchestrated by the CNS. These responses are the result of the complex interaction of the immune system and the CNS. This constellation of stereotyped responses is mediated in large part by the hypothalamus, and includes coordinated autonomic, endocrine, and behavioral components with adaptive consequences to restore homeostasis. It is now clear that cytokines produced by white blood cells of the immune system mediate the CNS responses. Early evidence supporting this hypothesis was provided by the seminal observations that cytokines such as IL-1β can activate the HPA axis.[182-184] Neuroimmunology, the discipline arising from the study of reciprocal interactions between the neuroendocrine

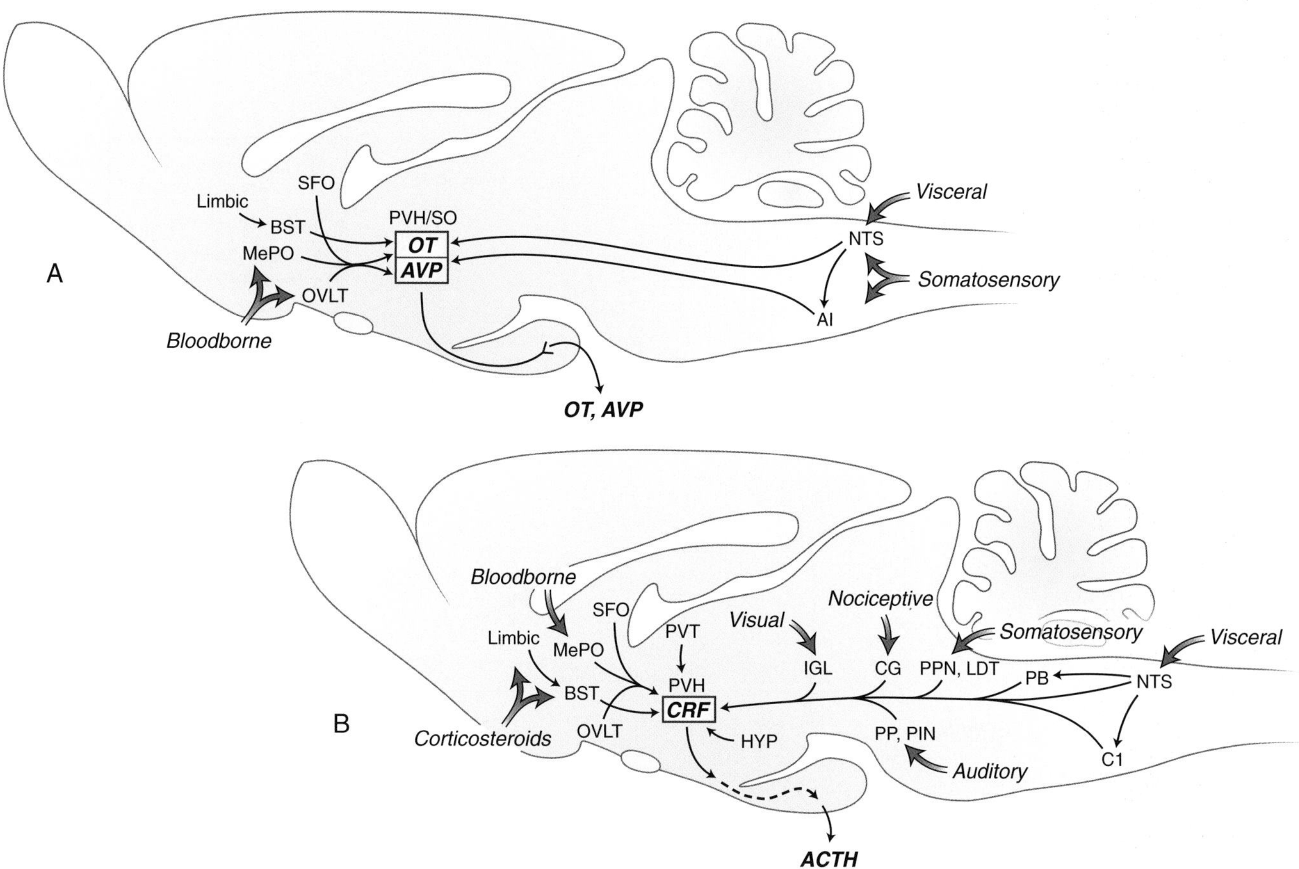

Figure 7–17 ■ Neuronal inputs to magnicellular **(A)** and parvicellular **(B)** neurons of the paraventricular nucleus. *AVP,* Arginine vasopressin; *BST,* bed nucleus of the stria terminalis; *CG,* central gray; *IGL,* intergeniculate leaf; *LDT,* laterodorsal tegmental nucleus; *MePO,* medial preoptic nucleus; *NTS,* nucleus of the tractus solitarius; *OT,* oxytocin; *OVLT,* organum vasculosum of the lamina terminalis; *PB,* parabrachial nucleus; *PIN,* posterior intralaminar nucleus; *PP,* peripeduncular nucleus; *PPN,* pedunculopontine nucleus; *SFO,* subfornical organ. (From Sawchenko PE, Brown ER, Chan RK, et al. The paraventricular nucleus of the hypothalamus and the functional neuroanatomy of visceromotor responses to stress. Prog Brain Res 1996;107:201-222.)

and immune systems, and particularly the role of cytokines in mediating cachexia is covered fully in Chapter 34.

This section focuses on cytokines and activation of the HPA axis. The resultant glucocorticoid secretion acts as a classic negative feedback to the immune system to dampen its response. In general, glucocorticoids inhibit most limbs of the immune response, including lymphocyte proliferation, production of immunoglobulins, cytokines, and cytotoxicity. These inhibitory reactions form the basis of the antiinflammatory actions of glucocorticoids.

Glucocorticoid feedback on immune responses is regulatory and beneficial because loss of this function makes animals with adrenal insufficiency vulnerable to inflammation. Moreover, this feedback response can have pathophysiologic consequences, as chronic activation of the HPA axis can certainly be detrimental.[185,186] Indeed, it is well established that chronic stress can lead to immunosuppression. The fact that products of inflammation such as IL-1β can activate the HPA axis suggests the operation of a negative feedback control loop to regulate the intensity of inflammation. The role of the hypothalamus in regulating pituitary-adrenal function is an excellent example of neuroimmunomodulation. Proposed models to explain how immune system signals might act upon the CNS to modulate homeostatic circuits by the integration of vagal input, peripheral cytokine interactions with receptors in the CVOs and cerebral blood vessels, and local production of cytokines within the CNS are explored in Chapter 34.

Other Factors Influencing Secretion of Corticotropin

Circadian Rhythms

Levels of ACTH and cortisol (in humans) peak in the early morning, fall during the day to reach a nadir at about midnight, and begin to rise between 1 AM and 4 AM (see Fig. 7–7). Within the circadian cycle, approximately 15 to 18 pulses of ACTH can be discerned, their height varying with the time of day.[187] The set-point of feedback control by glucocorticoids also varies in a circadian pattern. Pituitary-adrenal rhythms are entrained to the light-dark cycle and can be changed over several days by exposure to an altered light schedule. It has long been assumed that the rhythm of ACTH secretion is driven by CRH rhythms, and CRH knockout mice were found to exhibit no circadian rhythm in corticosterone production. Remarkably, however, a diurnal rhythm in corticosterone was restored by a constant infusion of CRH to the CRH knockout mouse,[188] suggesting that CRH is necessary to permit pituitary or adrenal responsiveness to another diurnal rhythm generator.

Corticotropin Release-Inhibiting Factor

Disconnection of the pituitary from the hypothalamus in several species leads to increased basal levels of ACTH, and certain responses to physical stress (in contrast to psychological stress) are retained in such animals. These observations have led several investigators to postulate the existence of an ACTH

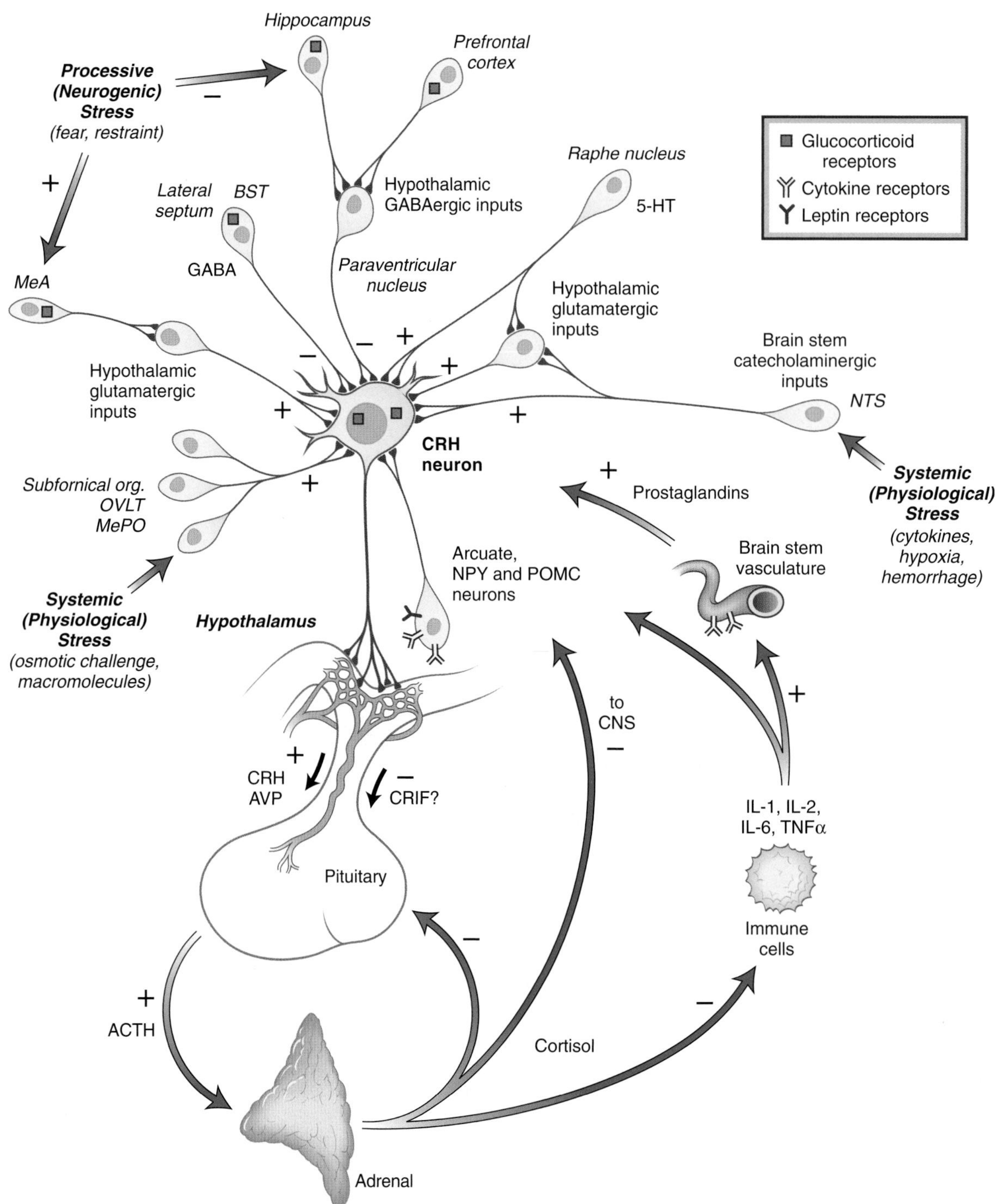

Figure 7–18 ▪ Regulation of the hypothalamic-pituitary-adrenal axis. *ACTH,* Adrenocorticotropic hormone; *AVP,* arginine vasopressin; *BST,* bed nucleus of the stria terminalis; *CNS,* central nervous system; *CRH,* corticotropin-releasing hormone; *CRIF,* corticotropin release-inhibiting factor; *GABA,* γ-aminobutyric acid; *5-HT,* 5-hydroxytryptamine; *IL-1,* interleukin-1; *MeA,* medial amygdala; *MePO,* medial preoptic; *NPY,* neuropeptide Y; *NTS,* nucleus of the tractus solitarius; *OVLT,* organum vasculosum of the lamina terminalis; *POMC,* pro-opiomelanocortin.

inhibitory factor analogous to dopamine in the control of PRL secretion and to somatostatin in the control of GH secretion. Candidate hypothalamic peptides to inhibit ACTH release at the level of the pituitary include atrial natriuretic peptide, activins and inhibins, and sequence 178 to 199 of the TRH prohormone.[189] There is not yet a consensus on the existence of a physiologically relevant ACTH release-inhibiting factor or on its identity.

Growth Hormone–Releasing Hormone

Chemistry and Evolution

Evidence for neural control of GH secretion came from studies of its regulation in animals with lesions of the hypothalamus[190] and from the demonstration that hypothalamic extracts stimulate the release of GH from the pituitary. When it was shown that GH is released episodically, follows a circadian rhythm, responds

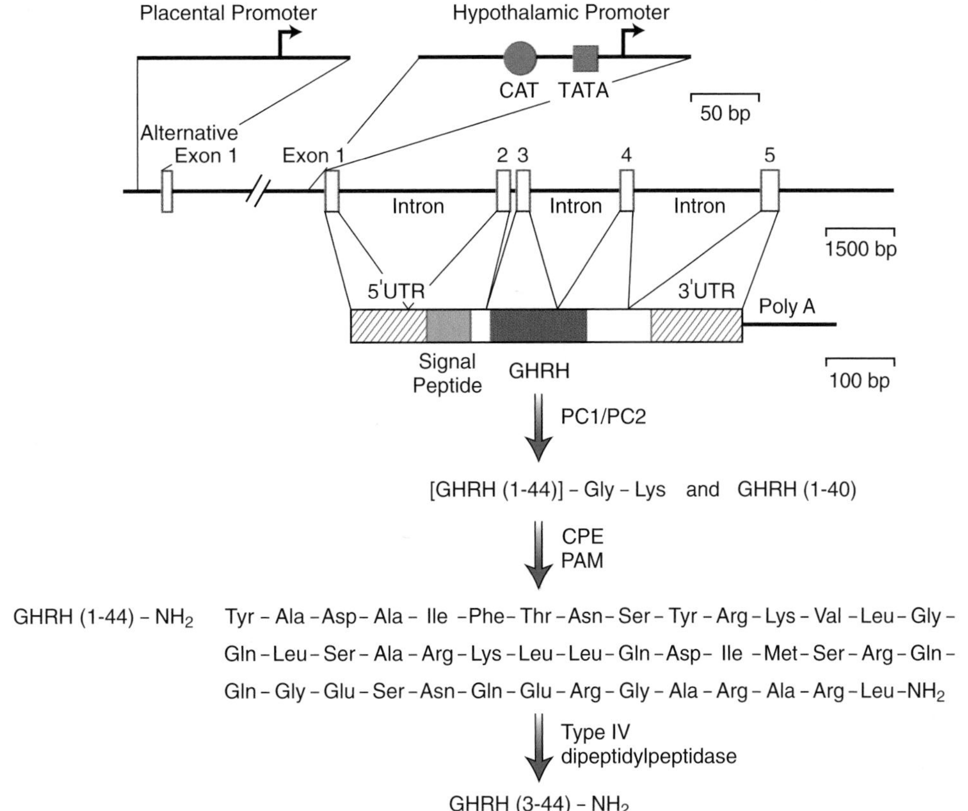

Figure 7–19 ■ Diagram illustrating the genomic organization, mRNA structure, and posttranslational processing of the human growth hormone–releasing hormone (GHRH) prohormone. Few details are known about the transcriptional regulation of the GHRH gene except that distinct promoter sequences and alternative 5′ exons are utilized by hypothalamic neurons and extrahypothalamic tissues. All of the amino acid residues required for bioactive GHRH peptides are encoded by exon 3. An amino-terminal exopeptidase that cleaves the Tyr-Ala dipeptide is primarily responsible for the inactivation of GHRH peptides in extracellular compartments. *CPE,* Carboxypeptidase E; *PAM,* peptidylglycine α-amidating monooxygenase; *PC1/PC2,* prohormone convertases 1 and 2; *UTR,* untranslated region. (Compiled from data of Mayo KE, Cerelli GM, Lebo RV, et al. Gene encoding human growth hormone-releasing factor precursor: structure, sequence, and chromosomal assignment. Proc Natl Acad Sci U S A 1985;82:63-67; Frohman LA, Downs TR, Chomczynski P, et al. Growth hormone-releasing hormone: structure, gene expression and molecular heterogeneity. Acta Paediatr Scand [suppl] 1990;367:81-86; and González-Crespo S, Boronat A. Expression of the rat growth hormone-releasing hormone gene in placenta is directed by an alternative promoter. Proc Natl Acad Sci U S A 1991;88:8749-8753.)

rapidly to stress, and is blocked by pituitary stalk section, the concept of neural control of GH secretion became a certainty. However, it was only with the discovery of the paraneoplastic syndrome of ectopic GHRH secretion by pancreatic adenomas in humans that sufficient starting material became available for peptide sequencing and subsequent cloning of a complementary deoxyribonucleic acid (cDNA).[191-194]

Two principal molecular forms of GHRH occur in human hypothalamus: GHRH(1-44)-NH_2 and GHRH(1-40)-OH (Fig. 7–19).[195] As with other neuropeptides, the various forms of GHRH arise from post-translational modification of a larger prohormone.[191,196] The NH_2-terminal tyrosine of GHRH (or histidine in rodent GHRHs) is essential for bioactivity, but a COOH-terminal NH_2 group is not. Fragments as short as (1-29)-NH_2 are active, but GHRH(1-27)-NH_2 is inactive. A circulating type IV dipeptidylpeptidase potently inactivates GHRH to its principal and more stable metabolite, GHRH(3-44)-NH_2,[197] which accounts for most of the immunoreactive peptide detected in plasma. As in the case of GnRH, there are species differences among GHRHs; the peptides from seven species range in sequence homology with the human peptide from 93% in the pig to 67% in the rat.[195] The COOH-terminal end of GHRH exhibits the most sequence diversity among species, consistent with the exon arrangement of the gene and dispensability of these residues for GHRH receptor binding.

Despite its importance for the elucidation of GHRH structure, ectopic secretion of the peptide is a rare cause of acromegaly. Fewer than 1% of acromegalic patients have elevated plasma levels of GHRH (see Chapter 8).[198] Approximately 20% of pancreatic adenomas and 5% of carcinoid tumors contain immunoreactive GHRH, but most are clinically silent.[199,200]

In addition to expression in the hypothalamus, the GHRH gene is expressed eutopically in human ovary, uterus, and placenta,[201] although its function in these tissues is not known. Studies in rat placenta indicate that an alternative transcriptional start site 10 kilobases upstream from the hypothalamic promoter is utilized together with an alternatively spliced exon 1a.[202]

Growth Hormone–Releasing Hormone Receptor

The GHRH receptor is a member of a subfamily of G protein–coupled receptors that includes receptors for VIP, pituitary adenylyl cyclase-activating peptide, secretin, glucagon, glucagon-

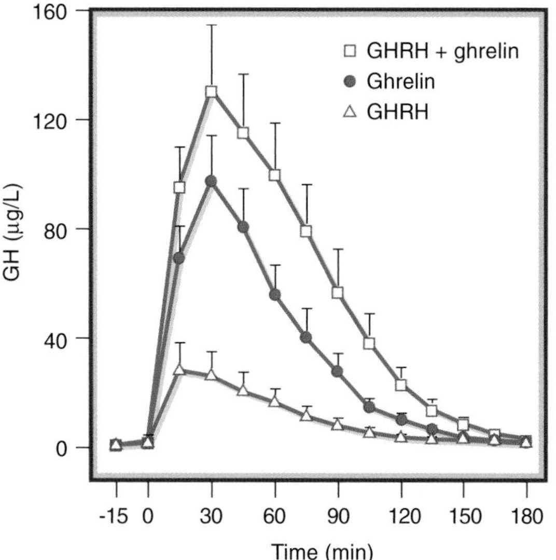

Figure 7–20 ▪ Response of normal men to growth hormone–releasing hormone (GHRH)(1-29) (1 μg/kg), ghrelin (1 μg/kg), or the combination of GHRH(1-29) and ghrelin administered by intravenous injection. Note the prompt release of GH, followed by a rather prolonged fall in hormone level in response to both secretagogues. Ghrelin alone was more efficacious than GHRH(1-29), and there was an additive effect from the two peptides administered simultaneously. (From Arvat E, Macario M, Di Vito L, et al. Endocrine activities of ghrelin, a natural growth hormone secretagogue (GHS), in humans: comparison and interactions with hexarelin, a nonnatural peptidyl GHS, and GH-releasing hormone. J Clin Endocrinol Metab 2001;86:1169-1174.)

like peptide 1, calcitonin, parathyroid hormone or parathyroid hormone–related peptide, and gastric inhibitory polypeptide.[203,204] GHRH elevates intracellular cAMP by its receptor coupling to a G_s, which activates adenylyl cyclase, increases intracellular free Ca^{2+}, releases preformed GH, and stimulates GH mRNA transcription and new GH synthesis (see Chapter 8).[205] GHRH also increases pituitary phosphatidylinositol turnover. Nonsense mutations in the human GHRH receptor gene are the cause of rare familial forms of GH deficiency[206,207] and indicate that no other gene product can fully compensate for the specific receptor in pituitary.

Effects on the Pituitary and Mechanism of Action

Intravenous administration of GHRH to individuals with normal pituitaries caused a prompt, dose-related increase in serum GH that peaked between 15 and 45 minutes, followed by a return to basal levels by 90 to 120 minutes (Fig. 7–20).[208] A maximally stimulating dose of GHRH is approximately 1 μg/kg, but the response differs considerably between individuals and within the same individual tested on different occasions, presumably because of cosecretagogue and somatostatin tone that exists at the time of GHRH injection. Repeated bolus administration or sustained infusions of GHRH over several hours cause a modest decrease in the subsequent GH secretory response to acute GHRH administration. However, unlike the marked desensitization of the GnRH receptor and decline in circulating gonadotropins that occur in response to continuous GnRH exposure, pulsatile GH secretion and insulin-like growth factor I (IGF-I) production are maintained by constant GHRH in the human.[208] This response suggests the involvement of additional factors that mediate the intrinsic diurnal rhythm of GH, and these factors are addressed in the following sections.

The pituitary effects of a single injection of GHRH are almost completely specific for GH secretion, and there is minimal evidence for any interaction between GHRH and the other classic hypophyseotropic releasing hormones.[208] GHRH has no effect on gut peptide hormone secretion. The GH secretory response to GHRH is enhanced by estrogen administration, glucocorticoids, and starvation. Major factors known to blunt the response to GHRH in humans are somatostatin, obesity, and advancing age.

In addition to its role as a GH secretagogue, GHRH is a physiologically relevant growth factor for somatotrophs. Transgenic mice expressing a GHRH cDNA coupled to a suitable promoter developed diffuse somatotroph hyperplasia and eventually pituitary macroadenomas.[209,210] The intracellular signal transduction pathways mediating the mitogenic action of GHRH are not known with certainty but probably involve an elevation of adenylyl cyclase activity. Several lines of evidence support this conclusion, including the association of activating mutations of the $G_{s\alpha}$ polypeptide in many human somatotroph adenomas.[211]

Extrapituitary Functions

GHRH has few known extrapituitary functions. The most important may be its activity as a sleep regulator. The administration of nocturnal GHRH boluses to normal men significantly increased the density of slow wave sleep, as also shown in other species.[212] Furthermore, there is a striking correlation between the age-related declines in slow wave sleep and daily integrated GH secretion in healthy men.[213] These and other data suggest that central GHRH secretion is under circadian entrainment and nocturnal elevations in GHRH pulse amplitude or frequency directly mediate sleep stage and sleep-induced increases in GH secretion.

GHRH has been reported to stimulate food intake in rats and sheep, but the effect is dependent on route of administration, time of administration, and macronutrient composition of the diet.[203] The neuropeptide's physiologic relevance to feeding in humans is unknown, although a study indicated that GHRH stimulated food intake in patients with anorexia nervosa but reduced it in patients with bulimia or in normal female control subjects.[214]

Growth Hormone–Releasing Peptides

In studies of the opioid control of GH secretion, several peptide analogues of met-enkephalin were found to be potent GH secretagogues. These include the GH-releasing peptide GHRP-6 (Fig. 7–21), hexarelin (His-D2MeTrp-Ala-Trp-DPhe-Lys-NH_2), and other more potent analogues including cyclic peptides and modified pentapeptides.[203,215] Subsequently, a series of nonpeptidyl GHRP mimetics were synthesized with greater oral bioavailability, including the spiropiperidine MK-0677 and the shorter acting benzylpiperidine L-163,540 (see Fig. 7–21). Common to all these compounds, and the basis of their differentiation from GHRH analogues in pharmacologic activity screens, is their activation of phospholipase C and inositol 1,4,5-trisphosphate. This property was exploited in a cloning strategy that led to the identification of a G protein–coupled receptor GHS-R that is highly selective for the GH secretagogue class of ligands.[216] The GHS-R is unrelated to the GHRH receptor and is highly expressed in the anterior pituitary gland and multiple brain areas, including the medial basal hypothalamus, the hippocampus, and the mesencephalic nuclei that are centers of dopamine and serotonin production.

Peptidyl and nonpeptidyl GHSs are active when administered by intranasal and oral routes, are more potent on a weight basis than GHRH itself, are more effective in vivo than in vitro, synergize with coadministered GHRH and are almost ineffective in the absence of GHRH, and do not suppress somatostatin secretion.[203,208] Prolonged infusions of GHRP amplify pulsatile GH secretion in normal men. GHRP administration, like that of GHRH, facilitates slow wave sleep. Patients with hypothalamic disease leading to GHRH deficiency have low or no response to

GHRP-6: His-DTrp-Ala-Trp-DPhe-Lys-NH_2

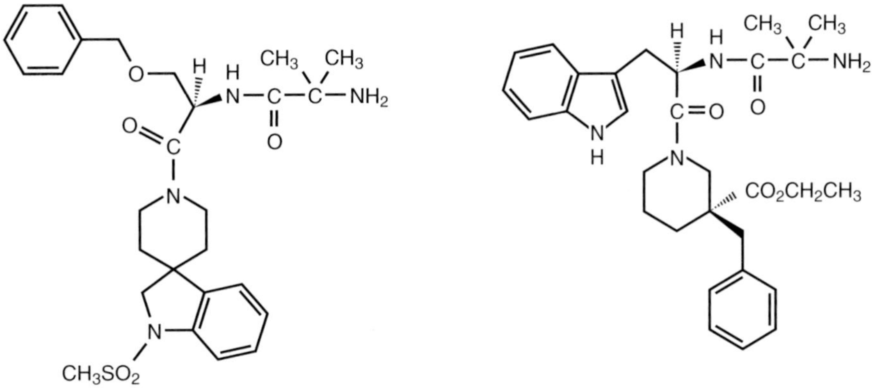

MK-0677 L-163,540

$O = C - (CH_2)_6 - CH_3$

Ghrelin: Gly - Ser - Ser - Phe - Leu - Ser - Pro - Glu - His - Gln - Arg - Val - Gln - Gln - Arg - Lys - Glu - Ser - Lys - Lys - Pro - Pro - Ala - Lys - Leu - Gln - Pro - Arg

Figure 7–21 ▪ Structure of a nonnatural peptidyl (GHRP-6) and nonpeptidyl (MK-0677 and L-163,540) growth hormone secretagogues and a natural ligand (ghrelin) that all bind and activate the growth hormone secretagogue receptor. Ghrelin is an acylated 28-amino-acid peptide. The O-n-octanoylation at Ser3 is essential for biologic activity and is a unique posttranslational modification among the known neuropeptides. (Adapted from Smith RG, Feighner S, Prendergast K, et al. A new orphan receptor involved in pulsatile growth hormone release. Trends Endocrinol Metab 1999;10:128-135; Kojima M, Hosoda H, Date Y, et al. Ghrelin is a growth hormone-releasing acylated peptide from stomach. Nature 1999;402:656-660.)

hexarelin; similarly, pediatric patients with complete absence of the pituitary stalk have no GH secretory response to hexarelin.[217]

The potent biologic effects of GHRPs and the identification of the GHS-R suggested the existence of a natural ligand for the receptor that is involved in the physiologic regulation of GH secretion. A probable candidate for this ligand is the acylated peptide ghrelin, produced and secreted into the circulation from the stomach (Fig. 7–22).[13] The effects of ghrelin on GH secretion in humans are identical to or more potent than those of the non-natural GHRPs (see Fig. 7–20).[218] In addition, ghrelin acutely increases circulating PRL, ACTH, cortisol, and aldosterone levels.[218] There is debate concerning the extent and localization of ghrelin expression in the brain that must be resolved before the implications of gastric-derived ghrelin in the regulation of pituitary hormone secretion are fully understood. A proposed role for ghrelin in appetite and the regulation of food intake is discussed in Chapter 34.

Clinical Applications

GHRH stimulates growth in children with intact pituitaries, but the optimal dosage, route, and frequency of administration, as well as possible usefulness by the nasal route, have not been determined. The availability of recombinant hGH (which requires less frequent injections than GHRH) and the development of the more potent GHSs with improved oral bioavailability have reduced enthusiasm for the clinical use of GHRH or its analogues. GHRH is not useful for the differential diagnosis of hypothalamic and pituitary causes of GH deficiency in children. However, in adults a combined GHRH-GHRP challenge test may be ideal for the diagnosis of GH reserve. GH release in response to the combined secretagogues is not influenced by age, gender, or body mass index, and the test has a wider margin of safety than an insulin tolerance test.[219,220]

The potential clinical applications of GHSs including MK-0677 are still being explored.[203,215] An area of intense interest is the normal decline in GH secretion with age. GH administration in healthy older individuals has been associated with increased lean body mass, increased muscle strength, and decreased fat mass, although there is a high incidence of adverse side effects. The physiologic GH profile induced by MK-0677 may be better tolerated than GH injections. However, unlike treatment with GHRH, chronic administration of GHSs leads to significant desensitization of the GHS-R and attenuation of the GH response. The release of pituitary hormones other than GH may also limit the applicability of GHS therapy. Finally, apart from actions on GH secretion, both GHRH and GHSs are being investigated for the treatment of sleep disorders commonly associated with aging.

Neuroendocrine Regulation of Growth Hormone Secretion

GH secretion is regulated by hypothalamic GHRH and somatostatin interacting with circulating hormones and additional modulatory peptides at the level of both the pituitary and the hypothalamus (see Fig. 7–22).[203,208] Additional background on somatostatin and its functions other than control of GH secretion are presented in a later section (see Somatostatin).

Feedback Control

Negative feedback control of GH release is mediated by GH itself and by IGF-I, which is synthesized in the liver under control of GH. Direct GH effects on the hypothalamus are produced by short-loop feedback, whereas those involving IGF-I and other circulating factors influenced by GH, including free fatty acids and glucose, are long-loop systems analogous to the pituitary-thyroid and pituitary-adrenal axes. Control of GH secretion thus includes two closed-loop systems (GH and IGF-I) and one open-loop regulatory system (neural).

Although most of the evidence for a direct role of GH in its own negative feedback has been derived from animals, an elegant study in normal men demonstrated that GH pretreatment blocks the subsequent GH secretory response to GHRH by a mechanism that is dependent on somatostatin.[221] The mechanism responsible for GH feedback through the hypothalamus has been largely elucidated in rodent models. GH receptors are selectively expressed on somatostatin neurons in the hypothalamic periventricular nucleus and on NPY neurons in the arcuate nucleus. C-Fos gene expression is acutely elevated in both populations of GH receptor-positive neurons by GH administration, indicating an activation of hypothalamic circuitry that includes

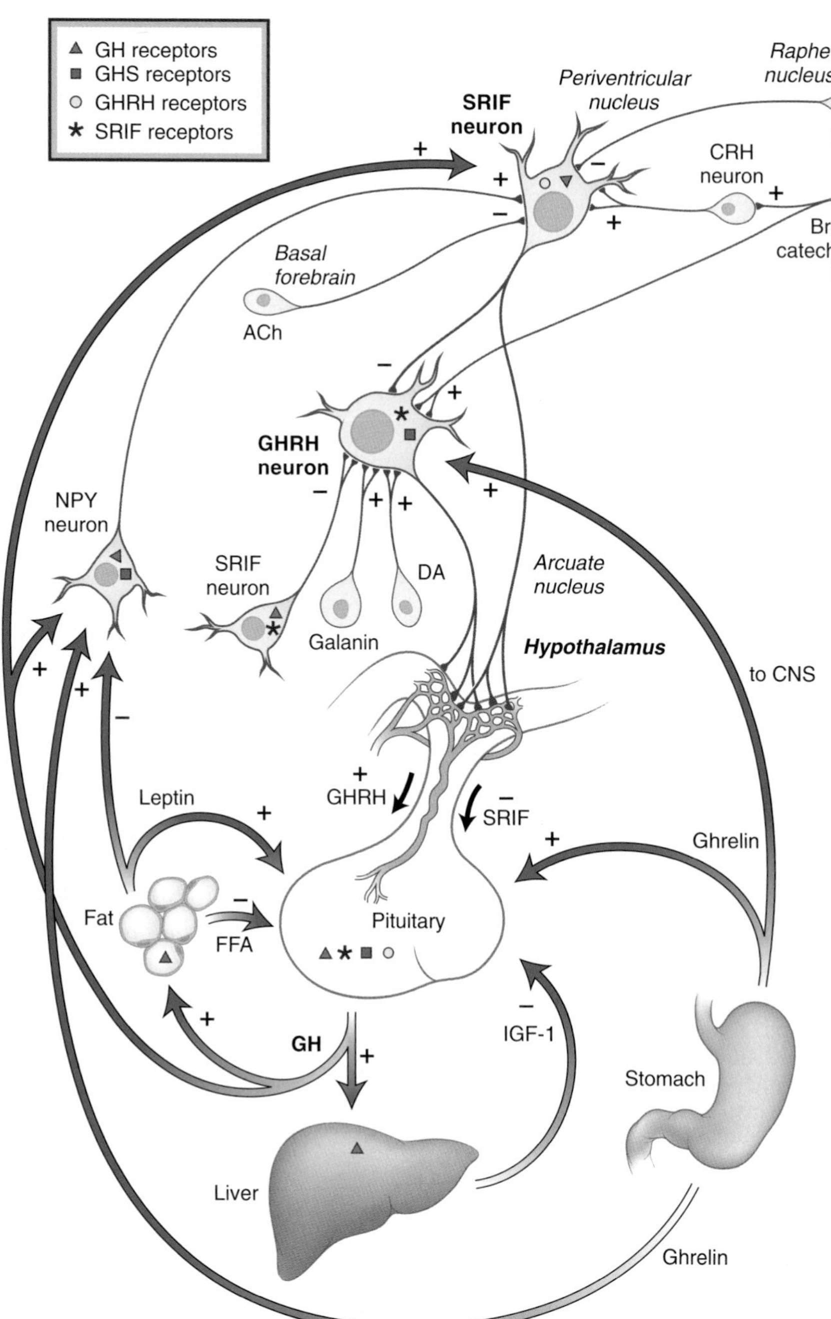

Figure 7–22 ■ Regulation of the hypothalamic-pituitary-growth hormone (GH) axis. GH secretion by the pituitary is stimulated by GH-releasing hormone (GHRH) and is inhibited by somatostatin (SRIF). Negative feedback control of GH secretion is exerted at the pituitary level by insulin-like growth factor I (IGF-I) and by free fatty acids (FFA). GH itself exerts a short-loop negative feedback by the activation of SRIF neurons in the hypothalamic periventricular nucleus. These SRIF neurons directly synapse on arcuate GHRH neurons and project to the median eminence. Neuropeptide Y (NPY) neurons in the arcuate nucleus also indirectly modulate GH secretion by integrating peripheral GH, leptin, and ghrelin signals and projecting to periventricular SRIF neurons. Ghrelin is secreted from the stomach and is a putative natural ligand for the GH secretagogue receptor that stimulates GH secretion at both the hypothalamic and pituitary levels. On the basis of indirect pharmacologic data, it appears that release of GHRH is stimulated by galanin, γ-aminobutyric acid (GABA), and α_2-adrenergic and dopaminergic stimuli and inhibited by somatostatin. Secretion of somatostatin is inhibited by acetylcholine (muscarinic receptors) and 5-HT (type 1D receptors), and increased by β_2-adrenergic stimuli and corticotropin-releasing hormone (CRH). *ACh,* Acetylcholine; *CNS,* central nervous system; *DA,* dopamine.

these neurons. Similarly, GHRH neurons in the arcuate nucleus are acutely activated by MK-0677 because of their selective expression of the GHS-R. Zheng and colleagues[222] showed in the latter group of neurons that c-Fos induction after MK-0677 administration was blocked by pretreatment of mice with GH (Fig. 7–23). The effect must be indirect because there are no GH receptors on GHRH neurons. However, there are type 2 somatostatin receptors expressed on GHRH neurons, and the somatostatin analogue octreotide also significantly blocked c-Fos activation in the arcuate nucleus by MK-0677. The inhibitory effects of either GH or octreotide pretreatment were abolished in knockout mice lacking the specific somatostatin receptor (see Fig. 7–23). Together with data from many other experiments, these results strongly support a model of GH-negative feedback regulation that involves the primary activation of periventricular somatostatin neurons by GH. These tuberoinfundibular neurons then inhibit GH secretion directly by release of somatostatin in the median eminence, but they also indirectly inhibit GH secretion by way of collateral axonal projections to the arcuate nucleus that synapse on and inhibit GHRH neurons (see Fig. 7–22). It is probable from evidence in rodents that NPY and galanin also play a part in the short-loop feedback of GH secretion, but a definitive mechanism in humans is not yet established.

IGF-I has a major inhibitory action on GH secretion at the level of the pituitary gland.[203] IGF-I receptors are expressed on human somatotroph adenoma cells and inhibit both spontaneous and GHRH-stimulated GH release. In addition, gene expression of both GH and the pituitary-specific transcription factor PIT1 is inhibited by IGF-I. Conflicting data among species suggest that circulating IGF-I may also regulate GH secretion by actions within the brain. The feedback effects of IGF-I account for the fact that in conditions in which circulating levels of IGF-I are low, such as anorexia nervosa, protein-calorie starvation,[223] and

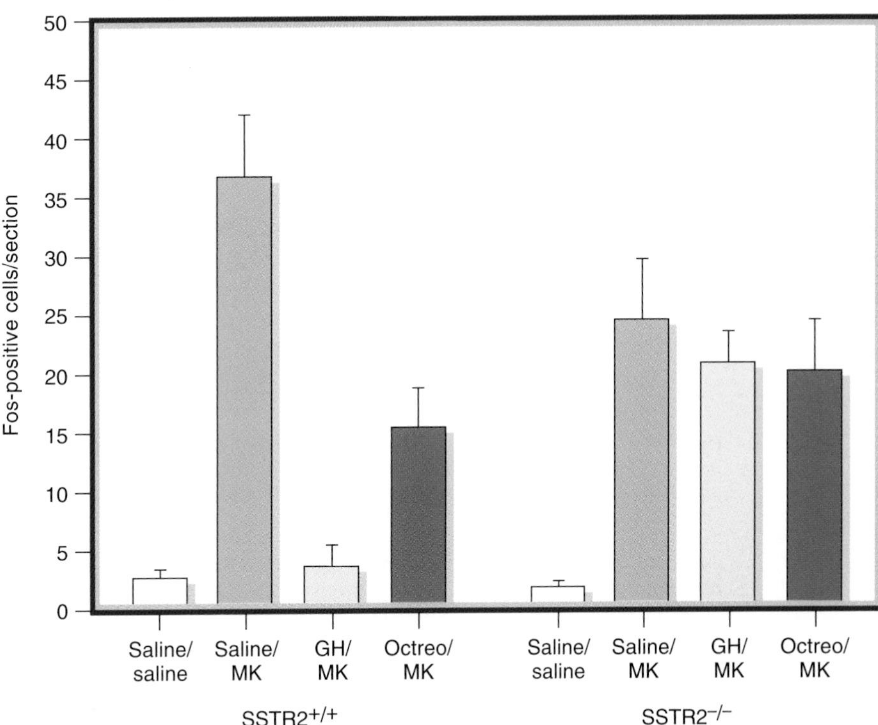

Figure 7–23 ▪ Somatostatin and the somatostatin receptor 2 subtype are involved in the short-loop inhibitory feedback of growth hormone (GH) on arcuate neurons. Activation of neurons in the arcuate nucleus was determined by the quantification of immunoreactive c-Fos–positive cells after administration of the growth hormone secretagogue MK-0677 (MK). Preliminary treatment of wild-type mice ($SSTR2^{+/+}$) with either GH or the somatostatin analogue octreotide (Octreo) significantly attenuated the neuronal activation by MK-0677. In contrast, GH and octreotide had no effect on MK-0677 neuronal activation in somatostatin receptor 2–deficient mice ($SSTR2^{-/-}$). (Adapted from Zheng H, Bailey A, Jian M-H, et al. Somatostatin receptor subtype 2 knockout mice are refractory to growth hormone-negative feedback on arcuate neurons. Mol Endocrinol 1997;11:1709-1717.)

Laron dwarfism (the result of a defect in the GH receptor), serum GH levels are elevated.

Neural Control

The predominant hypothalamic influence on GH release is stimulatory, and section of the pituitary stalk or lesions of the basal hypothalamus cause reduction of basal and induced GH release. When the somatostatinergic component is inactivated (e.g., by antisomatostatin antibody injection in rats), basal GH levels and GH responses to the usual provocative stimuli are enhanced.

GHRH-containing nerve fibers that terminate adjacent to portal vessels in the external zone of the median eminence arise principally from within, above, and lateral to the infundibular nucleus in human hypothalamus, corresponding to rodent arcuate and ventromedial nuclei.[224] Perikarya of the tuberoinfundibular somatostatin neurons are located almost completely in the medial periventricular nucleus and parvocellular component of the anterior PVH. Neuroanatomic and functional evidence suggests a bidirectional synaptic interaction between the two peptidergic systems.[203]

Multiple extrahypothalamic brain regions provide efferent connections to the hypothalamus and regulate GHRH and somatostatin neuronal activity (Fig. 7–24; see Fig. 7–22). Somatosensory and affective information is integrated and filtered through the amygdaloid complex. The basolateral amygdala provides an excitatory input to the hypothalamus, and the central extended amygdala, which includes the central and medial nuclei of the amygdala together with the bed nucleus of the stria terminalis, provides a GABAergic inhibitory input. Many intrinsic neurons of the hypothalamus also release GABA, often with a peptide cotransmitter. Excitatory cholinergic fibers arise to a small extent from forebrain projection nuclei but mostly from hypothalamic cholinergic interneurons, which densely innervate the external zone of the median eminence. Similarly, the origin of dopaminergic and histaminergic neurons is local with their cell bodies located in the hypothalamic arcuate and tuberomammillary bodies, respectively. Two important ascending pathways to the medial basal hypothalamus regulate GH secretion and originate from serotoninergic neurons in the raphe nuclei and adrenergic neurons in the nucleus of the tractus solitarius and ventral lateral nucleus of the medulla.

Both GHRH and somatostatin neurons express presynaptic and postsynaptic receptors for multiple neurotransmitters and peptides (Table 7–5). The α_2-adrenoreceptor agonist clonidine reliably stimulates GH release, and for this reason a clonidine test was a standard diagnostic tool in pediatric endocrinology. The stimulatory effect is blocked by the specific α_2-antagonist yohimbine and appears to involve a dual mechanism of action, inhibition of somatostatin neurons and activation of GHRH neurons. In addition, partial attenuation of the effects of clonidine by mixed 5-HT1 and 5-HT2 antagonists suggests that some of the relevant α_2-receptors are located presynaptically on serotoninergic nerve terminals and increase serotonin release. Both norepinephrine and epinephrine play physiologic roles in the adrenergic stimulation of GH secretion. The α_1-agonists have no effect on GH secretion in humans, but β_2-agonists such as the bronchodilator salbutamol inhibit GH secretion by stimulating the release of somatostatin from nerve terminals in the median eminence. These effects are blocked by propranolol, a nonspecific β-antagonist. Dopamine generally has a net effect to stimulate GH secretion, but the mechanism is not clear because of multiple dopamine receptor subtypes and the apparent activation of both GHRH and somatostatin neurons.

Serotonin's effect on GH release in humans was difficult to decipher because of the large number of receptor subtypes. However, clinical studies with the receptor-selective agonist sumatriptan clearly implicated the 5-HT1D receptor subtype in the stimulation of basal GH levels.[225] The drug also potentiates the effect of a maximal dose of GHRH, suggesting the recurring theme of GH disinhibition by inhibition of hypothalamic somatostatin neurons in its mechanism of action. Histaminergic pathways acting through H1 receptors play only a minor, conditional stimulatory role in GH secretion in humans.

Acetylcholine appears to be an important physiologic regulator of GH secretion.[226] Blockade of acetylcholinergic muscarinic receptors reduces or abolishes GH secretory responses to

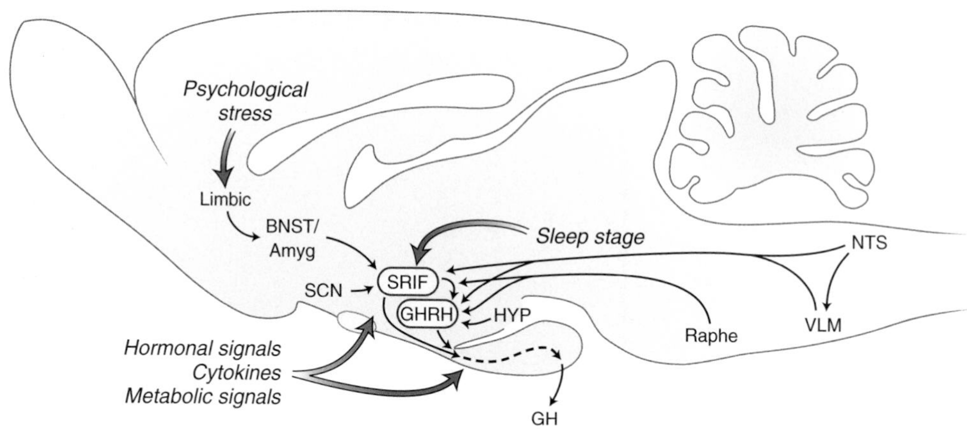

Figure 7–24 ■ Neural pathways involved in growth hormone (GH) regulation. This diagram illustrates the varied pathways by which impulses from the limbic system and brain stem ultimately impinge on the hypothalamic periventricular and arcuate nuclei to stimulate GH release through the mediation of somatostatin (SRIF) and growth hormone–releasing hormone (GHRH). Psychological stress modulates hypothalamic function indirectly through the bed nucleus of the stria terminalis (BNST) and amygdalar complex (Amyg). Circadian rhythms are entrained in part by projections from the suprachiasmatic nucleus (SCN). Complex reciprocal interactions between sleep stage and GHRH release involve cortex and subcortical nuclei, but the detailed mechanisms are not known. Dopaminergic and histaminergic input are from neurons located in the arcuate and mammillary nuclei, respectively, of the hypothalamus (HYP). Ascending catecholaminergic projections arise in both the nucleus of the tractus solitarius (NTS) and ventral lateral medulla (VLM). Serotoninergic (5-HT) afferents are from the raphe nuclei. In addition to these neural pathways, a variety of peripheral hormonal and metabolic signals and cytokines influence GH secretion by actions within the medial basal hypothalamus and pituitary gland.

GHRH, glucagon and arginine, morphine, and exercise. In contrast, drugs that potentiate cholinergic transmission increase basal GH levels and enhance the GH response to GHRH in normal individuals or in subjects with obesity or Cushing's disease. In vitro acetylcholine inhibits somatostatin release from hypothalamic fragments, and acetylcholine can act directly on the pituitary to inhibit GH release. There even may be a paracrine cholinergic control system within the pituitary. However, the sum of evidence suggests that the primary mechanism of action of M1 agonists is inhibition of somatostatin neuronal activity or the release of peptide from somatostatinergic terminals. Short-term cholinergic blockade with the M1 muscarinic receptor antagonist pirenzepine reduced the GH excess of patients with poorly controlled diabetes mellitus.[227] However, in the long term, cholinergic blockade did not prevent complications associated with the hypersomatotropic state.

Many neuropeptides in addition to GHRH and somatostatin are involved in the modulation of GH secretion in humans (see Table 7–5).[203,208] Among these, the evidence is most compelling for a stimulatory role of galanin acting in the human hypothalamus by a GHRH-dependent mechanism.[228] Many GHRH neurons are immunopositive for galanin as well as neurotensin and tyrosine hydroxylase. Galanin's actions may be explained, in part, by presynaptic facilitation of catecholamine release from nerve terminals and subsequent direct adrenergic stimulation of GHRH release.[229] Opioid peptides also stimulate GH release, probably by disinhibition of GHRH neurons, but under normal circumstances endogenous opioid tone in the hypothalamus is presumed to be low because opioid antagonists have little acute effect on GH secretion.

A larger number of neuropeptides are known or suspected to inhibit GH secretion in humans, at least under certain circumstances.[208] The list includes NPY, CRH, calcitonin, oxytocin, neurotensin, VIP, and TRH. Inhibitory actions of NPY are well established in the rat. The effect on GH secretion is secondary to stimulation of somatostatin neurons and is of particular interest because of the presumed role in GH autofeedback (discussed earlier) and the integration of GH secretion with regulation of energy intake and expenditure (discussed in a later section see External and Metabolic Signals). Finally, TRH has the well-established paradoxical effect of increasing GH secretion in patients with acromegaly, type 1 diabetes mellitus, hypothyroidism, or hepatic and renal failure.

Factors Influencing Secretion of Growth Hormone

Human Growth Hormone Rhythms

The deciphering of rhythmic GH secretion has relied on a combination of technical innovations in sampling and GH assay, and sophisticated mathematical modeling including deconvolution analysis and the calculation of approximate entropy as a measure of orderliness or regularity in minute-to-minute secretory patterns.[208] At least three distinct categories of GH rhythms, which differ markedly in their time scales, can be considered here. The daily GH secretion rate varies over two orders of magnitude from a maximum of nearly 2.0 mg/day in late puberty to a minimum of 20 μg/day in older or obese adults. The neonatal period is characterized by markedly amplified GH secretory bursts followed by a prepubertal decade of stable, moderate GH secretion of 200 to 600 μg/day. There is a marked increase in daily GH secretion during puberty that is accompanied by a commensurate rise in plasma IGF-I to levels that constitute a state of physiologic hypersomatotropism. This pubertal increase in GH secretion is due to increased GH mass per secretory burst and not to increased pulse frequency. Although the changes are clearly related to the increases in gonadal steroid hormones and can be mimicked by administration of estrogen or testosterone to hypogonadal children, the underlying neuroendocrine mechanisms are not fully understood. One hypothesis is that decreased sensitivity of the hypothalamic-pituitary axis to negative feedback of GH and IGF-I leads to increased GHRH release and action. Young adults have a return of daily GH secretion to prepubertal levels despite continued gonadal steroid elevation. The so-called somatopause is defined by an exponential decline in GH secretory rate with a half-life of 7 years starting in the third decade of life.

GH secretion in young adults exhibits a true circadian rhythm over a 24-hour period, characterized by a greater noc-

TABLE 7–5 FACTORS THAT CHANGE GROWTH HORMONE SECRETION IN HUMANS

Physiologic	Hormones and Neurotransmitters	Pathologic
	STIMULATORY FACTORS	
Episodic, spontaneous release	Insulin hypoglycemia	Acromegaly
Exercise	2-Deoxyglucose	TRH
Stress	Amino acid infusions	GnRH
Physical	Arginine, lysine	Glucose
Psychological	Neuropeptides	Arginine
Slow wave sleep	GHRH	Interleukins 1, 2, 6
Postprandial glucose decline	Ghrelin	Protein depletion
Fasting	Galanin	Starvation
	Opioids (μ-receptors)	Anorexia nervosa
	Melatonin	Renal failure
	Classical neurotransmitters	Liver cirrhosis
	α_2-Adrenergic agonists	Type 1 diabetes mellitus
	β-Adrenergic antagonists	
	M1-cholinergic agonists	
	5-HT1D-serotonin agonists	
	H1-histamine agonists	
	GABA (basal levels)	
	Dopamine (? D2 receptor)	
	Estrogen	
	Testosterone	
	Glucocorticoids (acute)	
	INHIBITORY FACTORS*	
Postprandial hyperglycemia	Glucose infusion	Acromegaly
Elevated free fatty acids	Neuropeptides	L-Dopa
Elevated GH levels	Somatostatin	D2R DA agonists
Elevated IGF-I (pituitary)	Calcitonin	Phentolamine
Rapid eye movement (REM) sleep	Neuropeptide Y (NPY†)	Galanin
Senescence, aging	CRH†	Obesity
	Classical neurotransmitters	Hypothyroidism
	$\alpha_{1/2}$-Adrenergic antagonists	Hyperthyroidism
	β_2-Adrenergic agonists	
	H1-Histamine antagonists	
	Serotonin antagonist	
	Nicotinic cholinergic agonists	
	Glucocorticoids (chronic)	

*In many instances, the inhibition can be demonstrated only as a suppression of GH release induced by a pharmacologic stimulus.

†The inhibitory actions of NPY and CRH on GH secretion are firmly established in the rodent and are secondary to increased somatostatin tone. Contradictory evidence exists in the human for both peptides and further studies are required.

CRH, Corticotropin-releasing hormone; *DA,* dopamine; *GHRH,* growth hormone-releasing hormone; *GnRH,* gonadotropin-releasing hormone; *IGF-I,* insulin-like growth factor I; *TRH,* thyrotropin-releasing hormone.

turnal secretory mass that is independent of sleep onset.[230] However, as discussed earlier, GH release is further facilitated when slow wave sleep coincides with the normal circadian peak. Under basal conditions, GH levels are low most of the time, with an ultradian rhythm of about 10 (men) or 20 (women) secretory pulses per 24 hours as calculated by deconvolution analysis.[231] Both sexes have an increased pulse frequency during the nighttime hours, but the fraction of total daily GH secretion associated with the nocturnal pulses is much greater in men. Overall, women have more continuous GH secretion and more frequent GH pulses that are of more uniform size than men.[231] A complementary study using approximate entropy analysis concluded that the nonpulsatile regularity of GH secretion is also significantly different in men and women.[232] These sexually dimorphic patterns in the human are actually quite similar to those in the rat, although the sex differences are not as extreme in humans.[208,232] The neuroendocrine basis for sex differences in the ultradian rhythm of GH secretion is not fully understood. Gonadal sex steroids play both an organizational role during development of the hypothalamus and an activational role in the adult, regulating expression of the genes for many of the peptides and receptors central to GH regulation.[203,208] In the human, unlike the rat, the hypothalamic actions of testosterone appear to be predominantly due to its aromatization to 17β-estradiol and interaction with estrogen receptors. Hypothalamic somatostatin appears to play a more prominent role in men than in women in the regulation of pulsatile GH secretion, and this difference is postulated to be a key factor in producing the sexual dimorphism.[231,233,234]

External and Metabolic Signals

The various peripheral signals that modulate GH secretion in humans are summarized in Table 7–5 (also see Figs. 7–22 and 7–24). Of particular importance are factors related to energy intake and metabolism because they provide a common signal between the peripheral tissues and hypothalamic centers regulating nonendocrine homeostatic pathways in addition to the classical hypophyseotropic neurons. It is also in this complex arena that species-specific regulatory responses are particularly prominent, making extrapolations between rodent experimental models and human GH regulation less reliable.[203,208]

Important triggers of GH release include the normal decrease in blood glucose level after intake of a carbohydrate-rich meal, absolute hypoglycemia, exercise, physical and emotional stress, and high intake of protein (mediated by amino acids). Some of the pathologic causes of elevated GH represent extremes of these physiologic signals and include protein-calorie starvation, anorexia nervosa, liver failure, and type 1 diabetes mellitus. A critical concept is that many of these GH triggers work through the same final common mechanism of somatostatin withdrawal and consequent disinhibition of GH secretion. In contrast, postprandial hyperglycemia, glucose infusion, elevated plasma free fatty acids, type 2 diabetes mellitus (with obesity and insulin resistance), and obesity are all associated with inhibition of GH secretion. The role of leptin in mediating either increases or decreases in GH release is complicated by its multiple sites of action and coexistent secretory environment. Similarly, other members of the cytokine family including IL-1, IL-2, IL-6, and endotoxin have been inconsistently shown to stimulate GH in humans.

The actions of steroid hormones on GH secretion are complex because of their multiple loci of action within the proximal hypothalamic-pituitary components in addition to secondary effects on other neural and endocrine systems. Glucocorticoids in particular produce opposite responses that are dependent on the chronicity of administration. Moreover, glucocorticoid effects follow an inverted U-shaped dose-response curve. Both low and high glucocorticoid levels reduce GH secretion, the former because of decreased GH gene expression and somatotroph responsiveness to GHRH and the latter because of increased hypothalamic somatostatin tone and decreased GHRH. Similarly, physiologic levels of thyroid hormones are necessary to maintain GH secretion and promote GH gene expression. Excessive thyroid hormone is also inhibitory to the GH axis, and the mechanism is speculated to be a combination of increased hypothalamic somatostatin tone, GHRH deficiency, and suppressed pituitary GH production.

Somatostatin

Chemistry and Evolution

A factor that potently inhibited GH release from pituitary in vitro was unexpectedly identified during early efforts to isolate GHRH from hypothalamic extracts.[235] Somatostatin, the peptide responsible for this inhibition of GH secretion and the inhibition of insulin secretion by a pancreatic islet extract, was eventually isolated from hypothalamus and sequenced by Brazeau and colleagues in 1973.[236] The term *somatostatin* was originally applied to a cyclic peptide containing 14 amino acids (somatostatin-14 [SST-14]; Fig. 7–25). Subsequently, a second form, N-extended somatostatin-28 (SST-28), was identified as a secretory product. Both forms of somatostatin are derived by independent cleavage of a common prohormone by prohormone convertases.[237] In addition, the isolation of SST-28(1-12) in some tissues suggests that SST-14 can be secondarily processed from SST-28. SST-14 is the predominant form in the brain (including the hypothalamus), whereas SST-28 is the major form in the gastrointestinal tract, especially the duodenum and jejunum.

The name *somatostatin* is descriptively inadequate because the molecule also inhibits TSH secretion from the pituitary and has nonpituitary roles including activity as a neurotransmitter or neuromodulator in the central and peripheral nervous systems and as a regulatory peptide in gut and pancreas. As a pituitary regulator, somatostatin is a true neurohormone, that is, a neuronal secretory product that enters the blood (hypophyseal-portal circulation) to affect cell function at remote sites. In the gut, somatostatin is present in both the myenteric plexus, where it acts as a neurotransmitter, and epithelial cells, where it influences the function of adjacent cells as a paracrine secretion. Somatostatin can influence its own secretion from delta cells (an autocrine function) in addition to acting as a paracrine factor in pancreatic islets. Gut exocrine secretion can be modulated by intraluminal action, so it is also a lumone. Because of its wide distribution, broad spectrum of regulatory effects, and evolutionary history, this peptide can be regarded as an archetypical pan-system modulator.

The genes that encode somatostatin in humans[238] (see Fig. 7–25) and a number of other species exhibit striking sequence homology, even in primitive fish such as the anglerfish. Furthermore, the amino acid sequence of SST-14 is identical in all vertebrates. Formerly, it was accepted that all tetrapods have a single gene encoding both SST-14 and SST-28 whereas teleost fish have two nonallelic pre-prosomatostatin genes (PPSI and PPSII), each of which encodes only one form of the mature somatostatin peptides. This situation implied that a common ancestral gene underwent a duplication event after the split of teleosts from the descendants of tetrapods.

However, both lampreys and amphibians, which predate and postdate the teleost evolutionary divergence, respectively, have now been shown to have at least two PPS genes.[239] A more distantly related gene has been identified in mammals that encodes cortistatin, a somatostatin-like peptide that is highly expressed in cortex and hippocampus.[240,241] Cortistatin-14 differs from SST-14 by three amino acid residues but has high affinity for all known subtypes of somatostatin receptors (see next section). The human gene sequence predicts a tripeptide-extended cortistatin-17 and a further N-terminally extended cortistatin-29.[242] A revised evolutionary concept of the somatostatin gene family is that a primordial gene underwent duplication at or before the advent of chordates and the two resulting genes underwent mutation at different rates to produce the distinct pre-prosomatostatin and pre-procortistatin genes in mammals.[239] A second gene duplication probably occurred in teleosts to generate PPSI and PPSII from the ancestral somatostatin gene.

Apart from its expression in neurons of the periventricular and arcuate hypothalamic nuclei and involvement in GH secretion discussed earlier, somatostatin is highly expressed in the cortex, lateral septum, extended amygdala, reticular nucleus of the thalamus, hippocampus, and many brain stem nuclei. Cortistatin is present in the brain at a small fraction of the levels of somatostatin and in a more limited distribution primarily confined to cortex and hippocampus. The molecular mechanisms underlying the developmental and hormonal regulation of somatostatin gene transcription have been most extensively studied in pancreatic islet cells.[243-245] Less is known concerning the regulation of somatostatin gene expression in neurons except that activation is strongly controlled by binding of the phosphorylated transcription factor cAMP response element-binding protein to its cognate cAMP response element contained in the promoter sequence.[246,247] Enhancer elements in the somatostatin gene promoter that bind complexes of homeodomain-containing transcription factors (PAX6, PBX, PREP1) and up-regulate gene expression in pancreatic islets may actually represent gene silencer elements in neurons (see Fig. 7–25, pro-

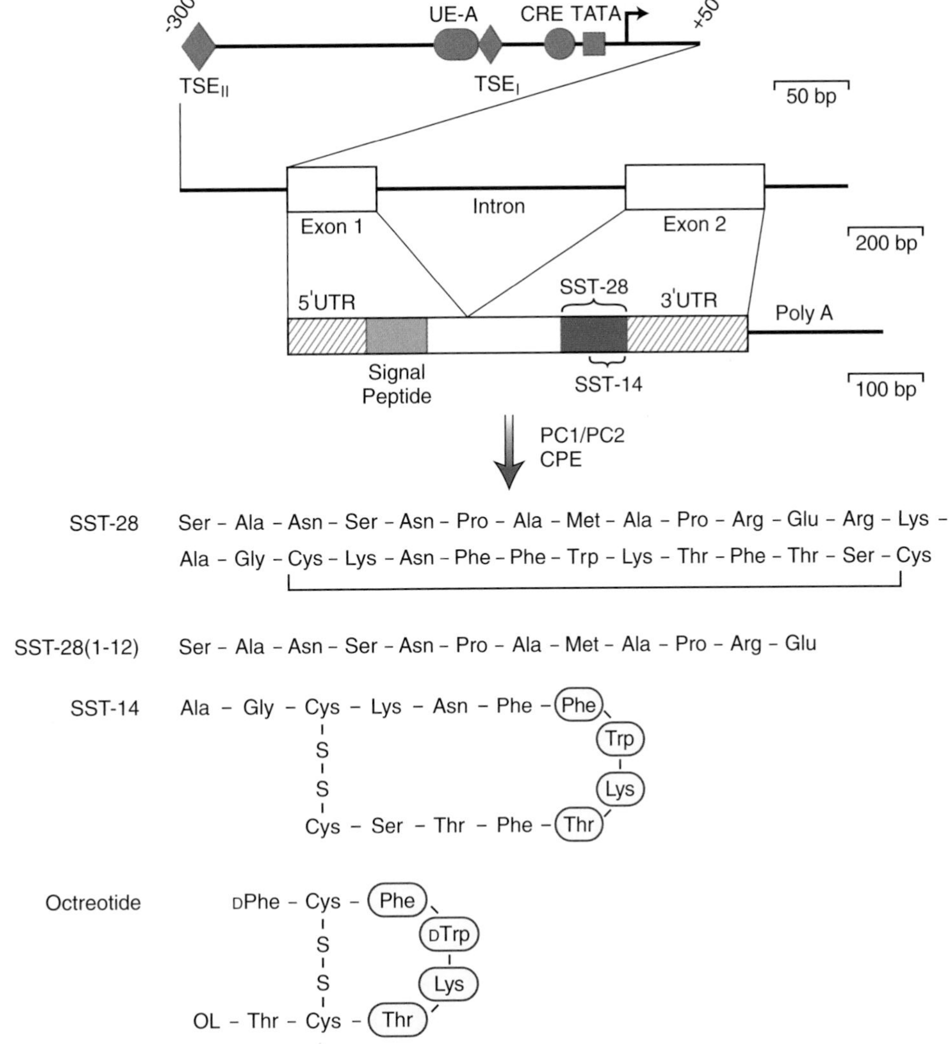

Figure 7–25 ▪ Diagram illustrating the genomic organization, mRNA structure, and posttranslational processing of the human somatostatin prohormone. Transcriptional regulation of the somatostatin gene, including the identification of tissue-specific elements (TSE), upstream elements (UE), and the cyclic adenosine monophosphate (cAMP) response element (CRE) that are binding sites for specific factors, has been studied extensively in pancreatic islet cell lines. It is not known whether all or some of these factors are also involved in the neural-specific expression of somatostatin. SST-28 and SST-14 are cyclic peptides containing a single covalent disulfide bond between a pair of Cys residues. A β turn containing the tetrapeptide Phe-Trp-Lys-Thr is stabilized by hydrogen bonds to produce the core receptor binding epitope. This minimal structure has been the model for conformationally restrained analogues of somatostatin including octreotide. *CPE,* Carboxypeptidase E; *PC1/PC2,* prohormone convertases 1 and 2; *UTR,* untranslated region. (Compiled from data by Shen LP, Rutter WJ. Sequence of the human somatostatin 1 gene. Science 1984;224:168-171; Goudet G, Delhalle S, Biemar F, et al. Functional and cooperative interactions between the homeodomain PDX1, Pbx, and Prep1 factors on the somatostatin promoter. J Biol Chem 1999;274:4067-4073; and Milner-White EJ. Predicting the biologically active conformations of short polypeptides. Trends Pharmacol Sci 1989;10:70-74.)

moter elements TSE$_{II}$ and UE-A).[245] Conversely, another related *cis* element in the somatostatin gene (see Fig. 7–25, promoter element TSE$_{I}$) apparently binds a homeodomain transcription factor PDX1 (also called STF1/IDX1/IPF1) that is common to developing brain, pancreas, and foregut and regulates gene expression in both the CNS and gut.[248]

The function of somatostatin in GH and TSH regulation is considered earlier in this chapter. Its actions in the extrahypothalamic brain and diagnostic and therapeutic roles are considered in the remainder of this section and in Chapter 8. An additional function of somatostatin in pancreatic islet cell regulation is described in Chapter 33, and the manifestations of somatostatin excess as in somatostatinoma are described in Chapter 38.

Somatostatin Receptors

Five somatostatin receptor subtypes (SSTR1 to SSTR5) have been identified by gene cloning techniques and one of these (SSTR2) is expressed in two alternatively spliced forms.[249] These subtypes are encoded by separate genes located on different chromosomes, are expressed in unique or partially overlapping distributions in multiple target organs, and differ in their coupling to second messenger signaling molecules and therefore in their range and mechanism of intracellular actions.[249,250] The subtypes also differ in their binding affinity to specific somatostatin analogues. Certain of these differences have important implications for the use of somatostatin analogues in therapy and in diagnostic imaging.

All SSTR subtypes are coupled to pertussis toxin–sensitive G proteins and bind SST-14 and SST-28 with high affinity in the low nanomolar range, although SST-28 has a uniquely high affinity for SSTR5. SSTR1 and SSTR2 are the two most abundant subtypes in brain and probably function as presynaptic autoreceptors in the hypothalamus and limbic forebrain, respectively, in addition to their postsynaptic actions. SSTR4 is most prominent in hippocampus. All the subtypes are expressed in pituitary, but SSTR2 and SSTR5 are the most abundant on somatotrophs. These two subtypes are also the most physiologically important in pancreatic islets, with SSTR5 responsible for inhibition of insulin secretion from bata cells and SSTR2 responsible for inhibition of glucagon from alpha cells.[251]

Binding of somatostatin to its receptor leads to activation of one or more plasma membrane-bound inhibitory G proteins ($G_{i/o}$), which in turn inhibit adenylyl cyclase activity and lower intracellular cAMP. Other G protein–mediated actions common to all SSTRs are activation of a vanadate-sensitive phosphotyrosine phosphatase and modulation of mitogen-activated protein kinase (MAPK). Different subsets of SSTRs are also coupled to inwardly rectifying K^+ channels, voltage-dependent Ca^{2+} channels, a Na^+/H^+ exchanger, α-amino-3-hydroxy-5-methyl-4-isoxazole proprionic acid (AMPA)-kainate glutamate receptors,

TABLE 7–6 BIOLOGIC ACTIONS OF SOMATOSTATIN OUTSIDE THE CENTRAL NERVOUS SYSTEM

Inhibits Hormone Secretion by	Inhibits Other Gastrointestinal Actions
Pituitary gland	Gastric acid secretion
GH, thyrotropin, ACTH, prolactin	Gastric and jejunal fluid secretion
Gastrointestinal tract	Gastric emptying
Gastrin	Pancreatic bicarbonate secretion
Secretin	Pancreatic enzyme secretion
Gastrointestinal polypeptide	(Stimulates intestinal absorption of water and electrolytes)
Motilin	
Glicentin (enteroglucagon)	Gastrointestinal blood flow
VIP	AVP-stimulated water transport
Pancreas	Bile flow
Insulin	
Glucagon	**Extragastrointestinal Actions**
Somatostatin	Inhibits the function of activated immune cells
Genitourinary tract	
Renin	Inhibition of tumor growth

ACTH, Adrenocorticotropic hormone; *AVP,* arginine vasopressin; *GH,* growth hormone; *VIP,* vasoactive intestinal peptide.

phospholipase C, and phospholipase A_2.[249] The lowering of intracellular cAMP and Ca^{2+} is the most important mechanism for the inhibition of hormone secretion, and actions on phosphotyrosine phosphatase and MAPK are postulated to play a role in somatostatin's antiproliferative effect on tumor cells.

Effects on Target Tissues and Mechanism of Action

In the pituitary, somatostatin inhibits secretion of GH and TSH and, under certain conditions, of PRL and ACTH as well. It exerts inhibitory effects on virtually all endocrine and exocrine secretions of the pancreas, gut, and gallbladder (Table 7–6). Somatostatin inhibits secretion by the salivary glands and, under some conditions, the secretion of parathyroid hormone and calcitonin. Somatostatin blocks hormone release in many endocrine-secreting tumors, including insulinomas, glucagonomas, VIPomas, carcinoid tumors, and some gastrinomas.

The physiologic actions of somatostatin in extrahypothalamic brain remain the subject of investigation.[252] In the striatum, somatostatin increases the release of dopamine from nerve terminals by a glutamate-dependent mechanism. It is widely expressed in GABAergic interneurons of limbic cortex and hippocampus, where it modulates the excitability of pyramidal neurons. Temporal lobe epilepsy is associated with a marked reduction in somatostatin-expressing neurons in the hippocampus consistent with a putative inhibitory action on seizures.[253] A wealth of correlative data has linked reduced forebrain and CSF concentrations of somatostatin with Alzheimer's disease, major depression, and other neuropsychiatric disorders, raising speculation about the role of somatostatin in modulating neural circuits underlying cognitive and affective behaviors.[254]

Clinical Applications of Somatostatin Analogues

An extensive pharmaceutical discovery program has produced somatostatin analogues with receptor subtype selectivity and improved pharmacokinetics and oral bioavailability compared with the native peptide. Initial efforts focused on the rational design of constrained cyclic peptides that incorporated D-amino acid residues and included the Trp^8-Lys^9 dipeptide of somatostatin, which was shown by structure-function studies to be necessary for high-affinity binding to its receptor (see Fig. 7–25). Many such analogues have been studied in clinical trials including octreotide, lanreotide, vapreotide, and the hexapeptide MK-678. These compounds are agonists with similarly high-affinity binding to SSTR2 and SSTR5, moderate binding to SSTR3, and no (or low) binding to SSTR1 and SSTR4. A combinatorial chemistry approach has led to a new generation of nonpeptidyl somatostatin agonists that bind selectively and with subnanomolar affinity to each of the five SSTR subtypes.[255,256] In contrast to the marked success in development of potent and selective somatostatin agonists, there is a relative paucity of useful antagonists.[249]

The actions of octreotide (SMS 201-995 or Sandostatin) illustrate the general potential of somatostatin analogues in therapy.[257,258] Octreotide controls excess secretion of GH in acromegaly in most patients and shrinks tumor size in about one third. It is also indicated for the treatment of TSH-secreting adenomas that recur after surgery. It is used to treat other functioning metastatic neuroendocrine tumors, including carcinoid, VIPoma, glucagonoma, and insulinoma, but is seldom of use for the treatment of gastrinoma. Octreotide is also useful in the management of many forms of diarrhea (acting on salt and water excretion mechanisms in the gut) and in reducing external secretions in pancreatic fistulae (thus permitting healing). A decrease in blood flow to the gastrointestinal tract is the basis for its use in bleeding esophageal varices, but it is not effective in the treatment of bleeding from a peptic ulcer.

The only major undesirable side effect of octreotide is reduction of bile production and of gallbladder contractility, leading to "sludging" of bile and an increased incidence of gallstones. Other common adverse effects including nausea, abdominal cramps, diarrhea secondary to malabsorption of fat, and flatulence usually subside spontaneously within 2 weeks of continued treatment. Impaired glucose tolerance is not associated with long-term octreotide therapy, despite an inhibitory effect on insulin secretion, because of compensating reductions in carbohydrate absorption and GH and glucagon secretion that are caused by the drug.

Somatostatin analogues labeled with a radioactive tracer have been used as external imaging agents for a wide range of disorders.[257,258] A ^{111}In-labeled analogue of octreotide (OctreoScan) has been approved for clinical use in the United States and several other countries (Fig. 7–26). The majority of neuroendocrine tumors and many pituitary tumors that express somatostatin receptors are visualized by external imaging techniques after administration of this agent; a variety of nonendocrine tumors and inflammatory lesions are also visualized, all of which have in common the expression of somatostatin receptors. Such tumors include non–small cell cancer of the lung (100%), meningioma (100%), breast cancer (74%), and astrocytomas (67%). Because activated T cells of the immune system display somatostatin receptors, inflammatory lesions that take up the tracer include sarcoidosis, Wegener's granulomatosis, tuberculosis, and many cases of Hodgkin's disease and non-Hodgkin's lymphoma. Although the tracer lacks specificity in differential diagnosis, its ability to identify the presence of abnormality and the extent of the lesion provides important information for management, including tumor staging. The use of a small handheld radiation detector in the operating room makes it possible to ensure the completeness of removal of medullary thyroid carcinoma metastases.[259] New developments in the synthesis of tracers chelated to octreotide for positron emission tomography have allowed the sensitive detection of meningiomas only 7 mm in diameter and located beneath osseous structures at the base of the skull.[260]

The ability of somatostatin to inhibit the growth of normal and some neoplastic cell lines and to reduce the growth of experimentally induced tumors in animal models has stimu-

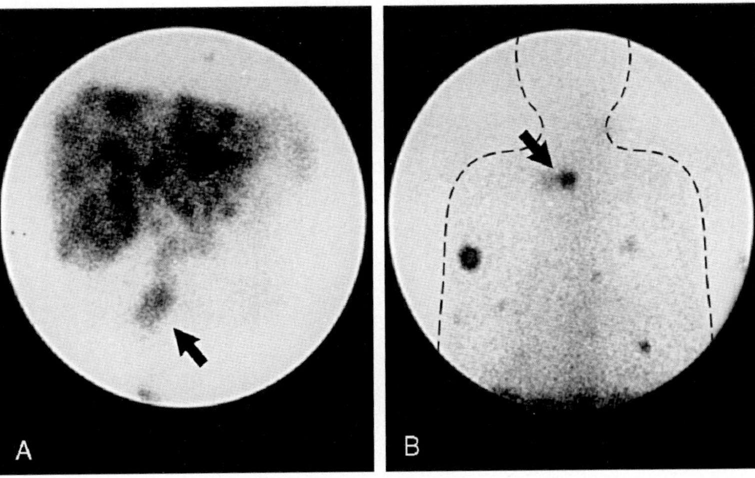

Figure 7–26 ■ The use of ^{111}In-labeled diethylenetriamine-pentaacetic acid (DTPA)-octreotide (radioactive somatostatin analogue) and external imaging techniques to localize a carcinoid tumor expressing somatostatin receptors. Pictures were taken 24 hours after administration of labeled tracer. **A,** Anterior view of the abdomen showing nodular metastases in an enlarged liver and the primary carcinoid tumor (*arrow*) in the wall of the jejunum of a patient with severe flushing and diarrhea. **B,** Posterior view of the chest and neck showing a metastasis in a lymph node on the left side of the neck (*arrow*) and multiple metastases in the ribs and pleura. (Reprinted with modifications from Lamberts SWJ, Krenning EP, Reubi J-C. The role of somatostatin and its analogs in the diagnosis and treatment of tumors. Endocrine Rev 1991;12:450-482. Copyright 1991, The Endocrine Society.)

lated interest in somatostatin analogues for the treatment of cancer. Somatostatin's tumoristatic effects may be a combination of direct actions on tumor cells related to inhibition of growth factor receptor expression, inhibition of MAPK, and stimulation of phosphotyrosine phosphatase. SSTR1, SSTR2, SSTR4, and SSTR5 can all promote cell cycle arrest associated with induction of the tumor suppressor retinoblastoma and p21, and SSTR3 can trigger apoptosis accompanied by induction of the tumor suppressor p53 and the proapoptotic protein Bax.[249] In addition, somatostatin has indirect effects on tumor growth by its inhibition of circulating, paracrine, and autocrine tumor growth-promoting factors and it can modulate the activity of immune cells and influence tumor blood supply. Despite this promise, the therapeutic utility of octreotide as an antineoplastic agent remains controversial.

Two new treatment approaches in preclinical trials may yet effectively utilize somatostatin receptors in the arrest of cancer cells.[257] The first is receptor-targeted radionuclide therapy using octreotide chelated to a variety of γ- or β-emitting radioisotopes. Theoretical calculations and empirical data suggest that radiolabeled somatostatin analogues can deliver a tumoricidal radiotherapeutic dose to some tumors after receptor-mediated endocytosis. A variation on this theme is the chelation of a cytotoxic chemotherapeutic agent to a somatostatin analogue. A second approach involves somatic cell gene therapy to transfect SSTR-negative pancreatic cancer cells with an SSTR gene.[261] Therapeutic results can be obtained with the creation of autocrine or paracrine inhibitory growth effects or the addition of targeted radionuclide treatments.

Prolactin-Regulating Factors

Dopamine

It is well known that PRL secretion, unlike the secretion of other pituitary hormones, is primarily under tonic inhibitory control by the hypothalamus (Fig. 7–27).[262] Destruction of the stalk median eminence or transplantation of the pituitary gland to ectopic sites causes a marked constitutive increase in PRL secretion, in contrast to a decrease in the release of GH, TSH, ACTH, and the gonadotropins. Many lines of evidence indicate that dopamine is the principal, physiologic prolactin-inhibiting factor (PIF) released from the hypothalamus.[263] Dopamine is present in hypophyseal-portal vessel blood in sufficient concentration to inhibit PRL release,[264] dopamine inhibits PRL secretion from lactotrophs both in vivo and in vitro,[265] and dopamine D2 receptors are expressed on the plasma membrane of lactotrophs.[266,267] Mutant mice with a targeted disruption of the D2 receptor gene uniformly developed lactotroph hyperplasia, hyperprolactinemia, and eventually lactotroph adenomas, further emphasizing the importance of dopamine in the physiologic regulation of lactotroph proliferation in addition to hormone secretion.[268]

The intrinsic dopamine neurons of the medial-basal hypothalamus constitute a dopaminergic population with regulatory properties that are distinct from those in other areas of the brain. Notably, they lack D2 autoreceptors but express PRL receptors, which are essential for positive feedback control as discussed in detail later (see Feedback Control). In the rat, these neurons are subdivided by location into the A12 group within the arcuate nucleus and the A14 group in the anterior periventricular nucleus. The caudal A12 dopamine neurons are further classified as tuberoinfundibular (TIDA) because of their axonal projections to the external zone of the median eminence.

Tuberohypophyseal (THDA) neuronal soma are located more rostrally in the arcuate nucleus and project to both the neural lobe and intermediate lobe through axon collaterals that are found in the internal zone of the median eminence. Finally, the A14 periventricular hypophyseal (PHDA) neurons send their axons only to the intermediate lobe of the pituitary gland.

Although the TIDA neurons are generally considered to be the major source of dopamine to the anterior lobe through the long portal vessels originating in the median eminence, dopamine can also reach the anterior lobe from the neural and intermediate lobes by the interconnecting short portal veins.[269] Consistent with this pathway for dopamine access to the anterior lobe, surgical removal of the neurointermediate lobe in rats caused a significant increase in basal PRL levels.[270] In addition to direct actions of dopamine on lactotrophs, central dopamine can indirectly affect PRL secretion by altering the activity of inhibitory interneurons that in turn synapse on the TIDA neurons. These effects are complicated by opposing intracellular signaling pathways linked to D1 and D2 receptors located on different populations of interneurons.[271]

The binding of dopamine or selective agonists such as bromocriptine to the D2 receptor has multiple effects on lactotroph function. D2 receptors are coupled to pertussis toxin-sensitive G proteins and inhibit adenylyl cyclase and decrease intracellular cAMP levels. Other effects include activation of an inwardly rectifying K^+ channel, increase of voltage-activated K^+ currents, decrease of voltage-activated Ca^{2+} currents, and inhibition of inositol phosphate production. Together, this spectrum of intracellular signaling events decreases free Ca^{2+} concentrations and inhibits exocytosis of PRL secretory granules.[272] Dopamine also has a modest effect on thyrotrophs to inhibit the secretion of TSH.

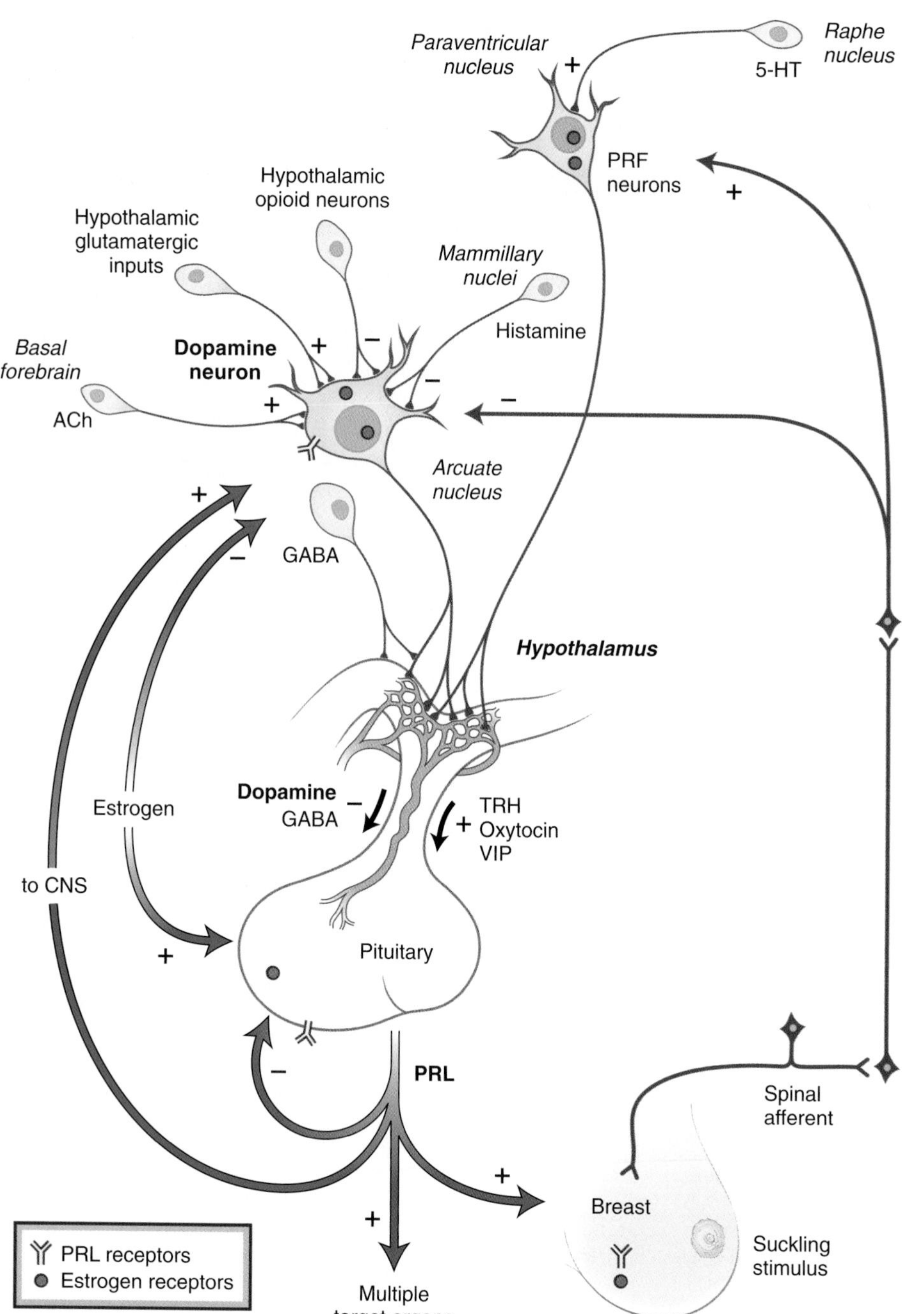

Figure 7–27 ▪ Regulation of the hypothalamic-pituitary-prolactin (PRL) axis. The predominant effect of the hypothalamus is inhibitory, an effect mediated principally by dopamine secreted by the tuberohypophyseal dopaminergic neuron system. The dopamine neurons are stimulated by acetylcholine (ACh) and glutamate and inhibited by histamine and opioid peptides. One or more prolactin-releasing factors (PRFs) probably mediate acute release of PRL as in suckling and stress. There are several candidate PRFs, including thyrotropin-releasing hormone (TRH), vasoactive intestinal polypeptide (VIP), and oxytocin. PRF neurons are activated by serotonin (5-HT). Estrogen sensitizes the pituitary to release PRL, which feeds back on the pituitary to regulate its own secretion (ultrashort-loop feedback) and also influences gonadotropin secretion by suppressing the release of luteinizing hormone-releasing hormone (LHRH). Short-loop feedback is also mediated indirectly by prolactin receptor regulation of hypothalamic dopamine synthesis, secretion, and turnover. *CNS,* Central nervous system; *GABA,* γ-aminobutyric acid.

There is continuing debate concerning the mechanism by which D2 receptor activation inhibits transcription of the PRL gene. Likely pathways involve the inhibition of MAPK or protein kinase C, with a resultant reduction in the phosphorylation of Ets family transcription factors. Ets factors are important for the stimulatory responses of TRH, insulin, and epidermal growth factor on PRL expression[273-275] and they interact cooperatively with the pituitary-specific POU protein Pit1, which is essential for cAMP-mediated PRL gene expression.[276]

The second messenger pathways used by the D2 receptor to inhibit lactotroph cell division are also unsettled. A study using primary pituitary cultures from rats demonstrated that forskolin treatment, which activates protein kinase A and elevates intracellular cAMP, or insulin treatment, which activates a potent receptor tyrosine kinase, were both effective mitogenic stimuli for lactotrophs. Bromocriptine competitively antagonized the proliferative response caused by elevated cAMP. Furthermore, inhibition of MAPK signaling by PD98059 markedly suppressed the mitogenic action of both insulin and forskolin, suggesting an interaction of MAPK and protein kinase A signaling.[277]

Another study used immortalized mammosomatotroph tumor cells that were transfected with a D2 receptor expression vector and concluded that stimulation of a phosphotyrosine phosphatase activity was an important component of dopamine's antiproliferative action.[278] Therefore, it is clear that dopamine actions on lactotrophs involve multiple different intracellular signaling pathways linked to activation of the D2 receptor, but different combinations of these pathways are relevant for the inhibitory effects on PRL secretion, PRL gene transcription, and lactotroph proliferation.

The other major action of dopamine in the pituitary is the inhibition of hormone secretion from the POMC-expressing cells of the intermediate lobe, although, as noted earlier, the adult human differs from most other mammals in the rudimentary nature of this lobe. THDA and PHDA axon terminals provide a dense plexus of synaptic-like contacts on melanotrophs. Dopamine release from these terminals is inversely correlated with serum MSH levels[279] and also regulates POMC gene expression and melanotroph proliferation.[280]

Other hypothalamic factors probably play a role secondary to that of dopamine as additional PIFs.[262] The primary reason to conjecture the existence of these PIFs is the frequent inconsistency between portal dopamine levels and circulating PRL in different rat models. GABA is the strongest candidate and most likely acts through $GABA_A$ inotropic receptors in the anterior pituitary. Melanotrophs, like lactotrophs, are inhibited by both dopamine and GABA but with the principal involvement of G protein–coupled, metabotropic $GABA_B$ receptors.[281] Because basal dopamine tone is high, the measurable inhibitory effects of GABA on PRL release are generally small under normal circumstances. Other putative PIFs include somatostatin and calcitonin.

Prolactin-Releasing Factors

Although tonic suppression of PRL release by dopamine is the dominant effect of the hypothalamus on PRL secretion, a number of stimuli promote PRL release, not merely by disinhibition of PIF effects but by causing release of one or more neurohormonal PRFs (see Fig. 7–27). The most important of the putative PRFs are TRH, oxytocin, and VIP, but vasopressin, angiotensin II, NPY, galanin, substance P, bombesin-like peptides, and neurotensin can also trigger PRL release under different physiologic circumstances.[262] TRH is discussed in a previous section of this chapter. In humans there is an imperfect correlation between pulsatile PRL and TSH release, suggesting that TRH cannot be the sole physiologic PRF under basal conditions.[282]

Like TRH, oxytocin, vasopressin, and VIP fulfill all the basic criteria for a PRF. They are produced in paraventricular hypothalamic neurons that project to the median eminence. Concentrations of the hormones in portal blood are much higher than in the peripheral circulation and are sufficient to stimulate PRL secretion in vitro. Moreover, there are functional receptors for each of the neurohormones in the anterior pituitary gland and either pharmacologic antagonism or passive immunization against each hormone can decrease PRL secretion, at least under certain circumstances.[283-287]

Vasopressin is released during stress and hypovolemic shock, as is PRL, suggesting a specific role for vasopressin as a PRF in these contexts. Similarly, another candidate PRF, peptide histidine isoleucine, may be specifically involved in the secretion of PRL in response to stress. Peptide histidine isoleucine and the human homologue PHM are structurally related to VIP and synthesized from the same prohormone precursor in their respective species.[288] Both peptides are coexpressed with CRH in parvocellular paraventricular neurons and presumably released by the same stimuli that cause release of CRH into the hypophyseal-portal vessels.[289]

There is evidence suggesting that dopamine itself may also act as a PRF, in contrast to its predominant function as a PIF.[262] At concentrations three orders of magnitude lower than that associated with maximal inhibition of PRL secretion, dopamine was shown to be capable of stimulating secretion from primary cultures of rat pituitary cells.[290] These studies were extended to an in vivo model by Arey and colleagues,[291] who demonstrated that low-dose dopamine infusion in cannulated rats caused a further increase in circulating PRL above the already elevated baseline produced by pharmacologic blockade of endogenous dopamine biosynthesis. The physiologic relevance of these findings to humans has yet to be established.

Finally, reports of "new" PRFs continue to be published. Much excitement was generated by the isolation of a mammalian RFamide peptide from bovine hypothalamus named *prolactin-releasing peptide* (PrRP).[292,293] PrRP binds with high affinity to its G protein–coupled receptor expressed specifically in human pituitary and selectively stimulates PRL release from rat pituitary cells with a potency similar to that of TRH. However, PrRP is expressed predominantly in a subpopulation of noradrenergic neurons in the medulla and a small population of non-neurosecretory neurons of the VMH, raising the serious question of whether PrRP reaches the anterior pituitary and actually causes PRL secretion. Subsequent studies found no direct evidence for release of PrRP in the arcuate nucleus-median eminence, further suggesting that the peptide is not a hypophyseotropic neurohormone. However, PrRP probably does function as a neuromodulator within the CNS at sites expressing its receptor and may be involved in the neural circuitry mediating satiety.[293]

Intrapituitary Regulation of Prolactin Secretion

Probably more than that of any other pituitary hormone, the secretion of PRL is regulated by autocrine-paracrine factors within the anterior lobe and by neurointermediate lobe factors that gain access to venous sinusoids of the anterior lobe by way of the short portal vessels. The wealth of local regulatory mechanisms within the anterior lobe has been reviewed extensively[262,294] and is also discussed in Chapter 8. Galanin, VIP, endothelin-like peptides, angiotensin II, epidermal growth factor, basic fibroblast growth factor, GnRH, and the cytokine IL-6 are among the most potent local stimulators of PRL secretion. Locally produced inhibitors include PRL itself, acetylcholine, transforming growth factor β, and calcitonin. Although none of these stimulatory or inhibitory factors plays a dominant role in the regulation of lactotroph function and much of the research in this area has not been directly confirmed in human pituitary, it seems apparent that the local milieu of autocrine and paracrine factors plays an essential modulatory role in determining the responsiveness of lactotrophs to hypothalamic factors in different physiologic states.

As noted earlier, a proportion of the inhibitory dopamine tone to the anterior lobe lactotrophs is derived from the neurointermediate lobe. It was therefore unanticipated that surgical removal of this structure in rats would block suckling-induced PRL release over the moderate basal increase attributed to partial dopamine disinhibition.[295] Further studies showed that exposure of the anterior pituitary to intermediate lobe extracts (devoid of VIP, vasopressin, and other known PRFs) stimulated PRL secretion. At least two kinds of PRF activity have been isolated from intermediate lobe tumors of the mouse, but the specific molecules involved have yet to be identified.[296] Other researchers have suggested a more passive role for the neurointermediate lobe in the regulation of PRL secretion. Melanotroph-derived N-acetylated MSH appears to act as a lactotroph responsiveness factor by recruiting nonsecretory cells to an active state and sensitizing secreting lactotrophs to the actions of other direct PRFs.[297] However, the relevance of the neurointermediate lobe for PRL regulation in primates (including humans) is not clear because of its attenuated structure in these species.

Neuroendocrine Regulation of Prolactin Secretion

Secretion of PRL, like that of other anterior pituitary hormones, is regulated by hormonal feedback and neural influences from the hypothalamus.[262,263,298] Feedback is exerted by PRL itself at the level of the hypothalamus. PRL secretion is regulated by many physiologic states including the estrous and menstrual cycles, pregnancy, and lactation. Furthermore, PRL is stimulated by several exteroceptive stimuli including light, ultrasonic vocalization of rodent pups, olfactory cues, and various modalities of stress. Expression and secretion of PRL are also influenced strongly by estrogens at the level of both the lactotrophs and TIDA neurons[299] (see Fig. 7–27) and by paracrine regulators within the pituitary such as galanin and VIP.

Feedback Control

Negative feedback control of PRL secretion is mediated by a unique short-loop mechanism within the hypothalamus.[300] PRL activates PRL receptors, which are expressed on all three subpopulations of A12 and A14 dopamine neurons, leading to increased tyrosine hydroxylase expression and dopamine synthesis and release.[299,301] Ames dwarf mice that secrete virtually no PRL, GH, or TSH have decreased numbers of arcuate dopamine neurons and this hypoplasia can be reversed by neonatal administration of PRL, suggesting a trophic action on the neurons.[302] However, another mouse model of isolated PRL deficiency generated by gene targeting appears to have normal numbers of hypofunctioning dopamine neurons secondary to the loss of PRL feedback.[303]

Neural Control

Lactotrophs have spontaneously high secretory activity, and therefore the predominant effect of the hypothalamus on PRL secretion is tonic suppression, which is mediated by regulatory hormones synthesized by tuberohypophyseal neurons. Secretory bursts of PRL are caused by the acute withdrawal of dopamine inhibition, stimulation by PRFs, or combinations of both events. At any given moment, locally produced autocrine and paracrine regulators further modulate the responsiveness of individual lactotrophs to neurohormonal PIFs and PRFs.

Multiple neurotransmitter systems impinge on the hypothalamic dopamine and PRF neurons to regulate their neurosecretion[262] (see Fig. 7–27). Nicotinic cholinergic and glutamatergic afferents activate TIDA neurons, whereas histamine, acting predominantly through H2 receptors, inhibits these neurons. An inhibitory peptidergic input to TIDA neurons of major physiologic significance is that associated with the endogenous opioid peptides enkephalin and dynorphin and their cognate μ- and κ-receptor subtypes.[304] Opioid inhibition of dopamine release has been associated with increased PRL secretion under virtually all physiologic conditions, including the basal state, different phases of the estrous cycle, lactation, and stress.

Ascending serotoninergic inputs from the dorsal raphe nucleus are the major activator of PRF neurons in the PVH.[305] There is still debate concerning the identity of the specific 5-HT receptors involved in this activation.

The PRL regulatory system and its monoaminergic control have been scrutinized in detail because of the frequent occurrence of syndromes of PRL hypersecretion (see Chapter 8). Both the pituitary and the hypothalamus have dopamine receptors, and unfortunately the response to dopamine receptor stimulation and blockade does not distinguish between central and peripheral actions of the drug. Many commonly used neuroleptic drugs influence PRL secretion. Reserpine (a catecholamine depletor) and phenothiazines such as chlorpromazine and haloperidol enhance PRL release by disinhibition of dopamine action on the pituitary, and the PRL response is an excellent predictor of the antipsychotic effects of phenothiazines because of its correlation with D2 receptor binding and activation.[306] The major antipsychotic neuroleptic agents act on brain dopamine receptors in the mesolimbic system and in the pituitary-regulating tuberoinfundibular system. Consequently, treatment of such patients with dopamine agonists such as bromocriptine can reverse the psychiatric benefits of such drugs. A report of three patients with psychosis and concomitant prolactinomas recommended the combination of clozapine and quinagolide as the treatment of choice to manage both diseases simultaneously.[307]

Factors Influencing Secretion

Circadian Rhythm

PRL is detectable in plasma at all times during the day but is secreted in discrete pulses superimposed on basal secretion and exhibits a diurnal rhythm with peak values in the early morning hours.[308] There is a true circadian rhythm in humans because it is maintained in a constant environment independently of the sleep rhythm.[309] The combined body of data examining TIDA neuronal activity, dopamine concentrations in the median eminence, and manipulations of the SCN suggests that endogenous diurnal alterations in dopamine tone that are entrained by light constitute the major neuroendocrine mechanism underlying the circadian rhythm of PRL secretion.

External Stimuli

The suckling stimulus is the most important physiologic regulator of PRL secretion. Within 1 to 3 minutes of nipple stimulation, PRL levels rise and remain elevated for 10 to 20 minutes.[310] This reflex is distinct from the milk let-down, which involves oxytocin release from the neurohypophysis and contraction of mammary alveolar myoepithelial cells. These reflexes provide a mechanism by which the infant regulates both the production and the delivery of milk. The nocturnal rise in PRL secretion in nursing women and in nonnursing women may have evolved as a mechanism of milk maintenance during prolonged nonsuckling periods at night.

Pathways involved in the suckling reflex arise in nerves innervating the nipple, enter the spinal cord by way of spinal afferent neurons, ascend the spinal cord through spinothalamic tracts to the midbrain, and enter the hypothalamus by way of the median forebrain bundle (see Fig. 7–27). In most of the pathway, neurons regulating the oxytocin-dependent milk let-down response accompany those involved in PRL regulation and then separate at the level of the paraventricular nuclei. The suckling reflex brings about an inhibition of PIF activity and a release of PRFs, although the identity of an undisputed suckling-induced PRF is unsettled.

Although the significance for PRL regulation in humans is not certain, environmental stimuli from seasonal changes in light duration and auditory and olfactory cues are clearly of great importance to many mammalian species.[262] Seasonal breeders, such as the sheep, exhibit a reduction in PRL secretion in response to shortened days. The specific ultrasound vocalization of rodent pups is among the most potent stimuli for PRL secretion in lactating and virgin female rats. Olfactory stimuli from pheromones also have potent actions in rodents. A prime example is the Bruce effect or spontaneous abortion induced by exposure of a pregnant female rat to an unfamiliar male. It is mediated by a well-studied neural circuitry involving the vomeronasal nerves, corticomedial amygdala, medial preoptic area of the hypothalamus, and finally activation of TIDA neurons and a reduction in circulating PRL that is essential for maintenance of luteal function in the first half of pregnancy.

Stress in many forms dramatically affects PRL secretion, although the teleologic significance is uncertain. It may be related to actions of PRL on cells of the immune system or some other aspect of homeostasis. Different stressors are associated with either a reduction or an increase in PRL secretion, depending on the local regulatory environment at the time of the stress. However, whereas well-documented changes in PRL are associated with relatively severe forms of stress in laboratory animal models, a study of academic stress in college students failed to show any significant correlation among the time periods before, during, or after final examinations and diurnal PRL levels.[311]

Gonadotropin-Releasing Hormone and Control of the Reproductive Axis

Chemistry and Evolution

The hypothalamic neuropeptide that controls the function of the reproductive axis is GnRH. GnRH is a 10-amino-acid peptide that is synthesized as part of a larger precursor molecule and is then enzymatically cleaved to remove a signal peptide from the N-terminus and GnRH-associated peptide (GAP) from the C-terminus (Fig. 7–28).[312] All forms of the decapeptide have a pyroGlu at the N-terminus and Gly-amide at the C-terminus, indicating the functional importance of the terminal regions throughout evolutionary biology.

Within mammals, two genes encoding GnRH have been identified.[313,314] The first encodes a 92-amino-acid precursor protein. This form of GnRH is now referred to as GnRH-I and is the form found in hypothalamic neurons that serves as a releasing factor to regulate pituitary gonadotroph function.[315] The second GnRH gene, GnRH-II, encodes a decapeptide that differs from the first by three amino acids.[316] This form of GnRH is found in the midbrain region and serves as a neurotransmitter rather than as a pituitary releasing factor. Both GnRH-I and GnRH-II are found in phylogenetically diverse species, from fish to mammals, suggesting that these multiple forms of GnRH diverged from one another early in vertebrate evolution.[315] A third form of GnRH, GnRH-III, has been identified in neurons of the telencephalon in teleost fish. GnRH is also found in cells outside the brain. The roles of GnRH peptides produced outside the brain are not well understood but are an area of current investigation.

All GnRH genes have the same basic structure, with the pre-prohormone mRNA encoded in four exons. Exon 1 contains the 5′ untranslated region of the gene; exon 2 contains the signal peptide, GnRH, and the N-terminus of GAP; exon 3 contains the central portion of GAP; and exon 4 contains the C-terminus of GAP and the 3′ untranslated region (see Fig. 7–28).[315] Among species, the nucleotide sequences encoding the GnRH decapeptide are highly homologous. In this chapter, we focus on the hypothalamic GnRH that is derived from GnRH-1 mRNA and that plays an important role in the regulation of the hypothalamic-pituitary-gonadal axis.

Two transcriptional start sites have been identified in the rat GnRH-1 gene at +1 and −579, with the +1 promoter being active in hypothalamic neurons and the other promoter active in placenta. The first 173 base pairs of the promoter are highly conserved among species. In the rat, this promoter region has been shown to contain two OCT1 binding sites; three regions that bind the POU domain family of transcription factors, SCIP, OCT6, and TST1; and three regions that can bind the progesterone receptor.[317] In addition, a variety of hormones and second messengers have been shown to regulate GnRH gene expression, and the majority of the *cis*-acting elements thus far character-

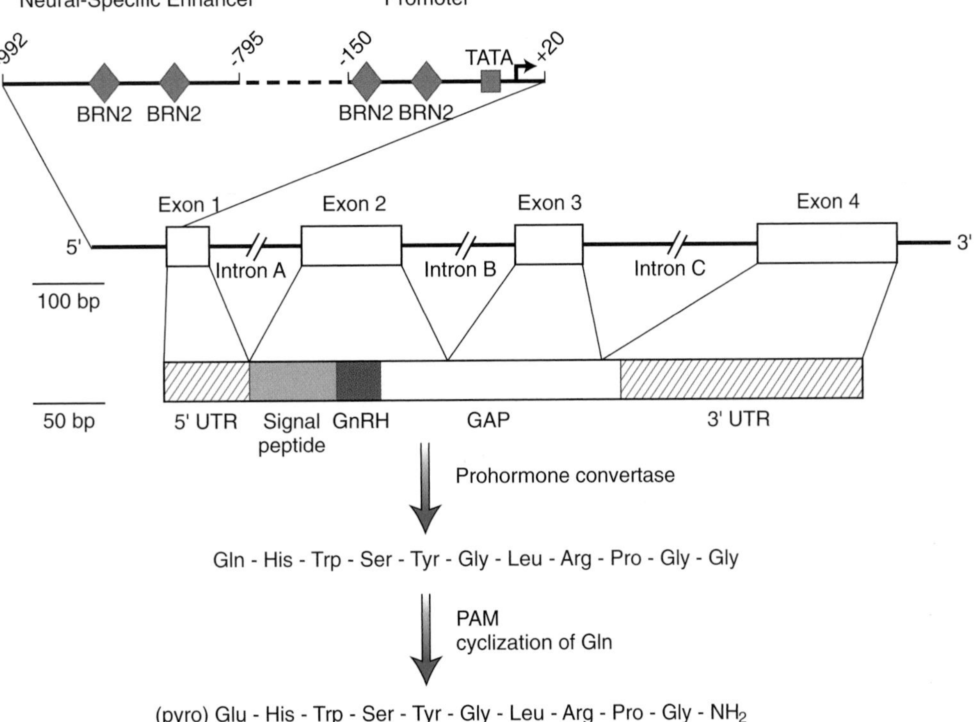

Figure 7–28 ▪ Schematic diagram of the human gene for gonadotropin-releasing hormone-I (GnRH-I), the hypothalamic cDNA, and posttranslational processing of the GnRH peptide. A cluster of binding sites for the homeodomain transcription factor BRN2 is present in both the proximal promoter and a distal enhancer region and is important for neuron-specific expression of the gene. Phylogenetically conserved homologous regions have been identified in the rat GnRH-I gene, however, in this species the OCT1 transcription factor has been implicated in neuron-specific expression. The cDNA for GnRH-1 isolated from human placenta has a longer 5′UTR because of differential splicing of the hnRNA and inclusion of intron A sequences. *GAP,* GnRH-associated peptide; *PAM,* peptidylglycine α-amidating monooxygenase; *UTR,* untranslated region. (Compiled from data of Cheng CK, Leung PCK. Molecular biology of gonadotropin-releasing hormone (GnRH)-I, GnRH-II, and their receptors in humans. Endocr Rev 2005;26:283-306; Wolfe A, Kim HH, Tobet S, et al. Identification of a discrete promoter region of the human GnRH gene that is sufficient for directing neuron-specific expression: a role for POU homeodomain transcription factors. Mol Endocrinol 2002;16:435-449.)

ized for hormonal control of GnRH transcription have been localized to the proximal promoter region.[318,319] The 5′ flanking region of the rodent and human GnRH-1 genes also contain a distal 300-base-pair enhancer region that is 1.8 or 0.9 kb, respectively, upstream of the transcription start site.[319,320] Recent studies implicate the homeodomain transcription factors OCT1, MSX, and DLX in the specification of neuron expression and developmental activation.[320,321]

Anatomic Distribution

GnRH neurons are small, diffusely located cells that are not concentrated in a discrete nucleus. They are generally bipolar and fusiform in shape, with slender axons projecting predominantly to the median eminence and infundibular stalk. The location of hypothalamic GnRH neurons is species-dependent. In the rat, hypothalamic GnRH neurons are concentrated in rostral areas including the medial preoptic area, the diagonal band of Broca, the septal areas, and the anterior hypothalamus. In humans and nonhuman primates, the majority of hypothalamic GnRH neurons are located more dorsally in the medial basal hypothalamus, the infundibulum, and periventricular region. Throughout the hypothalamus, neurohypophyseal GnRH neurons are interspersed with nonneuroendocrine GnRH neurons, which extend their axons to other regions of the brain including other hypothalamic regions and various regions of the cortex. GnRH secreted from nonneuroendocrine neurons has been implicated in the control of sexual behavior in rodents but not in higher primates.[322]

Embryonic Development

GnRH neuroendocrine neurons are an unusual neuronal population in that they originate outside the CNS, from the epithelial tissue of the nasal placode (reviewed in reference 323). During embryonic development, GnRH neurons migrate across the surface of the brain and into the hypothalamus, with the final hypothalamic location differing somewhat among species. Migration is dependent on a scaffolding of neurons and glial cells along which the GnRH neurons move, with neural cell adhesion molecules playing a critical role in guiding the migration process. In contrast to this widely accepted view of GnRH development, recent data have suggested an alternative embryonic origin of GnRH neurons from the anterior pituitary placode and cranial neural crest.[29]

Failure of GnRH neurons to migrate properly leads to a clinical condition, Kallmann's syndrome, in which GnRH neuroendocrine neurons do not reach their final destination and thus do not stimulate pituitary gonadotropin secretion.[324] Patients with Kallmann's syndrome do not enter puberty spontaneously. X-linked Kallmann's syndrome results from a deficiency of the KAL1 gene, which encodes a putative protein of 680 amino acids and contains four fibronectin type III repeats and a four-disulfide core motif. Loss of function mutations in the fibroblast growth factor receptor type 1 gene (FGFR1) produce an autosomal dominant form of Kallman's syndrome. However, these known genetic mechanisms together account for a minority of cases, and other lesions are yet to be characterized.[325] Administration of exogenous GnRH effectively treats this form of hypothalamic hypogonadism. Patients with Kallmann's syndrome often have other congenital midline defects, including anosmia, which results from hypoplasia of the olfactory bulb and tracts.

Action at the Pituitary

Receptors

GnRH binds to a membrane receptor on pituitary gonadotrophs and stimulates both LH and FSH synthesis and secretion. The GnRH receptor is a seven-transmembrane-domain G protein–coupled receptor, but it lacks a typical intracellular C-terminal cytoplasmic domain.[319] Under physiologic conditions, GnRH receptor number varies and is usually directly correlated with the gonadotropin secretory capacity of pituitary gonadotrophs. For example, across the rat estrous cycle, a rise in GnRH receptors is seen just before the surge of gonadotropins that occurs on the afternoon of proestrus. GnRH receptor message levels are regulated by a variety of hormones and second messengers including steroid hormones (estradiol can both suppress and stimulate, and progesterone suppresses), gonadotropins (which suppress), and calcium and protein kinase C (which stimulate).[319]

$G_{q/11}$ is the primary guanosine triphosphate–binding protein mediating GnRH responses; however, there is evidence that GnRH receptors can couple to other G proteins including G_s and G_i.[319] With activation, the GnRH receptor couples to a phosphoinositide-specific phospholipase C, which leads to increases in calcium transport into gonadotrophs and calcium release from internal stores through a diacylglycerol-protein kinase C pathway. Increased calcium entry is a critical step in GnRH-stimulated release of gonadotropin secretion. However, the MAPK cascade is also stimulated by GnRH.

When there is a decline in GnRH stimulation to the pituitary, as occurs in a variety of physiologic conditions including states of lactation, undernutrition, or seasonal periods of reproductive quiescence, the number of GnRH receptors on pituitary gonadotrophs declines dramatically. Subsequent exposure of the pituitary to pulses of GnRH restores receptor number by a Ca^{2+}-dependent mechanism that requires protein synthesis.[326] The effect of GnRH to induce its own receptor is termed up-regulation or self-priming. Only certain physiologic frequencies of pulsatile GnRH can augment GnRH receptor production, and these frequencies appear to differ among species.[327] Up-regulation of GnRH receptors after a period of low GnRH stimulation to the pituitary can take hours to days of exposure to pulsatile GnRH, depending on the duration and extent of the prior decrease in GnRH. The self-priming effect of GnRH to up-regulate its own receptors also plays a crucial role in the production of the gonadotropin surge that occurs at midcycle in females of spontaneously ovulating species and triggers ovulation. Just before the gonadotropin surge, two factors, the increased frequency of pulsatile GnRH release and a sensitization of the pituitary gonadotrophs by rising levels of estradiol, make the pituitary exquisitely sensitive to GnRH and allow an output of LH that is an order of magnitude greater than the release seen during the rest of the female reproductive cycle. This surge of LH triggers the ovulatory process at the ovary.

In contrast to up-regulation of GnRH receptors by pulsatile regimens of GnRH, continuous exposure to GnRH leads to down-regulation of GnRH receptors and an accompanying decrease in LH and FSH synthesis and secretion, termed desensitization.[328] Down-regulation does not require calcium mobilization or gonadotropin secretion. It involves a rapid uncoupling of receptor from G proteins and sequestration of the receptors from the plasma membrane, followed by internalization and proteolytic degradation of the receptors.

The concept of down-regulation has a number of clinical applications. For example, the most common current therapy for precocious puberty of hypothalamic origin (i.e., precocious GnRH secretion) is to treat the child with a long-acting GnRH agonist, which down-regulates pituitary GnRH receptors and effectively turns off the reproductive axis.[327,329] Children with precocious puberty can be maintained with long-acting GnRH agonists for years to suppress the premature activation of the reproductive axis, and at the normal age of puberty agonist treatment can be withdrawn, allowing a reactivation of pituitary gonadotrophs and a downstream increase in gonadal steroid hormone production (also see Chapter 24). Long-acting GnRH agonists are also used in the treatment of forms of breast cancer that are estrogen-dependent as well as other gonadal steroid-dependent cancers.[327] Long-acting antagonists of GnRH have been developed that can also be used for these therapies.[330] Antagonists have the advantage of not having a flare effect, that is, an acute stimulation of gonadotropin secretion that is seen during the initial treatment of individuals with superagonists.

Pulsatile Gonadotropin-Releasing Hormone Stimulation

Because a single pulse of GnRH stimulates the release of both LH and FSH and chronic exposure of the pituitary to pulsatile GnRH supports the synthesis of both LH and FSH, it is generally believed that there is only one releasing factor regulating the synthesis and secretion of LH and FSH. However, in a number of physiologic conditions there are divergent patterns of LH and FSH secretion, and thus a second FSH-releasing peptide has been proposed, but such a peptide has not been isolated to date. Other mechanisms, discussed in more detail later, are likely to account for the differential regulation of LH and FSH release.

The ensemble of GnRH neurons in the hypothalamus that send axons to the portal blood system in the median eminence fire in a coordinated, repetitive, episodic manner, producing distinct pulses of GnRH in the portal bloodstream.[331] The pulsatile nature of GnRH stimulation to the pituitary leads to the release of distinct pulses of LH into the peripheral bloodstream. In experimental animals, in which it is possible to collect blood samples simultaneously from the portal and peripheral bloodstream, GnRH and LH pulses have been found to correspond in about a one-to-one ratio at most physiologic rates of secretion.[332] Because the portal bloodstream is generally inaccessible in humans, the collection of frequent blood samples from the peripheral bloodstream is used to define the pulsatile nature of LH secretion (i.e., frequency and amplitude of LH pulses), and pulsatile LH is used as an indirect measure of the activity of the GnRH secretory system. Indirect assessment of GnRH secretion by monitoring the rate of pulsatile LH secretion also is used in many animal studies examining the factors that govern the regulation of the pulsatile activity of the reproductive neuroendocrine axis. Unlike LH secretion, FSH secretion is not always pulsatile, and even when it is pulsatile, there is only partial concordance between LH and FSH pulses.

It is possible to place multiple unit recording electrodes in the medial basal hypothalamus of monkeys and other species and find spikes of electrical activity that are concordant with the pulsatile secretion of LH secretion.[333] It is unknown, however, whether these bursts of electrical activity reflect the activity of GnRH neurons themselves or the activity of neurons that impinge on GnRH neurons and govern their firing. With the development of mice in which the gene for green fluorescent protein has been put under the regulation of the GnRH promoter, it has been possible to identify GnRH neurons in hypothalamic tissue slices using fluorescence microscopy and record from them intracellularly.[14] These studies have shown that many, but not all, GnRH neurons show a bursting pattern of electrical activity. A central, unsolved question in the field of reproductive neuroendocrinology is what causes GnRH neurons to pulse in a coordinated manner. Studies using a line of clonal GnRH neurons have shown that these neurons grown in culture can release GnRH in a pulsatile pattern, suggesting that the pulse-generating capacity of GnRH neurons may be intrinsic.[334] The term *GnRH pulse generator* is often used to acknowledge the fact that GnRH secretion occurs in pulses and to refer to the central mechanisms responsible for pulsatile GnRH release.

A critical factor governing LH and FSH secretion and release is the rate of pulsatile GnRH stimulation of the gonadotrophs. Experimental studies in which the hypothalamus was lesioned and GnRH was replaced by pulsatile administration of exogenous GnRH showed that different frequencies of GnRH can lead to differential ratios of LH to FSH secretion from the pituitary. Figure 7–29 shows that in a monkey with a hypothalamic lesion, replacement of one pulse of GnRH per hour led to a relatively low ratio of FSH to LH secretion. Subsequent institution of a slower pulse frequency of one pulse of GnRH every 3 hours led to a decrease in LH secretion but an increase in FSH secretion such that the ratio of FSH to LH secretion was greatly elevated. It is likely that this effect of pulse frequency on the ratio of FSH to LH secretion accounts, at least in part, for the clinical finding that at times when the GnRH pulse generator is just turning on, such as at the onset of puberty and during recovery from chronic undernutrition, the ratio of FSH to LH is higher than when it is measured in adults experiencing regular reproductive function. As discussed subsequently, steroid hormones act at both the hypothalamus and pituitary to influence strongly the rate of pulsatile GnRH release and amount of LH and FSH secreted from the pituitary.

GnRH pulse frequency not only influences the rate of pulsatile gonadotropin release and the ratio of FSH to LH secretion but also plays an important role in modulating the structural makeup of the gonadotropins. LH and FSH are structurally similar glycoprotein hormones. Each of these hormones is made up of an α and a β subunit. LH, FSH, and TSH share a common

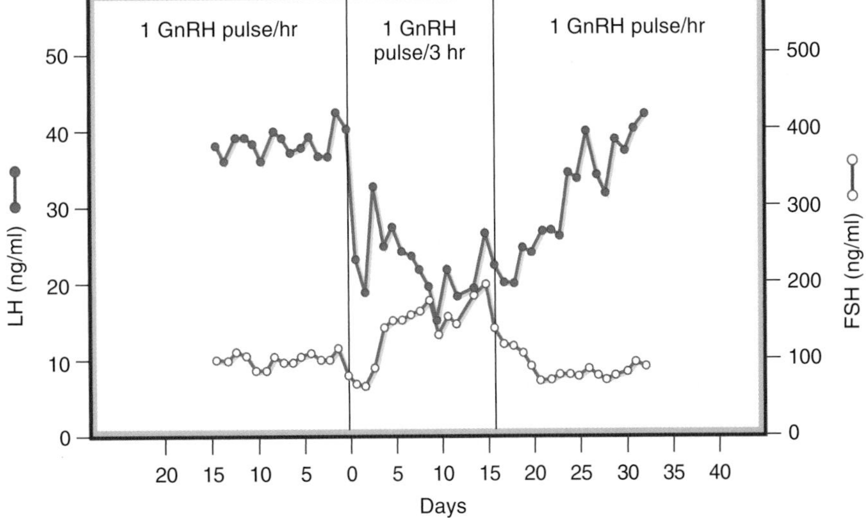

Figure 7–29 ▪ The influence of gonadotropin-releasing hormone (GnRH) pulse frequency on luteinizing hormone (LH) and follicle-stimulating hormone (FSH) secretion in a female rhesus monkey with an arcuate nucleus lesion ablating endogenous GnRH support of the pituitary. Decreasing GnRH pulse frequency from 1 pulse/hour to 1 pulse/3 hours leads to a decrease in plasma LH concentrations but an increase in plasma FSH concentrations. (Redrawn from Wildt L, Haulser A, Marshall G, et al. Frequency and amplitude of gonadotropin-releasing hormone stimulation and gonadotropin secretion in the rhesus monkey. Endocrinology 1981;109:376-385.)

α subunit, and each has a unique β subunit that conveys receptor specificity to the intact hormone. Before secretion of gonadotropins, terminal sugars are attached to each gonadotropin molecule.[112] The sugars include sialic acid, galactose, N-acetylglucosamine, and mannose, but the most important is sialic acid. The extent of glycosylation of LH and FSH is important for the physiologic function of these hormones.[112] Forms of gonadotropin with more sialic acid have a longer half-life because they are protected from degradation by the liver. Forms of gonadotropin with less sialic acid can have more potent effects at their biologic receptors. Both the rate of GnRH stimulation and ovarian hormone feedback at the level of the pituitary regulate the degree of LH and FSH glycosylation. For example, slow frequencies of GnRH, seen during follicular development, are associated with greater degrees of FSH glycosylation, which would provide sustained FSH support to growing follicles. In contrast, faster frequencies of GnRH, seen just before the midcycle gonadotropin surge, are associated with lesser degrees of FSH glycosylation, providing a more potent but shorter lasting form of FSH at the time of ovulation.[335]

Regulatory Systems

Many neurotransmitter systems from the brain stem, limbic system, and other areas of the hypothalamus convey information to GnRH neurons (Fig. 7–30). These afferent systems include neurons that contain norepinephrine, dopamine, serotonin, GABA, glutamate, endogenous opiate peptides, NPY, galanin, and a number of other peptide neurotransmitters. Glutamate and norepinephrine play important roles in providing stimulatory drive to the reproductive axis, whereas GABA and endogenous opioid peptides provide a substantial portion of the inhibitory drive to GnRH neurons. Influences of specific neurotransmitter systems are discussed where appropriate in later sections on the physiologic regulation of GnRH neurons.

GnRH neurons are surrounded by glial processes, and only a small percentage of their surface area is available to receive dendritic contacts from afferent neurons. Changes in the steroid hormone milieu influence the degree of glial sheathing and may play important roles in regulating afferent input to GnRH neurons by this mechanism.[41,43] Some glial cells also secrete substances

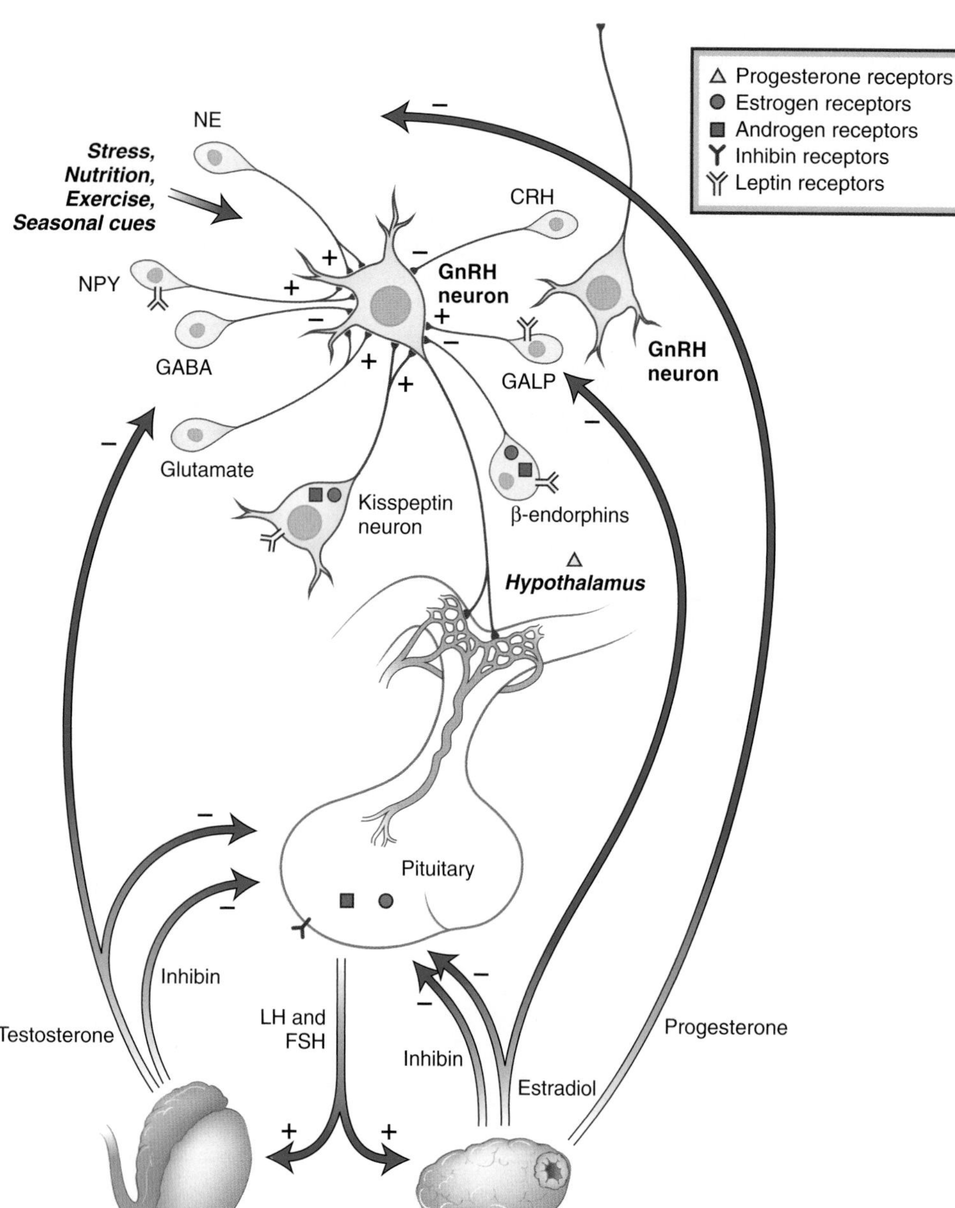

Figure 7–30 ▪ Regulation of the hypothalamic-pituitary-gonadal axis. Schematic diagram of the hypothalamic-pituitary-gonadal axis showing neural systems that regulate GnRH secretion and feedback of gonadal steroid hormones at the level of the hypothalamus and pituitary. *CRH,* Corticotropin-releasing hormone; *FSH,* follicle-stimulating hormone; *GABA,* γ-aminobutyric acid; *GALP,* galanin-like peptide; *LH,* luteinizing hormone; *NPY,* neuropeptide Y.

including transforming growth factor α and PGE_2 that can modulate the activity of GnRH neurons.

Feedback Regulation

Steroid hormone receptors are abundant in the hypothalamus and in many neural systems that impinge on GnRH neurons, including noradrenergic, serotoninergic, β-endorphin–containing, and NPY neurons. Early studies identifying regions of the brain that bound labeled estrogens showed that in rodents the preoptic area and ventromedial hypothalamus had the highest concentrations of estrogen receptors in the brain. Further localization studies, identifying estrogen receptors by immunocytochemistry or in situ hybridization, confirmed the abundance of estrogen receptors in the hypothalamus and in brain areas with strong connections to the hypothalamus, including the amygdala, septal nuclei, bed nucleus of the stria terminalis, medial part of the nucleus of the solitary tract, and lateral portion of the parabrachial nucleus.[336] In 1986, a new member of the steroid hormone receptor superfamily with high sequence homology to the classical estrogen receptor (now referred to as *estrogen receptor* α) was isolated from rat prostate and named *estrogen receptor* β. This novel estrogen receptor was shown to bind estradiol and to activate transcription by binding to estrogen response elements.[337]

In situ hybridization studies examining the localization of estrogen receptor β mRNA have shown that these receptors are present throughout the rostral-caudal extent of the brain, with a high level of expression in the preoptic area, bed nucleus of the stria terminalis, paraventricular and supraoptic nuclei, amygdala, and laminae II to VI of the cerebral cortex.[338] Specific receptors for progesterone are induced by estrogen in hypothalamic regions of the brain, including the preoptic area, the ventromedial and ventrolateral nuclei, and the infundibular-arcuate nucleus, although there is also evidence for constitutive expression of progesterone receptors in some regions.[339] Androgen receptor mapping studies have shown considerable overlap in the distribution of androgen and estrogen receptors throughout the brain. The highest density of androgen receptors was found in hypothalamic nuclei known to participate in the control of reproduction and sexual behaviors, including the arcuate nucleus, PVH, medial preoptic nucleus, VMH, and brain regions with strong connections to the hypothalamus including the amygdala, nuclei of the septal region, bed nucleus of the stria terminalis, nucleus of the solitary tract, and lateral division of the parabrachial nucleus.[336] The anterior pituitary also contains receptors for all of the gonadal steroid hormones.

Steroid hormones can dramatically alter the pattern of pulsatile release of GnRH and of the gonadotropins through actions at both the hypothalamus and the pituitary. At the hypothalamus, estradiol, progesterone, and testosterone can all act to slow the frequency of GnRH release into the portal bloodstream as part of a closed negative feedback loop.[340] Because GnRH neurons have generally been shown to lack steroid hormone receptors, it is likely that the effects of steroid hormones on the firing rate of GnRH neurons are mediated by steroid hormone actions on other neural systems that provide afferent input to GnRH neurons. For example, progesterone-mediated negative feedback on GnRH secretion in primates appears to be regulated by β-endorphin-containing neurons in the hypothalamus, acting primarily through μ-opioid receptors. If a μ-receptor antagonist, such as naloxone, is administered along with progesterone, the negative feedback action of progesterone on GnRH secretion can be blocked.

Negative feedback of steroid hormones can also occur directly at the level of the pituitary. For example, estradiol has been shown to be capable of binding to the pituitary, decreasing LH and FSH synthesis and release, and decreasing the sensitivity of pituitary gonadotrophs to the actions of GnRH such that less LH and FSH are released when a pulse of GnRH stimulates the pituitary. Evidence for such a direct pituitary action of estradiol came from studies with rhesus monkeys that had been rendered deficient in endogenous GnRH by a lesion in the arcuate nucleus and showed a decline in endogenous gonadotropin secretion. When these monkeys received a pulsatile regimen of GnRH gonadotropin secretion, subsequent estradiol infusions dramatically suppressed the responsiveness of the pituitary to GnRH and suppressed the gonadotropin secretion that was being driven by the pulsatile administration of GnRH.[341] Steroid hormones can have direct negative feedback actions at the pituitary; however, the extent of hypothalamic versus pituitary negative feedback actions is species-specific. In primate species including humans, there is considerable feedback of estradiol at the pituitary, but most of the progesterone and testosterone negative feedback occurs at the level of the hypothalamus.[340]

Most of the time, the hypothalamic-pituitary axis is under the negative feedback influence of gonadal steroid hormones. If the gonads are removed surgically or their normal secretion of steroid hormones is suppressed pharmacologically, there is a dramatic increase (10- to 20-fold) in circulating levels of LH and FSH secretion.[340] This type of "castration response" occurs normally at the menopause in women, when ovarian follicular development and thus ovarian production of large quantities of estradiol and progesterone decrease and eventually cease.

In addition to negative feedback, estradiol can have a positive feedback action at the level of the hypothalamus and pituitary to lead to a massive release of LH and FSH from the pituitary. This massive release of gonadotropins occurs once each menstrual cycle and is referred to as the LH-FSH surge. The positive feedback action of estradiol occurs as a response to the rising tide of estradiol that is produced during the process of dominant follicle development in the late follicular phase of the menstrual cycle. In women, elevated estradiol levels are generally maintained at about 300–500 pg/mL for about 36 hours prior to stimulation of the gonadotropin surge.

Experiments have shown that both a critical concentration of plasma estradiol and a critical duration of elevated estradiol are necessary to achieve positive feedback and a resulting gonadotropin surge. Moreover, the duration of estrogen elevation that is required to trigger a surge depends on the concentration of circulating estrogen. If supraphysiologic doses of estradiol are administered, the surge can occur as early as 18 hours after their administration. Because the ovary is responsible for the production of estradiol and the time course and magnitude of estradiol release control the rate of positive feedback, the ovary has been referred to as the zeitgeber of the menstrual cycle. The dependence of the positive feedback system on the magnitude of estradiol production helps explain the fact that the portion of the menstrual cycle that varies most in length is the follicular phase. Production of higher levels of estradiol by a dominant follicle in one cycle would lead to a more rapid positive feedback action with earlier ovulation and thus a shorter follicular phase compared with a cycle in which the dominant follicle produced lower levels of estradiol.

As with negative feedback in response to estradiol, the positive feedback actions of estradiol occur both at the hypothalamus, to increase GnRH secretion, and at the pituitary, to enhance greatly pituitary responsiveness to GnRH. At the pituitary, estradiol increases pituitary sensitivity to GnRH by increasing the synthesis of new GnRH receptors and by enhancing the responsiveness to GnRH at a postreceptor site of action. At the level of the hypothalamus in rodent species, estradiol appears to act at a "surge center" to induce the ovulatory surge of GnRH. Lesions in areas adjacent to the medial preoptic area, near the anterior commissure and septal complex, block the ability of estradiol

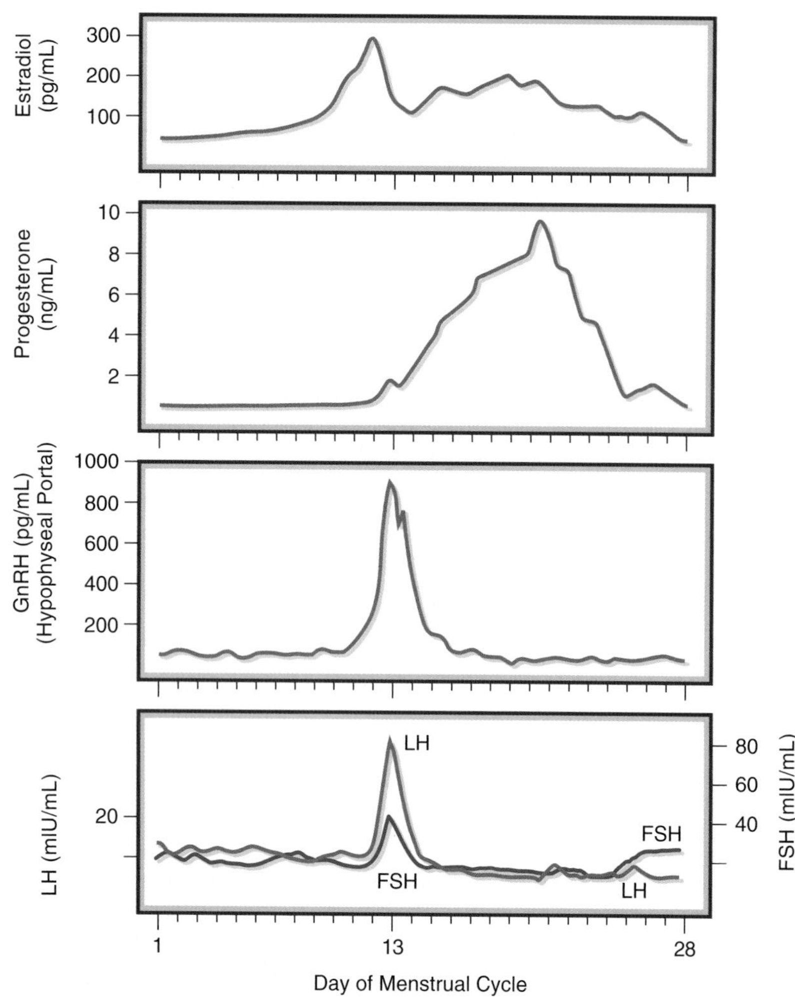

Figure 7–31 ■ Diagrammatic representation of changes in plasma levels of estradiol, progesterone, luteinizing hormone (LH), and follicle-stimulating hormone (FSH), and of portal levels of gonadotropin-releasing hormone (GnRH) over the human menstrual cycle.

to induce a surge in these species without blocking negative feedback effects of estradiol.[342] In primate species, there does not appear to be a separate surge center mediating the positive feedback actions of estradiol.

The cellular mechanisms that mediate the switch from negative to positive feedback of estrogen are not fully understood, but there is support for the concept that estrogen induction of various transcription factors and receptors (notably progesterone receptors) may play an important role in mediating this switch.[343] Alternatively, estrogen has been shown to have biphasic actions on hypothalamic GABAergic neurons that impinge on GnRH neurons and are strong regulators of their activity, with the switch in action dependent on the duration of estradiol exposure. The molecular mechanisms by which estradiol influences GnRH gene expression are not well understood, but it is likely that these influences also occur through actions of neural systems afferent to GnRH neurons.

Regulation of the Ovarian Cycle

Cyclic activity in the ovary is controlled by an interplay between steroid hormones produced by the ovary and the hypothalamic-pituitary neuroendocrine components of the reproductive axis. The duration of each phase of the ovarian cycle is species-dependent, but the general mechanisms controlling the cycle are similar in all species that have spontaneous ovarian cycles. In the human menstrual cycle, day 1 of the cycle is designated as the first day of menstrual bleeding. At this time, small and medium-sized follicles are present in the ovaries and only small amounts of estradiol are produced by the follicular cells. As a result, there is a low level of negative feedback to the hypothalamic-pituitary axis, LH pulse frequency is relatively fast (one pulse about every 60 minutes), and FSH concentrations are slightly elevated compared with much of the rest of the cycle (Fig. 7–31). FSH acts at the level of the ovarian follicles to stimulate development and causes an increase in follicular estradiol production, which in turn provides increased negative feedback to the hypothalamic-pituitary unit.

A result of the increased negative feedback is a slowing of pulsatile LH secretion over the course of the follicular phase to a rate of about one pulse every 90 minutes. However, as the growing follicle (or follicles, depending on the species) secretes more estradiol, a positive feedback action of estradiol is triggered that leads to an increase in GnRH release and a surge release of LH and FSH. The surge of gonadotropins acts at the fully developed follicle to stimulate the dissolution of the follicular wall and leads to ovulation of the matured ovum into the nearby fallopian tube, where fertilization takes place if sperm are present. Ovulation results in a reorganization of the cells of the follicular wall, which undergo hypertrophy and hyperplasia and start to secrete large amounts of progesterone and some estradiol. Progesterone and estradiol have a negative feedback effect at the level of the hypothalamus and pituitary, and thus LH pulse frequency becomes very slow during the luteal phase of the menstrual cycle. The corpus luteum has a fixed life span, and without additional stimulation in the form of chorionic gonadotropin from a developing embryo, the corpus luteum regresses spontaneously after about 14 days and progesterone and estradiol secretion diminishes. This reduces the negative feedback signals to the hypothalamus and pituitary and allows an increase in FSH and LH secretion. The fall in progesterone is also a withdrawal of steroid hormone support to the endometrial lining of the uterus, and as a result the endometrium is shed as menses and a new cycle begins.

In other species, the interplay between the neuroendocrine and ovarian hormones is similar but the timing of events is different and other factors, such as circadian and seasonal regulatory factors, play a role in regulating the cycle. The rat has a 4- or 5-day ovarian cycle with no menses (the endometrial lining is absorbed rather than shed). The rat also shows strong circadian rhythmicity in the timing of the LH-FSH surge, with the surge always occurring in the afternoon of the day of proestrus. Sheep are an example of a species that has a strongly seasonal pattern of ovarian cyclicity. During the breeding season they have 15-day cycles, with a very short follicular phase and an extended luteal phase; during the nonbreeding season signals relaying information about day length through the visual system, pineal, and SCN cause a dramatic suppression of GnRH neuronal activity, and cyclic ovarian function is prevented by a decrease in trophic hormonal support from the pituitary.

Early Development and Puberty

Neuroendocrine stimulation of the reproductive axis is initiated during fetal development, and in primates in midgestation circulating levels of LH and FSH reach values similar to those in castrated adults.[344] Later in gestational development, gonadotropin levels decline, restrained by rising levels of circulating gonadal steroids. The steroids that have this effect are probably placental in origin in that after parturition there is a rise in circulating gonadotropin levels that is apparent for variable periods of the first year of life, depending on the species.[345] The decline in reproductive hormone secretion in the postnatal period appears to be due to a decrease in GnRH stimulation of the reproductive axis because it occurs even in the castrated state and gonadotropin and gonadal steroid secretion can be supported by administration of pulses of GnRH.[346]

Pubertal reawakening of the reproductive axis occurs in late childhood and is marked initially by nighttime elevations in gonadotropin and gonadal steroid hormone levels.[346,347] The mechanisms controlling the pubertal reawakening of the GnRH pulse generator have been an area of intense investigation for the past 2 decades.[346] Although the mechanisms are not fully understood, significant progress has been made in identifying central changes in the hypothalamus that appear to play a role in this process. There appear to be both a decrease in transsynaptic inhibition to the GnRH neuronal system at puberty and an increase in stimulatory input to GnRH neurons at this time.[346] One of the major inhibitory inputs to the GnRH system is provided by GABAergic neurons. Studies in rhesus monkeys have shown that hypothalamic levels of GABA decrease during early puberty and that blocking GABAergic input before puberty, by intrahypothalamic administration of antisense oligodeoxynucleotides against the enzymes responsible for GABA synthesis, results in premature activation of the GnRH neuronal system.

It has been suggested, on the basis of findings that a subset of glutamate receptors (i.e., kainate receptors) increase in the hypothalamus at puberty, that the pubertal decrease in GABA tone may be caused by an increase in glutamatergic transmission. Further evidence for a role for glutamate comes from studies showing that administration of N-methyl-DL-aspartic acid (NMDA) to prepubertal rhesus monkeys can drive the reawakening of the reproductive axis.[348] Increased stimulatory drive to the GnRH neuronal system also appears to come from increases in norepinephrine and NPY at the time of puberty.[346] Furthermore, as discussed earlier, there is evidence that growth factors act through release of prostaglandin from glial cells at puberty to play a role in stimulating GnRH neurons.[349]

Despite an increased understanding of the neural changes occurring at puberty, the question of what signals trigger the pubertal awakening of the reproductive axis is unanswered at this time.[350] However, recent descriptions of two novel neuropeptide systems have shed further light on this area. The first was the isolation of a novel mammalian RFamide peptide named *kisspeptin* or *metastin* that is the natural ligand for the orphan G protein–coupled receptor GPR54.[293] Loss of function mutations in GPR54 cause hypogonadotropic hypogonadism, kisspeptin is expressed in subpopulations of arcuate and anteroventral periventricular neurons that project to GnRH neurons, kisspeptin expression is regulated by estradiol and testosterone and is upregulated at the time of puberty, and intracerebroventricular administration of kisspeptin causes the secretion of GnRH and gonadotropins.[351,352] The second discovery was galanin-like peptide (GALP), which is expressed specifically in the arcuate nucleus and binds with high affinity to galanin receptors. GALP is a potent central stimulator of gonadotropin release and sexual behavior in the rat and can reverse the decreased reproductive function associated with diabetes mellitus and hypoinsulinemia.[353] Both kisspeptin and GALP neurons are targets of leptin and are hypothesized to be involved in the well-known modulation of puberty and reproductive function by food availability and nutritional status (see the following section).

Reproductive Function and Stress

Many forms of physical stresses, such as energy restriction, exercise, temperature stress, infection, pain, and injury, as well as psychological stresses, such as being subordinate in a dominance hierarchy or being acutely psychologically stressed, can suppress the activity of the reproductive axis.[354,355] If the stress exposure is brief, there may be acute suppression of circulating gonadotropins and gonadal steroid hormones and in females disruption of normal menstrual cyclicity, but fertility is unlikely to be impaired.[354] In contrast, prolonged periods of significant stress exposure can lead to complete impairment of reproductive function, also characterized by low circulating levels of gonadotropins and gonadal steroids.[355] Stress appears to decrease the activity of the reproductive axis by decreasing GnRH drive to the pituitary because in all cases in which it has been examined, administration of exogenous GnRH can reverse the effects of the stress-induced decline in reproductive hormone secretion. Although we do not know the neural circuits through which many forms of stress suppress GnRH neuronal activity, some forms of stress-induced suppression of reproductive function are better understood.

In the case of foot shock stress in rats[356] and immune stress (i.e., injection of IL-1α) in primates,[357] the suppression of gonadotropin secretion that occurs has been shown to be reversible by administration of a CRH antagonist, implying that endogenous CRH secretion mediates the effects of these stresses on GnRH neurons. In other studies, naloxone, a μ-opiate receptor antagonist, has been shown to be capable of reversing restraint stress-induced suppression of gonadotropin secretion in monkeys; however, naloxone is ineffective in reversing the suppression of gonadotropin secretion that occurs during insulin-induced hypoglycemia.[358,359] In the case of metabolic stresses, multiple regulators appear to mediate changes in the neural drive to the reproductive axis.

Various metabolic fuels including glucose and fatty acids can regulate the function of the reproductive axis, and blocking cellular utilization of these fuels can lead to suppression of gonadotropin secretion and decreased gonadal activity.[360] Leptin, a hormone produced by fat cells, can also modulate the activity of the reproductive axis. Mutant mice deficient in leptin or leptin receptors are infertile, and fertility can be restored to *ob/ob* mice by administration of leptin.[361] Moreover, leptin administration has been shown to reverse the suppressive effects of undernutrition on the reproductive axis in some situations.[362] Leptin receptors are found in several populations that are known to have a strong influence on the reproductive axis, particularly NPY and kisspeptin neurons.

In summary, it appears that a number of neural circuits can mediate effects of stress on the GnRH neuronal system and that the neural systems involved are at least somewhat specific to the type of stress that is experienced.

NEUROENDOCRINE DISEASE

Disease of the hypothalamus can cause pituitary dysfunction, neuropsychiatric and behavioral disorders, and disturbances of autonomic and metabolic regulation. In the diagnosis and treatment of suspected hypothalamic or pituitary disease, four issues must be considered: the extent of the lesion, the physiologic impact, the specific cause, and the psychosocial setting. The etiology of hypothalamic neuroendocrine disorders categorized by age and syndrome is summarized in Tables 7–7 and 7–8.

Manifestations of pituitary insufficiency secondary to hypothalamic or pituitary stalk damage are not identical to those of primary pituitary insufficiency. Hypothalamic injury causes decreased secretion of most pituitary hormones but can cause hypersecretion of hormones normally under inhibitory control by the hypothalamus, as in hypersecretion of PRL after damage to the pituitary stalk and precocious puberty caused by loss of the normal restraint over gonadotropin maturation. Impairment of inhibitory control of the neurohypophysis can lead to the syndrome of inappropriate vasopressin secretion (SIADH) (see Chapter 9). More subtle abnormalities in secretion can result from impairment of the control system. For example, loss of the normal circadian rhythm of ACTH secretion may occur before loss of pituitary-adrenal secretory reserve and responses to physiologic stimuli may be paradoxical. Because hypophyseo-

TABLE 7–7 ETIOLOGY OF HYPOTHALAMIC DISEASE BY AGE

Premature Infants and Neonates

- Intraventricular hemorrhage
- Meningitis: bacterial
- Tumors: glioma, hemangioma
- Trauma
- Hydrocephalus, kernicterus

1 mo to 2 yr

- Tumors
  - Glioma, especially optic glioma
  - Histiocytosis X
  - Hemangioma
- Hydrocephalus
- Meningitis
- Familial disorders
  - Laurence-Moon-Biedl syndrome
  - Prader-Willi syndrome

2 to 10 yr

- Neoplasms
  - Craniopharyngioma
  - Glioma, dysgerminoma, hamartoma
  - Histiocytosis X, leukemia
  - Ganglioneuroma, ependymoma
  - Medulloblastoma
- Meningitis
  - Bacterial mening it is
  - Tuberculous mening it is
- Encephalitis
  - Viral
  - Exanthematous demyelinating
- Familial
  - Diabetes insipidus
- Radiation therapy
- Diabetic ketoacidosis
- Moyamoya disease, circle of Willis

10 to 25 yr

- Tumors
  - Craniopharyngioma
  - Glioma, hamartoma, dysgerminoma
  - Histiocytosis X, leukemia
  - Dermoid, lipoma, neuroblastoma
- Trauma
- Vascular
  - Subarachnoid hemorrhage
  - Aneurysm
  - Arteriovenous malformation
- Inflammatory disease
  - Meningitis
  - Encephalitis
  - Sarcoidosis
  - Tuberculosis
- Structural brain defect
  - Chronic hydrocephalus
  - Increased intracranial pressure

25 to 50 yr

- Nutritional: Wernicke's disease
- Tumors
  - Glioma, lymphoma, meningioma
  - Craniopharyngioma, pituitary tumors
  - Angioma, plasmacytoma, colloid cysts
  - Ependymoma, sarcoma, histiocytosis X
- Inflammatory disease
  - Sarcoidosis
  - Tuberculosis, viral encephalitis
- Vascular
  - Aneurysm, subarachnoid hemorrhage
  - Arteriovenous malformation
- Damage from pituitary radiation therapy

50 yr and Older

- Nutritional: Wernicke's disease
- Tumors: pituitary tumors, sarcoma, glioblastoma, ependymoma, meningioma, colloid cysts, lymphoma
- Vascular disease
  - Infarct, subarachnoid hemorrhage
  - Pituitary apoplexy
- Inflammatory disease: encephalitis, sarcoidosis, meningitis
- Damage from radiation therapy for ear-nose-throat carcinoma, pituitary tumors

Adapted from Plum F, Van Uitert R. Nonendocrine diseases and disorders of the hypothalamus. In Reichlin S, Baldessarini RJ, Martin JB, eds. The Hypothalamus, Vol 56. New York: Raven Press, 1978:415-473.

TABLE 7–8 ETIOLOGY OF ENDOCRINE SYNDROMES OF HYPOTHALAMIC ORIGIN

Hypophyseotropic Hormone Deficiency
Surgical pituitary stalk section
Inflammatory disease: Basilar meningitis and granuloma, sarcoidosis, tuberculosis, sphenoid osteomyelitis, eosinophilic granuloma
Craniopharyngioma
Hypothalamic tumor: Infundibuloma, teratoma (ectopic pinealoma), neuroglial tumor, particularly astrocytoma
Maternal deprivation syndrome, psychosocial dwarfism
Isolated growth hormone-releasing hormone (GHRH) deficiency
Hypothalamic hypothyroidism
Panhypophyseotropic failure
Disorders of Regulation of Gonadotropin-Releasing Hormone Secretion
Female
Precocious puberty: GnRH-secreting hamartoma, hCG-secreting germinoma
Delayed puberty
Neurogenic amenorrhea
Pseudocyesis
Anorexia nervosa
"Functional" amenorrhea and oligomenorrhea
Drug-induced amenorrhea
Male
Precocious puberty
Fröhlich's syndrome
Olfactory-genital dysplasia (Kallmann's syndrome)
Disorders of Regulation of Prolactin-Regulating Factors
Tumor
Sarcoidosis
Drug-induced
Reflex
Herpes zoster of chest wall
Post-thoracotomy
Nipple manipulation
Spinal cord tumor
"Psychogenic"
Hypothyroidism
Carbon dioxide narcosis
Disorders of Regulation of Corticotropin-Releasing Hormone
Paroxysmal corticotropin discharge (Wolff's syndrome)
Loss of circadian variation
Depression
CRH-secreting gangliocytoma

CRH, corticotropin-releasing hormone; *GnRH*, gonadotropin-releasing hormone; *hCG*, human chorionic gonadotropin.

tropic hormone levels cannot be measured directly and pituitary hormone secretion is regulated by complex, multilayered controls, assay of pituitary hormones in blood does not necessarily give a meaningful picture of events at hypothalamic and higher levels. Rarely, tumors secrete excessive amounts of releasing peptides and cause hypersecretion of hormones from the pituitary.

Disorders of the hypothalamic-pituitary unit can result from lesions at several levels. Defects can arise from destruction of the pituitary (as by tumor, infarct, inflammation, or autoimmune disease) or from a hereditary deficiency of a particular hormone as in rare cases of isolated FSH, GH, or POMC deficiency. Selective loss of thyroid hormone receptors in the pituitary can give rise to increased TSH secretion and thyrotoxicosis. Furthermore, disorders can arise through disruption of the stalk-median eminence contact zone, the stalk itself, or the nerve terminals of the tuberohypophyseal system; such disruption occurs after surgical stalk section, with tumors involving the stalk, and in some inflammatory diseases. At a higher level, tonic inhibitory and excitatory inputs can be lost as manifested by absence of circadian rhythms or the development of precocious puberty. Physical stress, cytokine products of inflammatory cells, toxins, and reflex inputs from peripheral homeostatic monitors also impinge on the tuberoinfundibular system. At the highest level of control, emotional stress and psychological disorders can activate the pituitary-adrenal stress response and suppress gonadotropin secretion (e.g., psychogenic amenorrhea) or inhibit GH secretion (e.g., psychosocial dwarfism) (see Chapter 23). Intrinsic disease of the anterior pituitary is reviewed in Chapter 8, and disturbances in neurohypophyseal function are discussed in Chapter 9. This chapter considers diseases of the hypothalamic-pituitary unit.

Pituitary Isolation Syndrome

Destructive lesions of the pituitary stalk, as occur with head injury, surgical transection, tumor, or granuloma, produce a characteristic pattern of pituitary dysfunction.[363-365] Central diabetes insipidus (DI) develops in a large percentage of patients, depending on the level at which the stalk has been sectioned. If the cut is close to the hypothalamus, DI is almost always produced, whereas if the section is low on the stalk, the incidence is lower. The extent to which nerve terminals in the upper stalk are preserved determines the clinical course. The classic triphasic syndrome of initial polyuria followed by normal water control and then by vasopressin deficiency over a period of 1 week to 10 days occurs in less than half of the patients. The sequence is attributed to an initial loss of neurogenic control of the neural lobe, followed by autolysis of the neural lobe with release of vasopressin into the circulation and finally by complete loss of vasopressin. However, full expression of polyuria requires adequate cortisol levels; if cortisol is deficient, vasopressin deficiency may be present with only minimal polyuria. DI can also develop after stalk injury without an overt transitional phase. When DI occurs after head injury or operative trauma, varying degrees of recovery can be seen even after months or years. Sprouting of nerve terminals in the stump of the pituitary stalk may give rise to sufficient functioning tissue to maintain water balance. In contrast to the effects of stalk section, nondestructive injury to the neurohypophysis or stalk, as during surgical resection of optic chiasmatic astrocytomas, can sometimes give rise to transient SIADH.[366]

Although head injury, granulomas, and tumors are the most common causes of acquired DI, other cases develop in the absence of a clear-cut cause.[367] Some cases may be due to autoimmune disease of the hypothalamus as suggested by the finding of autoantibodies to neurohypophyseal cells in a third of cases of "idiopathic" DI in one series.[368] However, autoantibodies were also frequently found in association with histiocytosis-X. Later reports suggest the importance of continued vigilance in cases of idiopathic DI because a definite cause is frequently uncovered in time, including a high proportion of occult germinomas whose detection by magnetic resonance imaging may be preceded by elevated levels of human chorionic gonadotropin (hCG) in CSF.[369,370] Congenital DI can be part of a hereditary disease. DI in the Brattleboro rat is due to an autosomal recessive genetic defect that impairs production of vasopressin but not of oxytocin. In contrast, inherited forms of DI in humans have been attributed to mutations in the vasopressin V2 receptor gene or less frequently in the aquaporin or vasopressin genes.[371-374]

Menstrual cycles cease after stalk section although gonadotropins may still be detectable, unlike the situation after hypophysectomy. Plasma glucocorticoid levels and urinary excretion of cortisol and 17-hydroxycorticoids decline after hypophysectomy and stalk section, but the change is slower after stalk section. A transient increase in cortisol secretion after stalk section is believed to be due to release of ACTH from preformed stores. The ACTH response to the lowering of blood cortisol is markedly reduced but ACTH release after stress may be normal, possibly because of CRH-independent mechanisms. Reduction in thyroid function after stalk section is similar to that seen with hypophysectomy. The fall in GH secretion is said to be the most sensitive indication of damage to the stalk; however, the insidious nature of this endocrinologic change in adults who have suffered traumatic brain injuries may cause it to be overlooked and therefore contribute to delayed rehabilitation.[375]

Humans with stalk sections or with tumors of the stalk region have widely varying levels of hyperprolactinemia and may have galactorrhea.[376] PRL responses to hypoglycemia and to TRH are blunted, in part because of loss of neural connections with the hypothalamus. PRL responses to dopamine agonists and antagonists in the pituitary isolation syndrome are similar to those in patients with prolactinomas. Interestingly, PRL secretion continues to show a diurnal variation in patients with either hypothalamopituitary disconnection or microprolactinoma.[308] Both forms of hyperprolactinemia are characterized by a similarly increased frequency of PRL pulses and a marked rise in nonpulsatile or basal PRL secretion, although the disruption is greater in the tumoral hyperprolactinemia.

An incomplete pituitary isolation syndrome may occur with the empty sella syndrome, intrasellar cysts, or pituitary adenomas.[377-379] Anterior pituitary failure after stalk section is in part due to loss of specific neural and vascular links to the hypothalamus and in part due to pituitary infarction.

Hypophyseotropic Hormone Deficiency

Selective pituitary failure can be due to a deficiency of specific pituitary cell types or a deficiency of one or more hypothalamic hormones. Isolated GnRH deficiency is the most common hypophyseotropic hormone deficiency. In Kallmann's syndrome (gonadotropin deficiency commonly associated with hyposmia),[324] hereditary agenesis of the olfactory lobe may be demonstrable by magnetic resonance imaging.[380] Abnormal development of the GnRH system is due to defective migration of the GnRH-containing neurons from the olfactory nasal epithelium in early embryologic life (see the earlier section on GnRH). Other malformations of the cranial midline structures, such as absence of the septum pellucidum in septo-optic dysplasia (De Morsier's syndrome), can cause hypogonadotropic hypogonadism (HH) or, less commonly, precocious puberty. A surprisingly large percentage of children with septo-optic dysplasia who otherwise have multiple hypothalamic-pituitary abnormalities actually retain normal gonadotropin function and enter puberty spontaneously.[381] The genetic basis of HH has now been established in approximately 10% of patients.[325,382] Mutations in the KAL1 (Kallmann's syndrome) gene and the AHC-DAX1 (adrenal hypoplasia congenita-HH) gene cause X-linked recessive disease. Autosomal recessive HH has been associated with mutations in the GnRH receptor, leptin, leptin receptor, FSH, LH, PROP-1 (combined pituitary deficiency), and HESX (septo-optic dysplasia) genes while deficient FGFR1 function causes an autosomal dominant form of HH.

The GnRH response test is of little value in the differential diagnosis of hypothalamic hypogonadism. Most patients with GnRH deficiency show little or no response to an initial test dose, but normal responses are seen after repeated injection. This slow response has been attributed to down-regulation of GnRH receptors in response to prolonged GnRH deficiency. Furthermore, with intrinsic pituitary disease the response to GnRH may be absent or normal. Consequently, it is not possible to distinguish between hypothalamic and pituitary disease with a single injection of GnRH. Prolonged infusions or repeated administration of GnRH agonists after hormone replacement therapy priming may aid in the diagnosis or provide therapeutic options for women with Kallmann's syndrome wishing to become pregnant.[383,384]

Deficiency of TRH secretion gives rise to hypothalamic hypothyroidism, also called tertiary hypothyroidism, which can occur in hypothalamic disease or more rarely as an isolated defect.[385] Molecular genetic analyses have revealed infrequent autosomal recessive mutations in the TRH and TRH receptor genes in the etiology of central hypothyroidism.[386] Hypothalamic and pituitary causes of TSH deficiency are most readily distinguished by imaging methods. Although theoretically reasonable, the TRH stimulation test for the differentiation of hypothalamic disease from pituitary disease is of limited value. The typical pituitary response to TRH administration in patients with TRH deficiency is an enhanced and somewhat delayed peak, whereas the response with pituitary failure is subnormal or absent. The hypothalamic type of response has been attributed to an associated GH deficiency that sensitizes the pituitary to TRH (possibly through suppression of somatostatin secretion), but GH also affects T_4 metabolism and may alter pituitary responses as well.[387] In practice, the responses to TRH in hypothalamic and pituitary disease overlap so much that they cannot be used reliably for a differential diagnosis. Persistent failure to demonstrate responses to TRH is good evidence for the presence of intrinsic pituitary disease, but the presence of a response does not mean that the pituitary is normal. Deficient TRH secretion leads to altered TSH biosynthesis by the pituitary, including impaired glycosylation. Poorly glycosylated TSH has low biologic activity, and dissociation of bioactive and immunoreactive TSH can lead to the paradox of normal or elevated levels of TSH in hypothalamic hypothyroidism.[385,388]

GHRH deficiency appears to be the principal cause of hGH deficiency in children with idiopathic dwarfism.[389] This condition is frequently associated with abnormal electroencephalograms, a history of birth trauma, and breech delivery, although a cause and effect relationship has not been established. Magnetic resonance imaging scans show that most children with isolated, idiopathic hGH deficiency have a normal sized or only slightly reduced anterior pituitary; less common findings are ectopic posterior pituitary, anterior pituitary hypoplasia, or empty sella.[390] In contrast, children with idiopathic combined pituitary hormone deficiency are significantly more likely to have evidence of moderate to severe anterior pituitary hypoplasia, ectopic posterior pituitary, complete agenesis of the pituitary stalk (both nervous and vascular components), and a variety of associated midline cerebral malformations.[390] Human GH is the most vulnerable of the anterior pituitary hormones when the pituitary stalk is damaged. It can be difficult to differentiate between primary pituitary disease and GHRH deficiency by standard tests of GH reserve. However, a substantial GH secretory response to a single administration of hexarelin occurs only in the presence of at least a partially intact vascular stalk (Fig. 7–32).[217]

In many children with dwarfism, the anatomic abnormalities of the intrasellar contents and pituitary stalk together with the frequent occurrence of other midline defects, such as those in septo-optic dysplasia, are consistent with the alternative hypothesis of a developmental defect occurring in embryogenesis.[390] There has been a remarkable advance in our understanding of the molecular ontogeny of the hypothalamic-pituitary unit, much of it based on mutant mouse models.[26] Parallel genetic analyses have been conducted in children with isolated GH deficiency or combined pituitary hormone deficiencies. These

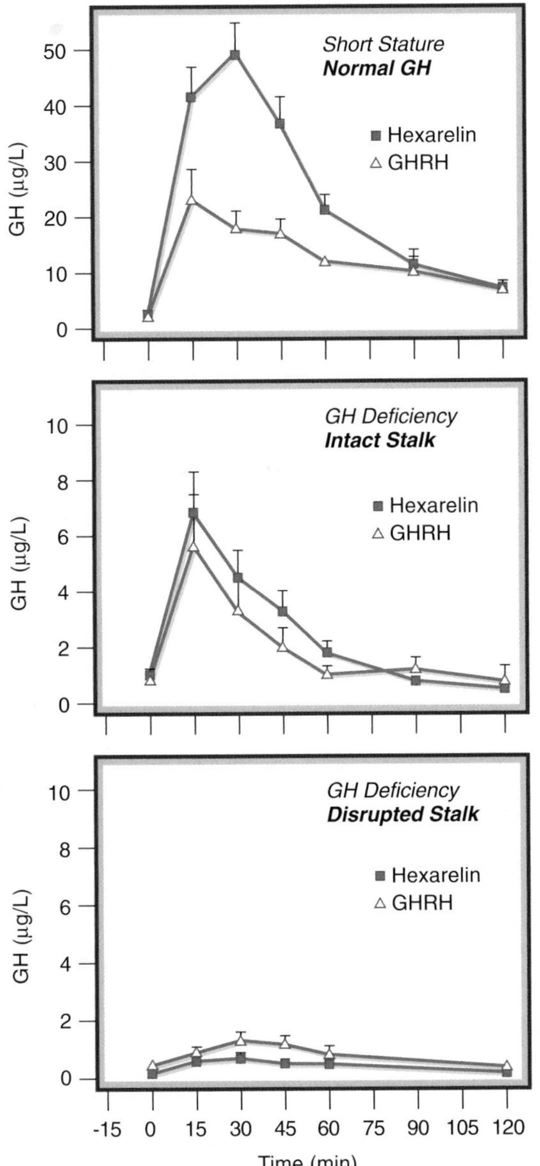

Figure 7–32 ▪ Effect of hypothalamic-pituitary disconnection on the growth hormone (GH) secretory responses to GH-releasing hormone (GHRH) (1 µg/kg) and hexarelin (2 µg/kg) administered intravenously to children with GH deficiency. (*Top*) Mean responses in a group of 24 prepubertal children with short stature secondary to familial short stature or constitutional growth delay. Children with GH deficiency and an intact vascular pituitary stalk as visualized by dynamic magnetic resonance imaging exhibited a clear, but blunted, GH response to both secretagogues (*middle*). In contrast, children with pituitary stalk agenesis (both vascular and neural components) had no or a markedly attenuated response to both peptides (*bottom*). (From Maghnie M, Spica-Russotto V, Cappa M, et al. The growth hormone response to hexarelin in patients with different hypothalamic-pituitary abnormalities. J Clin Endocrinol Metab 1998;83:3886-3889.)

studies have identified autosomal recessive mutations in both structural and regulatory genes including the GHRH receptor, PIT1, PROP1, HESX1, LHX3, and LHX4 that are responsible for a sizable proportion of congenital hypothalamic-pituitary disorders once considered idiopathic.[206,207,389,390]

Adrenal insufficiency is another manifestation of hypothalamic disease and rarely is due to CRH deficiency.[391] Isolated ACTH deficiency is uncommon, but there is suggestive evidence in at least one family of genetic linkage to the CRH gene locus.[392] More recent investigations have revealed mutations in the TPIT gene, a T box transcription factor expressed only in pituitary corticotrophs and melanotrophs, associated with the majority of cases of isolated ACTH deficiency in neonates.[393] The CRH stimulation test does not reliably distinguish hypothalamic from pituitary failure as a cause of ACTH deficiency.[394]

Apart from intrinsic diseases of the hypothalamus such as tumors and granulomas, two environmental causes of central hypophyseotropic deficiencies are of increasing clinical importance. These are trauma to the brain,[364,365,375] particularly from motor vehicle accidents, and the sequelae of chemotherapy and radiation therapy for intracranial lesions in children and adults.[388,395,396] Improved short-term survival from head injuries associated with coma and CNS malignancies has greatly increased the prevalence of long-term neuroendocrine consequences.

Craniopharyngioma

Craniopharyngioma is the most common pediatric tumor occurring in the sellar and parasellar area (see Table 7–7). Because of their location these benign neoplasms frequently cause significant neuroendocrine dysfunction. The more common adamantinomatous tumors in children usually contain both a cystic component filled with a turbid, cholesterol-rich fluid and a solid component characterized by organized epithelial cells.[397] Roughly 25% of craniopharyngiomas are diagnosed in patients older than age 25 and this subset of tumors is more typically papillary in nature, solid, and less likely to be calcified or cystic.[397] Both forms of craniopharyngioma probably result from metaplastic changes in vestigial epithelial cell rests that originate in Rathke's pouch and the craniopharyngeal duct during fetal development.

Common presenting symptoms are those due to a mass intracranial lesion and increased intracranial pressure. Visual field defects, papilledema, and optic atrophy can occur from compression of the optic chiasm or nerves. Eighty percent to 90% of affected children have signs and symptoms of endocrine dysfunction, although these are not usually the chief complaint. The most frequent hormone deficiencies are GH and gonadotropin. The latter is almost universal in adolescents and adults and likely also present, but undetected, in prepubertal children. TSH and ACTH deficiency are also common. Even if not present at initial diagnosis, endocrine dysfunction often occurs subsequently to treatment and necessitates long-term follow-up and retesting.[398]

Magnetic resonance imaging (MRI) is the imaging modality of choice in cases of suspected craniopharyngioma.[399] A recommended examination includes T1-weighted thin sagittal and coronal sections both precontrast and postcontrast through the sella and suprasellar regions. T2 and fluid attenuation inversion recovery (FLAIR) images are useful to further delineate cysts, which are hyperintense. Computed tomography (CT) scans can be useful to determine the presence of calcification.

■ Hypophyseotropic Hormone Hypersecretion

Pituitary hypersecretion is occasionally caused by tumors of the hypothalamus. GnRH-secreting hamartomas can cause precocious puberty.[400] CRH-secreting gangliocytomas can cause Cushing's syndrome,[401] and GHRH-secreting gangliocytomas of the hypothalamus can cause acromegaly.[402] Although they do not arise from the hypothalamus, paraneoplastic syndromes can also cause pituitary hypersecretion, as with CRH-secreting tumors and GHRH-secreting tumors of the bronchi and pancreas. Bronchial carcinoids and pituitary islet cell tumors are the usual causes of this phenomenon.

Neuroendocrine Disorders of Gonadotropin Regulation

Precocious Puberty

The term precocious puberty is used when physiologically normal pituitary-gonadal function appears at an early age (see also Chapter 24).[403] By convention, the onset of androgen secretion and spermatogenesis must occur before the age of 9 or 10 in boys and the onset of estrogen secretion and cyclic ovarian activity before age 7 or 8 in girls.[404,405] Central precocious puberty is due to disturbed CNS function, which may or may not have an identifiable structural basis. Pseudoprecocious puberty refers to premature sexual development resulting from excessive secretion of androgens, estrogens, or hCG caused by tumors (both gonadal and extragonadal), administration of exogenous gonadal steroids, or genetically determined activation of gonadotropin receptors (see Chapter 24). Central precocious puberty with neurogenic causes and pineal gland disease is discussed in this chapter.

Idiopathic Sexual Precocity

Familial occurrence is uncommon, but there is a hereditary form of idiopathic sexual precocity that is largely confined to males. Abnormal electroencephalograms and behavioral disturbances, suggesting the presence of brain damage, have been reported occasionally in girls with idiopathic precocious puberty. The pathogenesis may be related to the rate of hypothalamic development or other as yet undetermined nutritional, environmental, or psychosocial factors. Many cases previously thought to be idiopathic are due to small hypothalamic hamartomas discussed in more detail in the following section. It has been argued that localized activation of discrete cellular subsets connected to GnRH neurons may be sufficient to initiate puberty.[406]

Neurogenic Precocious Puberty

Approximately two thirds of hypothalamic lesions that influence the timing of human puberty are located in the posterior hypothalamus, but in the subset of patients who come to autopsy, damage is extensive. Specific lesions known to cause precocity include craniopharyngioma (although delayed puberty is far more common), astrocytoma, pineal tumors, subarachnoid cysts, encephalitis, miliary tuberculosis, tuberous sclerosis or neurofibromatosis type 1, the Sturge-Weber syndrome, porencephaly, craniostenosis, microcephaly, hydrocephalus, empty sella syndrome, and Tay-Sachs disease.[407,408]

Hamartoma of the hypothalamus is an exception to the generalization that tumors of the brain cause precocious puberty by impairment of gonadotropin secretion (although hamartomas on occasion cause hypothalamic damage). A hamartoma is a tumor-like collection of normal-appearing nerve tissue lodged in an abnormal location. The parahypothalamic type consists of an encapsulated nodule of nerve tissue attached to the floor of the third ventricle or suspended from the floor by a peduncle and typically less than 1 cm in diameter. The intrahypothalamic or sessile type is enveloped by the posterior hypothalamus and can distort the third ventricle. These tend to be larger than the pedunculated variety, grow in the interpeduncular cistern, and are frequently accompanied by seizures, mental retardation, developmental delays, and roughly half the incidence of precocious puberty associated with the parahypothalamic lesions.[409,410] Before the development of high-resolution scanning techniques, this tumor was considered rare, but small ones can now be visualized. Miniature hamartomas of the tuber cinereum are common at autopsy. Precocious puberty occurs when the hamartoma makes connections with the median eminence and thus serves as an accessory hypothalamus. Peptidergic nerve terminals containing GnRH have been found in the tumors.[400] Early pubertal development is presumably due to unrestrained GnRH secretion, although the hamartomas almost certainly have an intrinsic pulse generator of GnRH secretion because pulsatility is required for stimulation of gonadotropin secretion (see earlier section on GnRH).

Manifestations of premature puberty in patients with hamartomas are similar to those associated with other central causes of precocity. Hamartomas occur in both sexes and may be present as early as age 3 months. In the past most cases were thought to be fatal by age 20, but many hamartomas cause no brain damage and need not be excised.[409] The interpeduncular fossa of the brain is difficult to approach, and surgical experience is somewhat limited. Early in the course of illness, epilepsy manifested as "brief, repetitive, stereotyped attacks of laughter"[411] may provide a clue to the disease. Late in the course, hypothalamic damage can cause severe neurologic defects and intractable seizures.

Hypothyroidism

Hypothyroidism can cause precocious puberty in girls that is reversible with thyroid therapy. Hyperprolactinemia and galactorrhea may be present. One possibility is that elevated TSH levels (in children with thyroid failure) cross-react with the FSH receptor.[412] Alternatively, low levels of thyroid hormone might simultaneously activate release of LH, FSH, and TSH. A third possibility is that hypothyroidism causes hypothalamic encephalopathy that impairs the normal tonic suppression of gonadotropin release by the hypothalamus. The high PRL levels that sometimes accompany this disorder may be due to a deficiency in PIF secretion, increased secretion of TRH, or increased sensitivity of the lactotrophs to TRH secretion.

Tumors of the Pineal Gland

Pineal gland tumors account for only a small percentage of intracranial neoplasms. They occur as a central midline mass with an enhancing lesion on magnetic resonance imaging frequently accompanied by hydrocephalus. Pinealomas cause a variety of neurologic abnormalities. Parinaud's syndrome, which consists of paralysis of upward gaze, pupillary areflexia (to light), paralysis of convergence, and a wide-based gait, occurs with about half of pinealomas. Gait disturbances can also occur because of brain stem or cerebellar compression. Additional neurologic signs occurring with moderate frequency include spasticity, ataxia, nystagmus, syncope, vertigo, cranial nerve palsies other than VI and VIII, intention tremor, scotoma, and tinnitus.

Several discrete cytopathologic entities account for mass lesions in the pineal region (Table 7–9).[413] The most common nonneoplastic conditions are degenerative pineal cysts, arachnoid cysts, and cavernous hemangioma. Pinealocytes give rise to primitive neuroectodermal tumors, the so-called small blue cell tumors that are immunopositive for the neuronal marker synaptophysin and negative for the lymphocyte marker CD45. True pinealomas can be relatively well-differentiated pineocytomas, intermediate mixed forms, or the less differentiated pineoblastomas,[413,414] which are essentially identical to medul-

TABLE 7–9 CLASSIFICATION OF TUMORS OF THE PINEAL REGION

A. **Germ Cell Tumors**
  1. Germinoma
    a. Posterior third ventricle and pineal lesions
    b. Anterior third ventricle, suprasellar or intrasellar lesions
    c. Combined lesions in anterior and posterior third ventricle, apparently noncontiguous, with or without foci of cystic or solid teratoma
  2. Teratoma
    a. Evidencing growth along two or three germ lines in varying degrees of differentiation
    b. Dermoid and epidermoid cysts with or without solid foci of teratoma
    c. Histologically malignant forms with or without differentiated foci of benign, solid, or cystic teratoma-teratocarcinoma, chorioepithelioma, embryonal carcinoma (endodermal-sinus tumor or yolk-sac carcinoma); combinations of these with or without foci of germinoma, chemodectoma

B. **Pineal Parenchymal Tumors**
  1. Pinealocytes
    a. Pineocytoma
    b. Pineoblastoma
    c. Ganglioglioma and chemodectoma
    d. Mixed forms exhibiting transitions between these
  2. Glia
    a. Astrocytoma
    b. Ependymoma
    c. Mixed forms and other less frequent gliomas (e.g., glioblastoma, oligodendroglioma)

C. **Tumors of Supporting or Adjacent Structures**
  1. Meningioma
  2. Hemangiopericytoma

D. **Nonneoplastic Conditions of Neurosurgical Importance**
  1. "Degenerative" cysts of pineal gland lined by fibrillary astrocytes
  2. Arachnoid cysts
  3. Cavernous hemangioma

From DeGirolami U. Pathology of tumors of the pineal region. In Schmidek HH, ed. Pineal Tumors. New York: Masson, 1977:1-19.

loblastomas, neuroblastomas, and oat cell carcinomas of the lung.

The most common tumors of the pineal gland are actually germinomas (a form of teratoma), so designated because of their presumed origin in germ cells. Germinomas may also occur in the anterior hypothalamus or the floor of the third ventricle, where they are often associated with the clinical triad of DI, pituitary insufficiency, and visual abnormalities.[408] Identical tumors can be found in the testis and anterior mediastinum. Intracranial germinomas have a tendency to spread locally, infiltrate the hypothalamus, and metastasize to the spinal cord and CSF. Extracranial metastases (to the skin, lung, or liver) are rare. Teratomas derived from two or more germ cell layers also occur in the pineal region. Chorionic tissue in teratomas and germinomas may secrete hCG in sufficient amounts to cause gonadal maturation, and some of these tumors have histologic and functional characteristics of choriocarcinomas. Diagnosis is confirmed by the combination of a mass lesion, cytologic analysis of CSF, and radioimmunoassay detection of hCG in the CSF.

Precocious puberty is a relatively unusual manifestation of pineal gland disease. When it occurs, neuroanatomic studies suggest that the cause is secondary to pressure or destructive effects of the pineal tumor on the function of the adjacent hypothalamus or to the secretion of hCG. Most patients have other evidence of hypothalamic involvement such as DI, polyphagia, somnolence, obesity, or behavioral disturbance. Choriocarcinoma of the pineal gland is associated with high plasma levels of hCG. The hCG can stimulate testosterone secretion from the testes but not estrogen secretion by the ovaries and hence causes premature puberty almost exclusively in boys. The prevalence of elevated hCG levels in children with premature puberty related to tumors in the pineal region is unknown, but the fact that this phenomenon occurs further challenges the theory that nonparenchymal tumors cause precocious puberty by damaging the normal pineal gland. Rarely, pinealomas cause delayed puberty, raising speculation about a role of melatonin in inhibiting gonadotropin secretion in these cases.

Management of tumors in the pineal region is not straightforward.[413,415] Operative mortality rates can be high, but the rationale for an aggressive approach to the pineal region is based on the need to make a histologic diagnosis, the variety of lesions found in this region, the possibility of cure of an encapsulated lesion, and the effectiveness of chemotherapeutic agents for germinomas and choriocarcinoma. Stereotaxic biopsy of the pineal region provided diagnosis in 33 of 34 cases in one series, suggesting that this is a useful alternative to open surgical exploration for diagnostic purposes.[416] Long-term palliation or cure of many pineal region tumors is possible by combinations of surgery, radiation, gamma knife, or chemotherapy, depending on the nature of the lesion.[417]

Approach to the Patient with Precocious Puberty

Several groups have reviewed the diagnostic approach to suspected central precocious puberty (see also Chapter 24).[418,419] Although guidelines differ, the index of suspicion is clearly inversely proportional to the age of the patient. A GnRH stimulation test to assess gonadotropin release and thereby differentiate between primed and inactive gonadotrophs is probably the single most important endocrinologic measure. If LH and FSH levels are not stimulated and there is no evidence of gonadal germ cell maturation, the cause of precocious puberty lies outside the hypothalamic-pituitary axis and the diagnostic process should focus on the adrenal glands and gonads (see Chapters 14 and 18). Magnetic resonance imaging studies are central to the work-up for exclusion or characterization of organic lesions in the areas of the sella, optic chiasm, suprasellar hypothalamus, and interpeduncular cistern.[420]

Management of Sexual Precocity

Structural lesions of the hypothalamus are treated by surgery, radiation, chemotherapy, or combinations of these as indicated by the pathologic diagnosis and extent of disease. Endocrinologic manifestations of precocious puberty are best treated by GnRH agonists with the therapeutic goals of delaying sexual maturation to a more appropriate age and achieving optimal linear growth and bone mass, possibly with the combined use of GH treatment.[421,422] Other approaches include the use of cyproterone acetate, testolactone, or spironolactone to antagonize or inhibit gonadal steroid biosynthesis.[423,424] Precocious puberty is stressful to both the child and the parents, and it is essential that psychological support be provided.

Psychogenic Amenorrhea

Menstrual cycles can cease in young nonpregnant women with no demonstrable abnormalities of the brain, pituitary, or ovary in several situations,[425,426] including pseudocyesis (false pregnancy), anorexia nervosa, excessive exercise, psychogenic disorders, and hyperprolactinemic states (see Chapter 16). Psychogenic amenorrhea, the most common cause of secondary amenorrhea except for pregnancy, can occur with major psychopathology or minor psychic stress and is often temporary. Psychogenic amenorrhea is probably mediated by excessive endogenous opioid activity because naloxone or naltrexone (opiate receptor blockers) can induce ovulation in some patients with this disorder.[426]

Exercise-induced amenorrhea may be a variant of psychogenic amenorrhea or may result from loss of body fat.[425,427] The syndrome is associated with intense and prolonged physical exertion such as running, swimming, or ballet dancing. Such women are always below ideal body weight and have low stores of fat. If the activity is begun before puberty, normal sexual maturation can be delayed for many years. Fat mass may be a regulator of gonadotropin secretion with adipocyte-derived leptin as the principal mediator between peripheral energy stores and hypothalamic regulatory centers.[428] Studies in nonhuman primates showed a direct role of caloric intake in the pathogenesis of amenorrhea associated with long-distance running.[429] Exercise and psychogenic amenorrhea can have adverse effects because of the associated estrogen deficiency and accompanying osteopenia.[430]

Neurogenic Hypogonadism in Males

A discussion of neurogenic hypogonadism in males should begin with an account of Fröhlich's syndrome (adiposogenital dystrophy), originally characterized as delayed puberty, hypogonadism, and obesity associated with a tumor that impinges on the hypothalamus.[1] It was subsequently recognized that either hypothalamic or pituitary dysfunction can induce hypogonadism and the presence of obesity indicates that the appetite-regulating regions of the hypothalamus have been damaged. Several organic lesions of the hypothalamus can cause this syndrome, including tumors, encephalitis, microcephaly, Friedreich's ataxia, and demyelinating diseases. Other important causes of hypogonadotropic hypogonadism are Kallmann's syndrome, a disorder caused by failure of GnRH-containing neurons to migrate normally (see earlier in the section on GnRH and hypophyseotropic hormone deficiency), and a subset of the Prader-Willi syndrome.[431]

However, most males with delayed sexual development do not have serious neurologic conditions. Furthermore, most obese boys with delayed sexual development have no structural damage to the hypothalamus but have constitutional delayed puberty, which is commonly associated with obesity. It is not known whether there is a functional disorder of the hypothalamus in this condition. It is generally believed that psychosexual development of brain maturation depends on the presence of androgens within a critical developmental window corresponding to puberty and therefore hypogonadism in boys (regardless of cause) should be treated by the middle teen years (15 years at the latest).

In adult men, hypogonadism (including reduced spermatogenesis) can be induced by emotional stress or severe exercise,[432] but this abnormality is seldom diagnosed because the symptoms are more subtle than menstrual cycle changes in similarly stressed women. Prolonged physical stress and sleep and energy deficiency can also decrease testosterone and gonadotropin levels.[433] Chronic intrathecal administration of opiates for the control of intractable pain syndromes is strongly associated with hypogonadotropic hypogonadism, and to a lesser extent hypocorticism and GH deficiency, in both men and women.[434] Finally, critical illness with multiple causes is well known to be associated with hypogonadism and ineffectual altered pulsation of GnRH.[435]

Neurogenic Disorders of Prolactin Regulation

Neurogenic causes of hyperprolactinemia include irritative lesions of the chest wall (herpes zoster, thoracotomy), excessive tactile stimulation of the nipple, and lesions within the spinal cord such as ependymoma.[436] Prolonged mechanical stimulation of the nipples by suckling or the use of a breast pump can initiate lactation in some women who are not pregnant, and neurologic lesions that interrupt the hypothalamic-pituitary connection can cause hyperprolactinemia, as discussed earlier. Hyperprolactinemia also occurs after certain forms of epileptic seizures. In one series, six of eight patients with temporal lobe seizures had a marked increase in PRL, whereas only one in eight with frontal lobe seizures progressed to hyperprolactinemia.[437] Agents that block D2-like dopamine receptors (e.g., the phenothiazines and later generation atypical antipsychotics) or prevent dopamine release (e.g., reserpine and methyldopa) must be excluded in all cases.

Because the nervous system exerts such profound effects on PRL secretion, patients with hyperprolactinemia (including those with adenomas) may have a deficit of PIF or an excess of PRF activity. In studies of PRL secretion in patients apparently cured of hyperprolactinemia by removal of a pituitary microadenoma, regulatory abnormalities persisted in some but not all patients. Persistence of regulatory abnormalities may be due to incomplete removal of tumor, abnormal function of the remaining part of the gland, or underlying hypothalamic abnormalities.[438]

Neurogenic Disorders of Growth Hormone Secretion

Hypothalamic Growth Failure

Loss of the normal nocturnal increase in GH secretion and loss of GH secretory responses to provocative stimuli occur early in the course of hypothalamic disease and may be the most sensitive endocrine indicator of hypothalamic dysfunction. As noted earlier, anatomic malformations of midline cerebral structures are associated with abnormal GH secretion, presumably related to failure of the development of normal GH regulatory mechanisms. Such disorders include optic nerve dysplasia and midline prosencephalic malformations (absence of the septum pellucidum, abnormal third ventricle, and abnormal lamina terminalis). Certain complex genetic disorders including Prader-Willi syndrome also commonly involve reduced GH secretory capacity.[439] Idiopathic hypopituitarism with GH deficiency was considered earlier in this chapter.

Maternal Deprivation Syndrome and Psychosocial Dwarfism

Infant neglect or abuse can impair growth and cause failure to thrive (the maternal deprivation syndrome). Malnutrition interacts with psychological factors to cause growth failure in children with the maternal deprivation syndrome, and each case should be carefully evaluated from this point of view. Older children with growth failure in a setting of abuse or severe emotional disturbance (termed psychosocial dwarfism) may also have abnormal circadian rhythms and deficient hGH release after insulin-induced hypoglycemia or arginine infusion (see Chapter 23).[440] Deficient release of ACTH and gonadotropins may also be present. A new variant termed hyperphagic short stature has been identified.[441] These disorders are reversible by placing the child in a supportive milieu where growth and neuroendocrine hGH responses rapidly return to normal.[442] The pathogenesis of altered GH secretion in children in response to deprivation is unknown. In the adult human, furthermore, physical or emotional stress usually causes an increase in hGH secretion, as noted earlier.

Neuroregulatory Growth Hormone Deficiency

The availability of biosynthetic hGH for treatment of short stature has brought into focus a group of patients who grow at low rates (below the third percentile) and have low levels of serum IGF-I but a normal hGH secretory reserve. Studies of 24-hour hGH secretion profiles indicate that many of these children do not have normal spontaneous hGH secretion (abnormal ultradian and circadian rhythms and decreased number or amplitude of secretory bursts, or both). These children with idiopathic short stature may have a functional regulatory disturbance of the hypothalamus and appear to grow normally when given exogenous hGH.[443]

There is considerable uncertainty about the criteria for the diagnosis of neuroregulatory hGH deficiency. Many normally growing children have profiles of hGH secretion that are indistinguishable from those in children with the postulated syndrome.[444] Patterns of hGH secretion do not predict which child will benefit from therapy, and there is a poor correlation between hGH secretion and growth. Furthermore, the results of repeated tests in children show considerable variability. It has been suggested that specific genetic defects may underlie the pathogenesis of a subset of children with this heterogeneous syndrome of growth failure.[445] The prevalence of an hGH neuroregulatory deficiency syndrome is thus unclear, and the decision to treat short children with hGH should be made cautiously.[446,447]

Neurogenic Hypersecretion of Growth Hormone

Diencephalic Syndrome

Children and infants with tumors in and around the third ventricle frequently become cachectic, which is often associated with elevated hGH levels and paradoxical GH secretory responses to glucose and insulin.[448] GH hypersecretion may be due to a hypothalamic abnormality or to malnutrition. Deficits of pituitary-adrenal regulation are less common. A striking feature is an alert appearance and seeming euphoria despite the profound emaciation. A variety of associated neurologic abnormalities may be present including nystagmus, irritability, hydrocephalus, optic atrophy, tremor, and excessive sweating. CSF abnormalities include increased protein and the presence of abnormal cells. Most cases are due to chiasmatic-hypothalamic gliomas, with the majority classified as astrocytomas.[448] Treatment options include surgical resection, radiation therapy, and chemotherapy.[449]

Growth Hormone Hypersecretion Associated with Metabolic Disturbances

Apparently inappropriate hGH hypersecretion (the syndrome of inappropriate somatotropin secretion) occurs with uncontrolled diabetes mellitus, hepatic failure, uremia, anorexia nervosa, and protein-calorie malnutrition. Nutritional factors are probably important in this response because in normal persons obesity inhibits and fasting stimulates episodic GH hypersecretion.[450] In diabetes mellitus cholinergic blockers reverse the abnormality,[227] possibly by inhibiting hypothalamic somatostatin secretion (see earlier in the section on neurotransmitter regulation of GH). Loss of inhibition of GH secretion by IGF-I may also play a role because most disorders in which this syndrome occurs are associated with low IGF-I levels.

Neurogenic Disorders of Corticotropin Regulation

Hypothalamic CRH hypersecretion is the likely cause of sustained pituitary-adrenal hyperfunction in at least two situations: Cushing's syndrome caused by the rare CRH-secreting gangliocytomas of the hypothalamus[451] and severe depression. Severe depression is associated with pituitary-adrenal abnormalities, including inappropriately elevated ACTH levels, abnormal cortisol circadian rhythms, and resistance to dexamethasone suppression.[155,159,166,452] The dexamethasone suppression test has, in fact, been used as an aid to the diagnosis of depressive illness. Another possible example of disordered neurogenic control of CRH associated with stress is the metabolic syndrome.[453,454] This syndrome is characterized by mild hypercortisolism, blunted dexamethasone suppression of the HPA axis, visceral obesity, and hypertension and may be strongly associated with greater risks for cardiovascular disease and stroke.

A unique syndrome of ACTH hypersecretion termed periodic hypothalamic discharge (Wolff's syndrome) has been described in one young man. The patient had a recurring cyclic disorder characterized by high fever, paroxysms of glucocorticoid hypersecretion, and electroencephalographic abnormalities.[455]

Nonendocrine Manifestations of Hypothalamic Disease

The hypothalamus is involved in the regulation of diverse functions and behaviors (Table 7–10). Psychological abnormalities in hypothalamic disease include antisocial behavior; attacks of rage, laughing, and crying; disturbed sleep patterns; excessive sexuality; and hallucinations. Both somnolence (with posterior lesions) and pathologic wakefulness (with anterior lesions) occur, as do bulimia and profound anorexia. The abnormal eating patterns are analogous to the syndromes of hyperphagia produced in rats by destruction of the VMH or of connections to the PVH. Lateral hypothalamic damage causes profound anorexia. A more complete discussion of imbalance in energy homeostasis (both obesity and cachexia) associated with hypothalamic dysfunction and neuropeptides is presented in Chapter 34.

Patients with hypothalamic damage may experience hyperthermia, hypothermia, unexplained fluctuations in body temperature, and poikilothermy. Disturbances of sweating, acrocyanosis, loss of sphincter control, and diencephalic epilepsy are occasional manifestations. Hypothalamic damage also causes loss of recent memory, believed to be due to damage of the mammillothalamic pathways. Severe memory loss, obesity, and personality changes (apathy, loss of ability to concentrate, aggressive antisocial behavior, severe food craving, inability to work or attend school) may occur with suprasellar extension of pituitary tumors, hypothalamic radiation, or damage incurred from surgical removal of parasellar tumors. Hypothalamic tumors grow slowly and may reach a large size while producing minimal disturbance of behavior or visceral homeostasis, whereas surgery of limited extent can produce striking functional abnormalities. Presumably, this is because slowly growing lesions permit compensatory responses to develop. These potential consequences should be weighed carefully by the neurosurgeon, patient, and patient's family in planning the therapeutic approach. Adverse effects of treatment have led to more conservative surgical guidelines for the treat-

TABLE 7–10 NEUROLOGIC MANIFESTATIONS OF NONENDOCRINE HYPOTHALAMIC DISEASE

Disorders of Temperature Regulation
Hyperthermia
Hypothermia
Poikilothermia

Disorders of Food Intake
Hyperphagia (bulimia)
Anorexia nervosa, aphagia
Cachexia

Disorders of Water Intake
Compulsive water drinking
Adipsia
Essential hypernatremia

Disorders of Sleep and Consciousness
Narcolepsy/cataplexy
Somnolence
Sleep rhythm reversal
Akinetic mutism
Coma
Delirium

Periodic Disease of Hypothalamic Origin
Diencephalic epilepsy
Kleine-Levin syndrome
Periodic discharge syndrome of Wolff

Disorders of Psychic Function
Rage behavior
Hallucinations
Hypersexuality

Disorders of Autonomic Nervous System
Pulmonary edema
Cardiac arrhythmias
Sphincter disturbance

Congenital Hypothalamic Disease
Prader-Willi syndrome
Laurence-Moon-Biedl syndrome

Miscellaneous
Diencephalic syndrome of infancy
Cerebral gigantism

ment of craniopharyngioma. A recent review from the University of Pittsburgh summarizes their individualized treatment program that includes microsurgical tumor resection, intracavitary ^{32}P radiotherapy, and gamma knife stereotactic radiosurgery to produce maximal benefit with minimal morbidity.[456]

Narcolepsy

A convergence of functional genomics from two animal species, the dog and mouse, has dramatically refocused attention on neuropeptide circuits of the hypothalamus in the control of sleep and wakefulness. Positional cloning was used to identify mutations in the hypocretin-orexin receptor 2 as a cause of canine narcolepsy.[457] Subsequently knockout of the gene encoding the hypocretin-orexin peptide precursor produced an equivalent narcoleptic syndrome in mice,[458] further establishing this neuropeptide system as a major component of sleep-modulating neural circuits. The additional role of hypocretin-orexin in coordinating arousal states and feeding behavior is discussed in Chapter 34. These new discoveries add to the list of other hypothalamic neuropeptides including GHRH, somatostatin, and cortistatin with established functions in modulation of the sleep cycle.

Histaminergic neurons of the tuberomammillary nucleus express both forms of the orexin receptor and make reciprocal synaptic connections with orexin neurons in the lateral hypothalamus. Furthermore, orexin is an excitatory transmitter for the histamine neurons, suggesting that the two populations cooperate in the regulation of rapid eye movement sleep.[459] Targeted ablation of orexin neurons in the lateral hypothalamus of rats by means of a hypocretin receptor 2-saporin conjugate produced narcoleptic-like sleep behavior,[460] closely paralleling the clinical findings and profound reduction in the numbers of hypocretin-orexin neurons in the lateral hypothalamus of humans with narcolepsy.[461] Therefore most cases of spontaneous narcolepsy with cataplexy result from a degenerative hypothalamic disorder, most likely autoimmune in pathogenesis, resulting in a selective destruction of neuropeptidergic neurons. The absence of immunoreactive hypocretin-orexin in CSF is a sensitive diagnostic test for the disease. Future development of bioavailable, hypocretin-orexin receptor selective compounds may provide a specific treatment alternative or adjunct to the stimulant and antidepressant drugs currently used for management of symptoms. More generally, these recent discoveries suggest the possibility that other cryptic hypothalamic disorders are caused by selective disturbances to other neuropeptidergic circuits.

ACKNOWLEDGMENTS

The author is highly indebted to Dr. Seymour Reichlin, not only for material he shared from the ninth edition of this text, but also for the inspiration and mentorship he provided to the current generation of neuroendocrinologists. Thanks are also due to Drs. Roger Cone, Joel Elmquist, and Judy Cameron for their respective contributions to the tenth edition of this text.

REFERENCES

1. Fröhlich A. Ein Fall von Tumor der Hypophysis cerebri ohne Akromegalie. Wein Klin Rundsch 1901;15:883.
2. Crowe S, Cushing H, Homans J. Experimental hypophysectomy. Bull Johns Hopkins Hosp 1910;21:128-169.
3. Aschner B. Über die Funktion der Hypophyse. Pflügers Arch Physiol 1912;146:1.
4. Hetherington AW, Ranson SW: Hypothalamic lesions and adiposity in the rat. Anat Rec 1940;78:149-172.
5. Popa G, Fielding U. A portal circulation from the pituitary to the hypothalamic region. J Anat 1930;65:88.
6. Wislocki GB, King LS. Permeability of the hypophysis and hypothalamus to vital dyes, with study of hypophyseal blood supply. Am J Anat 1936;58:421-472.
7. Harris G. Neural control of the pituitary. Physiol Rev 1948;28:139-179.
8. Schally AV, Redding TW, Bowers CY, et al. Isolation and properties of porcine thyrotropin-releasing hormone. J Biol Chem 1969;244:4077-4088.
9. Burgus R, Dunn TF, Desiderio D, et al. Characterization of ovine hypothalamic hypophysiotropic TSH-releasing factor. Nature 1970;226:321-325.
10. Schally AV. Aspects of hypothalamic regulation of the pituitary gland (Nobel lecture). Science 1978;202:18-28.
11. Guillemin R. Peptides in the brain: the new endocrinology of the neuron (Nobel lecture). Science 1978;202:390-402.
12. Zhang Y, Proenca A, Maffei M, et al. Positional cloning of the mouse obese gene and its human homologue. Nature 1994;372:425-434.
13. Kojima M, Hosoda H, Date Y, et al. Ghrelin is a growth-hormone-releasing acylated peptide from stomach. Nature 1999;402:656-660.
14. Spergel DJ, Kruth U, Hanley DF, et al. GABA- and glutamate-activated channels in green fluorescent protein-tagged gonadotropin-releasing hormone neurons in transgenic mice. J Neurosci 1999;19:2037-2050.

15. Cowley MA, Smart JL, Rubinstein M, et al. Leptin activates anorexigenic POMC neurons through a neural network in the arcuate nucleus. Nature 2001;411:480-484.
16. Scharrer B. Neurosecretion: beginnings and new directions in neuropeptide research. Annu Rev Neurosci 1987;10:1-17.
17. Sawyer CH: History of the neurovascular concept of hypothalamo-hypophysial control. Biol Reprod 1978;18:325-328.
18. Hokfelt T, Johansson O, Ljungdahl A, et al. Peptidergic neurons. Nature 1980;284:515-521.
19. Harris GW. Structure and function of the median eminence. Am J Anat 1970;129:245-246.
20. Loewy AD. Anatomy of the autonomic nervous system: an overview. New York: Oxford University Press, 1990.
21. Hokfelt T, Lundberg J, Schultzberg M, et al. Coexistence of peptides and putative transmitters in neurons. Adv Biochem Psychopharmacol 1980;22:1-23.
22. Ahren B. Autonomic regulation of islet hormone secretion—implications for health and disease. Diabetologia 2000;43:393-410.
23. Berthoud HR, Fox EA, Powley TL. Localization of vagal preganglionics that stimulate insulin and glucagon secretion. Am J Physiol 1990;258:R160-R168.
24. Saltiel AR. New perspectives into the molecular pathogenesis and treatment of type 2 diabetes. Cell 2001;104:517-529.
25. Levin BE, Dunn-Meynell AA, Routh VH. Brain glucose sensing and body energy homeostasis: role in obesity and diabetes. Am J Physiol 1999;276:R1223-R1231.
26. Zhu X, Lin CR, Prefontaine GG, et al. Genetic control of pituitary development and hypopituitarism. Curr Opin Genet Dev 2005; 15:332-340.
27. Koutcherov Y, Mai JK, Paxinos G. Hypothalamus of the human fetus. J Chem Neuroanat 2003;26:253-270.
28. McClellan KM, Parker KL, Tobet S. Development of the ventromedial nucleus of the hypothalamus. Front Neuroendocrinol 2006;27: 193-209.
29. Whitlock KE. Origin and development of GnRH neurons. Trends Endocrinol Metab 2005;16:145-151.
30. Caqueret A, Yang C, Duplan S, et al. Looking for trouble: a search for developmental defects of the hypothalamus. Horm Res 2005;64:222-230.
31. Forger NG. Cell death and sexual differentiation of the nervous system. Neuroscience. 2006;138:929-938.
32. Simerly RB. Wired on hormones: endocrine regulation of hypothalamic development. Curr Opin Neurobiol 2005;15:81-85.
33. Fujisawa I. Magnetic resonance imaging of the hypothalamic-neurohypophyseal system. J Neuroendocrinol 2004;16:297-302.
34. Braak H, Braak E. Anatomy of the human hypothalamus (chiasmatic and tuberal region). Prog Brain Res 1992;93:3-14; discussion 14-16.
35. Evans VR, Manning AB, Bernard LH, et al. Alpha-melanocyte-stimulating hormone and N-acetyl-beta-endorphin immunoreactivities are localized in the human pituitary but are not restricted to the zona intermedia. Endocrinology 1994;134:97-106.
36. Lincoln DW, Paisley AC. Neuroendocrine control of milk ejection. J Reprod Fertil 1982;65:571-586.
37. Burstein R, Cliffer KD, Giesler GJ Jr. Direct somatosensory projections from the spinal cord to the hypothalamus and telencephalon. J Neurosci 1987;7:4159-4164.
38. Knigge KM, Scott DE. Structure and function of the median eminence. Am J Anat 1970;129:223-243.
39. Trandafir T, Dionisie C, Repciuc E. The development of the hypothalamo-hypophysial portal system in human fetus. Endocrinologie 1982;20:127-134.
40. Page RB. Pituitary blood flow. Am J Physiol 1982;243:E427-E442.
41. Rodriguez EM, Blazquez JL, Pastor FE, et al. Hypothalamic tanycytes: a key component of brain-endocrine interaction. Int Rev Cytol 2005;247:89-164.
42. Clarke I, Jessop D, Millar R, et al. Many peptides that are present in the external zone of the median eminence are not secreted into the hypophysial portal blood of sheep. Neuroendocrinology 1993;57:765-775.
43. King JC, Rubin BS. Dynamic alterations in luteinizing hormone-releasing hormone (LHRH) neuronal cell bodies and terminals of adult rats. Cell Mol Neurobiol 1995;15:89-106.
44. Koutcherov Y, Mai JK, Ashwell KW, et al. Organization of the human paraventricular hypothalamic nucleus. J Comp Neurol 2000;423:299-318.
45. Johnson AK, Gross PM. Sensory circumventricular organs and brain homeostatic pathways. Faseb J 1993;7:678-686.
46. Ganong WF. Circumventricular organs: definition and role in the regulation of endocrine and autonomic function. Clin Exp Pharmacol Physiol 2000;27:422-427.
47. Ferguson AV, Bains JS. Actions of angiotensin in the subfornical organ and area postrema: implications for long term control of autonomic output. Clin Exp Pharmacol Physiol 1997;24:96-101.
48. Rodriguez EM, Rodriguez S, Hein S. The subcommissural organ. Microsc Res Tech 1998;41:98-123.
49. Banks WA, Kastin AJ, Huang W, et al. Leptin enters the brain by a saturable system independent of insulin. Peptides 1996;17:305-311.
50. Tatro JB, Entwistle ML. Identification of a specific mammalian melanocortin receptor antagonist. Ann N Y Acad Sci 1994;739: 315-319.
51. Schwartz MW, Seeley RJ, Campfield LA, et al. Identification of targets of leptin action in rat hypothalamus. J Clin Invest 1996;98: 1101-1106.
52. Elias CF, Aschkenasi C, Lee C, et al. Leptin differentially regulates NPY and POMC neurons projecting to the lateral hypothalamic area. Neuron 1999;23:775-786.
53. Blatteis CM. Role of the OVLT in the febrile response to circulating pyrogens. Prog Brain Res 1992;91:409-412.
54. Oka T, Oka K, Scammell TE, et al. Relationship of EP(1-4) prostaglandin receptors with rat hypothalamic cell groups involved in lipopolysaccharide fever responses. J Comp Neurol 2000;428: 20-32.
55. Oldfield BJ, Bicknell RJ, McAllen RM, et al. Intravenous hypertonic saline induces Fos immunoreactivity in neurons throughout the lamina terminalis. Brain Res 1991;561:151-156.
56. Standaert DG, Saper CB. Origin of the atriopeptin-like immunoreactive innervation of the paraventricular nucleus of the hypothalamus. J Neurosci 1988;8:1940-1950.
57. Saper CB, Levisohn D. Afferent connections of the median preoptic nucleus in the rat: anatomical evidence for a cardiovascular integrative mechanism in the anteroventral third ventricular (AV3V) region. Brain Res 1983;288:21-31.
58. Simpson JB, Routtenberg A. Subfornical organ: a dipsogenic site of action of angiotensin II. Science 1978;201:379-381.
59. Miller AD, Leslie RA. The area postrema and vomiting. Front Neuroendocrinol 1994;15:301-320.
60. Merchenthaler I, Lane M, Shughrue P. Distribution of pre-proglucagon and glucagon-like peptide-1 receptor messenger RNAs in the rat central nervous system. J Comp Neurol 1999;403:261-280.
61. Moran TH, Robinson PH, Goldrich MS, et al. Two brain cholecystokinin receptors: implications for behavioral actions. Brain Res 1986;362:175-179.
62. Osborn JW, Collister JP, Carlson SH. Angiotensin and osmoreceptor inputs to the area postrema: role in long-term control of fluid homeostasis and arterial pressure. Clin Exp Pharmacol Physiol 2000;27:443-449.
63. Reppert SM. Melatonin receptors: molecular biology of a new family of G protein-coupled receptors. J Biol Rhythms 1997;12: 528-531.
64. Dubocovich ML, Markowska M. Functional MT1 and MT2 melatonin receptors in mammals. Endocrine 2005;27:101-110.
65. Moore RY, Lenn NJ. A retinohypothalamic projection in the rat. J Comp Neurol 1972;146:1-14.
66. Watts AG, Swanson LW. Efferent projections of the suprachiasmatic nucleus: II. Studies using retrograde transport of fluorescent dyes and simultaneous peptide immunohistochemistry in the rat. J Comp Neurol 1987;258:230-252.
67. Leak RK, Moore RY. Topographic organization of suprachiasmatic nucleus projection neurons. J Comp Neurol 2001;433:312-334.
68. Saper CB, Loewy AD, Swanson LW, et al. Direct hypothalamo-autonomic connections. Brain Res 1976;117:305-312.
69. Rando TA, Bowers CW, Zigmond RE. Localization of neurons in the rat spinal cord which project to the superior cervical ganglion. J Comp Neurol 1981;196:73-83.

70. Borjigin J, Li X, Snyder SH. The pineal gland and melatonin: molecular and pharmacologic regulation. Annu Rev Pharmacol Toxicol 1999;39:53-65.
71. Boutin JA, Audinot V, Ferry G, et al. Molecular tools to study melatonin pathways and actions. Trends Pharmacol Sci 2005;26:412-419.
72. Foulkes NS, Borjigin J, Snyder SH, et al. Rhythmic transcription: the molecular basis of circadian melatonin synthesis. Trends Neurosci 1997;20:487-492.
73. Nakazawa K, Marubayashi U, McCann SM. Mediation of the short-loop negative feedback of luteinizing hormone (LH) on LH-releasing hormone release by melatonin-induced inhibition of LH release from the pars tuberalis. Proc Natl Acad Sci U S A 1991;88: 7576-7579.
74. Reiter RJ. The pineal and its hormones in the control of reproduction in mammals. Endocr Rev 1980;1:109-131.
75. Reiter RJ. Melatonin and human reproduction. Ann Med 1998;30:103-108.
76. Rea MS, Figueiro MG, Bullough JD, et al. A model of phototransduction by the human circadian system. Brain Res Brain Res Rev 2005;50:213-228.
77. Shibata S, Cassone VM, Moore RY. Effects of melatonin on neuronal activity in the rat suprachiasmatic nucleus in vitro. Neurosci Lett 1989;97:140-144.
78. Liu C, Weaver DR, Jin X, et al. Molecular dissection of two distinct actions of melatonin on the suprachiasmatic circadian clock. Neuron 1997;19:91-102.
79. Jin X, von Gall C, Pieschl RL, et al. Targeted disruption of the mouse Mel(1b) melatonin receptor. Mol Cell Biol 2003;23: 1054-1060.
80. Arendt J. Melatonin, circadian rhythms, and sleep. N Engl J Med 2000;343:1114-1116.
81. Buscemi N, Vandermeer B, Hooton N, et al. The efficacy and safety of exogenous melatonin for primary sleep disorders. A meta-analysis. J Gen Intern Med 2005;20:1151-1158.
82. Buscemi N, Vandermeer B, Hooton N, et al. Efficacy and safety of exogenous melatonin for secondary sleep disorders and sleep disorders accompanying sleep restriction: meta-analysis. Br Med J 2006;332:385-393.
83. Houk JC. Control strategies in physiological systems. FASEB J 1988;2:97-107.
84. Yates F. Modeling periodicities in reproductive, adrenocortical and metabolic systems. In Ferin M, Hakberg F, Richart RM, eds. Biorhythms and Human Reproduction. New York: John Wiley & Sons, 1974:133-142.
85. DiStefano JI, Stubberud A, Williams I. Theory and Problems of Feedback and Control Systems. New York: Schaum Publishing, 1967.
86. Moore RY. The fourth C.U. Ariens Kappers lecture. The organization of the human circadian timing system. Prog Brain Res 1992;93:99-115; discussion 115-117.
87. Saper CB, Lu J, Chou TC, et al. The hypothalamic integrator for circadian rhythms. Trends Neurosci 2005;28:152-157.
88. Reppert SM, Weaver DR. Coordination of circadian timing in mammals. Nature 2002;418:935-941.
89. Richter CP. Sleep and activity: their relation to the 24-hour clock. Res Publ Assoc Res Nerv Ment Dis 1967;45:8-29.
90. Perreau-Lenz S, Pevet P, Buijs RM, et al. The biological clock: the bodyguard of temporal homeostasis. Chronobiol Int 2004;21:1-25.
91. Gachon F, Nagoshi E, Brown SA, et al. The mammalian circadian timing system: from gene expression to physiology. Chromosoma 2004;113:103-112.
92. Welsh DK, Logothetis DE, Meister M, et al. Individual neurons dissociated from rat suprachiasmatic nucleus express independently phased circadian firing rhythms. Neuron 1995;14:697-706.
93. Reppert SM. Pre-natal development of a hypothalamic biological clock. Prog Brain Res 1992;93:119-131; discussion 132.
94. Yamada M, Radovick S, Wondisford FE, et al. Cloning and structure of human genomic DNA and hypothalamic cDNA encoding human prepro thyrotropin-releasing hormone. Mol Endocrinol 1990;4:551-556.
95. Lee SL, Stewart K, Goodman RH. Structure of the gene encoding rat thyrotropin releasing hormone. J Biol Chem 1988;263: 16604-16609.
96. Nillni EA, Sevarino KA. The biology of pro-thyrotropin-releasing hormone-derived peptides. Endocr Rev 1999;20:599-648.
97. Jackson IM. Thyrotropin-releasing hormone. N Engl J Med 1982;306:145-155.
98. Gautvik KM, Tashjian AH Jr, Kourides IA, et al. Thyrotropin-releasing hormone is not the sole physiologic mediator of prolactin release during suckling. N Engl J Med 1974;290:1162-1165.
99. Yamada M, Satoh T, Mori M. Mice lacking the thyrotropin-releasing hormone gene: what do they tell us? Thyroid 2003;13:1111-1121.
100. Straub RE, Frech GC, Joho RH, et al. Expression cloning of a cDNA encoding the mouse pituitary thyrotropin-releasing hormone receptor. Proc Natl Acad Sci U S A 1990;87:9514-9518.
101. Sun Y, Lu X, Gershengorn MC. Thyrotropin-releasing hormone receptors—similarities and differences. J Mol Endocrinol 2003; 30:87-97.
102. Gary KA, Sevarino KA, Yarbrough GG, et al. The thyrotropin-releasing hormone (TRH) hypothesis of homeostatic regulation: implications for TRH-based therapeutics. J Pharmacol Exp Ther 2003;305:410-416.
103. Callahan AM, Frye MA, Marangell LB, et al. Comparative antidepressant effects of intravenous and intrathecal thyrotropin-releasing hormone: confounding effects of tolerance and implications for therapeutics. Biol Psychiatry 1997;41:264-272.
104. Takeuchi Y, Takano T, Abe J, et al. Thyrotropin-releasing hormone: role in the treatment of West syndrome and related epileptic encephalopathies. Brain Dev 2001;23:662-667.
105. Morley JE: Neuroendocrine control of thyrotropin secretion. Endocr Rev 1981;2:396-436.
106. Dyess EM, Segerson TP, Liposits Z, et al. Triiodothyronine exerts direct cell-specific regulation of thyrotropin-releasing hormone gene expression in the hypothalamic paraventricular nucleus. Endocrinology 1988;123:2291-2297.
107. Schreiber G, Southwell BR, Richardson SJ. Hormone delivery systems to the brain-transthyretin. Exp Clin Endocrinol Diabetes 1995;103:75-80.
108. Lechan RM, Kakucska I. Feedback regulation of thyrotropin-releasing hormone gene expression by thyroid hormone in the hypothalamic paraventricular nucleus. Ciba Found Symp 1992; 168:144-158; discussion 158-164.
109. Lechan RM, Fekete C. Role of thyroid hormone deiodination in the hypothalamus. Thyroid 2005;15:883-897.
110. Arimura A, Schally AV. Increase in basal and thyrotropin-releasing hormone (TRH)-stimulated secretion of thyrotropin (TSH) by passive immunization with antiserum to somatostatin in rats. Endocrinology 1976;98:1069-1072.
111. Brabant G, Prank K, Ranft U, et al. Physiological regulation of circadian and pulsatile thyrotropin secretion in normal man and woman. J Clin Endocrinol Metab 1990;70:403-409.
112. Fares F. The role of O-linked and N-linked oligosaccharides on the structure-function of glycoprotein hormones: development of agonists and antagonists. Biochim Biophys Acta 2006;1760:560-567.
113. Arancibia S, Rage F, Astier H, et al. Neuroendocrine and autonomous mechanisms underlying thermoregulation in cold environment. Neuroendocrinology 1996;64:257-267.
114. Sánchez E, Uribe RM, Corkidi G, et al. Differential responses of thyrotropin-releasing hormone (TRH) neurons to cold exposure or suckling indicate functional heterogeneity of the TRH system in the paraventricular nucleus of the rat hypothalamus. Neuroendocrinol 2001;74:407-422.
115. Toni R, Jackson IM, Lechan RM. Neuropeptide-Y-immunoreactive innervation of thyrotropin-releasing hormone-synthesizing neurons in the rat hypothalamic paraventricular nucleus. Endocrinology 1990;126:2444-2453.
116. Wartofsky L, Burman KD. Alterations in thyroid function in patients with systemic illness: the "euthyroid sick syndrome." Endocr Rev 1982;3:164-217.
117. Kakucska I, Qi Y, Lechan RM. Changes in adrenal status affect hypothalamic thyrotropin-releasing hormone gene expression in parallel with corticotropin-releasing hormone. Endocrinology 1995;136:2795-2802.
118. Cintra A, Fuxe K, Wikstrom AC, et al. Evidence for thyrotropin-releasing hormone and glucocorticoid receptor-immunoreactive neurons in various preoptic and hypothalamic nuclei of the male rat. Brain Res 1990;506:139-144.

119. Shi ZX, Levy A, Lightman SL. Hippocampal input to the hypothalamus inhibits thyrotrophin and thyrotrophin-releasing hormone gene expression. Neuroendocrinology 1993;57:576-580.
120. Spencer CA, Lum SM, Wilber JF, et al. Dynamics of serum thyrotropin and thyroid hormone changes in fasting. J Clin Endocrinol Metab 1983;56:883-888.
121. Blake NG, Eckland DJ, Foster OJ, et al. Inhibition of hypothalamic thyrotropin-releasing hormone messenger ribonucleic acid during food deprivation. Endocrinology 1991;129:2714-2718.
122. Ahima RS, Prabakaran D, Mantzoros C, et al. Role of leptin in the neuroendocrine response to fasting. Nature 1996;382:250-252.
123. Legradi G, Emerson CH, Ahima RS, et al. Leptin prevents fasting-induced suppression of prothyrotropin-releasing hormone messenger ribonucleic acid in neurons of the hypothalamic paraventricular nucleus. Endocrinology 1997;138:2569-2576.
124. Lechan RM, Fekete C. Feedback regulation of thyrotropin-releasing hormone (TRH): mechanisms for the non-thyroidal illness syndrome. J Endocrinol Invest 2004;27:105-119.
125. Lechan RM, Fekete C. Role of melanocortin signaling in the regulation of the hypothalamic-pituitary-thyroid (HPT) axis. Peptides 2006;27:310-325.
126. Harris M, Aschkenasi C, Elias CF, et al. Transcriptional regulation of the thyrotropin-releasing hormone gene by leptin and melanocortin signaling. J Clin Invest 2001;107:111-120.
127. Montague CT, Farooqi IS, Whitehead JP, et al. Congenital leptin deficiency is associated with severe early-onset obesity in humans. Nature 1997;387:903-908.
128. Farooqi IS, Yeo GS, Keogh JM, et al. Dominant and recessive inheritance of morbid obesity associated with melanocortin 4 receptor deficiency. J Clin Invest 2000;106:271-279.
129. Dubuis JM, Dayer JM, Siegrist-Kaiser CA, et al. Human recombinant interleukin-1 beta decreases plasma thyroid hormone and thyroid stimulating hormone levels in rats. Endocrinology 1988;123: 2175-2181.
130. Scarborough DE, Lee SL, Dinarello CA, et al. Interleukin-1 beta stimulates somatostatin biosynthesis in primary cultures of fetal rat brain. Endocrinology 1989;124:549-551.
131. Pang XP, Hershman JM, Mirell CJ, et al. Impairment of hypothalamic-pituitary-thyroid function in rats treated with human recombinant tumor necrosis factor-alpha (cachectin). Endocrinology 1989;125:76-84.
132. Koenig JI, Snow K, Clark BD, et al. Intrinsic pituitary interleukin-1 beta is induced by bacterial lipopolysaccharide. Endocrinology 1990;126:3053-3058.
133. Spath-Schwalbe E, Schrezenmeier H, Bornstein S, et al. Endocrine effects of recombinant interleukin 6 in man. Neuroendocrinology 1996;63:237-243.
134. Shibahara S, Morimoto Y, Furutani Y, et al. Isolation and sequence analysis of the human corticotropin-releasing factor precursor gene. EMBO J 1983;2:775-779.
135. Lovejoy DA, Balment RJ. Evolution and physiology of the corticotropin-releasing factor (CRF) family of neuropeptides in vertebrates. Gen Comp Endocrinol 1999;115:1-22.
136. Hsu SY, Hsueh AJ. Human stresscopin and stresscopin-related peptide are selective ligands for the type 2 corticotropin-releasing hormone receptor. Nat Med 2001;7:605-611.
137. Chen R, Lewis KA, Perrin MH, et al. Expression cloning of a human corticotropin-releasing-factor receptor. Proc Natl Acad Sci U S A 1993;90:8967-8971.
138. Chang CP, Pearse RV 2nd, O'Connell S, et al. Identification of a seven transmembrane helix receptor for corticotropin-releasing factor and sauvagine in mammalian brain. Neuron 1993;11:1187-1195.
139. Stenzel P, Kesterson R, Yeung W, et al. Identification of a novel murine receptor for corticotropin-releasing hormone expressed in the heart. Mol Endocrinol 1995;9:637-645.
140. Valdenaire O, Giller T, Breu V, et al. A new functional isoform of the human CRF2 receptor for corticotropin-releasing factor. Biochim Biophys Acta 1997;1352:129-132.
141. Kostich WA, Chen A, Sperle K, et al. Molecular identification and analysis of a novel human corticotropin-releasing factor (CRF) receptor: the CRF2 gamma receptor. Mol Endocrinol 1998;12:1077-1085.
142. Takahashi K, Totsune K, Sone M, et al. Regional distribution of urocortin-like immunoreactivity and expression of urocortin mRNA in the human brain. Peptides 1998;19:643-647.
143. Iino K, Sasano H, Oki Y, et al. Urocortin expression in the human central nervous system. Clin Endocrinol (Oxf) 1999;50:107-114.
144. Chalmers DT, Lovenberg TW, De Souza EB. Localization of novel corticotropin-releasing factor receptor (CRF2) mRNA expression to specific subcortical nuclei in rat brain: comparison with CRF1 receptor mRNA expression. J Neurosci 1995;15:6340-6350.
145. Lovenberg TW, Chalmers DT, Liu C, et al. CRF2 alpha and CRF2 beta receptor mRNAs are differentially distributed between the rat central nervous system and peripheral tissues. Endocrinology 1995;136:4139-4142.
146. Linton EA, Wolfe CD, Behan DP, et al. Circulating corticotropin-releasing factor in pregnancy. Adv Exp Med Biol 1990;274:147-164.
147. Behan DP, Linton EA, Lowry PJ. Isolation of the human plasma corticotrophin-releasing factor-binding protein. J Endocrinol 1989; 122:23-31.
148. Orth DN, Mount CD. Specific high-affinity binding protein for human corticotropin-releasing hormone in normal human plasma. Biochem Biophys Res Commun 1987;143:411-417.
149. Bale TL, Vale WW. CRF and CRF receptors: role in stress responsivity and other behaviors. Annu Rev Pharmacol Toxicol 2004;44:525-557.
150. Rivier J, Rivier C, Vale W. Synthetic competitive antagonists of corticotropin-releasing factor: effect on ACTH secretion in the rat. Science 1984;224:889-891.
151. Maecker H, Desai A, Dash R, et al. Astressin, a novel and potent CRF antagonist, is neuroprotective in the hippocampus when administered after a seizure. Brain Res 1997;744:166-170.
152. Habib KE, Weld KP, Rice KC, et al. Oral administration of a corticotropin-releasing hormone receptor antagonist significantly attenuates behavioral, neuroendocrine, and autonomic responses to stress in primates. Proc Natl Acad Sci U S A 2000;97:6079-6084.
153. Broadbear JH, Winger G, Rivier JE, et al. Corticotropin-releasing hormone antagonists, astressin B and antalarmin: differing profiles of activity in rhesus monkeys. Neuropsychopharmacology 2004;29:1112-1121.
154. Ruhmann A, Bonk I, Lin CR, et al. Structural requirements for peptidic antagonists of the corticotropin-releasing factor receptor (CRFR): development of CRFR2beta-selective antisauvagine-30. Proc Natl Acad Sci U S A 1998;95:15264-15269.
155. Claes SJ. Corticotropin-releasing hormone (CRH) in psychiatry: from stress to psychopathology. Ann Med 2004;36:50-61.
156. Keck ME, Holsboer F, Muller MB. Mouse mutants for the study of corticotropin-releasing hormone receptor function: development of novel treatment strategies for mood disorders. Ann N Y Acad Sci 2004;1018:445-457.
157. Gravanis A, Margioris AN. The corticotropin-releasing factor (CRF) family of neuropeptides in inflammation: potential therapeutic applications. Curr Med Chem 2005;12:1503-1512.
158. Smagin GN, Heinrichs SC, Dunn AJ. The role of CRH in behavioral responses to stress. 2001;Peptides 2001;22:713-724.
159. Modell S, Lauer CJ, Schreiber W, et al. Hormonal response pattern in the combined DEX-CRH test is stable over time in subjects at high familial risk for affective disorders. Neuropsychopharmacology 1998;18:253-262.
160. Nemeroff CB, Widerlov E, Bissette G, et al. Elevated concentrations of CSF corticotropin-releasing factor-like immunoreactivity in depressed patients. Science 1984;226:1342-1344.
161. Parkes DG, Weisinger RS, May CN. Cardiovascular actions of CRH and urocortin: an update. Peptides 2001;22:821-827.
162. Coste SC, Kesterson RA, Heldwein KA, et al. Abnormal adaptations to stress and impaired cardiovascular function in mice lacking corticotropin-releasing hormone receptor-2. Nat Genet 2000;24: 403-409.
163. Bale TL, Contarino A, Smith GW, et al. Mice deficient for corticotropin-releasing hormone receptor-2 display anxiety-like behaviour and are hypersensitive to stress. Nat Genet 2000;24:410-414.
164. Jessop DS, Harbuz MS, Lightman SL. CRH in chronic inflammatory stress. Peptides 2001;22:803-807.
165. Newell-Price J, Grossman AB: The differential diagnosis of Cushing's syndrome. Ann Endocrinol (Paris) 2001;62:173-179.

166. Nemeroff CB, Vale WW. The neurobiology of depression: inroads to treatment and new drug discovery. J Clin Psychiatry 2005; 66(suppl 7):5-13.
167. Seymour PA, Schmidt AW, Schulz DW. The pharmacology of CP-154,526, a non-peptide antagonist of the CRH1 receptor: a review. CNS Drug Rev 2003;9:57-96.
168. Kunzel HE, Zobel AW, Nickel T, et al. Treatment of depression with the CRH-1-receptor antagonist R121919: endocrine changes and side effects. J Psychiatr Res 2003;37:525-533.
169. Zobel AW, Nickel T, Kunzel HE, et al. Effects of the high-affinity corticotropin-releasing hormone receptor 1 antagonist R121919 in major depression: the first 20 patients treated. J Psychiatr Res 2000;34:171-181.
170. Kunzel HE, Ising M, Zobel AW, et al. Treatment with a CRH-1-receptor antagonist (R121919) does not affect weight or plasma leptin concentration in patients with major depression. J Psychiatr Res 2005;39:173-177.
171. Keller-Wood ME, Dallman MF. Corticosteroid inhibition of ACTH secretion. Endocr Rev 1984;5:1-24.
172. Arriza JL, Simerly RB, Swanson LW, et al. The neuronal mineralocorticoid receptor as a mediator of glucocorticoid response. Neuron 1988;1:887-900.
173. de Kloet ER, Oitzl MS, Joels M. Functional implications of brain corticosteroid receptor diversity. Cell Mol Neurobiol 1993;13:433-455.
174. Sapolsky RM, Krey LC, McEwen BS. The neuroendocrinology of stress and aging: the glucocorticoid cascade hypothesis. Endocr Rev 1986;7:284-301.
175. Watts AG. Glucocorticoid regulation of peptide genes in neuroendocrine CRH neurons: a complexity beyond negative feedback. Front Neuroendocrinol 2005;26:109-130.
176. Malcher-Lopes R, Di S, Marcheselli VS, et al. Opposing crosstalk between leptin and glucocorticoids rapidly modulates synaptic excitation via endocannabinoid release. J Neurosci 2006;26:6643-6650.
177. Dallman MF. Fast glucocorticoid actions on brain: back to the future. Front Neuroendocrinol 2005;26:103-108.
178. Herman JP, Figueiredo H, Mueller NK, et al. Central mechanisms of stress integration: hierarchical circuitry controlling hypothalamo-pituitary-adrenocortical responsiveness. Front Neuroendocrinol 2003;24:151-180.
179. Sawchenko PE, Li HY, Ericsson A. Circuits and mechanisms governing hypothalamic responses to stress: a tale of two paradigms. Prog Brain Res 2000;122:61-78.
180. Ziegler DR, Cullinan WE, Herman JP. Organization and regulation of paraventricular nucleus glutamate signaling systems: N-methyl-D-aspartate receptors. J Comp Neurol 2005;484:43-56.
181. Roland BL, Sawchenko PE. Local origins of some GABAergic projections to the paraventricular and supraoptic nuclei of the hypothalamus in the rat. J Comp Neurol 1993;332:123-143.
182. Sapolsky R, Rivier C, Yamamoto G, et al. Interleukin-1 stimulates the secretion of hypothalamic corticotropin-releasing factor. Science 1987;238:522-524.
183. Berkenbosch F, van Oers J, del Rey A, et al. Corticotropin-releasing factor-producing neurons in the rat activated by interleukin-1. Science 1987;238:524-526.
184. Besedovsky H, del Rey A, Sorkin E, et al. Immunoregulatory feedback between interleukin-1 and glucocorticoid hormones. Science 1986;233:652-654.
185. Reichlin S. Neuroendocrinology of infection and the innate immune system. Recent Prog Horm Res 1999;54:133-181; discussion 181-183.
186. Reichlin S. Neuroendocrine-immune interactions. N Engl J Med 1993;329:1246-1253.
187. Gudmundsson A, Carnes M. Pulsatile adrenocorticotropic hormone: an overview. Biol Psychiatry 1997;41:342-365.
188. Muglia LJ, Jacobson L, Weninger SC, et al. Impaired diurnal adrenal rhythmicity restored by constant infusion of corticotropin-releasing hormone in corticotropin-releasing hormone-deficient mice. J Clin Invest 1997;99:2923-2929.
189. Engler D, Redei E, Kola I. The corticotropin-release inhibitory factor hypothesis: a review of the evidence for the existence of inhibitory as well as stimulatory hypophysiotropic regulation of adrenocorticotropin secretion and biosynthesis. Endocr Rev 1999;20:460-500.
190. Reichlin S. Growth and the hypothalamus. Endocrinology 1960; 67:760-773.
191. Mayo K, Vale W, Rivier J, et al. Expression-cloning and sequence of a cDNA encoding human growth hormone-releasing factor. Nature 1983;306:86-88.
192. Rivier J, Speiss J, Thorner M, et al. Characterisation of a growth hormone-releasing factor from a human pancreatic islet tumour. Nature 1982;300:276-278.
193. Guillemin R, Barazeau P, Bohlen P, et al. Growth hormone-releasing factor from a human pancreatic tumor that caused acromegaly. Science 1981;218:585-587.
194. Frohman L, Szabo M, Berelowitz M, et al. Partial purification and characterization of a peptide with growth hormone-releasing activity from extrapituitary tumors in patients with acromegaly. J Clin Invest 1980;65:43-54.
195. Frohman LA, Downs TR, Chomczynski P, et al. Growth hormone-releasing hormone: structure, gene expression and molecular heterogeneity. Acta Paediatr Scand Suppl 1990;367:81-86.
196. Mayo KE, Cerelli GM, Lebo RV, et al. Gene encoding human growth hormone-releasing factor precursor: structure, sequence, and chromosomal assignment. Proc Natl Acad Sci U S A 1985;82: 63-67.
197. Frohman LA, Downs TR, Heimer EP, et al. Dipeptidylpeptidase IV and trypsin-like enzymatic degradation of human growth hormone-releasing hormone in plasma. J Clin Invest 1989;83:1533-1540.
198. Thorner M, Frohman L, Leong D, et al. Extrahypothalamic growth hormone-releasing factor (GRF) is a rare cause of acromegaly: plasma GRF levels in 177 acromegalic patients. J Clin Endocrinol Metab 1984;59:846-849.
199. Asa S, Kovacs K, Thorner M, et al. Immunohistological localization of growth hormone-releasing hormone in human tumors. J Clin Endocrinol Metab 1985;60:423-427.
200. Dayal Y, Lin H, Tallberg K, et al. Immunocytochemical demonstration of growth hormone-releasing factor in gastrointestinal and pancreatic endocrine tumors. Am J Clin Pathol 1986;85:13-20.
201. Khorram O, Garthwaite M, Grosen E, et al. Human uterine and ovarian expression of growth hormone-releasing hormone messenger RNA in benign and malignant gynecologic conditions. Fertil Steril 2001;75:174-179.
202. Gonzalez-Crespo S, Boronat A. Expression of the rat growth hormone-releasing hormone gene in placenta is directed by an alternative promoter. Proc Natl Acad Sci U S A 1991;88:8749-8753.
203. Muller EE, Locatelli V, Cocchi D. Neuroendocrine control of growth hormone secretion. Physiol Rev 1999;79:511-607.
204. Gaylinn BD, Harrison JK, Zysk JR, et al. Molecular cloning and expression of a human anterior pituitary receptor for growth hormone-releasing hormone. Mol Endocrinol 1993;7:77-84.
205. Mayo KE, Godfrey PA, Suhr ST, et al. Growth hormone-releasing hormone: synthesis and signaling. Recent Prog Horm Res 1995; 50:35-73.
206. Baumann G, Maheshwari H. The Dwarfs of Sindh: severe growth hormone (GH) deficiency caused by a mutation in the GH-releasing hormone receptor gene. Acta Paediatr Suppl 1997;423:33-38.
207. Wajnrajch MP, Gertner JM, Harbison MD, et al. Nonsense mutation in the human growth hormone-releasing hormone receptor causes growth failure analogous to the little (lit) mouse. Nat Genet 1996;12:88-90.
208. Giustina A, Veldhuis JD. Pathophysiology of the neuroregulation of growth hormone secretion in experimental animals and the human. Endocr Rev 1998;19:717-797.
209. Stefaneanu L, Kovacs K, Horvath E, et al. Adenohypophysial changes in mice transgenic for human growth hormone- releasing factor: a histological, immunocytochemical, and electron microscopic investigation. Endocrinology 1989;125:2710-2718.
210. Mayo KE, Hammer RE, Swanson LW, et al. Dramatic pituitary hyperplasia in transgenic mice expressing a human growth hormone-releasing factor gene. Mol Endocrinol 1988;2:606-612.
211. Vallar L, Spada A, Giannattasio G. Altered Gs and adenylate cyclase activity in human GH-secreting pituitary adenomas. Nature 1987;330:566-568.
212. Steiger A, Guldner J, Hemmeter U, et al. Effects of growth hormone-releasing hormone and somatostatin on sleep EEG and nocturnal hormone secretion in male controls. Neuroendocrinology 1992;56: 566-573.

213. Van Cauter E, Leproult R, Plat L. Age-related changes in slow wave sleep and REM sleep and relationship with growth hormone and cortisol levels in healthy men. JAMA 2000;284:861-868.
214. Vaccarino FJ, Kennedy SH, Ralevski E, et al. The effects of growth hormone-releasing factor on food consumption in anorexia nervosa patients and normals. Biol Psychiatry 1994;35:446-451.
215. Smith RG, Feighner S, Prendergast K, et al. A new orphan receptor involved in pulsatile growth hormone release. Trends Endocrinol Metab 1999;10:128-135.
216. Howard AD, Feighner SD, Cully DF, et al. A receptor in pituitary and hypothalamus that functions in growth hormone release. Science 1996;273:974-977.
217. Maghnie M, Spica-Russotto V, Cappa M, et al. The growth hormone response to hexarelin in patients with different hypothalamic-pituitary abnormalities. J Clin Endocrinol Metab 1998;83:3886-3889.
218. Arvat E, Maccario M, Di Vito L, et al. Endocrine activities of ghrelin, a natural growth hormone secretagogue (GHS), in humans: comparison and interactions with hexarelin, a nonnatural peptidyl GHS, and GH-releasing hormone. J Clin Endocrinol Metab 2001; 86:1169-1174.
219. Baldelli R, Otero XL, Camina JP, et al. Growth hormone secretagogues as diagnostic tools in disease states. Endocrine 2001;14: 95-99.
220. Gasperi M, Aimaretti G, Scarcello G, et al. Low dose hexarelin and growth hormone (GH)-releasing hormone as a diagnostic tool for the diagnosis of GH deficiency in adults: comparison with insulin-induced hypoglycemia test. J Clin Endocrinol Metab 1999;84: 2633-2637.
221. Ross RJ, Tsagarakis S, Grossman A, et al. GH feedback occurs through modulation of hypothalamic somatostatin under cholinergic control: studies with pyridostigmine and GHRH. Clin Endocrinol (Oxf) 1987;27:727-733.
222. Zheng H, Bailey A, Jiang MH, et al. Somatostatin receptor subtype 2 knockout mice are refractory to growth hormone-negative feedback on arcuate neurons. Mol Endocrinol 1997;11:1709-1717.
223. Soliman AT, ElZalabany MM, Salama M, et al. Serum leptin concentrations during severe protein-energy malnutrition: correlation with growth parameters and endocrine function. Metabolism 3000;49:819-825.
224. Bloch B, Gaillard RC, Brazeau P, et al. Topographical and ontogenetic study of the neurons producing growth hormone-releasing factor in human hypothalamus. Regul Pept 1984;8:21-31.
225. Mota A, Bento A, Penalva A, et al. Role of the serotonin receptor subtype 5-HT1D on basal and stimulated growth hormone secretion. J Clin Endocrinol Metab 1995;80:1973-1977.
226. Muller EE. Cholinergic function and neural control of GH secretion. A critical reappraisal. Eur J Endocrinol 1997;137:338-342.
227. Atiea J, Creagh F, Page M, et al. Early morning hyperglycemia in insulin-dependent diabetes: acute and sustained effects of cholinergic blockage. J Clin Endocrinol Metab 1989;69:390-395.
228. Giustina A, Licini M, Schettino M, et al. Physiological role of galanin in the regulation of anterior pituitary function in humans. Am J Physiol 1994;266:E57-E61.
229. Cella SG, Locatelli V, De Gennaro V, et al. Epinephrine mediates the growth hormone-releasing effect of galanin in infant rats. Endocrinology 1988;122:855-859.
230. Van Cauter E, Kerkhofs M, Caufriez A, et al. A quantitative estimation of growth hormone secretion in normal man: reproducibility and relation to sleep and time of day. J Clin Endocrinol Metab 1992;74:1441-1450.
231. Jaffe CA, Ocampo-Lim B, Guo W, et al. Regulatory mechanisms of growth hormone secretion are sexually dimorphic. J Clin Invest 1998;102:153-164.
232. Pincus SM, Gevers EF, Robinson IC, et al. Females secrete growth hormone with more process irregularity than males in both humans and rats. Am J Physiol 1996;270:E107-E115.
233. Low MJ, Otero-Corchon V, Parlow AF, et al. Somatostatin is required for masculinization of growth hormone-regulated hepatic gene expression but not of somatic growth. J Clin Invest 2001;107: 1571-1580.
234. Wagner C, Caplan SR, Tannenbaum GS. Genesis of the ultradian rhythm of GH secretion: a new model unifying experimental observations in rats. Am J Physiol 1998;275:E1046-E1054.
235. Krulich L, Dhariwal A, McCann S. Stimulatory and inhibitory effects of purified hypothalamic extracts on growth hormone release from rat pituitary in vitro. Endocrinology 1968;83: 783-790.
236. Brazeau P, Vale W, Burgus R, et al. Hypothalamic polypeptide that inhibits the secretion of immunoreactive pituitary growth hormone. Science 1973;179:77-79.
237. Galanopoulou AS, Kent G, Rabbani SN, et al. Heterologous processing of prosomatostatin in constitutive and regulated secretory pathways. Putative role of the endoproteases furin, PC1, and PC2. J Biol Chem. 1993;268:6041-6049.
238. Shen LP, Rutter WJ. Sequence of the human somatostatin I gene. Science 1984;224:168-171.
239. Conlon JM, Tostivint H, Vaudry H. Somatostatin- and urotensin II-related peptides: molecular diversity and evolutionary perspectives. Regul Pept 1997;69:95-103.
240. de Lecea L, Criado JR, Prospero-Garcia O, et al. A cortical neuropeptide with neuronal depressant and sleep-modulating properties. Nature 1996;381:242-245.
241. Spier AD, de Lecea L. Cortistatin: a member of the somatostatin neuropeptide family with distinct physiological functions. Brain Res Brain Res Rev 2000;33:228-241.
242. Fukusumi S, Kitada C, Takekawa S, et al. Identification and characterization of a novel human cortistatin-like peptide. Biochem Biophys Res Commun 1997;232:157-163.
243. Andersen FG, Jensen J, Heller RS, et al. Pax6 and Pdx1 form a functional complex on the rat somatostatin gene upstream enhancer. FEBS Lett 1999;445:315-320.
244. Goudet G, Delhalle S, Biemar F, et al. Functional and cooperative interactions between the homeodomain PDX1, Pbx, and Prep1 factors on the somatostatin promoter. J Biol Chem 1999;274: 4067-4073.
245. Schwartz PT, Vallejo M. Differential regulation of basal and cyclic adenosine 3′,5′- monophosphate-induced somatostatin gene transcription in neural cells by DNA control elements that bind homeodomain proteins. Mol Endocrinol 1998;12:1280-1293.
246. Capone G, Choi C, Vertifuille J. Regulation of the preprosomatostatin gene by cyclic-AMP in cerebrocortical neurons. Brain Res Mol Brain Res 1998;60:247-258.
247. Montminy M, Brindle P, Arias J, et al. Regulation of somatostatin gene transcription by cyclic adenosine monophosphate. Metabolism 1996;45:4-7.
248. Schwartz PT, Perez-Villamil B, Rivera A, et al. Pancreatic homeodomain transcription factor IDX1/IPF1 expressed in developing brain regulates somatostatin gene transcription in embryonic neural cells. J Biol Chem 2000;275:19106-19114.
249. Patel YC. Somatostatin and its receptor family. Front Neuroendocrinol 1999;20:157-198.
250. Thoss VS, Perez J, Probst A, et al. Expression of five somatostatin receptor mRNAs in the human brain and pituitary. Naunyn Schmiedebergs Arch Pharmacol 1996;354:411-419.
251. Strowski MZ, Parmar RM, Blake AD, et al. Somatostatin inhibits insulin and glucagon secretion via two receptors subtypes: an in vitro study of pancreatic islets from somatostatin receptor 2 knockout mice. Endocrinology 2000;141:111-117.
252. Blake AD, Badway AC, Strowski MZ. Delineating somatostatin's neuronal actions. Curr Drug Targets CNS Neurol Disord 2004;3: 153-160.
253. Mathern GW, Babb TL, Pretorius JK, et al. Reactive synaptogenesis and neuron densities for neuropeptide Y, somatostatin, and glutamate decarboxylase immunoreactivity in the epileptogenic human fascia dentata. J Neurosci 1995;15:3990-4004.
254. Bissette G, Myers B. Somatostatin in Alzheimer's disease and depression. Life Sci 1992;51:1389-1410.
255. Yang L, Berk SC, Rohrer SP, et al. Synthesis and biological activities of potent peptidomimetics selective for somatostatin receptor subtype 2. Proc Natl Acad Sci U S A 1998;95:10836-10841.
256. Rohrer SP, Birzin ET, Mosley RT, et al. Rapid identification of subtype-selective agonists of the somatostatin receptor through combinatorial chemistry. Science 1998;282:737-740.
257. Slooter GD, Mearadji A, Breeman WA, et al. Somatostatin receptor imaging, therapy and new strategies in patients with neuroendocrine tumours. Br J Surg 2001;88:31-40.
258. Lamberts SW, van der Lely AJ, de Herder WW, et al. Octreotide. N Engl J Med 1996;334:246-254.
259. Schirmer WJ, O'Dorisio TM, Schirmer TP, et al. Intraoperative localization of neuroendocrine tumors with 125I-TYR(3)-octreotide

and a hand-held gamma-detecting probe. Surgery 1993;114:745-751; discussion 751-742.
260. Henze M, Schuhmacher J, Hipp P, et al. PET imaging of somatostatin receptors using [^{68}Ga]DOTATOC. J Nucl Med 2001;42: 1053-1056.
261. Rochaix P, Delesque N, Esteve JP, et al. Gene therapy for pancreatic carcinoma: local and distant antitumor effects after somatostatin receptor sst2 gene transfer. Hum Gene Ther 1999; 10:995-1008.
262. Freeman ME, Kanyicska B, Lerant A, et al. Prolactin: structure, function, and regulation of secretion. Physiol Rev 2000;80: 1523-1631.
263. Ben-Jonathan N, Hnasko R. Dopamine as a prolactin (PRL) inhibitor. Endocr Rev 2001;22:724-763.
264. Ben-Jonathan N. Dopamine: a prolactin-inhibiting hormone. Endocr Rev 1985;6:564-589.
265. MacLeod RM, Fontham EH, Lehmeyer JE. Prolactin and growth hormone production as influenced by catecholamines and agents that affect brain catecholamines. Neuroendocrinology 1970;6:283-294.
266. Caron MG, Beaulieu M, Raymond V, et al. Dopaminergic receptors in the anterior pituitary gland. Correlation of [3H]dihydroergocryptine binding with the dopaminergic control of prolactin release. J Biol Chem 1978;253:2244-2253.
267. Goldsmith PC, Cronin MJ, Weiner RI. Dopamine receptor sites in the anterior pituitary. J Histochem Cytochem 1979;27:1205-1207.
268. Asa SL, Kelly MA, Grandy DK, et al. Pituitary lactotroph adenomas develop after prolonged lactotroph hyperplasia in dopamine D2 receptor-deficient mice. Endocrinology 1999;140:5348-5355.
269. Lerant A, Herman ME, Freeman ME. Dopaminergic neurons of periventricular and arcuate nuclei of pseudopregnant rats: semicircadian rhythm in Fos-related antigens immunoreactivities and in dopamine concentration. Endocrinology 1996;137:3621-3628.
270. Peters LL, Hoefer MT, Ben-Jonathan N. The posterior pituitary: regulation of anterior pituitary prolactin secretion. Science 1981; 213:659-661.
271. Durham RA, Johnson JD, Eaton MJ, et al. Opposing roles for dopamine D1 and D2 receptors in the regulation of hypothalamic tuberoinfundibular dopamine neurons. Eur J Pharmacol 1998;355: 141-147.
272. Vallar L, Meldolesi J. Mechanisms of signal transduction at the dopamine D2 receptor. Trends Pharmacol Sci 1989;10:74-77.
273. Wang YH, Maurer RA. A role for the mitogen-activated protein kinase in mediating the ability of thyrotropin-releasing hormone to stimulate the prolactin promoter. Mol Endocrinol 1999;13: 1094-1104.
274. Yonehara T, Kanasaki H, Yamamoto H, et al. Involvement of mitogen-activated protein kinase in cyclic adenosine 3′,5′-monophosphate-induced hormone gene expression in rat pituitary GH(3) cells. Endocrinology 2001;142:2811-2819.
275. Jacob KK, Wininger E, DiMinni K, et al. The EGF response element in the prolactin promoter. Mol Cell Endocrinol 1999;152:137-145.
276. Day RN, Liu J, Sundmark V, et al. Selective inhibition of prolactin gene transcription by the ETS-2 repressor factor. J Biol Chem 1998;273:31909-31915.
277. Suzuki S, Yamamoto I, Arita J. Mitogen-activated protein kinase-dependent stimulation of proliferation of rat lactotrophs in culture by 3′,5′-cyclic adenosine monophosphate. Endocrinology 1999;140:2850-2858.
278. Florio T, Pan MG, Newman B, et al. Dopaminergic inhibition of DNA synthesis in pituitary tumor cells is associated with phosphotyrosine phosphatase activity. J Biol Chem 1992;267:24169-24172.
279. Lindley SE, Gunnet JW, Lookingland KJ, et al. Effects of alterations in the activity of tuberohypophysial dopaminergic neurons on the secretion of alpha-melanocyte stimulating hormone. Proc Soc Exp Biol Med 1988;188:282-286.
280. Chronwall BM, Millington WR, Griffin WS, et al. Histological evaluation of the dopaminergic regulation of proopiomelanocortin gene expression in the intermediate lobe of the rat pituitary, involving in situ hybridization and [3H]thymidine uptake measurement. Endocrinology 1987;120:1201-1211.
281. Chronwall BM, Davis TD, Severidt MW, et al. Constitutive expression of functional GABA(B) receptors in mIL-tsA58 cells requires both GABA(B(1)) and GABA(B(2)) genes. J Neurochem 2001;77: 1237-1247.
282. Samuels MH, Veldhuis J, Ridgway EC. Copulsatile release of thyrotropin and prolactin in normal and hypothyroid subjects. Thyroid 1995;5:369-372.
283. Nagy GM, Gorcs TJ, Halasz B. Attenuation of the suckling-induced prolactin release and the high afternoon oscillations of plasma prolactin secretion of lactating rats by antiserum to vasopressin. Neuroendocrinology 1991;54:566-570.
284. Arey BJ, Freeman ME. Oxytocin, vasoactive-intestinal peptide, and serotonin regulate the mating-induced surges of prolactin secretion in the rat. Endocrinology 1990;126:279-284.
285. Samson WK, Lumpkin MD, McCann SM. Evidence for a physiological role for oxytocin in the control of prolactin secretion. Endocrinology 1986;119:554-560.
286. Shimatsu A, Kato Y, Ohta H, et al. Involvement of hypothalamic vasoactive intestinal polypeptide (VIP) in prolactin secretion induced by serotonin in rats. Proc Soc Exp Biol Med 1984;175: 414-416.
287. Kjaer A. Vasopressin as a neuroendocrine regulator of anterior pituitary hormone secretion. Acta Endocrinol (Copenh) 1993;129: 489-496.
288. Itoh N, Obata K, Yanaihara N, et al. Human preprovasoactive intestinal polypeptide contains a novel PHI-27-like peptide, PHM-27. Nature 1983;304:547-549.
289. Hokfelt T, Fahrenkrug J, Tatemoto K, et al. The PHI (PHI-27)/corticotropin-releasing factor/enkephalin immunoreactive hypothalamic neuron: possible morphological basis for integrated control of prolactin, corticotropin, and growth hormone secretion. Proc Natl Acad Sci U S A 1983;80:895-898.
290. Denef C, Manet D, Dewals R. Dopaminergic stimulation of prolactin release. Nature 1980;285:243-246.
291. Arey BJ, Burris TP, Basco P, et al. Infusion of dopamine at low concentrations stimulates the release of prolactin from alpha-methyl-p-tyrosine-treated rats. Proc Soc Exp Biol Med 1993;203: 60-63.
292. Hinuma S, Habata Y, Fujii R, et al. A prolactin-releasing peptide in the brain. Nature 1998;393:272-276.
293. Fukusumi S, Fujii R, Hinuma S. Recent advances in mammalian RFamide peptides: the discovery and functional analyses of PrRP, RFRPs and QRFP. Peptides 2006;27:1073-1086.
294. Schwartz J, Van de Pavert S, Clarke I, et al. Paracrine interactions within the pituitary gland. Ann N Y Acad Sci 1998; 839:239-243.
295. Murai I, Ben-Jonathan N. Posterior pituitary lobectomy abolishes the suckling-induced rise in prolactin (PRL): evidence for a PRL-releasing factor in the posterior pituitary. Endocrinology 1987;121: 205-211.
296. Allen DL, Low MJ, Allen RG, Ben-Jonathan N. Identification of two classes of prolactin-releasing factors in intermediate lobe tumors from transgenic mice. Endocrinology 1995;136:3093-3099.
297. Ellerkmann E, Porter TE, Nagy GM, et al. N-acetylation is required for the lactotrope recruitment activity of alpha-melanocyte-stimulating hormone and beta-endorphin. Endocrinology 1992;131:566-570.
298. Voogt JL, Lee Y, Yang S, et al. Regulation of prolactin secretion during pregnancy and lactation. Prog Brain Res 2001;133:173-185.
299. DeMaria JE, Livingstone JD, Freeman ME. Ovarian steroids influence the activity of neuroendocrine dopaminergic neurons. Brain Res 2000;879:139-147.
300. Milenkovic L, Parlow AF, McCann SM. Physiological significance of the negative short-loop feedback of prolactin. Neuroendocrinology 1990;52:389-392.
301. Arbogast LA, Voogt JL. Prolactin (PRL) receptors are colocalized in dopaminergic neurons in fetal hypothalamic cell cultures: effect of PRL on tyrosine hydroxylase activity. Endocrinology 1997;138:3016-3023.
302. Phelps CJ, Hurley DL. Pituitary hormones as neurotrophic signals: update on hypothalamic differentiation in genetic models of altered feedback. Proc Soc Exp Biol Med 1999;222:39-58.
303. Phelps CJ, Horseman ND. Prolactin gene disruption does not compromise differentiation of tuberoinfundibular dopaminergic neurons. Neuroendocrinology 2000;72:2-10.
304. Callahan P, Klosterman S, Prunty D, et al. Immunoneutralization of endogenous opioid peptides prevents the suckling-induced prolactin increase and the inhibition of tuberoinfundibular dopaminergic neurons. Neuroendocrinology 2000;71:268-276.

305. Van de Kar LD, Bethea CL. Pharmacological evidence that serotonergic stimulation of prolactin secretion is mediated via the dorsal raphe nucleus. Neuroendocrinology 1982;35:225-230.
306. Creese I, Burt DR, Snyder SH. Dopamine receptor binding predicts clinical and pharmacological potencies of antischizophrenic drugs. Science 1976;192:481-483.
307. Melkersson K, Hulting AL. Prolactin-secreting pituitary adenoma in neuroleptic treated patients with psychotic disorder. Eur Arch Psychiatry Clin Neurosci 2000;250:6-10.
308. Veldman RG, Frolich M, Pincus SM, et al. Basal, pulsatile, entropic, and 24-hour rhythmic features of secondary hyperprolactinemia due to functional pituitary stalk disconnection mimic tumoral (primary) hyperprolactinemia. J Clin Endocrinol Metab 2001;86: 1562-1567.
309. Waldstreicher J, Duffy JF, Brown EN, et al. Gender differences in the temporal organization of prolactin (PRL) secretion: evidence for a sleep-independent circadian rhythm of circulating PRL levels-a clinical research center study. J Clin Endocrinol Metab 1996;81: 1483-1487.
310. Diaz S, Seron-Ferre M, Cardenas H, et al. Circadian variation of basal plasma prolactin, prolactin response to suckling, and length of amenorrhea in nursing women. J Clin Endocrinol Metab 1989;68:946-955.
311. Malarkey WB, Hall JC, Pearl DK, et al. The influence of academic stress and season on 24-hour concentrations of growth hormone and prolactin. J Clin Endocrinol Metab 1991;73:1089-1092.
312. Seeburg PH, Adelman JP. Characterization of cDNA for precursor of human luteinizing hormone releasing hormone. Nature 1984;311:666-668.
313. Urbanski HF, White RB, Fernald RD, et al. Regional expression of mRNA encoding a second form of gonadotropin-releasing hormone in the macaque brain. Endocrinology 1999;140:1945-1948.
314. Sherwood NM, Lovejoy DA, Coe IR. Origin of mammalian gonadotropin-releasing hormones. Endocr Rev 1993;14:241-254.
315. Fernald RD, White RB. Gonadotropin-releasing hormone genes: phylogeny, structure, and functions. Front Neuroendocrinol 1999;20:224-240.
316. Pawson AJ, Morgan K, Maudsley SR, et al. Type II gonadotrophin-releasing hormone (GnRH-II) in reproductive biology. Reproduction 2003;126:271-278.
317. Nelson SB, Eraly SA, Mellon PL. The GnRH promoter: target of transcription factors, hormones, and signaling pathways. Mol Cell Endocrinol 1998;140:151-155.
318. Hapgood JP, Sadie H, van Biljon W, et al. Regulation of expression of mammalian gonadotrophin-releasing hormone receptor genes. J Neuroendocrinol 2005;17:619-638.
319. Cheng CK, Leung PC. Molecular biology of gonadotropin-releasing hormone (GnRH)-I, GnRH-II, and their receptors in humans. Endocr Rev 2005;26:283-306.
320. Givens ML, Kurotani R, Rave-Harel N, et al. Phylogenetic footprinting reveals evolutionarily conserved regions of the gonadotropin-releasing hormone gene that enhance cell-specific expression. Mol Endocrinol 2004;18:2950-2966.
321. Givens ML, Rave-Harel N, Goonewardena VD, et al. Developmental regulation of gonadotropin-releasing hormone gene expression by the MSX and DLX homeodomain protein families. J Biol Chem 2005;280:19156-19165.
322. Phoenix CH, Chambers KC. Sexual performance of old and young male rhesus macaques following treatment with GnRH. Physiol Behav 1990;47:513-517.
323. Wray S. Development of luteinizing hormone releasing hormone neurones. J Neuroendocrinol 2001;13:3-11.
324. MacColl G, Quinton R, Bouloux PM. GnRH neuronal development: insights into hypogonadotrophic hypogonadism. Trends Endocrinol Metab 2002;13:112-118.
325. Sato N, Katsumata N, Kagami M, et al. Clinical assessment and mutation analysis of Kallmann syndrome 1 (KAL1) and fibroblast growth factor receptor 1 (FGFR1, or KAL2) in five families and 18 sporadic patients. J Clin Endocrinol Metab 2004;89:1079-1088.
326. Clayton RN. Mechanism of GnRH action in gonadotrophs. Hum Reprod 1988;3:479-483.
327. Conn PM, Crowley WF Jr. Gonadotropin-releasing hormone and its analogs. Annu Rev Med 1994;45:391-405.
328. Rispoli LA, Nett TM. Pituitary gonadotropin-releasing hormone (GnRH) receptor: structure, distribution and regulation of expression. Anim Reprod Sci 2005;88:57-74.
329. Lahlou N, Carel JC, Chaussain JL, et al. Pharmacokinetics and pharmacodynamics of GnRH agonists: clinical implications in pediatrics. J Pediatr Endocrinol Metab 2000;13(suppl 1):723-737.
330. Reissmann T, Schally AV, Bouchard P, et al. The LHRH antagonist cetrorelix: a review. Hum Reprod Update 2000;6:322-331.
331. Carmel PW, Araki S, Ferin M. Pituitary stalk portal blood collection in rhesus monkeys: evidence for pulsatile release of gonadotropin-releasing hormone (GnRH). Endocrinology 1976;99:243-248.
332. Clarke IJ, Cummins JT. The temporal relationship between gonadotropin releasing hormone (GnRH) and luteinizing hormone (LH) secretion in ovariectomized ewes. Endocrinology 1982;111:1737-1739.
333. Mori Y, Nishihara M, Tanaka T, et al. Chronic recording of electrophysiological manifestation of the hypothalamic gonadotropin-releasing hormone pulse generator activity in the goat. Neuroendocrinology 1991;53:392-395.
334. Martinez de la Escalera G, Choi AL, Weiner RI. Generation and synchronization of gonadotropin-releasing hormone (GnRH) pulses: intrinsic properties of the GT1-1 GnRH neuronal cell line. Proc Natl Acad Sci U S A 1992;89:1852-1855.
335. Chappel SC, Ulloa-Aguirre A, Coutifaris C. Biosynthesis and secretion of follicle-stimulating hormone. Endocr Rev 1983;4:179-211.
336. Simerly RB, Chang C, Muramatsu M, et al. Distribution of androgen and estrogen receptor mRNA-containing cells in the rat brain: an in situ hybridization study. J Comp Neurol 1990;294:76-95.
337. Kuiper GG, Shughrue PJ, Merchenthaler I, et al. The estrogen receptor beta subtype: a novel mediator of estrogen action in neuroendocrine systems. Front Neuroendocrinol 1998;19:253-286.
338. Shughrue PJ, Lane MV, Merchenthaler I. Comparative distribution of estrogen receptor-alpha and -beta mRNA in the rat central nervous system. J Comp Neurol 1997;388:507-525.
339. Bethea CL, Brown NA, Kohama SG. Steroid regulation of estrogen and progestin receptor messenger ribonucleic acid in monkey hypothalamus and pituitary. Endocrinology 1996;137:4372-4383.
340. Plant TM. Gonadal regulation of hypothalamic gonadotropin-releasing hormone release in primates. Endocr Rev 1986;7:75-88.
341. Nakai Y, Plant TM, Hess DL, et al. On the sites of the negative and positive feedback actions of estradiol in the control of gonadotropin secretion in the rhesus monkey. Endocrinology 1978;102: 1008-1014.
342. Bishop W, Kalra PS, Fawcett CP, et al. The effects of hypothalamic lesions on the release of gonadotropins and prolactin in response to estrogen and progesterone treatment in female rats. Endocrinology 1972;91:1404-1410.
343. Levine JE, Chappell PE, Schneider JS, et al. Progesterone receptors as neuroendocrine integrators. Front Neuroendocrinol 2001;22: 69-106.
344. Kaplan SL, Grumbach MM, Aubert ML. The ontogenesis of pituitary hormones and hypothalamic factors in the human fetus: maturation of central nervous system regulation of anterior pituitary function. Recent Prog Horm Res 1976;32:161-243.
345. Winter JS, Faiman C, Hobson WC, et al. Pituitary-gonadal relations in infancy. I. Patterns of serum gonadotropin concentrations from birth to four years of age in man and chimpanzee. J Clin Endocrinol Metab 1975;40:545-551.
346. Plant TM. Neurobiological bases underlying the control of the onset of puberty in the rhesus monkey: a representative higher primate. Front Neuroendocrinol 2001;22:107-139.
347. Boyar RM, Rosenfeld RS, Kapen S, et al. Human puberty. Simultaneous augmented secretion of luteinizing hormone and testosterone during sleep. J Clin Invest 1974;54:609-618.
348. Gay VL, Plant TM. Sustained intermittent release of gonadotropin-releasing hormone in the prepubertal male rhesus monkey induced by *N*-methyl-DL-aspartic acid. Neuroendocrinology 1988; 48:147-152.
349. Ojeda SR, Ma YJ, Lee BJ, et al. Glia-to-neuron signaling and the neuroendocrine control of female puberty. Recent Prog Horm Res 2000;55:197-223; discussion 223-224.
350. Ebling FJ. The neuroendocrine timing of puberty. Reproduction 2005;129:675-683.

351. Seminara SB. Metastin and its G protein-coupled receptor, GPR54: critical pathway modulating GnRH secretion. Front Neuroendocrinol 2005;26:131-138.
352. Dungan HM, Clifton DK, Steiner RA. Minireview: kisspeptin neurons as central processors in the regulation of gonadotropin-releasing hormone secretion. Endocrinology 2006;147:1154-1158.
353. Stoyanovitch AG, Johnson MA, Clifton DK, et al. Galanin-like peptide rescues reproductive function in the diabetic rat. Diabetes 2005;54:2471-2476.
354. Cameron JL. Stress and behaviorally induced reproductive dysfunction in primates. Semin Reprod Endocrinol 1997;15:37-45.
355. Lachelin GC, Yen SS. Hypothalamic chronic anovulation. Am J Obstet Gynecol 1978;130:825-831.
356. Rivier C, Rivier J, Vale W. Stress-induced inhibition of reproductive functions: role of endogenous corticotropin-releasing factor. Science 1986;231:607-609.
357. Feng YJ, Shalts E, Xia LN, et al. An inhibitory effect of interleukin-1a on basal gonadotropin release in the ovariectomized rhesus monkey: reversal by a corticotropin-releasing factor antagonist. Endocrinology 1991;128:2077-2082.
358. Chen MD, O'Byrne KT, Chiappini SE, et al. Hypoglycemic "stress" and gonadotropin-releasing hormone pulse generator activity in the rhesus monkey: role of the ovary. Neuroendocrinology 1992;56:666-673.
359. Norman RL, Smith CJ. Restraint inhibits luteinizing hormone and testosterone secretion in intact male rhesus macaques: effects of concurrent naloxone administration. Neuroendocrinology 1992;55:405-415.
360. Wade GN, Schneider JE. Metabolic fuels and reproduction in female mammals. Neurosci Biobehav Rev 1992;16:235-272.
361. Chehab FF, Lim ME, Lu R. Correction of the sterility defect in homozygous obese female mice by treatment with the human recombinant leptin. Nat Genet 1996;12:318-320.
362. Schneider JE, Zhou D, Blum RM. Leptin and metabolic control of reproduction. Horm Behav 2000;37:306-326.
363. Honegger J, Buchfelder M, Fahlbusch R. Surgical treatment of craniopharyngiomas: endocrinological results. J Neurosurg 1999;90:251-257.
364. Yuan XQ, Wade CE. Neuroendocrine abnormalities in patients with traumatic brain injury. Front Neuroendocrinol 1991;12:209-230.
365. Benvenga S, Campenni A, Ruggeri RM, et al. Clinical review 113: hypopituitarism secondary to head trauma. J Clin Endocrinol Metab 2000;85:1353-1361.
366. Daaboul J, Steinbok P. Abnormalities of water metabolism after surgery for optic/chiasmatic astrocytomas in children. Pediatr Neurosurg 1998;28:181-185.
367. Maghnie M, Cosi G, Genovese E, et al. Central diabetes insipidus in children and young adults. N Engl J Med 2000;343:998-1007.
368. Scherbaum WA, Wass JA, Besser GM, et al. Autoimmune cranial diabetes insipidus: its association with other endocrine diseases and with histiocytosis X. Clin Endocrinol (Oxf) 1986;25:411-420.
369. Al-Agha AE, Thomsett MJ, Ratcliffe JF, et al. Acquired central diabetes insipidus in children: a 12-year Brisbane experience. J Paediatr Child Health 2001;37:172-175.
370. Mootha SL, Barkovich AJ, Grumbach MM, et al. Idiopathic hypothalamic diabetes insipidus, pituitary stalk thickening, and the occult intracranial germinoma in children and adolescents. J Clin Endocrinol Metab 1997;82:1362-1367.
371. Nagasaki H, Ito M, Yuasa H, et al. Two novel mutations in the coding region for neurophysin-II associated with familial central diabetes insipidus. J Clin Endocrinol Metab 1995;80:1352-1356.
372. Morello JP, Bichet DG. Nephrogenic diabetes insipidus. Annu Rev Physiol 2001;63:607-630.
373. Birnbaumer M. The V2 vasopressin receptor mutations and fluid homeostasis. Cardiovasc Res 2001;51:409-415.
374. Nielsen S, Frokiaer J, Marples D, et al. Aquaporins in the kidney: from molecules to medicine. Physiol Rev 2002;82:205-244.
375. Lieberman SA, Oberoi AL, Gilkison CR, et al. Prevalence of neuroendocrine dysfunction in patients recovering from traumatic brain injury. J Clin Endocrinol Metab 2001;86:2752-2756.
376. Smith MV, Laws ER Jr. Magnetic resonance imaging measurements of pituitary stalk compression and deviation in patients with non-prolactin-secreting intrasellar and parasellar tumors: lack of correlation with serum prolactin levels. Neurosurgery 1994;34:834-839; discussion 839.
377. Voelker JL, Campbell RL, Muller J. Clinical, radiographic, and pathological features of symptomatic Rathke's cleft cysts. J Neurosurg 1991;74:535-544.
378. Zucchini S, Ambrosetto P, Carla G, et al. Primary empty sella: differences and similarities between children and adults. Acta Paediatr 1995;84:1382-1385.
379. Bjerre P. The empty sella. A reappraisal of etiology and pathogenesis. Acta Neurol Scand Suppl 1990;130:1-25.
380. Klingmuller D, Dewes W, Krahe T, et al. Magnetic resonance imaging of the brain in patients with anosmia and hypothalamic hypogonadism (Kallmann's syndrome). J Clin Endocrinol Metab 1987;65:581-584.
381. Nanduri VR, Stanhope R. Why is the retention of gonadotrophin secretion common in children with panhypopituitarism due to septo-optic dysplasia? Eur J Endocrinol 1999;140:48-50.
382. Bhagavath B, Podolsky RH, Ozata M, et al. Clinical and molecular characterization of a large sample of patients with hypogonadotropic hypogonadism. Fertil Steril 2006;85:706-713.
383. Chryssikopoulos A, Gregoriou O, Vitoratos N, et al. The predictive value of double Gn-RH provocation test in unprimed Gn-RH-primed and steroid-primed female patients with Kallmann's syndrome. Int J Fertil Womens Med 1998;43:291-299.
384. Hayes FJ, Seminara SB, Crowley WF Jr. Hypogonadotropic hypogonadism. Endocrinol Metab Clin North Am 1998;27:739-763, vii.
385. Samuels MH, Ridgway EC. Central hypothyroidism. Endocrinol Metab Clin North Am 1992;21:903-919.
386. Winter WE, Signorino MR. Review: molecular thyroidology. Ann Clin Lab Sci 2001;31:221-244.
387. Jorgensen JO, Pedersen SA, Laurberg P, et al. Effects of growth hormone therapy on thyroid function of growth hormone-deficient adults with and without concomitant thyroxine-substituted central hypothyroidism. J Clin Endocrinol Metab 1989;69:1127-1132.
388. Rose SR. Cranial irradiation and central hypothyroidism. Trends Endocrinol Metab 2001;12:97-104.
389. Argente J, Abusrewil SA, Bona G, et al. Isolated growth hormone deficiency in children and adolescents. J Pediatr Endocrinol Metab 2001;14(suppl 2):1003-1008.
390. Maghnie M, Ghirardello S, Genovese E. Magnetic resonance imaging of the hypothalamus-pituitary unit in children suspected of hypopituitarism: who, how and when to investigate. J Endocrinol Invest 2004;27:496-509.
391. Nishihara E, Kimura H, Ishimaru T, et al. A case of adrenal insufficiency due to acquired hypothalamic CRH deficiency. Endocr J 1997;44:121-126.
392. Kyllo JH, Collins MM, Vetter KL, et al. Linkage of congenital isolated adrenocorticotropic hormone deficiency to the corticotropin releasing hormone locus using simple sequence repeat polymorphisms. Am J Med Genet 1996;62:262-267.
393. Vallette-Kasic S, Brue T, Pulichino AM, et al. Congenital isolated adrenocorticotropin deficiency: an underestimated cause of neonatal death, explained by TPIT gene mutations. J Clin Endocrinol Metab 2005;90:1323-1331.
394. Fukata J, Shimizu N, Imura H, et al. Human corticotropin-releasing hormone test in patients with hypothalamo-pituitary-adrenocortical disorders. Endocr J 1993;40:597-606.
395. Gleeson HK, Shalet SM. Endocrine complications of neoplastic diseases in children and adolescents. Curr Opin Pediatr 2001;13:346-351.
396. Arlt W, Hove U, Muller B, et al. Frequent and frequently overlooked: treatment-induced endocrine dysfunction in adult long-term survivors of primary brain tumors. Neurology 1997;49:498-506.
397. Prabhu VC, Brown HG. The pathogenesis of craniopharyngiomas. Childs Nerv Syst 2005;21:622-627.
398. Halac I, Zimmerman D. Endocrine manifestations of craniopharyngioma. Childs Nerv Syst 2005;21:640-648.
399. Curran JG, O'Connor E. Imaging of craniopharyngioma. Childs Nerv Syst 2005;21:635-639.
400. Hochman HI, Judge DM, Reichlin S. Precocious puberty and hypothalamic hamartoma. Pediatrics 1981;67:236-244.

401. Asa SL, Kovacs K, Tindall GT, et al. Cushing's disease associated with an intrasellar gangliocytoma producing corticotrophin-releasing factor. Ann Intern Med 1984;101:789-793.
402. Asa SL, Scheithauer BW, Bilbao JM, et al. A case for hypothalamic acromegaly: a clinicopathological study of six patients with hypothalamic gangliocytomas producing growth hormone-releasing factor. J Clin Endocrinol Metab 1984;58:796-803.
403. Lee PA. Central precocious puberty. An overview of diagnosis, treatment, and outcome. Endocrinol Metab Clin North Am 1999;28: 901-918, xi.
404. De Sanctis V, Corrias A, Rizzo V, et al. Etiology of central precocious puberty in males: the results of the Italian Study Group for Physiopathology of Puberty. J Pediatr Endocrinol Metab 2000; 13(suppl 1):687-693.
405. Cisternino M, Arrigo T, Pasquino AM, et al. Etiology and age incidence of precocious puberty in girls: a multicentric study. J Pediatr Endocrinol Metab 2000;13(suppl 1):695-701.
406. Ojeda SR, Heger S. New thoughts on female precocious puberty. J Pediatr Endocrinol Metab 2001;14:245-256.
407. Virdis R, Sigorini M, Laiolo A, et al. Neurofibromatosis type 1 and precocious puberty. J Pediatr Endocrinol Metab 2000;13(suppl 1):841-844.
408. Rivarola MA, Belgorosky A, Mendilaharzu H, et al. Precocious puberty in children with tumours of the suprasellar and pineal areas: organic central precocious puberty. Acta Paediatr 2001;90: 751-756.
409. Arita K, Ikawa F, Kurisu K, et al. The relationship between magnetic resonance imaging findings and clinical manifestations of hypothalamic hamartoma. J Neurosurg 1999;91:212-220.
410. Debeneix C, Bourgeois M, Trivin C, et al. Hypothalamic hamartoma: comparison of clinical presentation and magnetic resonance images. Horm Res 2001;56:12-18.
411. Berkovic SF, Andermann F, Melanson D, et al. Hypothalamic hamartomas and ictal laughter: evolution of a characteristic epileptic syndrome and diagnostic value of magnetic resonance imaging. Ann Neurol 1988;23:429-439.
412. Anasti JN, Flack MR, Froehlich J, et al. A potential novel mechanism for precocious puberty in juvenile hypothyroidism. J Clin Endocrinol Metab 1995;80:276-279.
413. Fauchon F, Jouvet A, Paquis P, et al. Parenchymal pineal tumors: a clinicopathological study of 76 cases. Int J Radiat Oncol Biol Phys 2000;46:959-968.
414. Jouvet A, Saint-Pierre G, Fauchon F, et al. Pineal parenchymal tumors: a correlation of histological features with prognosis in 66 cases. Brain Pathol 2000;10:49-60.
415. Baumgartner JE, Edwards MS. Pineal tumors. Neurosurg Clin North Am 1992;3:853-862.
416. Popovic EA, Kelly PJ. Stereotactic procedures for lesions of the pineal region. Mayo Clin Proc 1993;68:965-970.
417. Dahlborg SA, Petrillo A, Crossen JR, et al. The potential for complete and durable response in nonglial primary brain tumors in children and young adults with enhanced chemotherapy delivery. Cancer J Sci Am 1998;4:110-124.
418. Chalumeau M, Chemaitilly W, Trivin C, et al. Central precocious puberty in girls: an evidence-based diagnosis tree to predict central nervous system abnormalities. Pediatrics 2002;109:61-67.
419. Iughetti L, Predieri B, Ferrari M, et al. Diagnosis of central precocious puberty: endocrine assessment. J Pediatr Endocrinol Metab 2000;13(suppl 1):709-715.
420. Argyropoulou MI, Kiortsis DN. MRI of the hypothalamic-pituitary axis in children. Pediatr Radiol 2005;35:1045-1055.
421. Klein KO, Barnes KM, Jones JV, et al. Increased final height in precocious puberty after long-term treatment with LHRH agonists: the National Institutes of Health experience. J Clin Endocrinol Metab 2001;86:4711-4716.
422. Tato L, Savage MO, Antoniazzi F, et al. Optimal therapy of pubertal disorders in precocious/early puberty. J Pediatr Endocrinol Metab 2001;14(suppl 2):985-995.
423. Laron Z, Kauli R. Experience with cyproterone acetate in the treatment of precocious puberty. J Pediatr Endocrinol Metab 2000; 13(suppl 1):805-810.
424. Feuillan P, Merke D, Leschek EW, et al. Use of aromatase inhibitors in precocious puberty. Endocr Relat Cancer 1999;6:303-306.
425. Warren MP, Fried JL. Hypothalamic amenorrhea. The effects of environmental stresses on the reproductive system: a central effect of the central nervous system. Endocrinol Metab Clin North Am 2001;30:611-629.
426. Yen SS. Female hypogonadotropic hypogonadism. Hypothalamic amenorrhea syndrome. Endocrinol Metab Clin North Am 1993; 22:29-58.
427. Cannavo S, Curto L, Trimarchi F. Exercise-related female reproductive dysfunction. J Endocrinol Invest 2001;24:823-832.
428. Moschos S, Chan JL, Mantzoros CS. Leptin and reproduction: a review. Fertil Steril 2002;77:433-444.
429. Williams NI, Helmreich DL, Parfitt DB, et al. Evidence for a causal role of low energy availability in the induction of menstrual cycle disturbances during strenuous exercise training. J Clin Endocrinol Metab 2001;86:5184-5193.
430. Hobart JA, Smucker DR. The female athlete triad. Am Fam Physician 2000;61:3357-3364.
431. Goldstone AP: Prader-Willi syndrome: advances in genetics, pathophysiology and treatment. Trends Endocrinol Metab 2004;15: 12-20.
432. Hackney AC. Endurance exercise training and reproductive endocrine dysfunction in men: alterations in the hypothalamic-pituitary-testicular axis. Curr Pharm Des 2001;7:261-273.
433. Opstad K. Circadian rhythm of hormones is extinguished during prolonged physical stress, sleep and energy deficiency in young men. Eur J Endocrinol 1994;131:56-66.
434. Abs R, Verhelst J, Maeyaert J, et al. Endocrine consequences of long-term intrathecal administration of opioids. J Clin Endocrinol Metab 2000;85:2215-2222.
435. Vanhorebeek I, Van den Berghe G. The neuroendocrine response to critical illness is a dynamic process. Crit Care Clin 2006;22: 1-15, v.
436. Biller BM, Luciano A, Crosignani PG, et al. Guidelines for the diagnosis and treatment of hyperprolactinemia. J Reprod Med 1999;44:1075-1084.
437. Meierkord H, Shorvon S, Lightman S, et al. Comparison of the effects of frontal and temporal lobe partial seizures on prolactin levels. Arch Neurol 1992;49:225-230.
438. Molitch ME. Diagnosis and treatment of prolactinomas. Adv Intern Med 1999;44:117-153.
439. Burman P, Ritzen EM, Lindgren AC. Endocrine dysfunction in Prader-Willi syndrome: a review with special reference to GH. Endocr Rev 2001;22:787-799.
440. Gohlke BC, Khadilkar VV, Skuse D, et al. Recognition of children with psychosocial short stature: a spectrum of presentation. J Pediatr Endocrinol Metab 1998;11:509-517.
441. Gilmour J, Skuse D. A case-comparison study of the characteristics of children with a short stature syndrome induced by stress (hyperphagic short stature) and a consecutive series of unaffected "stressed" children. J Child Psychol Psychiatry 1999;40:969-978.
442. Albanese A, Hamill G, Jones J, et al. Reversibility of physiological growth hormone secretion in children with psychosocial dwarfism. Clin Endocrinol (Oxf) 1994;40:687-692.
443. Bercu BB, Diamond FB Jr. Growth hormone neurosecretory dysfunction. Clin Endocrinol Metab 1986;15:537-590.
444. Lin TH, Kirkland RT, Sherman BM, et al. Growth hormone testing in short children and their response to growth hormone therapy. J Pediatr 1989;115:57-63.
445. Attie KM. Genetic studies in idiopathic short stature. Curr Opin Pediatr 2000;12:400-404.
446. Voss LD. Short normal stature and psychosocial disadvantage: a critical review of the evidence. J Pediatr Endocrinol Metab 2001;14:701-711.
447. Mehta A, Hindmarsh PC. The use of somatropin (recombinant growth hormone) in children of short stature. Paediatr Drugs 2002;4:37-47.
448. Poussaint TY, Barnes PD, Nichols K, et al. Diencephalic syndrome: clinical features and imaging findings. AJNR Am J Neuroradiol 1997;18:1499-1505.
449. Gropman AL, Packer RJ, Nicholson HS, et al. Treatment of diencephalic syndrome with chemotherapy: growth, tumor response, and long term control. Cancer 1998;83:166-172.
450. Ho KY, Veldhuis JD, Johnson ML, et al. Fasting enhances growth hormone secretion and amplifies the complex rhythms of growth hormone secretion in man. J Clin Invest 1988; 81:968-975.

451. Saeger W, Puchner MJ, Ludecke DK. Combined sellar gangliocytoma and pituitary adenoma in acromegaly or Cushing's disease. A report of 3 cases. Virchows Arch 1994;425:93-99.
452. Posener JA, DeBattista C, Williams GH, et al. 24-Hour monitoring of cortisol and corticotropin secretion in psychotic and nonpsychotic major depression. Arch Gen Psychiatry 2000;57:755-760.
453. Chrousos GP. The role of stress and the hypothalamic-pituitary-adrenal axis in the pathogenesis of the metabolic syndrome: neuro-endocrine and target tissue-related causes. Int J Obes Relat Metab Disord 2000;24(suppl 2):S50-S55.
454. Bjorntorp P, Rosmond R. The metabolic syndrome—a neuroendocrine disorder? Br J Nutr 2000;83(Suppl 1):S49-S57.
455. Wolff S, Adler R, Buskirk E, et al. A syndrome of periodic hypothalamic discharge. Am J Med 1964;36:956-967.
456. Albright AL, Hadjipanayis CG, Lunsford LD, et al. Individualized treatment of pediatric craniopharyngiomas. Childs Nerv Syst 2005;21:649-654.
457. Lin L, Faraco J, Li R, et al. The sleep disorder canine narcolepsy is caused by a mutation in the hypocretin (orexin) receptor 2 gene. Cell 1999;98:365-376.
458. Chemelli RM, Willie JT, Sinton CM, et al. Narcolepsy in orexin knockout mice: molecular genetics of sleep regulation. Cell 1999;98:437-451.
459. Eriksson KS, Sergeeva O, Brown RE, et al. Orexin/hypocretin excites the histaminergic neurons of the tuberomammillary nucleus. J Neurosci 2001;21:9273-9279.
460. Gerashchenko D, Kohls MD, Greco M, et al. Hypocretin-2-saporin lesions of the lateral hypothalamus produce narcoleptic-like sleep behavior in the rat. J Neurosci 2001;21:7273-7283.
461. Thannickal TC, Moore RY, Nienhuis R, et al. Reduced number of hypocretin neurons in human narcolepsy. Neuron 2000;27:469-474.

CHAPTER 8

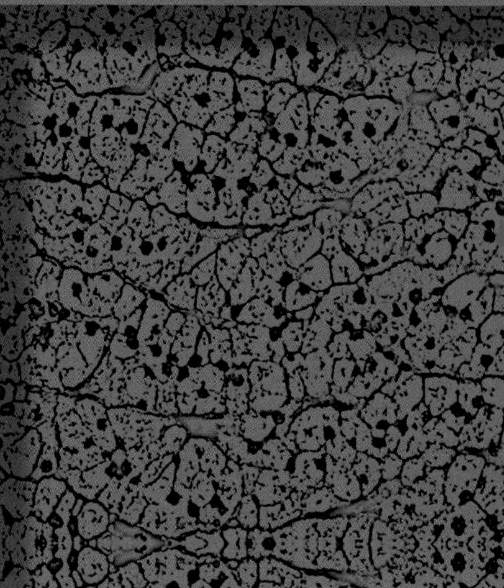

ANTERIOR PITUITARY

Shlomo Melmed and David Kleinberg

DEVELOPMENT, ANATOMY, AND OVERVIEW OF CONTROL OF HORMONE SECRETION

The pituitary gland, situated within the sella turcica, derives its name from the Greek *ptuo* and Latin *pituita,* "phlegm," reflecting its nasopharyngeal origin. Galen hypothesized that nasal phlegm originated from the brain and drained via the pituitary gland. It is now clear that together with the hypothalamus, the pituitary orchestrates the structural integrity and function of endocrine glands including the thyroid, adrenal, and gonads, in addition to target tissues including cartilage and breast. The pituitary stalk serves as an anatomic and functional connection to the hypothalamus. Preservation of the hypothalamic-pituitary unit is critical for integration of anterior pituitary control of sexual function and fertility, linear and organ growth, lactation, stress responses, energy, appetite, and temperature regulation and secondarily for carbohydrate and mineral metabolism.

Integration of vital body functions by the brain was first proposed by Descartes in the 17th century. In 1733, Morgagni recorded the absence of adrenal glands in an anencephalic neonate, providing early evidence for a developmental and functional connection between the brain and the adrenal glands. In 1849, Claude Bernard set the stage for the subsequent advances in neuroendocrinology by demonstrating that central lesions to the area of the fourth ventricle resulted in polyuria.[1] Subsequent studies led to the identification and chemical isolation of pituitary hormones, and astute clinical observations led to the realization that pituitary tumors were associated with functional hypersecretory syndromes, including acromegaly and Cushing's disease.[2-4] In 1948, Geoffrey Harris, the father of modern neuroendocrinology, in reviewing anterior pituitary gland hormone control, proposed their hypothalamic regulation, predicting the subsequent discovery of specific hypothalamic regulating hormones.[5]

Anatomy

The pituitary gland comprises the predominant anterior lobe, the posterior lobe, and a vestigial intermediate lobe (Fig. 8–1). The gland is situated within the bony sella turcica and is overlaid by the dural diaphragma sella, through which the stalk connects to the median eminence of the hypothalamus. The adult pituitary weighs about 600 mg (range 400-900 mg) and measures about 13 mm in the longest transverse diameter, 6 to 9 mm vertically, and about 9 mm anteroposteriorly. Structural variation can occur in multiparous women, and gland volume also changes during the menstrual cycle. During pregnancy these measurements may be increased in either dimension, with pituitary weight increasing up to 1 gram. Recently, normal pituitary hypertrophy without evidence for the presence of an adenoma was described in seven eugonadal women with pituitary height greater than 9 mm and a convex upper gland boundary observed on magnetic resonance imaging (MRI).[6]

The sella turcica, located at the base of the skull, forms the thin bony roof of the sphenoid sinus. The lateral walls comprising, either bony or dural tissue, abut the cavernous sinuses, which are traversed by the third, fourth, and sixth cranial nerves and the internal carotid arteries (Fig. 8–2). Thus, the cavernous sinus contents are vulnerable to increased intrasellar expansion. The dural roofing protects the gland from compression by fluctuant cerebrospinal fluid (CSF) pressure. The optic chiasm, located anterior to the pituitary stalk, is directly above the diaphragma sella. The optic tracts and central structures are therefore vulnerable to pressure effects by an expanding pituitary mass, which likely follows the path of least tissue resistance by lifting the diaphragma sella (Fig. 8–3). The intimate relationship of the pituitary and chiasm is borne out in optic chiasmic hypoplasia associated with developmental pituitary dysfunction seen in patients with septo-optic dysplasia. The posterior pituitary gland, in contrast to the anterior pituitary, is directly innervated by supraopticohypophyseal and tuberohypophyseal nerve tracts of the posterior stalk. Hypothalamic neuronal lesions, stalk disruption, or direct systemically derived metasta-

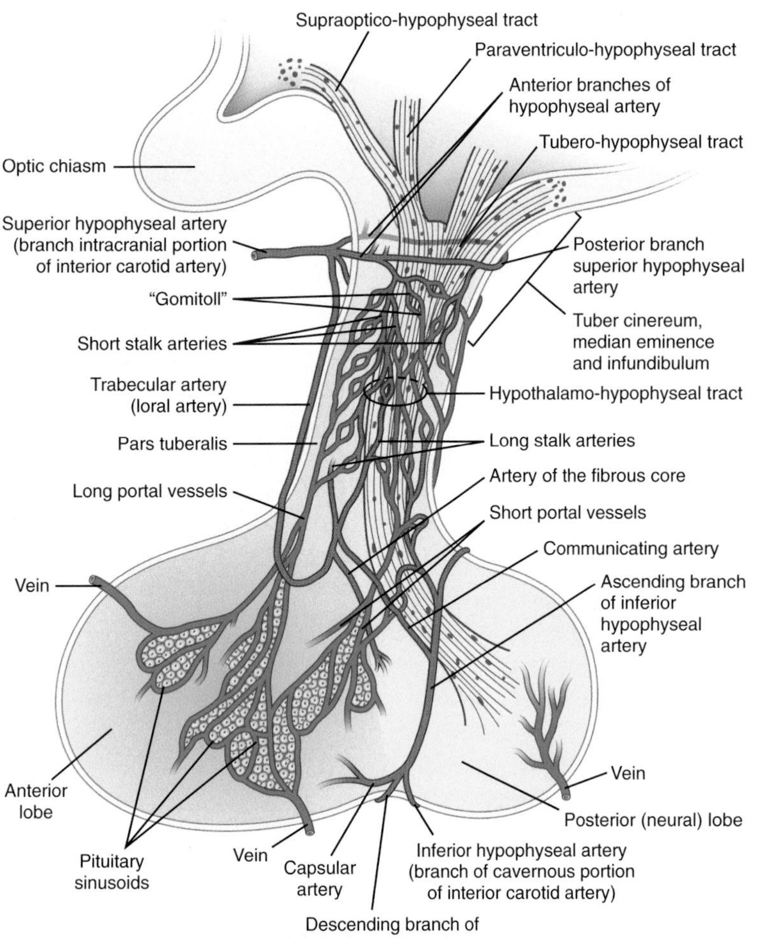

Figure 8–1 ▪ Schematic representation of the blood supply of the hypothalamus and pituitary (From Scheithauer BW. The hypothalamus and neurohypophysis. In Kovacs K, Asa SL, eds. Functional Endocrine Pathology. Boston: Blackwell Science, 1991:170-244.)

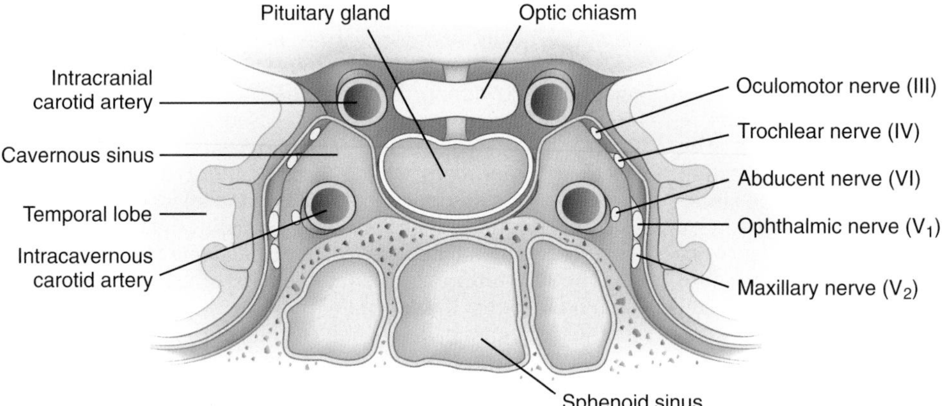

Figure 8–2 ▪ Coronal section of the sellar structures and cavernous sinus showing the relationship of the oculomotor (III), trochlear (IV), trigeminal ophthalmic and maxillary divisions (V_1 and V_2), and abducent (VI) cranial nerves to the pituitary gland. (From Stiver SI, Sharpe JA. Neuro-ophthalmologic evaluation of pituitary tumors. In Thapar K, Kovacs K, Scheithauer BW, Lloyd RV, eds. Diagnosis and Management of Pituitary Tumors Totowa, NJ: Humana Press, 2001:173-200).

ses therefore are often associated with attenuated vasopressin (AVP) (diabetes insipidus) or oxytocin secretion, or both.

The hypothalamus contains nerve cell bodies that synthesize hypophysiotropic releasing and inhibiting hormones, as well as the neurohypophyseal hormones of the posterior pituitary (AVP and oxytocin). Five distinct hormone-secreting cell types are present in the mature anterior pituitary gland. Corticotroph cells express pro-opiomelanocortin (POMC) peptides including adrenocorticotropic hormone (ACTH); somatotroph cells express growth hormone (GH); thyrotroph cells express the common glycoprotein α-subunit and the specific thyroid-stimulating hormone (TSH) β-subunit; gonadotrophs express the α and β subunits for both follicle-stimulating hormone (FSH) and luteinizing hormone (LH); the lactotroph expresses prolactin (PRL). Each cell type is under highly specific signal controls, which regulate their respective differentiated gene expression.

Pituitary Development

The pituitary gland arises from within the rostral neural plate. Rathke's pouch, a primitive ectodermal invagination anterior to the roof of the oral cavity, is formed by the fourth to fifth week of gestation and gives rise to the anterior pituitary gland (Fig.

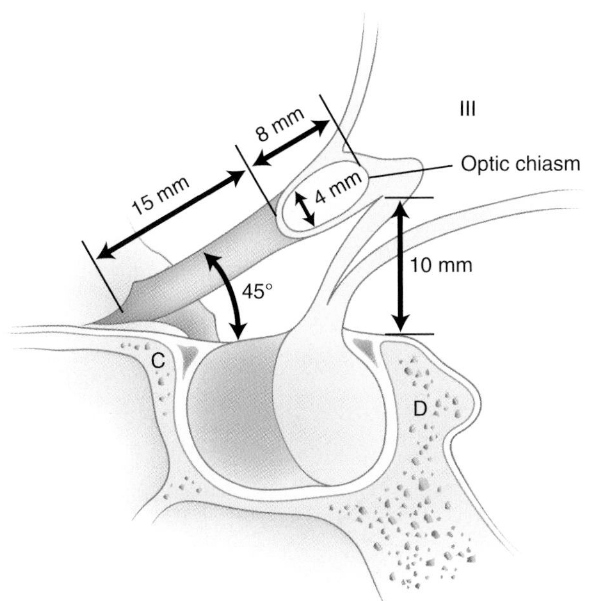

Figure 8–3 ▪ Relationship of the pituitary gland to the optic chiasm. The intracranial optic nerve/chiasmal complex lies up to 10 mm above the diaphragma sellae (*C* represents the anterior clinoid process and *D* represents the dorsum of the sella turcica). (From Miller NR. Walsh and Hoyt's Clinical Neuro-Opthalmology, 4th ed, Vol 1. Baltimore: Williams and Wilkins, 1985:60-69).

8–4).[7,8] The pouch is directly connected to the stalk and hypothalamic infundibulum, and it ultimately becomes distinct from the oral cavity and nasopharynx. Rathke's pouch proliferates toward the third ventricle, where it fuses with the diverticulum, and subsequently obliterates its lumen, which sometimes persists as Rathke's cleft. The anterior lobe is formed from Rathke's pouch, and the diverticulum gives rise to the adjacent posterior lobe. Remnants of pituitary tissue can persist in the nasopharyngeal midline, and they rarely give rise to functional ectopic hormone-secreting tumors in the nasopharynx. The neurohypophysis arises from neural ectoderm associated with third ventricle development.[9]

Functional development of the anterior pituitary cell types involves complex spatiotemporal regulation of cell lineage–specific transcription factors expressed in pluripotential pituitary stem cells, as well as dynamic gradients of locally acting soluble factors.[10,11,12] Critical neuro-ectodermal signals for organizing the dorsal gradient of pituitary morphogenesis include infundibular bone morphogenetic protein 4 (BMP4) required for the initial pouch invagination,[8] fibroblast growth factor 8 (FGF-8), Wnt 5, and Wnt 4. Subsequent ventral developmental patterning and transcription factor expression is determined by spatial and graded expression of BMP2 and sonic hedgehog protein (shh) which appears critical for directing early patterns of cell proliferation.[13]

The human fetal Rathke's pouch is evident at 3 weeks, and the pituitary grows rapidly in utero. By 7 weeks, the anterior pituitary vasculature begins to develop, and by 20 weeks, the entire hypophyseal-portal system is already established. The anterior pituitary undergoes major cellular differentiation during the first 12 weeks, by which time all the major secretory cell compartments are structurally and functionally intact, except for lactotrophs. Totipotential pituitary stem cells give rise to acidophilic (mammosomatotroph, somatotroph, and lactotroph) and basophilic (corticotroph, thyrotroph, and gonadotroph) differentiated pituitary cell types, which appear at clearly demarcated developmental stages. At 6 weeks, corticotroph cells are morphologically identifiable, and immunoreactive ACTH is detectable by 7 weeks. At 8 weeks, somatotroph cells are evident, with abundant immunoreactive cytoplasmic GH expression. Glycoprotein hormone–secreting cells express a common α-subunit for TSH, and at 12 weeks, differentiated thyrotrophs and gonadotrophs express immunoreactive β-subunits LH and FSH, respectively. Interestingly, in female fetuses, LH- and FSH-expressing gonadotrophs are equally distributed, whereas in the male fetus, LH-expressing gonadotrophs predominate.[14] Fully differentiated PRL-expressing lactotrophs are only evident late in gestation (after 24 weeks). Before then, immunoreactive PRL is only detectable in mixed mammosomatotrophs, also expressing GH, reflecting the common genetic origin of these two hormones.[15]

Pituitary Transcription Factors

Determination of anterior pituitary cell type lineages results from a temporally regulated cascade of homeodomain transcription factors. Although most pituitary developmental information has been acquired from murine models,[16] histologic and pathogenetic observations in human subjects have largely corroborated these developmental mechanisms (see Fig. 8–4). Early cell differentiation requires intracellular Rpx and Ptx expression. Rathke's pouch expresses several transcription factors of the LIM homeodomain family, including Lhx3, Lhx4, and Isl-1,[17] which are early determinants of functional pituitary development. Pitx1 is expressed in the oral ectoderm, and subsequently in all pituitary cell types, particularly those arising ventrally.[18] Rieger's syndrome, characterized by defective eye, tooth, umbilical cord, and pituitary development, is caused by defective related Pitx2.[19,20]

Ptx behaves as a universal pituitary regulator and activates transcription of the α-glycoprotein subunit (α-GSU), POMC, and LHβ (Ptx1) and GH (Ptx2). Lhx3 determines GH-, PRL-, and TSH-cell diffentiation, and Prop-1 behaves as a prerequisite for Pit-1, which activates GH, PRL, TSH, and growth hormone–releasing hormone (GHRH) receptor transcription. TSH and gonadotropin-expressing cells share a common α-subunit (αGSU) expression under developmental control of GATA-2.[11] These specific anterior pituitary transcription factors participate in a highly orchestrated cascade leading to the commitment of the five differentiated cell types (see Fig. 8–4). The major proximal determinant of pituitary cell lineage derived from a totipotential stem cell is thus Prop-1 expression, which determines subsequent development of PIT-1–dependent and gonadotroph cell lineages.[21]

POU1F1, the renamed Pit-1, is a POU-homeodomain transcription factor, which determines development and appropriate temporal and spatial expression of cells committed to GH-, PRL-, TSH-, and GHRH-receptor expression. POU1F1 binds to specific DNA motifs and activates and regulates somatotroph, lactotroph, and thyrotroph development and mature secretory function. Signal-dependent coactivating factors also cooperate with Pit-1 to determine specific hormone expression. Thus, in POU1F1-containing cells, high estrogen receptor levels induce a commitment to express PRL, whereas thyrotroph embryonic factor (TEF) favors TSH expression. Selective pituitary cell-type specificity is also perpetuated by binding of POU1F1 to its own DNA regulatory elements as well as those contained within the GH, PRL, and TSH genes. Steroidogenic factor (SF-1) and DAX-1 determine subsequent gonadotroph development.[22,23] Corticotroph cell commitment, although occurring earliest during fetal development, is independent of POU1F1-determined lineages, and T-pit protein appears to be a prerequisite for POMC expression.[24] Hereditary mutations arising within these transcription factors can result in isolated or combined pituitary hormone failure syndromes (see later).

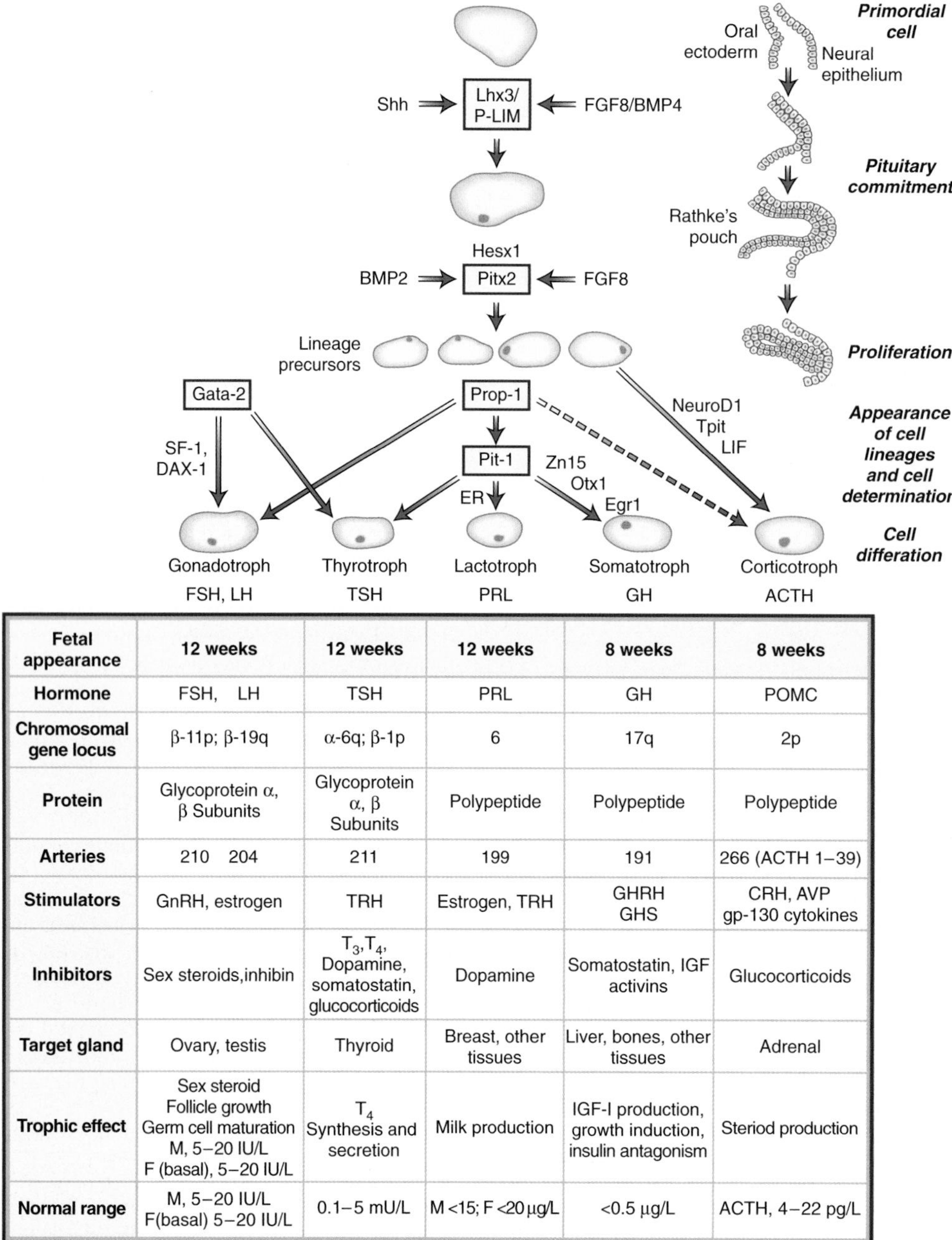

Fetal appearance	12 weeks	12 weeks	12 weeks	8 weeks	8 weeks
Hormone	FSH, LH	TSH	PRL	GH	POMC
Chromosomal gene locus	β-11p; β-19q	α-6q; β-1p	6	17q	2p
Protein	Glycoprotein α, β Subunits	Glycoprotein α, β Subunits	Polypeptide	Polypeptide	Polypeptide
Arteries	210 204	211	199	191	266 (ACTH 1–39)
Stimulators	GnRH, estrogen	TRH	Estrogen, TRH	GHRH GHS	CRH, AVP gp-130 cytokines
Inhibitors	Sex steroids,inhibin	T_3,T_4, Dopamine, somatostatin, glucocorticoids	Dopamine	Somatostatin, IGF activins	Glucocorticoids
Target gland	Ovary, testis	Thyroid	Breast, other tissues	Liver, bones, other tissues	Adrenal
Trophic effect	Sex steroid Follicle growth Germ cell maturation M, 5–20 IU/L F (basal), 5–20 IU/L	T_4 Synthesis and secretion	Milk production	IGF-I production, growth induction, insulin antagonism	Steriod production
Normal range	M, 5–20 IU/L F(basal) 5–20 IU/L	0.1–5 mU/L	M <15; F <20 μg/L	<0.5 μg/L	ACTH, 4–22 pg/L

Figure 8–4 ▪ Model for development of the human anterior pituitary gland and cell lineage determination by a cascade of transcription factors. Trophic cells are depicted with transcription factors known to determine cell-specific human or murine gene expression. ACTH, adrenocorticotropic hormone; BMP, bone morphogenetic protein; FSH, follicle-stimulating hormone; GH, growth hormone; FGF, fibroblast growth factor; LH, luteinizing hormone; PRL, prolactin; TSH, thyroid-stimulating hormone. (Adapted from Melmed S. Anterior Pituitary. In Conn P, Melmed S, eds. Scientific Basis of Endocrinology. Totowa, NJ: Humana Press, 1996:30-48; Amselem S. Perspectives on the molecular basis of developmental defects in the human pituitary region. In Rappaport R, Amselem S, eds. Hypothalamic-Pituitary Development. Basel: Karger, 2001:30-47; Dasen JS, Rosenfeld MG. Signaling mechanisms in pituitary morphogenesis and cell fate determination. Curr Opin Cell Biol 1999;11:669-677.)

Pituitary Blood Supply

The pituitary gland enjoys an abundant blood supply derived from several sources (see Fig. 8–1). The superior hypophyseal arteries branch from the internal carotid arteries to supply the hypothalamus, where they form a capillary network in the median eminence, external to the blood-brain barrier. Both long and short hypophyseal portal vessels originate from infundibular plexuses and the stalk, respectively. These vessels form the hypothalamic-portal circulation, the predominant blood supply to the anterior pituitary gland. They deliver hypothalamic releasing and inhibiting hormones to the trophic hormone-producing cells of the adenohypophysis, without significant systemic dilution, allowing the pituitary cells to be sensitively regulated by timed hypothalamic hormone secretion. Vascular transport of hypothalamic hormones is also locally regulated by a contractile internal capillary plexus (gomitoli) derived from stalk branches of the superior hypophysial arteries.[25] Retrograde blood flow toward the median eminence also occurs, facilitating bidirectional functional hypothalamic-pituitary interactions.[26] Systemic arterial blood supply is maintained by inferior hypophysial arterial branches, which predominantly supply the posterior pituitary. Disruption of stalk integrity can lead to compromised pituitary portal blood flow, depriving the anterior pituitary cells of hypothalamic hormone access.

Pituitary Control

Three levels of control subserve the regulation of anterior pituitary hormone secretion (Fig. 8–5). Hypothalamic control is mediated by adenohypophysiotropic hormones, which are secreted into the portal system and impinge directly upon anterior pituitary cell surface receptors. G-protein–linked cell surface membrane binding sites are highly selective and specific for each of the hypothalamic hormones, and they elicit positive or negative signals mediating pituitary hormone gene transcription and secretion. Peripheral hormones also participate in mediating pituitary cell function, predominantly by negative feedback regulation of trophic hormones by their respective target hormones. Intrapituitary paracrine and autocrine soluble growth factors and cytokines act to locally regulate neighboring cell development and function.

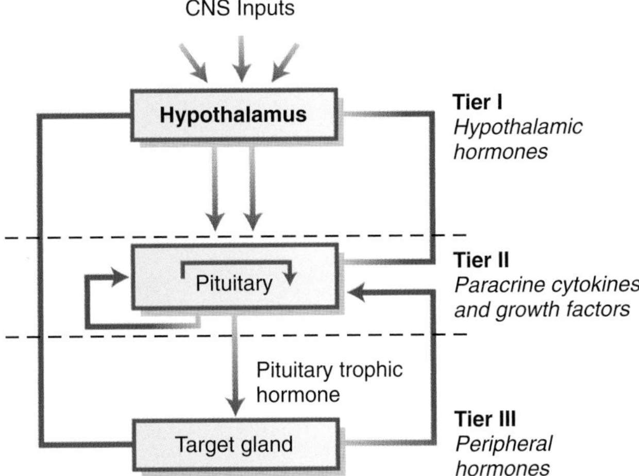

Figure 8–5 ▪ Model for regulation of anterior pituitary hormone secretion by three tiers of control. Hypothalamic hormones traverse the portal system and impinge directly upon their respective target cells. Intrapituitary cytokines and growth factors regulate tropic cell function by paracrine and autocrine control. Peripheral hormones exert negative feedback inhibition of respective pituitary trophic hormone synthesis and secretion. CNS, central nervous system. (From Ray D, Melmed S. Pituitary cytokine and growth factor expression and action. Endocr Rev 1997;18:206-228.)

The net result of these three tiers of complex intracellular signals is the controlled pulsatile secretion of the six pituitary trophic hormones, ACTH, GH, PRL, TSH, FSH, and LH, through the cavernous sinus, petrosal veins, and ultimately the systemic circulation via the superior vena cava (Fig. 8–6). The temporal and quantitative control of pituitary hormone secretion is critical for physiologic integration of peripheral hormonal systems, such as the menstrual cycle, which relies on complex and precisely regulated pulse control.

PITUITARY MASSES

Mass Effects

An expanding pituitary mass can inexorably alter the sellar size and shape by bony erosion and remodeling (Fig. 8–7). Although the exact time course for this process is unknown, it appears to be slowly progressive over years or decades. The tumor can invade soft tissue, and the dorsal sellar roof presents the least resistance to expansion from within the confines of the bony sella. Nevertheless, both suprasellar and parasellar compression and invasion can occur with an enlarging mass, with resultant clinical manifestations (Table 8–1).

As tumors impinge upon the optic chiasm they interfere with vision. Because of the anatomy of the chiasm, pressure from below affects temporal visual fields, starting superiorly

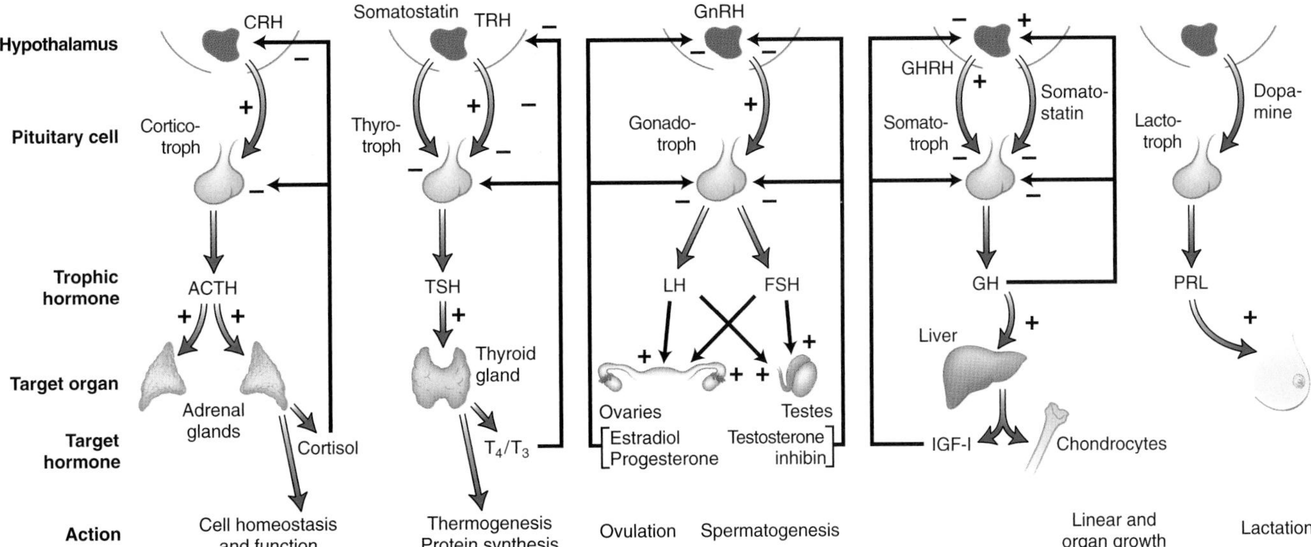

Figure 8–6 ▪ Control of hypothalamic-pituitary target organ axes. ACTH, adrenocorticotropic hormone; CRH, corticotropin-releasing hormone; FSH, follicle-stimulating hormone; GH, growth hormone; GHRH, growth hormone–releasing hormone; GnRH, gonadotropin-releasing hormone; IGF, insulin-like growth factor; LH, luteinizing hormone; T_3, triiodothyronine; T_4, thyroxine; TRH, thyrotrophin-releasing hormone; TSH, thyroid-stimulating hormone. Adapted from Melmed S, Mechanisms for pituitary tumorigenesis. The plastic pituitary. J Clin Investigation 2003 112:1603-1618.

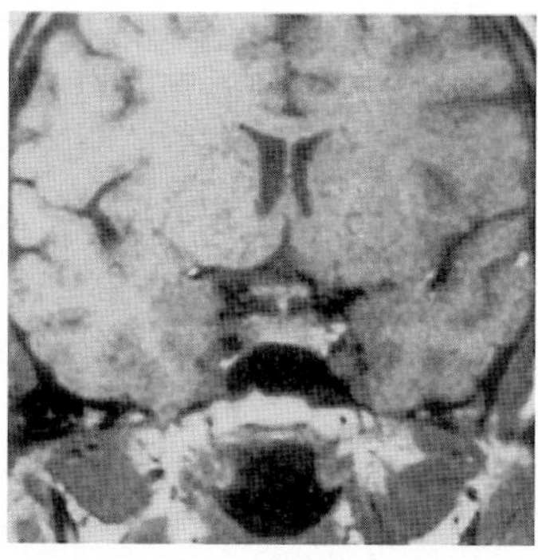

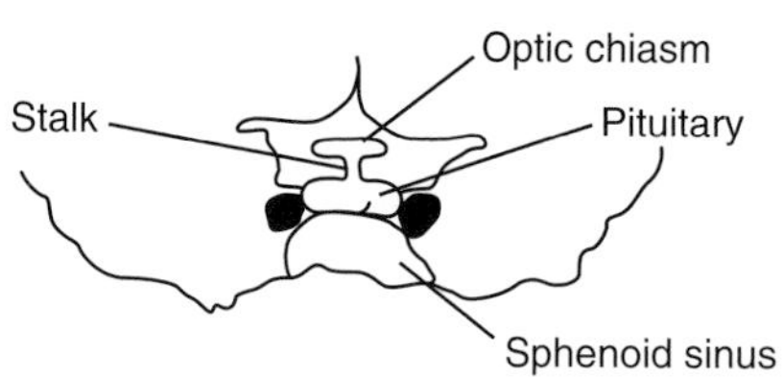

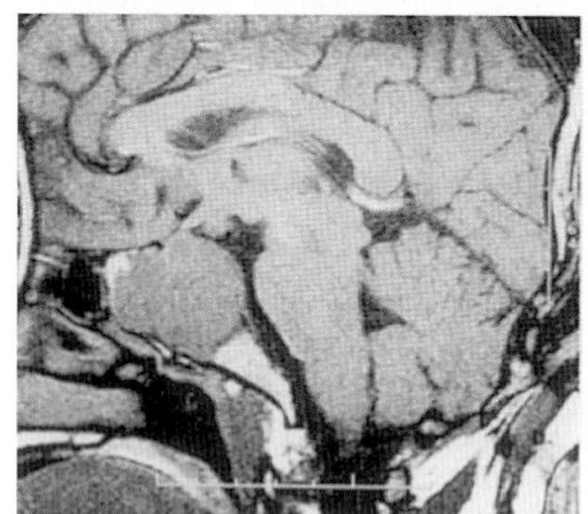

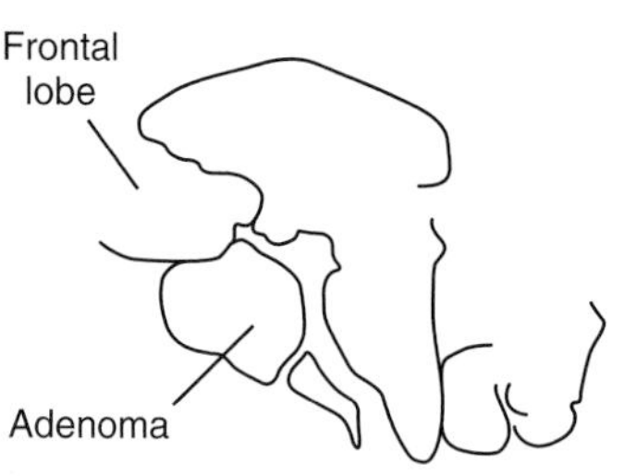

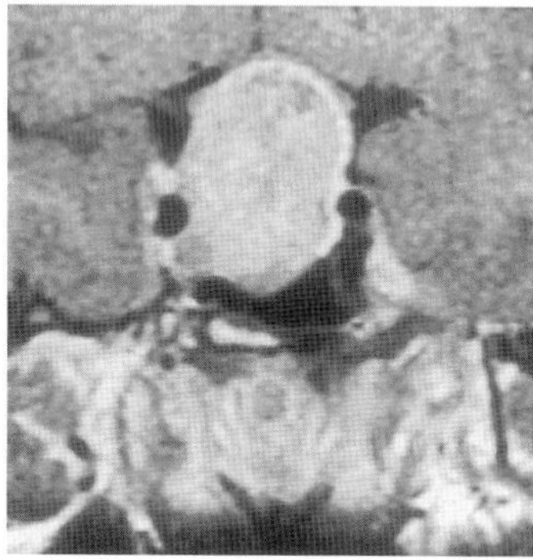

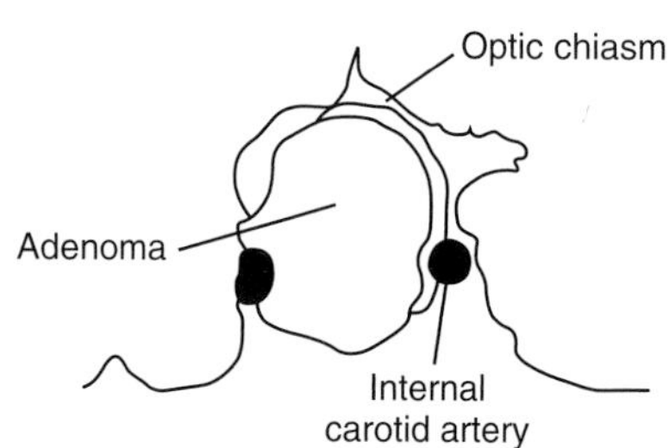

Figure 8–7 ▪ Magnetic resonance coronal section of a normal pituitary gland *(top)*. A large pituitary adenoma is seen lifting and distorting the optic chiasm *(arrow)* and also invading the sphenoid sinus *(middle)*. A sagittal section of a large macroadenoma with bone invasion and impinging brain structures *(bottom)*.

and ultimately extending to the entire temporal field. Continued growth and pressure on the optic apparatus can extend vision loss to the nasal field and can result in blindness. Long-standing optic chiasmal pressure results in optic disc pallor. Lateral invasion of pituitary lesions can invade the dural wall of the cavernous sinus, affecting the third, fourth, and sixth cranial nerves as well as the ophthalmic and maxillary branches of the fifth cranial nerve and can surround the internal carotid artery. Varying degrees of diplopia, ptosis, ophthalmoplegia, and decreased facial sensation infrequently occur, depending on the extent of the neural involvement by the cavernous sinus mass.

Downward extension into the sphenoid sinus indicates that the parasellar mass has eroded the bony sellar floor. Aggressive tumors can invade the roof of the palate and cause nasopharyngeal obstruction, infection and CSF leakage. Infrequently temporal or frontal lobes may be invaded causing uncinate seizures, personality disorders and anosmia. In addition to the anatomical lesions caused by the expanding mass direct hypothalamic involvement of the encroaching mass can lead to important metabolic sequelae discussed in Chapter 7.

Intrasellar tumors commonly manifest with headaches, even in the absence of demonstrable suprasellar extension. Small changes in intrasellar pressure caused by a microadenoma within the confined sella are sufficient to stretch the dural plate, with resultant headache. Headache severity does not correlate with the size of the adenoma or the presence of suprasellar extension.[27] Relatively minor diaphragmatic distortions or dural impingement may be associated with persistent headache. Successful medical management of small functional pituitary tumors with dopamine agonists or somatostatin analogues is often accompanied by a remarkable headache improvement or disappearance.

Regardless of their etiology or size, pituitary masses, including adenomas, may be associated with compression of surrounding healthy tissue and resultant hypopituitarism. In 49 patients undergoing transsphenoidal resection of pituitary adenomas, mean intrasellar pressure was elevated two- to threefold in patients with pituitary failure. Furthermore, prevalence of headache and elevated PRL levels correlated positively with intrasellar pressure levels,[28] suggesting interrupted portal delivery of hypothalamic hormones. Thus, surgical decompression of a sellar mass can lead to recovery of compromised anterior pituitary function. In patients who do not recover pituitary function postoperatively, ischemic necrosis is likely to have occurred. Stalk compression can result in pituitary failure caused by encroachment of the portal vessels that normally provide pituitary access to the hypothalamic hormones. Stalk compression also usually leads to hyperprolactinemia and concomitant failure of other pituitary trophic hormones.

TABLE 8–1 LOCAL EFFECTS OF AN EXPANDING PITUITARY OR HYPOTHALAMIC MASS

PITUITARY	CENTRAL
Adult hyposomatotrophism Growth failure Hypoadrenalism Hypogonadism Hypothyroidism	Dementia Headache Hydrocephalus Laughing seizures Psychosis
OPTIC TRACT	**NEURO-OPHTHALMOLOGIC TRACT**
Bitemporal hemianopia Blindness Loss of red perception Scotoma Superior or bitemporal field defect **HYPOTHALAMUS** Appetite, behavioral, and autonomic nervous system dysfunctions Temperature dysregulation, obesity, diabetes insipidus Thirst, sleep **CAVERNOUS SINUS** Diplopia Facial numbness Ophthalmoplegia Ptosis **TEMPORAL LOBE** Uncinate seizures **FRONTAL LOBE** Anosmia Personality disorder	**Field Defects** Bitemporal hemianopia (50%), amaurosis with hemianopia (12%), contralateral or monocular hemianopia (7%) Homonymous hemianopia Scotomas: Hemianopic; junctional; monocular central, arcuate, altitudinal **Acuity Loss** Color vision Contrast sensitivity Snellen Visual evoked potential **Pupillary Abnormality** Afferent defect Impaired light reactivity **Optic Atrophy** Cranial nerve palsy: Abducens, oculomotor, sensory trigeminal, trochlear Nystagmus Papilledema Postfixation blindness Visual hallucinations

Adapted from Melmed S. Acromegaly. In DeGroot LJ, Jameson JL, Burger H, et al (eds). Endocrinology, 4th Edition. Philadelphia: WB Saunders, 2001:300-312; and Arnold AC. Neuro-ophthalmologic Evaluation of Pituitary Disorders. In Melmed S. The Pituitary. Malden, MA: Blackwell, 2002:687-708.

Pituitary Adenomas

Pathogenesis

Pituitary tumors account for about 15% of all intracranial neoplasms and are commonly encountered at autopsy. The Brain Tumor Registry of Japan reports that 15.8% of 28,424 cases were histologically confirmed pituitary adenomas.[29,30] They are benign monoclonal adenomas that can express and secrete hormones autonomously, leading to hyperprolactinemia, acromegaly, and Cushing's disease, or they may be functionally silent and initially diagnosed as a sellar mass. Although invariably benign, the neoplastic features of these adenomas represent a unique tumor biology that is reflected in their important local and systemic manifestations. These monoclonal neoplasms have a slow doubling time, and if small, rarely resolve spontaneously. Nevertheless, they can be aggressive and locally invasive or compressive to vital central structures. They usually express a single gene product, but polyhormonal expression might reflect a primitive stem cell or mature bimorphous cellular origin.

Hypothalamic factors might have a specific role in the pathogenesis of pituitary tumors in addition to regulating pituitary hormone gene expression and secretion (Table 8–2). Ectopic GHRH-secreting tumors (bronchial carcinoids, pancreatic islet-cell tumors, or small-cell lung carcinomas) result in GH hypersecretion, acromegaly, somatotroph hyperplasia, and occasionally somatotroph adenoma formation.[31,32] In transgenic mice overexpressing a GHRH transgene, the pituitary size increases dramatically due to somatotroph hyperplasia, and older mice develop GH-secreting adenomas.[33] However, adenomatous hormonal secretion is usually independent of physiologic hypothalamic control, and the surgical resection of small well-defined adenomas usually results in definitive cure of hormonal hypersecretion. These observations imply that these tumors do not arise because of excessive polyclonal pituitary cell proliferation due to generalized hypothalamic stimulation. However, hypothalamic factors can promote and maintain growth of already transformed pituitary adenomatous cells.

Normal and hyperplastic pituitary tissues are polyclonal, and pituitary adenomas arise as the result of monoclonal pituitary cell proliferation. Using X-chromosomal inactivation analysis, the monoclonal origin of GH-secreting, PRL-secreting,[34] and ACTH-secreting adenomas,[35,36] and nonfunctioning pituitary tumors was confirmed in female patients heterozygous for variant alleles of the X-linked genes hypoxanthine

TABLE 8–2 FACTORS INVOLVED IN PITUITARY TUMOR PATHOGENESIS

HEREDITARY
MEN-1 Transcription factor defect (e.g., Prop-1 excess) Carney's complex AIP mutation
HYPOTHALAMIC
Excess GHRH or CRH production Receptor activation Dopamine deprivation
PITUITARY
Signal transduction mutations (e.g., gsp, CREB) Disrupted paracrine growth factor or cytokine action (e.g., FGF-2, FGF-4, LIF, EGF, NGF) Activated oncogene or cell cycle disruption (e.g., PTTG; ras; p27) Intrapituitary paracrine hypothalamic hormone action (e.g., GHRH, TRH) Loss of tumor suppressor gene function (11q13; 13)
ENVIRONMENTAL
Estrogens Irradiation
PERIPHERAL
Target failure (ovary, thyroid, adrenal)

CREB, cyclic adenosine monophosphate response element–binding protein; CRH, corticotropin-releasing hormone; EGF, epidermal growth factor; FGF, fibroblast growth factor; GHRH, growth hormone–releasing hormone; LIF, leukemia growth factor; MEN-1, multiple endocrine neoplasia type 1; NGF, nerve growth factor; PTTG, pituitary tumor transforming gene; TRH, thyrotropin-releasing hormone.

Compiled from Melmed S. Pituitary tumorigenesis: the plastic pituitary. J Clin Inv 2003;112:1602-1618.

phosphoribosyl transferase *(HPRT)* and phosphoglycerate kinase *(PGK)*. Thus, an intrinsic somatic pituitary cell genetic alteration likely gives rise to clonal expansion of a single cell, resulting in adenoma formation (Table 8–3).

Activating *gsp* mutations are present in up to 40% of human GH-secreting adenomas.[37-39] These somatic heterozygous activating point mutations of the G protein α-subunit ($G_s\alpha$) gene involving either arginine 201 (replaced by cysteine or histidine) or glutamine 227 (replaced with arginine or leucine) constitutively activate the $G_s\alpha$ protein and convert it into an oncogene *(gsp)*. This G protein activation increases cyclic adenosine monophosphate (cAMP) levels and activates protein kinase A (PKA), which in turn phosphorylates the cAMP response element-binding protein (CREB) and leads to sustained constitutive GH hypersecretion and cell proliferation. The *gsp*-bearing adenomas are smaller, have mildly lower GH levels and enhanced intratumoral cAMP, do not respond briskly to GHRH, and are extremely sensitive to the inhibitory effect of somatostatin.[39] The *gsp*-activating mutations do not occur in PRL-secreting and in TSH-producing adenomas and are rarely present in nonfunctioning pituitary tumors or ACTH-secreting tumors (<10%).

Similar early postzygotic somatic mutations in codon 201 of the $G_s\alpha$ were identified in tissues derived from patients with McCune-Albright syndrome, including GH-producing pituitary adenomas.[40] Transgenic mice overexpressing inactive pituitary CREB mutant exhibit a dwarf phenotype and somatotroph hypoplasia.[41] Thus, cAMP probably stimulates somatotroph proliferation by CREB phosphorylation. This was borne out by the observation that 15 human GH-secreting pituitary adenomas contained elevated levels of phosphorylated CREB.[42] However, only four of these tumors also contained the mutant *gsp* oncogene, and CREB phosphorylation was also demonstrated in adenomas overexpressing wild-type $G_s\alpha$ protein, suggesting a role of CREB that is independent of G-protein actions.

Very rarely, pituitary tumors metastasize either outside the central nervous system or as a separate focus within it.[43] Because no cell markers clearly distinguish aggressive invasiveness from malignancy, demonstration of extracranial metastasis is a prerequisite for diagnosis. When they occur, these malignancies most often secrete either ACTH or PRL. Ras mutations are rare in pituitary adenomas. H-ras gene mutations were identified in invasive prolactinoma[44] and in distant metastatic pituitary carcinomas, but not in their respective primary pituitary tumors or in noninvasive adenomas.[45,46] Thus, ras genetic alterations may be important in the very rare progression to metastatic formation and growth.

Pituitary tumor transforming gene (PTTG) was isolated from experimental pituitary tumors and shown to be highly abundant in all pituitary tumor types, especially prolactinomas.[47,48] PTTG, a mammalian securin homolog, also induces FGF production and angiogenesis and is up-regulated by estrogen.[49] PTTG overexpression can lead to dysregulated separation and cell aneuploidy.[50,51]

Multiple endocrine neoplasia type 1 (MEN-1), an autosomal dominant hereditary disorder characterized by combined tumor formation or hyperfunction of pancreatic islets, anterior pituitary, and, less commonly, carcinoid, thyroid, and adrenal tumors. The MEN-1 syndrome is fully described in Chapter 40. Unlike pituitary tumors comprising the MEN-1 syndrome, MEN-1 gene mutations were not identified in familial pituitary adenomas.[52,53] Patients with sporadic pituitary adenomas do not demonstrate germline or somatic pathogenic changes in the coding sequence of the MEN-1 gene, even in tumors with loss of heterozygosity of 11q13, and only two cases of sporadic pituitary adenomas (of 94 tumors studied) had specific MEN-1 mutations.[54] Thus, MEN-1 gene mutations do not appear to play a role in pituitary tumorigenesis in most sporadic adenomas.

Loss of heterozygosity for chromosomes 9, 11q13, and 13 are observed in about 15% of spontaneous pituitary adenomas, often correlating with tumor size and invasiveness. However, no distinct tumor suppressor gene has been identified for sporadic pituitary tumors. Loss of heterozygosity in proximity to the Rb locus on chromosome 13q14 was detected in malignant or highly invasive pituitary tumors and in their metastases, but immunohistochemical studies have shown the presence of Rb protein in these malignant tumors with 13q14 allelic loss,[55] suggesting that the Rb gene itself is not involved in pituitary adenoma development, and another suppressor gene located adjacent to the Rb locus can play a role in invasive or malignant pituitary tumorigenesis. No *p53* gene mutations were detected in secreting and nonsecreting pituitary tumors or in pituitary carcinomas and their metastases.[46,56]

Although mutations in the GHRH, corticotropin-releasing hormone (CRH), thyrotropin-releasing hormone (TRH), or gonadotropin-releasing hormone (GnRH) receptor have not been identified in pituitary adenomas[57,58] several GH-secreting adenomas express an alternatively spliced truncated GHRH receptor.[59] The insulin-like growth factor (IGF)-I receptor β-subunit in GH-cell adenomas exhibited intact regions of the receptor critical for signal transduction.[60] Dopamine D2 receptor gene appears intact in PRL- and TSH-producing or nonfunc-

TABLE 8–3 CANDIDATE GENES IN PITUITARY TUMORIGENESIS

Gene	Tumor Type	Mechanism of Overexpression or Inactivation	Function or Defect
		ACTIVATING	
gsp	40% GH-secreting tumors	Point mutation at codon 221 or 227	Elevated cAMP
CREB	GH-secreting	Increased ser-phosphorylated CREB	Dimerizes with cAMP-response elements
PTTG	All	Unknown, estrogen	Chromatid separation, regulates βFGF, disrupted cell cycle
H-ras	Metastatic pituitary carcinoma	Point mutation at codon 12, 13, or 61	Tyrosine kinase activation
FGFR	Prolactinomas	Truncated isoform	Constitutive phosphorylation
Galectin-3	All		Mediates progression
		INACTIVATING	
13q14	Highly invasive tumors	13q14 LOH	Inconsistent Rb protein loss, disrupted cell cycle regulation; epigenetic defect
CDKN2A	All tumor types	Gene methylation leading to absent p16, allowing Rb phosphorylation and cell cycle progression	Absent p16 leading to disrupted cell cycle regulation
C1P1/KIP1	Transgenic mouse models	Gene methylation leading to absent p27	Regulate CDK enzymes including CDK4/6-cyclin Ds
GADD45γ	Adenoma	Gene methylation	Growth arrest

cAMP, cyclic adenosine monophosphate; CDK, cyclin-dependent kinase; CREB, cAMP response element–binding protein; FGFR, fibroblast growth factor receptor; GH, growth hormone; LOH, loss of heterozygosity; Rb, retinoblastoma.

Adapted from Heaney AP, Melmed S: Molecular pathogenesis of pituitary tumors. In Wass JAH, Shalet SM (eds): Oxford Textbook of Endocrinology. New York: Oxford University Press, 2002:109-120.

TABLE 8–4 GENETIC SYNDROMES INVOLVING PITUITARY TUMORS

Syndrome	Clinical Features	Chromosome Location	Gene	Protein	Proposed Function or Defect
Multiple endocrine neoplasia type I (MEN-1)	Parathyroid, endocrine pancreas, anterior pituitary tumors (mostly prolactinomas)	11q13	Men1	Menin	Nuclear, tumor suppressor protein interacts with *junD*
Familial acromegaly	GH-cell adenomas, acromegaly/gigantism	11q13 and other loci	Not men1	—	—
McCune-Albright syndrome	Polyostotic fibrous dysplasia, pigmented skin patches; endocrine abnormalities: precocious puberty, GH-cell adenomas, acromegaly/gigantism; Cushing's syndrome	20q13.2 (mosaic)	GNAS1 (gsp)	$G_s\alpha$	Signal transduction/inactive GTPase results in constitutive cAMP elevation independent of GHRH
Carney's syndrome	Skin and cardiac myxomas, Cushing's syndrome, acromegaly	2p16	—	—	Protein kinase A signaling defect for activating GH

cAMP, cyclic adenosine monophosphate; GH, growth hormone; GHRH, growth hormone–releasing hormone; GTP, guanosine triphosphate.

Adapted from Prezant TR, Melmed S 1998 Pituitary oncogenes. In Webb SM (ed): Pituitary tumors. Bristol: Bioscientifica, 1998:81-91.

tioning adenomas.[61] Therefore, there is no apparent role of pituitary cell surface receptor mutations of hypothalamic releasing and inhibitory factors in pituitary tumorigenesis.

FGF-2 (basic FGF) and a truncated FGF receptor isoform are expressed in pituitary tissues, and they induce basal and stimulated PRL secretion from normal and pituitary adenoma cells.[62] Human pituitary adenomas express FGF-4, and transfected FGF-4 enhances PRL secretion[63,64] and tumor vascularity. FGF-4 is immunodetected in about a third of prolactinomas and is undetectable in normal pituitaries and other adenoma types.

Carney's complex is an autosomal dominant disorder comprising benign mesenchymal tumors including cardiac myxomas, schwannomas, thyroid adenomas, and pituitary adenomas associated with spotty skin pigmentation (Table 8–4).[65] The disorder has been mapped to chromosome 17q24 and results from a mutated RIα regulatory subunit of the cAMP-dependent PKA (PRKARIA), an apparent tumor suppressor gene.[66]

In summary, multifactorial mechanisms subserve the multistep pathogenetic process of pituitary adenoma formation, including early initiating chromosomal mutations that result in mutated pituitary stem cells (see Table 8–2). The transformed pituitary cell is subjected to signals facilitating clonal expansion, and several permissive factors, including hypothalamic hormone receptor signals, intrapituitary growth factors, and disordered cell cycle regulation, can determine the ultimate biologic fate of the tumor. Autonomous anterior pituitary hormone production and secretion and cell proliferation, which are the hallmarks of pituitary adenomas, result. However, the subcellular events initiating the formation of most secreting and nonfunctional pituitary adenomas have not yet been elucidated.[30]

Classification

Pituitary tumors arise from hormone-secreting adenohypophyseal cells, and their secretory products depend upon the cell of origin (Table 8–5). Previously clinically unapparent pituitary adenomas are found in about 11% of autopsies (Table 8–6). They localize to unique areas of the gland, reflecting relative cell type abundance and intragland distribution (Fig. 8–8). Although 46% of a subset of these immunostain for PRL,[67] expectant management may still be indicated.[68]

In a study on 100 normal volunteers, 10 were found to have focal abnormalities on MRI consistent with microadenomas; the abnormalities measured from 3 to 6 mm in diameter.[67,69,70] Such tumors have been called "incidentalomas." In a survey of 506 patients harboring incidentalomas, 20% were nonfunctioning, and of these, 20% increased in size during a mean follow-up of 50 months.[71]

When larger, particularly nonfunctioning tumors are encountered inadvertently, pituitary function should be assessed, including measuring PRL, IGF-I, LH, FSH, and sex steroids. A 24-hour urinary free cortisol or salivary cortisol might help exclude Cushing's disease.[72] Radiologic and surgical classifications are based upon tumor localization, size, and degree of invasiveness (Fig. 8–9). Microadenomas are intrasellar and generally less than 10 mm in widest diameter. Macroadenomas are greater than 10 mm and usually impinge upon adjacent sellar structures. Specific tumor types are considered later for each respective cell type.

Immunocytochemistry detects pituitary cell gene products at both the light and electron microscopic level and allows classification of pituitary tumors based on their function. Unlike the corticotroph, somatotroph, lactotroph, and thyrotroph cell tumors, which hypersecrete their respective hormones,[73] gonadotroph cell tumors are usually clinically silent and do not efficiently secrete their gene products.[74] Double immunostaining identifies mixed tumors expressing combinations of hormones, are often macroadenomas secreting GH concomitantly with PRL or TSH or ACTH. Generally, immunohistochemical identification of pituitary hormones correlates with tumor-specific mRNA markers measured either in whole tissue extracts by Northern analysis or at the single-cell level by in situ hybridization techniques.

With the exception of the glycoprotein α-subunit, immunohistochemical positivity of more than 5% of cells in the tumor usually reflects peripheral circulating hormone levels. Quantification of immunostaining intensity is subjective, and a scale of intensity should also include a description of the extent of staining, namely whether occasional, scattered, or most tumor cells express the immunodetectable protein. Electron microscopy is useful for assessing the ultrastructure of hormone secretory granules and their size and distribution. Other subcellular features important for diagnosis include visualizing large mitochondria in nonfunctioning oncocytomas and the secretory nature of the Golgi complex and endosplasmic reticulum, especially for prolactinomas. Peroxidase or colloid gold particles of different diameters are also sensitive electron microscopic markers for identifying and localizing intracellular hormone signals. Because even invasive pituitary tumors are slow growing, use of mitotic markers, including PCNA (proliferate cell nucleus antigen) and Ki-67, is of limited utility.[75]

Other Parasellar Masses

Hypothalamic masses are fully described in Chapter 7, and parasellar masses (Table 8–7) are described here.[76]

Rathke's Cyst

The anterior and intermediate lobes of the pituitary gland arise embryologically from Rathke's pouch. Inadequate pouch oblit-

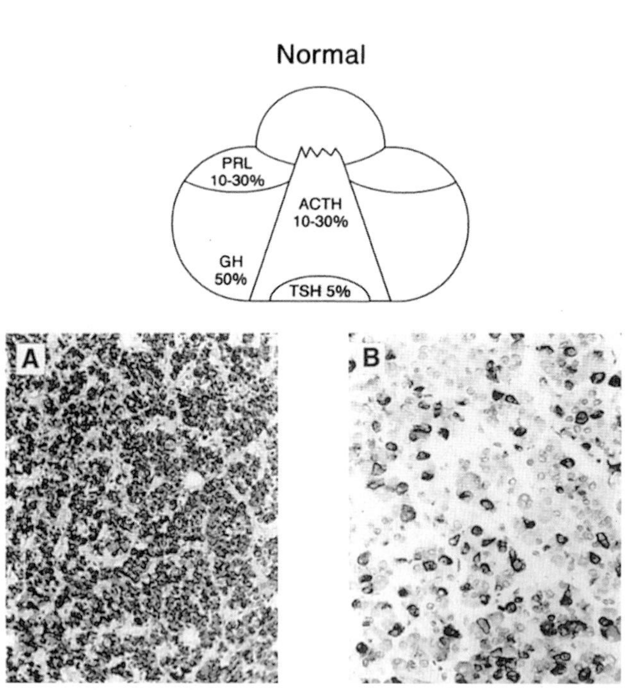

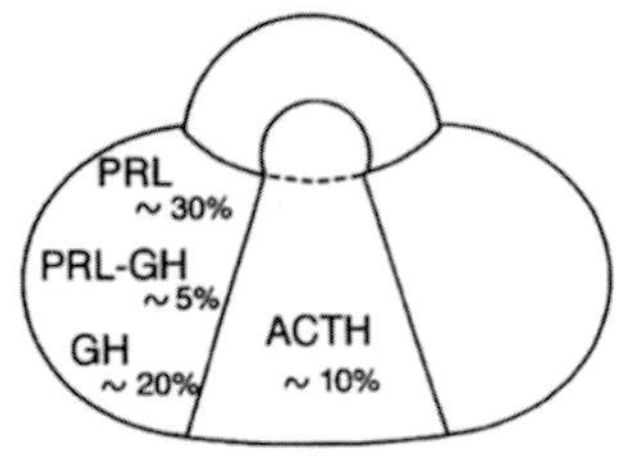

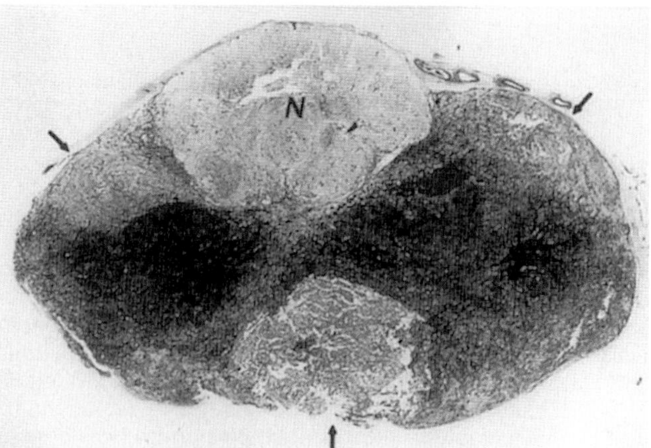

Figure 8–8 ▪ Schematic of the distribution of normal adenohypophyseal cells is reflected in that of pituitary adenomas. Nonfunctioning tumors, however, are typically macroadenomas that efface pituitary landmarks. The localization and frequency of functioning microadenomas reflects the maximum concentration of their corresponding normal pituitary cells. (From Scheithauer BW, Horvath E, Lloyd RV, Kovacs K. Pathology of pituitary adenomas and pituitary hyperplasia. In Thapar K, Kovacs K, Scheithauer BW, Lloyd RV, eds. Diagnosis and Management of Pituitary Tumors. Totawa, NJ: Humana Press, 2001:91-154.)

TABLE 8–5 CLINICAL AND PATHOLOGIC CHARACTERISTICS OF PITUITARY ADENOMAS

Adenoma Type	INCIDENCE (%)			Prevalence (total/10^6)	mRNA Expression	Immunohistochemistry	EM Secretory Granules (nm)	Clinical Syndrome
	Pathological	Clinical	Incidence (new cases/10^6/yr)					
LACTOTROPH								
All		29	6-10	60-100				
Sparsely granulated	28				PRL	PRL	150-500	Hypogonadism, galactorrhea
Densely granulated	1				PRL	PRL	400-1200	
SOMATOTROPH								
All		15	4-6	40-60				
Sparsely granulated	5				GH	GH	100-250	Acromegaly or gigantism
Densely granulated	5				GH	GH	300-700	
GH/PRL CELLS								
Combined		8						
Mixed	5				GH/PRL	GH/PRL	100-600	
MAMMOSOMATOTROPH								
All	1				GH/PRL	GH/PRL	350-2000	Hypogonadism, acromegaly, galactorrhea
Acidophil stem cell	3				GH/PRL	GH/PRL	50-300	
CORTICOTROPH								
All			2-3	20-30				
Cushing's	10	10			POMC	ACTH	250-700	Cushing's disease
Silent	3	6			POMC	ACTH	Variable	None
Nelson's	2				POMC	ACTH	250-700	Local signs
NONFUNCTIONING, NULL CELL, GONADOTROPH								
All		27	7-9	70-90				
Nononcocytic	14				FSH/LH αSU	Glycoprotein	<25% of cells 100-250	Silent or pituitary failure
Oncocytic	6				FSH/LH αSU	Glycoprotein	<25% of cells 100-250, many mitochondria	Pituitary failure
Gonadotroph	7-15				FSH/LH	FSH/LH	50-200	Silent or pituitary failure
OTHER								
Thyrotroph	1	0.9			TSH	TSH	50-250	Hyperthyroidism
Plurihormonal	10	4			GH/PRL	GH/PRL/Glycoprotein	Mixed	Mixed

FSH, follicle-stimulating hormone; GH, growth hormone; LH, luteinizing hormone; PRL, prolactin; αSU, α-subunit; TSH, thyroid-stimulating hormone.

Data are derived from studying a relatively stable 1 million catchment population surrounding Stoke-on-Trent, UK, reported in Clayton RN. Sporadic pituitary tumours: from epidemiology to use of databases. Baillieres Best Pract Res Clin Endocrinol Metab 1999;13:451-460; Asa SL. Pituitary neoplasms. In Mazzaferri EL, Samaan NA (eds): Endocrine Tumors. Boston: Blackwell Scientific, 1993:77-112.

TABLE 8–6 FREQUENCY OF PITUITARY ADENOMAS FOUND AT AUTOPSY

Study	Number of Pituitaries Examined	Number of Adenomas Found	Frequency (%)
Susman	260	23	9
Costello	1,000	225	23
Sommers	400	26	7
McCormick	1,600	140	9
Kovacs	152	20	13
Landolt	100	13	13
Mosca	100	24	24
Burrow	120	32	27
Parent	500	42	8
Muhr	205	3	2
Schwezinger	5,100	485	9
Coulon	100	10	10
Chambers	100	14	14
Siqueira	450	39	9
El-Hamid	486	97	20
Scheithauer	251	41	16
Marin	210	35	16
Mosca	111	13	11
Sano	166	15	9
Teramoto	1,000	51	5
Buurman	3,048	334	11
TOTAL	**15,459**	**1,742**	**11**

Modified from: Molitch ME. Pituitary incidentalomas. In de Herder WW (ed): Functional and Morphological Imaging of the Endocrine System. Norwell, MA: Kluwer Academic, 2000:59-70; and Buurman H, Saeger W. Subclinical adenomas in postmortem pituitaries: classification and correlations to clinical data. Eur J Endocrinol 2006;154:753-758.

eration results in cysts or cystic remnants at the interface between the anterior and posterior pituitary lobes, which are found in about 20% of pituitary glands at autopsy (Fig. 8–10).[77] Pituitary adenomas also occasionally contain small cleft cysts. They are lined by cuboidal or columnar ciliated epithelium surrounding mucoid cyst fluid. They arise from midline rudiments of failed Rathke's cyst invagination and account for about 3% of pituitary mass lesions.[78] In contrast, pituitary epidermoid cysts are lined by squamous epithelium, which rarely becomes malignant.

Rathke's cysts vary in size and can also extend to the suprasellar region. Cyst formation is associated with sellar enlargement. These lesions rarely manifest with panhypopituitarism with or without diabetes insipidus.[75] Most, however, are not symptomatic and should be followed expectantly. The extent of headache or visual disturbance is determined by the size and location of the cyst.

These lesions have heterogeneous MRI characteristics. MRI reveals hyperdense or hypodense masses on either T1 or T2 images, and computed tomography (CT) scan shows homogenous hypodense areas that can be distinguished from pituitary adenomas.[75] These patients should all be evaluated for hypopituitarism. After surgical resection or drainage, MRI should be performed during long-term follow-up for signs of cyst recurrence.[77,78]

Arachnoid, epidermoid, and dermoid cysts develop mainly in the cerebellopontine angle, but they can also arise in the suprasellar region. Dermoid cysts containing greasy sebaceous products or hair follicles are rarely encountered in the pituitary, and the cyst lining may be calcified. Acquired pituitary cysts can arise secondarily to intrapituitary hemorrhage, usually associated with an underlying adenoma, and these rarely cause

TABLE 8–7 PARASELLAR MASSES

GENETIC
Transcription factor mutations (e.g., PROP-1)
CYSTS
Arachnoid Dermoid Epidermoid Rathke's
TUMORS
Chordoma Craniopharyngioma Germ cell tumor Glioma Granular cell tumor Hormone-secreting or nonfunctional pituitary adenoma Meningioma Sarcoma Schwannoma Solid or hematological metastases Vascular tumor
MALFORMATIONS AND HAMARTOMAS
Ectopic pituitary, neurohypophyseal, or salivary tissue Gangliocytoma Hypothalamic hamartoma
MISCELLANEOUS LESIONS
Aneurysms Giant cell granuloma Histiocytosis X Hypophysitis Infections Sarcoidosis

PROP-1, prophet of Pit1 (paired-like homeodomain transcription factor).

pituitary failure.[79] Cyst compression causes internal hydrocephalus, visual disturbances, growth hormone or ACTH deficiency, hyperprolactinemia, and diabetes insipidus. Rarely squamous cell carcinoma arises in the cyst.[80]

Granular Cell Tumors

Pituitary choristomas, or schwannomas, usually manifest only after the age of 20 years. Their abundant cytoplasmic granules do not contain pituitary hormones, but these lesions can manifest with diabetes insipidus. Pituitary adenomas are occasionally coincidentally associated with these tumors.[81]

Chordomas

These slow-growing cartilaginous tumors arise from midline notochord remnants, are locally invasive, and can metastasize.[82] Most arise from the vertebrae and about one third involve the clivus region. Chordomas contain a mucin-rich matrix that allows diagnosis by fine-needle aspiration. They manifest with headaches, asymmetrical visual disturbances, hormone deficiency, and occasional nasopharyngeal obstruction. The tumor mass is associated with osteolytic bony erosion and calcification. MRI can allow the normal pituitary gland to distinguish it from the very heterogeneous and often flocculent tumor mass.

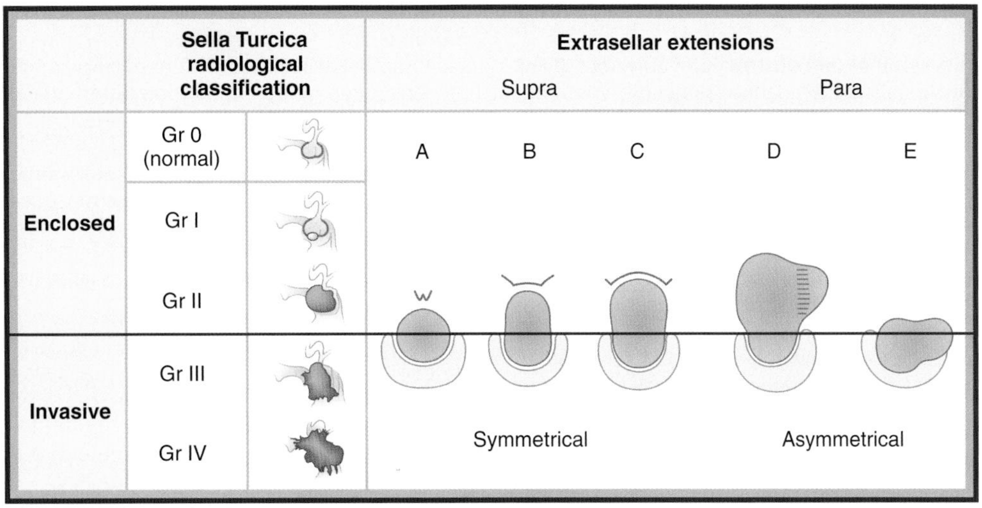

	Sella Turcica radiological classification		Extrasellar extensions				
			Supra			Para	
Enclosed	Gr 0 (normal)		A	B	C	D	E
	Gr I						
	Gr II		W				
Invasive	Gr III						
	Gr IV		Symmetrical			Asymmetrical	

Hardy classification of pituitary tumors			Extrasellar extensions
Radiologic	Anatomic	Surgical	***Suprasellar*** *(symmetrical)* A Supresellar cistern B Recesses of III ventricle C Whole anterior III ventricle
Grade 0	Intact, normal contour	Micro enclosed	***Parasellar*** *(asymmetrical)*
Grade I	Intact, focal bulging	Micro enclosed	D Intracranial intradural
Grade II	Intact, enlarged	Macro enclosed	Anterior
Grade III	Destroyed, partially	Macro invasive	Midline
Grade IV	Destroyed, totally	Macro invasive	Posterior
Grade V	Distant spread via CSF or blood	Macro carcinoma	E Extracranial extradural (lateral cavernous sinus)

Figure 8–9 ▪ Classification of pituitary tumors. CSF, cerebrospinal fluid; Gr, grade. (Adapted from Thapar K, Laws ER. Growth hormone–secreting pituitary tumors: operative management. In Krisht AF, Tindall GT, eds. Pituitary Disorders. Philadelphia: Lippincott Williams & Wilkins, 1999:243-258; Asa SL. In Tumors of the Pituitary Gland. Atlas of Tumor Pathology. Washington, DC: Armed Forces Institute of Pathology, 1997:51.)

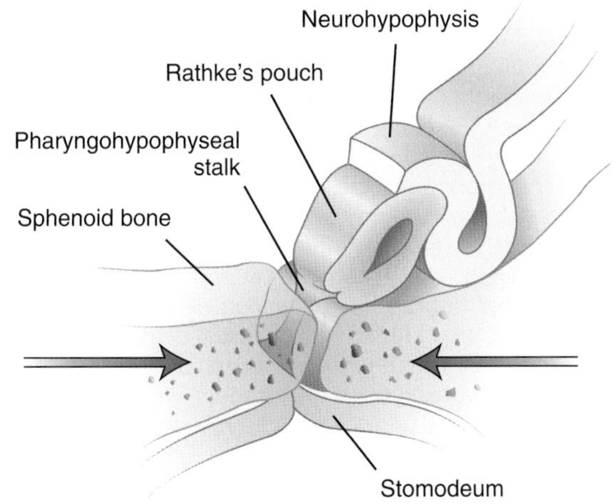

Figure 8–10 ▪ Pathogenesis of Rathke's cysts. Schematic of the embryologic progenitors of sellar and parasellar structures. Rathke's pouch arises from an outpocketing of stomodeum (ectoderm) and gives rise to the adenohypophysis. The pharyngohypophyseal stalk, which connects the stomadeum and Rathke's pouch, is divided by the sphenoid bone as it grows together *(arrows),* isolating Rathke's pouch and the neurohypophysis within the sella. (From Harrison MJ, Morgello S, Post KD. Epithelial cystic lesions of the sellular and parasellular region: a continuum of ectodermal derivates? J Neurosurg 1994;80:1018-1025.)

At surgery, the tumors are rough, heterogeneous, and lobular. Markers for epithelial cells, including cytokeratin and vimentin, are present. Recurrences commonly occur after surgical excision, and mean patient survival is about 5 years. Rarely, chordomas undergo sarcomatous transformation with an aggressive natural history and require extensive surgical dissection.[83]

Craniopharyngiomas

The craniopharyngioma is a parasellar tumor that constitutes about 3% of all intracranial tumors and up to 10% of childhood brain tumors. The tumor is commonly diagnosed during childhood and adolescence. Tumors arise from embryonic squamous remnants of Rathke's pouch extending dorsally toward the diencephalon. They may be large (>10 cm in diameter) and invade the third ventricle and associated brain structures. More than 60% arise from within the sella, and others arise from parasellar cell rests.[84-87] They rarely undergo malignant transformation.

Intrasellar tumors can often be distinguished from pituitary adenomas by the separate visible rim of normal pituitary tissue seen on MRI. The cystic mass is usually filled with cholesterol-rich viscous fluid, which can leak into the CSF, causing aseptic meningitis. They can also contain calcifications and immunoreactive human chorionic gonadotropin (hCG). Histology shows these tumors comprising two cell populations. Cysts are lined with a squamous epithelium containing islands characterized by columnar cells, and a mixed inflammatory reaction can also occur with calcification.

Large craniopharyngiomas can obstruct CSF flow. Increased intracranial pressure results in headache, projectile vomiting, papilledema, and somnolence, especially in children. Only about one third of patients are older than 40 years of age, and they commonly present with asymmetrical visual disturbances, including papilledema, optic atrophy, and field deficits. If cavernous sinus invasion is present, other cranial nerves may also be involved. On CT imaging, most children and about half of all adults exhibit characteristic flocculent or convex calcifications. Rarely, however, pituitary adenomas, other parasellar tumors, and vascular lesions within the sella are also calcified. In contrast to pituitary adenomas, which rarely cause diabetes insipidus, this disorder is often the earliest feature of craniopharyngioma. These patients can also develop partial or complete pituitary deficiency. Growth hormone deficiency, with short stature, diabetes insipidus, and gonadal failure are common. Pituitary stalk compression or damage to hypothalamic dopaminergic neurons results in hyperprolactinemia. Thus, craniopharyngioma can mimic a prolactinoma by intrapituitary imaging, presence of hyperprolactinemia, and favorable biochemical response to dopamine agonists.

The treatment of these lesions can involve radical surgery, radiation therapy, or a combination of these modalities.[87] More recently, transsphenoidal surgery has been successfully employed when possible.[88] Stereotactic irradiation has some success. Regardless of the form of therapy chosen, ablation of the mass invariably results in anterior or posterior (or both) pituitary hormone deficits. Tumors recur postoperatively in about 20% of patients undergoing radical surgical excision, but no difference in outcome occurs in those who undergo a subtotal surgical excision followed by radiation therapy. Pure papillary squamous cellular elements in the tumor can portend a higher surgical recurrence rate. Long-term effects of childhood irradiation for these tumors are considered in Chapter 24.

Meningiomas

Meningiomas arise from arachnoid and meningioendothelial cells, and those occurring in the sellar and parasellar region account for about one fifth of all meningiomas.[89] Sellar meningiomas are usually well circumscribed and do not attain the size of craniopharyngiomas. Suprasellar meningiomas can invade the pituitary ventrally, and intrasellar tumor origins are rare.[90] Coexisting functional pituitary adenomas have been described in patients with parasellar meningiomas. Secondary hyperprolactinemia occurs in up to half of patients, who usually present with local mass effects including headache and progressive visual disturbances accompanied by optic atrophy.

Distinguishing a suprasellar meningioma with downward extension from an upwardly extending pituitary adenoma may be difficult. On MRI, meningiomas are isodense on both T1 and T2 imaging, in contrast to other parasellar lesions, which are usually hyperdense on T2 imaging. Dural calcification may be evident on CT scanning.

Because of their rich vascularization, these tumors pose an intraoperative risk for hemorrhage and a resultant higher surgical mortality rate than usually encountered for pituitary adenoma resection.

Gliomas

Optic gliomas and low-grade astrocytomas arise from within the optic chiasm or optic tract and often infiltrate the optic nerve. Less than one third are intraorbital. Von Recklinghausen's disease is the underlying cause in about one third of these patients. Occasionally these tumors are associated with growth retardation, delayed or precocious puberty, and mass effects including visual disturbances, diencephalic syndrome, diabetes insipidus, and hydrocephalus. Rarely, gliomas arise within the sella and are associated with hyperprolactinemia; these should be considered in the uncommon differential diagnosis of a PRL-secreting pituitary adenoma.[91] Important distinguishing features include the young age of these patients (80% are younger than 10 years old), relatively intact pituitary function, gross visual disturbances, and localization of the mass as visualized on MRI. Gliomas, unlike hamartomas, usually enhance after contrast injection.

Mucocele

Mucoceles are expanding accumulations of fluid within the sphenoid sinus and can compress parasellar structures. Headaches, visual disturbances (usually unilateral), and exophthalmos are characteristic features. On MRI, the homogenous sphenoid mass may be quite prominent, but it may be distinguished from the pituitary gland dorsally.

Parasellar Aneurysms

Parasellar aneurysms can mimic a pituitary adenoma, and intraoperative rupture may be catastrophic, underlining the absolute need for preoperative diagnosis. Differentiating features of aneurysms from other pituitary masses may be subtle, including eye pain, very intense headaches, and relatively sudden onset of cranial nerve palsies. Although imaging techniques usually distinguish blood and hemorrhage from solid tumor or tissue, a highly vascular meningioma may be confused with an aneurysm.

Pituitary Infections

Acute pituitary abscesses and perisellar arachnoiditis are encountered with sinus infections, especially after transsphenoidal surgery. Pituitary abscess can develop from hematogenous or direct local spread of infectious agents.[92] Abscesses can arise within a preexisting pituitary adenoma,[93] and they can be difficult to distinguish from an adenoma, because these patients might not have fever or signs of meningitis.[94] On MRI imaging, an isointense central cavity with surrounding ring enhancement is characteristic for an abscess.[95]

Gram-positive streptococci or staphylococci can originate from nasopharyngeal passages.[94] Disseminated *Entamoeba histolytica* and *Pneumocystis jiroveci* can also seed to the pituitary.[96] Immunosuppressed patients can develop pituitary infections including CMV, toxoplasmosis, aspergillosis, histoplasmosis, and coccidiosis. Syphilitic gumma can lead to pituitary damage and insufficiency. Common viral infections, including influenza, measles, mumps, and herpes are rarely associated with pituitary damage and insufficiency.

Tuberculosis is rarely confined to the pituitary gland, but most of the fewer than 20 reported patients with pituitary tuberculosis exhibited suprasellar extension of the pituitary mass, compromised pituitary function, and visual defects.[97-99] Although evidence for systemic tuberculosis is usually present, isolated sellar tuberculoma have been described.[100]

Hematologic Malignancies

Primary central nervous system lymphomas are usually B-cell non-Hodgkin's types, and fewer than 20 such patients with pituitary lymphoma have been described.[101,102] The pituitary mass may be an isolated presentation of the underlying disease. The disorder is usually diagnosed by histology of tissue obtained by excision biopsy. Six of nine patients had headache, and five had cranial nerve abnormalities with varying degrees of hypopituitarism. MRI reveals cavernous sinus invasion and isodense T1-T2 weighted images that enhance after gadolinium. Patients with solitary pituitary plasmacytomas have been reported who do not develop classical multiple myeloma. Acute lymphoblastic leukemia may be associated with periglandular pituitary infiltrates with minimal pituitary dysfunction.

Pituicytoma

Pituicytoma is a rare benign suprasellar glial cell tumor that manifests with mass effects or hypopituitarism.[103,104] It arises from cells in the neurohypophysis and stains for vimentin, S100 protein, and glial fibrillary acidic protein.[105]

Pituitary Granulomas

Sarcoidosis

Infiltrative sarcoidosis of the hypothalamic pituitary region occurs in most patients with central nervous system sarcoid involvement. These patients can present with varying degrees of anterior pituitary failure with or without diabetes insipidus.[106] Hypothalamic granulomatous involvement is commonly encountered in patients with central nervous system sarcoidosis and may be the sole manifestation of the disease.[107] The hypothalamus, pituitary stalk, and posterior pituitary are diffusely invaded by noncaseating granulomas consisting of giant cells, macrophages, and lymphocytes.[108] Sarcoidosis may be progressive and eventually result in pituitary damage and even an empty sella. Onset of diabetes insipidus with no obvious features of a pituitary disorder should alert the physician to exclude hypothalamic sarcoid deposits, especially in the face of a thickened stalk on MRI.[109] Systemic steroids have been used in treating CNS sarcoid. Cladripine, an antimetabolite agent reverses diabetes indipidus caused by sarcoid.[110]

Hand-Schüller-Christian Disease

Hand-Schüller-Christian disease (histiocytosis X) can comprise sleep disorders, adypsia, and morbid obesity. Other features of granulomatous involvement, including axillary skin rash, history of recurrent pneumothorax, and classic bony lesions, should be sought, especially in young patients with new-onset diabetes insipidus.[111] The disorder may be associated with granulomatous damage to the hypothalamus or posterior pituitary (or both), with characteristic diabetes insipidus.[112] The pituitary lesions are composed of dendritic Langerhans cells, and pituitary MRI can reveal stalk thickening or a diminished posterior pituitary bright spot.[113] Adults with the disorder should be carefully evaluated for anterior pituitary hormone deficits, and hormones should be appropriately replaced.

While surgery and radiation were, for many years, the mainstay treatments for this disorder, a chemotherapeutic approach using cladripine has been advocated.

Metastases to the Pituitary Region

Pituitary metastases are found in up to 3.5% of cancer patients,[114-116] especially in older patients with diffuse malignant disease. Because the vascular supply to the posterior pituitary is derived directly from the systemic circulation via the internal carotid arteries, the posterior pituitary is the preferred site for bloodborne metastatic spread. Carcinomas that metastasize to the pituitary include breast, lung, and gastrointestinal tract. Up to one quarter of patients with metastatic breast cancer have pituitary metastases. Symptomatic pituitary metastases (usually diabetes insipidus) may be the presenting sign of occult malignancy and of malignancy of unknown origin. Rarely, isolated metastatic stalk deposits manifest with pituitary failure. If extensive bony erosion is present and disease onset is rapid, the diagnosis is more readily apparent. However, pituitary imaging might not clearly distinguish metastatic deposits from a pituitary adenoma, and these lesions can masquerade as adenoma; in this case, the diagnosis is only made by histologic study of the resected specimen.[117] When the diagnosis is clear-cut in the presence of a primary cancer, relatively low dose pituitary radiation may be sufficient to shrink the metastasis and improve morbidity.

Iron-storage diseases, including hemochromatosis and hemosiderosis, result in predominantly gonadotroph cell damage. Idiopathic retroperitoneal fibrosis can also be associated with a suprasellar mass and hypothalamic panhypopituitarism.[118]

Primary Hypophysitis

Pituitary mass lesions composed of inflammatory cells can arise as primary disorders of the anterior and posterior pituitary glands or the neurohypophysis.[119] At least three clinicopathologic forms have been described.

Lymphocytic Hypophysitis

This apparently autoimmune inflammatory disorder occurs during or shortly after parturition,[120] but it has also been reported after menopause,[119] and about 15% of reported cases occur in male patients.[121] Of the 57% of patients developing the disorder in association with pregnancy, most occur during the last month of pregnancy or during the first 2 months postpartum.[119,122] The disorder is characterized by a lymphocytic and plasma cell pituitary infiltrate that may be isolated or may be associated with other recognized endocrinopathies. Circulating antipituitary antibodies have occasionally been reported, and the presence of isolated pituitary hormone deficiency can imply a selectively targeted autoimmune process to pituitary cell types. Although the natural history is often short lived, the few comprehensive pathologic evaluations suggest that secondary adenohypophyseal cell atrophy, with a resultant empty sella, is a common outcome.

Pathologic criteria for diagnosis include islands of anterior pituitary cells surrounded by diffuse lymphocytic (T and B cell) infiltrates. More than 268 histologically confirmed cases have been reported.[119] The defining feature is lymphocytic infiltration comprising T and B lymphocytes. Caturegli and colleagues have reported that plasma cells were found in 53%, eosinophils in 12%, and macrophage histiocytes and neutrophils in 6% of cases.[119] Mast cells have also been identified in hypophysitis.[123]

Clinical Features

More than half the patients with lymphocytic hypophysitis present with headache, visual field impairment, and hyperprolactinemia,[119] and pituitary deficiency accounts for the remaining cases (Table 8–8). Fifty-six percent of patients have secondary hypoadrenalism, followed in frequency by hypothyroidism, hypogonadism, and growth hormone or PRL deficiency. This contrasts with hypopituitarism caused by pituitary adenomas. Hypothyroidism and hypothyroid can occur later, even after 9 months. MRI reveals a pituitary mass, often indistinguishable from an adenoma. Associated partially empty sella and contrast enhancement of the pituitary mass may be helpful distinguishing MRI features.[124] The inflammatory process often resolves with time, and initially abnormal pituitary function may be restored or can remain chronically compromised.

Limited numbers of patients have been reported with histologically proven lymphocytic hypophysitis and documented

TABLE 8–8 FEATURES OF LYMPHOCYTIC HYPOPHYSITIS

Feature	Percentage
Pituitary enlargement	80-95
Headache, visual disturbances	55-70
Hypopituitarism	63-68
Hyperprolactinemia	20-38
Associated autoimmune disease	30
Diabetes insipidus	14-19

spontaneous regression of pituitary mass on follow-up imaging. There can be intra- and suprasellar pituitary enlargement, and the pituitary stalk may be thickened, especially when diabetes insipidus is present.[115] In two patients with histologically proven hypophysitis, spontaneous resolution of the pituitary mass was followed by subsequent successful pregnancies.[125,126] Diabetes insipidus encountered in 20% of patients may be attributed to posterior pituitary or stalk infiltration.[127] In one third of patients, other autoimmune conditions, including thyroiditis, hypoadrenalism, parathyroid failure, atrophic gastritis, systemic lupus erythematosus, or Sjögren's syndrome are also present.[128]

The differential diagnosis includes prolactinoma and other sellar masses, and careful history and demonstrated loss of the posterior pituitary bright spot on MRI are useful for supporting the diagnosis.

Laboratory Evaluation

The erythrocyte sedimentation rate (ESR) is often elevated; antibodies to a 49-kd cytosolic protein were detected in 70% of patients with histologically confirmed lymphocytic hypophysitis and in 10% of controls.[129] Although the specificity of this and two additional antibodies to 68-kd and 43-kd human pituitary membrane antigens is high, all three were only detected in five of 13 patients with lymphocytic hypophysitis and one of 12 patients with infundibuloneurohypophysitis.[130] Similar results were obtained using radioligand assays for pituitary proteins.[119,131] Prolactin levels are usually elevated in both female and male patients, hyperprolactinemia is expected during pregnancy and during the early postpartum period, and the mass effect of the infiltrate can also contribute to stalk compression and secondary hyperprolactinemia. GH and ACTH responses to hypothalamic hormone challenges may be blunted. Rarely, isolated ACTH or TSH deficiencies have been reported.[132]

Treatment

If the diagnosis is convincingly supported, and in the absence of compressive visual field disturbances, surgical therapy should be withheld, pituitary hormone deficits appropriately replaced, and spontaneous resolution of the inflammatory mass expectantly followed. Treatment with adrenal steroids is advocated, often resolving the sellar mass and improving endocrine dysfunction. Steroids are also indicated if adrenal reserve is compromised. Transsphenoidal surgery may be required to confirm a tissue diagnosis and can also relieve compression symptoms,[133] but the degree of surgical resection should be constrained by the need to conserve viable pituitary tissue, particularly in view of common spontaneous resolution.

Granulomatous Hypophysitis

Granulomatous hypophysitis is not usually associated with pregnancy and has an equal female-to-male incidence. Rarely, the condition can coexist with lymphocytic hypophysitis in the same gland.[133] Pituitary histology shows histiocytes, multinucleated giant cells, and other features of chronic inflammation and granuloma.[134] Patients present with headache and can have aseptic meningitis. MRI imaging can reveal a thickened pituitary stalk or a characteristic tongue-shaped extension of the lesion under the hypothalamus. Granulomatous hypophysitis can reflect an underlying systemic disorder such as sarcoidosis[135] or Takayasu's disease.[136]

Xanthomatous Hypophysitis

Xanthomatous hypophysitis is the least common primary pituitary inflammatory process. t also occurs at equal frequency in both sexes and consists of lipid-laden macrophages, which resemble postinfectious cell debris. MRI often reveals a highly cystic lesion, leading to the suggestion that this entity reflects an inflammatory response to a damaged or ruptured pituitary cyst.[137]

Hemorrhage and Infarction

Intrapituitary hemorrhage and infarction is usually caused by ischemic damage to the hypophyseal-portal system and may be catastrophic. These acute events cause significant damage to the pituitary gland, and small clinically silent microinfarcts are found in up to 5% of unselected autopsies. Pituitary cells are relatively resilient to vascular insult, and pituitary insufficiency is only clinically apparent when about 75% of the gland is ischemically damaged. Ten percent residual functional pituitary cell mass appears sufficient to mask complete pituitary failure. Ischemic damage is limited to the anterior lobe, and posterior pituitary function usually remains intact, reflecting the predominant neural control of oxytocin and antidiuretic hormone ADH secretion. Acute intrapituitary hemorrhage can cause significant life-threatening damage to the pituitary and its surrounding vital structures.[138]

Postpartum Pituitary Infarction

During pregnancy, the pituitary gland normally enlarges in response to estrogen stimulation. The hypervascular gland is thus particularly vulnerable to arterial pressure changes and prone to hemorrhage. Sheehan's syndrome, classically described after severe postpartum hemorrhage, is now less commonly encountered with the advent of modern obstetric care,[139] but it occurs much more commonly in developing countries.[140] The presentation varies from development of hypovolemic shock, resulting in adenohypophyseal vessel vasospasm and pituitary necrosis,[141] to the gradual onset of partial to complete pituitary insufficiency over months to years. Most prominent among symptoms are inability to nurse and postpartum amenorrhea.[140] Pituitary autoimmunity has been implicated in gland failure after postpartum hemorrhage.[142]

Pituitary Apoplexy

Pituitary apoplexy can result from spontaneous hemorrhage into a pituitary adenoma or can occur after head trauma or skull base fracture. Pituitary apoplexy has been found in association with hypertension, diabetes mellitus, sickle cell anemia, and acute hypovolemic shock.[143,144]

Clinical Features

Pituitary apoplexy is an endocrine emergency.[145] The condition can evolve over 1 to 2 days, usually manifesting with severe headache and ocular palsies or visual field defects. Cardiovascular collapse, change in consciousness, neck stiffness, and sometimes hypoglycemia can occur. Acute adrenal insufficiency is a common occurrence due to loss of ACTH. It can also be superimposed due to disordered intravascular clotting disorders, heparin administration, or acute effects of central nervous system hemorrhage. Pituitary imaging without contrast (CT or MRI) usually reveals signs of intrapituitary or intra-adenoma hemorrhage, stalk deviation, and compression of normal pituitary tissue and, in severe cases, signs of parasellar hemorrhage.[146]

In a study of 13 consecutive acutely ill patients with pituitary apoplexy, baseline serum cortisol was less than 5 μg/dL in seven patients, 5-15 μg/dL in four, and greater than 15 μg/dL in only two. Five of the 13 also had low thyroxine (T_4), and all 13 had evidence of gonadal dysfunction. Thus, these pituitary tumor patients likely had preexisting pituitary insufficiency. They also had an increase in intrasellar pressure that was inversely related to serum PRL.[147] This, like Sheehan's syndrome, is one of the few pituitary tumor presentations in which hyperprolactinemia is not a feature unless the infarction occurs within a prolactinoma. Patient characteristics, signs and symptoms, and outcomes in 112 patients in three series are shown in Table 9.[145]

Management

Patients with visual field compromise require emergency transsphenoidal surgery. Others recover spontaneously but can develop long-term pituitary insufficiency. Patients who are fully alert and conscious and have no visual symptoms may be observed. The decision to initiate therapy with high-dose glucocorticoids depends on the clinical status,[138] but the high incidence of adrenal dysfunction either before or after treatment indicates a need for replacement or stress doses of cortisone in most. Ophthalmoplegia, which is common, can resolve spontaneously over time.[138] Postoperative recovery of visual function correlates inversely with the time that has elapsed subsequent to the acute hemorrhage.[148] Cranial nerve palsies, however, often improve whether or not surgery is undertaken. Pituitary function does not commonly recover after resolution of the acute hemorrhage, and patients require adrenal, thyroid, or gonadal steroid hormone replacement.[149] The subsequent atrophy of infarcted pituitary tissue often results in the development of a complete or partially empty sella evident on MRI.

TABLE 8–9 FEATURES OF PITUITARY APOPLEXY

Features	Bills DC et al (1993)	Randeva HS et al (1999)	Lubina et al (2005)
	PATIENTS		
Total number	37	35	40
Male	25	21	27
Female	12	14	13
Mean age (yr)	56.6	49.8	51.2
Not operated	1	4	6
	SYMPTOMS		
Headache	95%	97%	63%
Visual defects	64%	71%	61%
Ophthalmoplegia	78%	69%	40%
	ADENOMA TYPE		
NFPA	52%	61%	63%
PRL cell	17%	5.5%	31%
Visual fields improvement		76%	81%
Ocular palsy improvement		91%	71%
	HORMONE DEFICIENCY		
Central hypocortisol	82%	58%	40%
Central hypothyroid	89%	45%	54%
Hypogonadism	64%	43%	79%
Diabetes insipidus	11%	6%	8%

NFPA, nonfunctioning pituitary adenoma; PRL, prolactin.

Cocaine-Associated Hypopituitarism

Cocaine can cause hypopituitarism through its effect on the vasculature. Panhypopituitarism with or without diabetes insipidus can occur. It is usually associated with severe sinus disease.[150]

Evaluation

Approach to the Patient Harboring a Pituitary Mass

Masses in 91% of 1120 patients undergoing transsphenoidal surgery for sellar masses were diagnosed as pituitary adenomas.[95] Thus, the differential diagnosis of a pituitary mass should be aimed at excluding the diagnosis of a pituitary adenoma before considering other rare sellar lesions. The management and prognosis of anterior pituitary adenomas differs markedly from other nonpituitary masses, and an important diagnostic challenge is to effectively distinguish a pituitary adenoma from other parasellar masses.

Several physiologic states are associated with pituitary enlargement. Lactotroph hyperplasia is seen during pregnancy, and thyrotroph or gonadotroph hyperplasias occur in the presence of long-standing primary thyroid or gonadal failure, respectively. Pituitary enlargement can also occur as a result of ectopic GHRH or CRH secretion from carcinoid tumors or hypothalamic gangliocytomas, with resultant hyperplasia of somatotroph or corticotroph cells. Autopsy series show that up to 20% of subjects harbor an incidental, clinically silent pituitary adenoma. Incidental pituitary cysts, hemorrhages, and infarctions are also discovered at autopsy. With the widespread use of sensitive imaging techniques for nonpituitary indications, including head trauma, chronic sinusitis, or headaches, previously unapparent pituitary lesions are being identified with increasing frequency. Pituitary abnormalities compatible with the diagnosis of microadenoma are detectable in about 10% of the normal adult population undergoing MRI imaging.[69] Recognizing that about 90% of observed pituitary lesions represent pituitary adenomas, initial assessment should determine whether the mass is hormonally functional and whether local mass effects are apparent at the time of diagnosis or likely to develop in the future.

Because the onset of clinical features associated with disordered hormone secretion are insidious and may be unnoticed for years or decades, endocrine function should always be tested (Table 8–10). Clinical evaluation for changes compatible with hyper- or hyposecretion of GH, gonadotropins, PRL, or ACTH can reveal unique long-term sequelae requiring distinct therapies. In the absence of clinical features of a humoral hypersecretory syndrome, cost-effective laboratory screening should be performed. Serum PRL levels greater than 200 μg/L strongly suggest the presence of a micro- or macroprolactinoma. Any

TABLE 8–10 SCREENING TESTS FOR FUNCTIONAL PITUITARY ADENOMAS

Disorder	Test	Comments
Acromegaly	IGF-I	Interpret IGF-I relative to age- and gender-matched controls
	OGTT with GH obtained at 0, 30, and 60 min	Normal subjects should suppress growth hormone to <1 μg/L
Prolactinoma	Exclude medications	MRI of the sella should not be ordered unless prolactin is elevated
	Serum PRL level	
Cushing's disease	24-hr urinary free cortisol	Ensure urine collection is total and accurate
	Dexamethasone (1 mg) at 11 PM and fasting plasma cortisol measured at 8 AM	Normal subjects suppress to <5 μg/dL)
	ACTH assay	Distinguishes adrenal adenoma from ectopic ACTH or Cushing's disease

ACTH, adrenocorticotropic hormone; GH, growth hormone; IGF, insulin-like growth factor; MRI, magnetic resonance imaging; OGTT, oral glucose tolerance test; PRL, prolactin.

elevation in serum PRL from minimal to high can occur when a microadenoma is present. A minimal to moderate elevation can also indicate secondary stalk interruption by a pituitary mass (usually a macroadenoma). A PRL greater than 200 ng/mL used to be considered pathognomonic of a prolactinoma, but it has become apparent that similar elevations can be seen from other causes, such as treatment with risperidol. It might now be safe to say that a PRL greater than 1000 ng/mL is pathognomonic of a prolactinoma.

Elevated age- and gender-matched IGF-I levels indicate the presence of GH-secreting adenoma, and a high 24-hour urinary free cortisol level is an effective screen for most patients with Cushing's disease, although nighttime salivary cortisol is useful for screening. Nevertheless, the incidence of functional hormone-secreting tumors in asymptomatic subjects with incidentally discovered pituitary masses is low. The presence of, or the potential for, local compressive effects must also be considered. Because the risk of microadenoma enlargement toward a compressive macroadenoma is low, no direct intervention may be warranted. For parasellar masses of uncertain origin, histologic tissue examination may be the best approach to yield an accurate diagnosis. Although MRI or CT imaging features may be helpful in diagnosing a nonpituitary sellar mass, the final diagnosis can remain elusive until pathologic confirmation is obtained.

Parasellar masses include neoplastic and nonneoplastic lesions and manifest clinically by local compression of surrounding vital structures or as a result of metabolic or hormonal derangements. Rarely, sellar masses are the presenting feature of a previously undiagnosed systemic disorder such as lymphoma or tuberculosis.[151] Fever with or without associated sterile or septic meningitis is rarely caused by fluid leakage into the subarachnoid space from Rathke's cleft, dermoid and epidermoid cysts, and craniopharyngioma and apoplexy.[138,152-154,145] Pituitary masses can manifest with hemorrhage and infarction, especially during pregnancy (see earlier), when there is a pituitary tumor or when elderly patients with unsuspected pituitary tumors become hypotensive because of another illness. Rarely, these adenomas manifest with CSF leak, which can predispose to meningitis.

Pituitary masses can also undergo silent infarction, leading to development of a partial or totally empty pituitary sella with normal pituitary reserve, implying that the surrounding rim of pituitary tissue is fully functional. Large sellar cysts may be mistaken for an empty sella. Rarely, functional pituitary adenomas can arise within the remnant pituitary tissue, and these tumors might not be visible by sensitive MRI (i.e. <2 mm in diameter), despite their endocrine hyperactivity. More than one kind of tumor may be found in the same patient, (e.g. a pituitary tumor and a meningioma.[155] Acute or chronic infection with abscess formation rarely occurs within the mass. Compromised pituitary hormone hyposecretion can result from direct pressure effects of the expanding mass on hormone-secreting cells or parasellar pressure effects that attenuate synthesis or secretion of hypothalamic hormones, with resultant pituitary failure.

Imaging

Magnetic Resonance Imaging

Tumors of the pituitary gland are best diagnosed with magnetic resonance imaging (MRI), because it has better resolution than other radiologic modalities for identifying soft tissue changes (see Fig. 8–7).

When a pituitary tumor or other parasellar mass is suspected, an MRI specifically focused on the pituitary should be requested, because more widely spaced cuts during a routine brain MRI are often inadequate to visualize relatively small pituitary tumors.[156,157] This technique permits high-contrast, detailed visualization of tumor mass effects on neighboring soft tissue structures, including the cavernous sinus[158] or optic chiasm. A pituitary MRI includes images of the optic chiasm, hypothalamus, pituitary stalk, and cavernous and sphenoid sinuses.[159,160] High-resolution T1-weighted sections in the coronal and sagittal plane both before and after gadolinium pentetic acid contrast administration distinguish most pituitary masses.[161] Slice thickness should be less than 3 mm to obtain a pixel of 1 mm. Contiguous sections are therefore required to diagnose lesions of 1 to 3 mm.[162] If necessary, especially for diagnosing high signaling hemorrhage, T2-weighted images provide additional diagnostic information.

MRI clearly delineates the pituitary gland, stalk, optic tracts and surrounding soft tissues. The gland may be concave, convex, or flat. The posterior pituitary lobe exhibits a discrete bright spot of high signal intensity on T1-weighted images, which declines with age and is absent in diabetes insipidus and most posterior pituitary lesions. This T1 shortening can reflect the presence of ADH localized within neurosecretory vesicles.[163] The pituitary gland can transiently enlarge during adolescence and pregnancy and postpartum. Teenage girls exhibit increasing gland convexity during the menstrual cycle.[164,165] During pregnancy, the gland should normally not exceed 10 to 12 mm, and the stalk should not exceed 4 mm in diameter. Thickened stalk can indicate the presence of hypophysitis, granuloma, or atypical chordomas.

After gadolinium, microadenomas are usually hypodense as compared to the normal gland, especially when multiple thin section echo sequences are examined in the first few minutes after contrast injection. It has been suggested that this hypointensity can reflect compromised microadenoma vasculature.[166] Microadenomas can also cause gland asymmetry or stalk deviation. In contrast, macroadenomas, which are significantly more vascular than microadenomas, have a higher affinity for gadolinium. They often enlarge the sella turcica by remodeling the bony fossa, suggesting a gradual long-term process. These tumors can grow upward toward the optic apparatus and cause draping of the nerves over the tumor, which is often accompanied by visual field abnormalities. Tumors can also extend into the sphenoid sinus and can invade connective tissue separating the pituitary from the cavernous sinus.

Radiologically, visible tumor tissue surrounding the carotid artery confirms cavernous sinus invasion. Infrequently, these patients develop palsies of the third, fourth, or sixth cranial nerves. MRI can readily distinguish pituitary adenomas from other masses, including hyperplasias, craniopharyngiomas, meningiomas, chordomas, cysts, and metastatic lesions. Secondary distinguishing features such as visualization of distinct noninvolved pituitary tissue, mass consistency, calcification, hemorrhage, and suprasellar involvement usually allow an imaging diagnosis of these masses, but these can often only be confirmed by direct tissue histology. Preoperative localization of carotid artery aneurysms can also be confirmed by MRI or magnetic resonance angiography (MRA).

Computed Tomography

Pituitary CT allows visualization of bony structures including the sellar floor and clinoid bones, and their invasion. CT also recognizes calcifications that characterize craniopharyngiomas, meningiomas and, rarely, aneurysms that are not evident on MRI. Occasionally, pituitary adenomas can calcify. Pituitary CT scan is indicated for discovery of hemorrhagic lesions, metastatic deposits, chordomas, and evidence of calcification.

Receptor Imaging

Because prolactinomas express D2 receptors, they can be imaged with a radiolabeled D2 receptor antagonist by using ^{123}I-iodobenzamine single photon emission scanning. Failure to visualize nonfunctioning tumors by this technique has led some to advocate its use to distinguish the two tumor types.[167] Radiolabeled indium-pentetreotide has been used for in vivo tumor imaging. Most pituitary adenomas express somatostatin receptor subtypes to a varying degree, thus limiting the specificity of the procedure. The sensitivity of single photon emission CT (SPECT) is about 1 cm, which detects normal pituitary tissue receptor expression. Because most adenomas as well as normal tissue are identified by this technique, its utility is limited for tumor detection, but it may be helpful for imaging ectopic ACTH-secreting tumors.

Neuro-ophthalmologic Assessment of Pituitary Masses

The optic tracts are particularly vulnerable to compression by expanding pituitary masses. Accurate neuro-ophthalmologic evaluation is helpful for diagnosing tumors, determining pretreatment baseline visual status for post-treatment monitoring, or detecting recurrence of a mass.[168] The relationship of the optic chiasm and the intracranial components of the optic nerves with the pituitary gland and surrounding vessels are depicted in Fig. 8–2. A 10-mm posteriorly angled gap separates the optic chiasm and diaphragma sellae (see Fig. 8–3). Therefore, extensive suprasellar mass extension is required before visual function is compromised. Decussation of neural fibers originating from the nasal half of each retina occurs at the chiasm, and those originating from the temporal retinal halves are situated ipsilaterally.[169] Fibers from the superior and inferior retinal aspect are segregated in the corresponding chiasmal regions. Local vascular compromise or chiasmal stretching contribute to the pathogenesis of selective visual compromise. Reversibility of visual effects can correlate inversely with acuteness of the compressive insult.

Visual Symptoms

An abnormal visual examination can unmask the presence of a pituitary mass in an asymptomatic patient. Prior to the availability of sophisticated assay and imaging techniques, virtually all pituitary masses manifested with vision loss.[170] Currently, less than 10% of patients present with vision loss,[171] and most of these harbor clinically nonfunctioning pituitary adenomas often detected by incidental imaging. Unilateral or bilateral temporal or central vision loss is usually asymmetric and may be quite insidious, remitting or recurring. Rarely, sudden vision loss occurs in a previously asymptomatic patient. Other symptoms include diplopia, impaired depth perception, and, very rarely, visual hallucinations (Fig. 8–11).[172]

Clinical Signs

Impingement of the inferior crossing chiasmal fibers leads to bitemporal vision loss, especially in the superior field portions, accounting for most pituitary-related visual defects. Rarely, tumors can compress the optic chiasm from above and cause inferior temporal compromise. As damage to the optic chiasm becomes more extreme, field cuts can extend into the nasal field and also cause optic atrophy. Isolated impairment of nasal visual fields is mostly seen in patients with glaucoma. Pituitary-related defects preferentially marginate at the vertical field midline,[168] in contrast to other causes of bitemporal defects, which tend to occur away from the midline (Fig. 8–12).

Despite prominent field defects, many of which can be directly correlated with defined tumor location by MRI, visual acuity in the remaining fields is invariably normal in more than 95% of patients.[173] Anterior tumor extension can damage central visual acuity, and this is detected using the Snellen chart or by loss of color discrimination, especially in the red-green spectrum. Rarely, pupillary abnormalities, optic atrophy, papilledema, cranial nerve palsies and nystagmus may be encountered.

Visual fields are assessed by bedside confrontational testing, Goldmann perimetry the Amsler grid, and automated quantitative perimetry. Because red vision is lost before white, a small pin (<10 mm diameter) with the two colors can be employed. The patient should be asked to cover one ye so that the examiner can evaluate both temporal and nasal fields without compromise,

Management

The goals of therapy for masses are to alleviate local compressive mass effects and to suppress hormone hypersecretion or relieve hormone hyposecretion while maintaining intact pituitary trophic function. Three modes of available therapy include surgical, radiotherapeutic, and medical approaches. In general, the benefits of each therapy should be weighed against their respective risks, and comprehensive physician and patient awareness is required to individualize treatment approaches.

Surgical Management of Pituitary Tumors and Sellar Masses

Pituitary surgery is indicated for excision of mass lesions causing central pressure effects, including visual compromise, primary

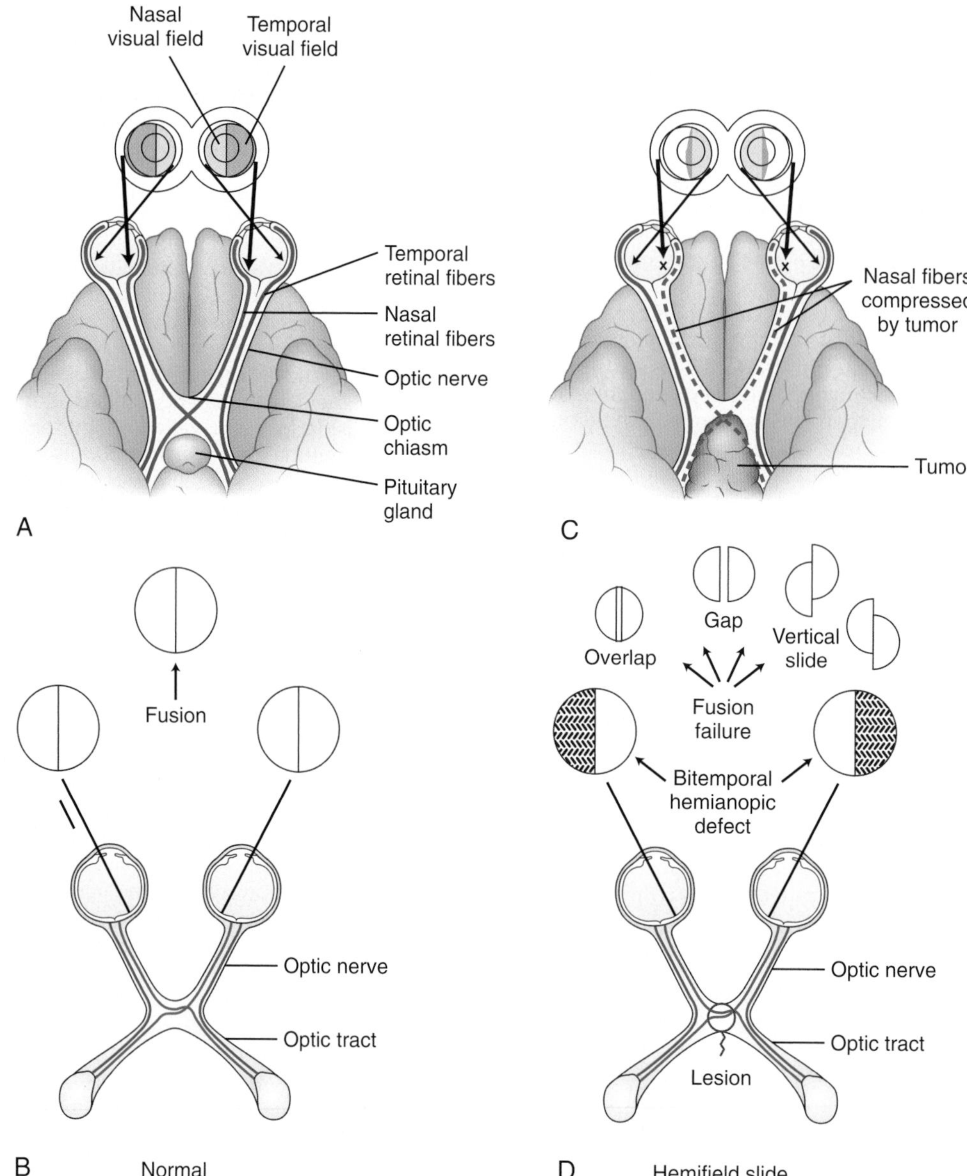

Figure 8–11 ■ Local effects of an expanding pituitary tumor causing visual field defects. **A** and **B,** Normal vision. **C,** Bitemporal hemianopia. **D,** Hemifield slide phenomena arising in the setting of bitemporal hemianopia from fusion instability. The nasal and temporal fields lose their linkage, resulting in overlap of the preserved visual fields. (**A** and **C** from Newell-Price J. Endocrine assessment. In Sheaves R, Jenkins PJ, Wass J, eds. Clinical Endocrine Oncology. Malden, MA: Blackwell Science, 1997:152-157; **B** and **D** from Stiver SI, Sharpe JA. Neuro-ophthalmologic evaluation of pituitary tumors. In Thapar K, Kovacs K, Scheithauer BW, Lloyd RV, eds. Diagnosis and Management of Pituitary Tumors. Totowa, NJ: Humana Press, 2001:173-200. Copyright © The Mayo Clinic, 2000.)

correction of hormonal hypersecretion, or functional tumor resection in patients resistant or not immediately responsive to medical treatment. Unusual sellar lesions can require diagnostic tissue evaluation, and, rarely, primary or secondary parasellar malignancies require excessive excision.

In 1904, Horsley reported the surgical resection of a pituitary tumor by a lateral middle fossa approach.[4] The first successful transsphenoidal approach for pituitary tumor resection was reported by Schloffer in 1907[174] and subsequently refined by Cushing, who between 1910 and 1925 operated on 231 patients harboring pituitary tumors with a remarkably low mortality rate of 5.6%.[4,170] Cushing used a sublabial incision to enable an endonasal approach for removing the septum, and he improved visualization by using Kanavel's headlight. Hardy later improved the technique by using the operating microscope and intraoperative fluoroscopy, resulting in markedly reduced morbidity and mortality usually encountered with craniotomy. Hardy's became the mainstay surgical technique for resecting these tumors.

The transsphenoidal approach precludes invasion of the cranial cavity and removes the need for brain tissue manipulation required during a subfrontal surgical approach (Fig. 8–13). A ventral sphenoid approach for resection of pituitary masses likewise does not violate the cranial fossa. Thus, transsphenoidal surgery is associated with minimal morbidity and mortality, most patients are ambulatory within 6 to 9 hours, and the hospital stay is generally about 3 days.

The transsphenoidal approach allows a clearly visible operative field with high magnification and internal illumination.

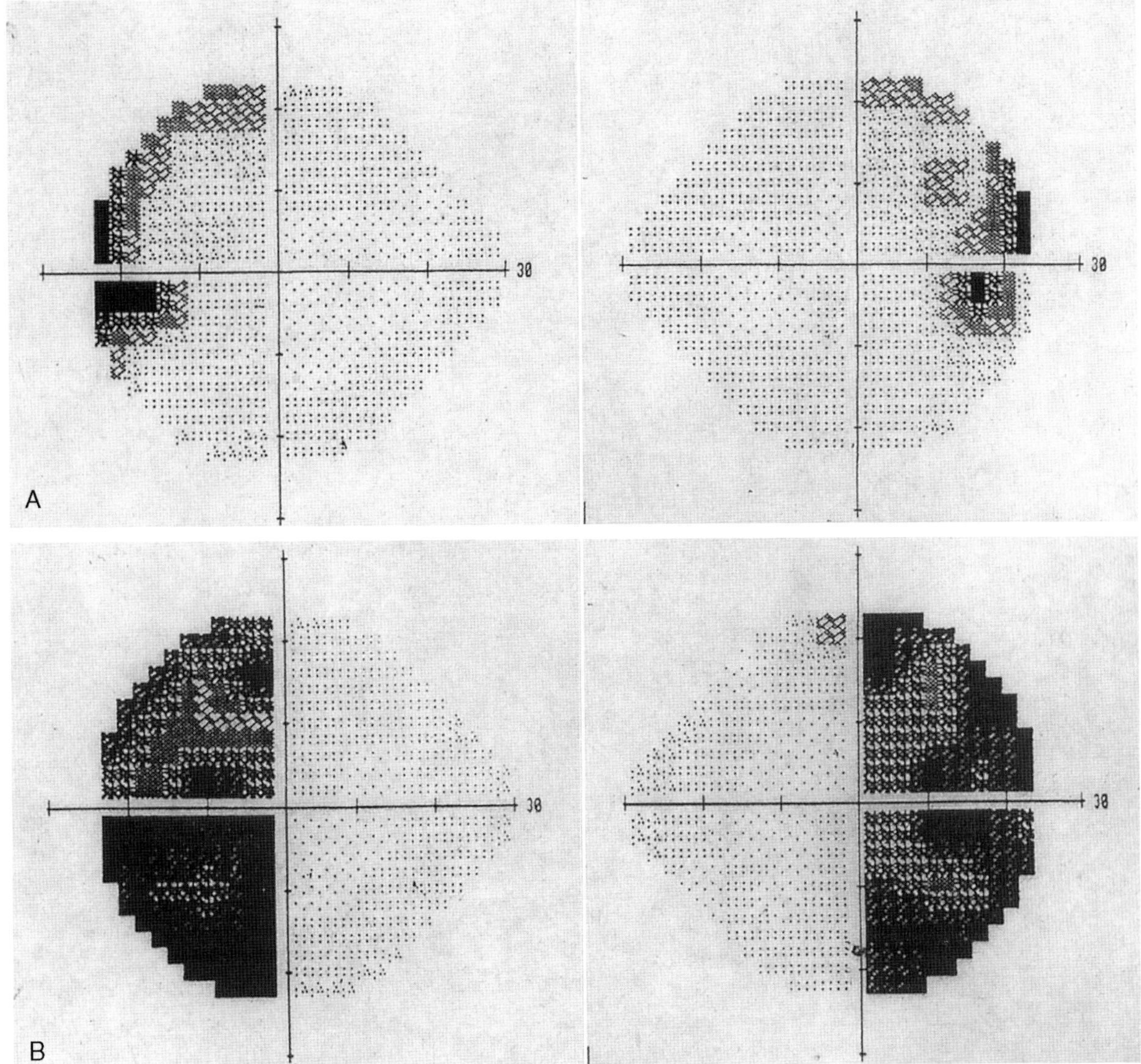

Figure 8–12 ■ Threshold field test showing bitemporal hemianopia in a patient with a pituitary tumor compressing the optic chiasm **(A)** and superior bitemporal field cuts **(B)**.

Normal pituitary can be clearly distinguished from tumor tissue, facilitating microdissection and small tumor resection (Fig. 8–14). The utility of the transsphenoidal approach has been greatly enhanced by several technologic advances including head-immobilization techniques, microinstrumentation development, and novel angled endoscopes. Enhanced MRI sensitivity and precision as well as intraoperative MRI allows clear delineation of tumor location, size, and invasiveness, all critical determinants of surgical success.

Craniotomy is indicated for the rare invasive suprasellar masses extending into the frontal or middle cranial fossa, optic nerves, or extensive posterior clival invasion. Suprasellar extension contained by a small diaphragmatic aperture (hourglass configuration) also can require a transcranial approach. Rarely, tumors that are too firm to be removed transsphenoidally can require a combination of transsphenoidal and intracranial surgery.

Goals of Surgery

The goal of pituitary surgery is total resection limited to the lesion, without compromising postoperative endogenous pituitary function. Careful selective mass resection may be difficult for poorly encapsulated lesions, those embedded deeply within the gland body, and those extending into the wall or the body of the cavernous sinuses or suprasellar lesions. However, many more suprasellar tumors (e.g. craniopharyngiomas) have been successfully removed via a transnasal approach than previously thought possible. Poor operative field visibility also limits resection precision.

Normal tissue excision or even gland manipulation should be avoided, unless it is critical for effective dissection. Occasionally, hemihypophysectomy or even nonselective total gland resection is indicated for multifocal tumors if the surrounding normal gland is necrotic or if no mass lesion is discernible despite an accurate clinical and biochemical diagnosis (especially for ACTH-cell tumors). Successful surgery should decompress central visual defects and compromised trophic hormone secretion. For children and young adults the consideration of adequate normal tissue for subsequent growth patterns and reproductive function is an important determinant for intraoperative decision making. Nevertheless, especially for functional tumors, small residual remnants attached to the dura are difficult to access but remain hypersecretory, with persistent clinical

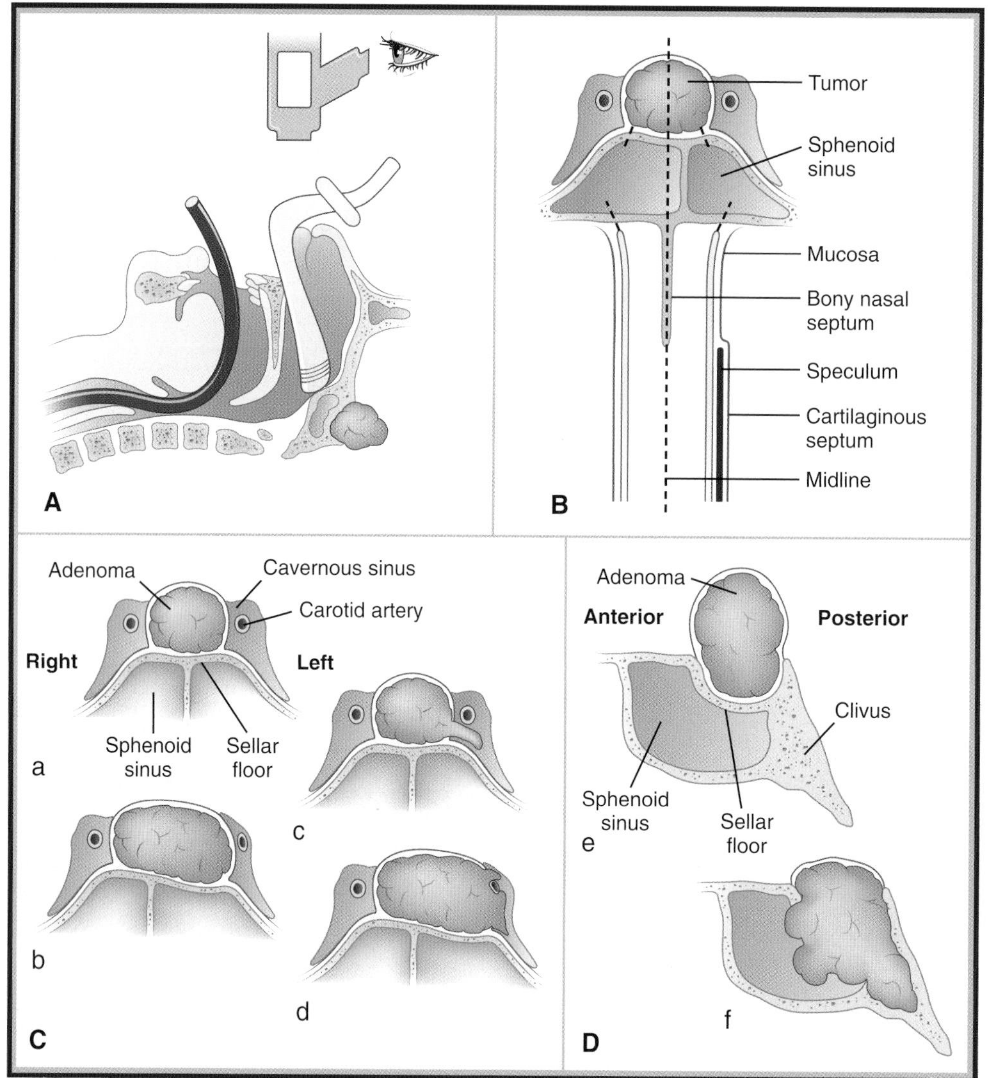

Figure 8–13 ▪ Transsphenoidal pituitary surgery. **A,** Route of the transsphenoidal approach (lateral view) and surgical corridor of the transsphenoidal approach and positioning of the retractor. **B,** The extent of removal of bone structures is indicated *(gray)*. **C,** Parasellar extensions of pituitary adenomas (coronal sections): *a,* intrasellar adenoma; *b,* displacement of the cavernous sinus; *c,* focal invasion of the cavernous sinus; *d,* diffuse invasion of the cavernous sinus by the adenoma. **D,** Extensions of a pituitary adenoma (sagittal sections): *e,* suprasellar extension; *f,* invasion of the sphenoid sinus and of the clivus. (Adapted from Honegger J, Buchfelder M, Fahlbusch R. Surgery for pituitary tumors. In Sheaves R, Jenkins PJ, Wass J, eds. Clinical Endocrine Oncology. Malden, MA: Blackwell Science, 1997:176-184).

progression. Thus, the skilled neurosurgeon carefully balances maximally effective tumor removal with the requirement to preserve nontumorous pituitary trophic function.

Recent advances have enabled improved surgical results, although long-term outcomes using these new techniques have not yet been rigorously compared to standard operations performed by skilled surgeons. Image-guided approaches enable intraoperative surgical neuronavigation by three-dimensional imaging. Intraoperative ultrasound and MRI technologies allow real-time assessment of the dimensions and extent of the pituitary mass and the progress of surgery. Intraoperative MRI is performed while the surgical field is still open, thus allowing the surgeon to directly assess the need for further dissection, and it also provides an excellent baseline for postoperative follow-up.[175] In contrast, postoperative image stabilization might not be evident for months after surgery.

Endonasal transsphenoidal endoscopy avoids use of a retractor or speculum, does not require nasal packing, and sometimes leads to a shorter operating time, allowing improved postoperative morbidity and a shorter hospital stay (Fig. 8–15). The advantages of the technique include a clear panoramic view of bony landmarks and the ability to access suprasellar and parasellar tumor extensions into the cavernous sinuses. Disadvantages of this relatively new approach include the management of perioperative intrasellar bleeding and CSF leaks, as well as the added requirement for a preoperative CT scan. Sometimes combining the transsphenoidal approach with use of an endoscope allows the advantages of both approaches.

Indications for Transsphenoidal Surgery

A pituitary mass that might or might not be compressing local vital structures should be evaluated for surgical resection (Table 8–11). Although surgical resection offers a rapid resolution of hormone hypersecretion and many of the resultant clinical features of functioning adenomas, indications for the procedure

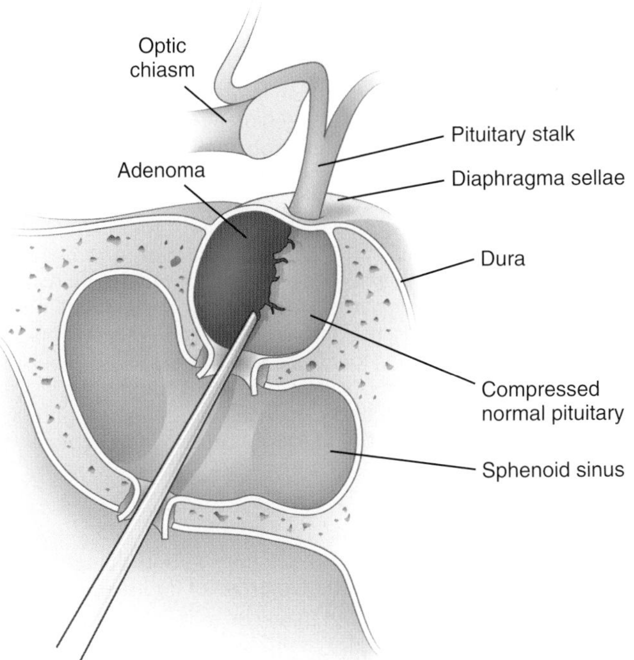

Figure 8–14 ▪ Transsphenoidal resection of pituitary adenoma.

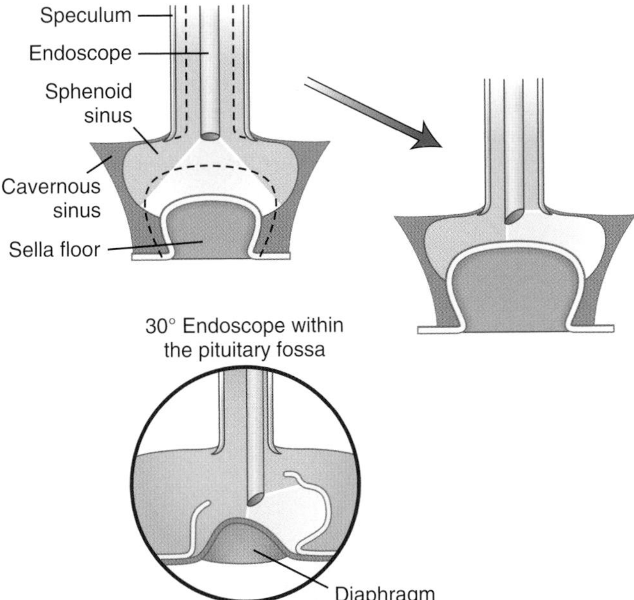

Figure 8–15 ▪ Endoscope-assisted microsurgery provides a panoramic view of the sphenoid sinus. Using a 30-degree endoscope, a view around the corner is possible. Parasellar structures can be visualized and residual tumor detected and resected. (From Fahlbush R, Buchfelder M, Kreutzer J, Nomikos P. Surgical management of acromegaly. In Wass J, ed. Handbook of Acromegaly. Bristol, UK: BioScientifica, 2001:34-48.)

TABLE 8–11 TRANSSPHENOIDAL PITUITARY SURGERY

PRIMARY INDICATIONS
General
Cerebrospinal fluid leak
Desire for immediate pregnancy with macroadenoma
Intolerance of medical therapy
Personal choice
Pituitary hemorrhage
Relief of compressive hypopituitarism by presenting, residual, or recurrent tumor tissue
Requirement for diagnostic tissue histology
Resistance to medical therapy
Tumor recurrence after surgery or radiation
Visual tract or central nervous compression arising from within the sella
Specific
Acromegaly
Clinically nonfunctioning macroadenoma
Cushing's disease
Nelson's syndrome
Prolactinoma
TSH-secreting adenoma
SIDE EFFECTS
Transient
Arachnoiditis
Arterial wall damage
Cerebrospinal fluid leak and rhinorrhea
Diabetes insipidus
Epistaxis
Inappropriate ADH secretion
Local abscess
Local hematoma
Meningitis
Narcolepsy
Postoperative psychosis
Pulmonary embolism
Permanent (Up to 10%)
CNS damage: Encephalopathy, hemiparesis, oculomotor palsy
Diabetes insipidus
Inappropriate ADH secretion
Nasal septum perforation
Total or partial hypopituitarism
Vascular occlusion
Visual loss
Surgery-Related Mortality (Up to 1%)
Acute cardiopulmonary disease
Anesthetic
Brain, hypothalamic injury
Cerebrospinal leak
Postoperative meningitis
Pneumocephalus
Seizure
Vascular damage

ADH, antidiuretic hormone; TSH, thyroid-stimulating hormone.

differ, depending on tumor type (see later). In general, patients who are intolerant or resistant to medical therapy require surgery. Surgery is primarily indicated for patients with well-circumscribed GH-secreting adenomas, TSH-secreting tumors, all ACTH-secreting tumors, and nonfunctioning macroadenomas that require surgery.

Surgery can also be indicated when tissue histology is required for diagnosing the nature of an enigmatic sellar mass. Progressive compressive features including visual field loss, compromised pituitary function, or other central nervous system functional change are indications for surgical debulking and sellar decompression. Hemorrhage into the encased bony sella turcica, usually occurring within a known or previously unknown adenoma, can require immediate surgical decompression. Urgent surgical decompression is required for acute pituitary hemorrhage, especially in patients who have developed sudden visual field compromise.

When pituitary function after surgery was assessed in 234 patients, 52 patients developed new trophic hormone dysfunction, and 45 of 93 patients with preoperative evidence of hypopituitarism recovered between one and three previously suppressed axes. Significant factors determining restoration of postoperative pituitary function were no visible tumor remnants as assessed by MRI ($P = 0.001$) and no tumor invasion as determined by the neurosurgeon and by pathologic examination of surrounding tissue ($P < 0.049$).[176] Therefore, because about half of all patients with preoperative pituitary failure recover function, depending on the clinical circumstance, patients should be considered for retesting before initiating postoperative substitution therapy, except for adrenal steroid replacement, which requires greater caution. Indications for second surgery in the same patient include tumor recurrence, persistent hormonal hypersecretion by tumor remnants, or repair of a CSF leak.

After surgery, patients should be kept on bedrest at an angle of 30 to 45 degrees, and urine and serum osmolality and serum electrolytes should be measured every 6 hours. Indications for postoperative vasopressin replacement include polyuria, especially with serum osmolality greater than 285 mOsm/L, elevated serum sodium concentrations, and inappropriately low urine osmolality. Postoperative polyuria alone is not an indication for vasopressin replacement, unless it is a reflection of compromised posterior pituitary function. Often excess fluid given intraoperatively can manifest as postoperative polyuria.

Side Effects

The success of surgery is largely determined by the skill and experience of the neurosurgeon. Tumor size, degree of invasiveness, preoperative hormone levels, or previous pituitary surgery are all determinants of surgical outcome. High-volume experienced surgeons report shorter postoperative lengths of stay.[177] CSF leakage, transient diabetes insipidus, and inappropriate ADH secretion (SIADH) are the most commonly encountered transient side effects, occurring in up to 20% of patients (see Table 8–11). Local damage can also result in arachnoiditis, vascular bleeding, hematoma formation, and epistaxis. Rarely, pulmonary embolism, narcolepsy, and local abscess have been reported. Iatrogenic hypopituitarism, diabetes insipidus, or SIADH are reported in up to 10% of patients. Rarely, the central nervous system is permanently damaged, with hemiparesis, cranial nerve palsies, or encephalopathy.

A triphasic phase of postoperative diabetes insipidus has been described, when the transient disorder is followed by an interphase on days 6 to 11 with no polydipsia or polyuria. During this later phase, hyponatremia with features of SIADH have also been reported.[178-180] Cognitive dysfunction, including deficits of anterograde memory and executive function, have been reported in several retrospective studies after transsphenoidal surgery.[181,182] Mortality has been reported in less than 1% of patients undergoing pituitary surgery and may be related to direct hypothalamic or cerebrovascular damage, meningitis, pneumocephalus formation, or anesthetic complications. Surgical failure can result from a nonpituitary-related event including anesthesia-related complication or bleeding disorder. Incomplete tumor removal may also be due to inaccurate preoperative MRI localization or identification. Rarely, a previously undiagnosed functioning pituitary tumor or ectopic source of ACTH is unmasked after initially unsuccessful pituitary surgery.

Pituitary Radiation

Principles

High-energy ionizing radiation can be delivered to deep tissues by megavoltage techniques. The challenge of this approach is to provide maximal localized necrotizing radiation to the pituitary lesion while minimally exposing surrounding normal structures to radiation damage. Several advances have improved efficacy and safety, including highly precise tumor localization, a high-voltage (6 to 15 MeV) linear accelerator, and accurate simulation models with isocentric rotational arcing, which allow repeat head positioning at the same exact points for each recurrent patient visit. Up to a maximum of 5000 rad are administered as 180-rad daily fractions for about 5 to 6 weeks. High-precision techniques such as stereotactic conformal radiotherapy[183] and gamma knife[164] allow delivery of high energy to the pituitary lesion while minimizing the mass of normal brain exposed to radiation (Fig. 8–16).

Indications

The use of radiation for treating pituitary tumors is highly individualized and depends on the expertise of the treating center, conviction of the treating physician in weighing the potential benefits and risks of the procedure, and patient preference based upon informed choice (Table 8–12). In general, radiation techniques are indicated for persistent hormone hypersecretion or residual mass effects after surgery or when surgery of a compressive mass is contraindicated. Because GH-secreting and PRL-secreting tumors are generally amenable to medical therapy, indications for their irradiation are rare. Most indications for radiation are adjuvant to either surgical or medical treatment. Radiation may be indicated after resection of a potentially recurring or inadequately resected pituitary mass, such as nonfunctioning pituitary adenoma, craniopharyngioma, or chordoma. In acromegaly, use of radiation as primary treatment is generally not recommended,[184] but for resistant, aggressively

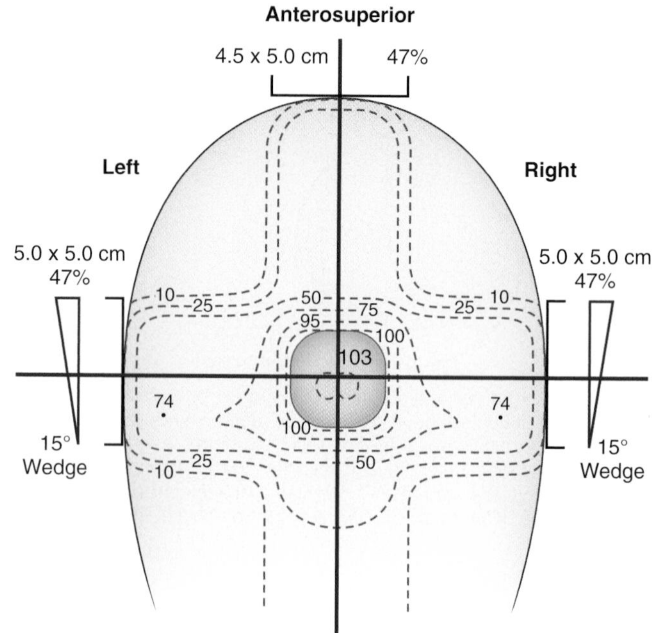

Figure 8–16 ▪ Pituitary radiotherapy. 8 mV x-ray isodosimetric plan. The three fields restrict high-dose volume to the target. (From Plowman PN. Pituitary radiotherapy: techniques and potential complications. In Sheaves R, Jenkins PJ, Wass J, eds. Clinical Endocrine Oncology. Malden, MA: Blackwell Science, 1997:185-188).

TABLE 8–12 PITUITARY RADIATION

INDICATIONS					
Craniopharyngioma Hormone hypersecretion recurrence Nelson's syndrome Nonadenomatous invasive sellar mass Pituitary adenoma: Acromegaly, Cushing's disease, nonfunctioning adenoma, prolactinoma Tumor recurrence					
SIDE EFFECTS					
Hypopituitarism: Deficient GH, gonadotropin, TSH, and ACTH reserve Eye: Visual loss, optic neuritis Brain: Brain necrosis, temporal lobe deficits, cognitive dysfunction					
RELATIVE RISK OF SECOND BRAIN TUMOR					
Second Tumor	**INCIDENCE**		**SIR**	**95% CI**	**Refs**
	Observed	**Expected**			
Astrocytoma (2) Meningioma (1) Meningeal Sarcoma (1)	5	0.53	9.4	3.05-21.98	Brada et al
Gliomas	4	0.25	16	4.4-41	Tsang et al
Astrocytoma (2) Meningioma (1)	3	1.13	2.7	0.55-7.76	Erfurth et al*
Meta-analysis	12	1.96	6.1	3.16-10.69	

*Excludes patients with acromegaly.

ACTH, adrenocorticotropic hormone; CI, confidence interval; GH, growth hormone; Refs, references; SIR, standardized incidence ratio for person-years at risk; TSH, thyroid-stimulating hormone.

Brada M, Ford D, Ashley S, et al. Risk of second brain tumour after conservative surgery and radiotherapy for pituitary adenoma. BMJ 1992;304:1343-1346.

Erfurth EM, Bulow B, Mikoczy Z, Hagmar L. Incidence of a second tumor in hypopituitary patients operated for pituitary tumors. J Clin Endocrinol Metab 2001;86:659-662.

Tsang RW, Laperriere NJ, Simpson WJ, et al. Glioma arising after radiation therapy for pituitary adenoma. A report of four patients and estimation of risk. Cancer 1993;72:2227-2233.

Adapted from Erfurth EM, Bulow B, Mikoczy Z, Hagmar L. Incidence of a second tumor in hypopituitary patients operated for pituitary tumors. J Clin Endocrinol Metab 2001;86:659-662.

growing prolactinomas, the procedure can prevent further local invasion. Recurrent pituitary-dependent Cushing's disease appears to be particularly suited for radiation, especially in younger patients.

Side Effects

Hypopituitarism

Pituitary failure occurs commonly in patients who have received pituitary irradiation. Within 10 years after radiation, up to 80% of patients have gonadotroph, somatotroph, thyrotroph, or corticotroph deficits.[184-187] The mechanism for hypopituitarism appears to involve damage to hypothalamic-releasing cells, as well as direct pituitary damage. These patients require lifelong endocrine follow-up for pituitary reserve testing and hormone replacement when appropriate.

Second Brain Tumors

Thirty-two cases of glioma occurring after conventional pituitary irradiation for adenomas and craniopharyngioma have been reported with a mean latency period of 11.5 years from initial diagnosis.[188] In patients irradiated for pituitary tumors, it appears that the SIR for second brain tumors is about 6 (CI, 3.16-10.69). This is based upon diagnosed second tumors with a latency of 6 to 24 years in separate cohorts.[189-191,192] Because patients harboring pituitary tumors are more likely to undergo routine brain imaging during follow-up, it is not clear whether observed meningiomas are coincidental findings.

Because this complication, which occurs in less than 5% of patients, also appears dose related, fractionated doses not exceeding 5000 rad should be given. Conformal radiation techniques to irradiate a smaller tissue volume, including radiosurgery, fractionated stereotactic radiotherapy, and proton beam can minimize this adverse effect. Nevertheless, prospectively controlled surveillance studies are required to rigorously evaluate this critical question.

Cerebrovascular Disease

The mortality from cerebrovascular disease appears higher in previously irradiated pituitary-deficient patients.[193,194] The direct cause of this relationship is as yet unclear.

Visual Damage

About 2% of patients develop impaired vision from optic nerve damage.[195] The risk of visual damage is minimized by fractionating dosages to less than 200 rad per treatment session. Although consequent blindness has been reported in two patients who received 4500 rad in 180-rad fractions,[196] the incidence of reported visual damage in patients undergoing radiosurgery is negligible.[164]

Brain Necrosis

Dose-related radiation-induced brain necrosis was documented by MRI in 14 of 45 patients, with temporal lobe atrophy, cystic atrophy, and diffuse cerebral atrophy.[197] Cognitive dysfunction, especially memory loss, has also been reported.[198]

Radiosurgery

Proton beam therapy, gamma knife using focused cobalt-60 emissions, and linear accelerator deliver high-dose radiation while sparing surrounding tissue. The delivery of high energy by gamma knife directly targeted at the pituitary tumor minimizes radiation exposure to surrounding tissues. Early reports indicate a more rapid reduction of hormone hypersecretion, with similar long-term efficacy and improved safety outcomes.[199] This procedure is best suited for intrasellar and cavernous lesions distant from the optic nerves. Review of 1621 patients undergoing radiosurgery reported from 35 independent centers emphasizes the heterogeneous efficacy rates, as well as the need for controlled prospective comparative trials, especially to assess efficacy and safety in comparison to surgery and medical therapy.[164]

Medical Management

Pituitary tumors often express receptors mediating hypothalamic control of hormone secretion, and appropriate ligands for the dopamine (D2) receptor and the somatostatin (SRIF) receptor subtype 2 are employed to effectively suppress PRL or GH hypersecretion (or both) to block tumor growth and often to shrink tumor size. Recently, a novel approach has employed a peripheral receptor antagonist to block GH action without targeting the pituitary tumor source. Medical ablation of target glands, including thyroid and adrenal, can also be useful in mitigating the deleterious impact of pituitary tumor hypersecretion. Each of these medical approaches is fully considered later.

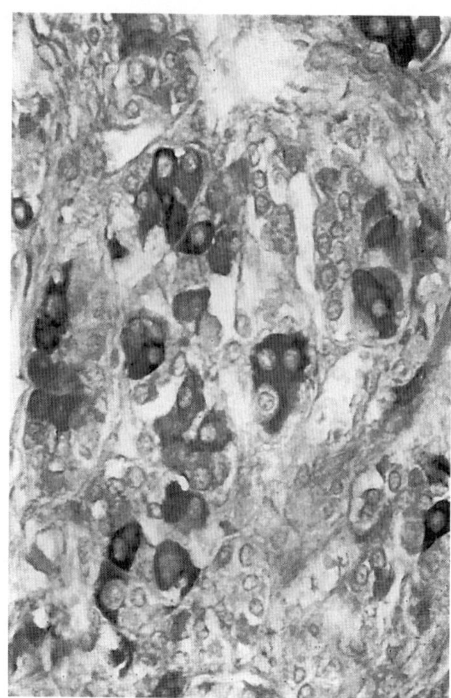

Figure 8–17 ▪ Lactotroph cell. Normal prolactin-secreting cells express strong positivity for prolactin within the cytoplasm of polyhedral cells, which have elongated cell processes. Some processes surround adjacent immunonegative cells that correspond to gonadotrophs. (From Asa SL. In Tumors of the Pituitary Gland. Atlas of Tumor Pathology. Washington, DC: Armed Forces Institute of Pathology, 1997:15.)

PHYSIOLOGY AND DISORDERS OF PITUITARY HORMONE AXES

Prolactin

Lactotroph Cells

Lactotroph cells comprise about 15 to 25% of functioning anterior pituitary cells (Fig. 8–17). Although their absolute number does not change with age, lactotroph hyperplasia does occur during pregnancy and lactation[200] and resolves within several months of delivery (Fig. 8–18). Most PRL-expressing cells appear to arise from GH-producing cells. Ablation of somatotrophs by expression of GH-diphtheria toxin and GH-thymidine kinase fusion genes inserted into the germ line of transgenic mice eliminates most lactotrophs, suggesting that the majority of PRL-producing cells arose from postmitotic somatotrophs.[201]

Two cell forms expressing the PRL gene include large polyhedral cells, which are found throughout the gland, and smaller angulated or elongated cells, which are clustered mainly in the lateral wings and median wedge. Large PRL secretory granules (250-800 nm) are present in the evenly distributed cells, and the laterally localized cells are sparsely populated by smaller (200-350 nm) granules (Fig. 8–19). Occasional mammosomatotroph cells also cosecrete both PRL and GH, often stored within the same granule (Fig. 8–20).

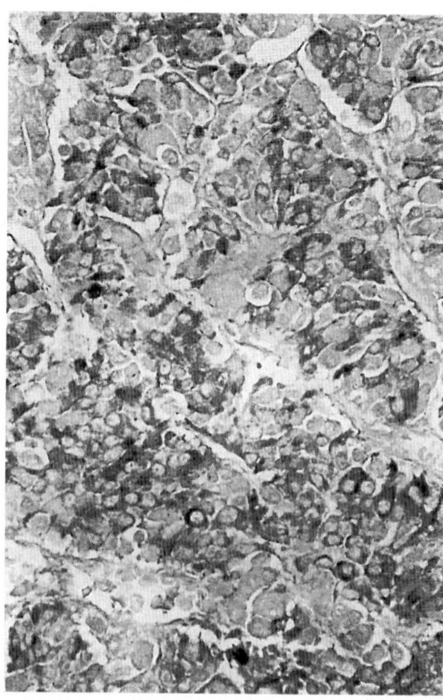

Figure 8–18 ▪ Prolactin cell hyperplasia. In the third trimester of pregnancy, prolactin cell hyperplasia occurs. Cells containing immunoreactive prolactin make up almost 50% of the cell population of the gland. (From Asa SL. In Tumors of the Pituitary Gland. Atlas of Tumor Pathology. Washington, DC: Armed Forces Institute of Pathology, 1997:15.)

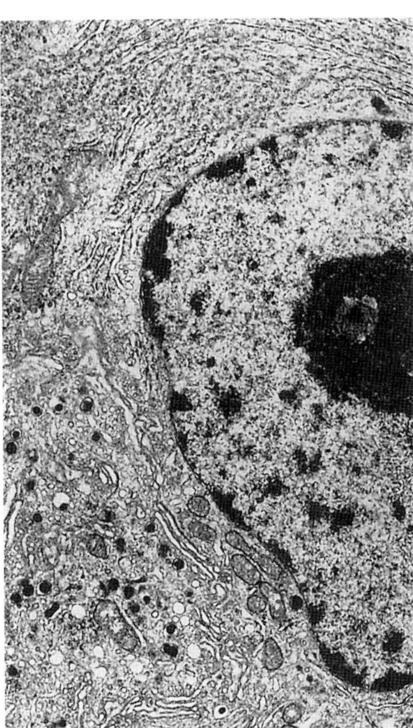

Figure 8–19 ▪ Electron micrograph of a normal lactotroph has a well-developed rough endoplasmic reticulum that forms concentric whorls. A prominent Golgi complex is seen in a juxtanuclear location and harbors forming pleomorphic secretory granules. The cytoplasm is otherwise sparsely granulated. (From Asa SL. In Tumors of the Pituitary Gland. Atlas of Tumor Pathology. Washington, DC: Armed Forces Institute of Pathology, 1997:16.)

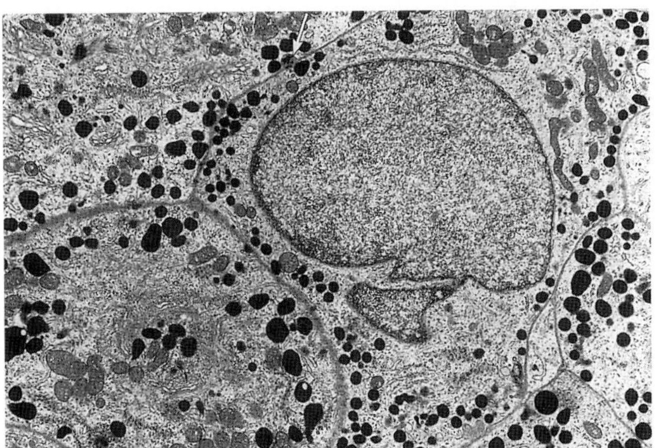

Figure 8–20 ▪ Normal mammosomatotroph. Occasional cells resembling densely granulated somatotrophs exhibit atypical features consistent with prolactin secretion. The secretory granules are highly pleomorphic, and there is misplaced exocytosis, that is, extrusion of secretory material along the lateral cell border *(arrow)*. (From Asa SL. In Tumors of the Pituitary Gland. Atlas of Tumor Pathology. Washington, DC: Armed Forces Institute of Pathology, 1997:17.)

In animal models, lactotroph cell function is heterogeneous. Thus, dopamine or TRH responsiveness and shifting proportions of PRL-secreting versus GH-secreting cells can depend on cell localization within the pituitary as well as the surrounding hormonal milieu, especially that of estrogen.[202]

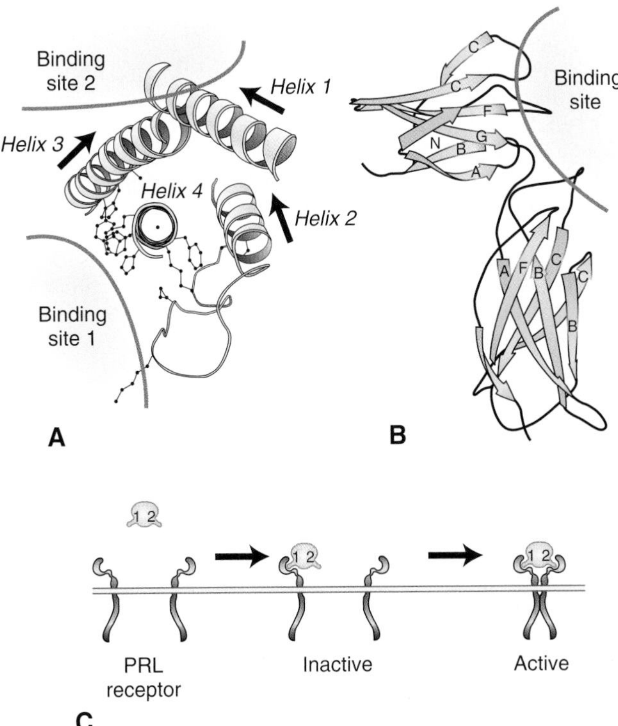

Figure 8–21 ▪ Molecular structure of prolactin (PRL) and its interaction with the receptor dimeric. (From Molitch ME. Prolactin. In Melmed S, ed. The Pituitary, 2nd ed. Malden, MA: Blackwell Science, 2002:119-171.)

Prolactin History

Shortly after its discovery and partial characterization,[203-205] PRL was prominently featured in The *New York Times* on December 3, 1937, in an article indicating that it held the "key to peace in the world." The article, based on a lecture delivered by Prof. C.R. Stockard, proposed that "higher forms of life" were "governed by a "glandocracy," with the glands of internal secretion as the supreme rulers (in this instance PRL) "exerting absolute control not only over the functioning of the individual from conception to death but also over the relationship of men and other vertebrate animals to each other."

The identification of PRL in humans was elusive until 1970, because human GH is highly lactogenic and active in bioassays used to isolate and measure PRL.[206] Furthermore, GH is present in human pituitary glands in much higher concentrations (5-10 mg per gland) than PRL (approximately 100 μg).[207,208] To distinguish human PRL from GH, lactogenic activity was neutralized with GH antiserum; sera from postpartum women and patients with galactorrhea had high lactogenic activity in the presence of GH antibodies.[209,210] Human PRL, bioassayed by stimulating pregnant mouse mammary milk production,[211] was elevated in patients with nonpuerperal galactorrhea due to pituitary tumors, exposure to phenothiazines, and withdrawal from oral contraceptives. The purification and isolation of PRL by Friesen and development of a specific radioimmunoassay underscored the new place of PRL in understanding human disease.[212,213]

Prolactin Structure

The human PRL gene, located on chromosome 6,[214] apparently arose from a single common ancestral gene giving rise to the relatively homologous PRL, GH, and placental lactogen-related proteins (Fig. 8–21).[215] Several factors influence PRL gene expression, including estrogen, dopamine, TRH, and thyroid hormones.[216]

PRL is a 199–amino acid polypeptide containing three intramolecular disulfide bonds. It circulates in blood in various sizes: monomeric PRL (little PRL; 23 kd), dimeric PRL (big PRL; 48-56 kd), and polymeric forms (big, big PRL; >100 kd).[217-219] The monomeric form is the most bioactive PRL. In response to TRH, the proportion of the more active monomeric form increases. A glycosylated form of PRL identified in pituitary extracts is less biologically active than little PRL.[220] Monomeric PRL is cleaved into 8- and 16-kd forms,[221] and the 16-kd variant is antiangiogenic.[222,223] A circulating PRL-binding protein corresponds to the extracellular domain of the PRL receptor.[224]

Regulation of Prolactin Secretion

Prolactin secretion is under the inhibitory control of dopamine, which is largely produced by the tuberoinfundibular (TIDA) cells, and the hypothalamic tuberohypophyseal dopaminergic system.[225,226] Dopamine reaches the lactotrophs via the hypothalamic pituitary portal system and inhibits PRL secretion by binding to the type 2 dopamine (D2) receptors on pituitary lactotrophs.[227] Prolactin, in turn, participates in negative feedback to control its release by increasing tyrosine hydroxylase activity in the TIDA neurons.[226] In PRL-deficient animals, dopamine is decreased in the median eminence.[228] Mice lacking the D2 receptor develop hyperprolactinemia and lactotroph proliferation.[227] Factors other than dopamine inhibit PRL secretion, including endothelin-1 and transforming growth factor (TGF)-β1, which act as paracrine PRL inhibitors,[229,230] and calcitonin, which may be derived from the hypothalamus.[231]

Several substances act as PRL-releasing factors. Basic FGF and epidermal growth factor (EGF) induce PRL synthesis and secretion. Vasoactive intestinal polypeptide (VIP) stimulates PRL synthesis via cAMP.[232] A hypothalamic PRL-releasing peptide (PrRP) produced in the hypothalamus acts through a specific receptor[233] in normal pituitary glands and in a subset of PRL-secreting tumors.[234] Oxytocin and pituitary adenylate cyclase activating protein also release PRL.[226] TRH stimulates PRL[235] but does not likely play an important role in PRL secretion. Estrogen stimulates PRL gene transcription and secretion,[236] explaining why women have higher PRL levels and why cycling women have a higher PRL pulse frequency than do postmenopausal women and men.[237] Galanin is synthesized in both the pituitary and hypothalamus and can act as a PRL-releasing factor.[238] The physiologic role of γ-aminobutyric acid (GABA), neurotensin, substance P, bombesin, and cholecystokinin (CCK) in regulating human PRL secretion is unresolved.[226]

Serotonin may be additive with VIP in releasing PRL, and infusion of 5-hydroxytryptophan (5-HT), a serotonin precursor, elicits PRL release. Nocturnal PRL secretion is attenuated by cyproheptadine. Thus, serotonin may mediate nocturnal PRL secretion and also participate with VIP in the suckling reflex. Opiates acutely induce PRL release, although naloxone does not consistently suppress PRL levels. GHRH, when administered at high doses, moderately induces PRL secretion, and patients harboring ectopic GHRH-producing tumors have mild to moderate hyperprolactinemia. GnRH also stimulates PRL in women, especially during the periovulatory menstrual phase. Although posterior pituitary hormones have been shown to regulate rat PRL secretion,[239] the role of vasopressin or oxytocin or other neurohypophyseal molecules in regulating human PRL remains unresolved. Histamine may act on the hypothalamus to regulate PRL, and H_2 blockers induce PRL secretion.

A short loop feedback of PRL has been proposed and transgenic mice with deleted PRL have decreased hypothalamic dopamine content.[240] In humans, the existence of this regulatory loop has been difficult to prove.

Prolactin Action

Prolactin Receptor

The PRL receptor gene is a member of the cytokine receptor superfamily.[241] It localizes to chromosome 5p13 and comprises 10 exons. The receptor gene has two 5′ promoters that direct transcription of a 598–amino acid peptide[242] comprising an extracellular domain, a hydrophobic transmembrane domain, and an intracytoplasmic region homologous to the GH receptor.[243] Similarly, PRL receptor dimerization occurs with ligand binding and subsequent phosphorylation of intracellular JAK/STAT molecules. Two binding sites encompassing helices 1 and 4 and 1 and 3 on the PRL molecule are critical for formation of the trimeric ligand-receptor complex and subsequent signaling (see Fig. 8–21).[244,245] PRL receptor induces protein tyrosine phosphorylation and activation of JAK2 kinase and STATS 1-5.[246,247] STAT5 phosphorylation mediates transcriptional activation of the β-case in the gene.[248]

PRL receptors are expressed in breast, pituitary, liver, adrenal cortex, kidneys, prostate, ovary, testes, intestine, epidermis, pancreatic islets, lung, myocardium, brain, and lymphocytes. Estrogen also induces liver PRL-receptor expression.[244] Regulation of milk production occurs via a cascade of intracellular events. Homozygous mice in whom the PRL receptor has been inactivated are infertile,[244] and heterozygous animals are fertile but unable to nurse their first litters, presumably because of inadequate PRL receptor expression after the first but not subsequent pregnancies.

Functions of Prolactin

PRL is essential for human species survival by milk production during pregnancy and lactation. Additional biologic functions ascribed to PRL include reproductive and metabolic effects, mammary development, pigeon crop sac activity, fresh water survival, melanin synthesis, water-seeking behavior of newt, molting, and parental behavior.[204] Although PRL and its receptor are clearly crucial in lower animals,[249] the impact of PRL on maternal behavior in humans has not been fully delineated.

Mammary Gland Development and Lactation

Puberty

Prolactin is not essential for pubertal mammary development, which appears to require GH, the action of which is mediated by IGF-I.[250-254] Studies on mammary development have, for the most part, been carried out in rodents.[255]

At birth, the mammary gland consists of a fat pad with small areas of ductal anlagen, which differentiate into pubertal mammary glandular elements under the influence of estrogen, GH, and IGF-I. At puberty, a surge of estrogen begins the process. Terminal end buds (TEBs) form and lead the process of mammary development by branching and extending into the substance of the mammary fat pad, leaving in its wake a network of ducts that virtually fill the mouse mammary fat pad.[255,256] Neither estrogen nor progesterone can act in the absence of GH and IGF-I.[257,258] These hormones are also responsible for most of ductal morphogenesis. Thus, GH acts on the mammary stromal compartment to produce IGF-I, which in turn stimulates formation of TEBs and ducts in synergy with estrogen.[252,259]

Parathyroid hormone–related protein is essential for fetal mammary development,[260] and epidermal growth is essential for pubertal mammary development,[261] but their relationships to other hormones are as yet unclear. Once fully developed, the pubertal mammary gland remains quiescent until pregnancy, although cyclical changes occur during the menstrual cycle. Progesterone, possibly in association with GH and PRL, causes formation of lobular decorations along ducts, which are precursors to true glands, and progestins have similar effects.[262]

Pubertal mammary development begins in girls between the ages of 8 and 13 years (see Tanner's developmental scale in Chapter 24).

Pregnancy

During pregnancy, the normal pituitary gland can double or more in size,[200] the result of a marked increase in the number of PRL-producing cells and a relative decrease in other hormone-secreting cells. Serum PRL concentrations rise to a mean of 207 μg/L during pregnancy,[263] and amniotic fluid PRL concentrations are 100 times those of maternal or fetal blood.[263]

In pregnancy, alveolar elements proliferate and begin to produce milk proteins and colostrum. At 3 to 4 weeks of gestation, terminal ductal sprouting occurs, followed by lobular-alveolar formation. Epithelial buds invade and replace the surrounding fat pad, and true alveoli form at the end of the first trimester. Glandular elements proliferate further, and secretory products appear in the alveolar lumina. During the third trimester, fat droplets are seen within alveolar cells, and the glands fill with colostrum.[264] A combination of estrogen, PRL, and progesterone (and possibly IGF-I) is largely responsible for this phase of mammary development.[265] Placental protein hormones (PRL, placental GH [GH-V], human placental lactogen [hPL])[266] can contribute to mammary development and milk formation. In the absence of PRL, formation of alveolar structures is impaired, as demonstrated in mice with targeted disruption of the PRL gene.[227] Likewise, women with isolated PRL deficiency are unable to lactate.[267]

Alveolar formation and milk production also requires progesterone, and lobular-alveolar formation does not occur in mice lacking the progesterone receptor.[268] Interestingly, only a minority of women have expressible milk during pregnancy, most likely due to inhibitory effects of estradiol[269] and progesterone[270] on PRL-induced milk production. Hormone perturbations during pregnancy also act on fetal mammary gland, causing prominent neonatal nipples and secretion of "witch's milk."

Lactation

Mechanisms of milk production are similar in all mammals, but milk composition differs.[271] Active lactation is due in part to a falloff in estrogen and progesterone and elevation of PRL levels after delivery.

Suckling increases milk production after parturition and is essential for continued lactation because of its distal effect on pituitary hormone production and because it empties the mammary gland of milk.[272] Milk accumulation further inhibits milk synthesis, explaining why a certain level of nursing activity is necessary for successful breastfeeding. In the absence of suckling, PRL concentrations, which rise throughout gestation, return to normal by 7 days postpartum.[263] Suckling increases serum PRL levels approximately 8.5-fold in actively nursing mothers,[273,274] and the milk letdown phenomenon is not associated with increased PRL. As nursing continues, PRL concentrations fall, but each suckling episode continues to cause a subsequent episodic rise in serum PRL. In one study, mean serum concentrations were 162 μg/L at 2 to 4 weeks postpartum, 130 μg/L at 5 to 14 weeks, and 77 μg/L at 15 to 24 weeks.[275] It is unclear why active milk production continues despite progressively lower PRL levels following parturition. Although PRL is essential for milk production, the milk yield does not closely correlate with serum PRL levels.[276]

In addition to its effects on PRL, suckling also stimulates posterior pituitary oxytocin release. Unlike PRL, oxytocin responses to suckling do not decline for up to 6 months as nursing continues. Mothers who breastfed exclusively had mean stimulated oxytocin levels significantly higher during late versus early lactation.[275] Oxytocin induces myoepithelial cell contraction, thereby causing milk ejection.[277] Oxytocin also has important effects on alveolar proliferation.[278] Mice deficient in oxytocin are unable to nurse their young, and oxytocin replacement permits dams to nurse.

Lactational Amenorrhea

Lactational amenorrhea is a form of contraception that depends upon the frequency and duration of breastfeeding. The !Kung hunter-gatherer women suckle approximately four times an hour and at will during the night and bear a mean of 4.7 children during their reproductive years.[279] In contrast, the Hutterites of North America bear a mean of 10.6 children during their lifetimes, presumably because they nurse according to a rigid schedule, use supplemental feedings, and wean at 1 year. In Edinburgh, resumption of menses, albeit anovulatory, occurs in 28 weeks, and the first ovulation occurs at a mean of 34 weeks postpartum due to persistently abnormal LH pulsatile secretion.[280]

Immune Function

Several lines of evidence indicate that PRL is a lymphocyte growth factor and stimulates immune responsiveness.[281] PRL levels change in concert with immune disease as seen in patients with lupus erythematosus. In immunosuppressed mice, PRL stimulates immune cell functions.[282] Although PRL has been suggested as an immunomodulatory hormone,[283] evidence indicates that PRL might not be important for immune function,[284] because innate immunity is not altered in mice that lack either the PRL receptor ($PRLR^{-/-}$) or the PRL gene ($PRL^{-/-}$).[227,284,285]

Effects on Reproductive Function

In mice with disrupted PRL receptor expression, both ovulation and the number of primary follicles are reduced.[228,286] These findings underscore the luteotrophic function of PRL but do not explain suppressed gonadal function observed in patients with hyperprolactinemia.[287] These include short luteal phase, reduced central FSH and LH levels, decreased granulosa cells, decreased estradiol levels, and ultimately amenorrhea (Fig. 8–22). Clearly, attenuated gonadotropin secretion is also a major determinant of ovarian dysfunction in these patients. Male mice with disrupted PRL receptor are fertile, with low gonadotropin and normal testosterone levels. In male subjects with hyperprolactinemia, LH and FSH pulsatility is attenuated, testosterone levels are suppressed, and sperm counts and motility are low.

Prolactin Assays

The PRL radioimmunoassay (RIA) is highly specific and clearly distinguishes PRL from GH. PRL measurements are standardized using reference preparations provided by the National Institute for Biological Standards and Control in London and the National Hormone and Pituitary Program in the United States. Improved assay efficiency, turnaround time, reproducibility, and sensitivity have been achieved by immunoradiometric (IRMA) and chemiluminescent (ICMA) PRL assays. Because these samples are usually assayed at a single dilution, extremely high PRL concentrations can saturate their ability to detect very high PRL levels, resulting in a falsely low value being reported.[288] This hook effect can result in PRL-secreting macroadenomas diagnosed as clinically nonfunctioning adenomas, with falsely normal PRL levels reported in about 5% of patients. In patients harboring macroadenomas with clear-cut clinical features of hyperprolactinemia, serum samples should be subjected to at least 1:100 dilution before assay.

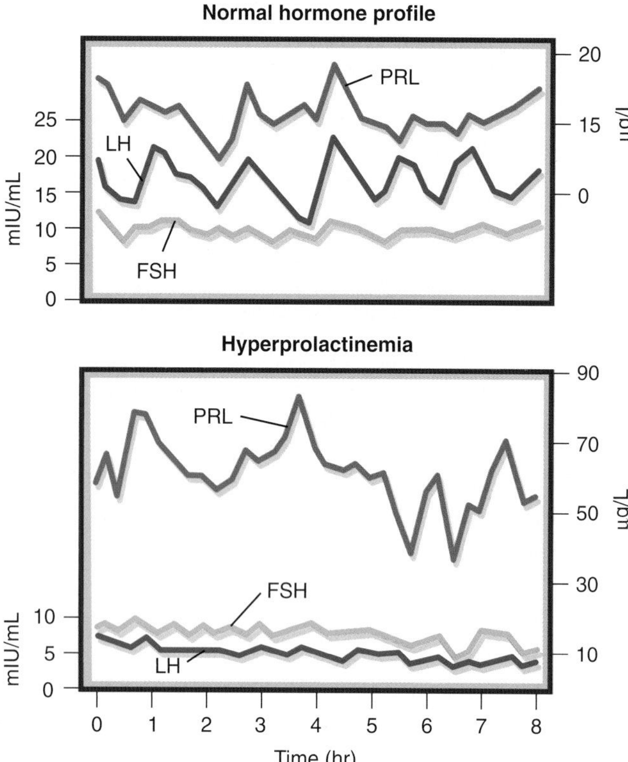

Figure 8–22 ▪ Effect of hyperprolactinemia on suppressing follicle-stimulating hormone (FSH) and luteinizing hormone (LH) secretory patterns leading to hypogonadotrophism in a female patient. PRL, prolactin. (Adapted from Tolis G. Prolactin: physiology and pathology. Hosp Pract 1980;15:85-95.)

Prolactin Secretion

The calculated production rate of PRL ranges from 200 to 536 µg/day per square meter, and the metabolic clearance rate ranges from 40 to 71 mL/min per square meter.[289] PRL is cleared rapidly, with a calculated disappearance half-life ranging from 26 to 47 minutes. PRL secretion occurs episodically in 4 to 14 secretory pulses each lasting 67 to 76 minutes over 24 hours.[290-292]

PRL is secreted episodically during the day, with highest levels achieved during sleep and lowest occurring between 10 AM and noon.[293] The nocturnal elevation is sleep entrained, and a temporal relationship exists between rapid eye movement (REM) and non-REM sleep cycles.[294] PRL can cause periods of REM sleep. VIP stimulates both REM sleep and PRL, and when VIP was given to rats together with a PRL antiserum, REM sleep was inhibited.

PRL levels fall with age in both men and women. In older men, less PRL is produced with each secretory burst than in younger men.[295] Likewise, postmenopausal women have lower mean serum PRL levels and PRL pulse frequency than do premenopausal women or men, suggesting a stimulatory effect of estrogen on both these parameters.[237]

Hyperprolactinemia

In the absence of a prolactinoma, hyperprolactinemia may be caused by other pituitary or sellar tumors that inhibit dopamine because of pressure on the pituitary stalk or interruption of the vascular connections between the pituitary and hypothalamus (Table 8–13).

Idiopathic Hyperprolactinemia

An elevated circulating PRL level in patients in whom no cause is identified is considered idiopathic, and these patients are relatively resistant to dopamine. Mean serum PRL levels in patients with idiopathic hyperprolactinemia is usually less than 100 µg/L.[296]

Macroprolactinemia

Prolactin is a 23-kd single chain polypeptide, but it may also be produced in higher molecular weight forms (50 kd and 150 kd). Macroprolactinemia reflects a predominant larger circulating PRL molecule, (particularly the 150 kd variety) with markedly reduced bioactivity, and few of the expected clinical abnormalities usually associated with hyperprolactinemia (sexual dysfunction, galactorrhea, osteoporosis) occur.[297] The high molecular weight PRL variant may represent 85% or more of the total PRL, but under usual circumstances the 22 kd variety predominates. Screening for macroprolactinemia can be accomplished by polyethylene glycol precipitation of serum samples. In a recent survey, macroprolactinemia was detected in 22% of 2089 hyperprolactinemia samples.[298]

Mild hyperprolactinemia occurs in up to 30% of women with polycystic ovarian syndrome (PCOS).[299] No definite cause-and-effect relationship between the two disorders is apparent.[300] Dopamine agonists reduce PRL and LH levels in patients with PCOS with or without the presence of hyperprolactinemia, and indeed a subset of patients with amenorrhea experiences a return of menses following treatment with these drugs.[301]

Breast stimulation has only a minimal effect on serum PRL levels. In 18 normal women, serum PRL rose from a mean of 10 µg/L to 15 µg/L during breast pump stimulation,[273] and no increase was observed in men.

Up to 20% of patients with hypothyroidism have elevated PRL levels.[302] Although the cause for this elevation is not known, studies in hypothyroid animals suggest increased pituitary TRH.[303] Treatment of hypothyroidism with thyroid hormone normalizes serum PRL if the hyperprolactinemia is due to thyroid hormone deprivation.[304]

Prolactin is moderately elevated (mean 28 µg/L) in patients with chronic renal failure and those on dialysis.[305] The increase is largely a result of an increase in little PRL, due in part to decreased glomerular filtration rate. A specific pituitary defect is also suggested by the observation that TRH fails to evoke PRL in these patients.[306] Sexual dysfunction is common, and reducing PRL with dopamine agonists improves sexual function in men on dialysis,[307] but dopamine agonists do not normalize menses.[308] Side effects of dopamine agonists in patients with renal failure may be exacerbated because of fluid shifts and multiple medication interactions.

PRL levels rise in response to stress, correlate with the degree of stress, and generally return to normal as stress abates. Mean peak serum PRL in 19 women undergoing general anesthesia was 39 µg/L immediately prior to surgery, was 173 µg/L at surgery, and was still elevated 24 hours after surgery at 47 µg/L.[309] Severe head trauma also results in hyperprolactinemia, often accompanied by diabetes insipidus or SIADH and other anterior pituitary hormone deficiencies. Fifty percent of patients develop moderate hyperprolactinemia after cranial and hypothalamic radiation.[310]

A variety of medications cause minimal or moderate PRL elevations and can cause galactorrhea, amenorrhea, or reduced male sexual function. Neuroleptic drugs elevate PRL because of their dopamine-antagonist properties. Chlorpromazine stimulates PRL acutely after an intramuscular injection[211] and chronically during oral administration.[311] Neuroleptics that act by antagonizing both serotonin and dopamine receptors, including clozapine and olanzapine, weakly induce PRL, but others, such

TABLE 8–13 ETIOLOGY OF HYPERPROLACTINEMIA

PHYSIOLOGIC
Coitus
Exercise
Lactation
Pregnancy
Sleep
Stress
PATHOLOGIC
Hypothalamic-Pituitary Stalk Damage
Granulomas
Infiltrations
Irradiation
Rathke's cyst
Trauma: Pituitary stalk section, suprasellar surgery
Tumors: Craniopharyngioma, dysgerminoma, hypothalamic metastases, meningioma, suprasellar pituitary mass extension
Pituitary
Acromegaly
Idiopathic
Lymphocytic hypophysitis or parasellar mass
Macroadenoma (compressive)
Macroprolactinemia
Plurihormonal adenoma
Prolactinoma
Surgery
Trauma
Systemic Disorders
Chest: Neurogenic chest wall trauma, surgery, herpes zoster
Chronic renal failure
Cirrhosis
Cranial radiation
Epileptic seizures
Polycystic ovarian disease
Pseudocyesis
PHARMACOLOGIC
Anesthetics
Anticonvulsants
Phenytoin
Antidepressants
Selective serotononin reuptake inhibitors: Fluoxetine
Tricyclic antidepressants: Amitriptyline, chlorimipramine
Antihistamines (H_2)
Cimetidine
Ranitidine
Antihypertensives
Labetolol
Reserpine
Verapamil
Cholinergic Agonists
Physostigmine
Drug-Induced Hypersecretion
Catecholamine depletors
Reserpine
Dopamine receptor blockers
Butyrophenones: Haloperidol
Phenothiazines: Chlorpromazine, perphenazine
Metoclopramide
Thioxanthenes
Dopamine synthesis inhibitors
α-Methyldopa
Estrogens
Oral contraceptives
Oral contraceptive withdrawal
Neuroleptics
Butaperazine
Chlorpromazine
Fluphenazine
Haloperidol
Molindone
Perphenazine
Pimozide
Promazine
Promethazine
Thiethylperazine
Thioridazine
Thiothixene
Trifluoperazine
Neuropeptides
Thyrotropin-releasing hormone
Opiates and Opiate Antagonists
Apomorphine
Heroin
Methadone
Morphine

as risperidone, are potent stimulators of PRL and have also been associated with enhanced incidence of reported prolactinomas.[312]

Treatment of Drug-Induced Hyperprolactinemia

Unless patients exhibit sexual dysfunction, related osteoporosis, or troublesome galactorrhea, no treatment may be advised. It should not always be assumed that hyperprolactinemia in patients on drugs known to elevate PRL is, in fact, due to those medications. Prolactinoma, other pituitary or hypothalamic lesions, hypothyroidism, or renal failure should be considered. In patients taking neuroleptic medications, if the clinical situation permits, temporary drug withdrawal might be considered to determine if PRL levels normalize. If not, a pituitary MRI should be performed. When neuroleptics elevate PRL, olanzapine may be tried because it does not elevate PRL.[313]

In determining to discontinue a drug or use an alternative medication, the benefits should be weighed against the risks of drug replacement or cessation. Although combined use of dopamine antagonists and dopamine agonists is not usually advised because of increased risk of side effects, such as postural hypotension and a worsening of psychosis, some advocate the use of both simultaneously.[314,315]

Galactorrhea

The Talmud describes a man who nursed his baby after his wife's untimely death, likely representing the first recorded case of male galactorrhea. Galactorrhea and amenorrhea were reported in the 19th century by Chiari,[316] and only in the 1950s did Argonz and colleagues[317] and Forbes and colleagues[318] associate galactorrhea and amenorrhea with pituitary tumors and PRL.

Galactorrhea, inappropriate secretion of milk-like substances from the nipples of either men or women[254] can persist after childbirth or discontinuation of nursing for as long as 6 months. Thereafter, continued milk production is considered abnormal, and other etiologies for galactorrhea should be investigated. Galactorrhea can occur either unilaterally or bilaterally, be profuse or sparse, and vary in color and thickness. If blood is present in the galactorrhea fluid, it could be the harbinger of an underlying pathologic process, such as a ductal papilloma or carcinoma, and mammography or sonography is indicated. Blood can also appear in galactorrhea fluid with no underlying tumor, such as during pregnancy. Conversely, the absence of blood does not rule out an underlying tumor, particularly when galactorrhea is unilateral and emanates from a single duct.

The most common cause of galactorrhea is hyperprolactinemia.[302] It is likely that most patients who have so-called idiopathic galactorrhea with amenorrhea harbor microprolactinomas. Fifty percent of patients with acromegaly also have hyperprolactinemia. Even in the absence of hyperprolactinemia, human GH is a potent lactogen and can cause galactorrhea when elevated.[319] Twenty-nine of 48 patients with pituitary tumors and galactorrhea had PRL concentrations less than 200 µg/L, suggesting that they had pituitary tumors other than prolactinomas on the basis of stalk compression.

Idiopathic Galactorrhea with Regular Menses

The diagnosis of idiopathic galactorrhea with regular menses represents the largest single cause of galactorrhea. In two thirds of patients, galactorrhea begins after parturition, persists despite the resumption of menses, and likely does not represent a pathologic entity. Normal PRL levels can still permit milk production, because treatment of such patients with dopamine agonists alleviates galactorrhea.

Chiari-Frommel Syndrome

The syndrome first described by Chiari and later in the 19th century by Frommel[316] consists of postpartum galactorrhea, amenorrhea, and utero-ovarian atrophy in patients not nursing. Eighteen such patients had galactorrhea and amenorrhea for up to 11 years after parturition.[302] The mean PRL level was 45 µg/L. This disorder is usually self-limiting, and patients eventually become spontaneously fertile, sometimes without having had an intervening menstrual period. Individual patients with postpartum amenorrhea, hyperprolactinemia, and galactorrhea have also subsequently been found to harbor prolactinomas.

Management

Treating the underlying cause of galactorrhea is usually effective. Treating prolactinomas with dopamine agonists reduces tumor size and PRL, normalizes abnormal sexual function, and alleviates galactorrhea. If a pituitary tumor is not PRL-secreting, high PRL levels are normalized and galactorrhea is reduced by dopamine agonists, but the underlying disorder is not addressed. For medication-induced galactorrhea, an alternative medication might be tried. Galactorrhea due to hypothyroidism should be treated with thyroid hormone replacement. If the galactorrhea is entirely due to inadequate thyroid hormone, thyroxine therapy should normalize both TSH and PRL secretion and suppress nonpuerperal galactorrhea. If hyperprolactinemia persists after thyroxine therapy, the possibility of two coexisting disorders is likely. It might not be necessary to treat all patients who have galactorrhea unless it is profuse or troublesome to the patient or is associated with sexual dysfunction.[320]

Prolactin-Secreting Adenomas

With development of a human PRL assay in 1970,[210,212] it became apparent that prolactinomas were the most commonly encountered secretory pituitary tumor, occurring with an annual incidence of approximately 6/100,000. This incidence would be much higher if the estimate included the microadenomas discovered in approximately 11% of pituitaries at autopsy, 46% of which immunostain positively for PRL.[67] The female-to-male ratio for microprolactinomas is 20:1, but for macroadenomas, the gender ratio is roughly equivalent.[321] Both PRL levels and tumor size generally remain stable when followed prospectively.[322,323] In some patients, PRL levels fall over time, and microadenomas sometimes disappear on MRI and do not return after discontinuing dopamine agonist therapy, but 7% to 14 % of microadenomas continue to grow.[324,325]

Macroprolactinomas have a greater propensity to grow and are typically larger in men than in women. Tumor size correlates positively with serum PRL levels, so that a PRL level greater than 200 ng/mL strongly indicates a PRL-secreting pituitary tumor. In 45 men and 51 women with prolactinomas, mean serum PRL was 2789 ± 572 ng/mL versus 292 ± 74 ng/mL, respectively. Tumor size was also larger in men than women (26 ± 2 mm vs. 10 ± 1 mm) (Fig. 8–23). Tumors in men are more invasive and show histologic evidence of more rapid growth.[326] However, PRL levels greater than 200 ng/mL do not always indicate a prolactinoma and might reflect use of a drug such as risperidol.

In contrast, a PRL concentration of less than 200 ng/mL in a patient harboring a macroadenoma indicates that the tumor is likely not producing PRL. In that case, PRL elevation likely occurs as a result of mass pressure on the pituitary stalk or portal circulation, presumably interrupting inhibitory control by dopamine.[327] However, when a clinician sees a patient with a small macroadenoma and a PRL slightly below or above 200 ng/mL, it is prudent to first treat medically. If the tumor is indeed a prolactinoma, cabergoline treatment should lower PRL levels and shrink the tumor. If the tumor does not shrink, the likelihood is that the tumor is not secretory and that the hyperprolactinemia is caused by stalk effect.

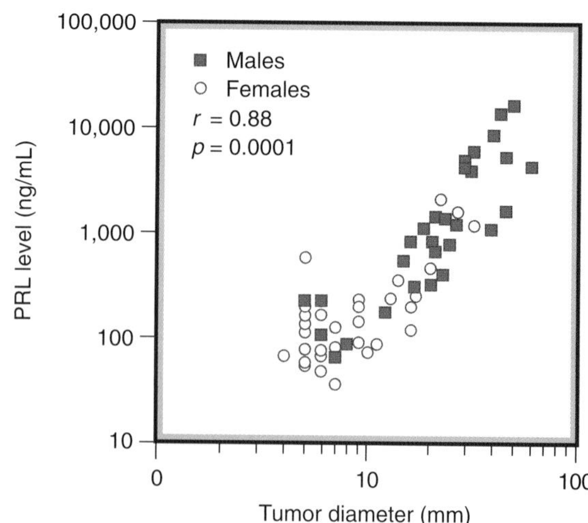

Figure 8–23 ▪ Prolactin-secreting tumors are more often macroadenomas in men (n = 31) than in women (n = 45). Serum prolactin levels highly correlate with tumor size. (Adapted with permission from Danila DC, Klibanski A. Prolactin secreting pituitary tumors in men. Endocrinologist 2001;11:105-111.)

Pathology and Pathogenesis

Although more than 99% of prolactinomas are benign and often sharply demarcated without evidence of invasion, about half invade local structures,[328] as evidenced by pathologic examination (Fig. 8–24).[329] Invasive tumors might have higher mitotic activity and are more cellular and pleomorphic. Invasion into adjacent dura, bone, or venous structures can represent an intermediate form of prolactinoma between the sharply demarcated benign variety and the exceedingly rare malignant tumor. Invasive tumors that do not metastasize are considered benign.[330] Immunostaining for PRL confirms the diagnosis of prolactinoma, which is usually distinct from the adjacent normal pituitary but is not truly encapsulated. These tumors have a pseudocapsule composed of compressed adenohypophyseal cells and a reticulin fiber network.[330] A prolactinoma is only malignant if a distant extracranial metastasis is demonstrated.[331,332]

For the most part, prolactinomas are slow growing, arise sporadically, usually occur singly, and are monoclonal.[34] Often, more than one prolactinoma arises within the gland.[333] Prolactinomas are the most common pituitary tumors associated with MEN-1, occurring in approximately 20 % of a large kindred,[334] although the occurrence of prolactinomas is not evenly distributed. Familial prolactinomas have been described with no other features of MEN-1.[335]

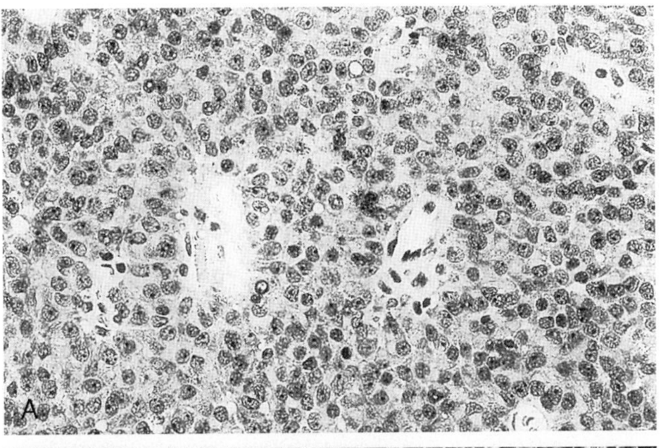

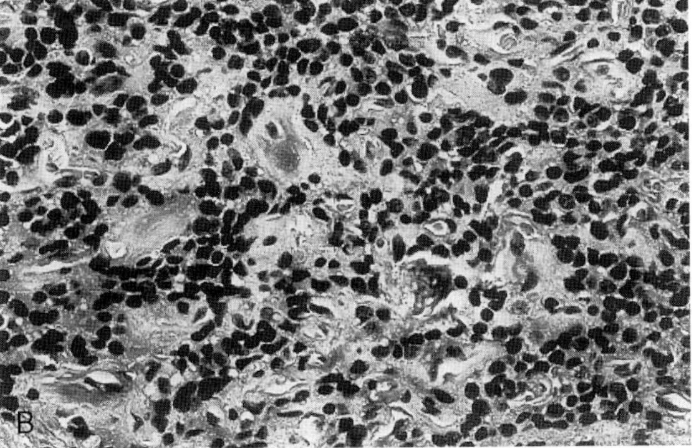

Figure 8–24 ▪ *Top,* A prolactin-secreting adenoma removed at surgery with no preoperative dopamine agonist therapy. *Bottom,* Prolactin-producing pituitary adenoma removed at surgery from a patient treated with a dopamine agonist in the preoperative period. The adenoma cells are small and have dark nuclei and a narrow rim of cytoplasm. Mild accumulation of interstitial connective tissue is apparent. (Hematoxylin-eosin stain; original magnification × 400.) (Courtesy of Kalman Kovacs.)

Clinical Features

Prolactinomas usually come to attention because of symptoms or signs associated with either hyperprolactinemia or tumor size or invasiveness (Table 8–14).

Hyperprolactinemia

Both large and small PRL-secreting tumors can manifest with signs and symptoms of hyperprolactinemia. Menstrual irregularities, sexual dysfunction, galactorrhea,[302] and osteopenia[320] are attributable to elevated PRL levels. Elevated PRL causes sexual dysfunction via a short-loop feedback effect on gonadotropin pulsatilty,[336] presumably inhibiting gonadotropin-releasing hormone (GnRH)[337] (see Fig. 8–22). In oophorectomized rats, high PRL decreases LH pulse frequency and amplitude.[338] High PRL also directly inhibits ovarian and testicular function. Increased opioid LH inhibition has also been implicated as a cause of amenorrhea in hyperprolactinemic patients.[339]

Women with prolactinomas can present with primary or secondary amenorrhea, oligomenorrhea, menorrhagia, delayed menarche, or regular menses with a short luteal phase that can cause infertility. Patients may also report changes in libido and vaginal dryness. Sexual dysfunction in men usually manifests as loss of or decrease in libido, impotence, premature ejaculation or loss of erection, or oligospermia or azoospermia.[340]

Up to 50% of women and 35% of men with prolactinomas have galactorrhea.[208] This gender difference might occur because male mammary tissue is less susceptible to lactogenic effects of hyperprolactinemia.[254] Galactorrhea can be overlooked unless actively elicited. Bone density can decrease in both men and women as a result of hyperprolactinemia-induced sex steroid deficiency.[341]

Tumor Mass Effects

Prolactinomas can manifest as a result of tumor size or invasiveness. Microadenomas can be entirely asymptomatic tumors found at autopsy that are as small as 2 to 3 mm in diameter or larger ones that are still less than 10 mm in diameter. These tumors can be invasive despite their small size. The incidence of headache in microadenoma patients is double that of normal controls.[342]

In contrast, macroadenomas range in size from noninvasive or diffuse tumors approximately 1 cm in diameter to huge

TABLE 8–14 SIGNS AND SYMPTOMS OF PROLACTINOMAS

SIGNS AND SYMPTOMS ASSOCIATED WITH TUMOR MASS
Blurred vision or decreased visual acuity
Cranial nerve palsies
Headaches
Hydrocephalus (rare)
Pituitary apoplexy
Seizures (temporal lobe)
Symptoms of hypopituitarism
Unilateral exophthalmos (rare)
Visual field abnormalities
SIGNS AND SYMPTOMS ASSOCIATED WITH HYPERPROLACTINEMIA
Amenorrhea, oligomenorrhea, primary amenorrhea, infertility
Decreased libido, impotence, premature ejaculation, erectile dysfunction, oligospermia
Galactorrhea
Osteoporosis

tumors that can impinge upon parasellar structures. Signs and symptoms caused by large or invasive tumors are often related to compressive effects on visual structures. The most common ophthalmic complaint in a series of 1000 patients with tumors was loss of vision.[343] The most common objective findings were bitemporal hemianopia, superior bitemporal defects, and decreased visual acuity. Headaches are common, but seizures (a result of extension into the temporal lobe) and hydrocephalus[344] are rare, as is unilateral exophthalmos.[345] Many tumors invade the cavernous sinuses, and yet cranial nerve palsies are only rarely encountered. A sudden insult, such as pituitary apoplexy, is the more common cause of such palsies and may be a presenting symptom. Prolactinomas can also be found inadvertently on an MRI or CT performed for another purpose.

Evaluation

Patients with pituitary tumors should all have serum PRL levels measured. Patients with elevated serum PRL levels not fully explicable by an obvious cause (such as pregnancy or exposure to neuroleptic medications) should be evaluated for the presence of a pituitary tumor. Prolactinomas can coexist with another cause of hyperprolactinemia, such as neuroleptic drug administration. Even minimal to moderate PRL elevations are important to investigate because they can indicate the presence of a large pituitary tumor that does not secrete PRL. PRL levels correlate strongly with tumor size and are usually higher in male patients (see Fig. 8–23). Very occasionally, a patient with a very high serum PRL level might be found to have a normal result reported if dilutions of the patient's serum are not assayed, a phenomenon called the *high-dose hook effect.*[288]

A careful history often unmasks symptoms or signs of a space-related mass such as visual field abnormalities, impaired visual acuity, blurred or double vision, CSF rhinorrhea, headaches, diabetes insipidus, rare hydrocephalus,[344] and hypopituitarism. Patients should also be questioned carefully about sexual history including onset of menarche, regularity of menses, fertility, libido, potency, and ability to maintain an erection. A history of galactorrhea should also be ascertained. The coexistence of galactorrhea and amenorrhea should lead the physician to make a diagnosis of pituitary adenoma until otherwise proved. A change in posture or a history of bony fracture should be elucidated.

Prolactin is elevated in up to 50% of patients with acromegaly.[302] Patients in the early stages of acromegaly or with mild disease and patients harboring acidophil stem cell adenomas might have few obvious signs of GH excess.

Because human GH is as lactogenic as PRL by weight,[346] signs and symptoms of a prolactinoma may be mimicked by a purely GH-secreting tumor. Therefore, serum IGF-I should be measured. Elevated PRL levels are occasionally encountered in patients with TSH-secreting tumors. Other pituitary hormone functions should be ascertained to determine the presence of hypopituitarism. An MRI is required to make a definitive diagnosis of a prolactinoma.

Treatment

Optimal treatment outcomes for a prolactinoma include normalization of PRL levels (and associated signs and symptoms) and complete tumor removal or shrinkage with a reversal of tumor-mass effects (Table 8–15). Specifically, previously abnormal sexual function and fertility should be restored, galactorrhea stopped, impaired bone density improved, tumor eliminated or reduced in size without impairing pituitary or hypothalamic function, and vision normalized, if it is impaired.[347]

TABLE 8–15 DOPAMINE AGONIST TREATMENT OF PROLACTINOMAS (% OF PATIENTS)

Disorder	Bromocriptine (2.5-7.5 mg/day)	Cabergoline (0.5-1 mg twice weekly)
	MICROADENOMAS	
PRL normalized	70	80
Menses resumed	70	80
	MACROADENOMAS	
PRL normalized	65	70
Menses resumed	85	80
	TUMOR SHRINKAGE	
None	20	20
Up to 50%	40	55
50% or more	40	25
Visual field improvement	90	70
	OTHER	
Drug intolerance	15	5

PRL, prolactin.

Long-acting cabergoline has improved patient compliance and has fewer gastrointestinal side effects. For fertility, bromocriptine is preferred because it is short-acting and can be discontinued immediately on pregnancy confirmation.

Values derived from Webster J, Piscitelli G, Polli A, et al. A comparison of cabergoline and bromocriptine in the treatment of hyperprolactinemic amenorrhea. Cabergoline Comparative Study Group. N Engl J Med 1994;331:904-909; and Verhelst J, Abs R, Maiter D, et al. Cabergoline in the treatment of hyperprolactinemia: a study in 455 patients. J Clin Endocrinol Metab 1999;84:2518-2522.

Medical Management

Medical management of prolactinomas with dopamine-agonist drugs has been widely recommended as the treatment of choice.

Dopamine Agonists

Bromocriptine. Bromocriptine, a semisynthetic ergot alkaloid dopamine agonist, lowers elevated PRL levels, restores abnormal menstrual function in 80% to 90% of patients[348,349] shrinks prolactinomas, restores impaired sexual function, and improves galactorrhea.[350,351] Improvement in visual field abnormalities occurs in approximately 90% of affected patients.[352-354] Drug withdrawal can result in rapid tumor expansion.[355] In contrast, occasional tumors that have shrunk during bromocriptine therapy do not enlarge following drug withdrawal.[356] In a subset of patients, hyperprolactinemia disappears spontaneously after long-term observation.[357] Very occasionally, bromocriptine lowers PRL despite continued tumor expansion,[358] although when tumors grow during dopamine agonist therapy there is usually a simultaneous PRL elevation.

Despite high doses of bromocriptine, some patients are entirely or partially resistant to its effects as well as those of cabergoline.[359] Not infrequently, it is difficult to completely normalize PRL levels in patients with initially very high levels, although these patients have impressive tumor shrinkage and sometimes improved in sexual function. Although higher doses or a change in the form of dopamine agonist has been reported to further normalize PRL in some cases,[360,269] many such patients continue to have elevated PRL levels regardless of treatment employed.

Bromocriptine shrinks prolactinomas by shrinking tumor cell size, including cytoplasmic, nuclear, and nucleolar areas.[361-363] Histologic sections appear very dense as a result of small cell size and clumping of nuclei (see Fig. 8–24). Prolactin mRNA and synthesis is inhibited, exocytoses are reduced, PRL secretory granules decrease, and rough endoplasmic reticulum and Golgi apparatus involute. The net effect is reduced cell volume. Tumor necrosis can also occur.[364]

Perivascular fibrosis was noted in prolactinomas derived from patients treated with bromocriptine[365] and caused difficulty in tumor removal. However, others found no effect of prior treatment with bromocriptine on surgical success rates.[366,367] In contrast, bromocriptine was a helpful adjunct to transsphenoidal microsurgery for macroprolactinomas.[368] Even the largest tumors or those with the highest PRL levels respond well to treatment with 2.5 mg bromocriptine three times daily. Higher doses are often not more effective.[208] Once positive effects on tumor size and amenorrhea and galactorrhea are established, some patients can be satisfactorily maintained with smaller doses[369] although rarely without medication.

Cabergoline. Cabergoline has a longer duration of action than other available dopamine agonists and is usually administered once or twice weekly. Since its introduction, it has surpassed bromocriptine as the first-line therapeutic choice for most patients unless pregnancy is desired.[370] The long half-life of cabergoline is a result of its high affinity for D2 receptors on lactotrophs and a greater propensity of the drug to remain in pituitary tissue.[371]

In pharmacokinetic studies, cabergoline lowered PRL in a dose-related manner.[372,373] Prolactin levels were normalized in 83% of 459 women with hyperprolactinemia treated with cabergoline (0.5 to 1 mg twice weekly) and in 52 % of women on bromocriptine (2.5 to 5 mg twice daily). Cabergoline was also more effective than bromocriptine in restoring ovulatory cycles and fertility (72% vs. 52%; $P < 0.001$), was better tolerated than bromocriptine, and caused fewer but similar side effects (Fig. 8–25). Tumor size decreased in 11 of 15 patients with macroadenomas, and menses resumed in three of four premenopausal women.[374] In 85 patients with macroprolactinomas treated with cabergoline (0.25 mg to 10.5 mg per week), PRL concentrations were normalized in 61% of patients and decreased by at least 75% in an additional 24 patients, and tumor size decreased in 66% of patients (see Table 8–15). Nine patients were resistant to cabergoline despite doses of up to 7 mg per week.[350,375] Despite

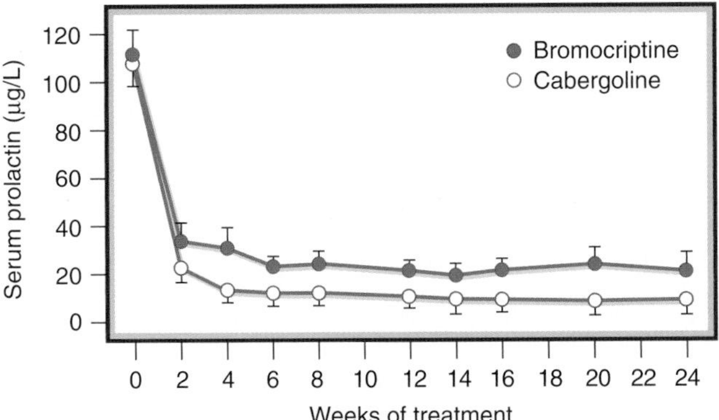

Figure 8–25 ▪ Comparison of bromocriptine and cabergoline in suppressing PRL levels in women with hyperprolactinemia. (From Webster J, Piscitelli G, Polli A, et al. A comparison of cabergoline and bromocriptine in the treatment of hyperprolactinemic amenorrhea. Cabergoline Comparative Study Group. N Engl J Med 1994;331:904-909.)

the continued experience that a subset of hyperprolactinemic patients is resistant to dopamine agonists, a report indicated that cabergoline normalized PRL in 15 of 19 patients with macroprolactinomas previously resistant to other dopamine agonists.[360] Cabergoline also can result in dramatic improvement of prolactinoma-associated headache.[376]

Prolactinomas completely or substantially resistant to medication are uncommon. Most "resistant" patients have only partial resistance, in that tumors shrink and PRL levels fall considerably lower but do not normalize. With the tumor growth controlled, one must overcome the still-elevated PRL levels by specifically addressing the specific disorders caused by hyperprolactinemia (Fig. 8–26).

Pergolide Mesylate. Pergolide, a long-acting ergot derivative with dopamine-agonist properties, has an estimated potency 100 times that of bromocriptine.[377] Pergolide is administered at 50 µg/day, with gradual dose escalation depending upon the extent of serum PRL normalization. Menses resumed in 76% of women and serum testosterone increased in 10 of 14 men not receiving testosterone, and tumor size decreased in 10 of 13 patients with macroadenomas.[269] In 22 patients with macroadenomas, pergolide lowered PRL from a mean of 2938 ng/mL to 59 ng/mL. Prolactin was normalized in 15 of 22 patients, and tumor shrinkage was observed in 95%.[378] The efficacy and side-effect profile of pergolide and bromocriptine were similar in a study of 96 patients with prolactinomas.[379]

Quinagolide. This nonergot dopamine agonist (CV 205-502), administered once daily (mean daily dose of 0.09 mg), normalized PRL in 5 of 10 patients previously intolerant of or resistant to bromocriptine.[380] Side effects, principally nausea, occurred in 6 of 10 women. In 26 patients similarly evaluated[381] quinagolide normalized PRL levels in 13, but the post-treatment mean remained above normal (30 ng/mL). Thirteen had return of menses, and galactorrhea was reduced in 12 of 15 women. The effect of this medication on tumor shrinkage is similar to that of other dopamine antagonists, but it is not available in the United States.

Administration

Attention to administration of dopamine agonists helps avoid or minimize potential adverse effects. Usual starting doses are 1.25 mg bromocriptine (daily), 0.025 mg pergolide (daily), or 0.25 mg cabergoline (weekly). Doses of medication are either increased gradually, as tolerated, or decreased depending on tolerability and should be initiated with a small dose with food before bedtime. Patients should initially avoid activities that cause peripheral vasodilation (e.g., hot showers or baths), thereby decreasing the risk of postural hypotension. If side effects are troublesome, the next dose should be halved, and subsequent doses should be increased gradually to reach effective levels. Switching from one medication to another may be beneficial,[319] as evidenced by the success of pergolide in patients intolerant of bromocriptine. Intravaginal bromocriptine administration has been used to reduce adverse events with some success.[382]

Adverse Events

Side effects of dopamine agonists are common. Nausea occurs in 31% to 50% of patients. Nasal stuffiness, depression, and digital vasospasm also occur, the latter more frequently with higher doses, in patients with Parkinson's disease. The most serious side effect, postural hypotension, which can cause loss of consciousness, occurs infrequently and can often be avoided by careful dosing.

Signs and symptoms of psychosis or exacerbation of preexisting psychosis can be encountered in up to 1.3% of patients taking bromocriptine.[383] Psychosis also occurs with other

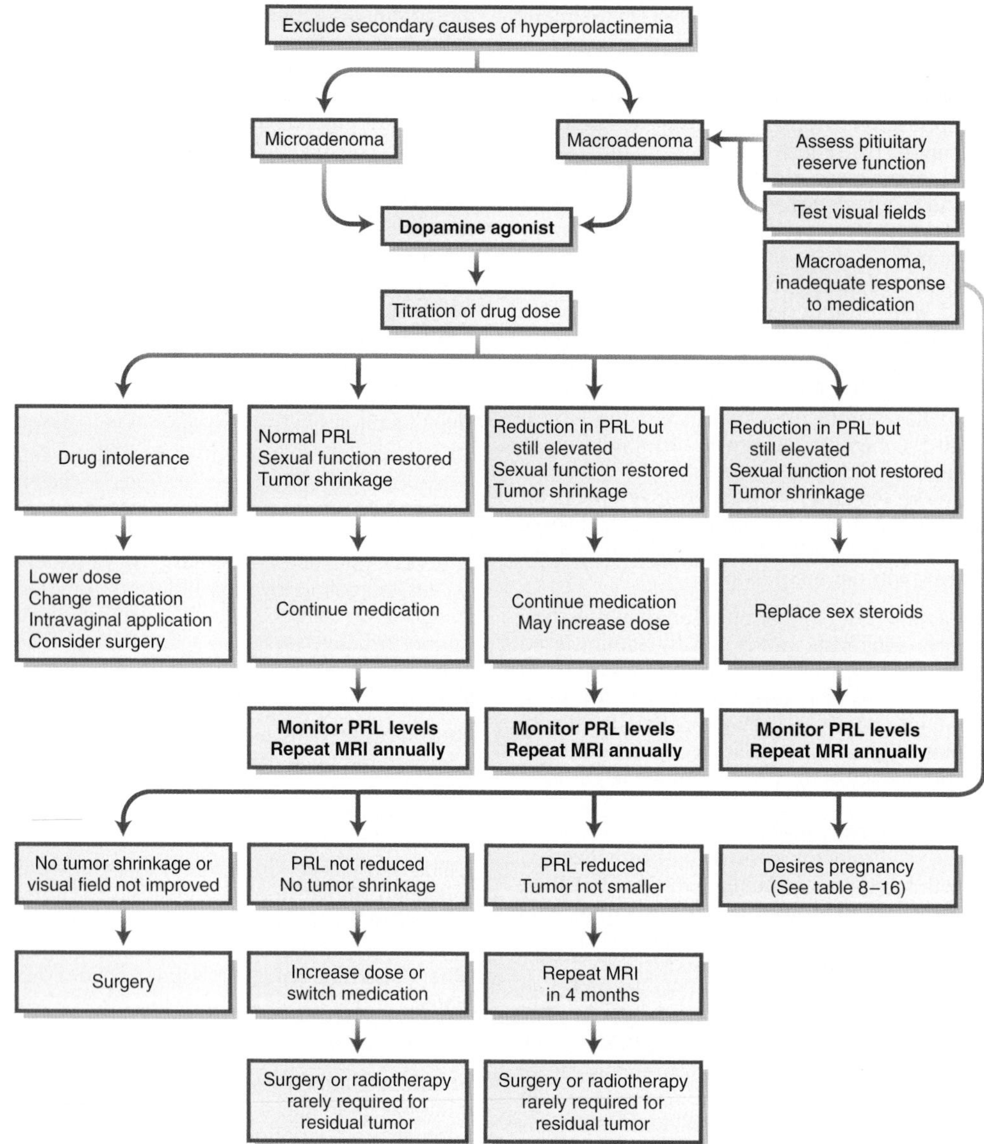

Figure 8–26 ▪ Prolactinoma management. After secondary causes of hyperprolactinemia have been excluded, subsequent management decisions are based on clinical imaging and biochemical criteria. MRI, magnetic resonance imaging; PRL, prolactin.

dopamine agonists, including cabergoline (personal experience). A history of present or past psychotic symptoms should raise concerns about using these medications. If psychosis occurs in a patient in whom dopamine agonists are clearly the treatment of choice, the judicious combination of this agent and antipsychotic medication can be effective. A neuroleptic that is not a potent PRL stimulator, such as olanzapine, is preferred.

The combined use of dopamine agonists and antagonists might increase the occurrence of side effects, particularly postural hypotension. Other rarely reported serious side effects include CSF rhinorrhea,[384] hepatic dysfunction[269] and cardiac arrythmias.[319] Retroperitoneal fibrosis and pleural effusions have been reported with high bromocriptine doses[385] and cardiac valve regurgitation with high cabergoline doses.[386]

Radiation Therapy

Linear accelerator radiotherapy is effective in controlling or reducing the size of prolactinomas.[387,388] However, this therapy takes years to achieve maximal effect. The usual recommended radiation dose is 4500 to 4600 cGy, and higher doses are associated with a greater complication rate.[389] Normalization of PRL was achieved in 7 of 12 patients during 3 to 8 years after radiotherapy[387] and in 18 of 36 patients at a mean of 7.3 years after treatment in another study.[390]

Hypopituitarism occurs as a side effect of radiation. In 165 patients after radiotherapy (3750-4250 cGy),[391] by 5 years, all patients were GH deficient, 91% were gonadotropin deficient, 77% were ACTH deficient, and 42% were TSH deficient. Of 36 patients with prolactinomas, of whom 83% had normal GH responses to insulin-induced hypoglycemia before therapy, 34 were GH deficient at 9 to 12 years after radiotherapy.[390] The incidence of other forms of hypopituitarism was lower.

Thus, although radiotherapy is useful for controlling tumor growth, it is not nearly as effective as dopamine agonists are on endocrine function. Stereotactic conformal radiotherapy with a linear accelerator can provide greater tumor focus and a smaller radiation field.[183] There are as yet no large-scale reports on treatment of prolactinomas with gamma knife radiotherapy.

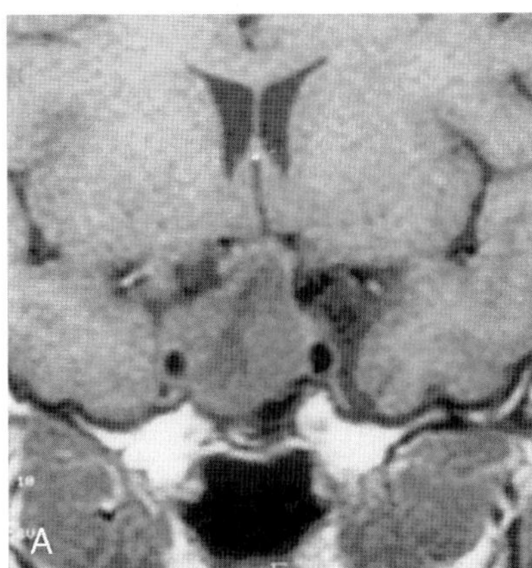

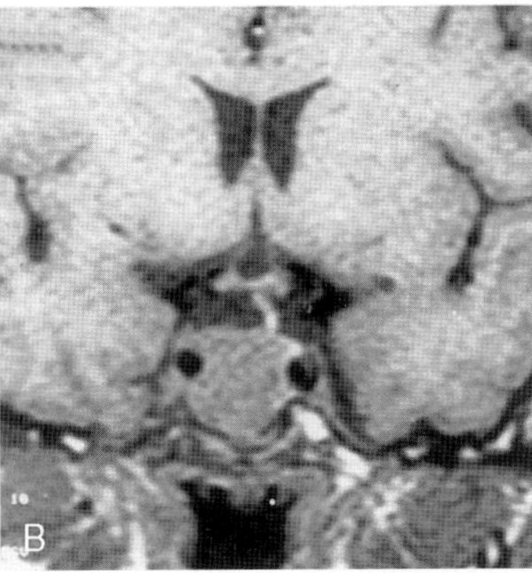

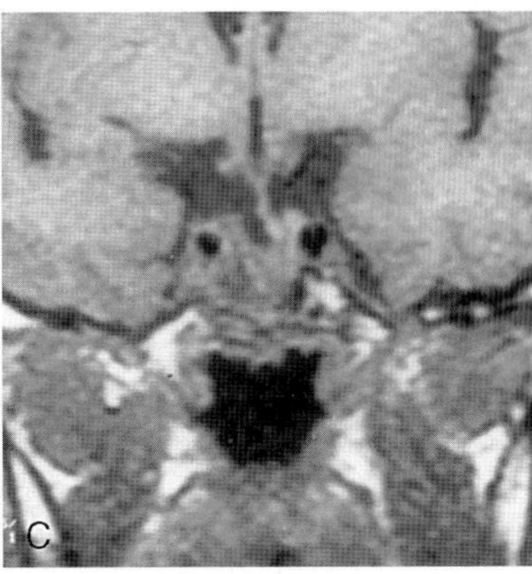

Figure 8–27 ▪ Shrinkage of macroadenoma by cabergoline in a woman harboring a macroadenoma **(A)** at 22 weeks' gestation when prolactin was 488 µg/L **(B)**, and further reduction at 3 weeks postpartum **(C)**. (From Liu C, Tyrell JB. Successful treatment of large macroprolactinoma with cabergoline during pregnancy. Pituitary 2002;4:3.)

Surgery

Surgical removal of prolactinomas by the transsphenoidal route was repopularized in the early 1970s.[392] As with other functioning pituitary tumors, the success rate of surgery correlates inversely with tumor size and serum PRL concentrations.[366,393] In a compilation of results in 31 published surgical series, serum PRL was normalized in 71% of 1224 patients with microprolactinomas. Although surgical cure rates for microprolactinomas are high, the rate of hyperprolactinemia recurrence is also relatively high,[394] now estimated to occur in 17% of patients initially considered cured.[395] In contrast, complete tumor removal of macroprolactinomas, especially large invasive ones, is difficult to achieve, with postoperative serum PRL normalized in only 32% of patients with macroadenomas, with a recurrence rate of 19%. The experience of the surgeon is of major importance, because the cure rate is not nearly as favorable in the hands of neurosurgeons who perform a limited number of these procedures.[396]

Although results of medical therapy are better than those of surgery, there remains a role for surgery in these patients. Patients with prolactinomas that are resistant to dopamine-agonist therapy are particularly well suited for surgery. If tumor removal is only partial, adjunctive radiation therapy should be considered. Prophylactic transsphenoidal surgery should also be considered in women whose prolactinomas are large enough to potentially threaten vision during pregnancy. A subset of patients cannot tolerate available dopamine agonists, and others prefer surgery and refuse medication (see Fig. 8–26).

Pregnancy

The normal pituitary enlarges during pregnancy so that by the end of pregnancy it can increase in size by 136%.[397] Prolactinomas can also increase in size during pregnancy.[398] The incidence of pregnancy-associated tumor enlargement, as determined by development of abnormal visual fields, has been estimated to occur in 1.4% of women with microadenomas and 16% of women with macroadenomas.[399] In other reports, the risk of macroadenoma enlargement has been estimated to be as high as 36%. In a prospective analysis in which 57 patients with microprolactinomas were followed by formal visual field examinations during pregnancy, none developed visual disturbances. In contrast, 6 of 8 primiparous women with macroadenomas developed vision loss.[400] The results on patients with macroadenomas are likely skewed because these patients were recommended for surgery prior to pregnancy.

Although dopamine agonists have been used during pregnancy to prevent tumor growth (Fig. 8–27),[401,402] it seems prudent to reduce fetal exposure to medication if possible. It is recommended that menstrual periods be allowed to occur naturally for a period of time (3-4 months) long enough to predict that a missed period might be a result of pregnancy (Table 8–16). Barrier contraception is recommended during this period. Within several days to a week of obtaining a positive hCG test, medication should be discontinued. Of 6239 pregnancies in patients managed in this manner, bromocriptine therapy was not associated with increased abortions or terminations, prematurity, multiple births, or infant malformations greater than that expected in the control population.

There is no evidence that other dopamine agonists are any less safe, but pregnancy exposure to the other agonist forms are less comprehensively documented. Treatment options for patients who are harboring prolactinomas and whose vision becomes impaired during pregnancy include bromocriptine during pregnancy, high-dose steroids, or surgery.[399,403] One study reported that of 53 pregnant women receiving bromocriptine, mean offspring birth weight was normal, congenital abnormalities occurred in four babies, and physical and intellectual development of children was normal for up to 9 years.

TABLE 8–16 MANAGEMENT OF PATIENTS WITH PROLACTINOMAS PLANNING PREGNANCIES

MICROADENOMA
Discontinue dopamine agonist when pregnancy test is positive Periodic visual field exams during pregnancy Postpartum MRI after 6 weeks*
MACROADENOMA
Consider surgery prior to pregnancy Ensure bromocriptine sensitivity prior to pregnancy Follow visual fields expectantly and frequently Administer bromocriptine if vision becomes compromised, or continue bromocriptine throughout pregnancy if tumor previously affected vision Consider high-dose steroids or surgery during pregnancy if vision or threatened or if the adenoma hemorrhages Postpartum MRI after 6 weeks*

*Pituitary MRI may be required during pregnancy if deemed necessary.
MRI, magnetic resonance imaging.

To avoid neurologic complications of tumor enlargement during pregnancy, it is recommended that women with prolactinomas be tested for sensitivity to dopamine agonists before proceeding with a pregnancy. If tumors are insensitive to dopamine agonist–related tumor shrinkage, prophylactic surgery would be appropriate. If the tumor is a macroadenoma approximating the optic chiasm, the likelihood of visual difficulties is greater, and therefore surgery would be prudent prior to pregnancy.[404]

Gonadotropins

Gonadotroph cells secreting FSH and LH compose about 10% to 15% of the functional anterior pituitary cells. Two classes of electrodense secretory granules are evident; large granules 350 to 450 nm and smaller granules 150 to 250 nm are packaged in vesicles (Figs. 8–28 and 8–29). They contain large round cell bodies with prominent rough endoplasmic reticulum and Golgi apparatus. LH secretory granules often accumulate peripherally, and their Golgi apparatus may be less prominent. Steroidogenic factor I (SF-I) and DAX-I orphan nuclear receptor determine gonadotroph-specific gene expression.

Biosynthesis

FSH and LH regulate gonadal steroid hormone biosynthesis and initiate and maintain germ cell development in concert with peripheral hormones and paracrine soluble factors. The four glycoprotein hormones, LH, FSH, TSH, and hCG, share structural homology, having evolved from a common ancestral gene. Although both the homologous LH and FSH molecules are cosecreted by the single gonadotroph cell, their regulatory mechanisms are not uniformly concordant. The α and β subunits are encoded by different genes located on chromosomes 6, 11, and 19 (Fig. 8–30). The heterodimeric structure of the common α and unique β subunit is essential for their biologic activity. Disulfide linkages maintain noncovalent subunit linkage, which also determine the ultrastructure of the mature folded molecule.[405] After processing of hormonal protein precursors, glycosylation occurs by transferring oligosaccharide complexes to asparaginyl residues.[406] Post-translational processing of carbohydrate side chains is critical for hormone signaling, and it may be

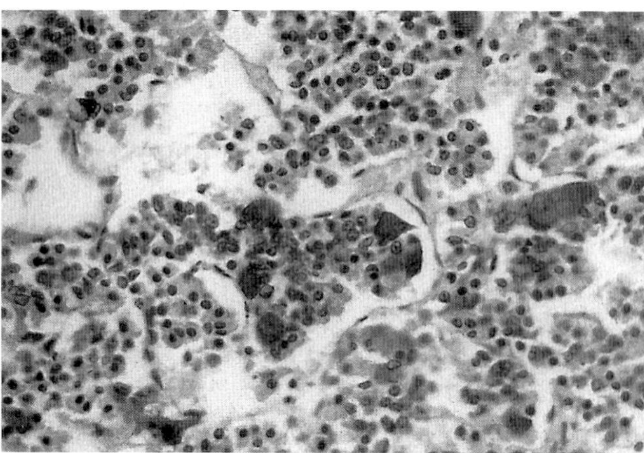

Figure 8–28 ■ Normal gonadotroph cells contain immunoreactive β-follicle-stimulating hormone scattered throughout acini of the nontumorous pituitary. These round cells have evenly dispersed cytoplasmic immunoreactivity for α and β gonadotrophic subunits. (From Asa SL. In Tumors of the Pituitary Gland. Atlas of Tumor Pathology. Washington, DC: Armed Forces Institute of Pathology, 1997:26.)

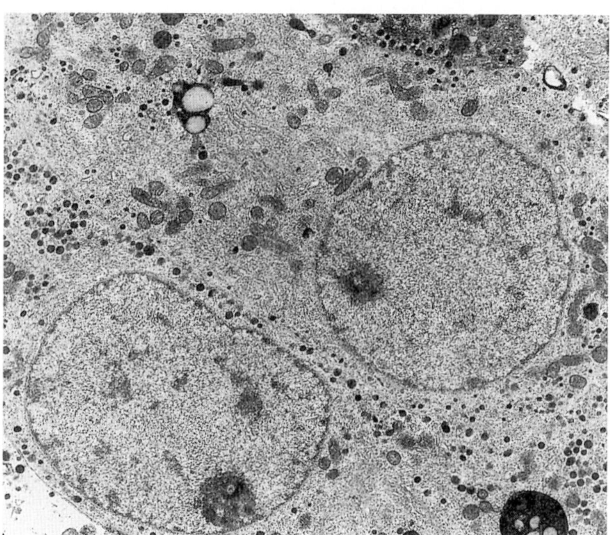

Figure 8–29 ■ Electron micrograph of gonadotroph cell showing large round to elongated cells with ovoid nuclei with occasional nucleoli. Short profiles of rough endoplasmic reticulum are scattered throughout the cytoplasm. Thse are dilated and frequently contain electron-lucent material. The Golgi complex is usually well developed and in a juxtanuclear location. Secretory granules are highly variable in size, shape, and electron density, and lysosomes are prominent. (From Asa SL. In Tumors of the Pituitary Gland. Atlas of Tumor Pathology. Washington, DC: Armed Forces Institute of Pathology, 1997:26.)

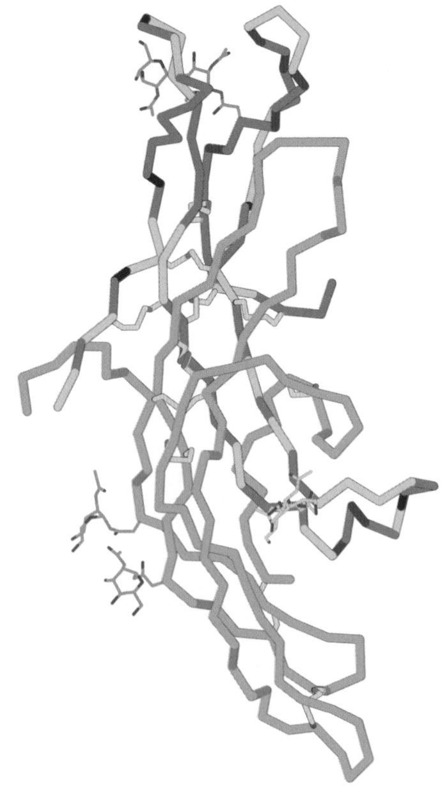

Figure 8–30 ■ Schematic depiction of the subunit structure and glycosylation sites of the four glycoprotein hormone heterodimers (α-subunit, *blue;* β-subunit, *green*). (From University of Glasgow Department of Chemistry. Glycoprotein hormones. Available at http://www.chem.gla.ac.uk/protein/glyco/GPH.html [accessed March 7, 2007].)

species specific and not uniformly similar for both human LH and FSH.

The complex human LHβ gene cluster comprises seven CG-like genes, one of which encodes LHβ, whose promoter and transcriptional start site differ from that of hCG.[407,408] The three exons and two introns encode a 24–amino acid leader peptide and a 121–amino acid mature protein. Unlike LHβ, hCG is only present in primate and equine species, and the hCG peptide product contains a 24–amino acid carboxy-terminal extension.[409] The cell-specific LH gene expression and GnRH-responsiveness of LH are subserved by different transcriptional mechanisms.[410,411] GnRH induces LHβ transcription, as does steroidogenic factor-1.[412] The rat LHβ promoter contains an estrogen-responsive motif and an NF-Y binding site that appears to be important for basal, but not GnRH-mediated, trancription.[410] The FSHβ gene comprises three exons and two introns located on chromosome 11.[413] The gene promoter is dissimilar from that of LHβ, and structure-function mechanisms for transcriptional regulation of the human gene by GnRH and sex steroids are not well clarified.[414]

Gonadotropin Assays

Because of the high homology of the glycoprotein hormones, development of highly specific assays, especially distinguishing free α-subunit from intact hormones, has been challenging. Heterogeneity of circulating LH and FSH molecules, insufficient assay sensitivity (especially for normal healthy measurements), and lack of rigorously pure reference preparations have hampered assay development. Immunofluorometric assays detect LH with a sensitivity of 0.1 mIU/mL.[415] Differences in carbohydrate moieties result in isoelectric charge heterogeneity for LH, accounting for some of the observed disparities in biologic and immunoreactive LH ratios observed after GnRH agonist treatment, acute critical illness, or aging.

LH bioassays include assessing testosterone generation by cell cultures,[416] and FSH bioassays include measuring granulosa cell or Sertoli cell aromatase generation.[417] Because only intact molecules, but not free α- or β-subunits, are biologically active, these cumbersome assays nevertheless are useful for measuring bioactive hormone without potential cross-reaction of free subunits.

α-Subunit Secretion

Both GnRH and TRH increase circulating levels of free α-subunit derived from either gonadotrophs or thyrotrophs, especially in patients with hypothyroidism, after castration and during the menopause. GnRH agonist treatment, TSH-secreting tumors, or nonfunctioning pituitary adenomas can result in discordant ratios of free α-subunit from intact LH dimer secretion.

Regulation of Follicle-Stimulating Hormone and Luteinizing Hormone Secretion

FSH and LH secretion patterns reflect the integration of sensitive complex hypothalamic, pituitary, and peripheral signals. GnRH pulse amplitude and frequency determine the physiologic patterns of LH and FSH secretion (Fig. 8–31).[418] In patients with hypothalamic GnRH deficiency, intravenous GnRH injections (25 ng/kg) that achieve GnRH levels similar to those present in primate hypophyseal-portal blood replicate the physiologic pattern of LH secretion.[419] The magnitude of the LH response exceeds that of FSH. Decreasing GnRH pulse frequency enhances LH pulse amplitudes, and increasing GnRH pulse frequency to more than every 2 hours down-regulates the subsequent LH response. The interpulse LH secretory interval is 55 minutes, and the pulse amplitude is about 40% of basal tonic secretion. Changes in gonadotropin secretion during infancy, childhood, puberty, and aging are described in Chapter 24 (Fig. 8–32). A log-linear relationship is evident between the GnRH dose and the quantity of LH, FSH, and free α-subunit pituitary secretion.

Pituitary and hypothalamic targets for testosterone signals mediate FSH and LH regulation, and in male subjects testosterone attenuates gonadotropin secretion Thus, after castration, elevated gonadotropin levels can be partially overcome by testosterone replacement. Mechanisms for these phenomena are complex, because testosterone also exerts a stimulatory effect

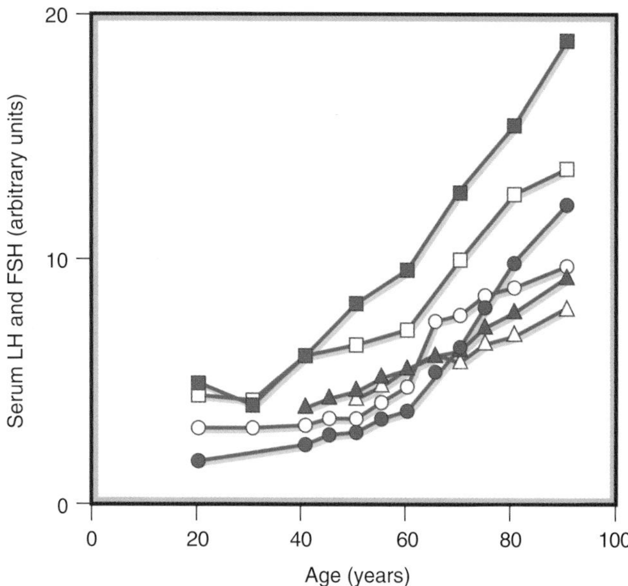

Figure 8–31 ▪ Serum luteinizing hormone (LH) levels *(open symbols)* and follicle-stimulating hormone (FSH) levels *(solid symbols)* in men as a function of age from three studies. (From Tenover JL, Male hormone replacement therapy including "andropause." Endocrinol Metab Clin North Am 1998;27:969-987; Bhasin S, Fisher CE, Sverdloff RS. Follicle-stimulating hormone and luteinizing hormone. In Melmed S, ed. The Pituitary, 2nd ed. Malden, MA: Blackwell Science, 2002:216-278.)

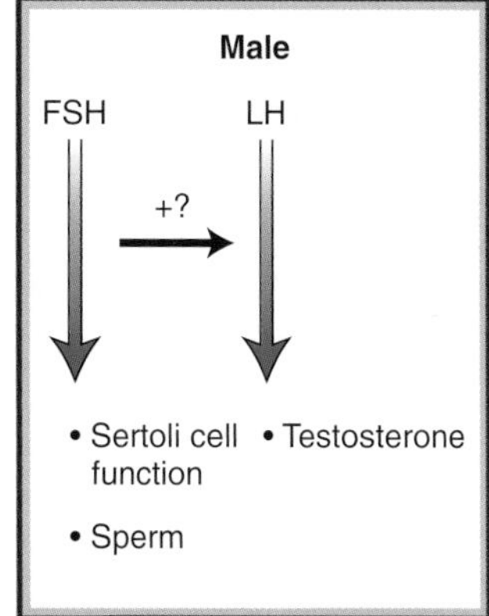

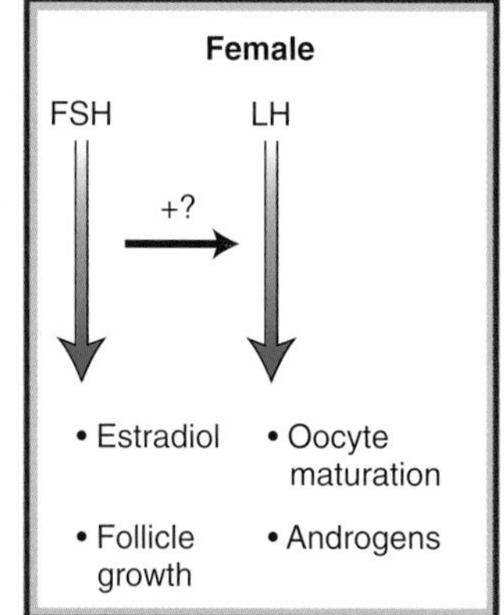

Figure 8–32 ▪ Functions of follicle-stimulating hormone (FSH) in male and female humans. *Plus signs* and *horizontal arrows* indicate potentially unrecognized new functions of FSH since the discovery of FSHβ gene mutations. LH, luteinizing hormone. (Modified from Layman LC. Genetics of human hypogonadotropic hypogonadism. Am J Med Genet [Semin Med Genet] 1999;89:240-248; Bhasin S, Fisher CE, Sverdloff RS. Follicle-stimulating hormone and luteinizing hormone. In Melmed S, ed. The Pituitary, 2nd ed. Malden, MA: Blackwell Science, 2002:216-278.).

on FSHβ mRNA levels. Although estrogen administration decreases LH pulse amplitude in normal and GnRH-deficient male subjects,[420,421] depending upon the clinical situation, estrogen can either stimulate or inhibit pituitary gonadotropin synthesis and secretion, and it also inhibits GnRH synthesis or action, or both. This pattern is manifest in the cyclical control of gonadotropin secretion during the menstrual cycle and during puberty.

LH, FSH, free α-subunit, and testosterone pulses are usually concordant in male subjects.[422] Deconvolution pulse analysis allows estimation of real-time hormone secretion rates, with an assumed disappearance rate constant. The characteristic secretory episodes characterized for LH and FSH indicate daily production rates of 1000 IU and 200 IU, respectively, and a disappearance half-life of 90 and 500 minutes for each respective β subunit.[289,423]

Gonadal Peptides

Pituitary gonadotropin secretion is regulated by gonadal peptides—including inhibin A, an α:βA heterodimer, and inhibin B, an α:βB heterodimer—and follistatin peptides. The activin A (βA), and activin AB (βB) homodimers stimulate in vitro FSH secretion.[424] These proteins, related to TGF-β and müllerian-inhibiting factor, are fully described in Chapter 16.

Follicle-Stimulating Hormone and Luteinizing Hormone Action

Female

Luteal cell LH receptors signal to enhance cAMP levels and induce cholesterol availability for ovarian steroidogenesis (see Fig. 8–32). The StAR (steroidogenic acute regulatory) protein[425] is induced by LH and mediates cholesterol delivery to the inner membrane. LH enhances cytochrome P450-linked enzyme activity to synthesize pregnenolone and induces 3β-hydroxysteroid dehydrogenase, 17α-hydroxylase, and 17,20-lyase synthesis. The FSH receptor, a G protein–linked seven-transmembrane molecule, shares 50% extracellular domain and 80% transmembrane homology with the LH receptor.[426] FSH regulates ovarian estrogen synthesis by inducing 17β-hydroxysteroid dehydrogenase and aromatase, and it induces follicular growth. Estrogens are also permissive for FSH action and enhance FSH-induced cAMP levels.[427]

Male

Leydig cell LH receptor signaling induces intratesticular testosterone synthesis mediated by enhanced cAMP production. FSH function in male subjects is not readily apparent, but it probably mediates spermatozoa development from spermatids in concert with testosterone, especially because failed spermatogenesis leads to elevated FSH levels.

GnRH Stimulation Test

A single bolus of GnRH (25-100 μg) dose-dependently evokes serum LH and FSH levels within 20 to 30 minutes. LH rises more abundantly than FSH, and peak values range from 8 to 34 mU/mL; patients with low testosterone levels exhibit more exuberant responses.[428] In contrast, patients who have hypogonadotropic hypogonadism and no demonstrable hypothalamic-pituitary lesion have blunted LH responses and reversal of the LH/FSH ratio. The test however, cannot adequately distinguish hypothalamic from pituitary lesions, and similar patterns are observed in patients with anorexia nervosa. Repetitive GnRH pulses can in fact normalize responses, as would be expected from an intact hypothalamic-pituitary unit. GnRH responses can vary during the stages of puberty, reflecting altered pituitary sensitivity.

Clomiphene (100 mg) administered daily for up to 4 weeks usually doubles LH levels, and FSH increases about 50% over baseline levels. Because an abnormal or absent response does not distinguish hypothalamic from pituitary lesions, the utility of this test is limited.

Gonadotropin Deficiency

Gonadotropin deficiency causes hypogonadism with decreased sex steroid production of varying degree, depending upon the severity of the insult (Table 8–17). This disorder can occur at any stage of life. In its complete form (e.g., panhypopituitarism, Kallman's syndrome), primary amenorrhea or total failure of male sexual development can occur. Later in life a varying spectrum of sexual dysfunction develops; in women these range from luteal abnormalities or oligomenorrhea to amenorrhea, and in men they include absence of libido, potency and fertility. Women exhibit secondary amenorrhea, vaginal dryness, hot flushes, decreased bone density, decreased breast tissue, and infertility. Men have impotence, testicular hypoplasia or atrophy, decreased libido, low energy, infertility, loss of secondary sexual characteristics, decreased muscle strength and mass, decreased bone mass, decreased body hair growth, and fine facial wrinkling. In men and women, serum gonadotropin levels are inappropriately low in the face of decreased sex steroids and sexual dysfunction.

In women with amenorrhea or oligomenorrhea, serum LH, FSH, and estradiol levels should be measured. Vaginal cytology is helpful in determining the adequacy of gonadotropin function. Endogenous estrogen sufficiency can also be assessed by the response to a progesterone challenge (100 mg IM or 10 mg provera orally daily for 5 days). Men should have serum gonadotropin and testosterone levels measured.

TABLE 8–17 CLINICAL FEATURES OF HYPOGONADOTROPHISM

PREPUBERTAL ONSET
Decreased or absent body hair
Eunuchoidal body proportions
Female escutcheon
High-pitched voice
Penile length <5 cm
Small prostate
Smooth scrotum with no rugae
Terminal facial hair
Testicular length <2.5 cm
Testicular volume <6 cm^3, hypoplastic
POSTPUBERTAL ONSET
Abnormal
Decreased body hair
Decreased libido
Decreased muscle and bone mass
Normal voice pitch
Slow beard growth
Testes atrophic if longstanding
Normal
Penis length
Prostate size
Scrotal rugae
Skeletal proportions

Hypogonadotropic Hypogonadism

Hypogonadotropic hypogonadism can result from hypothalamic or pituitary defects. Hypothalamic damage including Kallman's syndrome, radiation, anorexia nervosa, and excessive stress result in deficient GnRH secretion and action. Pituitary damage from tumors, infarction, or hyperprolactinemia can directly or indirectly attenuate FSH and LH secretion patterns. These acquired causes of central hypogonadism are considered fully in Chapter 16, and genetic causes are listed in Table 8–18.

Because FSH is required for quantitatively normal spermatogenesis, isolated FSH deficiency is associated with oligospermia or azoospermia in normally androgenized men in the face of normal testosterone and LH levels.[429] Isolated LH deficiency can manifest with eunuchoid body proportions and low testosterone levels. Low LH level in these patients leads to low intratesticular testosterone concentrations, with resultant decreased spermatogenesis.[430] Serum testosterone levels are restored in this fertile eunuch syndrome by hCG administration. Isolated hypogonadotropic hypogonadism[431] occurring after apparently normal puberty manifests with relatively mature secondary sex characteristics or even secondary infertility. These patients have abundant gonadotropin responses to pulsatile GRH therapy, which restores reproductive function and fertility.

Evaluation

In evaluating hypogonadal patients in the absence of an obvious pituitary or gonadal disorder, the primary diagnostic challenge is to distinguish constitutional pubertal delay from other causes of hypogonadotrophism.[432] When puberty is delayed after 14 years of age, a primary developmental disorder, hypogonadotropic hypogonadism, or acquired disorders of reproductive function should be considered. The presence of midline defects, pituitary mass lesion, anosmia, history of radiation or pituitary damage, drug ingestion, or other systemic illness should be excluded. Importantly, chronic liver disease or sickle cell disease can manifest with impaired pituitary reserve as well as primary testicular dysfunction. No single test clearly distinguishes constitutional delayed puberty and true hypogonadotropism, and expectant follow-up is often helpful because many patients enter puberty spontaneously.

To provide androgenization, testosterone replacement should be intermittently provided until age 18 years, with periodic interruptions to unmask physiologic pubertal advance. In adults presenting with features of hypogonadotropic hypogonadism, hyperprolactinemia, hemochromatosis, and sarcoidosis should also be excluded prior to the diagnosis of the idiopathic variety. Pituitary MRI and GH, TSH, and ACTH reserve testing should be performed.

Management

Sex steroid replacement therapy is required for inducing and maintaining primary and secondary sexual functions, for minimizing cardiovascular risk factors, and for maintaining normal body composition and integrity of bone mineral density and muscle mass. For patients not desiring fertility, sex steroid therapy is warranted to correct central hypogonadism. However, monitoring of LH and FSH responses does not accurately reflect adequate steroid hormonal replacement, because basal gonadotropin levels are already low or undetectable.

Women

Estrogens are administered as a tablet, patch, gel, or implant. For premenopausal women with pituitary deficiency, a combined oral contraceptive (20-35 μg ethinyl estradiol) may be used. Conjugated equine estrogens (0.625) or estradiol valerate (2 mg) provides relatively physiologic steroid replenishment. Estrogen patches or transcutaneous gels usually allow daily absorption of 50 to 100 μg estradiol. Concomitant cyclical progesterone therapy is indicated for women with an intact uterus to prevent unopposed endometrial proliferation and bleeding. Although early replacement lessens the risk of developing osteoporosis, effects of estrogen replacement on cardiovascular function are unresolved.

In patients with hypopituitarism, estrogen replacement should be maintained at least until the age of 50 years, whereafter continuation should be determined on an individual basis by assessing risks and benefits especially in terms of bone mineral integrity, cardiovascular function, and cancer risk. In women with ovarian deficiency, combined estrogen and testosterone replacement can improve libido and sexual function. Estrogen treatment may be associated with thromboembolic

TABLE 8–18 MUTATIONS AFFECTING GENES OF THE HYPOTHALAMIC-PITUITARY-GONADAL AXIS

HYPOTHALAMUS		ANTERIOR PITUITARY		OVARY		TESTES	
Gene	**Phenotype**	**Gene**	**Phenotype**	**Gene**	**Phenotype**	**Gene**	**Phenotype**
Kal-1	HH Anosmia	GnRH-R	Partial or complete HH	FSH-R	Primary or secondary amenorrhea Delayed puberty	FSH-R	Defective spermatogenesis
Dax-1	HH AHC	Dax-1	HH AHC	LH-R	Normal puberty	LH-R	Pseudo-hermaphroditism
PC-1	HH Amenorrhea Obesity	FSH-β	Primary amernorrhea Defective spermatogenesis			DAX-1	Genital ambiguity Defective spermatogenesis
Lep	HH	LH-β	Delayed puberty			AR	Androgen insensitivity
Lep-R	HH Obesity Short stature					DAZ RBM	OTA OTA

AR, Androgen receptor; DAZ, deleted in azoospermia; HH, hypogonadotrophic hypogonadism; OTA, oligoteratoazoospermia; RBM, RNA binding motif protein.

Adapted from Pralong FP. Genetic basis of hypothalamic-pituitary hypogonadism. In Rappaport R, Amselem S, eds. Hypothalamic-Pituitary Development. Genetic and Clinical Aspects. Basel: Karger, 2001:122-129.

disease, breast tenderness, and possibly enhanced risk of breast cancer.

Men

For men not desiring fertility, intramuscular injection of testosterone 17α-hydroxyl esters (testosterone enanthate and testosterone cyprionate) 200 mg every 2 or 3 weeks is effective, but it may be associated with fluctuations in sexual potency, energy level, and mood, reflecting dynamic changes in circulating testosterone concentrations.[433] Administration of lower doses, albeit on a more frequent basis (e.g., 100 mg weekly or 150 mg every 14 days) can stabilize hormone fluctuations. Elderly men require lower doses, as do boys with delayed puberty.

Scrotal and nonscrotal transdermal testosterone patch systems deliver 4 to 6 mg and sustain testosterone profiles. These preparations require adequate shaved scrotal skin for application. Nonscrotal patch sites can develop skin irritation, blisters, and vesicles in about 25% of patients.[434] Some patients require combined patches and low-dose injection to maintain adequate potency and energy levels.[435,436] There is no apparent cost-to-benefit advantage of patch delivery over intramuscular injection.

Oral androgen replacement therapy with 17α-hydroxyl ester testosterone undecanoate requires frequent dosing (two to four times daily), and because absorption is not uniform, testosterone levels might not be adequately maintained. Oral 17α-methyltestosterone is associated with hepatotoxicity and is not recommended.

Testosterone can cause acne, gynecomastia, rarely urinary retention due to prostatic obstruction, and polycythemia. Although, there is no compelling evidence that testosterone replacement causes prostate cancer, benign prostatic hypertrophy could be exacerbated, especially in elderly patients. Testosterone replacement should not be administered to men with diagnosed prostate cancer.

Fertility

In patients with hypogonadotropic hypogonadism, fertility may be achieved with gonadotropin or GnRH therapy. In male patients, coexistence of primary testicular dysfunction precludes the success of direct gonadotropin replacement or GnRH; however, the relatively low sperm counts induced may be adequate for impregnation when fertility is induced by gonadotropin or GnRH. Because testosterone therapy can suppress spermatogenesis, the steroid should be discontinued before initiating treatment. hCG is administered SC or IM (1000-2000 IU two or three times weekly) to induce spermatogenesis. Lower doses may also be effective.[437] If necessary, after 6 months, human menopausal gonadotropin (hMG) or purified FSH (75 IU 3 times weekly) should be added to improve sperm quantity, and doses may be doubled after a further 6 months. If testosterone levels are increased, subsequent conversion to estradiol may be enhanced, resulting in gynecomastia. Gonadotropin therapy can also cause androgenized oily skin and acne. Therefore, testosterone and estradiol levels should be monitored.

Pulsatile GnRH therapy is indicated for patients with normal pituitary function, that is, those with idiopathic hypogonadotropic hypogonadism or Kallman's syndrome. GnRH is infused subcutaneously by continuous minipump (5 mg every 2 hours), the dose titrated to maintain normal gonadotropin and testosterone levels. This method may be marginally more effective and cause less gynecomastia. These approaches require strong patient commitment, because adequate spermatogenesis might not be attained for 2 years or longer despite normalized testosterone levels. Aliquots of successfully generated sperm samples should be frozen for future impregnation.

In women with central hypogonadism, fertility may be effectively achieved by GnRH or gonadotropin therapy (fully discussed in Chapter 17). Although ovulation is often induced and pregnancy achieved by gonadotropin treatment, a high rate of multiple follicle development remains a concern. A pregnancy rate of 83% was achieved in 77 patients with hypogonadotropic hypogonadism treated by gonadotropins or pulsatile GnRH.[438] If residual pituitary gonadotroph reserve is sufficiently robust, GnRH therapy is more likely to result in ovulation of a single follicle rather than multiple follicles, thereby reducing the chances of multiple gestation.[439] The beneficial role of adding GH to these treatments remains unresolved,[440] except for women with known hypopituitarism and GH deficiency (see Chapter 17).

Producing-Producing Pituitary Tumors (Clinically Nonfunctioning Pituitary Tumors)

Nonfunctioning pituitary tumors constitute approximately 25% to 35% of pituitary tumors.[441] Most arise from gonadotroph cells, and they are monoclonal[34,36] and usually chromophobic. Although they most commonly manifest as clinically nonfunctioning masses and are not associated with elevated serum gonadotropins, they produce sufficient gonadotropin subunits detectable by immunohistochemistry. In one study, 13 of 14 nonfunctioning gonadotroph tumors produced gonadotropic hormone subunits detected by immunohistochemistry.[442] In another series of nonfunctioning adenomas, 42% of tumors immunostained for TSHβ, 83% for LHβ, 75% for FSHβ, and 2% for α-subunit.[292] Some also express chromogranin A.[443] Although LH, FSH, and α-subunit are released from these nonfunctioning tumors when maintained in culture, production is usually not sufficient to elevate blood levels.[74] In the past, when immunochemistry was unavailable, these tumors were often classified as null cell adenomas, which do not express glycoprotein subunits.[444] A small subset of tumors secrete sufficient hormone to elevate serum gonadotropin or α-subunit levels, which occasionally causes clinical syndromes.

Presentation

Clinically Nonfunctioning Gonadotroph Tumors

Clinically nonfunctioning tumors generally come to attention because of their large size or are detected incidentally (incidentaloma) (Table 8–19).[445] Of 506 incidentally discovered pituitary masses, 324 were clinically nonfunctioning tumors, and the

TABLE 8–19 PRESENTATION OF GONADOTROPH ADENOMAS

COMMON
Clinically nonfunctioning macroadenomas Immunostain for gonadotrophin subunits (usually more than one) Pituitary deficiency Usually discovered because of space-occupying effects, or inadvertently
UNCOMMON
Can cause clinical syndrome due to hormone overproduction Immunostain for subunits or intact hormone being hypersecreted Intact gonadotrophin overproduction Other pituitary hormones may be deficient Usually discovered because of space-occupying effects, or inadvertently

remainder were cystic or parasellar masses.[71] A gradual visual deficit arising from optic chiasmal compression is common, and patients are often unaware of the disturbance. Recognition of visual field deficits is often delayed because formal visual fields are not routinely evaluated unless a defect is suspected clinically. In the absence of associated space-occupying lesions or hormonal disorders, these large tumors can go unrecognized for many years and can be inadvertently detected on scans or x-rays performed for other purposes (incidentaloma). Sinusitis evaluation, pituitary apoplexy, or performance of a brain MRI for an unrelated indication (e.g., head trauma) can bring these tumors to clinical attention. Although hormone deficiency is not often the initial presenting complaint, these patients are commonly deficient in one or more pituitary hormones,[176] as was noted in two thirds of 56 patients with nonfunctioning macroadenomas.[176] The most common endocrine symptoms are related to gonadotropin deficiency.

Functioning Gonadotroph Tumors

The small subset of gonadotroph adenomas producing elevated serum FSH, LH, or α-subunit concentrations are considered functioning adenomas but are not often associated with specific endocrine syndromes. High serum FSH, usually with low LH levels, is usually the only sign that a pituitary tumor secretes FSH. Paradoxically, these patients can present with hypogonadism due to gonadal down-regulation. However, female patients with such tumors can present with pelvic pain caused by ovarian hyperstimulation.[446] High gonadotropin levels associated with menopause or testicular failure can complicate interpretation of gonadotropin levels, but LH and FSH are high in primary gonadal failure. LH-producing tumors are exceedingly rare and in male patients cause elevations in serum testosterone with acne and skin oiliness.

Evaluation

MRI, visual field examination, and pituitary hormones should be evaluated, the latter not only to detect hypopituitarism but also to exclude hormone overproduction that might not be clinically apparent. LH, FSH, α-subunit, PRL, T_4, T_3, TSH, cortisol, and IGF-I levels should be measured. A serum cortisol at 8 AM, cortisol response to cosyntropin, or an insulin tolerance test (ITT) can be helpful in excluding secondary adrenal insufficiency. The extent of hormone evaluation requires clinical judgment. When LH or FSH is elevated, the values must be interpreted in light of the patient's physiologic state. Elevated serum FSH in a woman with regular menstrual cycles would be interpreted differently from those detected in a menopausal patient. Gonadotropin elevations in patients with primary gonadal failure are not generally limited to one hormone, and circulating α-subunit elevation is consistent with a pituitary tumor but not gonadal failure. TRH stimulation can differentiate elevated gonadotropin levels ascribed to end organ failure or to independent tumor production. In patients harboring gonadotroph adenomas, increased FSH, LH, LHβ subunit, or α-subunit are evoked in response to TRH.[447] Calculating the molar ratio of LH or FSH to α-subunit can assist in the diagnosis.

Treatment

Clinical judgment should be used in determining appropriate therapy including surgery, surgery followed by radiation therapy, radiation therapy alone, or expectant observation (Fig. 8–33). Unfortunately, no reliable tumor marker predicts mass growth or recurrence.

Surgery and Radiation Therapy

If tumors threaten vision or are macroadenomas whose size threatens vital structures, transsphenoidal surgery is recommended. Vision improves in approximately 75% of patients whose vision is impaired.[448,449,450] In 100 patients undergoing transsphenoidal surgery, 72 had visual disturbances, 61 had hypopituitarism, and 36 had headache. Vision improved in 53 of 72 patients after surgery, and headache improved in all.

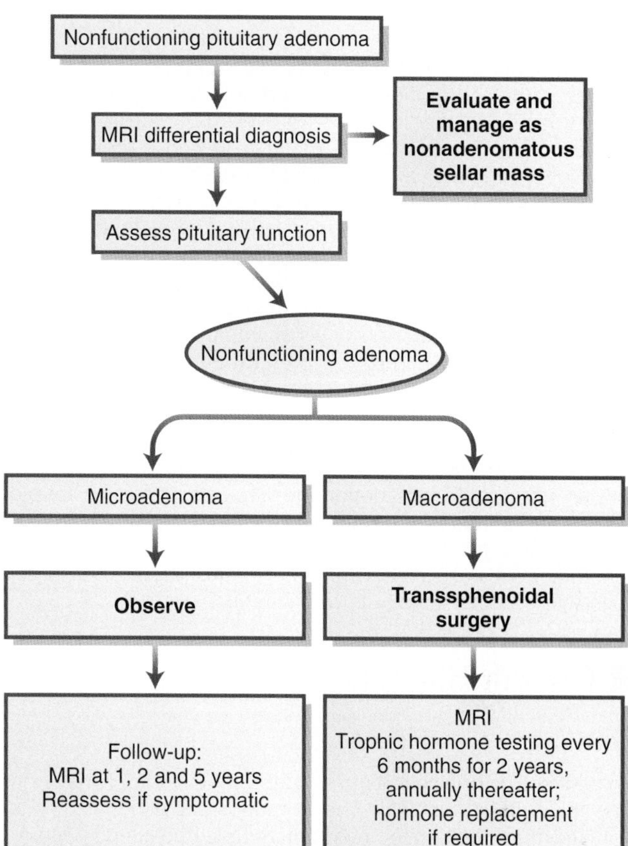

Figure 8–33 ▪ Management of nonfunctioning pituitary adenomas. Skilled interpretation of magnetic resonance imaging (MRI) is crucial to diagnose a nonadenomatous mass (e.g., meningioma, aneurysm, or other sellar lesion).

Of 50 patients who underwent surgery followed by radiation therapy, nine had tumor recurrences at a mean of 73 months after radiation therapy, and five recurrences were documented in 42 patients who did not receive radiation therapy.[451] An expectant follow-up of 65 patients after pituitary surgery for nonfunctioning adenomas showed that 32% of tumors grew during a mean follow-up period of 76 months.[452] In a retrospective comparison of 126 patients undergoing surgery alone, or surgery with radiation, early postoperative radiation therapy (within 12 months) significantly reduced the risk of tumor regrowth by about 15% at 10 years.[453] Despite the relatively high incidence of postoperative tumor regrowth, even after apparently complete resection, most neurosurgeons avoid routine postoperative radiation therapy. Radiation can be offered if the tumor mass re-expands.[449]

The role of gamma knife surgery appears more promising than that of fractionated radiation therapy, inasmuch as early reports indicate a lower incidence of resultant hypopituitarism.[454] This approach requires advising careful follow-up with periodic annual MRIs and vision evaluations. Because patients experience tumor regrowth even after radiation therapy, all should undergo periodic post-treatment MRIs, albeit less frequently.[455]

Expectant Observation

For nonfunctioning microadenomas or small macroadenomas (incidentalomas), patients may be followed expectantly.[456] Some tumors do not grow over years or even decades.[71] However, regular follow-up with MRIs is essential because these tumors can grow insidiously and are usually asymptomatic until they are large enough to affect vision. Periodic, but less frequent, endocrine evaluation is also suggested according to the clinical situation. Microadenomas only very rarely impair vision during pregnancy, as opposed to macroadenomas, which do so with greater frequency.[400] Because macroadenomas do not respond to medical therapy, the risks of vision impairment arising during a pregnancy must be weighed carefully, and resection prior to pregnancy may be indicated.

Medications

Medications are not effective in reducing tumor size and visual compromise. Although dopamine agonists,[457] GnRH antagonists[458] and somatostatin analogues[459] modestly shrink tumors in a very few patients, they are not sufficiently effective to be recommended as therapy. Dopamine agonists can attenuate the regrowth of tumor remnants after surgery.[457]

Growth Hormone

Somatotroph Cells

Mammosomatroph cells expressing both PRL and GH arise from the acidophilic stem cell and immunostain mainly for PRL. Somatotrophs are located predominantly in the lateral wings of the anterior pituitary gland and account for 35% to 45% of pituitary cells (Fig. 8–34). These ovoid cells contain prominent secretory granules up to 700 μm in diameter. Juxtanuclear Golgi bodies are particularly prominent, with secretory granules in formation. The gland contains a total of 5 to 15 mg of GH.[460]

Growth Hormone Biosynthesis

The human GH genome locus spans approximately 66 kb and contains a cluster of five highly conserved genes located on the long arm of human chromosome 17q22-24.[461] These include hGH-N, hCS-L, human chorionic somatomammotropin (hCS)-A, hGH-V, and hCS-B,[462] all of which consist of five exons separated by four introns. The hGH-N gene is selectively transcribed in pituitary somatotrophs and codes for a 22-kd (191–amino acid) protein. The hCS-A and hCS-B genes are expressed in placental trophoblasts.[463] Approximately 10% of pituitary GH is a 20-kd variant lacking amino acid residues 32-46. hGH-V, expressed in placental syncytiotrophoblasts, encodes a 22-kd protein detected in maternal circulation from midpregnancy as well as a minor form, hGH-V2. Elevated maternal hGH-V serum concentrations are accompanied by a decline in hGH-N, suggesting feedback regulation of the maternal hypothalamic pituitary axis. Postpartum circulating GH-V levels drop rapidly and are undetectable after 1 hour.[464]

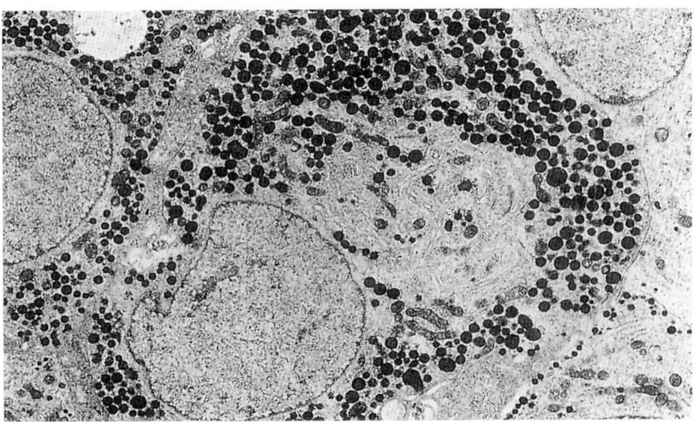

Figure 8–34 ▪ Normal somatotroph. A somatotroph in the nontumorous pituitary is large, is round to ovoid, and contains numerous electron-dense secretory granules that range from 250 to 700 μm in diameter. Short profiles of rough endoplasmic reticulum are scattered throughout the cytoplasm. The juxtanuclear Golgi complex is prominent and harbors forming secretory granules. (From Asa SL. In Tumors of the Pituitary Gland. Atlas of Tumor Pathology. Washington, DC: Armed Forces Institute of Pathology, 1997:14.)

The *hGH* promoter region contains *cis*-elements that mediate pituitary-specific and hormone-specific signaling. The POUIFI transcription factor confers tissue-specific GH expression, and a second, ubiquitous factor binds to a distal Pit-1 site containing a consensus sequence for the Sp1 transcription factor. Pit-1 and Sp1 contribute to GH promoter activation, because mutation of the Sp1 binding site attenuates promoter activity.[465] DNase hypersensitive sites of a locus control region (LCR) of the hGH gene determine somatotroph and lactotroph GH expression and involve regulation of a chromatin domain in these pituitary cells.[466] GH synthesis and release is under control of a variety of hormonal agents, including GHRH, somatostatin, ghrelin, IGF-I, thyroid hormone, and glucocorticoids. GHRH stimulates GH synthesis and release mediated by cAMP. CREB-binding protein (CBP) is phosphorylated by PKA and is a cofactor for Pit-1–dependent human GH activation. IGF-I attenuates basal and stimulated GH gene expression.

The GH molecule, a single-chain polypeptide hormone consisting of 191 amino acids, is synthesized, stored, and secreted by somatotroph cells. The crystal structure of human GH reveals four α-helices.[467] Circulating GH molecules consist of several heterogeneous forms: 22- and 20-kd monomers, acetylated 22-kd, and two desamido GH molecules. The 22-kd peptide is the major physiologic GH component, accounting for 75% of pituitary GH secretion. Amino acids 32 to 46 are deleted by alternative splicing of the GH gene to yield 20-kd GH, accounting for about 10% of pituitary GH. The 20-kd GH has a slower metabolic clearance,[468] accounting for the plasma 20:22 ratio being higher than the ratio in the pituitary gland. The 22-kd peptide retains growth-promoting activity but lacks diabetogenic effects, which are more pronounced with the 20-kd form.

GHRH and SRIF Interaction in Regulating Growth Hormone Secretion

The somatotroph cell expresses specific receptors for GHRH,[469] GH secretagogues, and SRIF receptor subtypes 2 and 5, which mediate GH secretion.[470,471] Hypothalamic SRIF and GHRH are secreted in independent waves and interact together with additional GH secretagogues to generate pulsatile GH release. GHRH selectively induces GH gene transcription and hormone release and does not induce other anterior pituitary or gut hormones.[472,473] SRIF suppresses basal and GHRH-stimulated GH pulse amplitude and frequency, but it does not affect GH biosynthesis. GHRH administered to normal adults elicits a prompt rise in serum GH levels, with higher levels occurring in female subjects.[474] Although mature GHRH comprises 44 amino acids, GH-releasing activity resides in shorter proteolyzed 1-37 and 1-40 forms and the N-terminus. GHRH is also a determinant of somatotroph mitotic activity.

The rat hypothalamus releases GHRH and SRIF 180 degrees out of phase every 3 to 4 hours, resulting in pulsatile GH levels. SRIF antibody administration elevates GH levels, with intact intervening GH pulses,[475] implying that hypothalamic SRIF secretion generates GH troughs. Similarly, GHRH antibodies eliminate spontaneous GH surges. In humans, GH pulsatility persists when GHRH is tonically elevated, as in ectopic tumor GHRH production, or during GHRH infusion,[381] suggesting that hypothalamic SRIF is largely responsible for GH pulsatility. Pre-exposure to SRIF enhances somatotroph sensitivity to GHRH stimulation. Hence, during a normal GH trough period, the high SRIF level probably primes the somatotroph to respond maximally to a subsequent GHRH pulse, thus optimizing GH release. SRIF also inhibits central GHRH release via direct synaptic connections with hypothalamic SRIF-containing neurons.

Chronic GHRH stimulation, either by continuous infusion or repeated bolus administration, eventually desensitizes GH release in vitro and in vivo, possibly due to depletion of a GHRH-sensitive pool of GH. GHRH pretreatment also decreases somatotroph GHRH binding sites.[476] GH stimulates hypothalamic SRIF, GHRH and SRIF also autoregulate their own respective secretion, and GHRH also stimulates SRIF release.[477-479] GH secretion is further regulated by its target growth factor, IGF-I, which participates in a hypothalamic pituitary peripheral regulatory feedback system.[480] GH stimulates IGF-I, which exerts a negative-feedback effect on the hypothalamus and pituitary. IGF-I stimulates hypothalamic SRIF release and inhibits pituitary GH gene transcription and secretion.

Growth Hormone Secretagogues and Ghrelin

Isolation of ghrelin implicates an additional control system for regulating GH secretion (see Chapter 34). Ghrelin is a 28–amino acid peptide that binds the GH secretagogue (GHS) receptor[481] to induce hypothalamic GHRH and pituitary GH.[482] A unique *n*-octanoylated serine 3 residue confers GH-releasing activity to the molecule. Ghrelin is synthesized in peripheral tissues, especially gastric mucosal neuroendocrine cells, as well as centrally in the hypothalamus.

Ghrelin administration dose-dependently evokes GH release and also induces food intake and obesity development (Fig. 8–35). Hypothalamic ghrelin likely controls GH secretion, and peripheral sources can have additional nutritional effects requiring further elucidation (see Chapter 34). Current evidence suggests that the dual control of GH secretion postulated for GHRH/SRIF should be expanded to incorporate ghrelin.[483] Synthetic hexapeptides (artificial GH secretagogues) recognize the GHS receptor, induce potent and reproducible GH release, and are useful for diagnosing GH deficiency.[484] GHSs stimulate GH secretion,[485] and GHRH and GHS act though distinct receptors and via different intracellular signaling pathways on somatotroph subpopulations. GHSs require the presence of a functional hypothalamus to evoke GH, as evidenced in patients with intact pituitary but disordered hypothalamic function, where GHS does not induce GH.[486] GHSs potentiate GH release in response to a maximum stimulating dose of exogenous GHRH[487] and after a saturating dose of GHRH, although subsequent GHRH administration is ineffective, GHS remain fully effective.[488]

Functional GHS receptors are expressed in the human fetal pituitary by the fifth week of gestation.[350] GHS-mediated GH release is demonstrable at birth, continues through infancy, increases at puberty, and decreases thereafter. Estrogen and testosterone increase GHS-mediated GH release in childhood.[489] Because GHS-evoked GH secretion is minimally altered by age, sex, or adiposity and is devoid of potential side effects (unlike insulin-induced hypoglycemia), GHSs may become a useful diagnostic tool in the diagnosis of adult GH deficiency. Slight PRL and ACTH or cortisol increases have been reported, and some GHSs lead to the development of novel GH secretagogues with more selective somatotroph actions.[490]

Regulation of Growth Hormone Secretion

Multiple factors regulate the integrated secretion of GH (Fig. 8–36). Major GH secretory pulses accounting for up to 70% of daily GH secretion occurs with the first episode of slow-wave sleep.[491] The decline in slow-wave sleep from early adulthood to midlife is paralleled by a major decline in GH secretion, suggesting that age-related GH axis alterations can partially reflect decreased sleep quality.[492] Jet lag transiently increases GH peak amplitude, resulting in a transient increase of 24-hour GH secretion. Exercise and physical stress, including trauma with hypovolemic shock and sepsis, increase GH levels.[493] Emotional deprivation is associated with suppressed GH secretion, and attenuated GH responses to provocative stimuli occur in endogenous depression.[494]

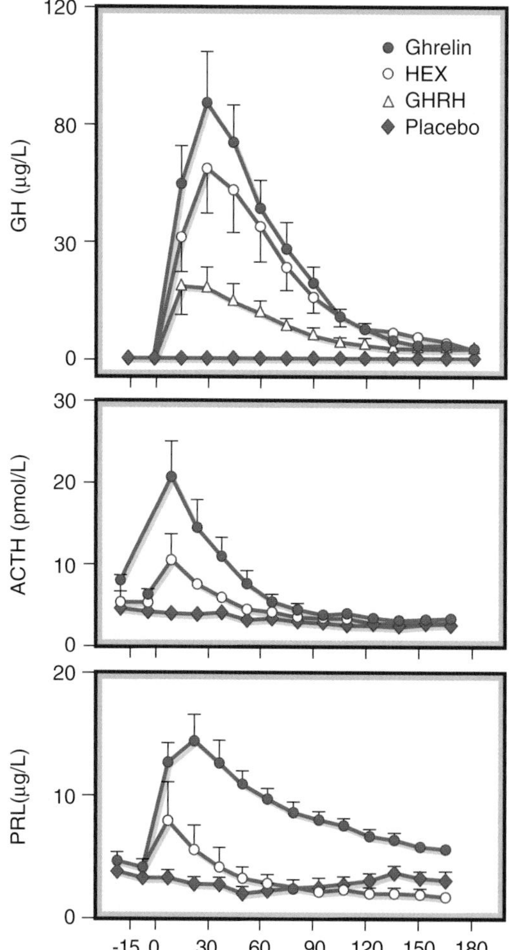

Figure 8–35 ■ Effect of GH secretagogues on GH, ACTH, and PRL secretion in healthy subjects. Mean (+ SEM) curve responses after administration of ghrelin (1.0 µg/kg), hexarelin (1.0 µg/kg), GHRH (1.0 µg/kg), or placebo. ACTH, adrenocorticotropic hormone; GH, growth hormone; GHRH, growth hormone–releasing hormone; HEX, hexarelin; PRL, prolactin; SEM, standard error of the mean. (Adapted from Arvat E, Maccario M, Di Vito L, et al. Endocrine activities of ghrelin, a natural growth hormone secretagogue (GHS), in humans: comparison and interactions with hexarelin, a nonnatural peptidyl GHS, and GH-releasing hormone. J Clin Endocrinol Metab 2001;86:1169-1174.)

Chronic malnutrition and prolonged fasting are associated with elevated GH pulse frequency and amplitude (Fig. 8–37).[495] Obesity decreases basal and stimulated GH secretion, insulin-induced hypoglycemia stimulates GH, and hyperglycemia inhibits GH secretion. Chronic hyperglycemia, is however, not associated with low GH levels, and in fact, poorly controlled diabetes is associated with increased basal and exercise-induced GH levels.[496] Central glucoreceptors appear to sense

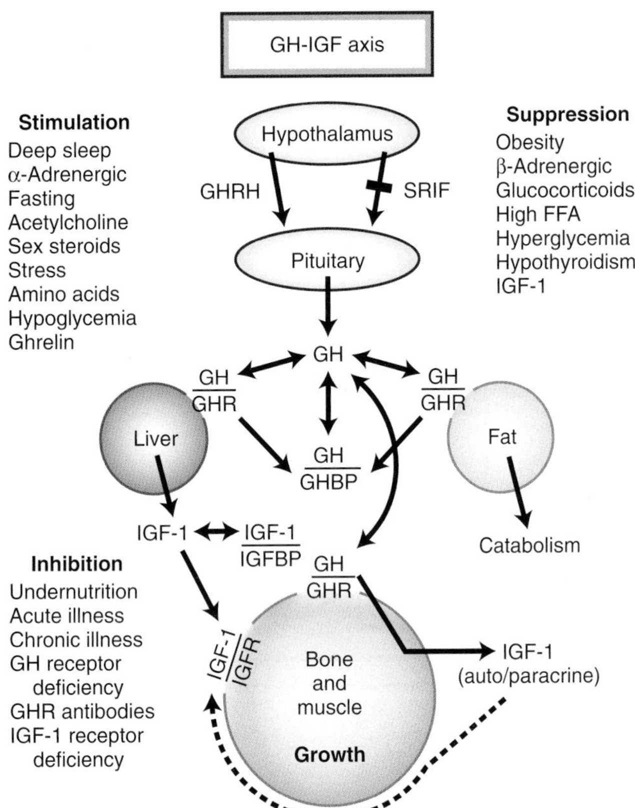

Figure 8–36 ▪ Growth hormone axis. Simplified diagram of GH–IGF-I axis involving hypophysiotropic hormones controlling pituitary GH release, circulating GH-binding protein and its GH receptor source, IGF-I and its largely GH-dependent binding proteins, and cellular responsiveness to GH and IGF-I interacting with their specific receptors. FFA, free fatty acid; GH, growth hormone; GHR, growth hormone receptor; GHRH, growth hormone–releasing hormone; IGF, insulin-like growth factor; IGFBP, insulin-like growth factor binding protein; IGFR, -I receptor; SRIF, somatostatin. (From Rosenbloom A. Growth hormone insensitivity: physiologic and genetic basis, phenotype and treatment. J Pediatr 1999;135:280-289.)

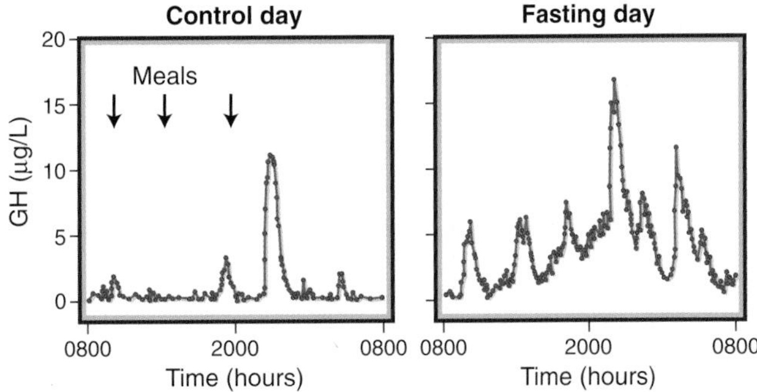

Figure 8–37 ▪ Effect of fasting on growth hormone secretion patterns in a healthy male subject. (FromHartman ML, Veldhuis JD, Johnson ML, et al. Augmented growth hormone [GH] secretory burst frequency and amplitude mediate enhanced GH secretion during a two-day fast in normal men. J Clin Endocrinol Metab 1992;74:757-765.)

glucose fluctuations, rather than absolute levels. High-protein meals, and intravenous single amino acids (including arginine and leucine) stimulate GH secretion. Increased serum free fatty acids blunt the effects of arginine infusion, sleep, L-dopa, and exercise on GHRH-stimulated GH release.[497]

Leptin plays a key role in regulating body fat mass,[498] food intake, and energy expenditure, and it can act as a metabolic signal to regulate GH secretion. Leptin and neuropeptide Y–producing hypothalamic neurons synapse with somatostatin neurons, and antisera to neuropeptide Y and somatostatin reverse starvation-induced GH release.[499] In GH-deficient hypopituitary adults, leptin concentrations are higher than would be expected from their body fat mass.[500]

Neuropeptides, neurotransmitters, and opiates impinge on the hypothalamus and modulate GHRH and SRIF release. Integrated effects of these complex neurogenic influences determine the final secretory pattern of GH. Apomorphine, a central dopamine receptor agonist, stimulates GH secretion,[501] as does levodopa treatment. Oral L-dopa administration evokes a brisk serum GH response within an hour in healthy young subjects. Norepinephrine increases GH secretion via α-adrenergic pathways and inhibits GH release via β-adrenergic pathways. Insulin-induced hypoglycemia, clonidine, arginine, exercise, L-dopa, and antidiuretic hormone (ADH) facilitate GH secretion by α-adrenergic effects.[502] β-Adrenergic blockade increases GHRH-induced GH release, possibly due to a direct pituitary action or by decreasing hypothalamic somatostatin release. Endorphins and enkephalins stimulate GH and can account for GH release during severe physical stress and extreme exercise.[502] Galanin, a 29–amino acid neuropeptide, induces GH release and responses to GHRH. Cholinergic and serotoninergic neurons and several neuropeptides stimulate GH including neurotensin, vasoactive intestinal polypeptide, motilin, cholecystokinin, and glucagon.

Other Hormones Facilitating Growth Hormone Secretion

Acute glucocorticoid administration stimulates GH secretion, and chronic steroid treatment inhibits GH. Three hours after acute glucocorticoid administration, GH levels rise and remain elevated for 2 hours.[503] However, supraphysiologic glucocorticoid exposure retards growth, and Cushing's disease is also associated with growth retardation, decreased serum GH, and decreased pituitary GH content surrounding the adenoma.[504] Glucocorticoids administered to normal subjects dose-dependently inhibit GHRH-simulated GH secretion, similar to that seen in Cushing's syndrome.[503] Furthermore, cortisol antagonizes peripheral GH action. In hyperthyroid patients, GH levels are decreased, but they normalize when patients are rendered euthyroid, suggesting that thyroid hormone suppresses GH secretion. Elevated circulating gonadal steroids observed during puberty can also account for higher pubertal GH levels. Estrogen stimulates GH secretory rates, and testosterone increases GH secretory mass per pulse, with resultant IGF-I induction.[502] TRH does not stimulate GH secretion in normal subjects but does induce GH secretion in about 70% of patients with acromegaly.[505] Discordant GH responses to TRH are evoked in patients with liver disease, renal disease, ectopic GHRH-releasing carcinoid tumors,[31] anorexia nervosa, and depression. Intravenous CRH modestly increases GH in some patients with acromegaly or chronic depression. GnRH stimulates GH secretion in about one third of patients with acromegaly.

Growth Hormone Binding Proteins

Two high- and low-affinity circulating GHBPs include a 20-kd low-affinity binding protein (BP) and a 60-kd high-affinity BP, which corresponds to the extracellular domain of the hepatic GH receptor and binds half of the circulating 22-kd GH form.[506,507] 20-kd GH binds preferentially to the low-affinity BP, which is unrelated to the GH receptor. The GHBPs function to dampen acute oscillations in serum GH levels associated with pulsatile pituitary GH secretion, and plasma GH half-life is prolonged by decreased renal GH clearance of bound GH. The high-affinity BP also prevents GH binding to surface GH receptors by competing for the GH ligand. Patients with either hypopituitarism or acromegaly have normal BP concentrations. GH resistance, as demonstrated in malnutrition, chronic liver disease, short stature, Laron dwarfism, and some African pygmies, is characterized by decreased plasma BP levels. High BP levels are encountered in obese and pregnant subjects and in those receiving estrogens or undergoing refeeding.[508]

Peripheral Growth Hormone Action

GH acts to mediate growth and metabolic functions (Fig. 8–38). GH elicits intracellular signaling though a peripheral receptor and initiates a phosphorylation cascade involving the JAK/STAT pathway.[509] The liver contains abundant GH receptors, and several peripheral tissues also express modest amounts of receptor, including muscle and fat (Fig. 8–39).[510] The GH receptor (GHR) is a 620–amino acid, 70-kd protein of the class I cytokine/hematopoietin receptor superfamily consisting of an extracellular ligand-binding domain, a single membrane-spanning domain, and a cytoplasmic signaling component.[511] The GH receptor superfamily is homologous with receptors for PRL, interleukin (IL)-2 to IL-7, erythropoietin, interferon, and colony-stimulating factor.

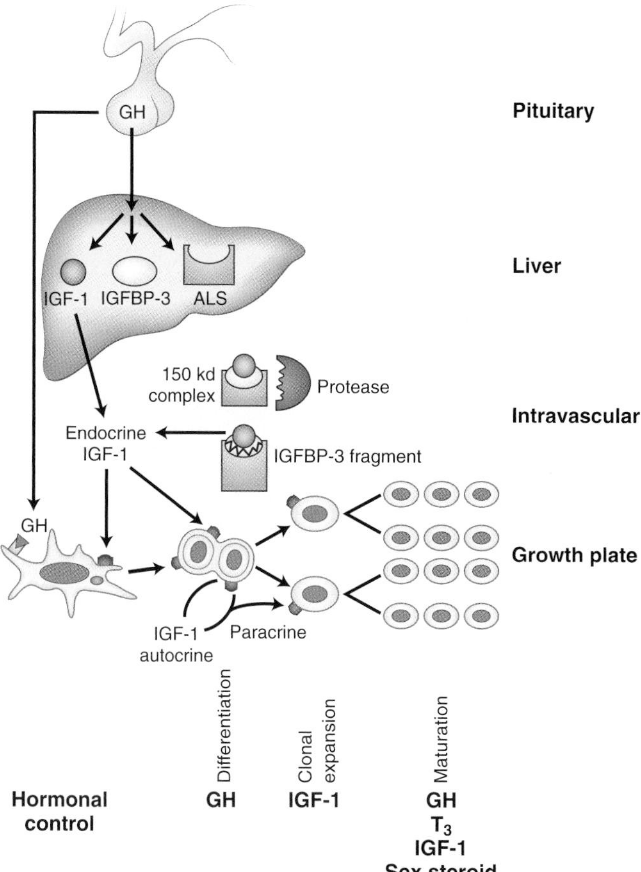

Figure 8–38 ▪ Integrated model of the GH-IGFBP-IGF axis in the growth process. Three mechanisms are proposed: (1) GH stimulates IGF-I production; circulating IGF-I (endocrine IGF-I) acts at the growth plate. (2) GH regulates hepatic production of IGFBP-3 and ALS: IGF-I binds to IGFBP-3 and thereafter with ALS, forming the 150-kd ternary complex; proteases cleave into fragments that release IGFBP-3 into fragments that release IGF-I in the intravascular space and at the growth plate. (3) GH induces differentiation local IGF-I production, and IGF-I acts via an autocrine and paracrine mechanism to stimulate cell division. ALS, acid-labile subunit; GH, growth hormone; IGF, insulin-like growth factor; IGFBP, insulin-like growth factor binding protein; T_3,triiodothyronine. (From Spagnoli A, Rosenfeld RG. The mechanism by which GH brings about growth. The relative contributions of GH and insulin-like growth factors. Endocrinol Metab Clin North Am 1996;25:615-631; 681. Clemmons DR, Van Wyk JJ, Ridgway EC, et al. Evaluation of acromegaly by radioimmunoassay of somatomedin-C. N Engl J Med 1979;301:1138-1142.)

GH complexes with two dimerized GHR components critical for subsequent GH signaling, followed by rapid JAK2 tyrosine kinase activation, leading to phosphorylation of intracellular signaling molecules, including the signal transducing activators of transcription proteins (STATs) 1, 3, and 5, critical signaling components for GH action.[512] Phosphorylated STAT proteins are directly translocated to the cell nucleus, where they elicit GH-specific target gene expression by binding to nuclear DNA. STAT1 and STAT5 can also interact directly with the GH receptor molecule.[512] GH also induces c-fos induction, insulin-receptor substrate (IRS)-1 phosphorylation, and insulin synthesis. Additional intracellular signaling pathways induced by GH include mitogen-activated protein (MAP) kinase, PKC, SH2-Bβ, SHP-2, SIRPα, Shc, FAK, CrKII, C-Src, paxillin, and tensin. How these seemingly overlapping pathways converge to integrate the net cellular effects of GH are at present unclear.[509]

IGF-I, a critical growth factor induced by GH, is likely responsible for most growth-promoting activities of GH[480] and also directly regulates GH receptor function.[511] Paracrine IGF-I produced in extrahepatic tissues appears critical for growth because growth persists even when hepatic IGF-I is deleted in mice.[513] GH receptor mutations are associated with partial or complete GH insensitivity and growth failure. These syndromes are associated with normal or high circulating GH levels, decreased circulating GHBP levels, and low levels of circulating IGF-I. Multiple homozygous or heterozygous exonic and intronic GHR mutations have been described. These occur mostly in the extracellular ligand-binding receptor domain (see Chapter 23). Tissue responses to GH signaling are also determined by the pattern of GH secretion, in addition to the absolute amount of circulating hormone.

Gender-specific patterns of GH secretion profiles determine sex-specific expression of cytochrome P450 enzymes. In turn, circulating steroids regulate neuroendocrine release of GH. SRIF, by suppressing interpulse GH levels, serves to masculinize the ultradian GH rhythm. In mice harboring a disrupted SRIF gene, plasma GH secretory patterns are elevated, and liver enzyme induction loses its gender-specific dimorphism, but these animals retain sexually dimorphic growth patterns.[514] Linear growth patterns and liver enzyme induction are phenotypically gender-specific due to higher GH pulse frequency rates and also show gender-specific STAT5b activity.[515] Sexually dimorphic patterns of GH secretion and tissue targeting appear to be determined by STAT5b, which is sensitive to repeated pulses of injected GH,[516] unlike other GH-induced responses, which are desensitized by repeated GH administration. Disruption of STAT5b in transgenic mice causes impaired male pattern body growth[517] associated with female pattern IGF-1 and testosterone levels. Appropriate GH pulsatility is also required to determine body growth mediated by STAT5b[518,519] but not for metabolic effects of GH on carbohydrate metabolism. A STAT mutation has been described as a cause of short stature.[520]

Intracellular GH signaling is abrogated by SOCS proteins, which disrupt the JAK/STAT pathway and thus disrupt GH action.[521] In transgenic mice with deletion of SOCS-2, gigantism develops, presumably due to unrestrained GH action. Because SOCS proteins are also induced by proinflammatory cytokines, critically ill patients, or those with renal failure, can develop GH

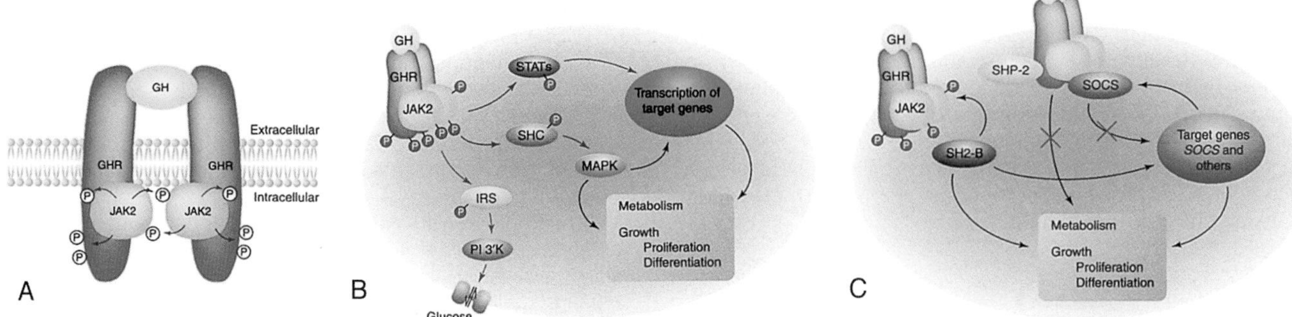

Figure 8–39 ▪ Growth hormone receptors. **A,** Model of GH activation of JAK2 tyrosine kinase. GH binding to two GH receptors increases the affinity to each receptor for JAK2. The two receptor-associated JAK2 molecules are in close proximity, so that each JAK2 can phosphorylate the activating tyrosine of the other JAK2 molecule *(blue arrows),* thereby activating it. Activated JAK2 then phosphorylates itself *(red arrow)* and the cytoplasmic domain of the GH receptor *(purple arrows)* on tyrosines. These phosphotyrosines within the GH receptor and JAK2 form binding sites for signaling proteins. **B,** Regulation of GH receptor-JAK2 signaling. SH2 enhances GH receptor signaling by increasing the activity of JAK2. GH-induced expression of SOCS proteins inhibits further GHR signaling by decreasing the activity of JAK2. Tyrosine phosphatases, such as SHP-2, might also contribute to inhibiting GH receptor signaling by dephosphorylating tyrosines in the GH receptor and/or JAK2. **C,** GH receptors signaling pathways. Some of the signaling pathways initiated by GH activation of JAK2 are shown. JAK2 phosphorylates SHC, leading to activation of MAPK *(blue arrows).* JAK2 also phosphorylates STAT transcription factors. MAPK and STATs are important for GH regulation of gene transcription *(purple arrows).* JAK2 phosphorylates IRS proteins, which are thought to lead to activation of PI3′-kinase (PI3K: *red arrows*). GH activation of PI3′ kinase via IRS protein might be important for GH stimulation of glucose transport. GH, growth hormone; GHR, growth hormone receptor; IRS, insulin receptor substrates; JAK2, Janus kinase 2; MAPK, mitogen-activated protein kinase; P, phosphate; PI3′K, phosphatidylinositol 3-kinase; SHP-2, src homology 2 domain-containing protein tyrosine phosphatase 2; SOCS, suppressor of cytokine signaling.STAT, signal transducers and activators of transcription. (From Herrington J, Carter-Su C. Signaling pathway activated by the growth hormone receptor. Trends Endocrinol Metab 2001;12:252-257.)

resistance due to cytokine-induced SOCS.[522] Unraveling STAT/SOCS regulation in syndromes associated with disordered GH signaling will likely yield mechanistic insights for dysregulated GH action. The impact of GH on growth is fully reviewed in Chapter 23.

Extrapituitary GH and GH secretagogues can complement the classic endocrine action among the GH-releasing factors, GH, and target tissues. Although GH immunoreactivity and mRNA expression have been documented in placenta, mammary gland, muscle, spleen, and lymphocytes,[523] the physiologic role of these findings is not yet apparent.

Metabolic Actions of Growth Hormone

GH continues to be secreted in adulthood after growth cessation, implying important metabolic functions for GH in adult life. Although acute transient insulin-like effects of GH have been demonstrated, chronic GH exposure exerts potent anti-insulin effects at hepatic and peripheral sites, resulting in decreased glucose utilization, increased lipolysis, and tissue refractoriness of the acute insulin-like effects of GH. Endogenous GH concentrations antagonize insulin action. GH secretion increases 3 to 5 hours after glucose ingestion, resulting in decreased disposal of a subsequent oral glucose challenge, associated with hyperinsulinemia occurring 2 hours after the GH peak. GH-deficient children have decreased fasting glucose levels, decreased insulin secretion, increased insulin sensitivity with increased glucose utilization, and blunted hepatic glucose release. GH replacement increases fasting glucose and insulin levels and restores hepatic glucose production.

GH-deficient adults have elevated fasting insulin levels and enhanced visceral fat mass, suggesting insulin resistance, which has been confirmed by hyperinsulinemic euglycemic clamp studies.[524]

TABLE 8–20 ADULT GH SECRETION*

Interval	Young Adult (μg/24 h)	Fasting	Obesity	Middle Age
24-hr secretion	540 ± 44	2171 ± 333	77 ± 20	196 ± 65
Secretory bursts	12 ± 1	32 ± 2	3 ± 0.5	10 ± 1
GH burst	45 ± 4	64 ± 9	24 ± 5	10 ± 6

GH, growth hormone.
*Deconvolution analysis of growth hormone (GH) secretion in men.
From Thorner MO, Vance ML, Horvath E, Kovacs K. The anterior pituitary. In Wilson JD, Foster DW, eds. Williams Textbook of Endocrinology. Philadelphia: WB Saunders, 1992:221-310.

GH is anabolic and causes urinary nitrogen retention, decreased plasma urea levels, and increased muscle mass. GH increases fat mobilization, decreases fat deposition, and activates hormone-sensitive lipase, resulting in increased triglyceride hydrolysis to free fatty acids and glycerol (lipolysis), as well as decreased fatty acid re-esterification. GH replacement to GH-deficient adults leads to decreased body fat and decreased adipocyte size and lipid content. As GH is degraded in the kidney, GH levels are elevated in patients with chronic renal failure, and GH rises paradoxically in response to a glucose load in these patients.

Growth Hormone Secretion Patterns

Frequent serum sampling for serum measurements of GH concentrations has revealed a pattern of pulsatile secretion separated by troughs, during which GH is undetectable (<0.4 μg/L) (Table 8–20). Using currently available assays, random GH levels are undetectable in 50% of samples obtained from healthy subjects. GH secretion is high in the fetal circulation, peaking at about 150 μg/L at midgestation. Neonatal levels are lower (about 30 μg/L), possibly reflecting the negative feedback control by rising levels of circulating IGF. GH levels during childhood (up to 7 μg/L) are characterized by enhanced pubertal GH pulse amplitude and mass, with unchanged GH pulse frequency. GH pulse amplitudes decline inexorably with age, such that GH levels in middle age are about 15% of pubertal levels. Healthy men produce about 0.25 to 0.52 mg GH/m^2 per 24 hours.[479] Obesity is associated with decreased GH pulse frequency and blunted evoked GH responses to secretagogues. In contrast, fasting is associated with enhanced GH pulse frequency and amplitude, possibly reflecting altered feedback regulation by nutritionally mediated changes in IGF binding protein concentrations and free IGF-I availability.

Measurement of Spontaneous Growth Hormone Secretion

Because pituitary GH secretion occurs episodically, accurate quantification of integrated GH secretion requires continuous measurement of secretion over 24 hours. This procedure requires insertion of a continuous withdrawal pump or patent indwelling catheter with unrestricted food intake and physical activity. Increasing sampling frequencies from every 20 minutes to every 5 minutes or every 30 seconds enhances the threshold for detecting more pulses per hour. Although cumbersome and expensive, this method eliminates the error of isolated peak or trough measurements that might otherwise be obtained by single or multiple random GH samplings.

The discriminating power of continuous 24-hour GH measurement in diagnosing GH deficiency in children has been disputed.[525] With no clear diagnostic advantage over GH stimulation tests, integrated GH levels in young healthy subjects can overlap those in patients with organic hypopituitary disorders and therefore limits its utility in diagnosing acquired adult GH deficiency. However, fasted subjects can exhibit a clear distinction of deficient integrated GH levels measured over 8 hours.[526]

Urinary Growth Hormone Measurement

Immunoassay methods for urinary GH measurement do not reliably reflect pharmacologic GH testing or adequately discriminate between normal and abnormal GH secretion. Clinical utility of urinary GH measurements requires rigorous age-and gender-matched controls and standardized expression of GH concentrations relative to body weight or creatinine excretion.[527]

Variability of Growth Hormone Assays

Plasma GH is measured by polyclonal or monoclonal RIA or by dual monoclonal IRMA, but comparative GH measurements obtained using 11 commercial immunoassays varied by a factor of three.[528] Measured GH concentrations are antibody dependent, and different antibodies bind to a heterogeneous spectrum of GH isoforms.[529] Furthermore, GH isoform patterns vary among individual subjects, and all circulating GH forms are not routinely detectable in GH assays, adding further variation to comparison of results from different GH immunoassays.

Monomeric 22-kd GH, the most abundant circulating form, is the only GH standard of sufficient purity and quantity, and it is used as the basis for GH measurement; however, it accounts for only about 25% of circulating immunoreactivity.[530] Other GH forms are recognized to varying and largely unknown degrees. Polyclonal antibodies used in earlier RIAs recognized several molecular forms of GH, as compared to newer immunometric assays employing highly specific monoclonal antibodies.[531] GH standards also affect comparison of GH values. In 1994, the first WHO international standard for somatotropin, IRP (international reference protein) 88/624,[532] used recombinant technology, in contrast to previous standards prepared from pituitary extracts. GH-binding proteins (GHBPs) can also interfere because approximately 50% of GH is complexed to GHBP, and noncompetitive immunometric assays can lead to low estimates of GH. In competitive assays, employing antibodies directed against GH molecular epitopes, which bind GHBP, spuriously high GH values may be reported.[533]

The heterogeneity of GH immunoassay results poses a challenge in the definition of accepted standards for diagnosis of GH deficiency. However the RIA is now infrequently used, and clinicians should be aware of the nature of the GH assay employed and how values compare to those previously obtained by polyclonal RIA. New GH assays based on measuring GH bioactivity have been developed, including eluted stain assay (ESTA) and immunofunctional assay (IFA). Growth hormone exclusion assay (GHEA) also measures circulating GH isoforms.[531]

Growth Hormone Deficiency

Growth hormone deficiency in adults is recognized as a distinct adult syndrome (Table 8–21).[534] GH is the most commonly deficient of the pituitary hormones in patients with pituitary disease, and GH deficiency causes negative effects on body composition, cardiovascular risk factors, and quality of life.[535,536] Life expectancy is reduced in hypopituitary patients with GH deficiency[193,537,538] largely as a consequence of cardiovascular and cerebrovascular events, especially in female subjects.[539] Although neither estrogen nor thyroid deficiency account for these risk factors and reduced survival, it is not yet rigorously confirmed that the observed increased mortality and morbidity occurs solely as a result of GH deficiency.

Pathophysiology

Adult GH deficiency is most often encountered in patients with pituitary or hypothalamic disease.[540] Although pituitary tumors and craniopharyngiomas are associated with GH deficiency, these patients can also develop GH deficiency as a result of head or neck radiation therapy. GH deficiency in children typically results from isolated GH deficiency, rare genetic causes (see Chapter 23), or other central structural abnormalities. Isolated GH deficiency may be complete or partial, and up to 67 % of children whose GH deficiency was initially diagnosed as "idiopathic" had normal GH responses when subsequently retested for GH deficiency following cessation of GH treatment as adults.[541] Children with GH deficiency should be retested before GH treatment is continued into adulthood unless they have clearly documented panhypopituitarism or a defined genetic or developmental abnormality that causes complete and irreversible GH deficiency. Mutations in the GH[542] and GHRH receptor genes,[543] and GH insensitivity as a result of primary GH receptor dysfunction,[544] result in GH deficiency. Other genetic abnormalities such as Prop1 or POU1F1 mutations cause GH deficiency, with concomitant deficiency in other pituitary hormones.[545]

Evaluation

Because GH is secreted in a pulsatile manner,[502] the diagnosis of GH deficiency requires tests of evoked GH sufficiency in response to specific GH secretagogues. The ITT has remained the gold standard test for GH deficiency. Although some GH secretagogues reliably differentiate normal GH reserve and GH deficiency, others are not as effective in clearly distinguishing normal from deficient levels because of overlapping GH values

TABLE 8–21 ADULT SOMATOTROPHIN DEFICIENCY

Effects of Deficiency	Effects of GH Replacement
CLINICAL	
Quality of Life	
Decreased energy and drive	Mood and energy uplift
Poor concentration	Enhanced vitality
Low self-esteem	Improved physical mobility
Social isolation	Improved social isolation
Body Composition	
Increased body fat mass with altered distribution	Increased lean body mass
Increased waist-to-hip ratio	Decreased fat mass
Decreased lean body mass	Increased bone mass
Exercise Capacity	
Reduced maximum O_2 uptake	Increased maximum O_2 uptake
Impaired cardiac function	Increased maximum power
Reduced muscle mass	
Cardiovascular Risk Factors	
Impaired cardiovascular structure and function	Increased stroke volume
Abnormal lipid profile	Increased diastolic volume
Decreased fibrinolytic activity	Increased LV wall mass
Atherosclerosis	Atherosclerosis impact
Omental obesity	
Insulin resistance	
Increased sialic acid	
Lower exercise frequency and duration	
IMAGING	
Mass or structural damage to pituitary	Decreased adipocyte size
Reduced bone density	Increased lipolysis
Excess omental adiposity	Decreased lipogenesis
LABORATORY	
Evoked GH <3 μg/L	Increased IGF-I levels
IGF-I and IGFBP3 low or normal	Increased BMR
Lipid disorders	Decreased LDL with probable increased HDL
Concomitant gonadotrophin, TSH, and/or ACTH reserve deficits	Transient hyperglycemia
	Increased T_3 levels
	Salt and water retention

ACTH, adrenocorticotropic hormone; BMR, basal metabolic rate; BP3, binding-protein 3; GH, growth hormone; HDL, high-density lipoprotein; IGF, insulin-like growth factor; IGFBP, insulin-like growth factor binding protein; LDL, low-density lipoprotein; LV, left ventricular; T_3, triiodothyronine; TSH, thyroid-stimulating hormone.

(Table 8–22). Differences in published responses can also be accounted for by subject gender, weight, or possibly age. For example, mean peak GH response to arginine plus GHRH in controls was 70 μg/L. In contrast, the peak response in older and more obese men was 18 μg/L. In normal control subjects, much higher GH responses have been noted when arginine plus GHRH, GHRH plus hexarelin, or GHRH plus GHRP-6 are administered than when insulin-induced hypoglycemia has been employed.[546] Although a GH response of less than 3 μg/L has been considered consistent with GH deficiency, according to current consensus[547,548] the recent recommended cut-off points below which adult patients should be considered GH deficient vary according to the test employed (Fig. 8–40).[484] Not unexpected is the fact that patients with pituitary disease with no or one pituitary hormone deficiency have a lower incidence of GH deficiency than do patients with multiple hormone deficiencies.

Ghrelin, an endogenous ligand for the GHRP receptor,[482] may also be proposed as a test for GH deficiency because it is a potent GH secretagogue.[549] The requirement to test patients who have proven panhypopituitarism has been questioned, because virtually all patients with more than two trophic hormone deficiencies are also GH deficient (see Fig. 8–40).[550] Although mean serum IGF-I levels are low in GH-deficient adults, and very low IGF-I levels can indicate GH deficiency, IGF-I is not a good screening test in adults, because about 60% of GH-deficient adults have normal age- and gender-matched IGF-I levels.[551] Forty percent of GH-deficient patients older than 60 years in fact had IGF-I concentrations that were normal for their age.[552] Measurement of IGF binding-protein 3 (IGFBP3) is also not a reliable screening procedure for adult GH deficiency.[553]

Presentation

Symptoms of GH deficiency are nonspecific and can include fatigue, lack of energy, social isolation, poor concentration and memory loss.[554] Signs include increased fat mass (especially abdominal and visceral),[555] decreased lean body mass, decreased body water,[534] decreased bone density (particularly in patients with more severe GH deficiency),[556] and long-standing childhood-onset GH deficiency.[557] Other features include hyperlipidemia,[558,559] reduced exercise capacity,[535] and increase in cardiovascular risk factors[539] including abdominal adiposity, insulin resistance,[560] and increased carotid intimal thickness.[561,562] GH deficiency might also be associated with heart abnormalities including reduced left ventricular mass.[554,563-565] Cardiovascular parameters of GH deficiency are often more pronounced in adults with childhood GH deficiency onset than in those who acquire the deficiency during adulthood who have more pronounced disordered quality of life, lipids, and body composition.[526,554,566,567]

Because many symptoms of GH deficiency are nonspecific, clinical judgment should be exercised in selecting patients for testing. Patients with pituitary or hypothalamic disease should be considered for diagnosis of GH deficiency and replacement with GH, even in the absence of other pituitary hormone deficiencies. Deficiencies in sex hormones also lead to body composition changes similar to those observed in GH deficiency. For example, testosterone deficiency causes decreased lean body and bone mass and increased fat mass, each of which can be partially improved when testosterone is administered.[568] That GH provides additional positive effects on body composition is suggested by observations that many patients with GH deficiency who improved body composition parameters after GH replacement were already receiving sex steroids. A study in healthy volunteers also demonstrated inhibition of catabolic effects when hGH was given along with prednisone.[569]

Growth Hormone Replacement Therapy

Treatment of GH-deficient adults with recombinant hGH for 4 to 6 months increased lean body mass and decreased fat mass (Figs. 8–41 to Fig. 8–43).[534] In a composite review of 9 placebo-controlled trials, hGH (in doses ranging from 2.6-26 μg/kg/day) increased lean body mass by a mean of 3.4 kg and reduced fat mass by 4.4%.[554] GH also increased bone density,[570] and parameters of bone formation and bone resorption were also increased.[571] GH-induced reduction in abdominal and visceral fat suggests an associated improvement in cardiovascular risk factors. The effect of hGH replacement on lipid abnormalities is

TABLE 8–22 RESPONSES TO GROWTH HORMONE STIMULATION TESTS

Study	Test	NUMBER		SEX		AGE (MEAN)		BMI (MEAN)		DOSE		Serum Sampling (All)	PEAK MEAN (RANGE) µg/L	
		Con	GHD	Con	GHD	Con	GHD	Con	GHD	Con	GHD		Con	GHD
Gasperi et al	ITT	33	19	M: 12 F: 21	M: 10 F: 9	34.1	39.99	N/A	24.5	0.1-0.15 U/kg IV	0.1-0.15 U/kg IV	q5min from −15 min to 90 min	22.1 (3-84)	0.6 (0.1-1.8)
Gasperi et al	Arginine-GHRH	77	19	M: 40 F: 37	M: 10 F: 9	28.1	39.9	N/A	24.5	.5 g/kg IV over 30 min	1 µg/kg IV over 30 min	q15min from −15 min to 90 min	69.5 (13.8-171)	3.6 (0.1-16.5)
Biller et al	ITT	34	39	M: 20 F: 14	M: 26 F: 13	47.2	48.9	30.3	30.5	0.1-0.15 U/kg IV	0.1-0.15 U/kg IV	20-30 min for 2.5 hr	17.8 (0.025-52)	0.95 (0.025-79)
Biller et al	Arginine-GHRH	34	39	M: 20 F: 14	M: 26 F: 13	47.2	48.9	30.3	30.5	30 g over 30 min IV	1 µg/kg IV	q30min for 2.5 h	18.4 (1.2-127)	1.44 (0.025-7.7)
Gasperi et al	Hexarelin-GHRH	25	19	M: 18 F: 7	M: 10 F: 9	28.5	39.9	N/A	24.5	0.25 µg/kg IV	1 µg/kg IV	q15min from −15 min to 90 min	83.6 (49-124)	2.6 (0.1-11.1)
Popovic et al	GHRH-GHRP-6	125	125	M: 65 F: 60	M: 73 F: 52	39.9	39.6	23.5	26.9	1 µg/kg IV	1 µg/kg IV	q15-30min from −30 min to 120 min	59.2 (15-139)	4.1 (0.01-15)

RECOMMENDED TEST SENSITIVITY (95% CL) TO DIAGNOSE ADULT GH DEFICIENCY

Test	Value < µg/L	References
ITT	5.1	Biller et al
Arginine + GHRH	4.1	Biller et al
Arginine + L-Dopa	1.7	Biller et al
Hexarelin + GHRH	3.0	Gasperi et al
GHRH + GHRP-6	15.0	Popovic et al

Results from studies on the effects of insulin-induced hypoglycemia and the combination of arginine and GHRH illustrate the effect of body weight on GH responses.

BMI, body mass index (kg/m^2); CL, confidence limits; Con, control subjects; GH, growth hormone; GHD, growth hormone–deficient subjects; GHRH, growth hormone–releasing hormone; GHRP, growth hormone releasing peptide; ITT, insulin tolerance test.

Biller BM, Vance ML, Kleinberg DL, et al. Clinical and reimbursement issues in growth hormone use in adults. Am J Manag Care 2000;6:S817-827.

Gasperi M, Aimaretti G, Scarcello G, et al. Low dose hexarelin and growth hormone (GH)-releasing hormone as a diagnostic tool for the diagnosis of GH deficiency in adults: comparison with insulin-induced hypoglycemia test. J Clin Endocrinol Metab 1999;84:2633-2637.

Popovic V, Leal A, Micic D, et al. GH-releasing hormone and GH-releasing peptide-6 for diagnostic testing in GH-deficient adults. Lancet 2000;356:1137-1142.

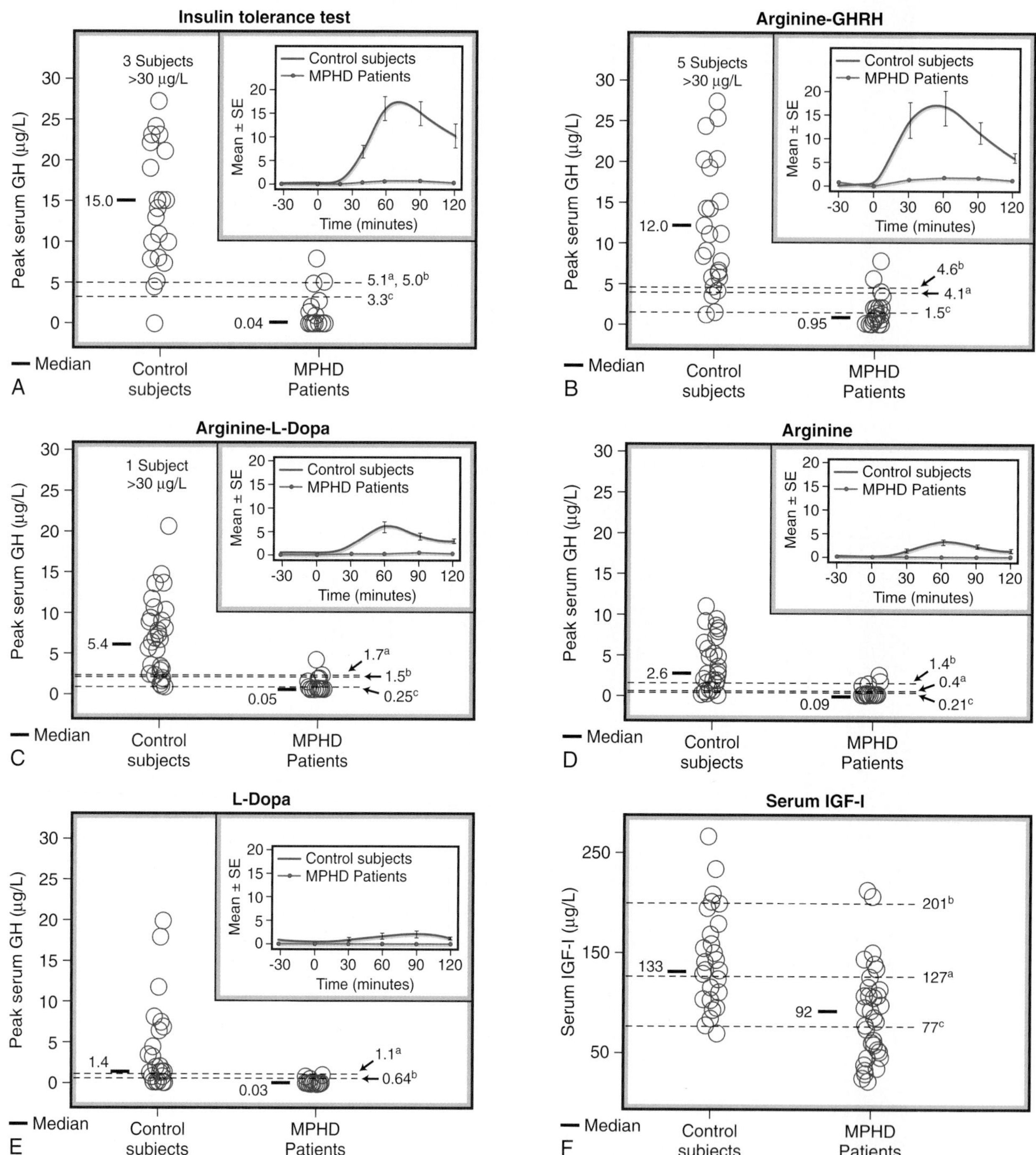

Figure 8–40 ▪ Effect of various GH secretagogues on GH in patients with 0 or 1 deficiency in a pituitary hormone. GHRH, growth hormone–releasing hormone; IGF, insulin-like growth factor; MPHD, multiple pituitary hormone deficiency. (From Biller BM, Samuels MH, Zagar A, et al. Sensitivity and specificity of six tests for the diagnosis of adult GH deficiency. J Clin Endocrinol Metab 2002;87:2067-2079.)

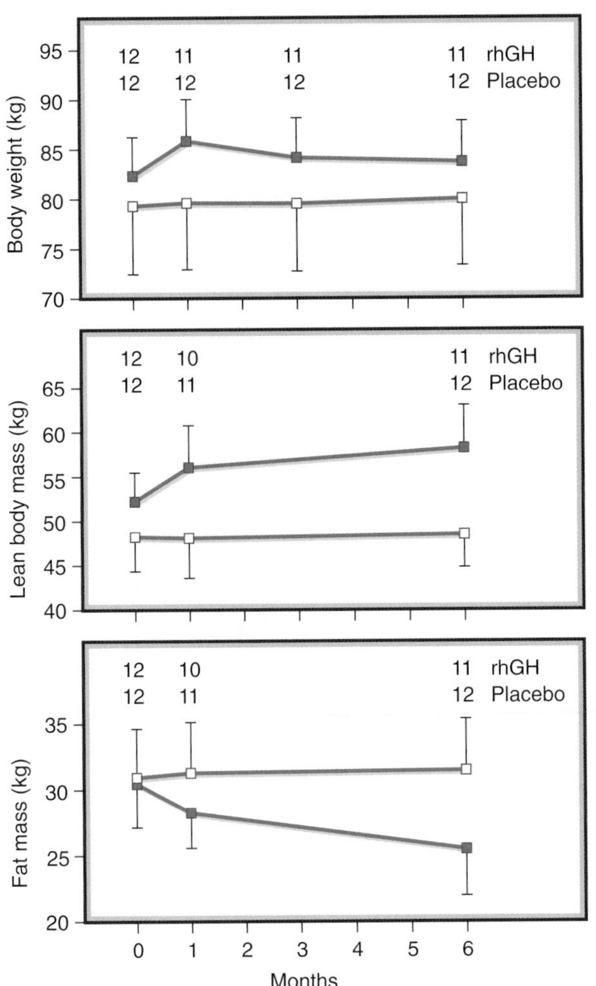

Figure 8–41 ▪ Effects of recombinant human growth hormone (rhGH) replacement on lean body mass and fat mass in adult GH deficiency. (Reproduced from Salomon F, Cuneo RC, Hesp R, Sonksen PH. The effects of treatment with recombinant human growth hormone on body composition and metabolism in adults with growth hormone deficiency. N Engl J Med 1989;321:1797-803.)

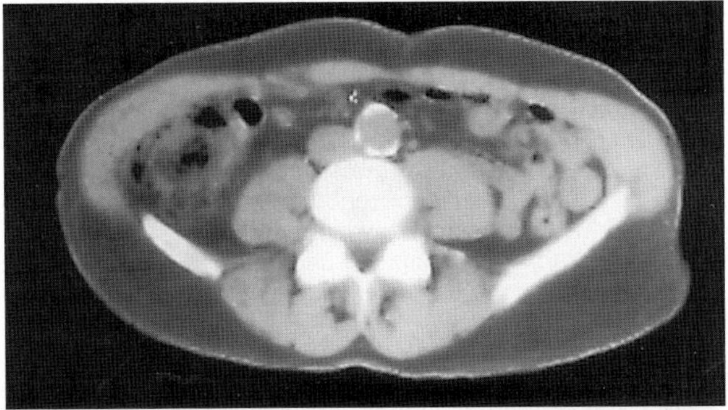

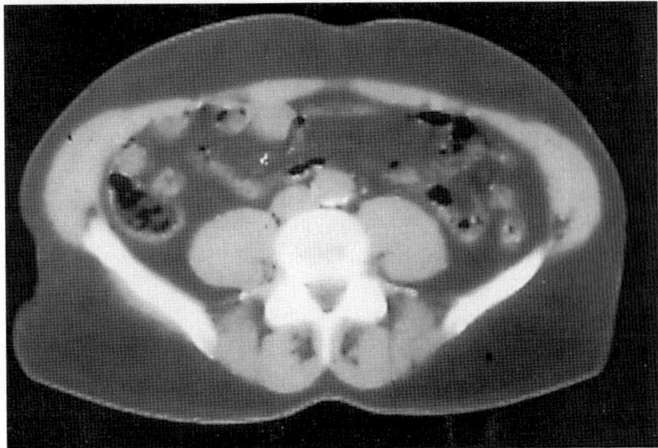

Figure 8–43 ▪ Computed tomographic scan through the abdomen before *(top)* and after *(bottom)* treatment with human growth hormone (hGH) in a GH-deficient patient. (Courtesy of B.A. Bengtsson.)

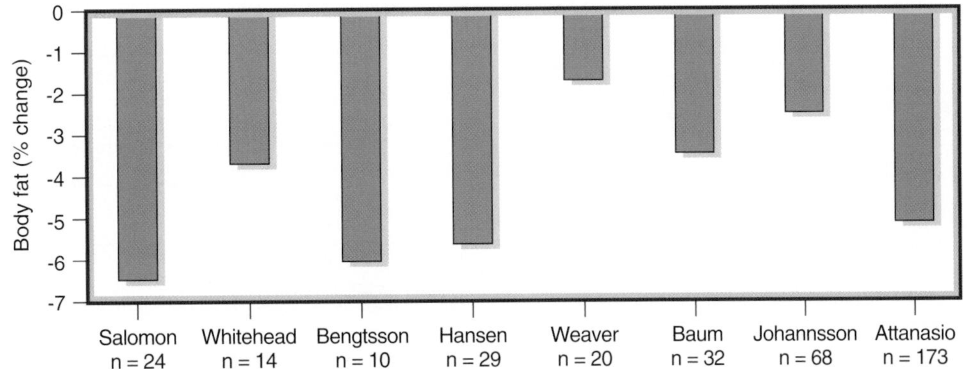

Figure 8–42 ▪ Effect of treatment with human growth hormone (hGH) on body fat in eight studies. (Adapted from Newman CB, Kleinberg DL. Adult growth hormone deficiency. Endocrinologist 1998;8:178-186.)

variable.[572] hGH had a significant effect on raising HDL cholesterol,[559] and overall, the most consistent change has been an improvement in the cholesterol-to-HDL cholesterol ratio. Some have reported increases in cardiac output,[573,574] reduction in intima media thickness,[561] and improved energy, mood, and quality of life,[575] but not all investigators concur.[576] A latency period up to 3 months can occur before patients recognize the benefits of hGH replacement, which are most obvious in those with the most profound symptoms and signs of GH deficiency.[550] Beneficial effects of GH replacement persist for at least 10 years.[577]

Growth Hormone Administration

GH is administered by nightly subcutaneous injection. The recommended adult dose is much lower than for children.[578] Side effects of GH in children are considerably less than those observed in adults. Men, particularly older ones, are more sensitive to GH and require lower GH doses than do women. The maintenance dose of hGH in 665 adult patients with GH deficiency was 0.43 mg/day for men and 0.53 mg/day for women.[540] Women with GH deficiency require higher doses of hGH with oral rather than transdermal estrogen (Fig. 8–44).[579,580] It is recommended that replacement be initiated with relatively low doses.[566] Most adults tolerate a starting dose of 300 μg/day or lower, which is then titrated according to serum IGF-I concentrations and side effects of the medication.[581] If side effects occur, the dose should be reduced, and if no side effects are reported, the therapeutic goal is to maintain IGF-I levels in the normal age- and gender-matched range, while avoiding levels in the upper quintile or above (Fig. 8–45).

Precautions and Caveats of Treating with hGH

The most common side effects of hGH are edema, arthralgias, and myalgias, which occur in up to one third of patients when the drug is administered as a weight-based dosage (Table 8–23). Using total daily doses titrated for IGF-I levels, the incidence of side effects is much lower.[559] Patients with active malignancies should not be treated with GH, nor should patients with active carpal tunnel syndrome or other fluid-retention disorders.

The possibility that hGH might initiate new cancers or stimulate growth of preexisting benign tumors is an important theoretical issue. An epidemiologic association between higher, albeit normal, IGF-I levels and later risk of developing prostate cancer,[582] breast cancer in premenopausal women,[583] and colon and lung cancer[584] has been reported. In contrast, patients with acromegaly, who have very high serum levels of IGF-I, do not

TABLE 8–23 SIDE EFFECTS OF GH ADULT TREATMENT

Arthralgias
Atrial fibrillation
Benign intracranial hypertension
Carpal tunnel syndrome
Edema
Headache
Hyperglycemia
Hypertension
Iatrogenic acromegaly
Increase in melanocytic nevi
Muscle stiffness
Myalgias
Paresthesias
Tinnitus

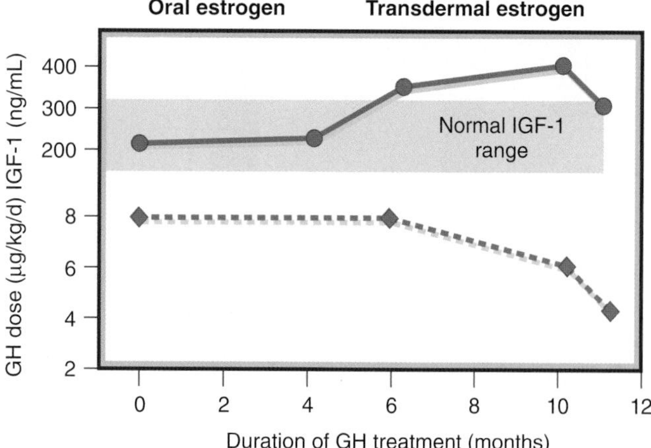

Figure 8–44 ▪ Time course of GH dose and serum IGF-I concentration in a representative patient (38-year-old woman) who was switched from oral to transdermal estrogen therapy during the course of GH replacement. GH, growth hormone; IGF, insulin-like growth factor. (From Cook DM, Ludlam WH, Cook MB. Route of estrogen administration helps to determine growth hormone (GH) replacement dose in GH-deficient adults. J Clin Endocrinol Metab 199984:3956-3960.)

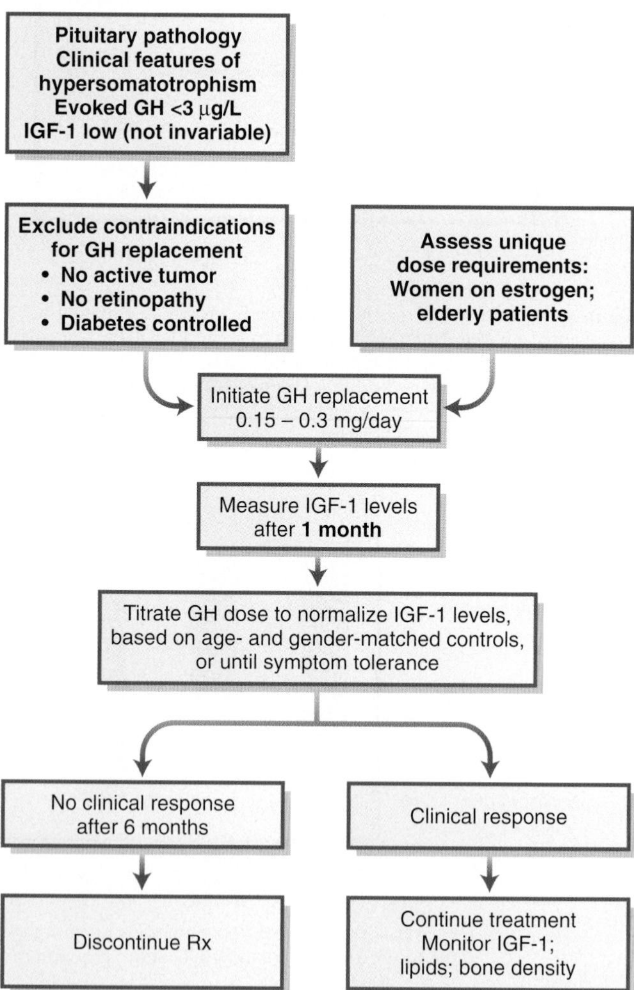

Figure 8–45 ▪ Management of adult somatotropin deficiency. Patients older than 60 years require lowoer maintenance doses. Women receiving transdermal estrogen require lower doses than those receiving oral estrogen preparations. GH, growth hormone; IGF-I insulin-like growth factor I; Rx, treatment.

have an increased incidence of either breast or prostate cancer or cancer in general. In fact the overall risk of cancer in acromegaly is lower than expected. However, these patients have a significantly increased mortality from colon cancer.[585-587]

The possibility that hGH treatment might cause new or recurrent malignancies has been best examined in children who developed GH deficiency as a result of treating their malignancies.[588] When comparing the relative risk of brain tumor recurrence in 180 children treated with hGH versus 891 who did not receive hGH, the risk of recurrence after a mean of 6.4 years was lower in the treated group than those not receiving hGH.[589] GH treatment does, however, increase the risk of radiation-induced second tumor, especially meningioma.[590]

Nevertheless, long-term surveillance with adequate control groups, and avoidance of high IGF-I levels in adults being treated for adult GH deficiency, are required to ensure that adult GH replacement does not increase the incidence of new cancers or growth of existing benign tumors. Blood glucose levels should also be monitored carefully, especially in patients also being treated for diabetes (see Fig. 8–45).

Growth Hormone Treatment of Catabolic States

The well-recognized anabolic actions of GH have prompted use of GH in catabolic states including surgery, trauma, burns, parenteral nutrition, and organ failure. These potential indications for GH are not approved in the United States. The negative nitrogen balance in critically ill patients is partly attributable to GH resistance as well as to decreased IGF-1 production and action.[591] GH administered to postsurgical patients as well as to normal subjects receiving hypocaloric intravenous alimentation results in reversion to positive nitrogen balance. Beneficial effects of GH have been reported in patients with extensive burns, patients receiving chronic high-dose glucocorticoid treatment, patients with chronic obstructive pulmonary disease, in cancer patients, and in patients with cardiac failure. Nevertheless, published endpoints for these studies have not been definitive. When GH was administered to elderly malnourished patients, it was found to be an effective adjuvant for dietary augmentation.[592] A study in which critically ill patients received very high doses of GH (up to 7 mg/day) was prematurely terminated due to enhanced unexplained mortality.[593] It has been suggested that GH might have had an adverse effect on acute phase protein synthesis in these patients.[594] Caution is advised for nonapproved uses of GH in adults.[595]

Growth Hormone Treatment for Osteoporosis

Because declining GH secretion has been implicated in the pathogenesis of osteoporosis, GH was administered to otherwise healthy subjects with idiopathic osteoporosis in an attempt to decrease bone loss. GH increased indices of bone formation and resorption, but a modest increase in spine bone mineral density was only observed in male subjects. A longer study in osteoporotic female subjects showed that GH together with calcitonin increased spine and total hip bone mineral density[596] after 2 years of treatment, although the response was less marked than that observed with estrogen or bisphosphonate therapy. Limited proven efficacy, as yet unclear side effects, and lack of comparative studies with other beneficial therapies for osteoporosis necessitate the need for further study of potential use of GH in treating osteoporosis.

Growth Hormone Treatment in HIV Infection

GH is FDA-approved for administration to adult patients with HIV-associated cachexia. It results in positive nitrogen balance, increased lean body mass, decreased body fat, and improved work output.[597] Ten HIV-infected subjects with fat redistribution syndrome associated with protease inhibitor therapy received 6 mg of GH subcutaneously daily for 12 weeks and showed decreased weight-to-hip ratios and enhanced mid-thigh circumference.[598,599] However, long-term beneficial effects of GH on survival and quality of life in HIV infection have not yet been reported.

Growth Hormone Use in Competitive Sports

The public policy issues of GH abuse in competitive sports have received much attention. GH has been used by athletes to enhance muscle mass.[600] Whether or not persistent GH use is accompanied by increased muscle strength is unclear. Continued use of pharmacologic GH doses by athletes could result in adverse effects of acromegaly, which would in fact decrease performance.

Decreased 1GF-1 Levels

Short-term fasted normal healthy subjects have moderately elevated basal GH levels, and protein-calorie malnutrition, starvation, and anorexia nervosa are associated with low IGF-I and markedly elevated GH levels.[568] This observation might reflect uncoupling of IGF-I feedback regulation of GH secretion. Low IGF-I levels in normal fasting subjects are normalized on caloric refeeding to a greater degree than by protein intake alone.[601]

Acromegaly

Overview

In 1886, Pierre Marie published the first clinical description of disordered somatic growth and proportion and proposed the name *acromegaly*. He also recognized cases previously described by others.[2] When relation of this syndrome to a pituitary tumor was later recognized, Benda showed in 1900 that these tumors comprise mainly adenohypophyseal eosinophilic cells, which he proposed to be hyperfunctioning.[602] Cushing, Davidoff, and Bailey documented the clinicopathologic features of acromegaly and demonstrated clinical remission of soft tissue signs after adenoma resection.[3] Evans and Long induced gigantism in rats injected with anterior pituitary extracts, confirming the association of a pituitary factor with somatic growth.[603] Establishment of the unequivocal pathophysiologic link between hyperfunctioning adenoma and acromegaly was the earliest example of a pituitary disorder to be clinically and pathologically recognized and appropriately managed by surgical excision of a hypersecreting source.

Incidence

The prevalence of acromegaly is estimated to range from 38 to 69 cases/million, and the annual incidence of new patients is 3 or 4 per million.[604-606] Based upon these largely Western European studies, it is apparent that more than 1000 new cases of acromegaly are diagnosed annually in the United States.

Pathogenesis

GH and IGF-I act both independently and dependently in inducing features of hypersomatotrophism. Acromegaly is caused by pituitary tumors secreting GH or very rarely by extrapituitary disorders (Fig. 8–46).[607] Regardless of the etiology, the disease is characterized by elevated levels of GH and IGF-I, with resultant signs and symptoms of hypersomatotrophism.

Pituitary Acromegaly

More than 95% of patients with acromegaly harbor a GH-secreting pituitary adenoma (Table 8–24). Pure GH-cell adenomas

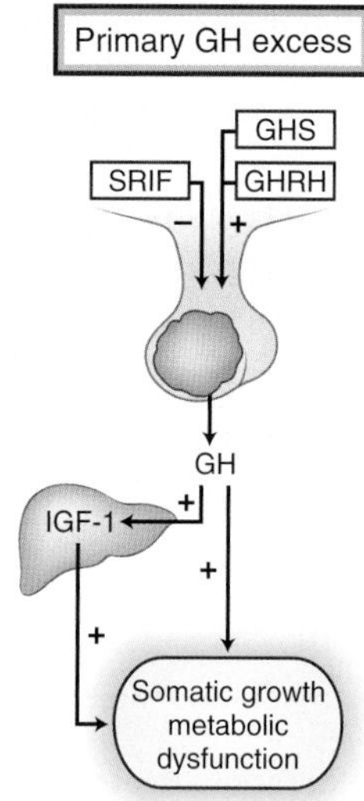

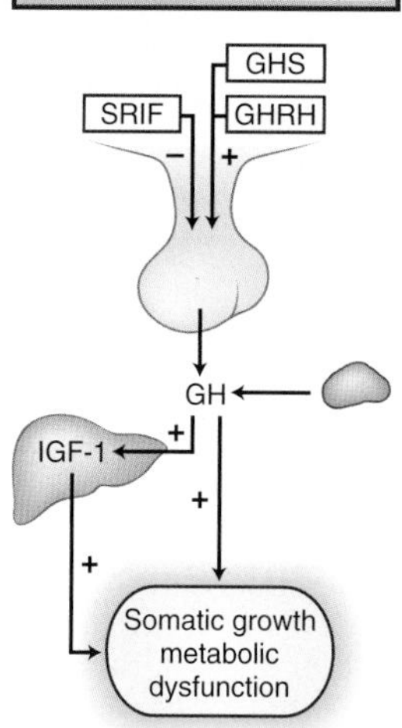

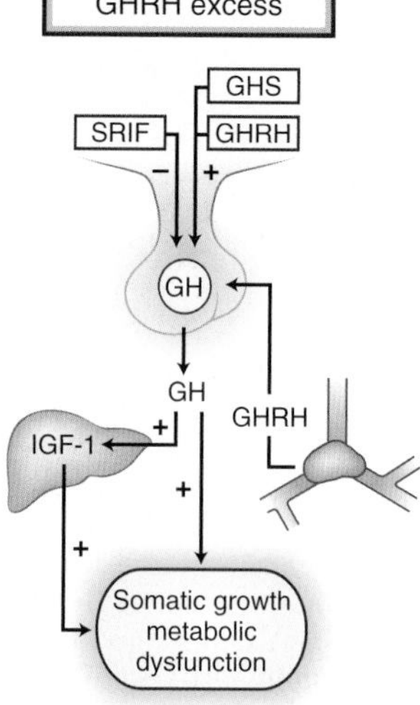

Pituitary adenoma
Densely granulated GH cell
Sparsely granulated
Mixed GH cell and PRL
Mammosomatotroph cell
Acidophil stem cell
Plurihormonal
Silent somatotroph

Pituitary carcinoma

Ectopic

Familial syndromes
Multi-endocrine neoplasia-type I
McCune-Albright syndrome
Familial acromegaly
Carney's syndrome

Pancreatic islet cell tumor
Lymphoma

Iatrogenic

Central
Hypothalamic tumor

Peripheral
Bronchial carcinoid,
pancreatic islet cell tumor,
small cell lung cancer,
adrenal adenoma,
medullary thyroid carcinoma,
pheochromocytoma

Figure 8–46 ▪ Pathogenesis of acromegaly. GH, growth hormone; GHRH, growth hormone–releasing hormone; IGF, insulin-like growth factor type I; PRL, prolactin; SRIF, somatostatin. (From Melmed S. Medical progress: acromegaly. N Engl J Med 2006;355:2558-2573. Erratum in N Engl J Med 2007;356:879.)

contain either densely or sparsely staining cytoplasmic GH granules, and these two variants are either slow growing (densely granulated) or rapidly growing (sparsely granulated).[608,609] The former arise insidiously and manifest during or after middle age; the latter arise in younger subjects with more florid disease. Mixed GH-cell and PRL-cell adenomas are composed of distinct somatotrophs expressing GH and lactotrophs expressing PRL. Monomorphous acidophil stem cell adenomas arise from the common GH and PRL stem cell and also often contain giant mitochondria and misplaced GH granule exocytosis. They grow rapidly, are invasive, and manifest with predominant features of hyperprolactinemia.[610]

Monomorphous mammosomatotroph cell adenomas express both GH and PRL from a single cell, and plurihormonal tumors can express GH with any combination of PRL, TSH, ACTH, or α-subunit.[611] These patients present with clinical features of acromegaly as well as hyperprolactinemia, Cushing's disease, or rarely hyperthyroxinemia. Somatotroph hyperplasia is difficult to distinguish from a GH-cell adenoma, and silver staining displays a well-preserved reticulin network without a surrounding pseudocapsule. The rigorous morphologic diagnosis of GH cell hyperplasia is usually associated with stimulation by ectopic GHRH derived from an extrapituitary tumor, causing acromegaly. Silent somatotroph adenomas immunostain positively for GH and are apparently clinically nonfunctional, although GH or PRL levels (or both) might in fact be modestly elevated in more than half these patients.

Pathogenesis of Somatotroph Cell Adenomas

Pituitary and hypothalamic factors influence pituitary tumor pathogenesis.[612,613] Even when exhibiting marked nuclear pleomorphism, mitotic activity, and invasiveness, these tumors are usually benign.

Disordered GHRH Secretion or Action

Adenomas express receptors for GHRH, ghrelin,[481] and SRIF[614] but activating mutations of either the GHRH or SRIF receptor have not been reported. GHRH directly stimulates GH gene expression and also induces somatotroph mitotic activity. Transgenic GHRH expression causes somatotroph hyperplasia and ultimately adenoma. Clinically, GHRH production by hypothalamic, abdominal, or chest neuroendocrine tumors causes somatotroph hyperplasia and occasionally adenoma, with resultant unrestrained GH secretion and acromegaly.[32] However, histologic examination of most pituitary GH-cell adenoma tissue specimens does not show hyperplastic somatotroph tissue surrounding the adenoma, implying no generalized hypothalamic overstimulation. Failure to down-regulate GH secretion during prolonged GHRH stimulation also points to a role for GHRH in maintaining persistent GH hypersecretion. Furthermore, a GHRH antagonist was found to reduce hGH production in 50 patients with acromegaly, suggesting a role for endogenous

TABLE 8–24 CAUSES OF ACROMEGALY

Cause	Prevalence (%)	Hormonal Product(s)	Clinical Features	Pathologic Characteristics
		EXCESS GROWTH HORMONE SECRETION		
Pituitary	98	GH	Slow-growing	Resemble normal somatotrophs,
Densely granulated GH cell adenoma	30		Clinically insidious	Numerous large secretory granules
Sparsely granulated adenoma	30	GH	Rapidly growing Often invasive	Cellular pleomorphism Characteristic ultrastructure
Mixed GH-cell and PRL-cell adenoma	25	GH and PRL	Variable	Densely granulated somatotrophs Sparsely granulated lactotrophs
Mammosomatotroph cell adenoma	10	GH and PRL	Common in children Gigantism Mild hyperprolactinemia	Both GH and PRL in same cell, often same secretory granule
Acidophil stem cell adenoma		PRL and GH	Rapidly growing/invasive hyperprolactinemia dominant	Distinctive ultrastructure Giant mitochondria
Plurihormonal adenoma		GH (PRL w/αGSU, FSH/LH, TSH, or ACTH	Often secondary hormonal products are clinically silent	Variable: either monomorphous or plurimorphous
GH-cell carcinoma or metastases		GH	Usually aggressive	Documented metastasis
MEN-1 (adenoma)				
McCune-Albright syndrome (rarely-adenoma)		GH, PRL	Classic triad	
Ectopic sphenoid or parapharyngeal sinus pituitary adenoma		GH	Ectopic mass	Adenoma
Familial acromegaly (adenoma)		GH		
Carney's syndrome (adenoma)		GH		
		EXTRAPITUITARY TUMOR		
Pancreatic islet-cell tumor	<1			
		EXCESS GHRH SECRETION		
Central				
Hypothalamic hamartoma, choristoma, ganglioneuroma	<1		Hypothalamic mass	Somatotroph hyperplasia
Peripheral				
Bronchial carcinoid, pancreatic islet-cell tumor, small cell lung cancer, adrenal adenoma, medullary thyroid carcinoma, pheochromocytoma	1	GH, PRL	Systemic features	Somatotroph hyperplasia Rarely adenoma

GH, growth hormone; GHRH, growth hormone–releasing hormone; MEN, multiple endocrine neoplasia.

Adapted from Melmed S. Acromegaly [see comments]. N Engl J Med 1990;322:966-977; and Melmed S, Braunstein GD, Horvath E, et al. Pathophysiology of acromegaly. Endocr Rev 1983;4:271-290.

GHRH.[615] Expression of intra-adenomatous GHRH correlates with tumor size and activity, implying a paracrine role for GHRH in mediating adenoma pathogenesis.[616] GHRH modestly stimulates PRL secretion, and up to 40% of patients with acromegaly also have hyperprolactinemia. Complete surgical resection of well-defined GH-secreting microadenomas usually results in a definitive cure of excess hormone secretion with very low postoperative tumor recurrence rates, strongly suggesting intact hypothalamic function in these patients. Although basal GH levels are usually high in acromegaly, the episodic pulsatile pattern of GH release is intact, and the nocturnal GH surge usually preserved.[617] Patients treated with SRIF analogues also retain GH pulsatility, and GH pulse amplitude and sensitivity to GHRH appear intact.

Disordered Somatotroph Cell Function

A somatotroph mutation may be a prerequisite for the abnormal growth response to disordered GHRH secretion or action. Monoclonal origin of somatotroph adenomas was determined by X-chromosome inactivation analysis of somatotroph tumor DNA.[618] An altered $G_s\alpha$ protein identified in a subset of GH-secreting pituitary adenomas leads to high levels of intracellular cAMP and GH hypersecretion.[619,620] Point mutations in two critical sites, Arg201, the site for ADP-ribosylation, and Gly227, the GTP-binding domain of $G_s\alpha$ proteins, prevent GTPase activity and result in constitutive adenyl cyclase activation. This dominant *gsp* mutant mimics GHRH effects, resulting in elevated cAMP levels, and is present in about 30% of GH-secreting tumors. Loss of heterozygosity has been observed for chromosomes 11, 13, and 9,[46,55,614] especially in larger, more invasive macroadenomas. However, no defined tumor-suppressor gene has been isolated for these sporadic nonfamilial tumors. An activating transforming gene, PTTG, isolated from pituitary tumors, is overexpressed in GH-secreting tumors, and its abundance correlates with tumor size and invasiveness.[47-49] PTTG participates as a securin protein, regulating sister chromatid separation during the cell cycle, and its overexpression can lead to cell aneuploidy.[50]

The sequence of events leading to somatotroph clonal expansions appears multifactorial. An activated oncogene may be required for initiating tumorigenesis, and promotion of tumor growth can require GHRH and other growth factor stimulation. The cellular mutation might not by itself be sufficient to provide a growth advantage for a GH-secreting adenoma without additional disordered hypothalamic or paracrine growth factor signaling.

Extrapituitary Acromegaly

The source of excess GH secretion in acromegaly is not necessarily pituitary in origin.[621] Because management of ectopic acromegaly differs from that for pituitary GH hypersecretion, rigorous clinical and biochemical criteria should be fulfilled to confirm the diagnosis of ectopic acromegaly.[622] These include demonstration of elevated circulating GHRH or GH levels in the absence of a primary pituitary lesion, a significant arteriovenous hormone gradient across the ectopic tumor source, biochemical and clinical cure of acromegaly after resection of the ectopic hormone-producing tumor, and normalization of the GHRH–GH–IGF-I axis. GHRH or GH gene product expression should be shown. Nonconclusive images or biochemical or clinical features of pituitary acromegaly can inadvertently be misdiagnosed as a nonpituitary source of excess GH secretion and these patients might be inappropriately treated.

GHRH Hypersecretion

Hypothalamic tumors, including hamartomas, choristomas, gliomas, and gangliocytomas, can produce GHRH with subsequent somatotroph hyperplasia, or even a pituitary GH-cell adenoma and resultant acromegaly.[32] Primary mammosomatotroph hyperplasia with no evidence of pituitary adenoma or an extrapituitary tumor source of GHRH has been described in gigantism.[623] The structure of hypothalamic GHRH was in fact elucidated from material extracted from pancreatic GHRH-secreting tumors in patients with acromegaly.[31] GHRH immunoreactivity is detectable in about 25% of carcinoid tumor samples. Acromegaly in these patients, however, is uncommon. In a retrospective survey of 177 patients with acromegaly, only a single patient was identified with elevated plasma GHRH levels.[473]

Most tumors associated with ectopic GHRH secretion are bronchial carcinoids. Rare pancreatic cell tumors, small cell lung cancers, adrenal adenoma, pheochromocytoma, medullary thyroid tumors, endometrial cancer, and breast cancer have been described that express GHRH and cause acromegaly.[624,625] Surgical resection of the tumor secreting ectopic GHRH should reverse the GH hypersecretion, and pituitary surgery is not required in these patients. Carcinoid syndrome with ectopic GHRH secretion can also be managed with somatostatin analogues, which lower GH and IGF-I levels and also suppresses ectopic tumor elaboration of GHRH.[626,627]

Ectopic Pituitary Adenomas

GH-secreting adenomas can arise from ectopic pituitary remnants in the sphenoid sinus, petrous temporal bone, or nasopharyngeal cavity.[628,629] Very rarely, pituitary carcinoma can spread to the meninges, CSF, or cervical lymph nodes, resulting in functional GH-secreting metastases that may be diagnosed by radiolabeled octreotide imaging (octreoscan).[456]

Peripheral GH-Secreting Tumors

Lung adenocarcinoma, breast cancer, and ovarian tissues contain immunoreactive GH without clinical evidence of acromegaly. Rarely, GH-secreting intramesenteric pancreatic islet cell tumor[593] or a non-Hodgkin's lymphoma[630] causes acromegaly. These patients have a normal-sized or small pituitary gland on MRI, no GH response to TRH injection, and normal levels of circulating plasma GHRH.[622]

Acromegaloidism

Rarely, patients exhibit soft tissue and skin changes usually associated with acromegaly, normal baseline; dynamic GH and IGF-I levels with no demonstrable pituitary or extrapituitary tumor have been termed *acromegaloid.* Pachydermoperiostosis should be considered in the differential diagnosis. Insulin resistance and defective IGF-I binding have been demonstrated in cells derived from some patients with acanthosis nigricans, and treatment is symptomatic.

McCune-Albright Syndrome

This rare hypersecretory syndrome consists of polyostotic fibrous dysplasia, cutaneous pigmentation, sexual precocity, hyperthyroidism, hypercortisolism, hyperprolactinemia, and acromegaly due to somatotroph hyperplasia.[631] Although few patients have definitive evidence for a pituitary adenoma, $G_s\alpha$ mutations have been detected in endocrine and nonendocrine tissues.[632] GH hypersecretion can be controlled by somatostatin analogues or pituitary irradiation.

Multiple Endocrine Neoplasia

GH-cell pituitary adenoma is a well-documented component of the autosomal dominant multiple endocrine neoplasia type 1 (MEN-1) syndrome, which also includes parathyroid and pancreatic tumors (see Chapter 40). MEN-1, associated with germ cell inactivation of the *MENIN* tumor suppressor gene located on chromosome 11q13,[633] appears intact in sporadic GH-cell adenomas.[54,634] Rarely, functional pancreatic tumors in patients with MEN-I also express GHRH.

Familial Acromegaly

Familial acromegaly can occur in association with the Carney complex, which maps to chromosome 2p.[635] Several families with isolated familial acromegaly comprise related cases of acromegaly and gigantism and harbor loss of heterozygosity in chromosome 11q13, distinct from *MENIN* (see Table 8–4).[636]

Clinical Features

Manifestations of acromegaly are caused by either central pressure effects of the pituitary mass or peripheral actions of excess GH and IGF-I. Central features of the expanding pituitary mass are common to all pituitary masses[321] and are described earlier. In acromegaly, headache is often severe and debilitating. Local signs are especially important presenting features because a higher preponderance of macroadenomas (>65%) is encountered in acromegaly, as compared to mostly microadenomas for PRL-secreting tumors.[637]

Gigantism

Tall stature may be caused by a GH-secreting pituitary tumor or hyperplasia. About 20% of patients have the McCune-Albright syndrome, with somatotroph hyperplasia or rarely pituitary adenomas. Somatotroph hyperplasia and acidophilic stem cell adenomas can cause gigantism in infancy or early childhood, suggesting early hypersecretion of GHRH or disordered pituicyte cell differentiation.[623,638] Pituitary gigantism should be considered in children who are more than 3 standard deviations (SD) above normal mean height for age, or more than 2 SDs over their adjusted mean parental height. The biochemical diagnosis is similar to that for acromegaly, namely, GH levels are in excess of 1 μg/L after a glucose load and serum IGF-I concentrations are elevated. In children undergoing pubertal growth spurts, GH responses to glucose may be paradoxical, and serum IGF-I concentrations are often physiologically elevated. Thus, the diagnosis requires clear-cut MRI evidence for a pituitary lesion. The differential diagnosis includes familial tall stature, redundancy of Y chromosomes, Marfan's syndrome, and homocystinuria.

Clinical Features

Effects of hypersomatotrophism on acral and soft tissue growth, and metabolic function, occur insidiously over several years (Table 8–25, Figs. 8–47 and 8–48).[639] The slow onset and elusive symptomatology often results in delayed diagnosis ranging from 6.6 to 10.2 years, with a mean delay of almost 9 years.[640] Patients might seek care for dental, orthopedic, rheumatologic, or cardiac disorders. Only 13% of 256 patients whose acromegaly was diagnosed during a 20-year period presented with primary symptoms of altered facial appearance or enlarged extremities.[641] In a review of several hundred patients presenting with acromegaly worldwide, 98% had acral enlargement, and hyperhidrosis was prominent in 70%.[639] When patients present early, facial and peripheral features are usually not obvious and serial review of old photographs often accentuates the progress of subtle physical changes.

Characteristic features include large fleshy lips and nose, spade-like hands, frontal skull bossing, and cranial ridges. Enlarged tongue, bones, salivary glands, thyroid, heart, liver, and spleen are the effects of generalized visceromegaly. Clinically apparent hepatosplenomegaly, however, is rare. Increase in shoe, ring, or hat size is commonly reported. Progressive acral changes can lead to facial coarsening and skeletal disfigurement, especially if excess GH secretion begins prior to epiphyseal closure.[642] These include mandibular overgrowth with prognathism, maxillary widening, teeth separation, jaw malocclusion, overbite, large nose, and coarse, oily skin with large pores.[643] Sonorous voice deepening occurs in association with laryngeal hypertrophy and enlarged paranasal sinuses.

Up to half of patients experience joint symptoms severe enough to limit daily activities. Arthropathy occurs in about 70% of patients, most of whom exhibit joint swelling, hypermobility, and cartilaginous thickening.[644] These problems often persist

TABLE 8–25 CLINICAL FEATURES OF ACROMEGALY

LOCAL TUMOR EFFECTS	VISCEROMEGALY
Cranial nerve palsy Headache Pituitary enlargement Visual field defects	Kidney Liver Prostate Salivary gland Spleen Thyroid Tongue
SOMATIC EFFECTS	**ENDOCRINE AND METABOLIC EFFECTS**
Acral Enlargement Thickness of hand and feet soft tissue **Cardiovascular** Asymmetric septal hypertrophy Cardiomyopathy Congestive heart failure Hypertension Left-ventricular hypertrophy **Colon** Polyps **Musculoskeletal** Acroparesthesia Arthralgias and arthritis Carpal tunnel syndrome Gigantism Hypertrophy of frontal bones Jaw malocclusion Prognathism Proximal myopathy **Pulmonary** Narcolepsy Sleep apnea—central and obstructive Sleep disturbances **Skin** Hyperhidrosis Oiliness Skin tags	**Carbohydrate** Diabetes mellitus Impaired glucose tolerance Insulin resistance and hyperinsulinemia **Electrolytes** Increased aldosterone Low renin **Lipids** Hypertriglyceridemia **Minerals** Hypercalciuria, increased 1,25$(OH)_2D_3$ Urinary hydroxproline **Multiple endocrine neoplasia type 1** Hyperparathyroidism Pancreatic islet cell tumors **Reproduction** Decreased libido, impotence, low sex hormone–binding globulin Galactorrhea Menstrual abnormalities **Thyroid** Goiter Low thyroxine-binding globulin

Most soft tissue and metabolic changes are reversible by tight hormonal control. Bone changes, hypertension, and central sleep apnea are generally not reversible.

Modified from Bonert V, Melmed S. Acromegaly. In Bar RS, ed. Early Diagnosis and Treatment of Endocrine Disorders (Contemporary Endocrinology). Totowa, NJ: Humana Press, 2002:201-228.

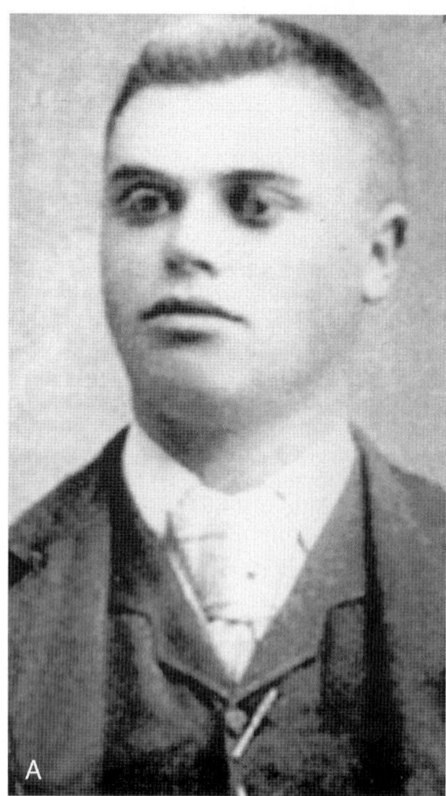

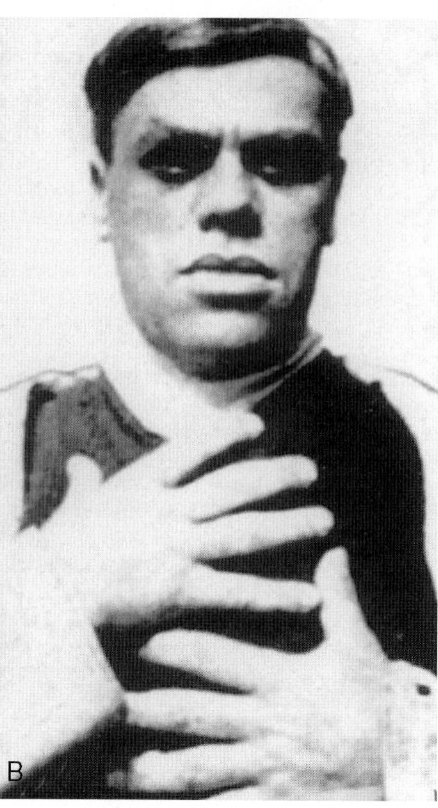

Figure 8–47 ▪ Harvey Cushing's first acromegaly patient. **A,** Some years before presentation. **B,** At admission. (From Jane JA, Laws ER. History of acromegaly. In Wass J, ed. Handbook of Acromegaly. Bristol, UK: BioScientifica, 2001:3-15.)

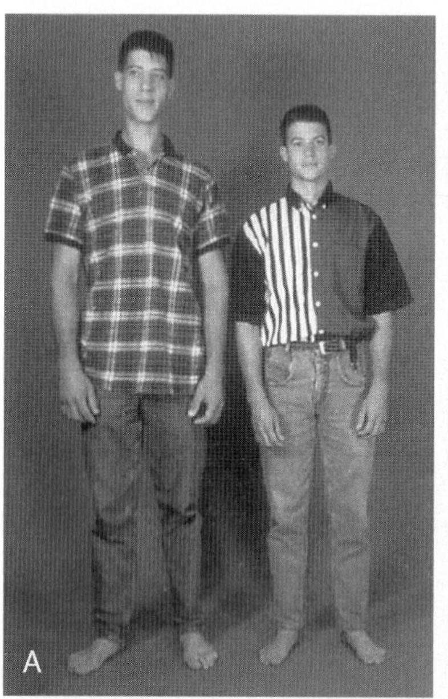

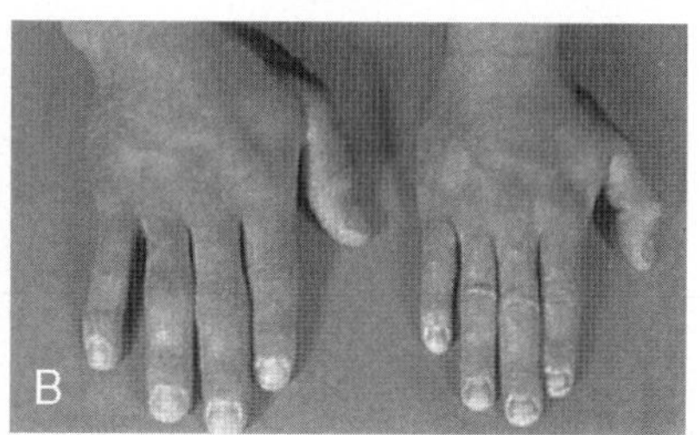

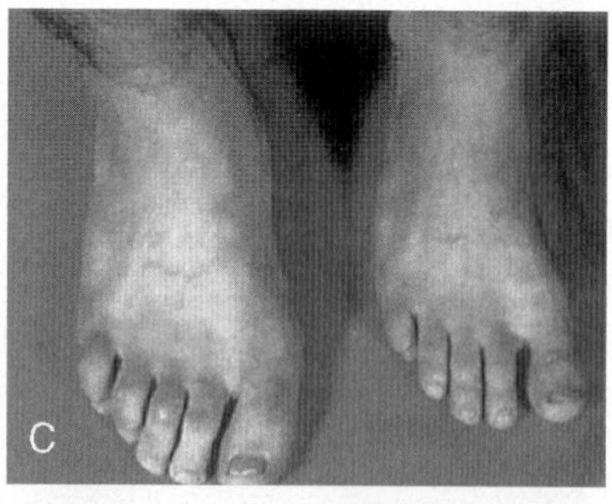

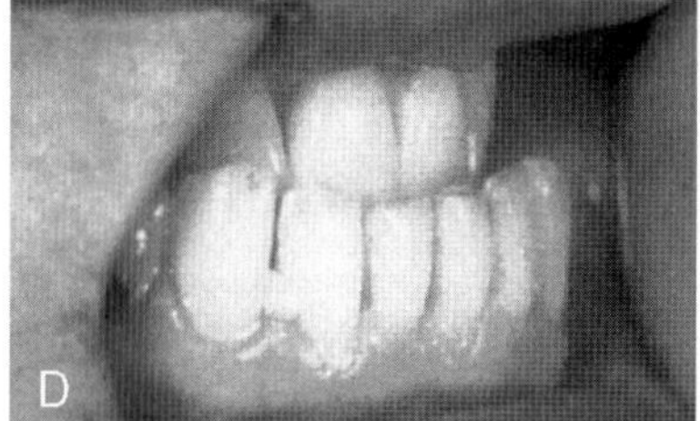

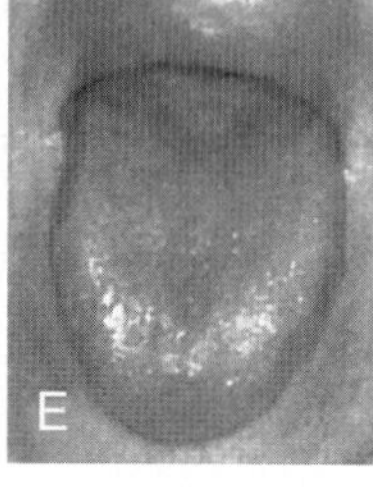

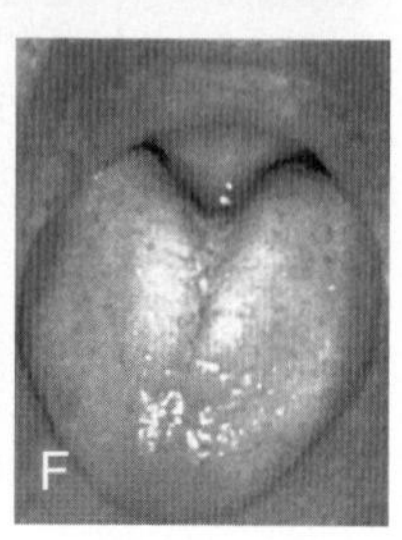

Figure 8–48 ▪ Clinical features of acromegaly. Features of acromegaly and gigantism in two identical twins. A 22-year-old man with gigantism due to excess growth hormone is shown to the left of his identical twin. The increase height and prognathism **(A)** and enlarged hand **(B)** and foot **(C)** of the affected twin are apparent. Their clinical features began to diverge at the age of approximately 13 years. Increased incisor spacing and prognathism **(D)**; macroglossia **(E)** and a normal tongue **(F)**. (**A** to **C** from Gagel R, McCutcheon IE. Images in clinical medicine: pituitary gigantism. N Engl J Med 1999;324:524; **D** to **F** from Turner HE. Clinical features, investigation and complications of acromegaly. In Wass J, ed. Handbook of Acromegaly. Bristol, UK: BioScientifica, 2001:19-28).

after complete remission.[645] Local periarticular fibrous tissue thickening can cause joint stiffening, deformities, and nerve entrapment. Knees, hips, shoulders, lumbosacral joints, elbows, and ankles are affected as mono- or polyarticular arthritides, but joint effusions rarely develop.[646] Spinal involvement includes osteophytosis, disc space widening, and increased anteroposterior vertebral length, which can result in dorsal kyphosis. Neural enlargement and wrist tissue swelling can lead to carpal tunnel syndrome in up to half of all patients. Chondrocyte proliferation with increased joint space occurs early, and ulcerations and fissures of weight-bearing cartilage areas are often accompanied by new bone formation. Debilitating osteoarthritis can result in bone remodeling, osteophyte formation, subchondral cysts, narrowed joint spaces, and lax periarticular ligaments. Osteophytes commonly occur at the phalangeal tufts and over the anterior aspects of spinal vertebrae. Ligaments can ossify, and periarticular calcium pyrophosphate deposition occurs. Although the duration of hypersomatotrophism correlates with clinical severity of the joint changes, it is unclear whether higher GH levels correlate with increased articular disease activity.

Therapeutic responses usually depend upon the degree of irreversible bony changes already in place. Hyperhidrosis and malodorous oily skin are common early signs, occurring in up to 70% of patients. Facial wrinkles, nasolabial folds, and heel pads thicken, and body hair may become coarsened,[647] attributed to glycosaminoglycan deposition and increased connective tissue collagen production.[648] Skin tags are common and may be markers for the adenomatous colonic polyps.[649] Raynaud's phenomenon is reported in up to one third of patients.

Symptomatic cardiac disease is present in about 20% of patients and is a major cause of morbidity and mortality.[650,651] Hypertension is present in about 50% of patients with active acromegaly, and half of these have evidence of left ventricular dysfunction.[652] Left ventricular hypertrophy is also observed in about half of normotensive patients with acromegaly. Asymmetric septal hypertrophy is common, and cardiac failure can occur with early or mild cardiomegaly. Subclinical left ventricular diastolic dysfunction is due to myocardial hypertrophy, interstitial fibrosis, and lymphocytic myocardial infiltrates. Resting electrocardiograms are abnormal in about 50% of patients, with S-T segment depression, T-wave abnormalities, conduction defects, and arrhythmias. Plasma renin levels are suppressed and endogenous plasma digitalis-like activity with chronic volume expansion has been identified in acromegaly.[653] Cardiovascular disease accounts for about 60% of deaths in patients with acromegaly,[654] and the presence of cardiovascular disease at the time of diagnosis portends high mortality rates, despite improved cardiac function after effective GH and IGF-I control.[375]

Prognathism, thick lips, macroglossia, and hypertrophied nasal structures can obstruct airways.[655,656] Irregular laryngeal mucosa, cartilage hypertrophy, tracheal calcification, and cricoarytenoid joint arthropathy lead to unilateral or bilateral vocal cord fixation or laryngeal stenosis with voice changes. Tracheal intubation may be particularly difficult in patients undergoing anesthesia and tracheostomy may be required. Central respiratory depression and airway obstruction leads to paroxysmal daytime sleep (narcolepsy), sleep apnea, and habitual excessive snoring. Obstructive sleep apnea, characterized by excessive daytime sleepiness with at least five episodes of apnea per hour of sleep causes daytime somnolence, especially in men with acromegaly, who also might have a ventilation-perfusion defect with hypoxemia. Sleep apnea may also be central in origin and associated with higher GH and IGF-I levels.[656]

Synovial edema leads to hyperplastic wrist ligaments and tendons that contribute to painful median nerve compression. Peripheral acroparesthesias and symmetrical peripheral neuropathy should be distinguished from diabetic neuropathy, which can occur secondary to acromegaly.[657] Proximal myopathy can also be accompanied by myalgias, cramps, and nonspecific electromyogram myopathic changes. Exophthalmos may be present, but it may be masked by frontal bossing. Hypertrophied tissue surrounding the canal of Schlemm can impede aqueous filtration, leading to open-angle glaucoma. Progressive face and body disfigurement often leads to lowered self-esteem. Depression, mood swings, and apathy can occur secondary to physical deformity.[658]

Growth Hormone and Tumor Formation

The early practice of hypophysectomy for managing metastatic carcinoma was based on evidence implicating GH as a factor in tumor development. GH or IGF-I (or both) might possess direct or indirect mitogenic effects on mammalian cells and act as permissive growth stimulators of cells previously exposed to other growth factors.[659] IGFBP3, also induced by GH (see Chapter 23), inhibits cell proliferation and promotes apoptosis.[660,661] Thus, the ultimate impact of elevated GH levels on cell proliferation reflects a balance of apoptotic versus growth-promoting signals.[586]

A compelling cause-and-effect relationship of acromegaly with cancer has not been established.[585,662-664] Benign colon polyps have been reported in 45% of 678 patients in 12 prospective studies (Table 8–26). A recent controlled study in 161 patients revealed no increase in polyp incidence in acromegaly.[587] More than three skin tags in patients older than 50 years may be peripheral markers for the presence of adenomatous colon polyps unrelated to GH or IGF-I serum levels.[665] Hypertrophic mucosal folds and colonic hypertrophy are commonly present; colonoscopy is warranted every 3 to 5 years after diagnosis, depending on the presence of other risk factors. Mortality from colon cancer is largely related to GH levels, rather than enhanced incidence of the disease in acromegaly (Table 8–27).

Analysis of nine retrospective reports (1956-1998) encompassing 21,470 person-years at risk, yielded no significant increased cancer incidence.[586] Cancer incidence was in fact lower than expected in 1362 patients with acromegaly in the United Kingdom, and enhanced colon cancer mortality observed in this study correlated with GH levels.[585] Thus, although disordered cell proliferation and increased risk for promotion of coexisting neoplasms could be anticipated, little evidence favors a significantly enhanced cancer incidence in acromegaly (Table 8–28). Colon cancer appears to be of particular concern, and screening colonoscopy should be performed at diagnosis in all patients. Although elevated IGF-I levels might correlate with colon polyp prevalence when patients are retested,[662] a controlled prospective study shows no increased colon polyp incidence in acromegaly.[586,587] Because patients are now living longer as a result of improved biochemical control, long-term prospective controlled studies are required to resolve this question in an aging population.

Endocrine Complications

About 30% of patients exhibit elevated serum PRL levels (up to 100 μg/L or more), with or without galactorrhea.[666] Functional pituitary stalk compression by a pituitary mass prevents lactotroph access of hypothalamic dopamine, releasing the cell from tonic hypothalamic inhibition. GH-secreting adenoma subtypes might also concomitantly secrete PRL. Because GH behaves as an agonist for breast PRL binding sites, the tumor can cause galactorrhea in the face of normal PRL levels. Tumor mass compressing surrounding normal pituitary tissue can also cause hypopituitarism. More than half of all patients have amenorrhea

TABLE 8–26 COLON POLYPS IN ACROMEGALY

Reference Number	NUMBER OF PATIENTS			Mean Age	Adenoma	Hyperplastic	Total	Carcinoma
	Total	Male	Female					
587	115	63	69	54.8*	27	18	45	3
662	66†	N/a	N/A	32.7	25	18	43	1
663	103	49	54	51	23	25	48	0
664	54	26	28	47	5	11	19	0
665	23	12	11	47	8	1	9	0
728	50	25	25	25-70	11	12	23	1
893	17	10	7	49	5	3	8	2
894	12	11	11	56	2	1	3	2
895	29	N/A	N/A	N/A	4	0	4	2
896	49	30	19	54	11	5	16	0
897	31	11	20	52	11	8	16	0
898	129	68	60	57	33	42	75	6
Totals	678				165(24%)	144 (21%)	309 (45%)	17 (2.5%)

*Median age.
†Repeat colonoscopy.
Incidence of colonic lesions in 678 patients prospectively evaluated in 12 studies. Up to 45% of asymptomatic men older than 50 years harbor colon adenomas.

Derived from Melmed S. Acromegaly and cancer: not a problem? J Clin Endocrinol Metab 2001;86:2929-2934, and Lieberman, DA. Use of colonoscopy to screen asymptomatic adults for colorectal cancer. N Engl J Med 2000;343:162-168.

TABLE 8–27 POST-TREATMENT GROWTH HORMONE LEVELS AND MORTALITY IN ACROMEGALY

POST-TREATMENT GH		MORTALITY			
Dose (ng/mL)	No. of Patients	Overall ($P < 0.0001$)		Cancer Related ($P < 0.05$)	
		%	Range	%	Range
<2.5	541	1.10	0.89-1.15	0.966	0.63-1.41
2.5-9.9	493	1.41	1.16-1.69	0.81	0.50-1.24
>10	207	2.12	1.70-2.62	1.81	1.13-2.74

Post-treatment growth hormone levels correlate with mortality in acromegaly. Standardized mortality ratios are depicted for overall mortality and for cancer-related mortality.

Adapted from Orme S, McNally RJQ, Cartwright RA, Belchetz PE. Mortality and cancer incidence in acromegaly: a retrospective cohort study. J Clin Endo Metab 1998;83:2730-2734.

TABLE 8–28 ACROMEGALY AND CANCER INDICENCE

Subjects	Number	Person-Years at Risk	CANCERS		*P*
			Observed	O/E	
MULTICENTER ANALYSIS*					
Female	95	1,351	8	1.33	NS
Male	128	1,630	5	1.30	NS
Total	223	2,981	13	1.3	
META-ANALYSIS†					
All	4,822	21,740	178	0.76-3.4	NA

*Multicenter analysis of cancer incidence in patients with acromegaly ranging in age from 1 to 79 years. Adapted from Mustacchi P, Shimkin MB. Occurrence of cancer in acromegaly and in hypopituitarism. Cancer 1957;10:100-104.
†Analysis of retrospective published reports (1956-1998) of cancer incidence in patients with acromegaly. Included are data from references 585, 604,605,641, 899, 900, 901, 902, and 903 and from Mustacchi 1956. Mustacchi P, Shimkin MB. Occurrence of cancer in acromegaly and in hypopituitarism. Cancer 1957;10:100-104.

NA, not applicable; NS, not significant; O/E, ratio of observed cancers to expected cancers.

or impotence,[637,667,668] and secondary thyroid or adrenal failure is present in about 20% of patients. Gonadal dysfunction can result in reduced bone.[669]

The direct anti-insulin effects of GH causes carbohydrate intolerance, and patients can also develop insulin-requiring diabetes mellitus. Carbohydrate intolerance and insulin requirements improve rapidly on lowering GH after surgery or somatostatin analogue therapy. Hypertriglyceridemia (type IV), hypercalciuria, and hypercalcemia also occur.

Thyroid dysfunction in acromegaly may be caused by diffuse or nodular toxic or nontoxic goiter or Graves' disease, especially because IGF-I is a major determinant of thyroid cell growth.[670] Associated MEN-1 features may be present in affected patients, including hypercalcemia with hyperparathyroidism or pancreatic tumors. Benign prostatic hypertrophy has been documented in acromegaly with no apparent increase in prostate cancer rates.[671,672]

Morbidity and Mortality

Cardiovascular disease, respiratory disorders, diabetes, and malignancy account for enhanced (threefold) mortality in acromegaly.[585,604,605,654,673-677] In a retrospective study reported in 1966, cardiovascular disease was the leading cause of death and 50%

of patients who died before the age of 50 years. In 194 patients with acromegaly, life expectancy was reduced, and cardiovascular disorders accounted for 24% of deaths, followed by respiratory (18%) and cerebrovascular disease (14%). Diabetes mellitus, occurring in 20% of patients, was associated with 2.5 times the predicted mortality, and hypertension was present in about half of all patients.[654] The most significant mortality determinants are GH levels and the presence of coexisting cardiac disease. Moreover, control of GH levels to less than 2.5 μg/L after surgery or medical treatments significantly reduces morbidity and mortality (Fig. 8–49).

Diagnosis

Measurement of Growth Hormone Levels

The diagnosis of acromegaly requires measurement of a random GH greater than 0.4 μg/L or a GH nadir during an oral glucose tolerance test (OGTT) of greater than 1 μg/L.[678] Using more sensitive newer assays, the GH cut-off may be even lower.[679] In healthy subjects, serum GH levels initially fall after receiving oral glucose and subsequently increase as plasma glucose declines. However, in patients with acromegaly, oral glucose fails to suppress GH; GH levels increase in one third of patients, remain unchanged in one third, or fall modestly in one third.

Basal morning (AM) and random GH levels are usually elevated in acromegaly. Because of the episodic nature of GH secretion, however, serum concentrations can normally fluctuate from undetectable up to 30 μg/L. Unlike the largely undetectable nadir GH levels in normal subjects, those with acromegaly sampled over 24 hours contain detectable levels of GH (>2 μg/L).[680]

Evoked GH responses to GHRH administration are not useful for diagnosis. A higher episodic GH pulse frequency occurs, and it often persists after surgical adenoma resection. Random GH levels measured with sensitive assays in acromegaly may be as low as 0.37 μg/L, with persistently elevated postoperative IGF-I levels.[676] Serum IGF-I levels are high[681] and correlate with the log of serum GH determinations. Age-and gender-matched IGF-I elevations can persist for several months after GH levels are biochemically controlled after treatment.[682] Elevated IGF-I levels are also encountered during pregnancy and late puberty. A high IGF-I level is thus highly specific for acromegaly and correlates with clinical indices of disease activity. IGFBP-3 levels are also elevated, but have little diagnostic value. GH-secreting adenomas exhibit discordant GH responses to TRH and GnRH administration in up to 50% of patients, but these adjunctive tests are rarely required to confirm the diagnosis.

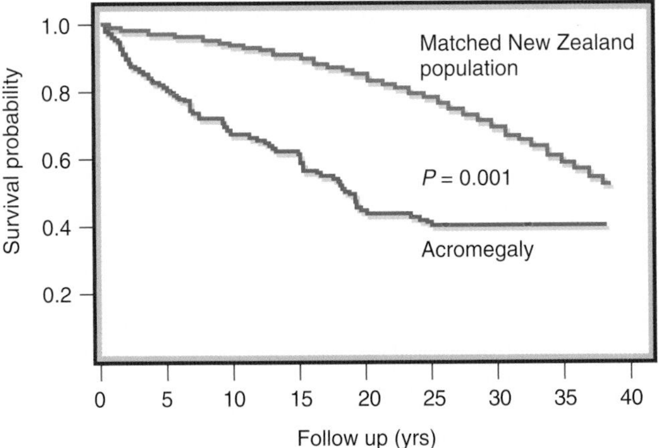

Figure 8–49 ▪ Mortality in acromegaly. Documented determinants of mortality outcome in retrospective studies of acromegaly. (Data integrated from Holdaway IM, Rajasoorya RC, Wong J, et al. The natural history of treated functional pituitary adenomas. In Webb SM, ed. Pituitary Tumors. Bristol, UK: BioScientifica, 1998:31-42.

Differential Diagnosis

The overwhelming majority of patients with acromegaly harbor a GH-cell pituitary adenoma; rarely extrapituitary acromegaly should be considered. Nevertheless, distinguishing pituitary versus extrapituitary acromegaly is important for planning effective management. Regardless of the cause of unrestrained GH secretion, IGF-I levels are invariably elevated, and GH levels fail to fall (<1 μg/L) after an oral glucose load.[683] When clinical features of acromegaly are associated with normal GH and IGF-I levels, burned out or silent acromegaly associated with an infarcted pituitary adenoma, often with a secondary empty sella, should be considered.[684]

About 5% of consecutive patients with proven GH-cell adenomas have normal GH and elevated IGF-I levels. It is likely that improved GH assay sensitivity will unmask abnormal GH secretion in these patients. Dynamic pituitary testing (TRH, dopamine) does not distinguish patients with pituitary adenomas from those harboring extrapituitary tumors. Plasma GHRH levels are invariably elevated in patients with peripheral GHRH-secreting tumors but are normal or low in patients with pituitary adenomas.[685] GHRH plasma level measurement is precise and cost-effective for diagnosis of ectopic acromegaly. Peripheral GHRH levels are not elevated in patients with hypothalamic GHRH-secreting tumors, presumably because eutopic hypothalamic GHRH secretion into the hypophyseal portal system does not appreciably enter the systemic circulation.

Unique or unexpected clinical features, including respiratory wheezing or dyspnea, facial flushing, peptic ulcers, or renal stones sometimes indicate the diagnosis of a nonpituitary endocrine tumor. Hypoglycemia, hyperinsulinemia, hypergastrinemia, and rarely hypercortisolism, all not usually encountered in pituitary acromegaly, should justify an evaluation for an extrapituitary source of GH excess. MRI and CT scanning are employed to localize pituitary or extrapituitary tumor. Routine abdominal or chest imaging of all patients yields a very low incidence of true positive cases of ectopic tumor, and such screening is not recommended as cost effective.

A normal or small-sized pituitary gland, or clinical and biochemical features of other tumors known to be associated with extrapituitary acromegaly and elevated circulating GHRH levels, are indications for extrapituitary imaging. An enlarged pituitary is, however, often present in patients with peripheral GHRH-secreting tumors, and the radiologic diagnosis of a pituitary adenoma may be difficult to exclude.

The McCune-Albright syndrome should be considered after definitive exclusion of pituitary and extrapituitary tumors.

Treatment

Aims

A comprehensive strategy for treating patients with acromegaly should aim to manage the pituitary mass, suppress GH and IGF-I hypersecretion, and prevent long-term clinical sequelae of hypersomatotrophism while maintaining normal anterior pituitary function.[678,686] Because elevated GH levels per se are associated with threefold increased morbidity and account for the single most important determinant of mortality,[654,673-675,677,687] it is important to reverse the mortality rate to that of age-matched healthy subjects by aiming for tight GH control.[677,686] Serum GH levels should be suppressed to at least less than 1 μg/L or less after an oral glucose load, and age- and gender-matched serum IGF-I levels should be normalized. A patient with controlled GH should also have a normal 24-hour integrated secretion of GH (<2.5 μg/L). GH might not be measurable for most of the day and yet the tumor might still be hypersecreting as reflected by elevated IGF-I levels. Current therapeutic modes for acromegaly management, including surgery, irradiation, and medical treatment, do not comprehensively fulfill these goals (Fig. 8–50).

Surgical Management

Well-circumscribed somatotroph cell adenomas should preferably be resected by transsphenoidal surgery.[688-695] Successful resection alleviates preoperative compression effects and compromised trophic hormone secretion, and the skilled surgeon balances the extent of maximal tumor tissue removal while preserving anterior pituitary function.

Outcomes

Within 2 hours of successful resection, metabolic dysfunction and soft tissue swelling start improving and GH levels are often controlled within 1 hour.

Surgical outcome correlates well with adenoma size and preoperative serum GH levels, and particularly with the experience of the surgeon. Smaller tumors (less than 5 mm), tumors totally confined within the sella, and preoperative serum GH levels less than 40 μg/L portend a favorable surgical outcome. Up to 90% of patients with microadenomas achieve postoperative GH levels less than 2.5 μg/L, but less than 50% of all-sized macroadenomas had postoperative GH levels less than 2 μg/L after

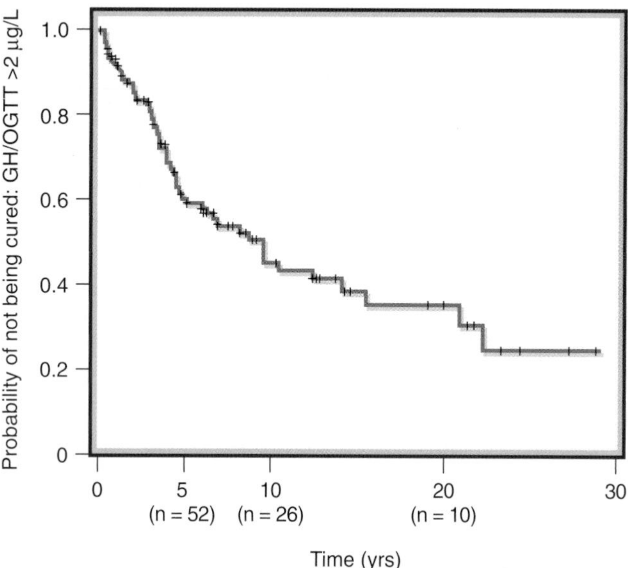

Figure 8–50 ▪ Radiation treatment of acromegaly. Long-term effects of radiation therapy on growth hormone (GH) secretion using a GH nadir after oral glucose load less than 2 μg/L as the cure criterion, and the probability of not being cured with time after radiotherapy. The numbers of patients not cured at 5, 10, and 20 years after pituitary irradiation are indicated in parentheses. Each step represents one cure; each cross (+) denotes a patient not cured at the latest follow-up. (From Barrande G, Pittino-Lungo M, Coste J, et al. Hormonal and metabolic effects of radiotherapy in acromegaly: long-term results in 128 patients followed in a single center. J Clin Endocrinol Metab 2000;85:3779-3785.)

glucose administration.[692] GH is controlled in less than one third of all patients after resection of adenomas larger than 10 mm. About 75% of patients with preoperative GH less than 5 μg/L have normalized IGF-I. Overall, in 17 studies of 1284 patients published between 1995 and 1999, 82% of patients harboring microadenomas have normalized IGF-I levels, and GH is controlled in 47% of those with macroadenomas (Table 8–29).

A review of 2665 patients from a single center showed that 72% of patients with microadenomas and 50% harboring macroadenomas had GH levels less than 1.0 μg/L during glucose loading and normal serum IGF-I levels.[696] Tumors recurred in 8% of these patients after 10 years. Endoscopic transnasal surgery offers promise as a less invasive procedure for resection of pituitary tumors[697] and accessing cavernous sinus tumor mass, although long-term comparative results are not yet available. Difficulties in endotracheal intubation due to macroglossia or severe kyphosis can necessitate tracheostomy for anesthesia.

Side Effects

Although surgical complications are often transient, they can require lifelong pituitary hormone replacement. New hypopituitarism develops in up to about 20% of patients, reflecting operative damage to the surrounding normal pituitary tissue.[698] Permanent diabetes insipidus, CSF leaks, hemorrhage, and meningitis occur in up to 10% of patients (see Table 8–10). The extent and prevalence of local complications depend upon tumor size and invasiveness. Experienced pituitary surgeons report more favorable postoperative complication rates.[699] Biochemical or anatomic recurrence (about 7% over 10 years) or postoperative tumor persistence might indicate incomplete resection of adenomatous tissue, surgically inaccessible cavernous sinus tissue, or nesting of functional tumor tissue within the dura.

Radiation

Primary or adjuvant radiation of GH-secreting tumors may be achieved by conventional external deep X-ray therapy as well as heavy-particle (proton beam)[184,187,700-702] or gamma knife radiation surgery.[703] Maximal tumor radiation should ideally be attained with minimal soft tissue damage. Precise MRI localization, accurate simulation and isocentral rotational techniques, and high voltage (6-15 MeV) delivery have improved radiation efficacy

Radiation is a highly individualized choice, depending upon the expertise and experience of the treating radiation therapist and upon the physician's and patient's choice of the benefits of therapy weighed against potential risks.

Outcomes

Up to 5000 rad are administered in split doses of 180 rad fractions divided over 6 weeks. Radiation arrests tumor growth, and most pituitary adenomas ultimately shrink.[187] GH levels fall gradually during the first year after treatment, and after 10 years, levels are less than 10 μg/L in 70% of patients. After 20 years, the National Institutes of Health experience is that more than 90% of patients have GH levels of less than 5 μg/L (Fig. 8–51).[700] When pretreatment GH levels were greater than 100 μg/L, only 60% of patients had GH less than 5 μg/L after 18 years. During the first 7 years after irradiation, less than 5% of patients normalize IGF-I levels,[701] but about 70% of patients exhibit normal IGF-I levels when tested during longer follow-up.[702]

Radiation therapy does not normalize GH secretory patterns, probably accounting for persistently elevated IGF-I levels in the face of apparently controlled GH levels.[704] Thus, during the initial years after irradiation, most patients are still exposed to unacceptably high levels of circulating GH and IGF-I. Promising stereotactic pituitary tumor ablation by the gamma-knife has been reported.[705]

TABLE 8–29 PRIMARY TRANSSPHENOIDAL SURGERY FOR GH-SECRETING PITUITARY ADENOMAS

Series	Number of Cases	Total Cure Rate (%)	Microadenomas (%)	Macroadenomas (%)	Definition of Cure
Abosch et al, 1998	254	76	75	71	GH <5 μg/L (<10 mU/l)
Ahmed et al, 1999	97	—	90	56	Basal GH ≤2.5 μg/L (<5 mU/l), OGTT GH <1 μg/L (<2 mU/l), normal IGF-I levels
Davis et al, 1993	174	52	N/A	N/A	GH ≦2 μg/L (<4 mU/l; basal or OGTT)
Fahlbusch et al, 1992	222	57	72	49	GH <2 μg/L (<4 mU/l) after OGTT
		71	81	65	GH <5 μg/L (<10 mU/l)
Fahlbusch, 2001	490	56	78	50	Basal GH ≦5 μg/l (<10 mU/l), OGTT GH <2 μg/L (≦4 mU/l), normal IGF-I levels
Freda et al, 1998	115	61	88	53	GH <2 μg/L (<4 mU/l) after OGTT or normal IGF-I levels
Laws et al, 2000	117	67	87	51	Basal GH <2.5 μg/L (<5 mU/l), OGTT GH <1 μg/L (<2 mU/l), normal IGF-levels)
Lissett et al, 1998	73	18	39	12	GH <5 μg/L after OGTT
Losa et al, 1989	29	55	N/A	N/A	GH <1 μg/L (<2 mU/l) and normal IGF-I levels
Ross and Wilson, 1988	153	56	N/A	N/A	GH <5 μg/L (<10 mU/l)
Sheaves et al, 1996	100	42	61	23	GH ≦2.5 μg/L (<5 mU/l)
Swearingen et al, 1998	162	57	91	48	Normal IGF-I levels
Tindall et al, 1993	91	82	N/A	N/A	GH <5 μg/L (<10 mU/l) and/or normal IGF-I levels

GH, growth hormone; IGF, insulin-like growth factor; N/A, not available; OGTT, oral glucose tolerance test.

Abosch A, Tyrrell JB, Lamborn KR, et al. Transsphenoidal microsurgery for growth hormone–secreting pituitary adenomas: initial outcome and long-term results. J Clin Endocrinol Metab 1998;83:3411-3418.

Ahmed S, Elsheikh M, Stratton IM, et al. Outcome of transphenoidal surgery for acromegaly and its relationship to surgical experience. Clin Endocrinol (Oxf) 1999;50:561-567.

Davis DH, Laws ER, Ilstrup DM. Results of surgical treatment for growth hormone-secreting pituitary adenomas. J Neurosurg 1993;79:70-75.

Fahlbusch R, Honegger J, Buchfelder M. Surgical management of acromegaly. Endocrinol Metab Clin North Am 1992;21:669-692.

Fahlbusch R, Buchfelder M, Kreutzer J, Nomikos P. Surgical management of acromegaly. In Wass J, ed. Handbook of Acromegaly. Bristol, UK: BioScientifica, 2001:41-47.

Freda PU, Post KD, Powell JS, Wardlaw SL. Evaluation of disease status with sensitive measures of growth hormone secretion in 60 postoperative patients with acromegaly. J Clin Endocrinol Metab 1998;83:3808-3816.

Laws ER, Vance ML, Thapar K. Pituitary surgery for the management of acromegaly. Horm Res 2000;53(suppl 3):71-75.

Lissett CA, Peacey SR, Laing I, et al. The outcome of surgery for acromegaly: the need for a specialist pituitary surgeon for all types of growth hormone (GH) secreting adenoma. Clin Endocrinol (Oxf) 1998;49:653-657.

Losa M, Oeckler R, Schopohl J, et al. Evaluation of selective transsphenoidal adenomectomy by endocrinological testing and somatomedin-C measurement in acromegaly. J Neurosurg 1989;70:561-567.

Ross DA, Wilson CB. Results of transsphenoidal microsurgery for growth hormone–secreting pituitary adenoma in a series of 214 patients. J Neurosurg 1988;68:854-867.

Sheaves R, Jenkins P, Blackburn P, et al. Outcome of transsphenoidal surgery for acromegaly using strict criteria for surgical cure. Clin Endocrinol (Oxf) 1996;45:407-413.

Swearingen B, Barker FG, Katznelson L, et al. Long-term mortality after transsphenoidal surgery and adjunctive therapy for acromegaly. J Clin Endocrinol Metab 1998;83:3419-3426.

Tindall GT, Oyesiku NM, Watts NB, et al. Transsphenoidal adenomectomy for growth hormone-secreting pituitary adenomas in acromegaly: outcome analysis and determinants of failure. J Neurosurg 1993;78:205-215.

Compiled from Fahlbusch R, Buchfelder M, Kreutzer EJ, Nomikos P. Surgical management of acromegaly. In Wass J, ed. Handbook of Acromegaly. Bristol, UK: BioScientifica, 2001:44; Lissett CA, Peacey SR, Laing I, et al. The outcome of surgery for acromegaly: the need for a specialist pituitary surgeon for all types of growth hormone (GH) secreting adenoma. Clin Endocrinol (Oxf) 1998;49:653-657; Swearingen B, Barker FG, Katznelson L, et al. Long-term mortality after transsphenoidal surgery and adjunctive therapy for acromegaly. J Clin Endocrinol Metab 1998;83:3419-3426.

Side Effects

After 10 years, about half of all patients receiving radiation therapy have signs of pituitary trophic hormone disruption, and this prevalence increases annually thereafter,[706] requiring gonadal steroids, thyroid hormone, cortisone replacement, or some combination of these. Side effects of conventional radiation including hair loss, cranial nerve palsies, tumor necrosis with hemorrhage, and loss of vision or pituitary apoplexy (both rare) have been documented in up to 2% of patients.[706] Lethargy, impaired memory, and personality changes can also occur.[707] The incidence and extent of local complications have been markedly diminished by use of highly reproducible simulators, precise rotational isocentric arc capability, and doses of less than 5000 rad.

Proton-beam therapy (Bragg Peak) is contraindicated in patients with suprasellar tumor extension due to unacceptable optic tract exposure to the radiation field. The rare development of second brain tumors in these patients has been reported at a cumulative risk frequency of 1.9% over 20 years.[191,192] Experience using gamma knife radiation surgery is scant, but 50% of patients with acromegaly achieved glucose-induced GH suppression to less than 1 ng/mL and normal IGF-I levels within 66 months of treatment.[703]

Radiation therapy effectively shrinks GH-cell adenomas and lowers GH levels over 20 years in more than 90% of patients.[708] In fact, GH deficiency can result from radiation.[709] Because of side effects, it should be employed as an adjuvant therapy for patients whose GH levels are not controlled by surgery or medical management and for those who refuse these therapies.

Dopamine Agonists

Because dopamine attenuates GH secretion in about one-third of patients with acromegaly, D2 receptor agonists, including

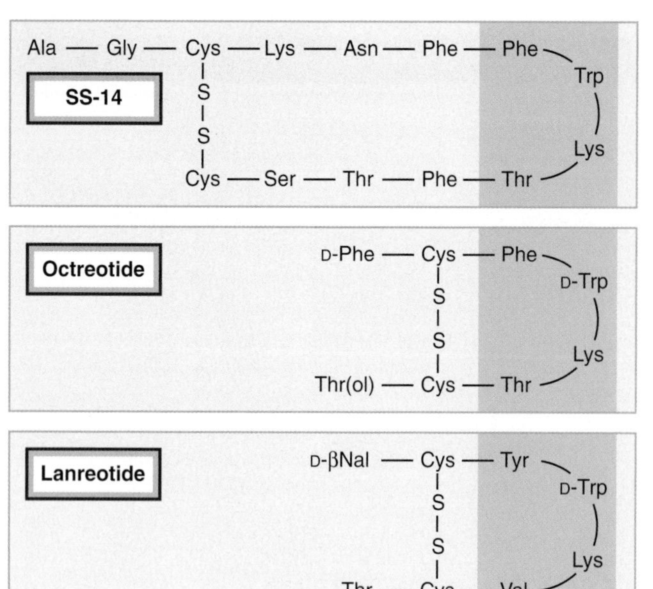

Figure 8–51 ▪ Amino acid sequences of somatostatin (SRIF) receptor ligands. Animo acid sequences of the three available somatostatin analogues, compared to endogenous somatostatin-14. (From van der Lely AJ, Lamberts SWJ. Medical therapy for acromegaly. In Wass J, ed. Handbook of Acromegaly. Bristol, UK: BioScientifica, 2001:51-64)

bromocriptine and cabergoline, have been used as either primary or adjuvant therapy for acromegaly.[360] Patients with hyperprolactinemia and minimal GH elevation might benefit most from dopamine agonist treatment.

Usually, bromocriptine up to 20 mg/day lowers GH, a dose higher than that required to suppress PRL in patients harboring prolactinomas. About 15% of patients worldwide have been reported to suppress GH levels less than 5 μg/L when taking the medication (7.5-80 mg/day)[710] and IGF-I is normalized in 10% of patients. The drug causes minimal tumor shrinkage, but most patients experience subjective clinical improvement and report reduced perspiration, decreased soft tissue swelling, and improved fatigue and headache, despite persistently elevated serum GH and/or IGF-I levels. Side effects of bromocriptine are more marked, especially because high doses are required. These include gastrointestinal upset, transient nausea and vomiting, headache, transient postural hypotension with dizziness, nasal stuffiness, and, rarely, cold-induced peripheral vasospasm (see above).

Cabergoline, a long-acting dopamine agonist, is highly effective in suppressing PRL hypersecretion and shrinking prolactinomas. In an open study, the drug has been reported to suppress GH to less than 2 μg/L, and normalize IGF-I in up to a third of patients with acromegaly.[711] Side effects include gastrointestinal symptoms, dizziness, headache, and mood disorders.

SRIF Receptor Ligands

Of the five SRIF receptor subtypes, SSTR2 and SSTR5 are preferentially expressed on somatotroph and thyrotroph cell surfaces and mediate suppression of GH and TSH secretion.[350,712] Several SRIF ligands have been employed as approved or investigational drugs for acromegaly (see Fig. 8–51). Since the 1980s, these analogues have proved safe and effective for controlling acromegaly.

Octreotide (D-Phe-Cys-Phe-D-Trp-LysThr-Cys-Thr-OH), an octapeptide SRIF analogue, binds predominantly to SSTR2 and SSTR5 and[713] inhibits GH secretion with a potency 45 times greater than native SRIF, although its potency for inhibiting insulin release is only 1.3-fold that of SRIF. The in vivo half-life of the analogue is prolonged (up to 2 hours) because of its relative resistance to enzymatic degradation. Rebound GH hypersecretion seen following SRIF infusion does not occur following octreotide injection. These properties are highly advantageous for long-term use in acromegaly.[714] A single subcutaneous administration (50 or 100 μg) suppresses GH secretion for up to 5 hours. In patients harboring microadenomas, integrated GH and IGF-I levels are almost invariably normalized,[715] although the response in larger tumors is less pronounced. In a double-blind, placebo-controlled trial, octreotide (injections every 8 hours) significantly attenuated GH and IGF-I levels overall in more than 90% of patients.[715] A combination of octreotide and bromocriptine or cabergoline may provide added efficacy.

In vivo octreoscan imaging visualizing SRIF receptors demonstrates that GH responsiveness directly correlates with the abundance of pituitary receptors, and patients resistant to octreotide do not have visible receptor binding sites.[716] Efficacy of octreotide action is determined by frequency of drug administration, total daily dose, tumor size, densely granulated tumors,[717] and pretreatment GH levels. Smaller tumors secreting less GH may in fact harbor more abundant SRIF receptors. Increasing the frequency of administration more effectively suppresses GH levels,[718] and continuous subcutaneous infusion (up to 600 μg/day) provides sustained GH control.[718] Total daily doses of 300 to 1500 μg of octreotide are optimal, and further dose increases are usually not beneficial for resistant patients. Elderly male patients are particularly sensitive to the GH-lowering effects of octreotide, and in the long-term, desensitization does not occur.[719]

Long-acting somatostatin analogue formulations are convenient, enhance compliance, and allow sustained biochemical control (Fig. 8–52). Serum levels of Sandostatin LAR (20-30 mg IM) a sustained-release octreotide depot preparation[720] peak at 28 days, with integrated GH levels effectively suppressed for up to 49 days. Monthly injections for 9 years reduced integrated serum GH levels to less than 2 μg/L in more than 75% of patients.[721] In an open-label study of 151 patients responsive to octreotide, the analogue suppressed serum GH levels to less than 2.5 μg/L in about 70% of all patients.[722,723] Overall, IGF-I levels are normalized in 60% to 70% of patients.[724]

Lanreotide is a slow-release, long-acting depot preparation, administered as a fixed 30-mg injectable dose every 7, 10 or 14 days. GH levels less than 2.5 μg/L were achieved in 60% of 56 patients treated for 48 weeks. Levels less than 2.5 μg/L were achieved in about one third of 22 patients treated for up to 3 years and IGF-I levels were normalized in almost two thirds of patients.[725] Lanreotide is not yet approved for use in the United States.

Effects of SRIF Receptor Ligands on Pituitary Adenoma

Tumors rarely grow while patients receive depot preparations of SRIF analogues. Significant tumor size decrease has been reported in 52% of patients on primary therapy.[726] A critical analysis of 14 studies reported that 37% of patients treated primarily by SRL experience significant tumor shrinkage.[727] Fifty-nine patients undergoing pituitary surgery were randomized, and 22 who received preoperative octreotide for 3 to 6 months demonstrated improved postoperative biochemical control and reduced hospital length of stay.[728,729]

Effects of SRIF Receptor Ligands on Clinical Features

More than 70% of patients experience improved general well-being, and soft tissue swelling dissipates within several days of treatment.[715] Headache, a common symptom in acromegaly, usually resolves within minutes of injection,[730] reflecting a specific central analgesic effect. Short-acting octreotide is prefera-

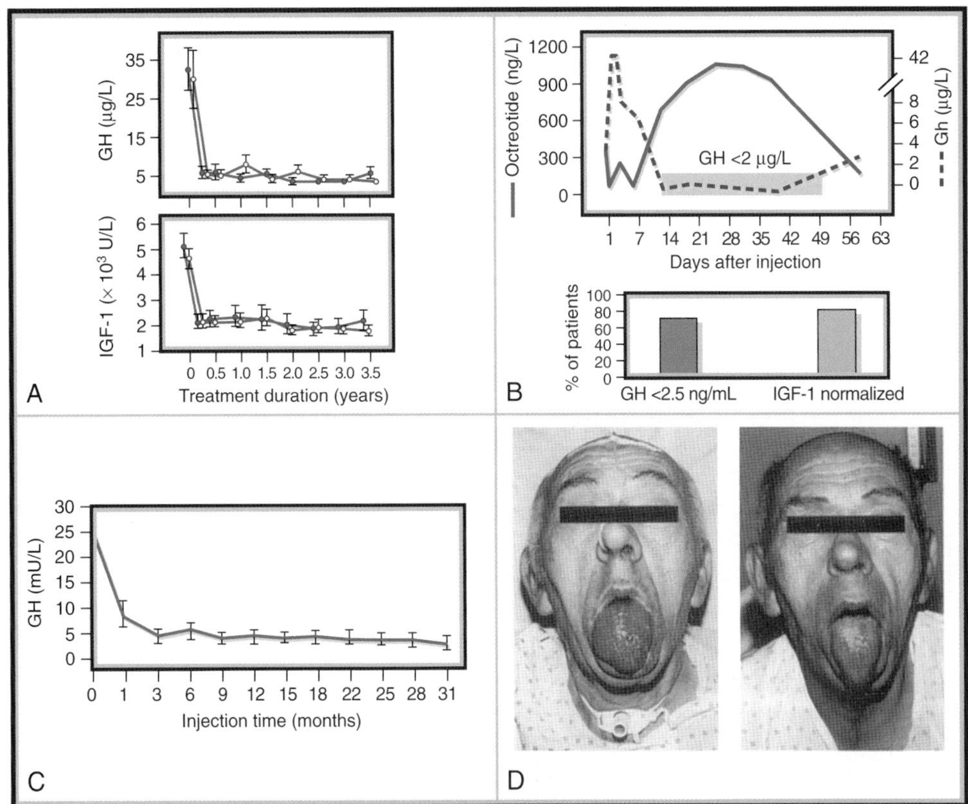

Figure 8–52 ▪ **A,** Growth hormone (GH) and insulin-like growth factor-1 (IGF-I) concentrations with long-term octreotide treatment. Comparison of primary octreotide treatment in 25 previously untreated patients and in 80 patients who had previously undergone surgical resection and/or irradiation. **B,** Pharmacodynamics of octreotide long-acting release (LAR). Twelve-hour mean serum octreotide and GH concentrations in a representative patient treated with a single 30-mg injection of Sandostatin LAR and followed for 60 days. After injection, drug levels peak at 28 days, and nadir GH levels are sustained for 4 weeks. **C,** Mean GH concentration with octreotide LAR long-term treatment. Serum GH levels in acromegaly following monthly octreotide LAR injections in 12 patients for 1 year and in 8 patients for 31 months. **D,** Clinical impact of octreotide in reducing soft tissue swelling. Acromegaly in a patient suffering from obstructive sleep apnea before octreotide. Note the macroglossia, tracheotomy for airway obstruction, and intranasal feeding tube. After 6 months of treatment with octreotide, tongue size was reduced by half. Tracheotomy and nasal tube have been removed and sleep apnea has resolved. (**A** from Newman CB, Melmed S, George A, et al. Octreotide as primary therapy for acromegaly. J Clin Endocrinol Metab 1998;83:3034-3040; **B** adapted from Lancranjan I, Bruns C, Grass P, et al. Sandostatin LAR: a promising therapeutic tool in the management of acromegalic patients. Metabolism 1996;45:67-71; **C** from Davies PH, Stewart SE, Lancranjan L, et al: Long-term therapy with long-acting octreotide (Sandostatin-LAR) for the management of acromegaly. Clin Endocrinol [Oxf] 1998;48:311-316; erratum in Clin Endocrinol [Oxf] 1998;48:673; **D** courtesy of S. Reichlin.)

ble to long-acting for acute headache resolution. Asymptomatic patients experience a significant decrease of blood pressure, heart rate, and left ventricular (LV) wall thickness.[731] In patients with cardiac failure, octreotide reversibly reduces systemic arterial resistance, oxygen consumption, and fluid volume and restores functional activity. In 30 patients, improved left ventricular ejection fraction and unchanged diastolic filling were associated with octreotide-induced GH suppression to less than 2.5 µg/L. Persistently elevated GH levels after 1 year were associated with increased systolic blood pressure.[732] Control of IGF-I and GH levels is associated with improved LV ejection function, but in patients whose IGF-I and GH levels were not controlled, cardiac performance worsened.[733] Joint function and crepitus improve, ultrasound shows evidence of bone or cartilage repair, and after several months, sleep apnea improves.[643]

Side Effects

SRLs are generally safe and well tolerated. Gastrointestinal side effects predominate and include transient loose stools, nausea, mild malabsorption, and flatulence in about one third of patients. Hypoglycemia or hyperglycemia are not commonly encountered, and insulin requirements in diabetic patients with acromegaly are dramatically reduced within hours of receiving octreotide, concomitant with GH lowering.

Octreotide attenuates gallbladder contractility, delays emptying, and leads to reversible sludge formation evidenced by ultrasonography in up to 25% of patients.[734] Frank cholecystitis is very rarely reported in these patients. The incidence of gallbladder sludge or stones is geographically variable, with higher rates reported in China, Australia and the United Kingdom. In the United States, up to 30% of patients have demonstrable evidence of echogenic gallbladder deposits within the first 18 months of treatment. Thereafter, further sludge formation is not usually encountered.[720]

Octreotide can interact with several drugs including cyclosporine, enhancing transplant rejection risk. SRL dose adjustments should be carefully titrated in patients requiring insulin or oral hypoglycemic agents, calcium channel blockers, and β-blockers. Asymptomatic sinus bradycardia has also been recognized.

Growth Hormone Receptor Antagonists

GH action through the surface membrane GH receptor is mediated by ligand-induced receptor signaling.[735] The postreceptor GH signal is not elicited if the receptor is bound by pegvisomant, a GH-receptor antagonist, which blocks subsequent IGF-I generation (Fig. 8–53).[735] The pegylated molecule also binds to the GH receptor dimer and interacts with GHBP.[736] Daily injections (20 mg) normalize IGF-I levels in more than 90% of patients and therapy dose-dependently improves fatigue, decreases soft tissue swelling as assessed by ring size, and diminishes perspiration.[735] The drug may be particularly useful in patients resistant to SRIF receptor ligand therapy, because it effectively normalizes IGF-I levels in these patients.[737] One study showed IGF-I

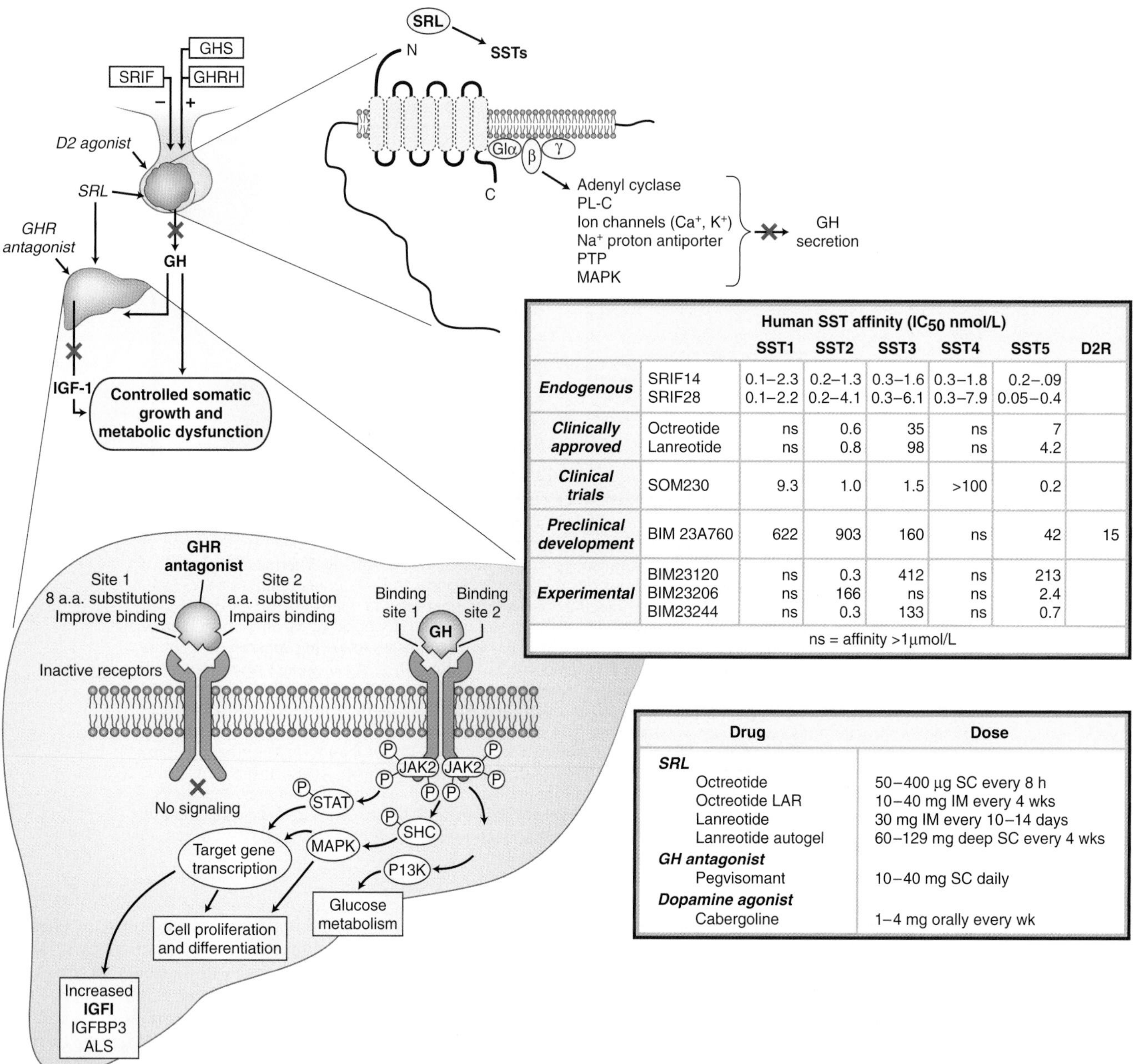

		Human SST affinity (IC_{50} nmol/L)					
		SST1	SST2	SST3	SST4	SST5	D2R
Endogenous	SRIF14	0.1–2.3	0.2–1.3	0.3–1.6	0.3–1.8	0.2–.09	
	SRIF28	0.1–2.2	0.2–4.1	0.3–6.1	0.3–7.9	0.05–0.4	
Clinically approved	Octreotide	ns	0.6	35	ns	7	
	Lanreotide	ns	0.8	98	ns	4.2	
Clinical trials	SOM230	9.3	1.0	1.5	>100	0.2	
Preclinical development	BIM 23A760	622	903	160	ns	42	15
Experimental	BIM23120	ns	0.3	412	ns	213	
	BIM23206	ns	166	ns	ns	2.4	
	BIM23244	ns	0.3	133	ns	0.7	

ns = affinity >1 μmol/L

Drug	Dose
SRL	
Octreotide	50–400 μg SC every 8 h
Octreotide LAR	10–40 mg IM every 4 wks
Lanreotide	30 mg IM every 10–14 days
Lanreotide autogel	60–129 mg deep SC every 4 wks
GH antagonist	
Pegvisomant	10–40 mg SC daily
Dopamine agonist	
Cabergoline	1–4 mg orally every wk

Figure 8–53 ▪ Action of GH receptor antagonist, somatostatin receptor ligands (SRLs), and dopamine agonists. Normally a single molecule of GH binds two GH receptors through sites 1 and 2, and the GH signal transduction pathway is activated. Pegvisomant increases binding of GH receptor to site 1 and blocks binding at site 2 to prevent functional GH-receptor dimerization, initiation of GH action, and induction of IGF-I synthesis and secretion. The peripheral effects of excess GH are antagonized at the cellular level, independent of the presence of somatostatin or dopamine receptors on the pituitary tumor. SRLs inhibit GH secretion and IGF-I synthesis and suppress pituitary tumor growth. GH-secreting adenomas express predominantly SST2 and SST5. BIM, bisindolylmaleimide; D2R, dopamine D2 receptor; GH, growth hormone; GHR, growth hormone receptor; GHRH, growth hormone–releasing hormone; GHS, growth hormone secretagogue; IGF, insulin-like growth factor; JAK2, Janus kinase 2; MAPK, mitogen-activated protein kinase; P, phosphate; PI3′K, phosphatidylinositol 3-kinase; SHC, Src homology-containing protein; SOM, somatostatin; SRIF, somatostatin; STAT, signal transducers and activators of transcription; SST, somatostatin. (Adapted from Melmed S. Medical progress: acromegaly. N Engl J Med 2006;355:2558-2573. Erratum in N Engl J Med 2007;356:879; Heaney AP, Melmed S. Molecular targets in pituitary tumors. Nat Rev Cancer. 2004;4:285-295.)

normalization in 12 of 16 patients. However, rebound tumor enlargement after discontinuing somatostatin analogues, and tumor growth while receiving pegvisomant, should be carefully monitored.[738]

Because elevated hepatic transaminases have been reported,[739] liver enzymes should be measured every 6 months. Local inflammation at the injection site and lipodystrophy have been reported. Long-term impact of the drug on pituitary tumor growth is not yet evident, and periodic MRI should be performed. Levels of GH rise as IGF-I negative feedback is lost, and patients should be monitored by IGF-I measurements.[740]

SRIF Receptor Ligand and Growth Hormone Receptor Antagonist Combination

Combination treatment for acromegaly is most effective in patients in whom there has been tumor shrinkage on somatostatin analogue with reduction, albeit inadequate, in GH or IGF-I levels. Dual blockade of the GH axis with pegvisomant and Sandostatin LAR has been shown to have greater efficacy than for either drug alone in 11 patients whose GH and IGF-I levels were not controlled.[741] Another group has employed monthly doses of long-acting somatostatin analogue and weekly doses of pegvisomant with some success.[742]

Choice of Therapy

Tight control of GH secretion should be achieved, because adverse mortality rates correlate strongly with GH levels. Each treatment modality has respective advantages and disadvantages that should be weighed in order to individualize patient care (Fig. 8–54 and Table 8–30).

Selective surgical excision of a well-defined pituitary microadenoma is recommended for most patients. Remission rates are unacceptably low for patients with macroadenomas and locally invasive tumors. Attempted medical debulking of the sellar mass prior to surgery would be desirable, although controlled prospective studies are required to confirm the validity of this approach to improve surgical morbidity and possibly enhance subsequent postoperative outcomes, especially for patients with surgically inaccessible tumor tissue and cavernous sinus invasion.

Postoperatively, patients whose GH and IGF-I levels are uncontrolled can be treated with cabergoline; although the efficacy of this drug is low, it is relatively inexpensive and free of major side effects. An SRIF analogue should be administered and GH and IGF-I measured after 2 hours; Sandostatin LAR (10, 20, or 30 mg) should be initiated if patients are shown to be responsive. However, the utility of an initial test dose of short-acting octreotide has been questioned.[743] More frequent dosing schedules, rather than increased in total drug dose, may be more efficacious and beneficial. Some patients benefit by addition of bromocriptine or cabergoline with octreotide. Gallbladder ultrasonography should only be performed in symptomatic patients, and those with demonstrable sludge or gallstones may require prophylactic anticholelilithogenic agents or laparoscopic cholecystectomy if symptoms develop.

Primary therapy with SRIF receptor ligands may be offered to patients in whom complete tumor removed is not likely or in those who refuse surgery or in whom the risks of surgery or anesthesia are unacceptable. Invasive macroadenomas invariably hypersecrete GH postoperatively and require somatostatin analogue treatment. In patients whose pituitary lesion does not compress vital structures, primary medical management may therefore be an appropriate therapeutic option.[744,745]

Radiation should be administered to patients who are resistant to or cannot tolerate the medication, patients who prefer not to receive long-term injections, or patients who cannot afford the medication. After irradiation, medications are required for several years until GH levels are effectively controlled. Recurring tumors despite medical therapy or irradiation rarely require reoperation. Although tight GH control is critical, these patients also require counseling for anxiety engendered by disfigurements and interpretation of laboratory test results.

Patients should be followed quarterly until biochemical control is achieved. Thereafter, hormone evaluation is performed semiannually. Patients who are biochemically in remission and in whom no residual tumor tissue is present, should have MRI every 1 to 2 years.[350] Follow-up evaluation includes documenting and treating new skin tag and lipoma growth, nerve entrapments, and jaw overbites; rheumatologic, dental, and cardiac evaluations; and metabolic assessment. Visual field perimetry and pituitary reserve testing should be repeated semiannually, and pituitary MRI should be performed annually, especially in patients with residual tumor or in those requiring hormone replacement or medical treatment. Mammography and colonoscopy should be performed as clinically indicated for patients older than 50 years or those harboring polyps. Maximal and sustained long-term GH and IGF-I control should ameliorate the deleterious effects of these hormones by judicious use of available treatment modalities.

Adrenocorticotropin

Corticotroph Cells

Corticotroph cells make up about 20% of functional anterior pituitary cells and are the earliest detectable human fetal pituitary cell type, appearing by the eighth week of gestation. Corticotrophs are clustered mainly in the central median pituitary wedge and are readily identified by immunostaining with ACTH or β-lipotropin antibodies. They are large irregular cells, and their ultrastructural features include prominent neurosecretory granules (150-400 nm), endoplasmic reticulum, and Golgi bodies (Figs. 8–55 and 8–56).[746] These cells produce the POMC gene products including ACTH(1-39), β-lipotropin, and endorphins. Because of the rich carbohydrate moiety of these molecules, the cells are strongly positive for periodic acid–Schiff (PAS). In the presence of excess glucocorticoid, characteristic hyaline deposits are evident (see Fig. 8–56).

ACTH Biosynthesis

The 8-kb human POMC gene, located on chromosome 2p23,[747] consists of three exons interspersed with two intervening introns (Fig. 8–57) The first exon encodes a leader sequence, the second encodes the signal initiation sequence and the N-terminal portion of the POMC peptide, and the third exon encodes most of the mature peptide sequences including ACTH and β-lipotropin.[748] A pituitary-selective promoter region for POMC generates an approximately 1200-nucleotide POMC mRNA transcript; an upstream promoter generates a longer (about 1350 nucleotides) transcript. A downstream promoter generates a shorter 800-nucleotide transcript arising from the 5′ end of exon 3, predominantly in extrapituitary tissues, including the gonads, placenta, gastrointestinal tissues, liver, kidney, adrenal medulla, lung, and lymphocytes. Elements of the promoter regions mediate POMC regulation by glucocorticoids, cAMP, AP-1, and STAT signaling molecules.[522] A corticotroph-specific factor, T-pit, has been described.[24]

POMC is the precursor for ACTH, which acts on the adrenal glands to induce synthesis and secretion of adrenal steroids. The primary translation product of POMC is a 266–amino acid proopiomelanocortin pre-prohormone molecule encoding corticotrophic, opioid, and melanotrophic peptides. The peptide contains a leader sequence and multiple dibasic proteolytic

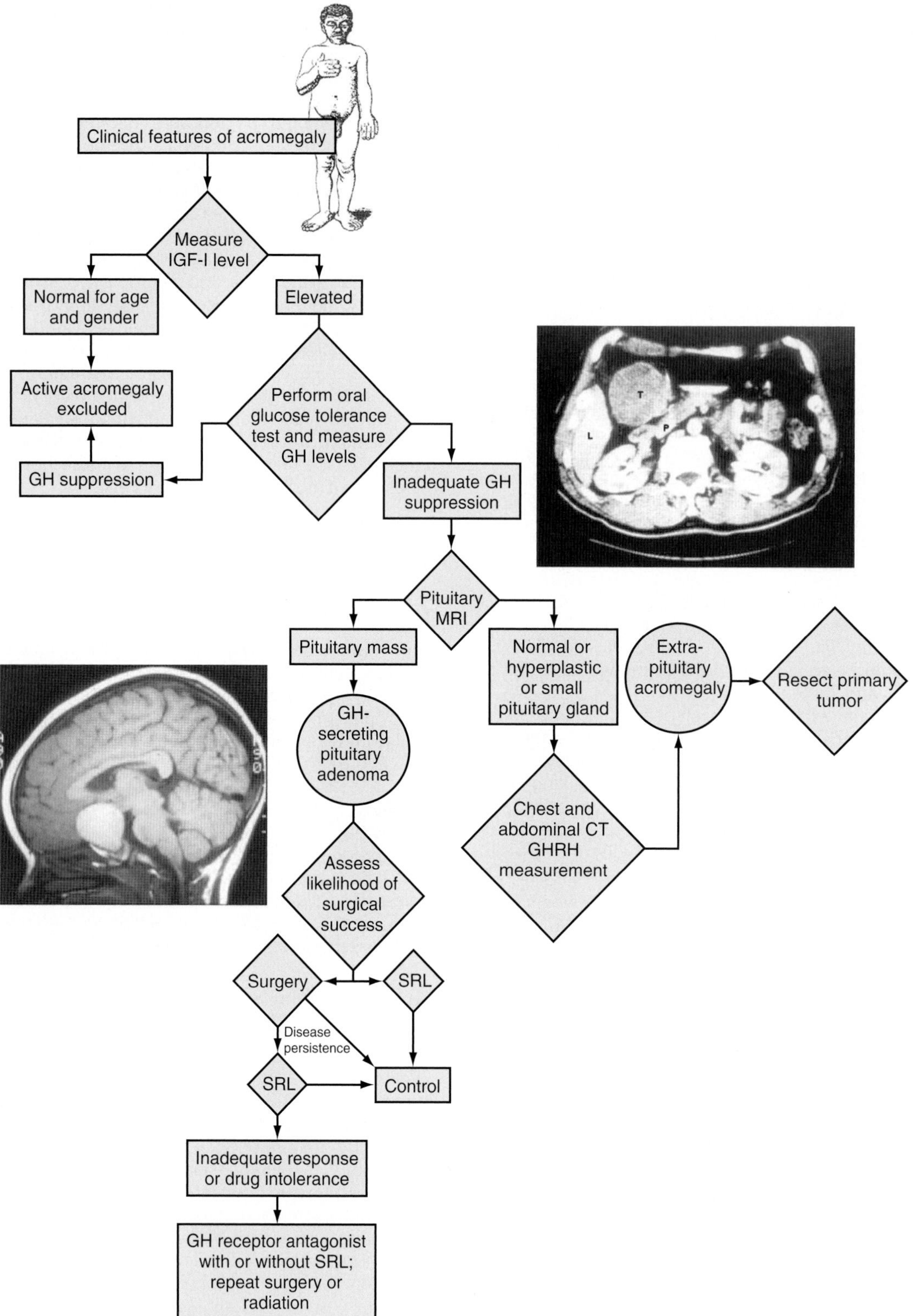

Figure 8–54 ▪ Diagnosis and treatment of acromegaly. Oral glucose tolerance test (OGTT) is performed with 75 g glucose; GH is measured over 2 hours. Disease control implies nadir GH level of less than 1 μg/L after OGTT, plus age- and gender-matched normal IGF-I level. GH, growth hormone; L, liver; MRI, magnetic resonance imaging; P, pancreas; SRL; somatostatin receptor ligand; T, tumor (secreting GH). (Clinical features figure from Minkowski O. Ueber einen Fall von Akromegalie. Berliner Klinische Wochenschrift 1887;21:371-374; from Melmed S. Medical progress: acromegaly. N Engl J Med 2006;355:2558-2573. Erratum in N Engl J Med 2007;356:879).

TABLE 8–30 ACROMEGALY MANAGEMENT

GOALS

Control GH and IGF-I secretion.
Control tumor growth.
Relieve central compressive effects.
Preserve or restore pituitary trophic hormone function.
Treat comorbidities (hypertension, cardiac failure, hyperglycemia, sleep apnea, arthritis).
Normalize mortality rates.
Prevent biochemical recurrence.

TREATMENTS

Characteristic	Surgery	Radiation Therapy	SRL	GHR Antagonist	Dopamine Agonist
Advantages					
Mode	Transsphenoidal resection	Noninvasive	Monthly injection	Daily injection	Oral
GH <2.5 μg/L	Macros <50% Micros >80%	~35% in 10 yr	~80%	increases	<15%
IGF-I normalized		<30%	~70%	>90%	<15%
Onset	Rapid	Slow (years)	Rapid	Rapid	Slow (weeks)
Patient compliance	Onetime consent	Good	Must be sustained	Must be sustained	Good
Tumor mass	Debulked or resected	Ablated	Growth constrained or shrinks ~50%	Unknown	Unchanged
Disadvantages					
Cost	One time	One time	Ongoing	Ongoing	Ongoing
Hypopituitarism	~10%	>50%	None	Very low IGF-I if overtreated	None
Other	Tumor persistence or recurrence 6% Diabetes insipidus 3% Local complications 5%	Local nerve damage 2nd brain tumor Visual and CNS disorders, ~2% cerebrovascular risk	Gallstones 20% Nausea, diarrhea	Elevated liver enzymes (rare)	Nausea ~30% Sinusitis High dose required

OUTCOMES

Feature	Evaluation	Treatment
Safe Biochemical Activity		
Nadir GH <1 μg/L Age- and gender-matched normal IGF-I Asymptomatic No comorbidities	Assess GH/IGF-I axis Evaluate adrenal, thyroid, and gonadal axes Periodic MRI	None or no change in current treatment
Unsafe Biochemical Activity		
Nadir GH >1 μg/L Elevated IGF-I Discordant GH and IGF-I Asymptomatic No comorbidities	Assess GH/IGF-I axis Evaluate pituitary function Periodic MRI	Weigh treatment benefit vs risks Consider new treatment if being treated
Unsafe Biochemical and Clinical Activity		
Nadir GH >1 μg/L Elevated IGF-I Clinically active tumor growing	Assess GH/IGF-I axis Evaluate pituitary function Assess cardiovascular, metabolic, and tumoral comorbidity Periodic MRI	Actively treat or change treatment

CNS, central nervous system; GH, growth hormone; GHR, growth hormone receptor; IGF, insulin-like growth factor; macros, macrotumors; micros, microtumors; MRI, magnetic resonance imaging; SRL, slow-release lanreotide.

From Melmed S. Medical progress: acromegaly. N Engl J Med 2006;355:2558-2573. Erratum in N Engl J Med 2007;356:879.

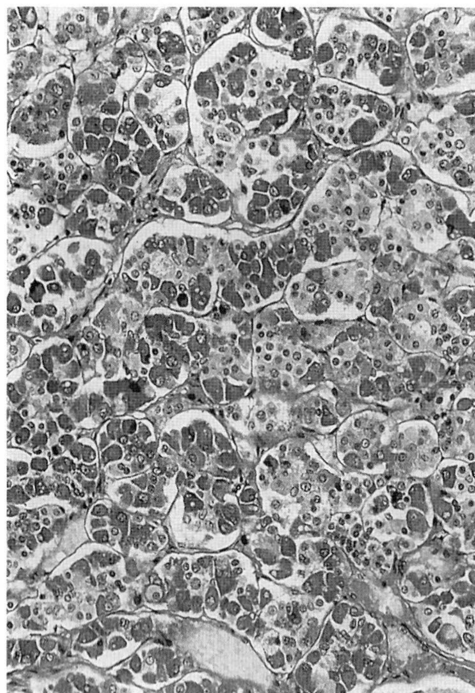

Figure 8–55 ▪ Corticotroph cell. The periodic acid–Schiff stain documents the presence of corticotrophs in the normal pituitary, reflecting glycosylation of the adrenocorticotropic hormone peptide. Some cells have clear cytoplasmic vacuoles corresponding to the enigmatic body. (From Asa SL. In Tumors of the Pituitary Gland. Atlas of Tumor Pathology. Washington, DC: Armed Forces Institute of Pathology, 1997:21.)

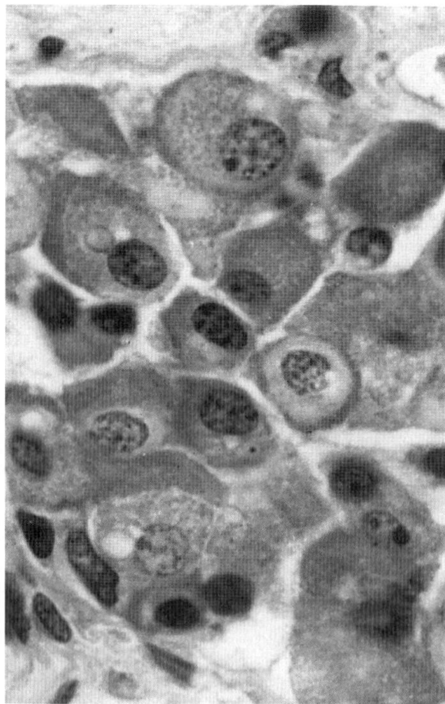

Figure 8–56 ▪ Crooke's hyalinization. Pituitary corticotrophs subjected to glucocorticoid excess develop cytoplasmic hyalinization that displaces adrenocorticotropic hormone–positive secretory material to the cell periphery. The clear vacuoles correspond to complex lysosomes known as *enigmatic bodies*. (From Asa SL. In Tumors of the Pituitary Gland. Atlas of Tumor Pathology. Washington, DC: Armed Forces Institute of Pathology, 1997:23.)

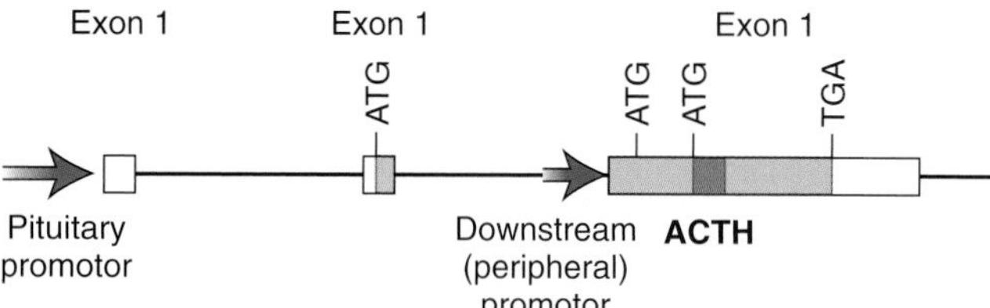

Figure 8–57 ▪ Structure of the *POMC* gene. Exon 1 encodes the RNA leader sequence, exon 2 encodes the initiator methionine (ATG), the signal peptide, and several N-terminal residues of the precursor peptide, the remainder of which is encoded by exon 3. Corticotroph expression is determined by the upstream pituitary promoter *(longer arrowhead)*, whereas peripheral expression of the short POMC mRNA is determined by the downstream promoter *(shorter arrowhead)*. Translation of these shorter transcripts initiates from the initiator methionines (ATG) indicated in exon 3. The precursor peptide coding region is shaded *lavender* and the ACTH coding region is *purple*. ACTH, adrenocortictropic hormone. (From Clark AJL, Swords FM. Molecular pathology of corticotroph function. In Rappaport R, Amselem S, eds. Hypothalamic-Pituitary Development. Basel: Karger, 2001:140-161)

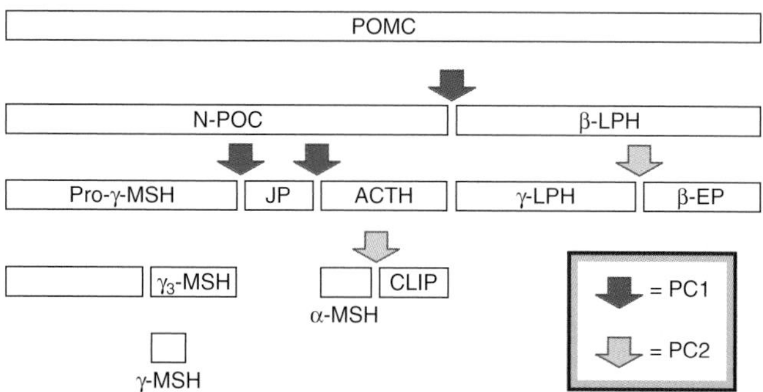

Figure 8–58 ▪ Processing and cleavage of POMC. The mature POMC precursor peptide is sequentially cleaved by PCI in the anterior pituitary corticotroph. In the neurointermediate lobe and other cell types, cleavage by PC2 allows release of β-MSH and/or β-endorphin. Carboxypeptidase H (not shown) removes residual basic amino acids at cleavage sites. ACTH, adrenocorticotropic hormone; CLIP, corticotropin-like intermediate lobe peptide; EP, endorphin; JP, joining peptide; β-LPH, β-lipotropin; γ-LPH, γ-lipotropin; MSH, melanocyte-stimulating hormone; N-POC, N-terminal pro-opiomelanocortin fragment; PC, prohormone convertase; POMC, pro-opiomelanocortin. (From Clark AJL, Swords FM. Molecular pathology of corticotroph function. In Rappaport R, Amselem S, eds. Hypothalamic-Pituitary Development. Basel: Karger, 2001:140-161)

cleavage sites for glycosylation, acetylation and amidation. Products of this processing include ACTH(1-39) and β-lipotropin, which in turn give rise to α-lipotropin and β-endorphin, also containing metenkephalin. ACTH itself can also be cleaved to α-MSH(1-13) and CLIP(18-39). The neuro-intermediate pituitary lobe is not developed in humans and is not normally a source of circulating POMC-derived peptides. (Fig. 8–58).

Multiple signals act in synergy to activate POMC gene expression. These include CRH, cytokines, AVP, catecholamines and VIP. Glucocorticoids inhibit POMC gene expression. The CRH type 1 receptor is predominantly expressed on the corticotroph,[749,750] and receptor activation increases cyclic AMP, protein kinase A, and CREB induction of CRH binding protein (CRHBP) binding to the promoter, leading to POMC transcription.[751] CRH also activates an AP-1 site within the first exon by a MAP kinase–mediated pathway. In addition to mediating ACTH secretion, this receptor also appears critical for fear and anxiety responses, possibly by a related ligand, urocortin.[752] The CRH type 2 receptor is predominantly important for cardiovascular function.[753]

Leukemia inhibitory factor (LIF), a proinflammatory cytokine also expressed in the pituitary and hypothalamus, signals via the JAK-STAT pathway and acts in synergy with CRH and induces direct STAT3 binding to POMC.[754] Glucocorticoid receptor activation leads to transcriptional suppression via two cooperative binding sites. The intracellular glucocorticoid receptor binds directly to 5′-regulatory elements to suppress POMC transcription.[755] CRH action is also potentiated by vasopressin (acting via phospholipase C) and β-adrenergic catecholamines, either by enhancing POMC mRNA levels or by increasing ACTH secretion, or both. The net effects of these intracellular signals are to regulate POMC gene transcription, peptide synthesis, and ACTH secretion for mediating appropriate neuroendocrine responses.[756]

POMC Processing

Several post-translational POMC modification steps are required for ultimate polypeptide hormone secretion (see Fig. 8–58). First, the N-terminal signal sequence is removed, followed by glycosylation via an O-linkage to Thr-45 and N-linkage to Asn-65.[757] Serine-phosphorylation then occurs within the Golgi apparatus. After being transported to secretory vesicles, the constituent peptides are cleaved at dibasic amino acid residues, and ACTH-related peptides are stored in dense secretory granules for ultimate regulated release. Some POMC products also undergo C-terminal amidation mediated by peptidylglycine-amidating monooxygenase (PAM), peptidyl-hydroxyglycine-amidating lyase (PAL),[758] and N-terminal acetylation. POMC proteolytic processing occurs at Lys-Arg or Arg-Arg residues. Prohormone convertase 1 (PC1) or prohormone convertase 2 (PC2), related to the subtilisin/kexin proteinases, exerts tissue-specific cleavage activities at dibasic sites. PC1 is most abundant in the pituitary and hypothalamus; PC2 is present in the CNS and pancreatic islets but is absent in the pituitary. Heterozygous mutations of the PC1 gene have been associated with childhood obesity, adrenal insufficiency, hyperproinsulinemia, and postprandial hypoglycemia[759] with elevated levels of plasma ACTH precursors.

Extrapituitary Tumor ACTH Synthesis

Tissue POMC is also expressed in the gonads, lung, gastrointestinal and adrenal medullary neuroendocrine cells, and white blood cells. Nevertheless, the overwhelming source of circulating ACTH is derived from the anterior pituitary or from neuroendocrine tumor ectopic production. Extrapituitary neuroendocrine tumors associated with ectopic ACTH secretion do not process the prohormone efficiently. Because ACTH is synthesized in nontumorous neuroendocrine cells, ectopic tumor hormone production might in fact reflect inappropriate ACTH processing. These patients also exhibit a higher ratio of circulating ACTH precursors, as well as smaller peptides, including CLIP.

ACTH Secretion

The complex control of ACTH secretion patterns are critical for maintenance of adrenal cortex function and reflects the neuroendocrine control of stress homeostasis. Essential metabolic and endocrine functions require a sensitively controlled nonstress pattern of hypothalamic-pituitary-adrenal (HPA) axis function. This baseline pattern allows the axis to mount an appropriate stress response, with a well-buffered reserve capacity to counteract life-threatening insults. The ACTH is a 39–amino acid polypeptide with a molecular weight of 4.5 kd. The highly conserved 12 N-terminal amino acid residues are critical for adrenal gland steroid synthesis.

Several variables characterize the central and peripheral control of ACTH secretion. The ACTH circadian rhythm is generated in the suprachiasmatic nucleus, which signals CRH release. The hormone is secreted with both circadian periodicity and ultradian pulsatility, and this centrally controlled pattern is influenced by peripheral corticosteroids. ACTH pulse amplitudes can vary by 40% over 24 hours, and the circadian pattern of ACTH secretion typically begins at about 4:00 AM and peaks before 7 AM, with both ACTH and adrenal steroid levels reaching their nadir between 11 PM and 3:00 AM. Within this overall 24-hour diurnal cycle, periodic ACTH secretory bursts occur at a frequency of 40 pulses per 24 hours, with changing pulse amplitudes throughout the day.[760] Each pulse contains an average of 24 ng/L of ACTH. Pulse amplitude changes, rather than frequency, appear to predominantly determine ACTH circadian rhythm.[761] ACTH circadian rhythm is entrained by visual cues and the light-dark cycle, and it is centrally controlled by CRH and other factors.[762]

Although continuous CRH administration desensitizes the ACTH response, prolonged pulsatile CRH administration restores cortisol secretion without depleting the pituitary ACTH pool.[763] 24-hour ACTH but not cortisol secretion is higher in male subjects, who also exhibit higher pulse frequency and peak amplitudes,[764] possibly reflecting gender-specific set points for cortisol feedback or a relative male adrenal insensitivity to ACTH. Endogenous and exogenous stress, including hypoglycemia, act centrally to increase ACTH pulse amplitude, and corticosteroids directly suppress basal or stimulated corticotroph ACTH pulse amplitude.[765]

ACTH Action

The primary action of ACTH is to maintain adrenal gland size, structure, and function; ACTH induces adrenal steroidogenesis by activating ACTH receptors situated on the adrenal cortex cell surface. ACTH signals via adenyl cyclase to regulate P450 enzyme transcription, cortisol aldosterone (10%), 17-OH-progesterone, and, to a lesser extent, adrenal androgen synthesis and secretion.[766] ACTH stimulates mitochondrial cholesterol transport and regulates the rate-limiting side-chain cleavage of cholesterol to pregnenolone.[767] Secretory cortisol pulses follow ACTH pulses within 5 to 10 minutes, with a linear dose-dependency, which is especially evident after physiologic CRH stimulation.[768] However, circulating cortisol levels plateau after attaining pharmacologic levels of ACTH by Cortrosyn injection.

Adrenal cortisol response to ACTH is sensitive to the background ambient ACTH milieu. In states of chronic ACTH deficiency, adrenal reserve is compromised, and during ongoing ACTH hypersecretion, the gland is primed such that a given ACTH bolus elicits a higher cortisol response. Basal and stimulated (e.g., by CRH) ACTH secretion are blunted by glucocorticoids. Conversely, low or absent circulating glucocorticoids (e.g., after adrenalectomy) result in exaggerated ACTH secretion.[769,770] and in corticotroph cell hyperplasia.[771]

The HPA axis is inhibited by a long feedback inhibition, whereby cortisol rapidly inhibits hypothalamic CRH and pituitary ACTH. These effects can also be delayed by 30 to 60 minutes by inhibition of ACTH release rather than synthesis,[772] especially after a single glucocorticoid bolus. After chronic glucocorticoid exposure (>24 hr), HPA suppression can persist for days or longer. In a short feedback loop, pituitary ACTH inhibits hypothalamic CRH, and in an ultrashort loop, it can also suppress the corticotroph itself.

Physiologic ACTH Regulation

Exercise enhances ACTH and β-endorphin levels, especially if it is exhausting and of short duration. Exercising up to 90% of maximum oxygen capacity causes a significant elevation of ACTH, similar to levels observed during surgery or hypoglycemia.[773] Levels can remain elevated for up to 6 minutes after exercise cessation. Lower-intensity exercise does not evoke ACTH.[774] Well-trained athletes exhibit hypercortisolism, possibly due to decreased adrenal ACTH sensitivity. Other causes of elevated ACTH include acute hemorrhage, surgery, and emotional stress. Acute illness is associated with increased ACTH and cortisol levels, with loss of diurnal secretory patterns.

Stress Response

Both exogenous and endogenous stress stimuli activate the HPA axis to produce sufficient glucocorticoid in an attempt to counteract the respective insult. The HPA stress response occurs in the context of a wide variety of peripheral and central adaptors to stress, including vasovagal and catecholamine activation, and cytokine secretion and action. A tightly controlled immunoneuroendocrine interface regulates the ACTH response to peripheral stressors, which include pain, infection, inflammation, hypovolemia, trauma, psychological stress, and hypoglycemia. These signals vary in their ability to generate ACTH secretion and to sensitize the ACTH response to glucocorticoids. In addition to CRH, peripheral and centrally released proinflammatory cytokines potently induce POMC transcription and ACTH secretion.[522] Sensitive intracellular signals within the corticotroph also serve to override the ACTH response to stress, thus preventing persistent and chronic hypercortisolemia.

Cytokines such as IL-6 and LIF activate the HPA axis and enhance glucocorticoid production, protecting the organism against lethality by constraining the inflammatory response.[522] Thus, mice with inactivated CRH or LIF genes mount an inadequate neuroendocrine response to stress, inflammation, or endotoxins.[522] During stress, glucocorticoid inhibition of ACTH is also prevented by NFκB activation, which interferes with pituitary glucocorticoid receptor function, thus further exaggerating enhanced ACTH secretion.[775]

Integrated Regulation of ACTH Secretion

Similar to other anterior pituitary hormones, ACTH regulation is subserved by at least three tiers of control. First, the brain and hypothalamus release regulatory molecules (including CRH, vasopressin, and other peptides), which traverse the portal system and directly signal to corticotroph secretory and mitotic activity. Second, intrapituitary cytokines and growth factors act locally to regulate ACTH either in concert with hypothalamic factors or independently. These paracrine controls often overlap and are redundant, and they have also recently been shown to induce sensitive intracellular molecules that limit the ACTH response and prevent chronic ACTH hypersecretion. Third, peripheral hormones, especially glucocorticoids, maintain a potent feedback inhibition control of corticotroph secretion and replication.

Measurement of ACTH

RIA and immunoradiometric (IRMA) assays employ antisera specifically directed against intact ACTH(1-39) or other POMC fragments. Generally, the IRMA is more sensitive, reproducible, and rapid.[776] Most IRMAs have a sensitivity of less than 0.5 ng/L, with precise variations of less than 10%. Intact ACTH or POMC precursor peptides are detectable, depending upon the sequence specificity of the assay employed. Awareness of the peptide specificity may be especially critical when evaluating ectopic POMC products secreted by lung tumors. ACTH precursors are assessed by a specific IRMA employing unique monoclonal antibodies to ACTH, N-POMC, β-LPH or β-endorphin.[777]

Ideally, nonstressed resting subjects should have venous blood withdrawn between 6:00 AM and 9:00 AM. Because ACTH is relatively unstable at room temperature and has a propensity to adhere to glass, plasma samples should immediately be separated in iced siliconized glass tubes containing EDTA (ethylenediaminetetraacetic acid) and stored at less than −20°C for transport. Normal 8 AM plasma ACTH levels range from 8 to 25 ng/L as measured by IRMA. Episodic secretion and short plasma half-life result in wide and rapid fluctuation of plasma measurements. Cortisol values at 4 PM are about half of morning levels, and at 11 PM, levels are usually less than 5 μg/dL. Altered corticosteroid binding protein (CBG) levels and stress can influence measured cortisol values.

Random ACTH values do not on their own provide an accurate assessment of HPA function unless concurrent cortisol levels are obtained. Thus, an integrated assessment of both hormone levels is required for interpreting the significance of an appropriately obtained ACTH value. Measurement of cortisol levels alone often provide a useful surrogate end point for ACTH action and HPA axis integrity. Plasma ACTH levels fluctuate broadly within the same person, and are highly sensitive to stress, time of collection, and gender. Male subjects exhibit greater ACTH pulse frequency and amplitude,[764] and pregnant subjects have higher ambient ACTH levels, possibly due to placental CRH secretion.[778]

Dynamic Testing for ACTH Reserve

Hypothalamic Testing

Insulin

Insulin hypoglycemia is a potent endogenous stressor that evokes ACTH secretion.[779] Thus insulin (0.1-0.15 U/kg) is injected intravenously after an overnight fast to achieve symptomatic hypoglycemia and a blood glucose level of less than 40 mg/dL. This test correlates well with other indices of ACTH reserve. Normal HPA response to this stressor evokes cortisol levels greater than 20 μg/dL. Because hypoglycemia acts centrally, a normal response implies integrity of all three tiers of HPA axis control. Up to 20% of patients require up to 0.3 U/kg insulin (or more) to achieve symptoms of glucopenia including sweating, hunger, palpitations, and tremors.[780] Venous samples are collected at −15, 0, 15, 30, 45, 60, 90, and 120 minutes for measurement of glucose, ACTH, and cortisol levels. GH can also be measured. After the test, oral glucose should be administered.

Intraindividual variations in blood glucose levels attained by a given dose of insulin, as well as fluctuations in central sensitivity to glucose and activation of catecholamines, can lead to difficulties in reproducibility. The test is contraindicated in subjects who have a history of seizures, who have active coronary or cerebral ischemia, or who are pregnant. If pronounced adrenal insufficiency is likely, insulin injection can provoke an adrenal crisis due to inadequate adrenal reserve, and hydrocortisone (100 mg) should be available for urgent intravenous use, if required.

Metyrapone

Metyrapone blocks cortisol synthesis by inhibiting adrenal 11-β-hydroxylase. Thus, the drug releases the HPA axis from negative feedback by cortisol, normally resulting in an ACTH surge and elevated levels of 11-deoxycortisol (compound S). A single oral dose (2-3 g) is given at midnight, and serum levels of ACTH, 11-deoxycortisol, and cortisol measured at 8 AM the following morning. The test is only valid in the face of documented suppressed cortisol levels to less than 10 μg/dL. In normal subjects, peak ACTH values greater than 200 ng/L are achieved. Side-effects include nausea, gastrointestinal upset, and insomnia.[781] False positive results may be obtained when phenytoin is being administered because the drug prevents adequate enzymatic blockade. This test should be performed under observation in the hospital because acute adrenal insufficiency can ensue.

Pituitary Stimulation

Pituitary ACTH secretion may be evoked by injecting either CRH or AVP. Ovine or human CRH (100 μg or 1 μg/kg) is administered intravenously, and cortisol and ACTH are measured at −5, −1, 0, 15, 30, 60, 90, and 120 minutes. Normally, maximal ACTH responses (two- to fourfold above baseline) are evoked at 30 minutes,[782] and cortisol levels peak (>20 μg/dL) at 60 minutes, or increase greater than 10 μg/dL above baseline.

Although CRH readily induces ACTH secretion and demonstrates ACTH deficiency or ACTH excess, the wide variation of responses observed has limited its utility. A useful application of the CRH test is in making the diagnosis of Cushing's disease with or without dexamethasone pretreatment and in the context of petrosal venous sampling for diagnosing ACTH-secreting pituitary adenoma. CRH injection allows a sensitive and specific ACTH gradient to be established that effectively distinguishes peripheral from pituitary sources of excessive ACTH secretion.[783]

Because of the suppressive impact of circulating glucocorticoids on pituitary CRH responsiveness, it may be difficult to distinguish a corticotroph adenoma from pseudo-Cushing's disease because hypercortisolism is associated with both conditions. In these circumstances, combining this test with dexamethasone suppression may be useful. The combined dexamethasone CRH test administers dexamethasone 0.5 mg every 6 hours for 48 hours starting at noon and ending at 6 AM, and then CRH is administered intravenously at 8 AM.[784] In normal subjects or those with pseudo-Cushing's disorder, cortisol levels do not rise and are less than 1.4 μg/dL. If cortisol levels elicited at 15 minutes exceed 4 μg/dL, the presence of an ACTH-secreting pituitary tumor is invariable, with 100% sensitivity and specificity.[784] CRH responsiveness (at least a 35% cortisol rise) is usually retained in ACTH-secreting adenomas, but it is not apparent in greater than 90% of ectopic ACTH-producing tumors, when ACTH increases of less than 35% above baseline are usually encountered. Although this approach has 100% specificity, only 90% sensitivity is achieved, and the test does not distinguish ACTH-secreting adenomas from pseudo-Cushing's disorder.[785]

Adrenal Stimulation

The acute response of the adrenal gland to a bolus ACTH injection reflects ambient ACTH concentrations to which the gland has been exposed. Thus, the cortisol response to an acute ACTH injection is blunted if the subject has had chronic pituitary ACTH hyposecretion, with resultant adrenal atrophy and diminished cortisol reserve. Conversely, persistently elevated ACTH levels lead to adrenal hypertrophy and augmented cortisol responses.[782] The utility of this test in diagnosing diminished pituitary ACTH reserve has been challenged, because the commonly employed dose of Cortrosyn (ACTH 1-24, 250 μg) or Synacthen is high and can evoke a normal cortisol response in hypopituitary subjects. An unacceptably high false negative rate (about 65%) has been determined in a large series,[786] although peak cortisol levels at 30 minutes do in fact correlate well with peak responses to ITT.[787]

A normal cortisol response is greater than 20 μg/dL, or a doubling of baseline values. Basal cortisol levels correlate inversely with the incremental response to ACTH.[788] Low-dose stimulation with 1 μg Synacthen evokes maximal serum cortisol levels at 30 minutes, and these correlate well with values observed after insulin or high-dose ACTH administration.[787] A cut-off of greater than 500 nM/L provides almost 100% sensitivity and a specificity of 80% to 100%.[789] Failure to respond to low-dose ACTH should be corroborated by a standard-dose insulin or ACTH test stimulation.

Adrenal Stimulation Test

For the test, 250 μg Cortrosyn (ACTH 1-24) is injected intramuscularly or intravenously. Cortisol levels are measured before the injection and 30 and 60 minutes after injection. Cortisol values greater than 20 μg/dL reflect a normal adrenal reserve response.

Interpretation

Fluctuation of CBG levels can confound interpretation of cortisol values. Cirrhosis and hyperthyroidism lower CBG and cortisol levels, whereas estrogens elevate CBG concentrations.

Secondary Adrenal Insufficiency

ACTH deficiency is usually reflective of already profound pituitary insufficiency with disordered GH, gonadotropin, and TSH reserve. Rarely, isolated ACTH deficiency manifests later in life. It is more common in male patients but can occur postpartum associated with autoimmune thyroiditis and diabetes mellitus. Two families with recessive mutations in the corticotroph-specific *TPIT* gene have been described with congenital adrenal insufficiency and ACTH deficiency.[24]

Insufficient ACTH secretion leads to attenuated adrenal corticosteroid production, with relative mineralocorticoid preservation. Patients present with slowly progressive weight and appetite loss, anorexia, and generalized fatigue. Because adrenal mineralocorticoid is largely unimpaired, salt wasting, volume contraction, and hyperkalemia, commonly encountered features in Addison's disease, are not manifest. Furthermore, hyperpigmentation usually associated with exuberant ACTH-related peptide secretion in the face of adrenal damage does not occur.

Morning serum cortisol levels of less than 3 μg/dL suggest ACTH deficiency, and basal AM cortisol levels greater than 18 μg/dL usually indicate normal ACTH reserve. Patients with ACTH deficiency have low-to-normal serum cortisol levels and low-to-normal plasma ACTH levels. Blunted responses to provocative tests such as insulin-induced hypoglycemia or metyrapone are required to document a partial deficiency.

Treatment

Hydrocortisone is used to directly replace deficient glucocorticoid hormone. The normal secretory rate of cortisol is about 20 mg/day, which is the recommended total daily dose for correcting hypoadrenalism and maintaining blood pressure. The plasma circulating half-life of cortisol is less than 2 hours, and twice-daily dosing regimens can result in very low cortisol levels in the late afternoon, with impaired quality of life. Three-times-daily hydrocortisone dosing of a total daily requirement of 20 mg (10 mg in the morning, 5 mg at noon, and 5 mg in the evening) is most effective for starting replacement.[550] Excessive dosing leads to iatrogenic Cushing's syndrome. Doses should be increased during stress or prior to operative procedures.

Cortisone acetate is metabolized to cortisol and has a slower onset of action and longer biologic activity than hydrocortisone. Other synthetic glucocorticoids, including prednisolone and dexamethasone, are less useful because they are difficult to monitor biochemically. Even modest cortisol overreplacement can result in bone mineral loss.[790]

Mineralocorticoid replacement is rarely required. Central diabetes insipidus is rarely unmasked after initial glucocorticoid replacement.

ACTH-Secreting Tumors

The evaluation and management of patients with Cushing's disease is fully described in Chapter 14.

Briefly, the diagnosis of an ACTH-secreting pituitary tumor is suggested by features of hypercortisolism, elevated 24-hour urinary free cortisol levels, and failure to suppress morning cortisol levels to less than 3 μg/dL after 1 mg dexamethasone administered at 11 PM. In healthy subjects, glucocorticoid feedback suppresses CRH and ACTH, attenuating cortisol secretion.

Surgical resection of an ACTH-secreting adenoma is the treatment of choice. Because these tumors are usually small, sometimes less than 2 mm in diameter, they may be localized incorrectly, or not at all, by venous sampling for ACTH (see earlier) and sensitive MRI. Therefore, these tumors pose a significant challenge even for the experienced surgeon. Furthermore, the disorder is also characterized by venous hypertension leading to turgid venous sinuses,[791] requiring control by the anesthetist.

Bilateral petrosal venous sampling for ACTH levels and cavernous sinus venography should ideally be performed before surgery. However, if sellar venous sinus drainage is predominately unilateral, left-right ACTH gradients might not reliably lateralize the lesion. Cavernous sinus venography can also outline a filling defect representing the tumor.[792]

If an ACTH gradient is indeed detected with normal venous drainage patterns, hemihypophysectomy is curative in 80% of such patients with clearly defined biochemical features of ACTH-dependent Cushing's disease. Meticulous surgical exploration of anterior and posterior lobes is required for these tiny tumors, which are often off-white and speckled by petechiae and may be inadvertently suctioned. Unfortunately, even carefully performed preoperative lateralization is not infallible, and the apparently normal side should also be carefully explored.

Assessment of Surgical Outcome

Transsphenoidal adenoma resection is the preferred treatment for these adenomas. After selective adenomectomy of a clearly identifiable adenoma, remission was achieved in 75% of 295 patients. However, partial hypophysectomy performed in 31 patients in whom an adenoma could not be identified resulted in biochemical remission in only 10 patients.[793] On the third postoperative day, 1 mg dexamethasone can be given at 10 PM, and cortisol levels can be measured the following morning before initiating hydrocortisone therapy. If the immediate postoperative cortisol level is less than 3 μg/dL, a 95% 5-year remission rate can be expected. In 21 of 27 patients tested before glucocorticoid administration, postoperative cortisol levels less 10 mg/dL, or less than those obtained from preoperative midnight sampling, predicted remission.[794]

Silent Corticotroph Adenoma

These basophilic tumors are generally nonfunctional and yet exhibit POMC, β-lipotropin, and β-endorphin immunoreactivity. ACTH secretion is apparently unaltered, with no associated clinical or biochemical features of hypercortisolism, although these tumors are morphologically indistinguishable from adenomas associated with Cushing's disease. They can represent up to 7% of all surgically removed adenomas[746] and are usually hemorrhagic and invariably macroadenomas. Unlike Cushing's disease, they have a 2:1 male preponderance and often manifest with mass effects. About one third have preoperative evidence for pituitary insufficiency. About half exhibit cavernous sinus or bony invasion, hemorrhage, necrosis, and cyst formation. These tumors often recur, and postoperative radiation and reoperation are required to eradicate tumor regrowth or residual mass.[795] Unless appropriate immunostaining is performed, many of these tumors remain undiagnosed and are classified as recurrent nonfunctioning macroadenomas.

Thyroid-Stimulating Hormone

Thyrotroph cells make up about 5% of the functional anterior pituitary cells and are situated predominantly in the anteromedial areas of the gland. They are smaller than the other cell types and are irregularly shaped, with flattened nuclei and relatively small secretory granules ranging from 120 to 150 μm (Fig. 8–59 and 8–60).

Biosynthesis

TSH is a glycoprotein hormone comprising a heterodimer of two noncovalently linked α and β subunits.[796] The α-subunit is common to TSH, LH, FSH and hCG, and the β-subunit is unique and confers specificity of action.[797] The α-subunit is the earliest hormone gene expressed embryonically; activation of the β-subunit gene occurs later under the influence of GATA-2 and Pit-1.[11] The 13.5-kb α-subunit gene is located on chromosome 6 and comprises 4 exons and 3 introns.[798] Although the α-subunit gene is expressed in thyrotroph, gonadotroph, and placental cells, its regulation is uniquely cell-specific. The downstream promoter region (–200 and below) is required for placental expression, intermediate sequences are required for gonadotroph expression, and upstream promoter elements are required for thyrotroph-specific expression.[799] α-Subunit transcription is inhibited by triiodothyronine (T_3) at regions close to the transcriptional initiation site, in concert with other nuclear corepressors.[800] The 4.9 kb TSH β-subunit gene located on chromosome 1 comprises 3 exons and two introns.[801] Pit-1 binds directly to the gene promoter to confer tissue-specific expression.[802] TSH-β gene transcription is suppressed by the thyroid hormone receptor acting directly on exon 1.[803]

This potent suppression is evident within 30 minutes of T_3 exposure and is a critical determinant of TSH synthesis and ultimate secretion. Both α and β TSH subunit gene transcription are induced by TRH, and depletion of cAMP by dopamine leads to suppressed gene transcription.[804] Intrapituitary TSH is stored

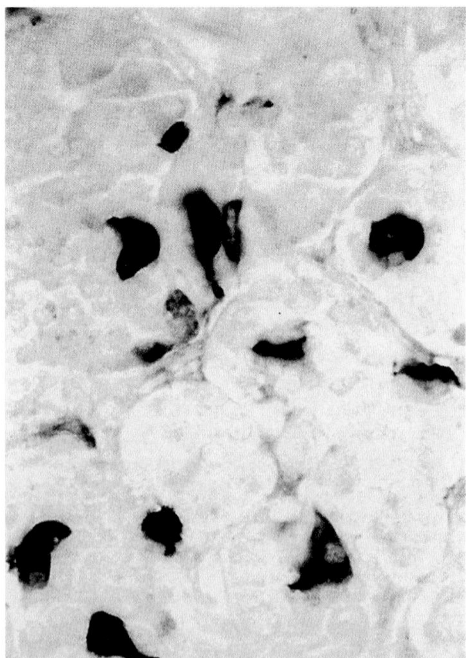

Figure 8–59 ▪ Normal thyrotrophs have angular cell bodies with elongated processes. (From Asa SL. In Tumors of the Pituitary Gland. Atlas of Tumor Pathology. Washington, DC: Armed Forces Institute of Pathology, 1997:19.)

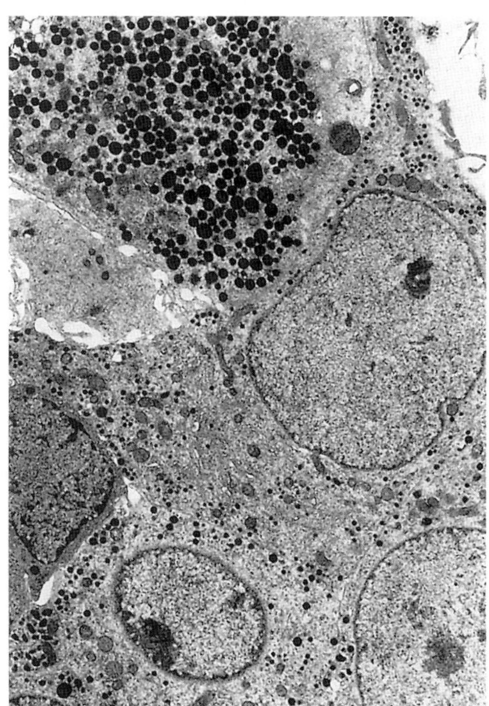

Figure 8–60 ▪ Electron micrograph of normal thyrotrophs showing angular cell bodies with elongated processes. (From Asa SL. In Tumors of the Pituitary Gland. Atlas of Tumor Pathology. Washington, DC: Armed Forces Institute of Pathology, 1997:19.)

in secretory granules, and the mature hormone (28 kd) is released into the venous circulation primarily in response to hypothalamic TRH. The predicted structural model of the TSH molecule is that of a cystine knot growth factor. The tertiary TSH structure comprises three hairpin loops separated by central disulfide bonds, with the longer loop straddling one side.[805,806]

Production of the mature heterodimeric TSH molecule requires complex cotranslational glycosylation and folding of nascent α- and β-subunits.[797] After subunit translation and signal peptide cleavage, glycosylation occurs at asparagine 23 on the β-subunit and at two asparagine residues, 52 and 78, on the α-subunit.[807] Appropriate glycosylation is required for accurate molecular folding and subsequent combination of α- and β-subunits within the rough endoplasmic reticulum and Golgi apparatus. TRH and T_3 regulate TSH glycosylation, albeit in opposite directions. TRH administration or T_3 deprivation as occurs in hypothyroidism or T_3 resistance enhances oligosaccharide addition to the TSH molecule.[808]

Secretion

TSH production rate is normally 100 to 400 mU/day[809] and the calculated circulating half-life is about 50 minutes. Secretion rates are enhanced up to 15-fold in hypothyroid subjects and are suppressed in states of hyperthyroidism. The degree of TSH glycosylation determines metabolic clearance rate and bioactivity, and in hypothyroidism, the molecule appears highly sialylated.[807] Immunoreactive fetal pituitary TSH is detectable by 12 weeks. Immediately after full-term birth, there is a brisk rise in TSH, which remains elevated for up to 5 days before stabilizing at adult levels.[810] Although TSH secretion is pulsatile, the low pulse amplitudes and long TSH half-life result in modest circulating variances. Secretory pulses every 2 to 3 hours are interspersed with periods of tonic, nonpulsatile TSH secretion.[292] Circadian TSH secretion peaks between 11 PM and 5 AM, mainly due to increased pulse amplitude, which does not appear to be sleep-entrained.[811] Pulsatile and circadian TSH secretory patterns are largely determined by ambient thyroid hormone levels, TRH release, dopamine, and cortisol. Primary hypothyroidism is associated with enhanced TSH pulse amplitudes occurring throughout the day, and nocturnal TSH surges are abrogated in patients with critical illness.[812]

Thyroid-Releasing Hormone and Thyroid Hormone Regulation

Because feedback control of TSH secretion by peripheral thyroid hormones is so sensitive, most thyrotroph disorders can be diagnosed by measuring basal TSH and thyroid hormone levels. However, evoked dynamic TSH measurements may be required to fully assess the integrity of the hypothalamic-pituitary-thyroid axis.[813] TRH (200-500 μg) is administered intravenously and TSH levels measured at 15 minutes before and at 0, 15, 30, 60, and 120 minutes after injection. In euthyroid subjects, peak TSH levels (up to 22-fold higher than basal) are observed after 30 minutes.[814] Because feedback suppression by elevated thyroid hormone levels on TSH overrides positive hypothalamic signals, hyperthyroid subjects have undetectable basal TSH levels that do not respond to TRH. In subjects with primary thyroid failure, the TSH response is exuberant, and in those with secondary thyroid failure due to pituitary disease, TSH levels do not change in response to TRH.

Sustained TRH infusions for up to 4 hours result in biphasic TSH increases, reflecting early release of preformed TSH, followed later by newly synthesized hormone. Further prolonged TRH infusions elevate thyroid hormone levels, which subsequently suppress pituitary TSH synthesis and release.[815] Within hours of T_3 administration, basal TSH levels suppress, and TRH-evoked TSH levels are attenuated. Thyroid hormones suppress tonic TSH secretion and pulse amplitude, but they do not appear to regulate TSH pulse frequency. T_3 also suppresses hypothalamic TRH synthesis and decreases pituitary TRH receptor number, thus further limiting TSH biosynthesis.

Other Factors

SRIF inhibits TSH pulse amplitude and blocks the nocturnal TSH surge[816] directly at the pituitary level. It might also suppress TRH release and possibly TRH receptor abundance.[817] Although SRIF analogues are used to treat TSH-secreting pituitary adenomas (see later), long-term SRIF treatment for acromegaly does not lead to hypothyroidism in adult subjects. T_4 levels may be lowered within the normal range,[719] but dopamine inhibits TSH β-subunit gene expression. Dopamine infusions suppress TSH pulse amplitude by 70% and abrogate the nocturnal TSH surge.[818] Prolonged use of dopamine agonists, however, does not result in hypothyroidism. Glucocorticoids suppress TSH secretion, and in patients with adrenal failure without autoimmune thyroid damage, TSH levels may be elevated. Sex steroids and cytokines alter TSH secretion in animal models, but their contribution to human TSH physiology is as yet unclear. Nonsteroidal antiinflammatory agents, especially meclofenamate and fenclofenac, decrease serum TSH levels, albeit still within the normal range. The mechanism for this effect might involve displacement of thyroid hormone ligands from their binding proteins or a direct inhibition of pituitary TSH.[819]

Action

TSH acts on the thyroid gland to induce thyroid hormone synthesis and release and to maintain trophic thyroid cell integrity.[820] The TSH GPC receptor is located on the thyrocyte plasma membrane and is encoded by a gene on chromosome 11q31. Its regulation is comprehensively described in Chapter 10.

Assays

The challenge of a clinically compelling robust TSH assay is to readily distinguish circulating TSH levels in euthyroid subjects from hyperthyroid and hypothyroid patients. The development of immunoradiometric TSH assays has provided high specificity with little or no cross-reactivity with other glycoprotein hormones. These assays detect quantifiable TSH levels in euthyroid control subjects with no overlap with the low values associated with hyperthyroidism.[814,821] Currently, the most sensitive commercially available third-generation assays have a functional sensitivity of 0.01-0.02 mU/L, and the newer fourth-generation assays portend greatly enhanced sensitivity (0.001-0.002 mU/L). Levels of free α-subunit (normal range 0.1-1.6 μg/L) are elevated in patients harboring TSH-secreting or nonfunctional pituitary adenomas, choriocarcinoma, and several other malignancies.

Deficiency

TSH deficiency results in childhood mental and/or growth retardation, and hypothyroidism in adults is associated with a broad spectrum of clinical features including hypothermia, fluid retention, voice and skin changes, and ultimately frank myxedema and death. Pituitary damage can result in functional TSH deficiency, often without a clearly demonstrable reduction in serum TSH levels. Although impractical to measure, nocturnal TSH pulse amplitudes may be attenuated in patients with pituitary dysfunction.[822] TSH deficiency should be diagnosed by measuring free T_4 levels, because TSH measurements are not helpful in diagnosing central hypothyroidism. In fact, only about one third of patients with secondary hypothyroidism have abnormally low basal TSH levels.[823] TSH deficiency is thus associated with low T_4 levels concomitant with low, normal, or even minimally elevated TSH levels. This biochemical profile may also be encountered in critically ill patients who have low TSH and T_4 levels but no evidence of pituitary disease.

Treatment

L-Thyroxine is used for replacement therapy, and dosing variables are similar to those required for treating primary hypothyroidism. Hypothyroid features are effectively ameliorated by T_4 (0.075-0.25 mg/day). The molecule is converted peripherally into the active T_3 and has a 7-day half-life with stable blood levels. The dose of levothyroxine in hypopituitary patients is titrated to achieve mid-normal clinically euthyroid serum free T_4 levels because serum TSH levels are low or undetectable in patients with damaged pituitary function. Measurement of TSH levels is not useful in determining thyroid hormone replacement because the damaged thyrotroph is unlikely to adequately reflect appropriate feedback suppression. Because many women with pituitary failure also likely receive estrogen replacement, measuring free T_4 levels is required due to increased TBG levels. T_4 overdosing can also lead to osteopenia and cardiac arrhythmias. Some patients might have associated ACTH deficiency, and thyroid hormone replacement should not be initiated until adrenal reserve has been evaluated and, if necessary, treated. Thyroid hormone replacement can also accelerate cortisol metabolism or requirements (or both) and can therefore exacerbate primary hypoadrenalism or precipitate adrenal crisis in patients with perturbed adrenal function.

Thyrotropin-Secreting Tumors

TSH-producing pituitary tumors are rare. Most older series indicate that they represent less than 1% of pituitary tumors.[568,824,825] From 1979 to 1992, Mindermann and Wilson analyzed tumor type by immunohistochemistry and found that the overall prevalence of TSH-secreting tumors was 19 or 2225 (0.85%). Between 1989 and 1991, the same group found a prevalence of 2.8%.[824] It is not clear whether the incidence of this tumor type is increasing or whether tumors are now more readily recognized, perhaps as a result of development of high-sensitivity TSH assays that distinguish normal TSH levels that are in fact inappropriately elevated for thyroid hormone level in some patients with TSH-producing tumors, and frankly low ones. TSH-secreting tumors can also cosecrete other hormones including growth hormone, PRL, and rarely ACTH.[826]

Pathology

These tumors are invasive, but for the most part benign, and distant metastases are extremely rare. The secretory pattern is determined by a panel of antibodies to TSH-β, α-subunit, GH, PRL, and ACTH. TSH-secreting tumors exhibit positive immunostaining for α-subunit and TSHβ in 20% to 75% of cells and for Pit-1.[827,828]

Presentation

Patients with TSH-secreting tumors present with symptoms that result from tumor size (e.g. visual field abnormalities, cranial nerve palsies, headache) or hormone overproduction. Signs and symptoms of hyperthyroidism, including palpitations, arrhythmias, weight loss, tremor and nervousness, or a goiter, are common. A case of periodic paralysis has been reported.[829] Serum TSH is often, but not invariably elevated; the combination of abnormally high thyroid hormone and a TSH within the normal range points to a TSH-producing pituitary tumor. A relatively long period of hyperthyroidism, initially thought to be Graves' disease and treated accordingly, often predates the realization that the hyperthyroidism is indeed a result of a TSH-secreting pituitary tumor. Alternatively, thyroid hormone insensitivity can also manifest with similar laboratory profiles.[830,831]

TSH-secreting tumors are usually large. Review of six reports indicates that 88% of TSH-secreting tumors are macroadenomas and 12% are microadenomas. More than 60% are also locally invasive.[832] From analysis of 10 reports on a total of 153 patients, we estimate that TSH is frankly elevated in 58 % of patients, and the remainder have normal albeit inappropriately elevated levels. Patients previously treated with radioactive iodine for presumed Graves' disease present with significantly higher TSH levels than patients not previously treated with radiation-ablation (mean, 56 mU/L vs. 9 mU/L, respectively).[823] An ectopic TSH-producing tumor has also been reported.[833] Serum T_4 is high in the majority of patients, as is the glycoprotein hormone α-subunit. Approximately two thirds[823] of patients with TSH-producing pituitary tumors have a goiter with elevated radioactive iodine uptakes. Signs or symptoms of acromegaly or hyperprolactinemia can also be presenting complaints.

Evaluation

T_4, T_3, TSH (by high-sensitivity assay), and α-subunit should be measured. The combination of high T_4, T_3, and α-subunit, high or inappropriately normal TSH, and a pituitary tumor strongly confirms the diagnosis of a TSH-producing pituitary adenoma. TRH stimulation differentiates between TSH overproduction by a TSH-secreting tumor and thyroid hormone insensitivity. In TSH-secreting tumors, the TSH response to TRH is blunted. In contrast, TSH usually rises in response to TRH in thyroid hormone insensitivity and in normal subjects. Concomitant measurement of α-subunit at each point during the TRH test is helpful because the molar ratio of α-subunit to TRH is high (>1) in almost 85% of patients with TSH-secreting tumors. Ratios greater than 1 can also be seen in normal subjects.[834]

A T_3 suppression test is helpful in that complete inhibition of TSH does not occur in patients with TSH-secreting tumors. This test can also differentiate subclinical hypothyroidism in a patient who was treated with radioactive iodine for hyperthyroidism in the past but is found to have an incidental pituitary tumor. TSH elevation can also result from inadequate thyroid hormone replacement. A pituitary MRI should be performed, and IGF-I and PRL levels determined to exclude acromegaly or hyperprolactinemia. The presence of other pituitary hormones in immunostained histologic sections does not necessarily imply that the serum levels are elevated.

The degree of hyperthyroidism should be assessed to determine whether control of these signs and symptoms should be undertaken prior to further evaluation or treatment of the pituitary tumor. One report characterized the hyperthyroidism in this condition as being severe in 14 of 25 patients and as having been present in most patients for years before the diagnosis was made.[832] Perioperative deaths in patients with TSH-secreting tumors have been reported, which might be attributed to poorly controlled hyperthyroidism.

Management

Surgery

Surgery is recommended as first-line treatment,[208] but surgical cures occur in no more than 40% of patients (Table 8–31).[835,836] However, the rarity of this tumor type has precluded large controlled studies. Fourteen of 22 patients had cavernous or sphenoid sinus invasion, and tumors were fibrous and unusually hard. Eight patients were considered cured after surgery.[826] In another study, surgery normalized T_4 in 15 patients and normalized parameters of cure in 7 of 17 patients. More than half the patients, when assessed by MRI 6 months after surgery, exhibited evidence of residual tumor.[837]

TABLE 8–31 MANAGEMENT OF TSH-SECRETING TUMORS

Study	Total Patients	Histology Stain	FEATURES				Cured by Surgery	RADIATION	
			Micro	Macro	Extrasellar Extension	Visual Field Deficit		Treated	Cured
Beckers, 1991	7	2/7 pure TSH 1/7 TSH, PRL 1/7 TSH, PRL, GH	1/7	6/7	—	—	3/4	—	—
Brucker-Davis, 1999	25	5/25 GH 4/25 PRL 3/25 FSH	2/25	23/25	20/25	7/18	8/22	11	—
Chanson, 1993	52	—	—	—	—	—	—	9/52	0/9
Chanson, 1992	37	—	2/37	35/37	—	—	—	8/37	0/8
Gesundheit, 1989	9	5/7 TSH 3/7 α-subunit	2/9	7/9	—	—	3/5	3/8	0/3
Grisoli, 1987	6	4/4 TSH 2/4 TSH, PRL	0/6	6/6	4/6	3/6	2/5	3/6	1/3
Kuhn, 2000	16		5/16	11/16	8/11	—	—	—	—
Losa, 1996	17	14 TSH 2 GH 3 PRL 1LH 13/14 a-subunit	3/17	14/17	10/14	3/17	7/17	—	—
McCutcheon, 1990	8	6/7 TSH 2/7 PRL	1/8	7/8	6/7	4/8	4/8	3/8	0/3
Mindermann, 1993	19	6/14 pure TSH 4/14 TSH, GH, PRL, ACTH 1/14 TSH, GH, PRL 1/14 TSH, PRL 1/14 TSH, GH 1 /14 TSH, ACTH	0/19	19/19	12/19	6/19	NA	9/19 E	NA
Total (%)	164	—	15/136 (11%)	121/136 (89%)	60/82 (73%)	23/66 (35%)	24/56 (43%)		

Beckers A, Abs R, Mahler C, et al. Thyrotropin-secreting pituitary adenomas: report of seven cases. J Clin Endocrinol Metab 1991;72:477-483.

Brucker-Davis F, Oldfield EH, Skarulis MC, et al. Thyrotropin-secreting pituitary tumors: diagnostic criteria, thyroid hormone sensitivity, and treatment outcome in 25 patients followed at the National Institutes of Health. J Clin Endocrinol Metab 1999;84:476-486.

Chanson P, Weintraub BD, Harris AG. Octreotide therapy for thyroid-stimulating hormone–secreting pituitary adenomas. A follow-up of 52 patients. Ann Intern Med. 1993;119:236-240.

Chanson P, Warnet A. Treatment of thyroid-stimulating hormone-secreting adenomas with octreotide. Metabolism 1992;41:62-65.

Gesundheit N, Petrick PA, Nissim M, et al. Thyrotropin-secreting pituitary adenomas: clinical and biochemical heterogeneity. Ann Intern Med 1989;111:827-835.

Kuhn JM, Arlot S, Lefebvre H. Evaluation of the treatment of thyrotropin-secreting pituitary adenomas with a slow release formulation of the somatostatin analog lanreotide. J Clin Endocrinol Metab 2000;85:1487-1491.

Losa M, Giovanelli M, Persani L, et al. Criteria of cure and follow-up of central hyperthyroidism due to thyrotropin-secreting pituitary adenomas. J Clin Endocrinol Metab 1996;81:3084-3090.

McCutcheon IE, Weintraub BD, Oldfield EH. Surgical treatment of thyrotropin-secreting pituitary adenomas. J Neurosurg 1990;73:674-683.

Mindermann T, Wilson CB. Thyrotropin-producing pituitary adenomas. J Neurosurg 1993;79:521-527.

Radiation Therapy

There are no large series reporting treatment of TSH-secreting tumors with radiotherapy alone. Radiation has mostly been employed as adjunctive therapy to surgery, especially when surgery was not curative.

Somatostatin Analogues

Octreotide, used as either primary or adjunctive treatment. normalizes T_4 and T_3 and reduces TSH levels by half.[838] In 25 patients treated with octreotide (100 to 500 μg daily) for up to 61 months, 84% had controlled thyroid function. However, tachyphylaxis developed in five patients, and three escaped the effect of the drug. Overall, tumor shrinkage occurs in about a third of patients. In 18 patients with TSH-secreting adenomas, lanreotide (30 mg every 10 or 14 days), significantly decreased TSH levels from 2.72 to 1.89 mU/L and decreased T_4 levels, but it did not shrink tumors. Octreotide LAR (up to 30 mg monthly) responsiveness appeared similar to that observed for the subcutaneous preparation in seven patients.[839]

Unless vision is threatened, patients should be evaluated to determine whether the clinical signs of hyperthyroidism warrant immediate treatment (Fig. 8–61). Propranolol, radioactive iodine thyroid ablation, thyroidectomy, antithyroid medications including tapazol and propylthiouracil, and somatostatin analogues are employed.[840] Radioactive iodine and antithyroid medications are targeted to the thyroid gland rather than the pituitary seat of the disorder. Both also inhibit the remaining negative feedback of T_3 on TSH and lead to increased tumor TSH production.[838] Surgery and somatostatin analogues simultaneously treat hyperthyroidism and tumor TSH hypersecretion. Propranolol is important for inhibiting peripheral hyperthyroid manifestations.[831,841] Somatostatin analogues lower TSH, α-subunit, and T_4 and are recommended as first-line drugs in the initial control of hyperthyroidism due to TSH-secreting tumors because their onset of action is faster than other therapeutic approaches and tumor shrinkage occurs in up to 40% of patients. If these drugs are ineffective or only partially effective, other therapeutic modalities should be undertaken. Thus, no single treatment is expected to cure patients with TSH-secreting adenomas. Surgery is curative in only a minority of patients, and although tumor bulk removal can normalize thyroid function when invasive tumor tissue persists, patients continue to have abnormal TSH responses to TRH and require somatostatin analogue therapy (see Fig. 8–61).

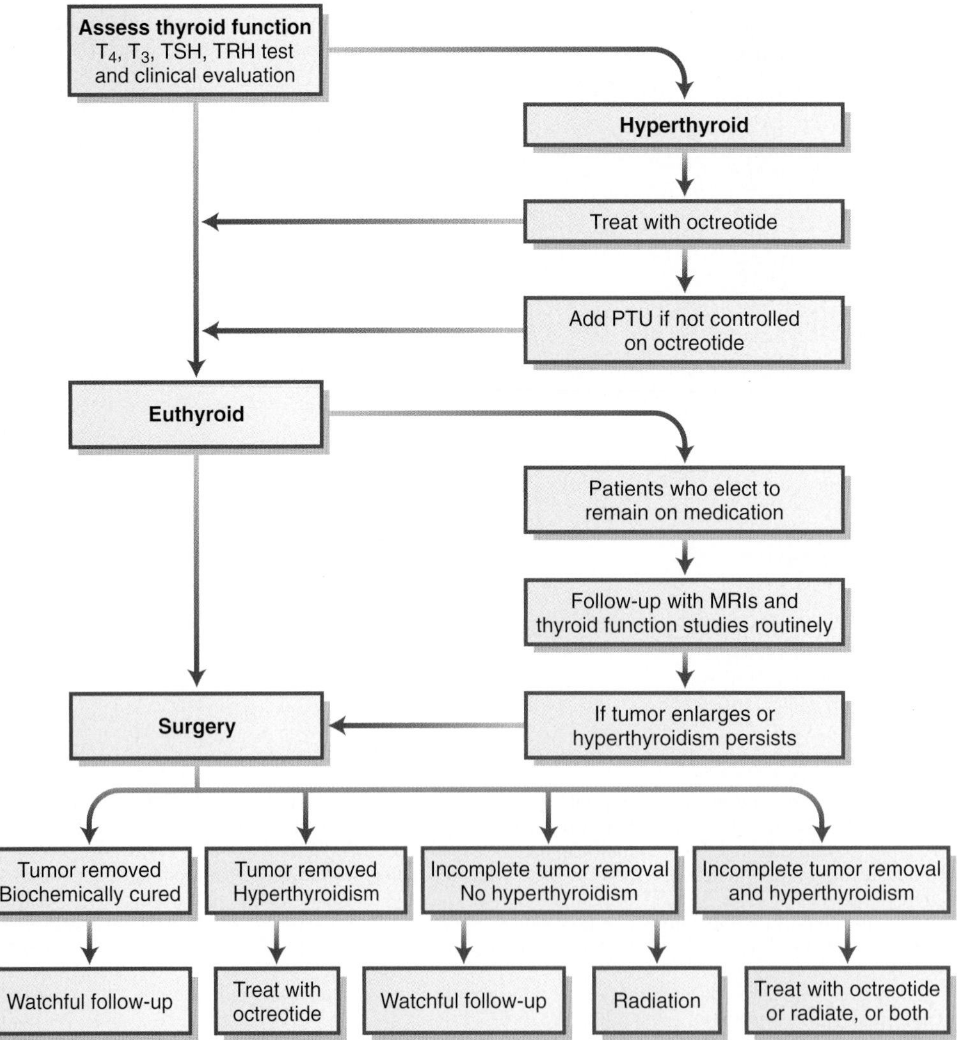

Figure 8–61 ▪ Management of thyroid-stimulating hormone (TSH)-secreting pituitary tumors. MRI, magnetic resonance imaging; PTU, propyltiouracil; T_3, triiodothyronine; T_4, thyroxine; TRH, thyrotrophin-releasing hormone.

PITUITARY FAILURE

Impaired synthesis of one or more anterior pituitary hormones can result from heritable genetic factors, acquired anatomic insults, inflammation, or vascular damage (Tables 8–32 and 8–33). Because of its close anatomic contiguity, impaired hypothalamic hormone synthesis or secretion can also occur as a component of the pituitary gland insult, especially following external radiation. Furthermore, distinct hypothalamic lesions can result in diminished pituitary hormone secretion by abrogating hypothalamic hypophysiotropic signals.

TABLE 8–32 ETIOLOGY OF INHERITED PITUITARY DEFICIENCY (CENTRAL)

	Hormone Deficit
GENETIC	
KAL mutation	FSH, LH
Lawrence-Moon-Biedl Syndrome	FSH, LH
Prader-Willi Syndrome	FSH, LH
RECEPTOR	
CRH receptor	ACTH
GHRH receptor	GH
GnRH Receptor	FSH, LH
Leptin and leptin receptor defect	LH, FSH
Melanocortin receptor	
STRUCTURAL	
CNS masses; encephalocele	Any
Pituitary aplasia	Any
Pituitary hypoplasia	Any
TRANSCRIPTION FACTOR DEFECT	
DAX1	Adrenal, LH, FSH
HESX1	GH, PRL, TSH, LH, FSH, ACTH
LHX3/4	GH, PRL, TSH, LH, FSH
Pit1	PRL, GH, TSH
PITX2	
Prop1	GH, PRL, TSH, LH, FSH, ACTH
T-Pit	ACTH
HORMONE MUTATION	
Bioinactive GH	GH
GH-1	GH
FSHβ	FSH
LHβ	LH
POMC	ACTH
POMC processing defect	ACTH
TSHβ	TSH

Developmental defects may be hypothalamic and/or pituitary.
ACTH, adrenocorticotropic hormone; CNS, central nervous system; CRH, corticotropin-releasing hormone; FSH, follicle-stimulating hormone; GH, growth hormone; GHRH, growth hormone–releasing hormone; GnRH, gonadotropin-releasing hormone; LH, luteinizing hormone; POMC, pro-opiomelanocortin; PRL, prolactin; TSH, thyroid-stimulating hormone.

Developmental and Genetic Causes of Pituitary Failure

Developmental Pituitary Dysfunction

Congenital pituitary gland absence (aplasia), partial hypoplasia, or ectopic tissue rudiments are rarely encountered. Pituitary development follows midline cell migration from Rathke's pouch. Impaired midline anomalies, including failed forebrain cleavage and anterior commissure and corpus callosum defects, lead to structural pituitary anomalies. Craniofacial developmental anomalies, including anencephaly, result in cleft lip and palate, basal encephalocele, hypertelorism, and optic nerve hypoplasia, with varying degrees of pituitary dysplasia and aplasia. If these infants survive, lifelong appropriate pituitary hormone replacement is required. Children with mild forms of midline anomalies are also more prone to GH deficiencies.

With sensitive MRI techniques for pituitary visualization, several anatomic features characteristic of hypopituitarism are now apparent. Evidence for acquired pituitary gland damage or destruction is often clearly visible on MRI, and patients presenting with hypopituitarism of undetermined etiology can exhibit decreased gland volume, partial or complete empty sella, disturbed sella turcica architecture, absent or transected pituitary stalk, and an absent or ectopic posterior pituitary bright intensity signal.[842] An absent infundibulum noted on MRI is associated with pituitary hormone deficits, and about 40% of patients with GH deficiency of unclear cause show imaging evidence of mild stalk defects, reflecting a midline developmental anomaly. Congenital basal encephalocele can cause the pituitary to herniate through the sphenoid sinus roof, resulting in pituitary failure and diabetes insipidus.

Heritable Disorders of Pituitary Failure

Mutations of transcription factors that determine anterior pituitary development can lead to pituitary deficiency syndromes (Table 8–34). Patients heretofore with diagnoses of idiopathic isolated or polyhormonal pituitary failure might in fact harbor such a mutation, and as the genetic control of pituitary development is clarified, increasing numbers of mutant genes have become apparent (Chapter 23).

PROP-1

PROP1 (OMIM601538) gene expression is required for subsequent Pit-1 activation. The gene, located on chromosome 5q, encodes a 223–amino acid protein expressed in GH-, PRL-, and TSH-secreting cells.[843] The Ames dwarf mouse harbors a missense *prop1* mutation (Ser83Pro) and exhibits a hypoplastic pituitary gland with combined GH, PRL, and TSH deficiency. This mutation abrogates Pit-1 activation and results in failed development of Pit-1–dependent cell lineages.[844] Several human mutations have been associated with GH, PRL, TSH, and gonadotropin deficiencies. The most commonly encountered mutation is a 2-bp deletion at position 296 (301-302delAG), resulting in early translational termination and a nonfunctional protein product. The clinical spectrum of combined pituitary hormone deficiency associated with PROP-1 mutations varies with the type of mutation and the age of the patient.[845]

Human *PROP1* mutations are associated with deficiencies in Pit-1–dependent lineages (GH, PRL, and TSH) and impaired FSH, LH, and ACTH reserve function.[545] Because development and mature function of these latter cell types are not Pit-1 dependent, it appears that additional critical developmental factors are disrupted in these patients, leading to the clinical phenotype. More than 50 patients with PROP-1 mutations leading to combined pituitary hormone deficiency have been described

TABLE 8–33 EVALUATION OF HEREDITARY PITUITARY DEFICIENCY

Gene	Pituitary Deficiency	MRI	Associated Malformations	Inheritance Mode	Mutation
HESX1	GH, PRL, TSH, LH, FSH, ACTH Posterior defects	Hypoplastic or hyperplastic anterior pituitary; normal or ectopic posterior pituitary	Septo-optic dysplasia	Recessive	
LHX3	GH, PRL, TSH, LH, FSH	Hypoplastic or hyperplastic anterior pituitary	Stubby neck with rigid cervical spine		
POU1F1	GH, PRL, ± TSH	Normal or hypoplastic anterior pituitary		Recessive Dominant	
PROP-1	GH, PRL, TSH, LH, FSH, ± ACTH	Normal, hypoplastic, hyperplastic or cystic anterior pituitary		Recessive	
T-Pit	ACTH	Normal	Red hair, obesity		

These genes are involved in pituitary development or in maintaining integrity of the GH axis. Functional defects include missense or frame shifts leading to truncated or deleted protein, DNA binding abnormality, inactivated protein, or impaired coactivation. *HESX-1* is critical for corpus development and is associated with structural brain defects. *POU1F1* mutations result in varying phenotype of early growth failure with or without hypothyroidism. *PROP-1* mutations may only be fully manifest in adulthood.

ACTH, adrenocorticotropic hormone; FSH, follicle-stimulating hormone; GH, growth hormone; LH, luteinizing hormone; MRI, magnetic resonance imaging; POMC, pro-opiomelanocortin; PRL, prolactin; TSH, thyroid-stimulating hormone.

Adapted from Netchine I, Léger J, Rappaport R. Magnetic resonance imaging of the hypothalamic-pituitary region in nontumoral hypopituitarism. In Rappaport R, Amselem S, eds. Hypothalamic-Pituitary Development. Genetic and Clinical Aspects. Basel: Karger, 2001:94-108.

since the original report in 1996,[846] and this disorder appears to be the most common heritable cause of combined pituitary hormone deficiency.

Molecular Analysis

Inheritance modes of *PROP1* mutations usually reflect autosomal recessive patterns. Thus, patients are usually homozygous for either deletion or missense frameshift mutations, leading to truncated PROP-1 protein products devoid of functional activity.[545,847] A hot spot in *PROPI* has been identified at a GA repeat in exon 2. Combination of a GA or AG deletion in this repeat results in a coding frameshift and premature termination at codon 109. Nonafflicted siblings are either heterozygous or bear a normal *PROP1* sequence on both alleles. Mutations in the transactivation domain at codon 582 lead to features of hypogonadism as the presenting phenotype.[848]

Clinical Features

The frequency of PROP1 gene mutations in patients with combined pituitary hormone deficiency is high, occurring in about 50% of affected subjects. However, in families with multiple affected subjects, *PROPI* mutations account for virtually all affected patients. Patients harboring *PROP1* mutations exhibit a predominantly hypogonadal phenotype. Puberty is often delayed, or absent, with markedly attenuated LH and FSH responses to GnRH stimulation.[465] Some patients enter puberty spontaneously and develop subsequent features of central hypogonadism akin to an acquired presentation.[847] A broad spectrum of variable time of onset and degree of pituitary loss is characteristic of the syndrome. Some older patients also exhibit blunted cortisol responses to cortrosyn administration, and others present with panhypopituitarism.[849]

Although the pituitary gland size is small or normal, patients have been described with grossly hyperplastic pituitary glands with cystic changes and development of a secondary empty sella. Slowing of linear growth usually becomes apparent after the age of 3 years, and these patients usually do not enter puberty. Height standard deviation score (SDS) may be severely impaired and can range to −10 with eunuchoidal proportions and reduced upper-to-lower body ratios. Affected adults are short, with infantile external genitalia. The onset of clinically evident pituitary failure usually is GH deficiency (about 80%) and thyroid failure (TSH deficiency, about 20%), followed by hypogonadism and later subclinical or overt adrenal insufficiency.[850]

PROP-1 excess has been described in a mouse model.[851] These animals have hypothyroidism, hypogonadism, and persistent Rathke's cleft cysts. After one year they develop pituitary adenomas.

Evaluation

Combined hypothalamic hormone stimulation (GnRH, TRH, CRH, and GHRH) or insulin-evoked hypoglycemia reveals blunted responses consistent with varying degrees of pituitary hormone deficiencies. Serum IGF-I and IGFBP3 levels are usually low, while peripheral thyroid hormone levels are low or at the lower limits of normal ranges. In the face of low or absent TSH responses, these findings are consistent with secondary hypothyroidism. Most older patients also exhibit blunted cortisol responses to CRH or ACTH (or both) or insulin stimulation.[848]

Pituitary Size

Heterogeneous changes in pituitary size can reflect a combination of apoptotic signals for the Pit-1 lineage, compensatory cystic expansion of nonaffected pituitary cell types with subsequent autoinfarction, and the absence of other unknown factors required for mature pituitary function.[852]

POU1F1

The *POU1F1* gene (Pit-1) is located on chromosome 3p11 (OMIM173110) and encodes a 290–amino acid protein. The N-terminal POU-specific domain activates gene transcription, and 2 DNA-binding domains recognize a TATNCAT consensus sequence present in the GH, PRL, and TSH hormones and the GHRH receptor gene.[853] The Pit-1 nuclear protein activates transcription of the GH, PRL, and TSH genes and the GHRH receptor gene and also partners with coactivators including thyroid hormone, estrogen, and retinoic acid receptors, as well as other transcription factors including CREB, P-Lim, Ptx-1, HESX-1, and Zn-15. Pit-1 autoregulates its own expression, rendering Pit-1 critical for maintaining appropriate Pit-1 expression. Because of the absolute requirement of Pit-1 for GH, PRL, and TSH cell development and specific gene expression, inactivating muta-

TABLE 8–34 ETIOLOGY OF ACQUIRED PITUITARY INSUFFICIENCY

INFECTION
Cytomegalovirus
Fungal (histoplasmosis, aspergillosis)
Parasites (toxomplasmosis)
Pneumocystis jiroveci
Tuberculosis
INFILTRATIVE/INFLAMMATORY
Hemochromatosis
Primary Hypophysitis
Granulomatous
Lymphocytic
Xanthomatous
Secondary Hypophysitis
Histiocytosis X
Infections
Sarcoidosis
Takayasu's disease
Wegener's granulomatosis
NEOPLASTIC
Parasellar Mass
Dermoid cyst
Ependymoma
Germinoma
Glioma
Meningioma
Pituitary metastatic deposits
Rathke's cyst
Hematologic Malignancy
Leukemia
Lymphoma
Other
Craniopharyngioma
Hypothalamic hamartoma, gangliocytoma
Pituitary adenoma
TRAUMA
Radiation damage
Surgical resection
Traumatic brain injury
VASCULAR
Aneurysm
Apoplexy
Arteritis
Diabetes
Hypotension
Pregnancy-related
Sickle cell disease

FUNCTIONAL
Critical Illness
Acute illness
Chronic kidney failure
Chronic liver failure
Drugs
Anabolic steroids
Dopamine
Estrogen
Glucocorticoid excess
GnRH agonists
Somatostatin analogue
Thyroid hormone excess
Hormones
Hyperprolactinemia
Hypothyroidism
Post-treatment of Cushing's disease
Nutrition
Caloric restriction
Malnutrition
Other
Excessive exercise

CAUSES OF ACQUIRED GROWTH HORMONE DEFICIENCY IN 1034 HYPOPITUITARY ADULT PATIENTS	
Cause	**%**
Pituitary tumor	53.9
Craniopharyngioma	12.3
Idiopathic	10.2
CNS tumor	4.4
Empty sella syndrome	4.2
Sheehan's syndrome	3.1
Head trauma	2.4
Hypophysitis	1.6
Surgery other than for pituitary treatment	1.5
Granulomatous diseases	1.3
Irradiation other than for pituitary treatment	1.1
CNS malformation	1.0
Perinatal trauma or infection	0.5
Other	2.5

CNS, central nervous system; GnRH, gonadotropin-releasing hormone.

Causes of acquired deficiency from Abs R, Bengtsson BA, Hernberg-Stahl E, et al. GH replacement in 1034 growth hormone deficient hypopituitary adults: demographic and clinical characteristics, dosing and safety. Clin Endocrinol (Oxf) 1999;50(6):703-713.

tions of the gene result in a spectrum of pituitary hormone deficiencies.[12]

Two dwarf mouse strains harbor *POU1F1* gene mutations. The Snell dwarf mouse harbors a tryptophan → cysteine missense mutation (Trp261Cys).[854] The Jackson mouse, although also a dwarf, harbors a truncated POU1F-1 protein with defective DNA binding.

Several *POU1F1* mutations exhibit characteristic clinical phenotypes.[855] Arg172Tyr mutants are associated with neonatal hypothyroidism and GH and PRL deficiency. Sporadic patients and multiplex families with multiple pituitary hormone defects have been described, and at least 10 recessive and three dominant Pit-1 mutations have been identified so far. Recessive mutations result in a varied spectrum of loss of DNA binding or transcriptional activation of TSH, GH, or PRL, or some combination of these.

Impaired retinoic acid activation of the Pit-1 distal enhancer has been described for a Pit-1 Lys261Glu mutation. This mutant protein also behaves as a dominant negative inhibitor of Pit-1 activation. A sporadic mutation (Arg271Try) binds well to DNA but dominantly inhibits pituitary gene transcription. Compound heterozygosity for a 1-bp deletion (747delA) and a missense mutation (Trp193Arg) cause defective DNA binding and transcriptional activation with severe combined GH, PRL, and TSH deficiencies.[856] CBP1p300 protein recruitment and Pit-1 dimerization are required for appropriate Pit-1 activation of target hormone genes.[857] *LHX4* appears to activate *POU1F1,* and mutations of *LHX4* also lead to growth retardation.[858]

HESX1

HESX1 (Rpx) is an early transcriptional marker of the primitive pituitary, with expression restricted to Rathke's pouch.[859] Coincidentally with appearance of specific pituitary cell types, *HESX1* expression declines and is extinguished in the mature anterior pituitary.[860] The gene is located on chromosome 3p212, encodes a 185–amino acid protein, and competes with PROP-1 protein for DNA binding. The heterogeneous syndrome of septo-optic dysplasia (hypoplastic optic nerves, absent corpus callosum and septum pellucidum, and panhypopituitarism) is associated with a homozygous Arg53Cys homeodomain mutation. Although the mutant molecule exhibits reduced DNA binding, no specific hormonal target gene is yet apparent, and panhypopituitarism may in fact occur secondarily to the profound anatomic defects in midline development. The reason for GH deficiency in these patients is not apparent.

LHX3

Missense and deletion mutations of *LHX3* are associated with panhypopituitarism except for intact ACTH reserve. These patients also exhibit defective neck rotation ability due to a rigid cervical spine.[861] PtX2 Rieger's syndrome (anterior eye, teeth, and umbilical maldevelopment) may be associated with GH deficiency and haploinsufficiency of the *RIEG* (PtX2) homeobox gene.

T-Pit

T-Pit mutations result in early-onset isolated ACTH deficiency and hypocortisolism.[24] Associated phenotypes including those for POMC deficiency include obesity, red hair pigmentation, and other associated pituitary deficiencies.

Heritable pituitary hormone deficiencies due to transcription factor defects are rare. Nevertheless, within this cohort of patients, *PROP1* mutations appear to be the most prevalent, accounting for well over 50% of retrospective reports and more than 90% of patients with more than one affected sibling. *Pit-1* mutations are less commonly encountered. Patients with a family history of pituitary dysfunction, and those who exhibit blunted hormonal response to TRH, GHRH, or GnRH stimulation, should be subjected to molecular screening for PROP-1 or Pit-1 defects. The pronounced clinical phenotype of *HESX1* mutations determines the need for further molecular analysis.

Lawrence-Moon-Biedl Syndrome

This autosomal recessive disorder is characterized by hypogonadotropic hypogonadism, mental retardation, obesity, retinitis pigmentosa, and hexadactyly, brachydactyly, or syndactyly. By age 30 years, most patients are blind.[862] Although most patients have evidence of GnRH deficiency, about 25% of afflicted male patients have primary testicular failure.

Prader-Willi Syndrome

Prader-Willi syndrome patients have marked hyperphagia and obesity, with retarded mental development, muscle hypotonia, and diabetes mellitus. Related conditions include micrognathia, absent auricular cartilage, and acromicria.[863] The condition has been ascribed to deletion or translocation of chromosome 15. In hypogonadal patients, bilateral cryptorchidism and absent scrotal folds are accompanied by evidence of attenuated GnRH secretion.[864] LH and FSH levels have been restored in some patients with chronic GnRH treatment. Defective oxytocin and vasopressin synthesis have also been reported.

Kallman's Syndrome

Kallman's syndrome consists of defective GnRH synthesis, with olfactory nerve agenesis or hypoplasia and variable anosmia. Associated developmental disorders include optic atrophy, color blindness, VIIIth nerve deafness, cleft palate, renal agenesis, cryptorchidism, and movement disorders.[865] This X-linked recessive disorder has been ascribed to a defective *KAL* gene located on chromosome Xp22.3.[866] The KAL protein mediates hypothalamic migration of GnRH cells from the primitive olfactory placode, and its absence therefore leads to defective GnRH synthesis and anosmia.[867,868] Autosomal recessive and dominant forms of the disorder have been described, indicating the involvement of FGF-1 receptor mutations in the pathogenesis of the disorder.[869]

Clinical Features

These patients are exposed to low or absent sex steroids from birth. Consequently, female patients are tall and present with primary amenorrhea and absent secondary sexual development and male patients have delayed puberty and micropenis.[870]

Laboratory

Absent GnRH secretory pulses result in characteristically low LH and FSH levels in the face of very low concentrations of estradiol or testosterone. Because the nonprimed normal pituitary might not respond initially to GnRH (25-100 μg IV) stimulation, this test is of little value in distinguishing the hypothalamic defect. In some patients, repetitive GnRH priming might elicit normal pituitary LH and FSH responses, indicating a hypothalamic defect in GnRH secretion.

The differential diagnosis of congenital hypogonadotropic hypogonadism includes Kallman's syndrome (*KAL* gene mutation), congenital adrenal hypoplasia (*DAX1* mutation),[871] GnRH receptor mutations, leptin and leptin receptor mutations, *PROP1* gene mutations, and mutations of the LH or FSH molecules themselves. These conditions are characterized by absent or low GnRH-mediated LH secretory patterns in the presence of a structurally normal pituitary gland. Importantly, the cause of hypogonadotropic hypogonadism still remains elusive in more than 80% of patients (see earlier). In the absence of a structural pituitary defect, genetic evaluation of these patients should be undertaken.

Acquired Pituitary Failure

Causes

In the absence of demonstrable hypothalamic-pituitary anatomic damage, and after excluding genetic and syndromic causes of pituitary insufficiencies, acquired, often transient, causes of pituitary failure should be considered (see Table 8–34). Causes of pituitary insufficiency including pituitary tumors, parasellar masses, hypophysitis, aneurysms, and pituitary apoplexy are discussed earlier. Hypothalamic damage reflected by the presence of a large parasellar mass leading to decreased GnRH production is associated with hyperphagia, obesity, and central hypogonadism, with low levels of FSH and LH (Fröhlich's syndrome).

Marked caloric restriction, anorexia,[872,873] weight loss from other etiologies, and strenuous exercise can attenuate GnRH secretion or action, or both. Hypogonadotropic hypogonadism can occur in men and women (see Chapter 7). Exogenous anabolic steroid and glucocorticoid therapy suppress the reproductive and adrenal axes, respectively.

Patients with severe critical illnesses or chronic debilitating disease (including cirrhosis) may have impaired GH-IGF-I and impaired adrenal and gonadal axes. Hyperprolactinemia causes sexual dysfunction by inhibiting GnRH pulsatility via a short feedback loop. Hypothyroidism, hypoadrenalism, or hypogonadism cause hyperplasia of specific trophic cells due to lack of negative feedback and sometimes actual pituitary tumor formation.[874] AIDS is associated with suppressed pituitary function independently of other associated infections.[874a] Drugs such as estrogens, which suppress FSH and LH, and GnRH analogues used for treating prostate cancer inhibit gonadotropin action. In addition to pituitary apoplexy, other vascular accidents such as aneurysms, strokes, cavernous sinus thrombosis, and arteritis can cause pituitary hormone insufficiency. Isolated pituitary hormone deficiencies can also occur as a manifestation of vascular abnormalities including arteritis.

Head Trauma

The pituitary may be partially or totally damaged by birth trauma, cranial hemorrhage, fetal asphyxia, or breech delivery. Head trauma can lead to direct pituitary damage by a sella turcica fracture, pituitary stalk section, trauma-induced vasospasm, or ischemic infarction following blunt trauma.[875] The most common traumatic cause of compromised pituitary function in the adult is iatrogenic neurosurgical trauma. Advertent or inadvertent pituitary manipulation or damage during surgery leads to transient or permanent diabetes insipidus and varying degrees of anterior pituitary dysfunction.

Although hypopituitarism following head trauma usually appears within a year after the insult, some patients only develop overt signs of pituitary failure after several decades. About 75% of patients with post-traumatic pituitary failure are men younger than 40 years who were involved in a motor vehicle accident within a year of diagnosis. Virtually all patients with subsequent pituitary failure have a history of loss of consciousness following trauma, and half of all such patients have documented skull fracture.[875] One third of these patients have demonstrable signs of hypothalamic or posterior pituitary hemorrhage (or both) or anterior lobe infarction on MRI. Diabetes insipidus is the most common endocrine disorder, encountered in about 30% of these patients. Gonadotropin failure, amenorrhea, and hyperprolactinemia can occur in the months following trauma or can even manifest years later.[876,877]

Pituitary testing performed within the first 48 hours of hospital admission shows that about 75% of patients have evidence of hypopituitarism,[878] and the degree of pituitary failure correlates with severity of head trauma. When retested after 12 months, worsening of pituitary function has been documented in prospective studies, despite improvement in some trophic hormone axes. About 20% of patients developed posterior pituitary dysfunction (either diabetes insipidus, or SIADH) after traumatic brain injury.[879]

Radiation

Pituitary irradiation, usually indicated for pituitary adenoma therapy, directly causes atrophy of the gland, in addition to the damaging impact of irradiation on hypothalamic synthesis of hypophysiotropic hormones. Pituitary function in children and adolescents is particularly sensitive to head and neck therapeutic irradiation.[880] Radiation dose exposure, time interval after completion of radiation therapy, and distance of the pituitary or hypothalamus from the central energy field correlate with development of pituitary hormone deficits (Figs. 8–62 and 8–63). After a median dose of 5000 rad directed at the skull base, nasopharynx, or cranium, up to 75% of patients develop pituitary insufficiency within 10 years.[881] Later manifestations of pituitary failure usually reflect hypothalamic damage rather than atrophy of irradiated pituitary cells. Although the degree of hormone loss after radiation is variable, the pattern of loss usually occurs sequentially: GH greater than FSH and LH, followed by ACTH and TSH.[882] Thus, evidence for secondary thyroid or adrenal failure usually implies that the GH and gonadotropin axes are also compromised. Previously irradiated patients should therefore undergo lifelong periodic anterior pituitary hormone testing. Ideally, rigorous long-term screening should unmask incipient pituitary failure prior to onset of morbidity.[883]

Empty Sella Syndrome

Damage to the sellar diaphragm can lead to arachnoid herniation into the sellar space. An empty sella can develop as a consequence of a primary congenital weakness of the diaphragm in patients in whom no secondary cause is evident. Up to 50% of patients with primary empty sella have associated benign intracranial hypertension.[884] A secondary empty sella can

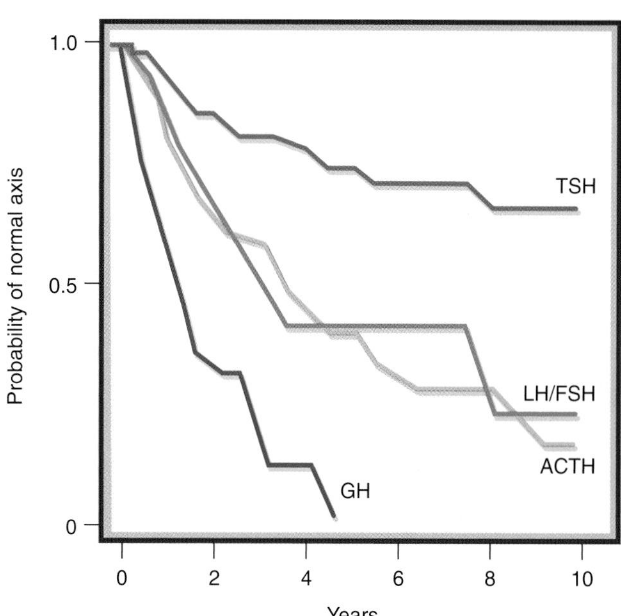

Figure 8–62 ■ Life-table analysis indicating probabilities of initially normal hypothalamic-pituitary-target gland axes remaining normal after radiotherapy (3750-4250 cGy). Browth hormone (GH) secretion is the most sensitive of the anterior pituitary hormones to the effects of external radiotherapy, and thyroid-stimulating hormone (TSH) secretion is the most resistant. In two thirds of patients, gonadotropin deficiency develops before adrenocorticotropic hormone (ACTH) deficiency. The reverse occurs in the remaining third. FSH, follicle-stimulating hormone; LH, luteinizing hormone. (From Littley MD, Shalet SM, Beardwell CG, et al. Hypopituitarism following external radiotherapy for pituitary tumors in adults. QJM 1989;70:145-160).

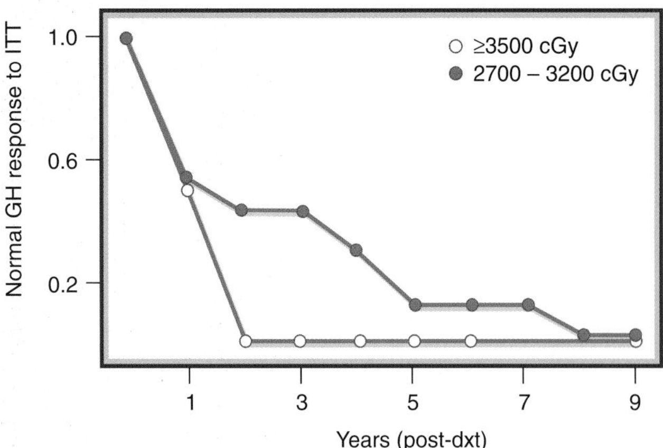

Figure 8–63 ▪ The incidence of growth hormone (GH) deficiency in children receiving 27 to 32 Gy or 35 Gy of cranial irradiation for a brain tumor in relation to time from irradiation (dxt). This illustrates that the speed at which individual pituitary hormone deficits develop is dose-dependent; the higher the radiation dose, the earlier GH deficiency occurs. (Courtesy of the Department of Medical Illustrations, Wilkington Hospital, Manchester, England. From Jöstel A, Shalet S. Hypopituitarism. In DeGroot LJ, Jameson JL, eds. Endocrinology, 5th ed. Philadelphia: WB Saunders, 2006:397-409).

develop subsequent to infarction of a pituitary adenoma or to surgical or radiation-induced damage to the sellar diaphragm. On MRI, these patients usually exhibit demonstrable pituitary tissue compressed against the sellar floor, with lateral stalk deviation. Although an empty sella is usually an incidental finding, if greater than 90% of pituitary tissue is compressed or atrophied, pituitary failure occurs. About 10% of patients develop small GH- or PRL-secreting adenomas within the rim of compressed pituitary tissue.

Clinical Features of Hypopituitarism

Patients with pituitary failure, regardless of course, were found to have excess mortality (SMR1187) primarily due to respiratory and vascular disease.[193] Age at diagnosis, female gender, and history of craniopharyngioma were the most striking determinants of increased mortality. The spectrum of clinical features of pituitary insufficiency depends on several factors. In acquired pituitary insufficiency the clinical spectrum depends upon the degree of hormone deficiency, the number of hormones impaired, and the rapidity of onset. In congenital forms, the earlier the age of onset, the greater the severity of thyroid, gonadal, adrenal, growth, or water disturbances.

Heritable genetic disorders invariably exhibit the most severe phenotypic changes, although later changes can also occur in these disorders, as seen with PROP-1 mutations. The resilience of the individual pituitary cell lineages to compressive, inflammatory, vascular, radiation, or invasive insults also differs. The lactotroph cell is often hyperfunctional as a result of decreased tonic inhibitory signals.

PRL deficiency is thus exceedingly rare, except for complete pituitary destruction or genetic syndromes. The order of diminished trophic hormone reserve function by pituitary compression usually follows the order GH > FSH > LH > TSH > ACTH. The corticotroph cell appears particularly resistant to hypothalamic or pituitary destruction and is usually the last cell to lose function. The qualitative phenotypic manifestations of pituitary failure are determined by which specific trophic hormones are lost (see earlier for descriptions of individual hormone deficiencies) (Table 8–35).

Adrenocorticotropic Hormone

Clinical symptoms and signs of ACTH deficiency are most profound and life-threatening. With acute pituitary failure, such as can occur with pituitary apoplexy, ACTH deficiency can manifest with hypotension, shock, hypoglycemia, nausea and vomiting, extreme fatigue and asthenia, and dilutional hyponatremia. Serum potassium is normal because these patients are only deficient in glucocorticoids and usually not mineralocorticoids. When acute ACTH deficiency is suspected clinically, treatment with steroids should not be withheld. Serum cortisol and ACTH should be drawn before glucocorticoid administration, and both ACTH and cortisol would be expected to be low.

In an acute setting, such as sudden apoplexy, responses to tetracosactrin (Synacthen) stimulation might be normal and misleading, because the blunted response of cortisol usually seen in secondary adrenal insufficiency is caused by loss of glucocorticoid-producing cells, which requires at least several weeks after the onset of ACTH deficiency. When ACTH deficiency occurs gradually, features are more insidious and include weight loss, asthenia, weakness, fatigue, nausea, and dilutional hyponatremia. This can result from corticotroph dysfunction arising as a result of an enlarging pituitary tumor, delayed effects of radiation, damage due to pituitary tumor surgery, or removal of parasellar masses. In these cases, tests for ACTH reserve are likely blunted. If not suspected or untreated, this form of adrenal insufficiency can also lead to death.

Caution must be exercised in performing an ITT or metyrapone test because the metyrapone test can cause worsening of adrenal insufficiency and the ITT can cause seizures and nausea. These tests should only be done in a hospital setting under supervision with available intravenous cortisone and glucose.

Steroid replacement doses should be appropriate to the clinical situation. Under conditions of major stress, such as pituitary apoplexy or pituitary surgery, maximum cortisone requirements range from 200 to 300 mg daily. Because the adrenal glands are incapable of increasing cortisol production during stress in the presence of deficient ACTH, initial IV dose of 100 mg solucortef in acute adrenal insufficiency, or an IV infusion of the same dose during pituitary surgery, is followed by 50 mg IV every 6 hours for the first day. Similar doses are employed during other forms of major stress in patients with established secondary adrenal insufficiency. Clinical judgment must be used in determining how long patients should be exposed to supraphysiologic doses of steroids. In our view, doses should be lowered to maintenance as soon as it is clinically feasible without endangering the patient. We employ replacement doses of 10 to 20 mg hydrocortisone daily, usually 10 mg in the morning and 5 mg in the evening. An additional 5 mg is administered in the afternoon if needed clinically. Because surgical decompression can lead to recovery of hormone deficiencies,[176,327] a clinical decision should be made postoperatively whether or not to wean patients off hormonal replacement therapy and retest them hormone by hormone. Great care must be taken when secondary adrenal insufficiency has been previously documented.

Thyroid-Stimulating Hormone

Because the half-life of serum T_4 is 6.8 days, hypothyroidism might not become apparent for several weeks in patients with acute pituitary insufficiency; therefore, thyroid function should be tested expectantly. TSH is not elevated in secondary hypothyroidism, and it cannot be used to assess adequacy of thyroid hormone replacement, nor is a TRH test helpful. Severity of symptoms of hypothyroidism depends on the degree of hypothyroidism and the length of time it has been present. Even in the absence of symptoms, T_4 should be administered if thyroid function studies are consistent with hypothyroidism. Glucocor-

TABLE 8–35 ASSESSMENT OF ANTERIOR PITUITARY FUNCTION

Test	Dose	Normal Response	Side Effects
		ADRENOCORTICOTROPIC HORMONE	
ACTH stimulation	250 μg IV or IM or 1 μg IV	Peak cortisol ≥20 μg/dL	Rare
CRH stimulation	100 μg IV	Peak ACTH ≥2-4-fold Peak cortisol ≥20 μg/dL	Flushing
Insulin tolerance	0.1-0.15 U/kg IV	Peak cortisol response >18 μg/dL, or increase by 7 μg/dL	Sweating, palpitation, tremor
Metyrapone	Oral administration of 30 mg/kg at 11 PM	Peak 11-DOC ≥7 μg/dL Peak cortisol ≤7 μg/dL Peak ACTH >75 pg/mL	Nausea, insomnia, adrenal crisis
		THYROID-STIMULATING HORMONE	
TRH stimulation Total T_3 Serum T_4 (free T_4)	200-500 μg IV	Peak TSH ≥2.5-fold or ↑ ≥5-6 mU/L (female) ↑ ≥2-3 mU/L (male)	Flushing, nausea, urge to micturate
		PROLACTIN	
Serum PRL TRH stimulation	200-500 μg IV	PRL ≥2.5-fold	Flushing, nausea, urge to micturate
		LUTEINIZING HORMONE AND FOLLICLE-STIMULATING HORMONE	
Serum LH and FSH Serum testosterone	100 μg IV	Elevated in menopause and in men with primary testicular failure (otherwise normal) 300-900 ng/mL LH ≥2-3-fold, or by 10 IU/L	Rare
GnRH stimulation		FSH 1.5-2-fold, or by 2 IU/L	
		GROWTH HORMONE	
Insulin tolerance	0.1-0.15 U/kg	GH peak >3 μg/L	Sweating, palpitations, tremor
L-Arginine	0.5 g/kg (max 30 g) IV over 30-120 min		Nausea
with			
GHRH	1-5 μg/kg	GH peak >5 μg/L	Flushing

ACTH, adrenocorticotropic hormone; CRH, corticotropin-releasing hormone; 11-DOC, 11-deoxycortisol; FSH, follicle-stimulating hormone; GH, growth hormone; GHRH, growth hormone–releasing hormone; LH, luteinizing hormone; PRL, prolactin; TRH, thyroid-releasing hormone; TSH, thyroid-stimulating hormone;

ticoids should be replaced before thyroid hormone, because thyroid hormone in hypothyroid patients increases the requirement for glucocorticoids in stressful situations.

Gonadotropins

Sexual dysfunction due to gonadotropin deficiency is far more common in patients with pituitary disease than is hypothyroidism or hypoadrenalism. Its presence is established by the constellation of abnormal menses or amenorrhea with no elevated LH and FSH levels in women and sexual dysfunction in men with low testosterone and normal or low gonadotropin levels. Because even mild hyperprolactinemia can cause sexual dysfunction, it should be determined whether PRL is causing hypogonadism. Treatment with dopamine agonists might normalize sexual function without the need for replacing sex steroids. A GnRH stimulation test rarely differentiates causes of gonadotropin deficiency and is usually not indicated.

Sex steroid replacement in deficient patients has important effects on body composition in addition to normalizing sexual function. Testosterone replacement might not be as effective in normalizing sexual function in men with longstanding secondary hypogonadism and loss of libido as it is when the sexual dysfunction is recent. Osteoporosis is common in women deficient in estrogen and men deficient in testosterone,[885] and replacement improves bone density. Testosterone reduces abdominal and visceral fat and improves muscle mass in deficient men.[886] Therefore, sex hormone replacement is important even though sexual function might not be normalized or is not desired.

Growth Hormone

Growth hormone deficiency is comprehensively discussed earlier. It is invariably present when two or more other trophic hormones are deficient.[887]

Prolactin

Prolactin deficiency is extremely rare, because it only occurs when the anterior pituitary is completely destroyed, as in patients after apoplexy or in patients with congenital causes of PRL deficiency. PRL deficiency prevents lactation.[254] In fact, PRL is often elevated in most forms of pituitary insufficiency. For

TABLE 8–36 REPLACEMENT THERAPY FOR ADULT HYPOPITUITARISM

ADRENOCORTICOTROPIC HORMONE
Hydrocortisone 10-20 mg daily in divided doses Cortisone acetate 15-25 mg daily in divided doses
FOLLICLE-STIMULATING HORMONE/LUTEINIZING HORMONE
Female Patients Conjugated estrogen 0.65 mg/day Micronized estradiol 1 mg/day Estradiol valerate 2 mg/day Piperazine estrone sulfate 1.25 mg/day Ethinyl estradiol 0.02-0.05 mg/day Estradiol skin patch 4-8 mg twice weekly Estradiol plus testosterone All of the above with progesterone or progestin sequentially or in combination if the uterus is present Oral contraceptives For fertility: Menopausal gonadotropin and hCG or GnRH **Male Patients** Testosterone enanthate 200 mg IM every 2-3 wk Testosterone skin patch 2.5-5.0 mg/day; can increase dose up to 7.5 mg/day Testosterone gel 3-6 g daily For fertility: hCG three times a week, or hCG plus FSH or menopausal gonadotropin or GnRH
GROWTH HORMONE
Adults Somatotropin 0.2-1.0 mg SC daily **Children** Somatotropin 0.02-0.05 mg/kg/day
THYROID-STIMULATING HORMONE
L-Thyroxine 0.05-0.2 mg daily according to T_4 levels
VASOPRESSIN
Intranasal desmopressin-rhinal tube 5-20 μg twice daily Oral DDAVP 300-600 μg daily, usually in divided doses

DDAVP, desmopressin; FSH, follicle-stimulating hormone; GnRH; gonadotropin-releasing hormone; hCG, human chorionic gonadotropin.

Doses shown should be individualized and reassessed during stress, surgery, or pregnancy. Male and female fertility management are fully discussed in Chapter 17.

example, many patients with preoperative hyperprolactinemia due to tumor pressure on stalk structures continue to have hyperprolactinemia even after tumors are surgically debulked. Likewise, hyperprolactinemia occurs in 50% of patients treated with whole brain radiation, the most common endocrine disturbance.[880]

Posterior Pituitary

Diabetes insipidus occurs commonly after pituitary surgery, and hyponatremia can also develop as the second of three phases of postoperative diabetes insipidus, or it can develop without evidence of diabetes insipidus after surgery. This subject is comprehensively covered in Chapter 9.

Screening for Pituitary Failure

Because the onset of hypopituitarism may be extremely slow, subclinical pituitary failure is often not apparent to the patient or physician. Screening for pituitary dysfunction should be undertaken in patients with hypothalamic or pituitary mass lesions, developmental craniofacial abnormalities, inflammatory disorders, brain granulomatous disease, prior head or neck irradiation, head trauma, prior skull base surgery, patients with newly discovered empty sella, and those who have previously experienced pregnancy-associated hemorrhage or blood pressure changes.[888]

Because hypopituitarism can develop insidiously and is often not readily clinically apparent, screening of appropriate patients is important to prevent long-term morbidity. Therefore, all patients harboring hypothalamic or pituitary masses should be screened for hypopituitarism. PRL should be measured because many patients with hypopituitarism also present with secondary hyperprolactinemia. Up to two thirds of patients harboring pituitary macroadenomas, craniopharyngiomas, and other parasellar lesions have compromised pituitary reserve function. Less commonly, patients with intrasellar aneurysms, pituitary metastases, parasellar meningiomas, optic gliomas, and hypothalamic astrocytomas also have pituitary failure. Although about a third of patients with hypopituitarism undergoing pituitary surgery recover function after decompression, about 25% of patients experience further loss of pituitary function after surgery and therefore should be screened annually. Treatment of pituitary failure is fully described above (Table 8–36).

REFERENCES

1. Bernard C. Physiologie; chiens rendus diabetiques. C R Soc Biol 1849;1:60.
2. Marie P. On two cases of acromegaly: marked hypertrophy of the upper and lower limbs and the head. Rev Med 1886;6:297-333.
3. Cushing H. Partial hypophysectomy for acromegaly: with remarks on the function of the hypophysis. Ann Surg 1909;50:1002-1017.
4. Cushing H. Surgical experiences with pituitary disorders. JAMA 1914;63:1515-1525.
5. Harris GW. Neural control of pituitary gland. Physiol Rev 1948;28: 139-179.
6. Chanson P, Daujat F, Young J, et al. Normal pituitary hypertrophy as a frequent cause of pituitary incidentaloma: a follow-up study. J Clin Endocrinol Metab 2001;86:3009-3015.
7. Etchevers HC, Vincent C, Le Douarin NM, Couly GF. The cephalic neural crest provides pericytes and smooth muscle cells to all blood vessels of the face and forebrain. Development 2001; 128:1059-1068.
8. Takuma N, Sheng HZ, Furuta Y, et al. Formation of Rathke's pouch requires dual induction from the diencephalon. Development 1998;125:4835-4840.
9. Gleiberman AS, Fedtsova NG, Rosenfeld MG. Tissue interactions in the induction of anterior pituitary: role of the ventral diencephalon, mesenchyme, and notochord. Dev Biol 1999;213:340-353.
10. Sheng HZ, Westphal H. Early steps in pituitary organogenesis. Trends Genet 1999;15:236-240.
11. Dasen JS, O'Connell SM, Flynn SE, et al. Reciprocal interactions of Pit1 and GATA2 mediate signaling gradient—induced determination of pituitary cell types. Cell 1999;97:587-598.
12. Andersen B, Rosenfeld MG. POU domain factors in the neuroendocrine system: lessons from developmental biology provide insights into human disease. Endocr Rev 2001;22:2-35.
13. Treier M, Gleiberman AS, O'Connell SM, et al. Multistep signaling requirements for pituitary organogenesis in vivo. Genes Dev 1998;12:1691-1704.
14. Asa SL, Kovacs K, Laszlo FA, Domokos I, Ezrin C. Human fetal adenohypophysis. Histologic and immunocytochemical analysis. Neuroendocrinology 1986;43:308-316.
15. Dubois PM, Hemming FJ. Fetal development and regulation of pituitary cell types. J Electron Microsc Tech 1991;19:2-20.

16. Zhu X, Lin CR, Prefontaine GG, Tollkuhn J, Rosenfeld MG. Genetic control of pituitary development and hypopituitarism. Curr Opin Genet Dev 2005;15:332-340.
17. Sheng HZ, Zhadanov AB, Mosinger B Jr, et al. Specification of pituitary cell lineages by the LIM homeobox gene *Lhx3*. Science 1996;272:1004-1007.
18. Lanctot C, Gauthier Y, Drouin J. Pituitary homeobox 1 *(Ptx1)* is differentially expressed during pituitary development. Endocrinology 1999;140:1416-1422.
19. Semina EV, Datson NA, Leysens NJ, et al. Exclusion of epidermal growth factor and high-resolution physical mapping across the Rieger syndrome locus. Am J Hum Genet 1996;59:1288-1296.
20. Lu MF, Pressman C, Dyer R, Johnson RL, Martin JF. Function of Rieger syndrome gene in left-right asymmetry and craniofacial development. Nature 1999;401:276-278.
21. Martin D, Camper, S. Genetic regulation of forebrain and pituitary development. In Rapaport R, Amselem S (eds). Hypothalamic-Pituitary Development: Genetic and Clinical Aspects. Basel: Karger, 2001:1-12.
22. Muscatelli F, Strom TM, Walker AP, et al. Mutations in the *DAX-1* gene give rise to both X-linked adrenal hypoplasia congenita and hypogonadotropic hypogonadism. Nature 1994;372:672-676.
23. Tabarin A, Achermann JC, Recan D, et al. A novel mutation in *DAX1* causes delayed-onset adrenal insufficiency and incomplete hypogonadotropic hypogonadism. J Clin Invest 2000;105: 321-328.
24. Lamolet B, Pulichino AM, Lamonerie T, et al. A pituitary cell-restricted T box factor, Tpit, activates POMC transcription in cooperation with Pitx homeoproteins. Cell 2001;104:849-859.
25. Stanfield JP. The blood supply of the human pituitary gland. J Anat 1960;94:257-273.
26. Bergland RM, Page RB. Pituitary-brain vascular relations: a new paradigm. Science 1979;204:18-24.
27. Musolino NR, Marino Junior R, Bronstein MD. Headache in acromegaly: dramatic improvement with the somatostatin analogue SMS 201-995. Clin J Pain 1990;6:243-245.
28. Arafah BM, Prunty D, Ybarra J, Hlavin ML, Selman WR. The dominant role of increased intrasellar pressure in the pathogenesis of hypopituitarism, hyperprolactinemia, and headaches in patients with pituitary adenomas. J Clin Endocrinol Metab 2000;85: 1789-1793.
29. Brain Tumor Registry of Japan. Neurol Med Chir (Tokyo) 1992;32(7 spec no):381-547.
30. Melmed S. Mechanisms for pituitary tumorigenesis: the plastic pituitary. J Clin Invest 2003;112:1603-1618.
31. Thorner MO, Perryman RL, Cronin MJ, et al. Somatotroph hyperplasia. Successful treatment of acromegaly by removal of a pancreatic islet tumor secreting a growth hormone-releasing factor. J Clin Invest 1982;70:965-977.
32. Sano T, Asa SL, Kovacs K. Growth hormone–releasing hormone–producing tumors: clinical, biochemical, and morphological manifestations. Endocr Rev 1988;9:357-373.
33. Mayo KE, Hammer RE, Swanson LW, Brinster RL, Rosenfeld MG, Evans RM. Dramatic pituitary hyperplasia in transgenic mice expressing a human growth hormone–releasing factor gene. Mol Endocrinol 1988;2:606-612.
34. Herman V, Fagin J, Gonsky R, Kovacs K, Melmed S. Clonal origin of pituitary adenomas. JClin Endocrinol Metab 1990;71:1427-1433.
35. Schulte HM, Oldfield EH, Allolio B, et al. Clonal composition of pituitary adenomas in patients with Cushing's disease: determination by X-chromosome inactivation analysis. J Clin Endocrinol Metab 1991;73:1302-1308.
36. Alexander JM, Biller BM, Bikkal H, et al. Clinically nonfunctioning pituitary tumors are monoclonal in origin. J Clin Invest 1990;86: 336-340.
37. Spada A, Vallar L. G-protein oncogenes in acromegaly. Horm Res 1992;38:90-93.
38. Zhang X, Sun H, Danila DC, et al. Loss of expression of GADD45 gamma, a growth inhibitory gene, in human pituitary adenomas: implications for tumorigenesis. J Clin Endocrinol Metab 2002;87: 1262-1267.
39. Levy A, Lightman S. Molecular defects in the pathogenesis of pituitary tumours. Front Neuroendocrinol 2003;24:94-127.
40. Dotsch J, Kiess W, Hanze J, et al. $G_s\alpha$ mutation at codon 201 in pituitary adenoma causing gigantism in a 6-year-old boy with McCune-Albright syndrome. J Clin Endocrinol Metab 1996;81: 3839-3842.
41. Struthers RS, Vale WW, Arias C, Sawchenko PE, Montminy MR. Somatotroph hypoplasia and dwarfism in transgenic mice expressing a non-phosphorylatable CREB mutant. Nature 1991;350: 622-624.
42. Bertherat J, Chanson P, Montminy M. The cyclic adenosine 3′,5′-monophosphate-responsive factor CREB is constitutively activated in human somatotroph adenomas. Mol Endocrinol 1995;9: 777-783.
43. Kaltsas GA, Nomikos P, Kontogeorgos G, et al. Clinical review: Diagnosis and management of pituitary carcinomas. J Clin Endocrinol Metab 2005;90:3089-3099.
44. Karga HJ, Alexander JM, Hedley-Whyte ET, et al. Ras mutations in human pituitary tumors. J Clin Endocrinol Metab 1992;74: 914-919.
45. Pei L, Melmed S, Scheithauer B, et al. H-ras mutations in human pituitary carcinoma metastases. J Clin Endocrinol Metab 1994;78: 842-846.
46. Herman V, Drazin NZ, Gonsky R, Melmed S. Molecular screening of pituitary adenomas for gene mutations and rearrangements. J Clin Endocrinol Metab 1993;77:50-55.
47. Pei L, Melmed S. Isolation and characterization of a pituitary tumor-transforming gene (PTTG). Mol Endocrinol 1997;11: 433-441.
48. Zhang X, Horwitz GA, Heaney AP, et al. Pituitary tumor transforming gene (PTTG) expression in pituitary adenomas. J Clin Endocrinol Metab 1999;84:761-767.
49. Heaney AP, Horwitz GA, Wang Z, Singson R, Melmed S. Early involvement of estrogen-induced pituitary tumor transforming gene and fibroblast growth factor expression in prolactinoma pathogenesis. Nat Med 1999;5:1317-1321.
50. Zou H, McGarry TJ, Bernal T, Kirschner MW. Identification of a vertebrate sister-chromatid separation inhibitor involved in transformation and tumorigenesis. Science 1999;285:418-422.
51. Yu R, Heaney AP, Lu W, et al. Pituitary tumor transforming gene causes aneuploidy and p53-dependent and p53-independent apoptosis. J Biol Chem 2000;275:36502-36505.
52. Tanaka C, Kimura T, Yang P, et al. Analysis of loss of heterozygosity on chromosome 11 and infrequent inactivation of the *MEN1* gene in sporadic pituitary adenomas. J Clin Endocrinol Metab 1998;83:2631-2634.
53. Tanaka C, Yoshimoto K, Yamada S, et al. Absence of germ-line mutations of the multiple endocrine neoplasia type 1 (MEN1) gene in familial pituitary adenoma in contrast to MEN1 in Japanese. J Clin Endocrinol Metab 1998;83:960-965.
54. Prezant TR, Levine J, Melmed S. Molecular characterization of the *MEN1* tumor suppressor gene in sporadic pituitary tumors. J Clin Endocrinol Metab 1998;83:1388-1391.
55. Pei L, Melmed S, Scheithauer B, et al. Frequent loss of heterozygosity at the retinoblastoma susceptibility gene (RB) locus in aggressive pituitary tumors: evidence for a chromosome 13 tumor suppressor gene other than RB. Cancer Res 1995;55:1613-1616.
56. Levy A, Hall L, Yeudall WA, Lightman SL. p53 gene mutations in pituitary adenomas: rare events. Clin Endocrinol (Oxf) 1994;41: 809-814.
57. Faccenda E, Melmed S, Bevan JS, Eidne KA. Structure of the thyrotrophin-releasing hormone receptor in human pituitary adenomas. Clin Endocrinol (Oxf) 1996;44:341-347.
58. Kaye PV, Hapgood J, Millar RP. Absence of mutations in exon 3 of the GnRH receptor in human gonadotroph adenomas. Clin Endocrinol (Oxf) 1997;47:549-554.
59. Hashimoto K, Koga M, Motomura T, et al. Identification of alternatively spliced messenger ribonucleic acid encoding truncated growth hormone–releasing hormone receptor in human pituitary adenomas. J Clin Endocrinol Metab 1995;80:2933-2939.
60. Greenman Y, Prager D, Melmed S. The IGF-I receptor sub-membrane domain is intact in GH-secreting pituitary tumours. Clin Endocrinol (Oxf) 1995;42:169-172.
61. Friedman E, Adams EF, Hoog A, et al. Normal structural dopamine type 2 receptor gene in prolactin-secreting and other pituitary tumors. J Clin Endocrinol Metab 1994;78:568-574.
62. Ezzat S, Zheng L, Zhu XF, et al. Targeted expression of a human pituitary tumor–derived isoform of FGF receptor-4 recapitulates pituitary tumorigenesis. J Clin Invest 2002;109:69-78.

63. Shimon I, Huttner A, Said J, et al. Heparin-binding secretory transforming gene *(hst)* facilitates rat lactotrope cell tumorigenesis and induces prolactin gene transcription. J Clin Invest 1996;97: 187-195.
64. Gonsky R, Herman V, Melmed S, Fagin J. Transforming DNA sequences present in human prolactin-secreting pituitary tumors. Mol Endocrinol 1991;5:1687-1695.
65. Casey M, Vaughan CJ, He J, et al. Mutations in the protein kinase A R1α regulatory subunit cause familial cardiac myxomas and Carney complex. J Clin Invest 2000;106:R31-R38.
66. Kirschner LS, Carney JA, Pack SD, et al. Mutations of the gene encoding the protein kinase A type I-α regulatory subunit in patients with the Carney complex. Nat Genet 2000;26:89-92.
67. Molitch ME. Pituitary incidentalomas. Endocrinol Metab Clin North Am 1997;26:725-740.
68. Chanson P, Young, J. Pituitary incidentalomas. Endocrinologist 2003;13:124-135.
69. Hall WA, Luciano MG, Doppman JL, Patronas NJ, Oldfield EH. Pituitary magnetic resonance imaging in normal human volunteers: occult adenomas in the general population. Ann Intern Med 1994;120:817-820.
70. Howlett TA, Como J, Aron DC. Management of pituitary incidentalomas. A survey of British and American endocrinologists. Endocrinol Metab Clin North Am 2000;29:223-230, xi.
71. Sanno N, Oyama K, Tahara S, et al. A survey of pituitary incidentaloma in Japan. Eur J Endocrinol 2003;149:123-127.
72. Sam S, Molitch ME. The pituitary mass: diagnosis and management. Rev Endocr Metab Disord 2005;6:55-62.
73. Kovacs K, Horvath E, Stefaneanu L, et al. Pituitary adenoma producing growth hormone and adrenocorticotropin: a histological, immunocytochemical, electron microscopic, and in situ hybridization study. Case report. J Neurosurg 1998;88:1111-1115.
74. Saccomanno K, Bassetti M, Lania A, et al. Immunodetection of glycoprotein hormone subunits in nonfunctioning and glycoprotein hormone–secreting pituitary adenomas. J Endocrinol Invest 1997;20:59-64.
75. Mukherjee JJ, Islam N, Kaltsas G, et al. Clinical, radiological and pathological features of patients with Rathke's cleft cysts: tumors that may recur. J Clin Endocrinol Metab 1997;82:2357-2362.
76. Saeki N, Tamaki K, Murai H, et al. Long-term outcome of endocrine function in patients with neurohypophyseal germinomas. Endocr J 2000;47:83-89.
77. el-Mahdy W, Powell M. Transsphenoidal management of 28 symptomatic Rathke's cleft cysts, with special reference to visual and hormonal recovery. Neurosurgery 1998;42:7-16; discussion 16-17.
78. Freda PU, Wardlaw SL, Post KD. Unusual causes of sellar/parasellar masses in a large transsphenoidal surgical series. J Clin Endocrinol Metab 1996;81:3455-3459.
79. Cohen JE, Abdallah JA, Garrote M. Massive rupture of suprasellar dermoid cyst into ventricles. Case illustration. J Neurosurg 1997; 87:963.
80. Lewis AJ, Cooper PW, Kassel EE, Schwartz ML. Squamous cell carcinoma arising in a suprasellar epidermoid cyst. Case report. J Neurosurg 1983;59:538-541.
81. Schaller B, Kirsch E, Tolnay M, Mindermann T. Symptomatic granular cell tumor of the pituitary gland: case report and review of the literature. Neurosurgery 1998;42:166-170; discussion 170-161.
82. Volpe R, Mazabraud A. A clinicopathologic review of 25 cases of chordoma (a pleomorphic and metastasizing neoplasm). Am J Surg Pathol 1983;7:161-170.
83. Rosenberg AE, Nielsen GP, Keel SB, et al. Chondrosarcoma of the base of the skull: a clinicopathologic study of 200 cases with emphasis on its distinction from chordoma. Am J Surg Pathol 1999;23:1370-1378.
84. Karavitaki N, Brufani C, Warner JT, et al. Craniopharyngiomas in children and adults: systematic analysis of 121 cases with long-term follow-up. Clin Endocrinol (Oxf) 2005;62:397-409.
85. Weiner HL, Wisoff JH, Rosenberg ME, et al. Craniopharyngiomas: a clinicopathological analysis of factors predictive of recurrence and functional outcome. Neurosurgery 1994;35:1001-1010; discussion 1010-1001.
86. Fahlbusch R, Honegger J, Paulus W, Huk W, Buchfelder M. Surgical treatment of craniopharyngiomas: experience with 168 patients. J Neurosurg 1999;90:237-250.
87. Honegger J, Buchfelder M, Fahlbusch R. Surgical treatment of craniopharyngiomas: endocrinological results. J Neurosurg 1999;90: 251-257.
88. Maira G, Anile C, Albanese A, et al. The role of transsphenoidal surgery in the treatment of craniopharyngiomas. J Neurosurg 2004;100:445-451.
89. Nozaki K, Nagata I, Yoshida K, Kikuchi H. Intrasellar meningioma: case report and review of the literature. Surg Neurol 1997;47:447-452; discussion 452-444.
90. Beems T, Grotenhuis JA, Wesseling P. Meningioma of the pituitary stalk without dural attachment: case report and review of the literature. Neurosurgery 1999;45:1474-1477.
91. Collet-Solberg PF, Sernyak H, Satin-Smith M, et al. Endocrine outcome in long-term survivors of low-grade hypothalamic/chiasmatic glioma. Clin Endocrinol (Oxf) 1997;47:79-85.
92. Gokalp HZ, Deda H, Baskaya MK, et al. Pituitary abscesses. Report of three cases. Neurosurg Rev 1994;17:199-203.
93. Wolansky LJ, Gallagher JD, Heary RF, et al. MRI of pituitary abscess: two cases and review of the literature. Neuroradiology 1997;39:499-503.
94. Jain KC, Varma A, Mahapatra AK. Pituitary abscess: a series of six cases. Br J Neurosurg 1997;11:139-143.
95. Freda PU, Post KD. Differential diagnosis of sellar masses. Endocrinol Metab Clin North Am 1999;28:81-117, vi.
96. Telzak EE, Cote RJ, Gold JW, et al. Extrapulmonary *Pneumocystis carinii* infections. Rev Infect Dis 1990;12:380-386.
97. Ashkan K, Papadopoulos MC, Casey AT, et al. Sellar tuberculoma: report of two cases. Acta Neurochir 1997;139:523-525.
98. Berger SA, Edberg SC, David G. Infectious disease in the sella turcica. Rev Infect Dis 1986;8:747-755.
99. Gazioglu N, Ak H, Oz B, et al. Silent pituitary tuberculoma associated with pituitary adenoma. Acta Neurochir 1999;141: 785-786.
100. Dutta P, Bhansali A, Singh P, Bhat MH. Suprasellar tubercular abscess presenting as panhypopituitarism: a common lesion in an uncommon site with a brief review of literature. Pituitary 2006;9: 73-77.
101. Capra M, Wherrett D, Weitzman S, et al. Pituitary stalk thickening and primary central nervous system lymphoma. J Neurooncol 2004;67:227-231.
102. Giustina A, Gola M, Doga M, Rosei EA. Clinical review 136: primary lymphoma of the pituitary: an emerging clinical entity. J Clin Endocrinol Metab 2001;86:4567-4575.
103. Brat DJ, Scheithauer BW, Staugaitis SM, et al. Pituicytoma: a distinctive low-grade glioma of the neurohypophysis. Am J Surg Pathol 2000;24:362-368.
104. Figarella-Branger D, Dufour H, Fernandez C, et al. Pituicytomas, a mis-diagnosed benign tumor of the neurohypophysis: report of three cases. Acta Neuropathol (Berl) 2002;104:313-319.
105. Chen KT. Crush cytology of pituicytoma. Diagn Cytopathol 2005; 33:255-257.
106. Newman LS, Rose CS, Maier LA. Sarcoidosis. N Engl J Med 1997; 336:1224-1234.
107. Bell NH. Endocrine complications of sarcoidosis. Endocrinol Metab Clin North Am 1991;20:645-654.
108. Sharma OP. Neurosarcoidosis: a personal perspective based on the study of 37 patients. Chest 1997;112:220-228.
109. Pitale SU, Camacho PM, Gordon DL. Central nervous sysstem involvement in sarcoidosis presenting as a recurrent pituitary mass. Endocrinologist 2000;10:429-431.
110. Tikoo RK, Kupersmith MJ, Finlay JL. Treatment of refractory neurosarcoidosis with cladribine. N Engl J Med 2004;350: 1798-1799.
111. Kaltsas GA, Powles TB, Evanson J, et al. Hypothalamo-pituitary abnormalities in adult patients with langerhans cell histiocytosis: clinical, endocrinological, and radiological features and response to treatment. J Clin Endocrinol Metab 2000;85:1370-1376.
112. Braunstein GD, Kohler PO. Pituitary function in Hand-Schüller-Christian disease. Evidence for deficient growth-hormone release in patients with short stature. N Engl J Med 1972;286: 1225-1229.
113. Vadakekalam J, Stamos T, Shenker Y. Sometimes the hooves do belong to zebras! An unusual case of hypopituitarism. J Clin Endocrinol Metab 1995;80:17-20.

114. Komninos J, Vlassopoulou V, Protopapa D, et al. Tumors metastatic to the pituitary gland: case report and literature review. J Clin Endocrinol Metab 2004;89:574-580.
115. Rivera JA. Lymphocytic hypophysitis: disease spectrum and approach to diagnosis and therapy. Pituitary 2006;9:35-45.
116. Losa M, Grasso M, Giugni E, et al. Metastatic prostatic adenocarcinoma presenting as a pituitary mass: shrinkage of the lesion and clinical improvement with medical treatment. Prostate 1997; 32:241-245.
117. Schubiger O, Haller D. Metastases to the pituitary-hypothalamic axis. An MR study of 7 symptomatic patients. Neuroradiology 1992;34:131-134.
118. Braun J, Schuldes H, Berkefeld J, et al. Panhypopituitarism associated with severe retroperitoneal fibrosis. Clin Endocrinol (Oxf) 2001;54:273-276.
119. Caturegli P, Newschaffer C, Olivi A, et al. Autoimmune hypophysitis. Endocr Rev 2005;26:599-614.
120. Leung GK, Lopes MB, Thorner MO, et al. Primary hypophysitis: a single-center experience in 16 cases. J Neurosurg 2004;101: 262-271.
121. Bellastella A, Bizzarro A, Coronella C, et al. Lymphocytic hypophysitis: a rare or underestimated disease? Eur J Endocrinol 2003;149: 363-376.
122. Cheung CC, Ezzat S, Smyth HS, Asa SL. The spectrum and significance of primary hypophysitis. J Clin Endocrinol Metab 2001; 86:1048-1053.
123. Vidal S, Rotondo F, Horvath E, Kovacs K, Scheithauer BW. Immunocytochemical localization of mast cells in lymphocytic hypophysitis. Am J Clin Pathol 2002;117:478-483.
124. Unluhizarci K, Bayram F, Colak R, et al. Distinct radiological and clinical appearance of lymphocytic hypophysitis. J Clin Endocrinol Metab 2001;86:1861-1864.
125. Gagneja H, Arafah B, Taylor HC. Histologically proven lymphocytic hypophysitis: spontaneous resolution and subsequent pregnancy. Mayo Clin Proc 1999;74:150-154.
126. Ishihara T, Hino M, Kurahachi H, et al. Long-term clinical course of two cases of lymphocytic adenohypophysitis. Endocr J 1996; 43:433-440.
127. Lee YJ, Lin JC, Shen EY, et al. Loss of visibility of the neurohypophysis as a sign of central diabetes insipidus. Eur J Radiol 1996; 21:233-235.
128. Muir A, Maclaren NK. Autoimmune diseases of the adrenal glands, parathyroid glands, gonads, and hypothalamic-pituitary axis. Endocrinol Metab Clin North Am 1991;20:619-644.
129. Crock PA. Cytosolic autoantigens in lymphocytic hypophysitis. J Clin Endocrinol Metab 1998;83:609-618.
130. Nishiki M, Murakami Y, Ozawa Y, Kato Y. Serum antibodies to human pituitary membrane antigens in patients with autoimmune lymphocytic hypophysitis and infundibuloneurohypophysitis. Clin Endocrinol (Oxf) 2001;54:327-333.
131. Tanaka S, Tatsumi KI, Kimura M, et al. Detection of autoantibodies against the pituitary-specific proteins in patients with lymphocytic hypophysitis. Eur J Endocrinol 2002;147:767-775.
132. Burke CW, Moore RA, Rees LH, et al. Isolated ACTH deficiency and TSH deficiency in the adult. J R Soc Med 1979;72:328-335.
133. Honegger J, Fahlbusch R, Bornemann A, et al. Lymphocytic and granulomatous hypophysitis: experience with nine cases. Neurosurgery 1997;40:713-722; discussion 722-713.
134. Shimizu C, Kubo M, Kijima H, et al. Giant cell granulamatous hypophysitis with remarkable uptake on gallium-67 scintigraphy. Clin Endocrinol (Oxf) 1998;49:131-134.
135. Hayashi H, Yamada K, Kuroki T, et al. Lymphocytic hypophysitis and pulmonary sarcoidosis. Report of a case. Am J Clin Pathol 1991;95:506-511.
136. Toth M, Szabo P, Racz K, et al. Granulomatous hypophysitis associated with Takayasu's disease. Clin Endocrinol (Oxf) 1996;45: 499-503.
137. Tauber JP, Babin T, Tauber MT, et al. Long term effects of continuous subcutaneous infusion of the somatostatin analog octreotide in the treatment of acromegaly. J Clin Endocrinol Metab 1989;68: 917-924.
138. Maccagnan P, Macedo CL, Kayath MJ, Nogueira RG, Abucham J. Conservative management of pituitary apoplexy: a prospective study. J Clin Endocrinol Metab 1995;80:2190-2197.
139. Kovacs K. Sheehan syndrome. Lancet 2003;361:520-522.
140. Kelestimur F. Sheehan's syndrome. Pituitary 2003;6:181-188.
141. Yen SSC. Chronic anovulation due to CNS-hypothalamic-pituitary dysfunction. In Yen SSC, Jaffe RB, eds. Reproductive endocrinology, 3rd ed. Philadelphia: Saunders, 1991:631-689.
142. Goswami R, Kochupillai N, Crock PA, et al. Pituitary autoimmunity in patients with Sheehan's syndrome. J Clin Endocrinol Metab 2002;87:4137-4141.
143. Arafah BM, Harrington JF, Madhoun ZT, Selman WR. Improvement of pituitary function after surgical decompression for pituitary tumor apoplexy. J Clin Endocrinol Metab 1990;71:323-328.
144. Wakai S, Fukushima T, Teramoto A, Sano K. Pituitary apoplexy: its incidence and clinical significance. J Neurosurg 1981;55: 187-193.
145. Lubina A, Olchovsky D, Berezin M, et al. Management of pituitary apoplexy: clinical experience with 40 patients. Acta Neurochir (Wien) 2005;147:151-157; discussion 157.
146. Elsasser Imboden PN, De Tribolet N, Lobrinus A, et al. Apoplexy in pituitary macroadenoma: eight patients presenting in 12 months. Medicine (Baltimore) 2005;84:188-196.
147. Zayour DH, Selman WR, Arafah BM. Extreme elevation of intrasellar pressure in patients with pituitary tumor apoplexy: relation to pituitary function. J Clin Endocrinol Metab 2004;89:5649-5654.
148. Ayuk J, McGregor EJ, Mitchell RD, Gittoes NJ. Acute management of pituitary apoplexy—surgery or conservative management? Clin Endocrinol (Oxf) 2004;61:747-752.
149. Turgut M. Spinal congenital dermal sinus associated with thoracic meningocele. Neurosurg Focus 2004;16:1 p following ECP1.
150. Insel JR, Dhanjal N. Pituitary infarction resulting from intranasal cocaine abuse. Endocr Pract 2004;10:478-482.
151. Lam KS, Sham MM, Tam SC, et al. Hypopituitarism after tuberculous meningitis in childhood. Ann Intern Med 1993;118:701-706.
152. Case records of the Massachusetts General Hospital. Weekly clinicopathological exercises. Case 17-1980. N Engl J Med 1980;302: 1015-1023.
153. Van Hilten BJ, Roos RA, De Bakker HM, De Beer FC. Periodic fever: an unusual manifestation of a recurrent Rathke's cleft. J Neurol Neurosurg Psychiatry 1990;53:533.
154. Bills DC, Meyer FB, Laws ER Jr, et al. A retrospective analysis of pituitary apoplexy. Neurosurgery 1993;33:602-608; discussion 608-609.
155. Rehman HU, Atkin SL. Growth hormone–secreting pituitary macroadenoma and meningioma in a woman—a case report and review of the literature. Endocrinologist 2001;11:335-337.
156. Macpherson P, Hadley DM, Teasdale E, Teasdale G. Pituitary microadenomas. Does gadolinium enhance their demonstration? Neuroradiology 1989;31:293-298.
157. Witte RJ, Mark LP, Daniels DL, Haughton VM. Radiographic evaluation of the pituitary and anterior hypothalamus. In DeGroot LJ, Jameson JL, eds. Endocrinology, 4th ed. Philadelphia: WB Saunders, 2001:257-268.
158. Kucharczyk W, Peck WW, Kelly WM, et al. Rathke cleft cysts: CT, MR imaging, and pathologic features. Radiology 1987;165: 491-495.
159. Elster AD, Chen MY, Williams DW III, Key LL. Pituitary gland: MR imaging of physiologic hypertrophy in adolescence [see comments]. Radiology 1990;174:681-685.
160. Wolpert SM, Molitch ME, Goldman JA, Wood JB. Size, shape, and appearance of the normal female pituitary gland. AJR Am J Roentgenol 1984;143:377-381.
161. FitzPatrick M, Tartaglino LM, Hollander MD, et al. Imaging of sellar and parasellar pathology. Radiol Clin North Am 1999;37:101-121, x.
162. Pressman BD. Pituitary imaging. In Melmed S, ed. The Pituitary. Malden, MA: Blackwell Science, 2001:663-686.
163. Kucharczyk W, Lenkinski RE, Kucharczyk J, Henkelman RM. The effect of phospholipid vesicles on the NMR relaxation of water: an explanation for the MR appearance of the neurohypophysis? AJNR Am J Neuroradiol 1990;11:693-700.
164. Sheehan JP, Niranjan A, Sheehan JM, et al. Stereotactic radiosurgery for pituitary adenomas: an intermediate review of its safety, efficacy, and role in the neurosurgical treatment armamentarium. J Neurosurg 2005;102:678-691.
165. Elster AD, Sanders TG, Vines FS, Chen MY. Size and shape of the pituitary gland during pregnancy and post partum: measurement with MR imaging. Radiology 1991;181:531-535.

166. Turner HE, Nagy Z, Gatter KC, et al. Angiogenesis in pituitary adenomas and the normal pituitary gland. J Clin Endocrinol Metab 2000;85:1159-1162.
167. de Herder WW, Reijs AE, Kwekkeboom DJ, et al. In vivo imaging of pituitary tumours using a radiolabelled dopamine D_2 receptor radioligand. Clin Endocrinol (Oxf) 1996;45:755-767.
168. Arnold AC. Neuroophthalmologic evaluation of pituitary disorders. In Melmed S, ed. The Pituitary. Malden, MA: Blackwell Science, 2001:687-708.
169. Hoyt WF. Correlative functional anatomy of the optic chiasm. 1969. Clin Neurosurg 1970;17:189-208.
170. Henderson WR. The pituitary adenomata. A follow-up study of the surgical results in 338 cases. Br J Surg 1939;26:811-921.
171. Anderson D, Faber P, Marcovitz S, et al. Pituitary tumors and the ophthalmologist. Ophthalmology 1983;90:1265-1270.
172. Poon A, McNeill P, Harper A, O'Day J. Patterns of visual loss associated with pituitary macroadenomas. Aust N Z J Ophthalmol 1995;23:107-115.
173. Ikeda H, Yoshimoto T. Visual disturbances in patients with pituitary adenoma. Acta Neurol Scand 1995;92:157-160.
174. Schloffer H. Erfolgreiche operation eines hypohysentumors auf nasalen wege. Wein Klin Wochenschr 1907;20(6):621-624.
175. Steinmeier R, Fahlbusch R, Ganslandt O, et al. Intraoperative magnetic resonance imaging with the magnetom open scanner: concepts, neurosurgical indications, and procedures: a preliminary report. Neurosurgery 1998;43:739-747; discussion 747-738.
176. Webb SM, Rigla M, Wagner A, et al. Recovery of hypopituitarism after neurosurgical treatment of pituitary adenomas. J Clin Endocrinol Metab 1999;84:3696-3700.
177. Barker FG 2nd, Klibanski A, Swearingen B. Transsphenoidal surgery for pituitary tumors in the United States, 1996-2000: mortality, morbidity, and the effects of hospital and surgeon volume. J Clin Endocrinol Metab 2003;88:4709-4719.
178. Jane JA Jr, Dumont AS, Sheehan JP, Laws ER Jr. Surgical techniques in transsphenoidal surgery: what is the standard of care in pituitary adenomas surgery? Curr Opin Endocrinol Diabetes 2004;14: 264-270.
179. Olson BR, Rubino D, Gumowski J, Oldfield EH. Isolated hyponatremia after transsphenoidal pituitary surgery. J Clin Endocrinol Metab 1995;80:85-91.
180. Nemergut EC, Dumont AS, Barry UT, Laws ER. Perioperative management of patients undergoing transsphenoidal pituitary surgery. Anesth Analg 2005;101:1170-1181.
181. Guinan EM, Lowy C, Stanhope N, et al. Cognitive effects of pituitary tumours and their treatments: two case studies and an investigation of 90 patients. J Neurol Neurosurg Psychiatry 1998;65: 870-876.
182. Peace KA, Orme SM, Padayatty SJ, et al. Cognitive dysfunction in patients with pituitary tumour who have been treated with transfrontal or transsphenoidal surgery or medication. Clin Endocrinol (Oxf) 1998;49:391-396.
183. Jalali R, Brada M, Perks JR, et al. Stereotactic conformal radiotherapy for pituitary adenomas: technique and preliminary experience. Clin Endocrinol (Oxf) 2000;52:695-702.
184. Barrande G, Pittino-Lungo M, Coste J, et al. Hormonal and metabolic effects of radiotherapy in acromegaly: long-term results in 128 patients followed in a single center. J Clin Endocrinol Metab 2000;85:3779-3785.
185. McCord MW, Buatti JM, Fennell EM, et al. Radiotherapy for pituitary adenoma: long-term outcome and sequelae. Int J Radiat Oncol Biol Phys 1997;39:437-444.
186. Brada M, Rajan B, Traish D, et al. The long-term efficacy of conservative surgery and radiotherapy in the control of pituitary adenomas. Clin Endocrinol (Oxf) 1993;38:571-578.
187. Biermasz NR, van Dulken H, Roelfsema F. Long-term follow-up results of postoperative radiotherapy in 36 patients with acromegaly. J Clin Endocrinol Metab 2000;85:2476-2482.
188. Simmons NE, Laws ER Jr. Glioma occurrence after sellar irradiation: case report and review. Neurosurgery 1998;42:172-178.
189. Erfurth EM, Bulow B, Mikoczy Z, Hagmar L. Incidence of a second tumor in hypopituitary patients operated for pituitary tumors. J Clin Endocrinol Metab 2001;86:659-662.
190. Brada M, Ford D, Ashley S, et al. Risk of second brain tumour after conservative surgery and radiotherapy for pituitary adenoma. BMJ 1992;304:1343-1346.
191. Tsang RW, Laperriere NJ, Simpson WJ, et al. Glioma arising after radiation therapy for pituitary adenoma. A report of four patients and estimation of risk. Cancer 1993;72:2227-2233.
192. Minniti G, Traish D, Ashley S, et al. Risk of second brain tumor after conservative surgery and radiotherapy for pituitary adenoma: update after an additional 10 years. J Clin Endocrinol Metab 2005;90:800-804.
193. Tomlinson JW, Holden N, Hills RK, et al. Association between premature mortality and hypopituitarism. West Midlands Prospective Hypopituitary Study Group. Lancet 2001;357:425-431.
194. Erfurth EM, Bulow B, Svahn-Tapper G, et al. Risk factors for cerebrovascular deaths in patients operated and irradiated for pituitary tumors. J Clin Endocrinol Metab 2002;87:4892-4899.
195. Millar JL, Spry NA, Lamb DS, Delahunt J. Blindness in patients after external beam irradiation for pituitary adenomas: two cases occurring after small daily fractional doses. Clin Oncol (R Coll Radiol) 1991;3:291-294.
196. Jones JI, D'Ercole AJ, Camacho-Hubner C, Clemmons DR. Phosphorylation of insulin-like growth factor (IGF)-binding protein 1 in cell culture and in vivo: effects on affinity for IGF-I. Proc Natl Acad Sci U S A 1991;88:7481-7485.
197. al-Mefty O, Kersh JE, Routh A, Smith RR. The long-term side effects of radiation therapy for benign brain tumors in adults. J Neurosurg 1990;73:502-512.
198. Peace KA, Orme SM, Sebastian JP, et al. The effect of treatment variables on mood and social adjustment in adult patients with pituitary disease. Clin Endocrinol (Oxf) 1997;46:445-450.
199. Landolt AM, Haller D, Lomax N, et al. Stereotactic radiosurgery for recurrent surgically treated acromegaly: comparison with fractionated radiotherapy. J Neurosurg 1998;88:1002-1008.
200. Scheithauer BW, Sano T, Kovacs KT, et al. The pituitary gland in pregnancy: a clinicopathologic and immunohistochemical study of 69 cases. Mayo Clin Proc 1990;65:461-474.
201. Burrows HL, Birkmeier TS, Seasholtz AF, Camper SA. Targeted ablation of cells in the pituitary primordia of transgenic mice. Mol Endocrinol 1996;10:1467-1477.
202. Boockfor FR, Hoeffler JP, Frawley LS. Estradiol induces a shift in cultured cells that release prolactin or growth hormone. Am J Physiol 1986;250:E103-E105.
203. Stricker S, Grueter F. Action du lobe anterieur de l'hypophyse sur la montée laiteuse. Compt Rend Soc Biol 1928;99:1978-1980.
204. Riddle O. Prolactin in vertebrate function and organization. J Nat Cancer Inst 1963;31:1039-1110.
205. Riddle O, Bates RW, Dykshorn SW. The preparation, identification, and assay of prolactin—a hormone of the anterior pituitary. Am J Physiol 1933;105:191-216.
206. Wilhelmi AE. Fractionation of human pituitary glands. Can J Bichem 1961;39:1659-1668.
207. Suganuma N, Seo H, Yamamoto N, et al. Ontogenesis of pituitary prolactin in the human fetus. J Clin Endocrinol Metab 1986; 63:156-161.
208. Thorner MO, Vance ML, Laws ER Jr, et al. The anterior pituitary. In Wilson JD, Foster DW, eds. Williams Textbook of Endocrinology, 9th ed. Philadelphia: WB Saunders, 1998:249-340.
209. Kleinberg DL, Frantz AG. A sensitive in vitro assay for prolactin. Program of the 51st Meeting of the Endocrine Society 1969:32-32.
210. Frantz AG, Kleinberg DL. Prolactin: evidence that it is separate from growth hormone in human blood. Science 1970;170:745-747.
211. Kleinberg DL, Frantz AG. Human prolactin: measurement in plasma by in vitro bioassay. J Clin Invest 1971;50:1557-1568.
212. Hwang P, Guyda H, Friesen H. A radioimmunoassay for human prolactin. Proc Natl Acad Sci U S A 1971;68:1902-1906.
213. Friesen HG. The discovery of human prolactin: a very personal account. Clin Invest Med 1995;18:66-72.
214. Owerbach D, Rutter WJ, Cooke NE, et al. The prolactin gene is located on chromosome 6 in humans. Science 1981;212:815-816.
215. Cooke NE, Coit D, Weiner RI, et al. Structure of cloned DNA complementary to rat prolactin messenger RNA. J Biol Chem 1980; 255:6502-6510.
216. Lamberts SW, Macleod RM. Regulation of prolactin secretion at the level of the lactotroph. Physiol Rev 1990;70:279-318.
217. Farkouh NH, Packer MG, Frantz AG. Large molecular size prolactin with reduced receptor activity in human serum: high proportion in basal state and reduction after thyrotropin-releasing hormone. J Clin Endocrinol Metab 1979;48:1026-1032.

218. Sinha YN. Structural variants of prolactin: occurrence and physiological significance. Endocr Rev 1995;16:354-369.
219. Suh HK, Frantz AG. Size heterogeneity of human prolactin in plasma and pituitary extracts. J Clin Endocrinol Metab 1974;39: 928-935.
220. Lewis UJ, Singh RN, Sinha YN, VanderLaan WP. Glycosylated human prolactin. Endocrinology 1985;116:359-363.
221. Mittra I. A Novel "cleaved prolactin" in the rat pituitary: Part I. Biosynthesis, characterization and regulatory control. Biochem Biophys Res Comm 1980;95(4):1750-1759.
222. Lee H, Struman I, Clapp C, et al. Inhibition of urokinase activity by the antiangiogenic factor 16K prolactin: activation of plasminogen activator inhibitor 1 expression. Endocrinology 1998;139: 3696.
223. Ferrara N, Clapp C, Weiner R. The 16K fragment of prolactin specifically inhibits basal or fibroblast growth factor stimulated growth of capillary endothelial cells. Endocrinology 1991;129: 896-900.
224. Kline JB, Clevenger CV. Identification and characterization of the prolactin-binding protein in human serum and milk. J Biol Chem 2001;276:24760-24766.
225. Liu JW, Ben Jonathan N. Prolactin-releasing activity of neurohypophysial hormones: structure-function relationship. Endocrinology 1994;134:114-118.
226. Horseman ND. Prolactin. In DeGroot LJ, Jameson JL, eds. Endocrinology, 4th ed. Philadelphia: WB Saunders, 2001:209-220.
227. Horseman ND, Zhao W, Montecino-Rodriguez E, et al. Defective mammopoiesis, but normal hematopoiesis, in mice with targeted disruption of the prolactin gene. EMBO J 1997;16:6926-6935.
228. Steger RW, Chandrashekar V, Zhao W, et al. Neuroendocrine and reproductive functions in male mice with targeted disruption of the prolactin gene. Endocrinology 1998;139:3691-3695.
229. Kanyicska B, Lerant A, Freeman ME. Endothelin is an autocrine regulator of prolactin secretion. Endocrinology 1998;139: 5164-5173.
230. Sarkar DK, Kim KH, Minami S. Transforming growth factor-β1 messenger RNA and protein expression in the pituitary gland: its action on prolactin secretion and lactotropic growth. Mol Endocrinol 1992;6:1825-1833.
231. Shah GV, Pedchenko V, Stanley S, et al. Calcitonin is a physiological inhibitor of prolactin secretion in ovariectomized female rats. Endocrinology 1996;137:1814-1822.
232. Ben Jonathan N. Regulation of prolactin secretion. In Imura H, ed. The Pituitary Gland, 2nd ed. New York: Raven Press, 1994: 261-283.
233. Hinuma S, Habata Y, Fujii R, et al. A prolactin-releasing peptide in the brain [see comments] [published erratum appears in Nature 1998 Jul 16;394(6690):302]. Nature 1998;393:272-276.
234. Rubinek T, Hadani M, Barkai G, et al. Prolactin (PRL)-releasing peptide stimulates PRL secretion from human fetal pituitary cultures and growth hormone release from cultured pituitary adenomas. J Clin Endocrinol Metab 2001;86:2826-2830.
235. Reichlin S. TRH: historical aspects. Ann N Y Acad Sci 1989; 553:1-6:1-6.
236. Cooke NE. Prolactin: normal synthesis, regulation, and actions. In DeGroot LJ, Besser GM, Cahill GFJ, eds. Endocrinology. Philadelphia: WB Saunders, 1989:384-407.
237. Katznelson L, Riskind PN, Saxe VC, Klibanski A. Prolactin pulsatile characteristics in postmenopausal women. J Clin Endocrinol Metab 1998;83:761-764.
238. Bredow S, Kacsoh B, Obal F Jr, et al. Increase of prolactin mRNA in the rat hypothalamus after intracerebroventricular injection of VIP or PACAP. Brain Res 1994;660:301-308.
239. Peters LL, Hoefer MT, Ben-Jonathan N. The posterior pituitary: regulation of anterior pituitary prolactin secretion. Science 1981; 213:659-661.
240. Asa SL, Kelly MA, Grandy DK, Low MJ. Pituitary lactotroph adenomas develop after prolonged lactotroph hyperplasia in dopamine D2 receptor–deficient mice. Endocrinology 1999;140:5348-5355.
241. Bazan JF. Structural design and molecular evolution of a cytokine receptor superfamily. Proc Natl Acad Sci U S A 1990;87: 6934-6938.
242. Arden KC, Boutin JM, Djiane J, et al. The receptors for prolactin and growth hormone are localized in the same region of human chromosome 5. Cytogenet Cell Genet 1990;53:161-165.
243. Hu ZZ, Zhuang L, Meng J, et al. The human prolactin receptor gene structure and alternative promoter utilization: the generic promoter hPIII and a novel human promoter hP(N). J Clin Endocrinol Metab 1999;84:1153-1156.
244. Bole-Feysot C, Goffin V, Edery M, et al. Prolactin (PRL) and its receptor: actions, signal transduction pathways and phenotypes observed in PRL receptor knockout mice. Endocr Rev 1998;19: 225-268.
245. de Vos AM, Ultsch M, Kossiakoff AA. Human growth hormone and extracellular domain of its receptor: Crystal structure of the complex. Science 1992;255:306-312.
246. Gao J, Hughes JP, Auperin B, et al. Interactions among JANUS kinases and the prolactin (PRL) receptor in the regulatation of a PRL response element. Mol Endocrinol 1996;10:847-856.
247. Hynes NE, Cella N, Wartmann M. Prolactin mediated intracellular signaling in mammary epithelial cells. J Mammary Gland Biol Neopl 1997;2:19-27.
248. Goffin V, Kelly PA. The prolactin/growth hormone receptor family: structure/function relationships. J Mammary Gland Biol Neopl 1997;2:7-17.
249. Lucas BK, Ormandy CJ, Binart N, et al. Null mutation of the prolactin receptor gene produces a defect in maternal behavior. Endocrinology 1998;139:4102-4107.
250. Kleinberg DL, Ruan W, Catanese V, et al. Non-lactogenic effects of growth hormone on growth and insulin-like growth factor-I messenger ribonucleic acid of rat mammary gland [published erratum appears in Endocrinology 1990 Oct;127(4):1977]. Endocrinology 1990;126:3274-3276.
251. Feldman M, Ruan WF, Cunningham BC, et al. Evidence that the growth hormone receptor mediates differentiation and development of the mammary gland. Endocrinology 1993;133:1602-1608.
252. Ruan W, Catanese V, Wieczorek R, et al. Estradiol enhances the stimulatory effect of insulin-like growth factor-I (IGF-I) on mammary development and growth hormone–induced IGF-I messenger ribonucleic acid. Endocrinology 1995;136:1296-1302.
253. Ruan W, Newman CB, Kleinberg DL. Intact and aminoterminally shortened forms of insulin-like growth factor I induce mammary gland differentiation and development. Proc Natl Acad Sci U S A 1992;89:10872-10876.
254. Kleinberg DL. Endocrinology of mammary development, lactation and galactorrhea. In DeGroot LJ, Jameson JL, eds. Endocrinology, 4th ed. Philadelphia: WB Saunders, 2000:2464-2475.
255. Cunha GR. Role of mesenchymal-epithelial interactions in normal and abnormal development of the mammary gland and prostate. Cancer 1994;74:1030-1044.
256. Daniel CW, Silberstein GB. Postnatal development of the rodent mammary gland. In Neville MC, Daniel CW, eds. The Mammary Gland. New York: Plenum Press, 1987:3-36.
257. Ruan W, Kleinberg DL. Insulin-like growth factor I is essential for terminal end bud formation and ductal morphogenesis during mammary development. Endocrinology 1999;140:5075-5081.
258. Ruan W, Monaco ME, Kleinberg DL. Progesterone stimulates mammary gland ductal morphogenesis by synergizing with and enhancing insulin-like growth factor-I action. Endocrinology 2005;146:1170-1178.
259. Walden PD, Ruan W, Feldman M, Kleinberg DL. Evidence that growth hormone acts on stromal tissue to stimulate pubertal mammary gland development. 79th Annual Meeting of the Endocrine Society, Minneapolis, MN, 1997, Abstract P1-120.
260. Wysolmerski JJ, Stewart AF. The physiology of parathyroid hormone–related protein: an emerging role as a developmental factor. Annu Rev Physiol 1998;60:431-60:431-460.
261. Wiesen JF, Young P, Werb Z, Cunha GR. Signaling through the stromal epidermal growth factor receptor is necessary for mammary ductal development. Development 1999;126:335-344.
262. Anderson TJ, Battersby S, King RJB, et al. Oral contraceptive use influences resting breast proliferation. Hum Pathol 1989;20: 1139-1144.
263. Tyson JE, Hwang P, Guyda H. Studies of prolactin secretion in human pregnancy. Am J Obstet Gynecol 1972;113:14-20.
264. Vorherr H. Hormonal and biochemical changes of pituitary and breast during pregnancy. Semin Perinat 1979;3:193-198.
265. Richert MM, Wood TL. The Insulin-like growth factors (IGF) and the IGF type I receptor during postnatal growth of the murine

mammary gland: sites of messenger ribonucleic acid expression and potential functions. Endocrinology 1999;140:454-461.
266. Pepe GJ, Albrecht ED. Actions of placental and fetal adrenal steroid hormones in primate pregnancy. Endocr Rev 1995;16: 608-648.
267. Falk RJ. Isolated prolactin deficiency: a case report. Fertil Steril 1992;58:1060-1062.
268. Humphreys RC, Lydon J, O'Malley BW, Rosen JM. Mammary gland development is mediated by both stromal and epithelial progesterone receptors. Mol Endocrinol 1997;11:801-811.
269. Kleinberg DL, Boyd AE II, Wardlaw S, et al. Pergolide for the treatment of pituitary tumors secreting prolactin or growth hormone. N Engl J Med 1983;309:704-709.
270. Graham JD, Clarke CL. Physiological action of progesterone in target tissues. Endocr Rev 1997;18:502-519.
271. Neville MC. Mammary gland biology and lactation: a short course. Presented at the International Society for Research in Human Milk and Lactation, Plymouth, MA, 1997.
272. Vorherr H. Galactopoiesis, galactosecretion, and onset of lactation. In Vorherr H, ed. The Breast. New York: Academic Press, 1974:71-127.
273. Noel GL, Suh HK, Frantz AG. Prolactin release during nursing and breast stimulation in postpartum and nonpostpartum subjects. J Clin Endocrinol Metab 1974;38:413-423.
274. Diaz S, Seron-Ferre M, Cardenas H, et al. Circadian variation of basal plasma prolactin, prolactin response to suckling, and length of amenorrhea in nursing women. J Clin Endocrinol Metab 1989;68:946-955.
275. Johnston JM, Amico JA. A prospective longitudinal study of the release of oxytocin and prolactin in response to infant suckling in long term lactation. J Clin Endocrinol Metab 1986;62:653-657.
276. Howie PW, McNeilly AS, McArdle T, et al. The relationship between suckling-induced prolactin response and lactogenesis. J Clin Endocrinol Metab 1980;50:670-673.
277. Leite V, Cowden EA, Friesen HG. Endocrinology of lactation and nursing: disorders of lactation. In DeGroot LJ, ed. Endocrinology, 3rd ed. Philadelphia: WB Saunders, 1995:2224-2233.
278. Wagner KU, Young WS, Liu X, Furth PA, Hennighausen L. Oxytocin and milk removal are required for post partum mammary-gland development. Genes Funct 1997;1:233-244.
279. Short RV. Breast feeding. Sci Am 1984;250:35-41.
280. Glasier A, McNeilly AS. Physiology of lactation. Bailliere Clin Endocrinol Metab 1990;4:379-395.
281. Walker SE, Allen SH, McMurray RW. Prolactin and autoimmune disease. Trends Endocrinol Metab 1993;4:147-151.
282. Zellweger R, Zhu XH, Wichmann MW, et al. Prolactin administration following hemorrhagic shock improves macrophage cytokine release capacity and decreases mortality from subsequent sepsis. J Immunol 1996;157:5748-5754.
283. Richards SM, Murphy WJ. Use of human prolactin as a therapeutic protein to potentiate immunohematopoietic function. J Neuroimmunol 2000;109:56-62.
284. Dorshkind K, Horseman ND. The roles of prolactin, growth hormone, insulin-like growth factor-I, and thyroid hormones in lymphocyte development and function: insights from genetic models of hormone and hormone receptor deficiency. Endocr Rev 2000 Jun;21(3):292-312..
285. Ormandy CJ, Camus A, Barra J, et al. Null mutation of the prolactin receptor gene produces multiple reproductive defects in the mouse. Genes Dev 1997;11:167-178.
286. Clement-Lacroix P, Ormandy C, Lepescheux L, et al. Osteoblasts are a new target for prolactin: analysis of bone formation in prolactin receptor knockout mice. Endocrinology 1999;140:96-105.
287. Demura R, Ono M, Demura H, et al. Prolactin directly inhibits basal as well as gonadotropin-stimulated secretion of progesterone and 17β-estradiol in the human ovary. J Clin Endocrinol Metab 1982; 54:1246-1250.
288. Barkan AL, Chandler WF. Giant pituitary prolactinoma with falsely low serum prolactin: the pitfall of the "high-dose hook effect": case report. Neurosurgery 1998;42:913-915.
289. Cooper DS, Ridgway EC, Kliman B, et al. Metabolic clearance and production rates of prolactin in man. J Clin Invest 1979;64: 1669-1680.
290. Veldhuis JD, Johnson ML. Operating characteristics of the hypothalamo-pituitary-gonadal axis in men: circadian, ultradian, and pulsatile release of prolactin and its temporal coupling with luteinizing hormone. J Clin Endocrinol Metab 1988;67:116-123.
291. Greenspan SL, Klibanski A, Rowe JW, Elahi D. Age alters pulsatile prolactin release: influence of dopaminergic inhibition. Am J Physiol 1990;258:E799-804.
292. Samuels MH, Henry P, Kleinschmidt-DeMasters BK, et al. Pulsatile glycoprotein hormone secretion in glycoprotein-producing pituitary tumors. J Clin Endocrinol Metab 1991;73:1281-1288.
293. Sassin JF, Frantz AG, Weitzman ED, Kapen S. Human prolactin: 24-hour pattern with increased release during sleep. Science 1972;177:1205-1207.
294. Parker DC, Rossman LG, Vanderlaan EF. Relation of sleep-entrained human prolactin release to REM-nonREM cycles. J Clin Endocrinol Metab 1974;38:646-651.
295. Iranmanesh A, Mulligan T, Veldhuis JD. Mechanisms subserving the physiological nocturnal relative hypoprolactinemia of healthy older men: dual decline in prolactin secretory burst mass and basal release with preservation of pulse duration, frequency, and interpulse interval—a General Clinical Research Center study. J Clin Endocrinol Metab 1999;84:1083-1090.
296. Berinder K, Stackenas I, Akre O, et al. Hyperprolactinaemia in 271 women: up to three decades of clinical follow-up. Clin Endocrinol (Oxf) 2005;63:450-455.
297. Kleinberg DL. Pharmacologic therapies and surgical options in the treatment of hyperprolactinemia. Endocrinologist 1997;7(suppl): 379-384.
298. Gibney J, Smith TP, McKenna TJ. The impact on clinical practice of routine screening for macroprolactin. J Clin Endocrinol Metab 2005;90:3927-3932.
299. Franks S. Polycystic ovary syndrome [published erratum appears in N Engl J Med 1995 Nov 23;333(21):1435] [see comments]. N Engl J Med 1995;333:853-861.
300. Bracero N, Zacur HA. Polycystic ovary syndrome and hyperprolactinemia. Obstet Gynecol Clin North Am 2001;28:77-84.
301. Falaschi P, Rocco A, del Pozo E. Inhibitory effect of bromocriptine treatment on luteinizing hormone secretion in polycystic ovary syndrome. J Clin Endocrinol Metab 1986;62:348-351.
302. Kleinberg DL, Noel GL, Frantz AG. Galactorrhea: a study of 235 cases, including 48 with pituitary tumors. N Engl J Med 1977;296:589-600.
303. Lam KS, Lechan RM, Minamitani N, et al. Vasoactive intestinal peptide in the anterior pituitary is increased in hypothyroidism. Endocrinology 1989;124:1077-1084.
304. Biller BM, Sesmilo G, Baum HB, et al. Withdrawal of long-term physiological growth hormone (GH) administration: differential effects on bone density and body composition in men with adult-onset GH deficiency. J Clin Endocrinol Metab 2000;85: 970-976.
305. Travaglini P, Moriondo P, Togni E, et al. Effect of oral zinc administration on prolactin and thymulin circulating levels in patients with chronic renal failure. J Clin Endocrinol Metab 1989;68: 186-190.
306. LeRoith D, Danovitz G, Trestan S, Spitz IM. Dissociation of prolactin response to thyrotropin-releasing hormone and metoclopramide in chronic renal failure. J Clin Endocrinol Metab 1979;49:815-817.
307. Ramirez G, Butcher DE, Newton JL, et al. Bromocriptine and the hypothalamic hypophyseal function in patients with chronic renal failure on chronic hemodialysis. Am J Kidney Dis 1985;6: 111-118.
308. Lim VS, Henriquez C, Sievertsen G, Frohman LA. Ovarian function in chronic renal failure: evidence suggesting hypothalamic anovulation. Ann Intern Med 1980;93:21-27.
309. Noel GL, Suh HK, Stone JG, Frantz AG. Human prolactin and growth hormone release during surgery and other conditions of stress. J Clin Endocrinol Metab 1972;35:840-851.
310. Agha A, Sherlock M, Brennan S, et al. Hypothalamic-pituitary dysfunction after irradiation of nonpituitary brain tumors in adults. J Clin Endocrinol Metab 2005;90:6355-6360.
311. Kleinberg DL, Noel GL, Frantz AG. Chlorpromazine stimulation and L-dopa suppression of prolactin. J Clin Endocrinol Metab 1971;33:873-876.
312. Szarfman A, Tonning JM, Levine JG, Doraiswamy PM. Atypical antipsychotics and pituitary tumors: a pharmacovigilance study. Pharmacotherapy 2006;26:748-758.

313. Crawford AM, Beasley CMJ, Tollefson GD. The acute long-term effect of olanzapine compared with placebo and haloperidol on serum prolactin concentrations. Schizophr Res 1997;26:41-54.
314. Perovich RM, Lieberman JA, Fleischhacker WW, Alvir J. The behavioral toxicity of bromocriptine in patients with psychiatric illness. J Clin Psychopharmacol 1989;9:417-422.
315. Tollin SR. Use of the dopamine agonists bromocriptine and cabergoline in the management of risperidone-induced hyperprolactinemia in patients with psychotic disorders. J Endocrinol Invest 2000;23:765-770.
316. Sharp EA. Historical review of a syndrome embracing utero-ovarian atrophy with persistent lactation (Frommel's disease). Am J Obstet Gynecol 1935;30:411-414.
317. Argonz J, del Castillo EB. A syndrome characterized by estrogenic insufficiency, galactorrhea and decreased urinary gonadotropin. J Clin Endocrinol Metab 1953;13:79-87.
318. Forbes AP, Henneman PH, Griswold GC, Albright F. Syndrome characterized by galactorrhea, amenorrhea and low urinary FSH: comparison with acromegaly and normal lactation. J Clin Endocrinol Metab 1954;14:265-271.
319. Kleinberg DL, Lieberman A, Todd J, et al. Pergolide mesylate: a potent day-long inhibitor of prolactin in rhesus monkeys and patients with Parkinson's disease. J Clin Endocrinol Metab 1980;51:152-154.
320. Klibanski A, Neer RM, Beitins IZ, et al. Decreased bone density in hyperprolactinemic women. N Engl J Med 1980;303:1511-1514.
321. Melmed S, Braunstein GD, Chang RJ, Becker DP. Pituitary tumors secreting growth hormone and prolactin. Ann Intern Med 1986;105:238-253.
322. Koppelman MCS, Jaffe MJ, Rieth KG, et al. Hyperprolactinemia, amenorrhea, and galactorrhea. Ann Intern Med 1984;100:115-121.
323. Sisam DA, Sheehan JP, Sheeler LR. The natural history of untreated microprolactinomas. Fertil Steril 1987;48:67-71.
324. Schlechte J, Dolan K, Sherman B, et al. The natural history of untreated hyperprolactinemia: a prospective analysis. J Clin Endocrinol Metab 1989;68:412-418.
325. Colao A, Di Sarno A, Cappabianca P, et al. Withdrawal of long-term cabergoline therapy for tumoral and nontumoral hyperprolactinemia. N Engl J Med 2003;349:2023-2033.
326. Delgrange E, Trouillas J, Maiter D, et al. Sex-related difference in the growth of prolactinomas: a clinical and proliferation marker study. J Clin Endocrinol Metab 1997;82:2102-2107.
327. Arafah BM, Nekl KE, Gold RS, Selman WR. Dynamics of prolactin secretion in patients with hypopituitarism and pituitary macroadenomas. J Clin Endocrinol Metab 1995;80:3507-3512.
328. Kovacs K, Horvath E. Pathology of pituitary tumors. Endocrinol Metab Clin North Am 1987;16:529-551.
329. Kovacs K, Horvath E, Asa SL. Classification and pathology of pituitary tumors. In Wilkins RH, Rengachary SS, eds. Neurosurgery. New York: McGraw Hill, 1985:834-842.
330. Scheithauer BW, Kovacs KT, Laws ER Jr, Randall RV. Pathology of invasive pituitary tumors with special reference to functional classification. J Neurosurg 1986;65:733-744.
331. Pernicone PJ, Scheithauer BW, Sebo TJ, et al. Pituitary carcinoma: a clinicopathologic study of 15 cases. Cancer 1997;79:804-812.
332. Hurel SJ, Harris PE, McNicol AM, et al. Metastatic prolactinoma: effect of octreotide, cabergoline, carboplatin and etoposide; immunocytochemical analysis of proto-oncogene expression. J Clin Endocrinol Metab 1997;82:2962-2965.
333. Kontogeorgos G, Kovacs K, Horvath E, Scheithauer BW. Multiple adenomas of the human pituitary. A retrospective autopsy study with clinical implications. J Neurosurg 1991;74:243-247.
334. Burgess JR, Shepherd JJ, Parameswaran V, et al. Spectrum of pituitary disease in multiple endocrine neoplasia type 1 (MEN 1): clinical, biochemical, and radiological features of pituitary disease in a large MEN 1 kindred. J Clin Endocrinol Metab 1996;81:2642-2646.
335. Berezin M, Karasik A. Familial prolactinoma. Clin Endocrinol (Oxf) 1995;42:483-486.
336. Sauder SE, Frager M, Case GA, et al. Abnormal patterns of pulsatile luteinizing hormone secretion in women with hyperprolactinemia and amenorrhea: responses to bromocriptine. J Clin Endocrinol Metab 1984;59:941-948.
337. Milenkovic L, D'Angelo G, Kelly PA, Weiner RI. Inhibition of gonadotropin hormone–releasing hormone release by prolactin from GT1 neuronal cell lines through prolactin receptors. Proc Natl Acad Sci U S A 1994;91:1244-1247.
338. Cohen-Becker IR, Selmanoff M, Wise PM. Hyperprolactinemia alters the frequency and amplitude of pulsatile luteinizing hormone secretion in the ovariectomized rat. Neuroendocrinology 1986;42:328-333.
339. Matera C, Freda PU, Ferin M, Wardlaw SL. Effect of chronic opioid antagonism on the hypothalamic-pituitary-ovarian axis in hyperprolactinemic women. J Clin Endocrinol Metab 1995;80:540-545.
340. Ciccarelli A, Guerra E, De Rosa M, et al. PRL secreting adenomas in male patients. Pituitary 2005;8:39-42.
341. Klibanski A, Biller BMK, Rosenthal DI, Saxe V. Effects of prolactin and estrogen deficiency in amenorrheic bone loss. J Clin Endocrinol Metab 1988;67:124-130.
342. Kemmann E, Jones JR. Hyperprolactinemia and headaches. Am J Obstet Gynecol 1983;145:668-671.
343. Hollenhorst RW, Younge BR. Ocular manifestations produced by adenomas of the pituitary gland: analysis of 1000 cases. In Kohler PO, Ross GT, eds. Diagnosis and Treatment of Pituitary Tumors. New York: Elsevier, 1973:53-64.
344. Zikel OM, Atkinson JL, Hurley DL. Prolactinoma manifesting with symptomatic hydrocephalus. Mayo Clin Proc 1999;74:475-477.
345. Krassas GE, Pontikides N, Kaltsas T. Giant prolactinoma presented as unilateral exophthalmos in a prepubertal boy: response to cabergoline. Horm Res 1999;52:45-48.
346. Kleinberg DL, Todd J. Evidence that human growth hormone is a potent lactogen in primates. J Clin Endocrinol Metab 1980;51:1009-1015.
347. De Rosa M, Ciccarelli A, Zarrilli S, et al. The treatment with cabergoline for 24 months normalizes the quality of seminal fluid in hyperprolactinaemic males. Clin Endocrinol (Oxf) 2006;64:307-313.
348. Thorner MO, Martin WH, Rogol AD, et al. Rapid regression of pituitary prolactinomas during bromocriptine treatment. J Clin Endocrinol Metab 1980;51:438-445.
349. Besser GM, Thorner MO. Bromocriptine in the treatment of the hyperprolactinaemia-hypogonadism syndromes. Postgrad Med J 1976;52(suppl 1):64-70.
350. Shimon I, Melmed S. Management of pituitary tumors. Ann Intern Med 1998;129:472-483.
351. Bevan JS, Webster J, Burke CW, Scanlon MF. Dopamine agonists and pituitary tumor shrinkage. Endocr Rev 1992;13:220-240.
352. Colao A, Vitale G, Cappabianca P, et al. Outcome of cabergoline treatment in men with prolactinoma: effects of a 24-month treatment on prolactin levels, tumor mass, recovery of pituitary function, and semen analysis. J Clin Endocrinol Metab 2004;89:1704-1711.
353. Weiss MH. Treatment options in the management of prolactin-secreting pituitary tumors. Clin Neurosurg 1986;33:547-552.
354. Vance ML, Evans WS, Thorner MO. Drugs five years later. Bromocriptine. Ann Intern Med 1984;100:78-91.
355. Thorner MO, Perryman RL, Rogol AD, et al. Rapid changes of prolactinoma volume after withdrawal and reinstitution of bromocriptine. J Clin Endocrinol Metab 1981;53:480-483.
356. Kovacs K, Stefaneanu L, Horvath E, et al. Effect of dopamine agonist medication on prolactin producing pituitary adenomas. A morphological study including immunocytochemistry, electron microscopy and in situ hybridization. Virchows Arch A Pathol Anat Histopathol 1991;418:439-446.
357. Jeffcoate WJ, Pound N, Sturrock ND, Lambourne J. Long-term follow-up of patients with hyperprolactinaemia. Clin Endocrinol (Oxf) 1996;45:299-303.
358. Kupersmith MJ, Kleinberg DL, Warren A, et al. Growth of prolactinoma despite lowering of serum prolactin by bromocriptine. Neurosurgery 1989;24:417-423.
359. Molitch ME. Pharmacologic resistance in prolactinoma patients. Pituitary 2005;8:43-52.
360. Colao A, Di Sarno A, Sarnacchiaro F, et al. Prolactinomas resistant to standard dopamine agonists respond to chronic cabergoline treatment. J Clin Endocrinol Metab 1997;82:876-883.
361. Tindall GT, Kovacs K, Horvath E, Thorner MO. Human prolactin-producing adenomas and bromocriptine: a histological, immunocytochemical, ultrastructural, and morphometric study. J Clin Endocrinol Metab 1982;55:1178-1183.

362. Bassetti M, Spada A, Pezzo G, Giannattasio G. Bromocriptine treatment reduces the cell size in human macroprolactinomas: a morphometric study. J Clin Endocrinol Metab 1984;58:268-273.
363. Saitoh Y, Mori S, Arita N, et al. Cytosuppressive effect of bromocriptine on human prolactinomas: stereological analysis of ultrastructural alterations with special reference to secretory granules. Cancer Research 1986;46:1507-1512.
364. Hallenga B, Saeger W, Ludecke DK. Necroses of prolactin-secreting pituitary adenomas under treatment with dopamine agonists: light microscopical and morphometric studies. Exp Clin Endocrinol 1988;92:59-68.
365. Landolt AM, Osterwalder V. Perivascular fibrosis in prolactinomas: is it increased by bromocriptine? J Clin Endocrinol Metab 1984;58:1179-1183.
366. Tyrrell JB, Lamborn KR, Hannegan LT, et al. Transsphenoidal microsurgical therapy of prolactinomas: initial outcomes and long-term results. Neurosurgery 1999;44:254-261.
367. Hubbard JL, Scheithauer BW, Abboud CF, Laws ER Jr. Prolactin-secreting adenomas: the preoperative response to bromocriptine treatment and surgical outcome. J Neurosurg 1987;67:816-821.
368. Fahlbusch R, Buchfelder M, Schrell U. Short-term preoperative treatment of macroprolactinomas by dopamine agonists. J Neurosurg 1987;67:807-815.
369. Biswas M, Smith J, Jadon D, et al. Long-term remission following withdrawal of dopamine agonist therapy in subjects with microprolactinomas. Clin Endocrinol (Oxf) 2005;63:26-31.
370. Cook DM. Long-term management of prolactinomas—use of long-acting dopamine agonists. Rev Endocr Metab Disord 2005;6:15-21.
371. Di Salle E, Ornati G, Giudici D. A comparison of the in vivo and in vitro duration of prolactin lowering effect in rats of FCE 21336, pergolide and bromocriptine. Presented at the Fourth International Congress on Prolactin, Charlottesville, SC, June 27-29, 1984, abstract 142.
372. Andreotti AC, Pianezzola E, Persiani S, et al. Pharmacokinetics, pharmacodynamics, and tolerability of cabergoline, a prolactin-lowering drug, after administration of increasing oral doses (0.5, 1.0, and 1.5 milligrams) in healthy male volunteers. J Clin Endocrinol Metab 1995;80:841-845.
373. Webster J, Piscitelli G, Polli A, et al. A comparison of cabergoline and bromocriptine in the treatment of hyperprolactinemic amenorrhea. N Engl J Med 1994;331:904-909.
374. Biller BM, Molitch ME, Vance ML, et al. Treatment of prolactin-secreting macroadenomas with the once-weekly dopamine agonist cabergoline. J Clin Endocrinol Metab 1996;81:2338-2343.
375. Colao A, Di Sarno A, Landi ML, et al. Long-term and low-dose treatment with cabergoline induces macroprolactinoma shrinkage. J Clin Endocrinol Metab 1997;82:3574-3579.
376. Negoro K, Kawai M, Tada Y, et al. A case of postprandial cluster-like headache with prolactinoma: dramatic response to cabergoline. Headache 2005;45:604-606.
377. Goldstein M, Lieberman A, Lew JY, et al Interaction of pergolide with central dopaminergic receptors. Proc Natl Acad Sci U S A 1980;77:3725-3728.
378. Freda PU, Andreadis CI, Khandji AG, et al. Long-term treatment of prolactin-secreting macroadenomas with pergolide. J Clin Endocrinol Metab 2000;85:8-13.
379. Lamberts SWJ, Quik RFP. A comparison of the efficacy and safety of pergolide and bromocriptine in the treatment of hyperprolactinemia. J Clin Endocrinol Metab 1991;72:635-641.
380. Newman CB, Hurley AM, Kleinberg DL. Effect of CV 205-502 in hyperprolactinemic patients intolerant of bromocriptine. Clin Endocrinol 1989;31:391-400.
381. Vance ML, Cragun JR, Reimnitz C, et al. CV205-502 treatment of hyperprolactinemia. J Clin Endocrinol Metab 1989;68:336-339.
382. Kletzky OA, Vermesh M. Effectiveness of vaginal bromocriptine in treating women with hyperprolactinemia. Fertil Steril 1989;51:269-272.
383. Turner TH, Cookson JC, Wass JA, et al. Psychotic reactions during treatment of pituitary tumours with dopamine agonists. Br Med J (Clin Res Ed) 1984;289:1101-1103.
384. Leong KS, Foy PM, Swift AC, et al. CSF rhinorrhoea following treatment with dopamine agonists for massive invasive prolactinomas. Clin Endocrinol (Oxf) 2000;52:43-49.
385. Melmed S, Braunstein GD. Bromocriptine and pleuropulmonary disease. Arch Intern Med 1989;149:258-259.
386. Schude et al. Dopamine agonists and risk of cardiac valve regurgitation. N Engl J Med 2007;356:29–38.
387. Rush SC, Newall J. Pituitary adenoma: the efficacy of radiotherapy as the sole treatment [see comments]. Int J Radiat Oncol Biol Phys 1989;17:165-169.
388. Halberg FE, Sheline GE. Radiotherapy of pituitary tumors. Endocrinol Metab Clin 1987;16:667-684.
389. Littley MD, Shalet SM, Beardwell CG, et al. Radiation-induced hypopituitarism is dose-dependent. Clin Endocrinol 1989;31:363-373.
390. Tsagarakis S, Grossman A, Plowman PN, et al. Megavoltage pituitary irradiation in the management of prolactinomas: long-term follow-up. Clin Endocrinol (Oxf) 1991;34:399-406.
391. Littley MD, Shalet SM, Beardwell CG, et al. Hypopituitarism following external radiotherapy for pituitary tumours in adults. Q J Med 1989;70:145-160.
392. Hardy J. Transphenoidal hypophysectomy. J Neurosurg 1971;34:582-591.
393. Randall RV, Laws ER Jr, Abboud CF, et al. Transsphenoidal microsurgical treatment of prolactin-producing pituitary adenomas. Results in 100 patients. Mayo Clin Proc 1983;58:108-121.
394. Serri O, Rasio E, Beauregard H, et al. Recurrence of hyperprolactinemia after selective transsphenoidal adenomectomy in women with prolactinoma. N Engl J Med 1983;309:280-283.
395. Molitch ME. Management of prolactinomas. Annu Rev Med 1989;40:225-232.
396. Clayton RN, Stewart PM, Shalet SM, Wass JA. Pituitary surgery for acromegaly. Should be done by specialists. BMJ 1999;319(7210):588-589.
397. Gonzalez JG, Elizondo G, Saldivar D, et al. Pituitary gland growth during normal pregnancy: an in vivo study using magnetic resonance imaging. Am J Med 1988;85:217-220.
398. Molitch ME, Thorner MO, Wilson C. Management of prolactinomas. J Clin Endocrinol Metab 1997;82:996-1000.
399. Molitch ME, Elton RL, Blackwell RE, et al. Bromocriptine as primary therapy for prolactin-secreting macroadenomas: results of a prospective multicenter study. J Clin Endocrinol Metab 1985;60:698-705.
400. Kupersmith MJ, Rosenberg C, Kleinberg D. Visual loss in pregnant women with pituitary adenomas. Ann Int Med 1994;121:473-477.
401. Liu C, Tyrrell JB. Successful treatment of a large macroprolactinoma with cabergoline during pregnancy. Pituitary 2001;4(3):179-185.
402. Krupp P, Turkalj I. Surveillance of Parlodel (bromocriptine) in pregnancy. In Jacobs HS, Harrison RF, Bonnar J, eds. Prolactinomas and Pregnancy. Lancaster, UK: MTP Press, 1983:45-50.
403. Maeda T, Ushiroyama T, Okuda K, et al. Effective bromocriptine treatment of a pituitary macroadenoma during pregnancy. Obstet Gynecol 1983;61:117-121.
404. Laws ER Jr, Fode NC, Randall RV, et al. Pregnancy following transsphenoidal resection of prolactin-secreting pituitary tumors. J Neurosurg 1983;58:685-688.
405. Gharib SD, Wierman ME, Shupnik MA, Chin WW. Molecular biology of the pituitary gonadotropins. Endocr Rev 1990;11:177-199.
406. Sairam MR, Bhargavi GN. A role for glycosylation of the α subunit in transduction of biological signal in glycoprotein hormones. Science 1985;229:65-67.
407. Albanese C, Colin IM, Crowley WF, et al. The gonadotropin genes: evolution of distinct mechanisms for hormonal control. Recent Prog Horm Res 1996;51:23-58.
408. Shupnik MA. Gonadotropin gene modulation by steroids and gonadotropin-releasing hormone. Biol Reprod 1996;54:279-286.
409. Ezashi T, Hirai T, Kato T, et al. The gene for the β subunit of porcine LH: clusters of GC boxes and CACCC elements. J Mol Endocrinol 1990;5:137-146.
410. Keri RA, Bachmann DJ, Behrooz A, et al. An NF-Y binding site is important for basal, but not gonadotropin-releasing hormone–stimulated, expression of the luteinizing hormone β subunit gene. J Biol Chem 2000;275:13082-13088.
411. Duan WR, Shin JL, Jameson JL. Estradiol suppresses phosphorylation of cyclic adenosine 3′,5′- monophosphate response element binding protein (CREB) in the pituitary: evidence for indirect

action via gonadotropin-releasing hormone. Mol Endocrinol 1999; 13:1338-1352.
412. Halvorson LM, Ito M, Jameson JL, Chin WW. Steroidogenic factor-1 and early growth response protein 1 act through two composite DNA binding sites to regulate luteinizing hormone β-subunit gene expression. J Biol Chem 1998;273:14712-14720.
413. Glaser T, Lewis WH, Bruns GA, et al. The β-subunit of follicle-stimulating hormone is deleted in patients with aniridia and Wilms' tumour, allowing a further definition of the WAGR locus. Nature 1986;321:882-887.
414. Brown P, McNeilly AS. Transcriptional regulation of pituitary gonadotrophin subunit genes. Rev Reprod 1999;4:117-124.
415. Jaakkola T, Ding YQ, Kellokumpu-Lehtinen P, et al. The ratios of serum bioactive/immunoreactive luteinizing hormone and follicle-stimulating hormone in various clinical conditions with increased and decreased gonadotropin secretion: reevaluation by a highly sensitive immunometric assay. J Clin Endocrinol Metab 1990;70:1496-1505.
416. Lucky AW, Rich BH, Rosenfield RL, et al. LH bioactivity increases more than immunoreactivity during puberty. J Pediatr 1980; 97:205-213.
417. Jia XC, Hsueh AJ. Granulosa cell aromatase bioassay for follicle-stimulating hormone: validation and application of the method. Endocrinology 1986;119:1570-1577.
418. Knobil E. The neuroendocrine control of the menstrual cycle. Recent Prog Horm Res 1980;36:53-88.
419. Crowley WF Jr, Whitcomb RW, Jameson JL, et al. Neuroendocrine control of human reproduction in the male. Recent Prog Horm Res 1991;47:27-62.
420. Finkelstein JS, O'Dea LS, Whitcomb RW, Crowley WF Jr. Sex steroid control of gonadotropin secretion in the human male. II. Effects of estradiol administration in normal and gonadotropin-releasing hormone–deficient men. J Clin Endocrinol Metab 1991;73: 621-628.
421. Finkelstein JS, Whitcomb RW, O'Dea LS, et al. Sex steroid control of gonadotropin secretion in the human male. I. Effects of testosterone administration in normal and gonadotropin- releasing hormone-deficient men. J Clin Endocrinol Metab 1991;73: 609-620.
422. Bhasin S, Fisher CE, Sverdloff RS. Follicle-stimulating hormone and luteinizing hormone. In Melmed S, ed. The Pituitary, 2nd ed. Malden, MA: Blackwell Science, 2002:216-278.
423. Veldhuis JD, Pincus SM, Garcia-Rudaz MC, et al. Disruption of the synchronous secretion of leptin, LH, and ovarian androgens in nonobese adolescents with the polycystic ovarian syndrome. J Clin Endocrinol Metab 2001;86:3772-3778.
424. Vale W, Rivier C, Hsueh A, et al. Chemical and biological characterization of the inhibin family of protein hormones. Recent Prog Horm Res 1988;44:1-34.
425. Stocco DM. Tracking the role of a star in the sky of the new millennium. Mol Endocrinol 2001;15:1245-1254.
426. Sprengel R, Braun T, Nikolics K, et al. The testicular receptor for follicle stimulating hormone: structure and functional expression of cloned cDNA. Mol Endocrinol 1990;4:525-530.
427. Hsueh AJ, Adashi EY, Jones PB, Welsh TH Jr. Hormonal regulation of the differentiation of cultured ovarian granulosa cells. Endocr Rev 1984;5:76-127.
428. Mortimer CH, Besser GM, McNeilly AS, et al. Luteinizing hormone and follicle stimulating hormone–releasing hormone test in patients with hypothalamic-pituitary-gonadal dysfunction. BMJ 1973;4:73-77.
429. Zirkin BR, Awoniyi C, Griswold MD, et al. Is FSH required for adult spermatogenesis? J Androl 1994;15:273-276.
430. McCullagh DR. Dual endocrine activity of the testes. Science 1932;76:19-23.
431. Nachtigall LB, Boepple PA, Pralong FP, Crowley WF Jr. Adult-onset idiopathic hypogonadotropic hypogonadism—a treatable form of male infertility. N Engl J Med 1997;336:410-415.
432. Anawalt BD, Bremner, W.J. Diagnosis and treatment of male gonadotropin insufficiency. In Lamberts SW, ed. The diagnosis and treatment of pituitary insufficiency. Bristol: BioScientifica Ltd, 1997:163-207.
433. Snyder PJ, Lawrence DA. Treatment of male hypogonadism with testosterone enanthate. J Clin Endocrinol Metab 1980;51: 1335-1339.
434. Handelsman DJ, Conway AJ, Boylan LM. Pharmacokinetics and pharmacodynamics of testosterone pellets in man. J Clin Endocrinol Metab 1990;71:216-222.
435. Whitsel EA, Boyko EJ, Matsumoto AM, et al. Intramuscular testosterone esters and plasma lipids in hypogonadal men: a meta-analysis. Am J Med 2001;111:261-269.
436. Anawalt BD, Bebb RA, Bremner WJ, Matsumoto AM. A lower dosage levonorgestrel and testosterone combination effectively suppresses spermatogenesis and circulating gonadotropin levels with fewer metabolic effects than higher dosage combinations. J Androl 1999;20:407-414.
437. Bhasin S, Salehian B. Gonadotropin therapy of men with hypogonadotropic hypogonadism. Curr Ther Endocrinol Metab 1997;6: 349-352.
438. Balen AH, Braat DD, West C, et al. Cumulative conception and live birth rates after the treatment of anovulatory infertility: safety and efficacy of ovulation induction in 200 patients. Hum Reprod 1994;9:1563-1570.
439. Martin KA, Hall JE, Adams JM, Crowley WF Jr. Comparison of exogenous gonadotropins and pulsatile gonadotropin-releasing hormone for induction of ovulation in hypogonadotropic amenorrhea. J Clin Endocrinol Metab 1993;77:125-129.
440. Suikkari A, MacLachlan V, Koistinen R, et al. Double-blind placebo controlled study: human biosynthetic growth hormone for assisted reproductive technology. Fertil Steril 1996;65:800-805.
441. Horvath E, Kovacs K. Ultrastructural diagnosis of human pituitary adenomas. Microsc Res Tech 1992;20:107-135.
442. Jameson JL, Klibanski A, Black PM, et al. Glycoprotein hormone genes are expressed in clinically nonfunctioning pituitary adenomas. J Clin Invest 1987;80:1472-1478.
443. Nobels FR, Kwekkeboom DJ, Coopmans W, et al. A comparison between the diagnostic value of gonadotropins, α-subunit, and chromogranin-A and their response to thyrotropin-releasing hormone in clinically nonfunctioning, α-subunit-secreting, and gonadotroph pituitary adenomas. J Clin Endocrinol Metab 1993;77:784-789.
444. Kovacs K, Horvath E, Ryan N, Ezrin C. Null cell adenoma of the human pituitary. Virchows Arch A Pathol Anat Histol 1980;387: 165-174.
445. Chaidarun SS, Klibanski A. Gonadotropinomas. Semin Reprod Med 2002;20:339-348.
446. Valimaki MJ, Tiitinen A, Alfthan H, et al. Ovarian hyperstimulation caused by gonadotroph adenoma secreting follicle-stimulating hormone in 28-year-old woman. J Clin Endocrinol Metab 1999; 84:4204-4208.
447. Daneshdoost L, Gennarelli TA, Bashey HM, et al. Recognition of gonadotroph adenomas in women. N Engl J Med 1991;324: 589-594.
448. Snyder PJ. Clinically nonfunctioning pituitary adenomas. Endocrinol Metab Clin North Am 1993;22:163-175.
449. Boelaert K, Gittoes NJ. Radiotherapy for non-functioning pituitary adenomas. Eur J Endocrinol 2001;144:569-575.
450. Minniti G, Traish D, Ashley S, Gonsalves A, Brada M. Fractionated stereotactic conformal radiotherapy for secreting and nonsecreting pituitary adenomas. Clin Endocrinol (Oxf) 2006;64:542-548.
451. Ebersold MJ, Quast LM, Laws ER Jr, et al. Long-term results in transsphenoidal removal of nonfunctioning pituitary adenomas. J Neurosurg 1986;64:713-719.
452. Turner HE, Stratton IM, Byrne JV, et al. Audit of selected patients with nonfunctioning pituitary adenomas treated without irradiation—a follow-up study. Clin Endocrinol (Oxf) 1999;51:281-284.
453. Gittoes NJ. Radiotherapy for non-functioning pituitary tumors—when and under what circumstances? Pituitary 2003;6:103-108.
454. Losa M, Valle M, Mortini P, et al. Gamma knife surgery for treatment of residual nonfunctioning pituitary adenomas after surgical debulking. J Neurosurg 2004;100:438-444.
455. Dekkers OM, Pereira AM, Roelfsema F, et al. Observation alone after transsphenoidal surgery for nonfunctioning pituitary macroadenoma. J Clin Endocrinol Metab 2006;91:1796-1801.
456. Greenman Y, Melmed S. Diagnosis and management of nonfunctioning pituitary tumors. Annu Rev Med 1996;47:95-106.
457. Greenman Y, Tordjman K, Osher E, et al. Postoperative treatment of clinically nonfunctioning pituitary adenomas with dopamine agonists decreases tumour remnant growth. Clin Endocrinol (Oxf) 2005;63:39-44.

458. McGrath GA, Goncalves RJ, Udupa JK, et al. New technique for quantitation of pituitary adenoma size: use in evaluating treatment of gonadotroph adenomas with a gonadotropin-releasing hormone antagonist. J Clin Endocrinol Metab 1993;76:1363-1368.
459. Plockinger U, Reichel M, Fett U, et al. Preoperative octreotide treatment of growth hormone–secreting and clinically nonfunctioning pituitary macroadenomas: effect on tumor volume and lack of correlation with immunohistochemistry and somatostatin receptor scintigraphy. J Clin Endocrinol Metab 1994;79:1416-1423.
460. Frohman LA, Burek L, Stachura MA. Characterization of growth hormone of different molecular weights in rat, dog and human pituitaries. Endocrinology 1972;91:262-269.
461. Ho Y, Liebhaber SA, Cooke NE. Activation of the human GH gene cluster: roles for targeted chromatin modification. Trends Endocrinol Metab 2004;15:40-45.
462. Miller WL, Eberhardt NL. Structure and evolution of the growth hormone gene family. Endocr Rev 1983;4:97-130.
463. Lewis UJ, Dunn JT, Bonewald LF, et al. A naturally occurring structural variant of human growth hormone. J Biol Chem 1978;253: 2679-2687.
464. Frankenne F, Closset J, Gomez F, et al. The physiology of growth hormones (GHs) in pregnant women and partial characterization of the placental GH variant. J Clin Endocrinol Metab 1988;66: 1171-1180.
465. Parks JS, Brown MR, Hurley DL, et al. Heritable disorders of pituitary development. J Clin Endocrinol Metab 1999;84:4362-4370.
466. Bennani-Baiti IM, Asa SL, Song D, et al. DNase I-hypersensitive sites I and II of the human growth hormone locus control region are a major developmental activator of somatotrope gene expression. Proc Natl Acad Sci U S A 1998;95:10655-10660.
467. Cunningham BC, Ultsch M, De Vos AM, et al. Dimerization of the extracellular domain of the human growth hormone receptor by a single hormone molecule. Science 1991;254:821-825.
468. Baumann G, MacCart JG, Amburn K. The molecular nature of circulating growth hormone in normal and acromegalic man: evidence for a principal and minor monomeric forms. J Clin Endocrinol Metab 1983;56:946-952.
469. Mayo KE, Miller T, DeAlmeida V, et al. Regulation of the pituitary somatotroph cell by GHRH and its receptor. Recent Prog Horm Res 2000;55:237-266.
470. Shimon I, Taylor JE, Dong JZ, et al. Somatostatin receptor subtype specificity in human fetal pituitary cultures. Differential role of SSTR2 and SSTR5 for growth hormone, thyroid-stimulating hormone, and prolactin regulation. J Clin Invest 1997;99:789-798.
471. Shimon I, Yan X, Taylor JE, et al. Somatostatin receptor (SSTR) subtype-selective analogues differentially suppress in vitro growth hormone and prolactin in human pituitary adenomas. Novel potential therapy for functional pituitary tumors. J Clin Invest 1997;100:2386-2392.
472. Barinaga M, Yamonoto G, Rivier C, et al. Transcriptional regulation of growth hormone gene expression by growth hormone–releasing factor. Nature 1983;306:84-85.
473. Thorner MO, Frohman LA, Leong DA, et al. Extrahypothalamic growth-hormone-releasing factor (GRF) secretion is a rare cause of acromegaly: plasma GRF levels in 177 acromegalic patients. J Clin Endocrinol Metab 1984;59:846-849.
474. Gelato MC, Pescovitz O, Cassorla F, et al. Effects of a growth hormone releasing factor in man. J Clin Endocrinol Metab 1983;57:674-676.
475. Tannenbaum GS, Ling N. The interrelationship of growth hormone (GH)-releasing factor and somatostatin in generation of the ultradian rhythm of GH secretion. Endocrinology 1984;115:1952-1957.
476. Bilezikjian LM, Seifert H, Vale W. Desensitization to growth hormone–releasing factor (GRF) is associated with down-regulation of GRF-binding sites. Endocrinology 1986;118:2045-2052.
477. Kineman RD, Teixeira LT, Amargo GV, et al. The effect of GHRH on somatotrope hyperplasia and tumor formation in the presence and absence of GH signaling. Endocrinology 2001;142:3764-3773.
478. Gaykema RP, Compaan JC, Nyakas C, et al. Long-term effects of cholinergic basal forebrain lesions on neuropeptide Y and somatostatin immunoreactivity in rat neocortex. Brain Res 1989; 489:392-396.
479. Pombo M, Pombo CM, Garcia A, et al. Hormonal control of growth hormone secretion. Horm Res 2001;55:11-16.
480. LeRoith D, Buler, A. What is the role of circulating IGF-I? Trends Endocrinol Metab 2001;12:48-52.
481. Howard AD, Feighner SD, Cully DF, et al. A receptor in pituitary and hypothalamus that functions in growth hormone release. Science 1996;273:974-977.
482. Kojima M, Hosoda H, Date Y, et al. Ghrelin is a growth-hormone-releasing acylated peptide from stomach. Nature 1999;402: 656-660.
483. Tannenbaum GS, Epelbaum J, Bowers CY. Interrelationship between the novel peptide ghrelin and somatostatin/growth hormone–releasing hormone in regulation of pulsatile growth hormone secretion. Endocrinology 2003;144:967-974.
484. Popovic V, Leal A, Micic D, et al. GH-releasing hormone and GH-releasing peptide-6 for diagnostic testing in GH-deficient adults. Lancet 2000;356:1137-1142.
485. Chang CH, Rickes EL, McGuire L, et al. Growth hormone (GH) and insulin-like growth factor I responses after treatments with an orally active GH secretagogue L-163,255 in swine. Endocrinology 1996;137:4851-4856.
486. Popovic V, Damjanovic S, Micic D, et al. Blocked growth hormone–releasing peptide (GHRP-6)–induced GH secretion and absence of the synergic action of GHRP-6 plus GH-releasing hormone in patients with hypothalamopituitary disconnection: evidence that GHRP- 6 main action is exerted at the hypothalamic level. J Clin Endocrinol Metab 1995;80:942-947.
487. Penalva A, Pombo M, Carballo A, et al. Influence of sex, age and adrenergic pathways on the growth hormone response to GHRP-6. Clin Endocrinol (Oxf) 1993;38:87-91.
488. Jaffe CA, Friberg RD, Barkan AL. Suppression of growth hormone (GH) secretion by a selective GH- releasing hormone (GHRH) antagonist. Direct evidence for involvement of endogenous GHRH in the generation of GH pulses. J Clin Invest 1993;92: 695-701.
489. Loche S, Colao A, Cappa M, et al. The growth hormone response to hexarelin in children: reproducibility and effect of sex steroids. J Clin Endocrinol Metab 1997;82:861-864.
490. Raun K, Hansen BS, Johansen NL, et al. Ipamorelin, the first selective growth hormone secretagogue. Eur J Endocrinol 1998;139: 552-561.
491. Van Cauter E, Plat L, Copinschi G. Interrelations between sleep and the somatotropic axis. Sleep 1998;21:553-566.
492. Van Cauter E. Slow wave sleep and release of growth hormone. JAMA 2000;284:2717-2718.
493. Vigas M, Malatinsky J, Nemeth S, Jurcovicova J. α-Adrenergic control of growth hormone release during surgical stress in man. Metabolism 1977;26:399-402.
494. Sachar EJ, Mushrush G, Perlow M, et al. Growth hormone responses to L-dopa in depressed patients. Science 1972;178:1304-1305.
495. Ho KY, Veldhuis JD, Johnson ML, et al. Fasting enhances growth hormone secretion and amplifies the complex rhythms of growth hormone secretion in man. J Clin Invest 1988;81:968-975.
496. Vigneri R, Squatrito S, Pezzino V, et al. Growth hormone levels in diabetes. Correlation with the clinical control of the disease. Diabetes 1976;25:167-172.
497. Casanueva FF, Dieguez C. Neuroendocrine regulation and actions of leptin. Front Neuroendocrinol 1999;20:317-363.
498. Carro E, Senaris R, Considine RV, et al. Regulation of in vivo growth hormone secretion by leptin. Endocrinology 1997; 138:2203-2206.
499. Okada K, Sugihara H, Minami S, Wakabayashi I. Effect of parenteral administration of selected nutrients and central injection of gamma-globulin from antiserum to neuropeptide Y on growth hormone secretory pattern in food-deprived rats. Neuroendocrinology 1993;57:678-686.
500. al-Shoumer KA, Anyaoku V, Richmond W, Johnston DG. Elevated leptin concentrations in growth hormone–deficient hypopituitary adults. Clin Endocrinol (Oxf) 1997;47:153-159.
501. Lal S, Martin JB, De la Vega CE, Friesen HG. Comparison of the effect of apomorphine and L-dopa on serum growth hormone levels in normal men. Clin Endocrinol (Oxf) 1975;4:277-285.
502. Giustina A, Veldhuis JD. Pathophysiology of the neuroregulation of growth hormone secretion in experimental animals and the human. Endocr Rev 1998;19:717-797.
503. Casanueva FF, Burguera B, Muruais C, Dieguez C. Acute administration of corticoids: a new and peculiar stimulus of growth

hormone secretion in man. J Clin Endocrinol Metab 1990;70: 234-237.
504. Suda T, Demura H, Demura R, et al. Anterior pituitary hormones in plasma and pituitaries from patients with Cushing's disease. J Clin Endocrinol Metab 1980;51:1048-1053.
505. Irie M, Tsushima T. Increase of serum growth hormone concentration following thyrotropin-releasing hormone injection in patients with acromegaly or gigantism. J Clin Endocrinol Metab 1972;35: 97-100.
506. Herington AC, Ymer S, Stevenson J. Identification and characterization of specific binding proteins for growth hormone in normal human sera. J Clin Invest 1986;77:1817-1823.
507. Leung DW, Spencer SA, Cachianes G, et al. Growth hormone receptor and serum binding protein: purification, cloning and expression. Nature 1987;330:537-543.
508. Baumann G, Shaw MA, Amburn K. Regulation of plasma growth hormone–binding proteins in health and disease. Metabolism 1989;38:683-689.
509. Carter-Su C, Schwartz J, Smit LS. Molecular mechanism of growth hormone action. Annu Rev Physiol 1996;58:187-207.
510. Brown RJ, Adams JJ, Pelekanos RA, et al. Model for growth hormone receptor activation based on subunit rotation within a receptor dimer. Nat Struct Mol Biol 2005;12:814-821.
511. Leung KC, Waters MJ, Markus I, et al. Insulin and insulin-like growth factor-I acutely inhibit surface translocation of growth hormone receptors in osteoblasts: a novel mechanism of growth hormone receptor regulation. Proc Natl Acad Sci U S A 1997;94: 11381-11386.
512. Xu BC, Wang X, Darus CJ, Kopchick JJ. Growth hormone promotes the association of transcription factor STAT5 with the growth hormone receptor. J Biol Chem 1996;271:19768-19773.
513. Yakar S, Liu JL, Stannard B, et al. Normal growth and development in the absence of hepatic insulin-like growth factor I. Proc Natl Acad Sci U S A 1999;96:7324-7329.
514. Low MJ, Otero-Corchon V, Parlow AF, et al. Somatostatin is required for masculinization of growth hormone–regulated hepatic gene expression but not of somatic growth. J Clin Invest 2001;107: 1571-1580.
515. Udy GB, Towers RP, Snell RG, et al. Requirement of STAT5b for sexual dimorphism of body growth rates and liver gene expression. Proc Natl Acad Sci U S A 1997;94:7239-7244.
516. Ram PA, Park SH, Choi HK, Waxman DJ. Growth hormone activation of Stat 1, Stat 3, and Stat 5 in rat liver. Differential kinetics of hormone desensitization and growth hormone stimulation of both tyrosine phosphorylation and serine/threonine phosphorylation. J Biol Chem 1996;271:5929-5940.
517. Teglund S, McKay C, Schuetz E, et al. Stat5a and Stat5b proteins have essential and nonessential, or redundant, roles in cytokine responses. Cell 1998;93:841-850.
518. Davey HW, Park SH, Grattan DR, McLachlan MJ, Waxman DJ. STAT5b-deficient mice are growth hormone pulse–resistant. Role of STAT5b in sex-specific liver p450 expression. J Biol Chem 1999;274:35331-35336.
519. Park SH, Liu X, Hennighausen L, et al. Distinctive roles of STAT5a and STAT5b in sexual dimorphism of hepatic P450 gene expression. Impact of STAT5a gene disruption. J Biol Chem 1999;274: 7421-7430.
520. Eugster EA, Pescovitz OH. New revelations about the role of STATs in stature. N Engl J Med 2003;349:1110-1112.
521. Starr R, Hilton DJ. SOCS: suppressors of cytokine signalling. Int J Biochem Cell Biol 1998;30:1081-1085.
522. Greenhalgh CJ, Rico-Bautista E, Lorentzon M, et al. SOCS2 negatively regulates growth hormone action in vitro and in vivo. J Clin Invest 2005;115:397-406.
523. Harvey S, Hull KL. Growth hormone. A paracrine growth factor? Endocrine 1997;7:267-279.
524. Johansson JO, Fowelin J, Landin K, et al. Growth hormone–deficient adults are insulin-resistant. Metabolism 1995;44:1126-1129.
525. Rose SR, Ross JL, Uriarte M, et al. The advantage of measuring stimulated as compared with spontaneous growth hormone levels in the diagnosis of growth hormone deficiency. N Engl J Med 1988;319:201-207.
526. Aimaretti G, Colao A, Corneli G, et al. The study of spontaneous GH secretion after 36-h fasting distinguishes between GH-deficient and normal adults. Clin Endocrinol (Oxf) 1999;51:771-777.
527. Rosenfeld RG, Albertsson-Wikland K, Cassorla F, et al. Diagnostic controversy: the diagnosis of childhood growth hormone deficiency revisited. J Clin Endocrinol Metab 1995;80:1532-1540.
528. Granada ML, Sanmarti A, Lucas A, et al. Assay-dependent results of immunoassayable spontaneous 24-hour growth hormone secretion in short children. Acta Paediatr Scand Suppl 1990;370:63-70.
529. Reiter EO, Morris AH, MacGillivray MH, Weber D. Variable estimates of serum growth hormone concentrations by different radioassay systems. J Clin Endocrinol Metab 1988;66:68-71.
530. Baumann G, Shaw M, Amburn K, et al. Heterogeneity of circulating growth hormone. Nucl Med Biol 1994;21:369-379.
531. Strasburger CJ, Dattani MT. New growth hormone assays: potential benefits. Acta Paediatr Suppl 1997;423:5-11.
532. Bristow AF, Gaines-Das R, Jeffcoate SL, Schulster D. The First International Standard for Somatropin: report of an international collaborative study. Growth Regul 1995;5:133-141.
533. Fisker S, Orskov H. Factors modifying growth hormone estimates in immunoassays. Horm Res 1996;46:183-187.
534. Salomon F, Cuneo RC, Hesp R, Sonksen PH. The effects of treatment with recombinant human growth hormone on body composition and metabolism in adults with growth hormone deficiency. N Engl J Med 1989;321:1797-1803.
535. de Boer H, Blok GJ, van der Veen EA. Clinical aspects of growth hormone deficiency in adults. Endocr Rev 1995;16:63-86.
536. Molitch ME, Clemmons DR, Malozowski S, et al. Evaluation and treatment of adult growth hormone deficiency: an Endocrine Society Clinical Practice Guideline. J Clin Endocrinol Metab 2006;91:1621-1634.
537. Rosen T, Bengtsson BA. Premature mortality due to cardiovascular disease in hypopituitarism. Lancet 1990;336:285-288.
538. Bates AS, Van't Hoff W, Jones PJ, Clayton RN. The effect of hypopituitarism on life expectancy. J Clin Endocrinol Metab 1996;81:1169-1172.
539. Bulow B, Hagmar L, Eskilsson J, Erfurth EM. Hypopituitary females have a high incidence of cardiovascular morbidity and increased prevalence of cardiovascular risk factors. J Clin Endo Metab 2000;85:574-584.
540. Abs R, Bengtsson BA, Hernberg-Stahl E, et al. GH replacement in 1034 growth hormone deficient hypopituitary adults: demographic and clinical characteristics, dosing and safety. Clin Endocrinol (Oxf) 1999;50:703-713.
541. Tauber M, Moulin P, Pienkowski C, et al. Growth hormone retesting and auxological data in 131 GH-deficient patients after completion of treatment. J Clin Endocrinol Metab 1997;82:352-356.
542. Cogan JD, Phillips JA, Schenkman SS, et al. Familial growth hormone deficiency: a model of dominant and recessive mutations affecting a monomeric protein. J Clin Endocrinol Metab 1994;79:1261-1265.
543. Baumann G. Mutations in the growth hormone releasing hormone receptor: a new form of dwarfism in humans. Growth Horm IGF Res 1999;9(suppl B):24-29.
544. Rosenfeld RG, Rosenbloom AL, Guevara-Aguirre J. Growth hormone (GH) insensitivity due to primary GH receptor deficiency. Endocr Rev 1994;15:369-390.
545. Wu W, Cogan JD, Pfaffle RW, et al. Mutations in PROP1 cause familial combined pituitary hormone deficiency. Nature Gen 1998;18:147-149.
546. Sesmilo G, Biller BM, Llevadot J, et al. Effects of growth hormone (GH) administration on homocyst(e)ine levels in men with GH deficiency: a randomized controlled trial. J Clin Endocrinol Metab 2001;86:1518-1524.
547. Consensus guidelines for the diagnosis and treatment of adults with growth hormone deficiency: summary statement of the Growth Hormone Research Society Workshop on Adult Growth Hormone Deficiency. J Clin Endocrinol Metab 1998;83:379-381.
548. Carroll PV, Christ ER, Bengtsson BA, et al. Growth hormone deficiency in adulthood and the effects of growth hormone replacement: a review. Growth Hormone Research Society Scientific Committee. J Clin Endocrinol Metab 1998;83:382-395.
549. Arvat E, Di Vito L, Broglio F, et al. Preliminary evidence that ghrelin, the natural GH secretagogue (GHS)-receptor ligand, strongly stimulates GH secretion in humans. J Endocrinol Invest 2000;23:493-495.
550. Drake WM, Howell SJ, Monson JP, Shalet SM. Optimizing GH therapy in adults and children. Endocr Rev 2001;22:425-450.

551. Marzullo P, Di Somma C, Pratt KL, et al. Usefulness of different biochemical markers of the insulin-like growth factor (IGF) family in diagnosing growth hormone excess and deficiency in adults. J Clin Endocrinol Metab 2001;86:3001-3008.
552. Hilding A, Hall K, Wivall-Helleryd IL, et al. Serum levels of insulin-like growth factor I in 152 patients with growth hormone deficiency, aged 19-82 years, in relation to those in healthy subjects. J Clin Endocrinol Metab 1999;84:2013-2019.
553. Gill MS, Toogood AA, O'Neill PA, et al. Urinary growth hormone (GH), insulin-like growth factor I (IGF-I), and IGF-binding protein-3 measurements in the diagnosis of adult GH deficiency. J Clin Endocrinol Metab 1998;83:2562-2565.
554. Newman CB, Kleinberg DL. Adult growth hormone deficiency. Endocrinologist 1998;8:178-186.
555. Rosen T, Bosaeus I, Tolli J, Lindstedt G, Bengtsson BA. Increased body fat mass and decreased extracellular fluid volume in adults with growth hormone deficiency. Clin Endocrinol (Oxf) 1993; 38:63-71.
556. Colao A, Di Somma C, Pivonello R, et al. Bone loss is correlated to the severity of growth hormone deficiency in adult patients with hypopituitarism. J Clin Endocrinol Metab 1999;84:1919-1924.
557. Vance ML, Mauras N. Growth hormone therapy in adults and children. N Engl J Med 1999;341:1206-1216.
558. Sesmilo G, Biller BM, Llevadot J, et al. Effects of growth hormone administration on inflammatory and other cardiovascular risk markers in men with growth hormone deficiency. A randomized, controlled clinical trial. Ann Intern Med 2000;133:111-122.
559. Attanasio AF, Lamberts SWJ, Matranga AMC, et al. Adult growth hormone (GH)-deficient patients demonstrate heterogeneity between childhood onset and adult onset before and during human GH treatment. J Clin Endocrinol Metab 1997;82:82-88.
560. Svensson J, Fowelin J, Landin K, et al. Effects of seven years of GH-replacement therapy on insulin sensitivity in GH-deficient adults. J Clin Endocrinol Metab 2002;87:2121-2127.
561. Pfeifer M, Verhovec R, Zizek B, et al. Growth hormone (GH) treatment reverses early atherosclerotic changes in GH-deficient adults. J Clin Endocrinol Metab 1999;84:453-457.
562. Borson-Chazot F, Serusclat A, Kalfallah Y, et al. Decrease in carotid intima-media thickness after one year growth hormone (GH) treatment in adults with GH deficiency. J Clin Endocrinol Metab 1999;84:1329-1333.
563. Merola B, Cittadini A, Colao A, et al. Cardiac structural and functional abnormalities in adult patients with growth hormone deficiency. J Clin Endocrinol Metab 1993;77:1658-1661.
564. Amato G, Carella C, Fazio S, et al. Body composition, bone metabolism, and heart structure and function in growth hormone (GH)-deficient adults before and after GH replacement therapy at low doses. J Clin Endocrinol Metab 1993;77:1671-1676.
565. Klibanski A. Growth hormone and cardiovascular risk markers. Growth Horm IGF Res 2003;13(suppl A):S109-S115.
566. Murray RD, Skillicorn CJ, Howell SJ, et al. Dose titration and patient selection increases the efficacy of GH replacement in severely GH deficient adults. Clin Endocrinol (Oxf) 1999;50: 749-757.
567. Murray RD, Skillicorn CJ, Howell SJ, et al. Influences on quality of life in GH deficient adults and their effect on response to treatment. Clin Endocrinol (Oxf) 1999;51:565-573.
568. Wang TC, Koh TJ, Varro A, et al. Processing and proliferative effects of human progastrin in transgenic mice. J Clin Invest 1996;98:1918-1929.
569. Horber FF, Haymond MW. Human growth hormone prevents the protein catabolic side effects of prednisone in humans. J Clin Invest 1990;86:265-272.
570. Baum HB, Biller BM, Finkelstein JS, et al. Effects of physiologic growth hormone therapy on bone density and body composition in patients with adult-onset growth hormone deficiency. A randomized, placebo-controlled trial. Ann Intern Med 1996;125: 883-890.
571. Kotzmann H, Riedl M, Bernecker P, et al. Effect of long-term growth-hormone substitution therapy on bone mineral density and parameters of bone metabolism in adult patients with growth hormone deficiency. Calcif Tissue Int 1998;62:40-46.
572. Cuneo RC, Judd S, Wallace JD, et al. The Australian Multicenter Trial of Growth Hormone (GH) Treatment in GH-Deficient Adults. J Clin Endocrinol Metab 1998;83:107-116.
573. Boger RH, Skamira C, Bode-Boger SM, et al. Nitric oxide may mediate the hemodynamic effects of recombinant growth hormone in patients with acquired growth hormone deficiency. A double-blind, placebo-controlled study. J Clin Invest 1996;98:2706-2713.
574. Colao A, Marzullo P, Di Somma C, Lombardi G. Growth hormone and the heart. Clin Endocrinol (Oxf) 2001;54:137-154.
575. Rosilio M, Blum WF, Edwards DJ, et al. Long-term improvement of quality of life during growth hormone (GH) replacement therapy in adults with GH deficiency, as measured by questions on life satisfaction—hypopituitarism (QLS-H). J Clin Endocrinol Metab 2004;89:1684-1693.
576. Baum HB, Katznelson L, Sherman JC, et al. Effects of physiological growth hormone (GH) therapy on cognition and quality of life in patients with adult-onset GH deficiency. J Clin Endocrinol Metab 1998;83:3184-3189.
577. Gibney J, Wallace JD, Spinks T, et al. The effects of 10 years of recombinant human growth hormone (GH) in adult GH-deficient patients. J Clin Endocrinol Metab 1999;84:2596-2602.
578. Blethen S. Dosing, monitoring, and safety of growth hormone–replacement therapy in adults with growth hormone deficiency. Endocrinologist 1998;8:36S-40S.
579. Cook DM, Ludlam WH, Cook MB. Route of estrogen administration helps to determine growth hormone (GH) replacement dose in GH-deficient adults. J Clin Endocrinol Metab 1999;84:3956-3960.
580. Hoffman DM, Pallasser R, Duncan M, et al. How is whole body protein turnover perturbed in growth hormone- deficient adults? J Clin Endocrinol Metab 1998;83:4344-4349.
581. de Boer H, Blok GJ, Popp-Snijders C, et al. Monitoring of growth hormone replacement therapy in adults, based on measurement of serum markers. J Clin Endocrinol Metab 1996;81:1371-1377.
582. Chan JM, Stampfer MJ, Giovannucci E, et al. Plasma insulin-like growth factor-I and prostate cancer risk: A prospective study. Science 1998;279:563-566.
583. Hankinson SE, Willett WC, Colditz GA, et al. Circulating concentrations of insulin-like growth factor-I and risk of breast cancer. Lancet 1998;351:1393-1396.
584. Yu H, Rohan T. Role of the insulin-like growth factor family in cancer development and progression. J Natl Cancer Inst 2000; 92:1472-1489.
585. Orme S, McNally RJQ, Cartwright RA, Belchetz PE. Mortality and cancer incidence in acromegaly: a retrospective cohort study. J Clin Endo Metab 1998;83:2730-2734.
586. Melmed S. Acromegaly and cancer: not a problem? J Clin Endocrinol Metab 2001;86:2929-2934.
587. Renehan AG, Bhaskar P, Painter JE, et al. The prevalence and characteristics of colorectal neoplasia in acromegaly. J Clin Endocrinol Metab 2000;85:3417-3424.
588. Sklar C. Paying the price for cure—treating cancer survivors with growth hormone. J Clin Endocrinol Metab 2000;85:4441-4443.
589. Swerdlow AJ, Reddingius RE, Higgins CD, et al. Growth hormone treatment of children with brain tumors and risk of tumor recurrence. J Clin Endocrinol Metab 2000;85:4444-4449.
590. Ergun-Longmire B, Mertens AC, Mitby P, et al. Growth hormone treatment and risk of second neoplasms in the childhood cancer survivor. J Clin Endocrinol Metab 2006;91(9):3494-3498.
591. Jenkins RC, Ross RJ. Growth hormone therapy for protein catabolism. QJM 1996;89:813-819.
592. Chu LW, Lam KS, Tam SC, et al. A randomized controlled trial of low-dose recombinant human growth hormone in the treatment of malnourished elderly medical patients. J Clin Endocrinol Metab 2001;86:1913-1920.
593. Takala J, Ruokonen E, Webster NR, et al. Increased mortality associated with growth hormone treatment in critically ill adults. N Engl J Med 1999;341:785-792.
594. Hoiden-Guthenberg I, Flores-Morales A, Norstedt G, Fryklund L. Anabolic actions of growth hormone in catabolic states: analysis of differential gene expression in rats treated with GH and LPS using cDNA microarrays. Presented at the Endocrine Society's 83rd Annual Meeting, Denver, Colorado, June 22-25, 2001.
595. Perls TT, Reisman NR, Olshansky SJ. Provision or distribution of growth hormone for "antiaging": clinical and legal issues. JAMA 2005;294:2086-2090.
596. Holloway L, Kohlmeier L, Kent K, Marcus R. Skeletal effects of cyclic recombinant human growth hormone and salmon calcito-

nin in osteopenic postmenopausal women. J Clin Endocrinol Metab 1997;82:1111-1117.
597. Schambelan M, Mulligan K, Grunfeld C, et al. Recombinant human growth hormone in patients with HIV-associated wasting. A randomized, placebo-controlled trial. Serostim Study Group. Ann Intern Med 1996;125:873-882.
598. Grinspoon S, Carr A. Cardiovascular risk and body-fat abnormalities in HIV-infected adults. N Engl J Med 2005;352:48-62.
599. Lo JC, Mulligan K, Noor MA, et al. The effects of recombinant human growth hormone on body composition and glucose metabolism in HIV-infected patients with fat accumulation. J Clin Endocrinol Metab 2001;86:3480-3487.
600. Sonksen PH. Insulin, growth hormone and sport. J Endocrinol 2001;170:13-25.
601. Isley WL, Underwood LE, Clemmons DR. Dietary components that regulate serum somatomedin-C concentrations in humans. J Clin Invest 1983;71:175-182.
602. Benda C. Beitrage zur normalen und pathologischen histologic der menschhchen hypophysis cerebri. Klin Wochenschr 1900;36:1205.
603. Evans HM, Long, J.A. The effect of the anterior lobe of the pituitary administered intra-peritoneally upon growth, maturity and oestrus cycle of the rat. Anat Rev 1921;21:62.
604. Alexander L, Appleton D, Hall R, et al. Epidemiology of acromegaly in the Newcastle region. Clin Endocrinol (Oxf) 1980;12:71-79.
605. Bengtsson BA, Eden S, Ernest I, et al. Epidemiology and long-term survival in acromegaly. A study of 166 cases diagnosed between 1955 and 1984. Acta Med Scand 1988;223:327-335.
606. Ritchie CM, Atkinson AB, Kennedy AL, et al. Ascertainment and natural history of treated acromegaly in Northern Ireland. Ulster Med J 1990;59:55-62.
607. Melmed S. Acromegaly [see comments]. N Engl J Med 1990;322: 966-977.
608. Asa SL, Kovacs K. Pituitary pathology in acromegaly. Endocrinol Metab Clin North Am 1992;21:553-574.
609. Lloyd RV, Cano M, Chandler WF, et al. Human growth hormone and prolactin secreting pituitary adenomas analyzed by in situ hybridization. Am J Pathol 1989;134:605-613.
610. Maheshwari HG, Prezant TR, Herman-Bonert V, et al. Long-acting peptidomimergic control of gigantism caused by pituitary acidophilic stem cell adenoma. J Clin Endocrinol Metab 2000;85: 3409-3416.
611. Kovacs K, Horvath E, Asa SL, et al. Pituitary cells producing more than one hormone. Trends Endocrinol Metab 1989;1:104-108.
612. Melmed S. Pituitary function and neoplasia. In Jameson JL, ed. Principles of Molecular Medicine. Totowa, NJ: Humana Press, 1998:443-449.
613. Heaney AP, Melmed S. Molecular pathogenesis of pituitary tumors. Wass JAH, Shalet SM, eds. Oxford Textbook of Endocrinology. Oxford: Oxford University Press, 2002:109-120.
614. Shimon I, Melmed S. Genetic basis of endocrine disease: pituitary tumor pathogenesis. J Clin Endocrinol Metab 1997;82:1675-1681.
615. Dimaraki EV, Chandler WF, Brown MB, et al. The role of endogenous growth hormone–releasing hormone in acromegaly. J Clin Endocrinol Metab 2006;91:2185-2190.
616. Thapar K, Kovacs K, Stefaneanu L, et al. Overexpression of the growth-hormone-releasing hormone gene in acromegaly-associated pituitary tumors. An event associated with neoplastic progression and aggressive behavior. Am J Pathol 1997;151:769-784.
617. Thorner MO, Vance ML. Growth hormone, 1988. J Clin Invest 1988;82:745-747.
618. Herman I, Gonsky R, Fagin J. Clonal origin of secretory and nonsecretory pituitary tumors. Clin Res 1990;38:296A-296A.
619. Vallar L, Spada A, Giannattasio G. Altered Gs and adenylate cyclase activity in human GH-secreting pituitary adenomas. Nature 1987;330:566-568.
620. Landis CA, Harsh G, Lyons J, et al. Clinical characteristics of acromegalic patients whose pituitary tumors contain mutant Gs protein. J Clin Endocrinol Metab 1990;71:1416-1420.
621. Frohman LA, Jansson JO. Growth hormone–releasing hormone. Endocr Rev 1986;7:223-253.
622. Melmed S, Ezrin C, Kovacs K, et al. Acromegaly due to secretion of growth hormone by an ectopic pancreatic islet-cell tumor. N Engl J Med 1985;312:9-17.
623. Moran A, Asa SL, Kovacs K, et al. Gigantism due to pituitary mammosomatotroph hyperplasia. N Engl J Med 1990;323: 322-327.
624. Faglia G, Arosio M, Bazzoni N. Ectopic acromegaly. Endocrinol Metab Clin North Am 1992;21:575-595.
625. Frohman LA, Szabo M, Berelowitz M, Stachura ME. Partial purification and characterization of a peptide with growth hormone–releasing activity from extrapituitary tumors in patients with acromegaly. J Clin Invest 1980;65:43-54.
626. Drange MR, Melmed S. Long-acting lanreotide induces clinical and biochemical remission of acromegaly caused by disseminated growth hormone–releasing hormone–secreting carcinoid [see comments]. J Clin Endocrinol Metab 1998;83:3104-3109.
627. Barkan AL, Shenker Y, Grekin RJ, Vale WW. Acromegaly from ectopic growth hormone–releasing hormone secretion by a malignant carcinoid tumor. Successful treatment with long-acting somatostatin analogue SMS 201-995. Cancer 1988;61:221-226.
628. Lloyd RV, Chandler WF, Kovacs K, et al. Ectopic pituitary adenomas with normal anterior pituitary glands. Am J Surg Pathol 1986;10:546-552.
629. Madonna D, Kendler A, Soliman AM. Ectopic growth hormone–secreting pituitary adenoma in the sphenoid sinus. Ann Otol Rhinol Laryngol 2001;110:99-101.
630. Beuschlein F, Strasburger CJ, Siegerstetter V, et al. Acromegaly caused by secretion of growth hormone by a non-Hodgkin's lymphoma. N Engl J Med 2000;342:1871-1876.
631. Misaki M, Shima T, Ikoma J, et al. Acromegaly and hyperthyroidism associated with McCune-Albright syndrome. Horm Res 1988; 30:26-27.
632. Weinstein LS, Shenker A, Gejman PV, et al. Activating mutations of the stimulatory G protein in the McCune-Albright syndrome. N Engl J Med 1991;325:1688-1695.
633. Chandrasekharappa SC, Guru SC, Manickam P, et al. Positional cloning of the gene for multiple endocrine neoplasia-type 1. Science 1997;276:404-407.
634. Teh BT, Kytola S, Farnebo F, et al. Mutation analysis of the *MEN1* gene in multiple endocrine neoplasia type 1, familial acromegaly and familial isolated hyperparathyroidism. J Clin Endocrinol Metab 1998;83:2621-2626.
635. Stratakis CA, Carney JA, Lin JP, et al. Carney complex, a familial multiple neoplasia and lentiginosis syndrome. Analysis of 11 kindreds and linkage to the short arm of chromosome 2. J Clin Invest 1996;97:699-705.
636. Gadelha MR, Prezant TR, Une KN, et al. Loss of heterozygosity on chromosome 11q13 in two families with acromegaly/gigantism is independent of mutations of the multiple endocrine neoplasia type I gene. J Clin Endocrinol Metab 1999;84:249-256.
637. Drange MR, Fram NR, Herman-Bonert V, Melmed S. Pituitary tumor registry: a novel clinical resource. J Clin Endocrinol Metab 2000;85:168-174.
638. Daughaday WH. Pituitary gigantism. Endocrinol Metab Clin North Am 1992;21:633-647.
639. Molitch ME. Clinical manifestations of acromegaly. Endocrinol Metab Clin North Am 1992;21:597-614.
640. Jadresic A, Banks LM, Child DF, et al. The acromegaly syndrome. Relation between clinical features, growth hormone values and radiological characteristics of the pituitary tumours. Q J Med 1982;51:189-204.
641. Nabarro JD. Acromegaly. Clin Endocrinol (Oxf) 1987;26:481-512.
642. Colao A, Marzullo P, Vallone G, et al. Reversibility of joint thickening in acromegalic patients: an ultrasonography study. J Clin Endocrinol Metab 1998;83:2121-2125.
643. Colao A, Ferone D, Marzullo P, Lombardi G. Systemic complications of acromegaly: epidemiology, pathogenesis, and management. Endocr Rev 2004;25:102-152.
644. Lieberman SA, Bjorkengren AG, Hoffman AR. Rheumatologic and skeletal changes in acromegaly. Endocrinol Metab Clin North Am 1992;21:615-631.
645. Biermasz NR, Pereira AM, Smit JW, et al. Morbidity after long-term remission for acromegaly: persisting joint-related complaints cause reduced quality of life. J Clin Endocrinol Metab 2005;90: 2731-2739.
646. Dons RF, Rosselet P, Pastakia B, et al. Arthropathy in acromegalic patients before and after treatment: a long- term follow-up study. Clin Endocrinol (Oxf) 1988;28:515-524.

647. Ben-Shlomo A, Melmed S. Skin manifestations in acromegaly. Clin Dermatol 2006;24:256-259.
648. Verde GG, Santi I, Chiodini P, et al. Serum type III procollagen propeptide levels in acromegalic patients. J Clin Endocrinol Metab 1986;63:1406-1410.
649. Leavitt J, Klein I, Kendricks F, et al. Skin tags: a cutaneous marker for colonic polyps. Ann Intern Med 1983;98:928-930.
650. Lombardi G, Colao A, Marzullo P, et al. Is growth hormone bad for your heart? Cardiovascular impact of GH deficiency and of acromegaly. J Endocrinol 1997;155 Suppl 1:S33-S37; discussion S39.
651. Colao A, Cuocolo A, Marzullo P, et al. Impact of patient's age and disease duration on cardiac performance in acromegaly: a radionuclide angiography study. J Clin Endocrinol Metab 1999;84: 1518-1523.
652. Lopez-Velasco R, Escobar-Morreale HF, Vega B, et al. Cardiac involvement in acromegaly: specific myocardiopathy or consequence of systemic hypertension? J Clin Endocrinol Metab 1997;82:1047-1053.
653. Deray G, Rieu M, Devynck MA, et al. Evidence of an endogenous digitalis-like factor in the plasma of patients with acromegaly. N Engl J Med 1987;316:575-580.
654. Rajasoorya C, Holdaway IM, Wrightson P, et al. Determinants of clinical outcome and survival in acromegaly. Clin Endocrinol (Oxf) 1994;41:95-102.
655. Rosenow F, Reuter S, Deuss U, et al. Sleep apnoea in treated acromegaly: relative frequency and predisposing factors. Clin Endocrinol (Oxf) 1996;45:563-569.
656. Grunstein RR, Ho KK, Sullivan CE. Effect of octreotide, a somatostatin analog, on sleep apnea in patients with acromegaly. Ann Intern Med 1994;121:478-483.
657. Jenkins PJ, Sohaib SA, Akker S, et al. The pathology of median neuropathy in acromegaly. Ann Intern Med 2000;133:197-201.
658. Furman K, Ezzat S. Psychological features of acromegaly. Psychother Psychosom 1998;67:147-153.
659. Stewart CE, Rotwein P. Growth, differentiation, and survival: multiple physiological functions for insulin-like growth factors. Physiol Rev 1996;76:1005-1026.
660. Grinspoon S, Clemmons D, Swearingen B, Klibanski A. Serum insulin-like growth factor–binding protein-3 levels in the diagnosis of acromegaly. J Clin Endocrinol Metab 1995;80:927-932.
661. Cohen P, Peehl DM, Graves HC, Rosenfeld RG. Biological effects of prostate specific antigen as an insulin-like growth factor binding protein-3 protease. J Endocrinol 1994;142:407-415.
662. Jenkins PJ, Frajese V, Jones AM, et al. Insulin-like growth factor I and the development of colorectal neoplasia in acromegaly. J Clin Endocrinol Metab 2000;85:3218-3221.
663. Delhougne B, Deneux C, Abs R, et al. The prevalence of colonic polyps in acromegaly: a colonoscopic and pathological study in 103 patients. J Clin Endocrinol Metab 1995;80:3223-3226.
664. Ladas SD, Thalassinos NC, Ioannides G, Raptis SA. Does acromegaly really predispose to an increased prevalence of gastrointestinal tumours? Clin Endocrinol (Oxf) 1994;41:597-601.
665. Ezzat S, Strom C, Melmed S. Colon polyps in acromegaly. Ann Intern Med 1991;114:754-755.
666. Barkan AL, Stred SE, Reno K, et al. Increased growth hormone pulse frequency in acromegaly. J Clin Endocrinol Metab 1989; 69:1225-1233.
667. Katznelson L, Kleinberg D, Vance ML, et al. Hypogonadism in patients with acromegaly: data from the multi-centre acromegaly registry pilot study. Clin Endocrinol (Oxf) 2001;54:183-188.
668. Kaltsas GA, Mukherjee JJ, Jenkins PJ, et al. Menstrual irregularity in women with acromegaly. J Clin Endocrinol Metab 1999;84: 2731-2735.
669. Lesse GP, Fraser WD, Farquharson R, et al. Gonadal status is an important determinant of bone density in acromegaly. Clin Endocrinol (Oxf) 1998;48:59-65.
670. Kasagi K, Shimatsu A, Miyamoto S, et al. Goiter associated with acromegaly: sonographic and scintigraphic findings of the thyroid gland. Thyroid 1999;9:791-796.
671. Colao A, Marzullo P, Ferone D, et al. Prostatic hyperplasia: an unknown feature of acromegaly. J Clin Endocrinol Metab 1998; 83:775-779.
672. Colao A, Marzullo P, Spiezia S, et al. Effect of growth hormone (GH) and insulin-like growth factor I on prostate diseases: an ultrasonographic and endocrine study in acromegaly, GH deficiency, and healthy subjects. J Clin Endocrinol Metab 1999;84: 1986-1991.
673. Jenkins D, O'Brien I, Johnson A, et al. The Birmingham pituitary database: auditing the outcome of the treatment of acromegaly. Clin Endocrinol (Oxf) 1995;43:517-522.
674. Swearingen B, Barker FG, Katznelson L, et al. Long-term mortality after transsphenoidal surgery and adjunctive therapy for acromegaly. J Clin Endocrinol Metab 1998;83:3419-3426.
675. Abosch A, Tyrrell JB, Lamborn KR, et al. Transsphenoidal microsurgery for growth hormone–secreting pituitary adenomas: initial outcome and long-term results. J Clin Endocrinol Metab 1998;83: 3411-3418.
676. Freda PU, Post KD, Powell JS, Wardlaw SL. Evaluation of disease status with sensitive measures of growth hormone secretion in 60 postoperative patients with acromegaly. J Clin Endocrinol Metab 1998;83:3808-3816.
677. Holdaway IM, Rajasoorya RC, Gamble GD. Factors influencing mortality in acromegaly. J Clin Endocrinol Metab 2004;89: 667-674.
678. Giustina A, Barkan A, Casanueva FF, et al. Criteria for cure of acromegaly: a consensus statement. J Clin Endocrinol Metab 2000;85:526-529.
679. Freda PU, Reyes CM, Nuruzzaman AT, et al. Basal and glucose-suppressed GH levels less than 1 μg/L in newly diagnosed acromegaly. Pituitary 2003;6:175-180.
680. Duncan E, Wass JA. Investigation protocol: acromegaly and its investigation. Clin Endocrinol (Oxf) 1999;50:285-293.
681. Clemmons DR, Van Wyk JJ, Ridgway EC, et al. Evaluation of acromegaly by radioimmunoassay of somatomedin-C. N Engl J Med 1979;301:1138-1142.
682. Costa AC, Rossi A, Martinelli CE Jr, et al. Assessment of disease activity in treated acromegalic patients using a sensitive GH assay: should we achieve strict normal GH levels for a biochemical cure? J Clin Endocrinol Metab 2002;87:3142-3147.
683. Melmed S, Ho K, Klibanski A, et al. Clinical review 75: Recent advances in pathogenesis, diagnosis, and management of acromegaly. J Clin Endocrinol Metab 1995;80:3395-3402.
684. Dimaraki EV, Jaffe CA, DeMott-Friberg R, et al. Acromegaly with apparently normal GH secretion: implications for diagnosis and follow-up. J Clin Endocrinol Metab 2002;87:3537-3542.
685. Frohman LA. Ectopic hormone production by tumors. Clin Neuroendocr Perspect 1984;3:201–224.
686. Melmed S, Jackson I, Kleinberg D, Klibanski A. Current treatment guidelines for acromegaly. J Clin Endocrinol Metab 1998;83: 2646-2652.
687. Freda PU, Wardlaw SL, Post KD. Long-term endocrinological follow-up evaluation in 115 patients who underwent transsphenoidal surgery for acromegaly. J Neurosurg 1998;89:353-358.
688. Lissett CA, Peacey SR, Laing I, et al. The outcome of surgery for acromegaly: the need for a specialist pituitary surgeon for all types of growth hormone (GH) secreting adenoma. Clin Endocrinol (Oxf) 1998;49:653-657.
689. Ahmed S, Elsheikh M, Stratton IM, et al. Outcome of transphenoidal surgery for acromegaly and its relationship to surgical experience. Clin Endocrinol (Oxf) 1999;50:561-567.
690. Sheaves R, Jenkins P, Blackburn P, et al. Outcome of transsphenoidal surgery for acromegaly using strict criteria for surgical cure. Clin Endocrinol (Oxf) 1996;45:407-413.
691. Ross DA, Wilson CB. Results of transsphenoidal microsurgery for growth hormone–secreting pituitary adenoma in a series of 214 patients. J Neurosurg 1988;68:854-867.
692. Fahlbusch R, Honegger J, Buchfelder M. Surgical management of acromegaly. Endocrinol Metab Clin North Am 1992;21:669-692.
693. Gittoes NJ, Bates AS, Tse W, et al. Radiotherapy for non-function pituitary tumours. Clin Endocrinol (Oxf) 1998;48:331-337.
694. Laws ER, Thapar K. Pituitary surgery. Endocrinol Metab Clin North Am 1999;28:119-131.
695. Fahlbusch R, Keller B, Ganslandt O, et al. Transsphenoidal surgery in acromegaly investigated by intraoperative high-field magnetic resonance imaging. Eur J Endocrinol 2005;153:239-248.
696. Shimon I, Cohen ZR, Ram Z, Hadani M. Transsphenoidal surgery for acromegaly: endocrinological follow-up of 98 patients. Neurosurgery 2001;48:1239-1243; discussion 1244-1235.

697. Cappabianca P, de Divitiis E. Image guided endoscopic transnasal removal of recurrent pituitary adenomas. Neurosurgery 2003;52: 483-484; author reply 484.
698. Kreutzer J, Vance ML, Lopes MB, Laws ER Jr. Surgical management of GH-secreting pituitary adenomas: an outcome study using modern remission criteria. J Clin Endocrinol Metab 2001;86: 4072-4077.
699. Gittoes NJ, Sheppard MC, Johnson AP, Stewart PM. Outcome of surgery for acromegaly—the experience of a dedicated pituitary surgeon. QJM 1999;92:741-745.
700. Eastman RC, Gorden P, Glatstein E, Roth J. Radiation therapy of acromegaly. Endocrinol Metab Clin North Am 1992;21:693-712.
701. Barkan AL, Halasz I, Dornfeld KJ, et al. Pituitary irradiation is ineffective in normalizing plasma insulin-like growth factor I in patients with acromegaly. J Clin Endocrinol Metab 1997;82:3187-3191.
702. Powell JS, Wardlaw SL, Post KD, Freda PU. Outcome of radiotherapy for acromegaly using normalization of insulin-like growth factor I to define cure. J Clin Endocrinol Metab 2000;85: 2068-2071.
703. Jezkova J, Marek J, Hana V, et al. Gamma knife radiosurgery for acromegaly—long-term experience. Clin Endocrinol (Oxf) 2006; 64:588-595.
704. Peacey SR, Toogood AA, Veldhuis JD, et al. The relationship between 24-hour growth hormone secretion and insulin- like growth factor I in patients with successfully treated acromegaly: impact of surgery or radiotherapy. J Clin Endocrinol Metab 2001;86:259-266.
705. Castinetti F, Taieb D, Kuhn JM, et al. Outcome of gamma knife radiosurgery in 82 patients with acromegaly: correlation with initial hypersecretion. J Clin Endocrinol Metab 2005;90: 4483-4488.
706. van der Lely AJ, de Herder WW, Lamberts SW. The role of radiotherapy in acromegaly. J Clin Endocrinol Metab 1997;82: 3185-3186.
707. Alexander MJ, DeSalles AA, Tomiyasu U. Multiple radiation-induced intracranial lesions after treatment for pituitary adenoma. Case report. J Neurosurg 1998;88:111-115.
708. Jenkins PJ, Bates P, Carson MN, Stewart PM, Wass JA. Conventional pituitary irradiation is effective in lowering serum growth hormone and insulin-like growth factor-I in patients with acromegaly. J Clin Endocrinol Metab 2006;91:1239-1245.
709. Murray RD, Darzy KH, Gleeson HK, Shalet SM. GH-deficient survivors of childhood cancer: GH replacement during adult life. J Clin Endocrinol Metab 2002;87:129-135.
710. Jaffe CA, Barkan AL. Treatment of acromegaly with dopamine agonists. Endocrinol Metab Clin North Am 1992;21:713-735.
711. Abs R, Verhelst J, Maiter D, et al. Cabergoline in the treatment of acromegaly: a study in 64 patients. J Clin Endocrinol Metab 1998;83:374-378.
712. Weckbecker G, Lewis I, Albert R, et al. Opportunities in somatostatin research: biological, chemical and therapeutic aspects. Nat Rev Drug Discov 2003;2:999-1017.
713. Lamberts SW, van der Lely AJ, de Herder WW, Hofland LJ. Octreotide. N Engl J Med 1996;334:246-254.
714. Lamberts SW, Uitterlinden P, Verschoor L, et al. Long-term treatment of acromegaly with the somatostatin analogue SMS 201-995. N Engl J Med 1985;313:1576-1580.
715. Ezzat S, Snyder PJ, Young WF, et al. Octreotide treatment of acromegaly. A randomized, multicenter study. Ann Intern Med 1992;117:711-718.
716. Ur E, Mather SJ, Bomanji J, et al. Pituitary imaging using a labelled somatostatin analogue in acromegaly. Clin Endocrinol (Oxf) 1992;36:147-150.
717. Bhayana S, Booth GL, Asa SL, et al. The implication of somatotroph adenoma phenotype to somatostatin analog responsiveness in acromegaly. J Clin Endocrinol Metab 2005;90:6290-6295.
718. Wang C, Lam KS, Arceo E, Chan FL. Comparison of the effectiveness of 2-hourly versus 8-hourly subcutaneous injections of a somatostatin analog (SMS 201-995) in the treatment of acromegaly. J Clin Endocrinol Metab 1989;69:670-677.
719. Newman CB, Melmed S, Snyder PJ, et al. Safety and efficacy of long-term octreotide therapy of acromegaly: results of a multicenter trial in 103 patients—a clinical research center study. J Clin Endocrinol Metab 1995;80:2768-2775.
720. Gillis JC, Noble S, Goa KL. Octreotide long-acting release (LAR). A review of its pharmacological properties and therapeutic use in the management of acromegaly. Drugs 1997;53:681-699.
721. Cozzi R, Montini M, Attanasio R, et al. Primary treatment of acromegaly with octreotide LAR: a long-term (up to nine years) prospective study of its efficacy in the control of disease activity and tumor shrinkage. J Clin Endocrinol Metab 2006;91:1397-1403.
722. Lancranjan I, Atkinson AB. Results of a European multicentre study with Sandostatin LAR in acromegalic patients. Sandostatin LAR Group. Pituitary 1999;1:105-114.
723. Baldelli R, Colao A, Razzore P, et al. Two-year follow-up of acromegalic patients treated with slow release lanreotide (30 mg). J Clin Endocrinol Metab 2000;85:4099-4103.
724. Colao A, Ferone D, Marzullo P, et al. Long-term effects of depot long-acting somatostatin analog octreotide on hormone levels and tumor mass in acromegaly. J Clin Endocrinol Metab 2001;86: 2779-2786.
725. Caron P, Morange-Ramos I, Cogne M, Jaquet P. Three year follow-up of acromegalic patients treated with intramuscular slow-release lanreotide. J Clin Endocrinol Metab 1997;82:18-22.
726. Bevan JS. Clinical review: The antitumoral effects of somatostatin analog therapy in acromegaly. J Clin Endocrinol Metab 2005;90: 1856-1863.
727. Melmed S, Sternberg R, Cook D, et al. A critical analysis of pituitary tumor shrinkage during primary medical therapy in acromegaly. J Clin Endocrinol Metab 2005;90:4405-4410.
728. Colao A, Ferone D, Cappabianca P, et al. Effect of octreotide pretreatment on surgical outcome in acromegaly. J Clin Endocrinol Metab 1997;82:3308-3314.
729. Biermasz NR, van Dulken H, Roelfsema F. Direct postoperative and follow-up results of transsphenoidal surgery in 19 acromegalic patients pretreated with octreotide compared to those in untreated matched controls. J Clin Endocrinol Metab 1999;84:3551-3555.
730. Pascual J, Freijanes J, Berciano J, Pesquera C. Analgesic effect of octreotide in headache associated with acromegaly is not mediated by opioid mechanisms. Case report. Pain 1991;47:341-344.
731. Colao A, Marzullo P, Ferone D, et al. Cardiovascular effects of depot long-acting somatostatin analog Sandostatin LAR in acromegaly. J Clin Endocrinol Metab 2000;85:3132-3140.
732. Colao A, Cuocolo A, Marzullo P, et al. Effects of 1-year treatment with octreotide on cardiac performance in patients with acromegaly. J Clin Endocrinol Metab 1999;84:17-23.
733. Colao A, Cuocolo A, Marzullo P, et al. Is the acromegalic cardiomyopathy reversible? Effect of 5-year normalization of growth hormone and insulin-like growth factor I levels on cardiac performance. J Clin Endocrinol Metab 2001;86:1551-1557.
734. Melmed S, Dowling, R.H., Frohman, L., et al. Consensus statement: benefits vs. risks of medical therapy for acromegaly. Am J Med 1994;97:468.
735. Trainer PJ, Drake WM, Katznelson L, et al. Treatment of acromegaly with the growth hormone–receptor antagonist pegvisomant. N Engl J Med 2000;342:1171-1177.
736. Ross RJ, Leung KC, Maamra M, et al. Binding and functional studies with the growth hormone receptor antagonist, B2036-PEG (pegvisomant), reveal effects of pegylation and evidence that it binds to a receptor dimer. J Clin Endocrinol Metab 2001;86: 1716-1723.
737. Herman-Bonert VS, Zib K, Scarlett JA, Melmed S. Growth hormone receptor antagonist therapy in acromegalic patients resistant to somatostatin analogs. J Clin Endocrinol Metab 2000;85: 2958-2961.
738. Colao A, Pivonello R, Auriemma RS, et al. Efficacy of 12-month treatment with the GH receptor antagonist pegvisomant in patients with acromegaly resistant to long-term, high-dose somatostatin analog treatment: effect on IGF-I levels, tumor mass, hypertension and glucose tolerance. Eur J Endocrinol 2006;154:467-477.
739. Biering H, Saller B, Bauditz J, et al. Elevated transaminases during medical treatment of acromegaly: a review of the German pegvisomant surveillance experience and a report of a patient with histologically proven chronic mild active hepatitis. Eur J Endocrinol 2006;154:213-220.
740. van der Lely AJ, Muller A, Janssen JA, et al. Control of tumor size and disease activity during cotreatment with octreotide and the growth hormone receptor antagonist pegvisomant in an acromegalic patient. J Clin Endocrinol Metab 2001;86:478-481.

741. Jorgensen JO, Feldt-Rasmussen U, Frystyk J, et al. Cotreatment of acromegaly with a somatostatin analog and a growth hormone receptor antagonist. J Clin Endocrinol Metab 2005;90:5627-5631.
742. Feenstra J, de Herder WW, ten Have SM, et al. Combined therapy with somatostatin analogues and weekly pegvisomant in active acromegaly. Lancet 2005;365:1644-1646.
743. de Herder WW, Taal HR, Uitterlinden P, et al. Limited predictive value of an acute test with subcutaneous octreotide for long-term IGF-I normalization with Sandostatin LAR in acromegaly. Eur J Endocrinol 2005;153:67-71.
744. Newman CB, Melmed S, George A, et al. Octreotide as primary therapy for acromegaly. J Clin Endocrinol Metab 1998;83: 3034-3040.
745. Sheppard MC. Primary medical therapy for acromegaly. Clin Endocrinol (Oxf) 2003;58:387-399.
746. Scheithauer BW, Horvath, E, Lloyd RV, Kovacs, K. Pathology of pituitary adenomas and pituitary hyperplasia. In Thapar K, Kovacs, K, Scheithauer BW, Lloyd RV, eds. Diagnosis and Management of Pituitary Tumors. Totowa, NJ: Humana Press, 2001:91-154.
747. Zabel BU, Naylor SL, Sakaguchi AY, et al. High-resolution chromosomal localization of human genes for amylase, proopiomelanocortin, somatostatin, and a DNA fragment (D3S1) by in situ hybridization. Proc Natl Acad Sci U S A 1983;80:6932-6936.
748. Cochet M, Chang AC, Cohen SN. Characterization of the structural gene and putative 5′-regulatory sequences for human proopiomelanocortin. Nature 1982;297:335-339.
749. Chen WY, Wight DC, Wagner TE, Kopchick JJ. Expression of a mutated bovine growth hormone gene suppresses growth of transgenic mice. Proc Natl Acad Sci U S A 1990;87:5061-5065.
750. Arai M, Assil IQ, Abou-Samra AB. Characterization of three corticotropin-releasing factor receptors in catfish: a novel third receptor is predominantly expressed in pituitary and urophysis. Endocrinology 2001;142:446-454.
751. Jin WD, Boutillier AL, Glucksman MJ, et al. Characterization of a corticotropin-releasing hormone–responsive element in the rat proopiomelanocortin gene promoter and molecular cloning of its binding protein. Mol Endocrinol 1994;8:1377-1388.
752. Weninger SC, Dunn AJ, Muglia LJ, et al. Stress-induced behaviors require the corticotropin-releasing hormone (CRH) receptor, but not CRH. Proc Natl Acad Sci U S A 1999;96:8283-8288.
753. Coste SC, Kesterson RA, Heldwein KA, et al. Abnormal adaptations to stress and impaired cardiovascular function in mice lacking corticotropin-releasing hormone receptor-2. Nat Genet 2000;24: 403-409.
754. Bousquet C, Zatelli MC, Melmed S. Direct regulation of pituitary proopiomelanocortin by STAT3 provides a novel mechanism for immuno-neuroendocrine interfacing. J Clin Invest 2000;106: 1417-1425.
755. Eberwine JH, Roberts JL. Glucocorticoid regulation of pro-opiomelanocortin gene transcription in the rat pituitary. J Biol Chem 1984;259:2166-2170.
756. Loeffler JP, Kley N, Pittius CW, Hollt V. Calcium ion and cyclic adenosine 3′,5′-monophosphate regulate proopiomelanocortin messenger ribonucleic acid levels in rat intermediate and anterior pituitary lobes. Endocrinology 1986;119:2840-2847.
757. Seidah NG, Chretien M. Complete amino acid sequence of a human pituitary glycopeptide: an important maturation product of pro-opiomelanocortin. Proc Natl Acad Sci U S A 1981;78:4236-4240.
758. Fenger M, Johnsen AH. Alpha-amidated peptides derived from pro-opiomelanocortin in normal human pituitary. Biochem J 1988;250:781-788.
759. Jackson RS, Creemers JW, Ohagi S, et al. Obesity and impaired prohormone processing associated with mutations in the human prohormone convertase 1 gene. Nat Genet 1997;16:303-306.
760. Veldhuis JD, Iranmanesh A, Johnson ML, Lizarralde G. Twenty-four-hour rhythms in plasma concentrations of adenohypophyseal hormones are generated by distinct amplitude and/or frequency modulation of underlying pituitary secretory bursts. J Clin Endocrinol Metab 1990;71:1616-1623.
761. Veldhuis JD, Iranmanesh A, Johnson ML, Lizarralde G. Amplitude, but not frequency, modulation of adrenocorticotropin secretory bursts gives rise to the nyctohemeral rhythm of the corticotropic axis in man. J Clin Endocrinol Metab 1990;71:452-463.
762. Gomez MT, Magiakou MA, Mastorakos G, Chrousos GP. The pituitary corticotroph is not the rate limiting step in the postoperative recovery of the hypothalamic-pituitary-adrenal axis in patients with Cushing syndrome. J Clin Endocrinol Metab 1993;77:173-177.
763. Desir D, Van Cauter E, Beyloos M, et al. Prolonged pulsatile administration of ovine corticotropin-releasing hormone in normal man. J Clin Endocrinol Metab 1986;63:1292-1299.
764. Horrocks PM, Jones AF, Ratcliffe WA, et al. Patterns of ACTH and cortisol pulsatility over twenty-four hours in normal males and females. Clin Endocrinol (Oxf) 1990;32:127-134.
765. Dorin RI, Ferries LM, Roberts B, et al. Assessment of stimulated and spontaneous adrenocorticotropin secretory dynamics identifies distinct components of cortisol feedback inhibition in healthy humans. J Clin Endocrinol Metab 1996;81:3883-3891.
766. Keeney DS, Waterman MR. Regulation of steroid hydroxylase gene expression: importance to physiology and disease. Pharmacol Ther 1993;58:301-317.
767. Ilvesmaki V, Voutilainen R. Interaction of phorbol ester and adrenocorticotropin in the regulation of steroidogenic P450 genes in human fetal and adult adrenal cell cultures. Endocrinology 1991;128:1450-1458.
768. Orth DN. Corticotropin-releasing hormone in humans. Endocr Rev 1992;13:164-191.
769. Debold CR, Jackson RV, Kamilaris TC, et al. Effects of ovine corticotropin-releasing hormone on adrenocorticotropin secretion in the absence of glucocorticoid feedback inhibition in man. J Clin Endocrinol Metab 1989;68:431-437.
770. Sonino N, Zielezny M, Fava GA, Fallo F, Boscaro M. Risk factors and long-term outcome in pituitary-dependent Cushing's disease. J Clin Endocrinol Metab 1996;81:2647-2652.
771. Kubota T, Hayashi M, Kabuto M, et al. Corticotroph cell hyperplasia in a patient with Addison disease: case report. Surg Neurol 1992;37:441-447.
772. Keller-Wood ME, Dallman MF. Corticosteroid inhibition of ACTH secretion. Endocr Rev 1984;5:1-24.
773. Kanaley JA, Weltman JY, Pieper KS, et al. Cortisol and growth hormone responses to exercise at different times of day. J Clin Endocrinol Metab 2001;86:2881-2889.
774. Luger A, Deuster PA, Kyle SB, et al. Acute hypothalamic-pituitary-adrenal responses to the stress of treadmill exercise. Physiologic adaptations to physical training. N Engl J Med 1987;316: 1309-1315.
775. Urban RJ, Kaiser DL, van Cauter E, et al. Comparative assessment of objective pulse detection algorithms. II. Studies in men. Am J Physiol 1988;254:E113-E119.
776. White A, Smith H, Hoadley M, et al. Clinical evaluation of a two-site immunoradiometric assay for adrenocorticotrophin in unextracted human plasma using monoclonal antibodies. Clin Endocrinol (Oxf) 1987;26:41-51.
777. Crosby SR, Stewart MF, Ratcliffe JG, White A. Direct measurement of the precursors of adrenocorticotropin in human plasma by two-site immunoradiometric assay. J Clin Endocrinol Metab 1988;67: 1272-1277.
778. Allolio B, Gunther RW, Benker G, et al. A multihormonal response to corticotropin-releasing hormone in inferior petrosal sinus blood of patients with Cushing's disease. J Clin Endocrinol Metab 1990;71:1195-1201.
779. Erturk E, Jaffe CA, Barkan AL. Evaluation of the integrity of the hypothalamic-pituitary-adrenal axis by insulin hypoglycemia test. J Clin Endocrinol Metab 1998;83:2350-2354.
780. Abdu TA, Elhadd TA, Neary R, Clayton RN. Comparison of the low dose short synacthen test (1 μg), the conventional dose short synacthen test (250 μg), and the insulin tolerance test for assessment of the hypothalamo-pituitary-adrenal axis in patients with pituitary disease. J Clin Endocrinol Metab 1999;84:838-843.
781. Hartzband PI, Van Herle AJ, Sorger L, Cope D. Assessment of hypothalamic-pituitary-adrenal (HPA) axis dysfunction: comparison of ACTH stimulation, insulin-hypoglycemia and metyrapone. J Endocrinol Invest 1988;11:769-776.
782. l'Allemand D, Penhoat A, Lebrethon MC, et al. Insulin-like growth factors enhance steroidogenic enzyme and corticotropin receptor messenger ribonucleic acid levels and corticotropin steroidogenic responsiveness in cultured human adrenocortical cells. J Clin Endocrinol Metab 1996;81:3892-3897.
783. Oldfield EH, Doppman JL, Nieman LK, et al. Petrosal sinus sampling with and without corticotropin-releasing hormone for the

differential diagnosis of Cushing's syndrome. N Engl J Med 1991;325:897-905.
784. Yanovski JA, Cutler GB Jr, Chrousos GP, Nieman LK. Corticotropin-releasing hormone stimulation following low-dose dexamethasone administration. A new test to distinguish Cushing's syndrome from pseudo-Cushing's states. JAMA 1993;269:2232-2238.
785. Nieman LK, Oldfield EH, Wesley R, et al. A simplified morning ovine corticotropin-releasing hormone stimulation test for the differential diagnosis of adrenocorticotropin-dependent Cushing's syndrome. J Clin Endocrinol Metab 1993;77:1308-1312.
786. Hurel SJ, Thompson CJ, Watson MJ, et al. The short Synacthen and insulin stress tests in the assessment of the hypothalamic-pituitary-adrenal axis. Clin Endocrinol (Oxf) 1996;44:141-146.
787. Rasmuson S, Olsson T, Hagg E. A low dose ACTH test to assess the function of the hypothalamic- pituitary-adrenal axis. Clin Endocrinol (Oxf) 1996;44:151-156.
788. Kukreja SC, Williams GA. Corticotrophin stimulation test: inverse correlation between basal serum cortisol and its response to corticotrophin. Acta Endocrinol (Copenh) 1981;97:522-524.
789. Shankar RR, Jakacki RI, Haider A, et al. Testing the hypothalamic-pituitary-adrenal axis in survivors of childhood brain and skull-based tumors. J Clin Endocrinol Metab 1997;82:1995-1998.
790. Peacey SR, Guo CY, Robinson AM, et al. Glucocorticoid replacement therapy: are patients over treated and does it matter? Clin Endocrinol (Oxf) 1997;46:255-261.
791. Wilson CB. Surgical management of pituitary tumors. J Clin Endocrinol Metab 1997;82:2381-2385.
792. Wilson CB, Mindermann T, Tyrrell JB. Extrasellar, intracavernous sinus adrenocorticotropin-releasing adenoma causing Cushing's disease. J Clin Endocrinol Metab 1995;80:1774-1777.
793. Fahlbusch R, Thapar K. New developments in pituitary surgical techniques. Baillieres Best Pract Res Clin Endocrinol Metab 1999;13:471-484.
794. Simmons NE, Alden TD, Thorner MO, Laws ER Jr. Serum cortisol response to transsphenoidal surgery for Cushing disease. J Neurosurg 2001;95:1-8.
795. Baldeweg SE, Pollock JR, Powell M, Ahlquist J. A spectrum of behaviour in silent corticotroph pituitary adenomas. Br J Neurosurg 2005;19:38-42.
796. Pierce JG, Parsons TF. Glycoprotein hormones: structure and function. Annu Rev Biochem 1981;50:465-495.
797. Grossmann M, Weintraub BD, Szkudlinski MW. Novel insights into the molecular mechanisms of human thyrotropin action: structural, physiological, and therapeutic implications for the glycoprotein hormone family. Endocr Rev 1997;18:476-501.
798. Fiddes JC, Goodman HM. The gene encoding the common α subunit of the four human glycoprotein hormones. J Mol Appl Genet 1981;1:3-18.
799. Sarapura VD, Strouth HL, Wood WM, et al. Activation of the glycoprotein hormone α-subunit gene promoter in thyrotropes. Mol Cell Endocrinol 1998;146:77-86.
800. Tagami T, Madison LD, Nagaya T, Jameson JL. Nuclear receptor corepressors activate rather than suppress basal transcription of genes that are negatively regulated by thyroid hormone. Mol Cell Biol 1997;17:2642-2648.
801. Wondisford FE, Radovick S, Moates JM, et al. Isolation and characterization of the human thyrotropin β-subunit gene. Differences in gene structure and promoter function from murine species. J Biol Chem 1988;263:12538-12542.
802. Steinfelder HJ, Hauser P, Nakayama Y, et al. Thyrotropin-releasing hormone regulation of human TSHB expression: role of a pituitary-specific transcription factor (Pit-1/GHF-1) and potential interaction with a thyroid hormone–inhibitory element. Proc Natl Acad Sci U S A 1991;88:3130-3134.
803. Bodenner DL, Mroczynski MA, Weintraub BD, et al. A detailed functional and structural analysis of a major thyroid hormone inhibitory element in the human thyrotropin β-subunit gene. J Biol Chem 1991;266:21666-21673.
804. Ross DS, Downing MF, Chin WW, et al. Changes in tissue concentrations of thyrotropin, free thyrotropin β, and α-subunits after thyroxine administration: comparison of mouse hypothyroid pituitary and thyrotropic tumors. Endocrinology 1983;112:2050-2053.
805. Abel ED, Kaulbach HC, Campos-Barros A, et al. Novel insight from transgenic mice into thyroid hormone resistance and the regulation of thyrotropin. J Clin Invest 1999;103:271-279.
806. Beck-Peccoz P, Persani L. Variable biological activity of thyroid-stimulating hormone. Eur J Endocrinol 1994;131:331-340.
807. Lania A, Persani L, Ballare E, et al. Constitutively active $G_s\alpha$ is associated with an increased phosphodiesterase activity in human growth hormone–secreting adenomas. J Clin Endocrinol Metab 1998;83:1624-1628.
808. Papandreou MJ, Persani L, Asteria C, et al. Variable carbohydrate structures of circulating thyrotropin as studied by lectin affinity chromatography in different clinical conditions. J Clin Endocrinol Metab 1993;77:393-398.
809. Ridgway EC, Weintraub BD, Maloof F. Metabolic clearance and production rates of human thyrotropin. J Clin Invest 1974;53: 895-903.
810. Vanhole C, Aerssens P, Naulaers G, et al. L-Thyroxine treatment of preterm newborns: clinical and endocrine effects. Pediatr Res 1997;42:87-92.
811. Goichot B, Weibel L, Chapotot F, et al. Effect of the shift of the sleep-wake cycle on three robust endocrine markers of the circadian clock. Am J Physiol 1998;275:E243-248.
812. Van den Berghe G, de Zegher F, Veldhuis JD, et al. Thyrotrophin and prolactin release in prolonged critical illness: dynamics of spontaneous secretion and effects of growth hormone- secretagogues. Clin Endocrinol (Oxf) 1997;47:599-612.
813. Faglia G. The clinical impact of the thyrotropin-releasing hormone test. Thyroid 1998;8:903-908.
814. Spencer CA, Schwarzbein D, Guttler RB, et al. Thyrotropin (TSH)-releasing hormone stimulation test responses employing third and fourth generation TSH assays. J Clin Endocrinol Metab 1993;76: 494-498.
815. Samuels MH, Henry P, Luther M, Ridgway EC. Pulsatile TSH secretion during 48-hour continuous TRH infusions. Thyroid 1993;3: 201-206.
816. Samuels MH, Henry P, Ridgway EC. Effects of dopamine and somatostatin on pulsatile pituitary glycoprotein secretion. J Clin Endocrinol Metab 1992;74:217-222.
817. Siler TM, Yen SC, Vale W, Guillemin R. Inhibition by somatostatin on the release of TSH induced in man by thyrotropin-releasing factor. J Clin Endocrinol Metab 1974;38:742-745.
818. Cooper DS, Klibanski A, Ridgway EC. Dopaminergic modulation of TSH and its subunits: in vivo and in vitro studies. Clin Endocrinol (Oxf) 1983;18:265-275.
819. Wang R, Nelson JC, Wilcox RB. Salsalate administration—a potential pharmacological model of the sick euthyroid syndrome. J Clin Endocrinol Metab 1998;83:3095-3099.
820. Rapoport B, Chazenbalk GD, Jaume JC, McLachlan SM. The thyrotropin (TSH) receptor: interaction with TSH and autoantibodies. Endocr Rev 1998;19:673-716.
821. Nicoloff JT, Spencer CA. Clinical review 12: The use and misuse of the sensitive thyrotropin assays. J Clin Endocrinol Metab 1990; 71:553-558.
822. Adriaanse R, Romijn JA, Brabant G, et al. Pulsatile thyrotropin secretion in nonthyroidal illness. J Clin Endocrinol Metab 1993;77: 1313-1317.
823. Beck-Peccoz P, Persani L. TSH-producing adenomas. In DeGroot LJ, Jameson JL, eds. Endocrinology, 4th ed. Philadelphia: W.B Saunders, 2001:321-328.
824. Mindermann T, Wilson CB. Thyrotropin-producing pituitary adenomas. J Neurosurg 1993;79:521-527.
825. Saeger W, Ludecke DK. Pituitary adenomas with hyperfunction of TSH. Frequency, histological classification, immunocytochemistry and ultrastructure. Virchows Arch A Pathol Anat Histol 1982;394:255-267.
826. McCutcheon IE, Weintraub BD, Oldfield EH. Surgical treatment of thyrotropin-secreting pituitary adenomas. J Neurosurg 1990;73: 674-683.
827. Sanno N, Teramoto A, Matsuno A, et al. GH and PRL gene expression by nonradioisotopic in situ hybridization in TSH-secreting pituitary adenomas. J Clin Endocrinol Metab 1995;80:2518-2522.
828. Sanno N, Teramoto A, Matsuno A, et al. Clinical and immunohistochemical studies on TSH-secreting pituitary adenoma: its multihormonality and expression of Pit-1. Mod Pathol 1994;7: 893-899.
829. Alings AM, Fliers E, de Herder WW, et al. A thyrotropin-secreting pituitary adenoma as a cause of thyrotoxic periodic paralysis. J Endocrinol Invest 1998;21:703-706.

830. Weintraub BD, Gershengorn MC, Kourides IA. Inappropriate secretion of thyroid-stimulating hormone. Ann Intern Med 1981;95: 339-351.
831. Beck-Peccoz P, Brucker-Davis F, Persani L, et al. Thyrotropin-secreting pituitary tumors. Endocr Rev 1996;17:610-638.
832. Brucker-Davis F, Oldfield EH, Skarulis MC, et al. Thyrotropin-secreting pituitary tumors: diagnostic criteria, thyroid hormone sensitivity, and treatment outcome in 25 patients followed at the National Institutes of Health. J Clin Endocrinol Metab 1999;84: 476-486.
833. Cooper DS, Wenig BM. Hyperthyroidism caused by an ectopic TSH-secreting pituitary tumor. Thyroid 1996;6:337-343.
834. Kourides IA, Ridgway EC, Weintraub BD, et al. Thyrotropin-induced hyperthyroidism: use of α and β subunit levels to identify patients with pituitary tumors. J Clin Endocrinol Metab 1977; 45:534-543.
835. Beckers A, Abs R, Mahler C, et al. Thyrotropin-secreting pituitary adenomas: report of seven cases. J Clin Endocrinol Metab 1991; 72:477-483.
836. Chanson P, Weintraub BD, Harris AG. Octreotide therapy for thyroid-stimulating hormone–secreting pituitary adenomas. A follow-up of 52 patients. Ann Intern Med 1993;119:236-240.
837. Losa M, Giovanelli M, Persani L, et al. Criteria of cure and follow-up of central hyperthyroidism due to thyrotropin-secreting pituitary adenomas. J Clin Endocrinol Metab 1996;81:3084-3090.
838. Beck-Peccoz P, Mariotti S, Guillausseau PJ, et al. Treatment of hyperthyroidism due to inappropriate secretion of thyrotropin with the somatostatin analog SMS 201-995. J Clin Endocrinol Metab 1989;68:208-214.
839. Caron P, Arlot S, Bauters C, et al. Efficacy of the long-acting octreotide formulation (octreotide-LAR) in patients with thyrotropin-secreting pituitary adenomas. J Clin Endocrinol Metab 2001;86: 2849-2853.
840. Samuels MH, Wood WM, Gordon DF, et al. Clinical and molecular studies of a thyrotropin-secreting pituitary adenoma. J Clin Endocrinol Metab 1989;68:1211-1215.
841. Warnet A, Timsit J, Chanson P, et al. The effect of somatostatin analogue on chiasmal dysfunction from pituitary macroadenomas. J Neurosurg 1989;71:687-690.
842. Root AW. Neonatal screening for 21-hydroxylase deficient congenital adrenal hyperplasia—the role of CYP21 analysis. J Clin Endocrinol Metab 1999;84:1503-1504.
843. Duquesnoy P, Roy A, Dastot F, et al. Human Prop-1: cloning, mapping, genomic structure. Mutations in familial combined pituitary hormone deficiency. FEBS Lett 1998;437:216-220.
844. Sornson MW, Wu W, Dasen JS, et al. Pituitary lineage determination by the Prophet of Pit-1 homeodomain factor defective in Ames dwarfism. Nature 1996;384:327-333.
845. Fofanova O, Takamura N, Kinoshita E, et al. Compound heterozygous deletion of the PROP-1 gene in children with combined pituitary hormone deficiency. J Clin Endocrinol Metab 1998;83: 2601-2604.
846. Cohen LE, Radovick S. Molecular basis of combined pituitary hormone deficiencies. Endocr Rev 2002;23:431-442.
847. Deladoey J, Fluck C, Bex M, et al. Aromatase deficiency caused by a novel P450arom gene mutation: impact of absent estrogen production on serum gonadotropin concentration in a boy. J Clin Endocrinol Metab 1999;84:4050-4054.
848. Reynaud R, Barlier A, Vallette-Kasic S, et al. An uncommon phenotype with familial central hypogonadism caused by a novel PROP1 gene mutant truncated in the transactivation domain. J Clin Endocrinol Metab 2005;90:4880-4887.
849. Agarwal G, Bhatia V, Cook S, Thomas PQ. Adrenocorticotropin deficiency in combined pituitary hormone deficiency patients homozygous for a novel PROP1 deletion. J Clin Endocrinol Metab 2000;85:4556-4561.
850. Rosenbloom AL, Almonte AS, Brown MR, et al. Clinical and biochemical phenotype of familial anterior hypopituitarism from mutation of the PROP1 gene. J Clin Endocrinol Metab 1999;84: 50-57.
851. Cushman LJ, Watkins-Chow DE, Brinkmeier ML, et al. Persistent Prop1 expression delays gonadotrope differentiation and enhances pituitary tumor susceptibility. Hum Mol Genet 2001;10:1141-1153.
852. Reynaud R, Saveanu A, Barlier A, et al. Pituitary hormone deficiencies due to transcription factor gene alterations. Growth Horm IGF Res 2004;14:442-448.
853. Voss JW, Rosenfeld MG. Anterior pituitary development: short tales from dwarf mice. Cell 1992;70:527-530.
854. Li S, Crenshaw EB 3rd, Rawson EJ, et al. Dwarf locus mutants lacking three pituitary cell types result from mutations in the POU-domain gene pit-1. Nature 1990;347:528-533.
855. Turton JP, Reynaud R, Mehta A, et al. Novel mutations within the POU1F1 gene associated with variable combined pituitary hormone deficiency. J Clin Endocrinol Metab 2005;90:4762-4770.
856. Hendriks-Stegeman BI, Augustijn KD, Bakker B, et al. Combined pituitary hormone deficiency caused by compound heterozygosity for two novel mutations in the POU domain of the Pit1/POU1F1 gene. J Clin Endocrinol Metab 2001;86:1545-1550.
857. Cohen RN, Brue T, Naik K, et al. The role of CBP/p300 interactions and Pit-1 dimerization in the pathophysiological mechanism of combined pituitary hormone deficiency. J Clin Endocrinol Metab 2006;91:239-247.
858. Machinis K, Amselem S. Functional relationship between LHX4 and POU1F1 in light of the LHX4 mutation identified in patients with pituitary defects. J Clin Endocrinol Metab 2005;90: 5456-5462.
859. Dattani MT, Martinez-Barbera JP, Thomas PQ, et al. Mutations in the homeobox gene *HESX1/Hesx1* associated with septo-optic dysplasia in human and mouse. Nat Genet 1998;19:125-133.
860. Thomas PQ, Dattani MT, Brickman JM, et al. Heterozygous *HESX1* mutations associated with isolated congenital pituitary hypoplasia and septo-optic dysplasia. Hum Mol Genet 2001;10:39-45.
861. Netchine I, Sobrier ML, Krude H, et al. Mutations in *LHX3* result in a new syndrome revealed by combined pituitary hormone deficiency. Nat Genet 2000;25:182-186.
862. Green JS, Parfrey PS, Harnett JD, et al. The cardinal manifestations of Bardet-Biedl syndrome, a form of Laurence-Moon-Biedl syndrome. N Engl J Med 1989;321:1002-1009.
863. Bray GA, Dahms WT, Swerdloff RS, et al. The Prader-Willi syndrome: a study of 40 patients and a review of the literature. Medicine (Baltimore) 1983;62:59-80.
864. Ledbetter DH, Mascarello JT, Riccardi VM, et al. Chromosome 15 abnormalities and the Prader-Willi syndrome: a follow-up report of 40 cases. Am J Hum Genet 1982;34:278-285.
865. Kallmann F, Schonfeld WA, Barrera WS. Genetic aspects of primary eunuchoidism. Am J Ment Defic 1944;48:203.
866. Rugarli EI, Ballabio A. Kallmann syndrome. From genetics to neurobiology. JAMA 1993;270:2713-2716.
867. Hardelin JP, Levilliers J, Young J, et al. Xp22.3 deletions in isolated familial Kallmann's syndrome. J Clin Endocrinol Metab 1993;76: 827-831.
868. Prager D, Braunstein GD. X-chromosome-linked Kallmann's syndrome: pathology at the molecular level. J Clin Endocrinol Metab 1993;76:824-826.
869. Pitteloud N, Acierno JS Jr, Meysing A, et al. Mutations in fibroblast growth factor receptor 1 cause both Kallmann syndrome and normosmic idiopathic hypogonadotropic hypogonadism. Proc Natl Acad Sci U S A 2006;103:6281-6286.
870. Lieblich JM, Rogol AD, White BJ, Rosen SW. Syndrome of anosmia with hypogonadotropic hypogonadism (Kallmann syndrome): clinical and laboratory studies in 23 cases. Am J Med 1982;73: 506-519.
871. Zhang YH, Guo W, Wagner RL, et al. *DAX1* mutations map to putative structural domains in a deduced three- dimensional model. Am J Hum Genet 1998;62:855-864.
872. Stoving RK, Veldhuis JD, Flyvbjerg A, et al. Jointly amplified basal and pulsatile growth hormone (GH) secretion and increased process irregularity in women with anorexia nervosa: indirect evidence for disruption of feedback regulation within the GH-insulin-like growth factor I axis. J Clin Endocrinol Metab 1999; 84:2056-2063.
873. Stoving RK, Hangaard J, Hansen-Nord M, Hagen C. A review of endocrine changes in anorexia nervosa. J Psychiatr Res 1999;33:139-152.
874. Kleinberg DL. Pituitary tumors and failure of endocrine target organs. Arch Intern Med 1979;139:969-970.

874a. Mulroney SE, McDonnell KJ, Pert CB, et al. HIV gp120 inhibits the somatotropic axis: a possible GH-releasing hormone receptor mechanism for the pathogenesis of AIDS wasting. Proc Natl Acad Sci U S A 1998;95:1927–1932.
875. Benvenga S, Campenni A, Ruggeri RM, Trimarchi F. Clinical review 113: Hypopituitarism secondary to head trauma. J Clin Endocrinol Metab 2000;85:1353-1361.
876. Schneider HJ, Schneider M, Saller B, et al. Prevalence of anterior pituitary insufficiency 3 and 12 months after traumatic brain injury. Eur J Endocrinol 2006;154:259-265.
877. Agha A, Rogers B, Sherlock M, et al. Anterior pituitary dysfunction in survivors of traumatic brain injury. J Clin Endocrinol Metab 2004;89:4929-4936.
878. Aimaretti G, Ambrosio MR, Di Somma C, et al. Residual pituitary function after brain injury–induced hypopituitarism: a prospective 12-month study. J Clin Endocrinol Metab 2005;90:6085-6092.
879. Agha A, Thornton E, O'Kelly P, et al. Posterior pituitary dysfunction after traumatic brain injury. J Clin Endocrinol Metab 2004;89: 5987-5992.
880. Constine LS, Woolf PD, Cann D, et al. Hypothalamic-pituitary dysfunction after radiation for brain tumors. N Engl J Med 1993;328:87-94.
881. Clayton PE, Shalet SM. Dose dependency of time of onset of radiation-induced growth hormone deficiency. J Pediatr 1991;118: 226-228.
882. Rose SR, Lustig RH, Pitukcheewanont P, et al. Diagnosis of hidden central hypothyroidism in survivors of childhood cancer. J Clin Endocrinol Metab 1999;84:4472-4479.
883. Toogood AA. Endocrine consequences of brain irradiation. Growth Horm IGF Res 2004;14(suppl A):S118-S124.
884. De Marinis L, Bonadonna S, Bianchi A, et al. Primary empty sella. J Clin Endocrinol Metab 2005;90:5471-5477.
885. Finkelstein JS, Klibanski A, Neer RM, et al. Increases in bone density during treatment of men with idiopathic hypogonadotropic hypogonadism. J Clin Endocrinol Metab 1989;69:776-783.
886. Wang C, Eyre DR, Clark R, et al. Sublingual testosterone replacement improves muscle mass and strength, decreases bone resorption, and increases bone formation markers in hypogonadal men—a clinical research center study. J Clin Endocrinol Metab 1996;81:3654-3662.
887. Hartman ML, Crowe BJ, Biller BM, et al. Which patients do not require a GH stimulation test for the diagnosis of adult GH deficiency? J Clin Endocrinol Metab 2002;87:477-485.
888. Prabhakar VK, Shalet SM. Aetiology, diagnosis, and management of hypopituitarism in adult life. Postgrad Med J 2006;82:259-266.
889. Webster J, Piscitelli G, Polli A, et al. A comparison of cabergoline and bromocriptine in the treatment of hyperprolactinemic amenorrhea. Cabergoline Comparative Study Group. N Engl J Med 1994;331:904-909.
890. Thorner MO, Vance ML, Horvath E, Kovacs K. The anterior pituitary. In Wilson JD, Foster DW, eds. Williams Textbook of Endocrinology. Philadelphia: WB Saunders, 1992:221-310.
891. Gasperi M, Aimaretti G, Scarcello G, et al. Low dose hexarelin and growth hormone (GH)-releasing hormone as a diagnostic tool for the diagnosis of GH deficiency in adults: comparison with insulin-induced hypoglycemia test. J Clin Endocrinol Metab 1999; 84:2633-2637.
892. Biller BM, Vance ML, Kleinberg DL, et al. Clinical and reimbursement issues in growth hormone use in adults. Am J Manag Care 2000;6:S817-827.
893. Klein I, Parveen G, Gavaler JS, Vanthiel DH. Colonic polyps in patients with acromegaly. Ann Intern Med 1982;97:27-30.
894. Ituarte EA, Petrini J, Hershman JM. Acromegaly and colon cancer. Ann Intern Med 1984;101:627-628.
895. Brunner JE, Johnson CC, Zafar S, et al. Colon cancer and polyps in acromegaly: increased risk associated with family history of colon cancer. Clin Endocrinol (Oxf) 1990;32:65-71.
896. Vasen HF, van Erpecum KJ, Roelfsema F, et al. Increased prevalence of colonic adenomas in patients with acromegaly. Eur J Endocrinol 1994;131:235-237.
897. Terzolo M, Tappero G, Borretta G, et al. High prevalence of colonic polyps in patients with acromegaly. Influence of sex and age. Arch Intern Med 1994;154:1272-1276.
898. Jenkins PJ, Fairclough PD, Richards T, et al. Acromegaly, colonic polyps and carcinoma. Clin Endocrinol (Oxf) 1997;47:17-22.
899. Wright AD, Hill DM, Lowy C, Fraser TR. Mortality in acromegaly. Q J Med 1970;39:1-16.
900. Cheung NW, Boyages SC. Increased incidence of neoplasia in females with acromegaly. Clin Endocrinol (Oxf) 1997;47:323-327.
901. Popovic V, Damjanovic S, Micic D, et al. Increased incidence of neoplasia in patients with pituitary adenomas. The Pituitary Study Group. Clin Endocrinol (Oxf) 1998;49:441-445.
902. Barzilay J, Heatley GJ, Cushing GW. Benign and malignant tumors in patients with acromegaly. Arch Intern Med 1991;151:1629-1632.
903. Ron E, Gridley G, Hrubec Z, et al. Acromegaly and gastrointestinal cancer. Cancer 1991;68:1673-1677.
904. Dasen JS, Rosenfeld, M.G. Signaling mechanisms in pituitary morphogenesis and cell fate determination. Curr Opin Cell Biol 1999;11:669-677.
905. Hartman ML, Veldhuis JD, Johnson ML, et al. Augmented growth hormone (GH) secretory burst frequency and amplitude mediate enhanced GH secretion during a two-day fast in normal men. J Clin Endocrinol Metab 1992;74:757-765.

CHAPTER 9

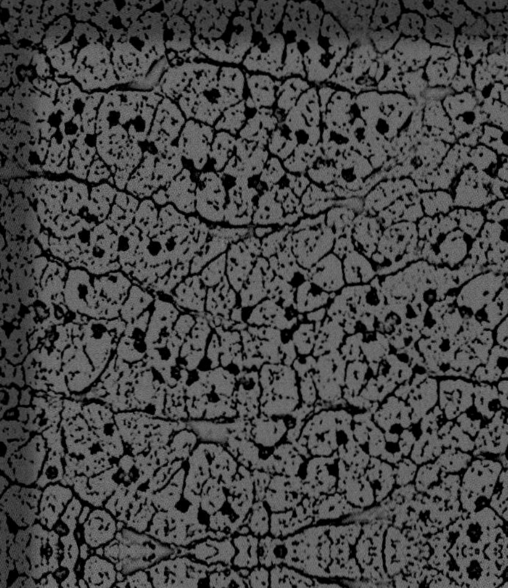

POSTERIOR PITUITARY

Alan G. Robinson and Joseph G. Verbalis

ANATOMY

Normal

The posterior pituitary is neural tissue and consists only of the distal axons of the hypothalamic magnocellular neurons that make up the neurohypophysis. The perikarya (cell bodies) of these axons are located in paired supraoptic nuclei and the paired paraventricular nuclei of the hypothalamus. During embryogenesis,[1] neuroepithelial cells of the lining of the third ventricle mature into magnocellular neurons while migrating laterally to and above the optic chiasm to form the supraoptic nucleus and to the walls of the third ventricle to form the paraventricular nuclei. In the posterior pituitary, the axon terminals of the magnocellular neurons contain neurosecretory granules, membrane-bound packets of hormones stored for subsequent release. The blood supply for the anterior pituitary is via the hypothalamic-pituitary portal system, but the posterior pituitary blood supply is directly from the inferior hypophyseal arteries, which are branches of the posterior communicating and internal carotid arteries. The drainage is into the cavernous sinus and internal jugular vein.

The hormones of the posterior pituitary—oxytocin and vasopressin—are synthesized in individual hormone-specific magnocellular neurons. The supraoptic nucleus is relatively simple with 80% to 90% of the neurons producing vasopressin[2] and virtually all axons projecting to the posterior pituitary.[1] The organization of the paraventriculer nucleus (PVN), however, is much more complex and varies among species. In the human there are five subnuclei[2] and parvocellular (smaller cells) divisions that synthesize other peptides, such as corticotropin-releasing hormone (CRH), thyrotropin-releasing hormone (TRH), and somatostatin,[3] and opioids.[4] The parvocellular neurons project to the median eminence, brain stem, and spinal cord[5] where they play a role in a variety of neuroendocrine autonomic functions. The suprachiasmatic nucleus, which is located in the midline at the base of and anterior to the third ventricle, also synthesizes vasopressin and controls circadian rhythms as well as seasonal rhythms.[2]

Numerous neurotransmitters have been described in the pathway to stimulation or inhibition of secretion of vasopressin and oxytocin. The major stimulatory input is glutamate, with noradrenergic stimulatory inputs acting by stimulation of glutamate.[6,7] Glutamate receptors account for 25% of synapsis on magnocellular neurons.[7] The major inhibitory input is γ-aminobutyric acid (GABA), which accounts for 50% of the synaptic input to the magnocellular neurons.[6] Steroid hormone actions on the magnocellular neurons are mediated by GABA or glutamate receptors.[8]

One of the most remarkable aspects of the magnocellular system is the plasticity of the system in response to prolonged stimulation. Plasticity is demonstrated in animals by prolonged osmotic stimulation with hypertonic saline but are probably most often of import in humans during parturition and lactation.[6] During prolonged stimulation the perikarya themselves enlarge and the glia retracts, diminishing astrocyte coverage of the neurons. These two events interact to increase the contact between cells, which enhances the synchrony and the pulsatile secretion, which for oxytocin is especially important during parturition and milk let-down of lactation. Secretion of oxytocin or vasopressin by dendrites of the respective neurons produces a positive feedback in a paracrine/autocrine fashion to enhance the further secretion of that hormone. Neurotransmitter numbers may increase on the neuron and the astrocytes themselves contribute to the plasticity, not just by altering their shape but also because they function to clear neurotransmitters from the extracellular space and release active substances themselves. This structural plasticity during stimulation is enabled by the continued presence in the supraoptic and paraventricular nuclei of cytoskeleton proteins and cell adhesion molecules that are present elsewhere in the brain only during embryogenesis.[9]

Ectopic Posterior Pituitary

With the development of magnetic resonance imaging (MRI) scans of the brain, it was discovered that T1-weighted images with MRI produced a bright signal in the posterior pituitary.[10] This new diagnostic imaging technology (described in detail later) allowed the identification of a group of patients in whom there was abnormal anatomy of the posterior pituitary and the "bright spot" was recognized in the base of the hypothalamus. These cases are referred to as *ectopic posterior pituitary.* Most of these cases are recognized in children with growth retardation and anterior pituitary deficiency rather than posterior pituitary deficiency. The degree of anterior pituitary deficit depends on the persistence of a pituitary stalk and a retained portal vasculature from the hypothalamus to the anterior pituitary.[11-13] Most authors believe this is not traumatic but represents a congenital abnormality with an "undescended"[13] posterior pituitary that may be at any level along the pituitary stalk.[13]

SYNTHESIS AND RELEASE OF NEUROHYPOPHYSEAL HORMONES

Vasopressin and oxytocin are nonapeptides consisting of a 6-amino-acid ring with a cysteine-to-cysteine bridge and a 3-amino-acid tail (Fig. 9–1). All mammals have arginine vasopressin and oxytocin, as illustrated in the figure, with the exception of the pig. In the pig, a lysine is substituted for arginine in position 8 of vasopressin, producing lysine vasopressin.

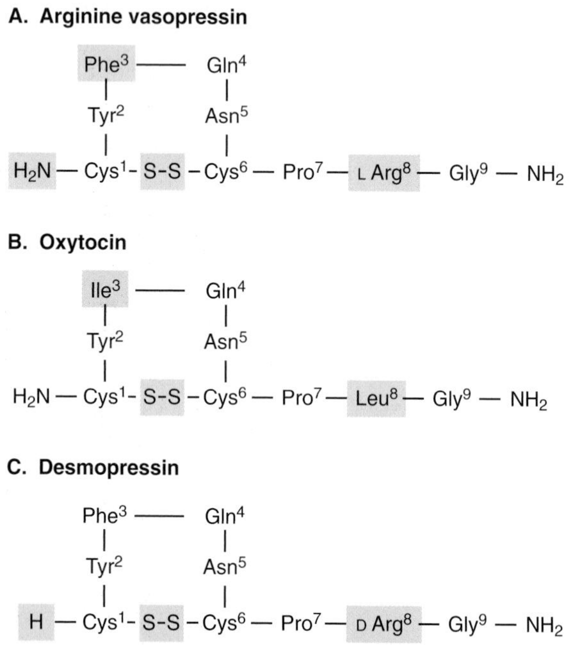

A. Arginine vasopressin

Phe³ — Gln⁴ | Tyr² | Asn⁵

H_2N — Cys¹ - S-S - Cys⁶ — Pro⁷ — L Arg⁸ — Gly⁹ — NH_2

B. Oxytocin

Ile³ — Gln⁴ | Tyr² | Asn⁵

H_2N — Cys¹ - S-S - Cys⁶ — Pro⁷ — Leu⁸ — Gly⁹ — NH_2

C. Desmopressin

Phe³ — Gln⁴ | Tyr² | Asn⁵

H — Cys¹ - S-S - Cys⁶ — Pro⁷ — D Arg⁸ — Gly⁹ — NH_2

Figure 9–1 ▪ Comparison of the chemical structure of arginine vasopressin, oxytocin, and desmopressin. The differences are illustrated by the shaded areas. Oxytocin differs from vasopressin in position 3 (Ile for Phe), and position 8 (Leu for Arg). Desmopressin differs from arginine vasopressin in that the terminal cystine is deanimated and the arginine in position 8 is a D rather than an L isomer. (From Robinson AG. UCLA, Los Angeles, CA, with permission.)

Both genes are found on chromosome 20,[14] although they are situated in a tail-to-tail position and transcribed in opposite directions.[15] The hormones are synthesized as part of a precursor molecule consisting of the nonapeptide and a hormone-specific neurophysin and for vasopressin a glycopeptide.[16]

When a stimulus for secretion of vasopressin or oxytocin acts on the appropriate magnocellular cell body, an action potential is generated and propagates down the long axon to the posterior pituitary. The action potential causes an influx of calcium, which induces neurosecretory granules to fuse with the cell membrane and extrude the entire contents of the neurosecretory granule into the perivascular space and subsequently into the capillary system of the posterior pituitary. At physiologic pH of plasma, there is no binding of hormone, vasopressin, or oxytocin to their respective neurophysins, so each peptide circulates independently in the bloodstream.

The control of hormone synthesis is at the level of transcription. Stimuli for secretion of vasopressin or oxytocin also stimulate transcription and increase the mRNA content in the magnocellular neurons. This has been studied in most detail in rats, in which dehydration[17] accelerates transcription and increases the levels of vasopressin (and oxytocin) mRNA[18-20] and, in which hypoosmolality produces a decrease in the content of vasopressin mRNA.[21]

The transport of neurosecretory vesicles from the site of synthesis to the posterior pituitary along microtubule tracks[22] is also regulated. When synthesis is turned off, transport stops; when synthesis is increased, transport is up-regulated.[22] Thus, there is coordination of stimulated release of hormone, transport of hormone, and synthesis of new hormone. There is, however, asynchrony in the timing of these events. The asynchrony is demonstrated by changes in the content of vasopressin stored in the posterior pituitary. The absolute content varies considerably among species but is quite a remarkable store, generally equivalent to the amount of hormone required to sustain basal release for 30 to 50 days or maximum release for 5 to 10 days.[23] In animals, prolonged and intense stimulation of vasopressin release (e.g., dehydration or salt-loading) produces a depletion of stored hormone in the posterior pituitary.[20,24,25] When animals are returned to normal water intake, in 7 to 14 days there is a gradual recovery of pituitary content back to baseline (or above). This phenomenon has been modeled by Fitzsimmons who provided experimental evidence that a long half-life of the vasopressin message, approximately 2 days,[26] is (from a minimalist point of view) a plausible explanation of the events. When a strong and/or sustained stimulus releases vasopressin, there is an immediate stimulus to transcription of new mRNA. But, it requires several days for the peak level of mRNA to be reached, so translation increases slowly. When the stimulus is removed, the elevated mRNA synthesizes hormone to replete the store in the posterior pituitary. The mRNA slowly declines to the previous baseline and synthesis of vasopressin returns to a basal rate.

PHYSIOLOGY OF SECRETION OF VASOPRESSIN AND THIRST

The physiologic regulation of vasopressin synthesis and secretion involves two systems: osmotic and pressure/volume (Fig. 9–2). Functions of these two systems are so distinct that historically it was thought there were two hormones—an antidiuretic hormone and a vasopressor hormone. Hence, the two names that are used interchangeably for (8-arginine) vasopressin. There are separate systems at the level of the receptors on the end organs of response. The V1 receptors on blood vessels are

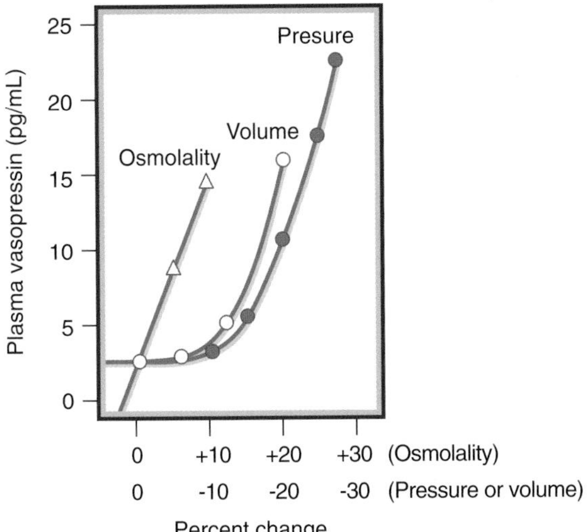

Figure 9–2 ▪ Comparison in humans of the release of vasopressin in response to percentage change of osmolality (increase) and to pressure or volume (decrease). *Note:* To increase plasma vasopressin the change in osmolality is much more sensitive, responding to as little as a 1% increase in osmolality, whereas volume and pressure require greater than a 10% to 15% change to stimulate release of vasopressin. (Redrawn from Robertson GL, Berl T. In Brenner B, Rector F Jr eds. Water Metabolism in the Kidney, 3rd ed., Vol 1 1986:385. Figure by Robinson AG. Los Angeles, CA: UCLA, with permission.)

distinct from V2 receptors on renal collecting duct epithelia. A third receptor is responsible for the nontraditional biologic action of vasopressin to stimulate adrenocorticotropic hormone (ACTH) secretion from the anterior pituitary and also V2 receptors regulate the nontraditional action of vasopressin to stimulate factor VIII production. Vasopressin is the main hormone involved in the regulation of water homeostasis and osmolality of body fluids. On the other hand, blood pressure and volume in humans is largely regulated by body sodium content, which is controlled by the renin-angiotensin-aldosterone system (RAAS). Therefore, the pathology of disorders of the neurohypophysis is primarily expressed as abnormalities of osmolality produced by abnormal excretion or retention of water. In the case of osmoregulation, vasopressin secretion is relatively uncomplicated, with small decreases in osmolality causing a parallel decrease in vasopressin secretion and small increases in osmolality causing a parallel increase in vasopressin secretion. The regulation of volume and blood pressure is significantly more complicated (see review by Thrasher[27]), and experimental models of vasopressin and baroreceptor regulation in animals often involve inhibiting and/or measuring other concurrent sympathetic inputs to the system in order to ascertain direct effects of any stimulus on secretion of vasopressin (see Fig. 9–2). Other influences on secretion of vasopressin such as the inhibiting influence of glucocorticoids and the potent stimulus of nausea and vomiting are less important as physiologic regulators of vasopressin, but they may be important in pathologic situations.

Volume and Pressure Regulation

High pressure arterial baroreceptors are located in the carotid sinus and aortic arch and low pressure volume receptors are located in the atria and pulmonary venous system.[27] The afferent signals from these receptors are carried from the chest to the brain stem through cranial nerves IX and X. Interruption of the vagal input by vagotomy or vagal cold block in dogs[28-30] and destruction of the A1 area of the medulla in rabbits, which receives input from cranial nerves IX and X,[31-33] leads to an increase in vasopressin secretion. These and other data led to the concept that baroreceptors and volume receptors normally inhibit the magnocellular neurons and that decreases in this tonic inhibition result in release of vasopressin. Arterial and venous constriction induced by vasopressin action on V1a receptors will contract the vessels around the existing plasma volume to effectively "increase" plasma volume and reestablish the inhibition of secretion of vasopressin. Vasopressin's action at the kidney to retain water will help replace volume but, in fact, the major hormonal regulation to control volume is the RAAS, which stimulates sodium reabsorption in the kidney (see chapter 14). The concept of tonic inhibition of vasopressin secretion by baroreceptors has been questioned,[27,34] but there is agreement that the volume/baroreceptor responses leading to an increase in vasopressin in humans are much less sensitive than are the osmoreceptors (see Fig. 9–2). The lesser response has been interpreted to be attributable to the fact that changes in blood volume and central venous pressure have little effect to increase vasopressin in humans as long as arterial pressure can be maintained by alternative regulatory mechanisms such as RAAS and sympathetic reflexes.[27] When the hypovolemia is sufficient to cause a decrease in blood pressure, there is a sudden and exponential increase in the level of vasopressin in plasma (see Fig. 9–2).[27,35] There is also agreement that changes in volume or pressure that are insufficient to cause direct increases in vasopressin can nonetheless modify the response of the vasopressin system to osmoregulatory inputs.[35,36] Increases in pressure and central volume will decrease the secretion of vasopressin,[37] but again, the response of the RAAS to cause sodium excretion is much more sensitive to small to moderate increases of pressure and volume than is the response to decrease secretion of vasopressin.[27] Consequently, changes in blood pressure and volume involve both excitatory and inhibitory influences from the brain stem to magnocellular neurons, with the dominant influence depending on the physiologic circumstances.

Osmotic Regulation

The primary receptors for sensing changes in osmolality are located in the brain. Most of the brain is within the blood-brain barrier, which is generally impermeable to polar solutes. The osmostat is insensitive to urea and glucose, which readily cross cellular membranes but not the blood-brain barrier, providing evidence that the osmoreceptors must be outside the blood-brain barrier. Experimental brain lesions in animals have strongly implicated cells in the organum vasculosum of the lamina terminalis (OVLT) and in areas of the adjacent anterior hypothalamus near the anterior wall of the third cerebral ventricle as the primary osmoreceptors. Because these and other circumventricular organs are perfused by fenestrated capillaries, they are, therefore, outside the blood-brain barrier. Surgical destruction of the OVLT abolishes vasopressin secretion and thirst responses to hyperosmolality but not their responses to other stimuli such as hypovolemia.[38] Essentially the same occurs in humans with brain damage that destroys the region around the OVLT and the patients are often unable to maintain normal plasma osmolalities even under basal conditions.[39] In contrast, destruction of the magnocellular neurons of the supraoptic nuclei (SON) and paraventricular nuclei (PVN) eliminates dehydration-induced secretion of vasopressin but does not alter thirst, clearly indicating that osmotically stimulated thirst must be generated at a site proximal to the magnocellular cells.

Extracellular fluid osmolality (predominantly determined by sodium concentration) varies from 280 to 295 mOsm/kg H_2O

in normal subjects but in any individual is maintained within a narrow range. The ability to maintain this narrow range is dependent upon the sensitive response of plasma vasopressin to changes in plasma osmolality; the sensitive response of urine osmolality to changes in plasma vasopressin; and the gain in the system by the response of urine volume to change in plasma vasopressin (Fig. 9–3). Basal plasma vasopressin is in the range of 0.5 to 2 pg/mL. As little as a 1% increase or decrease in plasma osmolality will cause a rapid increase in plasma vasopressin by release of vasopressin from the store of hormone in the posterior pituitary.[35] To rapidly decrease levels of vasopressin in plasma requires a rapid metabolism of vasopressin, which is also characteristic of the hormone that circulates in plasma with a short half-life of approximately 15 minutes. Thus, small increases in osmolality produce a concentrated urine and small decreases in osmolality produce a water diuresis. Figure 9–3 illustrates the linear relationship between plasma osmolality and plasma vasopressin that has been described in humans.[35] This linear relationship for osmolalities persists well above the normal excursion of osmolalities as demonstrated when the increase is induced either by infusion of hypertonic saline or is observed during dehydration of patients with nephrogenic diabetes insipidus.[40] Similarly, Figure 9–3 illustrates that there is a sensitive and linear relationship between the level of vasopressin in plasma and the induced osmolality of the urine. In this case, however, although plasma vasopressin may increase out of the normal physiologic range, the urine osmolality plateaus at approximately 1000 to 1200 mOsm/kg H_2O. This is because the maximum concentration that can be reached by the fluid in the renal collecting duct is limited by the osmolality of the inner medulla. Figure 9–3 also shows the relationship of plasma vasopressin to urine volume. This is a calculated relationship based on the urine volume necessary to excrete a fixed quantity of osmolytes (800 mOsm) at the urine osmolality produced by the change in plasma vasopressin. These graphs demonstrate the gain in the system when considering the changes in urine volume relative to plasma vasopressin. When vasopressin is absent, 18 to 20 L/day are excreted, but with an increase to as little as 0.5 to 1 pg/mL, urine volume is reduced to less than 4 L/day. This illustrates the important point that small changes at low plasma levels of vasopressin are much larger determinants of clinically significant polyuria than are greater changes at higher plasma levels.

In the kidney, water is conserved by the combined functions of the loop of Henle and the collecting duct. The loop of Henle generates a high osmolality in the renal medulla via the countercurrent multiplier system. Vasopressin acts in the collecting duct to increase water (and urea) permeability, thereby allowing osmotic equilibration between the urine and the hypertonic medullary interstitium. The net effect of this process is to extract water from the urine into the medullary interstitial blood vessels (vasa recta), resulting in increased urine concentration and decreased urine volume (antidiuresis). Vasopressin produces antidiuresis by its effects on the epithelial principal cells of the collecting tubule, which possess vasopressin receptors of the V2 type. Aquaporins, a widely expressed family of water channels are the intracellular organelles that mediate rapid water transport across collecting duct cell membranes.[41] Aquaporin-2 is regulated by vasopressin and mediates water transport across

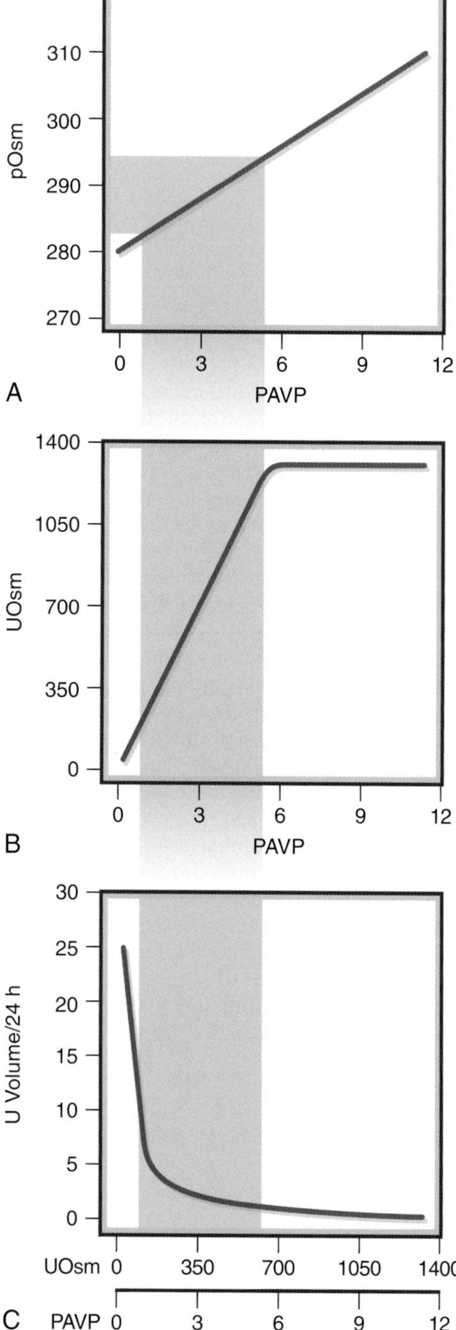

Figure 9–3 ▪ Relationship of plasma osmolality (mOsm/kg of H_2O) to plasma vasopressin (pg/mL) to urine osmolality (mOsm/kg of H_2O) to urine volume (L/day). **A,** Small changes in osmolality induce changes in vasopressin from less than 0.5 to 5 to 6 pg/mL. **B,** These small relation of plasma arginine vasopressin (PAVP) to plasma osolality urine osmolatity, and urine volume. changes in plasma vasopressin induce changes in urine osmolality through the full range from maximally dilute to maximally concentrated urine. Plasma vasopressin can rise to higher levels than 6 pg/mL as illustrated in **A,** but this does not translate into increased urine osmolality, which has a maximum determined by the osmolality of an inner medulla of the kidney. **C,** The relationship of volume to urine osmolality is logarithmic assuming a constant osmolar load and the urine volume that would excrete that osmolar load at the urine osmolality indicated. The interrelationships between the three graphs is illustrated by the shaded area that represents the normal range. Urine volume changes relatively little with small changes in the other parameters until there is nearly complete absence of vasopressin, and then the urine volume increases dramatically. (Calculated from formula presented in Robertson G, Shelton R, Athar S. Kidney Int 1976;10:25-37. Figure by Robinson AG. Los Angeles, CA: UCLA, with permission MacMilan Publishers, Ltd.)

the apical plasma membrane of the principal cells of the collecting ducts.[42] Aquaporin-3 and -4 are expressed at high levels in the basolateral plasma membranes of principal cells and are responsible for the constitutively high water permeability of the basolateral plasma membrane.[41,42] Vasopressin binding to the V2 receptor increases intracellular cyclic adenosine monophosphate (cAMP) levels by activating adenylate cyclase. cAMP activates protein kinase A (PKA), which phosphorylates aquaporin-2 and induces a fusion of aquaporin-2–containing intracytoplasmic vesicles with the apical plasma membranes of the principal cells—a process that increases apical water permeability by markedly increasing the number of water-conducting pores in the apical plasma membrane. Dissociation of vasopressin from the V2 receptor allows intracellular cAMP levels to decrease, and the water channels are then reinternalized into the intracytoplasmic vesicles, thereby terminating the increased water permeability. The aquaporin-containing vesicles remain just below the apical membrane and can be quickly "shuttled" into and out of the membrane in response to changes in intracellular cAMP levels. This mechanism therefore allows minute-to-minute regulation of renal water excretion in response to changes in ambient levels of vasopressin in plasma. There is also long-term regulation of collecting duct water permeability in response to prolonged high levels of circulating vasopressin. This response requires at least 24 hours to elicit and is not as rapidly reversible. The long-term effect is due to the ability of vasopressin to induce large increases in the abundance of aquaporin-2 and aquaporin-3 water channels in the collecting duct principal cells via increased synthesis. Greater total expression of the number of aquaporin-2 and -3 water channels, when combined with the short-term effect of vasopressin to insert aquaporin-2 into the apical plasma membrane, allows the collecting ducts to achieve extremely high water permeabilities during conditions of prolonged dehydration, thereby further enhancing the ability to conserve water in response to stimulated levels of circulating vasopressin.[41,42]

Thirst

Urine volume can be reduced to a minimum but not completely eliminated and insensible water loss is a continuous unregulated process. To maintain water homeostasis, water must also be consumed to replace the obligate urinary and insensible fluid losses. This is regulated by thirst. Thirst represents the body's defense mechanism and water consumption is increased in response to perceived deficits of body fluids. As with to vasopressin, increases in osmolality of the extracellular fluid (ECF) or decreases in intravascular volume can stimulate thirst. Furthermore, there is evidence that the receptors are similar, that is, osmoreceptors in the anterior hypothalamus and low- and/or high-pressure baroreceptors in the chest (with a likely contribution from circulating angiotensin II to stimulate thirst during more severe degrees of intravascular hypovolemia and hypotension).[43] Studies in humans using quantitative estimates of subjective symptoms of thirst have confirmed that increases in plasma osmolality of 2% to 3% are necessary to produce an unequivocal sensation described as "thirst."[39] Similar to vasopressin secretion, the threshold for producing thirst by hypovolemia is significantly higher.

Although osmotic changes clearly are effective stimulants of thirst, it is not likely that changes in plasma osmolality are responsible for the major part of day-to-day fluid intake. Most humans consume the bulk of their ingested water as a result of the relatively unregulated components of fluid intake, such as the consumption of beverages in association with food intake, for reasons of palatability or for desired secondary effects (e.g., caffeine), or for social or habitual reasons (e.g., sodas or alcoholic beverages); as a result, both animals and humans generally ingest volumes in excess of what can be considered to be an actual "need" for fluid. Consistent with this observation is the fact that under most conditions plasma osmolalities in humans remain within 1% to 2% of basal levels, and these relatively small changes in plasma osmolality are generally below the threshold levels that have been found to stimulate thirst. This suggests that despite the obvious vital importance of thirst during pathologic situations of hyperosmolality and hypovolemia, under normal physiologic conditions water balance in humans is accomplished more by free water excretion regulated by vasopressin than by water intake regulated by thirst. This also explains why water intake must be consciously restricted in cases of persistent unregulated secretion of vasopressin. (See later section, "The Syndrome of Inappropriate Antidiuretic Hormone Secretion".)

Clinical Consequences of Osmotic and Volume Regulation

In most physiologic situations there is concurrence and synergy between the effect of increased osmolality and decreased volume to stimulate release of vasopressin. For example, with dehydration, osmolality increases and volume decreases, and each stimulates the release of vasopressin. Furthermore, there is good evidence that a decrease in volume shifts the plasma vasopressin/plasma osmolality response curve to the left, resulting in a greater release of vasopressin at any given osmolality.[27,44] Similarly, excess of fluid produces a decrease in osmolality and an increase in volume, and both will cause a decrease in vasopressin secretion.

The physiology of the relationships between plasma osmolality, plasma vasopressin, and especially urine volume determines some of the pathophysiology of decreased or increased secretion of vasopressin. Note in Figure 9–3 that a regular loss of vasopressin neurons that might decrease the secretory capacity of the neurohypophysis from that able to produce a blood level of 10 to 20 pg/mL of vasopressin down to a secretory capacity only sufficient to maintain a blood level 5 pg/mL would not cause any significant change in the ability to attain a maximum urine osmolality. Below 5 pg/mL there is a linear decrease in the ability to maximally concentrate the urine. However, from the volume curve it can be seen that this results in only a modest increase in urine volume. Then, only when the last few vasopressinergic neurons are lost and the ability to maintain a maximum vasopressin drops from 1 to 0.5 pg/mL would there be a large increase in urine volume. These responses, therefore, allow water conservation even with minimal ability to secrete vasopressin and may explain why patients with diabetes insipidus that has persisted for a relatively long period of time (e.g., after surgery or head injury) may eventually be able to come off vasopressin treatment. The number of vasopressinergic neurons that need to recover to maintain an asymptomatic urine *volume* is small. The same pathophysiology is important in considering the syndrome of inappropriate secretion of antidiuretic hormone (SIADH). In this situation, however, one might consider the consequences to be an inability to suppress vasopressin to less that 1 pg/mL. Note that the maximum urine volume with a standard osmolar load might be as little as 2 L/day at vasopressin levels of 1 pg/mL. If a patient increases fluid intake greater than that which can be excreted with the fixed level of vasopressin of 1 pg/mL then the extra fluid will be retained and the sequence of events that causes hyponatremia in SIADH is initiated.

An analysis of what is presently known about the regulation of thirst and secretion of vasopressin in humans contributes to our understanding of this simple but elegant system to maintain water balance. Under normal physiologic conditions, the sensitivity of the osmoregulatory system for secretion of vasopressin accounts for maintenance of plasma osmolality (pOsm) within narrow limits by adjusting renal water excretion to small changes in osmolality. Stimulated thirst does not represent a major regulatory mechanism under these conditions, and unregulated fluid ingestion and water from metabolized food supplies water in excess of true "need." Excess water is excreted using osmoregulated secretion of vasopressin. However, when unregulated water intake does not supply body needs even with maximal antidiuresis, then plasma osmolality rises to levels that stimulate thirst, which produces water intake proportional to the elevation of osmolality. This arrangement has the advantage of freeing animals and humans from frequent episodes of thirst that would require a diversion of activities toward behavior oriented to seeking water when the water deficiency is sufficiently mild to be compensated for by renal water conservation, yet it does stimulate water ingestion when water deficiency reaches a potentially harmful level.

There are major shifts of fluid during pregnancy that produce a decreased pOsm of about 10 mmol/kg and an increase in plasma volume.[45] This decrease in osmolality is a normal consequence of pregnancy and is the best example of a true resetting of the osmostat. The shift in osmotic threshold appears at about 5 to 8 weeks' gestation and persists throughout pregnancy, returning to normal by 2 weeks after delivery.[45] The physiology of the reset osmostat has been considered in relation to the expanded plasma volume. Total body water in pregnant women is increased by 7 to 8 L due to profound vasodilation.[46] This volume is sensed as normal and vasopressin responds normally to decreases and increases of the expanded volume.[47,45] Both the changes in volume and the changes in regulation of osmolality have been reproduced by infusion of relaxin (a normal hormone of pregnancy that is a member of the insulin-like growth factor (IGF) family into virgin female and normal male rats[48,49] and reversed in pregnant rats by immunoneutralization of relaxin[50]; thus, relaxin is the proposed mediator of the effect.

In women, the placenta produces an enzyme, cysteine aminopeptidase, which is released into the plasma and is known as *oxytocinase*.[45,51] This enzyme is equally potent in degrading vasopressin. The activity of oxytocinase (vasopressinase) increases markedly around 20 weeks of gestation and increases further to 40 weeks, returning slowly to normal over a few weeks after delivery.[52]

Numerous studies have reported that elderly humans are at risk for both hypernatremia and hyponatremia.[53,54] In older subjects there is a decrease in glomerular filtration rate[54] and the collecting duct in the aged kidney may be less responsive to vasopressin-stimulated increases in aquaporin-2 water channels, thus limiting the ability to excrete free water.[55] Many other abnormalities of fluid and electrolyte balance in the elderly are due to comorbid conditions and/or the numerous pharmacologic agents to which these patients are often exposed. Studies of responses to dehydration, osmolar stimulation, or volume stimulation in the elderly are complicated by the fact that by age 75 to 80, there is a decline in total body water to 50% of the level of normal young adults.[56] The elderly have decreased thirst with dehydration and a lesser fluid intake to return their volume to normal during recovery from dehydration.[57-59] At the other end of the spectrum, elderly patients have been found to excrete a water load less well than younger subjects and at least part of this is due decreased suppression of vasopressin.[60] In summary, there are age-related changes in body volumes and renal function that predispose the elderly to abnormalities in water and electrolyte balance. Diseases that are more common in the elderly aggravate this phenomenon; furthermore, the therapy for these diseases affect water balance. Healthy elderly humans probably have at least a normal (or increased) ability to secrete vasopressin but a decreased appreciation for thirst and a decreased ability to achieve either a maximum concentration of urine to retain water or a maximum dilution of urine to excrete water. This demonstrates the necessity of paying attention to fluid balance problems in the elderly as undetected hypernatremia or hyponatremia can lead to increased morbidity and mortality.[61]

DIABETES INSIPIDUS

Diabetes insipidus is a disorder of a large volume of urine (diabetes) that is hypotonic, dilute, and tasteless (insipid). This is opposed to the hypertonic and sweet urine of diabetes mellitus (honey). Four pathophysiologic mechanisms related to vasopressin produce large volumes of dilute urine and polydipsia:

1. Hypothalamic (central or neurohypophyseal) diabetes insipidus with inability to secrete and usually to synthesize vasopressin in the neurohypophyseal system
2. Nephrogenic diabetes insipidus wherein there is an inappropriate renal response to vasopressin
3. Transient diabetes insipidus of pregnancy produced by the accelerated metabolism of vasopressin
4. Primary polydipsia wherein the initial pathophysiology is the ingestion of fluid rather than the excretion of fluid

Differential Diagnosis

To determine whether there is a large volume of urine one can measure a 24-hour urine or the patient can keep a diary for 24 hours recording the volume and the time of each voided urine. Simultaneously, there is a determination of whether polyuria is due to an osmotic agent such as glucose or to intrinsic renal disease. Usually routine laboratory studies and the clinical setting will distinguish these disorders from consideration of diabetes insipidus. If the thirst mechanism is intact, most patients present with a normal serum sodium and no evidence of dehydration. There is universal agreement that the diagnosis of diabetes insipidus is made by a dehydration test that stimulates the normal release of vasopressin but less than normal concentration of the urine. The most common test used clinically is a dehydration test in a controlled environment followed by measure of vasopressin in plasma and response to administered vasopressin or the analogue desmopressin. If the patient has mild polyuria, the test may begin in the evening with the major portion of dehydration carried out overnight. If the patient gives a history of large volumes of urine during the night it is best to perform the test during the day when the patient can be observed. The patient voids at the beginning of the test and the starting weight is recorded. A serum sodium measurement is obtained and nothing is allowed by mouth (certainly no fluid) during the test. Each voided urine is then recorded and urine osmolality measured. The patient is weighed after each liter of urine is excreted. When two consecutive measures of urine osmolality differ by no more than 10% and the patient has lost 2% of the body weight, plasma for Na^+, osmolality and vasopressin is drawn and the patient is given 2 μg of desmopressin intravenously or intramuscularly and urine output and osmolality is recorded hourly for an additional 2 hours.[62,63] The dehydration is stopped if the patient loses more than 3% of the body weight or if at any time the Na^+ is elevated above the normal range. The duration of the test varies among patients, with complete diabetes insipidus reaching a maximum and low urine osmolality being detected within a few hours, and with the test taking up to 18 hours in patients with other disorders. There is no difficulty determining the diagnosis in severe hypothalamic diabetes insipidus or severe nephrogenic diabetes insipidus. In the former, urine osmolality will have minimal concentration despite dehydration and there is a marked increase in urine osmolality in response to administered desmopressin, at least a 50% increase but often increasing 200% to 400%. At the end of the test, these patients will have undetectable vasopressin in plasma. In nephrogenic diabetes insipidus, there is also little concentration of the urine despite achieving dehydration, but the urine osmolality will also show little or no response to the administered desmopressin. These patients are unequivocally distinguished from patients with hypothalamic diabetes insipidus by high levels of vasopressin in plasma, often greater than 5 pg/μL at the end of the dehydration.

The difficulty is in differentiating partial hypothalamic diabetes insipidus from primary polydipsia. In both of these disorders, the urine shows some concentration with dehydration, often above plasma osmolality, but the urine osmolality does not approach 800 to 1000 mOsm/kg, which is characteristic in normal subjects. In response to the administered desmopressin, patients with partial hypothalamic diabetes insipidus usually have a further concentration of the urine—at least 10%—whereas patients with primary polydipsia have no further increase. The reliability of the response to desmopressin is debated. Some patients with primary polydipsia may achieve a plateau level in urine osmolality before reaching their maximum urine osmolality and hence respond to desmopressin. Alternatively, some patients with partial hypothalamic diabetes insipidus may, with severe dehydration, secrete sufficient vasopressin to achieve the maximum attainable urine osmolality and not respond with a further increase to administered desmopressin. Investigators who use a highly sensitive radioimmunoassay for vasopressin are able to distinguish between partial hypothalamic diabetes insipidus and primary polydipsia by the measure of vasopressin at the end of the dehydration phase[64,65]; these investigators further report that patients with one of these disorders may be inappropriately diagnosed with the other disorder when the standard dehydration test is used.[65,64] However, a longitudinal clinical study of patients with autoimmune hypothalamic diabetes insipidus reported good correlation between results of the dehydration test and measured vasopressin to diagnose partial diabetes insipidus.[66] When the diagnosis is in doubt, patients should have adequate follow-up to ensure that a good therapeutic response is obtained and that the patients do not develop hyponatremia. This clinical follow-up and response has been considered a continuation of the diagnosis with the trial of desmopressin as a test agent. If a standard dose of desmopressin produces a decrease in polyuria, a decrease in thirst, and no reduction of sodium, then the patient almost certainly has partial hypothalamic diabetes insipidus. However, if the polydipsia does not improve and the patient develops hyponatremia, then the patient has some abnormality of thirst and primary polydipsia.[64,67]

The clinical presentation is often helpful in the differential diagnosis. In a patient with onset of polyuria or polydipsia immediately after surgery in the hypothalamic/pituitary area or after head trauma (especially with skull fracture and loss of consciousness), the diagnosis of hypothalamic diabetes insipidus is highly likely. Sometimes diuresis after surgery is the result of water retention during the procedure. Vasopressin is released during surgical procedures and administered fluid may be retained. When the stress of surgery abates, the vasopressin level falls and administered fluid is excreted. If an attempt is made to match the urine output with further fluid infusion, persistent polyuria will occur and might be mistaken for diabetes insipidus. If in doubt, fluid can be withheld until there is a modest increase in sodium, then urine osmolality may be measured and the response to administered desmopressin noted. If the urine output decreases when the fluid is withheld and the serum sodium remains normal, then the polyuria was excretion of physiologically retained fluid. If the serum sodium begins to rise and there is a response to desmopressin, then the diagnosis of diabetes insipidus can be established.[68]

Patients with hypothalamic diabetes insipidus often have a sudden onset of symptoms and persistent thirst throughout the day and night associated with a desire for cold liquids.[69] Patients with diabetes insipidus usually have serum sodium in the high range of normal while patients with primary polydipsia have serum sodium in the low range of normal. Blood urea nitrogen concentration is often low in both hypothalamic diabetes insipidus and in primary polydipsia because of the high renal clearance, but there is a difference in serum uric acid concentrations. Serum uric acid is elevated in hypothalamic diabetes insipidus both because of modest volume contraction and because of absence of the normal action of vasopressin on V1 receptors in the kidney to increase urate clearance. A value greater than 5 μg/dL was reported to separate hypothalamic diabetes insipidus from primary polydipsia. Presumably in patients with primary polydipsia, there is modest volume expansion and intermittent secretion of vasopressin to act on V1 receptors to clear serum urate.[70] Urine volume greater than 18 L is highly suggestive of primary polydipsia because this exceeds the amount of urine delivered to the collecting duct. Most patients with hypothalamic diabetes insipidus have modest dehydration, decreased glomerular filtration rate, and excrete urine volumes in the range of 6 to 12 L/day.

Imaging of the Neurohypophysis

On T1-weighted images, MRI produces a bright spot in the sella[10] due to stored hormone in neurosecretory granules in the posterior pituitary.[25,71-74] The bright spot is present in approximately 80% of normal subjects[75,76] and is absent in most patients with diabetes insipidus. The intensity of posterior pituitary bright spot might vary with the physiologic state of water balance and decrease with a prolonged stimulus to vasopressin secretion.[77] Some studies have reported the presence of a bright spot in patients with clinical evidence of diabetes insipidus.[78] In patients with familial hypothalamic diabetes insipidus (see later), the posterior pituitary bright spot may be seen early in the disease (especially when the diabetes insipidus is partial), but usually disappears with increasing severity of the diabetes insipidus.[79] The role of stored oxytocin as a source of the pituitary bright spot has been ignored and it is possible that a persistent bright spot in patients with diabetes insipidus is due to pituitary content of oxytocin.

The presence of a positive posterior pituitary bright spot has been variably reported in other polyuric disorders. In primary polydipsia, the bright spot usually is seen.[73,80] In nephrogenic diabetes insipidus, the bright spot has been reported to be absent in some patients[73] but present in others.[73,81] These patients have high levels of vasopressin in plasma and are chronically dehydrated, so the posterior pituitary might be depleted of content of vasopressin. Similarly, with the osmotic stress of untreated diabetes mellitus or the transient diabetes insipidus of pregnancy, the posterior pituitary may be depleted and the bright spot lost during the event, but may return with recovery.[77,82]

Imaging of the hypothalamus is also an important diagnostic tool for diseases of the neurohypophysis. As noted earlier, the hormones of the neurohypophysis are synthesized in the paired paraventricular nuclei located bilaterally in the walls of the third ventricle and supraoptic nuclei located at the extremes of the optic chiasm. When this anatomic information is coupled with the knowledge that 90% of the vasopressinergic neurons must be destroyed to produce symptomatic diabetes insipidus,[83,84] it is apparent that for a mass lesion or a destructive lesion to produce diabetes insipidus it must destroy a large area of the hypothalamus, that is, 90% of the cell bodies, and/or be specifically located where the tracks converge in the base of the hypothalamus at the origin of the pituitary stalk. The hormones are synthesized in cells bodies quite distant from the site of release in the posterior lobe and with section of the axons or pressure on the axons at the level of the posterior lobe, there is a reaccumulation of neurosecretory material and regeneration of a posterior lobe above the site of injury.[85,77] Thus, tumors confined to the sella do not cause diabetes insipidus,[84] and the area of interest is the discrete area immediately above the diaphragm sella at the base of the hypothalamus. The pituitary stalk can also be readily identified on MRI, which is an additional tool used in the differential diagnosis of diseases of the neurohypophysis. Enlargement of the stalk is reported with the diseases listed in Table 9–1. When there is a diagnosis of diabetes insipidus, thickening of the stalk is usually associated with absence of the posterior pituitary bright spot and a search for systemic diseases is indicated.[86] When a diagnosis is still in doubt, repeat MRI should be done every 3 to 6 months, especially in children in whom enlargement may indicate a germinoma.[87,88] When follow-up shows a decrease in size of the stalk, a likely diagnosis is infundibulolymphohypophysitis.[89]

Clinical Syndromes of Hypothalamic Diabetes Insipidus

Hereditary Hypothalamic Diabetes Insipidus

Hereditary hypothalamic (central or neurohypophyseal) diabetes insipidus is characterized by the onset of classic diabetes insipidus, thirst, polydipsia, and polyuria in childhood,[90,91] but during infancy those who carry the genetic defect may be asymptomatic. This is in contrast to cases of familial nephrogenic diabetes insipidus in which the defect is expressed as a polyuric disease at birth (see later description). The relatively late onset of hereditary hypothalamic diabetes insipidus is also supported by MRI findings, which, while variable, may include a positive bright spot indicative of vasopressin stores early in the disease but a loss of signal or greatly decreased bright spot late in the disease.[81,92,93] Most reported cases are expressed as autosomal dominant hypothalamic (neurohypophyseal) diabetes insipidus, and the genetic defect is usually in the biologically inactive neurophysin part of the prohormone or in the signal peptide of the pre-prohormone. Disruption of the cleavage of the signal peptide from the prohormone and abnormalities of the folding of the vasopressin neurophysin precursor moiety are thought to produce abnormal trafficking and accumulation of mutant prohormone in the endoplasmic reticulum, which by unknown mechanisms leads to cell death and the delayed onset in the dominant genetic phenotype.[94-96] Autopsy studies have confirmed neuronal cell death.[97] In Wolfram's syndrome, diabetes insipidus is associated with diabetes mellitus, optic atrophy, and deafness (DIDMOAD). The genetic defect has been localized to the short arm of chromosome 4[98,99] and is usually unique to the family,[100] with variable phenotypes in different families, but usually with expression of diabetes mellitus before diabetes insipidus.

TABLE 9–1 DISEASES ASSOCIATED WITH ENLARGED INFUNDIBULAR STALK

1. Germinoma
2. Craniopharyngioma
3. Metastases to the hypothalamus and long portal vessels (e.g., carcinoma of the breast or lung)
4. Granulomatosis diseases
   a. Langerhans cell histiocytosis
   b. Sarcoidosis
   c. Wegener's granulomatosis
   d. Non–Langerhans cell histiocytosis (e.g., Erdheim-Chester disease)
5. Tuberculosis
6. Lymphocytic infundibulohypophysitis

Diabetes Insipidus Produced by Solid Tumors or Hematologic Malignancies

Some tumors such as craniopharyngioma and suprasellar germinoma or pinealoma characteristically occur in a suprasellar basal hypothalamic area and are regularly associated with diabetes insipidus.[101,102] It is not uncommon in craniopharyngioma, pinealomas, and suprasellar germinomas for diabetes insipidus to be the presenting complaint, although other evidence of hypopituitarism is often present. MRI often shows a thickened stalk[103] and may show a hypothalamic mass.

Metastatic disease involving the pituitary is usually found in association with widespread metastatic disease and may only be reported at autopsy, being asymptomatic during life. Metastases are twice as likely to involve the posterior pituitary as the anterior pituitary,[104,105] which is thought to be due to a more direct arterial blood supply to the posterior pituitary.[106] Most primary tumors in the hypothalamic-pituitary area that cause diabetes insipidus are relatively slow growing, and any tumor in this area that shows rapid growth in a short period of time should be considered to be a possible metastatic tumor.[107,108]

Diabetes insipidus is reported with lymphomas in the hypothalamic/pituitary area.[109] There may be some increased incidence of lymphoma presenting with diabetes insipidus due to the increased incidence of lymphoproliferative disease with human immunodeficiency virus (HIV) and hepatitis C infection.[110] Diabetes insipidus is also associated with leukemia. The mechanism is thought to be infiltration of the hypothalamus, thrombosis, or infection.[111,112] Diabetes insipidus is distinctly more common in nonlymphocytic leukemia.[113-116] MRI studies in leukemia may show infiltration or an infundibular mass,[114] but often results are normal even when leukemic cells are found in the cerebrospinal fluid (CSF).[113]

Response of the Neurohypophyseal System to Surgery or Trauma

Although diabetes insipidus is well known to occur after hypothalamic/pituitary surgery, this diagnosis should be made with caution.[68,117] Vasopressin is normally secreted in the stress of surgical procedures and fluid may be retained, which is then normally excreted after surgery (see "Differential Diagnosis"). Stress of surgery may also induce insulin resistance and exacerbate diabetes mellitus, producing an osmotic diuresis from glucose. The patterns of diabetes insipidus after surgery have been described in detail.[84] As many as 50% to 60% of patients will have some transient diabetes insipidus within 24 hours of pituitary surgery; this usually resolves, especially with transsphenoidal surgery in which the resection of a tumor is confined to the sella. If there is complete stalk section, patients may exhibit a pattern known as *triphasic diabetes insipidus* (Fig. 9–4). The first phase is diabetes insipidus with onset within the first 24 hours of surgery; this is thought to be due to axon shock

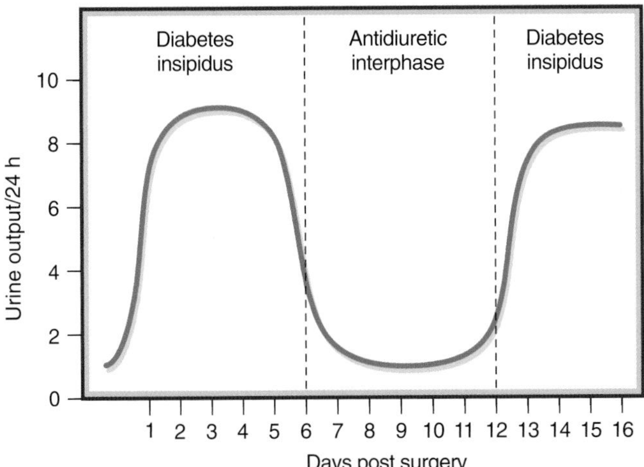

Figure 9–4 ▪ Typical triphasic response of urine volume following sectioning of the pituitary stalk induced by surgery or head trauma. The first phase of diabetes insipidus occurs immediately postoperatively and continues to day 6. The second phase of antidiuresis occurs from day 7 and continues to day 12. The third stage is the reocurrence of diabetes insipidus on day 13. (Durations vary. See text for discussion.) (From Robinson AG. Los Angeles, CA: UCLA, with permission.)

and inability of action potentials to be propagated from the cell body to the axon terminals in the posterior pituitary. The second phase is an antidiuretic phase that was originally described as a "normal interphase" but is not normal and is thought to be due to unregulated release of vasopressin from the store of hormone in the axons of the posterior pituitary as these axons degenerate. Because the release of vasopressin in this phase is unregulated, excess administration of fluids produces hyponatremia as in other SIADHs. When all the hormone has been released from the posterior pituitary, the third phase, the return of diabetes insipidus, occurs. The course of diabetes insipidus may be permanent, or it may subsequently resolve to partial or clinically unapparent disease.

An important observation is that the second phase of the triphasic response, that is, uncontrolled release of vasopressin due to axon trauma, may occur without preceding or subsequent diabetes insipidus.[118,119] This has been reported clinically and has been produced experimentally in the rat by a unilateral lesion of the supraopticohypophyseal tract.[119] The interpretation is that if the trauma is only to some of the axons coursing to the posterior pituitary, then the remaining intact axons will have sufficient vasopressin function to avoid clinically apparent diabetes insipidus characteristic of the first and third phase of the triphasic response. However, the store of hormone in the posterior pituitary is sufficiently large that degeneration and necrosis of even a fraction of these vasopressin neurons will cause enough uncontrolled release of vasopressin to produce hyponatremia if excess fluid is administered. The hyponatremia becomes apparent because it is often symptomatic with new-onset headache, nausea and emesis, or seizure.[120] When all the vasopressin from the damaged neurons has been secreted, the stimulus for water retention resolves and the retained water is excreted, producing recovery from the hyponatremia. Thus, the clinical picture is one of hyponatremia occurring around 7 days after pituitary surgery, persisting for a few days and then returning to normal. This syndrome of transient hyponatremia has been referred to as "isolated second phase"[119] to emphasize the pathophysiologic etiology. Isolated hyponatremia has been reported in 10% to 25% of patients after pituitary surgery.[121,122]

The same patterns of diabetes insipidus as occur after surgery can be seen in patients after closed-head trauma.[84,123] Three fourths of these cases are due to motor vehicle accidents[84,123,124] and there is a great preponderance of male patients, usually young men with a mean age in the 20s. Computed tomography (CT) or MRI in a large group of patients with posttraumatic hypopituitarism including diabetes insipidus reported hemorrhage in the hypothalamus or posterior pituitary in 55% of patients and approximately 5% of patients had stalk resection or infarction of the posterior pituitary.[123] There are several important clinical points to be made with regard to diabetes insipidus induced by head trauma. First, these patients are virtually always unconscious and will not have the normal ability to sense thirst. Second, it is a situation in which large volumes of fluid might be given because of blood loss or other volume deficits and this fluid loss or stress might induce diabetes mellitus and an osmotic diuresis (see "Differential Diagnosis"). Third, there may be a greater risk if the second phase is unrecognized because hyponatremia will produce cerebral edema and may aggravate any edema due to trauma. Therefore, in administering desmopressin, the effect of one dose should be allowed to wane before administering another dose to ensure that the patient has not entered the second phase. There is a high incidence of anterior pituitary deficiency in association with diabetes insipidus induced by head trauma.[123] The possibility of cortisol deficiency should be considered immediately because it may be life threatening in these patients. Cortisol deficiency should also be considered subsequently if diabetes insipidus appears to "improve" because of decrease of water excretion in the absence of an administered antidiuretic agent.[84] Finally, in a long-term follow-up of these patients, partial diabetes insipidus may be found,[125,126] but there may be return of sufficient vasopressin function such that the patient no longer has symptomatic diabetes insipidus.[84,125]

Granulomatous Diseases

In most cases of diabetes insipidus caused by granulomatus diseases, there is clear evidence of characteristic disease elsewhere in the body.[86,127,128] MRI will show involvement of the hypothalamus and absence of a posterior pituitary bright spot on T1-weighted images with widening of the stalk, Table 9–1. Although there are occasional reports of resolution of the diabetes insipidus with appropriate therapy, in most cases, once established, diabetes insipidus is permanent.[129-131]

When obvious causes of diabetes insipidus are not present, most cases of diabetes insipidus will be "idiopathic." As in other endocrine systems wherein loss of function is not associated with a specific etiology, the possibility of an autoimmune process is considered. A now well-recognized cause of autoimmune diabetes insipidus is lymphocytic infundibulohypophysitis.[132] Since the advent of MRI, lymphocytic infundibulohypophysitis has been diagnosed based on the appearance of a thickened stalk and/or enlargement of the posterior pituitary mimicking a pituitary tumor. In these cases, the characteristic bright spot on MRI T1-weighted images is lost.[133] Treatment of these patients with prednisone may be associated with decrease in size of the stalk, but this may also occur spontaneously.[134] Some cases have coexistence of infundibulohypophysitis and adenohypophysitis.[135,136]

Diabetes Insipidus in Pregnancy

There are two types of transient diabetes insipidus in pregnancy, both caused by the enzyme cysteine aminopeptidase (oxytocinase) described earlier.[137] In the first type, the activity of cysteine aminopeptidase (which is also a vasopressinase) is extremely and abnormally elevated. This syndrome has been referred to as *vasopressin-resistant diabetes insipidus of pregnancy.*[138] The concurrence of preeclampsia, acute fatty liver, and coagulopathies have been noted.[46,139,140] Usually subsequent pregnancies by these women are uncomplicated by either diabetes insipidus or acute fatty liver. In the second type, the accelerated metabolic clearance of vasopressin produces diabetes insipidus in a patient with borderline vasopressin function from a specific disease, such as mild nephrogenic diabetes insipidus or partial hypothalamic diabetes insipidus.[51,141] Vasopressin is rapidly destroyed and the neurohypophysis is unable to keep up with the increased demand. Desmopressin is clearly the treatment of choice for diabetes insipidus in pregnant women (see "Treatment"). Labor and parturition usually proceed normally and patients have no trouble with lactation.[142] There is the threat of chronic and severe dehydration when diabetes insipidus is unrecognized, which this may pose a threat to a pregnant woman.[143]

Essential Hypernatremia

A variant of diabetes insipidus is the syndrome of absent osmostat with intact baroreceptors,[144] also referred to as *adipsic hypernatremia* or *adipsic diabetes insipidus*.[145] Because of the dysfunction of the osmostat, the patients do not sense thirst and do not drink water. Unlike normal subjects, as the serum sodium rises, there is no (or markedly subnormal) release of vasopressin, so a hypotonic polyuria continues. Even when the patients are made euvolemic with the infusion of normal saline and the serum sodium is allowed to rise to high levels, there is not appropriate secretion of vasopressin. Vasopressin is, however, synthesized and stored because maneuvers to stimulate baroreceptors cause secretion of vasopressin and concentration of the urine.[146,147] The proposed pathophysiologic mechanism is that the inadequate water intake and excess water excretion produces a degree of dehydration with hypernatremia. When the dehydration is sufficient to stimulate the baroreceptors, vasopressin is released, urine is concentrated, and the patients remain in a steady-state of hypernatremia with modest dehydration. The increased concentration of sodium per se also causes sodium excretion to help maintain the new steady-state.[148] The disorder may be associated with a variety of insults to the hypothalamus and has been specifically described in clipping of anterior communicating artery aneurysm.[145]

Diabetes Insipidus and Brain Death

Diabetes insipidus is virtually universal in animal models of brain death[149] and is extremely common in clinical series, ranging in occurrence in 50% to 90% of cases.[150,151] Important clinical considerations are whether coexistent anterior pituitary deficiency exists, especially whether steroids should be administered, and whether the diabetes insipidus should be treated. This is controversial. Although there is no firm evidence that treating the diabetes insipidus affects the quality of donor organs,[152-154] there also is no evidence that treating the diabetes insipidus results in any complications.[155] Diabetes insipidus in brain death can be treated similarly to acute head injury.

Primary Polydipsia

Primary polydipsia and subsequent polyuria must be differentiated from diabetes insipidus and may also contribute to SIADH. Primary polydipsia may be induced by organic structural lesions in the hypothalamus identical to any of the disorders described as causes of diabetes insipidus, and may be especially associated with sarcoidosis of the hypothalamus.[156] It may also be produced by drugs that cause a dry mouth or by any peripheral disorder causing an elevation of renin and/or angiotensin.[157] Where there is not an identifiable pathologic etiology, the disorder may be habitual throughout a lifetime or more commonly is associated with psychiatric syndromes. Series of polydipsic patients in psychiatric hospital have shown an incidence as high as 42% of patients with some form of polydipsia; for more than half of those, there was no obvious explanation for the polydipsia.[158,159] Usually the patients are refractory to attempts to restrict fluid.[157] Propanolol has been used with some success, presumably because of its ability to inhibit the renin-angiotensin system.[160]

Clinical Syndromes of Nephrogenic Diabetes Insipidus

Congenital Nephrogenic Diabetes Insipidus

Babies with nephrogenic diabetes insipidus present with vomiting, constipation, failure to thrive, fever, and polyuria. Symptoms usually appear during the first week of life,[161-163] and upon testing, the patients will be found to have hypernatremia and a low urine osmolality. The diagnosis is established by high levels of vasopressin in the plasma in the presence of hypotonic polyuria and then the absence of response to administered desmopressin. There are two causes, mutation in the V2 receptor and mutations in the aquaporin-2 water channels, but the presentation of diabetes insipidus is independent of the genotype.[161-163]

Nephrogenic Diabetes Insipidus Caused by Mutation of the V2 Receptor

More than 90% of cases of congenital nephrogenic diabetes insipidus are an X-linked disorder occurring in males and caused by one of more than 155 individually different V2 receptor mutations.[164] Most mutations occur in the transmembrane domain of the receptor. In type 1 disorder, the receptor reaches the membrane surface but has abnormal hormone binding or signal transduction. More common is type 2, with defective transport of receptor in the endoplasmic reticulum due to abnormal folding.[164] In clinical series, approximately 10% of the V2 receptor defects causing congenital nephrogenic diabetes insipidus are thought to be de novo. This high incidence of de novo cases coupled with the large number of mutations that have been identified hinders the clinical use of genetic identification because it is necessary to sequence the entire open reading frame of the receptor gene rather than short sequences of DNA. Even though most female carriers of the X-linked V2 receptors defect have no clinical disease, some female carriers may have a decreased maximum urine osmolality in response to the plasma level of vasopressin that they obtain.[165] Rarely, girls have a defect as severe as boys, which is thought to be due to inactivation of the normal X chromosome.[163,166,167]

Nephrogenic Diabetes Insipidus Caused By Mutation of Aquaporin-2

When the proband is a girl it is likely the defect is a mutation of the aquaporin-2 water channel gene on chromosome 12, region q12-13, producing an autosomal recessive disease.[168,169] This should be especially considered where consanguinity is known in the family and the family history has expressed disease in men and women. The patients may be heterozygous for two different recessive mutations[170] or be homozygous for the same abnormality from both parents.[171] In some mutations, the aquaporin is not properly processed in the endoplasmic reticulum nor released into the cytoplasm[172] whereas with other mutations, aquaporins are processed but are not appropriately inserted in the cell membrane. Mutations of the aquaporin-2 protein may produce an autosomal dominant nephrogenic diabetes insipidus when the mutant aquaporin-2 protein associates with the wild type protein to inhibit normal intracellular routing and function of the wild type.[173-175]

Acquired Nephrogenic Diabetes Insipidus

The ability to produce a concentrated urine depends upon maintaining hyperosmolality of the inner medulla of the kidney. Producing and maintaining hyperosmolality of the inner medulla requires that the kidney architecture be intact with an intact tubular structure of a descending limb of the loop of Henle and an ascending limb essential to the development of the countercurrent multiplier and then a normal anatomy of the collecting duct to pass back through the inner medulla. The vascular structure must be anatomically intact so the hyperosmolality of the inner medulla is not washed away by normal blood flow. The broad definition of nephrogenic diabetes insipidus includes numerous chronic renal diseases that distort the architecture of the kidney such as polycystic kidney disease, renal infarcts with neovascularization such as produced by sickle cell anemia, infiltrative disease of the kidney, and washout of the medullary gradient or low-protein diet with reduced medullary urea concentration. Vascular anatomic causes of reduced concentration of urine are not considered diabetes insipidus by those who include only those disorders caused by abnormal function of vasopressin.[169] The polyuria associated with hypokalemia, hypercalcemia, and release of bilateral urinary tract obstruction are associated with down-regulation of aquaporin-2.[41,175]

Drug-Induced Nephrogenic Diabetes Insipidus

Administration of lithium to treat psychiatric disorders is the most common cause of drug-induced nephrogenic diabetes insipidus and illustrates the mechanisms.[175-177] Lithium produces a dramatic reduction in aquaporin-2 levels.[178] There is as much as a 95% decrease in aquaporin-2 content and even the 5% of aquaporin-2 that persists is not normally transported to the collecting duct membrane.[177] The defect of aquaporins is slow to correct both in experimental animals and in humans and may be permanent.[175,179] Demeclocycline is another commonly recognized drug to cause nephrogenic diabetes insipidus and is used clinically to treat SIADH (see later text). See the review by Bendz and Aurell[180] for a list of drugs that cause nephrogenic diabetes insipidus.

TREATMENT OF DIABETES INSIPIDUS

Patients with diabetes insipidus and inadequate thirst can rapidly become dehydrated and develop severe hypernatremia with devastating effects on the central nervous system (CNS). Hypertonic encephalopathy with obtundation, coma, and seizures may be produced by brain shrinkage. A decreased volume of brain in the skull may lead to subarachnoid hemorrhage, intracerebral bleeding, or petechial hemorrhage.[181] Fortunately these problems associated with severe hypernatremia are usually not observed in patients with diabetes insipidus who have an intact thirst mechanism; also, they are usually not a part of the syndromes of adipsic hypernatremia (essential hypernatremia), probably because of the chronic and slower onset of hypernatremia. Hypernatremic encephalopathy is a risk when the patients are unable to respond to thirst, either because of age or level of consciousness.

The absence of vasopressin per se does not produce pathology, and a major goal of therapy is to decrease the thirst and polyuria to an acceptable level to allow the patient to maintain a normal lifestyle. The therapeutic regimen should be easy for the patient to accommodate, and the timing and quantity of dosage should be individually prescribed. The safety of the prescribed agent and a regimen that avoids any detrimental effects of overtreatment are primary considerations because of the relatively benign course of diabetes insipidus and the adverse consequences of hyponatremia. The therapeutic agents to treat diabetes insipidus are listed in Table 9–2. Water is considered a therapeutic agent for diabetes insipidus because when taken in sufficient quantity there is no metabolic abnormality. As noted, therapy is designed to reduce the necessary water intake (and polyuria) to an acceptable level, but occasional lapses in pharmacologic therapy are not detrimental, may avoid overtreatment producing hyponatremia, and allow recognition of any spontaneous recovery.

Treatment in Different Clinical Situations

Hypothalamic Diabetes Insipidus

The drug of choice is desmopressin.[64,182] In this synthetic analogue, the substitution of D-arginine markedly reduces pressor activity and removing the terminal amine increases the half-life (see Fig. 9–1). The two changes produce an agent nearly 2000 times more specific for antidiuresis than naturally occurring L-arginine vasopressin.[183] Most patients would prefer to use the desmopressin tablets (0.1 and 0.2 mg), although many patients continue to be successfully treated with the desmopressin intranasal spray. Because of the variability among patients, it is desirable to determine the duration of action of individual doses in each patient.[184,185] The patient is first allowed to escape from the effects of any previous medication then for each voided urine the time can be recorded and the volume and (if possible osmolality) measured. The patient is allowed to drink fluid ad libitum. A decrease in urine volume is noted in 1 to 2 hours after an administered dose, and the total duration of action will usually range from 6 to 18 hours. Usually a satisfactory schedule can be determined with a modest dose, and the maximum dose needed is rarely more than 0.2 µg orally or 20 µg (two sprays) given two or three times a day (usually twice).[184,185] Using the tablets allows considerable flexibility in dosage by using either whole or split tablets. For the intranasally administered desmopressin, there is less flexibility with the metered spray, which is fixed at 10 µg in 100 µL. If greater flexibility is necessary, the patient should be taught to use the rhinal catheter. Specific directions are described elsewhere.[182] When a dose is sufficient to elicit a stable therapeutic response, further increasing the dose (e.g., doubling the dose) produces only a moderate increase in duration of a few hours,[184,185] consistent with the half-life of desmo-

TABLE 9–2 THERAPEUTIC AGENTS FOR TREATMENT OF DIABETES INSIPIDUS

1. Water
2. Water-retaining agents
   a. L-Arginine vasopressin
   b. Desmopressin, 1-(3 mercaptopropionic acid) 8-D-arginine vasopressin
   c. Chlorpropamide
   d. Carbamazepine*
   e. Clofibrate*
   f. Indomethacin
3. Natriuretic agents
   a. Thiazide diuretics
   b. Amiloride
   c. Indapamide

*Not recommended.

pressin in plasma.[185] Rarely is it necessary to resort to parenterally administered desmopressin (2-mL vials of 4 µg/mL) for ambulatory patients. If an intercurrent illness or allergy makes this desirable, a dose of 0.5 to 2.0 µg can be administered subcutaneously using an insulin (low-dose if necessary) syringe and needle.[184] Parenterally administered desmopressin gives virtually identical therapeutic response when given as an intravenous bolus, intramuscularly or subcutaneously,[184] and the parenteral administration is 5 to 20 times as potent as an intranasally administered dose.[184,182]

Therapeutic agents such as chlorpropamide or thiazide diuretics are especially useful when only a modest decrease in urine volume will make the patients asymptomatic, such as in "partial" diabetes insipidus, in which patients have some residual vasopressin secretion. The major action of chlorpropamide is on the renal tubule to increase the hydroosmotic action of vasopressin,[186] but the agent can also produce significant antidiuresis even in patients with severe hypothalamic diabetes insipidus.[64] The usual dose is 250 to 500 mg/day with a response noted in 1 to 2 days and a maximum antidiuresis in 4 days.[64,182] This is an off-label use of the drug. This agent should not be used in pregnancy and is not recommended in children, especially those with concurrent hypopituitarism because of the possibility of severe hypoglycemia. It is important to recognize that in patients with diabetes insipidus when the therapeutic agents listed in Table 9–2 are administered for specific indications, there might be some augmentation of the effect of administered desmopressin, exposing patients with diabetes insipidus to the possibility of excess water retention and hyponatremia.

Hyponatremia is a rare complication of desmopressin therapy and only occurs if the patient is continually antidiuretic while maintaining a fluid intake sufficient to become volume expanded and natriuretic. Thirst may be protective, but most patients with diabetes insipidus on standard therapy are not continuously maximally antidiuretic.

Diabetes Insipidus with Inadequate Thirst

This is a difficult management problem. With the lack of thirst, severe hypernatremia can develop; then if an antidiuretic agent is administered and the patient is encouraged to drink, hyponatremia can develop. Thus, these patients are subject to wide swings in osmolality but most characteristically persistent hypernatremia. The spectrum of disorders includes that described as "essential hypernatremia." The first therapeutic agent to try is chlorpropamide because it is useful to treat diabetes insipidus and has been reported to increase the thirst response.[187,188] If chlorpropamide does not produce adequate control, the appropriate therapy is a fixed dose of desmopressin and a prescribed quantity of water. These patients usually require encouragement to drink. A constant antidiuresis is maintained by a rigid regimen of desmopressin, and water intake is prescribed for every 6 to 8 hours during a 24-hour period. Regular follow-up with measurement of serum sodium is essential to ensure that these patients do not develop water intoxication with hyponatremia or recurrent dehydration with hypernatremia.

Diabetes Insipidus in Pregnancy

Desmopressin is the only therapy recommended for treatment of diabetes insipidus during pregnancy. Desmopressin has 2% to 25% the oxytocic activity of lysine vasopressin or arginine vasopressin[183] and can be used with minimal stimulation of the oxytocin receptors in the uterus.[142,189] The physician must note the naturally occurring volume expansion and reset osmostat that occurs in pregnancy as described earlier and give sufficient therapy to satisfy thirst and to maintain a serum sodium at the low level that is normal during pregnancy. Desmopressin is not destroyed by the cysteine aminopeptidase (oxytocinase) in the plasma of pregnant women[142,190,191] and is reported to be safe for both the mother and the child.[192,193] During delivery, these patients can maintain adequate oral intake and continued administration of desmopressin. Physicians should be cautious about overadministration of fluid parenterally during delivery because these patients will not be able to excrete the fluid and may develop water intoxication and hyponatremia. After delivery, oxytocinase decreases in plasma and the disorder may disappear or the patient may become asymptomatic with regard to fluid intake and urine volume.

Diabetes Insipidus after Hypothalamic-Pituitary Surgery and after Head Injury

The surgeon often knows how severely the posterior pituitary or stalk was injured. The difficulty in making the diagnosis in this clinical setting is discussed under "Differential Diagnosis". Sometimes the duration of diabetes insipidus is transient and the surgeon may prefer to treat this only with fluid replacement parenterally or orally (if the patient is awake and able to respond to thirst). To treat diabetes insipidus, 0.5 to 2 µg of desmopressin may be given parenterally subcutaneously, intramuscularly, or intravenously. The intravenous route may be preferable because there is no question about absorption. Urine output is reduced in 1 to 2 hours and the duration of effect is 6 to 24 hours. If the patient is alert, thirst is a good guide to fluid replacement. Because diabetes insipidus may be transient and because some patients may develop the triphasic pattern described previously, it is desirable to allow polyuria to return before administering subsequent doses of desmopressin.

Acute diabetes insipidus after blunt trauma to the head can be treated similarly to that in the postoperative situation except that the patient with head injury is more likely to be comatose and unable to respond to thirst, so hypernatremia is more likely to develop. Because a comatose patient must be given fluids parenterally, some clinicians prefer to use a continuous infusion of low-dose vasopressin. The vasopressin can be either added directly to the crystalloid solution that is being administered[194] or infused separately to maintain a constant antidiuresis while adjusting the fluid intake appropriate to any persistent polyuria and to cover insensible water loss. Doses of 0.25 to 2.7 mU/kg/hr have been described.[195-197] If this method is used, there is a potential to produce hyponatremia[194,197] and serum sodium must be checked regularly; with continuous replacement, one does not know whether there is return of normal function or whether a patient might be entering the second of a triphasic pattern.

Nephrogenic Diabetes Insipidus

Adequate water intake should always be maintained and, indeed, appropriate water intake may be lifesaving in congenital nephrogenic diabetes insipidus. By definition these forms of diabetes insipidus do not respond to vasopressin or desmopressin, although rarely there may be some partial defects with some response to high doses of desmopressin.[198] In congenital nephrogenic diabetes insipidus, therapy is aimed at reducing symptomatic polyuria by reducing the volume of urine output. This is done primarily by causing some element of volume contraction with a low-sodium diet and a thiazide diuretic. The antidiuretic effect has been interpreted as due to extracellular fluid volume contraction, decreased glomerular filtration rate, proximal sodium and water reabsorption, and decreased delivery of fluid to the collecting duct resulting in a decreased volume of urine.[199] However, studies have demonstrated that thiazide diuretics may increase aquaporin-2 independent of vasopressin.[200] All the thiazide diuretics appear to have similar effects.

Potassium replacement and/or coadministration of a potassium-sparing antidiuretic may be desirable. There is an added effect obtained by coadministration of indomethacin,[201] but duodenal ulcer and gastrointestinal hemorrhage may be produced by nonsteroidal antiinflammatory agents. Drug-induced nephrogenic diabetes insipidus should be treated by stopping the offending agent if possible. Persistence of nephrogenic diabetes insipidus can be similarly treated by hydrochlorothiazide and amiloride. With the induced volume contraction, these patients should be closely followed up for the development of renal or other toxicity of the drug causing the diabetes insipidus.[202] For example, volume contraction produced by thiazide diuretics when used to treat lithium-induced nephrogenic diabetes insipidus may decrease lithium excretion and predispose the patient to lithium toxicity.[180,203] Amiloride blocks Na^+ channels in the luminal membrane of the collecting duct cells and inhibits lithium reabsorption, a unique advantage in treating lithium-induced nephrogenic diabetes insipidus.[175]

In autosomal dominant nephrogenic diabetes insipidus in which the mutant V2 receptor protein or the mutant aquaporin-2 protein binds and inactivates the normal wild type protein, future therapy may be directed toward rescuing the wild type protein. For example, small V_2 receptor antagonists may penetrate the cell membrane, bind to the misfolded V2 receptor, change the folding, and allow the receptor to be inserted in the luminal membrane.[169,204] Similarly, chemical chaperones may rescue wild type aquaporin-2 protein.[205]

Diabetes Insipidus in Association with Other Therapeutic Decisions

Routine Surgical Procedures

For most routine surgical procedures, the patient is not unconscious for a sufficiently long period of time to require anything more than administration of the usual dose of desmopressin and careful monitoring of fluids during the surgery to ensure against overhydration. If the patient is on desmopressin given orally and is given nothing by mouth (NPO), a nasal or a parenteral dose can be administered before the procedure.

Panhypopituitarism

As hypothyroidism and adrenal insufficiency have a direct action on the kidney to inhibit the ability to excrete water, any patient who has anterior pituitary deficiency in association with diabetes insipidus is at risk to develop hyponatremia if he or she continues treatment for diabetes insipidus while stopping treatment with thyroid hormone and (more dramatically) hydrocortisone. It is important that such patients maintain treatment of all anterior and posterior pituitary deficiencies continuously because the balance among these replacements is essential.

Promoting a Saline Diuresis

In some clinical situations such as chemotherapy or use of some contrast agents, a diuresis is desirable to minimize renal toxicity. If desmopressin is continued and a large volume of normal saline is given, this will induce a prompt natriuresis and hyponatremia. Withholding desmopressin and replacing with D_5W may lead to hyperglycemia, while replacing with normal saline may lead to hypernatremia. It has been reported that very low-dose vasopressin administered continuously intravenously (similar to that described for comatose patients) can be used. In this case, the dose of vasopressin is even lower (e.g., 0.08 to 0.1 mU/kg/hr) to allow a moderate and controlled diuresis.[206] As with any situation in which vasopressin is given continuously, serum sodium must be checked regularly and the amount of fluids infused must be monitored carefully.

Hypertonic Encephalopathy

Conditions other than diabetes insipidus are the more common causes of hypernatremia with coma and hypernatremic encephalopathy. In patients with severe hypernatremia and hypernatremic encephalopathy, overaggressive treatment of the hypernatremia may cause cerebral edema and worsen the neurologic condition.[181,207-209] Sodium is mainly an extracellular action, and hypernatremia invariably leads to movement of water out of cells and cellular dehydration. Studies indicate that, in the brain, "idiogenic" osmoles are generated intracellularly so the degree of cell shrinkage is less than would be accounted for based on the degree of hypernatremia. These idiogenic osmoles are three organic classes: polyols, trimethylamines, and amino acids and their derivatives. The increase in these organic osmoles occurs within 1 to 2 hours in experimental animals,[207,210] but it may be somewhat slower in humans.[181] When fluid is replaced, these organic osmoles decrease much slower intracellularly than the decrease in osmolality of extracellular fluid. This asynchrony increases the potential for cerebral edema and worsening of the neurologic condition with overzealous treatment of hypernatremia.[181,210,211] In most cases of diabetes insipidus seen immediately after surgery or diagnosed promptly after head injury, the diagnosis is made within a few hours and therapy may be instituted promptly. When the duration of the hypernatremia is not known, the degree of correction of hypernatremia should not exceed 0.5 mEq/L/hr to prevent cerebral edema and convulsions.[181,211]

Organ Donors

As noted earlier, diabetes insipidus is a common accompaniment to brain death. Because these patients may be candidates for organ donation, it has been suggested that maintaining fluid homeostasis is desirable for maintenance of the health of the organs. Even though this is a controversial practice, some treatment of the diabetes insipidus is not unreasonable. This may be a situation in which continuous administration of vasopressin in a low dose is easier than maintaining antidiuresis with intermittent doses of desmopressin.

THE SYNDROME OF INAPPROPRIATE ANTIDIURETIC HORMONE SECRETION

SIADH results when plasma levels of arginine vasopressin are elevated at times when the physiologic secretion of vasopressin from the posterior pituitary would normally be suppressed. The clinical abnormality is a decrease in the osmotic pressure of body fluids, so the hallmark of SIADH is hypoosmolality, which led to the identification of the first well-described cases of this disorder in 1957.[212] Subsequent clinical investigations resulted in delineation of the essential characteristics of the syndrome.[213] It is therefore necessary to review hypoosmolality and hyponatremia before discussing details that are specific to SIADH.

Hypoosmolality and Hyponatremia

Incidence

Hypoosmolality is the most common disorder of fluid and electrolyte balance encountered in hospitalized patients. The incidence and prevalence of hypoosmolar disorders depend on the nature of the patient population studied as well as on the laboratory methods and criteria used to diagnose hyponatremia. Most investigators have used the serum sodium concentration ([Na^+]) to determine the clinical incidence of hypoosmolality. When hyponatremia is defined as a serum [Na^+] of less than 135 mEq/L, incidences as high as 15% to 30% have been observed in studies of both acutely and chronically hospitalized patients. However, incidences decrease to the range of 1% to 4% when only patients with serum [Na^+] less than 130 to 131 mEq/L are included, which represents a more appropriate level at which to define the occurrence of clinically significant cases of this disorder. Even using these more stringent criteria, incidences from 7% to 53% have been reported in institutionalized geriatric patients.[214] All studies to date have noted a high proportion of iatrogenic or hospital-acquired hyponatremia, which has accounted for as many as 40% to 75% of all patients studied.[215] Therefore, although hyponatremia and hypoosmolality are common, the majority of cases are relatively mild and most are acquired during the course of hospitalization. Nonetheless, hyponatremia is important clinically for the following reasons:

1. Severe hypoosmolality (serum [Na^+] levels <120 mEq/L) is associated with substantial morbidity and mortality.[216]
2. Even relatively mild hypoosmolality can quickly progress to more dangerous levels during the course of therapeutic management of other disorders.
3. Overly rapid correction of hyponatremia can itself cause severe neurologic morbidity and mortality.[217]
4. It has been observed that mortality rates are much higher, from 3- to 60-fold higher, in patients with even asymptomatic degrees of hypoosmolality compared with normonatremic patients.[218]

Osmolality, Tonicity, and Serum [Na^+]

As discussed previously, the osmolality of body fluid normally is maintained within narrow limits by osmotically regulated vasopressin secretion and thirst. Although basal plasma osmolality can vary appreciably among individuals, the range in the general population under conditions of normal hydration is between 280 and 295 mOsm/kg H_2O. Plasma osmolality can be determined directly by measuring the freezing-point depression or the vapor pressure of plasma. Alternatively, it can be calculated indirectly from the concentrations of the three major solutes in plasma:

$$\text{pOsm (mOsm/kg } H_2O) = 2 \times [Na^+] \text{ (mEq/L)} + \text{glucose (mg/dL)}/18 + \text{blood urea nitrogen (mg/dL)}/2.8$$

Both methods produce comparable results under most conditions. However, while either of these methods produce valid measures of *total* osmolality, this is not always equivalent to the *effective* osmolality, which is commonly referred to as the *tonicity* of the plasma. Only solutes such as Na^+ and Cl^- that are impermeable to the cell membrane and remain relatively compartmentalized within the ECF space are "effective" solutes, because these solutes create osmotic gradients across cell membranes and regulate the osmotic movement of water between the intracellular fluid (ICF) compartment and the ECF compartment. Solutes that readily permeate cell membranes (e.g., urea, ethanol, methanol) are not effective solutes. Therefore, only the concentrations of effective solutes in plasma should be used to ascertain whether clinically significant hyperosmolality or hypoosmolality is present.

Sodium and its accompanying anions represent the major effective plasma solutes, so hyponatremia and hypoosmolality are usually synonymous. However, there are two situations in which hyponatremia will not reflect true hypoosmolality. The first is *pseudohyponatremia,* which is produced by marked elevations of either lipids or proteins in plasma. If serum [Na^+] is measured by flame photometry, the concentration of sodium per liter of plasma is artifactually decreased because of the larger relative proportion of plasma volume that is occupied by the excess lipids or proteins.[219] However, the increased protein or lipid will not appreciably change the total number of solute particles in solution, so the directly measured plasma osmolality will not be significantly affected. Measurement of serum [Na^+] by ion-specific electrodes, which is now commonly employed by most clinical laboratories, is less influenced by high concentrations of lipids or proteins than is measurement of serum [Na^+] by flame photometry. The second situation in which hyponatremia does not reflect true plasma hypoosmolality occurs when high concentrations of effective solutes other than Na^+ are present in the plasma. The initial hyperosmolality produced by the additional solute causes an osmotic shift of water from the ICF to the ECF, which in turn produces a dilutional decrease in serum [Na^+]. Once equilibrium between both fluid compartments is achieved, the total effective osmolality remains relatively unchanged. This situation most commonly occurs with hyperglycemia and represents a frequent cause of hyponatremia in hospitalized patients, accounting for up to 10% to 20% of all cases.[218] Misdiagnosis of true hypoosmolality in such cases can be avoided by measuring plasma osmolality directly or, alternatively, by correcting the measured serum [Na^+] for the glucose elevation (traditionally this correction factor has been 1.6 mEq/L for each 100 mg/dL increase in serum glucose concentration above normal levels,[220] but recent studies have shown a more complex relation between hyperglycemia and serum [Na^+] and have suggested that a more accurate correction factor is closer to 2.4 mEq/L).[221] When the plasma contains significant amounts of unmeasured solutes, such as osmotic diuretics, radiographic contrast agents, and some toxins (ethanol, methanol, and ethylene glycol), plasma osmolality cannot be calculated accurately, and in these situations osmolality must be ascertained by direct measurement, although even this method does not yield an accurate measure of the true effective osmolality if the unmeasured solutes are noneffective solutes that freely permeate cell membranes (e.g., ethanol).

Pathogenesis of Hypoosmolality

Because water moves freely between the ICF and ECF, osmolality will always be equivalent in both of these fluid compartments. Because the bulk of body solute is composed of electrolytes, namely, the exchangeable Na^+ (Na^+_E) in the ECF and the exchangeable K^+ (K^+_E) in the ICF along with their associated anions, total body osmolality will largely be a function of these parameters[222]:

$$\begin{aligned} OSM_{ECF} = OSM_{ICF} &= \text{total body osmolality} \\ &= (\text{ECF solute} + \text{ICF solute}) \,/\, \text{body water} \\ &= (2 \times Na^+_E + 2 \times K^+_E + \text{non-electrolyte solute}) \,/\, \text{body water} \end{aligned}$$

According to this definition, the presence of plasma hypoosmolality indicates a relative excess of water to solute in the ECF. This can be produced either by an excess of body water, resulting in a *dilution* of remaining body solute, or by a *depletion* of body solute, either Na^+ or K^+, relative to body water. This classification is an oversimplification, because most hypoosmolar states involve significant components of both solute depletion and water retention. Nonetheless, it is conceptually useful for understanding the mechanisms underlying the pathogenesis of hypoosmolality and as a framework for therapy of hypoosmolar disorders.

Solute Depletion

Depletion of body solute can result from any significant losses of ECF. Body fluid losses by themselves rarely cause hypoosmolality because excreted or secreted body fluids are usually isotonic or hypotonic relative to plasma and therefore tend to increase plasma osmolality. When hypoosmolality accompanies ECF losses, it is the result of replacement of body fluid losses by more hypotonic solutions either by drinking or by infusion, thereby diluting the remaining body solutes. If the solute losses are marked, these patients show signs of volume depletion (e.g., addisonian crisis). However, such patients often have a more deceptive clinical presentation because the volume deficits have been partially replaced. Moreover, they may not manifest signs or symptoms of cellular dehydration because osmotic gradients will draw water into the relatively hypertonic ICF. Therefore, clinical evidence of hypovolemia strongly supports solute depletion as the cause of plasma hypoosmolality, but absence of clinically evident hypovolemia never completely eliminates this as a possibility. Although ECF solute losses are responsible for most cases of depletion-induced hypoosmolality, ICF solute loss can also cause hypoosmolality as a result of osmotic water shifts from the ICF into the ECF. This mechanism likely contributes to some cases of diuretic-induced hypoosmolality in which depletion of total body K^+ often occurs.[223]

Water Retention

Despite the importance of solute depletion in some patients, most cases of clinically significant hypoosmolality are caused by increases in total body water rather than by primary losses of extracellular solute. This can occur because of either impaired renal free water excretion or excessive free water intake. However, the former accounts for most hypoosmolar disorders because normal kidneys have sufficient diluting capacity to allow excretion of up to approximately 18 L/day of free water. Intakes of this magnitude are occasionally seen in some psychiatric patients but not in most patients with SIADH in whom fluid intakes average only 2 to 3 L/day.[224] Consequently, dilutional hypoosmolality usually is the result of an abnormality of renal free water excretion. The renal mechanisms responsible for impairments in free water excretion can be subgrouped according to whether the *major* impairment in free water excretion occurs in proximal or distal parts of the nephron, or both. Any disorder that leads to a decrease in glomerular filtration rate causes increased reabsorption of both Na^+ and water in the proximal tubule. As a result, the ability to excrete free water is limited because of decreased delivery of tubular fluid to the distal nephron. Disorders causing solute depletion through nonrenal mechanisms (e.g., gastrointestinal fluid losses) also produce this effect. Disorders that cause a decreased glomerular filtration rate in the absence of significant ECF fluid losses are, for the most part, edema-forming states associated with decreased effective arterial blood volume (EABV) and secondary hyperaldosteronism.[225] Even though these conditions are characterized by increased proximal reabsorption of both Na^+ and fluid, water retention also results from increased distal reabsorption caused by non-osmotic baroreceptor-mediated stimulated increases in plasma vasopressin levels. Distal nephron impairments in free water excretion are characterized by an inability to dilute tubular fluid maximally. These disorders are usually associated with abnormalities in the secretion of vasopressin from the posterior pituitary. However, just as depletion-induced hypoosmolar disorders usually include an important component of secondary impairments of free water excretion, so do most dilution-induced hypoosmolar disorders involve significant degrees of secondary solute depletion (see later discussion).

Some dilutional disorders do not fit well into either category, specifically the hyponatremia that sometimes occurs in patients who ingest large volumes of beer with little food intake for prolonged periods, called "beer potomania."[226] Even though the volume of fluid ingested may not seem sufficiently excessive to overwhelm renal diluting mechanisms, free water excretion is limited by very low urinary solute excretion, thereby causing water retention and dilutional hyponatremia.

Adaptation to Hyponatremia: ICF and ECF Volume Regulation

Many past studies have intimated that the combined effects of water retention plus urinary solute excretion cannot adequately explain the degree of plasma hypoosmolality observed in patients.[213,227] This observation led to the theory of "cellular inactivation of solute," which suggested that as ECF osmolality falls, water moves into cells along osmotic gradients, thereby causing the cells to swell. At some point during this volume expansion, the cells osmotically "inactivate" some of their intracellular solutes as a defense mechanism to prevent continued cellular swelling and subsequent detrimental effects on cell function and survival. This decreases the intracellular osmolality and water then shifts back out of the ICF into the ECF, further worsening the dilution-induced hypoosmolality. Despite the appeal of this theory, its validity has never been demonstrated conclusively in either human or animal studies. An alternative theory is that cell volume is maintained under hypoosmolar conditions by extrusion of potassium.[228] Whole brain volume regulation via electrolyte losses was first described by Yannet[229] and has long been recognized as the mechanism by which the brain is able to adapt to hyponatremia and limit brain edema to sublethal levels.[230] Following the recognition that low-molecular-weight organic compounds, called *organic osmolytes,* also constituted a significant osmotic component of a wide variety of cell types, studies demonstrated the accumulation of these compounds in response to hyperosmolality in both kidney[231] and brain[232] tissue (see earlier discussion of hypernatremic encephalopathy), and conversely that the brain also loses organic osmolytes in addition to electrolytes during volume regulation to hypoosmolar conditions in experimental animals[233,234] and human patients.[235] These losses occur relatively quickly (within 24 to 48 hours in rats) and can account for as much as one third of the brain solute losses during hyponatremia.[236] Such coordinate losses of both electrolytes and organic osmolytes from brain cells allow effective regulation of brain volume during chronic hyponatremia.

Although recent studies of volume regulation during hyponatremia have focused on the brain, all cells regulate volume by cellular losses of both electrolyte and organic solutes to varying degrees. However, volume regulatory processes are not limited to cells. In most cases of hyponatremia induced by stimulated antidiuresis and water retention, natriuresis also regulates the volumes of the ECF and intravascular spaces. Many experimental and clinical observations are consistent with ECF volume regulation via secondary solute losses. First, the concentrations of most blood constituents other than Na^+ and Cl^- are not decreased in patients with SIADH, [237] suggesting that plasma volume is not nearly as expanded as would be predicted simply by the measured decreases in serum $[Na^+]$. Second, an increased incidence of hypertension has never been observed in patients with SIADH, again evidence against significant expansion of the arterial blood volume. Third, results of animal studies in both dogs[238] and rats[239] have indicated that a significant component of chronic hyponatremia is attributable to secondary Na^+ losses rather than water retention. Furthermore, the relative contributions from water retention versus sodium loss vary with the duration and severity of the hyponatremia: water retention was found to be the major cause of decreased serum $[Na^+]$ in the first 24 hours of induced hyponatremia in rats, but Na^+ depletion then became the predominant etiologic factor after longer periods (7 to 14 days) of sustained hyponatremia, particularly at very low ($<$115 mEq/L) serum $[Na^+]$.[239] Finally, multiple studies of body fluid compartment volumes in hyponatremic patients have not demonstrated either plasma or ECF expansion. For example, a report of body fluid space measurements using isotope dilution techniques in hyponatremic and normonatremic patients with small cell lung carcinoma showed no differences between the two groups with regard to exchangeable sodium space, ECF volume by $^{35}SO_4$ distribution, or total body water.[240] Such results have generally been explained by the relative insensitivity of isotope dilution techniques for measurement of body fluid compartment spaces, but an equally plausible explanation is that body fluid compartments have regulated back toward normal via a combination of extracellular (predominantly electrolyte) and intracellular (electrolyte and organic osmolyte) solute losses.[241] Figure 9–5 schematically illustrates volume regulatory processes that occur in response to water retention induced by inappropriate antidiuresis.

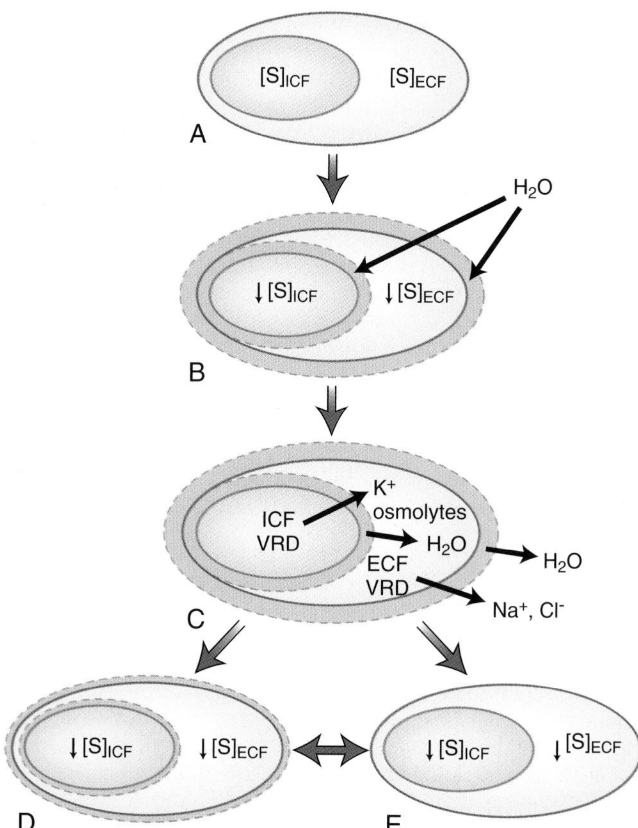

Figure 9–5 ▪ Schematic illustration of potential changes in whole body fluid compartment volumes at various times during adaptation to hyponatremia. **A,** Under basal conditions the concentrations of effective solutes in the extracellular fluid ($[S]_{ECF}$) and in the intracellular fluid ($[S]_{ICF}$) are in osmotic balance. **B,** During the first phase of water retention resulting from inappropriate antidiuresis, the excess water distributes across total body water, causing expansion of both ECF and ICF volumes *(dotted lines)* with equivalent dilutional decreases in $[S]_{ICF}$ and $[S]_{ECF}$. **C,** In response to the volume expansion, compensatory volume regulatory decreases (VRD) occur to reduce the effective solute content of both the ECF (via pressure diuresis and natriuretic factors) and ICF (via increased electrolyte and osmolyte extrusion mediated by stretch-activated channels and down-regulation of synthesis of osmolytes and osmolyte uptake transporters). **D** and **E,** If both processes go to completion, such as under conditions of fluid restriction, a final steady-state can be reached in which ICF and ECF volumes have returned to normal levels but $[S]_{ICF}$ and $[S]_{ECF}$ remain low. In most cases, this final steady-state is not reached, and moderate degrees of ECF and ICF expansion persist, but significantly less than would be predicted from the decrease in body osmolality **(D).** Consequently, the degree to which hyponatremia is due to dilution from water retention versus solute depletion from volume regulatory processes can vary markedly depending on which phase of adaptation the patient is in, and on the relative rates at which the different compensatory processes occur (e.g., delayed ICF VRD can worsen hyponatremia due to shifts of intracellular water into the extracellular fluid as intracellular organic osmolytes are extruded and subsequently metabolized, likely accounting for some component of the hyponatremia unexplained by the combination of water retention and sodium excretion in previous clinical studies). (From Verbalis JG. Hyponatremia: epidemiology, pathophysiology, and therapy. Curr Opin Nephrol Hyperten 1993;2:626-652.)

Differential Diagnosis of Hyponatremia and Hypoosmolality

Because of the multiplicity of disorders causing hypoosmolality and the fact that many involve more than one pathologic mechanism, a definitive diagnosis is not always possible at the time of initial presentation. Nonetheless, an approach based on clinical parameters of ECF volume status and urine sodium concentration generally allows a sufficient categorization for appropriate decisions regarding initial therapy and further evaluation (Table 9–3).

Decreased Extracellular Fluid Volume

Clinically detectable hypovolemia always signifies total body solute depletion. A low urine [Na^+] indicates a nonrenal cause and an appropriate renal response. A high urine [Na^+] indicates renal causes of solute depletion are more likely. Therapy with thiazide diuretics is the most common cause of renal solute losses,[223] particularly in the elderly,[242] but mineralocorticoid deficiency as a result of adrenal insufficiency or mineralocorticoid resistance[243] must be considered, as well as (less commonly) renal solute losses due to salt-wasting nephropathy (e.g., polycystic kidney disease, interstitial nephritis, or chemotherapy).

Increased Extracellular Fluid Volume

Clinically detectable hypervolemia always signifies total body Na^+ excess. In these patients hypoosmolality results from an even greater expansion of total body water caused by a marked reduction in the rate of water excretion (and sometimes an increased rate of water ingestion). The impairment in water excretion is secondary to a decreased EABV,[225] which increases the reabsorption of glomerular filtrate not only in the proximal nephron but also in the distal and collecting tubules by stimulated secretion of vasopressin. These patients generally have a low urine [Na^+] because of secondary hyperaldosteronism. However, under certain conditions urine [Na^+] may be elevated if there is concurrent diuretic therapy, a solute diuresis (e.g., glucosuria in diabetics), or after successful treatment of the underlying disease (e.g., improved cardiac output in patients with congestive heart failure).

Normal Extracellular Fluid Volume

Many different hypoosmolar disorders present with euvolemia, and measure of urinary [Na^+] is an especially important first step.[244] A high urine [Na^+] usually implies a distally mediated, dilution-induced hypoosmolality such as SIADH. However, glucocorticoid deficiency can mimic SIADH so closely that these two disorders are often indistinguishable in terms of water balance. Hyponatremia from diuretic use also can present without clinically evident hypovolemia, and the urine [Na^+] will usually be elevated.[223] A low urine [Na^+] suggests a depletion-induced hypoosmolality from ECF losses with subsequent volume replacement by water or other hypotonic fluids. The solute loss often is nonrenal, but an important exception is recent cessation of diuretic therapy, because urine [Na^+] can

TABLE 9–3 COMMON ETIOLOGIES OF SIADH

TUMORS
Pulmonary/mediastinal (bronchogenic carcinoma, mesothelioma, thymoma) Nonchest (duodenal carcinoma, pancreatic carcinoma, ureteral/prostate carcinoma, uterine carcinoma, nasopharyngeal carcinoma, leukemia)
CENTRAL NERVOUS SYSTEM DISORDERS
Mass lesions (tumors, brain abscesses, subdural hematoma) Inflammatory diseases (encephalitis, meningitis, systemic lupu erythematosus, acute intermittent porphyria, multiple sclerosis) Degenerative/demyelinative diseases (Guillain-Barré syndrome, spinal cord lesions) Miscellaneous (subarachnoid hemorrhage, head trauma, acute psychosis, delirium tremens, pituitary stalk section, transsphenoidal adenomectomy, hydrocephalus)
DRUG-INDUCED
Stimulated AVP release (nicotine, phenothiazines, tricyclics) Direct renal effects and/or potentiation of AVP antidiuretic effects (dDAVP, oxytocin, prostaglandin synthesis inhibitors) Mixed or uncertain actions (angiotensin-converting enzyme inhibitors, carbamazepine and oxcarbazepine, chlorpropamide, clofibrate, clozapine, cyclophosphamide, 3,4-methylenedioxymethamphetamine ["ecstasy"], omeprazole; serotonin reuptake inhibitors, vincristine)
PULMONARY DISEASES
Infections (tuberculosis, acute bacterial and viral pneumonia, aspergillosis, empyema) Mechanical/ventilatory (acute respiratory failure, COPD, positive pressure ventilation)
OTHER
Acquired immunodeficiency syndrome (AIDS) and AIDS-related complex Prolonged strenuous exercise (marathon, triathlon, ultramarathon, hot-weather hiking) Senile atrophy Idiopathic

decrease to low values within 12 to 24 hours after discontinuation of the drug. A low urine [Na^+] also can also be seen in some cases of hypothyroidism, in the early stages of decreased EABV before the development of clinically apparent salt retention and fluid overload, or during the recovery phase from SIADH. Hence, a low urine [Na^+] is less meaningful diagnostically than is a high value.

Clinical Syndrome of Inappropriate Antidiuretic Hormone Secretion

SIADH is the most common cause of euvolemic hypoosmolality, and it is also the single most common cause of hypoosmolality encountered in clinical practice, with prevalence rates from 20% to 40% among all hypoosmolar patients.[218,224] The clinical criteria necessary to diagnose SIADH remain basically as set forth by Bartter and Schwartz in 1967.[213]

1. Decreased effective osmolality of the extracellular fluid (P_{osm} <275 mOsm/kg H_2O). Pseudohyponatremia or hyperglycemia alone must be excluded.
2. Inappropriate urinary concentration at some level of hypoosmolality. This does not mean urine osmolality is greater than plasma osmolality, only less than maximally dilute (i.e., urine osmolality >100 mOsm/kg H_2O). Also, urine osmolality need not be elevated inappropriately at all levels of plasma osmolality, because in the reset osmostat variant form of SIADH, vasopressin secretion can be suppressed with resultant maximal urinary dilution if plasma osmolality is decreased to sufficiently low levels.[245]
3. Clinical euvolemia, as defined by the absence of signs of hypovolemia (orthostasis, tachycardia, decreased skin turgor, dry mucous membranes) or hypervolemia (subcutaneous edema, ascites). Hypovolemia or hypervolemia strongly suggest different causes of hypoosmolality. Patients with SIADH can become hypovolemic or hypervolemic for other reasons, but in such cases it is impossible to diagnose the underlying inappropriate antidiuresis until the patient is rendered euvolemic and is found to have persistent hypoosmolality.
4. Elevated urinary sodium excretion while on a normal salt and water intake. This criterion is included because of its utility in differentiating between hypoosmolality caused by a decreased EABV, in which case renal Na^+ conservation occurs, and distal dilution-induced disorders, in which urine Na^+ excretion is normal or increased secondary to ECF volume expansion. Patients with SIADH can have low urine Na^+ excretion if they subsequently become hypovolemic or solute-depleted, conditions that sometimes follow severe salt and water restriction. Consequently, a high urine Na^+ excretion is the rule in most patients with SIADH, its presence does not guarantee this diagnosis, and its absence does not rule out the diagnosis.
5. Absence of other potential causes of euvolemic hypoosmolality: hypothyroidism, hypocortisolism (Addison's disease or pituitary ACTH insufficiency) and diuretic use.

Several other criteria support, but are not essential for, a diagnosis of SIADH. Volume expansion and vasopressin acting on V1 receptors in the kidney increase the clearance of uric acid, so hypouricemia is found with SIADH. When patients are hyponatremic, values of uric acid are reported to be <4 mg/dL (<0.24 mmol/L).[246] A water-loading test is of value when there is uncertainty regarding the etiology of modest degrees of hypoosmolality in euvolemic patients, but it does not add useful information if the plasma osmolality is already less than 275 mOsm/kg H_2O. Inability to excrete a standard water load normally (with normal excretion defined as a cumulative urine output of at least 90% of the administered water load within 4 hours and suppression of urine osmolality to less than 100 mOsm/kg H_2O) confirms the presence of an underlying defect in free water excretion. However, water excretion is abnormal in almost all disorders that cause hypoosmolality, whether dilutional or depletion-induced with secondary impairments in free water excretion. Two exceptions are primary polydipsia, in which hypoosmolality can rarely be secondary to excessive water intake alone, and the reset osmostat variant of SIADH, in which normal excretion of a water load can occur once plasma osmolality falls below the new set-point for vasopressin secretion.

Another supportive criterion is an inappropriately elevated plasma vasopressin level in relation to plasma osmolality. With the development of sensitive vasopressin radioimmunoassays capable of detecting the small physiologic concentrations of this peptide that circulate in plasma,[247] there was hope that measurement of plasma vasopressin levels might become the definitive test for diagnosing SIADH. This has not occurred for several reasons. First, although plasma vasopressin levels are elevated in most patients with this syndrome, the elevations generally remain within the normal physiologic range and are abnormal only in relation to plasma osmolality (Fig. 9–6). Second, 10% to 20% of patients with SIADH do not have measurably elevated plasma vasopressin levels; as shown in Figure 9–7, and are at the limits of detection by radioimmunoassay.[248] Third, most disorders causing solute and volume depletion or decreased EABV are associated with elevations of plasma vasopressin levels secondary to non-osmotic hemodynamic stimuli.

Etiology

Although the list of disorders associated with SIADH is long (see Table 9–3), they can be divided into five etiologic groups: tumors, CNS disorders, drugs, pulmonary disorders, and other causes.

Tumors

The most common association of SIADH is with tumors. Although many different types of tumors have been associated with SIADH, bronchogenic carcinoma of the lung has been uniquely associated with SIADH since the first description of this disorder in 1957.[212] In virtually all cases, the bronchogenic carcinomas causing this syndrome have been of the small cell (or oat cell) variety. Incidences rates of hyponatremia as high as 11% of all patients with small cell carcinoma,[249] or 33% of cases with more extensive disease,[250] have been reported. The unusually high incidence of small cell carcinoma of the lung, together with the relatively favorable therapeutic response of this type of tumor, makes it imperative that all adult patients presenting with an otherwise unexplained SIADH be investigated thoroughly and aggressively for a possible lung tumor. The evaluation should include a chest CT scan or MRI scan and bronchoscopy with cytologic analysis of bronchial washings even if the results of routine chest radiography are normal, since several studies have reported hypoosmolality that predated radiographically abnormalities by 3 to 12 months. Head and neck cancers account for another group of malignancies associated with relatively higher incidences of SIADH,[251] and some of these tumors have clearly been shown to synthesize vasopressin.[252] A recent report from a large cancer hospital showed an incidence of hyponatremia for all malignancies combined of 3.7%, with approximately one third of these due to SIADH.[253]

Central Nervous System Disorders

A large number of different CNS disorders are associated with SIADH, but they lack a common denominator to link them. This is not surprising when one considers the neuroanatomy described earlier. Magnocellular vasopressin neurons receive excitatory inputs from osmoreceptive cells located in the anterior hypothalamus, but also a major innervation from brain stem cardiovascular regulatory and emetic centers. Although various

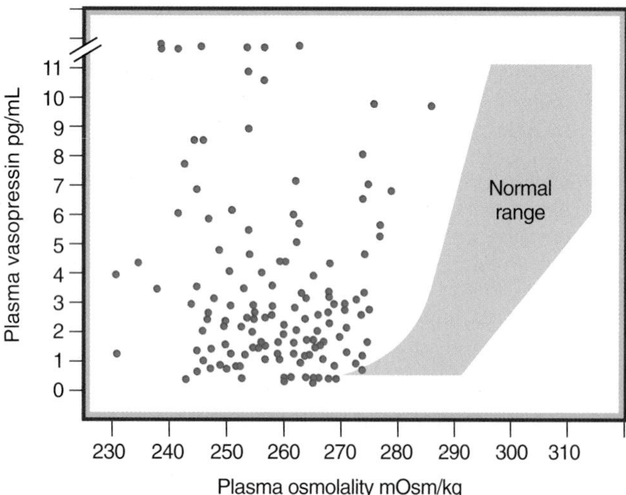

Figure 9–6 ▪ Plasma arginine vasopressin (AVP) levels in patients with syndrome of inappropriate antidiuretic hormone secretion as a function of plasma osmolality. Each point depicts one patient at a single point in time. The shaded area represents AVP levels in normal subjects over physiologic ranges of plasma osmolality. The lowest measurable plasma AVP levels using this radioimmunoassay was 0.5 pg/mL. (From Robertson GL, Aycinena P, Zerbe RL. Neurogenic disorders of osmoregulation. Am J Med 1982; 2:339-353.)

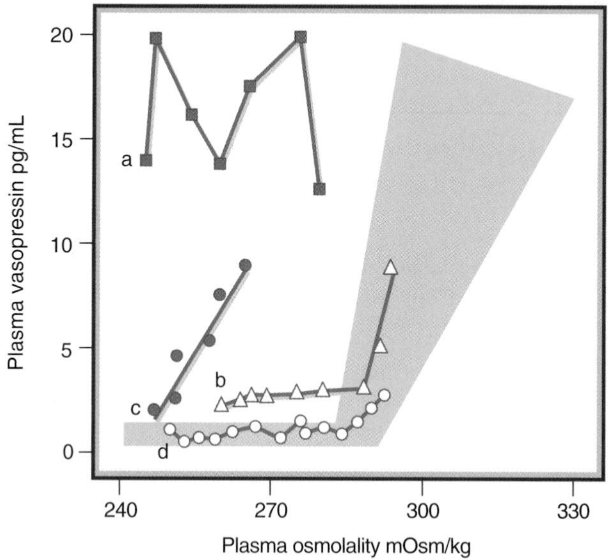

Figure 9–7 ▪ Schematic summary of different patterns of arginine vasopressin (AVP) secretion in patients with syndrome of inappropriate antidiuretic hormone secretion. Each line (a–d) represents the relation between plasma AVP and plasma osmolality of individual patients in whom osmolality was increased by infusion of hypertonic NaCl. The shaded area represents plasma AVP levels in normal subjects over physiologic ranges of plasma osmolality. (From Robertson GL. Thirst and vasopressin function in normal and disordered states of water balance. J Lab Clin Med 1983;101:351-371.)

components of these pathways have yet to be elucidated fully, many of them appear to have inhibitory as well as excitatory components. Consequently, any diffuse CNS disorder can potentially cause vasopressin hypersecretion either by nonspecifically exciting these pathways via irritative foci, or alternatively by disrupting them and thereby decreasing the level of inhibition. The wide variety of diverse CNS processes that can potentially cause SIADH stands in contrast to CNS causes of diabetes insipidus, which are limited to lesions of the suprasellar hypothalamus.

Drugs

Drug-induced hyponatremia is a common cause of hypoosmolality.[254] Table 9–3 lists some of the agents that have been associated with SIADH, but new drugs are added continually. Pharmacologic agents may stimulate secretion of vasopressin, activate renal V2 receptors, or potentiate the antidiuretic effect of vasopressin. However, not all of the drug effects are fully understood, and many appear to work through a combination of mechanisms. A particularly interesting, and clinically important, class of agents is the selective serotonin reuptake inhibitors (SSRIs). In studies in rats, serotonergic agents increase secretion of vasopressin,[255] whereas in humans SSRIs have generally failed to show significant effects on secretion of vasopressin.[256] Hyponatremia following SSRI administration has been reported almost exclusively in the elderly, with rates as high as 22% to 28%, although in larger series incidence was closer to 1 in 200.[257] A similar effect is likely also responsible for the recent reports of severe fatal hyponatremia caused by use of the recreational drug 3,4-methylenedioxymethamphetamine, or "ecstasy," which possesses substantial serotonergic activity.[258]

Pulmonary Disorders

A variety of pulmonary disorders have been associated with this syndrome, but other than tuberculosis, acute pneumonia, and advanced chronic obstructive lung disease, the occurrence of hypoosmolality has been noted only sporadically. Hypoxia stimulates secretion of vasopressin in animals,[259] but in humans hypercarbia is more associated with abnormal water retention. Elevated vasopressin may be limited to the initial days of hospitalization, when respiratory failure is most marked. Therefore, with SIADH in nontumor pulmonary disease, the pulmonary disease is obvious with severe dyspnea or extensive radiographically evident infiltrates and the inappropriate antidiuresis is usually limited to the period of respiratory failure. Mechanical ventilation can cause inappropriate secretion of vasopressin and can worsen SIADH caused by other factors. The mechanism is thought to be decreased venous return.

Other Causes

In acquired immunodeficiency syndrome (AIDS) or AIDS-related complex (ARC) and in patients with HIV infection, hyponatremia has been reported as high as 30% to 38% in adults[260] and children.[260] Although there are many potential etiologies, including dehydration, adrenal insufficiency, and pneumonitis, from 12% to 68% of AIDS patients who develop hyponatremia appear to meet criteria for a diagnosis of SIADH.[260] Not unexpectedly, some of the medications used to treat these patients may cause the hyponatremia, either via direct renal tubular toxicity or induced SIADH.[261]

Elderly patients often develop SIADH without any apparent underlying etiology, and the high incidence of hyponatremia in geriatric patients[214,262] suggests that the normal aging process may be accompanied by abnormalities of regulation of secretion of vasopressin. Such an effect could potentially account for the fact that drug-induced hyponatremia occurs much more frequently in elderly patients. In a recent series of 50 consecutive elderly patients meeting criteria for SIADH, 60% remained idiopathic despite rigorous evaluation, leading the authors to conclude that extensive diagnostic procedures were not warranted in such elderly patients if routine history, physical examination, and laboratory evaluation failed to suggest an underlying etiology.[263]

Pathophysiology

Sources of Vasopressin Secretion

Elevated plasma levels of vasopressin can be broadly divided into those associated with paraneoplastic ("ectopic") secretion of vasopressin or pituitary hypersecretion of vasopressin. There is substantial cumulative evidence that tumor tissue can, in fact, synthesize vasopressin,[264] but it is not certain that all tumors associated with SIADH do so, because only about half of small cell carcinomas have been found to contain vasopressin immunoreactivity, and many of the tumors listed in Table 9–3 have not been so studied.

Pituitary Vasopressin Secretion: Inappropriate versus Appropriate

In the majority of cases of SIADH, the vasopressin secretion originates from the posterior pituitary. This is also true of more than 90% of all cases of hyponatremia, including patients with hypovolemic and hypervolemic hyponatremia.[218] This raises the question of what is "inappropriate" secretion of vasopressin. Secretion of vasopressin in response to a hypovolemic stimulus is clearly physiologically "appropriate," but when it leads to symptomatic hyponatremia it could be considered "inappropriate" for the osmolality (see Fig. 9–6). Despite these semantic difficulties, the diagnosis of SIADH should rest on the original criteria and specifically exclude other clinical conditions that cause known impairments in free water excretion *even when* these are mediated by a secondary stimulation of vasopressin. Without maintaining these distinctions, arguable as some may be, the definition of SIADH becomes too broad to retain any practical clinical utility.

Patterns of Vasopressin Secretion

Studies of plasma vasopressin levels in patients with SIADH during graded increases in plasma osmolality produced by hypertonic saline administration have defined four patterns of secretion (Fig. 9–7): (a) random hypersecretion of vasopressin; (b) inappropriate nonsuppressible basal vasopressin release, but normal secretion in response to osmolar changes above basal plasma osmolality; (c) a "reset osmostat" system, whereby vasopressin is secreted at an abnormally low threshold of plasma osmolality but otherwise displays a normal response to relative changes in osmolality; and (d) low or even undetectable plasma vasopressin levels despite classic clinical characteristics of SIADH.[248] The first pattern, unregulated vasopressin secretion, is often observed in patients exhibiting paraneoplastic vasopressin production. Resetting of the osmotic threshold for vasopressin secretion has been well described with volume depletion[265] and edema-forming states with EABV,[225] but most patients with reset osmostat are clinically euvolemic[245] and may represent SIADH. The best physiologic example of a reset osmostat is pregnancy, as discussed earlier. Perhaps the most perplexing aspect of the reset osmostat pattern is its occurrence in patients with tumors, which suggests that in some of these cases a tumor-related mechanism may affect pituitary vasopressin secretion.[248] The pattern of SIADH that occurs without measurable vasopressin secretion is not yet well understood, but the positive response of one such patient to a vasopressin V2-

receptor antagonist would suggest that this may represent increased renal sensitivity to low circulating levels of vasopressin.[266] Recent studies of two pediatric patients with hyponatremia and unmeasurable plasma vasopressin levels led to the discovery of an activating mutation of the vasopressin V2 receptor as the cause of their inappropriate antidiuresis.[267] It is more appropriate to call these cases the *nephrogenic syndrome of inappropriate antidiuresis* (NSIAD), reserving SIADH only for those cases in which measured plasma vasopressin levels are really inappropriate. It is surprising that no correlation has been found between any of these patterns of secretion of vasopressin and the various etiologies of SIADH.[248] It seems likely that in many cases a heterogeneous group of CNS processes are involved, including osmotic and non-osmotic, stimulatory, and inhibitory pathways, rather than a single dominant cause.

Contribution of Natriuresis to the Hyponatremia of SIADH

Since the original cases studied by Schwartz and Bartter, increased renal Na^+ excretion has been one of the cardinal manifestations of SIADH, indeed one which later became embedded in the requirements for its diagnosis.[213] Demonstration that the natriuresis accompanying administration of antidiuretic hormone is not due to vasopressin itself but rather to the volume expansion produced as a result of water retention was unequivocally shown by Leaf even before the description of the disorder.[268] Although a negative Na^+ balance occurs during the development of hyponatremia in patients with SIADH, eventually urinary sodium excretion simply reflects daily sodium intake.[212] Thus, "renal sodium wasting" is continued excretion of sodium despite being hyponatremic, but in reality there is a new steady-state in which patients are in neutral sodium balance. Studies of long-term antidiuretic-induced hyponatremia in both dogs and rats have indicated that a large proportion of the hyponatremia was attributable to secondary Na^+ losses rather than to water retention,[238,239] but the natriuresis did not actually worsen the hyponatremia; rather, it allowed volume regulation of ECF. Because of the secondary natriuresis in patients with SIADH, expanded plasma or ECF volumes are not found using tracer dilution techniques.[240]

The degree to which hyponatremia might occur primarily as a result of natriuresis is controversial. Cerebral salt-wasting syndrome was first proposed by Peters in 1950[269] as an explanation for the natriuresis and hyponatremia that sometimes accompanies intracranial disease, particularly subarachnoid hemorrhage (SAH), in which up to one third of patients often develop hyponatremia. After the description of SIADH in 1957, such patients were generally assumed to have hyponatremia secondary to vasopressin hypersecretion with a secondary natriuresis. However, over the last decade, clinical and experimental data have suggested that some patients with SAH and other intracranial diseases indeed have a primary natriuresis leading to volume contraction rather than SIADH,[270,271] and the elevated plasma vasopressin levels may be physiologically appropriate for the degree of volume contraction. Some authors suggest there is insufficient evidence of hypovolemia despite ongoing natriuresis,[272] whereas others argue that the combined measures used to estimate ECF volume support hypovolemia in such patients.[273] With regard to the potential mechanisms of natriuresis, both plasma and CSF Atrial Natriuretic Peptide (ANP) levels are elevated in many patients with SAH, and they have been found to correlate variably with hyponatremia in patients with intracranial diseases.[274] However, SIADH also is frequently associated with elevated plasma ANP levels, so this finding does not prove causality. In other disorders of hyponatremia due to Na^+ wasting (e.g., Addison's disease) and diuretic-induced hyponatremia, infusion of saline restores normal ECF volume and plasma tonicity by shutting off the secondary vasopressin secretion. In SAH, however, large volumes of isotonic saline sufficient to maintain plasma volume did not change the incidence of hyponatremia.[275] It seems most likely that SAH and other intracranial diseases represent a mixed disorder in which some patients have *both* exaggerated natriuresis and inappropriate vasopressin secretion. Which mechanism predominates in the clinical presentation will depend on their relative intensities as well as the effects of concomitant therapy.

Renal Adaption

In addition to excreting osmoles to bring volumes back toward normal, there are adaptations that allow excretion of more water. As stated earlier, vasopressin stimulates water retention by increasing the activity and abundance of aquaporin-2 water channels in the renal collecting duct epithelium. Chronic stimulation by vasopressin in SIADH produces dramatic increases above normal of aquaporin-2 content and insertion into the epithelial cell membranes, which increases the efficiency of water retention and aggravates the pathology. However, the induced volume expansion and hypotonicity act on the tubular cells of the collecting duct to decrease the content and action of aquaporin-2, thus decreasing the amount of water resorbed despite high vasopressin. Recent studies have suggested that this may be due to down-regulation of vasopressin V2 receptor expression in the kidney.[276] This renal "escape" therefore represents another (in addition to natriuresis) adaptation that allows patients with persistent SIADH to come into a new steady-state of Na^+ and water balance despite low serum sodium concentrations.[277]

Clinical Manifestations of Hypoosmolar Disorders

Regardless of the etiology of hypoosmolality, most clinical manifestations are similar. Nonneurologic symptoms are relatively uncommon, but a number of cases of rhabdomyolysis have been reported, presumably secondary to osmotically induced swelling of muscle fibers. Hypoosmolality is associated primarily with a broad spectrum of neurologic manifestations, ranging from mild nonspecific symptoms (e.g., headache, nausea) to more significant disorders (e.g., disorientation, confusion, obtundation, focal neurologic deficits, and seizures).[215] This neurologic symptom complex has been termed *hyponatremic encephalopathy*[278] and primarily reflects brain edema resulting from osmotic water shifts into the brain because of decreased effective plasma osmolality. Significant neurologic symptoms generally do not occur until serum [Na^+] falls below 125 mEq/L, and the severity of symptoms are roughly correlated with the degree of hypoosmolality.[215,279] However, individual variability is marked, and for any single patient, the level of serum Na^+ at which symptoms appear cannot be predicted. Once the brain has volume-adapted via solute losses, thereby reducing brain edema, neurologic symptoms may even be virtually absent. From animal studies, the rate of fall of serum [Na^+] is often more strongly correlated with morbidity and mortality than is the actual magnitude of the decrease.[215] This is due to the fact that the volume-adaptation process takes a finite period of time to complete, and the more rapid the fall in serum [Na^+], the more brain edema will be accumulated before the brain is able to regulate volume. Thus, there is a much higher incidence of neurologic symptoms as well as a higher mortality in patients with acute hyponatremia than in those with chronic hyponatremia.[215] For example, the most dramatic cases of death due to hyponatremic encephalopathy have generally been reported in postoperative patients in whom hyponatremia develops rapidly as a result of intravenous infusion of hypotonic fluids.[216,280] In such cases, nausea and vomiting are frequently overlooked as potential early signs of increased intracranial pressure; but, hypoosmolality does not cause any direct effects on the gastrointestinal tract, so unexplained nausea or vomiting in a hypoosmolar patient should be assumed to be of CNS origin. Similarly, critically ill patients with unexplained seizures should be immediately evaluated for possible hyponatremia, because as many as one third of such patients have [Na^+] less than 125 mEq/L as the cause of the seizure activity.[281] Underlying neurologic disease and nonneurologic metabolic disorders (e.g., hypoxia,[282] acidosis, hypercalcemia) can raise the level of plasma osmolality at which CNS symptoms occur.

In the most severe cases of hyponatremic encephalopathy, death results from respiratory failure after tentorial cerebral herniation and brain stem compression. One fourth of patients with severe postoperative hyponatremic encephalopathy manifested hypercapnic respiratory failure, the expected result of brain stem compression; but, three fourths had pulmonary edema as the apparent cause of the hypoxia.[283] Furthermore, recent studies of acute hyponatremia after marathon races have shown hypoxia and pulmonary edema in association with brain edema.[284] These results therefore suggest the possibility that hypoxia from noncardiogenic pulmonary edema may represent an early sign of developing cerebral edema even before the brain stem compression and tentorial herniation. Clinical studies have also suggested that menstruating women[280] and young children[285] may be particularly susceptible to the development of neurologic morbidity and mortality during hyponatremia, especially in the acute postoperative setting.[278] However, other studies have failed to corroborate these findings.[286,287] Consequently, the true clinical incidence as well as the underlying mechanisms responsible for these sometime catastrophic cases is not certain.

Therapy of Hypoosmolar Disorders

Despite some areas of continuing controversy concerning correction of osmolality in hypoosmolar patients, a relative consensus has evolved regarding the most appropriate treatment of this disorder.

Initial Evaluation

The ECF volume status determines treatment of hyponatremia. If volume is expanded, the treatment of the underlying disease should take precedence over correction of plasma osmolality. Often this involves treatment with diuretics, which should simultaneously improve plasma tonicity by virtue of stimulating excretion of hypotonic urine. If hypovolemia is present, the patient must be considered to have depletion-induced hypoosmolality, in which case volume repletion with isotonic saline (0.9% NaCl) at a rate appropriate for the estimated fluid deficit should be initiated. If diuretic use is known or suspected, the isotonic saline should be supplemented with potassium (30 to 40 mEq/L) even if serum [K^+] is not low, because of the propensity of such patients to develop total body potassium depletion. Most often, the hypoosmolar patient is clinically euvolemic. However, a possibility of depletion-induced, rather than dilution-induced, hypoosmolality exists; it is most appropriate to treat the patient initially with isotonic saline, regardless of whether signs of hypovolemia are present. An improvement in, and eventual correction of, the hyponatremia verifies solute and volume depletion. On the other hand, if the patient has SIADH rather than solute depletion, the administration of a limited volume (e.g., 1 to 2 L) of isotonic saline will produce Na^+ and water excretion without significantly changing plasma osmolality.[212]

A patient who meets the essential criteria for SIADH but has a low urine osmolality should be observed on a trial of modest fluid restriction. If the hypoosmolality is attributable to transient SIADH or severe polydipsia, the urine will remain dilute and the plasma osmolality will be fully corrected as free water is excreted. If, however, the patient has the reset osmostat form of the disorder, then the urine will become concentrated at some point before the plasma osmolality and serum [Na^+] return to normal ranges. If either primary or secondary adrenal insufficiency is suspected, glucocorticoid replacement should be initiated immediately after the completion of a rapid adrenocorticotropic hormone stimulation test. A prompt water diuresis after initiation of glucocorticoid treatment supports a diagnosis of glucocorticoid deficiency, but absence of a quick response does not necessarily negate this diagnosis because several days of glucocorticoid replacement are sometimes required for normalization of plasma osmolality.[288] If hypothyroidism is suspected, thyroid function tests should be measured. Usually replacement therapy is withheld pending these results unless the patient is obviously myxedematous.

Acute Treatment

In any hyponatremic patient, one must decide how quickly the plasma osmolality should be increased and to what level. This decision depends on the risks of uncorrected hyponatremia and the risks of the correction. It has become clear that correcting severe hyponatremia too rapidly is dangerous because this can sometimes be associated with pontine and extrapontine myelinolysis, a brain demyelinating disease that causes severe neurologic morbidity and mortality.[217] Consequently, appreciation of the appropriate therapy of hyponatremia requires understanding this disease as well as the pathophysiology underlying hyponatremic encephalopathy.

Pontine and Extrapontine Myelinolysis

Over the last decade it has become apparent that the demyelinating disease of central pontine myelinolysis (CPM) occurs with a significantly higher incidence in patients with hyponatremia,[289] and in both animal[290] and human studies[217] brain demyelination has clearly been shown to be associated with the rapid correction of existing hyponatremia. In animal models of chronic hyponatremia, this pathologic disorder is likely precipitated by the brain dehydration that has been demonstrated to occur following correction of serum [Na^+] toward normal ranges.[291,292] Recent magnetic resonance studies in animals have shown that chronic hypoosmolality predisposes rats to opening of the blood-brain barrier following rapid correction of hyponatremia, and that disruption of the blood-brain barrier is highly correlated with subsequent demyelination.[293] Opening the blood-brain barrier might lead to subsequent myelinolysis via an influx of complement, which is toxic to the oligodendrocytes that manufacture and maintain myelin sheaths of neurons.[294]

Studies in both patients[295] and experimental animals[290] support the notion that both the rate of correction of hyponatremia and the total magnitude of the correction over the first few days determine the risk of demyelination. In rats an initial rate of correction of hyponatremia less than 20 mEq/L in 24 hours[296] has less risk, and clinical data indicate that the initial magnitude of correction represents the major risk factor related to subsequent neurologic morbidity and mortality. Initial reports implicated increases in serum [Na^+] greater than 25 mEq/L over the first 24 to 48 hours of treatment,[297] while later studies have suggested occurrence of CPM with even lesser increases in serum [Na^+] of more than 12 mEq/L in 24 hours or 18 mEq/hr in 48 hours.[298] Whereas overcorrection of hyponatremia to supranormal levels is clearly a risk factor for neurologic deterioration, both clinical and experimental studies have found that demyelination occurred following corrections to serum Na^+ levels still below normal ranges. Both experimental studies[290] and clinical reports[217,299,300] have demonstrated that demyelination occurs independently of the method used to correct the hyponatremia.

The susceptibility to demyelination following correction of hyponatremia is influenced importantly by the severity and the duration of the preexisting hyponatremia. The more severe the hyponatremia and the longer it has been maintained, the greater the degree of solute loss that will have occurred during the process of brain volume regulation, and the solute lost impairs the ability of the brain to buffer volume in response to subsequent increases in plasma osmolality. Clinical studies show that CPM rarely occurs in patients with a starting serum [Na^+] greater than 120 mEq/L, and it does not appear to occur in patients with psychogenic polydipsia who develop hyponatremia acutely from massive water ingestion and correct rapidly as they diurese the excess fluid.[301] Other independent risk factors for the occurrence of CPM are chronic alcoholism and malnutrition.[302] It seems likely that the threshold for increases in serum [Na^+] that increase the risk for CPM will be lower in alcoholic and malnourished patients, and a recent case report of myelinolysis in a patient with beer-potomania in whom the rate of correction stayed within the recommended guidelines supports this likelihood.[303] Interestingly, uremia appears to protect hyponatremic patients from myelinolysis following rapid correction of hyponatremia, purportedly because the urea acts as an intracellular osmolyte to stabilize intracellular volume and thereby reduces the degree of brain dehydration produced following rapid correction of hyponatremia.[304]

The term *central* pontine myelinolysis is historically correct but is anatomically too limited.[289] Demyelination following correction of hyponatremia frequently occurs in white matter areas of the brain other than the pons (which led to the term *osmotic demyelination syndrome* [ODS]).[217] In accordance with the widespread nature of the neuropathologic lesions, a much broader range of neurologic disorders is now being reported in patients following correction of hyponatremia, including cognitive, behavioral, and neuropsychiatric disorders, presumably as a result of demyelination in subcortical, corpus callosal and hippocampal white matter, and movement disorders, as a result of demyelination in the basal ganglia. Whereas the presence of positive MRI findings strongly supports a diagnosis of ODS, scans often fail to demonstrate the characteristic demyelinative lesions because scans are usually negative until sufficient time has passed (generally 3 to 4 weeks) after the correction of hyponatremia and the onset of neurologic symptoms.[305,306] Although most cases of osmotically induced ODS have been associated with rapid correction of hyponatremia, the disorder has also been reported with severe hypernatremia in both animal models[307] and human patients.[308] It is clear that one cannot predict with any degree of certainty which patients will develop demyelination. Many patients undergo very rapid and large change of their serum [Na^+] without subsequent neurologic complications as is clearly true of experimental animals as well.[290,296] Consequently, overly rapid correction of hyponatremia should be viewed as a factor that puts patients *at risk* for ODS, but does not inevitably precipitate this disorder

Individualization of Therapy

Based on the previous discussions of hyponatremic encephalopathy and pontine and extrapontine myelinolysis, it follows that optimal treatment of hyponatremic patients must entail balancing the risks of hyponatremia against the risks of correction for each patient individually.[309,310] Three factors should be taken into consideration when making a treatment decision in a hypoosmolar patient: (1) the severity of the hyponatremia, (2) the duration of the hyponatremia, and (3) the patient's neurologic symptoms.

Acute Hyponatremia

Cases of acute hyponatremia (arbitrarily defined as 48 hours in duration) are usually symptomatic if the hyponatremia is severe (i.e., <120 mEq/L). These patients are at greatest risk for neurologic complications from the hyponatremia, but rarely develop demyelination,[301] presumably because sufficient brain volume regulation has not yet occurred. Consequently, serum [Na^+] in such patients should be corrected relatively quickly. Hypoosmolar patients should always be evaluated quickly for the presence of neurologic symptoms so that appropriate therapy can be initiated, if indicated, even while other results of the diagnostic evaluation are still pending. Postoperative patients,[311] and particularly young women and children in some studies,[280,285] appear to be at somewhat greater risk for rapidly progressing hyponatremic encephalopathy. They should be treated especially promptly, and administration of hypotonic fluids should be avoided in such patients postoperatively.[278]

Chronic Asymptomatic Hyponatremia

Conversely, patients with chronic hyponatremia (arbitrarily defined as greater than 48 hours in duration) who have minimal neurologic symptoms are at little risk from complications of hyponatremia itself but can develop demyelination after rapid correction because of greater degrees of brain volume regulation through electrolyte and osmolyte losses.[236] There is no indication to correct these patients rapidly, regardless of the initial serum [Na^+], and they should be treated using slower-acting therapies, such as fluid restriction.

Chronic Symptomatic Hyponatremia

Although the first two extremes have clear treatment indications, most hypoosmolar patients have hyponatremia of indeterminate duration and varying degrees of neurologic symptoms. Such patients should be treated promptly because of their symptoms, but using methods that allow a *controlled and limited increase* of their hypoosmolality.[310] Some studies have suggested that correction parameters should consist of a maximal rate of correction of serum [Na^+] in the range of 1 to 2 mEq/L/hr so long as the total magnitude of correction does not exceed 25 mEq/L over the first 48 hours,[297] while others recommend that these parameters should be even more conservative, with maximal correction rates of 0.5 mEq/L/hr or less and magnitudes of correction that do not exceed 12 mEq/L in the first 24 hours and 18 in the first 48 hours.[298] A reasonable approach for treatment of individual patients would therefore entail choosing correction parameters within these limits depending on their symptoms. In patients who are only minimally symptomatic, one should proceed at the lower recommended limits of 0.5 mEq/L/hr or less, while in those who manifest more severe neurologic symptoms, an initial correction at a rate of 1 to 2 mEq/L/hr (or even 3 to 5 mEq/L/hr in comatose or seizing patients who are at risk for imminent tentorial herniation and respiratory arrest) would be more appropriate. Regardless of the initial rate of correction chosen, acute treatment should be interrupted once any of three end-points is reached: (1) the patient's symptoms are abolished, (2) a safe serum [Na^+] (generally greater than 125 mEq/L) is achieved, or (3) a total magnitude of correction of 18 mEq/L is achieved. Once any of these end-points is reached, the active correction should be stopped and the patient treated with slower-acting therapies, such as oral rehydration or fluid restriction, depending on the etiology of the hypoosmolality. It follows from these recommendations that serum Na^+ levels must be carefully monitored at frequent intervals (at least every 4 hours) during the active phases of treatment to adjust therapy to keep the correction within these guidelines.

Choice of Interventional (Active) Therapies for Acute Corrections

Controlled limited corrections can be accomplished with either isotonic or hypertonic saline infusions, depending on the etiology of the hypoosmolality. Patients with volume depletion hypoosmolality (e.g., clinical hypovolemia, diuretic use, or urine $[Na^+]$ less than 30 mEq/L) usually respond well to isotonic (0.9%) NaCl.[244] However, patients with diuretic-induced hyponatremia are especially susceptible to rapid corrections because (1) such patients are usually are only minimally volume depleted, (2) they are often small elderly women with correspondingly small plasma volumes, (3) with cessation of diuretic therapy these patients often develop a free water diuresis as their urinary diluting defect dissipates, and (4) the hypokalemia that frequently accompanies the hyponatremia in such patients appears to be an additional risk factor for demyelination after correction.[312] Consequently, in the absence of marked neurologic symptoms, such patients should simply be treated by institution of a regular sodium diet (4 to 6 g/day) and discontinuing the diuretics. If isotonic saline is infused, it should be done so judiciously (e.g., 50 to75 mL/hr), with K^+ replacement. Patients with euvolemic hypoosmolality (including patients with SIADH) generally will not respond to isotonic NaCl[212,244] and are best treated with hypertonic (3%) NaCl solution given by continuous infusion. An initial infusion rate can be estimated by multiplying the patient's body weight in kilograms by the desired rate of increase in serum $[Na^+]$ in milliequivalents per liter per hour (e.g., in a 70-kg patient, an infusion of 3% NaCl at 70 mL/hr will increase serum $[Na^+]$ by approximately 1 mEq/L/hr, while an infusion of 35 mL/hr will increase serum $[Na^+]$ by about 0.5 mEq/L/hr). In patients with known cardiovascular disease, furosemide can be used to treat volume overload.[313] It cannot be emphasized too strongly that it is necessary only to correct the plasma osmolality acutely to a safe range rather than completely to normonatremia.

Spontaneous (Passive) Correction

Rarely, patients may spontaneously correct their hyponatremia by means of a water diuresis. If the hyponatremia is acute, such as water intoxication from psychogenic polydipsia, spontaneous correction appears to be of little risk for subsequent demyelination.[301] In cases in which the hyponatremia has been chronic, patients are at risk for demyelination,[299,314] and one might consider intervention (e.g., administration of desmopressin or intravenous infusion of hypotonic fluid) to limit the rate and magnitude of correction of serum $[Na^+]$. In some cases, an overcorrection occurs spontaneously before it is noticed. Animal models of this situation have reported that a delayed lowering of the serum $[Na^+]$ can prevent subsequent brain damage from occurring,[315] which would be consistent with the occurrence of a delayed immunologic demyelination as a result of complement influx into the brain following a sustained blood-brain barrier disruption.[294] Recent experimental studies in rats indicate that treatment with pharmacologic doses of corticosteroids may prevent subsequent osmotic demyelination by stabilizing the blood-brain barrier.[316]

Long-Term Treatment

Fluid Restriction

The treatment of chronic SIADH entails a choice among several suboptimal therapeutic regimens. Any drugs known to be associated with SIADH should be discontinued or changed. Continued fluid restriction represents the least toxic treatment choice and is the preferred treatment for most cases of mild to moderate SIADH. Several points should be remembered with use of this approach: (1) all fluids, not only water, must be included in the restriction; (2) the degree of restriction required depends on urine output plus insensible fluid loss (in general, discretionary, i.e., nonfood, fluids should be limited to 500 mL a day below the average daily urine volume); (3) several days of restriction are usually necessary before a significant increase in plasma osmolality occurs, and (4) only fluid, not salt, should be restricted. Because of the ongoing natriuresis, patients with chronic SIADH often have a negative total body sodium balance and therefore should be maintained on relatively high NaCl intakes unless otherwise contraindicated. Failure to improve after several days of confirmed negative fluid balance prompts reconsideration of other possible causes, including solute depletion and clinically inapparent hypovolemia.

While not confirmed in humans, in animals the expanded volume and hypotonicity of SIADH down-regulates the vasopressin-induced increase of aquaporin-2 water channels in the collecting duct and this "escape" allows more water excretion.[277] Unfortunately, from a therapeutic standpoint, correction of expanded volume and hyponatremia by restriction of fluid would reduce this "escape" phenomenon. Consequently aquaporin content and action will increase again in response to the persistent elevated level of vasopressin and the efficiency of extracting free water will increase. This is a plausible explanation for the clinical observation that a patient with stable hyponatremia on modest fluid intake may require severe water restriction to permanently correct serum sodium.

Pharmacologic Therapy

Pharmacologic intervention is reserved for refractory cases in which the degree of fluid restriction required to avoid hypoosmolality is so severe that the patient is unable, or unwilling, to maintain it. Pharmacologic intervention should also be avoided initially in patients with SIADH that is secondary to tumors, because successful treatment of the underlying malignant lesion often eliminates or reduces the inappropriate vasopressin secretion. When pharmacologic management is necessary, the preferred drug is the tetracycline derivative demeclocycline.[317] This agent causes nephrogenic diabetes insipidus, thereby decreasing urine concentration even in the presence of high plasma vasopressin levels. Appropriate doses of demeclocycline range from 600 to 1200 mg/day administered in divided doses. Treatment must be continued for several days to achieve maximal diuretic effects and one should wait 3 to 4 days before deciding to increase the dose. Demeclocycline can cause reversible azotemia and sometimes nephrotoxicity, especially in patients with cirrhosis.[318] Renal function should therefore be monitored on a regular basis in patients treated with demeclocycline and the medication discontinued if increasing azotemia is noted.

Other agents, such as lithium, have similar renal effects but are less desirable because of inconsistent results and significant side effects.[319] Urea has also been described as an alternative mode of treatment for SIADH as well as other hyponatremic disorders.[320] Several other drugs have been described to decrease vasopressin hypersecretion in some cases (e.g., diphenylhydantoin, opiates, ethanol), but responses are erratic and unpredictable. One potential exception is the recent development of agonists selective for kappa opioid receptors, which appear to be more specific for inhibition of vasopressin hypersecretion in animal studies,[321] and in clinical trials successfully produced an aquaresis in patients with cirrhosis.[322]

Vasopressin Antagonists

An antagonist of the kidney, vasopressin V2 receptors would be the ideal agent for treatment of patients with dilutional hyponatremia. Previous attempts at using peptide vasopressin receptor antagonists in humans were frustrated by species variability with regard to partial agonistic effects of such compounds. Recently several nonpeptide V2 receptor antagonists have been described that appear to overcome these problems.[323-325] In December 2005, the Food and Drug Administration approved conivaptan as the first vasopressin receptor antagonist for the treatment of euvolemic hyponatremia, and several additional promising compounds are in the late phases of clinical trials.[326] We are therefore poised to begin a new era in both the evaluation and treatment of patients with SIADH. Clinical trials using selective V2 receptor antagonists will enable investigators to answer some longstanding questions about the role of vasopressin receptor activation in producing antidiuresis, as well as other potential effects, in various disease states (e.g., hyponatremic patients without measurable vasopressin levels). In cases in which correction with vasopressin receptor antagonists is too rapid, the patient will still be at risk for pontine and extrapontine myelinolysis, which has already been documented in animals,[327] but appropriate dosing and monitoring should allow successful adherence to the same guidelines for limited controlled correction that apply to other methods of treatment.

OXYTOCIN

Study of the normal physiologic regulation of oxytocin secretion and action is complicated by the fact that secretion and function of oxytocin varies markedly among different experimental mammals. There are varying sites of synthesis in the ovary and in tissues of the uterus that are different among species. It is difficult to study pregnant women and human tissue, so physiologic regulation of oxytocin secretion and function is less well known in humans than in other species. The classic roles of oxytocin are uterine myometrial contraction at parturition and smooth muscle activation promoting milk let-down with nursing.

Lactation

A characteristic of all mammals is lactation and all mammals secrete oxytocin to stimulate milk let-down associated with nursing.[328] The other hormone critical to lactation is prolactin. Each of these pituitary-hypothalamic hormones is importantly influenced and regulated by gonadal steroid hormones. The milk-producing unit of the breast is the alveolar system with multiple clusters of milk-producing cells surrounded by specialized myoepithelial cells. The alveoli are directly connected to ductules and then ducts converge and lead to the nipple. Milk is synthesized in the glandular cells of the alveoli.[329] Oxytocin receptors are localized on glandular cells and oxytocin in the systemic circulation acts on these receptors to cause myoepithelial contraction. Oxytocin also acts on myoepithelial cells along the duct to shorten and widen the ducts to enhance milk flow through the ducts to the nipple.[330]

When an infant begins sucking at the breast, an afferent signal is transmitted from the mechanoreceptors or tactile receptors in the breast to the spinal cord and from the spinal cord to the lateral cervical nucleus. These ascending fibers cross in the medulla and eventually ascend to the oxytocinergic magnocellular neurons in the supraoptic nucleus and the paraventricular nucleus.[330-332] Numerous neurotransmitters and neuropeptides are activated by different inputs to stimulate or inhibit the magnocellular neurons[330] to produce a synchronous pulsatile depolarization of oxytocin neurons.[333,334] The plasticity of the neurohypophysis to promote synchrony is described earlier with an emphasis on increased neuron-to-neuron apposition, which promotes signaling between cells. The pulsatile release of oxytocin by the posterior pituitary produces a pumping action on the alveoli, which promotes maximum emptying of milk from the alveoli.[329] Whereas the plastic changes are sufficient for synchrony within a single nuclear group, it does not explain the synchrony that must occur between the four nuclear groups (paired PVNs and paired SONs). Because there is no evidence of a central pacemaker, the synchrony among these nuclei must be due to the common suckling stimulus with some gating phenomenon of the neuro input. It is postulated that nitric oxide may be involved in regulation of the gating.[335] The importance of oxytocin in maintaining milk secretion is demonstrated by transgenic mice with a knockout that inhibits oxytocin synthesis. These animals deliver their young normally, and they have normal milk production, but there is no milk release despite normal suckling. The pups die of dehydration with no milk in the stomach.[336,337] Administration of oxytocin to these oxytocin-deficient mice rescues the ability to secrete milk and allows the pups to survive. Similarly oxytocin may promote successful lactation in women who have difficulty with lactation and milk production.[338]

In most species, suckling must occur for the sequence of events leading to milk let-down to occur and, indeed, let-down may not follow until several minutes of suckling.[339] In humans, suckling is not essential because oxytocin secretion and milk let-down are well known to occur by psychological stimuli such as preparing for nursing or hearing a baby cry.[340-342] However, if oxytocin is not secreted, only 20% to 30% of stored milk is released during nursing.[343]

The role of steroids in oxytocin secretion is complex. Estrogen stimulates oxytocin release by dendrites[344] and progesterone withdrawal in an estrogen primed animal stimulates oxytocin synthesis.[345,346] Changes in these steroid hormones at the time of parturition probably modulate the lactation response both by modulating oxytocin synthesis and secretion but also by modulating oxytocin receptors. As breastfeeding continues in humans, the basal levels of oxytocin decrease but pulses of oxytocin in response to suckling continue and may increase.[347] Women with diabetes insipidus have been able to successfully breastfeed infants, which has caused some to question the importance of oxytocin in humans.[348] However, oxytocin secretion may be preserved in the absence of vasopressin in patients with diabetes insipidus, even in those with traumatic section of the stalk.

Parturition

The isolation of oxytocin was followed quickly by the description of the ability of oxytocin to stimulate uterine contractions, which was followed shortly by clinical use of oxytocin as a uterotonic agent.[349]

In all mammals, oxytocin is secreted with the expulsive stage of parturition, but there is controversy about the role of oxytocin to initiate parturition. There is considerable variability among various species as to the timing of secretion and the mechanism by which oxytocin action may be increased during parturition. Knockout mice that are unable to synthesize oxytocin have normal delivery (but not lactation), but in the rat and baboon, oxytocin antagonists decrease uterine contraction.[335] Understanding the role of oxytocin in parturition is enhanced by thinking of changes in oxytocin levels and changes in oxytocin receptor as comparable events enhancing the action of oxytocin. In humans, changes in the oxytocin receptor may be more important than changes in oxytocin secretion, and oxytocin receptor function does increase at parturition.[350] In all species, oxytocin is the most powerful uterotonic stimulant for contractions and oxytocin secretion increases with the expulsive phase of parturition in multiple births or during secretion of the placenta in single births in humans via the Fergusson reflex, in which mechanical dilatation of the cervix produces an increased secretion of oxytocin.[350-352]

The uterine myometrial cells have intrinsic contractile activity so during pregnancy the uterus is maintained in a quiet state by the actions of progesterone and relaxin (produced by the corpus luteum and decidual tissue).[353-355] The initiation of labor is accomplished by a relative increase in estrogen activation and decrease in progesterone activation. Progesterone withdrawal may be an initiating factor of parturition is several species. The mechanism of the increase of the estrogen to progesterone ratio, however, may vary considerably among species. In some species such as the mouse and sheep, the corpus luteum is maintained throughout pregnancy and secretes progesterone. Luteolysis at the time of parturition causes an abrupt fall in progesterone. In the human and the nonhuman primate, the corpus luteum is only present during the first trimester[356] and estrogen and progesterone rise throughout pregnancy, although the rate of increase in estrogen is greater than progesterone as parturition approaches.[357] A decreasing effect of progesterone and increasing effect of estrogen in humans may be more important at a paracrine level in fetal membranes[358,359] where progesterone is inactivated and estrogen synthesis increased. It is also reported that estrogen receptor increases in human fetal membranes at parturition whereas progesterone receptor remains stable.[353,360] Thus, the cycle of events that are observed in plasma in some species may be reproduced distally as a paracrine action in primates.[358,361,362]

In the human there is a 200-fold increase in the responsiveness of the uterus to oxytocin as parturition approaches.[359] This is accompanied by an increase in oxytocin receptor density[363] and by the formation of gap junctions between myometrial cells.[364] Gap junctions are a prerequisite to synchronous contraction of the uterus and, like other events, gap junction formation is inhibited by progesterone and stimulated by estrogens.[363]

In various species, several other hormones play a role in initiation of and/or completion of parturition, including prostaglandins, endothelins, adrenergic agonists, glucocorticoids, and cytokines.[353,359,363,365] The role of oxytocin in the complex interplay of these various agents is not well understood in the human. A necessary accompaniment of myometrial contraction is softening and dilatation of the cervix, which is accomplished by biochemical events similar to an inflammatory reaction or proinflammatory reaction in which cytokines play an important role.[366,367] The predominant prostaglandin is PGF-2α. Prostaglandins promote a controlled inflammatory response in the cervix to assist in thinning and dilatation.[368]

In the nonhuman primate as parturition approaches, synchronized nocturnal contractions begin but then revert to asynchronous contractures during the day. These nocturnal synchronized contractions have been shown to correlate with plasma oxytocin levels[369] and are blocked by administration of an oxytocin antagonist. Similarly, the response of the uterus to administered oxytocin in the monkey is greater at night than during the day,[370] and fetal DHEAS (dehydroepiandrosterone) is also highest at night.[371] DHEAS secretion by the fetus may be an important source of estrogen because the DHEAS is converted to estradiol by the placenta. Estradiol stimulates oxytocin synthesis in decidua and also stimulates synthesis of PGF-2α in decidua. There is a feed-forward mechanism whereby increased PGF-2α stimulates oxytocin, which in turn stimulates increased production of PGF-2α. Teleologically it makes sense that the developing fetus when it reaches maturation would be a controlling factor in the initiation of labor. In the sheep there is an absolute requirement of the fetal hypothalamic pituitary adrenal axis to initiate labor and in the primate the interaction of fetal DHEAS, estrogen, oxytocin, and progesterone provide a potential similar mechanism.

A complicated cascade of events interact with each other at parturition and feed forward with cross-stimulation. It is not surprising that a physiologic event as important to the species as pregnancy and parturition would have many redundant systems to assure survival of the species. Additionally, the complicated interaction of these various redundant systems and the feed-forward nature of the responses makes it unlikely that interrupting any single hormonal response after parturition is initiated would be sufficient to inhibit completion of delivery.[372]

An obvious thing to note in all of these discussions is the lack of understanding of the role of cysteine aminopeptidase (oxytocinase) in the physiology of pregnancy in the human. If this enzyme developed as a protective mechanism, then one would assume that oxytocin secretion by the neurohypophysis was increased throughout pregnancy, but the very presence of this enzyme and the obvious inability to do studies of the hypothalamus in vivo makes this possibility uncertain. However, the presence of the oxytocin-associated neurophysin throughout pregnancy would support this point of view.[373] Furthermore, the presence of circulating cysteine aminopeptidase provides a teleologic explanation for the development of oxytocin synthesis and secretion in fetal membranes in a manner that serves a paracrine function possibly protected from the degradative activity of the cysteine aminopeptidase in plasma.

Behavior

In addition to the actions in the periphery to stimulate milk letdown and uterine contraction, oxytocin is reported to have numerous actions on the CNS. The separate functions, peripheral and central, are mirrored anatomically by two sets of neurons, the magnocellular neurons and smaller parvocellular neurons, respectively.[374] Because the role of oxytocin secreted peripherally is to regulate physiologic events surrounding reproduction, most of the emphasis regarding CNS effects has been on various aspects of maternal behavior.[328] Maternal behavior is coincident with parturition and lactation in most mammalian species and is not seen with other physiologic events that produce only changes in gonadal steroid secretion. Therefore, it is likely that something in addition to or in place of gonadal steroids is active in inducing maternal behavior.[375] Studies have found that oxytocin is increased in various areas of the brain that are thought to be sites of regulation of maternal behavior, such as in the olfactory lobes of rats.[375] Injection of oxytocin into the cerebral ventricles can, in some species, initiate maternal behavior and injection of oxytocin antagonists can inhibit such behavior. It should be noted, however, that the findings regarding oxytocin and reproductive behavior vary markedly among species and among strains within a given species.[328] In males, oxytocin has also been reported to play a role but this is much less certain. In rodents, oxytocin administered in the CNS will induce arousal and penile erection and in some species has been reported to increase sperm transport.[376,377]

REFERENCES

1. Makarenko I, Ugrumov M, Derer P, et al. Projections from the hypothalamus to the posterior lobe in rats during ontogenesis: 1,1′-dioctadecyl-3,3,3′,3′-tetramethylindocarbocyanine perchlorate tracing study. J.Comp Neurol 2000;422(3):327-337.

2. Sofroniew MV. Morphology of vasopressin and oxytocin neurones and their central and vascular projections. Prog Brain Res 1983;60:101-114.
3. Treier M, Rosenfeld R. The hypothalamic-pituitary axis: co-development of two organs. Curr Opin Cell Biol 1996;8(6): 833-843.
4. Sawchenko P, Swanson L. The organization and biochemical specificity of afferent projections to the paraventricular and supraoptic nuclei. Prog Brain Res 1983;60:19-29.
5. Swanson L, Sawchenko P. Paraventricular nucleus: a site for the integration of neuroendocrine and autonomic mechanisms. Neuroendocrinology 1980;31(6):410-417.
6. Theodosis D, Poulain D. Maternity leads to morphological synaptic plasticity in the oxytocin system. Prog Brain Res 2001;133:49-58.
7. Oliet S. Functional consequences of morphological neuroglial changes in the magnocellular nuclei of the hypothalamus. J Neuroendocrinol 2002;14(3):241-246.
8. Brussaard A, Koksma J. Conditional regulation of neurosteroid sensitivity of GABAA receptors. Ann N Y Acad Sci 2003; 1007:29-36.
9. Miyata S, Hatton G. Activity-related, dynamic neuron-glial interactions in the hypothalamo-neurohypophysial system. Microsc Res Tech 2002;56(2):143-157.
10. Mark L, Pech P, Daniels D, et al. The pituitary fossa: a correlative anatomic and MR study. Radiology 1984;153(2):453-457.
11. Ultmann M, Siegel S, Hirsch W, et al. Pituitary stalk and ectopic hyperintense T1 signal on magnetic resonance imaging. Implications for anterior pituitary dysfunction. Am J Dis Child 1993;147(6): 647-652.
12. Maghnie M, Genovese E, Villa A, et al. Dynamic MRI in the congenital agenesis of the neural pituitary stalk syndrome: the role of the vascular pituitary stalk in predicting residual anterior pituitary function. Clin Endocrinol (Oxf) 1996;45(3):281-290.
13. Chen S, Leger J, Garel C, et al. Growth hormone deficiency with ectopic neurohypophysis: anatomical variations and relationship between the visibility of the pituitary stalk asserted by magnetic resonance imaging and anterior pituitary function. J Clin Endocrinol Metab 1999;84(7):2408-2413.
14. Gainer H, Wray S. Cellular and molecular biology of oxytocin and vasopressin. In KnobilNeill, eds. The Physiology of Reproduction, 2nd ed. New York: Raven Press, 1994:1099-1129.
15. Chen L, Rose J, Breslow E, et al. Crystal structure of a bovine neurophysin II dipeptide complex at 2.8 A determined from the single-wavelength anomalous scattering signal of an incorporated iodine atom. Proc Natl Acad Sci U S A 1991;88(10):4240-4244.
16. Acher R. Evolution of neurohypophysial control of water homeostasis: integrative biology of molecular, cellular and organismal aspects. In Saito T, Kurokawa K, Yoshida S (eds). Neurohypophysis: Recent Progress of Vasopressin and Oxytocin Research. Amsterdam, Elsevier, 1995:39-54.
17. Herman J, Schafer M, Watson S, et al. In situ hybridization analysis of arginine vasopressin gene transcription using intron-specific probes. Mol Endocrinol 1991;5(10):1447-1456.
18. Majzoub J. Vasopressin biosynthesis. In Schrier, ed. Vasopressin. New York: Raven Press, 1985:465-474.
19. Sherman T, Akil H, Watson S. Vasopressin mRNA expression: a Northern and in situ hybridization analysis. In Schrier, ed. Vasopressin. New York: Raven Press, 1985:475-483.
20. Zingg H, Lefebvre D, Almazan G. Regulation of vasopressin gene expression in rat hypothalamic neurons. Response to osmotic stimulation. J Biol Chem 1986;261(28):12956-12959.
21. Robinson A, Roberts M, Evron W, et al. Hyponatremia in rats induces downregulation of vasopressin synthesis. J Clin Invest 1990;86(4): 1023-1029.
22. Roberts M, Robinson A, Hoffman G, et al. Vasopressin transport regulation is coupled to the synthesis rate. Neuroendocrinology 1991; 53(4):416-422.
23. Lederis K, Jayasena K. Storage of neurohypophysial hormones and the mechanism for their release. In Heller, Pickering, eds. Pharmacology of the Endocrine System and Related Drugs. London: Pergamon, 1970:111-154.
24. Sato N, Tanaka S, Tateno M, et al. Origin of posterior pituitary high intensity on T1-weighted magnetic resonance imaging. Immunohistochemical, electron microscopic, and magnetic resonance studies of posterior pituitary lobe of dehydrated rabbits. Invest Radiol 1995;30(10):567-571.
25. Kurokawa H, Fujisawa I, Nakano Y, et al. Posterior lobe of the pituitary gland: correlation between signal intensity on T1-weighted MR images and vasopressin concentration. Radiology 1998;207(1): 79-83.
26. Fitzsimmons M, Roberts M, Sherman T, et al. Models of neurohypophyseal homeostasis. Am J Physiol 1992;262(6 Pt 2): R1121-R1130.
27. Thrasher T. Baroreceptor regulation of vasopressin and renin secretion: low- pressure versus high-pressure receptors. Front Neuroendocrinol 1994;15(2):157-196.
28. Share L, Levy M. Cardiovascular receptors and blood titer of antidiuretic hormone. Am J Physiol 1962;203:425-428.
29. Thames M, Schmid P. Cardiopulmonary receptors with vagal afferents tonically inhibit ADH release in the dog. Am J Physiol 1979;237(3):H299-H304.
30. Bishop V, Thames M, Schmid P. Effects of bilateral vagal cold block on vasopressin in conscious dogs. Am J Physiol 1984;246(4 Pt 2): R566-R569.
31. Blessing W, Sved A, Reis D. Destruction of noradrenergic neurons in rabbit brainstem elevates plasma vasopressin, causing hypertension. Science 1982;217(4560):661-663.
32. Sved A, Blessing W, Reis D. Caudal ventrolateral medulla can alter vasopressin and arterial pressure. Brain Res Bull 1985; 14(3):227-232.
33. Blessing W, Sved A, Reis D. Arterial pressure and plasma vasopressin: regulation by neurons in the caudal ventrolateral medulla of the rabbit. Clin Exp Hypertens [A] 1984;6(1-2):149-156.
34. Schreihofer A, Stricker E, Sved A. Chronic nucleus tractus solitarius lesions do not prevent hypovolemia- induced vasopressin secretion in rats. Am J Physiol 1994;267(4 Pt 2):R965-R973.
35. Robertson G. Thirst and vasopressin function in health and disease. Recent Prog Horm Res 1977;33:333-385.
36. Callahan M, Ludwig M, Tsai K, et al. Baroreceptor input regulates osmotic control of central vasopressin secretion. Neuroendocrinology 1997;65(4):238-245.
37. Pump B, Gabrielsen A, Christensen N, et al. Mechanisms of inhibition of vasopressin release during moderate antiorthostatic posture change in humans. Am J Physiol 1999;277(1 Pt 2): R229-R235.
38. Johnson A, Thunhorst R. The neuroendocrinology of thirst and salt appetite: visceral sensory signals and mechanisms of central integration. Front Neuroendocrinol 1997;18(3):292-353.
39. Baylis P, Thompson C. Osmoregulation of vasopressin secretion and thirst in health and disease. Clin.Endocrinol (Oxf) 1988;29(5): 549-576.
40. Baylis P. Investigation of suspected hypothalamic diabetes insipidus. ClinEndocrinol (Oxf) 1995;43(4):507-510.
41. Nielsen S, Frokiaer J, Marples D, et al. Aquaporins in the kidney: from molecules to medicine. Physiol Rev 2002;82(1): 205-244.
42. Brown D. The ins and outs of aquaporin-2 trafficking. Am J Physiol Renal Physiol 2003;284(5):F893-F901.
43. Stocker S, Sved A, Stricker E. Role of renin-angiotensin system in hypotension-evoked thirst: studies with hydralazine. Am J Physiol Regul Integr Comp Physiol 2000;279(2):R576-R585.
44. Robertson G, Berl T. Water metabolism. In Brenner, Rector Jr, eds. The Kidney, 3rd ed. Philadelphia: WB Saunders, 1986:385-432.
45. Lindheimer M, Davison J. Osmoregulation, the secretion of arginine vasopressin and its metabolism during pregnancy. Eur J Endocrinol 1995;132(2):133-143.
46. Lindheimer M, Barron W. Water metabolism and vasopressin secretion during pregnancy. Baillieres Clin Obstet Gynaecol 1994;8(2): 311-331.
47. Barron W, Stamoutsos B, Lindheimer M. Role of volume in the regulation of vasopressin secretion during pregnancy in the rat. J Clin Invest 1984;73(4):923-932.
48. Danielson L, Sherwood O, Conrad. Relaxin is a potent renal vasodilator in conscious rats. J Clin Invest 1999;103(4):525-533.
49. Danielson L, Kercher L, Conrad K. Impact of gender and endothelin on renal vasodilation and hyperfiltration induced by relaxin in conscious rats. Am J Physiol Regul Integr Comp Physiol 2000;279(4): R1298-R1304.

50. Novak J, Danielson L, Kerchner L, et al. Relaxin is essential for renal vasodilation during pregnancy in conscious rats. J Clin Invest 2001;107(11):1469-1475.
51. Robinson A, Fitzsimmons M. Diabetes insipidus. In Mazzaferri, Bar, Kreisberg, eds. Advances in Endocrinology and Metabolism. St. Louis: Mosby, 1994:261-296.
52. Davison J, Sheills E, Barron W, et al. Changes in the metabolic clearance of vasopressin and in plasma vasopressinase throughout human pregnancy. J Clin Invest 1989;83(4):1313-1318.
53. Stout N, Kenny R, Baylis P. A review of water balance in ageing in health and disease. Gerontology 1999;45(2):61-66.
54. Davis P, Davis F. Water excretion in the elderly. Endocrinol Metab Clin North Am 1987;16(4):867-875.
55. Tian V, Serino R, Verbalis J. Downregulation of renal vasopressin V2 receptor and aquaporin-2 expression parallels age-associated defects in urine concentration. Am J Physiol Renal Physiol 2004;287(4):F797-F805.
56. Fulop T Jr, Worum I, Csongor J, et al. Body composition in elderly people. II. Comparison of measured and predicted body composition in healthy elderly subjects. Gerontology 1985;31(3):150-157.
57. Phillips P, Johnston C, Gray L. Disturbed fluid and electrolyte homoeostasis following dehydration in elderly people. Age Ageing 1993;22(1):S26-S33.
58. Takamata A, Ito T, Yaegashi K, et al. Effect of an exercise-heat acclimation program on body fluid regulatory responses to dehydration in older men. Am J Physiol 1999;277(4 Pt 2):R1041-R1050.
59. Phillips P, Bretherton M, Johnston J, et al. Reduced osmotic thirst in healthy elderly men. Am J Physiol 1991;261(1 Pt 2):R166-R171.
60. Crowe M, Forsling M, Rolls B, et al. Altered water excretion in healthy elderly men. Age Ageing 1987;16(5):285-293.
61. Roberts M, Robinson A. Hyponatremia in the elderly. Geriatric Nephrology and Urology 1993;3:43-50.
62. Miller M, Dalakos T, Moses A, et al. Recognition of partial defects in antidiuretic hormone secretion. Ann Intern Med 1970;73(5): 721-729.
63. Baylis P, Cheetham T. Diabetes insipidus. Arch Dis Child 1998;79(1):84-89.
64. Robertson G. Diabetes insipidus. Endocrinol Metab Clin North Am 1995;24(3):549-572.
65. Zerbe R, Robertson G. A comparison of plasma vasopressin measurements with a standard indirect test in the differential diagnosis of polyuria. N Engl J Med 1981;305(26):1539-1546.
66. De Bellis A, Colao A, Di Salle F, et al. A longitudinal study of vasopressin cell antibodies, posterior pituitary function, and magnetic resonance imaging evaluations in subclinical autoimmune central diabetes insipidus. J Clin Endocrinol Metab 1999;84(9): 3047-3051.
67. Baylis P. Diabetes insipidus [see comments]. J R Coll Physicians Lond 1998;32(2):108-111.
68. Bononi P, Robinson A. Central diabetes insipidus: management in the postoperative period. Endocrinologist 1991;1(3):180-185.
69. Salata R, Verbalis J, Robinson A. Cold water stimulation of oropharyngeal receptors in man inhibits release of vasopressin. J Clin Endocrinol Metab 1987;65(3):561-567.
70. Decaux C, Prospert F, Namias B, et al. Hyperuricemia as a clue for central diabetes insipidus (lack of V1 effect) in the differential diagnosis of polydipsia. Am J Med 1997;103(5):376-382.
71. Arslan A, Karaarslan E, Dincer A. High intensity signal of the posterior pituitary. A study with horizontal direction of frequency-encoding and fat suppression MR techniques. Acta Radiol 1999;40(2): 142-145.
72. Tien R, Kucharczyk J, Kucharczyk W. MR imaging of the brain in patients with diabetes insipidus [see comments]. AJNR Am J Neuroradiol 1991;12(3):533-542.
73. Moses A, Clayton B, Hochhauser L. Use of T1-weighted MR imaging to differentiate between primary polydipsia and central diabetes insipidus [comment] [see comments]. AJNR Am J Neuroradiol 1992;13(5):1273-1277.
74. Gudinchet F, Brunelle F, Barth M, et al. MR imaging of the posterior hypophysis in children. Am J Nucl Radiol 1989;10:511-514.
75. Brooks B, el Gammal T, Allison J, et al. Frequency and variation of the posterior pituitary bright signal on MR images. AJNR Am J Neuroradiol 1989;10(5):943-948.
76. Saeki N, Tokunaga H, Wagai N, et al. MRI of ectopic posterior pituitary bright spot with large adenomas: appearances and relationship to transient postoperative diabetes insipidus. Neuroradiology 2003; 45(10):713-716.
77. Fujisawa I. Magnetic resonance imaging of the hypothalamic-neurohypophyseal system. J Neuroendocrinol 2004;16(4):297-302.
78. Maghnie M, Genovese E, Bernasconi S, et al. Persistent high MR signal of the posterior pituitary gland in central diabetes insipidus. AJNR Am J Neuroradiol 1997;18(9):1749-1752.
79. Miyamoto S, Sasaki N, Tanabe Y. Magnetic resonance imaging in familial central diabetes insipidus. Neuroradiology 1991; 33(3):272-273.
80. Maghnie M, Villa A, Arico M, et al. Correlation between magnetic resonance imaging of posterior pituitary and neurohypophyseal function in children with diabetes insipidus. J Clin Endocrinol Metab 1992;74(4):795-800.
81. Kubota T, Yamamoto T, Ozono K, et al. Hyperintensity of posterior pituitary on MR T1WI in a boy with central diabetes insipidus caused by missense mutation of neurophysin II gene. Endocr J 2001;48(4):459-463.
82. Yamamoto T, Ishii T, Yoshioka K, et al. Transient central diabetes insipidus in pregnancy with a peculiar change in signal intensity on T1-weighted magnetic resonance images. Intern Med 2003;42(6): 513-516.
83. Heinbecker P, White H. Hypothalamico-hypophysial system and its relation to water balance in the dog. Am J Physiol 1944;133: 582-593.
84. Verbalis J, Robinson A, Moses M. Postoperative and post-traumatic diabetes insipidus. In Czernichowp, Robinson A eds. Diabetes insipidus in man. Karger, Basel, 1985:247-267.
85. Fujisawa I, Uokawa K, Horii N, et al. Bright pituitary stalk on MR T1-weighted image: damming up phenomenon of the neurosecretory granules. Endocr J 2002;49(2):165-173.
86. Prosch H, Grois N, Prayer D, et al. Central diabetes insipidus as presenting symptom of Langerhans cell histiocytosis. Pediatr Blood Cancer 2004;43(5):594-599.
87. Leger J, Velasquez A, Garel C, et al. Thickened pituitary stalk on magnetic resonance imaging in children with central diabetes insipidus. J Clin Endocrinol Metab 1999;84(6):1954-1960.
88. Czernichow P, Garel C, Leger J. Thickened pituitary stalk on magnetic resonance imaging in children with central diabetes insipidus. Horm Res 2000;53(suppl 3):61-64.
89. Maghnie M. Diabetes insipidus. Horm Res 2003;59(suppl 1): 42-54.
90. Siggaard C, Rittig S, Corydon T, et al. Clinical and molecular evidence of abnormal processing and trafficking of the vasopressin preprohormone in a large kindred with familial neurohypophyseal diabetes insipidus due to a signal peptide mutation. J Clin Endocrinol Metab 1999;84(8):2933-2941.
91. Baylis P, Robertson G. Vasopressin function in familial cranial diabetes insipidus. Postgrad Med J 1981;57(663):36-40.
92. Ozata M, Tayfun C, Kurtaran K, et al. Magnetic resonance imaging of posterior pituitary for evaluation of the neurohypophyseal function in idiopathic and autosomal dominant neurohypophyseal diabetes insipidus. Eur Radiol 1997;7(7):1098-1102.
93. Skordis N, Patsalis P, Hettinger J, et al. A novel arginine vasopressin-neurophysin II mutation causes autosomal dominant neurohypophyseal diabetes insipidus and morphologic pituitary changes. Horm Res 2000;53(5):239-245.
94. Baglioni S, Corona G, Maggi M, et al. Identification of a novel mutation in the arginine vasopressin-neurophysin II gene affecting the sixth intrachain disulfide bridge of the neurophysin II moiety. Eur J Endocrinol 2004;151(5):605-611.
95. Christensen J, Siggaard C, Corydon T, et al. Differential cellular handling of defective arginine vasopressin (AVP) prohormones in cells expressing mutations of the AVP gene associated with autosomal dominant and recessive familial neurohypophyseal diabetes insipidus. J Clin Endocrinol Metab 2004;89(9):4521-4531.
96. Rittig S, Siggaard C, Ozata M, et al. Autosomal dominant neurohypophyseal diabetes insipidus due to substitution of histidine for tyrosine(2) in the vasopressin moiety of the hormone precursor. J Clin Endocrinol Metab 2002;87(7):3351-3355.
97. Christensen J, Siggaard C, Rittig S. Autosomal dominant familial neurohypophyseal diabetes insipidus. APMIS Suppl 2003; 109:92-95.
98. Minton J, Rainbow L, Ricketts C, et al. Wolfram syndrome. Rev Endocr Metab Disord 2003;4(1):53-59.

99. ven Ouweland J, Cryns K, Pennings R, et al. Molecular characterization of WFS1 in patients with Wolfram syndrome. J Mol Diagn 2003;5(2):88-95.
100. Cryns K, Sivakumaran T, Van den Ouweland J, et al. Mutational spectrum of the WFS1 gene in Wolfram syndrome, nonsyndromic hearing impairment, diabetes mellitus, and psychiatric disease. Hum Mutat 2003;22(4):275-287.
101. Smith D, Finucane F, Phillips J, et al. Abnormal regulation of thirst and vasopressin secretion following surgery for craniopharyngioma. Clin Endocrinol (Oxf) 2004;61(2):273-279.
102. Karavitaki N, Brufani C, Warner J, et al. Craniopharyngiomas in children and adults: systematic analysis of 121 cases with long-term follow-up. Clin Endocrinol (Oxf) 2005;62(4):397-409.
103. Alter C, Bilaniuk L. Utility of magnetic resonance imaging in the evaluation of the child with central diabetes insipidus. J Pediatr Endocrinol Metab 2002;15(suppl 2):681-687.
104. Max M, Deck M, Rottenberg D. Pituitary metastasis: incidence in cancer patients and clinical differentiation from pituitary adenoma. Neurology 1981;31(8):998-1002.
105. Kovacs K. Metastatic cancer of the pituitary gland. Oncology 1983;27:533-542.
106. Basaria S, Westra W, Brem H, et al. Metastatic renal cell carcinoma to the pituitary presenting with hyperprolactinemia. J Endocrinol Invest 2004;27(5):471-474.
107. Komninos J, Vlassopoulou D, Protopapa V, et al. Tumors metastatic to the pituitary gland: case report and literature review. J Clin Endocrinol Metab 2004;89(2):574-580.
108. Fassett D, Couldwell W. Metastases to the pituitary gland. Neurosurg Focus 2004;16(4):E8.
109. Pascual J, Gonzalez-Llanos F, Roda J. Primary hypothalamic-third ventricle lymphoma. Case report and review of the literature. Neurocirugia (Astur) 2002;13(4):305-310.
110. Agarwal S, Gockerman J, Aldous M, et al. Primary central nervous system lymphoma, presenting as diabetes insipidus, as a sequela of hepatitis C [letter]. Am J Med 1999;107(3):303-304.
111. Castagnola C, Morra E, Bernasconi P, et al. Acute myeloid leukemia and diabetes insipidus: results in 5 patients. Acta Haematol 1995; 93(1):1-4.
112. Foresti V, Casati O, Villa A, et al. Central diabetes insipidus due to acute monocytic leukemia: case report and review of the literature. J Endocrinol Invest 1992;15(2):127-130.
113. Ra'anani P, Shpilberg O, Berezin M, et al. Acute leukemia relapse presenting as central diabetes insipidus. Cancer 1994;73(9): 2312-2316.
114. Dilek J, Uysal A, Demirer T, et al. Acute myeloblastic leukemia associated with hyperleukocytosis and diabetes insipidus. Leuk Lymphoma 1998;30(5-6):657-660.
115. Nieboer P, Vellenga E, Adriaanse R, et al. Central diabetes insipidus preceding acute myeloid leukemia with t(3;12)(q26;p12). Neth J Med 2000;56(2):45-47.
116. Kanabar D, Betts D, Gibbons B, et al. Monosomy 7, diabetes insipidus and acute myeloid leukemia in childhood. Pediatr Hematol Oncol 1994;11(1):111-114.
117. Buonocore C, Robinson A. The diagnosis and management of diabetes insipidus during medical emergencies. Endocrinol Metab Clin North Am 1993;22(2):411-423.
118. Cusick J, Hagen T, Findling J. Inappropriate secretion of antidiuretic hormone after transsphenoidal surgery for pituitary tumors. N Engl J Med 1984;311(1):36-38.
119. Ultmann M, Hoffman G, Nelson P, et al. Transient hyponatremia after damage to the neurohypophyseal tracts. Neuroendocrinology 1992;56(6):803-811.
120. Olson B, Rubino D, Gumowski J, et al. Isolated hyponatremia after transsphenoidal pituitary surgery. J Clin Endocrinol Metab 1995; 80(1):85-91.
121. Olson B, Gumowski J, Rubino D, et al. Pathophysiology of hyponatremia after transsphenoidal pituitary surgery. J Neurosurg 1997;87(4): 499-507.
122. Hensen J, Henig A, Fahlbusch R, et al.Prevalence, predictors and patterns of postoperative polyuria and hyponatraemia in the immediate course after transsphenoidal surgery for pituitary adenomas. Clin.Endocrinol (Oxf) 1999;50(4):431-439.
123. Benvenga S, Campenni A, Ruggeri R, et al. Clinical review 113: Hypopituitarism secondary to head trauma. J Clin Endocrinol Metab 2000;85(4):1353-1361.
124. Boughey J, Yost M, Bynoe R. Diabetes insipidus in the head-injured patient. Am.Surg 2004;70(6):500-503.
125. Agha A, Sherlock M, Phillips J, et al. The natural history of post-traumatic neurohypophysial dysfunction. Eur J Endocrinol 2005;152(3):371-377.
126. Agha A, Thornton E, O'Kelly P, et al. Posterior pituitary dysfunction after traumatic brain injury. J Clin Endocrinol Metab 2004;89(12): 5987-5992.
127. Kilborn T, Teh J, Goodman T. Paediatric manifestations of Langerhans cell histiocytosis: a review of the clinical and radiological findings. Clin Radiol 2003;58(4):269-278.
128. Donadieu J, Rolon M, Thomas C, et al. Endocrine involvement in pediatric-onset Langerhans' cell histiocytosis: a population-based study. J Pediatr 2004;144(3):344-350.
129. Garovic V, Clarke B, Chilson T, et al. Diabetes insipidus and anterior pituitary insufficiency as presenting features of Wegener's granulomatosis. Am J Kidney Dis 2001;37(1):E5.
130. Mahnel R, Tan K, Fahlbusch R, et al. Problems in differential diagnosis of non Langerhans cell histiocytosis with pituitary involvement: case report and review of literature. Endocr Pathol 2002; 13(4):361-368.
131. Tabuena R, Nagai S, Handa T, et al. Diabetes insipidus from neurosarcoidosis: long-term follow-up for more than eight years. Intern Med 2004;43(10):960-966.
132. Pivonello R, De Bellis A, Faggiano A, et al. Central diabetes insipidus and autoimmunity: relationship between the occurrence of antibodies to arginine vasopressin-secreting cells and clinical, immunological, and radiological features in a large cohort of patients with central diabetes insipidus of known and unknown etiology. J Clin Endocrinol Metab 2003;88(4): 1629-1636.
133. De Bellis A, Colao A, Bizzarro A, et al: Longitudinal study of vasopressin-cell antibodies and of hypothalamic-pituitary region on magnetic resonance imaging in patients with autoimmune and idiopathic complete central diabetes insipidus. J Clin Endocrinol Metab 2002;87(8):3825-3829.
134. Takahashi M, Otsuka F, Miyoshi T, et al. An elderly patient with transient diabetes insipidus associated with lymphocytic infundibulo-neurohypophysitis. Endocr J 1999;46(5):741-746.
135. Hashimoto K, Takao T, Makino S. Lymphocytic adenohypophysitis and lymphocytic infundibuloneurohypophysitis. Endocr J 1997; 44(1): 1-10.
136. Thodou E, Asa S, Kontogeorgos G, et al. Clinical case seminar: lymphocytic hypophysitis: clinicopathological findings. J Clin Endocrinol Metab 1995;80(8):2302-2311.
137. Oiso Y. Transient diabetes insipidus during pregnancy. Intern Med 2003;42(6):459-460.
138. Barron W, Cohen L, Ulland L, et al. Transient vasopressin-resistant diabetes insipidus of pregnancy. N Engl J Med 1984; 310(7):442-444.
139. Krege J, Katz V, Bowes W Jr. Transient diabetes insipidus of pregnancy. Obstet Gynecol Surv 1989;44(11):789-795.
140. Kennedy S, Hall P, Seymour A, et al. Transient diabetes insipidus and acute fatty liver of pregnancy. Br J Obstet Gynaecol 1994; 101(5):387-391.
141. Hashimoto M, Ogura T, Otsuka F, et al. Manifestation of subclinical diabetes insipidus due to pituitary tumor during pregnancy. Endocr J 1996;43(5):577-583.
142. Amico J. Diabetes insipidus and pregnancy. In Czernichow P, Robinson A, eds. Diabetes Insipidus in Man. Karger, Basel, 1985:266-277.
143. Sherer D, Cutler J, Santoso P, et al. Severe hypernatremia after cesarean delivery secondary to transient diabetes insipidus of pregnancy. Obstet Gynecol 2003;102(5 Pt 2):1166-1168.
144. Verbalis J. Diabetes insipidus. Rev Endocr Metab Disord 2003; 4(2):177-185.
145. Smith D, McKenna K, Moore K, et al. Baroregulation of vasopressin release in adipsic diabetes insipidus. J Clin Endocrinol Metab 2002;87(10):4564-4568.
146. DeRubertis F, Michelis M, Beck N, et al. "Essential" hypernatremia due to ineffective osmotic and intact volume regulation of vasopressin secretion. J Clin Invest 1971;50(1):97-111.
147. Halter J, Goldberg A, Robertson G, et al. Selective osmoreceptor dysfunction in the syndrome of chronic hypernatremia. J Clin Endocrinol Metab 1977;44(4):609-616.

148. Oh M, Carroll H. Essential hypernatremia: is there such a thing? Nephron 1994;67(2):144-145.
149. Bittner H, Kendall S, Chen E, et al. Endocrine changes and metabolic responses in a validated canine brain death model. J Crit Care 1995;10(2):56-63.
150. Dominguez-Roldan J, Garcia-Alfaro C, Diaz-Parejo P, et al. Risk factors associated with diabetes insipidus in brain dead patients. Transplant Proc 2002;34(1):13-14.
151. Saner F, Kavuk I, Lang H, et al. Organ protective management of the brain-dead donor. Eur J Med Res 2004;9(10):485-490.
152. Guesde R, Barrou B, Leblanc I, et al. Administration of desmopressin in brain-dead donors and renal function in kidney recipients. Lancet 1998;352(9135):1178-1181.
153. Howlett T, Keogh A, Perry L, et al. Anterior and posterior pituitary function in brain-stem-dead donors. A possible role for hormonal replacement therapy. Transplantation 1989;47(5):828-834.
154. Gramm H, Meinhold H, Bickel U, et al. Acute endocrine failure after brain death? Transplantation 1992;54(5):851-857.
155. Wong M, Chin N, Lew T. Diabetes insipidus in neurosurgical patients. Ann Acad Med Singapore 1998;27(3):340-343.
156. Bell N. Endocrine complications of sarcoidosis. Endocrinol Metab Clin North Am 1991;20(3):645-654.
157. Moses A. Clinical and laboratory observations in the adult with diabetes insipidus and related syndromes. In Czernichow P, Robinson A, eds. Diabetes Insipidus in Man. Karger, Basel, 1985:156-175.
158. De Leon J, Dadvand M, Canuso C, et al. Polydipsia and water intoxication in a long-term psychiatric hospital. Biol Psychiatry 1996; 40(1):28-34.
159. Siegel A, Baldessarini J, Klepser M, et al. Primary and drug-induced disorders of water homeostasis in psychiatric patients: principles of diagnosis and management. Harv Rev Psychiatry 1998;6(4): 190-200.
160. Kishi Y, Kurosawa H, Endo S. Is propranolol effective in primary polydipsia? Int J Psychiatry Med 1998;28(3):315-325.
161. van Lieburg A, Knoers N, Monnens L. Clinical presentation and follow-up of 30 patients with congenital nephrogenic diabetes insipidus. J Am Soc Nephrol 1999;10(9):1958-1964.
162. Bichet D. Nephrogenic diabetes insipidus. Am J Med 1998;105(5): 431-442.
163. Knoers N, Monnens L. Nephrogenic diabetes insipidus. Semin Nephrol 1999;19(4):344-352.
164. Thibonnier M. Genetics of vasopressin receptors. Curr Hypertens Rep 2004;6(1):21-26.
165. Schoneberg T, Schulz A, Biebermann H, et al. V2 vasopressin receptor dysfunction in nephrogenic diabetes insipidus caused by different molecular mechanisms. Hum Mutat 1998;12(3): 196-205.
166. Wildin R, Cogdell D. Clinical utility of direct mutation testing for congenital nephrogenic diabetes insipidus in families. Pediatrics 1999;103(3):632-639.
167. Chan Seem C, Dossetor J, Penney M. Nephrogenic diabetes insipidus due to a new mutation of the arginine vasopressin V2 receptor gene in a girl presenting with non-accidental injury. Ann Clin Biochem 1999;36(Pt 6):779-782.
168. Deen P, Knoers N. Vasopressin type-2 receptor and aquaporin-2 water channel mutants in nephrogenic diabetes insipidus. Am J Med Sci 1998;316(5):300-309.
169. Morello J, Bichet D. Nephrogenic diabetes insipidus. Annu Rev Physiol 2001;63:607-630.
170. Canfield M, Tamarappoo B, Moses A, et al. Identification and characterization of aquaporin-2 water channel mutations causing nephrogenic diabetes insipidus with partial vasopressin response. Hum Mol Genet 1997;6(11):1865-1871.
171. van Os C, Deen P. Aquaporin-2 water channel mutations causing nephrogenic diabetes insipidus. Proc Assoc Am Physicians 1998;110(5):395-400.
172. Tamarappoo B, Yang B, Verkman A. Misfolding of mutant aquaporin-2 water channels in nephrogenic diabetes insipidus. J Biol Chem 1999;274(49):34825-34831.
173. Kamsteeg E, Mulders S, Bichet D, et al. Consequences of aquaporin 2 tetramerization for genetics and routing. Nephrol Dial Transplant 2000;15(suppl 6):26-28.
174. de Mattia F, Savelkoul P, Bichet D, et al. A novel mechanism in recessive nephrogenic diabetes insipidus: wild-type aquaporin-2 rescues the apical membrane expression of intracellularly retained AQP2-P262L. Hum Mol Genet 2004;13(24):3045-3056.
175. Nguyen M, Nielsen S, Kurtz I. Molecular pathogenesis of nephrogenic diabetes insipidus. Clin Exp Nephrol 2003;7(1):9-17.
176. Peet M, Pratt J. Lithium. Current status in psychiatric disorders. Drugs 1993;46(1):7-17.
177. Marples D, Frokiaer J, Knepper M, et al. Disordered water channel expression and distribution in acquired nephrogenic diabetes insipidus. Proc Assoc Am Physicians 1998;110(5): 401-406.
178. Marples D, Christensen S, Christensen E, et al. Lithium-induced downregulation of aquaporin-2 water channel expression in rat kidney medulla. J Clin Invest 1995;95(4):1838-1845.
179. Bendz H, Sjodin I, Aurell M. Renal function on and off lithium in patients treated with lithium for 15 years or more. A controlled, prospective lithium-withdrawal study. Nephrol Dial Transplant 1996;11(3): 457-460.
180. Bendz H, Aurell M. Drug-induced diabetes insipidus: incidence, prevention and management. Drug Saf 1999;21(6):449-456.
181. Adrogue H, Madias N. Hypernatremia. N Engl J Med 2000;342(20): 1493-1499.
182. Robinson A, Verbalis J. Diabetes insipidus. Curr Ther Endocrinol Metab 1997;6:1-7.
183. Robinson A. DDAVP in the treatment of central diabetes insipidus. N Engl J Med 1976;294(10):507-511.
184. Richardson D, Robinson A. Desmopressin. Ann Intern Med 1985;103(2): 228-239.
185. Lam K, Wat M, Choi K, et al. Pharmacokinetics, pharmacodynamics, long-term efficacy and safety of oral 1-deamino-8-D-arginine vasopressin in adult patients with central diabetes insipidus. Br J Clin Pharmacol 1996;42(3):379-385.
186. Pokracki F, Robinson A, Seif S. Chlorpropamide effect: measurement of neurophysin and vasopressin in humans and rats. Metabolism 1981;30(1):72-78.
187. Nandi M, Harrington A. Successful treatment of hypernatremic thirst deficiency with chlorpropamide. Clin Nephrol 1978; 10(3):90-95.
188. Bode H, Harley B, Crawford J. Restoration of normal drinking behavior by chlorpropamide in patients with hypodipsia and diabetes insipidus. Am J Med 1971;51(3):304-313.
189. Edwards C, Kitau M, Chard T, et al. Vasopressin analogue DDAVP in diabetes insipidus: clinical and laboratory studies. BMJ 1973;3(876):375-378.
190. Davison J, Sheills E, Philips P, et al. Metabolic clearance of vasopressin and an analogue resistant to vasopressinase in human pregnancy. Am J Physiol 1993;264(2 Pt 2):F348-F353.
191. Burrow G, Wassenaar W, Robertson G, et al. DDAVP treatment of diabetes insipidus during pregnancy and the post- partum period. Acta Endocrinol (Copenh) 1981;97(1):23-25.
192. Ray J. DDAVP use during pregnancy: an analysis of its safety for mother and child. Obstet Gynecol Surv 1998;53(7):450-455.
193. Kallen B, Carlsson S, Bengtsson B. Diabetes insipidus and use of desmopressin (Minirin) during pregnancy. Eur J Endocrinol 1995; 132(2):144-146.
194. Ralston C, Butt W. Continuous vasopressin replacement in diabetes insipidus. Arch Dis Child 1990;65(8):896-897.
195. Lugo N, Silver P, Nimkoff L, et al. Diagnosis and management algorithm of acute onset of central diabetes insipidus in critically ill children. J Pediatr Endocrinol Metab 1997;10(6):633-639.
196. Lee Y, Yang D, Shyur S, et al. Neurogenic diabetes insipidus in a child with fatal Coxsackie virus B1 encephalitis. J Pediatr Endocrinol Metab 1995;8(4):301-304.
197. Chanson P, Jedynak C, Dabrowski G, et al. Ultralow doses of vasopressin in the management of diabetes insipidus. Crit Care Med 1987;15(1):44-46.
198. Postina R, Ufer E, Pfeiffer R, et al. Misfolded vasopressin V2 receptors caused by extracellular point mutations entail congential nephrogenic diabetes insipidus. Mol.Cell Endocrinol 2000;164(1-2): 31-39.
199. Magaldi A. New insights into the paradoxical effect of thiazides in diabetes insipidus therapy. Nephrol Dial Transplant 2000;15(12): 1903-1905.
200. Loffing J. Paradoxical antidiuretic effect of thiazides in diabetes insipidus: another piece in the puzzle. J Am Soc Nephrol 2004;15(11):2948-2950.

201. Hochberg Z, Even L, Danon A. Amelioration of polyuria in nephrogenic diabetes insipidus due to aquaporin-2 deficiency. Clin Endocrinol (Oxf) 1998;49(1):39-44.
202. Bendz H, Aurell M, Balldin J, et al. Kidney damage in long-term lithium patients: a cross-sectional study of patients with 15 years or more on lithium. Nephrol Dial Transplant 1994;9(9):1250-1254.
203. Singer I, Oster J, Fishman L. The management of diabetes insipidus in adults. Arch Intern Med 1997;157(12):1293-1301.
204. Morello J, Salahpour A, Laperriere A, et al. Pharmacological chaperones rescue cell-surface expression and function of misfolded V2 vasopressin receptor mutants. J Clin Invest 2000;105(7):887-895.
205. Tamarappoo B, Verkman A. Defective aquaporin-2 trafficking in nephrogenic diabetes insipidus and correction by chemical chaperones. J Clin Invest 1998;101(10):2257-2267.
206. Bryant W, O'Marcaigh A, Ledger G, et al. Aqueous vasopressin infusion during chemotherapy in patients with diabetes insipidus. Cancer 1994;74(9):2589-2592.
207. Lien Y, Shapiro J, Chan L. Effects of hypernatremia on organic brain osmoles. J Clin Invest 1990;85(5):1427-1435.
208. Brown W, Caruso J. Extrapontine myelinolysis with involvement of the hippocampus in three children with severe hypernatremia. J Child Neurol 1999;14(7):428-433.
209. Fall P. Hyponatremia and hypernatremia. A systematic approach to causes and their correction. Postgrad Med 2000;107(5):75-82.
210. Ayus J, Armstrong D, Arieff A. Effects of hypernatraemia in the central nervous system and its therapy in rats and rabbits. J Physiol (Lond) 1996;492(Pt 1):243-255.
211. Kahn A, Brachet E, Blum D. Controlled fall in natremia and risk of seizures in hypertonic dehydration. Intensive Care Med 1979; 5(1):27-31.
212. Schwartz W, Bennett S, Curelop S, et al. A syndrome of renal sodium loss and hyponatremia probably resulting from inappropriate secretion of antidiuretic hormone. Am J Med 1957; 23:529-542.
213. Bartter F, Schwartz W. The syndrome of inappropriate secretion of antidiuretic hormone. Am J Med 1967;42(5):790-806.
214. Miller M, Morley J, Rubenstein L. Hyponatremia in a nursing home population. J Am Geriatr Soc 1995;43(12):1410-1413.
215. Arieff A, Llach F, Massry S. Neurological manifestations and morbidity of hyponatremia: correlation with brain water and electrolytes. Medicine (Baltimore) 1976;55(2):121-129.
216. Arieff A. Hyponatremia, convulsions, respiratory arrest, and permanent brain damage after elective surgery in healthy women. N Engl J Med 1986;314(24):1529-1535.
217. Sterns R, Riggs J, Schochet S Jr. Osmotic demyelination syndrome following correction of hyponatremia. N Engl J Med 1986;314(24): 1535-1542.
218. Anderson R, Chung H, Kluge R, et al. Hyponatremia: a prospective analysis of its epidemiology and the pathogenetic role of vasopressin. Ann Intern Med 1985;102(2):164-168.
219. Weisberg L. Pseudohyponatremia: a reappraisal. Am J Med 1989;86(3):315-318.
220. Katz M. Hyperglycemia-induced hyponatremia—calculation of expected serum sodium depression. N Engl J Med 1973;289(16): 843-844.
221. Hillier T, Abbott R, Barrett E. Hyponatremia: evaluating the correction factor for hyperglycemia. Am J Med 1999;106(4):399-403.
222. Rose B. New approach to disturbances in the plasma sodium concentration. Am J Med 1986;81(6):1033-1040.
223. Spital A. Diuretic-induced hyponatremia. Am J Nephrol 1999; 19(4):447-452.
224. Gross P, Pehrisch H, Rascher W, et al. Pathogenesis of clinical hyponatremia: observations of vasopressin and fluid intake in 100 hyponatremic medical patients. Eur J Clin Invest 1987; 17(2):123-129.
225. Schrier R. Body fluid volume regulation in health and disease: a unifying hypothesis. Ann Intern Med 1990;113(2):155-159.
226. Demanet J, Bonnyns M, Bleiberg H, et al. Coma due to water intoxication in beer drinkers. Lancet 1971;2(7734):1115-1117.
227. Cooke C, Turin M, Walker W: The syndrome of inappropriate antidiuretic hormone secretion (SIADH): pathophysiologic mechanisms in solute and volume regulation. Medicine (Baltimore) 1979; 58(3):240-251.
228. Grantham J, Linshaw M. The effect of hyponatremia on the regulation of intracellular volume and solute composition. Circ Res 1984;54(5):483-491.
229. Yannet H. Changes in the brain resulting from depletion of extracellular electrolytes. Am J Physiol 1940;128:683-689.
230. Holliday A, Kalayci M, Harrah J. Factors that limit brain volume changes in response to acute and sustained hyper- and hyponatremia. J Clin Invest 1968;47(8):1916-1928.
231. Garcia-Perez A, Burg M. Renal medullary organic osmolytes. Physiol Rev 1991;71(4):1081-1115.
232. Heilig C, Stromski M, Blumenfeld J, et al. Characterization of the major brain osmolytes that accumulate in salt-loaded rats. Am J Physiol 1989;257(6 Pt 2):F1108-F1116.
233. Lien Y, Shapiro J, Chan L. Study of brain electrolytes and organic osmolytes during correction of chronic hyponatremia. Implications for the pathogenesis of central pontine myelinolysis. J Clin Invest 1991;88(1):303-309.
234. Verbalis J, Gullans S. Hyponatremia causes large sustained reductions in brain content of multiple organic osmolytes in rats. Brain Res 1991;567(2):274-282.
235. Videen J, Michaelis T, Pinto P, et al. Human cerebral osmolytes during chronic hyponatremia. A proton magnetic resonance spectroscopy study. J Clin Invest 1995;95(2):788-793.
236. Gullans S, Verbalis J. Control of brain volume during hyperosmolar and hypoosmolar conditions. Annu Rev Med 1993;44:289-301.
237. Graber M, Corish D. The electrolytes in hyponatremia. Am J Kidney Dis 1991;18(5):527-545.
238. Smith M Jr, Cowley M Jr, Guyton A, et al. Acute and chronic effects of vasopressin on blood pressure, electrolytes, and fluid volumes. Am J Physiol 1979;237(3):F232-F240.
239. Verbalis J. Pathogenesis of hyponatremia in an experimental model of the syndrome of inappropriate antidiuresis. Am J Physiol 1994;267(6 Pt 2):R1617-R1625.
240. Southgate H, Burke B, Walters G. Body space measurements in the hyponatraemia of carcinoma of the bronchus: evidence for the chronic "sick cell" syndrome? Ann Clin Biochem 1992;29(Pt 1):90-95.
241. Verbalis J. Hyponatremia: epidemiology, pathophysiology, and therapy. Curr Opin Nephrol Hypertens 1993;2(4):636-652.
242. Clark B, Shannon R, Rosa R, et al. Increased susceptibility to thiazide-induced hyponatremia in the elderly. J Am Soc Nephrol 1994; 5(4):1106-1111.
243. Zennaro M. Mineralocorticoid resistance. Steroids 1996;61(4): 189-192.
244. Chung H, Kluge R, Schrier R, et al. Clinical assessment of extracellular fluid volume in hyponatremia. Am J Med 1987; 83(5): 905-908.
245. Michelis M, Fusco R, Bragdon R, et al. Reset of osmoreceptors in association with normovolemic hyponatremia. Am J Med Sci 1974;267(5): 267-273.
246. Beck L. Hypouricemia in the syndrome of inappropriate secretion of antidiuretic hormone. N Engl J Med 1979;301(10):528-530.
247. Robertson G, Mahr E, Athar S, et al. Development and clinical application of a new method for the radioimmunoassay of arginine vasopressin in human plasma. J Clin Invest 1973; 52(9): 2340-2352.
248. Zerbe R, Stropes L, Robertson G. Vasopressin function in the syndrome of inappropriate antidiuresis. Annu Rev Med 1980; 31:315-327.
249. List A, Hainsworth J, Davis B, et al. The syndrome of inappropriate secretion of antidiuretic hormone (SIADH) in small-cell lung cancer. J Clin Oncol 1986;4(8):1191-1198.
250. Maurer L, O'Donnell J, Kennedy S, et al. Human neurophysins in carcinoma of the lung: relation to histology, disease stage, response rate, survival, and syndrome of inappropriate antidiuretic hormone secretion. Cancer Treat Rep 1983;67(11):971-976.
251. Ferlito A, Rinaldo A, Devaney K. Syndrome of inappropriate antidiuretic hormone secretion associated with head neck cancers: review of the literature. Ann Otol Rhinol Laryngol 1997;106(10 Pt 1):878-883.
252. Kavanagh B, Halperin E, Rosenbaum L, et al. Syndrome of inappropriate secretion of antidiuretic hormone in a patient with carcinoma of the nasopharynx. Cancer 1992;69(6):1315-1319.
253. Berghmans T, Paesmans M, Body J. A prospective study on hyponatraemia in medical cancer patients: epidemiology, aetiology

and differential diagnosis. Support Care Cancer 2000;8(3): 192-197.
254. Moses A, Miller M. Drug-induced dilutional hyponatremia. N Engl J Med 1974;291(23):1234-1239.
255. Gibbs D, Vale W. Effect of the serotonin reuptake inhibitor fluoxetine on corticotropin-releasing factor and vasopressin secretion into hypophysial portal blood. Brain Res 1983;280(1):176-179.
256. Faull C, Rooke P, Baylis P. The effect of a highly specific serotonin agonist on osmoregulated vasopressin secretion in healthy man. Clin Endocrinol (Oxf) 1991;35(5):423-430.
257. Wilkinson T, Begg E, Winter A, et al. Incidence and risk factors for hyponatraemia following treatment with fluoxetine or paroxetine in elderly people. Br J Clin Pharmacol 1999;47(2):211-217.
258. Burgess C, O'Donohoe A, Gill M. Agony and ecstasy: a review of MDMA effects and toxicity. Eur Psychiatry 2000;15(5):287-294.
259. Kelestimur H, Leach R, Ward J, et al. Vasopressin and oxytocin release during prolonged environmental hypoxia in the rat. Thorax 1997;52(1):84-88.
260. Tang W, Kaptein E, Feinstein E, et al. Hyponatremia in hospitalized patients with the acquired immunodeficiency syndrome (AIDS) and the AIDS-related complex. Am J Med 1993;94(2):169-174.
261. Yeung K, Chan M, Chan C. The safety of i.v. pentamidine administered in an ambulatory setting. Chest 1996;110(1):136-140.
262. Miller M, Hecker M, Friedlander D, et al. Apparent idiopathic hyponatremia in an ambulatory geriatric population. J Am Geriatr Soc 1996;44(4):404-408.
263. Hirshberg B, Ben Yehuda A. The syndrome of inappropriate antidiuretic hormone secretion in the elderly. Am J Med 1997; 103(4):270-273.
264. Ishikawa S, Kuratomi Y, Saito T. A case of oat cell carcinoma of the lung associated with ectopic production of ADH, neurophysin and ACTH. Endocrinol Jpn 1980;27(2):257-263.
265. Robertson G, Athar S. The interaction of blood osmolality and blood volume in regulating plasma vasopressin in man. J Clin Endocrinol Metab 1976;42(4):613-620.
266. Kamoi K. Syndrome of inappropriate antidiuresis without involving inappropriate secretion of vasopressin in an elderly woman: effect of intravenous administration of the nonpeptide vasopressin V2 receptor antagonist OPC-31260. Nephron 1997;76(1):111-115.
267. Feldman B, Rosenthal S, Vargas G, et al. Nephrogenic syndrome of inappropriate antidiuresis. N Engl J Med 2005; 352(18): 1884-1890.
268. Leaf A, Bartter F, Santos R, et al. Syndrome in man that urinary electrolyte loss induced by pitressin is a function of water retention. J Clin Invest 1953;32:868-878.
269. Peters J, Welt K, Sims E, et al. A salt-wasting syndrome associated with cerebral disease. Trans Ass Am Physiol 1950;63:57-64.
270. Nelson P, Seif S, Gutai J, et al. Hyponatremia and natriuresis following subarachnoid hemorrhage in a monkey model. J Neurosurg 1984;60(2):233-237.
271. Wijdicks E, Ropper A, Hunnicutt E, et al. Atrial natriuretic factor and salt wasting after aneurysmal subarachnoid hemorrhage. Stroke 1991;22(12):1519-1524.
272. Oh M, Carroll H. Cerebral salt-wasting syndrome. We need better proof of its existence. Nephron 1999;82(2):110-114.
273. Maesaka J, Gupta S, Fishbane S. Cerebral salt-wasting syndrome: does it exist? Nephron 1999;82(2):100-109.
274. Diringer M, Lim J, Kirsch J, et al. Suprasellar and intraventricular blood predict elevated plasma atrial natriuretic factor in subarachnoid hemorrhage. Stroke 1991;22(5):577-581.
275. Diringer M, Wu K, Verbalis J, et al. Hypervolemic therapy prevents volume contraction but not hyponatremia following subarachnoid hemorrhage. Ann Neurol 1992;31(5):543-550.
276. Tian Y, Sandberg K, Murase T, et al. Vasopressin V2 receptor binding is down-regulated during renal escape from vasopressin-induced antidiuresis. Endocrinology 2000;141(1):307-314.
277. Verbalis J, Murase T, Ecelbarger C, et al. Studies of renal aquaporin-2 expression during renal escape from vasopressin-induced antidiuresis. Adv Exp Med Biol 1998;449:395-406.
278. Fraser C, Arieff A. Epidemiology, pathophysiology, and management of hyponatremic encephalopathy. Am J Med 1997; 102(1):67-77.
279. Daggett P, Deanfield J, Moss F. Neurological aspects of hyponatraemia. Postgrad Med J 1982;58(686):737-740.
280. Ayus J, Wheeler J, Arieff A. Postoperative hyponatremic encephalopathy in menstruant women. Ann Intern Med 1992;117(11): 891-897.
281. Wijdicks E, Sharbrough F. New-onset seizures in critically ill patients. Neurology 1993;43(5):1042-1044.
282. Vexler Z, Ayus J, Roberts T, et al. Hypoxic and ischemic hypoxia exacerbate brain injury associated with metabolic encephalopathy in laboratory animals. J Clin Invest 1994;93(1):256-264.
283. Ayus J, Arieff A. Pulmonary complications of hyponatremic encephalopathy. Noncardiogenic pulmonary edema and hypercapnic respiratory failure. Chest 1995;107(2):517-521.
284. Ayus J, Varon J, Arieff A. Hyponatremia, cerebral edema, and noncardiogenic pulmonary edema in marathon runners. Ann Intern Med 2000;132(9):711-714.
285. Arieff A, Ayus J, Fraser C. Hyponatraemia and death or permanent brain damage in healthy children. BMJ 1992; 304(6836):1218-1222.
286. Wattad A, Chiang M, Hill L. Hyponatremia in hospitalized children. Clin Pediatr (Phila) 1992;31(3):153-157.
287. Wijdicks E, Larson T. Absence of postoperative hyponatremia syndrome in young, healthy females. Ann Neurol 1994;35(5): 626-628.
288. Carroll P, McHenry L, Verbalis J. Isolated adrenocorticotrophic hormone deficiency presenting as chronic hyponatremia. N Y State J Med 1990;90(4):210-213.
289. Wright D, Laureno R, Victor M. Pontine and extrapontine myelinolysis. Brain 1979;102(2):361-385.
290. Verbalis J, Martinez A. Neurological and neuropathological sequelae of correction of chronic hyponatremia. Kidney Int 1991;39(6): 1274-1282.
291. Verbalis J, Baldwin E, Robinson A. Osmotic regulation of plasma vasopressin and oxytocin after sustained hyponatremia. Am J Physiol 1986;250(3 Pt 2):R444-R451.
292. Sterns R, Thomas D, Herndon R. Brain dehydration and neurologic deterioration after rapid correction of hyponatremia. Kidney Int 1989;35(1):69-75.
293. Adler S, Martinez J, Williams D, et al. Positive association between blood brain barrier disruption and osmotically-induced demyelination. Mult Scler 2000;6(1):24-31.
294. Baker E, Tian Y, Adler S, et al. Blood-brain barrier disruption and complement activation in the brain following rapid correction of chronic hyponatremia. Exp Neurol 2000;165(2):221-230.
295. Sterns R. The management of symptomatic hyponatremia. Semin Nephrol 1990;10(6):503-514.
296. Soupart A, Penninckx R, Stenuit A, et al. Treatment of chronic hyponatremia in rats by intravenous saline: comparison of rate versus magnitude of correction. Kidney Int 1992;41(6): 1662-1667.
297. Ayus J, Krothapalli R, Arieff A. Treatment of symptomatic hyponatremia and its relation to brain damage. A prospective study. N Engl J Med 1987;317(19):1190-1195.
298. Sterns R, Cappuccio J, Silver S, et al. Neurologic sequelae after treatment of severe hyponatremia: a multicenter perspective. J Am Soc.Nephrol 1994;4(8):1522-1530.
299. Verbalis J. Hyponatremia. Endocrinologic causes and consequences of therapy. Trends Endocrinol Metab 1992;3:1-7.
300. Ellis S. Extrapontine myelinolysis after correction of chronic hyponatraemia with isotonic saline. Br J Clin Pract 1995;49(1):49-50.
301. Cheng J, Zikos D, Skopicki H, et al. Long-term neurologic outcome in psychogenic water drinkers with severe symptomatic hyponatremia: the effect of rapid correction. Am J Med 1990;88(6): 561-566.
302. Adams R, Victor M, Mancall E. Central pontine myelinolysis: a hitherto undescribed disease occurring in alcoholic and malnourished patients. Arch Neurol Psych 1959;81:154-172.
303. Kelly J, Wassif W, Mitchard J, et al. Severe hyponatraemia secondary to beer potomania complicated by central pontine myelinolysis. Int J Clin Pract 1998;52(8):585-587.
304. Soupart A, Penninckx R, Stenuit A, et al. Azotemia (48 h) decreases the risk of brain damage in rats after correction of chronic hyponatremia. Brain Res 2000;852(1):167-172.
305. Brunner J, Redmond J, Haggar A, et al. Central pontine myelinolysis and pontine lesions after rapid correction of hyponatremia: a prospective magnetic resonance imaging study. Ann Neurol 1990;27(1):61-66.

306. Kumar S, Mone A, Gray L, et al. Central pontine myelinolysis: delayed changes on neuroimaging. J Neuroimaging 2000;10(3): 169-172.
307. Soupart A, Penninckx R, Namias B, et al. Brain myelinolysis following hypernatremia in rats. J Neuropath Exp Neurol 1997;55:106-113.
308. McComb R, Pfeiffer R, Casey J, et al. Lateral pontine and extrapontine myelinolysis associated with hypernatremia and hyperglycemia. Clin Neuropathol 1989;8(6):284-288.
309. Berl T. Treating hyponatremia: damned if we do and damned if we don't. Kidney Int 1990;37(3):1006-1018.
310. Verbalis J. Adaptation to acute and chronic hyponatremia: implications for symptomatology, diagnosis, and therapy. Semin Nephrol 1998;18(1):3-19.
311. Ayus J, Arieff A. Brain damage and postoperative hyponatremia: the role of gender. Neurology 1996;46(2):323-328.
312. Lohr J. Osmotic demyelination syndrome following correction of hyponatremia: association with hypokalemia. Am J Med 1994;96(5):408-413.
313. Hantman D, Rossier B, Zohlman R, et al. Rapid correction of hyponatremia in the syndrome of inappropriate secretion of antidiuretic hormone. An alternative treatment to hypertonic saline. Ann Intern Med 1973;78(6):870-875.
314. Tanneau R, Henry A, Rouhart F, et al. High incidence of neurologic complications following rapid correction of severe hyponatremia in polydipsic patients. J Clin Psychiatry 1994;55(8):349-354.
315. Soupart A, Penninckx R, Stenuit A, et al. Reinduction of hyponatremia improves survival in rats with myelinolysis-related neurologic symptoms. J Neuropathol Exp Neurol 1996;55(5):594-601.
316. Sugimura Y, Murase T, Takefuji S, et al. Protective effect of dexamethasone on osmotic-induced demyelination in rats. Exp Neurol 2005;192(1):178-183.
317. De Troyer A. Demeclocycline. Treatment for syndrome of inappropriate antidiuretic hormone secretion. JAMA 1977;237(25): 2723-2726.
318. Miller P, Linas S, Schrier R. Plasma demeclocycline levels and nephrotoxicity. Correlation in hyponatremic cirrhotic patients. JAMA 1980;243(24):2513-2515.
319. Forrest J Jr, Cox M, Hong C, et al. Superiority of demeclocycline over lithium in the treatment of chronic syndrome of inappropriate secretion of antidiuretic hormone. N Engl J Med 1978; 298(4):173-177.
320. Decaux G, Mols P, Cauchi P, et al. Use of urea for treatment of water retention in hyponatraemic cirrhosis with ascites resistant to diuretics. Br Med J (Clin Res Ed) 1985;290(6484):1782-1783.
321. Brooks D, Valente M, Petrone G, et al. Comparison of the water diuretic activity of kappa receptor agonists and a vasopressin receptor antagonist in dogs. J Pharmacol Exp Ther 1997; 280(3):1176-1183.
322. Gadano A, Moreau R, Pessione F, et al. Aquaretic effects of niravoline, a kappa-opioid agonist, in patients with cirrhosis. J Hepatol 2000;32(1):38-42.
323. Yamamura Y, Ogawa H, Yamashita H, et al. Characterization of a novel aquaretic agent, OPC-31260, as an orally effective, nonpeptide vasopressin V2 receptor antagonist. Br J Pharmacol 1992; 105(4):787-791.
324. Serradeil-Le Gal C, Lacour C, Valette G, et al. Characterization of SR 121463A, a highly potent and selective, orally active vasopressin V2 receptor antagonist. J Clin Invest 1996;98(12): 2729-2738.
325. Tahara A, Tomura Y, Wada K, et al. Pharmacological profile of YM087, a novel potent nonpeptide vasopressin V1A and V2 receptor antagonist, in vitro and in vivo. J Pharmacol Exp Ther 1997;282(1): 301-308.
326. Greenberg A, Verbalis J. Vasopressin receptor antagonists. Kidney Int 2006;12:2124-2130.
327. Verbalis J, Martinez A. Determinants of brain myelinolysis following correction of chronic hyponatremia in rats. In Jamison, Jard, eds. Vasopressin. Paris: John Libbey, 1991:539-547.
328. Insel T, Gingrich B, Young L. Oxytocin: who needs it? Prog Brain Res 2001;133:59-66.
329. Glasier A, McNeilly A. Physiology of lactation. Baillieres Clin Endocrinol Metab 1990;4(2):379-395.
330. Crowley W, Armstrong W. Neurochemical regulation of oxytocin secretion in lactation. Endocr Rev 1992;13(1):33-65.
331. Giraldi A, Enevoldsen A, Wagner G. Oxytocin and the initiation of parturition. A review. Dan Med Bull 1990;37(4):377-383.
332. Uvnas-Moberg K, Eriksson M. Breastfeeding: physiological, endocrine and behavioural adaptations caused by oxytocin and local neurogenic activity in the nipple and mammary gland. Acta Paediatr 1996;85(5):525-530.
333. Brown D, Moos F. Onset of bursting in oxytocin cells in suckled rats. J Physiol (Lond) 1997;503(Pt 3):625-634.
334. McKenzie D, Leng G, Dyball R. Electrophysiological evidence for mutual excitation of oxytocin cells in the supraoptic nucleus of the rat hypothalamus. J Physiol (Lond) 1995;485(Pt 2):485-492.
335. Higuchi T, Okere C. Role of the supraoptic nucleus in regulation of parturition and milk ejection revisited. Microsc Res Tech 2002;56(2):113-121.
336. Young III W, Shepard E, DeVries A, et al. Targeted reduction of oxytocin expression provides insights into its physiological roles. Adv Exp Med Biol 1998;449:231-240.
337. Wagner K, Young III W, Liu X, et al. Oxytocin and milk removal are required for post-partum mammary-gland development. Genes Funct 1997;1(4):233-244.
338. Renfrew M, Lang S, Woolridge M. Oxytocin for promoting successful lactation. Cochrane Database Syst Rev 2000;2:CD000156.
339. Crowley W, Parker S, Armstrong, et al. Neurotransmitter and neurohormonal regulation of oxytocin secretion in lactation. Ann N Y Acad Sci 1992;652:286-302.
340. Lindow S, Hendricks M, Nugent F, et al. Morphine suppresses the oxytocin response in breast-feeding women. Gynecol Obstet Invest 1999;48(1):33-37.
341. Jenkins J, Nussey S. The role of oxytocin: present concepts. Clin Endocrinol (Oxf) 1991;34(6):515-525.
342. Yokoyama Y, Ueda T, Irahara M, et al. Releases of oxytocin and prolactin during breast massage and suckling in puerperal women. Eur J Obstet Gynecol Reprod Biol 1994;53(1):17-20.
343. McNeilly A, Tay C, Glasier A. Physiological mechanisms underlying lactational amenorrhea. Ann N Y Acad Sci 1994;709:145-155.
344. Wang H, Ward A, Morris J. Oestradiol acutely stimulates exocytosis of oxytocin and vasopressin from dendrites and somata of hypothalamic magnocellular neurons. Neuroscience 1995;68(4): 1179-1188.
345. Thomas A, Crowley R, Amico J. Effect of progesterone on hypothalamic oxytocin messenger ribonucleic acid levels in the lactating rat. Endocrinology 1995;136(10):4188-4194.
346. Leng G. Steroidal influences on oxytocin neurones [comment]. J Physiol (Lond) 2000;524(Pt 2):315.
347. Johnston J, Amico J. A prospective longitudinal study of the release of oxytocin and prolactin in response to infant suckling in long term lactation. J Clin Endocrinol Metab 1986;62(4):653-657.
348. De Coopman J. Breastfeeding after pituitary resection: support for a theory of autocrine control of milk supply? J Hum Lact 1993;9(1):35-40.
349. Robinson A, Amico J. Remarks on the history of oxytocin. In Amico, Robinson, eds. Oxytocin: clinical and laboratory studies. Proceedings of the Second International Conference on Oxytocin, Lac Beauport, Quebec, Canada, June 29 to July 1, 1984, xvii-xxiv. Amsterdam, Excerpta Medica, 1985.
350. Mitchell B, Schmid B. Oxytocin and its receptor in the process of parturition. J Soc Gynecol Investig 2001;8(3):122-133.
351. Russell J, Leng G, Douglas A. The magnocellular oxytocin system, the fount of maternity: adaptations in pregnancy. Front Neuroendocrinol 2003;24(1):27-61.
352. Blanks A, Thornton S. The role of oxytocin in parturition. Br J Obstet Gynaecol 2003;110(suppl 20):46-51.
353. Olson D, Mijovic J, Sadowsky D. Control of human parturition. Semin Perinatol 1995;19(1):52-63.
354. Evans J. Oxytocin in the human—regulation of derivations and destinations. Eur J Endocrinol 1997;137(6):559-571.
355. Hertelendy F, Zakar T. Prostaglandins and the myometrium and cervix. Prostaglandins Leukot Essent Fatty Acids 2004; 70(2):207-222.
356. Muglia L. Genetic analysis of fetal development and parturition control in the mouse. Pediatr Res 2000;47(4 Pt 1):437-443.
357. Moran D, McGarrigle H, Lachelin G. Lack of normal increase in saliva estriol/progesterone ratio in women with labor induced at 42 weeks' gestation. Am J Obstet Gynecol 1992;167(6): 1563-1564.

358. Mitchell B, Chibbar R. Synthesis and metabolism of oxytocin in late gestation in human decidua. Adv Exp Med Biol 1995;395:365-380.
359. Russell J, Leng G. Sex, parturition and motherhood without oxytocin? J Endocrinol 1998;157(3):343-359.
360. Mitchell B, Chibbar R, Miller F, et al. Estrogen regulates oxytocin gene expression in term human fetal membranes and decidua. Presented at the meeting of the Society for Gynecologic Investigation, Toronto, 1992.
361. Chibbar R, Miller F, Mitchell B. Synthesis of oxytocin in amnion, chorion, and decidua may influence the timing of human parturition. J Clin Invest 1993;91(1):185-192.
362. Mitchell B, Fang X, Wong S. Oxytocin: a paracrine hormone in the regulation of parturition? Rev Reprod 1998;3(2):113-122.
363. Keelan J, Coleman M, Mitchell M. The molecular mechanisms of term and preterm labor: recent progress and clinical implications. Clin Obstet Gynecol 1997;40(3):460-478.
364. McLean M, Smith R. Corticotrophin-releasing hormone and human parturition. Reproduction 2001;121(4):493-501.
365. Steer P. The endocrinology of parturition in the human. Baillieres Clin Endocrinol Metab 1990;4(2):333-349.
366. Mohan A, Loudon J, Bennett P. Molecular and biochemical mechanisms of preterm labour. Semin Fetal Neonatal Med 2004;9(6):437-444.
367. Weiss G. Endocrinology of parturition. J Clin Endocrinol Metab 2000;85(12):4421-4425.
368. Uozumi N, Kume K, Nagase T, et al. Role of cytosolic phospholipase A2 in allergic response and parturition. Nature 1997;390(6660):618-622.
369. Hirst J, Haluska G, Cook M, et al. Comparison of plasma oxytocin and catecholamine concentrations with uterine activity in pregnant rhesus monkeys. J Clin Endocrinol Metab 1991;73(4):804-810.
370. Honnebier M, Myers T, Figueroa J, et al. Variation in myometrial response to intravenous oxytocin administration at different times of the day in the pregnant rhesus monkey. Endocrinology 1989;125(3):1498-1503.
371. Walsh S, Stanczyk F, Novy M. Daily hormonal changes in the maternal, fetal, and amniotic fluid compartments before parturition in a primate species. J Clin Endocrinol Metab 1984;58(4):629-639.
372. Nathanielsz P. A time to be born: implications of animal studies in maternal-fetal medicine. Birth 1994;21(3):163-169.
373. Robinson A, Archer D, Tolstoi L. Neurophysin in women during oxytocin-related events. J Clin Endocrinol Metab 1973;37(5):645-652.
374. De Wied D, Diamant M, Fodor M. Central nervous system effects of the neurohypophyseal hormones and related peptides. Front Neuroendocrinol 1993;14(4):251-302.
375. Pedersen C. Oxytocin control of maternal behavior. Regulation by sex steroids and offspring stimuli. Ann N Y Acad Sci 1997;807:126-145.
376. Argiolas A, Gessa G. Central functions of oxytocin. Neurosci Biobehav Rev 1991;15(2):217-231.
377. Insel T, Young L, Wang Z. Central oxytocin and reproductive behaviours. Rev Reprod 1997;2(1):28-37.

SECTION III

Thyroid

CHAPTER 10

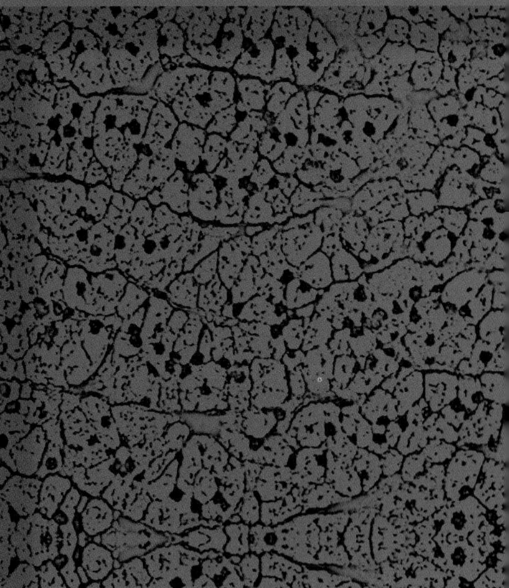

THYROID PHYSIOLOGY AND DIAGNOSTIC EVALUATION OF PATIENTS WITH THYROID DISORDERS

P. Reed Larsen, Terry F. Davies, Martin-Jean Schlumberger, and Ian D. Hay

Dysfunction and anatomic abnormalities of the thyroid are among the most common diseases of the endocrine glands. This chapter provides an up-to-date physiologic and biochemical background and describes the various tests for evaluating patients with suspected thyroid disease based on the pathophysiology of these conditions.

PHYLOGENY, EMBRYOLOGY, AND ONTOGENY

Phylogeny

The phylogeny, embryogenesis, and certain aspects of thyroid function are closely interlinked with the gastrointestinal tract. The capacity of the thyroid to metabolize iodine and incorporate it into a variety of organic compounds occurs widely throughout the animal and plant kingdoms. Monoiodotyrosine (3′-monoiodo-L-tyrosine [MIT]) and diiodotyrosine (3,5′-diiodo-L-tyrosine [DIT]) are present in a variety of invertebrate species, including mollusks, crustaceans, coelenterates, annelids, insects, and certain marine algae (Fig. 10–1). In these lower forms, however, no recognizable thyroid tissue is present. Thyroid tissue is confined to, and is present in, all vertebrates. A close link to the thyroid of higher vertebrates is evident in the ammocoete, the larval form of the lamprey. Here the endostyle is capable of carrying out iodinations, but prior to metamorphosis, a protease is expressed in the endostyle that can hydrolyze the iodoprotein formed. Presumably this permits the endostyle to lose its connection with the pharynx during metamorphosis and to assume its adult function as an endocrine organ that secretes iodothyronines, including 3,5,3′,5′-tetraiodo-L-thyronine (thyroxine, T_4) and 3,5,3′-triiodo-L-thyronine (T_3) (see Fig. 10–1).

The phylogenetic association of the thyroid gland and the gastrointestinal tract is evident in several functions. The salivary and gastric glands, like the thyroid, are capable of concentrating iodide in their secretions, although iodide transport in these

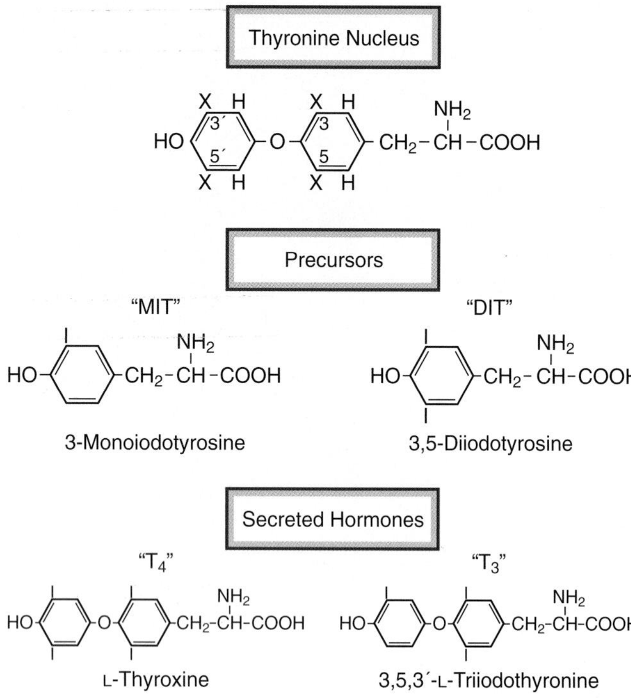

Figure 10–1 ▪ Structure of thyroid hormone and related compounds. The thyronine nucleus, the precursor iodinated amino acids, and the secreted hormones, T_4 and T_3. Iodinated thyronines are formed by the oxidative coupling of the precursor iodotyrosines monoiodotyrosine and diiodotyrosine (MIT and DIT) in the thyroglobulin molecule.

sites is not responsive to stimulation by thyrotropin (TSH). The salivary gland contains enzymes that are capable of iodinating tyrosine in the presence of hydrogen peroxide, although it forms insignificant quantities of iodoproteins under normal circumstances.

Structural Embryology

The human thyroid anlage is first recognizable at E16-17. The primordium begins as a thickening of epithelium in the pharyngeal floor, which later forms a diverticulum adjacent to the developing myocardial cells. With continuing development, the median diverticulum is displaced caudally following the myocardial cells in their descent. The primitive stalk connecting the primordium with the pharyngeal floor elongates into the thyroglossal duct. During its caudal displacement, the primordium assumes a bilobate shape, coming into contact and fusing with the ventral aspect of the fourth pharyngeal pouch when it reaches its final position at about E50. Normally the thyroglossal duct undergoes dissolution and fragmentation by about the second month after conception, leaving at its point of origin a small dimple at the junction of the middle and posterior thirds of the tongue, the *foramen caecum.* Cells of the lower portion of the duct differentiate into thyroid tissue, forming the pyramidal lobe of the gland. At this time the lobes contact the ultimobranchial glands, leading to the incorporation of C cells into the thyroid. Concomitantly, histologic alterations occur throughout the gland. Complex interconnecting cordlike arrangements of cells interspersed with vascular connective tissue replace the solid epithelial mass and become tubule-like structures at about the third month of fetal life; shortly thereafter, follicular arrangements devoid of colloid appear, and by 13 to 14 weeks the follicles begin to fill with colloid. Investigations of thyroid gland development in mice using gene targeting techniques are beginning to identify the critical factors which are required for normal thyroid gland development.[1,2] The role of these various homeobox proteins is currently being evaluated with respect to the potential for defects in the synthesis or formation of the thyroid gland (see Chapter 12).

Functional Ontogeny

The ontogeny of thyroid function and its regulation in the human fetus are fairly well defined.[3] Future follicular cells acquire the capacity to form thyroglobulin (Tg) as early as the 29th day of gestation, whereas the capacities to concentrate iodide and synthesize thyroxine (T_4) are delayed until about the 11th week. Radioactive iodine inadvertently given to the mother would be accumulated by the fetal thyroid soon thereafter. Early growth and development of the thyroid do not seem to be TSH-dependent, because the capacity of the pituitary to synthesize and secrete TSH is not apparent until the 14th week. Subsequently, rapid changes in pituitary and thyroid function take place. Probably as a consequence of hypothalamic maturation and increasing secretion of thyrotropin-releasing hormone (TRH), the serum TSH concentration increases between 18 and 26 weeks' gestation, after which levels remain higher than those in the mother.[3,4] The higher levels may reflect a higher set-point of the negative feedback control of TSH secretion during fetal life than at maturity. Thyroxine-binding globulin (TBG), the major thyroid hormone–binding protein in plasma, is detectable in the serum by the 10th gestational week and increases in concentration progressively to term. This increase in TBG concentration accounts in part for the progressive increase in the serum T_4 concentration during the second and third trimesters, but increased secretion of T_4 must also play a role because the concentration of or free T_4 also rises.

Several aspects of thyroid development are of note from the clinical standpoint.[5] Rarely, thyroid tissue may develop from remnants of the thyroglossal duct near the base of the tongue. Such lingual thyroid tissue may be the sole functioning thyroid present and, thus, its surgical removal will lead to hypothyroidism. More commonly, elements of the thyroglossal duct may persist and later give rise to thyroglossal duct cysts, or ectopic thyroid tissue may be present at any location in the mediastinum or, rarely, even in the heart.

ANATOMY AND HISTOLOGY

The thyroid is one of the largest of the endocrine organs, weighing approximately 15 to 20 g in North American adults. Moreover, the potential of the thyroid for growth is tremendous. The enlarged thyroid, commonly termed a *goiter,* can weigh many hundreds of grams. The normal thyroid is made up of two lobes joined by a thin band of tissue, the isthmus. The latter is approximately 0.5 cm thick, 2 cm wide, and 1 to 2 cm high. The individual lobes normally have a pointed superior pole and a poorly defined blunt inferior pole that merges medially with the isthmus. Each lobe is approximately 2.0 to 2.5 cm in thickness and width at its largest diameter and is approximately 4.0 cm in length. Occasionally, especially when the remainder of the gland is enlarged, a pyramidal lobe is discernible as a finger-like projection directed upward from the isthmus, generally just lateral to the midline, usually on the left. The right lobe is normally more vascular than the left, is often the larger of the two, and tends to enlarge more in disorders associated with a diffuse increase in gland size. Two pairs of vessels constitute the major arterial blood supply, the superior thyroid artery, arising from the external carotid artery, and the inferior thyroid artery, arising from the subclavian artery. Estimates of thyroid blood flow range from 4 to 6 mL/min/g, well in excess of the blood flow to the kidney (3 mL/min/g). In diffuse toxic goiter due to Graves' disease, blood flow may exceed 1 L/min and be associated with an audible bruit or even a palpable thrill.

The gland is composed of closely packed spherical units termed *follicles*, which are invested with a rich capillary network. The interior of the follicle is filled with the clear proteinaceous colloid that normally is the major constituent of the total thyroid mass. On cross section, thyroid tissue appears as closely packed ring-shaped structures consisting of a single layer of thyroid cells surrounding a lumen. The diameter of the follicles varies considerably, even within a single gland, but averages about 200 μm. The follicular cells vary in height with the degree of glandular stimulation, becoming columnar when active and cuboidal when inactive. The epithelium rests on a basement membrane that is rich with glycoproteins separating the follicular cells from the surrounding capillaries. From 20 to 40 follicles are demarcated by connective tissue septa to form a lobule supplied by a single artery. The function of a given lobule may differ from that of its neighbors.

On electron microscopy, the thyroid follicular epithelium has many features in common with other secretory cells and some peculiar to the thyroid. From the apex of the follicular cell, numerous microvilli extend into the colloid. It is at or near this surface of the cell that iodination, exocytosis, and the initial phase of hormone secretion, namely colloid resorption, occur (Fig. 10–2).[6] The nucleus has no distinctive features and the cytoplasm contains an extensive endoplasmic reticulum laden with microsomes. The endoplasmic reticulum is composed of a network of wide irregular tubules that contain the precursor of Tg. The carbohydrate component of Tg is added to this precursor in the Golgi apparatus which is located apically. Lysosomes and mitochondria are scattered throughout the cytoplasm. Stimulation by TSH results in enlargement of the Golgi apparatus, formation of pseudopodia at the apical surface, and the appearance in the apical portion of the cell of many droplets that contain colloid taken up from the follicular lumen (see Fig. 10–2).

The thyroid also contains parafollicular cells, or C cells, that are the source of calcitonin. These cells arise during embryonic development from the last pair of pharyngeal pouches but ultimately come to rest either among the cells of the follicular epithelium or in the thyroid interstitium. They differ from the cells of the follicular epithelium in never bordering on the follicular lumen and in being rich in mitochondria. The C cells undergo hyperplasia early in the syndrome of familial medullary carcinoma of the thyroid (MEN2) and give rise to this tumor in both its familial and its sporadic forms (see Chapter 40).

IODINE AND THE SYNTHESIS AND SECRETION OF THYROID HORMONES

Overview

The function of the thyroid is to generate the quantity of thyroid hormone necessary to meet the demands of the peripheral tissues. This requires the daily thyroidal cell transport by the sodium-iodide symporter (NIS) of sufficient iodide, its transfer to the colloid and its oxidation by thyroid peroxidase (TPO) to allow the synthesis of approximately 110 nmoles (85 μg) of T_4, which is 65% iodine by weight. This requires the synthesis of a 660-kd glycoprotein homodimer, thyroglobulin (Tg). Specific tyrosine residues of thyroglobulin are then iodinated at the apical margin of the thyroid cell to form diiodotyrosine and monotyrosine (see Figs. 10–1 and 10–2). This requires formation of H_2O_2 by Duox1 and 2 and TPO, which catalyzes the oxidation of iodide and its transfer to tyrosine. TPO also catalyzes the coupling of two molecules of DIT or one of DIT and one of MIT leading to formation of T_4 and T_3, respectively, which are then stored as colloid, still as part of the Tg molecule. Pinocytosis of stored colloid leads to the formation of phagolysosomes, the colloid droplets in which Tg is digested by specific proteases to release T_4, T_3, DIT, and MIT as the droplet is translocated toward the basal portion of the cell. Thyroxine and T_3 are transported out of the phagolysomes and across the basolateral cell membrane exit the cell into the capillaries and the DIT and MIT are deiodinated by the iodotyrosine halogenase to allow recycling of the iodide to iodinate newly synthesized Tg. The synthesis of thyroid hormones requires the expression of a number of thyroid cell–specific proteins. In addition to Tg and TPO, the TSH receptor is also required to transduce the effects of extracellular TSH

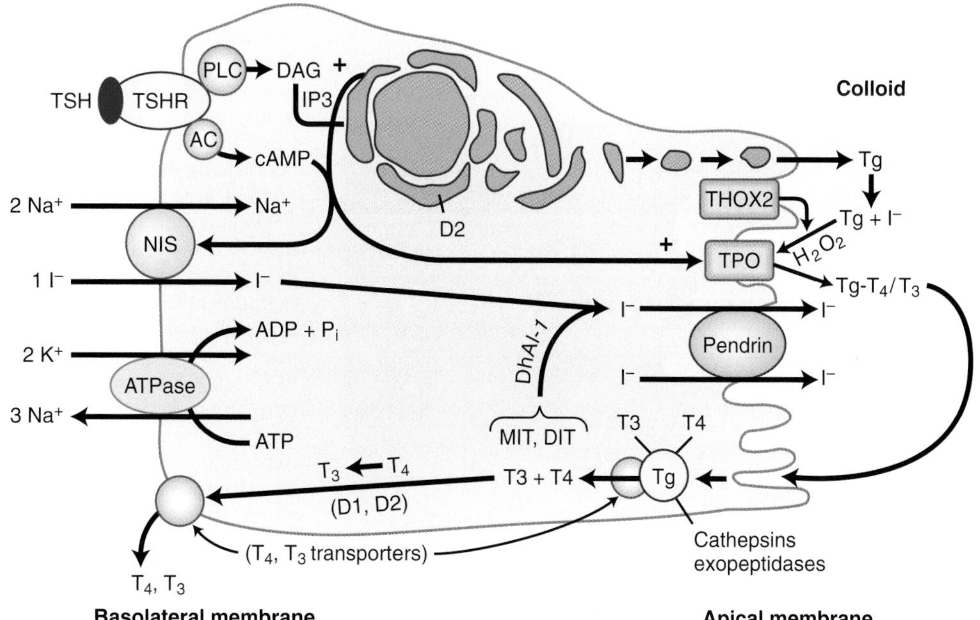

Figure 10–2 ▪ Schematic illustration of a follicular cell showing the key aspects of thyroid iodine transport and thyroid hormone synthesis. *NIS,* Sodium-iodide symporter; *T_3,* triiodothyronine; *T_4,* thyroxine; *Tg,* thyroglobulin; *TPO,* thyroid peroxidase *TSHR,* thyrotropin receptor. (Modified from Spitzweg C, Heufelder AE, Morris JC. Thyroid iodine transport. Thyroid 2000;10(4):321-330.)

for efficient hormone synthesis. A number of transcription factors are required for synthesis of these various hormonogenic enzymes including NkX2-1 (Ttf-1), Pax8, Foxel (Ttf-2), Foxe2 (HNF-3), as well as TSH.[1,2,7] Several thyroid cell–specific proteins, thyroid transcription factors 1 and 2 (TTF 1 and 2) and PAX8, stimulate transcription of the Tg and TPO genes. While the biochemical details of these processes are beyond the scope of this discussion, those aspects with clinical relevance are reviewed in greater detail in the following section.

Dietary Iodine

Formation of normal quantities of thyroid hormone requires the availability of adequate quantities of exogenous iodine to allow thyroidal uptake of approximately 60 to 75 μg daily, taking into account the fecal losses of about 10 to 20 μg iodine of iodothyronines as glucuronides and about 100 to 150 μg as urinary iodine in iodine-sufficient populations. Plasma iodide (I^-), the form of the element in biologic solutions, is completely filterable with about 60% to 70% of the filtered load reabsorbed passively. At least 100 μg of iodine per day is required to eliminate all signs of iodine deficiency (Table 10–1). In North America, the daily dietary iodine intake is in the range of 150 to 300 μg daily, largely owing to the iodination of salt, whereas in Japan, where large quantities of foods rich in iodine are consumed, intakes may be as high as several milligrams per day. Notably, iodine intake in the United States is decreasing due to a reduction in salt intake, with median urinary iodine of 15 μg/dL but a low urinary iodine (<5 μg/dL) in 12% of the population.[8-10] The daily dietary intake of iodine varies widely throughout the world, depending on the iodine content of soil and water and on dietary practice (see Table 10–1). Even in a single area, iodine intake varies among different individuals and in the same individual from day to day. Iodine may also enter the body via medications, diagnostic agents, dietary supplements and food additives. As discussed more extensively under "Regulation of Thyroid Function," iodine deficiency is common, especially in mountainous and formerly glaciated regions of the earth.[11] An estimated 1 billion individuals live in iodine-deficient areas of the world and they often develop TSH-induced compensatory enlargement of the thyroid *(endemic goiter)*. If iodine deficiency is severe during pregnancy, fetal thyroid hormone production falls with irreparable damage to the developing central nervous system (CNS). This is manifested by varying degrees of mental retardation and is termed *endemic cretinism.* Thus, iodine-deficiency disorders (IDDs), including endemic goiter and cretinism, are the most common thyroid-related human illnesses, indeed, the most common endocrine disorders worldwide.

TABLE 10–1 RECOMMENDED AND TYPICAL VALUES FOR DIETARY IODINE INTAKE

	μg /day
RECOMMENDED DAILY INTAKE	
Adults	150
During pregnancy	200
Children	90-120
TYPICAL IODINE INTAKES	
North America (1992)	75-300
Chile (1981)	<50-150
Belgium (1993)	50-60
Germany (1993)	20-70
Switzerland (1993)	130-160

Plasma iodide is partly replenished by that lost from the thyroid into the blood and by iodide liberated through deiodination of iodothyronines in peripheral tissues. Ultimately, however, the diet is its most important source. Iodine is ingested in both inorganic and organically bound forms. Iodide per se is rapidly and efficiently absorbed from the gastrointestinal tract (within 30 minutes), and little is lost in the stool. In the body, iodide is confined largely to the extracellular fluid. It is also found, however, in red blood cells and is concentrated in the intraluminal fluids of the gastrointestinal tract, notably the saliva and gastric juice, from which it is reabsorbed, thus reentering the extracellular fluid. Iodide is also concentrated in milk. Until oxidized and bound to tyrosyl residues in Tg, iodide entering the thyroid by active transport is in rapid equilibrium with the main iodide pool. The concentration of iodide in the extracellular fluid is normally 10 to 15 μg/L ($\sim 10^{-7}$ M), and the content of the peripheral pool is approximately 250 μg. The thyroid contains the largest pool of body iodine, under normal circumstances approximately 8000 μg, most of which is in the form of DIT and MIT. Normally this pool of iodine turns over slowly (about 1% per day).

Iodide Metabolism by the Thyroid Cell

Because the concentration of iodide in plasma is so low, a mechanism is required for the thyroid cell to concentrate the required amounts of this element. This process, iodide trapping, is accomplished by a membrane protein, the *sodium-iodide symporter (NIS or SLC5A)*.[12] Human NIS is a 643-amino-acid glycoprotein with 13 membrane-spanning domains. The transport of iodide is an active process dependent on the presence of sodium gradient across the basal membrane of the thyroid cell such that downhill transport of 2 Na^+ ions results in the entry of one iodide atom against an electrochemical gradient (see Fig. 10–2). In addition to being expressed in the basolateral membrane of the thyroid cell, NIS has also been identified in other iodide-concentrating cells, including salivary and mammary glands, choroid plexus, and gastric mucosa and in the cytotrophoblast and syncytiotrophoblast.[13-15] The iodide transport system generates an iodide gradient of 20 to 40 over the cell membrane and NIS will also transport TcO_4^-, ClO_4^-, and SCN^-, accounting for the utility of radioactive TcO_4^- as a thyroid scanning tool and the capacity of $KClO_4^-$ to block iodide uptake.[16,17] On the other hand, the affinity of NIS for iodide is much higher than it is for the other inorganic anions, such as bromide and chloride, accounting for the selectivity of the thyroid transport mechanism. Transcription of the NIS gene is increased by TSH, and TSH also prolongs NIS protein half-life and targets the protein to the cell membrane. That the iodide-concentrating mechanism is required for normal thyroid function has been known for decades in that its absence is associated with congenital hypothyroidism and goiter unless large quantities of inorganic iodide are provided.[18] A number of families have now been identified in which various mutations in the NIS gene are associated with congenital hypothyroidism and an iodide transport defect.[12] Importantly, several studies have documented decreases in NIS expression in human thyroid adenomas and carcinomas which contribute to the loss of iodine uptake in neoplastic thyroid cells which, therefore, present as "cold" nodules on radioisotopic imaging.[19,20] However, changes in the subcellular location of NIS may also explain this phenomenon. Pendrin is a highly hydrophobic membrane glycoprotein with 12 putative transmembrane domains expressed in the thyroid cell. It is also found in the endolymphatic system of the inner ear and at lower levels in other tissues.[21] It is found in the apical border of the thyroid follicular cell and its capacity to catalyze the transport of iodide as well as the deficiency in iodide organification found in patients with *Pendred's syndrome* have suggested that it may function to facilitate the apical transfer of iodide into the follicular lumen.[22] Pendred's syndrome itself is a hereditary condition in which sensorineural hearing loss is combined with a mild impairment thyroid hormone synthesis. In the inner ear, pendrin is required for ion and fluid transport in the cochlear apparatus. A deficiency in that process accounts for enlargement of the endolymphatic system and the deafness that is the major phenotypic manifestation of in Pendred's syndrome. Curiously, targeted inactivation of the PDS gene does not result in thyroid dysfunction in mice. This argues against a rate-limiting role for this protein for apical follicular transport at least in this animal. A second recently identified iodide transporter termed human *apical iodide transporter* may facilitate that process.[23] This protein is a transporter of short chain fatty acids, but the relationship between fatty acid and apical iodide transport is still not clear.

In addition to the active transport of iodide from the extracellular fluid, intracellular iodide is also generated by the action of the iodotyrosine dehalogenase (Dhal) enzymes. Two genes have been identified, *Dhal1* and *Dhal1b*, encoding similar isoenzymes.[24] *Dhal1* transcription is stimulated by cyclic AMP and encodes a membrane protein concentrated at the apical cell surface, which catalyzes NADPH-dependent deiodination of monotyrosine and diodotyrosine. The iodide thereby released is immediately reconjugated to newly synthesized thyroglobulin after exiting the apical membrane of the cell. This process is interrupted by the thiourea class of antithyroid drugs which inhibit thyroid peroxidase (TPO) such as methimazole (MMI), carbimazole (CBZ), and propylthiouracil (PTU), thus causing intrathyroidal iodine deficiency in patients receiving these agents.[25]

Iodide Oxidation and Organification

Within the thyroid, iodide participates in a series of reactions that lead to the synthesis of the active thyroid hormones. The first of these involves oxidation of iodide and incorporation of the resulting intermediate into the hormonally inactive iodotyrosines MIT and DIT, a process termed *organification*. Iodide is normally oxidized rapidly, immediately appearing in organic combination in Tg. The iodinations that lead to formation of iodotyrosines occur within Tg, rather than on the free amino acids. Oxidation of thyroidal iodide is mediated by the heme-containing protein *thyroid peroxidase* (TPO) and requires the H_2O_2 generated by the calcium dependent Duox1 and 2 enzymes. The protein contains a membrane-spanning region near the COOH terminus, and it is oriented in the apical membrane of the thyroid cell with residues 1-844 in the follicular lumen where iodination occurs (see Fig. 10–2).[26] TPO is the major thyroid microsomal antigen, and recombinant human TPO is now used for the detection of antithyroid microsomal antibodies commonly present in the serum of patients with Hashimoto's thyroiditis. The evanescent product of the peroxidation of iodide, i.e., the active iodinating form, may be free hypoiodous acid, I_2 or iodinium (I^+).[27] The Duox1 and 2 genes (also termed THOX1 and THOX2) encode glycoflavoproteins predominantly expressed at the apical thyrocyte membrane (see Fig. 10–2).[28] They are Ca^{2+}, NADPH-dependent oxidases that catalyze the formation of the H_2O_2 required for TPO-catalyzed thyroglobulin iodination. Iodide excess inhibits DUOX2 glycosylation, which may be an additional mechanism for the Wolff-Chaikoff effect.[29]

The rate of organic iodinations is dependent on the degree of thyroid stimulation by TSH (see below). Congenital defects in the organic binding mechanism cause goitrous congenital hypothyroidism or, if less severe, goiter without hypothyroidism. In some families, the thyroidal TPO is absent.[30] In others, the defect may reside in inadequate production of hydrogen peroxide by DUOX2 or abnormalities in Tg that render it less readily iodinated (see Chapter 12).[31,32]

Iodothyronine Synthesis

The MIT and DIT formed via oxidation and organic binding of iodide are precursors of the hormonally active iodothyronines T_4 and T_3. Because non-iodinated thyronine cannot be demonstrated in Tg, T_4 and T_3 must arise from iodinated tyrosine precursors. Synthesis of T_4 from DIT requires the TPO-catalyzed fusion of two DIT molecules to yield a structure with two diiodinated rings linked by an ether bridge (the coupling reaction). Concomitantly, a residual dehydroalanine is formed at the site of the DIT residue contributing the phenolic hydroxyl group.[33]

Efficient synthesis of T_4 and T_3 in the thyroid requires Tg. The Tg mRNA is ~8.5 kb in length and encodes a 330-kd (12S) subunit that is 10% carbohydrate by weight. There are 134 tyrosyl residues in the 660-kd homodimer. Only 25 to 30 of these are iodinated, but only residues 5, 1290, and 2553 form T_4 and residue 2746, T_3.[34,35] The T_4-forming, readily iodinated, and iodothyronine-forming acceptor residues of Tg from different species are in a Glu/AspTyr or a Thr/SerTyrSer sequence, suggesting an important role of primary sequence in these reactions. There are three to four T_4 molecules in each molecule of human Tg under conditions of normal iodination (~25 atoms per Tg molecule, approximately 0.5% iodine by weight), but only about one in five molecules of human Tg contains a T_3 residue. In Tg from patients with untreated Graves' disease, the content of T_4 residues remains approximately the same, but the number of T_3 residues doubles to an average of 0.4 per molecule.[36] This difference is independent of the iodination state of the Tg and is a consequence of thyroidal stimulation. Because the coupling reaction is catalyzed by TPO, virtually all agents that inhibit organic binding (e.g., the thiourea drugs) also inhibit coupling.

Storage and Release of Thyroid Hormone

The thyroid is unique among the endocrine glands by virtue of the large store of hormone it contains and the low rate at which the hormone turns over (1% per day). This aspect of thyroid hormone economy has homeostatic value in that the reservoir provides prolonged protection against depletion of circulating hormone in case synthesis ceases. In normal humans, the administration of antithyroid agents for as long as 2 weeks has little effect on serum T_4 concentrations. There are approximately 250 μg T_4 per gram of wet weight in normal human thyroid or 5000 μg of T_4 in a 20-g gland.[25] This is sufficient to maintain a euthyroid state for at least 50 days. When released rapidly in an uncontrolled fashion during subacute or painless thyroiditis, this quantity of T_4 will cause significant transient thyrotoxicosis. Thyroglobulin is present in the plasma of normal individuals at concentrations up to 80 ng/mL, probably leaving the thyroid through the lymphatics. However, peripheral hydrolysis of Tg does not contribute significantly to the thyroid hormones in the circulation, even during thyroiditis when large quantities of this protein are present.

The first step in thyroid hormone release is the endocytosis of colloid from the follicular lumen by two processes: macropinocytosis by pseudopods formed at the apical membrane and micropinocytosis by small coated vesicles that form at the apical surface (see Fig. 10–2). Both processes are stimulated by TSH, but the relative importance of the two pathways varies among species, with micropinocytosis thought to predominate in humans. Following endocytosis, endocytotic vesicles fuse with lysosomes, and proteolysis is catalyzed by cathepsin D and D-like thiol proteases, all of which are active at the acidic pH of the lysosome.[37] The iodotyrosines released from Tg are rapidly deiodinated by an NADPH-dependent iodotyrosine deiodinase, and the released iodine is recycled. Thyroid hormones are released from Tg in the lysosome, but it is not clear how their transfer into the cytosol and subsequently the plasma is effected. Given the expression of the thyroid hormone transporter MCT8 in the thyroid gland (see later), it is possible that this transporter could be involved in the exit of T_4 and/or T_3 from the phagolysosome or thyroid cell. It has been shown that T_4 can be released from thyroglobulin within the thyroid cell with minimal disruption of its molecular weight.[38] This presumably is a consequence of selective proteolysis, which is facilitated by the fact that the major hormonogenic peptides of the thyroglobulin molecule are located at the amino- and carboxytermini of the thyroglobulin monomer.

Presumably the T_4 becomes accessible to the thyroidal type 1 and 2 deiodinases (D1 and D2) present therein as basal and TSH-stimulated conversion of T_4 to T_3 is readily demonstrated in the perfused dog thyroid.[39] Because this conversion is inhibited by PTU, it is catalyzed by D1. The contribution of thyroidal T_4 deiodination to T_3 secretion in humans under physiologic conditions is not known. The fact that the ratio of T_4 to T_3 in human Tg is 15 : 1 while estimates of the molar ratio of T_4 to T_3 in thyroid secretion is approximately 10 : 1 suggests that this does occur. Stimulation of D1- and D2-catalyzed 5′-deiodination of T_4 in Graves' thyroid may enhance that pathway and contribute to the marked increase of the ratio of T_3 to T_4 production in that condition.[40] An inhibition of the D1-catalyzed T_4 to T_3 conversion may contribute to the rapid effect of PTU to reduce T_3 production in the Graves' patient (see Chapter 11).[40,41] That thyroid cell deiodinases can modulate the systemic conversion of T_4 to T_3 has been shown in several patients with metastatic thyroid carcinoma. The high expression of D2 in one large mediastinal tumor mass was associated with a high normal T_3 and reduced T_4 with a normal TSH. Removal of the tumor reversed these abnormalities.[42]

T_4 release from the thyroid cells is inhibited by several agents, the most important of which is iodide. Inhibition of hormone release is responsible for the rapid improvement that iodide causes in hyperthyroid patients. The mechanism by which this effect is mediated is uncertain, but iodide inhibits the stimulation of thyroid adenylate cyclase by TSH and by the stimulatory immunoglobulins of Graves' disease. Increasing iodination of Tg also increases its resistance to hydrolysis by acid proteases in the lysosomes. Lithium inhibits thyroid hormone release, although its mechanism of action is poorly understood and may differ from that of iodide.[43,44]

Role and Mechanism of Thyrotropin (TSH) Effects

All steps in the formation and release of thyroid hormones are stimulated by TSH secreted by the pituitary thyrotrophs (see Chapter 8). Thyroid cells express the TSH receptor (TSHR), a member of the glycoprotein G protein–coupled receptor family. The deduced amino acid sequence of this protein predicts a large extracellular NH_2-terminal domain, seven membrane-spanning domains, and an intracellular domain that transduces the signal by promoting exchange of GDP for GTP on the a subunit of G proteins.[1,2,45] In fact, the TSHR has been reported to couple to 11 different G protein α subunits in vitro and, therefore, much remains to be learned about signaling through it.[46] Although the TSHR mainly couples to Gs, when activated by high concentrations of TSH (100-fold physiologic) it couples also to Gq/11, activating the inositol-phosphate diacylglycerol cascade. The induction of signal via the phospholipase C (PLC) and intracellular Ca^{2+} pathways regulates iodide efflux, H_2O_2 production, and Tg iodination while the signal via the protein kinase A (PKA) pathways mediated by cAMP regulates iodine uptake and transcription of Tg, TPO, and the sodium-iodide symporter (NIS) mRNAs leading to thyroid hormone production (Table 10–2).[47,48] Although the discovery that different mutations in various regions of the TSHR molecule resulted in intrinsic activation and the identification of important domains for intramolecular TSHR signal transduction (see Chapter 11), the precise mechanisms of receptor activation and the early events of TSHR signal transduction are not fully understood.[45] Studies using mutational analyses have suggested that the interactions between the ectodomain and the extracellular loops of the transmembrane domains in the TSHR may be critical for the maintenance of an inactive state with no constitutive activity. When these constraints are removed, an "open" conformation ensues. Therefore, it has been proposed that the TSHR exists in both a "closed" (inactive) and "open" (active) format. This model predicts that only the "open" format of the receptor would be able to bind ligand and become activated.[49] Further support for this model came from the development of constitutive activation when the TSHR ectodomain was truncated, suggesting that its presence dampened a constitutively active β subunit.

The TSHR, in addition to TSH, also binds thyroid-stimulating antibody (TSAb), thyroid-blocking antibodies (TBAb), and neutral antibodies to the TSHR (see Chapter 11). The closely

TABLE 10–2 THYROID CELL FUNCTIONS STIMULATED BY THYROTROPIN

Function Affected	General Mechanism
IODIDE METABOLISM	
Increase I^- in follicular lumen	PL-C
Delayed increased in NIS expression	cAMP
Increase thyroid blood flow	↑ Nitric oxide synthesis (↓ cellular iodide)
Increase in I^- efflux from thyroid cell	?
THYROID HORMONE SYNTHESIS	
↑ Hydrogen peroxide	PL-C
↑ Thyroglobulin and TPO synthesis	cAMP
↑ NADPH via pentose-phosphate pathway	?
THYROID HORMONE SECRETION	
↑ Pinocytosis of thyroglobulin	cAMP
↑ Release of thyroglobulin into plasma via basolateral membrane	cAMP (?)
Mitogenesis	cAMP, PL-C, and IGF-I– and FGF-mediated kinase activation

cAMP, Cyclic adenosine monophosphate; *FGF,* follicular growth factor; *IGF-I,* insulin-like growth factor I; *NIS,* sodium-iodide symporter; *PL-C,* phospholipase C; *TPO,* thyroid peroxidase.

related luteinizing hormone (LH) and chorionic gonadotropin (CG) also bind to and activate TSHR signaling.[45] The latter accounts for the physiologic hyperthyroidism of early pregnancy.

Besides the thyrocyte, the TSHR is also expressed in a variety of tissues such as osteoclasts, fibroblasts, and adipocytes, as well as retroorbital adipocytes.[45] As discussed earlier, certain activating and inactivating mutations, either germline or somatic, have been identified in the membrane-spanning or intracellular portions of the TSHR molecule that cause generalized or nodular hyperfunction and congenital hypofunction.[45,50]

THYROID HORMONES IN PERIPHERAL TISSUES

Plasma Transport

The metabolic transformations of thyroid hormones in peripheral tissues determine their biologic potency and regulate their biologic effects. Consequently, an understanding of thyroid physiopathology requires a knowledge of the pathways of thyroid hormone metabolism. A wide variety of iodothyronines and their metabolic derivatives exist in plasma. Of these, T_4 is highest in concentration and the only one that arises solely from direct secretion by the thyroid gland. In normal humans, T_3 is also released from the thyroid but approximately 80% is derived from the peripheral tissues by the enzymatic removal of a single 5′ iodine atom (outer ring or 5′ monodeiodination) from T_4.[51] The remaining iodothyronines and their derivatives are generated in the peripheral tissues from T_4 and T_3. Principal among them are 3,3′,5′-triiodothyronine (reverse T_3, or rT_3) and 3,3′-diiodo-L-thyronine (3,3′-T_2) (Fig. 10–3). Trace concentrations of other diiodothyronines, monoiodothyronines, and conjugates thereof with glucuronic or sulfuric acid are also present.[52,53] Deaminated derivatives of T_4 and T_3 that bear an acetic acid rather than an alanine side chain (tetrac and triac) are also present in low concentrations (see Fig. 10–3). The major iodothyronines are poorly soluble in water and thus bind reversibly to plasma proteins. The plasma proteins with which T_4 is mainly associated are thyroxine-binding globulin (TBG) and transthyretin (TTR; formerly termed T_4-binding prealbumin [TBPA]) and albumin (Table 10–3). About 75% to 80% of T_3 is bound by TBG, and the remainder by TTR and albumin.

Thyroxine-Binding Globulin (TBG). TBG is a glycoprotein with a molecular mass of about 54 kd, about 20% of which is carbohydrate. The gene encoding the protein is found on the X chromosome.[54] The protein sequence of TBG resembles that of the SERPIN family of serine antiproteases.[55] Because there is one iodothyronine binding site per TBG molecule, the T_4 or T_3 binding capacity of TBG in normal human serum is equivalent to its concentration, which is approximately 270 nmol/L (1.5 μg/

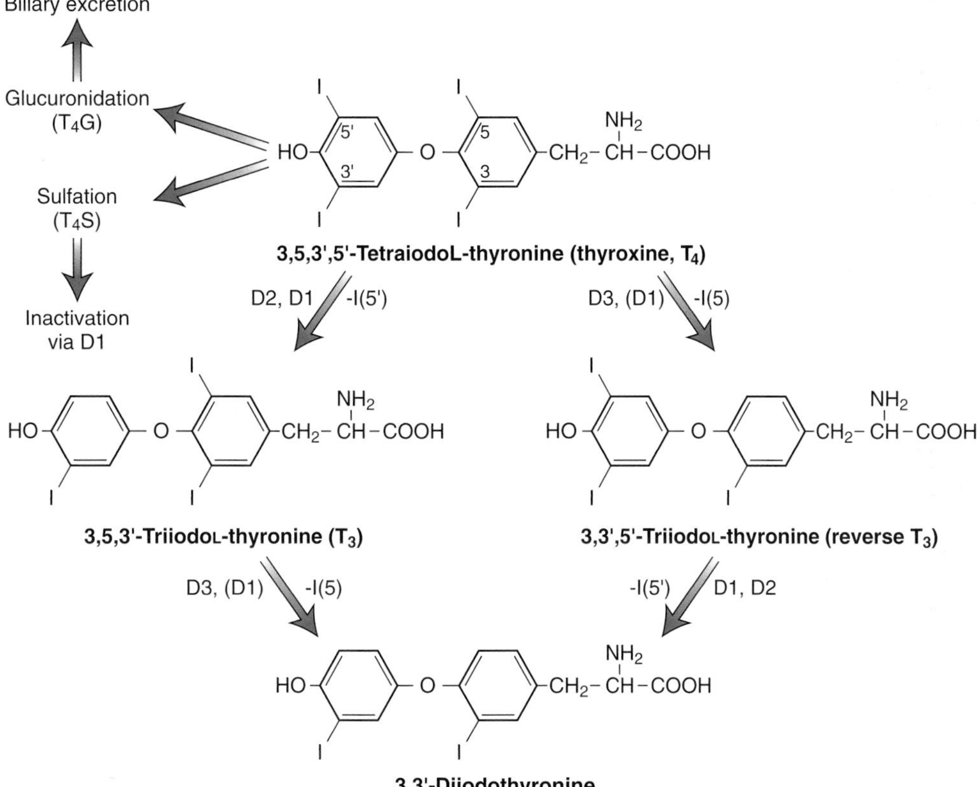

Figure 10–3 ▪ Major deiodinative and non-deiodinative pathways of thyroid hormone metabolism. The iodothyronine deiodinases are abbreviated D1, D2, and D3 for type 1, 2, and 3 deiodinases, respectively. *Arrows* refer to monodeiodination of the outer or inner ring of the iodothyronine nucleus, which are termed 5′ or 5 by convention. T_4 is activated by monodeiodination of the phenolic thyronine ring by D1 or D2 to form T_3. Deiodination of the tyrosyl ring by D1 or D3 inactivates T_4 and T_3. This inactivation pathway is markedly favored by sulfation of the phenolic hydroxyl to form T_4SO_4 (T_4S) or T_3SO_4 (T_3S). Glucuronidated T_4 and T_3 (T_4G and T_3G) are excreted into the bile but may be partially reabsorbed after deglucuronidation in the intestine. (From Zavacki AM, Larsen PR. CARs and DRUGs: a risky combination. Endocrinology 2005;146:992.)

TABLE 10–3 COMPARISON OF THE MAJOR HUMAN THYROID HORMONE-BINDING PROTEINS

	Thyroxine-Binding Globulin	Transthyretin	Albumin
Mol wt of holoprotein (kd)	54,000	54,000 (4 subunits)	66,000
Plasma concentrations (μmol/L)	0.27	4.6	640
T_4 binding capacity as μg T_4/dL	21	350	50,000
Association constants of the major binding site (L/M)			
T_4	1×10^{10}	7×10^7	7×10^5
T_3	5×10^8	1.4×10^7	1×10^5
Fraction of sites occupied by T_4 in euthyroid plasma	0.31	0.02	<0.001
Distribution volume (L)	7	5.7	7.8
Turnover rate (% day)	13	59	5
Distribution of iodothyronines (% protein)			
T_4	68	11	20
T_3	80	9	11

dL). The half-life of the protein in plasma is about 5 days. A congenital deficiency of TBG is common, occurring in 1/5000 newborns, and is associated with the complete absence of the protein in males. L-Asparaginase blocks the synthesis of TBG, which accounts for the low TBG concentrations in patients receiving this agent.[56]

The glycosylation of TBG influences its clearance from the plasma and its behavior during isoelectric focusing.[57] In estrogen-treated patients, there is an increase in the prevalence of the more acidic bands of TBG. The more highly sialylated TBG is cleared more slowly from plasma than is the more positively charged TBG, because sialylation inhibits the hepatic uptake of glycoproteins. Sera from pregnant patients, women receiving oral contraceptives, and patients with acute hepatitis have increased fractions of acidic TBG. Patients with inherited TBG excess have normal amounts of highly sialylated TBG, as do men and nonpregnant women. Because TBG is the principal T_4- and T_3-binding protein, changes in TBG or its binding are paralleled by changes in total plasma T_4 and T_3 even though T_4 and T_3 production is little changed.

Another posttranslational modification affecting TBG occurs in septic patients or following cardiopulmonary bypass surgery.[58] TBG is subjected to cleavage by a serine protease released from polymorphonuclear leukocytes resulting in the release of a 5-kd COOH terminal loop with a consequent decrease in affinity for T_4. An analogous reaction has been described for CBG, which releases cortisol at the site of inflammation.[59] It has been postulated that the released T_4 might play a critical role in the response to injury perhaps by providing a supply of iodine for antibacterial purposes.[58] The cleaved TBG of approximately 49 kd circulates and, because it binds T_4 with lower avidity, it may explain the increased ratio of free to bound T_4 in acute illness, even when TBG saturation studies or immunoassays indicate TBG concentration is normal (later section, "Thyroid Function during Fasting or Illness").

Transthyretin (TTR). Transthyretin exists in part as a complex with retinol (vitamin A)-binding protein, hence its name. It consists of four identical polypeptide chains with a total molecular mass of approximately 55 kd and it is not glycosylated. Its concentration in plasma is approximately 4 mmol/L (250 μg/mL). Each mole of TTR binds 1 mole of T_4 with high affinity, and a second T_4 molecule is bound with lower affinity at high concentrations of T_4.[60] Its half-life in plasma is normally about 2 days, but this decreases during illness.[61] TTR is expressed in the choroid plexus and it is the major thyroid hormone-binding protein in the cerebrospinal fluid (CSF).[62] Targeted TTR gene disruption in mice shows that there is no impairment of uptake of T_4 into the brain, leaving the role of TTR in CSF undefined in regard to thyroid physiology.[63,64]

Variant forms of TTR are associated with familial amyloidotic polyneuropathy.[60,65] In affected families, the TTR monomer has one of several different point mutations, and TTR accumulates in the amyloid tissue deposits. Neither thyroid dysfunction nor altered vitamin A metabolism has been reported, although there is altered affinity of some of the mutant proteins for T_4. Families with both high-affinity TTR and a few with increased TTR levels have been reported.[66]

Competition for T_4 and T_3 Binding to TBG and TTR by Therapeutic Agents. The TBG binding site has an affinity for T_3 that is about 20-fold less than that for T_4 (see Table 10–3). Binding of T_4 and T_3 by TBG are inhibited by phenytoin,[67] salicylate,[68] salsalate,[69] furosemide, fenclofenac, and mitotane. The affinity of these compounds for TBG is much weaker than are those of the iodothyronines but their concentration in plasma is sufficiently high to compete with T_4 and T_3 binding and reduce total hormone levels although free T_4 remains normal. Because all methods used for estimating the free fractions of T_4 and T_3 in human serum except ultrafiltration dilute the serum, euthyroid patients receiving these drugs may appear to have low total and free T4 or whereas in vivo, the free T_4 is normal.

Albumin. The affinity of albumin for T_4 and T_3 binding is much lower than that of either TBG or TTR, but the high concentration of this protein results in the binding of 10% of the plasma thyroid hormones (see Table 10–3). Changes in albumin concentration per se have little influence on the total hormone levels, unless accompanied by alterations in TBG and TTR, all three of which are synthesized in the liver. Hepatic failure or nephrotic syndrome leads to decreases in the plasma concentration of all three, and the serum albumin concentration in patients with these illnesses may serve as a surrogate for estimating TBG concentrations.

The role of albumin in thyroid physiology becomes clinically important in patients with familial dysalbuminemic hyperthyroxinemia (FDH).[70,71] In this autosomal dominant disorder, the plasma contains high amounts of a usually minor albumin variant that binds T_4 but not T_3, with increased avidity. This increases total T_4, but free T_4 and total and free T_3 remain normal in an otherwise euthyroid patient. However, such patients may have a confusing pattern of test results especially when analogue methods or labeled T_3 are used to estimate the free T_4 or T_3 (see Chapter 6).

Other Plasma Thyroid Hormone–Binding Proteins. Between 3% and 6% of plasma T_4 and T_3 are bound to lipoproteins. The T_4-binding lipoprotein is a 27-kd homodimer with an affinity for T_4, which is lower than that of TBG. This binding is of uncertain physiologic significance but could play a role in targeting T_4 delivery to specific tissues.

Free Thyroid Hormones

Because most of the circulating T_4 and T_3 is bound to TBG, its concentration and degree of saturation are the major determinants of the free fraction of T_4. Binding of the thyroid hormones to the plasma proteins alters their metabolism. The negligible urinary excretion of T_3 and T_4 is due to the limited filterability of the hormone-binding protein complexes at the glomerulus. The volume of distribution and rate of turnover of the hormones are also affected by their protein associations. In vitro, the interaction between the thyroid hormones and their binding proteins conforms to a reversible binding equilibrium that can be expressed by conventional equilibrium equations. For the formulations that follow, T_4 is used as the prototype, with the understanding that similar interactions apply in the case of T_3. The interaction between T_4 and TBG can be expressed as follows:

$$T_4 + TBG \xrightarrow{k_a} T_4 \cdot TBG$$

Here TBG represents the *unoccupied* binding protein, k_a the equilibrium association constant for the interaction; T_4 the concentration of *free* T_4; $T_4 \cdot TBG$ is T_4 bound to TBG (~68% of total T_4 is bound to TBG).

Rearranging,

$$\frac{T_4 \cdot TBG}{(T_4)(TBG)} = k_a$$

$$\frac{T_4}{T_4 \cdot TBG} = \frac{1}{(TBG)k_a}$$

Thus, the free fraction of T_4 ($T4/T4 \cdot TBG$) is inversely proportional to the concentration of *unoccupied* TBG binding sites. Estimates of the free T_4 concentration in serum can be generated by direct or indirect assays. For example, with the aid of radiolabeled T_4, the proportion of T_4 that is free can be determined by dialysis, and the concentration of free T_4 can be calculated as the product of the total hormone concentration and the free fraction. In normal serum, the free T_4 is approximately 0.02% of the total (about 20 pmol/L, 1.5 ng/dL). The approximately 20-fold lower affinity of TBG for T_3 results in a higher proportion of unbound T_3 (0.30%) (see Table 10–3).

It is the free hormone that is available to the tissues for intracellular transport and feedback regulation, that induces its metabolic effects, and that undergoes deiodination or degradation. The bound hormone acts merely as a reservoir. It follows that the concentration of the free hormone is the determinant of the metabolic state and it is this concentration that is defended by homeostatic mechanisms. If an increase in TBG occurs, the free T_4 concentration and T3 concentrations can be maintained at normal levels only if the bound hormone increases. The plasma concentration of T_4 is determined by its rate of entry into, and exit from, the plasma. The metabolic clearance rate relates the quantity of T_4 removed from the plasma per unit time to the quantity available for removal, that is, its plasma concentration. Thus,

$$MCR = D/[P]$$

where MCR is the metabolic clearance rate (volume/time), D is the absolute disposal or removal rate (amount/time), and [P] is the plasma concentration (amount/volume). Transposing,

$$[P] = D/MCR$$

However, under steady-state conditions, the production rate of T_4 (PR) and the disposal rate (D) are equal. Hence,

$$[P] = PR/MCR$$

Thus, for any level of T_4 production, be it increased, normal, or decreased, the total plasma T_4 level varies inversely with its MCR. However, if only the free T_4 enters the cells while the bound T_4 is confined largely to the intravascular space, then reducing the fraction of total T_4 that is free, that is, changing the amount that is available to the tissues, changes the MCR in a parallel manner. When TBG concentrations are increased by administration of excess estrogen, the free T_4 reduction reduces T_4 clearance allowing an increase in the plasma total T_4 concentration. This is an iterative process that eventually would normalize the free T_4 at a new equilibrium without a change in T_4 secretion rate. The transient decrease in free thyroid hormones also slightly reduces the negative feedback on the hypothalamic-pituitary-thyroid axis, which probably does cause an increase in thyroid hormone production as an additional compensation.[72,73] Whether the slight increase in TSH when estrogen is introduced in patients on stable levothyroxine dose reflects a failure of this internal compensation or a change in thyroxine requirements due, for example, to an increase in the type 3 (the inactivating) deiodinase, remains to be seen.

The above formulation is termed the *free thyroid hormone hypothesis.*[74,75] If it is free hormone that is available for cellular entry, what is the role, if any, of the hormone-binding proteins? Protein binding facilitates the distribution of the hydrophobic thyroid hormones throughout the vascular system. For example, if a protein-free solution containing tracer T_3 is perfused through rat liver via the portal vein, there is a steep concentration gradient with a decreasing quantity of T_3 in the solution as the distance from the center of the portal lobule increases.[76] In fact, virtually all of the T_3 is taken up by the first cells to be contacted by the bolus. In contrast, if albumin is added to the perfusate, the distribution of tracer is uniform throughout the lobule. Both influx and efflux of thyroid hormone from tissues is rapid. Thus, intracellular free T_3 and T_4 are in equilibrium with the free hormone pool in plasma although transporter activity and metabolism will influence the magnitude of the ratio. In the steady-state, the rate of T_3 and T_4 metabolism, not the dissociation rate from plasma proteins or its intracellular concentration, is rate-limiting in the exit of hormones from the plasma.

T_4 and T_3 Transport across Cell Membranes and Intracellular T_3 Binding

The progress in the field of transmembrane thyroid hormone transport in recent years has been truly astonishing. Recently a defect in a single thyroid hormone transporter molecule, MCT8, has been shown to cause a severe developmental neurologic phenotype.[77,78] MCT8 is a T-type amino acid transporter belonging to the monocarboxylate transporter family and facilitates transport of T_3, T_4, rT_3 and T_2 across cell membranes in vitro.[79] It is expressed in the brain, heart, kidney, liver, and skeletal muscle and is encoded on the X chromosome. The Allan-Herndon-Dudley syndrome (AHDS) is an X-linked condition characterized by severe mental retardation, dysarthria, athetoid movements, muscle hypoplasia, and spastic paraplegia. All patients tested with this syndrome have mutations in the MCT8 gene.[73,74,76] Animal studies show high expression of this protein in the choroid plexus, cerebral cortex, hippocampus, and medulla with a distribution suggesting that the protein is expressed in neurons rather than glial cells.[80] The type 2 iodothyronine deiodinase (D2) is predominantly expressed in astrocytes and tanycytes. The tanycytes are specialized ependymal cells that line the inferior portion of the third ventricle with extensive processes extending into the adjacent hypothalamus and median eminence.[81,82] Another transporter specific for T_4, OATP1C1 (a member of the organic anion transporting polypeptide family) is expressed in capillaries throughout the brain suggesting it may be involved in the transport of T_4 across the blood-brain barrier.[83] Taken together, these results suggest that the supply of T_3 to neurons may occur according to the schema shown in Figure 10–4.[84] T_4 is transferred into the choroid plexus or into tanycytes via the action of OATP1C1, which is negatively regulated in brain capillaries by thyroid hormone.[85] In the tanycyte or astrocyte, T_4 is converted to T_3 by D2 and exits the cell, possibly via the MCT8 transporter, where it becomes available for neuronal uptake, also via MCT8. Neurons express the type 3 deiodinase, which prevents activation of T_4 and catalyzes degradation of T_3. (See "Iodothyronine Deiodination.")

This would provide a logical explanation of the association of the mutations in MCT8 with the ADH syndrome although it still remains puzzling why the neurologic manifestations of this condition are so different from those seen in patients with untreated congenital hypothyroidism or severe iodine deficiency (see Chapter 12). In the latter individuals, the principal abnormalities are growth retardation, spasticity, and mental retardation. It still remains conceivable that MCT8 also transfers an additional substance that is required for the normal development of neurons though that seems remote.

The transport field has become more complex as evidence accumulates of tissue-specific as well as generalized iodothyronine transporters belonging to a number of different transporter protein families. Each of these has many members with small variations in structure which alter the specificity of the target

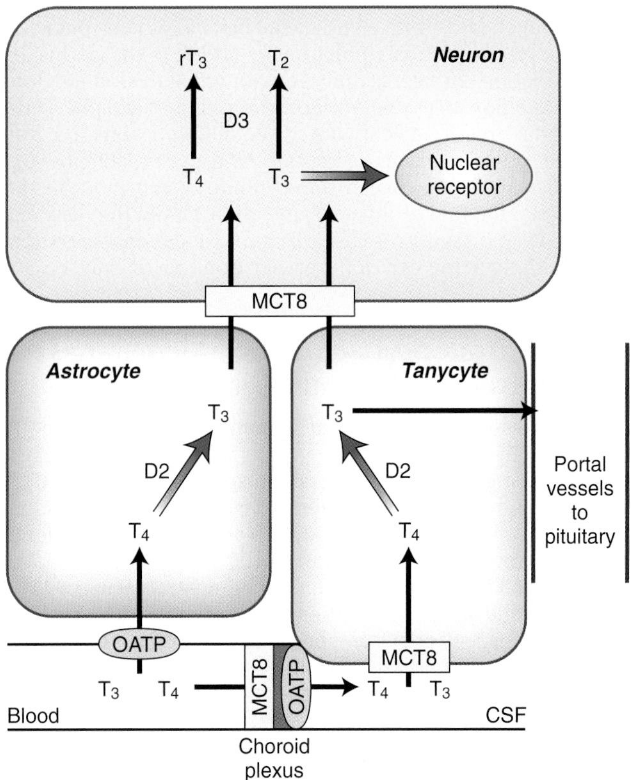

Figure 10–4 ▪ Potential pathways for entry of T_3 into the central nervous system. Thyroid hormones are transported through the blood-brain barrier (OATP) or the blood-CSF barrier (OATP and MCT8). In the astrocytes and tanycytes, T_4 is converted to T_3, which then enters the neurons, possibly through MCT8. In the neurons, both T_4 and T_3 are degraded by D3. T_3 from the tanycytes may reach the portal vessels in the median eminence. Other transporters may be present on the astrocyte or tanycyte membranes. In most cases the transport could be bidirectional, although only one direction is shown. *CSF,* cerebrospinal fluid; *D2 and D3,* type 2 and type 3 iodothyronine deiodinases; *MCT8,* the monocarboxylate transporter 8; *OATP,* organic anion transporting polypeptide. (From Bernal J. The significance of thyroid hormone transporters in the brain. Endocrinology 2005;146:1698.)

substance. A thorough review of this topic is beyond the scope of this chapter and the interested reader is referred to excellent reviews for further information.[83]

In most cells, about 90% of the intracellular T_3 is located in the cytosol. The known exception is in the pituitary, where approximately 50% of the intracellular T_3 is present in the nucleus.[86] The mechanisms determining this distribution are still unknown but it would not be surprising if there were active transport of thyroid hormones in and out of the nucleus and between other intracellular compartments. An intracellular T_3-inding protein (CTPB) has been identified which is expressed at high levels in human brain and heart, but is widely distributed.[87] This protein or similar proteins may also play a role in the subcellular localization of the active hormone.

Iodothyronine Deiodination

The most important pathway for T_4 metabolism is its outer ring (5′) monodeiodination to the active thyroid hormone, T_3. This reaction is catalyzed by the type 1 and 2 deiodinases (D1 and D2) and is the source of more than 80% of the circulating T_3 in humans (see Fig. 10–3). Inner ring deiodination, an inactivating step, is catalyzed primarily by the type 3 (D3) deiodinase, which inactivates T_3 and prevents activation of T_4 by converting it to reverse T_3 (see Fig. 10–3).[51,88] The structures of the three human deiodinases are similar, all being homodimers and integral membrane proteins. They contain the rare amino acid selenocysteine in the active catalytic center (Table 10–4). Selenocysteine has nucleophilic properties that make it ideal for catalysis of oxidoreductive reactions such as iodothyronine deiodination and the reduction of H_2O_2 by another family of selenoenzymes, the glutathione peroxidases.[89,90] Selenium is thought to be the iodine acceptor during deiodination reactions. Mutagenesis of selenocysteine in D1 to cysteine, that is, replacing selenium with sulfur, reduces the enzyme velocity by approximately 100-fold. Synthesis of selenoproteins is a complex process in that the normal "STOP" translation function of its UGA codon must be overridden by the cell. This is accomplished by a combination of a specific structural feature, the SECIS element, in the 3′ untranslated region of the mRNAs encoding these proteins together with a specific group of selenocysteine incorporating gene products.[91,92]

Enzymology and Regulation of the Selenodeiodinases. While both D1 and D2 activate T_4, they have several important differences (see Table 10–4). D1 catalyzes both 5′ and 5 deiodination of T_4 to form T_3 and rT_3, respectively, although the Km for these reactions is approximately 3 orders of magnitude greater than that of D2 and D3 for this substrate. In fact, the preferred substrates of D1 are rT_3 (5′ deiodination) and T_3-SO4 (5 deiodination). Type 1–catalyzed reactions are susceptible to inhibition by PTU unlike those catalyzed by D2 and D3. D1 also differs from D2 in being markedly increased by excess thyroid hormone through increased gene transcription, whereas D2 mRNA and protein are reduced by thyroid hormones. D2 has a half-life of only 20 to 30 minutes while that of D1 and D3 is more than 12 hours. This is due to the rapid ubiquitination of D2, a process that is accelerated by interaction with its substrate T_4 or rT_3.[51] D1 and D3 are not thought to be ubiquitinated.

The cellular location of D2 close to the nucleus gives the T_3 formed by its catalytic action better access to the nucleus than that formed by D1.[93] For this reason D2 has principally been thought of as an enzyme that provides intracellular T_3 but there is increasing evidence that it is also an important source of plasma T_3 in humans. In fact, its widespread distribution in skeletal muscle and its greater catalytic efficiency compared with D1 at physiologic free T_4 and cofactor concentrations suggest it may be as important as D1 as a source of circulating T_3 in the euthyroid human.[93] On the other hand, in thyrotoxico-

TABLE 10–4 HUMAN IODOTHYRONINE SELENODEIODINASES

Parameter	Type 1 (Outer and Inner ring)	Type 2 (Outer Ring)	Type 3 (Inner Ring)
Physiologic role	rT_3 and T_3S degradation, the source of plasma T_3 in thyrotoxic patients	Provide intracellular T_3 in specific tissues, a source of plasma T_3	Inactivate T_3 and T_4
Tissue location	Liver, kidney, thyroid, pituitary (?) (not CNS)	CNS, pituitary, BAT, placenta thyroid, skeletal muscle, heart	Placenta, CNS, hemangiomas, fetal or adult liver, skeletal muscle
Subcellular location	Plasma membrane	Endoplasmic reticulum	Plasma membrane
Preferred substrates (position deiodinated)	rT_3 (5′), T_3S (5)	T_4, rT_3 (5′)	T_3, T_4 (5)
Km	rT_3, 10^{-7}; T_4, 10^{-6}	10^{-9}	10^{-9}
Susceptibility to PTU	High	Absent	Absent
Response to increased T_4	↑	↓	↑

BAT, brown adipose tissue; CNS, central nerrous system; PTU, 6-n propylthiouraci T_3S, T_3SO_4.

sis, the threefold to fourfold increase in D1, particularly in the thyroid and the reduced D2 make D1 the major extrathyroidal source of T_3. This can account for why PTU causes a much more rapid fall in circulating T_3 than does methimazole (Tapazole) in the Graves' patient.[40,41] The important paracrine role of D2 in astrocytes and tanycytes as a source of T_3 for neurons is discussed earlier (see Fig. 10–4).

Type 3 deiodinase is highly expressed in placenta and uterine endometrium as well as in the CNS where it is primarily in neurons. The highest expression identified to date occurs in infantile hemangiomas. In infants with extensive hepatic lesions, D3 may overwhelm the secretory capacity of the infant's thyroid, causing hypothyroidism, a syndrome termed *consumptive hypothyroidism.*[94] D3 expression is increased by thyroid hormone at a transcriptional level.[95]

Gene targeting studies have begun to provide further insights into the physiologic roles of the deidodinases in mammals.[96] Inactivation of the *Dio2* gene results in a phenotypically normal mouse with an elevated serum T_4, normal serum T_3, and elevated serum TSH. These animals have hypothalamic-pituitary resistance to T_4, impaired auditory function, impaired thermogenesis in response to cold stress, and relatively subtle defects in neurologic function. These are all consistent with the expectations based on earlier studies indicating an especially important role for D2 in brown fat cell function, cochlear maturation, and neurologic development. Mice with targeted inactivation of *Dio1* are phenotypically normal but also have an elevated serum T_4, and a normal serum T_3 and but TSH is normal.[97] The most striking finding in the D1-deficient mouse is a marked shift in the T_4 clearance pathway from deiodination to biliary/fecal clearance. Mice with inactivation of the *Dio3* gene show profound abnormalities. They have impaired fertility and develop central hypothyroidism in adult life, presumably due to hypothalamic thyrotoxicosis during developmental programming.[98] These problems have precluded more extensive studies at this time.

Quantitative and Qualitative Aspects of Thyroid Hormone Metabolism

Thyroid Hormone Turnover. In the normal adult, T_4 has a distribution volume of approximately 10 L (Table 10–5). Because the concentration of total T_4 in plasma is approximately 100 nmol/L (~8 μg/dL), the extrathyroidal T_4 pool is approximately 1 μmol (~800 μg). In the adult, the fractional rate of turnover of T_4 in the periphery is about 10% per day (halftime, 6.7 days). Thus, about 1.1 L of the peripheral T_4 distribution

TABLE 10–5 COMPARISON OF TRIIODOTHYROXINE (T_3) AND THYROXINE (T_4) IN HUMANS

	T_3	T_4
Production rate (nmol/day)	50	110
Fraction from thyroid	0.2	1.0
Relative metabolic potency	1.0	0.3
Serum concentration		
Total (nmol/L)	1.8	100
Free (pmol/L)	5	20
Fraction of total hormone in free form ($\times 10^{-2}$)	0.3	0.02
Distribution volume (L)	40	10
Fraction intracellular	0.64	0.15
Half-life (days)	0.75	6.7

To convert T_4 from nmol/L to μg/dL (total) or pmol/L to ng/dL (free), divide by 12.87. To convert T_3 from nmol/L to ng/dL (total) or pmol/L to pg/dL (free), multiply by 65.1.

space is cleared of hormone daily, a volume containing approximately 110 nmol (85 μg) of T_4.

The kinetics of T_3 metabolism differ from those of T_4, partly because of its 10- to 15-fold lower affinity for TBG. The volume of distribution of T_3 in the normal adult is about 40 L, about four times that of T_4, and its fractional turnover rate is approximately 60% per day. At a mean normal serum T_3 concentration of 1.8 nmol/L (120 ng/dL), 50-fold lower than T_4, the daily production of T_3 is approximately 50 nmol (33 μg) or about 46% that of T_4 (see Table 10–5). The rapid metabolic clearance rate of the product of inner ring T_4 deiodination rT_3, and the low concentration in plasma (0.25 nmol/L, 15 ng/dL) combine to yield daily production rates for rT_3 of about 45 nmol. Thus, 80% to 85% of T_3 and all of rT_3 production in humans can be accounted for by peripheral deiodination of T_4, findings consonant with the high ratio of T_4 to T_3 (15 : 1) and rT_3 (>100 : 1) in human Tg. Of the T_3 generated via T_4 5′ deiodination in euthyroid humans, only 20% to 25% is inhibited by PTU consistent with a significant contribution of D2-dependent T_3 production.[93,99,100] Although much of the T_3 and rT_3 produced from T_4 in peripheral tissues exits those tissues and enters the blood, an uncertain fraction of both are degraded intracellularly before their exit. As discussed below, in some D2-containing tissues such as the pituitary, a significant fraction of T_3 in the cell nucleus is derived from intracellular T_4 deiodination to T_3 production, rather than from the plasma. This is particularly true in the thyrotroph.[101]

Other pathways are also involved in T_4 and T_3 metabolism. In humans, T_4, but minimal amounts of T_3, undergo glucuronidation of the phenolic hydroxyl by the UDP-glucuronyltransferases (UDPGT) (see Fig. 10–3). This pathway is clinically significant because certain pharmacotherapeutic agents may enhance glucuronide conjugation through induction of uridine diphosphate glucuronyl transferase (UDPGT), leading to biliary excretion of T_4-glucuronide (T_4-G) into the intestine.[102] These agents include phenobarbital, phenytoin, rifampin, and, possibly, certain of the synaptosomal serotonin reuptake inhibitors, such as sertraline. Because T_4-G may not be easily reabsorbed from intestinal contents, the significance of this pathway is that therapy with such agents will generally increase levothyroxine requirements. In patients with an intact thyroid, this will not be apparent because internal adjustments will increase the T_4 production rate to compensate for the accelerated biliary excretion. In patients with hypothyroidism, however, an increase in levothyroxine dosage will often be required. Deamination and decarboxylation reactions that produce tetrac and triac and sulfation of T_4 and T_3 at the phenolic hydroxyl account for an as yet unidentified fraction of T_4 and T_3 metabolism in humans.

Sources of Intracellular T_3. In view of the differential tissue distribution of the various deiodinases, their different K_m values and differential regulation, it is not surprising that tissues may derive intracellular T_3 via different pathways (Fig. 10–5). In rat kidney and liver, D1-expressing tissues, most of the nuclear T_3 is derived from plasma T_3. In the rat cerebral cortex, pituitary, and brown fat, all of which express D2, half or more of intracellular T_3 is generated locally from T_4 within the tissue. This may be due in part to the differences in the subcellular localization between D2 and D1 mentioned earlier. In the CNS, the D2-generated T_4 in neurons is likely to derive from paracrine sources in tanycytes and astrocytes (see Fig. 10–4). In the rat, the tissues that depend on D2 for nuclear T_3 are those in which a constant supply of thyroid hormone is critical for either normal development (cerebral cortex), thyroid gland regulation (pituitary), or survival during cold stress (brown adipose tissue). These tissues are also characterized by a high degree of saturation of the nuclear T_3 receptors in comparison to tissues such as liver and kidney in which nuclear T_3 receptor sites are only about 50% occupied at normal serum T_3 concentrations (see Fig. 10–5). This arrangement allows multiple levels of regulation of thyroid hormone action.

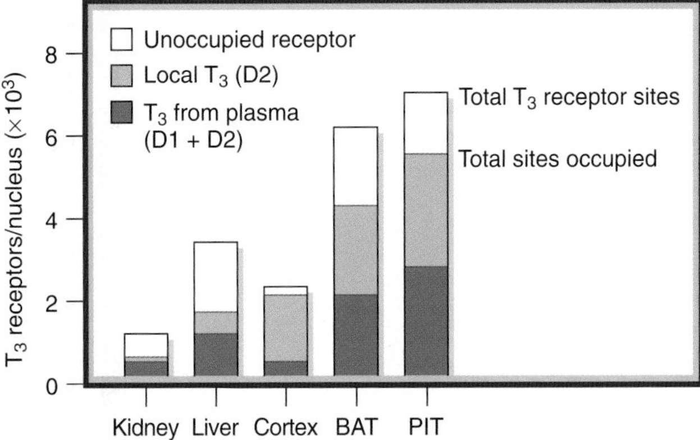

Figure 10–5 ▪ Schematic diagram of the origin of the specifically bound nuclear T_3 in various rat tissues. Data are derived from studies in which the sources of specifically bound nuclear T_3 in rat tissues were estimated using double-isotope labeling techniques. In tissues in which the receptor saturation is significantly greater than 50%, the additional T_3 is provided by D2-catalyzed T_4 to T_3 conversion. T_3 in rat plasma is derived from thyroid secretion (~40%) with the remainder from D1- and D2-catalyzed T_4 to T_3 conversion. *BAT,* Brown adipose tissue; *PIT,* pituitary.

Intracellular D2-catalyzed T_3 production has important implications for thyroid hormone physiology. First, because the T_3 produced from T_4 occupies a significant fraction of the receptors in those tissues, changes in either serum T_4 or T_3 can change receptor occupancy. However, because a fall in T_4 will also increase D2 protein half-life by decreasing the rate of ubiquitination and its proteasomal degradation, a rise in D2 activity mitigates the impact of a reduction of serum T_4 in D2-expressing tissues, helping to maintain T_3 homeostasis.[51] The requirement for both T_3 and T_4 for normal saturation of pituitary and CNS T_3 receptors permits a response of the hypothalamic-pituitary axis to a reduction in plasma T_4, which is the earliest manifestation of iodine deficiency or primary hypothyroidism (see "Regulation of Thyroid Function"). Because the *Dio2* gene is positively regulated by cyclic AMP, D2 activity and T_3 production increase rapidly in brown adipose tissue under stimulation by the sympathetic nervous system during cold exposure.[103] This response is critical to adaptive thermogenesis during cold exposure in the human neonate and lifelong in the rodent.[104]

Pharmacologic Agents Inhibiting Thyroid Hormone Deiodination. A number of commonly used pharmacologic agents have significant effects on thyroid hormone deiodination. Propylthiouracil inhibition of D1 is mentioned earlier. The antiarrhythmic drug amiodarone shares sufficient structural similarity with T_4 that it can inhibit deiodination of T_4 and reverse T_3 by D1 and possibly by D2 (Fig. 10–6). This causes an increase in plasma T_4 to maintain serum T_3 in the normal range. There is also an increase in TSH within the first weeks of therapy, which gradually returns to normal as the thyroid axis reequilibrates.[105] The T_4 and rT_3 metabolic clearance rates are reduced by 20% to

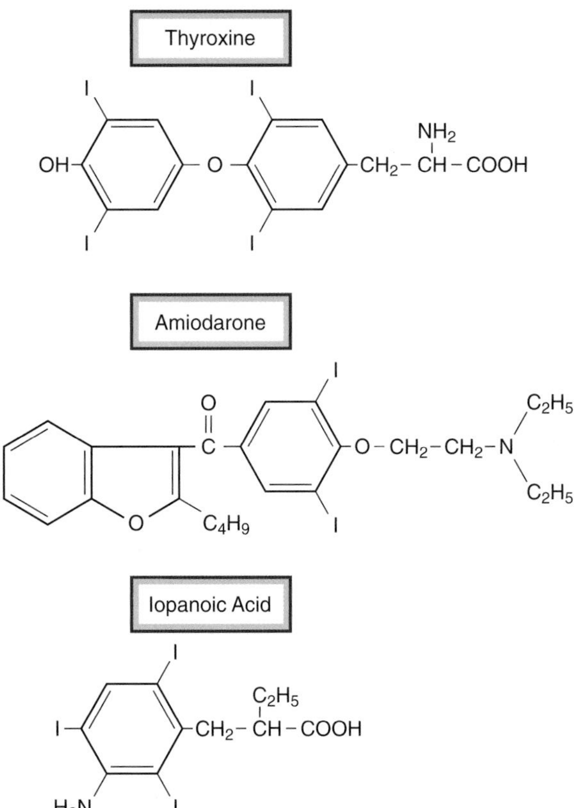

Figure 10–6 ▪ Comparison of the chemical structure of thyroxine with those of two agents that block the deiodination of the iodothyronines. The inhibition of T_4 to T_3 conversion, which occurs in patients receiving amiodarone, may be due to the drug itself or to a metabolic product. Iopanoic acid and related iodoanilines are competitive inhibitors of all three iodothyronine deiodinases.

25%, with a reduction in the fractional T_4 to T_3 conversion rate of about 50%. The mechanism is likely to be due to competitive inhibition either by the drug or by one of its metabolites but inactivation of D1 and accelerated D2 degradation may also occur. Amiodarone also inhibits the active transport of T_4 and T_3 into hepatocytes[106] and the drug or one of its products may interfere with T_3 binding to thyroid hormone receptors.

The effects of amiodarone resemble those observed with the iodoaniline derivatives formerly used for gallbladder visualization (see Fig. 10–6). Iopanoic and iopodipic acid inhibit the deiodinases by competing with the iodothyronine substrates.[51] This makes these agents useful in the acute treatment of patients with severe hyperthyroidism although they are no longer available for clinical use in the United States.[107]

High dosages of glucocorticoids (10 times replacement) will acutely reduce the ratio of T_3 to T_4 in plasma, suggesting that T_4 to T_3 conversion is blocked. The ratio of rT_3 to T_4 increases, raising the possibility that D3 action is also increased.[108] These effects resolve during long-term therapy such that thyroid function is little affected nor are thyroid hormone requirements increased by chronic glucocorticoid therapy.

Recombinant growth hormone increases circulating T_3/T_4 and reduces rT_3/T_4 ratios.[109] This also occurs in patients with hypothyroidism receiving levothyroxine, indicating it is a peripheral effect. Growth hormone deficiency is associated with a decrease the ratio of T_3 to T_4 in serum possibly associated with a decrease in outer ring deiodination. Dietary selenium deficiency also inhibits synthesis of D1 in humans.[110]

Mechanism of Thyroid Hormone Action

Thyroid hormone acts by binding to a specific nuclear thyroid hormone receptor (TR), which, in turn, binds to DNA usually as a heterodimer with retinoid X receptor at specific sequences (thyroid hormone response elements, or TREs) dictated by the DNA binding-site preferences of the RXR-TR (or TR-TR) complex (Fig. 10–7). The general mechanism by which nuclear receptor-activating ligands such as T_3 produce their effects is discussed in Chapter 4. Triiodothyronine has a 15-fold higher binding affinity for TRs than does T_4, explaining its function as the active thyroid hormone. In humans, there are two TR genes, α and β, found on different chromosomes (TRα, chromosome 17; TRβ, chromosome 3). There are several alternatively spliced gene products from each of these genes forming both active and inactive gene products. The active proteins are $TR\alpha_1$, and TRs β_1, β_2, and β_3.[111] The structure of the TRs conforms to a protein with three major functional domains, one binding DNA, one binding ligand, and a major transcriptional activation domain in the carboxy-terminus.

There are tissue-specific preferences in expression of the various TRs suggesting that they subserve different functions in different tissues.[112] In general, TRβ, particularly $TR\beta_2$, is thought to be important in the hypothalamus and pituitary where regulation of thyroid function occurs.[113] In addition to differences in the amino-terminus between $TR\beta_1$ and $TR\beta_2$, the two proteins are under the regulation of different promoters, which can function in tissue-specific patterns. $TR\beta_2$ is down-regulated by T_3, whereas $TR\beta_1$ mRNA expression is not affected.[114] $TR\beta_2$ is also expressed in the cochlea. $TR\alpha_1$ is expressed in all tissues, although its mRNA is especially highly expressed in the kidney, liver, brain and heart. $TR\alpha_1$ mRNA is expressed in the brain and at lower levels in skeletal muscle, lungs, and heart. $TR\beta_3$ mRNA is expressed at very low levels but is more abundant in the liver or kidneys and lungs in comparison with other tissues.

Experiments in which TRα and TRβ have been inactivated illuminate their different physiologic roles.[115] Disruption of the

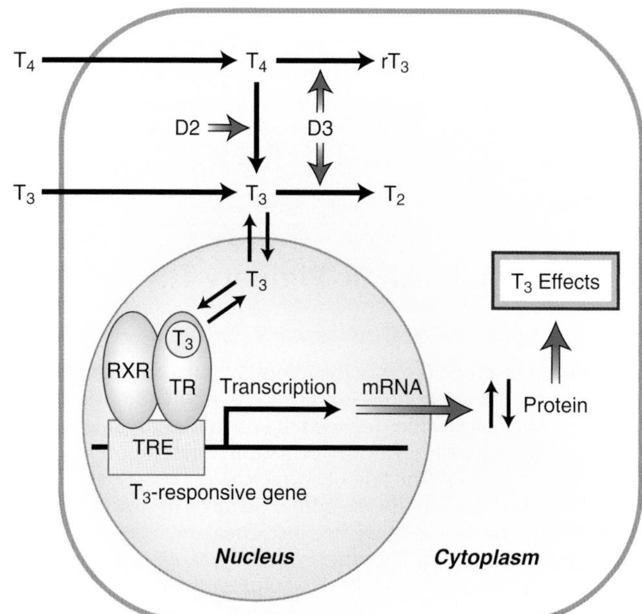

Figure 10–7 ▪ Schematic diagram of thyroid hormone activation and inactivation in a cell expressing D2 and D3. The T_3 that enters the cell can either be deiodinated to 3,3′-T_2 or enter the nucleus and bind to the thyroid hormone receptor. An additional source of T_3 is that generated by outer ring deiodination of T_4 within the cell. The interaction of T_3 with the thyroid hormone receptor (TR) bound as a heterodimer with retinoid X receptor (RXR) to the thyroid hormone–response element (TRE), usually in the 5′ flanking region of a T_3-responsive gene, causes either an increase or a decrease in the transcription of that gene. This leads to parallel changes in the concentrations of critical proteins, thus producing the thyroid hormone response characteristic of a given cell.

TRβ gene (both $TR\beta_1$ and $TR\beta_2$) in mice causes deafness, a marked reduction in feedback sensitivity of hypothalamic-pituitary-thyroid axis, and a decrease in hepatic D1. Thus, these mice have marked elevations in both TSH and thyroid hormones similar to that in families with *resistance to thyroid hormone* (RTH) in which TRβ mutations markedly reduce its binding affinity for T_3.[116,117] This binding defect produces a $TR\beta_1$ or $TR\beta_2$ protein which acts as a dominant negative inhibitor of the intact TRβ proteins encoded by the normal allele (see Chapters 4 and 12). Despite evidence of impaired feedback regulation, there is relatively little abnormality in the brain and heart of TRβ-deficient mice. The effect of a $TR\alpha_1$ disruption in the mouse is quite different. The predominant phenotypic effects are modest bradycardia and hypothermia.

These studies have led to the generalization that feedback regulation of thyroid hormone effects and cochlear development are functions of TRβ, whereas cardiac function and energy metabolism are more likely to be regulated by TRα. It is likely that small differences in the ligand-binding domains of TRα and TRβ will allow design of thyroid hormone analogues selective for one or the other of these receptors.[118] This may result in agents that could, for example, suppress TSH in patients with thyroid cancer, without inducing tachycardia, such as GC-1.[119]

Other potential mechanisms for thyroid hormone action by interaction with the membrane are under investigation. The pivotal role of T_3 in the activation of thyroid hormone–dependent genes argues that T_4 serves primarily as a prohormone. However, continuing investigations show T_4 and thyroid hormone analogues such as GC-1 can activate MAPK and have proangiogenic effects in a model system.[120] The MAPK signal results in serine phosphorylation of several nuclear proteins and occurs within minutes of exposure analogous to the effects of

17β-estradiol. The physiologic relevance of these effects is currently under investigation. The effect of T_4 *per se* to initiate the ubiquitination of D2 is also a nongenomic, epigenetic effect.[51]

REGULATION OF THYROID FUNCTION

The Hypothalamic-Pituitary-Thyroid Axis

The thyroid participates with the hypothalamus and pituitary in a classical feedback control loop (Fig. 10–8). In addition, there is an inverse relationship between the glandular organic iodine level and the rate of hormone formation. Such autoregulatory mechanisms stabilize the rate of hormone synthesis despite fluctuations in the availability of iodine. Stability in hormone production is achieved in part because the large intraglandular store of hormone buffers the effect of acute increases or decreases in hormone synthesis. Autoregulatory mechanisms within the gland, in turn, tend to maintain a constant thyroid hormone pool. Finally, the hypothalamic-pituitary feedback mechanism senses variations in the availability of free thyroid hormones, however small, and acts to correct them. There is a close relationship between the hypothalamus, the anterior pituitary, the thyroid gland, and still higher centers in the brain, the function of the entire complex being modified in a typical negative-feedback manner by the availability of the thyroid hormones. In addition, other hormones and neuropeptides also influence this axis (see Chapters 7 and 8).

Thyrotropin-Releasing Hormone (TRH) Synthesis and Secretion. TRH, a modified tripeptide (pyroglutamyl-histidyl-proline-amide), is derived from a large prepro-TRH molecule that contains five progenitor sequences. The TRH peptides are released from the prepro molecule by a peptidase that acts at flanking lysine/arginine residues. TRH is expressed in the hypothalamus, the brain, the C cells of the thyroid gland, the beta cells of the pancreas, the myocardium, the reproductive organs including prostate and testis, and the spinal cord. The parvocellular region of the paraventricular nuclei (PVN) of the hypothalamus is the source of the TRH that regulates TSH secretion.

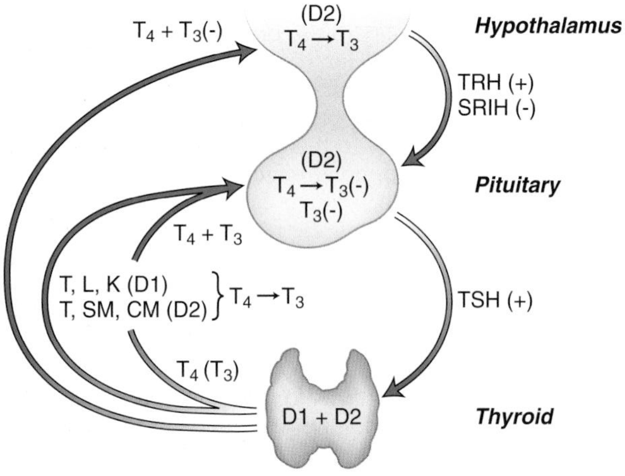

Figure 10–8 ■ Role of T_4 and T_3 in the feedback regulation of TRH and TSH secretion. Secreted T_4 must be converted to T_3 to produce its effects. This conversion may take place in tissues such as the liver (L), kidney (K), and thyroid (T) catalyzed by D1. D2 is present in human thyroid (T), skeletal muscle (SM), possibly cardiac muscle (CM) and the pituitary and hypothalamus.

The 5′ flanking region of the gene encoding TRH has sequences for mediating responses to glucocorticoids and cAMP. In addition, at least two elements in this region of the gene can confer negative regulation of thyroid hormone receptor complexes.[121] TRH travels in the axons of the peptidergic neurons through the median eminence and is released close to the hypothalamic-pituitary portal plexus. The neuron bodies producing TRH are innervated by catecholamine, leptin, neuropeptide Y, AgRP, NPY or MSH, and somatostatin-containing axons, all of which potentially influence the rate of synthesis of the prepro-TRH molecule (see Chapter 7).

There is an acute reduction of TSH in fasted humans, associated with a fall in leptin levels. This is due to a decrease in the amplitude of the TSH pulses.[122] Unlike in the rat, only administration of supraphysiologic amounts of leptin partially attenuates the reduced TSH, suggesting there may be some differences between humans and rats in its role in TRH-TSH regulation. Leptin does not normalize the reduced T_3 of fasting, suggesting the reduction in T_4 to T_3 conversion is not related to reductions in this adipokine.[122] Consistent with this, while a human leptin gene-inactivating mutation causes morbid obesity and hypogonadism, it does not cause central hypothyroidism, suggesting the system may differ from that in the rodent.[123]

T_3 suppresses the levels of prepro-TRH mRNA in the hypothalamus,[124,125] but normal feedback regulation of prepro-TRH mRNA synthesis by thyroid hormone requires a combination of T_3 and T_4 in the circulation, the latter giving rise to T_3 via T_4 5′ deiodination in the CNS in astrocytes and tanycytes (see Fig. 10–4). Thus, part of the negative feedback induced by T_4 may be generated at the median eminence/arcuate nucleus at a point where neuropeptides and T_3 enter the pituitary portal system.[126] In addition to inhibiting the synthesis of prepro-TRH mRNA, thyroid hormone also blocks the capacity of TRH to stimulate TSH release from the thyrotroph.

Thyrotropin (Thyroid-Stimulating Hormone) Synthesis and Secretion. TSH is the major regulator of the morphologic and functional states of the thyroid. It is a glycoprotein secreted by the thyrotrophs in the anteromedial portion of the adenohypophysis (see Chapter 8). TSH is composed of an α-subunit of 14 kd (92 amino acids) that is common to luteinizing hormone (LH), follicle-stimulating hormone (FSH), and human chorionic gonadotropin (hCG) and a specific β-subunit synthesized in thyrotrophs, which is a 112-amino-acid protein. In normal thyrotrophs and in thyrotroph tumors, synthesis of α-subunit is in excess, indicating that the quantity of β-subunit is rate-limiting for TSH secretion. Levels of α-subunit in serum range from 0.5 to 5 μg/L but are increased in postmenopausal women and patients with pituitary tumors. TRH increases and thyroid hormone suppresses the transcription of both subunits; these are the two most important influences on TSH synthesis.

The physiologic glycosylation of TSH involves addition of preformed asparagine-linked oligosaccharides in the rough endoplasmic reticulum, modifications in proximal and distal Golgi apparatus, and the appearance of the intact folded hormone in the secretory granules.[127] TRH is required for this process. The glycosylation of the subunits protects them from intracellular degradation and permits normal folding of the protein chains so that internal disulfide linkages are correctly formed. Glycosylation is required for full biologic activity.[128,129] The biologic activity of the TSH in the serum of patients with pituitary tumors or hypothalamic disorders is inappropriately low compared with immunologic activity due to TRH deficiency.[130]

In normal serum, TSH is present at concentrations between 0.4 and 4.2 mU/L. The level is increased in primary hypothyroidism and reduced in thyrotoxicosis. The plasma TSH half-life is about 30 minutes, and production rates in humans are 40 to

150 mU/day. Circulating TSH displays both pulsatile and circadian variations. The former are characterized by fluctuations at 1- to 2-hour intervals. As mentioned, the magnitude of TSH pulsations is decreased during fasting, illness, or after surgery.[122] The circadian variation is characterized by a nocturnal surge that precedes the onset of sleep and appears to be independent of the cortisol rhythm and fluctuations in the serum and T_4 and T_3 concentrations.[131,132] When the onset of sleep is delayed, the nocturnal TSH surge is enhanced and prolonged, and the early onset of sleep results in a surge of lesser magnitude and shorter duration.

The degree of thyroid hypofunction after destruction of the hypothalamus is less severe than that which follows hypophysectomy, and residual thyroid function in the former circumstance can be altered by raising or lowering the concentration of thyroid hormones in the blood. Thus, both T_4 and T_3 mediate the feedback regulation of TSH secretion, and TRH determines its set-point (see Fig. 10–8). There is a linear inverse relationship between the serum free T_4 concentration and the log of the TSH (Fig. 10–9), making the serum TSH concentration an exquisitely sensitive indicator of the thyroid state of patients with an intact hypothalamic-pituitary axis. Recent gene targeting studies show that TRH secretion is likely to be the dominant factor mediating the thyroid hormone feedback regulation of TSH secretion because the markedly elevated TSH secretion of mice with inactivation of the TRβ cannot be sustained in mice lacking the TRH gene.[133] This is somewhat surprising given the less severe hypothyroidism associated with hypothalamic, as opposed to primary hypothyroidism, but may be explained by the absolute nature of the TRH deficiency achieved by the genetic manipulation as opposed to the clinical situation in humans with central hypothyroidism wherein the TRH deficiency is not likely to be complete.

Somatostatin (somatotropin release–inhibiting hormone, SRIH), acting through inhibitory G protein (G_i), decreases TSH secretion in vitro and in vivo, but prolonged treatment with a somatostatin analogue does not cause hypothyroidism.[134,135] Similar acute effects occur during dopamine infusion and the administration of bromocriptine, a dopamine agonist. Both of these agents inhibit adenylate cyclase. Conversely, blockade of the dopamine receptor by metoclopramide increases the basal serum TSH concentration in both euthyroid and hypothyroid patients. These findings indicate that dopamine is a regulator of TSH secretion, but chronic administration of dopamine agonists, for example, for the treatment of prolactinoma, do not cause central hypothyroidism, indicating that compensatory mechanisms negate these acute effects.[136]

A number of drugs or hormones may suppress TSH secretion (Table 10–6). Glucocorticoids given in high doses transiently suppress TSH secretion, although prolonged therapy is not associated with central hypothyroidism.[137] Patients with Cushing's disease have subnormal TSH production but with minimal effects on T_4 production.[137,138] Bexarotene, a retinoid X receptor agonist used for treatment of T-cell lymphoma, suppresses TSH sufficiently to cause central hypothyroidism, presumably by reducing TSH-β gene transcription.[139,140]

A recently identified agonist of the TSH receptor is *thyrostimulin*. It is a noncovalent heterodimer of two glycoprotein hormone-like proteins, alpha2 and beta5. It is synthesized in the corticotrophs and placenta, has high affinity for TSH receptors, and increases thyroid hormones in rats with a suppressed TSH.[141] Studies are currently underway to determine whether this protein is present in the circulation and how it is regulated.

Iodine Deficiency

The response of vertebrates to iodine deficiency is designed to conserve this limited resource and improve the efficiency of its

TABLE 10–6 ENDOGENOUS AND EXOGENOUS AGENTS THAT MAY SUPPRESS THYROTROPIN SECRETION

Thyroid hormones and analogues
Dopamine and dopamine agonists
Somatostatin and somatostatin analogues
Dobutamine
Glucocorticoids (acute, high-dose)
Interleukin-1β, interleukin-6
Tumor necrosis factor-α
Bexarotene (retinoid X receptor agonist)
Phenytoin

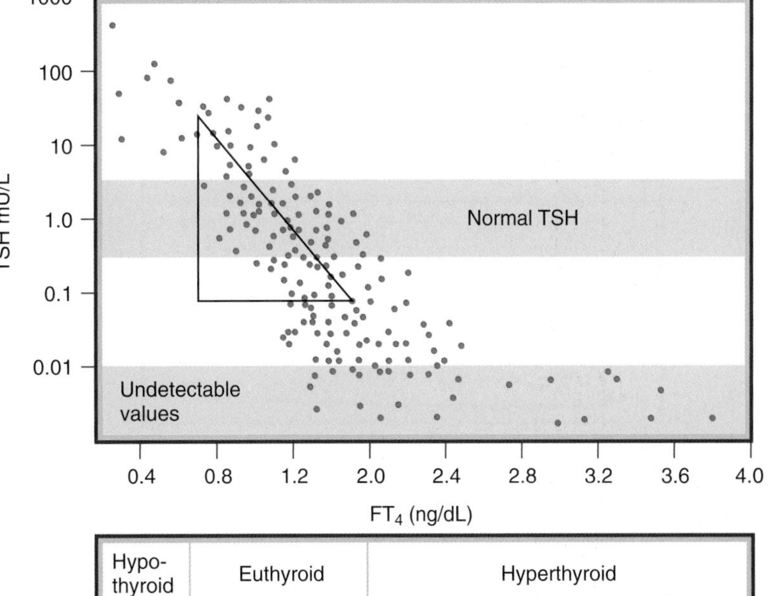

Figure 10–9 ▪ The log/linear relationship between TSH (on the vertical axis) and the free T_4 concentrations (FT_4). Typical free T_4 concentrations in hypothyroid, euthyroid, and hyperthyroid patients are shown. (Modified from Spencer CA, LoPresti JS, Patel A, et al. Applications of a new chemiluminometric thyrotropin assay to subnormal measurement. J Clin Metab 1990;70:453-460.)

utilization. These adjustments occur at the hypothalamic, pituitary, thyroid, and peripheral tissue levels. Removal of iodine from the diet causes a rapid decrease in serum T_4 concentrations and a simultaneous increase in serum TSH (Fig. 10–10).[142] Interestingly, no detectable decrease in T_3 occurs, suggesting that the signal to increase TSH must derive from a decrease in the T_3 generated intracellularly from T_4 in the pituitary, the hypothalamus, or both. TSH increases NIS, Tg, and TPO synthesis and iodine organification and Tg turnover (see Fig. 10–2). Because of the decrease in iodide supply and the ratio of DIT/MIT, the ratio of T_4 to T_3 in Tg decreases and the rate of thyroidal T_3 secretion may increase despite a fall in T_4 secretion. TSH also stimulates cell division, leading to goiter. In the rat model, the fall in plasma T_4 increases D2 from 5- to 20-fold in the CNS, hypothalamus, and pituitary, increasing the efficiency of T_4 conversion to T_3. With moderately severe iodine deficiency, D3 in the CNS is also reduced, prolonging the mean residence time of T_3 in that organ.[143,144] This permits serum T_3 to remain normal and the CNS T_3 to be only moderately reduced despite up to a 10-fold decrease in circulating T_4.[145] Supporting an important role for D2 in humans is the positive association between mental retardation in an iodine-deficient region of China and two common SNPs in the *Dio2* gene.[146]

Despite the TSH elevation and nearly undetectable serum T_4 in acutely iodine-deficient rodents, growth, O_2 consumption, and thermal homeostasis can be maintained.[147,148] However, if iodine deficiency is prolonged and severe, hypothyroidism will supervene. In humans, these compensatory alterations in thyroid function come into operation when total iodine intake falls below 75 μg/d (see Table 10–1). This situation can occur in some countries in Europe and South America as well as affecting several hundred million individuals in China, India, Indonesia, and Africa.[149,150] It makes the recent 50% decrease in iodine intake found in NHANES III in the United States worrisome.[8]

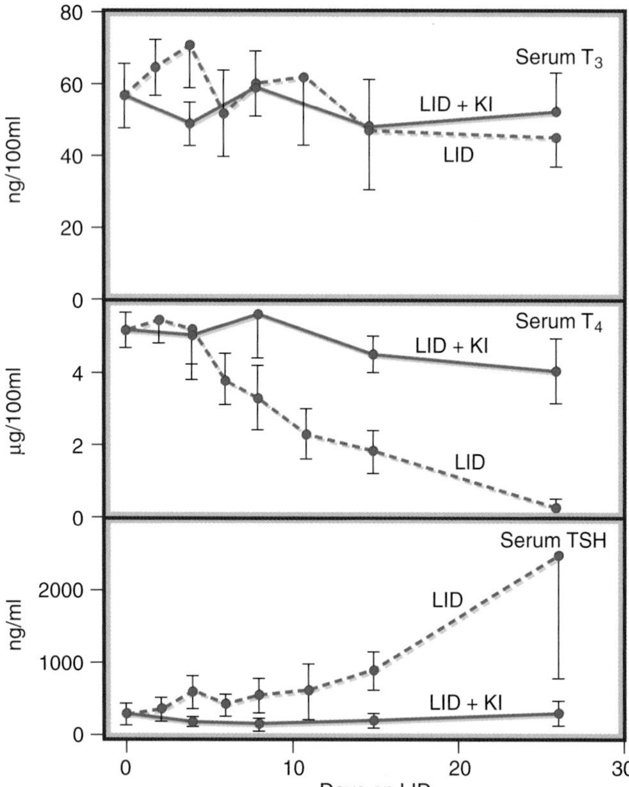

Figure 10–10 ▪ Effects of acute depletion of dietary iodine on serum T_3, T_4, and TSH in rats. Animals received a low iodine diet (LID) without or with supplementation of potassium iodide (KI) in drinking water. (From Riesco G, Taurog A, Larsen PR, et al. Acute and chronic responses to iodine deficiency in rats. Endocrinology 1977;100:303-313).

Changes in serum hormones seen in experimental animals have been well documented in humans in areas of iodine deficiency and in patients with NIS mutations.[18,151] However, they may not be seen in older members of the population when thyroid autonomy often develops. The physiologic response to iodine deficiency is similar to that which occurs during the development of primary hypothyroidism in humans.[152] It is also reproduced when the efficiency of iodide trapping and organification is reduced in Hashimoto's disease or in the patient with Graves' disease receiving thiourea drugs.[25,36] The physiologic effects of this series of events are clear. Triiodothyronine has approximately three times the potency of the prohormone T_4 and contains only three iodine atoms. This results in a fourfold more efficient use of the iodine atom. Maintenance of normal circulating T_3 independent of serum T_4 concentrations should provide hormone for those tissues in which the nuclear T_3 is completely derived from the plasma such as liver, kidney, and heart (see Fig. 10–5.)

Iodine Excess

The thyroid is also protected against an excess of iodide that might otherwise lead to hyperthyroidism. As with the response to iodine deficiency, there are multiple levels of defense against this eventuality. The usual source of excess iodine is pharmaceutical, with radiographic dyes, amiodarone, and povidone-iodine being the most common sources (Table 10–7).

Effects of Increased Iodine Intake on Thyroid Hormone Synthesis. The quantity of iodine organified in thyroglobulin which includes T_4 and T_3 displays a biphasic response to increasing doses of iodide, at first increasing and then decreasing as a result of a relative blockade of organic binding. This decreasing yield of organic iodine from increasing doses of iodide, termed the *Wolff-Chaikoff effect*, results from a high concentration of inorganic iodide within the thyroid cell.[153-155] The susceptibility to the *Wolff-Chaikoff effect* can be increased either by stimulation of iodide trapping, as occurs in patients with Graves' disease, or during persistent TSH stimulation, by impairment of iodine organification in the human fetus, in patients with Hashimoto's disease, or in thyroids previously irradiated by either ^{131}I or external beam therapy. In such situations, goiter and hypo-

TABLE 10–7 IODINE CONTENT OF VARIOUS IODINATED PHARMACEUTICALS*

Saturated solution of potassium iodide	38 mg/drop
Lugol's solution	6 mg/drop
Iodized salt (1 part KI/10,000 NaCl)	760 μg/10 g
Amiodarone	75–200 mg tablet
Iopanoate, ipodate	350 mg/tablet
Angiographic and CT dyes	400–4000 mg/dose
Povidone-iodine	10 mg/mL
Kelp tablets	150 μg/tablet
Prenatal vitamins	150 μg/tablet
Iodinated glycerol	25 mg/mL
Quantity of iodine required to suppress radioactive iodine to <2%	>30 mg/day

CT, Computed tomography; *KI*, potassium iodide; *NaCl*, sodium chloride.
*Typical iodide intake in the United States is 100 to 400 μg/day.

thyroidism (iodide myxedema) can develop if excess iodide is given for long periods.[156] The mechanism for organification inhibition may involve inhibitory effects of high iodide concentrations on TPO and THOX2.

In normal subjects given iodide, the inhibition of iodothyronine formation is reduced over time. This "escape" or "adaptation" phenomenon occurs because iodide transport activity decreases probably through a decrease in NIS expression. Consequently, thyroidal iodide falls to levels insufficient to maintain the full *Wolff-Chaikoff effect.*[157,158] Importantly, it does *not* occur in the third trimester fetus, so chronic high iodine intake during pregnancy must be avoided because it will cause fetal hypothyroidism and compensatory potentially obstructive goiter (Fig. 10–11).

Effects on Thyroid Hormone Release. An important practical effect of pharmacologic doses of iodine is the prompt inhibition of thyroid hormone release. This occurs to some extent normally but is especially apparent in patients with Graves' disease or toxic nodules (see Chapter 11). The mechanism is unknown, but the effect is mediated at the thyroid cell level, rather than through an action on TSH. Iodine also diminishes the hypervascularity and hyperplasia that characterize the diffuse toxic goiter of Graves' disease. This effect facilitates surgical therapy for the disorder.[159]

Thyroid Function in Pregnancy and in the Fetus and Newborn

Pregnancy affects virtually all aspects of thyroid hormone economy (Table 10–8).[3,160,161] The total serum T_4 and T_3 concentrations rise to levels about 1.5-fold those of nonpregnant women owing to the increase in TBG concentration in the first trimester (Fig. 10–12). Free T_4 levels also increase during the first trimester, but return to normal by about 20 weeks' gestation and decrease modestly thereafter until term. The increase in free T_4 is due to hCG, which is a weak agonist for the TSH receptor.[162] The decrease in serum TSH in the first trimester is all the more surprising in that it coincides with a number of events that act to increase maternal requirements for thyroid hormone. In addition to the increase in serum TBG, there is also an increased plasma volume as well as accelerated inactivation of T_3 and T_4 by D3 expression in the fetal-placental-uterine unit.[163-165] Based on the changes in requirements for levothyroxine during gestation in women with primary hypothyroidism, the estimated increase in thyroxine production required during this period is 40% to 50%.

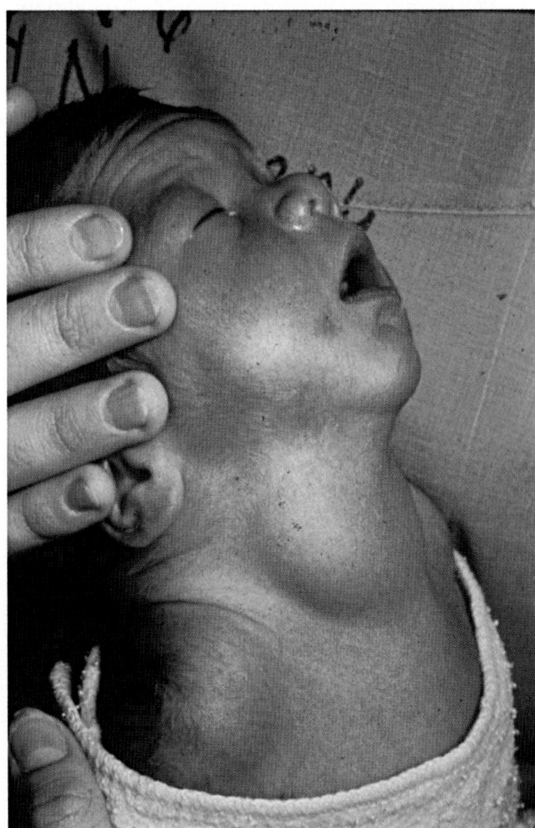

Figure 10–11 ▪ Newborn infant with iodide-induced goiter due to Lugol's solution treatment of the mother during the third trimester. This illustrates the danger of chronic excess iodide administration during gestation.

TABLE 10–8 EFFECTS OF PREGNANCY ON THYROID PHYSIOLOGY

Physiologic Change	Thyroid-Related Consequences
↑ Serum thyroxine-binding globulin	↑ Total T_4 and T_3; ↑ T_4 production
↑ Plasma volume	↑ T_4 and T_3 pool size; ↑ T_4 production; ↑ cardiac output
D3 expression in placenta and (?) uterus	↑ T_4 production
First trimester ↑ in hCG	↑ Free T_4; ↓ basal thyrotropin; ↑ T_4 production
↑ Renal I^- clearance	↑ Iodine requirements
↑ T_4 production; fetal T_4 synthesis during second and third trimesters	
↑ Oxygen consumption by fetoplacental unit, gravid uterus, and mother	↑ Basal metabolic rate; ↑ cardiac output

hCG, Human chorionic gonadotropin.

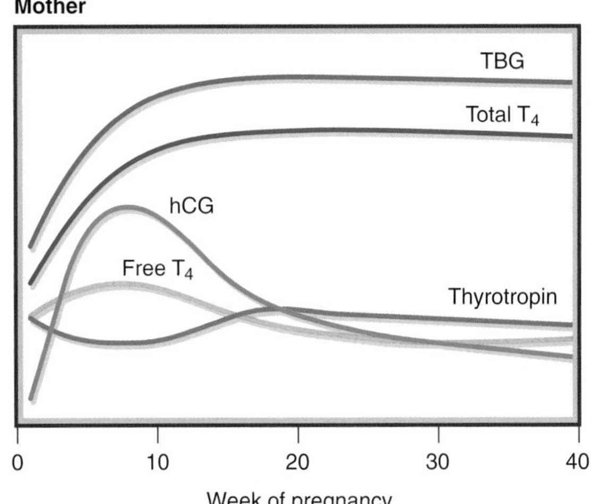

Figure 10–12 ▪ Changes in various critical components of the thyroid-pituitary axis during pregnancy. Note the early increase in free T_4, probably due to thyroidal stimulation by hCG, which causes a reciprocal modest suppression of serum TSH during the late first trimester. (From Burrow GN, Fisher DA, Larsen PR. Mechanisms of disease: maternal and fetal thyroid function. N Engl J Med 1994;331: 1072-1078.)

The requirement for increased T_4 secretion increases iodine requirements during pregnancy. This need is compounded by the fact that the higher glomerular filtration rate during gestation enhances renal iodide clearance, leading to higher fractional urinary excretion of circulating iodide. In addition, maternal iodine intake must be increased to supply the requirements of the fetal thyroid during the second and third trimesters (see Table 10–8). If these increased requirements for iodide are not met, serum T_4 falls and TSH rises. This series of events is well-documented in areas of endemic iodine deficiency or borderline iodine supply, such as Brussels.[9] In that city, 70% of pregnant women carefully followed up throughout pregnancy had a 20% or greater increase in thyroid volume during gestation due to increased TSH.[166] This contrasts with the lack of goiter during pregnancy in studies in North America.[167] After delivery, the changes in thyroid function gradually return to normal and serum TBG values reach normal levels 6 to 8 weeks postpartum.

During pregnancy, autoimmunity is suppressed, affecting patients with Graves' and Hashimoto's diseases (see Chapters 11 and 12).[168] In general, TSH receptor antibody (TRAb)-mediated thyroid stimulation in the Graves' patient is exacerbated during the first trimester and is attenuated during the second and third trimesters only to exacerbate in the first several months postpartum. Thyroid autoantibody titers fall during gestation in patients with Hashimoto's disease only to rise sharply postpartum in association with a phase of acute T-cell–mediated thyroid cell destruction, postpartum thyroid disease (PPTD), which occurs in about 30% of Hashimoto's patients with significant residual thyroid tissue.[169]

The basal metabolic rate (BMR) increases during the second trimester owing to the increase in the total mass of body tissue consequent to the pregnancy. The changes of pregnancy, together with the decreased peripheral vascular resistance, vasodilatation, and modest tachycardia, may suggest thyrotoxicosis (see Table 10–8). It is important to appreciate that such changes are physiologic in pregnancy, especially when managing the hyperthyroid pregnant patient.

Fetal Thyroid Function. The peripheral metabolism of T_4 in the human fetus differs markedly from that in the adult, both quantitatively and qualitatively. Overall, rates of production and degradation of T_4 in unit per body mass exceed those in the adult by 10-fold. In addition, D1 catalysis is reduced and D3 is enhanced, favoring the formation of the inactive rT_3 already introduced at the expense of T_3. D3 is highly expressed in fetal tissues including the liver, skin, tracheobronchial, urothelial, and gastrointestinal epithelia.[165] This results in a persistently subnormal serum T_3 concentration and an elevated serum rT_3. This permits the highly regulable T_4 to T_3 conversion by D2 to be the major pathway for generating tissue T_3.[170]

Fetal thyroid function begins at about the end of the first trimester. Thereafter, there are steady increases in fetal TBG, and total T_4 and T_3.[171,172] Throughout gestation, the serum TSH values are greater than are present in maternal circulation and higher than would be expected in adults with normal thyroid function. This indicates that there is increasing hypothalamic-pituitary resistance to T_4 during fetal development which is speculated to be a consequence of increased TRH secretion.[172,173] Despite the low circulating T_3, the fetal free T_4 concentrations approximate those in the maternal circulation from gestational age of 28 weeks and onward.

Maternal-Fetal Interactions. The fetal pituitary-thyroid axis functions as a unit that is essentially independent of the mother.[3,4,173] Transplacental passage of TSH from mother to fetus is negligible but the same is not true of maternal T_4. In infants with congenital hypothyroidism caused either by genetic TPO deficiency or athyreosis, serum concentrations of T_4 in cord blood are usually one third to one half of normal.[30] Thus, at least when the maternal-fetal concentration gradient is high, significant transfer of maternal T_4 to the fetal circulation can occur. This transfer may be significant, given the capacity of the fetal brain to increase the efficiency of T_4 to T_3 conversion.[174] Furthermore, T_4 can be found in coelemic and amniotic fluids before the onset of thyroid function.[175] The major factor limiting T_4 and T_3 transfer from mother to fetus is the D3 expressed in the uterus, placenta and fetal epithelium.

Thyroid Function in the Newborn. Mean total T_4 levels in cord sera are 150 nmol/L (12 µg/dL). Serum TBG concentrations are elevated, but not as high as in the maternal serum. At term, free T_4 concentrations are slightly lower than those in the mother. Cord serum T_3 concentrations are low ($\sim 0.8 \times 10^{-9}$ M, 50 ng/dL), and rT_3 and T_3SO_4 are elevated.[3,173,176] After delivery, the serum TSH level in the neonate increases rapidly to a peak at about 2 to 4 hours after birth, returning to its initial value within 48 hours.[177] Levels above 60 mU/L are typical. This neonatal TSH surge is thought to occur in response to the rapid reduction in environmental temperature after delivery. In response, the serum T_4, T_3, and Tg concentrations increase rapidly during the first few hours after delivery and are in the hyperthyroid range by 24 hours of life.[178] The TSH surge doubtless contributes to the increase in serum T_3 concentration, but enhancement of extrathyroidal conversion of T_4 to T_3 by D1 or D2 is thought to be a major factor as well.[51] The adrenergic stimulation of the *Dio2* gene as well as the reactivation of D2 by its deubiquitination in brown adipose tissue are likely to be major contributors to this increase.[179]

Premature infants have an immature hypothalamic-pituitary-thyroid axis with low T_4, T_3, and TSH.[180] Serum T_4, TBG, and free T_4 all tend to correlate with gestational age. Preterm infants also have an attenuated TSH surge postdelivery. In addition, when prematurity is accompanied by complications, such as respiratory distress syndrome or nutritional problems, serum T_4, and especially T_3, may fall to low levels due to a combination of reduced TBG production, immaturity of the thyroid gland, suppression of the hypothalamic-pituitary axis due to illness, impairment of T_4 to T_3 conversion and increases in D3 activity.[181] These changes are, in many respects, similar to those in adults with severe illness. All of these issues need to be taken into account when evaluating the thyroid status of the preterm infant, particularly given the increased prevalence of congenital hypothyroidism in this age group.[182]

Thyroid hormone production rates are higher per unit of body weight in neonatal infants and children than in adults. The daily levothyroxine requirement is about 10 µg/kg in the newborn, decreasing progressively to about 1.6 µg/kg in the adult.[172]

Aging and the Thyroid

In the healthy elderly patient, there is a normal free T_4 but a relatively lower serum TSH than in younger individuals. In addition, while there is still some disagreement, it appears that serum T_3 is lower.[183] Individuals in the eighth and ninth decades also have a reduction in serum T_3 to T_4 ratio as well and, in addition, there is a reduction in the daily secretion rate of TSH.[184] The requirement for complete levothyroxine replacement is reduced about 20% by the eighth decade.

Thyroid Function during Fasting or Illness

A number of changes take place in thyroid function during nutritional deprivation or illness. These consist of a central reduction in TSH secretion and a decrease in T_4 activation in the periphery and in serum T_4 and T_3 binding in serum. The pattern of changes in circulating thyroid hormones and TSH during fasting and illness are quite similar. During fasting, there is a reduction of 50% or more in serum T_3 and an increase in serum reverse T_3 without initial changes in serum total or free T_4 (Table 10–9).[122,185] While the role of specific deiodinases in causing these changes has not been documented at a tissue level in humans during fasting, several lines of evidence suggest they reflect decreases in peripheral T_4 to T_3 conversion by both D1 and D2 and a reduced clearance of reverse T_3 by D1. A role for impaired D2-catalyzed T_4 to T_3 conversion in skeletal muscle seems likely based on recent evidence suggesting an important role for this enzyme in peripheral T3 production in humans and the complete absence of D2 in skeletal muscle in individuals dying in an intensive care unit.[93] While the reduction in D1- and D2-catalyzed deiodination can explain the low T_3 and high rT_3, the inactivating enzyme, D3, is found in the liver and skeletal muscle of patients dying in an intensive care unit.[186] Deiodination by D3 increases the generation of rT_3 from T_4 and converts T_3 to 3,3′ diiodothyronine (see Fig. 10–3), which would exaggerate the changes resulting from the decrease in outer ring deiodination. It is not yet known if such an increase in D3 also occurs during caloric restriction. The attenuation of TSH secretion despite a fall in serum T_3 levels during fasting is discussed earlier (see "The Hypothalamic-Pituitary-Thyroid Axis").

During fasting, basal oxygen consumption and heart rate decline and nitrogen balance, initially negative, returns toward normal.[187] In some studies, these changes in overall metabolism are partially reversed by replacement of exogenous T_3 while fasting continues. Thus, the decrease in T_3 during fasting (and presumably illness) can be viewed as a beneficial energy and nitrogen sparing adaptation. Chronic malnutrition such as occurs in anorexia nervosa is also associated with a reduction in serum T_3 and rarely free T_4.[188,189] TSH concentrations remain in the normal range, although again they are inappropriately low in the context of the reductions in circulating T_3. In contrast, overfeeding, particularly with carbohydrate, increases T_3 production rates and the serum T_3 concentration, reduces serum rT_3, and increases basal thermogenesis.[190]

During illness, decreases in T_3 and pulsatile TSH release and increases in reverse T_3 also occur.[191] This constellation of findings is termed the *low T_3 syndrome, the euthyroid sick syndrome,* or *nonthyroid illness.* If illness progresses, the hypothalamic-pituitary-thyroid axis is even further suppressed with a consequent reduction in the free T_4. This is associated with a decrease in TRH mRNA in the human PVN.[192] An increase in T_3 production by D2-catalyzed T_4 to T_3 conversion in the tanycytes lining the third ventricle during illness may contribute to the blunted response of TSH to the reduced serum T_3, particularly during infections.[193] Cytokines, such as interleukin-6, also increase during illness and parallel the decrease in circulating T_3, although it is not clear whether this is the cause of the hypothalamic changes.[194] These endogenous changes may be further exaggerated by agents such as dopamine or glucocorticoids, which will also, at least transiently, suppress the TRH-TSH axis[195,196] The changes in thyroid function are a continuum with the abnormalities becoming progressively more severe paralleling the patient's clinical condition (see Table 10–9). Mild to moderate changes are observed in patients with illnesses such as mild myocardial infarction, with elective surgical procedures, or during infections such as pyelonephritis or pneumonia in an otherwise healthy individual. In these circumstances, the serum free T_3 is reduced up to 50% and the total rT_3 concentration is increased twofold to threefold. The total serum T_4 concentration remains normal, as does TSH. As illness becomes more severe, the fall in T_3 and increase in rT_3 becomes more marked, but the free T_4 paradoxically may not decrease as TSH begins to fall. This is due to an increase in the free fraction of T_4 in part due to release of free fatty acids and other unidentified substeances into the circulation which reduce the binding of T_4 to TBG. There is often a paradoxical increase in free T_4 early in illness due to such changes.[197] During prolonged critical illness, serum free T_4 and TSH are markedly reduced, and T_3 is reduced in plasma and in tissues to barely detectable levels.[198] It is the patients in the latter condition that postmortem studies show hepatic D1 activity reduced about 50%, skeletal muscle D2 absent, and the presence of D3 in liver and skeletal muscle.[186] Tissue T_3 is reduced in these individuals in parallel with the decrease in the serum hormone concentration. No differences have been found in the T_3 transporter MCT8 in skeletal muscle or liver, although possible abnormalities in other thyroid hormone transporters have not been evaluated.

Interestingly, the same global pattern of changes during acute medical illness has been described in patients with primary hypothyroidism receiving levothyroxine.[199] In such patients, serum T_4, T_3, and TSH concentrations all fell about 50% over the first 3 days, presumably due to a disruption of T_4 binding due to a decrease in TBG, TTR, and albumin, as well as to blockade of T_4-protein interactions due to endogenous interfering substances.[200] Contributing to this may be the translational modification of TBG due to a serpin-catalyzed release of a carboxy-terminal fragment of TGB in inflamed tissues discussed earlier (see "Thyroxine-Binding Globulin").[54,58]

Therapies have been introduced in an attempt to ameliorate certain of the illness-related central abnormalities in the hypothalamic-pituitary axis (including decreases in growth hormone and gonadotropins). One of these, infusions of growth-releasing hormone peptide 2 (GHRP-2), combined with TRH have resulted in increases in TSH, T_3, and T_4 as well as IGF-1, insulin, and the IgF BPs 1, 3, and 5.[201] While the biochemical improvements were significant, the clinical state did not change. Neither T_3 nor T_4 administration improves the outcomes in sick patients, and insulin-mediated improvements in hyperglycemia have not altered the abnormalities in thyroid-related parameters in critically ill patients.[202]

Although serum TSH concentrations in severely ill patients are reduced, an increase in TSH above the normal range may appear during recovery, with the elevation in TSH concentration persisting until circulating free T_4 and T_3 levels return to

TABLE 10–9 CHANGES IN THYROID HORMONE DURING ILLNESS

	Hormone				
Severity of Illness	**Free T_3**	**Free T_4**	**Reverse T_3**	**TSH**	**Probable Cause**
Mild	↓	N	↑	N	↓ D2, D1
Moderate	↓↓	N, ↑ ↓	↑↑	N, ↓	↓↓ D2, D1, ?↑ D3
Severe	↓↓↓	↓	↑	↓↓	↓↓ D2, D1, ↑ D3
Recovery	↓	↓	↑	↑	?

normal.[203] This pattern can be confusing if the elevated TSH concentration is associated with the still-reduced concentrations of free T4. Such patients meet all laboratory criteria for primary hypothyroidism with the exception of the clinical context. Follow-up generally reveals a normalization of TSH and T_4 within 1 to 2 months (see Table 10–9).

Despite the severity of the abnormalities, particularly in serum T_3, there is still disagreement as to whether or not therapeutic intervention should be initiated even in the most severely ill patients. This is because most controlled studies have not shown beneficial effects of T_4 or T_3 supplementation in such individuals.[202,204] The one exception is the possible beneficial effect of T_3 therapy in patients after coronary artery bypass grafting, with one study showing a positive effect and a second, no beneficial effect.[205,206]

The Thyroid Axis and Neuropsychiatric Illness. Patients with neuropsychiatric disease can present with any of a number of abnormalities in thyroid function. Patients with bipolar disorders may show slight elevations in serum TSH and reductions in free T_4, whereas patients with severe depression have slight elevation in serum T_4 and reduced serum TSH.[207] Other acutely psychotic patients may have either high or low serum TSH concentrations and tend to have elevations in free T_4.[208,209] The etiology of these minor abnormalities is not clear but such patients may have thyroid function test results resembling those in patients with primary thyroid disease from whom they must be differentiated.

Effects of Hormones on Thyroid Function

Glucocorticoids. The acute administration of pharmacologic doses of glucocorticoid eliminates pulsatile release of serum TSH concentrations in normal patients presumably by reducing TRH release.[210] With continued administration, there is an escape from this suppression (Table 10–10). Pharmacologic doses of glucocorticoid decrease the serum T_3 concentration in normal and hyperthyroid patients as well as in hypothyroid patients maintained on levothyroxine. The latter finding and the accompanying increase in rT_3 production suggest that glucocorticoids may increase D3 activity.[108]

Primary adrenal insufficiency may be associated with reduced serum T_4 and elevated serum TSH concentrations, suggesting the coexistence of primary hypothyroidism. However, treatment of the adrenal insufficiency can lead to complete resolution of these abnormalities, suggesting that in some patients they are a consequence of glucocorticoid deficiency rather than primary thyroid disease.[211] Nevertheless, the prevalence of primary hypothyroidism is increased in patients with autoimmune hypoadrenalism, so the two causes must be differentiated (see Chapter 14). Likewise, patients successfully treated for Cushing's disease can develop thyroid autoimmunity.[212]

Gonadal Steroids. Estrogen increases TBG by mechanisms already mentioned.[57] Estrogen administration to postmenopausal women causes an increase of 15% to 20% in TSH.[72] Presumably this increases T_4 secretion, in that total T_4 increases and free T_4 is unchanged. Estrogen also increases the levothyroxine requirement in patients with primary hypothyroidism.[213] In contrast, administration of androgens to women decreases TBG and decreases T_4 turnover and levothyroxine requirements in patients with primary hypothyroidism.[214]

Growth Hormone. Growth hormone increases the serum free T_3 and decreases free T_4 in both levothyroxine-treated and normal individuals, suggesting either suppression of D3 activity or increased T_4 to T_3 conversion.[109]

TABLE 10–10 EFFECTS OF HORMONES ON THYROID FUNCTION

GLUCOCORTICOIDS
Excess
Decrease TSH, TBG, TTR (high-dose)
Decrease serum T_3/T_4 and increase rT_3/T_4 ratios
Increase rT_3 production (? ↑ D3)
Decrease T_4 and T_3 secretion in Graves' disease
Deficiency
Increase TSH
ESTROGEN
Increase TBG sialylation and half-life in serum
Increase TSH in postmenopausal women
Increase T_4 requirement in hypothyroid patients
ANDROGEN
Decrease TBG
Decrease T_4 turnover in women and reduce T_4 requirements in hypothyroid patients
GROWTH HORMONE
Decrease D3 activity

D3, Type 3 deiodinase; *rT_3*, reverse T_3 *TBG*, thyroxine-binding globulin; *TSH*, thyrotropin; *TTR*, transthyretin.

PHYSICAL EVALUATION OF THE THYROID GLAND

Manifestations of thyroid disease are usually due to excessive or insufficient production of thyroid hormone, local symptoms in the neck (principally goiter but occasionally pain or compression of adjacent structures), or, in the case of Graves' disease, ophthalmopathy or dermopathy. A functional diagnosis of thyroid disease is based on a carefully taken history, a thorough search for the physical signs of hypothyroidism or thyrotoxicosis, and an appraisal of the results of laboratory tests. Although conditioned by the functional diagnosis, the anatomic diagnosis depends largely on the physical examination of the thyroid gland itself. The typical symptoms of an excess or a deficiency of thyroid hormone are discussed in Chapters 11 and 12.

Physical Examination. Examination of the neck is best accomplished with the patient seated in good light with the neck relaxed. The patient should be provided with a cup of water to facilitate swallowing. The physician should first inspect the neck, especially while the patient swallows, with the neck slightly extended. The presence of old surgical scars, distended veins, and redness or fixation of the overlying skin should be noted. The position of the trachea should be noted. If a mass is present, a determination should be made as to whether it moves with swallowing. A midline mass high in the neck, which rises further when the patient extends the tongue, is typical of a thyroglossal duct remnant or cyst. Movement on swallowing is a characteristic of the thyroid gland because it is ensheathed in the pretracheal fascia; this feature distinguishes a goiter from most other neck masses. However, if the thyroid is so large that it occupies all the available space in the neck movement on swallowing may be lost. The physician should also inspect the posterior dorsum of the tongue, which is the origin of the thyroglossal duct and the location of lingual thyroid tissue.

Except when the thyroid enlargement is extreme, the thyroid examination can be readily performed with the physician facing the seated patient. The physician should use gentle pressure with his or her thumb to locate the thyroid isthmus just caudal to the cricoid cartilage. This provides a convenient starting point for the palpation of the lobes of the gland but an increase in the thickness of the isthmus or a firm texture will already suggest the presence of some generalized thyroid enlargement due to Hashimoto's or Graves' disease. To examine the right lobe, the right thumb is then moved laterally, without release of gentle pressure, to locate the lobe of the thyroid by pressing it against the trachea as the patient swallows sips of water. This strategy allows the palpating thumb to laterally displace the medial border of the sternocleidomastoid muscle, allowing direct access to the entire thyroid lobe. As the patient swallows with the thumb pressing the lobe against the trachea with sufficient tension to displace it slightly over the midline, it will slide up and down under the ball of the thumb. This permits an appreciation of the size and texture of the gland as well as the presence or absence of nodules. A similar strategy with the left thumb is employed for the left lobe. The thyroid may also be examined with the physician standing behind the seated patient palpating with the fingertips of both hands.

The examiner should note the shape of the gland, its size in relation to normal, and its consistency, which is usually slightly greater than adipose tissue but less than muscle. The normal thyroid lobe has approximately the same size in frontal projection as the terminal phalanx of the patient's thumb. Whereas a diffuse goiter and the hyperplastic gland of the hyperthyroid patient with Graves' disease may be softer than normal, the gland of Hashimoto's disease is usually firm. Irregularities of the surface, variations in consistency, and tender areas should be noted. If nodules are palpated, their shape, size, position, translucency, and consistency in relation to the surrounding tissue should be determined. It is counterintuitive, but a firm nodule is more likely to be a cyst than a malignancy. A search should be made for the pyramidal lobe; this is a thin band of tissue extending upward from the isthmus to the thyroid cartilage to the right or left of the midline. A hypertrophied pyramidal lobe may be mistaken for a pretracheal lymph node that sometimes accompanies thyroid carcinoma or thyroiditis. It is usually palpable in patients with generalized thyroid disease, such as Hashimoto's or Graves' disease. During palpation, a vascular thrill may be felt that, in the absence of cardiac disease, is suggestive of hyperthyroidism. Finally, palpation should always include examination of the regional lymph nodes along the jugular vein, posterior to the sternocleidomastoids and in the supraclavicular region.

Auscultation of the neck may confirm the increased vascularity of an enlarged, hyperactive gland suggesting Graves' disease. A systolic or continuous bruit is sometimes heard over a hyperplastic gland. Care should be taken to distinguish a thyroid bruit from a murmur transmitted from the base of the heart or from a venous hum that can be obliterated by gentle compression of the external jugular vein or by turning the head. A venous hum is generally found in younger patients with high cardiac output, such as occurs in Graves' disease or with severe anemia.

An arm-raising test is useful when a retrosternal goiter is suspected. The basis for this maneuver is that if the size of the thoracic inlet is already reduced by such a goiter, raising both arms until they touch the sides of the head further narrows the thoracic inlet and causes congestion and venous engorgement of the face and sometimes respiratory distress *(Pemberton's sign)* or even (rarely) syncope.

In addition to examination of the thyroid gland and regional lymph nodes, evidence of compression or displacement of adjacent structures should be sought. Hoarseness may indicate compression of the recurrent laryngeal nerve, usually by a malignant thyroid neoplasm, and this should be confirmed by laryngoscopy. Displacement of the trachea may be evident, usually associated with a large nodule or nodules and inspiratory stridor may indicate its compression.

It is likely that an ultrasound device will become a common instrument in the endocrinologist's office or clinic in the coming years due to its superior sensitivity for the detection of thyroid nodules. This should enhance, not replace, the physical examination of the thyroid, the only endocrine gland accessible to physical examination

LABORATORY ASSESSMENT OF THYROID STATUS

In considering the laboratory assessment of the patient with known or suspected thyroid disease, the physician should seek to arrive at both functional and, when appropriate, an anatomic diagnosis. Laboratory determinations will confirm whether there is an excess, normal, or insufficient supply of thyroid hormone to verify the inferences from the clinical history and physical examination. Laboratory tests can be divided into five major categories: (1) those that assess the state of the hypothalamic-pituitary-thyroid axis; (2) estimates of the T_4 or T_3 concentrations in the serum; (3) tests that reflect the impact of thyroid hormone on tissues; (4) tests for the presence of autoimmune thyroid disease; and (5) tests that provide information about thyroidal iodine metabolism. The use of iodine and other isotopes for scintiscanning is discussed in Chapter 13.

Tests of the Hypothalamic-Pituitary-Thyroid Axis

TSH. While an inherently indirect reflection of thyroid hormone supply, tests that assess the state of the hypothalamic-pituitary-thyroid axis play a critical role in the diagnosis of thyroid disease. This is because the rate of TSH secretion is exquisitely sensitive to the plasma concentrations of free thyroid hormones thus providing a precise and specific barometer of the thyroid status of the patient (see Figs. 10–8 and 10–9). The rare exceptions to this rule are discussed below. Immunometric assay technology now makes it possible to define the normal range for serum TSH and hence to ascertain both when thyroid function is inadequate or when the hormone supply is excessive (see Chapter 6). This assay uses the TSH molecule as a link between a TSH antibody bound to an inert surface (e.g., particles, the side of a test tube) and a second antibody directed against a different TSH epitope that is labeled with a detectable marker (^{125}I, an enzyme, or a chemiluminescent reagent). Thus, the signal generated is proportional to the concentration of TSH in the serum. This technique is more specific, sensitive, and rapid than radioimmunoassay.

The normal range of the serum TSH concentration by immunometric assay varies slightly in different laboratories but is most commonly 0.4 to 4.2 mU/L. There has been discussion of adopting an even lower upper limit for the normal range but the 4.2 value includes 96% of the disease- and risk-free population.[215,216] The lower limit of 0.4 is too high for pregnancy due to hCG-induced hyperthyroidism as discussed earlier.[217] It should be kept in mind that there is a diurnal variation of TSH secretion with peak values in the early evening and a nadir in the afternoon. A borderline abnormal value should always be repeated within a period of a week or so to be certain that it is representative. A minimally suitable TSH assay should be able to quantitate concentrations of TSH of 0.1 mU/L with a coefficient of variation of less than 20%. Potential artifacts of these assays are discussed in Chapter 6.

The free α-subunit common to TSH, FSH, LH, and hCG is generally detectable in serum with a normal range of 1 to 5 μg/L,[218] but the TSH β-subunit is not. When FSH and LH production are increased, as in postmenopausal women, or when TSH production is increased, as in primary hypothyroidism, the free α-subunit level is also increased. The α-subunit level may also be increased in patients with glycoprotein-producing tumors of the anterior pituitary (see Chapter 8). Its measurement may be useful in the rare patient with hyperthyroidism and a normal or elevated TSH to differentiate between neoplastic and nonneoplastic causes of TSH excess.[218,219]

TSH in Patients with Thyroid Dysfunction. Patients with hyperthyroidism (excess thyroid hormone secretion) and/or thyrotoxicosis (excess thyroid hormone from any cause) will virtually always have a subnormal TSH. The values fall into two general categories: those between the lower limit of normal and 0.1 mU/L, and those less than 0.1 mU/L. Individuals in the former category are asymptomatic *(subclinical hyperthyroidism)*, whereas the latter usually have symptomatic thyrotoxicosis and a significant elevation in free T_4. Patients with hypothalamic or pituitary hypothyroidism often have normal or even slightly elevated serum TSH. The circulating TSH generally has reduced biologic activity due to abnormal glycosylation, reflecting the impaired access of TRH to the thyrotroph.[128,129] Patients with primary hypothyroidism have serum TSH concentrations that range from minimally elevated to 1000 mU/L. In general, the degree of TSH elevation correlates with the clinical severity of the hypothyroidism. Patients with serum TSH values in the range of 5 to 15 mU/L have few if any symptoms,[220] and the serum free T_4 or free T_4 index (F T_4I) is typically low-normal while serum free T_3 concentrations are normal.[152,221] Such individuals with modest TSH elevation are said to have *subclinical hypothyroidism* if the serum free T_4 is in the normal range. These findings indicate minor thyroidal decompensation with a compensatory increase in TSH secretion. A detailed discussion of the various conditions associated with abnormal serum TSH concentrations follows that describing the quantitation of serum thyroid hormones.

An elevation in both serum TSH and free T_4 is unusual and indicates either autonomous TSH production as with a TSH-secreting pituitary tumor, *resistance to thyroid hormone* (RTH), or hyperthyroidism with an artifactual elevation in TSH. Differentiating between these diagnoses may require magnetic resonance imaging (MRI) of the hypothalamic-pituitary region or consultation with the clinical chemistry laboratory to rule out an assay artifact (see Chapter 6).

QUANTITATION OF SERUM THYROID HORMONE CONCENTRATIONS

Total T_4 and T_3. Quantitation of the circulating thyroid hormone concentrations is essential to confirm that the thyroid status abnormality suggested by an abnormal TSH result is accurate as well as documenting its severity. Sensitive and specific radioimmunoassays are available for measuring the total concentrations of T_4 and T_3 and some of their metabolic by-products (see Chapter 6). Because the thyroid status correlates with the free, rather than with the total, hormone concentration, the physician must also obtain some estimate of that (see below). The degree of abnormality in the free T_4 generally correlates with the severity of the hormone excess or deficiency, whereas the serum TSH concentration is an indication of the impact of this abnormality in that specific patient. The normal range for total T_4 in healthy, euthyroid adults with a normal circulating TBG concentration is 64 to 142 nmol/L (5 to 11 μg/dL). Normal serum T_3 concentrations are 1.1 to 2.9 nmol/L (70 to 190 ng/dL). At birth (cord serum), T_3 concentrations are about 50% of those in normal adults, but within a few hours T_3 rises abruptly, peaking at about 24 hours at concentrations in the low thyrotoxic range for adults.

Radioimmunoassays for rT_3, T_3SO_4, triac, tetrac, and the diiodothyronines are of primary interest in the research setting because these iodothyronines are derived from the circulating T_4 or T_3, both of which can be easily quantitated. An exception to this may be "compound W," an as yet unidentified product of T_4 metabolism in the fetal circulation which appears in maternal sera.[102] If validated, measurements of compound W could serve as a much needed index of the state of fetal thyroid function to monitor the effects of maternal antithyroid drug therapy on fetal thyroid function.

Concentrations of Free T_4 and T_3. The most accurate and direct measurements of the concentrations of free T_4 and free T_3 in serum are performed by assay of these hormones in a dialysate or ultrafiltrate of serum.[222,223] This is not practical for clinical purposes and alternative strategies have been developed to estimate free thyroid hormone concentrations. In one method, serum is enriched with tracer amounts of the labeled hormone and the concentration of the isotope in the dialysate or ultrafiltrate is expressed as a fraction of that in undiluted serum. The absolute concentration of free hormone is the product of the total hormone concentration and the fraction that is dialyzable or ultrafiltrable. As mentioned, about 0.02% of T_4 and 0.3% of T_3 is free or unbound (see Table 10–5). The normal ranges for free T_4 and T_3 are 9 to 30 pmol/L (0.7 to 2.5 ng/dL) and for free T_3, 3 to 8 pmol/L (0.2 to 0.5 ng/dL).

Because T_4 is the major secretory product of the thyroid and correlates most closely with the serum TSH, in most situations, a free T_4 estimate is all that is required to ascertain the state of thyroid secretion or supply. An array of methods is used to quantitate free T_4 (or T_3) in whole serum using automated methods.[224] Even though many such automated tests imply that they quantitate free T_4 directly, they do not, and results in sera with abnormal binding proteins are not generally absolute.[224-226] There are two general categories of methods: comparative free T_4 methods and so-called free T_4 index methods. Three general approaches are used: (1) two-step labeled hormone methods, (2) one-step labeled analogue methods, and (3) labeled antibody approaches (see Chapter 6). In general, two-step labeled hormone back titration methods are less subject to artifacts due to abnormal binding proteins, changes in albumin, TBG, or increases in free fatty acids than are one-step hormone analogue methods.[222,223,227] All general approaches are subject to artifacts from endogenous antibodies to T_4 , abnormal binding proteins, or illness.[224,228] Thus, the clinician must be wary if the free T_4 result by *any* method does not agree with the clinical state and the TSH. In such cases, another method should be used to estimate the free T_4, such as quantitation of T_4 in a dialysate or ultrafiltrate, the free T_4 index should be measured, or the result should be ignored. For pregnant or severely ill patients, the automated methods typically give falsely low results, particularly if these are performed using one-step procedures. A reasonable alternative for pregnancy is to use the normal range for the serum T_4 concentration multiplied by 1.5 in lieu of an automated free T_4 assay.[161,229]

The Free T_4 Index (FT_4 I). Particularly useful in estimating the free T_4 in severely ill patients is the determination of the thyroid hormone–binding ratio (THBR), multiplying this result by the total T_4 (or T_3) to obtain a free hormone index (FT_4I or FT_3I). In this test, a tracer quantity of labeled T_4 (or T_3) is added to serum, which is then exposed to a solid phase matrix coated with T_4 or T_3 antibody or to an inert matrix that binds the iodothyronine irreversibly. The proportion of labeled T_4 or T_3 bound by the solid phase is then quantitated. This value, like the free fraction of T_4 quantitated directly in a dialysate, varies inversely with the concentration of unoccupied TBG sites in the serum. Where tracer T_3 is used, its binding to TBG is determined by the ratio of T_4, not T_3, to TBG in that T_4 is present in 50- to 60-fold higher concentrations than T_3, has a much higher affinity for TBG than does T_3 and, therefore, determines the ratio of unoccupied to occupied TBG.

The results of such assays are normalized by comparing them with those obtained simultaneously for standard control sera with normal TBG and serum T_4 concentrations. This is generally done by dividing the result for the unknown sample by that obtained for control sera in the same assay. The quotient is the THBR, which typically has a normal range of 0.85 to 1.10.[225] Because the THBR is proportional to the free fraction of the endogenous thyroid hormones in the serum, it can be multiplied by the total T_4 (or T_3) concentration to estimate the free thyroid hormone concentration, termed the *free T_4* or *free T_3 index* (FT_4I or FT_3I). Because the normal THBR is 1.0, the FT_4I has a normal range in units that is identical to that of the total T_4 (or T_3), for example, 64 to 142 for SI units and 5 to 11 in gravimetric terms. A schematic demonstration of the relationships between total and free T_4, occupied and unoccupied TBG binding sites, and the THBR is shown in Figure 10–13 for euthyroid individuals with variations in TBG concentrations and in Figure 10–14 for subjects with a constant TBG and alterations in serum thyroid hormone production rates.

Estrogen, pregnancy, and severe illness are more common causes of changes in total T_4 concentrations than are hyperthyroidism and hypothyroidism (Table 10–11). In the euthyroid person, only about one third of the available binding sites on TBG are occupied by T_4, and the free T_4 fraction is 2×10^{-4} of the total. During pregnancy, the TBG binding capacity, the serum T_4, and the number of unoccupied TBG binding sites approximately double, leading to an approximately 50% reduction of the free T_4 fraction. This is reflected in a reduced THBR. If the reduced THBR (or free fraction) is multiplied by the increased total T_4, the FT_4I estimate is normal, an accurate reflection of the free T_4 concentration. In patients in whom the serum T_4 concentration is reduced owing to a low TBG, the concentration of unoccupied binding sites is reduced to an even greater extent. This reduction leads to an increase in the free T_4 (and T_3) fractions and the THBR, and both the free T_4 and the FT_4I remain in the normal range.

There is one caution when calculating the FT_4I index using the product of the total T_4 and the THBR. The THBR is not linearly related to the free fraction of thyroid hormones at the extremes of its range. Therefore, it is important to consider both the calculated FT_4I and the pattern of the deviations of total hormone and THBR from normal to derive the maximum information. When concentrations of TBG are altered, the deviation of the total T_4 measurements from normal is in the opposite direction to that of the THBR (central panels of Fig. 10–13). On the other hand, when the T_4 level is elevated due to increased T_4 secretion or overreplacement, the concentration of unoccupied TBG binding sites is reduced, and both the free fraction and the total T_4 are altered in the same direction (see Fig. 10–14). The changes in hypothyroidism are both in the opposite direction, although of lower magnitude. The reduced FT_4I of hypothyroidism is due predominantly to the decrease in T_4 rather than to a decrease in its free fraction.

TABLE 10–11 CIRCUMSTANCES ASSOCIATED WITH ALTERED BINDING OF THYROXINE BY THYROXINE-BINDING GLOBULIN

Increased Binding	Decreased Binding
Pregnancy	Androgens
Neonatal state	Large doses of glucocorticoids
Estrogens and hyperestrogenemic states	Active acromegaly
Tamoxifen	Nephrotic syndrome
Oral contraceptives	Major systemic illness
Acute intermittent porphyria	Genetic factors
Infectious and chronic active hepatitis	Asparaginase
Biliary cirrhosis	
Genetic factors	
Perphenazine	
HIV infection	

HIV, Human immunodeficiency virus.

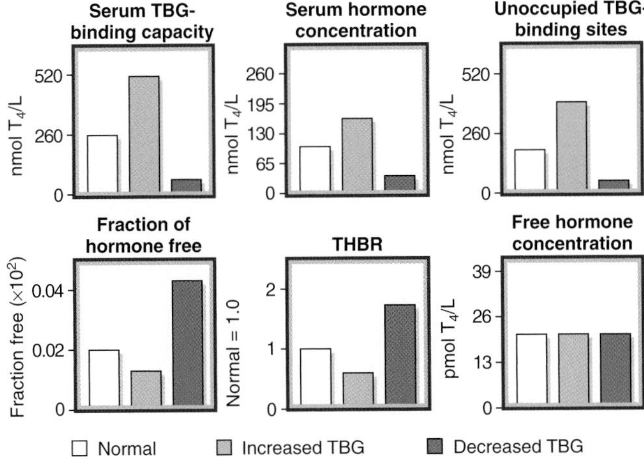

Figure 10–13 ▪ Pattern of changes in total serum T_4 concentrations and the thyroid hormone–binding ratio (THBR) in euthyroid patients with alterations in the circulating concentrations of thyroxine-binding globulin (TBG). To convert T_4 from nmol/L to μg/dL (total) or pmol/L (free), divide by 12.87.

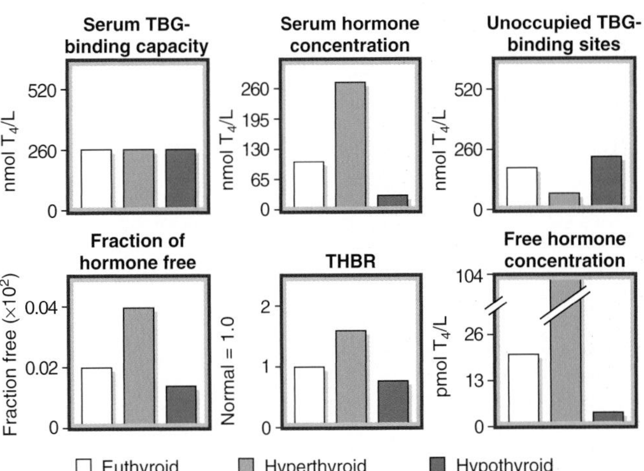

Figure 10–14 ▪ Pattern of changes in total serum T_4 concentration and thyroid hormone binding ratio (THBR) in patients with hyperthyroidism or hypothyroidism with normal serum thyroxine-binding globulin (TBG) concentration.

Simultaneous abnormalities in both TBG and thyroid hormone production may also occur. One should suspect hyperthyroidism during pregnancy when the T_4 concentration is very high and the THBR is not *subnormal.* Likewise, a serum T_4 concentration in the lower portion of normal range for a nonpregnant individual accompanied by a significant reduction in the THBR indicates hypothyroidism. For pregnant patients, the best strategy may be to use the normal range for total T_4 for the assay being used multiplied by 1.5.[230]

Several caveats should be kept in mind in the interpretation of these results. The use of labeled T_3 in some assays can produce difficulties in three situations: in cases of familial dysalbuminemic hyperthyroxinemia (FDH); in the presence of endogenous antibodies directed against T_3; and in sick patients, as already discussed. In FDH, the abnormal albumin binds T_4, but *not* T_3, with increased avidity. Therefore, these patients have an elevated total T_4 and reduced free fraction of T_4, *but not* T_3.[70]

An alternative approach to assessing the FT_4I is to measure TBG either by saturation analysis or radioimmunoassay. Normal concentrations of TBG by radioimmunoassay are about 270 nmol/L (1.0 to 1.5 mg/dL) and are only slightly higher in women than in men. However, it should be recalled (see TBG) that the elastase released from leukocytes during infection may reduce the binding affinity of TBG for T_4 (and T_3) but not change its immunoreactivity or its binding capacity.[231] In such patients, the gravimetric TBG concentration is not paralleled by its binding affinify for T_4 or T_3. With this proviso, the serum TBG concentration result can be employed in one of two ways. First, normalization of the T_4/TBG (or T_3/TBG) ratio yields values that correlate reasonably well with the FT_4I or FT_3I. Second, an FT_4I can be derived from the concentrations of TBG, total T_4, and the association constant for the interaction between the two. In most instances, values calculated in this manner correlate with the FT_4I determined by other techniques, although the T_4/TBG ratio suggests a subnormal FT_4I in some euthyroid patients with an elevated TBG.[227]

Causes of Abnormal TSH or Thyroid Hormone Concentrations

Many causes of an abnormal TSH should be considered by the clinician (Table 10–12). The clinical status and free T_4 or FT_4I results allow assignment of the etiology for these. Assay of the FT_3I is rarely required but is included for completeness.

Causes of a Suppressed TSH. The most common cause of a reduction in serum TSH is an excess supply of thyroid hormone due to either increased endogenous thyroid hormone production or excessive exogenous thyroid hormone. Because the concentration of TSH is inversely proportional to the degree of thyroid hormone excess, patients with clinical symptoms almost invariably have serum TSH concentrations below 0.1 mU/L. Such patients nearly always have an increase in the serum free T_4. In rare patients with low iodine intake, with clinical thyrotoxicosis, the FT_4I is only high-normal despite a suppressed TSH. An FT_3I is required in those patients to establish a diagnosis of T_3 thyrotoxicosis. When thyroid hormone supply is only slightly in excess of the requirement for that patient, serum TSH is sup-

TABLE-10–12 THYROID STATUS AND FREE THYROID HORMONE LEVELS IN CLINICAL STATES ASSOCIATED WITH ABNORMAL SERUM THYROTROPIN (TSH) CONCENTRATIONS

	Expected TSH (mU/L)	Clinical Thyroid Status	Free T_4 Index	Free T_3 Index
	THYROTROPIN REDUCED			
Hyperthyroidism of any cause	<0.1	↑	↑	↑
"Euthyroid" Graves' disease	0.2-0.5	N, (↑)	N	N, (↑)
Autonomous nodule or multinodular goiter	0.2-0.5	N, (↑)	N	↑
Exogenous thyroid hormone excess	<0.1-0.5	N, ↑	N, ↑	↑
Thyroiditis (subacute or painless)	<0.1-0.5	N, ↑	N, ↑	↑, (N)
Recent thyrotoxicosis due to any cause	<0.1-0.5	↑, N, ↓	N, ↓	N, ↓
Illness with or without dopamine infusion	<0.1-5.0	N	↑, N, ↓	↓
First trimester of pregnancy	0.2-0.5	N, (↑)	N, (↑)	↑
Hyperemesis gravidarum	0.2-0.5	N, (↑)	↑, (N)	↑
Hydatidiform mole	0.1-0.4	↑	↑	↑
Acute psychosis or depression (rare)	0.4-10	N	N, (↑)	N, (↓ or ↑)
Elderly (small fraction)	0.2-0.5	N	N	N
Glucocorticoids (acute, high dose)	0.1-0.5	N	N	↓
Congenital TSH deficiency				
a. PITI deficiency	0	↓	↓	↓
b. CAGYC mutant	0	↓	↓	↓
	THYROTROPIN ELEVATED			
Primary hypothyroidism	6-500	↓	↓	N, ↓
Recovery from severe illness	5-30	N, (?)	N, ↓	N, ↓
Iodine deficiency	6-150	N, ↓	↓	N
Thyroid hormone resistance	1-20	↑, N, ↓	↑	↑
Thyrotroph tumor	0.5-50	↑	↑	↑
Hypothalamic-pituitary disease	1-20	↓	↓	N, ↓
Psychiatric illnesses	0.4-10	N	N	N, ↓
Adrenal insufficiency	5-30	N	N	N, ↓
Artifact (endogenous antimouse γ-globulin antibodies)	10-500	N	N	N

Arrows indicate the nature of the abnormality in the T_4 or T_3 index. Parentheses indicate that such a result is unusual but may occur.

pressed, but clinical manifestations are subtle or absent and the FT_4I (and FT_3I) are in the high-normal range. Such minimal changes can occur with "euthyroid" Graves' disease, autonomous thyroid hormone-producing adenomas, multinodular goiters, subacute or painless thyroiditis, and the ingestion of an amount of exogenous thyroid hormone slightly greater than that required for metabolic needs. This condition is termed *subclinical hyperthyroidism.*

The hypothalamic-pituitary axis may remain suppressed for up to 3 months after complete resolution of the thyrotoxic state.[232,233] The best test for assessing the physiologic state in such patients is the free T_4 or FT_4I. A common scenario for this pattern is during follow-up of patients receiving antithyroid drugs or ^{131}I for Graves' disease. With time, the TSH feedback regulatory loop will normalize, and TSH secretion will return and become appropriate for the circulating free thyroid hormone concentration.

In severe illnesses, with or without dopamine infusion or excess glucocorticoid, TSH is suppressed, making assessment of thyroid functional status difficult (see earlier discussion). Because the FT_4I may also be reduced in such patients, astute clinical judgment is required to assign thyroid status.

Because hCG can activate the TSH receptor, conditions in which hCG is elevated, such as in the first trimester of pregnancy, with twin pregnancies, during severe *hyperemesis gravidarum,* and in patients with hydatidiform mole or choriocarcinoma, the TSH concentration is often suppressed.[217] TSH returns to normal in the second and third trimesters in the euthyroid patient. A persistently suppressed TSH (<0.1 mU/L) in the pregnant patient after the first trimester suggests that the hyperthyroidism is due to autonomous thyroid function.

Changes in thyroid tests results in patients with psychosis or depression, in the geriatric population, and in use of long-term glucocorticoids are discussed earlier.

If the serum TSH is suppressed *and* the serum free T_4 is low, one should be suspicious that liothyronine (triiodothyronine) is being ingested. Desiccated thyroid also has a high T_3/T_4 ratio and if given in excess may cause a similar abnormality.[234]

Causes of an Elevated TSH. Elevations in TSH nearly always imply a reduction in the supply of T_4 or T_3, which may be permanent or transient. Primary hypothyroidism is far and away the usual explanation. Other causes include acutely ill patients as in renal insufficiency[235] or the asynchronous return of the hypothalamic-pituitary and thyroid axes to normal as critically ill patients recover.[236] Iodine deficiency is the most common cause of an elevation in TSH worldwide, but this does not occur in North America. The rare patient with *resistance to thyroid hormone* (RTH) may be clinically hyperthyroid, euthyroid, or hypothyroid. The most common laboratory pattern is a serum TSH that is "normal" in absolute terms but inappropriately high for the elevated free T_4. Individuals with a more marked "pituitary" than "general" resistance to thyroid hormone (sometimes termed pituitary RTH or PRTH) have symptoms suggesting hyperthyroidism, an elevated FT_4I, and a normal or even elevated serum TSH.[237,238] They must be differentiated from the patient with a thyrotroph tumor in whom the persistent secretion of TSH causes hyperthyroidism (see Chapters 8 and 11).[219]

Patients with hypothalamic-pituitary dysfunction may have clinical and chemical hypothyroidism, but low, normal, or even elevated serum TSH concentrations. The explanation for this paradox is that the biologic effectiveness of the circulating TSH is impaired due to abnormal glycosylation secondary to reduced TRH stimulation of the thyrotrophs. Nonetheless, the abnormal TSH is a suitable antigen in the immunometric assay. In adrenal insufficiency, TSH may be modestly elevated but returns to normal with glucocorticoid replacement.[211] This may reflect glucocorticoid mediated amelioration of Hashimoto's thyroiditis.

Despite the utility and general efficacy of the serum TSH measurement alone as a screening tool for identifying patients with thyroid dysfunction, a patient should not receive treatment for this dysfunction solely on the basis of an abnormal TSH. The TSH assay is an *indirect reflection* of thyroid hormone supply and does not, by itself, permit a conclusive diagnosis of a specific disorder of thyroid hormone production. Accordingly, the TSH abnormality must be verified and an alteration in thyroid hormone concentrations verified before initiating treatment.

Tests That Assess the Metabolic Impact of Thyroid Hormones

Abnormalities in the supply of thyroid hormone to the peripheral tissues are associated with alterations in a number of metabolic processes that can be quantitated. Some of these may be useful in the rare patient in whom serum TSH is not an accurate barometer of thyroid status, such as those with RTH. These tests may be the sole means of evaluating the metabolic response of the peripheral tissues to thyroid hormones in such patients.

Basal Metabolic Rate. Thyroid hormones increase energy expenditure and heat production, as manifested by weight loss, increased caloric requirement, and heat intolerance. Because it is impractical to measure heat production directly, the based metabolic rate (BMR) measures oxygen consumption under specified conditions of fasting, rest, and tranquil surroundings. Under these conditions, the energy equivalent of 1 L of oxygen is 4.83 kcal.

Under basal conditions, approximately 25% of oxygen consumption is due to energy expenditure in visceral organs, including the liver, kidneys, and heart; 10% in the brain; 10% in respiratory activity; and the remainder in skeletal muscle. Because energy expenditure is related to functioning tissue mass, oxygen consumption is related to some index thereof, most often body surface area. Calculated in this way, basal oxygen consumption (resting energy expenditure) is higher in men than in women and declines rapidly from infancy to the third decade, and more slowly thereafter. Values in patients, calculated as a percentage of established normal means for gender and age, normally range from −15% to +5%. In severely hypothyroid patients, values may be as low as −40%, and in thyrotoxic patients, these may reach +25% to +50%. Abnormal, usually elevated, values are seen during recovery in burn patients and in systemic disorders, such as febrile illnesses, pheochromocytoma, myeloproliferative disorders, anxiety, and disorders associated with involuntary muscular activity. Resting energy expenditure correlates very well with the free T_4 and TSH in hypothyroid patients given varying doses of exogenous levothyroxine.[239]

Biochemical Markers of Altered Thyroid Status. Occasionally a diagnosis of thyroid dysfunction is first suspected due to an abnormality in a laboratory result performed during an evaluation for an unrelated medical problem. Classic examples are a markedly elevated creatine kinase MM isoenzyme or low-density lipoprotein (LDL) cholesterol leading to the recognition of hypothyroidism.[240] Other similar markers are listed in Table 10–13. These tests are not useful in the diagnosis of thyroid disease, but some, such as sex hormone–binding globulin (SHBG), ferritin, or LDL cholesterol, have been used as endpoints in clinical studies of the responsivity of the liver to thyroid hormone in patients with thyroid hormone resistance.[241,242]

Serum Thyroglobulin

The sensitivity of modern thyroglobulin (Tg) assays is 1 ng/mL or even less.[243] The results can be artifactually altered by serum

TABLE 10–13 BIOCHEMICAL MARKERS OF THYROID STATUS

THYROTOXICOSIS
Increased
Osteocalcin
Urine pyridinium collagen cross-links
Alkaline phosphatase (bone or liver)
Atrial natriuretic hormone
Sex hormone–binding globulin
Ferritin
von Willebrand's factor
Decreased
Low-density-lipoprotein cholesterol
Lp(a)
HYPOTHYROIDISM
Increased
Creatine kinase (MM isoform)
Low-density-lipoprotein cholesterol
Lp(a)
Plasma norepinephrine
Decreased
Vasopressin

Lp(a), Lipoprotein a.

anti-Tg antibodies, and serum should be screened for Tg antibodies with a sensitive Tg-antibody immunoassay or for interferences with a recovery test. In immunoradiometric assays, interferences lead to underestimations of Tg or false-negative values with radioimmunoassays relatively unaffected especially if the antibody titer is low. Tg is normally present in the serum, the concentration ranging up to 90 pmol/L (50 ng/mL); mean normal values vary with the assay used but are on the order of 30 pmol/L (20 ng/mL).[244,245] Concentrations are somewhat higher in women than in men and are several-fold elevated in pregnant women and in the newborn. Levels are elevated in three types of thyroid disorders: goiter and thyroid hyperfunction, inflammatory or physical injury to the thyroid, and differentiated follicular-cell derived thyroid tumors. Values are elevated in both endemic and sporadic nontoxic goiter, and the degree of elevation correlates with the thyroid size. Transient elevations occur in patients with subacute thyroiditis and as a result of trauma to the gland during thyroid surgery or after ^{131}I therapy.[246,247] Subnormal or undetectable concentrations are found in patients with thyrotoxicosis factitia and aid in differentiating this disorder from other causes of thyrotoxicosis with a low thyroid radioiodine uptake (RAIU).[248] Antithyroglobulin antibodies interfere with measurements of the Tg concentration precluding its use in patients with Hashimoto's disease.[245]

A major clinical value of measuring the level of serum Tg is in the management, but not in the diagnosis, of differentiated thyroid carcinoma.[243,245] Serum Tg concentrations are increased in patients with both benign and differentiated malignant follicular-cell derived tumors of the thyroid and do not serve to distinguish between the two. After total thyroid ablation for papillary or follicular thyroid carcinoma, Tg should not be detectable, and its subsequent appearance signifies the presence of persistent or recurrent disease.[249] Secretion of Tg is TSH-dependent. Therefore, the serum Tg level may rise when suppressive therapy is withdrawn or after injections of rhTSH,[250,251] which will increase the sensitivity of the marker for the detection of persistent or recurrent thyroid carcinoma, even when ^{131}I scans are negative (see Chapter 13). Supersensitive assays of thyroglobulin with a functional sensitivity less than 0.1 ng/mL

TABLE 10–14 PREVALENCE OF THYROID AUTOANTIBODIES (Ab)

Group	TSHrAb (%)	hTgAb (%)	hTPOAb (%)
General population	0	5-20	8-27
Graves' disease	80-95	50-70	50-80
Autoimmune thyroiditis	10-20	80-90	90-100
Relatives of patients	0	40-50	40-50
Patients with IDDM	0	40	40
Pregnant women	0	14	14

IDDM, Insulin-dependent diabetes mellitus; *Tg,* thyrogobulin; *TPO,* thyroid peroxidase.

improve the sensitivity during thyroid hormone treatment but at the expense of a decreased specificity.[245] In the hypothyroid newborn, serum Tg is undetectable in patients with thyroid agenesis and is usually elevated in those with ectopic thyroid tissue or goiter.

Tests for Thyroid Autoantibodies

Graves' disease and Hashimoto's thyroiditis are well-characterized and interrelated *autoimmune thyroid disorders* (AITDs) with a variety of clinical manifestations. The diagnostic hallmark of the AITDs are circulating antibodies and reactive T cells against one or another thyroid antigen, which are present in the vast majority of patients.[252] Three varieties of thyroid autoantibodies are in common use and widely available in clinical diagnostic laboratories (Table 10–14). In this section, antibodies to thyroglobulin (Tg) and thyroid peroxidase (TPO) are discussed. Antibodies directed against the TSH receptor, the cause of hyperthyroidism in patients with Graves' disease, are covered in detail in Chapter 11.

Autoantibodies to Thyroid Peroxidase and Thyroglobulin. Modern assay techniques for thyroid autoantibodies have good precision because they depend on the direct measurement of the interaction between autoantibody and autoantigen (i.e., the interaction between labeled thyroid antigen and the patient's serum). In general, the more sensitive an assay, the more precise and antigen-specific it is. However, many euthyroid individuals in our population exhibit low levels of autoantibodies and, therefore, the specificity of the more sensitive tests is reduced and the absolute concentration becomes more important; the higher the concentration of autoantibody, the greater the clinical specificity (see Table 10–14).[253]

To compare levels of thyroid antibodies from one office visit to the next and to compare results between patients and among laboratories, assays for thyroid autoantibodies have been standardized. Antibody results can then be expressed as standard units/mL. Of course, the actual standard serum preparation cannot be included in every assay. Instead, a serum pool is usually compared and normalized to the original standard. Yet autoantibodies differ considerably in their affinity and epitope recognition of antigen. Hence, despite this attempt at standardization, assay results from different commercial assays may still vary considerably. Hence, when following antibody titers (e.g., after the treatment of thyroid cancer), it is important to use the same autoantibody assay.

Do Thyroglobulin and Thyroid Peroxidase Antibodies Have a Pathogenic Role? Tg and TPO autoantibodies appear to be a secondary response to thyroid injury and are not thought to cause disease themselves, although they may contribute to its development and chronicity. Both types of antibodies are polyclonal, and although they are of the IgG class, they are not restricted to one particular IgG subclass. Polyclonality mitigates against a primary role in disease pathogenesis.[254,255] For example, these thyroid antibodies cannot transfer disease from mother to fetus or between animals although many pass across the placenta. Both of these antibodies, however, may contribute to disease mechanisms. For example, TPO-Ab on the surface of B cells may be involved in antigen presentation, thus activating thyroid specific T cells.[256] Others may have complement-fixing cytotoxic activity. TPOAb autoantibodies, in particular, correlate with thyroidal damage and lymphocytic infiltration.

Thyroid Autoantibodies in Hashimoto's Thyroiditis and Graves' Disease. The disease widely most associated with TgAb and TPOAb is *autoimmune thyroiditis*, or Hashimoto's disease (terms that embrace both goitrous thyroiditis, as first described by Hashimoto, and atrophic thyroid failure previously referred to as *primary myxedema*). Both TgAb and TPOAb are found in almost 100% of such patients, but TPO antibodies are of higher affinity and in higher concentrations and are the best choice if only a single test is ordered.

Antibodies to Tg and TPO are also detectable in 50% to 90% of patients with Graves' disease, indicative of the associated thyroiditis that is evident histologically as a heterogeneous lymphocytic infiltration. Although the presence of such autoantibodies favors a diagnosis of an autoimmune cause for the hyperthyroidism over other causes, the tests are neither sensitive nor specific in this setting and are interpretable only as part of the clinical scenario. TSH receptor antibodies remain the test of choice in such patients.

Thyroid Autoantibodies in Nonautoimmune Thyroid Disorders. Antibodies to Tg and TPO are more common in patients with sporadic goiter, multinodular goiter, and isolated thyroid nodules and cancer than in the general population. This finding usually represents an associated thyroiditis on histologic examination. Low levels of thyroid autoantibodies may occur transiently in patients with subacute (de Quervain's) thyroiditis but correlate poorly with disease course and are probably a nonspecific response to thyroid injury. There is also a higher prevalence of thyroid autoantibodies in other autoimmune diseases, particularly insulin-dependent diabetes mellitus (IDDM).

The "Normal" Population. Although the prevalence of thyroid autoantibodies depends on the technique used for detection, autoantibodies to Tg and TPO are common in the general population (see Table 10–14) and, at all ages, are almost 5 times more common in women than in men.[253] Selected groups at risk include younger women and relatives of patients with an AITD, in whom the incidence is higher. The low levels of autoantibodies to TPO and Tg found in many individuals are of uncertain significance in the presence of normal thyroid function; however, within a family with AITD, they remain a significant risk factor.[257]

Radioiodine Uptake

The only direct test of thyroid function employs a radioactive isotope of iodine as a tag for the body's stable form of iodine, ^{127}I. Most often the test involves the measurement of the fractional uptake by the thyroid of a tracer (chemically inconsequential) dose of radioiodine. However, several factors make this test less frequently used than in the past. The first is the improvement in indirect methods for assessing thyroid status. The second is the decrease in normal values for thyroid RAIU consequent to the widespread increase in daily dietary iodine intake,[258] reducing the utility of the test in the diagnosis of thyroid disorders.

^{131}I (half-life 8.1 days) and ^{123}I (half-life 0.55 day) both emit gamma radiation, which permits their external detection and quantitation at sites of accumulation, such as the thyroid. These isotopes (abbreviated I* hereafter) are physiologically indistinguishable, not only from one another but also from the naturally occurring ^{127}I, which permits their use as valid tracers. The shorter half-life of ^{123}I is preferable because the radiation delivered to the thyroid per amount of administered ^{123}I is only about 1% of that delivered by ^{131}I.

Physiologic Basis. When tracer quantities of inorganic radioiodine are administered orally or intravenously, the isotope quickly mixes with the endogenous stable iodide in the extracellular fluid and begins to be removed by the two major sites of clearance, the thyroid and the kidneys. As this process continues, the plasma level of tracer iodide I* decreases exponentially. Low levels are reached by 24 hours, and inorganic I* is virtually undetectable in the plasma 72 hours after its administration. The thyroid content of I* increases rapidly during the early hours, then at a decreasing rate until a plateau is approached. The proportion of administered I* ultimately accumulated by the thyroid is a function of the clearance of iodide by the thyroid and kidneys. The relation is simply expressed as follows:

$$\text{RAIU at plateau} = \frac{C_T}{C_T + C_K}$$

where C_T represents the thyroid iodide clearance rate, and C_K the renal iodide clearance rate. The normal thyroid iodide clearance rate is approximately 0.4 L/hr, and the renal iodide clearance rate is 2.0 L/hr, so the uptake of I* normally approximates 20% of the administered dose.

Measurements of RAIU are generally made at 24 hours, both as a matter of convenience and because the value at 24 hours is usually near the plateau but can be measured at 6 hours with appropriate determination of a normal range. The RAIU usually indicates the rate of thyroid hormone synthesis and, by inference, the rate of thyroid hormone release into the blood.

Radioactive Iodine Uptake (RAIU). Little difference will be noted if the uptake is measured at any time during the day following that on which the isotope was administered, and for the calculation of therapeutic radioiodine doses in treating thyrotoxic Graves' disease an early uptake at 3 to 6 hours may produce results comparable to those found at 20 to 28 hours.[259] With the use of this modified early RAIU measurement, diagnosis and treatment of thyrotoxic Graves' disease can be accomplished on the same day. In general, the range of normal values in North America is approximately 5% to 25%. Higher values are found in iodine-deficient regions or in patients with thyroid hyperfunction, but as with other procedures, patients with mild hyperthyroidism may display values at or just above the upper limit of the normal range (Table 10–15).

The Perchlorate Discharge Test. In normal individuals, more than 90% of thyroidal radioiodine is present as iodotyrosine and iodothyronine within minutes of its entry into the thyroid. It is then no longer in the intracellular iodide pool. In patients with Pendred's syndrome or with other disorders that inhibit the iodination of tyrosine, such as Hashimoto's thyroiditis, or those receiving thiourea drugs, this process is delayed, as shown by the exit (discharge) of more than 10% of the thyroidal radioiodine within 2 hours of administration of 500 mg of $KClO_4$.[16] Perchlorate inhibits NIS function by competing with iodide for NIS, eliminating the iodide gradient that is required for maintaining the radioiodide in the gland. This illustrates that both iodide transport by NIS at the basal pole of the thyrocyte and its efflux across the apical membrane by pendrin are required for thyroid hormone synthesis.

TABLE 10–15 FACTORS THAT INFLUENCE 24-HOUR THYROID IODIDE UPTAKE

FACTORS THAT INCREASE UPTAKE
Increased hormone synthesis
Hyperthyroidism
Response to glandular hormone depletion
Recovery from thyroid suppression
Recovery from subacute thyroiditis
Antithyroid agents
Excessive hormone losses
Nephrotic syndrome
Chronic diarrheal states
Soybean ingestion
Normal hormone synthesis
Iodine deficiency
Dietary insufficiency
Excessive loss (dehalogenase defect, pregnancy)
Hormone biosynthetic defects
FACTORS THAT DECREASE UPTAKE
Decreased hormone synthesis
Primary hypofunction
Primary hypothyroidism
Antithyroid agents
Hormone biosynthetic defects
Hashimoto's disease
Subacute thyroiditis
Secondary hypofunction
Exogenous thyroid hormones
Not reflecting decreased hormone synthesis
Increased availability of iodine
Diet or drugs
Cardiac or renal insufficiency
Increased hormone release
Very severe hyperthyroidism (rare)

States Associated with Increased RAIU

Hyperthyroidism. Hyperthyroidism causes increased RAIU unless body iodide stores are increased. Such increases in uptake are always evident except in patients with severe thyrotoxicosis, in whom release of hormone can be so rapid that the thyroid content of I* has decreased to the normal range by the time the measurement is made. This condition is rare and is usually associated with obvious thyrotoxicosis.

Aberrant Hormone Synthesis. RAIU can be increased in the absence of hyperthyroidism in disorders in which iodine accumulation is normal but the secretion of hormone is impaired, such as in patients with abnormal thyroglobulin synthesis.[260] The magnitude of the increase in uptake and the time at which the plateau is achieved vary with the nature and severity of the disorder. Differentiation of the foregoing states from hyperthyroidism is generally not difficult, because in the former, clinical findings and laboratory evidence of hyperthyroidism are lacking, and indeed hypothyroidism may be present.

Iodine Deficiency. RAIU is increased in acute or chronic iodine deficiency, as demonstrated by measurement of urinary iodine excretion, with urinary iodine values lower than 100 μg/day, indicating deficiency. Chronic iodine deficiency is usually the result of an inadequate content of iodine in the food and water (endemic iodine deficiency). Patients with cardiac, renal, or hepatic disease may develop iodine deficiency if given diets severely restricted in salt, especially if diuretic agents are administered.

Response to Thyroid Hormone Depletion. Rebound increases in RAIU are seen after withdrawal of antithyroid therapy, after subsidence of transient or subacute thyroiditis, and after recovery from prolonged suppression of thyroid function by exogenous hormone. A striking increase in uptake occurs in patients with iodide-induced myxedema after cessation of iodide administration. The duration of the rebound depends on the time required to replenish thyroid hormone stores.

Excessive Hormone Losses. In nephrotic syndrome, excessive losses of hormone in the urine occurring in association with urinary loss of binding protein cause a compensatory increase in hormone synthesis and RAIU. A similar sequence may occur when losses of hormone via the gastrointestinal tract are abnormal, as in chronic diarrheal states or during ingestion of agents, such as soybean protein and cholestyramine, that bind T_4 in the gut.

States Associated with Decreased RAIU. A general increase in iodine intake has made values of the RAIU in hypothyroidism indistinguishable from those at the lower end of the normal range. Therefore, the major indication for measuring the RAIU is to establish whether thyrotoxicosis is due to hyperthyroidism (high RAIU) or thyroiditis (low RAIU).

Exogenous Thyroid Hormone: Thyrotoxicosis Factitia. Except in disorders in which homeostatic control is disrupted or overridden (e.g., Graves' disease or autonomously functioning thyroid nodules), administration of exogenous thyroid hormone suppresses TSH secretion and reduces the RAIU, usually to values below 5%.

Low values of the RAIU in a patient who is clinically thyrotoxic may also indicate the presence of *thyrotoxicosis factitia,* the syndrome produced by the ingestion of excess thyroid hormone. The unmeasurably low level of Tg in serum differentiates thyrotoxicosis factitia from other causes of thyrotoxicosis with decreased RAIU.[248]

Disorders of Hormone Storage. The RAIU is usually low in the early phase of subacute thyroiditis and in chronic thyroiditis with transient hyperthyroidism. Here, inflammatory follicular disruption leads to loss of the normal storage function of the gland and leakage of hormone into the blood. In the early stage of subacute thyroiditis, leakage of hormone is usually sufficient to suppress TSH secretion and the RAIU. Transient hypothyroidism often occurs late in both diseases, when stores of preformed hormone are depleted; the RAIU may return to normal or increased values at that time.

Exposure to Excessive Iodine. Exposure to excessive iodine is a common cause of a subnormal RAIU. Such decreases are spurious in the clinical sense because they do not indicate decreased absolute iodine uptake or decreased hormone production but can be produced by the introduction of excessive iodine in any form of inorganic, organic, or elemental. Common offenders are organic iodinated dyes used as x-ray contrast media and amiodarone (see Table 10–7). The duration of suppression of the uptake varies among individuals and with the compound administered. In general, dyes used for pyelography or CT scanning are cleared within a few months, whereas amiodarone may influence the uptake for up to 12 months due to its storage in fat. A single large dose of inorganic iodide can decrease uptake for several days, and chronic ingestion of iodide may depress the uptake for many weeks. Excessive quantities of iodine may also be present in vitamin and mineral preparations, vaginal or rectal suppositories, and iodinated antiseptics such as povidone (see Table 10–7).

The measurement of urinary iodine excretion is an invaluable means of establishing or excluding the existence of excessive body iodide stores; the 24-hour iodine excretion can be extrapolated from the iodide-to-creatinine ratio in a random urine sample. Values in excess of 2 mg/day can account for a low RAIU value, whereas values less than 1 mg/day suggest that a low RAIU value is due to one of the other disorders discussed in this section.

REFERENCES

1. De Felice M, Di Lauro R. Thyroid development and its disorders: genetics and molecular mechanisms. Endocr Rev 2004;25: 722-746.
2. Park SM, Chatterjee VK. Genetics of congenital hypothyroidism. J Med Genet 2005;42:379-389.
3. Burrow GN, Fisher DA, Larsen PR. Mechanisms of disease: maternal and fetal thyroid function. N Engl J Med 1994;331:1072-1078.
4. Thorpe-Beeston JG, Nicolaides KH, Felton CV, et al. Maturation of the secretion of thyroid hormone and thyroid-stimulating hormone in the fetus. N Engl J Med 1991;324:532-536.
5. Mansberger AR, Wei JP. Surgical embryology and anatomy of the thyroid and parathyroid glands. Surg Clin North Am 1993;73: 727-746.
6. Ericson LE. Exocytosis and endocytosis in the thyroid follicle cell. Mol Cell Endocrinol 1981;22:1-24.
7. De Felice M, Postiglione MP, Di Lauro R. Minireview: thyrotropin receptor signaling in development and differentiation of the thyroid gland: insights from mouse models and human diseases. Endocrinology 2004;145:4062-4067.
8. Hollowell JG, Staehling NW, Hannon WH, et al. Iodine nutrition in the United States. Trends and public health implications: iodine excretion data from National Health and Nutrition Examination Surveys I and III (1971-1974 and 1988-1994). J Clin Endocrinol Metab 1998;83:3401-3408.
9. Glinoer D. Maternal and fetal impact of chronic iodine deficiency. Clin Obstet Gynecol 1997;40:102-116.
10. Glinoer D, Delange F. The potential repercussions of maternal, fetal, and neonatal hypothyroxinemia on the progeny. Thyroid 2000;10:871-887.
11. de Benoist B, Andersson M, Takkouche B, et al. Prevalence of iodine deficiency worldwide. Lancet 2003;362:1859-1860.
12. Dohan O, De la Vieja A, Paroder V, et al. The sodium/iodide symporter (NIS): characterization, regulation, and medical significance. Endocr Rev 2003;24:48-77.
13. Bidart JM, Lacroix L, Evain-Brion D, et al. Expression of Na^+/I^- symporter and Pendred syndrome genes in trophoblast cells. J Clin Endocrinol Metab 2000;85:4367-4372.
14. Kosugi S, Inoue S, Matsuda A, et al. Novel, missense and loss-of-function mutations in the sodium/iodide symporter gene causing iodide transport defect in three Japanese patients. J Clin Endocrinol Metab 1998;83:3373-3376.
15. De La Vieja A, Dohan O, Levy O, et al. Molecular analysis of the sodium/iodide symporter: impact on thyroid and extrathyroid pathophysiology. Physiol Rev 2000;80:1083-1105.
16. Wolff J. Perchlorate and the thyroid gland. Pharmacol Rev 1998;50:89-105.
17. Van Sande J, Massart C, Beauwens R, et al. Anion selectivity by the sodium iodide symporter. Endocrinology 2003;144:247-252.
18. Wolff J. Congenital goiter with defective iodide transport. Endocrinol Rev 1983;4:240.
19. Filetti S, Bidart JM, Arturi F, Caillou B, et al. Sodium/iodide symporter: a key transport system in thyroid cancer cell metabolism. Eur J Endocrinol 1999;141:443-457.
20. Spitzweg C, Heufelder AE, Morris JC. Thyroid iodine transport. Thyroid 2000;10:321-330.
21. Gillam MP, Sidhaye AR, Lee EJ, et al. Functional characterization of pendrin in a polarized cell system. Evidence for pendrin-mediated apical iodide efflux. J Biol Chem 2004;279:13004-13010.
22. Porra V, Bernier-Valentin F, Trouttet-Masson S, et al. Characterization and semiquantitative analyses of pendrin expressed in normal and tumoral human thyroid tissues. J Clin Endocrinol Metab 2002;87:1700-1707.
23. Lacroix L, Pourcher T, Magnon C, et al. Expression of the apical iodide transporter in human thyroid tissues: a comparison study with other iodide transporters. J Clin Endocrinol Metab 2004; 89:1423-1428.
24. Gnidehou S, Caillou B, Talbot M, et al. Iodotyrosine dehalogenase 1 (DEHAL1) is a transmembrane protein involved in the recycling of iodide close to the thyroglobulin iodination site. FASEB J 2004;18:1574-1576.
25. Larsen PR. Thyroidal triiodothyronine and thyroxine in Graves' disease: correlation with presurgical treatment, thyroid status, and iodine content. J Clin Endocrinol Metab 1975;41:1098-1104.
26. Yokoyama N, Taurog A. Porcine thyroid peroxidase: relationship between the native enzyme and an active, highly purified tryptic fragment. Mol Endocrinol 1988;2:838-844.
27. Taurog A, Dorris ML, Doerge DR. Mechanism of simultaneous iodination and coupling catalyzed by thyroid peroxidase. Arch Biochem Biophys 1996;330:24-32.
28. Lacroix L, Nocera M, Mian C, et al. Expression of nicotinamide adenine dinucleotide phosphate oxidase flavoprotein DUOX genes and proteins in human papillary and follicular thyroid carcinomas. Thyroid 2001;11:1017-1023.
29. Morand S, Chaaraoui M, Kaniewski J, et al. Effect of iodide on nicotinamide adenine dinucleotide phosphate oxidase activity and Duox2 protein expression in isolated porcine thyroid follicles. Endocrinology 2003;144:1241-1248.
30. Vulsma T, Gons MH, DeVijlder JMM. Maternal fetal transfer of thyroxine in congenital hypothyroidism due to a total organification defect of thyroid dysgenesis. N Engl J Med 1989;321:13-16.
31. Bakker B, Bikker H, Vulsma T, et al. Two decades of screening for congenital hypothyroidism in The Netherlands: TPO gene mutations in total iodide organification defects (an update). J Clin Endocrinol Metab 2000;85:3708-3712.
32. Gerard AC, Daumerie C, Mestdagh C, et al. Correlation between the loss of thyroglobulin iodination and the expression of thyroid-specific proteins involved in iodine metabolism in thyroid carcinomas. J Clin Endocrinol Metab 2003;88:4977-4983.
33. Ohmiya Y, Hayashi H, Kondo T, et al. Location of dehydroalanine residues in the amino acid sequence of bovine thyroglobulin. Identification of "donor" tyrosine sites for hormonogenesis in thyroglobulin. J Biol Chem 1990;265:9066-9071.
34. Gentile F, Ferranti P, Mamone G, et al. Identification of hormonogenic tyrosines in fragment 1218-1591 of bovine thyroglobulin by mass spectrometry. Hormonogenic acceptor TYR-12donor TYR-1375. J Biol Chem 1997;272:639-646.
35. Dunn AD, Corsi CM, Myers HE, et al. Tyrosine 130 is an important outer ring donor for thyroxine formation in thyroglobulin. J Biol Chem 1998;273:25223-25229.
36. Izumi M, Larsen PR. Triiodothyronine, thyroxine, and iodine in purified thyroglobulin from patients with Graves' disease. J Clin Invest 1977;59:1105-1112.
37. Dunn JT, Dunn AD. Update on intrathyroidal iodine metabolism. Thyroid 2001;11:407-414.
38. Rousset B, Selmi S, Bornet H, et al. Thyroid hormone residues are released from thyroglobulin with only limited alteration of the thyroglobulin structure. J Biol Chem 1989;264:12620-12626.
39. Laurberg P. Selective inhibition of the secretion of triiodothyronines from the perfused canine thyroid by propylthiouracil. Endocrinology 1978;103:900-905.
40. Abuid J, Larsen PR. Triiodothyronine and thyroxine in hyperthyroidism. Comparison of the acute changes during therapy with antithyroid agents. J Clin Invest 1974;54:201-208.
41. Laurberg P, Torring J, Weeke J. A comparison of the effects of propylthiouracil and methimazol on circulating thyroid hormones and various measures of peripheral thyroid hormone effects in thyrotoxic patients. Acta Endocrinol (Copenh) 1985; 108:51-54.
42. Kim BW, Daniels GH, Harrison BJ, et al. Overexpression of type 2 iodothyronine deiodinase in follicular carcinoma as a cause of low circulating free thyroxine levels. J Clin Endocrinol Metab 2003;88:594-598.
43. Berens SC, Bernstein RS, Robbins J, et al. Antithyroid effects of lithium. J Clin Invest 1970;49:1357-1856.
44. Lazarus JH. The effects of lithium therapy on thyroid and thyrotropin-releasing hormone. Thyroid 1998;8:909-913.
45. Davies TF, Ando T, Lin RY, et al. Thyrotropin receptor-associated diseases: from adenomata to Graves' disease. J Clin Invest 2005;115:1972-1983.
46. Uyttersprot N, Allgeier A, Baptist M, et al. The cAMP in thyroid: from the TSH receptor to mitogenesis and tumorigenesis. Adv Second Messenger Phosphoprotein Res 1997;31:125-140.
47. Vassart G, Desarnaud F, Duprez L, et al. The G protein-coupled receptor family and one of its members, the TSH receptor. Ann N Y Acad Sci 1995;766:23-30.

48. Saavedra AP, Tsygankova OM, Prendergast GV, et al. Role of cAMP, PKA and Rap1A in thyroid follicular cell survival. Oncogene 2002;21:778-788.
49. Vlaeminck-Guillem V, Ho SC, Rodien P, et al. Activation of the cAMP pathway by the TSH receptor involves switching of the ectodomain from a tethered inverse agonist to an agonist. Mol Endocrinol 2002;16:736-746.
50. Van Sande J, Parma J, Tonacchera M, et al. Somatic and germline mutations of the TSH receptor gene in thyroid diseases. J Clin Endocrinol Metab 1995;80:2577-2585.
51. Bianco AC, Salvatore D, Gereben B, et al. Biochemistry, cellular and molecular biology and physiological roles of the iodothyronine selenodeiodinases. Endocr Rev 2002;23:38-89.
52. Curran PG, DeGroot LJ. The effect of hepatic enzyme-inducing drugs on thyroid hormones and the thyroid gland. Endocr Rev 1991;12:135-150.
53. Findlay KA, Kaptein E, Visser TJ, et al. Characterization of the uridine diphosphate-glucuronosyltransferase-catalyzing thyroid hormone glucuronidation in man. J Clin Endocrinol Metab 2000;85:2879-2883.
54. Schussler GC. The thyroxine-binding proteins. Thyroid 2000;10: 141-149.
55. Buettner C, Grasberger H, Hermansdorfer K, et al. Characterization of the thyroxine-binding site of thyroxine-binding globulin by site-directed mutagenesis. Mol Endocrinol 1999;13:1864-1872.
56. Garnick MB, Larsen PR. Acute deficiency of thyroxine-binding globulin during L-asparaginase therapy. N Engl J Med 1979; 301(5):252-253.
57. Ain KB, Mori Y, Refetoff S. Reduced clearance rate of thyroxine-binding globulin (TBG) with increased sialylation: a mechanism for estrogen-induced elevation of serum TBG concentration. J Clin Endocrinol Metab 1987;65:689-696.
58. Jirasakuldech B, Schussler GC, Yap MG, et al. A characteristic serpin cleavage product of thyroxine-binding globulin appears in sepsis sera. J Clin Endocrinol Metab 2000;85:3996-3999.
59. Pemberton PA, Stein PE, Pepys MB, et al. Hormone binding globulins undergo serpin conformational change in inflammation. Nature 1988;336:257-258.
60. Bartalena L. Recent achievements in studies on thyroid hormone-binding proteins. Endocr Rev 1990;11:47-64.
61. Surks MI, Oppenheimer JH. Postoperative changes in the concentration of thyroxine-binding prealbumin and serum free thyroxine. J Clin Endocrinol 1964;24:794-801.
62. Dickson PW, Aldred AR, Marley PD, et al. Rat choroid plexus specializes in the synthesis and secretion of transthyretin (prealbumin). J Biol Chem 1985;261:3475.
63. Palha JA, Episkopou V, Maeda S, et al. Thyroid hormone metabolism in a transthyretin-null mouse strain. J Biol Chem 1994; 269:32767.
64. Palha JA, Fernandes R, de Escobar GM, et al. Transthyretin regulates thyroid hormone levels in the choroid plexus, but not in the brain parenchyma: study in a transthyretin-null mouse model. Endocrinology 2000;141:3267-3272.
65. Bartalena L. Thyroid hormone-binding proteins: update 1994. Endocr Rev 1994;3:140-142.
66. Rosen HN, Moses AC, Murrell JR, et al. Thyroxine interactions with transthyretin: a comparison of 10 different naturally occurring human transthyretin variants. J Clin Endocrinol Metab 1993; 77:370-374.
67. Chin W, Schussler GC. Decreased serum free thyroxine concentration in patients treated with diphenylhydantoin. J Clin Endocrinol 168;28:181-186.
68. Larsen PR. Salicylate-induced increases in free triiodothyronine in human serum. Evidence of inhibition of triiodothyronine binding to thyroxine-binding globulin and thyroxine-binding prealbumin. J Clin Invest 1972;51:1125-1134.
69. Wang R, Nelson JC, Wilcox RB. Salsalate and salicylate binding to and their displacement of thyroxine from thyroxine-binding globulin, transthyretin, and albumin. Thyroid 1999;9: 359-364.
70. Docter R, Bos G, Krenning EP, et al. Inherited thyroxine excess: a serum abnormality due to an increased affinity for modified albumin. Clin Endocrinol 1981;15:363-371.
71. Mendel CM, Cavalieri RR. Thyroxine distribution and metabolism in familial dysalbuminemic hyperthyroxinemia. J Clin Endocrinol Metab 1984;59:499-504.
72. Marqusee E, Braverman LE, Lawrence JE, et al. The effect of droloxifene and estrogen on thyroid function in postmenopausal women. J Clin Endocrinol Metab 2000;85:4407-4410.
73. Arafah BM. Increased need for thyroxine in women with hypothyroidism during estrogen therapy. N Engl J Med 2001;344: 1743-1749.
74. Robbins J, Rall JE. The interaction of thyroid hormones and protein in biological fluids. Rec Progr Horm Res 1957;13:161.
75. Mendel CM. The free hormone hypothesis: a physiologically based matematical model. Endocr Rev 1989;10(3):232-274.
76. Mendel CM, Weisiger RA, Jones AL, et al. Thyroid hormone-binding proteins in plasma facilitate uniform distribution of thyroxine withing tissues: a perfused rat liver study. Endocrinology 1987;120:1742-1749.
77. Friesma EC, Jansen J, Hever H, Trajkovic M, Bauer K, Visser TJ. Mechanisms of disease: psychomotor retardation and high T_3 levels caused by mutations in monocarboxylate transporter 8. N Clin Pract Endocrinol Metab 2006;2:512-523.
78. Brockmann K, Dumitrescu AM, Best TT, et al. X-linked paroxysmal dyskinesia and severe global retardation caused by defective MCT8 gene. J Neurol 2005;252:663-666.
79. Friesema EC, Ganguly S, Abdalla A, et al. Identification of monocarboxylate transporter 8 as a specific thyroid hormone transporter. J Biol Chem 2003;278:40128-40135.
80. Heuer H, Maier MK, Iden S, et al. The monocarboxylate transporter 8 linked to human psychomotor retardation is highly expressed in thyroid hormone-sensitive neuron populations. Endocrinology 2005;146:1701-1706.
81. Tu HM, Kim SW, Salvatore D, et al. Regional distribution of type 2 thyroxine deiodinase messenger ribonucleic acid in rat hypothalamus and pituitary and its regulation by thyroid hormone. Endocrinology 1997;138:3359-3368.
82. Guadano-Ferraz A, Escamez MJ, Rausell E, et al. Expression of type 2 iodothyronine deiodinase in hypothyroid rat brain indicates an important role of thyroid hormone in the development of specific primary sensory systems. J Neurosci 1999;19: 3430-3439.
83. Jansen J, Friesema EC, Milici C, et al. Thyroid hormone transporters in health and disease. Thyroid 2005;15:757-768.
84. Bernal J. The significance of thyroid hormone transporters in the brain. Endocrinology 2005;146:1698-1700.
85. Sugiyama D, Kusuhara H, Taniguchi H, et al. Functional characterization of rat brain-specific organic anion transporter (Oatp14) at the blood-brain barrier: high affinity transporter for thyroxine. J Biol Chem 2003;278:43489-43495.
86. Oppenheimer JH, Schwartz HL. Stereospecific transport to triiodothyronine from plasma to cytosol and from cytosol to nucleus in rat liver, kidney, brain and heart. J Clin Invest 1985;75:147-154.
87. Nishii Y, Hashizume K, Ichikawa K, et al. Induction of cytosolic triiodo-L-thyronine (T3) binding protein (CTBP) by T3 in primary cultured rat hepatocytes. Endocr J 1993;40:399-404.
88. St. Germain DL, Galton VA. The deiodinase family of selenoproteins. Thyroid 1997;7:655-668.
89. Berry MJ, Banu L, Larsen PR. Type I iodothyronine deiodinase is a selenocysteine-containing enzyme. Nature 1991;349:438-440.
90. Berry MJ, Larsen PR. The role of selenium in thyroid hormone action. Endocr Rev 1992;13:207-219.
91. Berry MJ, Banu L, Chen YY, et al. Recognition of UGA as a selenocysteine codon in type I deiodinase requires sequences in the 3′ untranslated region. Nature 1991;353:273-276.
92. Hoffmann PR, Berry MJ. Selenoprotein synthesis: a unique translational mechanism used by a diverse family of proteins. Thyroid 2005;15:769-775.
93. Maia AL, Kim BW, Huang SA, et al. Type 2 iodothyronine deiodinase is the major source of plasma T3 in euthyroid humans. J Clin Invest 2005;115:2524-2533.
94. Huang SA, Tu HM, Harney JW, et al. Severe hypothyroidism caused by type 3 iodothyronine deiodinase in infantile hemangiomas. N Engl J Med 2000;343:185-189.
95. Hernandez A. Structure and function of the type 3 deiodinase gene. Thyroid 2005;15:865-874.
96. St. Germain DL, Hernandez A, Schneider MJ, et al. Insights into the role of deiodinases from studies of genetically modified animals. Thyroid 2005;15:905-916.
97. Schneider MJ, Fiering SN, Thai B, et al. Targeted disruption of the type 1 selenodeiodinase gene (dio1) results in marked changes in

thyroid hormone economy in mice. Endocrinology 2006;147: 580-589.
98. Hernandez A, Martinez ME, Fiering S, et al. Type 3 deiodinase is critical for the maturation and function of the thyroid axis. J Clin Invest 2006;116:476-484.
99. Saberi M, Sterling FH, Utiger RD. Reduction in extrathyroidal triiodothyronine production by propylthiouracil in man. J Clin Invest 1975;55:218-223.
100. Geffner DL, Azukizawa M, Hershman JM. Propylthiouracil blocks extrathyroidal conversion of thyroxine to triiodothyronine and augments thyrotropin secretion in man. J Clin Invest 1975;55: 224-229.
101. Christoffolete MA, Ribeiro R, Singru P, et al. Atypical expression of type 2 iodothyronine deiodinase in thyrotrophs explains the thyroxine-mediated pituitary TSH feedback mechanism. Endocrinology 2006;147:1735-1743.
102. Wu SY, Green WL, Huang WS, et al. Alternate pathways of thyroid hormone metabolism. Thyroid 2005;15:943-958.
103. Silva JE, Larsen PR. Adrenergic activation of triiodothyronine production in brown adipose tissue. Nature 1983;305:712-713.
104. Ribeiro MO, Carvalho SD, Schultz JJ, et al. Thyroid hormone-sympathetic interaction and adaptive thermogenesis are thyroid hormone receptor isoform-specific. J Clin Invest 2001;108:97-105.
105. Martino E, Bartalena L, Bogazzi F, et al. The effects of amiodarone on the thyroid. Endocr Rev 2001;22:240-254.
106. Krenning EP, Docter R, Bernard HF, et al. Decreased transport of thyroxine (T4), 3,3′,5-triiodothyronine (T3) and 3,3′,5′-triiodothyronine (rT3) into rat hepatocytes in primary culture due to a decrease of cellular ATP contnent and various drugs. FEBS Lett 1982;140:229-233.
107. Wu SY, Chopra IJ, Solomon DH, et al. The effect of repeated administration of ipodate (Oragrafin) in hyperthyroidism. J Clin Endocrinol Metab 1978;47:1358-1362.
108. LoPresti JS, Eigen A, Kaptein E, et al. Alterations in 3,3′5′-triiodothyronine metabolism in response to propylthiouracil, dexamethasone, and thyroxine administration in man. J Clin Invest 1989;84:1650-1656.
109. Jorgensen JOL, Pedersen SA, Laurberg P, et al. Effects of growth hormone therapy on thyroid function of growth hormone-deficient adults with and without concomitant thyroxine-substituted central hypothyroidism. J Clin Endocrinol Metab 1989;69: 1127-1132.
110. Kohrle J. Selenium and the control of thyroid hormone metabolism. Thyroid 2005;15:841-853.
111. Lazar MA. Thyroid hormone action: a binding contract. J Clin Invest 2003;112:497-499.
112. Amma LL, Campos-Barros A, Wang Z, et al. 2001. Distinct tissue-specific roles for thyroid hormone receptors beta and alpha1 in regulation of type 1 deiodinase expression. Mol Endocrinol 2001;15:467-475.
113. Abel ED, Kaulbach HC, Campos-Barros A, et al. Novel insight from transgenic mice into thyroid hormone resistance and the regulation of thyrotropin. J Clin Invest 1999;103:271-279.
114. Forrest D, Golarai G, Connor J, et al. Genetic analysis of thyroid hormone receptors in development and disease. Rec Progr Hormone Res 1996;51:1-22.
115. Forrest D, Vennstrom B. Functions of thyroid hormone receptors in mice. Thyroid 2000;10:41-52.
116. Usala SJ. New developments in clinical and genetic aspects of thyroid hormone resistance syndromes. Endocrinologist 1995;5: 68-76.
117. Beck-Peccoz P, Chatterjee VKK. The variable clinical phenotype in thyroid hormone resistance syndrome. Thyroid 1994;4: 225-231.
118. Wagner RL, Apriletti JW, McGrath ME, et al. A structural role for hormone in the thyroid hormone receptor. Nature 1995;378: 690-697.
119. Trost SU, Swanson E, Gloss B, et al.. The thyroid hormone receptor-beta-selective agonist GC-1 differentially affects plasma lipids and cardiac activity. Endocrinology 2000;141:3057-3064.
120. Mousa SA, O'Connor LJ, Bergh JJ, et al.. The proangiogenic action of thyroid hormone analogue GC-1 is initiated at an integrin. J Cardiovasc Pharmacol 2005;46:356-360.
121. Hollenberg AN, Monden T, Flynn TR, et al. The human thyrotropin-releasing hormone gene is regulated by thyroid hormone through two distinct classes of negative thyroid hormone response elements. Mol Endocrinol 1995;9:540-550.
122. Chan JL, Heist K, DePaoli AM, et al. The role of falling leptin levels in the neuroendocrine and metabolic adaptation to short-term starvation in healthy men. J Clin Invest 2003;111:1409-1421.
123. Ozata M, Ozdemir IC, Licinio J. Human leptin deficiency caused by a missense mutation: multiple endocrine defects, decreased sympathetic tone, and immune system dysfunction indicate new targets for leptin action, greater central than peripheral resistance to the effects of leptin, and spontaneous correction of leptin-mediated defects. J Clin Endocrinol Metab 1999;84:3686-3695.
124. Segerson TP, Kauer J, Wolfe H, et al. Thyroid hormone regulates TRH biosynthesis in the paraventricular nucleus of the rat hypothalamus. Science 1987;238:78-80.
125. Dyess EM, Segerson TP, Liposits Z, et al. Triiodothyronine exerts direct cell-specific regulation of thyrotropin-releasing hormone gene expression in the hypothalamic paraventricular nucleus. Endocrinology 1988;123:2291-2297.
126. Lechan RM, Fekete C. Role of thyroid hormone deiodination in the hypothalamus. Thyroid 2005;15:883-897.
127. Magner JA. Thyroid-stimulating hormone: biosynthesis, cell biology and bioactivity. Endocr Rev 1990;11:354.
128. Beck-Peccoz P, Amir S, Menezes-Ferreira MM, et al. Decreased receptor binding of biologically inactive thyrotropin in central hypothyroidism: effect of treatment with thyrotropin-releasing hormone. N Engl J Med 1985;312:1085-1090.
129. Gesundheit N, Petrick PA, Nissim M, et al. Thyrotropin-secreting pituitary adenomas: clinical and biochemical heterogeneity. Ann Intern Med 1989;11:827-835.
130. Persani L, Ferretti E, Borgato S, et al. Circulating thyrotropin bioactivity in sporadic central hypothyroidism. J Clin Endocrinol Metab 2000;85:3631-3635.
131. Adriaanse R, Romijn JA, Brabant G, et al. Pulsatile thyrotropin secretion in nonthyroidal illness. J Clin Endocrinol Metab 1993;77:1313-1317.
132. Brabant G, Frank K, Ranft U. Physiological regulation of circadian and pulsatile thyrotropin secretion in normal man and woman. J Clin Endocrinol Metab 1990;70:403.
133. Nikrodhanond AA, Ortiga-Carvalho TM, Shibusawa N, et al. Dominant role of thyrotropin-releasing hormone in the hypothalamic-pituitary-thyroid axis. J Biol Chem 2005;285:5000-5007.
134. Morley JE. Neuroendocrine control of thyrotropin secretion. Endocr Rev 1981;2:396-436.
135. Beck-Peccoz P, Brucker-Davis F, Persani L, et al. Thyrotropin-secreting pituitary tumors. Endocr Rev 1996;17:610-638.
136. Biller BM, Molitch ME, Vance ML, et al. Treatment of prolactin-secreting macroadenomas with the once-weekly dopamine agonist cabergoline. J Clin Endocrinol Metab 1996;81:2338-2343.
137. Brabant A, Brabant G, Schuermeyer T, et al. 1989. The role of glucocorticoids in the regulation of thyrotropin. Acta Endocrinol (Copenh) 1989;121:95-100.
138. Adriaanse R, Brabant G, Endert E, et al. Pulsatile thyrotropin secretion in patients with Cushing's syndrome. Metabolism 1994;43: 782-786.
139. Sherman SI, Gopal J, Haugen BR, et al. Central hypothyroidism associated with retinoid X receptor-selective ligands. N Engl J Med 1999;340:1075-1079.
140. Sharma V, Hays WR, Wood WM, et al. Effects of rexinoids on thyrotrope function and the hypothalamic-pituitary-thyroid axis. Endocrinology 2006;147:1438-1451.
141. Nakabayashi K, Matsumi H, Bhalla A, et al. Thyrostimulin, a heterodimer of two new human glycoprotein hormone subunits, activates the thyroid-stimulating hormone receptor. J Clin Invest 2002;109:1445-1452.
142. Riesco G, Taurog A, Larsen R, et al. Acute and chronic responses to iodine deficiency in rats. Endocrinology 1997;100:303-313.
143. Peeters R, Fekete C, Goncalves C, et al. Regional physiological adaptation of the central nervous system deiodinases to iodine deficiency. Am J Physiol Endocrinol Metab 2001;281:E54-E61.
144. Meinhold H, Campos-Barros A, Walzog B, et al. Effects of selenium and iodine deficiency on type I, type II and type III iodothyronine deiodinases and circulating thyroid hormones in the rat. Exp Clin Endocrinol 1993;101:87-93.
145. Campos-Barros A, Meinhold H, Walzog B, et al. Effects of selenium and iodine deficiency on thyroid hormone concentrations in the

central nervous system of the rat. Eur J Endocrinol 1997; 136:316-323.
146. Guo TW, Zhang FC, Yang MS, et al. Positive association of the DIO2 (deiodinase type 2) gene with mental retardation in the iodine-deficient areas of China. J Med Genet 2004;41:585-590.
147. Silva E. Disposal rates of thyroxine and triiodothyronine in iodine-deficient rats. Endocrinology 1972;91:1430-1435.
148. Pazos-Moura CC, Moura EG, Dorris ML, et al. Effect of iodine deficiency and cold exposure on thyroxine 5′-deiodinase activity in various rat tissues. Am J Physiol 1991;260:E175-E182.
149. Boyages SC. Clinical review 49: iodine deficiency disorders. J Clin Endocrinol Metab 1993;77:587-591.
150. Delange F. The disorders induced by iodine deficiency. Thyroid 1994;4:107-128.
151. Gershengorn MC, Wolff J, Larsen PR Thyroid-pituitary feedback during iodine repletion. J Clin Endocrinol 1976;43:601-605.
152. Bigos ST, Ridgway EC, Kourides IA, et al. Spectrum of pituitary alterations with mild and severe thyroid impairment. J Clin Endocrinol Metab 1978;46:317.
153. Wolff J, Chaikoff IL. Plasma inorganic iodide as a homeostatic regulator of thyroid function. J Biol Chem 1948;174:555.
154. Wolff J. Iodide goiter and the pharmacologic effects of excess iodide. Am J Med 1969;47:101-124.
155. Wolff J. Physiological aspects of iodide excess in relation to radiation protection. J Mol Med 1980;4:151-165.
156. Vagenakis AG, Downs P, Braverman LE, et al. Control of thyroid hormone secretion in normal subjects receiving iodides. J Clin Invest 1973;52:528-532.
157. Uyttersprot N, Pelgrims N, Carrasco N, et al. Moderate doses of iodide in vivo inhibit cell proliferation and the expression of thyroperoxidase and Na^+/I^- symporter mRNAs in dog thyroid. Mol Cell Endocrinol 1997;131:195-203.
158. Eng PH, Cardona GR, Fang SL, et al. Escape from the acute Wolff-Chaikoff effect is associated with a decrease in thyroid sodium/iodide symporter messenger ribonucleic acid and protein. Endocrinology 1999;140:3404-3410.
159. Chang DC, Wheeler MH, Woodcock JP, et al. The effect of preoperative Lugol's iodine on thyroid blood flow in patients with Graves' hyperthyroidism. Surgery 1987;102:1055-1061.
160. Glinoer D. The regulation of thyroid function in pregnancy: pathways of endocrine adaptation from physiology to pathology. Endocr Rev 1997;18:404-433.
161. LeBeau SO, Mandel SJ. Thyroid disorders during pregnancy. Endocrinol Metab Clin North Am 2006;35:117-136, vii.
162. Kimura M, Amino N, Tamaki H, et al. Physiologic thyroid activation in normal early pregnancy is induced by circulating hCG. Obstet Gynecol 1990;75:775-778.
163. Galton VA, Martinez E, Hernandez A, et al. Pregnant rat uterus expresses high levels of the type 3 iodothyronine deiodinase. J Clin Invest 1999;103:979-987.
164. Alexander EK, Marqusee E, Lawrence J, et al. Time of onset and magnitude of increase in levothyroxine requirements during pregnancy in women with hypothyroidism. In 75th Annual Meeting of the American Thyroid Association, Palm Beach, FL, 2003: A91:82.
165. Huang SA, Dorfman DM, Genest DR, et al. Type 3 iodothyronine deiodinase is highly expressed in the human uteroplacental unit and in fetal epithelium. J Clin Endocrinol Metab 2003;88: 1384-1388.
166. Glinoer D, Delange F, Laboureur I, et al. Maternal and neonatal thyroid function at birth in an area of marginally low iodine intake. J Clin Endocrinol Metab 1992;75:800-805.
167. Nelson M, Wickus GG, Caplan RH, et al. Thyroid gland size in pregnancy: an ultrasound and clinical study. J Reprod Med 1987;32:888-890.
168. Weetman AP. The immunology of pregnancy. Thyroid 1999;9:643-646.
169. Weetman AP. Prediction of post-partum thyroiditis. Clin Endocrinol (Oxf) 1994;41:7-8.
170. Dentice M, Bandyopadhyay A, Gereben B, et al. The hedgehog-inducible ubiquitin ligase subunit WSB-1 modulates thyroid hormone activation and PTHrP secretion in the developing growth plate. Nat Cell Biol 2005;7:698-705.
171. Thorpe-Beeston JG, Nicolaides KH, McGregor AM. Fetal thyroid function. Thyroid 1992;2:207-217.
172. Fisher DA, Schoen EJ, La Franchi S, et al. The hypothalamic-pituitary-thyroid negative feedback control axis in children with treated congenital hypothyroidism. J Clin Endocrinol Metab 2000;85:2722-2727.
173. Fisher DA, Nelson JC, Carlton EI, et al. Maturation of human hypothalamic-pituitary-thyroid function and control. Thyroid 2000; 10:229-234.
174. Larsen PR. Ontogenesis of thyroid function, thyroid hormone and brain development, diagnosis and treatment of congenital hypothyroidism. In DeGroot LJ, Larsen PR, Hennemann G, eds. The Thyroid and Its Diseases. New York: Churchill Livingstone, 1996:541-567.
175. Contempre B, Jauniaux E, Calvo R, et al. Detection of thyroid hormones in human embryonic cavities during the first trimester of pregnancy. J Clin Endocrinol Metab 1993;77:1719-1722.
176. Abe T, Kakyo M, Sakagami H, et al. Molecular characterization and tissue distribution of a new organic anion transporter subtype (oatp3) that transports thyroid hormones and taurocholate and comparison with oatp2. J Biol Chem 1998;273:22395-22401.
177. Fisher DA, Odell WD. Acute release of thyrotropin in the newborn. J Clin Invest 1969;48:1670-1677.
178. Abuid J, Stinson DA, Larsen PR. 1973. Serum triiodothyronine and thyroxine in the neonate and the acute increases in these hormones following delivery. J Clin Invest 1973;52:1195-1199.
179. de Jesus LA, Carvalho SD, Ribeiro MO, et al. The type 2 iodothyronine deiodinase is essential for adaptive thermogenesis in brown adipose tissue. J Clin Invest 2001;108:1379-1385.
180. Adams LM, Emery JR, Clark SJ, et al. Reference ranges for newer thyroid function tests in premature infants. J Pediatr 1995;126: 122-127.
181. LaFranchi S. Thyroid function in the preterm infant. Thyroid 1999;9:71-78.
182. Frank JE, Faix JE, Hermos RJ, et al. Thyroid function in very low birth weight infants: effects on neonatal hypothyroidism screening. J Pediatr 1996;128:548-554.
183. Mariotti S, Barbesino G, Caturegli P, et al. Complex alteration of thyroid function in healthy centenarians. J Clin Endocrinol Metab 1993;77:1130-1134.
184. Mariotti S, Franceschi C, Cossarizza A, et al. The aging thyroid. Endocr Rev 1995;16:686-715.
185. Chan JL, Bullen J, Stoyneva V, et al. Recombinant methionyl human leptin administration to achieve high physiologic or pharmacologic leptin levels does not alter circulating inflammatory marker levels in humans with leptin sufficiency or excess. J Clin Endocrinol Metab 2005;90:1618-1624.
186. Peeters RP, Wouters PJ, Kaptein E, et al. Reduced activation and increased inactivation of thyroid hormone in tissues of critically ill patients. J Clin Endocrinol Metab 2003;88:3202-3211.
187. Byerley LO, Heber D. Metabolic effects of triiodothyronine replacement during fasting in obese subjects. J Clin Endocrinol Metab 1996;81:968-976.
188. Kiyohara K, Tamai H, Takaichi Y, et al. Decreased thyroidal triiodothyronine secretion in patients with anorexia nervosa: influence of weight recovery. Am J Clin Nutr 1989;50:767-772.
189. Onur S, Haas V, Bosy-Westphal A, et al. L-Tri-iodothyronine is a major determinant of resting energy expenditure in underweight patients with anorexia nervosa and during weight gain. Eur J Endocrinol 2005;152:179-184.
190. Danforth JE, Horton ES, O'Connell M, et al. Dietary-induced alterations in thyroid hormone metabolism during overnutrition. J Clin Invest 1979;64:1336-1347.
191. Van den Berghe G. Novel insights into the neuroendocrinology of critical illness. Eur J Endocrinol 2000;143:1-13.
192. Alkemade A, Friesema EC, Unmehopa UA, et al. Neuroanatomical pathways for thyroid hormone feedback in the human hypothalamus. J Clin Endocrinol Metab 2005;90:4322-4334.
193. Fekete C, Sarkar S, Christoffolete MA, et al. Bacterial lipopolysaccharide (LPS)-induced type 2 iodothyronine deiodinase (D2) activation in the mediobasal hypothalamus (MBH) is independent of the LPS-induced fall in serum thyroid hormone levels. Brain Res 2005;1056:97-99.
194. Boelen A, Platvoet-Ter Schiphorst MC, Wiersinga WM. Association between serum interleukin-6 and serum 3,5,3′-triiodothyronine in nonthyroidal illness. J Clin Endocrinol Metab 1993;77: 1695-1699.

195. Van den Berghe G, de Zegher F, Veldhuis JD, et al. Thyrotrophin and prolactin release in prolonged critical illness: dynamics of spontaneous secretion and effects of growth hormone- secretagogues. Clin Endocrinol (Oxf) 1997;47:599-612.
196. Van den Berghe G, de Zegher F, Baxter RC, et al. Neuroendocrinology of prolonged critical illness: effects of exogenous thyrotropin-releasing hormone and its combination with growth hormone secretagogues. J Clin Endocrinol Metab 1998;83:309-319.
197. Kaplan MM, Larsen PR, Crantz FR, et al. Prevalence of abnormal thyroid function test results in patients with acute medical illnesses. Am J Med 1982;72:9-16.
198. Franklyn JA, Black EG, Betteridge J, et al. Comparison of second and third generation methods for measurement of serum thyrotopin in patients with overt hyperthyroidism, patients receiving thyroxine therapy, and those with nonthyroidal illness. J Clin Endocrinol Metab 1994;78:1368-1371.
199. Wadwekar D, Kabadi UM. Thyroid hormone indices during illness in six hypothyroid subjects rendered euthyroid with levothyroxine therapy. Exp Clin Endocrinol Diabetes 2004;112:373-377.
200. Vos RA, DeJong M, Bernard BF, et al. Impaired T_4 and T_3 handling by rat hepatocytes in the presence of serum of patients with nonthyroidal illness (NTI). J Clin Endocrinol Metab 1995;80: 2364-2370.
201. Van den Berghe G, Wouters P, Weekers F, et al. Reactivation of pituitary hormone release and metabolic improvement by infusion of growth hormone-releasing peptide and thyrotropin-releasing hormone in patients with protracted critical illness. J Clin Endocrinol Metab 1999;84:1311-1323.
202. Brent GA, Hershman JM. Thyroxine therapy in patients with severe nonthyroidal illness and low serum thyroxine concentrations. J Clin Endocrinol Metab 1986;63:1-8.
203. Hamblin PS, Dyer SA, Mohr VS, et al. Relationship between thyrotropin and thyroxine changes during the recovery from severe hypothyroxinemia of critical illness. J Clin Endocrinol Metab 1986;62:717-722.
204. Becker RA, Vaughan GM, Ziegler MG, et al. Hypermetabolic low triiodothyronine syndrome of burn injury. Crit Care Med 1982; 10:870-875.
205. Bennett-Guerrero E, Jimenez JL, White WD, et al. Cardiovascular effects of intravenous triiodothyronine in patients undergoing coronary artery bypass graft surgery. A randomized, double-blind, placebo-controlled trial. Duke T_3 Study Group. JAMA 1996; 275:687-692.
206. Klein I, Ojamaa K. Thyroid hormone and the cardiovascular system. N Engl J Med 2001;344:501-509.
207. Kirkegaard C, Faber J. The role of thyroid hormones in depression. Eur J Endocrinol 1998;138:1-9.
208. Jackson IM. The thyroid axis and depression. Thyroid 1998;8: 951-956.
209. Nader S, Warner MD, Doyle S, et al. Euthyroid sick syndrome in psychiatric inpatients. Biol Psychiatry 1996;40:1288-1293.
210. Brabant G, Brabant A, Ranft U. Circadian and pulsatile thyrotropin secretion in euthyroid man under the influence of thyroid hormone and glucocorticoid administration. J Clin Endocrinol Metab 1987;65:83.
211. Topliss DJ, White EL, Stockigt JR. Significance of thyrotropin excess in untreated primary adrenal insufficiency. J Clin Endocrinol Metab 1980;50:52-56.
212. Colao A, Pivonello R, Faggiano A, et al. Increased prevalence of thyroid autoimmunity in patients successfully treated for Cushing's disease. Clin Endocrinol (Oxf) 2000;53:13-19.
213. Arafah BM. Increased need for thyroxine in women with hypothyroidism during estrogen therapy. N Engl J Med 2001;344: 1743-1749.
214. Arafah BM. Decreased levothyroxine requirement in women with hypothyroidism during androgen therapy for breast cancer. Ann Intern Med 1994;121:247-251.
215. Surks MI, Goswami G, Daniels GH. The thyrotropin reference range should remain unchanged. J Clin Endocrinol Metab 2005;90:5489-5496.
216. Wartofsky L, Dickey RA. The evidence for a narrower thyrotropin reference range is compelling. J Clin Endocrinol Metab 2005;90:5483-5488.
217. Dashe JS, Casey BM, Wells CE, et al. Thyroid-stimulating hormone in singleton and twin pregnancy: importance of gestational age-specific reference ranges. Obstet Gynecol 2005;106:753-757.
218. Kuzuya N, Kinji I, Ishibashi M. Endocrine and immunohistochemical studies on thyrotropin (TSH)-secreting pituitary adenomas: responses of TSH, α-subunit, and growth hormone to hypothalamic releasing hormones and their distribution in adenoma cells. J Clin Endocrinol Metab 1990;71:1103-1111.
219. Brucker-Davis F, Oldfield EH, Skarulis MC, et al. Thyrotropin-secreting pituitary tumors: diagnostic criteria, thyroid hormone sensitivity, and treatment outcome in 25 patients followed at the National Institutes of Health. J Clin Endocrinol Metab 1999; 84:476-486.
220. Nystrom E, Caidahl K, Fager G, et al. A double-blind cross-over 12-month study of L-thyroxine treatment of women with "subclinical" hypothyroidism. Clin Endocrinol 1988;29:63-76.
221. Bell GM, Todd WTA, Forfar JC, et al. End-organ responses to thyroxine therapy in subclinical hypothyroidism. Clin Endocrinol 1985;22:83-89.
222. Nelson JC, Weiss RM, Wilcox RB. Underestimates of serum free thyroxine (T_4) concentrations by free T_4 immunoassays. J Clin Endocrinol Metab 1994;79:76-79.
223. Nelson JC, Wilcox RB, Pandian MR. Dependence of free thyroxine estimates obtained with equilibrium tracer dialysis on the concentration of thyroxine-binding globulin. Clin Chem 1992;38: 1294-1300.
224. Wang R, Nelson JC, Weiss RM, et al. Accuracy of free thyroxine measurements across natural ranges of thyroxine binding to serum proteins. Thyroid 2000;10:31-39.
225. Hay ID, Bayer MF, Kaplan MM, et al. American Thyroid Association assessment of current free thyroid hormone and thyrotropin measurements and guidelines for future clinical assays. The Committee on Nomenclature of the American Thyroid Association. Clin Chem 1991;37:2002-2008.
226. Steele BW, Witte DL, Whitley RJ, et al. The effects of modifying proficiency testing materials on thyroid function test results. A College of American Pathologists Ligand Assay Survey Study. Arch Pathol Lab Med 1997;121:1241-1246.
227. Faix JD, Rosen HN, Velazquez FR. Indirect estimation of thyroid hormone-binding proteins to calculate free thyroxine index: comparison of nonisotopic methods that use labeled thyroxine ("T-uptake"). Clin Chem 1995;41:41-47.
228. Nelson JC, Weiss RM. The effect of serum dilution on free thyroxine (T_4) concentrations in the low T_4 syndrome of nonthyroidal illness. J Clin Endocrinol Metab 1985;61:239-246.
229. Demers LM, Spencer CA. Laboratory medicine practice guidelines: laboratory support for the diagnosis and monitoring of thyroid disease. Clin Endocrinol (Oxf) 2003;58:138-140.
230. Mandel SJ, Spencer CA, Hollowell JG. Are detection and treatment of thyroid insufficiency in pregnancy feasible? Thyroid 2005; 15:44-53.
231. Afandi B, Vera R, Schussler GC, et al. Concordant decreases of thyroxine and thyroxine binding protein concentrations during sepsis. Metabolism 2000;49:753-754.
232. Toft AD, Irvine WJ, Hunter WM, et al.. Anomalous plasma TSH levels in patients developing hypothyroidism in the early months after ^{131}I therapy for thyrotoxicosis. J Clin Endocrinol Metab 1974;39:607.
233. Davies P, Franklyn JA, Daykin J, et al. The significance of TSH values measured in a sensitive assay in the follow-up of hyperthyroid patients treated with radioiodine. J Clin Endocrinol Metab 1992;74:1189-1194.
234. Rees-Jones RW, Larsen PR. Triiodothyronine and thyroxine content of desiccated thyroid tablets. Metabolism 1977;26:1213-1218.
235. Kaptein EM. Thyroid hormone metabolism and thyroid diseases in chronic renal failure. Endocr Rev 1996;17:45-63.
236. Bacci V, Schussler GC, Kaplan TB. The relationship between serum triiodothyronine and thyrotropin during systemic illness. J Clin Endocrinol Metab 1982;54:1229.
237. Weiss RE, Refetoff S. Treatment of resistance to thyroid hormone—primum non nocere. J Clin Endocrinol Metab 1999;84:401-404.
238. Refetoff S, Weiss RE, Usala SJ. The syndromes of resistance to thyroid hormone. Endocr Rev 1993;14:348-399.
239. al-Adsani H, Hoffer LJ, Silva JE. Resting energy expenditure is sensitive to small dose changes in patients on chronic thyroid

hormone replacement. J Clin Endocrinol Metab 1997;82: 1118-1125.
240. Becker C. Hypothyroidism and atherosclerotic heart disease: pathogenesis, medical management, and the role of coronary artery bypass surgery. Endocr Rev 1985;6:432-440.
241. Brenta G, Schnitman M, Gurfinkiel M, et al. Variations of sex hormone-binding globulin in thyroid dysfunction. Thyroid 1999;9:273-277.
242. Smallridge RC, Parker RA, Wiggs EA, et al. Thyroid hormone resistance in a large kindred: physiologic, biochemical, pharmacologic, and neuropsychologic studies. Am J Med 1989;86:289-296.
243. Mazzaferri EL, Robbins RJ, Spencer CA, et al. A consensus report of the role of serum thyroglobulin as a monitoring method for low-risk patients with papillary thyroid carcinoma. J Clin Endocrinol Metab 2003;88:1433-1441.
244. Spencer CA, Wang CC. Thyroglobulin measurement. Techniques, clinical benefits, and pitfalls. Endocrinol Metab Clin North Am 1995;24:841-863.
245. Spencer CA, Bergoglio LM, Kazarosyan M, et al. Clinical impact of thyroglobulin (Tg) and Tg autoantibody method differences on the management of patients with differentiated thyroid carcinomas. J Clin Endocrinol Metab 2005;90:5566-5575.
246. Izumi M, Larsen PR. Correlation of sequential changes in serum thyroglobulin, triiodothyronine, and thyroxine in patients with Graves' disease and subacute thyroiditis. Metabolism 1978;27: 449-460.
247. Spencer CA. Serum thyroglobulin measurements: clinical utility and technical limitations in the management of patients with differentiated thyroid carcinomas. Endocr Pract 2000;6:481-484.
248. Mariotti S, Martino E, Cupini C, et al. Low serum thyroblobulin as a clue to the diagnosis of thyrotoxicosis factitia. N Engl J Med 1982;307:410-412.
249. Tenenbaum F, Corone C, Schlumberger M, et al. Thyroglobulin measurement and postablative iodine-131 total body scan after total thyroidectomy for differentiated thyroid carcinoma in patients with no evidence of disease. Eur J Cancer 1996;32A:1262.
250. Schneider AB, Ikekubo K. Sequential serum thyroglobulin determinations, ^{131}I scans, and ^{131}I uptakes after triiodothyronine withdrawal in patients with thyroid cancer. J Clin Endocrinol Metab 1981;53:1199-1206.
251. Haugen BR, Pacini F, Reiners C, et al. A comparison of recombinant human thyrotropin and thyroid hormone withdrawal for the detection of thyroid remnant or cancer. J Clin Endocrinol Metab 1999;84:3877-3885.
252. Rapoport B, McLachlan SM. Thyroid autoimmunity. J Clin Invest 2001;108:1253-1259.
253. Hollowell JG, Staehling NW, Flanders WD, et al. Serum TSH, T(4), and thyroid antibodies in the United States population (1988 to 1994): National Health and Nutrition Examination Survey (NHANES III). J Clin Endocrinol Metab 2002;87:489-499.
254. Martin A, Barbesino G, Davies TF. T-cell receptors and autoimmune thyroid disease—signposts for T-cell-antigen driven diseases. Int Rev Immunol 1999;18:111-140.
255. Latrofa F, Pichurin P, Guo J, et al. Thyroglobulin-thyroperoxidase autoantibodies are polyreactive, not bispecific: analysis using human monoclonal autoantibodies. J Clin Endocrinol Metab 2003;88:371-378.
256. Guo J, Wang Y, Rapoport B, et al. Evidence for antigen presentation to sensitized T cells by thyroid peroxidase (TPO)-specific B cells in mice injected with fibroblasts co-expressing TPO and MHC class II. Clin Exp Immunol 2000;119:38-46.
257. Vanderpump MPJ, Tunbridge WMG, French JM, et al. The incidence of thyroid disorders in the community: a twenty-year follow-up of the Whickham survey. Clin Endocrinol 43:55-68.
258. Pittman JA Jr, Dailey GE III, Beschi RJ. Changing normal values for thyroidal radioiodine uptake. N Engl J Med 1969;280:1431-1441.
259. Hayes AA, Akre CM, Gorman CA. Iodine-131 treatment of Graves' disease using modified early iodine-131 uptake measurements in therapy dose calculations. J Nucl Med 1990;31:519-522.
260. Medeiros-Neto G, Kim PS, Vono J, et al. Congenital hypothyroid goiter with deficient thyroglobulin. J Clin Invest 1996;98: 2838-2844.

CHAPTER 11

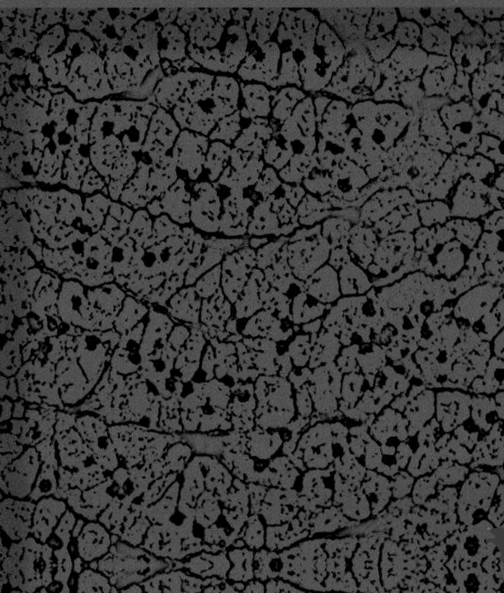

THYROTOXICOSIS

Terry F. Davies and P. Reed Larsen

INTRODUCTION

The term *thyrotoxicosis* refers to the classic physiologic manifestations of excessive quantities of the thyroid hormones that are so characteristic of this condition. The term *thyrotoxicosis* rather than *hyperthyroidism* should be used for this disorder, because it need not be associated with hyperfunction of the thyroid gland. The term *hyperthyroidism* is reserved for disorders that result from sustained overproduction of hormone by the thyroid itself, Graves' disease being the most common (Table 11–1). The other common conditions causing thyrotoxicosis inflammation of the thyroid gland, or thyroiditis, which is usually autoimmune or postviral multimoded or goiter. Hyperthyroidism and thyroiditis must be differentiated from thyrotoxicosis caused by exogenous thyroid hormone, whether this is iatrogenic or self-administered. For most patients with thyrotoxicosis, it is the symptoms or signs caused by an excess of the thyroid hormone, whatever its source, that lead to medical attention. Others may have surprisingly few symptoms and are referred because of a suppressed thyroid-stimulating hormone (TSH).

We begin with a brief review of the symptoms and signs of thyrotoxicosis and their pathophysiologic basis. The appropriate use of the laboratory tests described in Chapter 10 is presented to show how these can focus the search for a diagnosis.

CLINICAL MANIFESTATIONS OF THYROTOXICOSIS

Overview

One very important clinical clue to the cause of the patient's thyrotoxicosis is the duration of the symptoms. Patients with hyperthyroidism have generally had manifestations for many months before presentation but because the week-to-week increases in thyroid hormones are so small, they may become rather extreme, even though unnoticed by the patient. In addition, patients will often attribute the symptoms to other causes, such as their fatigue to family and/or work responsibilities, heat intolerance to the weather, weight loss to an effective diet, and dyspnea and palpitations to a lack of regular exercise. On the other hand, patients with thyrotoxicosis due to thyroiditis can often date the onset of their symptoms precisely, usually to within a month or so of their seeking medical attention, as might be expected from the effects of the release of the equivalent of 30 to 60 days' supply of thyroid hormone into the circulation over a few days to weeks. Thus, ascertaining the chronology as well as the spectrum of symptoms is a critical goal of the interview process. Another general characteristic is that the symptoms and signs of thyrotoxicosis are more readily recognized in

TABLE 11-1 CAUSES OF THYROTOXICOSIS

SUSTAINED HORMONE OVERPRODUCTION (HYPERTHYROIDISM)
Low TSH, High RAIU
Graves' disease (von Basedow's disease)
Toxic multinodular goiter
Toxic adenoma
Chorionic gonadotropin–induced
Gestational hyperthyroidism
Physiologic hyperthyroidism of pregnancy
Familial gestational hyperthyroidism due to TSH receptor mutations
Trophoblastic tumors
Inherited nonimmune hyperthyroidism associated with TSH receptor or G protein mutations
Low TSH, Low RAIU
Iodide-induced hyperthyroidism (Jod Basedow)
Amiodarone-associated hyperthyroidism due to iodide release
Struma Ovarii
Metastatic functioning thyroid carcinoma
Normal or Elevated TSH
TSH-secreting pituitary tumors
Thyroid hormone resistance with pituitary predominance
TRANSIENT HORMONE EXCESS (THYROTOXICOSIS)
Low TSH, Low RAIU
Thyroiditis
Autoimmune
Lymphocytic thyroiditis (silent thyroiditis, painless thyroiditis, postpartum thyroiditis)
Acute exacerbation of Hashimoto's disease
Viral or postviral
Subacute (granulomatous, painful, postviral) thyroiditis
Drug-induced or associated thyroiditis
Amiodarone
Lithium, interferon-α, interleukin-2, GM-CSF
Infectious thyroiditis
Exogenous Thyroid Hormone
Iatrogenic overreplacement
Thyrotoxicosis factitia
Ingestion of natural products containing thyroid hormone
"Hamburger" thyrotoxicosis
Natural foodstuffs
Thyromimetic compounds (e.g., Tiracol)
Occupational exposure to thyroid hormone (e.g., pill manufacturing, veterinary occupations)

GM-CSF, Granulocyte-macrophage colony-stimulating factor; *RAIU,* radioactive iodine uptake; *TSH,* thyroid-stimulating hormone.

the young than in the older patient.[1] The term *masked* or *apathetic* thyrotoxicosis is used to describe the syndrome sometimes seen in the elderly, which may present as congestive heart failure with arrhythmia or as unexplained weight loss without the increased appetite typical of the younger patient.

At present, the ready availability of the sensitive serum TSH assay, a reliable indicator of excess thyroid hormone in the ambulatory patient (see Chapter 10), has made the more classical and severe manifestations of longstanding thyrotoxicosis less prevalent. In fact, a current area of controversy is how aggressively to treat the condition termed *subclinical hyperthyroidism,* a biochemical diagnosis in which a subnormal serum TSH level is accompanied by normal free thyroid hormone concentrations in an asymptomatic patient. Nonetheless, the classical presentation is still common, serves to illustrate the pleiotropic physiologic effects of excess thyroid hormones, and, if not recognized, can progress to life-threatening severity even though hyperthyroidism is a benign condition. The next sections review the pathophysiology of the most important manifestations of excess thyroid hormone.

Cardiovascular System

Alterations in cardiovascular function in the thyrotoxic patient are, in part, due to increased circulatory demands that result from the hypermetabolism and the need to dissipate the excess heat produced.[2] At rest, peripheral vascular resistance is decreased, and cardiac output is increased as a result of an increase first in heart rate and, with more severe disease, in stroke volume. Thyroid hormones in excess also have a direct ionotropic effect on cardiac contraction mediated by an increase in the ratio of α to β myosin heavy chain expression. Tachycardia is virtually always present due to a combination of increased sympathetic and decreased vagal tone.[3] Widening of the pulse pressure is due to the increase in systolic and decrease in diastolic pressure due to reduced resistance.[4,5] The decreased resistance is due to increased nitric oxide production.[6] The increased systolic force is often felt by the patient as a "palpitation" and is evident on inspection or palpation of the precordium. Because of the diffuse and forceful nature of the apex beat, the heart may seem enlarged and echocardiography may show an increased ventricular mass. In addition, the preejection period is shortened and the ratio of preejection period to left ventricular ejection time is decreased.[5] The heart sounds are enhanced, particularly S_1, and a scratchy systolic sound along the left sternal border, resembling a pleuropericardial friction rub *(Means-Lerman scratch),* may also be heard. These manifestations abate when a normal metabolic state is restored. Mitral valve prolapse occurs more frequently with Graves' or Hashimoto's disease than in the normal population.[7,8] Cardiac arrhythmias are almost invariably supraventricular, especially in younger patients.[9] Between 2% and 20% of patients with thyrotoxicosis have atrial fibrillation, and about 15% of patients with otherwise unexplained atrial fibrillation are thyrotoxic.[2] In a study of more than 2000 individuals 60 years of age or older, 28% of those with a suppressed TSH developed atrial fibrillation.[10]

The increased cardiovascular cost of a standard workload or metabolic challenge is adequately met if the thyrotoxic patient is not or has not previously been in heart failure. Thus, in most patients without underlying heart disease, cardiac competence is maintained. Mild peripheral edema may occur in the absence of heart failure. Heart failure per se usually occurs in patients with preexisting heart disease, and therefore typically in the elderly, but it may not be possible to determine whether underlying heart disease is present until after thyrotoxicosis is relieved. Atrial fibrillation decreases the efficiency of the cardiac response to any increased circulatory demand and may play a role in causing cardiac failure.[11] Attempts to convert atrial fibrillation to sinus rhythm are not indicated while thyrotoxicosis is present and about 60% of patients revert spontaneously to sinus rhythm after treatment, most within 4 months.[12] For this reason and because thromboembolism is rare in patients younger than 50 years of age with thyrotoxicosis, routine anticoagulation is not recommended for younger patients without a history of underlying heart disease or prior history of thrombotic disorder.[13,14] Medical or electrical cardioversion of patients with thyrotoxicosis-induced atrial fibrillation is often successful even after a year has passed.[15]

Protein, Carbohydrate, and Lipid Metabolism

The stimulation of metabolism and heat production is reflected in the increased basal metabolic rate, increased appetite, and heat intolerance, but only rarely by elevated basal body temperature.[16] Despite an increased food intake, a state of chronic caloric and nutritional inadequacy often ensues, depending on the degree of increased metabolism. Both synthesis and degradation rates of proteins are increased, the latter to a greater extent than the former, with the result that in severe thyrotoxicosis there is a net decrease in tissue protein, as indicated by loss of weight, muscle wasting, proximal muscle weakness, and even mild hypoalbuminemia. Preexisting diabetes mellitus may be aggravated, one cause being accelerated turnover of insulin. Both lipogenesis and lipolysis are increased in thyrotoxicosis, but the net effect is lipolysis, as reflected by an increase in the plasma concentration of free fatty acids and glycerol and a decrease in serum cholesterol level; triglyceride levels are usually slightly decreased. The enhanced mobilization and oxidation of free fatty acids in response to fasting or catecholamines are due to enhancement of lipolytic pathways by thyroid hormones.[16]

Sympathetic Nervous System and Catecholamines

Many of the manifestations of thyrotoxicosis and of sympathetic nervous system activation are similar. Nonetheless, the plasma concentrations of epinephrine and norepinephrine, as well as their urinary excretion and that of their metabolites, is not increased in patients with thyrotoxicosis, and thyroid hormones exert effects separate from, but similar and additive to, those of the catecholamines.[17] The improvement in cardiac function in patients with hyperthyroidism by β blockade has led to the concept that there is increased sympathetic tone or increased cardiac sensitivity to the sympathetic nervous system.[18] The latter is supported by results in the transgenic mouse in which overexpression of type 2 deiodinase in the heart increases myocardial T_3 and by the cyclic adenosine monophosphate (cAMP) response to norepinephrine in the cardiac myocytes due to alterations in G proteins.[19,20] In addition, adipocytes from thyrotoxic patients have threefold increases in norepinephrine-induced lipolysis, 15-fold increases in response to β_2-adrenergic receptor agonists and threefold increases in response to forskolin or cAMP.[21] Thus, thyroid hormones increase sensitivity to catecholamines in both cardiomyocytes and adipocytes by a variety of mechanisms.

Nervous System

Alterations in the function of the nervous system in thyrotoxicosis are manifested by nervousness, emotional lability, and hyperkinesia. Fatigue may be due to both the muscle weakness and the insomnia that are commonly present. Emotional lability is common and in rare cases mental disturbance may be severe; manic depressive, schizoid, or paranoid reactions may emerge. The hyperkinesia of the thyrotoxic patient is characteristic. During the interview, the patient shifts positions frequently, and movements are quick, jerky, exaggerated, and often purposeless. In children, in whom such manifestations tend to be more severe, inability to focus may lead to deterioration of school performance, suggesting attention deficit hyperactivity disorder. A fine tremor of the hands, tongue, or lightly closed eyelids may appear and mimic that of parkinsonism. The electroencephalogram reveals an increase in fast wave activity, and in patients with convulsive disorders, the frequency of seizures is increased.

Muscle

Weakness and fatigability are usually not accompanied by objective evidence of muscle disease except for the generalized wasting associated with weight loss. The weakness is most prominent in the proximal muscles of the limbs, causing difficulty in climbing stairs or fatigue from minimal exertion such as using a blow-dryer or lifting an infant. Proximal muscle wasting may be out of proportion to the overall loss of weight *(thyrotoxic myopathy)*. Myopathy affects men with thyrotoxicosis more commonly than women and may overshadow the other manifestations of the syndrome. In the most severe forms, the myopathy may involve the more distal muscles of the extremities and the muscles of the trunk and face. Although myopathy of ocular muscles is unusual, the disorder may mimic myasthenia gravis or ophthalmic myasthenia.[22] Muscular strength returns to normal when a normal metabolic state is restored, but muscle mass takes longer to recover.

Graves' disease occurs in about 3% to 5% of patients with myasthenia gravis, and about 1% of the patients with Graves' disease develop myasthenia gravis. Antibodies and T cells specific for the TSH and acetylcholine receptors are involved in the pathogenesis of the two diseases.[23] Unlike in thyrotoxic myopathy, the association of myasthenia gravis with Graves' disease has a distinct female preponderance. The effect of both thyrotoxicosis and its alleviation on the course of myasthenia gravis is variable, but in most cases, myasthenia is accentuated during the thyrotoxic state and improves when a normal metabolic state is restored.

Periodic paralysis of the hypokalemic type may occur together with thyrotoxicosis, and its severity is accentuated by the latter disorder. The coincidence of the two disorders is particularly common in Asian and Latino males.[24-26]

Eyes

Retraction of the upper and/or lower eyelids, evident as the presence of a rim of sclera between either lid and the limbus, is frequent in all forms of thyrotoxicosis, regardless of the underlying cause, and is responsible for the typical "stare" of the patient. Also common is either lid lag, a phenomenon in which the upper lid lags behind the globe when the patient is asked to shift the gaze slowly downward, or globe lag, which becomes evident when the eye lags behind the upper lid when the patient looks up. These ocular manifestations appear to be the result of increased adrenergic tone. *It is important to differentiate these signs, which may occur in all forms of thyrotoxicosis, from those of infiltrative orbitopathy, which are associated with Graves' disease and are described later.*

Skin and Hair

The most characteristic change in the patient with longstanding thyrotoxicosis is the warm, moist feel of the skin that results from cutaneous vasodilation and excessive sweating. The elbows may be smooth and pink, the complexion is rosy, and the patient blushes readily. Palmar erythema may resemble "liver palms," and telangiectasia may be present. The hair is fine and friable, and hair loss may increase. The nails are often soft and friable. A characteristic but uncommon finding is *Plummer's nails,* onycholysis typically involving the fourth and fifth fingers.

Vitiligo, another autoimmune disease, is more common in patients with autoimmune thyroid disease.

Respiratory System

Dyspnea is common in severe thyrotoxicosis, and several factors may contribute to this condition. Vital capacity is commonly reduced, with this reduction resulting mainly from weakness of the respiratory muscles. During exercise, ventilation is increased out of proportion to the increase in oxygen uptake, but the diffusing capacity of the lung is normal.

Alimentary System

An increase in appetite is common but is usually not seen in patients with mild disease. In more severe disease, the increased intake of food is inadequate to meet the increased caloric requirements, and weight is lost at a variable rate. More often, the patient reports a gratifying success with a previously frustrated attempt at weight control. The frequency of bowel movements is increased, but diarrhea is rare. The increased gastric emptying and intestinal motility in thyrotoxicosis appear to be responsible for slight malabsorption of fat, and these functions return to normal when a normal metabolic state has been restored. Celiac and Graves' diseases may coexist, and there is an increased prevalence of pernicious anemia.

Hepatic dysfunction occurs, particularly when thyrotoxicosis is severe; hypoproteinemia and increases in serum alanine aminotransferase (ALT) and bone and/or liver alkaline phosphatase levels may be elevated.[27] Hepatomegaly and jaundice can develop with severe, prolonged disease, and liver failure was a cause of death before the development of successful treatment for Graves' patients. Splanchnic oxygen consumption is increased in proportion to the metabolic rate, but splanchnic blood flow is not proportionately increased. As a result, the arteriovenous oxygen difference across the splanchnic bed is increased, and hypoxia may contribute to hepatic dysfunction.[28] A reduction in cardiac output by pulse rate reduction due to β-adrenergic blockade may exacerbate that process in that it does not reduce the hepatic hypermetabolism.

Skeletal System: Calcium and Phosphorus Metabolism

Thyrotoxicosis is generally associated with increased excretion of calcium and phosphorus in urine and stool; with demineralization of bone, as demonstrated by routine bone densitometry; and occasionally with pathologic fractures, especially in older women.[29-32] In such instances, the pathologic changes are variable and may include osteitis fibrosa, osteomalacia, or osteoporosis. Urinary excretion of collagen breakdown products is increased in thyrotoxicosis. Kinetic studies indicate an increase in the exchangeable calcium pool and acceleration of both bone resorption and accretion, particularly the former. The changes lead to a transient decreased bone density. As the thyrotoxicosis is treated, bone density will normalize in younger patients.[33] Postmenopausal women, however, may have a permanent reduction in bone density that requires treatment (see Chapter 27), although some long-term follow-up studies show fracture risk is not increased.[34] Much controversy has existed over the induction of decreased bone density by TSH-suppression therapy in patients with thyroid cancer. Suffice it to say that postmenopausal, but not premenopausal, women given a TSH-suppressive dosage of thyroid hormones are at risk of osteopenia and require prophylaxis with calcium and vitamin D.[35,36]

Hypercalcemia may occur in patients with severe thyrotoxicosis. The total serum calcium concentration is increased in as many as 27% of patients, and the ionized serum calcium is elevated in 47%. The concentrations of heat-labile serum alkaline phosphatase and osteocalcin are also frequently elevated. These findings resemble those of primary hyperparathyroidism, but the concentration of parathyroid hormone in serum is low-normal in most.[37] True primary hyperparathyroidism and thyrotoxicosis sometimes coexist. Plasma 25-hydroxycholecalciferol levels are decreased in thyrotoxic patients; this alteration could contribute to the decreased intestinal absorption of calcium and osteomalacia noted in some.

Renal Function: Water and Electrolyte Metabolism

Thyrotoxicosis produces no symptoms referable to the urinary tract except mild polyuria, which may lead to nocturia. Nevertheless, renal blood flow, glomerular filtration, and tubular reabsorptive and secretory maxima are increased. Total exchangeable potassium is decreased, possibly due to a decrease in lean body mass, but electrolytes are normal, except when hypokalemic periodic paralysis occurs.

Hematopoietic System

The red blood cells are usually normal, as judged by the usual indices, but red blood cell mass is increased. The increase in erythropoiesis is due to both the direct effect of thyroid hormones on the erythroid marrow and the increased production of erythropoietin. A parallel increase in plasma volume also occurs, resulting in normal hematocrit.

Approximately 3% of patients with Graves' disease have pernicious anemia, and a further 3% have antibodies to intrinsic factor but normal absorption of vitamin B_{12}. Autoantibodies against gastric parietal cells may also be present in patients with Graves' disease, and the requirements for vitamin B_{12} and folic acid appear to be increased. The total white blood cell count is often low because of a decrease in the number of neutrophils. The absolute lymphocyte count is normal or increased, leading to a relative lymphocytosis. The numbers of monocytes and eosinophils may also be increased. Splenic enlargement occurs in about 10% of the patients, and thymic and lymph node enlargement is common. The latter may manifest as a mediastinal mass. Thymic hyperplasia is also due to thyrotoxicosis in that it is sometimes seen in patients receiving excess exogenous thyroxine for TSH suppression.[38,39]

Platelet levels and the intrinsic clotting mechanism are normal, but the concentration of factor VIII is often increased and returns to normal when the thyrotoxicosis is treated. *Despite this increase, there is an enhanced sensitivity to warfarin because of the accelerated clearance of the vitamin K–dependent clotting factors.* Somewhat paradoxically then, the dosage of warfarin needs to be reduced in thyrotoxic patients.[40] This must be kept in mind if initiating anticoagulant treatment for atrial fibrillation.[41] Coincidental autoimmune thrombocytopenia may also occur.

Pituitary and Adrenocortical Function

The thyrotoxic state imposes several challenges on pituitary and adrenocortical function. The hepatic inactivation of cortisol is accelerated including 5α/5β-reductases and 11β-hydroxysteroid dehydrogenase. As a result of these changes, the disposal of cortisol is accelerated, but its rate of secretion is also increased, so the plasma cortisol concentration remains normal. The concentration of corticosteroid-binding globulin in plasma is also normal. The urinary excretion of free cortisol is normal or slightly increased (see Chapter 14).[42]

Reproductive Function

Thyrotoxicosis in early life may cause delayed sexual maturation, although physical development is normal and skeletal growth may be accelerated. Thyrotoxicosis after puberty influences reproductive function, especially in women. The intermenstrual interval may be prolonged or shortened, and menstrual flow is initially diminished and ultimately ceases. Fertility may be reduced, and if conception takes place, there is an increased risk of miscarriage. An association of thyroid autoantibodies and increased pregnancy loss is not related to changes in thyroid function; the thyroid autoantibodies are thought to represent a marker of immune instability.[43]

In some patients, menstrual cycles are predominantly anovulatory with oligomenorrhea, but in most, ovulation occurs, as indicated by a secretory endometrium. In the former, a subnormal midcycle surge of luteinizing hormone (LH) may be responsible. In premenopausal women with thyrotoxicosis, basal plasma concentrations of LH and follicle-stimulating hormone (FSH) are reportedly normal but may display enhanced responsiveness to gonadotropin-releasing hormone (GnRH).

Thyrotoxicosis, whether spontaneous or induced by exogenous hormone, is accompanied by an increase in the concentration of sex hormone–binding globulin (SHBG) in plasma.[44] As a result, the plasma concentrations of total testosterone, dihydrotestosterone, and estradiol are increased, but their unbound fractions are normal or transiently decreased. The increased binding in plasma may be responsible for the decreased metabolic clearance rate of testosterone and dihydrotestosterone. In the case of estradiol, however, the metabolic clearance rate is normal, suggesting that tissue metabolism of the hormone is increased. Conversion rates of androstenedione to testosterone, estrone, and estradiol, and of testosterone to dihydrotestosterone are increased.[45] The increased rate of conversion of androgens to estrogenic by-products may be the mechanism for gynecomastia and erectile dysfunction in approximately 10% of thyrotoxic men and one mechanism for menstrual irregularities in women. Another likely mechanism for menstrual changes is the disruption in amplitude and frequency of LH/FSH pulses due to thyroid hormone influences on GnRH signaling.

LABORATORY DIAGNOSIS OF THYROTOXICOSIS

The effects of thyrotoxicosis on the major organ systems are the same regardless of the underlying etiology. Their frequency and intensity and the other findings with which they are associated are influenced by the cause of the excess thyroid hormone. To a large extent, the same is true of laboratory test results. However, the patient with thyrotoxic symptoms will virtually always have a serum TSH concentration less than 0.1 mU/L and an elevated serum free T_4. In general, when thyrotoxicosis is due to hyperthyroidism, serum free T_3 is more elevated than is the free T_4 but this measurement is rarely required for an accurate diagnosis. If the possibility of exogenous thyroid hormone can be eliminated, the primary differential is between hyperthyroidism and thyroiditis (Fig. 11–1). Often this differentiation can be made on the basis of the history and physical, but the most critical differentiating test is the radioiodine uptake (RAIU), which is elevated or high normal in hyperthyroidism and very low in patients with thyroiditis.

If the physical examination or thyroid ultrasonography indicates the presence of a nodular thyroid, scintigraphy should accompany the uptake to differentiate diffuse from nodular hyperfunction. In the absence of that indication, the extra expense and patient inconvenience is not justified. In patients with iodine-induced hyperthyroidism, such as may occur with amiodarone, the uptake is usually undetectable in iodine-sufficient regions, which is the major exception to this strategy. The association of thyrotoxicosis with an elevated TSH is rare and suggests a TSH-producing pituitary tumor (see Fig. 11–1). The possibility of an artifactually elevated TSH in a patient with Graves' disease should be ruled out by repeating the assay by a different method in another laboratory (see Chapter 6). Exceptions to these general guidelines are discussed below within the appropriate subsection.

GRAVES' DISEASE

Background

Robert Graves' disease, although first described by Parry in 1825,[46] is best known as Graves' disease in the English-speaking world and as von Basedow's disease on the continent of Europe because of the prominence of the disease reports by these eminent physicians. It is the most enigmatic and, in areas of iodine abundance, one of the most common thyroid diseases.

Presentation

Graves' disease is characterized by diffuse goiter and thyrotoxicosis and may be accompanied by an infiltrative orbitopathy and ophthalmopathy, and occasionally infiltrative dermopathy. In the individual patient, thyroid disease and the infiltrative phenomena may occur singly or together but run courses that may be largely independent. The thyroid component is closely related to autoimmune thyroiditis (Hashimoto's disease) in its pathogenesis and clinical course. In Graves' disease, hyperthyroidism occurs in the presence of some degree of chronic thyroiditis and may ultimately be replaced, in the long term, by thyroid hypofunction. Conversely, hyperthyroidism may occasionally supervene in patients with preexisting Hashimoto's thyroiditis. Both of these diseases may occur within the same family.

Autoimmune Characteristics

Autoimmune thyroid disease is characterized by the occurrence in the serum of antibodies against thyroid peroxidase (TPO) (still incorrectly called the "microsomal" antigen by many physicians), thyroglobulin (Tg), and the TSH receptor (TSHR). T cell–mediated autoimmunity can also be demonstrated against the three primary thyroid antigens, as judged by a variety of criteria, including the ability of the T cells to elaborate various lymphokines and to exhibit a mitogenic response when exposed to thyroid antigens or to peptide sequences from the antigens.[47] Autoimmune thyroid disease is also characterized by lymphocytic infiltration of the thyroid gland—intense in autoimmune thyroiditis and heterogeneous in Graves' disease. In patients and their relatives, there is an increased frequency of other disorders of autoimmune origin, such as insulin-dependent diabetes mellitus, pernicious anemia, myasthenia gravis, adrenal

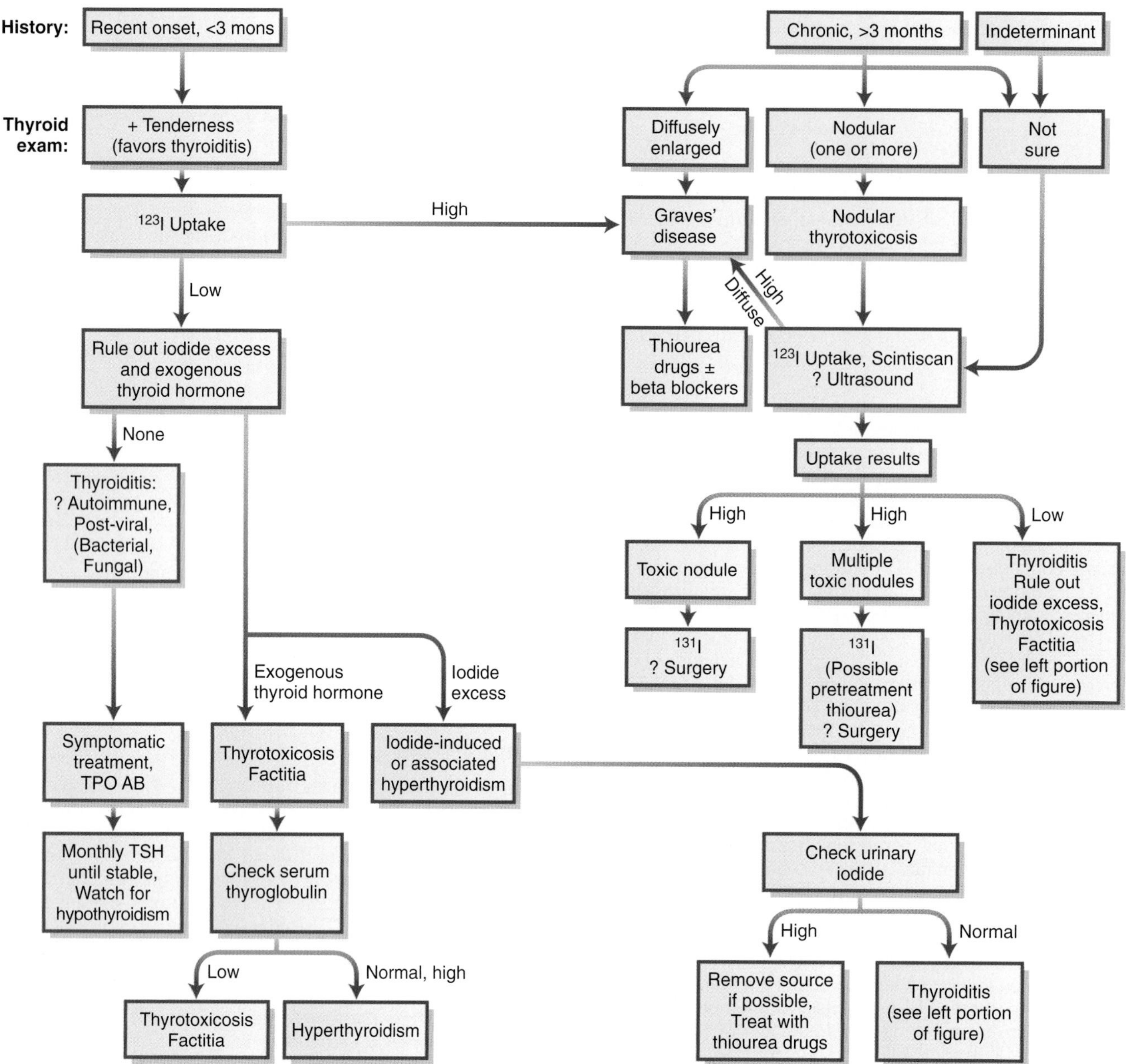

Figure 11–1 ▪ Algorithm for determining the cause of thyrotropin-independent thyrotoxicosis. TPO AB, thyroid peroxidase antibody; TSH, thyrotropin.

atrophy, Sjögren's syndrome, lupus erythematosus, rheumatoid arthritis, and idiopathic thrombocytopenic purpura (see Chapter 41).

The circulating autoantibodies specific to hyperthyroid Graves' disease are directed against the TSHR (TSHRAbs) and behave as thyroid-stimulating antibodies.[48] These antibodies can compete for the binding of TSH to its specific receptor site in the cell membrane and can activate adenylate cyclase. Similar but distinct autoantibodies in the sera of some patients with autoimmune thyroiditis also compete for TSH binding but do not stimulate the thyroid cell and may block the ligand-binding site and act as TSH antagonists while others are neutral in their bioactivity, neither blocking TSH activity nor stimulating the receptor (Fig. 11–2).

The thyroid gland itself is the major site of thyroid autoantibody secretion in autoimmune thyroid disease via the B cells that form part of the intrathyroidal infiltrate. Transplantation of Graves' thyroid tissue into T cell–deficient and B cell–deficient mice with severe combined immunodeficiency (scid mice) results in the appearance of human thyroid autoantibodies, including TSHRAb, in the serum.[49] Additional evidence for a role of the thyroid itself in antibody production comes from animal models of thyroiditis and from the decline in thyroid autoantibody levels after antithyroid drug treatment,[50] thyroidectomy, or radioiodine ablation.[51] After thyroidectomy and radioiodine treatment, however, some patients show no loss of autoantibody secretion, which suggests extrathyroidal sources of continued production.

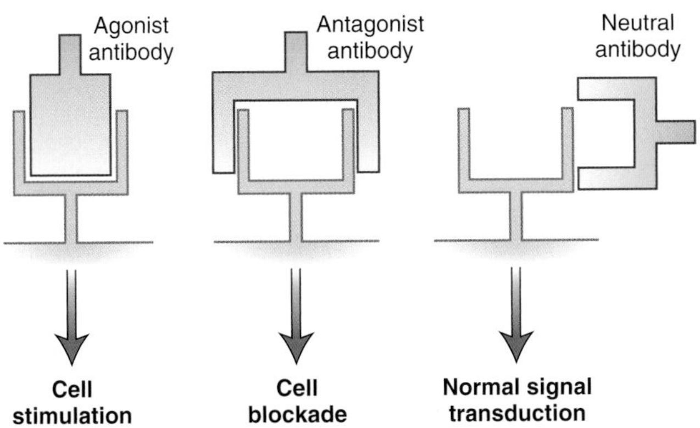

Figure 11–2 ▪ Schematic diagram of thyroid cell stimulation and blockade by antibodies to the thyrotropin-stimulating hormone receptor. Such autoantibodies may act as agonists or antagonists, or may be neutral, depending on how they interact with the receptor binding site.

Pathology

In patients with Graves' disease, the thyroid gland is characterized by a nonhomogeneous lymphocytic infiltration with an absence of follicular destruction (Fig. 11–3). Antithyroid drug treatment may reduce the degree of infiltration influencing the commonly observed histology in such patients. Although the intrathyroidal lymphocyte population is mixed, most are T lymphocytes (both Th1 and Th2 types along with CD25+ regulatory T cells); while B-cell germinal centers are much less common than in autoimmune thyroiditis. However, both intraepithelial T cells and plasma cells can be seen in peripolesis within the thyroid follicles. Follicular epithelial cell size correlates with the intensity of the local infiltrate, suggesting local thyroid cell stimulation by TSHRAb. Memory T cells may predominate within the T-cell population, but this finding can vary from patient to patient. Activated B-cell and T-cell markers are more frequent in intrathyroidal lymphocyte cultures than in peripheral blood cultures.

Prevalence

The prevalence of hyperthyroidism varies with the degree of iodine sufficiency in the population under study. The National Health and Nutrition Examination Survey (NHANES III) data[52] from the United States and a detailed epidemiologic survey in the United Kingdom[53] demonstrated the female preponderance of thyroid patients and the lower prevalence of hyperthyroidism compared with hypothyroidism. The results have indicated a prevalence of approximately 1% to 2%, in women, and in men, the prevalence is about one tenth that much. Overall, in women the incidence was estimated to be 1 case per 1000 per year over a 20-year follow-up. Graves' disease is the most common cause of spontaneous hyperthyroidism in patients younger than 40 years of age, and the risk does not change with age. The overall prevalence of autoimmune thyroid disease, comprising Graves' disease and autoimmune thyroiditis, approaches or exceeds that of diabetes mellitus and, when mild thyroid disease is included, the prevalence may be much greater.

Pathogenesis

The Major Antigen of Graves' Disease—The Thyrotropin Receptor

The TSHR is G protein–linked with seven transmembrane domains and employs cAMP and the phosphoinositol pathways

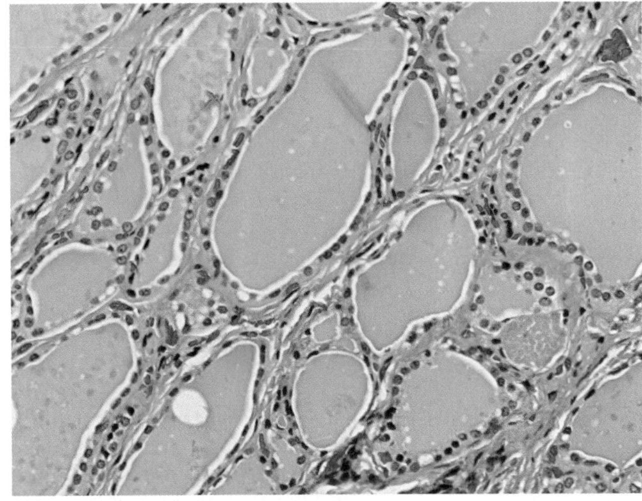
A

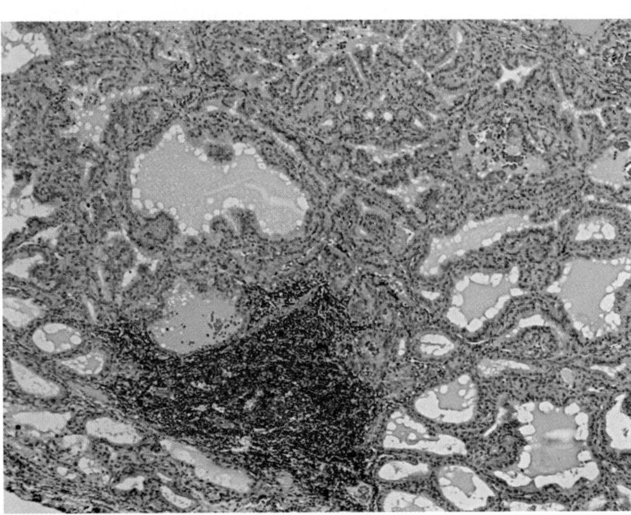
B

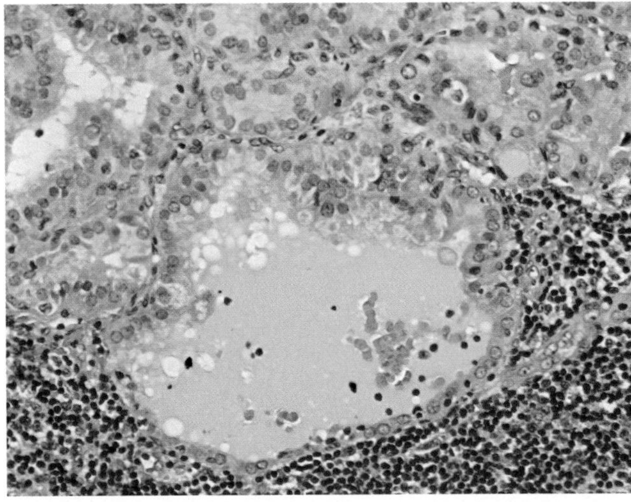
C

Figure 11–3 ▪ Histopathology of the Graves' thyroid. Sections of thyroid glands from normal tissue (**A**) and from a patient with Graves' disease (**B** and **C**). (Courtesy of Dr. Pamela Unger, Mount Sinai School of Medicine, New York, NY.)

for signal transduction. The human TSHR (hTSHR) is the primary autoantigen of Graves' disease, as shown by the development of hyperthyroidism in mice and hamsters after exposure to normal hTSHR antigen.[54-56] Extrathyroidal TSHR messenger RNA (mRNA) and protein have been reported in many other tissues, including fibroblasts, adipocytes, muscle cells, lymphocytes, osteoclasts, osteoblasts, and pituitary cells. While the physiologic role of TSH receptors in these sites is slowly being revealed, their role in autoimmune thyroid disease remains mostly unclear.

Molecular Structure of the Human Thyrotropin Receptor

Cloning of human TSHR complementary DNA (cDNA) made it possible to define the structure of the hTSHR gene and its chromosomal location (14q31). Seven hydrophobic transmembrane spanning regions in the hTSHR indicate that it is a member of the G protein–coupled receptor gene superfamily, and those receptors with large extracellular domains have been designated subgroup B. The TSH holoreceptor consists of a 100-kd, glycosylated, 744-amino-acid sequence and a 20–amino acid signal peptide. ProTSHR is cleaved into two subunits, α (or A) and β (or B), which are linked by disulfide bonds to form the physiologic receptor (Fig. 11–4).[57,58] The 50-kd α subunit is water-soluble and has TSH-binding activity. TSH is thought to bind to the leucine-rich repeat region of the α subunit.[59] The 30-kd β subunit is water-insoluble, contains the membrane-spanning domain with its three extracellular loops and three cytoplasmic loops, and is 70% to 75% homologous with the LH/human chorionic gonadotropin (hCG) receptor. Shedding of the α subunit has been shown in vitro and has been suggested to also occur in vivo. The TSHR forms dimers and multimeric complexes on the thyroid cell surface, which appear to reduce the random cleavage of the receptor into its constituent subunits.[48]

Autoantibodies to the Thyrotropin Receptor

In Graves' disease, TSHRAbs, discovered by Adams and Purves[61,62] bind to the TSH receptor, activate adenylate cyclase, induce thyroid growth, increase vascularity, and cause an increased rate of thyroid hormone production and secretion. As shown earlier, TSHRAbs in patients with Graves' disease are referred to as thyroid-stimulating antibodies. Other varieties of TSHRAbs may also be present—namely, a receptor antibody that acts as a TSH antagonist and is referred to as *blocking TSHRAbs* or a neutral form of antibody with no functional effect on the receptor.[48] Blocking TSHRAbs may be coincident with the stimulating type and may also predominate in certain patients after treatment with radioiodine, antithyroid drugs, or surgery (see Fig. 11–2). Blocking TSHRAbs can also be found in 15% of patients with autoimmune thyroiditis, particularly in patients without a goiter (the atrophic variety).[63] TSHRAbs are not detectable in the normal population with the use of currently available methods.

Bioactivity of Thyrotropin Receptor Autoantibody

The self-infusion of sera from patients with Graves' disease caused thyroid stimulation and was the first demonstration of the role of TSHRAbs in the induction of human hyperthyroidism.[64] Another example of the in vivo effects of TSHRAbs came from studies in neonates demonstrating the transplacental stimulation of the fetal thyroid in mothers with high titers of TSHRAbs.[65] TSHRAbs show light chain restriction in many patients with Graves' disease, and TSHRAbs that exhibit TSH agonist bioactivity are in the immunoglobulin G_1 (IgG_1) subclass; both observations suggest oligoclonality.[66,67] TSHR autoantibodies, like TSH, are thought to bind to conformational epitopes in the leucine-rich repeat region of the extracellular

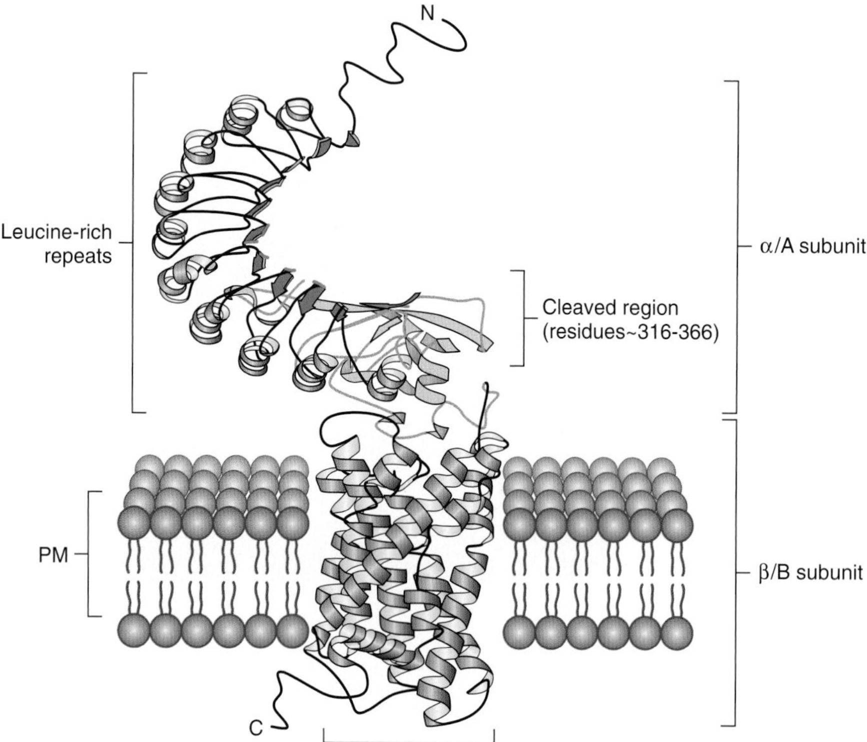

Figure 11–4 ▪ A current model of the human thyrotropin (TSH) receptor structure. The TSH receptor has seven transmembrane domains, a large extracellular domain, and a small intracellular domain. The receptor is cleaved, probably after activation, into α (or A) and β (or B) subunits. The α subunit is thought to be shed from the cell surface. PM, plasma membrane; TM, transmembrane domain. (Adapted from Nunez MR, Sanders J, Jeffreys J, et al. Analysis of the thyrotropin receptor-thyrotropin interaction by comparative modeling. Thyroid 2004;14:991-1011.)

domain of the TSHR. Further complicating this issue is the fact that many patients have all three antibodies: TSHR-stimulating, TSHR-blocking, and neutral antibodies. Hence, the degree of thyroid stimulation depends on the relative concentration and bioactivity of the different autoantibodies.

Prevalence of Thyrotropin Receptor Autoantibodies in Graves' Disease

The fact that TSHRAbs are detectable only in patients with autoimmune thyroid disease indicates that the autoantibodies are disease-specific, in contrast with the high prevalence of Tg antibodies and TPO antibodies in the population. Furthermore, TSHRAbs are unique human autoantibodies and do not occur in natural animal disease. A total of 90% to 100% of untreated hyperthyroid patients with Graves' disease have detectable TSHRAbs with thyroid-stimulating activity when using a sensitive assay.[68-70] The levels of TSHRAbs are decreased by treatment of the disease and, when they persist, may predict recurrence.[71,72] With time, TSHR-blocking autoantibodies may become the more prevalent type after treatment of Graves' disease causing hypothyroidism.

Intrathyroidal T Cells

T cells in patients with autoimmune thyroid disease are reactive to thyroid antigens and to peptides derived from these antigens[73,74] and are oligoclonal. About 10% of activated T cells infiltrating the thyroid gland in patients with autoimmune thyroid disease proliferate in response to thyroid cell antigens. Intrathyroidal T cells from patients with Graves' disease exhibit characteristics of both the helper T-cell subset 1 (Th_1) (which are recognized by their secretion of interleukin-2 (IL-2) and interferon γ and helper T-cell subset 2 (Th_2) (which are recognized by their secretion of IL-4).[75]

Regulation of the Immune Response in Autoimmune Thyroid Disease

Although thyroid hormone excess itself may give rise to changes in T-cell numbers, the immune system continues to exert its overall peripheral control. This is achieved by secretion of T-cell cytokines, the suppressive influence of "anergized" T cells, and by the presence of regulatory cells, which are a subset of CD4+ T cells (D25+Fox3p+) that have now been extensively characterized.[76] Such regulatory cells can suppress experimental thyroiditis in a variety of models,[77] although there are no data, to date, in patients with Graves' disease. In addition to these regulatory influences, another important mechanism of control is central tolerance caused by positive and negative selection of T cells and B cells in the thymus, where thyroid antigens are expressed.[78,79] Certain human leukocyte antigen (HLA)-DR haplotypes may be associated with reduced regulatory T-cell function, accounting for their association with AITD. Such mechanisms for the development of pathology must be distinguished from those risk factors that initiate disease and which are discussed separately.

Mechanisms in the Development of Autoimmune Thyroid Disease

The Consequences of an Insult

Initiation of autoimmune thyroid disease is thought to occur with an insult that leads to an immune response (Fig. 11–5). This may take the form of a direct insult to the thyroid gland by a viral infection or another external influence, including trauma,

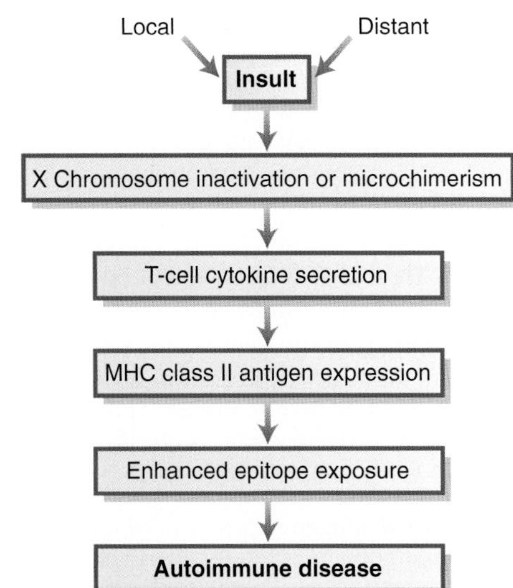

Figure 11–5 ▪ An overview of the most likely mechanisms involved in the cause and/or precipitation of Graves' disease. *MHC,* Major histocompatibility complex.

leading to activation of T cells.[80,81] Alternatively, it may be initiated elsewhere in the body. In the latter case, the arrival of activated T cells in the thyroid gland would start the process. Such an arrival may be nonspecific because the same T cells may arrive in many glands but the patient has a particular susceptibility to autoimmune thyroid disease. Initiation of disease may be mediated by bystander activation, molecular mimicry, or cryptic antigen presentation as described below, but the importance of these different mechanisms in Graves' disease remains uncertain.

Mechanism #1—Bystander Activation

Evidence has mounted that bystander activation of local resident antigen-specific and nonspecific T cells may initiate autoimmunity.[82,83] The presence of activated T cells within the thyroid gland following an insult may induce, via cytokine secretion, the activation of local thyroid-specific and non–thyroid-specific T cells as seen in animal models of thyroiditis. This series of events can occur only in a susceptible individual with the right immune repertoire. Bystander activation would arise from any activated T cells within the thyroid gland, which may be activated by many different infections and antigens unrelated to the thyroid gland itself. The attractiveness of this model is that many different types of infections would lead to the same clinical disease phenotype. There is much evidence for residual thyroid-resident T cells in the glands of patients with Graves' disease which could have been activated by this mechanism at the time of disease onset.[84]

Mechanism #2—Molecular Mimicry (Specificity Crossover)

In addition to the effects of the direct release of cytokines from T cells activated elsewhere via the bystander effect, intrathyroidal T cells may become activated in another nonspecific way. Structural or conformational similarity (i.e., sequence or shape, or both) between different antigens can lead to specificity crossover (or molecular mimicry).[85] Antigenic similarity between bacteria, viruses, and human proteins is common, and in one study 4% of monoclonal antibodies raised against a variety of viruses cross-reacted with antigens in tissues.[86] Furthermore, mice infected with reovirus type 1 developed an autoimmune polyendocrinopathy with autoantibodies directed against normal pancreas, pituitary, thyroid, and gastric mucosa, suggesting molecular mimicry between a reoviral antigen and a common tissue antigen.[87] Molecular mimicry has also been reported between *Yersinia enterocolitica* and the TSHR based on the observed cross-reaction between sera from patients with *Yersinia* infection and sera from patients with Graves' disease.[88,89] Similar evidence has been presented on the basis of structural similarities between *Borrelia* and retroviral sequences and the TSH receptor.[90]

Mechanism #3—Thyroid Cell Involvement by Aberrant Expression of Class II HLA Antigens

Normal thyroid epithelial cells do not express HLA class II antigens, but they are markedly expressed in thyroid glands from patients with autoimmune thyroid disease (Fig. 11–6).[91] A local insult, whether trauma or infection of the thyroid gland, may cause an inflammatory infiltrate and the production of interferon γ or other cytokines in the thyroid gland, which are able to induce HLA class II antigen expression. HLA class II antigens are used to present antigen to the immune system (see earlier text) and overexpression on the thyroid cell would lead to enhanced presentation of thyroid autoantigens and activation of local autoreactive thyroid-specific T cells in a susceptible individual. Support for this concept comes from the in vivo induction of such molecules on mouse thyrocytes by interferon γ that also induced autoimmune thyroiditis[92] and the demonstration of the necessity for such molecules on TSH receptor expressing fibroblasts used in the induction of Graves' disease in mice.[54] A number of viruses may also induce thyroid cell expression of such antigens "independent" of immune cell cytokine secretion, including reovirus types 1 and 3 and cytomegalovirus.

Mechanism #4—Cryptic Antigens

T-cell tolerance depends on the visualization of self-antigens by the immune system in sufficient amounts to initiate continuous T-cell deletion, anergy induction, and regulatory T-cell activation. However, many molecules are not seen in sufficient concentrations to cause the removal of T cells that may react to them. These molecules contain what are sometimes called cryptic epitopes.[93] Hence, T cells specific for these cryptic epitopes may be present in the immune repertoire. They may then induce autoaggressive T cells if such an epitope is uncovered or increased in concentration by a local insult. HLA class II antigen expression in a situation where it normally does not occur, such as the thyroid epithelial cell, would then allow the presentation of these normally cryptic thyroid antigens to local autoreactive T cells if they are present.

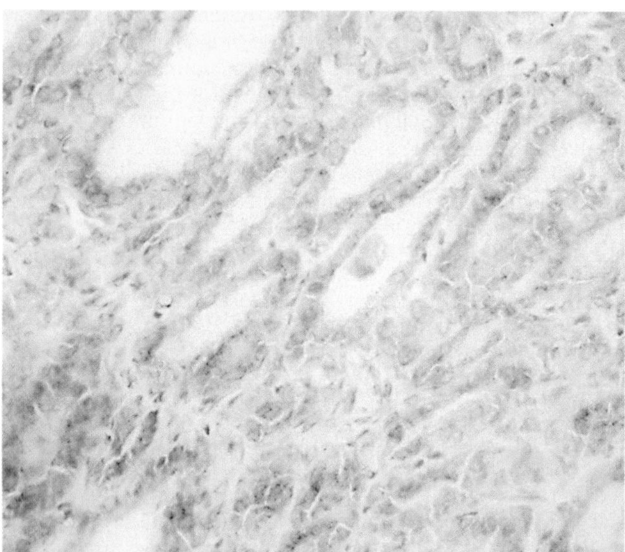

Figure 11–6 ▪ Photomicrograph of Graves' thyroid tissue stained for HLA class II (DR) antigen expression using the immunoperoxidase technique. Note the brown thyroid epithelial cells indicating the presence of DR antigen. Note also the relative absence of lymphocytic infiltration in this region.

Potential Risk Factors for Graves' Disease

Risk Factor #1—Genetic Susceptibility

The development and the subsequent course of Graves' disease are greatly influenced by heredity.[94] The role of hereditary factors is evidenced by the increased incidence of other autoimmune disorders in members of patients' families, such as Graves' and Hashimoto's disease, insulin-dependent diabetes (type 1), or pernicious anemia. Additionally, autoantibodies against endocrine tissues, gastric parietal cells, and intrinsic factor in some families suggests a hereditary influence. Hence, the high risk of a sibling being affected is shown by a sibling recurrence rate (Δ) of 11.6.[95] Indeed, the propensity for development of thyroid autoantibodies appears to be an autosomal dominant trait linked to the CTLA-4 gene that codes for a modulator of the second signal to T cells.[96] In addition, monozygotic twins have a higher concordance rate of Graves' disease than do dizygotic twins,[97] despite the rearrangement of B-cell and T-cell V genes that cause the immune repertoires of identical twins to differ (see also Chapter 41).

Because there are a number of genetic loci that may contribute to Graves' disease susceptibility, it is often referred to as a polygenic or complex disorder. There is a much investigated association with the HLA gene region (e.g., increased frequency of the HLA DR3 and DQA10501 haplotypes in Caucasians) but the HLA region provides less than 5% of the genetic susceptibility and gives a risk ratio of only threefold to fourfold.[98,99] The remaining nonspecifc genetic susceptibility after the HLA and CTLA-4 contributions remain to be clarified, but the gene for lymphoid tyrosine phosphatase (LYP) may also be important. However, the search for thyroid specific genetic susceptibility has led to only small influences exerted by polymorphisms in the thyroglobulin gene and the TSH receptor gene. More remains to be learned about thyroid disease specificity in genetic susceptibility.

Risk Factor #2—Infection

Much has been written about the possible role of infection in the development of autoimmunity acting via bystander effects or molecular mimicry.[100,101] It is not known whether a specific infection initiates Graves' disease.[80] If infection is the cause of Graves' disease, an identifiable agent should be present in most patients, and transfer of the agent to susceptible recipients should transfer the disease. As discussed earlier, it has been long suggested that Graves' disease is "associated" with infectious agents (e.g., *Y. enterocolitica*), but no studies meet the necessary criteria to prove this. Infections of the thyroid gland itself (e.g., subacute thyroiditis, congenital rubella) are associated with thyroid autoimmune phenomena.[80] Nevertheless, a causative role of infectious agents has not been definitively demonstrated in Graves' disease, despite observing thyroid disease induced in experimental animals by certain viral infections.[102] Reports of retroviral sequences in the thyroid glands of patients with Graves' disease have failed to be reproduced although clinical HTLV-1 has recently been reported to be associated with the development of autoimmune thyroid disease.[103]

Risk Factor #3—Stress

Graves' disease commonly appears to become evident either after severe emotional stress, such as the actual or threatened separation from a loved one, or after an acute fright, such as an automobile accident. There are, in fact, many clinical experiences and reports associating major stress with the onset of Graves' disease, including data on the high incidence of thyrotoxicosis among refugees from Nazi prison camps, which may have been more directly related to iodine status. Some data suggest that stress induces an overall state of immune suppression by nonspecific mechanisms,[104,105] perhaps secondary to the effects of cortisol and corticotropin-releasing hormone action at the level of the immune cell. More patients with Graves' disease give a history of major stress in the 12 months before disease onset compared with control groups.

Following the acute immune suppression by stress, there is presumably an overcompensation by the immune system when the suppression is released. This would then precipitate autoimmune thyroid disease, as seen after the release from the immunosuppression of pregnancy where in the postpartum period either thyroiditis or Graves' disease may develop.[106] The rebound phenomenon would result in greater immune activity than normal and would initiate disease if the individual were genetically susceptible.

Risk Factor #4—Gender

Graves' disease is more common in women than in men (7 to 10 : 1) and tends to become more prevalent after puberty. The female preponderance and the fact that the disorder is uncommon before puberty have suggested that female sex steroids may be responsible for this difference. Indeed, androgens may actually suppress autoimmune thyroiditis.[107,108] In contrast, estrogen has been shown to influence the immune system, particularly the B-cell repertoire, and has often been suggested as the reason for female susceptibility. However, Graves' disease continues to occur after the menopause and it is seen in many men. In fact, when the disease develops in men, it tends to occur at a later age, to be more severe, and to be accompanied more often by ophthalmopathy. Such observations have suggested that perhaps it is the X chromosome rather than sex steroids that is the responsible element in female susceptibility. Women have two X chromosomes and therefore would receive twice the gene dose. Genetic studies first identified a locus on the X chromosome linked to Graves' disease, but this has not been confirmed in larger studies.[109] The phenomenon of X chromosome inactivation (XCI) has also been invoked in autoimmune disease.[110] Female cells may inactivate different X chromosomes to different degrees in different tissues, leading to potentially differing immune responses. Evidence for XCI being important has been described in Graves' disease.[111]

Risk Factor #5–Pregnancy

Severe Graves' disease is uncommon during pregnancy because hyperthyroidism is associated with reduced fertility. For those women with milder disease who successfully conceive, hyperthyroidism endows an increased risk of pregnancy loss and established pregnancy complications[112] as exemplified by the influence of high thyroid hormone levels in normal pregnancy seen in thyroid hormone resistance.[113] Such data indicate that excess thyroid hormone has a direct toxic effect on the fetus. However, pregnancy is a time of immunosuppression, so that the disease tends to improve as pregnancy progresses. Both T-cell and B-cell functions are diminished as pregnancy progresses under the influence of both local placental factors and regulatory T cells (see later discussion).[114] Rebound from this immunosuppression after delivery may contribute to the development of postpartum thyroid disease.[115] As many as 30% of young women give a history of pregnancy in the 12 months before the onset of Graves' disease,[116] indicating that postpartum Graves' disease is a surprisingly common presentation and that pregnancy is a major risk factor for development of the disease in susceptible women (see later section on Graves' disease in pregnancy).

Risk Factor #6—Iodine and Drugs

Iodine and iodine-containing drugs, such as amiodarone, and iodine-containing contrast media may precipitate Graves' disease or its recurrence in a susceptible individual.[117,118] Iodine is most likely to precipitate thyrotoxicosis in an iodine-deficient population simply by allowing TSHRAbs to effectively stimulate the formation of more thyroid hormone. Whether there is any other precipitating event is unclear. Iodine may also damage thyroid cells directly and release thyroid antigens to the immune system.

Risk Factor #7—Irradiation

There is no evidence that radiation exposure itself is a risk factor for Graves' disease although Graves' disease is well known to be precipitated in some patients treated with radioactive iodine for multinodular goiter.[119,120] There is also evidence that thyroid autoantibodies are more prevalent in a radiation-exposed population and claims of increased autoimmune thyroiditis in such populations have been made.[121-123] In addition, radioactive iodine treatment may cause the onset or worsening of clinical ophthalmopathy, but often this is transient (see later discussion).[124]

Pathogenesis and Risk Factors for Graves' Orbitopathy and Dermopathy

The pathogenesis of the orbitopathy and dermopathy is now better understood than ever before. The extraocular muscle and adipose tissue are swollen by the accumulation in the extracellular matrix of glycosaminoglycans that are secreted by fibroblasts under the influence of cytokines such as interferon γ from local lymphocytes (see Fig. 11–6).[125] This accumulation disrupts and impairs the function of muscle. As the disease runs its course and inflammation decreases, the damaged muscles become fibrosed. Hence, histologic examination of the extraocular muscles shows disrupted muscle fibrils and a patchy lymphocytic infiltrate, predominantly of T cells, and some muscle cells exhibit HLA class II antigen as seen within the thyroid gland. Such T cells react in vitro with retroorbital tissue.[126,127] Transplantation of extraocular muscle into mice deficient in B cells and T cells (scid/scid mice) causes TSHRAbs to appear in the murine serum, showing accumulation of TSH receptor reactive cells within the muscle samples.[128] Evidence of TSH receptor expression in retroorbital and pretibial tissues such as fibroblasts and adipocytes have strengthened the notion that it is the TSH receptor itself that is responsible for the immune response.[125] The fact that retroorbital fibroblasts may be distinct from other similar cells[129] and may express more TSH receptor than seen at other sites also supports the TSH receptors as the primary antigen of Graves' orbitopathy.

In keeping with this hypothesis, patients with the most severe orbitopathy have the highest titers of TSHRAbs, and the level of TSHRAbs often correlates with the severity of the eye disease. There is currently no convincing evidence that specific antibodies against orbital tissue contents play a primary pathogenic role. More likely, antigen-specific T cells have the major role in initiating the disorder. However, non–eye-specific antibodies may serve as markers of extraocular muscle inflammation and recently antibodies to the IGF-1 receptor, expressed on many cells, have been shown to be present in such patients and may synergize with TSHR-Abs.[130]

Risk Factors

There is no evidence that a separate and distinct genetic risk can be ascribed to severe ophthalmic Graves' disease, suggesting that it is mainly environmental factors that lead to the enhanced retroorbital inflammation in some patients.[131] All of the same risk factors (e.g., infection, stress, gender, gonadal steroids, pregnancy, drugs, and irradiation) apply to the onset of both thyroid and eye involvement in Graves' disease.

There are three additional distinct risk factors that deserve attention. The first is smoking, which has increased the risk for ophthalmic involvement in many studies, perhaps by causing anoxia or simply direct inflammation.[132] The second is radioiodine, which in controlled clinical trials accentuates ophthalmic Graves' disease.[124] However, this worsening may be mild and transient and can be ameliorated with corticosteroid treatment for the subsequent 3 to 4 months. Nevertheless, some physicians are reluctant to prescribe radioiodine to a patient with severe eye disease unless the patient is receiving corticosteroids. Lastly, the role of trauma in the initiation of thyroid and retroorbital inflammation is well recognized.[79,81,131]

Natural History and Course of Graves' Disease

The course of the thyrotoxic component of Graves' disease is variable and often erratic. In some patients, thyrotoxicosis persists, although it may vary in severity. In others, the course may be cyclic, exhibiting remissions of varying frequency, intensity, and duration. This cyclic feature has an important bearing on treatment. With the passage of months or years, thyrotoxicosis tends to give way to euthyroidism. Approximately one third of patients become hypothyroid within 20 years of treatment with antithyroid agents.[133]

The orbitopathy may or may not commence together with the thyrotoxic component. Thus, thyrotoxic patients may initially be free of eye disease but are affected by it months or years later, or not at all. Conversely, Graves' disease may begin with orbitopathy and only later, if at all, be associated with thyrotoxicosis. In euthyroid patients with orbitopathy, so-called euthyroid Graves' disease, evidence of a thyroid abnormality, as judged from thyroid function tests and tests for TSHRAbs and other thyroid autoantibodies is common. Some such patients become hypothyroid within a few years, some become hyperthyroid, and a few remain euthyroid. Many such euthyroid patients do have evidence of chronic thyroiditis. The course of thyroid function in many of these patients is therefore unpredictable.

Histopathology

Thyroid Gland

The older designation for Graves' disease, *diffuse toxic goiter,* denoted that the gland was both enlarged and uniformly affected. The gland may vary in consistency from softer than normal to firm and rubbery. The outer surface is usually smooth but may be somewhat lobular; less commonly, the gland is grossly nodular before treatment. The cut surface is red and glistening. Microscopically, the follicles are small and lined with hyperplastic columnar epithelium and contain scant colloid that displays much marginal scalloping and vacuolization (see Fig. 11–3). Nuclei are vesicular and basally located and exhibit occasional mitoses. Papillary projections of the hyperplastic epithelium extend into the lumina of the follicles. Vascularity is increased, and there is a varying heterogeneous infiltration by lymphocytes and plasma cells that collect in aggregates and may form infrequent germinal centers. In such regions, thyroid epithelial cells express HLA class II antigens not seen in normal thyroid glands and are large, perhaps due to local stimulation by TSHRAbs. When the patient is given iodine or antithyroid drugs, the thyroid gland may undergo involution if TSHRAbs decrease. Then hyperplasia and vascularity regress, papillary projections recede, and follicles enlarge and become filled with colloid once again.

Eyes

In patients with infiltrative orbitopathy, the volume of orbital contents is enlarged because of an increase both in retrobulbar connective tissue and adipose tissue and in the total extraocular muscle mass (Fig. 11–7). Some of the increase in connective tissue is due to edema resulting from accumulation in the ground substance of hyaluronic acid and chondroitin sulfates,

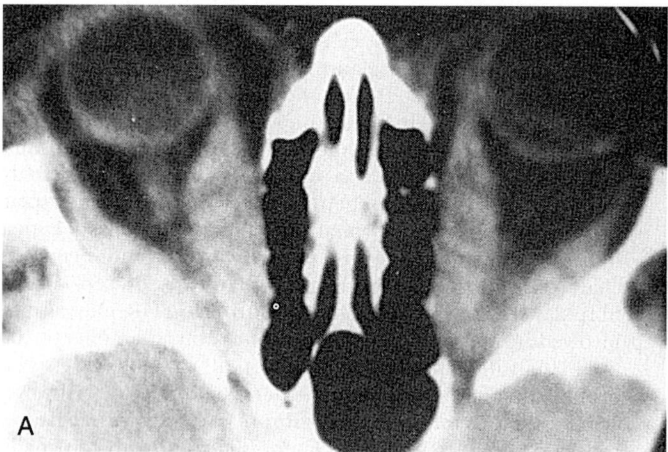

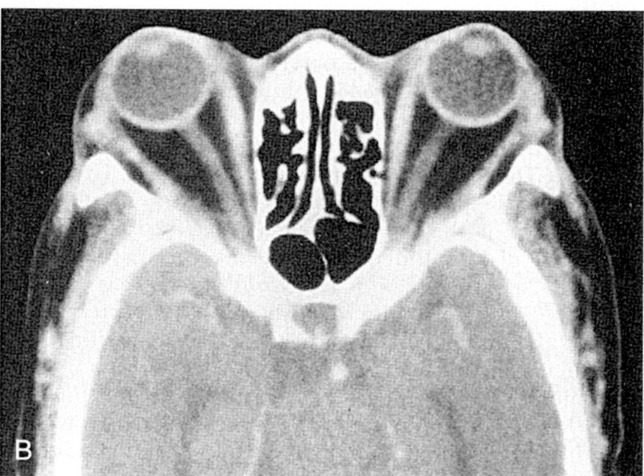

Figure 11–7 ▪ Computed tomography scans of orbits in two patients with Graves' orbitopathy. **A,** Note the obviously grossly swollen medial rectus extraocular muscles in both orbits and the resulting proptosis. **B,** The patient shows considerable proptosis with only minimal muscle enlargement, suggesting the presence of a large amount of retroorbital fat. (Courtesy of Dr. Peter Som, New York, NY.)

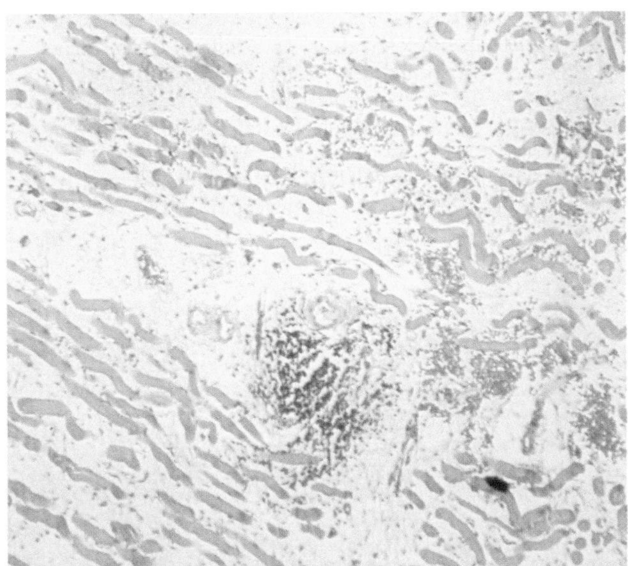

Figure 11–8 ▪ Section of extraocular muscle from a biopsy taken from a patient with severe Graves' orbitopathy. Note that within the muscle fibers is a patch of lymphocytic infiltration. (Courtesy of Dr. D. Kendler, University of British Columbia, Vancouver, Canada.)

which are hydrophilic. The extraocular muscles are swollen, and some fibers exhibit loss of striation, fragmentation, and lymphocytic infiltration. The lacrimal glands may also be involved. Ultimately, the tissues fibrose (Fig. 11–8).

Skin

The most uncommon of the Graves' manifestations, dermopathy (Fig. 11–9), usually appears later, and 99% of patients with infiltrative dermopathy have Graves' orbitopathy.[133a] The content of hyaluronic acid and chondroitin sulfates in the dermis is increased, presumably by lymphokine activation of fibroblasts. This causes compression of the dermal lymphatics and nonpitting edema: the collagen fibers are separated and fragmented, and early lesions contain a lymphocytic infiltrate. As discussed earlier, TSH receptor expression can be demonstrated in fibroblasts and adipocytes,[125] and TSHRAbs are very high in such patients. Nodule and plaque formation may occur in chronic lesions.

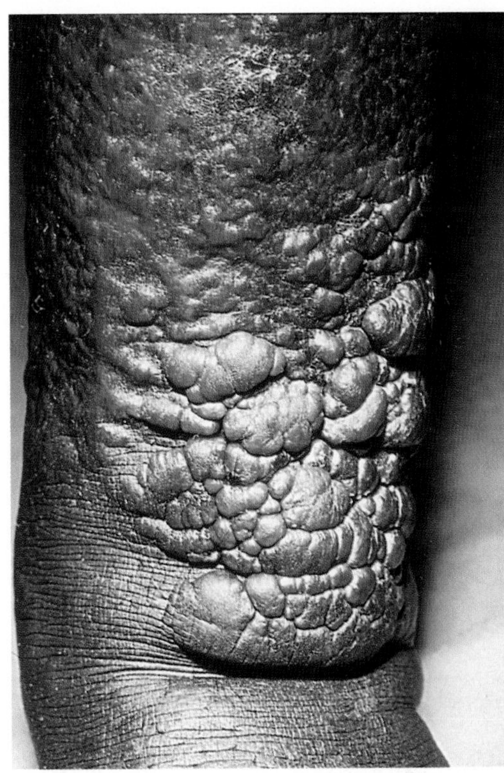

Figure 11–9 ▪ Chronic pretibial myxedema in a patient with Graves' disease and orbitopathy. The lesions are firm and nonpitting, with a clear edge to palpation. (Courtesy of Dr. Andrew Werner, New York, NY.)

Pathophysiology

In Graves' disease, normal regulatory mechanisms are overridden by the action of TSHRAbs of the stimulating variety. The resulting hyperfunction of the thyroid gland leads to suppression of TSH secretion that is reflected in undetectable serum TSH. In this context, the term functional autonomy is often misused when the intent is to imply that thyroid function is independent of TSH stimulation. True functional autonomy occurs when the thyroid gland is capable of functioning at a normal or an increased pace in the absence of both TSH and any other circulating thyroid stimulator (e.g., in congenital hyperthyroidism secondary to constitutively activated TSH receptors). In Graves' disease, the thyroid gland is controlled by an abnormal stimulator, the TSHRAbs (as in molar pregnancy, in which hCG is responsible). When that stimulator is withdrawn (i.e., when the disease enters remission), hyperfunction subsides, and the nonautonomous nature of thyroid function becomes evident in the reemergence of normal TSH secretion and control of thyroid function.

The molar ratio of T_3 to thyroxine (T_4) in thyroglobulin (Tg) is about twice normal, reflective of chronic hyperstimulation of the gland. The major product of glandular secretion is still T_4 but the ratio of T_3 to T_4 in the thyroid secretion is increased in proportion to the overproduction of T_3. In some instances, especially where there is iodine deficiency, T_3 appears to be the major secretory product, so that the serum T_3 level is increased while serum T_4 concentration is within the normal range (T_3 *thyrotoxicosis*). The proportion of total plasma T_4 and T_3 in the free (or unbound) state is increased, both because of a decrease in concentration of thyroxine-binding globulin (TBG) and because of the increase in the concentration of T_4.

Clinical Picture

The Thyroid Gland

Graves' disease is most common in the third and fourth decades of life, is rare before age 10 years, and occurs in the elderly, sometimes in an apathetic form. The features include diffuse goiter, thyrotoxicosis, infiltrative orbitopathy, and occasionally infiltrative dermopathy. Because the orbitopathy and dermopathy may be independent of other manifestations, they are discussed separately. In other respects, the symptoms and signs of thyrotoxicosis are the same in Graves' disease as in patients with other causes of hyperthyroidism.

In most patients, the thyroid gland is enlarged; but hyperthyroidism in Graves' disease occurs in a gland of normal size in a minority of patients, and in the older patient, goiter may be absent in 20%. The size of the thyroid gland is most often two or three times normal but may be massively enlarged. The consistency varies from soft to firm and rubbery. The enlargement is usually symmetrical. The surface is generally smooth but may feel lobular. In severe cases, a thrill may be felt, usually over the upper poles, and a thrill is always accompanied by an audible bruit. The thrills and bruits are due to increased blood flow and are usually continuous but sometimes are present only in systole. The bruit is most easily detected at the upper or lower poles and should not be confused with a venous hum or murmur arising from the base of the heart. Mitral valve prolapse is more common than in the normal population and may account for a cardiac murmur.[134]

Manifestations of Infiltrative Orbitopathy and Dermopathy

Objective Assessment of Eye Disease

The American Thyroid Association has classified the eye changes of Graves' disease by using a mnemonic system in which the first letters of each category constitute the term NOSPECS (see Table 11–2). "NO" connotes the absence or a mild degree of involvement. "SPECS" represents the more serious degrees of involvement. NOSPECS and the numerical indices derived from it are useful as a memory tool for physical examination. The system is less satisfactory for objective assessment of orbital changes.[135]

TABLE 11–2 AMERICAN THYROID ASSOCIATION CLASSIFICATION OF EYE CHANGES IN GRAVES' DISEASE: "NO SPECS"

Class	Definition
0	No physical signs or symptoms
1	Only signs, no symptoms (signs limited to upper lid retraction, stare, lid lag, and proptosis to 22 mm)
2	Soft tissue involvement (symptoms and signs)
3	Proptosis >22 mm
4	Extraocular muscle involvement
5	Corneal involvement
6	Sight loss (optic nerve involvement)

An overall activity score is helpful in the follow-up of such patients and can be determined by assigning 1 point each for the presence of spontaneous retrobulbar pain, pain on eye movement, eyelid erythema, conjunctival injection, chemosis, swelling of the caruncle, or eyelid edema or fullness. The range is thus 0 to 7. More sophisticated orbitopathy indices are also available. In clinical practice, the objective measurements of markedly affected patients should include the following for each eye separately:

1. Degree of proptosis using an exophthalmometer (Hertel or Luedde)
2. Documentation of maximum lid fissure width
3. Assessment of exposure keratitis with rose bengal or fluorescein
5. Quantitation of extraocular muscle function (with the use of the Hess chart or Maddox rod test)
6. Measurement of intraocular pressure
7. Measurements of visual acuity, fields, and color vision

Signs and Symptoms

Spasm and retraction of the eyelids lead to widening of the palpebral fissures so that the sclera are exposed above the superior margin of the limbus (Fig. 11–10). Lid retraction may be asymmetrical. When the patient looks downward, the upper lid lags behind the globe, exposing more sclera. When the patient gazes upward, often with difficulty, the globe lags behind the lid (lid lag and globe lag). The movements of the lids are jerky and spasmodic, and the lightly closed lids may show a tremor. Simple lid retraction and globe and lid lag are often a manifestation of the thyrotoxicosis per se. These manifestations will often abate when the thyrotoxicosis is relieved. On the other hand, significant swelling and inflammation of the muscles and orbital contents (so-called infiltrative orbitopathy) may occur. The disease symptoms and signs of infiltrative ophthalmopathy may appear in varying combinations. Early symptoms and signs include a sense of irritation in the eyes, resembling that caused by a foreign body, and excessive tearing that is often made worse by exposure to air or wind, especially if exophthalmos is present. The conjunctivae may be injected. Exophthalmos is frequently asymmetrical and may cause a feeling of pressure

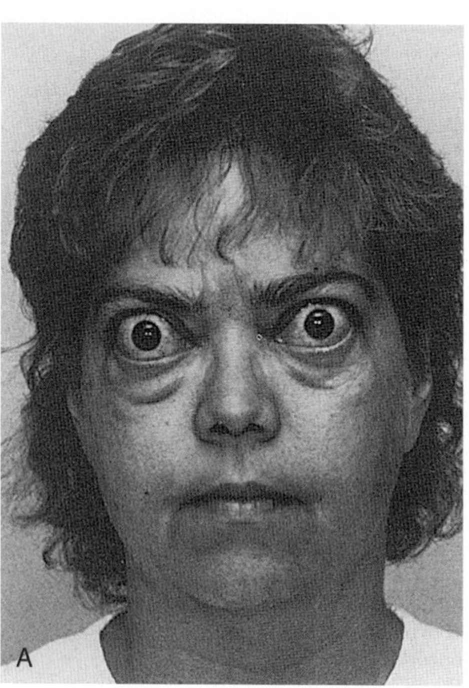

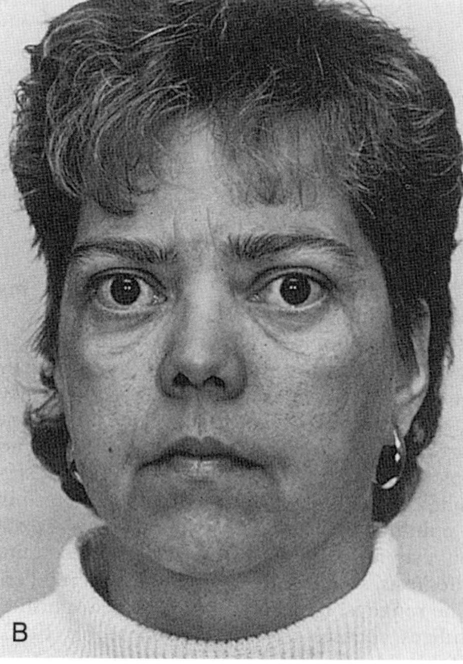

Figure 11–10 ▪ Characteristic signs of Graves' orbitopathy **(A)** subsequently corrected by orbital decompression surgery **(B).** Note the thyroid stare, the asymmetry, the proptosis, and the periorbital edema before correction. (Courtesy of Dr. Jack Rootman, University of British Columbia, Vancouver, Canada.)

behind the globes. When exophthalmos is pronounced, the eyes may not close during sleep, a condition termed *lagophthalmos*. Exophthalmos may be masked by periorbital edema, which is a common accompaniment and source of complaint. Patients frequently describe blurred vision and easy tiring of the eyes. Double vision may occur in combination with the foregoing symptoms or alone. In severe cases, color vision, and then visual acuity, may be decreased or lost and the corneas may ulcerate or become infected. The manifestations of extreme orbitopathy can be catastrophic and include subluxation of the globe. Blindness may result from ulceration or infection of the cornea secondary to incomplete apposition of the lids or to optic nerve ischemia due to reduced blood flow caused by increased intraocular and intraorbital pressure. In the most severe cases, which should now be unusual, ophthalmoscopic examination may reveal venous congestion and papilledema; these may be accompanied by visual field defects.

Infiltrative orbitopathy may follow an independent course from the thyrotoxic manifestations and is often uninfluenced by their treatment. Infiltrative orbitopathy is evident in about 50% of patients. However, ultrasonography,[136] computed tomography (CT), or magnetic resonance imaging (MRI) of the orbits reveals changes, such as swelling of extraocular muscles and increased retroorbital fat, in virtually all patients with Graves' disease, including those in whom the clinical changes are minimal or absent. Occasionally, infiltrative ophthalmopathy occurs in the absence of hyperthyroidism (so-called euthyroid Graves' ophthalmopathy).

Infiltrative Dermopathy

Dermopathy now occurs in less than 5% of patients with Graves' disease and is almost always accompanied by infiltrative orbitopathy, usually of a severe degree. These lesions cause hyperpigmented, nonpitting induration of the skin of the legs, commonly over the pretibial area (pretibial myxedema) and the dorsa of the feet, usually in the form of individual nodules and plaques but occasionally becoming confluent with a smooth characteristic edge or shoulder (see Fig. 11–9). Rarely, lesions develop on the face, elbows, or dorsa of the hands. Clubbing of the digits is occasionally associated with longstanding thyrotoxicosis (thyroid acropachy), which is now uncommon with early treatment (Fig. 11–11). The cause of the characteristic pretibial location of the dermopathy is unclear but most likely depends on trauma to the exposed areas. Indeed, surgical trauma to such tissues aggravates the disease dramatically.[81]

Laboratory Tests

In moderate or severe Graves' disease, laboratory findings are consistent with the pathophysiology previously discussed. The serum TSH level, when measured by a sensitive immunoassay, is almost totally suppressed, and serum T_4 and T_3 levels are elevated. (See Chapter 10 and Fig. 11–1.) The free T_4 and T_3 are increased more than are the total T_4 and T_3 levels. The serum T_3 concentration may be proportionally more elevated than the serum T_4 level. The increase in thyroid iodide uptake and clearance rate is often, but not always, reflected in the increased radioactive iodine uptake (RAIU) usually measured at 24 hours. However, in patients with severe accompanying illness, conversion of T_4 to T_3 may be impaired, permitting the return to normal of the free T_3 concentration but usually not the free T_4 (*T_4 thyrotoxicosis*). Occasionally, the discrepancy between T_4 and T_3 levels is exaggerated, with the serum T_4 concentration being normal and the serum T_3 concentration alone being elevated (*T_3 thyrotoxicosis*).

Because there are other causes of suppressed serum TSH, such as depression and hypothalamic-pituitary disease (see Table 10–12), and to exclude the possibility that an increase in serum T_4 concentration is the result of an increase in hormone binding in the blood, either the free T_4 concentration or the free T_4 index should also be measured.

The diagnostic accuracy of the RAIU in hyperthyroidism does not approach that of the serum TSH plus free T_4 measurement. Therefore, determining the RAIU is not useful in the diagnosis of straightforward Graves' disease but is useful in excluding thyrotoxicosis not caused by hyperthyroidism. Very low values of the RAIU in association with thyrotoxicosis signal the presence of factitious thyrotoxicosis, ectopic thyroid tissue, subacute "viral" thyroiditis, or the thyrotoxic phase of autoimmune (silent) thyroiditis (see Fig. 11–1). A low value may also alert one to unsuspected iodine-induced hyperthyroidism in which production of hormone by the thyroid gland is increased, for example, following contrast medium or amiodarone administration.

Mild (Subclinical) Graves' Disease

In subtle or mild cases of thyrotoxicosis, laboratory tests are most important, particularly when values are only slightly abnormal. A TSH concentration below 0.2 mU/L (normal range, 0.4 to 4.2 mU/L) is typically associated with symptoms of an excessive thyroid hormone supply. A value between 0.1 and 0.4 mU/L sug-

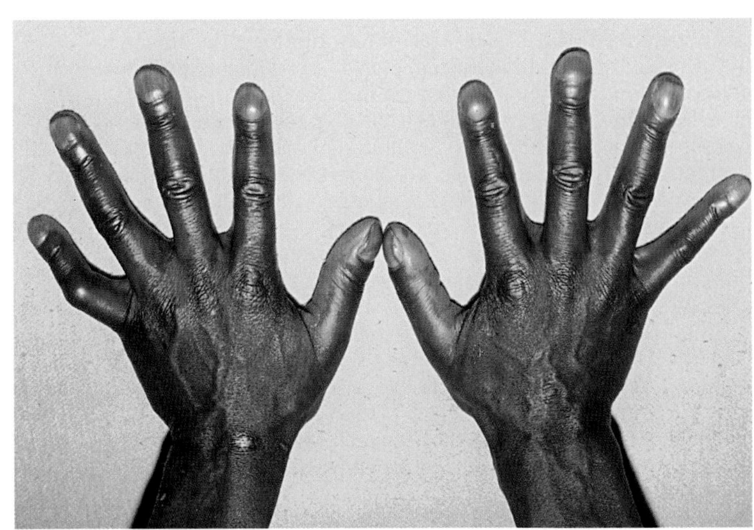

Figure 11–11 ▪ Rare thyroid acropachy in a patient with Graves' disease. The hypermetabolic state leads to axial bone destruction, presumably secondary to enhanced osteoclast activity. Acropachy is not to be confused with clubbing, which is usually painless. (Courtesy of Dr. Andrew Werner, New York, NY.)

gests a supranormal exposure to thyroid hormones but not a condition likely to be associated with significant clinical manifestations. Treatment of such patients is discussed later (see "Subclinical Thyrotoxicosis").

Measuring Thyrotropin Receptor Autoantibodies

Two types of tests are usually employed for the detection of TSHRAbs and both are available commercially. The first test assesses the capacity of patient serum or IgG to inhibit the binding of labeled TSH to solubilized TSH receptors. This protein-binding inhibition assay is of low cost and good precision, and the frequency of positive results in patients with active and untreated disease has increased as the sensitivity of the assay has improved and is now greater than 90%. Most recently, a human monoclonal antibody to the TSHR has been claimed to provide an even more sensitive binding inhibition assay than using labeled TSH as the probe.

The second type of test is a bioassay that assesses the capacity of patient's serum or IgG to stimulate adenylate cyclase in thyroid epithelial cells or mammalian cells expressing recombinant TSHR. Tests of this type, which measure the biologic action of the antibodies, are much more expensive, have relatively poor precision, and are positive in 80% to 90% of the patients with active untreated Graves' disease. Because of the proliferation of acronyms describing these antibodies, the authors encourage the designation of the specific assay used.

Standardization

As with all autoantibody tests, it is important to use an internationally accepted standard to allow comparison of results from different laboratories. A TSHRAb standard from the Medical Research Council (MRC) is often employed and reported in MRC units. Alternatively, results have been reported in terms of equivalent TSH units. However, the hTSHRAbs from different patients may not give parallel results with the MRC standards or TSH standards when measured in different dilutions. This means that the conversion of hTSHRAb data into MRC units or TSH units can be erroneous.

Indications for Measuring Thyrotropin Receptor Autoantibodies

Quantitation of TSHRAbs may be a useful indicator of the degree of disease activity in an individual patient and can confirm the clinical diagnosis of Graves' disease in a scientific manner. A bioassay is not needed in a hyperthyroid patient because the patient is already demonstrating antibody bioactivity. Demonstration of TSHRAbs may also be of diagnostic value in the euthyroid patient with exophthalmos, especially when it is unilateral. High TSHRAbs in a pregnant woman with Graves' disease increase the likelihood that neonatal thyrotoxicosis will be present in her offspring, and in this situation a bioassay late in pregnancy is preferred.

Another use of TSHRAb testing is in the prognosis of patients with Graves' disease who are treated with antithyroid agents. A persisting high level of TSHRAbs is a useful predictor of relapse on cessation of the drug.[72,137] Unfortunately, in patients with low or negative titers, the test is much less helpful. Furthermore, the presence of iodine deficiency may also interrupt the development of hyperthyroidism despite the presence of TSHRAbs.[138]

Differential Diagnosis

The patient with major manifestations of Graves' disease—namely, thyrotoxicosis, goiter, and infiltrative orbitopathy—does not pose a diagnostic problem. In some patients, however, one of the major manifestations either dominates the clinical picture or is present alone, and the disorder may mimic another disease. All of these issues can be resolved by appropriate laboratory testing.

Thyroid Differential

The diffuse goiter of Graves' disease may rarely be confused with that of other thyroid diseases if thyrotoxicosis is present. In subacute thyroiditis, particularly the painless variant, asymmetry of the gland, tenderness, and systemic evidence of inflammation assist in the diagnosis. The very low RAIU distinguishes this disease from Graves' disease (see Fig. 11–1). When Graves' disease is in a latent or inactive phase and thyrotoxicosis is absent, the goiter may require differentiation from Hashimoto's thyroiditis or simple nontoxic goiter as possible diagnoses. The goiter of Hashimoto's disease is somewhat lobulated and firmer and rubbery compared with that of Graves' disease. Serum levels of thyroid antibodies are generally higher in Hashimoto's disease but may not be helpful in distinguishing individual patients. In the absence of thyrotoxicosis, the diffuse goiter of Graves' disease cannot be distinguished from nontoxic, or simple, goiter. An abnormal serum TSH concentration and the presence of TSHRAbs indicate underlying Graves' disease, but their absence does not exclude quiescent disease.

Eye Disease Differential

The orbitopathy of Graves' disease, if bilateral and associated with thyrotoxicosis past or present, does not require differentiation from exophthalmos of any other origin such as is seen in morbid obesity. However, unilateral exophthalmos, even when associated with thyrotoxicosis, should alert the physician to the possibility of a local cause. Rare diseases that may produce either unilateral or bilateral exophthalmos include orbital neoplasms, carotid-cavernous sinus fistulae, cavernous sinus thrombosis, infiltrative disorders affecting the orbit, and pseudotumor of the orbit. Mild bilateral exophthalmos, generally without infiltrative signs, is occasionally present on a familial basis and also sometimes occurs in patients with Cushing's syndrome, cirrhosis, uremia, chronic obstructive pulmonary disease, and superior vena cava syndrome.

Ophthalmoplegia as the sole manifestation of the orbitopathy of Graves' disease requires exclusion of diabetes mellitus and other disorders affecting the brain stem and its connections. The demonstration of swelling of the extraocular muscles by orbital ultrasonography, CT, or MRI is diagnostic of Graves' orbitopathy, as is the detection of TSHRAbs in serum and/or the demonstration of a suppressed TSH level.

Treatment

It is not yet possible to treat the basic pathogenetic factors in Graves' disease. Existing therapies for both the thyrotoxic and the ophthalmic manifestations are only palliative. The lack of general agreement as to which therapy is the best is due to the fact that none is ideal.[139] Because the therapeutic problems posed by thyrotoxicosis and orbitopathy differ, and because they run independent courses, their treatments are discussed separately. Treatment of thyrotoxicosis is designed to impose restraint on hormone secretion either by means of chemical agents that inhibit hormone synthesis or release or by reducing the quantity of thyroid tissue.

Antithyroid Agents

Thionamides

The major agents for treating thyrotoxicosis are drugs of the thionamide class, most commonly propylthiouracil, methimazole, and carbimazole.[140] These agents inhibit the oxidation and organic binding of thyroid iodide and, therefore, produce intrathyroidal iodine deficiency that further increases the ratio of T_3 to T_4 in the thyroid secretion, as reflected in the high T_3/T_4 ratio in the serum. In addition, large doses of propylthiouracil, but not methimazole, impair the conversion of T_4 to T_3 by type 1 deiodinase (D1) in the peripheral tissues and thyroid itself.[141] The PTU-sensitive D1 is the major source of peripheral T_3 production in the hyperthyroid patient.[142] Because of this additional action, large doses of propylthiouracil may provide rapid alleviation of severe thyrotoxicosis.[143]

The half-life in plasma of methimazole is about 6 hours, whereas that of propylthiouracil is about 1.5 hours, and both drugs are accumulated by the thyroid gland.[140] A single dose of methimazole may exert an antithyroid effect for longer than 24 hours. This provides a rational basis for the single daily dose regimen of methimazole for mild or moderate thyrotoxicosis. The propylthiouracil concentration in serum correlates with the extent of blockade of organic binding of iodine within the thyroid gland. Both these drugs cross the placenta and can inhibit thyroid function in the fetus but both drugs have been used highly effectively in pregnancy (see later discussion of hyperthyroidism in pregnancy).

Immunosuppressive Action of Thionamides

Thionamide drugs may also directly influence the immune response in patients with autoimmune thyroid disease.[50] This action occurs within the thyroid gland, where the drugs are concentrated. The action on the thyroid cells themselves decreases thyroid antigen expression and decreases prostaglandin and cytokine release from thyroid cells. Thionamides also inhibit the generation of oxygen radicals in T cells, B cells, and particularly antigen-presenting cells and hence may cause a further decline in antigen presentation. More recently, it has been shown that methimazole induces the expression of Fas ligand on the thyroid epithelial cell, thus inducing apoptosis of infiltrating lymphocytes such as T cells that express FasL and decreasing the lymphocytic infiltration.[144,145]

The clinical importance of immunosuppression and induction of apoptosis compared with inhibition of thyroid hormone formation is unclear. However, the decrease in the immune infiltration of patients on such drugs and the fall in autoantibody levels after their introduction to a patient is powerful evidence of their effect.

Use of Thionamides

Based on their half-lives, methimazole can be prescribed on a once-daily basis while PTU is best given more often, usually three times a day. However, the initial dose of methimazole commonly employed in significant thyrotoxicosis is 10 to 15 mg twice a day (or the equivalent of carbimazole) until the patient is euthyroid. An equivalent dose of propylthiouracil is 150 to 200 mg every 8 hours. These doses are effective in most patients. Higher doses are required in patients with severe thyrotoxicosis and large thyroid glands, or possibly because of more rapid degradation of the drug within the gland or extrathyroidally. When large amounts are required, propylthiouracil should be administered at 4- to 6-hour intervals, although this agent is only available in 50-mg tablets.

The therapeutic response to effective antithyroid therapy invariably occurs after a latent period because the agents inhibit the synthesis but not the release of hormone; hence reduction in the supply of hormone to the tissues does not occur until glandular hormone stores are depleted. Although propylthiouracil differs from methimazole in having the additional effect of inhibiting the peripheral conversion of T_4 to T_3, there appears to be little difference in the duration of the latent period when either of these agents is employed alone in the usual dosage. This is because the extrathyroidal effect of propylthiouracil on conversion of T_4 to T_3 is more apparent at dosages greater than 600 mg/day. This effect may be an advantage in the acute treatment of severe hyperthyroidism.[141,143]

As would be expected, the period taken to achieve a therapeutic effect is shortened by administration of larger doses (more than 600 mg daily of propylthiouracil), but such doses should only be given when a more rapid therapeutic response is required. Generally, improvement within the first 2 weeks includes decreased nervousness and palpitations, increased strength, and weight gain. Usually, the metabolic state becomes normal within about 6 weeks. At this time, the dosage can often be reduced substantially to maintain a normal metabolic state.

During treatment, the size of the thyroid gland decreases in one third to one half of the patients. In the remainder, it may remain unchanged or even enlarge. In the latter situation, the change signals either an intensification of the disease process, which often requires that the dosage of drug be increased, or the production of hypothyroidism and increased TSH secretion as a result of excessive dosage. It is important to differentiate between these causes. Clinical criteria are not the main guidelines by which the adequacy of treatment is judged, and confirmation should be sought in the serum T_4 and T_3 levels and, with chronic therapy, the serum TSH concentration. Mild thyrotoxicosis may persist despite a serum T_4 concentration in the normal range because the serum T_3 concentration may still be elevated typically due to intrathyroidal iodine deficiency[146] and the increased T_3/T_4 ratio in Graves' thyroglobulin.[147] The latter phenomenon may also account for maintenance of a normal metabolic state in the setting of a subnormal serum T_4 level. Importantly, the serum TSH concentration may remain subnormal for many months, presumably secondary to accelerated conversion of T_4 to T_3 in the pituitary thyrocytes. An enlarging thyroid gland in a treated patient with Graves' disease may also indicate the presence of a neoplasm and should be investigated appropriately.

Antithyroid agents can cause hypothyroidism if given in excessive amounts over long periods. When this occurs, the patient often complains of gain in weight, sluggishness, and fatigue, and signs of mild hypothyroidism may be present. As suggested earlier, one major sign of incipient hypothyroidism is enlargement of the thyroid gland secondary to increased TSH. The hypothyroidism can be reversed by reducing the dosage of the antithyroid drug or by administering supplemental thyroid hormone. To forestall this development, which may also have adverse effects on preexisting orbitopathy, some physicians employ supplemental thyroid hormone routinely, the "block-and-replace" approach.

Block-and-Replace Regimens

The logic behind prescribing a full dose of a thionamide drug and adding T_4 supplements to prevent the patient from becoming hypothyroid is twofold. First, a few patients are difficult to keep euthyroid with thionamide therapy alone, and a block-and-replace regimen can be helpful and requires fewer office visits. Second, the immunosuppressive action of the thionamides may be helpful in attenuating the natural history of the autoimmune thyroid diseases directly.

Although some investigators found the relapse rate after the block-and-replace approach to be much reduced,[148] others have found no difference.[149] One explanation for such disparities may be the iodine status of the different patient groups. One group has also reported that continuing levothyroxine replacement after withdrawal of antithyroid drugs also increased the remission rate, possibly because suppression of pituitary TSH-inhibited expression of thyroid antigens and reduced immune stimulation (an effect influenced by the level of TSHRAbs). Such studies have also not been reproduced,[150] and this approach is not recommended.

Predicting the Response to Drug Withdrawal

A central question in the treatment of Graves' disease patients with antithyroid drugs is how to determine the appropriate duration of antithyroid drug treatment. As discussed earlier, antithyroid therapy may alter the course of the underlying autoimmune process, but remission after withdrawal of treatment will persist only if the disorder has been eradicated or has entered an inactive phase. This latter transition and the natural decline in the levels of TSHRAbs are more likely to occur the longer the course of treatment. This reasoning is the basis for the traditional practice of continuing antithyroid treatment for 6 to 12 months or longer. However, persistence of high levels of circulating TSHRAbs during treatment of Graves' disease portends recurrence after withdrawal of antithyroid drugs. This is helpful in the management of the individual patient who remains TSHR-Ab positive (see later discussion).[151]

Factors preventing a recurrence include (1) a change from stimulating TSHRAbs to blocking antibodies, which occurs rarely, (2) the progression of concomitant autoimmune thyroiditis, and (3) iodine deficiency itself, which may prevent the recurrence of Graves' disease. These factors may explain why some authors have been unable to confirm the predictive value of TSHRAb measurement. However, most patients do not have persisting high levels of TSHRAb, and predicting their outcome is more difficult. Additional factors associated with the likelihood of long-term remission after withdrawal of therapy include (1) the initial presence of T_3 toxicosis, (2) a small thyroid gland (less than twice normal), (3) a decrease in the size of the thyroid gland, (4) return of the TSH concentration to normal during treatment, (5) the return of serum thyroglobulin to normal, and (6) a diet low in iodine content. Genetic typing—for example, using HLA—is still not helpful in such predictions when examining the individual patient. However, the results of combining HLA with thyroglobulin haplotyping are beginning to look impressive in a small number of patients.[152]

Hence, treatment should generally be continued for about 6 to 12 months and then withdrawn if the TSHRAbs disappear and serum TSH returns to normal. About 75% of relapses occur in the first 3 months after withdrawal of therapy, and most of the remainder occur during the subsequent 6 months. Suppression of the TSH concentration below normal levels is the first signal of relapse even in the presence of a normal serum T_4 level.

Long-Term Remission

Although there are no very recent data, it seems clear that the frequency with which long-term remission occurs after withdrawal of antithyroid therapy has decreased over the past 30 years,[153] in part because of the increase in dietary iodine intake. However, this decrease has also occurred in geographic regions where iodine intake has remained constant and low. Nevertheless, about one third of patients experience a lasting remission. This fact alone indicates that antithyroid agents have a significant role as a sole therapy in the initial treatment of thyrotoxicosis.

Adverse Reactions

Adverse reactions occur in only a small number of patients taking thionamide drugs, although some may be severe if left treated (Table 11–3). Mild side effects include skin reactions, arthralgias, gastrointestinal symptoms, an abnormal sense of taste, and occasional sialadenitis. Of the more serious side effects, the one most talked about is agranulocytosis. In fact, this occurs in fewer than 1% of the patients, generally within the first few weeks or months of treatment. It is accompanied by fever and sore throat.[140] When therapy with a thionamide is begun, the patient should be instructed to discontinue the drug and to notify the physician immediately if these symptoms develop. This precaution is more important than the frequent measurement of white blood cell counts because agranulocytosis may develop within a day or two. Because of the high frequency of lymphopenia in hyperthyroidism itself, a complete blood count with differential is recommended before antithyroid drug therapy is started. If the absolute neutrophil count falls below 1500 cells/μL, the drug should be withdrawn. Similarly, if agranulocytosis occurs, the drug should be discontinued immediately and the patient treated with antibiotics as appropriate. Granulocyte colony-stimulating factor may speed the recovery that invariably takes place. Lymphocytes of patients who have developed agranulocytosis while taking propylthiouracil undergo blast transformation when exposed in vitro to propylthiouracil or methimazole and consequently they should not be given a thionamide drug again. Granulocytopenia occurs during antithyroid therapy and is sometimes a forerunner of agranulocytosis, but as already mentioned, it can also be a manifestation of thyrotoxicosis itself. Granulocytopenia that develops during the first few weeks of therapy may be difficult to interpret. In this circumstance, serial measurements of the leukocyte count should be made. If they display a downward trend, the antithyroid drugs should be discontinued. When serial measurements of the white blood cell count remain constant or return to normal, treatment need not be interrupted.

Sometimes, myalgia, neuritis, hepatitis (with propylthiouracil) or cholestasis (with methimazole) are seen, and rarely liver necrosis may necessitate transplantation if left unchecked. Other effects include thrombocytopenia, enlargement of lymph nodes or salivary glands, edema, a lupus-like syndrome includ-

TABLE 11–3 INCIDENCE OF MAJOR TOXIC REACTIONS WITH ANTITHYROID DRUGS IN ADULTS

Side Effect	Frequency	Comments
Polyarthritis	1% to 2%	—
ANCA+ vasculitis	Rare	Mostly PTU
Agranulocytosis	0.1% to 0.5%	May be more common with PTU
Hepatitis	0.1% to 0.2%	PTU only
Cholestasis	Rare	Methimazole only

ANCA+, Antineutrophil cytoplasmic antibody–positive; *PTU*, propylthiouracil.

Adapted from Cooper DS. Antithyroid drugs. N Engl J Med 2005;352:905-917.

ing the development of antineutrophil cytoplasmic antibody (ANCA)-positive vasculitis,[154] and toxic psychoses. The mechanisms underlying these reactions are not known, although some reactions disappear with continuance of treatment. It is critical to have a baseline complete blood count and helpful to have liver function studies before initiation of antithyroid drugs to help interpret the possibility of some of these side effects. We believe that the suspicion of any serious manifestation should be an indication for abandonment of antithyroid therapy and a recourse to surgery or ^{131}I therapy.

Iodide Transport Inhibitors

Both thiocyanate and perchlorate inhibit thyroid iodide transport. Theoretical and practical disadvantages, such as frequent side effects, preclude their use except in special circumstances.

Iodine and Iodine-Containing Agents

Iodine may be administered directly or may be contained in contrast media used therapeutically. However, iodine is now rarely used as a sole therapy. The mechanism of action of iodine in relieving thyrotoxicosis differs from that of the thionamides. Although quantities of iodine in excess of several milligrams can acutely inhibit organic binding (acute Wolff-Chaikoff effect), this transient phenomenon probably does not contribute to the therapeutic effect. Instead, the major action of iodine is to inhibit hormone release. Administration of iodine increases glandular stores of organic iodine, but the beneficial effect of iodine is evident more quickly than the effects of even large doses of agents that inhibit hormone synthesis. In patients with Graves' disease, iodine acutely retards the rate of secretion of T_4, an effect that is rapidly lost when iodine is withdrawn. These features of iodine action provide both disadvantages and advantages. The enrichment of glandular organic iodine stores that occurs when this agent is given alone may retard the clinical response to subsequently administered thionamide, and the decrease in RAIU produced by iodine prevents the use of radioiodine as treatment for several weeks. Furthermore, if iodine is withdrawn, resumption of accelerated release of hormone from an enriched glandular hormone pool may exacerbate the disorder.

Another reason for not using iodine alone is that the therapeutic response on occasion is either incomplete or absent. Even if initially effective, iodine treatment may lose its effect with time. (This phenomenon, which has been termed *iodine escape*, should not be confused with the escape from the acute Wolff-Chaikoff effect [see Chapter 10].)[155] Nevertheless, the rapid slowing of hormone release by iodine makes it more effective than the thionamide drugs when prompt relief of thyrotoxicosis is mandatory. Therefore, aside from its use in preparation for thyroid surgery, iodine is useful mainly in patients with actual or impending thyrotoxic crisis, severe thyrocardiac disease, or acute surgical emergencies.

If iodide is used in these circumstances, it should be administered with large doses of a thionamide, as the severity of the thyrotoxicosis itself indicates. The dose of iodine required for control of thyrotoxicosis is approximately 6 mg daily, a quantity much less than that usually given. Six milligrams of iodine is present in one eighth of a drop of saturated solution of potassium iodide (SSKI) or approximately 1 drop of Lugol's solution; many physicians, however, prescribe 5 to 10 drops of one of these agents three times daily. Although it is advisable to administer amounts larger than the suggested minimal effective dose, huge quantities of iodine are more likely to produce adverse reactions, including iodide myxedema. We recommend the use of a maximum of 2 to 3 drops of SSKI twice daily.

In patients who are so ill that medications cannot be taken by mouth, antithyroid agents can be triturated and administered by stomach tube; iodine can be given by the same route or can be absorbed through the oral mucosa. When use of a stomach tube is contraindicated, thionamide drugs cannot be administered because there are no parenteral preparations available. Here, the disadvantages attendant on administration of iodine may be accepted if the clinical situation is sufficiently serious. Iodine appears to be particularly effective after administration of a therapeutic dose of ^{131}I for the rapid alleviation of thyrotoxicosis.

Reactions to Iodine

Adverse reactions to iodine are unusual and are generally not serious but may include rash, which may be acneiform; drug fever; sialadenitis; conjunctivitis and rhinitis; vasculitis; and a leukemoid eosinophilic granulocytosis. Sialadenitis may respond to reduction of dosage and the addition of lemon-lime candies to increase salivary flow; in the case of the other reactions, iodine should be stopped.

Other Antithyroid Agents

Cholecystographic Agents

In doses of 1 g daily, the iodine-containing cholecystographic contrast agent sodium ipodate (or iopanoate) causes a prompt decrease in serum T_4 and serum T_3 concentrations in patients with hyperthyroidism.[156] These effects are the result of both the release of iodine and the ability of the agent to inhibit peripheral T_3 production from T_4, a combination that can be useful in the seriously ill patient. As with iodine itself, however, withdrawal of the drug carries the risk of an exacerbation. Supplies of this compound are no longer readily available in the United States.

Lithium

Lithium carbonate also inhibits thyroid hormone secretion, but, unlike iodine, it does not interfere with the accumulation of radioiodine. Lithium, 300 to 450 mg every 8 hours, is employed only to provide temporary control of thyrotoxicosis in patients who are allergic to both thionamide and iodide. This is because the blocking effect is often lost with time. The goal is to maintain a serum lithium concentration of 1 mEq/L.[157] Another short-term use for lithium has been as an adjunct to radioiodine therapy in that the drug slows the release of iodine from the thyroid.

Dexamethasone

Dexamethasone, 8 mg/day, inhibits the glandular secretion of hormone, may inhibit the peripheral conversion of T_4 to T_3, and has immunosuppressive effects. The inhibitory effect of dexamethasone on the conversion of T_4 to T_3 is additive to that of propylthiouracil, suggesting a different mechanism of action. Concurrent administration of propylthiouracil, SSKI, and dexamethasone to the patient with severe accelerating thyrotoxicosis effects a rapid reduction in serum T_3 concentration, often to within the normal range in 24 to 48 hours.[137]

β-Blocking Agents

Drugs that block the response to catecholamines at the receptor site (e.g., propranolol) ameliorate some of the manifestations of thyrotoxicosis and are often used as adjuncts in management. Tremulousness, palpitations, excessive sweating, eyelid retraction, and heart rate decrease; effects are rapidly manifested and appear to be mediated largely through modulating the increased sensitivity to the sympathetic nervous system induced by excess thyroid hormone mentioned earlier.[19,21] Propranolol (but not other β-adrenergic agents) may also weakly block the conversion of T_4 to T_3 via a mechanism independent of its effect on catecholamine signaling.

Adrenergic antagonists are most useful in the interval before the response to thionamide or radioiodine therapy occurs. They are of limited usefulness in patients with mild to moderate disease but are useful in patients with thyrotoxic symptoms and those with impending or actual thyrotoxic crisis (see "Thyroid Storm"). Adrenergic antagonists are especially useful when tachycardia is contributing to cardiac insufficiency. However, the fact that β-adrenergic blockade can reduce cardiac output without altering oxygen consumption can have adverse effects in some organs, such as the liver, where the arteriovenous oxygen difference is already elevated in the hyperthyroid state.[28] Moreover, thyroid hormone also has a direct effect on the myocardium independent of the adrenergic nervous system.

Propranolol is the most widely used agent because it is relatively free from adverse effects and has a short half-life, allowing for easy control. It can be given orally in a dose of 20 to 60 mg every 6 or 8 hours. For intravenous use, a shorter-acting agent may be preferable (see "Thyroid Storm"). Propranolol may be contraindicated in patients with asthma or chronic obstructive pulmonary disease because it aggravates bronchospasm. Because of its myocardial depressant action, it is also contraindicated in patients with heart block and in patients with congestive failure, unless severe tachycardia is a contributory factor. β-Blocking agents such as atenolol or metoprolol are longer-acting drugs that allow a once-a-day regimen when treatment is likely to be prolonged.

Surgery

Both types of ablative therapy—surgery and radioiodine—ameliorate thyrotoxicosis by permanent removal or destruction of thyroid tissue, impairing the capacity of the gland to synthesize hormone. Antithyroid therapy, aimed at preserving the thyroid gland, and ablative therapy are different, and their opposite properties may be advantageous or disadvantageous, depending on one's point of view. The impermanence of antithyroid therapy leads to a relatively frequent recurrence, whereas recurrence is uncommon with ablative therapy. However, antithyroid therapy causes less permanent hypothyroidism, whereas the frequency of permanent hypothyroidism is very high with ablative therapy.

The surgical procedure of choice for the treatment of Graves' disease has been a bilateral subtotal thyroidectomy, leaving approximately 2 g of tissue (0.5%), to avoid the dangers of hypoparathyroidism and recurrent laryngeal nerve injury. With the increasing sophistication of surgery, there has been a trend toward total thyroidectomy in Graves' disease because of the recurrence rate after subtotal removal (at least 2% and often much higher in children).[158] In experienced hands this has proved to cause no more complications than a subtotal approach and with zero recurrence (Table 11–4).

Complications of Surgery

Because the hazards of thyroidectomy are inversely related to the experience and skill of the surgical team, it is impossible to generalize about the frequency of complications (Table 11–4). Unless circumstances are otherwise compelling, thyroidectomy should not be performed by surgeons who do the operation only occasionally. Bleeding into the operative site, the most serious postoperative complication, can rapidly produce death by asphyxia and requires immediate evacuation of the blood and ligation of the bleeding vessel. Even with subtotal surgery, the recurrent laryngeal nerve can be damaged. If such damage is unilateral, it causes dysphonia that usually decreases in a few weeks but that may leave the patient slightly hoarse.

TABLE 11–4 COMPLICATIONS OF SURGERY IN 322 PATIENTS WITH GRAVES' HYPERTHYROIDISM IN EXPERIENCED HANDS (1986-1995)

Complication	%
Recurrent hyperthyroidism	2.0
Vocal cord paralysis	
Transient	2.5
Permanent	0.3
Prolonged postoperative hypocalcemia (>7 days)	3.7
Permanent hypoparathyroidism	0.6

Adapted from Werga-Kjellman P, Zedenius J, Tallstedt L, et al. Surgical treatment of hyperthyroidism: a ten-year experience. Thyroid 2001;11:187-192.

TABLE 11–5 COMPLICATIONS OF HYPERTHYROIDISM IN PREGNANCY

Increased and recurrent pregnancy loss
Preterm delivery
Preeclampsia
Fetal growth restriction
Fetal thyroid hyperfunction or hypofunction caused by TSHRAbs
Fetal goiter from excessive antithyroid drug treatment
Neonatal thyrotoxicosis
Increased perinatal and maternal mortality
Decreased IQ of offspring because of excessive use of antithyroid drugs

Hypoparathyroidism can be either transient or permanent. Transient hypoparathyroidism results from inadvertent removal of some parathyroids and impairment of blood supply to those that remain. Depending on the severity of these insults, symptoms and signs of hypocalcemia appear, usually within 1 to 7 days after surgery. The earliest evidence of hypoparathyroidism may be anxiety and mental depression, followed by paresthesias and heightened neuromuscular excitability, such as Chvostek's and Trousseau's signs and carpopedal spasm. The serum calcium level is subnormal, and the serum inorganic phosphate level is increased.

Severe hypoparathyroidism should be treated with intravenous calcium gluconate. Milder cases can be treated with oral calcium carbonate in a dose of 1 g three times daily. It is impossible at the onset to predict whether hypoparathyroidism will be permanent or will regress within a few weeks, as usually occurs. Some surgeons insist on prophylactic calcium and prophylactic 1,25-dihydroxycholecalciferol before thyroidectomy. Of course, this approach may hide any developing deficiency. With the increasing use of ambulatory thyroid surgery, it is likely that this approach will be taken more often.

However, the hypocalcemia that occurs immediately after surgery for thyrotoxicosis may not be due to transient hypoparathyroidism, because it occurs more frequently in the Graves' patient than after surgery for other thyroid disorders. Instead, it may be due to "hungry bones" because of the demineralization of bone that occurs in hyperthyroidism. This begins to be reversed after cure of the hyperthyroid state and may contribute to the modest elevation in alkaline phosphatase during recovery unless the patient has been rendered euthyroid for some time before surgery. The treatment of hypoparathyroidism is discussed in Chapter 27, but many surgeons who fear that they have caused damage to the parathyroid glands at total thyroidectomy may reimplant the apparent parathyroid tissue into local muscles.

Hypothyroidism after Subtotal Thyroidectomy for Graves' Disease

Another major advantage of subtotal surgery, as opposed to total thyroidectomy and RAI, was thought to be the avoidance of thyroid failure, which was inevitable after a total procedure. It was previously assumed that overt hypothyroidism usually developed within 1 year after operation, but long-term studies have indicated a progressive increase in the cumulative incidence with time after subtotal thyroidectomy (to more than 40%) similar to that produced by radioiodine but of lesser magnitude. The frequency of mild hypothyroidism (as revealed by small increases in serum TSH with normal free T_4 levels) is even higher. Therefore, many physicians start early thyroid hormone replacement even after a subtotal thyroidectomy.

This increasing frequency of hypothyroidism over time may result from progressive loss of stimulating antibodies, from a restriction of blood supply, or from autoimmune destruction of the thyroid remnant to an appearance of autoimmune thyroiditis.[133] If eventual thyroid failure is a frequent consequence of the Graves' disease process itself, the increase in the cumulative frequency with time of hypothyroidism after either subtotal surgery or radioiodine therapy is to be expected and is unavoidable. Treatment that destroys thyroid tissue would accelerate the emergence of hypothyroidism resulting from the disease process itself.

There is an inverse relationship between the frequency of recurrence after surgery and that of the development of hypothyroidism, and both partly depend on the amount of thyroid tissue left in place. When one considers that thyroid glands vary in size and degree of hyperfunction and that the techniques of surgeons vary to a considerable extent, it is remarkable that a normal metabolic state is restored for long periods in many patients. The reason for this favorable outcome may be that the amount of tissue remaining after operation is insufficient to sustain a normal metabolic state and hence becomes stimulated by endogenous TSH. In this way, the patient's endogenous homeostatic mechanism provides the adjustment in thyroid function that surgery alone could not. This hypothesis is supported by the return of serum TSH levels to normal in patients restored to a normal metabolic state by surgery. However, this explanation would suffice only in the absence of TSHRAbs, which rapidly decrease and disappear in many patients after surgery. How the autoimmune disease is suppressed following surgery is unclear, but clearly the release of thyroid antigen during the procedure must induce apoptosis of many of the clones of TSHR-specific T cells and B cells.

Preparation for Surgery

Preoperative use of antithyroid agents has greatly decreased the morbidity and mortality rates of surgery for Graves' disease because these drugs deplete glandular hormone stores and restore the metabolic state to normal. However, these agents do not improve the hyperplasia and hypervascularity of the gland in the short term unless TSHRAb levels fall. Iodine, however, is reported to cause a decrease in height of the follicular cells, enlargement of follicles with retention of colloid, and reduction of hypervascularity. Hence, the aim of preoperative management is to restore the metabolic state to normal with antithyroid agents and then to induce involution of the gland with iodine.[159,160]

Patients who are to undergo subtotal thyroidectomy are first given antithyroid therapy in the manner described earlier. Often, relatively large doses are given in order to hasten the clinical response and because surgical candidates are often patients with severe disease or large goiters. After the metabolic state is restored to normal, SSKI is added (2 to 3 drops twice daily) for a further 7 to 10 days. During this period, a preexisting bruit or thrill may decrease in intensity or disappear entirely and the gland may become firm.

Several cautions should be observed: No date for surgery should be set until a normal metabolic state has been restored. Much too often, the operation is planned well in advance and the patient is given a standardized regimen independent of the clinical progress. Therapy with iodine should not be started until a normal metabolic state has been restored; iodine should not be relied upon to complete an as yet incomplete response to antithyroid therapy because iodine will enrich glandular hormone stores if the antithyroid drug is not entirely effective. Antithyroid agents should not be withdrawn when iodine therapy is begun.

β-Blockade Alone before Thyroid Surgery

Propranolol may be a useful adjunct in controlling signs and symptoms (see earlier discussion) while the patient is being prepared for surgery. However, propranolol has been used alone in preoperative preparation of the patient in whom surgery is to be undertaken.[161] Although this mode of therapy is probably safe and effective in many patients with mild disease, thyroid crises can still occur when patients receive propranolol alone. However, there is no compelling indication for the use of propranolol alone. Restoration of the patient to a eumetabolic state, as outlined earlier, is appropriate before subjecting the patient to the stress of surgery.

Radioiodine

Radioiodine (RAI) produces thyroid ablation without the complications of surgery. Previously, there was concern that this form of therapy might also produce thyroid carcinoma, leukemia, or an increase in thyroid cell mutation rates. However, during the half-century in which radioiodine has been in use, no increased prevalence of thyroid or other carcinoma in adult treated patients has been noted.[162] The prevalence of leukemia is also no greater in adults treated with radioiodine, and the frequency of genetic damage in the offspring of patients treated earlier with radioiodine does not appear to be increased. As long as hypothyroidism is treated appropriately, there is no increase in mortality.[163] In view of the lack of evidence of serious toxicity from radioiodine in doses generally employed for treating adults with hyperthyroidism, the age limit for the use of radioiodine has been lowered progressively by some physicians from the initial lower limit of 40 years of age to 10 years of age or younger.[164]

Radioiodine Dosing

Attempts have been made to standardize the radiation delivered to the thyroid gland by varying the dose of radioiodine according to the size of the gland, the uptake of ^{131}I, and its subsequent rate of release (dosimetry). However, such calculations do not provide uniform results, probably because of variations in individual sensitivity determined, perhaps by stimulating TSHRAbs. A dose of 20 mCi achieves thyroid ablation in almost all patients and results in 75% to 90% hypothyroidism.[165] Some physicians have settled on an arbitrary dose calculated to result in the delivery of 300 MBq (~8 mCi) of ^{131}I to the thyroid gland 24 hours after administration.[166] Others aim to deliver 50 to 100 Gy (5000 to 10,000 rad) to the gland. No data support an advantage of dosimetry over a fixed dose regimen.

Treatment before Radioiodine Therapy

The use of antithyroid drugs before RAI treatment is widely used to theoretically decrease a post-RAI increase in thyroid hormone release. This is considered especially dangerous in older age groups with ischemic heart disease in which cardiac deaths have been reported. Antithyroid drugs may also prevent the post-RAI increase in thyroid autoantibodies that may affect ophthalmopathy.[167] Clearly, it is important to monitor T_4 and T_3 levels in at-risk patients and to consider β-adrenergic blockade whether or not antithyroid drugs are used before RAI treatment. There is no convincing evidence that pretreatment with antithyroid drugs affects the outcome of radioiodine therapy. Normally, such drugs are withdrawn 3 to 77 days before treatment and, if needed, can then be reintroduced 7 days after treatment. Drug-induced radioresistance has been the subject of much discussion, particularly in relation to PTU, but it is not a major issue.[165,168] Treatment with antithyroid drugs after radioiodine therapy should be avoided for approximately 1 week because they also reduce the success of treatment, particularly when nonablative doses are used, via their acceleration of ^{131}I release.[169] Indeed, lithium has been used to enhance radioiodine trapping in the thyroid gland in metastatic thyroid cancer. There is no need for this in Graves' disease in which uptake and trapping are more than adequate.

Complications from Radioiodine Therapy

#1—The Danger of Low-Level Exposure

There is no increase in thyroid cancer following the diagnostic use of radioiodine in adults.[170] There remain concerns, however, about a potential increased prevalence of thyroid carcinoma in patients treated with low amounts of radiation in childhood or adolescence as exemplified by the increased prevalence of thyroid cancer in children exposed to the Chernobyl radiation.[171,172] However, in Chernobyl the exposure for most of the children who developed thyroid carcinoma was to relatively low doses of radiation rather than the thyrodestructive doses prescribed in hyperthyroidism.[173] Nevertheless, many physicians think that the use of radioactivity in children should be avoided when possible.

#2—Late Hypothyroidism

Many reports have documented that the incidence of hypothyroidism is significant during the first year or two after treatment with RAI, even after dosimetry to avoid such an outcome. This continues to increase at a rate of approximately 5% per year thereafter. This incidence depends upon the dose of radioiodine prescribed and may be seen in patients treated with calculated doses (i.e., dosimetry) but also where a modest standard dose has been used.[174] The incidence of postradioiodine hypothyroidism at 1 year is approximately 25% and continues to increase with time. When the dose delivered is an ablative dose, then permanent hypothyroidism will ensue in almost all patients by 6 months. Because of the high incidence of hypothyroidism after lower doses, many physicians opt for this approach for all their patients once they are euthyroid with antithyroid drugs.

#3—Radiation Thyroiditis

The beneficial effect of radioiodine and the early induction of hypothyroidism are both consequences of radiation-induced destruction of thyroid parenchyma. With the larger doses of radioactive iodine, a tender radiation thyroiditis may develop within the first week of treatment, as evidenced by epithelial swelling and necrosis, disruption of follicular architecture, edema, and infiltration with mononuclear cells. Resolution of the acute phase is followed by fibrosis, vascular narrowing, and further lymphocytic infiltration. These changes account for the early response to radioiodine, be it favorable or excessive. In some studies, the likelihood of hypothyroidism is increased by the presence of high levels of thyroid antibodies and, presumably, of thyroid-specific T cells, at the time of treatment and with increasing age of the patient. The two predisposing factors may be related to one another. If this is true, it is unlikely that the early ablative effects can be obtained free from subsequent late effects, and calculated doses of radioiodine sufficient to exert an early therapeutic action will inevitably be associated with a high frequency of delayed hypothyroidism.

Radiation thyroiditis may lead to an exacerbation of thyrotoxicosis 10 to 14 days after radioiodine is administered, with occasionally serious consequences, including precipitation of a thyrotoxic crisis and aggravation of patients with severe thyrotoxicosis or cardiac insufficiency. In thyrocardiac disease, therefore, antithyroid drugs should always be given for several months before radioiodine is given to deplete glandular hormone stores and an adrenergic β-blocking regimen initiated to limit any potential arrhythmias, if this is appropriate. Antithyroid drugs prevent an outpouring of hormone if severe radiation thyroiditis occurs. The antithyroid agent should be withdrawn 3 to 5 days before administration of the radioiodine; if the clinical condition warrants, the agent can be started again 1 week later.

#4—The Therapeutic Dosing Dilemma

As discussed earlier, there is no definitive recommendation as to ablative dosing of radioiodine versus calculated dosing and no definite recommendations as to dosimetry versus a single standard modest dose such as 7 mCi.[174] The therapeutic dilemma with respect to the dosing of radioiodine therapy is handled differently in different practices. Some clinicians continue to administer the "conventional" calculated dose because of its effectiveness and because of their belief that late hypothyroidism, if it occurs, can be easily treated. A disadvantage of such a "conventional" approach is that the onset and progression of hypothyroidism will be insidious, that prolonged follow-up of patients may not be possible, and that patients may not associate symptoms arising long after therapy with a complication. The advantage of using an ablative dose is that it minimizes the dangers of persistent or recurrent thyrotoxicosis, which may be hazardous, especially in the elderly, and it allows the early initiation of long-term thyroxine replacement therapy. For these reasons, an increasing number of physicians advocate an ablative approach to treatment.[166]

#5—Orbitopathy and Radioiodine

As discussed earlier, Graves' orbitopathy is probably the result of a crossover specificity between retroorbital and thyroid antigens, perhaps the TSH receptor itself. Any worsening of the autoimmune thyroid response may therefore worsen the orbital immune response. Following radioiodine therapy, the levels of circulating TSHRAbs are elevated strikingly,[51,175] perhaps secondary to impairment of immune restraint caused by the intrathyroidal irradiation where regulatory cells may be more sensitive. This change is in keeping with exacerbation of pretibial myxedema after radioiodine administration.[176] Similarly, carefully conducted studies indicate that significant eye disease worsens in about 10% of patients with Graves' orbitopathy who are treated with radioiodine (Fig. 11–12)[177,178] although this may not apply in mild disease.[179] If there is any deterioration, it is usually mild and temporary but on occasion can involve a dramatic worsening.

Some physicians advocate the use of glucocorticoids at the time of radioiodine treatment to prevent such effects.[124,180] One regimen involves prednisone, 0.4 to 0.5 mg/kg 1 month before ^{131}I treatment, with a gradual tapering over 3 to 4 months. However, maneuvers such as careful control of thyroid function before and after therapy and cessation of smoking by the patient may also help minimize ocular changes. We do not advocate the use of radioiodine in patients with severe Graves' ophthalmopathy unless steroid therapy is provided.

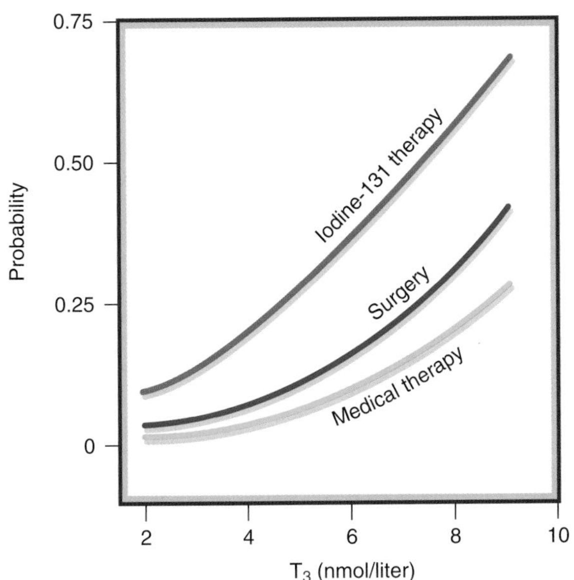

Figure 11–12 ▪ Probability of the development of worsening of orbitopathy in patients with Graves' disease. The serum triiodothyronine (T_3) levels are shown before treatment, and the type of therapy is shown as a variable. (From Tallestedt L, Lundell G, Torring O, et al. Occurrence of ophthalmopathy after treatment for Graves' disease. N Engl J Med 1992;326:1733-1738.)

#6—Other Side Effects of Radioiodine

Additional hazards may attend the use of radioiodine, particularly large doses. The parathyroid glands are exposed to radiation in patients treated with radioiodine. Although parathyroid reserve may be diminished in some patients, development of overt hypoparathyroidism is rare. The effect of radioiodine on other tissues that concentrate iodide (e.g., the salivary glands, the gastric glands, and the breasts) has often had attention, but such effects are not likely to be a problem with the relatively low doses prescribed for Graves' disease when compared with the treatment of thyroid cancer.

Because ^{131}I administration is contraindicated during pregnancy, a pregnancy test should be carried out in women of childbearing age before ^{131}I therapy is initiated if there is any possibility of pregnancy.[181]

Choice of Therapy

The choice of therapy for thyrotoxicosis is influenced by emotional attitudes, economic considerations, and family and personal issues. Our choice of therapy takes into account the natural history of the disease, the advantages and disadvantages of the available therapies, and the features of the population group in which the patient falls. Apart from patients directly requesting surgery, this procedure is recommended only when the shortcomings of other modes of therapy are of particular importance (e.g., patients with antithyroid drug allergy, a coincident cold nodule, patients with very large goiters, and patients with the need for a rapid return to normal). Occasionally, in young adults, it is necessary to remove a diffuse toxic goiter because of obstructive symptoms or cosmetic disfigurement. Nevertheless, only a small percentage of patients with Graves' disease are now recommended for surgery in the United States. The choice, therefore, is among antithyroid drugs, RAI, or a mixture of both.

In one common approach to therapy in adults, the physician initiates treatment with antithyroid drugs in all patients to produce a euthyroid state before reaching a final decision regarding a definitive therapeutic strategy. This allows the patient to return to a euthyroid status as rapidly as possible and provides an estimate of the antithyroid drug dose requirement. The magnitude of the drug requirement and the size of the thyroid gland are two of a number of factors considered in the evaluation of the patient with regard to the likelihood of a remission. The options for treatment are explained to the patient during these first months of contact, and individual recommendations are then formulated. This approach allows the establishment of a workable physician-patient relationship, which is especially important in addressing anxieties about the use of radioiodine. Such concerns lead many patients, especially those younger than 50 years of age, to elect a prolonged trial of antithyroid drugs before definitive therapy with ^{131}I.

In patients with a large thyroid gland, a maintenance thionamide dose requirement of more than 10 mg of methimazole (or carbimazole equivalent) or 100 mg/day of propylthiouracil, and/or high titers of TSHRAbs require prolonged antithyroid treatment and are advised that the chance of spontaneous remission is less than 30%. A therapeutic trial is generally pursued for 6 to 12 months if long-term thionamide therapy is selected. One can, in theory, treat forever unless side effects occur. When a decision in favor of radioiodine is made, ^{131}I may be prescribed at a dose designed to result in the retention of about 300 MBq (8 mCi) ^{131}I in the thyroid gland at 24 hours or an ablative dose (>20 mCi) may be prescribed. The former treatment follows an ^{123}I uptake test performed immediately before radioiodine administration and at 3 to 5 days after stopping thionamides. Patients with a larger goiter (more than four times normal) or those who have received large doses of propylthiouracil usually require more radioiodine.[166] Because ^{131}I is best given when the patient is euthyroid, no additional therapy is required immediately after treatment except for patients in whom a recurrence of hyperthyroidism poses a medical risk (e.g., patients with coronary artery disease or congestive heart failure).

Patients are seen at 4-week intervals after ^{131}I administration, monitored by serum T_4 and TSH levels, and hypothyroidism is treated when it appears with an elevated TSH level, generally within 3 months. Women planning to become pregnant are advised to wait for an arbitrary period of 4 to 6 months after ^{131}I therapy to allow for resolution of any transient effects of gonadal radiation. If, after a period of 6 months, hyperthyroidism is still present and the patient is symptomatic, the treatment is repeated, generally with about 1.5 times the initial dose of ^{131}I or an ablative amount.

Hypothyroidism in the Recently Hyperthyroid Patient

The early onset of hypothyroidism may cause distinct symptoms in the previously thyrotoxic patient after ^{131}I or surgical treatment or even with high doses of thionamide drugs. Such patients may develop severe muscle cramps, often in large muscle groups, such as the trapezius or latissimus dorsi, or the proximal extremity muscles. Such symptoms can develop even when the serum hormone levels are only low-normal or slightly decreased and before the serum TSH concentration has risen. It is possible to mistake a symptom such as back pain for an unrelated illness and the patient should be warned in advance. It is also not unusual for patients to complain of hypothyroid symptoms when thyroid function test results return to within the normal range. Such patients appear to have trouble adjusting to the normal thyroid hormone levels after being exposed to excessive amounts for long periods. Weight gain is a frequent complaint after recovery from chronic thyrotoxicosis and patients should be cautioned regarding their diet.[182]

Treatment of Infiltrative Orbitopathy

Infiltrative orbitopathy varies in severity from the common mild form to a severe form that threatens vision. The latter type is rare and remains difficult to treat. The natural course of the disorder, which is variable and characterized by exacerbations and remissions, makes conclusions about the efficacy of any treatment difficult.[183-185] A further source of confusion is the variable terminology for describing the manifestations of orbitopathy and the lack of rigid criteria for defining their severity. Use of the American Thyroid Association NOSPECS classification and its expanded indices, described earlier, is strongly recommended for everyday clinical practice (see Table 11–2).

Effect of Treatment of the Thyroid Gland on Orbitopathy

The first question that arises is whether different treatments for thyrotoxicosis affect the course of the eye disease differently. Subtotal thyroidectomy and thionamide drug therapy do not influence ophthalmopathy unless they lead to the development of hypothyroidism. Hypothyroidism has an adverse effect on the disorder and should be treated fully when it occurs. However, exogenous thyroid hormone in the absence of hypothyroidism does not improve the ophthalmopathy.

As discussed earlier, controlled studies suggest that radioiodine treatment may lead to a slight but significant worsening of orbitopathy (see earlier discussion), and it may be best to avoid radioiodine in patients with severe eye disease. Alternatively, as mentioned earlier, coincidental glucocorticoid therapy may prevent deterioration of orbitopathy after radioiodine but may itself cause significant side effects.[186,186a]

Symptomatic Treatment

Treatment modalities can be those that are largely symptomatic (useful mainly in the mild form) and those that attempt to arrest or reverse the progression of the disorder. With milder forms, little treatment is required. The patient who experiences photophobia and sensitivity to wind or cold air can benefit by wearing dark glasses, which also afford protection from foreign bodies. Elevation of the head of the bed at night and instillation of lubricants, such as 1% methylcellulose, may help when the eyelids do not appose completely during sleep. Artificial tears can be used during the day. Because the ophthalmic manifestations tend to be self-limited and the progression to a more severe form is uncommon, such measures usually suffice to tide over the patient until the disorder regresses spontaneously.

Glucocorticoids

The appearance of increasing proptosis with inability to appose the eyelids or of severe infiltrative manifestations such as chemosis warrants the use of more vigorous therapeutic measures. Such changes, even when severe, may respond favorably and rapidly to glucocorticoids. Some physicians use massive doses of prednisone (120 to 140 mg/day). If improvement occurs, the dose is decreased to the lowest level at which improvement is maintained. The latter dose is still likely to be large, but it is hoped that a halt to the progression or actual regression of the disease will occur before untoward effects make withdrawal of the drug necessary. Other physicians find that much smaller doses of prednisone (20 to 30 mg/day) can be highly effective with rapid reduction to a longer term maintenance dose (10 to 15 mg/day). Intravenous hydrocortisone pulse therapy is said to have the advantage of fewer side effects than high doses of prednisone.[186a] It is important to protect the patient's bones during corticosteroid treatment, especially with a postmenopausal woman, and this can be achieved with a bisphosphonate drug such as alendronate, given at 70 mg once a week in combination with calcium/vitamin D supplements.

External Radiation

The value of external radiation to the orbits has been established in some, but not all, clinical trials.[187-190] In fact, this treatment is steroid-sparing rather than steroid-replacing therapy and is said by some clinicians to work best in combination.[124] Whether it is even more effective than prednisone therapy is unclear. The safe administration of highly collimated supervoltage radiation to the retroorbital space requires experienced personnel and should, in our opinion, be reserved for the early treatment of severe disease. While periorbital edema may be helped, exophthalmos and ophthalmoparesis are usually affected minimally. There is a clear need for a reliable disease marker to monitor the effects of such treatment.

Orbital Decompression

If glucocorticoid therapy and external radiation do not halt progression of the disease and if loss of vision is threatened either by ulceration or infection of the cornea or by changes in the retina or optic nerve, orbital decompression can be performed by a variety of techniques.[191,192] In some patients, a desire for a nearly complete cosmetic correction may be such that decompression surgery is also the only satisfactory route. This procedure usually involves removal of either the lateral wall or the roof of the orbit or resection of the lateral wall of the ethmoid sinus and the roof of the maxillary sinus. However, the operation often causes or worsens diplopia, and even in the best of hands corrective muscle surgery is necessary later. However, overall results are usually good in 95% of patients and up to a 5-mm reduction in proptosis can be achieved. Whenever possible, such surgery should be delayed until the disease becomes less active.

An Approach to the Treatment of Orbitopathy

There are no controlled trials to support the suggestion that infiltrative orbitopathy is benefited or that its progression is retarded by total ablation of the thyroid gland, whether by surgery, radioiodine, or a combination of the two, although some experts think otherwise.[193] Nor is there any difference in the outcome after total thyroidectomy versus subtotal thyroidectomy.[194] Hence, we recommend a trial of oral or intravenous glucocorticoid therapy for patients with severe or progressive orbitopathy. If a positive effect is not seen within a few weeks, a course of external radiation may be attempted if edema predominates. During oral glucocorticoid therapy, however, may be an opportune time to treat with radioiodine or to remove the goiter.

Along with these major forms of treatment, local measures should be employed. Ulceration and infection of the cornea should be treated with antibiotics, lubricants, and protective shields. An attempt to appose the eyelids by means of sutures (tarsorrhaphy) should be performed only by an experienced ophthalmologist because sutures may tear loose and cause scarring.

The management of severe orbitopathy should never be undertaken by the endocrinologist or by the ophthalmologist acting alone. Close, coordinated observation of the effects of medical therapy and the progress of the disease is necessary to determine whether and when surgery is appropriate. Surgery almost invariably halts the progress of the disease and preserves vision if it is performed in time. This decision is influenced by the ability of the available surgical team because the degree of success of such procedures is proportional to experience.

Treatment of Infiltrative Dermopathy

Treatment of infiltrative dermopathy is necessary as soon as the condition is recognized. The application of a topical, high-potency glucocorticoid preparation with an occlusive dressing may cause regression or disappearance of the lesion.[195,196] Long-standing untreated dermopathy is more resistant to treatment.

Thyroid Storm (Accelerated Hyperthyroidism)

Accelerated hyperthyroidism or *thyroid storm* is an extreme accentuation of thyrotoxicosis. It is an uncommon but serious complication, usually occurring in association with Graves' disease but sometimes with toxic multinodular goiter. Before the availability of adequate means for achieving full preoperative control, crisis frequently followed thyroidectomy in hyperthyroid patients.

Presentation

Thyrotoxic crisis is usually of abrupt onset and occurs in patients in whom preexisting thyrotoxicosis has been treated incompletely or has not been treated at all. Crisis is usually precipitated by infection, trauma, surgical emergencies, or operations and, less commonly, by radiation thyroiditis, diabetic ketoacidosis, toxemia of pregnancy, or parturition. The mechanism by which such factors worsen thyrotoxicosis may be related to cytokine release and acute immunologic disturbance caused by the precipitating condition. The serum thyroid hormone levels in crisis are not appreciably greater than those in severe uncomplicated thyrotoxicosis, but the patient can no longer adapt to the metabolic stress.

The clinical picture is one of severe hypermetabolism. Fever is almost invariable and may be severe; sweating is profuse. Marked tachycardia of sinus or ectopic origin and arrhythmias may be accompanied by pulmonary edema or congestive heart failure. Tremulousness and restlessness are present; delirium or frank psychosis may supervene. Nausea, vomiting, and abdominal pain may occur early in the course. As the disorder progresses, apathy, stupor, and coma may supervene, and hypotension can develop. If unrecognized, the condition may be fatal. This clinical picture in a patient with a history of preexisting thyrotoxicosis or with goiter or exophthalmos, or both, is sufficient to establish the diagnosis, and emergency treatment should not await laboratory confirmation.

There are no foolproof criteria by which severe thyrotoxicosis complicated by some other serious disease can be distinguished from thyrotoxic crisis induced by that disease. In any event, the differentiation between these alternatives is of no great significance because treatment of the two is the same.

Treatment of Thyroid Storm

Treatment aims to correct both the severe thyrotoxicosis and the precipitating illness and to provide general support. The patient thought to have thyroid storm should be monitored in a medical intensive care unit during the initial phases of therapy. The therapy itself is designed to inhibit hormone synthesis and release and to antagonize the adrenergically mediated aspects of peripheral thyroid hormone action and to combat the hyperpyrexia.

Large doses of an antithyroid agent (300 to 400 mg of propylthiouracil every 4 to 6 hours) are given by mouth, by stomach tube, or, if necessary, per rectum. Propylthiouracil is preferable to methimazole because it has the additional action of inhibiting the peripheral generation of T_3 from T_4 by type 1 iodothyronine deiodinase both in peripheral tissues and in the thyroid itself, which is, together with direct thyroid secretion, the source of the T_3 (Fig. 11–13).[141-143,197,197a] Administration of propylthiouracil initiates therapy for the postcrisis period and prevents enrichment of glandular hormone stores by the iodide, whose administration is of more immediate importance. The latter agent, administered either as SSKI (three drops twice daily) or the equivalent as Lugol's solution (10 drops twice daily). SSKI (see Table 10–7) acutely retards the release of hormone from the thyroid gland.

Theoretically, propylthiouracil should be administered before iodine to inhibit the synthesis of additional thyroid hormone from the administered iodide. Nonetheless, because iodide is the only agent that will block release of preformed thyroid hormones from the thyroid gland and it blocks its own organification through the Wolff-Chaikoff effect, its administration should not be delayed or omitted in the severely toxic patient if propylthiouracil (or methimazole) is not immediately available.

Large doses of dexamethasone (8 mg orally once daily) should be given to support the response to stress, inhibit both the release of hormone from the gland and the peripheral generation of T_3 from T_4, synergizing with iodide and propylthiouracil, respectively, in these actions. Indeed, the combined use of propylthiouracil, iodide, and dexamethasone can restore the concentration of T_3 to normal within 24 to 48 hours.[198] In the absence of cardiac insufficiency or asthma, a β-adrenergic blocking agent should be given to ameliorate the hyperadrenergic state. Most experience has been with propranolol given at a dose of 40 to 80 mg orally every 6 hours, but a very short-acting β-adrenergic blocker such as labetalol or esmolol may be safer than propranolol in this situation. High-output congestive heart failure can develop in patients with severe thyrotoxicosis, and a β-adrenergic antagonist may further reduce cardiac output. If β-adrenergic blocking agents are contraindicated, a calcium channel blocker (diltiazem) may be used to slow the heart rate.

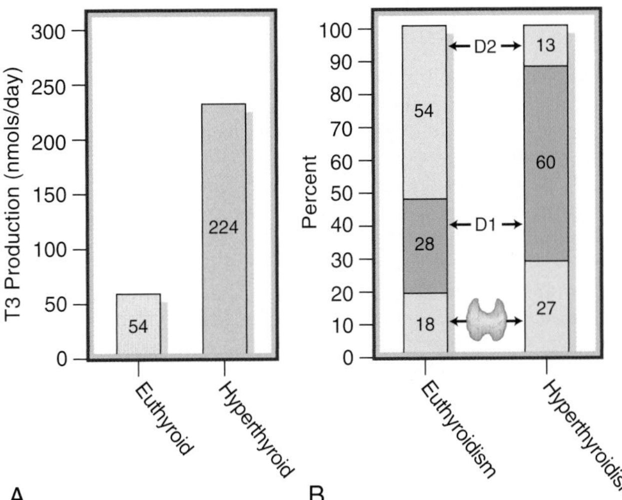

Figure 11–13 ▪ Comparisons of the amount **(A)** and sources **(B)** of T_3 in euthyroid individuals with those in patients with severe hyperthyroidism due to Graves' disease. With thyroid stimulation, T_4 and T_3 increase, suppressing type 2 deiodinase and increasing type 1 deiodinase activity in liver, kidneys, and thyroid, making the latter the most important enzyme for peripheral T_3 production in the thyrotoxic patient. Thus, the combination of iodide to inhibit thyroid hormone release and large doses of propylthiouracil to block T_4 to T_3 conversion results in a 60% to 80% decrease in serum T_3 concentrations within 24 hours.

Supportive measures include correction of dehydration and hypernatremia, if present, and administration of glucose. Hyperpyrexia should be treated vigorously. In mild cases, acetaminophen may suffice, but a cold blanket or ice packs may be required. Salicylates should be avoided because they compete with T_3 and T_4 for binding to TBG and transthyretin (TTR) and therefore increase the free hormone levels.[199] In addition, high doses of salicylates increase the metabolic rate. If heart failure or pulmonary congestion is present, appropriate diuretics are indicated. In patients with atrial fibrillation, the rapid ventricular response requires appropriate blockade of atrioventricular node conduction.

When treatment is successful, improvement is usually manifested within 1 or 2 days and recovery occurs within a week. At this time, iodide and dexamethasone can be withdrawn and plans for long-term management are made.

Graves' Disease in Pregnancy and the Postpartum Period

Although seen regularly in clinical practice, a truly overactive thyroid gland is uncommon in established pregnancy, affecting approximately 0.2% of women. This low rate is because the immune system tends to suppress autoimmune responses during pregnancy and Graves' disease, an autoimmune disorder, is the most common cause of hyperthyroidism in young women.[114,200] Furthermore, while hyperthyroidism has a variety of negative influences on fertility itself, it is also associated with increased pregnancy loss and serious medical complications if it persists (see Table 11–5).[201,202]

Difficulty in conception and fetal wastage are increased in women with Graves' disease, but occasional patients become pregnant despite antecedent untreated hyperthyroidism. More commonly, a woman under treatment for hyperthyroidism becomes pregnant. Whatever the sequence, pregnancy complicates the diagnosis and treatment of hyperthyroidism in Graves' disease and influences its severity and course.

Influence of Pregnancy on the Immune System

The development of pregnancy and the growth of the placenta have profound influences on the immune system as discussed earlier (see "Risk Factor #5"). The overall suppression of autoimmune reponses that occurs is designed to allow the fetus with its 50% paternal antigens to survive immune assault.[200,203] The mechanisms invoked in pregnancy are multiple and include peripheral tolerance mechanisms that deplete fetal reactive cells and the inhibition of pathways capable of causing damage after immune activation (Table 11–6). These changes promote maternofetal tolerance but the role of regulatory T cells (which increase in number in pregnancy) and their suppression of maternal responses to the fetus appear to be predominant and long lived.[204] It has been shown that a major shift in such T-cell control reduces the effectiveness of all inflammatory T cells.

TABLE 11–6 MECHANISMS OF IMMUNOSUPPRESSION IN PREGNANCY LEADING TO IMMUNE PRIVILEGE

MATERNAL PERIPHERAL IMMUNE SYSTEM
Regulatory T cells suppress fetal-reactive immune cells. Sex steroids affect the immune system and negatively regulate B cells.
MATERNAL-FETAL INTERFACE (TROPHOBLAST–IMMUNE CELL INTERACTION)
Apoptosis is induced in activated T cells by Fas expression on trophoblast cells. T-cell proliferation is inhibited by local cytokines and chemokines. Natural killer cells are inhibited by HLA-G expression. Complement system is inactivated.

Fetal Microchimerism

In normal pregnancy, cells pass from mother to child and from child to mother. The presence of fetal microchimerism in parous women has been shown to persist for more than 20 years,[205] indicating complete tolerance for the fetal cells. This is an exaggerated and long-lasting form of the immunosuppression of pregnancy described earlier. Whether such cells can ever stimulate an immune response as tolerance fades has been the subject of much speculation, fueled by the apparent accumulation of fetal cells at sites of inflammation, but the idea remains unproven.[206] However, fetal microchimerism has also been associated with Graves' disease–susceptible HLA haplotypes,[207] and a failure of fetal tolerance remains a likely contributing mechanism to postpartum thyroid disease.[208]

Thyroid Antibodies in Pregnant Patients with Graves' Disease

The hallmark of the immune effects initiated by the placenta is the fall in thyroid autoantibody secretion, TPOAb, TgAb, and TSHRAbs, that is seen in almost all patients.[209] This is now considered secondary to enhanced regulatory T-cell activity[210] and precedes a rapid increase in autoantibody levels after the immunosuppression is lost. Assays for TSHRAbs in the serum of pregnant women with Graves' disease may be of clinical value in selected cases because a failure of this immunosuppression may indicate potential fetal problems.[65,211-213] Because maternal antibodies cross the placenta, there is a correlation between the maternal level of stimulatory TSHRAbs, as measured by bioassay, and the development of fetal thyrotoxicosis. Although thyrotoxicosis occurs in only 1% of infants of mothers with Graves' disease, it is helpful to know the level of maternal TSHRAbs by competition assay, and in those women in whom the level remains high in the third trimester, a formal bioassay should be obtained to estimate the stimulatory capacity of the TSHRAbs. Pregnant women at risk for failure to suppress thyroid autoantibodies include those with more severe hyperthyroidism and those with significant Graves' orbitopathy or infiltrative dermopathy. In addition, the prior ablative treatment of the mother with either surgery or radioiodine may not always be accompanied by a reduction in TSHRAbs. Thus, the fetus of a treated patient with Graves' disease may still be at risk for development of neonatal thyrotoxicosis and the mother may need antithyroid drug treatment and the fetus monitored by umbilical cord blood testing and ultrasonography.[214]

Differential Diagnosis

When mild thyrotoxicosis is present during early pregnancy, it may be due to gestational thyrotoxicosis (GTT) secondary to hCG stimulation of the thyroid gland (see later discussion).[215-217] When it is more severe it is usually due to Graves' disease in that toxic multinodular goiters and hot nodules are uncommon in this age group.

Diagnosis

Pregnancy and hyperthyroidism are both accompanied by thyroid stimulation, a hyperdynamic circulation, and hypermetabolism. Note that amenorrhea may occur in thyrotoxicosis not associated with pregnancy. In pregnancy, serum TBG levels are increased by estrogen-induced changes in glycosylation, which lengthen the half-life, and thus in both conditions, the total serum T_4 and T_3 levels are elevated. Serum TSH is suppressed in hyperthyroidism during pregnancy; however, there is sometimes a modest suppression of TSH (between 0.1 and 0.4 mU/L) during the 8th to 14th weeks of normal pregnancy because of stimulation of the thyroid gland by hCG during this interval (GTT) as discussed above. A serum TSH below 0.1 mU/L and an elevated free T_4 level strongly suggests coexistent hyperthyroidism. Detection of TSHRAbs can confirm the diagnosis, which may or may not be obvious from the clinical history and examination.

Treatment during Pregnancy

The management of hyperthyroidism during pregnancy can be an even greater problem than the diagnosis; however, as discussed earlier, pregnancy has an attenuating influence on the hyperthyroid state because of the immunosuppression associated with pregnancy, manifested here by a decrease in the level of thyroid autoantibodies (including levels of TSHRAbs). Pregnancy is also one of the few clinical situations in which the biologic activity of the TSHRAbs is helpful by predicting its effect on the newborn.

Antithyroid Drugs

Because antithyroid drug treatment poses no greater risk to the mother or fetus than does surgery and possibly involves less risk, medical therapy is the method of choice in pregnancy. Yet because of the usual improvement in the disease, the dosage of antithyroid drug required to control the disease in the latter phases of pregnancy is generally much less than that which would be required in the same patient if she were not pregnant. Overtreatment of the hyperthyroid pregnant woman remains a common clinical problem with potentially severe consequences for the fetus.[214,218-220]

Certain aspects of placental physiology are relevant to the use of antithyroid drugs. Propylthiouracil and methimazole, which readily and equally cross the placenta, are concentrated in the fetal thyroid, and in excess quantity can cause goitrous hypothyroidism in the fetus.[221] The administration of as little as 150 mg/day of propylthiouracil to the mother may decrease the fetal serum T_4 concentration and elevate the TSH level in neonates.[219] The long-term complication of this mild hypothyroidism is unknown but should be kept in mind in view of the observations of reduced childhood intelligence when mothers have increased TSH levels during gestation.[222] Although maternal T_4 crosses the placenta (as evidenced by infants born with significant circulating serum T_4 concentrations despite congenital hypothyroidism), placental transfer is not efficient and varies from patient-to-patient. For these reasons, the flux of antithyroid agent to the fetus should be limited by giving the mother the smallest dosage of antithyroid agent that induces a physiologic state consistent with normal pregnancy. The authors believe that propylthiouracil in excess of 200 mg (15 mg of methimazole) is undesirable, especially in the third trimester. It may cause fetal goiter and neonatal respiratory distress. A "block-and-replace" strategy is therefore not appropriate for thionamide therapy in the pregnant patient.

The serum free T_4 level should be maintained in the upper normal range and no attempt made to normalize the serum TSH concentration. However, the concentration of serum T_4 must not override consideration of the clinical status of the patient. A modest tachycardia is a physiologic response to the increased metabolic demands of pregnancy; and pulse rates of 90 to 100 beats/minute are well tolerated without evidence of myocardial decompensation during delivery. The natural amelioration of Graves' disease in the third trimester should be kept in mind and repeated attempts made to reduce the thioamide dose made as the delivery date approaches to avoid TSH-induced fetal/newborn goiter, which may cause asphyxia (see Fig. 10–11).

In most cases, the daily maintenance dose of propylthiouracil should be 200 mg or less in early pregnancy, although higher maintenance doses may occasionally be required. Propylthiouracil has been generally preferred to methimazole because of claims for more fetal side effects with methimazole, in particular a scalp defect—aplasia cutis.[218,223,224] However, both drugs have proven safe in millions of pregnancies throughout the world and both accumulate equally in the breast. Larger studies have failed to demonstrate such an embryopathy.[225] Nevertheless, reports emerging of a "carbimazole embryopathy" have aroused concern and propylthiouracil has become the drug of choice.[218]

All pregnant patients with significant Graves' disease should be managed in close cooperation with obstetricians experienced with modern techniques for monitoring the fetus for intrauterine thyroid dysfunction. These techniques normally include fetal heart rate monitoring and ultrasonographic assessment of fetal growth rate. With advanced ultrasonography, it is usually possible to examine the fetus for the presence of goiter. Convincing evidence of fetal hyperthyroidism may be an indication to consider another approach. In a compliant patient, a dose requirement in excess of 200 mg/day of propylthiouracil is a reasonable threshold for considering subtotal thyroidectomy, preferably in the second trimester. However, transplacental passage of TSHRAb may continue to stimulate the fetal thyroid, although 50 to 100 mg of propylthiouracil is generally sufficient to treat this condition due to its transplacental transfer.[226]

Iodide and β-Blockers

Obviously, radioiodine is contraindicated in pregnancy, although no harm has been shown by diagnostic doses.[181] Iodide itself should also not be used as therapy for any length of time in the pregnant woman because it readily crosses the placenta and can induce in the fetus an extremely large goiter that may cause airway obstruction and even death (see Fig. 10–11). Whether propranolol or other β-blockers should be used in the pregnant woman with hyperthyroidism has been a matter of debate. In the experience of some, it can cause intrauterine growth retardation, delayed lung development, and neonatal hypoglycemia or depression,[227] but large studies have suggested that it can be employed with safety for short periods or at very low doses.[228,229]

Surgery

Surgery during the first and third trimesters is not desirable because of the possible induction of early pregnancy loss and later premature labor. Surgery may be successful during the middle trimester but it is always best to avoid major surgery during pregnancy if possible. Nevertheless, if antithyroid drug requirements are very high or cannot be used, and surgery may be required. Short term (<2 weeks) SSKI may be used to help prepare the pregnant patient.

Consequences of Overtreatment

The influence of maternal hypothyroidism on fetal brain development and the subsequently reduced IQ of the children of hypothyroid mothers is discussed elsewhere (see Chapter 12).[230] Needless to say, the overuse of antithyroid drugs in pregnancy may lead to the same consequences. There is considerable evidence that many pregnant patients with Graves' disease are overtreated as far as the fetus is concerned as evidenced by transiently elevated serum TSH levels on newborn screening tests[231]; this is another reason why it is better to maintain pregnant women as slightly hyperthyroid rather than slightly hypothyroid.

Graves' Disease in the Postpartum Period

Postpartum thyroiditis with transient thyrotoxicosis due to thyroid cell destruction may occur with some frequency (approximately 5% to 10%) during the postpartum period (4 to 12 months) (see later discussion).[232] The onset of hyperthyroidism is less common.

Changes in the Immune Response in the Postpartum Period

As discussed earlier, pregnancy induces a variety of immune changes that are responses to the paternal foreign antigens so that the fetus is not rejected. These include enhanced regulatory T cell influences and a T-cell shift from Th_1 to Th_2, resulting in an overall decrease in all autoimmune responses as evidenced by marked decreases in thyroid autoantibodies. Following delivery, these immune changes are slowly lost and a return to normal is observed but only after a period of exacerbated autoimmune reactivity in which large increases in T-cell and autoantibody activity occur. It is at this time—3 to 12 months' postpartum—that new-onset or recurrent thyroid disease is seen. Such thyroid dysfunction may be transient or permanent.

Presentation of Postpartum Graves' Disease

A high percentage of women in the 20- to 35-year age group give a history of pregnancy in the 12 months before the onset of Graves' disease.[116,233] Pregnancy and the postpartum state also apparently influence the course of preexisting Graves' disease. Patients in clinical remission during pregnancy are prone to postpartum relapse. In 41 pregnancies in 35 patients in remission, 78% were followed by development of thyrotoxicosis during the postpartum period. The patients with Graves' disease and postpartum thyrotoxicosis were classified into three categories: (1) Some patients had persistent recurrent hyperthyroidism with an elevated RAIU (classic Graves' disease). (2) Some patients had a transient disorder associated with a normal or an elevated RAIU (transient Graves' disease). (3) Some patients, especially those with the highest titers of TPOAb, experienced a transient thyrotoxicosis with a decreased RAIU (the thyrotoxic phase of postpartum thyroiditis). This phase, in turn, may be followed by a hypothyroid phase (see later discussion).[106]

The Desire for Pregnancy

A special problem related to hyperthyroidism and pregnancy occurs in the patient who is in early remission after a course of antithyroid drug treatment or is being treated with antithyroid agents and wants to become pregnant in the near future. Management with antithyroid agents can be continued through pregnancy or reinstituted if hyperthyroidism recurs, but in such instances definitive therapy (radioiodine or surgery) should be considered to forestall the complexities of managing hyperthyroidism during pregnancy. As with the therapy of Graves' disease in general, such decisions must involve education of the patient so that the risks and benefits of the various alternatives are clearly appreciated.

Nursing and Antithyroid Drugs

Older studies suggested that relatively more methimazole than propylthiouracil appeared in breast milk of women receiving these drugs but more recent evidence shows little difference between them.[221,225] However, it is often recommended that women who take antithyroid drugs be advised not to nurse their infants because of the difficulty in monitoring thyroid function in infants. No serious drug side effects have been reported in neonates whose mothers were taking antithyroid drugs, although periodic tests of neonatal thyroid function may be appropriate in women taking very high doses.[234]

INHERITED NONIMMUNE HYPERTHYROIDISM

Toxic diffuse thyroid hyperplasia without the pathologic characteristics of autoimmune disease has been reported in families and appears to be inherited as an autosomal dominant condition.[48,235,236] Polymorphic genomic mutations in the *TSHR* gene have been reported to cause constitutively activated TSHRs differing from family to family. Recessive mutations on both chromosomes have also been described as causing hyperthyroidism while the parents remained euthyroid. These gain-of-function mutations, mostly in the transmembrane regions of the *TSHR*, are similar to those somatic mutations seen in toxic adenomas but are in the germline.[237] Treatment is by radioiodine ablation or thyroidectomy, depending on the age of the patient.

TOXIC MULTINODULAR GOITER

Toxic multinodular goiter is a disorder in which hyperthyroidism arises in a multinodular goiter, usually of long standing, and is the result of one of several pathogenetic factors.[238]

Pathogenesis

The pathogenesis of toxic multinodular goiter cannot be considered apart from that of its invariable forerunner, nontoxic multinodular goiter, from which it emerges slowly and surreptitiously. Two hallmarks of the disorder, structural and functional heterogeneity and functional autonomy, evolve over time; the increase in the extent of autonomous function causes the disease to move from the nontoxic to the toxic phase, but the mechanisms of this change in all cases are uncertain. The somatic mutations in the *TSHR* gene demonstrated in toxic adenomas have been demonstrated in some cases of toxic multinodular goiter and appear to differ from nodule to nodule.[239] However, only about 60% of toxic nodules have TSHR mutations and only a very few have G protein mutations. Hence there are many nodules with autonomy of undetermined cause.[240]

Radioiodine scintiscans show localization of isotope in one or more discrete nodules, while iodine accumulation in the remainder of the gland is usually suppressed. No further suppression is produced by exogenous thyroid hormone, but TSH stimulates iodine uptake in the previously inactive areas, indicating that the suppression is due to the lack of TSH. Histopathologically, the functioning areas resemble adenomas in being reasonably well demarcated from surrounding tissue. They generally consist of large follicles, sometimes with hyperplastic epithelium, but here, too, architecture correlates poorly with functional state. The remaining tissue appears inactive, and zones of degeneration are present in both functioning and nonfunctioning areas. Hence from the pathophysiologic standpoint, these thyroids harbor multiple solitary hyperfunctioning and hypofunctioning adenomas interspersed by suppressed normal thyroid tissue.

Clinical Presentation

The overproduction of thyroid hormone in toxic multinodular goiter is usually less than that in Graves' disease. First, the clinical manifestations of thyrotoxicosis are rarely flagrant. Second, the serum T_4 and T_3 concentrations may be only marginally increased, and a suppressed TSH may be the major abnormality. Finally, the total RAIU is only slightly increased or within the normal range. The mildness of the hyperthyroidism is consistent with either of its presumed pathogenetic origins. Toxic multinodular goiter is a common complication of nontoxic multinodular goiter, but its precise incidence is unknown. Toxic multinodular goiter usually occurs after the age of 50 in patients who have had nontoxic multinodular goiter for many years, often in regions of iodine deficiency.[241] Like its forerunner, toxic multinodular goiter is many times more common in women than in men. Sometimes, hyperthyroidism develops abruptly, usually after exposure to increased quantities of iodine, which permits autonomous foci to increase hormone secretion to excessive levels and which may simply exacerbate already established mild hyperthyroidism (see Iodide-Induced Hyperthyroidism). In addition, Graves' disease may either initially manifest or develop in a multinodular gland as confirmed by the presence of TSHRAb of the stimulating variety. Toxic multinodular goiter is almost never accompanied by infiltrative ophthalmopathy, and when the two coexist, it represents the emergence of Graves' disease.

Cardiovascular manifestations tend to predominate, possibly because of the age of the patients, and include atrial fibrillation or tachycardia, with or without heart failure. Weakness and wasting of muscles are common, the so-called "apathetic" or "masked" thyrotoxicosis. The nervous manifestations are less prominent than in younger patients with thyrotoxicosis, but emotional lability may be pronounced. Because of the physical characteristics of the thyroid gland and its frequent retrosternal extension, obstructive symptoms are more common than in Graves' disease. On palpation, the characteristics of the goiter are the same as those of the more common nontoxic multinodular goiter. In as many as 20% of elderly patients with thyrotoxicosis, the thyroid gland is firm and irregular but not distinctly enlarged. Ultrasound examination will confirm the diagnosis as toxic multinodular goiter rather than a single toxic adenoma or Graves' disease.

Laboratory Tests and Differential Diagnosis

All patients with a multinodular goiter should be screened annually with a serum TSH. If suppressed, the free T_4 (or if normal, the free T_3) should be determined. Serum TSH levels intermediate between 0.1 and 0.4 mU/L are not usually associated with significant symptoms. Such patients have thyroid autonomy, but are not thyrotoxic (see "Subclinical Thyrotoxicosis"). For patients with established thyrotoxicosis, an RAIU study with scintiscan will help in gauging the dose of ^{131}I to be administered as well as identify the autonomously functioning nodules. The latter can then be followed after ^{131}I therapy.

Treatment

Radioiodine is the treatment of choice for most patients with toxic multinodular goiter despite disagreement about the size and number of doses required to achieve a therapeutic response.[238,242] We attempt to deposit about 12 to 14 mCi into the gland at 24 hours based on a pretreatment RAIU test. Because many patients with this disorder have underlying heart disease, the administration of radioiodine should be preceded by a course of antithyroid therapy until a eumetabolic state is achieved. Medication is then discontinued for at least 3 days before radioiodine is administered. Seven days thereafter, the antithyroid drug is reinstituted so that the thyrotoxicosis is controlled until radioiodine takes effect, which typically requires 3 to 4 months. A decrease in size of the hyperfunctioning nodules is a positive sign. At that time, the antithyroid drug can be tapered, but if the TSH falls a second course of therapy can be given. In some patients, despite hyperthyroidism, the 24-hour RAIU is low.

Surgery

Surgical therapy may be often recommended after adequate preoperative preparation in patients with obstructive manifestations. In these patients, a CT or MRI is recommended to define the extent of the goiter and the adequacy of the tracheal walls. Respiratory function studies may also be helpful in assessing the need for surgery. Patients with fixed, especially partially retrosternal, goiter should be considered for therapy due to the risk of more complete obstruction in case hemorrhage into a nodule occurs. When surgery is contraindicated, even significant obstructive symptoms can be relieved by adequate radioiodine therapy.[243]

TOXIC ADENOMA

A third, less common form of hyperthyroidism is caused by one or more autonomous adenomas of the thyroid gland. As herein employed, the term *toxic adenoma* refers to a tumor in a thyroid that is otherwise intrinsically normal. The disorder is usually caused by a single adenoma that is palpable as a solitary nodule and hence is sometimes referred to as *hyperfunctioning solitary nodule* or *toxic nodule*. Occasionally, two or three adenomas of similar character are present.

Pathogenesis

Toxic adenomas are true follicular adenomas (for histopathologic characteristics, see Chapter 13). The basic pathogenesis of a large fraction of them is one of several somatic point mutations in the TSHR gene, commonly in the third transmembrane loop. These single nucleotide substitutions cause amino acid changes which lead to constitutive activation of the TSHR in the absence of TSH.[244] It appears, therefore, that the TSHR is "tripped" from an "off state" to an "on state." Similarly, loss-of-function rather than gain-of-function mutations may also occur in the *TSHR* gene and cause hypothyroidism (see later discussion). A small number of autonomous adenomas have mutations in the G protein genes that lead to a similar state of constitutive activation.[240]

Clinical Presentation

The toxic adenoma often presents as a nodule in a patient with a suppressed TSH which appears in a radioiodine thyroid scan as a localized area of increased radioiodine accumulation (Fig. 11–14). This condition occurs in a younger age group than does toxic multinodular goiter, typically in patients in their 30s or 40s. Frequently there is a history of a longstanding, slowly growing

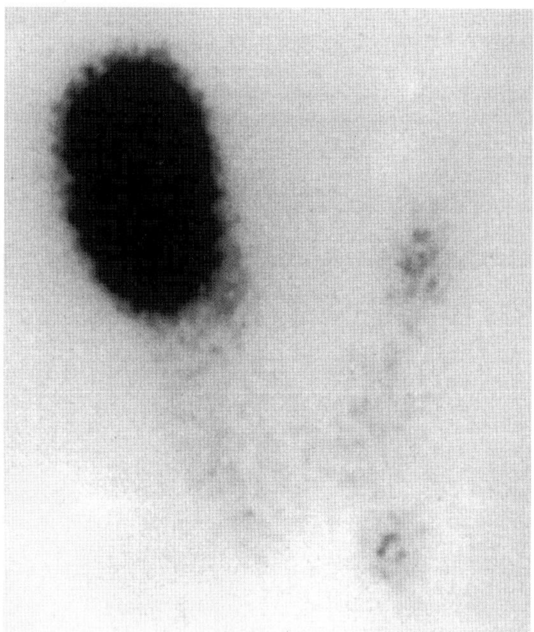

Figure 11–14 ▪ ^{123}I scanning of a hyperfunctioning hot nodule corresponding to physical findings with a faint outline of the remaining suppressed gland. In this unusual case, Graves' disease developed a few months later after an oral contrast agent load. (From Soule J, Mayfield R. Graves' disease after ^{131}I therapy for toxic nodule. Thyroid 2001;11:91-92.)

lump in the neck. It is unusual for adenomas to produce thyrotoxicosis until they have achieved a diameter of more than 3 cm and, up to that point, patients have subclinical hyperthyroidism.[238] The adenoma can undergo central necrosis and hemorrhage, spontaneously relieving the thyrotoxicosis, the remainder of the thyroid may resume its function, and the adenoma may appear on scintiscan as a cold area or a doughnut-shaped image with a central cold area. Calcification in the area of hemorrhage may take place and may be evident on sonogram examination. Such calcification is usually macroscopic and irregular and does not resemble the finely stippled calcification observed in papillary cancers. The peripheral clinical manifestations of a toxic adenoma are generally milder than those of Graves' disease and are notable for the absence of infiltrative orbitopathy and myopathy, although cardiovascular manifestations may occur. The nodule is generally easily visible and is palpable as smooth, well-defined and firm and moves freely on swallowing. The remainder of the gland may be difficult to feel.

Laboratory Tests

The results of laboratory tests depend on the stage and function of the adenoma. At first, serum thyroid hormone concentrations are normal except for borderline suppression of the serum TSH. This, together with ultrasound examination to exclude multiple nodules, confirms the diagnosis. Later a thyroid scan may show localization of radioisotope in the palpated nodule, but this does not occur until TSH secretion is suppressed. If the nodule continues to grow, frank hyperthyroidism is accompanied by elevation of serum thyroid hormone levels. When the nodule is small, the RAIU is normal but the lesion remains functional when TSH is suppressed by exogenous levothyroxine, evidence of its true autonomy. Occasionally, the serum free T_4 concentration is normal, and only the serum T_3 level is increased (T_3 thyrotoxicosis). Incidental thyroid carcinoma may rarely coexist within a gland exhibiting a hyperfunctioning adenoma, although autonomous malignant nodules causing functional hyperthyroidism are very rare.

Treatment

Although hyperfunctioning adenomas may eventually cause clinical hyperthyroidism, many do so slowly and others not at all.[238] Therefore treatment of asymptomatic patients with functional adenomas is decided on an individual basis. Euthyroid subjects can be followed with an annual TSH. Suppression below normal indicates that an evaluation for hyperthyroidism is in order and that therapy may be warranted. Two definitive therapies are available: radioiodine and surgery.

Radioiodine

In terms of the specificity of treatment, functioning thyroid nodules are ideal candidates for radioiodine therapy. The radiation should, in theory, be directed almost exclusively to the diseased tissue. This is because TSH is suppressed and the normal thyroid tissue surrounding the nodule does not take up radioiodine. However, this suppression may be incomplete and a significant fraction of patients receiving ^{131}I develop thyroid failure. For the patient older than age 18 with a nodule 5 cm in diameter or smaller, ^{131}I is an appropriate treatment if the risk of eventual hypothyroidism is acceptable to the patient. For such lesions, doses of radioiodine are given sufficient to result in the presence of 300 to 370 MBq (8 to 10 mCi) in the nodule at 24 hours based on the uptake.[238] Because of the potential for hypothyroidism, prolonged follow-up is mandatory. Complete suppression of TSH by exogenous levothyroxine (~100 μU/day for 2 weeks) may be used in appropriate patients to reduce TSH and thus ^{131}I uptake by the normal thyroid tissue during therapy.[242]

Surgery

Large nodules with concomitant physical symptoms are most readily treated with surgical excision. Surgical excision is also used in patients younger than 18 years of age to avoid significant irradiation to the perinodular tissue. The toxic adenoma is not diffusely hypervascular, and consequently preoperative preparation with iodine is not required. In the patient with overt thyrotoxicosis, however, a normal metabolic state should be restored with an antithyroid drug before surgery.

IODIDE-INDUCED HYPERTHYROIDISM

Administration of supplemental iodine to subjects with endemic iodine-deficiency goiter can result in iodine-induced Graves' disease. This response, termed *iodide-induced hyperthyroidism* or the *Jod Basedow* effect, occurs in only a small fraction of individuals at risk. The term Jod Basedow specifically refers to iodine-induced Basedow's (Graves') disease but is often used to refer to iodine-induced hyperthyroidism of any type. There are two major patterns of the underlying thyroid disorder.[245] In the first, which is common in older individuals, a nodular goiter with areas of autonomous function is present, and TSHRAbs are not detectable in the blood. The second pattern occurs in younger individuals with diffuse goiter in whom stimulating TSHRAbs are often present. These findings indicate that jod-Basedow occurs in thyroid glands in which thyroid function is independent of TSH stimulation. The occurrence of Jod Basedow is not a contraindication to treat endemic iodine deficiency.

Apart from the many other benefits that accrue from iodine treatment and prophylaxis, over the long run the frequency of spontaneous hyperthyroidism due to toxic nodular goiter is diminished.[241]

Iodide-induced hyperthyroidism is an important disorder in areas of the world in which dietary iodine intake is high.[246] In regions in which iodine intake is marginal but overt iodine deficiency is absent, moderate increments in iodine intake may induce hyperthyroidism in patients with autonomous thyroid nodules. Consequently, the physician must be alert to the possibility of inducing hyperthyroidism when administering iodine in expectorants, x-ray contrast media, medications containing iodine (e.g., amiodarone), povidone-iodine, or any other form to patients with nodular goiter.[247,248] Because nodular goiter is generally a disease of the elderly, induction of the Jod Basedow phenomenon can have serious consequences, particularly because enrichment of the thyroid with iodine forestalls administration of ^{131}I and delays the response to antithyroid agents. In these patients, serum T_3 concentration is sometimes normal, although total and free T_4 concentrations are increased and TSH is suppressed (T_4 thyrotoxicosis). Prevention of an acute exacerbation may be achieved by pretreatment of at-risk subjects with methimazole or perchlorate starting before exposure and for several weeks afterward.[249,250]

Although the Jod Basedow phenomenon can occur only when the thyroid is partially autonomous, patients with iodine-induced hyperthyroidism have been reported in whom thyroid function was normal and normally suppressible after iodine was withdrawn and a euthyroid state restored. The mechanism by which iodine induces thyrotoxicosis in such instances is unknown. The treatment of these individuals may be difficult. Even after discontinuation of exogenous iodide, the uptake of ^{131}I by the thyroid gland may remain low, not adequate for conventional doses of radioiodine. The elevated thyroid hormone content secondary to the iodide level also makes thiourea drugs less effective. It may be necessary to treat such individuals for prolonged periods (6 to 9 months) before administering radioiodine. On the other hand, if uptake is detectable, larger doses of radioiodine may be given to destroy thyroid tissue.

Amiodarone

Arguably, the most common drug associated with iodine-induced thyrotoxicosis is amiodarone. This iodine-rich drug has become increasingly popular because of its effectiveness in combating severe cardiac arrhythmias. The drug has complex effects on the thyroid, although a majority (~80%) of patients remain euthyroid.[251] Structurally, the drug resembles T_4 (see Fig. 10–6) and contains 37% iodine by weight. About 6 mg of iodide is released per day of the 75 mg of iodine present in a 200-mg tablet compared with the typical daily iodine supply of about 150 to 200 µg in North America. Amiodarone has a half-life of 50 to 60 days and therefore remains available for a long period even after drug withdrawal. In addition to providing huge amounts of iodide, amiodarone inhibits the type 1 and probably the type 2 deiodinases and may compete with T_3 for binding to the thyroid hormone receptor. Amiodarone also has a direct cytotoxic effect on thyroid cells via induction of apoptosis.[252] In addition, the iodine load, the drug or its metabolites, may precipitate autoimmune thyroid disease in susceptible individuals.

Clinical Presentation

In all patients receiving this drug, its effects, particularly the inhibition of the deiodinases, cause a compensatory increase in TSH secretion. This increases serum free T_4 30% to 50% with the serum T_3 and TSH concentrations remaining normal after equilibrium occurs.[253] This pattern is identical to that observed in mouse models with low D1 activity due to *Dio 1* gene inactivation or genetic D1 deficiency and should not be confused with that of thyrotoxicosis in which TSH is suppressed.[254,255] The pathologic effects on the thyroid may result in iodide-induced hypothyroidism (the most common thyroid complication in iodine-sufficient regions; see Chapter 12), hyperthyroidism in susceptible individuals due to the Jod Basedow effect in iodine-deficient regions, or thyrotoxicosis due to a thyroiditis-type damage to the thyroid gland. The hyperthyroidism and thyroiditis-like syndromes have also been referred to as type I and type II amiodarone-induced thyrotoxicosis, respectively.[217] Amiodarone-induced thyrotoxicosis may develop at the outset of exposure or not until after several years of treatment. It commonly presents as an exacerbation of the underlying cardiac pathology that was the indication for its use in the first instance. This serious complication can sometimes be anticipated by its early recognition due to a progressive decrease in serum TSH. Monitoring of TSH is a worthwhile precaution, particularly in areas of borderline or deficient iodine supply so that thionamide prophylaxis can be initiated before severe manifestations occur.

Diagnosis

All patients with amiodarone-induced thyrotoxicosis will have a suppressed TSH with the degree of suppression proportional to the clinical severity. Serum free T_4 will be elevated but the elevation in serum free T_3 will be less than that in typical thyrotoxic states due to the blockade of T_4 to T_3 conversion by the drug. Distinction between the two causes of thyrotoxicosis may not be possible, although many strategies have been suggested. In North America, the cause of thyrotoxicosis is usually thyroiditis, whereas a more evenly divided mix of the two causes occurs in Europe.[251,256,257] Doppler flow ultrasonography showing hypervascularity accompanied by an enlarged gland favors iodide-induced hyperthyroidism, whereas a normal-sized gland and "normal" or reduced vascularity points to thyroiditis, but results can be equivocal.[251,256] RAIU values are virtually always low except in areas of low iodine intake.

Treatment

If possible, amiodarone should be discontinued. In patients with thyroiditis, a spontaneous resolution may occur but in most a combination of methimazole or carbimazole (20 to 40 mg/day) and prednisolone/prednisone 20 to 40 mg/day is given to cover both diagnostic possibilities.[258] The latter may be tapered after 4 to 6 weeks to see if a remission has occurred. In patients with iodide-induced hyperthyroidism, perchlorate, 500 mg twice a day for 1 to 2 weeks, may accelerate the resolution of the condition although this agent has potential significant renal and bone marrow toxicities precluding long-term use.[251,259] In patients who remain unstable or whose cardiac condition is likely to require lifelong amiodarone therapy, thyroid surgery is appropriate. Opinions are divided as to whether amiodarone can be restarted in patients who have recovered from thyroiditis but most patients remain euthyroid when this is done.[217,260]

HYPERTHYROIDISM DUE TO THYROTROPIN SECRETION

Excess thyrotropin is an exceedingly rare cause of hyperthyroidism. However, pituitary thyrotroph tumors cause this condition and may present as a Graves'-like syndrome with diffuse goiter and substantial thyrotoxicosis. Laboratory studies demonstrating an inappropriately detectable or somewhat elevated TSH in the presence of thyrotoxic symptoms alert the clinician to this as the most likely possibility once assay artifacts are eliminated. This condition, discussed in depth in Chapter 8, must be differentiated from the rare patient who has *familial resistance to thyroid hormone (RTH)*.[261-263]

Thyroid Hormone Resistance

In some patients with familial thyroid hormone resistance due to mutations in the β isoform of the thyroid hormone receptor, the hypothalamic-pituitary feedback mechanism is more resistant to the effects of thyroid hormone than are peripheral tissues such as the heart, which expresses the thyroid receptor α isoform.[261-263] These patients may therefore present with a hyperthyroid appearance with tachycardia, nervousness, and goiter associated with an elevated free T_4. However, because the thyroid hormone hyperproduction is TSH-driven, serum TSH concentrations are detectable (>0.1 mU/L) or even elevated inappropriately for the high serum thyroid hormone levels. In general, the manifestations are not due to to excessive hormone action, but rather to inadequate thyroid hormone action, and these individuals may require treatment with thyroid hormone or thyroid hormone analogues and/or β adrenergic receptor-blocking agents rather than antithyroid drugs (see Chapter 12 for a more extensive discussion of RTH). The critical historical point in such patients is a family history because RTH is inherited in an autosomal dominant pattern.

CHORIONIC GONADOTROPIN–INDUCED HYPERTHYROIDISM

Overview

Human chorionic gonadotropin is a glycoprotein heterodimer composed of an α subunit identical to that of TSH, LH, and FSH and a specific β subunit which has similarity to TSH β. This glycoprotein binds to the human TSH receptor, with an in vitro potency of about 1 U hCG = 0.7 μU of human TSH. In high concentrations this will cause hyperthyroidism characterized by a diffuse goiter, elevated free T_4, and suppressed TSH. This is readily recognized in the late first trimester of normal pregnancy in which a physiologic mild *transient gestational thyrotoxicosis* or *hyperthyroidism* occurs (see Chapter 10).

Transient Gestational Thyrotoxicosis

This syndrome is an exaggeration of the physiologic increase in thyroid stimulation in the first trimester as it is associated with high levels of hCG (100,000 to 200,000 U/L), such as those found in twin pregnancies, and is often accompanied by hyperemesis.[264,265] In most patients, the condition is self-limited but in rare circumstances low doses of propylthiouracil (100 mg day or less) may be required for a few weeks until the hCG falls spontaneously. It may be difficult to separate this syndrome from early Graves' disease and a TSHRAb test may be helpful.

A rare inherited variant of gestational thyrotoxicosis has been reported in which a mutation in the TSH receptor gene resulted in a receptor protein with an increased responsiveness to hCG.[266] Such patients develop hyperthyroidism with each pregnancy due to physiologic serum hCG concentrations.

Hyperthyroidism Associated with Trophoblastic Tumors

Thyroid hyperfunction may accompany hydatidiform mole, choriocarcinoma, or metastatic embryonal carcinoma of the testis.[217] Such neoplasms, particularly hydatidiform mole, elaborate differentially glycosylated hCG molecules that exhibit crossover specificity for binding to the TSH receptor and can induce thyroid overactivity.[267] Some patients have clinically overt thyrotoxicosis; however, clinical manifestations are usually not prominent, and goiter is absent or minimal despite laboratory evidence of a hyperthyroid state. The free T_4 and/or free T_3 levels are increased, and TSH values are suppressed. The reason for this discordance between the clinical and the laboratory indices is not known but may be due to the relatively short duration of thyroid hormone excess. The possibility of a molar pregnancy should be considered in a young woman with hyperthyroidism and amenorrhea because the appropriate therapy is evacuation of the uterus.

TRANSIENT THYROTOXICOSIS

Overview

As mentioned at the outset of this chapter, *transient thyrotoxicosis* must be differentiated from the *sustained hyperthyroidism* of Graves' disease and other causes of hyperthyroidism. Transient thyrotoxicosis is caused by thyroid cell breakdown and the hyperthyroid symptoms are of abrupt onset and short duration. This process may be followed by recovery of thyroid function or the development of transient or permanent thyroid failure. The discussion in this chapter focuses on thyroiditis as the most common cause of transient thyrotoxicosis and this disorder is covered more completely in Chapter 12 because *Hashimoto's disease* most commonly causes hypothyroidism after the phase of transient hyperthyroidism. Unfortunately, transient thyrotoxicosis has a confusing nomenclature that can be clarified as follows:

1. In the autoimmune forms *(Hashimoto's thyroiditis)*, there are often no local symptoms of thyroid inflammation leading to the terms *silent* or *painless thyroiditis* and also referred to as *lymphocytic thyroiditis* or *"Hashitoxicosis"* but this may also present with thyroid tenderness.
2. In the form of postviral thyroiditis (also termed *subacute, de Quervain's*, or *granulomatous thyroiditis*), thyroid tenderness may be the most prominent symptom.
3. Acute thyroiditis due to bacterial or fungal infections is only rarely accompanied by thyrotoxicosis and the local symptoms predominate (see Chapter 12).
4. Thyroiditis may also be drug-induced, with the principal offender being amiodarone but lithium and perhaps some of the new small molecule kinase inhibitors (sunitinib) may also cause this.[267a]

Transient Thyrotoxicosis Due to Autoimmune (Hashimoto's) Thyroiditis

As described earlier, Hashimoto's disease causes two different thyrotoxicosis-associated transient syndromes. The most common is the *painless* form in which the symptoms of thyrotoxicosis, usually mild, predominate and the more uncommon form has a painful form of presentation probably secondary to a more acute onset. Histopathology in such patients with thy-

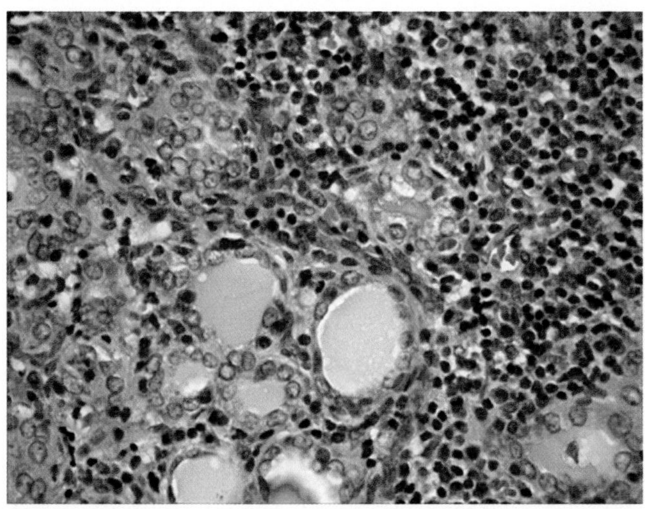

Figure 11–15 ▪ Lymphocytic thyroiditis in a patient with transient thyrotoxicosis (painless thyroiditis) secondary to autoimmune (Hashimoto's) thyroiditis. Note the diffuse lymphocytic invasion of the tissue including the follicular epithelium and the loss of follicles. (Courtesy of Dr. Vania Nosé, Brigham and Women's Hospital, Boston, MA.)

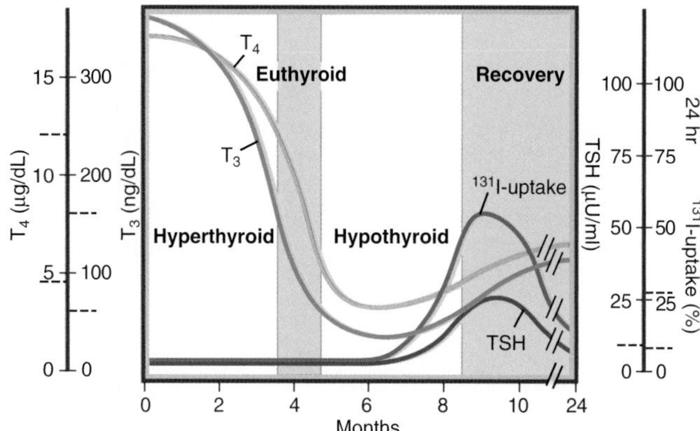

Figure 11–16 ▪ The typical course in patients with lymphocytic (painless) thyroiditis with transient thyrotoxicosis. The duration of each phase may vary, and some patients do not experience a discernible hyperthyroid or hypothyroid phase. (From Woolf PD. Transient painless thyroiditis with hyperthyroidism: a variant of lymphocytic thyroiditis? Endocr Rev 1980;1:411-420.)

roiditis shows diffuse or local lymphocytic infiltration, varying degrees of fibrosis, and disruption of the follicular architecture (Fig. 11–15).

Thyrotoxicosis from Painless Autoimmune Thyroiditis

This presentation may occur postpartum or spontaneously. *Postpartum thyroiditis* is the most common example and its pathophysiology, postpartum enhancement of thyroid-directed autoimmunity, is analogous to the postpartum exacerbation of Graves' disease (see Graves' Disease in the Postpartum Period). The incidence of postpartum thyroiditis varies but may occur in as many as 10% of women and in more than 30% of those with positive TPO autoantibodies and even a larger fraction in patients with type 1 diabetes mellitus.[201] In women found to be TPOAb-positive prenatally, postpartum assessment of thyroid function is recommended at 3, 6, and 12 months. As expected, there is a strong association with the HLADR3 and HLADR5 haplotypes, which are also associated with autoimmune thyroid disease.[268] *Thyrotoxicosis from autoimmune thyroiditis* has all the same characteristics as postpartum thyroiditis and is seen in patients early in their development of classic Hashimoto's disease and before the onset of hypothyroidism.

Thyrotoxicosis from Painful Autoimmune Thyroiditis

While some patients may present with local thyroid tenderness this is uncommon. Such tender episodes, which may be unilateral, may recur until the thyroid gland is completely destroyed by the disease process.

Clinical Presentation of Transient Autoimmune Thyrotoxicosis

More than 75% of patients are women who present with the acute onset of symptoms of thyrotoxicosis, usually nervousness, palpitations, and irritability, and they can often pinpoint the time of recent onset. In the postpartum syndrome, symptoms present 3 to 6 months after delivery but may be mild and overlooked in the myriad of events involved in the care of the newborn. After 1 to 2 months, the thyrotoxic symptoms fade but are often replaced by those suggesting hypothyroidism (Fig. 11–16).

In a significant number of postpartum patients, the thyrotoxic phase is too mild to be noticed and the patient presents somewhat later after delivery with hypothyroid symptoms. The physical examination shows mild signs of thyrotoxicosis, tachycardia being the most prominent, without the specific eye signs or dermopathy associated with Graves' disease. The thyroid gland is normal in size but may be firm if the Hashimoto's disease is chronic.

Diagnosis

Thyrotoxicosis is usually mild and is reflected in the degree of suppression of the serum TSH level and elevation of the serum free T_4. Significant elevation of the TPO antibodies is typical. Systemic manifestations of inflammation are lacking, and the erythrocyte sedimentation rate is normal or nearly normal, but the ultrasound may indicate the heterogeneity of an inflamed gland. If true hyperthyroidism cannot be eliminated as a diagnosis on clinical grounds, the RAIU study should be performed unless the patient is nursing. The classic decreased RAIU is due partly to feedback suppression of TSH secretion but also to thyroid follicular cell destruction. The tendency of the disorder to pass through a hypothyroid phase is not surprising in view of the extensive depletion of thyroglobulin, which is processed to thyroxine and not replaced by the dysfunctional cells.

Natural History

The duration of the thyrotoxic phase, typically not severe enough to require treatment, averages about 1 to 2 months. About one half of the patients return to a euthyroid phase and remain well in the short term. In the remaining half, a hypothyroid phase may follow and may last from 2 to 9 months. In most, there is eventual restoration of euthyroidism, but some develop permanent hypothyroidism years later.[269] About one third retain a goiter, usually with persistence of thyroid autoantibodies in the serum. The opposite sequelae, recurrence of thyrotoxicosis, may also occur months or years after restoration of a euthyroid state or particularly after pregnancy.

Treatment

The thyrotoxic phase may require alleviation of the peripheral manifestations through the use of β blockers. Prednisone (20 to 40 mg/day) may decrease the duration of the thyrotoxic phase, but is typically not needed except when the painful form of the disease is present. If mild and brief, the hypothyroid phase may also not require treatment. When treatment with levothyroxine is required, it should be withdrawn slowly approximately 6 months later, because the hypothyroidism is often not permanent.

Subacute Thyroiditis

Subacute thyroiditis (also termed *granulomatous, giant cell,* or *de Quervain's' thyroiditis*) is thought to be caused directly or indirectly by a viral infection of the thyroid gland and often follows an upper respiratory illness. A tendency to appear in the spring in the northern latitudes has been noted and again it predominates in the female. The mumps virus has been implicated in some cases, and coxsackievirus, influenza virus, echovirus, and adenoviruses may also be etiologic agents. Positive TPO antibodies are present transiently during the active phase of the disease, although some patients may retain evidence of thyroid autoimmunity for many years. A small number of patients eventually develop autoimmune thyroid disease. Subacute thyroiditis is uncommon, but mild cases may be mistakenly diagnosed as pharyngitis.

Pathology

The histopathologic changes are different from those in Hashimoto's disease. The lesions are patchy in distribution and vary in their stage of development from area to area. Affected follicles are infiltrated predominantly with mononuclear cells and show disruption of epithelium, partial or complete loss of colloid, and fragmentation and duplication of the basement membrane (Fig. 11–17).

To this extent, the histopathologic appearance may resemble that in Hashimoto's disease. A characteristic feature is the well-developed follicular lesion that consists of a central core of colloid surrounded by the multinucleated giant cells, from which stems the designation *giant cell thyroiditis.* Colloid may be found in the interstitium or within the giant cells. The follicular changes progress to form granulomas. Interfollicular fibrosis and an interstitial inflammatory reaction are present to varying degrees. When the disease subsides, an essentially normal histologic appearance is restored.

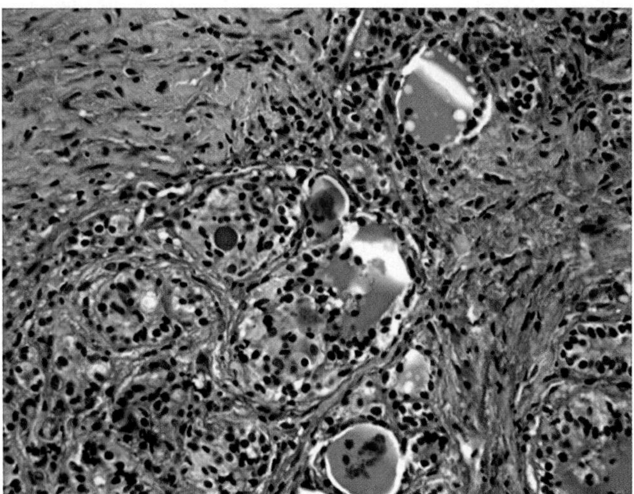

Figure 11–17 ▪ Subacute (viral or postviral) thyroiditis. Diffuse neutrophilic invasion with active destruction of follicles and a multinucleated giant cell are present. Fibrosis and near complete loss of follicles have occurred. (Courtesy of Dr. Vania Nosé, Brigham and Women's Hospital, Boston, MA.)

Pathophysiology

Apoptosis of follicular epithelium and loss of follicular integrity are the primary events in the pathophysiology. Thyroglobulin, T_4, and iodinated thyroglobulin fragments are released into the circulation often in quantities sufficient to elevate not just the serum Tg level but also the serum free T_4, producing clinical thyrotoxicosis and suppressing TSH secretion. As a result, the RAIU decreases to low levels, and hormone synthesis ceases. Later in the disease, when stores of pre-formed hormone are depleted, serum T_4 and T_3 concentrations decline, sometimes into the hypothyroid range, and the serum TSH level rises, often to elevated values exactly as occurs in silent thyroiditis (Fig. 11–18).

As the disease becomes inactive, the RAIU may be greater than normal for a time as hormone stores are repleted. Ultimately, when hormone secretion resumes, serum T_4 and T_3 concentrations rise, and serum TSH concentration decreases to normal values.

Clinical Picture

The characteristic feature is the gradual or sudden appearance of pain in the region of the thyroid gland with or without fever. The pain, which is aggravated by turning the head or swallowing, characteristically radiates to the ear, jaw, or occiput and may mimic disorders arising in these areas. The absence of pain does not exclude the diagnosis, because biopsy-proven painless subacute thyroiditis occurs, but it must be distinguished from acute autoimmune thyroiditis. Hoarseness and dysphagia may be present, and patients may complain of palpitations, in view of nervousness, and lassitude. The lassitude can be extreme, considering the local nature of the disease, suggesting a systemic component. Although acute manifestations are present in severe cases, in milder disease, often overlooked, symptoms may be present for months.

On palpation, at least part of the thyroid is slightly to moderately enlarged, firm, often nodular, and usually exquisitely tender, with one lobe frequently being more severely affected than the other. Indeed the symptoms may be truly unilateral. The overlying skin may be warm and erythematous. Occasionally the locus of maximal involvement migrates over the course of a few weeks to other parts of the gland. The disease usually subsides within a few months, leaving no residual deficiency of thyroid function in 90% of patients. In rare patients, the disease smolders, with repeated exacerbations over many months and hypothyroidism sometimes being the final result.

Diagnosis

The laboratory findings vary with the phase of the disease. During the active phase, the erythrocyte sedimentation rate is increased, often to a remarkable extent (>100 mm/hr). Indeed a diagnosis of active subacute thyroiditis is hardly tenable when the sedimentation rate is normal. The white blood cell count is normal or, at most, moderately increased. The serum Tg level is characteristically high, in keeping with the degree of thyroid destruction.

Subacute thyroiditis must be differentiated from acute hemorrhagic degeneration in a preexisting thyroid nodule, Hashimoto's disease with painful recurrence (see earlier text), and

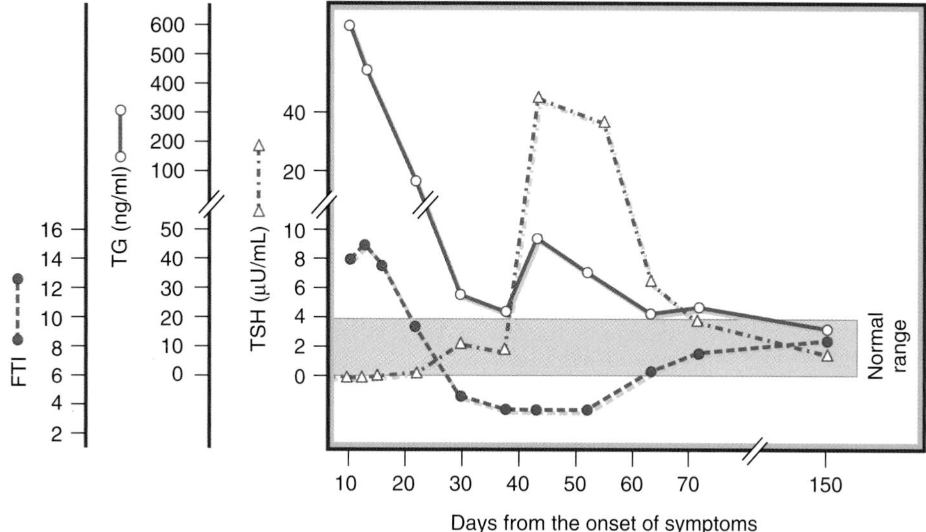

Figure 11–18 ▪ Thyroid function in a patient during the course of subacute (viral or postviral) thyroiditis. During the thyrotoxic phase (days 10 to 20), the serum thyroglobulin (TG) concentration was greatly elevated, the FT_4I was high, and TSH was suppressed; the erythrocyte sedimentation rate was 86 mm/hr, and the thyroidal RAIU was 2%. The TG level and FT_4I declined in parallel. During the phase of hypothyroidism (days 30 to 63), when the FT_4I was below normal, a modest transient increase in the serum TG level occurred in parallel with the increase in serum TSH. All parameters of thyroid function were normal by day 150, five months after the onset of symptoms. FT_4I, free thyroxine index, RAIU, radioactive iodine uptake; TSH, thyrotropin. (From DeGroot LJ, Larsen PR, Henneman G. Acute and subacute thyroiditis. In The Thyroid and Its Diseases, 6th ed. New York: Churchill Livingstone, 1996:705.)

acute pyogenic or fungal thyroiditis and rarely thyroid malignancy with painful nodules. Acute painful exacerbations of Hashimoto's disease may be difficult to distinguish from subacute thyroiditis. Lack of elevation of the erythrocyte sedimentation rate and high titers of thyroid autoantibodies strongly suggest the former. Acute pyogenic thyroiditis is distinguished by the presence of a septic focus elsewhere, by a greater inflammatory reaction in the tissues adjacent to the thyroid, and by much greater leukocytic and febrile responses (see Chapter 12). The RAIU and thyroid function are usually preserved in acute pyogenic thyroiditis. Rarely, widespread infiltrating cancer of the thyroid can present with a clinical and laboratory picture almost indistinguishable from that of subacute thyroiditis.[270] Ultrasound and fine-needle aspiration should be performed if this is a consideration.

Treatment

In mild cases, aspirin or nonsteroidal antiinflammatory drugs cyclooxygenase-2 (COX-2) may control the symptoms. With more severe pain, glucocorticoids (e.g., prednisone up to 40 mg/day) is the only solution for the extreme discomfort. This may be required for several months and should then be withdrawn gradually. If the TSH is not suppressed, TSH-suppressive therapy with levothyroxine may decrease the size of the gland, relieving the pressure on the thyroid capsule. TSH is needed for thyroid cell regeneration, so such therapy should be decreased as the symptoms subside.

Drug-Associated Thyroiditis

Thyroiditis is an uncommon complication of pharmacotherapy. Amiodarone is an important exception and is discussed earlier. Most cases of thyroiditis associated with various therapeutic agents appear to be due to drug-induced exacerbation of underlying autoimmune disease. This is understandable for those agents that are specifically administered to modify the immune system. They include interleukin-2, interferon-α, and granulocyte-macrophage colony-stimulating factor (GM-CSF), all of which can precipitate silent thyroiditis.[271] This has also been described with lithium and the gonadotropin-releasing hormone (GnRH) agonist leuprolide but the pathophysiology is obscure.[272-274]

We have recently observed a previously undescribed form of thyroiditis in association with therapy in patients with gastrointestinal stromal tumors with a multitargeting kinase inhibitor sunitinib (Sutent) given for gastrointestinal stromal tumors and renal cell carcinoma. This may present as subacute thyroiditis with a suppressed TSH as the major manifestation of the early phase but then progress to destruction of the gland through an unclear mechanism. Even though imatinib (Gleevec) has been associated with an increase in levothyroxine requirements in hypothyroid patients (analogous to the effects of phenytoin acid and rifampin), those changes are independent of thyroid function.[275]

OTHER CAUSES OF THYROTOXICOSIS ASSOCIATED WITH A LOW RADIOIODINE UPTAKE

Overview

In addition to silent and subacute thyroiditis, there are several other entities that should be considered in the patient with thyrotoxicosis in whom the thyroid gland is either not palpable or not enlarged and in whom biochemical findings of thyrotoxicosis are accompanied by a low RAIU.

Thyrotoxicosis Factitia

Thyrotoxicosis that arises from the ingestion, usually chronic, of excessive quantities of thyroid hormone usually occurs in individuals with a background of underlying psychiatric disease, especially in paramedical personnel who have access to thyroid hormone or in patients for whom thyroid hormone medication has been prescribed in the past. Generally the patient is aware of taking thyroid hormone but may adamantly deny it. In other instances, large doses of thyroid hormone or other thyroactive material may be given without the knowledge of the patient, usually as part of a regimen for weight reduction. Some "natural" products for weight reduction stated not to contain thyroid hormone nonetheless do. Symptoms are typical of thyrotoxicosis and may be severe.

In the absence of preexisting disease of the thyroid, the diagnosis is made from the combination of typical thyrotoxic manifestations, together with thyroid atrophy and hypofunction. Infiltrative ophthalmopathy never occurs, but lid lag, stare, and other "thyrotoxic" eye signs may be present. TSH levels are suppressed. Serum T_4 concentrations are increased unless the patient is taking T_3, in which case they will be subnormal. Serum T_3 concentrations are increased in either case. Hypofunction of the thyroid gland is evidenced by the subnormal values of the RAIU test. The presence of low, rather than elevated, values of serum Tg is a clear indication that the thyrotoxicosis results from exogenous hormone rather than thyroid hyperfunction.

This disorder may be confused with other varieties of thyrotoxicosis associated with a subnormal RAIU and absence of goiter, including silent thyroiditis, ectopic thyroid tissue, and hyperfunctioning metastatic follicular carcinoma. Evidence for the two latter disorders can be obtained by demonstration of the ectopic focus or foci by external radioiodine scanning or the presence of normal to elevated serum Tg concentrations. Differentiation from silent thyroiditis may be difficult. The presence of TPOAb points to painless chronic autoimmune thyroiditis, whereas a firm thyroid and brief history suggest the painless variant of subacute thyroiditis. Treatment of *thyrotoxicosis factitia* consists of withdrawing the offending medication. Psychiatric consultation is often required.

Hamburger Thyrotoxicosis

An unusual form of exogenous thyrotoxicosis occurred in the midwestern portion of the United States in 1984 and 1985. The source was the inclusion of large quantities of bovine thyroid in ground beef preparations.[276] When the slaughtering practices were changed, this condition disappeared. Such a possibility, although remote, should be considered, especially if the clinician is confronted with epidemic exogenous thyrotoxicosis.

Thyrotoxicosis Due to Extrathyroidal Tissue

Struma Ovarii

Thyroid tissue may be present in 5% to 10% of ovarian teratomas and occasionally such foci are hyperfunctional.[277,278] About 5% to 10% of these tumors are bilateral. While thyrotoxicosis is unusual, it may occur in as many as 8% to 10% of all patients. Rarely, males with germ cell tumors may also develop hCG-induced hyperthyroidism.[279]

Clinical Presentation

Patients present with variable degrees of thyrotoxicosis but without goiter and generally have lower abdominal symptoms such as a pain or a mass. Rarely, ascites is present. Laboratory studies show reduced TSH and increased free T_4 of a variable degree, but the RAIU is low. The thyroglobulin may be elevated, particularly if the teratoma is malignant and has metastasized to the peritoneum. Abdominal CT or MRI shows a multilocular ovarian mass or masses. Rarely, a struma ovarii is accompanied by Graves' disease.[280]

Treatment

The patient should be rendered euthyroid if thyrotoxicosis is significant, followed by removal of the involved ovary or ovaries. Therapeutic radioiodine will be required for metastatic disease after ablation of the normal thyroid gland.[281,282]

Metastatic Thyroid Carcinoma

In general, thyroid carcinomas are made up of poorly functioning tissue. On occasion, follicular thyroid carcinomas will have sufficient function that, when combined with the total mass of the metastases, results in an elevation in serum free T_4 or T_3. Typically, such a course is a complication of a previously diagnosed lesion (see Chapter 13).[283] The symptoms of thyrotoxicosis will vary and the metastatic disease is usually obvious from radiologic studies. On occasion, the presentation may be confusing if the patient is receiving TSH-suppressive therapy and diagnosis will require its discontinuation. Even so, TSH remains suppressed and the serum free T_4 is elevated. Treatment of this condition is typical for that of thyroid carcinoma and is described in Chapter 13. In patients with thyrotoxicosis due to metastatic tumor, serum thyroglobulin is quite elevated indicating that the thyrotoxicosis is caused by thyroidal tissue that is not located in the neck. An RAIU study during the thyrotoxic phase will show no neck uptake due to TSH suppression even if the thyroid is still present.

SUBCLINICAL (MILD) HYPERTHYROIDISM

Definition

As mentioned in Chapter 10, the availability of sensitive assays for TSH have allowed recognition of a syndrome, *subclinical thyrotoxicosis,* in which there are no signs or symptoms of thyrotoxicosis but the serum TSH is subnormal despite normal serum free thyroid hormone concentrations. Although the term is somewhat of a misnomer, in that it is defined by biochemical characteristics, all endocrinologists have a concept of what is meant by the term. Nonetheless, it is still not clear whether the fact that a patient is classified as having subclinical thyrotoxicosis is because our ability to detect physiologic evidence of excess thyroid hormone on a chronic basis is less sensitive than is our capacity to measure TSH. This is further complicated by the fact that the hypothalamic-pituitary axis is sensitive to both serum free T_4 and T_3, whereas the peripheral tissues such as the heart primarily sense the free T_3 (see Chapter 10).[284,285] It is easy to assume, given the wide normal range for free thyroid hormone concentrations, that an individual with a low normal free T_4 set-point for TSH secretion would have a reduced TSH if that concentration were increased by 50% but still remained within the normal range. In fact, in patients with primary hypothyroidism but normal TSH levels, small additional quantities of levothyroxine will decrease TSH below normal without a supranormal free T_4.[284] On the other hand, in the now classic studies in the Framingham population older than 60 years of age, the cumulative incidence of atrial fibrillation over 10 years was 28% in patients with a serum TSH concentration of 0.1 mU/L or less, whereas it was only 11% in those with serum TSH concentrations falling between 0.1 and 0.4 mU/L. The latter was only slightly higher than that in the normal population.[10,286] Other studies have shown similar results.[287,288]

Bone density is another end-point for such studies because it is well known that excess thyroid hormone causes a net resorption of cortical bone. Several studies demonstrate lower bone density in patients with *subclinical thyrotoxicosis*, although others do not.[36] These results illustrate the conundrum of the term *subclinical* because, by definition, such patients should not have any clinical abnormalities associated with thyrotoxicosis.[289] Hence, we prefer the term "mild."

This is a subject of considerable interest in that the condition is much more common than overt thyrotoxicosis (e.g., 0.7% of the population in NHANES III) and has broad implications with respect to the cost of diagnosis, treatment, and follow-up.[52] In general, normalization of thyroid function in postmenopausal women with subclinical thyrotoxicosis seems to improve bone density and certain aspects of cardiac function.[290-292] These data would generally favor treatment in the older population but unfortunately there are no large, long-term, randomized studies to allow evidence-based conclusions as to the risk/benefit ratio.

Diagnosis

The diagnosis of subclinical thyrotoxicosis requires tests revealing several subnormal TSH concentration results spaced months apart in the presence of normal free thyroid hormone concentrations. Several studies show that suppressed TSH can normalize spontaneously over several years, particularly in patients without nodular goiter.[293,294] As with overt thyrotoxicosis, there are two sources of excess thyroid hormones: endogenous and exogenous. In a study of more than 25,000 individuals attending health fairs in Colorado, 58% of those with a TSH less than 0.3 mU/L were receiving thyroid hormones.[295] If this is not being done intentionally for the treatment of persistent thyroid carcinoma, it is easily treated by more careful monitoring of the levothyroxine dosage using serum TSH concentrations. Endogenous subclinical thyrotoxicosis has the same causes as for overt thyrotoxicosis (see earlier text). In the population older than 60 years of age, multinodular goiter is a more likely cause of thyrotoxicosis than it is in younger individuals.

Treatment

There are insufficient data to conclude that individuals with serum TSH concentrations greater than 0.1 mU/L will benefit from treatment.[296] In evaluating the decision for or against treatment of individuals with persistently subnormal TSH concentrations less than 0.1 mU/L (with normal free thyroid hormones), the patient should be evaluated for the conditions that may benefit from this (Table 11–7) as well as determining its cause.

TABLE 11–7 INDICATIONS FOR TREATMENT OF PERSISTENT SUBCLINICAL HYPERTHYROIDISM

Postmenopausal osteoporosis
Rheumatic valvular disease with left atrial enlargement or atrial fibrillation
Recent-onset atrial fibrillation or recurrent cardiac arrhythmias
Congestive heart failure
Angina pectoris
Infertility or menstrual disorders
Nonspecific symptoms such as fatigue, nervousness, depression, or gastrointestinal disorders, especially in patients older than 60 years of age (consider therapeutic trial)

In the elderly, postmenopausal osteoporosis and various cardiac diseases are the primary indications for which treatment should be considered. Infertility or menstrual disorders are important in young women.

Identifying the cause of the hyperthyroidism allows assessment of the potential risks of treatment. At one extreme, the treatment of mild Graves' disease with radioiodine usually causes hypothyroidism, whereas this typically does not occur in patients with multinodular toxic goiter. Thus in an asymptomatic patient with mild Graves' disease, watchful waiting for several years, awaiting a possible spontaneous remission, may be one course of action.[294] On the other hand, patients with subclinical thyrotoxicosis due to toxic nodular goiter or a solitary hyperfunctioning adenoma can often be treated with a single dose of radioactive iodine with a low risk of subsequent hypothyroidism. As always, the rationale for treatment, its risks and benefits, should be carefully discussed with the patient and one should be guided by common sense and not by the principle of simply treating an abnormal test result.[297-299]

REFERENCES

1. Davis PJ, Davis FB. Hyperthyroidism in patients over the age of 60 years—clinical features in 85 patients. Medicine 1974;53:161-181.
2. Kahaly GJ, Dillmann WH. Thyroid hormone action in the heart. Endocr Rev 2005;26:704-728.
3. Burggraaf J, Tulen JH, Lalezari S, et al. Sympathovagal imbalance in hyperthyroidism. Am J Physiol Endocrinol Metab 2001;281: E190-E195.
4. Kahaly GJ, Wagner S, Nieswandt J, et al. Stress echocardiography in hyperthyroidism. J Clin Endocrinol Metab 1999;84:2308-2313.
5. Fazio S, Palmieri EA, Lombardi G, et al. Effects of thyroid hormone on the cardiovascular system. Recent Prog Horm Res 2004; 59:31-50.
6. Napoli R, Biondi B, Guardasole V, et al. Impact of hyperthyroidism and its correction on vascular reactivity in humans. Circulation 2001;104:3076-3080.
7. Brauman A, Rosenberg T, Gilboa Y, et al. Prevalence of mitral valve prolapse in chronic lymphocytic thyroiditis and nongoitrous hypothyroidism. Cardiology 1988;75:269-273.
8. Alvarado A, Ribeiro JP, Freitas FM, et al. Lack of association between thyroid function and mitral valve prolapse in Graves' disease. Braz J Med Biol Res 1990;23:133-139.
9. Northcote RJ, MacFarlane P, Kesson CM, et al. Continuous 24-hour electrocardiography in thyrotoxicosis before and after treatment. Am Heart J 1986;112:339-344.
10. Sawin CT, Geller A, Wolf PA, et al. Low serum thyrotropin concentrations as a risk factor for atrial fibrillation in older persons. N Engl J Med 1994;331:1249-1252.
11. Trivalle C, Doucet J, Chassagne P, et al. Differences in the signs and symptoms of hyperthyroidism in older and younger patients. J Am Geriatr Soc 1996;44:50-53.
12. Nakazawa HK, Sakurai K, Hamada N, et al. Management of atrial fibrillation in the post-thyrotoxic state. Am J Med 1982; 72:903-906.
13. Kahaly GJ, Nieswandt J, Mohr-Kahaly S. Cardiac risks of hyperthyroidism in the elderly. Thyroid 1998;8:1165-1169.
14. Petersen P, Hansen JM. Stroke in thyrotoxicosis with atrial fibrillation. Stroke 1988;19:15-18.
15. Nakazawa H, Lythall DA, Noh J, et al. Is there a place for the late cardioversion of atrial fibrillation? A long-term follow-up study of patients with post-thyrotoxic atrial fibrillation. Eur Heart J 2000;21:327-333.
16. Silva JE. The thermogenic effect of thyroid hormone and its clinical implications. Ann Intern Med 2003;139:205-213.
17. Coulombe P, Dussault JH, Walker P. Plasma catecholamine concentrations in hyperthyroidism and hypothyroidism. Metabolism 1976;25:973-979.
18. Palmieri EA, Fazio S, Palmieri V, et al. Myocardial contractility and total arterial stiffness in patients with overt hyperthyroidism: acute effects of betal-adrenergic blockade. Eur J Endocrinol 2004; 150:757-762.

19. Carvalho-Bianco SD, Kim B, Harney JW, et al. Chronic cardiac-specific thyrotoxicosis increases myocardial beta-adrenergic responsiveness. Mol Endocrinol 2004;18:1840-1849.
20. Ojamaa K, Klein I, Sabet A, et al. Changes in adenylyl cyclase isoforms as a mechanism for thyroid hormone modulation of cardiac beta-adrenergic receptor responsiveness. Metabolism 2000;49: 275-279.
21. Hellstrom L, Wahrenberg H, Reynisdottir S, et al. Catecholamine-induced adipocyte lipolysis in human hyperthyroidism. J Clin Endocrinol Metab 1997;82:159-166.
22. Marino M, Barbesino G, Pinchera A, et al. Increased frequency of euthyroid ophthalmopathy in patients with Graves' disease associated with myasthenia gravis. Thyroid 2000;10:799-802.
23. Yu Wai Man CY, Chinnery PF, Griffiths PG. Extraocular muscles have fundamentally distinct properties that make them selectively vulnerable to certain disorders. Neuromuscul Disord 2005; 15:17-23.
24. Ober KP. Thyrotoxic periodic paralysis in the United States. Report of 7 cases and review of the literature. Medicine (Baltimore) 1992;71:109-120.
25. Kodali VR, Jeffcote B, Clague RB. Thyrotoxic periodic paralysis: a case report and review of the literature. J Emerg Med 1999;17: 43-45.
26. Dias Da Silva MR, Cerutti JM, Arnaldi LA, et al. A mutation in the KCNE3 potassium channel gene is associated with susceptibility to thyrotoxic hypokalemic periodic paralysis. J Clin Endocrinol Metab 2002;87:4881-4884.
27. Gurlek A, Cobankara V, Bayraktar M. Liver tests in hyperthyroidism: effect of antithyroid therapy. J Clin Gastroenterol 1997;24: 180-183.
28. Myers JD, Brannon ES, Holland BC. A correlative study of the cardiac output and the hepatic circulation in hyperthyroidism. J Clin Invest 1950;29:1069-1077.
29. Wakasugi M, Wakao R, Tawata M, et al. Bone mineral density in patients with hyperthyroidism measured by dual energy X-ray absorptiometry. Clin Endocrinol (Oxf) 1993;38:283-286.
30. Wakasugi M, Wakao R, Tawata M, et al. Change in bone mineral density in patients with hyperthyroidism after attainment of euthyroidism by dual energy X-ray absorptiometry. Thyroid 1994;4: 179-182.
31. Bassett JH, Williams GR. The molecular actions of thyroid hormone in bone. Trends Endocrinol Metab 2003;14:356-364.
32. Mohan HK, Groves AM, Fogelman I, et al. Thyroid hormone and parathyroid hormone competing to maintain calcium levels in the presence of vitamin D deficiency. Thyroid 2004;14:789-791.
33. Wejda B, Hintze G, Katschinski B, et al. Hip fractures and the thyroid: a case-control study. J Intern Med 1995;237:241-247.
34. Hallengren B, Elmstahl B, Berglund J, et al. No increase in fracture incidence in patients treated for thyrotoxicosis in Malmo during 1970-74. A 20-year population-based follow-up. J Intern Med 1999;246:139-144.
35. Faber J, Galloe AM. Changes in bone mass during prolonged subclinical hyperthyroidism due to L-thyroxine treatment: a meta-analysis. Eur J Endocrinol 1994;130:350-356.
36. Bauer DC, Ettinger B, Nevitt MC, et al. Risk for fracture in women with low serum levels of thyroid-stimulating hormone. Ann Intern Med 2001;134:561-568.
37. Iqbal AA, Burgess EH, Gallina DL, et al. Hypercalcemia in hyperthyroidism: patterns of serum calcium, parathyroid hormone, and 1,25-dihydroxyvitamin D_3 levels during management of thyrotoxicosis. Endocr Pract 2003;9:517-521.
38. Godart V, Weynand B, Coche E, et al. Intense 18-fluorodeoxyglucose uptake by the thymus on PET scan does not necessarily herald recurrence of thyroid carcinoma. J Endocrinol Invest 2005;28:1024-1028.
39. Montella L, Caraglia M, Abbruzzese A, et al. Mediastinal images resembling thymus following 131-I treatment for thyroid cancer. Monaldi Arch Chest Dis 2005;63:114-117.
40. Erem C, Ersoz HO, Karti SS, et al. Telatar M. Blood coagulation and fibrinolysis in patients with hyperthyroidism. J Endocrinol Invest 2002;25:345-350.
41. Kurnik D, Loebstein R, Farfel Z, et al. Complex drug-drug-disease interactions between amiodarone, warfarin, and the thyroid gland. Medicine (Baltimore) 2004;83:107-113.
42. Taniyama M, Honma K, Ban Y. Urinary cortisol metabolites in the assessment of peripheral thyroid hormone action: application for diagnosis of resistance to thyroid hormone. Thyroid 1993;3: 229-233.
43. Stagnaro-Green A, Roman SH, Cobin RH, et al. Detection of at-risk pregnancy by means of highly sensitive assays for thyroid autoantibodies. JAMA 1990;264:1422-1426.
44. Meikle AW. The interrelationships between thyroid dysfunction and hypogonadism in men and boys. Thyroid 2004;14(suppl 1): S17-S25.
45. Tagawa N, Takano T, Fukata S, et al. Serum concentration of androstenediol and androstenediol sulfate in patients with hyperthyroidism and hypothyroidism. Endocr J 2001;48:345-354.
46. Parry CH. Collections from the Unpublished Medical Writings of the Late Caleb Hillier Parry. Diseases of the Heart. Enlargement of the Thyroid Gland in connection with Enlargement or Palpitation of the Heart. London: Underwoods Fleet-Street, 1825:111-129.
47. Rapoport B, McLachlan SM. Thyroid autoimmunity. J Clin Invest 2001;108:1253-1259.
48. Davies TF, Ando T, Lin RY, et al. Thyrotropin receptor-associated diseases: from adenomata to Graves disease. J Clin Invest 2005;115:1972-1983.
49. Martin A, Valentine M, Unger P, et al. Engraftment of human lymphocytes and thyroid tissue into Scid and Rag2-deficient mice: absent progression of lymphocytic infiltration. J Clin Endocrinol Metab 1994;79:716-723.
50. Weetman AP. The immunomodulatory effects of antithyroid drugs. Thyroid 1994;4:145-146.
51. McGregor AM, Petersen MM, Capiferri R, et al. Effects of radioiodine on thyrotrophin binding inhibiting immunoglobulins in Graves' disease. Clin Endocrinol 1979;11:437-444.
52. Hollowell JG, Staehling NW, Flanders WD, et al. Serum TSH, T(4), and thyroid antibodies in the United States population (1988 to 1994): National Health and Nutrition Examination Survey (NHANES III). J Clin Endocrinol Metab 2002;87:489-499.
53. Vanderpump MPJ, Tunbridge WMG, French JM, et al. The incidence of thyroid disorders in the community: a twenty-year follow-up of the Whickham survey. Clin Endocrinol 1995;43 55-68.
54. Shimojo N, Kohno Y, Yamaguchi K, et al. Induction of Graves-like disease in mice by immunization with fibroblasts transfected with the thyrotropin receptor and a class II molecule. Proc Natl Acad Sci U S A 1996;93:11074-11079.
55. Kita M, Ahmad L, Marians RC, et al. Regulation and transfer of a murine model of thyrotropin receptor antibody mediated Graves' disease. Endocrinology 1999;140:1392-1398.
56. Nagayama Y, Kita-Furuyama M, Ando T, et al. A novel murine model of Graves' hyperthyroidism with intramuscular injection of adenovirus expressing the thyrotropin receptor. J Immunol 2002;168:2789-2794.
57. Parkes AB, Kajita Y, Buckland PR, et al. Immunoprecipitation of TSH-TSH receptor complexes. Clinical Endocrinology 1985;22: 511-520.
58. Rees Smith B, McLachlan SM, Furmaniak J. Autoantibodies to the thyrotropin receptor. Endocr Rev 1988;9:106-121.
59. Costagliola S, Bonomi M, Morgenthaler NG, et al. Delineation of the discontinuous-conformational epitope of a monoclonal antibody displaying full in vitro and in vivo thyrotropin activity. Mol Endocrinol 2004;18:3020-3034.
60. Nunez MR, Sanders J, Jeffreys J, et al. Analysis of the thyrotropin receptor-thyrotropin interaction by comparative modeling. Thyroid 2004;14:991-1011.
61. Adams DD, Purves HD. Abnormal responses in the assay of thyrotropin. Proceedings of the University of Otago Medical School 1956;34:11-12.
62. Adams DD. The presence of an abnormal thyroid-stimulating hormone in the serum of some thyrotoxic patients. J Clin Endocrinol Metab 1958;18:699-712.
63. Kraiem Z, Lahat N, Glaser B, et al. Thyrotropin receptor blocking antibodies: incidence, characterization and in-vitro synthesis. Clin Endocrinol 1987;27:409-421.
64. Adams DD, Fastier FN, Howie JB, et al. Stimulation of the human thyroid by infusions of plasma containing LATS protector. J Clin Endocrinol Metab 1974;39:826-832.

65. Munro DS, Dirmikis SM, Humphries H, et al. The role of thyroid-stimulating immunoglobulins of Graves' disease in neonatal thyrotoxicosis. Br J Obstet Gynaecol 1978;85:837-843.
66. Zakarija MJ. Immunochemical characterization of the thyroid-stimulating antibody (TSab) of Graves' disease: evidence for restricted heterogeneity. J Clin Lab Immunol 1983;10:77-85.
67. Weetman AP, Yateman ME, Ealey PA, et al. Thyroid-stimulating antibody activity between different immunoglobulin G subclasses. J Clin Invest 1990;86:723-727.
68. Bolton J, Sanders J, Oda Y, et al. Measurement of thyroid-stimulating hormone receptor autoantibodies by ELISA. Clin Chem 1999;45:2285-2287.
69. Costagliola S, Morgenthaler NG, Hoermann R, et al. Second generation assay for thyrotropin receptor antibodies has superior diagnostic sensitivity for Graves' disease. J Clin Endocrinol Metab 1999;84:90-97.
70. Smith BR, Bolton J, Young S, et al. A new assay for thyrotropin receptor autoantibodies. Thyroid 2004;14:830-835.
71. Davies TF, Yeo PP, Evered DC, et al. Value of thyroid-stimulating-antibody determinations in predicting short-term thyrotoxic relapse in Graves' disease. Lancet 1977;1:1181-1182.
72. Davies TF. Thyroid-stimulating antibodies predict hyperthyroidism. J Clin Endocr Metab 1998;83:3777-3781.
73. Mackenzie WA, Schwartz AE, Friedman EW, et al. Intrathyroidal T cell clones from patients with autoimmune thyroid disease. J Clin Endocrinol Metab 1987;64:818-824.
74. Dayan CM, Londei M, Corcoran AE, et al. Autoantigen recognition by thyroid-infiltrating T cells in Graves disease. Proc Natl Acad Sci U S A 1991;88:7415-7419.
75. Grubeck Loebenstein B, Turner M, Pirich K, et al. CD4+ T-cell clones from autoimmune thyroid tissue cannot be classified according to their lymphokine production. Scand J Immunol 1990;32:433-440.
76. Valmori D, Merlo A, Souleimanian NE, et al. A peripheral circulating compartment of natural naive CD4 Tregs. J Clin Invest 2005;115:1953-1962.
77. Verginis P, Li HS, Carayanniotis G. Tolerogenic semimature dendritic cells suppress experimental autoimmune thyroiditis by activation of thyroglobulin-specific CD4+CD25+ T cells. J Immunol 2005;174:7433-7439.
78. Li HS, Carayanniotis G. Detection of thyroglobulin mRNA as truncated isoform(s) in mouse thymus. Immunology 2005;115:85-89.
79. Murakami M, Hosoi Y, Negishi T, et al. Thymic hyperplasia in patients with Graves' disease. Identification of thyrotropin receptors in human thymus. J Clin Invest 1996;98:2228-2234.
80. Tomer Y, Davies TF. Infection, thyroid disease and autoimmunity. Endocr Rev 1993;14:107-120.
81. Rapoport B, Alsabeh R Aftergood D, et al. 2000. Elephantiasic pretibial myxedema: insight into and a hypothesis regarding the pathogenesis of the extrathyroidal manifestations of Graves' disease. Thyroid 2000;10:685-692.
82. Horwitz MS, Bradley LM, Harbertson J, et al. Diabetes induced by Coxsackie virus: initiation by bystander damage and not molecular mimicry [see comments]. Nat Med 1998;4:781-785.
83. Wen L, Wong FS. How can the innate immune system influence autoimmunity in type 1 diabetes and other autoimmune disorders? Crit Rev Immunol 2005;25:225-250.
84. De Riu A, Martin A, Valentine M, et al. Graves' disease thyroid transplants in Scid mice: persistent selectivity in hTcR V alpha gene family use. Autoimunity 1994;19:271-277.
85. Wickham S, Carr DJ. Molecular mimicry versus bystander activation: herpetic stromal keratitis. Autoimmunity 2004;37:393-397.
86. Srinivasappa J, Saegusa J, Prabhakar BS, et al. Molecular mimicry: frequency of reactivity of monoclonal antiviral antibodies with normal tissues. J Virol 1986;57:397-401.
87. Haspel MV, Onodrera T, Prabhakar BS, et al. Multiple organ-reactive monoclonal autoantibodies. Nature 1983;304:73-76.
88. Wenzel BE, Strieder TM, Gaspar E, et al. Chronic infection with *Yersinia enterocolitica* in patients with clinical or latent hyperthyroidism. Adv Exp Med Biol 2003;529:463-466.
89. Gangi E, Kapatral V, El-Azami El-Idrissi, et al. Characterization of a recombinant *Yersinia enterocolitica* lipoprotein; implications for its role in autoimmune response against thyrotropin receptor. Autoimmunity 2004;37:515-520.
90. Benvenga S, Guarneri F, Vaccaro M, et al. Homologies between proteins of *Borrelia burgdorferi* and thyroid autoantigens. Thyroid 2004;14:964-966.
91. Mirakian R, Hammond LJ, Bottazzo GF. Pathogenesis of thyroid autoimmunity: the Bottazzo-Feldmann hypothesis. Immunol Today 1998;19:97-98.
92. Kawakami Y, Kuzuya N, Watanabe T, et al. Induction of experimental thyroiditis in mice by recombinant interferon gamma administration. Acta Endocrinol (Copenh) 1990;122:41-48.
93. Moudgil KD, Sercarz EE. Understanding crypticity is the key to revealing the pathogenesis of autoimmunity. Trends Immunol 2005;26:355-359.
94. Davies TF, Greenberg D, Tomer Y. The genetics of the autoimmune thyroid diseases. Annales D Endocrinologie 2003;64:28-30.
95. Villanueva R, Greenberg DA, Davies TF, et al. Sibling recurrence risk in autoimmune thyroid disease. Thyroid 2003;13:761-764.
96. Tomer Y, Greenberg DA, Barbesino G, et al. CTLA-4 and not CD28 is a susceptibility gene for thyroid autoantibody production. J Clin Endocrinol Metab 2001;86:1687-1693.
97. Brix TH, Christensen K, Holm NV, et al. A population-based study of Graves' disease in Danish twins. Clinical Endocrinology 1998; 48:397-400.
98. Barbesino G, Tomer Y, Concepcion ES, et al. Linkage analysis of candidate genes in autoimmune thyroid disease: 1. Selected immunoregulatory genes. J Clin Endocrinol Metab 1998;83: 1580-1584.
99. Ban Y, Concepcion ES, Villanueva R, et al. Analysis of immune regulatory genes in familial and sporadic Graves' disease. J Clin Endocrinol Metab 2004;89:4562-4568.
100. Samarkos M, Vaiopoulos G. The role of infections in the pathogenesis of autoimmune diseases. Curr Drug Targets Inflamm Allergy 2005;4:99-103.
101. Olson JK, Croxford JL, Miller SD. Virus-induced autoimmunity: potential role of viruses in initiation, perpetuation, and progression of T-cell-mediated autoimmune disease. Viral Immunol 2001; 14:227-250.
102. Carter JK, Smith RE. Rapid induction of hypothyroidism by an avian leukosis virus. Infect Immun 1983;40:795-805.
103. Matsuda T, Tomita M, Uchihara JN, et al. Human T cell leukemia virus type I-infected patients with Hashimoto's thyroiditis and Graves' disease. J Clin Endocrinol Metab 2005;90:5704-5710.
104. Irwin M. Stress-induced immune suppression: role of brain corticotropin releasing hormone and autonomic nervous system mechanisms. Adv Neuroimmunol 1994;4:29-47.
105. Marshall GD. Neuroendocrine mechanisms of immune dysregulation: applications to allergy and asthma. Ann Allergy Asthma Immunol 2004;93:S11-S17.
106. Amino N, Tada H, Hidaka Y, et al. Therapeutic controversy: screening for postpartum thyroiditis. J Clin Endocrinol Metab 1999;84: 1813-1821.
107. Ansar AS, Young PR, Penhale WJ. Beneficial effect of testosterone in the treatment of chronic autoimmune thyroiditis in rats. J Immunol 1986;136:143-147.
108. Fassler R, Dietrich H, Kromer G, et al. The role of testosterone in spontaneous autoimmune thyroiditis of Obese strain (OS) chickens. J Autoimmun 1988;1:97-108.
109. Tomer Y, Davies TF. Searching for the autoimmune thyroid disease susceptibility genes: From gene mapping to gene function. Endocr Rev 2003;24:694-717.
110. Chow JC, Yen Z, Ziesche SM, et al. Silencing of the mammalian X chromosome. Annu Rev Genomics Hum Genet 2005;6:69-92.
111. Heiberg BT, Knudsen GP, Kristiansen M, et al. High frequency of skewed X chromosome inactivation in females with autoimmune thyroid disease: a possible explanation for the female predisposition to thyroid autoimmunity. J Clin Endocrinol Metab 2005;90: 6332-6333.
112. Mestman JH. Hyperthyroidism in pregnancy. Endocrinol Metab Clin North Am 1998;27:127-149.
113. Anselmo J, Cao D, Karrison T, et al. Fetal loss associated with excess thyroid hormone exposure. JAMA 2004;292:691-695.
114. Aluvihare VR, Kallikourdis M, Betz AG. Tolerance, suppression and the fetal allograft. J Mol Med 2005;83:88-96.
115. Stagnaro-Green A, Roman SH, Cobin RH, et al. A prospective study of lymphocyte-initiated immunosuppression in normal pregnancy:

evidence of a T-cell etiology for postpartum thyroid dysfunction. J Clin Endocrinol Metab 1992;74:645-653.
116. Jansson R, Dahlberg PA, Winsa B, et al. The postpartum period constitutes an important risk for the development of clinical Graves' disease in young women. Acta Endocrinol 1987;116: 321-325.
117. Bartalena L, Bogazzi F, Martino E. Amiodarone-induced thyrotoxicosis: a difficult diagnostic and therapeutic challenge. Clin Endocrinol (Oxf) 2002;56:23-24.
118. Basaria S, Cooper DS. Amiodarone and the thyroid. Am J Med 2005;118:706-714.
119. DeGroot L. Effects of irradiation on the thyroid gland. Adolesc Endocrinol 1993;22:607.
120. Huysmans D, Hermus A, Edelbrook M, et al. Autoimmune hyperthyroidism occurring late after radioiodine treatment for volume reduction of large multinodular goiters. Thyroid 1997;7:535-539.
121. Pacini F, Vorontsova T, Molinaro E, et al. Prevalence of thyroid autoantibodies in children and adolescents from Belarus exposed to the Chernobyl radioactive fallout. Lancet 1998;352:763-766.
122. Vermiglio F, Castagna MG, Volnova E, et al. Post-Chernobyl increased prevalence of humoral thyroid autoimmunity in children and adolescents from a moderately iodine-deficient area in Russia. Thyroid 1999;9:781-786.
123. Vykhovanets EV, Chernyshov VP, Slukvin I, et al. 131-I dose-dependent thyroid autoimmune disorders in children living around Chernobyl. Clin Immunol Immunopathol 1997;84:251-259.
124. Bartalena L, Marcocci C, Tanda ML, et al. An update on medical management of Graves' ophthalmopathy. J Endocrinol Invest 2005;28:469-478.
125. Prabhakar BS, Bahn RS, Smith TJ. Current perspective on the pathogenesis of Graves' disease and ophthalmopathy. Endocr Rev 2003;24:802-835.
126. Feldon SE, Park DJ, O'Loughlin CW, et al. Autologous T-lymphocytes stimulate proliferation of orbital fibroblasts derived from patients with Graves' ophthalmopathy. Invest Ophthalmol Vis Sci 2005;46:3913-3921.
127. Grubeck-Loebenstein B, Trieb K, Holter W, et al. Retrobulbar T cells from patients with Graves' ophthalmopathy are CD8+ and specifically autologous fibroblasts. J Clin Invest 1993;93: 2738-2743.
128. Mori S, Yoshikawa N, Tokoro T, et al. Studies of retroorbital tissue xenografts from patients with Graves' ophthalmopathy in severe combined immunodeficient (SCID) mice: detection of thyroid-stimulating antibody. Thyroid 1996;6:275-281.
129. Sanders J, Allen F, Jeffreys J, et al. Characteristics of a monoclonal antibody to the thyrotropin receptor that acts as a powerful thyroid-stimulating autoantibody antagonist. Thyroid 2005;15: 672-682.
130. Gianoukakis AG, Douglas RS, King CS, et al. IgG from patients with Graves' disease induces IL-16 and RANTES expression in cultured human thyrocytes: a putative mechanism for T cell infiltration of the thyroid in autoimmune disease. Endocrinology 2006;147: 1941-1949.
131. Villanueva R, Inzerillo AM, Tomer Y, et al. Limited genetic susceptibility to severe Graves' ophthalmopathy: no role for CTLA-4 but evidence for an environmental etiology. Thyroid 2000;10:791-798.
132. Bertelsen JB, Hegedus L. Cigarette smoking and the thyroid. Thyroid 1994;4:327-331.
133. Wood LC, Ingbar SH. Hypothyroidism as a late sequela in patients with Graves' disease treated with antithyroid agents. J Clin Invest 1979;64:1429-1436.
133a. Fatourechi V, Pajouhi M, Fransway AF. Dermopathy of Graves disease (pretibial myxedema). Review of 150 cases. Medicine (Baltimore) 1994;1:1-7.
134. Marks AD, Bertram BJ, Channick J, et al. Chronic thyroiditis and mitral valve prolapse. Ann Intern Med 1995;102:479-483.
135. Wartofsky L. Classification of eye changes of Graves' disease. Thyroid 1992;3:235-236.
136. Fledelius HC, Zimmermann-Belsing T, Feldt-Rasmussen U. Ultrasonically measured horizontal eye muscle thickness in thyroid associated orbitopathy: cross-sectional and longitudinal aspects in a Danish series. Acta Ophthalmol Scand 2003;81:143-150.
137. Mechanick JI, Davies TF. Medical management of hyperthyroidism: theoretical and practical aspects. In Falk SA, editor. Thyroid Disease: Endocrinology, Surgery, Nuclear Medicine and Radiotherapy. New York: Lippincott-Raven, 1997:253-296.
138. Feldt-Rasmussen U, Schleusner H, Carayon P. Meta-analysis evaluation of the impact of thyrotropin receptor antibodies on long term remission after medical therapy of Graves' disease. J Clin Endocrinol Metab 1994;78:98-102.
139. Singer PA, Cooper DS, Levy E, et al. Treatment guidelines for patients with hyperthyroidism and hypothyroidism. JAMA 1995; 273:808-812.
140. Cooper DS. Antithyroid drugs. N Engl J Med 2005;352:905-917.
141. Abuid J, Larsen PR. Triiodothyronine and thyroxine in hyperthyroidism. Comparison of the acute changes during therapy with antithyroid agents. J Clin Invest 1974;54:201-208.
142. Maia AL, Kim BW, Huang SA, et al. Type 2 iodothyronine deiodinase is the major source of plasma T3 in euthyroid humans. J Clin Invest 2005;115:2524-2533.
143. Laurberg P, Vestergaard H, Nielsen S et al. Sources of circulating 3,5,3′—triiodothyronine in hyperthyroidism estimated after blocking of type 1 and type 2 iodothyronine deiodinases. J Clin Endocrinol Metab 2007; 92:2149–2156.
144. Stassi G, Zeuner A, Di Liberto, et al. Fas-FasL in Hashimoto's thyroiditis. J.Clin.Immunol. 2001;21:19-23.
145. Mitsiades N, Poulaki V, Tseleni-Balafouta S, et al. Fas ligand expression in thyroid follicular cells from patients with thionamide-treated Graves' disease. Thyroid 2001;11:605-606.
146. Larsen PR. Thyroidal triiodothyronine and thyroxine in Graves' disease: correlation with presurgical treatment, thyroid status, and iodine content. J Clin Endocrinol Metab 1975;41:1098-1104.
147. Izumi M, Larsen PR. Triiodothyronine, thyroxine, and iodine in purified thyroglobulin from patients with Graves' disease. J Clin Invest 1977;59:1105-1112.
148. Romaldini JH, Bromberg N, Werner RS, et al. Comparison of effects of high and low dosage regimens of antithyroid drugs in the management of Graves' hyperthyroidism. J Clin Endocrinol Metab 1983;57:563-570.
149. McIver B, Rae P, Beckett G, et al. Lack of effect of thyroxine in patients with Graves' hyperthyroidism who are treated with an antithyroid drug. N Engl J Med 1996;334:220-224.
150. Rittmaster RS, Abbott EC, Douglas R, et al. Effect of methimazole with or without L-thyroxine, on remission rates in Graves' disease. J Clin Endocrinol Metab 1998;83:814-818.
151. Davies TF, Roti E, Braverman LE, et al. Thyroid controversy—stimulating antibodies. J Clin Endocrinol Metab 1998;83: 3777-3785.
152. Ban Y, Greenberg DA, Concepcion E, et al. Amino acid substitutions in the thyroglobulin gene are associated with susceptibility to human and murine autoimmune thyroid disease. Proc Natl Acad Sci U S A 2003;100:15119-15124.
153. Schleusener H, Peters H, Fischer C, et al. [What is the recurrence rate for Basedow's disease treated with thyrostatic agents. Answers from a prospective study.] Schweiz Med Wochenschr 1990;120: 769-771.
154. Harper L, Chin L, Daykin J, et al. Propylthiouracil and carbimazole associated-antineutrophil cytoplasmic antibodies (ANCA) in patients with Graves' disease. Clin Endocrinol (Oxf) 2004;60: 671-675.
155. Emerson CH, Anderson AJ, Howard WJ, et al. Serum thyroxine and triiodothyronine concentrations during iodide treatment of hyperthyroidism. J Clin Endocrinol Metab 1975;40:33-36.
156. Braga M, Cooper DS. Clinical review 129: oral cholecystographic agents and the thyroid. J Clin Endocrinol Metab 2001;86: 1853-1860.
157. Lazarus JH, Richards AR, Addison GM, et al. Treatment of thyrotoxicosis with lithium carbonate. Lancet 1974;2:1160-1163.
158. Werga-Kjellman P, Zedenius J, Tallstedt L, et al. Surgical treatment of hyperthyroidism: a ten-year experience. Thyroid 2001;11: 187-192.
159. Chang DC, Wheeler MH, Woodcock JP, et al. The effect of preoperative Lugol's iodine on thyroid blood flow in patients with Graves' hyperthyroidism. Surgery 1987;102:1055-1061.
160. Rangaswamy M, Padhy AK, Gopinath PG, et al. Effect of Lugol's iodine on the vascularity of thyroid gland in hyperthyroidism. Nucl Med Commun 1989;10:679-684.

161. Toft AD, Irvine WJ, Sinclair I, et al. Thyroid function after surgical treatment of thyrotoxicosis. A report of 100 cases treated with propranolol before operation. N Engl J Med 1978;298:643-647.
162. Franklyn JA, Maisonneuve P, Sheppard M, et al. Cancer incidence and mortality after radioiodine treatment for hyperthyroidism: a population-based cohort study. Lancet 1999;353:2111-2115.
163. Franklyn JA, Sheppard MC, Maisonneuve P. Thyroid function and mortality in patients treated for hyperthyroidism. JAMA 2005;294:71-80.
164. Cheetham TD, Wraight P, Hughes IA, et al. Radioiodine treatment of Graves' disease in young people. Horm Res 1998;49:258-262.
165. Razvi S, Basu A, McIntyre EA, et al. Low failure rate of fixed administered activity of 400 MBq ^{131}I with pre-treatment with carbimazole for thyrotoxicosis: the Gateshead Protocol. Nucl Med Commun 2004;25:675-682.
166. Alexander EK, Larsen PR. High dose of (131)I therapy for the treatment of hyperthyroidism caused by Graves' disease. J Clin Endocrinol Metab 2002;87:1073-1077.
167. Nakazato N, Yoshida K, Mori K, et al. Antithyroid drugs inhibit radioiodine-induced increases in thyroid autoantibodies in hyperthyroid Graves' disease. Thyroid 1999;9:775-779.
168. Tuttle RM, Patience T, Budd S. Treatment with propylthiouracil before radioactive iodine therapy is associated with a higher treatment failure rate than therapy with radioactive iodine alone in Graves' disease. Thyroid 1995;5:243-247.
169. Sabri O, Zimny M, Schreckenberger M, et al. Radioiodine therapy in Graves' disease patients with large diffuse goiters treated with or without carbimazole at the time of radioiodine therapy. Thyroid 1999;9:1181-1188.
170. Dickman PW, Holm LE, Lundell G, et al. Thyroid cancer risk after thyroid examination with 131I: a population-based cohort study in Sweden. Int J Cancer 2003;106:580-587.
171. Moysich KB, Menezes RJ, Michalek AM. Chernobyl-related ionising radiation exposure and cancer risk: an epidemiological review. Lancet Oncol 2002;3:269-279.
172. Nikiforov Y, Heffess C, Korzenko A, et al. Characteristics of follicular tumors and nonneoplastic thyroid lesions in children and adolescents exposed to radiation as a result of the Chernobyl disaster. Cancer 1995;76:900.
173. Gavrilin Y, Khrouch V, Shinkarev S, et al. Individual thyroid dose estimation for a case-control study of Chernobyl-related thyroid cancer among children of Belarus—Part I: I-131, short-lived radioiodines (I-132, I-133, I-135), and short-lived radiotelluriums (Te-131M and Te-132). Health Physics 2004;86:565-585.
174. Metso S, Jaatinen P, Huhtala H, et al. Long-term follow-up study of radioiodine treatment of hyperthyroidism. Clin Endocrinol (Oxf) 2004;61:641-648.
175. Rubio IG, Perone BH, Silva MN, et al. Human recombinant TSH preceding a therapeutic dose of radioiodine for multinodular goiters has no significant effect in the surge of TSH-receptor and TPO antibodies. Thyroid 2005;15:134-139.
176. Harvey RD, Metclafe RA, Morteo C, et al. Acute pre-tibial myxedema following radioiodine therapy for thyrotoxic Graves' disease. Clin Endocrinol 1995;42:657-660.
177. Bartalena L, Marcocci C, Bogazzi F, et al. Use of corticosteroids to prevent progression of Graves' ophthalmopathy after radioiodine therapy for hyperthyroidism. N Engl J Med 1989;321:1349-1352.
178. Tallestedt L, Lundell G, Torring O, et al. Occurrence of ophthalmopathy after treatment for Graves' disease. N Engl J Med 1992;326:1733-1738.
179. Gorman CA. Therapeutic controversies. Radioiodine therapy does not aggravate Graves' ophthalmopathy. J Clin Endocrinol Metab 1995;80:340-342.
180. Wartofsky L. Therapeutic controversies. Summation, commentary, and overview: concerns over aggravation of Graves' ophthalmopathy by radioactive iodine treatment and the use of retrobulbar radiation therapy. J Clin Endocrinol Metab 1995;80:347-349.
181. Gorman CA. Radioiodine and pregnancy. Thyroid 1999;9: 721-726.
182. Dale J, Daykin J, Holder R, et al. Weight gain following treatment of hyperthyroidism. Clin Endocrinol (Oxf) 2001;55:233-239.
183. Wiersinga WM, Bartalena L. Epidemiology and prevention of Graves' ophthalmopathy. Thyroid 2002;12:855-860.
184. Perros P, Crombie AL, Kendall-Taylor P. Natural history of thyroid associated ophthalmopathy. Clin Endocrinol 1995;42:45-50.
185. Bartley GB, Fatourechi V, Kadrmas EF, et al. Chronology of Graves' ophthalmopathy in an incidence cohort. Am J Ophthalmol 1996;121:426-434.
186. Wiersinga WM, Prummel MF. An evidence-based approach to the treatment of Graves' ophthalmopathy. Endocrinol Metab Clin North Am 2000;29:297-319, vi-vii.
186a. Kahaly GJ, Pitz S, Hommel G, Dittmar M. Randomized, single blind trial of intravenous versus oral steroid monotherapy in Graves' orbitopathy. J Clin Endocrinol Metab 2005;90:5234-5240.
187. Beckendorf V, Maalouf T, George JL, et al. Place of radiotherapy in the treatment of Graves' orbitopathy. Int J Radiat Oncol Biol Phys 1999;43:805-815.
188. Perros P, Krassas GE. Orbital irradiation for thyroid-associated orbitopathy: conventional dose, low dose or no dose? Clin. Endocrinol.(Oxf) 2002;56:689-691.
189. Gorman CA, Garrity JA, Fatourechi V, et al. The aftermath of orbital radiotherapy for Graves' ophthalmopathy. Ophthalmology 2002;109:2100-2107.
190. Gorman CA, Garrity JA, Fatourechi V, et al. A prospective, randomized, double-blind, placebo-controlled study of orbital radiotherapy for Graves' ophthalmopathy. Ophthalmology 2001;108: 1523-1534.
191. Rose JG Jr, Burkat CN, Boxrud CA. Diagnosis and management of thyroid orbitopathy. Otolaryngol Clin North Am 2005;38: 1043-1074.
192. Boulos PR, Hardy I. Thyroid-associated orbitopathy: a clinicopathologic and therapeutic review. Curr Opin Ophthalmol 2004;15: 389-400.
193. Sridama V, DeGroot LJ. Treatment of Graves' disease and the course of ophthalmopathy. Am J Med 1989;87:70-73.
194. Jarhult J, Rudberg C, Larsson E, et al. Graves' disease with moderate-severe endocrine ophthalmopathy-long term results of a prospective, randomized study of total or subtotal thyroid resection. Thyroid 2005;15:1157-1164.
195. Fatourechi V. Pretibial myxedema: pathophysiology and treatment options. Am J Clin Dermatol 2005;6:295-309.
196. Chung-Leddon J. Pretibial myxedema. Dermatol Online J 2001; 7:18.
197. Bianco AC, Salvatore D, Gereben B, et al. Biochemistry, cellular and molecular biology and physiological roles of the iodothyronine selenodeiodinases. Endocr Rev 2002;23:38-89.
197a. Laurberg P, Vestergaard H, Nielsen S, Christensen SE, Seefeldt T, Helleberg K. Sources of circulating T3 in hyperthyroidism estimated after blocking of type 1 and type 2 iodothyronine deiodinases. J Clin Endocrinol Metab 2007: (in press).
198. Croxson MS, Hall TD, Nicoloff JT. Combination drug therapy for treatment of hyperthyroid Graves' disease. J Clin Endocrinol Metab 1977;45:623-630.
199. Larsen PR. Salicylate-induced increases in free triiodothyronine in human serum. Evidence of inhibition of triiodothyronine binding to thyroxine-binding globulin and thyroxine-binding prealbumin. J Clin Invest 1972;51:1125-1134.
200. Davies TF. The thyroid immunology of the postpartum period. Thyroid 1999;9:675-684.
201. Lazarus JH. Thyroid disease in pregnancy and childhood. Minerva Endocrinol 2005;30:71-87.
202. Stagnaro-Green A, Glinoer D. Thyroid autoimmunity and the risk of miscarriage. Best Pract Res Clin Endocrinol Metab 2004;18: 167-181.
203. Weetman AP. The immunology of pregnancy. Thyroid 1999;9: 643-646.
204. Somerset DA, Zheng Y, Kilby MD, et al. Normal human pregnancy is associated with an elevation in the immune suppressive CD25+ CD4+ regulatory T-cell subset. Immunology 2004;112:38-43.
205. Evans PC, Lambert N, Maloney S, et al. Long-term fetal microchimerism in peripheral blood mononuclear cell subsets in healthy women and women with scleroderma. Blood 1999;93:2033-2037.
206. Ando T, Davies TF. Clinical review 160: postpartum autoimmune thyroid disease: the potential role of fetal microchimerism. J Clin Endocrinol Metab 2003;88:2965-2971.
207. Lambert NC, Evans PC, Hashizumi TL, et al. Cutting edge: persistent fetal microchimerism in T lymphocytes is associated with HLA-DQA1*0501: implications in autoimmunity. J Immunol 2000; 164:5545-5548.

208. Ando T, Davies TF. Self-recognition and the role of fetal microchimerism. Best Pract Res Clin Endocrinol Metab 2004;18:197-211.
209. Amino N, Kuro R, Tanizawa O, et al. Changes of serum antithyroid antibodies during and after pregnancy in autoimmune thyroid diseases. Clin Exp Immunol 1978;31:30-37.
210. Aluvihare VR, Kallikourdis M, Betz AG. Regulatory T cells mediate maternal tolerance to the fetus. Nat Immunol 2004;5:266-271.
211. Zakarija M, McKenzie JM. Pregnancy-associated changes in thyroid-stimulating antibody of Graves' disease and the relationship to neonatal hyperthyroidism. J Clin Endocrinol Metab 1983;57:1036-1040.
212. Mejias-Heredia A, Litchfield WR, Zurakowski D. Assessing the risk of neonatal Graves' disease using TSI measurements. 77th Meeting of the Endocrine Society 1995;P3:460.
213. Tamaki H, Amino N, Aozasa M, et al. Universal predictive criteria for neonatal overt thyrotoxicosis requiring treatment. Am J Perinatol 1988;5:152-158.
214. Luton D, Le Gac I, Vuillard E, et al. Management of Graves' disease during pregnancy: the key role of fetal thyroid gland monitoring. J Clin Endocrinol Metab 2005;90:6093-6098.
215. Glinoer D, De Nayer P, Bourdoux P, et al. Regulation of maternal thyroid during pregnancy. J Clin Endocrinol Metab 1990;71: 276-287.
216. Amino N, Tanizawa O, Mori H, et al. Aggravation of thyrotoxicosis in early pregnancy and after delivery in Graves' disease. J Clin Endocrinol Metab 1982;55:108-112.
217. Hershman JM. Human chorionic gonadotropin and the thyroid: hyperemesis gravidarum and trophoblastic tumors. Thyroid 1999;9:653-657.
218. LeBeau SO, Mandel SJ. Thyroid disorders during pregnancy. Endocrinol Metab Clin North Am 2006;35:117-136, vii.
219. Cheron RG, Kaplan M, Reed Larsen P, et al. Neonatal thyroid function after propylthiouracil therapy for maternal Graves' disease. N Engl J Med 1981;304:525-528.
220. Ochoa-Maya MR, Frates MC, Lee-Parritz A, et al. Resolution of fetal goiter after discontinuation of propylthiouracil in a pregnant woman with Graves' hyperthyroidism. Thyroid 1999;9:1111-1114.
221. Mortimer RH, Cannell GR, Addison RS, et al. Methimazole and propylthiouracil equally cross the perfused human term placental lobule. J Clin Endocrinol Metab 1997;82:3099-3102.
222. Haddow JE, Palomaki GE, Allan WC, et al. Maternal thyroid deficiency during pregnancy and subsequent neuropsychological development of the child. N Engl J Med 1999;341:549-555.
223. Milham S Jr. Scalp defects in infants of mothers treated for hyperthyroidism with methimazole or carbimazole during pregnancy. Teratology 1985;32:321.
224. Foulds N, Walpole I, Elmslie F, et al. Carbimazole embryopathy: an emerging phenotype. Am J Med Genet A 2005;132:130-135.
225. Mandel SJ, Cooper DS. The use of antithyroid drugs in pregnancy and lactation. J Clin Endocrinol Metab 2001;86:2354-2359.
226. Fisher DA. Fetal thyroid function: diagnosis and management of fetal thyroid disorders. Clin Obstet Gynecol 1997;40:16-31.
227. Petit KP, Nielsen HC. Chronic in utero beta-blockade alters fetal lung development. Dev Pharmacol Ther 1992;19:131-140.
228. Ray JG, Vermeulen MJ, Burrows EA, et al. Use of antihypertensive medications in pregnancy and the risk of adverse perinatal outcomes: McMaster Outcome Study of Hypertension in Pregnancy 2 (MOS HIP 2). BMC Pregnancy Childbirth 2001;1:6.
229. Momotani N, Hisaoka T, Noh J, et al. Effects of iodine on thyroid status of fetus versus mother in treatment of Graves' disease complicated by pregnancy. J Clin Endocrinol Metab 1992;75:738-744.
230. Klein RZ, Sargent JD, Larsen PR, et al. Relation of severity of maternal hypothyroidism to cognitive development of offspring. J Med Screen 2001;8:18-20.
231. Lamberg BA, Konen EI, Teramo K, et al. Treatment of maternal hyperthyroidism with antithyroid agents and changes in thyrotropin and thyroxine in the newborn. Acta Endocrinol 1981;97: 186-195.
232. Stagnaro-Green A. Recognizing, understanding, and treating postpartum thyroiditis. Endocrinol Metab Clin North Am 2000;29:417-430, ix.
233. Rochester DB, Davies TF. Increased risk of Graves' disease after pregnancy. Thyroid 2005;15:1287-1290.
234. Momotani N, Yamashita R, Makino F, et al. Thyroid function in wholly breast-feeding infants whose mothers take high doses of propylthiouracil. Clin Endocrinol (Oxf) 2000;53:177-181.
235. Refetoff S. Resistance to thyrotropin. J Endocrinol Invest 2003; 26:770-779.
236. Duprez L, Parma J, Van Sande J, et al. Germline mutations in the thyrotropin receptor gene cause non-autoimmune autosomal dominant hyperthyroidism. Nat Genet 1994;7:396-401.
237. Parma J, Duprez L, Van Sande J, et al. Somatic mutations of the thyrotropin receptor gene cause hyperfunctioning thyroid adenomas. Nature 1993;365:649-651.
238. Hegedus L, Bonnema SJ, Bennedbaek FN. Management of simple nodular goiter: current status and future perspectives. Endocr Rev 2003;24:102-132.
239. Tonacchera M, Agretti P, Chiovato L, et al. Activating thyrotropin receptor mutations are present in nonadenomatous hyperfunctioning nodules of toxic or autonomous multinodular goiter. J Clin Endocrinol Metab 2000;85:2270-2274.
240. Krohn K, Fuhrer D, Bayer Y, et al. Molecular pathogenesis of euthyroid and toxic multinodular goiter. Endocr Rev 2005;26:504-524.
241. Baltisberger BL, Minder CE, Burgi H. Decrease of incidence of toxic nodular goitre in a region of Switzerland after full correction of mild iodine deficiency. Eur J Endocrinol 1995;132:546-549.
242. Nygaard B, Hegedus L, Nielsen KG, et al. Long-term effect of radioactive iodine on thyroid function and size in patients with solitary autonomously functioning toxic thyroid nodules. Clin Endocrinol (Oxf) 1999;50:197-202.
243. Huysmans DA, Hermus AR, Corstens FH, et al. Large, compressive, goiters treated with radioiodine. Ann Intern Med 1994;121: 757-762.
244. Tonacchera M, Agretti P, Rosellini V, et al. Sporadic nonautoimmune congenital hyperthyroidism due to a strong activating mutation of the thyrotropin receptor gene. Thyroid 2000;10:859-863.
245. Roti E, Uberti ED. Iodine excess and hyperthyroidism. Thyroid 2001;11:493-500.
246. Fradkin JE, Wolff J. Iodide-induced thyrotoxicosis. Medicine 1983;62:1-20.
247. Martin FI, Tress BW, Colman PG, et al. Iodine-induced hyperthyroidism due to nonionic contrast radiography in the elderly. Am J Med 1993;95:78-82.
248. Conn JJ, Sebastian MJ, Deam D, et al. A prospective study of the effect of nonionic contrast media on thyroid function. Thyroid 1996;6:107-110.
249. Nolte, MR, Siggelkow H, et al. Prophylactic application of thyrostatic drugs during excessive iodine exposure in euthyroid patients with thyroid autonomy: a randomized study. Eur J Endocrinol 1996;134:337-341.
250. Lawrence JE, Lamm SH, Braverman LE. The use of perchlorate for the prevention of thyrotoxicosis in patients given iodine rich contrast agents. J Endocrinol Invest 1999;22:405-407.
251. Martino E, Bartalena L, Bogazzi F, et al. The effects of amiodarone on the thyroid. Endocr Rev 2001;22:240-254.
252. Smyrk TC, Goellner JR, Brennan MD, et al. Pathology of the thyroid in amiodarone-associated thyrotoxicosis. Am J Surg Pathol 1987; 11:197-204.
253. Melmed S, Nademanee K, Reed AW, et al. Hyperthyroxinemia with bradycardia and normal thyrotropin secretion after chronic amiodarone administration. J Clin Endocrinol Metab 1981;53:997-1001.
254. Berry MJ, Grieco D, Taylor BA, et al. Physiological and genetic analyses of inbred mouse strains with a type I iodothyronine 5′ deiodinase deficiency. J Clin Invest 1993;92:1517-1528.
255. St. Germain DL, Hernandez A, Schneider MJ, et al. Insights into the role of deiodinases from studies of genetically modified animals. Thyroid 2005;15:905-916.
256. Eaton SE, Euinton HA, Newman CM, et al. Clinical experience of amiodarone-induced thyrotoxicosis over a 3-year period: role of colour-flow Doppler sonography. Clin Endocrinol (Oxf) 2002; 56:33-38.
257. Osman F, Franklyn JA, Sheppard MC, et al. Successful treatment of amiodarone-induced thyrotoxicosis. Circulation 2002;105: 1275-1277.
258. Pearce EN, Farwell AP, Braverman LE. Thyroiditis. N Engl J Med 2003;348:2646-2655.
259. Daniels GH. Amiodarone-induced thyrotoxicosis. J Clin Endocrinol Metab 2001;86:3-8.

260. Ryan LE, Braverman LE, et al. Can amiodarone be restarted after amiodarone-induced thyrotoxicosis? Thyroid 2004;14:149-153.
261. Refetoff S, Weiss RE, Usala SJ. The syndromes of resistance to thyroid hormone. Endocr Rev 1993;14:348-399.
262. Refetoff S, Weiss RE, Usala SJ, et al. The syndromes of resistance to thyroid hormone: update. Endocr Rev 1994;3:336-342.
263. Beck-Peccoz P, Mannavola D, Persani L. Syndromes of thyroid hormone resistance. Ann Endocrinol (Paris) 2005;66:264-269.
264. Grun JP, Meuris S, De Nayer P, et al. The thyrotrophic role of human chorionic gonadotrophin (hCG) in the early stages of twin (versus single) pregnancies. Clin Endocrinol (Oxf) 1997;46: 719-725.
265. Goodwin TM, Montoro M, Mestman JH, et al. The role of chorionic gonadotropin in transient hyperthyroidism of hyperemesis gravidarum. J Clin Endocrinol Metab 1992;75:1333-1337.
266. Rodien P, Bremont C, Sanson ML, et al. Familial gestational hyperthyroidism caused by a mutant thyrotropin receptor hypersensitive to human chorionic gonadotropin. N Engl J Med 1998;339: 1823-1826.
267. Pekary AE, Jackson IM, Goodwin TM, et al. Increased in vitro thyrotropic activity of partially sialated human chorionic gonadotropin extracted from hydatidiform moles of patients with hyperthyroidism. J Clin Endocrinol Metab 1993;76:70-74.
267a. Desai J, Yassa L, Marqusee E, George S, Frates MC, Chen MH, Morgan JA, Dychter SS, Larsen PR, Demetri GD, Alexander EK. Hypothyroidism after sunitinib treatment for patients with gastrointestinal stromal tumors. Ann Intern Med 2006;145:660-664.
268. Tachi J, Amino N, Tamaki H, et al. Long term followup and HLA association in patients with postpartum hyperthyroidism. J Clin Endocrinol Metab 1988;66:480-484.
269. Sarvghadi F, Hedayati M, Mehrabi Y, et al. Follow up of patients with postpartum thyroiditis: a population-based study. Endocrine 2005;27:279-282.
270. Rosen IB, Strawbridge HG, Walfish PG, et al. Malignant pseudothyroiditis: a new clinical entity. Am J Surg 1978;136:445-449.
271. Koh LK, Greenspan FS, Yeo PP. Interferon-alpha induced thyroid dysfunction: three clinical presentations and a review of the literature. Thyroid 1997;7:891-896.
272. Doi F, Kakizaki S, Takagi H, et al. Long-term outcome of interferon-alpha-induced autoimmune thyroid disorders in chronic hepatitis C. Liver Int 2005;25:242-246.
273. Miller KK, Daniels GH. 2001. Association between lithium use and thyrotoxicosis caused by silent thyroiditis. Clin Endocrinol (Oxf) 2001;55:501-508.
274. Baethge C, Blumentritt H, Berghofer A, et al. Long-term lithium treatment and thyroid antibodies: a controlled study. J Psychiatry Neurosci 2005;30:423-427.
275. de Groot JW, Zonnenberg BA, Plukker JT, et al. Imatinib induces hypothyroidism in patients receiving levothyroxine. Clin Pharmacol Ther 2005;78:433-438.
276. Hedberg CW, Fishbein DB, Janssen RS, et al. An outbreak of thyrotoxicosis caused by the consumption of bovine thyroid gland in ground beef. N Engl J Med 1987;316:993-998.
277. DeSimone CP, Lele SM, Modesitt SC. Malignant struma ovarii: a case report and analysis of cases reported in the literature with focus on survival and I131 therapy. Gynecol Oncol 2003; 89:543-548.
278. Dunzendorfer T, deLas Morenas A, Kalir T, et al. Struma ovarii and hyperthyroidism. Thyroid 1999;9:499-502.
279. Giralt SA, Dexeus F, Amato R, et al. Hyperthyroidism in men with germ cell tumors and high levels of beta-human chorionic gonadotropin. Cancer 1992;69:1286-1290.
280. Bayot MR, Chopra IJ. Coexistence of struma ovarii and Graves' disease. Thyroid 1995;5:469-471.
281. Berghella V, Ngadiman S, Rosenberg H, et al. Malignant struma ovarii. A case report and review of the literature. Gynecol Obstet Invest 1997;43:68-72.
282. Volpi E, Ferrero A, Nasi PG, et al. Malignant struma ovarii: a case report of laparoscopic management. Gynecol Oncol 2003;90: 191-194.
283. Als C, Gedeon P, Rosler H, et al. Survival analysis of 19 patients with toxic thyroid carcinoma. J Clin Endocrinol Metab 2002; 87:4122-4127.
284. Carr K, Mcleod DT, Parry G, et al. Fine adjustment of thyroxine replacement dosage: comparison of the thyrotrophin releasing hormone tests using a sensitive thyrotrophin assay with measurement of free thyroid hormones and clinical assessment. Clin Endocrinol 1988;28:325-333.
285. Bell GM, Sawers JS, Forfar JC, et al. The effect of minor increments in plasma thyroxine on heart rate and urinary sodium excretion. Clin Endocrinol 1983;18:511-516.
286. Cappola AR, Fried LP, Arnold AM, et al. Thyroid status, cardiovascular risk, and mortality in older adults. JAMA 2006;295: 1033-1041.
287. Tenerz A, Forberg R, Jansson R. Is a more active attitude warranted in patients with subclinical thyrotoxicosis? J Intern Med 1990;228:229-233.
288. Monreal M, Lafoz E, Foz M, et al. Occult thyrotoxicosis in patients with atrial fibrillation and an acute arterial embolism. Angiology 1988;39:981-985.
289. Biondi B, Palmieri EA, Klain M, et al. Subclinical hyperthyroidism: clinical features and treatment options. Eur J Endocrinol 2005; 152:1-9.
290. Faber J, Jensen IW, Petersen L, et al. Normalization of serum thyrotrophin by means of radioiodine treatment in subclinical hyperthyroidism: effect on bone loss in postmenopausal women. Clin Endocrinol (Oxf) 1998;48:285-290.
291. Sgarbi JA, Villaca FG, Garbeline B, et al. The effects of early antithyroid therapy for endogenous subclinical hyperthyroidism in clinical and heart abnormalities. J Clin Endocrinol Metab 2003;88:1672-1677.
292. Faber J, Wiinberg N, Schifter S, et al. Haemodynamic changes following treatment of subclinical and overt hyperthyroidism. Eur J Endocrinol 2001;145:391-396.
293. Sawin CT, Geller A, Kaplan MM, et al. Low serum thyrotropin (thyroid-stimulating hormone) in older persons without hyperthyroidism. Arch Intern Med 1991;151:165-168.
294. Woeber KA. Observations concerning the natural history of subclinical hyperthyroidism. Thyroid 2005;15:687-691.
295. Canaris GJ, Manowitz NR, Mayor G, et al. The Colorado thyroid disease prevalence study. Arch Intern Med 2000;160:526-534.
296. Surks MI, Ortiz E, Daniels GH, et al. Subclinical thyroid disease: scientific review and guidelines for diagnosis and management. JAMA 2004;291:228-238.
297. Marqusee E, Haden ST, Utiger RD. Subclinical thyrotoxicosis. Endocrinol Metab Clin North Am 1998;27:37-49.
298. Toft AD. Clinical practice. Subclinical hyperthyroidism. N Engl J Med 2001;345:512-516.
299. Col NF, Surks MI, Daniels GH. Subclinical thyroid disease: clinical applications. JAMA 2004;291:239-243.

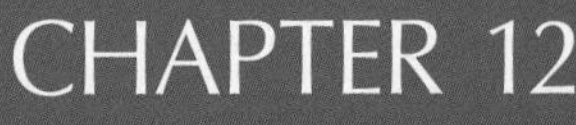

CHAPTER 12

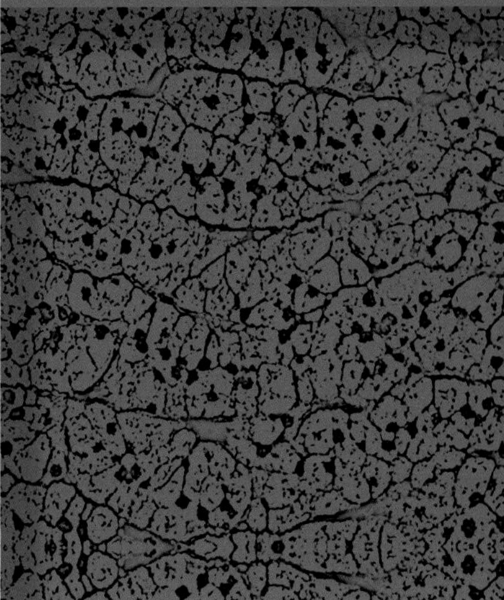

HYPOTHYROIDISM AND THYROIDITIS

Gregory A. Brent, P. Reed Larsen, and Terry F. Davies

HYPOTHYROIDISM

Reduced production of thyroid hormone is the central feature of the clinical state termed *hypothyroidism.*[1,2] Permanent loss or destruction of the thyroid, through processes such as autoimmune destruction or irradiation injury, is described as *primary hypothyroidism* (Table 12–1). Hypothyroidism due to transient or progressive impairment of hormone biosynthesis is typically associated with compensatory thyroid enlargement. Central or secondary hypothyroidism, due to insufficient stimulation of a normal gland, is the result of hypothalamic or pituitary disease or defects in the thyroid-stimulating hormone (TSH) molecule. Transient or temporary hypothyroidism can be observed as a phase of subacute thyroiditis. Primary hypothyroidism is the etiology in approximately 99% of cases of hypothyroidism, with less than 1% being due to TSH deficiency or other causes. Central hypothyroidism is discussed in Chapters 7 and 8.

Reduced action of thyroid hormone at the tissue level, despite normal or increased thyroid hormone production from the thyroid gland, can also be associated with clinical hypothyroidism. Conditions associated with reduced thyroid hormone action are rare and include abnormalities of thyroid hormone metabolism and defects in nuclear signaling. Consumptive hypothyroidism, identified in an increasing number of clinical settings, is the result of accelerated inactivation of thyroid hormone by the type 3 iodothyronine deiodinase. Defects of activation of the prohormone, thyroxine (T_4), to the active form, triiodothyronine (T_3), have also been identified. Resistance to thyroid hormone (RTH), the result of defects in the thyroid hormone nuclear receptor (TR) or nuclear cofactors, is associated with elevated circulating levels of thyroid hormone. Some tissues, depending on the level of expression of the mutant receptor and other forms of local compensation, have evidence of reduced thyroid hormone action.

Estimates of the incidence of hypothyroidism vary depending on the population studied.[3-5] In the United States, 0.3% have overt hypothyroidism, defined as an elevated serum TSH concentration and reduced free thyroxine concentration (fT_4), and 4.3% have what has been described as subclinical or mild hypothyroidism.[5] Although a number of clinical manifestations have been associated with this early or mild phase of hypothyroidism, we will use the term "subclinical" to describe this group as is used in most clinical studies. Subclinical hypothyroidism is

TABLE 12–1 CAUSES OF HYPOTHYROIDISM

Primary Hypothyroidism
Acquired
Hashimoto's thyroiditis
Iodine deficiency (endemic goiter)
Drugs blocking synthesis or release of T_4 (e.g., lithium, ethionamide, sulfonamides, iodide)
Goitrogens in foodstuffs or as endemic substances or pollutants
Cytokines (interferon-α, interleukin-2)
Thyroid infiltration (amyloidosis, hemochromatosis, sarcoidosis, Riedel's struma, cystinosis, scleroderma)
Postablative due to ^{131}I, surgery, or therapeutic irradiation for nonthyroidal malignancy
Congenital
Iodide transport or utilization defect (NIS or pendrin mutations)
Iodotyrosine dehalogenase deficiency
Organification disorders (TPO* deficiency or dysfunction)
Defects in thyroglobulin synthesis or processing
Thyroid agenesis or dysplasia
TSH receptor* defects
Thyroidal Gs protein abnormalities (pseudohypoparathyroidism type 1a)
Idiopathic TSH unresponsiveness

Transient (Post-thyroiditis) Hypothyroidism
Following subacute, painless, or postpartum thyroiditis

Consumptive Hypothyroidism
Rapid destruction of thyroid hormone due to D3 expression in large hemangiomas or hemangioendotheliomas

Defects of Thyroxine to Triiodothyronine Conversion
Selenocysteine insertion sequence–binding protein (SECIS-BP2) defect

Drug-Induced Thyroid Destruction
Tyrosine kinase inhibitor (sunitinib)

Central Hypothyroidism
Acquired
Pituitary origin (secondary)
Hypothalamic disorders (tertiary)
Bexarotene (retinaid X receptor agonist)
Dopamine and/or severe illness
Congenital
TSH deficiency or structural abnormality
TSH receptor defect

Resistance to Thyroid Hormone
Generalized
"Pituitary" dominant

NIS, sodium-iodide symporter; TPO, thyroid peroxidase; TSH, thyroid-stimulating hormone.

defined as an elevated serum TSH level with a normal serum (fT_4) concentration.[6] Subclinical hypothyroidism can progress to overt hypothyroidism,[7] as well as being associated with manifestations that, in some patients, may benefit from treatment.[6-9] The incidence of hypothyroidism is higher among women, the elderly, and in some racial and ethnic groups.[5] Neonatal screening programs for congenital hypothyroidism identify hypothyroidism (almost all primary) in almost 1 in 3500 newborns.[10]

CLINICAL PRESENTATION

Hypothyroidism can affect all organ systems, and these manifestations are largely independent of the underlying disorder but are a function of the degree of hormone deficiency. The following sections discuss the pathophysiology of each organ system at various levels of thyroid hormone deficiency, from mild to severe. The term *myxedema,* formerly used as a synonym for hypothyroidism, refers to the appearance of the skin and subcutaneous tissues in the patient in a severely hypothyroid state (Fig. 12–1). Hypothyroidism of this severity is rarely seen today, and the term should be reserved to describe the physical signs.

Skin and Appendages

Hypothyroidism causes an accumulation of hyaluronic acid that alters the composition of the ground substance in the dermis and other tissues.[11] This material is hygroscopic, producing the mucinous edema that is responsible for the thickened features and puffy appearance (myxedema) with full-blown hypothyroidism. Myxedematous tissue is characteristically boggy and nonpitting and is apparent around the eyes, on the dorsa of the hands and feet, and in the supraclavicular fossae (see Fig. 12–1). It causes enlargement of the tongue and thickening of the pharyngeal and laryngeal mucous membranes.

A histologically similar deposit may occur in patients with Graves' disease, usually over the pretibial area (infiltrative dermopathy or pretibial myxedema). In addition to having a puffy appearance, the skin is pale and cool as a result of cutaneous vasoconstriction. Anemia may contribute to the pallor; hypercarotenemia gives the skin a yellow tint but does not cause scleral icterus (see Fig. 12–1). The secretions of the sweat glands and sebaceous glands are reduced, leading to dryness and coarseness of the skin, which in extreme cases may resemble that in ichthyosis.

Wounds of the skin tend to heal slowly. Easy bruising is due to an increase in capillary fragility. Head and body hair is dry and brittle, lacks luster, and tends to fall out. Hair may be lost from the temporal aspects of the eyebrows, although this is not specific for hypothyroidism (see Fig. 12–1B). Growth of hair is retarded so that haircuts and shaves are required less often. The nails are brittle and grow slowly. Topical T_3 has been shown to accelerate wound healing and stimulate hair growth in a euthyroid mouse model, demonstrating a role for thyroid hormone in these processes.[12]

Histopathologic examination of the skin reveals hyperkeratosis with plugging of hair follicles and sweat glands. The dermis is edematous, and the connective tissue fibers are separated by an increased amount of metachromatically staining, periodic acid–Schiff (PAS)–positive mucinous material. This material consists of protein complexed with two mucopolysaccharides: hyaluronic acid and chondroitin sulfate B. The hygroscopic glycosaminoglycans are mobilized early during treatment with thyroid hormone, leading to an increase in urinary excretion of nitrogen and hexosamine as well as tissue water.[11]

Patients with hypothyroidism due to Hashimoto's thyroiditis may also have skin lesions with loss of pigmentation characteristic of the autoimmune skin condition vitiligo. This is not a manifestation of reduced thyroid hormone action, but reflects the common association of autoimmune endocrine disease and this skin condition, recognized as a component of autoimmune polyendocrine syndromes.[13]

Cardiovascular System

The cardiac output at rest is decreased because of reduction in both stroke volume and heart rate, reflecting loss of the inotropic and chronotropic effects of thyroid hormones. Peripheral vascular resistance at rest is increased, and blood volume is reduced. These hemodynamic alterations cause narrowing of

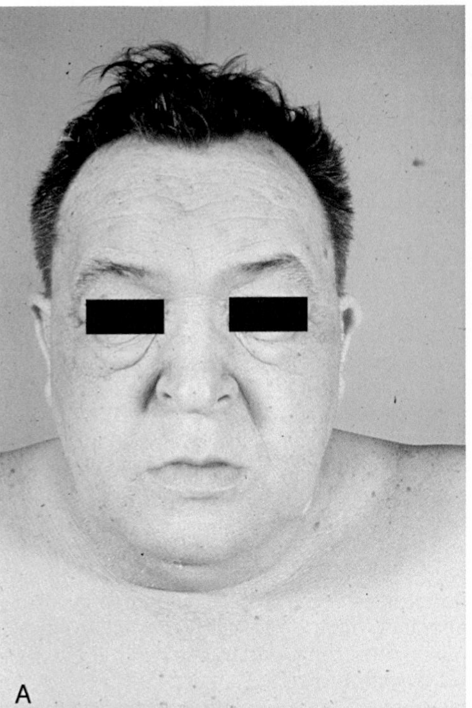

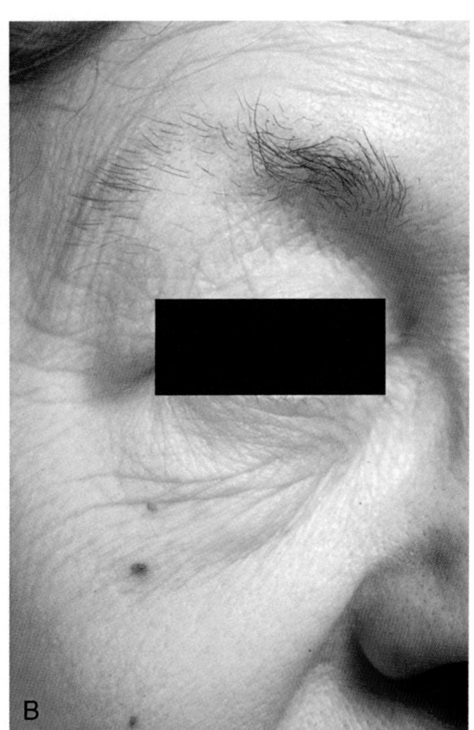

Figure 12–1 ▪ Typical appearance with moderately severe primary hypothyroidism or myxedema. Note dry skin and sallow complexion; the absence of scleral pigmentation differentiates the carotenemia from jaundice. Both individuals demonstrate periorbital myxedema. The patient in **B** illustrates the loss of the lateral aspect of the eyebrow, sometimes termed *Queen Anne's sign.* That finding is not unusual in the age group that is commonly affected by severe hypothyroidism and should not be considered to be a specific sign of the condition.

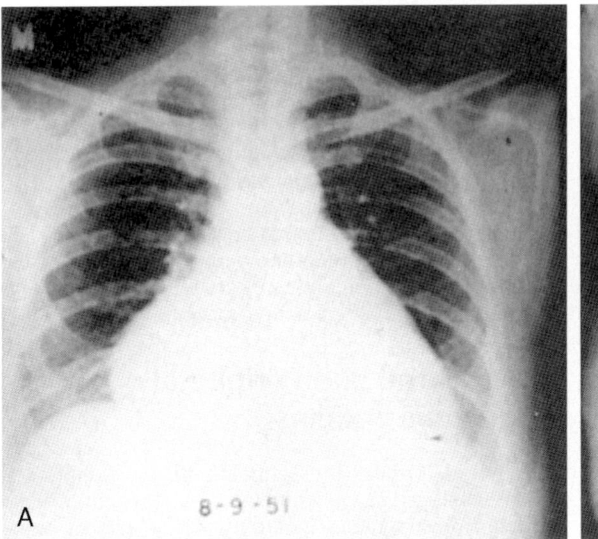

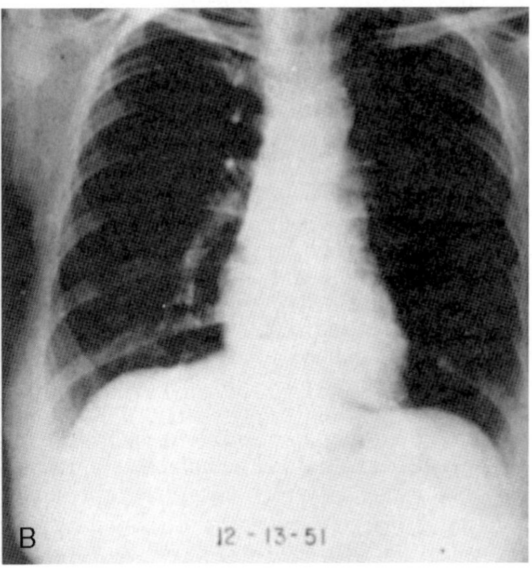

Figure 12–2 ▪ **A** and **B,** Chest roentgenograms in a patient with myxedema heart disease. The patient had signs of severe congestive heart failure and was given thyroid hormone alone. Within 4 months, the heart had returned to normal size **(B)** and there was no evidence of underlying heart disease.

pulse pressure, prolongation of circulation time, and decrease in blood flow to the tissues.[14-17] The reduction in cutaneous circulation is responsible for the coolness and pallor of the skin and the sensitivity to cold. In most tissues, the decrease in blood flow is proportional to the decrease in oxygen consumption, so the arteriovenous oxygen difference remains normal. The hemodynamic alterations at rest resemble those of congestive heart failure. However, in hypothyroidism, cardiac output increases and peripheral vascular resistance decreases normally in response to exercise unless the hypothyroid state is severe and of long standing.

In severe primary hypothyroidism the cardiac silhouette is enlarged (Fig. 12–2), and the heart sounds are diminished in intensity.[18] These findings are the result largely of effusion into the pericardial sac of fluid rich in protein and glycosaminoglycans, but the myocardium may also be dilated. Pericardial effusion is rarely of sufficient magnitude to cause tamponade.

Angina pectoris may first appear or worsen during treatment of the hypothyroid state with thyroid hormone, although most patients with hypothyroidism and coronary artery disease have no change, or improvement, in anginal symptoms with thyroxine treatment.[19] Electrocardiographic changes include sinus bradycardia, prolongation of the PR interval, low amplitude of the P wave and QRS complex, alterations of the ST segment, and flattened or inverted T waves. Pericardial effusion is probably responsible for the low amplitude in severe hypothyroidism. Systolic time intervals are altered; the preejection period is prolonged, and the ratio of preejection period to left ventricular ejection time is increased. Echocardiographic studies have revealed resting left ventricular diastolic dysfunction in overt, and in some studies, subclinical hypothyroidism.[17] These findings normalize when the hypothyroidism is treated.

Serum levels of homocysteine, creatine kinase, aspartate aminotransferase, and lactate dehydrogenase may be increased in hypothyroidism.[14,20] Typically, the isoenzyme patterns suggest that the source of the increased creatine kinase and lactate dehydrogenase is skeletal, not cardiac, muscle. All levels return to normal with therapy. Sequential cardiac biopsies in a hypothyroid patient with heart failure showed that mRNA levels from genes regulated by thyroid hormone and important for the strength of myocardial contraction were normalized after thyroxine treatment.[21]

The combination of large heart, hemodynamic and electrocardiographic alterations, and the serum enzyme changes has been termed *myxedema heart.* In the absence of coexisting organic heart disease, treatment with thyroid hormone corrects the hemodynamic, electrocardiographic, and serum enzyme alterations of myxedema heart and restores heart size to normal (see Fig. 12–2).

Hypothyroidism is consistently associated with elevations of total and low-density lipoprotein (LDL) cholesterol, which improve with thyroxine replacement.[22] The magnitude of reduction in LDL cholesterol after thyroxine therapy is greater the higher the original serum TSH concentration and elevation of serum LDL. Some subsets of hypothyroid patients may have elevated serum triglycerides and C-reactive protein that improve with thyroxine treatment.[23] Serum high-density lipoprotein (HDL) levels are not influenced by thyroid status.

Hypothyroidism has been shown to be a risk factor for atherosclerosis and cardiovascular disease by several studies, although others have not shown this association. In the Rotterdam study, 1149 Dutch postmenopausal women with TSH greater than 4.0 μU/L, and a normal free thyroxine were followed prospectively. There was an increased prevalence of aortic atherosclerosis (odds ratio, 1.7; confidence interval, 1.1 to 2.6) and myocardial infarction (odds ratio, 2.3; confidence interval, 1.3 to 4.0), even after controlling for lipid levels and body weight.[24] A prospective study from Japan showed an increase risk of ischemic heart disease in men, but not women, with subclinical hypothyroidism.[25] The Whickham Study showed no increase in cardiovascular mortality in patients with subclinical hypothyroidism followed up for more than 20 years.[4] A prospective study in the United States, following up men and women age 65 or older for more than 10 years, showed no influence of hypothyroidism (overt or subclinical), on cardiovascular outcome or mortality.[26]

Respiratory System

Pleural effusions usually are evident only on radiologic examination but in rare instances may cause dyspnea. Lung volumes are usually normal, but maximal breathing capacity and diffusing capacity are reduced. In severe hypothyroidism, myxedematous involvement of respiratory muscles and depression of both the hypoxic and the hypercapnic ventilatory drives may cause alveolar hypoventilation and carbon dioxide retention, which in turn can contribute to the development of myxedema coma. Obstructive sleep apnea is common but is reversible with restoration of a euthyroid state.

Alimentary System

Although most patients experience a modest gain in weight, appetite is usually reduced. The weight gain that occurs is caused partly by retention of fluid by the hydrophilic glycoprotein deposits in the tissues, but does not exceed 10% of body weight. Peristaltic activity is decreased and, together with the decreased food intake, is responsible for the frequent complaint of constipation. The latter may lead to fecal impaction (myxedema megacolon). Gaseous distention of the abdomen (myxedema ileus), if accompanied by colicky pain and vomiting, may mimic mechanical ileus.[27]

Elevations in the serum levels of carcinoembryonic antigen, which may occur on the basis of hypothyroidism alone, add to the impression that an organic obstruction is present. Ascites in the absence of another cause is unusual in hypothyroidism, but it can occur, usually in association with pleural and pericardial effusions. Like pericardial and pleural effusions, the ascitic fluid is rich in protein and glycosaminoglycans.

Achlorhydria after maximal histamine stimulation may be present in patients with primary hypothyroidism. Circulating antibodies against gastric parietal cells have been found in about one third of patients with primary hypothyroidism and may be secondary to atrophy of the gastric mucosa. Overt pernicious anemia is reported in about 12% of patients with primary hypothyroidism. The coexistence of pernicious anemia and other autoimmune diseases, such as gluten enteropathy, with primary hypothyroidism reflects the fact that autoimmunity plays the central role in the pathogenesis of these diseases (see Chapter 41).

Hypothyroidism has complex effects on intestinal absorption. Although the rates of absorption for many substances are decreased, the total amount absorbed may be normal or even increased because the decreased bowel motility may allow more time for absorption. Malabsorption is occasionally overt.

Liver function test results are usually normal, but levels of aminotransaminases may be elevated, probably because of impaired clearance. The gallbladder contracts sluggishly and may be distended, but whether these changes predispose to the development of gallstones is unknown.[28]

Atrophy of the gastric and intestinal mucosa and myxedematous infiltration of the bowel wall may be demonstrated on histologic examination. The colon may be greatly distended, and the volume of fluid in the peritoneal cavity is usually increased. The liver and pancreas are normal.

Central and Peripheral Nervous Systems

Thyroid hormone is essential for the development of the central nervous system. Deficiency in fetal life or at birth impair neurologic development, including hypoplasia of cortical neurons with poor development of cellular processes, retarded myelination, and reduced vascularity.[10,29] If the deficiency is not corrected in early postnatal life, the damage is irreversible. Deficiency of thyroid hormone beginning in adult life causes less severe manifestations that usually respond to treatment with the hormone. Cerebral blood flow is reduced, but cerebral oxygen consumption is usually normal; this finding is in accord with the conclusion that the oxygen consumption of isolated brain tissue in vitro, unlike that of most other tissues, is not stimulated by administration of thyroid hormones. In severe cases, decreased cerebral blood flow may lead to cerebral hypoxia.

All intellectual functions, including speech, are slowed in thyroid hormone deficiency. Loss of initiative is present, slow-wittedness and memory defects are common, lethargy and somnolence are prominent, and dementia in elderly patients may be mistaken for senile dementia. Psychiatric disorders are common and are usually of the paranoid or depressive type and may induce agitation (myxedema madness).[30] Headaches are frequent. Cerebral hypoxia due to circulatory alterations may predispose to confusional attacks and syncope, which may be prolonged and lead to stupor or coma. Other factors predisposing to coma in hypothyroidism include exposure to severe cold, infection, trauma, hypoventilation with carbon dioxide retention, and depressant drugs.

Epileptic seizures have been reported and tend to occur in myxedema coma. Night blindness is due to deficient synthesis of the pigment required for dark adaptation. Hearing loss of the perceptive type is frequent due to myxedema of the eighth cranial nerve and serous otitis media. Perceptive deafness may also occur in association with a defect in the organic binding of thyroidal iodide (Pendred's syndrome) (see Chapter 10), but in these instances it is not due to hypothyroidism per se.

Thick, slurred speech and hoarseness are due to myxedematous infiltration of the tongue and larynx, respectively. Body movements are slow and clumsy, and cerebellar ataxia may occur. Numbness and tingling of the extremities are frequent; in the fingers these symptoms may be due to compression by glycosaminoglycan deposits in and around the median nerve in the carpal tunnel (carpal tunnel syndrome).[31] The tendon reflexes are slow, especially during the relaxation phase, producing the characteristic "hung-up reflexes"; this phenomenon is due to a decrease in the rate of muscle contraction and relaxation rather than a delay in nerve conduction.

The presence of extensor plantar responses or diminished vibration sense should alert the physician to the possibility of coexisting pernicious anemia with combined system disease. Electroencephalographic changes include slow alpha-wave activity and general loss of amplitude. The concentration of protein in the cerebrospinal fluid is often increased, but cerebrospinal pressure is normal.

Histopathologic examination of the brain in patients with untreated hypothyroidism reveals that the nervous system is edematous with mucinous deposits in and around nerve fibers. In patients with cerebellar ataxia, neural myxedematous infiltrates of glycogen and mucinous material are present in the cerebellum. There may be foci of degeneration and an increase in glial tissue. The cerebral vessels show atherosclerosis, but this is much more common if the patient has had coexistent hypertension.

Hypothyroidism has been associated with several neurologic conditions, although a strong etiologic link has not been established. Epidemiologic studies have shown an association between Alzheimer's disease and hypothyroidism. It is difficult to convincingly demonstrate this association, because the incidence of thyroid disease in the elderly population is high and like dementia, increases with age. A mechanistic link is suggested by the observation of amyloid deposition in Down's syndrome, a condition associated with an increased incidence of Hashimoto's disease, and thyroid hormone regulates amyloid gene processing in a number of cellular and animal models. Subclinical hyperthyroidism, however, has also been associated with Alzheimer's disease.[32] There is an increase in cerebrospinal fluid reverse T_3 levels in Alzheimer's disease patients, all with normal circulating thyroid hormone levels, suggesting the potential for altered thyroid hormone metabolism in the brain.[33] The impact of normalizing T_3 levels in the brain, however, is not known. A corticosteroid-responsive encephalopathy is associated with chronic Hashimoto's thyroiditis, but may be linked to autoimmunity rather than a process mediated specifically by low thyroid hormone levels or thyroid autoantibodies.[34]

Muscular System

Stiffness and aching of muscles are common and are worsened by cold temperatures. Delayed muscle contraction and relaxation cause the slowness of movement and delayed tendon jerks. Muscle mass may be reduced or enlarged due to interstitial myxedema. Muscle mass may be slightly increased, and the muscles tend to be firm. Rarely, a profound increase in muscle mass with slowness of muscular activity may be the predominant manifestation (the *Kocher-Debré-Sémélaigne, or Hoffmann,* syndrome). Myoclonus may be present. The electromyogram may be normal or may exhibit disordered discharge, hyperirritability, and polyphasic action potentials.

On histopathologic examination, the muscles appear pale and swollen. The muscle fibers may show swelling, loss of normal striations, and separation by mucinous deposits. Type I muscle fibers tend to predominate.

Skeletal System: Calcium and Phosphorus Metabolism

Thyroid hormone is essential for normal growth and maturation of the skeleton, and growth failure is due both to impaired general protein synthesis and to a reduction in growth hormone, but especially of insulin-like growth factor I (Fig. 12–3).[35] Before puberty, thyroid hormone plays a major role in the maturation of bone. Deficiency of thyroid hormone in early life leads to both a delay in the development of, and an abnormal, stippled appearance of the epiphyseal centers of ossification (epiphyseal dysgenesis) (Fig. 12–4). Impairment of linear growth leads to dwarfism in which the limbs are disproportionately short in

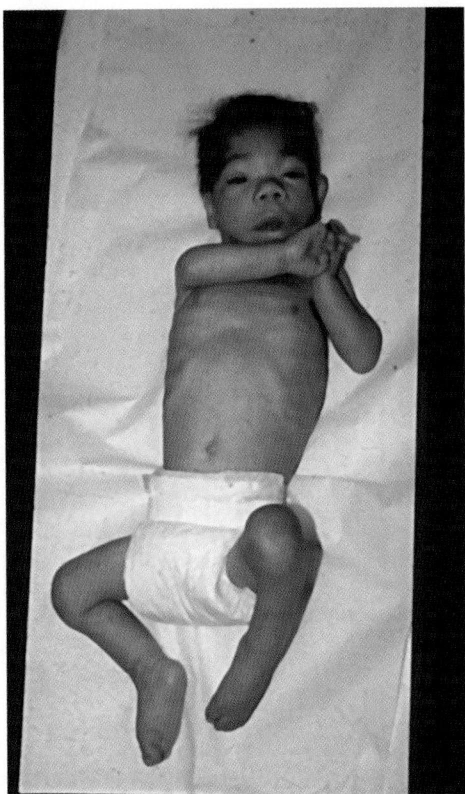

Figure 12–3 ▪ The consequences of untreated congenital hypothyroidism are demonstrated in this 17-year-old girl. Her condition had been diagnosed at birth but, through a series of misunderstandings, was not treated with thyroid hormone. Note her size, the poorly developed nasal bridge, the wide-set eyes, and the ears, which are larger than are appropriate for head size. Her tongue is enlarged, and her extremities are inappropriately short in relation to her trunk. (Courtesy of Dr. Ronald B. Stein.)

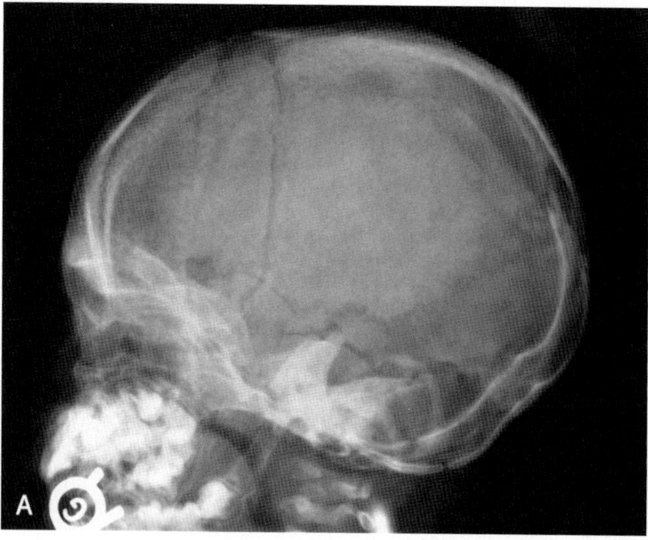

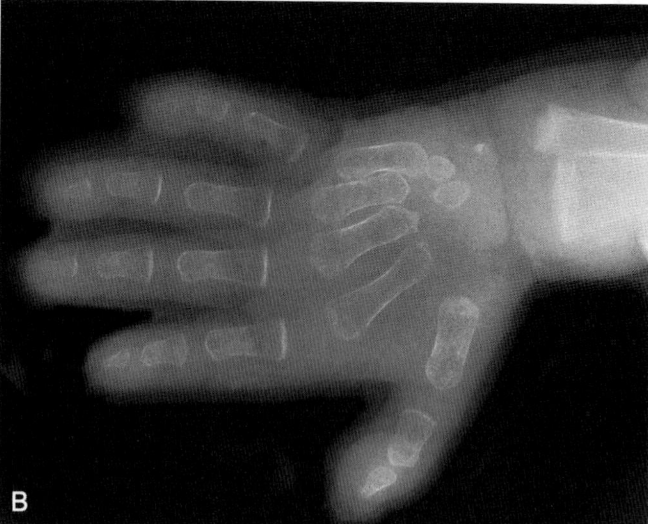

Figure 12–4 ▪ X-ray films of the skull and hand of the 17-year-old patient illustrated in Figure 12–3. **A,** Skull film showing that the posterior and anterior fontanelles are open and that the sutures are not fused. The deciduous and permanent teeth are present. **B,** Radiograph of the wrist and hand showing the delayed appearance of the epiphyseal centers of the bones of the hand and the absence of the distal radial epiphysis. The estimated bone age is 9 months. (Courtesy of Dr. Ronald B. Stein.)

relation to the trunk but cartilage growth is unaffected (see Fig. 12–3). Children with prolonged hypothyroidism, even after adequate treatment, do not reach predicted height based on mid-parental height calculations.[36]

Urinary excretion of calcium is decreased, as is the glomerular filtration rate, whereas fecal excretion of calcium and both urinary and fecal excretion of phosphorus are variable. Calcium balance is also variable, and any changes are slight. The exchangeable pool of calcium and its rate of turnover are reduced, changes that reflect decreased bone formation and resorption.[37] Because levels of parathyroid hormone are often slightly increased, some degree of resistance to its action may be present; levels of $1{,}25(OH)_2D$ are also increased.

Levels of calcium and phosphorus in serum are usually normal, but calcium may be slightly elevated. The alkaline phosphatase level is usually below normal in infantile and juvenile hypothyroidism. Bone density may be increased. The radiologic appearance of the skeleton in cretinism and juvenile hypothyroidism are discussed subsequently.

Renal Function: Water and Electrolyte Metabolism

Renal blood flow, glomerular filtration rate, and tubular reabsorptive and secretory maxima are reduced. Blood urea nitrogen and serum creatinine levels are normal, but uric acid levels may be increased. Urine flow is reduced, and delay in the excretion of a water load may result in reversal of the normal diurnal pattern of urine excretion. The delay in water excretion appears to be due to decreased volume delivery to the distal diluting segment of the nephron as a result of the diminished renal perfusion; evidence supporting inappropriate secretion of vasopressin (syndrome of inappropriate antidiuretic hormone secretion) is less compelling.[38] These changes are reversed by treatment with thyroid hormone. The ability to concentrate urine may be slightly impaired. Mild proteinuria may occur.

The impaired renal excretion of water and the retention of water by the hydrophilic deposits in the tissues result in an increase in total body water, even though plasma volume is reduced. This increase accounts for the hyponatremia occasionally noted because the level of exchangeable sodium is increased. The amount of exchangeable potassium is usually normal in relation to lean body mass. Serum magnesium concentration may be increased, but exchangeable magnesium levels and urinary magnesium excretion are decreased.

Hematopoietic System

In response to the diminished oxygen requirements and decreased production of erythropoietin, the red blood cell mass is decreased; this is evident in the mild normocytic, normochromic anemia that often occurs. Less commonly, the anemia is macrocytic, sometimes from deficiency of vitamin B_{12}. Reference has already been made to the high incidence of pernicious anemia (and of achlorhydria and vitamin B_{12} deficiency without overt anemia) in primary hypothyroidism (see Chapter 41). Conversely, overt and subclinical hypothyroidism is present in 12% and 15% of patients, respectively, with pernicious anemia. Folate deficiency from malabsorption or dietary inadequacy may also cause macrocytic anemia. The frequent menorrhagia and the defective absorption of iron resulting from achlorhydria may contribute to a microcytic, hypochromic anemia.

The total and differential white blood cell counts are usually normal, and platelets are adequate, although platelet adhesiveness may be impaired. If pernicious anemia or significant folate deficiency is present, the characteristic changes in peripheral blood and bone marrow will be found. The intrinsic clotting mechanism may be defective because of decreased concentrations in plasma of factors VIII and IX, and this, together with an increase in capillary fragility and the decrease in platelet adhesiveness, may account for the bleeding tendency that sometimes occurs.[27]

Pituitary and Adrenocortical Function

In longstanding primary hypothyroidism, hyperplasia of the thyrotropes may cause the pituitary gland to be enlarged. This feature can be detected radiologically as an increase in the volume of the pituitary fossa.[39] Rarely, the pituitary enlargement compromises the function of other pituitary cells and causes pituitary insufficiency or visual field defects. Patients with severe hypothyroidism may have increased serum prolactin levels, stimulated by the elevation in TRH and proportional to the level of serum TSH elevation, and galactorrhea may develop in some patients. Treatment with thyroid hormone normalizes the serum prolactin and TSH levels and causes disappearance of galactorrhea, if present.

In rodents, thyroid hormone directly regulates growth hormone synthesis.[35] Growth hormone is not directly regulated by thyroid hormone in humans, but thyroid status influences the growth hormone axis. Hypothyroid children have delayed growth and the response of growth hormone to provocative stimuli may be subnormal.[35]

As a result of the decreased rate of turnover of cortisol due to decreased hepatic 11β-hydroxysteroid dehydrogenase type 1 (11β-HSD-1), the 24-hour urinary excretion of cortisol and 17-hydroxycorticosteroids is decreased but the plasma cortisol level is usually normal (see Chapter 14). The responses of urinary 17-OH-corticosteroid to exogenous adrenocorticotropic hormone and metyrapone are usually normal but may be decreased. The response of plasma cortisol to insulin-induced hypoglycemia may be impaired.

In severe, longstanding primary hypothyroidism, pituitary and adrenal function may be secondarily decreased and adrenal insufficiency may be precipitated by stress or by rapid replacement therapy with thyroid hormone.[40] The rate of turnover of aldosterone is decreased, but the plasma level is normal. Plasma renin activity is decreased, and sensitivity to angiotensin II is increased (see Chapter 15).

Reproductive Function

In both sexes, thyroid hormones influence sexual development and reproductive function.[41] Infantile hypothyroidism, if untreated, leads to sexual immaturity, and juvenile hypothyroidism causes a delay in the onset of puberty followed by anovulatory cycles. Paradoxically, primary hypothyroidism may also rarely cause precocious sexual development and galactorrhea, presumably due to "spillover" of elevated TSH stimulating the LH receptor.[42]

In adult women, severe hypothyroidism may be associated with diminished libido and failure of ovulation. Secretion of progesterone is inadequate, and endometrial proliferation persists, resulting in excessive and irregular breakthrough menstrual bleeding. These changes may be due to deficient secretion of luteinizing hormone and/or pulse frequency and amplitude. Rarely, in primary hypothyroidism, secondary depression of pituitary function may lead to ovarian atrophy and amenorrhea. Fertility is reduced, and there is an increase in spontaneous abortion and preterm delivery, although many pregnancies are successful.[43,44] Pregnancy complications are associated with overt and subclinical hypothyroidism, although the impact has varied among different studies.[45] A randomized prospective study of levothyroxine treatment in pregnant women with subclinical hypothyroidism has shown that the increased incidence of preterm delivery and spontaneous abortions are reversed by treatment.[46] Primary ovarian failure can also be seen in patients with Hashimoto's thyroiditis as part of an autoimmune polyendocrine syndrome.[13] Hypothyroidism in men may cause diminished libido, impotence, and oligospermia.

Values for plasma gonadotropins are usually in the normal range in primary hypothyroidism; in postmenopausal women, levels are usually somewhat lower than in euthyroid women of the same age but are nevertheless within the menopausal range. This provides a valuable means of differentiating primary from secondary hypothyroidism.

The metabolism of both androgens and estrogens is altered in hypothyroidism. Secretion of androgens is decreased, and the metabolism of testosterone is shifted toward etiocholanolone rather than androsterone. With respect to estradiol and estrone, hypothyroidism favors metabolism of these steroids via 16α-hydroxylation over that via 2-oxygenation, with the result that formation of estriol is increased and that of 2-hydroxyestrone and its derivative, 2-methoxyestrone, is decreased. The sex hormone–binding globulin in plasma is decreased, with the result that the plasma concentrations of both testosterone and estradiol are decreased, but the unbound fractions are increased. The alterations in steroid metabolism are corrected by restoration of the euthyroid state.[47]

Catecholamines

The plasma cyclic adenosine monophosphate (cAMP) response to epinephrine is decreased in hypothyroidism, suggesting a state of decreased adrenergic responsiveness. The fact that the responses of plasma cAMP to glucagon and parathyroid hormone are also decreased suggests that thyroid hormones have a general modulating influence on cAMP generation.[48] The reduced adrenergic responsiveness associated with hypothyroidism has been linked to all steps of catecholamine signaling, including receptor and postreceptor actions, resulting in an impaired cAMP response. Direct measurement of norepinephrine in abdominal fat of hypothyroid patients shows reduced levels and there is reduced production of glycerol in response to adrenergic agonist stimulation.[49] Augmentation of α2-receptor signaling has also been proposed as a factor reducing catecholamine responsiveness.

Energy Metabolism: Protein, Carbohydrate, and Lipid Metabolism

The decrease in energy metabolism and heat production is reflected in the low basal metabolic rate, decreased appetite, cold intolerance, and slightly low basal body temperature. Both the synthesis and the degradation of protein are decreased, the latter especially so, with the result that nitrogen balance is usually slightly positive. The decrease in protein synthesis is reflected in retardation of both skeletal and soft tissue growth.

Permeability of capillaries to protein is increased, accounting for the high levels of protein in effusions and in cerebrospinal fluid. In addition, the albumin pool is increased because of the greater decrease in albumin degradation compared to albumin synthesis. A greater than normal fraction of exchangeable albumin is in the extravascular space. The total concentration of serum proteins may be increased.

Hypothyroidism is associated with a reduction in glucose disposal to skeletal muscle and adipose tissue.[50] Thyroid hormone has been shown to stimulate expression of the insulin sensitive glucose transporter (GLUT-4), and the levels of this transporter are reduced in hypothyroidism. Hypothyroidism is also, however, associated with reduced gluconeogenesis.[50] The net effect of these influences is usually a minimal effect of hypothyroidism on serum glucose levels. Thyroid hormone down-regulates expression of prohormone processing enzymes, which, therefore, have increased activity in hypothyroidism.[51] Degradation of insulin, therefore, is slowed and the sensitivity to exogenous insulin may be increased. In a patient with preexisting diabetes mellitus who develops hypothyroidism, insulin requirements may be reduced. A further influence on glucose uptake may occur at the tissue level. Polymorphisms in the 5′-deiodinase type 2 (D2) gene, which may affect local T_3

production, have shown to be associated with impaired glucose disposal.[50]

Both the synthesis and the degradation of lipid are depressed in hypothyroidism. Degradation, however, is reduced to a greater extent, with a net effect of accumulation of LDL and triglycerides.[52] The decrease in the lipid degradation rate may reflect the decrease in post-heparin lipolytic activity, as well as reduced LDL receptors.[53] HDL concentrations are reduced. Plasma free fatty acid levels are decreased, and the mobilization of free fatty acids in response to fasting, catecholamines, and growth hormone is impaired. Impaired lipolysis of white fat in hypothyroid patients at baseline and in response to catecholamine, reflects impaired free fatty acid mobilization.[49] All of these abnormalities are relieved by treatment.

There was a correlation shown between total cholesterol and serum TSH levels in hypothyroid individuals identified from among 25,862 participants in a health fair, including those not aware of being hypothyroid and those on thyroxine replacement.[54] An elevation in serum LDL cholesterol has been associated, in most studies, with overt and subclinical hypothyroidism.[22] According to most studies, serum HDL and triglycerides levels, are not influenced by hypothyroidism.[22,55] The reduction in LDL with thyroxine therapy is generally related to the original magnitude of LDL and TSH elevation, the higher the initial levels, the greater reduction in LDL is observed.[22,55] A typical reduction in LDL is 5% to 10% of the original level.

The role of adipocytokines, such as leptin, adiponectin, and resistin, in metabolic regulation has been increasingly recognized as well as the potential for interaction with thyroid hormone.[56] Rodent studies have shown that leptin regulates central adaptation between the starved and fed state, and that falling leptin levels, associated with starvation, lead to a suppression of the thyroid axis. Hypothyroidism in rodents is associated with reduced leptin and increased resistin levels. Leptin infusion into the cerebral ventricles reverses some of the metabolic changes seen with hypothyroidism, including improved glucose disposal and reduced skeletal muscle fat.[56] Human studies, however, have not shown consistent changes in adipocytokines in hypothyroidism.[57]

CURRENT CLINICAL PICTURE

In the adult, the onset of hypothyroidism is usually so insidious that the typical manifestations may take months or years to appear and go unnoticed by family and friends. The gradual development of the hypothyroid state is due to slow progression both of thyroid hypofunction and of the clinical manifestations after thyroid failure is complete. This course is in contrast with the more rapid development of the hypothyroid state when replacement therapy is discontinued in a patient with treated primary hypothyroidism or when the thyroid gland of a normal subject is surgically removed. In such patients, manifestations of frank hypothyroidism are usually present by 6 weeks and myxedema appears by 3 months.

Hypothyroidism continues to be diagnosed at earlier stages. Based on the most recent data, subclinical or early hypothyroidism is seen approximately 14 times more commonly than overt hypothyroidism. Scales for assessment of clinical symptoms suggesting hypothyroidism have been developed, reflecting the more typical earlier identification (Fig. 12–5).[58] In general, many of the symptoms are similar but are much less prevalent than they were and do not effectively discriminate the hypothyroid from the euthyroid patient (e.g., cold intolerance or pulse rate). Early symptoms are variable and relatively nonspecific. The reason for the increased prevalence of hypothyroid patients presenting with minimal symptoms is largely the availability of

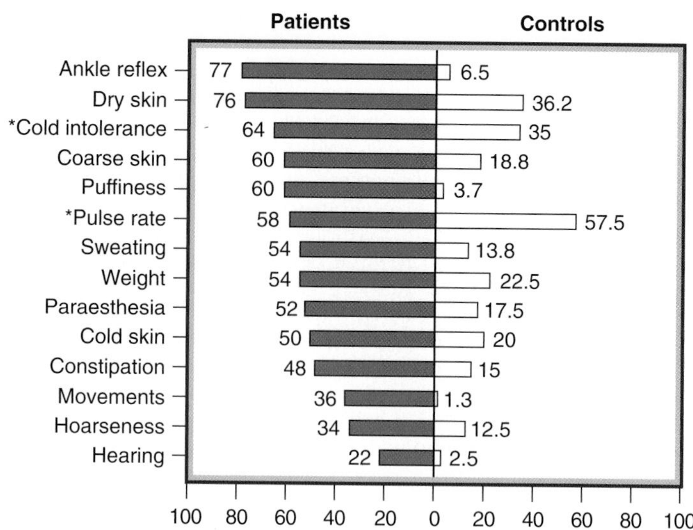

Figure 12–5 ▪ Frequency of hypothyroid symptoms and signs (percentage) in 50 patients with overt hypothyroidism and in 80 euthyroid controls. Two symptoms (pulse rate and cold intolerance, marked by asterisks) showed positive and negative predictive values of less than 70% and were thus excluded from the new score. (From Zulewski H, Müller B, Exer P, et al. Estimation of tissue hypothyroidism by a new clinical score: evaluation of patients with various grades of hypothyroidism and controls. J Clin Endocrinol Metab 1997;82:771-776.)

sensitive and specific laboratory tests that allow recognition of the primary form of the disease long before severe symptoms have developed. There should, therefore, be a low threshold to test patients for suspected primary hypothyroidism with a TSH determination. Patients with significant biochemical abnormalities of hypothyroidism may well not score high on indices of symptoms and signs.[58]

With respect to physical signs of hypothyroidism, the presence of coarse skin, periorbital puffiness that obscures the curve of the malar bone (see Fig. 12–1), cold skin, and delayed ankle reflex relaxation phase are all signs that should lead to appropriate diagnostic tests.

Acute hypothyroidism in the previously hyperthyroid patient seen after radioiodine therapy is characterized by painful cramping of large muscle groups is discussed under "Treatment of Graves' Disease" in Chapter 11.

Hypothyroidism in Infants and Children

Severe hypothyroidism is seldom apparent at birth, hence the requirement for systematic screening for congenital hypothyroidism.[10] Congenital hypothyroidism can be due to complete thyroid agenesis, ectopic thyroid, or incomplete thyroid development.[10] Mutations in genes important for thyroid development have been identified in a number of patients, and in some cases may explain associated abnormalities in development of other structures, such as the heart. The age at which symptoms appear depends on the degree of impairment of thyroid function (see Figs. 12–3 and 12–4). Severe hypothyroidism in infancy is termed *cretinism.* As the age at onset increases, the clinical picture of cretinism merges imperceptibly with that of juvenile hypothyroidism. Retardation of mental development and growth, the hallmark of cretinism, becomes manifest only in later infancy and the former is largely irreversible. Consequently, early recognition is crucial and has been achieved by universal population screening in the developed world by measuring serum T_4 or TSH concentrations routinely in blood spots taken from neonates.

During the first few months of life, symptoms of hypothyroidism include feeding problems, failure to thrive, constipation, a hoarse cry, and somnolence. In succeeding months, especially in severe cases, protuberance of the abdomen, dry skin, poor growth of hair and nails, and delayed eruption of the deciduous teeth become evident. Retardation of mental and physical development is manifested by delay in reaching the normal milestones of development, such as holding up the head, sitting, walking, and talking.

Thyroid hormone plays a major role in bone development and thyroid hormone receptors are expressed in osteoclasts and osteoblasts.[59] The primary targets of thyroid hormone have been identified in the epiphyseal plates. Impairment of linear growth in congenital hypothyroidism results in dwarfism, with the limbs disproportionately short in relation to the trunk (see Fig. 12–3). Delayed closure of the fontanelles causes the head to be large in relation to the body. The naso-orbital configuration remains infantile. Maldevelopment of the femoral epiphyses results in a waddling gait. The teeth are malformed and susceptible to caries. The characteristic appearance includes a broad, flat nose; widely set eyes; periorbital puffiness; large protruding tongue; sparse hair; rough skin; short neck; and protuberant abdomen with an umbilical hernia. Mental deficiency is usually severe.

Radiologic examination of the skeleton is diagnostic. The skull shows a poorly developed base; delayed closure of the fontanelles; widely set orbits; and a short, flat nasal bone. The pituitary fossa may be enlarged. Shedding of deciduous teeth and eruption of permanent teeth are delayed (see Fig. 12–4).

The radiologic picture of epiphyseal dysgenesis is virtually pathognomonic of hypothyroidism in infancy and childhood and may involve any center of endochondral ossification, depending on the age at onset of the hypothyroid state; it is usually best seen in the femoral and humeral heads and the navicular bone of the foot. The centers of ossification appear late, so bone age is retarded in relation to chronologic age, and when they eventually appear, instead of a single center, multiple small centers are scattered through a misshapen epiphysis (see Fig. 12–4). These small centers of ossification eventually coalesce and form a single center with an irregular outline and a stippled appearance (stippled epiphysis). Epiphyseal dysgenesis is evident only in centers that normally ossify at a time after the onset of the hypothyroidism. After a normal metabolic state is restored by treatment, centers destined to ossify at a later age develop normally.

Hypothyroidism that begins in childhood is usually Hashimoto's disease and can be transient in this age group. The clinical manifestations are intermediate, between those of infantile and those of adult hypothyroidism, in that the developmental retardation is not as severe as that of cretinism and the manifestations of full-blown adult myxedema are rarely seen. Growth and sexual development are affected predominantly. If left untreated, linear growth is severely retarded and sexual maturation and the onset of puberty are delayed.[35,36] On radiologic examination, epiphyseal dysgenesis may be present and epiphyseal union is always delayed, resulting in a bone age that is younger relative to chronologic age.

LABORATORY EVALUATION

Primary and Central Hypothyroidism

A decrease in secretion of the thyroid hormones is common to all varieties of hypothyroidism, except for disorders of thyroid hormone metabolism or action, such as *consumptive hypothyroidism* and *resistance to thyroid hormone* (see later). In patients with primary thyroid disease, the cause of hypothyroidism in more than 99% of the patients, there is a significant increase in basal serum TSH concentration. A strategy for evaluating the patient suspected of hypothyroidism involves a TSH determination (Table 12–2). If the suspicion of hypothyroidism is strong, if a goiter is present, or if central hypothyroidism is part of the differential diagnosis, a free T_4 assay should be included (see Chapter 10). If hypothyroidism is thought to be unlikely but must be excluded, only a TSH determination is required because primary hypothyroidism is almost always the cause. If TSH is elevated, a free T_4 assay can be added to the same determination (Fig. 12–6). As hypothyroidism progresses, the serum TSH increases further, the serum free T_4 falls, and finally at the most severe stage, serum triiodothyronine (T_3) concentrations may become subnormal (see Table 12–2). The persistence of a normal serum T_3 is, in part, due to preferential synthesis and secretion of T_3 by residual functioning thyroid tissue under the influence of the increased plasma TSH. In addition, the efficiency of conversion of T_4 to T_3 by D2 is increased as the serum T_4 level falls.[60] Consequently, the serum T_3 concentration may remain within the normal range.

The principal differential diagnosis is between primary and central hypothyroidism (see Chapter 8). The serum TSH concentration is the critical laboratory determination that, in general, allows recognition of the cause of the disease when the serum free thyroxine is reduced. An exception is the individual with a recent history of thyrotoxicosis (and suppressed TSH) in whom a low free T_4 level may be associated with a reduced TSH level for several months after treatment of the thyrotoxicosis. In patients with primary hypothyroidism, the absence of thyroid peroxidase (TPO) antibodies raises a possible diagnosis of transient hypothyroidism following an undiagnosed episode of subacute or postviral thyroiditis.

The differentiation of hypothyroidism due to intrinsic thyroid failure from hypothyroidism due to diminished TSH secretion from hypothalamic or pituitary disease (central or secondary hypothyroidism) is the most critical decision point in this pathway (see Fig. 12–6). A low thyroid hormone level with a normal or low TSH level should lead to an evaluation for the possibility of failure of other endocrine systems that require trophic pituitary hormones for normal function (see Table 12–1) (see Chapters 7 and 8). The only exception to this is the early stages of *post-hyperthyroid* hypothyroidism, in which TSH levels may remain suppressed for several months even though hypothyroidism, as revealed by a low free T_4 level, has been induced by ^{131}I, surgery, or antithyroid drugs (see Table 12–2). In some patients with central hypothyroidism, the basal serum TSH concentration (and the response to TRH) may even be somewhat elevated, but the TSH has reduced biologic potency even though it is immunologically reactive.[61]

In patients with an elevated TSH level and a reduced free T_4, the presence or absence of thyroid peroxidase (TPO) antibodies should be ascertained (see Fig. 12–6). The presence of TPO antibodies generally points to autoimmune thyroid disease (Hashimoto's disease) as the cause of the hypothyroidism. On the other hand, the absence of TPO antibodies requires a search for less common causes of hypothyroidism such as transient hypothyroidism, infiltrative thyroid disorders, and external irradiation, as discussed later (see Table 12–1), although some patients with Hashimoto's disease, approximately 10%, will not have detectable TPO antibodies.

Measurement of radioactive iodine uptake (RAIU) is rarely required in the evaluation of hypothyroidism. Tests that employ radioiodine to assess the function of the thyroid gland display a variable pattern, depending on the underlying thyroid disorder. The diagnostic value of a low RAIU is limited because of

TABLE 12–2 LABORATORY EVALUATION OF PATIENTS WITH SUSPECTED HYPOTHYROIDISM OR THYROID ENLARGEMENT

Initial Tests: Serum TSH, Serum Free T_4, TPO* or TgAb**

TSH, Free T_4	TPO Ab	Diagnosis
TSH >10 mU/L		
Free T_4		
Low	+	primary hypothyroidism due to autoimmune thyroid disease
Low normal	+	primary "subclinical" hypothyroidism (autoimmune)
Low or low normal	–	recovery from systemic illness
		external irradiation, drug-induced, congenital hypothyroidism
		iodine deficiency
		seronegative autoimmune thyroid disease
		rare thyroid disorders (amyloidosis, sarcoidosis, etc.)
		recovery from subacute granulomatous thyroiditis
Normal	+, –	consider TSH or T_4 assay artifacts
Elevated	–	thyroid hormone resistance
		blockade of T_4 to T_3 conversion (amiodarone) or a congenital 5′-deiodinase deficiency
		consider assay artifacts
TSH 5-10 mU/L		
Free T_4		
Low, low normal	+	early primary autoimmune hypothyroidism
Low, low normal	–	milder forms of non-autoimmune hypothyroidism (see above)
		central hypothyroidism with impaired TSH bioactivity
Elevated	– (+)	consider thyroid hormone resistance
		T_4 to T_3 conversion blockade (e.g., amiodarone)
TSH 0.5-5 mU/L		
Free T_4		
Low, low normal	– (+)	central hypothyroidism
		salicylate or phenytoin therapy
		desiccated thyroid or T_3 replacement
TSH <0.5 μU/L		
Free T_4		
Low, low normal	– (+)	"post hyperthyroid" hypothyroidism (^{131}I or surgery)
		central hypothyroidism
		T_3 or desiccated thyroid excess
		post excess levothyroxine withdrawal

*TSH, thyroid-stimulating hormone; TPOAb, thyroid peroxidase autoantibody; TgAb, anti-thyroglobulin antibody.

the relatively high dietary iodine intake in North America, reducing uptake of the tracer dose of radioiodine, and variation in iodine intake from day to day in the same individual. National surveys of dietary iodine intake had shown a progressive reduction in iodine intake over the last several decades,[62] but a recent survey indicates that the intake has not continued to fall, but has remained relatively stable.[63] The RAIU may be normal or even increased when hypothyroidism results primarily from a biochemical defect in thyroid hormone synthesis rather than thyroid cell destruction leading to compensatory thyroid enlargement. Specific functional patterns in relation to the causes of hypothyroidism are discussed later. Nonetheless, measurement of RAIU is almost never required in the diagnostic evaluation of the hypothyroid patient.

Differential Diagnosis

The clinical picture of fully developed hypothyroidism is quite characteristic, but the abnormalities can be overlooked, even by experienced clinicians, if the diagnosis is not considered. Despite the availability of inexpensive and specific tests, it is still surprising how often what is retrospectively obvious, severe, primary hypothyroidism is not recognized. A high index of suspicion is required to avoid this oversight.

For the milder forms of hypothyroidism, the clinical presentation overlaps to a significant extent with other conditions. The fact that these disorders often occur in older patients is partly responsible for the diagnostic uncertainty.[64] In some cases, slowing of mental and physical activity, dry skin, and loss of hair may mimic similar findings in hypothyroidism. Furthermore, older people often become hypothermic with cold exposure. In patients with chronic renal insufficiency, anorexia, torpor, periorbital puffiness, sallow complexion, and anemia (e.g., see Fig. 12–1) may suggest hypothyroidism and may call for specific testing. Distinguishing nephrotic states from hypothyroidism by clinical examination alone may be even more difficult. In this disorder, waxy pallor, edema, hypercholesterolemia, and hypometabolism may suggest hypothyroidism. In addition, the total serum T_4 concentration may be decreased if significant thyroid binding globulin is lost in the urine but the free T_4 and TSH would be normal.

In patients with pernicious anemia, psychiatric abnormalities, pallor, and numbness and tingling of the extremities may mimic similar findings in hypothyroidism. Although there is a clinical and immunologic overlap between primary hypothyroidism and pernicious anemia, this association is not invariable (see Chapter 41). The presence of hypothyroidism is often suspected in patients who are severely ill, especially in the elderly.[64] In such patients, the total T_4 concentration may be decreased, often markedly so, but the free T_4 is generally normal

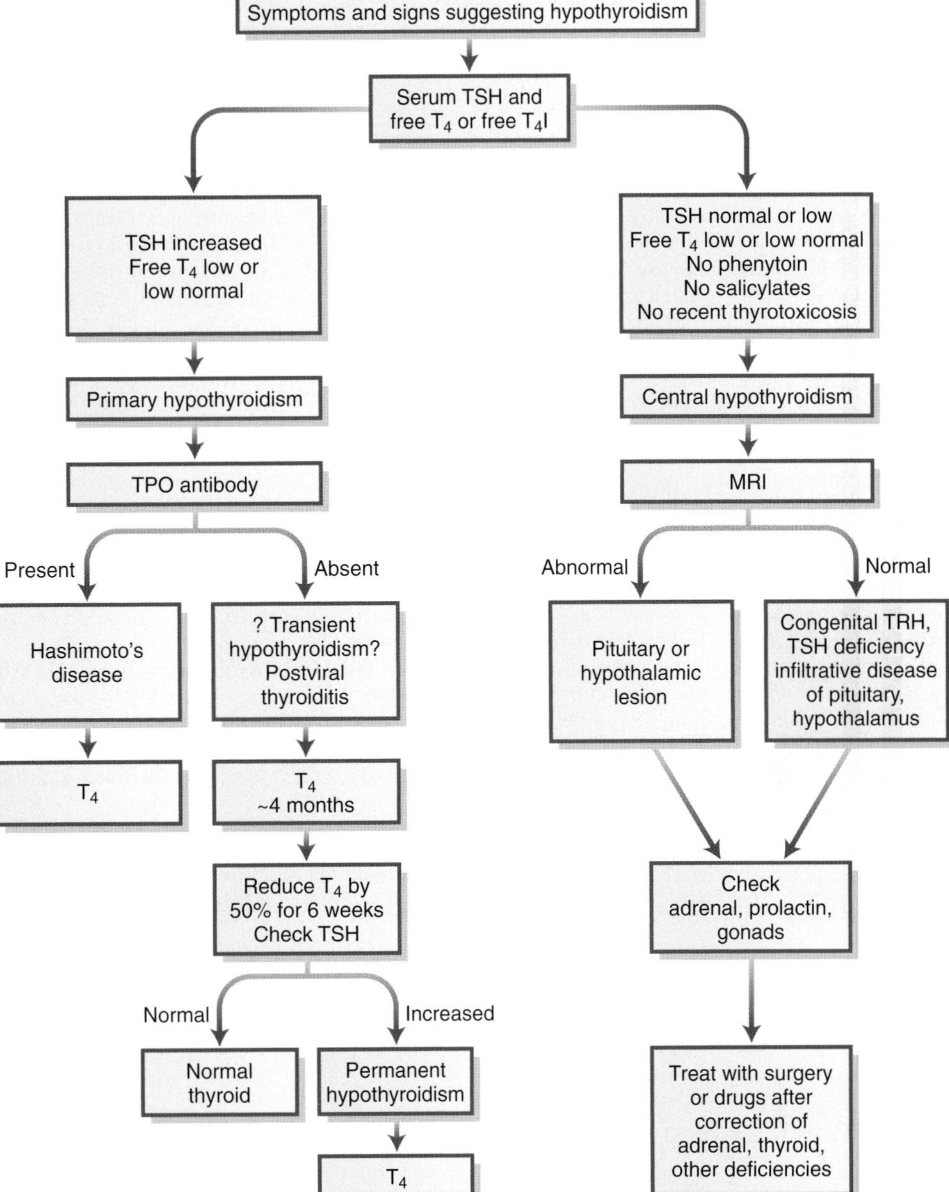

Figure 12–6 ▪ Strategy for the laboratory evaluation of patients with suspected hypothyroidism. The principal differential diagnosis is between primary and central hypothyroidism (see Chapter 8). The serum thyrotropin (TSH) concentration is the critical laboratory determination that, in general, allows recognition of the cause of the disease. An exception is the individual with a recent history of thyrotoxicosis (and suppressed TSH) in whom a low free thyroxine (T_4) level may be associated with a reduced TSH level for several months after relief of the thyrotoxicosis. In patients with primary hypothyroidism, the absence of thyroid peroxidase (TPO) antibodies raises a possible diagnosis of transient hypothyroidism following an undiagnosed episode of subacute or postviral thyroiditis. In such patients, a trial of levothyroxine in reduced dosage after 4 months may reveal recovery of thyroid function, thus avoiding permanent levothyroxine replacement. *MRI,* Magnetic resonance imaging.

unless the patient is severely ill (see Chapter 10). These features, together with the absence of an elevation of serum TSH, usually serve to differentiate the ill euthyroid patient from one with primary hypothyroidism. The serum TSH, however, can be transiently increased (up to 20 mU/L) during recovery from severe illness.

Hypothyroidism may develop either because of some extrinsic factor or acquired condition or because of a congenital defect impairing thyroid hormone biosynthesis (see Table 12–1). Inadequate synthesis of hormone leads to hypersecretion of TSH, which in turn produces both goiter and stimulation of all steps in hormone biosynthesis capable of response. In some instances, however, the compensatory TSH response overcomes the impairment in hormone biosynthesis, and the patient is euthyroid with a goiter. The latter condition is discussed in Chapter 13 under "Simple or Nontoxic Goiter." Less commonly, hypothyroidism is associated with an atrophic gland or, in the case of a congenital abnormality, one that never developed properly.

CLASSIFICATION

Acquired Causes

Hashimoto's Thyroiditis

Hashimoto's disease is the most common cause of hypothyroidism in areas of the world in which dietary iodine is sufficient. The terminology used to classify *autoimmune thyroid diseases* does not reflect our current understanding of the pathophysiology of these disorders and suggests that Hashimoto's disease and Graves' disease are distinct entities. In pathologic terms, thyroiditis implies the presence of both a mononuclear cell infiltrate and destruction of thyroid follicles. However, these are arbitrary criteria. The term *chronic thyroiditis* is more appropriately defined simply as evidence of "intrathyroidal lymphocytic infiltration" without the necessity of follicular damage. Because, by this definition, patients with both Graves' disease and Hashimoto's disease have thyroiditis, replacement of the term *autoimmune thyroid disease* with the more correct term *autoimmune thyroiditis* allows a simple classification for autoimmune thyroid disease.[65] Most classification systems, however, use the term *autoimmune thyroiditis* as synonymous with *transient or chronic inflammation,* associated with follicular destruction.[1,2]

Autoantibodies to the TSH receptor that act as TSH antagonists may be the cause of some cases of the atrophic form of Hashimoto's disease (in the past referred to as primary myxedema).[66] Both Graves' disease and Hashimoto's disease may occur within the same families and may share human leukocyte antigen (HLA) and other genetic susceptibility haplotypes.[66,67] Furthermore, thyroid failure occurs in some patients with Graves' disease, and hyperthyroidism and even orbitopathy develop in some patients with Hashimoto's disease. Both types of patients may have autoantibodies to thyroglobulin, TPO, and the TSH receptor. Hence, the diseases must be closely related, and autoimmune thyroid disease can be viewed as a spectrum from hyperthyroidism to hypothyroidism.

Until the demonstration of circulating thyroid antigen–specific T cells and thyroid autoantibodies, the diagnosis of Hashimoto's disease could be confirmed only by biopsy of the thyroid. The ease with which we can now demonstrate high levels of circulating antibodies and thyroid antigen–specific T cells in most patients with Hashimoto's disease led to the use of the term *autoimmune thyroiditis,* which, as explained earlier, we prefer to use for any mononuclear infiltrate.

Hashimoto's disease is common and may be increasing in frequency. The mean incidence in women is in the order of 3.5 cases per 1000 people per year and in men is 0.8 case per 1000 people per year.[3-5] No age group is exempt, although the prevalence increases with age in both women and men. Hashimoto's disease is the most common cause of goitrous hypothyroidism in areas of iodine sufficiency.

Pathophysiology

Impairment of hormone synthesis is due to apoptotic destruction of the thyroid cells. The sick cells exhibit a defect in organic binding of thyroid iodide, as evidenced by a positive perchlorate discharge test (see Chapter 10). In addition, release of iodoproteins, mostly thyroglobulin, is enhanced by cell lysis. Approximately 90% of the thyroid gland must be destroyed before hypothyroidism develops. The presence of lymphocytic infiltration of the thyroid (hence the older term *lymphocytic thyroiditis*), circulating thyroid autoantibodies, and clinical or immunologic overlap with other diseases with autoimmune components indicate that Hashimoto's disease is an autoimmune thyroid disorder.

The current understanding of autoimmune mechanisms has been discussed earlier in Chapter 11. However, autoimmune thyroiditis is characterized by thyroid cell apoptosis leading to follicular destruction rather than thyroid stimulation and thyroid cell hyperplasia. Although both autoantibodies to thyroid peroxidase (TPOAb) and thyroglobulin (TgAb) may be complement-fixing and cytotoxic, the thyroid gland is infiltrated by both B cells and T cells; the latter are armed with Fas ligand and capable of destroying thyroid cells expressing Fas via apoptosis (Fig. 12–7).[68,69] In addition, other cell death pathways may

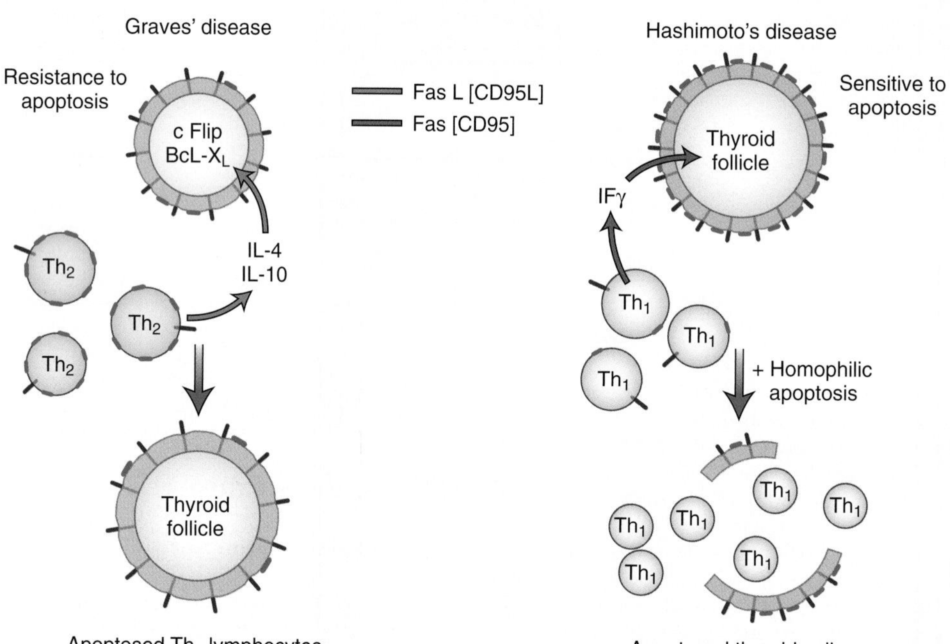

Figure 12–7 ▪ Possible involvement of Fas-Fas L in the apoptosis of Hashimoto's thyroiditis. In Graves' disease, the thyroid follicles thrive because the thyroid cells do not express many functional Fas molecules (shown in red) and therefore, the thyroid cells are resistant to the Fas L (Fas ligand) both on the thyroid cells themselves and on the Th_2 T cells (shown in blue). Further apoptotic resistance may be driven by Th_2 cytokines, such as interleukin-4 (IL-4) and IL-10. However, the Th_2 cells express Fas and may themselves be deleted by the Fas L constitutively expressed on the thyroid cells. The result is thyroid cell survival with T-cell destruction. In contrast, in Hashimoto's disease, the thyroid cell expresses many functional Fas molecules, perhaps induced by gamma interferon from the Th_1 type T cells associated with this disease. The expression of thyroid cell Fas may lead to self (homophilic) apoptosis via thyroid cell Fas L, or apoptosis may result from attack by the Fas L–armed Th_1 cells. The result is thyroid follicle destruction and T-cell proliferation.

be involved.[70] Fas expression on thyroid cells may be secondary to elaboration of a variety of cytokines from T cells that undergo blast transformation when exposed to thyroid antigens (thyrotropin receptor, TPO, and thyroglobulin), suggesting that cell-mediated autoimmune mechanisms are pathogenetically involved.[71]

These manifestations of autoimmunity in Hashimoto's disease and other autoimmune thyroid disorders reflect a hereditary susceptibility to thyroid disease that allows the survival and persistence of B cells and T cells directed against thyroid antigens.[72] The fact that infusion of interleukin-2 and lymphokine-activated killer cells causes progression or development of hypothyroidism in patients with detectable TPOAb is additional evidence of the autoimmune nature of this disease.[72] Animal models and increasing use of interferon-α use in chronic liver disease have demonstrated a role of cytokines in initiating thyroid destruction in the setting of lymphocytic infiltration of the thyroid.[74,75]

Histopathology

The thyroid gland is pale and firm and has a rubbery texture (Fig. 12–8A). Histopathologic changes vary in type and extent but usually consist of diffuse lymphocytic infiltration with germinal center formation and obliteration of thyroid follicles by widespread apoptosis (see Fig. 12–8B). In most cases, there is destruction of epithelial cells and degeneration and fragmentation of the follicular basement membrane. The remaining epithelial cells may be larger and show oxyphilic changes in the cytoplasm; these so-called Askanazy cells are virtually pathognomonic. In some cases, colloid is sparse. Fibrosis is generally present in the more longstanding tissues but not to the extent seen in Riedel's thyroiditis (see Fig. 12–8C).

In the past, the diagnosis of Hashimoto's disease required the presence of Askanazy cells or lymphoid follicles, but now the primary observation should be follicular destruction, often with mononuclear cell invasion of the follicular spaces. The degree of lymphocytic infiltration usually correlates with the levels of circulating thyroid autoantibodies. In Graves' disease, the heterogeneous lymphocytic infiltration and associated antibodies may favor the development of hypothyroidism in the long term, accelerated by partial thyroidectomy or radioiodine therapy.

Risk Factors

Genetic Susceptibility

We have already referred to the familial predisposition to autoimmune disease in patients with autoimmune thyroid disease. As with Graves' disease, there is a significant but weak association between Hashimoto's disease and HLA-DR3, perhaps also HLA-DR5, and certain DQ alleles.[66,67] Unlike the situation of diabetes mellitus, formal linkage of specific histocompatibility antigens with autoimmune thyroid disease has been difficult to demonstrate.

Hashimoto's disease occurs with increased frequency in Down's syndrome and (probably) gonadal dysgenesis.[66] The fact that thyroid cells can express HLA-DR antigens, at least as a secondary phenomenon, indicates the potential role of these

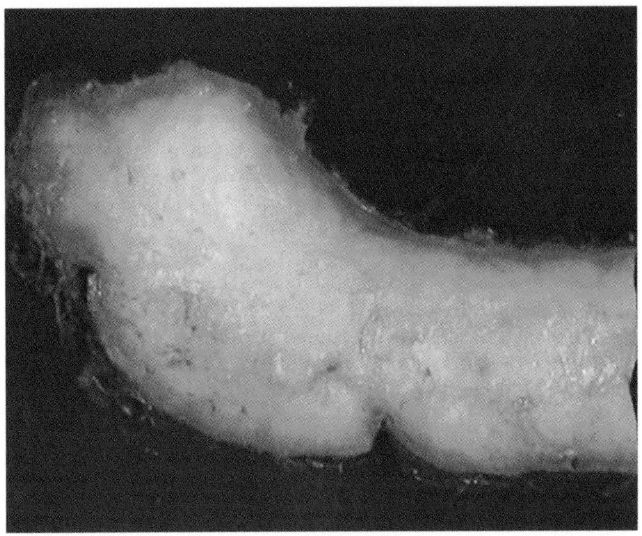

A

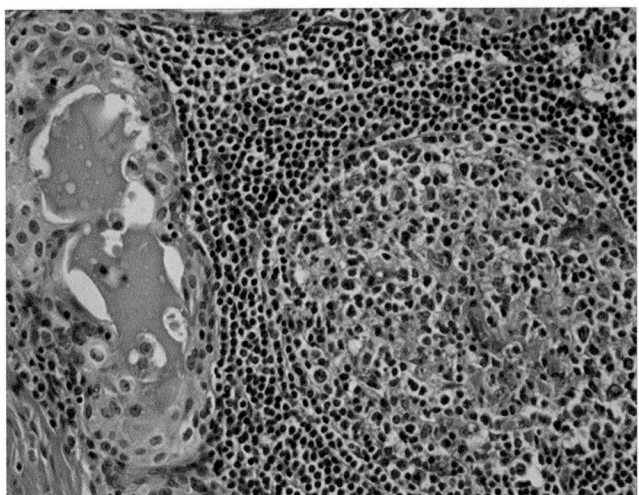

B

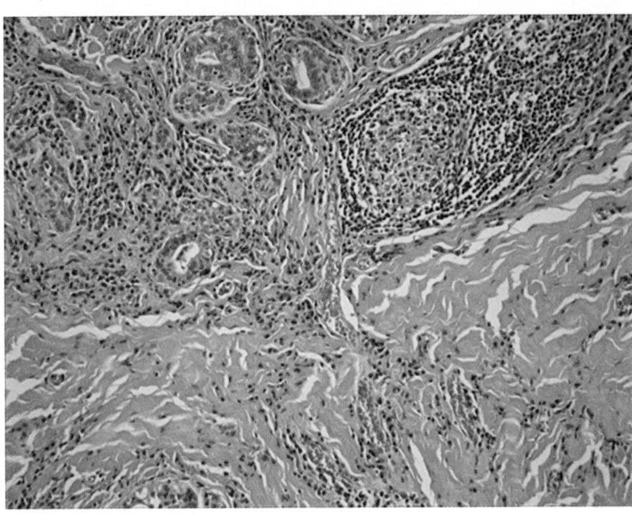

C

Figure 12–8 ▪ Hashimoto's thyroiditis. **A,** Gross appearance of a cut section of the thyroid lobe demonstrating the pale color of the tissue due to lymphocytic infiltration, fibrosis, and loss of follicles. **B,** Typical histologic appearance illustrating a germinal center, heavy lymphocytic infiltration, and a partially disrupted thyroid follicle. **C,** Fibrous variant showing extensive fibrosis and loss of follicles. (Courtesy of Dr. Vania Nosé, Department of Pathology, Brigham and Women's Hospital, Boston, MA.)

cells in perpetuating the immune response and may be related to the propensity of autoimmune disease for certain HLA-DR subgroups. Hashimoto's disease almost certainly is associated with a polygenetic susceptibility, HLA being one gene involved. Efforts are under way to identify non-HLA susceptibility genes in families with autoimmune thyroid disease. In this regard, polymorphisms in the *CTLA4* gene have been linked to the propensity to secrete thyroid autoantibodies and may, in turn, be an important risk factor for disease itself.[66]

Nongenetic Risk Factors

Many of the factors that have been identified as increasing the risk for Graves' disease (pregnancy, drugs, age and sex, infection, and irradiation) apply equally to autoimmune thyroiditis. These are detailed in Chapter 11 and are briefly considered here.

Pregnancy

The recognition of transient postpartum thyroiditis as an important clinical entity has also provided an example of the immune manipulation of thyroid disease with a predictable onset and recovery (see Chapter 11). Maternal microchimerism may be an important component of this risk analysis.[76] The disease is essentially postpartum Hashimoto's disease except for its transient nature. Data suggest that 8% to 10% of women experience thyroiditis in the postpartum period with a variety of consequences (see later).[77] Pregnancy is, therefore, an important risk factor, with transient postpartum thyroiditis developing in some patients and thyroid failure developing permanently or in the early years after pregnancy in a significant proportion.

Iodine and Drugs

Iodine and iodine-containing drugs (such as amiodarone) precipitate autoimmune thyroiditis in susceptible populations.[78-80] This form should be distinguished from direct blockade and destruction of the thyroid gland by iodine. The mechanism of this precipitation is unknown. However, much evidence accumulated in animal models suggests that increased iodination of thyroglobulin enhances its immunoreactivity.[81]

Cytokines

Treatment of patients with interleukin-2 or interferon-α may precipitate the appearance of autoimmune thyroid disease.[73,74] Destructive thyrotoxicosis may appear suddenly, but persistent Graves' disease may also develop in such patients. Autoimmune thyroid disease is more common in patients with preexisting TPOAbs.

Irradiation

Radiation exposure has been shown to induce thyroid autoantibodies and autoimmune thyroid disease in a number of studies. These include radiation from the atomic bomb detonation in Japan,[82] the Chernobyl disaster,[83] and therapeutic radiation for Hodgkin's, disease.[84] Hodgkin's disease survivors have a 17-fold relative risk of developing hypothyroidism.[85] A long-term follow-up of Japanese atomic bomb survivors after over 55 years, however, showed a persistent effect on an increased risk of thyroid nodules, but not thyroid autoantibodies.[86] It is postulated that the specific effect of radiation on thyroid autoantibody expression may diminish with longer-term follow-up as the incidence of autoimmune thyroid disease in the general population increases with age.

Age

Autoimmune thyroid failure continues to occur throughout adult life, so that the prevalence of the disease increases markedly with age.[3-5] This is similar to other markers of autoimmunity and may reflect an increasing loss of tolerance to self.

Infection

There is no direct evidence that infection causes autoimmune thyroiditis in humans. A number of viral infections in animals, however, do precipitate thyroid autoimmunity.[87] In addition, there is evidence from long-term follow-up of patients with subacute thyroiditis (see later), thought to be a reaction to a viral infection, that persisting signs of thyroid autoimmune disease can be found. Infection remains a likely cause of a local or distant insult that is considered to be needed to precipitate autoimmune disease in susceptible individuals (see "Mechanisms in Graves' Disease," Chapter 11).

Clinical Picture

Goiter, the hallmark of classic Hashimoto's disease, usually develops gradually and may be found during routine examination or by ultrasonography. On occasion, the thyroid gland enlarges rapidly and, when accompanied by pain and tenderness, may mimic de Quervain's or subacute thyroiditis (see Chapter 11). Some patients, particularly those with the fibrous variant, are hypothyroid when first seen. The goiter is generally moderate in size and firm in consistency and moves freely on swallowing. The surface is either smooth or bumpy, but well-defined nodules are unusual. Both lobes are enlarged, but the gland may be asymmetrical. The pyramidal lobe may also be enlarged, and adjacent structures, such as the trachea, esophagus, and recurrent laryngeal nerves, may be compressed. Enlargement of regional lymph nodes is unusual.

Other patients with hypothyroidism present without a goiter (atrophic hypothyroidism) (see later), which is thought to be the end result of autoimmune destruction of the thyroid. The progression of goitrous Hashimoto's disease to the atrophied state is not commonly seen in the individual patient. The atrophic thyroid is likely the reflection of rapid large-scale apoptosis early in the onset of Hashimoto's disease. Indeed, the histopathologic picture tends to remain rather static except for an increase in fibrous tissue.

Clinically, the untreated goiter remains unchanged or enlarges gradually over many years. The manifestations of hypothyroidism may develop over several years in patients who are initially euthyroid. Thyroid lymphoma occurs almost exclusively in patients with underlying Hashimoto's disease and should be suspected if there is rapid, usually painful, enlargement of the thyroid gland.[88] As mentioned earlier, the presence of coexistent Hashimoto's disease may be a favorable prognostic factor in patients with papillary carcinoma.[89]

Occasionally, hyperthyroidism due to Graves' disease develops in patients with Hashimoto's disease. In other patients with early autoimmune thyroiditis, transitory thyrotoxicosis (painless or silent thyroiditis with thyrotoxicosis) occurs as the result of thyroid cell destruction. In such cases, evidence of ongoing thyroid hyperfunction is lacking because the thyroid RAIU is depressed. As described earlier, a phase of transient hypothyroidism begins 3 to 6 months post partum in 30% of women with autoimmune thyroiditis, as evidenced by the presence of TPOAb.[77] The history may suggest earlier mild thyrotoxicosis (see syndromes associated with transient hyperthyroidism in Chapter 11).

Laboratory Tests

The results of the common tests of thyroid function depend on stage of disease (see Table 12–2). Rarely, the tests may suggest thyroid hyperfunction with a suppressed TSH but without overproduction of hormone. The RAIU may be increased in these rare patients, but serum T_4 and T_3 levels remain normal. At this stage, the patient may be eumetabolic. As the TSH level rises, the glandular response at first compensates for the impairment of hormone biosynthesis. With time, the ability of the thyroid to respond to TSH diminishes, and the RAIU and serum T_4 level decline to subnormal values. The serum T_3 concentration, however, remains normal, probably reflecting maximal stimulation of the failing thyroid by the increased serum TSH. The early phases of the foregoing sequence, when the serum TSH is increased but T_4 and T_3 are still normal is termed *subclinical hypothyroidism* (see Table 12–2).

The diagnosis of Hashimoto's disease is confirmed by the presence of thyroid autoantibodies in the serum, usually in high levels. TPO autoantibodies are more common and in higher concentrations than thyroglobulin autoantibodies. Sometimes part of a gland with autoimmune thyroiditis may look and feel like a firm thyroid nodule, and ultrasonography should be performed to resolve the issue.

Differential Diagnosis

Differentiation of Hashimoto's disease from other uncomplicated disorders of the thyroid is facilitated by the demonstration that high levels of thyroid autoantibodies occur more commonly in Hashimoto's disease than in other thyroid disorders. The frequent coexistence of hypothyroidism and Hashimoto's disease serves to distinguish this disease from nontoxic goiter and thyroid neoplasia.

Differentiation of euthyroid Hashimoto's disease from a multinodular goiter is often difficult, although diffuse nontoxic goiter tends to be softer than that of Hashimoto's disease and ultrasound examination may reveal the heterogeneous echotexture characteristic of Hashimoto's disease. In adolescents, differentiation of Hashimoto's disease from diffuse nontoxic goiter is even more difficult because in this age group Hashimoto's disease may not be accompanied by such high levels of thyroid autoantibodies. The presence of well-defined nodules usually distinguishes nontoxic multinodular goiter from Hashimoto's disease.

Differentiation between euthyroid Hashimoto's disease and thyroid carcinoma can sometimes be made on clinical grounds and ultrasound examination. Thyroid carcinoma is usually nodular and firm or hard and the gland may be fixed to adjacent structures. Compression of the recurrent laryngeal nerve with hoarseness is virtually pathognomonic of thyroid neoplasia but occurs late in the disease progression. A history of a recent enlargement of the goiter is more common in thyroid malignancies (either carcinoma or lymphoma) than in Hashimoto's disease. Enlargement of regional lymph nodes also suggests thyroid malignancy. In thyroid carcinoma, ultrasound examination or radioiodine scanning of the thyroid may reveal only the isolated lesion. In Hashimoto's disease, activity is usually heterogeneous.

Treatment

In many patients, no treatment is required because the goiter is small and the disease is asymptomatic, with the TSH level remaining in the normal range. In other patients, treatment with thyroid hormone is directed at alleviating goiter, hypothyroidism, or both.

Levothyroxine treatment is indicated in patients when the goiter presses on adjacent structures or is unsightly, and it is most effective in goiters of recent onset. In longstanding goiter, treatment with thyroid hormone is usually ineffective, possibly because of fibrosis.

Glucocorticoids may cause regression of the goiter and decrease autoantibody levels, but these agents are not recommended in the usual patient because of untoward side effects and the return of activity after treatment is withdrawn.

Full-replacement doses of thyroid hormone should be given when hypothyroidism supervenes. Surgery is justified if pressure symptoms or unsightly enlargement persists after a trial of suppressive therapy. Administration of levothyroxine should be continued after surgery because hypothyroidism is inevitable. The importance of maintaining the serum TSH level within the normal range is discussed later.

Iodine Deficiency (Endemic Goiter)

The term *endemic goiter* denotes any goiter occurring in a region where goiter is prevalent.[90] As mentioned, endemic goiter almost always occurs in areas of environmental iodine deficiency. Although this condition is estimated to affect more than 200 million people throughout the world and is of major public health significance, it is most common in mountainous areas, such as the Alps, Himalayas, and Andes, or in the Great Lakes and Mississippi Valley regions of the United States, owing to the depletion of iodine consequent to the persistent glacial run-off in these regions.

The causative role of iodine deficiency in the genesis of endemic goiter is supported by the inverse correlation between the iodine content of soil and water and the incidence of goiter, the kinetics of iodine metabolism in patients with the disorder, and a decrease in incidence after iodine prophylaxis. The latter accounts for its absence in the population residing in the Great Plains region of the United States.

The occurrence of endemic goiter can vary, even within an area of known iodine deficiency; the role of dietary minerals or naturally occurring goitrogens and of pollution of water supplies has been suggested in instances of this type. For example, in the Cauca Valley of Colombia, waterborne goitrogens have been implicated, and in many areas of endemic iodine deficiency, consumption of cassava meal, which gives rise to thiocyanate, aggravates the iodine-deficient state by inhibiting thyroid iodide transport. Familial clustering of goiters within iodine insufficient areas, usually with an autosomal dominant inheritance, suggest an important genetic component.[91]

Most abnormalities in iodine metabolism in patients with endemic goiter are consistent with the expected effects of iodine deficiency (see Chapter 10, "Iodine Metabolism"). Thyroid iodide clearance rates and RAIU are increased in proportion to the decrease in the urinary excretion of stable iodine. The absolute iodine uptake is normal or low. In areas of moderate iodine deficiency, the serum T_4 concentration is usually in the lower range of normal; in areas of severe deficiency, however, values are decreased. Nevertheless, most patients in these areas do not appear to be in a hypothyroid state because of an increase in the synthesis of T_3 at the expense of T_4 and because of an increase in the activity of thyroidal D1 and D2. TSH levels are typically in the upper range of normal.

The incidence and severity of endemic goiter and the metabolic state of the goitrous patient depend mainly on the degree of iodine deficiency. In the absence of hypothyroidism, the effects of the goiter are mainly cosmetic. When the goiter becomes nodular, however, hemorrhage into a nodule may cause acute pain and swelling, mimicking subacute thyroiditis or neoplasia. The goiter may also compress adjacent structures, such as the trachea, esophagus, and recurrent laryngeal nerves. The borderline nature of the iodine supply in many countries of Western Europe is exemplified by the development in Belgium of compensatory maternal and fetal goiter during pregnancy due to the increased requirement for thyroid hormone during gestation.[92]

The incidence of endemic goiter has been greatly reduced in many areas by the introduction of iodized salt. In the United States, table salt is enriched with potassium iodide to a concentration of 0.01%, which, if the intake of salt is average, would provide an iodine intake of approximately 150–300 μg/day, the desired amount in an adult (see Table 10–1). The use of iodine-containing flour in bread products and iodized salt in commercially produced food has been markedly reduced.[93] Iodine content of bread and infant formula is variable within a given product and often does not match the measured content.[93] As mentioned, iodine intake in the United States has been decreasing in recent decades, likely due to reduced iodine in commercial food products, although iodine intake has now stabilized.[63] It is now theoretically possible that some pregnant patients in the United States may have an inadequate iodine supply. An annual injection of iodized oil is another effective means of administering iodine, and endemic goiter can be treated by the addition of iodine to communal drinking water.

Administration of iodine has little, if any, effect on a long-standing endemic goiter, but it causes the early endemic hyperplastic goiter of iodine deficiency to regress.[94] Similarly, thyroid hormone usually has no effect on long-standing goiter or on established mental or skeletal changes, but it should be given in full-replacement doses if there is evidence of hypothyroidism. This is of paramount importance in pregnant women. Surgical treatment is indicated if the adjacent structures are compressed or if the goiter is either very large or is enlarging rapidly.

Endemic Cretinism

Endemic cretinism is a developmental disorder that occurs in regions of severe endemic goiter.[95,96] Both parents of an endemic cretin are usually goitrous, and in addition to the features of sporadic cretinism described earlier, endemic cretins often have deaf-mutism, spasticity, motor dysfunction, and abnormalities in the basal ganglia demonstrable by magnetic resonance imaging.[97]

Three types of cretins can be discerned: (1) hypothyroid cretins, (2) neurologic cretins, and (3) cretins with combined features of the two. The pathogenesis of neurologic cretinism is obscure but may be due to severe thyroid hormone deficiency during a critical early phase of central nervous system development in utero.[29] Some cretins are goitrous, but the thyroid may also be atrophic, possibly as a consequence of exhaustion atrophy from continuous overstimulation or the lack of iodine.

Iodide Excess

Goiter and hypothyroidism, either alone or in combination, are sometimes induced by chronic administration of large doses of iodine in either organic or inorganic form (see Table 10–7).[79,80,98] Iodide-induced goiter was formerly seen in patients with chronic respiratory disease, who were given potassium iodide as an expectorant. The development of iodide goiter has also been reported after a single administration of radiographic contrast medium from which iodide is released slowly over a long period and may also occur during amiodarone administration.[80] Iodide goiter without hypothyroidism may occur endemically, such as on the island of Hokkaido, Japan, where seaweed products are consumed in large quantities.

From an analysis of reported cases and from the fact that only a small percentage of patients who receive iodides chronically develop goiter, it appears that the disorder evolves on a background of underlying thyroid dysfunction. Categories of susceptible individuals include the following: patients with Hashimoto's disease, patients with Graves' disease, especially after its treatment with radioiodine, and patients with cystic fibrosis.

Among these groups, many individuals display a positive iodide-perchlorate discharge test, indicating a defect in the thyroidal organic iodine-binding mechanism (see Chapter 10, "Iodine Metabolism"). However, intrinsic thyroid disease need not be present because a propensity to develop iodide goiter and hypothyroidism has also been demonstrated in patients who have undergone hemithyroidectomy for a solitary thyroid nodule in whom the remaining lobe was histologically normal. In these patients, as in those with Hashimoto's disease or Graves' disease studied prospectively, individuals with the highest basal serum TSH concentrations, even within the normal range, were those who developed iodide goiter. Iodinated contrast material, amiodarone and povidone-iodine are common sources.[98]

Goiter and hypothyroidism commonly occur in newborn infants born to women given large quantities of iodine during pregnancy, and death from neonatal asphyxia has been reported (see Fig. 10–11). In such cases, the mother is usually free from goiter. Pregnant women should not receive large doses of iodine (>1 mg/day) over prolonged periods (>10 days), especially near term. Maternal amiodarone therapy causes thyroidal dysfunction in up to 20% of newborns.[80] It is not known whether iodide goiter in newborns results from an inherent hypersensitivity of the fetal thyroid or from the fact that the placenta concentrates iodide several-fold, or both.

As discussed earlier (see Chapter 10, "Regulation of Thyroid Function"), large doses of iodine cause an acute inhibition of organic binding that abates in the normal individual, despite continued iodine administration (acute Wolff-Chaikoff effect and escape).[99] Iodide goiter appears to result from a more pronounced inhibition of organic binding and the failure of the escape phenomenon. As a consequence of decreased hormone synthesis and the consequent increase in TSH, iodide transport is enhanced. Because inhibition of organic binding is a function of the intrathyroidal concentration of iodide, a vicious circle, augmented by this increase in serum TSH, is set in motion.

The disorder usually appears as a goiter with or without hypothyroidism, although in rare instances iodine may produce hypothyroidism unaccompanied by goiter. Usually the thyroid gland is firm and diffusely enlarged, often greatly so. Histopathologic examination reveals intense hyperplasia. The free T_4 concentration is low, TSH concentration is increased, and the 24-hour urinary iodine excretion and the serum inorganic iodide concentration are increased. The disorder regresses after iodine is withdrawn. Thyroid hormone may also be given to relieve severe symptoms.

Drugs Blocking Thyroid Hormone Synthesis or Release, Causing Goiter Formation

Ingestion of compounds that block thyroid hormone synthesis or release may cause goiter with or without hypothyroidism. Apart from the agents used in the treatment of hyperthyroidism, antithyroid agents may be encountered either as drugs for the treatment of disorders unrelated to the thyroid gland or as natural agents in foodstuffs.[79]

Goiter with or without hypothyroidism can occur in patients given lithium, usually for bipolar manic-depressive psychosis.[79] Like iodide, lithium inhibits thyroid hormone release, and in high concentrations can inhibit organic binding reactions. At least acutely, iodide and lithium act synergistically in the latter respect. The mechanisms underlying the several effects of lithium are uncertain; what differentiates patients who develop goiter during lithium therapy from those who do not is also unclear. Underlying autoimmune thyroiditis may be at least one factor because many patients with this combination have autoimmune thyroid disease.

Other drugs that occasionally produce goitrous hypothyroidism include paraaminosalicylic acid, phenylbutazone, aminoglutethimide, and ethionamide. Like the thionamides, these drugs interfere with both the organic binding of iodine and perhaps in later steps in hormone biosynthesis. Although soybean flour is not an antithyroid agent, soybean products in feeding formulas formerly resulted in goiter in infants by enhancing fecal loss of hormone, which, together with the low iodine content of soybean products, produced a state of iodine deficiency. Feeding formulas containing soybean products are now enriched with iodine.

Cigarette smoking increases the risk of hypothyroidism in patients with underlying autoimmune thyroid disease. Although the mechanism is unclear, certain components of cigarette smoke, including thiocyanate, hydroxypyridine, and benzopyrene derivatives, may be responsible. These components of smoke may also interfere with thyroid hormone action.[100]

Both the goiter and the hypothyroidism usually subside after the antithyroid agent is withdrawn. If continued administration of pharmacologic goitrogens is required, however, replacement therapy with thyroid hormone causes the goiter to regress.

Goitrogens in Foodstuffs or as Endemic Substances or Pollutants

Antithyroid agents also occur naturally in foods. These are widely distributed in the family Cruciferae or Brassicaceae, particularly in the genus *Brassica,* including cabbages, turnips, kale, kohlrabi, rutabaga, mustard, and various plants that are not eaten by humans but that serve as animal fodder. It is likely that some thiocyanate is present in such plants (particularly cabbage). Cassava meal, a dietary staple in many regions of the world, contains linamarin, a cyanogenic glycoside, the preparation of which leads to the formation of thiocyanate. Ingestion of cassava can accentuate goiter formation in areas of endemic iodine deficiency. Except for thiocyanate, dietary goitrogens influence thyroid iodine metabolism in the same manner as do the thionamides, which they resemble chemically; their role in the induction of disease in humans is uncertain. Waterborne, sulfur-containing goitrogens of mineral origin are believed to contribute to the development of endemic goiter in certain areas of Colombia.

A number of synthetic chemical pollutants have been implicated as a cause of goitrous hypothyroidism, including polychlorinated biphenyls and resorcinol derivatives.[101,102] Perchlorate has also been noted in high concentrations in geographic regions in which explosives and rocket fuel were made.[103] Perchlorate has been detected in water, food, and breast milk, although the amount does not appear to be sufficient to disrupt thyroid function.[103] In an area of Chile with a high level of natural perchlorate contamination in the water, thyroid function in pregnant women was not different from that in a region with no perchlorate.[104]

Cytokines

Patients with chronic hepatitis C or various malignancies may be given interferon-α or interleukin-2.[73,74] Such patients may experience hypothyroidism, which is usually transient but may persist. These agents activate the immune system and can induce a clinical picture suggesting an exacerbation of underlying autoimmune disease such as occurs during postpartum thyroiditis (see Chapter 11). Graves' disease with hyperthyroidism may also develop, and ablative therapy may be required to treat this condition. Patients with preexisting evidence of autoimmune thyroid disease who have positive TPO antibodies are probably at higher risk for this complication and should be monitored carefully during and after a course of treatment with either of these cytokines.

Congenital Causes of Goiter

Inherited defects in hormone biosynthesis are rare causes of goitrous hypothyroidism and account for only about 10% to 15% of the 1 in 3500 newborns with congenital hypothyroidism.[10] In most instances, the defect appears to be transmitted as an autosomal recessive trait. Individuals with goitrous hypothyroidism are believed to be homozygous for the abnormal gene, whereas euthyroid relatives with slightly enlarged thyroids are presumably heterozygous. In the latter group, appropriate functional testing may disclose a mild abnormality of the same biosynthetic step that is defective in the homozygous individual. In contrast with nontoxic goiter, which is more common in females than in males, these defects, as a group, affect females only slightly more commonly than males.

Although goiter may be present at birth, it usually does not appear until several years later. Therefore, the absence of goiter in a child with functioning thyroid tissue does not exclude the presence of hypothyroidism. The goiter is initially diffusely hyperplastic, often intensely so, suggesting papillary carcinoma, but eventually becomes nodular. In general, the more severe the biosynthetic defect, the earlier the goiter appears, the larger it is, and the greater the likelihood of early development of hypothyroidism or even cretinism. Five specific defects in the pathways of hormone synthesis have been identified.

Iodide Transport Defect

An iodide transport defect, a result of impaired iodide transport by the sodium/iodide symporter (NIS) protein mechanism, is rare and is reflected in defective iodide transport in the thyroid, salivary gland, and gastric mucosa.[105] Some mutations in such patients produce reduced activity, and others completely inactivate NIS by preventing the protein from being transported and inserted into the membrane. With the milder NIS mutations, administration of iodide raises the plasma and intrathyroidal iodide concentration, permitting the synthesis of normal quantities of hormone.

Defects in Expression or Function of Thyroid Peroxidase

TPO is a protein that is required for normal synthesis of iodothyronines. Quantitative or qualitative abnormalities of TPO have been identified in 1 in 66,000 infants in the Netherlands.[106] The most common of the 16 mutations identified in 35 families was a GGCC insertion in exon 8, leading to a premature stop codon.

Pendred's Syndrome

The most common presentation in patients with Pendred's syndrome is a defect in iodine organification accompanied by sensory nerve deafness.[107] The abnormality is in the *PDS* gene encoding pendrin, which is involved in the apical secretion of iodide into the follicular lumen (see Fig. 10–2 and Chapter 10, "Iodine Metabolism"). Thyroid function is only mildly impaired in this disorder.

Defects in Thyroglobulin Synthesis

Defects in the synthesis of thyroglobulin due to genetic causes are rare, having been identified only in a small number of families with congenital hypothyroidism.[108] Some defects lead to premature termination of translation, whereas another defect causes deficiency in endoplasmic reticulum processing of the thyroglobulin molecule. The complex regulation and huge size of this gene makes screening for mutations a difficult task, and considerable work is still required to unravel the extent of the defects in this gene.

Iodotyrosine Dehalogenase Defect

The pathogenesis of goiter and hypothyroidism in the iodotyrosine dehalogenase defect is complex. The major abnormality is an impairment of both intrathyroidal and peripheral deiodination of iodotyrosines, presumably because of the dysfunction of the iodotyrosine *Dehal1b* gene (see "Iodide Metabolism" in Chapter 10).

As a consequence of intense thyroid stimulation and lack of intrathyroidal recycling of iodide derived from dehalogenation, iodide is rapidly accumulated by the thyroid gland and is rapidly released; monoiodotyrosine (MIT) and diiodotyrosine (DIT) are elevated in plasma and, together with their deaminated derivatives, in the urine. Hypothyroidism is presumed to result from the loss of large quantities of MIT and DIT in the urine and to secondary iodine deficiency. The goiter and hypothyroidism are relieved by administration of high doses of iodine.

Thyroid Infiltration Causing Hypothyroidism and Goiter

A number of infiltrative or fibrosing conditions may cause hypothyroidism. Some are often associated with goiter, such as Riedel's struma (see later).[109] Others, such as amyloidosis,[110] hemochromatosis,[111] or scleroderma,[112] may not be. Although the other manifestations of these conditions are usually obvious and hypothyroidism is only a complication, the presence of significant hypothyroidism without evidence of autoimmune thyroiditis should lead to a consideration of these rare causes of this condition.

Postablative Hypothyroidism

Postablative hypothyroidism is a common cause of thyroid failure in adults. One type follows total thyroidectomy usually performed for thyroid carcinoma. Although functioning remnants may be present, as indicated by foci of radioiodine accumulation, hypothyroidism invariably develops. Another etiologic mechanism is subtotal resection of the diffuse goiter of Graves' disease or multinodular goiter. Its frequency depends on the amount of tissue remaining, but continued autoimmune destruction of the thyroid remnant in patients with Graves' disease may be a factor because some studies suggest a correlation between the presence of circulating thyroid autoantibodies in thyrotoxicosis and the development of hypothyroidism after surgery.[113] Hypothyroidism can be manifested during the first year after surgery, but, as with postradioiodine hypothyroidism, the incidence increases with time to approach 100%. In some patients, mild hypothyroidism appears during the early postoperative period and then may occasionally remit, as also occurs after radioiodine treatment.

Hypothyroidism after destruction of thyroid tissue with radioiodine is common and is the one established disadvantage of this form of treatment for hyperthyroidism in adults. Its frequency is determined, in large part, by the dose of radioiodine and radioiodine uptake, but is also influenced by other factors including age, thyroid gland size, magnitude of thyroid hormone elevations, and use of antithyroid drugs.[114] The incidence of postradioiodine hypothyroidism increases with time, approaching 100%. Although the free T_4 is low in patients with postablative hypothyroidism, serum TSH levels may be anomalously low for several months after either surgical or ^{131}I-induced hypothyroidism if TSH synthesis has been suppressed for a long period prior to treatment.

Primary atrophic thyroid failure may also develop in patients with Hodgkin's disease after treatment with mantle irradiation or after high-dose neck irradiation for other forms of lymphoma or carcinoma.[84,85] Surgical, radioiodine, or external beam therapy may also lead to a state of subclinical hypothyroidism (see Table 12–2).

Congenital Causes

Thyroid Agenesis or Dysplasia

Developmental defects of the thyroid are often responsible for the hypothyroidism that occurs in 1 in 3500 newborns.[10,115] These defects may take the form of complete absence of thyroid tissue or failure of the thyroid to descend properly during embryologic development. Thyroid tissue may then be found anywhere along its normal route of descent from the foramen caecum at the junction of the anterior two thirds and posterior third of the tongue (lingual thyroid) to the normal site or below. Absence of thyroid tissue or its ectopic location can be ascertained by scintiscanning.

As indicated, a number of proteins are known to be crucial for normal thyroid gland development.[115] These include the thyroid-specific transcription factor PAX8, as well as thyroid transcription factors 1 and 2 (TTF1 and 2). It might be anticipated that defects in one or more of these proteins may explain abnormalities in thyroidal development. These have been identified in several patients with *PAX8* mutations, and a mutation in the human *TTF2* gene was associated with thyroid agenesis, cleft palate, and choanal atresia. Despite a specific search, no mutations have been found in the *TTF1* gene in infants with congenital hypothyroidism.

Thyroid Aplasia Due to Thyrotropin Receptor Unresponsiveness

Several families exist in which thyroid hypoplasia, high TSH concentrations, and a low free T_4 level are associated with loss-of-function mutations in the TSH receptor.[115,116] The thyroid glands were in the normal location but did not trap pertechnetate (TCO_4^-). Somewhat surprisingly, thyroglobulin levels were still detectable. The molecular details of these patients are still under study.

A second type of abnormality that may cause TSH unresponsiveness is a mutation in the Gs protein that occurs in pseudohypoparathyroidism type 1A. These patients have inactivating mutations in the α-subunit of the Gs protein and, consequently, mild hypothyroidism.[117] Other as yet unexplained patients with elevated TSH levels and hypothyroidism in which the molecular nature of the defect has not been defined have been reported.[118]

Transient Hypothyroidism

Transient hypothyroidism is defined as a period of reduced free T_4 with suppressed, normal, or elevated TSH levels that are eventually followed by a euthyroid state. This form of hypothyroidism usually occurs in the clinical context of a patient with subacute (postviral), lymphocytic (painless), or postpartum thyroiditis. These conditions are reviewed in detail in Chapter 11.

The patient reports mild to moderate symptoms of hypothyroidism of short duration, and serum TSH concentrations are typically elevated, although not greatly so. The patient often has a preceding episode of symptoms consistent with mild or moderate thyrotoxicosis. If these symptoms cannot be elucidated from the history, it may be difficult to distinguish such patients from those with a permanent form of hypothyroidism. In the early phases of post-thyroiditis hypothyroidism, TSH concentrations may still be suppressed even though the free T_4 is low because of the delayed recovery of pituitary TSH synthesis, such as in patients with Graves' disease or with toxic nodules who have undergone surgery and who have experienced rapid relief of hypothyroidism (see Table 12–2). In that situation, the TSH response to hypothyroidism may be suppressed for many months; in post-thyroiditis hypothyroidism, this period is rarely longer than 3 to 4 weeks.

A significant fraction (~33%) of women with autoimmune thyroiditis but normal thyroid function have episodes of hypothyroidism during the postpartum period.[77] In some, the preceding hyperthyroidism is relatively asymptomatic, which can make an accurate clinical diagnosis difficult. Patients who have had an episode of typical subacute postviral thyroiditis with pain, tenderness, and hyperthyroidism are not difficult to recognize.

Diagnostic evaluation should include a determination of TSH, free T_4, and TPOAbs. Negative or low antibodies argue strongly for a nonautoimmune cause. This is significant, in that it may be possible for the patient to be treated only temporarily for hypothyroidism. In such patients, a trial of a lower levothyroxine dosage after 3 to 6 months may reveal that thyroid function has recovered (see Fig. 12–6). This may also occur in patients with hypothyroidism that follows acute autoimmune thyroiditis (e.g., in the postpartum period), but it is somewhat less likely to occur because of the underlying progressive nature of the autoimmune thyroiditis.

In patients with hypothyroidism due to postviral thyroiditis, the thyroid gland is usually relatively small and atrophic. In patients with hypothyroidism that follows an episode of subacute thyroiditis, the gland is usually slightly enlarged and somewhat firm, reflecting the underlying scarring and infiltration associated with that condition.

Consumptive Hypothyroidism

Consumptive hypothyroidism is the term given to an unusual cause of hypothyroidism that has been identified in infants with visceral hemangiomas or related tumors.[119] The first patient reported with this syndrome presented with abdominal distention caused by a large hepatic hemangioma with respiratory compromise secondary to upward displacement of the diaphragm. However, clinical signs suggested hypothyroidism, which was confirmed by finding a markedly elevated TSH level and undetectable T_4 and T_3 levels. The infant's response to an initial IV infusion of liothyronine (T_3) was transient, leading to the decision to use parenteral thyroid hormone replacement to relieve the clinical hypothyroidism. The accelerated degradation of thyroid hormone was apparent from the fact that it required 96 µg of liothyronine plus 50 µg of levothyroxine to normalize the TSH level. The equivalent dosage as levothyroxine alone is roughly nine times that ordinarily required for treatment of infants with congenital hypothyroidism. The infant succumbed to complications of the hemangioma, and a postmortem tumor biopsy showed type 3 iodothyronine deiodinase (D3) activity in the tumor at levels eightfold higher than those normally present in term placenta. The serum reverse T_3 was extremely elevated (400 ng/dL), and the serum thyroglobulin was greater than 1000 ng/mL indicating the presence of a highly stimulated thyroid gland.

Retrospective search revealed two other patients with similar pathophysiology in whom the cause of the hypothyroidism had not been recognized. Significant D3 expression has subsequently been noted in all proliferating cutaneous hemangiomas studied to date. The cutaneous hemangiomas of infancy, although they express D3, are not associated with hypothyroidism owing to their small size. Because a significant fraction of hemangiomas remit with glucocorticoid and interferon α therapy, it is important to treat such patients with adequate doses of thyroid hormone to prevent the permanent neurologic complications associated with untreated hypothyroidism during the critical phase of neurologic development. Subsequent reports have identified a similar syndrome in adults, including a 21-year-old with epithelioid hemangioendothelioma[120] and an individual with a fibrous tumor.[121]

Defects in Activation of Thyroxine to Triiodothyronine

The enzymes that convert the precursor T_4 to the active form, T_3, are 5′-deiodinase 1 (D1) and 5′-deiodinase 2 (D2), both of which contain selenocysteine in their active site.[60] A stem loop structure in the 3′-untranslated region of the mRNA, termed *SECIS element,* directs insertion of selenocysteine at the UGA codon, rather then allowing it to function as a stop codon. Defects in a SECIS-binding protein (SECISBP2) were found in two families with an elevated free T_4, reduced T_3, and elevated TSH.[121] Affected individuals have growth retardation, compared with unaffected family members.

Polymorphisms in genes associated with thyroid hormone metabolism have been associated with patterns of thyroid function studies as well as obesity. The D2 polymorphism resulting in a change from threonine (Thr) to alanine (Ala) at codon 92 (Thr92Ala) has been associated with obesity, reduced glucose disposal, and lower D2 activity in skeletal muscle.[122] This polymorphism also has a higher frequency in groups with a high incidence of obesity and type 2 diabetes: Mexican Americans and Pima Indians.[122]

Hypothyroidism due to Drug-Induced Thyroid Destruction

Thyroid inflammation or activation of autoimmune thyroid destruction has been associated with a number of drugs.[71] The tyrosine kinase inhibitor, sunitinib, however, has been associated with a high incidence of hypothyroidism due to thyroid destruction.[123] Sunitinib is used to treat renal cell carcinoma and gastrointestinal stromal tumors and inhibits multiple cellular pathways including KIT, PDGF, VEGF, and RET. An abnormal TSH was found in 62% of patients on sunitinib followed up for 37 weeks. Patients studied by ultrasound demonstrated no thyroid tissue. Although 40% of hypothyroid patients initially had a suppressed TSH, suggesting thyroiditis, the long-term course was most consistent with sunitinib-induced follicular cell apoptosis. These findings indicate that it is important to monitor thyroid function in patients on sunitinib and perhaps other tyrosine kinase inhibitors. Such agents may in future be useful to destroy malignant thyroid cells.

Central Hypothyroidism

Central hypothyroidism is due to TSH deficiency caused by either acquired or congenital hypothalamic or pituitary gland disorders (see Chapters 7 and 8). The causes of TSH deficiency may be classified as those of pituitary (*secondary* hypothyroidism) and hypothalamic (*tertiary* hypothyroidism) origins, but this distinction is not necessary in the initial separation of primary from central hypothyroidism.

In many cases, hyposecretion of TSH is accompanied by decreased secretion of other pituitary hormones, with the result that evidence of somatotroph, gonadotroph, and corticotroph failure is also present. Hyposecretion of TSH as the sole demonstrable abnormality (monotropic deficiency) is less common but does occur in both acquired and congenital forms. Hypothyroidism due to pituitary insufficiency varies in severity from instances in which it is mild and overshadowed by features of gonadal and adrenocortical failure to those in which the features of the hypothyroid state are predominant. Because a small but significant fraction of thyroid gland function is independent of TSH (~10% to 15%), hypothyroidism due to central causes is less severe than primary hypothyroidism.

The causes of central hypothyroidism are both acquired and congenital. The general subject is discussed in Chapters 7 and 8, and those causes with relatively specific thyroid-related deficiencies are mentioned here for completeness. In addition to pituitary tumors, hypothalamic disorders, and the like, an unusual cause of secondary hypothyroidism occurs in individuals given bexarotene (a retinoid X receptor [RXR] agonist) for T-cell lymphoma.[124] This drug suppresses the activity of the human TSH β-subunit promoter in vitro. Serum T_4 concentrations are reduced about 50%, and patients experience clinical benefit from thyroid hormone replacement. Dopamine, dobutamine, high-dose glucocorticoids, or severe illness may suppress TSH release transiently, leading to a pattern of thyroid hormone abnormalities suggesting central hypothyroidism. As discussed earlier (see Chapter 10, "Changes in Thyroid Function during Severe Illness"), this severe state of hypothalamic-pituitary-thyroid suppression is a manifestation of stage 3 illness (see Table 10–10). Although these agents might be expected to have similar effects when given long term, they do not; nor does somatostatin have a similar effect when given for acromegaly, although it does block the response of TSH to TRH and it has been administered to patients with thyrotropin-secreting pituitary adenomas.[125]

Congenital defects in either the stimulation or the synthesis of TSH or in its structure have been identified as rare causes of congenital hypothyroidism.[115] These include the consequences of defects in several of the homeobox genes, including *POU1F1* (formerly termed *Pit-1*), *PROP1,* and *HESX1.* The last gene encodes a factor necessary for the development of the hypothalamus, pituitary, and olfactory portions of the brain. Defects in *POU1F1* and *PROP1* cause hereditary hypothyroidism, usually accompanied by deficiencies in growth hormone and prolactin.[126] One patient has been identified with a familial defect in the TRH receptor gene.[127] All of these conditions are associated with the typical pattern of reduced free T_4 and TSH.

Structural defects in TSH have also been described. These include those with a mutation in the CAGYC peptide sequence of the β-subunit, thought to be necessary for its association with the α-subunit,[128] and defects that produce premature termination of the TSH β-subunit gene.[129] As mentioned, some of these abnormalities may be associated with elevations in TSH, suggesting the diagnosis of primary hypothyroidism, but the TSH molecule is immunologically, but not biologically, intact.

Resistance to Thyroid Hormone

The clinical manifestations of resistance to thyroid hormone (RTH) depend on the nature of the mutation.[130,131] The majority of patients with RTH have a mutation in the *TR-beta (TRβ)* gene that interferes with the capacity of that receptor to respond normally to T_3, usually by reducing its T_3-binding affinity (see Fig. 10–7).

Alternatively, patients with RTH may have hyperthyroidism if the resistance is more severe in the hypothalamic-pituitary axis than in the remainder of the tissues. In clinical terms, patients in the former group are said to have *generalized resistance to thyroid hormone,* whereas patients in the latter group are said to have *pituitary resistance to thyroid hormone.* The mutations in the TRβ gene causing RTH cluster in three areas of the thyroid hormone receptor, which have been recognized to have important contacts with the hydrophobic ligand-binding domain cavity of TRβ as recognized from its crystal structure.[132] The mutations do not interfere with the function of the DNA-binding domain, its co-repressor binding domain, or its region of heterodimerization with RXR. Some mutations affect the activation domain in the carboxy-terminus of the TRβ receptor.[133]

RTH is probably produced by the heterodimerization of the mutant TRβ with RXR or homodimerization with a normal TRβ or TRα. These mutant TRβ-containing dimers compete with wild-type TR-containing dimers for binding to the thyroid hormone response elements (TREs) of thyroid hormone–dependent genes (see Fig. 10–8).[134] Because these complexes bind co-repressor molecules that cannot be released in the absence of T_3 binding, genes containing these TREs are more repressed than they would be normally at the prevailing concentrations of circulating thyroid hormones. Receptors that contain mutations in the activation domain may have a combination of both decreased affinity for T_3 as well as impaired activating potential.

Thus, the mutant TRβ complex can interfere with the function of the three normal TR-expressing genes, producing a pattern termed *dominant negative inhibition* with an autosomal dominant pattern of inheritance. At least 400 families have been identified with this condition, and there are probably many more unreported cases. The gene frequency estimate is about 1 : 50,000, and the study of the function of the mutant receptors in this disorder has provided valuable insights into the mechanism of thyroid hormone action.[130,131]

Patients with RTH usually are recognized because of thyroid enlargement, which is present in about two thirds of these individuals. Despite one's expectations, patients usually report a peculiar mixture of symptoms of hyperthyroidism and hypothyroidism. With respect to the heart, palpitations and tachycardia are more common than a reduced heart rate; however, patients may also demonstrate growth retardation and retarded skeletal maturation.[135] This has been attributed to the fact that thyroid hormone effects in the heart appear to be primarily dependent on TRα rather than TRβ, whereas the hypothalamic-pituitary axis is primarily regulated through TRβ, particularly TRβ2.

Abnormalities in neuropsychological development exist, with an increased prevalence of attention deficit hyperactivity disorder, which is found in approximately 10% of such individuals.[136] Other neuropsychological abnormalities have also been described.[137] Deafness in patients with RTH reflects the important role of TRβ and thyroid hormone in the normal development of auditory function. The mixture of symptoms, some suggesting hypothyroidism and others suggesting hyperthyroidism, may even differ in individuals within the same family, despite the identical mutation, thus confusing the clinical picture.

Because patients may present with symptoms suggesting hyperthyroidism, it is important to keep this diagnosis in mind in a patient with tachycardia, goiter, and elevated thyroid hormones. RTH is discussed here because a reduced response to thyroid hormone is the biochemical basis for the condition. However, the laboratory results may be the first clear evidence that a patient, otherwise thought to have hyperthyroidism, has RTH. These tests show the unusual combination of an increased free T_4 accompanied by normal or slightly *increased* TSH levels (see Table 12–2). Thus, the principal differential diagnosis is between a TSH-secreting pituitary tumor causing hyperthyroidism and RTH.[137,138]

Factors that may assist in the differential diagnosis are as follows: absence of a family history in patients with TSH-producing tumors, normal thyroid hormone levels in family members of individuals with TSH-induced hyperthyroidism due to pituitary tumor and the presence of an elevated glycoprotein α-subunit in patients with pituitary tumor but not in those with thyroid hormone resistance.

A definitive diagnosis requires sequencing of the *TRβ* gene demonstrating the abnormality. Mutations in the *TRβ* gene are found in about 90% of individuals with a clinical diagnosis. In a few individuals this is not the case, suggesting that there may be mutations in coactivator proteins or one of the RXR receptors, which can also present in a similar fashion.[139]

Treatment is difficult because thyroid hormone analogues designed to suppress TSH, thereby relieving the hyperthyroxinemia, may lead to worsening of the cardiovascular manifestations of the condition.[140] Therapy with 3,5,3′-triiodothyroacetic acid (TRIAC) has been used in several patients.[141] The development of analogues of thyroid hormone with TRβ, as opposed to mixed or TRα preferential effects, as well as analogues that selectively bind mutant TRs, may eventually prove useful in treatment.[142]

TREATMENT

Hypothyroidism, either primary or central, is gratifying to treat because of the ease and completeness with which it responds to thyroid hormone. Treatment is nearly always with levothyroxine, and the proper use of this medication has been reviewed extensively.[143-145] A primary advantage of levothyroxine therapy is that the peripheral deiodination mechanisms can continue to produce the amount of T_3 required in tissues under the normal physiologic control. If one accepts the principle that replicating the natural state is the goal of hormone replacement, it is logical to provide the "prohormone" and allow the peripheral tissues to activate it by physiologically regulated mechanisms.

Pharmacologic and Physiologic Considerations

Levothyroxine has a 7-day half-life; about 80% of the hormone is absorbed relatively slowly and equilibrates rapidly in its distribution volume, therefore avoiding large postabsorptive perturbations in free T_4 levels. With its long half-life, omission of a single day's tablet has no significant effect and the patient may safely take an omitted tablet the following day. In fact, the levothyroxine dosage can be calculated almost as satisfactorily on a weekly, as on a daily, basis.

According to the U.S. Pharmacopeia, the levothyroxine content of replacement tablets must be between 90% and 110% of the stated amount, and the Food and Drug Administration (FDA) has issued standards for single dose bioequivalence studies in normal volunteers to assess and compare thyroxine products in the United States.[146] The AUC (area under the curve) confidence interval must fall within 80% to 125% of the comparison product for a preparation to be considered equivalent. The desirability of a pharmacotherapeutic measurement, such as TSH as an end-point has been suggested by many professional organizations[146] but, to date, rejected by the FDA. This means that, in patients with a history of thyroid cancer, in whom precise degrees of suppression of TSH are the desired therapeutic result, brand name products should be prescribed as opposed to generics. The availability in many countries of a multiplicity of tablet strengths with content ranging from 25 to 300 μg allows precise titration of the daily levothyroxine dosage for most patients with a single tablet, improving compliance significantly.

The typical dose of levothyroxine, approximately 1.6 to 1.8 μg/kg ideal body weight per day (0.7 to 0.8 μg/pound), generally results in the prescription of between 75 and 112 μg/day for women and 125 to 200 μg/day for men. Replacement doses need not be adjusted upward in obese patients and should be based on lean body mass.[147] This dosage is about 20% greater than the T_4 production rate owing to incomplete absorption of the levothyroxine. In patients with primary hypothyroidism, these amounts usually result in serum TSH concentrations that are within the normal range. Because of the 7-day half-life, approximately 6 weeks is required before there is complete equilibration of the free T_4 and the biologic effects of levothyroxine. Accordingly, assessments of the adequacy of a given dose or the effects of a change in dosage, with rare exception such as pregnancy, should not be made until this interval has passed.

By and large, levothyroxine products are clinically equivalent, although problems do occur.[148] However, the variation permitted by the FDA in tablet content can result in slight variations in serum TSH in patients with primary hypothyroidism even when the same brand is used. Although the serum TSH level is an *indirect reflection* of the levothyroxine effect in patients with primary hypothyroidism, it is superior to any other readily available method of assessing the adequacy of therapy. Return of the serum TSH level to normal is therefore the goal of levothyroxine therapy in the patient with primary hypothyroidism. Some patients may require slightly higher or lower doses than generally used, owing to individual variations in absorption, and a number of conditions or associated medications may change levothyroxine requirements in patients with established hypothyroidism (see later).

In decades past, desiccated thyroid was successfully employed for the treatment of hypothyroidism and still accounts for a small fraction of the prescriptions written for thyroid replacement in the United States. Although this approach was successful, desiccated thyroid preparations contain thyroid hormone derived from animal thyroid glands that have significantly higher ratios of T_3 to T_4 than the 1 : 11 value in normal human thyroid gland.[149] Accordingly, these unnatural preparations may lead to supraphysiologic levels of T_3 in the immediate postabsorptive period (2 to 4 hours) owing to the rapid release of T_3 from thyroglobulin, its immediate and nearly complete absorption, and the 1-day period required for T_3 to equilibrate with its 40-L volume of distribution (see Table 10–5).[150]

Mixtures of liothyronine and levothyroxine *(liotrix)* contain in a 1-grain (64-mg) equivalent tablet (Thyrolar-1 in the United States) the amounts of T_3 (~12.5 μg) and T_4 (~50 μg) present in the most popular desiccated thyroid tablet.[151] The levothyroxine equivalency of a 1-grain desiccated thyroid tablet or its liotrix equivalent can be estimated as follows. The 12.5 μg of liothyronine (T_3) is completely absorbed from desiccated thyroid or from liotrix tablets.[150] Levothyroxine is approximately 80% absorbed,[152] and about 36% of the 40 μg of levothyroxine absorbed is converted to T_3, with the molecular weight of T_3 (651) being 84% that of T_4 (777). Accordingly, a 1-grain tablet should provide about 25 μg of T_3,[12.5+12.1] which would be approximately equivalent to that obtained from 100 μg of levothyroxine. This equivalency ratio can be used as an initial guide in switching patients from desiccated thyroid or liotrix to levothyroxine. Although levothyroxine is absorbed in the stomach and small intestine, normal gastric acid secretion is required for complete absorption.[153] Patients with impaired acid secretion on levothyroxine therapy require a 22% to 34% higher dose of levothyroxine to maintain the desired serum TSH. In those patients in whom acid secretion was normalized therapeutically, the levothyroxine dose returned to baseline.[153]

As indicated earlier, the use of levothyroxine as thyroid hormone replacement is a compromise with the normal pathway of T_3 production, in which about 80% of T_3 is derived from T_4 3′-monodeiodination and approximately 20% (~6 μg) is secreted directly from the thyroid gland.[60] Studies in thyroidectomized rats, for example, show that it is not possible to normalize T_3 simultaneously in all tissues by an intravenous infusion of T_4.[154] However, it should be recalled from the earlier discussion of T_4 deiodination that the ratio of T_3/T_4 in the human thyroid gland is about 0.09 but is 0.17 in the rat thyroid gland.[60] Thus, about 40% of the rat's daily T_3 production is derived from the thyroid versus about 20% in humans.[60] Accordingly, the demonstration that T_4 alone cannot provide normal levels of T_3 in all tissues in the rat is of interest but is not strictly applicable to thyroid hormone replacement in humans. Nonetheless, the ratio of T_3 to T_4 in the serum of a patient receiving levothyroxine as the only source of T_3 must be about 20% lower than that in a normal individual.

Similarly, the quantity of levothyroxine required to normalize TSH in an athyreotic patient results in a slightly higher serum free T_4 concentration than is present in normal individuals. Although this may, to some extent, compensate for the lack of T_3 secretion, the fact that T_4 has an independent mechanism for TSH suppression owing to the intracellular generation of T_3 in the hypothalamic-pituitary-thyroid axis results in a portion of the feedback regulation being independent of the plasma T_3 concentration.

Does this slightly lower T_3 concentration in patients receiving levothyroxine make any difference physiologically? Probably not, although the question is difficult to answer definitively because the most readily measurable end-point, TSH, cannot be used. Although the concept of combined T_4/T_3 therapy has been recognized for many years, a positive study generated a great deal of interest in this approach.[155] Patients received 12.5 μg of T_3 as a substitution for 50 μg of their levothyroxine preparation and scored, on average, somewhat higher on tests of mood than when they were taking levothyroxine alone. The dosage of thyroid hormone used in these studies was excessive, as judged by the fact that 20% of the group had serum TSH values below normal on either regimen and the test period was only a few months. A large number of subsequent studies using a wide range of replacement strategies and relative T_4/T_3 content were performed in different populations, and none has shown an advantage of combination therapy over thyroxine alone.[156]

On the other hand, another study showed that the free T_4 index correlated as closely with the resting energy expenditure, as did TSH levels, in a group of patients in whom small supplements or decrements in their ideal replacement levothyroxine dosage were made.[157] The correlation with serum T_3 was not statistically significant, suggesting that in humans, perhaps as a result of differences in the peripheral metabolism of T_4 from that in rodents, the free T_4 index may be as accurate as the TSH value as an index of satisfactory thyroid hormone replacement. The practical difficulty with the design of tablets providing combinations of T_3 and T_4 is that the approximate dose of 6 μg of T_3 provided would need to be released in a sustained fashion over 24 hours, which is quite different from the rapid absorption of T_3 with a peak at 2 to 4 hours when given in its conventional form. Thus, for the present, it appears that the current approach to thyroid replacement using levothyroxine alone, although not a perfect replication of the normal physiology, is satisfactory for most patients. A sustained-release T_3 preparation has been developed and produces more stable levels of serum T_3.[158] The clinical consequence of this more "physiologic" replacement profile is not known.

Institution of Replacement Therapy

The initial dose of levothyroxine prescribed depends on the degree of hypothyroidism and the age and general health of the patient. Patients who are young or middle-aged and otherwise healthy with no associated cardiovascular or other abnormalities and mild to moderate hypothyroidism (TSH concentrations 5 to 50 mU/L) can be given an initial complete replacement dose of about 1.7 μg/kg of ideal body weight. The resulting increase in serum T_4 concentration to normal requires 5 to 6 weeks, and the biologic effects of T_3 are sufficiently delayed that these patients do not experience adverse effects. At the other extreme, the elderly patient with heart disease, particularly angina pectoris, without reversible coronary lesions, should be given a small initial dose of levothyroxine (25 μg/day), and the dosage should be increased in 12.5-μg increments at 2- to 3-month intervals with careful clinical and laboratory evaluation.

The goal in the patient with primary hypothyroidism is to return serum TSH concentrations to normal, reflecting normalization of that patient's thyroid hormone supply. This usually results in a mid to high-normal serum free T_4. The serum TSH should be evaluated 6 weeks after a theoretically complete replacement dose has been instituted to allow minor adjustments to optimize the individual dose.[159] In patients with central hypothyroidism, serum TSH is not a reliable index of adequate replacement and the serum free T_4 should be restored to a concentration in the upper half of the normal range. Such patients should also be evaluated and treated for glucocorticoid deficiency before institution of thyroid replacement (see Chapter 8).

Although the adverse effects of the rapid institution of therapy are unusual, pseudotumor cerebri has been reported in profoundly hypothyroid juveniles between ages 8 and 12 years who were given even modest initial levothyroxine replacement.[160] This complication appears 1 to 10 months after initiation of treatment and responds to acetazolamide and dexamethasone.

The interval between the initiation of treatment and the first evidence of improvement depends on the strength of dose given and the degree of the deficit. An early clinical response in moderate to severe hypothyroidism is a diuresis of 2 to 4 kg. The serum sodium (Na^+) level increases even sooner if hyponatremia was present initially. Thereafter, pulse rate and pulse pressure increase, appetite improves, and constipation may disappear. Later, psychomotor activity increases and the delay in the deep tendon reflex disappears. Hoarseness abates slowly, and changes in skin and hair do not disappear for several months. In individuals started on a complete replacement dose, the serum free T_4 level should normalize after 6 weeks; a somewhat longer period may be necessary for serum TSH levels to return to normal, perhaps up to 3 months.

In some cases (e.g. myxedema coma [see later]), it is clinically appropriate to alleviate hypothyroidism rapidly. For example, patients with severe hypothyroidism withstand acute infections or other serious illnesses poorly and myxedema coma may develop as a complication. In such circumstances, rapid near repletion of the peripheral hormone pool in the average adult can be accomplished by a single intravenous dose of 500 μg of levothyroxine. Alternatively, by virtue of its rapid onset of action, liothyronine (25 μg orally every 12 hours) can be administered if the patient can take medication by mouth. With both approaches, an initial biological effect is achieved within 24 hours. Parenteral therapy with levothyroxine is then continued with a dose that is 80% of the appropriate oral dose but not in excess of 1.4 μg/kg of ideal body weight. Because of the possibility that rapid increases in metabolic rate will overtax the existing pituitary-adrenocortical reserve, supplemental glucocorticoid (intravenous hydrocortisone 5 mg/hour) should also be given to patients with severe hypothyroidism receiving high initial doses of thyroid hormones. Finally, in view of the tendency of hypothyroid patients to retain free water, intravenous fluids containing only dextrose should not be given.

When replacement therapy is withdrawn for short periods (4 to 6 weeks) for purposes of evaluating therapy for thyroid cancer, rapid reinstitution of levothyroxine using a loading dose of three times the daily replacement dose for 3 days can usually be given unless there are other complicating medical illnesses.

When hypothyroidism results from administration of iodine-containing or antithyroid drugs, withdrawal of the offending agent usually relieves both the hypothyroidism and the accompanying goiter, although it is appropriate to provide interim replacement until the gland recovers its function. This is especially true for amiodarone, which may remain in tissues for up to a year.

Infants and Children

In infants with congenital hypothyroidism, the determining factor for eventual intellectual attainment is the age at which adequate treatment with thyroid hormone is begun.[10] The therapy for infants with congenital hypothyroidism should consist initially of raising the serum T_4 level to more than 130 nmol/L (10 μg/dL) as rapidly as possible and maintaining it at that level for the first 3 to 4 years of life. This is usually accomplished by administering an initial levothyroxine dose of 50 μg/day, which is higher than the adult dose on a weight basis and in keeping with the higher metabolic clearance of the hormone in the infant.[161] The serum TSH concentration may not return to normal even with this high dose because of residual reset of the pituitary feedback mechanism. After 2 years of age, however, a TSH level in the normal range is an index of optimal therapy as it is in adults.[162]

Monitoring Replacement Therapy

Monitoring the adequacy of, and compliance with, thyroid hormone therapy in patients with primary hypothyroidism is easily done by measurement of serum TSH. This value should be within the normal range for an assay sufficiently sensitive to measure, with confidence, the lower limit of the normal range. The normal serum TSH concentration varies between 0.5 and 4.0 mU/L in most second-generation and third-generation assays, and results within this range are associated with the elimination of all clinical and biochemical manifestations of primary hypothyroidism, except in patients with RTH. Based on analysis of the NHANES III reference group,[5] a reference TSH range with an upper limit of 2.5 mU/L has been suggested. This adjustment, however, would identify a large number of individuals as having abnormal thyroid function, without a clear indication of the clinical significance of TSH levels in this range.[163]

After the first 6 months of therapy, the dose should be reassessed because restoration of euthyroidism increases the metabolic clearance of T_4. A dose that was adequate during the early phases of therapy may not be adequate when the same patient is euthyroid owing to an acceleration in the clearance of thyroid hormone.

Under normal circumstances, the finding of a normal serum TSH level on an annual basis is adequate to ensure that the proper levothyroxine dose is being taken by the patient. If the serum TSH level is above the normal range and noncompliance is not the explanation, small adjustments, usually in 12-μg increments, can be made with reassessment of TSH concentrations after the 6 weeks required for full equilibration have passed. In North America, this strategy is simplified by the availability of multiple tablet strengths, many of which differ by only 12 μg. Most patients can receive the same dose until they reach the seventh or eighth decade, at which point a downward adjustment of 20% to 30% is indicated because thyroid hormone clearance decreases in the elderly.

Thyroid hormone requirements may be altered in several situations (Table 12–3). A reduction in replacement dosage may be required in women who are receiving androgen therapy for adjuvant treatment of breast carcinoma.[164] Most other conditions or medications increase the levothyroxine requirement in patients receiving maintenance therapy. During pregnancy, the levothyroxine requirement is increased by 25% to 50% in most hypothyroid women,[165] and prospective study demonstrated that the increased requirement occurs early in the first trimester.[166] Athyreotic patients who are planning a pregnancy should be advised to increase the dose by around 30% as soon as the diagnosis is confirmed because the change in requirement appears soon after implantation. The increased requirement is probably due to a combination of factors, including increases in thyroxine-binding globulin and the volume of distribution of T_4, an increase in body mass, and an increase in D3 in placenta and perhaps the uterus.[167,168] The increased requirement persists throughout pregnancy but returns to normal within a few weeks after delivery. Therefore, the dose should be reduced to the original pre-pregnancy level at the time of delivery. Maternal T_4 is critically important to the athyreotic fetus, and in the normal fetus in the first trimester before the thyroid gland develops.[169] Maternal hypothyroidism has been associated with fetal loss, preterm delivery, and intellectual deficit in the offspring.[43,44,170] These findings are not seen in hypothyroid women on thyroxine replacement sufficient to normalize their TSH, suggesting that these associations are directly related to maternal thyroid hormone status. A randomized prospective study in pregnant women with subclinical hypothyroidism demonstrated the benefit of levothyroxine treatment to prevent these complications.[46]

Other conditions in which levothyroxine requirements are increased (see Table 12–3)[79] include malabsorption due to bowel disease, impaired gastric acid secretion,[153] or adsorption of levothyroxine to coadministered medications such as sucralfate, aluminum hydroxide, and calcium carbonate,[171] ferrous sulfate,[172] lovastatin,[173] or various resins.[174] Certain medications, notably rifampin,[175] carbamazepine,[176] phenytoin,[177] and sertraline,[178] increase the clearance of levothyroxine by inducing

TABLE 12–3 CONDITIONS THAT ALTER LEVOTHYROXINE REQUIREMENTS

Increased Levothyroxine Requirements
Pregnancy
Gastrointestinal Disorders
Mucosal diseases of the small bowel (e.g., sprue)
After jejunoileal bypass and small bowel resection
Impaired gastric acid secretion (e.g., atrophic gastritis)
Diabetic diarrhea
Therapy with Certain Pharmacologic Agents
Drugs That Interfere with Levothyroxine Absorption
Cholestyramine
Sucralfate
Aluminum hydroxide
Calcium carbonate
Ferrous sulfate
Drugs That Increase the Cytochrome P450 Enzyme (CYP3A4)
Rifampin
Carbamazepine
Estrogen
Phenytoin
Sertraline
? Statins
Drugs That Block T_4 to T_3 Conversion
Amiodarone
Conditions That May Block Deiodinase Synthesis
Selenium deficiency
Cirrhosis
Decreased Levothyroxine Requirements
Aging (65 years and older)
Androgen therapy in women

T_4, Thyroxine; T_3, triiodothyronine.

CYP3A4 in the liver. Estrogen given to postmenopausal women may act in the same way, although the changes in thyroglobulin and distribution volume make the exact resolution of the cause of the increased levothyroxine requirement uncertain.[179] Soy protein and soybean isoflavones have been proposed to interfere directly with thyroid hormone action as well as synthetic thyroxine absorption.[180] There is no evidence that soy interferes with thyroid function in euthyroid individuals who are iodine sufficient, and the effect of soy on thyroxine absorption in hypothyroid patients is modest.[180] Amiodarone increases levothyroxine requirements by blocking conversion of T_4 to T_3 and perhaps by interfering with T_3–thyroid hormone receptor binding.[181] Selenium deficiency is rare, but because it is rate-limiting in the synthesis of D1 (see Fig. 10–6),[60] a deficiency, such as may occur in patients receiving diets restricted in protein, may increase levothyroxine requirements.[182]

Occasionally, in patients who have been treated with radioactive iodine for Graves' disease or toxic nodular goiter, some degree of thyroid hormone secretion persists and, although inadequate, is autonomous. Such patients may have a suppressed TSH on what otherwise would be considered a replacement dose of levothyroxine. The levothyroxine dose in these individuals should be reduced until TSH levels rise to normal, keeping in mind that several months may be required before TSH secretion recovers after its prolonged suppression. Because of either the delayed effects of radioiodine or the natural history of Graves' disease, per se, this autonomous T_4 secretion may decrease with time, leading to an increase in levothyroxine requirements in subsequent years. Rarely, the opposite occurs; that is, a patient treated with radioiodine develops an increased TSH level, but, after several months of therapy, the requirement for such replacement is either reduced or eliminated. This may reflect transient impairment of thyroid function by a combination of pre-irradiation antithyroid drug therapy and immediate, but transient, effects of irradiation on the thyroid. In such patients, frequent monitoring of levothyroxine replacement is required to avoid overreplacement.

In North America, based on the recent previously discussed changes in assessment of levothyroxine bioequivalence, the possibility of a difference in tablet levothyroxine content should be considered if a new preparation changes the biologic or biochemical effects of the same dosage. Although the difference in preparation is unlikely to cause a significant difference in most patients, the change in manufacturer introduces another potential source of variability.[183]

Adverse Effects of Levothyroxine Therapy

Although the administration of excessive doses of levothyroxine causes accelerated bone loss in postmenopausal patients, most authorities believe that returning thyroid status to normal does not have adverse effects on bone density.[184,185] Administration of excessive doses also increases cardiac wall thickness and contractility and, in elderly patients, increases the risk of atrial fibrillation.[14,17]

In some patients, TSH levels remain elevated despite the prescription of adequate replacement doses. This is most often a consequence of poor compliance. The combination of normal or even elevated serum free T_4 values and elevated TSH levels can occur if the patient does not take levothyroxine regularly but ingests several pills the day before testing. The integrated dose of levothyroxine over prior weeks is best reflected in the serum TSH level, and noncompliant patients require careful education as to the rationale for treatment. Subtle changes in dietary habits, such as increasing the ingestion of bran-containing products, soy, or calcium, may decrease levothyroxine absorption, and their recognition requires a careful history.[171,180]

Patients with Hypothyroid Symptoms despite Restitution of Normal Thyroid Function

In patients taking levothyroxine replacement with a normal range serum TSH concentration, symptoms consistent with hypothyroidism may persist. A survey of hypothyroid patients on levothyroxine with normal range serum TSH and control patients included questions about symptoms that might be associated with thyroid hormone deficiency. Although a significant fraction of both groups reported such symptoms, a greater fraction of patients on levothyroxine replacement had these symptoms. Such patients should be educated as to the relationship between symptoms of hypothyroidism and the role of thyroid hormone in relieving these, and other causes should be sought for the symptomatology. In rare cases, hypothyroid symptoms are associated with hypometabolism despite normal levels of serum thyroid hormones and TSH.[187] Such patients may have RTH in peripheral but not central tissues, a situation that has been documented only rarely.

SPECIAL ASPECTS OF HYPOTHYROIDISM

Subclinical Hypothyroidism

The term *subclinical hypothyroidism* was originally used to describe the patient with a low-normal free T_4 but a slightly elevated serum TSH level. Other terms for this condition are *mild hypothyroidism early thyroid failure, preclinical hypothyroidism,* and *decreased thyroid reserve* (see Table 12–2). The TSH elevation in such patients is modest, with values typically between 4 and 15 mU/L, although patients with a TSH above 10 mU/L more often have a reduced free T_4 and may have some hypothyroid symptoms. The definition of this syndrome depends significantly on the reference range for a normal TSH concentration. This syndrome is most often seen in patients with early Hashimoto's disease and is a common phenomenon, occurring in 7% to 10% of older women.[3,5,6]

A number of studies on the effects of thyroid hormone treatment in such patients have used physiologic end-points (e.g., measurements of various serum enzymes, systolic time intervals, serum lipids, psychometric testing), and results have been variable. In the most carefully controlled studies, one or another of the parameters has returned to normal in about 25% to 50% of patients.[6,8,16,17] In general, free T_4 and TSH levels normalize, but free T_3, usually normal at the outset, does not change. In one study that employed a double-blind, crossover approach, the 4 of 17 women who improved could be differentiated from the remainder only by a somewhat lower serum free T_3 at the start of the study.[188] Modest improvements in cardiac indices and lipid profiles have been noted in most, but not all studies.[6,8,16,17,22] The association of mild hypothyroidism with an increase in risk for atherosclerotic heart disease has been shown by some,[23,24,25] but not other studies.[8,26] The impact of treatment to reduce the risk of atherosclerotic heart disease, other than reduction in risk factors such as cholesterol and C-reactive protein, have not yet been studied.

One factor favoring a decision to recommend levothyroxine therapy is the likelihood of developing overt hypothyroidism.

The risk of progression from *subclinical* to *overt* hypothyroidism (elevated serum TSH concentration and reduced serum free T_4 concentration) is most closely related to the magnitude of serum TSH elevation and the presence of anti-TPO antibodies. Prospective studies of women with subclinical hypothyroidism have shown rates of progression from approximately 3% to 8% per year, with the higher rates seen in individuals with initial TSH concentration greater than 10 and those with positive anti-TPO antibodies.[7] Although most individuals progress slowly to overt hypothyroidism, rapid progression over weeks to months has been reported.[189] Factors that may predispose to rapid progression include being elderly, high levels of TPO antibody, intercurrent systemic infection or inflammation, iodine contrast agents, and medications such as amiodarone and lithium. The decision to treat with levothyroxine must also take into account the expense and inconvenience of a daily medication, not acceptable to some patients, and the possibility that overdosage with levothyroxine may exacerbate osteoporosis or cause cardiac arrhythmias. Ultimately, the decision to treat must depend on a careful consideration of the individual clinical situation and patient preference.[9] If a therapeutic trial is performed, the TSH concentration should be monitored carefully and should not be reduced below normal. If no therapy is given, such patients should be monitored at intervals of 6 to 12 months both clinically and by measurements of serum TSH.

Metabolic Insufficiency

Nonspecific symptoms of true hypothyroidism include mild lassitude, fatigue, slight anemia, constipation, apathy, cold intolerance, menstrual irregularities, loss of hair, and weight gain (see Fig. 12–5). For this reason, some patients with such complaints but with normal laboratory results for thyroid function have been considered candidates for levothyroxine therapy. The response to thyroid hormone therapy is sometimes gratifying, at least initially, but symptomatic improvement usually disappears after a time unless the dose is increased. Eventually, even larger doses fail to alleviate the symptoms, confirming that they do not arise from a deficiency of thyroid hormone.

Thus, thyroid hormone therapy should be avoided in patients with no biochemical documentation of impaired thyroid function. Furthermore, even in patients with subclinical hypothyroidism, symptoms may be out of proportion to abnormalities in the free T_4. It is unwise to raise a patient's expectations that such symptoms will be relieved by correction of mild biochemical abnormalities.

Thyroid Function Testing in Patients Receiving Replacement Therapy for Unclear Reasons

Physicians are frequently confronted with patients receiving levothyroxine in whom the basis for the diagnosis cannot be established. It is often difficult to obtain previous clinical findings or laboratory data to determine whether thyroid hormone replacement is indicated. If serum TSH is in the normal range and primary hypothyroidism is suspected, a simple way of assessing the need for levothyroxine therapy is to switch levothyroxine to an every-other-day dosage or to reduce the daily dose by 50% and to reevaluate TSH and free T_4 after 4 weeks. If there has been no significant increase in TSH concentration and free T_4 remains constant during that period, residual thyroid function is present, although it may still not be completely normal. To answer this question, levothyroxine can then be withdrawn and blood tests repeated 4 to 8 weeks later.

If the initial TSH level is suppressed, indicating overreplacement, the levothyroxine dose should be reduced until TSH becomes detectable before this trial is instituted. If central hypothyroidism is suspected, the free T_4 must be monitored during these procedures.

Emergent Surgery in the Hypothyroid Patient

The perioperative course of patients with untreated hypothyroidism has been evaluated in several studies. In general, such patients were not recognized to be hypothyroid or did not require surgery despite the presence of significant hypothyroidism. Complications were uncommon. Perioperative hypotension, ileus, and central nervous system disturbances were more common in hypothyroid patients, and patients with major infections had fewer episodes of fever than did euthyroid control subjects.[190] Other complications were delayed recovery from anesthesia and abnormal hemostasis, possibly owing to an acquired form of von Willebrand's disease.[27]

From these studies, one may conclude that emergent surgery should not be postponed in hypothyroid patients but that such patients should be rigorously monitored for evidence of carbon dioxide retention, bleeding, infection, and hyponatremia. These findings are also relevant to the treatment of hypothyroid individuals with symptomatic coronary artery disease. Considering the lack of significant increase in perioperative complications in the hypothyroid patient, the option of surgery for remediable coronary artery lesions is open to hypothyroid individuals without the risk of a myocardial infarction in association with restitution of the euthyroid state (see later).[191]

HEART DISEASE AND THYROID HORMONE THERAPY

Coexisting Coronary Artery Disease and Hypothyroidism

In many patients with coronary artery disease and primary hypothyroidism, cardiac function is improved in response to levothyroxine therapy because of a decrease in peripheral vascular resistance and improvement in myocardial function.[14,15] However, patients with preexisting angina pectoris should be evaluated for correctable lesions of the coronary arteries and treated appropriately before levothyroxine is administered.[191-193] Retrospective studies indicate that this approach is safer than the institution of replacement therapy prior to angiography and angioplasty or even coronary artery bypass grafting.[191,192]

In a few patients, lesions may not be remediable or small-vessel disease is severe even after bypass grafting, so that complete replacement cannot be instituted. Such patients must receive optimal antianginal therapy combined with β-adrenergic receptor blockers in judicious quantities, and complete restitution of the euthyroid state may not be possible.

Thyroid Hormone for Compromised Cardiovascular Function

In addition to the issues raised in patients with combined hypothyroidism and coronary artery disease, there is interest in the potential therapeutic use of thyroid hormone in the treatment of patients with either cardiomyopathy or status post–coronary artery bypass grafting (CABG) or other cardiac procedures.[14,15,92,194] As expected, T_3 levels are reduced in patients with advanced congestive heart failure, as with any illness.[195] In one report, 23 patients with advanced heart failure (mean ejection fraction, 22%) were given up to 2.7 μg/kg of liothyronine over 6 hours with an increase in cardiac output and decrease in systemic vascular resistance but without increase in heart or metabolic rate.[194] Similar effects were seen with a dose of liothyronine, 110 μg, over 6 hours after CABG.[193]

Liothyronine has also been given postoperatively for congenital heart disease and, again, an improvement in cardiac output and decrease in vascular resistance occurred without adverse side effects.[196] These results suggest that, in certain selected circumstances, liothyronine may be useful as adjunctive therapy in patients with congestive heart failure because of its effect of relaxing vascular smooth muscle.

Although most therapeutic trials of thyroid hormone treatment have used T_3, thyroid hormone analogs have also been utilized.[197] The most extensively studied is 3,5-diiodothyropropionic acid (DITPA), an analogue that binds both TR α and β with low affinity. Preliminary studies suggest enhancement of cardiac performance without increasing heart rate.

SCREENING FOR PRIMARY HYPOTHYROIDISM

The utility of screening for hypothyroidism has been addressed by a number of studies, but remains controversial.[8,198] The conclusions depend, to a great extent, on assumptions regarding the effectiveness and economic value of identifying and treating patients with subclinical hypothyroidism.[8,197,199] One study concluded that the cost of an every-5-year TSH determination for women and men would be approximately $9000 per quality-adjusted life-year in women.[199] An evidenced-based medicine review of the literature by an expert panel concluded that there was insufficient evidence to support population-based screening.[8] Aggressive "case finding," based on identification of risk factors such as family history, was advocated for pregnant women, women older than 60 years, and others at high risk. The fraction of patients with hypothyroidism missed when a "case finding" strategy is utilized, however, is not known. A report from the U.S. Preventive Services Task Force also concluded that population screening for hypothyroidism in nonpregnant adults was not justified.[198] Large, randomized, prospective studies of levothyroxine treatment in patients with subclinical hypothyroidism to establish benefit, however, have not yet been performed. Given the very high incidence of hypothyroidism in older women and the absence of robust clinical symptoms, an assessment of TSH levels at 5-year intervals in women older than age 50 years seems justified until more extensive studies have been performed.

A second complex issue involves whether women planning pregnancy should be screened for the presence of hypothyroidism as a routine part of a prenatal visit. This question is raised because of increasing association of adverse outcomes in pregnancy, even with subclinical hypothyroidism including impairment of mental development in infants of mothers, fetal loss, and preterm delivery.[44,45,170] The prevalence of overt hypothyroidism during pregnancy is approximately 2%,[200] and screening of all patients has been advocated by several professional organizations.

Maternal free T_4 concentrations in the lowest 10% of the normal range, even with normal TSH levels, have also been suggested as a risk factor for impaired neuropsychological development of the fetus.[201] It is not clear why this is a risk factor for impaired fetal neuropsychological development, because such patients are not hypothyroid.

A number of questions are raised regarding the appropriate timing of testing, whether thyroid autoantibodies should be measured, the relative importance of TSH and free T_4, the influence of trimester on the normal ranges, and the threshold for intervention.[202] The association of maternal subclinical hypothyroidism and preterm delivery[46] is a much more proximal and defined end-point to study compared to intellectual performance in offspring. The morbidity and mortality from preterm delivery is significant for the newborn, and these findings are likely to allow for more focused intervention studies to determine the response to thyroxine treatment.

For the moment, it appears that any patient with a family history of autoimmune thyroid disease, with symptoms suggesting hypothyroidism, or with thyroid enlargement should be tested for thyroid dysfunction prior to pregnancy or as soon after conception as is feasible. Optimization of levothyroxine therapy for women known to have hypothyroidism prior to conception, when possible, may be the most effective intervention to prevent hypothyroid-related complications of pregnancy. Although the data do not yet reach the threshold to mandate universal screening, the ease of testing, associated adverse outcomes, and demonstrated benefit of intervention make thyroid testing of pregnant women a reasonable choice based on clinical judgement.

MYXEDEMA COMA

Myxedema coma is the ultimate stage of severe longstanding hypothyroidism.[203,204] This state, which almost invariably affects older patients, occurs most commonly during the winter months and is associated with a high mortality rate. It is usually accompanied by a subnormal temperature. Values as low as 23° C have been recorded. The external manifestations of severe myxedema, bradycardia, and severe hypotension are invariably present. The characteristic delay in deep tendon reflexes may be lacking if the patient is areflexic. Seizures may accompany the comatose state. Although the pathogenesis of myxedema coma is not clear, factors that predispose to its development include exposure to cold, infection, trauma, and central nervous system depressants or anesthetics. Alveolar hypoventilation, leading to carbon dioxide retention and narcosis, and dilutional hyponatremia resembling that seen with inappropriate secretion of arginine vasopressin (AVP) may also contribute to the clinical state.

From the foregoing, it appears that myxedema coma should be readily recognized from its clinical signs, but this is not the case. After a brain stem infarction, elderly patients with features suggestive of hypothyroidism may be both comatose and hypothermic. In addition, hypothermia of any cause, due for example to exposure to cold, may cause changes suggestive of myxedema, including delayed relaxation of deep tendon reflexes. The importance of the difficulty in diagnosing myxedema coma is that a delay in therapy worsens the prognosis. Consequently, the diagnosis should be made on clinical grounds, and, after sending serum for thyroid function tests, therapy should be initiated without awaiting the results of confirmatory tests because mortality may be 20% or higher.

Treatment consists of administration of thyroid hormone and correction of the associated physiologic disturbances.[203-205] Because of the sluggish circulation and severe hypometabolism, absorption of therapeutic agents from the gut or from subcutaneous or intramuscular sites is unpredictable, and medications should be administered intravenously if possible. Administration of levothyroxine as a single intravenous dose of 500 to

does loss of parathyroid function. The RAIU may be normal or low. Circulating thyroid autoantibodies are less common and are found in lower titers than in Hashimoto's disease.

Surgery may be required to preserve tracheal and esophageal function. If extensive involvement of perithyroid tissues is present, resection of the isthmus may relieve some symptoms. Treatment with thyroid hormone relieves the hypothyroidism but has no effect on the primary process, which may progress inexorably. Immunosuppressive treatment and even chemotherapy has been tried in individual cases. Glucocorticoids have been used for treatment with sporadic improvement. The use of tamoxifen has been successful in some patients.[221]

MISCELLANEOUS CAUSES

Only a few causes of generalized inflammation of the thyroid gland have been reported. These include inflammation arising after ^{131}I treatment for Graves' disease, a residual thyroid lobe in a patient with thyroid cancer of the contralateral lobe, and thyroiditis arising from external beam therapy for conditions such as Hodgkin's or non-Hodgkin's lymphoma, breast carcinoma, or other lesions of the oropharynx. Anaplastic thyroid carcinoma has been reported as associated with a diffuse thyroiditis and elevation of thyroid hormone levels. In general, only radioiodine-induced thyroiditis is associated with pain, and glucocorticoid treatment may be useful in symptomatic therapy.

REFERENCES

1. Dayan CM, Daniels GH. Chronic autoimmune thyroiditis. N Engl J Med 1996;335:99-107.
2. Pearce EN, Farwell AP, Braverman LE. Thyroiditis. N Engl J Med 2003;348:2646-2655.
3. Tunbridge WMG, Evered DC, Hall R, et al. The spectrum of thyroid disease in the community: the Whickham Survey. Clin Endocrinol 1977;7:481-493.
4. Vanderpump MP, Tunbridge WM, French JM, et al. The incidence of thyroid disorders in the community: a twenty year follow-up of the Whickham Survey. Clin Endocrinol (Oxf). 1995;43:55-68.
5. Hollowell JG, Stehling NW, Flanders D, et al. Serum TSH, T4, and thyroid antibodies in the United States population (1988 to 1994): National Health and Nutrition Examination Survey (NHANES III). J Clin Endocrinol Metab 2002;87:489-499.
6. Cooper DS. Subclinical hypothyroidism. N Engl J Med 2001; 345:260-265.
7. Huber G, Staub J-J, Meier C, et al. Prospective study of the spontaneous course of subclinical hypothyroidism: prognostic value of thyrotropin, thyroid reserve, and thyroid antibodies. J Clin Endocrinol Metab 2002;87:3221-3226.
8. Surks MI, Ortiz E, Daniels GH, et al. Subclinical thyroid disease: scientific review and guidelines for diagnosis and management. JAMA 2004;291:228-238.
9. Col NF, Surks MI, Daniels GH. Subclinical thyroid disease: clinical applications. JAMA 2004;291:239-243.
10. LaFranchi S. Congenital hypothyroidism: etiologies, diagnosis, and management. Thyroid 1999;9:735-740.
11. Smith TJ, Bahn RS, Gorman CA. Connective tissue, glycosaminoglycans, and diseases of the thyroid. Endocr Rev 1989;10: 366-391.
12. Safer JD, Crawford TM, Holick MF. Topical thyroid hormone accelerates wound healing in mice. Endocrinology 2005; 146:4425-4430.
13. Eisenbarth GS, Gottlieb PA. Autoimmune polyendocrine syndromes. N Engl J Med 2004;50:2068-2079.
14. Klein I, Ojamaa K. Thyroid hormone and the cardiovascular system. N Engl J Med 2001;344:501-509.
15. Kahaly GJ, Dillmann WH. Thyroid hormone action and the heart. Endocr Rev 2005;26:704-728.
16. Kahaly GJ. Cardiovascular and atherogenic aspects of subclinical hypothyroidism. Thyroid 2000;10:665-679.
17. Biondi B, Palmieri EA, Lombardi G, et al. Subclinical hypothyroidism and cardiac function. Thyroid 2002;12:505-510.
18. Hardisty CA, Naik DR, Munro DS. Pericardial effusion in hypothyroidism. Clin Endocrinol (Oxf) 1980;13:349-354.
19. Keating FR, Parkin TW, Selby JB, et al. Treatment of heart disease associated with myxedema. Prog Cardiovasc Dis 1961;3:364-381.
20. Hussein WI, Green R, Jacobsen DW, et al. Normalization of hyperhomocysteinemia with L-thyroxine in hypothyroidism. Ann Intern Med 1999;131:348-351.
21. Ladenson PW, Sherman SI, Baughman KL, et al. Reversible alterations in myocardial gene expression in a young man with dilated cardiomyopathy and hypothyroidism. Proc Natl Acad Sci U S A 1992;89:5251-5255.
22. Danese MD, Ladenson PW, Meinert CL, et al. Clinical review 115: effect of thyroxine therapy on serum lipoproteins in patients with mild thyroid failure: a quantitative review of the literature. J Clin Endocrinol Metab 2000;85:2993-3001.
23. Kvetny J, Heldgaard PE, Bladbjerg EM, et al. Subclinical hypothyroidism is associated with a low-grade inflammation, increased triglyceride levels and predicts cardiovascular disease in males below 50 years. Clin Endocrinol (Oxf.) 2004;61:232-238.
24. Hak AE, Pols HA, Visser TJ, et al. Subclinical hypothyroidism is an independent risk factor for atherosclerosis and myocardial infarction in elderly women: the Rotterdam Study. Ann Intern Med 2000;132:270-278.
25. Imaizumi M, Akahoshi M, Ichimaru S, et al. Risk for ischemic heart disease and all-cause mortality in subclinical hypothyroidism. J Clin Endocrinol Metab 2004;89:3365-3370.
26. Cappola AR, Fried LP, Arnold AM, et al. Thyroid status, cardiovascular risk, and mortality in older adults. JAMA 2006;295: 1033-1041.
27. Tachman ML, Guthrie GP Jr. Hypothyroidism: diversity of presentation. Endocr Rev 1984;5:456-465.
28. Malik R, Hodgson H. The relationship between the thyroid gland and the liver. Q J Med 2002;95:559-569.
29. Porterfield SP, Hendrich CE. The role of thyroid hormones in prenatal and neonatal neurological development: current perspectives. Endocr Rev 1993;14:94-106.
30. Esposito S, Prange AJ Jr, Golden RN. The thyroid axis and mood disorders: overview and future prospects. Psychopharmacol Bull 1997;33:205-217.
31. Bland JH, Frymoyer JW. Rheumatic syndromes of myxedema. N Engl J Med 1970;282:1171-1174.
32. Kalmijn S, Mehta KM, Pols HA, et al. Subclinical hyperthyroidism and the risk of dementia: the Rotterdam study. Clin Endocrinol (Oxf.) 2000;53:733-777.
33. Sampaolo S, Campos-Barros A, Mazziotti G, et al. Increased cerebrospinal fluid levels of 3,3′,5′-triiodothyronine in patients with Alzheimer's disease. J Clin Endocrinol Metab 2005;90: 198-202.
34. Sawka AM, Fatourechi V, Boeve BF, et al. Rarity of encephalopathy associated with autoimmune thyroiditis: a case series from Mayo Clinic from 1950-1996. Thyroid 2002;12:393-398.
35. Brent GA. Regulation of gene expression by thyroid hormones; relation to growth and development. In Kostyo JL, ed. Hormonal Control of Growth: Handbook of Physiology. New York: Oxford University Press, 1999:757-782.
36. Rivkees SA, Bode HH, Crawford JD. Long-term growth in juvenile acquired hypothyroidism: the failure to achieve normal adult stature. N Engl J Med 1988;31:599-602.
37. Greenspan SL, Greenspan FS. The effect of thyroid hormone on skeletal integrity. Ann Intern Med 1999;130:750-758.
38. Iwasaki Y, Oiso Y, Yamauchi K, et al. Osmoregulation of plasma vasopressin in myxedema. J Clin Endocrinol Metab 1990;70: 534-539.
39. Lecky BRF, Williams TDM, Lightman SL, et al. Myxoedema presenting with chiasmal compression: resolution after thyroxine replacement. Lancet 1987;1:1347-1350.
40. Kamilaris TC, DeBold CR, Pavlou SN, et al. Effect of altered thyroid hormone levels on hypothalamic-pituitary-adrenal function. J Clin Endocrinol Metab 1987;65:994-999.
41. Redmond GP. Thyroid dysfunction and women's reproductive health. Thyroid 2004;14(suppl):S5-S15.
42. Yoshimura M, Hershman JM. Thyrotropic action of human chorionic gonadotropin. Thyroid 1995;5:425-434.

43. Abalovich M, Gutierrex S, Alcaraz G, et al. Overt and subclinical hypothyroidism complicating pregnancy. Thyroid 2002;12:63-68.
44. Casey BM, Dashe JS, Wells CE, et al. Subclinical hypothyroidism and pregnancy outcomes. Obstet Gynecol 2005;105:239-245.
45. La Franchi SH, Haddow JE, Hollowell JG. Is thyroid inadequacy during gestation a risk factor for adverse pregnancy and developmental outcomes? Thyroid 2005;15:60-71.
46. Negro R, Formoso G, Mangieri T, et al. Levothyroxine treatment in euthyroid pregnant women with autoimmune thyroid disease: effects on obstetrical complications. J Clin Endocrinol Metab 2006;91:2587-2591.
47. Brenta G, Schnitman M, Gurfinkiel M, et al. Variations of sex hormone-binding globulin in thyroid dysfunction. Thyroid 1999; 9:273-277.
48. Michel-Reher MB, Gross G, Jasper JR, et al. Tissue- and subunit-specific regulation of G-protein expression by hypo- and hyperthyroidism. Biochem Pharmacol 1993;45:1417-1423.
49. Haluzik M, Nedvidkova J, Bartak V, et al. Effects of hypo- and hyperthyroidism on noradrenergic activity and glycerol concentrations in human subcutaneous abdominal adipose tissue assessed with microdialysis. J Clin Endocrinol Metab 2003; 88:5605-5608.
50. Chidakel A, Mentuccia D, Celi FS. Peripheral metabolism of thyroid hormone and glucose homeostasis. Thyroid 2005;15:899-903.
51. Li Q-L, Jansen E, Brent GA, et al. Regulation of prohormone convertase 1 (PC1) by thyroid hormone. Am J Physiol 2001;280: E160-170.
52. O'Brien T, Katz K, Hodge D, et al. The effect of the treatment of hypothyroidism and hyperthyroidism on plasma lipids and apolipoproteins AI, AII, and E. Clin Endocrinol (Oxf) 1997;46:17-20.
53. Scarabottolo L, Trezzi E, Roma P, et al. Experimental hypothyroidism modulates the expression of the low-density lipoprotein receptor by the liver. Atherosclerosis 1986;59:329-333.
54. Canaris GJ, Manowitz NR, Mayor G, et al. The Colorado thyroid disease prevalence study. Arch Intern Med 2000;160:526-534.
55. Caraccio N, Ferrannini E, Monzani F. Lipoprotein profile in subclinical hypothyroidism: respone to levothyroxine replacement, a randomized placebo-controlled study. J Clin Endocrinol Metab 2002;87:1533-1538.
56. Vettor R. The metabolic actions of thyroid hormone and leptin: a mandatory interplay or not? Diabetologia 2005;48:621-623.
57. Iglesias P, Alvarez Fidalgo P, Codoceo R, et al. Serum concentrations of adipocytokines in patients with hyperthyroidism and hypothyroidism before and after control of thyroid function. Clin Endocrinol (Oxf) 2003;59:621-629.
58. Zulewski H, Müller B, Exer P, et al. Estimation of tissue hypothyroidism by a new clinical score: evaluation of patients with various grades of hypothyroidism and controls. J Clin Endocrinol Metab 1997;82:771-776.
59. Murphy E, Williams GR. The thyroid and the skeleton. Clin Endocrinol (Oxf) 2004;61:285-298.
60. Bianco AC, Slavatore D, Gereben B, et al. Biochemistry, cellular and molecular biology, and physiological roles of the iodothyronine selenodeiodinases. Endocr Rev 2001;23:38-39.
61. Gesundheit N, Petrick PA, Nissim M, et al. Thyrotropin-secreting pituitary adenomas: clinical and biochemical heterogeneity. Ann Intern Med 1989;11:827-835.
62. Hollowell JG, Staehling NW, Hannon WH, et al. Iodine nutrition in the United States—trends and public health implications: iodine excretion data from National Health and Nutrition Examination Surveys I and III (1971-1974 and 1988-1994). J Clin Endocrinol Metab 1998;83:3401-3408.
63. Caldwell KL, Jones R, Hoolowell JG. Urinary iodine concentration: United States National Health and Nutrition Examination Survey 2001-2002. Thyroid 2005;15:692-699.
64. Mariotti S, Franceschi C, Cossarizza A, et al. The aging thyroid. Endocr Rev 1995;16:686-715.
65. Davies TF, Amino N. A new classification for human autoimmune thyroid disease. Thyroid 1993;3:331-333.
66. Tomer Y, Davies TF. Searching for the autoimmune thyroid disease susceptibility genes: from gene mapping to gene function. Endocr Rev 2003;23:694-717.
67. Dittmar M, Kahaly GJ. Immunoregulatory and susceptibility genes in thyroid and polyglandular autoimmunity. Thyroid 2005;15: 239-250.
68. Giordano C, Stassi G, De Maria R, et al. Potential involvement of Fas and its ligand in the pathogenesis of Hashimoto's thyroiditis. Science 1997;275:960-963.
69. Stassi G, Di Liberto D, Todaro M, et al. Control of target cell survival in thyroid autoimmunity by T-helper cytokines via regulation of apoptotic proteins. Nat Immunol 2000;1:483-488.
70. Phelps E, Wu P, Bretz J, et al. Thyroid cell apoptosis: a new understanding of thyroid autoimmunity. Endocrinol Metab Clin North Am 2000;29:375-388.
71. Doniach D, Botttazo GF, Russell RCG. Goitrous autoimmune thyroiditis. Clin Endocrinol (Oxf) 1979;8:63-80.
72. Martin A, Davies TF. T cells and human autoimmune thyroid disease: emerging data show lack of need to invoke suppressor T-cell problems. Thyroid 1992;2:247-261.
73. Atkins MB, Mier JW, Parkinson DR, et al. Hypothyroidism after treatment with interleukin-2 and lymphokine-activated killer cells. N Engl J Med 1988;318:1558-1563.
74. Prummel MF, Laurberg P. Interferon-α and autoimmune thyroid disease. Thyroid 2003;13:547-551.
75. Wang SH, Bretz JD, Phelps E, et al. A unique combination of inflammatory cytokines enhances apoptosis of thyroid follicular cells and transforms nondestructive to destructive thyroiditis in experimental autoimmune thyroiditis. J Immunol 2002;168: 2470-2474.
76. Ando T, Davies TF. Clinical review 160: postpartum autoimmune thyroid disease: the potential role of fetal microchimerism. J Clin Endocrinol Metab 2003;88:2965-2971.
77. Stagnaro-Green A. Clinical review 152: postpartum thyroiditis. J Clin Endocrinol Metab 2002;87:4042-4047.
78. Hall R, Lazarus JH. Changing iodine intake and the effect on thyroid disease. Br Med J 1987;294:721-722.
79. Surks MI, Sievert R. Drugs and thyroid function. N Engl J Med 1995;333:1688-1694.
80. Martino E, Bartalena L, Bogazzi F, et al. The effects of amiodarone on the thyroid. Endocr Rev 2001;22:240-254.
81. Sundick RS, Herdegen DM, Brown TR, et al. The incorporation of dietary iodine into thyroglobulin increases its immunogenicity. Endocrinology 1987;120:2078-2084.
82. Nagataki S, Shibata Y, Inoue S, et al. Thyroid diseases among atomic bomb survivors in Nagasaki. JAMA 1994;272:364-370.
83. Vermiglio F, Castagna MG, Volnova E, et al. Post-Chernobyl increased prevalence of humoral thyroid autoimmunity in children and adolescents from a moderately iodine-deficient area in Russia. Thyroid 1999;9:781-786.
84. Illes A, Biro E, Miltenyi Z, et al. Hypothyroidism and thyroiditis after therapy for Hodgkin's disease. Acta Haematol 2003;109: 11-17.
85. Skla C, Whitton J, Mertens A, et al. Abnormalities of the thyroid in survivors of Hodgkin's disease: data from the childhood cancer survivor study. J Clin Endocrinol Metab 2000;85: 3227-3232.
86. Imaizumi M, Usa T, Tominaga T, et al. Radiation dose-response relationships for thyroid nodules and autoimmune thyroid diseases in Hiroshima and Nagasaki atomic bomb survivors 55-58 years after radiation exposure. JAMA 2006;295:1011-1022.
87. Tomer Y, Davies TF. Infection, thyroid disease, and autoimmunity. Endocr Rev 1993;14:107-120.
88. Matsuzuka F, Miyauchi A, Katayama S, et al. Clinical aspects of primary thyroid lymphoma: diagnosis and treatment based on our experience of 119 cases. Thyroid 1993;3:93-99.
89. Baker J, Fosso CK. Immunological aspects of cancers arising from thyroid follicular cells. Endocr Rev 1993;14:729-746.
90. Boyages SC. Clinical review 49: iodine deficiency disorders. J Clin Endocrinol Metab 1993;77:587-591.
91. Bottcher Y, Eszlinger M, Tonjes A, et al. The genetics of euthyroid familial goiter. Trends Endocrinol Metab 2005;16:314-319.
92. Glinoer D. The regulation of thyroid function in pregnancy: pathways of endocrine adaptation from physiology to pathology. Endocr Rev 1997;18:404-433.
93. Pearce EN, Pino S, He X, et al. Sources of dietary iodine: bread, cows' milk, and infant formula in the Boston area. J Clin Endocrinol Metab 2004;89:3421-3424.
94. Wolff J. Physiology and pharmacology of iodized oil in goiter prophylaxis. Medicine (Baltimore) 2001;80:20-36.
95. Boyages SC, Halpern JP. Endemic cretinism: toward a unifying hypothesis. Thyroid 1993;3:59-69.

96. Delange F. The disorders induced by iodine deficiency. Thyroid 1994;4:107-128.
97. Halpern JP, Boyages SC, Maberly GF. The neurology of endemic cretinism. A study of two endemias. Brain 1991;114:825-841.
98. Silva JE. Effects of iodine and iodine-containing compounds on thyroid function. Med Clin North Am 1985;69:881-898.
99. Wolff J, Chaikoff IL. Plasma inorganic iodide as a homeostatic regulator of thyroid function. J Biol Chem 1948;174:555.
100. Muller B, Zulewski H, Huber P, et al. Impaired action of thyroid hormone associated with smoking in women with hypothyroidism. N Engl J Med 1995;333:964-969.
101. Brucker-Davis F. Effects of environmental synthetic chemicals on thyroid function. Thyroid 1998;8:827-856.
102. Porterfield SP. Thyroidal dysfunction and environmental chemicals—potential impact on brain development. Environ Health Perspect 2000;108(suppl 3):433-438.
103. Hershman JM. Perchlorate and thyroid function: what are the environmental issues? Thyroid 2005;15:427-431.
104. Tellez Tellez R, Michaud Chacon P, Reyes Abarca C, et al. Long-term environmental exposure to perchlorate through drinking water and thyroid function during pregnancy and the neonatal period. Thyroid 2005;15:963-974.
105. Dohan O, De la Vieja A, Paroder V, et al. The sodium/iodide symporter (NIS): characterization, regulation, and medical significance. Endocr Rev 2003;24:48-77.
106. Bakker B, Bikker H, Vulsma T, et al. Two decades of screening for congenital hypothyroidism in The Netherlands: TPO gene mutations in total iodide organification defects (an update). J Clin Endocrinol Metab 2000;85:3708-3712.
107. Kopp P. Pendred's syndrome and genetic defects in thyroid hormone synthesis. Rev Endocr Metab Disord. 2000;1:109-121.
108. Vono-Toniolo J, Rivolta CM, Targovnik HM, et al. Naturally occurring mutations in the thyroglobulin gene. Thyroid 2005;15: 1021-1033.
109. Best TB, Munro RE, Burwell S, et al. Riedel's thyroiditis associated with Hashimoto's thyroiditis, hypoparathyoidism, and retroperitoneal fibrosis. J Endocrinol Invest 1991;14:767-772.
110. Kimura H, Yamashita S, Ashizawa K, et al. Thyroid dysfunction in patients with amyloid goitre. Clin Endocrinol (Oxf) 1997;46: 769-774.
111. Oerter KE, Kamp GA, Munson PJ, et al. Multiple hormone deficiencies in children with hemochromatosis. J Clin Endocrinol Metab 1993;76:357-361.
112. Gordon MB, Klein I, Dekker A, et al. Thyroid disease in progressive systemic sclerosis: increased frequency of glandular fibrosis and hypothyroidism. Ann Intern Med 1981;95:431-435.
113. Rees Smith B, McLachlan SM, Furmaniak J. Autoantibodies to the thyrotropin receptor. Endocr Rev 1988;9:106-121.
114. Alexander EK, Larsen PR. High dose of (131)I therapy for the treatment of hyperthyroidism caused by Graves' disease. J Clin Endocrinol Metab 2002;87:1073-1077.
115. Kopp P. Perspective: genetic defects in the etiology of congenital hypothyroidism. Endocrinology 2002;143:2019-2024.
116. Biebermann H, Schoneberg T, Krude H, et al. Mutations of the human thyrotropin receptor gene causing thyroid hypoplasia and persistent congenital hypothyroidism. J Clin Endocrinol Metab 1997;82:3471-3480.
117. Spiegel AM, Shenker A, Weinstein LS. Receptor-effector coupling by G proteins: implications for normal and abnormal signal transduction. Endocr Rev 1992;13:536-565.
118. Xie J, Pannain S, Pohlenz J, et al. Resistance to thyrotropin (TSH) in three families is not associated with mutations in the TSH receptor or TSH. J Clin Endocrinol Metab 1997;82:3933-3940.
119. Huang SA, Tu HM, Harney JW, et al. Severe hypothyroidism caused by type 3 iodothyronine deiodinase in infantile hemangiomas. N Engl J Med 2000;343:185-189.
120. Huang SA, Fish SA, Dorfman DM, et al. A 21-year-old woman with consumptive hypothyroidism due to a vascular tumor expressing type 3 iodothyronine deiodinase. J Clin Endocrinol Metab 2002;87:4457-4461.
121. Dumitrescu AM, Lio X-H, Abdullah SY, et al. Mutations in SECISBP2 result in abnormal thyroid hormone metabolism. Nat Genet 2005;37:1247-1252.
122. Canani LH, Capp C, Dora JM, et al. Type 2 deiodinase Thr92Ala polymorphism is associated with decreased enzyme velocity and severe insulin resistance in type 2 diabetes mellitus patients. J Clin Endocrinol Metab 2005;90:3472-3478.
123. Desai J, Yassa L, Marqusee E, et al. Hypothyroidism after sunitinib treatment for patients with gastrointestinal stromal tumors. Ann Intern Med 2006;145:660-664.
124. Sherman SI, Gopal J, Haugen BR, et al. Central hypothyroidism associated with retinoid X receptor-selective ligands. N Engl J Med 1999;340:1075-1079.
125. Comi RJ, Gesundheit N, Murray L. Response of thyrotropin-secreting pituitary adenomas to a long-acting somatostatin analogue. N Engl J Med 1987;317:12-17.
126. Radovick S, Nations M, Du Y, et al. A mutation in the POU-homeodomain of Pit-1 responsible for combined pituitary hormone deficiency. Science 1992;257:1115-1118.
127. Collu R, Tang J, Castagne J, et al. A novel mechanism for isolated central hypothyroidism: inactivating mutations in the thyrotropin-releasing hormone receptor gene. J Clin Endocrinol Metab 1997; 82:1561-1565.
128. Hayashizaki Y, Hiraoka Y, Tatsumi K. Deoxyribonucleic acid analyses of five families with familial inherited thyroid stimulating hormone deficiency. J Clin Endocrinol Metab 1990;71:792.
129. Medeiros-Neto G, Herodotou DT, Rajan S, et al. A circulating, biologically inactive thyrotropin caused by a mutation in the beta subunit gene. J Clin Invest 1996;97:1250-1256.
130. Refetoff S, Weiss RE, Usala SJ. The syndromes of resistance to thyroid hormone. Endocr Rev 1993;14:348-399.
131. Refetoff S, Weiss RE, Usala SJ, et al. The syndromes of resistance to thyroid hormone: update 1994. Endocr Rev 1994;3:336-342.
132. Apriletti JW, Ribeiro RC, Wagner RL, et al. Molecular and structural biology of thyroid hormone receptors. Clin Exp Pharmacol Physiol Suppl 1998; 25:S2-S11.
133. Nagaya T, Seo H. Molecular basis of resistance to thyroid hormone (RTH). Endocr J 1998;45:709-718.
134. Zavacki AM, Harney JW, Brent GA, et al. Dominant negative inhibition by mutant thyroid hormone receptors is thyroid hormone response element and receptor isoform specific. Mol Endocrinol 1993;7:1319-1330.
135. Weiss RE, Refetoff S. Effect of thyroid hormone on growth. Lessons from the syndrome of resistance to thyroid hormone. Endocrinol Metab Clin North Am 1996;25:719-730.
136. Hauser PH, Zametkin AJ, Martinez P, et al. Attention deficit-hyperactivity disorder in people with generalized resistance to thyroid hormone. N Engl J Med 1993;328:997-1001.
137. Brucker-Davis F, Skarulis MC, Grace MB, et al. Genetic and clinical features of 42 kindreds with resistance to thyroid hormone. Ann Intern Med 1995;123:572-583.
138. Brucker-Davis F, Oldfield EH, Skarulis MC, et al. Thyrotropin-secreting pituitary tumors: diagnostic criteria, thyroid hormone sensitivity, and treatment outcome in 25 patients followed at the National Institutes of Health. J Clin Endocrinol Metab 1999; 84:476-486.
139. Reutrakul S, Sadow PM, Pannain S, et al. Search for abnormalities of nuclear corepressors, coactivators, and a coregulator in families with resistance to thyroid hormone without mutations in thyroid hormone receptor beta or alpha genes. J Clin Endocrinol Metab 2000;85:3609-3617.
140. Weiss RE, Refetoff S. Treatment of resistance to thyroid hormone-primum non nocere. J Clin Endocrinol Metab 1999;84:401-404.
141. Ueda S, Takamatsu J, Fukata S, et al. Differences in response of thyrotropin to 3,5,3′-triiodothyronine and 3,5,3′-triiodothyroacetic acid in patients with resistance to thyroid hormone. Thyroid 1996;6:563-570.
142. Trost SU, Swanson E, Gloss B, et al. The thyroid hormone receptor-beta-selective agonist GC-1 differentially affects plasma lipids and cardiac activity. Endocrinology 2000;141:3057-3064.
143. Roti E, Minelli R, Gardini E, et al. The use and misuse of thyroid hormone. Endocr Rev 1993;14:401-423.
144. Mandel SJ, Brent GA, Larsen PR. Levothyroxine therapy in patients with thyroid disease. Ann Intern Med 1993;119:492-502.
145. Toft AD. Thyroxine therapy. N Engl J Med 1994;331:174-180.
146. Hennessey JV. Levothyroxine a new drug? Since when? How could that be? Thyroid 2003;13:279-282.
147. Santini F, Pinchera A, Marsili A, et al. Lean body mass is a major determinant of levothyroxine dosage in the treatment of thyroid disease J Clin Endocrinol Metab 2005;90:124-127.

148. Olveira G, Almaraz MC, Soriguer F, et al. Altered bioavailability due to changes in the formulation of a commercial preparation of levothyroxine in patients with differentiated thyroid carcinoma. Clin Endocrinol (Oxf) 1997;46:707-711.
149. Rees-Jones RW, Larsen PR. Triiodothyronine and thyroxine content of desiccated thyroid tablets. Metabolism 1977;26:1213-1218.
150. LeBoff MS, Kaplan MM, Silva JE, et al. Bioavailability of thyroid hormones from oral replacement preparations. Metabolism 1982;31:900-905.
151. Blumberg KR, Mayer WJ, Parikh DK, et al. Liothyronine and levothyroxine in Armour thyroid. J Pharm Sci 1993;76:346-347.
152. Hays MT. Localization of human thyroxine absorption. Thyroid 1991;3:241-248.
153. Centanni M, Gargano L, Canettieri G, et al. Thyroxine in goiter, *Helicobacter pylori* infection, and chronic gastritis. N Engl J Med 2006;354:1787-1795.
154. Escobar-Morreale HF, Obregon MJ, Escobar del Ray F, et al. Replacement therapy for hypothyroidism with thyroxine alone does not ensure euthyroidism in all tissues, as studied in thyroidectomized rats. J Clin Invest 1995;96:2828-2838.
155. Bunevicius R, Kazanavicius G, Zalinkevicius R, et al. Effects of thyroxine as compared with thyroxine plus triiodothyronine in patients with hypothyroidism. N Engl J Med 1999;340:424-429.
156. Cooper DS. Combined T_4 and T_3 therapy—back to the drawing board. JAMA 2003;290:3002-3004.
157. al-Adsani H, Hoffer LJ, Silva JE. Resting energy expenditure is sensitive to small dose changes in patients on chronic thyroid hormone replacement. J Clin Endocrinol Metab 1997;82: 1118-1125.
158. Henneman G, Docter R, Visser TJ, et al. Thyroxine plus low-dose, slow-release triiodothyronine replacement in hypothyroidism: proof of principle. Thyroid 2004;14:271-275.
159. Carr K, Mcleod DT, Parry G, et al. Fine adjustment of thyroxine replacement dosage: comparison of the thyrotrophin releasing hormone tests using a sensitive thyrotrophin assay with measurement of free thyroid hormones and clinical assessment. Clin Endocrinol (Oxf) 1988;28:325-333.
160. Van Dop C, Conte FA, Koch TK, et al. Pseudotumor cerebri associated with initiation of levothyroxine therapy for juvenile hypothyroidism. N Engl J Med 1983;308:1076-1080.
161. Burrow GN, Fisher DA, Larsen PR. Mechanisms of disease: maternal and fetal thyroid function. N Engl J Med 1994;331:1072-1078.
162. Fisher DA, Schoen EJ, La Franchi S, et al. The hypothalamic-pituitary-thyroid negative feedback control axis in children with treated congenital hypothyroidism. J Clin Endocrinol Metab 2000;85:2722-2727.
163. Surks MI, Goswami G, Daniels GH. The thyrotropin reference range should remain unchanged. J Clin Endocrinol Metab 2005;90:5489-5496.
164. Arafah BM. Decreased levothyroxine requirement in women with hypothyroidism during androgen therapy for breast cancer. Ann Intern Med 1994;121:247-251.
165. Mandel SJ, Larsen PR, Seely EW, et al. Increased need for thyroxine during pregnancy in women with primary hypothyroidism N Engl J Med 1990;323:91-96.
166. Alexander EK, Marqusee E, Lawrence J, et al. Timing and magnitude of increases in levothyroxine requirements during pregnancy in women with hypothyroidism. N Engl J Med 2004;351:241-249.
167. Koopdonk-Kool JM, deVijlder JJM, Veenboer GJM, et al. Type II and type III deiodinase activity in human placenta as a function of gestational age. J Clin Endocrinol Metab 1996;81:2154-2158.
168. Galton VA, Martinez E, Hernandez A, et al. Pregnant rat uterus expresses high levels of the type 3 iodothyronine deiodinase. J Clin Invest 1999;103:979-987.
169. Vulsma T, Gons MH, DeVijlder JMM. Maternal fetal transfer of thyroxine in congenital hypothyroidism due to a total organification defect of thyroid dysgenesis. N Engl J Med 1989;321:13-16.
170. Haddow JE, Palomaki GE, Allan WC, et al. Maternal thyroid deficiency during pregnancy and subsequent neuropsychological development of the child. N Engl J Med 1999;341:549-555.
171. Singh N, Singh PN, Hershman JM. Effect of calcium carbonate on the absorption of levothyroxine. JAMA 2000;283:2822-2825.
172. Campbell NRC, Hasinoff BB, Stalts H, et al. Ferrous sulfate reduces thyroxine efficacy in patients with hypothyroidism. Ann Intern Med 1992;117:1010-1013.
173. Demke DM. Drug interaction between thyroxine and lovastatin. N Engl J Med 1989;321:1341-1342.
174. McLean M, Kirkwood I, Epstein M, et al. Cation-exchange resin and inhibition of intestinal absorption of thyroxine. Lancet 1993;341:1286.
175. Isley WL. Effect of rifampin therapy on thyroid function tests in a hypothyroid patient on replacement L-thyroxine. Ann Intern Med 1987;107:517-518.
176. DeLuca F, Arrigo T, Pandullo E, et al. Changes in thyroid function tests induced by 2-month carbamazepine treatment in L-thyroxine-substituted hypothyroid children. Eur J Pediatr 1986;145:77-79.
177. Faber J, Lumholtz IB, Kirkegaard C, et al. The effects of phenytoin on the extrathyroidal turnover of thyroxine, 3,5,3′-triiodothyronine, 3,3′,5′-triiodothyronine, and 3′,5′-diiodothyronine in man. J Clin Endocrinol Metab 1985;61:1093-1099.
178. McCowen KC, Garber JR, Spark R. Elevated serum thyrotropin in thyroxine-treated patients with hypothyroidism given sertraline. N Engl J Med 1997;337:1010-1011.
179. Arafah BM. Increased need for thyroxine in women with hypothyroidism during estrogen therapy. N Engl J Med 2001;344: 1743-1749.
180. Messina M, Redmond G. Effects of soy protein and soybean isoflavones on thyroid function in healthy adults and hypothyroid patients: a review of the relevant literature. Thyroid 2006;16:249-258.
181. Figge J, Dluhy RG. Amiodarone-induced elevation of thyroid stimulating hormone in patients receiving levothyroxine for primary hypothyroidism. Ann Intern Med 1990;113:553-555.
182. Jochum F, Terwolbeck K, Meinhold H, et al. Effects of a low selenium state in patients with phenylketonuria. Acta Paediatr 1997;86:775-777.
183. Abramowicz M [editor]. Generic levothyroxine. The Medical Letter of Drugs and Therapeutics 2004;46(1192):77-78.
184. Ross DS. Hyperthyroidism, thyroid hormone therapy, and bone. Thyroid 1994;4:319-326.
185. Marcocci C, Golia F, Bruno-Bosoro G, et al. Carefully monitored levothyroxine suppressive therapy is not associated with bone loss in premenopausal women. J Clin Endocrinol Metab 1994;78: 818-823.
186. Saravanan P, Chau WF, Roberts N, et al. Psychological well-being in patients on "adequate" doses of L-thyroxine: results of a large, controlled community-based questionnaire study. Clin Endocrinol (Oxf) 2002;57:577-585.
187. Kaplan MM, Swartz SL, Larsen PR. Partial peripheral resistance to thyroid hormone. Am J Med 1981;70:1115-1121.
188. Nystrom E, Caidahl K, Fager G, et al. A double-blind cross-over 12-month study of L-thyroxine treatment of women with "subclinical" hypothyroidism. Clin Endocrinol (Oxf) 1988;29:63-76.
189. Heymann R, Brent GA. Rapid progression from subclinical to symptomatic overt hypothyroidism. Endocr Prac 2005;11:115-119.
190. Sherman SI, Ladenson PW. Complications of surgery in hypothyroid patients. Am J Med 1991;90:367-370.
191. Hay ID, Duick DX, Vlietstra RE, et al. Thyroxine therapy in hypothyroid patients undergoing coronary revascularization: a retrospective analysis. Ann Intern Med 1981;95:456-457.
192. Sherman SI, Ladenson PW. Percutaneous transluminal coronary angioplasty in hypothyroidism. Am J Med 1991;90:367-370.
193. Klemperer JD, Klein I, Gomez M, et al. Thyroid hormone treatment after coronary artery bypass surgery. N Engl J Med 1995;333: 1522-1527.
194. Hamilton MA, Stevenson LW, Fonarow GC, et al. Safety and hemodynamic effects of intravenous triiodothyronine in advanced congestive heart failure. Am J Cardiol 1998;81:443-447.
195. Hamilton MA, Stevenson LW, Luu M, et al. Altered thyroid hormone metabolism in advanced heart failure. J Am Coll Cardiol 1990;16:91-95.
196. Chowdhury D, Parnell VA, Ojamaa K, et al. Usefulness of triiodothyronine (T3) treatment after surgery for complex congenital heart disease in infants and children. Am J Cardiol 1999;84:1107-1109, A10.
197. Morkin E, Ladenson P, Goldman S, et al. Thyroid hormone analogs for treatment of hypercholesterolemia and heart failure: past, present and future projects. J Mol Cell Cardiol 2004;37: 1137-1146.

198. Helfand M. Screening for subclinical thyroid dysfunction in nonpregnant adults: a summary of the evidence for the U.S. preventative services task force. Ann Intern Med 2004;140:128-141.
199. Danese MD, Powe NR, Sawin CT, et al. Screening for mild thyroid failure at the periodic health examination: a decision and cost-effectiveness analysis. JAMA 1996;276:285-292.
200. Klein RZ, Haddow JE, Faix JD, et al. Prevalence of thyroid deficiency in pregnant women. Clin Endocrinol (Oxf) 1991;35:41-46.
201. Pop VJ, Kuijpens JL, van Baar AL, et al. Low maternal free thyroxine concentrations during early pregnancy are associated with impaired psychomotor development in infancy. Clin Endocrinol (Oxf) 1999;50:149-155.
202. Mandel SJ, Spencer CA, Hollowell JG. Are detection and treatment of thyroid insufficiency in pregnancy feasible? Thyroid 2005;15:44-53.
203. Fliers E, Wiersinga WM. Myxedema coma. Rev Endocr Metab Discord 2003;4:137-141.
204. Reinhardt W, Mann K. Incidence, clinical picture, and treatment of hypothyroid coma: results of a survey. Med Klin 1997; 92:521-524.
205. Nicoloff JT, LoPresti JS. Myxedema coma: a form of decompensated hypothyroidism. Endocrinol Metab Clin North Am 1993; 22:279-290.
206. Miller KK, Daniels GH. Association between lithium use and thyrotoxicosis caused by silent thyroiditis. Clin Endocrinol (Oxf) 2001;55:501-508.
207. Szabo SM, Allen DB. Thyroiditis-differentiation of acute suppurative and subacute: case report and review of the literature. Clin Pediatr 1989;28:171-174.
208. Singer PA. Thyroiditis: acute, subacute, and chronic. Med Clin North Am 1991;75:61-77.
209. Das DK, Pant CS, Chachra KL, et al. Fine-needle aspiration cytology diagnosis of tuberculous thyroiditis: a report of eight cases. Acta Cytol 1992;36:517-522.
210. Chiovato L, Canale G, Maccherini D, et al. *Salmonella brandenburg:* a novel cause of acute suppurative thyroiditis. Acta Endocrinol (Copenh) 1993;128:439-442.
211. Gandhi RT, Tollin SR, Seely EW. Diagnosis of *Candida* thyroiditis by fine-needle aspiration. J Infect 1994;28:77-81.
212. Miyauchi A, Matsuzuka F, Kuma K, et al. Piriform sinus fistula: an underlying abnormality common in patients with acute suppurative thyroiditis. World J Surg 1990;14:400-405.
213. Lucaya J, Berdon WE, Enriquez G, et al. Congenital pyriform sinus fistula: a cause of acute left-sided suppurative thyroiditis and neck abscess in children. Pediatr Radiol 1990;21:27-29.
214. Bernard PJ, Som PM, Urken ML, et al. The CT findings of acute thyroiditis and acute suppurative thyroiditis. Otolaryngol Head Neck Surg 1988;99:489-493.
215. Hatabu H, Kasagi K, Yamamoto K, et al. Acute suppurative thyroiditis associated with piriform sinus fistula: sonographic findings. Am J Med 1990;155:845-847.
216. Bartholomew LG, Cain JC, Woolner LB, et al. Sclerosing cholangitis: its possible association with Riedel's struma and fibrous retroperitonitis—report of two cases. N Engl J Med 1963;269:8-13.
217. Chopra D, Wool MS, Grossen A, et al. Riedel's struma associated with subacute thyroiditis, hypothyroidism, and hypoparathyroidism. J Clin Endocrinol Metab 1978;46:869-871.
218. Zelmanovitz F, Zelmanovitz T, Beck M, et al. Riedel's thyroiditis associated with high titers of antimicrosomal and antithyroglobulin antibodies and hypothyroidism. J Endocrinol Invest 1994; 17:733-737.
219. Julie C, Vieillefond A, Desligneres S, et al. Hashimoto's thyroiditis associated with Riedel's thyroiditis and retroperitoneal fibrosis. Pathol Res Pract 1997;193:573-577.
220. Heufelder AE, Goellner JR, Bahn RS, et al. Tissue eosinophilia and eosinophil degranulation in Riedel's invasive fibrous thyroiditis. J Clin Endocrinol Metab 1996;81:977-984.
221. Jung YJ, Schaub CR, Rhodes R, et al. A case of Riedel's thyroiditis treated with tamoxifen: another successful outcome. Endocr Pract 2004;10:483-486.

CHAPTER 13

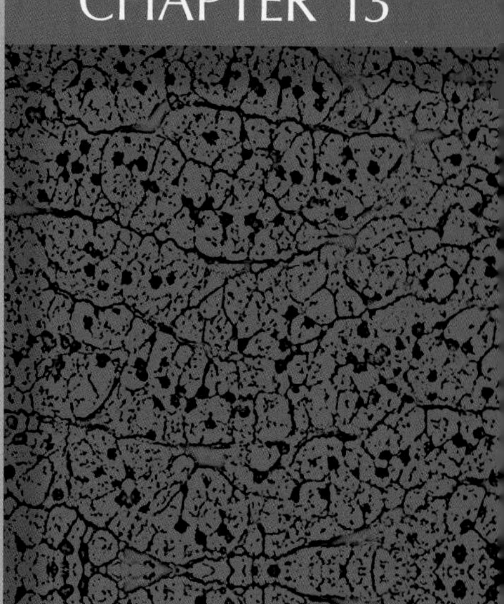

NONTOXIC DIFFUSE AND NODULAR GOITER AND THYROID NEOPLASIA

Martin-Jean Schlumberger, Sebastiano Filetti, and Ian D. Hay

In this chapter, we review the imaging techniques available for evaluating thyroid structural abnormalities; the units of measurement used in evaluation of the radiation dose and radioactivity are defined in Table 13–1.

Goiter resulting in thyrotoxicosis and other thyroid conditions arising from autoimmune thyroid disease are considered in Chapters 11 and 12.

This chapter deals with the increasingly recognized problem of nodular thyroid disease. Moreover, thyroid neoplasia, both benign and malignant, is discussed authoritatively. We consider an appropriate histologic classification and staging of thyroid cancer and present a management program for the most common thyroid cancer types.

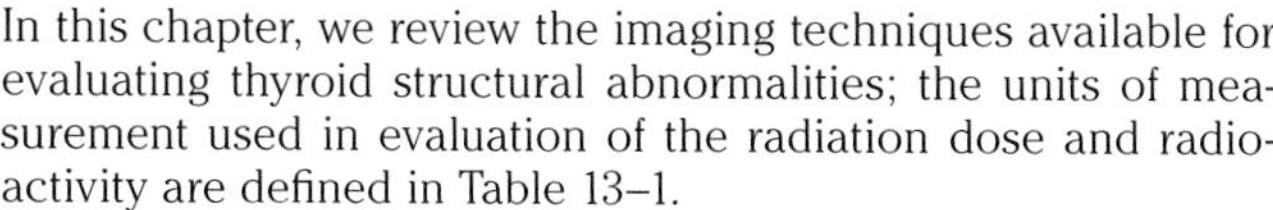

EVALUATION OF STRUCTURAL ABNORMALITIES BY IMAGING TECHNIQUES

External Scintiscanning

Localization of functioning or nonfunctioning thyroid tissue in the area of the thyroid gland or elsewhere is made possible by techniques of external scintiscanning. The underlying principle is that isotopes that are selectively accumulated by thyroid tissue can be detected by a gamma camera and the data transformed into a visual display. Radioactivity in specific areas can be quantified.[1-3]

Several radioisotopes are employed in thyroid imaging. Technetium 99m (^{99m}Tc) pertechnetate is a monovalent anion that is actively concentrated by the thyroid gland but undergoes negligible organic binding and diffuses out of the thyroid gland as its concentration in the blood decreases. The short physical half-life of ^{99m}Tc (6 hours), its low fractional uptake, and its transient stay within the thyroid make the radiation delivered to the thyroid gland by a standard activity very low. Consequently, the intravenous administration of large activities (>37 MBq [1 mCi]) permits, about 30 minutes later, adequate imaging of the thyroid.

Two radioactive isotopes of iodine have been used in thyroid imaging. Iodine 131 (^{131}I) was commonly used in the past. However, ^{131}I is a beta emitter, its physical half-life is 8.1 days, and the energy of its main gamma ray is high and thus poorly adapted for its detection.[3] ^{123}I is, in many respects, ideal but it is expensive. The energy of its main gamma ray is adapted for its detection by gamma cameras. Its short half-life (0.55 day) and the absence of beta radiation result in a radiation dose to the thyroid that is about 1% of that delivered by a comparable activity of ^{131}I.[4]

The most important use of scintigraphic imaging of thyroid tissue is to define areas of increased or decreased function ("hot" or "cold" areas, respectively) relative to the function of the remainder of the gland. Almost all malignant nodules are hypofunctioning, but more than 80% of benign nodules are also nonfunctioning. Conversely, functioning nodules (hot nodules),

TABLE 13–1 RADIATION NOMENCLATURE: TRADITIONAL AND INTERNATIONAL SYSTEM (SI) UNITS

Radioactivity (or Activity)	
Radiation Dose	**Abbreviation**
1 Gy = 100 rad = absorption of 1 joule/kg	Gy = gray
1 rad = 0.01 Gy = 1 cGy	rad = radiation absorbed dose
1 Sv = 100 rem	rem = roentgen-equivalent-man
	Sv = sievert
1 Bq = 1 disintegration per second	mCi = millicurie
1 mCi = 37 MBq	Bq = becquerel
1 GBq = 10^3 MBq =	kBq = kilobecquerel
10^6 kBq = 10^9 Bq	MBq = megabecquerel
	GBq = gigabecquerel

particularly if the function of the surrounding tissue is decreased or absent, are rarely malignant.

In the past, several nuclear medical tests were used to evaluate thyroid disorders (stimulation test after administration of exogenous thyroid-stimulating hormone [TSH] or suppression test by administration of thyroid hormone) but should no longer be used because the use of sensitive TSH assays and of scanning with a gamma camera permits the diagnosis of most hot nodules.

Scintiscanning with radioactive iodine can also be used to demonstrate that intrathoracic masses represent thyroid tissue, to detect ectopic thyroid tissue in the neck, and to detect functioning metastases of thyroid carcinoma.

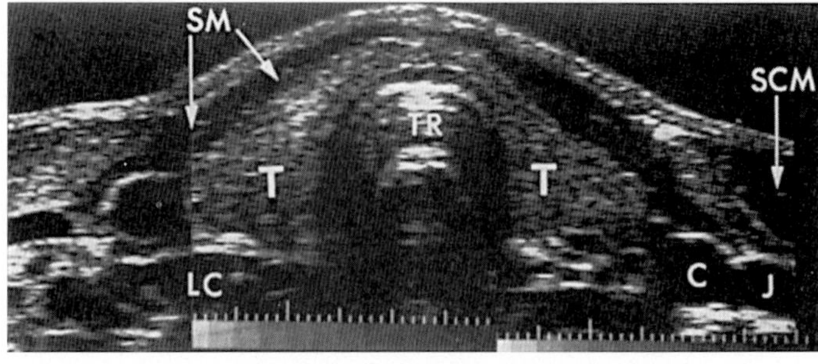

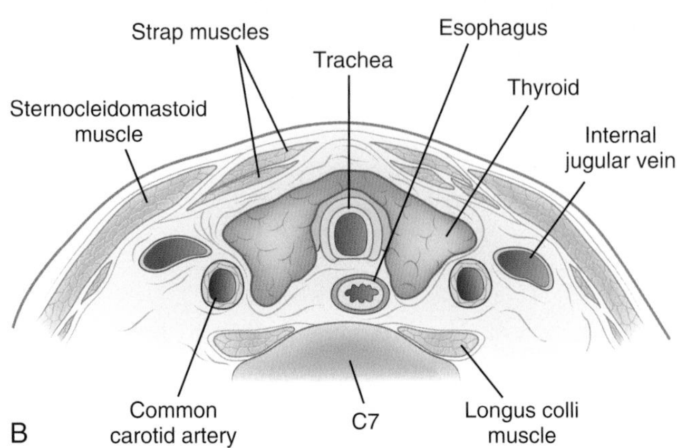

Figure 13–1 ■ Transverse composite sonogram **(A)** and corresponding anatomic map **(B)** of the normal thyroid gland. *C,* Common carotid artery; *LC,* longus colli muscle; *SM,* strap muscles; *SCM,* sternocleidomastoid muscle; *T,* thyroid; *TR,* trachea. (From Rifkin MD, Charboneau JW, Laing FC. Special course: ultrasound 1991. In Reading CC, ed. Syllabus: Thyroid, Parathyroid, and Cervical Lymph Nodes. Oak Brook, IL: Radiological Society of North America, 1991:363-377.)

Ultrasonography

Sonography is a noninvasive technique that is becoming an integral part of the clinical examination.[5] High-frequency sound waves are emitted by a transducer and reflected as they pass through the body, whereupon the returning echoes are received by the transducer, which also acts as a receiver. The amplitude of the reflections of the sound waves is influenced by differences in the acoustic impedance of the tissues encountered by the sound; for example, *fluid-filled* structures reflect few echoes and therefore have no or few internal echoes and well-defined margins; *solid* structures reflect varying amounts of sound and thus have various degrees of internal echoes and less well-defined margins; and *calcified* structures reflect virtually all incoming sound and yield pronounced echoes with an acoustic "shadow" posteriorly.

Intrathyroidal nodules as small as 3 mm in diameter and cystic nodules as small as 2 mm can be readily detected. Color flow Doppler ultrasonography allows visualization of very small vessels, so that vascularity of thyroid nodules can be assessed.

The thyroid gland must be examined thoroughly in transverse and longitudinal planes. Imaging should also include the region of the carotid artery and jugular vein to identify enlarged cervical lymph nodes.[6-8]

The normal thyroid parenchyma has a characteristic homogeneous medium-level echogenicity, with little identifiable internal architecture (Fig. 13–1). The surrounding muscles have the appearance of hypoechoic structures. The air-filled trachea in the midline gives a characteristic curvilinear reflecting surface with an associated reverberation artifact. The esophagus is usually hidden from sonographic visualization by the tracheal air shadow.

A diagrammatic representation of the neck showing the location or locations of any abnormal finding and their characteristics is a useful supplement to the routine film images recorded during an ultrasound examination. Such a cervical map (Fig. 13–2) can help communicate the anatomic relationships of the pathology more clearly to the referring clinician and serves as a reference for the sonographer on follow-up examinations.

Neck ultrasonography is clinically useful at each step of thyroid evaluation (Table 13–2). It may confirm the presence of a thyroid nodule when the findings on physical examination are equivocal and may reveal the presence of other nonpalpable nodules.

In patients with a thyroid nodule, gray-scale and color Doppler ultrasound are used to evaluate its sonographic features, including size, shape, echogenicity (hypoechoic or hyperechoic), and composition (cystic, solid, or mixed), as well as the presence of coarse or fine calcifications, a halo and margins, and internal blood flow. These technique will examine the rest of the thyroid gland and lymph node areas.

In patients with known thyroid cancer, sonography can be useful in evaluating the extent of disease, both preoperatively and postoperatively.[5-8] Thus, in patients who present with cervical lymphadenopathy caused by papillary thyroid carcinoma (PTC) but in whom the gland is palpably normal, sonography may be used preoperatively to detect an occult, primary intra-

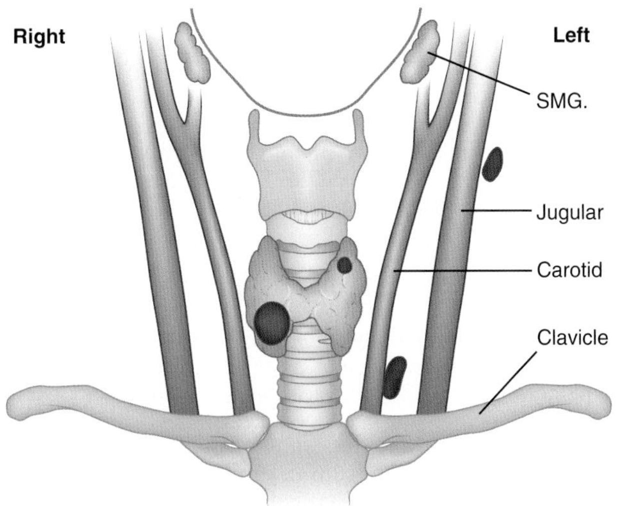

Figure 13–2 ■ Cervical map, derived from sonographic images, helps communicate anatomic relationships of pathology to clinicians and serves as a reference for follow-up examinations. *SMG,* submandibular gland. (From James EM, Charboneau JW, Hay ID. The thyroid. In Rumack CM, Wilson SR, Charboneau JW, eds. Diagnostic Ultrasound, Vol 1. St. Louis: Mosby–Year Book, 1991:507-528.)

TABLE 13–2 CLINICAL UTILITY OF NECK ULTRASOUND EXAMINATION

Map of the neck (thyroid and lymph node areas)
Thyroid gland: size, volume, characteristics
Nodules: number and characteristics of each nodule: diameter, shape, echogenicity, composition, limits, presence of calcifications, vascularization
Lymph node areas
Follow-up: number and diameters of nodules
Guidance for fine needle aspiration biopsy
Follow-up of thyroid cancer: thyroid bed and neck lymph node areas
Guidance for radiofrequency and ethanol ablation

thyroid focus. Some surgeons do regularly obtain a preoperative sonogram in patients with PTC or medullary thyroid carcinoma (MTC) in order to identify before surgery the anatomic locations of any sonographically suspicious regional lymph nodes and thereby permit planning of the extent of nodal dissection. Occasionally, a handheld ultrasound probe can be used intraoperatively to identify impalpable residual cancer that has been identified by preoperative ultrasonography and proved to be cytologically positive by ultrasound-guided fine needle aspiration biopsy (FNAB).

After surgery for thyroid cancer, sonography is the preferred method for detecting residual, recurrent, or metastatic disease in the neck.[6-8] In patients who have undergone less than a near-total thyroidectomy, the sonographic appearance of the remaining thyroid tissue may be an important factor in the decision whether to recommend completion thyroidectomy. Also, it is more sensitive than neck palpation in detecting recurrent disease within the thyroid bed and metastatic disease in cervical lymph nodes. However, benign lymph node hyperplasia is frequent and should be differentiated from lymph node metastases.

Sonography may also be useful to guide fine needle biopsy of thyroid bed masses and lymph nodes, especially when these abnormalities are not palpable.[5]

Computed Tomography

The computed tomography (CT) appearance of the anatomic structures depends on the attenuation of the tissue examined. The thyroid gland, because of its high concentration of iodine, has higher attenuation than that of the surrounding soft tissues. Recent advances with spiral CT and reconstruction algorithms improved the performance of the method.[9,10]

The diagnostic utility of CT in the evaluation of nodular thyroid disease is limited because thyroid masses, whether benign or malignant, may be hypodense, hyperdense, or isodense compared with adjacent normal thyroid tissue. In aggressive pathologic processes, such as anaplastic thyroid carcinoma, CT can define the extension of the tumor to the mediastinum and its relationships to surrounding structures.[9,10] CT imaging is less sensitive than neck ultrasonography for the detection of lymph node metastases. In patients with thyroid cancer, CT is used most frequently to search for lymph node metastases in the mediastinum and for lung metastases.

CT scanning can provide useful information regarding the presence and extent of intrathoracic (substernal) goiters. The CT findings of an intrathoracic mass in continuity with the thyroid gland, with high attenuation on non–contrast-enhanced images and marked enhancement after intravenous contrast material injection, all suggest intrathoracic goiter. Radioiodine scanning can also be performed in this clinical setting, but false-negative results can occur when little or no functional tissue is present in the intrathoracic goiter. Because of the necessity of infusing iodine-containing contrast agents, CT should be performed at least 4 weeks before any administration of radioiodine.

Magnetic Resonance Imaging

Because the hydrogen atoms of different tissues have different relaxation times (termed T1 and T2), a computer-assisted analysis of T1-weighted and T2-weighted signals is used to differentiate the thyroid gland from skeletal muscles, blood vessels, or regional lymph nodes. Normal thyroid tissue tends to be slightly more intense than muscles on a T1-weighted image, and tumors often appear more intense than normal thyroid tissue.

Magnetic resonance imaging (MRI) does not distinguish benign from malignant nodules and does not assess functional status; however, it can define the anatomic extent of large goiters with great clarity.

Recurrent neoplasms in the thyroid bed or regional lymph nodes can be detected with MRI; MRI is comparable in accuracy to CT. Recurrence is characterized by a mass with low to medium intensity on T1-weighted images and medium to high signal intensity on T2-weighted images. Conversely, scar tissue or fibrous tissue has low signal intensity on both T1-weighted and T2-weighted images.[9,10] Tumor invasion of adjacent skeletal muscle has high signal intensity on T2-weighted images. Edema or inflammation in the muscle can cause a similar appearance and can be difficult to differentiate from recurrent tumor.

MRI is useful for assessment of the extent of bone involvement in cases of bone metastases from follicular cell–derived and medullary thyroid carcinoma that are poorly visualized on bone scintigraphy.[11] CT and MRI with arterial phase are useful for the detection of liver metastases from medullary thyroid cancer.[12] However, MRI is less useful than CT for the diagnosis of lung metastases.

Positron Emission Tomography

Positron emission tomography (PET) is both quantitative and tomographic. The radionuclide used emits a positron that is converted into a pair of photons after a short path of a few millimeters in the tissue. The coincidence detection of the two photons, which travel on a line in opposite directions, permits the localization of the site of the radionuclide decay.

The agent most widely used with PET is [^{18}F]fluorodeoxyglucose (^{18}FDG). This agent is transported and phosphorylated as a glucose substitute but remains metabolically trapped inside tumor cells because of its inability to undergo glycolysis.

PET scanners permit in vivo images related to regional glucose metabolism, with high sensitivity and a spatial resolution less than 5 mm. Superimposition of CT and PET images greatly improves both the sensitivity and specificity of the technique and the anatomic localization of any focus of abnormal uptake. Elevated glucose metabolism in thyroid cancer tissue is increased following TSH stimulation.[13,14]

PET scanning should be performed in only selected patients with papillary and follicular thyroid carcinoma who have no tumoral radioiodine uptake, in patients with elevated serum thyroglobulin (Tg) and no other evidence of disease, and in those patients who are candidates for aggressive treatment to exclude the presence of other neoplastic foci. In these patients, PET scanning is useful for the detection of lymph node metastases in the mediastinum, or distant metastases. High FDG uptake in large metastases indicates a poor prognosis.[15]

High uptake has also been observed in several thyroid diseases, such as thyroiditis, but PET cannot be used to differentiate benign from malignant thyroid nodules. The discovery of thyroid uptake on a FDG PET scan performed for other reasons should lead to a complete workup, because one third of these nodules may prove to be malignant.[16]

In clinical research settings, PET scanning with ^{124}I has also been used for quantitation of uptake and for accurate dosimetry in distant metastases from thyroid cancer,[17] and with ^{18}F-DOPA, to visualize neoplastic foci of medullary thyroid carcinoma.[18]

NONTOXIC GOITER: DIFFUSE AND NODULAR

Nontoxic goiter may be defined as any thyroid enlargement characterized by uniform or selective (i.e., restricted to one or more areas) growth of thyroid tissue that is not associated with overt hyperthyroidism or hypothyroidism and that does not result from inflammation or neoplasia. A thyroid nodule is defined as a discrete lesion within the thyroid gland that is due to an abnormal focal growth of thyroid cells.

Epidemiology

The prevalence of goiter, diffuse or nodular, differs widely depending on the iodine intake by the population living in a given area. Thus, goiter may occur endemically, due mainly to iodine deficiency, or sporadically, depending whether the goiter prevalence in children is more or less than 5%, respectively. In general population, the Framingham survey indicates a 4.6% prevalence, being 6.4% in women and 1.5% in men, and the Whickham study displays a 3.2% prevalence (6.6 : 1 ratio women/men).[19,20] However, different variables (regional variation in the iodine intake, smoking habits, age and sex distribution and primarily the methodology used to determine thyroid volume, palpation vs sonography) may have biased many of these data. Thus, by using sonography as the screening method, a prevalence of up to 30% to 50% of an unselected adult population has been described as having a goiter. This prevalence is even higher in an iodine-deficient area and in older people. In this regard, a prevalence of thyroid nodules of up to 50% has been described in autopsy series[21] and of more than 60% in healthy adults screened with sonography.[22]

Etiology and Pathophysiology

Goiter has been traditionally regarded as the adaptive response of the thyroid follicular cell to any factor that impairs thyroid hormone synthesis. This classic concept no longer appears to encompass the many aspects of goiters. Indeed, goiter is characterized by a variety of clinical, functional, and morphologic presentations, and whether this heterogeneity represents different entities remains to be clarified. Also, iodine deficiency as the sole factor responsible for goiter appears to be an oversimplification. Thus, not all inhabitants in an iodine-deficient region develop goiter; moreover, endemic goiter has been observed in countries with no iodine deficiency, and even in some regions with iodine excess, and has not been observed in some regions with severe iodine deficiency. These findings suggest that other factors, both genetic and environmental, may play a role in the genesis of diffuse and nodular goiter, and some of these factors may act synergistically. Environmental factors include cigarette smoking, infections, drugs, and goitrogens.[23]

The role of genetic factors is suggested by several lines of evidence,[24] such as (1) the clustering of goiters within families; (2) the higher concordance rate for goiters in monozygotic than in dizygotic twins; (3) the female/male ratio (1 : 1 in endemic versus 7 : 1 to 9 : 1 in sporadic goiters); (4) the persistence of goiters in areas where a widespread iodine prophylaxis program has been properly implemented.

By studying families affected by goiter, researchers have been able to detect several gene abnormalities involving proteins related to thyroid hormone synthesis, such as mutations in thyroglobulin *(Tg)*, sodium/iodide symporter *(NIS)*, thyroid peroxidase *(TPO)*, pendrin syndrome *(PDS)*, and TSH receptor *(TSHR)* genes. In addition, three loci for this disorder have been identified that map to chromosomalregions 14q, Xp22, and 3q26.[25,26] Although an autosomal dominant inheritance has been demonstrated in several families, multiple genes may be involved in other families. This may explain why predisposing gene alterations remain unidentified in most patients with nontoxic goiter.

TSH has long been considered the major agent determining thyroid growth in response to any factor that impairs thyroid hormone synthesis. Indeed, in the rare clinical setting of functioning TSH-secreting pituitary tumor, the increased blood TSH levels typically cause an enlargement of the thyroid gland.[27] Similarly, goiter is also a typical feature of Graves' disease, in which a stimulatory growth effect on thyroid tissue is induced by thyroid-stimulating antibody through TSHR activation.[28] Moreover, thyroid enlargement may appear during the course of Graves' disease when increased TSH levels result from overtreatment with antithyroid drugs. In addition, toxic thyroid hyperplasia is usually present in nonautoimmune autosomal dominant hyperthyroidism, a disorder related to germline-activating mutations of the *TSHR* gene.[29] This clinical condition further emphasizes the role of TSH-TSHR system activation in the genesis of thyroid hyperplasia.[24]

Serum TSH concentration is normal in most patients with nontoxic goiter.[23] Experimentally, it has been demonstrated that in rats iodine depletion enhances the promotion of thyroid growth by normal level of TSH.[30] Hence, any factor that impairs intrathyroidal iodine levels may lead to gradual development of goiter in response to normal concentrations of TSH.

Indeed, a complex network of both TSH-dependent and TSH-independent pathways directs thyroid follicular cell growth and function and plays a role in the goitrogenic process. In particular, a variety of growth factors, derived either from the bloodstream or through autocrine or paracrine secretion, may serve to regulate thyroid cell proliferation and differentiation processes.[24]

Typically, early in the course of goiter formation, areas of microheterogeneity of structure and function are intermixed and include areas of functional autonomy and areas of focal hemorrhage.

Analysis of hyperplastic nodules by rigid criteria also indicated that morphologically indistinguishable hyperplastic thyroid nodules may be either monoclonal or polyclonal. Monoclonal adenomas within hyperplastic thyroid glands may reflect a stage in progression along the hyperplasia-neoplasia spectrum; accumulation of multiple somatic mutations may subsequently confer a selective growth advantage to this single-cell clone.[31]

Histologically, nodules contain irregularly enlarged, involuted follicles distended with colloid or clusters of smaller follicles lined by taller epithelium and containing small colloid droplets. The nodules tend to be incompletely encapsulated and are poorly demarcated from and merge with the internodular tissue, which also has an altered architecture. However, the nodules in some glands appear to be localized, with areas of apparently normal architecture elsewhere. Here, the distinction from a follicular adenoma may be difficult, and some pathologists apply terms such as *colloid* or *adenomatous* nodules to such lesions.

Natural History

Nontoxic goiter has a female preponderance. There appears to be no physiologic increase in thyroid volume during normal adolescence. Development of a goiter during adolescence, therefore, is a pathologic rather than a physiologic process.[32] However, as evidenced by sonographic measurement of thyroid volume in women living in an area of moderate iodine intake, normal pregnancy is goitrogenic, especially in women with preexisting thyroid disorders. The increased thyroid volume during pregnancy is associated with biochemical features of thyroid stimulation (i.e., an increased triiodothyronine/thyroxine [T_3/T_4] ratio) owing to slightly elevated serum TSH levels at delivery or a high human chorionic gonadotropin (hCG) concentration during the first trimester.[33] Repeated pregnancies may play a role in the development of later thyroid disorders, a relation that might explain the higher prevalence of thyroid disorders in women.[34] Natural outcome of nontoxic nodular goiter has been examined in adult population with two main findings: (1) benign thyroid nodules likely although slowly grow over time; (2) as a consequence, the concept that the growing nodules are malignant whereas the stable are benign should be discarded.[35]

Clinical Presentation

In an era when patients are advised on self-examination to detect cancer at an early stage, the finding of a palpable abnormality in such a superficial location as the thyroid gland can be disconcerting. The affected patient is likely to seek medical evaluation. At the end of an appropriate investigation, the clinician can usually reassure the patient that the goiter or the nodule is benign. Autonomous nodules or autonomous functional areas in the context of a multinodular goiter may result in an increased thyroid hormone secretion and subsequently a subclinical or overt thyrotoxicosis. However, in general, thyroid nodules are usually not associated with abnormal thyroid hormone secretion. Therefore, affected patients do not exhibit clinical symptoms or signs of thyroid dysfunction. The only clinical features of nontoxic goiter are those of thyroid enlargement. Nearly 70% of patients with sporadic nontoxic goiter complain of neck discomfort; the remainder have cosmetic concerns or a fear of possible malignancy.[23]

Large goiters, which may displace or compress the trachea, esophagus, and neck vessels, can be associated with symptoms and signs including inspiratory stridor, dysphagia, and a choking sensation. These obstructive symptoms may be accentuated by the so-called Pemberton maneuver (see Chapter 10). Compression of the recurrent laryngeal nerve, with hoarseness, suggests carcinoma rather than nontoxic goiter, but vocal cord paralysis can occasionally result from benign nodular goiters. Hemorrhage into a nodule or cyst produces acute, painful enlargement locally and may enhance or induce obstructive symptoms.[23]

Initial Investigation

Thyroid nodules are generally benign hyperplastic (or colloid) nodules or benign follicular adenomas, and only about 5% to 10% of nodules coming to medical attention are carcinomas. Differentiating true neoplasms from hyperplastic nodules and distinguishing between benign and malignant tumors are major challenges.

Moreover, with the widespread practice of medical checkups in healthy individuals and the increasing use of imaging technology, this problem is likely to become more common. High-resolution ultrasound studies suggest that the prevalence of nodular thyroid disease in healthy adults is above 60%.[22] However, during 2005 in the United States, only about 25,690 new cases of thyroid cancer were likely to be diagnosed.[36] Therefore, most of these so-called thyroid incidentalomas are obviously benign and do not progress to clinical tumors.[22]

In identifying the nodules that are likely to be malignant, a thorough history and a careful physical examination should be supplemented with laboratory testing, imaging procedures, and, most important, FNAB of the nodule in question. With the use of this approach, it is possible to assess the likelihood of malignancy and to advise appropriate treatment in the majority of patients.[23]

History and Physical Examination

Historical features that favor benign disease include the following: a family history of Hashimoto's thyroiditis, benign thyroid nodule, or goiter; symptoms of hypothyroidism or hyperthyroidism; a sudden increase in size of the nodule with pain or tenderness, suggesting a cyst or localized subacute thyroiditis.[23]

Historical features that suggest malignancy include the following: young age (younger than 20 years old) or old age (older than 60 years old); male sex; a history of external neck radiation during childhood or adolescence; rapid growth; recent changes in speaking, breathing, or swallowing; a family history of thyroid cancer or multiple endocrine neoplasia (MEN) type 2.[23]

On physical examination, manifestations of thyroid malignancy should be sought, including firm consistency of the nodule, irregular shape, fixation to underlying or overlying tissues, vocal cord paralysis, and suspicious regional lymphadenopathy.[23]

Many studies have shown that nodule size is not predictive of malignancy and that the incidence of cancer in incidentally identified or nonpalpable thyroid nodules is the same as in patients with palpable nodules. However, given the excellent

TABLE 13–3 CLINICAL AND ULTRASOUND FINDINGS IN FAVOR OF MALIGNANT THYROID NODULES

Clinical Features	Ultrasound Findings
HISTORICAL FEATURES	Hypoechoic lesions
Young (<20 years old) or old (>60 years old) age	Irregular margins
	Presence of calcifications
Male sex	Absence of halo
Neck irradiation during childhood or adolescence	Internal or central blood flow
Rapid growth	**LOW SUSPICION**
Recent changes in speaking, breathing, or swallowing	Echo-free (cystic) lesion
	Homogeneously hyperechoic lesions
Family history of thyroid malignancy or multiple endocrine neoplasia type 2	
PHYSICAL EXAMINATION	
Firm and irregular consistency of nodule	
Fixation to underlying or overlying tissues	
Vocal cord paralysis	
Regional lymph adenopathy	

prognosis of micropapillary thyroid carcinomas of less than 1 cm in diameter, most authors recommend to investigate only those nodules of more than 1 cm in diameter and those with clinical or sonographic suspicious findings.[5,22,37,38]

Recent evaluation of large groups of patients has shown that the presence of multiple nodules does not decrease the likelihood of thyroid cancer. In patients with multiple nodules, the rate per nodule decreases, but the decrease is approximately proportional to the number of nodules, so that the overall rate per patient is the same as in patients with a solitary nodule. Also, thyroid cancers are often in the dominant nodule, but in approximately one third of cases, the cancer is in a nondominant nodule.[35]

In both prospective and retrospective studies, the sensitivity and specificity rates for detecting thyroid malignancy by history and physical examination (Table 13–3) were about 60% and 80%, respectively.[39,40] In these historical series, only about 20% of patients with later confirmed malignancy had, when initially seen, neither suspicious historical features nor evidence of potential malignancy on neck examination.

Laboratory Tests

Serum TSH, measured in a highly sensitive immunometric assay and eventually combined with a single measurement of free thyroid hormone concentrations may be used as a first-line screening test.

An undetectable serum TSH, even associated with normal free thyroid hormone levels, should suggest the possibility of toxic, autonomously functioning nodular areas in the goiter and should lead to thyroid scintigraphy. Such a finding should prompt further cardiac investigation, especially in elderly patients, whose risk of atrial fibrillation may be increased as much as threefold when serum TSH levels are less than 0.1 mU/L.[41] Patients with thyroid cancer rarely have abnormalities in serum TSH levels.

Measurement of serum anti-TPO antibody and anti-Tg antibody levels may be helpful in diagnosis of chronic autoimmune thyroiditis, especially if the serum TSH level is elevated. Chronic thyroiditis has a typical hypoechoic appearance on sonography; the thyroid gland's size and consistency may simulate either a solitary nodule or bilateral nodules; hypoechoic nodules should be submitted to FNAB that will distinguish between foci of thyroiditis and nodules of epithelial origin.

Follicular cell–derived thyroid cancers (FCTCs) may release increased amounts of Tg into the bloodstream. Unfortunately, there is overlap of serum Tg levels in FCTCs and in a number of benign conditions, and measurement of serum Tg levels is not useful in the initial workup of nodular thyroid disease. Similarly, some investigators routinely measure calcitonin (CT) levels in all patients with nodular thyroid disease to identify cases of MTC. In fact, the calcitonin level is increased in virtually all patients with clinical MTC.[42] However, because of the rarity of unsuspected MTC, the high frequency of false-positive results that may prompt a thyroidectomy despite a reassuring cytologic result, and the unknown clinical relevance of medullary microcarcinomas, it is neither cost-effective nor necessary to measure calcitonin levels in patients with nodular thyroid disease in the absence of clinical suspicion of MTC or abnormal cytologic findings.[23]

The molecular abnormality in more than 95% of familial MTC cases is a germline mutation of the *RET* proto-oncogene that is located on the long arm of chromosome 10.[43] Many investigators advocate *RET* mutation testing in all patients with MTC, including apparently sporadic cases, because 4% to 6% of such patients have germline mutations of the gene (see Chapter 36).[44] If a mutation is found, family members at risk are then tested to identify affected individuals. A negative result obviates the need for any further testing, and individuals who harbor such mutations should undergo prophylactic total thyroidectomy to prevent later development of the multicentric MTC that occurs in this disorder.[44]

Imaging in Nodular Goiter Evaluation

Today, when a nodular goiter is clinically present, ultrasonography represents by far the more useful thyroid imaging technique by providing helpful information for disease management and treatment. Indeed, ultrasonography should be used to assess both morphology and size of the goiter and may assist in both screening and follow-up of thyroid nodules.[5,23] Ultrasonography is capable of detecting even minute thyroid nodules. In fact, of 1000 normal control subjects, 65% had detectable nodularity on high-resolution scanning.[22] Attempts have been made to develop criteria for distinguishing benign and malignant nodules (see Table 13–3). Echo-free (cystic) and homogeneously hyperechoic lesions are reputed to carry a low risk of malignancy.[5,23] Positive predictive criteria of malignancy include predominantly solid nodules and absence of cystic elements, hypoechoic nodules, presence of microcalcifications, irregular margins, and absence of halo. However, nodules that can be clearly identified as benign by sonography are uncommon. The color Doppler finding of predominantly internal or central blood flow appears to increase the risk that a nodule is malignant. However, as with other sonographic features, color Doppler cannot be used to diagnose or exclude malignancy with a high degree of confidence.[5,23]

Ultrasonography is useful in identifying hypoechoic solid nodules that should be submitted to FNAB, particularly in the presence of microcalcifications and in examining the rest of the thyroid gland and lymph node areas (Fig. 13–3).[5] It may also be used in the case of partially cystic nodules to direct the needle into the solid portions, and in the setting of nonpalpable nodules to guide FNAB, especially when the diameter of the nodule is

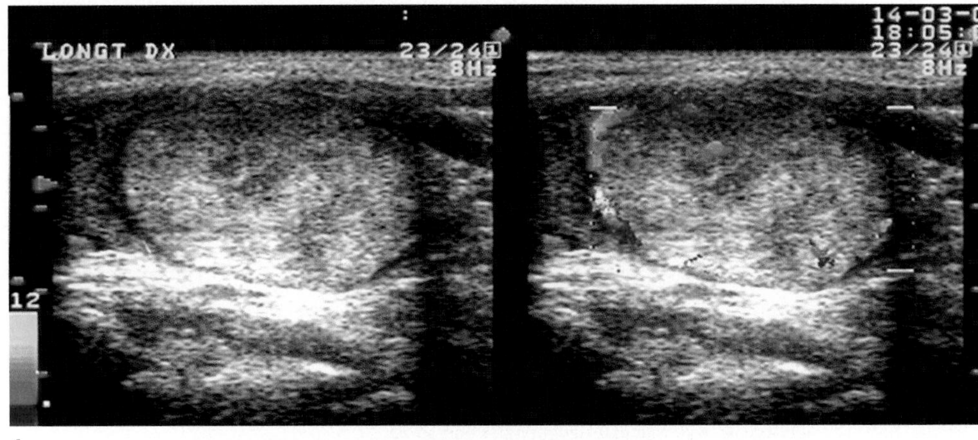

A

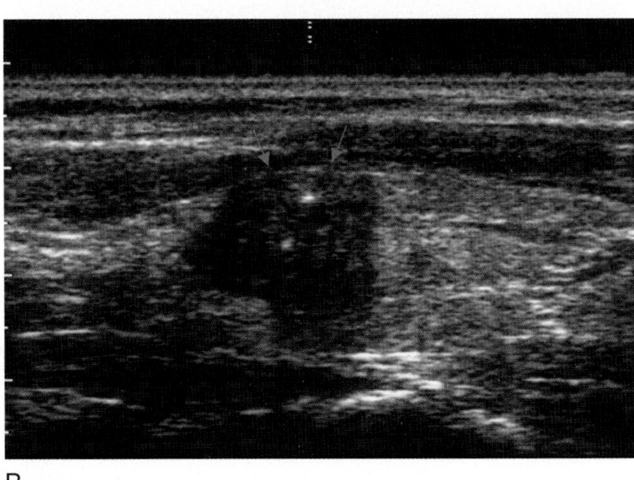

B

Figure 13–3 ▪ Conventional and color flow Doppler sonography. **A,** Benign lesion. Sonograms show well-defined, oval, hyperechoic nodule with perinodular and slight intranodular blood flow. **B,** Malignant lesion. Sonogram shows a nodule with inhomogeneous hypoechoic aspect, microcalcifications, and irregular borders, with invasion of the thyroid capsule *(arrows)*.

1 cm or more.[5] Cystic lesions may be treated by aspiration of the fluid and ethanol injection to avoid recurrence; this is optimally performed under ultrasonographic guidance.[45]

In patients with large goiters, conventional radiography of the neck and the upper mediastinum should be used to determine the presence of tracheal compression. CT and MRI are indicated in the presence of intrathoracic goiter to define the relationships with surrounding structures.

The traditional imaging procedure of the thyroid in past years has been scintigraphy using ^{131}I, ^{123}I, or ^{99m}Tc. Most thyroid carcinomas are inefficient in trapping and organifying iodine and appear on scans as areas of diminished isotope uptake, so-called cool or cold nodules. This feature reflects the early decrease of NIS expression during tumorigenesis. Unfortunately, most benign nodules also do not concentrate iodine and therefore are cold nodules. Furthermore, not all nodules with normal or slightly increased ^{99m}Tc uptake are benign and some may appear cold on a thyroid scan with radioactive iodine.[1,2]

The only situation in which an iodine scan can exclude malignancy with reasonable certainty is in the case of a toxic adenoma, which is characterized by significantly increased uptake within the nodule, so-called "hot" nodule, and markedly suppressed or absent uptake in the remainder of the gland. These lesions are suspected at clinical examination and are typically associated with a low or suppressed serum TSH level. They account for fewer than 10% of thyroid nodules and are almost invariably benign.[23] Thyroid scintigraphy should be used as a second-line technique to detect hyperfunctioning nodules in patients with suppressed serum TSH.

CT scanning and MRI in the initial diagnosis of thyroid malignancy do not provide higher quality images of the thyroid and cervical nodes than those of ultrasonography. CT examination of the lower central neck is preferable when tracheal or mediastinal invasion is suspected.[23]

Fine Needle Aspiration Biopsy

FNAB of thyroid nodules has eclipsed all other techniques for diagnosing thyroid cancer, with reported overall rates of sensitivity and specificity exceeding 90% in iodine-sufficient geographical areas.[5,23,38,46,47] The technique is easy to perform and safe, with only a handful of complications having been reported in the literature,[48] and causes little discomfort. However, care must be taken to obtain an adequate specimen; most authors recommend between three and six aspirations per nodule.[46,47] A satisfactory specimen contains at least five or six groups of 10 to 15 well-preserved cells. The cells are categorized by their cytologic appearances into *benign, indeterminate* or *suspicious,* and *malignant* (Table 13–4).

The diagnosis of PTC by FNAB on the basis of characteristic nuclear changes is particularly reliable and accurate, with sensitivity and specificity both approaching 100%. For follicular neoplasms, however, the usefulness of FNAB is lower. If strict criteria for malignancy are used, sensitivity may be as low as 8%.[40] If any follicular neoplasm that is not clearly benign on cytologic examination is classified as cancerous, sensitivity rises to about 90% or more. Unfortunately, this increase is asso-

TABLE 13–4 PROBABILITY OF MALIGNANCY AT HISTOLOGY BASED ON FINE NEEDLE ASPIRATION BIOPSY CYTOLOGY (SUMMARY OF THE LITERATURE)

Cytology	Results (%), Mean (Range)	Probability of Malignancy (%), Range
Inadequate/ nondiagnostic	16 (15-20)	10-20
Benign	70 (53-90)	1-2
Suspicious*	10 (5-23)	10-20
Malignant	4 (1-10)	>95

*The suspicious category includes follicular neoplasms (hyperplastic nodules, follicular adenomas, and follicular carcinomas) and some Hürthle cell tumors.

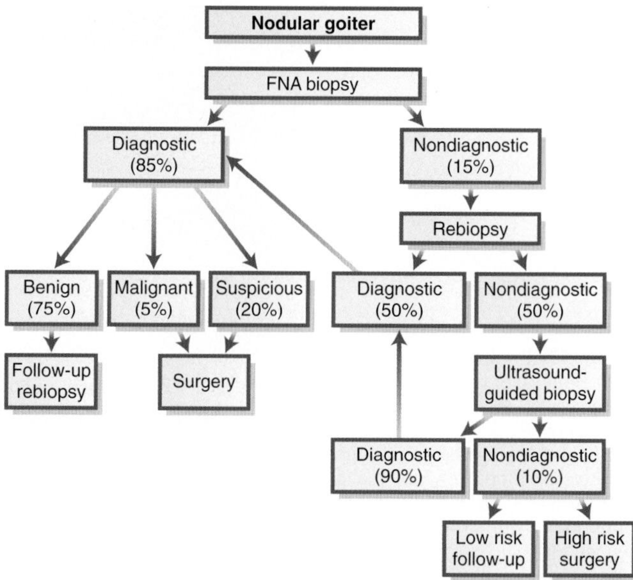

Figure 13–4 ▪ Management of nodular goiter based on fine needle aspiration (FNA) biopsy as the first diagnostic test. Subsequent management is based on cytologic results. Percentages in parentheses indicate satisfactory or unsatisfactory biopsy results. (From Gharib H. Fine-needle aspiration biopsy of thyroid nodules: advantages, limitations, and effect. Mayo Clin Proc 1994;69:44-49.)

ciated with a considerable drop in specificity to less than 50% (i.e., a large number of false-positive results).[46] This seriously limits the usefulness of FNAB in iodine-deficient regions, where the incidence of follicular thyroid carcinoma (FTC) approaches that of PTC and where both follicular adenomas and hyperplastic adenomatous nodules are prevalent.[49]

Attempts have been made to improve the accuracy of cytology and to decrease the percentage of indeterminate cases. TPO immunochemistry with a monoclonal antibody (MoAb 47) shows promise in improving the accuracy of FNAB for follicular lesions.[50] For 100% sensitivity, a specificity of almost 70% has been achieved with this technique. Galectin 3 has also been used, either alone or combined with TPO. They may be a valuable adjunct to the standard cytologic techniques in case of typical follicular lesions, either benign or malignant. However, these techniques did not reliably improve the accuracy of cytology in case of suspicious findings.[51] Other markers have recently been advocated such as telomerase, or a combination of markers identified with the microarray technology, but this needs independent confirmation of their usefulness.

The use of large-needle biopsy in addition to standard FNAB has improved diagnostic accuracy in difficult FNA cases, but the technique is more exacting than FNAB alone and is associated with increased morbidity.[52] Particularly for cystic thyroid nodules, sampling from the margin of the nodule, rather than from the cystic fluid and debris in the center, increases accuracy. Ultrasonographically guided FNA can be used for this purpose. Although such guided biopsies are sometimes helpful, routine use of ultrasound-guided biopsy for clinically palpable solid nodules is not any better than "freehand" aspiration.

In some centers, both preoperative FNAB and intraoperative frozen section are combined. In the hands of experienced surgeon-pathologist teams, this approach results in less than 5% misdiagnoses, as evidenced by subsequent review of paraffin-embedded specimens. The approach avoids unnecessarily extensive surgery in patients with benign tumors, achieves resection of nearly all malignant tumors, and rarely necessitates a second operation for completion thyroidectomy.[53] Such an approach is employed at the Mayo Clinic and at the Institut Gustave Roussy, where intraoperative frozen section is routine.

Apart from its limited utility in the evaluation of follicular neoplasms, the only other limitation of FNAB is nondiagnostic specimens, which may be obtained in up to 20% of cases.[46,47] Although repeated aspiration increases both the accuracy and the rate of diagnostic aspirations, even repeated attempts may sometimes fail. The rate of cancer in surgically resected nodules with nondiagnostic FNA is 10% to 20%. Hence, either close observation or surgical removal of the nodule is probably the best option. Some authorities recommend a trial of TSH suppression, which can sometimes shrink benign nodules. However, a significant proportion of benign nodules do not shrink, and some carcinomas do shrink; consequently, the diagnostic value of TSH suppression is doubtful. Whether ultrasound-guided FNAB can help overcome this problem in some patients is likely, but confirmation is required. Figure 13–4 is an algorithm for the management of nodular thyroid disease in which FNAB is the first diagnostic test and subsequent management is based on cytologic results.

The most expeditious way to diagnose thyroid malignancy is to obtain a thorough history and physical examination, followed by ultrasonography, FNAB, and evaluation of the sample by an experienced cytologist. In some cases, FNAB should be performed under ultrasound guidance. Imaging procedures, in addition to ultrasonography, and other tests may occasionally be helpful, but diagnostic thyroid scintiscanning, as traditionally practiced, is of little or no value and should be abandoned.[23]

In iodine-sufficient areas with a high relative prevalence of PTC, the combination of history and physical examination and FNAB is usually sufficient to confirm malignancy. Conversely, if history and physical examination, ultrasonography, and FNAB do not suggest malignancy, the chances of missing PTC are probably less than 1%.[46,47] In areas where the prevalence of follicular tumors is higher, more patients may require neck exploration because FNAB may not be conclusive[49]; in experienced hands, however, intraoperative frozen sections can limit the number of unnecessarily extensive bilateral procedures.

Surgery should also be considered for large tumors (>4 cm), especially in young subjects, in order to avoid repeated evaluations; in addition, because these tumors may be composed of various cell populations, results of FNAB may be less reliable.

Finally, micronodules less than 1 cm in diameter, found incidentally during imaging, do not need to be tested any further, unless there are sonographic features suggestive of PTC or MTC. The usual advice is to repeat ultrasonography of such lesions after an interval of 6 to 12 months.[22]

Management of Benign Nontoxic Diffuse and Nodular Goiter

Patients with small, asymptomatic goiters can be monitored by clinical examination and evaluated periodically with ultrasound measurements. In fact, goiter growth can be variable, and some patients have stable goiters for many years. For more than a century, thyroid "feeding" has been employed to reduce the size of nontoxic goiters. The 1953 report of Greer and Astwood, in which two thirds of patients' goiters regressed with thyroid therapy, led to widespread acceptance of suppressive therapy,[54] despite some doubts about the value of such therapy.[55] An overview of studies performed from 1960 to 1992 suggested that 60% or more of sporadic nontoxic goiters respond to suppressive therapy.[55] In a prospective placebo-controlled, double-blind, randomized clinical trial, 58% of the thyroxine-treated group had a significant response at 9 months, as measured by ultrasonography, in contrast with 5% after placebo.[56]

Nodular goiters appear to be less responsive than diffuse goiters. A recent meta-analysis failed to demonstrate a significant benefit of thyroxine therapy, which was found to carry a relative risk of nodule shrinkage of only 1.9 (95% confidence interval [CI], 0.95-3.81).[57] Statistical significance emerged from a multicenter, randomized, double-blind, placebo-controlled trial: after 18 months of follow-up the nodule shrinkage was significantly greater in the L-T_4 group than in the placebo group (P = .01), as well as the proportion of responders (P = .04).[58] It is likely that a subset of patients respond to thyroxine suppressive therapy, particularly younger patients with small or recently diagnosed nodules.[57] However, thyroid nodules rapidly return to the pretreatment size after discontinuation of therapy.[23] Therefore, maintainance of the size reduction may require continuous treatment.

A major concern in relation to long-term thyroxine suppression therapy is the possibility of detrimental effects on the skeleton and heart. It has been reported that TSH suppression therapy is associated with variable degrees of bone loss, particularly in postmenopausal women.[59,60] However, other studies did not demonstrate significant change in bone mass after long-term thyroxine therapy.[61] Furthermore, there is no evidence that levothyroxine per se is detrimental to the heart in young subjects when TSH is decreased to subnormal but still detectable values.[59]

Surgery for nontoxic goiter is physiologically unsound because it further restricts the ability of the thyroid to meet hormone requirements. Nevertheless, surgery may become necessary because of persistence of obstructive manifestations despite a trial of levothyroxine. Surgery should consist of a near-total or total thyroidectomy, but recurrence is seen in about 10% to 20% within 10 years.[61] Surgical complications have been reported in 7% to 10% of cases and are more common with large goiters and with reoperation.[62] Prophylactic treatment with levothyroxine after goiter resection probably does not prevent goiter recurrence.[63]

Traditionally, the role of ^{131}I therapy for nontoxic goiter was to reduce the size of a massive goiter in elderly patients who were poor candidates for surgery or to treat goiter that recurs after resection. However, several studies have demonstrated that primary treatment of nontoxic goiter with ^{131}I is followed by a reduction in thyroid volume.[64,65] In one study, thyroid volume (assessed by ultrasonography) was reduced by 40% after 1 year and 55% after 2 years with no further reduction thereafter, and 60% of the total reduction occurred within the first 3 months.[64]

A randomized trial comparing levothyroxine at suppressive doses with radioactive iodine treatment (120 μCi/g corrected for 24-hour thyroid uptake) showed impressive differences in outcome. After ^{131}I therapy, 97% of patients responded, with a mean decrease in goiter size of 39% at 1 year and 46% at 2 years; the initial side effects were neck tenderness and slight thyrotoxic symptoms in 12% of patients, and at 2 years 35% of patients were hypothyroid and 10% had subclinical thyrotoxicosis. In contrast, with levothyroxine therapy, 43% of patients responded with a mean decrease of 23% at 1 year and 22% at 2 years; the initial side effect was a mild thyrotoxicosis in 30% of patients and at 2 years a significant decrease in spine bone density.[65]

Considering its effectiveness in reducing the size of the thyroid gland, ^{131}I therapy has also been used for the treatment of nonautonomous thyroid nodules: a significant shrinkage has been observed, ranging from 31% to 60% (Fig. 13–5).[66,67]

It was formerly argued that treatment of large goiters or goiters with substernal extension with ^{131}I should be avoided because of the risks of acute swelling of the gland and consequent tracheal compression.[67] Ultrasonographic studies of thyroid volume after ^{131}I have failed to demonstrate significant early volume increase. Moreover, decreased tracheal deviation and increased tracheal lumen size were demonstrable by MRI in patients who had compression by nontoxic goiters with substernal extension.[64]

Therefore, it appears that ^{131}I treatment of nontoxic diffuse or multinodular goiter is effective and safe: hypothyroidism has been reported in 20% to 40%; transient thyrotoxicosis and mild pain can occur.[64] Regular follow-up, preferably by a systematic annual recall scheme, is necessary. The activities used are in the range of those used for ^{131}I treatment of hyperthyroidism, and thus radiation doses are comparable, and long-term thyroid and nonthyroidal cancer risk after ^{131}I treatment for hyperthyroidism are reassuring.[68] Stimulation with low doses of recombinant human TSH (rhTSH) (0.01 to 0.03 mg) increases the thyroid ^{131}I uptake and therefore may allow the administration of a lower dosage of ^{131}I, but it also increases thyroid hormone production, so overproduction of thyroid hormones should be excluded before its use.[69] Long-term randomized studies comparing the effects, side effects, and costs and benefits of surgery and ^{131}I treatment need to be performed.

Percutaneous ethanol injection should be used only for recurrent symptomatic cystic nodules.[45] Laser therapy is still an experimental procedure and can be proposed, in experienced centers, for selected patients with symptomatic nodular goiters when surgery is not possible.[70]

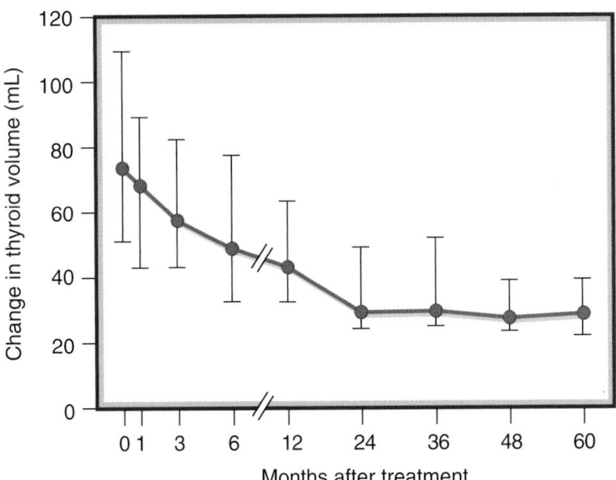

Figure 13–5 ■ Median changes in thyroid volume alterations after iodine 131 treatment in 39 patients with nontoxic multinodular goiter who remained euthyroid after a single dose. *Bars* represent quartiles. (From Nygaard B, Hegedus L, Gervil M, et al. Radioiodine treatment of multinodular nontoxic goiter. BMJ 1993;307:828-832.)

MANAGEMENT OF MALIGNANT NODULAR GOITER

Thyroid tumors are the most common endocrine neoplasms. The management of a patient with typical thyroid cancer is effective and usually consists of surgical resection, followed by medical therapy and regular surveillance.[37,71-73] Some degree of consensus has been achieved with regard to the initial management of differentiated thyroid cancer, but important clinical and biologic questions remain unanswered.[37,73] In the following discussion, we present a widely used scheme for classifying and staging tumors of the thyroid gland. We also review the features of the principal types of benign and malignant thyroid neoplasms and the controversies in the management of differentiated thyroid carcinoma.

Classification of Thyroid Tumors

Histologic Classification

Two monographs have had a major impact on the histologic classification of thyroid tumors. One is from the World Health Organization (WHO)[74]; the other is from the Armed Forces Institute of Pathology (AFIP).[75] The classification described in Table 13–5 is modified from the guidelines described by these organizations.

Lesions of follicular cell origin constitute more than 95% of the cases, and the remainder are largely made up of tumors exhibiting C-cell differentiation. Mixed medullary and follicular carcinomas, made up of cells with both C-cell and follicular differentiation, are rare and of uncertain histogenesis. Nonepithelial thyroid tumors mainly include malignant lymphomas, which may involve the thyroid gland as the only manifestation of the disease or as part of a systemic disease. True sarcomas and malignant hemangioendotheliomas are exceptional. Blood-borne metastases to the thyroid are not uncommon at autopsy in patients with widespread malignancy but rarely cause clinically detectable thyroid enlargement.

TABLE 13–5 CLASSIFICATION OF THYROID NEOPLASMS

PRIMARY EPITHELIAL TUMORS
Tumors of follicular cells
Benign: follicular adenoma
Malignant: carcinoma
Differentiated
Papillary
Follicular
Poorly differentiated
Insular
Others
Undifferentiated (anaplastic)
Tumors of C cells
Medullary carcinoma
Tumors of follicular and C cells
Mixed medullary-follicular carcinoma
PRIMARY NONEPITHELIAL TUMORS
Malignant lymphomas
Sarcomas
Others
SECONDARY TUMORS

Staging of Thyroid Carcinoma

In addition to the histologic classification of thyroid tumors developed by the WHO and AFIP groups, the International Union Against Cancer (UICC) and the American Joint Committee on Cancer (AJCC) have agreed on a staging system in thyroid cancer.[76,77] As stated by the AJCC, "the principal purpose served by international agreement on the classification of cancer cases by extent of disease was to provide a method of conveying clinical experience to others without ambiguity."

The AJCC based its system of classification on the TNM system, which relies on assessing three components: (1) extent of the primary tumor (T), (2) absence or presence of regional lymph node metastases (N), and (3) absence or presence of distant metastases (M).

The TNM system allows a reasonably precise description and recording of the anatomic extent of disease. The classification may be either *clinical* (cTNM), based on evidence (including biopsy) acquired before treatment, or *pathologic* (pTNM), by which intraoperative and surgical pathology data are available. Obviously, pTNM classification is preferable because a precise size can be assigned to the primary tumor, the histotype is identified, and extrathyroid invasion is demonstrated unequivocally.

Typically, in the 1992 classification,[76] the primary thyroid tumor (T) status is defined according to the size of the primary lesion: T1, greatest diameter 1 cm or smaller; T2, larger than 1 cm but not larger than 4 cm; T3, larger than 4 cm; T4, direct (extrathyroidal) extension or invasion through the thyroid capsule. A thyroid tumor with four degrees of T, two degrees of N, and two degrees of M can have 16 different TNM categories.

For purposes of tabulation and analysis, these categories have been condensed into a convenient number of TNM stage-groupings (Table 13–6). Whereas head and neck cancer is usually staged entirely on the basis of anatomic extent, in thyroid cancer staging both the histologic diagnosis and the age of the patient for PTC and FTC are included because of their importance in predicting the behavior and prognosis of thyroid cancer.

According to this staging scheme, all patients younger than age 45 years with PTC or FTC are in stage I, unless they have distant metastases (DM), in which case they would be in stage II. In young patients and especially in children, the risk of recurrence is high and may be underestimated by the TNM staging system.[78] Older patients (45 years of age and older) with node-negative papillary or follicular microcarcinoma (T1, N0, M0) are in stage I. Tumors between 1.1 and 4.0 cm are classified as stage II, and those with either nodal spread (N1) or extrathyroidal invasion (T4), stage III.

For MTC, the scheme is similar, in that microcarcinoma is stage I and a node-positive tumor is stage III. There is no age distinction for MTC, although age is a significant independent prognostic indicator in most multivariate analyses,[79-81] and local (extrathyroidal) invasion is grouped within stage II. For patients with MTC and older patients with PTC or FTC, stage IV denotes the presence of DM. Independent of age or tumor extent, all patients with undifferentiated (anaplastic) cancer are considered to be in stage IV.

The 2002 TNM classification is more complicated, and the definition of minimal or more extensive thyroid tumor extension may be difficult to define retrospectively.[77] Six lymph nodes need to be examined at histology to qualify for the definition of N0, and the prognostic difference between central lymph node metastases and other regional metastases has yet to be validated; in fact, the risk of persistent/recurrent disease appeared to be related with the involvement of the central neck compartment and the numbers of involved lymph nodes and of lymph

TABLE 13–6 THE TUMOR-NODE-METASTASES (TNM) SCORING SYSTEM: 1992 and 2002 Versions

DEFINITION OF TNM

	1992		2002
PRIMARY TUMOR (T)			
T0	No evidence of primary tumor		No evidence of primary tumor
T1	Tumor ≤1 cm limited to the thyroid		Tumor ≤2 cm limited to the thyroid
T2	Tumor >1 to ≤4 cm limited to the thyroid		Tumor >2 to ≤4 cm limited to the thyroid
T3	Tumor >4 cm limited to the thyroid		Tumor >4 cm limited to the thyroid or any tumor with minimal extrathyroid extension (e.g., extension to sternothyroid muscle or perithyroid soft tissues)
T4	Any size extending beyond the thyroid capsule	T4a	Tumor of any size with extension beyond the thyroid capsule and invades any of the following: subcutaneous soft tissues, larynx, trachea, esophagus, recurrent laryngeal nerve
		T4b	Tumor invades prevertebral fascia, mediastinal vessels, or encases carotid artery
REGIONAL LYMPH NODE (N)			
N0	No regional lymph node metastasis		No regional lymph node metastasis*
N1	Regional lymph node metastasis		Regional lymph node metastasis
		N1a	Metastases in pretracheal and paratracheal, including prelaryngeal and Delphian lymph nodes
		N1b	Metastases in other unilateral, bilateral, or contralateral cervical or upper mediastinal lymph nodes
DISTANT METASTASES (M)			
M0	No distant metastasis		No distant metastasis
M1	Distant metastasis		Distant metastasis

TNM STAGING

	1992	2002
Age <45 years		
Stage I	Any T, any N, M0	Any T, any N, M0
Stage II	Any T, any N, M1	Any T, any N, M1
Stage III	None None	
Stage IV	None None	
Age ≥45 years		
Stage I	T1, N0, M0T1, N0, M0	
Stage II	T2-T3, N0, M0	T2, N0, M0
Stage III	T4, N0, M0 or any T, N1, M0	T3, N0, M0 or any T1-3, N1a, M0
Stage IV	Any T, any N, M1	Stage IVA T1-3, N1b, M0 or T4a, any N, M0
		Stage IVB T4b, any N, M0
		Stage IVC Any T, any N, M1

*To classify as N0, at least six lymph nodes should be examined at histology. Otherwise, the disease is classified as Nx.
From Beahrs OH, Henson DE, Hutter RVP et al. Manual for staging of cancer. Philadelphia JB Lippincott, 1992. American Joint Committee on Cancer. Thyroid. In AJCC Cancer Staging Handbook, 6th ed. New York: Springer, 2002:89-98.

nodes with capsular extension.[82] Currently, it is not possible to ascertain whether the modifications included in the 2002 TNM classification will significantly improve its prognostic value and will have a clinical impact on therapeutic strategies. One risk is that some centers advocating lobectomy for tumors less than 1 cm (T1 of the previous classification) may extend this indication to the recently redefined T1 (i.e., tumors up to 2 cm). This attitude, based on cause-specific mortality, may lead to undertreatment of some patients, exposing them to a higher risk of recurrence.

Follicular Adenoma

Follicular adenoma is a benign, encapsulated tumor with evidence of follicular cell differentiation.[74,75] It is the most common thyroid neoplasm and may be found in 4% to 20% of glands examined at autopsy.[83] The tumor has a well-defined fibrous capsule that is grossly and microscopically complete. There is a sharp demarcation and distinct structural difference from the surrounding parenchyma. These adenomas vary in size, but most have a diameter of 1 to 3 cm at the time of excision. Degenerative changes, including necrosis, hemorrhage, edema, fibrosis, or calcification, are common features, particularly in larger tumors.

Follicular adenomas can be classified into subtypes according to the size or presence of follicles and degree of cellularity. Each adenoma tends to have a consistent architectural pattern. *Microfollicular, normofollicular,* and *macrofollicular* adenomas owe their names to the size of their follicles compared with follicles in the neighboring, nonneoplastic areas of the gland. *Trabecular adenomas* are cellular and consist of columns of cells arranged in compact cords. They show little follicle formation and rarely contain colloid. A variant, the *hyalinizing trabecular adenoma,* has unusually elongated cells and prominent hyaline changes in the extracellular space.[84]

The histologic differences between these subtypes are striking but of no clinical importance. The only practical value of the classification is that the more cellular a follicular nodule is, the more one should search for evidence of malignancy in the form of invasion of blood vessels and capsule, either singly or in combination.[74,75] Atypical adenomas are hypercellular or heterogeneous, or both, with gross and histologic appearances that suggest the possibility of malignancy but not invasion. They account for fewer than 3% of all follicular adenomas. Follow-up indicates that this lesion behaves in a benign fashion. The fact that the tumor does not recur or produce metastases after removal does not prove that it is actually benign; removal may have interrupted a natural history that would have culminated in invasion and metastases. This is the reason why they are classified as tumors of "undefined malignancy."

The most important cytologic variant is the *oxyphilic* or *oncocytic (Hürthle cell) adenoma,* which is composed predominantly (at least 75%) or entirely of large cells with granular, eosinophilic cytoplasm.[85] Ultrastructurally, the cells are rich in mitochondria and may exhibit nuclear pleomorphism with distinct nucleoli. Although all such neoplasms are thought by some to be potentially malignant,[86] the biologic behavior and clinical course of oncocytic tumors correlate closely with the histology and the size of the initial lesion. The absence of invasion predicts a benign outcome,[85] but larger tumors may rarely be associated with later recurrence or metastases, even in the absence of obvious microscopic evidence of invasion; fortunately, such an occurrence is rare, and generally a diagnosis of benign Hürthle cell adenoma can be reliable.[87,88]

Some normofollicular adenomas may contain pseudopapillary structures that can be confused with the papillae of papillary carcinoma. These structures are probably an expression of localized hyperactivity and are most common in adenomas that show autonomous function.

In the majority of hyperfunctioning follicular adenomas, activating point mutations have been identified in the TSHR or in the α subunit of the stimulatory guanyl nucleotide protein ($G\alpha_s$) (Fig. 13–6).[29,89] Such mutations may trap the G protein in a state

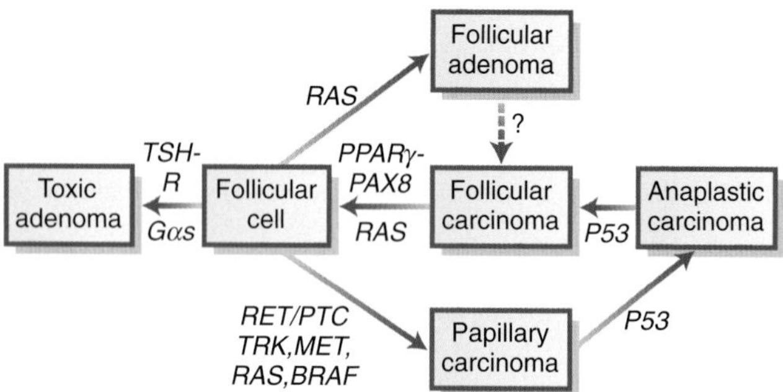

Figure 13–6 ▪ Genetic events in thyroid tumorigenesis. Activating point mutations of the *RAS* genes are found with a high frequency in both follicular adenomas and follicular carcinomas, and are considered an early event in follicular tumorigenesis. The PPARγ-PAX8 rearrangement is found only in follicular tumors. Rearrangements of transmembrane receptors with tyrosine kinase activity (*RET, TRK* genes) and activating point mutations of the *BRAF* gene are found only in papillary thyroid carcinomas. Inactivating point mutations of the *P53* gene are found only in poorly differentiated and anaplastic thyroid carcinomas. Activation of the cyclic adenosine monophosphate pathway, by point mutation of the thyrotropin receptor (TSH-R) or the a subunit of the G protein genes, leads to the appearance of hyperfunctioning thyroid nodules. $G\alpha_s$, Stimulatory guanyl nucleotide protein.

of constitutive activation, resulting in enhanced cyclic adenosine monophosphate (cAMP) production and constitutive hyperstimulation of the cells. Genetic abnormalities found in hypofunctioning adenomas are detailed later.

Papillary Thyroid Carcinoma

PTC has been defined as "a malignant epithelial tumor showing evidence of follicular cell differentiation, and characterized by the formation of papillae and/or a set of distinctive nuclear changes."[74,75] The most common thyroid malignancy, PTC, constitutes 50% to 90% of differentiated FCTCs worldwide.[90]

Papillary thyroid microcarcinoma (PTM) is defined by the WHO as a PTC 1.0 cm in diameter or smaller.[74,75,90-93] The incidence rates for clinically diagnosed PTC in the United States are approximately 5 per 100,000 for tumors larger than 1 cm in diameter and 1 per 100,000 for PTM. By contrast, the incidence of PTM in autopsy material from various continents ranges from 4% to 36%.[74,75] This is the basis for the apparent increasing incidence of PTM in recent years, that is at least in part related to more extensive screening.

PTCs appear as firm, unencapsulated or partially encapsulated tumors. PTCs may be partly necrotic and some are cystic. Typically, PTC shows a predominance of papillary structures, consisting of a fibrovascular core lined by a single layer of epithelial cells, but the papillae are usually admixed with neoplastic follicles having characteristic nuclear features.

The nuclei of PTC cells have a distinctive appearance that has a diagnostic significance comparable to that of the papillae. Indeed, the preoperative diagnosis of PTC can often be made on the basis of the characteristic nuclear changes seen in FNA material: Nuclei are larger than in normal follicular cells and overlap, they may be fissured like coffee beans, chromatin is hypodense (ground glass nuclei), limits are irregular, and they frequently contain an inclusion corresponding to a cytoplasmic invagination.

Psammoma bodies are often present in the core of papillae or in the tumor stroma; they are microscopic structures of calcified layers.

Several subtypes exist and account for about 20% of all PTCs: The tumor is designated a *follicular variant* of PTC when the lining cells of the neoplastic follicles have the same nuclear features as seen in typical PTC and the follicular predominance over the papillae is complete.[74,75] The *diffuse sclerosing variant* is characterized by diffuse involvement of one or both thyroid lobes, widespread lymphatic permeation, prominent fibrosis, and lymphoid infiltration. The *tall cell variant* is characterized by well-formed papillae that are covered by cells twice as tall as they are wide. The *columnar cell variant* differs from other forms of PTC because of the presence of prominent nuclear stratification of elongated cells. The tall cell and columnar cell variants are more aggressive, but controversy exists regarding outcome for the diffuse sclerosing variant.[90]

In children, tumor extension is usually substantial at diagnosis: tumors are large, unencapsulated, and invasive with solid trabecular features. Extension beyond the thyroid capsule, lymph node metastases, and lung metastases are frequently observed.[78]

Molecular Pathogenesis

The thyroid follicular cell may give rise to both benign and malignant tumors, and the malignancy can be of either papillary or follicular histotype. There is no evidence that human benign tumors ever undergo malignant transformation into classical PTC. Structural abnormalities of the chromosomes may occur in about 50% of PTCs, frequently involving the long arm of chromosome 10.[89,94-98] The *RET* proto-oncogene is located on chromosome 10q11-2. It encodes a transmembrane receptor with a tyrosine kinase domain. Its ligands, such as the glial cell line–derived neutrophilic factor (GDNF) binds to the GDNF receptor (the GFRα-1) and induces RET protein dimerization. *RET* activation was first demonstrated in transfection experiments and has been found only in PTC tumors. It was therefore called *RET/PTC*.

All activated forms of the *RET* proto-oncogene are the consequence of oncogenic rearrangements fusing the tyrosine kinase domain of the *RET* gene with the 5′ domain of different genes. The foreign gene is constitutively expressed, and its 5′ domain acts as a promoter, resulting in permanent expression of the *RET* gene. Furthermore, these genes have domains that induce *RET* activation by permanent dimerization. Because of this fusion, the chimeric protein is localized in the cytoplasm and not in the plasma cell membrane.

Three major classes of *RET/PTC* have been identified: *RET/PTC*$_1$ is formed by an intrachromosomal rearrangement fusing the *RET* tyrosine kinase domain to a gene designated *H4*, whose function is still unknown. *RET/PTC*$_2$ is formed by an interchromosomal rearrangement fusing the *RET* tyrosine kinase domain to a gene located on chromosome 17 encoding the RIα regulatory subunit of protein kinase A. *RET/PTC*$_3$ is formed by an intrachromosomal rearrangement fusing the *RET* tyrosine kinase domain to a gene designated *ELE1*, whose function is still unknown. Several variants of *RET/PTC* have been observed in post-Chernobyl thyroid tumors, including rearrangements formed by fusing the tyrosine kinase domain of the RET gene at other breakpoint sites or with other partners.

The frequency of *RET/PTC* rearrangements occurring in adult PTC patients without prior childhood neck irradiation varies between 2.5% and 35%. In these tumors, the frequencies of *RET/PTC*$_1$ and *RET/PTC*$_3$ were similar and that of *RET/PTC*$_2$ was lower. The *RET/PTC* rearrangements were more frequently found (in 60% to 80% of cases) in PTC cases occurring either in children even in the absence of radiation exposure or in subjects of any age after radiation exposure during childhood, either external irradiation or contamination after the Chernobyl accident.[89,98] *RET/PTC*$_3$ was more frequently found in aggressive tumors that occurred early after the accident and *RET/PTC*$_1$ in less aggressive tumors that occurred later. The finding of *RET/PTC* rearrangement in micropapillary thyroid carcinomas suggests that it constitutes an early event in thyroid carcinogenesis. On the other hand, *RET/PTC*-positive tumors lack evidence of progression to poorly or undifferentiated tumor phenotypes.

Several additional oncogenes may occasionally be involved in PTC, including *NTRK1* (also named *TRKA*), which codes for a neural growth factor receptor with a tyrosine kinase domain and which is activated by rearrangement in about 10% of PTCs. The receptor for hepatocyte growth factor is a transmembrane tyrosine kinase encoded by the *MET* oncogene; it is overexpressed in some patients with PTC, and low expression has been associated with the occurrence of DM.

An activating point mutation of the *RAS* genes is found in about 10% of PTCs, mostly in the follicular variant.[99] More recently, a single activating point mutation of the *BRAF* gene at codon 600 has been found in 40% (range, 29% to 69%) of PTCs occurring in adults in the absence of neck exposure to radiation during childhood.[100] Its presence did not overlap with *RET/PTC* and it was rarely found in PTC occurring in children or following neck exposure to radiation.[96] *BRAF* mutation is more frequently found in aggressive PTC and in the tall cell variant, but it has not been found in other thyroid tumor types. Finally, an intrachromosomal rearrangement of the *BRAF* gene with the *AKAP9* gene has recently been found in PTC occurring after the Chernobyl accident.[101]

In conclusion, the RET/PTC, RAS, BRAF, MAP kinase pathway is activated in approximately 80% of sporadic or radiation-induced PTCs, and mutations affecting this pathway are considered as initiating events of PTC and mediate mitogenic phenotype.[96,102]

A high incidence of PTC has been reported in patients with adenomatous polyposis coli that has a peculiar histologic appearance, with solid areas and elongated cells, and Cowden's disease (the multiple hamartoma syndrome), suggesting that the predisposing genes may play a role in the occurrence of papillary carcinoma. About 3% of cases of PTC are familial; their behavior is similar to or slightly more aggressive than that of nonfamilial cases.[103,104] The gene predisposing to familial thyroid tumors with cellular oxyphilia has been mapped to chromosome 19q13.2, and in a family with PTC and renal carcinoma, a separate gene was mapped to chromosome 1q21.

The expression of thyroid-specific genes has been studied at the messenger ribonucleic acid (mRNA) and protein levels in large series of human thyroid tumors. Expression of *NIS* was profoundly decreased in both benign and malignant thyroid hypofunctioning nodules; moreover, in malignant nodules, low expression of TPO, PDS, and Tg was also found.[105,106] These abnormalities clearly explain many of the metabolic defects typically observed in thyroid cancer tissues: a low iodine concentration, a low rate of iodine organification, low hormonal synthesis, and a short intrathyroidal half-life of iodine. NIS expression is heterogeneous among tumor cells.[105] However, Tg is expressed in variable amounts in almost all FCTCs and can be shown by immunohistochemistry, which can prove useful in cases with atypical histology. Also, TSH receptor is expressed in many FCTCs, and TSH may stimulate both their differentiation and growth.

Multiple other abnormalities have been found in follicular cell–derived tumors, including overexpression of VEGF and of VEGF receptors, which is in line with the hypervascularization observed in these tumors.[107]

Presenting Features

Although PTCs can occur at any age, most occur in patients between 30 and 50 years of age (mean age, 45 years). Women are affected more frequently (female predominance, 60% to 80%). Most primary tumors are 1 to 4 cm in size; they average about 2 to 3 cm in greatest diameter.[90,91] The increased incidence observed in recent years is mostly related to small PTC.[108] PTC is frequently multifocal when it occurs in a single lobe, and is bilateral in 20% to 80% of cases, depending on whether or not the thyroid was meticulously examined. Recent studies have suggested that contralateral PTC may have independent clonal origins.[109] Extrathyroidal invasion of adjacent soft tissues is present in about 15% (range, 5% to 34%) at primary surgery, and about one third of PTC patients have clinically evident lymphadenopathy at presentation.[90,91] About 35% to 50% of excised neck nodes have histologic evidence of involvement, and in patients 17 years of age or younger, nodal involvement may be present in up to 90%.[78,110] Only 1% to 7% of PTC patients have DM at diagnosis.[90,91] Spread to superior mediastinal nodes is usually associated with extensive neck nodal involvement.

The TNM classification is a widely used system for tumor staging.[111] Most PTC patients present with either stage I (60%) or stage II (22%). Patients 45 years of age or older with either nodal metastases or extrathyroidal extension (stage III) account for fewer than 20% of cases.[90,91] As already noted, few (1% to 7%) PTC patients present with DM and have stage IV disease. Figure 13–7 (upper left) illustrates the distribution of TNM stages in 2284 PTC cases seen at the Mayo Clinic, and Figure 13–8 demonstrates survival by TNM stage in this cohort of PTC patients treated from 1940 to 1997. In these and subsequent figures

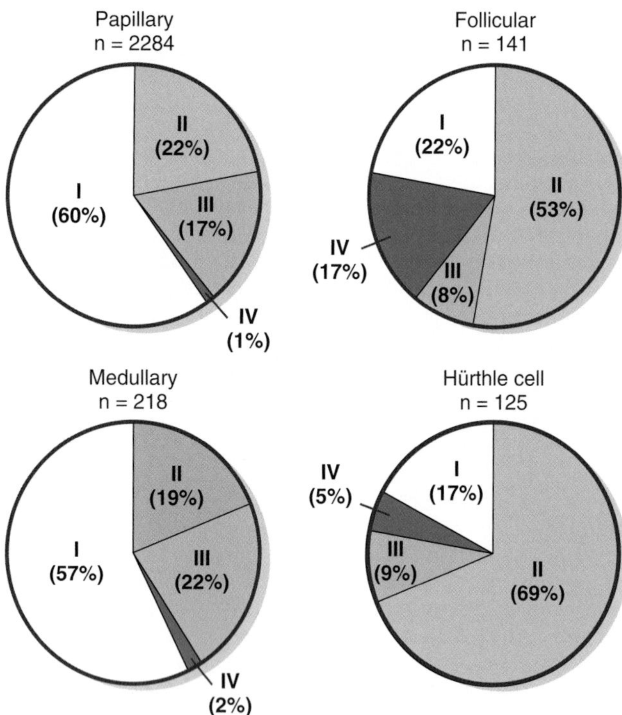

Figure 13–7 ▪ Distribution of pathologic tumor-node-metastases (pTNM) stages in 2284 patients with papillary thyroid carcinoma *(upper left)*, 218 patients with medullary thyroid cancer *(lower left)*, 141 patients with follicular thyroid cancer *(upper right)*, and 125 patients with Hürthle cell cancer *(lower right)* undergoing primary surgical treatment at the Mayo Clinic from 1940 to 1997.

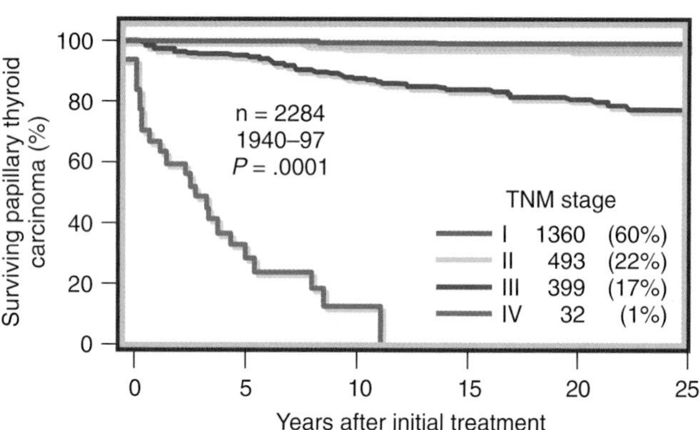

Figure 13–8 ▪ Cause-specific survival according to pathologic tumor-node-metastases (pTNM) stage in a cohort of 2284 patients with papillary thyroid carcinoma treated at the Mayo Clinic from 1940 to 1997. The numbers in parentheses represent the percentages of patients in each pTNM 1992 stage grouping.

shown in this chapter, and in illustrating outcome results from the Mayo Clinic from the 1940 to 1997 cohort of DTC patients, the pTNM stages are derived from the older (pre-2002) definition, in part because of the challenges in defining from available records the N1a versus N1b status and the exact location of the extrathyroidal extension necessary to ascribe T4a or T4b status to the tumor extent at surgery.

Recurrence and Mortality

Three types of tumor recurrence may occur with PTC: (1) postoperative *nodal metastases* (NM), (2) *local recurrence* (LR), and (3) postoperative *distant metastases* (DM).

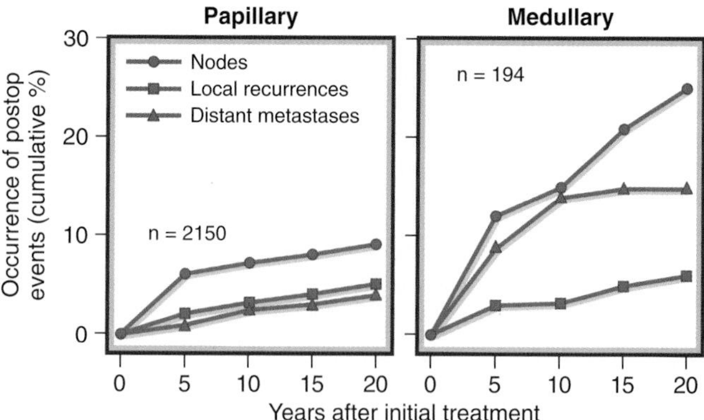

Figure 13–9 ▪ Development of neck nodal metastases, local recurrences, and distant metastases in the first 20 years after definitive surgery for papillary thyroid cancer (PTC) or medullary thyroid cancer (MTC) performed at the Mayo Clinic from 1940 to 1997. Figures are based on 2150 consecutive PTC *(left)* and 194 MTC *(right)* patients who had complete surgical resection (i.e., had no gross residual disease) and were without distant metastases on initial examination. *Postop,* Postoperative.

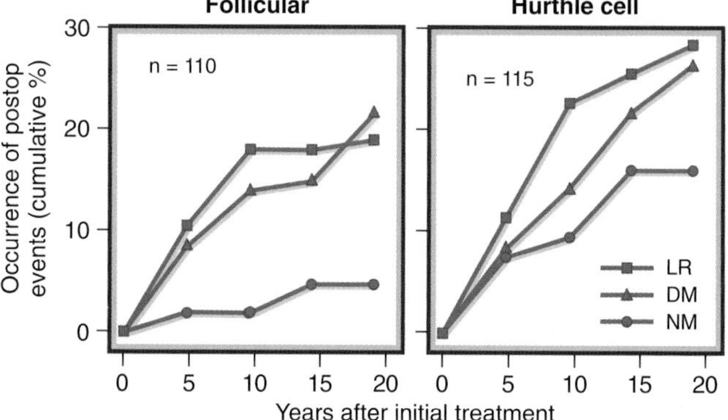

Figure 13–10 ▪ Development of neck nodal metastases (NM), local recurrences (LR), and distant metastases (DM) in the first 20 years after definitive surgery for follicular thyroid cancer (FTC) or Hürthle cell cancer (HCC) performed at the Mayo Clinic from 1940 to 1997. Figures are based on 110 consecutive FTC patients *(left)* and 115 HCC patients *(right)* who had complete surgical resection and were without distant metastases on initial examination. *Postop,* Postoperative.

LR may be defined as "histologically confirmed tumor occurring in the resected thyroid bed, thyroid remnant, or other adjacent tissues of the neck (excluding lymph nodes)" after complete surgical removal of the primary tumor.[112] Nodal or distant spread may be considered postoperative if the metastases are discovered within 180 or 30 days, respectively.[90] Ideally, tumor recurrence should be considered only as it occurs in patients without initial DM who had complete surgical resection of the primary tumors.

Figure 13–9 illustrates rates of PTC recurrence at local, nodal, and distant sites in 2150 patients with PTC treated at one institution from 1940 to 1997. After 20 years of follow-up, postoperative NM had been discovered in 9%, and LR and DM occurred in 5% and 4%, respectively. Both LR and DM are less common in PTC than in FTC (Fig. 13–10). However, postoperative cases of NM were more frequent in PTC than in FTC.

Cause-specific mortality (CSM) rates for differentiated thyroid cancer are shown in Figure 13–11. CSM rates for PTC were 2% at 5 years, 4% at 10 years, and 5% at 20 years. Among those with lethal PTC, 20% of deaths occurred in the first year after diagnosis, and 80% of the deaths occurred within 10 years. The 25-

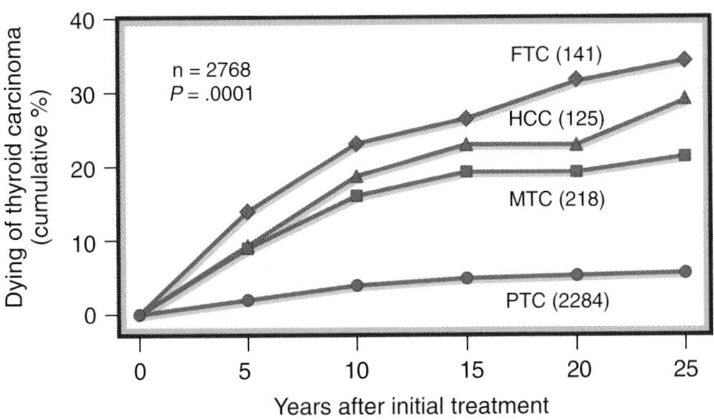

Figure 13–11 ▪ Cumulative cause-specific mortality rates for patients with differentiated thyroid carcinoma in the first 25 years after treatment with initial surgery performed at the Mayo Clinic from 1940 to 1997. Figures are based on 2768 consecutively treated patients (2284 with papillary thyroid carcinoma [PTC], 141 with follicular thyroid cancer [FTC], 125 with Hürthle cell cancer [HCC], and 218 with medullary thyroid cancer [MTC]).

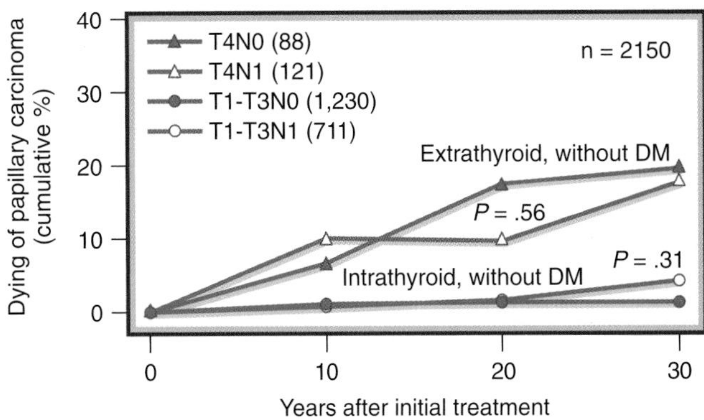

Figure 13–13 ▪ Lack of influence of nodal metastases at initial operation on cumulative mortality from papillary thyroid carcinoma in 1941 patients with pT1-3 intrathyroidal tumors (completely confined to the thyroid gland) and 209 pT4 patients with extrathyroidal (locally invasive) tumors. The pTNM 1992 clarification was used. All patients had initial surgical treatment at the Mayo Clinic from 1940 to 1997. *DM,* Distant metastases.

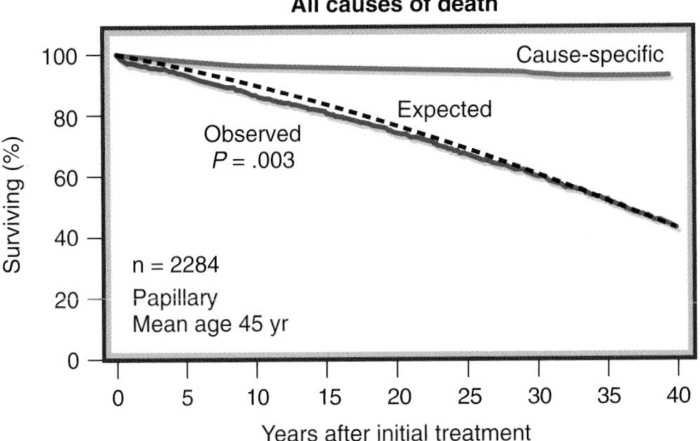

Figure 13–12 ▪ Survival to death from all causes and to death from thyroid cancer (cause-specific mortality) in 2284 consecutive patients with papillary thyroid carcinoma undergoing initial management at the Mayo Clinic from 1940 to 1997. Also plotted is the expected survival (all causes) of persons of the same age and sex and with the same date of treatment but living under mortality conditions of the northwest central United States.

year cause-specific survival rate of 95% for PTC was significantly higher than the 79%, 71%, and 66% rates seen with MTC, Hürthle cell cancer (HCC), and FTC, respectively.

Outcome Prediction

Only a fraction (~15%) of patients with PTC are likely to experience relapse of disease, and even fewer (~5%) have a lethal outcome. Exceptional patients, who have an aggressive course, tend to experience relapse early (Fig. 13–12), and the rare fatalities usually occur within 5 to 10 years of diagnosis.[90,91] Multivariate analyses have been used to identify variables predictive of CSM.[91,113-119] Increasing age of the patient and the presence of extrathyroidal invasion are independent prognostic factors in all studies.

The presence of initial DM and large size of the primary tumor are also significant variables in most studies,[91,113-115,118] and some groups[90,91,113,114,117] have reported that histopathologic grade (degree of differentiation) is an independent variable. The completeness of initial tumor resection (postoperative status) is also a predictor of mortality.[90,115,118] The presence of initial neck NM, although relevant to future nodal recurrence, does not influence CSM (Fig. 13–13).[90,91,118]

Several scoring systems based on these significant prognostic indicators have been devised. Each system allows one to assign the majority of PTC patients (80% or more) to a low-risk group, in which the CSM at 25 years is less than 2%, and the others (a small minority) to a high-risk group, in which almost all cancer-related deaths are observed. In general, these systems provide prediction of postoperative events comparable to that of the internationally accepted TNM staging system.[119]

A scoring index devised to assign PTC patients to prognostic risk groups[113] was named the AGES scheme after the four independent variables: patient's *a*ge, tumor *g*rade, tumor *e*xtent (local invasion, DM), and tumor *s*ize. With the use of such a scoring system, 86% of patients were in the minimal risk group (AGES score <4) and they experienced a 20-year CSM rate of only 1%.[90] By contrast, patients with AGES scores of 4+ (high-risk; 14% of the total) had a 20-year CSM of 36%.

Figure 13–14 compares the AGES scores with TNM stage and with two other subsequently introduced schemes designed to stratify PTC patients into groups at either minimal risk or high risk of cancer-related death. Such a prognostic scoring system makes it possible to counsel patients and to aid in the planning of individualized postoperative management programs in PTC.[113,118]

Although the AGES scheme had the potential for universal application, some academic centers could not include the differentiation (G) variable because their surgical pathologists did not recognize higher-grade PTC tumors.[119] Accordingly, a prognostic scoring system for predicting PTC mortality rates was devised with the use of candidate variables that included completeness of primary tumor resection but excluded histologic grade.[118] Cox model analysis and stepwise variable selection led to a final prognostic model that included five variables: *m*etastasis, *a*ge, *c*ompleteness of resection, *i*nvasion, and *s*ize (MACIS). The final score was defined as follows:

3.1 (age 39 years or younger)
or 0.08 × age (age 40 years or older)
+ 0.3 × tumor size (in centimeters)
+ 1 (if tumor not completely resected)
+ 1 (if locally invasive) + 3 (if DM present)

As illustrated by Figure 13–15, the MACIS scoring system permits identification of groups of patients with a broad range of risk of death from PTC. Twenty-year cause-specific survival

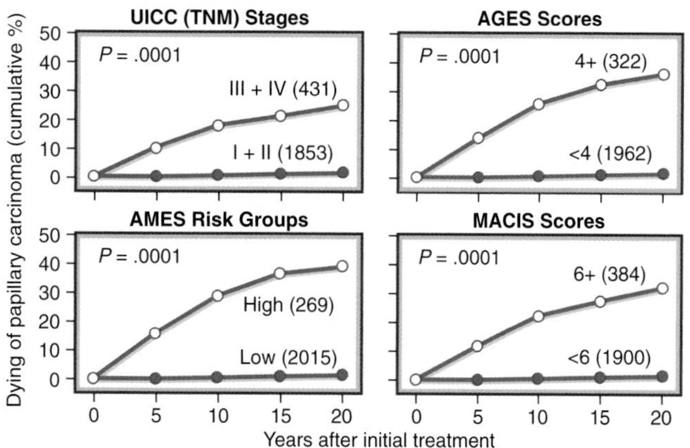

Figure 13–14 ▪ Cumulative mortality from papillary thyroid carcinoma in patients at either minimal risk or higher risk of cancer-related death as defined by International Union Against Cancer (UICC) pathologic tumor-node-metastases (pTNM) stages *(upper left)*, AGES scores *(upper right)*, AMES risk groups *(lower left)*, and MACIS scores *(lower right)*. The minimal risk group constitutes 81% of the 2284 patients when defined by pTNM stages I and II, 86% as defined by AGES scores less than 4, 88% as defined by AMES low risk, and 83% when defined by a MACIS score less than 6. The cause-specific mortality (CSM) rates at 20 years were 25% for stages III and IV, 36% for AGES scores of 4+, 39% for AMES high risk, and 32% for patients with MACIS scores of 6+. The CSM ratios between the high-risk and low-risk groups at 20 years were 19 for pTNM, 36 for AGES, 35 for AMES, and 40 for MACIS.

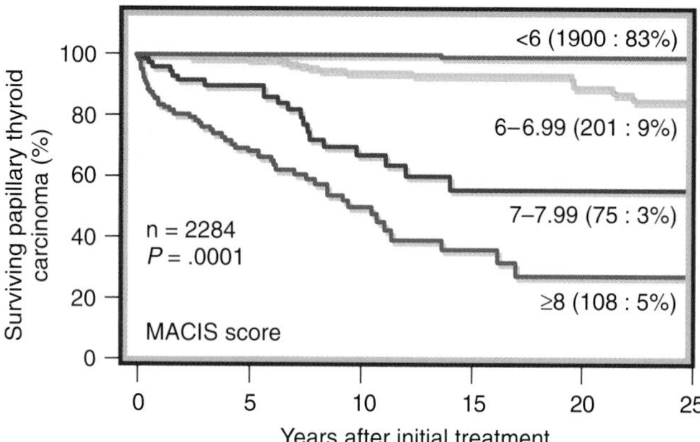

Figure 13–15 ▪ Cause-specific survival according to MACIS (*m*etastases, *a*ge, *c*ompleteness of resection, *i*nvasion, and *s*ize) scores of less than 6, 6 to 6.99, 7 to 7.99, and 8+ in a cohort of 2284 consecutive patients with papillary thyroid carcinoma (PTC) undergoing initial treatment at the Mayo Clinic from 1940 to 1997. The numbers in parentheses represent the numbers and percentages of PTC patients in each of the four risk groups.

rates for patients with MACIS scores of less than 6, 6 to 6.99, 7 to 7.99, and 8+ were 99%, 89%, 56%, and 27%, respectively ($P <$ .0001). When cumulative mortality from all causes of death was considered, approximately 85% of PTC patients with AGES scores below 4 or MACIS scores below 6 had no excess mortality over rates predicted for control subjects.[113,118]

It should be emphasized that the five variables in MACIS scoring are easy to define after primary operation; consequently, the system can be applied in any clinical setting. The MACIS system can be used for counseling individual PTC patients and can help guide decision making concerning the intensity of the postoperative tumor surveillance and the appropriateness of adjunctive radioiodine therapy. Because the CIS (*c*ompleteness of resection, *i*nvasion, and *s*ize) variables require information obtained at surgery, the system probably should not be used to decide the extent of primary surgery.

Follicular Thyroid Carcinoma

FTC is "a malignant epithelial tumor showing evidence of follicular cell differentiation but lacking the diagnostic features of papillary carcinoma."[74] Such a definition excludes the follicular variant of PTC, and it is also customary to exclude both the poorly differentiated insular carcinoma[120] and the rare mixed medullary and follicular carcinoma.[121] The correct classification of tumors with predominant oncocytic features (Hürthle cell carcinomas) is controversial.[85] The WHO committee has taken the stance that this tumor is an oxyphilic variant of FTC.[74] The AFIP monograph, by contrast, states that "the tumors made up of this cell type have gross, microscopic, behavioral, cytogenetic (and conceivably etiopathogenic) features that set them apart from all others and justify discussing them in a separate section."[75]

Thus categorized, FTC is a relatively rare neoplasm whose identification requires invasion of the capsule, blood vessel, or adjacent thyroid. In epidemiologic surveys, FTC constituted from 5% to 50% of differentiated thyroid cancers and tended to be more common in areas with iodine deficiency.[122] Owing to a combination of changing diagnostic criteria and an increase in the incidence of PTC associated with dietary iodine supplementation, the diagnosis of FTC has decreased in frequency; in one North American experience, minimally invasive non-oxyphilic FTC made up fewer than 2% of thyroid malignancies.[123]

The microscopic appearance of FTC varies from well-formed follicles to a predominantly solid growth pattern.[74,75] Poorly formed follicles and atypical patterns (e.g., cribriform) may occur, and multiple architectural types may coexist. Mitotic activity is not a useful indicator of malignancy.

FTC is best divided into two categories on the basis of degree of invasiveness: (1) minimally invasive or encapsulated and (2) widely invasive. There is little overlap between these two types.

Minimally invasive FTC is an encapsulated tumor whose growth pattern resembles that of a trabecular or solid, microfollicular, or atypical adenoma. The diagnosis of malignancy depends on the demonstration of blood vessel or capsular invasion, or both. The criteria for invasion must therefore be strict.[74,75] Blood vessel invasion is almost never seen grossly. Microscopically, the vessels "should be of venous caliber, be located in or immediately outside of the capsule and contain one or more clusters of tumor cells attached to the wall and protruding into the lumen."[75] Interruption of the capsule must involve the full thickness to qualify as capsular invasion. Penetration of only the inner half or the presence of tumor cells embedded in the capsule does not qualify for the diagnosis of FTC. Foci of capsular invasion must be distinguished from the capsular rupture that can result from FNA. The acronym WHAFFT (*w*orrisome *h*istologic *a*lterations *f*ollowing *F*NA of the *t*hyroid) is applied to such changes.[124] The diagnosis of malignancy of these tumors may be difficult and not reproducible among pathologists, and immunohistochemistry with markers such as TPO, Galectin 3 or HMBE1 may help for this purpose, but these techniques did not reliably improve the accuracy of pathology in case of suspicious findings.[51] Global gene expression studies with the microarray technology demonstrates different profiles between papillary carcinoma and follicular tumors,[125-127] but the reported distinction between follicular adenomas and minimally invasive follicular carcinoma with the expression study of a limited number of genes needs confirmation.[128]

In contrast, the rare *widely invasive* form of FTC can be distinguished easily from benign lesions. Although the tumor may be partially encapsulated, the margins are infiltrative even on gross examination and vascular invasion is often extensive. The structural features are variable, with solid and trabecular areas, but a follicular element is always present. When follicular differentiation is poor or absent, the tumor may be classified as a poorly differentiated (insular) carcinoma.[75]

Focal or extensive clear-cell changes can occur. A rare clear-cell variant of FTC has been described in which glycogen accumulation or dilatation of the granular endoplasmic reticulum is responsible for the clear cells.[129] When more than 75% of cells in an FTC exhibit Hürthle cell (or oncocytic) features, the tumor is classified as a Hürthle cell or an oncocytic carcinoma,[75,130] or an oxyphilic variant FTC.[74]

Molecular Pathogenesis

There is still no accepted paradigm for the pathogenesis of follicular thyroid cancer. A multistep adenoma-to-carcinoma pathogenesis, similar to that for colon cancer and other adenocarcinomas,[98] is not universally accepted because pathologists do not recognize follicular carcinoma in situ and documentation of the evolution of adenoma to carcinoma is rare. Nevertheless, several facts about the pathogenesis of FTC are firmly established.[89,94]

First, most follicular adenomas and all FTCs are probably of monoclonal origin. Second, oncogene activation, particularly by point mutation of the *RAS* oncogene, is common both in follicular adenomas (~20%) and in FTCs (~40%), supporting a role in early tumorigenesis.[89,99] Such *RAS* mutations are not specific for follicular tumors and also occur in approximately 10% of all PTCs, mostly in the follicular variant. The *RET* oncogene does not appear to be involved in follicular tumors.[89,94] Third, cytogenetic abnormalities and evidence of genetic loss are more common in FTC than in PTC and also occur in follicular adenomas.[97,131]

Of the cytogenetic abnormalities described in FTC, the most common are deletions, partial deletions, and deletion-rearrangements involving the p arm of chromosome 3. Loss of heterozygosity (LOH) on chromosome 3p appears to be limited to FTC because no evidence for 3p LOH has been found in follicular adenomas or PTC. A translocation, t(2;3)(q13;p25), resulting in the fusion of the deoxyribonucleic acid (DNA) binding domains of the thyroid transcription factor PAX-8 to domains of the peroxisome proliferator-activated receptor (PPARγ1, was detected in 30% (range, 11% to 63%) of FTCs and in 10% of follicular adenomas, but not in PTCs or multinodular hyperplasia.[132-134] The chimeric protein may retard growth inhibition and follicular differentiation normally induced by PPARγ1.[133] The two main genetic alterations found in follicular carcinomas may act through distinct molecular pathways.[134]

Presenting Features

FTC tends to occur in older people, with the mean age in most studies being more than 50 years, about 10 years older than that for typical PTC.[122] The average median age of patients with oxyphilic FTC (HCC) is about 60 years.[122,130] As in most thyroid malignancies, women outnumber men by more than 2 to 1. Most patients with FTC present with a painless thyroid nodule, with or without background thyroid nodularity, and they rarely (4% to 6%) have clinically evident lymphadenopathy at presentation.[122] Lymph node metastases to the neck in FTC are so exceptional that "wherever they are observed, the alternative possibilities of follicular variant papillary carcinoma, oncocytic carcinoma, and poorly differentiated (insular) carcinoma should be considered."[75]

In most series in which tumor sizes were reported, the average tumor in FTC (oxyphilic or non-oxyphilic) was larger than those seen with PTC.[122,130] Direct extrathyroidal extension, by definition, does not occur with minimally invasive FTC but is common in the rare patients with invasive FTC. Between 5% and 20% of patients may have DM at presentation.[122] The most common sites for DM in FTC are lung and bone.[75,122] The bones most often involved are long bones (e.g., femur), flat bones (particularly the pelvis, sternum, and skull), and vertebrae. When DM is the first manifestation of the disease, definitive proof of its thyroid origin should be obtained, usually by a biopsy of a metastasis, before performing any thyroid surgery. It is unusual for patients with FTC to have thyrotoxicosis caused by massive tumor burden.[135]

Most patients (53% to 69%) with FTC or HCC have pTNM stage II disease. Patients 45 years of age or older with nodal metastases or extrathyroidal extension (stage III) account for only 4% of FTCs and 9% of HCCs (see Fig. 13–7). About 5% of HCCs and 17% or more of non-oxyphilic FTCs have DM at the time of diagnosis (stage IV).

Recurrence and Mortality

Nodal metastases are rare in typical FTC, and the nodal recurrence rate at 20 postoperative years is the lowest in differentiated thyroid carcinoma, being around 2% (see Fig. 13–10). About 6% of patients with HCC have node involvement at presentation,[136] but within 25 years after primary surgery, about 17% of HCC patients have nodal recurrence.[122] When recurrences at either neck or distant sites are taken into consideration, patients with HCC (Fig. 13–16) have the highest numbers of tumor recurrences after 10 to 20 years. As illustrated by Figure 13–10, local recurrences at 20 years have occurred in 20% of FTCs and 30% of HCCs. Comparable DM rates are 23% and 28%, respectively.

CSM rates vary with the presenting TNM stage in both FTC (Fig. 13–17) and HCC. The death rates tend to parallel the curves for development of DM (see Fig. 13–10). In more than five decades of experience at the Mayo Clinic, the mortality rate for FTC initially exceeds that of HCC, but by 20 to 30 postoperative years there are no significant differences in cause-specific survival rates between FTC and HCC (Fig. 13–18), both being around 80% at 20 and 70% at 30 postoperative years.[122] Curves representing mortality from all causes differ in FTC and HCC. On average, patients with FTC are about 5 years younger, tend to die within the first 10 postoperative years, and have high all-cause mortality for 10 to 30 postoperative years (Fig. 13–19).

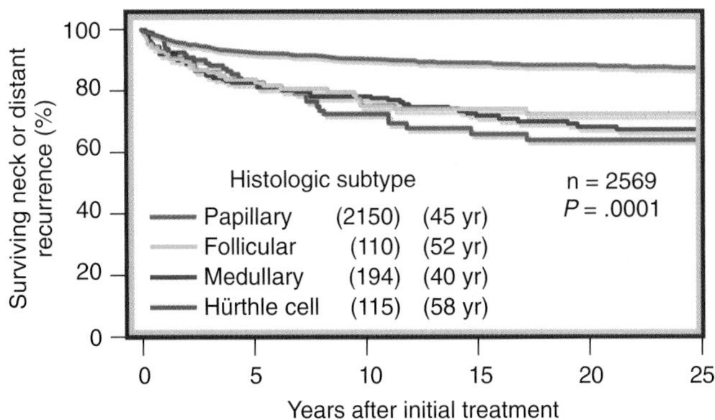

Figure 13–16 ▪ Postoperative recurrence (any site) in the first 20 years after definitive surgery for differentiated thyroid carcinoma performed at the Mayo Clinic from 1940 to 1997. Figures are based on 2569 consecutive patients (2150 papillary thyroid carcinoma, 110 follicular thyroid carcinoma, 115 Hürthle cell carcinoma, and 194 medullary thyroid carcinoma) who had complete tumor resection and had no distant metastases at presentation. The ages in parentheses represent the median age at diagnosis for each of the four histologic subtypes.

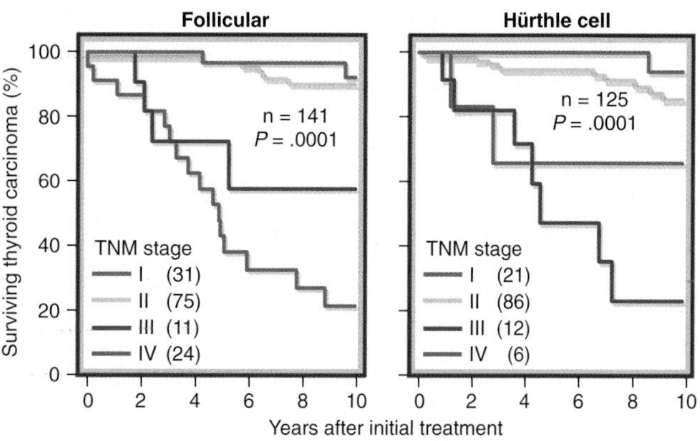

Figure 13–17 ▪ Cause-specific survival according to pathologic tumor-node-metastases (pTNM) stages in a cohort of 141 patients with follicular thyroid carcinoma *(left panel)* and 125 patients with Hürthle cell carcinoma *(right panel)* treated at the Mayo Clinic from 1940 to 1997. Numbers in parentheses represent the number of patients in each pTNM 1992 stage grouping.

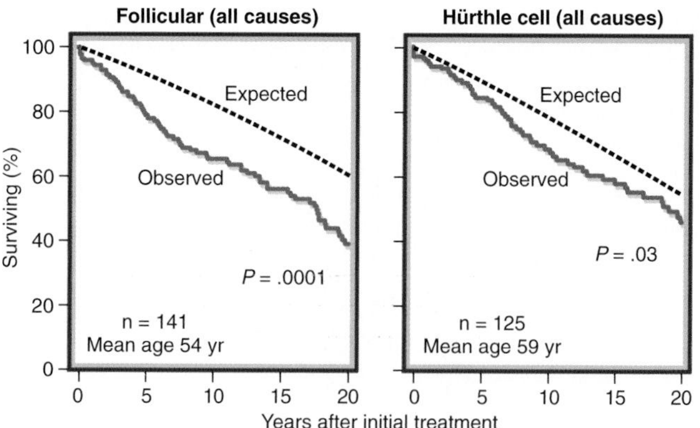

Figure 13–19 ▪ Survival to death from all causes in 141 consecutive patients with follicular thyroid carcinoma *(left)* and 125 patients with Hürthle cell cancer *(right)* undergoing initial management at the Mayo Clinic from 1940 to 1997. Also plotted is the expected survival (all causes) of persons of the same age and sex and with the same date of treatment but living under mortality conditions of the northwest central United States.

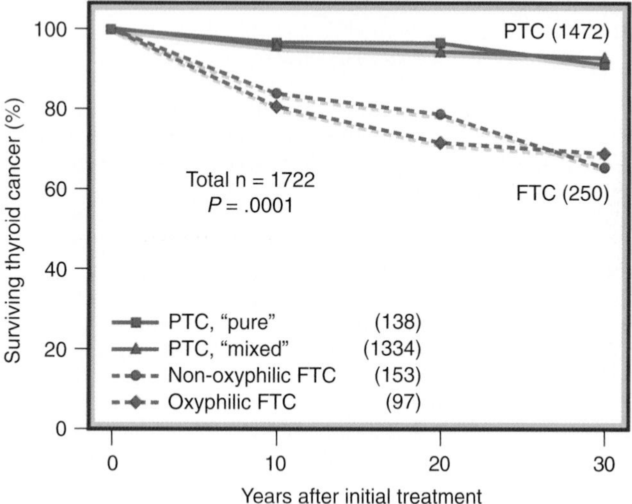

Figure 13–18 ▪ Comparison of cause-specific survival in 1472 papillary thyroid carcinoma (PTC) and 250 follicular thyroid carcinoma (FTC) patients treated at the Mayo Clinic from 1940 to 1990. One hundred and thirty-eight of the PTCs were "pure" papillary in histotype (no follicular elements); 97 of the FTC patients had predominantly oxyphilic tumors. There is a significant difference ($P = .0001$) between the PTC and the FTC survival curves. However, within either the PTC or FTC group, the two survival curves are insignificantly different. (From Grebe SKG, Hay ID. Follicular thyroid cancer. Endocrinol Metab Clin North Am 1995;24:761-801.)

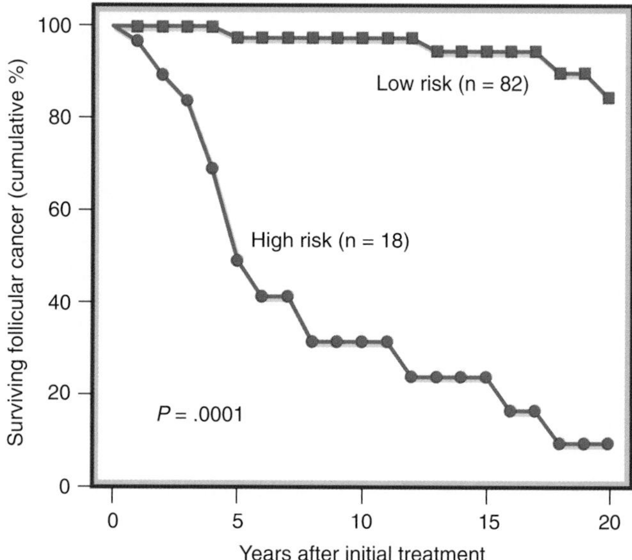

Figure 13–20 ▪ Cumulative cause-specific survival among 100 patients with non-oxyphilic follicular thyroid carcinoma treated at the Mayo Clinic from 1946 to 1970, plotted by high-risk and low-risk categories. *High risk* means that two or more of the following factors were present: age older than 50 years, marked vascular invasion, and metastatic disease at time of initial diagnosis. (From Brennan MD, Bergstralh EJ, van Heerden JA, et al. Follicular thyroid cancer treated at the Mayo Clinic, 1946 through 1970: initial manifestations, pathologic findings, therapy, and outcome. Mayo Clin Proc 1991;66:11-22.)

Deaths related to HCC occur gradually over the first 15 years; however, by 25 years, the average survivor of HCC is 84 years old, and by that time, almost 50% of the treated cohort would be predicted by the actuarial curve to have died from all causes.

Outcome Prediction

The risk factors that predict outcome in FTC are largely the same as in PTC: DM at presentation, increasing age of the patient, large tumor size, and the presence of local (extrathyroidal) invasion.[122,137-143] To a lesser degree, increased mortality is associated with male sex and higher grade (less well-differentiated) tumors. In addition, vascular invasiveness, lymphatic involvement at presentation, DNA aneuploidy, and oxyphilic histology are potential prognostic variables unique to FTC.[122] The importance of vascular invasion is underscored by a study showing that FTC patients with minimal capsular invasion and no evidence of vascular invasion had 0% CSM at 10-year follow-up.[137]

Prognostic scoring systems for FTC[122,138] allow stratification of patients into high-risk and low-risk categories. A multivariate analysis at the Mayo Clinic found that DM at presentation, patient's age older than 50 years, and marked vascular invasion predict a poor outcome.[122] As illustrated by Figure 13–20, if two or more of these factors are present, the 5-year survival rate is only 47%, and 20-year survival is 8%. By contrast, if only one

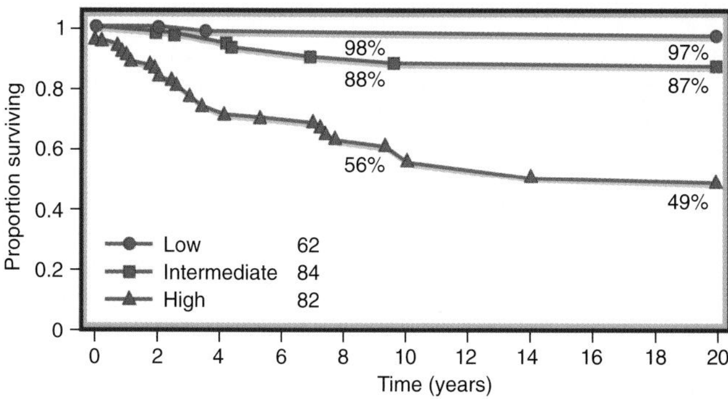

Figure 13–21 ▪ Survival differences in low-risk, intermediate-risk, and high-risk groups for 228 consecutive patients with follicular thyroid carcinoma who were seen and treated at the Memorial Sloan-Kettering Cancer Center during a period of 55 years from 1930 to 1985. (From Shaha AR, Loree TR, Shah JP. Prognostic factors and risk group analyses in follicular carcinoma of the thyroid. Surgery 1995;118:1131-1138.)

of these factors is present, 5-year survival is 99%, and 20-year survival is 86%.

Systems developed to predict outcome in either PTC or FTC have been applied to FTC patients. The pTNM as well as the AMES risk group categorization (*a*ge, *m*etastasis, *e*xtent, *s*ize) have proved to be useful in FTC.[139] Additionally, from a multivariate analysis of 228 patients with FTC treated at the Memorial Sloan Kettering Cancer Center, the independent adverse prognostic factors were identified as age older than 45 years, Hürthle cell histotype, extrathyroidal extension, tumor size exceeding 4 cm, and the presence of DM.[140] The prognostic importance in FTC of histologic grade was also confirmed,[140] and this factor was included in assignment of risk groups to low, intermediate, or high categories (Fig. 13–21).

The AGES scheme, originally developed for PTC, has also been successfully applied to FTC.[141,142] Additionally, it has recently been demonstrated that, when compared with the TNM, AGES, and AMES prognostic schemes, the MACIS classification was the most accurate predictor of survival in FTC.[143] It would therefore appear that scoring systems used in PTC may be cautiously applied to FTC as long as some of the unique features of this tumor, such as vascular invasiveness and the remarkable significance of DNA aneuploidy in HCC, are kept in mind.[122]

Poorly Differentiated (Insular, Solid, or Trabecular) Carcinoma

Poorly differentiated thyroid carcinoma has been defined as "a tumor of follicular cell origin with morphological and biologic attributes intermediate between differentiated and anaplastic carcinomas of the thyroid."[75] The most distinctive histologic feature is the presence of small cells with round nuclei and scant cytoplasm with a diffuse solid pattern or organized in round or oval nests (insulae) or in trabeculae. The predominant pattern of growth is solid, but microfollicles are also seen, some of which contain dense colloid. Extrathyroidal extension and blood vessel invasion are common. Most such tumors exhibit foci of necrosis, are larger than 5 cm in diameter at diagnosis, and have an invasive margin on gross examination.

The mean age at diagnosis is about 55 years, and the female-to-male ratio is about 2 : 1.[75] Poorly differentiated carcinoma is aggressive and often lethal. Metastases are common in regional nodes and distant sites (lung, bone, brain). In one series, 56% of patients died of their tumor within 8 years of initial therapy.[120] The tumor is viewed by the WHO committee[74] as a morphologic variant of FTC, but others view it as a poorly differentiated variant of either PTC or FTC.[75] Some tumors formerly classified as the compact form of undifferentiated small cell carcinoma probably belonged to this category.[75] The AFIP group also considers that a large proportion of "low-risk" young patients with aggressive PTC or FTC belong to this category of high-grade poorly differentiated FTC.[75]

Undifferentiated (Anaplastic) Carcinoma

Anaplastic carcinoma constitutes about 1% to 2% of all thyroid carcinomas, usually occurs after the age of 60 years, and is slightly more common in women (1.3 : 1 to 1.5 : 1).[144-146] This carcinoma is highly malignant, nonencapsulated, and extends widely. Evidence of invasion of adjacent structures, such as the skin, muscles, nerves, blood vessels, larynx, and esophagus, is common. DM occurs early in the course of the disease in lungs, liver, bones, and brain.

On histopathologic examination, the lesion is composed of atypical cells that exhibit numerous mitoses and form a variety of patterns. Spindle-shaped cells, multinucleate giant cells, and squamoid cells usually predominate. Areas of necrosis and polymorphonuclear infiltration are common, and the presence of PTC or FTC suggests that they may be the precursors of anaplastic carcinoma. Mutations of the *p53* gene are present in many undifferentiated carcinomas but may not be found in the residual well-differentiated component, suggesting that these mutations occurred after the development of the original tumor and may have played a key role in tumor progression.[89,94]

The usual clinical complaint is of a rapid, often painful enlargement of a mass that may have been present in the thyroid gland for many years. The tumor invades adjacent structures, causing hoarseness, inspiratory stridor, and difficulty in swallowing. On examination, the overlying skin is often warm and discolored. The mass is tender and is often fixed to adjacent structures. It is stony hard in consistency, but some areas may be soft or fluctuant. The regional lymph nodes are enlarged, and there may be evidence of DM. Anaplastic carcinomas do not accumulate iodine and do not typically produce thyroglobulin.

Treatment should be initiated rapidly to avoid death from locally infiltrative disease and possible suffocation. It consists of surgical resection of the tumor tissue present in the neck, when this is feasible, followed by a combination of external irradiation and chemotherapy.[145,146]

Medullary Thyroid Carcinoma

MTC accounts for less than 10% of thyroid malignancies (see Chapter 40). It arises from the parafollicular or C cells of the thyroid gland, and the tumor cells typically produce an early biochemical signal (hypersecretion of calcitonin). MTC readily invades the intraglandular lymphatics and spreads to other parts of the gland, in addition to the pericapsular and regional lymph nodes. It also regularly spreads through the bloodstream to the lungs, bone, and liver.[79-81,147]

MTC tumors are firm and usually unencapsulated. On histopathologic examination, the tumor is composed of cells that vary in morphologic features and arrangement. Round, polyhedral, and spindle-shaped cells form a variety of patterns, which may vary from solid, trabecular to endocrine or glandular-like structures. An amyloid stroma is commonly present.[74,75] Gross or microscopic foci of carcinoma may be present in other parts of the gland, and blood vessels may be invaded. The histopathologic appearance of the metastases resembles that of the primary lesion. In all cases, the diagnosis can be confirmed by positive immunostaining of tumor tissue for calcitonin and carcinoembryonic antigen (CEA).

MTC first appears either as a hard nodule or mass in the thyroid gland or as an enlargement of the regional lymph nodes. Occasionally, a metastatic lesion in a distant site is found first. The neck masses are frequently painful; they are sometimes bilateral and are often localized to the upper two thirds of each lobe of the gland, which reflects the anatomic location of the parafollicular cells.

The tumor occurs in both sporadic and hereditary forms, the latter making up about 20% of the total. The hereditary variety can be transmitted as a single entity, familial MTC, or it can arise as part of MEN syndrome type 2A or 2B. The hereditary form is typically bilateral and is usually preceded by a premalignant C-cell hyperplasia. Total thyroidectomy at this premalignant stage can cure the disease in more than 90% of cases.[43,44,147-149] *RET* proto-oncogene testing should be performed in all MTC patients. The finding of a germline mutation in this gene indicates a hereditary disease; the mutation should then be sought in all first-degree family members.

Early series of MTC mainly described sporadic cases, in which 80% of patients presented with TNM stage II or III. As more patients with familial MTC or MEN-2A have been diagnosed, more patients have curable (stage I) disease, and the survival rate has improved, a trend that should continue with widespread application of *RET* proto-oncogene testing.[147-149] Patients with MTC now have outcomes similar to or better than those of patients with nonpapillary FCTC (see Fig. 13–9). The cause-specific survival curves for 218 consecutive MTC cases treated from 1940 to 1997 at the Mayo Clinic, according to TNM stage, are presented in Figure 13–22.

Prognostic factors relevant to outcome in MTC include (1) age at diagnosis, (2) male gender, (3) initial extent of the disease, such as NM and DM, (4) tumor size, (5) extrathyroidal invasion, (6) vascular invasion, (7) calcitonin immunoreactivity and amyloid staining in tumor tissue, (8) postoperative gross residual disease, and (9) postoperative plasma calcitonin levels.[79-81]

In multivariate analysis, only the age of the patient at initial treatment and the stage of the disease remain significantly independent indicators of survival. This suggests that, in routine practice, clinicians attempting to predict outcome in MTC should take into account not only the presenting disease stage, as assessed by the pTNM system (see Fig. 13–22), but also the age of the patient at diagnosis.[79-81]

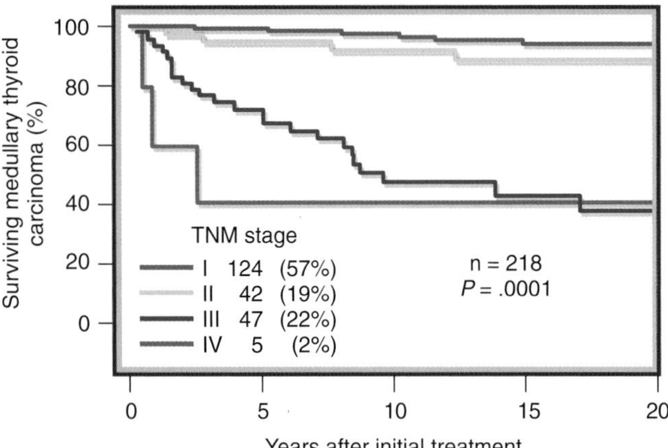

Figure 13–22 ▪ Cause-specific survival according to pathologic tumor-node-metastases (pTNM) stage in a cohort of 218 patients with medullary thyroid carcinoma treated at the Mayo Clinic from 1940 to 1997. Numbers in parentheses represent the percentages of patients in each pTNM 1992 stage grouping.

Cushing's syndrome may occur at an advanced stage of the disease, because of secretion of corticotropin by the tumor. Prostaglandins, serotonin, kinins, and vasoactive intestinal peptide may also be secreted and are variously responsible for flushing and for the attacks of watery diarrhea that about one third of patients experience, usually at an advanced stage of the disease.[79-81,147] In MEN-2A, hyperparathyroidism occurs late and is usually due to parathyroid hyperplasia rather than adenoma. Pheochromocytomas invariably occur later than MTC; they are often bilateral and may be clinically silent, and patients at risk should be screened with measurements of urinary metanephrine excretion. In MEN-2B, MTC and pheochromocytomas are associated with multiple mucosal neuromas *(bumpy lip syndrome)*, a marfanoid habitus, and typical facies, but such patients do not have hyperparathyroidism.[147]

Differentiation of sporadic MTC from other types of thyroid nodule on clinical grounds alone may be difficult. In patients with a family history of thyroid cancer associated with hypertension or hyperparathyroidism, the MEN-2A syndrome should be suspected. FNAB has made it possible to diagnose MTC before surgery. In some patients, however, cytologic findings may be misleading because the type of carcinoma is difficult to determine and HCC may occasionally be confused with MTC.[74,75,147]

Positive immunocytochemical staining for calcitonin allows confirmation of the diagnosis. Basal plasma calcitonin levels are elevated in virtually all patients with clinical MTC.[42] Infusions of pentagastrin or calcium elicit secretion of calcitonin, and the response may be exaggerated in patients with either MTC or the antecedent C-cell hyperplasia; its use should be restricted to patients with an undetectable or borderline plasma calcitonin level (see Chapter 40).

When the diagnosis of MTC is made from calcitonin measurements or FNAB, patients should be evaluated for hyperparathyroidism and for pheochromocytoma. If these diagnoses are satisfactorily excluded, a total thyroidectomy with removal of regional nodes can safely be performed.[150,151] In patients with MEN, surgery should be performed for pheochromocytomas before surgery for MTC is performed. First-degree relatives of patients with MEN or familial MTC should undergo DNA testing for the presence of the mutant *RET* gene (see Chapter 40). Gene carriers with the 634 RET mutation (the most frequent) should undergo a prophylactic total thyroidectomy between 5 and 7 years of age.[43,44,148,149]

Primary Malignant Lymphoma

Primary lymphomas of the thyroid are uncommon tumors, constituting fewer than 2% of all thyroid malignancies. The peak incidence is in the seventh decade, and the male-to-female ratio is 1 : 3.[152] Aggressive thyroid lymphomas are almost invariably seen as a rapidly enlarging, painless neck mass, fixed to surrounding tissues; they cause compressive symptoms and should be differentiated from anaplastic carcinoma. Unilateral or bilateral lymph node enlargement is present in about 50% of affected patients. Clinically evident distant disease is uncommon. The palpated mass is solid and, if studied by imaging, would be hypoechoic on ultrasonography and nonfunctioning on thyroid scintiscan. Most primary thyroid lymphomas arise in patients who have chronic autoimmune thyroiditis. Nonetheless, the disease is a rare complication of Hashimoto's thyroiditis.

Primary thyroid lymphomas should be distinguished from generalized lymphomas with thyroid involvement. FNAB can be useful in distinguishing lymphoid proliferation from epithelial tumors. However, differentiating lymphoma from chronic autoimmune thyroiditis by thyroid cytology may be difficult. Therefore, surgical specimens are needed for diagnosis. Immunohistochemical studies identify lymphoid proliferation if findings are positive for leukocyte common antigen. Monoclonality for light chain immunoglobulin is considered a strong indication of malignant lymphoma.

Because chronic autoimmune thyroiditis reproduces the exact features of a mucosa-associated lymphoid tissue (MALT), most cases of thyroid lymphoma are considered MALT lymphomas.[152] Those small cell lymphomas are characterized by a low grade of malignancy, slow growth, and a tendency for recurrence in other MALT sites, such as the gastrointestinal or respiratory tract, the thymus, or the salivary glands.

A large proportion of clinical cases are large cell lymphomas and have an aggressive course.[153] With immunohistochemistry, nearly all of them show B-cell markers. Usually, immunohistochemistry is positive for BCL2 in small cell and negative in large cell lymphomas.

Although accurate staging is very important for planning treatment, patients are often elderly, in poor condition, or may require urgent therapy to relieve symptoms, thus making a full staging investigation before treatment impractical. Staging includes physical examination; complete blood count; serum lactate dehydrogenase and β_2-microglobulin measurements; liver function tests; bone marrow biopsy; CT scanning of the neck, thorax, abdomen, and pelvis; FDG PET scan; and appropriate biopsies at sites where tumor is suspected. Involvement of Waldeyer's ring and of the gastrointestinal tract has been associated with thyroid lymphomas, and for this reason upper gastrointestinal radiography or endoscopy should be performed.

Disseminated disease necessitates chemotherapy. In patients with disease apparently confined to the neck, therapy is guided by the histologic features of the lymphoma.[152] Chemotherapy with an anthracycline-based regimen and involved-field radiotherapy should be given to all patients with large cell thyroid lymphoma and in some series has provided long-term survival rates of nearly 100%. For small cell MALT lymphomas, radiation alone may be adequate if the disease is determined to be localized after accurate staging.

SURGICAL TREATMENT OF THYROID CARCINOMA

The extent of surgery appropriate for thyroid malignancy is a matter of controversy.[112,113] Factors that influence this decision include the histologic diagnosis, the size of the original lesion, the presence of lymph node and distant metastases, the patient's age, and the risk group category. Obviously, the surgeon must be appropriately skilled in thyroid surgery, and the goal of surgery should be to remove all the malignant neoplastic tissue present in the neck. Therefore, the thyroid gland and affected neck lymph nodes should all be carefully identified and adequately resected.

In the case of PTC and FTC, although some debate still exists regarding the extent of thyroid surgery, many favor a near-total (leaving no more than 2 to 3 g of thyroid tissue) thyroidectomy for all patients.[37,71-73,90] Near-total thyroidectomy reduces the recurrence rate, compared with more limited surgery, because many PTCs are both multifocal and bilateral. Removal of most, if not all, of the thyroid gland facilitates postoperative remnant ablation with ^{131}I.

For extremely low-risk patients (i.e., those with unifocal intrathyroidal PTM and possibly small [<2 cm] FTC with only capsular invasion), a lobectomy may be an appropriate primary surgical procedure.[92,93,122] In patients who have undergone a previous unilateral lobectomy for a supposedly benign tumor that proves to be an angioinvasive FTC, a completion thyroidectomy is advisable because it facilitates future follow-up.

Surgery of lymph nodes is routinely performed in patients with PTC. It should include dissection of the central compartment (paratracheal and tracheoesophageal areas) and may also include dissection of the ipsilateral supraclavicular area and the lower third of the jugulocarotid chain. A modified ipsilateral neck dissection is performed if palpable lymph node metastases are present in the jugulocarotid chain or a preoperative ultrasound demonstrates biopsy-proven lateral neck nodal disease. Dissection is preferable to lymph node picking. Although this type of lymph node dissection has not been shown to improve the recurrence and survival rates,[82,136,154] several arguments support its routine use in patients with papillary carcinomas. These include the fact that histologic evidence of lymph node metastases is present in up to two thirds of PTC patients, of whom more than 80% have involvement of the central compartment, and metastases are difficult to detect by palpation in lymph nodes located behind the vessels or in the paratracheal groove. The knowledge of initial lymph node status, acquired by such a routine, is a requisite for TNM classification, is useful for the indication of postsurgical radioiodine treatment, and helps in the interpretation of any cervical abnormality identified during the subsequent postoperative follow-up. In the case of FTC, lymph node metastases are less frequent, but a lymph node dissection should be performed if FTC has already been diagnosed and palpable lymph nodes are present.

MTC is usually treated by total thyroidectomy, with a dissection of the central compartment of the neck and the jugulocarotid chains. A bipateral modified neck dissection is performed either routinely or for MTC affecting the lateral neck nodes.[148-151]

Ideally, patients with anaplastic carcinoma should be treated with near-total thyroidectomy and lymph node dissection, but lesions are frequently too extensive for any procedure but palliative surgery.[145,146] In these cases, surgery may be performed later in the case of tumor regression after a combination of chemotherapy and external radiotherapy.

In recommending surgery, the endocrinologist should discuss potential operative complications with the patient. Unilateral lobectomy virtually never causes permanent hypocalcemia but can cause temporary vocal cord paralysis in as many as 3% of patients. Near-total thyroidectomy causes temporary hypocalcemia in 7% to 10% of patients and permanent hypocalcemia in 0.5% to 1%; permanent vocal cord paralysis occurs in less than 1%, and may benefit from specific treatments.[155] The risk of hypoparathyroidism should be reduced by identifying parathyroid glands, possibly simplified by methylene blue staining, and certainly, if viability is in doubt, by autotransplanting the parathyroid glands at the time of initial neck exploration. The experience of the surgeon is important in terms of the finer technical points of thyroidectomy, including preservation of the external branch of the recurrent laryngeal nerve, which is important in the fine regulation of voice pitch.

A history of radiation in childhood increases the risk of both benign and malignant thyroid nodules in later life.[156] The risk increases with a younger age at exposure and larger radiation dose. Several issues are relevant for the thyroidologist. With respect to the extent of surgery, the protocol described previously should be applied to patients with a thyroid carcinoma.[156,157] In cases with benign lesions, individuals with bilateral nodular disease should have a near-total thyroidectomy; in infrequent patients, when the opposite lobe is normal at US and is macroscopically normal at surgery, one must weigh the relative risk of complications associated with a more extensive surgical procedure against the possibility of recurrence of thyroid nodules in the residual thyroid tissue.

In one irradiated population, both benign and malignant nodules recurred after previous subtotal thyroidectomy. The overall risk of recurrence in this study was approximately 20% and was lower in those who had more thyroid tissue removed than in those who had less extensive procedures. In those patients, suppression of TSH by thyroid hormone led to a reduction in recurrence from 35% to approximately 8%, but TSH suppression had no influence on the occurrence of malignant nodules.[156]

Thus, the recommendations for such patients must take into account the estimated risk of developing a thyroid nodule and the experience of the operating surgeon. All irradiated patients who have had thyroid nodules removed should receive TSH-suppressive doses of levothyroxine regardless of the extent of surgery. The appearance of new thyroid nodules is, however, fairly common, and such patients should be monitored indefinitely for this possibility.

It is not clear whether this experience should be extrapolated to prescribe routine TSH suppression therapy for all irradiated patients, even if nodularity is not present, because its beneficial effects have not been quantified and the risks of long-term TSH suppression in women, especially vis-à-vis osteoporosis, have not been clearly defined and may be significant. At present, this approach cannot be recommended for all irradiated patients but can be recommended for patients at high risk of developing a thyroid nodule.[156]

POSTOPERATIVE MANAGEMENT

In view of the foregoing uncertainties and the different needs of individual patients, postoperative treatment of thyroid carcinoma cannot always accord with a rigid algorithm.[37,158] One must consider the extent of disease at surgery, the histotype and differentiation of the tumor, the age of the patient, and the risk group category.

Iodine 131 Therapy

^{131}I is an effective agent for delivering high radiation doses to the thyroid tissue with low spillover to other portions of the body. The radiation dose to the thyroid tissue is related to the tissue concentration, the ratio between the total tissue uptake and the volume of functional tissue, and the effective half-life of ^{131}I in the tissue. Thyroid tissue is able to concentrate iodine only after TSH stimulation, but even after optimal TSH stimulation, iodine uptake in neoplastic tissue is always lower than in normal thyroid tissue and may not be detectable in about one third of cases.[105,159]

^{131}I therapy is given postoperatively for three reasons. First, it destroys normal thyroid remnants *(ablation)*, thereby increasing the sensitivity of subsequent ^{131}I total body scanning and the specificity of measurements of serum Tg for the detection of persistent or recurrent disease.[160] Second, it may destroy occult or known microscopic carcinoma, thereby potentially decreasing the long-term recurrence rate. Finally, it makes it possible to perform a postablative ^{131}I total body scan, a sensitive tool for detecting persistent carcinoma.

It cannot be emphasized too strongly that postoperative ^{131}I therapy should be used *selectively* and that not all patients with a diagnosis of FCTC benefit from routine postoperative radioiodine ablative therapy.[37,91,158] In very low-risk patients, the long-term prognosis after surgery alone is so favorable that ^{131}I ablation is not recommended. However, patients who are at high risk of recurrence (Table 13–7) are routinely treated with ^{131}I because such therapy can potentially decrease both recurrence and death rates. Young children are also usually candidates for postoperative radioiodine therapy because they may have extensive neck lymph node involvement and frequently harbor pulmonary metastases that may not be detectable with standard radiographs or even with CT imaging of the chest.[78,110] Finally, in the other patients, there is currently no evidence that it may improve the long term outcome; radioiodine is administered postoperatively when surgery has not been complete or doubtful.

Postoperatively, no levothyroxine treatment is given for 4 to 6 weeks but liothyronine can be substituted for at least 3 to 4 weeks and then discontinued for 2 weeks before radioiodine studies. At that time, the serum TSH level should be greater than an empirically determined level of 25 to 30 mU/L; undetectable serum Tg level indicates a very low risk of finding persistent disease or of subsequent recurrence.[161] In case of incomplete thyroidectomy, neck uptake may be measured with a tracer activity of ^{131}I or ^{123}I; the activity used should be small enough to avoid stunning, that is, a decrease of thyroid uptake with the subsequent high activity of radioiodine.[162,163] High uptake (>10%) and high risk of persistent disease should lead to completion surgery. ^{131}I therapy can be administered to the other patients, usually with 24-hour uptakes considerably less than 10%. A total body scan is performed 3 to 7 days after the treatment activity and is highly informative in patients with a low uptake (<1%) in the thyroid bed. Levothyroxine suppressive therapy is then initiated. Total ablation (defined as no visible uptake) may be verified by an ^{131}I total body scan 6 to 12 months later, typically with 2 to 5 mCi (74 to 185 MBq). However, control ^{131}I total body scan is not more routinely performed when postablation scan has

TABLE 13–7 INDICATIONS FOR ^{131}I TREATMENT IN PATIENTS WITH PAPILLARY, FOLLICULAR, OR HÜRTHLE CELL THYROID CARCINOMA AFTER INITIAL DEFINITIVE NEAR-TOTAL THYROIDECTOMY

NO INDICATION
Adult patients at very low risk of cause-specific mortality and of relapse: complete surgical resection and favorable histology and limited extent of the disease (e.g., PTC patients with MACIS scores <6 or patients with T <1 cm, N0, M0).
INDICATIONS
Definite
Distant metastasis at diagnosis
Or incomplete tumor resection
Or complete tumor resection but high risk for mortality or recurrence (e.g., PTC with MACIS 6+ and pTNM stage II/III FTC or HCC)
Probable
Incomplete surgery (less than near-total thyroidectomy, no lymph node dissection)
PTC or FTC in children <16 years
PTC: tall cell or columnar cell variant and diffuse sclerosing variant
FTC: widely invasive or poorly differentiated
Bulky nodal metastases

FTC, Follicular thyroid carcinoma; *HCC*, Hürthle cell carcinoma; *MACIS*, metastasis, age, completeness of resection, invasion, and size; *PTC*, papillary thyroid carcinoma; *pTNM*, pathologic tumor-node-metastasis.

been informative, because it does not afford any further information,[164,165] and total ablation is currently defined by an undetectable serum Tg level following rhTSH stimulation and a normal neck ultrasonography.[37,166]

Total ablation is achieved after administration of either 100 mCi (3700 MBq) or 30 mCi (1100 MBq) in more than 80% of patients who had at least a near-total thyroidectomy.[167,168] After less extensive surgery, ablation is achieved in only two thirds of patients with 30 mCi (1100 MBq). Therefore, a near-total thyroidectomy should be performed in all patients who are to be treated with ^{131}I. Also, in high-risk patients, a high activity (100 mCi or more) should be administered with the aims of ablating normal thyroid remnants and irradiating residual neoplastic tissue; in low-risk patients in whom the risk of residual disease is low, a lower activity (30 mCi) may be sufficient. Total ablation requires that a dose of at least 300 Gy (30,000 rad) is delivered to thyroid remnants, and a dosimetric study can allow a more precise estimate of the ^{131}I dose to be administered.[159] Some recent data suggest that intramuscular injections of rhTSH (0.9 mg for 2 consecutive days) given on LT4 treatment may achieve an effective stimulation of radioiodine uptake by normal thyroid remnant, and this is used in Europe in low-risk patients.[169] ^{131}I ablation therapy does not play a regular role in the management of patients with anaplastic thyroid cancer, MTC, or thyroid lymphoma.

External Radiotherapy

External radiotherapy to the neck and mediastinum is indicated only for older patients with extensive PTC in whom complete surgical excision is impossible and in whom the tumor tissue does not take up ^{131}I. Retrospective studies have shown that in these selected patients, external radiotherapy decreases the risk of neck recurrence.[170] The target volume encompasses the thyroid bed, bilateral neck lymph node areas, and the upper part of the mediastinum. Typically, 50 Gy (5000 rad) would be delivered in 25 fractions over 5 weeks, with a boost of 5 to 10 Gy on any residual macroscopic focus.

In patients with MTC, this protocol may be applied after incomplete resection of the tumor and after apparently complete surgery, when plasma calcitonin remains detectable in the absence of DM. In these patients, it may decrease the risk of neck recurrence by a factor of 2 to 4.[79,147]

In patients with anaplastic thyroid carcinoma, when the extent of disease is limited and surgery is feasible, accelerated external radiotherapy in combination with chemotherapy permits local control of the disease in two thirds of the patients and long-term survival in about 20%.[145,146]

Levothyroxine Treatment

The growth of thyroid tumor cells is controlled by TSH, and inhibition of TSH secretion with levothyroxine is thought to improve the recurrence and survival rates.[171] Therefore, levothyroxine should be given to all patients with FCTC, whatever the extent of thyroid surgery and other treatment. The initial effective dose is about 2 μg/kg body weight in adults; children require a higher dose and elderly patients a lower dose. The adequacy of therapy is monitored by measuring serum TSH 3 months after it is begun, with the initial goal being a serum TSH concentration of 0.1 mU/L. In some centers, the serum free T_3 concentration is also documented to be within the normal range.

In patients with anaplastic thyroid carcinoma, MTC, or thyroid lymphoma, a replacement dose of levothyroxine is given with the aim of obtaining a serum TSH level in the normal range.

FOLLOW-UP

In patients with PTC or FTC, the goals of follow-up after initial therapy are to maintain adequate levothyroxine therapy and to detect persistent or recurrent thyroid carcinoma. Most recurrences occur during the first years of follow-up, but some occur late. Therefore, follow-up is necessary throughout the patient's life.

Early Detection of Recurrent Disease

Clinical and Ultrasonographic Examinations

Palpation of the thyroid bed and lymph node areas is routinely performed at all follow-up visits in patients with thyroid cancer. Ultrasonography is more sensitive and may detect lymph nodes as small as 2 to 3 mm in diameter.[6-8] Metastatic lymph nodes should be differentiated from frequent benign lymph node hyperplasia and false-positive findings may have deleterious consequences and should be obviated. Lymph nodes that are small, thin, or oval; in the posterior neck chains; and especially if they decrease in size after an interval of 3 months are considered benign. By contrast, round shape, mass effect, hypoechogenicity and absence of a central echogenic line, microcalcifications, a cystic component, and peripheral hypervascularization on color Doppler ultrasonography are suspicious findings. These characteristics may be difficult to recognize in small lymph nodes, and such patients should be reassured and followed up at short intervals. The size is a less reliable criterion for malignancy, although the risk of malignancy increases as the size of the lymph node increases above 7 mm in the smallest diameter.

Serum Tg is undetectable in more than 20% of patients receiving levothyroxine treatment who have isolated lymph node metastases detected by palpation or ^{131}I total body scanning, and probably in a higher proportion of patients with lymph node metastases detected only by neck ultrasonography.[71,160] Therefore, undetectable values do not exclude metastatic lymph node disease. If in doubt, ultrasound-guided node biopsy for cytology and Tg measurement in the fluid aspirate may be performed.[172] Sensitive reverse transcriptase-polymerase chain reaction (RT-PCR) to amplify Tg mRNA in the fluid aspirate appears to be even more sensitive but is not yet being used by commercial laboratories.[173]

Radiographs

Bone and chest radiographs are no longer routinely obtained for patients with undetectable serum Tg concentrations. The reason is that virtually all patients with abnormal radiographs have readily detectable serum Tg concentrations.

Serum Thyroglobulin Determinations

Tg is a glycoprotein that is produced only by normal or neoplastic thyroid follicular cells. Methods used for serum Tg determination and serum interferences are detailed in Chapter 10.[174] It should not be detectable in patients who have had total thyroid ablation, which improves both the sensitivity and the specificity for the detection of persistent or recurrent disease.[160] In patients who are in complete remission after total thyroid ablation, serum Tg antibodies decline gradually to low or undetectable levels, with a median time of 3 years.[175] Their persistence or their reappearance during follow-up should be considered suspicious for persistent or recurrent disease.

There is a close relationship between tumor burden and the Tg level, both during levothyroxine and following TSH stimulation[174,176]; this explains why serum Tg may be undetectable in patients with isolated lymph node metastases in the neck or with small lung metastases not visible on X-ray films. The production of Tg by both normal and neoplastic thyroid tissue is in part TSH dependent. High serum TSH concentrations can be achieved by withdrawing levothyroxine for 4 to 6 weeks. However, the resulting hypothyroidism is poorly tolerated by some patients. This effect can be attenuated by substituting the more rapidly metabolized liothyronine for levothyroxine for 3 to 4 weeks and withdrawing it for 2 weeks or simply by reducing the dose of levothyroxine by 50%. The serum TSH concentration should be above an empirically determined value (>25 to 30 mU/L) in patients treated in this way; if it is not, withdrawal should be prolonged until it is. Intramuscular injections of rhTSH (0.9 mg for 2 consecutive days) are an alternative because levothyroxine treatment need not be discontinued and side effects are minimal. After rhTSH stimulation, the peak of serum Tg is usually obtained 3 days after the second injection.[177] Although the increase in serum Tg is frequently less following rhTSH than withdrawal, the diagnostic efficiency of rhTSH for stimulating Tg production in the serum is comparable to that of levothyroxine withdrawal in most patients.[160,177]

When serum Tg is detectable during levothyroxine treatment, it increases after TSH stimulation obtained either after the treatment is discontinued or with injections of rhTSH. When the serum Tg is undetectable during levothyroxine treatment in a blood test performed 3 months after initial treatment, it will increase in 14% to 20% following TSH stimulation at 9 to 12 months.[160,164,165] At that time, the serum Tg concentration is an excellent prognostic indicator. Most patients with undetectable serum Tg concentrations who were not receiving levothyroxine therapy remained free of relapse after more than 15 years of follow-up, and less than 1% had a neck lymph node recurrence that was detected by sonography.[160,164,165] Conversely, persistent or recurrent disease was found in one third of patients with detectable serum Tg concentrations and twice more frequently located in neck lymph nodes than at distant sites; in these patients, serum Tg levels increased with time or remained elevated. In the other patients, serum Tg obtained following TSH stimulation at subsequent blood tests performed some months or years later will decrease to low or undetectable levels, even in the absence of any further treatment; these patients can also be considered cured.[160,178,179] Persistent thyroid cells may produce Tg for several months after ^{131}I treatment and this may disappear during subsequent months. These data demonstrate that the trend in serum Tg level is probably much more relevant than the actual serum Tg level by itself.

Several researchers have developed sensitive RT-PCR assays to amplify circulating Tg mRNA. The technique appeared sensitive in that the test was positive in most patients with thyroid tissue, but results were not related to the extent of the disease.[180] It was positive in some patients who had no detectable thyroid tissue; due to its low specificity, this technique is not being used in routine practice.

Iodine 131 Total Body Scan

The results of a ^{131}I total body scan depend on the ability of neoplastic thyroid tissue to take up ^{131}I in the presence of high serum TSH concentrations, which are achieved by either withdrawing levothyroxine or administering intramuscular injections of rhTSH (0.9 mg for 2 consecutive days, with radioiodine administration on the day following the second injection).[177]

When ^{131}I scanning is planned, patients should be instructed to avoid iodine-containing medications and iodine-rich foods, and urinary iodine should be measured in doubtful cases. Pregnancy must be excluded in women of childbearing age. For routine diagnostic scans, from 2 to 5 mCi (74 to 185 MBq) of ^{131}I is given; higher activities may reduce the uptake of a subsequent therapeutic activity of ^{131}I.[162,163] The scan is done and uptake, if any, is measured 48 to 72 hours after the activity, preferably using a double-head gamma camera equipped with thick crystals and high-energy collimators. False-positive results are rare and are usually easily recognized (Table 13–8).

Post–Iodine 131 Therapy Total Body Scans

Assuming equivalent fractional uptake after administration of either a diagnostic or a therapeutic activity of ^{131}I, uptake too low to be detected with 2 to 5 mCi (74 to 185 MBq) may be detectable after the administration of 100 mCi (3700 MBq). Thus, a total body scan should be routinely performed 3 to 7 days after a high-activity dose (Fig. 13–23). This is also the rationale for administering a large activity of ^{131}I in patients with persistently elevated or increasing Tg levels (>10 ng/mL in the absence of levothyroxine treatment), even if the diagnostic scan is negative.[181]

Other Tests

These tests should be performed only in selected cases and may include spiral CT or MR imaging of the neck and chest, bone scintigraphy, MRI of bones, and PET scanning using ^{18}FDG.[13-15] The sensitivity of FDG PET scan may be improved by TSH stimulation, obtained following levothyroxine withdrawal or injections of rhTSH.[14] The FDG PET scan is more frequently positive in metastatic patients with no detectable ^{131}I uptake in the metastases and is particularly useful for the discovery of mediastinal lymph nodes (Fig. 13–24). Compared to FDG PET scan, neck ultrasonography is more sensitive for the detection of neck lymph node metastases and a spiral CT scan is more sensitive for the discovery of small lung metastases.

TABLE 13–8 NONTHYROIDAL CONDITIONS ASSOCIATED WITH ^{131}I ACCUMULATION

CONTAMINATION
Skin, hair, clothes
PHYSIOLOGIC ACCUMULATIONS
Salivary glands (mouth, esophagus), nose Stomach, colon (in hypothyroidism) Bladder Breast in young women Diffuse hepatic uptake (^{131}I-labeled iodoproteins)
INFLAMMATORY PROCESSES
Lung or bronchial, cutaneous, dental, sinusoidal
VARIOUS OTHER CONDITIONS
Nonthyroidal neoplasms: salivary glands, stomach, lung, meningioma Struma ovarii Cysts: renal, pleuropericardial, hepatic, salivary, mammary, testicular hydrocele Thymus: normal or hyperplastic Ectasia of the common carotid artery with stasis Esophagus: dilatation, hiatal hernia Pericardial effusion, cardiac insufficiency

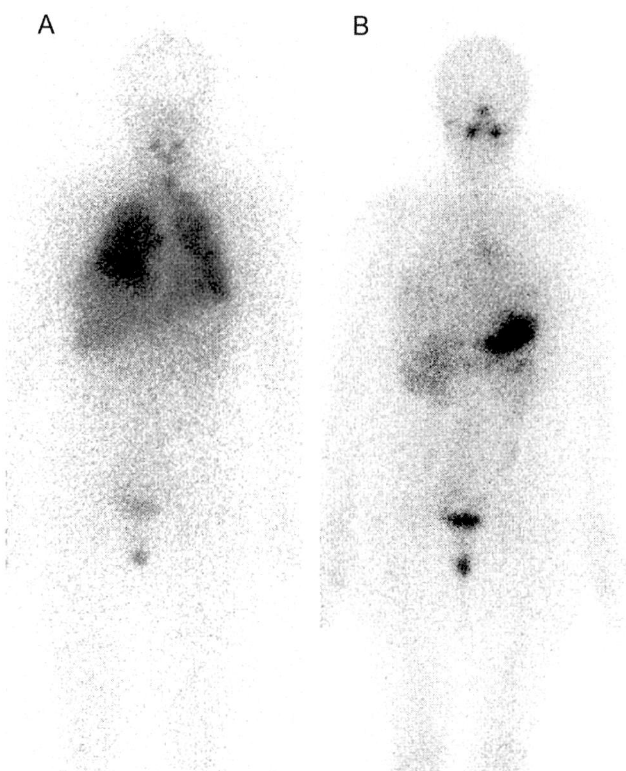

Figure 13–23 ▪ Asymptomatic 34-year-old patient who underwent surgery for a papillary thyroid carcinoma. Results of the chest radiograph were normal. **A,** Total body scan performed 4 days after the postoperative administration of 100 mCi (3700 MBq) of radioactive iodine (^{131}I). Note the presence of diffuse uptake in the lungs, and of uptake in the thyroid remnants. **B,** Total body scan performed 6 months later after the administration of a second treatment with 100 mCi of radioactive iodine that demonstrated the disappearance of all foci of uptake. The thyroglobulin level became undetectable during levothyroxine therapy and 6 years later the patient was still considered to be in complete remission.

Follow-up Strategy

If the total body scan performed after administration of ^{131}I to destroy the thyroid remnants is informative (when uptake in normal thyroid remnants is low, <1%) and does not show any uptake outside the thyroid bed, physical examination is performed and serum TSH and Tg are measured during levothyroxine treatment 3 months later (Fig. 13–25). In most centers, a neck ultrasonography is performed and the serum Tg level is measured after thyroid hormone withdrawal or rhTSH stimulation 6 to 12 months later.[37,166] A diagnostic ^{131}I total body scan is no longer routinely performed in low-risk patients with undetectable serum Tg, because the vast majority of patients with ^{131}I uptake in their metastases also have detectable serum Tg levels. Also, visible uptake in the thyroid bed that is too low to be quantified should not be considered evidence of disease in the absence of any other abnormality. Thus, ablation is currently established by an undetectable serum Tg level following TSH stimulation. Furthermore, neck ultrasonography can identify lymph node metastases that are too small to produce detectable serum Tg levels and that may be not seen on ^{131}I total body scan (Table 13–9).[6-8]

Patients with undetectable serum Tg following TSH stimulation and with normal neck ultrasonography, are considered cured, the risk of long-term recurrence being less than 1%.[164,165] The dose of levothyroxine is decreased to maintain a serum TSH

TABLE 13–9 SENSITIVITY OF VARIOUS METHODS AND OF THEIR COMBINATION FOR THE DETECTION OF LYMPH NODE METASTASES*

	STUDY INFORMATION N1/PATIENTS		
Methods	**Pacini[7] 27/340**	**Frasoldati[6] 51/494**	**Torlontano[8] 38/456**
Tg/TSH	85% (rhTSH)	57% (WD)	82% (WD)
^{131}I TBS	21%	45%	34%
Neck ultrasonography	70%	94%	100%
Tg/TSH + ultrasonography	96%	99.5%	100%

*Tg (serum thyroglobulin) and TBS (total body scan) were obtained following either withdrawal (WD) or rhTSH (••).
N1/Patients, Number of N, patients/Total number of patients.
From Schlumberger M, Berg G, Cohen O, et al. Follow-up of low-risk patients with differentiated thyroid carcinoma: a European perspective. Eur J Endocrinol 2004;50:105-112.

concentration within the normal range 0.5 to 2.5 mU/L. In high-risk patients, higher doses of levothyroxine are given, with the goal being a serum TSH concentration between 0.1 and 0.5 mU/L.[171,182] Clinical and biochemical evaluations are performed annually; neck ultrasonography is frequently performed in case of doubt or in high-risk patients, but any other testing is unnecessary as long as the patient's serum Tg concentration is undetectable and the patient does not produce an interfering anti-Tg autoantibody.

Suspicious abnormalities at neck ultrasonography should be submitted to FNAB, even if serum Tg remains undetectable following TSH stimulation. Lymph node metastases are indeed treated, but currently there is no evidence that treatment at a very early stage (when lymph nodes measure less than 5 mm in diameter) may improve the outcome as compared to treatment at a stage when they measure 5 to 10 mm in diameter.

At 9 to 12 months, serum Tg becomes detectable following TSH stimulation in 14% to 20% of patients. The discovery of any other abnormality will dictate specific treatments. In the absence of any other abnormalities, suppressive thyroxine treatment is maintained and another rhTSH is performed some months or years later depending on serum Tg level and the clinical context. Serum Tg will decrease or become undetectable in the absence of any further treatment in two thirds of patients who then will be considered cured. Serum Tg will increase in the remaining one third of patients who should then be submitted to an extensive workes up, which may include ultrasound examination of the neck, helical CT of the lungs, bone scintigraphy, FDG-PET/CT scanning and administration of a large activity of ^{131}I with total body scanning 3 to 5 days later; clinical recurrence will likely be found in time for curative measures in most of this third of patients treated for PTC or FTC.

In very low-risk PTC patients who have had a near-total thyroidectomy but who were not given ^{131}I postoperatively, the intensity of the follow-up strategy depends largely on the serum Tg level and on neck sonography. If the Tg is not detectable during levothyroxine treatment and a neck ultrasound is negative, ^{131}I total body scanning may be avoided. However, if despite adequate TSH suppression, the Tg is readily detectable and increases with time, an ablative ^{131}I treatment may be necessary or, if no neck uptake persists, the responsible neck nodes may be treated either surgically or by radiofrequency or percutaneous ultrasound-guided ethanol injections.[183,184] The follow-up protocol previously described is then applied on the basis of serum Tg determinations.

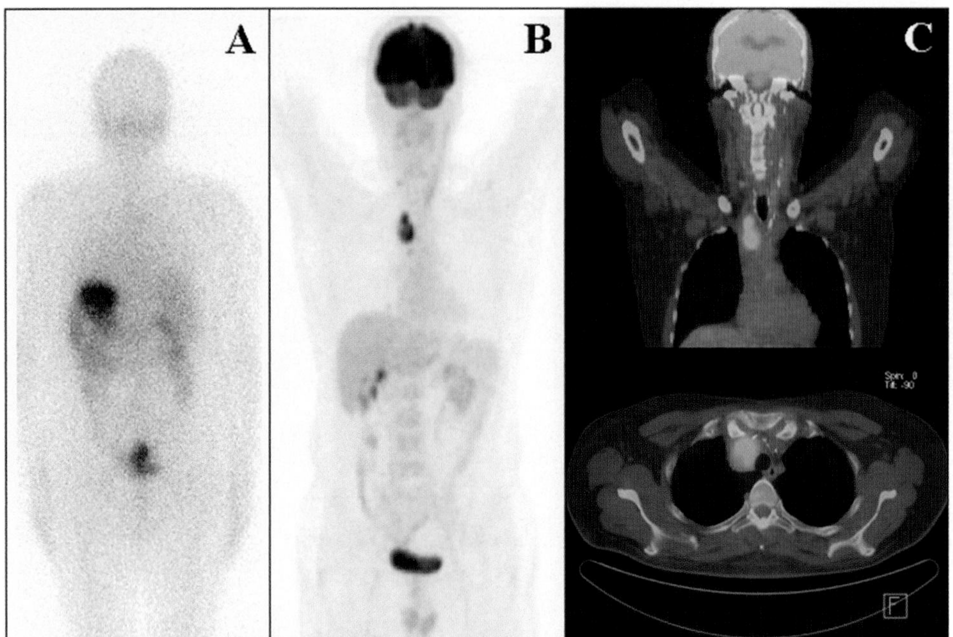

Figure 13–24 ▪ The patient was being monitored for a papillary thyroid carcinoma treated by total thyroidectomy and postoperative radioiodine. The serum thyroglobulin level was 45 ng/mL during levothyroxine suppressive treatment. **A,** Total body scan posterior view performed 3 days after administration of 100 mCi (3.7 GBq); there is no visible uptake in the neck and thorax; note accumulation of radioiodine in the stomach, colon, and bladder. **B,** Positron emission tomography scan using [^{18}F]fluorodeoxyglucose (^{18}FDG): maximal intensity projection demonstrating significant uptake in the upper mediastinum. **C,** Fusion images of ^{18}FDG-PET scan and CT scan: axial and coronal slices localizing the FDG uptake in the right paratracheal mediastinum and corresponding to a lymph node metastasis that was subsequently excised. Serum Tg became undetectable during thyroid hormone treatment.

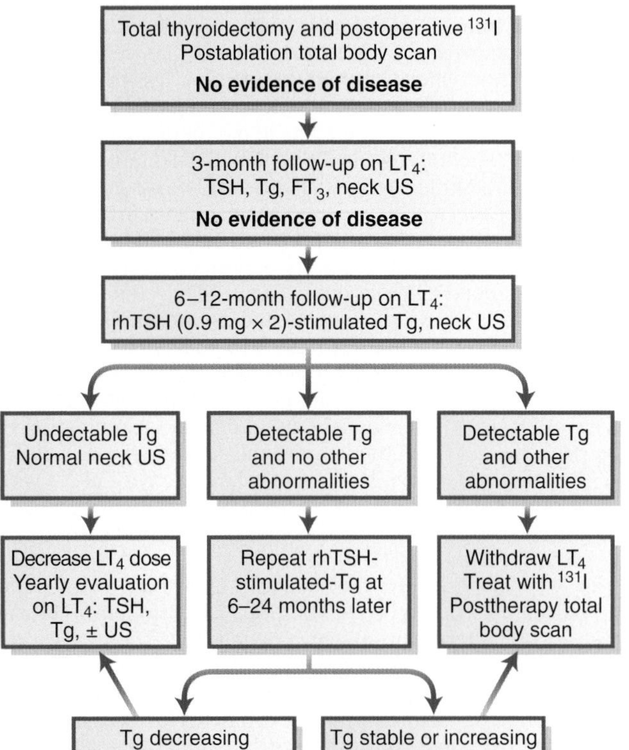

Figure 13–25 ▪ Follow-up of patients with PTC or FTC after near-total thyroidectomy and ^{131}I ablation, based on serum thyroglobulin (Tg) measurements and neck ultrasonography (US). *LT_4,* Levothyroxine; *TBS,* total body scan; *TSH,* thyrotropin; *Undetectable Tg,* Tg level below the detection limit of the assay. (From Schlumberger M, Berg G, Cohen O, et al. Follow-up of low-risk patients with differentiated thyroid carcinoma: a European perspective. Eur J Endocrinol 2004;50:105-112.)

In low-risk PTC patients who have initially undergone only a unilateral lobectomy for PTM, yearly follow-up should consist of a careful neck examination and serum Tg determination during levothyroxine treatment. With time, ultrasonography is likely to show focal nodular abnormalities in the remaining lobe in most patients with detectable Tg concentrations. Usually, biopsies of these lesions can be performed under sonographic guidance, and most prove to be cytologically benign. However, if recurrent PTC is found on biopsy, a completion thyroidectomy should be performed.

For MTC patients, the tumor marker for follow-up is the plasma calcitonin level. In about 90% of young patients whose disease is treated at a preclinical stage on the basis of a *RET* oncogene mutation, the postoperative calcitonin level returns to normal and peak levels after stimulation with either pentagastrin or calcium are absent.[148,149] Patients with a negative pentagastrin stimulation test after two follow-up evaluations are likely to be cured, even though approximately 5% of them have subsequent biologic recurrence of the disease.[81]

In adults with sporadic MTC, who most often present with TNM stage III (node-positive) disease, postoperative calcitonin levels are rarely normal.[183-185] In general, basal and stimulated calcitonin levels correlate with MTC tumor mass, but many MTC patients who have surgery with a curative intent still have postoperative elevations in calcitonin levels without clinical or imaging evidence of persistent disease. In these patients, the localization of neoplastic foci may be difficult and may require morphologic examinations with neck and liver ultrasonography, CT scan of the neck and chest, bone sintigraphy and MRI of bones and liver[11,12]; if tests are negative, a venous sampling catheterization with calcitonin measurements may be indicated.[184,185] Preliminary data of PET scanning with ^{18}F-DOPA are promising for localizing neoplastic MTC foci.[18] Reinterventions based on the results of selective venous sampling catheterization allow the removal of neoplastic foci in most patients, but they are not likely to improve the cure rate by more than 5% to 30%.[184,185] Such a situation may exist for several postoperative years, and slowly rising calcitonin levels may not necessarily imply a prognosis worse than that indicated by the presenting stage of disease.

A second major tumor marker for MTC is carcinoembryonic antigen (CEA). In general, serum CEA levels are higher in more malignant MTC, whereas the plasma calcitonin level is higher in those with better differentiated tumors, leading some authorities to suggest that a rising CEA level postoperatively correlates better with the emergence of a potentially aggressive tumor recurrence. The doubling times of calcitonin and CEA levels appear highly significant prognostic indicators for survival.[186]

Papillary and Follicular Thyroid Carcinoma

Locoregional Recurrences

Locoregional recurrences occur in 5% to 20% of patients with PTC and FTC. More than one third of reoperations for persistent or recurrent disease are related to inadequate initial thyroid surgery.[187] A recurrence that is palpable or easily visualized with ultrasonography or CT scanning should be excised.[188,189] Total excision may be facilitated by total body scanning 3 to 5 days after administration of 100 mCi (3700 MBq) of ^{131}I because additional tissue that should be excised may be identified. In some selected centers, surgery is performed 1 day later, typically using an intraoperative probe. The completeness of resection is verified 1 to 2 days after surgery by another total body scan, and in one series this was achieved in 92% of cases.[189] External radiotherapy is indicated only in FCTC patients with soft tissue recurrences that cannot be completely excised and that do not take up ^{131}I.

Recently, it has been reported that patients with PTC who were not eligible for further surgery or ^{131}I therapy have been treated for regional nodal recurrence with ultrasound-guided radiofrequency ablation or percutaneous ethanol injections (PEI).[190,191] Both techniques appear promising in selected PTC patients with recurrent nodal disease.

Distant Metastases

In a large group of patients with differentiated carcinoma (PTC, FTC, and HCC), only 9% developed DM.[192] Mortality rates at 5 and 10 years after the diagnosis of metastasis were 65% and 75% for all patients with DM, and nearly 80% of the deaths were due to thyroid cancer respectively.[192-194] Thus, the development of DM in FCTC portends an ominous prognosis. Lung metastases are more frequent in young patients with PTC, and the lung is almost the only site of distant spread in children. Bone metastases are more common in older patients and in those with FTC. Other less common sites are the brain, liver, and skin.[192-194]

Clinical symptoms of lung involvement are uncommon. By contrast, pain, swelling, or fracture occurs in more than 80% of patients with bone metastases. The pattern of lung involvement may vary from macronodular to diffuse infiltrates. The latter, when not detected by chest radiography, are usually diagnosed with ^{131}I total body scan and may be confirmed by helical CT; enlarged mediastinal lymph nodes are often present in patients with PTC, especially children. Bone metastases are osteolytic and are often difficult to visualize on radiographs; bone scintigraphy may show decreased or moderately increased uptake, and bone involvement is better visualized by MRI. Nearly all patients with DM have high serum Tg concentrations unless the lung metastases are not visible on radiographs, and two thirds of such patients have ^{131}I uptake in their sites of metastasis.

Palliative surgery is required for bone metastases when there are neurologic or orthopedic complications or a high risk of such complications. Surgery may also be performed with a curative intent in patients with a single or a few bone metastases.[195]

Patients with DM that take up ^{131}I are treated with 100 to 150 mCi (3700 to 5550 MBq) every 4 to 6 months during the first 2 years and then at longer intervals. Between ^{131}I treatments, suppressive doses of levothyroxine are given. The radiation dose to the tumor tissue and outcome of ^{131}I therapy are correlated.[159] A radiation dose higher than 80 Gy (8000 rads) should be delivered to obtain cure; with radiation doses less than 35 Gy (3500 rads), there is little chance for success. This is the rationale for using lithium salts in these patients, because their use may increase ^{131}I retention in tumor foci.[196] In patients with functioning metastases, PET scanning with ^{124}I showed that in a given patient, uptake may vary between metastases, and also within a given metastasis.[17] Finally, uptake may be heterogeneous at the cellular level.[105,106] This heterogeneity in the dose distribution in neoplastic foci may explain the ineffectiveness of ^{131}I treatment, despite significant uptake on total body scan. For treatment to be effective in this clinical setting, appropriate levels of TSH stimulation and absence of iodine contamination are essential. Prolonged withdrawal usually induces higher uptake than rhTSH, due to more prolonged stimulation and to longer body retention of ^{131}I, and should be the preferred method of TSH stimulation before radioiodine treatment in the absence of contraindication. Also, for this reason, higher activities (200 mCi [7400 MBq] or more) have been advocated in patients with bone metastases, but their effectiveness remains to be demonstrated. Lower doses (1 mCi [37 MBq]/kg body weight) are given to children. There is no limit to the cumulative dose of ^{131}I that can be given to patients with DM, although the risk of leukemia and of solid cancers rises significantly above a cumulative activity of 500 mCi (18,500 MBq); also, above this activity, further ^{131}I therapy may rarely provide significant benefit.[193]

External radiotherapy is given to bone metastases visible on radiographs, even in the presence of iodine uptake.[193] Alternatively, embolization or cement injection may be considered. Chemotherapy is poorly effective and should be given only to patients with progressing and nonfunctioning metastases.[197] Retinoic acid analogues increased iodine uptake by neoplastic tissue and decreased its growth rate in several in vitro models but are poorly effective in clinical settings. Molecular targeted therapies against tyrosine kinases and antiangiogenic drugs are promising.[198]

Disappearance of imaging abnormalities have been obtained overall in about 45% of patients with DM showing avidity for ^{131}I, and responses are even more frequent in younger patients and in those with small pulmonary metastases; complete responses may be obtained several years after initiation of therapy.[193,194] When response was judged to have been complete after ^{131}I therapy, subsequent relapse rarely occurred even though serum Tg levels were persistently detectable in some patients.[193]

Overall survival after the discovery of DM is more favorable in young patients with well-differentiated tumors that take up ^{131}I and have metastases that are small when discovered. When the tumor mass is considered, the location of the DM, be it in the lungs or bone, has no independent prognostic influence.[193] The poor prognosis of patients with bone metastases is linked to the large size of their lesions.[193-195] Large DMs with high FDG uptake on PET scanning almost never respond to ^{131}I therapy, confirming the clinical prognostic classification.[15] The prognostic importance of the small size of metastases at their discovery has led to the administration of 100 mCi (3700 MBq) activities of ^{131}I to patients who have elevated serum Tg concentrations that increase with time in the absence of obvious disease.[181] Some researchers believe that there is no conclusive evidence that ^{131}I treatment of these asymptomatic patients meaningfully prolongs life. Others have reported a 33% complete remission rate in treated patients who had a positive post-^{131}I therapy total body scan.

Complications of Treatment with Iodine 131

Acute side effects (nausea, sialadenitis, loss of taste) after treatment with ^{131}I are common but are typically mild and resolve rapidly. Radiation thyroiditis is usually trivial, but if the thyroid remnant is large, the patient may have enough pain to warrant corticosteroid therapy for a few days. Tumor in certain locations, such as the brain, spinal cord, and paratracheal region, may swell in response to TSH stimulation or after ^{131}I therapy, causing compressive symptoms. Xerostomia and obstruction of lacrimal ducts may occur in 5% to 10% of patients treated with ^{131}I.[199,200] Radiation fibrosis may develop in patients with diffuse lung metastases and can eventually prove fatal if high doses (>150 mCi [5550 MBq]) are administered at short intervals (<3 months).

Particular attention must be paid to avoid administration of ^{131}I to pregnant women. After ^{131}I treatment, spermatogenesis may be transiently depressed,[201] and women may have transient ovarian failure. Genetic damage induced by exposure to ^{131}I before conception has been a major subject of concern. However, the only anomaly reported to date is an increased frequency of miscarriages in women treated with ^{131}I during the year preceding the conception. Therefore, it is recommended that conception be postponed for 1 year after treatment with ^{131}I.[202] There is no evidence that pregnancy affects tumor growth in women receiving adequate levothyroxine therapy. In case of pregnancy in a patient treated with replacement dose of levothyroxine, the dose of levothyroxine is increased by 30% as soon as the pregnancy is confirmed and serum TSH level is measured every month during the first half of pregnancy.[203] In a patient treated with a suppressive dose of levothyroxine, serum TSH level is controlled every month, and the daily dose of levothyroxine is increased when serum TSH is found increased.

Mild pancytopenia may occur after repeated ^{131}I therapy, especially in patients with bone metastases also treated with external radiotherapy. The overall relative risk of leukemia and of solid tumors was found to be increased in patients treated with a high cumulative dose of ^{131}I (>500 mCi [18,500 MBq]) or in association with external radiotherapy.[204]

Medullary Thyroid Carcinoma

For patients with locoregional recurrence of MTC, a complete diagnostic work up should be obtained, principally to exclude DM. Surgery is performed when feasible and is typically followed by external radiotherapy.

DM is usually multifocal in each involved organ and frequently involve multiple organs, including liver, lungs, and bones. Metastasis may progress slowly and may be compatible with decades of survival. Systemic chemotherapy is poorly efficient and may be indicated only in cases of rapid tumor progression.[205] Symptomatic treatments are given, in particular against diarrhea. Chemoembolization with (Adriamycin) of liver metastasis provided a high response rate both on symptoms and on tumor masses.[206] Molecular targeted therapies directed against the RET or other tyrosine kinases are promising in this disease and are being evaluated in prospective clinical trials.[198]

REFERENCES

1. Price DC. Radioisotopic evaluation of the thyroid and the parathyroids. Radiol Clin North Am 1993;31:991-1015.
2. Meller J, Becker W. The continuing importance of thyroid scintigraphy in the era of high-resolution ultrasound. Eur J Nucl Med Mol Imaging 2002;29(suppl 2):S425-S438.
3. Robbins RJ, Schlumberger MJ. The evolving role of ^{131}I for the treatment of differentiated thyroid carcinoma. J Nucl Med 2005;46:28S-37S.
4. Loevinger R, Budinger TF, Watson EE. MIRD primer for absorbed dose calculations. New York: The Society of Nuclear Medicine, 1988.
5. Frates MC, Benson CB, Charboneau JW, et al. Management of thyroid nodules detected at US: Society of Radiologists in Ultrasound consensus conference statement. Radiology 2005;237:794-800.
6. Frasoldati A, Pesenti M, Gallo M, et al. Diagnosis of neck recurrences in patients with differentiated thyroid carcinoma. Cancer 2003;97:90-96.
7. Pacini F, Molinaro E, Castagna MG, et al. Recombinant human thyrotropin-stimulated serum thyroglobulin combined with neck ultrasonography has the highest sensitivity in monitoring differentiated thyroid carcinoma. J Clin Endocrinol Metab 2003;88:3668-3673.
8. Torlontano M, Attard M, Crocetti U, et al. Follow-up of low risk patients with papillary thyroid cancer: role of neck ultrasonography in detecting lymph node metastases. J Clin Endocrinol Metab 2004;89:3402-3407.
9. Phan TT, Jager PL, van Tol KM, Links TP. Thyroid cancer imaging. Cancer Treat Res 2004;122:317-343.
10. Alberico RA, Husain SH, Sirotkin I. Imaging in head and neck oncology. Surg Oncol Clin N Am 2004;13:13-35.
11. Mirallie E, Vuillez JP, Bardet S, et al. High frequency of bone/bone marrow involvement in advanced medullary thyroid cancer. J Clin Endocrinol Metab 2005;90:779-788.
12. Dromain C, de Baere T, Lumbroso J, et al. Detection of liver metastases from endocrine tumors: a prospective comparison of somatostatin receptor scintigraphy, computed tomography, and magnetic resonance imaging. J Clin Oncol 2005;23:70-78.
13. Dietlen M, Scheidhauer K, Voth E, et al. Fluorine-18-fluorodeoxyglucose positron emission tomography and iodine-131 whole-body scintigraphy in the follow-up of differentiated thyroid cancer. Eur J Nucl Med 1997;24:1342-1348.
14. Chin BB, Patel P, Cohade C, et al. Recombinant human thyrotropin stimulation of fluoro-D-glucose positron emission tomography uptake in well-differentiated thyroid carcinoma. J Clin Endocrinol Metab 2004;89:91-95.
15. Robbins RJ, Wan QW, Grewal RK, et al. Real-time prognosis for metastatic thyroid carcinoma based on 2-[^{18}F] fluoro-2-deoxy-D-glucose positron emission tomography. J Clin Endocrinol Metab 2006;91:498-505.
16. Van den Bruel A, Maes A, De Potter T, et al. Clinical relevance of thyroid fluorodeoxyglucose-whole body positron emission tomography incidentaloma. J Clin Endocrinol Metab 2002;87:1517-1520.
17. Sgouros G, Kolbert KS, Sheikh A, et al. Patient specific dosimetry for 131I thyroid cancer therapy using 124I PET and 3-dimensional-internal dosimetry (3D-ID) software. J Nucl Med 2004;45:1366-1372.
18. Gourgiotis L, Sarlis NJ, Reynolds JC, et al. Localization of medullary thyroid carcinoma metastasis in a multiple endocrine neoplasia type 2A patient by 6-(F-18)-fluorodopamine positron emission tomography. J Clin Endocrinol Metab 2003;88:637-641.
19. Vander JB, Gaston EA, Dawber TR. The significance of nontoxic thyroid nodules. Final report of a 15-year study of the incidence of thyroid malignancy. Ann Intern Med 1968;69:537-540.
20. Tunbridge WM, Evered DC, Hall R, et al. The spectrum of thyroid disease in a community: the Whickham survey. Clin Endocrinol (Oxf) 1977;7:481-493.
21. Mortensen JD, Woolner LB, Bennett WA. Gross and microscopic findings in clinically normal thyroid glands. J Clin Endocrinol Metab 1955;15:1270-1280.
22. Tan GH, Gharib H. Thyroid incidentalomas: management approaches to nonpalpable nodules discovered incidentally on thyroid imaging. Ann Intern Med 1997;126:226-231.
23. Hegedus L, Bonnema SJ, Bennedbaek FN. Management of simple nodular goiter: current status and future perspectives. Endocr Rev 2003;24:102-132.

24. Krohn K, Fuhrer D, Bayer Y, et al. Molecular pathogenesis of euthyroid and toxic multinodular goiter. Endocr Rev 2005;26:504-524.
25. Bignell GR, Canzian F, Shayeghi M, et al. Familial nontoxic multinodular thyroid goiter locus maps to chromosome 14q but does not account for familial nonmedullary thyroid cancer. Am J Hum Genet 1997;61:1123-1130.
26. Capon F, Tacconelli A, Giardina E, et al. Mapping a dominant form of multinodular goiter to chromosome Xp22. Am J Hum Genet 2000;67:1004-1007.
27. Abs R, Stevenaert A, Beckers A. Autonomously functioning thyroid nodules in a patient with a thyrotropin-secreting pituitary adenoma: possible cause-effect relationship. Eur J Endocrinol 1994;131:355-358.
28. Salvi M, Fukazawa H, Bernard N, et al. Role of autoantibodies in the pathogenesis and association of endocrine autoimmune disorders. Endocr Rev 1988;9:450-466.
29. Van Sande J, Parma J, Tonacchera M, et al. Genetic basis of endocrine disease. Somatic and germline mutations of the TSH receptor gene in thyroid diseases. J Clin Endocrinol Metab 1995: 80:2577-2585.
30. Bray GA. Increased sensitivity of the thyroid in iodine-depleted rats to the goitrogenic effects of thyrotropin. J Clin Invest 1968;47:1640-1647.
31. Apel RL, Ezzat S, Bapat BV, et al. Clonality of thyroid nodules in sporadic goiter. Diagn Mol Pathol 1995;4:113-121.
32. Foley TP. Goiter in adolescents. Endocrinol Metab Clin North Am 1993;22:593-606.
33. Glinoer D. The regulation of thyroid function during normal pregnancy: importance of the iodine nutrition status. Best Pract Res Clin Endocrinol Metab 2004;18:133-152.
34. Hennemann G. Goiter and pregnancy: a new insight into an old problem: comment. Thyroid 1992;2:71-72.
35. Alexander EK, Hurwitz S, Heering JP, et al. Natural history of benign solid and cystic thyroid nodules. Ann Intern Med 2003;138:315-318.
36. Anonymous. Cancer Fact and Figures. Atlanta: American Cancer Society, 2005.
37. Cooper DS, Doherty GM, Haugen BR, et al. Management guidelines for patients with thyroid nodules and differentiated thyroid cancer. Thyroid 2006;16:1-33.
38. Papini E, Guglielmi R, Bianchini A, et al. Risk of malignancy in nonpalpable thyroid nodules: predictive value of ultrasound and color-Doppler features. J Clin Endocrinol Metab 2002;87: 1941-1946.
39. Blum M, Rothschild M. Improved nonoperative diagnosis of the solitary "cold" thyroid nodule: surgical selection based on risk factors and three months of suppression. JAMA 1980;243: 242-245.
40. Okamoto T, Yamashita T, Harasawa A, et al. Test performances of three diagnostic procedures in evaluating thyroid nodules: physical examination, ultrasonography and fine needle aspiration cytology. Endocr J 1994;41:243-247.
41. Biondi B, Palmieri EA, Filetti S, et al. Mortality in elderly patients with subclinical hyperthyroidism. Lancet 2002;359:799-800.
42. Elisei R, Bottici V, Luchetti F, et al. Impact of routine measurement of serum calcitonin on the diagnosis and outcome of medullary thyroid cancer: experience in 10,864 patients with nodular thyroid disorders. J Clin Endocrinol Metab 2004;89:163-168.
43. Marx SJ. Molecular genetics of multiple endocrine neoplasia types 1 and 2. Nat Rev Cancer 2005;5:367-375.
44. Brandi ML, Gagel RF, Angeli A, et al. Guidelines for diagnosis and therapy of MEN type 1 and type 2. J Clin Endocrinol Metab 2001;86:5658-5671.
45. Zingrillo M, Torlontano M, Chiarella R, et al. Percutaneous ethanol injection may be a definitive treatment for symptomatic thyroid cystic nodules not treatable by surgery: five-year follow-up study. Thyroid 1999;9:763-767.
46. Hamburger JI. Diagnosis of thyroid nodules by fine needle biopsy: use and abuse. J Clin Endocrinol Metab 1994;79:335-339.
47. Gharib H. Changing concepts in the diagnosis and management of thyroid nodules. Endocrinol Metab Clin North Am 1997; 26:777-800.
48. Hales MS, Hsu FS. Needle tract implantation of papillary carcinoma of the thyroid following aspiration biopsy. Acta Cytol 1990;34:801-804.
49. Mikosch P, Gallowitsch HJ, Kresnik E, et al. Value of ultrasound-guided fine-needle aspiration biopsy of thyroid nodules in an endemic goitre area. Eur J Nucl Med 2000;27:62-69.
50. DeMicco C, Vasko V, Garcia S, et al. Fine needle aspiration of thyroid follicular neoplasm: diagnostic use of thyroid peroxidase immunochemistry with monoclonal antibody 47. Surgery 1994; 116:1031-1034
51. Mills LJ, Poller DN, Yiangou C. Galectin-3 is not useful in thyroid FNA. Cytopathology. 2005;16:132-138.
52. Carpi A, Nicolini A. The role of large-needle aspiration biopsy in the preoperative selection of palpable thyroid nodules: a summary of principal data. Biomed Pharmacother 2000;54:350-353.
53. Furlan JC, Bedard YC, Rosen IB. Role of fine-needle aspiration biopsy and frozen section in the management of papillary thyroid carcinoma subtypes. World J Surg 2004;28:880-885.
54. Greer MA, Astwood EB. Treatment of simple goiter with thyroid. J Clin Endocrinol 1953;13:1312-1331.
55. Ross DS. Thyroid hormone suppressive therapy of sporadic nontoxic goiter. Thyroid 1992;2:263-269.
56. Berghout A, Wiersinga WM, Drexhage HA, et al. Comparison of placebo with L-thyroxine alone or with carbimazole for treatment of sporadic nontoxic goitre. Lancet 1990;336:193-197.
57. Castro MR, Caraballo PJ, Morris JC. Effectiveness of thyroid hormone suppressive therapy in benign solitary thyroid nodules: a meta-analysis. J Clin Endocrinol Metab 2002;7:4154-4159.
58. Wemeau JL, Caron P, Schvartz C, et al. Effects of thyroid-stimulating hormone suppression with levothyroxine in reducing the volume of solitary thyroid nodules and improving extranodular nonpalpable changes: a randomized, double-blind, placebo-controlled trial by the French Thyroid Research Group. J Clin Endocrinol Metab 2002;87:4928-4934.
59. Surks MI, Ortiz E, Daniels GH, et al. Subclinical thyroid disease. Scientific review and guidelines for diagnosis and management. JAMA 2004;291:228-238.
60. Biondi B, Palmieri EA, Klain M, et al. Subclinical hyperthyroidism: clinical features and treatment options. Eur J Endocrinol 2005; 152:1-9.
61. Berghout A, Wiersinga WM, Drexhage HA, et al. The long-term outcome of thyroidectomy for sporadic nontoxic goitre. Clin Endocrinol (Oxf) 1989;31:193-199.
62. Agerback H, Pilegaard HK, Watt-Boolsen S, et al. Complications of 2,028 operations for benign thyroid disease. Ugeskr Laeger 1988;150:533-536.
63. Bistrup C, Nielsen JD, Gregersen G, et al. Preventive effect of levothyroxine in patients operated for nontoxic goitre: a randomized trial of one hundred patients with nine years follow-up. Clin Endocrinol (Oxf) 1994;40:323-327.
64. Bonnema SJ, Nielsen VE, Hegedus L. Long-term effects of radioiodine on thyroid function, size and patient satisfaction in non-toxic diffuse goitre. Eur J Endocrinol 2004:150:439-445.
65. Wesche MFT, Tiel-V Buul MCC, Lips P, et al. A randomized trial comparing levothyroxine with radioactive iodine in the treatment of sporadic nontoxic goiter. J Clin Endocrinol Metab 2001;86: 998-1005.
66. Manders JMB, Corstens FHM. Radioiodine therapy of euthyroid multinodular goiters. Eur J Nucl Med Mol Imaging 2002;29(suppl 2):S466-S40.
67. Nygaard B, Faber J, Hegedus L. Acute changes in thyroid volume and function following ^{131}I therapy of multinodular goiter. Clin Endocrinol (Oxf) 1994;41:715-718.
68. Holm LE, Hall P, Wiklund K, et al. Cancer risk after iodine-131 therapy for hyperthyroidism. J Natl Cancer Inst 1991;83: 1072-1077.
69. Huysmans DA, Nieuwlaat WA, Erdtsieck RJ, et al. Administration of a single low dose of recombinant human thyrotropin significantly enhances thyroid radioiodide uptake in nontoxic nodular goiter. J Clin Endocrinol Metab 2000;85:3592-3596.
70. Papini E, Guglielmi R, Bizzarri G, et al. Ultrasound-guided laser thermal ablation for treatment of benign thyroid nodules. Endocr Pract 2004;10:276-283.
71. Schlumberger MJ. Papillary and follicular thyroid carcinoma. N Engl J Med 1998;338:297-306.
72. Mazzaferri EL, Kloos RT. Current approaches to primary therapy for papillary and follicular thyroid cancer. J Clin Endocrinol Metab 2001;86:1447-1463.

73. Pacini F, Schlumberger M, Dralle H, et al. European consensus for the management of patients with differentiated thyroid cancer of the follicular epithelium. Eur J Endocrinol 2006;154: 783-803.
74. Hedinger C, Williams ED, Sobin LH. Histological typing of thyroid tumours, 2nd ed, no 11. In International Histological Classification of Tumours, World Health Organization. New York: Springer-Verlag, 1988:1-20.
75. Rosai J, Carganio ML, Delellis RA. Tumors of the Thyroid Gland. Washington, DC: Armed Forces Institute of Pathology, 1992.
76. Beahrs OH, Henson DE, Hutter RVP, et al. Manual for staging of cancer. Philadelphia: JB Lippincott, 1992.
77. American Joint Committee on Cancer. Thyroid. In AJCC Cancer Staging Handbook, 6th ed. New York: Springer, 2002:89-98.
78. Schlumberger M, de Vathaire F, Travagli JP, et al. Differentiated thyroid carcinoma in childhood: long term follow-up of 72 patients. J Clin Endocrinol Metab 1987;65:1088-1094.
79. Brierley J, Tsang R, Simpson WJ, et al. Medullary thyroid cancer: analyses of survival and prognostic factors and the role of radiation therapy in local control. Thyroid 1996;6:305-310.
80. Kebebew E, Ituarte PH, Siperstein AE, et al. Medullary thyroid carcinoma: clinical characteristics, treatment, prognostic factors, and a comparison of staging systems. Cancer 2000;88:1139-1148.
81. Modigliani E, Cohen R, Campos JM, et al. Prognostic factors for survival and for biochemical cure in medullary thyroid carcinoma: results in 899 patients. The GETC Study Group. Groupe d'Étude des Tumeurs á Calcitonine. Clin Endocrinol (Oxf) 1998;48:265-273.
82. Leboulleux S, Rubino C, Baudin E, et al. Prognostic factors for persistent or recurrent disease of papillary thyroid carcinoma with neck lymph node metastases and/or tumor extension beyond the thyroid capsule at initial diagnosis. J Clin Endocrinol Metab 2005;90:5723-5729.
83. Bisi H, Fernandes VS, Asato de Camargo RY, et al. The prevalence of unsuspected thyroid pathology in 300 sequential autopsies, with special reference to the incidental carcinoma. Cancer 1989;64:1888-1893.
84. Carney JA, Ryan J, Goellner JR. Hyalinizing trabecular adenoma of the thyroid gland. Am J Surg Pathol 1987;11:583-592.
85. Carcangiu ML, Bianchi S, Savino D, et al. Follicular Hürthle cell neoplasms of the thyroid gland: a study of 153 cases. Cancer 1991;68:1944-195.
86. Gundry SR, Burney RE, Thompson NW, et al. Total thyroidectomy for Hürthle cell neoplasm of the thyroid. Arch Surg 1983;118: 529-532.
87. Grant CS, Barr D, Goellner JR, et al. Benign Hürthle cell tumors of the thyroid: a diagnosis to be trusted? World J Surg 1988;12: 488-494.
88. Chen H, Nicol TL, Zeiger MA, et al. Hürthle cell neoplasms of the thyroid: are there factors predictive of malignancy? J Nucl Med 1998;34:1626-1631.
89. Suarez HG. Genetic alterations in human epithelial thyroid tumours. Clin Endocrinol (Oxf) 1998;48:531-546.
90. Hay ID. Papillary thyroid carcinoma. Endocrinol Metab Clin North Am 1990;19:545-576.
91. Hay ID, Thompson GB, Grant CS, et al. Papillary thyroid carcinoma managed at the Mayo Clinic during six decades (1940-1999): temporal trends in initial therapy and long-term outcome in 2444 consecutively treated patients. World J Surg 2002;26: 879-885.
92. Hay ID, Grant CS, van Heerden JA, et al. Papillary thyroid microcarcinoma: a study of 535 cases observed in a 50-year period. Surgery 1992;112:1139-1147.
93. Baudin E, Travagli J, Ropers J, et al. Microcarcinoma of the thyroid gland: the Gustave Roussy Institute experience. Cancer 1998;83: 553-559.
94. Fagin JA. Molecular pathogenesis. In Braverman LE, Utiger RD, eds. Werner & Ingbar's The Thyroid, A Fundamental and Clinical Text, 8th ed. Philadelphia: Lippincott Williams & Wilkins, 2000:886-898.
95. Pierotti MA, Bongarzone I, Borrello MG, et al. Cytogenetics and molecular genetics of carcinomas arising from thyroid epithelial follicular cells. Genes Chromosom Cancer 1996;16:1-14.
96. Fagin JA. Challenging dogma in thyroid cancer molecular genetics. Role of RET/PTC and BRAF in tumor initiation. J Clin Endocrinol Metab 2004;89:4264-4266.
97. Herrmann MA, Hay ID, Bartlet DH, et al. Cytogenetic and molecular genetic studies of follicular and papillary thyroid cancers. J Clin Invest 1991;88:1596-1603.
98. Williams ED. Cancer after nuclear fallout: lessons from the Chernobyl accident. Nat Rev 2002;2:543-549.
99. Vasko V, Ferrand M, Di Cristofaro J, et al. Specific pattern of RAS oncogene mutations in follicular thyroid tumors. J Clin Endocrinol Metab 2003;88:2745-2752.
100. Cohen Y, Xing M, Mambo E, et al. BRAF mutation in papillary thyroid carcinoma. J Natl Cancer Inst 2003;95:625-627.
101. Ciampi R, Knauf JA, Kerler R, et al. Oncogenic AKAP9-BRAF fusion is a novel mechanism of MAPK pathway activation in thyroid cancer. J Clin Invest 2005;115:20-23.
102. Melillo RM, Castellone MD, Guarino V, et al. The RET/PTC-RAS-BRAF linear signaling cascade mediates the motile and mitogenic phenotype of thyroid cancer cells. J Clin Invest 2005;115: 1069-1081.
103. Sturgeon C, Clark OH. Familial nonmedullary thyroid cancer. Thyroid 2005;15:588-593.
104. Harach HR. Familial nonmedullary thyroid neoplasia. Endocr Pathol 2002;12:97-112.
105. Schlumberger M, Lacroix L, Russo D, et al: Defects in iodine metabolism in thyroid caucer and implications for the follow-up and treatment of patients. Nat Clin Pract Endocrin of Metab 2007;3:260-269.
106. Lacroix L, Pourcher T, Magnon C, et al. Expression of the apical iodide transporter in human thyroid tissues: a comparison study with other iodide transporters. J Clin Endocrinol Metab 2004;89: 1423-1428.
107. Mitchell JC, Parangi S. Angiogenesis in benign and malignant thyroid disease. Thyroid 2005;15:494-510.
108. Colonna M, Grosclaude P, Remontet L, et al. Incidence of thyroid cancer in adults recorded by French cancer registries (1978-1997). Eur J Cancer 2002;38:1762-1768.
109. Shattuck TM, Westra WH, Ladenson PW, et al. Independent clonal origins of distinct tumor foci in multifocal thyroid carcinoma. N Engl J Med 2005;352:2406-2412.
110. Zimmerman D, Hay ID, Gough IR, et al. Papillary thyroid carcinoma in children and adults: long-term follow-up of 1,039 patients conservatively treated at one institution during three decades. Surgery 1988;104:1157-1166.
111. Kukkonen ST, Haapiainen RK, Fransila KO, et al. Papillary thyroid carcinoma: the new, age-related TNM classification system in a retrospective analysis of 199 patients. World J Surg 1990;14: 837-842.
112. Grant CS, Hay ID, Gough IR, et al. Local recurrence in papillary thyroid carcinoma: is extent of surgical resection important? Surgery 1988;104:954-962.
113. Hay ID, Grant CS, Taylor WF, et al. Ipsilateral lobectomy versus bilateral lobar resection in papillary thyroid carcinoma: a retrospective analysis of surgical outcome using a novel prognostic scoring system. Surgery 1987;102:1088-1095.
114. Tsang RW, Brierley JD, Simpson WJ, et al. The effects of surgery, radioiodine, and external radiation therapy on the clinical outcome of patients with differentiated thyroid carcinoma. Cancer 1998;82:375-388.
115. DeGroot LJ, Kaplan EL, McCormick M, et al. Natural history, treatment and course of papillary thyroid carcinoma. J Clin Endocrinol Metab 1990;71:414-424.
116. Shah JP, Loree TR, Dharker D, et al. Prognostic factors in differentiated carcinoma of the thyroid gland. Am J Surg 1992;164: 658-661.
117. Akslen LA, Livolsi VA. Prognostic significance of histologic grading compared with subclassification of papillary thyroid carcinoma. Cancer 2000;88:1902-1908.
118. Hay ID, Bergstralh EJ, Goellner JR, et al. Predicting outcome in papillary thyroid carcinoma: development of a reliable prognostic scoring system in a cohort of 1,779 patients surgically treated at one institution during 1940 through 1989. Surgery 1993;114: 1050-1058.
119. Brierley JD, Panzarella T, Tsang RW, et al. A comparison of different staging systems predictability of patient outcome: thyroid carcinoma as an example. Cancer 1997;79:2414-2423.
120. Carcangiu MC, Zempi G, Rosai J. Poorly differentiated ("insular") thyroid carcinoma: a reinterpretation of Langhans "wuchernde Struma." Am J Surg Pathol 1984;8:655-668.

121. Sobrinho-Simoes M. Mixed medullary and follicular carcinoma of the thyroid. Histopathology 1993;23:187-189.
122. Grebe SKG, Hay ID. Follicular thyroid cancer. Endocrinol Metab Clin North Am 1996;24:761-801.
123. Livolsi VA, Asa SL. The demise of follicular carcinoma of the thyroid gland. Thyroid 1994;4:233-236.
124. Livolsi VA, Merino MJ. Worrisome histologic alterations following fine-needle aspiration of the thyroid. Pathol Annu 1994;29: 99-120.
125. Chevillard S, Ugolin N, Vielh P, et al. Gene expression profiling of differentiated thyroid neoplasms: diagnostic and clinical implications. Clin Cancer Res 2004;10:6586-6597.
126. Cerutti JM, Delcelo R, Amadei MJ, et al. A preoperative diagnostic test that distinguishes benign from malignant thyroid carcinoma based on gene expression. J Clin Invest 2004;113:1234-1242.
127. Barden CB, Shister KW, Zhu B, et al. Classification of follicular thyroid tumors by molecular signature: results of gene profiling. Clin Cancer Res 2003;9:1792-1800.
128. Weber F, Shen L, Aldred MA, et al. Genetic classification of benign and malignant thyroid follicular neoplasia based on a three-gene combination. J Clin Endocrinol Metab 2005;90: 2512-2521.
129. Ishimaru Y, Fukuda S, Kurano R, et al. Follicular thyroid carcinoma with clear cell change showing unusual ultrastructural features. Am J Surg Pathol 1988;12:240-246.
130. Watson RG, Brennan MD, Goellner JR, et al. Invasive Hürthle cell carcinoma of the thyroid: natural history and management. Mayo Clin Proc 1984;59:851-855.
131. Roque L, Rodrigues R, Pinto A, et al. Chromosome imbalance in thyroid follicular neoplasms: a comparison between adenomas and carcinomas. Genes Chromosom Cancer 2003;36:292-302.
132. Kroll TG, Sarraf P, Pecciarini L, et al. *PAX8-PPARγ1* fusion oncogene in human thyroid carcinoma. Science 2000;289: 1357-1360.
133. Powell GJ, Wang X, Allard BL, et al. The PAX8/PPAR gamma fusion oncoprotein transforms immortalized human thyrocytes through a mechanism probably involving wild-type PPAR gamma inhibition. Oncogene 2004;23:3634-3641.
134. Nikiforova MN, Lynch RA, Biddinger PW, et al. RAS point mutations and PAX8-PPAR gamma rearrangement in thyroid tumors: evidence for distinct molecular pathways in thyroid follicular carcinoma. J Clin Endocrinol Metab 2003;88:2318-2326.
135. Paul SJ, Sisson JC. Thyrotoxicosis caused by thyroid cancer. Endocrinol Metab Clin North Am 1990;19:593-612.
136. Grebe SKG, Hay ID. Thyroid cancer nodal metastases: biologic significance and therapeutic considerations. Surg Oncol Clin North Am 1996;5:43-63.
137. van Heerden JA, Hay ID, Goellner JR, et al. Follicular thyroid carcinoma with capsular invasion alone: a non-threatening malignancy. Surgery 1992;112:1130-1136.
138. Mueller-Gaertner HW, Brzac HT, Rehpenning W. Prognostic indices for tumor relapse and tumor mortality in follicular thyroid carcinoma. Cancer 1991;67:1903-1908.
139. Cady R, Rossi R. An expanded view of risk-group definition in differentiated thyroid carcinoma. Surgery 1985;98:1171-1176.
140. Shaha AR, Loree TR, Shah JP. Prognostic factors and risk group analysis in follicular carcinoma of the thyroid. Surgery 1995;118:1131-1138.
141. Emerick GT, Duh QY, Siperstein AE, et al. Diagnosis, treatment, and outcome of follicular thyroid carcinoma. Cancer 1993;72: 3287-3294.
142. Davis NL, Bugis SD, McGregor GI, et al. An evaluation of prognostic scoring systems in patients with follicular thyroid cancer. Am J Surg 1995;170:476-480.
143. d'Avanzo A, Ituarte P, Treseler P, et al. Prognostic scoring systems in patients with follicular thyroid cancer: a comparison of different staging systems in predicting the patient outcome. Thyroid 2004;14:453-458.
144. McIver B, Hay ID, Giuffrida DF, et al. Anaplastic thyroid carcinoma: a 50-year experience at a single institution. Surgery 2001;130: 1028-1034.
145. De Crevoisier R, Baudin E, Bachelot A, et al. Combined treatment of anaplastic thyroid carcinoma with surgery, chemotherapy, and hyperfractionated accelerated external radiotherapy. Int J Radiation Oncology Biol Phys 2004;60:1137-1143.
146. Kebebew E, Greenspan FS, Clark OH, et al. Anaplastic thyroid carcinoma. Treatment outcome and prognostic factors. Cancer 2005;103:1330-1335.
147. Leboulleux S, Baudin E, Travagli JP, et al. Medullary thyroid carcinoma. Clin Endocrinol (Oxf) 2004;61:299-310.
148. Machens A, Niccoli-Sire P, Hoegel J, et al. Early malignant progression of hereditary medullary thyroid cancer. N Engl J Med 2003;349:1517-1525.
149. Skinner MA, Moley JA, Dilley WG, et al. Prophylactic thyroidectomy in multiple endocrine neoplasia type 2A. N Engl J Med 2005;353:1105-1113.
150. Moley JF, DeBenedetti MK. Patterns of nodal metastases in palpable medullary thyroid carcinoma. Recommendations for extent of node dissection. Ann Surg 1999;6:880-888.
151. Scollo C, Baudin E, Travagli JP, et al. Rationale for central and bilateral lymph node dissection in sporadic and hereditary medullary thyroid cancer. J Clin Endocrinol Metab 2003;88:2070-2075.
152. Thieblemont C, Mayer A, Dumontet C, et al. Primary thyroid lymphoma is a heterogeneous disease. J Clin Endocrinol Metab 2002;87:105-111.
153. Harris NL, Jaffe ES, Stein H, et al. A revised European-American classification of lymphoid neoplasms: a proposal from the International Lymphoma Study Group. Blood 1994;84:1361-1392.
154. Hay ID, Bergstralh EJ, Grant CS, et al. Impact of primary surgery on outcome in 300 patients with pathologic tumor-node-metastasis stage III papillary thyroid carcinoma treated at one institution from 1940 through 1989. Surgery 1999;126:1173-1181.
155. Hartl DM, Travagli JP, Leboulleux S, et al. Current concepts in the management of unilateral recurrent laryngeal nerve paralysis after thyroid surgery. J Clin Endocrinol Metab 2005;90: 3084-3088.
156. Schneider AB, Sarne DH. Long-term risks for thyroid cancer and other neoplasm after exposure to radiation. Nat Clin Pract Endocrinol Metab 2005;1:82-91.
157. Rubino C, Cailleux AF, Abbas M, et al. Characteristics of follicular cell-derived thyroid carcinomas occurring after external radiation exposure: results of a case control study nested in a cohort. Thyroid 2002;12:299-304.
158. Pacini F, Schlumberger M, Harmer C, et al. Post-surgical use of radioiodine (131I) in patients with papillary and follicular thyroid cancer and the issue of remnant ablation: a consensus report. Eur J Endocrinol 2005;153:651-659.
159. Maxon HR, Thomas SR, Hertzberg VS, et al. Relation between effective radiation dose and outcome of radioiodine therapy for thyroid cancer. N Engl J Med 1983;309:937-941.
160. Eustatia-Rutten CFA, Smit JWA, Romijn JA, et al. Diagnostic value of serum thyroglobulin measurements in the follow-up of differentiated thyroid carcinoma, a structured meta-analysis. Clin Endocrinol (Oxf) 2004;61:61-74.
161. Toubeau M, Touzery C, Arveux P, et al. Predictive value for disease progression of serum thyroglobulin levels measured in the post-operative period and after (^{131}I) ablation therapy in patients with differentiated thyroid cancer. J Nucl Med 2004;45:988-994.
162. Lassman M, Luster M, Hanscheid H, et al. The impact of I-131 diagnostic activities on the biokinetics of thyroid remnants. J Nucl Med 2004;45:619-625.
163. Postgard P, Jimmelman J, Lindencrona U, et al. Stunning of iodine transport by (131)I irradiation in cultured thyroid epithelial cells. J Nucl Med 2002;43:828-834.
164. Cailleux AF, Baudin E, Travagli JP, et al. Is diagnostic iodine-131 scanning useful after total thyroid ablation for differentiated thyroid cancer? J Clin Endocrinol Metab 2000;85:175-178.
165. Pacini F, Capezzone M, Elisei R, et al. Diagnostic 131-iodine whole-body scan may be avoided in thyroid cancer patients who have undetectable stimulated serum Tg levels after initial treatment. J Clin Endocrinol Metab 2002;87:1499-1501.
166. Schlumberger M, Berg G, Cohen O, et al. Follow-up of low-risk patients with differentiated thyroid carcinoma: a European perspective. Eur J Endocrinol 2004;50:105-112.
167. Bal CS, Kumar A, Pant GS. Radioiodine dose for remnant ablation in differentiated thyroid carcinoma: a randomized clinical trial in 509 patients. J Clin Endocrinol Metab 2004;89:1666-1673.
168. Sawka AM, Thephamongkhol K, Brouwers M, et al. A systemic review and metaanalysis of the effectiveness of radioactive iodine remnant ablation for well-differentiated thyroid cancer. J Clin Endocrinol Metab 2004;89:3668-3676.

169. Pacini F, Ladenson PW, Schlumberger M, et al. Radioiodine ablation of thyroid remnants after preparation with recombinant human thyrotropin in differentiated thyroid carcinoma: results of an international, randomized, controlled study. J Clin Endocrinol Metab 2006;91:926-932.
170. Farahati J, Reiners C, Stuschke M, et al. Differentiated thyroid cancer: impact of adjuvant external radiotherapy in patients with perithyroidal tumor infiltration (stage pT4). Cancer 1996;77:172-180.
171. Biondi B, Filetti S, Schlumberger M. Thyroid-hormone therapy and thyroid cancer: a reassessment. Nat Clin Pract Endocrinol Metab 2005;1:32-40.
172. Pacini F, Fugazzola L, Lippi F, et al. Detection of thyroglobulin in fine needle aspirates of nonthyroidal neck masses: a clue to the diagnosis of metastatic differentiated thyroid cancer. J Clin Endocrinol Metab 1992;74:1401-1404.
173. Arturi F, Russo D, Giuffrida D, et al. Early diagnosis by genetic analysis of differentiated thyroid cancer metastases in small lymph nodes. J Clin Endocrinol Metab 1997;82:1638-1641.
174. Balogh Z, Carayon P, Conte-Devolx B, et al: Laboratory medicine practice guidelines. Laboratory support for the diagnosis and monitoring of thyroid disease. Thyroid 2003;13:3-126.
175. Chiovato L, Latrofa F, Braverman LE, et al. Disappearance of humoral thyroid autoimmunity after complete removal of thyroid antigens. Ann Intern Med 2003;139:346-351.
176. Bachelot A, Cailleux AF, Klain M, et al. Relationship between tumor burden and serum thyroglobulin level in patients with papillary and follicular thyroid carcinoma. Thyroid 2002;12:707-711.
177. Haugen BR, Pacini F, Reiners C, et al. A comparison of recombinant human thyrotropin and thyroid hormone withdrawal for the detection of thyroid remnant or cancer. J Clin Endocrinol Metab 1999;84:3877-3885.
178. Baudin E, Do Cao C, Cailleux AF, et al. Positive predictive value of serum thyroglobulin levels, measured during the first year of follow-up after thyroid hormone withdrawal in thyroid cancer patients. J Clin Endocrinol Metab 2003;88:1107-1111.
179. Pacini F, Agate L, Elisel R, et al. Outcome of differentiated thyroid cancer with detectable serum Tg and negative diagnostic ^{131}I whole-body scan: comparison of patients treated with high ^{131}I activities versus untreated patients. J Clin Endocrinol Metab 2001;86:4092-4097.
180. Ringel MD, Balducci-Silano PL, Anderson JS, et al. Quantitative reverse transcription-polymerase chain reaction of circulating thyroglobulin messenger ribonucleic acid for monitoring patients with thyroid carcinoma. J Clin Endocrinol Metab 1999;84:4037-4042.
181. Schlumberger M, Mancusi F, Baudin E, et al. ^{131}I therapy for elevated thyroglobulin levels. Thyroid 1997;7:273-276.
182. Cooper DS, Specker B, Ho M, et al. Thyrotropin suppression and disease progression in patients with differentiated thyroid cancer: results from the National Thyroid Cancer Treatment Cooperative Registry. Thyroid 1998;8:737-744.
183. van Heerden JA, Grant CS, Gharib H, et al. Long-term course of patients with persistent hypercalcitoninemia after apparent curative primary surgery for medullary thyroid carcinoma. Ann Surg 1990;212:395-400.
184. Pellegriti G, Leboulleux S, Baudin E, et al. Long-term outcome of medullary thyroid carcinoma in patients with normal postoperative medical imaging. Br J Cancer 2003;88:1537-1542.
185. Kebebew E, Kikuchi S, Duh QY, et al. Long-term results of reoperation and localizing studies in patients with persistent or recurrent medullary thyroid cancer. Arch Surg 2000;135:895-901.
186. Barbet J, Campion L, Kraeber-Bodéré F, et al. Prognostic impact of serum calcitonin and carcinoembryonic antigen doubling-times in patients with medullary thyroid carcinoma. J Clin Endocrinol Metab 2005;90:6077-6084.
187. Kouvaraki MA, Lee JE, Shapiro SE, Sherman SI, et al. Preventable reoperations for persistent and recurrent papillary thyroid carcinoma. Surgery 2004;136:1183-1191.
188. Pacini F, Cetani F, Miccoli P, et al. Outcome of 309 patients with metastatic differentiated thyroid carcinoma treated with radioiodine. World J Surg 1994;18:600-604.
189. Travagli JP, Cailleux AF, Ricard M, et al. Combination of radioiodine (^{131}I) and probe-guided surgery for persistent or recurrent thyroid carcinoma. J Clin Endocrinol Metab 1998;83:2675-2680.
190. Dupuy DE, Monchik JM, Decrea C, et al. Radiofrequency ablation of regional recurrence from well-differentiated thyroid malignancy. Surgery 2001;130:971-977.
191. Lewis BD, Hay ID, Charboneau JW, et al. Percutaneous ethanol injection for treatment of cervical lymph node metastases in patients with papillary thyroid carcinoma. Am J Radiol 2002; 178:301-306.
192. Ruegemer JJ, Hay ID, Bergstralh EJ, et al. Distant metastases in differentiated thyroid carcinoma: a multivariate analysis of prognostic variables. J Clin Endocrinol Metab 1988;63:960-967.
193. Durante C, Haddy N, Baudin E, et al: Long term outcome of 444 patients with distant metastases from papillary and follicular thyroid carcinoma: benefits and limits of radioiodine therapy. J Clin Endocrinol Metab 2006;91:2892-2899.
194. Casara D, Rubello D, Saladini G, et al. Different features of pulmonary metastases in differentiated thyroid cancer: natural history and multivariate statistical analysis of prognostic variables. J Nucl Med 1993;34:1626-1631.
195. Bernier MO, Leenhardt L, Hoang C, et al. Survival and therapeutic modalities in patients with bone metastases of differentiated thyroid carcinomas. J Clin Endocrinol Metab 2001;86:1568-1573.
196. Koong S, Reynolds J, Movius E, et al. Lithium as a potential adjuvant to 131I therapy of metastatic, well-differentiated thyroid carcinoma. J Clin Endocrinol Metab 1999;84:912-916.
197. Shimaoka K, Schoenfeld DA, DeWys WD, et al. A randomized trial of doxorubicin versus doxorubicin plus cisplatin in patients with advanced thyroid carcinoma. Cancer 1985;56:2155-2160.
198. Baudin E, Schlumberger M: New therapeutic approaches for metastatic thyroid carcinoma. Lancet Oncol 2007;8:148-156.
199. Kloos RT, Duvuuri V, Jhiang SM, et al. Nasolacrimal drainage system obstruction from radioactive iodine therapy for thyroid carcinoma. J Clin Endocrinol Metab 2002;87:5817-5820.
200. Mandel SJ, Mandel L. Radioactive iodine and the salivary glands. Thyroid 2003;13:265-271.
201. Pacini F, Gasperi M, Fugazzola L, et al. Testicular function in patients with differentiated thyroid carcinoma treated with radioiodine. J Nucl Med 1994;35:1418-1422.
202. Schlumberger M, de Vathaire F, Ceccarelli C, et al. Exposure to radioactive iodine-131 for scintigraphy or therapy does not preclude pregnancy in thyroid cancer patients. J Nucl Med 1996; 37:606-612.
203. Alexander EK, Marqusee E, Lawrence J, et al. Timing and magnitude of increase in levothyroxine requirements during pregnancy in women with hypothyroidism. N Engl J Med 2004;351:241-249.
204. Rubino C, De Vathaire F, Dottorini ME, et al. Second primary malignancies in thyroid cancer patients. Br J Cancer 2003;89:1638-1644.
205. Nocera M, Baudin E, Pellegriti G, et al. Treatment of advanced medullary thyroid cancer with an alternating combination of doxorubicin-streptozocin and 5 FU-dacarbazine. Groupe d'Étude des Tumeurs a Calcitonine (GETC). Br J Cancer 2000;83:715-718.
206. Fromigué J, De Baere T, Baudin E, et al: Chemoembolization for liver metastases from meslullary thyroid carcinoma. J Clin Endocrinol Metab 2006;91:2496-2499.

SECTION IV

Adrenal Cortex and Endocrine Hypertension

CHAPTER 14

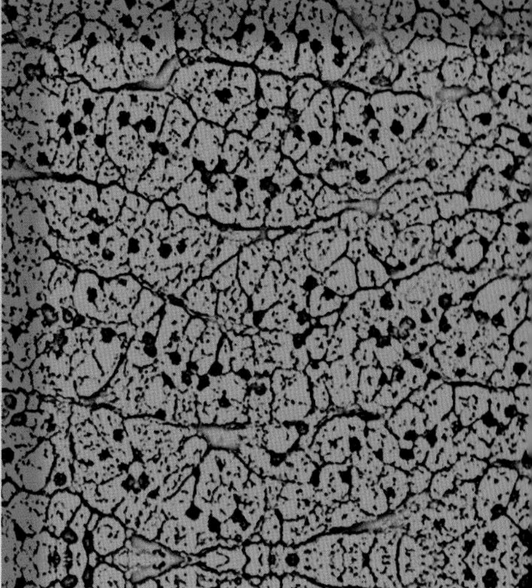

THE ADRENAL CORTEX

Paul M. Stewart

THE ADRENAL CORTEX—HISTORICAL MILESTONES

The anatomy of the adrenal glands was described almost 450 years ago by Bartholomeo Eustacius[1] and the zonation of the gland and its distinction from the medulla elucidated shortly thereafter. However, a functional role for the adrenal glands was not accurately defined until the pioneering work of Thomas Addison who described the clinical and autopsy findings in 11 cases of "Addison's disease" in his classical monograph in 1855.[2] Just a year later Brown-Séquard demonstrated that the adrenal glands were "organs essential for life" by performing adrenalectomies in dogs, cats, and guinea pigs.[3] In 1896, William Osler first administered adrenal extract to a patient with Addison's disease, a feat that was repeated by others in both animal and human studies over the next 40 years. As a consequence, between 1937 and 1955 the adrenocorticosteroid hormones were isolated, their structures defined and synthesised,[4] notable breakthroughs being the discovery of cortisone and the clinical evaluation of its antiinflammatory effect in patients with rheumatoid arthritis,[5] and the isolation of aldosterone.[6]

The control of adrenocortical function by a pituitary factor was demonstrated in the 1920s, which led to the isolation of sheep adrenocorticotropic hormone (ACTH) by Li, Evans, and Simpson in 1943.[7] Such a concept was supported through clinical studies, notably by Harvey Cushing in 1932 who associated his original clinical observations of 1912 (a "polyglandular syndrome" caused by pituitary basophilism) with adrenal hyperactivity.[8] The neural control of pituitary ACTH secretion by corticotropin-releasing factor was defined by Harris and other workers in the 1940s, but corticotropin-releasing factor (CRF) was not characterized and synthesized until 1981 in the laboratory of Wylie Vale.[9] Jerome Conn described primary aldosteronism in 1955[10] and the control of adrenal aldosterone secretion by angiotensin II was confirmed shortly afterward. Recent advances in radioimmunoassay and particularly molecular biology have facilitated an exponential increase in our understanding of adrenal physiology and pathophysiology (Table 14–1).

ANATOMY

The adrenal cortex derives from mesenchymal cells attached to the coelomic cavity lining adjacent to the urogenital ridge. The fetal adrenal is evident from 6 to 8 weeks' gestation and rapidly increases in size so that by midgestation it is larger than its adjacent kidney. In fetal life, and up to 12 months postpartum, two distinct zones are evident, an inner prominent fetal zone and an outer definitive zone that differentiates into the adult adrenal gland. Postpartum the fetal zone regresses and the definitive zone containing an inner zona fasciculata and outer glomerulosa proliferates.[11,12] The innermost zone, the zona reticularis is evident after 1 year of life. The differentiation of the adrenal cortex into distinct zones has important functional consequences and is thought to be dependent upon the temporal expression of transcription factors including Pref-1/ZOG, inner zone antigen, and steroidogenic factor-1.[13,14]

The adult gland is a pyramidal structure, approximately 4 g in weight, 2 cm wide, 5 cm long, and 1 cm thick lying immediately above the kidney on its posteromedial surface. Beneath the capsule, the zona glomerulosa comprises approximately 15% of the cortex (depending upon sodium intake) (Fig. 14–1). Cells are clustered in spherical nests and are small with smaller nuclei in comparison to other zones. The zona fasciculata comprises 75% of the cortex; cells are large and lipid-laden and form radial cords between the fibrovascular radial network. The

TABLE 14–1 HISTORY OF THE ADRENAL CORTEX: IMPORTANT MILESTONES

1563	Eustachius describes the adrenals (published by Lancisi in 1714).
1849	Thomas Addison, while searching for the cause of pernicious anemia, "stumbles" on a bronzed appearance associated with the adrenal glands—"melasma suprarenale."
1855	Thomas Addison describes the clinical features and autopsy findings of 11 cases of diseases of the suprarenal capsules, at least 6 of which were tuberculous in origin.
1856	In adrenalectomy experiments, Brown-Séquard demonstrates that the adrenal glands are essential for life.
1896	William Osler gives an oral glycerine extract derived from pig adrenals and demonstrates clinical benefit in patients with Addison's disease.
1905	Bulloch and Sequeria describe patients with congenital adrenal hyperplasia.
1929	Liquid extracts of cortical tissue are used to keep adrenalectomized cats alive indefinitely (Swingle and Pfiffner). Subsequently, this extract was used successfully to treat a patient with Addison's disease (Rowntree and Greene).
1932	Harvey Cushing associates the "polyglandular syndrome" of pituitary basophilism first described by him in 1912 with hyperactivity of the pituitary-adrenal glands.
1936	Concept of stress and its effect upon pituitary-adrenal function described by Seyle.
1937–1952	Isolation and structural characterisation of adrenocortical hormones (Kendall, Reichstein).
1943	Li and colleagues isolate pure adrenocorticotropic hormone from sheep pituitary.
1950	Hench, Kendall, and Reichstein share Nobel Prize in medicine for describing the anti-inflammatory effects of cortisone in patients with rheumatoid arthritis.
1953	Isolation and analysis of the structure of aldosterone (Simpson and Tait).
1956	Conn describes primary aldosteronism.
1981	Characterization and synthesis of corticotropin-releasing hormone (Vale).
1980–present	The "molecular era." Cloning and functional characterization of steroid receptors, steroidogenic enzymes, and adrenal transcription factors. Definition of the molecular basis for human adrenal diseases.

innermost zona reticularis is sharply demarcated from both the zona fasciculata and adrenal medulla. Cells here are irregular with little lipid content. The maintenance of normal adrenal size appears to involve a progenitor cell population lying between the zona glomerulosa and zona fasciculata; cell migration and differentiation occur within the fasciculata and senescence occurs within the reticularis, but the factors regulating this important aspect of adrenal regeneration are unknown. ACTH administration results in glomerulosa cells adopting a fasciculata phenotype and, in turn, the innermost fasciculata cells adopt a reticularis phenotype that is reversible upon withdrawal of ACTH.

The vasculature of the adrenal cortex is complex. Arterial supply is conveyed by up to 12 small arteries from the aorta, inferior phrenic, renal, and intercostal arteries. These branch to form a subcapsular arteriolar plexus from which radial capillaries penetrate deeper into the cortex. In the zona reticularis, a dense sinusoidal plexus is created, which empties into a central vein. The right adrenal vein is short, draining directly into the inferior vena cava while the longer left adrenal vein usually drains into the left renal vein.

ADRENAL STEROIDS AND STEROIDOGENESIS

Three main types of hormone are produced by the adrenal cortex—glucocorticoids (cortisol, corticosterone), mineralocorticoids (aldosterone, deoxycorticosterone), and sex steroids (mainly androgens). All steroid hormones are derived from the cyclopentanoperhydrophenanthrene structure, that is, three cyclohexane rings and a single cyclopentane ring (Fig. 14–2). Steroid nomenclature is defined in two ways: by trivial names (e.g., cortisol, aldosterone) or by the chemical structure as defined by the International Union of Pure and Applied Chemistry (IUPAC).[15] The IUPAC classification is inappropriate for clinical use, but does provide an invaluable insight into steroid structure. The basic structure, trivial, and IUPAC names of some common steroids are given in Fig. 14–2 and Table 14–2. Estrogens have 18 carbon atoms (C18 steroids) and androgens have 19 carbon atoms (C19), while glucocorticoids/progestogens are C21 steroid derivatives.

TABLE 14–2 IUPAC AND TRIVIAL NAMES OF SEVERAL NATURAL AND SYNTHETIC STEROIDS

Trivial Name	IUPAC Name
Aldosterone	4-Pregnen-11β,21-diol-3,18,20-trione
Androstenedione	4-Androsten-3,17-dione
Cortisol	4-Pregnen-11β,17α,21-triol-3,20-dione
Cortisone	4-Pregnen-17α,21-diol-3,11,20-trione
Dehydroepiandrosterone	5-Androsten-3β-ol-17-one
Deoxycorticosterone	4-Pregnen-21-ol-3,20-dione
Dexamethasone	1,4-Pregnadien-9α-fluoro-16α-methyl-11β,17α,21-triol-3,20-dione
Dihydrotestosterone	5α-Androstan-17β-ol-3-one
Estradiol	1,3,5(10)-Estratrien-3,17β-diol
Fludrocortisone	4-Pregnen-9α-fluoro-11β,17α,21-triol-3,20-dione
17-Hydroxyprogesterone	4-Pregnen-17α-ol-3,20-dione
Methylprednisolone	1,4-Pregnadien-6α-methyl-11β,17α,21-triol-3,20-dione
Prednisolone	1,4-Pregnadien-11β,17α,21-triol-3,20-dione
Prednisone	1,4-Pregnadien-17α,21-diol-3,11,20-trione
Pregnenolone	5-Pregnen-3β-ol-20-one
Progesterone	4-Pregnen-3,20-dione
Testosterone	4-Androsten-17β-ol-3-one
Triamcinolone	1,4-Pregnadien-9α-fluoro-11β,16α,17α,21-tetrol-3,20-dione

IUPAC, International Union of Pure and Applied Chemistry.

Cholesterol is the precursor for all adrenal steroidogenesis. The principal source of this cholesterol is provided from the circulation in the form of low-density lipoprotein (LDL) cholesterol.[16] Uptake is by specific cell surface LDL receptors present on adrenal tissue[17]; LDL is then internalized via receptor mediated endocytosis,[18] the resulting vesicles fuse with lysozymes,

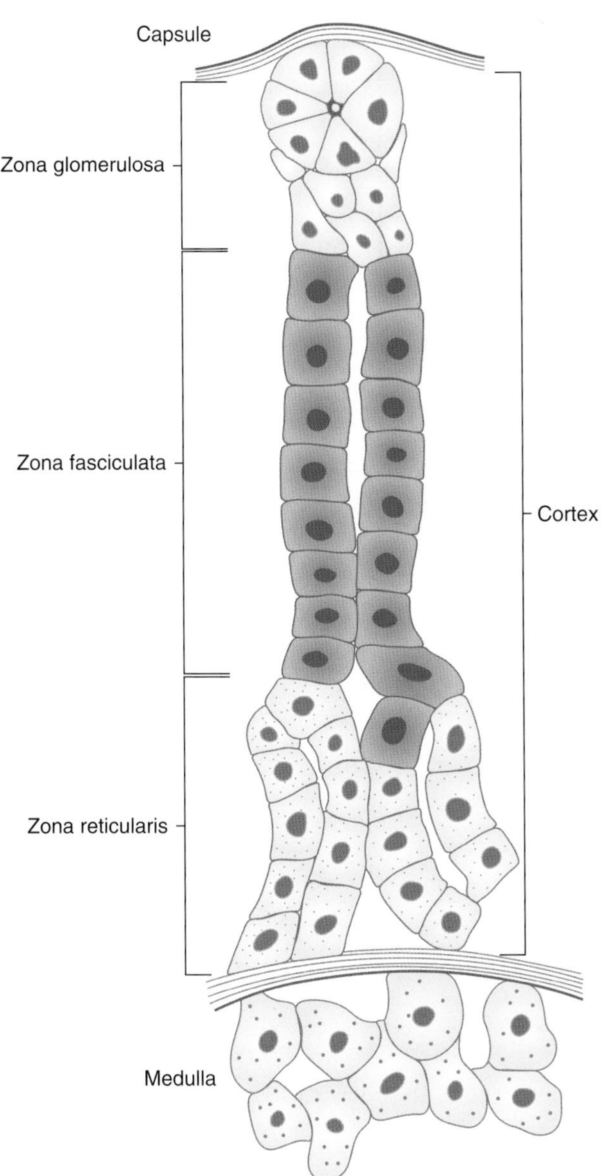

Figure 14–1 ▪ Schematic diagram of the structure of the human adrenal cortex, depicting the outer zona glomerulosa and inner zona fasciculata and zona reticularis.

and free cholesterol is produced following hydrolysis. However, it is clear that this cannot be the sole source of adrenal cholesterol; patients with abetalipoproteinemia who have undetectable circulating LDL and patients with defective LDL receptors in the setting of familial hypercholesterolemia still have normal basal adrenal steroidogenesis. Cholesterol can be generated de novo within the adrenal cortex from acetyl coenzyme A. In addition, there is evidence that the adrenal can utilize HDL cholesterol following uptake through the recently characterized putative HDL receptor, SR-B1.[19]

The biochemical pathways involved in adrenal steroidogenesis are shown in Fig. 14–3. The initial hormone-dependent rate-limiting step is the transport of intracellular cholesterol from the outer to inner mitochondrial membrane for conversion to pregnenolone by cytochrome P450scc. Human experiments of nature have confirmed the importance of a 30-kd protein, steroidogenic acute regulatory protein (StAR), in mediating this effect. StAR is induced by an increase in intracellular cyclic adenosine monophosphate (cAMP) following binding of

TABLE 14–3 NOMENCLATURE FOR ADRENAL STEROIDOGENIC ENZYMES AND THEIR GENES AND CHROMOSOMAL LOCALIZATION

Enzyme Name	Gene	Chromosome
Cholesterol side-chain cleavage (SCC) (desmolase)	*CYP11A1*	15q23-q24
3β-Hydroxysteroid dehydrogenase (3β-HSD) (type II isozyme)	*HSD3B2*	1p13.1
17α-Hydroxylase/17,20 lyase	*CYP17*	10q24.3
21-Hydroxylase	*CYP21A2*	6p21.3
11β-Hydroxylase	*CYP11B1*	8q24.3
Aldosterone synthase	*CYP11B2*	8q24.3

ACTH to its cognate receptor, providing the first important rate-limiting step in adrenal steroidogenesis.[20] Other transporters, including the peripheral benzodiazepine-like receptor, may be involved.[21]

Steroidogenesis involves the concerted action of several enzymes including a series of cytochrome P450 enzymes, all of which have been cloned and characterized (Table 14–3). Cholesterol side chain cleavage enzyme and the CYP11B enzymes are localized to the mitochondria and require an electron shuttle system—provided through adrenodoxin/adrenodoxin reductase to oxidise/oxidize steroids.[22,23] 17α-hydroxylase and 21-hydroxylase are localized to the microsomal/ER fraction and require electron transfer from NADPH by the enzyme P450 oxidoreductase (P450 OR).[23,24] In addition, the 17,20-lyase activity of P450 CYP17 is dependent upon a flavoprotein b5 that functions as an allosteric facilitator of the CYP17 and P450 OR interaction[25] (Fig. 14–4). Mutations in the genes encoding these enzymes result in human disease, so some understanding of the underlying pathways and steroid precursors is required.[26] After uptake of cholesterol to the mitochondrion, cholesterol is cleaved by the P450 enzyme cholesterol side chain cleavage to form pregnenolone.[27] In the cytoplasm, pregnenolone is converted to progesterone by the type II isozyme of 3β-hydroxysteroid dehydrogenase by a reaction involving dehydrogenation of the 3-hydroxyl group and isomerization of the double bond at C5.[28] Progesterone is hydroxylated to 17OH-progesterone through the activity of CYP 17α-hydroxylase. 17-Hydroxylation is an essential prerequisite for glucocorticoid synthesis and the zona glomerulosa does not express 17-hydroxylase. CYP17 also possesses 17,20 lyase activity, which results in the production of the C19 adrenal androgens, dehydroepiandrosterone and androstenedione.[29] In humans, however, 17-OH progesterone is not an efficient substrate for CYP17, and there is negligible conversion of 17-OH progesterone to androstenedione. Adrenal androstenedione secretion is dependent upon the conversion of dehydroepiandrosterone to androstenedione by 3β-HSD—this enzyme will also convert 17-OH pregnenolone to 17-OH progesterone but the preferred substrate is pregnenolone.

21-Hydroxylation of either progesterone (zona glomerulosa) or 17-OH-progesterone (zona fasciculata) is carried out by the product of the CYP21A2 gene, 21 hydroxylase, to yield deoxycorticosterone or 11-deoxycortisol, respectively.[30] The final step in cortisol biosynthesis takes place in the mitochondria and involves the conversion of 11-deoxycortisol to cortisol by the enzyme CYP11B1, 11β-hydroxylase.[31] In the zona glomerulosa, 11β-hydroxylase may also convert deoxycorticosterone to corticosterone. However, the enzyme CYP11B2 or aldosterone synthase may also carry out this reaction and, in addition, is required for the conversion of corticosterone to aldosterone via the intermediate 18-OH corticosterone.[32,33] Thus CYP11B2 can carry out 11β-hydroxylation, 18-hydroxylation, and 18 methyl

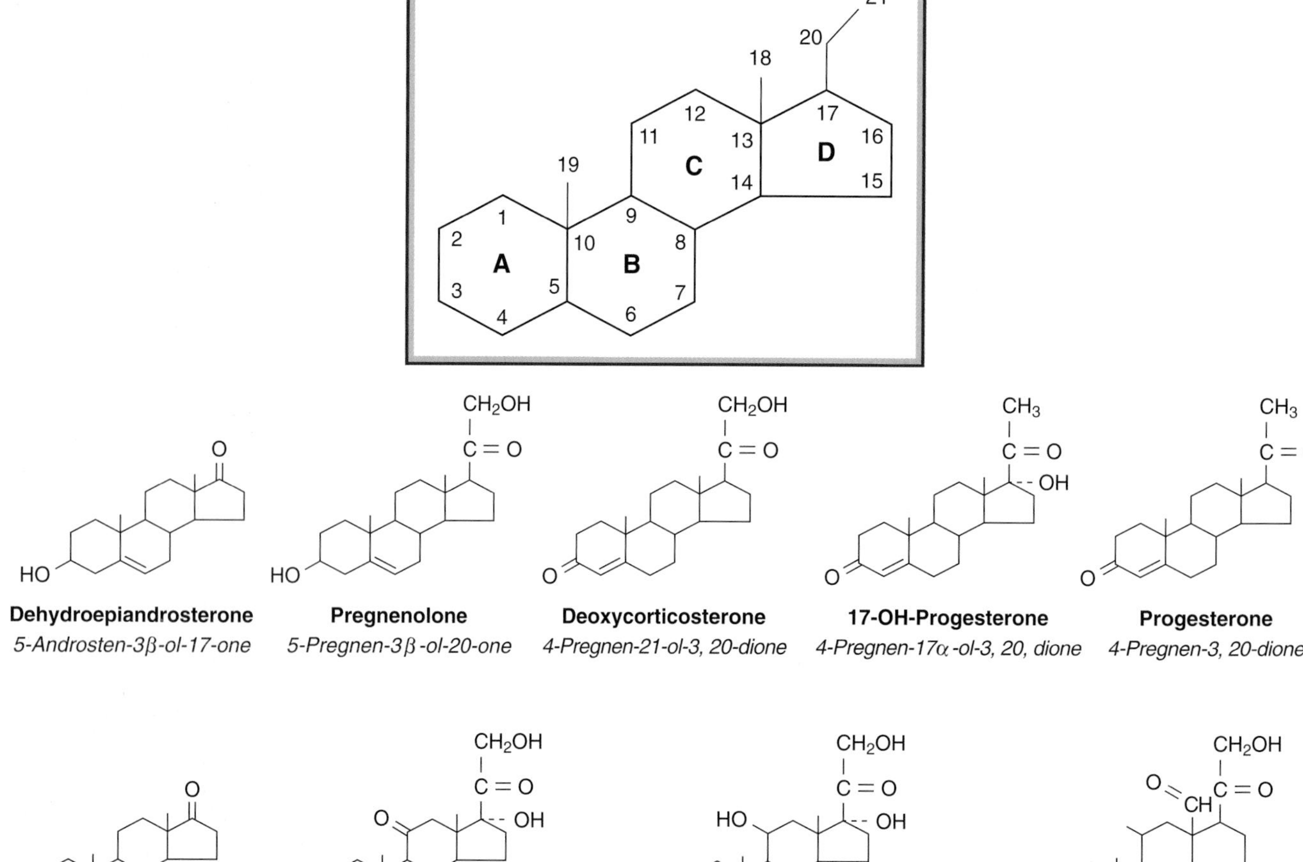

Figure 14–2 ▪ The cyclopentanoperhydrophenanthrene structure of corticosteroid hormones, highlighting the structure of some endogenous steroid hormones together with their nomenclature.

oxidation to yield the characteristic C11-18 hemi-acetyl structure of aldosterone.

Regulation of Adrenal Steroidogenesis

"Functional Zonation" of the Adrenal Cortex

Glucocorticoids are secreted in relatively high amounts (cortisol 10 to 20 mg/day) from the zona fasciculata under the control of ACTH, whereas mineralocorticoids are secreted in low amounts (aldosterone 100 to 150 μg/day) from the zona glomerulosa under the principal control of angiotensin II. As a class, adrenal androgens (dehydroepiandrosterone [DHEA], dehydroepiandrosterone sulfate [DHAS], androstenedione) are the most abundant steroids secreted from the adult adrenal gland (>20 mg/day). In each case, this is facilitated through the expression of steroidogenic enzymes in a specific "zonal" manner. The zona glomerulosa cannot synthesize cortisol because it does not express 17α-hydroxylase. In contrast, aldosterone secretion is confined to the outer zona glomerulosa through the restricted expression of CYP11B2. Although CYP11B1 and CYP11B2 share 95% homology, the 5′ promoter sequences differ and permit regulation of the final steps in glucocorticoid and mineralocorticoid biosynthesis by ACTH and angiotensin II, respectively. In the zona reticularis, high levels of cytochrome b5 confer 17,20-lyase activity upon CYP17 and androgen production. DHEA is sulfated in the zona reticularis by the DHEA sulfotransferase (*SULT2A1*) to form DHEAS.[34]

In the fetal adrenal, steroidogenesis occurs primarily within the inner fetal zone. Because of a relative lack of 3β-HSD and high sulfotransferase activity, the principal steroidogenic products are DHEA and DHAS, which are then aromatized by placental trophoblast to estrogens. Thus he majority of maternal estrogen across pregnancy is, indirectly, fetally derived.[35]

Classical endocrine feedback loops are in place to control the secretion of both hormones—cortisol inhibits the secretion of both corticotropin-releasing factor and ACTH from the hypothalamus and pituitary, respectively, and the aldosterone-induced sodium retention inhibits renal renin secretion.

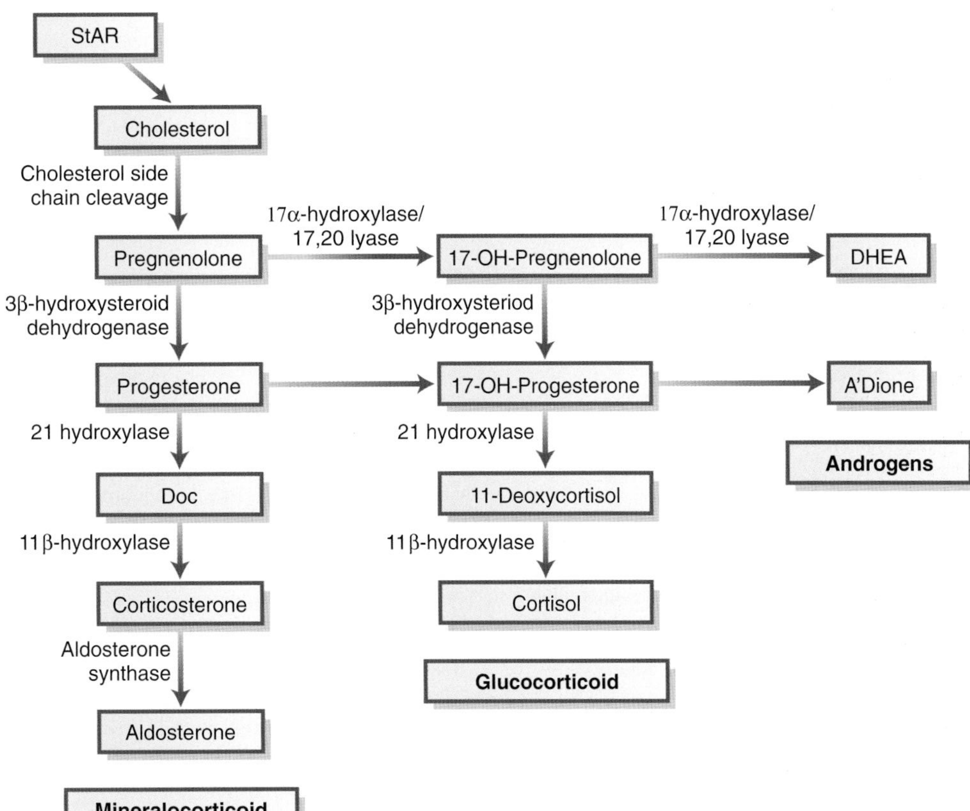

Figure 14–3 ▪ Adrenal steroidogenesis. After the steroidogenic acute regulatory (StAR) protein-mediated uptake of cholesterol into mitochondria within adrenocortical cells, aldosterone, cortisol, and adrenal androgens are synthesized through the coordinated action of a series of steroidogenic enzymes in a zone-specific fashion. *A'Dione*, Androstenedione; *DHEA*, dehydroepiandrosterone; *Doc*, deoxycorticosterone.

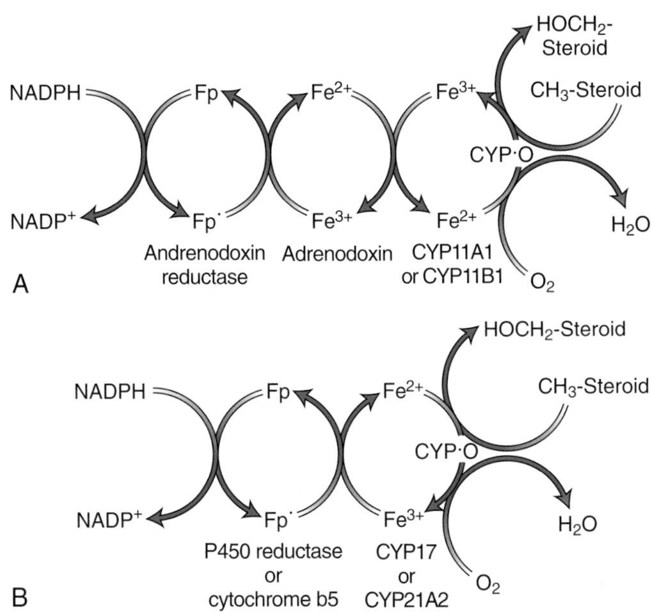

Figure 14–4 ▪ **A,** Electron shuttle system for the mitochondrial enzymes, CYP11A1 and CYP11B1. Adrenodoxin reductase receives electrons from reduced nicotinamide adenine dinucleotide phosphate (NADPH) and reduces adrenodoxin, which transfers reducing equivalents to the CYP enzyme. The enzyme then transfers electrons, by way of oxygen, to the steroid. *Fp*, Flavoprotein; Fp˙, reduced form of flavoprotein. **B,** Electron shuttle system for the microsomal enzymes, CYP17 and CYP21A2. P450 reductase, a flavoprotein, accepts electrons from NADPH and transfers them to the NADPH-P450 enzyme. The enzyme then transfers electrons, by way of oxygen, to the steroid. A second reducing equivalent may be supplied to CYP17 by NADPH-P450 reductase or cytochrome b_5.

Glucocorticoid Secretion—The Hypothalamus-Pituitary-Adrenal Axis

Pro-opiomelanocortin and ACTH

ACTH is the principal hormone stimulating adrenal glucocorticoid biosynthesis and secretion. ACTH has 39 amino acids but is synthesized within the anterior pituitary as part of a much larger 241 amino acid precursor, pro-opiomelanocortin (POMC). A transcription factor—Tpit—appears to be essential for the differentiation of POMC expressing cells within the anterior pituitary.[36] POMC is cleaved in a tissue-specific fashion to yield smaller peptide hormones. In the anterior pituitary, this results in the secretion of β-lipoprotein (β-LPH) and pro-ACTH, the latter being further cleaved to an N-terminal peptide, joining peptide and ACTH itself[37,38] (Fig. 14–5). Post secretion cleavage of Pro-γ-MSH by a serine protease (AsP) expressed in the outer adrenal cortex is thought to mediate the trophic action of "ACTH" on the adrenal cortex.[39] The first 24 aa of ACTH are common to all species and synthetic ACTH 1-24 (Synacthen) is available commercially for clinical testing of the hypothalamo-pituitary-adrenal (HPA) axis and assessing adrenal glucocorticoid reserve. Melanocyte stimulating hormones (a, β and γ) are also cleaved products from POMC but the increased pigmentation characteristic of Addison's disease is thought to arise directly from increased ACTH concentrations binding to the melanocortin-1 receptor rather than the result of α-MSH secretion.[40]

POMC is also transcribed in many extrapituitary tissues, notably brain, liver, kidney, gonad, and placenta.[37,41,42] In these normal tissues, POMC mRNA is usually shorter than the pituitary 1200-bp species due to lack of exons 1 and 2 and the 5′ region of exon 3.[43] As a result, it is probable that this POMC-like peptide is neither secreted nor active. However, in ectopic ACTH syn-

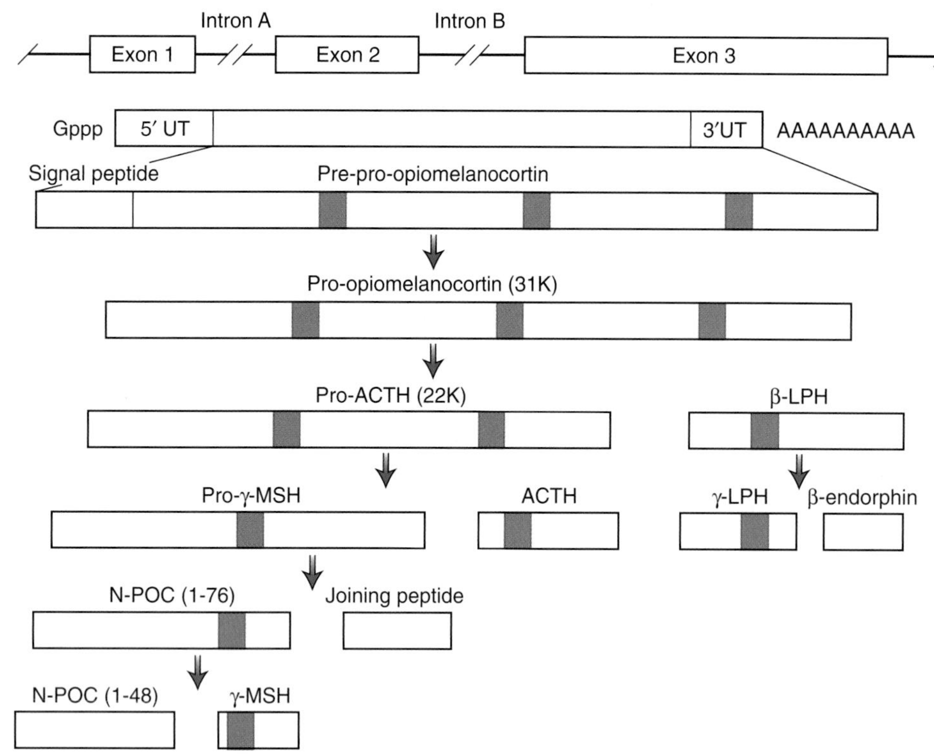

Figure 14–5 ▪ Synthesis and cleavage of pro-opiomelanocortin (POMC) within the human anterior pituitary gland. Prohormone convertase enzymes sequentially cleave POMC to adrenocorticotropic hormone (ACTH). *Shaded areas* represent melanocyte-stimulating hormone (MSH) structural units. *β-LPH*, β-Lipoprotein; *γ-LPH*, γ-lipoprotein; *N-POC*, amino-terminal pro-opiomelanocortin.

drome, additional POMC mRNA species are described, which are longer than normal pituitary 1200-bp POMC species (typically 1450 bp) due to the use of alternative promoters in the 5′ region of the gene.[44,45] This may in part explain the resistance of POMC secretion to glucocorticoid feedback in these tumors. Others factors, including interaction with tissue-specific transcription factors[46] and POMC methylation,[47] may explain the ectopic expression of ACTH in some malignant tissues. The cleavage of POMC is also tissue-specific,[48] and, at least in some cases of ectopic ACTH syndrome, it is possible that circulating ACTH precursors, notably pro-ACTH, may cross-react in current ACTH radioimmunoassays.[49,50] The biologic activity of POMC itself upon adrenal function is thought to be negligible.

POMC expression and processing within neurons in the hypothalamus, specifically the generation of α-MSH that interacts with MCR-4 receptors, appears to be of crucial importance in appetite control and energy homeostasis (see later).[51]

Corticotropin-Releasing Hormone and Arginine Vasopressin

POMC secretion is tightly controlled by numerous factors, notably corticotropin releasing hormone (CRH) and arginine vasopressin (AVP)[52,53] (Fig. 14–6). Additional control is provided through an endogenous circadian rhythm, stress and feedback inhibition by cortisol itself. CRH is a 41 amino acid peptide that is synthesized in neurones within the paraventricular nucleus of the hypothalamus.[9,54,55] Human and rat CRH are identical, but ovine CRH differs by 7 amino acids[56,57]; in humans, it is slightly more potent than human CRH in stimulating ACTH secretion but has a longer half-life and is therefore used diagnostically. CRH is secreted into the hypophyseal portal blood where it binds to specific type I CRH receptors on anterior pituitary corticotrophs[58] to stimulate POMC gene transcription through a process that includes the activation of adenylate cyclase. It is unclear whether hypothalamic CRH contributes in any way to circulating levels; CRH is also synthesized in other tissues and it is likely that circulating CRH reflects synthesis from testis, gastrointestinal tract, adrenal medulla, and particularly the placenta,[59] where the increased secretion across pregnancy results in a threefold increase in circulating CRH levels.[60] In the circulation, CRH is bound to CRH-binding protein (CRH-BP); levels of CRH-BP also increase during pregnancy so that cortisol secretion is not markedly elevated.[61] CRH is the principal stimulus for ACTH secretion,[62] but AVP is able to potentiate CRH-mediated secretion.[63] In this case, AVP acts through the V1B receptor to activate protein kinase C. The peak response of ACTH to CRH does not differ across the day, but it is affected by endogenous function of the HPA axis in that responsiveness is reduced in subjects treated with corticosteroids but increased in subjects with Cushing's disease. Other reported ACTH secretagogues, including angiotensin II, cholecystokinin, ANF, and vasoactive peptides, probably act to modulate the CRH control of ACTH secretion.[64]

The Stress Response and Immune-Endocrine Axis

The proinflammatory cytokines, notably interleukin 1 (IL-1), IL-6, and TNF-α also increase ACTH secretion either directly or by augmenting the effect of CRF.[65,66] Leukemia inhibitory factor (LIF), a cytokine of the IL-6 family, is a further activator of the HPA axis.[67] This explains the response of the HPA axis to an inflammatory stimulus and is an important immune-endocrine interaction (see Chapter 7). Physical stresses increase ACTH and cortisol secretion, again through central actions mediated via CRH and AVP. Thus, cortisol secretion rises in response to fever, surgery,[68] burn injury,[69] hypoglycemia,[70] hypotension, and exercise.[71] In all of these cases, this can be viewed as a normal counterregulatory response to the insult. Acute psychological stress will raise cortisol levels,[72] but secretion rates appear to be normal in patients with chronic anxiety states and underlying psychotic illness. However, depression is associated with high circulating cortisol concentrations and this is an important consideration in the differential diagnosis of Cushing's syndrome (see later).

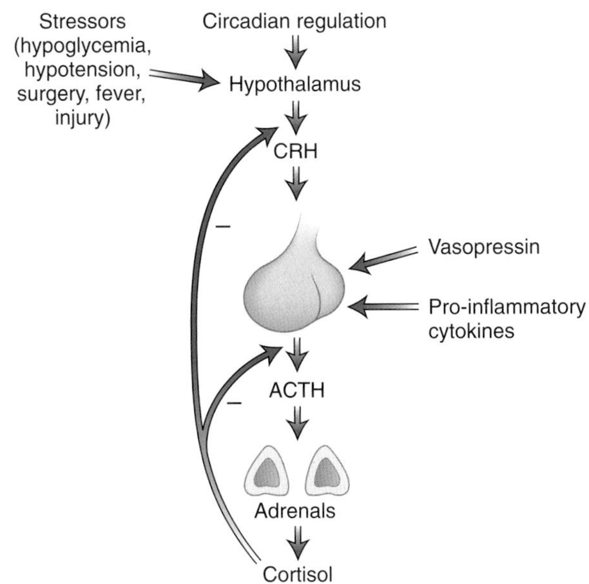

Figure 14–6 ▪ Normal regulation of adrenal glucocorticoid secretion. Adrenocorticotropic hormone (ACTH) is secreted from the anterior pituitary under the influence of two principal secretagogues, corticotropin-releasing hormone (CRH) and arginine vasopressin; other factors, including cytokines, also play a role. CRH secretion is regulated by an inbuilt circadian rhythm and additional stressors operating through the hypothalamus. Secretion of both CRH and ACTH is inhibited by cortisol, highlighting the importance of negative feedback control.

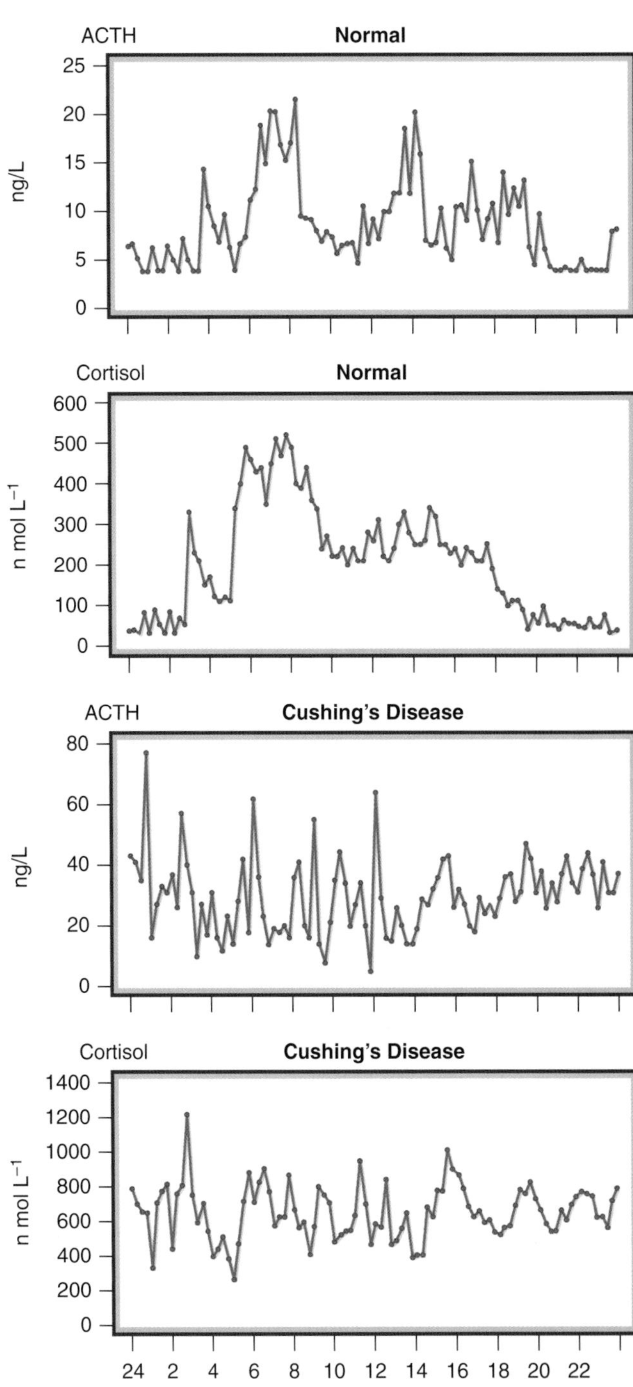

Figure 14–7 ▪ Circadian and pulsatile secretion of adrenocorticotropic hormone (ACTH) and cortisol in a normal subject *(top two panels)* and in a patient with Cushing's disease. In a normal subject, secretion of ACTH and cortisol is highest in early morning and falls to a nadir at midnight. ACTH pulse frequency and pulse amplitude are increased in Cushing's disease, and circadian rhythm secretion is lost.

Circadian Rhythm

ACTH is secreted in a pulsatile fashion with a circadian rhythm so that levels are highest on wakening and decline throughout the day, reaching nadir values in the evening[73] (Fig. 14–7). ACTH pulse frequency is higher in normal adult males compared with females (on average, 18 pulses versus 10 pulses/24 hours) and the circadian ACTH rhythm appears to be mediated principally by an increased ACTH pulse amplitude between 05.00–09.00h but also by a reduction in ACTH pulse frequency between 18.00–24.00h.[74,75] Food ingestion is a further stimulus to ACTH secretion. Circadian rhythm is dependent upon both day-night[76] and sleep-wake[77] patterns and is disrupted by alternating day-night shift working patterns and by long-distance travel across time zones.[78] It may take up to 2 weeks for circadian rhythm to reset to an altered day-night cycle.

Negative Feedback

An important aspect of CRH and ACTH secretion is the negative feedback control exerted by glucocorticoids themselves. Glucocorticoids inhibit POMC gene transcription in the anterior pituitary[52] and CRH and AVP mRNA synthesis and secretion in the hypothalamus.[79,80] This negative feedback effect is dependent upon the dose, potency, half-life, and duration of administration of the glucocorticoid and has important physiologic and diagnostic consequences. Suppression of the HPA axis by pharmacologic corticosteroids may persist for many months after cessation of therapy and adrenocortical insufficiency should be anticipated. Diagnostically, the feedback mechanism in Addison's disease explains ACTH hypersecretion, and undetectable ACTH levels in patients with a cortisol-secreting adrenal adenoma. Feedback inhibition is principally mediated via the glucocorticoid receptor (GR); patients with glucocorticoid resistance due to mutations in the GR[81] and mice lacking the GR gene[82] have ACTH and cortisol hypersecretion due to perceived lack of negative feedback.

The ACTH Receptor and ACTH Effects on the Adrenal

ACTH binds to a G-protein–coupled, melanocortin-2 receptor,[83] of which there are approximately 3500 on each adrenocortical cell. Signal transduction is mediated principally through the stimulation of adenylate cyclase and intracellular cAMP,[84] although both extracellular and intracellular Ca^{2+} play a role.[85]

Other factors synergize with or inhibit the effects of ACTH on the adrenal cortex, including angiotensin II, activin, inhibin, and cytokines (TNF-α and leptin).[86] Cell-to-cell communication via gap junctions is also important in mediating the effects of ACTH.[87] The effects of ACTH on the adrenal include both immediate and chronic effects; the end result is the stimulation of adrenal steroidogenesis and growth. Acutely, steroidogenesis is stimulated through a StAR-mediated increase in cholesterol delivery to the CYP11A1 enzyme in the inner mitochondrial membrane.[20] Chronically (within 24 to 26 hours of exposure), ACTH acts to increase the synthesis of all steroidogenic CYP enzymes (CYP11A1, CYP17, CYP21A2, CYP11B1) in addition to adrenodoxin,[88,89] effects which are mediated at the transcriptional level. ACTH also increases synthesis of the LDL and HDL receptors and possibly also HMG-CoA reductase, the rate-limiting step in cholesterol biosynthesis. ACTH increases adrenal weight by inducing both hyperplasia and hypertrophy. Adrenal atrophy is a feature of ACTH deficiency.

Mineralocorticoid Secretion—The Renin-Angiotensin-Aldosterone Axis

Aldosterone is secreted from the zona glomerulosa under the control of three principal secretagogues, angiotensin II, potassium, and to a lesser extent ACTH. Other factors, notably somatostatin, heparin, atrial natriuretic factor, and dopamine, can directly inhibit aldosterone synthesis. The secretion of aldosterone and its intermediary 18-hydroxylated metabolites is restricted to the zona glomerulosa because of the zonal-specific expression of CYP11B2—aldosterone synthase.[90] Corticosterone and deoxycorticosterone, while synthesized in both the zona fasciculata and glomerulosa, can act as mineralocorticoids, which becomes significant in some clinical disease, notably some forms of congenital adrenal hyperplasia and adrenal tumors. Similarly, it is now established that cortisol can act as a mineralocorticoid in the setting of impaired metabolism to cortisone carried out by the enzyme 11β-hydroxysteroid dehydrogenase; this is important in patients with hypertension, ectopic ACTH syndrome, and renal disease. The renin-angiotensin system is described in detail in Chapter 15.

Angiotensin II and potassium stimulate aldosterone secretion principally by increasing the transcription of *CYP11B2* through common intracellular signaling pathways. cAMP response elements in the 5′ region of the *CYP11B2* gene are activated following an increase in intracellular Ca^{2+} and activation of calmodulin kinases. The potassium effect is mediated through membrane depolarization and opening of calcium channels, and the AII effect following binding of AII to the surface AT_1 receptor and activation of phospholipase C.[90]

The effect of ACTH upon aldosterone secretion is modest and differs in the acute and chronic situation (see Chapter 15). An acute bolus of ACTH will increase aldosterone secretion, principally by stimulating the early pathways of adrenal steroidogenesis (see above) but circulating levels increase by no more than 10% to 20% above baseline values. ACTH has no effect upon *CYP11B2* gene transcription or enzyme activity. Chronic continual ACTH stimulation has either no effect or an inhibitory effect on aldosterone production, possibly because of receptor down-regulation or suppression of AII-stimulated secretion because of a mineralocorticoid effect of cortisol, DOC, or corticosterone. Dopamine and atrial natriuretic peptide inhibit aldosterone secretion, as does heparin.

The separate control of glucocorticoid biosynthesis through the HPA axis and mineralocorticoid synthesis via the renin-angiotensin system has important clinical consequences. Patients with primary adrenal failure invariably have both cortisol and aldosterone deficiency, whereas patients with ACTH deficiency due to pituitary disease have glucocorticoid deficiency, but aldosterone concentrations are normal because the renin-angiotensin system is intact.

Adrenal Androgen Secretion

Adrenal androgens represent an important component (>50%) of circulating androgens in premenopausal females.[91] In males, this contribution is much smaller because of the testicular production of androgens, but adrenal androgen excess even in males may be of clinical significance, notably in patients with congenital adrenal hyperplasia. The adult adrenal secretes approximately 4 mg/day of DHEA, 7 to 15 mg/day of DHEAS, 1.5 mg of androstenedione, and 0.05 mg/day of testosterone. DHEA is a crucial precursor of human sex steroid biosynthesis and exerts androgenic or estrogenic activity following conversion by the activities of 3β-HSD, a superfamily of β-HSD isozymes and aromatase, expressed in peripheral target tissues, which is of clinical importance in many diseases.[92] Only desulfated DHEA is converted downstream and biologically active. Serum DHEAS was previously thought to represent a circulating storage pool for DHEA regeneration. However, recent work has suggested that conversion of DHEAS to DHEA by steroid sulfatase plays a minor role in adult physiology and that the equilibrium between serum DHEA and DHEAS is mainly regulated by DHEA sulfotransferase (SULT2A1) activity. This would suggest that serum DHEAS may not always appropriately reflect the active DHEA pool, in particular if SULT2A1 activity is impaired, for example, in the inflammatory stress response.[93]

ACTH stimulates androgen secretion; DHEA (but not DHAS because of its increased plasma half-life) and androstenedione demonstrate a similar circadian rhythm to cortisol.[94] However, there are many discrepancies between adrenal androgen and glucocorticoid secretion, leading to to the suggestion of an additional "cortical androgen-stimulating hormone" (CASH). Many putative CASHs have been proposed, including POMC derivatives such as joining peptide, prolactin, and IGF-1, but conclusive proof is lacking. Efficient adrenal steroidogenesis toward androgen synthesis is crucially dependent upon the relative activities of 3β-HSD and 17α-hydroxylase and, in particular, upon the 17,20 lyase activity of 17α-hydroxylase. Factors that determine whether 17-hydroxylated substrates, 17-OH pregnenolone and 17-OH progesterone, undergo 21-hydroxylation to form glucocorticoid or side chain cleavage by 17α-hydroxylase to form DHEA and androstenedione are unresolved and seem likely to be important in defining the activity of any putative CASH (Table 14–4).

TABLE 14–4 DISSOCIATION OF ADRENAL ANDROGEN AND GLUCOCORTICOID SECRETION: EVIDENCE FOR AN ADRENAL-STIMULATING HORMONE

Dexamethasone studies: Complete cortisol suppression with chronic high-dose dexamethasone. DHEA falls by only 20%. Greater sensitivity of DHEA to acute low-dose dexamethasone administration.

Adrenarche: Rise in circulating DHEA at 6 to 8 years of age. Cortisol production unaltered.

Aging: Reduction in DHEA production, no change in cortisol.

Anorexia nervosa and illness: Fall in DHEA, no change (or increase) in cortisol.

DHEA, dehydroepiandrosterone.

CORTICOSTEROID HORMONE ACTION

Receptors and Gene Transcription

Both cortisol and aldosterone exert their effects following uptake of free hormone from the circulation and binding to intracellular receptors, termed the *glucocorticoid* and *mineralocorticoid receptors* (GR and MR).[95-97] These are both members of the thyroid/steroid hormone receptor superfamily of transcription factors comprising a C-terminal ligand–binding domain, a central DNA binding domain interacting with specific DNA sequences on target genes, and an N-terminal hypervariable region. In both cases, although there is only a single gene encoding the GR and MR, splice variants have been described; this together with tissue-specific posttranslational modification (phosphorylation, sumoylation, and ubiquitination) is thought to account for many of the diverse actions of corticosteroids[98,99] (Fig. 14–8).

Glucocorticoid hormone action has been studied in more depth than mineralocorticoid action. The binding of steroid to the GRa in the cytosol results in activation of the steroid-receptor complex through a process which involves the dissociation of heat-shock proteins (HSP 90 and HSP 70).[100] Following translocation to the nucleus, gene transcription is stimulated or repressed following binding of dimerized GR–ligand complexes to specific DNA sequences in the promoter regions of target genes.[101] This "glucocorticoid-response element" (GRE) is invariably a palindromic CGTACAnnnTGTACT sequence which binds with high affinity to two loops of DNA within the DNA binding domain of the GR ("zinc fingers"). This stabilizes the RNA polymerase II complex facilitating gene transcription. The GRα variant may act as a dominant negative regulator of GRa transactivation.[98] Naturally occurring mutations in the GR (as seen in patients with glucocorticoid resistance) and in vitro–generated GR mutants have highlighted critical regions of the receptor responsible for binding and transactivation,[102] but, in addition, numerous others factors are required (coactivators, corepressors[103]), which may confer tissue-specificity of response. This is a rapidly evolving field and beyond the scope of this chapter. However, the interaction between GR and two particular transcription factors are important in mediating the antiinflammatory effects of glucocorticoids and explain the effect of glucocorticoids upon genes that do not contain obvious GREs in their promoter regions. Activator protein-1 (AP-1) comprises Fos and Jun subunits and is a proinflammatory transcription factor induced by a series of cytokines and phorbol ester. The GR–ligand complex can bind to c-jun and prevent interaction with the AP-1 site, thereby mediating the so-called transrepressive effects of glucocorticoids.[104] Similarly, functional antagonism exists between the GR and nuclear factor-kappa B (NF-κB). NF-κB is a ubiquitously expressed transcription factor that activates a series of genes involved in lymphocyte development, inflammatory response, host defense, and apoptosis[105] (Fig. 14–9). In keeping with the diverse array of actions of cortisol, many hundred glucocorticoid-responsive genes have been identified. Some glucocorticoid-induced genes and repressed genes are depicted in Table 14–5.

In contrast to the diverse actions of glucocorticoids, mineralocorticoids have a more restricted role, principally to stimulate epithelial sodium transport in the distal nephron, distal colon, and salivary glands.[106] This is mediated through the induction of the apical sodium channel (comprising three subunits α, β, and γ)[107] and the α_1 and β_1 subunits of the basolateral Na^+,K^+,ATPase[108] through transcriptional regulation of serum and glucocorticoid-induced kinase (sgk).[109] Aldosterone binds to the MR, principally in the cytosol (although there is evidence for expression of the unliganded MR in the nucleus) followed by translocation of the hormone-receptor complex to the nucleus (Fig. 14–10). The MR and GR share considerable homology—57% in the steroid binding domain and 94% in the DNA binding domain. It is perhaps not surprising, therefore, that there is promiscuity of ligand binding with aldosterone (and the synthetic "mineralocorticoid" fludrocortisone) binding to the GR and cortisol binding to the MR. For the MR, this is particularly impressive—in vitro the MR has the same inherent affinity for aldosterone, corticosterone, and cortisol.[96] Specificity upon the MR is conferred through the "pre-receptor" metabolism of cortisol via the enzyme 11β-hydroxysteroid dehydrogenase type 2 (11β-HSD2), which inactivates cortisol and corticosterone to inactive 11-keto metabolites, enabling aldosterone to bind to the MR.[110,111] Mineralocorticoid hormone action has recently been extended beyond this "classical" action in sodium-transporting epithelia with the demonstration that aldosterone can induce cardiac fibrosis and inflammatory changes in renal vasculature. The underlying signaling pathways remain to be fully clarified but the effects are reversible with MR antagonists.[112]

Finally, for both glucocorticoids and mineralocorticoids there is accumulating evidence for so-called nongenomic effects

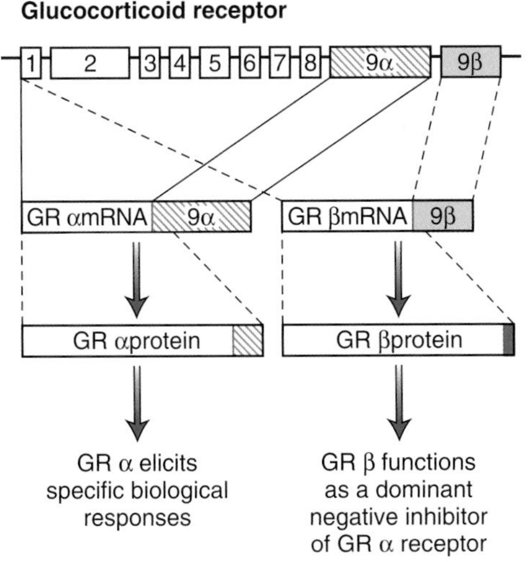

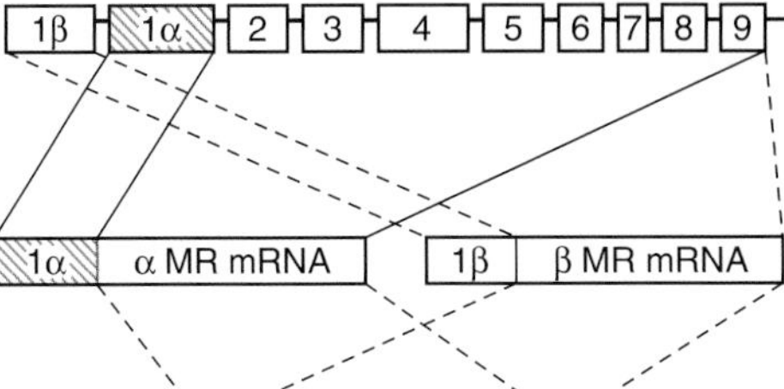

Figure 14–8 ▪ Schematic structure of the human genes encoding the glucocorticoid receptor (GR) and mineralocorticoid receptor (MR). In both cases, splice variants have been described; in the case of the GR, there is evidence that the GRβ isoform can act as a dominant negative inhibitor of GRα action. *mRNA,* Messenger ribonucleic acid.

TABLE 14–5 SOME OF THE GENES REGULATED BY GLUCOCORTICOIDS OR GLUCOCORTICOID RECEPTORS

Site of Action	Induced Genes	Repressed Genes
Immune system	IκB (NFκB inhibitor)	Interleukins
	Haptoglobin	TNF-α
	TCR ζ	IFN-γ
	p21, p27, and p57	E-selectin
	Lipocortin	ICAM-1
		Cyclooxygenase 2
		iNOS
Metabolic	PPAR-γ	Tryptophan hydroxylase
	Tyrosine aminotransferase	Metalloprotease
	Glutamine synthase	
	Glycogen synthase	
	Glucose-6-phosphatase	
	PEPCK	
	Leptin	
	γ-Fibrinogen	
	Cholesterol 7α-hydroxylase	
	C/EBP/β	
Bone	Androgen receptor	Osteocalcin
	Calcitonin receptor	Collagenase
	Alkaline phosphatase	
	IGF-BP-6	
Channels and transporters	Epithelial sodium channel (ENaC) α, β, γ	
	Serum and glucocorticoid–induced kinase (SGK)	
	Aquaporin 1	
Endocrine	bFGF	GR
	VIP	PRL
	Endothelin	POMC/CRH
	RXR	PTHrP
	GHRH receptor	Vasopressin
	Natriuretic peptide receptors	
Growth and development	Surfactant protein A, B, C	Fibronectin
		α-Fetoprotein
		NGF
		Erythropoietin
		G1 cyclins
		Cyclin-dependent kinases

Modified from McKay LI, Cidlowski JA. Molecular control of immune/inflammatory responses: interactions between nuclear factor–κB and steroid receptor–signalling pathways. Endocr Rev 1999;20:435-459.
bFGF, Basic fibroblast growth factor; *CRH,* corticotropin-releasing hormone; *C/EBP/β,* CAAT-enhancer binding protein-beta; *GR,* glucocorticoid receptor; *GHRH,* growth hormone–releasing hormone; ICAM, intercellular adhesion molecule; *IFN,* interferon; *IGF-BP,* insulin-like growth factor–binding protein; *IκB,* inhibitory kappa B; *iNOS,* inducible nitric oxide synthase; *NFκB,* nuclear factor κB; *NGF,* nerve growth factor; *PEPCK,* phosphoenolpyruvate carboxykinase; *POMC,* pro-opiomelanocortin; *PPAR,* peroxisome proliferator–activated receptor; *PTHrP,* parathyroid hormone–related protein; *RXR,* retinoid X receptor; *SGK,* serum and glucocorticoid-induced kinase; *TCR,* T-cell receptor; *TNF-α,* tumor necrosis factor-α; *VIP,* vasoactive intestinal peptide.

involving hormone response obviating the genomic GR or MR. A series of responses have been reported within seconds or minutes of exposure to corticosteroids and are thought to be mediated by as yet uncharacterized membrane-coupled receptors.[113,114]

Cortisol Binding Globulin and Corticosteroid Hormone Metabolism

More than 90% of circulating cortisol is bound, predominantly to the α_2-globulin, cortisol binding globulin (CBG).[115] This 383 amino acid protein is synthesized in the liver and binds cortisol with high affinity. Affinity for synthetic corticosteroids (except prednisolone, which has an affinity for CBG approximately 50% of that of cortisol) is negligible. Circulating CBG concentrations are approximately 700 nmol/L. Levels are increased by estrogens and in some patients with chronic active hepatitis but reduced by glucocorticoids and in patients with cirrhosis, nephrosis, and hyperthyroidism. The estrogen effect can be marked with levels increasing twofold to threefold across pregnancy, which should be taken into account when measuring plasma "total" cortisol in pregnancy and in women taking estrogens. Inherited abnormalities in CBG synthesis are much rarer than those described for thyroid-binding globulin but include patients with elevated CBG, partial and complete deficiency of CBG, or CBG variants with reduced affinity for cortisol.[116,117] In each case, alterations in CBG concentrations change total circulating cortisol concentrations accordingly but "free" cortisol concentrations are normal. Only this free circulating fraction is available for transport into tissues for biologic activity. The excretion of "free" cortisol through the kidneys is termed urinary free cortisol and represents only 1% of the total cortisol secretion rate.

The circulating half-life of cortisol varies between 70 and 120 minutes. The major steps for cortisol metabolism are depicted in Fig. 14–11.[118] These comprise the following:

- The interconversion of the 11-hydroxyl (cortisol, Kendall's compound F) to the 11-oxo group (cortisone, compound E) through the activity of 11β-hydroxysteroid dehydrogenase (EC 1.1.1.146).[119,120] The metabolism of cortisol and cortisone then follow similar pathways.
- Reduction of the C4-5 double bond to form dihydrocortisol (DHF) or DHE followed by hydroxylation of the 3-oxo group to form tetrahydrocortisone (THF) and THE. The reduction of the C4-5 double can be carried out by either tetrahydrocortisor 5β-reductase or 5α-reductase to yield, respectively, 5β-THF (THF) or 5α-THF (allo-THF). In normal subjects, the 5β metabolites predominate (5β : 5α-THF 2 : 1). THF, allo-THF and THE are rapidly conjugated with glucuronic acid and excreted in the urine.
- Further reduction of the 20-oxo group by either 20α or 20β-hydroxysteroid dehydrogenase to yield α and β-cortols and cortolones from cortisol and cortisone, respectively. Reduction of the C20 position may also occur without A ring reduction, giving rise to 20α- and 20β-hydroxycortisol.
- Hydroxylation at C6 to form 6β-hydroxycortisol.
- Cleavage of THF and THE to the C19 steroids 11 hydroxy or 11-oxo androsterone or etiocholanolone.
- Oxidation of the C21 position or cortols and cortolones to form the extremely polar metabolites, cortolic and cortolonic acids.

Approximately 50% of secreted cortisol appears in the urine as THF, allo-THF, and THE; 25% as cortols/cortolones; 10% as C19 steroids; and 10% as cortolic/cortolonic acids. The remaining metabolites are free, unconjugated steroids (cortisol, cortisone, 6β-, and 20α/20β-metabolites of F and E).

The principal site of cortisol metabolism has been considered to be the liver, but many of the above enzymes have been described in the mammalian kidney, notably the inactivation of cortisol to cortisone by 11β-hydroxysteroid dehydrogenase (11β-HSD). Quantitatively the interconversion of cortisol to cortisone by 11β-HSD is also the most important pathway. Furthermore,

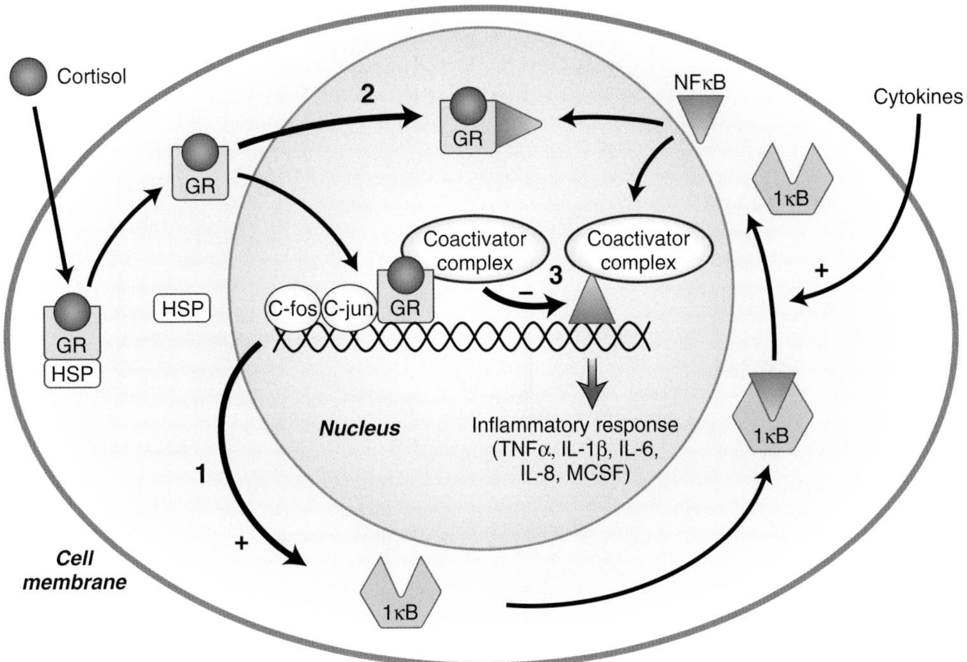

Figure 14–9 ▪ The antiinflammatory action of glucocorticoids. Cortisol binds to the cytoplasmic glucocorticoid receptor (GR). Conformational changes in the receptor-ligand complex result in dissociation from heat shock proteins (HSPs) 70 and 90 and migration to the nucleus. Binding occurs to specific DzNA motifs–glucocorticoid response elements in association with the activator protein-1 (AP-1) comprising c-fos and c-jun. Glucocorticoids mediate their antiinflammatory effects through several mechanisms: (1) The inhibitory protein 1κB, which binds and inactivates nuclear factor κB (NFκB), is induced. (2) The GR–cortisol complex is able to bind NFκB and thus prevent initiation of an inflammatory process. (3) Both GR and NFκB compete for the limited availability of coactivators, which include cyclic adenosine monophosphate response element binding protein (CREB) and steroid receptor coactivator-1.

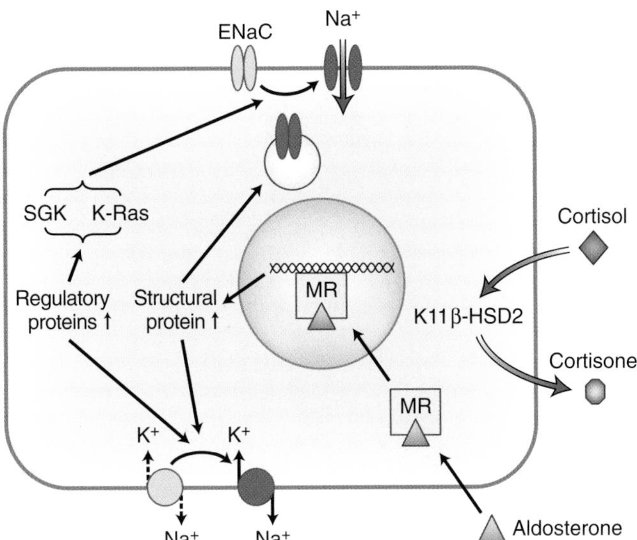

Figure 14–10 ▪ Mineralocorticoid hormone action. An epithelial cell is depicted in the distal nephron or distal colon, or both. The much higher concentrations of cortisol are inactivated by the type 2 isozyme of 11β-hydroxysteroid dehydrogenase (11β-HSD2) to cortisone, permitting the endogenous ligand, aldosterone, to bind to the mineralocorticoid receptor (MR). Relatively few mineralocorticoid target genes have been identified, but these include serum and glucocorticoid-induced kinase (SGK), subunits of the epithelial sodium channel (ENaC), and basolateral Na^+,K^+-adenosine triphosphatase.

the bioactivity of glucocorticoids is in part related to the hydroxyl group at C11; cortisone with a C11-oxo group is an inactive steroid, such that 11β-HSD expressed in peripheral tissues plays a crucial role in regulating corticosteroid hormone action. Two distinct 11β-HSD isozymes have been reported, a type 1, NADPH-dependent oxo-reductase expressed principally in the liver, which confers bioactivity upon orally administered cortisone by converting it to cortisol,[120] and a type 2, NAD-dependent dehydrogenase. It is 11β-HSD2, coexpressed with the MR in the kidney, colon, and salivary gland, that inactivates cortisol to cortisone and permits aldosterone to bind to the MR in vivo. If this “enzyme-protective mechanism” is impaired, cortisol is able to act as a mineralocorticoid; this explains some forms of endocrine hypertension (apparent mineralocorticoid excess, licorice ingestion) and the mineralocorticoid excess state that characterizes the ectopic ACTH syndrome.[119,121]

Hyperthyroidism results in increased cortisol metabolism and clearance and hypothyroidism the converse, principally due to an effect of thyroid hormone upon hepatic 11β-HSD1 and 5α/5β-reductases.[120] IGF-1 increases cortisol clearance by inhibiting hepatic 11β-HSD1 (conversion of cortisone to cortisol).[122] 6β-hydroxylation is normally a minor pathway but cortisol itself induces 6β-hydroxylase so that 6β-hydroxycortisol excretion is markedly increased in patients with Cushing's syndrome.[123] Furthermore, some drugs, notably rifampicin and phenytoin, increase cortisol clearance through this pathway.[124] Patients with renal disease have impaired cortisol clearance because of reduced renal cortisol to cortisone conversion.[125] These observations have clinical implications for patients with thyroid disease, acromegaly, and renal disease and for patients taking cortisol replacement therapy. Adrenal crisis has been reported in steroid-replaced Addisonian patients given rifampicin,[126] and hydrocortisone replacement therapy may need to be increased in treated patients who develop hyperthyroidism or reduced in patients with untreated growth-hormone deficiency.

Aldosterone is also metabolized in the liver and kidneys. In the liver it undergoes tetrahydro reduction and is excreted in the urine as a 3-glucuronide tetrahydroaldosterone derivative. However, glucuronide conjugation at the 18 position occurs directly in the kidney as does 3α and 5α/5β metabolism of the free steroid.[127] Because of the aldehyde group at the C18 position, aldosterone is not metabolized by 11β-HSD2.[128] Hepatic aldosterone clearance is reduced in patients with cirrhosis, ascites, and severe congestive heart failure.

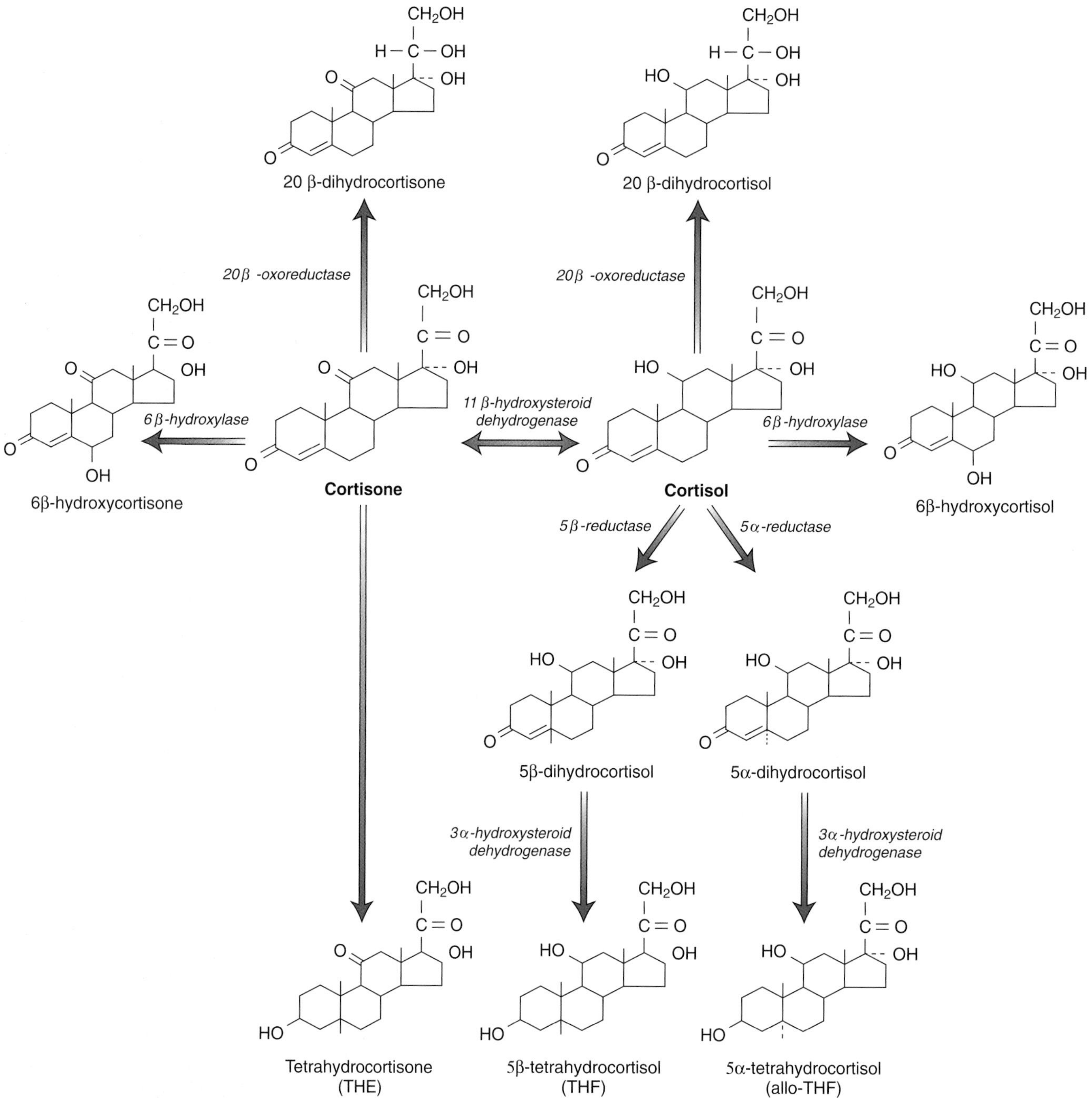

Figure 14–11 ▪ The principal pathways of cortisol metabolism. Interconversion of hormonally active cortisol to inactive cortisone is catalyzed by two isozymes of 11β-hydroxysteroid dehydrogenase (11β-HSD), with 11β-HSD1 principally converting cortisone to cortisol and 11β-HSD2 doing the reverse. Cortisol can be hydroxylated at the C6 and C20 positions. A ring reduction is undertaken by 5α-reductase or 5β-reductase and 3α-hydroxysteroid dehydrogenase.

Effects of Glucocorticoids (Fig. 14–12)

Carbohydrate, Protein, and Lipid Metabolism

Glucocorticoids increase blood glucose concentrations through their action on glycogen, protein, and lipid metabolism. In the liver, cortisol stimulates glycogen deposition by increasing glycogen synthase and inhibiting the glycogen-mobilizing enzyme, glycogen phosphorylase.[129] Hepatic glucose output increases through the activation of key enzymes involved in gluconeogenesis, principally glucose-6-phosphatase and phosphoenolpyruvate kinase (PEPCK).[130,131] In peripheral tissues (muscle, fat), cortisol inhibits glucose uptake and utilization.[132] In adipose tissue, lipolysis is activated, resulting in the release of free fatty acids into the circulation. An increase in total circulating cholesterol and triglycerides is observed but HDL cholesterol levels fall. Glucocorticoids also have a permissive effect upon other hormones including catecholamines and glucagon. The resultant effect is to cause insulin resistance and an increase in blood

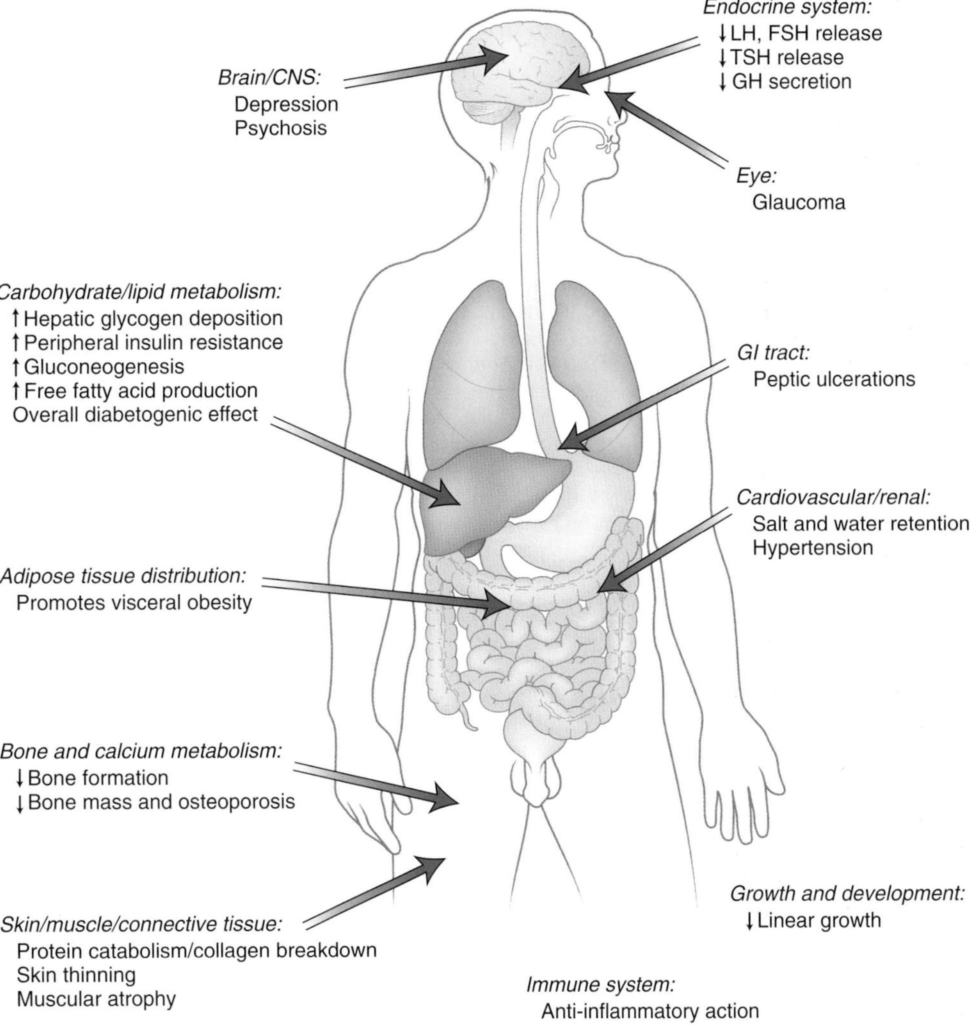

Figure 14–12 ▪ The principal sites of action of glucocorticoids in humans highlighting some of the consequences of glucocorticoid excess. *CNS*, Central nervous system; *GI*, gastrointestinal; *FSH*, follicle-stimulating hormone; *GH*, growth hormone; *LH*, luteinizing hormone; *TSH*, thyroid-stimulating hormone.

glucose concentrations, at the expense of protein and lipid catabolism.

Glucocorticoids stimulate adipocyte differentiation, promoting adipogenesis through the transcriptional activation of key differentiation genes, including lipoprotein lipase, glycerol-3-phosphate dehydrogenase, and leptin.[133] Long-term, the effects of glucocorticoid excess upon adipose tissue is more complex, at least in humans, where the deposition of visceral or central adipose tissue is stimulated,[134] providing a useful discriminatory sign for the diagnosis of Cushing's syndrome. The explanation for the predilection for visceral obesity may relate to the increased expression of both the GR[135] and 11β-HSD1 in omental compared with subcutaneous adipose tissue.[136]

Skin, Muscle, and Connective Tissue

In addition to inducing insulin-resistance in muscle tissue, glucocorticoids also cause catabolic changes in muscle, skin, and connective tissue. In the skin and connective tissue, glucocorticoids inhibit epidermal cell division and DNA synthesis, and reduce collagen synthesis and production.[137] In muscle, glucocorticoids cause atrophy (but not necrosis), which seems to be specific for type II or "phasic" muscle fibers. Muscle protein synthesis is reduced.

Bone and Calcium Metabolism

Glucocorticoids inhibit osteoblast function, which is thought to account for the osteopenia and osteoporosis that characterize glucocorticoid excess.[138] With up to 1% of Western populations taking long-term glucocorticoid therapy,[139] glucocorticoid-induced osteoporosis is becoming a prevalent health concern, affecting 50% of patients treated with corticosteroids for more than 12 months. However, the complication perhaps most feared by physicians is osteonecrosis. Osteonecrosis (also termed *avascular necrosis*) involves the rapid and focal deterioration in bone quality and primarily affects the femoral head, leading to pain and ultimately collapse of the bone, often requiring hip replacement. It can affect individuals of all ages and may occur with relatively low doses of glucocorticoids (e.g., during corticosteroid replacement therapy for adrenal failure).[140] Recent data implicate glucocorticoid-induced osteocyte apoptosis in the pathogenesis of the condition,[141] and the lack of a direct role for an interrupted blood supply suggests that the term *osteonecrosis* is preferable to *avascular femoral necrosis*. However, there is still no explanation for individual susceptibility.

Glucocorticoids also induce negative calcium balance by inhibiting intestinal calcium absorption and increasing renal calcium excretion. As a consequence, PTH secretion is usually increased. In children, glucocorticoids suppress growth but the increases in body mass index are thought to offset a deleterious effect on bone mineral density.[142]

Salt and Water Homeostasis, Blood Pressure Control

Glucocorticoids increase blood pressure by a variety of mechanisms involving actions on the kidney and vasculature.[143] In vascular smooth muscle, they increase sensitivity to pressor agents such as catecholamines and angiotensin II while reducing nitric oxide–mediated endothelial dilatation. Angiotensinogen synthesis is increased by glucocorticoids.[144] In the kidney, depending upon the activity 11β-HSD2, cortisol can act on the distal nephron to cause sodium retention and potassium loss (mediated via the MR).[121] Elsewhere across the nephron, glucocorticoids increase glomerular filtration rate, proximal tubular epithelial sodium transport, and free water clearance.[145] This latter effect involves antagonism of the action of vasopressin and explains the dilutional hyponatremia seen in patients with glucocorticoid deficiency.[146]

Antiinflammatory Actions and the Immune System

Glucocorticoids suppress immunologic responses, which has been the stimulus to develop a series of highly potent pharmacologic glucocorticoids to treat a variety of autoimmune and inflammatory conditions. The inhibitory effects are mediated at many levels. In the peripheral blood, glucocorticoids reduce lymphocyte counts acutely (T lymphocytes > B lymphocytes) by redistributing lymphocytes from the intravascular compartment to spleen, lymph nodes, and bone marrow. Conversely, neutrophil counts increase following glucocorticoid administration. Eosinophil counts rapidly fall, an effect that was historically used as a bioassay for glucocorticoids. The immunologic actions of glucocorticoids involve direct actions on both T and B lymphocytes, which include inhibition of immunoglobulin synthesis and stimulation of lymphocyte apoptosis. Inhibition of cytokine production from lymphocytes is mediated through inhibition of the action of NF-κB. NF-κB plays a crucial and generalized role in inducing cytokine gene transcription; glucocorticoids can bind directly to NF-κB to prevent nuclear translocation and, in addition, induce NF-κB inhibitor, which sequesters NF-κB in the cytoplasm thereby inactivating its effect.[105]

Additional antiinflammatory effects involve inhibition of monocyte differentiation into macrophages and macrophage phagocytosis and cytotoxic activity. Glucocorticoids reduce the local inflammatory response by preventing the action of histamine and plasminogen activators. Prostaglandin synthesis is impaired through the induction of lipocortins, which inhibit phospholipase A2 activity.[147]

Central Nervous System and Mood

Clinical observations on patients with glucocorticoid excess and deficiency reveal that the brain is an important target tissue for glucocorticoids, with depression, euphoria, psychosis, apathy, and lethargy being important manifestations. Both glucocorticoid and mineralocorticoid receptors are expressed in discrete regions of the rodent brain, including hippocampus, hypothalamus, cerebellum, and cortex.[148] Glucocorticoids cause neuronal death, notably in the hippocampus,[149] which may underlie the recent interest in glucocorticoids and cognitive function, memory, and neurodegenerative diseases such as Alzheimer's.[150] Local blockade of cortisol generation by 11β-HSD1 has been shown to improve cognitive function.[151] DHEA has been shown to have neuroprotective effects in the hippocampus region.[152] CYP7B, an enzyme metabolizing DHEA to its 7α-hydroxylated metabolite, is highly expressed in brain but expression was decreased in dentate neurons in the hippocampus.[153] In the eye, glucocorticoids act to raise intraocular pressure through an increase in aqueous humor production and deposition of matrix within the trabecular meshwork, which inhibits aqueous drainage. Steroid-induced glaucoma appears to have a genetic predisposition but the underlying mechanisms are unknown.[154]

Gut

Long-term but not acute administration of glucocorticoids increases the risk of developing peptic ulcer disease.[155] Pancreatitis with fat necrosis is reported in patients with glucocorticoid excess. The GR is expressed throughout the gastrointestinal tract, and the MR in the distal colon; these mediate the corticosteroid control of epithelial ion transport.

Gowth and Development

Although glucocorticoids stimulate GH gene transcription in vitro, glucocorticoids in excess inhibit linear skeletal growth,[142,156] probably as a result of catabolic effects on connective tissue, muscle, and bone and through inhibition of the effects of IGF-1. Experiments on mice lacking the GR gene,[82] emphasize the role of glucocorticoids in normal fetal development. In particular, glucocorticoids stimulate lung maturation through the synthesis of surfactant proteins (SP-A, SP-B, SP-C),[157] and mice lacking the GR die shortly after birth due to hypoxia from lung atelectasis. Glucocorticoids also stimulate the enzyme phenylethanolamine N-methyltransferase (PNMT), which converts noradrenaline to adrenaline in adrenal medulla and chromaffin tissue. Mice lacking the GR do not develop an adrenal medulla.[82]

Endocrine Effects

Glucocorticoids suppress the thyroid axis, probably through a direct action on TSH secretion. In addition, they inhibit 5′ deiodinase activity mediating the conversion of thyroxine to active triiodothyronine. Glucocorticoids also act centrally to inhibit GnRH pulsatility and LH FSH release.

Therapeutic Corticosteroids

Since the dramatic antiinflammatory effect of cortisone was first demonstrated in the 1950s, a series of synthetic corticosteroids have been developed for therapeutic purposes. These are used to treat a diverse variety of human diseases and principally rely on their antiinflammatory and immunologic actions (Table 14–6). The main corticosteroids used in clinical practice, together with their relative glucocorticoid and mineralocorticoid potencies, are listed in Table 14–7.

The structures of common synthetic steroids are depicted in Fig. 14–13. Biologic activity of a corticosteroid is dependent upon a 4-3-keto, 11β-hydroxy, 17α,21-trihydroxyl configuration.[158] Conversion of the C11 hydroxyl group to a C11 keto group (cortisol to cortisone) inactivates the steroid. The addition of a 1,2 unsaturated bond to cortisol results in prednisolone, which is four times more potent than cortisol in classical glucocorticoid bioassays such as hepatic glycogen deposition, suppression of eosinophils, and antiinflammatory actions. Prednisone, widely prescribed in the United States, is the "cortisone-equivalent" of prednisolone and relies upon conversion by 11β-HSD1 in the liver for bioactivity.[159] Potency is further increased by the

TABLE 14–6 THERAPEUTIC USE OF CORTICOSTEROIDS

Endocrine: Replacement therapy (Addison's disease, pituitary disease, congenital adrenal hyperplasia), Grave's ophthalmopathy
Skin: Dermatitis, pemphigus
Hematology: Leukemia, lymphoma, hemolytic anemia, idiopathic thrombocytopenic purpura
Gastrointestinal: Inflammatory bowel disease (ulcerative colitis, Crohn's disease)
Liver: Chronic active hepatitis, transplantation, organ rejection
Renal: Nephrotic syndrome, vasculitides, transplantation, rejection
Central nervous system: Cerebral edema, raised intracranial pressure
Respiratory: Angioedema, anaphylaxis, asthma, sarcoidosis, tuberculosis, obstructive airway disease
Rheumatology: Systemic lupus erythematosus, polyarteritis, temporal arteritis, rheumatoid arthritis
Muscle: polymyalgia rheumatica, myasthenia gravis

TABLE 14–7 RELATIVE BIOLOGIC POTENCIES OF SYNTHETIC STEROIDS IN BIOASSAY SYSTEMS

Steroid	Anti-inflammatory Action	Hypothalamic-Pituitary-Adrenal Suppression	Salt Retention
Cortisol	1	1	1
Prednisolone	3	4	0.75
Methylprednisolone	6.2	4	0.5
Fludrocortisone	12	12	125
Δ^1 Fludrocortisone	14		225
Triamcinolone	5	4	0
Dexamethasone	26	17	0

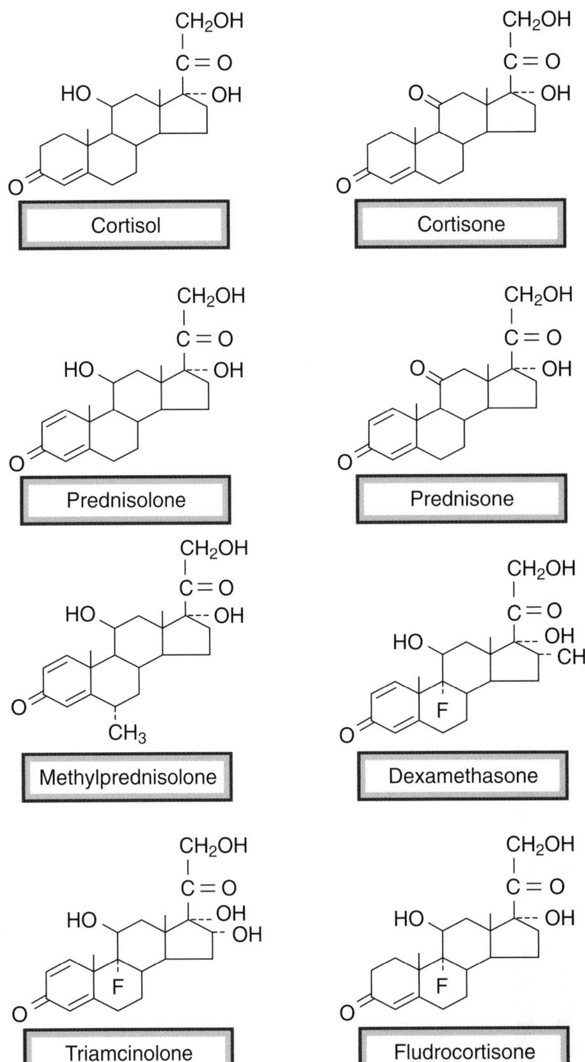

Figure 14–13 ▪ Structures of the natural glucocorticoid cortisol, some of the more commonly prescribed synthetic glucocorticoids, and the mineralocorticoid fludrocortisone. Note that triamcinolone is identical to dexamethasone except that a 16α-hydroxyl group is substituted for the 16α-methyl group. Betamethasone, another widely used glucocorticoid, has a 16β-methyl group.

addition of a 6α-methyl group to prednisolone (methylprednisolone). Fludrocortisone is a synthetic mineralocorticoid having 125-fold greater potency than cortisol in stimulating sodium reabsorption. This is achieved through the addition of a 9α-fluoro group to cortisol. Interestingly, fludrocortisone also has glucocorticoid potency (12-fold greater than cortisol) and the addition of a 16α-methyl group and 1,2, saturated bond to fludrocortisone results in dexamethasone, a highly potent glucocorticoid (25-fold that of cortisol) but with negligible mineralocorticoid activity.[158,160] Betamethasone has the same structure but with a 16β-methyl group and is widely used in respiratory and nasal aerosol sprays.

Corticosteroids are given orally, parenterally, and by numerous topical routes (e.g., eyes, skin, nose, inhalation, rectal suppositories).[160] Unlike hydrocortisone, which has a high affinity for CBG, most synthetic steroids have low affinity for this binding protein and circulate as free steroid (~30%) or bound to albumin (~70%). Circulating half-lives vary depending upon individual variability and underlying disease, particularly renal and hepatic impairment. Cortisone acetate should not be used parenterally as it requires metabolism by the liver to active cortisol.

It is beyond the remit of this chapter to describe which steroid should be given and by which route for the nonendocrine conditions listed in Table 14–6. The acute and long-term administration of corticosteroid therapy in patients with hypoadrenalism and congenital adrenal hyperplasia is discussed under these sections. In addition to the undoubted benefit that corticosteroids provide, there is increasingly a "misuse" of corticosteroid therapy, particularly in patients with respiratory or rheumatologic disease, to such an extent that up to 1% of the population is now prescribed long-term corticosteroid therapy.[139] Because of their established euphoric effect, corticosteroids often make patients feel better but without any objective measures of improvements in underlying disease parameters. In view of the long-term sequelae of chronic glucocorticoid excess, decisions regarding treatment should be evidence-based and subject to constant review based on efficacy and side effects. The endocrinologic consequences of this, notably suppression of the HPA axis, are an important aspect of modern clinical practice. Endocrinologists need to be aware of the effects of long-term therapy and of steroid withdrawal. Selective glucocorticoid receptor agonists (SEGRAs) are being developed with the aim of dissociating the transrepressive, antiinflammatory actions of glucocorticoids from the transactivating effects that, by and large, mediate deleterious side effects.[161]

Long-Term Corticosteroid Therapy, HPA Axis Suppression, and Steroid Withdrawal

The negative feedback control of the HPA axis by endogenous cortisol has been discussed. Synthetic corticosteroids similarly suppress the function of the HPA axis through a process that is dependent on both dose and duration of treatment. As a result, the sudden cessation of corticosteroid therapy may result in adrenal failure.[160] This may also occur following treatment with high doses of the synthetic progestogen, medroxyprogesterone acetate, which possesses glucocorticoid agonist activity.[162] In patients taking any steroid dose for less than 3 weeks' duration, clinically significant suppression of the HPA axis is rarely a problem and patients can withdraw from steroids suddenly with no ill-effect. The possible exception to this is the patient who receives frequent "short" courses of corticosteroid therapy, for example, patients with recurrent episodes of severe asthma. Conversely, suppression of the HPA axis is invariable in patients taking the equivalent of 15 mg/day or more of prednisolone long-term.[163] In patients taking lower doses of corticosteroid long-term (prednisolone 5 to 15 mg/day or equivalent), suppression of the HPA axis is variable. Defects in response of the HPA axis to insulin-induced hypoglycemia or exogenous ACTH have been reported in patients taking doses as low as 5 mg/day of prednisolone,[164] but clinically significant suppression at these doses is debatable. Alternate-day therapy has been associated with lesser suppression of the HPA axis.

All patients treated long-term with corticosteroids should be treated in a similar fashion to patients with chronic ACTH deficiency; they should carry steroid cards and be offered steroid alert bracelets or necklaces. In the event of an intercurrent stress (infection, surgery), supplemental steroid cover should be given, equivalent to 100 to 150 mg/day of hydrocortisone. If the patient is unable to take drugs orally, parenteral therapy is required.

Recovery from suppression may take 6 to 9 months. CRH secretion returns to normal and within a few weeks ACTH levels begin to increase and indeed rise above normal values until adrenal steroidogenesis recovers. In the interim, and without replacement therapy, patients may experience symptoms of glucocorticoid deficiency, including anorexia, nausea, weight loss, arthralgia, lethargy, skin desquamation, and postural dizziness[165] (see Adrenal Insufficiency). To avoid symptoms of glucocorticoid deficiency, steroids should be cautiously withdrawn over a period of months.[166] Assuming the underlying disease permits steroid reduction, doses should be reduced from pharmacologic levels to physiologic levels (equivalent to 7.5 mg/day prednisolone) over a few weeks. Thereafter, doses should be reduced by 1 mg/day of prednisolone every 2 to 4 weeks depending upon patient well-being. An alternative approach is to switch the patient to hydrocortisone 20 mg/day and reduce the daily dose by 2.5 mg/day every week to 10 mg/day. Doses at night should be avoided because this results in greater suppression of early morning ACTH secretion. After 2 to 3 months on these reduced doses of corticosteroids, endogenous function of the HPA axis can be assessed through a corticotropin (ACTH-Synacthen) stimulation test or an insulin-induced hypoglycemia test. A pass response to these tests indicates adequate function of the HPA axis and corticosteroid therapy can be safely withdrawn. In patients taking physiologic doses of prednisolone (less than 5 to 7.5 mg/day) or equivalent, a Synacthen stimulation test (SST) 12 to 24 hours having omitted steroid therapy will provide an immediate answer on whether sudden or gradual withdrawal of steroid therapy is indicated (Table 14–8).

Iatrogenic-induced Cushing's syndrome occurs in patients taking suppressive doses of corticosteroids for more than 3 weeks.[166] The rapidity of onset of clinical features is dependent upon the administered dose but can occur within 1 month of therapy.

Adrenocortical Diseases

Adrenocortical diseases are relatively rare but their importance lies in their morbidity and mortality if untreated, coupled with the relative ease of diagnosis and the availability of effective therapy. The diseases are most readily classified on the basis of whether there is hormone excess or deficiency (see Table 14–9).

Glucocorticoid Excess

In 1912, Harvey Cushing first described a 23-year-old female with obesity, hirsutism, and amenorrhea and 20 years later postulated that this "polyglandular syndrome" was due to a primary pituitary abnormality causing adrenal hyperplasia.[8] Adrenal tumors were shown to cause the syndrome in some cases,[167] but ectopic ACTH production was not characterized until much later in 1962.[168] The term Cushing's *syndrome* is used to describe all causes, whereas Cushing's *disease* is reserved for cases of pituitary-dependent Cushing's syndrome.

Cushing's syndrome comprises the symptoms and signs associated with prolonged exposure to inappropriately elevated levels of free plasma glucocorticoids. The use of the term *gluco-*

TABLE 14–8 SUGGESTED PLAN FOR STEROID REPLACEMENT IN PATIENTS WITHDRAWING FROM CHRONIC CORTICOSTEROID THERAPY

	Duration of Glucocorticoid Treatment			
Dose (mg pred/day)	**≤3 wk***	**>3 wk**		
≥7.5 mg	Can stop	Reduce rapidly e.g., 2.5 mg every 3-4 days THEN		
5-7.5 mg	Can stop	Reduce by 1 mg every 2-4 wk THEN	OR	Convert 5 mg pred to HC 20 mg and ↓ by 2.5 mg/wk to 10 mg for 2-3 mo ↓ SST/ITT ↙ ↘ Pass: Withdraw / Fail: Continue
<5 mg	Can stop	Reduce by 1 mg every 2-4 wk		

*Beware frequent steroid courses, e.g., in asthma.
pred, Prednisolone; *SST,* short Synacthen test; *ITT,* insulin tolerance test.

TABLE 14–9 ADRENOCORTICAL DISEASES

Glucocorticoid Excess
Cushing's syndrome
Pseudo-Cushing's syndromes

Glucocorticoid Resistance

Glucocorticoid Deficiency
Primary hypoadrenalism
Secondary hypoadrenalism
Post-chronic corticosteroid replacement therapy

Congenital Adrenal Hyperplasia
21-Hydroxylase, 3β-hydroxysteroid dehydrogenase, 17α-hydroxylase, 11β-hydroxylase, and StAR deficiencies

Mineralocorticoid Excess

Mineralocorticoid Deficiency
Defects in aldosterone synthesis
Defects in aldosterone action
Hyporeninemic hypoaldosteronism

Adrenal Incidentalomas, Adenomas, and Carcinomas

StAR, Steroidogenic acute regulatory (protein).

TABLE 14–10 PREVALENCE OF SYMPTOMS AND SIGNS IN CUSHING'S SYNDROME AND DISCRIMINANT INDEX COMPARED WITH PREVALENCE OF FEATURES IN PATIENTS WITH SIMPLE OBESITY

Findings	%	Discriminant Index
SYMPTOMS		
Weight gain	91	
Menstrual irregularity	84	1.6
Hirsutism	81	2.8
Psychiatric dysfunction	62	
Backache	43	
Muscle weakness	29	8.0
Fractures	19	
Loss of scalp hair	13	
SIGNS		
Obesity	97	
Truncal	46	1.6
Generalized	55	0.8
Plethora	94	3.0
Moon facies	88	
Hypertension	74	4.4
Bruising	62	10.3
Red-purple striae	56	2.5
Muscle weakness	56	
Ankle edema	50	
Pigmentation	4	
OTHER FINDINGS		
Hypertension	74	
Diabetes	50	
Overt	13	
Impaired glucose tolerance test	37	
Osteoporosis	50	
Renal calculi	15	

Data from Ross EJ, Linch DC. Cushing's syndrome–killing disease: discriminatory value of signs and symptoms aiding early diagnosis. Lancet 1982;2:646-649.

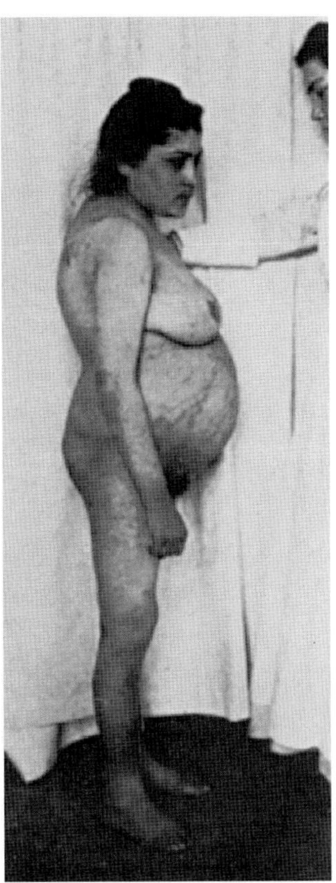

Figure 14–14 ▪ Minnie G., Cushing's index patient, at age 23 years. (From Cushing H. The basophil adenomas of the pituitary body and their clinical manifestations [pituitary basophilism]. Bull Johns Hopkins Hosp 1932;50:137-195.)

corticoid in the definition covers both endogenous (cortisol) and exogenous (e.g., prednisolone, dexamethasone) excess. Iatrogenic Cushing's syndrome is common,[160,166] occurring to some degree in the majority of patients taking long-term corticosteroid therapy. Endogenous causes of Cushing's syndrome are rare and result in loss of the normal feedback mechanism of the HPA axis and the normal circadian rhythm of cortisol secretion. The incidence of pituitary-dependent Cushing's syndrome is estimated to be 5 to 10 cases/million population/year. The incidence of ectopic ACTH syndrome parallels that of bronchogenic carcinoma, and although 0.5% of lung cancer patients have ectopic ACTH syndrome, the rapid progression of the underlying disease often precludes an early diagnosis. Cushing's disease and adrenal adenomas are four times more common in women, whereas ectopic ACTH syndrome is more common in men.

Clinical Features of Cushing's Syndrome

The classic features of Cushing's syndrome of centripetal obesity, moon face, hirsutism, and plethora are well known following Cushing's initial descriptions in 1912 and 1932 (Figs. 14–14, 14–15, and 14–16). However, this gross clinical picture is not always present and a high index of suspicion is required in many cases. Once the normal physiologic effects of glucocorticoids are appreciated (see Fig. 14–12), the clinical features of glucocorticoid excess are easier to define. These are summarized in Table 14–10 together with the most discriminatory features that will assist in distinguishing Cushing's syndrome from simple obesity.[169]

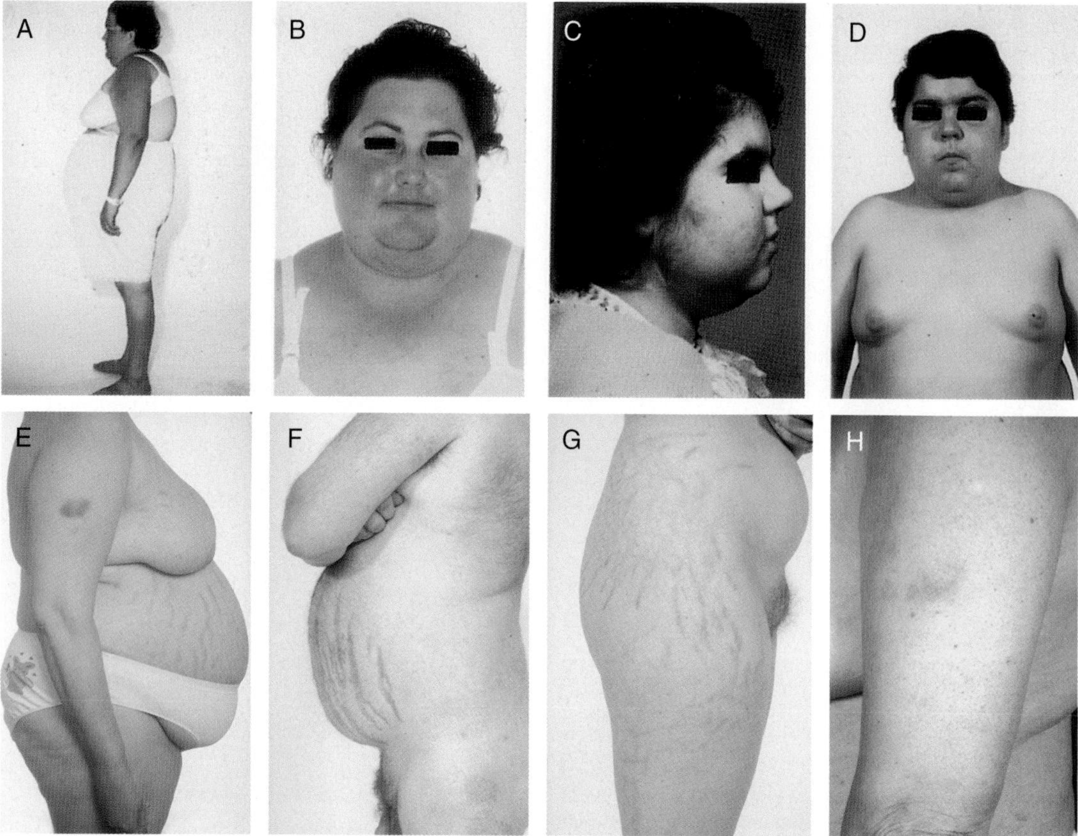

Figure 14–15 ▪ Clinical features of Cushing's syndrome. **A,** Centripetal and some generalized obesity and dorsal kyphosis in a 30-year-old woman with Cushing's disease. **B,** Same woman as in *A,* showing moon facies, plethora, hirsutism, and enlarged supraclavicular fat pads. **C,** Facial rounding, hirsutism, and acne in a 14-year-old girl with Cushing's disease. **D,** Central and generalized obesity and moon facies in a 14-year-old boy with Cushing's disease. **E** and **F,** Typical centripetal obesity with livid abdominal striae seen in a 41-year-old woman **(E)** and a 40-year-old man **(F)** with Cushing's syndrome. **G,** Striae in a 24-year-old patient with congenital adrenal hyperplasia treated with excessive doses of dexamethasone as "replacement" therapy. **H,** Typical bruising and thin skin of Cushing's syndrome. In this case, the bruising has occurred without obvious injury.

Obesity

Weight gain and obesity are the most common sign, and, at least in adults, this is invariably centripetal in nature.[134,170] Indeed generalized obesity is more common in the general population than it is in patients with Cushing's syndrome. One exception is in childhood wherein glucocorticoid excess may result in generalized obesity. In addition to centripetal obesity, patients develop fat depots over the thoracocervical spine ("buffalo" hump), in the supraclavicular region, and over the cheeks and temporal regions, giving rise to the rounded "moon-like" facies. The epidural space is another site of abnormal fat deposition, which may lead to neurologic deficits.

Reproductive

Gonadal dysfunction is common, with menstrual irregularity in females and loss of libido in both sexes. Hirsutism is frequently found in female patients, as is acne. The most common form of hirsutism is vellus hypertrichosis on the face, which should be distinguished from darker terminal differentiated hirsutism that may occur because of ACTH-mediated adrenal androgen excess. Hypogonadism occurs because of a direct inhibitory effect of cortisol upon GnRH pulsatility and LH/FSH secretion, and is reversible upon correction of the hypercortisolism.[171,172]

Psychiatric

Psychiatric abnormalities occur in approximately 50% of patients with Cushing's syndrome regardless of cause.[173,174] Agitated depression and lethargy are among the most common problems, but paranoia and overt psychosis are also well recognized. Memory and cognitive function may also be affected, and increased irritability may be an early feature. Insomnia is common and both rapid eye movement and delta wave sleep patterns are reduced.[175] Lowering of plasma cortisol by medical or surgical therapy usually results in a rapid improvement in the psychiatric state.

Bone

In childhood the most commont presentation is with poor linear growth and weight gain[140]; as discussed, glucocorticoids have profound effects on growth and development.[156] Many patients with longstanding Cushing's syndrome have lost height because of osteoporotic vertebral collapse. This can be assessed by measuring the patient's height and comparing it with their span; in normal subjects these measurements should be equal. Pathologic fractures, either spontaneous or after minor trauma, are not uncommon. Rib fractures, in contrast to those of the vertebrae, are often painless. The radiograph appearances are typical, with exuberant callus formation at the site of the healing

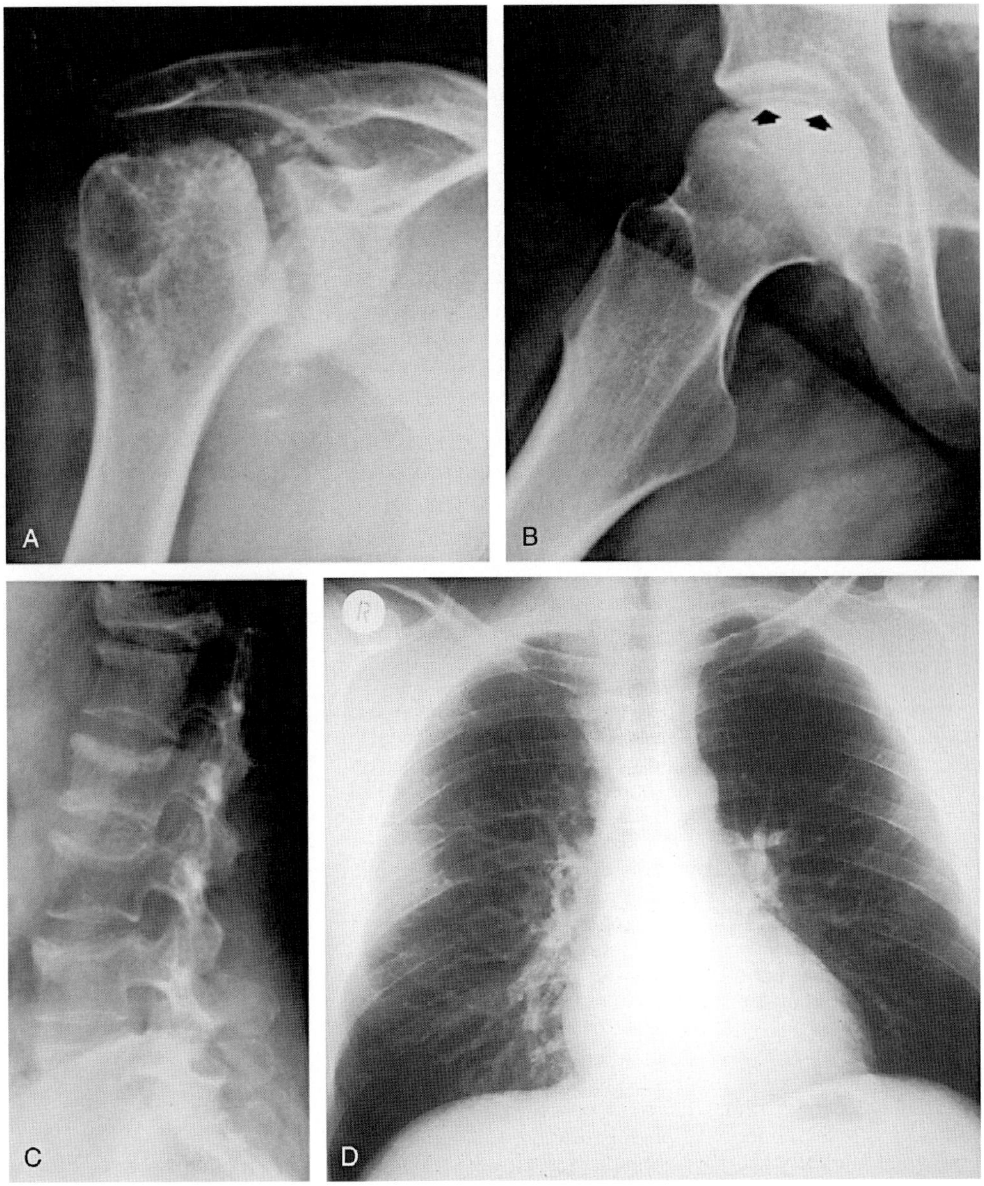

Figure 14–16 ▪ Bone abnormalities in Cushing's disease. **A,** Aseptic necrosis of the right humeral head of a 43-year-old woman with Cushing's disease of about 8 months' duration. **B,** Aseptic necrosis of the right femoral head in a 24-year-old woman with Cushing's disease of about $4^1/_2$ years' duration. The *arrows* indicate the crescent subchondral radiolucency, best seen in this lateral view. **C,** Diffuse osteoporosis, vertebral collapse, and subchondral sclerosis in the patient whose shoulder is shown in *A*. **D,** Rib fracture in a 38-year-old man with Cushing's disease. (*A-C,* From Phillips KA, Nance EP Jr, Rodriguez RM, et al. Avascular necrosis of bone: a manifestation of Cushing's disease. Reprinted from the Southern Medical Journal 1986;79: 825-829.)

fracture. In addition, osteonecrosis of the femoral and humeral heads is a recognized feature of endogenous Cushing's syndrome (see Fig. 14–16). Hypercalciuria may lead to renal calculi but hypercalcemia is not a feature.

Skin

Hypercortisolism results in skin thinning, separation and exposure of the subcutaneous vascular tissue. On examination, wrinkling of the skin on the dorsum of the hand may be seen, resulting in a "cigarette paper" appearance (Liddle's sign). Minimal trauma may result in bruising, which frequently resembles the appearance of "senile purpura." The plethoric appearance of the patient with Cushing's syndrome is secondary to the thinning of the skin[176] combined with loss of facial subcutaneous fat and is not due to true polycythemia. Acne and papular lesions may occur over the face, chest, and back.

The typical, almost pathognomic red-purple livid striae greater than 1 cm in diameter are most frequently found on the abdomen but may also be present on the upper thighs, breasts, and arms. They are very common in younger patients and less so in those older than 50 years of age. They must be differentiated from the paler, less pigmented striae that occur postpartum (striae gravidarum) or in association with rapid weight loss.

Skin pigmentation is rare in Cushing's disease but common in the ectopic ACTH syndrome, and arises because of overstimulation of melanocyte receptors by ACTH.

Muscle

Myopathy and bruising are two of the most discriminatory features of the syndrome.[169] The myopathy of Cushing's involves the proximal muscles of lower limb and shoulder girdle.[177] Complaints of weakness, such as inability to climb stairs or get up from a deep chair are relatively uncommon, but testing for proximal myopathy by asking the patient to rise from a crouching position often reveals the problem.

Cardiovascular

Hypertension is another prominent feature occurring in up to 75% of cases; even though epidemiologic data show a strong association between blood pressure and obesity, hypertension is much more common in patients with Cushing's syndrome than in those with simple obesity.[143] This together with the established metabolic consequences of the disease (diabetes, hyperlipidemia), is thought to explain the increased cardiovascular mortality in untreated cases.[178-180] Cardiovascular events are also more common in patients with presumed iatrogenic Cushing's due to prescribed corticosteroids.[181] In addition, thromboembolic events may be more common in Cushing's patients.

Infections

Infections are more common in Cushing's patients.[182,183] In many instances, these are asymptomatic and occur because the normal inflammatory response is suppressed. Reactivation of tuberculosis has been reported[184] and has even been the presenting feature in some cases. Fungal infections of the skin (notably tinea versicolor) and nails may occur, as may opportunistic fungal infections. Bowel perforation is more common in patients with extreme hypercortisolism and, in turn, the hypercortisolism may mask the usual symptoms and signs of the condition. Wound infections are more common and contribute to poor wound healing.

Metabolic and Endocrine

Glucose intolerance occurs and overt diabetes mellitus is present in up to one third of patients in some series. Hepatic lipoprotein synthesis is stimulated, and increases in circulating cholesterol and triglycerides may be found.[185] Hypokalemic alkalosis is found in 10% to 15% of patients with Cushing's disease but in more than 95% of patients with ectopic ACTH syndrome. Severe factors may contribute to this "mineralocorticoid excess state," including corticosterone and deoxycorticosterone excess, but the principal culprit is thought to be cortisol itself. Depending upon the prevailing cortisol production rate, cortisol swamps 11β-HSD2 in the kidney, to act as a mineralocorticoid. Hypokalemic alkalosis is more common in ectopic ACTH syndrome because cortisol production rates are higher than in patients with Cushing's disease.[121] This can be diagnosed by documenting an increase in the ratio of urinary cortisol/cortisone metabolites. In addition, hepatic 5α-reductase activity is inhibited, resulting in a greater excretion of 5β-cortisol metabolites.[186]

The function of both the pituitary-thyroid axis and pituitary-gonadal axis is suppressed in patients with Cushing's syndrome due to a direct effect of cortisol upon TSH and gonadotropin secretion.[187,188] Cortisol causes a reversible form of hypogonadotrophic hypogonadism but also directly inhibits Leydig cell function. Growth hormone secretion is reduced, possibly mediated through an increase in somatostatinergic tone.

Eye

Ocular effects include raised intraocular pressure[189] and exophthalmos[190] (in up to one third of patients in Cushing's original series), the latter occurring because of increased retroorbital fat deposition. Cataracts, a well-recognized complication of corticosteroid therapy, seem to be uncommon,[191] except as a complication of diabetes. In the author's experience, chemosis is a sensitive and underreported feature of Cushing's syndrome.

CLASSIFICATION AND PATHOPHYSIOLOGY OF CUSHING'S SYNDROME

The condition is most readily classified into ACTH-dependent and ACTH-independent causes (Table 14–11).

TABLE 14–11 CLASSIFICATION OF CAUSES OF CUSHING'S SYNDROME

ACTH-DEPENDENT
Cushing's disease (pituitary-dependent) Ectopic ACTH syndrome Ectopic CRH syndrome Macronodular adrenal hyperplasia Iatrogenic (treatment with ACTH 1-24)
ACTH-INDEPENDENT
Adrenal adenoma and carcinoma Primary pigmented nodular adrenal hyperplasia and Carney's syndrome. McCune-Albright syndrome Aberrant receptor expression (gastric inhibitory polypeptide, interleukin-1β). Iatrogenic (e.g., pharmacologic doses of prednisolone, dexamethasone)
PSEUDO-CUSHING'S SYNDROMES
Alcoholism Depression Obesity

ACTH, Adrenocorticotrophic hormone; *CRH*, corticotropin-releasing hormone.

ACTH-Dependent Causes

Cushing's Disease

When iatrogenic causes are excluded, the commonest cause of Cushing's syndrome is Cushing's disease, accounting for approximately 70 percent of cases. The adrenal glands in these patients show bilateral adrenocortical hyperplasia with widening of the zona fasciculata and reticularis.

Etiology

Cushing himself raised the question as to whether this disease was a primary pituitary condition or secondary to an abnormality in the hypothalamus, and there has been an ongoing debate on this issue ever since.[192] The hypothalamic theory states that ACTH-secreting adenomas arise because of dysfunctional regulation of corticotrophs through chronic stimulation by CRF (or arginine vasopressin), whereas other studies provide data to support a primary pituitary defect as the cause of the condition (Table 14–12).

The hypothalamus may have an initiating role, but the overwhelming evidence is that, at presentation, the condition is pituitary-dependent. In 85% to 90% cases, the disease is due to a pituitary adenoma of monoclonal origin[193,194]; basophil hyperplasia alone is found in 9% to 33% of pathologic series.[192] The majority of tumors are small "microadenomas" (<1 cm), but larger macroadenomas occur in up to 10% of cases and usually signify a more invasive tumor.[195] Selective surgical removal of a microadenoma results in cure with a very low recurrence rate. However, it is possible, particularly in cases with no identifiable pituitary adenoma, that Cushing's disease may be heterogeneous with different subtypes.

A key biochemical hallmark of the disease is a relative resistance of ACTH secretion to normal glucocorticoid feedback inhibition.[196] ACTH-secreting pituitary adenomas function at a higher than normal set-point for cortisol feedback. In Cush-

TABLE 14–12 HYPOTHALAMIC VERSUS PITUITARY THEORY UNDERPINNING THE ETIOLOGY OF CUSHING'S DISEASE

Hypothalamic Theory	Pituitary Theory
Neuroendocrine abnormalities[266,267] Loss of circadian rhythm, sleep disturbance, other "hypothalamic defects" (TSH, LH-FSH secretion)	Lack of "cure" after pituitary stalk section Circulating and CSF CRH levels are suppressed[268] Reversal of "hypothalamic defects" upon correction of hypercortisolism
Efficacy of centrally acting drugs[269,270] Bromocriptine, cyproheptadine, sodium valproate	
Recurrences after pituitary surgery	High surgical cure rate (recurrences resulting from regrowth of initial inadequately resected tumor rather than "real" recurrence)[271,272] Secondary hypoadrenalism after successful pituitary surgery (may be prolonged and associated with reduced ACTH expression in surrounding adjacent normal corticotrophs)[273]
Ectopic CRH-secreting tumors cause Cushing's disease,[265] but pathology shows basophil hyperplasia, not adenomas	Pituitary ACTH-secreting adenoma in almost 90% of cases are monoclonal in origin[274,275]

ACTH, Adrenocorticotropic hormone; *CRH*, corticotropin-releasing hormone; *CSF*, cerebrospinal fluid; *FSH*, follicle-stimulating hormone; *LH*, luteinizing hormone; *TSH*, thyroid-stimulating hormone.

ing's disease, the predominant finding is an increase in ACTH pulse amplitude with loss of normal circadian rhythm but ACTH pulse frequency is also increased in some cases (see Fig. 14–7).[197]

Ectopic ACTH Syndrome

In 15% of cases, Cushing's syndrome may be associated with nonpituitary tumors secreting ACTH—the ectopic ACTH syndrome.[198-202] On clinical grounds, this can be divided into two entities, cases occurring in the setting of highly malignant tumors such as small cell carcinoma of bronchus (Table 14–13) and more indolent cases occurring in patients with underlying neuroendocrine tumors such as bronchial carcinoids. In the former case, the clinical presentation more commonly resembles Addison's disease than Cushing's syndrome. Circulating ACTH concentrations and cortisol secretion rates can be extremely high. As a result, duration of symptoms from onset to presentation is short (<3 months); patients are commonly pigmented and the metabolic manifestations of glucocorticoid excess are often rapid and progressive. Weight loss, myopathy, and glucose intolerance are prominent symptoms and signs. The association of these features with hypokalemic alkalosis and peripheral edema should alert the clinician to the diagnosis.

Depending upon local referral practice, approximately 20% of cases of ectopic ACTH syndrome are explained by indolent tumors, such as benign bronchial carcinoids, which produce ACTH.[202,203] In these cases, symptoms and signs are commonly present for 18 months from onset to clinical presentation. Such patients present with the typical features of Cushing's syndrome and may be biochemically similar to patients with Cushing's disease. Thus, having established a diagnosis of Cushing's syndrome the principal diagnostic dilemma is in the distinction of pituitary-dependent Cushing's from these indolent causes of ectopic ACTH syndrome.[199,201]

Etiology

POMC is expressed in some normal extrapituitary tissues and many tumors (lung, testis) regardless of the presence of Cushing's syndrome, raising the appropriateness of the term *"ectopic" ACTH syndrome.*[204] Tumors most commonly associated with ectopic ACTH syndrome arise from neuroendocrine tissues, the cells of which possess the ability to uptake and decarboxylate amine precursors (APUD cells). However, in the case of small cell lung cancer, only 0.5% to 1% of tumors are associated with ectopic ACTH syndrome and the explanation for the development of ectopic ACTH secretion remains unclear. POMC mRNA transcripts are usually shorter in tumors not associated with ectopic ACTH syndrome, whereas those with the syndrome express larger POMC mRNA species in addition to the "pituitary" size transcript. In addition to aberrant transcriptional regulation of the POMC gene, interaction with tissue-specific transcription factors or methylation status of the POMC gene may be involved. Once secreted, POMC is cleaved in the pituitary by specific serine endoproteases to produce ACTH precursors; in ectopic ACTH syndrome, aberrant peripheral processing of POMC may lead to increased circulating ACTH precursor concentrations (pro-ACTH, N-POC) (Figure 14–5). In contrast to ACTH-secreting pituitary adenomas, ectopic POMC/ACTH production is not responsive to normal glucocorticoid feedback[204] due to a defective GR or GR signaling mechanism.[206] However, this sensitivity to glucocorticoid feedback is far from clear-cut, which is one reason why the differential diagnosis of ACTH-dependent Cushing's syndrome can be challenging.[199]

TABLE 14–13 TUMORS ASSOCIATED WITH THE ECTOPIC ADRENOCORTICOTROPIC HORMONE SYNDROME

Tumor Type	Approximate Incidence (%)
Small cell lung carcinoma	50
Non–small cell lung carcinoma	5
Pancreatic tumors (including carcinoids)	10
Thymic tumors (including carcinoids)	5
Lung carcinoids	10
Other carcinoids	2
Medullary carcinoma of thyroid	5
Pheochromocytoma and related tumors	3
Rare carcinomas of prostate, breast, ovary, gallbladder, colon	10

Ectopic Corticotropin Releasing Factor (CRF) Production

This is a very rare cause of pituitary-dependent Cushing's. A number of cases have now been described in which a tumor (usually bronchial carcinoid, medullary thyroid, or prostate carcinoma) has been shown to secrete CRF alone or in combination with ACTH.[202,207-209] Where available, pituitary histology reveals corticotroph hyperplasia but not adenoma formation. Biochemically these patients usually behave in a similar fashion to patients with ectopic ACTH syndrome with loss of the normal negative glucocorticoid feedback mechanism—50% are resistant to high-dose dexamethasone therapy. It has been suggested that ectopic CRF production may explain the suppression of cortisol secretion following high-dose dexamethasone found in some patients with the "ectopic" ACTH syndrome.

Macronodular Adrenal Hyperplasia

In 10% to 40% of patients with Cushing's disease, there is bilateral adrenocortical hyperplasia associated with one or more nodules, which may be up to several centimeters in diameter.[210-213] Patients tend to be older and have had symptoms for a longer time, but otherwise present with the classic clinical features of Cushing's syndrome. Pathologically the nodules are lobulated and can be markedly enlarged, but internodular hyperplasia is invariably found. Macronodular adrenal hyperplasia (MAH) is thought to result from longstanding adrenal ACTH stimulation, which leads to autonomous adrenal adenoma formation. Thus, as the adrenals in a patient with Cushing's disease become more hyperplastic, they secrete more cortisol for a given ACTH level, which ultimately may lead to "autosuppression." Individual clinical cases support this hypothesis, and MAH should be regarded as an ACTH-dependent form of Cushing's syndrome, even though ACTH levels may be relatively low and dexamethasone suppressibility less marked than in other cases of Cushing's disease.[214] The adenomas can be a trap for the unwary because they may be mistaken for primary adrenal tumours.

ACTH-Independent Causes

Cortisol-Secreting Adrenal Adenoma and Carcinoma

With the exclusion of iatrogenic Cushing's syndrome, adrenal adenomas are responsible for about 10% to 15% of cases and carcinomas for less than 5%. By contrast, in children, 65% of cases of Cushing's syndrome have an adrenal etiology (15% adenomas, 50% carcinomas).[212-214] Onset of clinical features is gradual in patients with adenomas, but often rapid in adrenal carcinoma. In addition to the features of hypercortisolism, patients may complain of loin or abdominal pain and a tumor may be palpable. The tumor may secrete other steroids, such as androgens or mineralocorticoids. Thus, in females, there may be features of virilization, with hirsutism, clitoromegaly, breast atrophy, deepening of the voice, temporal recession, and severe acne. In "pure" cortisol-secreting adenomas, hirsutism is uncommon. Subclinical Cushing's syndrome has been reported in patients with adrenal "incidentalomas" (see Incidentalomas).

Primary Pigmented Nodular Adrenal Hyperplasia (PPNAD) and Carney's Syndrome

About 100 cases of ACTH-independent Cushing's syndrome have been reported in association with bilateral, small pigmented adrenal nodules. Pathologically these nodules are usually 2 to 4 mm in diameter (although they can be larger) and black or brown on cut section. Adjacent adrenal tissue is atrophic, distinguishing this condition from MAH. Presentation is with typical features of Cushing's syndrome but is always in persons younger than 30 years of age and, in 50% of cases, in persons younger than 15 years of age.[217] Cases of PPNAD have been reported without Cushing's syndrome. Bilateral adrenalectomy is curative.

A familial autosomal dominant variant called *Carney's complex* (Table 14–14) comprises mesenchymal tumors (especially atrial myxomas), spotty skin pigmentation, peripheral nerve tumors, and various tumors including breast lesions, testicular tumors, and GH-secreting pituitary tumors.[218] Mutations of the gene encoding for protein kinase A (PKA) regulatory subunit type IA (PRKAR1A) lead to abnormal PKA signaling and explain the phenotype in some cases.[219] Other cases have been mapped to chromosome 2p16 but the underlying genetic mutation is unknown.

McCune-Albright Syndrome

In this condition, fibrous dysplasia and cutaneous pigmentation may be associated with pituitary, thyroid, adrenal, and gonadal hyperfunction. The most common manifestation is with sexual precocity and GH excess, but Cushing's syndrome has been reported.[220] The underlying abnormality is a somatic mutation in the α-subunit of the stimulatory G protein, which is linked to adenyl cyclase. The mutation results in the G protein being constitutively activated, mimicking constant ACTH stimulation at the level of the adrenal. ACTH levels are suppressed and adrenal adenomas may occur.

Macronodular Hyperplasia and Aberrant Receptor Expression

Although macronodular hyperplasia commonly occurs in patients with ACTH-dependent Cushing's syndrome, truly ACTH-independent macronodular hyperplasia (AIMAH) is also recognized as a distinct entity.[221] The nodules are nonpigmented and greater than 5 mm in diameter; occasionally the adrenals may be massively enlarged. The majority of cases are explained on the basis of aberrant receptor expression within the adrenal

TABLE 14–14 CLINICAL FEATURES OF THE CARNEY COMPLEX

Feature	Prevalence (%)
Skin lesions	80
Pigmented lesions	
Blue nevi	
Cutaneous myxomas	
Cardiac myxomas	72
Pigmented nodular adrenal hyperplasia	45
Breast lesions	
Bilateral fibroadenomas	45 (females only)
Testicular tumors	56 (males only)
Pituitary lesions, usually growth hormone–secreting	10
Neural lesions (gastric schwannomas)	<5
Miscellaneous	
Thyroid cancer	Rare
Acoustic neuromas	Rare
Hepatoma	Rare

cortex.[222] Food-induced hypercortisolism due to enhanced adrenal responsiveness to gastric inhibitory polypeptide (GIP) was the first cause of AIMAH described, due to expression of GIP receptors within the adrenal cortex, but aberrant expression of the vasopressin V1, β-adrenergic, LH, serotonin, and angiotensin (AT-1) receptors have also been linked to AIMAH. Protocols have been suggested for the further investigation of AIMAH.[222]

Iatrogenic Cushing's Syndrome

The basis for this condition is discussed under the section on therapeutic corticosteroids. Development of the features of Cushing's syndrome depends upon the dose, duration, and potency of corticosteroid used in clinical practice. ACTH is rarely prescribed but long-term will also result in cushingoid features. Some features such as an increase in intraocular pressure, cataracts, benign intracranial hypertension, aseptic necrosis of the femoral head, osteoporosis, and pancreatitis are more common in iatrogenic compared with endogenous Cushing's syndrome, whereas other features, notably hypertension, hirsutism, and oligorrhea/amenorrhea are more rare.

Special Features of Cushing's Syndrome

Cyclical Cushing's Syndrome

Of particular clinical interest has been a group of patients with cyclical Cushing's syndrome, characterized by periods of excess cortisol production, interspersed by intervals of normal cortisol production (Fig. 14–17). Some of these patients demonstrate a paradoxical rise in plasma ACTH and cortisol when treated with dexamethasone, and occasional patients show benefit with dopamine agonist (bromocriptine) or serotonin antagonist (cyproheptadine) therapy. The majority of cases have been thought to have pituitary-dependent disease and in many of these patients, basophil adenomas have been removed, some with long-term cure. However, cortisol secretion may show some evidence of cyclicity in patients with an ectopic source of ACTH syndrome.[223,224]

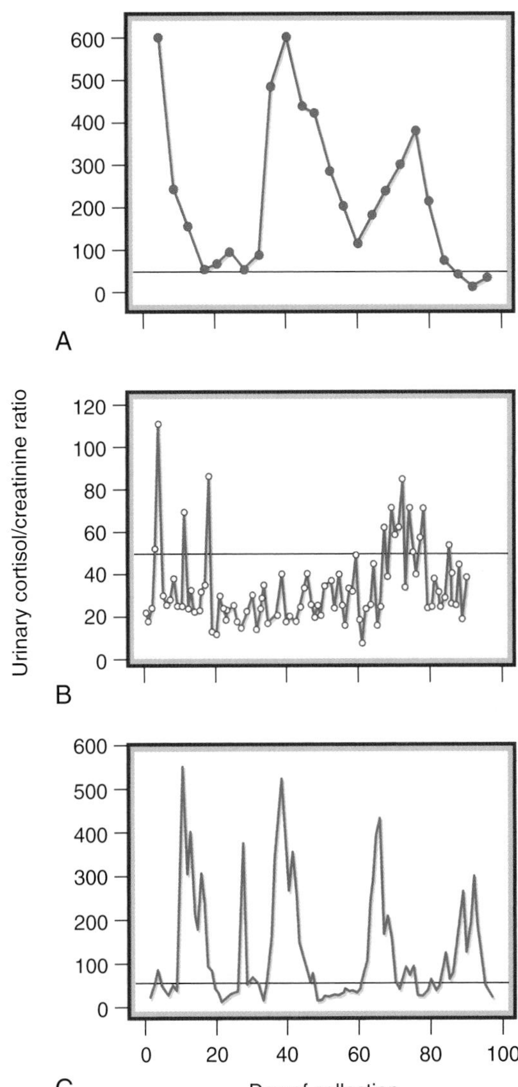

Figure 14–17 ▪ Patterns of cortisol secretion in three patients with cyclical Cushing's syndrome. In each case, ratios of early morning urinary cortisol (nmol/L) to creatinine (mmol/L) are plotted against time. Variable periodicity in cortisol hypersecretion is shown. (From Atkinson AB, McCance DR, Kennedy L, et al. Cyclical Cushing's syndrome first diagnosed after pituitary surgery: a trap for the unwary. Clin Endocrinol 1992;36:297-299.)

Children

In children, in addition to the previously mentioned features, growth arrest is almost invariable.[225] The dissociation between height and weight on the growth chart is obvious. If the patient is growing along the same centile line, then the diagnosis of Cushing's syndrome is highly unlikely. In addition to glucocorticoid-induced growth arrest, androgen excess may result in precocious puberty. Adrenal causes account for 65% of all cases.

Pregnancy

Pregnancy is rare in women with Cushing's syndrome because of associated amenorrhea due to androgen excess or hypercortisolism. However, approximately 100 such cases have been reported, 50% of which are due to adrenal adenomas.[226] A few cases of true pregnancy-induced Cushing's syndrome are described with regression postpartum.[227] In these cases, the etiology is unknown. Establishing a diagnosis and cause can be difficult; clinically striae, hypertension, and gestational diabetes are common features in pregnancy, yet hypertension and diabetes are the most common signs of Cushing's syndrome in a pregnant women (70% and 30% of all cases, respectively). Furthermore, biochemically normal pregnancy is associated with a threefold increase in plasma cortisol due to increased cortisol production rates and increases in cortisol-binding globulin. Urinary free cortisol also rises and dexamethasone does not suppress plasma cortisol to the same degree as the nonpregnant state. Left untreated, the condition has a high maternal and fetal morbidity and mortality. Adrenal and/or pituitary adenomas should be excised. Metyrapone, which is not teratogenic, has been effective in many cases in controlling the hypercortisolism.

Pseudo-Cushing's Syndromes

A pseudo-Cushing's state can be defined as some or all of the clinical features of Cushing's syndrome together with some evidence for hypercortisolism. Resolution of the underlying cause results in disappearance of the Cushingoid state. Several causes are described.

Alcohol

In the original description of this syndrome, urinary and plasma cortisol levels were elevated and failed to suppress with dexamethasone. Plasma ACTH has been found to be normal or suppressed. The condition is rare but should be suspected in a patient with an ongoing history of heavy alcohol intake and biochemical/clinical evidence of chronic liver disease.[228] The pathogenesis of this condition remains unknown but a "two-hit" hypothesis has been put forward to explain its etiology. Chronic liver disease regardless of the cause is associated with impaired cortisol metabolism, but in alcoholic patients this is associated with an increase in cortisol secretion rate, rather than concomitant suppression in the face of impaired metabolism.[229] In some studies, alcohol has directly stimulated cortisol secretion; alternatively, vasopressin levels are elevated in patients with decompensated liver disease and may stimulate the HPA axis. With abstinence from alcohol, the biochemical abnormalities rapidly revert to normal.

Depression

Although the cause is unknown, it is recognized that patients with depression may exhibit the hormonal abnormalities of patients with Cushing's syndrome.[230] These abnormalities are reversible on correction of the psychiatric condition. Conversely, patients with Cushing's syndrome are frequently depressed and a careful clinical and endocrinologic assessment is required.

Obesity

Although one of the most common referrals to a clinical endocrinologist is to exclude an underlying endocrine cause in a patient with obesity, the diagnosis of Cushing's syndrome in such patients should not cause difficulties. Patients with obesity have mildly increased cortisol secretion rates, and the data suggest that this is due to activation of the HPA axis.[231,232] However, circulating cortisol concentrations are invariably normal and urinary free cortisol concentrations are either normal or only slightly elevated. The stimulus to the increased secretion rate appears to be increased peripheral metabolism and hence clearance of cortisol (principally reduced hepatic conversion of cortisone to cortisol by 11β-HSD1 and increased conversion of cortisol to 5α-reduced derivatives).[232]

Investigation of Patients with Suspected Cushing's Syndrome

There are two stages in the investigation of a patient with suspected Cushing's syndrome. (1) Does this patient have Cushing's syndrome? (2) If the answer is "yes," then what is the cause? Unfortunately, many investigators fail to make this distinction and ill-advisedly use tests that are relevant to question (2) to try to answer question (1). In particular, it is essential that radiologic investigations are not undertaken until Cushing's syndrome has been confirmed biochemically. The major tests are listed in Table 14–15.[230,233,234]

TABLE 14–15 TESTS USED IN THE DIAGNOSIS AND DIFFERENTIAL DIAGNOSIS OF CUSHING'S SYNDROME

DIAGNOSIS
Does the patient have Cushing's syndrome?
Circadian rhythm of plasma cortisol
Urinary free cortisol excretion*
Low-dose dexamethasone suppression test*
DIFFERENTIAL DIAGNOSIS
What is the cause of the Cushing's syndrome?
Plasma ACTH
Plasma potassium, bicarbonate
High-dose dexamethasone suppression test
Metyrapone test
Corticotropin-releasing hormone
Inferior petrosal sinus sampling
CT, MRI scanning of pituitary, adrenals
Scintigraphy
Tumor markers

*Valuable outpatient screening tests (see text).
ACTH, Adrenocorticotropic hormone; *CT,* computed tomography; *MRI,* magnetic resonance imaging.

Question 1: "Does this patient have Cushing's syndrome?"

Circadian Rhythm of Plasma Cortisol

In normal subjects, plasma cortisol levels are at their highest first thing in the morning and reach a nadir at around midnight (<50 nmol/L [<2 μg/dL] in a nonstressed subject).[235] This circadian rhythm is lost in patients with Cushing's syndrome such that in the majority of patients the 09.00 hour plasma cortisol is normal but nocturnal levels are raised. Random morning plasma cortisol levels are therefore of little value in making the diagnosis, whereas a midnight cortisol of greater than 200 nmol/L (>7.5 μg/dL) indicates Cushing's syndrome. However, various factors such as stress of venepuncture, intercurrent illness, and admission to hospital may result in false-positive results. Ideally, patients should be hospitalized for 24 to 48 hours before measuring cortisol at midnight, but some centers have reported discriminant results from simply measuring midnight values as an outpatient. Very few laboratories have developed methods for the measurement of free levels of serum cortisol.[236] Because more than 90% of serum cortisol is protein bound, the results of the conventional assay will be affected by drugs or conditions that alter CBG levels. Thus, estrogen therapy or pregnancy may elevate CBG and total serum cortisol. Loss of circadian rhythm is a sensitive diagnostic test, but for the above reasons is not a widely used screening test.

Salivary Cortisol

CBG is absent from saliva and the use of salivary cortisol measurements offers a sensible alternative in that it does not require hospitalization. The diagnostic accuracy of a single midnight salivary cortisol has been established in several studies; a cortisol value over 2.0 ng/mL (5.5 nmol/L) having a 100% sensitivity and 96% specificity for diagnosing Cushing's syndrome.[233,237,238]

Urinary Free Cortisol Excretion

For many years the diagnosis of Cushing's syndrome was based on the measurement of urinary metabolites of cortisol (24-hour urinary 17-hydroxycorticosteroid or 17-oxogenic steroid excretion, depending on the method used). However, the sensitivity and specificity of these methods is poor and most centers have replaced these assays with the more sensitive measurement of urinary free cortisol excretion. Urinary free cortisol is an integrated measure of plasma free cortisol; as cortisol secretion increases, the binding capacity of CBG is exceeded and results in a disproportionate rise in urinary free cortisol. Normal values are less than 220 to 330 nmol/24 hours (80 to 120 μg/24 hours) depending upon the assay used. Patients should make two or three complete consecutive collections to account for patient error in collecting samples and episodic cortisol secretion, notably from adrenal adenomas. Simultaneous creatinine excretion (which differs by no more than 10% on a day-to-day basis) may be used to ensure adequacy of collection. Urinary free cortisol is a useful screening test, but even so, it is accepted that urinary free cortisol may be normal in up to 8% to 15% of patients with Cushing's syndrome.[233,234,239] Conversely, moderately elevated results should always be endorsed by further testing before making a diagnosis of Cushing's syndrome.

Measurement of the cortisol-to-creatinine ratio on the first urine specimen passed on waking obviates the need for a timed collection and has been used as a screening test, particularly if cyclical Cushing's syndrome is suspected.[240] Urine aliquots can be sent by post to the local endocrinology laboratory with ratios repeatedly over 25 nmol cortisol/mmol creatinine being indicative of hypercortisolism.

Low-Dose/Overnight Dexamethasone Suppression Tests

In normal subjects, the administration of a supraphysiologic dose of glucocorticoid results in suppression of ACTH and cortisol secretion. In Cushing's syndrome of whatever cause, there is a failure of this suppression when low doses of the synthetic glucocorticoid dexamethasone are given.[196]

The overnight test is a useful outpatient screening test.[230,233,241] Various doses of dexamethasone have been used, but 1 mg of dexamethasone is usually given at midnight. A normal response is a plasma cortisol less than 140 nmol/L (<5 μg/dL) between 08.00-09.00 hours the following morning. A dose of 1.5 or 2 mg gives a 30% false-positive rate, whereas after 1 mg this is reduced to 12.5% with a false-negative rate of less than 2%. In addition, sensitivity can be improved by reducing the plasma cortisol cut-off value—a post dexamethasone cortisol value of less than 50 nmol/L (<2 μg/dL) effectively excludes Cushing's syndrome. Thus, the outpatient overnight test has high sensitivity (95%) but low specificity, and further investigation is often required.[242,243]

In the 48-hour low-dose dexamethasone test, plasma cortisol is measured at 09.00 hours on day 0 and 48 hours later following dexamethasone given in a dose of 0.5 mg 6 hourly for 48 hours. Using a post dexamethasone plasma cortisol concentration of less than 50 nmol/L (<2 μg/dL), this test is reported as having a 97% to 100% true-positive rate and a false-positive rate of less than 1%.[230,242] Sensitivity is higher if plasma rather than urinary cortisol is measured.

Certain drugs (phenytoin, rifampicin) may increase the metabolic clearance rate of dexamethasone thereby giving false-positive results. Simultaneous measurement of plasma dexamethasone may be useful here and will also detect whether or not patients failed to take the drug.[243]

Pseudo-Cushing's or True Cushing's Syndrome?

In patients with depression, urinary free cortisol concentrations may be elevated and overlap with those seen in patients with true Cushing's syndrome. Compared with patients with Cushing's disease, depressed patients have greater suppressibility following dexamethasone and reduced response to CRF but neither of these tests is diagnostic.[230,244] However, by performing a CRF test after the standard 2-day low-dose dexamethasone suppression test, separation of true versus pseudo-Cushing's syndrome has been reported. In normal subjects and in patients with endogenous depression, insulin-induced hypoglycemia results in a rise in ACTH and cortisol levels, a response that is usually not seen in Cushing's syndrome. Finally, loperamide lowers cortisol values in patients with pseudo-Cushing's but not in true Cushing's syndrome.[230]

Question 2: Having Confirmed Cushing's Syndrome Clinically and Biochemically, "What is the cause?"

Once the biochemical diagnosis has been made, a series of investigations is required to determine the cause of the Cushing's syndrome.

09.00h Plasma ACTH

Ideally ACTH should be measured using a modern two-site immunoradiometric assay. This will differentiate ACTH-dependent from ACTH-independent causes. In Cushing's disease, 50% of patients have a 09.00h ACTH within the normal reference range (2 to 11 pmol/L or 9 to 52 pg/mL); in the remainder it is modestly elevated. ACTH levels in the ectopic ACTH syndrome are high (usually greater than 20 pmol/L [>90 pg/mL]); nevertheless, overlap values are seen in Cushing's disease in 30% of cases[245] and cannot therefore be used to differentiate these two conditions (Fig. 14–18). The most discriminatory time of day to measure ACTH is between 23.00 to 01.00 when ACTH/cortisol secretion is at a nadir; in our practice, ACTH is usually measured alongside cortisol in the circadian rhythm studies. A midnight ACTH result greater than 5 pmol/L (>22 pg/mL) in a

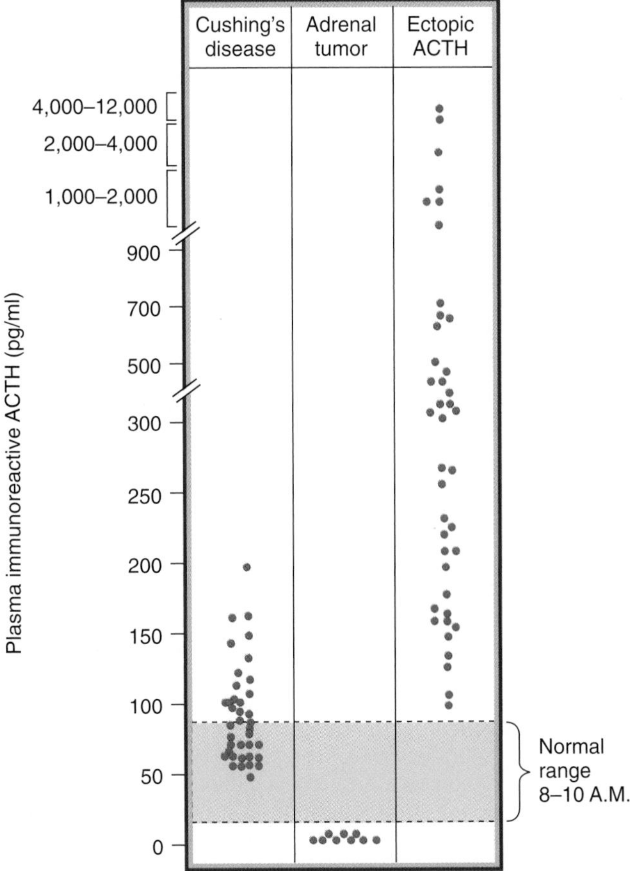

Figure 14–18 ■ Plasma adrenocorticotropic hormone (ACTH) concentrations in patients with Cushing's disease and Cushing's syndrome associated with adrenocortical tumors and ectopic ACTH syndrome. To convert values to pmol/L, multiply by 0.2202. (From Besser GM, Edwards CRW. Cushing's syndrome. Clin Endocrinol Metab 1972;1:451-490.)

patient with biochemical hypercortisolism confirms that the underlying disease is ACTH-dependent. The measurement of ACTH precursors (pro-ACTH, POMC) is not routinely available but may be more useful in detecting an ectopic source of ACTH; more data are required on patients with "occult" tumors causing the syndrome.

In patients with adrenal tumors, plasma ACTH is invariably undetectable (<1 pmol/L). This can also occur with degradation of ACTH; as a result, nonhemolyzed blood samples should be placed in ice and immediately separated.

"Problem patients" are those in whom plasma ACTH levels are low normal or intermittently detectable. This may occur in macronodular hyperplasia. The danger is that in some patients the asymmetry of the nodular hyperplasia may lead to a diagnosis of adrenal adenoma, the plasma ACTH is ignored, and an inappropriate adrenalectomy is performed. Conversely, in some patients with this syndrome, an autonomous adrenal tumor develops and, despite detectable ACTH, unilateral adrenalectomy is required.

Plasma Potassium

Hypokalemic alkalosis is present in more than 95% of patients with the ectopic ACTH syndrome, but is present in fewer than 10% of patients with Cushing's disease. The etiology of this mineralocorticoid excess state is now established. Patients with the ectopic syndrome usually have higher cortisol secretion rates, which saturate the renal protective 11β-HSD2 enzyme, resulting in cortisol-induced mineralocorticoid hypertension[121] (see Chapter 15). In addition, these patients have higher levels of the ACTH-dependent mineralocorticoid, deoxycorticosterone.

High-Dose Dexamethasone Suppression Test

The rationale for this test is that in Cushing's disease there is a resetting of the negative feedback control of ACTH to a higher level than normal. Thus, cortisol levels do not suppress with low-dose, but do so following high-dose dexamethasone. The original test introduced by Liddle was based on giving dexamethasone 2 mg 6 hourly for 48 hours and demonstrating a greater than 50% fall in urinary 17-hydroxycorticosteroids following dexamethasone.[196] In the modern test, plasma and/or urinary free cortisol is measured at 0 and +48 hours and a greater than 50% suppression of plasma cortisol in comparison to the basal sample has been used to define a positive response. In all cases, response is graded and dependent upon the original cortisol secretion rate; greater suppression is often observed in patients with lower basal cortisol values. In Cushing's disease, about 90% of patients have a positive 48-hour test in comparison with 10% with the ectopic ACTH syndrome. The robustness of the test can be improved by altering the cortisol cut-off value; thus the test has 100% specificity for diagnosing pituitary disease if more than 90% suppression in urinary free cortisol is used. Less commonly, 8 mg dexamethasone is given orally at 23.00 hours and plasma cortisol taken at 08.00 hours on the same day (basal sample) and at 08.00 hours on the following morning.[246] A further variation on this test is the timed (5- to 7-hour) infusion of dexamethasone (1 mg/hour).[247]

Up to 50% of patients with ectopic ACTH syndrome due to indolent bronchial carcinoid tumors exhibit some suppression following high-dose dexamethasone. Conversely, some patients with Cushing's disease, usually those with large invasive ACTH-secreting pituitary macroadenomas, may show no suppression following high-dose dexamethasone.[248]

Metyrapone Test

Metyrapone blocks the conversion of 11-deoxycortisol to cortisol and deoxycorticosterone to corticosterone by inhibiting 11β-hydroxylase (see Fig. 14–3). This lowers plasma cortisol and, via negative feedback control, increases plasma ACTH. This in turn stimulates an increase in the secretion of adrenal steroids proximal to the block. Given in doses of 750 mg 4 hourly for 24 hours, patients with Cushing's disease exhibit an exaggerated rise in plasma ACTH with 11-deoxycortisol levels at 24 hours exceeding 1000 nmol/L (35 μg/dL). In most patients with the ectopic ACTH syndrome there is little or no response, but occasional patients (possibly those producing both ACTH and CRF) have an 11-deoxycortisol response that may be similar to that observed in Cushing's disease.[249]

The metyrapone test was originally used to distinguish patients with Cushing's disease from those with a primary adrenal cause. However, these can be more reliably distinguished by measuring plasma ACTH and subsequent CT scanning of the adrenals. As indicated, the test does not reliably distinguish between Cushing's disease and the ectopic ACTH syndrome and the value of this test in modern endocrine practice has been questioned. It should be reserved for patients when the results of other tests are equivocal.

Corticotropin-Releasing Factor Test

CRF is a 41 amino acid peptide, identified by Vale in 1981 from ovine hypothalami. The ovine sequence differs by seven amino acid residues from that of the human; even so, it is slightly more effective in stimulating the release of ACTH in humans.[250] The test involves the intravenous injection of either ovine or human CRF in a dose of 1 μg/kg body weight or a single dose of 100 μg (Fig. 14–19). In some centers, CRF is combined with arginine vasopressin (AVP), which results in an augmented ACTH response. The test can be performed in the morning or afternoon, and, after basal sampling, blood samples for ACTH and cortisol are taken every 15 minutes for 1 to 2 hours following the administration of CRF.[240,242,251,252]

In normal subjects, CRF produces a rise in ACTH and cortisol (approximately 15% to 20%), but this response is exaggerated in Cushing's disease, where typically an ACTH increase greater than 50% and a cortisol rise greater than 20% over baseline values is seen. No response is seen in the ectopic ACTH syndrome, but false-positive results have been reported. In distinguishing pituitary-dependent Cushing's from the ectopic ACTH syndrome, the response of ACTH and cortisol to CRF has a specificity and sensitivity of approximately 90%. However, using an ACTH increase of 100% or a cortisol rise of 50% over baseline values, a positive response effectively eliminates a diagnosis of ectopic ACTH syndrome, which is the real benefit of this test. Up to 10% of patients with Cushing's disease do not respond to CRF.

Inferior Petrosal Sinus Sampling/Selective Venous Catheterization

The most robust test to distinguish Cushing's disease from the ectopic ACTH syndrome is inferior petrosal sinus sampling (IPSS).[201] As blood from each half of the pituitary drains into the ipsilateral inferior petrosal sinus, catheterization and venous sampling of both sinuses simultaneously can distinguish a pituitary from an ectopic source[248,253] (Fig. 14–20). In virtually all patients with the ectopic ACTH syndrome, the ratio of ACTH concentrations between the inferior petrosal sinus and simultaneously drawn peripheral venous level is less than 1.4 : 1. In contrast, in Cushing's disease this ratio is elevated at greater than 2.0. However, because of the problem of intermittent ACTH secretion, it is useful to make measurements before and at intervals (e.g., 2, 5, and 15 minutes), after intravenous injection of 100 μg synthetic ovine CRF.[254,255] Using this approach, an ACTH petrosal sinus/peripheral ratio greater than 3.0 post-CRF has a sensitivity of 97% and specificity of 100% in diagnosing

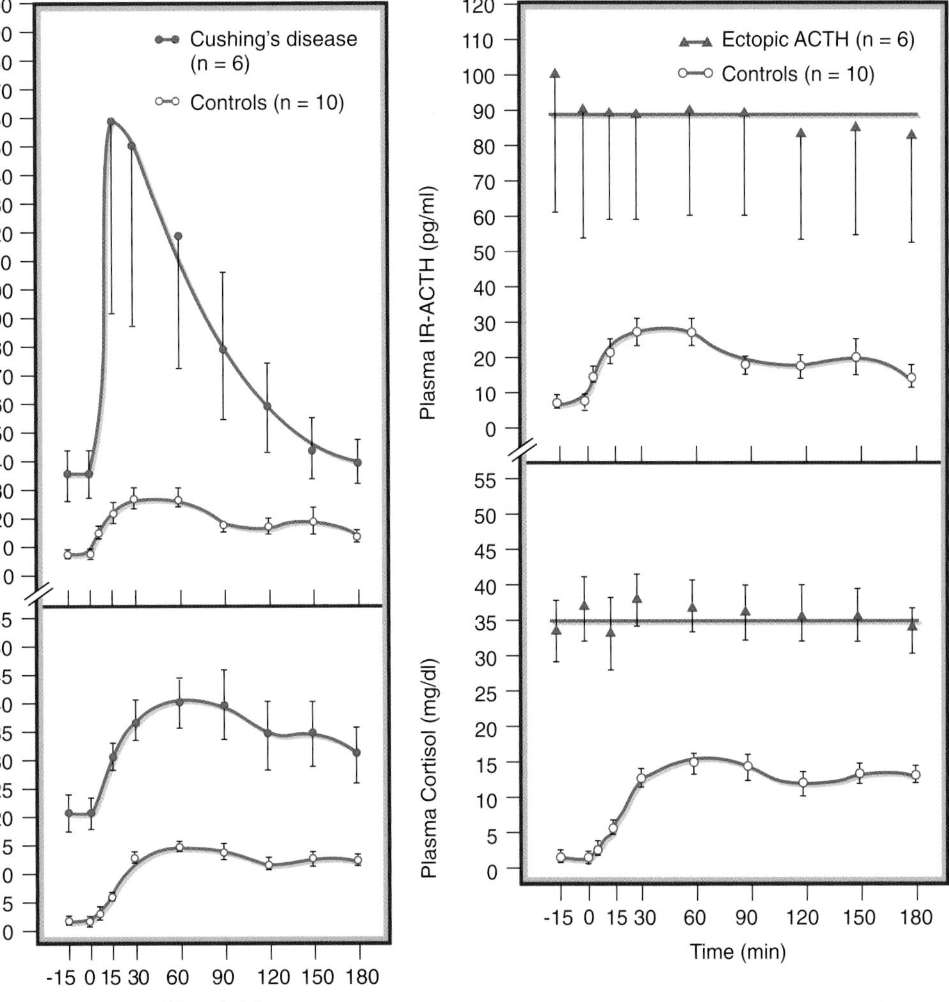

Figure 14–19 ▪ Comparison of the cortisol and adrenocorticotropic hormone (ACTH) responses to an intravenous injection of ovine corticotropin-releasing hormone (1 µg/kg) in normal subjects, patients with Cushing's disease, and patients with ectopic ACTH. (From Chrousos GP, Schulte HM, Oldfield EH, et al. The corticotropin-releasing factor stimulation test: an aid in the evaluation of patients with Cushing's syndrome. N Engl J Med 1984; 310:622-626.)

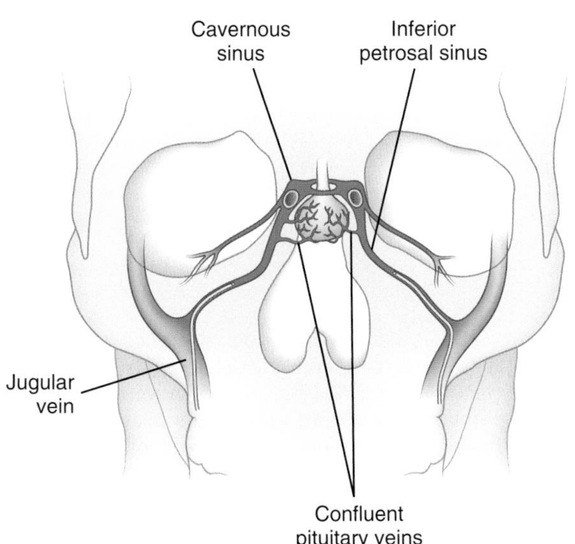

Figure 14–20 ▪ Anatomy of the venous drainage of the pituitary gland through the inferior petrosal venous sinuses. (From Oldfield EH, Chrousos GP, Schulte HM, et al. Preoperative lateralization of ACTH-secreting pituitary microadenomas by bilateral and simultaneous inferior petrosal sinus sampling. Reprinted from N Engl J Med 1985;312:100-103.)

Cushing's disease.[255] IPSS may also be of value in lateralizing a pituitary tumor in a patient in whom imaging techniques have failed to demonstrate a microadenoma, although other centers have found that this is of little value in predicting tumor location. Coadministration of desmopressin with CRF may help in localizing the tumor. However, it should be remembered that many tumors are central and may drain into both sinuses; current evidence suggests that it would unwise to base the surgical procedure on the results of IPSS studies alone.

IPSS is technically demanding; it has been associated with complications (referred aural pain, thrombosis) and should only be performed in an experienced tertiary referral center. In our practice we adopt a clinical diagnostic algorithm (Fig. 14–21) and use IPSS where the differential diagnosis remains in doubt (i.e., lack of adequate suppression following high-dose dexamethasone or CRF response or identified lesion on pituitary MRI scan).

Rarely, selective catheterization of vascular beds may be required to identify the source of ectopic ACTH secretion, for example, from a small pulmonary carcinoid or thymic tumor.

Tumor Markers

Many tumors responsible for the ectopic ACTH syndrome also produce peptide hormones other than ACTH or its precursors.

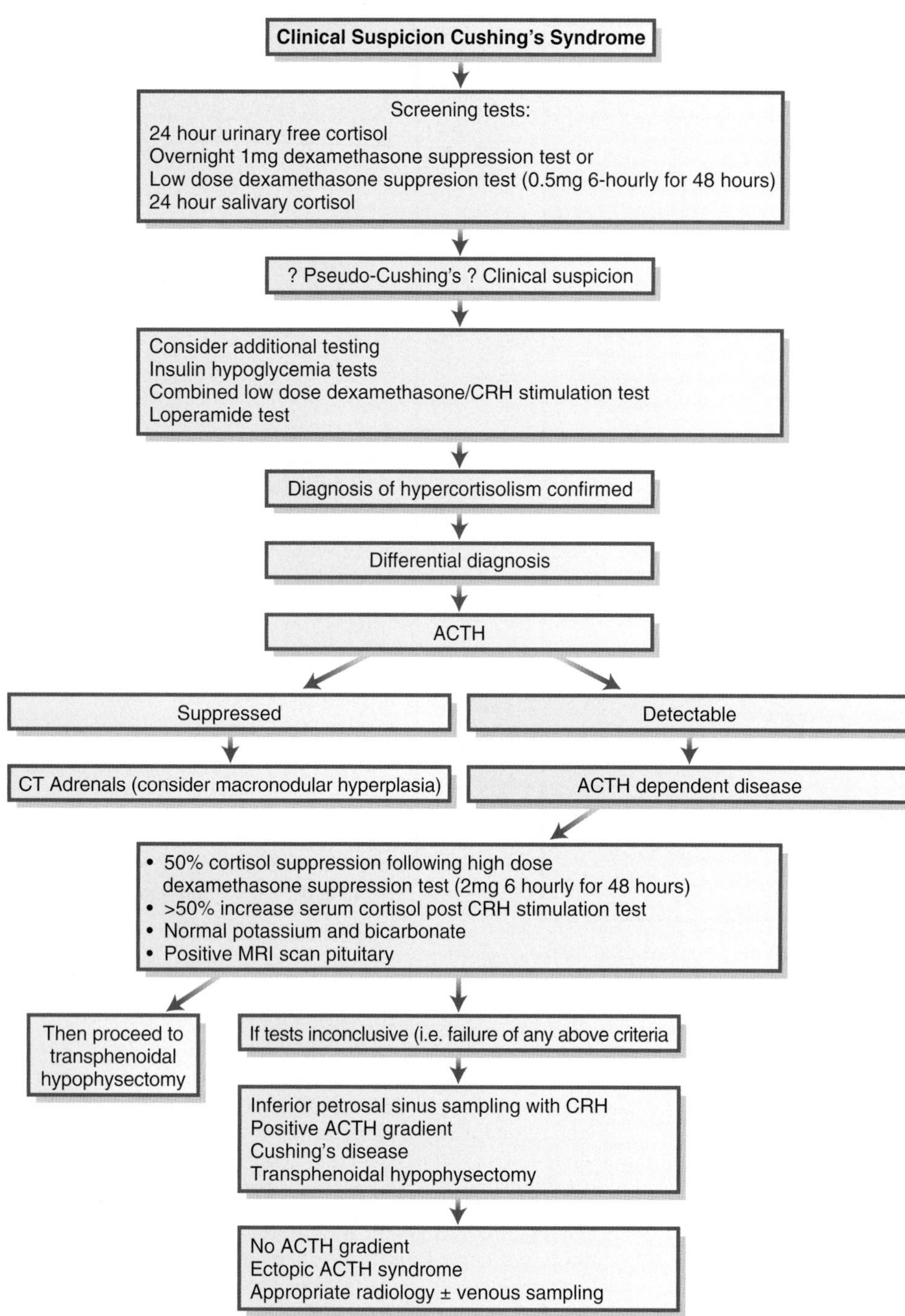

Figure 14–21 ▪ Investigation of a patient with suspected Cushing's syndrome. The laboratory diagnosis of Cushing's syndrome and the differential diagnosis of its cause are debatable and differ in any given center depending on many factors, including familiarity, turn-around time of hormone assays, and local expertise in techniques such as inferior petrosal sinus sampling (IPSS). Depicted here is an algorithm in use within many endocrine units based upon the reported sensitivity and specificity of each endocrine test.

Imaging

CT/MRI Scanning of Pituitary and Adrenals

High-resolution, thin-section contrast-enhanced imaging using either CT or MRI has revolutionized the investigation of Cushing's syndrome.[248,253] However, it is essential that the results of any imaging technique must always be interpreted alongside the biochemical results if mistakes are to be avoided. In imaging the adrenals, asymmetrical nodular hyperplasia may lead to a false diagnosis of adrenal adenoma. Due to the presence of "pituitary incidentalomas,"[256] pituitary CT/MRI scanning may produce false-positive results, particularly for lesions less than 5 mm in diameter.

Pituitary MRI is the investigation of choice once the biochemical tests suggest Cushing's disease, with a sensitivity of 70% and specificity of 87% (Fig. 14–22). About 90% of ACTH-secreting pituitary tumors are microadenomas (i.e., less than 10 mm in diameter). The classic features of a pituitary microadenoma are a hypodense lesion after contrast, associated with deviation of the pituitary stalk, and a convex upper surface of the pituitary gland (see Fig. 14–22). With such small tumors it is not surprising that the sensitivity of CT scanning is relatively low (20% to 60%) with a similar specificity.

By contrast, for adrenal imaging, CT rather than MRI is the investigation of choice offering better spatial resolution (Fig. 14–23),[257] but MRI scanning may provide diagnostic information in patients with suspected adrenal carcinoma. Once again, it is

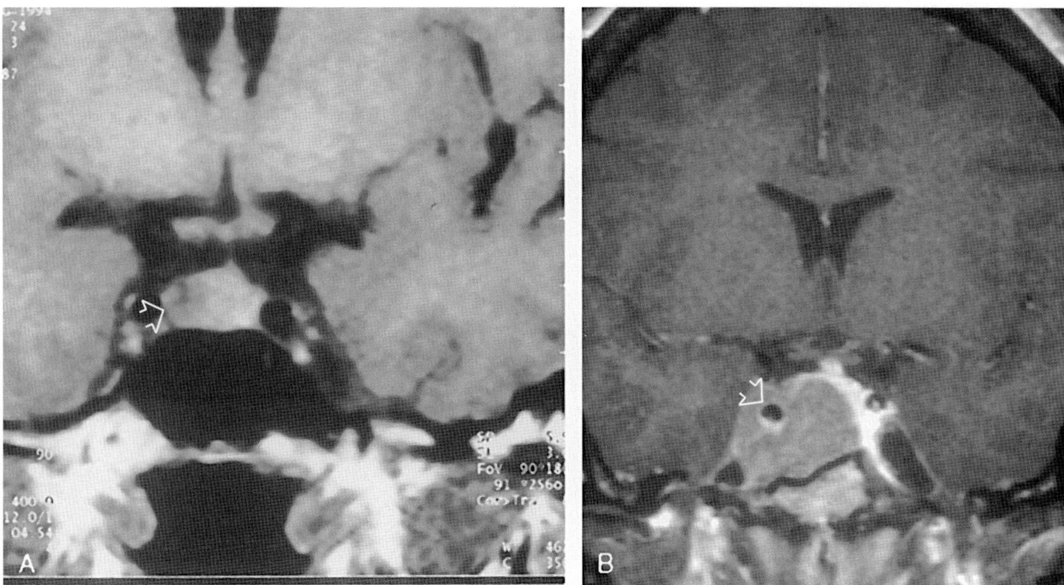

Figure 14–22 ▪ **A,** Magnetic resonance imaging (MRI) scan of pituitary demonstrating the typical appearance of a pituitary microadenoma. A hypodense lesion is seen in the right side of the gland with deviation of the pituitary stalk away from the lesion. After a biochemical diagnosis of Cushing's disease, this patient was cured following transsphenoidal hypophysectomy. **B,** MRI scan of the pituitary gland demonstrating a large macroadenoma in a patient with Cushing's disease. In contrast to smaller tumors, these tumors are invariably invasive and recur after surgery.

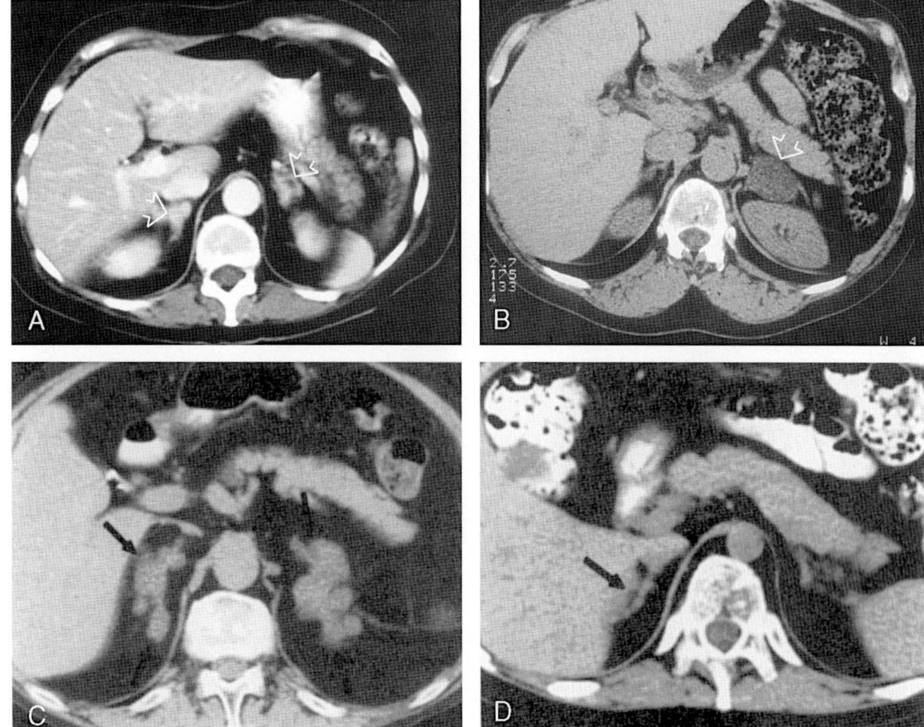

Figure 14–23 ▪ **A,** Adrenal computed tomographic (CT) scan demonstrating bilateral adrenal hyperplasia in a patient with Cushing's disease. **B,** CT scan of a typical solitary left adrenal adenoma causing Cushing's syndrome. **C,** Cushing's syndrome caused by massive macronodular hyperplasia. Adrenal glands are replaced by multiple nodules *(arrows)*. Combined weight of adrenal glands was over 100 g. **D,** Cushing's syndrome caused by surgically proven primary pigmented nodular adrenal disease in a 21-year-old patient. Notice the multiple small nodules with the relatively atrophic internodular adrenocortical tissue involving the medial limb of the right adrenal gland *(arrow)*. (*C* and *D* from Findling JW, Doppman JL. Biochemical and radiologic diagnosis of Cushing's syndrome. Endocrinol Metab Clin North Am 1994;23:511-537.)

stressed that "adrenal incidentalomas" are present in up to 5% of normal subjects, and thus adrenal imaging should not be performed unless biochemical investigation suggests a primary adrenal cause (undetectable ACTH concentrations). Adrenal carcinomas are large and often associated with metastatic spread at presentation (Fig. 14–24).

In patients with "occult" ectopic ACTH syndrome, high-definition CT/MRI scanning of thorax, abdomen, and pelvis with images every 0.5 cm may be required to detect small ACTH-secreting carcinoid tumors (Fig. 14–25).

Scintigraphy Studies

This is of value in certain patients with primary adrenal pathology. The most commonly used agent is ^{131}I-6β-iodomethyl-19-norcholesterol.[258] This is a marker of adrenocortical cholesterol

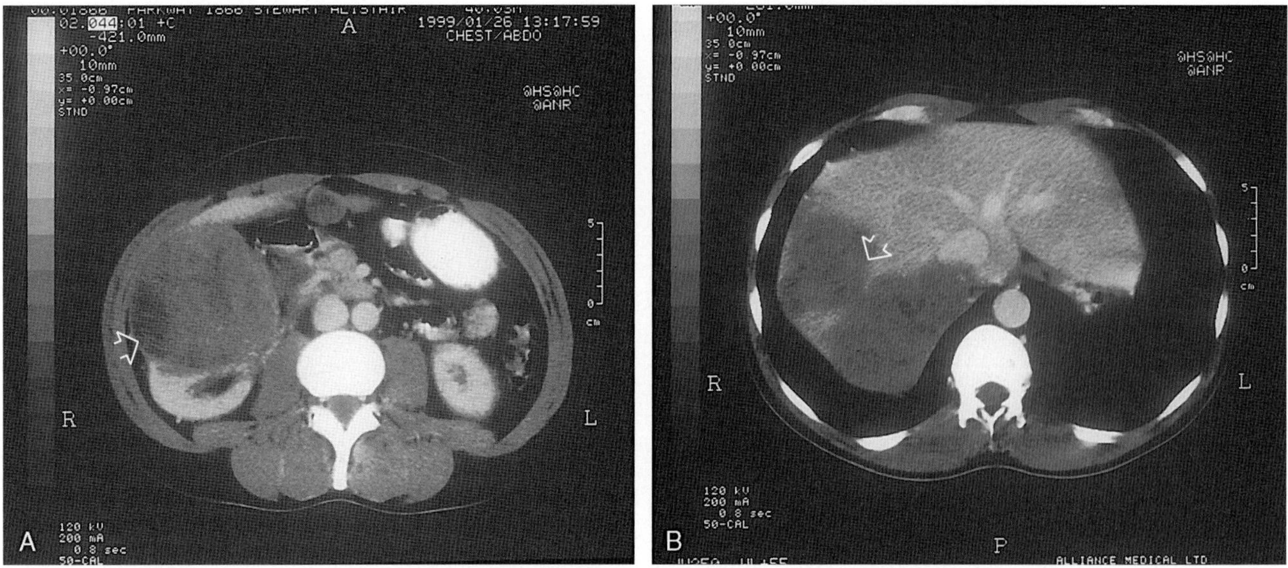

Figure 14–24 ▪ Computed tomographic scan of a patient with rapidly progressing Cushing's syndrome caused by an adrenal carcinoma. An irregular right adrenal mass is shown **(A)** with a large liver metastasis **(B).**

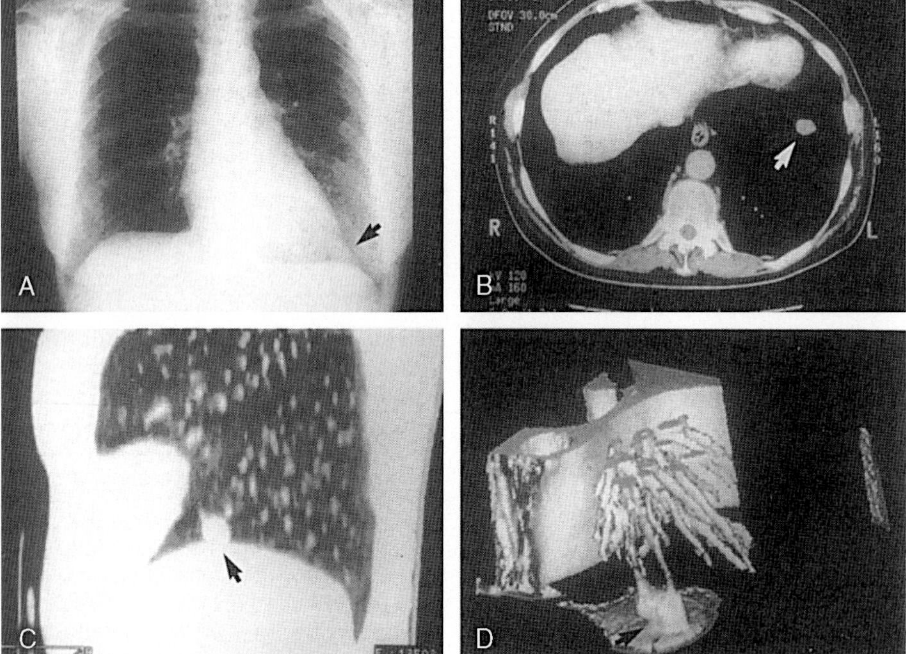

Figure 14–25 ▪ Imaging of the thorax in the ectopic adrenocorticotropic hormone (ACTH) syndrome. **A,** Plain chest radiograph demonstrating suspicious lesion behind the left heart border *(arrow)*. **B** and **C**, Axial and sagittal computed tomographic images demonstrating a bronchial carcinoid tumor *(arrow)* abutting the diaphragm. **D,** Three-dimensional reconstruction illustrating adherence of the tumor to the diaphragm *(arrow)*, which was confirmed at surgery. (From Newell-Prince J, Trainer P, Besser M, et al. The diagnosis and differential diagnosis of Cushing's syndrome and pseudo-Cushing's states. Endocr Rev 1998;19:647-672.)

uptake. In patients with adrenal adenomas, the isotope is taken up by the adenoma but not by the contralateral suppressed adrenal. Adrenal scintigraphy is useful in patients with suspected adrenocortical macronodular hyperplasia, in which CT scanning may be misleading by suggesting unilateral pathology, whereas with isotope scanning the bilateral adrenal involvement is identified.

Many neuroendocrine tumors giving rise to the ectopic ACTH syndrome express somatostatin receptors and can be imaged by administering radiolabeled analogues of somatostatin (most commonly ^{111}Indium-labeled octreotide). This technique can detect tumors only a few millimeters in diameter and should be considered in patients with ACTH-dependent Cushing's syndrome in whom pituitary disease has been excluded.[259]

Treatment of Cushing's Syndrome

Adrenal Causes

Adrenal adenomas should be removed by unilateral adrenalectomy, with a 100% cure rate.[260] With the increasing experience of laparoscopic adrenalectomy in most tertiary centers, this has now become the surgical treatment of choice for unilateral tumors, reducing surgical morbidity and postoperative hospital stay compared with traditional open approaches.[261] Following operation, it may take many months or even years for the contralateral suppressed adrenal to recover. It is wise, therefore, to give slightly suboptimal replacement therapy with dexamethasone 0.5 mg in the morning, with intermittent measurement of morning plasma cortisol before taking dexamethasone. When the morning plasma cortisol is above 180 nmol/L (6.5 µg/dL), dexamethasone can be stopped. A subsequent insulin tolerance test may then demonstrate whether the response to stress is normal. In the interim, all patients should carry a steroid alert card and increase their dose of replacement therapy in the event of an intercurrent illness.

Adrenal carcinomas have a very poor prognosis and most patients are dead within 2 years of diagnosis.[216] It is usual practice to try to remove the primary tumor even though metastases may be present so as to enhance the response to the adrenolytic agent *o,p′*-DDD[262] (Mitotane). Radiotherapy to the tumor bed and to some metastases, such as those in the spine, may be of limited value.

Pituitary-Dependent Cushing's Syndrome

The treatment of Cushing's disease has been significantly enhanced through transsphenoidal surgery conducted by an experienced surgeon. Before the selective removal of a pituitary microadenoma, the treatment of choice was bilateral adrenalectomy. This had an appreciable mortality even in the best centers (up to 4%) and significant morbidity. The major risk was the subsequent development of Nelson's syndrome (postadrenalectomy hyperpigmentation with a locally aggressive pituitary tumor) (Fig. 14–26), which was attributed to loss of any negative feedback following adrenalectomy.[263] In an attempt to avoid this, pituitary irradiation was often carried out at the time of bilateral adrenalectomy.[264] In addition, these patients required lifelong replacement therapy with hydrocortisone and fludrocortisone. Currently, bilateral adrenalectomy is rarely indicated for patients with Cushing's disease but may be performed when pituitary surgery has failed or when the condition has recurred.

The surgical outcome for transsphenoidal hypophysectomy is center-dependent and related to surgical expertise.[265] Because of the hazards of untreated Cushing's disease and potential complications of surgery, the endocrinologist should refer cases only to a recognized surgical specialist where outcome data have been established. In optimal centers, cure rates are 80% to 90% for microadenomas and 50% for macroadenomas.[266] Rates for hypopituitarism and permanent diabetes insipidus postoperatively depend upon how aggressive the surgeon has been in removing pituitary tissue. The ideal outcome is a cured patient with intact pituitary function, but this may not be possible in a patient with Cushing's disease in whom a pituitary adenoma was not identified preoperatively or during the operation itself.

At the time of surgery, patients should be treated with corticosteroids as for any other patient with potential or confirmed deficit of the HPA axis. Postoperatively, hydrocortisone can be withdrawn to maintenance replacement doses usually within 3 to 7 days. On day 5 postoperatively, a 09.00h plasma cortisol should be measured with the patient having omitted hydrocortisone for 24 hours. Following selective removal of a microadenoma, the surrounding corticotrophs are normally suppressed (Fig. 14–27). In these cases, plasma cortisol levels are less than 30 nmol/L (<1 µg/dL) postoperatively and glucocorticoid replacement therapy is required. Using the dexamethasone regimen described earlier after removal of an adrenal adenoma, there is usually (but not invariably) gradual recovery of the HPA axis (Fig. 14–28). A nonsuppressed plasma cortisol postoperatively suggests that the patient is not "cured," even though cortisol secretion may have fallen to normal or subnormal values.[267,268] The recurrence rate in patients with an established "cure" following pituitary surgery is 2%, but this value is higher in children (up to 40%).[269,270] A detailed assessment of residual pituitary function is required in each case and close follow-up of such individuals is warranted.

In the past, pituitary irradiation was often used in the treatment of Cushing's disease. However, the improvements in pituitary surgery have resulted in far fewer patients being so treated. In children, pituitary irradiation appears to be more effective.[271] Radiotherapy is not recommended as a primary treatment but is reserved for patients not responding to pituitary microsurgery or when bilateral adrenalectomy has been performed, or in patients with established Nelson's syndrome.

Ectopic ACTH Syndrome

Treatment of the ectopic ACTH syndrome depends on the cause. If the tumor can be found and has not spread, then its removal can lead to cure (e.g., bronchial carcinoid or thymoma). However, the prognosis for small cell lung cancer associated with the ectopic ACTH syndrome is poor. The cortisol excess and associated hypokalemic alkalosis and diabetes mellitus can be ameliorated by medical therapy. The treatment of the small cell tumor itself will also, at least initially, produce improvement. Sometimes, if the ectopic source of ACTH cannot be found, it may be necessary to perform bilateral adrenalectomy and then follow up the patient carefully (sometimes for several years) before the primary tumor becomes apparent.

Medical Treatment of Cushing's syndrome

Several drugs have been used in the treatment of Cushing's syndrome. Metyrapone inhibits 11β-hydroxylase and has been most commonly given, often to lower cortisol concentrations before definitive therapy, or while awaiting benefit from pituitary irradiation. The daily dose has to be determined by measuring either plasma or urinary free cortisol. The aim should be to achieve a mean plasma cortisol of about 300 nmol/L (11 µg/dL) during the day or a normal urinary free cortisol. The drug is usually given in doses ranging from 250 mg twice daily to 1.5 g every 6 hours. Nausea is a side effect that can be helped (if not due to adrenal insufficiency) by giving the drug with milk.[272]

Aminoglutethimide is a more toxic drug, which in high dose blocks earlier enzymes in the steroidogenic pathway and thus affects the secretion of steroids other than cortisol. In doses of 1.5 to 3 g daily (start with 250 mg 8 hourly) it commonly produces nausea, marked lethargy, and a high incidence of skin rash.[273] It is commonly prescribed as combination therapy with metyrapone.

Trilostane, a 3β-hydroxysteroid dehydrogenase inhibitor, is ineffective in Cushing's disease, as the block in steroidogenesis is overcome by the rise in ACTH. However, it can be effective in patients with adrenal adenomas.[274]

Ketoconazole is an imidazole that has been widely used as an antifungal agent but causes abnormal liver function tests in about 15% of patients. Ketoconazole blocks a variety of steroidogenic cytochrome P450–dependent enzymes and thus lowers plasma cortisol levels. For effective control of Cushing's syndrome, 400 to 800 mg daily have been required.[275]

Following the demonstration of the expression of the PPAR-γ receptor in ACTH-secreting pituitary tissue, a potentially novel therapy for treating Cushing's disease is the thiozolidinedione rosiglitazone.[276] Doses up to 8 mg/day are required to suppress cortisol secretion but the drug seems to have lasting benefit in approximately only 20% of cases studied.[277] Further studies are under way.

o,p′-DDD, or mitotane, is an adrenolytic drug that is taken up by both normal and malignant adrenal tissue causing adrenal atrophy and necrosis.[262] Because of its toxicity, it has been used mainly in the management of adrenal carcinoma. Doses of up

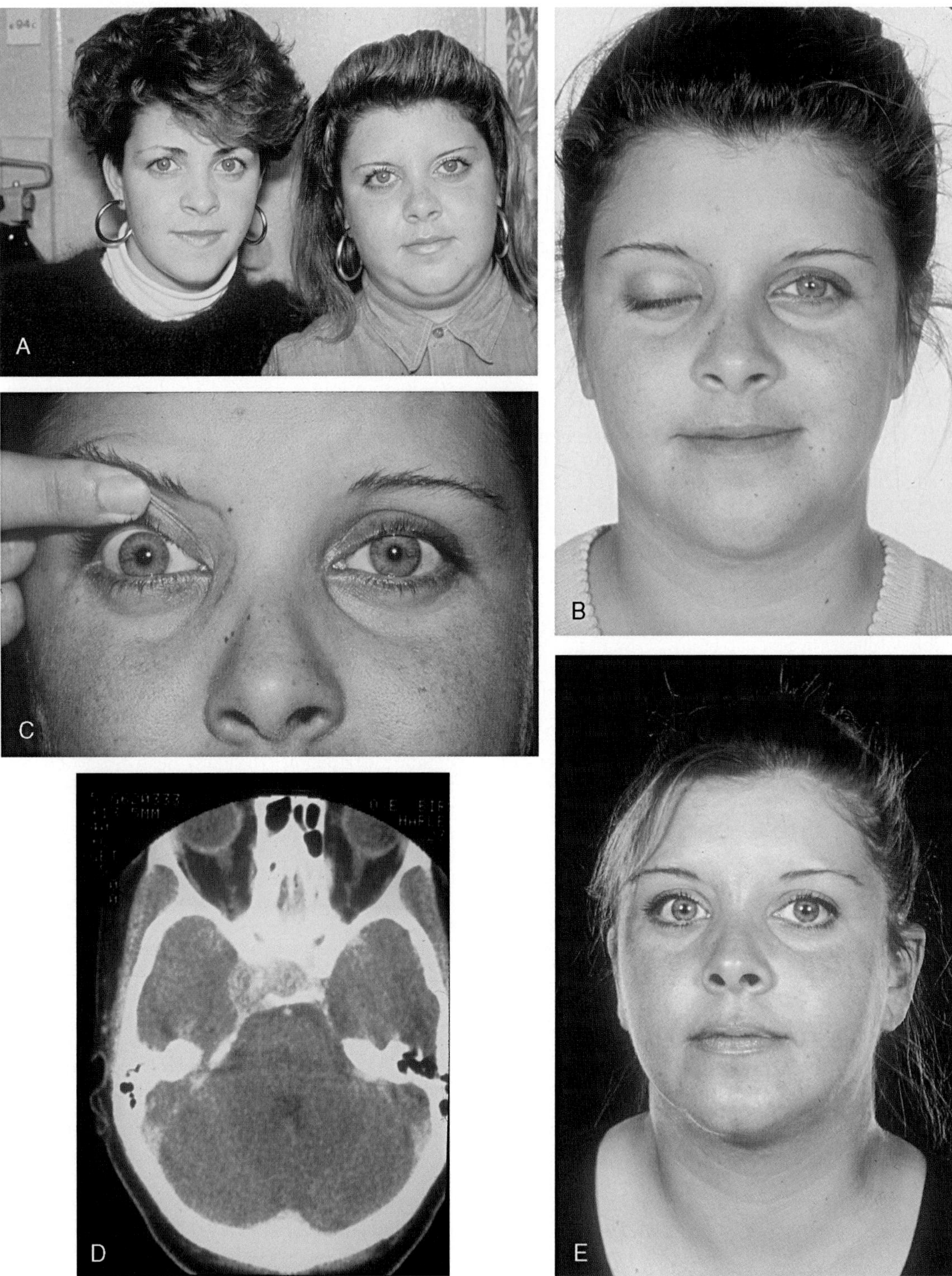

Figure 14–26 ■ A young woman with Cushing's disease, photographed initially beside her identical twin sister **(A)**. In this case, treatment with bilateral adrenalectomy was undertaken. Several years later, the patient presented with Nelson's syndrome and a right third cranial nerve palsy (**B** and **C**) related to cavernous sinus infiltration from a locally invasive corticotropinoma **(D)**. Hypophysectomy and radiotherapy were performed with reversal of the third nerve palsy **(E)**. Note the advancing skin pigmentation of Nelson's syndrome.

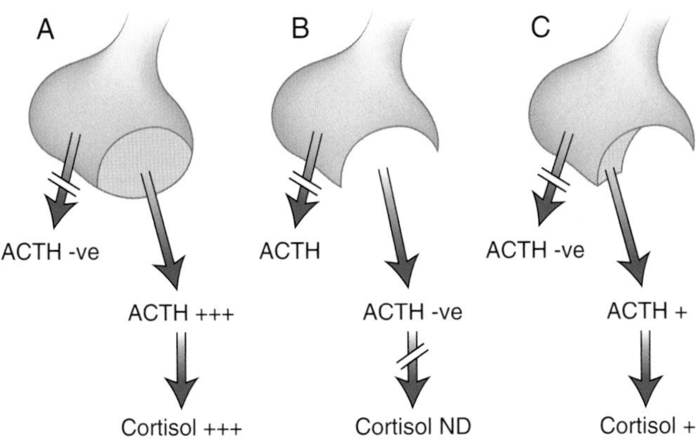

Figure 14–27 ▪ Selective removal of a microadenoma and its effect on the hypothalamic-pituitary-adrenal axis. Because the surrounding normal pituitary corticotrophs are suppressed in a patient with an adrenocorticotropic hormone (ACTH)-secreting pituitary adenoma, successful removal of the tumor results in ACTH and hence adrenocortical deficiency with an undetectable (<50 nmol/L [2 μg/dL]) plasma cortisol level. A plasma cortisol level higher than 50 nmol/L (2 μg/dL) postoperatively implies that the patient is not cured. (Courtesy of Dr. Peter Trainer.)

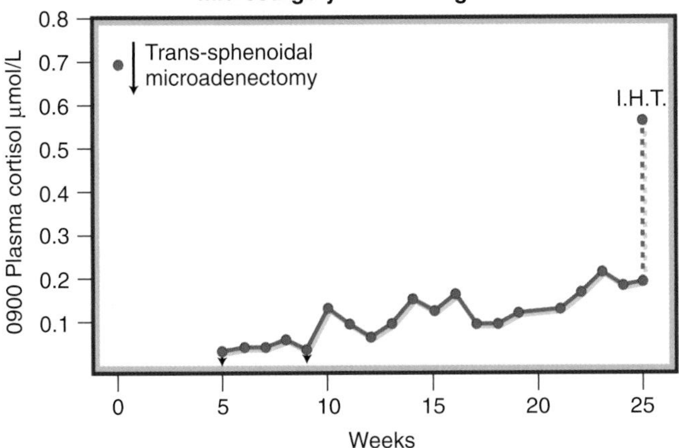

Figure 14–28 ▪ Gradual recovery of function of the hypothalamic-pituitary-adrenal axis after removal of a pituitary adrenocorticotropic hormone–secreting microadenoma. The insulin hypoglycemia test (I.H.T.) eventually demonstrated the return of a normal stress response.

to 5 g/day are required to control glucocorticoid excess, although evidence that it causes tumor shrinkage or improves long-term survival is lacking. The drug will also produce mineralocorticoid deficiency and concomitant glucocorticoid and mineralocorticoid replacement therapy may be required. Side effects are common and include fatigue, skin rashes, neurotoxicity, and gastrointestinal disturbance.

Prognosis of Cushing's Syndrome

Studies carried out before the introduction of effective therapy indicated that 50% of patients with untreated Cushing's syndrome died within 5 years, principally from vascular disease.[178] Even with modern management, an increased prevalence of cardiovascular risk factors persist for many years after an apparent "cure."[179,180] Paradoxically, upon correction of the hypercortisolism, patients can often feel worse. Skin desquamation, steroid-withdrawal arthropathy, profound lethargy, and mood changes may occur and take several weeks or months to resolve.[278] In the author's experience, these features, together with postural hypotension, are particularly severe in "cured" patients who may also be rendered vasopressin-deficient. They can usually be ameliorated by a transient increase in glucocorticoid replacement therapy. Patients are invariably GH-deficient and GH replacement therapy may produce clinical benefit.

Features of Cushing's syndrome disappear over a period of 2 to 12 months. Hypertension and diabetes mellitus improve, but as with other secondary causes may not resolve completely. The osteopenia of Cushing's syndrome improves rapidly in the first 2 years after treatment but resolves more slowly thereafter.[279] Vertebral fractures and osteonecrosis are irreversible and permanent deformity results. Visceral obesity and myopathy are both reversible features. Reproductive and sexual function return to normal within 6 months as long as anterior pituitary function was not compromised.

Glucocorticoid Resistance

A small number of patients have been described who have increased cortisol secretion but without the stigmata of Cushing's syndrome.[81,280] These patients are resistant to suppression of cortisol with low-dose dexamethasone but respond to high doses. ACTH levels are elevated and lead to increased adrenal production of androgens and deoxycorticosterone. Thus patients may present with the features of androgen and/or mineralocorticoid excess. Treatment with a dose of dexamethasone adequate to suppress ACTH (usually 3 mg/day) results in a fall in adrenal androgens and often returns plasma potassium and blood pressure to normal levels. Many of these patients have been found to have point mutations in the steroid-binding domain of the glucocorticoid receptor, with consequent reduction of glucocorticoid-binding affinity, but this is not invariable. A useful clinical discriminatory test to differentiate this condition from Cushing's syndrome is to measure bone mineral density—this is preserved in patients with glucocorticoid resistance or even increased in female cases because of the androgen excess. In addition, circadian rhythm for ACTH and cortisol is preserved in patients with glucocorticoid resistance.

GLUCOCORTICOID DEFICIENCY

Primary and Secondary Hypoadrenalism

Primary hypoadrenalism refers to glucocorticoid deficiency occurring in the setting of adrenal disease, whereas secondary hypoadrenalism arises because of deficiency of ACTH (Table 14–16). A major distinction between these two is that mineralocorticoid deficiency invariably accompanies primary hypoadrenalism, but this does not occur in secondary hypoadrenalism because only ACTH is deficient; the renin-angiotensin-aldosterone axis is intact. A further important cause of adrenal insufficiency where there may be dissociation of glucocorticoid and mineralocorticoid secretion is congenital adrenal hyperplasia.

TABLE 14–16 ETIOLOGY OF ADRENOCORTICAL INSUFFICIENCY (EXCLUDING CAH)

PRIMARY: ADDISON'S DISEASE
Autoimmune
Sporadic
Autoimmune polyendocrine syndrome type I (Addison's disease, chronic mucocutaneous candidiasis, hypoparathyroidism, dental enamel hypoplasia, alopecia, primary gonadal failure, see Chapter 41)
Autoimmune polyendocrine syndrome type II (Schmidt's syndrome) (Addison's disease, primary hypothyroidism, primary hypogonadism, insulin-dependent diabetes, pernicious anemia, vitiligo, Chapter 41)
Infections
Tuberculosis
Fungal infections
Cytomegalovirus
HIV
Metastatic tumor
Infiltrations
Amyloid
Hemochromatosis
Intra-adrenal hemorrhage (Waterhouse-Friderichsen syndrome) after meningococcal septicemia
Adrenoleukodystrophies
Congenital adrenal hypoplasia
DAX-1 mutations
SF-1 mutations
ACTH resistance syndromes
Mutations in *MC2-R*
Triple A syndrome
Bilateral adrenalectomy
SECONDARY
Exogenous glucocorticoid therapy
Hypopituitarism
Selective removal of ACTH-secreting pituitary adenoma
Pituitary tumors and pituitary surgery, craniopharyngiomas
Pituitary apoplexy
Granulomatous disease (tuberculosis, sarcoid, eosinophilic granuloma)
Secondary tumor deposits (breast, bronchus)
Postpartum pituitary infarction (Sheehan's syndrome)
Pituitary irradiation (effect usually delayed for several years)
Isolated ACTH deficiency
Idiopathic
Lymphocytic hypophysitis
TRIT gene mutations
POMC processing defect
POMC gene mutations

ACTH, Adrenocorticotropic hormone; *HIV,* human immunodeficiency virus; *POMC,* pro-opiomelanocortin.

Primary Hypoadrenalism

Addison's Disease

Thomas Addison described this condition in his classic monograph published in 1855.[2]

Etiology

This is a rare condition with an estimated incidence in the developed world of 0.8 cases per 100,000 and prevalence of 4 to 11 cases/100,000 population. Nevertheless, it is associated with significant morbidity and mortality but once the diagnosis is made it can be easily treated.[281,282] The causes of Addison's disease are listed in Table 14–16.

TABLE 14–17 INCIDENCE OF OTHER ENDOCRINE AND AUTOIMMUNE DISEASES IN PATIENTS WITH AUTOIMMUNE ADRENAL INSUFFICIENCY (N = 448)

Disease	Incidence (%)
Thyroid disease	
Hypothyroidism	8
Nontoxic goiter	7
Thyrotoxicosis	7
Gonadal failure	
Ovarian	20
Testicular	2
Insulin-dependent diabetes mellitus	11
Hypoparathyroidism	10
Pernicious anemia	5
None	53

Autoimmune Adrenalitis

In the Western world, autoimmune adrenalitis accounts for over 70% of all cases.[283] Pathologically, the adrenal glands are atrophic with loss of most of the cortical cells, but the medulla is usually intact. In 75% of cases, adrenal autoantibodies can be detected.[284] Fifty percent of patients with this form of Addison's disease have an associated autoimmune disease (Table 14–17), thyroid disease being the most common. Conversely only 1% to 2% of patients with more common autoimmune diseases such as insulin-dependent diabetes mellitus or thyrotoxicosis have antiadrenal autoantibodies and develop adrenal disease. This figure is higher in patients with autoimmune hypoparathyroidism (16%). These "polyglandular autoimmune syndromes" (PGA) have been classified into two distinct variants[284]; PGA type I or autoimmune polyendocrinopathy-candidiasis-ectodermal dysplasia (APECED), is a rare autosomal recessive condition comprising Addison's disease, chronic mucocutaneous candidiasis, and hypoparathyroidism and the more common PGA II, comprising Addison's disease, autoimmune thyroid disease, diabetes mellitus, and hypogonadism. Here, autoantibodies to 21-hydroxylase are usually present and are predictive for the development of adrenal destruction.[284] PGA syndromes are discussed in greater detail in Chapter 41.

Infections

Worldwide, infectious diseases are the most commont cause of primary adrenal insufficiency and comprise tuberculosis, fungal infections (histoplasmosis, cryptococcus), and cytomegalovirus. Adrenal failure may also occur in the acquired immunodeficiency syndrome.[285]

Tuberculous Addison's disease results from hematogenous spread of the infection from elsewhere in the body and extraadrenal disease is usually evident. The adrenals are initially enlarged with extensive epithelioid granulomas and caseation, and both the cortex and the medulla are affected. Fibrosis ensues and the adrenals become normal or smaller in size with calcification evident in 50% of cases. The adrenals are frequently involved in patients with acquired immunodeficiency syndrome[285,286]; adrenalitis may occur following infection with cytomegalovirus or atypical mycobacterium, and Kaposi's sarcoma may result in adrenal replacement. Onset is often insidious, but if tested, more than 10% of patients with AIDS will demonstrate a subnormal cortisol response following a short Synacthen test. Adrenal insufficiency may be precipitated through the concomitant administration of appropriate antiinfectives such as ketoconazole (inhibits cortisol synthesis) or rifampicin (increases cortisol metabolism). Rarely patients with AIDS and features of adrenal insufficiency are found to have elevated circulating ACTH and cortisol concentrations that fail to suppress normally following low-dose dexamethasone administration. This is thought to reflect an "acquired" form of glucocorticoid resistance due to reduced GR affinity, but the underlying cause remains unknown.[287]

Miscellaneous

With the exception of tuberculosis and autoimmune adrenal failure, other causes of Addison's disease are rare (see Table 14–16). Adrenal metastases (the most commont primary being lung and breast) are often found at postmortem examinations, but adrenal insufficiency from these is uncommon,[288] perhaps because more than 90% of the adrenal cortex needs to be compromised before symptoms and signs become apparent. Necrosis of the adrenals due to intraadrenal hemorrhage should be considered in any severely sick patient, particularly those with underlying infection, trauma, or coagulopathy.[289] Intraadrenal bleeding may be found in any cause of severe septicemia, particularly in children in whom a common cause is infection with *Pseudomonas aeruginosa*. When caused by meningococci, the association with adrenal insufficiency is known as the Waterhouse-Friederichsen syndrome. Adrenal replacement may also occur with amyloidosis and hemochromatosis.

Adrenal hypoplasia congenita is an X-linked disorder comprising congenital adrenal insufficiency and hypogonadotrophic hypogonadism. The condition is caused by mutations in the DAX-1 gene, a member of the nuclear receptor family of unknown function that is expressed in the adrenal cortex, gonads, and hypothalamus.[290,291] Mutations in another transcription factor—steroidogenic factor-1—may also result in adrenal insufficiency due to lack of development of a functional adrenal cortex.[292] The transcriptional regulation of many P450 steroidogenic enzymes is dependent upon SF-1.[14] Congenital adrenal hypoplasia may also occur in association with glycerol kinase deficiency and muscular dystrophy.[293]

Adrenoleukodystrophy has a prevalence rate of 1:20,000 and is a cause of adrenal insufficiency in association with demyelination within the nervous system due to a failure of β-oxidation of fatty acids within peroxisomes due to reduced activity of very long chain acyl-CoA synthetase.[294] Increased accumulation of very long chain fatty acids (VLCFA) occurs in many tissues, and serum assays can be used diagnostically. Only males have the fully expressed condition and carrier females are usually normal. Several forms are recognized; a childhood cerebral form (30% to 40% cases), adult adrenomyeloneuropathy (40% cases), and Addison's disease only (7% cases). The childhood onset form presents at 5 to 10 years of age with progression eventually to a blind, mute, and severely spastic tetraplegic state. Adrenal insufficiency is usually present but does not appear to correlate with the neurologic deficit. Nevertheless, this is the most commont form of adrenal insufficiency in a child younger than 7 years of age.[295] Adrenomyeloneuropathy, by contrast, presents later in life with the gradual development of spastic paresis and peripheral neuropathy. Both the childhood and the adult condition result from mutations in the ABCD1 gene on chromosome Xq28, which encodes for an ABC peroxisomal membrane protein involved in the import of VLCFA into the peroxisome. So far, more than 400 mutations have been reported in the ABCD1 gene with no relationship between genotype or phenotype.[297,298] Treatment is poor. Monounsaturated fatty acids, which block the synthesis of the saturated VLCFA have been used. A combination of erucic acid and oleic acid (Lorenzo's oil) has led to normal levels of VLCFA; treatment does not alter the rate of neurologic deterioration, but may prevent new neurologic damage in asymptomatic cases.[298] Bone marrow transplantation is a further possibility.

Familial glucocorticoid deficiency (FGD), or inherited unresponsiveness to ACTH, is a rare autosomal recessive cause of hypoadrenalism that usually presents in childhood. The renin-angiotensin-aldosterone axis is intact and children usually present either with neonatal hypoglycemia or later with increasing pigmentation, often with enhanced growth velocity. Patients have glucocorticoid deficiency with very high plasma ACTH levels. The type 1 variant accounts for approximately 25% of all cases and is explained upon inactivating mutations in the melanocortin-2 or ACTH-receptor (MC2-R).[299] FGD without MCR-2 mutations is termed the *type 2* variant—mutations in *MRAP*—a gene encoding melanocortin 2 receptor accessory protein that is thought to mediate intracellular trafficking of the MCR-2, have been reported in some families[300]; other loci are being defined.

A variant called the *Triple A* or *Allgrove's* syndrome refers to the triad of adrenal insufficiency due to ACTH resistance, achalasia, and alacrima. It is not caused by mutations in the MC2-R; recent studies have mapped this disease to chromosome 12q13 but the responsible gene is unknown.[301]

Secondary Hypoadrenalism (ACTH Deficiency)

This is a common clinical problem and is most often due to a sudden cessation of exogenous glucocorticoid therapy. Such therapy suppresses the HPA axis with consequent adrenal atrophy, which may last for months after stopping glucocorticoid treatment. Adrenal atrophy and subsequent deficiency should be anticipated in any subject who has taken more than the equivalent of 30 mg hydrocortisone per day orally (~7.5 mg/day prednisolone or 0.75 mg/day dexamethasone) for more than 3 weeks. In addition to the magnitude of the dose of glucocorticoid, the timing of administration of the dose may affect the degree of adrenal suppression. Thus, prednisolone in a dose of 5 mg given last thing at night and 2.5 mg in the morning will produce more marked suppression of the HPA axis compared with 2.5 mg at night and 5 mg in the morning, because the larger evening dose blocks the early morning surge of ACTH. Secondary hypoadrenalism may also occur following failure to give adequate glucocorticoid replacement therapy for intercurrent stress in a patient who has been on long-term glucocorticoid therapy.

Other causes of secondary adrenal insufficiency (see Table 14–16) reflect inadequate ACTH production from the anterior pituitary gland. In many of these, other pituitary hormones are deficient in addition to ACTH, so that the patient presents with partial or complete hypopituitarism. The clinical features of hypopituitarism make this a relatively easy diagnosis to make. Isolated ACTH deficiency is rare but a difficult diagnosis to make. It may occur in patients with lymphocytic hypophysitis. Mutations in the gene encoding Tpit, the product of which regulates POMC expression, have been reported in a few cases of isolated ACTH deficiency occurring in neonatal life.[302] A rare but fascinating cause relates to a defect in the normal posttranslational processing of POMC to ACTH by the prohormone convertase enzymes (PC1 and PC2).[303] Such patients may have more generalized defects in peptide processing (for example, cleavage or proinsulin to insulin) giving rise to diabetes mellitus.

Patients have also been described with mutations in the POMC gene, which interrupts the synthesis of ACTH and causes

ACTH deficiency. The elucidation of the phenotype of these cases has uncovered a novel role for POMC peptides in regulating appetite and hair color. A central role for α-MSH in regulating food intake via the hypothalamic melanocortin-4-receptor has been established.[51] Thus, in addition to adrenal insufficiency, mutations in the POMC gene result in severe obesity and red hair pigmentation.[304] In recombinant mice lacking the POMC gene, the obese phenotype can be reversed by giving an α-MSH agonist peripherally.[305]

Secondary hypoadrenalism is also observed in patients with Cushing's disease following successful and selective removal of the ACTH-secreting pituitary adenoma. The function of adjacent "normal" pituitary corticotrophs are suppressed and may remain so for many months after surgery.[267-269]

Hypoadrenalism during Critical Illness

Hypoadrenalism may also complicate critical illness even in individuals with a previously intact HPA axis.[306] This has been termed *functional adrenal insufficiency* to reflect the notion that hypoadrenalism is transient and not due to a structural lesion. Functional adrenal insufficiency has been difficult to define biochemically and is of uncertain etiology. An inability to mount an adequate and appropriate cortisol response to overwhelming stress and/or sepsis frequently encountered in intensive care units, substantially increases the risk of death during acute illness.[307] This has stimulated attempts to define functional adrenal insufficiency quantitatively and treat it with supplemental corticosteroids.

Clinical Features of Adrenal Insufficiency

Patients with primary adrenal failure usually have both glucocorticoid and mineralocorticoid deficiency. In contrast, those with secondary adrenal insufficiency have an intact renin-angiotensin-aldosterone system. This accounts for differences in salt and water balance in the two groups of patients, which in turn result in different clinical presentations. The most obvious feature that differentiates primary from secondary hypoadrenalism is skin pigmentation (Table 14–18), which is nearly always present in primary adrenal insufficiency (unless of short duration) and absent in secondary insufficiency. The pigmentation is seen in sun-exposed areas, recent rather than old scars, axillae, nipples, palmar creases, pressure points, and in mucous membranes (buccal, vaginal, vulval, anal). The cause of the pigmentation has long been debated but is thought to reflect increased stimulation of the melanocortin-1 receptor by ACTH itself. In autoimmune Addison's disease there may be associated vitiligo (Fig. 14–29).

The clinical features relate to the rate of onset and severity of adrenal deficiency.[281] In many cases, the disease has an insidious onset and a diagnosis is only made when the patient presents with an acute crisis during an intercurrent illness. Acute adrenal insufficiency or an adrenal or Addisonian crisis is a medical emergency manifesting as hypotension and acute circulatory failure (Table 14–19). Anorexia may be an early feature, which progresses to nausea, vomiting, diarrhea, and, sometimes abdominal pain. Fever may be present and hypoglycemia may occur. Patients presenting acutely with adrenal hemorrhage have hypotension, abdominal, flank or lower chest pain, anorexia, and vomiting. The condition is difficult to diagnose but evidence of occult hemorrhage (rapidly falling hemoglobin), progressive hyperkalemia, and shock should alert the clinician to the diagnosis.

Alternatively, the patient may present with vague features of chronic adrenal insufficiency—weakness, tiredness, weight loss, nausea, intermittent vomiting, abdominal pain, diarrhea or constipation, general malaise, muscle cramps, arthralgia, and symptoms suggestive of postural hypotension (see Table 14–18). Salt-craving may be a feature and there may be a low-grade fever. Supine blood pressure is usually normal but almost invariably there is a fall in blood pressure on standing. Adrenal androgen secretion is lost, which is clinically more apparent in women who may complain of loss of axillary and pubic hair and frequently suffer from dry and itchy skin. Psychiatric symptoms may occur in longstanding cases and include memory impairment, depression, and psychosis. Patients may be inappropriately diagnosed as suffering from chronic fatigue syndrome or anorexia nervosa. These features regress upon treatment with replacement corticosteroids.

TABLE 14–18 CLINICAL FEATURES OF PRIMARY ADRENAL INSUFFICIENCY

Symptom, Sign, or Laboratory Finding	Frequency (%)
SYMPTOM	
Weakness, tiredness, fatigue	100
Anorexia	100
Gastrointestinal symptoms	92
Nausea	86
Vomiting	75
Constipation	33
Abdominal pain	31
Diarrhea	16
Salt craving	16
Postural dizziness	12
Muscle or joint pains	6-13
SIGN	
Weight loss	100
Hyperpigmentation	94
Hypotension (<110 mm Hg systolic)	88-94
Vitiligo	10-20
Auricular calcification	5
LABORATORY FINDING	
Electrolyte disturbances	92
Hyponatremia	88
Hyperkalemia	64
Hypercalcemia	6
Azotemia	55
Anemia	40
Eosinophilia	17

TABLE 14–19 CLINICAL AND LABORATORY FEATURES OF AN ADRENAL CRISIS

- Dehydration, hypotension, or shock out of proportion to severity of current illness
- Nausea and vomiting with a history of weight lost and anorexia
- Abdominal pain, so-called acute abdomen
- Unexplained hypoglycemia
- Unexplained fever
- Hyponatremia, hyperkalemia, azotemia, hypercalcemia, or eosinophilia
- Hyperpigmentation or vitiligo
- Other autoimmune endocrine deficiencies, such as hypothyroidism or gonadal failure

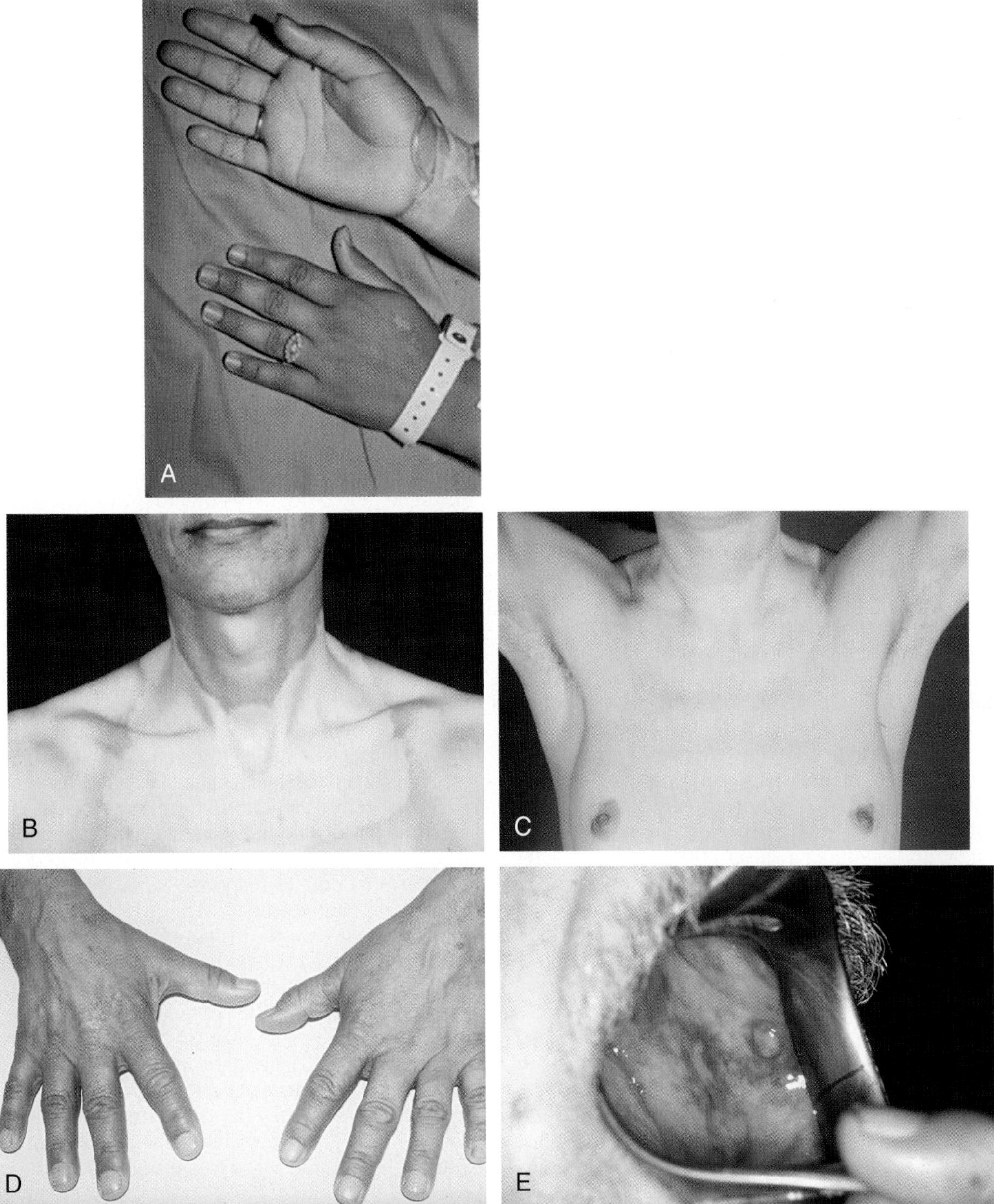

Figure 14–29 ▪ Pigmentation in Addison's disease. **A,** Hands of an 18-year-old woman with autoimmune polyendocrine syndrome and Addison's disease. Pigmentation in a patient with Addison's disease before **(B)** and after **(C)** treatment with hydrocortisone and fludrocortisone. Note the additional presence of vitiligo. **D**, Similar changes also seen in a 60-year-old man with tuberculous Addison's disease before and after corticosteroid therapy. **E,** Buccal pigmentation in the same patient. (*B* and *C* courtesy of Professor C.R.W. Edwards.)

In secondary adrenal insufficiency due to hypopituitarism, the presentation may relate to deficiency of hormones other than ACTH, notably LH/FSH (infertility, oligorrhea/amenorrhea, poor libido) and TSH (weight gain, cold intolerance). Fasting hypoglycemia occurs because of loss of the gluconeogenic effects of cortisol. It is rare in adults unless there is concomitant alcohol abuse or additional GH deficiency. However, hypoglycemia is a common presenting feature of ACTH/adrenal insufficiency in childhood.[308] In addition, patients with ACTH deficiency present with malaise, weight loss, and other features of chronic adrenal insufficiency. Rarely, presentation may be more acute in patients with pituitary apoplexy.

Investigation of Hypoadrenalism

Routine Biochemical Profile

In established primary adrenal insufficiency, hyponatremia is present in about 90% of cases and hyperkalemia in 65%. The blood urea concentration is usually elevated. Hyperkalemia occurs because of aldosterone deficiency and is usually absent, therefore, in patients with secondary adrenal failure. Hyponatremia may be depletional in an Addisonian crisis, but in addition vasopressin levels are elevated, resulting in increased free water retention.[309] Thus, in secondary adrenal insufficiency, there may be a dilutional hyponatremia with normal or low blood urea. Reversible abnormalities in liver transaminases frequently occur. Hypercalcemia occurs in 6% of all cases,[310] which may be particularly marked in patients with coexisting thyrotoxicosis. However, usually, free thyroxine concentrations are low or normal, but TSH values are frequently moderately elevated.[311] This is a direct effect of glucocorticoid deficiency and reverses with replacement therapy. Persistent elevation of TSH in association with positive thyroid autoantibodies suggests concomitant autoimmune thyroid disease.

Mineralocorticoid Status

In primary hypoadrenalism, mineralocorticoid deficiency usually occurs with elevated plasma renin activity and either low or low normal plasma aldosterone. The investigation of zona glomerulosa activity is frequently neglected in Addison's disease as compared with assessment of zona fasciculata function. In secondary adrenal insufficiency, the renin-angiotensin-aldosterone system is intact.

Assessing Adequacy of Function of the HPA Axis

Clinical suspicion of the diagnosis should be confirmed with definitive diagnostic tests. Basal plasma cortisol and urinary free cortisol levels are often in the low normal range and cannot be used to exclude the diagnosis. However, a basal cortisol value greater than 400 nmol/L (14.5 μg/dL) invariably indicates an intact HPA axis.[312] In practice, rather than wait for results of insensitive basal tests, all patients suspected of having adrenal insufficiency should have an ACTH stimulation test, although in patients with an Addisonian crisis, treatment should be instigated immediately and stimulation tests conducted at a later stage. The ACTH stimulation test or short Synacthen test (SST) involves the intramuscular or intravenous administration of 250 μg tetracosactin comprising the first 24 amino acids of normally secreted 1-39 ACTH.[313] Plasma cortisol levels are measured at 0 and 30 minutes after ACTH, and a normal response is defined by a peak plasma cortisol of greater than 550 nmol/L (>20 μg/dL).[314] This value equates to the 5th percentile response in normal subjects but is very much "assay" dependent, with different cortisol radioimmunoassays giving different results. Incremental responses (i.e., the difference between peak and basal values) are of no value in defining a "pass" response except in diagnosing relative adrenal insufficiency in patients with critical illness. Response is unaffected by the time of day of the test and the test can still be performed in patients who have commenced corticosteroid replacement therapy as long as this is of short duration and does not comprise hydrocortisone (which would cross-react in the cortisol assay). A prolonged ACTH stimulation test involving the administration of depot or intravenous infusions of tetracosactin for 24 to 48 hours will differentiate primary from secondary hypoadrenalism. In normal subjects, the plasma cortisol at 4 hours is greater than 1000 nmol/L (36 μg/dL); beyond this time, there is no further increase. Patients with secondary hypoadrenalism show a delayed response with usually a much higher value at 24 and 48 hours than at 4 hours, but in primary hypoadrenalism there is no response at either time. However, the test is rarely required if plasma ACTH has been appropriately measured at baseline. In primary adrenal insufficiency, the ACTH level is disproportionately elevated in comparison to plasma cortisol.[315]

Whereas there is agreement upon the investigation of suspected primary adrenal failure, the diagnosis of secondary hypoadrenalism, notably in patients with existing hypothalamic/pituitary disease, is contentious. Based on correlations with the response of circulating cortisol to surgery, the insulin-induced hypoglycemia test or insulin tolerance test (ITT) was introduced over 30 years ago as a laboratory test to assess integrity of the HPA axis and should be considered the "gold standard" in this regard.[316] It should not be performed in patients with ischemic heart disease (always check an ECG before the test), epilepsy, or severe hypopituitarism (i.e., 09.00h plasma cortisol less than 180 nmol/L [6.5 μg/dL]). The test involves the intravenous administration of soluble insulin in a dose of 0.1 to 0.15 U/kg body weight, with measurement of plasma cortisol at 0, 30, 45, 60, 90, and 120 minutes. Adequate hypoglycemia (blood glucose less than 2.2 mmol/L with signs of neuroglycopenia—sweating and tachycardia) is essential. In normal subjects, the peak plasma cortisol exceeds 500 nmol/L (18 μg/dL). However, the cortisol response to hypoglycemia can be reliably predicted by the SST; a safer, cheaper, and quicker test.[313,317] This relies on the principle that the cortisol response to an exogenous bolus of ACTH will be determined by the endogenous ACTH trophic drive to the adrenal cortex; impaired ACTH secretion from the anterior pituitary results in an impaired cortisol response following Synacthen. However, the ACTH test should not be used to diagnose secondary hypoadrenalism in patients with a recent pituitary insult (surgery, apoplexy). Total hypophysectomy would result in a failed cortisol response to ITT immediately thereafter, but it takes 2 to 3 weeks for the adrenal cortex to readjust to the reduced level of ACTH secretion; in the interim, a false-positive cortisol response would be seen. The SST should also be avoided in patients with a primary diagnosis of Cushing's disease in whom an exaggerated cortisol response to ACTH may persist. In clinical practice, if the ACTH test is normal, insulin hypoglycemia testing is not necessary in the vast majority of cases unless there is also a need to document endogenous GH reserve in a patient with pituitary disease. In our practice, an ITT is performed in a patient with suspected hypopituitarism when there is a subnormal response to ACTH. Some patients have an inadequate response to ACTH, but then respond normally to hypoglycemia.[317] They do not require corticosteroid replacement therapy. This approach is open to debate and even taking into account the above caveats, false-positive results have been reported for the SST[318]; although these are rare (<2% cases), this should be noted, particularly in patients with ongoing symptoms and signs indicative of hypoadrenalism.

A low-dose SST giving only 1 μg ACTH has been proposed as a screen for adequacy of function of the HPA axis with the suggestion that it may be more sensitive than the conventional 250-μg test.[319,320] Other researchers dispute this suggestion,[321] and further validation of this test is required to support such a concept.

Two other tests have been advocated to assess adequacy of function of the HPA axis, but their use in modern clinical practice should be restricted to difficult diagnostic cases. In the overnight metyrapone test, 30 mg/kg (maximum 3 g) metyrapone is given at midnight and plasma cortisol and 11-deoxycortisol measured at 08.00h the following morning. In patients with an intact axis, ACTH levels rise following the blockade of cortisol synthesis by metyrapone and a normal result is signified by a peak 11-deoxycortisol value of greater than 7 μg/dL.[322] The CRF stimulation test has been used to diagnose adrenal insufficiency, and, unlike the metyrapone test will differentiate primary from secondary causes. Patients with primary adrenal failure have high ACTH levels, which rise further following CRF stimulation. Conversely, patients with secondary adrenal failure have low ACTH levels that fail to respond to CRF. Patients with hypothalamic disease show a steady rise in ACTH levels following CRF.[323]

Testing the HPA Axis during Critical Illness

Many factors complicate investigation of the HPA axis during critical illness. Cortisol levels vary broadly with disease severity making it difficult to define appropriate responses. Additionally, CBG levels decrease substantially, leading to increases in the ratio of free to bound serum cortisol and tests that assess the whole axis, for example, the ITT, are not appropriate in the critical care setting. Investigations are thus limited to basal cortisol levels or the SST. Recent guidance has suggested that a random cortisol value of less than 400 nmod/L (15 μg/dL) is suggestive of corticosteroid insufficiency, whereas a level more than 900 nmol/L (33 μg/dL) would be unlikely to occur in patients with compromised HPA axis function. For individuals with intermediate cortisol levels, an SST should be performed—a cortisol increment of less than 250 nmol/L (9 μg/dL) is an independent prognostic marker for death in critically ill patients.[307] Multicenter randomizes trials of patients with septic shock with an increment less than 250 nmol/L had a significant improvement in mortality when given replacement corticosteroids.[324] We recommend that individuals with low basal cortisol levels or intermediate levels with a poor increment should be treated with replacement corticosteroids during critical illness with further testing after recovery to demonstrate return of normal HPA axis function. This is an evolving area—other studies (notably the use of "free" serum cortisol estimations[236]) and trials are under way that are likely to improve our evidence base for diagnosing and treating "relative" adrenal insufficiency in critically ill patients.

Other Tests

Radioimmunoassays to detect autoantibodies such as those against the 21-hydroxylase antigen are now available and should be analyzed in patients with primary adrenal failure. In autoimmune Addison's disease, it is also important to look for evidence of other organ-specific autoimmune disease. A CT scan may reveal enlarged or calcified adrenals suggesting an infective, hemorrhagic or malignant diagnosis (Fig. 14–30). Chest radiograph, tuberculin testing, and early morning urine samples cultured for *Mycobacterium tuberculosis* should be performed if tuberculosis is suspected. CT guided adrenal biopsy may reveal an underlying diagnosis in patients with suspected malignant deposits in the adrenal. Adrenoleukodystrophy can be diagnosed by measuring circulating levels of VLCFA. Finally, appropriate investigations, including pituitary MRI scans and an

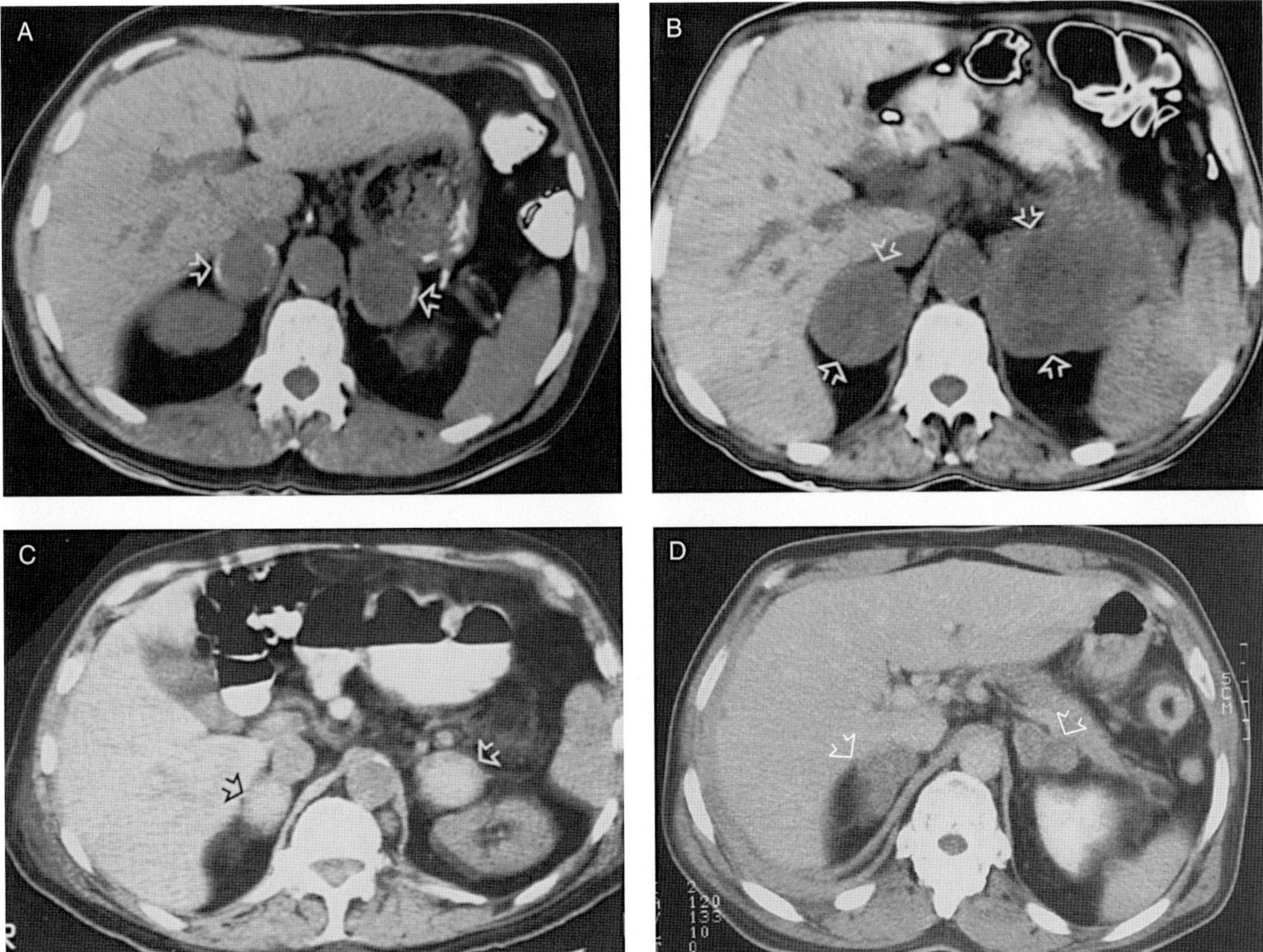

Figure 14–30 ▪ Computed tomographic (CT) scans of patients with primary adrenal insufficiency. The affected adrenal glands are indicated by *arrows*. **A,** CT scan of a 59-year-old man with histoplasmosis. Note the subcapsular calcium in both glands. **B,** CT scan of a 59-year-old man with metastatic melanoma. **C,** CT scan of an 80-year-old man with bilateral adrenal hemorrhage resulting from anticoagulation for pulmonary emboli. **D,** Bilateral adrenal tuberculomas in a 79-year-old man with tuberculosis affecting the urogenital tract. (*A* and *B* courtesy of Dr. William D. Salmon Jr; *C* courtesy of Dr. Craig R. Sussman.)

assessment of anterior function, are required in patients suspected with secondary hypoadrenalism who are not taking corticosteroid therapy.

Treatment of Acute Adrenal Insufficiency

This is a life-threatening emergency, and treatment should not be delayed while waiting for definitive proof of diagnosis (Table 14–20). However, in addition to measurement of plasma electrolytes and blood glucose, appropriate samples for ACTH and cortisol should be taken before giving corticosteroid therapy. If the patient is not critically ill, an acute ACTH stimulation test can be performed.

Intravenous hydrocortisone should be given in a dose of 100 mg 6-8 hourly. If this is not possible, then the intramuscular route should be used. In the shock patient, 1 L of normal saline should be given intravenously over the first hour. Because of possible hypoglycemia, it is normal to give 5% dextrose saline. Subsequent saline and dextrose therapy will depend upon biochemical monitoring and the patient's condition. Clinical improvement, especially in the blood pressure, should be seen within 4 to 6 hours if the diagnosis is correct. It is important to recognize and treat any associated condition, such as an infection, which may have precipitated the acute adrenal crisis.

After the first 24 hours, the dose of hydrocortisone can be reduced, usually to 50 mg intramuscularly 6 hourly and then, if the patient can take by mouth, to oral hydrocortisone, 40 mg in the morning and 20 mg at 18.00 hours. This can then be rapidly reduced to a more standard replacement dose of 20 mg on wakening and 10 mg at 18.00 hours.

Long-Term Replacement Therapy

The aim is to give replacement doses of hydrocortisone to mimic the normal cortisol secretion rate (Table 14–21). Initially this was thought to be approximately 25 to 30 mg/day, but stable isotope studies indicate lower normal cortisol production rates of 8 to 15 mg/day.[325] Increasingly most patients can cope with less than 30 mg/day (usually 15 to 25 mg/day in divided doses). Doses are usually given on wakening with a smaller dose at

TABLE 14–20 TREATMENT OF ACUTE ADRENAL INSUFFICIENCY (ADRENAL CRISIS)

EMERGENCY MEASURES
1. Establish intravenous access with a large-gauge needle.
2. Draw blood for stat serum electrolytes and glucose and routine measurement of plasma cortisol and ACTH. Do not wait for laboratory results.
3. Infuse 2 to 3 L of 154 mmol/L NaCl (0.9% saline) solution or 50 g/L (5%) dextrose in 154 mmol/L NaCl (0.9% saline) solution as quickly as possible. Monitor for signs of fluid overload by measuring central or peripheral venous pressure and listening for pulmonary rales. Reduce infusion rate if indicated.
4 Inject intravenous hydrocortisone (100 mg immediately and every 6 hr)
5. Use supportive measures as needed.
SUBACUTE MEASURES AFTER STABILIZATION OF THE PATIENT
1. Continue intravenous 154 mmol/L NaCl (0.9% saline) solution at a slower rate for next 24 to 48 hr.
2. Search for and treat possible infectious precipitating causes of the adrenal crisis.
3. Perform a short ACTH stimulation test to confirm the diagnosis of adrenal insufficiency, if patient does not have known adrenal insufficiency.
4. Determine the type of adrenal insufficiency and its cause if not already known.
5. Taper glucocorticoids to maintenance dosage over 1 to 3 days, if precipitating or complicating illness permits.
6. Begin mineralocorticoid replacement with fludrocortisone (0.1 mg by mouth daily) when saline infusion is stopped.

ACTH, Adrenocorticotropic hormone.

TABLE 14–21 TREATMENT OF CHRONIC PRIMARY ADRENAL INSUFFICIENCY

MAINTENANCE THERAPY
Glucocorticoid Replacement • Hydrocortisone 15 to 20 mg on awakening and 5 to 10 mg in early afternoon. • Monitor clinical symptoms and morning plasma ACTH.
Mineralocorticoid Replacement • Fludrocortisone 0.1 (0.05 to 0.2) mg orally. • Liberal salt intake. • Monitor lying and standing blood pressure and pulse, edema, serum potassium, and plasma renin activity. • Educate patient about the disease, how to manage minor illnesses and major stresses, and how to inject steroid intramuscularly. • Obtain MedicAlert bracelet/necklace, Emergency Medical Information Card.
TREATMENT OF MINOR FEBRILE ILLNESS OR STRESS
• Increase glucocorticoid dose twofold to threefold for the few days of illness; do not change mineralocorticoid dose. • Contact physician if illness worsens or persists for more than 3 days or if vomiting develops. • No extra supplementation is needed for most uncomplicated, outpatient dental procedures under local anesthesia. General anesthesia or intravenous sedation should not be used in the office.
EMERGENCY TREATMENT OF SEVERE STRESS OR TRAUMA
• Inject contents of prefilled dexamethasone (4-mg) syringe intramuscularly. • Get to physician as quickly as possible.
STEROID COVERAGE FOR ILLNESS OR SURGERY IN HOSPITAL
• For moderate illness give hydrocortisone 50 mg twice a day orally or intravenously. Taper rapidly to maintenance dose as patient recovers. • For severe illness give hydrocortisone 100 mg intravenously every 8 hr. Taper dose to maintenance level by decreasing by half every day. Adjust dose according to course of illness. • For minor procedures under local anesthesia and most radiologic studies, no extra supplementation is needed. • For moderately stressful procedures, such as barium enema, endoscopy, or arteriography, give a single 100 mg intravenous dose of hydrocortisone just before the procedure. • For major surgery, give hydrocortisone 100 mg intravenously just before induction of anesthesia and continue every 8 hr for first 24 hr. Taper dose rapidly, decreasing by half per day, to maintenance level.

18.00h, but some patients may feel better on three-a-day dosing. In primary adrenal failure, cortisol day curves with simultaneous ACTH measurements may provide some insight into adequacy of replacement therapy,[326] but there are no good objective tests in secondary adrenal failure. Decisions regarding doses of replacement therapy are largely based on crude yet important end-points such as weight, well-being, and blood pressure. Bone mineral density may be reduced on conventional doses of 30 mg/day hydrocortisone, highlighting the need to strive for minimally effective but safe doses.[327,328] Possibly because of the known action of IGF-1 to increase cortisol clearance,[122] it is the author's experience that glucocorticoid requirements are slightly lower in hypopituitary, GH-deficient subjects than in patients with primary adrenal insufficiency.

In primary adrenal failure, mineralocorticoid replacement is usually also required in the form of fludrocortisone (or 9a-fluorinated hydrocortisone) 0.05 to 0.2 mg/day. The mineralocorticoid activity of this is about 125 times that of hydrocortisone. After the acute phase has passed, the adequacy of mineralocorticoid replacement should be assessed by measuring electrolytes and supine and erect blood pressure and plasma renin activity (PRA)[329]; too little fludrocortisone may cause postural hypotension with elevated PRA, whereas too much causes the converse. Mineralocorticoid replacement therapy is all too frequently neglected in patients with adrenal failure.

Patients on glucocorticoid replacement therapy should be advised to double the daily dose in the event of intercurrent febrile illness, accident, or mental stress such as an important examination. If the patient is vomiting and cannot take medication by mouth, parenteral hydrocortisone must be given urgently. For minor surgery, 50 to 100 mg hydrocortisone hemisuccinate is given with the premedication. For major operations, this is then followed by the same regimen as for acute adrenal insufficiency (see Table 14–21). Pregnancy proceeds normally in patients taking replacement therapy, but daily doses of hydrocortisone are usually increased modestly (5 to 10 mg/day) in the last trimester. Progesterone is a mineralocorticoid antagonist and the rising levels across pregnancy may necessitate an increased dose of fludrocortisone. During labor, patients should be well hydrated with a saline drip and receive hydrocortisone 50 mg intramuscularly every 6 hours until delivery. Thereafter, doses can be rapidly tapered to pre-pregnancy levels.

Every patient on glucocorticoid therapy should be advised to register for a medical alert bracelet or necklace and must carry a "steroid card." Patients should receive regular education regarding the requirements of stress-related glucocorticoid dose adjustment, which should involve partner and family.

For patients with both primary and secondary adrenal failure, beneficial effects of adrenal androgen replacement therapy with 25 to 50 mg/day of DHEA have been reported. To date, reported benefit is principally confined to female patients and includes improvement in sexual function and well-being.[330]

CONGENITAL ADRENAL HYPERPLASIA

These inherited syndromes are caused by deficient adrenal corticosteroid biosynthesis.[331] In each case, there is reduced negative feedback inhibition of cortisol, and depending on the steroidogenic pathway involved, alteration in adrenal mineralocorticoid and androgen secretion (Table 14–22).

21-Hydroxylase Deficiency

Ninety percent of cases of congenital adrenal hyperplasia (CAH) are due to 21-hydroxylase deficiency.[332] In Western societies, the incidence varies from 1:5000 to 1:15,000 live births, but in isolated communities the incidence may be much higher (e.g., 1:300 in Alaskan Inuit). The condition arises because of defective conversion of 17α-hydroxyprogesterone to 11-deoxycortisol. Reduced cortisol biosynthesis results in reduced negative feedback drive and increased ACTH secretion; as a consequence, adrenal androgens are produced in excess (Fig. 14–31). Seventy-five percent of cases have mineralocorticoid deficiency because

TABLE 14–22 CONGENITAL ADRENAL HYPERPLASIA: FEATURES FOR EACH ENZYME DEFECT

Feature	21-Hydroxylase Deficiency	11β-Hydroxylase Deficiency	17α-Hydroxylase Deficiency	3β-Hydroxysteroid Deficiency	Lipoid Hyperplasia	Aldosterone Synthase Deficiency
Defective gene	*CYP21*	*CYP11B1*	*CYP17*	*HSD3B2*	*StAR*	*CYP11B2*
Chromosomal localization	6p21.3	8q24.3	10q24.3	1p13.1	8p11.2	8q24.3
Ambiguous genitalia	+(female)	+(female)	+(male) Absent puberty (female)	+(male) Mild in female	+(male) Absent puberty (female)	No
Acute adrenal insufficiency	+	Rare	No	+	+ +	Salt wasting only
Incidence	1:15,000	1:100,000	Rare	Rare	Rare	Rare
Hormones						
Glucocorticoids	Reduced	Reduced	Reduced	Corticosterone normal	Reduced	Normal
Mineralocorticoids	Reduced	Increased	Reduced	Increased	Reduced	Reduced
Androgens	Increased	Increased	Reduced	Reduced (male) Increased (female)	Reduced	Normal
Elevated metabolite	17-Hydroxy-progesterone	DOC, 11-deoxycortisol	B, DOC	DHEA, 17Δ^5-pregnenolone	None	B, 18-OHB
Blood pressure, sodium balance	Decreased	Increased	Decreased	Increased	Decreased	Decreased
Potassium	Increased	Decreased	Increased	Decreased	Increased	Increased

B, Corticosterone; *DHEA*, dehydroepiandrosterone; *DOC*, deoxycorticosterone; *18-OHB*, 18-hydroxycorticosterone.

of failure to convert progesterone to deoxycorticosterone in the zona glomerulosa. Clinically, several distinct variants of 21 hydroxylase deficiency have been recognized (Table 14–23).

Simple Virilizing Form

The enhanced ACTH drive to adrenal androgen secretion in utero leads to virilization of an affected female fetus. Depending on the severity, clitoral enlargement, labial fusion, and development of a urogenital sinus may occur, leading to sexual ambiguity at birth and even inappropriate sex assignment. Males are phenotypically normal at birth and are at risk of not being diagnosed; this explains the skewed female-to-male ratio of simple virilizing CAH diagnosed in the preneonatal screening era. Such cases may present in early childhood with signs of precocious pseudopuberty such as sexual precocity, pubic hair development, and/or growth acceleration due to premature androgen excess. If left untreated, this stimulates premature epiphyseal closure and final adult height is invariably diminished.[333,334]

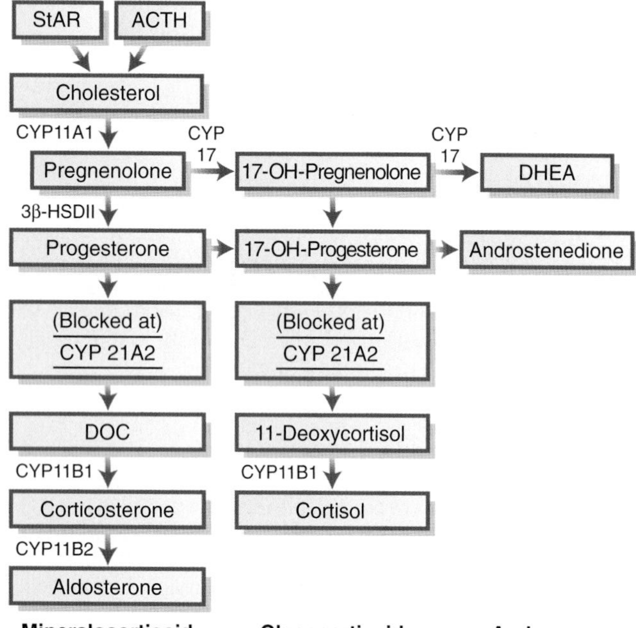

Figure 14–31 ■ Congenital adrenal hyperplasia related to 21-hydroxylase deficiency. The normal synthesis of cortisol is impaired, and adrenocorticotropic hormone (ACTH) levels increase because of loss of normal negative feedback inhibition, resulting in an increase in adrenal steroid precursors proximal to the block. The results are cortisol deficiency, variable mineralocorticoid deficiency, and excessive secretion of adrenal androgens. *DHEA*, Dehydroepiandrosterone; *DOC*, deoxycorticosterone; *HSD*, hydroxysteroid dehydrogenase; *StAR*, steroidogenic acute regulatory protein.

Salt-Wasting Form

Seventy-five percent of cases of both sexes also have concomitant deficiency of aldosterone deficiency. In addition to the described features, neonates may present within the first week of life with a salt-wasting crisis and hypotension. Indeed, this may alert the clinician to the diagnosis in a male, but unfortunately the diagnosis is still delayed in many cases and the condition carries a significant neonatal mortality rate.

Nonclassic or "Late-Onset" 21-Hydroxylase Deficiency

Patients present in childhood or early adulthood with premature pubarche or with a phenotype that may masquerade as polycystic ovary syndrome (PCOS).[332,335] Indeed, late-onset CAH is a recognized secondary cause of PCOS and appears to be more common than the classic variety. In some series from tertiary referral centers, late-onset 21 hydroxylase deficiency may account for up to 12% of all "PCOS" patients, but more realistic prevalence rates are probably 1% to 3%. Females present with hirsutism, primary or secondary amenorrhea, or anovulatory infertility.[335] Androgenic alopecia and acne may be other presenting features.

Heterozygote 21-Hydroxylase Deficiency

Salt-wasting, simple virilizing, and late-onset 21-hydroxylase deficiency are all caused by homozygous or compound heterozygote mutations in the human 21-hydroxylase gene (*CYP21A2*), whereas in the carrier, heterozygote state only one allele is

TABLE 14–23 DIFFERENT FORMS OF 21-HYDROXYLASE DEFICIENCY

Phenotype	Classical Salt Wasting	Simple Virilizing	Nonclassical
Age at diagnosis	Newborn to 6 mo	Newborn to 2 yr (female) 2 to 4 yr (male)	Child to adult
Genitalia	Males normal; females ambiguous	Males normal; females ambiguous	Males normal; females virilized
Incidence	1:20,000	1:60,000	1:1000
Hormones			
Aldosterone	Reduced	Normal	Normal
Renin	Increased	Normal or increased	Normal
Cortisol	Reduced	Reduced	Normal
17-Hydroxyprogesterone	>5000 nmol/L	2500 to 5000 nmol/L	500 to 2500 nmol/L (ACTH stimulation)
Testosterone	Increased	Increased	Variable, increased
Growth	–2 to –3 SD	–1 to –2 SD	Probably, normal
21-Hydroxylase activity (% of wild type)	0%	1%	20% to 50%
Typical *CYP21A2* mutations	Deletions, conversions, nt656g G110Δ8nt, R356W I236N, V237E, M239K, Q318X	I172N nt656g	V281L P30L

ACTH, Adrenocorticotropic hormone; *SD*, standard deviation.

mutated. The clinical significance of the heterozygote state is uncertain; it does not appear to disadvantage reproductive capability but may cause signs of hyperandrogenism in adult women.[332]

Molecular Genetics

The disorder is inherited as an autosomal recessive trait and the higher incidence of the condition in some ethnic communities almost certainly relates to consanguinity. The *CYP21A2* gene and its highly homologous pseudogene (*CYP21A1P*) are located on the short arm of chromosome 6 (6p21.3). Due to the genomic localization within the HLA locus, a region with a high frequency of genomic recombinations, most of the frequent 21-hydroxylase deficiency–causing mutations are generated by gene conversion events. Complete gene deletions or conversions of the *CYP21A2* gene, eight pseudogene-derived point mutations, and an 8-bp deletion are found in more than 95% of cases. Other rare pseudogen-independent *CYP21A2*-inactivating mutations occurring in single families or small populations have been reported. Approximately 65% to 75% of CAH patients are compound heterozygous for the disease-causing mutations. The genotype-phenotype correlation in CAH due to 21-hydroxylase deficiency is well established. The clinical phenotype correlates with the less severely mutated allele, and consequently, with the residual 21-hydroxylase activity[336,337] (Fig. 14–32). This correlation appears to be rather high, although divergence between genotype and phenotype has been observed.[38] The 21-hydroxylase activity measured by in vitro analysis provides a possibility for estimating the disease severity, albeit some phenotypic variability (e.g., salt-wasting, age of onset) seems likely to depend upon other interacting genes and maturation processes rather than *CYP21A2* itself.

A diagnosis of 21-hydroxylase deficiency should be considered in any newborn infant with genital ambiguity and salt-wasting, hypotension, or hypoglycemia. Hyponatremia, hyperkalemia with raised plasma renin activity, is found in salt-wasters. In later life, adrenal androgen excess (DHEAS, androstenedione) is found in patients presenting with sexual precocity or a "PCOS-like" phenotype. 17-hydroxyprogesterone (17-OHP) is invariably elevated and clinically useful nomograms have been developed comparing circulating concentrations of 17-OHP before and 60 minutes after exogenous ACTH.[339] This separates patients with classic and nonclassic 21-hydroxylase deficiency from heterozygote carriers and normal subjects, but there is some overlap between values seen in heterozygotes and normal subjects. 17-OHP is measured basally and then 60 minutes following 250 μg Synacthen. Stimulated values are invariably grossly elevated in patients with classical and nonclassical varieties (in excess of 35 nmol/L [11 μg/L]). Heterozygote patients usually have stimulated values between 10 and 30 nmol/L (3.3 and 10 μg/L) (Fig. 14–33). Stimulation tests are not always required to make a diagnosis; for example, a basal 17-OHP concentration of less than 5 nmol/L (<1.5 μg/L) in the follicular phase of the menstrual cycle effectively excludes late-onset 21-hydroxylase deficiency.[335] Increasingly, genotyping programs will form a useful adjunct to hormonal measurements. Androgen excess in 21-hydroxylase deficiency is readily suppressed following glucocorticoid administration.

Prenatal diagnosis of 21-hydroxylase deficiency has been advocated because treatment of an affected female may prevent masculinization in utero.[340] 17-OHP can be assayed in amniotic fluid but the most robust approach is the rapid genotyping of fetal cells obtained by chorionic villous sampling in early gestation. Unlike hydrocortisone, which is inactivated by placental 11β-hydroxysteroid dehydrogenase, maternally administered dexamethasone can cross the placenta to suppress the fetal HPA axis. One approach is to advocate dexamethasone therapy as soon as pregnancy is confirmed in high-risk cases and to continue this until the diagnosis is excluded in the female fetus. If the fetus is affected, only those of female sex require dexamethasone therapy across gestation. Therapy must be instigated at 6 to 7 weeks' gestation to be effective. However, because only 1 in 8 cases treated in this way will have an affected female fetus, the use of steroid therapy in this setting has been questioned.[341]

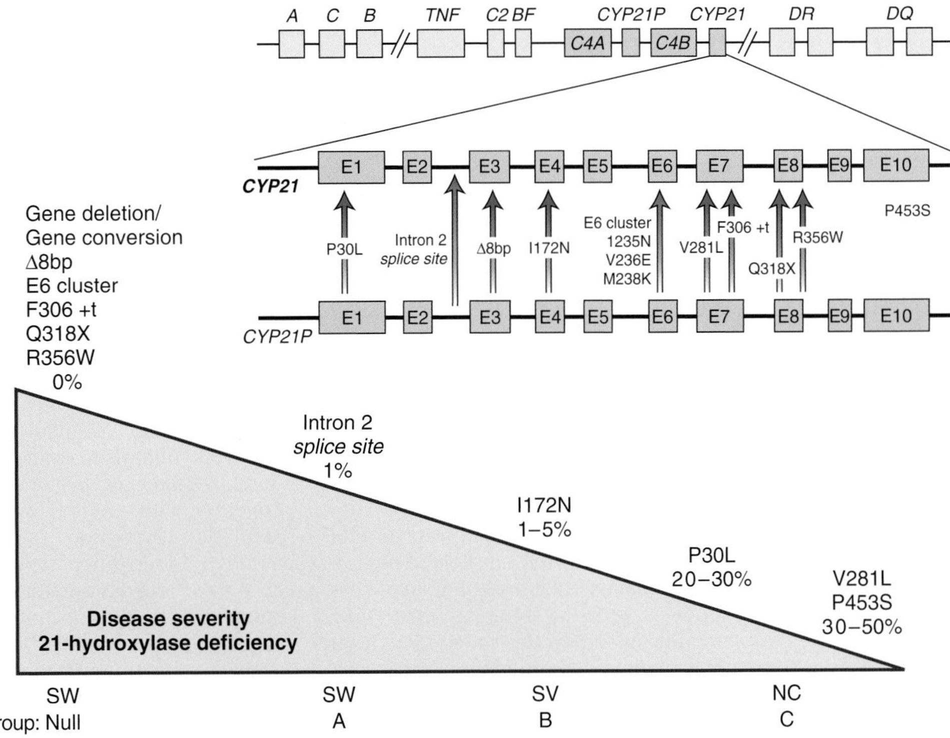

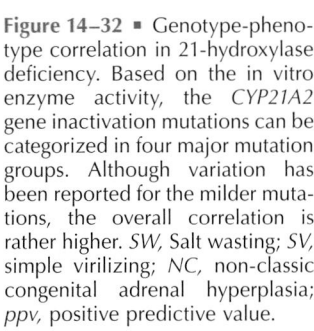

Figure 14–32 ▪ Genotype-phenotype correlation in 21-hydroxylase deficiency. Based on the in vitro enzyme activity, the *CYP21A2* gene inactivation mutations can be categorized in four major mutation groups. Although variation has been reported for the milder mutations, the overall correlation is rather higher. *SW*, Salt wasting; *SV*, simple virilizing; *NC*, non-classic congenital adrenal hyperplasia; *ppv*, positive predictive value.

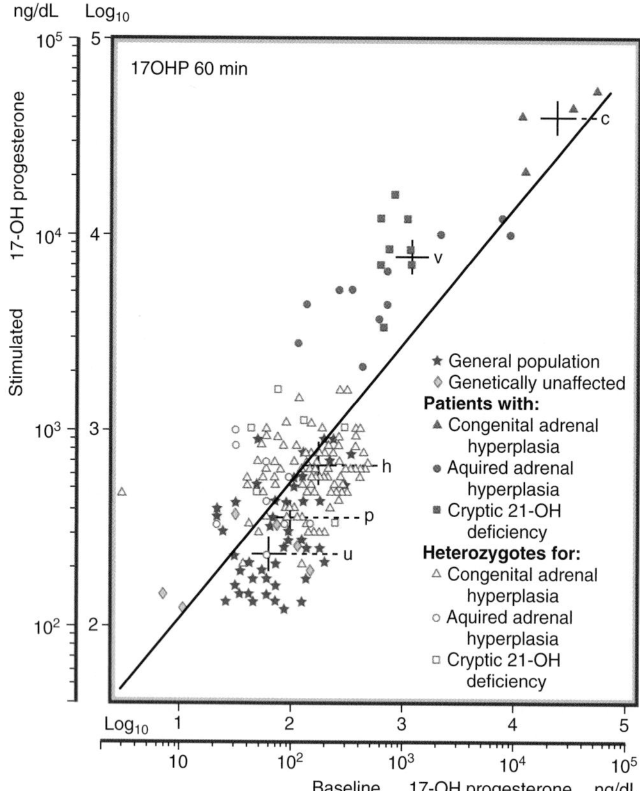

Figure 14–33 ■ Basal and stimulated plasma 17α-hydroxyprogesterone (17OHP) concentrations in patients with CYP21A2 (21-hydroxylase) deficiency. To convert values to nmol/L, multiply by 0.0303. The mean for each group is indicated by a large cross and the adjacent letter: *c*, patients with classical CYP21A2 deficiency; *v*, patients with nonclassical (acquired and cryptic) CYP21A2 deficiency; *h*, heterozygotes for all forms of CYP21A2 deficiency; *p*, general population; *u*, known unaffected persons (e.g., siblings of patients with CYP21A2 deficiency who carry neither affected parental haplotype as determined by human leukocyte antigen typing). (From White PC, New MI, Dupont B. Congenital adrenal hyperplasia: part 1. Reprinted from N Engl J Med 1987; 316:1519-1524.)

Dexamethasone can lead to maternal cushingoid effects in pregnancy[342] and may in turn have long-term, deleterious effects upon the fetus.

In known cases requesting fertility (either male or female), determination of 17-OHP levels across a Synacthen test in the partner before conception will uncover late-onset or heterozygote cases and provide the endocrinologist/geneticist with some assignment of risk before pregnancy.

Treatment

The objectives for treating 21-hydroxylase deficiency differ with age, but at all ages treatment and overall patient management can be fraught with difficulties. In childhood, the overall goal is to replace glucocorticoid and mineralocorticoid, thereby preventing further salt-wasting crises, but also to suppress adrenal androgen secretion so that normal growth and skeletal maturation can proceed. Accurate replacement is essential; in excess, glucocorticoids will suppress growth, whereas inadequate replacement will result initially in accelerated linear growth but ultimately short stature because of premature epiphyseal closure.[332] Response is best monitored through growth velocity and bone age, with biochemical markers from blood (17-OHP, DHEAS, testosterone), urine, and saliva (17-OHP, testosterone) being useful adjuncts. In difficult cases, a day curve study as described for patients with primary adrenal failure, but measuring the ACTH and 17-OHP response before and after corticosteroid replacement, may confirm overreplacement or underreplacement. Corrective surgery is frequently required (clitoral reduction, vaginoplasty) during childhood.

In late childhood and adolescence, appropriate replacement therapy is equally important. Overtreatment may result in obesity and delayed menarche/puberty with sexual infantilism, whereas underreplacement will result in sexual precocity. Compliance with regular medication is often an issue through adolescence.

Although much has been written about adequate control in childhood, adults with CAH often provide an ongoing dilemma for the endocrinologist. The follow-up of such patients should involve multidisciplinary clinics, initially with transition adolescence clinics to facilitate transfer from pediatric to adult care. Problems in adulthood relate to fertility concerns, hirsutism, and menstrual irregularity in women; obesity and impact of short stature; sexual dysfunction and psychological problems[332,343,344]; counseling is often required in addition to endocrine support. Males may develop enlargement of the testes due to "adrenal rests," that is, ectopic adrenal tissue, which regress after glucocorticoid suppression. These patients need adequate endocrine therapy rather than urologic referral with ensuing risk of removal of testis mistaken for a tumor.[345]

In the absence of any evidence-based data, there are no prescriptive steroid regimens to treat patients with CAH at any age and as a result many individualized regimens are used in clinical practice. Usual starting doses of hydrocortisone in childhood are 10 to 25 mg/m^2/day in three divided doses. "Reverse-phase" therapy may be appropriate, giving the largest dose of hydrocortisone at night to suppress early morning ACTH secretion. Long-acting steroids such as dexamethasone are more effective in this regard, but should not be given before end of puberty to avoid oversuppression and reduction in linear growth. Fludrocortisone is required for patients with salt-wasting (although this may spontaneously improve with age); doses of 0.1 to 0.2 mg/day should be given and blood pressure, electrolytes, and supine-erect plasma renin activity monitored to assess response. Fludrocortisone may improve linear growth in patients with simple virilizing CAH, even if they are not salt-wasters, and adequate fludrocortisone treatment may lead to hydrocortisone dose reduction. Adrenomedullary dysplasia is reported in the CAH adrenal, probably because of relative glucocorticoid deficiency, which results in epinephrine deficiency. Benefits of epinephrine replacement on the metabolic response to exercise are reported in children,[346] but further studies are required before advocating routine catecholamine replacement therapy. Bilateral adrenalectomy is effective but should be regarded as a "last resort"[347]; in addition to requiring lifelong corticosteroid replacement therapy, patients might also develop feedback ACTH-secreting pituitary tumours.[348]

In adult females with hyperandrogenism and untreated late-onset CAH, there is no evidence that final height is affected. In this setting, glucocorticoid suppression in isolation rarely controls hirsutism and additional antiandrogen therapy is often required (cyproterone acetate, spironolactone, flutamide together with an oral estrogen contraceptive pill). However, ovulation induction rates with gonadotropin therapy are improved following suppression of nocturnal ACTH levels with 0.25 to 0.5 mg dexamethasone. Once final height is achieved in adult males, strict control is only required for patients with adrenal rests within the testes or to ensure fertility; inadequate replacement therapy may result in adrenal androgen excess suppressing pituitary FSH secretion and lowering sperm counts.

11β-Hydroxylase Deficiency

11β-hydroxylase deficiency accounts for 7% of all cases of CAH with an incidence of 1:100,000 live births.[349] The incidence is higher in Israel (1:30,000), in particular in immigrants from Morocco. The condition arises because of mutations in the CYP11B1 gene, which result in loss of enzyme activity and a block in the conversion of 11-deoxycortisol to cortisol. There remains a poor correlation between genotype and phenotype, whereas some cases of late-onset 11-hydroxylase deficiency have been reported.[350] There is loss of negative cortisol feedback and enhanced ACTH-mediated adrenal androgen excess (Fig. 14–34). Clinical features therefore are very similar to those reported in the simple virilizing form of CAH (virilized female fetus, sexual ambiguity) and again milder cases can present later in childhood or even young adulthood. The principal difference to 21-hydroxylase deficiency is hypertension, which is thought to be secondary to the mineralocorticoid effect of deoxycorticosterone excess (Table 14–24). However, there is a poor correlation between DOC secretion and the presence of hypertension; furthermore, salt-wasting has been reported in few cases, which is unexplained.

On this clinical background, the diagnosis can be made by demonstrating a plasma ACTH-stimulated 11-deoxycortisol value, which is higher than three-times the 95th percentile for an age-matched normal group. Although established heterozygotes do not demonstrate an increase in 11-deoxycortisol above normal following Synacthen[351] (unlike the 17-OHP response observed in heterozygote 21 hydroxylase patients), exaggerated ACTH-stimulated responses have been observed in patients with hirsutism[352] and in patients with "essential" hypertension,[353] suggesting partial defects in 11β-hydroxylase activity. Treatment is with replacement glucocorticoid therapy; with suppression of DOC secretion, plasma renin activity (suppressed at baseline) increases into the normal range. In general, higher glucocorticoid doses are needed to suppress hyperandrogenism compared with patients suffering from 21-hydroxylase deficiency and add on antihypertensive therapy might be necessary in some cases.

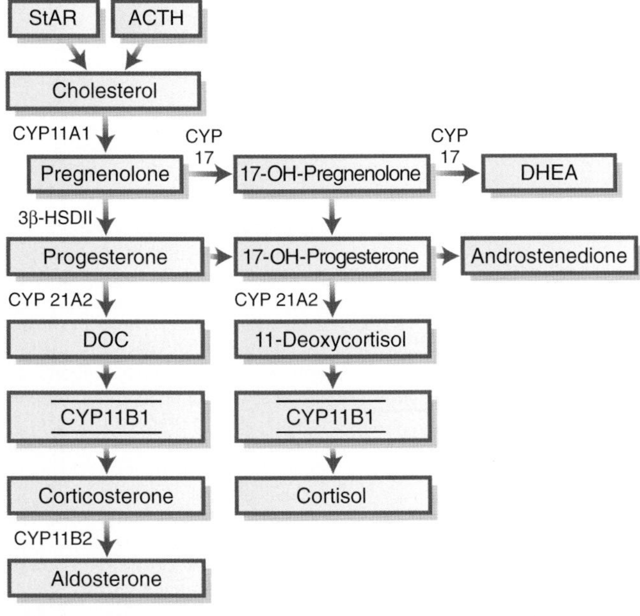

Figure 14–34 ▪ Congenital adrenal hyperplasia related to 11β-hydroxylase deficiency. The normal synthesis of cortisol is impaired, and adrenocorticotropic hormone (ACTH) levels increase because of loss of normal negative feedback inhibition resulting in an increase in adrenal steroid precursors proximal to the block. The results are cortisol deficiency, mineralocorticoid excess related to excessive deoxycorticosterone (DOC) secretion, and excessive secretion of adrenal androgens. *DHEA*, Dehydroepiandrosterone; *StAR*, steroidogenic acute regulatory protein.

17α-Hydroxylase Deficiency

Approximately 150 cases of 17α-hydroxylase deficiency have been reported.[354,355] Mutations within the CYP17 gene result in the failure to synthesize cortisol (17α-hydroxylase activity), adrenal androgens (17,20 lyase activity), and gonadal steroids (Fig. 14–35). Thus, in contrast to 21- and 11-hydroxylase deficiencies, 17α-hydroxylase deficiency results in adrenal and gonadal insufficiency. A single enzyme is expressed in adrenal and gonad and possesses both 17-hydroxylation and 17,20 lyase activities, but rarely patients with isolated deficiency in the hydroxylation of 17-OH progesterone or 17,20 lyase deficiency have been reported.[355] Loss of negative feedback results in increased secretion of steroids proximal to the block, and mineralocorticoid synthesis is enhanced. However, aldosterone levels are variable and the mineralocorticoid excess state that characterizes this condition is thought to be induced by DOC excess in more than 80% of cases. The genetic basis for the disease has been established in many cases involving point mutations, gene deletions, and conversions in the CYP17 gene.[356,357] Relative hydroxylase/lyase activities of mutant CYP17 cDNAs vary in vitro transfection assays, but correlations with clinical phenotype are lacking. Thus patients with clinically "pure" 17,20 lyase deficiency have mutant CYP17 cDNAs, selectively compromising 17,20 lyase activity.[358,359]

The diagnosis is usually made at the time of puberty when patients present with hypertension, hypokalemia, and hypogonadism, the latter occurring because of lack of CYP17 expression within the gonad and impaired gonadal steroidogenesis. As a result, LH and FSH levels are elevated. Female patients (XX) have primary amenorrhea with absent sexual characteristics whereas males (46XY) have complete pseudohermaphroditism with female external genitalia but absent uterus and fallopian tubes. The intraabdominal testes should be removed and such cases are usually reared as female.

Glucocorticoid replacement reverses the DOC-induced suppression of the renin-angiotensin system and lowers blood pressure. Additional sex steroid replacement is required from puberty onward.

Apparent Combined 17-Hydroxylase and 21-Hydroxylase Deficiency (P450 Oxidoreductase Deficiency)

Patients have been described with biochemical evidence of apparent combined 17α-hydroxylase and 21-hydroxylase deficiencies. Urinary GC/MS analysis reveals a typical pattern comprising increased pregnenolone and progesterone metabolites, slightly increased corticosterone metabolites, increased pregnanetriolone excretion, and low androgen metabolites. Cortisol baseline secretion may be normal but most if not all patients show an insufficient cortisol response to ACTH stimulation and thus require glucocorticoid replacement. Impaired 17,20 lyase activity results in deficient androgen synthesis and affected boys are often born undervirilized. However, conversely, most of the affected girls are born with virilized genitalia. After birth, however, virilization does not progress and circulating androgen concentrations are generally low. Some mothers develop

TABLE 14–24 CLINICAL AND BIOCHEMICAL CHARACTERISTICS OF REPORTED CASES OF APPARENT CORTISONE REDUCTASE DEFICIENCY

Age	Sex	Clinical Features	Serum Androgens	THF + allo THF: THE Ratio	Comments
28	F	Hirsuitism	↑ Testosterone ↑ DHEAS ↑ Androstenedione	—	Marked fall in serum androgens on treatment with dexamethasone
17	F	Oligomenorrhea, hirsutism, acne, obesity	↑ Testosterone ↑ DHEAS	0.039	Fall in androgens with dexamethasone treatment although developed cushingoid side effects
18	F	Oligomenorrhea, hirsutism, acne		0.045	Sibling of preceding patient Fall in androgens with treatment
30	F	Oligomenorrhea, hirsutism, infertility	↑ Testosterone	—	Fall in testosterone with treatment
	M	Excess body hair (sibling of preceding patient)		—	Sibling of preceding patient No mutations on genetic sequence analysis of *HSD11B1*
37	F	Obesity, oligomenorrhea, hirsutism	↑ Testosterone ↑ DHEAS ↑ Androstenedione	0.03 (0.5 to 1.15)	No mutations on genetic sequence analysis of *HSD11B1*
	F	Congenital adrenal hyperplasia diagnosed shortly after birth (21-hydroxylase deficiency). 17-Hydroxyprogesterone levels unresponsive to cortisone acetate		↓	17-OHP levels suppressed completely with prenisolone, indicative of an inability to activate cortisone acetate. No mutations on genetic sequence analysis of *HSD11B1*
55	F	Androgenetic alopecia, mild hirsutism	↑ Testosterone	0.04 (0.5 to 0.8)	No mutations on genetic sequence analysis of *HSD11B1*

DHEAS, Dehydroepiandrosterone sulfate; *allo-THF*, 5α-tetrahydrocortisol; *THE*, tetrahydrocortisone; *THF*, 5β-tetrahydrocortisol.

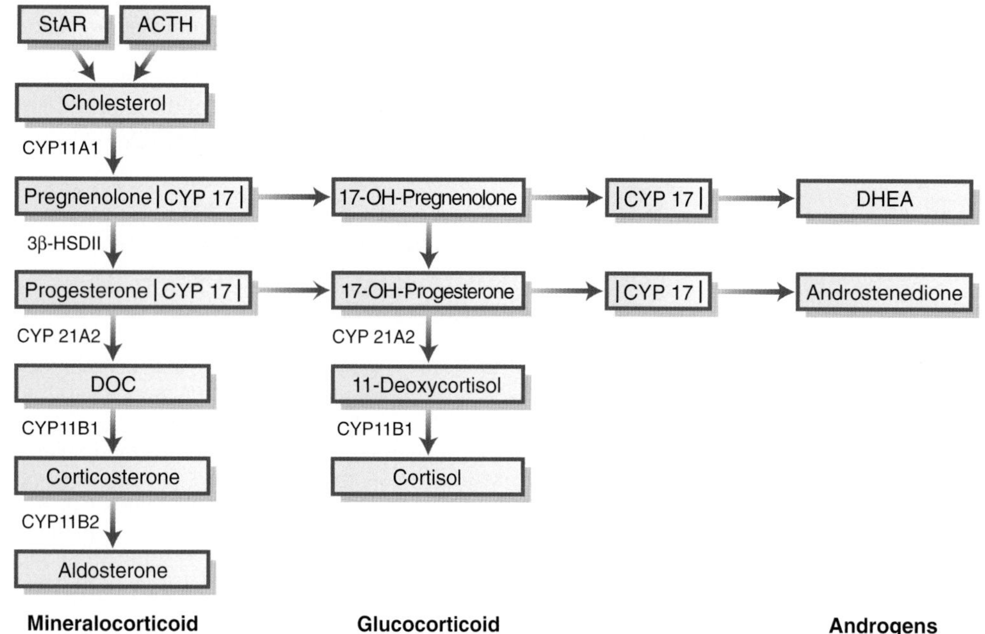

Figure 14–35 ■ Congenital adrenal hyperplasia related to 17-hydroxylase deficiency. The normal synthesis of cortisol is impaired, and adrenocorticotropic hormone (ACTH) levels increase because of loss of normal negative feedback inhibition resulting in an increase in adrenal steroid precursors proximal to the block. The result is cortisol deficiency and mineralocorticoid excess usually related to deoxycorticosterone (DOC) excess. Because gonadal 17-hydroxylase activity is also absent, sex steroid secretion in addition to adrenal androgen secretion is severely impaired, resulting in hypogonadism. *DHEA*, Dehydroepiandrosterone; *StAR*, steroidogenic acute regulatory protein.

signs of virilization during pregnancy with an affected child, resolving immediately after birth and thus further indicating intrauterine androgen excess. In addition to these features of congenital adrenal hyperplasia, affected children may also present with bone malformations, including midface hypoplasia, craniosynostosis, and radiohumeral synostosis, in some cases resembling the Antley-Bixler congenital malformation syndrome[24,360] (Fig. 14–36).

Having excluded mutations in the *CYP17* and *CYP21* genes, mutations in the gene encoding P450 oxidoreductase have been defined.[24,360] P450 OR provides electrons from NADPH to both 17-hydroxylase and 21-hydroxylase, but also to 14-lanosterol demethylase (CYP51), which is involved in sterol biosynthesis and has been shown to be linked to the bone phenotype in affected children. Furthermore, this variant of congenital adrenal hyperplasia may illustrate the presence of an alternative pathway in human androgen synthesis, present in fetal life only and explaining the apparently contradictory findings of prenatal androgen excess and postnatal androgen deficiency.[24] Considering the number of patients with P450 oxidoreductase deficiency reported within a short period after the initial description of the molecular cause of disease,[361] this variant may be the second most common cause of CAH.

3β-Hydroxysteroid Dehydrogenase Deficiency

In this rare form of CAH, the secretion of all classes of adrenal and ovarian steroids is impaired due to mutations within the HSD3B2 gene encoding 3β-HSDII.[362,363] Patients usually present in early infancy with adrenal insufficiency. Loss of mineralocorticoid secretion results in salt-wasting, although this is absent in 30% to 40% of cases (Fig. 14–37). As with 21-hydroxylase deficiency, absence of salt-wasting may delay the presentation into childhood or puberty. The correlation between genotype and phenotype is once again poor; identical mutations have been found in the HSD3B2 gene in both salt-wasters and non–salt-wasters.[362] The spectrum of genital development is variable in both sexes. In males, because the 3β-HSDII enzyme is also expressed within the gonad, male pseudohermaphroditism may occur with female external genitalia. In milder cases, hypospadias may be found or even normal male genitalia. In females, genital development can be normal, but usually there is evidence of mild virilization, presumably because of enhanced adrenal DHEA secretion, which is converted peripherally to testosterone. A late-onset form has been described in patients

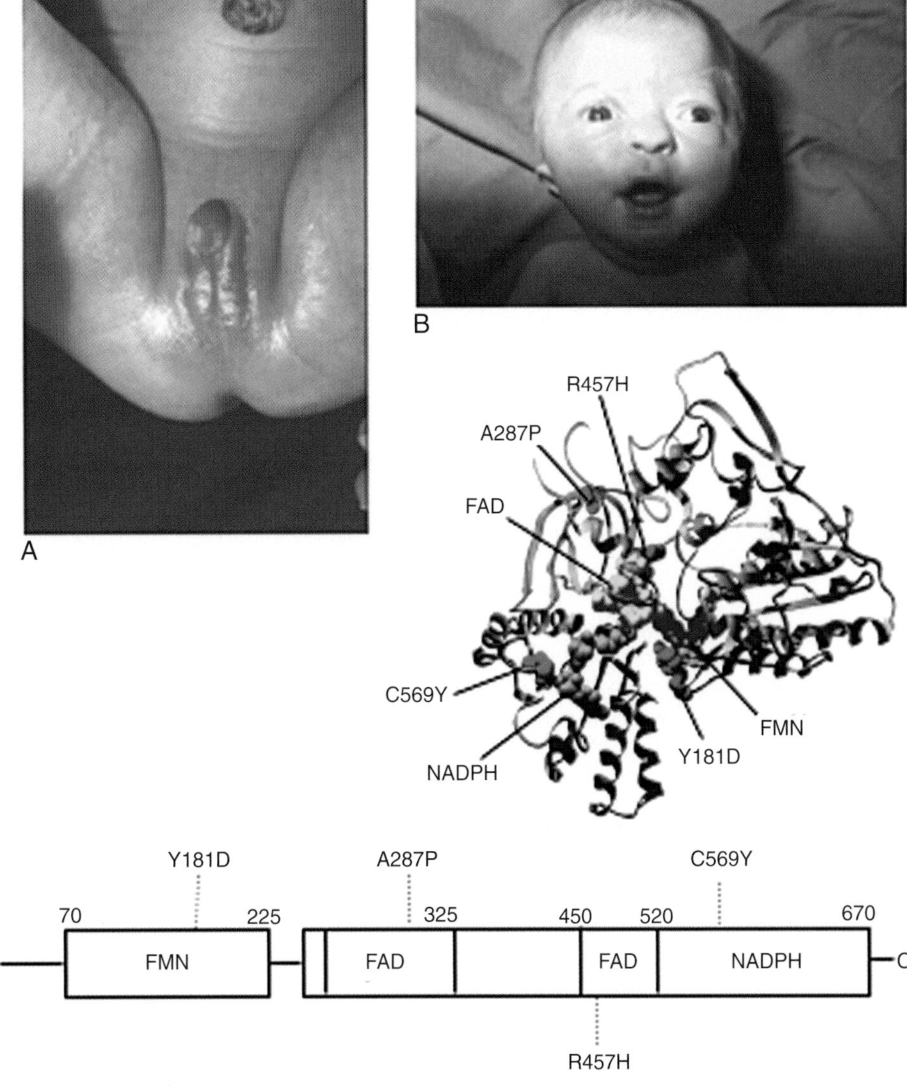

Figure 14–36 ▪ Congenital adrenal hyperplasia due to P450 oxidoreductase deficiency, also known as congenital adrenal hyperplasia with apparent combined CYP17 and CYP21 deficiency. Characteristic clinical features include ambiguous genitalia in both sexes and craniofacial malformations with pronounced frontal bossing and midface hypoplasia with a broad, depressed nasal bridge, pear-shaped nose, and low-set ears, as illustrated in an affected patient (46,XX) briefly after birth (**A** and **B**). Mutations in the P450 oxidoreductase gene are disease-causing. **C,** Four missense mutations[24] and their localization within the P450 oxidoreductase protein. Their location in immediate proximity to the binding domains of the central electron transfer chain (NADPH > FAD > FMN) disrupts the electron transfer from NADPH to electron-accepting P450 enzymes, such as CYP17 and CYP21. (Courtesy of Dr Christian Roth, Dept of Pediatrics, University Hospital Bonn, Germany, and of Dr Wiebke Arlt, University of Birmingham, United Kingdom.)

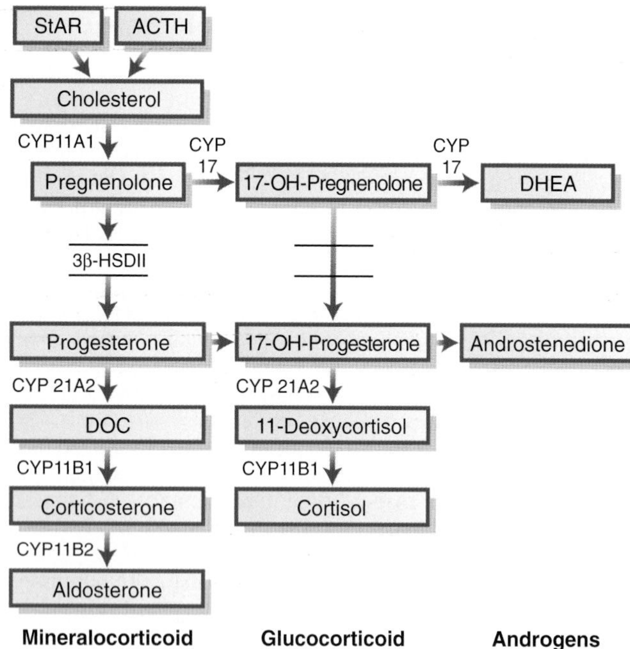

Figure 14–37 ▪ Congenital adrenal hyperplasia related to 3β-hydroxysteroid dehydrogenase (3β-HSD) deficiency resulting in cortisol deficiency and variable mineralocorticoid deficiency. Gonadal 3β-HSD activity is also absent, resulting in male pseudohermaphroditism and hypogonadism or primary amenorrhea in females. *ACTH*, Adrenocorticotropic hormone; *DOC*, deoxycorticosterone; *DHEA*, dehydroepiandrosterone; *StAR*, steroidogenic acute regulatory protein.

with premature pubarche[364] and a PCOS-like phenotype (hirsutism, oligorrhea/amenorrhea).[365]

Because activity of the 3β-HSDI enzyme, present in skin and other peripheral tissues, is intact, circulating Δ4 steroid levels (progesterone, 17α-hydroxyprogesterone, androstenedione) may be normal (or even increased). However, a diagnosis is established by demonstrating an increased ratio of Δ5 steroids (pregnenolone, 17α-hydroxy pregnenolone, DHEA) to Δ4 steroids in plasma or urine. ACTH stimulation may be required to detect a late-onset presentation. Treatment is with replacement glucocorticoids, fludrocortisone (if indicated), and sex steroids from puberty onward.

StAR Deficiency

Mutations in the gene encoding steroidogenic acute regulatory protein (StAR) results in a failure of transport of cholesterol from the outer to inner mitochondrial membrane in steroidogenic tissues. As a result, there is deficiency of all adrenal and gonadal steroid hormones.[20,366] Presentation is with acute adrenal insufficiency in the neonatal period and males exhibit pseudohermaphroditism due to absent gonadal steroids. The condition is fatal in infancy in two thirds of all cases. The adrenal glands are often massively enlarged and full of lipid; before the characterization of StAR, the condition was termed *congenital "lipoid" hyperplasia* and the putative candidate gene was thought to be cholesterol side chain cleavage (CYP11A1). In fact, to date, no mutations have been reported in the CYP11A1 gene; such mutations are thought to be lethal in utero. This clinical phenotype is endorsed by recombinant mouse models lacking the StAR gene.[367]

TABLE 14–25 CAUSES OF MINERALOCORTICOID DEFICIENCY

Addison's disease
Adrenal hypoplasia
Congenital adrenal hyperplasia (21-hydroxylase and 3β-hydroxysteroid dehydrogenase deficiencies)
Pseudohypoaldosteronism types I and II
Hyporeninemic hypoaldosteronism
Aldosterone biosynthetic defects
Drug induced

Cortisone Reductase Deficiency

In this condition, adrenal glands become "hyperplastic" because of ACTH stimulation from a defect in cortisol metabolism rather than an inherent defect within the gland itself.[120,368,369] Patients with cortisone reductase deficiency (CRD) have a defect in the conversion of cortisone to cortisol, suggesting inhibition of 11 oxo-reductase activity and by implication, inhibition of 11β-HSD1 (see Fig. 14–11). Cortisol clearance is increased and as a consequence ACTH secretion is elevated to maintain normal circulating cortisol concentrations but at the expense of adrenal androgen excess. As a consequence, patients described are usually adult and female who present with hirsutism, menstrual irregularity, and/or androgenic alopecia. Dexamethasone treatment to suppress ACTH has been used with some success to control the hyperandrogenism in these cases. Urinary tetrahydrometabolites of cortisol and cortisone show almost exclusively THE with little or no detectable THF or allo-THF (THF + allo-THF:THE ratio <0.05, reference range 0.8 to 1.3). Further studies have also shown impaired plasma cortisol concentrations following an oral dose of cortisone acetate. The molecular basis for CRD has been postulated to be secondary to coexisting mutations in two separate genes, first intronic mutations in the gene encoding 11β-HSD1, *HSD11B1*, and second inactivating mutations in hexose-6-phosphate dehydrogenase (H6PDH).[370] H6PDH, localized in the endoplasmic reticulum (ER), catalyses the conversion of glucose-6-phosphate to glucose-6-phosphogluconate, thereby generating NADPH that is crucial in conveying oxo-reductase activity upon 11β-HSD1. However, some of the H6PDH "mutations" described in CRD are also found in 3% to 4% of the normal population in subjects with normal urinary THF + allo-THF:THE ratios. Notwithstanding the importance of H6PDH in regulating the direction of 11β-HSD1 activity,[120] further sequencing studies are required to clarify the molecular basis for CRD.

Patients with polycystic ovary syndrome (PCOS) share many of the same clinical characteristics as those with CRD. Whereas there is evidence to support increased cortisol secretion rates in PCOS, perhaps indicative of a defect in cortisone to cortisol conversion, there remains to be a consensus with respect to THF + allo-THF:THE ratios. Association studies using single nucleotide polymorphic markers in the HSD11B1 and H6PDH genes have largely been negative.

Mineralocorticoid Deficiency

These syndromes are listed in Table 14–25. They can be divided into those that are congenital and others that are acquired. Mineralocorticoid deficiency may occur in some forms of congenital adrenal hyperplasia and with other causes of adrenal insufficiency (e.g., Addison's disease and congenital adrenal hypoplasia).

Primary Defects in Aldosterone Biosynthesis—Aldosterone Synthase Deficiency

Before the characterization of the CYP11B2 gene, the disease was termed *corticosterone methyl oxidase type I (CMO I) deficiency* and *corticosterone methyl oxidase type II (CMO II) deficiency.*[371] Subsequently both variants were shown to be secondary to mutations in aldosterone synthase and are now termed *type I and type II aldosterone synthase deficiency.*[372] Aldosterone synthase catalyses the three terminal steps of aldosterone biosynthesis, 11β-hydroxylation of deoxycorticosterone to corticosterone, 18-hydroxylation to 18-hydroxycorticosterone, and 18-oxidation to aldosterone. Patients with type I aldosterone synthase deficiency have low to normal levels of 18-hydroxycorticosterone, but undetectable levels of aldosterone (or urinary tetrahydroaldosterone), whereas patients with the type II variant have high levels of 18-hydroxycorticosterone and only subnormal or even normal levels of aldosterone. This suggests blockade of only the terminal 18-oxidation step with some residual aldosterone synthase activity. The explanation for the variable biochemical phenotype is unknown, particularly now that the same mutation in aldosterone synthase has been uncovered in both variants. It is possible that this may reflect polymorphic variants in the residual and normal product of the CYP11B1 gene, 11β-hydroxylase.

Both variants are rare and inherited as autosomal recessive traits.[372] The type II deficiency is found most frequently among Jews of Iranian origin. Presentation is usually in neonatal life as a salt-wasting crisis with severe dehydration, vomiting, and failure to grow and thrive. Hyperkalemia, metabolic acidosis, dehydration, and hyponatremia are found. The plasma renin activity is elevated, and plasma aldosterone levels are low. Plasma 18-hydroxycorticosterone levels and the ratio of plasma 18-hydroxycorticosterone to aldosterone and their urinary metabolites are used to differentiate the type I and II variants. In most infants, the disorders become less severe as the child ages—indeed in older children, adolescents, and adults, the abnormal steroid pattern described may be present and may persist throughout life without clinical manifestations. Mineralocorticoids are given (9α-fluorocortisone) during infancy and early childhood, but this therapy can be discontinued in the majority of adults. Spontaneous "normalization" of growth can occur in untreated patients. Rarely, presentation is in adulthood.[373]

Postadrenalectomy Hypoaldosteronism

In a patient with a unilateral aldosteronoma (Conn's syndrome), the contralateral zona glomerulosa is frequently suppressed. Without reversal of the chronic volume expansion preoperatively, postadrenalectomy patients may develop severe hyperkalemia and hypotension lasting several days to several weeks after surgery. This may be exacerbated by the use of spironolactone preoperatively. This drug has a long half-life and should be discontinued 2 to 3 days before surgery to minimize the risk of mineralocorticoid deficiency postoperatively.

Defects in Aldosterone Action: Pseudohypoaldosteronism

Pseudohypoaldosteronism (PHA) is a rare inherited salt-wasting disorder first described by Cheek and Perry in 1958 as a defective renal tubular response to mineralocorticoid in infancy. Patients present in the neonatal period with dehydration, hyponatremia, hypokalemia, metabolic acidosis, and failure to thrive despite normal glomerular filtration and normal renal and adrenal function.[374] Renin levels and plasma aldosterone are grossly elevated. When patients fail to respond to mineralocorticoid therapy, PHA is suspected as the underlying disorder.

PHA type I can be divided into two distinct disorders based on unique physiologic and genetic characteristics: the renal form of PHA, inherited as an autosomal dominant trait and a generalized autosomal recessive (AR) form of PHA. The autosomal dominant form is usually less severe with the patient's condition often improving spontaneously within the first several years of life, thus allowing discontinuation of therapy and treatment. By contrast, the AR form has a multiorgan disorder, with mineralocorticoid resistance seen in the kidney, sweat, and salivary glands, and the colonic mucosa. The condition does not spontaneously improve with age and is generally more severe.

The underlying basis for the AD form of PHA is explained on the basis of inactivating mutations in the mineralocorticoid receptor (MR).[374,375] By contrast, inactivating mutations in the α, and to a lesser extent the β and γ subunits of the ENaC account for the generalized AR form of mineralocorticoid resistance.[376,377] (In effect this represents the opposite of Liddle's syndrome—see Chapter 15). Generalized loss of ENaC activity leads to renal salt-wasting as seen in the renal form but in addition recurrent respiratory infections and neonatal respiratory distress, cholelithiasis, and polyhydramnios.

PHA I patients are resistant to mineralocorticoid therapy and thus standard treatment involves supplementation with sodium chloride (2 to 8 g/day) and cation exchange resins. This usually corrects the patient's biochemical imbalance. However, if a patient shows signs of severe hyperkalemia, peritoneal dialysis may be necessary. Hypercalciuria has been reported in some cases involving PHA I. In such cases, the recommended course of treatment usually involves either treatment with indomethacin or with hydrochlorothiazide. Indomethacin is thought to act by causing a reduction in the glomerular filtration rate or an inhibition of the effect of prostaglandin E_2 on renal tubules. Indomethacin has been shown to reduce polyuria, sodium loss, and hypercalciura. Hydrochlorothiazide has been used to diminish hyperkalemia and reduce hypercalciura in PHA I patients.

In patients with the autosomal dominant or renal form of PHA I, the signs and symptoms of PHA decrease with age; nevertheless, these patients usually require salt supplementation for the first 2 to 3 years of life. In patients with the autosomal recessive or multiorgan type of PHA I, however, resistance to therapy with sodium chloride or drugs that decrease serum potassium concentrations often occurs, and may even lead to death in infancy from hyperkalemia. Multiorgan PHA I patients often require very high amounts of salt in their diet (as high as 45 g NaCl per day). Carbenoxolone (CBX), a derivative of glycyrrhetinic acid in licorice, has been used with moderate success in helping reduce the high-salt diets for renal PHA I patients. CBX acts by inhibiting 11β-HSD2 activity and allows unmetabolized cortisol to bind to and activate mineralocorticoid receptors in a manner similar to that of aldosterone.[378] It was ineffective in patients with multiorgan PHA I.

Two other variants of PHA have been described—types II and III. Type II PHA, or Gordon's syndrome, is in retrospect a misnomer. Patients with Gordon's syndrome share some of the features of patients with PHA type I, notably hyperkalemia and metabolic acidosis, but exhibit salt retention with mild hypertension and suppressed plasma renin activity rather than salt-wasting. The condition is explained by mutations in a serine threonine kinase family, WNK1 and WNK4, resulting in increased expression of these proteins with activation of the thiazide-sensitive Na,Cl– cotransporter in the cortical and medullary collecting ducts.[379] The condition represents the exact opposite of Gitelman's syndrome but is not a true form of PHA.

Type III PHA is an acquired and usually transient form of mineralocorticoid resistance seen in patients with underlying renal pathologies including obstruction and infection and in patients with excessive loss of salt through the gut or skin. Reduced GFR is a hallmark of the condition. The cause is unknown, although increased TGF-β-mediated aldosterone resistance has been suggested to be an underlying factor.

Hyporeninemic Hypoaldosteronism

Angiotensin II is a key stimulus to aldosterone secretion, and damage or blockade of the renin-angiotensin system may result in mineralocorticoid deficiency. Various renal diseases have been associated with damage to the juxtaglomerular apparatus and hence renin deficiency. These include systemic lupus erythematosus (SLE), myeloma, amyloid, AIDS, and use of nonsteroidal antiinflammatory drugs, but the most common (>75% of cases) is diabetic nephropathy.[380,381]

The usual picture is of an elderly patient with hyperkalemia, acidosis, and mild to moderate impairment of renal function. Plasma renin activity and aldosterone are low and fail to respond to sodium depletion, the erect posture, or furosemide administration. In contrast to adrenal insufficiency, patients have normal or elevated blood pressure and no postural hypotension. Muscle weakness and cardiac arrhythmias may also occur. Other factors may contribute to the hyperkalemia, including the use of potassium-sparing diuretics, potassium supplementation, insulin deficiency, and β-adrenoceptor blocking drugs and prostaglandin synthetase inhibitors, which inhibit renin release.

Treatment of primary renin deficiency is with fludrocortisone in the first instance together with dietary potassium restriction. However, these patients are not salt depleted and may become hypertensive with fludrocortisone. In such a scenario, the addition of a loop-acting diuretic such as furosemide is appropriate. This will increase acid excretion and improve the metabolic acidosis.

ADRENAL ADENOMAS, INCIDENTALOMAS, AND CARCINOMAS

Adenomas

Cortisol-secreting adrenal adenomas have been discussed in detail, and aldosterone-secreting adenomas (Conn's syndrome) are discussed in Chapter 15.

Pure virilizing benign adrenal adenomas are rare, with approximately 50 cases reported in the literature. The majority of cases occur in women; male cases are restricted to childhood where presentation is with sexual precocity and accelerated bone age. In females, the majority of cases present before the menopause with marked hirsutism, deepening of the voice, and amenorrhea. Clitoromegaly is found in 80% of cases. Testosterone is usually strikingly elevated but gonadotropin levels may not be suppressed. By definition, urinary free cortisol is normal. Tumors vary in size and should be treated surgically. Postoperatively, clinical features invariably improve and normal menses return.[382]

Incidentalomas

Autopsy series had defined the prevalence of adrenal adenomas greater than 1 cm in diameter to be between 1.5% and 7%. It is perhaps not surprising, therefore, that with the advent of high-resolution imaging procedures (CT, MRI), incidentally discovered adrenal masses have become a common clinical problem. An adrenal mass will be uncovered in up to 4% of patients imaged for nonadrenal pathology.[383] Incidentalomas are uncommon in patients younger than 30 years of age but increase in frequency with age; they occur equally in males and females. In more than 85% of cases these lesions are nonfunctioning, benign adenomas. Occasionally they may represent myelolipomas, hamartomas, or granulomatous infiltrations of the adrenal and result in a characteristic CT/MRI appearance (Fig. 14–38). Functioning tumors (pheochromocytomas or those secreting cortisol, aldosterone, or sex steroids) and carcinomas comprise the remainder. In addition, it is established that some "incidentalomas" may cause abnormal hormone secretion without obvious clinical manifestations of a hormone excess state; the best example of this relates to "preclinical" Cushing's syndrome, which may occur in up to 20% of all cases.[383,384] This may explain why "incidentalomas" appear to be more common in patients with obesity and diabetes mellitus.[385] As a result, all patients with incidentally discovered adrenal masses should undergo appropriate endocrine screening tests. This should comprise 24-hour urinary catecholamine collection, 24-hour urinary free cortisol (and/or midnight salivary cortisol measurements) and overnight dexamethasone suppression tests. Because of the reported poor sensitivity of serum potassium measurements in detecting primary aldosteronism, our practice has been to measure supine circulating PRA/aldosterone levels. DHEAS should be measured as a marker of adrenal androgen secretion. Low levels may occur in patients with suppressed ACTH concentrations due to autonomous cortisol secretion from the adenoma,[386] and it is important that DHEAS is not measured during the overnight dexamethasone study. Some studies have also documented high levels of 17-OH progesterone following ACTH stimulation tests, suggesting partial defects in 21-hydroxylase in some tumors.

The possibility of malignancy should be considered in each case. In patients with a known extraadrenal primary, the incidence of malignancy is obviously much higher (up to 20% of patients with lung cancer, for example, have adrenal metastases on CT scanning). In those with no evidence of malignancy, adrenal carcinoma is rare—in one study only 26 of 630 incidentalomas were found to be adrenal carcinomas.[383] In true incidentalomas, size appears to be predictive of malignancy—a lesion less than 5 cm in diameter in size is most unlikely to be malignant. The majority of nonfunctioning lesions less than 5 cm can therefore be treated conservatively, and patients followed up with annual imaging. Even incidentalomas greater than 5 cm are more likely to be benign than malignant, but because of an increased risk of malignancy many centers recommend removal of tumors greater than 5 cm in diameter. Additional characteristic MRI appearances or scintigraphy studies may aid in differentiating malignant from nonmalignant lesions. If malignancy is suspected on imaging or clinical predictors, then open adrenalectomy rather than a laparoscopic approach is advised. CT-guided biopsy is useful in differentiating adrenal from nonadrenal tissue in the case of a suspected metastasis, but is poor in differentiating benign adenomas from malignant adrenal lesions.

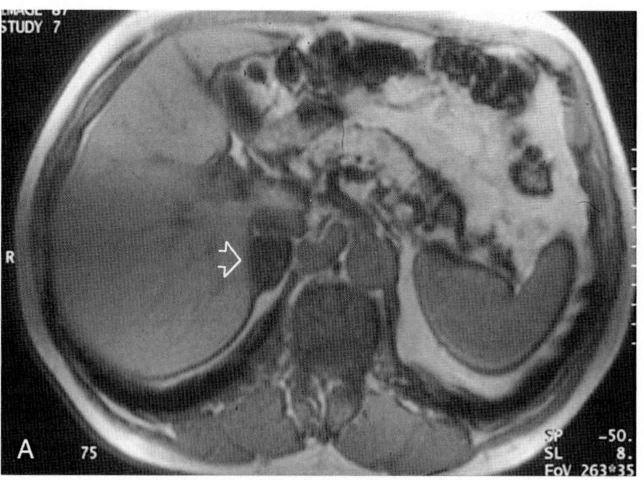

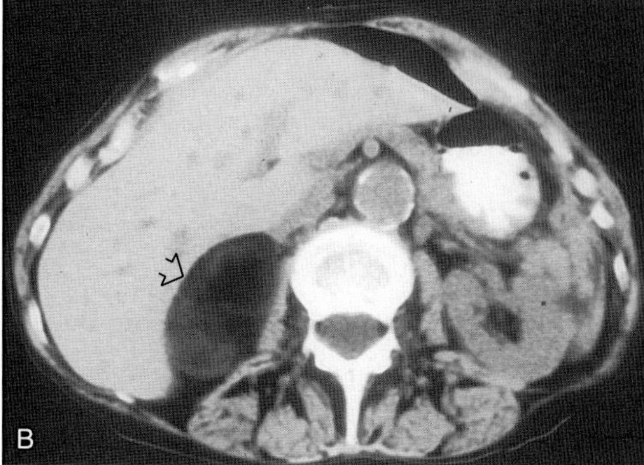

Figure 14–38 ■ **A,** Adrenal incidentaloma discovered in a woman undergoing investigation for abdominal pain. **B,** Incidentally discovered right adrenal myelolipoma.

Carcinomas

Primary adrenal carcinoma is very rare with an incidence of 1/ million population/year. Women are more commonly affected than men (2.5 : 1); mean age of onset is between 40 and 50 years of age, although males tend to be older at presentation. Eighty percent of tumors are functional, most commonly secreting glucocorticoids alone (45%), glucocorticoids and androgens (45%), or androgens alone (10%). Less than 1% of all cases secrete aldosterone. Patients present with features of the hormone excess state (glucocorticoid and/or androgen excess) but abdominal pain, weight loss, anorexia, and fever occur in 25% of cases. An abdominal mass may be palpable. Current treatments for what is often an aggressive tumor are poor. Surgery offers the only chance of cure for patients with local disease, but metastatic spread is evident in 75% of cases at presentation. Radiotherapy is ineffective, as are most chemotherapeutic regimens. Mitotane in high doses offers transient benefit in reducing tumor growth in 25% to 30% of cases and controlling hormonal hypersecretion in 75% of cases.[262] Overall, the prognosis is poor, with 5-year survival rates of less than 20%.

Etiology of Adrenal Tumors

The underlying basis for adrenal tumorigenesis is unknown. Clonal analysis suggests progression from a normal to adenomatous to carcinomatous lesion, but the molecular pathways involved remain obscure. Several factors have been associated with malignant transformation including genes encoding p53, p57 cyclin-dependent kinase, menin, IGF-II, MC2-R, and inhibin-α.[387] Mice lacking the inhibin-α gene develop adrenal tumors through a process that is also gonadotropin dependent.[388]

ACKNOWLEDGMENTS

Acknowledgments to Dr. W. Arlt, Dr. M. S. Cooper, Dr. N. Krone, Dr. J. W. Tomlinson, Dr. W. Young for assistance with parts of this chapter.

REFERENCES

1. Eustachius B. Tabulae Anatomicae. Lancisius B, ed. Amsterdam, 1774.
2. Addison T. On the Constitutional and Local Effects of Disease of the Supra-Renal Capsules. London: Highley, 1855.
3. Brown-Sequard CE. Recherches experimentales sur la physiologie et la pathologie des capsules surrenales. Arch Gen Med 1856; Ser 5, No 8: 385-401.
4. Medvei VC. A History of Clinical Endocrinology. Pearl River, NY: Parthenon, 1993.
5. Hench PS, Kendall EC, Slocumb CH, et al. The effect of a hormone of the adrenal cortex (17-hydroxy-11-dehydrocorticosterone: compound E) and of pituitary adrenocorticotropic hormone on rheumatoid arthritis. Mayo Clin Proc 1949;24:181-197.
6. Simpson SA, Tait JF. Recent progress in methods of isolation, chemistry, and physiology of aldosterone. Recent Prog Horm Res 1955;11:183-210.
7. Li CH, Simpson ME, Evans HM. Adrenocorticotrophic hormone. J Biol Chem, 1943;149:413-424.
8. Cushing H. The basophil adenomas of the pituitary body and their clinical manifestations (pituitary basophilism). Bull Johns Hopkins Hosp 1932;50:137-195.
9. Vale W, Spiess J, Rivier C, et al. Characterization of a 41-residue ovine hypothalamic peptide that stimulates secretion of corticotropin and β-endorphin. Science 1981;213:1394-1397.
10. Conn JW. Primary aldosteronism, a new clinical entity. J Lab Clin Med 1955;45:3-17.
11. Mesiano S, Jaffe RB. Developmental and functional biology of the primate fetal adrenal cortex. Endocr Rev 1997;18:378-404.
12. Jaffe RB, Mesiano S, Smith R, et al. The regulation and role of fetal adrenal development in human pregnancy. Endocr Res 1998; 24:919-926.
13. Okamoto M, Takemori H. Differentiation and zonation of the adrenal cortex. Curr Opin Endocrinol Diab 2000;7: 122-127.
14. Luo X, Ikeda Y, Parker KL. A cell-specific nuclear factor is essential for adrenal and gonadal development and sexual differentiation. Cell 1994;77:481-490.
15. International Union of Pure and Applied Chemistry. Definitive rules for the nomenclature of steroids. Pure Appl Chem 1972;31: 285-322.
16. Gwynne JT, Strauss JF III. The role of lipoprotein in steroidogenesis and cholesterol metabolism in steroidogenic glands. Endocr Rev 1982;3:299-329.
17. Faust JR, Goldstein JL, Brown MS. Receptor-mediated uptake of low density lipoprotein and utilization of its cholesterol for steroid synthesis in cultured mouse adrenal cells. J Biol Chem 1977;252: 4861-4871.
18. Goldstein JL, Anderson RGW, Brown MS. Coated pits, coated vesicles, and receptor-mediated endocytosis. Nature 1979;279: 679-685.
19. Landschulz KT, Pathak RK, Rigotti A, et al. Regulation of scavenger receptor, class B, type I, a high density lipoprotein receptor, in liver and steroidogenic tissues of the rat. J Clin Invest 1996;98: 984-995.

20. Stocco DM, Clark BJ. Regulation of the acute production of steroids in steroidogenic cells. Endocr Rev 1996;17:221-244.
21. Amri H, Li H, Culty M, et al. The peripheral-type benzodiazepine receptor and adrenal steroidogenesis. Curr Opin Endocrinol Diab 1999;6:179-184.
22. Bernhardt R. The role of adrenodoxin in adrenal steroidogenesis. Curr Opin Endocrinol Diab 2000;7:109-115.
23. Miller WL. Regulation of steroidogenesis by electron transfer. Endocrinology 2005;146:2544-2550.
24. Arlt W, Walker EA, Draper N, et al. Congenital adrenal hyperplasia caused by mutant P450 oxidoreductase and human androgen synthesis: analytical study. Lancet 2004;363:2128-2135.
25. Onoda M, Hall PF. Cytochrome b_5 stimulates purified testicular microsomal cytochrome P450 (C_{21} side-chain cleavage). Biochem Biophys Res Commun 1982;108:454-460.
26. Miller WL. Molecular biology of steroid hormone synthesis. Endocr Rev 1988;9:295-318.
27. John ME, John MC, Ashley P, et al. Identification and characterization of cDNA clones specific for cholesterol side-chain cleavage cytochrome P-450. Proc Natl Acad Sci U S A 1984;81:5628-5632.
28. Lorence MC, Murray BA, Trant JM, et al. Human 3β-hydroxysteroid dehydrogenase/Δ^5–Δ^4 isomerase from placenta: expression in nonsteroidogenic cells of a protein that catalyses the dehydrogenation/isomerization of C21 and C19 steroids. Endocrinology 1990;126:2493-2498.
29. Bradshaw KD, Waterman MR, Couch RT, et al. Characterization of complementary deoxyribonucleic acid for human adrenocortical 17α-hydroxylase: a probe for analysis of 17α-hydroxylase deficiency. Mol Endocrinol 1987;1:348-354.
30. White PC, New MI, Dupont B. Cloning and expression of cDNA encoding a bovine adrenal cytochrome P450 specific for steroid 21-hydroxylation. Proc Natl Acad Sci U S A 1984;81: 1986-1990.
31. Chua SC, Szabo P, Vitek A, et al. Cloning of cDNA encoding steroid 11β-hydroxylase (P450c11). Proc Natl Acad Sci U S A 1987;84: 7193-7197.
32. Mornet E, Dupont J, Vitek A, et al. Characterization of two genes encoding human steroid 11β-hydroxylase (P-450(11) β). J Biol Chem 1989;264:20961-20967.
33. Curnow KM, Tusie-Luna MT, Pascoe L, et al. The product of the CYP11B2 gene is required for aldosterone biosynthesis in the human adrenal cortex. Mol Endocrinol 1991;5:1513-1522.
34. Strott CA. Sulfonation and molecular action. Endocr Rev 2002; 23:703-732.
35. Siiteri PK, MacDonald PC. The utilization of dehydroisoandrosterone sulphate for estrogen synthesis during human pregnancy. Steroids 1963;2:713-730.
36. Lamolet B, Pulichino AM, Lamonerie T, et al. A pituitary cell-restricted T box factor, Tpit, activates POMC transcription in cooperation with Pitx homeoproteins. Cell 2001;104:849-859.
37. Smith AI, Funder JW. Proopiomelanocortin processing in the pituitary, central nervous system, and peripheral tissues. Endocr Rev 1988;9:159-179.
38. Donald RA. ACTH and related peptides. Clin Endocrinol (Oxf) 1980;12:491-524.
39. Bicknell AB, Lomthaisong K, Woods RJ, et al. Characterization of a serine protease that cleaves pro-gamma-melanotropin at the adrenal to stimulate growth. Cell 2001;105:903-912.
40. Suzuki I, Cone RD, Im S, et al. Binding of melanotropic hormones to the melanocortin receptor MC1R on human melanocytes stimulates proliferation and melanogenesis. Endocrinology 1996;137: 1627-1633.
41. DeBold CR, Nicholson WE, Orth DN. Immunoreactive proopiomelanocortin (POMC) peptides and POMC-like messenger ribonucleic acid are present in many rat nonpituitary tissues. Endocrinology 1988;122:2648-2657.
42. de Keyzer Y, Lenne F, Massias JF, et al. Pituitary-like proopimelanocortin transcripts in human Leydig cell tumours. J Clin Invest 1990;86:871-877.
43. Clark AJ, Lavender PM, Coates P, et al. In vitro and in vivo analysis of the processing and fate of the peptide products of the short proopiomelanocortin mRNA. Mol Endocrinol 1990;4:1737-1743.
44. de Keyzer Y, Bertagna X, Luton JP, Kahn A. Variable modes of proopiomelanocortin gene transcription in human tumors. Mol Endocrinol 1989;3:215-223.
45. Clark AJL, Lavender PM, Besser GM, et al. Pro-opiomelanocortin mRNA size heterogeneity in ACTH-dependent Cushing's syndrome. J Mol Endocrinol 1989;2:3-9.
46. Picon A, Bertagna X, de Keyzer Y. Analysis of the human proopiomelanocortin gene promoter in a small cell lung carcinoma cell line reveals an unusual role for E2F transcription factors. Oncogene 1999;18:22627-2633.
47. Newell-Price J, King P, Clark AJ. The CpG island promoter of the human proopiomelanocortin gene is methylated in nonexpressing normal tissue and tumors and represses expression. Mol Endocrinol 2001;15:338-348.
48. Zhou A, Bloomquist BT, Mains RE. The prohormone convertases PC1 and PC2 mediate distinct endoproteolytic cleavages in a strict temporal order during proopiomelancortin biosynthetic processing. J Biol Chem 1993;268(3):1763-1769.
49. Stewart PM, Gibson S, Crosby SR, et al. ACTH precursors characterize the ectopic ACTH syndrome. Clin Endocrinol (Oxf) 1994;40: 199-204.
50. Oliver RL, Davis JR, White A. Characterisation of ACTH related peptides in ectopic Cushing's syndrome. Pituitary 2003;6:119-126.
51. Coll AP, Farooqi IS, Challis BG, et al. Proopiomelanocortin and energy balance: insights from human and murine genetics. J Clin Endocrinol Metab 2004;89:2557-2562.
52. Lundblad JR, Roberts JL. Regulation of proopiomelanocortin gene expression in pituitary. Endocr Rev 1988;9:135-158.
53. Orth DN. Corticotropin-releasing hormone in humans. Endocr Rev 1992;13:164-191.
54. Taylor AL, Fishman LM. Corticotropin-releasing hormone. N Engl J Med 1988;319:213-222.
55. Antoni FA. Hypothalamic control of adrenocorticotropin secretion: advances since the discovery of 41-residue corticotropin-releasing factor. Endocr Rev 1986;7:351-378.
56. Shibahara S, Morimoto Y, Furutani Y, et al. Isolation and sequence analysis of the human corticotropin-releasing factor precursor gene. EMBO J 1983;2:775-779.
57. Furutani Y, Morimoto Y, Shibahara S, et al. Cloning and sequence analysis of cDNA for ovine corticotropin releasing factor precursor. Nature 1983;301:537-540.
58. Chen R, Lewis KA, Perrin MH, et al. Expression cloning of a human corticotropin-releasing-factor receptor. Proc Natl Acad Sci U S A 1993;90:8967-8971.
59. Sasaki A, Sato S, Murakami O, et al. Immunoreactive corticotropin-releasing hormone present in human plasma may be derived from both hypothalamic and extrahypothalamic sources. J Clin Endocrinol Metab 1987;65:176-182.
60. Campbell EA, Linton EA, Wolfe CD, et al. Plasma corticotropin-releasing hormone concentrations during pregnancy and parturition. J Clin Endocrinol Metab 1987;64:1054-1059.
61. Linton EA, Wolfe CD, Behan DP, et al. A specific carrier substance for human corticotrophin releasing factor in late gestational maternal plasma which could mask the ACTH-releasing activity. Clin Endocrinol (Oxf) 1988;28:315-324.
62. Rivier C, Rivier J, Vale W. Inhibition of adrenocorticotropic hormone secretion in the rat by immunoneutralization of corticotropin-releasing factor. Science 1982;218:377-379.
63. Hauger RL, Aguilera G. Regulation of pituitary corticotropin releasing hormone (CRH) receptors by CRH: interaction with vasopressin. Endocrinology 1993;133:1708-1714.
64. Watanabe T, Oki Y, Orth DN. Kinetic actions and interactions of arginine vasopressin, angiotensin-II, and oxytocin on adrenocorticotropin secretion by rat anterior pituitary cells in the microperifusion system. Endocrinology 1989;125:1921-1931.
65. Bateman A, Singh A, Kral T, et al. The immune-hypothalamic-pituitary-adrenal axis. Endocr Rev 1989;10:92-112.
66. Chrousos GP. The hypothalamo-pituitary-adrenal axis and immune-mediated inflammation. N Engl J Med 1998;332: 1351-1362.
67. Ray DW, Ren SG, Melmed S. Leukemia inhibitory factor (LIF) stimulates proopiomelanocortin (POMC) gene expression in a corticotroph cell line. Role of STAT pathway. J Clin Invest 1996;97: 1852-1859.
68. Udelsman R, Norton JA, Jelenich SE, et al. Responses of the hypothalamic-pituitary-adrenal and renin-angiotensin axes and the sympathetic system during controlled surgical and anesthetic stress. J Clin Endocrinol Metab 1987;64:986-994.

69. Vaughan GM, Becker RA, Allen JP, et al. Cortisol and corticotropin in burned patients. J Trauma 1982;22:263-272.
70. Fish HR, Chernow B, O'Brian JT. Endocrine and neurophysiologic responses of the pituitary to insulin-induced hypoglycemia: a review. Metabolism 1986;35:763-780.
71. Luger A, Deuster PA, Kyle SB, et al. Acute hypothalamic-pituitary-adrenal responses to the stress of treadmill exercise: physiologic adaptations to physical training. N Engl J Med 1987;316: 1309-1315.
72. Aguilera G. Regulation of pituitary ACTH secretion during chronic stress. Front Neuroendocrinol 1994;15:321-350.
73. Weitzman ED, Fukushima DK, Nogeire C, et al. Twenty-four hour pattern of the episodic secretion of cortisol in normal subjects. J Clin Endocrinol Metab 1971;33:14-22.
74. Veldhuis JD, Iranmanesh A, Johnson ML, et al. Amplitude, but not frequency, modulation of adrenocorticotropin secretory bursts gives rise to the nyctohemeral rhythm of the corticotropic axis in man. J Clin Endocrinol Metab 1990;71:452-463.
75. Horrocks PM, Jones AF, Ratcliffe WA, et al. Patterns of ACTH and cortisol pulsatility over twenty four hours in normal males and females. Clin Endocrinol (Oxf) 1990;32:127-134.
76. Boivin DB, Duffy JF, Kronauer RE, et al. Dose-response relationships for resetting of human circadian clock by light. Nature 1996;379:540-542.
77. Czeisler CA, Dumont M, Duffy JF, et al. Association of sleep-wake habits in older people with changes in output of circadian pacemaker. Lancet 1992;340:933-936.
78. Desir D, Van Cauter E, Fang VS, et al. Effects of "jet lag" on hormonal patterns: I. Procedures, variations in total plasma proteins, and disruption of adrenocorticotropin-cortisol periodicity. J Clin Endocrinol Metab 1981;52:628-641.
79. Davis LG, Arentzen R, Reid JM, et al. Glucocorticoid sensitivity of vasopressin mRNA levels in the paraventricular nucleus of the rat. Proc Natl Acad Sci U S A 1986;83:1145-1149.
80. Keller-Wood ME, Dallman MF. Corticosteroid inhibition of ACTH secretion. Endocr Rev 1984;5:1-24.
81. Lamberts SWJ, Koper JW, Biemond P, et al. Cortisol receptor resistance: the variability of its clinical presentation and response to treatment. J Clin Endocr Metab 1992;74:313-321.
82. Cole TJ, Blendy JA, Monaghan AP, et al. Targeted disruption of the glucocorticoid receptor gene blocks adrenergic chromaffin cell development and severely retards lung maturation. Genes Dev 1995;9:1608-1621.
83. Mountjoy KG, Robbins LS, Mortrud MT, et al. The cloning of a family of genes that encode the melanocortin receptors. Science 1992;257:1248-1251.
84. Cooke BA. Signal transduction involving cyclic ANP-dependent and cyclic AMP-independent mechanisms in the control of steroidogenesis. Mol Cell Endocrinol 1999;151:25-35.
85. Enyeart JJ, Mlinar B, Enyeart JA. T-type $Ca^{2}+$ channels are required for adrenocorticotropin-stimulated cortisol production by bovine adrenal zona fasciculata cells. Mol Endocrinol 1993;7:1031-1040.
86. Ehrhart-Bornstein M, Hinson JP, Bornstein SR, et al. Intraadrenal interactions in the regulation of adrenocortical steroidogenesis. Endocr Rev 1998;19:101-143.
87. Munari-Silem Y, Lebrethon MC, Morand I, et al. Gap junction-mediated cell-to-cell communication in bovine and human adrenal cells: a process whereby cells increase their responsiveness to physiological corticotropin concentrations. J Clin Invest 1995;95:1429-1439.
88. Simpson ER, Waterman MR. Regulation of the synthesis of steroidogenic enzymes in adrenal cortical cells by ACTH. Annu Rev Physiol 1988;50:427-440.
89. Waterman MR, Biscoff LJ. Cytochromes P450 12: diversity of ACTH (cAMP)-dependent transcription of bovine steroid hydroxylase genes. FASEB J 1997;11:419-427.
90. Rainey WE. Adrenal zonation: clues from 11beta-hydroxylase and aldosterone synthase. Mol Cell Endocrinol 1999:151:151-160.
91. Longcope C. Adrenal and gonadal secretion in normal females. Clin Endocrinol Metab 1986;15:213-228.
92. Labrie F, Belanger A, Simard J, et al. DHEA and peripheral androgen and oestrogen formation: intracrinology. Ann N Y Acad Sci 1995;774:16-28.
93. Hammer F, Subtil S, Lux P, et al. No evidence for hepatic conversion of dehydroepiandrosterone (DHEA) sulfate to DHEA: in vivo and in vitro studies. J Clin Endocrinol Metab 2005;90:3600-3605.
94. McKenna TJ, Fearon U, Clarke D, et al. A critical review of the origin and control of adrenal androgens. Balliere Clin Obstet Gynaecol 1997;11:229-248.
95. Weinberger C, Hollenberg SM, Rosenfeld MG, et al. Domain structure of the human glucocorticoid receptor and its relationship to the v-erb-A oncogene product. Nature 1985;318:670-672.
96. Arriza JL, Weinberger C, Cerelli G, et al. Cloning of human mineralocorticoid receptor complementary DNA: structural and functional kinship with the glucocorticoid receptor. Science 1987;237: 268-275.
97. Gustafsson J-AD, Carlstedt-Duke J, Poellinger L, et al. Biochemistry, molecular biology, and physiology of the glucocorticoid receptor. Endocr Rev 1987;70:185-234.
98. Zhou J, Cidlowski JA. The human glucocorticoid receptor: one gene, multiple proteins and diverse responses. Steroids 2005;5-7: 407-417.
99. Pascual-Le Tallec L, Lombes M. The mineralocorticoid receptor: a journey exploring its diversity and specificity of action. Mol Endocrinol 2005;9:2211-2221.
100. Pratt WB. The role of heat shock protein in regulating the function, folding and trafficking of the glucocorticoid receptor. J Biol Chem 1993;268:21455-21458.
101. Beato M, Sanchez-Pacheco A. Interaction of steroid hormone receptors with the transcription initiation complex. Endocr Rev 1996;17:587-609.
102. Bamberger CM, Schulte HM, Chrousos GP. Molecular determinants of glucocorticoid receptor function and tissue sensitivity to glucocorticoids. Endocr Rev 1996;17:245-261.
103. McKenna NJ, Lanz RB, O'Malley BW. Nuclear receptor coregulators: cellular and molecular biology. Endocr Rev 1999;20: 321-344.
104. Schule R, Rangarajan P, Kliewer S, et al. Functional antagonism between oncoprotein c-Jun and the glucocorticoid receptor. Cell 1990;62:1217-1226.
105. McKay LI, Cidlowski JA. Molecular control of immune/inflammatory responses: interactions between nuclear factor-kB and steroid receptor-signalling pathways. Endocr Rev 1999;20:435-459.
106. Funder JW. Aldosterone action. Annu Rev Physiol 1993;55: 115-130.
107. Rossier BC, Alpern RJ. Cell and molecular biology of epithelial transport. Curr Opin Nephrol Hypertens 1999;8:579-580.
108. Verrey F, Kraehenbuhl JP, Rossier BC. Aldosterone induces a rapid increase in the rate of Na,K-ATPase gene transcription in cultured kidney cells. Mol Endocrinol 1989;3:1369-1376.
109. Chen SY, Bhargava A, Mastroberardino L, et al. Epithelial sodium channel regulated by aldosterone-induced protein sgk. Proc Natl Acad Sci U S A 1999;93:6025-6030.
110. Edwards CRW, Stewart PM, Burt D, et al. Localisation of 11β-hydroxysteroid dehydrogenase—tissue specific protector of the mineralocorticoid receptor. Lancet 1988;ii:836-841.
111. Funder JW, Pearce PT, Smith R, et al. Mineralocorticoid action: target tissue specificity is enzyme, not receptor, mediated. Science 1988;242:583-585.
112. Funder JW. New biology of aldosterone, and experimental studies of the selective aldosterone blocker eplerenone. Am Heart J 2002;144:S8-S11.
113. Iwasaki Y, Aoki Y, Katahira M, et al. Non-genomic mechanisms of glucocorticoid inhibition of adrenocorticotropin secretion: possible involvement of GTP-binding protein. Biochem Biophys Res Commun 1997;235:295-299.
114. Funder JW. The nongenomic actions of aldosterone. Endocr Rev 2005;3:313-321.
115. Hammond GL. Molecular properties of corticosteroid binding globulin and the sex-steroid binding proteins. Endocr Rev 1990;11:65-79
116. Roitman A, Bruchis S, Bauman B, et al. Total deficiency of corticosteroid binding globulin. Clin Endocrinol (Oxf) 1984;21: 541-548.
117. Smith CL, Power SG, Hammond GL. A Leu-His substitution at residue 93 in human corticosteroid binding globulin results in reduced affinity for cortisol. J Steroid Biochem Mol Biol 1992;42: 671-676.

118. Fukushima DK, Bradlow HL, Hellman L, et al. Metabolic transformation of hydrocortisone ^{14}C in man. J Biol Chem 1960;235: 2246-2252.
119. White PC, Mune T, Agarwal AK. 11β-hydroxysteroid dehydrogenase and the syndrome of apparent mineralocorticoid excess. Endocr Rev 1997;18:135-136.
120. Tomlinson JW, Walker EA, Bujalska IJ, et al. 11beta-hydroxysteroid dehydrogenase type 1: a tissue-specific regulator of glucocorticoid response. Endocr Rev 2004;25:831-866.
121. Quinkler M, Stewart PM. Hypertension and the cortisol-cortisone shuttle. J Clin Endocrinol Metab 2003;88:2384-2392.
122. Moore JS, Monson JP, Kaltsas G, et al. Modulation of 11β-hydroxysteroid dehydrogenase isozymes by growth hormone and insulin-like growth factor: in vivo and in vitro studies. J Clin Endocr Metab 1999;84:4172-4177.
123. Voccia E, Saenger P, Peterson RE, et al. 6β-hydroxycortisol excretion in hypercortisolemic states. J Clin Endocrinol Metab 1979; 48:467-471.
124. Yamada S, Iwai K. Induction of hepatic cortisol-6-hydroxylase by rifampicin. Lancet 1976;2:366-367.
125. Whitworth JA, Stewart PM, Burt D, et al. The kidney is the major site of cortisone production in man. Clin Endocrinol (Oxf) 1989;31: 355-361.
126. Kyriazopoulou V, Parparousi O, Vagenakis AG. Rifampicin-induced adrenal crisis in Addisonian patients receiving corticosteroid replacement therapy. J Clin Endocrinol Metab 1984;59:1204-1206.
127. Morris DJ, Brem AS. Metabolic derivatives of aldosterone. Am J Physiol 1987;252:F365-F373.
128. Edwards C, Hayman A. Enzyme protection of the mineralocorticoid receptor: evidence in favour of the hemi-acetal structure of aldosterone. In Bonvalet JP, Farman N, Lombes M, et al, eds. Aldosterone Fundamental Aspects. Colloque INSERM/John Libbey Eurotext Ltd London, 1991;215:67-76.
129. Stalmans W, Laloux M. Glucocorticoids and hepatic glycogen metabolism. In Baxter JD, Rousseau GG, eds. Glucocorticoid Hormone Action. New York: Springer-Verlag, 1979:518-533.
130. Watts LM, Manchem VP, Leedom TA, et al. Reduction of hepatic and adipose tissue glucocorticoid receptor expression with antisense oligonucleotides improves hyperglycemia and hyperlipidemia in diabetic rodents without causing systemic glucocorticoid antagonism. Diabetes 2005;54:1846-1853.
131. Chakravarty K, Cassuto H, Reshef L, et al. Factors that control the tissue-specific transcription of the gene for phosphoenolpyruvate carboxykinase-C. Crit Rev Biochem Mol Biol 2005;40:129-154.
132. Olefsky JM. Effect of dexamethasone on insulin binding, glucose transport, and glucose oxidation of isolated rat adipocytes. J Clin Invest 1975;56:1499-1508.
133. Hauner H, Entenmann G, Wabitisch M, et al. Promoting effects of glucocorticoids on the differentiation of human adipocyte precursor cells cultured in a chemically defined medium. J Clin Invest 1989;84:1663-1670.
134. Rebuffe-Scrive M, Krotkiewski M, Elfverson J, et al. Muscle and adipose morphology and metabolism in Cushing's syndrome. J Clin Endocr Metab 1988;67:1122-1128.
135. Bronnegard M, Arner P, Hellstrom L, et al. Glucocorticoid receptor messenger ribonucleic acid in different regions of human adipose tissue. Endocrinology 1990;127:1689-1696.
136. Bujalska IJ, Kumar S, Stewart PM. Does central obesity reflect "Cushing's disease of the omentum?" Lancet 1997;349:1210-1213.
137. Leibovich SJ, Ross R. The role of the macrophage in wound repair: a study with hydrocortisone and antimacrophage serum. Am J Pathol 1975;78:71-100.
138. Canalis E. Clinical review 83: mechanisms of glucocorticoid action in bone: implications to glucocorticoid-induced osteoporosis. J Clin Endocrinol Metab 1996;81:3441-3447.
139. Van Staa TP, Leufkens HGM, Abenhaim L, et al. Use of oral corticosteroids in the United Kingdom. Q J Med 2000;93:105-111.
140. Williams PL, Corbett M. A vascular necrosis of bone complicating corticosteroid replacement therapy. Ann Rheum Dis 1983;42(3): 276-279.
141. Weinstein RS, Nicholas RW, Manolagas SC. Apoptosis of osteocytes in glucocorticoid-induced osteonecrosis of the hip. J Clin Endocrinol Metab 2000;85(8):2907-2912.
142. Leonard MB, Feldman HI, Shults J, et al. Long-term, high-dose glucocorticoids and bone mineral content in childhood glucocorticoid-sensitive nephrotic syndrome. N Engl J Med 2004;351: 868-875.
143. Fraser R, Davies DL, Connell JMC. Hormones and hypertension. Clin Endocrinol (Oxf) 1989;31:701-746.
144. Saruta T, Suzuki H, Handa M, et al. Multiple factors contribute to the pathogenesis of hypertension in Cushing's syndrome. J Clin Endocrinol Metab 1986;62:275-279.
145. Marver D. Evidence of corticosteroid action along the nephron. Am J Physiol 1984;246:F111-F123.
146. Raff H. Glucocorticoid inhibition of neurohypophysial vasopressin secretion. Am J Physiol 1987; 252:R635-R644.
147. Peers SH, Flowers RJ. The role of lipocortin in corticosteroid actions. Am Rev Respir Dis 1990;141:S18-S21.
148. McEwen BS, deKloet ER, Rostene W. Adrenal steroid receptors and action in the central nervous system. Physiol Rev 1986;66: 1121-1188.
149. Salpolsky RM, Krey LC, McEwen BS. Prolonged glucocorticoid exposure reduces hippocampal neuron number: implications for aging. J Neurosci 1985;5:1222-1227.
150. Lupien SJ, de Leon M, de Santi S, et al. Cortisol levels during human aging predict hippocampal atrophy and memory deficits. Nat Neurosci 1998;1:69-73.
151. Sandeep TC, Yau JL, MacLullich AM, et al. 11β-hydroxysteroid dehydrogenase inhibition improves cognitive function in healthy elderly men and type 2 diabetics. Proc Natl Acad Sci U S A 2004; 101:6329-6330.
152. Hajszan T, MacLusky NJ, Leranth C. Dehydroepiandrosterone increases hippocampal spine synapse density in ovariectomised female rats. Endocrinology 2004;145:1039-1041.
153. Yau JL, Rasumuson S, Andrew R, et al. Dehydroepiandrosterone 7-hydrozylase CYP7B: predominant expression in primate hippocampus and reduced expression in Alzheimer's disease. Neuroscience 2003;121:307-314.
154. Clark AF. Steroids, ocular hypertension, and glaucoma. J Glaucoma 1995;4:354-369.
155. Messer J, Reitman D, Sacks HS, et al. Association of adrenocorticosteroid therapy and peptic-ulcer disease. N Engl J Med 1983;309: 21-24.
156. Strickland AL, Underwood LE, Voina SJ. Growth retardation in Cushing's syndrome. Am J Dis Child 1972;123:207-213.
157. Ballard PL, Ertsey R, Gonzales LW, et al. Transcriptional regulation of human pulmonary surfactant proteins SP-B and SP-C by glucocorticoids. Am J Respir Cell Mol Biol 1996;14:599-607.
158. Dluhy RG, Newmark SR, Lauler DP, et al. Pharmacology and chemistry of adrenal glucocorticoids. In Azarnoff DL, ed. Steroid Therapy. Philadelphia: WB Saunders, 1975:1-14.
159. Meikle AW, Weed JA, Tyler FH. Kinetics and interconversion of prednisolone and prednisone studied with new radioimmunoassays. J Clin Endocrinol Metab 1975;41:717-721.
160. Axelrod L. Glucocorticoid therapy. Medicine (Baltimore) 1976; 55:39-65.
161. Schacke H, Schottelius A, Docke WD, et al. Dissociation of transactivation from transrepression by a selective glucocorticoid receptor agonist leads to separation of therapeutic effects from side effects. Proc Natl Acad Sci U S A 2004;101: 227-232.
162. Loprinzi CL, Jensen MD, Jiang N-S, et al. Effect of megestrol acetate on the human pituitary-adrenal axis. Mayo Clin Proc 1992;67: 1160-1162.
163. Christy NP. Corticosteroid withdrawal. In Bardin CW, ed. Current Therapy in Endocrinology and Metabolism, 3rd ed. New York: BC Decker, 1988:113-120.
164. Kane K, Emery P, Sheppard MC, et al. The insulin tolerance test versus the short synacthen test in assessing the hypothalamo-pituitary-adrenal axis in patients on long-term glucocorticoid therapy. Q J Med 1995;88:263-267.
165. Dixon RB, Christy NP. On the various forms of the corticosteroid withdrawal syndrome. Am J Med 1980;68:224-230.
166. Hopkins RL, Leinung MC. Exogenous Cushing's syndrome and glucocorticoid withdrawal. Endocrinol Metab Clin North Am 2005;34:371-384.
167. Walters W, Wilder RM, Kepler EJ. The suprarenal cortical syndrome with presentation of ten cases. Ann Surg 1934;100:670-688.
168. Meador CK, Liddle GW, Island DP, et al. Cause of Cushing's syndrome in patients with tumors arising from "nonendocrine" tissue. J Clin Endocrinol Metab 1962;22:693-703.

169. Ross EJ, Linch DC. Cushing's syndrome-killing disease: discriminatory value of signs and symptoms aiding early diagnosis. Lancet 1982;2:646-649.
170. Wajchenberg BL, Bosco A, Marone MM, et al. Estimation of body fat and lean tissue distribution by dual energy X-ray absorptiometry and abdominal body fat evaluation by computed tomography in Cushing's disease. J Clin Endocrinol Metab 1995;80:2791-2794.
171. Luton PJ, Thiebolt P, Valcke JC, et al. Reversible gonadotropin deficiency in male Cushing's disease. J Clin Endocrinol Metab 1977;45:488-495.
172. Lado Abeal J, Rodriguez Arnao J, Newell Price JD, et al. Menstrual abnormalities in women with Cushing's disease are correlated with hypercortisolemia rather than raised circulating androgen levels. J Clin Endocrinol Metab 1998;83:3083-3088.
173. Jeffcoate WJ, Silverstone JT, Edwards CRW, et al. Psychiatric manifestations of Cushing's syndrome: response to lowering of plasma cortisol. Q J Med 1979;48:465-472.
174. Dorn LD, Burgess ES, Dubbert B, et al. Psychopathology in patients with endogenous Cushing's syndrome: "atypical" or melancholic features. Clin Endocrinol (Oxf) 1995;43:433-442.
175. Friess E, Wiedemann K, Steiger A, et al. The hypothalamic-pituitary-adrenocortical system and sleep in man. Adv Neuroimmunol 1995;5:111-125.
176. Ferguson JK, Donald RA, Weston TS, et al. Skin thickness in patients with acromegaly and Cushing's syndrome and response to treatment. Clin Endocrinol (Oxf) 1983;18:347-353.
177. Pleasure DE, Engel WK. Atrophy of skeletal muscle in patients with Cushing's syndrome. Arch Neurol 1970;22:118-125.
178. Plotz CM, Knowlton AI, Ragan C. The natural history of Cushing's syndrome. Am J Med 1952;13:597-614.
179. Etxabe J, Vazquez JA. Morbidity and mortality in Cushing's disease: an epidemiological approach. Clin Endocrinol 1994;40:479-484
180. Colao A, Pivonello R, Spiezia S, et al. Persistence of increased cardiovascular risk factors in patients with Cushing's disease after five years of successful cure. J Clin Endocrinol Metab 1999; 84:2664-2672.
181. Wei L, MacDonald TM, Walker BR. Taking glucocorticoids by prescription is associated with subsequent cardiovascular disease. Ann Intern Med 2004;141:764-770.
182. Dale DC, Petersdorf RG. Corticosteroids and infectious diseases. Med Clin North Am 1973;57:1277-1287.
183. Graham BS, Tucker WS Jr. Opportunistic infections in endogenous Cushing's syndrome. Ann Intern Med 1984;101:334-338.
184. Hill AT, Stewart PM, Hughes EA, et al. Cushing's disease and tuberculosis. Respir Med 1998;92:604-605.
185. Taskinen MR, Nikkila EA, Pelkonen R, et al. Plasma lipoproteins, lipolytic enzymes, and very low density lipoprotein triglyceride turnover in Cushing's syndrome. J Clin Endocrinol Metab 1983; 57:619-626.
186. Stewart PM, Walker BR, Holder G, et al. 11β-hydroxysteroid dehydrogenase activity in Cushing's syndrome: explaining the mineralocorticoid excess state of the ectopic ACTH syndrome. J Clin Endocr Metab 1995;80:3617-3620.
187. Benker G, Raida M, Olbricht T, et al. TSH secretion in Cushing's syndrome: relation to glucocorticoid excess, diabetes, goiter and the "sick euthyroid syndrome." Clin Endocrinol 1990;33:777-786.
188. Saketos M, Sharma N, Santoro NF. Suppression of the hypothalamo-pituitary-ovarian axis in normal women by glucocorticoids. Biol Reprod 1993;49:1270-1276.
189. Sayegh F, Weigelin E. Intraocular pressure in Cushing's syndrome. Ophthalmic Res 1975;7:390-394.
190. Kelly W. Exophthalmos in Cushing's syndrome. Clin Endocrinol (Oxf) 1996;45:167-170.
191. Bouzas EA, Mastorakos G, Friedman G, et al. Posterior subcapsular cataract in endogenous Cushing syndrome: an uncommon manifestation. Invest Ophth Vis Sci 1993;34:3497-3500.
192. Biller BMK. Pathogenesis of pituitary Cushing's syndrome: pituitary versus hypothalamic. Endocrinol Metab Clin North Am 1994;23:547-554.
193. Gicquel C, Le Bouc Y, Luton J-P, et al. Monoclonality of corticotroph macroadenomas in Cushing's disease. J Clin Endocrinol Metab 1992;75:472-475.
194. Biller BMK, Alexander JM, Zervas NT, et al. Clonal origins of adrenocorticotropin-secreting pituitary tissue in Cushing's disease. J Clin Endocrinol Metab 1992;75:1303-1309.
195. Woo YS, Isidori AM, Wat WZ, et al. Clinical and biochemical characteristics of adrenocorticotropin-secreting macroadenomas. J Clin Endocrinol Metab 2005;90:4963-4969.
196. Liddle GW. Tests of pituitary-adrenal suppressibility in the diagnosis of Cushing's syndrome. J Clin Endocrinol Metab 1960;20: 1539-1560.
197. Stewart PM, Penn R, Gibson R, et al. Hypothalamic abnormalities in patients with pituitary-dependent Cushing's syndrome. Clin Endocrinol (Oxf) 1992;36:453-458.
198. Jex RK, van Heerden JA, Carpenter PC, et al. Ectopic ACTH syndrome, diagnostic and therapeutic aspects. Am J Surg 1985;149: 276-282.
199. Howlett TA, Drury PL, Perry L, et al. Diagnosis and management of ACTH-dependent Cushing's syndrome: comparison of the features in ectopic and pituitary ACTH production. Clin Endocrinol (Oxf) 1986;24:699-713.
200. Findling JW, Tyrrell JB. Occult ectopic secretion of corticotropin. Arch Intern Med 1986;146:929-933.
201. Ilias I, Torpy DJ, Pacak K. Cushing's syndrome due to ectopic corticotropin secretion: twenty years' experience at the National Institutes of Health. J Clin Endocrinol Metab 2005;90:4955-4962.
202. Wajchenberg BL, Mendonca B, Liberman B. Ectopic ACTH syndrome. J Steroid Biochem Mol Biol 1995;53:139-151.
203. Limper AH, Carpenter PC, Scheithauer B, et al. The Cushing syndrome induced by bronchial carcinoid tumours. Ann Intern Med 1992;117:209-214.
204. Odell WD. Ectopic ACTH secretion: a misnomer. Endocrinol Metab Clin North Am 1991;20:371-379.
205. Dichek HL, Nieman LK, Oldfield EH, et al. A comparison of the standard high dose dexamethasone suppression test for the differential diagnosis of adrenocorticotropin dependent Cushing's syndrome. J Clin Endocrinol Metab 1994;78:418-422.
206. Ray DW, Littlewood AC, Clark AJL, et al. Human small cell lung cancer cell lines expressing the proopiomelanocortin gene have aberrant glucocorticoid receptor function. J Clin Invest 1994; 93:1625-1630.
207. Carey RM, Varma SK, Drake CR Jr, et al. Ectopic secretion of corticotropin-releasing factor as a cause of Cushing's syndrome: a clinical, morphologic, and biochemical study. N Engl J Med 1984;311:13-20.
208. Mhller OA, Von Werder K. Ectopic production of ACTH and corticotropin-releasing hormone (CRH). J Steroid Biochem Mol Biol 1992;43:403-408.
209. Preeyasombat C, Sirikulchayanonta V, Mahachokelertwattana P, et al. Cushing's syndrome caused by Ewing's sarcoma secreting corticotropin releasing factor-like peptide. Am J Dis Child 1992; 146:1103-1105.
210. Aron DC, Findling JW, Fitzgerald PA, et al. Pituitary ACTH dependency of nodular adrenal hyperplasia in Cushing's syndrome: report of two cases and review of the literature. Am J Med 1981;71:302-306.
211. Doppman JL, Nieman LK, Travis WD, et al. CT and MR imaging of massive macronodular adrenocortical disease: a rare cause of autonomous primary adrenal hypercortisolism. J Comput Assist Tomogr 1991;15:773-779.
212. Samuels MH, Loriaux DL. Cushing's syndrome and the nodular adrenal gland. Endocrinol Metab Clin North Am 1994;23: 555-569.
213. Sturrock ND, Morgan L, Jeffcoate WJ. Autonomous nodular hyperplasia of the adrenal cortex: tertiary hypercortisolism? Clin Endocrinol (Oxf) 1995;43:753-758.
214. Hermus AR, Pieters GF, Smals AG, et al. Transition from pituitary-dependent to adrenal-dependent Cushing's syndrome. N Engl J Med 1988;318:966-970.
215. Luton J-P, Cerdas S, Billaud L, et al. Clinical features of adrenocortical carcinoma, prognostic factors, and the effect of mitotane therapy. N Engl J Med 1990;322:1195-1201.
216. Kasperlik-Zaluska AA, Migdalska BM, Zgliczynski S, et al. Adrenocortical carcinoma: a clinical study and treatment results of 52 patients. Cancer 1995;75:2587-2591.
217. Young WF Jr, Carney JA, Musa BU, et al. Familial Cushing's syndrome due to primary pigmented nodular adrenocortical disease: reinvestigation 50 years later. N Engl J Med 1989;321:1659-1664.
218. Stratakis CA, Kirschner LS, Carney JA. Clinical and molecular features of the Carney complex: diagnostic criteria and recommenda-

tions for patient evaluation. J Clin Endocrinol Metab 2001;86: 4041-4046.
219. Kirschner LS, Carney JA, Pack SD, et al. Mutations of the gene encoding the protein kinase A type I-alpha regulatory subunit in patients with the Carney complex. Nat Genet 2000;26:89-92.
220. Kirk JM, Brain CE, Carson DJ, et al. Cushing's syndrome caused by nodular adrenal hyperplasia in children with McCune-Albright syndrome. J Pediatr 1999;134:789-792.
221. Malchoff CD, MacGillivray D, Malchoff DM. Adrenocorticotropic hormone-independent adrenal hyperplasia. Endocrinologist 1996; 6:79-85.
222. Christopoulos S, Bourdeau I, Lacroix A. Aberrant expression of hormone receptors in adrenal Cushing's syndrome. Pituitary 2004;7:225-235.
223. Atkinson AB, Kennedy AL, Carson DJ, et al. Five cases of cyclical Cushing's syndrome. Br Med J 1985;291:1453-1457.
224. Mantero F, Scaroni CM, Albiger NM. Cycle Cushing's syndrome: an overview. Pituitary 2004;7:203-207.
225. Leinung MC, Zimmerman D. Cushing's disease in children. Endocr Metab Clin North Am 1994;23:629-639.
226. Lindsay JR, Jonklaas J, Oldfield EH, et al. Cushing's syndrome during pregnancy: personal experience and review of the literature. J Clin Endocrinol Metab 2005;90:3077-3083.
227. Wallace C, Toth EL, Lewanczuk RZ, et al. Pregnancy-induced Cushing's syndrome in multiple pregnancies. J Clin Endo Metab 1996;81:15-21.
228. Kirkman S, Nelson DH. Alcohol-induced pseudo-Cushing's disease: a study of prevalence with review of the literature. Metabolism 1988;37:390-394.
229. Stewart PM, Burra P, Shackleton CHL, et al. 11β-hydroxysteroid dehydrogenase deficiency and glucocorticoid status in patients with alcoholic and non-alcoholic chronic liver disease. J Clin Endocrin Metab 1993;76:748-751.
230. Newell-Price J, Trainer P, Besser M, et al. The diagnosis and differential diagnosis of Cushing's syndrome and pseudo-Cushing's states. Endocr Rev 1998;19:647-672.
231. Glass AR, Burman KD, Dahms WT, et al. Endocrine function in human obesity. Metabolism 1981;30:89-104.
232. Stewart PM, Boulton A, Kumar S, et al. Cortisol metabolism in human obesity: impaired cortisone–cortisol conversion in subjects with central obesity. J Clin Endocrinol Metab 1999;84: 1022-1027.
233. Arnaldi G, Angeli A, Atkinson AB, et al. Diagnosis and complications of Cushing's syndrome: a consensus statement. J Clin Endocrinol Metab 2003;88:5593-5602.
234. Findling JW, Raff H. Screening and diagnosis of Cushing's syndrome. Endocrinol Metab Clin North Am 2005;34:385-402.
235. Newell-Price J, Trainer P, Perry L, et al. A single sleeping midnight cortisol has 100% sensitivity for the diagnosis of Cushing's syndrome. Clin Endocrinol (Oxf) 1995;43:545-550.
236. Hamrahian AH, Oseni TS, Arafah BM. Measurements of serum free cortisol in critically ill patients. N Engl J Med 2004;350: 1629-1638.
237. Raff H, Raff JL, Findling JW. Late-night salivary cortisol as a screening test for Cushing's syndrome. J Clin Endocrinol Metab 1998; 83:2681-2686.
238. Yaneva M, Mosnier-Pudar H, Dugue M, et al. Midnight salivary cortisol for the initial diagnosis of Cushing's syndrome of various causes. J Clin Endocrinol Metab 2003;89:3345-3351.
239. Invitti C, Giraldi FP, Martin M, et al. Diagnosis and management of Cushing's syndrome: results of an Italian multicentre study. J Clin Endocrinol Metab 1999;84:440-448.
240. Corcuff JB, Tabarin A, Rashedi M, et al. Overnight urinary free cortisol determination: a screening test for the diagnosis of Cushing's syndrome. Clin Endocrinol (Oxf) 1998;48(4):503-508.
241. Cronin C, Igoe D, Duffy MJ, et al. The overnight dexamethasone test is a worthwhile screening procedure. Clin Endocrinol (Oxf) 1990;33:27-33.
242. Isidori AM, Kaltas GA, Mohammed S, et al. Discriminatory value of the low-dose dexamethasone suppression test in establishing the diagnosis and differential diagnosis of Cushing's syndrome. J Clin Endocrinol Metab 2003;88:5299-5306.
243. Meikle AW. Dexamethasone suppression tests: usefulness of simultaneous measurement of plasma cortisol and dexamethasone. Clin Endocrinol (Oxf) 1982;16:401-408.
244. Yanovski JA, Cutler GB Jr, Chrousos GP, et al. Corticotropin-releasing hormone stimulation following low-dose dexamethasone administration: a new test to distinguish Cushing's syndrome from pseudo-Cushing's states. JAMA 1993;269:2232-2238.
245. Findling JW. Clinical application of a new immunoradiometric assay for ACTH. Endocrinologist 1992;2:360-365
246. Tyrrell JB, Findling JW, Aron DC, et al. An overnight high-dose dexamethasone suppression test for rapid differential diagnosis of Cushing's syndrome. Ann Intern Med 1986;104:180-186.
247. Biemond P, de Jong FH, Lamberts SWJ. Continuous dexamethasone infusion for seven hours in patients with the Cushing syndrome: a superior differential diagnostic test. Ann Intern Med 1990;112:738-742.
248. Findling JW, Doppman JL. Biochemical and radiological diagnosis of Cushing's syndrome. Endocr Metab Clin North Am 1994;23: 511-537.
249. Avgerinos PC, Yanovski JA, Oldfield EH, et al. The metyrapone and dexamethasone suppression tests for the differential diagnosis of the adrenocorticotropin-dependent Cushing syndrome: a comparison. Ann Intern Med 1994;121:318-327.
250. Trainer PJ, Faria M, Newell-Price J, et al. A comparison of the effects of human and ovine corticotropin-releasing hormone on the pituitary-adrenal axis. J Clin Endocr Metab 1995;80: 412-417.
251. Chrousos GP, Schulte HM, Oldfield EH, et al. The corticotropin-releasing factor stimulation test: an aid in the evaluation of patients with Cushing's syndrome. N Engl J Med 1984;310:622-626.
252. Nieman LK, Oldfield EH, Wesley R, et al. A simplified morning ovine corticotropin-releasing hormone stimulation test for the differential diagnosis of adrenocorticotropin-dependent Cushing's syndrome. J Clin Endocrinol Metab 1993;77:1308-1312.
253. Lindsay JR, Nieman LK. Differential diagnosis and imaging in Cushing's syndrome. Endocrinol Metab Clin North Am 2005;34: 403-421.
254. Oldfield EH, Doppman LJ, Nieman LK, et al. Petrosal sinus sampling with and without corticotropin releasing hormone for the differential diagnosis of Cushing's syndrome. N Engl J Med 1991;325:897-905.
255. Kaltsas GA, Giannulis MG, Newell Price JD, et al. A critical analysis of the value of simultaneous inferior petrosal sinus sampling in Cushing's disease and the occult ectopic adrenocorticotropin syndrome. J Clin Endocr Metab 1999;84:487-492.
256. Hall WA, Luciano MG, Doppman JL, et al. Pituitary magnetic resonance imaging in normal human volunteers: occult adenomas in the general population. Ann Intern Med 1994;120:817-820.
257. Korobkin M, Francis IR. Adrenal imaging. Semin Ultrasound CT MR 1995;16:317-330.
258. Miles JM, Wahner HW, Carpenter PC, et al. Adrenal scintiscanning with NP-59, a new radioiodinated cholesterol agent. Mayo Clin Proc 1979;54:321-327.
259. de Herder WW, Krenning EP, Malchoff CD, et al. Somatostatin receptor scintigraphy: its value in tumor localization in patients with Cushing's syndrome caused by ectopic corticotropin or corticotropin-releasing hormone secretion. Am J Med 1994;96: 305-312.
260. Valimaki M, Pelkonen R, Porkka L, et al. Long-term results of adrenal surgery in patients with Cushing's syndrome due to adrenocortical adenoma. Clin Endocrinol (Oxf) 1984;20:229-236.
261. Young WF Jr, Thompson GB. Laparoscopic adrenalectomy for patients who have Cushing's syndrome. Endocrinol Metab Clin North Am 2005;34:489-499.
262. Allolio B, Hahner S, Weismann D, et al. Management of adrenocortical carcinoma. Clin Endocrinol (Oxf) 2004;60:273-287.
263. Assie G, Bahurel H, Coste J, et al. Corticotroph tumor progression after adrenalectomy in Cushing's Disease: A reappraisal of Nelson's Syndrome. J Clin Endo Met 2007;92(1):172-179.
264. Jenkins PJ, Trainer PJ, Plowman PN, et al. The long term outcome after adrenalectomy and prophylactic pituitary radiotherapy in adrenocorticotropin-dependent Cushing's syndrome. J Clin Endocrinol Metab 1995; 80:165-171.
265. Burch W. A survey of results with transsphenoidal surgery in Cushing's disease. N Engl J Med 1983;308:103-104.
266. Utz AL, Swearingen B, Biller BM. Pituitary surgery and postoperative management in Cushing's disease. Endocrinol Metab Clin North Am 2005;34:459-478.

267. Trainer PJ, Lawrie HS, Verhelst J, et al. Transsphenoidal resection in Cushing's disease: undetectable serum cortisol as the definition of successful treatment. Clin Endocrinol (Oxf) 1993;38:73-78.
268. McCance DR, Besser M, Atkinson AB. Assessment of cure after transsphenoidal surgery for Cushing's disease. Clin Endocrinol 1996;44:1-6.
269. Leinung MC, Kane LA, Scheithauer BW, et al. Long term follow-up of transsphenoidal surgery for the treatment of Cushing's disease in childhood. J Clin Endocrinol Metab 1995;80: 2475-2479.
270. Joshi SM, Hewitt RJ, Storr HL, et al. Cushing's disease in children and adolescents: 20 years of experience in a single neurosurgical center. Neurosurgery 2005;57:281-285.
271. Storr HL, Plowman PN, Carroll PV, et al. Clinical and endocrine responses to pituitary radiotherapy in paediatric Cushing's disease: an effective second-line treatment. J Clin Endocrinol Metab 2003;88:34-37.
272. Verhelst JA, Trainer PJ, Howlett TA, et al. Short and long-term responses to metyrapone in the medical management of 91 patients with Cushing's syndrome. Clin Endocrinol (Oxf) 1991;35: 169-178.
273. Child DF, Burke CW, Burley DM, et al. Drug control of Cushing's syndrome: combined aminoglutethimide and metyrapone therapy. Acta Endocrinol 1976;82:330-341.
274. Semple CG, Beastall GH, Gray CE, et al. Trilostane in the management of Cushing's syndrome. Acta Endocrinol 1983;102:107-110.
275. McCance DR, Hadden DR, Kennedy L, et al. Clinical experience with ketoconazole as a therapy for patients with Cushing's syndrome. Clin Endocrinol (Oxf) 1987;27:593-599.
276. Heaney AP, Fernando M, Young WH, et al. Functional PPAR-gamma receptor is a novel therapeutic target for ACTH-screening pituitary adenomas. Nat Med 2002;8:1281-1287.
277. Ambrosi B, Dall'Asta C, Cannavo S, et al. Effects of chronic administration of PPAR-gamma ligand rosiglitazone in Cushing's disease. Eur J Endocrinol 2004;151:173-178.
278. Bhattacharyya A, Kaushal K, Tymms DJ, et al. Steroid withdrawal syndrome after successful treatment of Cushing's syndrome: a reminder. Eur J Endocrinol 2005;153:207-210.
279. Hermus AR, Smals AG, Swinkels LM, et al. Bone mineral density and bone turnover before and after surgical cure of Cushing's syndrome. J Clin Endocrinol Metab 1995;80:2859-2865.
280. Charmandari E, Kino T, Souvatzoglou E, et al. Natural glucocorticoid receptor mutants causing generalized glucocorticoid resistance: molecular genotype, genetic transmission, and clinical phenotype. J Clin Endocrinol Metab 2004;89:1939-1949.
281. Oelkers W. Adrenal insufficiency N Engl J Med 1996;335: 1206-1212.
282. Arlt W, Allolio B. Adrenal insufficiency. Lancet 2003;361: 1881-1893.
283. Carey RM. The changing clinical spectrum of adrenal insufficiency. Ann Intern Med 1997;127:1103-1105.
284. Betterle C, Dal Pra C, Mantero F, et al. Autoimmune adrenal insufficiency and autoimmune polyendocrine syndromes: autoantibodies, autoantigens, and their applicability in diagnosis and disease prediction. Endocr Rev 2002;23:327-364.
285. Piedrola G, Casado JL, Lopez E, et al. Clinical features of adrenal insufficiency in patients with acquired immunodeficiency syndrome. Clin Endocrinol 1996;45:97-101.
286. Freda PU, Bilezikian JP. The hypothalamus-pituitary-adrenal axis in HIV disease. AIDS Read 1999;9:46-47.
287. Norbiato G, Galli M, Righini V, et al. The syndrome of acquired glucocorticoid resistance in HIV infection. Baillieres Clin Endocrinol Metab 1994;8:777-787.
288. Seidenwurm DJ, Elmer EB, Kaplan LM, et al. Metastases to the adrenal glands and the development of Addison's disease. Cancer 1984;54:552-557.
289. Xarli VP, Steele AA, Davis PJ, et al. Adrenal hemorrhage in the adult. Medicine (Baltimore) 1978;57:211-221.
290. Lalli E, Sassone-Corsi P. DAX-1 and the adrenal cortex. Curr Opin Endocrinol Metab 1999;6:185-190.
291. Taberin A, Achermann JC, Recan D, et al. A novel mutation in DAX-1 causes delayed-onset adrenal insufficiency and incomplete hypogonadotrophic hypogonadism. J Clin Invest 2000;105: 321-328.
292. Achermann JC, Ito M, Hindmarsh PC, Jameson JL. A mutation in the gene encoding steroidogenic factor 1 causes YY sex reversal and adrenal failure. Nat Genet 1999;22:125-126.
293. Scheuerle A, Greenberg F, McCabe ER. Dysmorphic features in patients with complex glycerol kinase deficiency. J Pediatr 1995;126:764-767.
294. Moser HW, Moser AE, Singh I, et al. Adrenoleukodystrophy: survey of 303 cases. Biochemistry, diagnosis, and therapy. Ann Neurol 1984;16:628-641.
295. Laureti S, Casucci G, Santeusanio F, et al. X-linked adrenoleukodystrophy is a frequent cause of idiopathic Addison's disease in young adult male patients. J Clin Endocrinol Metab 1996;81: 470-474.
296. Mosser J, Douar A-M, Sarde C-O, et al. Putative X-linked adrenoleukodystrophy gene shares unexpected homology with ABC transporters. Nature 1993;361:726-730.
297. Kemp S, Pujol A, Waterham HR, et al. ABCD1 mutations and the X-linked adrenoleukodystrophy mutation database: role in diagnosis and clinical correlations. Hum Mutat 2001;18:499-515.
298. Moser HW, Raymond GV, Lu SE, et al. Follow-up of 89 asymptomatic patients with adrenoleukodystrophy treated with Lorenzo's oil. Arch Neurol 2005;62:1073-1080.
299. Huebner A, Elias LL, Clark AJL. ACTH resistance syndromes. J Paediatr Endocrinol Metab 1999;12:277-293.
300. Metherell LA, Chapple JP, Cooray S, et al. Mutations in MRAP, encoding a new interacting partner of the ACTH receptor, cause familial glucocorticoid deficiency type 2. Nat Genet 2005;37:166-170.
301. Brooks BP, Kleta R, Stuart C, et al. Genotype heterogeneity and clinical phenotype in triple A syndrome: a review of the NIH experience 2000-2005. Clin Genet 2005;68:215-221.
302. Pulichino AM, Vallette-Kasic S, Couture C et al. Mouse Tpit gene mutations cause early onset pituitary ACTH deficiency. Genes Dev 2003;17:677-682.
303. O'Rahilly S, Gray H, Humphreys PJ, et al. Brief report: impaired processing of prohormones associated with abnormalities of glucose homeostasis and adrenal function. N Engl J Med 1995;333:1386-1390.
304. Krude H, Biebermann H, Luck W, et al. Severe early-onset obesity, adrenal insufficiency and red hair pigmentation caused by POMC mutations in humans. Nat Genet 1998;19:155-157.
305. Yaswen L, Diehl N, Brennan MB, et al. Obesity in the mouse model of pro-opiomelanocortin deficiency responds to peripheral melanocortin. Nat Med 1999;5:1066-1070.
306. Cooper MS, Stewart PM. Corticosteroid insufficiency in acutely ill patients. N Engl J Med 2003;348:727-734.
307. Annane D, Sebille V, Troche G, et al. A 3-level prognostic classification in septic shock based on cortisol levels and cortisol response to corticotrophin. JAMA 2000;283:1038-1045.
308. Artavia-Loria E, Chaussain JL, BougnPres PF, et al. Frequency of hypoglycemia in children with adrenal insufficiency. Acta Endocrinol 1986;279:275-278.
309. Laczi F, Janaky T, Ivanyi T, et al. Osmoregulation of arginine-8-vasopressin secretion in primary hypothyroidism and in Addison's disease. Acta Endocrinol 1987;114:389-395.
310. Muls E, Bouillon R, Boelaert J, et al. Etiology of hypercalcemia in a patient with Addison's disease. Calcif Tissue Int 1982;34: 523-526.
311. Topliss DJ, White EL, Stockigt JR. Significance of thyrotropin excess in untreated primary adrenal insufficiency. J Clin Endocrinol Metab 1980;50:52-55.
312. Hagg E, Asplund K, Lithner F. Value of basal plasma cortisol assays in the assessment of pituitary-adrenal insufficiency. Clin Endocrinol (Oxf) 1987;26:221-226.
313. Lindholm J, Kehlet H. Re-evaluation of the clinical value of the 30 min ACTH test in assessing the hypothalamic-pituitary-adrenocortical function. Clin Endocrinol (Oxf) 1987;26:53-69.
314. Clark PM, Neylon I, Raggatt PR, et al. Defining the normal cortisol response to the short synacthen test: Implications for the investigation of hypothalamic-pituitary disorders. Clin Endocrinol 1998;49: 287-292.
315. Oelkers W, Diederich S, Bahr V. Diagnosis and therapy surveillance in Addison's disease: rapid adrenocorticotropin (ACTH) test and measurement of plasma ACTH, renin activity, and aldosterone. J Clin Endocrinol Metab 1992;75:259-264.

316. Ertuck E, Jaffe CA, Barkan AL. Evaluation of the integrity of the hypothalamo-pituitary adrenal axis by insulin hypoglycaemia test. J Clin Endocrinol Metab 1998;83:2350-2354.
317. Stewart PM, Corrie J, Seckl JR, et al. A rational approach for assessing the hypothalamo-pituitary-adrenal axis. Lancet 1988;i: 1208-1210.
318. Streeten DHP, Anderson GH, Bonaventura MM. The potential for serious consequences from misinterpreting normal responses to the rapid adrenocorticotropin test. J Clin Endocrinol Metab 1996;81:285-290.
319. Oelkers W. Dose-response aspects in the clinical assessment of the hypothalamo-pituitary adrenal axis and the low dose adrenocorticotropin test. Eur J Endocrinol 1996;135:27-33.
320. Abdu TA, Elhadd TA, Neary R, et al. Comparison of the low dose short synacthen test (1 microg), the conventional dose short synacthen test (250 microg) and the insulin tolerance test for assessment of the hypothalamo-pituitary-adrenal axis in patients with pituitary disease. J Clin Endocrinol Metab 1999;84:838-843.
321. Suliman AM, Smith TP, Labib M, et al. The low-dose ACTH test does not provide a useful assessment of the hypothalamic-pituitary-adrenal axis in secondary adrenal insufficiency. Clin Endocrinol (Oxf) 2002;56:533-539.
322. Fiad TM, Kirby JM, Cunningham SK, et al. The overnight single-dose metyrapone test is a simple and reliable index of the hypothalamic-pituitary-adrenal axis. Clin Endocrinol (Oxf) 1994; 41:695-696.
323. Schlaghecke R, Kornley E, Santen RT, et al. The effect of long-term glucocorticoid therapy on pituitary-adrenal responses to exogenous corticotropin-releasing hormone. N Engl J Med 1992; 326:226-230.
324. Annane D, Sebille V, Charpentier C, et al. Effect of treatment with low doses of hydrocortisone and fludrocortisone on mortality in patients with septic shock. JAMA 2002;288:862-871.
325. Esteban NV, Loughlin T, Yergey AL, et al. Daily cortisol production rate in man determined by stable isotope dilution/mass spectrometry. J Clin Endocrinol Metab 1991;72:39-45.
326. Feek CM, Ratcliffe JG, Seth J, et al. Patterns of plasma cortisol and ACTH concentrations in patients with Addison's disease treated with conventional corticosteroid replacement. Clin Endocrinol (Oxf) 1981;14:451-458.
327. Peacy SR. Glucocorticoid replacement therapy: are patients over treated and does it matter? Clin Endocrinol 1997;46:255-261.
328. Howlett TA. An assessment of optimal hydrocortisone replacement therapy. Clin Endocrinol 1997;46:263-268.
329. Fiad TM, Conway JD, Cunningham SK, et al. The role of plasma renin activity in evaluating the adequacy of mineralocorticoid replacement in primary adrenal insufficiency. Clin Endocrinol 1996;45:529-534.
330. Arlt W, Callies F, van Vlijmen JC, et al. Dehydroepiandrosterone replacement in women with adrenal insufficiency. N Engl J Med 1999;341:1013-1020.
331. Merke DP, Bornstein SR. Congenital adrenal hyperplasia. Lancet 2005;365:2125-2136.
332. White PC, Speiser PW. Congenital adrenal hyperplasia due to 21-hydroxylase deficiency. Endocr Rev 2000;21:245-291.
333. Eugster EA, Dimeglio LA, Wright JC, et al. Height outcome in congenital adrenal hyperplasia caused by 21-hydroxylase deficiency: a meta-analysis. J Pediatr 2001;138:26-32.
334. Cabrera MS, Vogiatzi MG, New MI. Long term outcome in adult males with classic congenital adrenal hyperplasia. J Clin Endocrinol Metab 2001;86:3078-3078.
335. Azziz R, Dewailly D, Owerbach D. Nonclassic adrenal hyperplasia: current concepts. Clinical review 56. J Clin Endocrinol Metab 1996;78:810-815.
336. Speiser PW, Dupont J, Zhu D, et al. Disease expression and molecular genotype in congenital adrenal hyperplasia due to 21-hydroxylase deficiency. J Clin Invest 1992;90:584-595.
337. Krone N, Braun A, Roscher AA, et al. Predicting phenotype in steroid 21-hydroxylase deficiency? Comprehensive genotyping in 155 unrelated, well defined patients from southern Germany. J Clin Endocrinol Metab 2000;85:1059-1065.
338. Wilson RC, Mercado AB, Cheng KC, et al. Steroid 21-hydroxylase deficiency: genotype may not predict phenotype. J Clin Endocrinol Metab 1995;80:2322-2329.
339. New MI, Lorenzen F, Lerner AJ, et al. Genotyping steroid 21-hydroxylase deficiency: hormonal reference data. J Clin Endocrinol Metab 1983;57:320-326.
340. Forest MG, Betuel H, David M. Prenatal treatment in congenital adrenal hyperplasia due to 21-hydroxylase deficiency: update 88 of the French multicentric study. Endocr Res 1989;15:277-301.
341. Seckl JR, Miller WL. How safe is long-term prenatal glucocorticoid treatment? JAMA 1997;277:1077-1079.
342. Pang S, Clark AT, Freeman LC, et al. Maternal side effects of prenatal dexamethasone therapy for fetal congenital adrenal hyperplasia. J Clin Endocrinol Metab 1992;75:249-253.
343. Meyer-Bahlburg HF. What causes low rates of child-bearing in congenital adrenal hyperplasia? J Clin Endocrinol Metab 1999; 84:1844-1847.
344. Morgan JF, Murphy H, Lacey JH, et al. Long term psychological outcome for women with congenital adrenal hyperplasia: cross sectional survey. BMJ 2005;330:340-341.
345. Stikkelbroeck NM, Otten BJ, Pasic A, et al. High prevalence of testicular adrenal rest tumors, impaired spermatogenesis, and Leydig cell failure in adolescent and adult males with congenital adrenal hyperplasia. J Clin Endocrinol Metab 2001;86:5721-5728.
346. Weise M, Mehlinger SL, Drinkard B, et al. Patients with classic congenital adrenal hyperplasia have decreased epinephrine reserve and defective glucose elevation in response to high-intensity exercise. J Clin Endocrinol Metab 2004;89:591-597.
347. Van Wyk JJ, Ritzen EM. The role of bilateral adrenalectomy in the treatment of congenital adrenal hyperplasia. J Clin Endocrinol Metab 2003; 88:2993-2998.
348. Charmandari E, Chrousos GP, Merke DP. Adrenocorticotropin hypersecretion and pituitary microadenoma following bilateral adrenalectomy in a patient with classic 21-hydroxylase deficiency. J Pediatr Endocrinol Metab 2005;18:97-101.
349. White PC, Curnow KM, Pascoe L. Disorders of steroid 11β-hydroxylase isozymes. Endocr Rev 1994;15:421-438.
350. Joehrer K, Geley S, Strasser-Wozak EM, et al. CYP11B1 mutations causing non-classic adrenal hyperplasia due to 11 beta-hydroxylase deficiency. Hum Mol Genet 1997;6:1829-1834.
351. Pang S, Levine LS, Lorenzen F, et al. Hormonal studies in obligate heterozygotes and siblings of patients with 11β-hydroxylase deficiency congenital adrenal hyperplasia. J Clin Endocrinol Metab 1980;50:586-589.
352. Gabrilove JL, Sharma DC, Dorfman RI. Adrenocortical 11β-hydroxylase deficiency and virilism first manifest in an adult woman. N Engl J Med 1965;272:1189-1194.
353. Simone G, Tommaselli AP, Rossi R, et al. Partial deficiency of adrenal 11-hydroxylase. A possible cause of primary hypertension. Hypertension 1985;7:204-210.
354. Biglieri EG. 17α-hydroxylase deficiency: 1963-1966. J Clin Endocrinol Metab 1997;82:48-50.
355. Zachmann M, Werder EA, Prader A. Two types of male pseudohermaphroditism due to 17,20 desmolase deficiency. J Clin Endocrinol Metab 1982;55:487-
356. Yanase T, Simpson ER, Waterman MR. 17α-hydroxylase/17,20-lyase deficiency: from clinical investigation to molecular definition. Endocr Rev 1991;12:91-108.
357. Yamaguchi H, Nakazato M, Miyazato M, et al. A 5′ splice site mutation in the cytochrome P450 steroid 17α-hydroxylase gene in 17α-hydroxylase deficiency. J Clin Endocr Metab 1997;82:1934-1938.
358. Biason-Lauber A, Leiberman E, Zachmann M. A single amino acid substitution in the putative redox partner-binding site of P450c17 as cause of isolated 17,20-lyase deficiency. J Clin Endocrinol Metab 1997;82:3807-3812.
359. Sherbet DP, Tiosano D, Kwist KM, et al. CYP17 mutation E305G causes isolated 17,20-lyase deficiency by selectively altering substrate binding. J Biol Chem 2003;278:48563-48569.
360. Fluck CE, Tajima T, Pandey AV, et al. Mutant P450 oxidoreductase causes disordered steroidogenesis with and without Antley-Bixler syndrome. Nat Genet 2004;36:228-230.
361. Huang N, Pandey AV, Agrawal V, et al. Diversity and function of mutations in p450 oxidoreductase in patients with Antley-Bixler syndrome and disordered steroidogenesis. Am J Hum Genet 2005;76:729-749.
362. Rheaume E, Simard J, Morel Y, et al. Congenital adrenal hyperplasia due to point mutations in the type II 3β-hydroxysteroid dehydrogenase gene. Nat Genet 1992;1:239-245.

363. Simard J, Rheaume E, Mebarki F, et al. Molecular basis of human 3β-hydroxysteroid dehydrogenase deficiency. J Steroid Biochem Mol Biol 1995;53:127-138.
364. Marui S, Castro M, Latronico AC, et al. Mutations in the type II 3β-hydroxysteroid dehydrogenase (HSD3B2) gene can cause premature pubarche in girls. Clin Endocrinol 2000;52:67-75.
365. Pang S, Lerner AJ, Stoner E. Late-onset adrenal steroid 3β-hydroxysteroid dehydrogenase deficiency. I. A cause of hirsutism in pubertal and postpubertal women. J Clin Endocrinol Metab 1985;60: 428-439.
366. Bose HS, Sugawara T, Strauss JF III, et al. The pathophysiology and genetics of congenital lipoid adrenal hyperplasia. N Engl J Med 1996;335:1870-1878.
367. Caron KM, Soo SC, Wetsel WC, et al. Targeted disruption of the mouse gene encoding steroidogenic acute regulatory protein provides insights into congenital adrenal hyperplasia. Proc Natl Acad Sci USA, 1997;94:11540-11545
368. Phillipov G, Palermo M, Shackleton CH. Apparent cortisone reductase deficiency: a unique form of hypercortisolism. J Clin Endocrinol Metab 1996;81:3855-3860.
369. Jamieson A, Wallace AM, Andrew R, et al. Apparent cortisone reductase deficiency: a functional defect in 11beta-hydroxysteroid dehydrogenase type 1. J Clin Endocrinol Metab 1999;84: 3570-3574.
370. Draper N, Walker EA, Bujalska IJ, et al. Mutations in the genes encoding 11beta-hydroxysteroid dehydrogenase type 1 and hexose-6-phosphate dehydrogenase interact to cause cortisone reductase deficiency. Nat Genet 2003;34:434-439.
371. Veldhuis JD, Melby JC. Isolated aldosterone deficiency in man: acquired and inborn errors in the biosynthesis or action of aldosterone. Endocr Rev 1986;2:495-517.
372. White PC. Aldosterone synthase deficiency and related disorders. Mol Cell Endocrinol 2004;31:87-87.
373. Kayes-Wandover KM, Schindler RE, Taylor HC, et al. Type 1 aldosterone synthase deficiency presenting in a middle-aged man. J Clin Endocrinol Metab 2001;86:1008-1012.
374. Zennaro MC, Lombes M. Mineralocorticoid resistance. Trends Endocrinol Metab 2004;15:264-270.
375. Geller DS, Rodriguez-Soriano J, Vallo Boado A, et al. Mutations in the mineralocorticoid receptor gene cause autosomal dominant pseudohypoaldosteronism type 1. Nat Genet 1998;19:279-281.
376. Chang SS, Grunder S, Hanukoglu A, et al. Mutations in subunits of the epithelial sodium channel cause salt wasting with hyperkalaemic acidosis, pseudohypoaldosteronism type 1. Nat Genet 1996;12:248-253.
377. Strautnieks SS, Thompson RJ, Gardiner RM, et al. A novel splice site mutation in the gamma subunit of the epithelial sodium channel gene in three pseudohypoaldosteronism type I families. Nat Genet 1996;13:248-250.
378. Hanukoglu A, Joy O, Steinitz M, et al. Pseudohypoaldosteronism due to renal and multisystem resistance to mineralocorticoids respond differently to carbenoxolone. J Steroid Biochem Mol Bio 1997;60:105-112.
379. Wilson FH, Disse-Nicodeme S, Choate KA, et al. Human hypertension caused by mutations in WNK kinases. Science 2001;293: 1107-1112.
380. DeFronzo R. Hyperkalemia and hyporeninemic hypoaldosteronism. Kidney Int 1980;17:118-134.
381. Sunderlin FS, Anderson GH, Streeten DHP, et al. The renin-angiotensin-aldosterone system in diabetic patients with hyperkalaemia. Diabetes 1981;30:335-340.
382. Gabrilove JL, Seman AT, Sabet R, et al. Virilizing adrenal adenoma with studies on the steroid content of the adrenal venous effluent and a review of the literature. Endocr Rev 1981;2:462-470.
383. Kloos RT, Gross MD, Francis IR, et al. Incidentally discovered adrenal masses. Endocr Rev 1995;16:460-484.
384. Terzolo M, Bovio S, Reimondo G, et al. Subclinical Cushing's syndrome in adrenal incidentalomas. Endocrinol Metab Clin North Am 2005;34:423-439.
385. Catargi B, Rigalleau V, Poussin A, et al. Occult Cushing's syndrome in type-2 diabetes. J Clin Endocrinol Metab 2003;88:5808-5813.
386. Flecchia D, Mazza E, Carlini M, et al. Reduced serum levels of dehydroepiandrosterone sulphate in adrenal incidentalomas: a marker of adrenocortical tumour. Clin Endocrinol (Oxf) 1995;42: 129-134.
387. Gicquel C, Le Bouc Y, Luton JP, et al. Pathogenesis and treatment of adrenocortical carcinoma. Curr Opin Endocrinol Diab 1998;5:189-196.
388. Matzuk M, Finegold M, Mather J, et al. Development of cancer cachexia-like syndrome and adrenal tumours in inhibin-deficient mice. Proc Natl Acad Sci U S A 1994;91:8817-8821.

CHAPTER 15

ENDOCRINE HYPERTENSION

William F. Young, Jr.

Approximately 85 million people in the United States are estimated to be hypertensive.[1] In the majority, the hypertension is "essential" or "idiopathic," but a subgroup of approximately 15% has secondary hypertension. The secondary causes of hypertension can be divided into renal (e.g., renal parenchymal or renovascular disease) and endocrine causes. There are at least 14 endocrine disorders in which hypertension may be the initial clinical presentation (Table 15–1). An accurate diagnosis of endocrine hypertension provides the clinician with a unique treatment opportunity, that is, to render a surgical cure or to achieve a dramatic response with pharmacologic therapy. The diagnostic and therapeutic approaches to endocrine hypertension—ranging from the classic adrenal causes of hypertension (e.g., pheochromocytoma and primary aldosteronism) to pituitary-dependent hypertension (e.g., Cushing's syndrome and acromegaly)—are reviewed in this chapter.

ADRENAL MEDULLA AND CATECHOLAMINES

The adrenal medulla occupies the central portion of the adrenal gland and accounts for 10% of total adrenal gland volume. There is no clear demarcation between the adrenal cortex and medulla. The adrenal glands derive blood supply from the superior, middle, and inferior branches of the inferior phrenic artery, from the renal arteries, and directly from the aorta. The adrenal arteries branch and form a plexus under the capsule. This plexus supplies the cortex. Some of the plexus arteries penetrate the cortex and supply the medulla, as do capillaries draining the cortical cells, forming the corticomedullary portal system. The right adrenal vein is short and drains directly into the inferior vena cava. The left adrenal vein merges with the inferior phrenic vein, and this larger vein drains into the left renal vein.

Adrenomedullary cells are called *chromaffin cells* (stain brown with chromium salts) or *pheochromocytes*. Cytoplasmic granules turn dark when stained with chromic acid because of the oxidation of epinephrine and norepinephrine to melanin. Chromaffin cells differentiate in the center of the adrenal gland in response to cortisol; some chromaffin cells also migrate to form paraganglia, collections of chromaffin cells on both sides of the aorta. The largest cluster of chromaffin cells outside the adrenal medulla is near the level of the inferior mesenteric artery and is referred to as the *organ of Zuckerkandl*, which is quite prominent in the fetus and a major source of catecholamines in the first year of life. The preganglionic sympathetic neurons receive synaptic input from neurons within the pons, medulla, and hypothalamus, providing regulation of sympathetic activity by the brain. Axons from the lower thoracic and lumbar preganglionic neurons, via splanchnic nerves, directly innervate the cells of the adrenal medulla.

The term *catecholamine* refers to substances that contain catechol (ortho-dihydroxybenzene) and a side chain with an amino group—the *catechol nucleus* (Fig. 15–1).[2] Epinephrine is synthesized and stored in the adrenal medulla and released into the systemic circulation. Norepinephrine is synthesized and stored not only in the adrenal medulla, but also in the peripheral sympathetic nerves. Dopamine (DA), the precursor of norepinephrine found in the adrenal medulla and peripheral sympathetic nerves, acts primarily as a neurotransmitter in the central nervous system.

Catecholamines affect many cardiovascular and metabolic processes, including increasing the heart rate, blood pressure, myocardial contractility, and cardiac conduction velocity. Specific receptors mediate the biologic actions. The three types of adrenergic receptors (α, β, DA) and their receptor subtypes (α_1, α_2, β_1, β_2, β_3, DA_1, DA_2) have led to an understanding of the physiologic responses to exogenous and endogenous administration of catecholamines.[3] The α_1 subtype is a postsynaptic receptor that mediates vascular and smooth muscle contraction; stimulation causes vasoconstriction and increased blood pressure. The α_2 receptors are located on presynaptic sympathetic nerve endings and, when activated, inhibit release of norepinephrine; stimulation causes suppression in central sympathetic outflow and decreased blood pressure. There are three major β-receptor subtypes. The β_1 receptor mediates cardiac effects and is more responsive to isoproterenol than to epinephrine or norepinephrine; β_1 receptor stimulation causes positive inotropic and chronotropic effects are the heart, increased renin secretion in the kidney, and lipolysis in adipocytes. The β_2 receptor mediates bronchial, vascular, and uterine smooth muscle relaxation; stimulation causes bronchodilatation, vasodilatation in skeletal muscle, glycogenolysis, and increased release of norepinephrine from sympathetic nerve terminals. The β_3 receptor regulates energy expenditure and lipolysis. DA_1-receptors are localized to the cerebral, renal, mesenteric, and coronary vasculatures; stimulation causes vasodilatation in these vascular beds. DA_2-receptors are presynaptic and localized to sympathetic nerve endings, sympathetic ganglia, and brain; stimulation inhibits the release of norepinephrine, inhibits ganglionic transmission, and inhibits prolactin release, respectively.

Most cells in the body have adrenergic receptors. The pharmacologic development of selective α- and β-adrenergic agonists and antagonists has advanced the pharmacotherapy for various clinical disorders. For example, β_1-antagonists (e.g., atenolol and metoprolol) are considered standard therapies for angina pectoris, hypertension, and cardiac arrhythmias.[4] Administration of β_2-agonists (terbutaline and albuterol) causes bronchial smooth muscle relaxation; these agents are commonly prescribed in inhaled formulations for the treatment of asthma.[5]

TABLE 15–1 ENDOCRINE CAUSES OF HYPERTENSION

ADRENAL DEPENDENT

Pheochromocytoma
Primary aldosteronism
Hyperdeoxycorticosteronism
  Congenital adrenal hyperplasia
    11β-Hydroxylase deficiency
    17α-Hydroxylase deficiency
  Deoxycorticosterone-producing tumor
  Primary cortisol resistance
Cushing's syndrome

APPARENT MINERALOCORTICOID EXCESS (AME)/11β-HYDROXYSTEROID DEHYDROGENASE DEFICIENCY

Genetic
  Type 1 AME
  Type 2 AME
Acquired
  Licorice or carbenoxolone ingestion (type 1 AME)
  Cushing's syndrome (type 2 AME)

THYROID DEPENDENT
Hypothyroidism Hyperthyroidism
PARATHYROID DEPENDENT
Hyperparathyroidism
PITUITARY DEPENDENT
Acromegaly Cushing's syndrome

Catecholamine Synthesis

Catecholamines are synthesized from tyrosine by a process of hydroxylation and decarboxylation (see Fig. 15–1). Tyrosine is derived from ingested food or synthesized from phenylalanine in the liver, and it enters neurons and chromaffin cells by active transport. Tyrosine is converted to 3,4-dihydroxyphenylalanine (dopa) by tyrosine hydroxylase, the rate-limiting step in catecholamine synthesis. Increased intracellular levels of catechols down-regulate the activity of tyrosine hydroxylase; as catecholamines are released from secretory granules in response to a stimulus, cytoplasmic catecholamines are depleted and the feedback inhibition of tyrosine hydroxylase is released. Transcription of tyrosine hydroxylase is stimulated by glucocor-

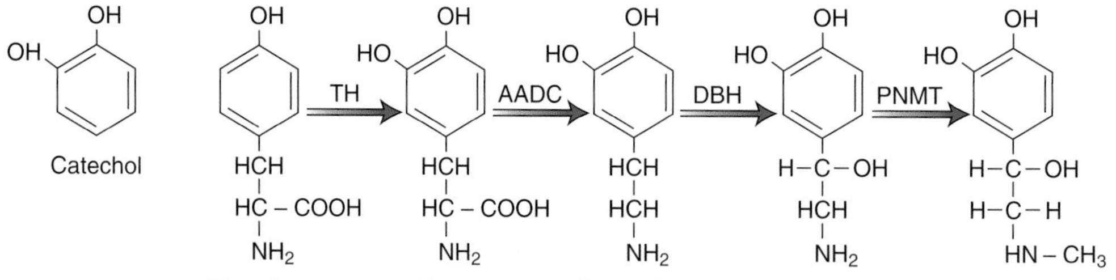

Figure 15–1 ▪ Biosynthetic pathway for catecholamines. The term *catecholamine* comes from the catechol (ortho-dihydroxybenzene) structure and a side chain with an amino group—the "catechol nucleus" (*left*). Tyrosine is converted to 3,4-dihydroxyphenylalanine (dopa) in the rate-limiting step by tyrosine hydroxylase (TH); this rate-limiting step provides the clinician with the option to treat patients with pheochromocytoma with a TH inhibitor, α-methyl-para-tyrosine (metyrosine). Aromatic L-amino acid decarboxylase (AADC) converts dopa to dopamine. Dopamine is hydroxylated to norepinephrine by dopamine β-hydroxylase (DBH). Norepinephrine is converted to epinephrine by phenylethanolamine *N*-methyltransferase (PNMT); cortisol serves as a cofactor for PNMT, which is why epinephrine-secreting pheochromocytomas are almost exclusively localized to the adrenal medulla. (Modified and redrawn from Dluhy RG, Lawrence JE, Williams GH. Endocrine hypertension. In Larsen PR, Kronenberg HM, Melmed S, Polonsky KS, eds. Williams Textbook of Endocrinology, 10th ed. Philadelphia: WB Saunders, 2003:555).

ticoids, cAMP-dependent protein kinases, calcium/phospholipid-dependent protein kinase, and calcium/calmodulin-dependent protein kinase. α-Methyl-paratyrosine (metyrosine) is a tyrosine hydroxylase inhibitor that may be used therapeutically in patients with catecholamine-secreting tumors.

Aromatic L-amino acid decarboxylase catalyzes the decarboxylation of dopa to dopamine (see Fig. 15–1). Dopamine is actively transported into granulated vesicles to be hydroxylated to norepinephrine by the copper-containing enzyme dopamine β-hydroxylase. Ascorbic acid is a cofactor and hydrogen donor. The enzyme is structurally similar to tyrosine hydroxylase and may share similar transcriptional regulatory elements; both are stimulated by glucocorticoids and cAMP-dependent kinases. These reactions occur in the synaptic vesicle of adrenergic neurons in the central nervous system, the peripheral nervous system, and the chromaffin cells of the adrenal medulla. The major constituents of the granulated vesicle are dopamine β-hydroxylase, ascorbic acid, chromogranin A, and adenosine triphosphate (ATP). In the adrenal medulla, norepinephrine is released from the granule into the cytoplasm, where the cytosolic enzyme phenylethanolamine *N*-methyltransferase (PNMT) converts it to epinephrine (see Fig. 15–1). Epinephrine is then transported back into another storage vesicle. The *N*-methylation reaction by PNMT involves *S*-adenosylmethionine as the methyl donor as well as oxygen and magnesium. PNMT expression is regulated by the presence of glucocorticoids, which are in high concentration in the adrenal medulla through the corticomedullary portal system. Thus, catecholamine-secreting tumors that secrete primarily epinephrine are localized to the adrenal medulla. In normal adrenal medullary tissue, approximately 80% of the catecholamine released is epinephrine.

Catecholamine Storage and Secretion

Catecholamines are found in the adrenal medulla and sympathetically innervated organs. Catecholamines are stored in electron-dense granules that also contain ATP, neuropeptides (e.g., adrenomedullin, adrenocorticotropin [ACTH], vasoactive intestinal polypeptide), calcium, magnesium, and chromogranins. Uptake into the storage vesicles is facilitated by active transport using vesicular monoamine transporters (VMATs).[6] The VMAT ATP-driven pump maintains a steep electrical gradient. For every monoamine transported, ATP is hydrolyzed and two hydrogen ions are transported from the vesicle into the cytosol. ^{123}I and ^{131}I-labeled metaiodobenzylguanidine (MIBG) are imported by VMATs into the storage vesicles in the adrenal medulla, which makes ^{123}I-MIBG useful for imaging localization of catecholamine-secreting tumors and ^{131}I-MIBG potentially useful in treating malignant catecholamine-secreting tumors.[7,8] Catecholamine uptake, as well as MIBG, is inhibited by reserpine.[9] The catecholamine stores are dynamic, with constant leakage and reuptake.[10]

Stressful stimuli (e.g., myocardial infarction, anesthesia, hypoglycemia) trigger adrenal medullary catecholamine secretion. Acetylcholine from preganglionic sympathetic fibers stimulates nicotinic cholinergic receptors and causes depolarization of adrenomedullary chromaffin cells. Depolarization leads to activation of voltage-gated calcium channels, which results in exocytosis of secretory vesicle contents. A calcium-sensing receptor appears to be involved in the process of exocytosis. During exocytosis, all the granular contents are released into the extracellular space. Norepinephrine modulates its own release by activating the α_2-receptors on the presynaptic membrane. Stimulation of the presynaptic α_2-receptors inhibits norepinephrine release (the mechanism of action of some antihypertensive medications such as clonidine and guanfacine). Catecholamines are among the shortest-lived signaling molecules in plasma; the initial biologic half-life of circulating catecholamines is between 10 and 100 seconds. Approximately one half of the catecholamines circulate in plasma in loose association with albumin. Thus, plasma concentrations of catecholamines fluctuate widely.

Catecholamine Metabolism and Inactivation

Catecholamines are removed from the circulation either by reuptake by sympathetic nerve terminals or by metabolism through two enzyme pathways (Fig. 15–2), followed by sulfate conjugation and renal excretion. Most of the metabolism of catecholamines occurs in the same cell in which they are synthesized.[10] Almost 90% of catecholamines released at sympathetic synapses are taken up locally by the nerve endings (uptake-1). Uptake-1 can be blocked by cocaine, tricyclic antidepressants, and phenothiazines. Extraneuronal tissues also take up catecholamines, termed *uptake-2*. Most of these catecholamines are metabolized by catechol-*O*-methyltransferase (COMT).

Although COMT is found primarily outside neural tissue, *O*-methylation in the adrenal medulla is the predominant source of metanephrine (COMT converts epinephrine to metanephrine) and a major source of normetanephrine (COMT converts norepinephrine to normetanephrine) by methylating the 3-hydroxy group.[10] *S*-Adenosylmethionine is used as the methyl donor, and calcium is required. Metanephrine and normetanephrine are oxidized by monoamine oxidase (MAO) to vanillylmandelic acid (VMA) by oxidative deamination. MAO may also oxidize epinephrine and norepinephrine to 3,4-dihydroxymandelic acid, which is then converted by COMT to VMA. MAO is located on the outer membrane of mitochondria. In the storage vesicle, norepinephrine is protected from metabolism by MAO. MAO and COMT metabolize dopamine to homovanillic acid (see Fig. 15–2).

PHEOCHROMOCYTOMA AND PARAGANGLIOMA

Catecholamine-secreting tumors that arise from chromaffin cells of the adrenal medulla and the sympathetic ganglia are referred to as *pheochromocytomas* and *extraadrenal catecholamine-secreting paragangliomas* (extraadrenal pheochromocytomas), respectively.[11] Because the tumors have similar clinical presentations and are treated with similar approaches, many clinicians use the term *pheochromocytoma* to refer to both adrenal pheochromocytomas and extraadrenal catecholamine-secreting paragangliomas. However, the distinction between pheochromocytoma and paraganglioma is an important one because of implications for associated neoplasms, risk for malignancy, and genetic testing. Catecholamine-secreting tumors are rare, with an annual incidence of 2 to 8 cases per million people.[12] From screening for secondary causes of hypertension in outpatients, the prevalence of pheochromocytoma has been estimated at 0.1% to 0.6%.[13-15] Nevertheless, it is important to suspect, confirm, localize, and resect these tumors because (1) the associated hypertension is curable with surgical removal of the tumor, (2) a risk of lethal paroxysm exists, (3) at least 10% of the tumors are malignant, and (4) 10% to 20% are familial and detection of this tumor in the proband may result in early diagnosis in other family members.

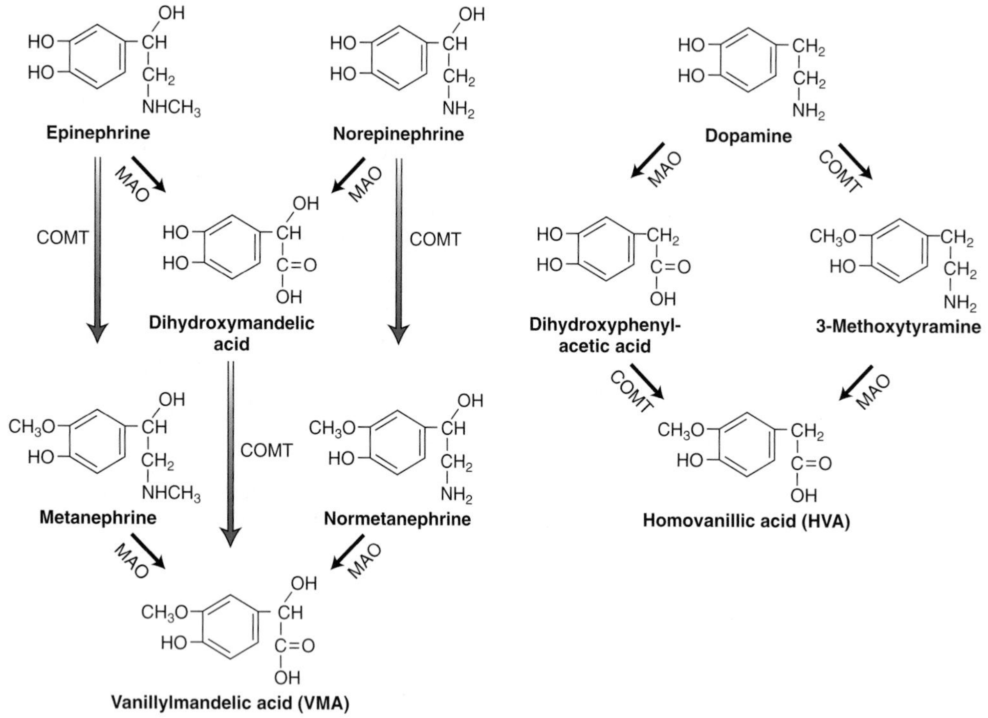

Epinephrine
Norepinephrine
Dopamine
Dihydroxymandelic acid
Dihydroxyphenyl-acetic acid
3-Methoxytyramine
Metanephrine
Normetanephrine
Homovanillic acid (HVA)
Vanillylmandelic acid (VMA)

Figure 15–2 ▪ Catecholamine metabolism. Metabolism of catecholamines occurs through two enzymatic pathways. Catechol-*O*-methyltransferase (COMT) converts epinephrine to metanephrine and converts norepinephrine to normetanephrine by meta-*O*-methylation. Metanephrine and normetanephrine are oxidized by monoamine oxidase (MAO) to vanillylmandelic acid (VMA) by oxidative deamination. MAO also may oxidize epinephrine and norepinephrine to dihydroxymandelic acid, which is then converted by COMT to VMA. Dopamine is also metabolized by MAO and COMT with the final metabolite homovanillic acid (HVA). (Modified and redrawn from Dluhy RG, Lawrence JE, Williams GH. Endocrine hypertension. In Larsen PR, Kronenberg HM, Melmed S, Polonsky KS, eds. Williams Textbook of Endocrinology, 10th ed. Philadelphia: WB Saunders, 2003:555.)

History

The association between adrenal medullary tumors and symptoms was first recognized by Fränkel in 1886.[16] He described Minna Roll, age 18, who had intermittent attacks of palpitation, anxiety, vertigo, headache, chest pain, cold sweats, and vomiting. She had a hard noncompressible pulse and retinitis. Despite champagne therapy and injections of ether, she died. At autopsy, bilateral adrenal tumors were initially thought to be angiosarcomas, but later a positive chromaffin reaction confirmed the pheochromocytoma lesion.

The term *paraganglioma*, introduced in 1908, was defined as an extraadrenal chromaffin tumor arising in a paraganglion.[17] The term *pheochromocytoma*, proposed by Pick in 1912,[18] comes from the Greek words *phaios* ("dusky"), *chroma* ("color"), *cytoma* ("tumor") because of the dark staining reaction that is caused by the oxidation of intracellular catecholamines when exposed to dichromate salts. In 1926, Roux in Lausanne, Switzerland, and Charles Mayo in Rochester, Minnesota, successfully surgically removed adrenal pheochromocytomas.[19] In 1929, it was discovered that a pheochromocytoma contains an excess amount of a pressor agent.[20] Subsequently, epinephrine (in 1936) and norepinephrine (in 1949) were isolated from pheochromocytoma tissue.[20] In 1950, it was found that patients with pheochromocytoma excreted increased amounts of epinephrine, norepinephrine, and dopamine in the urine.[21]

Clinical Presentation

Catecholamine-secreting tumors occur with equal frequency in men and women, primarily in the third, fourth, and fifth decades. These tumors are rare in children, and when discovered, they may be multifocal and associated with a hereditary syndrome. When symptoms are present, they are due to the pharmacologic effects of excess concentrations of circulating catecholamines (Table 15–2).[22] The resulting hypertension may be sustained (in approximately half of the patients) or paroxysmal (in approximately a third of the patients). The remaining patients have normal blood pressure. The lability in blood pressure can be attributed to episodic release of catecholamines, chronic volume depletion, and impaired sympathetic reflexes. In addition to volume depletion, altered sympathetic vascular regulation may have a role in the orthostasis frequently noted in patients with pheochromocytoma.[23] Symptoms (e.g., lightheadedness, presyncope, syncope) of orthostatic hypotension may dominate the presentation, especially in patients with epinephrine-predominant and dopamine-predominant tumors.[24-25]

Episodic symptoms may occur in spells, or paroxysms, that can be extremely variable in presentation but typically include forceful heartbeat, pallor, tremor, headache, and diaphoresis. The spell may start with a sensation of a "rush" in the chest and a sense of shortness of breath, followed by a "pounding" heartbeat in the chest that typically progresses to a throbbing headache. Peripheral vasoconstriction with a spell results in cool/cold hands and feet and facial pallor. Increased sense of body heat and sweating are common symptoms that occur toward the end of the spell. Spells may be either spontaneous or precipitated by postural change, anxiety, medications (e.g., metoclopramide, anesthetic agents), exercise, or maneuvers that increase intraabdominal pressure (e.g., change in position, lifting, defecation, exercise, colonoscopy, pregnancy, trauma). Although the types of spells experienced across the patient population are highly variable, spells tend to be stereotypical for each patient. Spells may occur multiple times daily or as infrequently as once monthly. The typical duration of a pheochromocytoma spell is 15 to 20 minutes, but it may be much shorter or last several hours. However, the clinician must recognize that most patients with spells do not have a pheochromocytoma (Table 15–3).[26]

Additional clinical signs of catecholamine-secreting tumors include hypertensive retinopathy, orthostatic hypotension, angina, nausea, constipation (megacolon may be the presenting symptom), hyperglycemia, diabetes mellitus, hypercalcemia, Raynaud's phenomenon, livedo reticularis, erythrocytosis, and mass effects from the tumor. Although the hypercalcemia may be a sign of multiple endocrine neoplasia type 2 (MEN-2), it is

TABLE 15–2 SIGNS AND SYMPTOMS ASSOCIATED WITH CATECHOLAMINE-SECRETING TUMORS

SPELL RELATED
Anxiety and fear of impending death Diaphoresis Dyspnea Epigastric and chest pain Headache Hypertension Nausea and vomiting Pallor Palpitation (forceful heartbeat) Tremor
CHRONIC
Anxiety and fear of impending death Cold hands and feet Congestive heart failure—dilated or hypertrophic cardiomyopathy Constipation Diaphoresis Dyspnea Ectopic hormone secretion–dependent symptoms (e.g., CRH/ACTH, GHRH, PTH-RP, VIP) Epigastric and chest pain Fatigue Fever General increase in sweating Grade II to IV retinopathy Headache Hyperglycemia Hypertension Nausea and vomiting Orthostatic hypotension Painless hematuria (associated with urinary bladder paraganglioma) Pallor Palpitation (forceful heartbeat) Tremor Weight loss
NOT TYPICAL OF PHEOCHROMOCYTOMA
Flushing

ACTH, Adrenocorticotropic hormone; *CRH*, corticotropin-releasing hormone; *GHRH*, growth hormone–releasing hormone; *PTH-RP*, parathyroid hormone–related peptide; *VIP*, vasoactive intestinal polypeptide.
Adapted from Young WF Jr. Pheochromocytoma: 1926-1993. Trends Endocrinol Metab 1993;4:122-127.

usually isolated and resolves with resection of the catecholamine-secreting tumor. Calcitonin secretion is a catecholamine-dependent process and serum calcitonin concentrations are frequently elevated in patients with a catecholamine-secreting tumors and usually unrelated to MEN 2. The fasting hyperglycemia and diabetes mellitus are caused in part by the α-adrenergic inhibition of insulin release. Painless hematuria and paroxysmal attacks induced by micturition and defecation are associated with urinary bladder paragangliomas. Some of the co-secreted hormones that may dominate the clinical presentation include ACTH (Cushing's syndrome), parathyroid hormone–related peptide (hypercalcemia), vasopressin (syndrome of inappropriate antidiuretic hormone secretion), vasoactive intestinal peptide (watery diarrhea), and growth hormone–releasing hormone (acromegaly).[27-29] Cardiomyopathy and congestive heart failure are the symptomatic presentations caused by pheochromocytoma that perhaps are most frequently unrecognized by clinicians.[30] The cardiomyopathy, whether dilated or hypertrophic, may be totally reversible with tumor resection. Myocarditis and myocardial infarction with normal coronary arteries seen on angiography are cardiac-based presentations that may not be recognized as pheochromocytoma.[31] The myocarditis is characterized by infiltration of inflammatory cells and focal contraction-band necrosis. Many physical examination findings can be associated with genetic syndromes that predispose to pheochromocytoma; these findings include retinal angiomas,

TABLE 15–3 DIFFERENTIAL DIAGNOSIS OF PHEOCHROMOCYTOMA-TYPE SPELLS

ENDOCRINE
Carbohydrate intolerance Hyperadrenergic spells Hypoglycemia Medullary thyroid carcinoma Pancreatic tumors (e.g., insulinoma) Pheochromocytoma Primary hypogonadism (menopausal syndrome) Thyrotoxicosis
CARDIOVASCULAR
Angina Cardiovascular deconditioning Labile essential hypertension Orthostatic hypotension Paroxysmal cardiac arrhythmia Pulmonary edema Renovascular disease Syncope
PSYCHOLOGICAL
Factitious (e.g., drugs, Valsalva) Hyperventilation Severe anxiety and panic disorders Somatization disorder
PHARMACOLOGIC
Chlorpropamide-alcohol flush Combination of a monoamine oxidase inhibitor and a decongestant Illegal drug ingestion (cocaine, phencyclidine, lysergic acid diethylamide) Sympathomimetic drug ingestion Vancomycin ("red man syndrome") Withdrawal of adrenergic-inhibitor
NEUROLOGIC
Autonomic neuropathy Cerebrovascular insufficiency Diencephalic epilepsy (autonomic seizures) Migraine headache Postural orthostatic tachycardia syndrome Stroke
OTHER
Carcinoid syndrome Mast cell disease Recurrent idiopathic anaphylaxis Unexplained flushing spells

marfanoid body habitus, café au lait spots, axillary freckling, subcutaneous neurofibromas, and mucosal neuromas on the eyelids and tongue. Some patients with pheochromocytoma may be asymptomatic despite high circulating levels of catecholamines, likely reflecting adrenergic receptor desensitization related to chronic stimulation.

A "rule of 10" has been quoted for describing the characteristics of catecholamine-secreting tumors: 10% are extraadrenal, 10% occur in children, 10% are multiple or bilateral, 10% recur after surgical removal, 10% are malignant, 10% are familial, and 10% of benign sporadic adrenal pheochromocytomas are found as adrenal incidentalomas.[20] None of these "rules" is precisely 10%. For example, recent studies have suggested that up to 20% of catecholamine-secreting tumors are familial.[32] Also, in a recent study, 19 of 33 patients (57.6%) with adrenal pheochromocytoma had tumors discovered incidentally on imaging.[33] Because of the increased use of computed imaging and familial testing, pheochromocytoma is diagnosed in many patients before any symptoms develop. Although typically these incidentally discovered tumors in asymptomatic patients are small (e.g., <3 cm), they may be up to 10-cm in size.

Pheochromocytomas are localized to the adrenal glands, with an average diameter of 4.5 cm (Fig. 15–3).[34] Paragangliomas are found where there is chromaffin tissue: along the para-aortic sympathetic chain, within the organs of Zuckerkandl (at the origin of the inferior mesenteric artery), in the wall of the urinary bladder, and along the sympathetic chain in the neck or mediastinum.[35] During early postnatal life, the extraadrenal sympathetic paraganglionic tissues are prominent, then they degenerate, leaving residual foci associated with the vagus nerves, carotid vessels, aortic arch, pulmonary vessels, and mesenteric arteries. Odd locations for paragangliomas include the intraatrial cardiac septum, spermatic cord, vagina, scrotum, and sacrococcygeal region. Paragangliomas in the head and neck region (e.g., carotid body tumors, glomus tumors, chemodectomas) usually arise from parasympathetic tissue and typically do not hypersecrete catecholamines and metanephrines. Whereas, paragangliomas in the mediastinum, abdomen, and pelvis usually arise from sympathetic chromaffin tissue and usually do hypersecrete catecholamines and metanephrines.

Genetic and Syndromic forms of Pheochromocytoma and Paraganglioma

Approximately 15% to 20% of patients with catecholamine-secreting tumors have germline mutations (inherited mutations present in all cells of the body) in genes associated with genetic disease (Table 15–4).[36,37] Hereditary catecholamine-secreting tumors typically present at a younger age than sporadic neoplasms.[32] Sporadic pheochromocytoma typically is diagnosed on the basis of symptoms or an incidental discovery on computed imaging, whereas syndromic pheochromocytoma is frequently diagnosed earlier in the course of disease because of biochemical surveillance or genetic testing.[38]

Multiple Endocrine Neoplasia Type 2A

Multiple endocrine neoplasia type 2A (MEN-2A) (Sipple's syndrome) is an autosomal dominant disorder with age-related penetrance.[39] The MEN-2A phenotype includes adrenal pheochromocytoma (usually bilateral and may be asynchronous), medullary carcinoma of the thyroid (MTC), and hyperparathyroidism. MTC is usually detected before pheochromocytoma. Pheochromocytoma occurs in approximately 50% of patients with MEN-2A. The prevalence of MEN-2A is approximately 1 in 35,000 people. Numerous activating mutations throughout the *RET* proto-oncogene have been documented in persons with MEN-2A. The *RET* proto-oncogene, located on chromosome 10q11.2, encodes a transmembrane receptor tyrosine kinase that is involved in the regulation of cell proliferation and apoptosis. Pheochromocytoma is associated most frequently with mutations in codon 634 (in exon 11).

Multiple Endocrine Neoplasia Type 2B

MEN type 2B (MEN-2B) is also an autosomal dominant disorder with age-related penetrance, and it represents approximately 5% of all MEN-2 cases.[39] The MEN-2B phenotype includes pheochromocytoma (usually bilateral), MTC, mucosal neuromas, thickened corneal nerves, intestinal ganglioneuromatosis, and

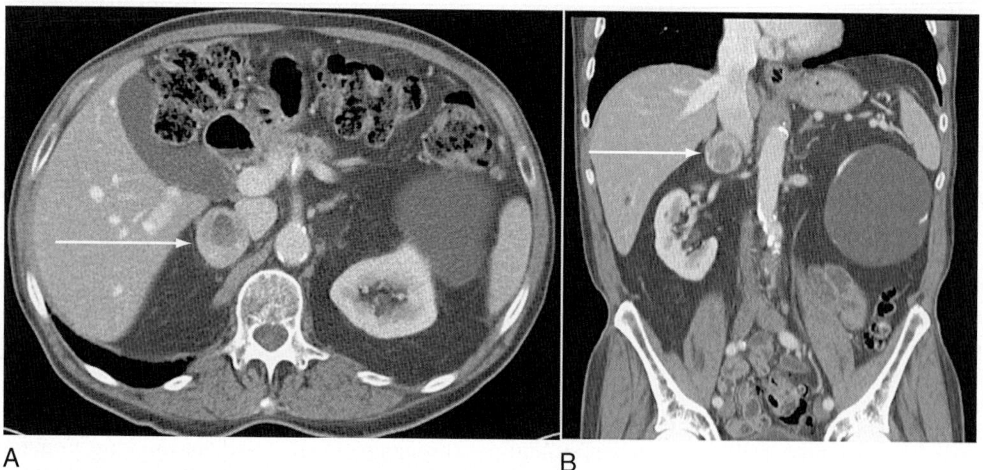

Figure 15–3 ▪ A computed tomographic (CT) scan of the abdomen with intravenous contrast agent of a 71-year-old man with an incidentally discovered right adrenal mass. The fractionated plasma free metanephrines were abnormal: metanephrine, 0.34 nmol/L (normal <0.5) and normetanephrine, 8.59 nmol/L (normal <0.9). The 24-hour urine studies were abnormal: norepinephrine, 455 μg (normal <170); epinephrine, 7.2 μg (normal <35); dopamine, 160 μg (normal <700); metanephrine, 173 μg (normal <400); and normetanephrine, 3147 μg (normal <900). **A,** The axial CT image shows a typical 3.8-cm heterogeneously enhancing right adrenal mass just lateral to the inferior vena cava and consistent with pheochromocytoma (*arrow*). **B,** Coronal view shows the location (*arrow*) of the mass superior to the right kidney and inferior and medial to the liver. After α- and β-adrenergic blockade, a 2.5 × 1.5 × 1.5-cm 20-g pheochromocytoma was removed laparoscopically.

TABLE 15–4 AUTOSOMAL DOMINANT SYNDROMES ASSOCIATED WITH PHEOCHROMOCYTOMA AND PARAGANGLIOMA

Syndrome	Gene	Gene Locus	Protein Product	Protein Function	Gene Mechanism	Typical Tumor Location
SDHD (familial paraganglioma type 1)*	*SDHD*	11q23	SDH D subunit	ATP production	Tumor suppressor	Head and neck, rarely adrenal medulla
Familial paraganglioma type 2*	Unknown	11q13.1	Unknown	ATP production	Unknown	Head and neck
SDHC (familial paraganglioma type 3)	*SDHC*	1q21	SDH C subunit	ATP production	Tumor suppressor	Head and neck
SDHB (familial paraganglioma type 4)	*SDHB*	1p36.1-35	SDH B subunit	ATP production	Tumor suppressor	Abdomen and pelvis, rarely adrenal medulla
MEN-1	*MENIN*	11q13	Menin	Transcription regulation	Tumor suppressor	Adrenal medulla
MEN-2A and -2B	*RET*	10q11.2	RET	Tyrosine kinase receptor	Proto-oncogene	Adrenal medulla bilaterally
Neurofibromatosis type 1	*NF1*	17q11.2	Neurofibromin	GTP hydrolysis	Tumor suppressor	Adrenal-periadrenal
von Hippel-Lindau disease	*VHL*	3p25–26	VHL	Transcription elongation suppression	Tumor suppressor	Adrenal medulla bilaterally, rarely paraganglioma

*Associated with maternal imprinting.
MEN, Multiple endocrine neoplasia; *SDH,* succinate dehydrogenase.

marfanoid body habitus. Overall, pheochromocytoma occurs in approximately 50% of patients with MEN-2. MEN-2B is associated with mutations in codon 918 (in exon 16) of the *RET* proto-oncogene.

Multiple Endocrine Neoplasia Type 2 Genetic Testing

More than 95% of patients with MEN-2A and more than 98% of those with MEN-2B have an identifiable mutation in the *RET* proto-oncogene. Genetic testing for mutations in the *RET* proto-oncogene is commercially available and should be considered for patients with bilateral pheochromocytoma, family history of pheochromocytoma, or co-phenotype disorders. Genetic counseling consultation should be considered before genetic testing is performed (see Chapter 40 for further discussion of MEN-2).

Multiple Endocrine Neoplasia Type 1

MEN-1 is an autosomal dominant disorder characterized by pituitary adenomas, primary hyperparathyroidism, pancreatic islet cells tumors, adrenal adenomas, carcinoid tumors, collagenomas, angiofibromas, lipomas, and rarely adrenal pheochromocytoma.[40,41] Pheochromocytoma has been documented in only a few patients with MEN-1.[42,43] The prevalence of MEN-1 is approximately 1 in 30,000 individuals.[40,41] MEN-1 is caused by inactivating mutations in the tumor suppressor gene *MEN1* located on chromosome 11q13. Genetic testing for mutations in *MEN1* is commercially available and should be considered only for patients with adrenal pheochromocytoma and MEN-1 co-phenotype disorders.

von Hippel-Lindau Disease

von Hippel-Lindau (VHL) disease is an autosomal dominant disorder characterized by pheochromocytoma (frequently bilateral), paraganglioma (rarely), retinal angiomas, cerebellar hemangioblastoma, epididymal cystadenoma, renal and pancreatic cysts, and renal cell carcinoma. Pheochromocytoma is reported to occur in about 10% to 20% of patients with VHL. The prevalence of VHL is approximately 1 in 35,000 people. The *VHL* tumor suppressor gene, located on chromosome 3p25-26, encodes a protein that regulates hypoxia-induced proteins.[44] More than 300 germline *VHL* mutations have been identified that lead to loss of function of the VHL protein. Nearly 100% of patients with VHL have an identifiable gene mutation. Genotype-phenotype correlations have been documented for this disorder, and specific mutations are associated with particular patterns of tumor formation.[45,46] In up to 98% of cases, pheochromocytoma is associated with missense mutations (rather than truncating or null mutations) in the *VHL* gene. Certain missense mutations appear to be associated with a "pheochromocytoma only" presentation of VHL. Genetic testing for VHL is commercially available and should be considered for patients with bilateral pheochromocytoma, family history of pheochromocytoma, diagnosis of pheochromocytoma at a young age (e.g., ≤20 years old), or co-phenotype disorders.

Pheochromocytomas occurring in patients with MEN 2 produce predominantly epinephrine and metanephrine, whereas pheochromocytomas occurring in patients with VHL produce predominately norepinephrine and normetanephrine. These biochemical phenotypes result from mutation-specific differential gene expression. PNMT is overexpressed in MEN 2-associated tumors (epinephrine and metanephrine profile) and underexpressed in VHL-associated tumors (norepinephrine and normetanephrine profile).[47] In addition, pheochromocytomas occurring in patients with MEN 2 have increased tyrosine hydroxylase activity compared with pheochromocytomas occurring in patients with VHL; this difference accounts for higher levels of catecholamines and metabolites in patients with MEN 2.

Neurofibromatosis Type 1

Neurofibromatosis type 1 (NF1) is an autosomal dominant disorder characterized by neurofibromas, café au lait spots, axillary and inguinal freckling, and iris hamartomas (Lisch nodules). Approximately 2% of patients with NF1 develop catecholamine-secreting tumors.[48] In these patients, the catecholamine-secreting tumor is usually a solitary benign adrenal pheochromocytoma, occasionally bilateral adrenal pheochromocytoma, and rarely an abdominal paraganglioma. The prevalence of NF1 is approximately 1 in 3000 people. The *NF1* tumor suppressor gene, located on chromosome 17q11.2, encodes neurofibromin, a GTPase-activating protein that inhibits Ras activity. Inactivating *NF1* mutations cause the disorder. More than 95% of *NF1* mutations can be identified with a multistep testing protocol. However, unless a patient with pheochromocytoma presents with additional clinical characteristics consistent with an NF1 diagnosis, genetic testing of the *NF1* gene is not recommended.

Familial Paraganglioma

Familial paraganglioma is an autosomal dominant disorder characterized by paragangliomas that are located most often in the head and neck but also in the thorax, abdomen, pelvis, and urinary bladder. The occurrence of catecholamine hypersecretion in a patient with familial paraganglioma depends on tumor location; approximately 5% of head and neck paragangliomas and more than 50% of abdominal paragangliomas produce hormones.[35] The mean age at diagnosis is 30 to 35 years, and it can vary greatly within a family (mean ± SD years difference, 14.3 ± 9.6; range, 0 to 37 years).[49] The prevalence of familial paraganglioma is unknown. Most cases of familial paraganglioma are caused by mutations in the succinate dehydrogenase (SDH; succinate:ubiquinone oxidoreductase) subunit genes (*SDHB, SDHC, SDHD*), which compose portions of mitochondrial complex II.[50,51] Mitochondrial complex II is a tumor suppressor gene involved in the electron transport chain and the tricarboxylic acid (TCA) cycle.

Inactivating germline mutations in *SDHD*, located on chromosome 11q23, have been identified in multigenerational families with head and neck parasympathetic paragangliomas that are usually nonfunctional.[52] However, catecholamine-secreting paragangliomas may occur when mutations are located in the 5′ portion of *SDHD*.[53] Adrenal pheochromocytomas may also be found in patients with *SDHD* mutations.[54] Before the gene was characterized, affected families were said to have paraganglioma syndrome type 1. In patients with *SDHD* mutations, penetrance depends on the mutation's parent of origin. Hence, the disease is not manifested when the mutation is inherited from the mother but is highly penetrant when inherited from the father.[52,54] This phenomenon is known as *maternal imprinting*.

Missense mutations in *SDHC*, located on chromosome 1q21, have been reported in families with head and neck parasympathetic paragangliomas that are usually nonfunctional.[55] Before the gene was characterized, affected families were said to have paraganglioma syndrome type 3. Genetic testing for *SDHC* should be considered for families with head and neck paragangliomas that are negative for mutations in *SDHD*.

The gene associated with paraganglioma syndrome type 2 has not been identified, although it has been mapped to chromosome 11q13.1. Like families with mutations in *SDHD*, families with paraganglioma syndrome type 2 also exhibit maternal imprinting.[56] Paraganglioma syndrome type 2 is associated with parasympathetic paragangliomas that typically occur in the head and neck.

Inactivating mutations in the tumor suppressor gene *SDHB*, located on chromosome 1p35-36, are associated with paragangliomas in the abdomen, pelvis, and mediastinum. Adrenal pheochromocytomas may also be found in patients with *SDHB* mutations.[54] Before the gene was characterized, affected families were said to have paraganglioma syndrome type 4. In families with *SDHB* mutations, imprinting has not been observed. Patients with *SDHB* mutations are at an increased risk for malignant paraganglioma.[54,57,58] In addition, in a population-based study patients with *SDHB* mutations appeared to be at an increased risk for renal cell carcinoma and papillary thyroid cancer,[54] but a referral center based study did not find this apparent association.[59]

The *SDH* gene mutation detection rate in persons with familial paraganglioma is not known. Genetic testing for *SDHB, SDHD,* and *SDHC* is available commercially and, because of the high prevalence among patients with paraganglioma, stepwise testing should be considered for all affected individuals (see below). In addition, large germline deletions of *SDHB* and *SDHD* have been identified in families with paraganglioma[60]; these large deletions are not detected with mutation analysis methods that molecular diagnostic laboratories currently use.

Other Neurocutaneous Syndromes

Additional neurocutaneous syndromes associated with catecholamine-secreting tumors include ataxia-telangiectasia, tuberous sclerosis, and Sturge-Weber syndrome. The Carney triad (gastric leiomyosarcoma, pulmonary chondroma, and catecholamine-secreting paraganglioma) is another syndrome associated with catecholamine-secreting tumors.[61] This syndrome is a rare, usually sporadic disorder of unknown etiology that primarily affects young women. The gastric stromal tumors are frequently multicentric and associated with early liver metastases. Despite the metastatic gastric stromal tumor, most affected patients have a very indolent course. The pulmonary chondromas are benign and, if asymptomatic, require no specific therapy. The paragangliomas may be catecholamine-secreting and should be resected when discovered. Additional features of the Carney triad include esophageal leiomyomas and adrenal cortical adenomas. The esophageal leiomyomas found incidentally at the time of esophagogastroduodenoscopy are benign and usually asymptomatic. The adrenal cortical adenomas may be nonfunctioning or secrete cortisol autonomously.

When and How to Order Genetic Testing

As previously outlined, genetic testing should be considered if a patient has one or more of the following: (1) paraganglioma; (2) bilateral adrenal pheochromocytoma; (3) unilateral adrenal pheochromocytoma and a family history of pheochromocytoma/paraganglioma; (4) unilateral adrenal pheochromocytoma onset at a young age (younger than 20 years); or (5) other clinical findings suggestive of one of the previously discussed syndromic disorders. An asymptomatic person at risk for disease on the basis of family history of pheochromocytoma/paraganglioma should have genetic testing only if an affected family member has a known mutation. Genetic testing can be complex; testing one family member has implications for related individuals. Genetic counseling is recommended to help families understand the implications of genetic test results; to coordinate testing of at-risk individuals; and to help families work through the psychosocial issues that may arise before, during, or after the testing process.

The clinician may obtain a list of clinically approved molecular genetic diagnostic laboratories at http://*www.genetests.org*. Given the considerable cost of genetic testing, using a stepwise approach based on each patient's clinical scenario is prudent. See the following examples:

- If a patient has a catecholamine-secreting abdominal paraganglioma, tests for mutations in the following genes should be ordered sequentially: *SDHB, SDHD, VHL*. If a mutation is identified at any point in the testing algorithm, no further testing should be performed.
- If a patient presents with bilateral adrenal pheochromocytoma but without a history of MTC or goiter, tests for

mutations in the following genes should be ordered sequentially: *VHL, RET.* If a *VHL* mutation is identified, do not order genetic testing of the *RET* proto-oncogene.

- If a patient 20 years of age or younger presents with apparent sporadic unilateral adrenal pheochromocytoma, tests for mutations in the following genes should be ordered sequentially: *VHL, RET, SDHB, SDHD.* If a mutation is identified at any point in the testing algorithm, no further testing should be performed.
- If a patient older than 20 years of age presents with apparent sporadic unilateral adrenal pheochromocytoma, tests for mutations in the following genes should be ordered sequentially: *SDHB, SDHD.* If a mutation is identified at any point in the testing algorithm, no further testing should be performed.

Diagnostic Investigation

Differential Diagnosis

Numerous disorders can cause signs and symptoms that may trigger the clinician to test for pheochromocytoma (see Table 15–3). The disorders span much of medicine and include endocrine disorders (e.g., primary hypogonadism), cardiovascular disorders (e.g., idiopathic orthostatic hypotension), psychological disorders (e.g., panic disorder), pharmacologic causes (e.g., withdrawal from an adrenergic inhibitor), neurologic disorders (e.g., postural orthostatic tachycardia syndrome), and miscellaneous disorders (e.g., mast cell disease) (see Table 15–3). Indeed, most patients tested for pheochromocytoma do not have it. In addition, fractionated catecholamines and metanephrine levels may be elevated in several clinical scenarios: withdrawal from medications or drugs (e.g., clonidine, alcohol), any acute illness (e.g., subarachnoid hemorrhage, migraine headache, preeclampsia), and many drugs and medications (e.g., cocaine, phencyclidine, lysergic acid diethylamide, amphetamines, ephedrine, pseudoephedrine, phenylpropanolamine, isoproterenol) (Table 15–5).

Case Finding

Pheochromocytoma should be suspected in patients who have one or more of the following:

- Hyperadrenergic spells (e.g., self-limited episodes of nonexertional palpitations, diaphoresis, headache, tremor, or pallor)
- Resistant hypertension
- A familial syndrome that predisposes to catecholamine-secreting tumors (e.g., MEN-2, NF1, VHL)
- A family history of pheochromocytoma
- An incidentally discovered adrenal mass
- Hypertension and diabetes
- Pressor response during anesthesia, surgery, or angiography
- Onset of hypertension at a young age (e.g., younger than 20 years)
- Idiopathic dilated cardiomyopathy
- A history of gastric stromal tumor or pulmonary chondromas (Carney triad).

TABLE 15–5 MEDICATIONS THAT MAY INCREASE MEASURED LEVELS OF CATECHOLAMINES AND METANEPHRINES

Tricyclic antidepressants
Levodopa
Drugs containing adrenergic receptor agonists (e.g., decongestants)
Amphetamines
Buspirone and most psychoactive agents
Prochlorperazine
Reserpine
Withdrawal from clonidine and other drugs
Ethanol
Acetaminophen (may increase measured levels of fractionated plasma metanephrines in some assays)

Measurement of Fractionated Metanephrines and Catecholamines in Urine and Blood

The diagnosis must be confirmed biochemically by the presence of increased concentrations of fractionated catecholamines and fractionated metanephrines in the urine or plasma (Fig. 15–4).[22] The majority of the metabolism of catecholamines is intratumoral, with formation of metanephrine and normetanephrine.[10] Most laboratories now measure fractionated catecholamines (dopamine, norepinephrine, and epinephrine) and metanephrines (metanephrine and normetanephrine) by high-performance liquid chromatography with electrochemical detection or tandem mass spectroscopy.[62] These techniques have overcome the problems with fluorometric analysis (e.g., false-positive results caused by α-methyldopa, labetalol, sotalol, and imaging contrast agents). At Mayo Clinic, the most reliable case-finding method for identifying catecholamine-secreting tumors is measuring metanephrines and catecholamines in a 24-hour urine collection (sensitivity = 98%, specificity = 98%).[63,64] If clinical suspicion is high, then fractionated plasma free metanephrines, which are products of intrapheochromocytoma catecholamine metabolism, should also be measured.[65] Some groups have advocated that fractionated plasma free metanephrines should be a first-line test for pheochromocytoma[65,66]; the predictive value of a negative test is extremely high, and normal fractionated plasma metanephrines excludes pheochromocytoma except in patients with early preclinical disease and those with strictly dopamine-secreting neoplasms.[64] A plasma test is also attractive because of simplicity. Although measurement of fractionated plasma metanephrines has a sensitivity of 96% to 100%,[64,65] the specificity is poor at 85% to 89%[64,65,67]; the specificity falls to 77% in patients older than 60 years.[64] It has been estimated that 97% of patients with hypertension seen in a tertiary care clinic who have a positive fractionated plasma metanephrine measurement will not have a pheochromocytoma.[67] This high rate of false-positive tests results in excessive health care expenditures because of subsequent imaging and potentially inappropriate surgery.[68] Thus, fractionated plasma free metanephrines lack the necessary specificity to be recommended as a first-line test; therefore, this measurement is reserved for cases for which the index of suspicion is high (see Fig. 15–4).

The index of suspicion should be high for the following scenarios: resistant hypertension; spells; a family history of pheochromocytoma; a genetic syndrome that predisposes to pheochromocytoma (e.g., MEN-2); a past history of resected pheochromocytoma and present history of recurrent hypertension or spells; or an incidentally discovered adrenal mass that has imaging characteristics consistent with pheochromocytoma (e.g., marked enhancement with intravenous contrast medium on computed tomography [CT], high signal intensity on T2-weighted magnetic resonance imaging [MRI], cystic and hemorrhagic changes, bilaterality, or larger size [e.g., >4 cm]). In addition, measuring fractionated plasma free metanephrines is a good first-line test for children because obtaining a complete 24-hour urine collection is difficult. Measurement of urinary dopamine or plasma methoxytyramine may be very useful in detecting the rare tumor with selective dopamine hypersecre-

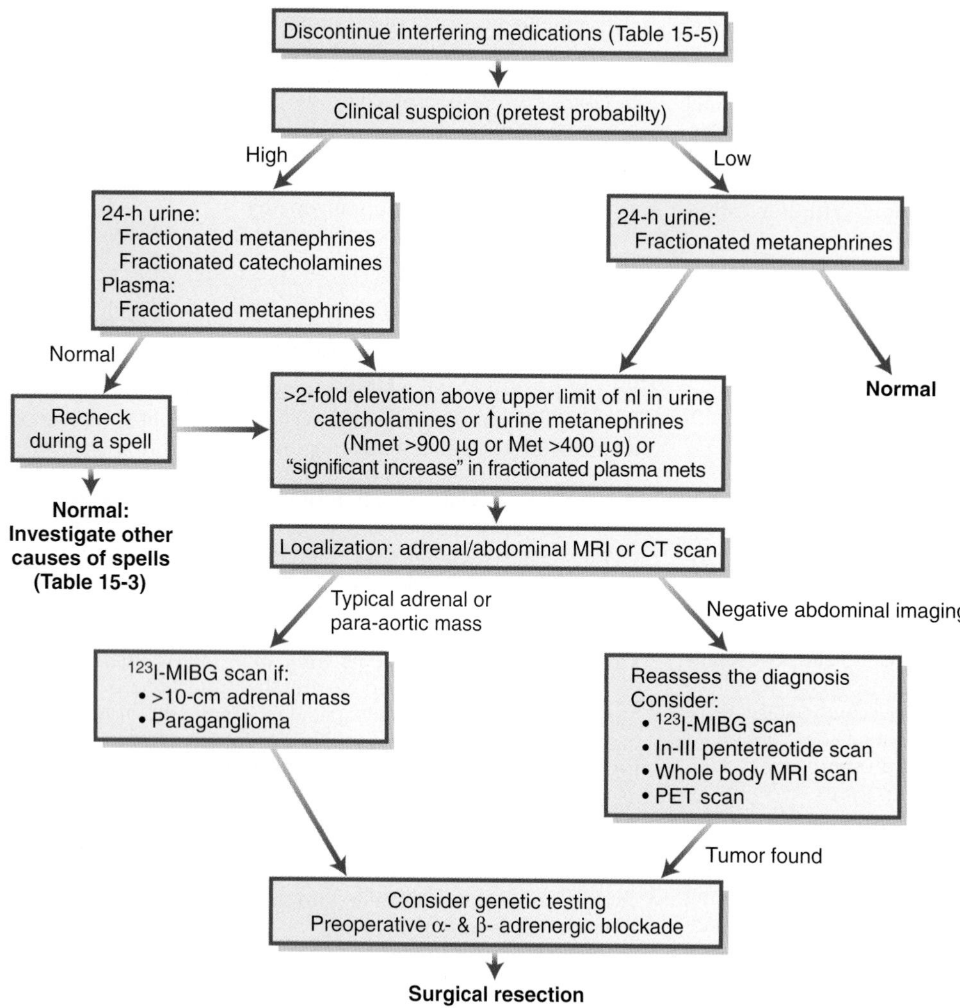

Figure 15–4 ■ Evaluation and treatment of catecholamine-secreting tumors. Clinical suspicion is triggered by the following: paroxysmal symptoms (especially hypertension); hypertension that is intermittent, unusually labile, or resistant to treatment; family history of pheochromocytoma or associated conditions; or incidentally discovered adrenal mass. The details are discussed in the text. *CT,* Computed tomography; *^{123}I-MIBG,* ^{123}I-metaiodobenzylguanidine; *mets,* metanephrines; *MRI,* magnetic resonance imaging; *nl,* normal; *Nmet,* normetanephrine; *PET,* positron emission tomography. (Modified from Young WF Jr. Pheochromocytoma: 1926-1993. Trends Endocrinol Metab 1993;4:122.)

tion because plasma metanephrine fractions are not direct metabolites of dopamine and may be normal in the setting of a dopamine-secreting tumor.[25,64]

The 24-hour urine collection for fractionated metanephrines and catecholamines should include measurement of urinary creatinine to verify an adequate collection. The normal ranges for plasma metanephrine and normetanephrine may be affected by the method used to obtain the blood sample. For example, the procedure of an indwelling cannula for 20 minutes following an overnight fast before the blood draw has resulted in lower diagnostic cutoffs (metanephrine <0.3 nmol/L, normetanephrine <0.66 nmol/L)[69] to exclude pheochromocytoma compared with venipuncture in a seated ambulant nonfasting patient (metanephrine <0.5 nmol/L, normetanephrine <0.9 nmol/L).[64] The diagnostic cutoffs for most fractionated 24-hour urinary metanephrine assays are based on normal ranges derived from a normotensive volunteer reference group, and this can result in excessive false-positive testing. For example, in normotensive laboratory volunteers, the 95th percentiles are 428 µg for normetanephrine and 200 µg for metanephrine; whereas the 95th percentiles in individuals being tested for pheochromocytoma (but who do not have the neoplasm) as part of routine clinical practice are 71% and 51% higher than those of normal volunteers, respectively.[70]

Although it is preferred that patients not receive any medication during the diagnostic evaluation, treatment with most medications may be continued. Tricyclic antidepressants interfere most frequently with the interpretation of 24-hour urinary catecholamines and metabolites. To effectively screen for catecholamine-secreting tumors, treatment with tricyclic antidepressants and other psychoactive agents listed in Table 15–5 should be tapered and discontinued at least 2 weeks before any hormonal assessments. There are certainly clinical situations for which it is contraindicated to discontinue certain medications (e.g., antipsychotics) and if case-finding testing is positive, then computed imaging would be needed to exclude a catecholamine-secreting tumor. Furthermore, catecholamine secretion may be appropriately increased in situations of physical stress or illness (e.g., stroke, myocardial infarction, congestive heart failure, obstructive sleep apnea). Therefore, the clinical circumstances under which catecholamines and metanephrines are measured must be assessed in each case.

Other Tests That Have Been Used to Test for Pheochromocytoma

Because of poor overall accuracy in testing for pheochromocytoma, measurement of plasma catecholamines no longer has a role.[69] Chromogranin A is stored and released from dense-core secretory granules of neuroendocrine cells and is increased in 80% of patients with pheochromocytoma.[71] Chromogranin A is not specific for pheochromocytoma and elevations may be seen with other neuroendocrine tumors. Plasma neuropeptide Y levels are increased in 87% of patients with pheochromocytoma,[72] but they also lack the accuracy of 24-hour urinary fractionated metanephrines and catecholamines. The 24-hour urinary VMA excretion has poor diagnostic sensitivity and specificity compared with fractionated 24-hour urinary metanephrines.

Clonidine Suppression Test

The high false-positive rate for plasma catecholamines and fractionated free metanephrines triggered the development of a confirmatory test, the clonidine suppression test. This test is intended to distinguish between pheochromocytoma and false-positive increases in plasma catecholamines and metanephrines. Clonidine is a centrally acting α_2-adrenergic receptor agonist that normally suppresses the release of catecholamines from neurons but does not affect the catecholamine secretion from a pheochromocytoma. Clonidine (0.3 mg) is administered orally, and plasma catecholamines or metanephrines are measured before and 3 hours after the dose.[73] In patients with essential hypertension, plasma catecholamine concentrations decrease (norepinephrine + epinephrine <500 pg/mL or >50% decrease in norepinephrine) as do plasma normetanephrine concentrations (into normal range or >40% decrease). However, these concentrations remain increased in patients with pheochromocytoma.[73,74]

Provocative Testing and Suppression Testing

Because of advances in the methodology for measuring catecholamines and metanephrines, phentolamine, glucagon, histamine, metoclopramide, and tyramine tests are rarely needed. From 1975 to 1994, we performed histamine and glucagon stimulation testing in 542 patients in whom pheochromocytoma was highly suspected despite normal 24-hour urinary excretion of total metanephrines or catecholamines; *not one patient* had a positive stimulation test in this setting.[75]

Renal Failure

Measurements of urinary catecholamines and metabolites may be invalid if the patient has advanced renal insufficiency.[76] Serum chromogranin A levels have poor diagnostic specificity in these patients.[77] In patients without pheochromocytoma who are receiving hemodialysis, plasma norepinephrine and dopamine concentrations are increased threefold and twofold above the upper limit of normal, respectively.[78,79] However, standard normal ranges can be used for interpreting plasma epinephrine concentrations.[80] Therefore, when patients with renal failure have plasma norepinephrine concentrations more than threefold above the upper normal limit or epinephrine concentrations more than the upper normal limit, pheochromocytoma should be suspected. The findings of one study suggested that plasma concentrations of free metanephrines are increased approximately twofold in patients with renal failure and may be useful in the biochemical evaluation of patients with marked renal insufficiency or renal failure.[81] However, the results of an earlier study suggested that concentrations of fractionated plasma free metanephrines could not distinguish between 10 patients with pheochromocytoma and 11 patients with end-stage renal disease who required long-term hemodialysis.[82]

Factitious Pheochromocytoma

As with other similar disorders, factitious pheochromocytoma can be very difficult to confirm.[83] The patient usually has a medical background. The patient may "spike" the 24-hour urine container or the catecholamines may be administered systemically.[84]

Localization

Localization studies should not be initiated until biochemical studies have confirmed the diagnosis of a catecholamine-secreting tumor (see Fig. 15–4). Computer-assisted imaging of the adrenal glands and abdomen with MRI or CT should be the first localization test (sensitivity, >95%; specificity, >65%) (see Fig. 15–4).[85-88] Approximately 85% of these tumors are found in the adrenal glands, and 95% are found in the abdomen. The most common locations of catecholamine-secreting paragangliomas include superior abdominal paraaortic region, 46%; inferior abdominal paraaortic region, 29%; urinary bladder, 10%; thorax, 10%; head and neck, 3%; and pelvis, 2%.[35]

CT, MRI, and "Imaging Phenotype"

Imaging phenotype refers to the characteristics of the mass on computed imaging (Table 15–6). Computed imaging is a powerful tool available to endocrinologists. The lipid-rich nature of cortical adenomas is helpful in distinguishing these benign neoplasms from pheochromocytoma. On CT scans, the density of the image (black = less dense) is attributed to X-ray attenuation. At the extremes of the CT density spectrum are air (black) and bone (white). The Hounsfield scale is a semiquantitative method of measuring X-ray attenuation. Typical Hounsfield unit (HU) values are air = 0 HU, adipose tissue = –20 to –50 HU, and kidney = 20 to 50 HU. If an adrenal mass is less than 10 HU on unenhanced CT, the likelihood that it is a benign adenoma is close to 100%.[89,90] Adrenal adenomas show a much earlier washout of contrast enhancement than do nonadenomas.[91] For example, Korobkin and colleagues[91] found that the mean percentage washout for adenomas was 51% at 5 minutes and 70% at 15 minutes, compared with 8% and 20%, respectively, for nonadenomas. The sensitivity and specificity for the diagnosis of adenoma were both 96% at a threshold attenuation value of less than 37 HU on the 15-minute postcontrast medium scan.

Although CT is still the primary adrenal imaging modality, MRI has advantages in certain clinical situations.[88] Several different MRI techniques have been used to characterize adrenal masses. Conventional spin-echo MRI was the first and remains the most frequently used technique. Early in the history of abdominal MRI, it became clear that with low or midfield-strength magnets T1- and T2-weighted imaging could be used to differentiate pheochromocytoma and malignancy from benign adenomas. On gadolinium-diethylenetriaminepenta-acetic acid (DPTA)-enhanced MRI, pheochromocytomas and malignant lesions show rapid and marked enhancement and a slower washout pattern, whereas adenomas demonstrate mild enhancement and a rapid washout of contrast.[92] Similar findings are made with CT.

Chemical shift MRI is a form of lipid-sensitive imaging. Chemical shift MRI is based on the principle that the hydrogen protons in water and lipid molecules resonate at different frequencies. Benign cortical adenomas contain approximately equal amounts of lipid and water, whereas the lipid content of pheochromocytomas is usually low. When the protons of water and lipid are aligned, they are "in-phase," and when opposite each other, they are "out-of-phase." When fat and water are in-phase on MRI, the signal intensity is maximized. When fat and water are out-of-phase, the signal intensity is reduced. This in-phase and out-of-phase process is the "chemical shift" technique. Benign adrenal cortical adenomas lose signal on out-of-phase images but appear relatively bright on in-phase images.[92] A recent modification of the chemical shift MRI technique uses gradient echo pulse sequences to produce a similar effect.

Imaging characteristics consistent with a benign cortical adenoma include round and homogeneous density, smooth contour and sharp margination, diameter usually less than 4 cm, unilateral location, low unenhanced CT attenuation values (<10 HU), limited enhancement on CT with intravenous contrast (<24 HU at 14 minutes, <37 HU at 30 minutes, and <30 HU at 60 minutes after administration of contrast medium),[91,93] isointen-

TABLE 15–6 TYPICAL IMAGING PHENOTYPES OF ADRENAL MASSES

Tumor Type	Size (cm)	Shape	Texture	Laterality	Contrast Enhancement	CT	MRI	Necrosis Hemorrhage Calcifications	Growth
Cortical adenoma	≤3	Round to oval smooth margins	Homogeneous	Usually unilateral	Limited	<10 HU precontrast >50% contrast washout at 10 min 30 min postcontrast	Isointense to liver on T2-weighted images	Rare	Slow
Cortical carcinoma	>4	Irregular with unclear margins	Inhomogeneous	Usually unilateral	Marked	>10 HU precontrast <50% contrast washout at 10 min	Hyperintense compared to liver on T2-weighted images	Common	Rapid
Pheochromocytoma	>3	Round to oval smooth margins	Inhomogeneous areas of cystic degeneration	Usually solitary and unilateral	Marked	>10 HU precont rast <50% contrast washout at 10 min	Hyperintense compared to liver on T2-weighted images	Common	1 cm/yr
Metastasis	Variable	Oval to irregular with unclear margins	Inhomogeneous	Often bilateral	Marked	>10 HU precontrast <50% contrast washout at 10 min	Hyperintense compared to liver on T2-weighted images	Common	Variable

CT, Computed tomography; *HU,* Hounsfield unit; *MRI,* magnetic resonance imaging.

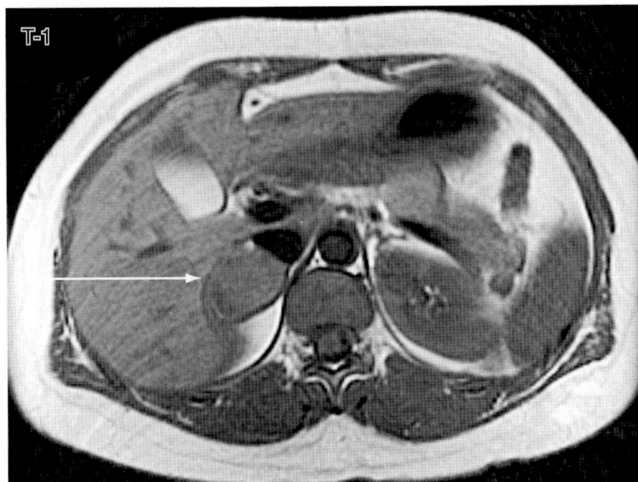

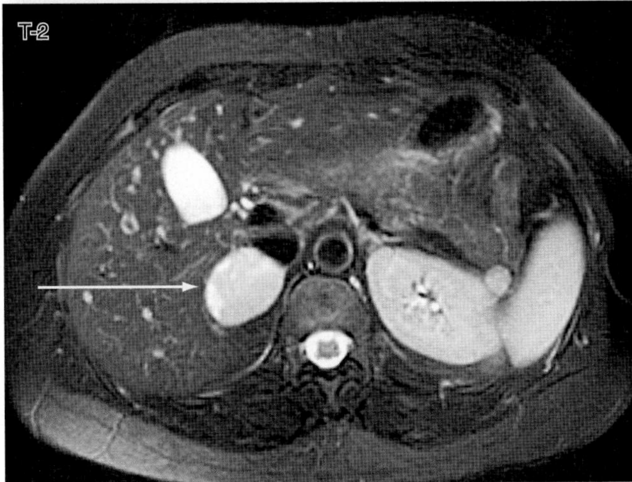

Figure 15–5 ▪ Magnetic resonance images of the abdomen of a 34-year-old woman with a recent onset of palpitations and hypertension. She presented with acute left ventricular failure following a single dose of a β-adrenergic blocker. The 24-hour urine test for total metanephrines and catecholamines showed total metanephrines, 3800 μg (normal <1000); norepinephrine, 37 μg (normal <170); epinephrine, 7.7 μg (normal <35); and dopamine, 147 μg (normal <700). The images show a 3.3 × 3.5 × 4.5-cm slightly heterogeneous right adrenal mass consistent with pheochromocytoma (*arrows*) that has increased signal intensity on T2-weighted images (*lower panel*). Following α-adrenergic blockade and restoration of normal left ventricular function, the patient had a laparoscopic adrenalectomy to remove a 5- × 4- × 3-cm 33-g pheochromocytoma. Postoperatively, the 24-hour urinary excretion of total metanephrines normalized.

sity with liver on both T1- and T2-weighted MRI sequences, and chemical shift evidence of lipid on MRI. The imaging phenotype consistent with pheochromocytoma includes enhancement with intravenous contrast medium on CT (see Fig. 15–3), high signal intensity on T2-weighted MRI (Fig. 15–5), cystic and hemorrhagic changes, and variable size; also the tumor may be bilateral. Although it has been suggested that patients with apparent simple adrenal cysts do not require hormonal evaluation, pheochromocytoma may mimic an adrenal cyst.

^{123}I-Metaiodobenzylguanidine Scintigraphy

If the results of abdominal imaging are negative, scintigraphic localization with ^{123}I-MIBG is indicated (Fig. 15–6). This radiopharmaceutical agent accumulates preferentially in catecholamine-producing tumors; however, this procedure is not as sensitive as initially hoped (sensitivity, 80%; specificity, 99%).[86-88] ^{123}I-MIBG is superior to ^{131}I-MIBG because the photon energy allows single photon emission computed tomographic (SPECT) images. However, the ^{123}I-MIBG is not approved by the U.S. Food and Drug Administration (FDA) and must be done in an institutional review board approved protocol. Thyroid uptake of ^{123}I should be blocked with the administration of an iodide preparation (e.g., Lugol's solution or SSKI) starting 24 hours before injection and for a total of 5 days. In a study of 282 patients with catecholamine-secreting tumors that were surgically confirmed, the overall sensitivity was 89% for CT, 98% for MRI, and 81% for ^{131}I-MIBG.[87] If a typical (<10 cm) unilateral adrenal pheochromocytoma is found on CT or MRI, ^{123}I-MIBG scintigraphy is superfluous and the results may even confuse the clinician.[94,95] Whereas, if the adrenal pheochromocytoma is greater than 10 cm in diameter or if a paraganglioma is identified on CT or MRI, then ^{123}I-MIBG scintigraphy is indicated because the patient has increased risk of malignant disease and additional paragangliomas (see Fig. 15–6). It is important for the clinician to recognize the medications that may interfere with ^{123}I-MIBG uptake (e.g., tricyclic antidepressants, labetalol, calcium channel blockers) because they should be discontinued before imaging is performed (Table 15–7).[96]

TABLE 15–7 DRUGS THAT MAY INTERFERE WITH METAIODOBENZYLGUANIDINE (MIBG) UPTAKE

UPTAKE-1 INHIBITION (SHOULD BE STOPPED AT LEAST 48 HOURS BEFORE MIBG ADMINISTRATION)
Antiemetic (e.g., prochlorperazine) Antipsychotics (e.g., chlorpromazine, haloperidol) Cocaine Labetalol Phenylpropanolamine Tricyclic antidepressants (e.g., amitriptyline, amoxapine, desipramine, doxepin, imipramine, nortriptyline)
DEPLETION OF STORAGE VESICLE CONTENTS (SHOULD BE STOPPED AT LEAST 72 HOURS BEFORE MIBG ADMINISTRATION)
Amphetamines (dextroamphetamine, fenfluramine, phentermine) Dopamine Labetalol Reserpine Sympathomimetics (e.g., ephedrine, phenylephrine, pseudoephedrine, salbutamol, terbutaline)
INHIBITION OF VESICULAR MONOAMINE TRANSPORTERS (SHOULD BE STOPPED AT LEAST 72 HOURS BEFORE MIBG ADMINISTRATION)
Reserpine
UNKNOWN MECHANISM (SHOULD BE STOPPED AT LEAST 48 HOURS BEFORE MIBG ADMINISTRATION)
Calcium channel blockers (e.g., diltiazem, nicardipine, nifedipine, nimodipine, verapamil)

Other Localizing Procedures

Localizing procedures that also can be used, but are rarely required, include computer-assisted imaging of the chest, neck, and head. Other localizing studies, such as somatostatin receptor imaging with ^{111}In-DTPA-pentetreotide, may also be considered. Although somatostatin receptors are usually expressed in pheochromocytomas and paragangliomas,[97] the sensitivity of somatostatin receptor imaging with ^{111}In-DTPA-pentetreotide is low. Although positron emission tomography (PET) scanning

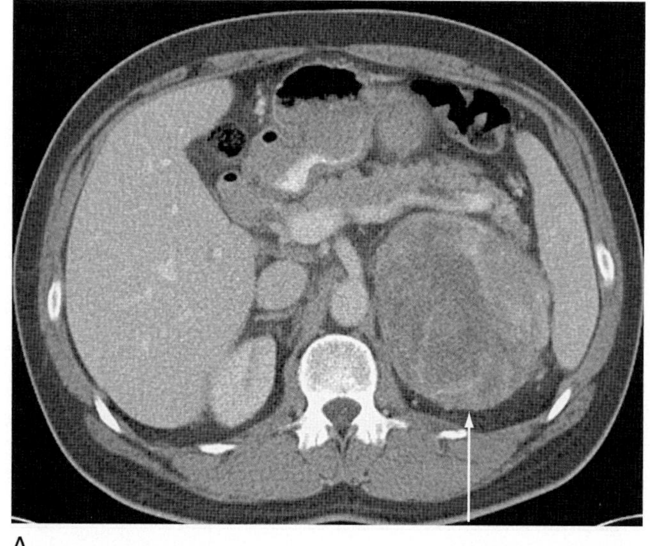

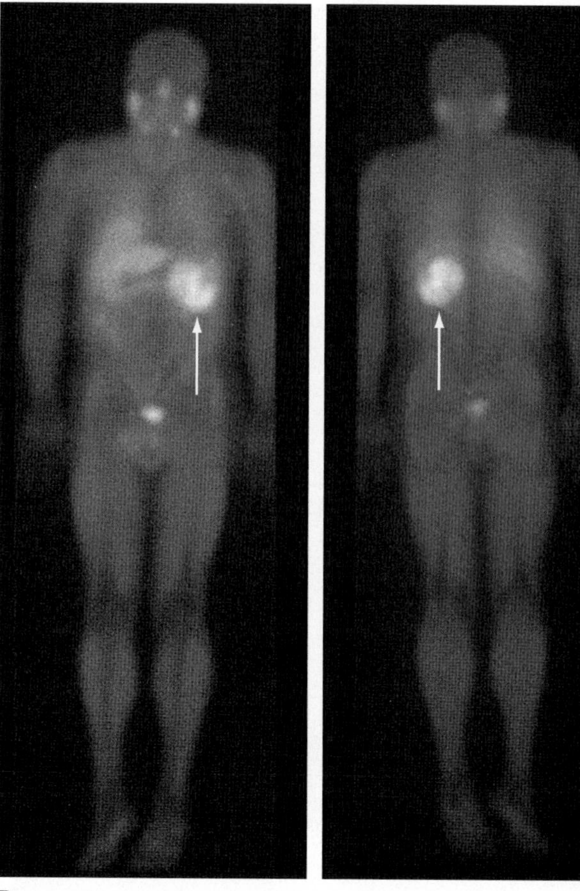

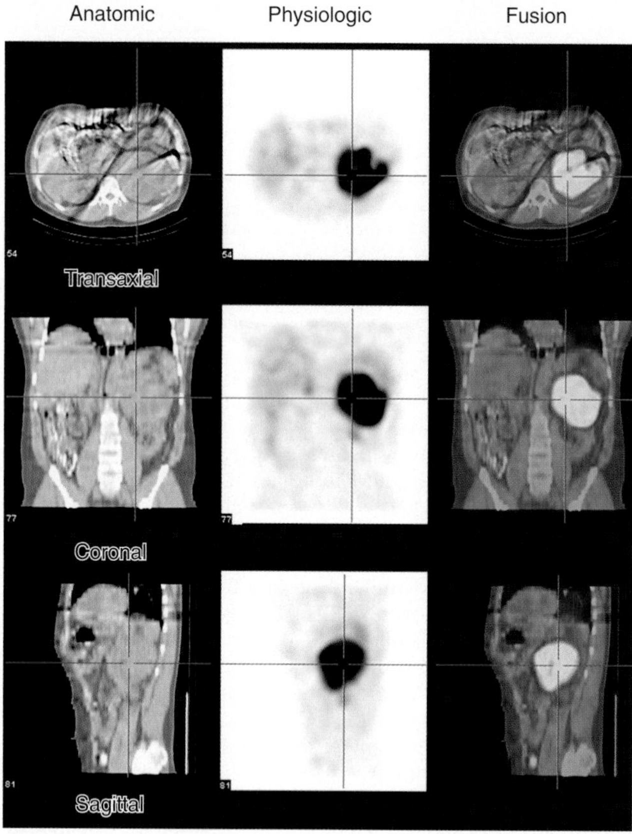

Figure 15–6 ▪ Computed tomography (CT) and ^{123}I-metaiodobenzylguanidine (^{123}I-MIBG) imaging of a 44-year-old man. He presented with a 9-year history of hypertension and recent onset of head throbbing, chest pressure, and abdominal pain. The 24-hour urine studies were abnormal: norepinephrine, 900 μg (normal <170); epinephrine, 28 μg (normal <35); dopamine, 468 μg (normal <700); and total metanephrines, 17,958 μg (normal <1000). **A,** Axial CT image with contrast shows a large partially vascular and partially necrotic left adrenal tumor (*arrow*). **B,** ^{123}I-MIBG whole body scan shows a large focus of increased radiotracer uptake in the left upper abdomen (*arrow*) that corresponds to the mass seen on the CT image; no other abnormal uptake is seen. **C,** ^{123}I-MIBG SPECT fusion CT images correlates the images seen on CT (anatomic) with those seen on ^{123}I-MIBG (physiologic) in the axial, coronal, and sagittal planes. After α- and β-adrenergic blockade, a 13.5 × 12 × 9-cm 680-g pheochromocytoma was removed.

with ^{18}F-fluorodeoxyglucose (FDG) or ^{11}C-hydroxyephedrine or 6-[^{18}F]fluorodopamine can identify paragangliomas,[86,88] these expensive techniques probably should be reserved for identifying sites of metastatic disease in patients with negative ^{123}I-MIBG scintigraphic results. Selective venous sampling for catecholamines is usually misleading and should be avoided.

Treatment

The treatment of choice for pheochromocytoma is complete surgical resection. Surgical survival rates are 98% to 100% and are highly dependent on the skill of the endocrinologist–endocrine surgeon–anesthesiologist team.[34,98] The most common adverse event following surgery is sustained hypertension. Careful preoperative pharmacologic preparation is crucial for successful treatment.[99] Most catecholamine-secreting tumors are benign and can be totally excised. Tumor excision usually cures hypertension.

Preoperative Management

Some form of preoperative pharmacologic preparation is indicated for all patients with catecholamine-secreting neoplasms.

However, no randomized controlled trials have compared the different approaches. Combined α- and β-adrenergic blockade is one approach to control blood pressure and prevent intraoperative hypertensive crises.[22] α-Adrenergic blockade should be started 7 to 10 days preoperatively to normalize blood pressure and expand the contracted blood volume. A longer duration of preoperative α-adrenergic blockade is indicated in patients with recent myocardial infarction, catecholamine cardiomyopathy, and catecholamine-induced vasculitis. Blood pressure should be monitored with the patient in the seated and standing positions twice daily. Target blood pressure is less than 120/80 mm Hg (seated), with systolic blood pressure greater than 90 mm Hg (standing); both targets should be modified on the basis of the patient's age and comorbid disease. On the second or third day of α-adrenergic blockade, patients are encouraged to start a diet high in sodium content (≥5000 mg daily) because of the catecholamine-induced volume contraction and the orthostasis associated with α-adrenergic blockade. This degree of volume expansion may be contraindicated in patients with congestive heart failure or renal insufficiency. After adequate α-adrenergic blockade has been achieved, β-adrenergic blockade is initiated, which typically occurs 2 to 3 days preoperatively.

α-Adrenergic Blockade

Phenoxybenzamine is the preferred drug for preoperative preparation to control blood pressure and arrhythmia. It is an irreversible, long-acting, nonspecific α-adrenergic blocking agent. The initial dosage is 10 mg once or twice daily, and the dose is increased by 10 to 20 mg in divided doses every 2 to 3 days as needed to control blood pressure and spells (Table 15–8). The final dosage of phenoxybenzamine is typically between 20 and 100 mg daily. The patient should be warned about the orthostasis and marked fatigue that occur in almost all patients. With their more favorable side-effect profiles, selective α_1-adrenergic blocking agents (e.g., prazosin, terazosin, or doxazosin) are preferable to phenoxybenzamine when long-term pharmacologic treatment is indicated (e.g., for metastatic pheochromocytoma). However, treatment with these agents is not routinely used preoperatively because of incomplete α-adrenergic blockade.

β-Adrenergic Blockade

The β-adrenergic antagonist should be administered only after α-adrenergic blockade is effective because with β-adrenergic blockade alone hypertension may be more severe from the unopposed α-adrenergic stimulation. Preoperative β-adrenergic blockade is indicated to control the tachycardia associated with both the high concentrations of circulating catecholamines and the α-adrenergic blockade. The clinician should exercise caution if the patient is asthmatic or has congestive heart failure. Chronic catecholamine excess can produce a myocardiopathy[30] that may become evident with the initiation of β-adrenergic blockade, resulting in acute pulmonary edema. Therefore, when the β-adrenergic blocker is administered, it should be used cautiously and at a low dose. For example, a patient is usually given 10 mg of propranolol every 6 hours to start. On the second day of treatment, the β-adrenergic blockade (assuming the patient tolerates the drug) is converted to a single long-acting dose. The dose is then increased as necessary to control the tachycardia (goal heart rate is 60 to 80 beats per minute).

Catecholamine Synthesis Inhibitor

α-Methyl-paratyrosine (metyrosine) should be used with caution and only when other agents have been ineffective or in patients where tumor manipulation or destruction (e.g., radiofrequency ablation of metastatic sites) will be marked. Although some centers advocate that this agent should be used routinely preoperatively, most reserve it primarily for patients who cannot be treated with the typical combined α- and β-adrenergic blockade

TABLE 15–8 ORALLY ADMINISTERED DRUGS USED TO TREAT PHEOCHROMOCYTOMA

Drug	Dosage, mg/day* Initial (maximum)	Side Effects
		α-ADRENERGIC BLOCKING AGENTS
Phenoxybenzamine	20† (100)†	Postural hypotension, tachycardia, miosis, nasal congestion, diarrhea, inhibition of ejaculation, fatigue
Prazosin	1 (20)‡	First-dose effect, dizziness, drowsiness, headache, fatigue, palpitations, nausea
Terazosin	1 (20)†	First-dose effect, asthenia, blurred vision, dizziness, nasal congestion, nausea, peripheral edema, palpitations, somnolence
Doxazosin	1 (20)	First-dose effect, orthostasis, peripheral edema, fatigue, somnolence
		COMBINED α- AND β-ADRENERGIC BLOCKING AGENT
Labetalol	200† (1200)†	Dizziness, fatigue, nausea, nasal congestion, impotence
		CALCIUM CHANNEL BLOCKERS
Nicardipine sustained release	30† (120)†	Edema, dizziness, headache, flushing, nausea, dyspepsia
		CATECHOLAMINE SYNTHESIS INHIBITOR
α-Methyl-p-L-tyrosine (Metyrosine)	1000‡ (4000)‡	Sedation, diarrhea, anxiety, nightmares, crystalluria, galactorrhea, extrapyramidal symptoms

*Given once daily unless otherwise indicated.
†Given in two doses daily.
‡Given in three or four doses daily.

protocol because of cardiopulmonary reasons. Metyrosine inhibits catecholamine synthesis by blocking the enzyme tyrosine hydroxylase.[100] The side effects of metyrosine can be disabling, and with long-term therapy, they include sedation, depression, diarrhea, anxiety, nightmares, crystalluria and urolithiasis, galactorrhea, and extrapyramidal signs. Metyrosine may be added to α- and β-adrenergic blockade when the resection will be difficult (e.g., malignant paraganglioma) or if destructive therapy is planned (e.g., radiofrequency ablation of hepatic metastases). Our typical protocol with short-term preprocedure preparation is to start with metyrosine 250 mg every 6 hours on day 1, then 500 mg every 6 hours on day 2, then 750 mg every 6 hours on day 3, and 1000 mg every 6 hours on the day before the procedure, with the last dose the morning of the procedure. With this short-course therapy, the main side effect is hypersomnolence.

Calcium Channel Blockers

Calcium channel blockers, which block norepinephrine-mediated calcium transport into vascular smooth muscle, have been used successfully at several medical centers to preoperatively prepare patients with pheochromocytoma.[101-103] Nicardipine is the most commonly used calcium channel blocker in this setting; the starting dose is 30 mg twice daily of the sustained release preparation (see Table 15–8). It is given orally to control blood pressure preoperatively and is given as an intravenous infusion intraoperatively (Table 15–9). Although there is less collective experience with calcium channel blockers than with α- and β-adrenergic blockade, when calcium channel blockers are used as the primary mode of antihypertensive therapy, they may be just as effective.[101,102] Clearly, the exclusive use of calcium channel blockers for the perioperative management of patients with catecholamine-secreting tumors does not prevent all hemodynamic changes; however, its use has been associated with low morbidity and mortality.[102] The main role for this class of drugs may be either to supplement the combined α- and β-adrenergic blockade protocol when blood pressure control is inadequate or to replace the adrenergic blockade protocol in patients with intolerable side effects.

Acute Hypertensive Crises

Acute hypertensive crises may occur before or during an operation, and they should be treated intravenously with sodium nitroprusside, phentolamine, or nicardipine. Sodium nitroprusside is an ideal vasodilator for intraoperative management of hypertensive episodes because of its rapid onset of action and short duration of effect. It is administered as an intravenous infusion at 0.5 to 5.0 μg/kg of body weight per minute and adjusted every few minutes for target blood pressure response; to keep the steady-state thiocyanate concentration below 1 mmol/L, the rate of a prolonged infusion should be no more than 3 μg/kg per minute (see Table 15–9). Phentolamine is a short-acting, nonselective α-adrenergic blocker available in lyophilized form in 5-mg vials. An initial test dose of 1 mg is administered and, if necessary, followed by repeat 5-mg boluses or continuous infusion (see Table 15–9). The response to phentolamine is maximal in 2 to 3 minutes after a bolus injection and lasts 10 to 15 minutes. Nicardipine can be started at an infusion rate of 5 mg/hr and titrated for blood pressure control (the infusion rate may be increased by 2.5 mg/hr every 15 minutes up to a maximum of 15.0 mg/hr) (see Table 15–9).

Anesthesia and Surgery

Surgical resection of a catecholamine-secreting tumor is a high-risk surgical procedure, and an experienced surgeon-anesthesiologist team is required. The last oral doses of α- and β-adrenergic blockers can be administered early in the morning on the day of the operation. Fentanyl, ketamine, and morphine should be avoided because they potentially can stimulate catecholamine release from a pheochromocytoma.[103] Also, parasympathetic nervous system blockade with atropine should be avoided because of the associated tachycardia. Anesthesia may be induced with intravenous injection of propofol, etomidate, or barbiturates in combination with synthetic opioids.[103] Most anesthetic gases can be used, but halothane and desflurane should be avoided. Cardiovascular and hemodynamic variables must be monitored closely. Continuous measurement of intraarterial pressure and heart rhythm is required. If the patient has

TABLE 15–9 INTRAVENOUSLY ADMINISTERED DRUGS USED TO TREAT PHEOCHROMOCYTOMA

Agent	Dosage Range
	FOR HYPERTENSION
Phentolamine	1 mg IV test dose, then 2- to 5-mg IV boluses as needed or continuous infusion
Nitroprusside	Infusion rates of 2 μg/kg of body weight per minute are suggested as safe, while rates greater than 4 μg/kg per minute may lead to cyanide toxicity within 3 hours. Doses exceeding 10 μg/kg per minute are rarely required and the maximal dose should not exceed 800 μg/min
Nicardipine	Initiate therapy at 5.0 mg/hr and the infusion rate may be increased by 2.5 mg/hr every 15 minutes up to a maximum of 15.0 mg/hr
	FOR CARDIAC ARRHYTHMIA
Lidocaine	Initiate therapy with a bolus of 1 to 1.5 mg/kg (75 to 100 mg); additional boluses of 0.5 to 0.75 mg/kg (25 to 50 mg) can be given every 5 to 10 minutes if needed up to a maximum of 3 mg/kg. Loading is followed by a maintenance infusion of 2 to 4 mg/min (30 to 50 μg/kg per minute) adjusted for effect and settings of altered metabolism (e.g., heart failure, liver congestion) and as guided by blood level monitoring.
Esmolol	An initial loading dose of 0.5 mg/kg is infused over a minute duration, followed by a maintenance infusion of 0.05 mg/kg per minute for the next 4 minutes. Depending on the desired ventricular response, the maintenance infusion may then be continued at 0.05 mg/kg per minute or increased stepwise (e.g., by 0.1 mg/kg per minute increments to a maximum of 0.2 mg/kg per minute) with each step being maintained for ≥4 minutes.

IV, Intravenous.

congestive heart failure or decreased cardiac reserve, monitoring of pulmonary capillary wedge pressure is indicated. The preoperative and perioperative treatment approach outlined here is the same for adults and children.[104,105]

In the past, an anterior midline abdominal surgical approach was generally used for resecting adrenal pheochromocytoma. However, the laparoscopic approach to the adrenal gland is currently the procedure of choice for patients with solitary intraadrenal pheochromocytomas less than 8 cm in diameter.[106] In a series of 39 patients with pheochromocytoma who had laparoscopic adrenalectomy, the mean hospitalization was 1.7 days[107] as opposed to the typical 5 to 7 days for open laparotomy. If the pheochromocytoma is in the adrenal gland, the entire gland should be removed. Laparoscopic adrenalectomy for pheochromocytoma should be converted to open adrenalectomy for difficult dissection, invasion, adhesions, or surgeon inexperience.[108] If the tumor is malignant, as much of the tumor should be removed as possible. If a bilateral adrenalectomy is planned preoperatively, the patient should receive glucocorticoid stress coverage while awaiting transfer to the operating room. Glucocorticoid coverage should be initiated in the operating room if unexpected bilateral adrenalectomy is necessary. Cortical-sparing bilateral adrenalectomies have been used to treat patients with VHL disease.

An anterior midline abdominal surgical approach is indicated for abdominal paragangliomas. The midline abdomen should be inspected carefully. Paragangliomas of the neck, chest, and urinary bladder require specialized approaches. "Unresectable" cardiac pheochromocytomas may require cardiac transplantation.

Hypotension may occur during and after surgical resection of the pheochromocytoma, and it should be treated with fluids and colloids and then intravenous pressor agents if necessary. Postoperative hypotension is less frequent in patients who have had adequate preoperative α-adrenergic blockade. If both adrenal glands were manipulated during surgery, adrenocortical insufficiency should be considered as a potential cause of postoperative hypotension. Because hypoglycemia can occur in the immediate postoperative period, blood glucose levels should be monitored and fluid given intravenously should contain 5% dextrose.

Blood pressure is usually normal by the time of hospital discharge. Some patients remain hypertensive for up to 4 to 8 weeks postoperatively. Longstanding, persistent hypertension does occur and may be related to accidental ligation of a polar renal artery, resetting of baroreceptors, hemodynamic changes, structural changes of the blood vessels, altered sensitivity of the vessels to pressor substances, functional or structural renal changes, or coincident primary hypertension.

Long-Term Postoperative Follow-Up

Approximately 1 to 2 weeks after surgery, fractionated catecholamines and metanephrines should be measured by collecting a 24-hour urine specimen. If the levels are normal, the resection of the pheochromocytoma should be considered complete. The survival rate after removal of a benign pheochromocytoma is nearly that of age-matched and sex-matched normal controls. Increased levels of catecholamines and metanephrines detected postoperatively are consistent with residual tumor due to either a second primary lesion or occult metastases. If bilateral adrenalectomy was performed, lifelong glucocorticoid and mineralocorticoid replacement therapy is prescribed. Twenty-four–hour urinary excretion of fractionated catecholamines and metanephrines or fractionated plasma metanephrines should be checked annually for life. Annual biochemical testing assesses for metastatic disease, tumor recurrence in the adrenal bed, or delayed appearance of multiple primary tumors. Recurrence rates are highest for patients with familial disease, right-sided adrenal pheochromocytoma, or a paraganglioma.[109] Follow-up CT or MRI is not needed unless the metanephrine and/or catecholamine levels become elevated or the original tumor was associated with minimal catecholamine excess.

Consider genetic testing for patients with one or more of the following: family history of pheochromocytoma, paraganglioma, or any sign that suggests a genetic cause (e.g., retinal angiomas, axillary freckling, café au lait spots, cerebellar tumor, MTC, hyperparathyroidism). In addition, all first-degree relatives of a patient with pheochromocytoma or paraganglioma should have biochemical testing (e.g., 24-hour urine for fractionated metanephrines and catecholamines). If mutation testing in a patient is positive, first-degree relatives (patient's parents, siblings, and children) should be offered genetic testing.

Malignant Pheochromocytoma and Paraganglioma

Distinguishing between benign and malignant catecholamine-secreting tumors is difficult on the basis of clinical, biochemical, or histopathologic characteristics. Malignancy is rare in patients with an adrenal familial syndrome, but is common in those with familial paraganglioma caused by mutations in *SDHB.* Patients with *SDHB* mutations are more likely to develop malignant disease and nonparaganglioma neoplasms (e.g., renal cell carcinoma).[54,57,58] Although the 5-year survival rate for patients with malignant pheochromocytoma is less than 50%, the prognosis is variable: approximately 50% of patients have an indolent form of the disease, with a life expectancy of more than 20 years, and the other 50% of patients have rapidly progressive disease, with death occurring within 1 to 3 years after diagnosis. The clinician should first assess the pace of the malignant disease and target the level of therapy to the aggressiveness of the tumor behavior. A multimodality multidisciplinary individualized approach is indicated to control catecholamine-dependent symptoms, local mass effect symptoms from the tumor, and overall tumor burden. Long-term pharmacologic therapy for the patient with metastatic pheochromocytoma is similar to that outlined for the preoperative preparation of the patient with a catecholamine-secreting tumor.

Metastatic sites include local tissue invasion, liver, bone, lung, omentum, and lymph nodes. Metastatic lesions should be resected if possible to decrease tumor burden. Skeletal metastatic lesions that are painful or threaten structural function can be treated with external radiotherapy or cryoablation. Thrombotic therapy for large unresectable liver metastases and radiofrequency ablation for small liver metastases are options to be considered. In selected cases, long-acting octreotide has been beneficial.[111] Because of the risk of massive catecholamine release, ablative therapy should be performed with great caution and only at centers with experience with these techniques; in addition to treatment with α- and β-adrenergic blockade, patients are usually treated with α-methyl-paratyrosine (metyrosine) before the procedure. External radiotherapy can also be used to treat unresectable soft tissue lesions.

Local tumor irradiation with therapeutic doses of ^{131}I-MIBG has produced partial and temporary responses in approximately one third of patients.[7,8,110] If the tumor is considered aggressive and the patient's quality of life is affected, combination chemotherapy may be considered. In a nonrandomized, single-arm trial, the efficacy of chemotherapy (CVD protocol: cyclophosphamide 750 mg/m^2 body surface area on day 1; vincristine, 1.4 mg/m^2 on day 1; and dacarbazine 600 mg/m^2 on days 1 and 2 and every 21 days) was studied in 14 patients with malignant pheochromocytoma.[112] The combination CVD protocol produced a complete and partial response rate of 57% (median duration, 21 months; range, 7 to more than 34 months). Complete and partial biochemical responses were seen in 79% of patients (median duration, more than 22 months; range, 6 to more than 35 months). All responding patients had objective improvement in performance status and blood pressure. CVD chemotherapy can be continued until the patient develops new lesions or there is a significant (e.g., >25%) increase in size of known tumor sites. Because CVD chemotherapy may induce massive catecholamine release, it is important that the patient is optimally α- and β-blocked just as if the patient were being prepared for surgery. In addition, the first cycle of CVD should be completed in the hospital and under close medical observation. Management of a patient who has malignant pheochromocytoma can be frustrating because curative options are limited. Clearly, innovative prospective protocols are needed to seek new treatment options for this neoplasm.[113]

Pheochromocytoma in Pregnancy

Pheochromocytoma in pregnancy can cause the death of both the fetus and the mother. The approach to the biochemical diagnosis is the same as for the nonpregnant patient. MRI is the preferred imaging modality and ^{123}I-MIBG is contraindicated. The treatment of hypertensive crises is the same as for nonpregnant patients except that use of nitroprusside should be avoided. Although the most appropriate management is debated,[114] adrenal pheochromocytomas should be removed promptly if diagnosed during the first two trimesters of pregnancy. The preoperative preparation is the same as for a nonpregnant patient. If the pregnancy is in the third trimester, one operation is recommended to perform a cesarean section and remove the adrenal pheochromocytoma at the same time. Spontaneous labor and delivery should be avoided. The management of catecholamine-secreting paragangliomas in pregnancy may require modification of these guidelines depending on tumor location.

RENIN-ANGIOTENSIN-ALDOSTERONE SYSTEM

The components of the renin-angiotensin-aldosterone system are shown in Figure 15–7.[115] Aldosterone is secreted from the zona glomerulosa under the control of three primary factors: angiotensin II, potassium, and ACTH. The secretion of aldosterone is restricted to the zona glomerulosa because of zonal-specific expression of aldosterone synthase (CYP11B2) (see Chapter 14). Dopamine, atrial natriuretic peptide, and heparin inhibit aldosterone secretion.

Renin and Angiotensin

Renin is an enzyme produced primarily in the juxtaglomerular apparatus of the kidney; it is stored in granules and released in response to specific secretagogues. The protein consists of 340 amino acids, of which the first 43 are a prosegment cleaved to produce the active enzyme. The release of renin into the circulation is the rate-limiting step in the renin-angiotensin-aldosterone system. Renal renin release is controlled by four factors: (1) the macula densa, a specialized group of distal convoluted tubular cells that function as chemoreceptors for monitoring the sodium and chloride loads present in the distal tubule; (2) juxtaglomerular cells acting as pressure transducers that sense stretch of the afferent arteriolar wall and thus renal perfusion pressure; (3) the sympathetic nervous system, which modifies the release of renin, particularly in response to upright posture in humans; and (4) humoral factors, including potassium, angiotensin II, and atrial natriuretic peptides. Thus, renin release is maximized in conditions of low renal perfusion pressure or low tubular sodium content (e.g., renal artery stenosis, hemorrhage, dehydration). Renin release is suppressed by elevated perfusion pressure at the kidney (hypertension) and high-sodium diets. Renin release is increased directly by hypokalemia and decreased by hyperkalemia.

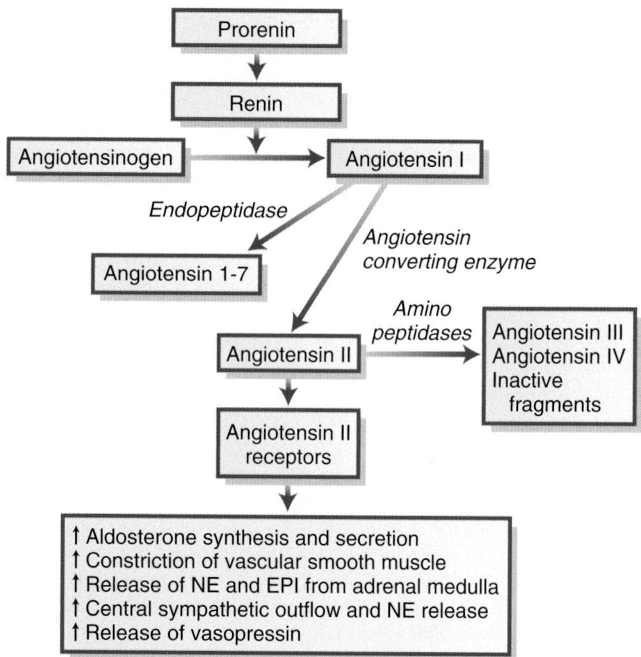

Figure 15–7 ▪ Components of the renin-angiotensin system. (Adapted and redrawn from Williams GH, Chao J, Chao L. Kidney hormones. In Conn PM, Melmed S, eds. Endocrinology: Basic and Clinical Principles. Totowa, NJ: Humana Press, 1997:393-404.) EPI, epinephrine; NE, nor epinephrine.

Angiotensinogen, an α_2-globulin synthesized in the liver, is the only known substrate for renin and is broken down into the angiotensin peptides. The protein consists of 485 amino acids, 33 of which constitute a presegment that is cleaved after secretion. The action of renin on angiotensinogen produces angiotensin I. Angiotensin I is composed of the first 10 amino acid sequence following the presegment and does not appear to have biologic activity. Angiotensin II, the main form of biologically active angiotensin, is formed by cleavage of the two carboxyl-terminal peptides of angiotensin I by angiotensin-converting enzyme (ACE) (see Fig. 15–7). ACE is localized to cell membranes in the lung and intracellular granules in certain tissues that produce angiotensin II. Amino peptidase A can remove the amino-terminal aspartic acid to produce the heptapeptide, angiotensin III. Angiotensin II and angiotensin III have equivalent efficacy in promoting aldosterone secretion and modifying renal blood flow. The half-life in the circulation of angiotensin II is short (<60 seconds). Elements of the renin-angiotensin-aldosterone system are present in the adrenal, the kidneys, the heart, and the brain. For example, the adrenal glomerulosa cells contain the proteins needed to produce and secrete angiotensin II. Other tissues contain one or more components of the renin-angiotensin system and require other cells or circulating components, or both, to generate angiotensin II.

Angiotensin II functions through the angiotensin receptor to maintain normal extracellular volume and blood pressure by (1) increasing aldosterone secretion from the zona glomerulosa by increasing transcription of CYP11B2, (2) constriction of vascular smooth muscle, thereby increasing blood pressure and reducing renal blood flow, (3) release of norepinephrine and epinephrine from the adrenal medulla, (4) enhancement of the activity of the sympathetic nervous system by increasing central sympathetic outflow, thereby increasing norepinephrine discharge from sympathetic nerve terminals, and (5) promotion of the release of vasopressin.

Aldosterone

Approximately 50% to 70% of aldosterone circulates bound to either albumin or weakly to corticosteroid-binding globulin; 30% to 50% of total plasma aldosterone is free. Thus, aldosterone has a relatively short half-life of 15 to 20 minutes. In the liver, aldosterone is rapidly inactivated to tetrahydroaldosterone. The classic functions of aldosterone are regulation of extracellular volume and control of potassium homeostasis. These effects are mediated by binding of free aldosterone to the mineralocorticoid receptor in the cytosol of epithelial cells, principally in the kidney. Mineralocorticoid receptors have a tissue-specific expression. For example, the tissues with the highest concentrations of these receptors are the distal nephron, colon, and hippocampus. Lower levels of mineralocorticoid receptors are found in the rest of the gastrointestinal tract and heart. Transport to the nucleus and binding to specific binding domains on targeted genes leads to their increased expression. Aldosterone-regulated kinase appears to be a key intermediary, and its increased expression leads to modification of the apical sodium channel, resulting in increased sodium ion transport across the cell membrane (see Chapter 14). The increased luminal negativity augments tubular secretion of potassium by the tubular cells and hydrogen ion by the interstitial cells. Glucocorticoids and mineralocorticoids bind equally to the mineralocorticoid receptor. Specificity of action is provided in many tissues by the presence of a glucocorticoid-degrading enzyme, 11β-hydroxysteroid dehydrogenase, which prevents glucocorticoids from interacting with the receptor (see Chapter 14). Mineralocorticoid "escape" refers to the counterregulatory mechanisms that are manifested after 3 to 5 days of excessive mineralocorticoid administration. Several mechanisms contribute to this escape, including renal hemodynamic factors and increased level of atrial natriuretic peptide.

In addition to the classic genomic actions mediated by aldosterone binding to cytosolic receptors, mineralocorticoids have acute, nongenomic actions due to activation of an unidentified cell surface receptor. This action involves a G protein signaling pathway and probably a modification of the sodium-hydrogen exchange activity. This effect has been demonstrated in both epithelial and nonepithelial cells.[116]

Aldosterone has additional, nonclassic effects primarily on nonepithelial cells.[117] These actions, although probably genomic and therefore mediated by activation of the cytosolic mineralocorticoid receptor, do not include modification of sodium-potassium balance. Aldosterone-mediated actions include the expression of several collagen genes; genes controlling tissue growth factors, such as transforming growth factor β, and plasminogen activator inhibitor type 1; or genes mediating inflammation.[118] The resultant actions lead to microangiopathy, necrosis (acutely), and fibrosis in various tissues such as the heart, the vasculature, and the kidney.[117] Increased levels of aldosterone are not necessary to cause this damage; an imbalance between the volume or sodium balance state and the level of aldosterone appears to be the critical factor.[117]

The action of angiotensin II on aldosterone involves a negative feedback loop that also includes extracellular fluid volume (Fig. 15–8).[119] The major function of this feedback loop is to modify sodium homeostasis and, secondarily, to regulate blood pressure. Thus, sodium restriction activates the renin-angiotensin-aldosterone axis. The effects of angiotensin II on both the adrenal cortex and the renal vasculature promote renal sodium conservation. Conversely, with suppression of renin release and suppression of the level of circulating angiotensin, aldosterone secretion is reduced and renal blood flow is increased, thereby promoting sodium loss. The renin-angiotensin-aldosterone loop is very sensitive to dietary sodium intake. Sodium excess enhances the renal and peripheral vasculature responsiveness and reduces the adrenal responsiveness to angiotensin II. Sodium restriction has the opposite effect. Thus, sodium intake modifies target tissue responsiveness to angiotensin II, a fine-tuning that appears to be critical to maintaining normal sodium homeostasis without a chronic effect on blood pressure.

Excess aldosterone secretion causes hypertension through two main mechanisms: (1) mineralocorticoid-induced expansion of plasma and extracellular fluid volume, and (2) increase in total peripheral vascular resistance.

PRIMARY ALDOSTERONISM

Hypertension, suppressed plasma renin activity (PRA), and increased aldosterone excretion characterize the syndrome of primary aldosteronism, first described in 1955.[120] Aldosterone-

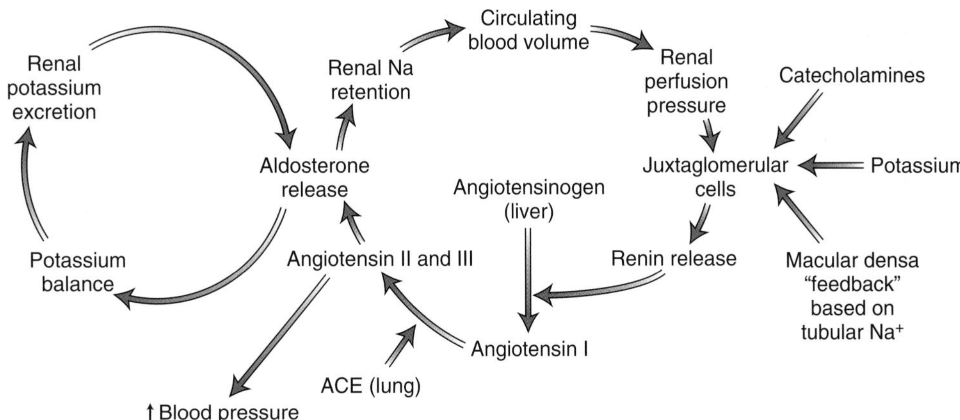

Figure 15–8 ▪ Renin-angiotensin-aldosterone and potassium-aldosterone negative feedback loops. Aldosterone production is determined by input from each loop. *ACE*, Angiotensin-converting enzyme; *Na*$^+$, sodium. (Adapted and redrawn from Williams GH, Dluhy RG. Diseases of the adrenal cortex. In Braunwald E, Fauci AD, Kasper D, et al, eds. Harrison's Principles of Internal Medicine, 15th ed. New York: McGraw-Hill, 2001:2087.)

TABLE 15–10 ADRENOCORTICAL CAUSES OF HYPERTENSION

LOW RENIN AND HIGH ALDOSTERONE
Primary Aldosteronism
Aldosterone-producing adenoma (APA)—35% of cases
Bilateral idiopathic hyperplasia (IHA)—60% of cases
Primary (unilateral) adrenal hyperplasia—2% of cases
Aldosterone-producing adrenocortical carcinoma—<1% of cases
Familial Hyperaldosteronism (FH)
Glucocorticoid-remediable aldosteronism (FH type I)—<1% of cases
FH type II (APA or IHA)—<2% of cases
Ectopic aldosterone-producing adenoma or carcinoma—<0.1% of cases
LOW RENIN AND LOW ALDOSTERONE
Hyperdeoxycorticosteronism
Congenital adrenal hyperplasia
11β-Hydroxylase deficiency
17α-Hydroxylase deficiency
Deoxycorticosterone-producing tumor
Primary cortisol resistance
Apparent Mineralocorticoid Excess (AME)/11β-Hydroxysteroid Dehydrogenase Deficiency
Genetic
Type 1 AME
Type 2 AME
Acquired
Licorice or carbenoxolone ingestion (type 1 AME)
Cushing's syndrome (type 2 AME)
Cushing's Syndrome
Exogenous glucocorticoid administration—most common cause
Endogenous
ACTH-dependent—85% of cases (pituitary, ectopic)
ACTH-independent—15% of cases (unilateral adrenal disease, bilateral adrenal disease: massive macronodular hyperplasia [rare]; primary pigmented nodular adrenal disease [rare])

ACTH, Adrenocorticotropic hormone.

producing adenoma (APA) and bilateral idiopathic hyperaldosteronism (IHA) are the most common subtypes of primary aldosteronism (Table 15–10). A much less common form, unilateral hyperplasia or primary adrenal hyperplasia (PAH), is caused by micronodular or macronodular hyperplasia of the zona glomerulosa of predominantly one adrenal gland. Familial hyperaldosteronism (FH) is also rare and two types have been described: FH type I and FH type II. FH type I, or glucocorticoid-remediable aldosteronism (GRA), is autosomal dominant in inheritance and associated with variable degrees of hyperaldosteronism, high levels of hybrid steroids (e.g., 18-hydroxycortisol and 18-oxocortisol), and suppression with exogenous glucocorticoids.[121] FH type II refers to the familial occurrence of APA or IHA or both.[122]

History

In his Presidential address at the Annual Meeting of the Central Society for Clinical Research, Chicago, Illinois, October, 29, 1954, Dr. Jerome W. Conn stated, "I have prepared no comprehensive review of my personal philosophy of clinical investigation. Instead, I plan to make a scientific report to you about a clinical syndrome, the investigation of which has been most exciting to me since I initiated it in April of this year."[120] Conn, a Professor of Medicine at the University of Michigan, had been active in government-funded research on the mechanisms of human acclimatization to humid heat. He established that the body's acclimatization response was to rapidly diminish renal salt and water loss and abruptly curtail the salt content of body sweat and saliva, and he suggested it was due to increased adrenocortical function with elaboration of salt-retaining steroids. He also showed that intramuscular administration of deoxycorticosterone acetate (DOCA) produced similar changes in the electrolyte composition of urine, sweat, and saliva.

In April 1954, he was asked to see M.W., a 34-year-old woman with a 7-year history of muscle spasms, temporary paralysis, tetany, and weakness and a 4-year history of hypertension. She was found to have a blood pressure of 176/104 mm Hg, severe hypokalemia (1.6 to 2.5 mEq/L), mild hypernatremia (146 to 151 mEq/L), and alkalosis (serum pH 7.62). Because there were no signs or symptoms of glucocorticoid or androgen excess, Conn suspected, based on his past research, that M.W.'s clinical presentation could result from excess secretion of the adrenal salt-retaining corticoid. Conn studied M.W. in the Metabolism Research Unit for 227 days. Using Streeten's bioassay technique to measure sodium retention in adrenalectomized rats after intraperitoneal injection of human urine, M.W. averaged 1333 μg DOCA equivalent per day compared with normotensive controls at 61.4 μg/d. In his presidential address, Conn stated, "It is believed that these studies delineate a new clinical syndrome which is designated temporarily as primary aldosteronism." (Note: the word "temporarily" was used because aldosterone was yet to be measured in any human bodily fluid.)[120] Conn planned for a bilateral adrenalectomy on December 10, 1954. In the 1995 Gittler and Fajans retelling of the surgical scene: "To the immense delight of Conn and those in the operating room, the surgeon, Dr. William Baum, encountered a right 13-g adrenal tumor which was removed while leaving the contralateral gland intact. The patient's postoperative studies showed an almost total reversal of the preoperative metabolic and clinical abnormalities. Conn had achieved irrefutable proof of the validity of his investigative conclusions and established for the first time the relationship among adrenal aldosterone-producing tumors, hypertension, and hypokalemia. A new era had arrived in the study of hypertension and adrenal mineralocorticoids."[123]

By 1964, Conn had collected 145 cases,[124] and he suggested that up to 20% of patients with essential hypertension might have primary aldosteronism.[125] This suggestion was downplayed by most as a gross overestimate.[126,127] Later, Conn decreased his predicted prevalence of primary aldosteronism to 10% of hypertensives[128]; a prediction that was substantiated nearly 40 years later.

Prevalence

In the past, clinicians would not consider the diagnosis of primary aldosteronism unless the patient presented with spontaneous hypokalemia, and then the diagnostic evaluation would require discontinuing antihypertensive medications for at least 2 weeks. The spontaneous "hypokalemia/no antihypertensive drug" diagnostic approach resulted in predicted prevalence rates of less than 0.5% of hypertensive patients.[126,127,129-133] However, it is now recognized that most patients with primary aldosteronism are not hypokalemic[134,135] and that screening can be completed with a simple blood test (plasma aldosterone concentration [PAC]-to-plasma renin activity [PRA] ratio) while the patient is taking antihypertensive drugs.[136-139] Using the PAC/

PRA ratio as a case-finding test, followed by aldosterone suppression confirmatory testing, has resulted in much higher prevalence estimates (5% to 13% of all patients with hypertension) for primary aldosteronism.[139-145]

Clinical Presentation

The diagnosis of primary aldosteronism is usually made in patients who are in the third to sixth decade of life. Few symptoms are specific to the syndrome. Patients with marked hypokalemia may have muscle weakness and cramping, headaches, palpitations, polydipsia, polyuria, nocturia, or a combination of these. Periodic paralysis is a very rare presentation in white patients, but it is not an infrequent presentation in patients of Asian decent.[146] For example, in a series of 50 patients with APA reported from Hong Kong, 21 (42%) presented with periodic paralysis.[146] Another rare presentation can be tetany associated with the decrease in ionized calcium with marked hypokalemic alkalosis. The polyuria and nocturia are a result of hypokalemia-induced renal concentrating defect and the presentation is frequently mistaken for prostatism in men. There are no specific physical findings. Edema is not a common finding because of "mineralocorticoid escape." The degree of hypertension is usually moderate to severe and may be resistant to usual pharmacologic treatments.[147] In the first 262 cases of primary aldosteronism diagnosed at Mayo Clinic (1957-1986), the highest blood pressure was 260/155 mm Hg; the mean (±SD) was 184/112 ± 28/16 mm Hg.[147] Patients with APA tend to have higher blood pressures than those with IHA.[148] Hypokalemia is frequently absent; thus, all patients with hypertension are candidates for this disorder. In other patients, the hypokalemia only becomes evident with addition of a potassium-wasting diuretic (e.g., hydrochlorothiazide, furosemide). In patients with chronic hypokalemia, deep-seated renal cysts are found in up to 60%.[149] Because of a reset osmostat, the serum sodium concentration tends to be high-normal or slightly above the upper limit of normal. This clinical clue is very useful when initially assessing the potential for primary aldosteronism.

Several studies have shown that patients with primary aldosteronism may be at higher risk than other patients with hypertension for target-organ damage of the heart and kidney.[150,151] When matched for age, blood pressure, and duration of hypertension, patients with primary aldosteronism have greater left ventricular mass measurements than patients with other types of hypertension (e.g., pheochromocytoma, Cushing's syndrome, or essential hypertension).[152] In patients with APA, the left ventricular wall thickness and mass decreases markedly after 1 year from the time of adrenalectomy.[153] A case control study of 124 patients with primary aldosteronism and 465 patients with essential hypertension (matched for age, sex, and systolic and diastolic blood pressure) found that patients presenting with either APA or IHA had a significantly higher rate of cardiovascular events (e.g., stroke, atrial fibrillation, and myocardial infarction) than the matched essential hypertension patients.[151] A negative effect of circulating aldosterone on cardiac function was found in young nonhypertensive subjects with GRA who had increased left ventricular wall thickness and reduced diastolic function compared with age- and sex-matched controls.[150]

Diagnosis

The diagnostic approach to primary aldosteronism can be considered in three phases: case-finding tests, confirmatory tests, and subtype evaluation tests.

Case-Finding Tests

Spontaneous hypokalemia is uncommon in patients with uncomplicated hypertension and, when present, strongly suggests associated mineralocorticoid excess. However, several studies have shown that most patients with primary aldosteronism have baseline serum levels of potassium in the normal range.[134,139,154-156] Therefore, hypokalemia is not and should not be the criterion used to make the diagnosis of primary aldosteronism. Patients with hypertension and hypokalemia (regardless of presumed cause), treatment-resistant hypertension (three antihypertensive drugs and poor control), severe hypertension (≥160 mm Hg systolic or ≥100 mm Hg diastolic), hypertension and an incidental adrenal mass, and onset of hypertension at a young age should undergo screening for primary aldosteronism (Fig. 15–9). In addition, primary aldosteronism should be tested for whenever considering a secondary hypertension evaluation (e.g., when a patient lacks a family history of hypertension or when testing for renovascular disease or pheochromocytoma).

In patients with suspected primary aldosteronism, screening can be accomplished by measuring a morning (preferably between 8 and 10 A.M.) ambulatory paired random PAC and PRA (see Fig. 15–9). This test may be performed while the patient is taking antihypertensive medications (with some exceptions [see below]) and without posture stimulation.[138,139157,158] Hypokalemia reduces the secretion of aldosterone, and it is optimal to restore the serum level of potassium to normal before performing diagnostic studies. Aldosterone receptor antagonists (e.g., spironolactone and eplerenone) are the only medications that absolutely interfere with interpretation of the ratio and should be discontinued at least 6 weeks before testing. ACE inhibitors have the potential to "falsely elevate" PRA. Therefore, in a patient treated with an ACE inhibitor, the finding of a detectable PRA level or a low PAC/PRA ratio does not exclude the diagnosis of primary aldosteronism. However, a very useful clinical point is that when a PRA level is undetectably low in a patient taking an ACE inhibitor, primary aldosteronism is likely. A second important clinical point is that

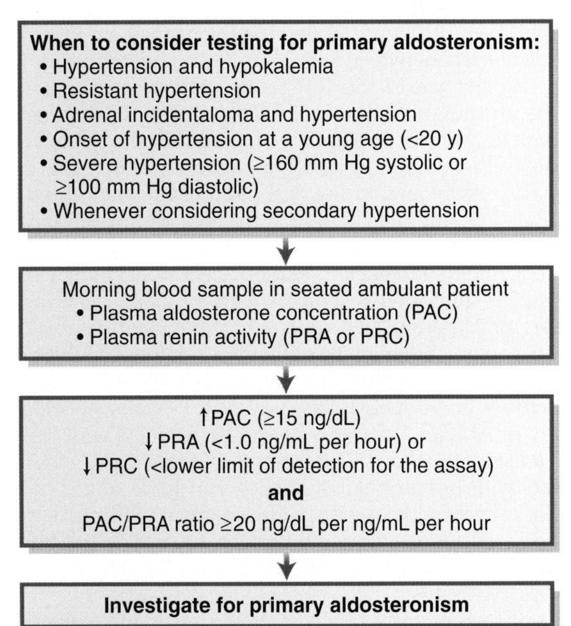

Figure 15–9 ▪ When to consider testing for primary aldosteronism and use of the plasma aldosterone concentration-to-plasma renin activity ratio as a case-finding tool. *PAC,* Plasma aldosterone concentration; *PRA,* plasma renin activity, *PRC,* plasma renin concentration.

the PRA is suppressed (<1.0 ng/mL/hr) in almost all patients with primary aldosteronism.

The PAC/PRA ratio, first proposed as a case-finding test for primary aldosteronism in 1981,[137] is based on the concept of paired hormone measurements. For example, in a hypertensive hypokalemic patient, (1) secondary hyperaldosteronism should be considered when both PRA and PAC are increased and the PAC/PRA ratio is less than 10 (e.g., renovascular disease), (2) an alternate source of mineralocorticoid receptor agonism should be considered when both PRA and PAC are suppressed (e.g., hypercortisolism), and (3) primary aldosteronism should be suspected when PRA is suppressed (<1.0 ng/mL/hr) and PAC is increased. At least 14 prospective studies have been published on the use of the PAC/PRA ratio in screening for primary aldosteronism.[159] Although there is some uncertainty about test characteristics and lack of standardization (see next), the PAC/PRA ratio is widely accepted as the screening test of choice for primary aldosteronism. It is important to understand that the lower limit of detection varies among different PRA assays and can have a dramatic effect on the PAC/PRA ratio. For example, if the lower limit of detection for PRA is 0.6 ng/mL/hr and the PAC is 16 ng/dL, then the PAC/PRA ratio would be 27; however, if the lower limit of detection for PRA is 0.1 ng/mL/hr and the PAC is 16 ng/dL, then the PAC/PRA ratio would be 160. Thus, the cutoff for a "high" PAC/PRA ratio is laboratory-dependent and, more specifically, PRA assay-dependent. In a retrospective study, the combination of a PAC/PRA ratio more than 30 and PAC more than 20 ng/dL had a sensitivity of 90% and a specificity of 91% for APA.[160] At Mayo Clinic, a PAC (in ng/dL)/PRA (in ng/mL/hr) ratio of 20 or more and PAC of at least 15 are found in more than 90% of patients with surgically confirmed APA. In patients without primary aldosteronism, most of the variation occurs within the normal range.[161] A high PAC/PRA ratio is a positive screening test result, a finding that warrants further testing.

It is critical for the clinician to recognize that the PAC/PRA ratio is only a case-finding tool, and all positive results should be followed by a confirmatory aldosterone suppression test to verify autonomous aldosterone production before treatment is initiated. In a systematic review of 16 studies, with a total of 3136 participants, the PAC/PRA cutoff levels used varied between 7.2 and 100 ng/dL per ng/mL/hr.[159] The sensitivity and specificity for APA varied between 64% and 100% and 87% and 100%, respectively. However, the description of the reference standard and the attribution of diagnosis at the end of the studies were incomplete, and there was a lack of standardization about origin of study cohort, ongoing antihypertensive medication, use of high-salt versus low-salt diet and circumstances during blood sampling. The authors concluded that none of the studies provided any valid estimates of the ratio test characteristics (sensitivity, specificity, and likelihood ratio at different cutoff levels).[159] In a recent study of 118 subjects with essential hypertension, neither antihypertensive medications nor acute variation of dietary sodium affected the accuracy of the PAC/PRA ratio adversely, with a sensitivity on and off therapy of 73% and 87%, respectively, and a specificity of 74% and 75%, respectively.[139] In a study of African-American and white subjects with resistant hypertension, the PAC/PRA ratio was elevated (>20) in 45 of 58 subjects with primary aldosteronism and in 35 of 207 patients without primary aldosteronism (sensitivity of 78% and specificity of 83%).[158] Furosemide and upright posture do not improve the posttest probability for APA more than the use of the baseline PAC/PRA ratio.[162]

The measurement of PRA is time consuming, shows poor interlaboratory variability, and requires special preanalytical prerequisites. To overcome these disadvantages, a monoclonal antibody against active renin is being used by several reference laboratories to measure plasma renin concentration (PRC) instead of PRA. However, few studies have focused on comparing the different methods in the testing for primary aldosteronism and these studies lack confirmatory testing.[163,164] In one study with 76 normotensive volunteers and 28 patients with confirmed primary aldosteronism, the PAC/PRC ratio performed as well as the PAC/PRA ratio in differentiating primary aldosteronism patients from normal volunteers.[165] Before a recommendation to replace PRA with PRC in the testing for primary aldosteronism can be made, more studies with larger cohorts are needed. Until such studies are completed it would be reasonable to consider a positive PAC/PRC test when the PAC is more than 15 ng/dL and the PRC is below the lower limit of detection for the assay (see Fig. 15–9).

Confirmatory Tests

An increased PAC/PRA ratio is not diagnostic by itself, and primary aldosteronism must be confirmed by demonstrating inappropriate aldosterone secretion. The list of drugs and hormones capable of affecting the renin-angiotensin-aldosterone axis is extensive, and frequently in patients with severe hypertension, a "medication-contaminated" evaluation is unavoidable. Calcium channel blockers and α_1-adrenergic receptor blockers do not affect the diagnostic accuracy in most cases. It is impossible to interpret data obtained from patients receiving treatment with aldosterone receptor antagonists (e.g., spironolactone, eplerenone) when PRA is not suppressed. Therefore, treatment with an aldosterone receptor antagonist should not be initiated until the evaluation has been completed and the final decisions about treatment have been made. If primary aldosteronism is suspected in a patient receiving treatment with spironolactone or eplerenone, the treatment should be discontinued for at least 6 weeks before further diagnostic testing. Aldosterone suppression testing can be performed with orally administered sodium chloride and measurement of urinary aldosterone or with intravenous sodium chloride loading and measurement of PAC.

Oral Sodium Loading Test

After hypertension and hypokalemia are controlled, patients should receive a high-sodium diet (supplemented with sodium chloride tablets if needed) for 3 days, with a goal sodium intake of 5000 mg of sodium (equivalent to 218 mEq of sodium or 12.8 g sodium chloride).[147] The risk of increasing dietary sodium in patients with severe hypertension must be assessed in each case.[166] Because the high-salt diet can increase kaliuresis and hypokalemia, vigorous replacement of potassium chloride may be needed and the serum level of potassium should be monitored daily. On the third day of the high-sodium diet, a 24-hour urine specimen is collected for measurement of aldosterone, sodium, and creatinine. To document adequate sodium repletion, the 24-hour urinary sodium excretion should exceed 200 mEq. Urinary aldosterone excretion more than 12 μg/24 hours in this setting is consistent with autonomous aldosterone secretion.[167] The sensitivity and specificity of the oral sodium loading test are 96% and 93%, respectively.[168]

Intravenous Saline Infusion Test

The intravenous saline infusion test has also been used widely for the diagnosis of primary aldosteronism.[169-171] Normal subjects show suppression of PAC after volume expansion with isotonic saline; subjects with primary aldosteronism do not show this suppression. The test is done after an overnight fast. Two liters of 0.9% sodium chloride solution are infused intravenously with an infusion pump over 4 hours into the recumbent patient. Blood pressure and heart rate are monitored during the infusion. At the completion of the infusion, blood is drawn for measurement of PAC. PAC levels in normal subjects decrease to less than 5 ng/dL; most patients with primary aldosteronism do not suppress to less than 10 ng/dL; post-saline infusion PAC values between 5 and 10 ng/dL are indeterminate and can be seen in patients with IHA.[131,169,170,172]

Fludrocortisone Suppression Test

In the fludrocortisone suppression test, fludrocortisone acetate is administered for 4 days (0.1 mg every 6 hour) in combination with sodium chloride tablets (2 g three times daily with food). Blood pressure and serum potassium need to monitored daily. In the setting of low PRA, failure to suppress the upright 10:00 AM PAC to less than 6 ng/dL on day 4 is diagnostic of PA.[173] It should be noted that an increased QT dispersion and deterioration of left ventricular function have been reported during fludrocortisone suppression tests.[166] Most centers no longer use the fludrocortisone suppression test.

Subtype Studies

Following case-finding and confirmatory testing, the third management issue guides the therapeutic approach by distinguishing APA and PAH from IHA and GRA. Unilateral adrenalectomy in patients with APA or PAH results in normalization of hypokalemia in all; hypertension is improved in all and is cured in approximately 30% to 60% of them.[174-176] In IHA and GRA, unilateral or bilateral adrenalectomy seldom corrects the hypertension.[147] IHA and GRA should be treated medically. APA is found in approximately 35% of cases and bilateral IHA in approximately 60% of cases (see Table 15–10). APAs are usually hypodense nodules (<2 cm in diameter) on CT and are golden yellow in color when resected. IHA adrenal glands may be normal on CT or show nodular changes. Aldosterone-producing adrenal carcinomas are almost always >4 cm in diameter and have an inhomogeneous phenotype on CT.

Adrenal Computed Tomography

Primary aldosteronism subtype evaluation may require one or more tests, the first of which is imaging the adrenal glands with CT. When a solitary unilateral hypodense (HU <10) macroadenoma (>1 cm) and normal contralateral adrenal morphology are found on CT in a young patient (younger than 40 years) with primary aldosteronism, unilateral adrenalectomy is a reasonable therapeutic option (Fig. 15–10). However, in many cases, CT may show normal-appearing adrenals, minimal unilateral adrenal limb thickening, unilateral microadenomas (≤1 cm), or bilateral macroadenomas (Fig. 15–11). In these cases, additional testing is required to determine the source of excess aldosterone secretion. Small APAs may be labeled incorrectly as "IHA" on the basis of CT findings of bilateral nodularity or normal-appearing adrenals. Also, apparent adrenal microadenomas may actually represent areas of hyperplasia, and unilateral adrenalectomy would be inappropriate. In addition, nonfunctioning unilateral adrenal macroadenomas are not uncommon, especially in older patients (older than 40 years).[177] Unilateral PAH may be visible on CT or the PAH adrenal may appear normal on CT. In general, patients with APAs have more severe hypertension, more frequent hypokalemia, higher plasma (>25 ng/dL) and urinary (>30 µg/24 hr) levels of aldosterone, and are younger (younger than 50 years) than those with IHA.[147,148] Patients fitting these descriptors are considered to have a "high probability of APA" regardless of the CT findings (see Fig. 15–10); 41% of patients with "high probability of APA" and a normal adrenal CT scan prove to have unilateral aldosterone hypersecretion.[178]

Adrenal CT is not accurate in distinguishing between APA and IHA. In one study, CT contributed to lateralization in only 59 of 111 patients with surgically proven APA; CT detected fewer than 25% of the APAs that were smaller than 1 cm in diameter.[179] In a another study of 203 patients with primary aldosteronism who were evaluated with both CT and adrenal vein sampling, CT was accurate in only 53% of patients[178]; based on CT findings, 42 patients (22%) would have been incorrectly excluded as candidates for adrenalectomy and 48 (25%) might have had unnecessary or inappropriate surgery.[178] Therefore, adrenal venous sampling is essential to direct appropriate therapy in patients with primary aldosteronism who have a high probability of APA and who seek a potential surgical cure.

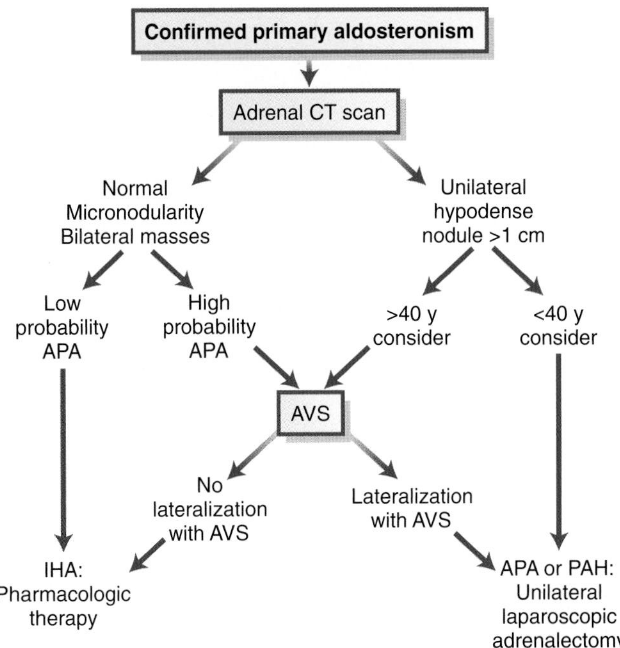

Figure 15–10 ■ Subtype evaluation of primary aldosteronism. See text for details. *APA*, Aldosterone-producing adenoma; *AVS*, adrenal venous sampling; *CT*, computed tomography; *IHA*, idiopathic hyperaldosteronism; *PAH*, primary adrenal hyperplasia. (Modified from Young WF Jr, Hogan MJ. Renin-independent hypermineralocorticoidism. Trends Endocrinol Metab 1994;5:97-106.)

Adrenal Venous Sampling

Adrenal venous sampling is the reference standard test to differentiate unilateral from bilateral disease in patients with primary aldosteronism.[178,179] Adrenal venous sampling is a difficult procedure because the right adrenal vein is small; the success rate depends on the proficiency of the angiographer. According to a review of 47 reports, the success rate for cannulating the right adrenal vein in 384 patients was 74%.[147] With experience, the success rate increased to 90% to 96%.[178,180,181] Some centers perform adrenal venous sampling in all patients who have the diagnosis of primary aldosteronism.[179] A more practical approach is the selective use of adrenal venous sampling outlined in Figure 15–10. To minimize stress-induced fluctuations in aldosterone secretion, an infusion of 50 µg of cosyntropin per hour is initiated 30 minutes before adrenal vein catheterization and continued throughout the procedure.[171,178,181] The adrenal veins are catheterized through the percutaneous femoral vein approach, and the position of the catheter tip is verified by gentle injection of a small amount of nonionic contrast medium and radiographic documentation. Blood is obtained from both adrenal veins and the inferior vena cava (IVC) below the renal veins and assayed for aldosterone and cortisol concentrations. To be sure there is no cross-contamination, the "IVC" sample should be obtained from an

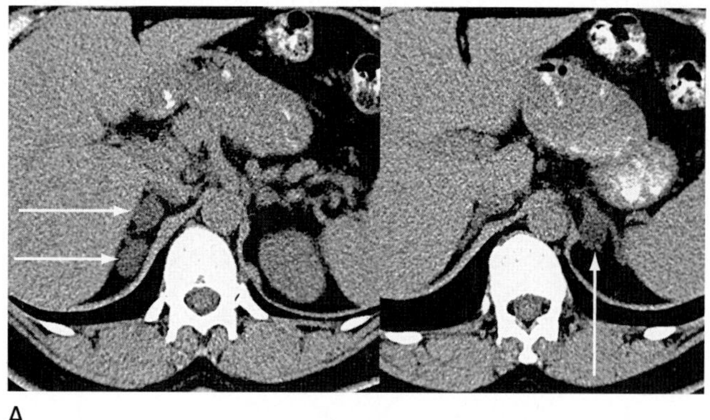

A

Results of bilateral adrenal venous sampling

Vein	Aldosterone (A), ng/dL	Cortisol (C), μg/dL	A/C ratio	Aldosterone ratio*
R adrenal vein	29,338	668	43.9	62.7
L adrenal vein	363	540	0.7	
Inferior vena cava	259	31	8.4	

*R adrenal vein A/C ratio divided by L adrenal vein A/C ratio.

B

Figure 15–11 ▪ A 43-year-old woman had a 2-year history of hypertension and hypokalemia. The screening test for primary aldosteronism was positive, with a plasma aldosterone concentration (PAC) of 37 ng/dL and low plasma renin activity (PRA) at less than 0.6 ng/mL/hr (PAC/PRA ratio >61). The confirmatory test for primary aldosteronism was also positive, with 24-hour urinary excretion of aldosterone of 53 μg on a high-sodium diet (urinary sodium, 196 mEq/24 hr). **A,** Adrenal computed tomography with a 12-mm low-density mass (*arrow,* right panel) in the medial limb of the left adrenal and two low-density 10-mm nodules (*arrows,* left panel) within the right adrenal gland. **B,** Adrenal venous sampling lateralized aldosterone secretion to the right, and two cortical adenomas (1.8 × 1.2 × 0.8 cm and 2.5 × 1.5 × 1.2 cm) were found at laparoscopic right adrenalectomy. The postoperative plasma aldosterone concentration was less than 1.0 ng/dL. Hypokalemia was cured and blood pressure was normal without the aid of antihypertensive medications.

iliac vein. The venous sample from the left side typically is obtained from the inferior phrenic vein immediately adjacent to the entrance of the adrenal vein. The right adrenal vein may be especially difficult to catheterize because it is short and enters the IVC at an acute angle.[181] The cortisol concentrations from the adrenal veins and IVC are used to confirm successful catheterization; the adrenal vein/IVC cortisol ratio is typically more than 10:1.

Dividing the right and left adrenal vein PACs by their respective cortisol concentrations corrects for the dilutional effect of the inferior phenic vein flow into the left adrenal vein; these are termed *cortisol-corrected ratios* (Fig. 15–12). In patients with APA, the mean cortisol-corrected aldosterone ratio (APA-side PAC/cortisol: normal adrenal PAC/cortisol) is 18:1.[178] A cutoff of the cortisol-corrected aldosterone ratio from high side to low side more than 4:1 is used to indicate unilateral aldosterone excess (see Fig. 15–12).[178] In patients with IHA, the mean cortisol-corrected aldosterone ratio is 1.8:1 (high side: low side); a ratio less than 3.0 to 1.0 is suggestive of bilateral aldosterone hypersecretion (see Fig. 15–12).[178] Therefore, most patients with a unilateral source of aldosterone will have cortisol-corrected aldosterone lateralization ratios greater than 4.0; ratios greater

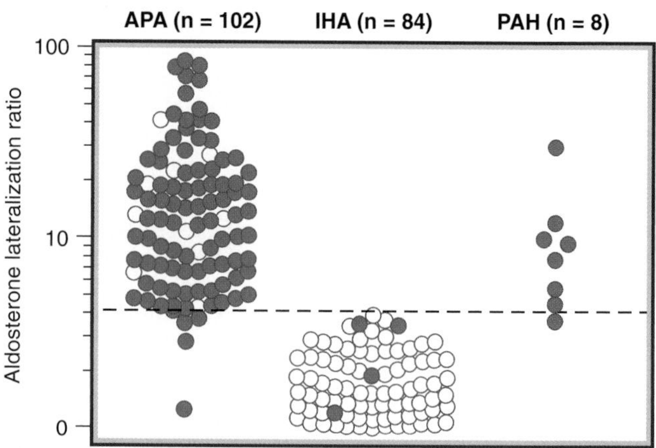

Figure 15–12 ▪ Adrenal vein aldosterone ratios for patients with unilateral aldosterone-producing adenomas (APA), bilateral idiopathic hyperplasia (IHA), and unilateral primary adrenal hyperplasia (PAH). The sensitivity and specificity of the cortisol-corrected plasma aldosterone concentration lateralization ratio greater than 4.0 for unilateral disease are 95.2% and 100%, respectively. *Shaded symbols,* the diagnosis was confirmed surgically. (From Young WF Jr, Stanson AW, Thompson GB, et al. Role for adrenal venous sampling in primary aldosteronism. Surgery 2004;136:1227-1235.)

than 3.0 but less than 4.0 represent a zone of overlap. Ratios no more than 3.0 are consistent with bilateral aldosterone secretion. The test characteristics of adrenal vein sampling for detecting unilateral aldosterone hypersecretion (APA or PAH) have sensitivity of 95% and a specificity of 100%.[178] At centers with experience with adrenal vein sampling, the complication rate is 2.5% or less.[178,180] Complications can include symptomatic groin hematoma, adrenal hemorrhage, and dissection of an adrenal vein. Adrenal venous sampling is essential to direct appropriate therapy for patients with primary aldosteronism who have a clinically high probability of APA and want to pursure surgical treatment.

Glucocorticoid-Remediable Aldosteronism (GRA—Familial Hyperaldosteronism Type I)

This syndrome is inherited in an autosomal dominant fashion and is responsible for fewer than 1% of cases of primary aldosteronism (see Table 15–10).[121] GRA is characterized by hypertension of early onset that is usually severe and refractory to conventional antihypertensive therapies, aldosterone excess, suppressed PRA, and excess production of 18-hydroxycortisol and 18-oxycortisol. GRA is caused by a chimeric gene duplication that results from unequal crossing over between the promoter sequence of *CYP11B1* gene (encoding 11β-hydroxylase) and the coding sequence of *CYP11B2* (encoding aldosterone synthase).[121] This chimeric gene contains the 3′ corticotropin-responsive portion of the promoter from the 11β-hydroxylase gene fused to the 5′ coding sequence of the aldosterone synthase gene. The result is ectopic expression of aldosterone synthase activity in the cortisol-producing zona fasciculata. Thus, mineralocorticoid production is regulated by corticotropin instead of the normal secretagogue, angiotensin II. Thus, aldosterone secretion can be suppressed by glucocorticoid therapy. In the absence of glucocorticoid therapy, this mutation results in overproduction of aldosterone and the hybrid steroids 18-hydroxycortisol and 18-oxycortisol, which can be measured in the urine to make the diagnosis.

Genetic testing is a sensitive and specific means of diagnosing GRA and obviates the need to measure the urinary levels of 18-oxyocortisol and 18-OH-cortisol or to perform dexamethasone suppression testing. Genetic testing for GRA should be considered for primary aldosteronism patients with a family history of primary aldosteronism or onset of primary aldosteronism at a young age (e.g., younger than 20 years), or in primary aldosteronism patients who have a family history of strokes at a young age.[182]

Familial Hyperaldosteronism Type II

FH type II is autosomal dominant and may be monogenic.[122] The hyperaldosteronism in FH type II does not suppress with dexamethasone and GRA mutation testing is negative. FH type II is more common than FH type I, but it still represents less than 2% of all patients with primary aldosteronism. The molecular basis for FH type II is unclear, although a recent linkage analysis study showed an association with chromosomal region 7p22.[122]

Historical Perspectives

One of the first methods used to differentiate unilateral from bilateral adrenal disease in patients with primary aldosteronism was adrenal venous sampling.[183] However, other diagnostic methods were sought because of the suboptimal catheter technology in the 1960s and 1970s and the difficulty with successfully sampling from both adrenal veins. [131I]-19-iodocholesterol scintigraphy[184] was first used in the early 1970s and an improved agent, [6-131I]iodomethyl-19-norcholesterol (NP-59), was introduced in 1977.[185] The sensitivity of this test depended heavily on the size of the adenoma.[186,187] In addition to its poor sensitivity, other reasons that NP-59 is rarely used in the United States include (1) NP-59 is not approved by the FDA and its use requires institutional review board approval, (2) dexamethasone is administered at 1 mg every 6 hours starting 7 days before NP-59 injection and continued throughout the scanning period, (3) imaging starts on day 4 after NP-59 injection and may continue daily through day 10, (4) a lateralizing scan can be seen in adrenal cortical adenomas that do not secrete aldosterone, and (5) only three or four centers in the United States currently offer NP-59 scintigraphy.

The posture stimulation test, also developed in the 1970s, was based on the finding that PAC in patients with APA showed diurnal variation and was relatively unaffected by changes in angiotensin II levels, whereas IHA was characterized by enhanced sensitivity to a small change in angiotensin II that occurred with standing.[188] In a review of 16 published reports, the accuracy of the posture stimulation test was 85% in 246 patients with surgically verified APA.[147] However, it became clear that some APAs were sensitive to angiotensin II and that some patients with IHA had diurnal variation in aldosterone secretion. Also, although the posture stimulation test may have predicted which patient had APA, it did not assist in localization.

18-Hydroxycorticosterone (18-OHB) is considered either the immediate precursor of aldosterone or a separate end product formed after 18-hydroxylation of corticosterone. Patients with APA generally have recumbent plasma 18-OHB levels greater than 100 ng/dL at 8:00 AM, whereas patients with IHA have levels that are usually less than 100 ng/dL.[189] 18-OHB actually proved to be a surrogate for PAC, which also tends to be higher in patients with APA than in those with IHA. However, the accuracy of supine morning 18-OHB and PAC in distinguishing between patients with APA and IHA is less than 80%.[147]

Principles of Treatment

The treatment goal is to prevent the morbidity and mortality associated with hypertension, hypokalemia, and cardiovascular damage.[190] The cause of the primary aldosteronism helps determine the appropriate treatment. Normalization of blood pressure should not be the only goal in managing a patient who has primary aldosteronism. In addition to the kidney and colon, mineralocorticoid receptors occur in the heart, brain, and blood vessels. Excessive secretion of aldosterone is associated with increased risk of cardiovascular disease and morbidity. Therefore, normalization of circulating aldosterone or aldosterone receptor blockade should be part of the management plan for all patients with primary aldosteronism.[154]

Surgical Treatment of Aldosterone-Producing Adenoma and Unilateral Hyperplasia

Unilateral laparoscopic adrenalectomy is an excellent treatment option for patients with APA or unilateral hyperplasia.[106] Although blood pressure control improves in nearly 100% of patients postoperatively, average long-term cure rates of hypertension after unilateral adrenalectomy for APA range from 30% to 60%.[174,176] Persistent hypertension following adrenalectomy is correlated directly with having more than one first-degree relative with hypertension, use of more than two antihypertensive agents preoperatively, older age, increased serum creatinine level, and duration of hypertension and is most likely due to coexistent primary hypertension.[174,176,191]

Laparoscopic adrenalectomy is the preferred surgical approach and is associated with shorter hospital stays and less long-term morbidity than the conventional open approach.[192,193] Because APAs are small and may be multiple, the entire adrenal gland should be removed.[194] To decrease the surgical risk, hypokalemia should be corrected with potassium supplements and/or a mineralocorticoid receptor antagonist preoperatively. The mineralocorticoid receptor-antagonist and potassium supplements should be discontinued postoperatively. PAC should be measured 1 to 2 days after the operation to confirm a biochemical cure. Serum potassium levels should be monitored weekly for 4 weeks after surgery and a generous sodium diet should be followed to avoid the hyperkalemia of hypoaldosteronism that may occur because of the chronic suppression of the renin-angiotensin-aldosterone axis. In approximately 5% of APA patients clinically significant hyperkalemia may develop after surgery and short-term fludrocortisone supplementation may be required. Typically, the hypertension resolves in 1 to 3 months postoperatively. It has been found that adrenalectomy for APA is significantly less expensive than long-term medical therapy.[195]

Pharmacologic Treatment

IHA and GRA should be treated medically. In addition, APA patients may be treated medically if the medical treatment includes mineralocorticoid receptor blockade.[196] A sodium-restricted diet (<100 mEq of sodium per day), maintenance of ideal body weight, tobacco avoidance, and regular aerobic exercise contribute significantly to the success of pharmacologic treatment. No placebo-controlled randomized trials have evaluated the relative efficacy of drugs in the treatment of primary aldosteronism.[197] Spironolactone has been the drug of choice to treat primary aldosteronism for more than three decades.[198] It is available as 25-, 50-, and 100-mg tablets. The dosage is 12.5 to 25 mg per day initially and is increased to 400 mg per day if necessary to achieve normokalemia without the aid of oral potassium chloride supplementation. Hypokalemia responds promptly, but hypertension may take as long as 4 to 8 weeks to be corrected. After several months of therapy, this dosage often can be decreased to as little as 25 to 50 mg per day; dosage titration is based on a goal serum potassium level in the high-normal range. Serum potassium and creatinine should be monitored frequently during the first 4 to 6 weeks of therapy (especially in patients with renal insufficiency or diabetes mellitus). Spironolactone has increased the half-life of digoxin, and for patients taking this drug, the dosage may need to be adjusted when treatment with spironolactone is started. Concomitant therapy with salicylates should be avoided because they interfere with the tubular secretion of an active metabolite and decrease the effectiveness of spironolactone. However, spironolactone is not selective for the aldosterone receptor. For example, antagonism at the testosterone receptor may result in painful gynecomastia, erectile dysfunction, and decreased libido in men; agonist activity at the progesterone receptor results in menstrual irregularity in women.[199]

Eplerenone is a steroid-based antimineralocorticoid that acts as a competitive and selective aldosterone receptor antagonist and was approved by the FDA for the treatment of uncomplicated essential hypertension in late 2003.[198] The 9,11-epoxide group in eplerenone results in a marked reduction of the molecule's progestational and antiandrogenic actions compared with spironolactone; eplerenone has 0.1% of the binding affinity to androgen receptors and less than 1% of the binding affinity to progesterone receptors compared with spironolactone. Treatment trials comparing the efficacy of eplerenone versus spironolactone for the treatment of primary aldosteronism have not been published. Presumably, eplerenone will be the superior drug if it is shown to be as effective as spironolactone for the treatment of mineralocorticoid-dependent hypertension and if it lacks the limiting antiandrogen side effects of spironolactone. Eplerenone is available as 25-mg and 50-mg tablets. It is approximately five times more expensive than spironolactone. For primary aldosteronism, it is reasonable to start with a dose of 25 mg twice daily (twice daily because of the shorter half-life of eplerenone compared to spironolactone) and titrated upward for normokalemia and blood pressure effect. The maximum dose approved by the FDA for hypertension is 100 mg daily. Potency studies with eplerenone show equal or 25% to 50% less milligram per milligram potency when compared with spironolactone. As with spironolactone, it is important to follow blood pressure, serum potassium, and serum creatinine levels closely. Eplerenone is contraindicated in the setting of hyperkalemia (serum potassium >5.5 mEq/L), clinically significant renal insufficiency (serum creatinine >2.0 mg/dL in men and >1.8 mg/dL in women), diabetes mellitus with microalbuminuria, concomitant administration of strong CYP3A4 inhibitors (e.g., ketoconazole, itraconazole), or concomitant treatment with potassium sparing diuretics. Side effects include dizziness, headache, fatigue, diarrhea, hypertriglyceridemia, and elevated liver enzymes.

Patients with IHA frequently require a second antihypertensive agent to achieve good blood pressure control. Hypervolemia is a major reason for resistance to drug therapy, and low doses of a thiazide (e.g., 12.5 to 50 mg of hydrochlorothiazide daily) or a related sulfonamide diuretic are effective in combination with the aldosterone receptor antagonist. Because these agents often lead to further hypokalemia, serum potassium levels should be monitored.

Before initiating treatment for GRA, it should be confirmed with genetic testing. In the GRA patient, chronic treatment with physiologic doses of a glucocorticoid normalizes blood pressure and corrects hypokalemia. The clinician should be cautious about iatrogenic Cushing's syndrome with excessive doses of glucocorticoids, especially with the use of dexamethasone in children. The smallest effective dose of shorter acting agents such as prednisone or hydrocortisone should be prescribed in relation to body surface area (e.g., hydrocortisone, 10 to 12 mg/m^2 per day). Target blood pressure in children should be guided by age-specific blood pressure percentiles.[200] Children should be monitored by pediatricians with expertise in glucocorticoid therapy, with careful attention paid to preventing retardation of linear growth by overtreatment. Treatment with mineralocorticoid receptor antagonists in these patients may be just as effective and avoids the potential disruption of the hypothalamic-pituitary-adrenal axis and risk of iatrogenic side effects. In addition, glucocorticoid therapy or mineralocorticoid receptor blockade may even have a role in normotensive GRA patients.[150]

OTHER FORMS OF MINERALOCORTICOID EXCESS OR EFFECT

The medical disorders associated with excess mineralocorticoid effect from 11-deoxycorticosterone (DOC) and cortisol are listed in Table 15–10. These diagnoses should be considered when PAC and PRA are low in patients with hypertension and hypokalemia.

Hyperdeoxycorticosteronism

Congenital Adrenal Hyperplasia

Congenital adrenal hyperplasia (CAH) is caused by enzymatic defects in adrenal steroidogenesis that result in deficient secretion of cortisol (see Chapter 14).[201] The lack of inhibitory feedback by cortisol on the hypothalamus and pituitary produces an ACTH-driven buildup of cortisol precursors proximal to the enzymatic deficiency. A deficiency of both 11β-hydroxylase (CYP11B) and 17α-hydroxylase (CYP17) causes hypertension and hypokalemia because of hypersecretion of the mineralocorticoid DOC. The mineralocorticoid effect of increased circulating levels of DOC also decreases PRA and aldosterone secretion. These defects are autosomal recessive in inheritance and typically are diagnosed in childhood. However, partial enzymatic defects have been shown to cause hypertension in adults.

11β-Hydroxylase Deficiency

Approximately 5% of all cases of CAH are due to 11β-hydroxylase deficiency; the prevalence in white patients is 1 in 100,000.[201] More than 40 mutations have been described in *CYP11B1*, the gene encoding 11β-hydroxylase.[202] There is an increased prevalence among Sephardic Jews from Morocco, suggestive of a founder effect. The impaired conversion of 11-DOC to corticosterone results in high levels of DOC and 11-deoxycortisol; the substrate mass effect results in increased levels of adrenal androgens. Females present in infancy or childhood with hypertension, hypokalemia, acne, hirsutism, and virilization, and males present with pseudoprecocious puberty. Approximately two thirds of patients have mild to moderate hypertension. Markedly increased levels of DOC, 11-deoxycortisol, and adrenal androgens confirm the diagnosis. Glucocorticoid replacement normalizes the steroid abnormalities and hypertension.

17α-Hydroxylase Deficiency

The 17α-hydroxylase deficiency form of CAH is rare. 17α-Hydroxylase is essential for the synthesis of cortisol and gonadal hormones, and deficiency results in decreased production of cortisol and sex hormones. Genetic 46,XY males present with either pseudohermaphroditism or as phenotypic females, and 46,XX females present with primary amenorrhea. Therefore, a person with this form of CAH may not come to medical attention until puberty. The biochemical findings include low concentrations of plasma adrenal androgens, plasma 17α-hydroxyprogesterone, aldosterone, and cortisol. The plasma concentrations of DOC, corticosterone, and 18-hydroxycorticosterone are increased and PRA is suppressed. Although rare, there is an increased prevalence among Dutch Mennonites. As with 11β-hydroxylase deficiency, glucocorticoid replacement normalizes the steroid abnormalities and hypertension.

Deoxycorticosterone-Producing Tumor

DOC-producing adrenal tumors are usually large and malignant.[203] Some of them secrete androgens and estrogens in addition to DOC, which may cause virilization in women and feminization in men. A high level of plasma DOC or urinary tetrahydrodeoxycorticosterone and a large adrenal tumor seen on CT confirm the diagnosis. Aldosterone secretion in these patients is typically suppressed. Optimal treatment is complete surgical resection.

Primary Cortisol Resistance

Increased cortisol secretion and plasma cortisol concentrations without evidence of Cushing's syndrome are found in patients with primary cortisol resistance (or glucocorticoid resistance), a rare familial syndrome.[204] The syndrome is characterized by hypokalemic alkalosis, hypertension, increased plasma concentrations of DOC, and increased adrenal androgen secretion. The hypertension and hypokalemia are likely due to the combined effects of excess DOC and increased cortisol access to the mineralocorticoid receptor (high rates of cortisol production that overwhelm 11β-HSD2 activity—see next section). Primary cortisol resistance is caused by defects in glucocorticoid receptors and the steroid-receptor complex (only eight mutations [families] have been reported). The treatment for the mineralocorticoid-dependent hypertension is blockade of the mineralocorticoid receptor with a mineralocorticoid receptor-antagonist or suppression of ACTH secretion with dexamethasone (typical dose required is 1 to 3 mg daily).

Apparent Mineralocorticoid Excess Syndrome

Apparent mineralocorticoid excess is the result of impaired activity of the microsomal enzyme 11β-hydroxysteroid dehydrogenase type 2 (11β-HSD2), which normally inactivates cortisol in the kidney by converting it to cortisone. Cortisol can be a potent mineralocorticoid, and as a result of the enzyme deficiency, high levels of cortisol accumulate in the kidney.[205] Thus, 11β-HSD2 normally excludes physiologic glucocorticoids from the nonselective mineralocorticoid receptor by converting them to the inactive 11-keto compound, cortisone. The characteristic abnormal urinary cortisol-cortisone metabolite profile seen in apparent mineralocorticoid excess reflects decreased 11β-HSD2 activity (ratio of cortisol to cortisone increased 10-fold from normal).[205]

Decreased 11β-HSD2 activity may be hereditary or secondary to pharmacologic inhibition of enzyme activity by glycyrrhizic acid, the active principle of licorice root (*Glycyrrhiza glabra*) and some chewing tobaccos. The congenital forms are rare (less than 50 patients have been identified worldwide) autosomal recessive disorders, and children present with low birth weight, failure to thrive, hypertension, polyuria and polydipsia, and poor growth.[202] The clinical phenotype of patients with apparent mineralocorticoid excess includes hypertension, hypokalemia, metabolic alkalosis, low PRA, low PAC, and normal plasma cortisol levels. The diagnosis is confirmed by demonstrating an abnormal ratio of cortisol to cortisone in a 24-hour urine collection. Treatment includes blockade of the mineralocorticoid receptor with a mineralocorticoid receptor-antagonist or suppression of endogenous cortisol secretion with dexamethasone.

The mineralocorticoid excess state caused by ectopic ACTH secretion, commonly seen in patients with Cushing's syndrome, is related to the high rates of cortisol production that overwhelm 11β-HSD2 activity. DOC levels may also be increased in severe ACTH-dependent Cushing's syndrome and contribute to the hypertension and hypokalemia in this disorder.

Liddle's Syndrome—Abnormal Renal Tubular Ionic Transport

In 1963, Liddle described an autosomal dominant renal disorder that appeared to be primary aldosteronism with hypertension, hypokalemia, and inappropriate kaliuresis.[206] However, PAC and PRA were very low in patients with Liddle's syndrome; thus, another name for this disorder is "pseudoaldosteronism." Liddle's syndrome is caused by mutations in the β or γ subunits of the amiloride-sensitive epithelial sodium channel.[202] This results in enhanced activity of the epithelial sodium channel increased sodium reabsorption, potassium wasting, hypertension, and hypokalemia. Clinical genetic testing is available (http://*www.genetests.org*). As would be predicted, amiloride and triamterene are very effective agents to treat the hypertension and hypokalemia. However, spironolactone is ineffective in these patients. Liddle's syndrome can easily be distinguished from apparent mineralocorticoid excess based on the basis of good clinical response to amiloride and triamterene, lack of efficacy of spironolactone and dexamethasone, and normal 24-hour urine cortisone/cortisol ratio.

Hypertension Exacerbated by Pregnancy

Hypertension exacerbated by pregnancy is a rare autosomal dominant disorder found in women with early-onset hypertension with suppressed levels of aldosterone and renin. During pregnancy, both the hypertension and hypokalemia are severely exacerbated. These patients have an activating mutation in the gene encoding the mineralocorticoid receptor, which allows progesterone and other mineralocorticoid antagonists to become agonists.[207]

OTHER ENDOCRINE DISORDERS ASSOCIATED WITH HYPERTENSION

Cushing's Syndrome

Hypertension occurs in 75% to 80% of patients with Cushing's syndrome (see Chapter 14).[208,209] The mechanisms of hypertension include increased production of DOC, enhanced pressor sensitivity to endogenous vasoconstrictors (e.g., norepinephrine and angiotensin II), increased cardiac output, activation of the renin-angiotensin system by increasing the hepatic production of angiotensinogen, and cortisol inactivation overload with stimulation of the mineralocorticoid receptor. The source of excess glucocorticoids may be exogenous (iatrogenic) or endogenous. Mineralocorticoid production is usually normal in endogenous Cushing's syndrome; aldosterone and renin levels are usually normal and DOC levels are normal or mildly increased. In adrenal carcinomas, DOC and aldosterone may be elevated.

The screening studies for endogenous cortisol excess include (1) midnight salivary cortisol, (2) 1-mg overnight dexamethasone suppression test, and (3) measurement of free cortisol in a 24-hour urine collection. Further studies to confirm Cushing's syndrome and to determine the cause of the cortisol excess state are outlined in Chapter 14.

The hypertension associated with Cushing's syndrome should be treated until a surgical cure is obtained. Mineralocorticoid receptor antagonists, at dosages used to treat primary aldosteronism, are effective in reversing the hypokalemia. Second-step agents (e.g., thiazide diuretics) may be added for optimal control of blood pressure. The hypertension associated with the hypercortisolism usually resolves over several weeks after a surgical cure, and antihypertensive agents can be tapered and withdrawn.

Thyroid Dysfunction

Hyperthyroidism

When excessive amounts of circulating thyroid hormones interact with thyroid hormone receptors on peripheral tissues, both metabolic activity and sensitivity to circulating catecholamines increase. Thyrotoxic patients usually have tachycardia, high cardiac output, increased stroke volume, decreased peripheral vascular resistance, and increased systolic blood pressure.[210] The initial management of patients with hypertension who have hyperthyroidism includes a β-adrenergic blocker to treat hypertension, tachycardia, and tremor. The definitive treatment of hyperthyroidism is cause-specific (see Chapter 11).

Hypothyroidism

The frequency of hypertension, usually diastolic, is increased threefold in hypothyroid patients and may account for as much as 1% of cases of diastolic hypertension in the population.[211] The mechanisms for the elevation in blood pressure include increased systemic vascular resistance and extracellular volume expansion. Treatment of thyroid hormone deficiency decreases blood pressure in most patients with hypertension and normalizes blood pressure in one third. Synthetic levothyroxine is the treatment of choice for hypothyroidism (see Chapter 12).

Primary Hyperparathyroidism

Hypercalcemia is associated with an increased frequency of hypertension. The most common cause of hypercalcemia is primary hyperparathyroidism. The frequency of hypertension in patients with primary hyperparathyroidism varies from 10% to 60%.[212] Most patients with primary hyperparathyroidism are asymptomatic, and the focus of the presentation may be the side effects of chronic hypercalcemia: polyuria and polydipsia, constipation, osteoporosis, renal lithiasis, peptic ulcer disease, and hypertension (see Chapter 27). The mechanisms are unclear because there is no direct correlation with the elevated parathyroid hormone or calcium levels. The hypertension associated with hyperparathyroidism can also result as a complication of hypercalcemia-induced renal impairment or when this disorder is part of MEN-2 (pheochromocytoma). The treatment of hyperparathyroidism is surgical; hypertension may or may not remit after successful parathyroidectomy.[213]

Acromegaly

Chronic growth hormone (GH) excess from a GH-producing pituitary tumor results in the clinical syndrome of acromegaly. The effects of chronic excess of GH include acral and soft tissue overgrowth, progressive dental malocclusion, degenerative arthritis related to chondral and synovial tissue overgrowth within joints, low-pitched sonorous voice, excessive sweating and oily skin, perineural hypertrophy leading to nerve entrapment (e.g., carpal tunnel syndrome), cardiac dysfunction, and hypertension (see Chapter 8). Hypertension occurs in 20% to 40% of the patients and is associated with sodium retention and extracellular volume expansion.[214] Pituitary surgery is the treatment of choice; if necessary, it is supplemented with medical therapy or irradiation or both. The hypertension of acromegaly is treated most effectively by curing the excess of GH. If a surgical cure is not possible, the hypertension usually responds well to diuretic therapy.

REFERENCES

1. Hajjar I, Kotchen TA. Trends in prevalence, awareness, treatment, and control of hypertension in the United States, 1988-2000. JAMA 2003;290:199-206.
2. Dluhy RG, Lawrence JE, Williams GH. Endocrine hypertension. In Larsen PR, Kronenberg HM, Melmed S, et al, eds. Williams Textbook of Endocrinology, 10th ed. Philadelphia: WB Saunders, 2003: 555.
3. Milligan G, Svoboda P, Brown CM. Why are there so many adrenoceptor subtypes? Biochem Pharmacol 1994;48:1059-1071.
4. Chobanian AV, Bakris GL, Black HR, et al. The Seventh Report of the Joint National Committee on Prevention, Detection, Evaluation, and Treatment of High Blood Pressure: the JNC 7 report. JAMA 2003;289:2560-2572.
5. Hospenthal MA, Peters JI. Long-acting beta(2)-agonists in the management of asthma exacerbations. Curr Opin Pulm Med 2005;11:69-73.
6. Flatmark T, Almas B, Ziegler MG. Catecholamine metabolism: an update on key biosynthetic enzymes and vesicular monoamine transporters. Ann N Y Acad Sci 2002;971:69-75.
7. Safford SD, Coleman RE, Gockerman JP, et al. Iodine-131 metaiodobenzylguanidine is an effective treatment for malignant pheochromocytoma and paraganglioma. Surgery 2003;134:956-963.
8. Rose B, Matthay KK, Price D, et al. High-dose 131I-metaiodobenzylguanidine therapy for 12 patients with malignant pheochromocytoma. Cancer 2003;98:239-248.
9. Erickson JD, Eiden LE, Hoffman BJ. Expression cloning of a reserpine-sensitive vesicular monoamine transporter. Proc Natl Acad Sci U S A 1992;89:10993-10997.
10. Eisenhofer G, Kopin IJ, Goldstein DS. Catecholamine metabolism: a contemporary view with implications for physiology and medicine. Pharmacol Rev 2004;56:331-349.
11. Lloyd RV, Tischer AS, Kimura N, et al. Adrenal tumors: introduction. In DeLellis RA, Lloyd RV, Heitz PU, et al, eds. World Health Organization Classification of Tumours: Pathology and Genetics of Tumours of Endocrine Organs. Lyon, France: IARC Press, 2004: 136-138.
12. Stenstrom G, Svardsudd K. Phaechromocytoma in Sweden, 1958-81. An analysis of the National Cancer Registry Data. Acta Med Scand 1986;220:225-232.
13. Sinclair AM, Isles CG, Brown I, et al. Secondary hypertension in a blood pressure clinic. Arch Intern Med 1987;147:1289-1293.
14. Anderson GH Jr, Blakeman N, Streeten DH. The effect of age on prevalence of secondary forms of hypertension in 4429 consecutively referred patients. J Hypertens 1994;12:609-615.
15. Omura M, Saito J, Yamaguchi K, et al. Prospective study on the prevalence of secondary hypertension among hypertensive patients visiting a general outpatient clinic in Japan. Hypertens Res 2004;27:193-202.
16. Fränkel F. Ein Fall von doppelseitigem, vollig latent verlaufenen nebennierentumor und gleichzeitiger nephritis mit veränderungen am circulationsapparat und retinitis. Virchows Arch Pathol

Anat Physiol 1886;103:244-263. Reprinted in 1984: Classics in oncology. A case of bilateral completely latent adrenal tumor and concurrent nephritis with changes in the circulatory system and retinitis: Felix Fränkel, 1886. CA Cancer J Clin 1984;34: 93-106.

17. Alezais, P. Un groupe nouveau de tumeurs epithéliales: les paraganglions. C R Seances Soc Biol Paris 1908;65:745-747.
18. Pick L. Das Ganglioma embryonale sympathicum (sympathoma embryonale), eine typische bösartige geschwuestform des sympathischen nervensystems. Berl Klin Wochenschr 1912;49:16-22.
19. Welbourn RB. Early surgical history of phaeochromocytoma. Br J Surg 1987;74:594-596.
20. Manger WM, Gifford RW. Background and importance and diagnosis. In Manger WM, Gifford RW, eds. Clinical and Experimental Pheochromocytoma, 2nd ed. Cambridge: Blackwell Science, 1996:1-7, 205-332.
21. Engel A, von Euler US. Diagnostic value of increased urinary output of noradrenaline and adrenaline in pheochromocytoma. Lancet 1950;2:387.
22. Young WF Jr. Pheochromocytoma: 1926-1993. Trends Endocrinol Metab 1993;4:122-127.
23. Munakata M, Aihara A, Imai Y, et al. Altered sympathetic and vagal modulations of the cardiovascular system in patients with pheochromocytoma: their relations to orthostatic hypotension. Am J Hypertens 1999;12:572-580.
24. Dubois LA, Gray DK. Dopamine-secreting pheochromocytomas: in search of a syndrome. World J Surg 2005;29:909-913.
25. Eisenhofer G, Goldstein DS, Sullivan P, et al. Biochemical and clinical manifestations of dopamine-producing paragangliomas: utility of plasma methoxytyramine. J Clin Endocrinol Metab 2005;90:2068-2075.
26. Young WF Jr, Maddox DE. Spells: in search of a cause. Mayo Clin Proc 1995;70:757-765.
27. O'Brien TO, Young WF Jr, Davila DG, et al. Cushing's syndrome associated with ectopic production of corticotrophin-releasing hormone, corticotrophin, and vasopressin by a phaeochromocytoma. Clin Endocrinol (Oxf) 1992;37:460-467.
28. Onozawa M, Fukuhara T, Minoguchi M, et al. Hypokalemic rhabdomyolysis due to WDHA syndrome caused by VIP-producing composite pheochromocytoma: a case in neurofibromatosis type 1. Jpn J Clin Oncol 2005;35:559-563.
29. Mune T, Katakami H, Kato Y, et al. Production and secretion of parathyroid hormone-related protein in pheochromocytoma: participation of an alpha-adrenergic mechanism. J Clin Endocrinol Metab 1993;76:757-762.
30. Schifferdecker B, Kodali D, Hausner E, et al. Adrenergic shock—an overlooked clinical entity? Cardiol Rev 2005;13:69-72.
31. Liao WB, Liu CF, Chiang CW, et al. Cardiovascular manifestations of pheochromocytoma. Am J Emerg Med 2000;18:622-625.
32. Neumann HP, Bausch B, McWhinney SR, et al. Germ-line mutations in nonsyndromic pheochromocytoma. N Engl J Med 2002; 346:1459-1466.
33. Motta-Ramirez GA, Remer EM, Herts BR, et al. Comparison of CT findings in symptomatic and incidentally discovered pheochromocytomas. AJR Am J Roentgenol 2005;185:684-688.
34. Kinney MA, Warner ME, vanHeerden JA, et al. Perianesthetic risks and outcomes of pheochromocytoma and paraganglioma resection. Anesth Analg 2000;91:1118-1123.
35. Erickson D, Kudva YC, Ebersold MJ, et al. Benign paragangliomas: clinical presentation and treatment outcomes in 236 patients. J Clin Endocrinol Metab 2001;86:5210-5216.
36. Elder EE, Elder G, Larsson C. Pheochromocytoma and functional paraganglioma syndrome: no longer the 10% tumor. J Surg Oncol 2005;89:193-201.
37. Gimm O, Koch CA, Januszewicz A, et al. The genetic basis of pheochromocytoma. Front Horm Res 2004;31:45-60.
38. Pawlu C, Bausch B, Reisch N, et al. Genetic testing for pheochromocytoma-associated syndromes. Ann Endocrinol (Paris) 2005; 66:178-185.
39. Peczkowska M, Januszewicz A. Multiple endocrine neoplasia type 2. Fam Cancer 2005;4:25-36.
40. Marx SJ. Molecular genetics of multiple endocrine neoplasia types 1 and 2. Nat Rev Cancer 2005;5:367-375.
41. Carling T. Multiple endocrine neoplasia syndrome: genetic basis for clinical management. Curr Opin Oncol 2005;17:7-12.
42. Schussheim DH, Skarulis MC, Agarwal SK, et al. Multiple endocrine neoplasia type 1: new clinical and basic findings. Trends Endocrinol Metab 2001;12:173-178.
43. Skogseid B, Rastad J, Gobl A, et al. Adrenal lesion in multiple endocrine neoplasia type 1. Surgery 1995;118:1077-1082.
44. Hes FJ, Hoppener JW, Lips CJ. Clinical review 155: pheochromocytoma in Von Hippel-Lindau disease. J Clin Endocrinol Metab 2003;88:969-974.
45. Friedrich CA. Genotype-phenotype correlation in von Hippel-Lindau syndrome. Hum Mol Genet 2001;10:763-767.
46. Bender BU, Gutsche M, Glasker S, et al. Differential genetic alterations in von Hippel-Lindau syndrome–associated and sporadic pheochromocytomas. J Clin Endocrinol Metab 2000;85: 4568-4574.
47. Eisenhofer G, Walther MM, Huynh TT, et al. Pheochromocytomas in von Hippel-Lindau syndrome and multiple endocrine neoplasia type 2 display distinct biochemical and clinical phenotypes. J Clin Endocrinol Metab 2001;86:1999-2008.
48. Walther MM, Herring J, Enquist E, et al. von Recklinghausen's disease and pheochromocytomas. J Urol 1999;162:1582-1586, 1999.
49. Young AL, Young WF Jr. Benign paragangliomas. In Linos D, van Heerden JA, eds. Adrenal Glands: Diagnostic Aspects and Surgical Therapy. New York: Springer-Verlag, 2005:201-209.
50. Baysal BE, Ferrell RE, Willett-Brozick JE, et al. Mutations in SDHD, a mitochondrial complex II gene, in hereditary paraganglioma. Science 2000;287:848-851.
51. Bayley JP, Devilee P, Taschner PE. The SDH mutation database: an online resource for succinate dehydrogenase sequence variants involved in pheochromocytoma, paraganglioma and mitochondrial complex II deficiency. BMC Med Genet 2005; 6:39.
52. Astuti D, Douglas F, Lennard TW, et al. Germline SDHD mutation in familial phaeochromocytoma. Lancet 2001;357:1181-1182.
53. Eng C, Kiuru M, Fernandez MJ, et al. A role for mitochondrial enzymes in inherited neoplasia and beyond. Nat Rev Cancer 2003;3:193-202.
54. Neumann HP, Pawlu C, Peczkowska M, et al. Distinct clinical features of paraganglioma syndromes associated with SDHB and SDHD gene mutations. JAMA 2004;292:943-951.
55. Schiavi F, Boedeker CC, Bausch B, et al. Predictors and prevalence of paraganglioma syndrome associated with mutations of the SDHC gene. JAMA 2005;294:2057-2063.
56. Mariman EC, van Beersum SE, Cremers CW, et al. Fine mapping of a putatively imprinted gene for familial non-chromaffin paragangliomas to chromosome 11q13.1: evidence for genetic heterogeneity. Hum Genet 1995;95:56-62.
57. Young AL, Baysal BE, Deb A, et al. Familial malignant catecholamine-secreting paraganglioma with prolonged survival associated with mutation in the succinate dehydrogenase B gene. J Clin Endocrinol Metab 2002;87:4101-4105.
58. Gimenez-Roqueplo AP, Favier J, Rustin P. Mutations in SDHB gene are associated with extra-adrenal and/or malignant pheochromocytomas. Cancer Res 2003;63:5615-5621.
59. Benn DE, Gimenez-Roqueplo AP, Reilly JR, et al. Clinical presentation and penetrance of pheochromocytoma/paraganglioma syndromes. J Clin Endocrinol Metab 2006;91:827-836.
60. McWhinney SR, Pilarski RT, Forrester SR, et al. Large germline deletions of mitochondrial complex II subunits SDHB and SDHD in hereditary paraganglioma. J Clin Endocrinol Metab 2004;89: 5694-5699.
61. Carney JA. Gastric stromal sarcoma, pulmonary chondroma, and extra-adrenal paraganglioma (Carney triad): natural history, adrenocortical component, and possible familial occurrence. Mayo Clin Proc 1999;74:543-552.
62. Taylor RL, Singh RJ. Validation of liquid chromatography-tandem mass spectrometry method for analysis of urinary conjugated metanephrine and normetanephrine for screening of pheochromocytoma. Clin Chem 2002;48:533-539.
63. Kudva YC, Sawka AM, Young WF Jr. Clinical review 164: the laboratory diagnosis of adrenal pheochromocytoma: the Mayo Clinic experience. J Clin Endocrinol Metab 2003;88:4533-4539.
64. Sawka AM, Jaeschke R, Singh RJ, et al. A comparison of biochemical tests for pheochromocytoma: measurement of fractionated plasma metanephrines compared with the combination of 24-hour

urinary metanephrines and catecholamines. J Clin Endocrinol Metab 2003;88:553-558.
65. Lenders JW, Pacak K, Walther MM, et al. Biochemical diagnosis of pheochromocytoma: which test is best? JAMA 2002;287: 1427-1434.
66. Raber W, Raffesberg W, Bischof M, et al. Diagnostic efficacy of unconjugated plasma metanephrines for the detection of pheochromocytoma. Arch Intern Med 2000;160:2957-2963.
67. Sawka AM, Prebtani AP, Thabane L, et al. A systematic review of the literature examining the diagnostic efficacy of measurement of fractionate plasma free metanephrines in the biochemical diagnosis of pheochromocytoma. BMC Endorc Disord 2004; 4:2.
68. Sawka AM, Gafni A, Thabane L, et al. The economic implications of three biochemical screening algorithms for pheochromocytoma. J Clin Endocrinol Metab 2004;89:2859-2866.
69. Lenders JW, Keiser HR, Goldstein DS, et al. Plasma metanephrines in the diagnosis of pheochromocytoma. Ann Intern Med 1995; 123:101-109.
70. Perry CG, Sawka AM, Singh R, et al. The diagnostic efficacy of fractionated urinary metanephrines measured by tandem mass spectrometry in detection of pheochromocytoma. The Endocrine Society's 87th Annual Meeting, OR42-1, Page 136, June 4-7, 2005, San Diego, CA.
71. Cotesta D, Caliumi C, Alo P, et al. High plasma levels of human chromogranin A and adrenomedullin in patients with pheochromocytoma. Tumori 2005;91:53-58.
72. Mouri T, Sone M, Takahashi K, et al. Neuropeptide Y as a plasma marker for phaeochromocytoma, ganglioneuroblastoma and neuroblastoma. Clin Sci (Lond) 1992;83:205-211.
73. Sjoberg RJ, Simcic KJ, Kidd GS. The clonidine suppression test for pheochromocytoma. A review of its utility and pitfalls. Arch Intern Med 1992;152:1193-1197.
74. Eisenhofer G, Goldstein DS, Walther MM, et al. Biochemical diagnosis of pheochromocytoma: how to distinguish true- from false-positive results. J Clin Endocrinol Metab 2003;88:2656-2666.
75. Young WF Jr. Phaeochromocytoma: how to catch a moonbeam in your hand. Eur J Endocrinol 1997;136:28-29.
76. Godfrey JA, Rickman OB, Williams AW, et al. Pheochromocytoma in a patient with end-stage renal disease. Mayo Clin Proc 2001; 76:953-957.
77. Canale MP, Bravo EL. Diagnostic specificity of serum chromogranin-A for pheochromocytoma in patients with renal dysfunction. J Clin Endocrinol Metab 1994;78:1139-1144.
78. Chauveau D, Martinez F, Houhou S, et al. Malignant hypertension secondary to pheochromocytoma in a hemodialyzed patient. Am J Kidney Dis 1993;21:52-53.
79. Stumvoll M, Radjaipour M, Seif F. Diagnostic considerations in pheochromocytoma and chronic hemodialysis: case report and review of the literature. Am J Nephrol 1995;15:147-151.
80. Morioka M, Yuihama S, Nakajima T, et al. Incidentally discovered pheochromocytoma in long-term hemodialysis patients. Int J Urol 2002;9:700-703.
81. Eisenhofer G, Huysmans F, Pacak K, et al. Plasma metanephrines in renal failure. Kidney Int 2005;67:668-677.
82. Marini M, Fathi M, Vallotton M. [Determination of serum metanephrines in the diagnosis of pheochromocytoma]. Ann Endocrinol (Paris) 1994;54:337-342.
83. Stern TA, Cremens CM. Factitious pheochromocytoma. One patient history and literature review. Psychosomatics 1998;39: 283-287.
84. Sawka AM, Singh RJ, Young WF Jr. False-positive biochemical testing for pheochromocytoma caused by surreptitious catecholamine addition to urine. The Endocrinologist 2001;11:421-423.
85. van Gils APG, Falke THM, van Erkel AR, et al. MR imaging and MIBG scintigraphy of pheochromocytomas and extraadrenal functioning paragangliomas. Radiographics 1991;11:37-57.
86. Ilias I, Pacak K. Current approaches and recommended algorithm for the diagnostic localization of pheochromocytoma. J Clin Endocrinol Metab 2004;89:479-491.
87. Jalil ND, Pattou FN, Combemale F, et al. Effectiveness and limits of preoperative imaging studies for the localisation of pheochromocytomas and paragangliomas: a review of 282 cases. French Association of Surgery (AFC), and The French Association of Endocrine Surgeons (AFCE). Eur J Surg 1998;164:23-28.
88. Brink I, Hoegerle S, Klisch J, et al. Imaging of pheochromocytoma and paraganglioma. Fam Cancer 2005;4:61-68.
89. Boland GWL, Lee MJ, Gazelle GS, et al. Characterization of adrenal masses using unenhanced CT: an analysis of the CT literature. AJR Am J Roentgenol 1998;171:201-204.
90. Teeger S, Papanicolaou N, Vaughan ED Jr. Current concepts in imaging adrenal masses. World J Urol 1999;17:3-8.
91. Korobkin M, Brodeur FJ, Francis IR, et al. CT time—attenuation washout curves of adrenal adenomas and nonadenomas. AJR Am J Roentgenol 1998;170:747-752.
92. Renken NS, Krestin GP. Magnetic resonance imaging of the adrenal glands. Semin Ultrasound CT MR 2005;26:162-171.
93. Szolar DH, Korobkin M, Reittner P, et al. Adrenocortical carcinomas and adrenal pheochromocytomas: mass and enhancement loss evaluation at delayed contrast-enhanced CT. Radiology 2005;234:479-485.
94. Miskulin J, Shulkin BL, Doherty GM, et al. Is preoperative iodine 123 meta-iodobenzylguanidine scintigraphy routinely necessary before initial adrenalectomy for pheochromocytoma? Surgery 2003;134:918-22.
95. Taieb D, Sebag F, Hubbard JG, et al. Does iodine-131 meta-iodobenzylguanidine (MIBG) scintigraphy have an impact on the management of sporadic and familial phaeochromocytoma? Clin Endocrinol (Oxf) 2004;61:102-108.
96. Solanki KK, Bomanji J, Moyes J, et al. A pharmacological guide to medicines which interfere with the biodistribution of radiolabelled meta-iodobenzylguanidine (MIBG). Nucl Med Commun 1992;13:513-521.
97. Mundschenk J, Unger N, Schulz S, et al. Somatostatin receptor subtypes in human pheochromocytoma: subcellular expression pattern and functional relevance for octreotide scintigraphy. J Clin Endocrinol Metab 2003;88:5150-5157.
98. Plouin PF, Duclos JM, Soppelsa F, et al. Factors associated with perioperative morbidity and mortality in patients with pheochromocytoma: analysis of 165 operations at a single center. J Clin Endocrinol Metab 2001;86:1480-1486.
99. Russell WJ, Metcalfe IR, Tonkin AL, et al. The preoperative management of phaeochromocytoma. Anaesth Intensive Care 1998;26:196-200.
100. Steinsapir J, Carr AA, Prisant LM, et al. Metyrosine and pheochromocytoma. Arch Intern Med 1997;157:901-906.
101. Combemale F, Carnaille B, Tavernier B, et al. Exclusive use of calcium channel blockers and cardioselective beta-blockers in the pre- and per-operative management of pheochromocytomas. 70 cases. Ann Chir 1998;52:341-345.
102. Lebuffe G, Dosseh ED, Tek G, et al. The effect of calcium channel blockers on outcome following the surgical treatment of phaeochromocytomas and paragangliomas. Anaesthesia 2005;60: 439-444.
103. Memtsoudis SG, Swamidoss C, Psoma M. Anesthesia for adrenal surgery. In Linos D, van Heerden JA, eds. Adrenal Glands: Diagnostic Aspects and Surgical Therapy. New York: Springer-Verlag, 2005:287-297.
104. Hack HA. The perioperative management of children with phaeochromocytoma. Paediatr Anaesth 2000;10:463-476.
105. Reddy VS, O'Neill JA Jr, Holcomb GW 3rd, et al. Twenty-five-year surgical experience with pheochromocytoma in children. Am Surg 2000;66:1085-1091.
106. Assalia A, Gagner M. Laparoscopic adrenalectomy. Br J Surg 2004;91:1259-1274.
107. Cheah WK, Clark OH, Horn JK, et al. Laparoscopic adrenalectomy for pheochromocytoma. World J Surg 2002;26:1048-1051.
108. Shen WT, Sturgeon C, Clark OH, et al. Should pheochromocytoma size influence surgical approach? A comparison of 90 malignant and 60 benign pheochromocytomas. Surgery 2004;136:1129-1137.
109. Amar L, Servais A, Gimeniz-Roqueplo AP, et al. Year of diagnosis, features at presentation, and risk of recurrence in patients with pheochromocytoma or secreting paraganglioma. J Clin Endocrinol Metab 2005;90:2110-2116.
110. Loh KC, Fitzgerald PA, Matthay KK, et al. The treatment of malignant pheochromocytoma with iodine-131 metaiodobenzylguanidine (131I-MIBG): a comprehensive review of 116 reported patients. J Endocrinol Invest 1997;20:648-658.
111. Lehnert H, Mundschenk J, Hahn K. Malignant pheochromocytoma. Front Horm Res 2004;31:155-162.

112. Averbuch SD, Steakley CS, Young RC, et al. Malignant pheochromocytoma: effective treatment with a combination of cyclophosphamide, vincristine, and dacarbazine. Ann Intern Med 1988; 109:267-273.
113. Eisenhofer G, Bornstein SR, Brouwers FM, et al. Malignant pheochromocytoma: current status and initiatives for future progress. Endocr Relat Cancer 2004;11:423-436.
114. Kamari Y, Sharabi Y, Leiba A, et al. Peripartum hypertension from pheochromocytoma: a rare and challenging entity. Am J Hypertens 2005;18:1306-1312.
115. Williams GH, Chao J, Chao L. Kidney hormones: the kallikrein kinin and renin-angiotensin systems. In Conn PM, Melmed S, eds. Endocrinology: Basic and Clinical Principles. Totowa, NJ: Humana Press, 1997:393-404.
116. Mihailidou AS, Funder JW. Nongenomic effects of mineralocorticoid receptor activation in the cardiovascular system. Steroids 2005;70:347-351.
117. Funder JW. The nongenomic actions of aldosterone. Endocr Rev 2005;26:313-321.
118. Brown NJ. Aldosterone and end-organ damage. Curr Opin Nephrol Hypertens 2005;14:235-241.
119. Williams GH, Dluhy RG. Diseases of the adrenal cortex. In Braunwald E, Fauci AD, Kasper D, et al, eds. Harrison's Principles of Internal Medicine, 15th ed. New York: McGraw-Hill, 2001: 2087.
120. Conn JW. Presidental address. Part I. Painting background. Part II. Primary aldosteronism, a new clinical syndrome. J Lab Clin Med 1955;45:3-17.
121. McMahon GT, Dluhy RG. Glucocorticoid-remediable aldosteronism. Cardiol Rev 2004;12:44-48.
122. So A, Duffy DL, Gordon RD, et al. Familial hyperaldosteronism type II is linked to the chromosome 7p22 region but also shows predicted heterogeneity. J Hypertens 2005;23:1477-1484.
123. Gittler RD, Fajans SS. Primary aldosteronism (Conn's syndrome). J Clin Endocrinol Metab 1995;80:3438-3441.
124. Conn JW, Knopf RF, Nesbit RM. Clinical characteristics of primary aldosteronism from analysis of 145 cases. Am J Surg 1964;107: 159-172.
125. Conn JW. Plasma renin activity in primary aldosteronism. Importance in differential diagnosis and in research of essential hypertension. JAMA 1964;190:222-225.
126. Fishman LM, Kuchel O, Liddle GW, et al. Incidence of primary aldosteronism uncomplicated "essential" hypertension. A prospective study with elevated aldosterone secretion and suppressed plasma renin activity used as diagnostic criteria. JAMA 1968; 205:497-502.
127. Kaplan NM. Hypokalemia in the hypertensive patient, with observations on the incidence of primary aldosteronism. Ann Intern Med 1967;66:1079-1090.
128. Conn JW. The evolution of primary aldosteronism: 1954-1967. Harvey Lect 1966;62:257-291.
129. Andersen GS, Toftdahl DB, Lund JO, et al. The incidence rate of phaeochromocytoma and Conn's syndrome in Denmark, 1977-1981. J Hum Hypertens 1988;2:187-189.
130. Berglund G, Andersson O, Wilhelmsen L. Prevalence of primary and secondary hypertension: studies in a random population sample. Br Med J 1976;2:554-556.
131. Streeten DH, Tomycz N, Anderson GH. Reliability of screening methods for the diagnosis of primary aldosteronism. Am J Med 1979;67:403-413.
132. Tucker RM, Labarthe DR. Frequency of surgical treatment for hypertension in adults at the Mayo Clinic from 1973 through 1975. Mayo Clin Proc 1977;52:549-545.
133. Sinclair AM, Isles CG, Brown I, et al. Secondary hypertension in a blood pressure clinic. Arch Intern Med 1987;147:1289-1293.
134. Mulatero P, Stowasser M, Loh KC, et al. Increased diagnosis of primary aldosteronism, including surgically correctable forms, in centers from five continents. J Clin Endocrinol Metab 2004;89: 1045-1050.
135. Gordon RD, Laragh JH, Funder JW. Low renin hypertensive states: perspectives, unsolved problems, future research. Trends Endocrinol Metab 2005;16:108-113.
136. Dunn PJ, Espiner EA. Outpatient screening tests for primary aldosteronism. Aust N Z J Med 1976;6:131-135.
137. Hiramatsu K, Yamada T, Yukimura Y, et al. A screening test to identify aldosterone-producing adenoma by measuring plasma renin activity. Results in hypertensive patients. Arch Intern Med 1981;141:1589-1593.
138. Gallay BJ, Ahmad S, Xu L, et al. Screening for primary aldosteronism without discontinuing hypertensive medications: plasma aldosterone-renin ratio. Am J Kidney Dis 2001;37:699-705.
139. Schwartz GL, Turner ST. Screening for primary aldosteronism in essential hypertension: diagnostic accuracy of the ratio of plasma aldosterone concentration to plasma renin activity. Clin Chem 2005;51:386-394.
140. Gordon RD, Stowasser M, Tunny TJ, et al. High incidence of primary aldosteronism in 199 patients referred with hypertension. Clin Exp Pharmacol Physiol 1994;21:315-318.
141. Loh KC, Koay ES, Khaw MC, et al. Prevalence of primary aldosteronism among Asian hypertensive patients in Singapore. J Clin Endocrinol Metab 2000;85:2854-2859.
142. Fardella CE, Mosso L, Gomez-Sanchez C, et al. Primary hyperaldosteronism in essential hypertensives: prevalence, biochemical profile, and molecular biology. J Clin Endocrinol Metab 2000;85: 1863-1867.
143. Lim PO, Dow E, Brennan G, et al. High prevalence of primary aldosteronism in the Tayside hypertension clinic population. J Hum Hypertens 2000;14:311-315.
144. Mosso L, Carvajal C, Gonzalez A, et al. Primary aldosteronism and hypertensive disease. Hypertension 2003;42:161-165.
145. Hamlet SM, Tunny TJ, Woodland E, et al. Is aldosterone/renin ratio useful to screen a hypertensive population for primary aldosteronism? Clin Exp Pharmacol Physiol 1985;12:249-252.
146. Ma JT, Wang C, Lam KS, et al. Fifty cases of primary hyperaldosteronism in Hong Kong Chinese with a high frequency of periodic paralysis. Evaluation of techniques for tumour localisation. Q J Med 1986;61:1021-1037.
147. Young WF Jr, Klee GG. Primary aldosteronism. Diagnostic evaluation. Endocrinol Metab Clin North Am 1988;17:367-395.
148. Blumenfeld JD, Sealey JE, Schlussel Y, et al. Diagnosis and treatment of primary hyperaldosteronism. Ann Intern Med 1994;121: 877-885.
149. Torres VE, Young WF Jr, Offord KP, et al. Association of hypokalemia, hypoaldosteronism, and renal cysts. N Engl J Med 1990;322:345-351.
150. Stowasser M, Sharman J, Leano R, et al. Evidence for abnormal left ventricular structure and function in normotensive individuals with familial hyperaldosteronism type I. J Clin Endocrinol Metab 2005;90:5070-5076.
151. Milliez P, Girerd X, Plouin PF, et al. Evidence for an increased rate of cardiovascular events in patients with primary aldosteronism. J Am Coll Cardiol 2005;45:1243-1248.
152. Tanabe A, Naruse M, Naruse K, et al. Left ventricular hypertrophy is more prominent in patients with primary aldosteronism than in patients with other types of secondary hypertension. Hypertens Res 1997;20:85-90.
153. Rossi GP, Sacchetto A, Visentin P, et al. Changes in left ventricular anatomy and function in hypertension and primary aldosteronism. Hypertension 1996;27:1039-1045.
154. Young WF Jr. Minireview: primary aldosteronism—changing concepts in diagnosis and treatment. Endocrinology 2003;144: 2208-2213.
155. Williams JS, Williams GH, Raji A, et al. Prevalence of primary hyperaldosteronism in mild to moderate hypertension without hypokalaemia. J Hum Hypertens 2006;20:129-136.
156. Calhoun DA, Nishizaka MK, Zaman MA, et al. Hyperaldosteronism among black and white subjects with resistant hypertension. Hypertension 2002;40:892-896.
157. Mulatero P, Rabbia F, Milan A, et al. Drug effects on aldosterone/plasma renin activity ratio in primary aldosteronism. Hypertension 2002;40:897-902.
158. Nishizaka MK, Pratt-Ubunama M, Zaman MA, et al. Validity of plasma aldosterone-to-renin activity ratio in African American and white subjects with resistant hypertension. Am J Hypertens 2005;18:805-812.
159. Montori VM, Young WF Jr. Use of plasma aldosterone concentration-to-plasma renin activity ratio as a screening test for primary

aldosteronism. A systematic review of the literature. Endocrinol Metab Clin North Am 2002;31:619-632.

160. Weinberger MH, Fineberg NS. The diagnosis of primary aldosteronism and separation of two major subtypes. Arch Intern Med 1993;153:2125-2129.
161. Young WF Jr. Primary aldosteronism: diagnosis. In Mansoor GA, ed. Secondary Hypertension: Clinical Presentation, Diagnosis, and Treatment. Totowa, NJ: Humana Press, 2004:119-137.
162. Hirohara D, Nomura K, Okamoto T, et al. Performance of the basal aldosterone to renin ratio and of the renin stimulation test by furosemide and upright posture in screening for aldosterone-producing adenoma in low renin hypertensives. J Clin Endocrinol Metab 2001;86:4292-4298.
163. Ferrari P, Shaw SG, Nicod J, et al. Active renin versus plasma renin activity to define aldosterone-to-renin ratio for primary aldosteronism. J Hypertens 2004;22:377-381.
164. Olivieri O, Ciacciarelli A, Signorelli D, et al. Aldosterone to renin ratio in a primary care setting: the Bussolengo study. J Clin Endocrinol Metab 2004;89:4221-4226.
165. Perschel FH, Schemer R, Seiler L, et al. Rapid screening test for primary hyperaldosteronism: ratio of plasma aldosterone to renin concentration determined by fully automated chemiluminescence immunoassays. Clin Chem 2004;50:1650-1655.
166. Lim PO, Farquharson CA, Shiels P, et al. Adverse cardiac effects of salt with fludrocortisone in hypertension. Hypertension 2001;37: 856-861.
167. Young WF Jr, Hogan MJ, Klee GG, et al. Primary aldosteronism: diagnosis and treatment. Mayo Clinic Proc 1990;65: 96-110.
168. Bravo EL, Tarazi RC, Dustan HP, et al. The changing clinical spectrum of primary aldosteronism. Am J Med 1983;74:641-651.
169. Kem DC, Weinberger MH, Mayes DM, Nugent CA: Saline suppression of plasma aldosterone in hypertension. Arch Intern Med 1971;128:380-386.
170. Holland OB, Brown H, Kuhnert L, et al. Further evaluation of saline infusion for the diagnosis of primary aldosteronism. Hypertension 1984;6:717-723.
171. Weinberger MH, Grim CE, Hollifield JW, et al. Primary aldosteronism: diagnosis, localization, and treatment. Ann Intern Med 1979;90:386-395.
172. Arteaga E, Klein R, Biglieri EG. Use of the saline infusion test to diagnose the cause of primary aldosteronism. Am J Med 1985;79:722-728.
173. Stowasser M, Gordon RD. Primary aldosteronism—careful investigation is essential and rewarding. Mol Cell Endocrinol 2004;217:33-39.
174. Sawka AM, Young WF, Thompson GB, et al. Primary aldosteronism: factors associated with normalization of blood pressure after surgery. Ann Intern Med 2001;135:258-261.
175. Meyer A, Brabant G, Behrend M. Long-term follow-up after adrenalectomy for primary aldosteronism. World J Surg 2005;29: 155-159.
176. Celen O, O'Brien MJ, Melby JC, Beazley RM. Factors influencing outcome of surgery for primary aldosteronism. Arch Surg 1996;131:646-650.
177. Kloos RT, Gross MD, Francis IR, et al. Incidentally discovered adrenal masses. Endocr Rev 1995;16:460-484.
178. Young WF, Stanson AW, Thompson GB, et al. Role for adrenal venous sampling in primary aldosteronism. Surgery 2004;136: 1227-1235.
179. Gordon RD, Stowasser M, Rutherford JC. Primary aldosteronism: are we diagnosing and operating on too few patients? World J Surg 2001;25:941-947.
180. Daunt N. Adrenal vein sampling: how to make it quick, easy, and successful. Radiographics 2005;25(suppl 1):S143-S158.
181. Doppman JL, Gill JR Jr. Hyperaldosteronism: sampling the adrenal veins. Radiology 1996;198:309-312.
182. Litchfield WR, Anderson BF, Weiss RJ, et al. Intracranial aneurysm and hemorrhagic stroke in glucocorticoid-remediable aldosteronism. Hypertension 1998;31:445-450.
183. Melby JC, Spark RF, Dale SL, et al. Diagnosis and localization of aldosterone-producing adenomas by adrenal-vein catheterization. N Engl J Med 1967;277:1050-1056.
184. Conn JW, Morita R, Cohen EL, et al. Primary aldosteronism. Photoscanning of tumors after administration of 131 I-19-iodocholesterol. Arch Intern Med 1972;129:417-425.
185. Sarkar SD, Cohen EL, Beierwaltes WH, et al. A new and superior adrenal imaging agent, 131I-6beta-iodomethyl-19-nor-cholesterol (NP-59): evaluation in humans. J Clin Endocrinol Metab 1977;45: 353-362.
186. Hogan MJ, McRae J, Schambelan M, et al. Location of aldosterone-producing adenomas with 131I-19-iodocholesterol. N Engl J Med 1976;294:410-414.
187. Nomura K, Kusakabe K, Maki M, et al. Iodomethylnorcholesterol uptake in an aldosteronoma shown by dexamethasone-suppression scintigraphy: relationship to adenoma size and functional activity. J Clin Endocrinol Metab 1990;71:825-830.
188. Ganguly A, Dowdy AJ, Luetscher JA, et al. Anomalous postural response of plasma aldosterone concentration in patients with aldosterone-producing adrenal adenoma. J Clin Endocrinol Metab 1973;36:401-404.
189. Biglieri EG, Schambelan M. The significance of elevated levels of plasma 18-hydroxycorticosterone in patients with primary aldosteronism. J Clin Endocrinol Metab 1979;49:87-91.
190. Young WF Jr. Primary aldosteronism—treatment options. Growth Horm IGF Res 2003;13(suppl A):S102-S108.
191. Proye CA, Mulliez EA, Carnaille BM, et al. Essential hypertension: first reason for persistent hypertension after unilateral adrenalectomy for primary aldosteronism? Surgery 1998;124:1128-1133.
192. Rossi H, Kim A, Prinz RA. Primary hyperaldosteronism in the era of laparoscopic adrenalectomy. Am Surg 2002;68:253-256, discussion 256-257.
193. Gonzalez R, Smith CD, McClusky DA 3rd, et al. Laparoscopic approach reduces likelihood of perioperative complications in patients undergoing adrenalectomy. Am Surg 2004;70:668-674.
194. Ishidoya S, Ito A, Sakai K, et al. Laparoscopic partial versus total adrenalectomy for aldosterone producing adenoma. J Urol 2005;174:40-43.
195. Sywak M, Pasieka JL. Long-term follow-up and cost benefit of adrenalectomy in patients with primary hyperaldosteronism. Br J Surg 2002;89:1587-1593.
196. Ghose RP, Hall PM, Bravo EL. Medical management of aldosterone-producing adenomas. Ann Intern Med 1999;131:105-108.
197. Lim PO, Young WF, MacDonald TM. A review of the medical treatment of primary aldosteronism. J Hypertens 2001;19:353-361.
198. Sica DA. Pharmacokinetics and pharmacodynamics of mineralocorticoid blocking agents and their effects on potassium homeostasis. Heart Fail Rev 2005;10:23-29.
199. Jeunemaitre X, Chatellier G, Kreft-Jais C, et al. Efficacy and tolerance of spironolactone in essential hypertension. Am J Cardiol 1987;60:820-825.
200. Morgenstern BZ. Hypertension in pediatric patients: current issues. Mayo Clin Proc 1994;69:1089-1097.
201. Merke DP, Bornstein SR. Congenital adrenal hyperplasia. Lancet 2005;365:2125-2136.
202. New MI, Geller DS, Fallo F, et al. Monogenic low renin hypertension. Trends Endocrinol Metab 2005;16:92-97.
203. Mussig K, Wehrmann M, Horger M, et al. Adrenocortical carcinoma producing 11-deoxycorticosterone: a rare cause of mineralocorticoid hypertension. J Endocrinol Invest 2005;28:61-65.
204. Kino T, Vottero A, Charmandari E, et al. Familial/sporadic glucocorticoid resistance syndrome and hypertension. Ann N Y Acad Sci 2002;970:101-111.
205. Stewart PM, Corrie JE, Shackleton CH. Syndrome of apparent mineralocorticoid excess. A defect in the cortisol-cortisone shuttle. J Clin Invest 1988;82:340-349.
206. Liddle GW, Blesdoe T, Coppage WS Jr. A familial renal disorder simulating primary aldosteronism but with negligible aldosterone secretion. Trans Assoc Am Physicians 1963;76:199-213.
207. Geller DS, Farhi A, Pinkerton N, et al. Activating mineralocorticoid receptor mutation in hypertension exacerbated by pregnancy. Science 2000;289:119-123.
208. Sacerdote A, Weiss K, Tran T, et al. Hypertension in patients with Cushing's disease: pathophysiology, diagnosis, and management. Curr Hypertens Rep 2005;7:212-218.
209. Baid S, Nieman LK. Glucocorticoid excess and hypertension. Curr Hypertens Rep 2004;6:493-499.

210. Danzi S, Klein I. Thyroid hormone and blood pressure regulation. Curr Hypertens Rep 2003;5:513-520.
211. Streeten DH, Anderson GH Jr, Howland T, et al. Effects of thyroid function on blood pressure: recognition of hypothyroid hypertension. Hypertension 1988;11:78-83.
212. Richards AM, Espiner EA, Nicholls MG, et al. Hormone, calcium and blood pressure relationships in primary hyperparathyroidism. J Hypertens 1988;6:747-752.
213. Sancho JJ, Rouco J, Riera-Vida R, et al. Long-term effects of parathyroidectomy for primary hyperparathyroidism on arterial hypertension. World J Surg 1992;16:732-736.
214. Terzolo M, Matrella C, Boccuzzi A, et al. Twenty-four hour profile of blood pressure in patients with acromegaly. Correlation with demographic, clinical and hormonal features. J Endocrinol Invest 1999;22:48-54.

SECTION V

Reproduction

CHAPTER 16

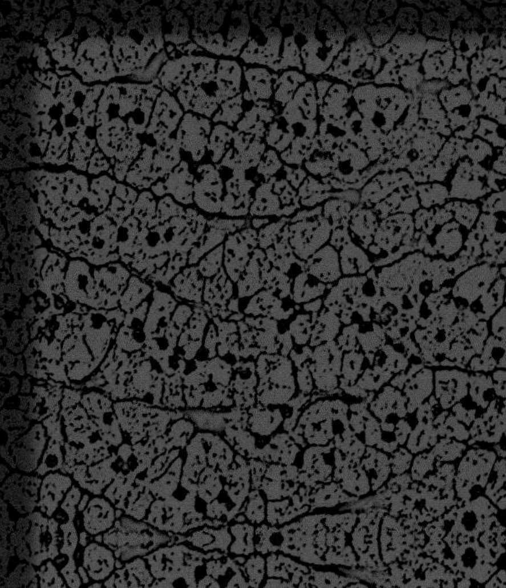

THE PHYSIOLOGY AND PATHOLOGY OF THE FEMALE REPRODUCTIVE AXIS

Serdar E. Bulun and Eli Y. Adashi

REPRODUCTIVE PHYSIOLOGY

Tightly coordinated functions of the hypothalamus, pituitary gland, ovaries, and endometrium give rise to cyclic, predictable menses that indicate regular ovulation. Regular ovulation also requires normal functioning of other endocrine units such as the thyroid and adrenal glands. For example, patients with hypothyroidism or hyperthyroidism, Cushing's syndrome, or glucocorticoid resistance may present with anovulation. Thus, it is imperative for the clinician to have a thorough knowledge of the functions of the hypothalamus, pituitary, ovaries, and uterus as well as interactions of these tissues with other systems in order to diagnose correctly reproductive disorders and generate treatment strategies.

The most obvious reproductive function of the hypothalamus is the pulsatile secretion of gonadotropin-releasing hormone (GnRH). Negative feedback effects of a number of factors, including ovarian steroids, regulate hypothalamic GnRH secretion into the portal vessels. Dopamine, norepinephrine, serotonin, and opioids produced in the brain may mediate the regulation of GnRH secretion by ovarian hormones or other stimuli. In response to GnRH, the anterior pituitary cells secrete follicle-stimulating hormone (FSH) and luteinizing hormone (LH). Steroids (estradiol and progesterone) and peptides (inhibin) of ovarian origin and activin and follistatin of pituitary origin modify secretion of FSH and LH. LH stimulates androstenedione production in theca cells of the ovary, whereas FSH regulates estradiol and inhibin B production in the granulosa cells and follicular growth. Release of an egg from the mature follicle is dependent on a sudden rise in LH levels in midcycle. After ovulation, the follicle transforms into a corpus luteum that secretes both estradiol and progesterone under the control of FSH and LH. LH also stimulates granulosa lutein cells of the corpus luteum to secrete inhibin A (Fig. 16–1A).

The endocrine effects of FSH, LH, estradiol, progesterone, inhibin A, and inhibin B have been deduced by changes in their serum levels throughout the menstrual cycle (see Fig. 16–1A). These postulated endocrine effects have been then demonstrated by cell-based and in vivo studies (see Fig. 16–1B). Activin and follistatin are produced both in the ovary and the pituitary. They appear to act on FSH in the pituitary by autocrine or paracrine but not endocrine pathways. Activin stimulates FSH production, whereas follistatin suppresses this action of activin.

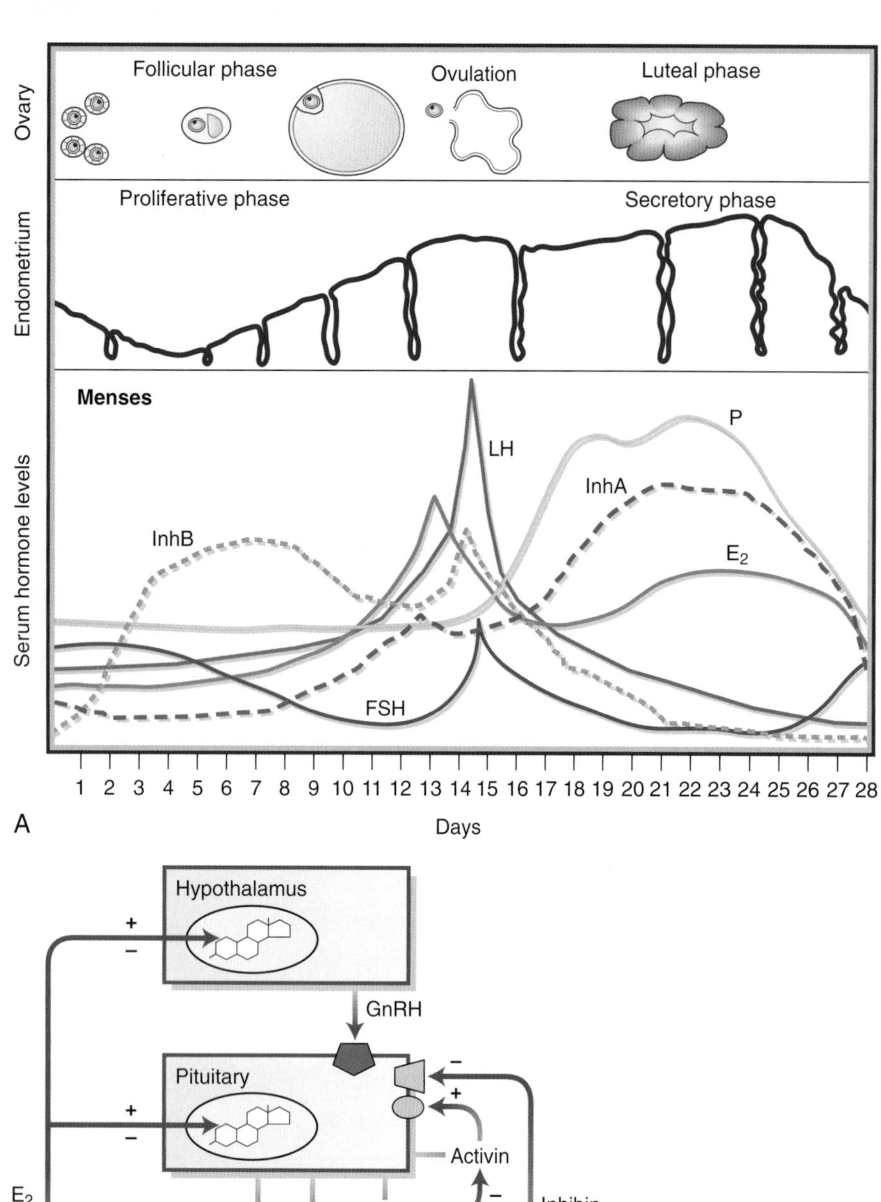

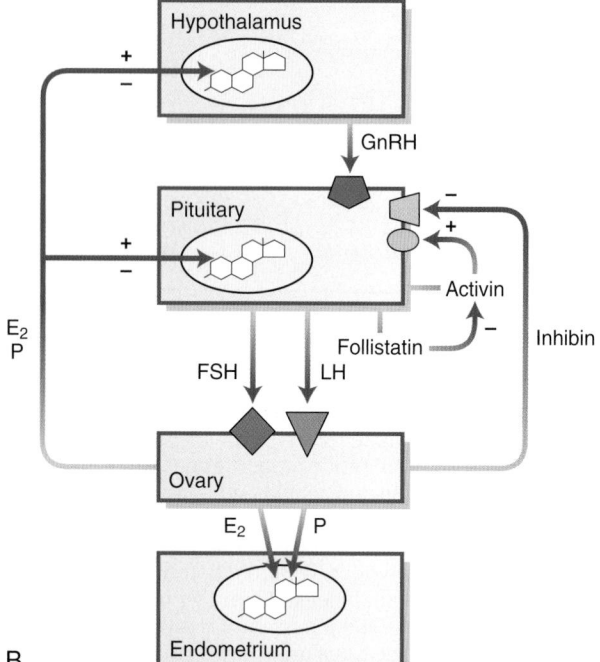

Figure 16–1 ▪ **A,** Changes in the ovarian follicle, endometrial thickness, and serum hormone levels during a 28-day menstrual cycle. Menses occur during the first few days of the cycle. **B,** Endocrine interactions in the female reproductive axis. Some of the well-characterized endocrine interactions between the hypothalamus, pituitary, ovary, and endometrium for regulation of the menstrual cycle are depicted. *E2,* Estradiol; *FSH,* follicle-stimulating hormone; *GnRH,* gonadotropin-releasing hormone; *InhA,* inhibin-A; *InhB,* inhibin-B; *LH,* luteinizing hormone; *P,* progesterone.

Endometrium, the mucosal lining of the uterine cavity, has extremely high concentrations of nuclear receptors for estrogen and progesterone and is extremely sensitive to these hormones. The biologically active estrogen estradiol induces the growth of endometrium, whereas progesterone limits this estrogenic effect and enhances differentiation. Sloughing off the functional portion (functionalis) of the endometrium follows withdrawal of estrogen or progesterone. The remaining basal layer (basalis) is capable of full regeneration in response to estrogen.

Ovaries remain quiescent until puberty because the hypothalamus is immature in prepubertal children, and FSH and LH do not stimulate the ovaries. The entire reproductive function and most of the endocrine function of the ovaries cease after menopause because ovaries have lost all oocytes and surrounding steroidogenic cells at this time. These prepubertal and postmenopausal states, characterized by the absence of ovarian function, are associated with the lack of menses.

In summary, the female reproductive function from puberty to menopause can be viewed as an extremely delicate ticking clock. The normal function of this apparatus is dependent on coordinate actions of the hypothalamus, pituitary, ovaries, and endometrium. The end result is regular menses every 24 to 35 days. Any disorder of these tissues or disorders of other systems that affect these reproductive units secondarily may result in anovulation and consequent irregular uterine bleeding.

REPRODUCTIVE FUNCTIONS OF THE HYPOTHALAMUS

Gonadotropin-Releasing Hormone

GnRH is a 10-amino-acid peptide that is synthesized primarily in specialized neuronal bodies of the arcuate nucleus of the medial basal hypothalamus.[1] Axons from GnRH neurons project to the median eminence and terminate in the capillaries that drain into the portal vessels.

The portal vein is a low-flow transport system that descends along the pituitary stalk and connects the hypothalamus to the anterior pituitary. The direction of the blood flow in this hypophyseal portal circulation is from the hypothalamus to the pituitary. Thus, GnRH originating in the neurons of the arcuate nucleus is secreted at the median eminence into the portal circulation, which delivers this hormone to the anterior pituitary (Fig. 16–2).[2]

The mature decapeptide GnRH is derived from the posttranslational processing of a large precursor molecule, pre-pro-GnRH (see Fig. 16–2).[3] This precursor peptide is the product of a gene located in the short arm of chromosome 8.[4] The pre-pro-GnRH consists of 92 amino acids and contains four parts (from the N-terminal to the C-terminal): (1) a 23-amino-acid signal domain,[5] (2) the GnRH decapeptide, (3) a 3-amino-acid proteolytic processing site, and (4) a 56-amino-acid domain called *GnRH-associated peptide*.[2,6] The cleavage products of this precursor, GnRH and GAP, are transported to the nerve terminals and secreted into the portal circulation (see Fig. 16–2).[3,7,8] A physiologic role of GAP has not been established.[7]

In humans, GnRH neurons are located primarily in the arcuate nucleus of the medial basal hypothalamus and the preoptic area of the anterior hypothalamus. The population of GnRH-producing neurons is relatively limited and is in the range of 1000 to 3000. The neurons that produce GnRH originate from the olfactory area during embryogenesis. These cells migrate during embryogenesis along cranial nerves connecting the nose and forebrain to the hypothalamus. A neuronal cell-surface glycoprotein that probably mediates cell-to-cell adhesion appears to be an important migratory determinant. Mutation of the gene that encodes this adhesion molecule is associated with X-linked isolated gonadotropin deficiency (Kallmann's syndrome) characterized by anosmia, GnRH deficiency, and hypogonadotropic hypogonadism.[9]

Knobil and colleagues demonstrated by a pioneering series of experiments that normal gonadotropin secretion requires pulsatile GnRH discharge within a critical frequency and amplitude.[10] The periodicity and amplitude of the pulsatile rhythm of GnRH and gonadotropin secretion are crucial in regulating gonadal activities and therefore the entire reproductive axis (Fig. 16–3). The self-priming effect of GnRH to up-regulate its receptors on pituitary gonadotropin-producing cells becomes manifest only at the physiologic periodicity (60 to 90 minutes).[11,12] Slower frequency causes anovulation and amenorrhea because of inadequate stimulation. Interestingly, higher frequency or constant exposure to GnRH also gives rise to anovulation by down-regulating expression of the GnRH receptor, thereby abolishing gonadotropin responses (see Fig. 16–3).

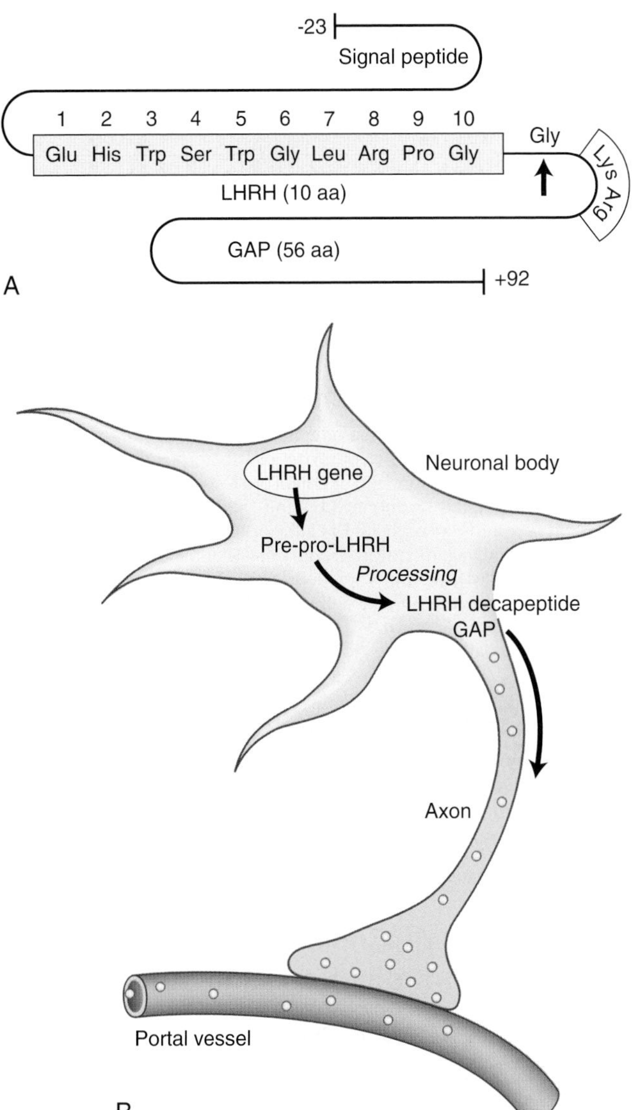

Figure 16–2 ▪ Gonadotropin-releasing hormone (GnRH) production. **A,** The GnRH gene encodes a precursor protein named pre-pro-GnRH in the neuronal body. GnRH is released from this protein by proteolytic processing, which gives rise to GnRH and GnRH-associated protein[2] within the neuronal body. Both GnRH and GAP are transported in an axon to the nerve terminal and secreted into the portal circulation. **B,** Pre-pro-GnRH is a 92-amino-acid (aa) protein. The biologically active decapeptide (aa 1 to 10) is sandwiched between the 23-aa signal peptide and the Gly-Lys-Arg sequence. The arrow indicates the site of proteolytic processing. The C-terminal 56-aa peptide is cleaved to produce GAP. (From Yen SSC. Endocrine regulation of the reproductive system. In Yen SSC, Jaffe RB, Barbieri RL, eds. Reproductive Endocrinology, 4th ed. Philadelphia: WB Saunders, 1999:44.)

The activation of gene expression for gonadotropin subunits including the common α subunit and specific β subunits for LH and FSH, dimerization of αβ subunits, and glycosylation are also governed by intermittency of GnRH inputs to pituitary gonadotrophs.[13] In humans, the measurement of LH pulses is commonly utilized as an indication of GnRH pulsatile secretion.[14] The LH pulse frequency is approximately 90 minutes during early follicular phase, 60 to 70 minutes during late follicular phase, 100 minutes during early luteal phase, and 200 minutes during late luteal phase.[15] This variation is responsible for changes in FSH and LH levels and ovarian steroid release during these phases of the menstrual cycle. The relationship of gonadotropin

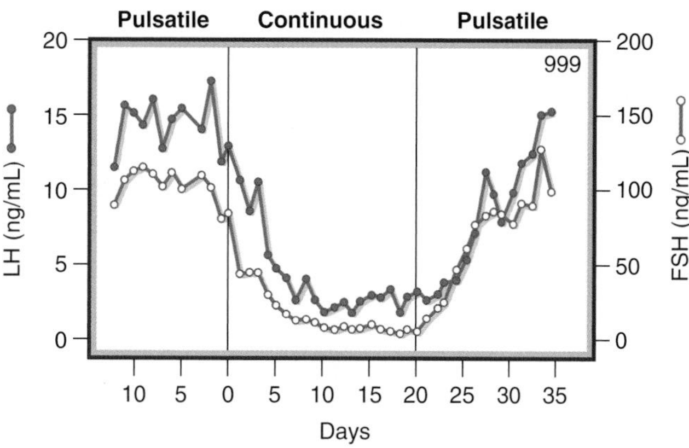

Figure 16–3 ▪ Effect of pulsatile or continuous administration of gonadotropin-releasing hormone (GnRH) to ovariectomized monkeys rendered them GnRH-deficient by placement of a lesion in the hypothalamus. Release of luteinizing hormone (LH) and follicle-stimulating hormone (FSH) was restored by hourly GnRH infusion, inhibited during a continuous infusion, and again restored after reinstitution of pulsatile GnRH administration. (Adapted from Belchetz PE, et al. Hypophysial responses to continuous and intermittent delivery of hypothalamic gonadotropin releasing hormone. Science 1978;202:631-633. Copyright © 1978 by American Association for the Advancement of Science.)

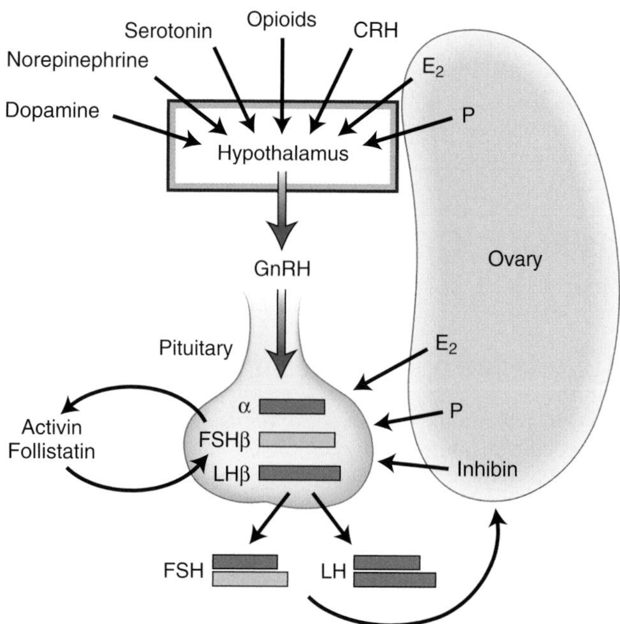

Figure 16–4 ▪ Regulation of gonadotropin-releasing hormone (GnRH), luteinizing hormone (LH), and follicle-stimulating hormone (FSH) secretion. Locally synthesized and systemic hormones regulate the pulsatile secretion of GnRH from the hypothalamus into the portal circulation. In turn, GnRH together with a number of steroid and peptide hormones regulate the synthesis of α and β gonadotropin subunits and the formation and secretion of FSH and LH. *CRH,* Corticotropin-releasing hormone; *E2,* estradiol; *P,* progesterone.

secretion to GnRH pulse pattern has been studied in hypophysectomized animals receiving exogenous GnRH as well as in numerous in vitro systems. In general, more rapid pulse frequencies favor LH secretion, whereas slower pulse frequencies favor FSH. It appears that variations in GnRH pulse frequency markedly influence both the absolute levels and the ratio of LH and FSH release.

Regulation of Gonadotropin-Releasing Hormone Secretion

Cyclic, predictable menses require the pulsatile release of GnRH within a critical range of frequencies as explained earlier. Pulsatile, rhythmic activity is an intrinsic property of GnRH neurons, and various hormones and neurotransmitters modulate this rhythm (Fig. 16–4).

The variations in GnRH pulse frequency are achieved, at least in part, by gonadal steroid feedback. Estradiol increases GnRH pulse frequency, whereas elevated progesterone levels decrease GnRH pulsatility.[13] Therefore, it is conceivable that increased progesterone levels may cause a decrease in GnRH pulse frequency and thereby lead to the preferential biosynthesis and secretion of FSH that is observed in the late luteal phase.[13]

Estrogen signaling to GnRH neurons appears to be critical for both suppressing FSH and LH and also coordinating the preovulatory surge release of LH. GnRH neurons are directly regulated by estradiol primarily through estrogen receptor-β, and indirectly through estradiol-sensitive afferent neurons. Direct treatment of GnRH neurons with estradiol generally represses GnRH gene expression but, in vivo, this repression is transiently overcome by indirect estradiol-dependent signals relayed by afferent neurons. Thus, estradiol can inhibit or stimulate GnRH secretion and coordinate both follicular maturation and the preovulatory surge release of LH.[16]

GnRH pulsatility is also modulated by the action of locally released neurotransmitters. Norepinephrine stimulates GnRH release, whereas dopamine exerts an inhibitory effect (see Fig. 16–4).[17] β-Endorphin and other opioids may also serve to suppress the hypothalamic release of GnRH.[18,19] The gonadal steroids modify endogenous opioid activity, and the negative feedback of steroids on gonadotropins appears to be mediated, at least in part, by endogenous opioids.[20] Thus, it was proposed that sex steroids enhance the activity of endogenous opioids that in turn exert an inhibitory effect on GnRH secretion.[21] The negative effect of opioids on GnRH secretion is also clinically explicable because the reduced GnRH secretion associated with hypothalamic amenorrhea may be mediated by an increase in endogenous opioid inhibitory tone.[22]

Kisspeptins, encoded by the Kiss1 gene, and their receptor, GPR54, play key roles in the regulation of GnRH secretion.[23] Mutations or targeted knockout of GPR54 produce isolated hypogonadotropic hypogonadism in humans and mice, indicating that signaling through this receptor is essential for sexual development and function.[24,25] Kisspeptins stimulate GnRH and gonadotropin secretion in prepubertal and adult animals.[26] Moreover, kisspeptin- and GPR54-expressing neurons are targets for the negative and positive feedback actions of sex steroids.[23]

Gonadotropin-Releasing Hormone Analogues

The half-life of GnRH is short (2 to 4 minutes) because it is degraded rapidly by peptidases in the hypothalamus and pituitary gland.[27] These peptidases cleave the bonds between amino acids 5 and 6, 6 and 7, and 9 and 10. Analogues of GnRH with different properties have been synthesized by altering amino acids at these positions. Thus far, many agonistic and antagonistic GnRH analogues with various biologic effects have been produced.

Gonadotropin-Releasing Hormone Agonists

A number of GnRH agonists were generated by substitution of amino acids at the 6 or 10 position. The increased biologic activity of agonistic peptides has been attributed to their high binding affinity to GnRH receptors and reduced susceptibility to enzymatic degradation. An amino acid substitution at position 6 gives rise to metabolic stability, whereas replacement of the C-terminal glycinamide residue by an ethylamide group increases strikingly the affinity for the receptors.[27-29] GnRH agonists are administered subcutaneously, intranasally, or intramuscularly. An initial agonistic action (i.e., the flare effect) is associated with an increase in the circulating levels of LH and FSH.

The most prominent agonistic response is observed during the early follicular phase, when the combined effects of GnRH agonist and elevated levels of estradiol create a large reserve pool of gonadotropins.[30] Desensitization and down-regulation of the pituitary produce hypogonadotropic hypogonadism. The administration of a long-acting depot formulation of a GnRH agonist gives rise eventually to down-regulation of the gonadotropin-gonadal axis within 1 to 3 weeks. The initial down-regulation effect is due to desensitization, whereas the sustained response is due to loss of receptors and the uncoupling of the receptor from its effector system. In addition, GnRH agonists may cause ovarian quiescence by the secretion of biologically inactive gonadotropins.

Thus far, the Food and Drug Administration (FDA) has approved the use of these agonists for the treatment of GnRH-dependent precocious puberty, endometriosis, and prostate cancer. Another indication is preoperative hematologic improvement of patients with anemia caused by uterine leiomyomas. Off-label indications of GnRH agonists include the down-regulation of the pituitary during ovulation induction, induction of endometrial atrophy before endometrial ablation surgery, and the prevention of menstrual bleeding in patients with coagulation defects. GnRH agonists have also been used to suppress ovarian steroidogenesis in hirsute patients.[31]

The most prominent side effects of long-term use of depot GnRH agonist formulations are caused by estrogen deficiency. Depot GnRH agonists induce a menopause-like state characterized by hot flashes, vaginal dryness, bone resorption, and osteopenia. Osteopenia is reversible in young women if treatment is maintained for no more than 6 months.[32,33] Therefore, the risk-benefit ratio must be considered carefully before GnRH agonist treatment is extended for longer durations. Add-back regimens employing low-dose estrogens or progestins, or both, administered along with GnRH agonists have provided a means to overcome these side effects and permit extending the length of agonist therapy.[34]

Gonadotropin-Releasing Hormone Antagonists

Multiple amino acid substitutions also permit the synthesis of GnRH antagonists. These include modifications of the pyroglutamic and glycine termini at positions 1 and 10 or deletion and substitution of hydrophobic amino acids at positions 2 and 3.[29] GnRH antagonists bind to the GnRH receptor and provide competitive inhibition for the naturally synthesized GnRH. GnRH antagonists have the advantage of inducing an immediate decrease in circulating gonadotropin levels with rapid reversal.[35] The early antagonists either lacked potency or were associated with undesirable side effects related to histamine release. Newer GnRH antagonists are at various stages of development.[36-41] These new antagonists are slightly more potent in the down-regulation of ovaries and do not cause histamine release. GnRH antagonists recently replaced GnRH agonists for the prevention of a natural LH surge during ovulation induction by injectable FSH.[42] Use of GnRH antagonists has especially become popular in ovulation induction protocols for in vitro fertilization (IVF).[42]

REPRODUCTIVE FUNCTIONS OF THE ANTERIOR PITUITARY

Gonadotroph

Gonadotrophs are specialized cell types of the anterior pituitary that synthesize and secrete LH and FSH. These cells constitute 7% to 15% of the total number of anterior pituitary cells and are detected in this location from early fetal life.[43] The majority of the gonadotrophs are capable of synthesizing both LH and FSH.[43,44] LH and FSH are each composed of two distinct, noncovalently associated protein subunits called α and β (see Fig. 16–4). In the gonadotroph, the subunit genes are transcribed into messenger ribonucleic acids (mRNAs), which are in turn translated into the subunit precursors. Gonadotrophs contain cell-surface GnRH receptors that mediate the action of GnRH. These receptors belong to the seven-transmembrane-domain and G protein–coupled receptor family.

Gonadotropin-Releasing Hormone Receptor

There are two G protein–coupled GnRH receptors in mammals.[45] Type I receptor in the gonadotroph has been well characterized in humans. Recent cloning of a second GnRH receptor subtype (type II GnRH receptor) in nonhuman primates revealed that it is structurally and functionally distinct from the mammalian type I receptor. However, the human type II receptor gene homolog carries a frameshift and a premature stop codon, suggesting that a full-length type II receptor does not exist in humans.[45] Thus, the following information is related to the type I GnRH receptor in humans.

In humans, hypothalamic GnRH regulates gonadotropin secretion through the pituitary GnRH type I receptor via activation of Gq/11.[46] Although the predominant coupling of the type I GnRH receptor in the gonadotroph is through Gq/11 stimulation, signal transduction can occur via other G proteins and potentially by G protein–independent means.[45,46] A number of downstream cascades are activated by GnRH. These include PKC-, Ca^{2+}-, and tyrosine kinase–dependent pathways.[45] In mouse pituitary gonadotrophs, the GnRH receptor was reported to activate several MAPK cascades including the ERK1/2, the c-Jun amino-terminal kinase (JNK), the p38 MAPK, and the big MAPK (BMK1/ERK5).[45] The cross-talk between these pathways remains to be clarified.

Activation of G protein–coupled receptors is typically followed by their desensitization and internalization, and these processes involve rapid agonist-induced receptor phosphorylation by both second messenger-dependent protein kinases and G protein–coupled receptor kinases. Because the serine and threonine residues that are phosphorylated by G protein–coupled receptor kinases are often located in the carboxyl-terminal tail, which is uniquely absent in the mammalian GnRH receptor, a number of studies have revealed that the tailless GnRH receptor neither undergoes rapid homologous desensitization nor exhibits agonist-induced receptor phosphorylation. In addition, the receptor internalizes slowly via clathrin-coated vesicles, and this process occurs independently of β-arrestin and dynamin.[45]

Luteinizing Hormone and Follicle-Stimulating Hormone

Each gonadotropin is a heterodimer. Both LH and FSH are made of two peptide subunits termed α and β (see Fig. 16–4). The subunits α and β are associated with noncovalent bonds. The α subunits of human LH, FSH, thyroid-stimulating hormone (TSH), and human chorionic gonadotropin (hCG) have an identical polypeptide structure. In contrast, the β subunit of each hormone has a unique amino acid sequence and confers the specific activity of the αβ heterodimer. Each subunit is cysteine-rich and contains multiple disulfide linkages. Each subunit also contains multiple carbohydrate moieties that play important roles in the biologic activity and metabolism of these hormones. The identical α subunit contains 92 amino acids. The β subunits of human FSH, LH, and hCG contain 117, 121, and 145 amino acids, respectively (Table 16–1).[47-50] Upon binding of GnRH to its receptor, the biosynthesis of the gonadotropins proceeds by transcription of the subunit genes, translation of the subunit mRNAs, posttranslational modifications of the precursor subunits and subunit folding and combination, mature hormone packaging, and hormone secretion (see Fig. 16–4).

The human α subunit gene is located on the short arm of chromosome 6. The encoded precursor polypeptide contains a 24-amino-acid leader sequence that is cleaved posttranslationally to produce the mature 92-amino-acid α subunit.

The human LH and hCG β subunit genes are located on chromosome 19q13.3, which contains a cluster of seven β subunit-like genes.[48] Five of these sequences are noncoding pseudogenes arranged in groups of tandem and inverted pairs. Only LH and hCG β subunit genes give rise to two distinct and functional mRNA species. The LH β subunit mRNA encodes a 145-amino-acid precursor protein that is later cleaved to produce a 24-amino-acid leader peptide and a 121-amino-acid biologically active mature peptide. The hCG β subunit mRNA also encodes a 145-amino-acid protein. This protein, however, is not processed posttranslationally and functions as the biologically active hCG β subunit. The amino acid sequences of the human LH and hCG β subunits are 82% homologous. These two β subunits confer identical biologic activities when associated with the α subunit.[48-50]

A single gene located on the short arm of chromosome 11 encodes FSH β subunit, which is 117 amino acids long.[51] Complementary DNA encoding human FSH-β, LH-β, or hCG-β in combination with the complementary DNA of α subunit was expressed in mammalian cells in culture. These cells can synthesize these proteins, modify them after translation, glycosylate and combine the subunits, and secrete them as intact FSH, LH, or hCG.[52] These recombinant gonadotropins are currently used clinically to stimulate gonadal function.

Regulation of Circulating Levels of Follicle-Stimulating Hormone and Luteinizing Hormone

The molecular mechanisms responsible for formation and combination of the α and β subunits of FSH and LH are not completely understood. Production rates of both α and β subunits are regulated at least in part by negative feedback by estrogen, which regulates the pulsatile release of GnRH from the hypothalamus.[52,53] The pituitary always contains more α subunit than β subunit mRNA, and readily detectable levels of free α subunit are present in serum. The free β subunit, on the other hand, is present at relatively low levels in pituitary and is rarely found in serum or urine. Thus, the specific β subunit may be the rate-limiting factor in the synthesis of these glycoprotein hormones.

Inhibin, activin, and follistatin were first identified as gonadal hormones that could exert selective effects on FSH secretion. Although the primary source of inhibin remains the ovary, both activin and follistatin are produced in extragonadal tissues and can exert effects on FSH through an autocrine-paracrine mechanism. Inhibin B is secreted by ovarian granulosa cells during the follicular phase (under the control of FSH) and inhibin A by the corpus luteum in the luteal phase under the control of LH. Inhibins act synergistically with estradiol to inhibit FSH secretion. Activin can directly stimulate FSH biosynthesis and release from the gonadotroph cells of the pituitary gland. Follistatin can negatively regulate these effects by binding activin and preventing it from interacting with the activin receptor at the cell membrane.[54]

Serum levels of gonadotropins are proportional to their secretion rates and serum half-lives, which are regulated by the number of carbohydrate residues. The higher the content of carbohydrate residues, especially the sialic acid residues, the lower the rate of metabolism and the higher the serum half-life.[55] The sialic acid content of gonadotropic hormones and other glycoproteins has a marked effect on their rate of clearance and also influences their apparent molecular size. The higher content of sialic acid in FSH compared with LH is responsible for slower clearance of FSH from the circulation; LH has the most rapid clearance rate. The hCG is highly sialylated and has the longest half-life (see Table 16–1).

TABLE 16–1 PROPERTIES OF GONADOTROPINS

Gonadotropins	Location of *β*-subunit gene	Size of *β*-subunit	Half-life in serum
FSH	Chromosome 11p13	117aa*	3-4h†
LH	Chromosome 19q13.3	121aa	20min‡
hCG	Chromosome 19q13.3	145aa	24h

*Aa, amino acid; †h, hour; ‡min, munute.

OVARY

The ovary is essential for periodic release of oocytes and the production of the steroid hormones, estradiol and progesterone. These activities are integrated into the cyclic repetitive process of follicular maturation, ovulation, and formation and regression of the corpus luteum. Thus, the ovary fulfills two major objectives: (1) the generation of a fertilizable ovum and (2) the preparation of the endometrium for implantation through the sequential secretion of estrogen and progesterone. The ovarian follicle comprising the egg and surrounding granulosa and theca cells constitutes the fundamental functional unit of the ovary.

Adult human ovaries are oval bodies with a length of 2 to 5 cm, a width of 1.5 to 3 cm, and a thickness of 0.5 to 1.5 cm. The combined weight of normal ovaries during the reproductive years is 10 to 20 g (average 14 g). The ovaries lie in approximation to the posterior and lateral pelvic wall and are attached to the posterior surface of the broad ligament by the peritoneal fold, termed the *mesovarium.* Blood vessels, nerves, and lymphatics traverse the mesovarium and enter the ovary at the hilum.[56]

The ovary consists of three structurally distinct regions: (1) an outer cortex containing the surface germinal epithelium and the follicles, (2) a central medulla consisting of stroma, and (3) a hilum around the area of attachment of the ovary to the mesovarium. The functional anatomy of the adult ovary is illustrated in Figure 16-5. The hilum is the point of attachment of the ovary to the mesovarium. It contains nerves, blood vessels, and hilus

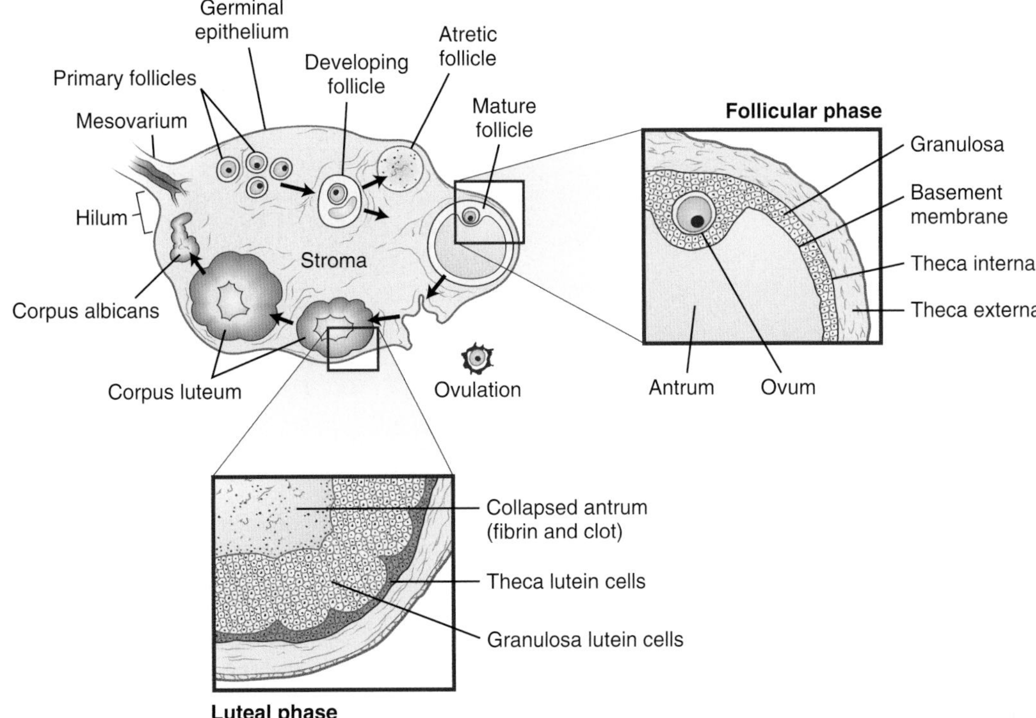

Figure 16–5 ■ Functional anatomy and developmental changes in the adult ovary during an ovarian cycle. (From Carr BR, Wilson JD. Disorders of the ovary and female reproductive tract. In Braunwald E, Isselbacher KJ, Petersdorf RG, et al, eds. Harrison's Principles of Internal Medicine, 11th ed. New York: McGraw-Hill, 1987:1818-1837.)

cells, which have the potential to become active in steroidogenesis or to form androgen-secreting tumors. These cells are similar to the testosterone-producing Leydig cells of the testes. The outermost portion of the cortex, called the *tunica albuginea*, is covered by a single layer of surface cuboidal epithelium termed the *germinal epithelium*. The oocytes, enclosed in complexes called *follicles*, are in the inner part of the cortex, embedded in stromal tissue (see Fig. 16–5). One dominant follicle is recruited for ovulation during each cycle. The preovulatory follicle transforms into a corpus luteum after ovulation (see Fig. 16–5). In the absence of pregnancy, the corpus luteum regresses to become corpus albicans (see Fig. 16–5). The stromal tissue is composed of connective tissue and interstitial cells, which are derived from mesenchymal cells and have the ability to respond to LH or hCG with the production of androstenedione. The central medullary area of the ovary is derived largely from mesonephric cells.

Genetic Determinants of Ovarian Differentiation and Folliculogenesis

Ovarian differentiation and folliculogenesis depend on coordinate expression and interaction of a multitude of genes.[57] Targeted gene disruption or insertion in mice has made it possible to inquire about the function of specific genes in ovarian differentiation and folliculogenesis. Figure 16-6 summarizes the biologic roles of some of these genes.[57] Genetically altered mice represent a first step in attempting to understand in vivo the various gene interactions that result in a functional ovary. Indeed, ovarian pathologic conditions in transgenic mice closely resemble disorders observed in mutant human homologues, as exemplified in cases involving the FSH-β subunit and FSH receptor. Many mouse models of ovarian pathologic conditions are available. In general, these can be divided into mice with prenatal ovarian failure with disordered gonad formation and diminished number of germ cells or absent germ cells and mice with postnatal ovarian failure as a result of defects at various stages of folliculogenesis (see Fig. 16–6).[57] These models should lead to the identification of genetic and molecular mechanisms responsible for the development and function of the human ovary.

In humans, certain gene defects may give rise to specific defects in folliculogenesis. This was exemplified by the discovery of a heterozygous mutation in the bone morphogenetic protein-15 (BMP15) gene, which caused ovarian dysgenesis. BMP15 is an oocyte-specific growth/differentiation factor that stimulates folliculogenesis and granulosa cell growth. In vitro, mutant BMP15 reduced granulosa cell growth, and antagonized the stimulatory activity of wild-type protein on granulosa cell proliferation. In vivo, this mutation was associated with familial ovarian dysgenesis, indicating that the action of BMP15 is required for the progression of human folliculogenesis.[58]

Ontogeny of the Ovary

The Oocyte

The primordial germ cells are known to originate outside the embryo proper, from the endoderm of the yolk sac. At this site, they can be identified as early as the end of the third week of gestation by alkaline phosphatase staining. Germ cells migrate to cross a remarkably long distance from the yolk sac to the genital ridge by ameboid movements with the aid of pseudopodia.[59] This long route of migration along the dorsal mesentery of the hindgut is interrupted only by the required lateral crossing of the coelomic angle at the level of the genital ridge (Fig. 16–7).

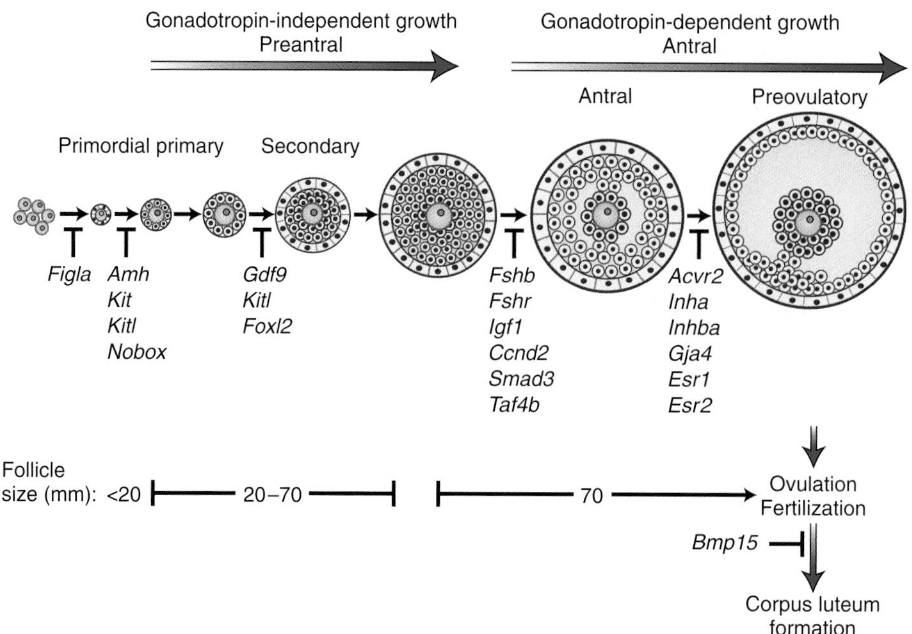

Figure 16–6 ▪ Diagram illustrating developmental stages at which certain murine genes affect oogenesis. Data from transgenic mice with disruption of various genes indicated critical roles of a number of genes during various phases of the follicular development. Preantral follicular growth is viewed to be gonadotropin-independent, whereas antrum formation and follicular maturation require action of follicle-stimulating hormone (FSH). *Acvr2,* Activin type II receptor; *Amh,* antimuellerian hormone; *Bmp15,* bone morphogenetic protein-15; *Ccnd2,* cyclin d2; *Esr1,* estrogen receptor-α; *Esr2,* estrogen receptor-β; *Figla,* factor in the germline-α; *Foxl2,* forkhead box L2; *Fshb,* FSH β subunit; *Fshr,* FSH receptor; *Gdf9,* growth differentiation factor-9; *Gja4,* gap junction protein connexin 37; *Igf1,* insulin-like growth factor I; *Inha,* inhibin α(alpha) subunit; *Inhba,* activin βA subunit; *Kit,* kit receptor, *Kitl,* kit-ligand; *Nobox,* newborn ovary homeobox gene; *Smad3,* Sma mothers against decapentaplegic-3; *Taf4b,* TATA-box-binding protein-associated factor-4b. (Modified from Simpson JL, Rajkovic A. Ovarian differentiation and gonadal failure. Am J Med Genet 1999;89:186-200 and Choi Y, Rajkovic A. Genetics of mammalian folliculogenesis. Cell Mol Life Sci 2006;63(5):579-590.)

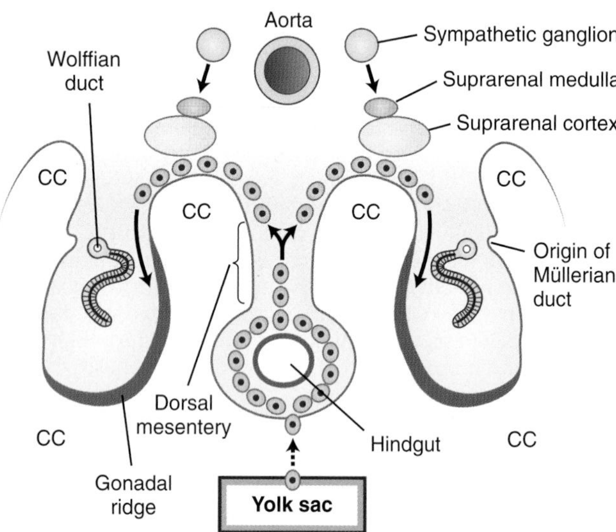

Figure 16–7 ▪ Transverse section of the caudal region of a 5-week embryo showing the location of gonadal ridges, the primordium of the adrenal glands, and the migration path of primordial germ cells. From the third week on, germ cells arising from the yolk sac cross the dorsal mesentery of the hindgut and migrate to the gonadal ridges. By the end of the fifth week, rapid division of primordial germ cells, gonadal epithelium, and mesenchyme starts the early gonad that differentiates subsequently into the ovary in a 46,XX fetus. *CC,* Coelomic cavity. (Modified from Moore K. The Developing Human. Philadelphia: WB Saunders, 1983.)

Some chemotaxis is operational, but the precise cellular mechanisms underlying the guidance of germ cells to the genital ridge remain uncertain. Germ cells appear unable to persist outside the genital ridge, which may thus be viewed as the only region competent to sustain gonadal development. By the same token, germ cells play an indispensable role in the induction of gonadal development. In fact, no functional gonad can form in the absence of germ cells.

On arrival at the genital ridge by the fifth week of gestation, the premeiotic germ cells are referred to as *oogonia.*[60] During the subsequent 2 weeks of intrauterine life (weeks 5 to 7 of gestation or the "indifferent" stage), the primordial gonadal structure constitutes no more than a bulge on the medial aspect of the urogenital ridge (see Fig. 16–7). This protuberance is created by proliferation of surface (coelomic) germinal epithelium, by growth of the underlying mesenchyme, and by oogonial multiplication. The oogonia total 10,000 by about 6 to 7 weeks of intrauterine life. Because meiosis and oogonial atresia are not occurring, the actual number of germ cells is dictated by mitotic division at this time.

It is during this indifferent phase that the gonadal cortex and medulla are first delineated. However, short of cytogenetic evidence, the precise sexual identity of the gonadal ridge cannot be ascertained at this point. Nevertheless, the absence of testicular development beyond 7 weeks of gestation is generally considered presumptive evidence of formation of the ovary. Additional clues to the sexual identity of the gonad can be derived from the detection of oogonial meiosis at about 8 weeks of gestation, because no comparable process is observed in the testis until puberty. The sexual identity of the gonadal ridge is histologically clear by 16 weeks of gestation, when the first primordial follicles can be visualized.

By about 8 weeks of intrauterine life, persistent mitosis increases the total number of oogonia to 600,000 (Fig. 16–8). From this point on, the oogonial endowment is subject to three simultaneous ongoing processes: mitosis, meiosis, and oogonial atresia. Stated differently, the onset of oogonial meiosis and oogonial atresia is now superimposed on oogonial mitosis. As a result of the combined impact of these processes, the number of germ cells peaks at 6 to 7×10^6 by 20 weeks of gestation (see Fig. 16–8). At this time, two thirds of the total germ cells are intrameiotic primary oocytes; the remaining third can still be viewed as oogonial. The midgestational peak and the postpeak decline are accounted for, if only in part, by the progressively decreasing rate of oogonial mitosis, a process destined to end entirely by about 7 months of intrauterine life. Equally relevant is the increasing rate of oogonial atresia, which peaks at about month 5 of gestation. During this period, regulation of the ovarian developmental process is complex and probably involves a diverse group of genes (see Fig. 16–6).[61,62]

From midgestation onward, relentless and irreversible attrition progressively diminishes the germ cell endowment of the gonad. Ultimately, some 50 years later, this is finally exhausted. For the most part, this is accomplished through follicular atresia rather than oogonial atresia, begins around month 6 of gestation, and continues throughout life (see Fig. 16–8). In contrast, oogonial atresia is destined to end at 7 months of intrauterine life as follicular atresia sets in. Follicular atresia has a profound effect on germ cell endowment, given that only 1 to 2×10^6 germ cells are present at birth (see Fig. 16–8).[63] Remarkably, this dramatic depletion of the germ cell mass occurs during a period as short as 20 weeks. No similar rate of depletion occurs earlier or subsequently. Consequently, newborn females enter life still far from realizing reproductive potential, having lost as much as 80% of their germ cell endowment. This decreases further to approximately 300,000 by the onset of puberty. Of these follicles, only 400 to 500 (i.e., less than 1% of the total) ovulate in the course of a reproductive life span.

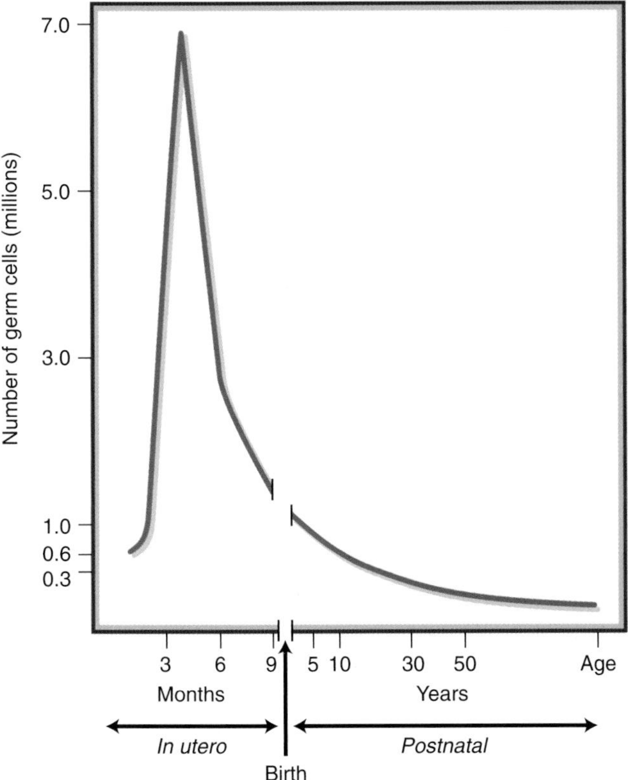

Figure 16–8 ▪ Age-dependent changes in germ cell number in the human ovary. The highest number of oocytes is found in the ovaries of a human fetus at midgestation. This number decreases sharply during the third trimester. After birth, the progressive decline in the number of ovarian follicles containing oocytes continues until complete depletion at the menopause. (From Baker TG. A quantitative and cytological study of germ cells in the human ovaries. Proc R Soc Biol Sci 1963;158:417-433.)

Between weeks 8 and 13 of fetal life, some of the oogonia depart from the mitotic cycle to enter the prophase of the first meiotic division. This change marks the conversion of these cells to primary oocytes well before actual follicle formation. Meiosis (beginning at about 8 weeks of gestation) provides temporary protection from oogonial atresia, thereby allowing the germ cells to invest themselves with granulosa cells and to form primordial follicles. Accordingly, oogonia that persist beyond the seventh month of gestation and have not entered meiosis are subject to oogonial atresia. Consequently, no oogonia are usually present at birth.

Once formed, the primary oocyte persists in prophase of the first meiotic division until the time of ovulation, when meiosis is resumed and the first polar body is formed and extruded (Fig. 16–9). Although the exact cellular mechanisms responsible for this meiotic arrest remain uncertain, it is generally presumed that a granulosa cell-derived putative meiosis inhibitor is in play. This hypothesis is based on the observation that denuded (granulosa-free) oocytes are capable of spontaneously completing meiotic maturation in vitro.

The primary oocyte is converted into a secondary oocyte by completion of the first meiotic metaphase and formation of the first polar body, before actual ovulation but after the LH surge. At ovulation, the secondary oocyte and the surrounding granulosa cells (cumulus oophorus) are extruded and enter the fallopian tube. If sperm penetration occurs, the secondary oocyte undergoes a second meiotic division, after which the second polar body is eliminated (see Fig. 16–9).

The Granulosa Cell Compartment

A basement lamina separates the oocyte and granulosa cells from the surrounding stromal cells.[64] Thus, the granulosa cells do not have direct access to the circulation (Fig. 16–10). The avascular nature of the granulosa cell compartment necessitates contact between neighboring cells. Thus, the granulosa cells are interconnected by extensive intercellular gap junctions, which result in their coupling to yield an expanded, integrated, and functional syncytium (see Fig. 16–10).[65,66] Gap junctions are composed of proteins called *connexins*. Connexin-37 is present in gap junctions in follicles, and gap junction protein connexin 37–deficient mice lack graafian follicles, fail to ovulate, and develop inappropriate corpora lutea (Gja4 in Fig. 16–6).[67] These specialized cell junctions may be important in metabolic exchange and in the transport of small molecules between neighboring granulosa cells. Moreover, the granulosa cells extend cytoplasmic processes that penetrate the zona pellucida to form gap junctions with the plasma membrane of the oocyte (see Fig. 16–10). In the gap junction protein connexin 37–deficient mice, the authors also found that oocyte development is arrested before meiotic competence.[67] Thus, gap junctions represent a crucial communication system that is needed for the tight control exerted by the cumulus granulosa cells on the resumption of meiosis by the enclosed primary oocyte.

The granulosa cells in the fully developed graafian follicle shortly before ovulation are stratified in a manner allowing the distinction of a number of populations of cells.[68,69] Distinct popu-

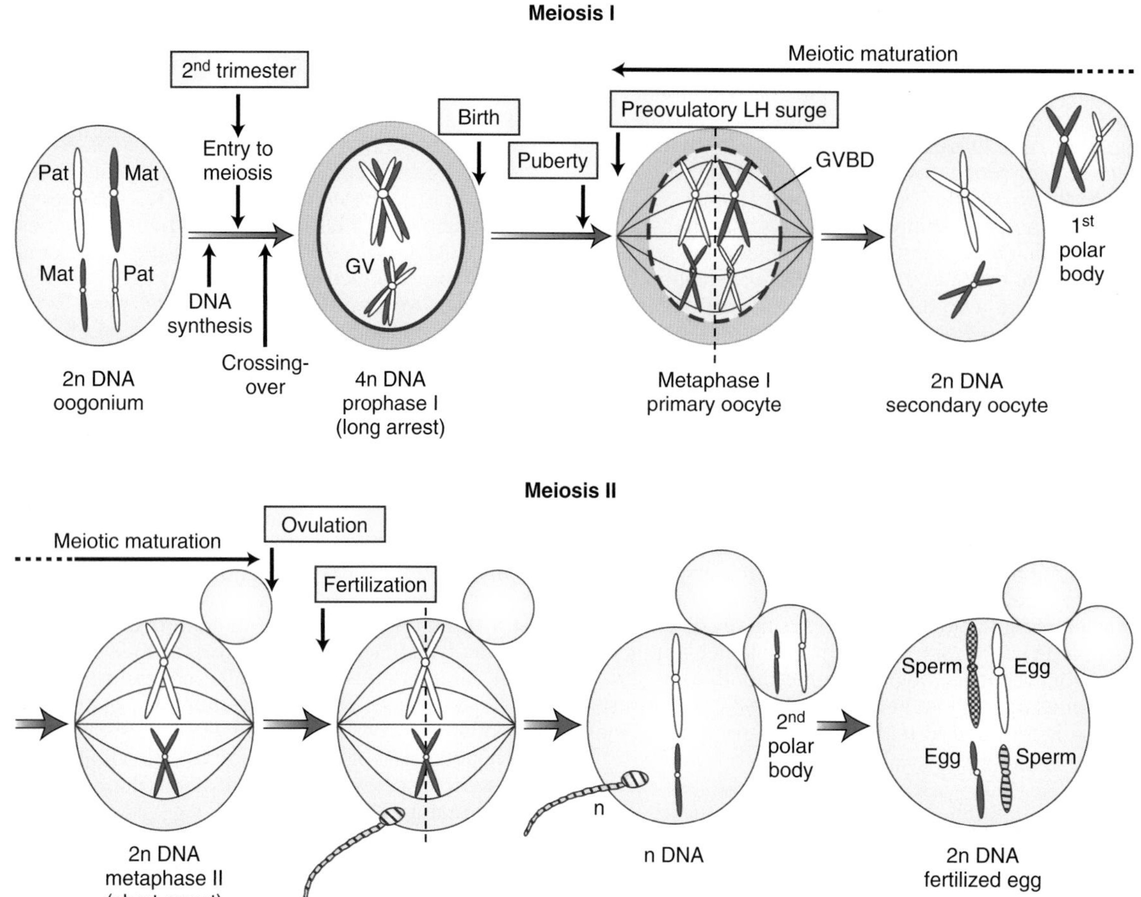

Figure 16–9 ▪ Meiotic cell division. Meiosis occurs exclusively in germ cells and serves two critical purposes: (1) generation of germ cells genetically distinct from the somatic cells and (2) generation of a mature egg with a reduction in the number of chromosomes from 46 to 23. Genetic recombination through crossing over of genes between homologous chromosomes and random assortment of (original) maternal and paternal chromosomes into daughter cells during the first meiotic division are responsible for the first function of meiosis, maintenance of genetic diversity. The second function is provided by a reduction in the number of chromosomes so that each daughter cell, or ovum, receives randomly one chromosome from each of the 23 pairs. During fertilization, the fusion of ovum and sperm, each of which has 23 chromosomes, produces a genetically novel individual with 46 chromosomes. The chromosome marked as white in the oogonium (upper left corner) originates from the father of the fetus, whereas the blue chromosome comes from the mother of the fetus. The random exchange of genes (alleles) between homologous chromosomes (crossing over) takes place before the meiotic arrest in the prophase I stage before birth. During postnatal life, these oocytes remain in meiotic arrest until puberty. In the developing oocyte in the graafian follicle, meiosis I is resumed immediately after the preovulatory luteinizing hormone (LH) surge during each ovulatory cycle. Meiotic maturation is defined as the period from the breakdown of the oocyte's nucleus (germinal vesicle, GV) until the oocyte reaches metaphase II (i.e., transition from oocyte to egg). A second and short meiotic arrest occurs at metaphase II until the oocyte is fertilized by a sperm. *DNA*, Deoxyribonucleic acid; *GVBD*, germinal vesicle breakdown; *mat*, maternal; *n*, the amount of DNA material in haploid number (23) of chromosomes; *pat*, paternal.

lations of granulosa cells exhibit specific, specialized functions.[70-72] Granulosa cells within the outermost layer adjacent to the basement layer contain high levels of gonadotropin hormone receptors and steroidogenic enzymes and thus account for most of the steroidogenesis in the follicle[68,69] (Fig. 16–11). The cumulus oophorus contains the egg and a surrounding mass of granulosa cells that have cell–cell interactions with the egg and thus seem to have critical roles in oocyte development[70-72] (see Fig. 16–11).

The Interstitial (Interfollicular) Compartment: Theca-Interstitial Cells

Ryan and Petro[73] demonstrated that the theca-interstitial cells produce C19-steroids, which serve primarily as precursors for estrogen and androgen. Rice and colleagues[74] noted the ability of the theca interna (see later) and interstitial tissue to undertake de novo synthesis of C19-steroids (Fig. 16–12). The C19-producing cells are located in the loose connective tissue of both the cortex and the medulla, arising in all likelihood from a population of unspecialized mesenchymal cells in the stromal compartment.

The cells making up the theca-interstitial compartment are heterogeneous in nature. One contemporary view of the dynamic alterations characteristic of this ovarian compartment is that of Erickson and colleagues.[75] Several classes of interstitial cells have been identified. Among these cell types, theca-interstitial cells represent the constant feature of all developing follicles (see Figs. 16-11 and 16-12). These cells are identified as theca interna, the stromal cell layer adjacent to the basal lamina

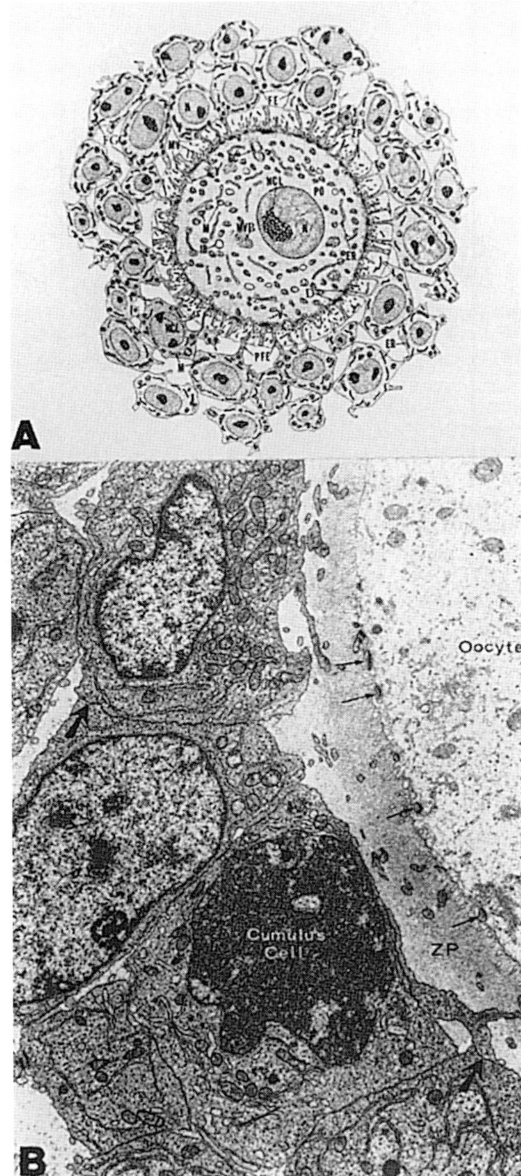

Figure 16–10 ▪ Structural relationship between the granulosa cell and the oocyte. **A,** Microvilli of an oocyte interdigitate with cytoplasmic extensions of granulosa cells, penetrating the zona pellucida. **B,** Note the penetration of the zona pellucida by cytoplasmic processes of granulosa cells. Small gap junctions (*thin arrows*) are observed between processes of the granulosa cell and the oocyte membrane. The thick arrow indicates a gap junction between granulosa cells. (From Erickson GF. An analysis of follicle development and ovum maturation. Semin Reprod Endocrinol 1986;4:233, Thieme Medical Publishers, New York, with permission.)

around granulosa cells, and theca externa, a less well-defined layer of stromal cells that make up the outermost layer of the follicle (see later, Figs. 16-11 and 16-12). Theca interstitial cells represent the main mature C19 steroid-producing component of the follicle.

Resident Ovarian White Blood Cells

Unlike the testicular seminiferous tubule, the ovary does not constitute an immunologically privileged site. Thus, resident ovarian mononuclear phagocytes (macrophages), lymphocytes, and polymorphonuclear granulocytes can be observed at various stages of the ovarian life cycle. For example, macrophages, but not other white blood cells, are known to constitute a major cellular component of the interstitial (i.e., interfollicular) ovarian compartment.[76] In part, these macrophages are present within the ovarian stroma near perifollicular capillaries. Lymphocytes and polymorphonuclear leukocytes, on the other hand, are observed in the follicle and corpus luteum in varying quantities during follicular development, corpus luteum formation, and follicular atresia.[77-79]

The significance of the preceding observations may be that resident ovarian representatives of the white blood cell series constitute potential in situ modulators of ovarian function, acting through the local secretion of regulatory cytokines.[80] Because the flow of information is probably multidirectional, the same cells are probably targeted for steroidal and peptidergic input. Moreover, immune cells are endowed with steroidogenic capabilities that could, in their own right, affect steroid economy.[81]

Follicles

The follicle represents the most important functional unit in the ovary with respect to germ cell development and steroid production. The follicles are embedded in loose connective tissue of the ovarian cortex and can be subdivided into two functional types: nongrowing (or primordial) and growing. The majority of follicles (90% to 95%) are nongrowing throughout reproductive life. Recruitment of a primordial follicle initiates dramatic changes in growth, structure, and function. The growing follicles are divided into four stages: primary, secondary, tertiary, and graafian (see Fig. 16–11). The first three stages of growth can occur in the absence of the pituitary and therefore appear to be controlled by intraovarian mechanisms (Fig. 16–13). The follicle destined to ovulate is recruited in the first few days of the current cycle.[82]

The early growth of follicles occurs over the time span of several preceding menstrual cycles, but the ovulatory follicle is one of a cohort recruited at the time of transition from the previous cycle's luteal phase and the current cycle's follicular phase (see Fig. 16–13).[83,84] The total time to achieve preovulatory status is approximately 85 days (see Fig. 16–13).[83,84] The majority of this period of development is FSH-independent. Eventually, this cohort of follicles reaches a stage at which, unless recruited by FSH, the next step is atresia. Thus, a cohort of follicles measuring 2 to 5 mm is continuously available for a response to FSH. The late luteal increase in FSH is the critical feature in rescuing this cohort of follicles from atresia, eventually allowing a dominant follicle to emerge and pursue a path to ovulation. In addition, maintenance of this increase in FSH for a critical duration of time is essential.[85]

Recruited primordial follicles either develop into dominant, mature graafian follicles destined to ovulate or degenerate as a result of atresia.[86] The average time for development of a selected follicle to the point of ovulation is 10 to 14 days (see Fig. 16–13). If a follicle is not recruited, it goes through a process called *atresia* during which the oocyte and granulosa cells within the basal lamina die and are replaced by fibrous tissue. In contrast, the thecal cells outside the basal lamina do not die but dedifferentiate and return to the pool of cells consisting of ovarian interstitial or stromal cells.[56] The process of atresia is generally thought to result from lack of the hormones or growth factors that are formed by the mature dominant follicle through intrinsic intraovarian mechanisms. There is general agreement that atresia of follicles is due to apoptosis.[87] Apoptosis is an active and regulated process triggered by a cascade of caspase proteases that lead to characteristic fragmentation of DNA and blebbing of membranes.

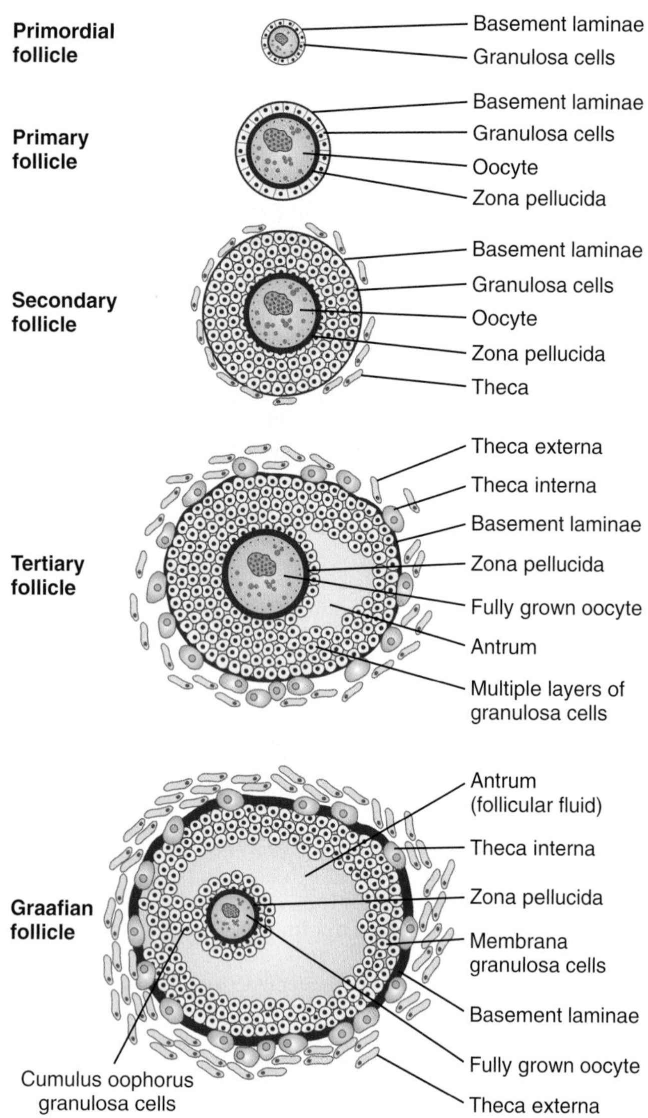

Figure 16–11 ▪ Developmental stages of the ovarian follicle. The primordial follicle is composed of a single layer of granulosa cells and a single immature oocyte arrested in the diplotene stage of the first meiotic division. The primordial follicle is separated from the surrounding stroma by a thin basal lamina (basement membrane). The oocyte and granulosa cells do not have a direct blood supply. The first sign of follicular recruitment is cuboidal differentiation in the spindle-shaped cells inside the basal lamina, which thereafter undergo successive mitotic divisions to form a multilayered granulosa cell zone. The oocyte enlarges and secretes a glycoprotein-containing mucoid substance called the *zona pellucida*, which surrounds the oocyte and separates the granulosa cells from the oocyte. This structure is a primary follicle. The secondary follicle is formed by further proliferation of granulosa cells and by the final phase of oocyte growth, in which the oocyte reaches 120 μm in diameter, coincident with proliferation of layers of cells immediately outside the basal lamina to constitute the theca. The portion of the theca adjacent to the basal lamina is termed the theca interna. Thecal cells that merge with the surrounding stroma are designated the theca externa. The secondary follicle acquires an independent blood supply consisting of one or more arterioles that terminate in a capillary bed at the basal lamina. Capillaries do not penetrate the basement membrane, and the granulosa and oocyte remain avascular. The tertiary follicle is characterized by further hypertrophy of the theca and the appearance of a fluid-filled space among the granulosa cells, named the *antrum*. The fluid in the antrum consists of a plasma transudate and secretory products of granulosa cells, some of which (estrogens) are found there in strikingly higher concentrations than in peripheral blood. The follicle rapidly increases in size under the influence of gonadotropins to form the mature or graafian follicle. In the graafian follicle, the granulosa and oocyte remain encased by the basal lamina and are devoid of direct vascularization. The antral fluid increases in volume, and the oocyte, surrounded by an accumulation of granulosa cells (the cumulus oophorus), occupies a polar, eccentric position within the follicle. The mature graafian follicle is ready to release the ovum by the process of ovulation. (Adapted from Erickson GF, Magoffin DA, Dyer CA. The ovarian androgen producing cells: a review of structure-function relations. Endocr Rev 1985;6:371-379. Copyright © 1985 by The Endocrine Society.)

Ovulation

There is a dramatic rise in circulating estradiol level as midcycle approaches (see later). This increase in estradiol is followed by a striking LH and, to a lesser extent, an FSH surge. This triggers the dominant follicle to ovulate. During each menstrual cycle, usually one follicle ovulates and gives rise to a corpus luteum. In the human, either LH or its surrogate hCG is essential to stimulate the rupture of the mature follicle. It was proposed that increased local prostaglandin biosynthesis in the follicle might mediate the ovulatory effect of LH.[88,89]

Ovulation consists of rapid follicular enlargement followed by protrusion of the follicle from the surface of the ovarian cortex. This is followed by the rupture of the follicle and extrusion of an egg–cumulus complex into the peritoneal cavity (Fig. 16–14). Follicular rupture or ovulation occurs predictably 34 to 36 hours from the start of the LH surge. Elevation of a conical "stigma" on the surface of the protruding follicle precedes rupture (see Fig. 16–14). Rupture of this stigma is accompanied by a gentle rather than explosive expulsion of the ovum and antral fluid. The gonadotropin-dependent production of proteases acting locally on protein substrates in the basal lamina may play an important role in stigma formation and follicular rupture.[90,91] In particular, plasminogen activator levels increase in the follicle before rupture.[92] Thus, plasminogen activator-mediated conversion of plasminogen to plasmin may contribute to the proteolytic digestion of the follicular wall, which is a prerequisite for follicular rupture.

Corpus Luteum

After ovulation, the dominant follicle reorganizes to become the corpus luteum (Fig. 16–15). After rupture of the follicle, capillaries and fibroblasts from the surrounding stroma proliferate and penetrate the basal lamina. This rapid vascularization of the corpus luteum may be guided by angiogenic factors, some of which are detected in the follicular fluid.[93] Vascular endothelial growth factor has been isolated from corpora lutea and has been postulated, along with basic fibroblast growth factor, to be a potential angiogenic agent in corpora lutea.[94] Concurrently, the granulosa and theca cells undergo morphologic changes collectively referred to as *luteinization*. The granulosa cells become granulosa-lutein cells (large cells), and the theca cells are transformed into theca-lutein cells (small cells; see Fig. 16–15B).[95] The so-called K cells, scattered throughout the corpus luteum, are believed to be macrophages.

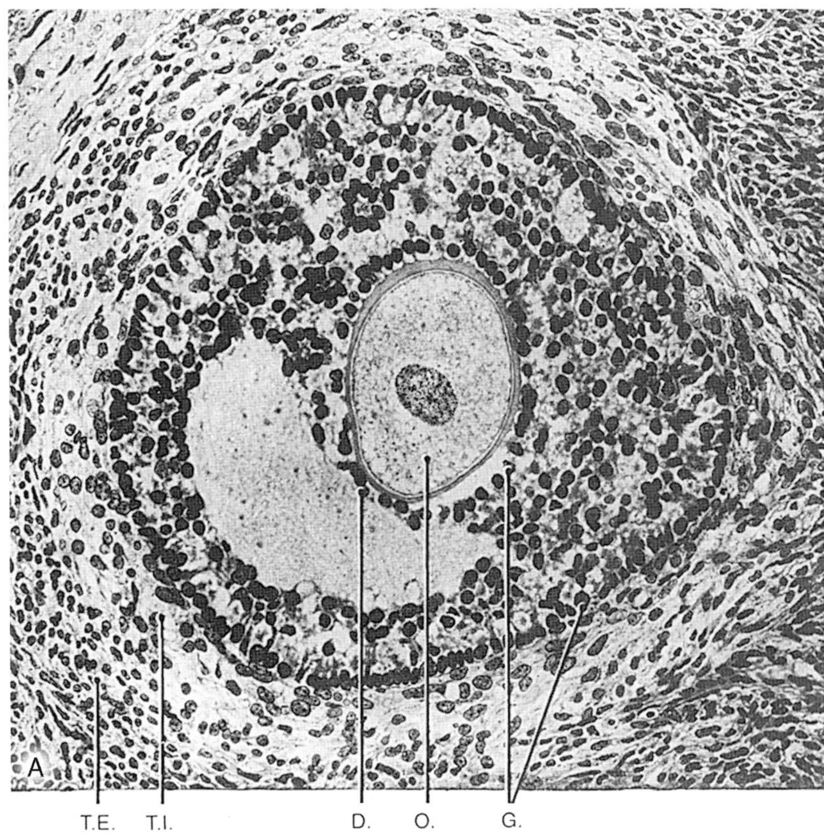

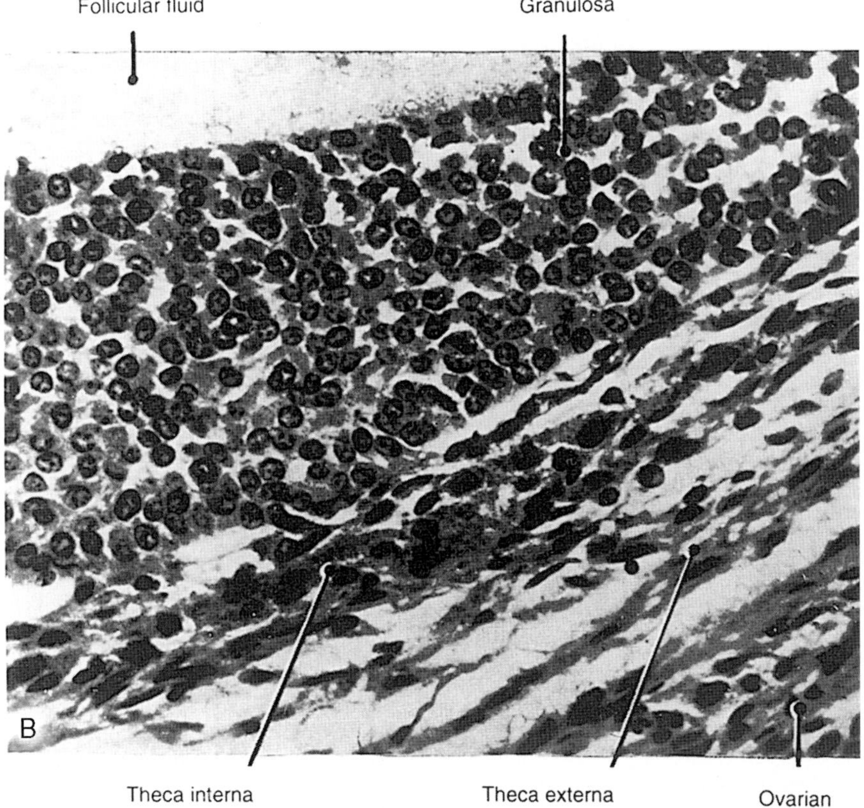

Figure 16–12 ▪ Histology of human graafian follicle. **A,** Cycle day 10 to 12 graafian follicle approaching maturity. *D.*, Discus proligerus (cumulus oophorus); *G.*, granulosa cell layer; *O.*, ovum; *T.E.*, theca externa; *T.I.*, theca interna. **B,** Section through the wall of a mature graafian follicle. (From Cunningham FG, et al. Pregnancy: overview and diagnosis; ovarian function and ovulation. In Williams Obstetrics, 19th ed. Stamford, CT: Appleton & Lange, 1993: 11-55.)

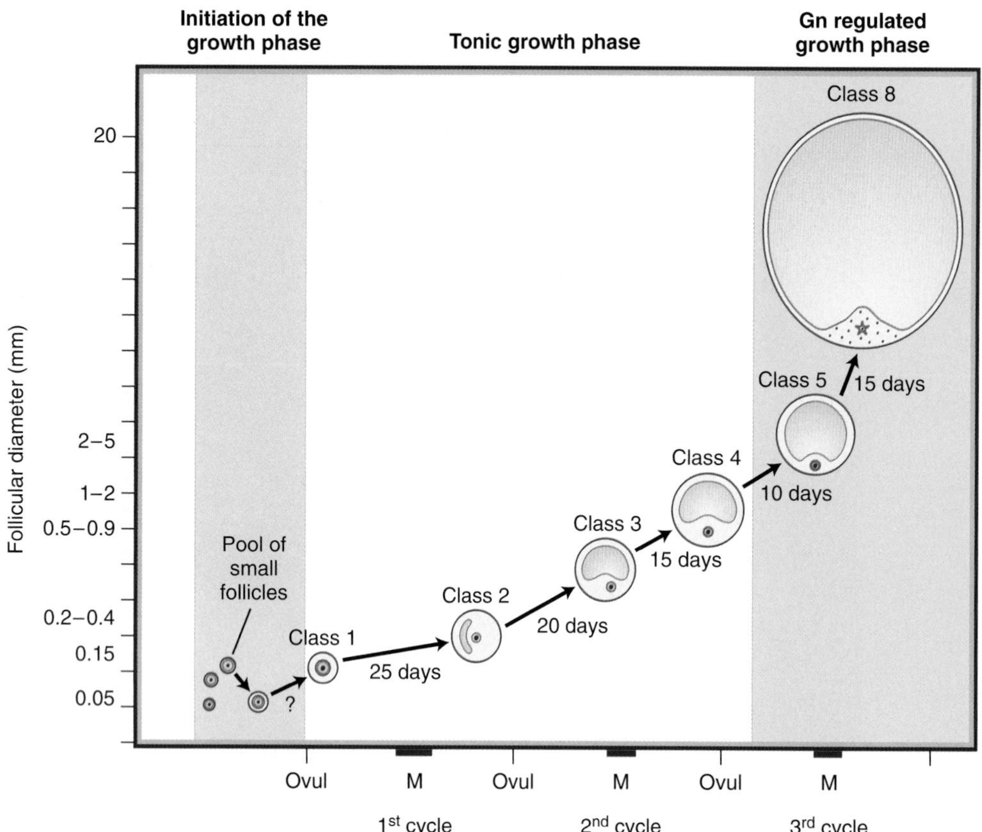

Figure 16–13 ▪ Complete follicular growth trajectory. Class 1 follicle is a secondary follicle with theca cells and is presumed to become responsive to gonadotropins. Although the tonic (early) stage of follicle development (class 1 to 4) is likely to be gonadotropin-dependent (albeit to a lesser extent), the final stages of follicular development (class 5 to 8) are the ones heavily dependent on gonadotropins. According to this view, late luteal phase, class 5 follicles constitute the cohort from which the follicle destined to ovulate in the following cycle is recruited. The exponential gonadotropin-dependent growth phase (class 5 to 8) takes place during the follicular phase of the cycle following the third menses from initiation of the growth phase. During this time, follicular selection and dominance are accomplished. The total duration of the process wherein a class 1 follicle is converted into preovulatory class 8 follicle is estimated to be 85 days and spans three ovulatory cycles. *Gn,* gonadotropin; *M,* menses; *Ovul,* ovulation. (Courtesy of A. Gougeon, Clamart, France.)

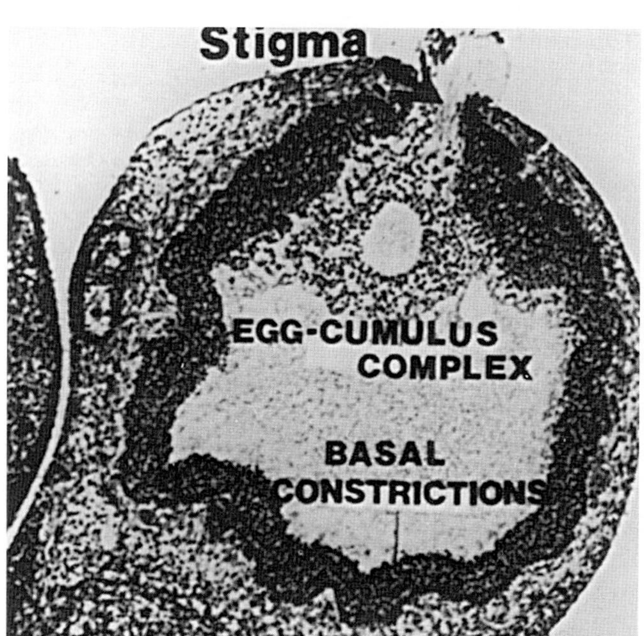

Figure 16–14 ▪ Ovulation of the cumulus–oocyte complex through the stigma. (From Erickson GF. An analysis of follicle development and ovum maturation. Semin Reprod Endocrinol 1986;4:233, Thieme Medical Publishers, New York, with permission.)

The corpus luteum is the endocrine gland that serves as the major source of sex steroid hormones secreted by the ovary during the postovulatory phase of the cycle. The human corpus luteum secretes as much as 40 mg of progesterone per day during the midluteal phase of the ovarian cycle.[96] In view of the small size of the corpus luteum, it is the most active steroidogenic tissue in humans. An important aspect of corpus luteum formation is the penetration of the follicle basement membrane by blood vessels, which provides the granulosa-lutein cells with low-density lipoprotein (LDL).[92] LDL cholesterol serves as the substrate for corpus luteum progesterone production.

A key regulator of steroidogenesis in the corpus luteum is LH. In humans, the LH receptor is maintained throughout the functional life span of corpora lutea and not down-regulated during the maternal recognition of pregnancy.[97] The rate-limiting step in LH-mediated progesterone formation in luteinized granulosa cells is the entry of cholesterol into the mitochondria, which is regulated by steroidogenic acute regulatory protein (StAR; see later).[98] Thus, the availability of LDL cholesterol and the StAR-mediated mitochondrial entry of cholesterol seem to be the two critical factors that account for the production of large amounts of progesterone in the corpus luteum.

The functional life span of the corpus luteum is normally 14 ± 2 days. Thereafter, the corpus luteum spontaneously regresses. It is replaced, unless pregnancy occurs, by an avascular scar referred to as the *corpus albicans.*

Factors that may regulate luteal life span include hormones such as hCG, maintenance of luteal vascularization, and immune cells.[99] There is little doubt about the central role of LH in the maintenance of corpus luteum function. Withdrawal of LH support in a variety of experimental circumstances has almost invariably resulted in luteal regression.[99] In pregnancy, however, the LH surrogate hCG, secreted by the gestational trophoblast, maintains the ability of the corpus luteum to elaborate progesterone; this stimulus helps to maintain the early gestation until the luteoplacental shift.[100] Accordingly, the corpus luteum doubles in size (compared with the pre-pregnancy size) during the first 6 weeks of gestation (see Fig. 16–15). This increase is due to proliferation of connective tissues and blood vessels, along with hypertrophy of the luteinized granulosa and theca cells. This early hypertrophy is later followed by regression. The

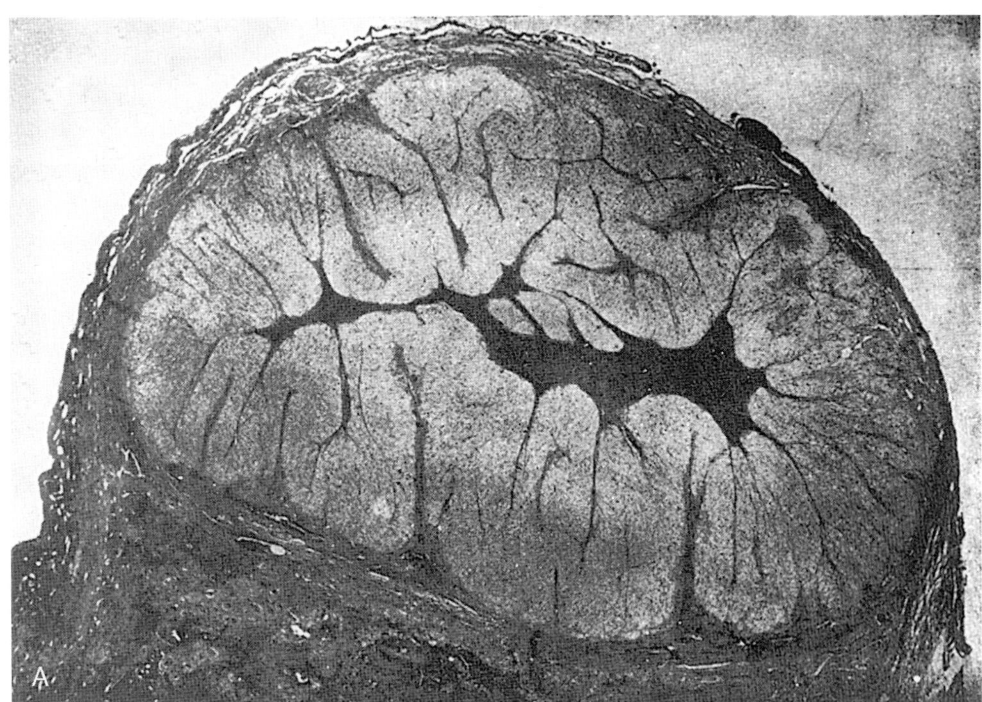

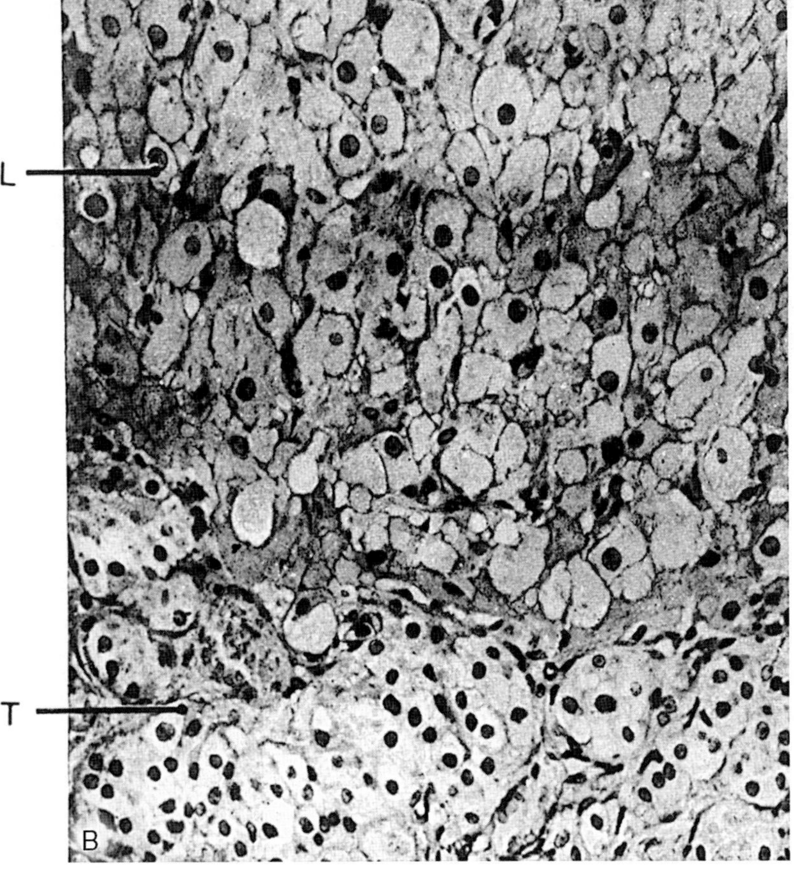

Figure 16–15 ▪ Corpus luteum of pregnancy. **A,** Lower power. **B,** High power. *L,* Granulosa lutein cells; *T,* theca lutein cells. (From Cunningham FG, MacDonald PC, Gant NF, et al. Pregnancy: overview and diagnosis; ovarian function and ovulation. In Williams Obstetrics, 19th ed. Stamford, CT: Appleton & Lange, 1993:11-55.)

corpus luteum at term is only half the size of that during the menstrual cycle.

Hormones such as estrogens and prostaglandins have been suggested as important factors in the promotion of luteal demise.[101,102] Immune factors may influence luteal life span because corpus luteal regression is associated with a progressive infiltration of lymphocytes and macrophages.[99]

Apoptosis may be the end-point mechanism by which human corpora lutea are deleted. Corpora lutea during the early luteal phase of the menstrual cycle and corpora lutea of early pregnancy show no evidence of apoptotic DNA fragmentation.[103] DNA fragmentation, on the other hand, is detected in midluteal and late luteal corpora.[103] Thus, it is hypothesized that apoptosis is a major mechanism for the demise of the corpus luteum. LH or hCG inhibits apoptosis in the corpus luteum. In the absence of these trophic factors, apoptosis ensues. The remaining corpus luteum is composed of dense connective tissue and is termed the *corpus albicans.*

Ovarian Follicle-Stimulating Hormone and Luteinizing Hormone Receptors

The FSH receptor is expressed exclusively by granulosa cells. The LH-hCG receptor is expressed primarily by the theca-interstitial cells of all follicles and by granulosa cells of large preovulatory follicles.

Granulosa cells in primary or secondary follicles that are in the early developmental stages before antrum formation (i.e., preantral follicles) primarily bind FSH but not LH. In these preantral follicles, the binding of LH and hCG is confined to theca-interstitial cells.[104] Granulosa cells in more mature tertiary follicles with an antrum appear capable of binding both LH and FSH. Thus, FSH receptors are found in granulosa cells from follicles of all sizes, but LH receptors are found only in granulosa cells of large preovulatory follicles.[105-107] These observations are consistent with the concept that the acquisition of LH receptors on granulosa cells is under the influence of FSH.[108,109]

The receptors for the glycoprotein hormones have related structures (Fig. 16–16). The receptors belong to the large family of G protein–coupled receptors, whose members all have a transmembrane domain that consists of seven membrane-traversing α-helices connected by three extracellular and three intracellular loops (see Fig. 16–16). The glycoprotein hormone receptors form a separate subgroup within this large family by virtue of their large extracellular hormone-binding domain at the N-terminus. FSH binds to the FSH receptor, and LH and hCG both bind to the same LH receptor. Both LH and FSH receptor genes are located on chromosome 2 at the p21 region.[51] The relationship of the glycoprotein hormone receptors to the other G protein–coupled receptors is indicated by their sequence homology in the C-terminal half of the receptor. This domain, encoded by a single, last exon, contains the seven transmembrane segments and the G protein–coupling domain. The unusually large extracellular domain of the glycoprotein hormone receptors is encoded by the first 9 or 10 exons (Fig. 16–17).

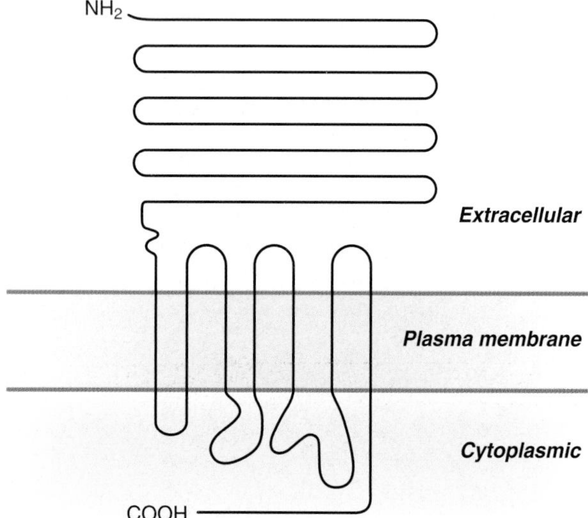

Figure 16–16 ▪ Gonadotropin receptor. The seven-transmembrane-domain, G protein–coupled receptors for luteinizing hormone and follicle-stimulating hormone located in the membranes of ovarian granulosa and theca cells typically have large extracellular domains. *NH_2,* amino-terminal; *COOH,* carboxyl-terminal. (From Bulun SE, Simpson ER, Mendelson CR. The molecular basis of hormone action. In Carr BR, Blackwell RE, eds. Textbook of Reproductive Medicine, 2nd ed. Stamford, CT: Appleton & Lange, 1998:137-156.)

Role of Follicle-Stimulating Hormone in Ovarian Function

As indicated by its name, FSH is the main promoter of follicular maturation. Given that FSH receptors have been exclusively localized to granulosa cells, it is generally presumed that FSH action in the ovary involves the granulosa cells. The ability of FSH to orchestrate follicular growth and differentiation depends on its ability to exert multiple actions concurrently.

Phenotypes of women with mutations that disrupt the function of the FSH-β subunit gene are in good agreement and demonstrate that FSH is necessary for normal follicular development, ovulation, and fertility.[51] Likewise, pubertal development is hampered in the absence of sufficient numbers of later stage follicles with the granulosa cells needed for adequate estrogen production. Treatment of at least one of these patients with exogenous FSH resulted in follicular maturation, ovulation, and normal pregnancy.[51] The presenting phenotype of FSH-β subunit deficiency is practically identical to that caused by inactivating mutations of the FSH receptor.[51] Women with FSH receptor mutations are clinically similar to patients with gonadal dysgenesis, with absent or poorly developed secondary sexual characteristics and high serum levels of FSH and LH. The notable difference was the presence of ovarian follicles in cases with FSH receptor mutation, consistent with the FSH independence of primordial follicle recruitment and early follicular growth and development. In contrast, total absence of all follicles, including those in the primordial stage, was observed in the cases in which the FSH receptor mutation could not be detected.[51] Thus, the ovarian phenotype of FSH receptor deficiency is distinct from the common form of gonadal dysgenesis as found in Turner's syndrome with streak gonads and absence of growing follicles.[51]

In vivo rodent studies suggest that FSH is capable of increasing the number of its own receptors in the granulosa cell. Whereas estradiol by itself may be without effect on the distribution, number, or affinity of granulosa cell FSH receptors, estrogens have been shown to synergize with FSH to enhance the overall number of granulosa cell FSH receptors.[110] Consequently, changes in the production of estradiol by preantral follicles could increase their response to FSH through the regulation of granulosa cell-surface FSH receptors. This interaction between FSH and estradiol in follicular development has been well established in rodents. It appears that both estrogen receptor α (ERα) and ERβ may mediate the estrogenic effect on ovarian development and follicular maturation in mice.[111] On the other hand, it is not clear at this time whether a similar relationship exists in the human ovary. ERα is not detected in the human ovary in significant quantities. The demonstration of ERβ in the human ovary, however, suggests an interaction between FSH and estrogen in the regulation of normal follicle development and ovulation in women.[112]

One of the major actions of FSH is the induction of granulosa cell aromatase activity.[113,114] Thus, little or no estrogen can be produced by FSH-unprimed granulosa cells even if they are supplied with aromatizable androgen precursors. On the other hand, treatment with FSH enhances the aromatization capability of granulosa cells, an effect related to enhancement of the granulosa cell aromatase content.[115,116]

Treatment with FSH has also been shown to induce LH receptors in granulosa cells. The ability of FSH to induce LH receptors is augmented by the concomitant presence of estrogens.[117] Furthermore, progestins, androgens, and LH itself may also induce

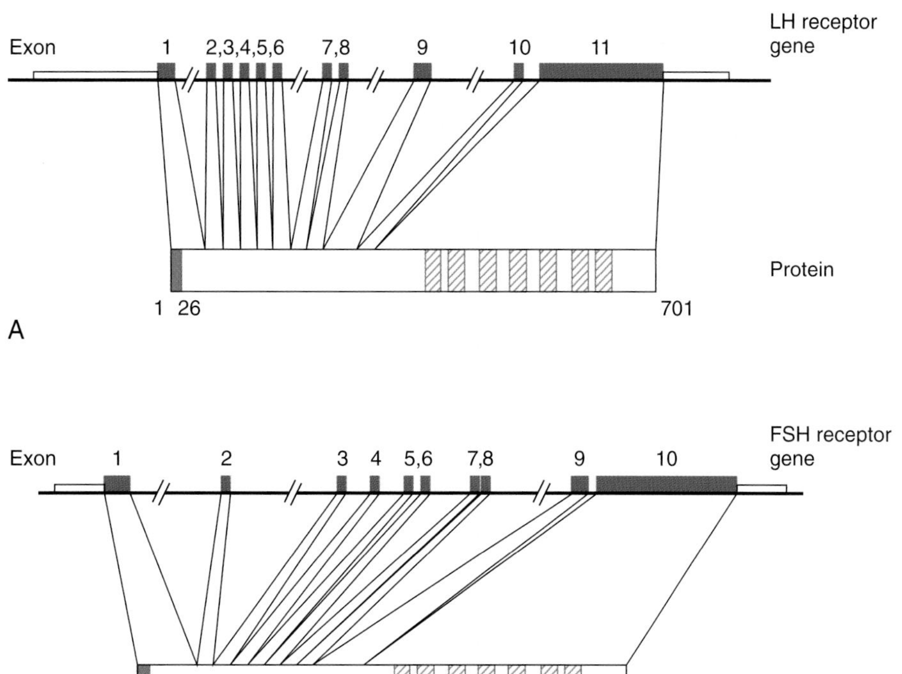

Figure 16–17 ■ Schematic representation of the human gonadotropin receptor genes. The structure of the genes is depicted at the top of the drawings. The open bars indicate sections of the exons that encode untranslated regions of the messenger ribonucleic acid; the closed bars indicate the sequences that encode the protein. Both genes are at least 80 kb in size. The relation between the intron-exon structure of the gene and the domains on the protein is indicated by the lines connecting the gene to the protein. The horizontally hatched part of the protein indicates the signal peptide, and the cross-hatched bars signify the seven segments of the transmembrane domain. The numbers below the protein indicate the start and end of the signal peptide and the length of the total protein product including the signal peptide. Note that the receptor genes are similar in structure with the exception of an additional exon in the luteinizing hormone (LH) receptor gene. Exon 1 encodes the signal peptide and a small part of the extracellular domain; the following eight or nine exons encode the rest of the extracellular domain, including the leucine-rich repeat motifs. In both receptor genes, the final exon is the largest and contains the information for the transmembrane signal transduction domain. *FSH*, Follicle-stimulating hormone. (From Themmen APN, Huhtaniemi IT. Mutations of gonadotropins and gonadotropin receptors: elucidating the physiology and pathophysiology of pituitary-gonadal function. Endocr Rev 2000;21:551-583. Copyright © 2000 by The Endocrine Society.)

LH receptors. Once induced, the granulosa cell LH receptor requires the continued presence of FSH for its maintenance.

Circumstantial evidence, as deduced from studies of women with disrupting mutations of the genes that encode FSH and LH receptors and aromatase P450 (P450arom), indicates that FSH action, but not estrogen or LH action, is essential for follicular growth in humans.[51,118] In women with deficient LH action or estrogen biosynthesis, follicular growth and development up to the antral stage were observed, although these individuals were anovulatory.[51,118] On the other hand, women with mutations of the FSH-β subunit or FSH receptor had only primordial follicles in their ovaries.[51] These data indicate that estrogen or LH is not critical for follicular development at least until the tertiary stage (see Figs. 16-11 and 16-13). It should be kept in mind, however, that FSH by itself is not sufficient to achieve normal follicular development and ovulation.

Role of Luteinizing Hormone in Ovarian Function

LH is essential for ovulation (follicular rupture) and the sustenance of corpus luteum function. In addition, LH plays other important roles in follicular function. First, it is likely that LH plays a major role in the promotion of theca interstitial cell androgen production. Moreover, LH may well synergize with FSH in the more advanced phases of follicular development. Last, small and sustained increments in the circulating levels of LH are both necessary and sufficient to cause small antral follicles to grow and develop to the preovulatory stage.[119,120]

It is presumed that LH acts on theca-interstitial cells of small follicles, where it promotes the biosynthesis of C19-steroids.[121] The consequent increase in estrogen production is presumed to contribute to the growth and development of the follicles. Treatment with small doses of LH also presumably results in an increase in LH receptor content as well as in induction of the key steroidogenic proteins such as StAR, side-chain cleavage P450 (P450scc), 3β-hydroxysteroid dehydrogenase type II (3β-HSD-II), and 17 hydroxylase (P450c17).

The role of LH action in human ovarian physiology was exemplified by the phenotype of a woman with a disrupting mutation of the LH receptor gene.[51] She presented with amenorrhea with normally developed secondary sexual characteristics, increased circulating FSH and LH levels, and low levels of estradiol and progesterone that were unresponsive to hCG treatment.[51] The ovary contained follicles that developed up to antral stage with a well-developed theca layer but no preovulatory follicles or corpora lutea. These observations collectively support the view that LH is essential for ovulation and sufficient estrogen production, whereas follicular development is initially autonomous and at later stages dependent on intact FSH action.

Ovarian Steroidogenesis

The steroid hormone contents of the ovarian vein effluents and peripheral venous blood were compared to distinguish steroids secreted by the ovary from those secreted by the adrenal and from those produced by peripheral conversion of precursors.[122] These studies revealed that the ovaries secrete pregnenolone, progesterone, 17α-hydroxyprogesterone, dehydroepiandrosterone (DHEA), androstenedione, testosterone, estrone, and estradiol.[123] Although such measurements provide insights into the steroidogenic pathways under study, they do not identify the specific ovarian cells involved. Studies using microdissected preovulatory follicles identified estrone and estradiol as the major steroid products (Fig. 16–18). Progesterone and 17α-hydroxyprogesterone, on the other hand, proved to be the major products of the corpus luteum (see Fig. 16–18).

The general steroidogenic pathway for the production of estrogens and androgens is depicted in Figure 16-18. The biologically active ovarian steroids are estradiol and progesterone (see Fig. 16–18). The major C19 steroid product of the ovary, androstenedione, is not biologically active. Androstenedione, however, acts as a dual precursor and contributes to circulating levels of estrone and testosterone through conversion in extraglandular tissues such as adipose tissue and skin (see later).[124-126] It is likely that estrogenically weak estrone is further converted to the potent estrogen estradiol, and testosterone is converted to the much more potent androgen dihydrotestosterone (DHT) locally in target tissues such as brain, breast, prostate, and genital skin in order to exert potent biologic effects.[126] The presence of multiple proteins with overlapping enzymatic activities (i.e., 17β-HSD and 5α-reductase) that catalyze these conversions in a large number of human tissues is supportive of this idea.[127]

The preovulatory follicle secretes estradiol during the first half of the menstrual cycle, whereas the corpus luteum secretes both estradiol and progesterone during the second half of the cycle (Fig. 16–19).[128-130] The production of these two biologically active steroids is orchestrated in the follicle and corpus luteum in a cell-specific manner under the control of LH and FSH.

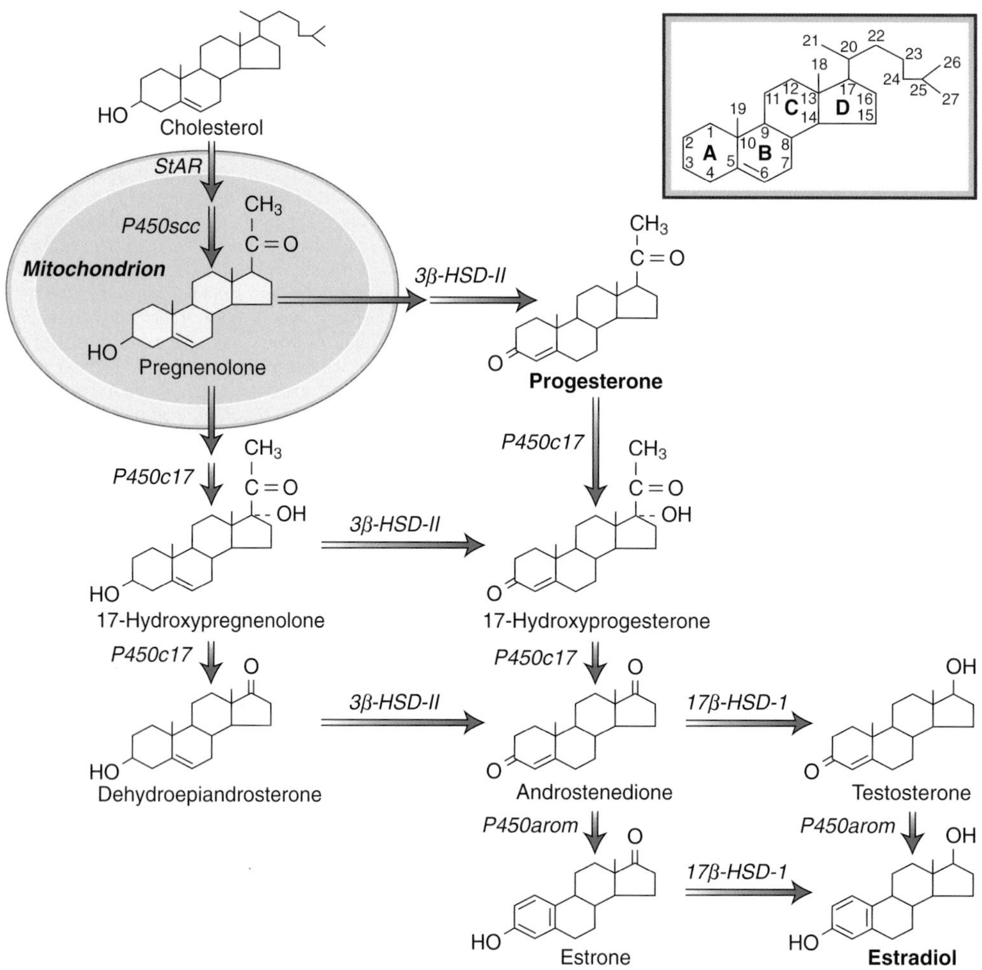

Figure 16–18 ▪ Steroidogenic pathway in the ovary. Biologically active steroids progesterone and estradiol are produced primarily in the ovary of a woman of reproductive age. Estradiol production requires the activity of six steroidogenic proteins including StAR and six enzymatic steps. P450c17, product of the CYP17 gene, catalyzes two enzymatic reactions. The four rings of the cholesterol molecule and its derivative steroids are identified by the first four letters in the alphabet, and the carbons are numbered in the sequence shown in the insert. *3β-HSD-II,* 3β-hydroxysteroid dehydrogenase Δ5, 4 isomerase type II; *17β-HSD-1,* 17β-hydroxysteroid dehydrogenase type 1; *P450arom,* aromatase; *P450c17,* 17α-hydroxylase/17,20-lyase; *StAR,* steroidogenic acute regulatory protein.

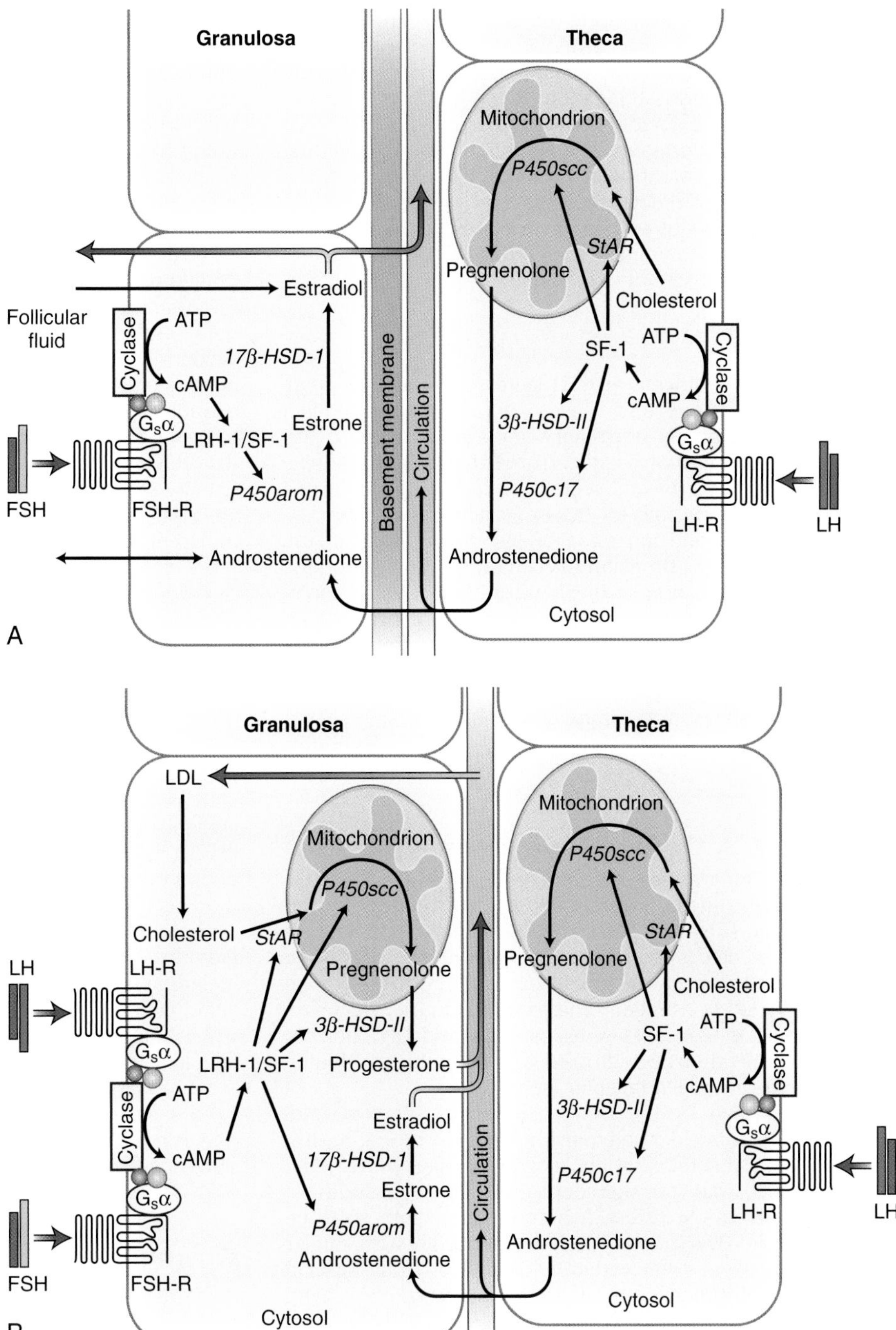

Figure 16–19 ▪ Two-cell hypothesis for ovarian steroidogenesis. **A,** The preovulatory follicle produces estradiol through a paracrine interaction between theca and granulosa cells. In response to stimulation with a gonadotropin, steroidogenic factor-1 (SF-1, a member of the nuclear receptor family) acts as a master switch to initiate transcription of a series of steroidogenic genes in theca cells. In follicular granulosa cells, another nuclear receptor, liver homologue receptor-1 (LRH-1), seems to primarily mediate the downstream effects of FSH in the rodent ovary.[128,129] In humans, the relative roles of SF-1 vs LRH-1 in steroidogenesis in preovulatory granulosa cells are not yet known. Because granulosa cells do not have a direct connection to the circulation, aromatase (P450arom) in granulosa cells is dependent for substrate on androstenedione that diffuses from theca cells. Two critical steps in estradiol formation seem to be the entry of cholesterol into mitochondria facilitated by steroidogenic acute regulatory protein (StAR) in theca cells and the conversion of androstenedione to estrone catalyzed by P450arom in granulosa cells. **B,** In the corpus luteum, granulosa lutein cells are heavily vascularized, which is critical for the entry of cholesterol into this cell type through primarily low-density lipoprotein receptors and for secretion of large amounts of progesterone into the circulation. The entry of cholesterol into mitochondria (by StAR) is likely to be the most critical steroidogenic step for progesterone formation in granulosa lutein cells. Androstenedione produced in theca lutein cells serves as a substrate for estradiol produced in granulosa lutein cells. Human data are suggestive that LRH-1 may mediate at least a portion of gonadotropin-dependent steroidogenesis in the corpus luteum.[130] Thus, gonadotropins, SF-1 and possibly LRH-1 play key roles for important steroidogenic steps in the ovary. *ATP,* Adenosine triphosphate; *cAMP,* cyclic adenosine monophosphate; *FSH-R,* follicle-stimulating hormone receptor; *HSD,* hydroxysteroid dehydrogenase; *LH-R,* luteinizing hormone receptor.

There are three major categories of ovarian steroids, as follows.

C18 Steroids

The naturally occurring estrogens are C18 steroids characterized by the presence of an aromatic A ring, a phenolic hydroxyl group at C-3, and either a hydroxyl group (estradiol) or a ketone group (estrone) at C-17. Aromatase is the key enzyme for estrogen production in the ovary (see Fig. 16–18). The protein aromatase P450 (P450arom) confers the specific activity of the aromatase–enzyme complex. P450arom production in the ovarian granulosa cell is regulated primarily by FSH.[131] The principal and most potent estrogen secreted by the ovary is estradiol. Although estrone is also secreted by the ovary, another important source of estrone is extraglandular conversion of androstenedione in peripheral tissues.[132] Estriol (16-hydroxyestradiol) is the most abundant estrogen in urine and is produced by the metabolism of estrone and estradiol in extraovarian tissues. All C18 steroids including estrone, estradiol, and estriol are commonly referred to as estrogens. It should be pointed out, however, that estrone and estriol are only weakly estrogenic and must be converted to estradiol to show full estrogenic action. There are at least seven enzymes in the 17β-HSD family with overlapping activities, which are capable of converting estrone to estradiol in the ovary and extraovarian tissues.[133]

Catechol estrogens are formed by hydroxylation of estrogens at the C-2 or C-4 position. The physiologic role of catechol estrogen, if any, is unclear. Low body weight and hyperthyroidism are associated with increased formation of catechol estrogens.[134] Estrone sulfate, formed by peripheral conversion of estradiol and estrone, is the most abundant estrogen in blood but is not physiologically active. Estrone sulfate is presumed to serve as a reservoir for estrone formation in a number of tissues, including those that are targets of estrogen. Estradiol regulates gonadotropin secretion and promotes development of the secondary sexual characteristics of women, uterine growth, thickening of the vaginal mucosa, thinning of the cervical mucus, and linear growth of the ductal system of the breast.

C21 Steroids

The principal progestogens are C21 steroids and include pregnenolone, progesterone, and 17-hydroxyprogesterone (see Fig. 16–18). Pregnenolone is of primary importance in the ovary because of its key position as precursor of all steroid hormones. Progesterone is the principal secretory product of the corpus luteum and is responsible for the progestational effects (i.e., cell differentiation and induction of secretory activity in the endometrium of the estrogen-primed uterus). Progesterone is required for implantation of the fertilized ovum and maintenance of pregnancy. It also induces decidualization of the endometrium, inhibits uterine contractions, increases the viscosity of cervical mucus, promotes lateral (alveolar) development of the breast glands, and increases basal body temperature. On the other hand, 17-hydroxyprogesterone, also secreted by the corpus luteum, has little, if any, biologic activity.

C19 Steroids

The ovary secretes a variety of C19 steroids, including DHEA, androstenedione, and testosterone (see Fig. 16–18). They are produced by the thecal cells and to a lesser degree by the ovarian stroma. The major C19 steroid is androstenedione, part of which is secreted directly into plasma, with the remainder converted to estrogen by the granulosa cells. Androstenedione can be converted to estrogen or testosterone in the ovary and in extraglandular tissues. Only testosterone and DHT but not androstenedione are true androgens with the capacity of interacting with the androgen receptor (see later).

Steroids formed by the ovary, as well as other steroid-producing organs, are derived from cholesterol (see Fig. 16–18). There are several sources of cholesterol that can provide the ovary with substrate for steroidogenesis. These include (1) plasma lipoprotein cholesterol, (2) cholesterol synthesized de novo within the ovary, and (3) cholesterol from intracellular stores of cholesterol esters within lipid droplets. In the human ovary, LDL cholesterol is an important source of cholesterol utilized for steroidogenesis.[96] LH stimulates the activity of adenylate cyclase, increasing production of cyclic adenosine monophosphate (cAMP), which serves as a second messenger to increase LDL receptor mRNA and the binding and uptake of LDL cholesterol as well as the formation of cholesterol esters.[95,96] LDL-derived cholesterol is particularly essential for normal levels of progesterone production in the granulosa lutein cells of the corpus luteum (see Fig. 16–19).[96]

The first and rate-limiting step in the synthesis of all ovarian steroid hormones is the movement of cholesterol into the mitochondrion, which is regulated by StAR (see Figs. 16-18 and 16-19).[135] This movement is followed by conversion of cholesterol to pregnenolone, catalyzed by the mitochondrial enzyme complex consisting of P450scc, adrenodoxin, and flavoprotein. LH induces steroidogenesis by increasing intracellular cAMP, which increases the conversion of cholesterol to pregnenolone in two distinct ways: (1) acute regulation, over minutes, occurs through the phosphorylation of preexisting StAR and rapid synthesis of new StAR protein, and (2) chronic stimulation, within hours to days, occurs through the induction of P450scc expression and consequent increased steroidogenesis (see Fig. 16–19). StAR increases the flow of cholesterol to mitochondria, thus regulating substrate availability to whatever amount of P450scc is available on the inner mitochondrial membrane.[135] In the absence of StAR, only 14% of the maximal StAR-induced level of steroidogenesis persists as StAR-independent steroidogenesis.[135]

StAR expression in the preovulatory graafian follicle is limited primarily to the thecal cells (see Fig. 16–19).[136] The most important product of the thecal cell during the follicular phase is the estrogen precursor androstenedione, whose production is controlled primarily by StAR (see Fig. 16–19). The biologically active steroid product of the ovary during the follicular phase is estradiol that arises from the granulosa cells located adjacent to theca cells (see Fig. 16–19). The rate-limiting step for granulosa cell estradiol production is regulated by the FSH-dependent activity of the aromatase enzyme in a cyclic fashion (see Fig. 16–19).[114] During the luteal phase, cells of the corpus luteum, including granulosa lutein cells, also show intense StAR immunoreactivity with a patchy distribution (see Fig. 16–19).[98,136] The delivery of cholesterol to the mitochondrial side-chain cleavage enzyme system in the corpus luteum is the rate-limiting step for progesterone biosynthesis and is regulated by StAR (see Fig. 16–19).[98] Thus, estradiol production seems to be regulated primarily by StAR and P450arom, whereas progesterone biosynthesis may be primarily under the control of StAR.

The ovarian granulosa, theca, and corpus luteum cells possess StAR plus five distinct proteins with specific enzyme activities for steroid hormone formation. These steroidogenic enzymes are P450scc, 3β-HSD-II, P450c17, P450arom, and 17β-HSD-1.[131] These enzymes are responsible for the conversion of cholesterol to the two major biologically active products estradiol and progesterone.[137]

Steroidogenesis dependent on LH and FSH in both theca and granulosa cells is mediated by common signaling molecules including cAMP and the specific transcription factors steroidogenic factor-1 (SF-1) and liver receptor homologue-1 (LRH-1), which belong to the nuclear receptor family (see Fig. 16–19).[138,139] SF-1 and LRH-1 regulate the expression of genes that encode StAR, P450scc, 3β-HSD-II, P450c17, and P450arom (see Fig. 16–19). Thus, SF-1 and possibly LRH-1 can be regarded as downstream master switches that orchestrate ovarian steroidogenesis.[139]

Summary of Updated Two-Cell Theory for Ovarian Steroidogenesis

The classical two-cell theory is supported by molecular findings in the following fashion. Ovarian steroidogenesis in the preovulatory follicle takes place through LH receptors on theca and FSH (possibly plus LH) receptors on granulosa cells (see Fig. 16–19). Cyclic AMP production and increased SF-1 binding to multiple steroidogenic promoters mediate LH action in theca cells. In particular, StAR is the primary regulator of production of androstenedione that subsequently diffuses into granulosa cells to serve as the estrogen precursor. In the preovulatory follicle, cholesterol in theca cells arises from circulating lipoproteins and de novo biosynthesis. FSH is responsible for follicular growth and also estrogen formation. FSH induces cAMP formation, increased LRH-1 and/or SF-1 binding activity, and P450arom expression in preovulatory granulosa cells to give rise to estradiol formation primarily through aromatization of androstenedione (see Fig. 16–19). The relative roles of SF-1 vs LRH-1 in human ovarian granulosa cells before ovulation is not known.

Rodent data suggest that LRH-1 might be the primary regulator.[128,129,140]

In the corpus luteum, large deposits of cholesterol (i.e., the yellow color) arise primarily from circulating lipoproteins to support production of extremely high quantities of progesterone. Other key anatomic events in formation of the corpus luteum are the disruption of the basement membrane between the granulosa and theca and strikingly increased vascularization of granulosa lutein cells (see Fig. 16–15). Theca lutein cells possess LH receptors and produce androstenedione. Cyclic AMP, SF-1, and StAR induced by LH remain as the key regulators for biosynthesis of thecal androstenedione, which serves as the estrogen precursor in neighboring granulosa lutein cells (see Fig. 16–19).

The granulosa lutein cell of the corpus luteum is both anatomically and functionally different from its counterpart in the preovulatory follicle. First, these cells are luteinized and heavily vascularized and contain large quantities of cholesterol. Second, granulosa lutein cells contain high levels of LH receptors in addition to FSH receptors. Third, they produce large quantities of progesterone that is regulated primarily by LH and StAR. Granulosa lutein cells also aromatize androstenedione of thecal origin and eventually give rise to estradiol formation through FSH action and P450arom. The common known mediators of LH and FSH in human granulosa lutein cells are cAMP and increased LRH-1 levels.[130] The relative roles of LRH-1 vs SF-1 for progesterone and estradiol production in granulose lutein cells are not clear. Specific functions of the two gonadotropins (i.e., differentiation, growth, and progesterone formation versus estradiol formation) are probably determined by as yet unidentified modifying factors (see Fig. 16–19).

Peptide Hormones Produced by the Ovary

The ovary produces a large number of peptides that can act in an intracrine, autocrine, paracrine, or endocrine fashion. These include numerous growth factors (e.g., insulin-like growth factors [IGFs]) and cytokines (e.g., interleukin-1β). IGFs crosstalk with the FSH-dependent signaling cascade to augment the effects of FSH in granulosa cells.

The group of peptides, including inhibin, activin, and follistatin, are produced in ovarian granulosa cells under the control of FSH and LH (Fig. 16–20). The production of inhibin and activin is not limited to the ovary. A number of other tissues, including the adrenal, pituitary, and placenta, synthesize these peptides. Two isoforms of inhibin have been isolated: inhibin-A and inhibin-B. Both contain an identical α subunit but distinct β subunits (βA and βB). Each subunit is encoded by a distinct gene. The heterodimers of inhibin, αβA and αβB, are termed *inhibin-A* and *inhibin-B*, respectively (see Fig. 16–20). Although inhibin is produced by a number of tissues in the body, most inhibin is derived from the gonads. In the ovary, the source of inhibin is granulosa cells. The main role of inhibin, for which it was discovered and named, is to suppress FSH production in the pituitary (see Figs. 16-1B and 16-4).

Although both isoforms of inhibin seem to have similar biologic properties, their synthesis is regulated differently during the follicular and luteal phases (see Fig. 16–1A). Under the influence of FSH, inhibin B is secreted mainly during the early follicular phase, with levels decreasing in midfollicular phase and becoming undetectable after the LH surge. LH-induced inhibin A levels, however, are low during the first half of the follicular phase but increase gradually during midfollicular phase with a peak during the luteal phase. All three subunits are detected in small antral follicles by immunohistochemistry and in situ hybridization.[141,142] The α and βA subunits are found in the dominant follicle and in the corpus luteum. All three subunits are expressed in response to gonadotropins or factors that increase intracellular cAMP.[143]

Activin is structurally related to inhibin but may exert opposite actions. Activin contains two subunits that are identical to the β subunits of inhibins A and B. Thus, the three activin isoforms are activin A (βAβA), activin B (βBβB), and activin AB (βAβB). In the pituitary, activin stimulates the release of FSH. In the ovarian follicle, activin enhances FSH action (see Fig. 16–20). As in the case of inhibin, activins are also produced both in ovarian granulosa cells and pituitary gonadotrophs. In contrast to inhibin, however, locally synthesized activin in the pituitary, rather than the ovarian-derived activin, is responsible for regulating FSH (see Fig. 16–4).

Follistatin is a single unit peptide produced in a number of human tissues including the pituitary and ovary (see Fig. 16–

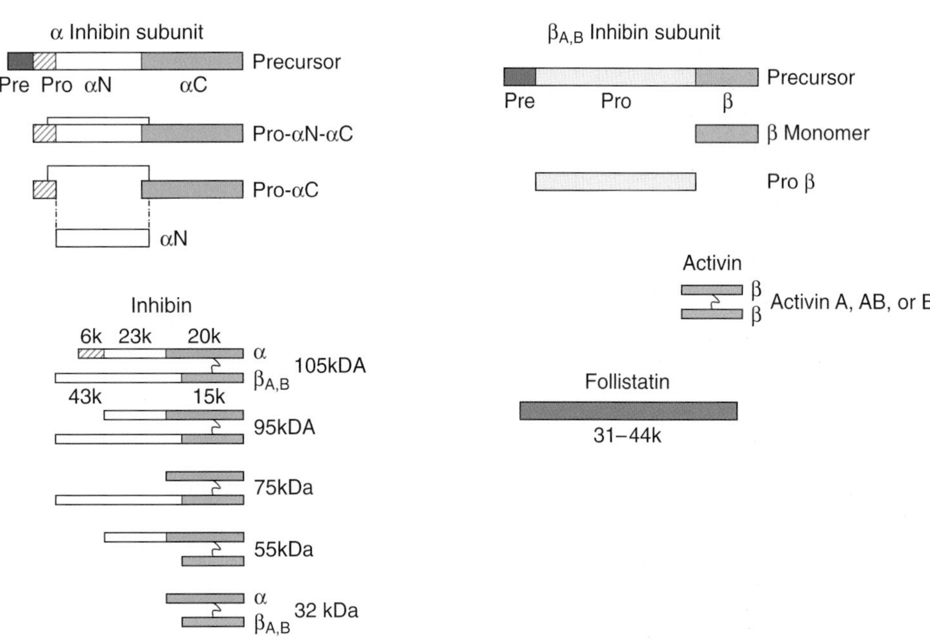

Figure 16–20 ▪ Diagrammatic presentation of the structures of inhibin subunit precursors and processed forms in serum, the activins, and the follistatins. The precise contribution of each molecular weight form of inhibin to the biological activity in serum is not known, but it has been established that the 55-kd and the 32-kd forms are biologically active. (Modified from Burger H. Inhibin, activin and neoplasia. In Yen SC, Jaffe RB, Barbieri RL, eds. Reproductive Endocrinology, 4th ed. Philadelphia: WB Saunders, 1999:669-675.)

20). It binds and neutralizes the biologic functions of activin. It appears that local follistatin levels in tissues modulate the effects of activin. This explains the inhibitory effect of follistatin on pituitary FSH secretion (see Fig. 16–4).

Overview of the Hormonal Changes During the Ovarian Cycle

FSH secretion is suppressed by negative feedback of the ovarian hormones estrogen, inhibin, and progesterone during the early and midluteal phase. Upon the regression of the corpus luteum during the late luteal phase, however, the sharp decline in estrogen, inhibin, and progesterone abolishes this negative feedback (see Fig. 16–1A). This permits increased secretion of FSH just before and during menses. This initial increase in FSH is essential for follicle recruitment and growth and steroidogenesis (see Fig. 16–1A). With continued growth of the follicle, autocrine and paracrine factors produced within the follicle maintain follicular sensitivity to FSH. Continuing and combined action of FSH and activin leads to the appearance of LH receptors on the granulosa cells, a prerequisite for ovulation and luteinization.

Ovulation is triggered by the rapid rise in circulating levels of estradiol. A positive feedback response at the level of the anterior pituitary and possibly at the hypothalamus results in the midcycle surge of LH necessary for expulsion of the egg and formation of the corpus luteum (see Fig. 16–1A). A rise in progesterone follows ovulation along with a second rise in estradiol, producing the 14-day-long luteal phase characterized by low FSH and LH levels. The demise of the corpus luteum concomitant with a fall in hormone (progesterone, estradiol, and inhibin A) levels allows FSH to increase again toward the end of the luteal phase, thus initiating a new cycle (see Fig. 16–1A). If pregnancy is established by the implantation of a blastocyst, however, the structural integrity and function (progesterone and estradiol production) of the corpus luteum are maintained by hCG that is secreted from the trophoblast. The hCG acts as a surrogate for LH on the corpus luteum.

In addition to FSH and LH, local factors (e.g., activin and inhibin) regulate follicular development and steroidogenesis. In the early follicular phase, activin produced by granulosa cells in immature follicles enhances the action of FSH on aromatase activity and FSH and LH receptor formation while simultaneously suppressing C19-steroid formation in theca cells. In the late follicular phase, increased production of inhibin by the granulosa cells and decreased activin promote the synthesis of C19 steroids in the theca layer in response to LH and local growth factors and cytokines to provide larger amounts of the precursor androstenedione for the production of estrone and ultimately estradiol in the granulosa cells.[144]

Both LH-mediated androstenedione production in theca cells and FSH-mediated estradiol production in granulosa cells are potentiated by IGFs.[145] The major endogenous IGF produced in the human ovarian follicle is IGF-II (versus IGF-I) in both granulosa and theca cells. The actions of both IGF-I and IGF-II are mediated by IGF receptor type I in both cells. IGF receptor type I is structurally similar to the insulin receptor. Thus, it appears that gonadotropin-related IGF action in the ovary is regulated primarily by IGF-II and IGF receptor type I.[145]

In summary, ovulation is under the control of substances functioning as classic hormones (FSH, LH, estradiol, and inhibin) transmitting messages between the ovary and the hypothalamic-pituitary axis and paracrine and autocrine factors such as IGF-II, inhibin, and activin, which coordinate sequential activities within the follicle destined to ovulate. The negative feedback relationship between corpus luteum products (estradiol, progesterone, and inhibin) and FSH results in the critical initial rise in FSH immediately before and during menses, and the positive feedback relationship between estradiol and LH is responsible for the ovulatory stimulus (see Fig. 16–1). Within the ovary, IGF-II, inhibin, and activin modify follicular responses necessary for growth and function. These endocrine, paracrine, and autocrine factors undoubtedly represent only a portion of a complete picture. The causes of anovulation are diverse and may be related to defects in cell-surface receptors, intracellular elements of signal transduction, or cell-cell interactions.[146]

Extraovarian Steroidogenesis

Estradiol formation takes place in a number of tissues in the woman of reproductive age. These tissues may be placed in three categories: (1) the ovary, (2) peripheral tissues such as subcutaneous fat and skin, and (3) physiologic and pathologic target sites such as the hypothalamus, breast cancer cells, and the cells of endometriosis (Fig. 16–21).[126] The latter two sources of estrogen are particularly critical in anovulatory premenopausal and postmenopausal women. Although small quantities of estrogen are produced by an individual adipose or skin fibroblast in a continuous fashion, these cell types contribute to circulating estradiol levels because of their relative abundance (see Fig. 16–21).[126] This effect is more pronounced in obese women because of increased mass of the adipose tissue and skin.[124]

P450arom in adipose and skin fibroblasts is responsible for peripheral aromatization of androstenedione that arises from both the ovary and adrenal in premenopausal women and primarily from the adrenal in postmenopausal women (see Fig. 16–21). The product of this reaction, estrone, is only weakly estrogenic, however. Estrone is further converted to estrone

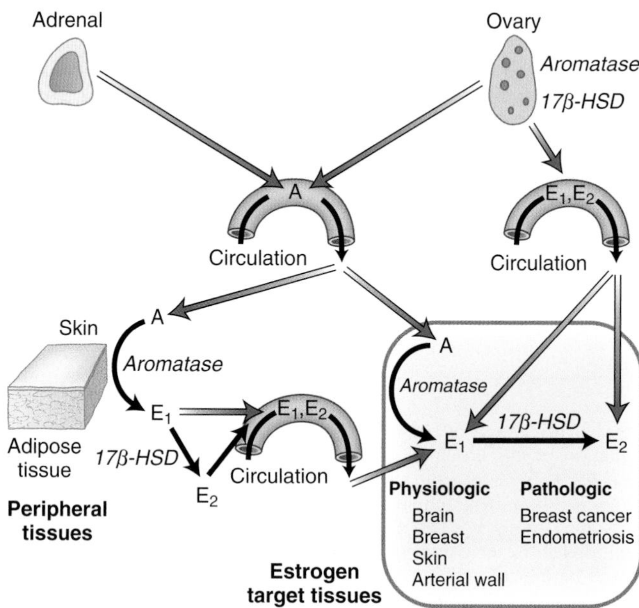

Figure 16–21 ▪ Estrogen biosynthesis in women. The biologically active estrogen estradiol (E2) is produced in at least three major sites: (1) by direct secretion from the ovary in reproductive-age women; (2) by conversion of circulating androstenedione (A) of adrenal or ovarian origins, or both, to estrone (E1) in peripheral tissues; and (3) by conversion of A to E1 in estrogen target tissues. In the latter two instances, estrogenically weak E1 is further converted to E2 within the same tissue. The presence of the enzyme aromatase and 17β-hydroxysteroid dehydrogenase (17β-HSD) is critical for E2 formation at these sites. E2 formation by peripheral and local conversion is particularly important in postmenopausal women and in estrogen-dependent diseases such as breast cancer, endometriosis, and endometrial cancer.

sulfate, which serves as a reservoir for estrone in blood and other tissues. Estrone (arising from androstenedione and estrone sulfate) is further converted to the biologically active estradiol in target tissues such as the endometrium and breast by a number of enzymatic proteins with overlapping reductive 17β-HSD activity (see Fig. 16–21).[133,147,148] It is likely that local P450arom expression in hypothalamus is critical for the regulation of gonadotropin secretion.[149] Finally, estrogen-dependent pathologic tissues such as those in breast cancer and endometriosis contain extremely high levels of P450arom that enhances tissue growth by increasing local estradiol concentrations (see Fig. 16–21).[150] Circulating androstenedione is the major substrate for aromatase activity in these physiologic and pathologic target tissues.[147,150]

Significant quantities of circulating androstenedione can also be converted to testosterone in peripheral tissues (see later). This is probably accomplished by the presence of multiple 17β-HSDs with overlapping reductive activities in peripheral tissues.[133] Androgenic action of testosterone is strikingly amplified by its conversion to DHT in peripheral and target tissues (e.g., skin and prostate). At least two distinct proteins encoded by two separate genes, 5α-reductase type 1 and type 2, catalyze the conversion of testosterone to DHT in the liver, prostate, and skin.[127] Local production of DHT in genital skin fibroblasts is critical for normal masculinization of external genitalia of male fetuses in utero.[127] DHT formation in the skin is also important in the etiology of hirsutism (see later).[151]

ENDOMETRIUM

The endometrium is the mucosal lining of the uterine cavity. The decidua is the highly modified and specialized endometrium of pregnancy. From the evolutionary perspective, the human endometrium is highly developed to accommodate the hemochorio-endothelial type of placentation, which requires the presence of spiral arteries (Fig. 16–22). Trophoblasts of the blastocyst invade spiral arteries during implantation and placentation in the establishment of uteroplacental vessels.

Spiral arteries of the human endometrium also confer another unique process termed *menstruation*. Menstruation is shedding of endometrial tissue with hemorrhage that is dependent upon sex steroid hormone-directed changes in blood flow in the spiral arteries. The presence of spiral arteries is essential for menstruation because only the human and a few other primates that have endometrial spiral arteries experience menstruation. With nonfertile but ovulatory ovarian cycles, menstruation affects desquamation of the endometrium. New endometrial growth and development must be initiated with each ovarian cycle, so that endometrial maturation corresponds rather precisely with the next opportunity for pregnancy. There seems to be a narrow window of endometrial receptivity to blastocyst implantation that corresponds to the period between days 20 and 24 during a 28-day menstrual cycle.[152]

Functional Anatomy of the Endometrium

The endometrium can be divided morphologically into an upper two-thirds functionalis layer and a lower one-third basalis layer (see Fig. 16–22). The purpose of the functionalis layer is to prepare for the implantation of the blastocyst; therefore, it is the site of proliferation, secretion, and degeneration. The purpose of the basalis layer is to provide the regenerative endometrium following menstrual loss of the functionalis.[153] Major histologic components of the endometrium include (1) stromal cells that constitute the skeleton of the tissue, (2) a single layer of epithelial cells that lines the lumen of the endometrial cavity and invaginations of the stroma, (3) blood vessels, and (4) resident immune cells. The epithelial cells that line the rather deep invaginations of the stroma are also referred to as glandular cells. It should be noted, however, that these deep crypts represent simply extensions of the intracavitary lumen and are not true glands. These invaginations lined by epithelial cells extend from the surface of the functionalis layer (i.e., luminal epithelium) deep into the basalis level (the so-called glandular epithelium). Thus, after the functionalis layer is shed at the time of menstruation, the basalis that contains both epithelial and stromal cells can give rise to a new functionalis layer for the upcoming cycle (Fig. 16–23).

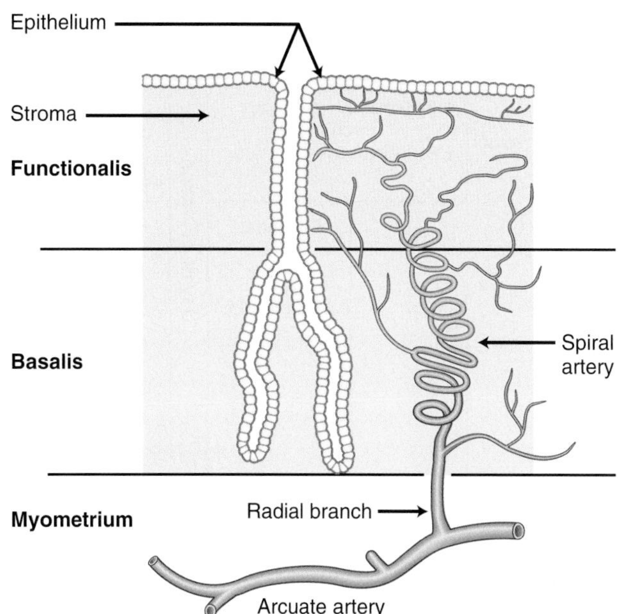

Figure 16–22 ▪ Functional anatomy of the endometrium. Endometrium is a multilayered mucosa specialized for implantation and support of pregnancy. A single, continuous layer of epithelial cells lines the surface of the stroma and penetrates the stroma with deep invaginations almost all the way down to the myometrium-endometrium junction. The entire thickness of the endometrium is penetrated by the spiral arteries and their capillaries. Spiral arteries originate from the radial branches of arcuate arteries, which in turn arise from uterine arteries. The superficial layer (functionalis) is shed during menstruation, whereas the permanent bottom layer (basalis) gives rise to the regeneration of endometrium after each menstruation. The striking changes in the spiral arteries (coiling, stasis, vasodilatation followed by intense vasoconstriction) are consistently observed before the onset of every menstruation episode. (Courtesy of Kristof Chwalisz, River Forest, IL.)

The cellular components of the functionalis layer undergo a striking progression during the menstrual cycle, whereas the basalis shows only modest alterations. The sequence of endometrial changes associated with an ovulatory cycle has been carefully studied by Noyes and colleagues in the human and Markee[154,155] and Bartelmez[156] in the subhuman primate and depicted diagrammatically in Figure 16–23.

Hormone-Induced Morphologic Changes of the Endometrium

The cyclic changes in endometrial histology are faithfully reproduced during each ovulatory ovarian cycle. These sex steroid hormone-induced modifications can be summarized as follows.

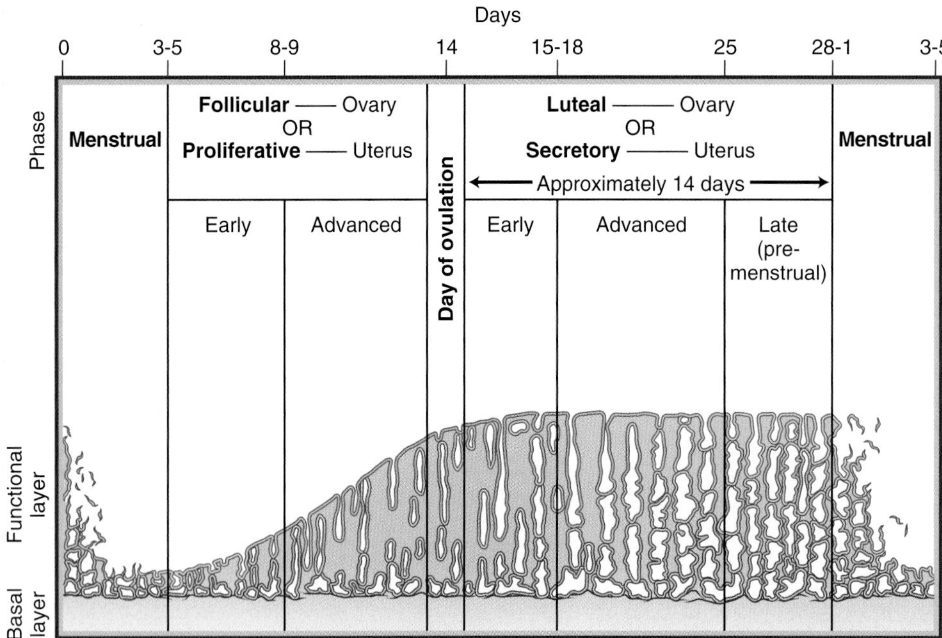

Figure 16–23 ▪ Cyclic changes in thickness and morphology of endometrium and the relation of these changes to those of the ovarian cycle. (From Cunningham FG, MacDonald PC, Gant NF, et al. The endometrium and decidua: menstruation and pregnancy. In Williams Obstetrics, 19th ed. Stamford, CT: Appleton & Lange, 1993:81-109.)

(1) During the preovulatory, or follicular, phase of the cycle, estradiol is secreted (principally by a single dominant follicle of one ovary) in increasing quantities until just before ovulation. (2) During the postovulatory, or luteal, phase of the cycle, progesterone is secreted by the corpus luteum in increasing amounts (up to 40 to 50 mg/day) until the midluteal phase. (3) Beginning about 7 to 8 days after ovulation, the rates of progesterone (and estrogen) secretion by the corpus luteum begin to decline and then diminish progressively before menstruation (see Fig. 16–1).

In response to these cyclic changes in the rates of ovarian sex steroid hormone secretion, there are five main stages of the corresponding endometrial cycle: (1) menstrual-postmenstrual reepithelialization; (2) endometrial proliferation in response to stimulation by estradiol; (3) abundant epithelial secretion, in response to the combined action of estradiol and progesterone; (4) premenstrual ischemia, the result of endometrial tissue volume involution, which causes stasis of blood in the spiral arteries; and (5) menstruation, which is preceded and accompanied by severe vasoconstriction of the endometrial spiral arteries and collapse and desquamation of all but the deepest layer of the endometrium. In the final analysis, menstruation is the consequence of the withdrawal of factors that maintain endometrial growth and differentiation (see Fig. 16–23).

Commonly, the initiation of menstruation is attributed to progesterone withdrawal. This concept was developed because the administration of estrogen to postmenopausal women and thence treatment with and then withdrawal of a progestin causes menstruation, even with continued estrogen treatment. Moreover, progesterone facilitates and permits decidualization of the endometrium and the maintenance of pregnancy, whereas progesterone withdrawal favors the initiation of menstruation, lactation, and parturition. There are probably multiple additional coordinated and interactive processes (other than progesterone withdrawal) that are operative and essential for the success of each of these events.

Both the preovulatory (follicular or proliferative) phase and the postovulatory (luteal or secretory) phase of the ovarian-endometrial cycles are customarily divided into early and late stages (see Fig. 16–1). The normal secretory phase of the endometrial (menstrual) cycle can be subdivided rather finely (almost day by day), by histologic criteria, from shortly after ovulation until the onset of menstruation. In fact, Noyes and other investigators have provided an extremely detailed description of the histologic features of the secretory phase endometrium, which permit accurate dating during the luteal phase. Gynecologists use the histologic dating of the endometrial biopsies obtained during the luteal phase to evaluate ovulation, progesterone production, or the degree of biologic response of the endometrium to progesterone. Normal endometrial development is assumed when the histologic and chronologic endometrial dating agree within 2 days. When they differ by more than 2 days, the endometrium is considered to be out of phase. Out-of-phase endometrial tissue may be a cause of implantation failure giving rise to infertility. Understanding the limitations of this test is important, if infertility treatments are based on biopsy results, because the sensitivity and the specificity of the dating of endometrial biopsy for the evaluation of infertility are unknown. For example, one important disadvantage of this test is interobserver variation in histologic interpretation of biopsies.

Effects of Ovarian Steroids on Endometrium

Estradiol or synthetic estrogens cause a striking thickening of endometrial tissue. Both stromal and epithelial cells of the endometrium proliferate rapidly under the influence of estradiol. Estrogen increases mitotic activity and DNA synthesis in both cell types strikingly (Fig. 16–24). While promoting growth, estrogen also renders endometrial tissue responsive to progesterone by inducing the expression of progesterone receptors (PRs) in this tissue because progesterone action is dependent on previous or concurrent estrogen exposure of the endometrium.[157]

In contrast to the proliferative effects of estrogen, progesterone action primarily gives rise to the differentiation of the endometrium. For example, progesterone can inhibit and even reverse the proliferative action of estrogen on the functionalis layer (see Fig. 16–24).[158-160] Moreover, progesterone action prepares the endometrium for implantation of the embryo through differentiation of both epithelial and stromal cells. Progesterone induces the production and secretion of a glycogen-rich substance from the epithelial cells. Progesterone also causes an

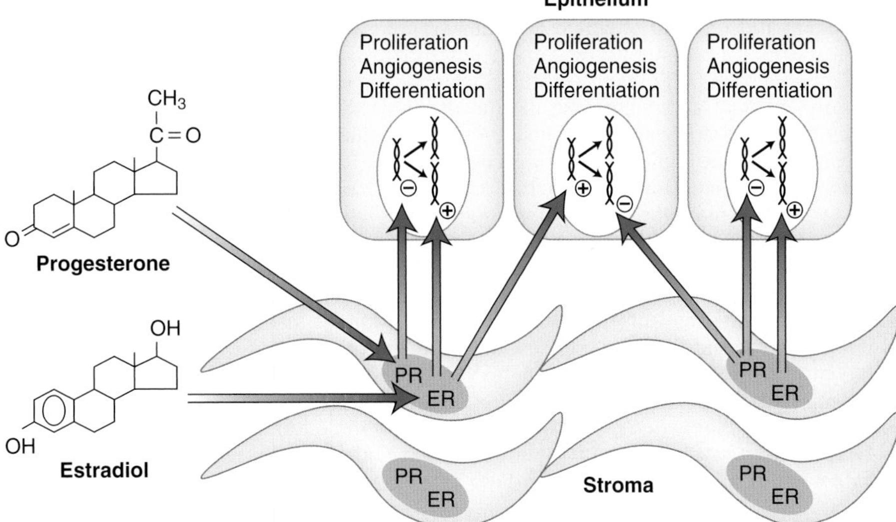

Figure 16–24 ▪ Critical epithelial effects of estrogen (e.g., DNA synthesis, proliferation, and gene expression) are mediated primarily by estrogen receptor α (ER) in stromal cells in a paracrine manner in the endometrium This was demonstrated in mice.[158] It was also shown in mice and humans that the antiestrogenic effects of progesterone on epithelial cells (e.g., decreased proliferation and enhanced differentiation) are mediated primarily by progesterone receptors (PRs) in stromal cells.[159,160]

increase in the stromal cell cytoplasm, a process called *pseudodecidualization.*

Estrogen Action

Estradiol, the biologically potent, naturally occurring estrogen, which is secreted by the granulosa cells of the dominant ovarian follicle, acts to promote responses of the endometrium via mechanisms similar to those used by other steroid hormones. Estradiol enters cells from blood by simple diffusion, but, in estrogen-responsive cells, binding to the ER sequesters estradiol. ERs are proteins with high affinity for estradiol and other biologically active estrogens, that is, synthetic estrogens. Although both ERα and ERβ are present in the endometrium, ERα seems to be the primary mediator of the estrogenic action in the endometrium.[161,162] The estradiol–receptor complex, after transformational changes, is a transcriptional factor that becomes associated with the estrogen response elements of specific genes. This interaction brings about ER-specific initiation of gene transcription, which promotes the synthesis of specific mRNAs and thereafter the synthesis of specific proteins.[163] Among the many proteins synthesized in most estrogen-responsive cells are additional ERs, as well as PRs. Thus, estradiol acts in the endometrium and in other estrogen-responsive tissues to promote the perpetuation of estrogen action and to promote the responsiveness of that tissue to progesterone.

The endometrial epithelial cells are estrogen-responsive but probably do not replicate as a result of the direct action of estradiol on the epithelial cells. Replication of human endometrial epithelial cells in culture is not increased appreciably, if at all, when estrogen is added to the medium. Further, estrogen acts on mouse uterine stromal cells to promote the synthesis of epithelial cell growth factors (see Fig. 16–24).[158] These growth factors operate in a paracrine manner to cause increased DNA synthesis and replication in the adjacent epithelial cells. This type of paracrine arrangement may be a common mechanism that mediates estrogen action in hormone-responsive tissues.

Progesterone Action

Progesterone also enters cells by diffusion and in responsive tissues becomes associated with PRs with high affinity for progesterone. The two PR isoforms, PR-A and PR-B, are both present in the human endometrium.[164] Because PR-B but not PR-A levels in the endometrium are tightly regulated during the human menstrual cycle, PR-B is presumed to play a more important biologic role.[164] Commonly, the cellular content of PRs is dependent on previous estrogen action. The progesterone–PR complex also promotes gene transcription, but the response to progesterone is strikingly different from that evoked by the estradiol–ER complex.

Progesterone actions include a decrease in the synthesis of ER molecules.[165] This is one means by which progesterone (and synthetic progestins) attenuates estrogen action. Progesterone also acts to increase the rate of enzymatic inactivation of estradiol to estrone through an increase in the activity of an oxidative type 17β-HSD enzyme. Progesterone-dependent transcription of a specific gene, namely 17β-HSD type 2, is responsible for this enzyme activity.[166] Progesterone also acts to increase sulfation of estrogens (estrogen sulfotransferase), another means of estrogen inactivation.[167] Therefore, progesterone acts as an antiestrogen in at least three ways: (1) by reducing the rate of synthesis of ERs, (2) by bringing about a decrease in the tissue levels of estradiol through conversion to estrone, and (3) by enhancing estrogen inactivation through sulfation. As in the case of estrogen action in the uterus, tissue recombination experiments using uteri of PR knockout and normal mice demonstrated that many effects of progesterone on epithelial cells are also mediated in a paracrine fashion by PRs in stromal cells but not by those in epithelial cells (see Fig. 16–24).[159] Progesterone-dependent 17β-HSD type 2 enzyme induction and consequent estradiol inactivation is also mediated primarily by stromal PRs in human endometrium.[160]

The most striking consequence of progesterone action is the differentiation of the endometrium. The histologic correlates of differentiation, stromal decidualization and epithelial secretion, are correlated with the presence of nuclear PRs and increased levels of circulating progesterone during the luteal phase. Molecular correlates of progesterone action with respect to differentiation include increased production of lactoferrin and glycodelin in epithelial cells and prolactin and IGF binding protein 1 in stromal cells of the endometrium.

The Receptive Phase of the Endometrium for Implantation

Unless the ovum is fertilized within 24 hours of ovulation, it does not survive. Fertilization takes place in the ampullary (one-third distal) portion of the oviduct. Over the next 2 days, the fertilized ovum remains unattached within the tubal lumen, utilizing tubal fluids and residual attached cumulus granulosa cells to sustain nutrition and energy for early cellular cleavage. After this stage, the solid ball of cells (morula), which is the embryo, leaves the oviduct and enters the uterine cavity. Fortunately, by this time endometrial secretions under the influence of luteal progesterone have filled the cavity and bathe the embryo in nutrients. This is the first of many neatly synchronized events that mark the conceptus-endometrial relationship. By 6 days after ovulation, the embryo (now a blastocyst) is ready to attach and implant. At this time, it finds an endometrial lining of sufficient depth, vascularity, and nutritional richness to sustain the important events of early placentation to follow. Just below the epithelial lining, a rich capillary plexus has been formed and is available for creation of the trophoblast-maternal blood interface. Later, the surrounding superficial portion of the functionalis zone, now occupying more and more of the endometrial cavity, provides a sturdy splint to retain endometrial architecture despite the invasive inroads of the burgeoning trophoblast.

Progesterone is essential for the maintenance of pregnancy. The blastocyst is dependent on progesterone produced by the corpus luteum at this time. The hCG that is secreted by the trophoblast prevents the regression of the corpus luteum by acting as a surrogate LH. This serves to maintain a continued supply of progesterone for the maintenance of pregnancy until the placental tissue itself starts to produce sufficient quantities of progesterone by 6 to 7 weeks after fertilization.

Studies in experimental and domestic animals have demonstrated that there must be synchronous development of the embryo and endometrium for normal implantation and development to occur. In laboratory animals, there is a discrete window for implantation, which in some species lasts only a matter of hours.

The receptive phase of the endometrium is the temporal window of endometrial maturation during which the trophectoderm of the blastocyst can attach to the endometrial epithelial cells and subsequently proceed to invade the endometrial stroma. In the study of human endometrial receptivity, a key question is the determination of the temporal window of implantation. Only factors expressed during this temporal window can be considered either markers or functional mediators of the receptive state.

The window of uterine receptivity can be inferred from what has been learned from transfer of embryos to uteri of women primed with exogenous estrogen and progesterone preparations (Fig. 16–25). There is a distinct window for embryo transfer leading to implantation, which spans endometrial cycle days 16 to 20. Presumably, the actual window of implantation follows this window of transfer because embryos need to develop further from the four-cell to eight-cell stage to the blastocyst stage before initiation of attachment and frank invasion.

The window of implantation in the humans was estimated to be between days 20 and 24 of the cycle using serial measurements of serum hCG as a marker of initial embryonic-maternal interaction.[168] Thus, it appears that the window of implantation in the human is relatively wide (approximately 4 days). These observations agree with the earlier morphologic data from Adams and colleagues.[169]

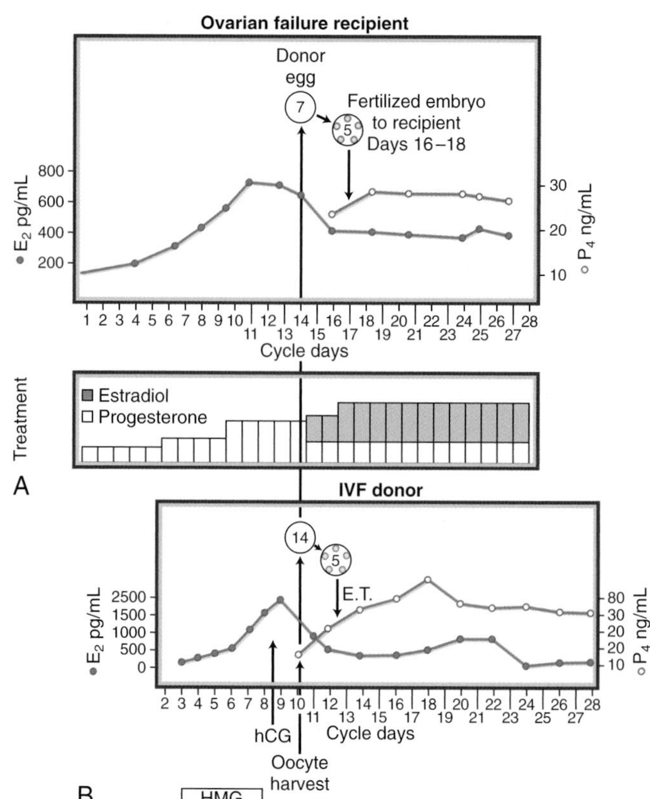

Figure 16–25 ▪ Diagrammatic representation of donation of excess oocytes by a woman undergoing in vitro fertilization (IVF) to a woman with ovarian failure treated with exogenous estrogen and progesterone. **A,** Woman with ovarian failure treated with increasing doses of estrogen during days 1 through 14 of the cycle. Exogenous progesterone was added to the estrogen treatment on days 15 through 28 and continued if pregnancy was diagnosed. Seven donor eggs were fertilized with sperm from the recipient's husband, and five embryos were transferred to the uterus on day 16 to 18. **B,** The IVF patient-donor was treated with human menopausal gonadotropin (hMG) until day 8, when human chorionic gonadotropin (hCG) was given, and oocytes were harvested 32 to 36 hours later. Half of the eggs were donated to the recipient, and the other half were fertilized with sperm from the donor's husband; the five fertilized eggs were transferred to the uterus of the IVF donor. Serum levels of E2 (estradiol) and P4 (progesterone) in both women are shown. To convert estradiol values to picomoles per liter, multiply by 3.671. To convert progesterone values to nanomoles per liter, multiply by 3.180. (Adapted from Rosenwaks Z. Donor eggs: their application in modern reproductive technologies. Fertil Steril 1987;47:895-909.)

Mechanism of Menstruation

In the absence of pregnancy, failure of the appearance of hCG, despite otherwise appropriate tissue reactions, leads to the vasomotor changes associated with estrogen-progesterone withdrawal and menstrual desquamation. A program of endometrial remodeling is initiated; alterations in the extracellular matrix and infiltration of leukocytes lead to hypoxia-reperfusion injury and sloughing of the functionalis, followed by activation of hemostatic and regenerative processes. The main histologic features of the premenstrual phase are degradation of the stromal reticular network, stromal infiltration by polymorphonuclear and mononuclear leukocytes, and secretory exhaustion of the endometrial glands, whose epithelial cells now have basal nuclei. The endometrium shrinks preceding menstruation, in part as a result of diminished secretory activity and the catabolism of extracellular matrix.

The most prominent and final effect of progesterone and estrogen withdrawal is menstruation (see Fig. 16–23). The classical studies of Markee[154] suggested that an ischemic phase caused by vasoconstriction of the arterioles and coiled arteries precedes the onset of menstrual bleeding by 4 to 24 hours. Bleeding occurs after the arterioles and arteries relax, leading to hypoxia-reperfusion injury. The superficial endometrial layers are distended by the formation of hematomas, and fissures subsequently develop, leading to the detachment of tissue fragments. Lysis and fragmentation of cells and apoptosis are evident. The menstrual efflux is composed of shed fragments of endometrium mixed with blood and liquefied by the fibrinolytic activity of the cellular debris (see Fig. 16–23). Clots of varying size may be present if blood flow is excessive.

Control of Endometrial Function Employing Synthetic Hormones

The fertility potential of a woman is primarily determined by the biologic quality of her oocytes, reflected in part by the capacity of the fertilized ovum to divide at an optimal rate and contain a normal chromosomal complement. This biologic quality of the oocyte declines sharply after the age of 35. The biologic potential of the endometrium for successful implantation, however, remains intact even at advanced ages.[170] Oocyte donation from a fertile woman and in vitro fertilization of these donor eggs with the recipient's male partner's sperm, followed by embryo transfer into the uterine cavity of the recipient woman who does not have functioning ovaries (e.g., premature ovarian failure), have been used successfully as a therapeutic strategy to treat infertility (see Fig. 16–25).[170,171] This clinical application has provided unique opportunities to examine the hormonal requirements for endometrial maturation. A number of hormone replacement protocols have been proposed, and many pregnancies have resulted from donor oocytes in women with ovarian failure (see Fig. 16–25). The success of these procedures has averaged about 50% (pregnancy rate) per embryo transfer.

The degree of endometrial differentiation in response to exogenous hormones has been evaluated by histologic analysis of endometrial biopsy specimens. The epithelial elements exhibit delayed maturation early during progesterone administration on days 20 to 22, but catch up by day 26. Despite this apparent dyssynchrony, the pregnancy rate in these patients with donor oocytes is higher than in conventional in vitro fertilization.[171]

The majority of infertility specialists currently use step-up administration of oral micronized estradiol in 2-, 4-, and 6-mg daily doses followed by 4 to 6 mg of estradiol combined with daily intramuscular progesterone (50 mg) to promote the secretory transformation. Serum estradiol in these subjects during the replacement "follicular" phase reaches sufficiently high levels to stimulate endometrial growth. Intramuscular injection of 50 mg/day of progesterone in oil generates serum levels of progesterone usually greater than 20 ng/mL. The length of exposure to progesterone, but not absolute plasma progesterone concentrations achieved after adequate priming of the endometrium with estrogen, is a key factor for the development of uterine receptivity. Thus, the exogenous administration of only estradiol and progesterone is sufficient to prepare the endometrium for implantation in the absence of ovarian function. This observation further underscores the essential roles of these steroids in uterine physiology.

APPROACH TO THE WOMAN WITH REPRODUCTIVE DYSFUNCTION

Reproductive dysfunction in an adult woman is most often manifest by disruption of cyclic, predictable menses. Efficient diagnosis of the underlying disorder requires a thorough understanding of female reproductive physiology and pathology and an accurate history and physical examination. Without a critical analysis of clinical findings based on thorough knowledge of normal and abnormal reproductive function, the application of predetermined algorithms of laboratory testing causes unnecessary use of hormone measurements or imaging studies and delays diagnosis.

History

An essential tool for the evaluation of a woman with a reproductive disorder is a carefully recorded history. The history should be obtained from the patient with the aim of assessing the biologic effects of each of the various hormones. Recording the details of pubertal development as a reference for the onset of particular symptoms provides critical clues to the etiology of certain reproductive disorders. For example, anovulation manifest by irregular uterine bleeding associated with the polycystic ovary syndrome (PCOS) most often begins during the pubertal years. The onset of gradually progressing hirsutism around puberty is suggestive of nonclassical adrenal hyperplasia or PCOS. In these cases, measurement of serum 17-hydroxyprogesterone may help differentiate nonclassical adrenal hyperplasia from PCOS (see later). The appearance of hirsutism before puberty or several years after normal pubertal development should alert the clinician to the possibility of ovarian or adrenal neoplasms. The sudden (versus gradual) onset of hirsutism at any age or the presence of virilization should prompt the physician to rule out steroid-secreting ovarian or adrenal tumors. Most women with symptomatic endometriosis suffer from severe episodes of painful menses (dysmenorrhea), which start during pubertal years.

Evaluation of female reproductive function depends upon a detailed history of the menses. For example, PCOS is unlikely without a longstanding history of irregular periods since the menarche. By the same token, history of a period of cyclic, predictable menses before the onset of menstrual irregularities should draw attention to hypothalamic or other causes of anovulation. The current frequency, regularity, length, and quantity of uterine bleeding should be carefully recorded for several reasons. First, this information reflects tightly regulated interactions of several tissues, including the hypothalamus, pituitary, ovaries, and endometrium. Second, regular, predictable menses imply ovulation. Third, defining the type of menstrual irregularity may help with the diagnosis of the underlying etiology. For example, prolonged amenorrhea in a thin and estrogen-deficient woman suggests anovulation of hypothalamic etiology. Infrequent periods of varying duration and amount of blood loss in a well-estrogenized overweight woman, on the other hand, suggest a primary ovarian dysfunction such as PCOS. It should be kept in mind that anovulation in a thin but well-estrogenized woman may also be due to PCOS. Regular but heavy and prolonged menses with intermittent spotting may be due to uterine anatomic disorders such as adenomyosis or leiomyomas. Finally, neoplastic disorders of the endometrium including endometrial polyps, hyperplasia, or malignancies may be manifest by any pattern of irregular bleeding. The combination of vaginal ultrasonography and endometrial biopsy is extremely sensitive for the diagnosis of endometrial neoplasia.[172]

Disruption of cyclic and predictable menses is a common and alarming symptom that initially brings the patient to the clinician. After a careful evaluation of the menstrual symptoms, the clinician should identify other obvious symptoms of endocrine disorder underlying irregular periods. Pregnancy is the most common cause of amenorrhea (and possibly any other menstrual irregularity) in a woman of reproductive age. In a woman presenting with amenorrhea or any other menstrual irregularity, normal pregnancy, ectopic pregnancy, or gestational trophoblastic disease must be excluded at the onset.

Careful evaluation of any past reproductive history, as well as of the patient's sexual activity and contraceptive practices, can provide useful indications of the likelihood of pregnancy. Furthermore, the reproductive history may suggest the possibility of Sheehan's syndrome of postpartum pituitary necrosis, if menses did not resume after a delivery complicated by significant hemorrhage.[173] In such instances, evidence of adrenal and thyroid insufficiency should be sought. A classical symptom of Sheehan's syndrome is the absence of lactation after delivery related to prolactin deficiency.

Amenorrhea is traditionally categorized as either primary (no history of menstruation) or secondary (cessation of menses after a variable time). The causes of primary amenorrhea are diverse and discussed extensively in Chapters 22 and 24. Although the distinction between primary and secondary amenorrhea is useful for identifying the mechanism of disease and differential diagnosis, the clinician should be aware that some disorders can initially present with either primary or secondary amenorrhea. For example, most women with gonadal dysgenesis have primary amenorrhea, but some patients have residual follicles and ovulate, and in these women with partial gonadal dysgenesis, some menstruation and rare pregnancies may occur before the cessation of ovarian function.[174,175] Patients with PCOS usually have secondary amenorrhea but occasionally have primary amenorrhea.

Secondary amenorrhea is most often due to chronic anovulation, which can be broadly categorized as (1) hypothalamic dysfunction, (2) galactorrhea-associated, (3) ovarian failure, (4) androgen excess, (5) chronic illness, and (6) primary uterine disease (e.g., intrauterine adhesion formation after a postpartum curettage).[176] Establishing any association of secondary amenorrhea with various life events is extremely useful. Strenuous exercise is often associated with amenorrhea. Weight loss often precedes or accompanies secondary amenorrhea and has been suggested as evidence of hypothalamic dysfunction. An unusual dietary history may be suggestive of bulimia or anorexia nervosa. A history of dilatation and curettage, postpartum endometritis, or disseminated tuberculosis with absent to scant menses should suggest the possibility of intrauterine adhesion.[177] The presence of any signs or symptoms of estrogen deficiency, including painful intercourse, atrophic vagina, emotional lability, and vasomotor instability, should suggest anovulation of a central nature with low concentrations of circulating gonadotropins (hypogonadotropic hypogonadism) or ovarian failure with elevated gonadotropins (hypergonadotropic hypogonadism).

Galactorrhea in the absence of a recent history of pregnancy is suggestive of a host of diagnostic possibilities and is frequently a manifestation of excessive prolactin secretion, although it may be a result of increased sensitivity of breast tissue to the hormones necessary for milk production. This history frequently reveals drug ingestion as the cause. Various drugs (including several psychotropic agents and antihypertensive agents as well as oral contraceptives) have been implicated. Primary hypothyroidism may be associated with precocious puberty with galactorrhea in the child and with amenorrhea, galactorrhea, or both in the adult woman. A history of excessive nipple manipulation or chest wall disease should be elicited and may well be the cause of galactorrhea. Prolactinomas, the prolactin-secreting adenomas of the pituitary, are a common etiology of galactorrhea related to abnormally high serum levels of prolactin.

Physical Examination

The quantity and distribution of excessive hair growth should be considered in light of the familial history. Hypertrichosis—excessive growth of hair on the extremities, the head, and the back—must be distinguished from true hirsutism, which is the development of facial hair, chest hair, and a male escutcheon with or without signs of virilization in response to increased production of or sensitivity to biologically active androgens. Some degree of hypertrichosis is not uncommon in women of Mediterranean descent, whereas the occurrence of any facial hirsutism in the relatively hairless Asian woman may require thorough investigation. Hirsutism is best documented and quantified with the help of photographs. Virilization is characterized as thickening of voice, severe cystic acne, hair loss, increased muscle mass, and clitoromegaly and implies a more severe degree of androgen excess than that found with hirsutism. The syndrome of complete androgen insensitivity is characterized by sparse to absent pubic and axillary hair because of resistance to androgen.

A careful inspection of the breasts is essential for a thorough physical examination. Classification of the stage of breast development according to the method of Marshall and Tanner[178] is a convenient and valuable adjunct. Whether the breasts appear to have decreased in size recently (e.g., severe androgen excess), whether the areolae are well formed and pigmented (as they are in pregnancy), and whether a discharge (e.g., galactorrhea) can be expressed should be assessed.

A woman with PCOS who has never ovulated or taken a progestin-containing medication may have Tanner stage 4 breast development related to adequate estrogen production, whereas the progression to Tanner stage 5 requires exposure to progesterone through either ovulation or ingesting a progestin (e.g., administration of oral contraceptives). See Chapter 24 for a detailed description and hormonal basis of Tanner staging of breast development.

The vulva, vagina, and cervix also represent sensitive indicators of sex steroid action. Because sensitivity of the genital skin and mucosa to androgen decreases with time from the early stages of fetal development to adulthood, the extent of any virilization can be helpful in suggesting the timing of androgen exposure. The most profound androgenic effects, such as posterior labial fusion with or without formation of a penile urethra, are generally observed in patients exposed to androgens during the first trimester (12 weeks) of pregnancy. Such findings have been described in patients with virilizing congenital adrenal hyperplasia, true hermaphroditism, and drug-induced virilization. Significant postnatal clitoromegaly, on the other hand, requires marked hormonal stimulation and, in the absence of significant exogenous steroids, strongly implicates an androgen-secreting tumor. Measurement of the base of the clitoris versus its length is a more accurate method for the determination of androgen-dependent clitoral growth. A clitoral index, defined as the product of the sagittal and transverse diameters at the base, greater than 35 mm^2 falls outside the 95% confidence interval (CI) for normality.

The vagina and uterine cervix are the most sensitive indicators of estrogen action. Under the influence of estrogen, the vaginal mucosa progresses during sexual maturation from a tissue with a shiny, bright red appearance with sparse, thin secretions to a tissue with a dull, gray-pink rugated surface with copious, thick secretions. Well-estrogenized vaginal mucosa with stretchable cervical mucus (spinnbarkeit) may be indicative of the proliferative phase of the menstrual cycle in an ovulatory woman or of extraovarian estrogen formation in an anovulatory woman with PCOS. The biologic activity of estrogen can also be quantified by vaginal cytology.

To summarize, irregular uterine bleeding is a common symptom that brings the woman with reproductive dysfunction to the physician's office. Various disorders of the hypothalamus, pituitary, ovaries, or uterus or other issues that affect reproductive function may be responsible for this alarming symptom. When pregnancy is ruled out, a detailed history and physical examination should be carefully recorded. In particular, the physician should pay attention to the salient features in the history and biologic indicators of hormone action at target tissues during the physical examination. An analysis of these findings most often leads to a tentative diagnosis. This diagnosis should then be confirmed with laboratory testing.

DISORDERS OF THE FEMALE REPRODUCTIVE SYSTEM

Chronic Anovulation

Chronic anovulation is one of the most common gynecologic problems encountered by the practitioner. These women may present with secondary amenorrhea, infrequent uterine bleeding (oligomenorrhea), or irregular episodes of excessive uterine bleeding. Infertility is an obvious consequence of chronic anovulation.

One group of anovulatory patients is estrogen-deficient. Common findings in this group include hypothalamic anovulation, galactorrhea-hyperprolactinemia (e.g., hypothyroidism, prolactinoma, nonfunctioning pituitary tumor), and premature ovarian failure in a woman of reproductive age. These patients are usually amenorrheic and deficient in estrogen. One serious consequence is bone loss giving rise to osteopenia and osteoporosis. If possible, the underlying cause should be corrected. Hormone replacement should be provided if ovulation cannot be restored.

Women with androgen excess constitute the second major group of anovulatory patients. A serious consequence of anovulation in this group is the greater risk for carcinoma of the endometrium because of unopposed action of estrogen formed continuously in extraovarian tissues. The most common disorder of the ovary associated with androgen excess and anovulation is PCOS. Insulin resistance plays a significant role in this condition and, along with hyperandrogenism, increases the risk of developing cardiovascular disease and diabetes mellitus.[146] The clinician must recognize the long-term impact of PCOS and undertake therapeutic management of these anovulatory patients to avoid unwanted consequences. The clinician should also develop a plan with the patient to address long-term complications of unopposed estrogen formation associated with PCOS (e.g., endometrial neoplasia). Oral contraceptives or periodic progestin supplementation may be provided to prevent endometrial hyperplasia and cancer.

For practical purposes, the following five broad categories include the majority of the etiologic factors giving rise to chronic anovulation in a woman of reproductive age:

1. Hypothalamic anovulation
2. Hyperprolactinemia
3. Androgen excess
4. Premature ovarian failure
5. Chronic illness (e.g., hepatic or renal failure, acquired immunodeficiency syndrome)

There may be multiple mechanisms responsible for anovulation in chronic illness. Effective treatment of the primary illness may restore normal menses. Alternatively, anovulatory bleeding may be managed by exogenous hormones in these chronically ill patients as outlined further subsequently. The following are detailed descriptions of specific disorders that cause chronic anovulation in a reproductive-age woman.

Hypothalamic Anovulation

Production of GnRH in the neurons of the arcuate nucleus in the hypothalamus and its secretion into the portal vessels in the median eminence in a pulsatile fashion are responsible for the production and secretion of FSH and LH from the pituitary.[10] GnRH neurons depolarize and release GnRH at critical pulse frequencies of 60 to 200 minutes during specific phases of the menstrual cycle to increase or decrease secretion of FSH and LH.[13,15] Variations in GnRH pulse frequency are achieved, at least partially, by gonadal steroid feedback. Local neuromodulators in the brain, including norepinephrine, dopamine, and β-endorphin, mediate the actions of gonadal steroids on the hypothalamus (see Fig. 16–4).[21] Any disorder of the central nervous system that interferes with this intricate process can thus cause anovulation. Some of these disorders may be demonstrated by defined genetic or anatomic evidence such as isolated gonadotropin deficiency (with or without anosmia), infection, suprasellar tumors (pituitary adenomas, craniopharyngioma), and head trauma.[10] These genetic and anatomic disorders affect the function of the hypothalamus, and some of them may be ruled out by history, physical examination, and imaging of the head (Table 16–2).

The most commonly observed form of hypothalamic anovulation, however, is not associated with a demonstrable neuroanatomic finding.[10] This common form is called *functional hypothalamic anovulation* because it is presumed to involve aberrant but reversible regulation of otherwise normal neuroendocrine pathways. Changes in lifestyle usually result in the return of normal ovulatory cycles. Functional hypothalamic anovulation may be associated with excessive exercise, abrupt weight loss, and emotional distress. It is hypothesized that these stress factors cause anovulation by affecting brain function and the GnRH pulse generator. Other causes of hypothalamic anovulation demonstrable by neuroanatomic or genetic evidence are relatively rare (see Table 16–2).

Functional Hypothalamic Anovulation

Anovulation of hypothalamic origin is characterized by estrogen deficiency and low levels of gonadotropins. No identifiable genetic or anatomic disorders are present in the majority of these patients. The concept of functional hypothalamic anovulation was first postulated in the 1940s as the failure of the hypothalamic-pituitary pathways to release LH from the anterior pituitary.[179] Since then, many clinical studies have confirmed this idea.[14] The data accumulated thus far suggest that the common underlying defect is an alteration in the pulsatile secretion of GnRH. Intriguingly, it has been shown in patients with this disorder that diverse etiologic factors such as malnutrition or caloric restriction, depression or psychogenic stress, excessive energy expenditure related to exercise, or combinations of these have preceded the onset of functional hypothalamic anovulation. Heightened awareness of diet and exercise and unrealistic expectations with respect to the body image of women have most likely contributed to the epidemic of this anovulatory disorder.

Diagnosis of Functional Hypothalamic Anovulation

Patients with functional hypothalamic anovulation most commonly present with secondary amenorrhea characterized by the absence of menstrual cycles for more than 6 months without evidence of an organic disorder. It should be emphasized once again that the diagnosis of hypothalamic anovulation is one of exclusion. There are many neuroanatomic or genetic disorders that can mimic functional hypothalamic anovulation (see Table 16–2). Thus, a careful and complete diagnostic evaluation is essential to make this diagnosis.

Women with functional hypothalamic anovulation usually present with a history of regular menses for a period of variable length after menarche. Thereafter, this period of normal ovulatory function (by history) is interrupted by anovulation usually

TABLE 16–2 CLASSIFICATION OF ANOVULATION CAUSED BY DISORDERS OF THE HYPOTHALAMIC-PITUITARY UNIT

FUNCTIONAL HYPOTHALAMIC ANOVULATION
Stress (psychogenic or physical) Dieting Vigorous exercise Chronic illness (e.g., chronic liver or renal failure, AIDS)
PSYCHIATRIC-MEDICAL EMERGENCIES
Anorexia nervosa
MEDICATIONS
Dopamine antagonists (e.g., haloperidol) Opiates Old antihypertensives (e.g., methyldopa, reserpine)
HYPOTHYROIDISM
ANATOMICALLY or GENETICALLY DEFINED PATHOLOGIES of the HYPOTHALAMIC-PITUITARY UNIT
Pituitary tumors Prolactinoma Clinically nonfunctioning adenoma GH-secreting adenoma (acromegaly) ACTH-secreting adenoma (Cushing's disease) Other pituitary tumors (e.g., metastasis, meningioma) Pituitary stalk section Hemorrhagic pituitary destruction, including pituitary apoplexy and Sheehan's syndrome Pituitary aneurysm Infiltrative disease of the pituitary (e.g., lymphocytic hypophysitis, sarcoidosis, histiocytosis X, tuberculosis) Empty sella syndrome Tumors that affect hypothalamic function (e.g., metastasis, craniopharyngioma) Infiltrative granulomatous disease of the hypothalamus (e.g., sarcoidosis, histiocytosis X, tuberculosis) Head trauma Irradiation to the head CNS infection Isolated gonadotropin deficiency (including Kallmann's syndrome) Other

ACTH, Adrenocorticotropic hormone; *AIDS*, acquired immunodeficiency syndrome; *CNS*, central nervous system; *GH*, growth hormone.

manifest by secondary amenorrhea. It should be emphasized that women with functional hypothalamic anovulation may occasionally present with primary amenorrhea.

Women with functional hypothalamic anovulation are typically normal to thin in body weight, driven, and involved in high-stress occupations. The occupation of the patient (e.g., a ballerina or competitive athlete) may be an extremely important clue. A detailed interview may reveal a variety of emotional crises or stressful events (e.g., divorce, death of a friend) preceding the onset of amenorrhea. During the interview, additional environmental and interpersonal factors may become evident, including academic pressure, social maladjustment, and psychosexual problems. When evaluating the patient, one should take note of the current diet regimen, the use of any sedatives or hypnotics, and the rigorousness of the patient's exercise habits. Despite a careful interview, a history of stress, excessive physical exercise, or an eating disorder may not be readily revealed in some women with functional hypothalamic anovulation. These women usually do not complain of hot flashes, which, on the other hand, are commonly observed in ovarian failure.

The physician should exclude a possible hyperprolactinemic etiology (e.g., prolactinoma, hypothyroidism) and evidence of androgen excess (e.g., PCOS) during the physical examination. These women have normal secondary sexual characteristics. The pelvic examination usually shows a thinning vaginal mucosa accompanied by scant to absent cervical mucus with a normal to small uterus, all evidence of estrogen deficiency. Signs of a well-estrogenized vagina and cervix observed during the physical examination make the diagnosis of hypothalamic anovulation unlikely.

Laboratory tests are obtained to exclude other causes of anovulation and secondary amenorrhea. LH and FSH levels should be obtained. Gonadotropin levels are usually lower than the normal values ordinarily found in the early follicular phase. TSH and prolactin levels are obtained to rule out hypothyroidism and hyperprolactinemia. The progestin challenge test (medroxyprogesterone acetate at 10 mg/day for 10 days) shows either a small spotting episode or absence of withdrawal uterine bleeding in most patients. This confirms that there is a scant or absent estrogenic effect on the endometrium because circulating estradiol levels are typically in the low or early follicular phase range. Measurement of the serum estradiol level is not necessary. Because a suprasellar or large pituitary tumor is in the differential diagnosis, a magnetic resonance imaging (MRI) scan of the head is necessary to rule this out. Imaging of the head is especially important if amenorrhea develops suddenly or is associated with a neurologic sign, both of which make the presence of a tumor more likely.

Pathophysiology of Functional Hypothalamic Anovulation

A key observation in functional hypothalamic anovulation is the absence of increased gonadotropin secretion despite the lack of inhibitory factors of ovarian origin, such as estradiol and inhibin. The secretory pattern of LH is abnormal. The causative factor in women with this type of anovulation is a slowdown in the frequency of pulsatile GnRH secretion.[14,180,181] Frequent peripheral blood samples were obtained from these patients to quantify the episodic secretion of LH, which provided an indirect assessment of endogenous GnRH secretion.[181]

There is considerable variability in the amplitude and frequency of the pulsatile LH secretion in functional hypothalamic anovulation. When the LH secretory patterns are compared with that of the follicular phase of the menstrual cycle, a characteristic abnormality in the LH pulse frequency and amplitude and on occasion a regression to a pronounced variability similar to what is seen in the prepubertal pattern are present.[14,180,181] In severe cases, the frequency and amplitude of LH pulses are markedly reduced. These LH patterns also suggest that GnRH pulsatile secretion is not altered to the same degree in each individual. During the recovery phase of hypothalamic anovulation, a reversal to a pattern of LH secretion seen early in puberty is often present, characterized by a sleep-associated increase in LH amplitude.

The response of the pituitary gland to GnRH with respect to production and release of gonadotropins is not impaired in functional hypothalamic anovulation. Intravenous pulsatile GnRH administration can restore normal levels of LH and FSH.[182,183]

Norepinephrine, dopamine, and serotonin produced in the brain have been shown to modulate GnRH or LH release in animal studies. Patients receiving medication that alters these neurotransmitters (e.g., sedatives, antidepressants, stimulants, and antipsychotics) have presented with abnormalities in their menstrual cycles. Thus, these responses to medications provide circumstantial evidence that disruptions of neural pathways can alter GnRH release in the human. From these observations, it appears that activation of the noradrenergic neurons principally stimulates release of GnRH,[184,185] whereas dopaminergic and serotoninergic neurons can stimulate or inhibit GnRH-LH secretion.[185]

A number of neuropharmacologic agents have been used as probes to determine whether GnRH-LH secretion can be normalized. For example, metoclopramide blocks the action of dopamine.[186] A metoclopramide injection results in a prompt increase in LH secretion in patients with functional hypothalamic anovulation. These studies suggest enhanced dopaminergic activity in functional hypothalamic anovulation. It should be emphasized, however, that chronic administration of dopamine antagonists (e.g., haloperidol, metoclopramide) may also cause anovulation.

Another group of substances that have inhibitory influences on GnRH secretion are endogenous opioid peptides.[187,188] Blockade of endogenous opiate receptors by the administration of naloxone, an opiate antagonist, to women with this disorder caused an increase in the frequency and amplitude of pulsatile LH release.[186] Gonadotropin secretion resumes if the activity of the opiate receptor is blocked by long-term naloxone use in these anovulatory patients, and ovulatory function may even be regained in some cases.[189] These studies suggest that there is an overall increase in endogenous opiate activity, which can reduce pulsatile GnRH secretion in functional hypothalamic anovulation.

Reproductive function may be disrupted by chronic exposure to stress.[179] In fact, activation of the pituitary-adrenocortical system is a common response in patients with chronic stress.[190] In functional hypothalamic anovulation, stressors such as exercise or emotional stress can chronically activate the hypothalamic-pituitary-adrenal axis. Daytime cortisol levels are markedly elevated, and the pituitary response to corticotropin-releasing hormone (CRH) is blunted.[183,191] The stress response is associated with increased secretion of CRH, adrenocorticotropic hormone (ACTH), cortisol, prolactin, oxytocin, vasopressin, epinephrine, and norepinephrine.

The association between emotional or physical stress and disruption of the reproductive function of the hypothalamus is complex and involves several mechanisms. In an animal model, CRH seems to be an important factor in the inhibition of GnRH pulsatility.[192,193] This inhibitory effect can be prevented by coadministration of a CRH antagonist or reversed by the opiate antagonist naloxone, which is suggestive of a cross-talk between the action of CRH and activation of the opioidergic system. Moreover, ACTH administration blocks the pituitary response to GnRH at the pituitary level.[194,195] In addition, another stress hormone, oxytocin, can inhibit hypothalamic GnRH secretion.[188] In summary, overproduction of CRH and other stress-related hormones in the brain and activation of the pituitary-adrenocortical system by chronic stress seem to play causative roles in the inhibition of gonadotropin secretion in functional hypothalamic anovulation.

Recently, the role of leptin deficiency was investigated as a cause of hypothalamic amenorrhea. In fact, leptin administration for the relative leptin deficiency in women with hypothalamic amenorrhea improved reproductive, thyroid, and growth hormone axes and markers of bone formation, suggesting that leptin, a peripheral signal reflecting the adequacy of energy stores, is required for normal reproductive and neuroendocrine function.[196]

Hypothalamic Anovulation and Exercise

Regular vigorous exercise can lead to menstrual disturbances, a delay in menarche, luteal phase dysfunction, and secondary amenorrhea. Thirty percent of adolescent ballet dancers have problems with the progression of puberty. The mean age of menarche is delayed until 15. In fact, advancement of pubertal stages seems to coincide with times of prolonged rest or following recovery from an injury.[197-202] The intensity, length, and type of the sport determine the severity of the disease. Activities associated with an increased frequency of reproductive dysfunction are those that favor a lower body weight and include middle-distance and long-distance running, competitive swimming, gymnastics, and ballet dancing.

Competitive athletes show endocrine abnormalities in the central nervous system consistent with those in other forms of functional hypothalamic anovulation. These include elevations in central CRH and β-endorphin levels.

The management of exercise-related anovulation is dependent on the patient's choices and expectations. Side effects such as osteoporosis and delay of puberty must be discussed at length with the patient.[203] Decrease in exercise level and behavioral modification may be sufficient for the return of ovulatory function. Hormone replacement should be provided if sufficient results are not achieved. A low-dose oral contraceptive is a suitable option for women of reproductive age.

Hypothalamic Anovulation Associated with Eating Disorders

Two common eating disorders associated with hypothalamic dysfunction are anorexia nervosa and bulimia. In anorexia nervosa, there is an extreme loss of weight (weight decrease of greater than 25% of original body weight) and a distorted body image accompanied by a striking fear of obesity. Bulimia is a related disorder characterized by alternating episodes of binge eating followed by periods of food restriction, self-induced vomiting, or excessive use of laxatives or diuretics. About 90% to 95% of these patients are female. Most patients with eating disorders are white and are from middle-class or upper-middle-class families. The incidence of classic anorexia nervosa is about 1 per 100,000 in the general population.[204] Among high school and college female students, bulimia, however, is fairly common.[5] The incidence of anorexia nervosa peaks twice during the teen years at ages 13 and 17. Bulimia usually begins at a later age, between 17 and 25 years. Anorexia nervosa has an extremely high mortality of 9% and is a true medical emergency. Death may be secondary to cardiac arrhythmia, which may be precipitated by diminished heart muscle mass and associated electrolyte abnormalities.[205] These patients are also at increased risk for suicide.[206]

Gonadotropin secretion in anorexic women exhibits a prepubertal pattern that is similar to that in other forms of hypothalamic anovulation. Transitional patterns of LH secretion are seen when there are moderate degrees of weight recovery and there is a normal or supranormal response to GnRH. Anovulation can persist in up to 50% of anorexic patients even after achieving normal weight. Both anorexic and bulimic patients exhibit hyperactivation of the hypothalamus-pituitary system. Although the diurnal variation is maintained, there is a persistent hypersecretion of cortisol throughout the day.[207] Cushingoid features, however, are not present, in part because of mild hypercortisolemia and also a reduction of peripheral glucocorticoid receptors. Levels of both CRH and β-endorphin are increased in the central nervous system.[208,209]

In anorexia nervosa, basal metabolism is decreased because peripheral conversion of thyroxine (T_4) to biologically potent triiodothyronine (T_3) is decreased. Instead, T_4 is converted to reverse T_3, an inactive isoform. This alteration is also observed in severely ill patients and during starvation.[210] Anorexics also have partial diabetes insipidus and are unable to concentrate urine appropriately because of the impaired secretion of vasopressin.[211]

Both anorexia nervosa and bulimia are extremely difficult to treat. The most accepted approaches include individual psychotherapy, group therapy, and behavior modification. Patients with eating disorders should have psychiatric consultation and follow-up. This helps with both the diagnosis and treatment. In patients who weigh less than 75% of their ideal body weight, immediate hospitalization and aggressive treatment are recommended. Chronic complications of anorexia nervosa include osteoporosis; other consequences are estrogen deficiency and generalized effects of malnutrition.[200] Hormone replacement in the form of an oral contraceptive should be provided until ovulatory function is achieved.

Treatment and Management of Functional Hypothalamic Anovulation

Treatment of chronic anovulation resulting from central nervous system–hypothalamic disorders should be directed at reversal of the primary cause (e.g., stress management, reduction of exercise, or correction of weight loss). The importance of successful treatment of this disease state is underscored because these women are prone to the development of osteoporosis. For a considerable number of patients, spontaneous recovery of menstrual function takes place after a modification of lifestyle, psychological guidance, or accommodation to environmental stress. Therefore, the initial treatment should be directed to a change in lifestyle and tailored to the individual patient. For individuals who remain amenorrheic, periodic assessment of reproductive status (every 4 to 6 months) is prudent.

If anovulation persists for more than 6 months or if reversal of the primary cause is not practical (e.g., professional athletes, ballerinas), a major concern is the long-term effect of hypoestrogenism, especially on bone metabolism. In addition to estrogen deficiency, IGF-I deficiency, hypercortisolism, or nutritional factors may all contribute to bone loss in this disorder.[212] Unfortunately, epidemiologic data on the risk of fractures and the benefits of hormone replacement are scant.[203,212] On the basis of studies of reproductive-age women who have been ovariectomized or who have undergone treatment with GnRH agonist for endometriosis, bone density would be expected to decrease significantly even within the first 6 months of amenorrhea. Because these patients are often reluctant to take medications, serial bone density studies of the lumbar spine and femur may be necessary to convince them of the necessity to begin estrogen replacement therapy. If the patient is not at risk for thromboembolism and does not smoke cigarettes, a low-dose combination oral contraceptive is a reasonable replacement option. Alternatively, a combination of conjugated estrogens (0.625 mg) and medroxyprogesterone acetate (2.5 mg) daily may be administered to provide estrogenic support. The progestin (medroxyprogesterone acetate) is added solely to prevent endometrial hyperplasia.

If the patient desires ovulation in order to achieve pregnancy, the most physiologic approach is ovulation induction with pulsatile GnRH. This is currently the best physiologic means of induction because the cause of the anovulatory state is the decrease in endogenous GnRH secretion. Pulsatile intravenous GnRH, 5 mcg every 90 minutes, was shown to be effective.[213] Monitoring of serum estradiol levels or follicular development can be minimized because the ovarian follicular response and gonadotropin output mimic the natural menstrual cycle. In these patients, either continuation of pulsatile GnRH or human chorionic gonadotropin, 1500 units intramuscularly every 3 days for a total of four doses, can support the function of the corpus luteum. The intravenous GnRH treatment results in ovulation rates of approximately 90%, pregnancy rates up to 30%, and hyperstimulation rates of less than 1% per treatment cycle.[213] Because the intravenous GnRH pump is not a practical choice for many women, an alternative strategy is the use of subcutaneous recombinant FSH for the development of one to three follicles and the induction of ovulation with intramuscular hCG followed by luteal support using either intramuscular hCG or progesterone in oil.

Chronic Anovulation Associated with Pituitary Disorders

The most common pituitary-related causes of anovulation are associated with hyperprolactinemia caused by either prolactinomas or other functional or anatomic disorders of the pituitary. These disorders are frequently associated with dysregulation of gonadotropin secretion. Hyperprolactinemia and other pituitary disorders and their relation to reproduction are discussed in detail in Chapter 8.

Chronic Anovulation Associated with Androgen Excess

The most common ovary-related disorder of chronic anovulation is the polycystic ovary syndrome (PCOS). Irregular periods and/or amenorrhea and androgen excess are the most commonly observed features of PCOS. Other causes of ovary-related anovulation include steroid-secreting ovarian tumors and premature ovarian failure. Androgen excess arising from extraovarian sources (e.g., adrenal disorders) is also associated with anovulation.

Approach to the Patient with Androgen Excess

Two natural androgens are testosterone, which is transported to target tissue by the circulation, and DHT, which is produced primarily by target tissues. Increased levels of these androgens can lead to hirsutism, which is excessive androgenic hair growth, or to virilization, a more severe form of androgen excess. Hirsutism is defined as the presence of terminal (coarse) hair in locations at which hair is not commonly found in women. It includes facial hair on the cheek, above the upper lip, and on the chin (Fig. 16–26A and B). The presence of midline chest hair is also significant (Fig. 16–26C). In addition, a male escutcheon, hair on the inner aspects of the thighs, and midline lower back hair entering the intergluteal area are hair growth patterns compatible with androgen excess. A moderate amount of hair on the forearms and lower legs by itself may not be abnormal, although it may be viewed by the patient as undesirable and may be mistaken for hirsutism. Numerous scoring systems are available for quantifying hirsutism. One of the most detailed scales was proposed by Ferriman, Gallwey, and Lorenzo.[214] A practical and clinically useful means of quantifying hirsutism is recording the hair growth in detail using simple drawings and photographs. In particular, photographs are invaluable for documenting hirsutism accurately.

In contrast to hirsutism, virilization is a more severe form of androgen excess and implies significantly higher rates of testosterone production. Its manifestations include temporal balding, deepening of voice, decreased breast size, increased muscle mass, loss of female body contours, and clitoral enlargement (Fig. 16–27). Even if testosterone levels are moderately increased (<1.5 ng/mL), temporal balding and clitoromegaly may be observed over a long period of time (>1 year) in the presence of persistent androgen excess. A marked increase in androgen secretion, as may occur from production by neoplasms, however,

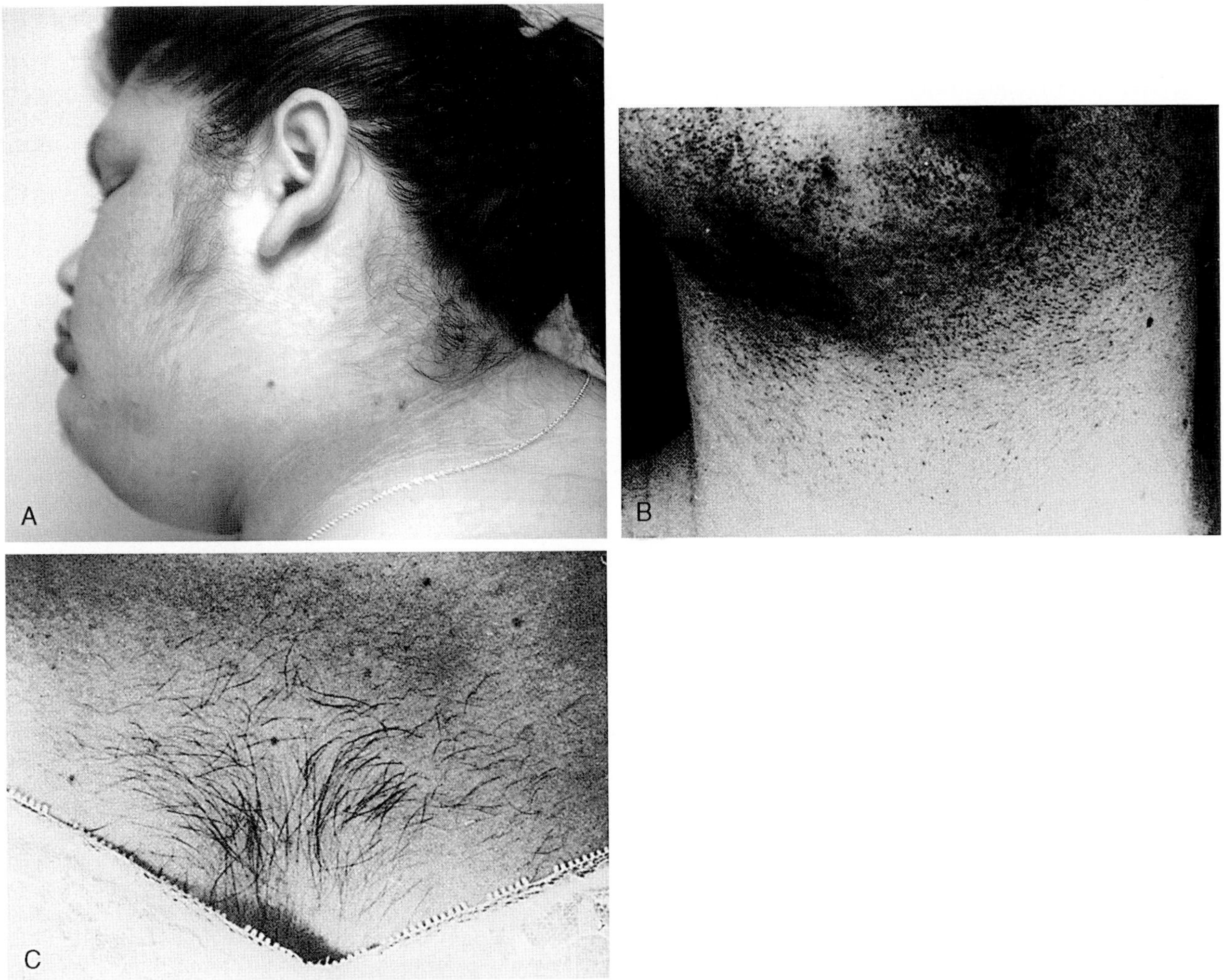

Figure 16–26 ▪ Hirsutism. **A,** Mild facial hirsutism. **B,** Severe facial hirsutism (chin), which requires regular shaving. **C,** Severe hirsutism on chest. (B and C from Dunaif A, Hoffman AR, Scully RE, et al. The clinical, biochemical and ovarian morphologic features in women with acanthosis nigricans and masculinization. Obstet Gynecol 1985;66:545-552.)

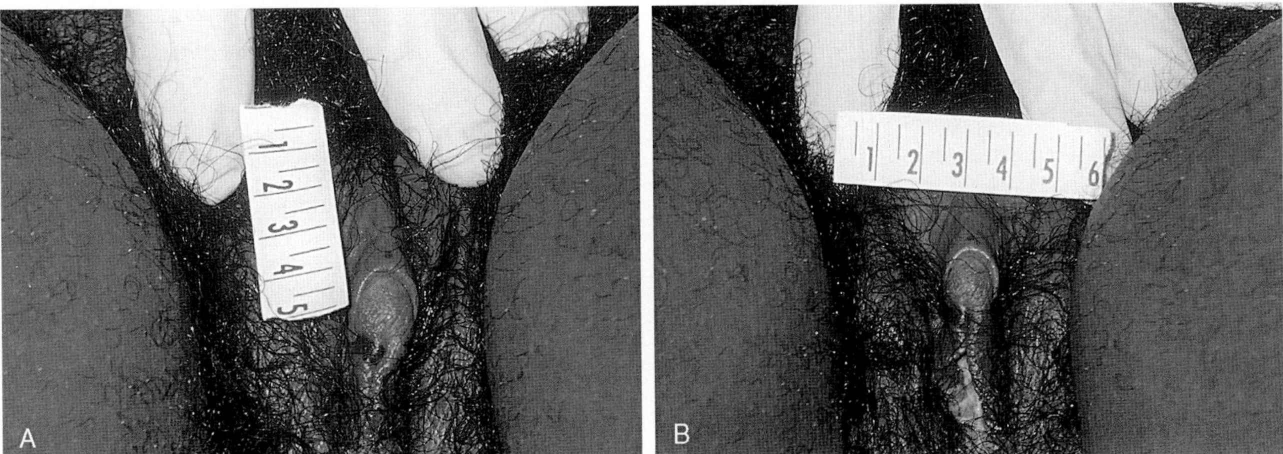

Figure 16–27 ▪ Severe clitoromegaly resulting from a testosterone-secreting ovarian tumor. **A,** The entire length of the clitoris is approximately 4 cm (normal <1 cm). **B,** The transverse diameter of the clitoris measures 1.5 cm (normal <0.7 cm).

leads to a more full-blown picture of virilization over a short duration of time (less than a few months).

Measurements of an enlarged clitoris may be used for the quantification of virilization. A clitoral length more than 10 mm is considered abnormal (see Fig. 16–27). Clitoral length is quite variable, however. An increase in clitoral diameter is a much more sensitive indicator of androgen action. Normal values for clitoral diameter are less than 7 mm at the base of the glans (see Fig. 16–27). The most accurate definition of clitoromegaly involves the use of the clitoral index (the product of the width and length of the glans clitoris). A clitoral index greater than 35 mm^2 is abnormal and correlates statistically with androgen excess.[215]

Origins of Androgens

Two natural C19 steroids are capable of acting as androgens on target organs: testosterone and dihydrotestosterone (DHT). In this chapter, the use of the term *androgen* refers to either of these steroids. Testosterone in reproductive-age women is produced by two major mechanisms: (1) direct secretion by the ovary, accounting for roughly one third of testosterone production, and (2) conversion of the precursor androstenedione to testosterone in the peripheral (extragonadal) tissues, accounting for two thirds of testosterone production (Fig. 16–28).[216,217] These peripheral tissues include the skin and adipose tissue. Androstenedione, the direct precursor of testosterone, is produced in both the ovary and the adrenal. The C19 steroids DHEAS and DHEA of adrenal origin and DHEA of ovarian origin indirectly contribute to testosterone formation by first being converted to androstenedione that is subsequently converted to testosterone (see Fig. 16–28).

Whereas testosterone is an androgen, DHEAS is a biologically inert steroid. Up to 20 mg of DHEAS are produced daily versus only 3 mg of androstenedione and 8 mg of DHEA per day. These C19 steroids of adrenal origin (DHEAS, DHEA) exert their effects after conversion to the potent androgen testosterone (see Fig. 16–28). Only androstenedione can be converted directly to testosterone. The conversion rate of circulating androstenedione to testosterone in extragonadal tissues is about 5% in both men and women.

Testosterone binds nuclear androgen receptors and activates androgen target genes. Testosterone, however, must be converted to an even more potent steroid, DHT, to exert full androgenic effects on target tissues such as hair follicles and external genitalia.[127,151] For example, intense androgen action in sex skin fibroblasts requires receptor occupancy by DHT. This conversion is catalyzed by the enzyme 5α-reductase and takes place in the liver and within androgen target cells such as sex skin fibroblasts (i.e., intracrine effect). The protein products of two genes (5α-reductase type 1 and type 2) exhibit this enzymatic activity.[127] The androgenic potential of DHT with respect to hair growth and virilization of external genitalia is markedly higher than that of testosterone.

Androgen action in target tissues is determined at least in part by the level of local 5α-reductase activity and the androgen receptor content. Androgen receptors mediate androgenic action in critical target tissues (see Fig. 16–28).[151,218] Local enzymes at target tissues other than 5α-reductase (e.g., aromatase and 17β-HSD or ketoreductase) also regulate androgen action by metabolizing testosterone to the androgenically inactive androstenedione or to estradiol, a potent estrogen. Thus, there appears to be a balance between the amplification of androgen action when DHT is formed and the reduction of androgenicity when inactive C19 steroids or estradiol is formed from testosterone in target tissues and other extragonadal tissues. In particular, the metabolism of testosterone to DHT versus androstenedione-estradiol in these tissues is relevant for androgen-dependent disorders (e.g., hirsutism, virilization) and estrogen-dependent disorders (e.g., malignancies of breast and endometrium) (see Figs. 16-21 and 16-28).

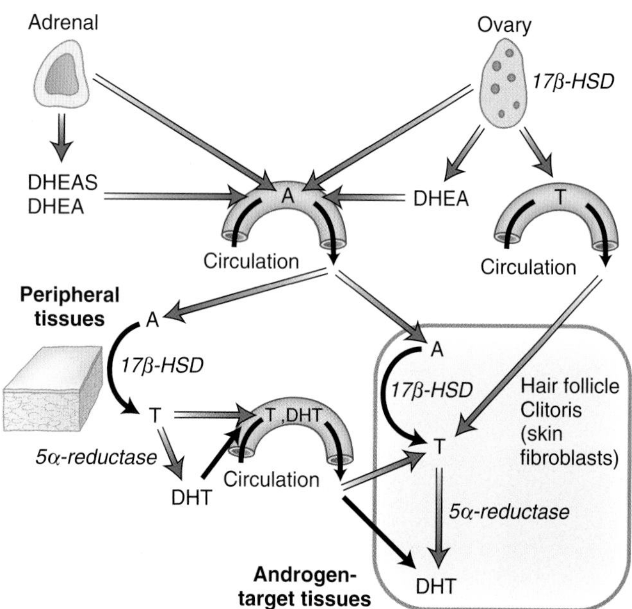

Figure 16–28 ▪ Androgen biosynthesis in women. There are two biologically active androgens, testosterone (T) and dihydrotestosterone (DHT). Depending on the menstrual cycle phase or postmenopausal status, 20% to 30% of T is secreted by the ovary. The rest of T production[217] is accounted for by the conversion of circulating androstenedione (A) to T in various peripheral tissues. Both the adrenal and ovary contribute to circulating A directly or indirectly depending on the cycle phase, reproductive-age versus postmenopausal status, and chronologic age. Moreover, T may also be formed locally in androgen target tissues. Finally, T is converted to the more potent androgen DHT within the target tissues and cells. For example, local conversion of T to DHT in sex skin fibroblasts and hair follicles amplifies androgenic action for clitoral enlargement and hirsutism. DHEA, dehydroepiandrosterone; *DHEAS,* dehydroepiandrosterone sulfate; *HSD,* hydroxysteroid dehydrogenase.

Laboratory Evaluation of Androgen Action

Testosterone circulates in three forms: that which is bound to sex hormone binding globulin (SHBG), the portion not bound to SHBG but rather loosely associated with albumin, and the fraction not bound by either SHBG or albumin, that is, free or dialyzable testosterone. Biologically active testosterone includes both the free and albumin-bound fractions. Thus, the blood testosterone available to diffuse into target tissues is referred to as bioavailable or non–SHBG-bound testosterone. The remainder is tightly bound to the protein SHBG.

SHBG is one of the primary regulators that determine the amounts of circulating bound and bioavailable testosterone available to act on target tissues. Conditions that decrease SHBG binding (e.g., androgen excess, obesity, acromegaly, hypothyroidism, and liver disease) also increase bioavailable testosterone, thus augmenting the effect of testosterone. SHBG also regulates the circulating amounts of bioavailable estradiol by binding a significant fraction of circulating estradiol. Hence, conditions that decrease SHBG levels also give rise to increased bioavailable (non–SHBG-bound) estradiol.

The measurement of non–SHBG-bound (bioavailable) forms of testosterone has been advocated in states of androgen excess to detect more accurately subtle forms of hirsutism. Although the diagnostic yield of this measurement is clearly superior to that of total serum testosterone, the correlation between total and non–SHBG-bound testosterone is excellent. Bioactive testosterone can usually be predicted from the total testosterone level.[219] The purpose of measuring serum testosterone is to establish the presence of circulating androgen excess and to detect extremely high values that might originate from an androgen-secreting neoplasm.

The normal serum levels of androgens, especially free testosterone determined by radioimmunoassay (RIA) vary from laboratory to laboratory. Therefore, a group of investigators compared serum free testosterone levels measured by equilibrium dialysis with those measured by a direct RIA and to those calculated from the free androgen index, 100 × testosterone/SHBG, a simple index that correlates with free testosterone.[220] Calculated values for free testosterone using the free androgen index correlated well with those obtained from equilibrium dialysis. In contrast, the direct RIA method had unacceptably high systematic bias and random variability and did not correlate as well with equilibrium dialysis values. Moreover, the lower limit of detection was higher for the direct RIA than for equilibrium dialysis or calculated free testosterone.[220] Thus, the clinician should be aware of limitations of RIAs performed without rigorous quality control.

For practical purposes, measuring the levels of all of these C19 steroids is not clinically necessary in the majority of patients presenting with androgen excess. The most useful initial test is a serum total testosterone level. An abnormal level in the presence of hirsutism or virilization may be associated with PCOS, hyperthecosis, nonclassic adrenal hyperplasia, or an androgen-secreting neoplasm. The majority of androgen-secreting tumors are of ovarian origin. The likelihood of a neoplasm correlates roughly with increasing testosterone levels. The following tests may be added on the basis of the clinical presentation: serum 17-hydroxyprogesterone (nonclassic adrenal hyperplasia, see below for details), serum prolactin and TSH (mild androgen excess associated with hyperprolactinemia), serum FSH and LH (elevated LH/FSH ratio in PCOS), serum DHEAS (adrenal tumors), and imaging of ovaries and adrenals (PCOS, tumors).

Causes of Androgen Excess

A variety of disorders give rise to androgen excess. These include unusual causes such as iatrogenic or drug-induced androgen excess, congenital genital ambiguity (e.g., excessive in utero androgen formation in female pseudohermaphroditism), and conditions unique to pregnancy (luteoma of pregnancy and hyperreactio luteinalis). These uncommon causes and relatively more prevalent disorders associated with androgen excess are listed in Table 16–3. The term *extraovarian steroid formation* is used synonymously with extraglandular, extragonadal, or peripheral steroid formation in this text.

Overall, the prevalence of androgen excess disorders was found to be as follows: PCOS, 72.1% (anovulatory patients, 56.6%; mildly affected, ovulatory patients, 15.5%), idiopathic hyperandrogenism, 15.8%; idiopathic hirsutism, 7.6%; 21-hydroxylase-deficient nonclassic adrenal hyperplasia, 4.3%; and androgen-secreting tumors, 0.2%.[221]

In most hyperandrogenic disorders, androgen originates from more than one source (see Fig. 16–28). For example, testosterone secretion is somewhat increased from the ovary in PCOS, but the bulk of testosterone comes from extraovarian conversion of significantly elevated circulating androstenedione of ovarian origin to testosterone. To add a further twist, patients with PCOS also show increased adrenal output of DHEAS, which (after peripheral conversion to DHEA that is further converted to androstenedione) contributes indirectly to extraovarian testosterone formation (see Fig. 16–28).

When androgen excess is associated with primary amenorrhea, abnormal in utero sexual differentiation should be strongly suspected. These disorders are covered in detail in Chapter 22. Furthermore, before embarking on a major workup for hirsutism or virilization, the clinician is well advised to rule out exogenous androgen use. It is best to ask the patient to list all prescriptions and over-the-counter medications that she takes on her own, including injections. This is usually more rewarding than simply asking the patient whether she takes any androgens. Medications that can cause hirsutism or virilization are related to testosterone. These include anabolic steroids and similar compounds.

The most common identifiable cause of androgen excess is PCOS. PCOS is discussed under a separate heading in this chapter. In this section, we first define some of the other disorders associated with hirsutism or virilization. This is followed by a simplified treatment strategy, which may be applied to the majority of hirsute patients within the categories PCOS, nonclassic adrenal hyperplasia, and idiopathic hirsutism.

TABLE 16–3 CAUSES OF ANDROGEN EXCESS IN A REPRODUCTIVE-AGE WOMAN

OVARIAN
PCOS, polycystic ovary syndrome Hyperthecosis (a severe PCOS variant) Ovarian tumor (e.g., Sertoli-Leydig cell tumor)
ADRENAL
Nonclassic adrenal hyperplasia Cushing's syndrome Glucocorticoid resistance Adrenal tumor (e.g., adenoma, carcinoma)
SPECIFIC CONDITIONS of PREGNANCY
Luteoma of pregnancy Hyperreactio luteinalis Aromatase deficiency in fetus
OTHER
Hyperprolactinemia, hypothyroidism Medications (danazol, testosterone, anabolizing agents) Idiopathic hirsutism (normal serum testosterone in an ovulatory woman) Idiopathic hyperandrogenism (patients who do not fall into any of the categories listed above)

Idiopathic Hirsutism

Excessive hair growth in the absence of demonstrable androgen excess in ovulatory women is also referred to as *idiopathic* or constitutional and occurs more frequently in certain ethnic populations, particularly in women of Mediterranean ancestry.[151] It is defined as hirsutism in conjunction with regular menstrual cycles and normal levels of serum testosterone. Idiopathic hirsutism is not associated with any sign of virilization. Its cause is not understood completely. It has been proposed that women with idiopathic hirsutism have significantly increased cutaneous 5α-reductase activity.[222] The presence or absence of such an association is not clear. Likewise, it is unclear which of the 5α-reductase isoenzymes (type 1 or 2), if any, is predominant in the development of idiopathic hirsutism.[151]

Idiopathic hirsutism is diagnosed in women who have (1) hirsutism, (2) normal ovulatory function, and (3) normal total or free testosterone levels. Overall, more than 80% of women with cyclic predictable menses are ovulatory. Ovulatory function may be verified by a luteal phase day 7 progesterone level, which should be at least 5 ng/mL. Luteal phase day 7 corresponds to cycle day 17 for 24-day intervals, cycle day 21 for 28-day intervals, and cycle day 28 for 35-day intervals. The presence of oligo-ovulation or anovulation in hirsute women after the exclusion of related disorders (e.g., hypothyroidism, hyperprolactinemia, or nonclassic adrenal hyperplasia) is consistent with the diagnosis of PCOS.[151] Thyroid dysfunction and hyperprolactinemia should be excluded by the measurements of TSH and prolactin. The follicular phase basal 17-hydroxyprogesterone level should be measured to exclude 21-hydroxylase–deficient, nonclassic adrenal hyperplasia. The use of exogenous androgens should also be excluded. In summary, the diagnosis of idiopathic hirsutism is one of exclusion, in which ovulatory dysfunction, elevated circulating testosterone, and other causes of androgen excess are ruled out.

Androgen-Secreting Tumors of the Ovary and Adrenal

The majority of androgen-secreting tumors arise from the ovary. These ovarian tumors secrete large quantities of testosterone or its precursor androstenedione. They include Sertoli-Leydig cell tumors, hilus cell tumors, lipoid cell tumors, and, infrequently, granulosa-theca tumors. Steroidogenically inert ovarian neoplasms such as epithelial cystadenomas or cystadenocarcinomas may produce factors that stimulate steroidogenesis in adjacent non-neoplastic ovarian stroma and induce production of sufficient amounts of androgen precursors such as androstenedione to give rise to clinically detectable androgen excess. Approximately 5% of androstenedione is converted to testosterone in extraovarian tissues to give rise ultimately to androgen excess (see Fig. 16–28).

Sertoli-Leydig cell tumors, which account for less than 1% of all solid ovarian tumors, tend to occur during the second to fourth decades of life, whereas hilus cell tumors occur more frequently in postmenopausal women. By the time the signs and symptoms of androgen excess cause the patient to seek medical assistance, Sertoli-Leydig cell tumors are usually so large that they are readily palpable on pelvic examination, whereas hilus cell tumors are still small. In women with either type of tumor, serum testosterone is markedly elevated. Granulosa-theca tumors primarily produce estradiol but may occasionally produce testosterone.

Rapidly progressing symptoms of androgen excess suggest the presence of an androgen-producing tumor unless proved otherwise. This rapid progression is typical of both ovarian and adrenal androgen-producing tumors. The progression is usually more from defeminizing signs (loss of female body contour, decrease in breast size) than from the androgenic signs. As the tumor continues to grow, more and more testosterone is produced, resulting in rapidly worsening hirsutism and progressive virilization. With all ovarian tumors, serum testosterone is characteristically elevated. This may be mediated by two mechanisms: (1) production and secretion of testosterone directly by the tumor[223] or (2) secretion of large quantities of androstenedione that is converted to testosterone in extragonadal tissues. The testosterone levels produced by certain ovarian tumors (e.g., the Sertoli-Leydig cell tumor) may be suppressed using a GnRH agonist.[224] Therefore, use of a GnRH agonist cannot be relied upon to distinguish a neoplasm from another functional state.

In interpreting testosterone levels, the clinician should first be familiar with the normal ranges of the clinical laboratory used. A value of three times the upper normal range (or >2 ng/mL) is suggestive of a neoplasm, particularly if the clinical history supports this diagnosis. It should be kept in mind that lower serum testosterone levels may occasionally be observed in association with virilizing ovarian tumors. When an androgen-secreting tumor is suspected, a measurement of androstenedione is also clinically useful. A severely elevated level of androstenedione is also consistent with an ovarian or adrenal tumor. When an elevated level of testosterone is found and confirmed by clinical history, meticulously performed transvaginal ultrasonography should be able to detect the ovarian tumor. Transvaginal ultrasonography is the most sensitive method for the detection of an ovarian tumor.

In contrast to testosterone-secreting tumors of the ovary, testosterone-secreting tumors of the adrenal are extremely rare. The cells of testosterone-producing adrenal tumors may resemble ovarian hilus cells, which are analogous to Leydig cells. These tumor cells produce testosterone and may be stimulated by both LH and hCG. Thus, in patients with testosterone-producing adrenal adenomas, testosterone secretion usually decreases after LH suppression and increases after hCG stimulation.

Virilizing adrenal tumors commonly secrete large quantities of DHEAS, DHEA, and androstenedione, whereas testosterone is usually produced by extraovarian conversion of these precursors. Levels of serum DHEAS are highly elevated in most virilizing adrenal tumors.[225] When DHEAS levels exceed 8 μg/mL, a scan by either computed tomography or MRI should be ordered unless the history is more suggestive of PCOS (longstanding history of symptoms and no virilization). In the latter case, a functional abnormality of the adrenal is likely to be present: either an enzymatic defect, such as congenital adrenal hyperplasia, or an unexplained hyperfunctional state that is commonly associated with PCOS. Under these circumstances, the scan can be deferred until further investigation has been carried out.

Levels of a variety of adrenal steroids including corticosteroids may be elevated in various combinations in the presence of an adrenal tumor. Thus, it is not possible to describe a particular pattern of hormones that defines an adrenal tumor.[225] In general, very high levels of serum DHEAS (>8 μg/mL) are suggestive of an adrenal tumor. Testosterone-secreting adrenal tumors are extremely rare. Virilizing ovarian tumors, on the other hand, are encountered much more frequently than those of an adrenal origin. If the presentation is compatible with an androgen-secreting tumor and the ovaries are normal by transvaginal ultrasonography, the adrenals should be evaluated next by imaging.

Testosterone levels three times the upper normal range (or >2 ng/mL) and DHEAS levels higher than 8 μg/mL have been used as guidelines to investigate further whether neoplasms of the ovary or adrenal are the sources of androgen excess. It should be emphasized that these numbers are provided only as guidelines and not as rules. The following exceptions to these guidelines must be pointed out. First, because tumors secrete androgens episodically, more than one value may be required to detect a significantly elevated level.[226] Second, other precursor steroids are often elevated as well (particularly androstenedione), and their measurement should be considered. Finally, the tumors may give rise to milder elevations of DHEAS and testosterone levels. In particular, even mild elevations in a postmenopausal woman are highly suspicious of an androgen-secreting tumor. By the same token, severely elevated serum testosterone levels may be observed in women with severe ovarian hyperthecosis (a severe variant of PCOS) in the absence of a tumor.

Virilization of recent onset and short duration should warrant further investigation, even if testosterone and DHEAS are mildly elevated. With improvements in scanning techniques—vaginal ultrasonography for the ovary; abdominal ultrasonography, computed tomography, and MRI for the adrenal—the diagnosis of even a small (ovarian or adrenal) tumor may be made.

However, if no neoplasm can be localized, imaging of the ovary or adrenal after intravenous administration of radiolabeled iodomethylnorcholesterol (NP-59), which detects active steroid-producing tumors, has proved useful.[227] These diagnostic studies should be pursued aggressively before the surgical exploration of a suspected tumor.

Nonneoplastic Adrenal Disorders and Androgen Excess

A number of adrenal disorders, such as classic congenital adrenal hyperplasia, Cushing's syndrome, and glucocorticoid resistance, give rise to androgen excess related to overproduction of testosterone precursors from the adrenal. These disorders are discussed in other chapters. Here, we discuss nonclassic adrenal hyperplasia.

The debate regarding the diagnosis and prevalence of nonclassic adrenal hyperplasia continues, although the disorder clearly exists. Other terms that have been used to describe this syndrome include late-onset, adult-onset, attenuated, incomplete, and cryptic adrenal hyperplasia. This form of adrenal hyperplasia is caused by a partial deficiency in 21-hydroxylase activity. Although deficiencies in 11β-hydroxylase and 3β-HSD may result in the disorder, defects in 21-hydroxylase account for more than 90% of cases.[228]

The clinical presentation is almost identical to that of patients with PCOS. The prevalence of this disorder varies according to ethnic background, and the prevalence reported by different investigators has varied widely. The characteristic presentation consists of anovulatory uterine bleeding and progressive hirsutism of pubertal onset. These individuals are born with normal genitalia, do not exhibit salt-wasting, and are symptom-free until puberty. Patients of northern European ancestry have a low frequency of this disorder, whereas Ashkenazi Jews, Hispanics, and patients of central European ancestry have a much higher prevalence.[229] Therefore, it is recommended that high-risk ethnic groups be screened.

Screening may first be carried out by obtaining an 8:00 AM serum 17-hydroxyprogesterone level in an anovulatory patient on any day. Although the majority of women with nonclassic adrenal hyperplasia are anovulatory, some women with this disorder present with regular periods and hirsutism of pubertal onset or with only unexplained infertility.[228] If nonclassic adrenal hyperplasia is suspected in an ovulatory patient on the basis of clinical presentation, an 8:00 AM serum 17-hydroxyprogesterone level should be obtained during the follicular phase because 17-hydroxyprogesterone levels are higher in the luteal phase versus the proliferative phase in affected or disease-free ovulatory women.[228] A level less than 2 ng/mL effectively rules out this diagnosis.[228]

The diagnosis of nonclassic adrenal hyperplasia can be made if the basal 17-hydroxyprogesterone level is higher than 8 ng/mL. No further testing is required in these cases. Values between 2 and 8 ng/mL are considered increased but not diagnostic of nonclassic adrenal hyperplasia. For example, disease-free women or patients with PCOS may also have basal 17-hydroxyprogesterone levels in this indeterminate range.[228] The only way to distinguish nonclassic adrenal hyperplasia from PCOS under these circumstances is with an ACTH stimulation test.[228] A rise of 17-hydroxyprogesterone to at least 10 ng/mL 60 minutes after intravenous injection of ACTH has been considered diagnostic of nonclassic adrenal hyperplasia.[230] It should be noted, however, that a higher basal 17-hydroxyprogesterone level within the 2 to 8 ng/mL range is associated with a higher likelihood of nonclassic adrenal hyperplasia. For example, an 8:00 AM 17-hydroxyprogesterone level higher than 4 ng/mL had a sensitivity of 90% for the diagnosis of nonclassic adrenal hyperplasia.[228]

In a patient with androgen excess who belongs to an ethnic group in which there is high prevalence, a baseline 17-hydroxyprogesterone level should be measured at 8:00 AM. In addition, the following patients should have a screening baseline 17-hydroxyprogesterone level obtained: patients with premature pubarche, those with androgen excess of early pubertal onset, women with progressive hirsutism or virilization, and patients with strong family histories of severe androgen excess.

Laboratory Testing to Aid the Differential Diagnosis of Androgen Excess

A number of algorithms exist for the differential diagnosis of anovulation associated with hirsutism or virilization, or both. Salient clinical features are of paramount importance to guide laboratory testing. The most important features include the onset and severity of the signs and the rapidity with which they progress. Rapidly progressing severe androgen excess implies an androgen-secreting tumor until proved otherwise. The possibility of a tumor is further underscored in a postmenopausal woman or in a reproductive-age woman with a recent history of cyclic, predictable periods. Ovarian hyperthecosis, a severe variant of PCOS, also gives rise to severe androgen excess that may progress rapidly, especially at the time of expected puberty. Androgen excess emerging at the time of puberty may be indicative of PCOS or nonclassic adrenal hyperplasia.

The most useful initial test to evaluate androgen excess is serum total testosterone (Table 16–4). Testosterone levels in most normal ovulatory women are below 0.6 ng/mL, although the value may vary from laboratory to laboratory. Women with idiopathic hirsutism have cyclic menses and normal testosterone levels. No further testing for androgen excess is required in this group.

If the testosterone level is elevated in an anovulatory woman, serum TSH and prolactin should be obtained next to rule out anovulation associated with hyperprolactinemia. Ultrasonography of the ovaries is also helpful at this time to assess the presence or absence of an ovarian tumor or polycystic ovaries. If the ethnic background of the patient (Ashkenazi Jews, Hispanics, and those of central European ancestry), onset of hirsutism (puberty), or family history is suggestive of nonclassic adrenal

TABLE 16–4 LABORATORY TESTS FOR THE DIFFERENTIAL DIAGNOSIS OF ANDROGEN EXCESS

INITIAL TESTING
Total testosterone Prolactin TSH
FURTHER TESTING BASED on CLINICAL PRESENTATION*
17-Hydroxyprogesterone (8:00 AM) 17-Hydroxyprogesterone 60 min after intravenous ACTH Cortisol (8:00 AM) after 1 mg dexamethasone at midnight DHEAS Androstenedione Imaging of ovaries (transvaginal ultrasonography) Imaging of adrenals (abdominal ultrasonography, CT scan, MRI) Nuclear imaging after intravenous administration of radiolabeled cholesterol

*See text.

ACTH, Adrenocorticotropic hormone; *CT*, computed tomography; *DHEAS*, dehydroepiandrosterone sulfate; *MRI*, magnetic resonance imaging; *TSH*, thyroid-stimulating hormone.

hyperplasia, a baseline serum 17-hydroxyprogesterone level should be obtained at 8:00 AM. Rare etiologies of androgen excess include an adrenal tumor, Cushing's syndrome, and glucocorticoid resistance. A serum DHEAS level and adrenal imaging are required to assess the presence or absence of an adrenal tumor. A computed tomographic scan, MRI scan, or abdominal ultrasonography may be used to assess the adrenals, depending on the expertise of the local radiology laboratory. A screening test for Cushing's syndrome and glucocorticoid resistance may be performed to explore rare adrenal causes of androgen excess (see Chapters 8 and 14).[231]

Most women with chronic anovulation and mild to moderate hirsutism of pubertal onset fall into the category of PCOS. These women have high normal or elevated testosterone levels and no other laboratory abnormalities. When other diagnoses are ruled out either by laboratory testing or on clinical grounds, a diagnosis of PCOS can be made.

Treatment of Hirsutism

Therapy for androgen excess should be directed toward its specific cause and suppression of abnormal androgen secretion. Specific treatments for hirsutism and virilization would be indicated for the following conditions: ovarian and adrenal tumors, hyperthecosis, Cushing's syndrome, and adrenal hyperplasia. Neoplasms warrant surgical intervention and are not discussed in greater detail. Suppression with a GnRH analogue may be tried initially for ovarian hyperthecosis. Unfortunately, bilateral oophorectomy is inevitable to control androgen excess arising from hyperthecosis in the majority of patients (see later). Patients with adrenal disease are treated specifically. For Cushing's syndrome, treatment is according to the source of hypercortisolism. For nonclassic adrenal hyperplasia, glucocorticoid replacement should be implemented as for adrenal insufficiency. When treating androgen excess associated with nonclassic adrenal hyperplasia, an antiandrogen (e.g., spironolactone) in combination with an oral contraceptive or a glucocorticoid may be used. The doses of glucocorticoids needed to suppress the adrenal, however, can often cause symptoms and signs of glucocorticoid excess during long-term treatment. Thus, a combination oral contraceptive plus spironolactone should be favored to treat androgen excess if the patient responds to this treatment with decreased hirsutism. Greater details of glucocorticoid therapy may be found in Chapters 14 and 22.

The general treatment of androgen excess is directed toward the prevention of abnormal hair growth and virilization. For practical purposes, the same approach is used for androgen excess associated with idiopathic hirsutism, PCOS, and nonclassic adrenal hyperplasia. The existing hair follicles and manifestations of virilization (e.g., thickening of voice, clitoromegaly, temporal balding) remain even after the elimination of excessive androgen production. Therefore, terminal hair should be removed by mechanical methods (e.g., electrolysis) at least 3 months after androgen suppression is achieved. Patients with clitoromegaly may be referred to a urologist for clitoral reduction surgery after the source of virilization is effectively eliminated. The following medications are available for the treatment of androgen excess and hirsutism.

Oral Contraceptives

Oral contraceptives reduce circulating testosterone and androgen precursors by suppression of LH and stimulation of SHBG levels and, thereby, reduce hirsutism in hyperandrogenic patients.[151] Oral contraceptives decrease circulating androgen in patients with PCOS and synergize with the effects of antiandrogens. It is possible that oral contraceptives may further improve the results of antiandrogen therapy in idiopathic hirsutism. It is advisable to use an oral contraceptive containing either 30 or 35 mcg of ethinyl estradiol to achieve effective suppression of LH.[151]

Spironolactone

The most common androgen blocker used for the treatment of hirsutism in the United States is spironolactone, an aldosterone antagonist structurally related to progestins. Spironolactone is effective for abnormal hair growth associated with PCOS or idiopathic hirsutism.

Because spironolactone acts through mechanisms different from that of oral contraceptives, the overall effectiveness is improved by combining these two medications, including patients with idiopathic hirsutism. Apart from the inhibition of steroidogenesis and acting as an androgen antagonist, spironolactone has a significant effect in inhibiting 5α-reductase activity.[151,232] Basic and several clinical studies clearly point to the efficacy of spironolactone for hyperandrogenism and suggest that the principal effect is related to its peripheral blocking ability of androgen production and action.[151]

Doses of spironolactone have varied in clinical studies from 50 to 400 mg daily. Although doses of 100 mg/day are generally effective for the treatment of hirsutism, higher doses (200 to 300 mg/day) may be preferable in extremely hirsute or markedly obese women.[151,232] Thus, it is recommended to start with 100 mg/day and gradually increase the dose by 25-mg/day increments every 3 months up to 200 mg/day on the basis of the response. This approach may be helpful to minimize side effects such as gastritis, dry skin, and anovulation.

In patients with normal renal function, hyperkalemia is almost never seen. Hypotension is rare except in older women. Monitoring, however, is imperative for electrolytes and blood pressure within the first 2 weeks at each dose level. Adjustments in dose should be made only after 3 to 6 months, as with other antiandrogens, to account for the slow changes in the hair cycle. Patients usually note an initial transient diuretic effect. Some women with normal cycles complain of menstrual irregularity with spironolactone. The latter complaint is remedied by either a downward dose adjustment or the addition of an oral contraceptive. The mechanism for abnormal bleeding is unclear. In women with oligomenorrhea, such as those with PCOS, resumption of normal menses may occur. In part, this may be due to an alteration in levels of circulating androgens, although LH levels have only occasionally been noted to decrease.[233] Another important consideration is the potential in utero feminizing effect of this antiandrogen on the genitalia of a 46,XY fetus. Thus, effective contraception should always be provided in women taking spironolactone.

Cyproterone Acetate

Cyproterone acetate is a 17-hydroxyprogesterone acetate derivative with strong progestagenic properties. Cyproterone acetate acts as an antiandrogen by competing with DHT and testosterone for binding to the androgen receptor. There is also some evidence that cyproterone acetate and ethinyl estradiol in combination can inhibit 5α-reductase activity in skin.[234] Cyproterone acetate is currently not available in the United States but has been used in other countries. The drug is mostly administered in doses of 50 to 100 mg from days 5 through 15 of the treatment cycle. Because of its slow metabolism, it is administered early in the treatment cycle, whereas ethinyl estradiol, when added, is usually used at 50-μg doses between days 5 and 26. This regimen is needed for menstrual control and is usually referred to as the reverse sequential regimen. Cyproterone acetate in doses of 50 to 100 mg/day, combined with ethinyl estradiol at 30 to 35 μg/day, is as effective as the combination of spironolactone, 100 mg/day, and an oral contraceptive in the treatment of hirsutism.[151] In smaller doses (2 mg), cyproterone acetate has been administered as an oral contraceptive in daily combination with 50 or 35 μg of ethinyl estradiol. This regimen is primarily suited for individuals with a milder form of hyperandrogenism.[151]

Finasteride

Finasteride inhibits 5α-reductase activity and has been used primarily for the treatment of prostatic hyperplasia. It can also be used in the treatment of hirsutism.[235,236] At a dose of 5 mg/day, a significant improvement of hirsutism is observed after 6 months of therapy, without significant side effects. In hirsute women, the decline in circulating DHT levels is small and cannot be used to monitor therapy. Although this treatment regimen increases testosterone levels, SHBG levels remain unaffected.[235]

Finasteride primarily inhibits 5α-reductase type 2. As hirsutism results from a combination of effects of type 1 and type 2, this agent is only partially effective. Although prolonged experience with finasteride is lacking, one of the potential advantages of this agent appears to be its benign side-effect profile. One study showed efficacy with 1 year of hirsutism treatment.[237] It was also reported that finasteride is less effective than spironolactone with respect to the reduction of hirsutism.[151] Nevertheless, finasteride represents a useful option for treating women with hirsutism at a dose of 5 mg/day for prolonged periods because of its benign side-effect profile and good tolerance by patients. As in the case of spironolactone, finasteride may also cause congenital genital ambiguity in a 46, XY fetus, and effective contraception should be provided during its use.

Flutamide

Flutamide is a potent antiandrogen used in the treatment of prostate cancer. It has been shown to be effective in the treatment of hirsutism.[238,239] Nevertheless, occasional severe hepatotoxicity makes this drug unsuitable for the indication of hirsutism.[240]

Summary

The preceding medications may be effective when administered as individual treatments. Patients with the most common form of hirsutism (i.e., PCOS) are often initially treated with a combination of two agents, one that suppresses the ovary (e.g., oral contraceptive) and another agent that suppresses the extraovarian (peripheral) action of androgens (e.g., spironolactone). Thus, an oral contraceptive containing 30 to 35 mcg of ethinyl estradiol combined with spironolactone, 100 mg/day, is the initial treatment of choice. Even in women with idiopathic hirsutism, the addition of an oral contraceptive to the antiandrogen spironolactone can improve efficacy and prevent abnormal bleeding. For women with only minor complaints of hirsutism, the use of an oral contraceptive alone may be an appropriate first approach.

Because the growth phase of body hairs lasts 3 to 6 months, one should not expect a response before 6 months from the onset of the treatment. Objective means should be used to assess changes in hair growth. Scoring systems and evaluation of anagen hair shafts are difficult; taking photographs is the simplest and most objective tool. Patients are often unaware that change is indeed taking place unless there is some objective measurement. Pictures of face and selected midline body areas before and during therapy are especially useful for the encouragement of the patient and compliance with the treatment.

Suppression of androgen production and action only inhibits new hair growth. Thus, existing coarse hair should be removed mechanically. Plucking, waxing, and shaving are ineffective for hair removal and cause irritation, folliculitis, and ingrown hairs. Electrolysis is still the method of choice. Laser epilation is relatively new and needs further evaluation.[151]

The majority of patients with PCOS and idiopathic hirsutism respond to this treatment within 1 year. Patients should be encouraged to continue treatment for at least 2 years. After this, depending on the wishes and clinical responses of patients, therapy can be stopped and the patient reevaluated. Many patients require continuous treatment for the suppression of hirsutism.

Polycystic Ovary Syndrome

PCOS is the most common form of chronic anovulation associated with androgen excess, perhaps occurring in 5% to 10% of reproductive-age women.[146] The diagnosis of PCOS is made by excluding other hyperandrogenic disorders (e.g., nonclassic adrenal hyperplasia, androgen-secreting tumors, and hyperprolactinemia) in women with chronic anovulation and androgen excess.

During the reproductive years, PCOS is associated with important reproductive morbidity including infertility, irregular uterine bleeding, and increased pregnancy loss. The endometrium of the patient with PCOS must be evaluated by biopsy because long-term unopposed estrogen stimulation leaves these patients at increased risk for endometrial cancer. PCOS is also associated with increased metabolic and cardiovascular risk factors.[241] These risks are linked to insulin resistance and compounded by the common occurrence of obesity, although insulin resistance is also present in non-obese women with PCOS.[146]

PCOS is viewed as a heterogeneous disorder of multifactorial etiology. PCOS risk is significantly increased with a positive family history of chronic anovulation and androgen excess, and this complex disorder may be inherited in a polygenic fashion.[242,243]

Historical Perspective

In their pioneering studies, Stein and Leventhal[244] described an association between the presence of bilateral polycystic ovaries and signs of amenorrhea, oligomenorrhea, hirsutism, and obesity (Fig. 16–29). At the time, these signs were strictly adhered to in the diagnosis of what was then known as Stein-Leventhal syndrome. These investigators also reported the results of bilateral wedge resection of the ovaries, removing at least one half of each ovary as a therapy for PCOS. Most of their patients resumed menses and achieved pregnancy after ovarian wedge resection. They postulated that removing the thickened capsule of the ovary would restore normal ovulation by allowing the follicles to reach the surface of the ovary (see Fig. 16–29). The exact mechanism responsible for the therapeutic effect of removing or destroying part of the ovarian tissue is still not well understood.

On the basis of Stein and Leventhal's work, a primary ovarian defect was inferred, and the disorder was commonly referred to as polycystic ovarian disease. Subsequent clinical, morphologic, hormonal, and metabolic studies have uncovered multiple underlying pathologies (see later). The term *polycystic ovary syndrome* was introduced to reflect the heterogeneity of this disorder.

One of the most significant discoveries regarding the pathophysiology of PCOS was the demonstration of a unique form of insulin resistance and associated hyperinsulinemia.[146] For the first time, Burghen and colleagues reported this finding in 1980.[245] The presence of insulin resistance in PCOS has since been confirmed by a number of groups worldwide.[146]

Diagnosis of Polycystic Ovary Syndrome and Laboratory Testing

One of the most prominent features of PCOS is the history of ovulatory dysfunction (amenorrhea, oligomenorrhea, or other

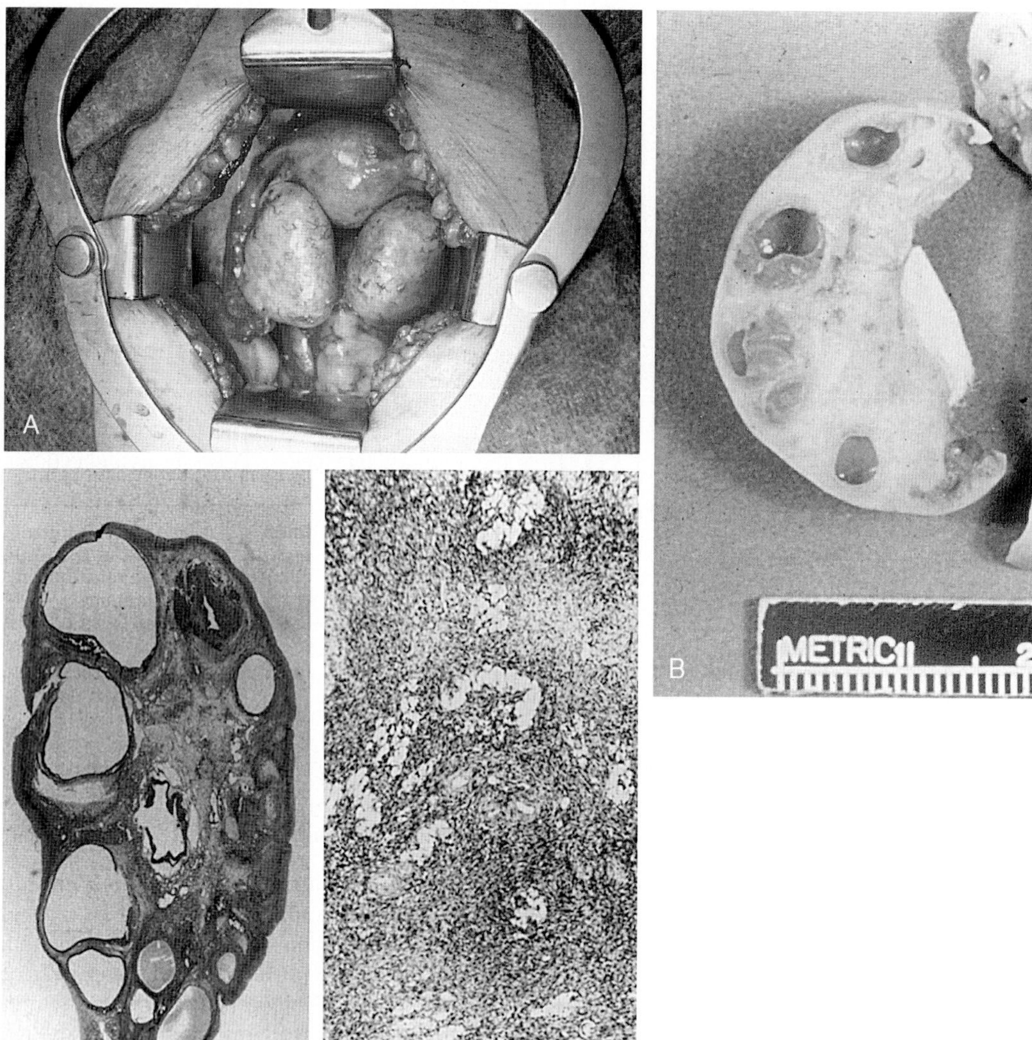

Figure 16–29 ▪ Polycystic ovaries. **A,** Operative findings of classical enlarged polycystic ovaries. The uterus is located adjacent to the two enlarged ovaries. **B,** Sectioned polycystic ovary with numerous follicles. **C,** Histologic section of a polycystic ovary with multiple subcapsular follicular cysts and stromal hypertrophy (low power, *left*). At higher power (×100), islands of luteinized theca cells are visible in the stroma (*right*). This morphologic change is called *stromal hyperthecosis* and appears to be directly correlated with circulating insulin levels. (C From Dunaif A. Insulin resistance and the polycystic ovary syndrome: mechanism and implications for pathogenesis. Endocr Rev 1997;18:774-800. Copyright © 1997 by The Endocrine Society.)

forms of irregular uterine bleeding) of pubertal onset. Thus, a clear history of cyclic predictable menses of menarchal onset makes the diagnosis of PCOS unlikely. Acquired insulin resistance associated with significant weight gain or an unknown cause, however, may occasionally induce the clinical picture of PCOS in a woman with a history of previously normal ovulatory function. Hirsutism may develop prepubertally or during adolescence, or it may be absent until the third decade of life. Seborrhea, acne, and alopecia are other common clinical signs of androgen excess. In extreme cases of ovarian hyperthecosis (a severe variant of PCOS), clitoromegaly may be observed. Nonetheless, rapid progression of androgenic symptoms and virilization are rare in ordinary PCOS. Some women may never have signs of androgen excess because of hereditary differences in target tissue sensitivity to androgens.[151] Infertility related to the anovulation may be the only presenting symptom.

During the physical examination, it is essential to search for and document signs of androgen excess (hirsutism or virilization or both), insulin resistance (acanthosis nigricans), and the presence of unopposed estrogen action (well-rugated vagina and stretchable clear cervical mucus) to support the diagnosis of PCOS (Fig. 16–30). It should be noted that none of these signs are specific for PCOS and may be associated with any of the conditions listed under the differential diagnosis of PCOS (Table 16–5).

PCOS has been defined until recently according to the proceedings of an expert conference sponsored by the National Institutes of Health[246] in 1990, which noted the disorder as having (1) hyperandrogenism and/or hyperandrogenemia, (2) oligo-ovulation, and (3) exclusion of known disorders of androgen excess and anovulation. Alternatively, another expert conference held in Rotterdam in 2003 defined PCOS, after the exclusion of related disorders, by two of the following three features: (1) oligo-ovulation or anovulation, (2) clinical and/or biochemical signs of hyperandrogenism, or (3) polycystic ovaries (Fig. 16–31). In essence, the Rotterdam 2003 criteria

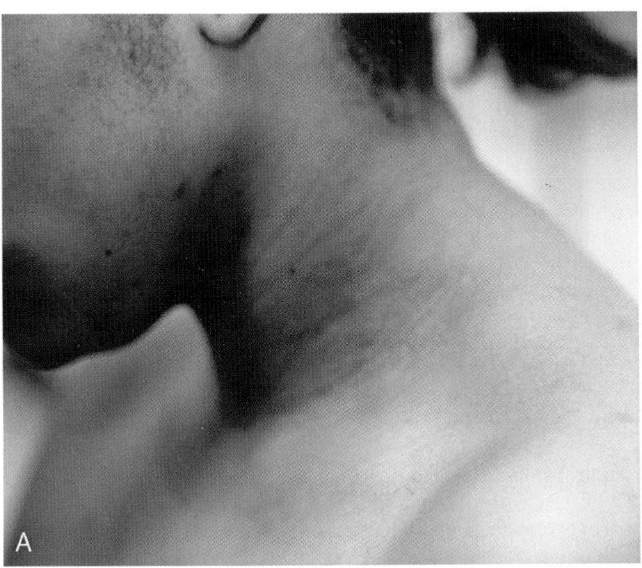

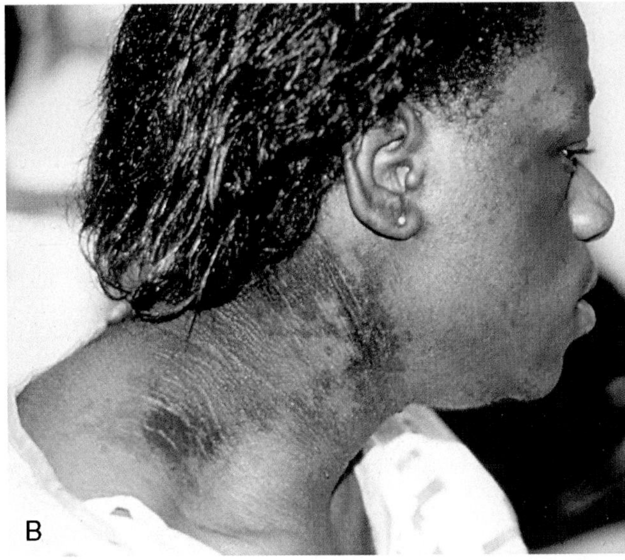

Figure 16–30 ▪ Acanthosis nigricans. **A,** Moderate acanthosis nigricans (darkening and thickening of skin) at the lateral lower fold of the neck. Note facial hirsutism (sideburns) in the same patient. **B,** Severe acanthosis nigricans in another patient with severe insulin resistance. (B Courtesy of Dr. R. Ann Word, Dallas, TX.)

TABLE 16–5 DIFFERENTIAL DIAGNOSIS OF POLYCYSTIC OVARY SYNDROME

Idiopathic hirsutism
Hyperprolactinemia, hypothyroidism
Nonclassic adrenal hyperplasia
Ovarian tumors
Adrenal tumors
Cushing's syndrome
Glucocorticoid resistance
Other rare causes of androgen excess

expanded the NIH 1990 definition by creating two new phenotypes: (1) ovulatory women with polycystic ovaries and hyperandrogenism and (2) oligoanovulatory women with polycystic ovaries, but without hyperandrogenism. The clinical usefulness of including these new groups with respect to increased risk of infertility, insulin resistance, and its long-term metabolic complications is not clear at this time.[247]

The exclusion of hyperprolactinemia, hypothyroidism, nonclassic adrenal hyperplasia, and tumors requires a careful history and physical examination as well as laboratory testing as detailed previously (see Table 16–4). Cushing's syndrome and glucocorticoid resistance may give rise to androgen excess and anovulation after a period of normal ovulatory function in teens. An 8:00 AM cortisol level after dexamethasone (1 mg) administration at midnight is a useful screening test for both conditions. Cushing's syndrome may be recognized by its typical signs, whereas 8:00 AM and 4:00 PM cortisol levels are essential to suspect the diagnosis of glucocorticoid resistance.[248] Glucocorticoid resistance is characterized by preserved diurnal rhythm despite significantly elevated cortisol, ACTH, and adrenal C19 steroid levels and absence of cushingoid symptoms and signs[248] (Table 16–6).[249,250]

As emphasized earlier, elevated total testosterone is the most direct evidence for androgen excess. Varying levels of testosterone are present in women with PCOS. Rarely, serum testosterone levels higher than 2 ng/mL may be encountered in association with the most severe form of PCOS, ovarian hyperthecosis. Overall, it is much more common to observe high normal levels or borderline elevations of testosterone in women with PCOS.

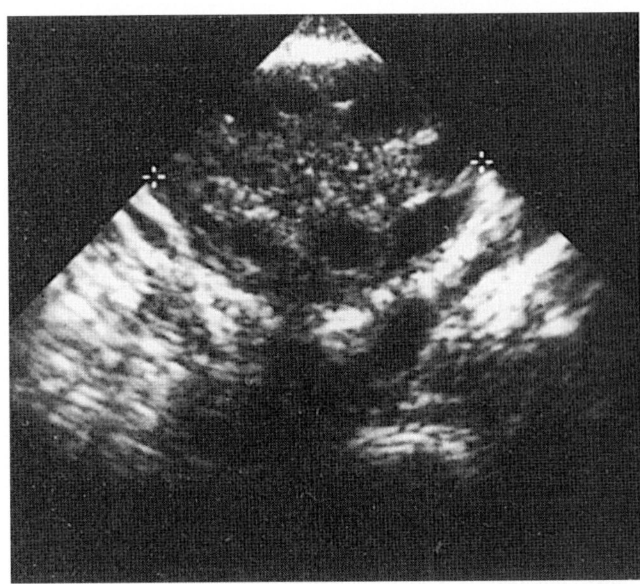

Figure 16–31 ▪ Transvaginal ultrasound image of a polycystic ovary. Note multiple midsized follicles in the periphery and increased solid area in the middle. (From Franks S. Medical progress: polycystic ovary syndrome. N Engl J Med 1995;333:853-861.)

Prolactin and TSH should be obtained routinely to rule out mild androgen excess and anovulation that may be associated with hyperprolactinemia. If basal LH levels are used as a marker for PCOS, a significant number of patients slip through the cracks because they do not all manifest elevated LH levels or increased LH/FSH ratios. The NIH-sponsored consensus conference on diagnostic criteria for PCOS in 1990 recommended that LH and the LH/FSH ratio are not required for the diagnosis of PCOS.[249,251] The heterogeneity of LH values in PCOS may be caused by the pulsatile nature of LH secretion and negative effects of obesity on LH levels. Thus, an elevated LH/FSH ratio

TABLE 16–6 CRITERIA FOR THE DEFINITION OF POLYCYSTIC OVARY SYNDROME

NIH, 1990[249]
To include all of the following: 1. Hyperandrogenism and/or hyperandrogenemia 2. Oligo-ovulation 3. Exclusion of related disorders*
ESHRE/ASRM (Rotterdam), 2003[250]
To include two of the following, in addition to exclusion of related disorders*: 1. Oligo-ovulation or anovulation (e.g., amenorrhea or irregular uterine bleeding) 2. Clinical and/or biochemical signs of hyperandrogenism (e.g., hirsutism and/or elevated serum total or free testosterone) 3. Polycystic ovaries (by ultrasound)

*Including but not limited to 21-hydroxylase deficient nonclassic adrenal hyperplasia, thyroid dysfunction, hyperprolactinemia, neoplastic androgen secretion, drug-induced androgen excess, Cushing's syndrome, or glucocorticoid resistance.
ASRM, American Society for Reproductive Medicine; *ESHRE*, European Society for Human Reproduction and Embryology.
(Modified from Azziz R. Diagnosis of Polycystic Ovarian Syndrome: The Rotterdam Criteria Are Premature J Clin Endocrinol Metab 2006;91:781-785. Copyright © 2006 by The Endocrine Society.)

is supportive of the diagnosis of PCOS and may be useful in differentiating mild cases of non-obese PCOS without prominent androgen excess from hypothalamic anovulation. Failure to exhibit an elevated LH level, however, is of no diagnostic value. By definition, nonclassic adrenal hyperplasia is not manifest as congenital virilization of external genitalia. Hyperandrogenic symptoms most commonly appear peripubertally or postpubertally. The clinical evaluation and laboratory-based diagnosis of nonclassic adrenal hyperplasia was discussed above under the subheading Non-Neoplastic Adrenal Disorders and Androgen Excess. Please refer to Chapters 8 and 14 for details of the ACTH stimulation test. A screening test for Cushing's syndrome or glucocorticoid resistance should be performed as clinically indicated (see Chapters 8 and 14).

Serum DHEAS levels may be increased (up to 8 μg/mL) in about 50% of anovulatory women with PCOS. DHEAS originates almost exclusively from the adrenal.[252] The etiology of adrenal hyperactivity in PCOS is not known. Obtaining a DHEAS level routinely in a patient with PCOS is not recommended because it does not change the diagnosis or management. On the other hand, if an adrenal tumor is suspected, a DHEAS level should be obtained. DHEAS levels above 8 μg/mL may be associated with steroidogenically active adrenal tumors, and imaging is then indicated.

The Rotterdam 2003 criteria include the use of ultrasound as a diagnostic tool. The use of ultrasonography in the diagnosis of PCOS must be tempered by an awareness of the broad spectrum of women with ultrasonographic findings characteristic of polycystic ovaries. The typical polycystic-appearing ovary emerges in a nonspecific fashion when a state of anovulation persists for any length of time (see Fig. 16–31). Whether diagnosis is by ultrasonography or by the traditional clinical and biochemical criteria, a cross-section of all anovulatory women at any point in time reveals that approximately 75% have polycystic-appearing ovaries as determined by ultrasonography.[253] Because there are numerous causes of anovulation, there are also numerous reasons for polycystic ovaries. A similar clinical picture and ovarian condition can reflect any of the dysfunctional states discussed previously. In other words, the polycystic-appearing ovary is the result of a functional derangement but not a specific central or local defect.

Biochemical evidence of insulin resistance or glucose intolerance is also not necessary for the diagnosis of PCOS. Glucose intolerance should nonetheless be investigated. Therefore, plasma glucose levels should be measured after a 75-g glucose load as a screen for glucose intolerance.

Women with PCOS commonly present with irregular uterine bleeding in the form of infrequent periods (oligomenorrhea) or amenorrhea. It is not necessary to document anovulation by ultrasonography, progesterone levels, or otherwise, especially if menstrual cycles are irregular with periods of amenorrhea. To confirm the diagnosis of chronic anovulation and unopposed estrogen exposure, most clinicians perform a progestin challenge test after a negative urine pregnancy test. Because endometrium is exposed to estradiol chronically in PCOS, these women respond to a challenge with a progestin (e.g., medroxyprogesterone acetate 10 mg/day orally for 10 days) by uterine bleeding within a few days after the last pill of progestin. The reasons for lack of uterine bleeding after a progestin challenge include pregnancy, insufficient prior estrogen exposure of the endometrium, or an anatomic defect. If uterine bleeding does not follow progestin challenge, pregnancy should be ruled out again along with other causes of chronic anovulation as described in this chapter. An anatomic defect such as intrauterine adhesions may be ruled out with a hysterosalpingogram or hysteroscopy.

Finally, during the initial workup, it is advisable to obtain an endometrial biopsy specimen using a plastic minisuction cannula (e.g., Pipelle) in the clinician's office. If chronic anovulation persists, endometrial biopsies should be repeated periodically. Pregnancy should be ruled out by a urine or serum pregnancy test before each biopsy. Response to oral contraceptives or periodic progestin treatment with predictable withdrawal bleeding episodes is reassuring, and these patients with predictable bleeding patterns do not need endometrial sampling during these treatments. In untreated patients, the risk of endometrial hyperplasia and malignancy is significantly increased even in young women with PCOS because of unopposed estrogen exposure.

Gonadotropin Production in Polycystic Ovary Syndrome

Women with PCOS have higher mean concentrations of LH but low or low-normal levels of FSH compared with levels found in normal women in the early follicular phase.[254] The elevated LH levels are partly due to increased sensitivity of the pituitary to GnRH stimulation manifest by increases in LH pulse frequency and, in particular, LH pulse amplitude.[255-257] Interestingly, an increased level of LH bioactivity accompanies high levels of LH in women with PCOS.[256]

The elevated LH levels in PCOS are presumed to be primarily due to accelerated GnRH-LH pulsatile activity.[257] Central opioid tone appears to be suppressed because the pattern of LH secretion does not change in response to naloxone.[258] Indeed, the enhanced pulsatile secretion of GnRH has been attributed to a reduction in hypothalamic opioid inhibition caused by the chronic absence of progesterone.[181] An increase in amplitude and frequency of LH secretion also correlates with the steady-state levels of circulating estrogen.

In obese women with PCOS, LH levels are not increased. The increase in LH pulse frequency is characteristic of the anovulatory state regardless of the body fat content.[259] LH pulse amplitude, however, is comparatively normal in overweight women with PCOS, whereas it is increased in non-obese women with

PCOS.[260] The overall LH reduction in obese women with PCOS may also be due to factors other than changes in LH pulse amplitude.[261] It should be noted again that a low LH value does not rule out the diagnosis of PCOS, whereas a high LH/FSH ratio is supportive of this diagnosis in an anovulatory woman.

Insulin has also been implicated as a potential regulator of LH secretion in PCOS. Insulin enhances the transcription of LHβ gene.[262,263] On the other hand, increased LH secretion in women with PCOS as well as in normal women was unaltered by prolonged insulin infusion.[264] Moreover, LH levels, LH pulse frequency and amplitude, as well as gonadotropin responses to GnRH were not influenced by pioglitazone, either with or without insulin infusion.[264] Thus, in vivo human studies do not support that insulin resistance or hyperinsulinemia is responsible for abnormal gonadotropin release.

Steroid Production in Polycystic Ovary Syndrome

Ovulatory cycles are characterized by cyclic fluctuating hormone levels that regulate ovulation and menses (see Fig. 16–1A). Anovulation in women with PCOS, on the other hand, is associated with steady-state levels of gonadotropins and ovarian steroids. In patients with persistent anovulation, the average daily production of estrogen and androgens is both increased and dependent on LH stimulation (Fig. 16–32).[265] This is reflected in higher circulating levels of testosterone, androstenedione, DHEA, DHEAS, 17-hydroxyprogesterone, and estrone.[266] Testosterone, androstenedione, and DHEA are secreted directly by the ovary, whereas DHEAS, elevated in about 50% of anovulatory women with PCOS, is almost exclusively an adrenal contribution.[252] Circulating levels of androstenedione, secreted by polycystic ovaries, are particularly high (see Fig. 16–32).

Estrone arises primarily from peripheral aromatization of androstenedione and, in part, from ovarian secretion (Fig. 16–33).[266] Estrone itself is not a potent estrogen but can be viewed as a precursor that must be converted to estradiol to exert full estrogenic action. The presence of a number of 17β-HSD isoenzymes with overlapping activities that catalyze the conversion of estrone to estradiol in peripheral (extraovarian) tissues is, in part, responsible for maintaining estradiol production in women with PCOS.[133,266] Increased androstenedione leads to a detectable increase in circulating levels of estradiol in women with PCOS compared with estradiol levels measured during the first few days of an ovulatory cycle. This occurs through aromatase and 17β-HSD activities in extraovarian tissues such as skin and subcutaneous adipose tissue. Also, local conversion of estrone to estradiol is an important physiologic process for certain estrogen target tissues such as disease-free breast and genital skin. Finally, local conversion can also promote the growth of pathologic estrogen-dependent tissues such as breast cancer and endometriosis (see Fig. 16–33).[133,267-269]

Overall, androstenedione of ovarian origin is the most strikingly elevated steroid in PCOS. Androstenedione is not biologically active but serves as a dual precursor for both androgen (testosterone that is further converted to the biologically far stronger androgen DHT) and estrogen (estrone that is further converted to biologically active estradiol in target tissues) (see Fig. 16–33).[124] Estradiol is an extremely potent steroid. Biologically effective circulating levels of estradiol are measured using units of pg/mL or pmol/L, whereas biologically effective levels of testosterone are measured in units of ng/mL or nmol/L and

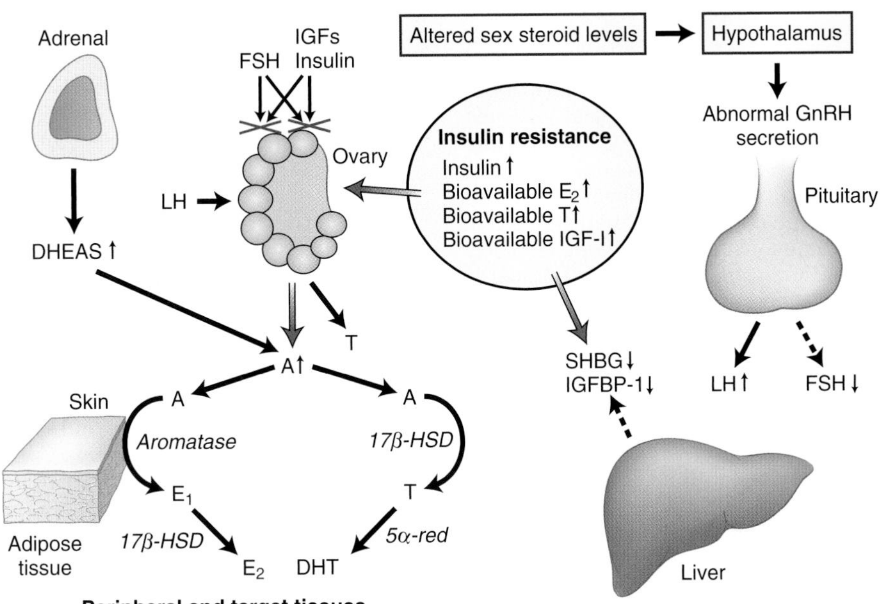

Figure 16–32 ▪ Pathologic mechanisms in polycystic ovary syndrome (PCOS). A deficient in vivo response of the ovarian follicle to physiologic quantities of follicle-stimulating hormone (FSH), possibly because of an impaired interaction between signaling pathways associated with FSH and insulin-like growth factors (IGFs) or insulin, may be an important defect in PCOS. This ovarian defect may be the key event responsible for anovulation in PCOS. Insulin resistance associated with increased circulating and tissue levels of insulin and bioavailable estradiol (E2), testosterone (T), and IGF-I gives rise to abnormal hormone production in a number of tissues. Oversecretion of luteinizing hormone (LH) and decreased output of FSH by the pituitary, decreased production of sex hormone–binding globulin (SHBG) and IGF-binding protein 1 (IGFBP-1) in the liver, increased adrenal secretion of dehydroepiandrosterone sulfate (DHEAS), and increased ovarian secretion of androstenedione (A) all contribute to the vicious circle that maintains anovulation and androgen excess in PCOS. Excessive amounts of E2 and T arise primarily from the conversion of A in peripheral and target tissues. *17β-HSD,* 17β-hydroxysteroid dehydrogenase; *5α-red,* 5α-reductase.

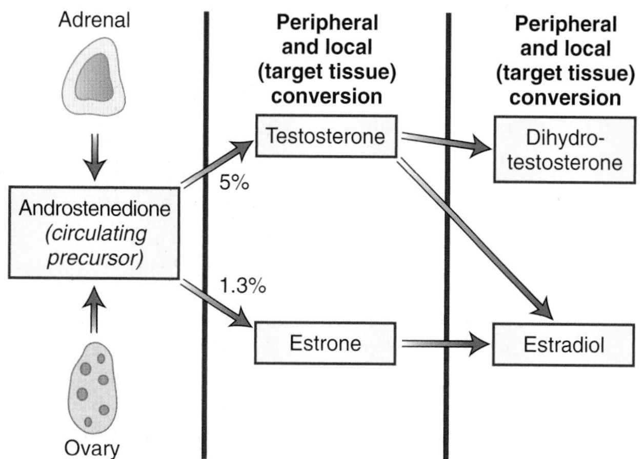

Figure 16–33 ▪ Extraovarian conversion of androstenedione to androgen and estrogen. Androstenedione of adrenal or ovarian origin, or both, acts as a dual precursor for androgen and estrogen. Five percent of circulating androstenedione is converted to circulating testosterone, whereas 1.3% of circulating androstenedione is converted to circulating estrone in peripheral tissues. Testosterone and estrone are further converted to biologically potent steroids, dihydrotestosterone and estradiol, in peripheral and target tissues. Biologically active amounts of estradiol in serum are measured in pg/mL (pmol/L), whereas biologically active levels of testosterone in serum are measured in ng/mL (nmol/L). Thus, 1.3% conversion of normal quantities of androstenedione to estrone may have a critical biologic impact in settings such as postmenopausal endometrial or breast cancer. Furthermore, significant androgen excess is observed in conditions with abnormally increased androstenedione formation (e.g., polycystic ovary syndrome).

circulate at 10 to 100 times the physiologic levels of estradiol. Thus, even small rates of conversion of androstenedione to estrone may have a significant biologic impact, whereas markedly elevated production of androstenedione is required to produce significant amounts of testosterone and manifestations of androgen excess (see Fig. 16–33). Because such elevated production of androstenedione does occur in PCOS, extraovarian production of testosterone is biologically significant in this disease. In contrast, in postmenopausal women, who have much lower levels of androstenedione, extraovarian production of testosterone is less important. On the other hand, relatively small quantities of estrone (and estradiol) produced primarily by peripheral aromatization of androstenedione have a biologic impact in men and postmenopausal women.[124]

Production of Sex Hormone–Binding Globulin in Polycystic Ovary Syndrome

SHBG binds both testosterone and estradiol and thus decreases the biologic activities of these critical steroids. In PCOS, there is an increase in the net production of androgen and estrogen. Increased estrogenic and androgenic effects in PCOS, however, are also due to a decrease in SHBG concentration giving rise to increased free or biologically active quantities of both estradiol and testosterone (see Fig. 16–32). The levels of SHBG are controlled by a balance of hormonal influences on its synthesis in the liver. Testosterone and insulin inhibit, whereas estrogen and T_4 stimulate, SHBG formation.[270] In anovulatory women with PCOS, circulating levels of SHBG are reduced approximately 50%; this may be a hepatic response to increased circulating levels of testosterone and insulin (see Fig. 16–33).[270] Circulating free estradiol and testosterone levels are increased because of the significant decrease in SHBG in patients with PCOS.

Thus, three mechanisms contribute to the presence of increased quantities of biologically available estradiol in PCOS: (1) increased production of estradiol from estrone in peripheral (extraovarian) tissues giving rise to increased levels of circulating estradiol, (2) increased biologically available circulating estradiol because of decreased SHBG, and (3) local conversion of estrone to estradiol at target tissues.[268] The last local mechanism is likely to be physiologically significant in estrogen targets such as the breast that proliferates in response to estrogen and in the central nervous system, which produces GnRH and gonadotropins under feedback regulation by estrogen (see Fig. 16–32).

In addition to giving rise to increased biologically available estradiol, decreased serum SHBG causes elevations in biologically available free testosterone levels. In turn, testosterone decreases serum SHBG levels, giving rise to a vicious feedback circle favoring low SHBG and high bioavailable testosterone levels (see Fig. 16–32). Insulin directly decreases serum SHBG concentrations in women with PCOS independent of any action of sex steroids.[270] Thus, insulin increases free testosterone in PCOS by two separate mechanisms: (1) by increasing ovarian secretion of testosterone precursors (e.g., androstenedione) and (2) by suppressing SHBG.[270]

Follicular Fate in Polycystic Ovary Syndrome

Under the influence of relatively low but constant levels of FSH, follicular growth is continuously stimulated, but not to the point of full maturation and ovulation.[271] Even though full growth potential is not realized, the follicular life span may extend several months in the form of multiple follicular cysts. Most of these follicles in polycystic ovaries are 2 to 10 mm in diameter, whereas some can be as large as 15 mm. Hyperplastic theca cells, often luteinized in response to the high LH levels, surround these follicles (see Fig. 16–29). The accumulation of follicles arrested at various stages of development allows increased and relatively constant production of steroids in response to steady-state levels of gonadotropins.

These follicles are also subject to atresia and are replaced by new follicles of similar limited growth potential. A steady-state of stromal cell turnover contributes to the stromal compartment of the ovary, and it is sustained by tissue derived from follicular atresia. A degenerating granulosa compartment, leaving the theca cells to contribute to the stromal compartment of the ovary, accompanies atresia (see Fig. 16–29). This functioning stromal tissue secretes significant amounts of androstenedione under the influence of increased LH. Androstenedione, by the mechanisms discussed above, leads to increases in free testosterone and free estradiol levels and decreases in SHBG (see Fig. 16–33). From the point of view of steroidogenesis and steroid action, the PCOS is the result of a complex vicious circle that includes a number of positive and negative feedback mechanisms (see Fig. 16–32).

Figure 16-32 depicts a summary of the currently postulated mechanisms underlying the PCOS. Because FSH and insulin/IGFs can synergize, it was postulated that this synergy does not occur in the presence of insulin resistance and might lead to relative resistance of the ovarian follicle to FSH. In vitro studies, however, do not support this view. Cultured granulosa cells obtained from the small follicles of polycystic ovaries produce negligible amounts of estradiol but show a dramatic increase in estrogen production when FSH or IGF-I is added to the culture medium. Moreover, when FSH and IGF-I were added together in vitro, they synergized to increase estrogen biosynthesis in granulosa cells from polycystic ovaries.[272]

Induction of ovulation in PCOS is achieved by increasing FSH levels that are hypothesized to overcome this postulated in vivo block to FSH at the granulosa cell level. Two currently popular treatments, oral clomiphene citrate and injectable recombinant

FSH, aim to provide increased levels of endogenous or exogenous FSH that may lead to ovulation at various doses. Some PCOS patients may require large doses of clomiphene citrate or FSH to achieve ovulation. Paradoxically, the polycystic ovary may overreact to pharmacologic levels of FSH by the recruitment of a large number of developing follicles at once, occasionally giving rise to the ovarian hyperstimulation syndrome (see below for the description and treatment of ovarian hyperstimulation syndrome).[273] The therapeutic window between ovarian nonresponsiveness and hyperreactivity is usually narrow. Thus, there are significant gaps of knowledge that do not permit reconciliation of clinical postulates with in vitro and in vivo findings related to the pathophysiology of PCOS.

Ovarian Hyperthecosis

Ovarian hyperthecosis is a severe variant of PCOS. The term refers to significantly increased stromal tissue with luteinized theca-like cells scattered throughout large sheets of fibroblast-like cells. Both clinical and histologic findings represent an exaggerated version of PCOS.[274] This diagnosis can be made on clinical grounds; an ovarian biopsy is not necessary except to rule out an ovarian tumor.

Increased androgen production leads to the clinical picture of more intense androgenization. The higher testosterone levels may also lower LH levels by blocking estrogen action at the hypothalamic-pituitary level.[261] Hyperthecosis seems to be an exaggerated version of the same process that gives rise to chronic ovulation in PCOS. A correlation exists between the severity of hyperthecosis and the degree of insulin resistance.[261] And in turn, because insulin and IGF-I stimulate proliferation of thecal interstitial cells, hyperinsulinemia may be an important pathophysiologic factor in the etiology of hyperthecosis.

It is not uncommon to encounter markedly high levels of testosterone, even above 2 ng/mL, in ovarian hyperthecosis. Virilization is common. These patients usually do not ovulate in response to clomiphene or recombinant FSH. It is usually difficult to suppress testosterone production even using a GnRH agonist. Bilateral oophorectomy should be used as the last resort but, unfortunately, may be necessary to control testosterone production in some of these patients.

Genetics of Polycystic Ovary Syndrome

The strong trend of PCOS to aggregate in families is suggestive of an underlying genetic basis.[275,276] It was previously emphasized that PCOS is of a multifactorial nature and that a similar pathology emerges from diverse mechanisms. These features are strongly suggestive of a polygenic pattern of inheritance. Efforts are ongoing to understand the genetic basis of PCOS. At least one group of patients with this condition has been described who inherited the disorder by means of X-linked dominant transmission. There was a twofold higher incidence of hirsutism and oligomenorrhea with paternal transmission but with marked variability of phenotypic expression. On the other hand, studies of large families were suggestive of inheritance in an autosomal dominant fashion, with premature balding as the phenotype in males.[277,278] In addition, the strong link between hyperinsulinemia and hyperandrogenism suggests that the stimulatory effect of insulin on ovarian androgen production is influenced by a genetic predisposition. In fact, women with hyperandrogenism, anovulation, and polycystic ovaries have a higher incidence of female relatives with hyperinsulinemia and male relatives with baldness.[279] Finally, familial aggregation of increased serum testosterone levels in PCOS suggests that androgen excess per se is a genetic trait. Genetic linkage studies are under way to identify individual gene defects that may be responsible for PCOS.[242,280,281]

Insulin Resistance and Polycystic Ovary Syndrome

Insulin resistance is a major factor in the pathogenesis of non-insulin-dependent diabetes mellitus (NIDDM). The term *insulin resistance* can be defined as impaired whole-body insulin-mediated glucose disposal, as determined using techniques such as the hyperinsulinemic glucose clamp technique.[146] Insulin resistance is defined clinically as the inability of a known quantity of exogenous or endogenous insulin to increase glucose uptake and utilization in an individual as much as it does in a normal population. Insulin resistance is frequently observed in both lean and obese women with PCOS. More severe degrees of insulin resistance or impaired glucose tolerance, however, are more common in obese women with PCOS.[146]

The association between a disorder of carbohydrate metabolism and androgen excess was first described in 1921 by Archard and Thiers and was called the "diabetes of bearded women." Since then, the association between PCOS and insulin resistance or impaired glucose tolerance has been well recognized.[146] This clinical association of insulin resistance and anovulatory hyperandrogenism is commonly found throughout the world and among different ethnic groups.[282] In addition, androgen excess and insulin resistance are often associated with acanthosis nigricans. Acanthosis nigricans is a gray-brown velvety discoloration and increased thickness of the skin, usually at the neck, groin, axillae, and under the breasts, and is a marker for insulin resistance (see Fig. 16–30). Hyperkeratosis and papillomatosis are the histologic characteristics of acanthosis nigricans. The presence of acanthosis nigricans in hyperandrogenic women is dependent on the presence and severity of hyperinsulinemia and insulin resistance.[283] The mechanism responsible for the development of acanthosis nigricans is uncertain. This abnormal growth response of the skin may be mediated through receptors for various growth factors, including those for insulin and IGF-I. Acanthosis nigricans is not specific for insulin resistance because it can be observed in the absence of insulin resistance or androgen excess.

Insulin resistance is characterized by an impaired glucose response to a specific amount of insulin. In many of these patients, normal glucose levels are maintained at the expense of increased circulating insulin to overcome the underlying defect. More severe forms of insulin resistance in PCOS range from impaired glucose tolerance to frank NIDDM. Resistance to insulin-stimulated glucose uptake is a relatively common phenomenon in the general population, sometimes referred to as *syndrome X* or *metabolic syndrome*. The fundamental abnormality leading to the manifestations that make up the metabolic syndrome is resistance to insulin-mediated glucose uptake in muscle and increased lipolysis giving rise to elevated circulating free fatty acid levels.[284] These individuals also have dyslipidemia, hypertension, and increased risk of developing cardiovascular disease. Not surprisingly, the incidences of dyslipidemia and cardiovascular risk are also increased significantly in women with PCOS.[285,286] The incidence of hypertension increases significantly after the menopause in women with a history of PCOS.[146] Thus, there is a significant clinical and pathologic overlap between the metabolic syndrome and PCOS.[287]

The clinical presentation of patients with insulin resistance depends on the ability of the pancreas to compensate for the target tissue resistance to insulin. During the first stages of the development of this condition, compensation is effective, and the only metabolic abnormality is hyperinsulinemia. In many patients, the beta cells of the pancreas eventually fail to meet the challenge, and declining insulin levels lead to impaired glucose tolerance and eventually frank diabetes mellitus. In fact, beta cell dysfunction is demonstrable in women with PCOS before the onset of glucose intolerance.[288]

Studies of well-characterized causes of hyperinsulinemia and androgen excess have illuminated various mechanisms of insulin resistance. Factors such as a decrease in insulin binding related to autoantibodies to insulin receptors, postreceptor defects, and a decrease in insulin receptor sites in target tissues are all involved in insulin resistance.[289] These rare syndromes, however, are found in an extremely small portion of women with anovulation, androgen excess, and insulin resistance, leaving the majority of PCOS patients without any demonstrable abnormalities in the number or quality of receptors or antibody formation. The exact nature of insulin resistance in the great majority of women with PCOS is not well understood.

In order to understand the molecular defect underlying insulin resistance in PCOS, Dunaif and colleagues[146] studied the differences between skin fibroblasts from women with and without PCOS with respect to insulin-dependent signal transduction. The fibroblasts of women with PCOS showed no change in insulin binding or receptor affinity. In half of the women with PCOS, however, a postreceptor defect was observed.[146] This defect is characterized by increased basal insulin receptor serine phosphorylation and a decrease in insulin-dependent tyrosine phosphorylation of the insulin receptor.[146] These abnormal patterns of phosphorylation of specific residues of the insulin receptor might represent a molecular mechanism responsible for the insulin resistance, anovulation, and androgen excess of PCOS.[146] The cause of this abnormal phosphorylation pattern and consequences for insulin action are important topics for future study.

Within the context of a unified hypothesis, insulin resistance seems to be a critical mechanism that explains the majority of the defects observed in PCOS (see Fig. 16–32). Insulin resistance is associated with the abnormal responses of the ovarian follicle to FSH, which leads to anovulation and androgen secretion. This results in noncyclic formation of estrogen from androgens in peripheral tissues. Estradiol together with increased androgen gives rise to abnormal gonadotropin secretion. This creates an anovulatory state favoring continuous formation of LH, steroid precursors, androgen and estrogen (see Fig. 16–32).

Role of Obesity in Insulin Resistance and Anovulation

Increased waist-to-hip ratio compounded by significantly increased body mass index is called *android obesity* because this type of adipose tissue distribution is observed more commonly in men. Overweight women with anovulatory androgen excess commonly have this particular body fat distribution.[290] Android obesity is the result of fat deposited in the abdominal wall and visceral mesenteric locations. This fat is more sensitive to catecholamines, less sensitive to insulin, and more active metabolically. Android obesity is associated with insulin resistance, glucose intolerance, diabetes mellitus, and an increase in androgen production rate resulting in decreased levels of SHBG and increased levels of free testosterone and estradiol.[290] Not surprisingly, android obesity is associated significantly with cardiovascular risk factors, including hypertension and dyslipidemia. It is also important to emphasize that android obesity has been tied to a notable increase in the risk of breast cancer, with a poor prognosis.[291,292] No direct association, however, has been reported between PCOS and breast cancer risk.[293]

Although the combination of insulin resistance and androgen excess is often observed in obese women overall, women with android-type obesity appear to be at a significantly higher risk for insulin resistance and androgen excess. However, insulin resistance and androgen excess are not confined to obese anovulatory women but also occur in non-obese anovulatory women.[259] Although obesity by itself causes insulin resistance, the combination of insulin resistance and androgen excess is a specific feature of PCOS. Not surprisingly, the combination of obesity and PCOS is associated with more severe degrees of insulin resistance than those found in non-obese women with PCOS.[259,294] Android-type obesity, in contrast to general obesity, is a much more specific risk factor for PCOS.

Diagnosis of Insulin Resistance

In everyday clinical practice, the criteria for diagnosing insulin resistance in an individual patient has not been standardized and present extremely complex issues. First, a quarter of the normal population has fasting and glucose-stimulated insulin levels that overlap those of insulin-resistant individuals[146] because of great variability of insulin sensitivity in normal subjects. Second, clinically available measures of insulin action, such as fasting or glucose-stimulated insulin levels, do not correlate well with more detailed measurements of insulin sensitivity in research settings.

In view of these constraints, it is reasonable to consider all women with PCOS at risk for insulin resistance and the associated abnormalities of the insulin resistance syndrome (metabolic syndrome)—dyslipidemia, hypertension, and cardiovascular disease.[287] A lipid profile should be obtained in all cases of PCOS. Especially obese women with PCOS should have fasting glucose levels and glucose levels 2 hours after a 75-g glucose load as a screen for glucose intolerance. The clinician should encourage the patient to take every possible measure (e.g., weight reduction and exercise) to reduce insulin resistance.

Use of Antidiabetic Drugs to Treat Anovulation and Androgen Excess

A logical approach to the management of PCOS includes the use of medications that improve insulin sensitivity in target tissues, thus achieving reductions in insulin secretion and stability of glucose tolerance. The antidiabetic medications metformin (a biguanide) and the thiazolidinediones, pioglitazone and rosiglitazone, have been used to reduce insulin resistance. Although metformin appears to influence ovarian steroidogenesis directly, this effect does not appear to be primarily responsible for the attenuation of ovarian androgen production in women with PCOS. Rather, metformin inhibits the output of hepatic glucose, necessitating a lower insulin concentration and thereby probably reducing the androgen production by theca cells.[295]

Metformin at a dose of 500 mg three times a day reduced hyperinsulinemia, basal and stimulated LH levels, and free testosterone concentrations in overweight women with PCOS.[296,297] A significant number of these anovulatory women ovulated and achieved pregnancy.[298] Among published studies of metformin in the PCOS, subject characteristics and control measures for effects of weight change, dose of metformin, and outcome vary widely. A meta-analysis of 13 studies in which metformin was administered to 543 participants reported that patients taking metformin had an odds ratio for ovulation of 3.88 (95% CI, 2.25 to 6.69) as compared with placebo and an odds ratio for ovulation of 4.41 (95% CI, 2.37 to 8.22) for metformin plus clomiphene as compared with clomiphene alone.[299] Metformin also improved fasting insulin levels, blood pressure, and levels of LDL cholesterol. These effects were judged to be independent of any changes in weight that were associated with metformin, but controversy persists as to whether the beneficial effects of metformin are entirely independent of the weight loss that is typically seen early in the course of therapy this time.[295,300]

The thiazolidinediones are pharmacologic ligands for the nuclear receptor peroxisome proliferator-activated receptor γ (PPARγ) and improve the action of insulin in the liver, skeletal muscle, and adipose tissue and have only a modest effect on hepatic glucose output. As with metformin, the thiazolidinediones are reported to affect ovarian steroid synthesis directly, although most evidence indicates that the reduction in insulin levels is responsible for decreased concentrations of circulating androgen.[295]

Women with PCOS who took troglitazone had consistent improvements in insulin resistance, hyperandrogenemia, and glucose tolerance.[301,302] In addition, troglitazone treatment was associated with relative improvement in pancreatic cell function.[301,302] These findings led to a double-blind, randomized, placebo-controlled study of troglitazone in PCOS.[303] Ovulation was significantly greater for women who received troglitazone than for those who received placebo; free testosterone levels decreased, and levels of SHBG increased in a dose-dependent fashion. Nearly all glycemic measures showed dose-related decreases with troglitazone treatment. Although troglitazone is no longer available because of its hepatotoxicity, subsequent studies using the more recently available compounds, rosiglitazone and pioglitazone, have had similar results.[304-306] Because of concern about using thiazolidinediones in pregnancy, the drugs have been less readily adopted for routine treatment of PCOS. The success of the strategy of reversing insulin resistance as a way to correct the critical abnormalities in PCOS argues for this defect as central to the pathogenesis of the disorder.

Management of Long-Term Deleterious Effects of Polycystic Ovary Syndrome

The long-term consequences of PCOS include irregular uterine bleeding, anovulatory infertility, androgen excess (hirsutism or virilization or both), chronically elevated free estrogen associated with an increased risk of endometrial cancer, and insulin resistance associated with an increased risk of cardiovascular disease and diabetes mellitus. Therefore, treatment must encompass the following: aid in achieving a healthy lifestyle and normal body weight, protection of the endometrium from unopposed estrogen effects, and a reduction in testosterone levels.

If the patient desires pregnancy, she is a candidate for the medical induction of ovulation. When pregnancy is achieved, patients with polycystic ovaries appear to have an increased risk of spontaneous miscarriage.[307] This increased risk may be related to elevated levels of LH that may produce an adverse environment for the oocyte and the endometrium. Therefore, LH levels should be suppressed with oral contraceptives before inducing ovulation. This suppression can be achieved in most patients with PCOS by the use of an oral contraceptive for 4 to 6 weeks before ovulation induction with clomiphene citrate or recombinant FSH.

If the patient does not wish to become pregnant, therapy is directed toward the interruption of unopposed effect of estrogen on the endometrium. Nonfluctuating levels of unopposed estradiol in the absence of progesterone cause irregular uterine bleeding, amenorrhea, and infertility and increase the risk of endometrial cancer. Anovulatory women with PCOS may develop endometrial cancer even in their early twenties.[308] Therefore, endometrial biopsy should be performed periodically in untreated women with PCOS regardless of age. Pregnancy should be ruled out before each endometrial biopsy. The uterine bleeding pattern should not influence the decision to perform an endometrial biopsy. The presence of amenorrhea does not rule out endometrial hyperplasia. The critical factor that determines the risk of endometrial neoplasia is the duration of anovulation and exposure to unopposed estradiol. Long-term treatment with a progestin or oral contraceptive significantly decreases the risk of endometrial cancer.

One of the simplest and most effective ways to administer a progestin in the long term is to use an oral contraceptive. Also, oral contraceptives provide two more benefits: reduction of androgen excess and contraception. Oral contraceptive pills reduce circulating androgen levels through suppression of circulating LH and stimulation of SHBG levels and have been shown to reduce hirsutism in hyperandrogenic patients.[151]

A concern regarding possible insulin-desensitizing effects of oral contraceptives has been raised.[146] Older oral contraceptives cause increased insulin resistance because of the high estrogen component.[309] Long-term follow-up studies, however, have failed to detect any increase in the incidence of diabetes mellitus in past or current users of high-dose pills.[310,311] In fact, more recent studies demonstrated that new oral contraceptives induced either no change or a significant decrease in insulin resistance in women with PCOS. The oral contraceptives that did not induce insulin resistance in women with PCOS contained an ethinyl estradiol dose of 30 μg or less and desogestrel, norgestimate, or gestodene as the progestin component.[312] Furthermore, past users of oral contraceptives have no increased cardiovascular risk.[313] Low-dose oral contraceptives have also been administered to women with gestational diabetes or insulin-dependent diabetes mellitus without an adverse impact.[314-316] Low-dose oral contraceptives have not increased the risk of retinopathy or nephropathy in diabetic patients, nor has there been any deterioration of lipid or biochemical markers.[314-316] It should be emphasized again that the major nongenetic contributing factor to hyperinsulinemia and insulin resistance in PCOS is obesity.[259,294] In summary, oral contraceptive treatment for anovulatory and hyperinsulinemic women with androgen excess does not increase cardiovascular risk.

For the patient who does not complain of hirsutism but is anovulatory and has irregular bleeding, treatment with a single progestin may be attempted as an alternative to oral contraceptives. Progestin therapy is directed toward interruption of the chronic exposure of endometrium to unopposed effects of estrogen. Medroxyprogesterone acetate may be administered intermittently (e.g., 10 mg daily for the first 10 days of every month) to ensure withdrawal bleeding and prevent endometrial hyperplasia. This treatment does not decrease androgen excess, nor does it provide contraception. Because new oral contraceptives (with an ethinyl estradiol content of 30 μg or less and a new progestin) suppress androgen excess of ovarian origin, provide contraception, protect the endometrium, and do not increase insulin resistance, a new low-dose oral contraceptive is the treatment of choice for nonsmokers with PCOS. An oral contraceptive together with the antiandrogen spironolactone, 100 mg/day, is the recommended starting treatment for a hirsute woman with PCOS. The dose of spironolactone can be increased in increments to suppress hair growth as previously described in this section.

Treatment with an oral contraceptive (plus or minus spironolactone) may not be effective in androgen suppression in severe cases of PCOS. In these patients resistant to oral contraceptives, suppression of the ovary with a GnRH agonist may be required. Because glucocorticoids increase insulin resistance, they should be used with caution in patients with hyperinsulinemia. Spironolactone does not affect insulin sensitivity in anovulatory women and can be used safely without causing adverse effects on carbohydrate or lipid metabolism.[317]

The clinician must counsel women with PCOS regarding their increased risk of future diabetes mellitus. The age of onset of non–insulin-dependent diabetes is significantly earlier in these women than in the general population.[241] Women with PCOS are more likely to experience gestational diabetes.[318] Long-term follow-up studies have shown a significantly increased risk for the development of frank diabetes mellitus in anovulatory patients with PCOS.[146] It is therefore important to monitor glucose tolerance with periodic glucose levels after fasting and after a 75-g glucose load.

Because insulin resistance contributes to the abnormal lipid profile and increased cardiovascular risk in women with PCOS, weight loss is a high priority for patients who are overweight.[319] Both insulin resistance and androgen excess can be reduced with a weight reduction of at least 5%.[320,321] Significant weight loss also resulted in ovulation and pregnancy in a number of patients with PCOS.[322] Therefore, long-term nutritional counseling and an emphasis on lifestyle changes are essential components of the long-term management of PCOS.

The place of insulin sensitizers, such as metformin and thiazolidinediones, in the long-term treatment of PCOS remains to be determined by data from future large clinical trials.[301,302,323] In long-term follow-up of women with PCOS, android obesity and hyperinsulinemia persisted during the postmenopausal years.[324] Thus, postmenopausal women who have previously been anovulatory, hyperandrogenic, and hyperinsulinemic are at risk for cardiovascular disease and diabetes mellitus. Preventive health care interventions that lower cardiovascular risk and other unfavorable consequences of PCOS are appropriate.[146]

The clinician should alert the patient with PCOS that up to half of first-degree relatives and sisters may be affected by PCOS or at least by androgen excess in the presence of regular menses.[243] These individuals may be at higher than average risk for cardiovascular disease and may benefit from preventive measures that reduce this risk.

Ovulation Induction in Polycystic Ovary Syndrome

Clomiphene Citrate

To induce ovulation in PCOS, FSH levels are increased through the use of, for example, clomiphene citrate or by injection of recombinant FSH. Presumably, pharmacologic levels of FSH overcome the ovarian defect responsible for anovulation in PCOS.

Clomiphene citrate is a nonsteroidal ovulation-inducing ER ligand with mixed agonistic-antagonistic properties.[325] Acting as an antiestrogen, clomiphene citrate is thought to displace endogenous estrogen from hypothalamic ERs, thereby removing the negative feedback effect exerted by endogenous estrogens. The resultant change in pulsatile GnRH release is thought to normalize the release of pituitary FSH and LH, followed by follicular recruitment and selection, assertion of dominance, and, ultimately, ovulation.[325]

Clomiphene citrate treatment can be started at any time in an amenorrheic and anovulatory patient as long as a pregnancy test is performed beforehand. Alternatively, uterine bleeding may be induced after a 21-day treatment with an oral contraceptive or 10-day treatment with medroxyprogesterone acetate (10 mg/day). Clomiphene citrate at 50 mg/day is started orally on day 3, 4, or 5 of the cycle and continued for 5 days. Over the past 20-some years, we have used a practical approach termed *triple-7* in order to monitor indicators of ovulation after the administration of clomiphene citrate.[325] The protocol is depicted in Figure 16-34. This approach is timed favorably to detect the preovulatory surge of serum estradiol 7 days after the last clomiphene citrate dose (arrow pointing up Figure 34) and a serum progesterone level 14 days after the last clomiphene citrate dose (arrow pointing down Figure 34) in order to document ovulation. A repeated office visit is scheduled 7 days after the progesterone determination, that is, 21 days after the last clomiphene citrate dose (see Fig. 16–34).[325] The patient should be encouraged to have intercourse every other day during the 10-day period following the last clomiphene citrate dose. Alternatively, measurement of urinary LH to detect an LH surge can be used to time intercourse. In this case, the couple should be instructed to have intercourse on the day of the LH surge.

If ovulation does not occur after the first course of therapy with clomiphene citrate at 50 mg/day, a second course of 100 mg

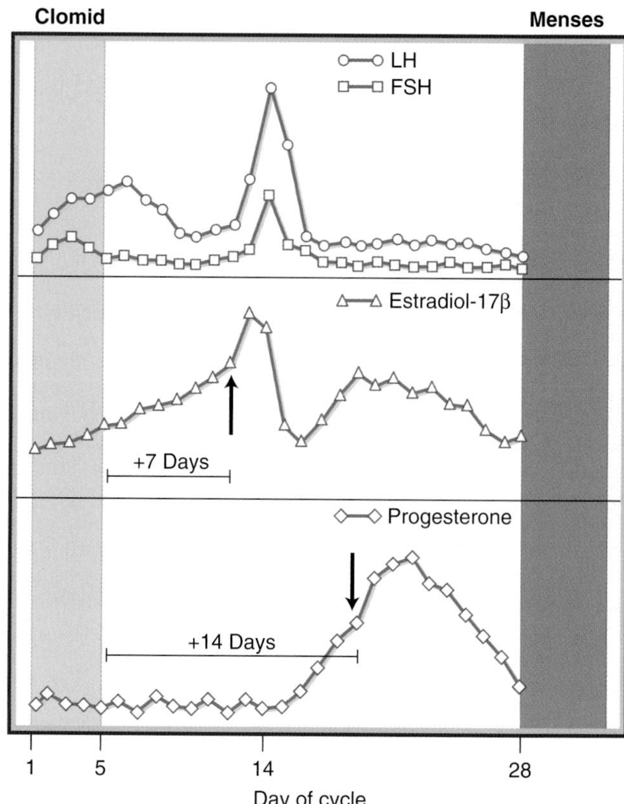

Figure 16–34 ■ Hormonal monitoring in clomiphene citrate–initiated ovulation: use of the triple-7 regimen. *Clomid,* clomiphere citrate. See text. (From Adashi EY. Clomiphene citrate-initiated ovulation: a clinical update. Semin Reprod Endocrinol 1986;4:255-276.)

daily for 5 days may be started. Lack of response at doses of 150 to 200 mg daily for 5 days should be an indication for a change of treatment. Most patients destined to conceive do so with the starting dose of clomiphene citrate (50 mg/day for 5 days). Most clomiphene citrate–initiated conceptions are likely to occur within the first six ovulatory cycles.[325] The incidence rate for multiple gestation in clomiphene citrate–induced pregnancies is 7.9%, of which 6.9% are twins.[325]

Aromatase Inhibitors

The aromatase inhibitors letrozole and anastrozole have been used as an experimental medication to induce ovulation.[326,327] The mechanism of action appears to be similar to that of clomiphene citrate. Oral administration of letrozole (2.5 mg/day) or anastrozole (1 mg/day) on days 3 to 7 after uterine bleeding is effective for ovulation induction in anovulatory infertility.[328] Ovulation induction by an aromatase inhibitor is presumed to be mediated by estrogen deficiency induced at the level of the hypothalamus.[118,326] Use of aromatase inhibitors may obviate the unfavorable effects on the endometrium frequently seen with the use of antiestrogens (e.g., clomiphene citrate) for ovulation induction. Clinical data regarding this experimental treatment are extremely scarce. There are few controlled studies, and the rest of the studies were pilot or preliminary comparisons.[328] Although worldwide experience with aromatase inhibitors for ovulation induction is increasing, definitive studies in the form of randomized controlled trials comparing clomiphene citrate with an aromatase inhibitor are lacking.[328]

Conventional-Dose Gonadotropin Therapy

For women who do not ovulate in response to clomiphene citrate, recombinant FSH is administered subcutaneously at a starting dose of two ampules (equivalent to 150 IU of FSH), starting on day 3 of spontaneous or progestin-induced uterine bleeding and increasing by 75 IU at 3- to 7-day intervals until serum estradiol concentrations begin to increase. The dose is then maintained until follicular rupture, which is induced by intramuscular administration of hCG (10,000 IU). Follicular growth is monitored by transvaginal ultrasonography and blood estradiol levels, which serve as biochemical markers for the granulosa cell mass in the growing follicle.[329] Three important complications of gonadotropin therapy in PCOS are significantly increased rates of multiple pregnancies, severe ovarian hyperstimulation syndrome, and spontaneous miscarriage.[329]

Ovarian hyperstimulation syndrome (OHSS) is a complication of ovarian stimulation. Milder forms are relatively common and are characterized by weight gain, abdominal discomfort, and enlarged ovaries. Home bed rest and oral intake of fluids are sufficient to manage this form. Severe OHSS occurs in 0.1% to 0.2% of stimulation attempts and is accompanied by severe ascites, pleural effusion, electrolyte imbalance, and hypovolemia with oliguria. The most dreaded complication is deep venous thrombosis and embolism. Its etiology is poorly understood. Large number of follicles, peak estradiol levels greater than 2000 pg/mL, and pregnancy are associated with a higher likelihood of OHSS. Its prevention includes withholding hCG injection and intrauterine insemination. Treatment of severe OHSS is hospitalization, maintenance of fluid and electrolyte balance, prophylaxis of thromboembolism by heparin, and drainage of severe ascites or pleural effusions. Frequently, supportive measures are sufficient to manage this self-limiting condition.

Low-Dose Gonadotropin Therapy

Conventional-dose gonadotropin therapy causes two important complications: (1) an alarming number of multiple pregnancies (range, 14% to 50% of treatment cycles) and (2) a significantly increased risk of severe ovarian hyperstimulation syndrome (range, 1.3% to 9.4% of treatment cycles).[329] Low-dose FSH regimens for induction of ovulation for women with PCOS have succeeded in reducing the rate of multiple pregnancies to as low as 6% in some series.[273] The low-dose regimen also practically eliminated the complication of severe ovarian hyperstimulation syndrome.[273] This has been achieved by reaching, but not exceeding, the threshold level of FSH, starting with a daily dose of 75 IU for more than 10 days and using small incremental dose increases when necessary. This regimen induces the development of a single follicle in 70% of cycles. Conception rates are comparable to those achieved with conventional therapy. The miscarriage rate remains somewhat higher than that after spontaneous conceptions (20% to 25%). The treatment time for the low-dose regimen is significantly longer than that required for conventional gonadotropin treatment. Recombinant FSH for a low-dose regimen, rather than urinary gonadotropins, shortens the treatment time.[330]

Premature Ovarian Failure

Premature ovarian failure, which is defined as early depletion of ovarian follicles before the age of 40, is a state of hypergonadotropic hypogonadism. These patients present with amenorrhea or oligomenorrhea. They go through a normal puberty and a variable period of cyclic menses followed by oligomenorrhea and amenorrhea. Therefore, premature ovarian failure should always be included in the differential diagnosis of chronic anovulation. History and physical examination may reveal menstrual irregularity or secondary amenorrhea accompanied by symptoms and signs of estrogen deficiency, such as hot flashes and urogenital atrophy. Elevated FSH levels (above the 95% confidence limits of the midcycle gonadotropin peak of the normal menstrual cycle, i.e., >40 IU/L) on at least two occasions confirm the diagnosis.[331]

On average, the menopause occurs at the age of 50 years, with 1% of women continuing to menstruate beyond the age of 60 years and another 1% whose menopause occurs before 40 years. Thus, premature menopause or ovarian failure has been arbitrarily defined as the cessation of menses before 40 years of age.[332] In most cases, the etiology of premature ovarian failure is not clear. The patient may be counseled that the disorder is probably a genetic one, causing ovarian follicles to disappear at a rate faster than normal. Specific sex chromosome anomalies may be identified in a subset of patients presenting with premature ovarian failure.[333] Among these, 45,X and 47,XXY are the most common, followed by mosaicism involving various combinations.[334]

The underlying ovarian defect may be manifest at varying ages, depending on the number of functional follicles left in the ovaries. The different symptoms may be regarded as phases in the process of perimenopausal change regardless of the actual age of the patient. If loss of follicles occurs rapidly before puberty, primary amenorrhea and lack of secondary sexual development ensue. The degree to which the adult phenotype develops and when the secondary amenorrhea actually occurs depend on whether follicle loss took place during or after puberty. In cases of primary amenorrhea associated with sexual infantilism, the ovarian remnants exist as streaks, and transvaginal ultrasonography usually cannot detect any ovaries.

Premature ovarian failure can be due to an autoimmune process, as this condition is frequently detected in association with autoimmune polyendocrine syndromes.[335] Other causes of premature failure can be related to the sudden destruction of the follicles through factors such as chemotherapy, radiation, or infections such as mumps oophoritis. The effect of radiation is dependent upon age and the x-ray dose.[336] Steroid levels begin to fall and gonadotropins rise within 2 weeks after radiation of the ovaries. Young women exposed to radiation are less likely to have permanent ovarian failure because of the higher number of oocytes present at younger ages. When the radiation field excludes the pelvis or the ovaries are transposed out of the pelvis by laparoscopic surgery before radiation, there is no risk of premature ovarian failure.[337] Most chemotherapeutic agents used for the eradication of malignancies are toxic to the ovaries and cause ovarian failure.[338] Resumption of menses and pregnancy have been reported after radiotherapy or chemotherapy.[339] By the same token, premature ovarian failure may occur years after chemotherapy or radiotherapy.[332]

Finally, gene defects may give rise to ovarian failure. These include mutations of FSH and LH receptors, fragile X premutations, and galactosemia.[340] Mutations of galactose-1-phosphate uridyltransferase, for example, can lead to ovarian failure because of the accumulation of galactose-1-phosphate at toxic levels.[5]

Diagnosis and Management of Premature Ovarian Failure

Premature ovarian failure should be suspected in a woman who is younger than 40 years who presents with amenorrhea, oligomenorrhea, or another form of menstrual irregularity. Menopausal serum FSH levels (40 IU/L) on at least two occasions are sufficient for the diagnosis of premature ovarian failure. Thus, these young women can be diagnosed with ovarian failure and infertility if gonadotropin levels are repeatedly elevated. There are, however, a number of case reports of pregnancies in affected women occurring during hormone replacement therapy.[341,342] A randomized trial of hormone replacement in this setting showed that folliculogenesis occurred often but was less frequently followed by ovulation and even less frequently by pregnancy (up to 14%); estrogen therapy did not improve the rate of folliculogenesis, ovulation, or pregnancy.[331] Therefore, the clinician should inform patients diagnosed with premature ovarian failure that there is a small but significant likelihood of spontaneous pregnancy in the future. Women desirous of achieving pregnancy are still best served by assisted reproductive technology employing donor oocytes because the probability of spontaneous pregnancy is low. Use of donor oocytes followed by in vitro fertilization with the partner's sperm and intrauterine embryo transfer after synchronization of the recipient patient's endometrium with the donor's cycle using exogenous estrogen and progesterone are offered to the patient who wishes to carry a pregnancy in her uterus (see Fig. 16–25). This approach offers an excellent chance of pregnancy (>50% per donor oocyte–in vitro fertilization cycle).

Patients with premature ovarian failure are at increased risk for having an abnormal complement of chromosomes.[333] The risk of having an abnormal karyotype increases with decreasing age of onset of the ovarian failure. A chromosomal analysis is recommended for some of these patients because of increased risk of a gonadal tumor associated with the presence of a Y chromosome.[343] The arbitrarily chosen age group for chromosomal analysis includes women 30 years of age or younger because it is extraordinarily rare to encounter a gonadal tumor in patients with premature ovarian failure after the age of 30.[344]

The presence of mosaicism including a Y chromosome has been associated with a high incidence of gonadal tumors.[343] These malignant tumors arise from germ cells and include gonadoblastomas, dysgerminomas, yolk sac tumors, and choriocarcinoma. In particular, the presence of secondary virilization in these patients with karyotypic abnormalities and premature ovarian failure significantly increases the risk of a dysontogenetic gonadal tumor. The precise risk of a tumor in various subsets of these patients is not well known because a significant number of women carrying a Y chromosome do not have symptoms of virilization. The frequency of Y-chromosome material determined by polymerase chain reaction is high in Turner's syndrome (12.2%), but the occurrence of a gonadal tumor among these Y-positive patients seems to be as low as 7% to 10%.[345]

Premature ovarian failure may also occur as an isolated autoimmune disorder or in association with hypothyroidism, diabetes mellitus, hypoadrenalism, hypoparathyroidism, or systemic lupus erythematosus.[346] Therefore, the tests listed in Table 16–7 should be performed every few years because premature ovarian failure can be part of an autoimmune polyendocrine syndrome.[335] Thyroid and adrenal insufficiency and diabetes mellitus are the endocrine disorders most frequently associated with premature ovarian failure. It should be noted, however, that overall it is fairly rare to encounter any endocrine disorder associated with premature ovarian failure.[347]

Treatment of premature ovarian failure should be directed toward its specific cause, if this is possible. In most cases, however, it is not possible to identify a specific etiology if there are no karyotypic anomalies. If the patient desires pregnancy, she should be offered ovum donation and in vitro fertilization using her partner's sperm (see Fig. 16–25). If pregnancy is not desired, she should be treated with an oral contraceptive or with estrogen and progestin replacement. Estrogen therapy promotes and maintains secondary sexual characteristics and prevents premature osteoporosis.

TABLE 16–7 LABORATORY EVALUATION OF PREMATURE OVARIAN FAILURE

FSH (to establish the diagnosis of premature ovarian failure)
Karyotype (<30 yr of age or sexual infantilism)
Cortisol after ACTH stimulation, antiadrenal antibodies (adrenal insufficiency)
TSH, antithyroid antibodies (hypothyroidism)
Glucose (fasting and 2 hr after 75-g glucose load, diabetes mellitus)
Calcium and phosphorus (hypoparathyroidism)
Sedimentation rate, complete blood count with differential, antinuclear antibody, rheumatoid factor (autoimmune disease)
Pregnenolone (to evaluate 17-hydroxylase deficiency in sexually infantile women)

ACTH, Adrenocorticotropic hormone; *FSH*, follicle-stimulating hormone; *TSH*, thyroid-stimulating hormone.
FSH (to establish the diagnosis of premature ovarian failure)

DIFFERENTIAL DIAGNOSIS AND MANAGEMENT OF ANOVULATORY UTERINE BLEEDING

Acyclic production of estrogen during anovulatory cycles gives rise to irregular shedding of the endometrium. These bleeding manifestations of anovulatory cycles in the absence of uterine pathology or systemic illness are commonly referred to as *dysfunctional uterine bleeding*. Anovulatory uterine bleeding is the most common cause of chronic menstrual irregularities and is a diagnosis of exclusion. Pregnancy, uterine leiomyomas, endometrial polyps, and adenomyosis should be ruled out as anatomic causes of irregular uterine bleeding. Malignancies of the vagina, cervix, endometrium, myometrium, fallopian tubes, and ovaries should also be ruled out before a diagnosis of anovulatory uterine bleeding is made. Finally, coagulation abnormalities should be excluded.

Anovulatory uterine bleeding can be managed without surgical intervention by either restoring ovulation or mimicking the ovulatory hormonal profile by providing exogenous steroids. The rationale for using exogenous steroids is based on the knowledge of predictable responses of the endometrium to estrogen and progesterone. Physiologic responses of the endometrium to natural ovarian steroids have been uncovered by observing the gross and microscopic changes in the endometrium during thousands of normal ovulatory cycles in humans and other primates.[154,156,348] The pharmacologic application of exogenous estrogens and progestins in women with anovulatory bleeding aims to correct the production of local tissue factors, which mediate physiologic steroid action, and thus reverse the excessive and prolonged flow typical of anovulatory cycles.

Clinical management of irregular uterine bleeding with exogenous hormones is a time-honored method and is also of diagnostic value. Failure to control vaginal bleeding with hormonal therapy, despite appropriate application and utilization, makes the diagnosis of anovulatory uterine bleeding considerably less likely. In this case, attention is directed to an anatomic pathologic entity within the reproductive axis as the cause of abnormal bleeding.

Heavy but regular menstrual bleeding (hypermenorrhea) can be encountered in ovulatory women. It may be due to anatomic causes such as a leiomyoma impinging on the endometrial cavity or the diffuse and pathologic presence of benign endometrial glands in the myometrium (adenomyosis). In the absence of a specific pathologic cause, however, it is presumed that hypermenorrhea reflects subtle disturbances in the endometrial tissue mechanism. In essentially all cases, evaluation and treatment are identical to the approach detailed in this section.

Characteristics of Normal Menses

Normal menstruation takes place about 14 days after each ovulation episode as a consequence of postovulatory estrogen-progesterone withdrawal. The quantity and duration of bleeding are quite reproducible. This predictability leads many women to expect a certain characteristic flow pattern. Any slight deviations, such as plus or minus 1 day in duration or minor deviation from expected tampon utilization, are causes for major concern in the patient. Most women of reproductive age can predict the timing of their flows so accurately that even some instances of minor variability may require reassurance by the clinician. Although variability of menstrual cycles is a common feature during teenage years and the perimenopausal transition, the characteristics of menstrual bleeding do not undergo appreciable change between ages 20 and 40.[349]

For ovulatory women, the changes in the length of menstrual cycles over the period of reproductive age are predictable. Between menarche and age 20, the cycle length for most ovulatory women is relatively longer. Between 20 and 40, there is increased regularity as cycles shorten. In the 40s, cycles begin to lengthen again. The highest incidence of anovulatory cycles occurs before age 20 and after age 40.[350] In this age group, the average length of a cycle is between 25 and 28 days. Among ovulatory women, the frequency of a cycle less than 21 days long or a cycle greater than 35 days is extremely rare (less than 2%).[351] Overall, most women have cycles that last from 24 to 35 days (Fig. 16–35).[349] Between ages 40 and 50, menstrual cycle length increases and anovulation becomes more prevalent.[352]

The average postovulatory bleeding lasts from 4 to 6 days. The normal volume of menstrual blood loss is 30 mL. More than 80 mL is considered abnormal. Most of the blood loss occurs during the first 3 days of a period, so excessive flow may exist without prolongation of flow.[353,354]

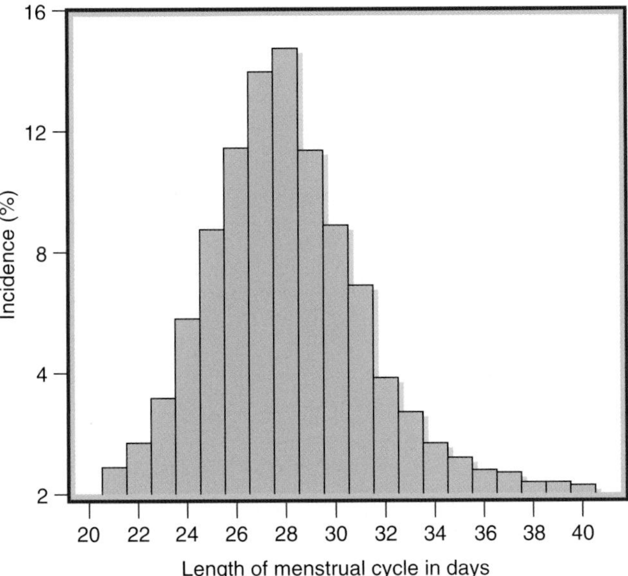

Figure 16–35 ▪ Variation of the duration of the menstrual cycle in women with regular cycles. (From Cunningham FG, MacDonald PC, Gant NF, et al. The endometrium and decidua: menstruation and pregnancy. In Williams Obstetrics, 19th ed. Stamford, CT: Appleton & Lange, 1993:81-109.)

During an ovulatory cycle, the duration from the ovulation to menses is relatively constant and averages 14 days (see Fig. 16–1A). Greater variability in the length of the proliferative phase, however, produces a distribution in the duration of a menstrual cycle. Menstrual bleeding more often than every 24 days or less often than every 35 days requires evaluation.[349,352] Flow that lasts 7 or more days also requires evaluation. A flow that totals more than 80 mL per month usually leads to anemia and should be treated.[355] In clinical practice, however, it is quite difficult to quantify menstrual flow because evaluation and treatment are based solely on the patient's perceptions regarding the duration, amount, and timing of her menstrual bleeding. Despite this difficulty in quantifying menstrual blood loss, the clinician should evaluate the cause of excessive uterine bleeding. Anemia should be ruled out by a complete blood count.[356] A low hemoglobin value accompanied by microcytic and hypochromic red blood cells suggests excessive blood loss during menses. These patients should be provided with iron supplementation. The likely presence of coagulation defects, uterine leiomyomas, or adenomyosis underlying prolonged menses should also be evaluated in anemic patients through a meticulous history and physical examination followed by relevant laboratory tests.

Terminology Describing Abnormal Uterine Bleeding

Oligomenorrhea is defined as intervals between episodes of uterine bleeding greater than 35 days, and the term *polymenorrhea* is used to describe intervals less than 24 days. *Hypermenorrhea* refers to regular intervals (24 to 35 days) but excessive flow or duration of bleeding, or both. *Hypomenorrhea* refers to diminution of the flow or shortening of the duration of regular menses, or both.

Uterine Bleeding in Response to Steroid Hormones

Estrogen Withdrawal Bleeding

Uterine bleeding follows acute cessation of estrogen support to the endometrium. Thus, this type of uterine bleeding can occur after bilateral oophorectomy, radiation of mature follicles, or administration of estrogen to a castrate and then discontinuation of therapy. Similarly, the bleeding that occurs after castration can be delayed by concomitant estrogen therapy. Flow occurs on discontinuation of exogenous estrogen. Thus, estrogen withdrawal by itself (in the absence of progesterone) almost invariably causes uterine bleeding.

Estrogen Breakthrough Bleeding

Long-term exposure to varying quantities of estrogen stimulates the growth of endometrium continuously in the absence of progesterone, as in the case of excessive extragonadal estrogen production in PCOS. After a certain point, the amount of estrogen produced in extraovarian tissue remains insufficient to maintain structural support for the endometrium. This gives rise to unpredictable episodes of shedding of the surface endometrium. Relatively low doses of estrogen yield intermittent spotting that may be prolonged but is generally light in quantity of flow. On the other hand, high levels of estrogen and sustained availability lead to prolonged periods of amenorrhea followed by acute, often profuse episodes of bleeding with excessive loss of blood.

Progesterone Withdrawal Bleeding

The typical progesterone withdrawal bleeding occurs after ovulation in the absence of pregnancy. Removal of the corpus luteum is another example that leads to endometrial desquamation. Pharmacologically, a similar event can be achieved by administration and discontinuation of progesterone or a synthetic progestin. Progesterone withdrawal bleeding occurs only if the endometrium is initially primed by endogenous or exogenous estrogen. If estrogen therapy is continued as progesterone is withdrawn, the progesterone withdrawal bleeding still occurs. Only if estrogen levels are increased markedly is progesterone withdrawal bleeding delayed.[357] Thus, progesterone withdrawal bleeding is quite predictable in the presence of previous or concomitant estrogen exposure.

Progestin Breakthrough Bleeding

This is a pharmacologic phenomenon that occurs in the presence of an unfavorably high ratio of progestin to estrogen. In the absence of sufficient estrogen, continuous progestin therapy leads to intermittent bleeding of variable duration, similar to the low-dose estrogen breakthrough bleeding noted previously. This type of bleeding is associated with the combination oral contraceptives that contain low-dose estrogen and the long-acting progestin-only contraceptive methods such as Norplant and Depo-Provera.[358] Progestin breakthrough bleeding is highly unpredictable and characterized by extensive variability between women.

Causes of Irregular Uterine Bleeding

Pregnancy and its complications represent one of the most common causes of irregular uterine bleeding (Table 16–8). Pregnancy should be ruled out by a urine test in any woman of reproductive age presenting with irregular bleeding (Table 16–9).

As pointed out earlier, anovulatory uterine bleeding arising from responses of the endometrium to inappropriate production of ovarian steroids has also been called *dysfunctional uterine bleeding* because treatments that restore ovulatory function potentially reverse the irregular bleeding pattern. Common examples of anovulatory bleeding include those associated with exercise-related anovulation, hyperprolactinemia, hypothyroidism, or PCOS.[359] In these cases, either restoring ovulatory menses by correction of the underlying disorder or use of exogenous hormones can achieve predictable uterine bleeding. On the other hand, various pathologic entities of the genital tract (ovaries, uterus, vagina, or vulva) or a coagulation abnormality may also cause deviation from normal menses (see Table 16–8).

Anovulatory uterine bleeding is a diagnosis of exclusion for the following reasons. Vulvar, vaginal, or uterine malignancies can give rise to irregular bleeding. Moreover, an estrogen- or androgen-secreting ovarian tumor may cause abnormal uterine bleeding (see Table 16–8). Pregnancy and pregnancy-related problems such as ectopic pregnancy or spontaneous miscarriage are extremely common causes of abnormal uterine bleeding. In fact, the most common cause of disruption of a normal menstrual pattern is pregnancy or a complication of pregnancy. Another common cause of irregular uterine bleeding is observed in oral contraceptive users in the form of progestin breakthrough bleeding. Progestin breakthrough bleeding during postmenopausal hormone replacement is also common (see later). Patients may be using other hormonal medications unknowingly with an impact on the endometrium. For example, the use of ginseng, an herbal root, has been associated with estrogenic

TABLE 16–8 CAUSES OF IRREGULAR UTERINE BLEEDING

COMPLICATIONS OF PREGNANCY
Threatened miscarriage
Incomplete miscarriage
Ectopic pregnancy
ANOVULATION
Physiologic
Uncomplicated pregnancy (amenorrhea)
Pubertal (postmenarchal) anovulation
Premenopausal anovulation
Medications (e.g., oral contraceptives, GnRH agonists, danazol)
Hypothalamic (frequently presents as amenorrhea)
Functional (e.g., diet, exercise, stress)
Anatomic (e.g., tumor, granulomatous disease, infection)
Medications
Other
Hyperprolactinemia, other pituitary disorders
Prolactinoma
Other pituitary tumors, granulomatous disease
Hypothyroidism
Medications
Other
Androgen excess
PCOS, hyperthecosis
Ovarian tumor (e.g., Sertoli-Leydig cell tumor)
Nonclassic adrenal hyperplasia
Cushing's syndrome
Glucocorticoid resistance
Adrenal tumor (e.g., adenoma, carcinoma)
Medications (e.g., testosterone, danazol)
Other
Premature ovarian failure (frequently presents as amenorrhea)
Chronic illness
Liver failure
Renal failure
AIDS
Other
ANATOMIC DEFECTS AFFECTING THE UTERUS
Uterine leiomyomas
Endometrial polyps
Adenomyosis (usually presents as hypermenorrhea)
Intrauterine adhesions (usually presents as amenorrhea)
Endometritis
Endometrial hyperplasia, cancer
Chronic estrogen exposure (e.g., PCOS, medication, liver failure)
Estrogen-secreting ovarian tumor (e.g., granulosa cell tumor)
Advanced cervical cancer
Other
COAGULATION DEFECTS (USUALLY PRESENT AS HYPERMENORRHEA)
Von Willebrand's disease
Factor XI deficiency
Other
EXTRAUTERINE GENITAL BLEEDING (MAY MIMIC UTERINE BLEEDING)
Vaginitis
Genital trauma
Foreign body
Vaginal neoplasia
Vulvar neoplasia
Other

AIDS, Acquired immunodeficiency syndrome; *GnRH*, gonadotropin-releasing hormone; *PCOS*, polycystic ovary syndrome.

TABLE 16–9 DIAGNOSTIC TESTS TO EVALUATE IRREGULAR UTERINE BLEEDING

COMMONLY USED TESTS
Urine hCG test Serum hCG level (incomplete miscarriage, ectopic pregnancy) Transvaginal pelvic ultrasonography (intrauterine or ectopic pregnancy, uterine leiomyoma, endometrial polyp or neoplasia, ovarian tumor) Serum FSH, LH (anovulation; ovarian failure) Serum prolactin, TSH (anovulation; hyperprolactinemia) Complete blood count, PT, PTT (coagulation defect) Liver and renal functions, HIV (anovulation; chronic disease) Endometrial biopsy (endometrial disease; polyp, neoplasia, endometritis)
LESS COMMONLY USED TESTS
Evaluation for PCOS, ovarian or adrenal tumor, nonclassic adrenal hyperplasia, Cushing's syndrome and glucocorticoid resistance (androgen excess) Head CT or MRI scan (hypothalamic anovulation, hyperprolactinemia) Pelvic MRI scan (adenomyosis, uterine leiomyoma) Hysterosonography with intrauterine saline installation (endometrial polyp, uterine leiomyoma) Hysteroscopy (endometrial polyp, uterine leiomyoma) Dilatation and curettage (endometrial disease not diagnosed by ultrasonography or biopsy)

CT, Computed tomography; *FSH*, follicle-stimulating hormone; *hCG*, human chorionic gonadotropin; *HIV*, human immunodeficiency virus; *LH*, luteinizing hormone; *MRI*, magnetic resonance imaging; *PCOS*, polycystic ovarian syndrome; *PT*, prothrombin time; *PTT*, partial thromboplastin time; *TSH*, thyroid-stimulating hormone.

activity and abnormal bleeding.[360] Although uterine bleeding is a common benign side effect of various long-term hormonal treatments, the clinician should always be convinced that no other pathology is present. Anatomically demonstrable pathologies of the menstrual outflow tract include endometrial hyperplasia and cancer, endometrial polyps, leiomyomata uteri, adenomyosis, and endometritis. Irregular, serious bleeding may also be associated with chronic illness, such as renal failure, liver failure, and acquired immunodeficiency syndrome. Finally, careful examination is worthwhile to discover genital injury or a foreign object (see Table 16–8).

At puberty, the most common cause of irregular uterine bleeding is anovulation. Approximately 20% of these adolescents with excessive irregular uterine bleeding, however, have a coagulation defect.[361,362] Among all women of reproductive age with hypermenorrhea, the prevalence of a coagulation disorder was reported to be 17%. Von Willebrand's disease was the most common defect, and factor XI deficiency was the second common diagnosis. Bleeding secondary to a coagulation defect is usually a heavy flow with regular, cyclic menses (hypermenorrhea), and the same pattern can be seen in patients being treated with anticoagulants.[363] Bleeding disorders are usually associated with hypermenorrhea since menarche and a history of bleeding with surgery or trauma. Hypermenorrhea may be the only sign of an inherited bleeding disorder.[364]

Early pregnancy or its complications should always be ruled out first by a sensitive urine hCG measurement in any reproductive-age woman presenting with irregular bleeding (see Table 16–9). Threatened or incomplete miscarriage and ectopic pregnancy are extremely common causes of irregular uterine bleeding. Other tests should be ordered if necessary on the basis of the initial clinical evaluation. These include tests to evaluate anovulatory disorders of various etiologies (see Table 9). In patients with a history of prolonged heavy menses (hypermenorrhea) of pubertal origin, coagulation studies (e.g., prothrombin time, partial thromboplastin time, and bleeding time) and a complete blood count should be obtained.

Pelvic ultrasonography through a vaginal probe is an extremely useful test for the evaluation of normal or abnormal pregnancy, uterine leiomyomas, endometrial neoplasia, and ovarian tumors (see Table 16–9). Other imaging studies may be used judiciously to rule out pathologies of the hypothalamus, pituitary, or adrenal (see earlier). Of note is the use of pelvic MRI to rule out adenomyosis, a uterine disorder characterized by the abnormal presence of diffuse endometrial tissue in the myometrial layer (see Table 16–9). Advanced adenomyosis is associated with diffuse enlargement of the uterus, hypermenorrhea, and anemia.

Endometrial histology should be determined by an endometrial biopsy performed in the clinician's office in patients at risk for the development of endometrial hyperplasia or cancer (e.g., PCOS, liver failure, obesity, diabetes mellitus, hormone replacement). A benign endometrial polyp or a uterine leiomyoma protruding into the uterine cavity can be diagnosed by hysterosonography using intrauterine saline installation or hysteroscopy. Hysterosonography and hysteroscopy are not appropriate tests to evaluate endometrial hyperplasia or cancer because these procedures may cause dissemination of malignant cells. If malignancy is suspected, it should be ruled out by an office endometrial biopsy (see Table 16–9). Occasionally, an office endometrial biopsy cannot be performed or is not diagnostic of endometrial neoplasia. In these rare instances, endometrial curettage under anesthesia is performed for a reliable tissue diagnosis.

Again, a careful history and physical examination eliminate the need for most of these diagnostic tests. A useful question to ask oneself before ordering a certain diagnostic study is whether that particular test will alter the ultimate clinical management.

Management of Anovulatory Uterine Bleeding

The terms *dysfunctional uterine bleeding* and *anovulatory bleeding* are used interchangeably and denote inappropriate stimulation of the endometrium during dysfunctional states of the reproductive system. If ovulatory function can be restored, anovulatory bleeding usually gives way to cyclic predictable periods. Because restoring ovulatory function may not be possible or practical in a large number of these women, exogenous estrogen and progestin are administered for a number of purposes. The indications for hormonal treatment of uterine bleeding include the need to stop acute uterine bleeding, to maintain predictable bleeding episodes, or to prevent endometrial hyperplasia. A number of hormonal treatments are used to stop anovulatory uterine bleeding and to induce predictable bleeding episodes. Again, anovulatory uterine bleeding is a diagnosis of exclusion. Various anatomically demonstrable pathologies of the genital tract as listed in Table 16–8 should be ruled out before administration of the following regimens.

Oral Contraceptives

Use of combination oral contraceptives in an acute or chronic fashion is the most common treatment for irregular uterine bleeding. The estrogen component of the combination pill stabilizes the endometrial tissue and stops shedding within hours and decreases ovarian secretion of sex steroids by suppression of gonadotropins within several days. The progestin component of the pill directly affects endometrial tissue to decrease shedding over days and potentiates ovarian suppression induced by estrogen. The progestin (in the presence of estrogen) induces differentiation of the endometrial tissue into a stable form termed pseudodecidua. Typically, a monophasic oral contraceptive preparation that contains 30 or 35 mcg of ethinyl estradiol is preferred. Triphasic oral contraceptives or those with less than 30 mcg of ethinyl estradiol are not suitable for the treatment of excessive anovulatory uterine bleeding. A combination oral contraceptive in high doses (two or three pills a day) can be used for short intervals (weeks) to treat an acute episode of excessive uterine bleeding. A usual dose (one pill per day) may be administered for years to manage chronic anovulatory bleeding associated with PCOS or hyperprolactinemia.

Oral Contraceptives and Acute Excessive Uterine Bleeding Associated with Anemia

Unopposed estrogen exposure in women with anovulatory uterine bleeding is commonly associated with chronic endometrial buildup and heavy bleeding episodes. Therapy is administered as one pill twice a day for 1 week. In obese women, the oral contraceptive may be given three times a day. This therapy is maintained despite cessation of flow within 2 days. If flow does not abate, other diagnostic possibilities (polyps, incomplete abortion, and neoplasia) should be reevaluated. In case of anovulatory bleeding, the flow does diminish rapidly within 2 days after the beginning of high-dose (one pill two or three times a day) oral contraceptive treatment. Specific causes of anovulation and possible coagulation disorders are evaluated during the following few days. At this time, the clinician also considers whether blood replacement or initiation of iron therapy is necessary. The high-dose estrogen-progestin combination has produced the structural rigidity intrinsic to the compact pseudodecidual reaction for the moment. Continued random breakdown of formerly fragile tissue is avoided and blood loss stopped. A large quantity of tissue, however, remains to react to estrogen-progestin withdrawal. The patient must be warned to anticipate a heavy flow with severely cramping flow a few days after stopping this therapy. The patient should also be warned of possible nausea that may be caused by high-dose oral contraceptive treatment.

At the end of a week of high-dose oral contraceptive treatment, the pill is stopped temporarily. A heavy flow usually starts within a few days. On the third day of this withdrawal bleeding, a regular dose of combination oral contraceptive medication (one pill a day) is started. This is repeated for several 3-week treatments interrupted by 1-week withdrawal intervals. A decrease in volume with each successive cycle is expected. Oral contraceptives reduce menstrual flow by more than half in most women.[365]

Early application of the estrogen-progestin combination limits growth and allows orderly regression of excessive endometrial height to normal levels. Because oral contraceptives do not treat the underlying cause of anovulation but provide symptomatic relief by directly affecting the endometrium, cessation of oral contraceptives results in the return of erratic uterine bleeding. Regardless of the requirement for contraception, oral contraceptives represent the best choice for hormonal management of heavy anovulatory bleeding and should be offered as long-term management.

Oral Contraceptives and Chronic Irregular Uterine Bleeding

PCOS is a common form of anovulation associated with chronic steady-state levels of unopposed estrogen that may give rise to endometrial hyperplasia and cancer (see earlier). Hypothalamic anovulation and hyperprolactinemia, on the other hand, are associated with low estrogen levels, insufficient to prevent bone loss. A combination oral contraceptive is a suitable long-term treatment for both forms of chronic anovulation.

Oral contraceptives represent the most suitable long-term symptomatic management option for any kind of anovulatory uterine bleeding, including oligomenorrhea. Before the administration of an oral contraceptive, pregnancy should be ruled out. For this purpose, one pill per day is ordinarily administered for 3-week periods interrupted by 1-week hormone-free intervals. Withdrawal bleeding is expected during the hormone-free interval. The progestin component serves to prevent endometrial hyperplasia associated with steady-state unopposed estrogen exposure in PCOS (see earlier). In cases of anovulation associated with hypoestrogenism (e.g., hypothalamic anovulation, hyperprolactinemia), on the other hand, the estrogen component of the pill provides sufficient replacement to prevent bone loss. The risk of thromboembolism, stroke, or myocardial infarction associated with long-term administration is extremely low in current nonsmokers and in the absence of a history of thromboembolism. Provided that an oral contraceptive controls the abnormal uterine bleeding effectively, a chronically anovulatory woman can continue this regimen until the menopause.

Synthetic Progestins

Synthetic progestins enhance endometrial differentiation and antagonize proliferative effects of estrogen on the endometrium (see Fig. 16–24).[165,366] The effects of progestins or natural progesterone include limitation of estrogen-induced endometrial growth and prevention of endometrial hyperplasia. The absence of naturally synthesized progesterone in anovulatory states is the rationale for administering a progestin.

The most common indication for long-term cyclic progestin administration is to prevent endometrial malignancy in a patient with PCOS and unopposed chronic estrogen exposure of the endometrium. A combination oral contraceptive is the treatment of choice in these cases. If the patient cannot use an oral contraceptive for some reason (e.g., history of thromboembolism), a progestin can be administered in a cyclic fashion to prevent endometrial hyperplasia. Before the administration of a progestin (or oral contraceptive), pregnancy should be ruled out. In the treatment of oligomenorrhea associated with PCOS, orderly limited withdrawal bleeding can be accomplished by administration of a progestin such as medroxyprogesterone acetate, 10 mg/day for at least 10 days every 2 months. Alternatively, norethindrone acetate at 5 mg/day or megestrol acetate at 20 mg/day may be administered for 10 days every 2 months. Absence of withdrawal bleeding requires further workup.

In the treatment of excessive uterine bleeding (hypermenorrhea or polymenorrhea), these progestins at higher daily doses (medroxyprogesterone acetate 20 mg/day, norethindrone acetate 10 mg/day, or megestrol acetate 40 mg/day) are prescribed for 2 weeks to induce predecidual stromal changes in the endometrium. A heavy progestin withdrawal flow usually follows within 3 days after the last dose. Thereafter, repeated progestin treatment (medroxyprogesterone acetate 10 mg/day, norethindrone acetate 5 mg/day, or megestrol acetate 20 mg/day) is offered cyclically for at least the first 10 days of every other month to ensure therapeutic effect. Failure of progestin to correct irregular bleeding requires diagnostic reevaluation such as endometrial biopsy. On the other hand, predictable withdrawal bleeding within several days after each cycle of progestin administration suggests the absence of endometrial malignancy.

High-Dose Estrogen for Acute Excessive Uterine Bleeding

As already outlined, an oral contraceptive given two or three times a day is the treatment of choice to stop heavy anovulatory bleeding. A high-dose oral contraceptive regimen should be offered to women with heavy uterine bleeding plus or minus asymptomatic anemia after an anatomically demonstrable pathology of the genital tract has been ruled out (see Table 16–8). On the other hand, a patient with acute and severe anovulatory bleeding accompanied by symptomatic anemia represents a medical emergency. These patients should be hospitalized immediately and offered a blood transfusion. When genital tract pathology has been ruled out by history, physical examination, and pelvic ultrasonography, intravenously administered high-dose estrogen is the treatment of choice to stop life-threatening bleeding. A well-established regimen is 25 mg of conjugated estrogen administered intravenously every 4 hours until bleeding markedly slows down or for at least 24 hours.[367] Estrogen most likely acts on the capillaries to induce clotting.[368] Before intravenous estrogen treatment is discontinued, an oral contraceptive pill is started three times a day. Oral contraceptive treatment is continued as described previously.

Because high-dose estrogen is a risk factor for thromboembolism, taking two or three oral contraceptives per day for a week or large doses of intravenous conjugated estrogens for 24 hours should also be regarded as significant risks. There are no data available, however, to evaluate any risk associated with this type of acute use of hormonal therapy for such short intervals. The clinician and patient should make a decision regarding high-dose hormone therapy after considering its risks and benefits. Alternative treatment options may be offered to patients with significant risk factors. In women with a past episode of idiopathic venous thromboembolism or a strong family history, exposure to high doses of estrogen should be avoided. High-dose hormone treatment should also be avoided in women with severe chronic illness such as liver failure or renal failure. One alternative for these patients is dilatation and curettage, followed by an oral contraceptive at one pill per day until the uterine bleeding is under control.

Gonadotropin-Releasing Hormone Analogues for Excessive Anovulatory Uterine Bleeding

A GnRH analogue may be given to women with excessive anovulatory bleeding or hypermenorrhea related to severe chronic illness such as liver failure or coagulation disorders. It should be pointed out that monthly depot injections of GnRH agonists are not effective for acute excessive uterine bleeding and may increase uterine bleeding for the first 2 weeks. GnRH antagonists, on the other hand, down-regulate FSH and LH without a delay and achieve amenorrhea more rapidly. The GnRH agonist leuprolide acetate depot, 3.75 mg intramuscularly monthly may be administered for 6 months or longer to control uterine bleeding due to chronic illness on a long-term basis. GnRH antagonists can probably be used to halt acute or chronic anovulatory bleeding; however, no sufficient published data are available to provide dose recommendations. Long-term side effects of GnRH analogues including osteoporosis make this an undesirable choice for long-term therapy. If long-term treatment with GnRH analogues is chosen, norethindrone acetate 2.5 mg daily should be added back. This add-back regimen is usually sufficient to prevent osteoporosis and does not ordinarily worsen the uterine bleeding.

HORMONE-DEPENDENT BENIGN GYNECOLOGIC DISORDERS

Endometriosis

Endometriosis is defined as the presence of endometrium-like tissue outside the uterine cavity, most often on the peritoneal surfaces of the pelvis and the ovaries. It is one of the most common causes of infertility and chronic pelvic pain and affects 1 in 10 women in the reproductive age group.[369] The incidence increases to 30% in patients with infertility and to 45% in patients with chronic pelvic pain.[370]

Reliable diagnosis of endometriosis can be made only by direct visualization of these peritoneal lesions by laparoscopy or laparotomy. As in other common chronic diseases such as diabetes mellitus and asthma, endometriosis is inherited in a polygenic manner.[369] Relatives of women with this disease have a sevenfold increase in the incidence of endometriosis compared with relatives of control subjects.[369] Sampson proposed the most widely accepted mechanism for the development of endometriosis on pelvic peritoneal surfaces as the implantation of endometrial tissue on the peritoneum through retrograde menstruation.[369] Because retrograde menstruation occurs in more than 90% of all women, endometriosis may be caused by genetic defects that favor survival and establishment of endometrial tissue in menstrual debris on the peritoneum.[269]

Endometriosis and normal endometrial tissues respond to estrogen and progesterone with similar histologic changes.[269] Estrogen favors the growth of endometriosis, whereas progesterone may limit this mitogenic action of estrogen. Some endometriotic implants undergo atrophy in response to prolonged oral contraceptive therapy just as the normal endometrium does, the so-called pregnancy state. Yet, endometriotic tissue does not respond to progestins or native progesterone as predictably as normal endometrium does.[269] Endometriotic tissue in ectopic locations such as the peritoneum or ovary is strikingly different from the eutopic endometrium within the uterus with respect to production of cytokines and prostaglandins, steroid biosynthesis and metabolism, steroid receptor content, and clinical response to progestins.[148,269,370]

Although current hormonal therapy for infertility associated with endometriosis is not of proven value, it is somewhat successful for pelvic pain associated with endometriosis.[369] The duration of relief provided by medical[371] treatment, however, is relatively short.[372] Various agents used are comparable in terms of efficacy. Most current medical treatments were designed to decrease estrogen secretion by the ovaries (e.g., GnRH agonists, oral contraceptives, danazol and progestins) or to antagonize the effects of estrogen on endometriotic implants (e.g., oral contraceptives, danazol and progestins). A possible alternative mechanism of action of the androgenic steroid danazol or a progestin is a direct antiproliferative effect on endometriotic tissue.

Many patients and clinicians do not favor danazol because of its anabolic and androgenic side effects of weight gain and muscle cramps and occasional irreversible virilization (e.g., clitoromegaly and voice changes).[373] In fact, up to 50% of patients with endometriosis fail to complete 6 months of treatment with danazol.[374] The rest of the hormonal agents—oral contraceptives, progestins, and GnRH agonists—show comparable efficacy for the control of endometriosis-associated pain.[375-377] A 6-month course using any one of these agents results in a significant reduction of pain in more than 50% of patients.[375-377] Induction of pain relief with a continuously administered oral contraceptive or progestin takes longer than with a GnRH agonist. There is, however, a high incidence of persistence of the disease after all of these medical therapies.[378] Six months after completion of a 6-month course of treatment with a progestin, oral contraceptive, or GnRH agonist, moderate to severe pain symptoms recurred in 50% of initial responders.[376] The recurrence rate of pain in the rest of the patients was approximately 5% to 20% per year during a 5-year follow-up.[378] A 6-month course of GnRH agonist treatment is currently the most popular regimen. The most serious side effect of the GnRH agonist treatment for endometriosis is bone loss related to estrogen deficiency, and oral estrogen-progestin preparations or bisphosphonates are usually added back to minimize bone loss.[34]

We are still far from the cure for endometriosis, and current treatments are not satisfactory for effective control of pain. The radical treatment is the removal of both ovaries, and even this was not found to be effective in a number of cases of postmenopausal endometriosis.[376] New strategies are needed to offer women with endometriosis a reasonable chance to live without suffering from chronic pelvic pain for decades. There are two important caveats, which are not addressed by the GnRH agonist treatment. First, large quantities of estrogen can be produced locally within the endometriotic cells. This represents an intracrine mechanism of estrogen action, in contrast to ovarian secretion, which is an endocrine means of supplying this steroid to target tissues (see Fig. 16–21).[269,376] Second, estradiol produced in peripheral tissue sites (e.g., adipose tissue and skin fibroblasts) may give rise to pathologically significant circulating levels of estradiol in a subset of women.[269] GnRH agonists do not inhibit peripheral estrogen formation or local estrogen production within the estrogen-responsive lesion. As a further twist, endometriosis is resistant to selective effects of progesterone and currently used progestins.[269] Thus, aromatase inhibitors and selective progesterone response modulators are candidate therapeutic agents for endometriosis.

Aromatase expression and local estrogen biosynthesis in endometriotic implants prompted pilot studies to target aromatase in endometriosis using its third-generation inhibitors. Among these inhibitors, anastrozole and letrozole were used successfully to treat endometriosis in both postmenopausal and premenopausal women.[379-383] These reports suggest the following. (1) Aromatase inhibitors effectively treat pelvic pain associated with endometriosis, even that, which is resistant to existing therapeutic modalities. (2) An aromatase inhibitor is the medical treatment of choice for persistent postmenopausal endometriosis. (3) Use of aromatase inhibitors in premenopausal women with endometriosis requires ovarian suppression via the addition of a GnRH analogue, progestin, or combination oral contraceptive. (4) Pilot data showed that side effect profiles were quite favorable and did not include bone loss in regimens that combined an aromatase inhibitor with an oral contraceptive or a progestin.[381,383] Thus, aromatase inhibitors represent one of the most promising new treatments of pain associated with endometriosis.

Uterine Leiomyomas

Uterine leiomyomas originate from the myometrium and are the most common solid tumor of the pelvis.[384] Leiomyomas are responsible for over 200,000 hysterectomies per year in the United States. They are almost invariably benign and represent clonal expansion of individual myometrial cells. Leiomyomas can cause a variety of symptoms including irregular and excessive uterine bleeding, pressure sensation in the lower abdomen, pain during intercourse, pelvic pain, recurrent pregnancy loss, infertility, and compression of adjacent pelvic organs, or they may be totally asymptomatic. The prevalence rate of uterine leiomyomas is estimated to be 25% to 30%.[384] Leiomyomas are more common in African-American women and have a polygenic inheritance pattern. Diagnosis can be made by abdominal and transvaginal ultrasonography. Transvaginal ultrasonography is a sensitive method for determining the size, number, and location of uterine leiomyomas.

Uterine leiomyomas appear during the reproductive years and regress after menopause, indicating their ovarian steroid-dependent growth potential. The role of steroids or other growth factors in the initiation and growth of these tumors, however, is not well understood. The neoplastic transformation of myometrium to leiomyoma probably involves somatic mutations of normal myometrium and the complex interactions of sex steroids and growth factors.[385] Traditionally, estrogen has been considered the major promoter of myoma growth. More recent biochemical, histologic, and clinical evidence suggests an important role for progesterone in the growth of uterine leiomyomas. Biochemical and clinical studies suggest that progesterone and progestins, acting through the PR, might enhance proliferative activity in leiomyomas.[385]

The therapeutic choices depend on the goals of therapy, with hysterectomy most often used for definitive treatment and myomectomy when preservation of childbearing is desired. Intracavitary and submucous leiomyomas can be removed by hysteroscopic resection. Laparoscopic myomectomy is now technically possible but apparently involves an increased risk of uterine rupture during pregnancy. The overall recurrence rate after myomectomy varies widely (10% to 50%). Although GnRH agonist-induced hypogonadism can reduce the overall volume of the uterus containing leiomyomas and tumor vascularity, the severe side effects and prompt recurrences make GnRH agonists useful only for short-term goals such as reducing anemia related to uterine bleeding or decreased tumor vascularity before hysteroscopic resection.[386]

MANAGEMENT OF THE MENOPAUSE

Consequences of the Menopause

The Climacteric

The menopause is the permanent cessation of menses as a result of the irreversible loss of a number of ovarian functions, including ovulation and estrogen production. The climacteric is a critical period of life during which striking endocrinologic, somatic, and psychological alterations occur in the transition to the menopause. The climacteric is also referred to as *the perimenopause*. The climacteric encompasses the change from ovulatory cycles to cessation of menses and is marked by irregularity of menstrual bleeding.

The most sensitive clinical indication of the climacteric is the progressively increasing occurrence of menstrual irregularities. The menstrual cycle for most ovulatory women lasts from 24 to 35 days, whereas approximately 20% of all reproductive-age women experience irregular cycles.[349] When women are in their 40s, anovulation becomes more prevalent; before anovulation, the menstrual cycle length increases, beginning several years before menopause.[352] The median age for the onset of the climacteric transition is 47.5 years.[387] Regardless of the age of its onset, the menopause (cessation of menses) is consistently preceded by a period of prolonged cycle intervals.[388] Elevated circulating FSH marks this menstrual cycle change before menopause and is accompanied by decreased inhibin levels, normal levels of LH, and slightly elevated levels of estradiol.[389]

These changes in serum hormone levels reflect a decreasing ovarian follicular reserve and can be detected more reliably on day 2 or 3 of the menstrual cycle.

During the climacteric, serum estradiol levels do not begin to decline until less than a year before menopause. The average circulating estradiol levels in perimenopausal women are estimated to be somewhat higher than those in younger women because of an increased follicular response to elevated FSH.[390] The decline in inhibin production by the follicle, allowing a rise in FSH, in the later reproductive years reflects diminishing follicular reserve and competence. Ovarian follicular output of inhibin begins to decrease after 30 years of age, and this decline becomes much more pronounced after age 40. These hormonal changes are parallel to a significant decrease in fecundity, which starts at age 35.

The climacteric is a transitional period during which postmenopausal levels of FSH can be observed despite continued menses, whereas LH levels still remain in the normal range. Pregnancy is still possible in the perimenopausal woman, because occasional ovulation and functional corpus luteum formation can occur. Thus, until complete cessation of menses is observed or FSH levels higher than 40 IU/L are measured on two separate occasions, some form of contraception should be recommended to prevent unwanted pregnancies.

The climacteric represents an optimal period to evaluate the general health of the mature woman and introduce the measures to prepare her for striking physiologic changes that come with the menopause. The patient and her clinician should attempt to achieve several important aims during the climacteric. The long-term goal is to maintain an optimal quality of physical and social life. Another immediate objective is the detection of any major chronic disorders that occur with aging. Finally, the clinician should counsel the perimenopausal woman about the symptoms and long-term consequences of menopause. The benefits and risks of hormone replacement should be discussed at great length at this time.

The Menopause

The median age of the menopause is approximately 51.[391] The age of menopause is probably determined in part by genetic factors because mothers and daughters tend to experience menopause at the same age.[392-394] A number of environmental factors may modify the age of menopause. For example, current smoking is associated with an earlier menopause, whereas alcohol consumption delays menopause.[391] Oral contraceptive use does not affect the age of menopause.

The symptoms frequently seen and related to decreased estrogen production in menopause include irregular frequency of menses followed by amenorrhea, vasomotor instability manifest as hot flashes and sweats, urogenital atrophy giving rise to pain during intercourse and a variety of urinary symptoms, and consequences of osteoporosis and cardiovascular disease. The combination and the extent of these symptoms differ widely for each patient. Some patients experience multiple severe symptoms that may be disabling, whereas others have no symptoms or mild discomfort associated with the climacteric.

Biosynthesis of Estrogen and Other Steroids in the Postmenopausal Woman

No follicular units can be detected histologically in the ovaries after the menopause.[395] In reproductive-age women, the granulosa cell of the ovulatory follicle is the major source of inhibin and estradiol. In the absence of these factors that inhibit gonadotropin secretion, both FSH and LH levels increase sharply after menopause. These levels peak a few years after menopause and decrease gradually and slightly thereafter.[396] The postmenopausal serum level of either gonadotropin may be more than 100 IU/L. FSH levels are usually higher than LH levels because LH is cleared from the blood strikingly more quickly and possibly because the low levels of inhibin in the menopause selectively lead to increased FSH secretion. Nevertheless, increased LH is a major factor that maintains significant quantities of androstenedione and testosterone secretion from the ovary, although the total production rates of both steroids decline after menopause.

The primary steroid products of the postmenopausal ovary are androstenedione and testosterone.[397] The average premenopausal rate of production of androstenedione of 3 mg/day is decreased by half to approximately 1.5 mg/day.[397] This decrease is primarily due to a substantial reduction in the ovarian contribution to the circulating androstenedione pool. Adrenal secretion accounts for most of the androstenedione production in the postmenopausal woman, with only a small amount secreted from the ovary.[398] Both DHEA and DHEAS originate almost exclusively from the adrenal and decline steadily with advancing age independent of the menopause. The serum levels of both DHEA and DHEAS after menopause are about one fourth of those in young adult women.[399]

Testosterone production is decreased by approximately one third after menopause.[397] Total testosterone production can be approximated by the sum of ovarian secretion and peripheral formation from androstenedione (see Fig. 16–28). In the premenopausal woman, significant amounts of testosterone are produced by reduction of androstenedione in extraovarian tissues. Because ovarian androstenedione secretion is substantially decreased after the menopause, the decrease in postmenopausal testosterone production is accounted for, in large measure, by a decrease in the relative contribution of extraovarian sources.[397] With the disappearance of follicles and decreased estrogen, the elevated gonadotropins drive the remaining stromal tissue in the ovary to maintain testosterone secretion at levels observed during the premenopausal years. Thus, the contribution of the postmenopausal ovary to the total testosterone production is increased in the presence of seemingly unaltered ovarian secretion.

The most dramatic endocrine alteration of the climacteric involves the decline in the circulating level and production rate of estradiol. The average menopausal level of circulating estradiol is less than 20 pg/mL. Both estradiol and estrone levels in postmenopausal women are usually slightly less than those in adult men. Circulating estradiol in postmenopausal women (and men) is derived from the peripheral conversion of androstenedione to estrone, which is, in turn, converted peripherally to estradiol (see Fig. 16–21).[386,400] The mean circulating level of estrone in postmenopausal women (37 pg/mL) is higher than that of estradiol. The average postmenopausal production rate of estrone is approximately 42 μg per 24 hours. After menopause, almost all estrone and estradiol are derived from the peripheral aromatization of androstenedione. Thus, there is a drastic change in the androgen-to-estrogen ratio because of the sharp decrease in estradiol levels and slightly reduced testosterone. The frequent onset of a mild hirsutism after menopause reflects this striking shift in the hormone ratio. During the postmenopausal years, DHEAS and DHEA levels continue to decline steadily with advancing age, whereas serum androstenedione, testosterone, estrone, and estradiol levels do not change significantly.[396]

The aromatization of androstenedione to estrone in extraovarian tissues correlates positively with weight and advancing age (see Figs. 16-21 and 16-33).[125] Body weight correlates positively with the circulating levels of estrone and estradiol. Because aromatase enzyme activity is present in significant quantities in adipose tissue, increased aromatization of androstenedione in overweight individuals may reflect the increased bulk of tissue containing the enzyme.[124] In addition, there is a twofold to fourfold increase in the specific activity of aromatase per cell with advancing age.[126] An increased overall number of adipose fibroblasts with aromatase activity and a decrease in the levels of SHBG cause an increased free estradiol level and contribute to the increased risk of endometrial cancer in obese women.[126] The production rate and circulating levels of estradiol after menopause are clearly insufficient to provide support for urogenital tissues and bone. Thus, osteoporosis and urogenital atrophy are some of the most dramatic and unwanted consequences of estradiol deficiency during the menopause.

Estrogen is also produced locally in pathologic tissues such as breast cancer through aromatase and reductive 17β-HSD (Fig. 16–36).[126,401] In postmenopausal women, androstenedione of adrenal origin is the most important substrate for aromatase in tumor tissue.[126,401] Estrone is produced primarily by aromatase that resides in undifferentiated adipose fibroblasts surrounding malignant epithelial cells (see Fig. 16–36).[126,401] Estrone then diffuses into malignant epithelial cells that contain reductive 17β-HSD activity and is converted to biologically active estradiol (see Fig. 16–36).[147] Thus, paracrine interactions in breast tumor tissue serve to produce estradiol in malignant epithelial cells to give rise to an effect such as proliferation. The clinical relevance of these findings was exemplified by the successful use of aromatase inhibitors as both first-line and second-line endocrine treatments for postmenopausal breast cancer.[402]

Postmenopausal Uterine Bleeding and its Management

Perimenopausal or postmenopausal bleeding can be due to hormone administration or excessive extra-ovarian estrogen formation. Irregular uterine bleeding is commonly observed during the perimenopausal transition as anovulatory cycles alternate with ovulatory cycles. Uterine bleeding after the menopause is less common if the patient is not receiving hormone replacement treatment.[403] Obese patients are more likely to experience postmenopausal bleeding because of increased peripheral aromatization of adrenal androstenedione. Patients receiving a continuous combination regimen of hormone replacement therapy (HRT) may experience unpredictable uterine bleeding (see later). The major objective in these circumstances is to rule out endometrial malignancy. This can be best achieved by tissue diagnosis through an office endometrial biopsy using a plastic cannula. Transvaginal ultrasonographic measurement of endometrial thickness may be used in postmenopausal women to avoid unnecessary biopsies.[172] A biopsy is required if an endometrial thickness greater than or equal to 5 mm is observed.

Before employing ultrasonography and endometrial biopsy to explore the etiology of bleeding that is assumed to arise from the intrauterine cavity, the clinician should rule out diseases of the vulva, vagina, and cervix as other potential causes of vaginal bleeding. Careful inspection of these organs and a normal cervical Pap smear within the past year are sufficient to rule out the vulva, vagina, and cervix as potential sources of bleeding. Postmenopausal uterine bleeding is the most common initial event that alerts the patient and her clinician to the possibility of endometrial cancer. On the other hand, the causes of postmenopausal uterine bleeding are benign most of the time. Endometrial malignancy is encountered in patients with bleeding in only about 1% to 2% of postmenopausal endometrial biopsies.[404] Approximately three fourths of these biopsies reveal either no pathology or an atrophic endometrium. Other histologic findings include hyperplasia (15%) and endometrial polyps (3%). Persistent unexplained uterine bleeding requires repeated evaluation, biopsy, hysteroscopy, or dilatation and curettage.

Unpredictable irregular uterine bleeding is observed in approximately 20% of postmenopausal women receiving a long-term (>1 year) continuous estrogen-progestin combination. This should also be evaluated with ultrasonography or biopsy, or both (see later).[172]

Hot Flash

The most frequent and striking symptom in the climacteric is the hot flash. The hot flash typically occurs at the time of transition from perimenopause to postmenopause, that is, the climacteric. The flash is also a major symptom of the postmenopause and can last up to 5 years after menopause.[405] More than four fifths of postmenopausal women experience hot flashes within 3 months after the cessation of ovarian function, whether natural or surgical in origin. Of these women, more than three fourths

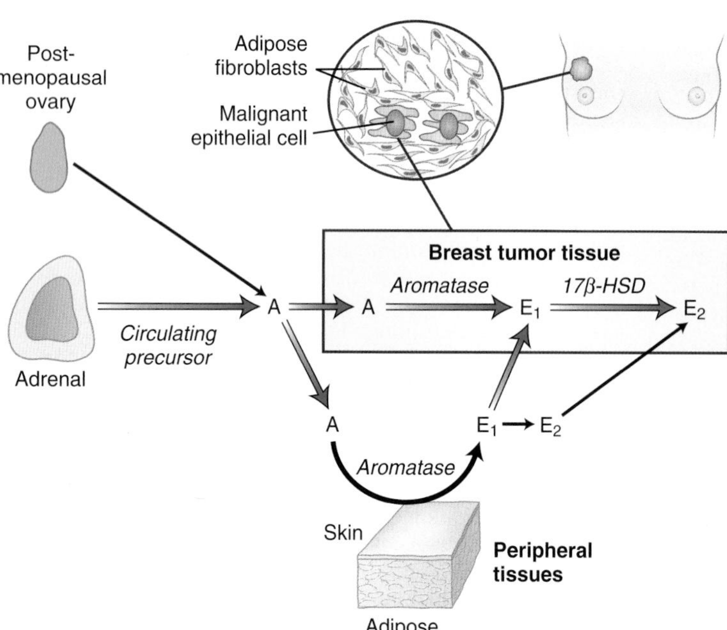

Figure 16–36 ▪ Tissue sources of estrogen in postmenopausal breast cancer. This figure exemplifies the important pathologic roles of extraovarian (peripheral) and local estrogen biosynthesis in an estrogen-dependent disease in postmenopausal women. The estrogen precursor androstenedione (A) originates primarily from the adrenal in the postmenopausal woman. Aromatase expression and enzyme activity in extraovarian tissues such as fat increase with advancing age. The aromatase activity in skin and subcutaneous adipose fibroblasts gives rise to formation of systemically available estrone (E1) and to a smaller extent estradiol (E2). The conversion of circulating A to E1 in undifferentiated breast adipose fibroblasts compacted around malignant epithelial cells and subsequent conversion of E1 to E2 in malignant epithelial cells provide high tissue concentrations of E2 for tumor growth. The clinical relevance of these findings is exemplified by the successful use of aromatase inhibitors to treat breast cancer.

have them for more than 1 year and approximately half for up to 5 years.[405] Hot flashes lessen in frequency and intensity with advancing age, unlike other sequelae of the menopause, which progress with time.

A hot flash is a subjective sensation of intense warmth of the upper body, which typically lasts for 4 minutes but may range in duration from 30 seconds to 5 minutes. It may follow a prodrome of palpitations or headache and is frequently accompanied by weakness, faintness, or vertigo. This episode usually ends in profuse sweating and a cold sensation. The frequency may vary from extremely rare to recurring every few minutes. At night, flashes are more frequent and severe enough to awaken a woman from sleep. They are also more intense during times of stress. In a cool environment, hot flashes are fewer, less intense, and shorter in duration than in a warm environment.[406]

The hot flash results from a sudden reduction of estrogen levels rather than from hypoestrogenism itself. Therefore, regardless of the cause of menopause, natural, surgical, or estrogen withdrawal caused by a long-acting GnRH agonist, hot flashes are associated with an acute and significant drop in estrogen level.

The consistent association between the onset of flashes and acute estrogen withdrawal is also supported by the effectiveness of estrogen therapy and the absence of flashes in prolonged hypoestrogenic states, such as gonadal dysgenesis. Hypogonadal women experience hot flashes only after estrogen is administered and withdrawn.[407] Not all hot flashes, however, are due to estrogen deficiency. Sudden episodes of sweating and flash may be due to catecholamine- or histamine-secreting tumors (e.g., pheochromocytoma, carcinoid), hyperthyroidism, or chronic infection (e.g., tuberculosis). The hot flash may also be psychosomatic in origin and not due to estrogen withdrawal. Under these circumstances of doubt, the clinician should obtain a serum FSH level to confirm the climacteric or menopause before initiating hormone replacement. Obese women tend to be less troubled by hot flashes. Asymptomatic women are found to have significantly increased weight compared with severely symptomatic women, even when matched for age, ovarian status, and years since menopause.[408] The lower frequency and intensity of hot flashes in obese women may result from the elevated circulating free estradiol concentrations.[409]

Urogenital Atrophy

The urogenital sinus gives rise to the development of the lower vagina, vulva, and urethra during embryonic development, and these tissues are estrogen-dependent. The decrease in estrogen at menopause causes the vaginal walls to become pale because of diminished vascularity and to thin down to only three to four cell layers. The vaginal epithelial cells in postmenopausal women contain less glycogen, which, prior to menopause, was metabolized by lactobacilli to create an acidic pH, thereby protecting the vagina from bacterial overgrowth. Loss of this protective mechanism leaves the thin, friable tissue vulnerable to infection and ulceration. The vagina also loses its rugae and becomes shorter and inelastic. Postmenopausal women may complain of symptoms secondary to vaginal dryness, such as pain during intercourse, vaginal discharge, burning, itching, or bleeding. Genitourinary atrophy leads to a variety of symptoms that affect the ease and quality of living.

Urethritis with dysuria, stress urinary incontinence, urinary frequency and dyspareunia are further results of mucosal thinning of the urethra and bladder. Intravaginal estrogen treatment can effectively alleviate recurrent urinary tract infections and vaginal symptoms in the postmenopausal patient.[410] Oral estrogen replacement also rapidly reverses vaginal atrophy and urethral symptoms caused by estrogen deficiency.

Postmenopausal Osteoporosis

Osteoporosis is a disease characterized by low bone mass and microarchitectural deterioration of bone tissue, leading to enhanced bone fragility and a consequent increase in fracture risk. The most frequent sites of fracture are the vertebral bodies, distal radius, and femoral neck. Osteoporosis has become a global health issue. It is currently at epidemic proportions in the United States, affecting over 20 million people.[411] The majority of osteoporotic patients are postmenopausal women.

Osteoporosis in postmenopausal women is a function of both advancing age and estrogen deficiency. Seventy-five percent or more of the bone loss in women during the first 15 years after menopause is attributed to estrogen deficiency rather than to aging itself.[412,413] For the first 20 years after the cessation of ovarian estrogen secretion, postmenopausal osteoporosis accounts for a 50% reduction in trabecular bone and 30% loss of cortical bone.[412,413] Vertebral bone is especially vulnerable because the trabecular bone of the vertebral bodies is metabolically very active and decreases dramatically in amount in response to estrogen deficiency. Vertebral bone mass is already significantly decreased in perimenopausal and early postmenopausal women who have rising FSH and decreasing estrogen levels, whereas bone loss from the radius is not detected until at least a year after menopause.[413]

The risk of fracture depends on two factors: the peak bone mass achieved at maturity (at approximately age 30) and the subsequent rate of bone loss. An accelerated rate of bone loss after menopause strongly predicts an increased risk of fracture. The combination of low premenopausal bone mass and accelerated loss of bone after menopause is additive, and these individuals are at the highest risk of fracture. An increased rate of average bone loss during menopause is an indicator of lower endogenous estrogen levels possibly because postmenopausal bone loss is considerably slower in women with increased adipose tissue mass and consequent increased peripheral estrogen formation.[267]

It has been shown conclusively by numerous studies that hormone replacement started at the climacteric prevents postmenopausal bone loss.[414] Hormone replacement started at any age in a postmenopausal woman has potential beneficial effects by at least preventing additional bone loss. It should be noted, however, that the incidence of fractures or rate of height loss was not reduced during a 4-year follow-up in women starting HRT at a mean age of 66.7 (±6.7) years. More recently, WHI results revealed a decreased number of vertebral and hip fractures in the group of postmenopausal women receiving estrogen/progestin or estrogen only; this important evidence was the first from randomized trials suggesting that estrogen prevents fractures.[415,416]

POSTMENOPAUSAL HORMONE REPLACEMENT

We should point out first that postmenopausal women who have undergone a hysterectomy are given hormone replacement therapy with estrogen only (HRT-E). A progestin is added to estrogen (HRT-EP) in the postmenopausal woman with a uterus in order to prevent endometrial hyperplasia or cancer. HRT-EP is much more commonly prescribed than is HRT-E. The risks and benefits of these two regimens are distinct. Therefore, we refer to each regimen distinctly in this section.

Until the late 1990s, the most common practice was to treat all women disturbed by the symptoms of hormone deprivation (hot flashes) with estrogen and to use long-term hormonal prophylaxis against osteoporosis. The notion that HRT was cardioprotective played an important role in encouraging postmenopausal women to stay on this regimen indefinitely. Estrogens and progestins used for postmenopausal hormone replacement were among the most commonly prescribed medications in the United States. A national survey suggested that there was a significant upward trend for the use of any forms of HRT from the 1970s till the 1990s. Many women started HRT at menopause or later and remained on it. At one point, 46% of women who have experienced a natural menopause and 71% of women who have had bilateral oophorectomy reported having used postmenopausal HRT.[417] The average duration of use in the United States as of 1992 was 6.6 years, but only 20% of users had maintained treatment for at least 5 years.

As of the early 2000s, after the publication of the principal results of the two large randomized trials, the Heart and Estrogen/Progestin Replacement Study (HERS) in 1998 and the Women's Health Initiative (WHI) trial in 2002, this trend has been changed drastically.[418-420] WHI results constituted the direct cause of discontinuation of HRT in approximately 30% of postmenopausal women.[420] Thus, a discussion of HERS and WHI and how they changed our practices is warranted here. Currently, there are a number of ongoing debates regarding the applicability of results of WHI and HERS to all or various subsets of postmenopausal women. While the use of HRT has dramatically decreased, these influential studies raise a number of important issues that will require further studies to address. We expect that more epidemiologic and experimental studies will clarify some of these debated issues by the next edition of this book.

WHI is a tremendously important contribution to our understanding of menopausal therapy. Most, although not all, earlier cohort, retrospective, and prospective observational studies have demonstrated significant, 40% to 60% reductions in coronary heart disease (CHD) in postmenopausal women taking HRT-E only or combined HRT-EP. These studies also showed reductions in all-cause mortality and osteoporotic fractures, but showed increases in risk of breast cancer on the order of 20% to 30%. Several similar studies have demonstrated reduced incidence of Alzheimer's-type dementia in women who had used HRT-EP versus women who did not. Given the inherent biases that confound observational studies, randomized clinical trials are needed to establish whether HRT protects against cardiovascular disease (CVD) or dementias. The HERS and other secondary prevention studies demonstrated no benefit in women with known CVD initiating HRT 8 to 23 years beyond the menopause. In the WHI hormone trials, in women with no prior history of clinical CVD, HRT-EP (combined conjugated equine estrogens [CEEs] and medroxyprogesterone acetate [MPA]) started an average of 12 years after menopause increased CHD risk slightly and nonsignificantly, whereas E-alone (CEEs given without MPA) did not increase CHD risk, but failed to significantly reduce it. There were modest increases in thromboembolic disease and stroke in both trials and a borderline statistically significant increase in breast cancer only in the E-plus-P arm of the WHI. Cognitive evaluation of women older than 65 in the WHI cohort demonstrated increases in incidence of new dementia and no difference in overall rates of cognitive decline. It was concluded that the overall risk/benefit ratio for HRT was unfavorable. Results from WHI indicate that the combined postmenopausal hormones CEEs, 0.625 mg/day, plus MPA, 2.5 mg/day, should not be initiated or continued for the primary prevention of CHD. In addition, the substantial risks for CVD and breast cancer must be weighed against the benefit for fracture protection in selecting from the available agents to prevent osteoporosis.

Historic Perspective of Scientific Studies Regarding HRT Use

As of the 1950s, a growing notion among physicians and their patients held that replacing the estrogen lost at menopause would prevent many of the manifestations of aging, including CHD, osteoporotic fractures, and a decline in cognitive and sexual function. This led to widespread use of HRT-E after menopause. Other evidence in support of CHD benefit was also consistent: observational studies showed less cases of heart disease among women taking estrogen, pathophysiologic mechanisms provided biologic plausibility, and clinical trials revealed improvements in blood lipid levels and other surrogate measures.[421]

The most commonly used form of HRT-E was CEEs. In the 1980s, it was recognized that postmenopausal HRT-E treatment was causing endometrial cancer. Although uncommon and usually curable, this cancer could be prevented by antagonizing the estrogen with a progestin, and several estrogen plus progestin combinations (HRT-EP) were explored in the search for one that preserved the benefits of estrogen. In the 1990s, after it was demonstrated that lipid effects remained largely favorable when conjugated estrogens were combined with medroxyprogesterone acetate (MPA), this particular estrogen plus progestin (CEEs + MPA) regimen became the most widely used in the United States for postmenopausal women with a uterus.[421]

In the late 1980s and 1990s, it also became apparent that HRT-EP increased the breast cancer incidence.[422] This increase, however, was significant but minimal. In view of HRT's perceived cardiovascular benefits and bone-protective effects, many women and their clinicians still considered the overall benefit largely to exceed the risk.[421]

In 1998, the HERS, the first major randomized trial of HRT unexpectedly found an increase in CHD events during the first year, and no overall cardiovascular benefit with longer follow-up, when HRT-EP was compared with placebo in 2763 women with prior coronary disease.[423] This trial also found that HRT-EP caused venous thromboembolism. In 2002, the WHI HRT-EP trial was interrupted prematurely because of a perceived net harm.[415] Among 16,608 healthy postmenopausal women with a uterus, HRT-EP caused an increased risk of coronary events, stroke, breast cancer, and pulmonary embolism. A global index formulated by the authors found these harmful outcomes to outweigh the decreased risk of hip fracture and colon cancer (Table 16–10). A following report showing a significant twofold increase in dementia among WHI women older than 65 years accentuated these concerns.[424] Results from HERS and WHI led the FDA to require a warning of potential harm and to recommend that estrogen preparations not be used to prevent CHD or be considered first-line therapy for prevention of osteoporosis. In view of these WHI study findings, a number of professional societies changed their guidelines to recommend that hormone therapy not be used for preventing disease, and when used for treating symptoms that it be at the lowest dose and for the shortest time possible.

Women and their clinicians anxiously awaited the results of the WHI HRT-E trial in 10,739 healthy women with hysterectomy who were randomly assigned to receive CEEs only or placebo.[416] As in the HERS and WHI HRT-EP trials, HRT-E did not reduce the risk of CHD, although early CHD harm, which may be a consequence of progestin, appeared less pronounced.[416] The risks from HRT as derived from the three randomized trials (HERS, WHI HRT-EP, and WHI HRT-E) may be summarized as the following. It should be underscored that these risks are statistically significant but minimal.

TABLE 16–10 HAZARD RATIOS FROM 3 HORMONE THERAPY TRIALS

Clinical Event	HAZARD RATIO (95% CONFIDENCE INTERVAL)		
	HERS (Estrogen + Progestin)	WHI (Estrogen + Progestin)	WHI Estrogen Alone
CHD events	0.99 (0.80-1.22)	1.29 (1.02-1.63)	0.91 (0.75-1.12)
Stroke	1.23 (0.89-1.70)	1.41 (1.07-1.85)	1.39 (1.10-1.77)
Pulmonary embolism	2.79 (0.89-8.75)	2.13 (1.39-3.25)	1.34 (0.87-2.06)
Breast cancer	1.30 (0.77-2.19)	1.26 (1.00-1.59)	0.77 (0.59-1.01)
Colon cancer	0.69 (0.32-1.49)	0.63 (0.43-0.92)	1.08 (0.75-1.55)
Hip fracture	1.10 (0.49-2.50)	0.66 (0.45-0.98)	0.61 (0.41-0.91)
Death	1.08 (0.84-1.38)	0.98 (0.82-1.18)	1.04 (0.88-1.22)
Global index†	. . .	1.15 (1.03-1.28)	1.01 (.91-1.12)

CHD, Coronary heart disease; *HERS*, Heart and Estrogen/Progestin Replacement Study; *WHI*, Women's Health Initiative.
*Data are based on the intent-to-treat analysis. For the primary CHD events, outcome (myocardial interaction plus CHD death), the three trials had similar numbers of events and thus similar power. For the other outcomes, the smaller HERS trial had fewer events and less precise hazard ratios.
†The global index was composed of the first occurrence of any of the events listed in the table.

Risks and Contraindications of Hormone Replacement Therapy

Coronary Heart Disease

Given the absence of evidence in all three trials that these hormone regimens prevent CHD in these populations, the previously available evidence in favor of HRT was probably misleading (see Table 16–10). HRT-EP or HRT-E does not prevent CHD as previously proposed. To the contrary, there may be a small but significant increase in CHD in women taking HRT-EP.[415,423] Both women with preexisting CHD and healthy women are at risk. HRT-E, on the other hand, does not increase the risk for healthy women.[416]

Stroke

Another outcome that is consistent across the three trials is the increased risk of stroke among women assigned to HRT-E or HRT-EP. Increased stroke is possibly attributable to the estrogen component of the hormone regimen, since it is the only statistically significant adverse effect of HRT-E.[415,416,423]

Pulmonary Embolism

A pattern of increased risk for pulmonary embolism was observed in all three studies, although the risk was attenuated and not statistically significant in the WHI HRT-E trial.[415,416,423]

Breast Cancer

The findings of the WHI HRT-E trial differed markedly from the findings of the HERS and WHI HRT-EP trials with respect to the breast cancer risk[415,416,423]. In the estrogen plus progestin trials (HERS and WHI HRT-EP), the risk for breast cancer was increased about 25%, and in the estrogen-only trial (WHI HRT-E) it was reduced by 23%. Numerous lines of evidence support an increased risk for breast cancer with estrogen exposure, including cell culture studies, animal models, many observational studies, and the fact that estrogen antagonists reduce the risk of developing breast cancer in healthy women. Thus, this discrepancy was somewhat surprising. Nonetheless, the higher risk for breast cancer observed in the estrogen plus progestin trials probably represents a harmful effect of the MPA. The increased risk was statistically significant in WHI HRT-EP. This was matched by a trend of the same magnitude in HERS and supported by evidence from large observational studies suggesting that the addition of MPA or another progestin to estrogen may significantly increase risk for breast cancer (see Table 16–10).

Ovarian Cancer

A retrospective 1979–1998 cohort study of 44,241 postmenopausal women revealed that HRT-E, particularly for 10 or more years, significantly increased risk for ovarian cancer. Relative risks for 10 to 19 years and 20 or more years were 1.8 (95% CI, 1.1 to 3.0) and 3.2 (95% CI, 1.7 to 5.7), respectively (*P*-value for trend <0.001). This study did not show an increased risk in women who used short-term HRT-EP, but authors suggested that risk associated with longer term HRT-EP warrants further investigation.[425] The WHI HRT-EP study found a trend for increased ovarian cancer risk, which was not significant.[416]

Dementia

In postmenopausal women 65 years of age or older, HRT-EP significantly increased risk and resulted in an additional 23 cases of probable dementia per 10,000 women per year.[426] Alzheimer's disease was the most common classification of dementia. A similar trend was observed in the HRT-E group, although this did not reach statistical significance.[426] When the data were pooled, HRT significantly increased probable dementia risk.[426]

Hyperlipidemia

This rare side effect is observed in patients with severe familial hypertriglyceridemia. An oral estrogen regimen can hasten severe hypertriglyceridemia or pancreatitis in women with severely elevated triglyceride levels.[427] Therefore, estrogen replacement is a relative contraindication in women with substantially increased triglyceride levels.

Gallbladder Disease

Both WHI trials (HRT-E and HRT-EP) trials showed greater risk of any gallbladder disease or surgery with estrogen.[428] Both trials indicated a higher risk for cholecystitis and for cholelithiasis. Also, these women undergoing either HRT regimen were more likely to receive cholecystectomy.[428] These data suggest an increase in risk of biliary tract disease among postmenopausal women using estrogen therapy. The morbidity and cost associated with these outcomes may need to be considered in decisions regarding the use of estrogen therapy. Preexisting gallbladder disease is a relative contraindication for estrogen replacement.

Benefits of Hormone Replacement Therapy

Hot Flash

HRT-E or HRT-EP reliably treats hot flashes in most women. Currently, hot flash is the most common indication of a short course of HRT (<5 years).

Fractures

Both HRT-EP and HRT-E significantly decreased hip, vertebral, and other osteoporotic fractures[415,416]. In this instance, results of observational studies of estrogen and fracture risk and trials using a surrogate end-point (bone mineral density) agree with the results of clinical trials of fracture prevention.

Colon Cancer

Colon cancer was significantly less common with hormone treatment in the WHI HRT-EP study but not in WHI HRT-E for reasons that are not clear.[415,416] It is possible that progestin is the protective hormone in this case.

Other Results

Negative WHI results relevant to previously postulated benefits of HRT. HRT-EP (WHI) resulted in no significant effects on general health, vitality, mental health, depressive symptoms, or sexual satisfaction.[429] The use of estrogen plus progestin was associated with a statistically significant but small and not clinically meaningful benefit in terms of sleep disturbance, physical functioning, and bodily pain after 1 year. At 3 years, there were no significant benefits in terms of any quality-of-life outcomes. Among women 50 to 54 years of age with moderate-to-severe vasomotor symptoms at baseline, HRT-EP improved hot flashes and resulted in a small benefit in terms of sleep disturbance but no benefit in terms of the other quality-of-life outcomes.[429] The group that received HRT-E (WHI) also did not have a meaningful improvement in health-related quality of life after 1 or 3 years.[430]

HRT-EP (WHI) did not improve cognitive function, as previously anticipated.[424] The group receiving HRT-E showed a trend for worsened mild cognitive impairment, although this was not significant[426]. Among postmenopausal women aged 65 years or older, HRT-EP did not improve cognitive function when compared with placebo, whereas HRT-E had an adverse effect on cognition, which was greater among women with low cognitive function at initiation of treatment.[431,432]

Interpretation of the Results of WHI and HERS in a Broader Perspective

The mean age of participants in all three randomized trials was in the mid-60s, raising the concern that these results may not apply to treatment begun early in menopause.[415,416,423] In this regard, the WHI HRT-E trial found that the subgroup of women in the youngest decade (50 to 59 years of age) appeared to respond to estrogen more favorably than older women for many of the outcomes, including the global index. However, the differences in hazard ratios among subgroups were statistically significant for only 1 of 23 tests and could well have occurred by chance.[416]

Even if hazard ratios are similar in women of all ages, the absolute risks differ substantially. In general, absolute risk for many diseases approximately doubles with each decade of age. Thus, women in their 50s have about half the risk of women in their 60s and one-fourth the risk of women in their 70s. This means that any effect of hormone therapy on these diseases will be less marked in younger than in older women. The possibility of more favorable findings in 50- to 59-year-old women and the low absolute risk of adverse outcomes in this age group both suggest that use of HRT-E to treat menopausal symptoms for a limited duration early in menopause is reasonable.

WHI trials suggest that HRT-E has advantages over HRT-EP for treating postmenopausal women—it has only one or two adverse outcomes (increased strokes and probably pulmonary emboli) rather than four (increased strokes, CHD, pulmonary emboli, and breast cancer), and both regimens have an important benefit (decreased fractures). However, this risk/benefit assessment does not take into account the dementia findings, and even in their absence, HRT-E produced no improvement in the overall global index. In addition, HRT-E in women with a uterus increases the risk of uterine cancer and rates of uterine bleeding, biopsy, and hysterectomy. As more deliberate and exhaustive analyses of these trials become available, they will likely contribute to new practice guidelines.

Finally, there is considerable debate regarding the type of estrogen and mode of administration. Estradiol might have advantages over CEEs and transdermal administration by avoiding high levels in the portal circulation, and delivery to the liver may have advantages over oral delivery.[433] New trials are under way employing transdermal estradiol.[434]

Post-WHI Recommendations for Hormone Replacement Therapy

HRT is effective for treating hot flashes, and for this indication HRT-E seems to be associated with less risk compared with HRT-EP. However, HRT-E does have adverse effects, and it remains prudent to keep the dose low and the duration of treatment short. A reasonable option may be continuous treatment with low-dose transdermal estradiol and administration of progestins periodically at long intervals (e.g., 15 days of progestin treatment every 3 to 6 months instead of monthly as conventionally administered). The long-term safety profile of this new regimen is unknown. Most postmenopausal women stop HRT within several years after the initiation of therapy because hot flashes may decrease or disappear at this time. Most clinicians believe that, upon the cessation of HRT that had lasted several years, hot flashes usually do not return or are less severe than during the climacteric.[435,436]

In the absence of evidence for an overall net benefit of postmenopausal treatment with HRT-E, and with the evidence that HRT-EP is harmful, neither therapy should be used for preventing cardiovascular disease (CVD) or improving mental function. Although it is possible that other forms or doses of hormones could be more beneficial, these benefits must be demonstrated in disease end-point trials before any hormone regimen can be recommended for disease prevention.

Target Groups for HRT

In women with gonadal dysgenesis and surgical menopause, the duration of estrogen deprivation is prolonged. Estrogen replacement is recommended for these patients for the reduction of hot flashes and for long-term prophylaxis against cardiovascular disease, osteoporosis, and target organ atrophy. A low-dose contraceptive may be offered to nonsmoking women until the age of 45. After this age, doses of estrogen equivalent to 0.625 mg of conjugated estrogens may be more appropriate because of a sharp age-related increase in risk for thromboembolic events. The clinician should recommend a continuous estrogen-progestin combination to those with a uterus and an estrogen-only regimen to women without a uterus.

During the climacteric, hot flashes can be suppressed with an estrogen-progestin combination. Because bone loss related to estrogen deprivation also begins during this period, a benefit for the women who take HRT to prevent hot flashes is that bone loss does not start for the few years of that therapy.[437] In climacteric women, unexplained uterine bleeding should be evaluated with an endometrial biopsy before the start of hormone replacement.

Estrogen Preparations and Beneficial Dose of Estrogen

The amount of estrogen that is effective for hot flashes varies. For this purpose, it is reasonable to start with CEEs 0.3 mg/day (or transdermal estradiol 0.025 mg/day) and gradually increase this dose to CEEs 0.625 mg/day (equivalent to transdermal estradiol 0.05 mg/day) and CEEs 1.25 mg/day (equivalent to transdermal estradiol 0.1 mg/day). If hot flashes in a postmenopausal woman are not alleviated by 1.25 mg/day CEEs or an equivalent transdermal estradiol dose, it is very unlikely that higher doses will be effective. In this case, alternative diagnoses (e.g., tuberculosis, depression) should be ruled out.

Low-dosage estrogen (CEEs 0.3 mg/day or transdermal estradiol 0.025 mg/day) maintains blood estradiol levels between 17 to 32 pg/mL (average 22 pg/mL) and may be sufficient for preserving bone density and for alleviating menopausal symptoms in early postmenopausal women.[438] The effect of estrogen on arterial thrombosis is probably dose-related.[438] For example, oral contraceptives with higher doses of estrogen are more likely to be associated with increased risks for myocardial infarction and stroke, especially in smokers. Thus, when choosing a dose for HRT, it is imperative to achieve and maintain the lowest beneficial levels of circulating estradiol and avoid higher levels to minimize the risk for thrombosis.

The addition of a progestin, either cyclically or continuously, to concomitant estrogen replacement reduces the risk for estrogen-induced endometrial hyperplasia or carcinoma but poses additional problems.[439] These problems include regular withdrawal bleeding in up to 90% of women treated with cyclic therapy and irregular spotting in 20% of women treated with continuous estrogen plus progestin. Furthermore, progestins appear to reduce the beneficial effects of estrogen on HDL and LDL cholesterol and increase the risks for pulmonary embolism, CHD, and breast cancer.[415,416,423]

A time-honored sequential regimen involves oral administration of 0.625 mg of CEEs or the equivalent doses of a variety of available products from day 1 to 25 of each month (Fig. 16–37). A daily dose of 10 mg of medroxyprogesterone acetate is added from day 12 to 25 or from day 16 to 25. Withdrawal bleeding is expected on or after day 26 of each month. Another common cyclic regimen involves continuous oral administration of 0.625 mg of conjugated estrogens or the equivalent daily dose (see Fig. 16–37). A daily dose of 5 to 10 mg of medroxyprogesterone acetate is added for the first 10 to 14 days of every month. One-year randomized trial data indicate that the 5-mg dose protects the endometrium as well as the 10-mg dose.[440] Progestin withdrawal bleeding occurs in 90% of women with a sequential or cyclic regimen.[441,442] These regimens can also cause adverse symptoms related to the relatively high daily doses of progestin, such as breast tenderness, bloating, fluid retention,

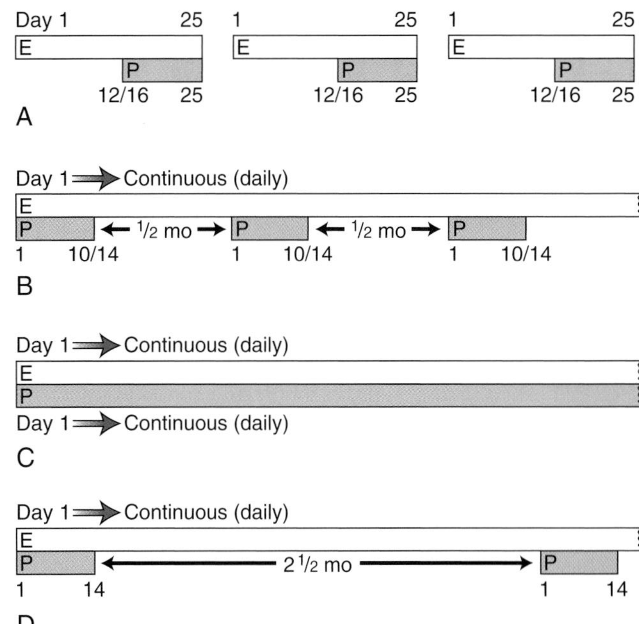

Figure 16–37 ■ Regimens of hormone replacement therapy.[403] Estrogen (E) is replaced in a postmenopausal woman to prevent osteoporosis, urogenital atrophy, and hot flashes. In the postmenopausal woman with a uterus, a progestin (P) needs to be added to estrogen to prevent endometrial hyperplasia and cancer. E and P can be administered in a number of ways. **A** and **B,** The postmenopausal women receiving hormone replacement have predictable withdrawal bleeding episodes after each P course. **C,** These women take E and P together continuously. After a year of continuous combination therapy, the rate of unpredictable breakthrough spotting is 20%. **D,** This is a relatively new regimen introduced to minimize the harmful effects of a progestin. Its long-term safety for endometrial hyperplasia/cancer risk is not known. Predictable bleeding after each progestin course every 3 months is presumed to be reassuring.

and depression. Thus, the lowest possible dose of a progestin is recommended.

The continuous combined method of treatment, on the other hand, has the potential benefit of reduced bleeding and amenorrhea but is occasionally complicated by breakthrough bleeding (see Fig. 16–37).[441,442] In this regimen, a combination of 0.625 mg of conjugated estrogens and 2.5 mg of medroxyprogesterone acetate is given orally every day. The continuous combination regimen is simple, convenient, and associated with a higher incidence of amenorrhea in 80% of patients after at least 6 months of use. The rest of the patients continue to experience some degree of unpredictable spotting. Thus, overall compliance is much better in users of the continuous combination regimen. Moreover, the lower daily dose of medroxyprogesterone acetate is associated with a lower incidence of breast tenderness with this regimen. Other estrogen-progestin combinations are also available for similar continuous use.

In addition to the continuous daily addition of progestin and addition of monthly cyclic progestin, cyclic progestin has been used at less frequent intervals—for example, every 3 to 6 months. When added to standard dosage estrogen, the addition of 10 mg of MPA every 3 months for 14 days produced a 1.5% rate of hyperplasia (a rate low enough to be interpreted as endometrial protection), and long-term use of MPA at 6-month intervals was associated with a low rate of endometrial cancer. However, clinicians have not determined the optimum progestin dosage and schedule to use together with low-dosage estrogen. Low-dosage estrogen use can reasonably be assumed to require less progestin for protecting the endometrium.

Most postmenopausal women can switch their HRT regimen from standard dosage HRT to low-dosage estrogen with MPA added at 3-month intervals or start HRT at this low-dose.[438] Although its long-term safety has not been proven with respect to endometrial hyperplasia, the following regimen appears to be a reasonable compromise for treating hot flashes and preventing osteoporosis while minimizing the harmful effects of progestins and high-dose estrogen:[438] CEEs 0.3 mg day or transdermal estradiol 0.025 mg are administered continuously. Every 3 months, a 14-day course of 5 mg of medroxyprogesterone acetate should be added to this regimen (see Fig. 16–37D). Endometrial biopsy is not required in the presence of withdrawal bleeding after each periodic progestin intake and in the absence of irregular bleeding. This regimen may be continued for up to 5 years. After discontinuation of HRT, the postmenopausal woman can be switched to a bisphosphonate or a selective estrogen receptor modulator (SERM) for bone protection.

Management of Breakthrough Bleeding during Postmenopausal Hormone Replacement

Approximately 90% of women receiving estrogen plus cyclic administration of a progestin have monthly progestin withdrawal bleeding in a predictable fashion, whereas continuous combined estrogen-progestin therapy causes breakthrough bleeding in approximately 40% of women during the first 6 months. (The rest of the women with a continuous combination regimen are amenorrheic.) The pattern of vaginal bleeding in the continuous regimen is unpredictable and causes anxiety in most patients. Fortunately, the incidence of breakthrough bleeding with the continuous combined regimen decreases to 20% after 1 year of treatment.[441-443] Breakthrough bleeding with the combined continuous regimen remains the most important reason for discontinuance of this therapy. Most patients find it unacceptable and prefer to switch to a cyclic progestin regimen or discontinue hormone replacement altogether. There is no effective pharmacologic method to manage the breakthrough bleeding associated with continuous combined estrogen-progestin regimens. One can only reassure the patient that the bleeding is likely to subside within a year from the start of HRT. If breakthrough bleeding continues beyond a year, the regimen should be changed to daily estrogen plus cyclic progestin.

HRT can be started in the amenorrheic postmenopausal patient at any time. Perimenopausal women with oligomenorrhea, hot flashes, or other associated symptoms can also be treated with HRT. In the oligomenorrheic patient, a hormone replacement regimen can be initiated on day 3 of one of the infrequent menses. If the candidate for hormone replacement does not have irregular uterine bleeding, it is not essential to perform endometrial biopsies routinely before beginning treatment. Studies indicate that asymptomatic postmenopausal women rarely have endometrial abnormalities.[443-445] Pretreatment biopsies using a thin plastic biopsy cannula in the office may be limited to patients at higher risk for endometrial hyperplasia (e.g., unpredictable uterine bleeding, history of PCOS or chronic anovulation, obesity, liver disease, and diabetes mellitus).

Giving a woman a combined estrogen-progestin regimen does not preclude the development of endometrial cancer.[446] It is, therefore, necessary to rule out endometrial malignancy in women receiving HRT who are experiencing irregular uterine bleeding. The important task is to differentiate breakthrough bleeding from bleeding induced by hyperplasia or cancer. Because breakthrough bleeding is extremely common, a large number of biopsies would have to be performed to detect a rare case of endometrial abnormality during HRT. In order to decrease the number of endometrial biopsies, a screening method using transvaginal ultrasonography has been introduced.[172] The thickness of the postmenopausal endometrium as measured by transvaginal ultrasonography in postmenopausal women correlates with the presence or absence of pathology.[172] Patients receiving either a cyclic or daily combination hormone replacement regimen who have an endometrial thickness less than 5 mm can be managed conservatively.[447-449] An endometrial thickness equal to or greater than 5 mm requires biopsy. Following this algorithm, it is estimated that 50% to 75% of bleeding patients receiving HRT and evaluated by ultrasonography require biopsy.[172]

Hormone Replacement Therapy after a Diagnosis of Breast Cancer

HRT is typically withheld from women with breast cancer because of concerns that estrogen may stimulate recurrence. Surprisingly, a number of relatively small studies showed either unaltered or lower risks of recurrence and mortality in women who used HRT after a diagnosis of breast cancer compared with nonusers.[450,451] HRT in most of these small studies was started after at least a 5-year disease-free interval.[450,451] On the basis of these insufficient but encouraging data, a decision to provide HRT is dependent on the choice of the individual patient. In these patients, tamoxifen, raloxifene, or a bisphosphonate represents a viable alternative to estrogen replacement for long-term prophylaxis against osteoporosis.

Selective Estrogen Receptor Modulators and Bisphosphonates as Alternatives to Hormone Replacement Therapy

(See Chapter 28)

Selective estrogen receptor modulators (SERMs) are compounds that act like estrogen in some target tissues but antagonize estrogenic effects in others.[452] One of the first SERMs was tamoxifen, for which estrogen-like agonist activity on bone was observed to occur simultaneously with estrogen antagonist activity on the breast.[453] An unwanted effect of tamoxifen is its estrogen-like action on the endometrium. Second-generation compounds have since been developed, most notably raloxifene, which has estrogen-like actions on bone, lipids, and the coagulation system; estrogen antagonist effects on the breast; and no detectable action in the endometrium.[454]

In randomized placebo-controlled studies involving postmenopausal women or patients with osteoporosis, raloxifene at 60 to 150 mg/day was effective in increasing bone mineral density over 12 to 36 months.[454] In another randomized study, raloxifene reduced the risk for invasive breast cancer.[455] Raloxifene also decreased the risk for vertebral fractures, but it had no effect on the risk for nonvertebral fractures.[455] Raloxifene is similar to placebo in its endometrial effects and similar to estrogen in causing a twofold to threefold increase in the risk for venous thromboembolism and stroke.[455,456] The propensity of raloxifene to cause hot flashes precludes its use in women with vasomotor symptoms.[457]

Another randomized study was performed to compare the tamoxifen with raloxifene with respect to breast cancer prevention. Raloxifene was as effective as tamoxifen in reducing the risk for invasive breast cancer and has a lower risk of thromboembolic events and cataracts but a nonstatistically significant higher risk for noninvasive breast cancer. The risk for other cancers (including uterine cancer), fractures, ischemic heart disease, and stroke is similar for both drugs.[458] Thus, both tamoxifen and raloxifene may be used to reduce the incidence of vertebral fractures and invasive breast cancer. The major drawbacks include hot flashes and increased thromboembolic events for both drugs.

The bisphosphonates are widely prescribed antiresorptive agents and are effective therapy for the treatment of postmenopausal osteoporosis. These agents suppress resorption by inhibiting the attachment of osteoclasts to bone matrix and enhancing programmed cell death in osteoclasts. First-generation bisphosphonates include etidronate and clodronate; neither drug is approved for the treatment of osteoporosis. Alendronate (5 to 10 mg/day or 35 to 70 mg/week) and risedronate (5 mg/day or 30 to 35 mg/week), two second-generation bisphosphonates, have been shown in randomized trials to increase bone mineral density in postmenopausal women with osteopenia or osteoporosis; in women with osteoporosis, they have been shown to reduce the incidence of hip, vertebral, and nonvertebral fractures by nearly 50%, particularly during the first year of treatment.[459] Both alendronate and risedronate have been approved by the FDA for the treatment or prevention of postmenopausal osteoporosis.[459]

Alendronate can be administered for at least 7 years without adversely affecting bone strength.[459] Moreover, discontinuation of long-term (5 years or more) alendronate therapy results in minimal bone loss over the ensuing 3 to 5 years. Alendronate or risedronate once weekly has been shown to reduce the rate of drug-induced esophagitis, as compared with daily doses.[460] In a recent 1-year head-to-head study, alendronate increased spine and hip bone mineral density slightly more than did risedronate, although the clinical significance of this finding is uncertain.[459,460] Recently, ibandronate, at a dose of 2.5 mg daily or 150 mg monthly, was approved by the FDA for both the prevention and treatment of postmenopausal osteoporosis.[461] Daily ibandronate has been shown to reduce significantly the incidence of vertebral fracture in women with osteoporosis and to reduce the incidence of nonvertebral fracture in women with severe osteoporosis.[461] Other intravenous bisphosphonates are available off-label for the treatment of osteoporosis. Intravenous pamidronate and zoledronate have been used to treat women who cannot tolerate oral bisphosphonates.[460]

REFERENCES

1. Seeburg PH, Adelman JP. Characterization of cDNA for precursor of human luteinizing hormone releasing hormone. Nature 1984;311(5987):666-668.
2. Berger SL, et al. Genetic isolation of ADA2: a potential transcriptional adaptor required for function of certain acidic activation domains. Cell 1992;70(2):251-265.
3. Seeburg PH, et al. The mammalian GnRH gene and its pivotal role in reproduction. Rec Prog Horm Res 1987;43:69-98.
4. Hayflick JS, et al. The complete nucleotide sequence of the human gonadotropin-releasing hormone gene. Nucleic Acids Res 1989;17(15):6403-6404.
5. Guerrero NV, et al. Risk factors for premature ovarian failure in females with galactosemia. J Pediatr 2000;137(6):833-841.
6. Nikolics K, et al. A prolactin-inhibiting factor within the precursor for human gonadotropin-releasing hormone. Nature 1985; 316(6028):511-517.
7. Ackland JF, et al. Molecular forms of gonadotropin-releasing hormone associated peptide (GAP): changes within the rat hypothalamus and release from hypothalamic cells in vitro. Neuroendocrinology 1988;48(4):376-386.
8. Ronnekleiv OK, et al. Combined immunohistochemistry for gonadotropin-releasing hormone (GnRH) and pro-GnRH, and in situ hybridization for GnRH messenger ribonucleic acid in rat brain. Mol Endocrinol 1989;3(2):363-371.
9. Bick D, et al. Brief report: intragenic deletion of the KALIG-1 gene in Kallmann's syndrome. N Engl J Med 1992;326(26):1752-1755.
10. Knobil E. The neuroendocrine control of the menstrual cycle. Rec Prog Horm Res 1980;36:53-88.
11. Van Vugt DA, et al. Gonadotropin-releasing hormone pulses in third ventricular cerebrospinal fluid of ovariectomized rhesus monkeys: correlation with luteinizing hormone pulses. Endocrinology 1985;117(4):1550-1558.
12. Gross KM, et al. Evidence for decreased luteinizing hormone-releasing hormone pulse frequency in men with selective elevations of follicle-stimulating hormone. J Clin Endocrinol Metab 1985;60(1):197-202.
13. Haisenleder DJ, et al. A pulsatile gonadotropin-releasing hormone stimulus is required to increase transcription of the gonadotropin subunit genes: evidence for differential regulation of transcription by pulse frequency in vivo. Endocrinology 1991; 128(1):509-517.
14. Reame NE, et al. Pulsatile gonadotropin secretion in women with hypothalamic amenorrhea: evidence that reduced frequency of gonadotropin-releasing hormone secretion is the mechanism of persistent anovulation. J Clin Endocrinol Metab 1985;61(5): 851-858.
15. Filicori M, et al. Characterization of the physiological pattern of episodic gonadotropin secretion throughout the human menstrual cycle. J Clin Endocrinol Metab 1986;62(6):1136-1144.
16. Petersen SL, et al. Direct and indirect regulation of gonadotropin-releasing hormone neurons by estradiol. Biol Reprod 2003;69(6): 1771-1778.
17. Herbison AE. Noradrenergic regulation of cyclic GnRH secretion. Rev Reprod 1997;2(1):1-6.
18. Gindoff PR, et al. Endogenous opioid peptides modulate the effect of corticotropin-releasing factor on gonadotropin release in the primate. Endocrinology 1987;121(3):837-842.
19. Rabinovici J, et al. Endocrine effects and pharmacokinetic characteristics of a potent new gonadotropin-releasing hormone antagonist (Ganirelix) with minimal histamine-releasing properties: studies in postmenopausal women. J Clin Endocrinol Metab 1992;75(5):1220-1225.
20. Shoupe D, et al. The effects of estrogen and progestin on endogenous opioid activity in oophorectomized women. J Clin Endocrinol Metab 1985;60(1):178-183.
21. Goodman RL, et al. Endogenous opioid peptides control the amplitude and shape of gonadotropin-releasing hormone pulses in the ewe. Endocrinology 1995;136(6):2412-2420.
22. Wildt L, et al. Treatment with naltrexone in hypothalamic ovarian failure: induction of ovulation and pregnancy. Hum Reprod 1993;8(3):350-358.
23. Gottsch ML, et al. Kisspeptin-GPR54 signaling in the neuroendocrine reproductive axis. Mol Cell Endocrinol 2006;254-255: 91-96.
24. Seminara SB, et al. The GPR54 gene as a regulator of puberty. N Engl J Med 2003;349(17):1614-1627.
25. de Roux N, et al. Hypogonadotropic hypogonadism due to loss of function of the KiSS1-derived peptide receptor GPR54. Proc Natl Acad Sci U S A 2003;100(19):10972-10976.
26. Messager S, et al. Kisspeptin directly stimulates gonadotropin-releasing hormone release via G protein-coupled receptor 54. Proc Natl Acad Sci U S A 2005;102(5):1761-1766.
27. Handelsman DJ, et al. Pharmacokinetics of gonadotropin-releasing hormone and its analogs. Endocr Rev 1986;7(1):95-105.
28. Galbiati M, et al. Transforming growth factor-beta and astrocytic conditioned medium influence luteinizing hormone-releasing hormone gene expression in the hypothalamic cell line GT1. Endocrinology 1996;137(12):5605-5609.
29. Karten MJ, et al. Gonadotropin-releasing hormone analog design. Structure-function studies toward the development of agonists and antagonists: rationale and perspective. Endocr Rev 1986;7(1): 44-66.
30. Lemay A, et al. Reversible hypogonadism induced by a luteinizing hormone-releasing hormone (LH-RH) agonist (Buserelin) as a new therapeutic approach for endometriosis. Fertil Steril 1984; 41(6):863-871.
31. Carr BR, et al. Oral contraceptive pills, gonadotropin-releasing hormone agonists, or use in combination for treatment of hirsutism: a clinical research center study. J Clin Endocrinol Metab 1995;80(4):1169-1178.
32. Cann CE, et al. Decreased spinal mineral content in amenorrheic women. JAMA 1984;251(5):626-629.

33. Matta WH, et al. Reversible trabecular bone density loss following induced hypo-oestrogenism with the GnRH analogue buserelin in premenopausal women. Clin Endocrinol (Oxf) 1988;29(1):45-51.
34. Surrey ES. Add-back therapy and gonadotropin-releasing hormone agonists in the treatment of patients with endometriosis: can a consensus be reached? Add-Back Consensus Working Group. Fertil Steril 1999;71(3):420-424.
35. Cetel NS, et al. The dynamics of gonadotropin inhibition in women induced by an antagonistic analog of gonadotropin-releasing hormone. J Clin Endocrinol Metab 1983;57(1):62-65.
36. Pavlou SN, et al. Single subcutaneous doses of a luteinizing hormone-releasing hormone antagonist suppress serum gonadotropin and testosterone levels in normal men. J Clin Endocrinol Metab 1986;63(2):303-308.
37. Pavlou SN, et al. Mode of suppression of pituitary and gonadal function after acute or prolonged administration of a luteinizing hormone-releasing hormone antagonist in normal men. J Clin Endocrinol Metab 1989;68(2):446-454.
38. Edelstein MC, et al. Single dose long-term suppression of testosterone secretion by a gonadotropin-releasing hormone antagonist (Antide) in male monkeys. Contraception 1990;42(2):209-214.
39. Behre HM, et al. High loading and low maintenance doses of a gonadotropin-releasing hormone antagonist effectively suppress serum luteinizing hormone, follicle-stimulating hormone, and testosterone in normal men. J Clin Endocrinol Metab 1997;82(5): 1403-1408.
40. Fujimoto VY, et al. Dose-related suppression of serum luteinizing hormone in women by a potent new gonadotropin-releasing hormone antagonist (Ganirelix) administered by intranasal spray. Fertil Steril 1997;67(3):469-473.
41. Andreyko JL, et al. Concordant suppression of serum immunoreactive luteinizing hormone (LH), follicle-stimulating hormone, alpha subunit, bioactive LH, and testosterone in postmenopausal women by a potent gonadotropin releasing hormone antagonist (detirelix). J Clin Endocrinol Metab 1992;74(2):399-405.
42. Gonzalez-Barcena D, et al. Treatment of uterine leiomyomas with luteinizing hormone-releasing hormone antagonist Cetrorelix. Hum Reprod 1997;12(9): 2028-2035.
43. Childs GV, et al. Heterogeneous luteinizing hormone and follicle-stimulating hormone storage patterns in subtypes of gonadotropes separated by centrifugal elutriation. Endocrinology 1983;113(6): 2120-2128.
44. Childs GV. Functional ultrastructure of gonadotropes: a review. Curr Top Neuroendocrinol 1986;(7):49-97.
45. Cheng CK, et al. Molecular biology of gonadotropin-releasing hormone (GnRH)-I, GnRH-II, and their receptors in humans. Endocr Rev 2005;26(2):283-306.
46. Millar RP, et al. Gonadotropin-releasing hormone receptors. Endocr Rev 2004;25(2):235-275.
47. Gharib SD, et al. Molecular biology of the pituitary gonadotropins. Endocr Rev 1990;11(1):177-199.
48. Talmadge K, et al. Evolution of the genes for the beta subunits of human chorionic gonadotropin and luteinizing hormone. Nature 1984;307(5946):37-40.
49. Jameson JL, et al. Human follicle-stimulating hormone beta-subunit gene encodes multiple messenger ribonucleic acids. Mol Endocrinol 1988;2(9):806-815.
50. Jameson L, et al. The gene encoding the beta-subunit of rat luteinizing hormone. Analysis of gene structure and evolution of nucleotide sequence. J Biol Chem 1984;259(24):15474-15480.
51. Themmen APN, et al. Mutations of gonadotropins and gonadotropin receptors: elucidating the physiology and pathophysiology of pituitary-gonadal function. Endocr Rev 2000;21(5):551-583.
52. Shupnik MA. Gonadotropin gene modulation by steroids and gonadotropin-releasing hormone. Biol Reprod 1996;54(2):279-286.
53. Abbud RA, et al. Chronic hypersecretion of luteinizing hormone in transgenic mice selectively alters responsiveness of the alpha-subunit gene to gonadotropin-releasing hormone and estrogens. Mol Endocrinol 1999;13(9):1449-1459.
54. Gregory SJ, et al. Regulation of gonadotropins by inhibin and activin. Semin Reprod Endocrinol 2004;22:253-267.
55. de Leeuw R, et al. Structure-function relationship of recombinant follicle stimulating hormone (Puregon). Mol Hum Reprod 1996;2(5):361-369.
56. Mossman KD. Comparative Morphology of the Mammalian Ovary. Wisconsin Press, Madison WI. 1973.
57. Simpson JL, et al. Ovarian differentiation and gonadal failure. Am J Med Genet 1999;89(4):186-200.
58. Di Pasquale E, et al. Hypergonadotropic ovarian failure associated with an inherited mutation of human bone morphogenetic protein-15 (BMP15) gene. Am J Hum Genet 2004;75(1):106-111.
59. Witschi E. Migration of the germ cells of human embryos from the yolk sac to the primitive gonadal folds. Carnegie Institute Contributions to Embryology No. 209 32:67-97. 1948.
60. Baker TG, et al. The fine structure of oogonia and oocytes in human ovaries. J Cell Sci 1967;2(2):213-224.
61. Shifren JL, et al. Human fetal ovaries and uteri: developmental expression of genes encoding the insulin, insulin-like growth factor I, and insulin-like growth factor II receptors. Fertil Steril 1993;59(5):1036-1040.
62. Bennett RA, et al. Immunohistochemical localization of transforming growth factor-alpha, epidermal growth factor (EGF), and EGF receptor in the human fetal ovary. J Clin Endocrinol Metab 1996;81(8):3073-3076.
63. Himelstein-Braw R, et al. Follicular atresia in the infant human ovary. J Reprod Fertil 1976;46(1):55-59.
64. Weakly JN, et al. Synaptic drive and postsynaptic inhibition: a physiological and pharmacological investigation. Proc West Pharmacol Soc 1966;9:42-44.
65. Albertini DF, et al. The appearance and structure of intercellular connections during the ontogeny of the rabbit ovarian follicle with particular reference to gap junctions. J Cell Biol 1974;63(1): 234-250.
66. Amsterdam A, et al. Hormonal regulation of cytodifferentiation and intercellular communication in cultured granulosa cells. Proc Natl Acad Sci U S A 1981;78(5):3000-3004.
67. Simon AM, et al. Female infertility in mice lacking connexin 37. Nature 1997;385(6616):525-529.
68. Zoller LC, et al. Identification of cytochrome P-450, and its distribution in the membrana granulosa of the preovulatory follicle, using quantitative cytochemistry. Endocrinology 1978;103(1):310-311.
69. Zoller LC, et al. A quantitative cytochemical study of glucose-6-phosphate dehydrogenase and delta 5-3 beta-hydroxysteroid dehydrogenase activity in the membrana granulosa of the ovulable type of follicle of the rat. Histochemistry 1979;62(2): 125-135.
70. Hillensjo T, et al. Gonadotropin releasing hormone agonists stimulate meiotic maturation of follicle-enclosed rat oocytes in vitro. Nature 1980;287(5778):145-146.
71. Lawrence TS, et al. Binding of human chorionic gonadotropin by rat cumuli oophori and granulosa cells: a comparative study. Endocrinology 1980;106(4):1114-1118.
72. Magnusson C, et al. Comparison between the progestin secretion responsiveness to gonadotrophins of rat cumulus and mural granulosa cells in vitro. Acta Endocrinol (Copenh) 1982;101(4): 611-616.
73. Ryan KJ, et al. Steroid biosynthesis by human ovarian granulosa and thecal cells. J Clin Endocrinol Metab 1966;26:46-52.
74. Rice B. Steroid hormone formation in the human ovary. IV Ovarian stromal compartment; formation of radioactive steroids. J Clin Endocrinol Metab 1966;26:593-609.
75. Erickson GF, et al. The ovarian androgen producing cells: a review of structure/function relationships. Endocr Rev 1985;6(3): 371-399.
76. Hume DA, et al. The mononuclear phagocyte system of the mouse defined by immunohistochemical localisation of antigen F4/80: macrophages associated with epithelia. Anat Rec 1984;210(3): 503-512.
77. Nakamura Y, et al. Increased number of mast cells in the dominant follicle of the cow: relationships among luteal, stromal, and hilar regions. Biol Reprod 1987;37(3):546-549.
78. Krishna A, et al. Histamine and increased ovarian blood flow mediate LH-induced superovulation in the cyclic hamster. J Reprod Fertil 1986;76(1):23-29.
79. Cavender JL, et al. Morphological studies of the microcirculatory system of periovulatory ovine follicles. Biol Reprod 1988;39(4): 989-997.
80. Takemura R, et al. Secretory products of macrophages and their physiological functions. Am J Physiol 1984;246(1 Pt 1): C1-9.

81. Reynolds H, et al. Release of estradiol from fetal bovine serum by rat thymus, spleen, kidney, lung and lung macrophage cultures. Endocrinology 1982;110(6):2213-2215.
82. Mais V, et al. The dependency of folliculogenesis and corpus luteum function on pulsatile gonadotropin secretion in cycling women using a gonadotropin-releasing hormone antagonist as a probe. J Clin Endocrinol Metab 1986;62(6):1250-1255.
83. Gougeon A. Regulation of ovarian follicular development in primates: facts and hypotheses. Endocr Rev 1996;17(2):121-155.
84. Gougeon A. Dynamics of follicular growth in the human: a model from preliminary results. Hum Reprod 1986;1(2):81-87.
85. Schipper I, et al. The follicle-stimulating hormone (FSH) threshold/window concept examined by different interventions with exogenous FSH during the follicular phase of the normal menstrual cycle: duration, rather than magnitude, of FSH increase affects follicle development. J Clin Endocrinol Metab 1998; 83(4):1292-1298.
86. Peters H, et al. The Ovary. Granada Publishing, London, Toronto, Sydney, New York. 1980:12-34.
87. Tilly JL, et al. Involvement of apoptosis in ovarian follicular atresia and postovulatory regression. Endocrinology 1991;129(5):2799-2801.
88. Bauminger A, et al. Periovulatory changes in ovarian prostaglandin formation and their hormonal control in the rat. Prostaglandins 1975;9(5):737-751.
89. Tsafriri A, et al. Physiological role of prostaglandins in the induction of ovulation. Prostaglandins 1972;2(1):1-10.
90. Espey LL. Ovarian proteolytic enzymes and ovulation. Biol Reprod 1974;10(2):216-235.
91. Bjersing L, et al. Ovulation and the mechanism of follicle rupture. IV. Ultrastructure of membrana granulosa of rabbit graafian follicles prior to induced ovulation. Cell Tissue Res 1974;153(1):1-14.
92. Beers WH, et al. Ovarian plasminogen activator: relationship to ovulation and hormonal regulation. Cell 1975;6(3):387-394.
93. Frederick JL, et al. Initiation of angiogenesis by human follicular fluid. Science 1984;224(4647):389-390.
94. Kamat BR, et al. Expression of vascular permeability factor/vascular endothelial growth factor by human granulosa and theca lutein cells. Role in corpus luteum development. Am J Pathol 1995;146(1):157-165.
95. Ohara A, et al. Functional differentiation in steroidogenesis of two types of luteal cells isolated from mature human corpora lutea of menstrual cycle. J Clin Endocrinol Metab 1987;65(6):1192-1200.
96. Carr BR, et al. The role of lipoproteins in the regulation of progesterone secretion by the human corpus luteum. Fertil Steril 1982;38:303-311.
97. Duncan WC, et al. Luteinizing hormone receptor in the human corpus luteum: lack of down-regulation during maternal recognition of pregnancy. Hum Reprod 1996;11(10):2291-2297.
98. Strauss JF 3rd, et al. Providing progesterone for pregnancy: control of cholesterol flux to the side-chain cleavage system. J Reprod Fertil Suppl 2000;55:3-12.
99. Bukovsky A, et al. Is irregular regression of corpora lutea in climacteric women caused by age-induced alterations in the "tissue control system?" Am J Reprod Immunol 1996;36(6):327-341.
100. Casper RF, et al. Induction of luteolysis in the human with a long-acting analog of luteinizing hormone-releasing factor. Science 1979;205(4404):408-410.
101. Schoonmaker et al. A receptive period for estradiol-induced luteolysis in the rhesus monkey. Endocrinology 1981;108(5): 1874-1877.
102. O'Gray J, et al. Inhibition of progesterone synthesis in vitro by prostaglandin F2a. J Reprod Fertil 1972;30(1):153-156.
103. Shikone T, et al. Apoptosis of human corpora lutea during cyclic luteal regression and early pregnancy. J Clin Endocrinol Metab 1996;81(6):2376-2380.
104. Bortolussi M, et al. Autoradiographic study of the distribution of LH(HCG) receptors in the ovary of untreated and gonadotrophin-primed immature rats. Cell Tissue Res 1977;183(3):329-342.
105. Nimrod A, et al. A specific FSH receptor in rat granulosa cells: properties of binding in vitro. Endocrinology 1976;98(1):56-64.
106. Nimrod A, et al. Appearance of LH-receptors and LH-stimulable cyclic AMP accumulation in granulosa cells during follicular maturation in the rat ovary. Biochem Biophys Res Commun 1977; 78(3):977-984.
107. Jaaskelainen K, et al. Internalization of receptor-bound human chorionic gonadotrophin in preovulatory rat granulosa cells in vivo. Acta Endocrinol (Copenh) 1983;103(3):406-412.
108. Uilenbroek JT, et al. Ovarian follicular development during the rat estrous cycle: gonadotropin receptors and follicular responsiveness. Biol Reprod 1979;20(5):1159-1165.
109. Zeleznik AJ, et al. Granulosa cell maturation in the rat: increased binding of human chorionic gonadotropin following treatment with follicle-stimulating hormone in vivo. Endocrinology 1974; 95(3):818-825.
110. Richards JS, et al. Ovarian follicular development in the rat: hormone receptor regulation by estradiol, follicle stimulating hormone and luteinizing hormone. Endocrinology 1976;99(6): 1562-1570.
111. Couse JF, et al. Estrogen receptor null mice: what have we learned and where will they lead us? Endocr Rev 1999;20(3):358-417.
112. Brandenberger AW, et al. Estrogen receptor alpha (ER-alpha) and beta (ER-beta) mRNAs in normal ovary, ovarian serous cystadenocarcinoma and ovarian cancer cell lines: down-regulation of ER-beta in neoplastic tissues. J Clin Endocrinol Metab 1998;83(3): 1025-1028.
113. Dorrington JH, et al. Estradiol-17beta biosynthesis in cultured granulosa cells from hypophysectomized immature rats; stimulation by follicle-stimulating hormone. Endocrinology 1975;97(5): 1328-1331.
114. Simpson ER, et al. Aromatase cytochrome P450, the enzyme responsible for estrogen biosynthesis. Endocr Rev 1994;15(3): 342-355.
115. Moon YS, et al. Stimulatory action of follicle-stimulating hormone on estradiol-17 beta secretion by hypophysectomized rat ovaries in organ culture. Endocrinology 1975;97(1):244-247.
116. Armstrong DT, et al. Stimulation of aromatization of exogenous and endogenous androgens in ovaries of hypophysectomized rats in vivo by follicle-stimulating hormone. Endocrinology 1976;99(4): 1144-1151.
117. Rani CS, et al. Follicle-stimulating hormone induction of luteinizing hormone receptor in cultured rat granulosa cells: an examination of the need for steroids in the induction process. Endocrinology 1981;108(4):1379-1385.
118. Bulun SE. Aromatase deficiency and estrogen resistance: from molecular genetics to clinic. Seminars in Reproductive Medicine. 18(1):31-39. 2000.
119. Richards JS, et al. Evidence that changes in tonic luteinizing hormone secretion determine the growth of preovulatory follicles in the rat. Endocrinology 1980;107(3):641-648.
120. Richards JS, et al. Effects of human chorionic gonadotropin and progesterone on follicular development in the immature rat. Endocrinology 1982;111(5):1429-1438.
121. Bogovich K, et al. Androgen biosynthesis in developing ovarian follicles: evidence that luteinizing hormone regulates thecal 17 alpha-hydroxylase and C17-20-lyase activities. Endocrinology 1982;111(4):1201-1208.
122. Barlow JJ, et al. Estradiol production after ovariectomy for carcinoma of the breast. N Engl J Med 1969;280(12):633-637.
123. Baird D, et al. Concentration of estrone and estradiol-17beta in follicular fluid and ovarian venous blood of women. Clin Endocrinol (Oxf) 1969;4(3):259-266.
124. Hemsell DL, et al. Plasma precursors of estrogen. II. Correlation of the extent of conversion of plasma androstenedione to estrone with age. J Clin Endocrin Metab 1974;38:476-479.
125. Bulun SE, et al. Competitive reverse transcription-polymerase chain reaction analysis indicates that levels of aromatase cytochrome P450 transcripts in adipose tissue of buttocks, thighs, and abdomen of women increase with advancing age. J Clin Endocrinol Metab 1994;78(2):428-432.
126. Bulun SE, et al. Aromatase in aging women. Semin Reprod Endocrinol 1999;17(4):349-358.
127. Mahendroo MS, et al. Male and female isoenzymes of steroid 5alpha-reductase. Rev Reprod 1999;4(3):179-183.
128. Hinshelwood MM, et al. Expression of LRH-1 and SF-1 in the mouse ovary: localization in different cell types correlates with differing function. Mol Cell Endocrinol 2003;207(1-2): 39-45.
129. Falender AE, et al. Differential expression of steroidogenic factor-1 and FTF/LRH-1 in the rodent ovary. Endocrinology 2003;144(8): 3598-3610.

130. Peng N, et al. The role of the orphan nuclear receptor, liver receptor homologue-1, in the regulation of human corpus luteum 3beta-hydroxysteroid dehydrogenase type II. J Clin Endocrinol Metab 2003;88(12):6020-6028.
131. Simpson ER, et al. Aromatase cytochrome P450, the enzyme responsible for estrogen biosynthesis. Endocr Rev 1994;15: 342-355.
132. Siiteri PK, et al. Role of extraglandular estrogen in human endocrinology. In Greep RO, Astwood EB, eds. Handbook of Physiology, Vol 2. Washington, DC: American Physiological Society, 1973:619-629.
133. Peltoketo H, et al. 17B- Hydroxysteroid dehydrogenase (HSD)/ 17-ketosteroid reductase (KSR) family; nomenclature and main characteristics of the 17HSD/KSR enzymes. J Mol Endocr 1999; 23:1-11.
134. Merriam GR, et al. Catechol estrogens and the control of gonadotropin and prolactin secretion in man. J Steroid Biochem 1983;19(1B):619-625.
135. Miller WL, et al. Molecular pathology and mechanism of action of the steroidogenic acute regulatory protein, StAR. J Steroid Biochem Mol Biol 1999;69:131-141.
136. Pollack SE, et al. Localization of the steroidogenic acute regulatory protein in human tissues. J Clin Endocrinol Metab 1997;82(12): 4243-4251.
137. Ying SY. Inhibins, activins, and follistatins: gonadal proteins modulating the secretion of follicle-stimulating hormone. Endocr Rev 1988;9(2):267-293.
138. Leers-Sucheta S, et al. Synergistic activation of the human type II 3beta-hydroxysteroid dehydrogenase/delta5-delta4 isomerase promoter by the transcription factor steroidogenic factor-1/adrenal 4-binding protein and phorbol ester. J Biol Chem 1997;272(12): 7960-7967.
139. Hanley NA, et al. Steroidogenic factor 1 (SF-1) is essential for ovarian development and function. Mol Cell Endocrinol 2000; 163(1-2):27-32.
140. Weck J, et al. Switching of NR5A proteins associated with the inhibin (alpha)-subunit gene promoter following activation of the gene in granulosa cells. Mol Endocrinol 2006;20(5):1090-1103.
141. Jaatinen TA, et al. Expression of inhibin alpha, beta A and beta B messenger ribonucleic acids in the normal human ovary and in polycystic ovarian syndrome. J Endocrinol 1994;143(1):127-137.
142. Roberts VJ, et al. Expression of inhibin/activin subunits and follistatin messenger ribonucleic acids and proteins in ovarian follicles and the corpus luteum during the human menstrual cycle. J Clin Endocrinol Metab 1993;77(5):1402-1410.
143. Eramaa M, et al. Regulation of inhibin alpha- and beta A-subunit messenger ribonucleic acid levels by chorionic gonadotropin and recombinant follicle-stimulating hormone in cultured human granulosa-luteal cells. J Clin Endocrinol Metab 1994;79(6): 1670-1677.
144. Groome NP, et al. Measurement of dimeric inhibin B throughout the human menstrual cycle. J Clin Endocrinol Metab 1996;81(4): 1401-1405.
145. Adashi EY. The IGF family and folliculogenesis. J Reprod Immunol 1998;39(1-2):13-19.
146. Dunaif A. Insulin resistance and the polycystic ovary syndrome: mechanism and implications for pathogenesis. Endocr Rev 1997;18(6):774-800.
147. Sasano H, et al. Aromatase and 17beta-hydroxysteroid dehydrogenase type 1 in human breast carcinoma. J Clin Endocrinol Metab 1996;81:4042-4046.
148. Zeitoun KM, et al. Deficient 17beta-hydroxysteroid dehydrogenase type 2 expression in endometriosis: failure to metabolize estradiol-17alpha. J Clin Endocrinol Metab 1998;83:4474-4480.
149. Bulun SE, et al. Expression of dioxin related trans-activating factors and target genes in human endometrium and endometriosis. Am J Obstet Gynecol 2000;182:767-775.
150. Bulun SE, et al. Endocrine disorders associated with inappropriately high aromatase expression. J Steroid Biochem Mol Biol 1997;61:133-139.
151. Azziz R, et al. Idiopathic hirsutism. Endocr Rev 2000;21(4): 347-362.
152. Psychoyos A. Uterine receptivity for nidation. Ann N Y Acad Sci 1986;476:36-42.
153. Wynn RM. Histology and ultrastructure of the human endometrium. In Wynn RM, ed. Biology of the Uterus. New York: Plenum Press, 1977:341-376.
154. Markee JE. Menstruation in intraocular endometrial transplants in the rhesus monkey. Carnegie Institute Coutributions to Embryology 1940;28:219-308.
155. Markee J. Morphological basis for menstrual bleeding: relation of regression to the initiation of bleeding. Bull N Y Acad Med 1948;24(253-268).
156. Bartelmez GW. The phases of the menstrual cycle and their interpretation in terms of the pregnancy cycle. Am J Obstet Gynecol 1957;74:931-955.
157. Eckert R, et al. Human endometrial cells in primary tissue culture: modulation of the progesterone receptor level by natural and synthetic estrogens in vitro. J Clin Endocrinol Metab 1981;52: 699-708.
158. Cooke PS, et al. Stromal estrogen receptors mediate mitogenic effects of estradiol on uterine epithelium. PNAS 1997;94: 6535-6540.
159. Kurita T, et al. Stromal progesterone receptors mediate the inhibitory effects of progesterone on estrogen-induced uterine epithelial cell deoxyribonucleic acid synthesis. Endocrinology 1998;139: 4708-4713.
160. Yang S, et al. Stromal progesterone receptors mediate induction of 17beta-hydroxysteroid dehydrogenase type 2 expression in human endometrial epithelium: a paracrine mechanism for inactivation of estradiol. Mol Endocrinol 2001;15:2093-2105.
161. Cooke P, et al. Mechanism of estrogen action: lessons from the estrogen receptor-alpha knockout mouse. Biol Reprod 1998;59: 470-475.
162. Matsuzaki S. Oestrogen receptor alpha and beta mRNA expression in human endometrium throughout the menstrual cycle. Mol Hum Reprod 1999;5:556-564.
163. Katzenellenbogen B. Estrogen receptors: bioactivities and interactions with cell signaling pathways. Biol Reprod 1996;54:287-293.
164. Attia GR, et al. Progesterone receptor isoform A but not B is expressed in endometriosis. J Clin Endocrinol Metab 2000;85: 2897-2902.
165. Tseng L, et al. Effects of progestins on estradiol receptor levels in human endometrium. J Clin Endocrinol Metab 1975;41:402-404.
166. Casey ML, et al. 17b-Hydroxysteroid dehydrogenase type 2: chromosomal assignment and progestin regulation of gene expression in human endometrium. J Clin Invest 1994;94:2135-2141.
167. Tseng L, et al. Stimulation of acylsulfotransferase activity by progestin in human endometrium in vitro. J Clin Endocrinol Metab 1981;53:418-421.
168. Bergh PA, et al. The impact of embryonic development and endometrial maturity on the timing of implantation. Fertil Steril 1992;58(3):537-542.
169. Adams EC, et al. A description of 34 human ova within the first 17 days of development. Am J Anat 1956;98(3):435-493.
170. Sauer MV, et al. Reversing the natural decline in human fertility. An extended clinical trial of oocyte donation to women of advanced reproductive age. JAMA 1992;268(10):1275-1279.
171. Rosenwaks Z. Donor eggs: their application in modern reproductive technologies. Fertil Steril 1987;47(6):895-909.
172. Langer RD, et al. Transvaginal ultrasonography compared with endometrial biopsy for the detection of endometrial disease. Postmenopausal Estrogen/Progestin Interventions Trial. N Engl J Med 1997;337(25):1792-1798.
173. Sheehan HL. The recognition of chronic hypopituitarism resulting from postpartum pituitary necrosis. Am J Obstet Gynecol 1971;111(6):852-854.
174. Simpson JL, et al. Gonadal dysgenesis in individuals with apparently normal chromosomal complements: tabulation of cases and compilation of genetic data. Birth Defects Orig Artic Ser 1971;7(6):215-228.
175. Hague WM, et al. 45 X Turner's syndrome in association with polycystic ovaries. Case report. Br J Obstet Gynaecol 1989;96(5): 613-618.
176. Division of Reproductive Sciences, O.R.P.R.C., Beaverton 97006. Progesterone-dependent expression of keratinocyte growth factor mRNA in stromal cells of the primate endometrium: keratinocyte growth factor as a progestomedin. J Cell Biol 1994;125(2): 393-401.

177. Asherman JG. Amenorrhea traumatica (atretica). J Obstet Gynecol Br Emp 1948;55:23-27.
178. Marshall W, et al. Variations in patterns of pubertal changes in girls. Arch Dis Child 1969;44:291-303.
179. Klinefelter HJ, et al. Experience with a quantitative test for normal or decreased amounts of follicle-stimulating hormone in urine in endocrinological diagnosis. J Clin Endocrinol Metab 1943; 3:529-544.
180. Khoury SA, et al. Diurnal patterns of pulsatile luteinizing hormone secretion in hypothalamic amenorrhea: reproducibility and responses to opiate blockade and an alpha 2-adrenergic agonist. J Clin Endocrinol Metab 1987;64(4):755-762.
181. Berga SL, et al. Neuroendocrine aberrations in women with functional hypothalamic amenorrhea. J Clin Endocrinol Metab 1989;68(2):301-308.
182. Yen SS, et al. Hypothalamic amenorrhea and hypogonadotropinism: responses to synthetic LRF. J Clin Endocrinol Metab 1973;36(5):811-816.
183. Loucks AB, et al. Alterations in the hypothalamic-pituitary-ovarian and the hypothalamic-pituitary-adrenal axes in athletic women. J Clin Endocrinol Metab 1989;68(2):402-411.
184. Wilson RC, et al. Central electrophysiologic correlates of pulsatile luteinizing hormone secretion in the rhesus monkey. Neuroendocrinology 1984;39(3):256-260.
185. Kalra SP. Catecholamine involvement in preovulatory LH release: reassessment of the role of epinephrine. Neuroendocrinology 1985;40(2):139-144.
186. Quigley ME, et al. Evidence for increased dopaminergic inhibition of secretion of thyroid-stimulating hormone in hyperprolactinemic patients with pituitary microadenoma. Am J Obstet Gynecol 1980;137(6):653-655.
187. Ropert JF, et al. Endogenous opiates modulate pulsatile luteinizing hormone release in humans. J Clin Endocrinol Metab 1981;52(3): 583-585.
188. Gambacciani M, et al. GnRH release from the mediobasal hypothalamus: in vitro inhibition by corticotropin-releasing factor. Neuroendocrinology 1986;43(4):533-536.
189. Genazzani AD, et al. Naltrexone treatment restores menstrual cycles in patients with weight loss-related amenorrhea. Fertil Steril 1995;64(5):951-956.
190. Selye H. The stress syndrome. Nature 1936;138:32.
191. Suh BY, et al. Hypercortisolism in patients with functional hypothalamic amenorrhea. J Clin Endocrinol Metab 1988;66(4): 733-739.
192. Xiao E, et al. Acute inhibition of gonadotropin secretion by corticotropin-releasing hormone in the primate: are the adrenal glands involved? Endocrinology 1989;124(4):1632-1637.
193. Rivier C, et al. Influence of corticotropin-releasing factor on reproductive functions in the rat. Endocrinology 1984;114(3): 914-921.
194. Matteri RL, et al. Adrenocorticotropin-induced changes in ovine pituitary gonadotropin secretion in vitro. Endocrinology 1986; 118(5):2091-2096.
195. Kamel F, et al. Modulation of gonadotropin secretion by corticosterone: interaction with gonadal steroids and mechanism of action. Endocrinology 1987;121(2):561-568.
196. Welt CK, et al. Recombinant human leptin in women with hypothalamic amenorrhea. N Engl J Med 2004;351(10):987-997.
197. Baranowska B, et al. The role of endogenous opiates in the mechanism of inhibited luteinizing hormone (LH) secretion in women with anorexia nervosa: the effect of naloxone on LH, follicle-stimulating hormone, prolactin, and beta-endorphin secretion. J Clin Endocrinol Metab 1984;59(3):412-416.
198. Atkinson RL. Naloxone decreases food intake in obese humans. J Clin Endocrinol Metab 1982;55(1):196-198.
199. Morley JE, et al. Stress-induced eating is mediated through endogenous opiates. Science 1980;209(4462):1259-1261.
200. Rigotti NA, et al. The clinical course of osteoporosis in anorexia nervosa. A longitudinal study of cortical bone mass. JAMA 1991;265(9):1133-1138.
201. Frisch RE, et al. Delayed menarche and amenorrhea in ballet dancers. N Engl J Med 1980;303(1):17-19.
202. Frisch RE, et al. Delayed menarche and amenorrhea of college athletes in relation to age of onset of training. JAMA 1981; 246(14):1559-1563.
203. Drinkwater BL, et al. Bone mineral content of amenorrheic and eumenorrheic athletes. N Engl J Med 1984;311(5):277-281.
204. Willi J, et al. Epidemiology of anorexia nervosa in a defined region of Switzerland. Am J Psychiatry 1983;140(5):564-567.
205. Schwartz DM, et al. Do anorectics get well? Current research and future needs. Am J Psychiatry 1981;138(3):319-323.
206. Swift WJ. The long-term outcome of early onset anorexia nervosa. A critical review. J Am Acad Child Psychiatry 1982;21(1):38-46.
207. Boyar RM, et al. Cortisol secretion and metabolism in anorexia nervosa. N Engl J Med 1977;296(4):190-193.
208. Gold PW, et al. Abnormal hypothalamic-pituitary-adrenal function in anorexia nervosa. Pathophysiologic mechanisms in underweight and weight-corrected patients. N Engl J Med 1986;314(21): 1335-1342.
209. Kaye WH, et al. Elevated cerebrospinal fluid levels of immunoreactive corticotropin-releasing hormone in anorexia nervosa: relation to state of nutrition, adrenal function, and intensity of depression. J Clin Endocrinol Metab 1987;64(2):203-208.
210. Moshang TJ. Low triiodothyronine euthyroidism in anorexia nervosa. In Vigersky RS, ed. Anorexia Nervosa. Raven Press, New York 1977:263-270.
211. Gold P, et al. Abnormalities in plasma and cerebrospinal fluid arginine vasopressin in patients with anorexia nervosa. N Engl J Med 1983;308:1117-1123.
212. Soyka LA, et al. The effects of anorexia nervosa on bone metabolism in female adolescents. J Clin Endocrinol Metab 1999;84(12): 4489-4496.
213. Liu JH, et al. The use of gonadotropin-releasing hormone for the induction of ovulation. Clin Obstet Gynecol 1984;27(4):975-982.
214. Hatch R, et al. Hirsutism: implications, etiology, and management. Am J Obstet Gynecol 1981;140(7):815-830.
215. Tagatz GE, et al. The clitoral index: a bioassay of androgenic stimulation. Obstet Gynecol 1979;54(5):562-564.
216. Bardin CW, et al. Testosterone and androstenedione blood production rates in normal women and women with idiopathic hirsutism or polycystic ovaries. J Clin Invest 1967;46(5):891-902.
217. Youngblood GL, et al. Isolation and characterization of the mouse P450$17\alpha$-hydroxylase/c17-20 lyase gene (CYP17): transcriptional regulation of the gene by cyclic adenosine 3′,5′-monophosphate in MA-10 Leydig cells. Mol Endocrinol 1992;6:927-934.
218. Mowszowicz I, et al. Androgen binding capacity and 5 alpha-reductase activity in pubic skin fibroblasts from hirsute patients. J Clin Endocrinol Metab 1983;56(6):1209-1213.
219. Schwartz U, et al. The diagnostic value of plasma free testosterone in non-tumorous and tumorous hyperandrogenism. Fertil Steril 1983;40(1):66-72.
220. Miller KK, et al. Measurement of free testosterone in normal women and women with androgen deficiency: comparison of methods. J Clin Endocrinol Metab 2004;89(2):525-533.
221. Carmina E, et al. Extensive clinical experience: relative prevalence of different androgen excess disorders in 950 women referred because of clinical hyperandrogenism. J Clin Endocrinol Metab 2006;91(1):2-6.
222. Paulson RJ, et al. Measurements of 3 alpha,17 beta-androstanediol glucuronide in serum and urine and the correlation with skin 5 alpha-reductase activity. Fertil Steril 1986;46(2):222-226.
223. Barbieri RL, et al. Presence of 17 beta-hydroxysteroid dehydrogenase type 3 messenger ribonucleic acid transcript in an ovarian Sertoli-Leydig cell tumor. Fertil Steril 1997;68(3):534-537.
224. Kennedy L, et al. Short term administration of gonadotropin-releasing hormone analog to a patient with a testosterone-secreting ovarian tumor. J Clin Endocrinol Metab 1987;64(6):1320-1322.
225. Derksen J, et al. Identification of virilizing adrenal tumors in hirsute women. N Engl J Med 1994;331(15):968-973.
226. Friedman CI, et al. Serum testosterone concentrations in the evaluation of androgen-producing tumors. Am J Obstet Gynecol 1985;153(1):44-49.
227. Taylor L, et al. Diagnostic considerations in virilization: iodomethyl-norcholesterol scanning in the localization of androgen secreting tumors. Fertil Steril 1986;46(6):1005-1010.
228. Azziz R, et al. Screening for 21-hydroxylase-deficient nonclassic adrenal hyperplasia among hyperandrogenic women: a prospective study. Fertil Steril 1999;72(5):915-925.
229. Speiser PW, et al. High frequency of nonclassical steroid 21-hydroxylase deficiency. Am J Hum Genet 1985;37(4):650-667.

230. New MI, et al. Genotyping steroid 21-hydroxylase deficiency: hormonal reference data. J Clin Endocrinol Metab 1983;57(2): 320-326.
231. Stratakis CA, et al. Glucocorticosteroid resistance in humans. Elucidation of the molecular mechanisms and implications for pathophysiology. Ann N Y Acad Sci 1994;746:362-374; discussion 374-376.
232. Lobo RA, et al. The effects of two doses of spironolactone on serum androgens and anagen hair in hirsute women. Fertil Steril 1985;43(2):200-205.
233. Evron S, et al. Induction of ovulation with spironolactone (Aldactone) in anovulatory oligomenorrheic and hyperandrogenic women. Fertil Steril 1981;36(4):468-471.
234. Mowszowicz I, et al. Androgen metabolism in hirsute patients treated with cyproterone acetate. J Steroid Biochem 1984;20(3): 757-761.
235. Rittmaster RS, Finasteride. N Engl J Med 1994;330(2):120-125.
236. Wong IL, et al. A prospective randomized trial comparing finasteride to spironolactone in the treatment of hirsute women. J Clin Endocrinol Metab 1995;80(1):233-238.
237. Castello R, et al. Outcome of long-term treatment with the 5 alpha-reductase inhibitor finasteride in idiopathic hirsutism: clinical and hormonal effects during a 1-year course of therapy and 1-year follow-up. Fertil Steril 1996;66(5):734-740.
238. Diamanti-Kandarakis E, et al. The effect of a pure antiandrogen receptor blocker, flutamide, on the lipid profile in the polycystic ovary syndrome. J Clin Endocrinol Metab 1998;83(8):2699-2705.
239. Moghetti P, et al. Flutamide in the treatment of hirsutism: long-term clinical effects, endocrine changes, and androgen receptor behavior. Fertil Steril 1995;64(3):511-517.
240. Wysowski DK, et al. Fatal and nonfatal hepatotoxicity associated with flutamide. Ann Intern Med 1993;118(11):860-864.
241. Legro RS, et al. Prevalence and predictors of risk for type 2 diabetes mellitus and impaired glucose tolerance in polycystic ovary syndrome: a prospective, controlled study in 254 affected women. J Clin Endocrinol Metab 1999;84(1):165-169.
242. Urbanek M, et al. Thirty-seven candidate genes for polycystic ovary syndrome: strongest evidence for linkage is with follistatin. Proc Natl Acad Sci U S A 1999;96(15):8573-8578.
243. Legro RS, et al. Evidence for a genetic basis for hyperandrogenemia in polycystic ovary syndrome. Proc Natl Acad Sci U S A 1998;95(25):14956-14960.
244. Stein I, et al. Amenorrhea associated with bilateral polycystic ovaries. Am J Obstet Gynecol 1935;29:181.
245. Burghen GA, et al. Correlation of hyperandrogenism with hyperinsulinism in polycystic ovarian disease. J Clin Endocrinol Metab 1980;50(1):113-116.
246. Tamura M, et al. Estrogen up-regulates cyclooxygenase-2 via estrogen receptor in human uterine microvascular endothelial cells. Fertil Steril 2004.81:1351-1356.
247. Azziz R. Controversy in clinical endocrinology: diagnosis of polycystic ovarian syndrome: the Rotterdam criteria are premature. J Clin Endocrinol Metab 2006;91(3):781-785.
248. Stratakis CA, et al. Glucocorticosteroid resistance in humans. Elucidation of the molecular mechanisms and implications for pathophysiology. Ann N Y Acad Sci 1994;746:362-374.
249. Zawadzki JK, et al. Diagnostic criteria for polycystic ovary syndrome: towards a rational approach. In Dunaif A, et al, eds. Polycystic Ovary Syndrome. Boston, MA, Blackwell 1992:377-384.
250. Revised 2003 consensus on diagnostic criteria and long-term health risks related to polycystic ovary syndrome. Fertil Steril 2004;81(1):19-25.
251. Dunaif A. Insulin resistance in polycystic ovarian syndrome. Ann N Y Acad Sci 1993;687:60-64.
252. Hoffman D, et al. The prevalence and significance of elevated dehydroepiandrosterone sulfate levels in anovulatory women. Fertil Steril 1980;42:853-861.
253. Franks S. Polycystic ovary syndrome. N Engl J Med 1995;333(13): 853-861.
254. Kletzky OA, et al. Clinical categorization of patients with secondary amenorrhea using progesterone-induced uterine bleeding and measurement of serum gonadotropin levels. Am J Obstet Gynecol 1975;121(5):695-703.
255. Venturoli S, et al. Episodic pulsatile secretion of FSH, LH, prolactin, oestradiol, oestrone, and LH circadian variations in polycystic ovary syndrome. Clin Endocrinol (Oxf) 1988;28(1):93-107.
256. Imse V, et al. Comparison of luteinizing hormone pulsatility in the serum of women suffering from polycystic ovarian disease using a bioassay and five different immunoassays. J Clin Endocrinol Metab 1992;74(5):1053-1061.
257. Hayes FJ, et al. Use of a gonadotropin-releasing hormone antagonist as a physiologic probe in polycystic ovary syndrome: assessment of neuroendocrine and androgen dynamics. J Clin Endocrinol Metab 1998;83(7):2343-2349.
258. Barnes RB, et al. Central opioid activity in polycystic ovary syndrome with and without dopaminergic modulation. J Clin Endocrinol Metab 1985;61(4):779-782.
259. Morales AJ, et al. Insulin, somatotropic, and luteinizing hormone axes in lean and obese women with polycystic ovary syndrome: common and distinct features. J Clin Endocrinol Metab 1996;81(8): 2854-2864.
260. Taylor AE, et al. Determinants of abnormal gonadotropin secretion in clinically defined women with polycystic ovary syndrome. J Clin Endocrinol Metab 1997;82(7):2248-2256.
261. Nagamani M, et al. Hyperinsulinemia in hyperthecosis of the ovaries. Am J Obstet Gynecol 1986;154(2):384-389.
262. Dorn C, et al. Insulin enhances the transcription of luteinizing hormone-beta gene. Am J Obstet Gynecol 2004;191(1):132-137.
263. Adashi EY, et al. Insulin enhancement of luteinizing hormone and follicle-stimulating hormone release by cultured pituitary cells. Endocrinology 1981;108(4):1441-1449.
264. Mehta RV, et al. Luteinizing hormone secretion is not influenced by insulin infusion in women with polycystic ovary syndrome despite improved insulin sensitivity during pioglitazone treatment. J Clin Endocrinol Metab 2005;90(4):2136-2141.
265. Chang RJ. Ovarian steroid secretion in polycystic ovarian disease. Semin Reprod Endocrinol 1984;2:244.
266. Wajchenberg BL, et al. The source(s) of estrogen production in hirsute women with polycystic ovarian disease as determined by simultaneous adrenal and ovarian venous catheterization. Fertil Steril 1988;49(1):56-61.
267. Bulun S, et al. Aromatase in aging women. Seminars in Reproductive Endocrinology 1999;17:349-358.
268. Reed MJ, et al. Regulation of estradiol 17beta-hydroxysteroid dehydrogenase in breast tissues: the role of growth factors. J Steroid Biochem Mol Biol 1991;39:791-798.
269. Bulun SE, et al. Regulation of aromatase expression in estrogen-responsive breast and uterine disease: from bench to treatment. Pharmacol Rev 2005;57(3):359-383.
270. Nestler JE. Obesity, insulin, sex steroids and ovulation. Int J Obes Relat Metab Disord 2000;24(suppl 2): S71-S73.
271. Fauser BC. Observations in favor of normal early follicle development and disturbed dominant follicle selection in polycystic ovary syndrome. Gynecol Endocrinol 1994;8(2):75-82.
272. Mason HD, et al. Insulin-like growth factor-I (IGF-I) inhibits production of IGF-binding protein-1 while stimulating estradiol secretion in granulosa cells from normal and polycystic human ovaries. J Clin Endocrinol Metab 1993;76(5):1275-1279.
273. Homburg R, et al. Low-dose FSH therapy for anovulatory infertility associated with polycystic ovary syndrome: rationale, results, reflections and refinements. Hum Reprod Update 1999;5(5): 493-499.
274. Judd HL, et al. Familial hyperthecosis: comparison of endocrinologic and histologic findings with polycystic ovarian disease. Am J Obstet Gynecol 1973;117(7):976-982.
275. Cooper HE, et al. Hereditary factors in the Stein-Leventhal syndrome. Am J Obstet Gynecol 1968;100(3):371-387.
276. Ferriman D, et al. The inheritance of polycystic ovarian disease and a possible relationship to premature balding. Clin Endocrinol (Oxf) 1979;11(3):291-300.
277. Carey AH, et al. Evidence for a single gene effect causing polycystic ovaries and male pattern baldness. Clin Endocrinol (Oxf) 1993;38(6):653-658.
278. Govind A, et al. Polycystic ovaries are inherited as an autosomal dominant trait: analysis of 29 polycystic ovary syndrome and 10 control families. J Clin Endocrinol Metab 1999;84(1):38-43.
279. Norman RJ, et al. Hyperinsulinemia is common in family members of women with polycystic ovary syndrome. Fertil Steril 1996;66(6):942-947.
280. Urbanek M, et al. Candidate gene region for polycystic ovary syndrome on chromosome 19p13.2. J Clin Endocrinol Metab 2005; 90(12):6623-6629.

281. Ho CK, et al. Increased transcription and increased messenger ribonucleic acid (mRNA) stability contribute to increased GATA6 mRNA abundance in polycystic ovary syndrome theca cells. J Clin Endocrinol Metab 2005;90(12):6596-6602.
282. Osei K, et al. Ethnic differences in secretion, sensitivity, and hepatic extraction of insulin in black and white Americans. Diabet Med 1994;11(8):755-762.
283. Dunaif A, et al. Acanthosis nigricans, insulin action, and hyperandrogenism: clinical, histological, and biochemical findings. J Clin Endocrinol Metab 1991;73(3):590-595.
284. Reaven GM, et al. Hypertension and associated metabolic abnormalities—the role of insulin resistance and the sympathoadrenal system. N Engl J Med 1996;334(6):374-381.
285. Mather KJ, et al. Hyperinsulinemia in polycystic ovary syndrome correlates with increased cardiovascular risk independent of obesity. Fertil Steril 2000;73(1):150-156.
286. Talbott E, et al. Coronary heart disease risk factors in women with polycystic ovary syndrome. Arterioscler Thromb Vasc Biol 1995;15(7):821-826.
287. Ehrmann DA, et al. Prevalence and predictors of the metabolic syndrome in women with polycystic ovary syndrome. J Clin Endocrinol Metab 2006;91(1):48-53.
288. Dunaif A, et al. Beta-cell dysfunction independent of obesity and glucose intolerance in the polycystic ovary syndrome. J Clin Endocrinol Metab 1996;81(3):942-947.
289. Reddy SS, et al. Epidermal growth factor receptor defects in leprechaunism. A multiple growth factor-resistant syndrome. J Clin Invest 1989;84(5):1569-1576.
290. Kirschner MA, et al. Androgen-estrogen metabolism in women with upper body versus lower body obesity. J Clin Endocrinol Metab 1990;70(2):473-479.
291. Schapira DV, et al. Abdominal obesity and breast cancer risk. Ann Intern Med 1990;112(3):182-186.
292. Kumar NB, et al. Android obesity at diagnosis and breast carcinoma survival: evaluation of the effects of anthropometric variables at diagnosis, including body composition and body fat distribution and weight gain during life span, and survival from breast carcinoma. Cancer 2000;88(12):2751-2757.
293. Anderson KE, et al. Association of Stein-Leventhal syndrome with the incidence of postmenopausal breast carcinoma in a large prospective study of women in Iowa. Cancer 1997;79(3): 494-499.
294. Campbell PJ, et al. Impact of obesity on insulin action in volunteers with normal glucose tolerance: demonstration of a threshold for the adverse effect of obesity. J Clin Endocrinol Metab 1990;70(4):1114-1118.
295. Ehrmann DA. Polycystic ovary syndrome. N Engl J Med 2005;352(12):1223-1236.
296. Velazquez EM, et al. Metformin therapy in polycystic ovary syndrome reduces hyperinsulinemia, insulin resistance, hyperandrogenemia, and systolic blood pressure, while facilitating normal menses and pregnancy. Metabolism 1994;43(5):647-654.
297. Nestler JE, et al. Decreases in ovarian cytochrome P450c17 alpha activity and serum free testosterone after reduction of insulin secretion in polycystic ovary syndrome. N Engl J Med 1996;335(9): 617-623.
298. Velazquez E, et al. Menstrual cyclicity after metformin therapy in polycystic ovary syndrome. Obstet Gynecol 1997;90(3):392-395.
299. Lord JM, et al. Insulin-sensitising drugs (metformin, troglitazone, rosiglitazone, pioglitazone, D-chiro-inositol) for polycystic ovary syndrome. Cochrane Database Syst Rev 2003(3):CD003053.
300. Crave JC, et al. Effects of diet and metformin administration on sex hormone-binding globulin, androgens, and insulin in hirsute and obese women. J Clin Endocrinol Metab 1995;80(7): 2057-2062.
301. Dunaif A, et al. The insulin-sensitizing agent troglitazone improves metabolic and reproductive abnormalities in the polycystic ovary syndrome. J Clin Endocrinol Metab 1996;81(9):3299-3306.
302. Ehrmann DA, et al. Troglitazone improves defects in insulin action, insulin secretion, ovarian steroidogenesis, and fibrinolysis in women with polycystic ovary syndrome. J Clin Endocrinol Metab 1997;82(7):2108-2116.
303. Azziz R, et al. Troglitazone improves ovulation and hirsutism in the polycystic ovary syndrome: a multicenter, double blind, placebo-controlled trial. J Clin Endocrinol Metab 2001;86(4): 1626-1632.
304. Ghazeeri G, et al. Effect of rosiglitazone on spontaneous and clomiphene citrate-induced ovulation in women with polycystic ovary syndrome. Fertil Steril 2003;79(3):562-566.
305. Belli SH, et al. Effect of rosiglitazone on insulin resistance, growth factors, and reproductive disturbances in women with polycystic ovary syndrome. Fertil Steril 2004;81(3):624-629.
306. Romualdi D, et al. Selective effects of pioglitazone on insulin and androgen abnormalities in normo- and hyperinsulinaemic obese patients with polycystic ovary syndrome. Hum Reprod 2003;18(6): 1210-1218.
307. Regan L, et al. Hypersecretion of luteinising hormone, infertility, and miscarriage. Lancet 1990;336(8724):1141-1144.
308. Gitsch G, et al. Endometrial cancer in premenopausal women 45 years and younger. Obstet Gynecol 1995;85(4):504-508.
309. Godsland IF, et al. Update on the metabolic effects of steroidal contraceptives and their relationship to cardiovascular disease risk. Am J Obstet Gynecol 1994;170(5 Pt 2):1528-1536.
310. Duffy TJ, et al. Oral contraceptive use: prospective follow-up of women with suspected glucose intolerance. Contraception 1984;30(3):197-208.
311. Hannaford PC, et al. Oral contraceptives and diabetes mellitus. BMJ 1989;299(6711):1315-1316.
312. Escobar-Morreale HF, et al. Treatment of hirsutism with ethinyl estradiol-desogestrel contraceptive pills has beneficial effects on the lipid profile and improves insulin sensitivity. Fertil Steril 2000;74(4):816-819.
313. Colditz GA. Oral contraceptive use and mortality during 12 years of follow-up: the Nurses' Health Study. Ann Intern Med 1994; 120(10):821-826.
314. Kjos SL, et al. Contraception and the risk of type 2 diabetes mellitus in Latina women with prior gestational diabetes mellitus. JAMA 1998;280(6):533-538.
315. Garg SK, et al. Oral contraceptives and renal and retinal complications in young women with insulin-dependent diabetes mellitus. JAMA 1994;271(14):1099-1102.
316. Petersen KR, et al. Effects of contraceptive steroids on cardiovascular risk factors in women with insulin-dependent diabetes mellitus. Am J Obstet Gynecol 1994;171(2):400-405.
317. Diamanti-Kandarakis E, et al. Insulin sensitivity and antiandrogenic therapy in women with polycystic ovary syndrome. Metabolism 1995;44(4):525-531.
318. Lanzone A, et al. Preconceptional and gestational evaluation of insulin secretion in patients with polycystic ovary syndrome. Hum Reprod 1996;11(11):2382-2386.
319. Wild RA, et al. Lipid and apolipoprotein abnormalities in hirsute women. I. The association with insulin resistance. Am J Obstet Gynecol 1992;166(4): 1191-1196; discussion 1196-1197.
320. Kiddy DS, et al. Improvement in endocrine and ovarian function during dietary treatment of obese women with polycystic ovary syndrome. Clin Endocrinol (Oxf) 1992;36(1):105-111.
321. Guzick DS, et al. Endocrine consequences of weight loss in obese, hyperandrogenic, anovulatory women. Fertil Steril 1994;61(4): 598-604.
322. Clark AM, et al. Weight loss results in significant improvement in pregnancy and ovulation rates in anovulatory obese women. Hum Reprod 1995;10(10):2705-2712.
323. Nestler JE, et al. Effects of metformin on spontaneous and clomiphene-induced ovulation in the polycystic ovary syndrome. N Engl J Med 1998;338(26):1876-1880.
324. Dahlgren E, et al. Women with polycystic ovary syndrome wedge resected in 1956 to 1965: a long-term follow-up focusing on natural history and circulating hormones. Fertil Steril 1992;57(3): 505-513.
325. Adashi EY. Clomiphene citrate-initiated ovulation: a clinical update. Semin Reprod Endocrinol 1986;4:225-276.
326. Mitwally MF, et al. Use of an aromatase inhibitor for induction of ovulation in patients with an inadequate response to clomiphene citrate. Fertil Steril 2001;75(2):305-309.
327. Al-Omari WR, et al. Comparison of two aromatase inhibitors in women with clomiphene-resistant polycystic ovary syndrome. Int J Gynaecol Obstet 2004;85(3):289-291.
328. Casper RF, et al. Review: aromatase inhibitors for ovulation induction. J Clin Endocrinol Metab 2006;91(3):760-771.
329. Hamilton-Fairley D, et al. Common problems in induction of ovulation. Baillieres Clin Obstet Gynaecol 1990;4(3):609-625.

330. Marci R, et al. A low-dose stimulation protocol using highly purified follicle-stimulating hormone can lead to high pregnancy rates in in vitro fertilization patients with polycystic ovaries who are at risk of a high ovarian response to gonadotropins. Fertil Steril 2001;75(6):1131-1135.
331. Taylor AE, et al. A randomized, controlled trial of estradiol replacement therapy in women with hypergonadotropic amenorrhea. J Clin Endocrinol Metab 1996;81(10):3615-3621.
332. Conway GS. Premature ovarian failure. Br Med Bull 2000;56(3):643-649.
333. Dewald G, et al. Sex chromosome anomalies associated with premature gonadal failure. Semin Reprod Endocrinol 1983;1:79.
334. Devi AS, et al. 45,X/46,XX mosaicism in patients with idiopathic premature ovarian failure. Fertil Steril 1998;70(1):89-93.
335. Myhre AG, et al. Autoimmune polyendocrine syndrome type 1 (APS I) in Norway. Clin Endocrinol (Oxf) 2001;54(2):211-217.
336. Wallace WH, et al. Ovarian failure following abdominal irradiation in childhood: natural history and prognosis. Clin Oncol (R Coll Radiol) 1989;1(2):75-79.
337. Morice P, et al. Fertility results after ovarian transposition for pelvic malignancies treated by external irradiation or brachytherapy. Hum Reprod 1998;13(3):660-663.
338. Bines J, et al. Ovarian function in premenopausal women treated with adjuvant chemotherapy for breast cancer. J Clin Oncol 1996;14(5):1718-1729.
339. Byrne J, et al. Effects of treatment on fertility in long-term survivors of childhood or adolescent cancer. N Engl J Med 1987;317(21):1315-1321.
340. Aittomaki K. The genetics of XX gonadal dysgenesis. Am J Hum Genet 1994;54(5):844-851.
341. Rebar RW, et al. Clinical features of young women with hypergonadotropic amenorrhea. Fertil Steril 1990;53(5):804-810.
342. Nelson LM, et al. Development of luteinized graafian follicles in patients with karyotypically normal spontaneous premature ovarian failure. J Clin Endocrinol Metab 1994;79(5):1470-1475.
343. Giltay JC, et al. Short stature as the only presenting feature in a patient with an isodicentric (Y)(q11.23) and gonadoblastoma. A clinical and molecular cytogenetic study. Eur J Pediatr 2001;160(3):154-158.
344. Manuel M, et al. The age of occurrence of gonadal tumors in intersex patients with a Y chromosome. Am J Obstet Gynecol 1976;124(3):293-300.
345. Gravholt CH, et al. Occurrence of gonadoblastoma in females with Turner syndrome and Y chromosome material: a population study. J Clin Endocrinol Metab 2000;85(9):3199-3202.
346. Nelson LM. Autoimmune ovarian failure: comparing the mouse model and the human disease. J Soc Gynecol Invest 2001;8(1 Suppl Proceedings):S55-S57.
347. Wheatcroft NJ, et al. Identification of ovarian antibodies by immunofluorescence, enzyme-linked immunosorbent assay or immunoblotting in premature ovarian failure. Hum Reprod 1997;12(12):2617-2622.
348. Markee J. Morphological basis for menstrual bleeding: relation of regression to the initiation of bleeding. Bull N Y Acad Med 1948;36:153.
349. Belsey EM, et al. Menstrual bleeding patterns in untreated women. Task Force on Long-Acting Systemic Agents for Fertility Regulation. Contraception 1997;55(2):57-65.
350. Chiazze L Jr, et al. The length and variability of the human menstrual cycle. JAMA 1968;203(6):377-380.
351. Munster K, et al. Length and variation in the menstrual cycle—a cross-sectional study from a Danish county. Br J Obstet Gynaecol 1992;99(5):422-429.
352. Treloar AE, et al. Variation of the human menstrual cycle through reproductive life. Int J Fertil 1967;12(1 Pt 2):77-126.
353. Rybo G. Menstrual blood loss in relation to parity and menstrual pattern. Acta Obstet Gynecol Scand 1966;45(suppl 7):25-45.
354. Haynes PJ, et al. Measurement of menstrual blood loss in patients complaining of menorrhagia. Br J Obstet Gynaecol 1977;84(10):763-768.
355. Higham JM, et al. Assessment of menstrual blood loss using a pictorial chart. Br J Obstet Gynaecol 1990;97(8):734-739.
356. Fraser IS, et al. A preliminary study of factors influencing perception of menstrual blood loss volume. Am J Obstet Gynecol 1984;149(7):788-793.
357. de Ziegler D, et al. Effects of luteal estradiol on the secretory transformation of human endometrium and plasma gonadotropins. J Clin Endocrinol Metab 1992;74(2):322-331.
358. Belsey EM. Vaginal bleeding patterns among women using one natural and eight hormonal methods of contraception. Contraception 1988;38(2):181-206.
359. Wilansky DL, et al. Early hypothyroidism in patients with menorrhagia. Am J Obstet Gynecol 1989;160(3):673-677.
360. Hopkins MP, et al. Ginseng face cream and unexplained vaginal bleeding. Am J Obstet Gynecol 1988;159(5):1121-1122.
361. Claessens EA, et al. Acute adolescent menorrhagia. Am J Obstet Gynecol 1981;139(3):277-280.
362. Smith YR, et al. Menorrhagia in adolescents requiring hospitalization. J Pediatr Adolesc Gynecol 1998;11(1):13-15.
363. van Eijkeren MA, et al. Measured menstrual blood loss in women with a bleeding disorder or using oral anticoagulant therapy. Am J Obstet Gynecol 1990;162(5):1261-1263.
364. Edlund M, et al. On the value of menorrhagia as a predictor for coagulation disorders. Am J Hematol 1996;53(4):234-238.
365. Nilsson L, et al. Treatment of menorrhagia. Am J Obstet Gynecol 1971;110(5):713-720.
366. Kirkland JL, et al. Progesterone inhibits the estrogen-induced expression of c-fos messenger ribonucleic acid in the uterus. Endocrinology 1992;130(6):3223-3230.
367. DeVore GR, et al. Use of intravenous Premarin in the treatment of dysfunctional uterine bleeding—a double-blind randomized control study. Obstet Gynecol 1982;59(3):285-291.
368. Livio M, et al. Conjugated estrogens for the management of bleeding associated with renal failure. N Engl J Med 1986;315(12):731-735.
369. Olive D, et al. Endometriosis. N Engl J Med 1993;328:1759-1769.
370. Vercellini P, et al. Progestins for symptomatic endometriosis: a critical analysis of the evidence. Fertil Steril 1997;68(3):393-401.
371. Collaborative Group on Hormonal Factors in Breast Cancer. Breast cancer and hormone replacement therapy: collaborative reanalysis of data from 51 epidemiological studies of 52,705 women with breast cancer and 108,411 women without breast cancer. Lancet 1997;350:1047-1059.
372. Waller KG, et al. Gonadotropin-releasing hormone analogues for the treatment of endometriosis: long-term follow-up. Fertil Steril 1993;59(3):511-515.
373. Shaw RW. An open randomized comparative study of the effect of goserelin depot and danazol in the treatment of endometriosis. Zoladex Endometriosis Study Team. Fertil Steril 1992;58(2):265-272.
374. Menopause. A decision tree for the use of estrogen replacement therapy or hormone replacement therapy in postmenopausal women: consensus opinion of the North American Menopause Society. 2000;7:76-86.
375. Vercellini P, et al. Progestins for symptomatic endometriosis: a critical analysis of the evidence. Fertil Steril 1997;68:393-401.
376. Takayama K, et al. Treatment of severe postmenopausal endometriosis with an aromatase inhibitor. Fertil Steril 1998;69(4):709-713.
377. Vercellini P, et al. A gonadotropin-releasing hormone agonist versus a low-dose oral contraceptive for pelvic pain associated with endometriosis. Fertil Steril 1993;60(1):75-79.
378. Waller KG, et al. Gonadotropin-releasing hormone analogues for the treatment of endometriosis: long-term follow-up. Fertil Steril 1993;59(3):511-515.
379. Takayama K, et al. Treatment of severe postmenopausal endometriosis with an aromatase inhibitor. Fertil Steril 1998;69:709-713.
380. Amsterdam L, et al. Treatment of endometriosis-related pelvic pain with a combination of an aromatase inhibitor (anastrozole) plus a combination oral contraceptive: a novel approach. Proceedings of the 85th Annual Endocrine Society Meeting 2003;1:360.
381. Ailawadi R, et al. Treatment of endometriosis and chronic pelvic pain with letrozole and norethindrone acetate: a pilot study. Fertil Steril 2004;81(2):290-296.
382. Soysal S, et al. The effects of post-surgical administration of goserelin plus anastrozole compared to goserelin alone in patients with severe endometriosis: a prospective randomized trial. Hum Reprod 2004;19:160-167.

383. Amsterdam L, et al. Anastrozole and oral contraceptives: a novel treatment for endometriosis. Fertil Steril 2005;84(2):300-304.
384. Stewart EA. Uterine fibroids. Lancet 2001;357(9252):293-298.
385. Maruo T, et al. Effects of progesterone on uterine leiomyoma growth and apoptosis. Steroids 2000;65(10-11):585-592.
386. Judd HL, et al. Endocrine function of the postmenopausal ovary: concentration of androgens and estrogens in ovarian and peripheral vein blood. J Clin Endocrinol Metab 1974;39(6):1020-1024.
387. McKinlay SM, et al. The normal menopause transition. Maturitas 1992;14(2):103-115.
388. den Tonkelaar I, et al. Menstrual cycle length preceding menopause in relation to age at menopause. Maturitas 1998;29(2): 115-123.
389. Buckler HM, et al. Gonadotropin, steroid, and inhibin levels in women with incipient ovarian failure during anovulatory and ovulatory rebound cycles. J Clin Endocrinol Metab 1991;72(1): 116-124.
390. Santoro N, et al. Characterization of reproductive hormonal dynamics in the perimenopause. J Clin Endocrinol Metab 1996;81(4):1495-1501.
391. McKinlay SM, et al. Smoking and age at menopause in women. Ann Intern Med 1985;103(3):350-356.
392. Torgerson DJ, et al. Factors associated with onset of menopause in women aged 45-49. Maturitas 1994;19(2):83-92.
393. Torgerson DJ, et al. Alcohol consumption and age of maternal menopause are associated with menopause onset. Maturitas 1997;26(1):21-25.
394. Cramer DW, et al. Family history as a predictor of early menopause. Fertil Steril 1995;64(4):740-745.
395. Gosden, et al. Follicular status at the menopause. Hum Reprod 1987;2(7):617-621.
396. Jiroutek MR, et al. Changes in reproductive hormones and sex hormone-binding globulin in a group of postmenopausal women measured over 10 years. Menopause 1998;5(2):90-94.
397. Adashi EY. The climacteric ovary as a functional gonadotropin-driven androgen-producing gland. Fertil Steril 1994;62(1):20-27.
398. Grodin JM, et al. Source of estrogen production in postmenopausal women. J Clin Endocrinol Metab 1973;36:207-214.
399. Labrie F, et al. Marked decline in serum concentrations of adrenal C19 sex steroid precursors and conjugated androgen metabolites during aging. J Clin Endocrinol Metab 1997;82(8):2396-2402.
400. Judd HL, et al. Origin of serum estradiol in postmenopausal women. Obstet Gynecol 1982;59:680-686.
401. Bulun SE, et al. Endocrine disorders associated with inappropriately high aromatase expression. J Steroid Biochem Mol Biol 1997;61(3-6):133-139.
402. Bonneterre J, et al. Anastrozole is superior to tamoxifen as first-line therapy in hormone receptor positive advanced breast carcinoma. Cancer 2001;92(9):2247-2258.
403. Kroman N, et al. Time since childbirth and prognosis in primary breast cancer: population based study. BMJ 1998;315:851-855.
404. Feldman S, et al. Two-year follow-up of 263 patients with post/perimenopausal vaginal bleeding and negative initial biopsy. Gynecol Oncol 1994;55(1):56-59.
405. Oldenhave A, et al. Impact of climacteric on well-being. A survey based on 5213 women 39 to 60 years old. Am J Obstet Gynecol 1993;168(3 Pt 1):772-780.
406. Kronnenberg F, et al. Modulation of menopausal hot flashes by ambient temperature. J Therm Biol 1992;17:43.
407. Yen SS. The biology of menopause. J Reprod Med 1977;18(6): 287-296.
408. Erlik Y, et al. Estrogen levels in postmenopausal women with hot flashes. Obstet Gynecol 1982;59(4):403-407.
409. Davidson BJ, et al. Free estradiol in postmenopausal women with and without endometrial cancer. J Clin Endocrinol Metab 1981;52(3):404-408.
410. Raz R, et al. A controlled trial of intravaginal estriol in postmenopausal women with recurrent urinary tract infections. N Engl J Med 1993;329(11):753-756.
411. Dempster DW, et al. Pathogenesis of osteoporosis. Lancet 1993;341(8848):797-801.
412. Richelson LS, et al. Relative contributions of aging and estrogen deficiency to postmenopausal bone loss. N Engl J Med 1984; 311(20):1273-1275.
413. Nilas L, et al. Bone mass and its relationship to age and the menopause. J Clin Endocrinol Metab 1987;65(4):697-702.
414. Christiansen C. Hormone replacement therapy and osteoporosis. Maturitas 1996;23(suppl):S71-S76.
415. Rossouw JE, et al. Risks and benefits of estrogen plus progestin in healthy postmenopausal women: principal results from the Women's Health Initiative randomized controlled trial. JAMA 2002;288(3):321-333.
416. Anderson GL, et al. Effects of conjugated equine estrogen in postmenopausal women with hysterectomy: the Women's Health Initiative randomized controlled trial. JAMA 2004;291(14):1701-1712.
417. Brett KM, et al. Use of postmenopausal hormone replacement therapy: estimates from a nationally representative cohort study. Am J Epidemiol 1997;145(6):536-545.
418. Ness J, et al. Use of hormone replacement therapy by postmenopausal women after publication of the Women's Health Initiative Trial. J Gerontol A Biol Sci Med Sci 2005;60(4):460-462.
419. Hoffmann M, et al. Changes in women's attitudes towards and use of hormone therapy after HERS and WHI. Maturitas 2005;52(1): 11-17.
420. Thunell L, et al. Scientific evidence changes prescribing practice—a comparison of the management of the climacteric and use of hormone replacement therapy among Swedish gynaecologists in 1996 and 2003. Br J Obstet Gyenaecol 2006;113(1):15-20.
421. Nicholson WK, et al. Hormone replacement therapy for African American women: missed opportunities for effective intervention. Menopause 1999;6(2):147-155.
422. Bergkvist L, et al. The risk of breast cancer after estrogen and estrogen-progestin replacement. N Engl J Med 1989;321:293-297.
423. Hulley S, et al. Randomized trial of estrogen plus progestin for secondary prevention of coronary heart disease in postmenopausal women. Heart and Estrogen/progestin Replacement Study (HERS) Research Group. JAMA 1998;280(7):605-613.
424. Shumaker SA, et al. Estrogen plus progestin and the incidence of dementia and mild cognitive impairment in postmenopausal women: the Women's Health Initiative Memory Study: a randomized controlled trial. JAMA 2003;289(20):2651-2662.
425. Lacey JV Jr, et al. Menopausal hormone replacement therapy and risk of ovarian cancer. JAMA 2002;288(3):334-341.
426. Shumaker SA, et al. Conjugated equine estrogens and incidence of probable dementia and mild cognitive impairment in postmenopausal women: Women's Health Initiative Memory Study. JAMA 2004;291(24):2947-2958.
427. Glueck CJ, et al. Severe hypertriglyceridemia and pancreatitis when estrogen replacement therapy is given to hypertriglyceridemic women. J Lab Clin Med 1994;123(1):59-64.
428. Cirillo DJ, et al. Effect of estrogen therapy on gallbladder disease. JAMA 2005;293(3):330-339.
429. Hays J, et al. Effects of estrogen plus progestin on health-related quality of life. N Engl J Med 2003;348(19):1839-1854.
430. Brunner RL, et al. Effects of conjugated equine estrogen on health-related quality of life in postmenopausal women with hysterectomy: results from the Women's Health Initiative Randomized Clinical Trial. Arch Intern Med 2005;165(17):1976-1986.
431. Rapp SR, et al. Effect of estrogen plus progestin on global cognitive function in postmenopausal women: the Women's Health Initiative Memory Study: a randomized controlled trial. JAMA 2003; 289(20):2663-2672.
432. Espeland MA, et al. Conjugated equine estrogens and global cognitive function in postmenopausal women: Women's Health Initiative Memory Study. JAMA 2004;291(24):2959-2968.
433. Reed SD, et al. Indications for hormone therapy: the post-Women's Health Initiative era. Endocrinol Metab Clin North Am 2004;33(4): 691-715.
434. Harman SM, et al. Is the estrogen controversy over? Deconstructing the Women's Health Initiative Study: a critical evaluation of the evidence. Annals of NY Acad Sci 2005;1052:43-56.
435. Speroff T, et al. A risk-benefit analysis of elective bilateral oophorectomy: effect of changes in compliance with estrogen therapy on outcome. Am J Obstet Gynecol 1991;164(1 Pt 1):165-174.
436. Berman R, et al. Compliance of women in taking estrogen replacement therapy. J Womens Health 1996:701(2):213.
437. Riis BJ, et al. Low bone mass and fast rate of bone loss at menopause: equal risk factors for future fracture: a 15-year follow-up study. Bone 1996;19(1):9-12.

438. Ettinger B, et al. Low-dosage esterified estrogens opposed by progestin at 6-month intervals. Obstet Gynecol 2001;98(2):205-211.
439. Lindheim SR, et al. A possible bimodal effect of estrogen on insulin sensitivity in postmenopausal women and the attenuating effect of added progestin. Fertil Steril 1993;60(4):664-647.
440. Woodruff JD, et al. Incidence of endometrial hyperplasia in postmenopausal women taking conjugated estrogens (Premarin) with medroxyprogesterone acetate or conjugated estrogens alone. The Menopause Study Group. Am J Obstet Gynecol 1994;170(5 Pt 1):1213-1223.
441. Archer DF, et al. Bleeding patterns in postmenopausal women taking continuous combined or sequential regimens of conjugated estrogens with medroxyprogesterone acetate. Menopause Study Group. Obstet Gynecol 1994;83(5 Pt 1):686-692.
442. The Writing Group for the PEPI Trial. (No authors Listed) Effects of estrogen or estrogen/progestin regimens in heart disease risk factors in postmenopausal women: the Postmenopausal Estrogen/Progestin Interventions (PEPI) trial. JAMA 1995;273:199-208.
443. Nand SL, et al. Bleeding pattern and endometrial changes during continuous combined hormone replacement therapy. The Ogen/Provera Study Group. Obstet Gynecol 1998;91(5 Pt 1):678-684.
444. Archer DF, et al. Endometrial morphology in asymptomatic postmenopausal women. Am J Obstet Gynecol 1991;165(2):317-320; discussion 320-322.
445. Korhonen MO, et al. Histologic classification and pathologic findings for endometrial biopsy specimens obtained from 2964 perimenopausal and postmenopausal women undergoing screening for continuous hormones as replacement therapy (CHART 2 Study). Am J Obstet Gynecol 1997;176(2):377-380.
446. McGonigle KF, et al. Development of endometrial cancer in women on estrogen and progestin hormone replacement therapy. Gynecol Oncol 1994;55(1):126-132.
447. Karlsson B, et al. Transvaginal ultrasonography of the endometrium in women with postmenopausal bleeding—a Nordic multicenter study. Am J Obstet Gynecol 1995;172(5):1488-1494.
448. Bakos O, et al. Transvaginal ultrasonography for identifying endometrial pathology in postmenopausal women. Maturitas 1994; 20(2-3):181-189.
449. Granberg S, et al. Endometrial sonographic and histologic findings in women with and without hormonal replacement therapy suffering from postmenopausal bleeding. Maturitas 1997;27(1):35-40.
450. O'Meara ES, et al. Hormone replacement therapy after a diagnosis of breast cancer in relation to recurrence and mortality. J Natl Cancer Inst 2001;93(10):754-762.
451. Col N, et al. Hormone replacement therapy after breast cancer: a systematic review and quantitative assessment of risk. J Clin Oncol 2001;19:2357-2363.
452. Dardes RC, et al. Novel agents to modulate oestrogen action. Br Med Bull 2000;56(3):773-786.
453. Diez JL. Skeletal effects of selective oestrogen receptor modulators (SERMs). Hum Reprod Update 2000;6(3):255-258.
454. Clemett D, et al. Raloxifene: a review of its use in postmenopausal osteoporosis. Drugs 2000;60(2):379-411.
455. Barrett-Connor E, et al. Effects of raloxifene on cardiovascular events and breast cancer in postmenopausal women. N Engl J Med 2006;355(2):125-137.
456. Burger HG. Selective oestrogen receptor modulators. Horm Res 2000;53(suppl 3):25-29.
457. Land SR, et al. Patient-reported symptoms and quality of life during treatment with tamoxifen or raloxifene for breast cancer prevention: the NSABP Study of Tamoxifen and Raloxifene (STAR) P-2 trial. JAMA 2006;295(23):2742-2751.
458. Vogel VG, et al. Effects of tamoxifen vs raloxifene on the risk of developing invasive breast cancer and other disease outcomes: the NSABP Study of Tamoxifen and Raloxifene (STAR) P-2 trial. JAMA 2006;295(23):2727-2741.
459. Bonnick S, et al. Comparison of weekly treatment of postmenopausal osteoporosis with alendronate versus risedronate over two years. J Clin Endocrinol Metab 2006;91(7): 2631-2637.
460. Epstein S. Update of current therapeutic options for the treatment of postmenopausal osteoporosis. Clin Ther 2006;28(2):151-173.
461. Close P, et al. Developments in the pharmacotherapeutic management of osteoporosis. Exp Opin Pharmacother 2006;7(12): 1603-1615.

CHAPTER 17

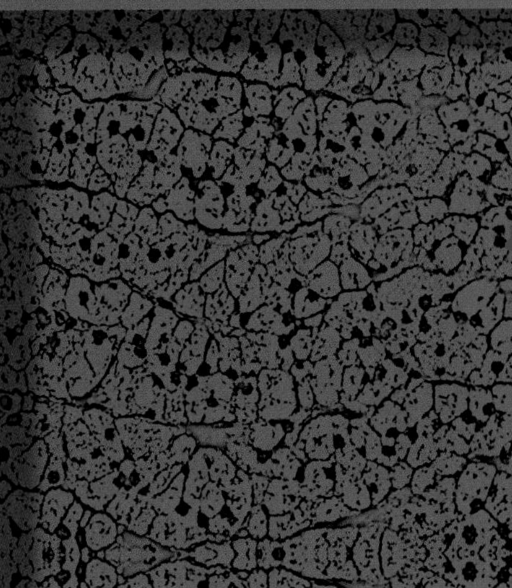

HORMONAL CONTRACEPTION

Philip D. Darney

Overview

Hormonal contraceptives using synthetic sex steroids remain the primary methods of nonsurgical birth control around the world. This chapter charts recent progress in delivering contraceptive doses of these steroids by the conventional oral route as well as new approaches using parenteral delivery through injections, transdermal and subdermal, and vaginal and uterine routes. Each route of delivery has particular advantages and disadvantages, but contraceptive success—defined as the avoidance of unintended pregnancy—depends mostly on the predilections and preferences of the user rather than special characteristics of the methods. The wider the selection, the more likely each woman and couple will find a method that will work well in particular circumstances. The proliferation of contraceptive methods over the past several years is a response to the individuality of contraceptive needs and accounts for declining numbers of unintended pregnancies in many places around the world. However, in some countries, such as the United States and most less-developed nations, at least half of pregnancies are unintended; therefore, the development, introduction, and successful use of modern contraceptives still has a long way to go.

Table 17–1 shows contraceptive failure rates achieved in clinical trials, which are the lowest that can be expected, and failure rates among typical users. The age and income of users strongly affect failure rates: users who are younger and those with lower incomes have more contraceptive failures. The intention of users to postpone or avoid additional births (as opposed to a first birth), also affects failure rates, with women who want to avoid additional births having fewer failures than women with no previous births.

ORAL CONTRACEPTION

The oral contraceptives (OCs) first introduced in the 1950s contained doses of estrogen and progestin nearly 10 times as high as those in today's pills. Over the years, old synthetic ovarian steroids like mestranol and chlormadinone were largely replaced by newer compounds with fewer adverse physiologic effects. More recently, pill administration schedules have been changed from the traditional and arbitrary 3 weeks on and 1 week off to a variety of regimens that increase efficacy and convenience and reduce side effects.

As birth control pill doses, steroids, and schedules evolved, knowledge of the physiologic and epidemiologic effects of pill use burgeoned. No drug has been as thoroughly evaluated as the combined oral contraceptive. Improved preparations and prescribing practices have dramatically reduced the morbidity and mortality associated with oral contraceptives so that today, on balance, the use of OCs has a substantial positive effect on public and individual health.

Mechanism of Action

The combination pill, consisting of estrogen and progestin, was the first hormonal contraceptive and was packaged to be taken daily for 3 out of every 4 weeks in order to mimic the menstrual cycle. Additional regimens, such as taking estrogen alone during the usual placebo week or taking a combination pill every day for 3 months, have been marketed more recently.

The combination pill prevents ovulation by inhibiting gonadotropin secretion via an effect on both pituitary and

TABLE 17–1 CONTRACEPTIVE FAILURE RATES DURING THE FIRST YEAR OF USE, UNITED STATES[1,2]

	PERCENTAGE OF WOMEN WITH PREGNANCY	
Method	**Lowest Expected**	**Typical**
None	85	85
PILLS		
Combination pill	0.1	7.6
Progestin only	0.5	3.0
IUDS		
Levonorgestrel IUD	0.1	0.1
Copper T 380A	0.6	0.8
IMPLANTS		
Six levonorgestrel capsules (Norplant)	0.05	0.2
Two levonorgestrel rods (Jadelle)	0.06	?
One etonogestrel rod (Implanon)	0.01	?
OTHER		
Injectable	0.3	3.0
Female sterilization	0.05	0.05
Male sterilization	0.1	0.15

hypothalamic centers. The progestational agent in the pill primarily suppresses luteinizing hormone (LH) secretion (preventing ovulation), and the estrogenic agent inhibits follicle-stimulating hormone (FSH) secretion (suppressing the emergence of a dominant follicle). Therefore, the estrogenic component significantly contributes to the contraceptive efficacy. However, even if follicular growth and development were not suppressed, the progestational component would prevent the surge-like release of LH necessary for ovulation.

The estrogen in the pill serves two other purposes. It provides stability to the endometrium so that irregular shedding and unwanted bleeding is minimized, and it potentiates the action of the progestational agents. The latter function of estrogen allows reduction of the progestational dose in the pill. The mechanism for this action is probably estrogen's effect in increasing the concentration of intracellular progesterone receptors. Therefore, a minimal pharmacologic level of estrogen is necessary to maintain the efficacy of the combination pill.

Because the effect of a progestational agent always takes precedence over estrogen unless the dose of estrogen is greatly increased, the endometrium, cervical mucus, and tubal function reflect progestational stimulation. The progestin in the combination pill produces an endometrium that is a decidualized bed with exhausted and atrophied glands and is therefore not receptive to ovum implantation. The cervical mucus becomes thick and impervious to sperm transport. It is possible that progestational influences on secretion and peristalsis within the fallopian tubes provide additional contraceptive effects. Even if there is some ovarian follicular activity as with the lowest dose products, these other actions serve to ensure good contraceptive efficacy.[3]

Efficacy

The contraceptive effectiveness of the new oral contraceptive regimens (multiphasic formulations and products with the lowest estrogen dose) is the same as that of older monophasic birth control pills in both the low-dose (<50 μg estrogen) and higher dose formulations.[3] Although carefully monitored studies with motivated subjects achieve an annual failure rate of 0.1%, typical use is associated with a 7.6% failure rate during the first year of use.[4] Contraceptive failure rates have been estimated using the data from the 1995 National Survey of Family Growth, correcting for the known underreporting of induced abortion.[2,4,5]

Patterns of Pill Taking

Effective contraception is present during the first cycle of pill use, provided the pills are started no later than the fifth day of the woman's cycle and that no pills are missed. Starting oral contraception on the first day of menses ensures immediate protection. In the United States, most clinicians and patients use the Sunday-start packages, beginning on the first Sunday following menstruation. This can be easier to remember, and it usually prevents menstrual bleeding on weekends. It is probable, but not totally certain, that even if a dominant follicle should emerge in occasional patients after a Sunday start, an LH surge and ovulation would still be prevented.[6]

The conventional approach to starting oral contraceptives, either with menses or on Sunday, carries with it a delay in achieving contraception for many women, so some clinicians advocate an immediate start on the day the patient receives her prescription, regardless of the patient's day in her cycle.[7] Combined with a backup method for the first week, preferably condoms, an immediate start can prevent unwanted pregnancies occurring during the delay before initiating oral contraception with the conventional methods. In some instances, a sensitive pregnancy test is a wise precaution. Women who use the immediate, or quick-start, method do not experience an increase in breakthrough bleeding.[8]

Postponement of a menstrual period can be easily achieved by omitting the 7-day hormone-free interval.

There is no rationale for recommending a pill-free interval to "rest," because this practice all too often results in unwanted pregnancies. The serious side effects are not eliminated by pill-free intervals.

Although the effects of fixed schedules are not well studied, there is reason to believe that precise pill taking minimizes breakthrough bleeding. In addition, compliance is improved by a fixed schedule that is habit forming.

Avoiding Menstrual Bleeding

More and more women are embracing the idea that fewer menstrual periods provide a welcome relief from bleeding and menstrual symptoms. A regimen (Seasonale) is available that supplies a package containing the number of pills required for 84 days of daily administration, reducing menstrual frequency to four menses per year.[9] However, clinicians for years have prescribed continuous daily oral contraceptives to treat conditions such as endometriosis, bleeding disorders, menstrual seizures, and menstrual migraine headaches, as well as to prevent bleeding in athletes and busy women. Many women do not require the periodic experience of vaginal bleeding to assure themselves they are not pregnant and can choose how frequently to have withdrawal bleeding.

Any combination OC can be used on a daily basis; even the lowest estrogen dose formulations provide acceptable bleeding and side effect profiles in a continuous regimen.[10,11] A further benefit of continuous use is simplification of the pill-taking schedule with the potential of better compliance and a lower failure rate. When breakthrough bleeding occurs, patients can be reassured that it is almost always temporary. When breakthrough bleeding is persistent, a 3- or 4-day interruption without pill taking has been reported to be helpful.[12]

Missed Pills

Irregular pill taking is a common occurrence. An electronic monitoring device demonstrates that consistency of pill taking is even worse than what patients report; only 33% of women were documented to have missed no pills in cycle 1, and by cycle 3, about one third of the women missed 3 or more pills with many episodes of consecutive days of missed pills.[13] These data indicate that women become less careful over time, emphasizing the importance of repeatedly reviewing with patients what to do when pills are missed.

Studies have questioned whether missing pills has an impact on contraception. One study demonstrated that skipping four consecutive pills at varying times in the cycle did not result in ovulation.[6] Studies in which women deliberately lengthen their pill-free interval up to 11 days have failed to show signs of ovulation.[14,15] So far, there is no evidence that moving to lower doses has had an impact on the margin of error. Despite greater follicular activity with the lowest-dose oral contraceptives, ovulation is still effectively prevented.[16] The progestational effects on endometrium and cervical mucus serve to ensure good contraceptive efficacy.[3]

The most prevalent identifiable problems associated with apparent oral contraceptive failures are vomiting and diarrhea.[17,18] Even if no pills have been missed, patients should be instructed to use a backup method for at least 7 days after an episode of gastroenteritis.

Clinical Problems Associated with Oral Contraceptive Use

Breakthrough Bleeding

There are two characteristic breakthrough bleeding problems: irregular bleeding in the first few months after starting oral contraception, and unexpected bleeding after many months of use. Effort should be made to manage the bleeding problem in a way that allows the patient to remain on low-dose oral contraception. There is no evidence that the onset of bleeding is associated with decreased efficacy, no matter what oral contraceptive formulation is used, even the lowest-dose products. Indeed, in a careful study, breakthrough bleeding did not correlate with changes in the blood levels of the contraceptive steroids.[19] On starting oral contraception, patients need to be fully informed about breakthrough bleeding.

The most commonly encountered breakthrough bleeding occurs in the first few months of use. The incidence is greatest in the first 3 months, ranging from 10% to 30% in the first month to less than 10% in the third month. Breakthrough bleeding rates are higher with the lowest-dose OCs, but not dramatically higher.[20,21] Breakthrough bleeding rates are higher in women who smoke and in smokers who use formulations with 20 μg ethinyl estradiol.[22] However, the differences among the various formulations currently available are of minimal clinical significance. The basic pattern is the same, highest in the first month and a greater prevalence in smokers, especially in later cycles.

Breakthrough bleeding that occurs after many months of oral contraceptive use is a consequence of the progestin-induced decidualization. This endometrium and the blood vessels within the endometrium tend to be fragile and prone to breakdown and asynchronous bleeding.

Two recognized factors (both preventable) are associated with a greater incidence of breakthrough bleeding. Inconsistent use and smoking increase spotting and bleeding, but inconsistency of pill taking is more important and has a greater effect in later cycles, whereas smoking exerts a general effect at any time.[23] Reinforcement of consistent pill taking can help minimize breakthrough bleeding. Cervical infection can be another cause of breakthrough bleeding; the prevalence of cervical chlamydial infections is higher among oral contraceptive users who report breakthrough bleeding.[24]

Thrombotic Complications

The administration of pharmacologic amounts of estrogen as in high-dose oral contraceptives causes an increase in the production of clotting factors such as factor V, factor VIII, factor X, and fibrinogen.[25] The progestin component also influences the clotting factor responses.[26] Some studies of the blood coagulation system have concluded that monophasic and multiphasic low-dose OCs have no significant clinical impact on the coagulation system. Slight increases in thrombin formation are offset by increased fibrinolytic activity.[27,28] Other studies of formulations containing 30 or 35 μg of ethinyl estradiol indicate an increase in clotting factors associated with an increase in platelet activity.[29] However, these changes are essentially all within normal ranges, and their clinical significance is unknown.[26]

Smoking produces a shift to hypercoagulability.[30] A 20-μg estrogen formulation has been reported to have no effect on clotting parameters, even in smokers.[30,31] One study comparing a 20-μg product with a 30-μg product found similar mild procoagulant and fibrinolytic activity, although there was a trend toward increased fibrinolytic activity with the lower dose.[32] These mixed reports make it essential to base clinical decisions on the epidemiologic studies of clinical events.

There is no evidence of an increase in risk of cardiovascular disease among past users of oral contraception.[33-35] In the Nurses' Health Study, the Royal College of General Practitioners' Study, and the Oxford Family Planning Association Study, long-term past use of oral contraceptives was not associated with an increase in overall mortality.[36-38] Part of the concern for a possible lingering effect of oral contraceptive use was based on a presumed adverse impact on the atherosclerotic process, which would then be added to the effect of aging and thus would be manifested later in life. Instead, the findings have been consistent with the contention that cardiovascular disease due to oral contraception is secondary to acute effects, specifically estrogen-induced thrombosis, a dose-related event.

Venous Thrombosis

Venous Thromboembolism

Older epidemiologic evaluations of oral contraceptives and vascular disease indicated that venous thrombosis was caused by estrogen, limited to current users, with a disappearance of the risk by 3 months after discontinuation.[39,40] Thromboembolic disease was believed to be a consequence of the pharmacologic administration of estrogen, and the level of risk was believed to be related to the estrogen dose.[41-43] Smoking was documented to produce an additive increase in the risk of arterial thrombosis,[44-46] but it had no effect on the risk of venous thromboembolism.[47,48]

In the first years of oral contraception, the available products, containing 80 and 100 μg ethinyl estradiol (extremely high doses), were associated with a sixfold increased risk of venous thrombosis, the same risk seen in pregnant women.[49] Because of the increased risks of venous thrombosis, myocardial infarction, and stroke, lower-dose formulations (<50 μg estrogen) came to dominate the market, and clinicians became more careful in their screening of patients and prescribing of oral contraception. Because of these two factors, the Puget Sound study in the United States documented a reduction in venous thrombosis risk to twofold.[50]

Venous Thromboembolism and the Factor V Leiden Mutation

A risk of idiopathic venous thrombosis persists with low-dose oral contraceptives at a level of approximately threefold to fourfold greater than the normal, general incidence.[51-55] However, an inherited resistance to activated protein C, the factor V Leiden mutation, might account for a significant portion of the patients who experience venous thrombosis while taking oral contraceptives (Table 17–2).

An inherited resistance to activated protein C, the factor V Leiden mutation, is the most common inherited coagulation problem transmitted in an autosomal-dominant fashion.[60,61] Heterozygotes have a 5- to 8-fold increased risk of venous thromboembolism, and homozygotes have an 80-fold increased risk. Oral contraceptive users who have this mutation have been reported to have a 30-fold increased risk of venous thrombosis.[62,63] Some have argued, however, that this increase has been overestimated, and it may be closer to 10- to 15-fold.[59,64] The risk of developing venous thrombosis is greatest in the initial months of use, and it has been suggested that venous thrombosis occurring in the first month of exposure should make the clinician suspect the presence of a clotting disorder.[65]

Combination oral contraception is contraindicated in women who have a history of idiopathic venous thromboembolism, as well as in women who have a close family history (parent or sibling) of idiopathic venous thromboembolism. These women will have a higher incidence of congenital deficiencies in important clotting measurements, especially antithrombin III, protein C, protein S, and resistance to activated protein C.[83] Such a patient who screens negatively for an inherited clotting deficiency might still consider using oral contraceptives, but this would be a difficult decision with unknown risks for both patient and clinician, and it is more prudent to consider other contraceptive options. Other risk factors for thromboembolism that should be considered by clinicians include an acquired predisposition, such as lupus anticoagulant or malignancy, and immobility or trauma. Varicose veins are not a risk factor unless they are very extensive.[49]

TABLE 17–2 RELATIVE RISK AND ACTUAL INCIDENCE OF VENOUS THROMBOEMBOLISM[56-59]

Population	Relative Risk	Incidence (no. per 100,000/year)
Young women (general population)	1	4-5
Pregnant women	12	48-60
High-dose oral contraceptives	6-10	24-50
Low-dose oral contraceptives	3-4	12-20
Leiden mutation carrier	5-8	20-40
Leiden carrier and oral contraceptives	10-30	40-150
Leiden mutation, homozygous	80	320-400

Arterial Thrombosis

The incidence of cerebral thrombotic attacks (thrombotic strokes and transient ischemic attacks) among young women is higher than that of venous thromboembolism and myocardial infarction, and death and disability are more likely. Because of the higher incidence and risk, cerebral arterial thrombosis is the most important possible side effect of oral contraceptives. A very low incidence of stroke in young women carries with it little increase in absolute risk. However, because the incidence of cerebral thrombotic attacks is higher in women older than 40 years, oral contraceptive users older than 40 years must be in good health and without significant risk factors for cardiovascular disease (especially hypertension, migraine with aura, and smoking).

The synergy of smoking and oral contraception in causing myocardial infarction is well documented (Table 17–3). It has been difficult to establish arterial thrombosis dose-response relationships with estrogen because these events are so rare. Nevertheless, the estrogen dose is an important factor for the risk of myocardial infarction and thrombotic strokes.[66,67]

Arterial Thrombosis—Stroke

Older case-control and cohort studies indicated an increased risk of cerebral thrombosis among current users of high-dose oral contraceptives.[70-72] However, thrombotic stroke did not appear to be increased in healthy, nonsmoking women who used oral contraceptives containing less than 50 μg ethinyl estradiol.[71,72] A case-control study of all 794 women in Denmark who suffered a cerebral thromboembolic attack during the period 1985 to 1989 concluded that there was an almost twofold increased relative risk associated with oral contraceptives containing 30 to 40 μg estrogen, and the risk was significantly influenced by both smoking and the dose of estrogen in additive (not synergistic) fashion.[46] A case-control analysis of data collected by the Royal College of General Practitioners' Oral Contraception Study concluded that current users were at increased risk for stroke (with a persisting effect in former users); however, this outcome was limited mainly to smokers and to formulations with 50 μg or more of estrogen.[72]

TABLE 17–3 INCIDENCE OF MYOCARDIAL INFARCTION IN REPRODUCTIVE-AGE WOMEN[68]

Population	Incidence (no. per 100,000/year)
Overall[69]	5
WOMEN YOUNGER THAN 35 YEARS	
Nonsmokers	4
Nonsmokers taking OCs	4
Smokers	8
Smokers taking OCs	43
WOMEN 35 YEARS AND OLDER	
Nonsmokers	10
Nonsmokers taking OCs	40
Smokers	88
Smokers taking OCs	485

OC, oral contraceptive.

Note: These incidences are estimates based on oral contraceptive use paired with cardiovascular risk factors prevalent in the general population. Effective screening would produce smaller numbers. The increased risks in the smokers and OC groups reflect the impact of undetected cardiovascular risk factors, especially hypertension.

TABLE 17–4 INCIDENCE OF STROKE IN REPRODUCTIVE-AGE WOMEN[69,73-75]

Population	Incidence (no. per 100,000/year)
ISCHEMIC STROKE	
Overall	5
Women < 35 y	1-3
Women ≥ 35 y	10
HEMORRHAGIC STROKE	
Overall	6
EXCESS DUE TO OC USE*	
Low-dose OC	2
Low-dose OC, <35 y	1
High-dose OC	8

*Includes women who smoke and women with hypertension.
OC, oral contraceptive.

A population-based, case-control study of 408 strokes from the California Kaiser Permanente Medical Care Program found no increase in risk for either ischemic stroke or hemorrhagic stroke.[73] The identifiable risk factors for ischemic stroke were smoking, hypertension, diabetes, elevated body weight, and low socioeconomic status. The risk factors for hemorrhagic stroke were the same plus greater body mass and heavy use of alcohol. Current users of low-dose oral contraceptives did not have an increased risk of ischemic or hemorrhagic stroke compared with former users and with never users. There was no evidence for an adverse effect of increasing age or for smoking (for hemorrhagic stroke, there was a suggestion of a positive interaction between current oral contraceptive use and smoking, but the numbers were small, and the result was not statistically significant). Table 17–4 summarizes current results.

Arterial Thrombosis—Current Assessment

There has been no evidence with respectable statistical power that the new (third generation) progestins have an appreciable difference in risk of arterial disease, an event not increased with low-dose older-type progestin oral contraceptives. It is possible that as these studies continue and acquire greater statistical power, a difference will emerge, but the difference will be minor and probably clinically insignificant even if this is the case.

Most importantly, the new studies fail to find any substantial risk of ischemic or hemorrhagic stroke with low-dose oral contraceptives in healthy young women. The WHO study did find evidence for an adverse impact of smoking in women younger than 35 years; the Kaiser study did not. This difference is explained by the confounding effect of hypertension, the major risk factor identified. In the WHO study, a history of hypertension was based on whether a patient reported ever having had high blood pressure (other than in pregnancy) and was not validated by medical records. In the Kaiser study, women were classified as having hypertension if they reported using antihypertensive medication (less than 5% of oral contraceptive users had treated hypertension, and there were no users of higher-dose products). In the WHO study, the effect of using oral contraceptives in the presence of a high-risk factor is apparent in the different odds ratios when European women who received good screening from clinicians were compared with women in developing countries who received little screening; therefore, more women with cardiovascular risk factors in developing countries were using oral contraceptives.

Oral contraceptives containing less than 50 μg ethinyl estradiol do not increase the risk of myocardial infarction or stroke in healthy nonsmoking women, regardless of age. The effect of smoking in women younger than 35 years is, as we have long recognized, not detectable in the absence of hypertension. After age 35 years, the subtle presence of hypertension makes analysis difficult, but the Kaiser study indicates that increasing age and smoking by themselves have little impact on the risk of stroke in low-dose oral contraceptive users. The screening of patients in the Kaiser program was excellent, resulting in few women with hypertension using oral contraceptives. The new studies indicate that hypertension should be a major concern, especially with regard to the risk of stroke.

Hypertension

Oral contraceptive–induced hypertension was observed in approximately 5% of users of higher-dose pills. More-recent evidence indicates that small increases in blood pressure can be observed even with 30-μg estrogen monophasic pills, including those containing the new progestins. However, an increased incidence of clinically significant hypertension has not been reported.[77-80] The lack of clinical hypertension in most studies may be due to the rarity of its occurrence. The Nurses' Health Study observed an increased risk of clinical hypertension in current users of low-dose oral contraceptives, providing an incidence of 41.5 cases per 10,000 women per year.[81] Therefore, an annual assessment of blood pressure is still an important element of clinical surveillance, even when low-dose oral contraceptives are used. Postmenopausal women in the Rancho Bernardo Study who had previously used oral contraceptives (probably high-dose products) had slightly higher (2 to 4 mm Hg) diastolic blood pressures.[82] Because past users do not demonstrate differences in incidence or risk factors for cardiovascular disease, it is unlikely this blood pressure difference has an important clinical effect.

Low-dose oral contraceptives are very safe for healthy young women. Screening for smoking and cardiovascular risk factors, especially hypertension, in women older than 35 years can nearly eliminate increased risk of arterial disease associated with low-dose oral contraceptives. There is no increased risk of cardiovascular events associated with duration of use (long term). In large cohort studies, the risk of overall mortality comparing users and nonusers of oral contraceptives is identical.[36-38]

Breast Cancer

Current and recent use of oral contraceptives, in case-control studies, may be associated with about a 20% increased risk of early (before age 35 years) premenopausal breast cancer, essentially limited to localized disease. This modest increase in relative risk is predicted to be associated with a very small increase in the actual number of cases (so small, there would be no major impact on incidence figures). The finding of a modest increase in relative risk in young women may be partly or entirely due to detection and surveillance bias and accelerated growth of already present malignancies, a situation similar to the effects of pregnancy and postmenopausal hormone therapy on the risk of breast cancer. Further comfort can be derived from the fact that the increase in breast cancer in American women was greater in older women from 1973 to 1994, those who did not have the opportunity to use oral contraception.[125] In women younger than 50 years, there was only a slight increase during this time period. The large American case-control study of women age 35 to 64 years was totally negative and very reassuring.

There is no effect of past use or duration of oral contraceptive use (up to 15 years of continuous use) on the risk of breast cancer, and there is no evidence indicating that higher-dose oral contraceptives increased the risk of breast cancer. In fact, previous oral contraceptive use may be associated with a reduced risk of metastatic breast cancer later in life and possibly with a reduced risk of postmenopausal breast cancer.

Oral contraceptive use does not further increase the risk of breast cancer in women with positive family histories of breast cancer or in women with proven benign breast disease. However, the clinician should not fail to take every opportunity to direct attention to all factors that affect breast cancer. Breastfeeding and control of alcohol intake are good examples and are also components of preventive health care. Especially important is this added motivation to encourage breastfeeding. The protective effect of breastfeeding is exerted mainly on premenopausal breast cancer, the cancer of concern to younger women using oral contraception.

Carbohydrate Metabolism

With the older high-dose oral contraceptives, many women had impaired glucose tolerance: plasma levels of insulin as well as the blood sugar were elevated in a glucose tolerance test. Generally, the effect of oral contraception is to produce an increase in peripheral resistance to insulin action. Most women can meet this challenge by increasing insulin secretion, and there is no change in the glucose tolerance test, although 1-hour values may be slightly elevated.

Insulin sensitivity is affected mainly by the progestin component of the pill.[84] The derangement of carbohydrate metabolism may also be affected by estrogen influences on lipid metabolism, hepatic enzymes, and elevation of unbound cortisol. The glucose intolerance is dose related: effects are less with the low-dose formulations. Insulin and glucose changes with low-dose monophasic and multiphasic oral contraceptives are so minimal that it is now believed they are of no clinical significance.[80,85-88] These studies include long-term evaluation with measurement of hemoglobin A1c (Hb_{A1c}).

Liver

The liver is affected in more ways and with more regularity and intensity by the sex steroids than any other extragenital organ. Estrogen influences the synthesis of hepatic DNA and RNA, hepatic cell enzymes, serum enzymes formed in the liver, and plasma proteins. Estrogenic hormones also affect hepatic lipid and lipoprotein formation, the intermediary metabolism of carbohydrates, and intracellular enzyme activity. Nevertheless, an extensive analysis of the prospective cohorts of women in the Royal College of General Practitioners' Oral Contraception Study and the Oxford Family Planning Association Contraceptive Study could detect no evidence of an increased incidence or risk of serious liver disease among oral contraceptive users.[89]

The active transport of biliary components is impaired by estrogens as well as some progestins. The mechanism is unclear, but cholestatic jaundice and pruritus were occasional complications of higher dose oral contraception. As in the recurrent jaundice of pregnancy, the cholestasis was benign and reversible. The incidence of this complication with lower dose oral contraception is unknown, but it must be very rare.

The only absolute hepatic contraindication to oral contraceptive use is acute or chronic cholestatic liver disease. Cirrhosis and previous hepatitis are not aggravated. Once recovered from the acute phase of liver disease, a woman can use oral contraception.

Oral Contraceptive Use and Medical Problems

Metabolic Disorders

Diabetes Mellitus

Oral contraception may be used by diabetic women younger than 35 years old who do not smoke and are otherwise healthy (especially an absence of diabetic vascular complications). A case-control study could find no evidence that oral contraceptive use by young women with insulin-dependent diabetes mellitus increased the development of retinopathy or nephropathy.[98] In a 1-year study of women with insulin-dependent diabetes mellitus who were using a low-dose oral contraceptive, no deterioration could be documented in lipoprotein or hemostatic biochemical markers for cardiovascular risk.[99] And finally, no effect of oral contraceptives on cardiovascular mortality could be detected in a group of women with diabetes mellitus.[100] Women with diabetes and vascular disease or major cardiovascular risk factors should avoid pharmacologic doses of exogenous estrogen.

Gallbladder Disease

Oral contraception use might precipitate a symptomatic attack in women known to have stones or a positive history for gallbladder disease and, therefore, should either be used very cautiously or not at all.

Hyperlipidemia

Because low-dose oral contraceptives have negligible impact on the lipoprotein profile, hyperlipidemia is not an absolute contraindication, with the exception of very high levels of triglycerides (which can be further elevated by estrogen). In women with triglyceride levels greater than 250 mg/dL, estrogen should be provided with great caution. If vascular disease is already present, oral contraception should be avoided. If other risk factors are present, especially smoking, oral contraception is not recommended. Dyslipidemic patients who begin oral contraception should have their lipoprotein profiles monitored monthly for a few visits to ensure no adverse impact. If the lipid abnormality cannot be controlled, an alternative method of contraception should be used.[108]

Oral contraceptives containing the less androgenic synthetic progestins—desogestrel, noregestimate, or gestodene—can increase high-density lipoprotein (HDL) levels, but it is not known if this change is clinically significant. If hypertriglyceridemia is the only concern, keep in mind that the triglyceride response to estrogen is rapid. A repeat level should be obtained in 2 to 4 weeks. A level greater than 750 mg/dL represents an absolute contraindication to estrogen treatment because of the risk of pancreatitis.

Hepatic Disease

Oral contraception may be used when liver function tests return to normal. Follow-up liver function tests should be obtained after 2 to 3 months of OC use.

Obesity

An obese woman who is otherwise healthy may use low-dose oral contraception. However, there are special considerations associated with obesity.

Obesity is an independent risk factor for venous thrombosis, and case-control studies have indicated that this risk adds to that associated with oral contraceptives.[109-111]

Recent evidence suggests that hormonal contraceptive failure is increased in overweight women (weight greater than 155 pounds).[112-114] Clinical trials have excluded women with high body weight, and for this reason, the effect of body weight on contraception was not well studied. Selecting a 50-μg estrogen product for overweight women might overcome the failure rate, but this would add the risks of venous thrombosis associated with a higher dose of estrogen to those already linked with obesity. Keep in mind that the conclusions regarding failure rates and weight were based on differences of only 2 to 4 pregnancies per 100 women per year. Efficacy in overweight women is still greater than that with barrier methods.

Polycystic Ovaries and Insulin Resistance

Because older, high-dose oral contraceptives increased insulin resistance, it has been suggested that this treatment should be avoided in anovulatory, overweight women. However, low-dose oral contraceptives have minimal effects on carbohydrate metabolism, and the majority of hyperinsulinemic, hyperandrogenic women can be expected to respond favorably to treatment with oral contraceptives.[115]

Insulin and glucose changes with low-dose (<50 μg ethinyl estradiol) oral contraceptives are so minimal that it is now believed that they are of no clinical significance.[87] Long-term follow-up studies have failed to detect any increase in the incidence of diabetes mellitus or impaired glucose tolerance (even in past and current users of high-dose pills).[116,117] Furthermore, there is no evidence of an increase in risk of cardiovascular disease among past users of oral contraceptives.[35,36] In addition, low-dose oral contraceptives have been administered to women with recent gestational diabetes without an adverse impact, and in women with insulin-dependent diabetes mellitus, low-dose oral contraceptives have not produced deterioration of lipid and biochemical markers for cardiovascular disease or increased the development of retinopathy or nephropathy.[96-99] The administration of a low-dose oral contraceptive to women with extreme obesity and very severe insulin resistance resulted in only a mild deterioration of glucose tolerance.[118]

Impressively, in a follow-up study (about 10 years) of women with polycystic ovaries and hyperinsulinism, comparing oral contraceptive users with nonusers, the metabolic parameters not only did not worsen in the users, but they actually improved, including body weight, glucose tolerance, insulin levels, and HDL-cholesterol levels, which was in striking contrast to the metabolic worsening observed in the nonusers.[119] This experience supports the safety of estrogen-progestin contraceptive treatment for anovulatory, hyperandrogenic, hyperinsulinemic women.

Eating Disorders

In patients with eating disorders, bone density correlates with body weight. The response of bone density to hormone therapy will be impaired as long as an abnormal weight is maintained.[120] The failure to respond to estrogen treatment with an increase in bone density may be due to the adverse bone effects of the hypercortisolism associated with stress disorders. Furthermore, because the pubertal gain in bone density is so significant, patients who fail to experience this adolescent increase can continue to have a deficit in bone mass despite hormone treatment. Reduced menstrual function for any reason early in life (even beyond adolescence) can leave a residual deficit in bone density that cannot be totally retrieved with resumption of menses or with hormone treatment.[121,122]

Cardiovascular Disorders

Hypertension

Low-dose oral contraception may be used in women younger than 35 years who have hypertension well controlled by medication and who are otherwise healthy and do not smoke. We recommend the lowest estrogen dose formulations. Nevertheless, a cross-sectional study in Brazil reported worse control of hypertension in users of oral contraceptives.[90] Certainly a woman with controlled hypertension who has additional medical problems or who smokes should not use estrogen-progestin contraceptives (including the transdermal and vaginal methods). In a young woman with controlled hypertension who is otherwise healthy, very frequent and close monitoring of the blood pressure is essential. Because myocardial infarction and stroke become more common after age 35 years, combined estrogen-progestin contraception should not be used by women who have controlled hypertension after age 35. Progestin-only methods are acceptable.

Mitral Valve Prolapse

Oral contraception use in women with mitral valve prolapse is limited to nonsmoking patients who are asymptomatic (no clinical evidence of mitral regurgitation). There is a small subset of patients with mitral valve prolapse who are at increased risk for thromboembolism. Patients with atrial fibrillation, migraine headaches, or clotting factor abnormalities should consider progestin-only methods or intrauterine contraception (prophylactic antibiotics should cover insertion if mitral regurgitation is present).

Smoking

Oral contraception is absolutely contraindicated in smokers older than 35 years. In patients 35 years and younger, heavy smoking (15 or more cigarettes per day) is a relative contraindication. The relative risk of cardiovascular events is increased for women of all ages who smoke and use oral contraceptives; however, because the actual incidence of cardiovascular events is so low at a young age, the absolute risk is very low for young women, although it increases with age. An ex-smoker (for at least 1 year) should be regarded as a nonsmoker. Risk is only linked to active smoking. In the absence of any other risk factors, low-dose oral contraceptives might be appropriate for a light smoker or the user of a nicotine patch. A 20-μg estrogen formulation may be a better choice for smoking women, regardless of age, because this dose of estrogen has no impact on clotting factors and platelet activation.[30,31]

Smoking continues to be a difficult problem, not only for patient management but also for analysis of data. In large U.S. surveys in 1982 and 1988, the decline in the prevalence of smoking was similar in users and nonusers of oral contraception; however, 24.3% of 35- to 45-year-old women who used oral contraceptives were smokers![76] In this group of smoking, oral contraceptive–using women, 85.3% smoked 15 or more cigarettes per day (heavy smoking). Despite the widespread teaching and publicity that smoking is a contraindication to oral contraceptive use in women older than 35 years, more older women who used oral contraceptives smoked and smoked heavily, compared with young women. This strongly suggests that older smokers are less than honest with clinicians when requesting oral contraception, and this further raises serious concern over how well this confounding variable can be controlled in case-control and cohort studies. A former smoker must have stopped smoking for at least 12 consecutive months to be regarded as a nonsmoker. Women who have nicotine in their bloodstream obtained from patches or gum should be regarded as smokers.

Congenital Heart Disease or Valvular Heart Disease

Oral contraception is contraindicated only if there is marginal cardiac reserve or a condition that predisposes to thrombosis.

Pregnancy-Associated Diseases

Pregnancy-Induced Hypertension

Women with pregnancy-induced hypertension may use oral contraception as soon as the blood pressure is normal in the postpartum period.

Gestational Diabetes

Low-dose formulations do not produce a diabetic glucose tolerance response in women with previous gestational diabetes, and there is no evidence that combined oral contraceptives increase the incidence of overt diabetes mellitus.[96,97] Women with previous gestational diabetes may use oral contraception with annual assessment of the fasting glucose level.

Cholestatic Jaundice in Pregnancy

Not all patients who have cholestatic jaundice in pregnancy will develop jaundice while taking oral contraception. Jaundice is especially unlikely with the low-dose formulations.

Benign Tumors

Uterine Leiomyoma

The risk of leiomyomas decreased by 31% in women who used higher dose oral contraception for 10 years.[91] However, case-control studies with lower-dose oral contraceptives have found neither a decrease nor an increase in risk, although the Nurses' Health Study reported a slightly increased risk when oral contraceptives were first used in early teenage years.[92-94] One case-control study indicated a decreasing risk of uterine myomas with increasing duration of oral contraceptive use.[95] The administration of low-dose oral contraceptives to women with leiomyomas does not stimulate fibroid growth, and it is associated with a reduction in menstrual bleeding.[95]

Benign Breast Disease

Benign breast disease is not a contraindication for oral contraception. With 2 years of use, the condition sometimes improves.

Pituitary Prolactin-Secreting Adenomas

Estrogen stimulates prolactin secretion and causes growth of pituitary lactotrophs, but oral contraceptives do not increase the risk of pituitary adenomas and may be used in the presence of microadenomas without affecting their rate of growth.

Neurologic and Psychiatric Disorders

Migraine Headaches

Some women report an improvement in their headaches with oral contraceptives. Low-dose oral contraception (the lowest estrogen dose formulations) may be used with careful surveillance in women with migraine headaches without aura. Daily administration can prevent menstrual migraine headaches. Oral contraception is best avoided in women with migraine headaches with aura or if additional risk factors for stroke are present (especially older age, smoking, and hypertension).

Seizure Disorders

Oral contraceptives do not exacerbate epilepsy, and in some women, seizure control has improved.[101,102] Antiepileptic drugs that affect liver metabolism, however, can decrease the effectiveness of oral contraception. Some clinicians advocate the use of higher -ose (50 μg estrogen) products; however, no studies have been performed to demonstrate that this higher dose is necessary. Another problem is that moving to a higher-dose product increases the estrogen dose (and the risk of side effects) but does not significantly change the progestin dose, the component that inhibits ovulation. A wiser course is to consider intrauterine contraception, long-acting progestin methods, or sterilization.

Depression

Low-dose oral contraceptives have minimal, if any, impact on mood.

Hematopoietic Disorders

Sickle Cell Disease

Women with sickle cell trait may use oral contraception. The potentiation of risk of thrombosis with sickle cell disease or sickle C diseases is a theoretical (and medicolegal) possibility. However, we believe effective protection against pregnancy in these patients warrants the use of low-dose oral contraception. In the only long-term (10 years) follow-up report of women with sickle cell disease using oral contraceptives at a time when higher dose products were prevalent, no apparent adverse effects were observed.[103] A study of erythrocyte deformability in women with sickle cell anemia could detect no adverse effects of contraceptive steroids.[104] Keep in mind that depot-medroxyprogesterone acetate (DMPA) used for contraception is associated with inhibition of sickling and improvement in anemia in patients with sickle cell disease.[105]

Hemorrhagic Disorders

Women with hemorrhagic disorders and women taking anticoagulants may use oral contraception. Inhibition of ovulation can prevent the serious problem of a hemorrhagic corpus luteum in these patients. A reduction in menstrual blood loss provides an additional benefit.

Inflammatory and Immune Conditions

Systemic Lupus Erythematosus

Oral contraceptive use can exacerbate systemic lupus erythematosus, and the vascular disease associated with lupus, when present, represents a contraindication to estrogen-containing contraceptives.[106] The progestin-only methods are a good choice. However, in patients with stable or inactive disease, without renal involvement or high antiphospholipid antibodies, low-dose oral contraception may be considered.[107]

Infectious Mononucleosis

Oral contraception may be used as long as liver function tests are normal.

Ulcerative Colitis

There is no association between oral contraception and ulcerative colitis. Women with this problem may use oral contraceptives.[123] Oral contraceptives are absorbed mainly in the small bowel.

Regional Enteritis (Crohn's Disease)

In a prospective cohort of women with Crohn's disease, no adverse impact of oral contraceptives could be detected on the clinical course, specifically on flare-ups.[124]

Elective Surgery

The recommendation that oral contraception should be discontinued 4 weeks before elective major surgery to avoid an increased risk of postoperative thrombosis is based on data derived from high-dose pills. If possible, it is safer to follow this recommendation when a period of immobilization is expected. With major surgery and immobilization, prophylactic anticoagulation should be considered for a current or recent user of oral contraceptives. It is prudent to maintain contraception right up to the performance of a sterilization procedure, and this short outpatient operation carries minimal risk.

Noncontraceptive Benefits of Oral Contraception

The noncontraceptive benefits of low-dose oral contraception can be grouped into two main categories: benefits that incidentally accrue when oral contraception is specifically used for contraceptive purposes and benefits that result from the use of oral contraceptives to treat problems and disorders. The noncontraceptive incidental benefits are listed in Table 17–5.

TABLE 17–5 NONCONTRACEPTIVE BENEFITS OF ORAL CONTRACEPTIVES
EFFECTIVE CONTRACEPTION
Less need for induced abortion
Less need for surgical sterilization
MORE REGULAR MENSES
Less flow
Less dysmenorrhea
Less anemia
OTHER
Less endometrial cancer
Less ovarian cancer
Fewer ectopic pregnancies
Less salpingitis
Increased bone density
Probably less endometriosis
Possibly less benign breast disease
Possibly less rheumatoid arthritis
Possibly protection against atherosclerosis
Possibly fewer fibroids
Possibly fewer ovarian cysts

Special Uses of Oral Contraception

The Progestin-Only Minipill

The minipill contains a small dose of a progestational agent and must be taken daily, in a continuous fashion.[126,127] There is no evidence for any major differences in clinical behavior among the available minipill products except that desogestrel suppresses ovulation more reliably than the others. All of them (listed in Table 17–6) could probably be used in high doses (10 to 20 pills) as emergency contraception, but only levonorgestrel has been proved effective.

Mechanism of Action

After taking a progestin-only minipill, the small amount of progestin in the circulation (about 25% of that in combined oral contraceptives) will have a significant effect only on tissues very sensitive to progesterone. The contraceptive effect is more dependent on effects on endometrial and cervical mucus because gonadotropins are not consistently suppressed. The cervical mucus becomes thick and impermeable to sperm, and the endometrium involutes and becomes hostile to implantation. Approximately 40% of patients ovulate normally.[128,129] Tubal physiology might also be affected, but this is speculative. The progestin-only minipill containing 0.075 mg desogestrel appears to be more effective, probably because it exerts a greater inhibition of ovulation than the other progestins.[130]

Because of the low dose, the minipill must be taken every day at the same time of day. The change in the cervical mucus requires 2 to 4 hours to take effect, and, most importantly, the impermeability diminishes 22 hours after administration, and by 24 hours sperm penetration is essentially unimpaired.

Ectopic pregnancy is not prevented as effectively as intrauterine pregnancy. Although the overall incidence of ectopic pregnancy is not increased (it is still much lower than the incidence in women not using a contraceptive method), when pregnancy occurs, the clinician must suspect that it is more likely to be ectopic. A previous ectopic pregnancy should not be regarded as a contraindication to the minipill; however, women at risk for subsequent ectopic pregnancy require the protection provided by methods, like the combined pill, that prevent fertilization.

There are no significant metabolic effects (lipid levels, carbohydrate metabolism, and coagulation factors remain unchanged),[84,131-133] and there is an immediate return to fertility on discontinuation, unlike the delay seen with the combination oral contraceptive.

Efficacy

Failure rates have been documented to range from 1.1 to 9.6 per 100 women in the first year of use.[134] The failure rate is higher in younger women (3.1 per 100 woman-years) compared with women older than 40 years (0.3 per 100 woman-years).[135] In motivated women, the failure rate is comparable to the rate (<1 per 100 woman-years) with combination oral contraception.[136,137]

TABLE 17–6 MINIPILLS AVAILABLE WORLDWIDE

Brand	Composition
Micronor, Nor-QD, Noriday, Norod	0.350 mg norethindrone
Microval, Noregeston, Microlut	0.030 mg levonorgestrel
Ovrette, Neogest	0.075 mg norgestrel (equivalent to 0.0375 mg levonorgestrel)
Exluton	0.500 mg lynestrenol
Femulen	0.500 mg ethynodial diacetate
Cerazette	0.075 mg desogestrel

Patterns of Pill Taking

The minipill should be started on the first day of menses, and a backup method must be used for the first 7 days because some women ovulate as early as 7 to 9 days after the onset of menses. Taking the pill should be keyed to a daily event to ensure regular administration at the same time of the day. If pills are forgotten or gastrointestinal (GI) illness impairs absorption, the minipill should be resumed as soon as possible, and a backup method should be used immediately and until the pills have been resumed for at least 2 days. If two or more pills are missed in a row and there is no menstrual bleeding in 4 to 6 weeks, a pregnancy test should be obtained. If the pill is taken more than 3 hours late, a backup method should be used for 48 hours.

Problems

In view of the unpredictable effect on ovulation, it is not surprising that irregular menstrual bleeding is the major clinical problem. The daily progestational impact on the endometrium also contributes to this problem. Patients can expect to have normal ovulatory cycles (40% to 50%); short, irregular cycles (40%); or a total lack of cycles ranging from irregular bleeding to spotting and amenorrhea (10%). Abnormal bleeding is the major reason women discontinue the minipill method of contraception.[137]

Women on progestin-only contraception develop more functional ovarian follicular cysts than those using methods that more profoundly suppress gonadotropins.[138,139] This is not a clinical problem because all or nearly all regress. Women who have experienced frequent ovarian cysts would be happier with methods that effectively suppress ovulation (combined oral contraceptives or DMPA).

The levonorgestrel minipill may be associated with acne. The mechanism is similar to that seen with Norplant (see later). The androgenic activity of levonorgestrel decreases the circulating levels of sex hormone–binding globulin (SHBG).[140] Therefore, free steroid levels (levonorgestrel and testosterone) will be increased despite the low dose. This is in contrast to the action of combined oral contraception, in which the effect of the progestin is countered by the estrogen-induced increase in SHBG.

Progestin-only minipills achieve efficacy comparable to combined pills in women older than 40 years and in women who are breastfeeding. There is no evidence for any adverse effect on breastfeeding as measured by milk volume and infant growth and development.[141-143] In fact, there is a modest positive effect; women using the minipill breastfeed longer and add supplementary feeding later.[144] Because of the slight positive impact on lactation, the minipill can be started immediately after delivery. A study investigating the effect of early initiation found no adverse effects on breastfeeding.[145]

The minipill is a good choice in situations where estrogen is contraindicated, such as patients with serious medical conditions (diabetes with vascular disease, severe systemic lupus erythematosus,[146] cardiovascular disease). The freedom from complications caused by estrogen, although likely, is presumptive. On the other hand, it is logical to conclude that any of the progestin effects associated with the combination oral contraceptives are found with the minipill, but a dose-response relationship should reduce adverse effects. The World Health Organization case-control study and the Transnational case-control study found no indication of increased risks of stroke, myocardial infarction, or venous thromboembolism with oral progestin-only contraceptives, but relatively small numbers have chosen to use this method of contraception and were included in these studies, which focused on combined OCs.[147,148] No impact can be measured on the coagulation system.[131,149] The minipill can probably be used in women with previous episodes of thrombosis, and the package insert in the United States was revised, eliminating vascular disease as a contraindication.

The minipill is a good alternative for the occasional woman who reports diminished libido on combination oral contraceptives, presumably due to decreased androgen levels. The minipill should also be considered for the few patients who report unacceptable levels of minor side effects (GI upset, breast tenderness, headaches) with the combination oral contraceptive.

Because of the relatively low doses of progestin administered, patients using medications that increase liver metabolism should avoid this method of contraception and other low-dose progestin methods, such as implants. These drugs include carbamazepine (Tegretol), felbamate, nevirapine, oxcarbazepine, phenobarbital, phenytoin (Dilantin), primidone (Mysoline), rifabutin, rifampicin (Rifampin), topiramate, St. John's wort, vigabatrin, and *possibly* ethosuximide, griseofulvin, and troglitazone. These medications can also limit the efficacy of combined pills.

Because of the relatively small numbers of users, we do not know if minipills confer the same benefits as combined oral contraceptives. The progestin impact on cervical mucus, endometrium, and ovulation leads one to think the benefits will be present (reduced risks of pelvic infection, endometrial cancer, and ovarian cancer). Although limited by small numbers, one case-control study indicated that protection against endometrial cancer was even greater with progestin-only pills than with combination oral contraceptives.[150]

Good efficacy with the minipill requires regularity of administration, taking the pill at the same time each day. There is less room for forgetting, and therefore the minipill is probably not a good choice for a disorganized adult or for the average adolescent.

Emergency Postcoital Contraception

The use of large doses of estrogen to prevent implantation was pioneered by Morris and van Wagenen at Yale in the 1960s. The initial work in monkeys led to the use of high doses of diethylstilbestrol (25 to 50 mg/day) and ethinyl estradiol in women.[151] It was quickly appreciated that these extremely large doses of estrogen were associated with a high rate of GI side effects. Albert Yuzpe developed a method using a combination oral contraceptive, resulting in an important reduction in dosage.[152] The following treatment regimens have been documented to be effective (Table 17–7):

- Ovral: 2 tablets followed by 2 tablets 12 hours later (0.5 mg norgestrel and 50 μg ethinyl estradiol per tablet)
- Alesse: 5 tablets followed by 5 tablets 12 hours later (100 μg levonorgestrel and 20 μg ethinyl estradiol per tablet)
- Lo Ovral, Nordette, Levlen, Triphasil (yellow tablets), Trilevlen (yellow tablets): 4 tablets followed by 4 tablets 12 hours later.

Levonorgestrel in a dose of 0.75 mg given twice, 12 hours apart, or in a single 1.5 mg dose, is more successful and better tolerated than the combination oral contraceptive method.[153,154] In many countries, special packages of two 0.75 mg levonorgestrel tablets (Plan B, Postinor, Norlevo, Vikela) are available for emergency contraception. In others, 20 levonorgestrel-containing mini pills are used to obtain an equivalent dose. Greater efficacy and fewer side effects make levonorgestrel alone the treatment of choice.[155,156]

This method has been commonly called *postcoital contraception* or the *morning after* treatment. *Emergency contraception* (EC) is a more accurate and appropriate name, indicating one-time protection. It is an important option for patients and should be considered when condoms break, when sexual assault occurs, when diaphragms or cervical caps dislodge, or with the lapsed use of any method. In studies at abortion units, 50% to

TABLE 17–7 EMERGENCY CONTRACEPTION

	DOSE PER TABLET				
Brand Name	**Ethinyl Estradiol**	**Levonorgestrel**	**Norgestrel**	**First Dose**	**Second Dose (12 hr Later)**
Alesse	20 µg	0.10 mg	—	5 tablets	5 tablets
Levlen	30 µg	0.15 mg	—	4 tablets	4 tablets
Lo Ovral	30 µg	—	0.3 mg	4 tablets	4 tablets
Nordette	30 µg	0.15 mg	—	4 tablets	4 tablets
Ovral	50 µg	—	0.5 mg	2 tablets	2 tablets
Plan B*	none	0.75 mg	—	1-2 tablets	0-1 tablets
Trilevlen	30 µg	0.125 mg	—	4 tablets	4 tablets
Triphasil	30 µg	0.125 mg	—	4 tablets	4 tablets
Ovrette, Neogest	none	—	0.075 mg	20 tablets	20 tablets

*Package only as emergency contraception; taken in one or two doses.

60% of the patients would have been suitable candidates for emergency contraception and would have used it if it were readily available.[157,158] In the United States, it is estimated that emergency contraception could annually prevent 1.7 million unintended pregnancies, and the number of induced abortions would decrease by about 40%.[159]

Many women do not know of this method, and it has been difficult to obtain.[158,160] Even if women are aware of it, accurate and detailed knowledge is lacking.[161] Women who have used emergency contraception are very satisfied with the method, and most importantly, they do not express an intention to substitute this method for regular contraception.[162] Information for patients and clinicians, including the latest available products, can be obtained from the web site and hotline maintained by the Office of Population Research at Princeton University: http://ec.princeton.edu; Telephone hotline: 1-888-NOT-2-LATE (1-888-668-2528).

Clinicians should consider providing emergency contraceptive kits to patients (a kit can simply be an envelope containing instructions and the appropriate number of oral contraceptives) to be taken when needed. In studies of self-administration, women in Scotland and young women in California increased the use of emergency contraception without adverse effects, such as increasing unprotected sex or contracting sexually transmitted disease.[163-167]

Progestin-only emergency contraception is now available without a prescription in many countries including the United States, where patients 18 and older can obtain it without first seeing a clinician. Younger patients, who are mostly likely to need it, must still have a prescription except in a few states that have more permissive laws.[168] Women are able to use this nonprescription access effectively and do not develop a reliance on emergency contraception as a regular method.[168] Adolescents use it in the same way as do older women.[167]

Mechanism and Efficacy

The mechanism of action is not known with certainty, but it is believed with justification that this treatment combines delay of ovulation with a local effect on the endometrium and prevention of fertilization.[169-173] How much a postfertilization effect contributes to efficacy is not known, but it is not believed to be the primary mechanism.[172,174]

Efficacy has been confirmed in large clinical trials and summarized in complete reviews of the literature.[175-177] Treatment with high doses of estrogen or with levonorgestrel yields a failure rate of approximately 1%; failure rate with the combination oral contraceptive is approximately 2% to 3%. The failure rate is lowest with high doses of ethinyl estradiol given within 72 hours (0.1%), but the negative side effects make this method a poor choice. In general clinical use, the method using oral contraceptives can reduce the risk of pregnancy by about 75%; this degree of reduction in probability of conception (given the relatively low chance, about 8%, for pregnancy associated with one act of coitus)[178] yields the 2% failure rate measured in clinical studies.[179-181]

Results with levonorgestrel are even better, approximately an 85% reduction in the risk of pregnancy; in the worldwide World Health Organization study, the risk of pregnancy was 60% lower with the levonorgestrel-only method compared with the oral contraceptive method, with less than half as much nausea and vomiting.[154]

Treatment Method

Treatment should be initiated as soon after exposure as possible, but no later than 120 hours. Careful assessment of the reported experience with emergency contraception indicates that the method is equally effective when started on the first, second, or third day after intercourse (which would allow user-friendly scheduling) and that efficacy might extend beyond 72 hours.[182,183] Data from the World Health Organization randomized clinical trial, however, support the importance of timing; this trial found a reduction in efficacy after 72 hours, and the greatest protection occurred when the medication was taken within 24 hours of intercourse.[184] Postponing the dose by 12 hours raises the chance of pregnancy by almost 50%. For this reason, the treatment should be initiated as soon as possible after sexual exposure, an important argument in favor of advance provision of emergency contraception.

In case the patient is already pregnant, there is no evidence that exposure to the amounts of estrogen and progestin in oral contraceptives is teratogenic.[185-187] Furthermore, emergency contraception will be ineffective in the presence of an established pregnancy. A delay in menses after treatment warrants testing for pregnancy and consideration of the possibility of an ectopic pregnancy.

When using combined oral contraceptives for emergency contraception, it is worth adding an antiemetic to the treatment; a long-acting nonprescription agent, 25 or 50 mg meclizine (Bonine, Dramamine II, Antivert) is recommended, to be taken 1 hour before the emergency contraception treatment. Side effects reflect the high doses used: nausea (50%), vomiting (20%), breast tenderness, headache, and dizziness. If a patient vomits within an hour after taking pills, additional pills must be administered as soon as possible. Nausea and vomiting with the levonorgestrel-only method is so uncommon that an antiemetic is not necessary.

The UK General Practice Research Database could find no evidence for an increased risk of venous thromboembolism with the short-term use of oral contraceptives for emergency contraception. Indeed, no cases were found for as long as 60 days after use in more than 100,000 episodes of use.[188,189]

A norethindrone–ethinyl estradiol combination was found to be equally effective to the levonorgestrel–ethinyl estradiol formulation, and it is likely that any combination oral contraceptive would be successful.[190] However, this is a moot point because the levonorgestrel-only method is now the treatment of choice.

The three major problems with the available methods of emergency contraception are the high rate of side effects, the need to start treatment promptly after intercourse, and the small, but important, failure rate. Use of the progesterone antagonist mifepristone in a single oral dose of 600 mg is associated with markedly less nausea and vomiting than is the use of combination oral contraceptives and has an efficacy rate of nearly 100%.[191,192] In randomized trials, 10 mg mifepristone was as effective as 25 mg, 50 mg, or 600 mg, preventing about 80% to 85% of expected pregnancies (the same efficacy as with the levonorgestrel method), with a slight decrease in efficacy when treatment was delayed to 5 days after intercourse.[155,193,194] Because the next menstrual cycle is delayed after mifepristone, contraception should be initiated immediately after treatment. Ironically, mifepristone, around which swirls the abortion controversy, can make an effective contribution to preventing unwanted pregnancies and induced abortions.

VAGINAL AND TRANSDERMAL STEROID CONTRACEPTION

Vaginal and transdermal steroid administration has the potential advantage of avoiding the first pass through the liver and the high initial serum concentrations that are associated with the oral intake of steroid hormones. For example, the impact on blood clotting may be reduced because acute stimulation of liver protein synthesis is avoided. Whether vaginal and transdermal administration of steroid hormones is safer than oral administration must await future epidemiologic assessment, but this remains a theoretical possibility. Another important possible advantage of vaginal and transdermal steroid contraception is an improvement in compliance achieved by the elimination of a daily regimen of treatment

Vaginal Steroid Contraception

The vaginal mucosa offers an excellent delivery site for steroid contraception. Absorption from the GI tract can be unpredictable and may be compromised by vomiting, drug-drug interference, or decreased intestinal absorption capacity. Avoidance of the first pass effect is particularly advantageous for compounds that undergo a high degree of hepatic metabolism; orally administered natural estrogens for example, are 95% metabolized by the liver. Oral administration results in marked fluctuations of contraceptive steroid serum concentrations that can lead to side effects like irregular bleeding and nausea. These daily changes are lower with vaginal than with oral or transdermal administration and lowest with implant and intrauterine methods.[195,196]

Vaginal contraceptive rings have been studied for 30 years. Six progestin-only and seven different progestin-estrogen (combined) vaginal contraceptive rings have been designed to provide 1 week to 1 year of contraception. Short-acting rings (1 week) contain weaker progestins like progesterone and medroxyprogesterone, and long-acting rings (up to 1 year) contain the more potent levonorgestrel and nesterone.

Only the NuvaRing vaginal combined steroid contraceptive is approved and available in the United States (Fig. 17–1). It is a flexible, soft, transparent ring made of ethylene vinyl acetate (EVA) copolymer (60%) in which are contained crystals of etonogestrel (the biologically active metabolite of desogestrel, previously known as 3-ketodesogestrel) and ethinyl estradiol. This ring is covered with a 2-µm thick membrane of EVA. The ring is available in only one size, 4 mm in thickness and 54 mm in diameter (smaller than a diaphragm). The NuvaRing releases 15 µg ethinyl estradiol and 120 µg etonogestrel per day.[197] The circulating estrogen levels reach a maximum level after 2 or 3 days and etonogestrel reaches maximum level after 7 days, and these levels remain stable for 35 days[196] (Fig. 17–2). The ring is inserted by the patient and worn for 3 weeks. Routine use requires the insertion of a new ring every 4 weeks to allow withdrawal bleeding, but continuous use is an appropriate option.

The ring produces circulating progestin and estrogen levels that are only 40% and 30%, respectively, of the *peak* levels associated with an oral contraceptive containing 150 µg desogestrel and 30 µg ethinyl estradiol.[196] These levels effectively inhibit ovulation, providing pregnancy rates of less than 1% in clinical trials.[197-199] Indeed, the ring contains enough steroid hormone to inhibit ovulation for at least a total of 5 weeks.[198] If the vaginal

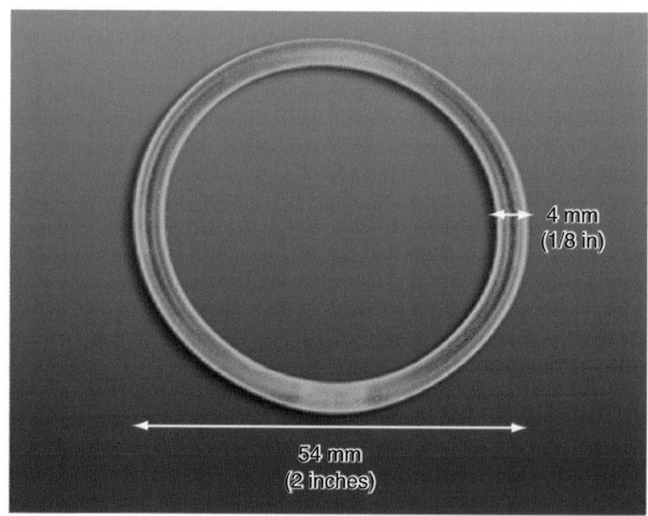

Figure 17–1 ▪ The vaginal ring with an estrogen/progestin combination.

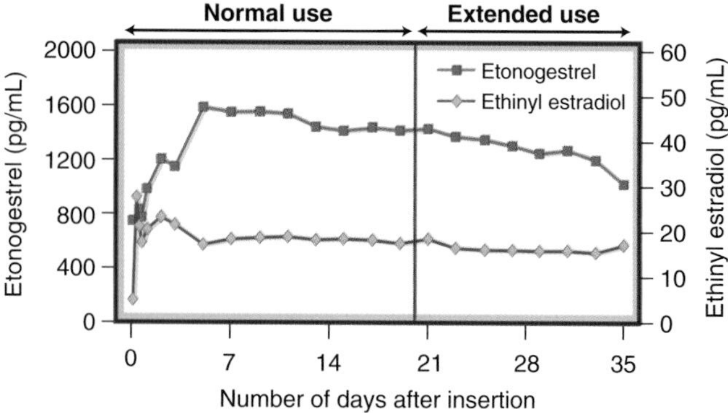

Figure 17–2 ▪ Pharmacokinetic profile of the ring during extended use. (From Timmer CJ, Mulders TM. Pharmacokinetics of etonogestrel and ethinylestradiol released from a combined contraceptive vaginal ring. Clin Pharmacokinet 2000;39:233-242.)

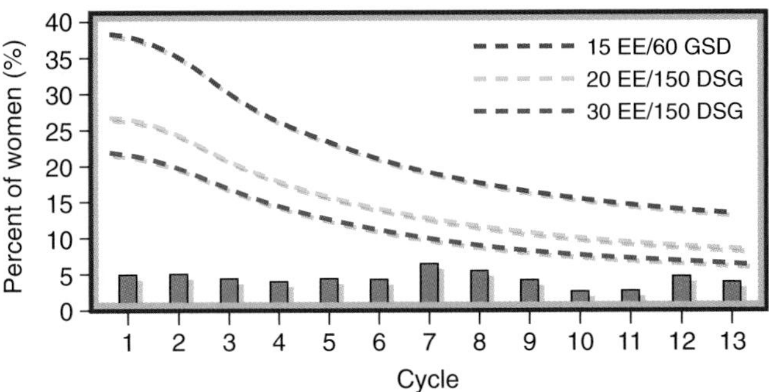

Figure 17–3 ▪ Irregular spotting with the ring. DSG, desogestrel; EE, ethinyl estradiol; GSD, gestodene. (From Roumen FJ, Apter D, Mulders TM, Dieben TO. Efficacy, tolerability and acceptability of a novel contraceptive vaginal ring releasing etonogestrel and ethinyl estradiol. Hum Reprod 2001;16:469-475.)

ring is removed and not replaced within 3 hours, the manufacturer recommends backup contraception until the ring has been in place for 7 days.

Taking into account bioavailability as influenced by protein binding, systemic exposure to etonogestrel is similar, comparing the vaginal ring to an oral contraceptive containing 150 μg desogestrel; however, the systemic exposure to ethinyl estradiol is about 50% of that of an oral contraceptive containing 30 μg ethinyl estradiol.[196] This might explain the low incidence of estrogen-related side effects such as nausea and breast tenderness.[197,199] Breakthrough bleeding and spotting rates are lower (around 6%) (Fig. 17–3) when compared with an oral contraceptive containing 30 μg of ethinyl estradiol and much lower than with 15- or 20-μg pills.[199,200]

It is not necessary to place the vaginal ring in a specific position; it need only be in contact with vaginal mucosa and need not surround the cervix. The vaginal ring is intended to be placed in a normal vagina; infections and anatomic abnormalities are reasons for clinicians and patients to consider other methods. The most common reasons for discontinuation (about 2% to 4% in the clinical trials) have been vaginal discomfort, unwanted awareness of the ring's presence, coital problems, or expulsion (during a year of use about 2% to 3% of women experience spontaneous expulsion). Women report that the ring is easy to insert and remove, and, although about 15% of women and 30% of partners report feeling the ring during intercourse, this is not a common reason for discontinuation.[199,201] Removal for sexual intercourse is not recommended, but efficacy is maintained if the ring is replaced within 3 hours. Cervical cytology and the vaginal flora are not affected by the presence of the ring.[199,202,203]

The spermicide, nonoxynol-9, has no effect on the release and absorption of the hormones in NuvaRing, as assessed by the measurement of serum levels of ethinyl estradiol and etonogestrel.[204] Combining a barrier method that contains nonoxynol-9 (in the widely advocated double method for protection against sexually transmitted diseases) should not affect the contraceptive efficacy of the ring. Vaginally applied antifungal agents (miconazole) likewise have no effect on absorption of contraceptive steroids released by NuvaRing, nor does the use of tampons.[204]

Transdermal Steroid Contraception

Method

The transdermal contraceptive patch (Ortho Evra) has an area of 20 cm^2 (4.5 cm × 4.5 cm) and three layers in a matrix-type arrangement. The backing outer polyester layer provides support for the middle layer that contains the adhesive and the hormones, and the inner layer is a polyester liner that is removed from the adhesive layer just before application. The size is that required to deliver an effective dose of the steroid hormones. The patch contains 750 μg ethinyl estradiol and 6.0 mg of norelgestromin and delivers 20 μg ethinyl estradiol and 150 μg norelgestromin each day when applied to discrete locations on the lower abdomen, upper outer arm, the buttock, or the upper torso (excluding the breast). Norelgestromin is the primary active metabolite of orally administered norgestimate and was previously known as 17-deacetylnorgestimate. Norelgestromin still undergoes liver metabolism with transdermal application; however, the resulting metabolite, levonorgestrel, is highly bound to sex hormone–binding globulin, limiting its biologic impact. About 97% of norelgestromin is bound to albumin and 3% is unbound.[205]

The patch is applied on the same day, but not on the exact same site, once each week for 3 weeks, followed by a week without use of the patch. Timing on the day of application need not be precise; the patch maintains adequate serum levels for 9 days. Instructions for first-day starts or Sunday starts of oral contraception are also recommended for the patch (backup contraception for 7 days unless the starting day is also day 1 of the menstrual period). As with oral contraceptives, patient and clinician may choose to use the contraceptive patch continuously, eliminating withdrawal bleeding but, perhaps, promoting irregular spotting.

Detachment occurs with about 5% of patches, and about half occur in cycle 1 with inexperienced patients.[206,207] In studies of at least a year's duration, about 2% to 5% of patches were replaced.[208,209] If the patch has been detached for more than 24 hours, a new patch is applied, initiating a new cycle and new change day (backup contraception for 7 days is recommended). Delay of a new patch cycle requires a new start with the usual 7-day backup. A delay within the patch cycle of no more than 2 days has no risk and does not change the cycle, but a delay of more than 2 days also requires the initiation of a new cycle and change day with backup. However, in a study that compared three treatment-free days in oral contraceptive and patch users, ovulation occurred significantly less with the patch compared with oral contraception.[210]

Effects

Serum hormonal concentrations are achieved rapidly after application: an average of about 0.7 ng/mL, which is within the range 0.6 to 1.2 ng/mL for norelgestromin, and an average of about 50 pg/mL, within the range of 25 to 75 pg/mL for ethinyl estradiol. These are ranges that are maintained by an oral formulation containing 250 μg norelgestromin and 35 μg ethinyl estradiol (Fig. 17–4).[211,212] However, the kinetics are not identical to orally administered hormones; daily fluctuations are avoided, but the area under the curve (AUC) over a week of use is greater with the patch than with daily oral administration of 35 μg of ethinyl estradiol. Whether this difference increases the risk of thrombosis in patch users has not been determined, with the only two studies in disagreement. Contraceptive blood levels are maintained even if patch replacement is delayed up to 2 days (9 days total).[213] Gonadotropin levels return to baseline values by 6 weeks after discontinuation.[210] Daily use has been well studied, and activities such as exercise, bathing, swimming, and the use of a sauna or hot tub do not cause detachment or changes in the blood levels of the hormones.[214]

Transdermal contraception produces the same spectrum of actions associated with oral contraceptives, achieving the same high level of efficacy in clinical trials. Therefore, the same considerations reviewed earlier about oral contraception apply to

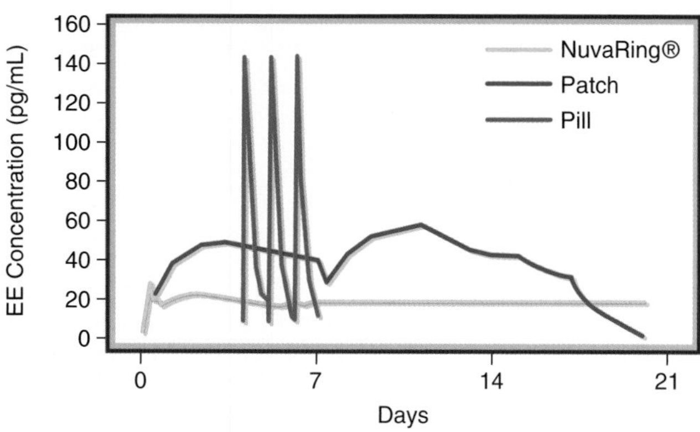

Figure 17–4 ■ Pharmacokinetic comparison of ethinyl estradiol levels provided by contraceptive ring, patch, and pill. (From Abrams LS, Skee DM, Natarajan J, et al. Multiple-dose pharmacokinetics of a contraceptive patch in healthy women participants. Contraception 2001;64: 287-294.)

transdermal contraception, including the same contraindications and noncontraceptive benefits. The avoidance of the liver first-pass effect offers the potential for less interaction with other drugs, but this is not known, and patients taking medications that affect liver metabolism should choose an alternative contraceptive. Tetracycline administration does not affect the blood concentrations of the steroid hormones with transdermal contraception, a neutral impact just as seen with oral contraceptives.[215]

Transdermal administration has effects on clotting proteins and lipoproteins like those seen with low-dose oral contraceptives. There are no clinically significant changes in coagulation parameters, triglycerides increase modestly, and the ratio of low-density lipoproteins to high-density lipoproteins (LDL/HDL ratio) declines slightly.[216] As with oral contraceptives, women who are at high risk for thrombosis due to genetic effects like factor V Leiden or protein C or S deficiencies or who have very high triglycerides should consider hormonal contraceptives that do not contain estrogen.

Clinical Responses

Ovulation suppression is comparable to that achieved with oral contraception, and failure rates in clinical studies are less than 1.0%.[113,206,208,209] Breakthrough bleeding and spotting rates with the transdermal method in randomized trials were comparable to those with monophasic and two triphasic formulations, except for a slightly higher incidence of spotting in the first two cycles.[206,208]

It is now well demonstrated that modern steroid contraception does not cause weight gain. The transdermal method is not an exception; body weight changes were identical in a randomized trial comparing the contraceptive patch with an identical placebo patch.[217] There were 15 pregnancies in the contraceptive patch clinical trials, and five of these were among women with body weights greater than 90 kg (198 pounds).[113] This is consistent with the greater failure rate reported in obese women taking oral contraceptives.[112] However, a high rate of overall contraceptive efficacy is still achieved in heavy women because only a 10% to 20% variability in hormone levels can be attributed to increased body weight.[113]

Poor compliance is a major contributor to the typical failure rate associated with oral contraception. The once-a-week schedule with transdermal contraception is simpler and less susceptible to delays and omissions. In randomized trials ranging from four cycles to 13 cycles, about 10% to 20% more of the participants demonstrated good compliance with the transdermal method compared with oral contraception.[206,208] In the clinical trials with transdermal contraception, lower overall pregnancy rates with the patch compared with oral contraception have been attributed to better compliance. Most importantly, young patients, especially those younger than 20 years, demonstrated greater compliance with transdermal contraception compared with oral contraceptives than did older patients.[218]

About 20% of patients experience some degree of skin reaction at the application site, and about 2% discontinue the method for this reason.[206,208,209,217] Breast discomfort is experienced during the first few months by 20% of users, more often with transdermal contraception compared with oral contraceptives, but it is usually not severe and resulted in discontinuation in only 1% of users.[217]

INJECTABLE CONTRACEPTION

Depot-Medroxyprogesterone Acetate

Depot-medroxyprogesterone acetate (DMPA or Depo-Provera) is the most thoroughly studied progestin-only contraceptive. Although its approval for contraception in the United States is recent (1992), it has been available in some countries since the mid-1960s. Much of our knowledge of the safety, efficacy, and acceptability of long-acting hormonal contraception comes from Indonesia, Sri Lanka, Thailand, and Mexico, where DMPA has been used and studied for decades. The long-delayed approval as a contraceptive in the United States was based on political and economic considerations rather than scientific ones.[219]

DMPA is formulated as microcrystals suspended in an aqueous solution. The approved dose for contraceptive purposes is 150 mg intramuscularly (gluteal or deltoid) every 3 months. A comparative trial established that the 100-mg IM dose is significantly less effective,[220] but a reformulation, introduced in 2005, of 104 mg administered subcutaneously every 3 months is as effective as the 150 mg IM formulation. The contraceptive level is maintained for at least 14 weeks, providing a safety margin. It is one of the most effective contraceptives available, with about 1 pregnancy per 100 women after 5 years of consistent use.[220,221]

DMPA is not a sustained-release system; it relies on high peaks of progestin to inhibit ovulation and thicken cervical mucus. The difference between low serum levels of progestins produced by sustained-release subdermal and intrauterine systems and a depot system like DMPA is as much as tenfold. Other widely used injectables are norethindrone enanthate, 200 mg every 2 months, and the monthly injectables, Lunelle (25 mg medroxyprogesterone acetate and 5 mg estradiol cypionate) and Mesigyna (50 mg norethindrone enanthate and 5 mg estradiol valerate).

The indications and contraindications for the clinical use of DMPA are summarized in Table 17–8.

Mechanism of Action

The mechanisms of action of DMPA are like those of other progestin-only methods: thickening of the cervical mucus, alteration of the endometrium, and blocking the LH surge to prevent ovulation.[222] Suppression of FSH is not as intense as with the combination oral contraceptive; therefore, follicular growth is maintained sufficiently to produce estrogen levels comparable to those in the early follicular phase of a normal menstrual cycle.[223] Symptoms of estrogen deficiency, such as vaginal

TABLE 17–8 INDICATIONS AND CONTRAINDICATIONS FOR USE OF DEPO-PROVERA

INDICATIONS
At least 1 year of birth spacing desired
Highly effective long-acting contraception not linked to coitus
Private, coitally independent method desired
Estrogen-free contraception needed
Breastfeeding
Sickle cell disease
Seizure disorder
CONTRAINDICATIONS
Absolute
Pregnancy
Unexplained genital bleeding
Severe coagulation disorders
Previous sex steroid–induced liver adenoma
Relative
Liver disease
Severe cardiovascular disease
Rapid return to fertility desired
Difficulty with injections
Severe depression

atrophy or a decrease in breast size, do not occur, but bone density can be lost.

Accidental pregnancies occurring at the time of the initial injection of DMPA have been reported to be associated with higher neonatal and infant mortality rates, probably due to an increased risk of intrauterine growth restriction.[224,225] The timing of the first injection is, therefore, very important. To ensure effective contraception, the first injection should be administered within the first 5 days of the menstrual cycle (before a dominant follicle emerges), or a backup method is necessary for 2 weeks.[226-228] The duration of action can be shortened if attention is not paid to proper administration. The injection must be given deeply in muscle by the Z-track technique and not massaged. It is prudent to avoid locations at risk for massage by daily activities.

Efficacy

The efficacy of this method is equal to that of sterilization and better than that of oral methods.[2,229] Because serum concentrations are relatively high, efficacy is not influenced by weight or by the use of medications that stimulate hepatic enzymes. On the contrary, DMPA is an excellent contraceptive choice for women taking antiepileptic drugs because the high progestin levels raise the seizure threshold.[230]

Advantages

Like sustained-release forms of contraception, DMPA does not require daily compliance and is not related to the coital event. Continuation rates are better and repeat pregnancy rates are reduced compared with oral contraceptive use in teenagers; however, continuation and repeat pregnancy rates are similar when adolescents begin these methods in the immediate postpartum period.[231,232] DMPA is useful for women whose ability to remember contraceptive requirements is limited. It should be considered for women who lead disorganized lives or who are mentally retarded, but it can be difficult for some women to plan a clinician visit for injection every 3 months. Self-injection with subcutaneous DMPA can provide a more convenient alternative in these cases.

The freedom from the side effects of estrogen allows DMPA to be considered for patients with congenital heart disease, sickle cell anemia, or a previous history of thromboembolism and for women older than 30 years who smoke or have other risk factors such as hypertension or diabetes mellitus. The absolute safety with regard to thrombosis is mainly theoretical; it has not been proved in a controlled study. However, an increased risk of thrombosis has not been observed in epidemiologic evaluation of DMPA users, and a World Health Organization (WHO) case-control study could find no evidence for increased risks of stroke, myocardial infarction, or venous thromboembolism.[147,221]

An important advantage exists for patients with sickle cell disease because evidence indicates an inhibition of in vivo sickling with hematologic improvement during treatment.[105] The frequency and the intensity of painful sickle cell crises are reduced.[233]

Another advantage is that DMPA increases the quantity of milk in nursing mothers, a direct contrast to the effect seen with combination contraception. The concentration of the drug in the breast milk is negligible, and no effects of the drug on infant growth and development have been observed.[234-236] In a careful study of male infants being breastfed by women treated with DMPA, no metabolites of DMPA could be detected in the infant's urine and no alterations could be observed in the infant levels of FSH, LH, testosterone, and cortisol.[237] Because of the slight positive impact on lactation, DMPA can be administered immediately after delivery. A study to investigate the impact of early initiation found no adverse effects on breastfeeding.[145]

DMPA should be considered in patients with seizure disorders; an improvement in seizure control can be achieved probably because of the sedative properties of progestins.[230]

Other benefits associated with DMPA use include a decreased risk of endometrial cancer, comparable with that observed with oral contraceptives,[238] and probably the same benefits found with the actions of the progestins in oral contraceptives: reduced menstrual flow and anemia, less pelvic inflammatory disease (PID), less endometriosis, fewer uterine fibroids,[239] and fewer ectopic pregnancies. A failure to document a reduced risk of ovarian cancer by the World Health Organization probably reflects the study's low statistical power and the high parity in the DMPA users.[240]

DMPA, like oral contraception, can reduce the risk of pelvic inflammatory disease; however, the only study was hampered by small numbers.[241] Suppression of ovulation means that ectopic pregnancies are abolished and ovarian cysts are rare.

The greater the number of choices that women have, the more likely they are to find a contraceptive that works well for them. For some women, the primary advantages of DMPA are privacy and ease of use. No one but the user needs know about the injection, and the 3-month schedule can be easy to maintain for women who do not mind injections. In some societies, injections are respected as efficacious; in these situations, DMPA is the most popular contraceptive despite bleeding changes and other side effects. The advantages of the use of DMPA are summarized in Table 17–9.

Problems

Major problems with DMPA are irregular menstrual bleeding, breast tenderness, weight gain, and depression.[220,221] By far, the most common problem is the change in menstrual bleeding. Up to 25% of patients discontinue in the first year because of irregular bleeding.[242] The bleeding is rarely heavy; in fact, hemoglobin

TABLE 17-9 ADVANTAGES OF THE USE OF DEPO-PROVERA

Easy to use, no daily or coital action required
Safe, no serious health effects
Very effective, as effective as sterilization, intrauterine contraception, and implant contraception
Free from estrogen-related problems
Private, use not detectable
Lactation is enhanced
Noncontraceptive benefits

values rise in DMPA users. The incidence of irregular bleeding is 70% in the first year and 10% thereafter. Bleeding and spotting decrease progressively with each reinjection, so that after 5 years, 80% of users are amenorrheic (compared with 10% of Norplant users).[243] Irregular bleeding can be disturbing and annoying, and, for many patients, it inhibits sexual activity; therefore, most users prefer the amenorrhea that comes with prolonged use.

If necessary, breakthrough bleeding can be treated with exogenous estrogen, 1.25 mg conjugated estrogens, or 2 mg estradiol, given daily for 7 days. A nonsteroidal antiinflammatory drug (NSAID) given for a week is also effective; another option is to administer an oral contraceptive for 1 to 3 months. Giving the DMPA injection earlier than 3 months does not change the bleeding pattern.[244] Most women can wait for amenorrhea without treatment if they know what to expect with time. Transdermal estrogen did not improve irregular bleeding enough to enhance continuation rates by young women who had had an abortion.[245]

About one third of patients discontinue DMPA by the end of 1 year, 50% by the end of 2 years, and about 80% by the end of 3 years.[246] The 1-year continuation rate in Texas public clinics was only 29%, much lower than reported elsewhere.[247] It was equally low among young women who requested an injection immediately after elective abortion.[245] In a large international study, the most common medical reasons for discontinuing DMPA during the first 2 years of use were headaches (2.3%), weight gain (2.1%), dizziness (1.2%), abdominal pain (1.1%), and anxiety (0.7%).[221]

In Western societies, depression, fatigue, decreased libido, and hypertension are also encountered. Whether medroxyprogesterone acetate causes these side effects is difficult to know because they are very common complaints in nonusers as well.[248] When DMPA users are studied closely, no increase in depressive symptoms can be observed, even in women with significant complaints of depression prior to treatment.[249,250]

Attempts to document weight gain specifically associated with DMPA have had mixed results, some finding no increase and others a small increase (e.g., about 4 kg over 5 years in one and 11 kg over 10 years in another).[251-254] In a placebo-controlled experiment, DMPA had no effects on food intake, energy expenditure, or body weight.[255] As with oral contraception, the weight gain may not be hormone-induced but reflect lifestyle and aging. On the other hand, specific patients and certain ethnic groups may be more susceptible to weight gain; for example, significant weight gain was reported in Navajo women using DMPA[256] and in already overweight African American teens. Those who were of normal weight at initiation of DMPA did not gain more than control subjects.[257]

If symptoms are truly due to the progestin, unlike pills, implants, rings, and patches, DMPA takes 6 to 8 months after the last injection to disappear. Clearance is slower in heavier women. Approximately half of women who discontinue DMPA can expect normal menses to return in 6 months after the last injection, but 25% will wait a year before resumption of a normal pattern.[243]

Cancer

Breast Cancer

A very large hospital-based case-control WHO study conducted over 9 years in three developing countries indicated that exposure to DMPA is associated with a very slightly increased risk of breast cancer in the first 4 years of use, but there was no evidence for an increase in risk with increasing duration of use.[258] The number of cases with recent use was not large, and the confidence intervals reflected this. A possible explanation for this finding is the combination of detection and surveillance bias and accelerated growth of an already present tumor, a situation similar to those described with oral contraceptives.

Other Cancers

An increased risk of cervical dysplasia cannot be documented even with long-term use (4 or more years).[259] No increase in adenocarcinoma or adenosquamous carcinoma could be detected in the WHO study.[260] The WHO study has not detected an increased risk of invasive squamous cell cancer of the cervix in DMPA users; however, the risk of cervical carcinoma *in situ* was slightly elevated in the WHO case-control study. It is not certain whether this is a real finding or a consequence of unrecognized biases, especially detection bias.[261,262]

Metabolic Effects

The impact of DMPA on the lipoprotein profile is uncertain. Although some studies fail to detect an adverse impact and claim that this is due to the avoidance of a first-pass effect in the liver, others have demonstrated a decrease in HDL cholesterol and increases in total cholesterol and LDL cholesterol.[263,264] In a multicenter clinical trial by the World Health Organization, a transient adverse impact was present only in the few weeks after injection when blood levels were high.[265] The clinical impact of these changes, if any, has yet to be reported.

There are no clinically significant changes in carbohydrate metabolism or in coagulation factors.[266,267] There are no studies available assessing the impact of DMPA in women with diabetes mellitus or in women with previous gestational diabetes.

Effect on Bone Density

Clinicians are concerned that the contraceptive use of DMPA is associated with the loss of bone, and the package insert announces this risk. It is attributed to the fact that blood levels of estrogen with DMPA are relatively lower over a period of time compared with a normal menstrual cycle, an idea that is supported by the demonstration that estrogen treatment prevents bone loss.[268] Lumbar and hip bone loss has been documented in cross-sectional studies.[269,270] An American cross-sectional study indicated a greater bone loss with increasing duration of use, especially in younger women, 18 to 21 years old.[271]

The degree of bone loss in these studies is not as severe as that observed in the early postmenopausal years. Furthermore, this amount of bone loss is not so great that at least a portion of it cannot be regained. Bone density measurements in women who stopped using DMPA indicated that the loss was largely regained in the lumbar spine but not in the femoral neck within 2 years even after long-term use, and in another cohort of past users, both spinal density and hip density were somewhat restored 30 months after discontinuation.[272,273] Most importantly, cross-sectional studies of postmenopausal women in New Zealand and in a large multicenter worldwide population could not detect a difference in bone density comparing former users of DMPA with never users, indicating that any loss of bone during use is likely to be modest.[274,275]

Bone density increases rapidly and significantly during adolescence. Almost all of the bone mass in the hip and the vertebral bodies is accumulated in girls by age 18, and the years immediately following menarche are especially important.[276,277] For this reason any drug that prevents this increase in bone density can increase the risk of osteoporosis later in life. A prospective study in 47 adolescents documented that DMPA (15 users) was associated with a loss of lumbar bone density (approximately 1.5% in 1 year) compared with the normal increases observed in users of Norplant (7 users) and oral contraceptives (9 users).[278]

The mixed results, the degree of bone loss, and evidence that some bone loss is regained all argue that the use of DMPA should not be limited by this concern and that supplemental estrogen treatment is not indicated (and would influence and complicate compliance). This concern will require ongoing surveillance of past users. However, at present, concern about bone loss should not be a reason to avoid this method of contraception. It is unlikely that bone loss occurs sufficiently to substantially raise the risk of osteoporosis later in life.

Effect on Future Fertility

The delay in becoming pregnant after ceasing use of DMPA is a problem unique to injectable contraception; all the other temporary methods allow a more prompt return to fertility.[279] However, medroxyprogesterone acetate does not permanently suppress ovarian function, and the concern that infertility with suppressed menstrual function may be caused by DMPA has not been supported by epidemiologic data. The pregnancy rate in women discontinuing the injections because of a desire to become pregnant is normal.[280] By 18 months after the last injection, 90% of DMPA users have become pregnant, the same proportion as for other methods.[281] The delay to conception is about 9 months after the last injection, and the delay does not increase with increasing duration of use. Because of this delay, women who want to conceive promptly after discontinuing their contraceptive should not use DMPA. Suppressed menstrual function persisting beyond 18 months after the last injection is not due to the drug and deserves evaluation.

Subcutaneous Administration of DMPA

Intramuscular DMPA has several disadvantages. Peak serum concentrations are higher than required for ovulation suppression and lead to decreased production of endogenous estradiol, so that bone density is lost. Prolonged release from muscle can delay return to ovulation for several months after the last IM injection. DMPA users must see a clinician every 3 months for repeat IM administration.

All of these problems are addressed by subcutaneous injection of 104 mg, rather than 150 mg, of DMPA suspended in 0.65 mL of excipients that differ from those used in IM DMPA. The peak DMPA concentrations are lower, but efficacy remains high; there were no pregnancies in the initial clinical trial among 1783 women, 11% of whom were obese. Bone density did not change over a year of use, and return to ovulation was faster than with the traditional IM formulation. Bleeding patterns are like those of IM DMPA, except that women become amenorrheic more slowly; at one year about 45% of users are amenorrheic, compared with 54% using IM DMPA.[282]

The needle packaged with subcutaneous DMPA is different from the one used for IM administration, making self-injection possible. A subset of women in the initial clinical trial were able to give their own injections without difficulty and had no pregnancies.

Short-Term Injectable Contraceptives

Monthly or every-other-month injectable combinations of estrogen and progestin are not new, having been developed over several decades.[283] This method of contraception is popular in China, Latin America, and eastern Asia. A preparation widely used in China consists of 250 mg 17-hydroxyprogesterone caproate and 5 mg estradiol valerate, known as Chinese Injectable No. 1.

Lunelle (Cyclofem)

Lunelle consists of 25 mg DMPA and 5 mg estradiol cypionate and is administered every 28 to 30 days (not to exceed 33 days) as a deep intramuscular injection. This method is as effective as Depo-Provera, but it avoids the problems of menstrual irregularity and heavy bleeding, as well as amenorrhea.[284-289] In addition, the method is rapidly reversible; fertility rates after discontinuation are similar to those with oral contraceptives.[290]

One disadvantage is the need for a monthly injection; another disadvantage is the likelihood that the combination of estrogen and progestin will inhibit lactation. The requirement for a monthly injection can be made more convenient by the use of an automatic device for self-administration.[291] Approximately 80% of women who are amenorrheic on Depo-Provera will develop vaginal bleeding if switched to Lunelle.[292] The same contraindications, concerns, problems, and probably benefits reported with oral contraception should apply to Lunelle, which is no longer sold in the United States but is available in many other countries.

Norethindrone Enanthate

Norethindrone enanthate is given in a dose of 200 mg intramuscularly every 2 months. This progestin acts in the same way as Depo-Provera and has the same problems.[221] A combination (Mesigyna) of norethindrone enanthate (50 mg) with estradiol valerate (5 mg) given monthly provides effective contraception with good cycle control.[293] Compared with Lunelle, use of Mesigyna is associated with fewer bleeding problems.[294] Fertility returns rapidly (within 1 month) after discontinuation.[290]

Dihydroxyprogesterone Acetophenide and Estradiol Enanthate

The combination of 150 mg dihydroxyprogesterone acetophenide with 10 mg estradiol enanthate (produced under various brand names) is the most widely used injectable contraceptive in Latin America. As with Mesigyna and Lunelle, the monthly regimen allows regular, and even reduced, cyclic bleeding.[295] A lower dose (90 mg dihydroxyprogesterone acetophenide and 6 mg estradiol enanthate) provides the same effective contraception as the higher dose with similar bleeding patterns.[296]

IMPLANT CONTRACEPTION

Subdermal contraceptive implants offer women long-acting controlled release of progestins. Since the 1980s, these implants have been approved in more than 60 countries and used by 11 million women worldwide. Their high efficacy, along with their ease of use, makes them a good contraceptive option for several groups of women: those who require progestin-only methods because they should not use estrogen, teens who find adherence to a contraceptive regimen difficult, and healthy adults who desire long-term protection. The levonorgestrel (LNG) implant, no longer marketed in the United States, garnered a million American users but was sometimes difficult to insert and remove. A highly effective and long-lasting single-rod etonogestrel (ENG) implant (Implanon) makes implant contraception available again in the United States.

Benefits of Implantable Contraception

Implants offer a variety of benefits to women. They provide long-term, effective prevention of pregnancy without the need for daily or weekly action, as with pills, rings or patches, or for regular injections. Implant contraception is cost-effective compared with short-acting methods or an unplanned pregnancy.[297] The sustained administration of a low dose of progestin and maintenance of stable serum levels provide high efficacy, a long duration of action, a short fertility recovery time, and no reported serious cardiovascular effects.[298]

Research and development of progestin-only subdermal implants began in the 1960s, but initial research with implants containing very low doses of progestins found that they were unsuccessful in preventing ectopic pregnancies. Development of the LNG implant, a 6-capsule implantable system using the potent progestin LNG, followed. In 1991 it became the first FDA-approved contraceptive implant. A million U.S. women chose the LNG implant as their contraceptive, and it proved highly effective: over a 7-year duration of use, only about 1% of users became pregnant.[299] Despite low rates of pregnancy and few serious side effects, limited supplies of the Silastic components and negative media coverage led to the LNG implant's withdrawal from distribution in 2002, which left no implant alternative for American women.[300]

The 15-year experience with the LNG implant instigated further development and improvements in implant design. A 2-rod LNG system was FDA approved in 1998 but never marketed in the United States, although it has many users in Europe and Asia. The FDA has reviewed a contraceptive implant containing 68 mg of etonogestrel (ENG), the active metabolite of desogestrel, in a single rod made of ethylene vinyl acetate (EVA). This 1-implant contraceptive, the most effective hormonal method of birth control yet developed, is now used by more than 2 million women in Europe and Asia.[301] In Australia, a quarter of all women practicing contraception in 2004 used this implant.

Progestin-Only Contraception

Levonorgestrel binds with high affinity to the progesterone, androgen, mineralocorticoid, and glucocorticoid receptors, but not to estrogen receptors. Etonogestrel has shown no estrogenic, antiinflammatory, or mineralocorticoid activity, but it has shown weak androgenic and anabolic activity and strong antiestrogenic activity. Unlike LNG, which is bound mainly to sex hormone–binding globulin, ENG is bound mainly to albumin, which is not significantly affected by varying endogenous or exogenous estradiol concentrations. The overall safety of ENG has been demonstrated through studies of combined estrogen-progestin OCs, the combined vaginal ring, and progestin-only OCs, all of which use desogestrel, a close relative of etonorgestrel, as a component.

Mechanisms of Action

Progestin-containing implants have two primary mechanisms of action: inhibition of ovulation and restriction of sperm penetration through cervical mucus.[305] The LNG implant disrupts follicular growth and inhibits the ovulatory process by exerting negative feedback on the hypothalamic-pituitary axis, causing a variety of changes that range from anovulation to insufficient luteal function. A small number of women using LNG implants will have quiescent ovaries, but most will begin to ovulate as blood concentrations of LNG gradually fall.[306] The ENG implant suppresses ovulation by altering the hypothalamic-pituitary-ovarian axis and down-regulating the luteinizing hormone surge, which is required to support the production, growth, and maturation of ovarian follicles.[307] Some women, especially those with higher endogenous estrogen, form ovarian cysts while using implants. These are not pathologic, are rarely painful and do not require treatment.

Even if follicles grow during use of progestin implants, oocytes are not fertilized. If the follicle ruptures, the abnormalities of the ovulatory process appear to prevent release of a viable egg. Antiestrogenic actions of the progestins affect the cervical mucus, making it viscous, scanty, and impenetrable by sperm.[308] These ovarian and cervical mechanisms of action provide high contraceptive efficacy and occur prior to fertilization. No signs of embryonic development have been found among implant users, a finding that indicates that progestin implants have no abortifacient properties.

The Single-Rod Etonogestrel Implant

Design

The high efficacy of this new device results from the capacity of a low dose of ENG to suppress ovulation and from its long duration of action. After subdermal insertion, users need do nothing more to have nearly complete protection from pregnancy for up to 3 years.[308] The one rod is a great improvement over the old six-capsule LNG implant system, both in time and in ease of insertion.[309,310] In the U.S. and European trials of the ENG implant system, which began in 1995, average insertion time was 1 minute and removal time was 3 minutes—much faster than with the LNG implant system.[301]

Its convenience is enhanced by other design features as well. The inserter is preloaded and disposable, and because only one rod is implanted, there is no chance that insertion of additional capsules will move previously placed capsules out of position.[311] In addition, EVA, the plastic from which it is fabricated, makes it is less likely than older Silastic implants to form a fibrous sheath that can make removal more difficult.[312] These differences likely simplify insertion and removal, which for patients means little discomfort, an unobtrusive implant, and almost no scarring. For clinicians it means faster and simpler insertion and removal procedures.

Pharmacology

The ENG implant (Implanon) consists of one nonbiodegradable rod of 40% EVA and 60% ENG (40 mm × 2 mm) covered with a rate-controlling EVA membrane 0.06 mm thick. The rod contains 68 mg ENG, initially absorbed by the body at a rate of 60 μg per day and slowly declining to 30 μg per day after 2 years of use. The high initial rate of absorption is probably due to a significant amount of ENG released from the uncovered ends of the implant. Peak serum concentrations (266 pg/mL) of ENG are achieved within 1 day after insertion, suppressing ovulation.[307,308] Like other contraceptive steroids, serum levels of ENG are reduced in women taking liver enzyme-inducing drugs such as carbamazepine, griseofulvin, phenytoin, and rifampicin but are not affected by antibiotics.

Steady release of ENG into the circulation avoids first-pass effects on the liver. Bioavailability of ENG remains nearly 100% throughout 2 years of use. The elimination half-life of ENG is 25 hours, compared with 42 hours for LNG. After implant removal, serum ENG concentrations become undetectable within 1 week. Return of ovulation occurs in 94% of women within 3 to 6 weeks after the method is discontinued.[307,308]

Efficacy

The efficacy of the single-rod ENG implant was established as greater than 99% in clinical trials of 1100 women for a total of 26,700 cycles of use.[313] Of these, 835 women completed 2 to 3 years and an additional 526 used the ENG implant for 3 years or longer. Neither intrauterine nor ectopic pregnancies were observed during these trials. Among the subjects were 365 women whose body weight was 154 pounds (70 kg) or more, none of whom became pregnant.[308]

Metabolic Effects

Published studies regarding the ENG implant indicate that metabolic effects are minimal and unlikely to be clinically significant. The ENG implant does not appear to have any clinically meaningful effect on lipid metabolism, carbohydrate metabolism, liver function, hemostatic factors, blood pressure, thyroid, or adrenal function.[314-317]

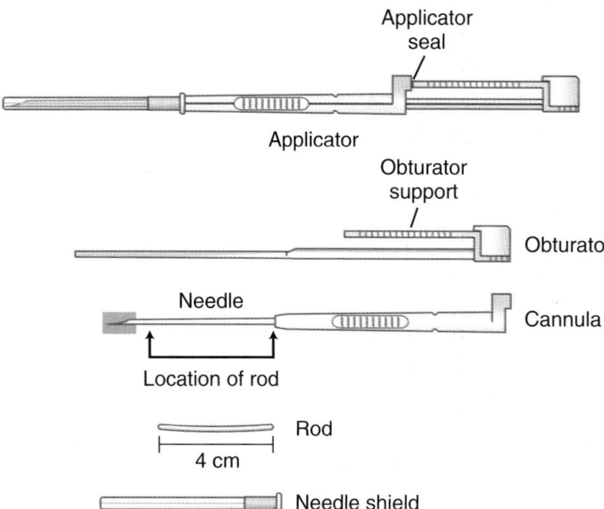

Figure 17–5 ▪ The etonogestrel rod insertion device.

Safety

Overall, implants, including the ENG implant, are regarded as safe, with rates of adverse events (including death, neoplastic disease, cardiovascular events, anemia, hypertension, bone density changes, diabetes, gall bladder disease, thrombocytopenia, and pelvic inflammatory disease) comparable with those in women not using implants.[318] The ENG implant reduced or eliminated menstrual pain in 88% of women previously experiencing dysmenorrhea; pain increased in only 2% of the ENG implant users.[318] In a study comparing 42 pairs of infants and lactating mothers using the ENG implant with 38 pairs using intrauterine devices, there were no significant differences between groups in milk volume, milk constituents, timing or amount of supplementary food, or infant growth rates.[304]

Low-dose progestin contraceptives have few contraindications. They may be less effective in obese women and in those using drugs that stimulate the liver's cytochrome metabolism of steroids, such as some antibiotics (e.g., rifampin) and some anticonvulsants (e.g., phenytoin).

Insertion and Removal

Although the ENG implant is designed to facilitate rapid and simple insertion and removal, clinicians should first be trained.[319] Insertion is less complex than with the six-capsule LNG implant, and average insertion time for the ENG implant is 1 to 2 minutes.[320] The disposable applicator comes preloaded.[321] The tip of the needle has two cutting edges, each with a different slope (Fig. 17–5). The extreme tip is more angulated than the remainder and is sharp to facilitate initial penetration of the skin. The upper portion is less angulated and unsharpened to reduce the risk of reperforating the skin during advancement of the implant after initial penetration.

For easy removal, the implant should be placed subdermally on the inner aspect of the nondominant arm, 6 to 8 cm above the elbow. After disinfecting the insertion site, a small amount (0.1 mL) of local anesthetic can be injected with a tuberculin syringe at the site of skin penetration, but this is not usually necessary because the 19-gauge insertion trocar is very sharp. After insertion, the implant might not be visible but should be palpable.

For women who either have not been using a contraceptive method or have been using a nonhormonal method, insertion should occur between days 1 and 5 of menses. For women changing from a combination or progestin-only OC or from intrauterine contraception, the ENG implant can be inserted during a hormone-free week. For women changing from injectable contraception, insertion should occur on the day the next injection is scheduled. No backup is necessary if timing of insertion occurs as detailed in the product information. If the ENG implant is the contraceptive method selected following an abortion or delivery, it can be inserted immediately; no additional contraceptive method is required. In all cases, pregnancy should be excluded before insertion, although there is no evidence that hormonal contraceptives cause birth defects.

The ENG implant can be removed at any time at the woman's discretion, but if left in place it remains effective for 3 years. Removal requires making a 2- to 3-mm incision at the distal tip of the implant and pushing the other end of the rod until it pops out. Mean removal time is commonly less than 5 minutes (2.6 to 5.4 minutes).[321] Pain, swelling, redness, and hematoma have been reported during insertion and removal. Because return to ovulation is rapid following removal, women still desiring contraception should begin another method immediately or have a new rod inserted through the removal incision.

Disadvantages

Although progestin-only contraceptives offer a safe and effective method of preventing pregnancy, they have some drawbacks. Implants require a minor surgical procedure by a trained clinician for insertion and removal. Cost-effectiveness of the method depends upon long-term use; early discontinuation negates this benefit.[297] Lack of protection against sexually transmitted infections (STIs) is a disadvantage of the ENG implants as well as of all hormonal contraceptive methods.

Side effects associated with the ENG implant include menstrual irregularities (infrequent bleeding (26.9%), amenorrhea (18.6%), prolonged bleeding (15.1%), frequent bleeding (7.4%)), weight gain (20.7%), acne (15.3%), breast pain (9.1%), and headache (8.5%), but these symptoms rarely provoked discontinuation.[301,318] Women using any of the progestin-only methods notice changes in bleeding patterns.[322,323] A comparative study of bleeding patterns in single-capsule ENG implant users and six-capsule LNG implant users found a statistically significant decrease in mean number of bleeding or spotting days in the ENG users (15.9 to 19.3 days versus 19.4 to 21.6 days; $P = .0169$).[324] Because total uterine blood loss is reduced, users of progestin-only contraceptives (as well as OCs) are less likely to be anemic.

TABLE 17–10 COMPARISON OF VAGINAL BLEEDING PATTERNS IN ENG AND LNG USERS[326,327]

Bleeding Pattern*	ENG Implant (%) (n = 169)	LNG Implant (%) (n = 163)	Statistically Significant
Amenorrhea	21	5	Yes
Infrequent bleeding	27	22	Yes
Frequent bleeding	6	4	No
Prolonged bleeding	12	9	No

*90-day reference periods.
ENG, etonogestrel; LNG, levonorgestrel.

However, the study also found that users of ENG implants had more variable bleeding patterns than users of the LNG implants.[324] Table 17–10 shows the differences in bleeding between implants, but it is impossible to predict which of these patterns a woman is likely to experience. Despite side effects and dependence on clinicians to insert implants, most women using implantable contraception are satisfied with the method and cite its long duration of use, convenience, and high efficacy.[325,326]

Discontinuation Rates

Discontinuation rates for the ENG implant have varied by area of use, ranging from 30.2% in Europe and Canada to 0.9% in Southeast Asia.[318,321] Bleeding irregularities are cited as the most common reason for discontinuation of the ENG implant. A meta-analysis of 13 studies published between 1989 and 1992 found that among 1716 women using the ENG implant, 5.3% discontinued in months 1 through 6, 6.4% discontinued in months 7 through 12, 4.1% discontinued in months 13 through 18, and 2.8% discontinued in months 19 through 24. Overall, 82% of women continued to use the ENG implant for up to 24 months.[301]

Counseling

Counseling women to expect bleeding irregularities reduces discontinuation of this system. Prospective users should receive complete information about bleeding irregularities so they can make informed decisions regarding the side effects they are willing to accept in order to benefit from high contraceptive efficacy. Preinsertion counseling and postinsertion follow-up are essential for continued use of implants. Satisfaction with the method increases with proper counseling and minimizes costly removals.

Sexually active women are exposed to the risk of pregnancy as well as to the risk of STIs, such as human immunodeficiency virus, hepatitis B, human papillomavirus, *Chlamydia trachomatis*, syphilis, and gonorrhea, whose sequelae may be life threatening. Implantable contraceptives neither increase the risk of nor offer protection against STIs.[326] Women counseled about contraception should also be informed about the risks of STIs and advised that use of condoms concomitantly with an effective method of pregnancy prevention is the best means of protection against unintended pregnancy and STIs. It seems likely that the ENG implant, like OCs and DMPA, reduces the risk of pelvic upper tract infection.

Clinical experience with the ENG implant has demonstrated that method effectiveness and satisfaction are closely associated with patient education and provider training. In the first 18 months after the ENG implant was introduced in Australia in May 2001, an unexpectedly high number of adverse incidents were reported, and 100 unintended pregnancies occurred. Almost all of these events were traced to improper insertion by untrained clinicians or to poor patient selection, timing, and counseling. Policies that adequately document the process, procedure, and patient consent were initiated by the Royal Australian College of General Practitioners and have corrected the problems.[327]

Intrauterine Hormonal Contraception

Both medicated and nonmedicated intrauterine devices have been used for contraception. Those containing copper or synthetic progestins are more effective and have fewer side effects than simple plastic or stainless steel devices, and they have largely replaced the earlier varieties. Much information about intrauterine contraception is outdated and irrelevant because it is based on studies of these old contraceptives.

The LNG-20 (Mirena), manufactured by Leiras-Schering AG in Finland, releases in vitro 20 μg of levonorgestrel per day.[328] The vertical arm of this T-shaped device has a collar that contains 52 mg levonorgestrel dispersed in polydimethylsiloxane. The LNG is released initially at a rate of 20 μg per day in vivo, progressively declining and reaching half of the initial rate after 5 years. The levonorgestrel intrauterine delivery system (IUS) is approved for 5 years, but it lasts up to 10 years, and reduces menstrual blood loss and pelvic infection rates.[329-331] Indeed, the levonorgestrel IUS is about as effective as endometrial ablation for the treatment of menorrhagia.[332] The local progestin effect directed to the endometrium can be used in patients taking tamoxifen,[333] patients with dysmenorrhea,[334] and postmenopausal women receiving estrogen therapy.[335,336] Smaller devices releasing 5 μg or 10 μg levonorgestrel have been developed in Europe for use for at least 5 years in postmenopausal women.[336,337]

The progestin-releasing IUS adds the endometrial action of the progestin to the foreign body reaction. The endometrium becomes decidualized with atrophy of the glands.[338] The progestin IUS probably has two mechanisms of action: inhibition of implantation and inhibition of sperm capacitation, penetration, and survival. The levonorgestrel IUS produces serum concentrations of the progestin about half those of Norplant so that ovarian follicular development and ovulation are also partially inhibited; after the first year, cycles are ovulatory in 50% to 75% of women, regardless of their bleeding patterns.[339] Finally, the progestin IUS thickens the cervical mucus, creating a barrier to sperm penetration. The progestin IUS decreases menstrual blood loss (about 40% to 50%) and dysmenorrhea; with the levonorgestrel IUS, bleeding can be reduced by 90% 1 year after insertion.[340] About 50% of women become amenorrheic 1 year after insertion of the levonorgestrel IUS.[341,342] Average hemoglobin and iron levels increase over time compared with preinsertion values.[343]

Efficacy

The copper-releasing intrauterine contraceptive (IUC) (TCu-380A or Paragard) is approved for use in the United States for 10 years. However, the TCu-380A has been demonstrated to maintain its efficacy over at least 12 years of use.[344] The TCu-200 is approved for 4 years and the Nova T for 5 years. The levonorgestrel IUS can be used for at least 7 years and probably 10 years.[345] The levonorgestrel device that releases 15 to 20 μg levonorgestrel per day is as effective as the new copper IUCs.[329,346-348]

The nonmedicated IUCs never have to be replaced. The deposition of calcium salts on the IUC can produce a structure that is irritating to the endometrium. If bleeding increases after a nonmedicated IUC has been in place for some time, it is worth replacing it. Some clinicians recommend replacing all older

TABLE 17–11 ECTOPIC PREGNANCY RATES PER 1000 WOMAN-YEARS[352,353]

Method	Rate
No contraceptive, all ages	3.00-4.50
Levonorgestrel IUS	0.20
TCu-380A IUC	0.20

IUC, intrauterine contraceptive; IUS, intrauterine delivery system.

IUCs with the new, more effective copper IUCs. This makes sense because newer IUCs are more effective.

The risk of ectopic pregnancy does not increase with increasing duration of use with the TCu-380A or the levonorgestrel IUS.[346,349] In a 7-year prospective study, not a single ectopic pregnancy was encountered with the levonorgestrel IUD, and in a 5-year study, only one.[346,350] In 8000 woman-years of experience in randomized multicenter trials, there has been only a single ectopic pregnancy reported with the TCu-380A (which is one-tenth the rate with the Lippes Loop or TCu-200).[346] Therefore, the risk of ectopic pregnancy during the use of the copper IUS or the levonorgestrel IUC is much lower compared with rates in noncontraceptive users; however, if pregnancy occurs, the likelihood of an ectopic pregnancy is high.[351]

The protection against ectopic pregnancy provided by the TCu-380A and the levonorgestrel IUD makes these IUDs acceptable choices for contraception in women with previous ectopic pregnancies (Table 17–11).

Side Effects

With effective patient screening and good insertion technique, the copper and medicated IUCs are not associated with an increased risk of infertility after their removal. Even if IUCs are removed for problems, subsequent fertility rates are normal.[348,354,355]

The symptoms most often responsible for IUC discontinuation are increased uterine bleeding and increased menstrual pain. Within 1 year, 5% to 15% of women discontinue IUC use because of these problems. Smaller copper and progestin IUDs have reduced the incidence of pain and bleeding considerably, but a careful menstrual history is still important in helping a woman consider an IUC. Women with prolonged, heavy menstrual bleeding or significant dysmenorrhea might not be able to tolerate copper IUCs but might benefit from a progestin IUC.[340] Because bleeding and cramping are most severe in the first few months after IUC insertion, treatment with an NSAID (which inhibits prostaglandin synthesis) during the first several menstrual periods can reduce bleeding and cramping and help a patient through this difficult time. Even persistent heavy menses can be effectively treated with NSAIDs.[356] NSAID treatment should begin at the onset of menses and be maintained for 3 days. A copper IUC is available in China that also releases a small amount of indomethacin; this device is associated with markedly less bleeding.[357]

It is not unusual to have a few days of intermenstrual spotting or light bleeding. Although aggravating, this does not cause significant blood loss. Such bleeding deserves the usual evaluation for cervical or endometrial pathology. These changes can be objectionable for women who are prevented from having intercourse while bleeding.

Following insertion of a modern copper IUC, menstrual blood loss increases by about 55%, and this level of bleeding continues for the duration of IUC use.[358] This is associated with a slight (1 to 2 days) prolongation of menstruation. Over a year's time, this amount of blood loss does not result in changes indicative of iron deficiency (e.g., serum ferritin). With longer use, however, ferritin levels are lower, suggesting a depletion of iron stores.[359] Assessment for iron depletion and anemia should be considered in long-term users and in women susceptible to iron deficiency anemia. In populations with a high prevalence of anemia, these changes occur more rapidly, and iron supplementation is recommended.[360]

Because of a decidualizing, atrophic impact on the endometrium, amenorrhea can develop over time with the progestin-containing IUS. With the levonorgestrel IUS, 70% of patients are oligomenorrheic and 30% to 40% are amenorrheic within 2 years.[342,361] In a group of women who used the levonorgestrel IUS for more than 12 years, 60% were amenorrheic; 12% experienced infrequent, scanty bleeding; and 28% had regular but light bleeding.[343] For some women, the lack of periods is so disconcerting that they request removal. On the other hand, this effect on menstruation is manifested by an increase in blood hemoglobin levels.[346,362]

The levonorgestrel IUS is very effective when used to treat menorrhagia.[340,363] This noncontraceptive benefit is of such a magnitude that this method of treatment achieves comparable results when compared to surgical methods such as endometrial ablation or hysterectomy.[332,364-366] Bleeding is even reduced in the presence of leiomyomas, along with a reduction in myoma size.[367] The levonorgestrel IUS has been used successfully to treat endometriosis, and especially dysmenorrhea associated with endometriosis.[368]

Sufficient progestin reaches the systemic circulation from the levonorgestrel-containing IUD so that androgenic side effects, such as acne and hirsutism, might occur; however, in one study no change could be detected in the circulating levels of sex hormone–binding globulin, and, therefore, clinical effects are unlikely.[140] More extensive clinical studies are needed to assess the impact of this IUS on the lipoprotein profile, but it is unlikely that the low dose of levonorgestrel has an important effect on cardiovascular risk.

Infections

IUC-related bacterial infection is now believed to be due to contamination of the endometrial cavity at the time of insertion. Mishell's classic study indicated that the uterus is routinely contaminated by bacteria at insertion.[369] Infections that occur 3 to 4 months after insertion are believed to be due to acquired STIs, not the direct result of the IUC. The early, insertion-related infections, therefore, are polymicrobial and are derived from the endogenous cervicovaginal flora, with a predominance of anaerobes.

A review of the World Health Organization database derived from all of the WHO IUC clinical trials concluded that the risk of pelvic inflammatory disease was six times higher during the 20 days after the insertion compared with later times during follow-up, but, most importantly, PID was extremely rare beyond the first 20 days after insertion.[370] In nearly 23,000 insertions, however, only 81 cases of PID were diagnosed, and a scarcity of PID was observed in those situations in which STIs are rare. There was no statistically significant difference comparing the copper IUC with the inert Lippes Loop or progestin-containing IUC. These data confirm earlier studies that the risk of infection is highest immediately after insertion and that PID risk does not increase with long-term use.[371,372] The problem of infection can be minimized with careful screening and the use of aseptic technique. Even women with type 1 diabetes mellitus do not have an increased risk of infection.[373,374]

Doxycycline (200 mg) or azithromycin (500 mg) administered orally one hour prior to insertion can provide protection against insertion-associated pelvic infection, but prophylactic antibiotics are probably of little benefit for women at low risk for STIs.

Compared with oral contraception, barrier methods, and hormonal IUCs, there is no reason to think that nonmedicated or copper IUCs can confer protection against STIs, specifically PID.[375] However, the levonorgestrel-releasing IUC has been reported to be associated with a protective effect against pelvic infection, and the copper IUC is associated with lower titers of antichlamydial antibody.[330,376] In vitro, copper inhibits chlamydial growth in endometrial cells.[377] Thus, the perception that IUC use is associated with pelvic infection (and infertility) is outmoded.[378] Women who use IUCs must be counseled to use condoms along with the IUC whenever they have intercourse with a partner who could be an STI carrier. Because sexual behavior is the most important modifier of the risk of infection, clinicians should ask prospective IUC users about numbers of partners, their partner's sexual practices, the frequency and age of onset of intercourse, and history of STIs.[379] Women at low risk are unlikely to have pelvic infections while using IUCs.[372]

REFERENCES

1. Trussell J. Contraceptive efficacy of the personal hormone monitoring system Persona. Br J Fam Plann 1999;25:178-179.
2. Fu H, Darroch JE, Haas T, Ranjit N. Contraceptive failure rates: new estimates from the 1995 National Survey of Family Growth. Fam Plann Perspect 1999;31:58-63.
3. Rossmanith WG, Steffens D, Schramm G. A comparative randomized trial on the impact of two low-dose oral contraceptives on ovarian activity, cervical permeability, and endometrial receptivity. Contraception 1997;56:23-30.
4. Trussell J, Vaughan B. Contraceptive failure, method-related discontinuation and resumption of use: results from the 1995 National Survey of Family Growth. Fam Plann Perspect 1999;31:64-72.
5. Trussell J. Contraceptive failure in the United States. Contraception 2004;70:89-96.
6. Letterie GS, Chow GE. Effect of "missed" pills on oral contraceptive effectiveness. Obstet Gynecol 1992;79:979-982.
7. Westhoff C, Kerns J, Morroni C, et al. Quick-start: a novel oral contraceptive initiation method. Contraception 2002;66:141-145.
8. Westhoff C, Morroni C, Kerns J, Murphy PA. Bleeding patterns after immediate vs. conventional oral contraceptive initiation: a randomized, controlled trial. Fertil Steril 2003;79:322-329.
9. Anderson FD, Hait H, and the Seasonale-301 Study Group. A multicenter, randomized study of an extended cycle oral contraceptive. Contraception 2003;68:89-96.
10. Kwiecien M, Edelman A, Nichols MD, Jensen JT. Bleeding patterns and patient acceptability of standard or continuous dosing regimens of a low-dose oral contraceptive: a randomized trial. Contraception 2003;67:9-13.
11. Miller L, Hughes JP. Continuous combination oral contraceptive pills to eliminate withdrawal bleeding: a randomized trial. Obstet Gynecol 2003;101:653-661.
12. Sulak PJ, Carl J, Gopalakrishnan I, et al. Outcomes of extended oral contraceptive regiments with a shortened hormone-free interval to manage breakthrough bleeding. Contraception 2004;70:281-287.
13. Potter L, Oakley D, de Leon-Wong E, Canamar R. Measuring compliance among oral contraceptive users. Fam Plann Perspect 1996;28:154-158.
14. Killick SR, Bancroft K, Oelbaum S, et al. Extending the duration of the pill-free interval during combined oral contraception. Adv Contracept 1990;6:33-40.
15. Elomaa K, Rolland R, Brosens I, et al. Omitting the first oral contraceptive pills of the cycle does not automatically lead to ovulation. Am J Obstet Gynecol 1998;179:41-46.
16. van Heusden AM, Fauser BC. Activity of the pituitary-ovarian axis in the pill-free interval during use of low-dose combined oral contraceptives. Contraception 1999;59:237-243.
17. Sparrow MJ. Pill method failures. N Z Med J 1987;100:102-105.
18. Hansen TH, Lundvall F. Factors influencing the reliability of oral contraceptives. Acta Obstet Gynecol Scand 1997;76:61-64.
19. Jung-Hoffmann C, Kuhl H. Intra- and interindividual variations in contraceptive steroid levels during 12 treatment cycles: no relation to irregular bleedings. Contraception 1990;42:423-438.
20. Endrikat J, Müller U, Düsterberg B. A twelve-month comparative clinical investigation of two low-dose oral contraceptives containing 20 μg ethinylestradiol/75 μg gestodene and 30 μg ethinylestradiol/75 μg gestodene, with respect to efficacy, cycle control, and tolerance. Contraception 1997;55:131-37.
21. Rosenberg MJ, Meyers A, Roy V Efficacy, cycle control, and side effects of low- and lower-dose oral contraceptives: a randomized trial of 20 micrograms and 35 micrograms estrogen preparations. Contraception 1999;60:321-329.
22. Rosenberg MJ, Waugh MS, Stevens CM. Smoking and cycle control among oral contraceptive users. Am J Obstet Gynecol 1996;174: 628-632.
23. Rosenberg MJ, Waugh MS, Higgins JE. The effect of desogestrel, gestodene, and other factors on spotting and bleeding. Contraception 1996;53:85-90.
24. Krettek JE, Arkin SI, Chaisilwattana P, Monif GR. Chlamydia trachomatis in patients who used oral contraceptives and had intermenstrual spotting. Obstet Gynecol 1993;81:728-731.
25. Meade TW. Oral contraceptives, clotting factors, and thrombosis. Am J Obstet Gynecol 1982;142:758-761.
26. The Oral Contraceptive and Hemostasis Study Group. The effect of seven monophasic oral contraceptive regimens on hemostatic variables: conclusions from a large randomized multicenter study. Contraception 2003;67:173-185.
27. Jespersen J, Petersen KR, Skouby SO. Effects of newer oral contraceptives on the inhibition of coagulation and fibrinolysis in relation to dosage and type of steroid. Am J Obstet Gynecol 1990;163:396-403.
28. Notelovitz M, Kitchens CS, Khan FY. Changes in coagulation and anticoagulation in women taking low-dose triphasic oral contraceptives: a controlled comparative 12-month clinical trial. Am J Obstet Gynecol 1992;167:1255-1261.
29. Schlit AF, Grandjean P, Donnez J, Lavenne E. Large increase in plasmatic 11-dehydro-TXB_2 levels due to oral contraceptives. Contraception 1995;51:53-58.
30. Fruzzetti F, Ricci C, Fioretti P. Haemostasis profile in smoking and nonsmoking women taking low-dose oral contraceptives. Contraception 1994;49:579-592.
31. Basdevant A, Conard J, Pelissier C, et al. Hemostatic and metabolic effects of lowering the ethinyl-estradiol dose from 30 μg to 20 μg in oral contraceptives containing desogestrel. Contraception 1993;48:193-204.
32. Winkler UH, Schindler AE, Endrikat J, Dusterberg B. A comparative study of the effects of the hemostatic system of two monophasic gestodene oral contraceptives containing 20 μg and 30 μg ethinylestradiol. Contraception 1996;53:75-84.
33. Croft P, Hannaford PC. Risk factors for acute myocardial infarction in women: evidence from the Royal College of General Practitioners' oral contraception study. BMJ 1989;298:165-168.
34. Rosenberg L, Palmer JR, Lesko SM, Shapiro S. Oral contraceptive use and the risk of myocardial infaraction. Am J Epidemiol 1990;131:1009-1016.
35. Stampfer MJ, Willett WC, Colditz GA, et al. Past use of oral contraceptives and cardiovascular disease: a meta-analysis in the context of the Nurses' Health Study. Am J Obstet Gynecol 1990;163:285-291.
36. Colditz GA. Oral contraceptive use and mortality during 12 years of follow-up: the Nurses' Health Study. Ann Intern Med 1994; 120:821-826.
37. Beral V, Hermon C, Kay C, et al. Mortality associated with oral contraceptive use: 25-year follow-up of cohort of 46,000 women from Royal College of General Practitioners' oral contraception study. BMJ 1999;318:96-100.
38. Vessey M, Painter R, Yeates D. Mortality in relation to oral contraceptive use and cigarette smoking. Lancet 2003;362: 185-191.
39. Bottiger LE, Boman G, Eklund G, Westerholm B. Oral contraceptives and thromboembolic disease: effects of lowering oestrogen content. Lancet 1980;1:1097-1101.
40. Gerstman BB, Piper JM, Tomita DK, et al. Oral contraceptive estrogen dose and the risk of deep venous thromboembolic disease. Am J Epidemiol 1991;133:32-37.

41. Vessey M, Mant D, Smith A, Yeates D. Oral contraceptives and venous thromboembolism: findings in a large prospective study. BMJ 1986;292:526-533.
42. Helmrich SP, Rosenberg L, Kaufman DW, et al. Venous thromboembolism in relation to oral contraceptive use. Obstet Gynecol 1987;69:91-95.
43. Thorogood M, Mann J, Murphy M, Vessey M. Risk factors for fatal venous thromboembolism in young women: a case-control study. Int J Epidemiol 1992;21:48-52.
44. Rosenberg L, Hennekens CH, Rosner B, et al. Oral contraceptive use in relation to nonfatal myocardial infarction. Am J Epidemiol 1980;11:59-66.
45. Royal College of General Practitioners' Oral Contraceptive Study. Incidence of arterial disease among oral contraceptive users. J R Coll Gen Pract 1983;33:75-82.
46. Lidegaard Ø. Oral contraception and risk of a cerebral thromboembolic attack: results of a case-control study. BMJ 1993;306: 956-963.
47. Lawson DH, Davidson JF, Jick H. Oral contraceptive use and venous thromboembolism: absence of an effect of smoking. BMJ 1977;2:729-730.
48. Petitti DB, Wingerd J, Pellegrin F, Ramcharan S. Oral contraceptives, smoking, and other factors in relation to risk of venous thromboembolic disease. Am J Epidemiol 1978;108:480-485.
49. Royal College of General Practitioners. Oral contraceptive study: oral contraceptives, venous thrombosis, and varicose veins. J R Coll Gen Pract 1978;28:393-399.
50. Porter JB, Hershel J, Walker AM. Mortality among oral contraceptive users. Obstet Gynecol 1987;70:29-32.
51. WHO Collaborative Study of Cardiovascular Disease and Steroid Hormone Contraception. Effect of different progestagens in low oestrogen oral contraceptives on venous thromboembolic disease. Lancet 1995;346:1582-1588.
52. Spitzer WO, Lewis MA, Heinemann LA, et al. Third generation oral contraceptives and risk of venous thromboembolic disorders: an international case-control study. BMJ 1996;312:83-88.
53. Jick H, Jick SS, Gurewich V, et al. Risk of idiopathic cardiovascular death and nonfatal venous thromboembolism in women using oral contraceptives with differing progestagen components. Lancet 1995;348:1589-1593.
54. Bloemenkamp KW, Rosendaal FR, Helmerhorst FM, et al. Enhancement by factor V Leiden mutation of risk of deep-vein thrombosis associated with oral contraceptives containing a third-generation progestagen. Lancet 1995;348:1593-1596.
55. Farmer RDT, Preston TD. The risk of venous thromboembolism associated with low estrogen oral contraceptives. J Obstet Gynaecol 1995;15:195-200.
56. Vandenbroucke JP, van der Meer FJ, Helmerhorst FM, Rosendaal FR. Factor V Leiden. BMJ 1996;313:1127-1130.
57. Ridker PM, Miletich JP, Hennekens CH, Buring JE. Ethnic distribution of factor V Leiden in 4047 men and women: implications for venous thromboembolism screening. JAMA 1997;277: 1305-1307.
58. Sidney S, Petitti DB, Soff GA, et al. Venous thromboembolic disease in users of low-estrogen combined estrogen-progestin oral contraceptives. Contraception 2004;70:3-10.
59. Emmerich J, Rosendaal FR, Cattaneo M, et al. Combined effect of factor V Leiden and prothrombin 20210A on the risk of venous thromboembolism-pooled analysis of 8 case-control studies including 2310 cases and 3204 controls. Study Group for Pooled-Analysis in Venous Thromboembolism. Thromb Haemost 2001;86:809-816.
60. Hajjar KA. Factor V Leiden: an unselfish gene? New Engl J Med 1994;331:1585-1587.
61. Vensson PJ, Dahlbäck B. Resistance to activated protein C as a basis for venous thrombosis. New Engl J Med 1994;330:517-522.
62. Hellgren M, Svensson PJ, Dahlbäck B. Resistance to activated protein C as a basis for venous thromboembolism associated with pregnancy and oral contraceptives. Am J Obstet Gynecol 1995;173:210-213.
63. Vandenbroucke JP, Koster T, Briet E, et al. Increased risk of venous thrombosis in oral-contraceptive users who are carriers of factor V Leiden mutation. Lancet 1994;344:1453-1457.
64. Spannagl M, Heinemann AJ, Schramm W. Are factor V Leiden carriers who use oral contraceptives at extreme risk for venous thromboembolism? Eur J Contracept Reprod Health Care 2000;5:105-112.
65. Bloemenkamp KW, Rosendaal FR, Helmerhorst FM, Vandenbroucke JP. Higher risk of venous thrombosis during early use of oral contraceptives in women with inherited clotting defects. Arch Intern Med 2000;160:49-52.
66. Lidegaard Ø, Kreiner S. Cerebral thrombosis and oral contraceptives. A case-control study. Contraception 1998;57:303-314.
67. Lidegaard Ø, Edström B. Oral contraceptives and myocardial infarction. A case-control study (abstract). Eur J Contracept Reprod Health Care 1996;1(suppl):72-73.
68. WHO Collaborative Study of Cardiovascular Disease and Steroid Hormone Contraception. Acute myocardial infarction and combined oral contraceptives: results of an international multicentre case-control study. Lancet 1997;349:1202-1209.
69. Petitti DB, Sidney S, Quesenberry CP Jr, Bernstein A. Incidence of stroke and myocardial infarction in women of reproductive age. Stroke 1997;28:280-283.
70. Jick H, Porter J, Rothman KJ. Oral contraceptives and nonfatal stroke in healthy young women. Ann Int Med 1978;89:58-60.
71. Vessey MP, Lawless M, Yeates D. Oral contraceptives and stroke: findings in a large prospective study. BMJ 1984;289:530-531.
72. Hannaford PC, Croft PR, Kay CR. Oral contraception and stroke: evidence from the Royal College of General Practitioners' Oral Contraception Study. Stroke 1994;25:935-942.
73. Petitti DB, Sidney S, Bernstein A, et al. Stroke in users of low-dose oral contraceptives. New Engl J Med 1996;335:8-15.
74. WHO Collaborative Study of Cardiovascular Disease and Steroid Hormone Contraception. Ischaemic stroke and combined oral contraceptives: results of an international, multicentre case-control study. Lancet 1996;348:498-405.
75. WHO Collaborative Study of Cardiovascular Disease and Steroid Hormone Contraception. Haemorrhagic stroke, overall stroke risk, and combined oral contraceptives: results of an international, multicentre, case-control study. Lancet 1996;348:505-510.
76. Barrett DH, Anda RF, Escobedo LG, et al. Trends in oral contraceptive use and cigarette smoking. Arch Fam Med 1994;3:438-443.
77. Kovacs L, Bartfai G, Apro G, et al. The effect of the contraceptive pill on blood pressure: a randomized controlled trial of three progestogen-oestrogen combinations in Szeged, Hungary. Contraception 1986;33:69-77.
78. Nichols M, Robinson G, Bounds W, et al. Effect of four combined oral contraceptives on blood pressure in the pill-free interval. Contraception 1993;47:367-376.
79. Shen Q, Lin D, Jiang X, et al. Blood pressure changes and hormonal contraceptives. Contraception 1994;50:131-141.
80. Darney P. Safety and efficacy of a triphasic oral contraceptive containing desogrestrel: results of three multicenter trials. Contraception 1993;48:323-337.
81. Chasan-Taber L, Willett WC, Manson JE, et al. Prospective study of oral contraceptives and hypertension among women in the United States. Circulation 1996;94:483-489.
82. Brady WA, Kritz-Silverstein D, Barrett-Connor E, Morales AJ. Prior oral contraceptive use is associated with higher blood pressure in older women. J Women's Health 1998;7:221-227.
83. Pabinger I, Schneider B, and the GTH Study Group. Thrombotic risk of women with hereditary antithrombin III, protein C, and protein S deficiency taking oral contraceptive medication. Thromb Haemost 1994;5:548-552.
84. Godsland IF, Crook D, Simpson R, et al. The effects of different formulations of oral contraceptive agents on lipid and carbohydrate metabolism. New Engl J Med 1990;323:1375-1381
85. van der Vange N, Kloosterboer HJ, Haspels AA. Effect of seven low-dose combined oral contraceptive preparations on carbohydrate metabolism. Am J Obstet Gynecol 1987;156:918-922.
86. Bowes WA Jr, Katta LR, Droegemueller W, Bright TG. Triphasic randomized clinical trial: Comparison of effects on carbohydrate metabolism. Am J Obstet Gynecol 1989;161:1402-1407.
87. Gaspard UJ, Lefebvre PJ. Clinical aspects of the relationship between oral contraceptives, abnormalities in carbohydrate metabolism, and the development of cardiovascular disease. Am J Obstet Gynecol 1990;163:334-343.
88. Troisi RJ, Cowie CC, Harris MI. Oral contraceptive use and glucose metabolism in a national sample of women in the United States. Am J Obstet Gynecol 2000;183:389-395.

89. Hannaford PC, Kay CR, Vessey MP, et al. Combined oral contraceptives and liver disease. Contraception 1997;55:145-151.
90. Lubianca JN, Faccin CS, Fuchs FD. Oral contraceptives: a risk factor for uncontrolled blood pressure among hypertensive women. Contraception 2003;67:19-24.
91. Ross RK, Pike MC, Vessey MP, et al. Risk factors for uterine fibroids: reduced risk associated with oral contraceptives. BMJ 1986; 293:359-362.
92. Parazzini F, Negri E, La Vecchia C, et al. Oral contraceptive use and risk of uterine fibroids. Obstet Gynecol 1992;79:430-433.
93. Samadi AR, Lee NC, Flanders WD, et al. Risk factors for self-reported uterine fibroids: a case-control study. Am J Public Health 1996;86:858-862.
94. Marshall LM, Spiegelman D, Goldman MB, et al. A prospective study of reproductive factors and oral contraceptive use in relation to the risk of uterine leiomyomata. Fertil Steril 1998;70:432-439.
95. Chiaffarino F, Parazzini F, La Vecchia C, et al. Use of oral contraceptives and uterine fibroids: results from a case-control study. Br J Obstet Gynaecol 1999;106:857-860.
96. Kjos SL, Shoupe D, Douyan S, et al. Effect of low-dose oral contraceptives on carbohydrate and lipid metabolism in women with recent gestational diabetes: results of a controlled, randomized, prospective study. Am J Obstet Gynecol 1990;163:1822-1827.
97. Kjos SL, Peters RK, Xiang A, et al. Contraception and the risk of type 2 diabetes in Latino women with prior gestational diabetes. JAMA 1998;280:533-538.
98. Garg SK, Chase HP, Marshall G, et al. Oral contraceptives and renal and retinal complications in young women with insulin-dependent diabetes mellitus. JAMA 1994;271:1099-1102.
99. Petersen KR, Skouby SO, Sidelmann J, et al. Effects of contraceptive steroids on cardiovascular risk factors in women with insulin-dependent diabetes mellitus. Am J Obstet Gynecol 1994;171: 400-405.
100. Klein BE, Klein R, Moss SE. Mortality and hormone-related exposures in women with diabetes. Diabetes Care 1999;22:248-252.
101. Mattson RH, Cramer JA, Darney PD, Naftolin F. Use of oral contraceptives by women with epilepsy. JAMA 1986;256:238-240.
102. Vessey M, Painter R, Yeates D. Oral contraception and epilepsy: findings in a large cohort study. Contraception 2002;66:77-79.
103. Lutcher CL, Milner PF. Contraceptive-induced vascular occlusive events in sickle cell disorders—fact or fiction? [abstract] Clin Res 1986;34:217A.
104. Yoong WC, Tuck SM, Yardumian A. Red cell deformability in oral contraceptive pill users with sickle cell anemia. Br J Haematol 1999;104:868-870.
105. De Ceulaer K, Gruber C, Hayes R, Serjeant GR. Medroxyprogesterone acetate and homozygous sickle-cell disease. Lancet 1982;2: 229-231.
106. Jungers P, Dougados M, Pelissier C, et al. Influence of oral contraceptive therapy on the activity of systemic lupus erythematosus. Arthritis Rheum 1982;25:618-623.
107. Petri M, Robinson C. Oral contraceptives and systemic lupus erythematosus. Arthritis Rheum 1997;40:797-703.
108. Knopp RH, LaRosa JC, Burkman RT Jr. Contraception and dyslipidemia. Am J Obstet Gynecol 1993;168:1994-2005.
109. WHO Collaborative Study of Cardiovascular Disease and Steroid Hormone Contraception. Venous thromboembolic disease and combined oral contraceptives: results of international multicentre case-control study. Lancet 1995;346:1575-1582.
110. Lidegaard Ø, Edström B, Kreiner S. Oral contraceptives and venous thromboembolism: a five-year national case-control study. Contraception 2002;65:187-196.
111. Abdollahi M, Cushman M, Rosendaal FR. Obesity: risk of venous thromboembolism and the interaction with coagulation factor levels and oral contraceptive use. Thromb Haemost 2003;89: 493-498.
112. Holt VL, Cushing-Haugen KL, Daling JR. Body weight and risk of oral contraceptive failure. Obstet Gynecol 2002;99:820-827.
113. Zieman M, Guillebaud J, Weisberg E, et al. Contraceptive efficacy and cycle control with the Ortho Evra/Evra transdermal system: the analysis of pooled data. Fertil Steril 2002;77(Suppl 2):S13-S18.
114. Norris PM, Kamat A, Estes C, et al. Contraceptive failure in overweight patients taking combination oral contraceptive pills. Presented at Association of Reproductive Health Professionals Annual Meeting, San Diego, Calif., 2003.
115. Azziz R. The hyperandrogenic-insulin-resistant acanthosis nigricans syndrome: therapeutic response. Fertil Steril 1994;61: 570-572.
116. Duffy TJ, Ray R. Oral contraceptive use: prospective follow-up of women with suspected glucose intolerance. Contraception 1984; 30:197-208.
117. Hannaford PC, Kay CR. Oral contraceptives and diabetes mellitus. BMJ 1989;299:1315-1316.
118. Nader S, Riad-Gabriel MG, Saad M. The effect of a desogestrel-containing oral contraceptive on glucose tolerance and leptin concentrations in hyperandrogenic women. J Clin Endocrinol Metab 1997;82:3074-3077.
119. Pasquali R, Gambineri A, Anconetani B, et al. The natural history of the metabolic syndrome in young women with the polycystic ovary syndrome and the effect of long-term oestrogen-progestogen treatment. Clin Endocrinol 1999;50:517-527.
120. Klibanski A, Biller BM, Schoenfeld DA, et al. The effects of estrogen administration on trabecular bone loss in young women with anorexia nervosa. J Clin Endocrinol Metab 1995;80:898-904.
121. Drinkwater BL, Bruemner B, Chesnut CH 3rd. Menstrual history as a determinant of current bone density in young athletes. JAMA 1990;263:545-548.
122. Jonnavithula S, Warren MP, Fox RP, Lazaro MI. Bone density is compromised in amenorrheic women despite return of menses: a 2-year study. Obstet Gynecol 1993;81:669-674.
123. Lashner BA, Kane SV, Hanauer SB. Lack of association between oral contraceptive use and ulcerative colitis. Gastroenterology 1990;99:1032-1036.
124. Cosnes J, Carbonnel F, Carrat F, et al. Oral contraceptive use and the clinical course of Crohn's disease: a prospective cohort study. Gut 1999;45:218-222.
125. American Cancer Society. Breast Cancer Facts and Figures 2003-2004. Available at http://www.cancer.org/docroot/STT/content/STT_1x_Breast_Cancer_Facts_Figures_2003-2004.asp (accessed December 9, 2006).
126. Chi I. The safety and efficacy issues of progestin-only oral contraceptives—an epidemiologic perspective. Contraception 1993;47: 1-21.
127. McCann MF, Potter LS. Progestin-only oral contraception: a comprehensive review. Contraception 1994;50(suppl 1):S9-S195.
128. Moghissi KS, Marks C. Effects of microdose progestogens on endogenous gonadotrophic and steroid hormones, cervical mucus properties, vaginal cytology and endometrium. Fertil Steril 1971;22:424-434.
129. Moghissi KS, Syner FN, McBride LC. Contraceptive mechanism of microdose norethindrone. Obstet Gynecol 1973;4:585-594.
130. Collaborative Study Group on the Desogestrel-Containing Progestogen-Only Pill. A double-blind study comparing the contraceptive efficacy, acceptability and safety of two progestogen-only pills containing desogestrel 75 μg/day or levonorgestrel 30 μg/day. Eur J Contracept Reprod Health Care 1998;3:169-178.
131. Fotherby K. The progestogen-only pill and thrombosis. Br J Fam Plann 1989;15:83-85.
132. Ball MJ, Ashwell E, Gillmer MD. Progestagen-only oral contraceptives: comparison of the metabolic effects of levonorgestrel and norethisterone. Contraception 1991;44:223-233.
133. Winkler UH. Blood coagulation and oral contraceptives. A critical review. Contraception 1998;57:203-209.
134. Trussell J, Kost K. Contraceptive failure in the United States: a critical review of the literature. Stud Fam Plann 1987;18:237-283.
135. Vessey MP, Lawless M, Yeates D, McPherson K. Progestogen-only contraception: findings in a large prospective study with special reference to effectiveness. Br J Fam Plann 1985;10:117-121.
136. Bisset AM, Dingwall-Fordyce I, Hamilton MJK. The efficacy of the progestogen-only pill as a contraceptive method. Br J Fam Plann 1990;16:84-94.
137. Broome M, Fotherby K. Clinical experience with the progestogen-only pill. Contraception 1990;42:489-495.
138. Tayob Y, Adams J, Jacobs HS, Guillebaud J. Ultrasound demonstration of increased frequency of functional ovarian cysts in women using progestogen-only oral contraception. Br J Obstet Gynaecol 1985;92:1003-1009.
139. Vessey M, Metcalfe A, Wells C, et al. Ovarian neoplasms, functional ovarian cysts, and oral contraceptives. BMJ 1987;294: 1518-1520.

140. Pakarinen P, Lahteenmaki P, Rutanen EM. The effect of intrauterine and oral levonorgestrel administration on serum concentrations of sex hormone-binding globulin, insulin and insulin-like growth factor binding protein-1. Acta Obstet Gynecol Scand 1999;78:423-428.
141. Tankeyoon M, Dusitsin N, Chalapati S, et al. Effects of hormonal contraceptives on milk volume and infant growth. WHO Special Programme of Research, Development and Research Training in Human Reproduction Task Force on Oral Contraceptives. Contraception 1984;30:505-522.
142. WHO Task Force for Epidemiological Research on Reproductive Health, Special Programme of Research, Development and Research Training in Human Reproduction. Progestogen-only contraceptives during lactation. I. Infant growth. Contraception 1994;50:35-53.
143. WHO Task Force for Epidemiological Research on Reproductive Health, Special Programme of Research, Development and Research Training in Human Reproduction. Progestogen-only contraceptives during lactation. II. Infant development. Contraception 1994;50:55-68.
144. McCann MF, Moggia AV, Higgins JE, et al. The effects of a progestin-only oral contraceptive (levonorgestrel 0.03 mg) on breastfeeding. Contraception 1989;40:635-648.
145. Halderman LD, Nelson AL. Impact of early postpartum administration of progestin-only hormonal contraceptives compared with nonhormonal contraceptives on short-term breast-feeding patterns. Am J Obstet Gynecol 2002;186:1250-1258.
146. Mintz G, Gutierrez G, Deleze M, Rodriguez E. Contraception with progestogens in systemic lupus erythematosus. Contraception 1984;30:29-38.
147. World Health Organization Collaborative Study of Cardiovascular Disease and Steroid Hormone Contraception. Cardiovascular disease and use of oral and injectable progestogen-only contraceptives and combined injectable contraceptives. Results of an international, multicenter, case-control study. Contraception 1998;57:315-324.
148. Heinemann LA, Assmann A, DoMinh T, Garbe E. Oral progestogen-only contraceptives and cardiovascular risk: results from the Transnational Study on Oral Contraceptives and the Health of Young Women. Eur J Contracept Reprod Health Care 1999;4:67-73.
149. Winkler UH, Howie H, Buhler K, et al. A randomized controlled double-blind study of the effects on hemostasis of two progestogen-only pills containing 75 μg desogestrel or 30 μg levonorgestrel. Contraception 1998;57:385-392.
150. Weiderpass E, Adami HO, Baron JA, et al. Risk of endometrial cancer following estrogen replacement with and without progestins. J Natl Cancer Inst 1999;91:1131-1137.
151. Morris JM, van Wagenen G. Compounds interfering with ovum implantation and development. III. The role of estrogens. Am J Obstet Gynecol 1966;96:804-815.
152. Yuzpe AA, Smith RP, Rademaker AW. A multicenter clinical investigation employing ethinyl estradiol combined with *dl*-norgestrel as a postcoital contraceptive agent. Fertil Steril 1982;37:508-513.
153. Ho PC, Kwan MSW. A prospective randomized comparison of levonorgestrel with the Yuzpe regimen in post-coital contraception. Hum Reprod 1993;8:389-392.
154. Task Force on Postovulatory Methods of Fertility Regulation. Randomised controlled trial of levonorgestrel versus the Yuzpe regimen of combined oral contraceptives for emergency contraception. Lancet 1998;352:428-433.
155. von Hertzen H, Piaggio G, Ding J; WHO Research Group on Post-ovulatory Methods of Fertility Regulation. Low dose mifepristone and two regimens of levonorgestrel for emergency contraception: a WHO multicentre randomised trial. Lancet 2002;360:1803-1810.
156. Arowojoulu AO, Okewole IA, Adekunie AO. Comparative evaluation of the effectiveness and safety of two regimens of levonorgestrel for emergency contraception in Nigerians. Contraception 2002;66:269-273.
157. Burton R, Savage W, Reader F. The "morning after pill." Is this the wrong name for it? Br J Fam Plann 1990;15:119-121.
158. Young L, McCowan LM, Roberts HE, Farquhar CM. Emergency contraception—why women don't use it. N Z Med J 1995;108:145-148.
159. Harper CC, Ellertson CE. The emergency contraceptive pill: a survey of knowledge and attitudes among students at Princeton. Am J Obstet Gynecol 1995;173:1438-1445.
160. Delbanco SF, Mauldon J, Smith MD. Little knowledge and limited practice: emergency contraceptive pills, the public, and the obstetrician-gynecologist. Obstet Gynecol 1997;89:1006-1011.
161. Trussell J, Stewart F, Guest F, Hatcher RA. Emergency contraceptive pills: a simple proposal to reduce unintended pregnancies. Fam Plann Perspect 1992;24:269-273.
162. Harvey SM, Beckman LJ, Sherman C, Petitti D. Women's experience and satisfaction with emergency contraception. Fam Plann Perspect 1999;31:237-240, 260.
163. Glasier A, Baird D. The effects of self-administering emergency contraception. New Engl J Med 1998;339:1-4.
164. Raine T, Harper C, Leon K, Darney P. Emergency contraception: advance provision in a young, high-risk clinic population. Obstet Gynecol 2000;96:1-7.
165. Jackson RA, Swarz EB, Freedman L, Darney P. Advance supply of emergency contraception: effect on use and usual contraception—a randomized trial. Obstet Gynecol 2003;102:8-16.
166. Raine TR, Harper CC, Rocca CH, et al. Direct access to emergency contraception through pharmacies and effect on unintended pregnancy and STIs: a randomized controlled trial. JAMA 2005;293(1):54-62.
167. Harper CC, Cheong M, Rocca CH, et al. The effect of increased access to emergency contraception among young adolescents. Obstet Gynecol 2005;106(3):483-491.
168. Gainer E, Blum J, Toverud EL, et al. Bringing emergency contraception over the counter: experiences of nonprescription users in France, Norway, Sweden and Portugal. Contraception 2003;68:117-124.
169. Young DC, Wiehle RD, Joshi SG, Poindexter AN 3rd. Emergency contraception alters progesterone-associated endometrial protein in serum and uterine luminal fluid. Obstet Gynecol 1994;84:266-271.
170. Swahn ML, Westlund P, Johannisson E, Bygdeman M. Effect of postcoital contraceptive methods on the endometrium and the menstrual cycle. Acta Obstet Gynecol Scand 1996;75:738-744.
171. Trussell J, Raymond EG. Statistical evidence about the mechanism of action of the Yuzpe regimen of emergency contraception. Obstet Gynecol 1999;93:872-876.
172. Marions L, Hultenby K, Lindell I, et al. Emergency contraception with mifepristone and levonorgestrel: mechanism of action. Obstet Gynecol 2002;100:65-71.
173. Croxatto HB, Fuentealba B, Brache V, et al. Effects of the Yuzpe regimen, given during the follicular phase, on ovarian function. Contraception 2002;65:121-128.
174. Trussell J, Ellertson C, Dorflinger L. Effectiveness of the Yuzpe regimen of emergency contraception by cycle day of intercourse: implications for mechanism of action. Contraception 2003;67:167-171.
175. Fasoli M, Parazzini F, Cecchetti G, La Vecchia C. Post-coital contraception: an overview of published studies. Contraception 1989;39:459-468.
176. Haspels AA. Emergency contraception: a review. Contraception 1994;50:101-108.
177. Glasier A. Emergency postcoital contraception. New Engl J Med 1997;337:1058-1064.
178. Wilcox AJ, Weinberg CR, Baird DD. Timing of sexual intercourse in relation to ovulation. Effects on the probability of conception, survival of the pregnancy, and sex of the baby. New Engl J Med 1995;333(23):1517-1521.
179. Trussell J, Ellertson C, Stewart F. The effectiveness of the Yuzpe regimen of emergency contraception. Fam Plann Perspect 1996;28:58-64.
180. Trussell J, Rodríguez G, Ellertson C. New estimates of the effectiveness of the Yuzpe regimen of emergency contraception. Contraception 1998;57:363-369.
181. Trussell J, Rodríguez C, Ellertson C. Updated estimates of the effectiveness of the Yuzpe regimen of emergency contraception. Contraception 1999;59:147-151.
182. Trussell J, Ellertson C, Rodriguez G. The Yuzpe regimen of emergency contraception: how long after the morning after? Obstet Gynecol 1996;88:150-154.

183. Rodrigues I, Grou F, Joly J. Effectiveness of emergency contraceptive pills between 72 and 120 hours after unprotected sexual intercourse. Am J Obstet Gynecol 2001;184:531-537.
184. Piaggio G, von Hertzen H, Grimes DA, Van Look PF. Timing of emergency contraception with levonorgestrel or the Yuzpe regimen. Lancet 1999;353:721.
185. Simpson JL, Phillips OP. Spermicides, hormonal contraception and congenital malformations. Adv Contraception 1990;6: 141-167.
186. Bracken MB. Oral contraception and congenital malformations in offspring: a review and meta-analysis of the prospective studies. Obstet Gynecol 1990;76:552-557.
187. Raman-Wilms L, Tseng AL, Wighardt S, et al. Fetal genital effects of first trimester sex hormone exposure: a meta-analysis. Obstet Gynecol 1995;85:141-149.
188. Vasilakis C, Jick SS, Jick H. The risk of venous thromboembolism in users of postcoital contraceptive pills. Contraception 1999;59:79-83.
189. Webb A, Taberner D. Clotting factors after emergency contraception. Adv Contracept 1993;9:75-82.
190. Ellertson C, Webb A, Blanchard K, et al. Modifying the Yuzpe regimen of emergency contraception: a multicenter randomized controlled trial. Obstet Gynecol 2003;101:1160-1167.
191. Webb AMC, Russell J, Elstein M. Comparison of Yuzpe regimen, danazol, and mifepristone (RU486) in oral postcoital contraception. BMJ 1992;305:927-931.
192. Glasier A, Thong KJ, Dewar M, et al. Mifepristone (RU 486) compared with high-dose estrogen and progestogen for emergency postcoital contraception. New Engl J Med 1992;327:1041-1044.
193. Task Force on Postovulatory Methods of Fertility Regulation. Comparison of three single doses of mifepristone as emergency contraception: a randomised trial. Lancet 1999;353:697-702.
194. Xiao BL, Von Hertzen H, Zhao H, Piaggio G. A randomized double-blind comparison of two single doses of mifepristone for emergency contraception. Hum Reprod 2002;17:3084-3089.
195. Alexander NJ, Baker E, Kaptein M, et al. Why consider vaginal drug administration? Fertil Steril 2004;82:1-12.
196. Timmer CJ, Mulders TM. Pharmacokinetics of etonogestrel and ethinylestradiol released from a combined contraceptive vaginal ring. Clin Pharmacokinet 2000;39:233-242.
197. Roumen FJ, Apter D, Mulders TM, Dieben TO. Efficacy, tolerability and acceptability of a novel contraceptive vaginal ring releasing etonogestrel and ethinyl estradiol. Hum Reprod 2001;16:469-475.
198. Mulders TM, Dieben TO. Use of the novel combined contraceptive vaginal ring NuvaRing for ovulation inhibition. Fertil Steril 2001;75:865-870.
199. Dieben TO, Roumen FJ, Apter D. Efficacy, cycle control, and user acceptability of a novel combined contraceptive vaginal ring. Obstet Gynecol 2002;100:585-593.
200. Bjarnadóttir RI, Tuppurainen M, Killick SR. Comparison of cycle control with a combined vaginal ring and oral levonorgestrel/ ethinyl estradiol. Am J Obstet Gynecol 2002;186:389-395.
201. Szarewski A. High acceptability and satisfaction with NuvaRing use. Eur J Contracept Reprod Health Care 2002;7:31-36.
202. Roumen FJ, Boon ME, van Velzen D, et al. The cervico-vaginal epithelium during 20 cycles' use of a combined contraceptive vaginal ring. Hum Reprod 1996;11:2443-2448.
203. Davies GC, Feng LX, Newton JR, et al. The effects of a combined contraceptive vaginal ring releasing ethinyloestradiol and 3-keto-desogestrel on vaginal flora. Contraception 1992;45:511-518.
204. Haring T, Mulders TM. The combined contraceptive ring NuvaRing and spermicide co-medication. Contraception 2003;67:271-272.
205. Hammond GL, Abrams LS, Creasy GW, et al. Serum distribution of the major metabolites of noregestimate in relation to its pharmacological properties. Contraception 2003;67:93-99.
206. Dittrich R, Parker L, Rosen JB, et al; Ortho Evra/Evra 001 Study Group. Transdermal contraception: evaluation of three transdermal norelgestromin/ethinyl estradiol doses in a randomized multicenter, dose-response study. Am J Obstet Gynecol 2002; 186:15-20.
207. Zacur HA, Hedon B, Mansour D, et al. Integrated summary of Ortho Evra/Evra contraceptive patch adhesion in varied climates and conditions. Fertil Steril 2002;77(Suppl 2):S32-S35.
208. Audet MC, Moreau M, Koltun WD, et al; Ortho Evra/Evra 004 Study Group. Evaluation of contraceptive efficacy and cycle control of a transdermal contraceptive patch vs an oral contraceptive. A randomized controlled trial. JAMA 2001;285:2347-2354.
209. Smallwood GH, Meador ML, Lenihan JP, et al; Ortho Evra/Evra 002 Study Group. Efficacy and safety of a transdermal contraceptive system. Obstet Gynecol 2001;98:799-805.
210. Pierson RA, Archer DF, Moreau M, et al. Ortho Evra/Evra versus oral contraceptives: follicular development and ovulation in normal cycles and after an intentional dosing error. Fertil Steril 2003;80:34-42.
211. Abrams LS, Skee DM, Natarajan J, et al. Multiple-dose pharmacokinetics of a contraceptive patch in healthy women participants. Contraception 2001;64:287-294.
212. Abrams LS, Skee DM, Natarajan J, et al. Pharmacokinetics of a contraceptive patch (Evra/Ortho Evra) containing norelgestromin and ethinyloestradiol at four application sites. Br J Clin Pharmacol 2002;53:141-146.
213. Abrams LS, Skee DM, Wong FA, et al. Pharmacokinetics of norelgestromin and ethinyl estradiol from two consecutive contraceptive patches. J Clin Pharmacol 2001;41:1232-1237.
214. Abrams LS, Skee DM, Natarajan J, et al. Pharmacokinetics of norelgestromin and ethinyl estradiol delivered by a contraceptive patch (Ortho Evra/Evra) under conditions of heat, humidity, and exercise. J Clin Pharmacol 2001;41:1301-1309.
215. Abrams LS, Skee D, Natarajan J, Wong FA. Pharmacokinetic overview of Ortho Evra/Evra. Fertil Steril 2002;77(Suppl 2): S3-S12.
216. Creasy GW, Fisher AC, Hall N, Shangold GA. Transdermal contraceptive patch delivering norelgestromin and ethinyl estradiol. Effects on the lipid profile. J Reprod Med 2003;48(3): 179-186.
217. Sibai BM, Odlind V, Meador ML, et al. A comparative and pooled analysis of the safety and tolerability of the contraceptive patch (Ortho Evra/Evra). Fertil Steril 2002;77(Suppl 2):S19-S26.
218. Archer DF, Bigrigg A, Smallwood GH, et al. Assessment of compliance with a weekly contraceptive patch (Ortho Evra/Evra) among North American women. Fertil Steril 2002;77(Suppl 2): S27-S31.
219. Rosenfield A, Maine D, Rochat R, et al. The Food and Drug Administration and medroxyprogesterone acetate: what are the issues? JAMA 1983;249:2922-2928.
220. Said S, Omar K, Koetsawang S, et al. A multicentered phase III comparative clinical trial of depot-medroxyprogesterone acetate given three-monthly at doses of 100 mg or 150 mg: I. Contraceptive efficacy and side effects. World Health Organization Task Force on Long-Acting Systemic Agents for Fertility Regulation. Special Programme of Research, Development and Research Training in Human Reproduction. Contraception 1986;34:223-235.
221. World Health Organization. Multinational comparative clinical evaluation of two long-acting injectable contraceptive steroids: norethisterone enanthate and medroxyprogesterone acetate. Final report. Contraception 1983;28:1-20.
222. Mishell DR Jr. Effect of 6 methyl-17-hydroxyprogesterone on urinary excretion of luteinizing hormone. Am J Obstet Gynecol 1967; 99:86-90.
223. Fraser IS, Weisberg EA. A comprehensive review of injectable contaception with special emphasis on depot medroxyprogesterone acetate. Med J Aust 1981;1(1 Suppl):3-19.
224. Pardthaisong T, Gray RH. In utero exposure to steroid contraceptives and outcome of pregnancy. Am J Epidemiol 1991;134: 795-803.
225. Gray RH, Pardthaisong. In utero exposure to steroid contraceptives and survival during infancy. Am J Epidemiol, 1991; 134:804-811.
226. Siriwongse T, Snidvongs W, Tantayaporn P, Leepipatpaiboon S. Effect of depot-medroxyprogesterone acetate on serum progesterone levels, when administered on various cycle days. Contraception 1982;26:487-493.
227. Petta CA, Faundes A, Dunson TR, et al. Timing of onset of contraceptive effectiveness in Depo-Provera users. I. Changes in cervical mucus. Fertil Steril 1998;69:252-257.
228. Petta CA, Faundes A, Dunson TR, et al. Timing of onset of contraceptive effectiveness in Depo-Provera users. II. Effects on ovarian function. Fertil Steril 1998;70:817-820.

229. Harlap S, Kost K, Forrest JD. Preventing Pregnancy, Protecting Health: A New Look at Birth Control Choices in the United States. New York: The Alan Guttmacher Institute, 1991.
230. Mattson RH, Cramer JA, Caldwell BV, Siconolfi BC. Treatment of seizures with medroxyprogesterone acetate: preliminary report. Neurology, 1984;34:1255-1258.
231. O'Dell CM, Forke CM, Polaneczky MM, et al. Depot medroxyprogesterone acetate or oral contraception in postpartum adolescents. Obstet Gynecol 1998;91:609-614.
232. Polaneczky M, Guarnaccia M, Alon J, Wiley J. Early experience with the contraceptive use of depo-medroxyprogesterone acetate in an inner-city population. Fam Plann Perspect 1996;28:174-178.
233. de Abood M, de Castillo Z, Guerrero F, et al. Effect of Depo-Provera or Microgynon on the painful crises of sickle-cell anemia patients. Contraception 1997;56:313-316.
234. Jimenez J, Ochoa M, Soler MP, Portales P. Long-term follow-up of children breast-fed by mothers receiving depot-medroxyprogesterone acetate. Contraception 1984;30:523-533.
235. Zacharias S, Aguilera E, Assenzo JR, Zanartu J. Effects of hormonal and non-hormonal contracepters on lactation and incidence of pregnancy. Contraception 1986;33:203-213.
236. Pardthaisong T, Yenchit C, Gray R. The long-term growth and development of children exposed to Depo-Provera during pregnancy or lactation. Contraception 1992;45:313-324.
237. Virutamasen P, Leepipatpaiboon S, Kriengsinyot R, et al. Pharmacodynamic effects of depot-medroxyprogesterone acetate (DMPA) administered to lactating women on their male infants. Contraception 1996;54:153-157.
238. Depot-medroxyprogesterone acetate (DMPA) and risk of endometrial cancer. The WHO Collaborative Study of Neoplasia and Steroid Contraceptives. Int J Cancer 1991;49:186-190.
239. Lumbiganon P, Rugpao S, Phandhu-fung S, et al. Protective effect of depot-medroxyprogesterone acetate on surgically treated uterine leiomyomas: a multicentre case-control study. Br J Obstet Gynaecol 1996;103:909-914.
240. Depot-medroxyprogesterone acetate (DMPA) and risk of epithelial ovarian cancer. The WHO Collaborative Study of Neoplasia and Steroid Contraceptives. Int J Cancer 1991;49:191-195.
241. Gray RH. Reduced risk of pelvic inflammatory disease with injectable contraceptives. Lancet 1985;1:1046-1049.
242. Cromer BA, Smith RD, Blair JM, et al. A prospective study of adolescents who choose among levonorgestrel implant (Norplant), medroxyprogesterone acetate (Depo-Provera), or the combined oral contraceptive pill as contraception. Pediatrics 1994;94: 687-694.
243. Gardner JM, Mishell DR Jr. Analysis of bleeding patterns and resumption of fertility following discontinuation of a long-acting injectable contraceptive. Fertil Steril 1970;21:286-291.
244. Harel Z, Biro FM, Kollar LM. Depo-Provera in adolescents: effects of early second injection or prior oral contraception. J Adolesc Health, 1995;16:379-384.
245. Goldberg AB, Cardenas LH, Hubbard AE, Darney PD. Post-abortion depot medroxyprogesterone acetate continuation rates: a randomized trial of cyclic estradiol. Contraception 2002; 66:215-220.
246. Smith RD, Cromer BA, Hayes JR. Medroxyprogesterone acetate (Depo-Provera) use in adolescents: uterine bleeding and blood pressure patterns, patient satisfaction, and continuation rates. Adolesc Pediatr Gynecol 19958:24-28.
247. Sangi-Haghpeykar H, Poindexter AN 3rd, Bateman L, Ditmore JR. Experiences of injectable contraceptive users in an urban setting. Obstet Gynecol 1996;88:227-233.
248. Westhoff C, Wieland D, Tiezzi L. Depression in users of depo-medroxyprogesterone acetate. Contraception 1995;51:351-354.
249. Westhoff C, Truman C, Kalmuss D, et al. Depressive symptoms and Depo-Provera. Contraception 1998;57:237-240.
250. Gupta N, O'Brien R, Jacobsen LJ, et al. Mood changes in adolescents using depot-medroxyprogesterone acetate for contraception: a prospective study. J Pediatr Adolesc Gynecol 2001; 14:71-76.
251. Moore LL, Valuck R, McDougall C, Fink W. A comparative study of one-year weight gain among users of medroxyprogesterone acetate, levonorgestrel implants, and oral contraceptives. Contraception 1995;52:215-219.
252. Mainwaring R, Hales HA, Stevenson K, et al. Metabolic parameters, bleeding, and weight changes in U.S. women using progestin only contraceptives. Contraception 1995;51:149-153.
253. Taneepanichskul S, Reinprayoon D, Khaosaad P. Comparative study of weight change between long-term DMPA and IUD acceptors. Contraception 1998;58:149-151.
254. Bahamondes L, Del Castillo S, Tabares G, et al. Comparison of weight increase in users of depot medroxyprogesterone acetate and copper IUD up to 5 years. Contraception 2001;64:223-225.
255. Pelkman CL, Chow M, Heinbach RA, Rolls BJ. Short-term effects of a progestational contraceptive drug on food intake, resting energy expenditure, and body weight in young women. Am J Clin Nutr 2001;73:19-26.
256. Espey E, Steinhart J, Ogburn T, Qualls C. Depo-provera associated with weight gain in Navajo women. Contraception 2000;62:55-58.
257. Cromer BA, Lazebnik R, Rome E, et al. Double-blinded randomized controlled trial of estrogen supplementation in adolescent girls who receive depot medroxyprogesterone acetate for contraception. Am J Obstet Gynecol 2005;192(1):42-47.
258. WHO Collaborative Study of Neoplasia and Steroid Contraceptives. Breast cancer and depot-medroxyprogesterone acetate: a multinational study. Lancet 1991;338:833-838.
259. The New Zealand Contraception and Health Study Group. History of long-term use of depot-medroxyprogesterone acetate in patients with cervical dysplasia; case-control analysis nested in a cohort study. Contraception 1994;50:443-449.
260. Thomas DB, Ray RM. Depot-medroxyprogesterone acetate (DMPA) and risk of invasive adenocarcinomas and adenosquamous carcinomas of the uterine cervix. WHO Collaborative Study of Neoplasia and Steroid Contraceptives. Contraception 1995;52: 307-312.
261. WHO Collaborative Study of Neoplasia and Steroid Contraception. Depot-medroxyprogesterone acetate (DMPA) and risk of invasive squamous cell cervical cancer. Contraception 1992;45:299-312.
262. Thomas DB, Ye Z, Ray RM. Cervical carcinoma in situ and use of depot-medroxyprogesterone acetate (DMPA). WHO Collaborative Study of Neoplasia and Steroid Contraceptives. Contraception 1995;51:25-31.
263. Garza-Flores J, De la Cruz DL, Valles de Bourges V, et al. Long-term effects of depot-medroxyprogesterone acetate on lipoprotein metabolism. Contraception 1991;44:61-71.
264. Enk L, Landgren BM, Lindberg UB, et al. A prospective, one-year study on the effects of two long acting injectable contraceptives (depot-medroxyprogesterone acetate and norethisterone enanthate) on serum and lipoprotein lipids. Horm Metab Res 1992;24:85-89.
265. Kongsayreepong R, Chutivongse S, George P, et al. A multicentre comparative study of serum lipids and apolipoproteins in long-term users of DMPA and a control group of IUD users. Contraception 1993;47:177-191.
266. Fahmy K, Khairy M, Allam G, et al. Effect of depo-medroxyprogesterone acetate on coagulation factors and serum lipids in Egyptian women. Contraception 1991;44:431-444.
267. Fahmy K, Abdel-Razik M, Shaaraway M, et al. Effect of long-acting progestagen-only injectable contraceptives on carbohydrate metabolism and its hormonal profile. Contraception 1991;44: 419-430.
268. Cundy T, Ames R, Horne A, et al. A randomized controlled trial of estrogen replacement therapy in long-term users of depot medroxyprogesterone acetate. J Clin Endocrinol Metab 2003;88:78-81.
269. Cundy T, Evans M, Roberts H, et al. Bone density in women receiving depot medroxyprogesterone acetate for contraception. BMJ 1991;303:13-16.
270. Cundy T, Cornish J, Roberts H, et al. Spinal bone density in women using depot medroxyprogesterone contraception. Obstet Gynecol 1998;92:569-573.
271. Scholes D, Lacroix AZ, Ott SM, et al. Bone mineral density in women using depot medroxyprogesterone acetate for contraception. Obstet Gynecol 1999;93:233-238.
272. Cundy T, Cornish J, Evans MC, et al. Recovery of bone density in women who stop using medroxyprogesterone acetate. BMJ 1994;308:247-248.
273. Scholes D, LaCroix AZ, Ichikawa LE, et al. Injectable hormone contraception and bone density: results from a prospective study. Epidemiology 2002;13:581-587.

274. Orr-Walker BJ, Evans MC, Ames RW, et al. The effect of past use of the injectable contraceptive depot medroxyprogesterone acetate on bone mineral density in normal post-menopausal women. Clin Endocrinol 1998;49:615-618.
275. Petitti DB, Piaggio G, Mehta S, et al. Steroid hormone contraception and bone mineral density: a cross-sectional study in an international population. Obstet Gynecol 2000;95:736-744.
276. Theintz G, Buchs B, Rizzoli R, et al. Longitudinal monitoring of bone mass accumulation in healthy adolescents: evidence for a marked reduction after 16 years of age at the levels of lumbar spine and femoral neck in female subjects. J Clin Endocrinol Metab 1992;75:1060-1065.
277. Matkovic V, Jelic T, Wardlaw GM, et al. Timing of peak bone mass in caucasian females and its implication for the prevention of osteoporosis: inference from a cross-sectional model. J Clin Invest 1994;93:799-808.
278. Cromer BA, Blair JM, Mahan JD, et al. A prospective comparison of bone density in adolescent girls receiving depot medroxyprogesterone acetate (Depo-Provera), levonorgestrel (Norplant), or oral contraceptives. J Pediatr 1996;129:671-676.
279. Garza-Flores J, Cardenas S, Rodriguez V, et al. Return to ovulation following the use of long-acting injectable contraceptives: a comparative study. Contraception 1985;31:361-366.
280. Pardthaisong T. Return of fertility after use of the injectable contraceptive Depo Provera: up-dated analysis. J Biosoc Sci 1984; 16:23-34.
281. Schwallie P, Assenzo J. The effect of depo-medroxyprogesterone acetate on pituitary and ovarian function, and the return of fertility following its discontinuation: a review. Contraception 1974; 10:181-202.
282. Darney P. Bleeding patterns shift to amenorrhea with continued use of subcutaneous or intramuscular depot medroxyprogesterone acetate. Obstet Gynecol 2005;105(4):54S.
283. Newton JR, d'Arcangues C, Hall PE. A review of "once-a-month" combined injectable contraceptives. J Obstet Gynaecol 1994; 14(Suppl 1):S1-S34.
284. World Health Organization Task Force on Long-Acting Systemic Agents for Fertility Regulation. A multicentered phase III comparative study of two hormonal contraceptive preparations given once-a-month by intramuscular injection. Contraception 1989;40:531-551.
285. Cuong DT, Huong M. Comparative phase III clinical trial of two injectable contraceptive preparations, depot-medroxyprogesterone acetate and Cyclofem in Vietnamese women. Contraception 1996;54:169-179.
286. Hall P, Bahamondes L, Diaz J, Petta C. Introductory study of the once-a-month, injectable contraceptive Cyclofem in Brazil, Chile, Columbia, and Peru. Contraception 1997;56:353-359.
287. Garza-Flores J, Moraks del Olmo A, Fuziwara JL, et al. Introduction of Cyclofem once-a-month injectable contraceptive in Mexico. Contraception 1998;58:7-12.
288. Kaunitz AM, Garceau RJ, Cromie MA. Comparative safety, efficacy, and cycle control of Lunelle monthly contraceptive injection (medroxyprogesterone acetate and estradiol cypionate injectable suspension) and Ortho-Novum 7/7/7 oral contraceptive (Norethindrone/ethinyl estradiol triphasic). Contraception 1999;60: 179-187.
289. Garceau RJ, Wajszczuk CJ, Kaunitz AM; Lunelle Study Group. Bleeding patterns of women using Lunelle monthly contraceptive injections (medroxyprogesterone aceate and estradiol cypionate injectable suspension) compared with those of women using Ortho-Novum 7/7/7 (norethindrone/ethinyl estradiol triphasic) or other oral contraceptives. Contraception 2000;62:289-295.
290. Bahamondes L, Lavin P, Ojeda G, et al. Return of fertility after discontinuation of the once-a-month injectable contraceptive Cyclofem. Contraception 1997;55:307-310.
291. Bahamondes L, Marchi NM, Nakagava HM, et al. Self-administration with UniJect of the once-a-month injectable contraceptive Cyclofem. Contraception 1997;56:301-304.
292. Piya-Anant M, Koetsawang S, Patrasupapong N, et al. Effectiveness of Cyclofem in the treatment of depot medroxyprogesterone acetate induced amenorrhea. Contraception 1998;57:23-28.
293. von Kesseru E, Aydinlik S, Etchepareborda JJ. Multicentered, phase III clinical trial of norethisteone enanthate 50 mg plus estradiol valerate 5 mg as a monthly injectable contraceptive; final three-year report. Contraception 1994;50:329-337.
294. Sang GW, Shao QX, Ge RS, et al. A multicentred phase III comparative clinical trial of Mesigyna, Cyclofem, and injectable no. 1 given monthly by intramuscular injection to Chinese women. I. Contraceptive efficacy and side effects. Contraception 1995;51:167-183.
295. Martínez GH, Castañeda A, Correa JE. Vaginal bleeding patterns in users of Perlutal, a once-a-month injectable contraceptive consisting of 10 mg estradiol enanthate combined with 150 mg dihydroxyprogesterone acetophenide. A trial of 5462 woman-months. Contraception 1998;58:21-27.
296. Coutinho EM, Spinola P, Barbosa I, et al. Multicenter, double-blind, comparative clinical study on the efficacy and acceptability of a monthly injectable contraceptive combination of 150 mg dihydroxyprogesterone acetophenide and 10 mg estradiol enanthate compared to a monthly injectable contraceptive combination of 90 mg dihydroxyprogesterone acetophenide and 6 mg estradiol enanthate. Contraception 1997;55:175-181.
297. Trussell J, Leveque JA, Koenig JD, et al. The economic value of contraception: a comparison of 15 methods. Am J Public Health 1995;85:494-503.
298. Diaz S, Pavez M, Cardenas H, Croxatto HB. Recovery of fertility and outcome of planned pregnancies after the removal of Norplant subdermal implants or Copper-T IUDs. Contraception 1987;35:569-579.
299. Sivin I, Mishell DR Jr, Darney P, et al. Levonorgestrel capsule implants in the United States: a 5-year study. Obstet Gynecol 1998;92:337-344.
300. Kuiper H, Miller S, Martinez E, et al. Urban adolescent females' views on the implant and contraceptive decision-making: a double paradox. Fam Plann Perspect 1997;29(4):167-172.
301. Croxatto HB, Urbancsek J, Massai R, et al. A multicentre efficacy and safety study of the single contraceptive implant Implanon. Implanon Study Group. Hum Reprod 1999;14:976-981.
302. Meirik O, Farley TM, Sivin I. Safety and efficacy of levonorgestrel implant, intrauterine device, and sterilization. Am J Obstet Gynecol 2001;97:539-547.
303. Diaz S, Herreros C, Juez G, et al. Fertility regulation in nursing women: influence of Norplant levonorgestrel implants upon lactation and infant growth. Contraception 1985;32:53-74.
304. Reinprayoon D, Taneepanichskul S, Bunyavejchevin S, et al. Effects of the etonogestrel-releasing contraceptive implant (Implanon) on parameters of breastfeeding compared to those of an intrauterine device. Contraception 2000;62:239-246.
305. Shaaban MM, Salem HT, Abdullah KA. Influence of levonorgestrel contraceptive implants, Norplant, initiated early postpartum, upon lactation and infant growth. Contraception 1985;32: 623-635.
306. Brache V, Faundes A, Johansson E, Alvarez F. Anovulation, inadequate luteal phase, and poor sperm penetration in cervical mucus during prolonged use of Norplant implants. Contraception 1985. 31:261-273.
307. Makarainen L, van Beek A, Tuomivaara L, et al. Ovarian function during the use of a single contraceptive implant: Implanon compared with Norplant. Fertil Steril 1998;69:714-721.
308. Croxatto HB, Mäkäräinen L. The pharmacodynamics and efficacy of Implanon. Contraception 1998;58:91S-97S.
309. Sivin I, Mishell DR Jr, Diaz S, et al. Prolonged effectiveness of Norplant capsule implants: a 7-year study. Contraception 2000;61(3):187-194.
310. Dunson TR, Amatya RN, Krueger SL. Complications and risk factors associated with the removal of Norplant implants. Obstet Gynecol 1995;85:543-548.
311. Zieman M, Klaisle C, Walker D, et al. Fingers versus instruments for removing levonorgestrel contraceptive implants (Norplant). J Gynecol Tech 1997;3: 213-217.
312. Meckstroth KR, Darney PD. Implant contraception. Semin Reprod Med 2001;19(4):339-354.
313. Meirik O, d'Arcangues C, for the WHO Consultation on Implantable Contraceptives for Women. Implantable contraceptives for women. Hum Reprod Update 2003;9:49-59.
314. Mascarenhas L, van Beek A, Bennink HC, Newton J. Twenty-four month comparison of apolipoproteins A-1, A-II and B in contraceptive implant users (Norplant and Implanon) in Birmingham, United Kingdom. Contraception 1998;58:215-219.

315. Biswas A, Viegas OA, Bennink HJ, et al. Effect of Implanon use on selected parameters of thyroid and adrenal function. Contraception 2000;62:247-251.
316. Biswas A, Viegas OA, Coeling Bennink HJ, et al. Implanon contraceptive implants: effects on carbohydrate metabolism. Contraception 2001;63:137-141.
317. Biswas A, Viegas OA, Roy AC. Effect of Implanon and Norplant subdermal contraceptive implants on serum lipids—a randomized comparative study. Contraception 2003;68:189-193.
318. Groxatto HB, Urbanesek J, Massai R, et al. A multicentren efficacy and safety study of the single contraceptive implant Implanon. Hum Repro 1999;14:976-981.
319. Bromham DR, Davey A, Gaffikin L, Ajello CA. Materials, methods and results of the Norplant training program. Br J Fam Plann 1995;10:256-262.
320. Mascarenhas L. Insertion and removal of Implanon: practical considerations. Eur J Contracept Reprod Health Care 2000;5(Suppl 2):29-34.
321. Smith A, Reuter S. An assessment of the use of Implanon in three community services. J Fam Plann Reprod Health Care 2002;28: 193-196.
322. Darney PD, Taylor RN, Klaisle C, et al. Serum concentrations of estradiol, progesterone, and levonorgestrel are not determinants of endometrial histology or abnormal bleeding in long-term Norplant implant users. Contraception 1996;53:97-100.
323. Alvarez-Sanchez F, Brache V, Thevenin F, et al. Hormonal treatment for bleeding irregularities in Norplant implant users. Am J Obstet Gynecol 1996;174:919-922.
324. Zheng SR, Zheng HM, Qian SZ, et al. A randomized multicenter study comparing the efficacy and bleeding pattern of a single-rod (Implanon) and a six-capsule (Norplant) hormonal contraceptive implant. Contraception 1999;60:1-8.
325. Darney PD, Atkinson E, Tanner S, et al. Acceptance and perceptions of Norplant among users in San Francisco, USA. Stud Fam Plann 1990;21:152-160.
326. Darney PD, Callegari LS, Swift A, et al. Condom practices of urban teens using Norplant contraceptive implants, oral contraceptives, and condoms for contraception. Am J Obstet Gynecol 1999;180: 929-937.
327. Harrison-Woolrych M, Hill R. Unintended pregnancies with the etonogestrel implant (Implanon): a case series from postmarketing experience in Australia. Contraception 2005;71(4):306-308.
328. Luukkainen T, Allonen H, Haukkamaa M, et al. Five years' experience with levonorgestrel-releasing IUDs. Contraception 1986; 33:139-148.
329. Sivin I, Stern J, Coutinho E, et al. Prolonged intrauterine contraception: a seven-year randomized study of the levonorgestrel 20 mcg/ day (LNg 20) and the copper T380 Ag IUDs. Contraception 1991;44:473-480.
330. Toivonen J, Luukkainen T, Allonen H. Protective effect of intrauterine release of levonorgestrel on pelvic infection: three years' comparative experience of levonorgestrel and copper-releasing intrauterine devices. Obstet Gynecol 1991;77:261-264.
331. Xiao BL, Zhou LY, Zhang XL, et al. Pharmacokinetic and pharmacodynamic studies of levonorgestrel-releasing intrauterine device. Contraception 1990;41:353-362.
332. Crosignani PG, Vercellini P, Mosconi P, et al. Levonorgestrel-releasing intrauterine device versus hysteroscopic endometrial resection in the treatment of dysfunctional uterine bleeding. Obstet Gynecol 1997;90:257-263.
333. Gardner FJE. Endometrial protection from tamoxifen-stimulated changes by a levonorgestrel-releasing intrauterine system: a randomised controlled trial. Lancet 2000;356:1711-1717.
334. Vercellini P, Aimi G, Panazza S, et al. A levonorgestrel-releasing intrauterine system for the treatment of dysmenorrhea associated with endometriosis: a pilot study. Fertil Steril 1999;72:505-508.
335. Varila E, Wahlstrom T, Rauramo I. A 5-year follow-up study on the use of a levonorgestrel intrauterine system in women receiving hormone replacement therapy. Fertil Steril 2001;76:969-973.
336. Raudaskoski T, Tapanainen J, Tomas E, et al. Intrauterine 10 microg and 20 microg levonorgestrel systems in postmenopausal women receiving oral oestrogen replacement therapy: clinical, endometrial and metabolic responses. BJOG 2002;109:136-144.
337. Wollter-Svensson LO, Stadberg E, Andersson K, et al. Intrauterine administration of levonorgestrel 5 and 10 μg/24 hours in perimenopausal hormone replacement therapy. A randomized clinical study during one year. Acta Obstet Gynecol Scand 1997;76: 449-454.
338. Critchley HO, Wang H, Jones RL, et al. Morphological and functional features of endometrial decidualization following long-term intrauterine levonorgestrel delivery. Hum Reprod 1998;13: 1218-1224.
339. Barbosa I, Olsson SE, Odlind V, et al. Ovarian function after seven years' use of levonorgestrel IUD. Adv Contraception 1995;11: 85-95.
340. Andersson J, Rybo G. Levonorgestrel-releasing intrauterine device in the treatment of menorrhagia. Br J Obstet Gynaecol 1990;97: 690-694.
341. Baldszti E, Wimmer-Puchinger B, Loschke K. Acceptability of the long-term contraceptive levonorgestrel-releasing intrauterine system (Mirena): a 3-year follow-up study. Contraception 2003;67: 87-91.
342. Hidalgo M, Bahamondes L, Perrotti M, et al. Bleeding patterns and clinical performance of the levonorgestrel-releasing intrauterine system (Mirena) up to two years. Contraception 2002;65:129-132.
343. Ronnerdag M, Odlind V. Health effects of long-term use of the intrauterine levonorgestrel-releasing system. A follow-up study over 12 years of continuous use. Acta Obstet Gynecol Scand 1999;78:716-721.
344. United Nations Development Programme/United Nations Population Fund/World Health Organization/World Bank, Special Programme of Research, and Development and Research Training in Human Reproduction. Long-term reversible contraception. Twelve years of experience with the TCu380A and TCu220C. Contraception 1997;56:341-352.
345. Chi, I.-c., The TCu-380A (AG), MLCu375, and Nova-T IUDs and the IUD daily releasing 20 μg levonorgestrel—four pillars of IUD contraception for the nineties and beyond? Contraception 1993;47: 325-347.
346. Sivin I, Stern J. Health during prolonged use of levonorgestrel 20 μg/d and the copper TCu 380 Ag intrauterine contraceptive devices: a multicenter study. International Committee for Contraception Research. Fertil Steril 1994;61:70-77.
347. Sivin I, Stern J, Diaz J, et al. Two years of intrauterine contraception with levonorgestrel and with copper: a randomized comparison of the TCu 380Ag and levonorgestrel 20 mcg/day devices. Contraception 1987;35:245-255.
348. Sivin I, Stern J, Diaz S, et al. Rates and outcomes of planned pregnancy after use of Norplant capsules, Norplant II rods, or levonorgestrel-releasing or copper TCu 380Ag intrauterine contraceptive devices. Am J Obstet Gynecol 1992;166:1208-1213.
349. WHO Special Programme of Research, Development and Research Training in Human Reproduction, and Task Force on the Safety and Efficacy of Fertility Regulating Methods. The TCu 380A, TCu 220C, Multiload 250, and Nova T IUDs at 3, 5, and 7 years of use. Contraception 1990;42:141-158.
350. Andersson K, Odlind V, Rybo G. Levonorgestrel-releasing and copper-releasing (Nova T) IUDs during five years of use: a randomized comparative trial. Contraception 1994;49(1):56-72.
351. Backman T, Rauramo I, Huhtala S, Koskenvuo M. Pregnancy during the use of levonorgestrel intrauterine system. Am J Obstet Gynecol 2004;190:50-54.
352. Sivin I. Dose- and age-dependent ectopic pregnancy risks with intrauterine contraception. Obstet Gynecol 1991;78:291-298.
353. Franks AL, Beral V, Cates W Jr, Hogue CJ. Contraception and ectopic pregnancy risk. Am J Obstet Gynecol 1990;163(4 Pt 1): 1120-123.
354. Wilson JC. A prospective New Zealand study of fertility after removal of copper intrauterine devices for conception and because of complications: a four-year study. Am J Obstet Gynecol 1989;160:391-396.
355. Skjeldestad FE, Bratt H. Fertility after complicated and non-complicated use of IUDs. A controlled prospective study. Adv Contracept 1988;4:179.
356. Cameron IT, Haining R, Lumsden MA, et al. The effects of mefenamic acid and norethisterone on measured menstrual blood loss. Obstet Gynecol 1990;76:85-88.
357. Zhao G, Li M, Zhu P, et al. A preliminary morphometric study on the endometrium from patients treated with indomethacin-

releasing copper intrauterine device. Hum Reprod 1997;12: 1563-1566.

358. Milsom I, Andersson K, Jonasson K, et al. The influence of the Gyne-T 380S IUD on menstrual blood loss and iron status. Contraception 1995;52:175-179.
359. Task Force for Epidemiological Research on Reproductive Health, United Nations Development Programme/United Nations Population Fund/World Health Organization/World Bank Special Programme of Research, and Develpment and Research Training in Human Reproduction. Effects of contraceptives on hemoglobin and ferritin. Contraception 1998;58:261-273.
360. Hassan EO, El-Husseini M, El-Nahal N. The effect of 1-year use of the CuT 380A and oral contraceptive pills on hemoglobin and ferritin levels. Contraception 1999;60:101-105.
361. Backman T, Huhtala S, Blom T, et al. Length of use and symptoms associated with premature removal of the levonorgestrel intrauterine system: a nation-wide study of 17,360 users. Br J Obstet Gynaecol 2000;107:335-339.
362. Sivin I, Schmidt F. Effectiveness of IUDs: a review. Contraception 1987;36:55-84.
363. Tang GW, Lo SS. Levonorgestrel intrauterine device in the treatment of menorrhagia in Chinese women: efficacy versus acceptability. Contraception 1995;51:231-235.
364. Crosignani PG, Vercellini P, Apolone G, et al. Endometrial resection versus vaginal hysterectomy for menorrhagia: long-term clinical and quality-of-life outcomes. Am J Obstet Gynecol 1997;177: 95-101.
365. Romer T. Prospective comparison study of levonorgestrel IUD versus Roller-Ball endometrial ablation in the management of refractory recurrent hypermenorrhea. Eur J Obstet Gynecol Reprod Biol 2000;90:27-29.
366. Istre O, Trolle B. Treatment of menorrhagia with the levonorgestrel intrauterine system versus endometrial resection. Fertil Steril 2001;76:304-309.
367. Fong YF, Singh K. Effect of the levonorgestrel-releasing intrauterine system on uterine myomas in a renal transplant patient. Contraception 1999;60:51-53.
368. Lockhat FB, Emembolu JO, Konje JC. The evaluation of the effectiveness of an intrauterine-administered progestogen (levonorgestrel) in the symptomatic treatment of endometriosis and in the staging of the disease. Hum Reprod 2004;19:179-184.
369. Mishell DR Jr, Bell JH, Good RG, Moyer DL. The intrauterine device: a bacteriologic study of the endometrial cavity. Am J Obstet Gynecol 1966;96:119-126.
370. Farley TM, Rosenberg MJ, Rowe PJ, et al. Intrauterine devices and pelvic inflammatory disease: an international perspective. Lancet 1992;339:785-788.
371. Lee NC, Rubin GL, Ory HW, Burkman RT. Type of intrauterine device and the risk of pelvic inflammatory disease. Obstet Gynecol 1983;62:1-6.
372. Lee NC, Rubin GL, Borucki R. The intrauterine device and pelvic inflammatory disease revisited: new results from the Womens' Health Study. Obstet Gynecol 1988;72:1-6.
373. Skouby SO, Molsted-Pedersen L, Kosonen A. Consequences of intrauterine contraception in diabetic women. Fertil Steril 1984; 42:568-572.
374. Kimmerle R, Weiss R, Berger M, Kurz KH. Effectiveness, safety, and acceptability of a copper intrauterine deivce (Cu Safe 300) in type I diabetic women. Diabetes Care 1993;16:1227-1230.
375. Buchan H, Villard-Mackintosh L, Vessey M, et al. Epidemiology of pelvic inflammatory disease in parous women with special reference to intrauterine device use. Br J Obstet Gynaecol 1990;97: 780-788.
376. Mehanna MT, Rizk MA, Ramadan M, Schachter J. Chlamydial serologic characteristics among intrauterine contraceptive device users: does copper inhibit chlamydial infection in the female genital tract? Am J Obstet Gynecol 1994;171:691-693.
377. Kleinman D, Insler V, Sarov I. Inhibition of *Chlamydia trachomatis* growth in endometrial cells by copper: possible relevance for the use of copper IUDs. Contraception 1989;39:665-676.
378. Mohllajee A, Curtis K, Peterson H. Does insertion and use of an intrauterine device increase the risk of pelvic inflammatory disease among women with sexually transmitted infection? A systematic review. Contraception 2006;73:145-153.
379. Lee NC, Rubin GL, Grimes DA. Measures of sexual behavior and the risk of pelvic inflammatory disease. Obstet Gynecol 1991;77: 425-430.

CHAPTER 18

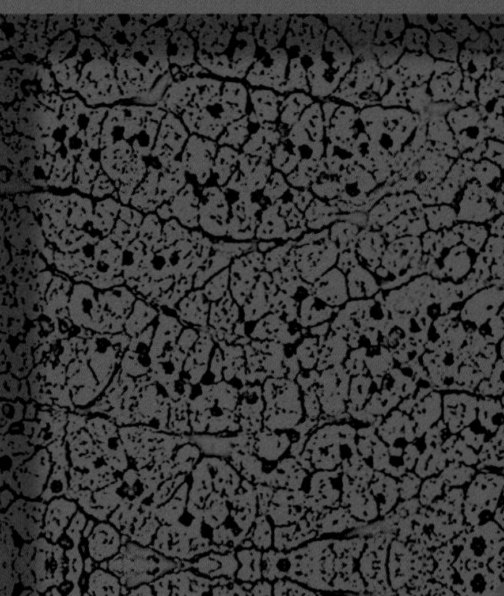

TESTICULAR DISORDERS

Shalender Bhasin

Although the testes are not essential for the survival of the individual, these organs are vital for survival of the species because of their crucial role in mammalian reproduction through production of sperm and sex-steroid hormones. Germ cell development in the testis is confined within the seminiferous tubules, and testosterone production by Leydig cells takes place in the interstitial compartment. Testicular size, contributed mostly by the germ cell compartment, varies considerably among mammals even after adjusting for body size, and it is unrelated to testicular location (abdominal or scrotal), body form, or locomotion.[1] In general, mammals with monogamous breeding systems have smaller testes than those with polygamous breeding, where several males may mate with a female during the same estrous cycle.[1] The larger testicular size in polygamous mammals has been ascribed to high mating frequency, the need for high sperm production rates, and competition among sperm of different males for fertilization of the ovum.[1]

PHYSIOLOGIC REGULATION OF TESTICULAR FUNCTION: SEX-STEROID PRODUCTION AND ACTION

Mammalian Sex-Steroid Production, Transport, and Metabolism

Testosterone, a 19-carbon steroid secreted by the testis, is the predominant androgen in most mammalian species. However, substantial amounts of Δ^4-androstenedione are secreted in the females of several mammalian species, including moles and spotted hyenas *(Crocuta crocuta)*.[2,3] The female spotted hyena has higher androstenedione levels, is heavier and more aggressive than the male hyena, and possesses a large, erectile pseudopenis.[2-5] In the pouch young of the tammar wallaby, 5-α-androstane-3α,17β diol is the principal androgen secreted by the testis during the period of prostate and phallus development.[6,7] In this species, during this period of differentiation, dihydrotestosterone (DHT) is formed by an alternate pathway from 5-α-androstane-3α,17β diol (5-androstanediol), which is derived from conversion of 17α hydroxyprogesterone to 5-α reduced progestogens, which are then converted to 5-androstanediol.

The importance of testosterone in regulating secondary sex characteristics, muscle growth, and sexual and nonsexual behavior in male mammals has long been recognized. In pioneering transplantation experiments, Adolph Berthold observed that chickens that were castrated during development became docile capons rather than roosters.[8] When testes from other chickens were implanted into the abdominal cavities of these capons, the animals developed into roosters, became aggressive, and demonstrated normal mating behavior. These early testicular transplantation experiments demonstrated that testes affect male development and behavior by secreting a potent hormone directly into the bloodstream.

Androgens directly or indirectly affect almost all body systems during fetal and pubertal development and in adult life. The sexual differentiation of the mammalian fetus requires not only the genetic information carried on the sex chromosomes but also the hormonal secretions of the fetal testis, namely testosterone and müllerian inhibiting hormone. Testosterone regulates the differentiation of the wolffian ducts into epididymis, vas deferens, and in some species seminal vesicles.[9] In humans, the conversion of testosterone to 5-α-dihydrotestosterone is required for the differentiation of urogenital tubercle and urogenital sinus into phallus, male urethra, and prostate.[10] In addition, increasing testosterone levels during puberty promote somatic growth and virilization of boys. Testosterone plays a critical role in mammalian reproduction; it is essential for maintaining sexual function, germ cell development, and accessory sex organs. In the adult animal, testosterone has additional effects on muscle, fat, bone, hematopoeisis, and coagulation;

lipid, protein, and carbohydrate metabolism; and psychosexual and cognitive behavior.

Androgen Production in the Human Male

In males of most mammalian species, 95% of circulating testosterone is derived from testicular secretion. In human males, 3 to 10 mg of testosterone is secreted daily by the testis; direct secretion of testosterone by the adrenal and the peripheral conversion of androstenedione secreted by the adrenal collectively account for another 500 μg of testosterone daily. In contrast, only a small amount of dihydrotestosterone (DHT, ~70 μg daily) is secreted directly by the human testis; most of the circulating DHT is derived from peripheral conversion of testosterone.

Testosterone is produced in the testis by a heterogeneous group of cells that includes the adult Leydig cells, Leydig cell precursors, and immature Leydig cells. Studies in hypogonadotropic *(hpg)* mice suggest that fetal development of both Sertoli and Leydig cells is independent of gonadotropins; however, normal differentiation and proliferation of the adult Leydig cell population requires the presence of gonadotropins. The number of Sertoli cells after birth is regulated by gonadotropins. 46,XY-Male humans with inactivating mutations of the luteinizing hormone (LH) receptor are characterized by Leydig cell agenesis or hypoplasia pointing to the important role of LH in regulation of Leydig cell development in humans. Leydig cells arise from poorly characterized mesenchymal precursor cells under the influence of LH, insulin-like growth factor I (IGF-I), transforming growth factor α (TGF-α), TGF-β, interleukin-1 (IL-1), and basic fibroblast growth factor. Leydig cells exist in two distinct generations in higher mammals, fetal and adult, that are separated by a prepubertal period during which the testis is devoid of Leydig cells.

Testosterone secretion by Leydig cells is under the control of LH, a pituitary glycoprotein hormone. LH binds to specific G-protein–coupled receptors on the Leydig cells and activates the cyclic adenosine monophosphate (cAMP) pathway.[11,12] Although LH also activates the phospholipase C pathway, it is unclear if this pathway is essential for LH-mediated stimulation of testosterone production. The major target of LH action is the side chain cleavage enzyme, CYP11A1. Prolactin receptor is not expressed on the Leydig cells in the human testis, and prolactin has not been shown to regulate testosterone production in men.[13]

Leydig cell production of testosterone is modulated by a number of paracrine growth factors, regulatory peptides, and cytokines within the seminiferous tubule and the interstitium of the testis, including IGF-I, IGF binding proteins, inhibins, activins, TGF-α, epidermal growth factor, IL-1, tumor necrosis factor α (TNF-α), basic fibroblast growth factor, gonadotropin releasing hormone (GnRH), and vasopressin.[14]

Cholesterol needed for testosterone biosynthesis can be imported into the cell from circulating cholesterol, or it can be synthesized within the cell either *de novo* from acetate or from cholesterol esters.[15] The rate-limiting step in testosterone biosynthesis is the delivery of cholesterol to the inner mitochondrial membrane, which is the site of the cholesterol side chain cleavage complex that converts cholesterol to pregnenolone (Fig. 18–1). A steroidogenesis acute regulatory protein (STAR) makes cholesterol available to the cholesterol side chain complex and regulates the rate of testosterone biosynthesis. Peripheral benzodiazepine receptor, a mitochondrial cholesterol-binding protein known to be involved in mediating cholesterol transport, is present in high concentration in the outer mitochondrial membrane; it has also been proposed as an acute regulator of Leydig cell steroidogenesis. In addition, another group of poorly characterized mitochondrial proteins has been implicated in control of steroidogenesis in Leydig cells.

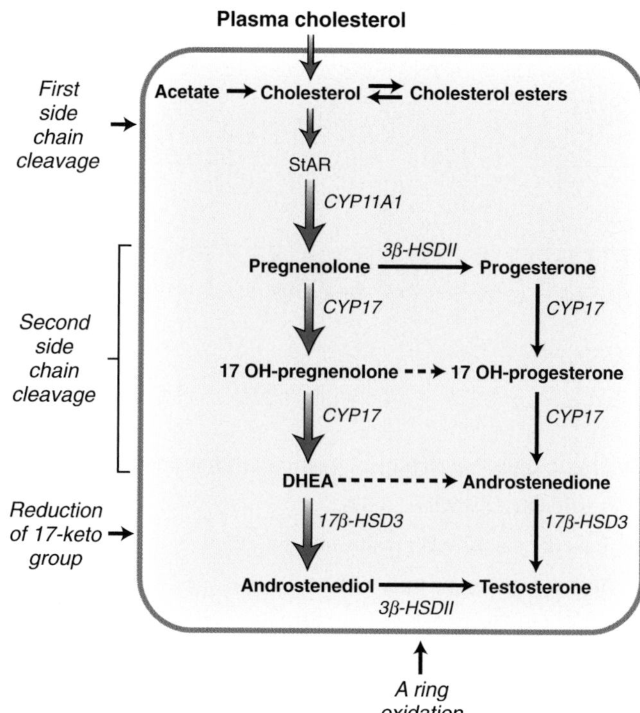

Figure 18–1 ▪ Testosterone biosynthetic pathways in the human testis. There are two pathways by which pregnenolone derived from cholesterol can be converted to testosterone. The Δ^5 pathway that goes through pregnenolone, 17-hydroxypregnenolone, DHEA, and androstenediol involves side chain cleavage and reduction of the 17-keto group before A-ring oxidation. The Δ^4 pathway involves A-ring oxidation of pregnenolone before side chain cleavage and the reduction of the 17-keto group. In the human testis, the Δ^5 pathway predominates. The delivery of cholesterol to the inner mitochondrial membrane for side chain cleavage, the rate-limiting step in testosterone biosynthesis, is under the control of luteinizing hormone (LH). As shown in the figure, cholesterol for testosterone biosynthesis can be synthesized de novo within the cell, or it can be derived from circulating cholesterol or from cholesterol esters. StAR, steroidogenic acute regulatory protein; CYP11A1, the side chain cleavage enzyme; 3βHSDII, 3-β hydroxysteroid dehydrogenase; CYP17, 17-α hydroxylase; 17β HSD3, 17-β hydroxysteroid dehydrogenase. (Reproduced from Griffin JE, Wilson JD. Disorders of the testis and the male reproductive tract. In Larsen PR, Kronenberg HM, Melmed S, Polonsky KS, eds.Williams Textbook of Endocrinology, 10th ed. Philadelphia: Saunders, 2003:709-763.)

The conversion of cholesterol into testosterone can occur through two biosynthetic pathways:[16] the Δ-5 pathway and the Δ-4 pathway. In the human testis, the Δ-5 pathway predominates and involves side chain cleavage of pregnenolone, reduction of the 17-keto group, and A-ring oxidation. In the Δ-4 pathway, A-ring oxidation precedes side chain cleavage and reduction of the 17-keto group.

Testosterone is the primary circulating androgen in the male human. The secretion of testosterone is regulated by feed-forward and feedback mechanisms that operate within the hypothalamic-pituitary-gonadal axis. Hypothalamic release of GnRH stimulates the anterior pituitary to release LH, which in turn stimulates the Leydig cells in the testes to synthesize testosterone. Testosterone secretion has pulsatile, diurnal, and circannual rhythms; the highest concentrations are observed in the hours after waking, and lower concentrations are observed in the afternoon and evening. Testosterone concentrations can vary considerably in a given patient due to the diurnal rhythm and the pulsatile nature of testosterone secretion.

Dehydroepiandrosterone (DHEA) and Δ^4-androstenedione are weak androgens[17]; Δ^4-androstenedione can be converted to estrogen in a number of extragonadal tissues. No biologic role has been ascribed to date to pregnenolone, 17-hydroxypregnenolone, and 17-hydroxyprogesterone.

Androgen Transport in the Body

Most of circulating testosterone is bound to two plasma proteins, the sex hormone binding globulin (SHBG) and albumin; only 0.5% to 3.0% of testosterone is unbound. Circulating testosterone is bound tightly with high affinity to SHBG and is loosely bound to albumin, with only 0.5% to 3% in the unbound form (Fig. 18–2). The binding affinity of testosterone and DHT to SHBG is at least four orders of magnitude higher than the binding affinity to albumin.[18] In men, testosterone is primarily bound to albumin (50% to 68%), and a smaller fraction is bound to SHBG (30% to 45%). In women, about 70% of circulating testosterone is bound to SHBG and 25% is bound to albumin. *Bioavailable testosterone* refers to free or unbound testosterone plus the albumin-bound fraction.

The free hormone hypothesis assumes that only the unbound fraction is biologically active[19] and that unbound testosterone, being lipophilic, enters the cell through free diffusion; however, a substantial body of evidence suggests that albumin-bound hormone might dissociate in the capillaries to varying extents and become bioavailable.[20] Sakiyama and colleagues[20] demonstrated that albumin- and SHBG-bound androgens represent the major circulating pool of bioavailable hormone for testis and prostate. Furthermore, some have argued that the SHBG–sex steroid complex may be available for influx through the blood-testis barrier or prostate-plasma membrane[21]; this view is not universally shared. Megalin, a member of the low-density lipoprotein receptor (LRP) family, has been shown to facilitate the endocytosis of SHBG-bound testosterone through endocytic pits.[22,23] Animals deficient in megalin demonstrated resistance to some, but not all, androgen actions.[22] These data have cast doubt on the validity of the free hormone hypothesis.

Sex-hormone binding globulin is a glycoprotein, synthesized in the liver, that possesses high-affinity binding for testosterone and estradiol.[18] Insulin, thyroid hormones, dietary factors, androgens, and estrogens regulate hepatic SHBG production. SHBG serves as the major transport protein for sex steroids in plasma, and its concentration largely determines their distribution between the protein-bound and unbound states, although its functional role in testosterone delivery to target organs has generated considerable debate.[18] Androgen administration, obesity, hyperinsulinemic states, and the nephrotic syndrome are associated with low SHBG concentrations.[18] Conversely, SHBG levels are increased in patients with hyperthyroidism, many types of chronic inflammatory states, hyperthyroidism, and aging. A locus that is associated with SHBG concentrations in African Americans and whites has been mapped to 1q44.[24] In addition, several other loci in blacks exhibit linkage with SHBG concentrations, suggesting that many genes likely regulate SHBG levels. Unlike humans and rats, mice do not have SHBG and express very low levels of androgen-binding protein in the testis, but they show no perturbations of fertility or mating behavior.[25]

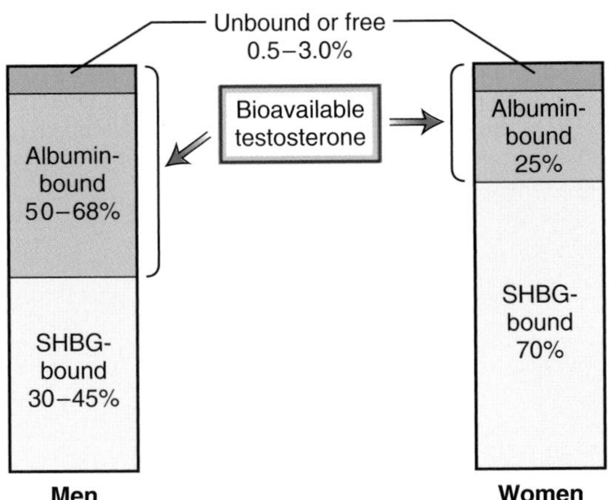

Figure 18–2 ▪ Binding of circulating testosterone to plasma proteins in men and women. Most of circulating testosterone is bound with high affinity to sex hormone–binding globulin and with low affinity to albumin. Only 0.5% to 3% of circulating testosterone is unbound or free and measured by the equilibrium dialysis method. The term *bioavailable testosterone* denotes the fraction of circulating testosterone that is unbound or bound to albumin and can be measured by the ammonium sulfate precipitation method. SHBG, steroid hormone–binding hormone; T, testosterone.

Testosterone Metabolism

Testosterone is metabolized predominantly in the liver (50% to 70%) although some degradation also occurs in peripheral tissues, particularly the prostate and the skin. Liver takes up testosterone from the blood and through a series of chemical reactions that involve 5-α and 5-β reductases, 3-β and 3-α hydroxysteroid dehydrogenases, and 17-hydroxysteroid dehydrogenase, converts it into androsterone and etiocholanolone (both inactive metabolites) and DHT and 3-androstanediol (Fig. 18–3). These compounds undergo glucaronidation or sulfation before their excretion by the kidneys. Free and conjugated androsterone and etiocholanolone are the predominant urinary metabolites of testosterone. Although a majority of these metabolites are inactive, some can be directly or indirectly active. For instance, 5-androstanediol potentially can be converted to 5-dihydrotestosterone (5-α DHT). Also, 5-β-androgen metabolites have been shown to stimulate hematopoeisis.[26]

Testosterone as a Prohormone: The Roles of Estradiol 17-β and 5-α DHT

Testosterone is converted in many peripheral tissues into its active metabolites, estradiol 17-β and 5-α DHT (Fig. 18–4). Aromatization of the A ring of testosterone converts it into 17-β estradiol. In addition, reduction of the 4,5 double bond converts testosterone into DHT. Testosterone actions in many tissues are mediated through these metabolites.

Testosterone effects on the trabecular bone resorption, plasma lipids, atherosclerosis progression, and the sexual differentiation of the brain require its aromatization to estradiol. Considerable insight into the role of estrogen in mammalian physiology has been gained from studies of natural mutations of estrogen receptor–α[27] and the CYP19 aromatase gene in humans and knockout mice harboring null mutations of estrogen receptor–α, estrogen receptor–β, and CYP19 aromatase genes. These models of estrogen deficiency exhibit significant disruption of spermatogenesis and fertility, elevated testosterone and LH levels, delayed epiphyseal fusion, decreased bone mass, and increased adiposity, indicating the important role of estrogens in regulation of bone mass, gonadotropin regulation, body composition, and spermatogenesis. A very small number of humans with inactivating mutations of the CYP19 aromatase gene have been reported.[28-31] Women with CYP19 gene mutations are masculinized, fail to undergo pubertal development, and have elevated levels of androgens and LH and follicle-stimulating hormone (FSH), polycystic ovaries, and tall stature.[28-31] Men with CYP19 aromatase mutations are characterized by elevated testosterone levels, low estradiol levels, osteoporosis,

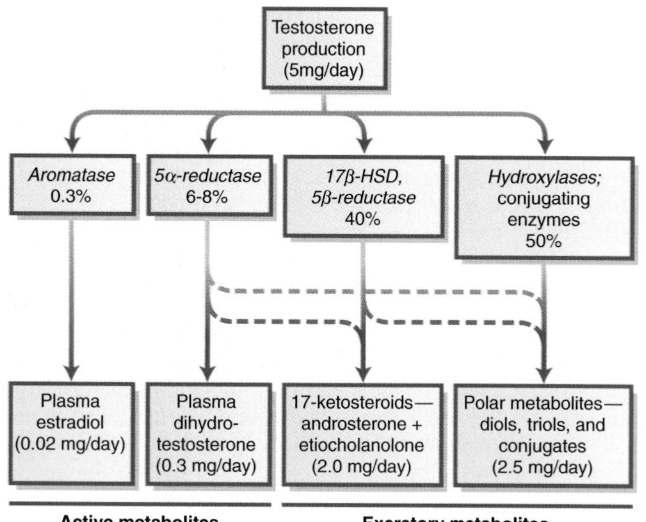

Figure 18–3 ▪ Testosterone is metabolized by a series of enzymatic reactions to active and inactive metabolites. Aromatization of A ring or 5-α reduction convert it into active metabolites, estradiol, and dihydrotestosterone. Additionally, through the action of a series of 5-α and 5-β reductases, 17-β hydroxysteroid dehydrogenases, and hydroxylases, testosterone is converted into a number of inactive metabolites that are conjugated and excreted in the urine. 17β HSD, 17-β hydroxysteroid dehydrogenase. (Reproduced from Griffin JE, Wilson JD. Disorders of the testis and the male reproductive tract. In Larsen PR, Kronenberg HM, Melmed S, Polonsky KS, eds.Williams Textbook of Endocrinology, 10th ed. Philadelphia: Saunders, 2003:709-763.)

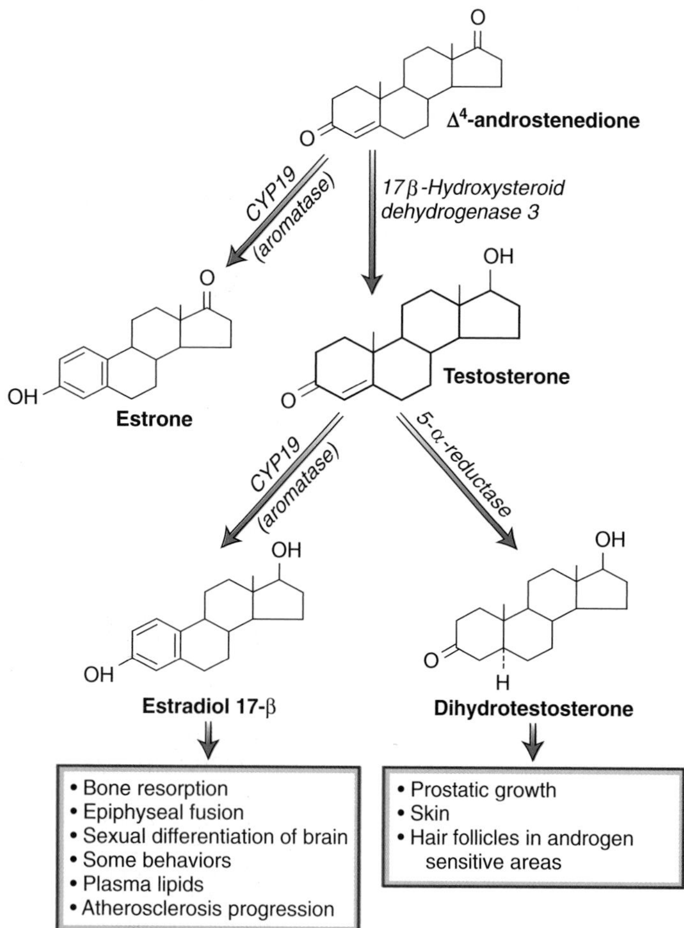

Figure 18–4 ▪ Testosterone as a prohormone. Testosterone can be converted by the action of steroid 5-α reductase to 5-α dihydrotestosterone or by the action of CYP19 aromatase into estradiol. Δ^4 androstenedione can also be aromatized to estrone. In addition, estriol can be formed by aromatization of 16-α-hydroxyprogesterone (not shown in this figure). Testosterone effects on the prostate, skin, and hair follicles in androgen sensitive areas require its obligatory 5-α reduction to 5-α-dihydrotestosterone. Testosterone's aromatization to estradiol 17-β is required for mediating its effects on bone resorption, epiphyseal fusion, sexual differentiation of the brain, some types of behavior, plasma lipids, and atherosclerosis progression.

increased bone turnover, delayed epiphyseal fusion and tall stature.[28-31]

At least two isoforms of steroid 5-α reductase (SRD5A) have been cloned and characterized.[32] Type 1 steroid 5-α reductase isoenzyme (SRD5A1) is expressed in many nongenital tissues, has been mapped to chromosome region 5p15, and has an optimal pH of 8. Type 2 steroid 5-α reductase isoenzyme (SRD5A2) is expressed in the prostate and other genital tissues, has been mapped to 2p23, and has an optimal pH of 5.0.[32] The biologic role of 5-α reductase type 1 has not been fully ascertained. The gene-targeting experiments suggest that the type 1 enzyme plays a role in progesterone metabolism at the end of pregnancy.[33] Mice that are null for SRD5A1 experience difficulties in cervical ripening and delivery.[33]

Testosterone effects on the prostate and sebaceous glands of the skin require its 5-α reduction to DHT by SRD5A2. SRD5A2 is the predominant form in the prostate and has been implicated in the pathophysiology of benign prostatic hypertrophy, hirsutism, and male-pattern baldness. During embryonic life, testosterone controls the differentiation of the wolffian ducts into epididymis, vasa deferentia, and seminal vesicles. The development of structures from the urogenital sinus and the genital tubercle such as the scrotum, penis, and penile urethra require the action of DHT. The role of 5-α reduction of testosterone in mediating its effects on the muscle and sexual function remains unclear. Although testosterone and DHT can both exert anabolic effects on the muscle, steroid 5-α reductase activity is very low or absent in the skeletal muscle,[34] and we do not know whether 5-α reduction of testosterone to DHT is obligatory for mediating androgen effects on the muscle. Published data also are unclear on whether androgen effects on sexual function in men are mediated through testosterone or its 5-α reduced metabolite, DHT.

Mechanism of Androgen Action

Most androgen actions are mediated through its binding to an intracellular androgen receptor that acts as a ligand-dependent transcription factor.[35-37] The androgen receptor has homology to other nuclear receptor proteins including the receptors for glucocorticoids, progesterone, and mineralocorticoids.[38-40] The predominant 919–amino acid, 110 kd androgen receptor protein has three conserved functional domains: the steroid-binding domain, the DNA-binding domain and the transcriptional activational domain (Fig. 18–5); of these, the central cysteine-rich DNA-binding domain is the most conserved.[38] The single copy androgen receptor gene spans a 90 kb region on chromosomal region Xq11-12. In the absence of its ligand, the androgen receptor protein is distributed in both the nucleus and the cytoplasm. However, androgen binding to the receptor causes it to translocate into the nucleus; amino acid sequences between 617 and 633 of the androgen receptor are important for its nuclear migration and *trans*-activation function.[35] Interaction of the binding complex with the appropriate sequence in the promoter region of the target gene changes the rate of transcription of the target gene.

Binding of androgens by the androgen receptor results in conformational change in this protein; the binding of androgen antagonist to androgen receptor might induce a different set of conformational changes than androgen agonists. The androgen receptor can use two *trans*-activation domains, AF1 and AF2. The *trans*-activation domain AF1 (including the 1 and 5 regions) is located in the aminoterminal part of the receptor protein, and AF2 is located in the carboxyterminal, ligand-dependent domain. In the intact receptor, both AF1 and AF2 are ligand-dependent and influenced by nuclear receptor coactivators. In contrast, in a truncated androgen receptor that is missing the ligand-binding domain, AF1 becomes constitutively active. Hormone binding to androgen receptor results in assembly of tissue-specific coactivators and corepressors that determine the specificity and tissue selectivity of hormone action.

In androgen target tissues, either testosterone or its 5-α-reduced metabolite, DHT, binds to the androgen receptor and regulates gene expression. Testosterone binds to the androgen receptor with half the affinity of DHT, although the maximal binding capacity is similar for both androgens. The DHT-androgen receptor complex has greater thermostability and slower dissociation rate than the testosterone-receptor complex.

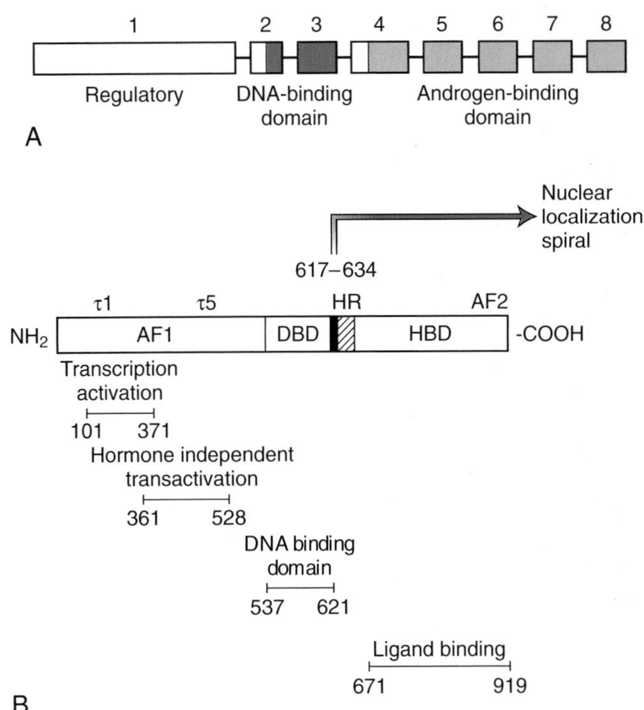

Figure 18–5 ▪ **A,** Schematic representation of the androgen receptor gene. Each box represents an exon. The androgen-binding domain comprises about 250 amino acids in the C-terminal region of the protein that are encoded by exons 4 to 8. The regulatory region is encoded by exon 1 and a part of exon 2, and the DNA-binding region is encoded by exon 3 and a part of exon 2. **B,** Functional domains of the androgen receptor protein. The N-terminal region of the androgen receptor protein contains the activation function 1 (AF1) domain with two *trans*-activation function T1 (101 to 371 aa) and T5 (361-528 aa). The DNA binding domain (DBD) resides in the middle and is followed by a nuclear localization signal (NLS) and the hinge region (HR). The hormone binding domain (HBD) is located at the carboxyterminal end of the protein and binds ligands and heat shock protein. (Adapted from Klocker H, Gromoll J, Cato ACB. Androgen receptor: molecular biology. In Nieschlag E, Behre HM, eds/ Testosterone: Action, Deficiency, Substitution. Cambridge, UK: Cambridge University Press, 2004:39-92.)

This might confer greater potency to DHT in mediating androgen effects in some androgen-sensitive tissues, such as the prostate. However, why 5-α reduction is necessary for mediating androgen effects in some tissues and not others is unclear. It is also unknown why this metabolic conversion step evolved for testosterone and not for other steroid hormones.

There is inconclusive evidence that some androgen effects may be mediated through nongenomic receptors on the cell membrane.

Pioneering investigations by Kochakian and others demonstrated that androgens promote nitrogen retention and stimulate muscle protein synthesis and hence increase muscle mass. Recent studies suggest that androgens increase skeletal muscle mass by promoting the differentiation of mesenchymal stem cells into myogenic lineage and inhibiting their adipogenic differentiation.[41,42] Androgens also might affect satellite cell entry into the cell cycle. Androgens also stimulate muscle protein synthesis.[43-48] Testosterone inhibits the differentiation of preadipocytes into adipocytes. Singh and colleagues[41] demonstrated that androgens promote the association of AR with β-catenin, stabilizing β-catenin and facilitating its translocation into the nucleus where the AR–β-catenin complex associates with TCF-4 and regulates a number of Wnt-target genes, thereby determining cell lineage, promoting myogenic differentiation, and inhibiting adipogenic differentiation.

Germ Cell Development in the Testis

Spermatogenesis, the process by which sperm are formed from spermatogonial stem cells in the seminiferous tubules of the testis, occurs in three stages (Fig. 18–6): spermatogonial replication, meiosis, and spermatogenesis. During the first stage, the spermatogonial stem cells divide mitotically several times to give rise to successive generations of spermatogonia, of which there are at least three main types in the human tubules: dark type A, pale type A, and type B. The type B spermatogonia proliferate to give rise to primary spermatocytes at the preleptotene stage of meiosis, in which DNA is actively synthesized.

During the second stage, primary spermatocytes that are diploid undergo meiosis, which consists of two successive divisions of the primary spermatocyte accompanied by only one duplication of chromosomes. At the completion of meiosis, four spermatids are produced, each containing a single, or haploid, set of chromosomes.

Spermiogenesis, the final stage of spermatogenesis, involves structural transformation and differentiation of the spermatid. During spermiogenesis, the chromatin of the spermatid condenses into a compact mass, the nucleus becomes invested by a membranous derivative of the Golgi apparatus, the acrosome, which contains enzymes that digest and enable the sperm to penetrate the outer vestments of the egg, and the cytoplasm elongates and surrounds the flagellum derived from a centriole. As sperm formation progresses, most of the cytoplasm is cast off in the form of a residual body.

The spermatid completes its metamorphosis into a spermatozoon by forming a complex tail by the axonemal complex of two inner singlet and nine outer doublet microtubules. In humans, the total duration of spermatogenesis is 74 days; the sperm spends an additional 21 days in the epididymis where it undergoes further maturation and capacitation.

Hormonal Regulation of Germ Cell Development

Normal spermatogenesis requires complex interactions between germ cells and Sertoli and Leydig cells, and the synergistic actions of the pituitary gonadotropins LH and FSH. LH, after binding to its G-protein–coupled receptor, stimulates testosterone production by the Leydig cells; high intratesticular testosterone concentrations are essential for the initiation and the maintenance of spermatogenesis within the testis. FSH acts on Sertoli cells and stimulates the secretion of a wide range of proteins and growth factors, such as androgen-binding protein, inhibin, activin, stem cell factor, plasminogen activator, transferrin, sulfated glycoproteins, and lactate, and the formation of the blood-testis barrier. During pubertal development, rising FSH concentrations sensitize the Leydig cells to stimulation by LH. Once spermatogenesis is established in the adult testis, Sertoli cells become less responsive to FSH.

The precise role of FSH in regulating human spermatogenesis is not fully understood. In adults who have spontaneous or experimentally induced hypogonadotropic hypogonadism and who have previously undergone pubertal maturation, LH or human chorionic gonadotropin (hCG) alone can reinitiate spermatogenesis. In men made hypogonadotropic by administration of testosterone enanthate, spermatogenesis can be reinitiated by hCG or FSH administered alone; combined administration of FSH and hCG is associated with higher sperm densities than hCG administration alone. Thus, in adults, addition of FSH is not

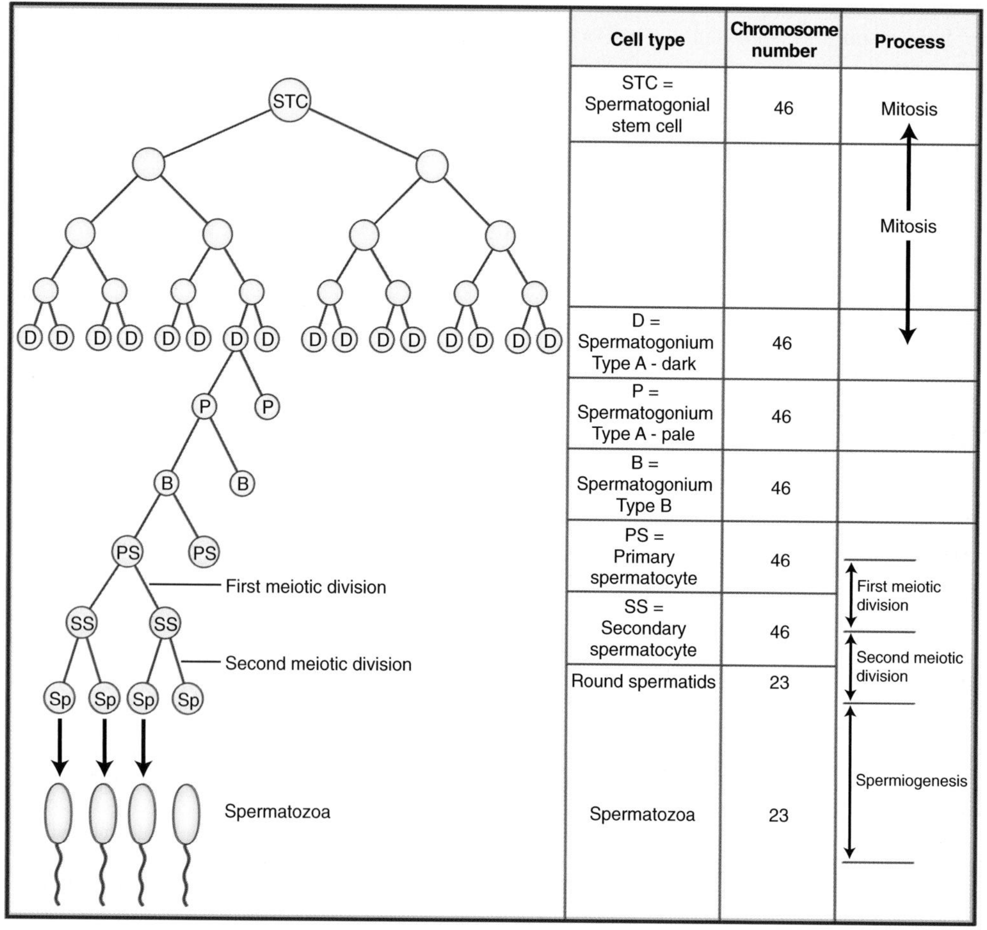

STC
D
P
B
PS
First meiotic division
SS
Second meiotic division
Sp
Spermatozoa
Cell type
Chromosome number
Process
STC = Spermatogonial stem cell
46
Mitosis
Mitosis
D = Spermatogonium Type A - dark
46
P = Spermatogonium Type A - pale
46
B = Spermatogonium Type B
46
PS = Primary spermatocyte
46
First meiotic division
SS = Secondary spermatocyte
46
Second meiotic division
Round spermatids
23
Spermiogenesis
Spermatozoa
23

Figure 18–6 ▪ A schematic representation of germ cell development during human spermatogenesis. The germ cell precursors are capable of self-renewal by mitotic division. After puberty, some spermatogonia undergo differentiation into primary spermatocytes, which underto two sets of meiotic divisions to form four haploid spermatids. The round spermatids by undergoing a series of differentiation steps, become elongated, develop a tail, and are transformed into sperm. The process of spermatogenesis takes 73 days in the human testis. Spermatogonial stem cells, spermatogonia, and primary spermatocytes are diploid (i.e. they carry 46 chromosomes), while spermatids and spermatozoa are haploid (i.e. they carry 23 chromosomes).

essential for reinitiating or maintaining spermatogenesis, but FSH augments spermatogenic response to LH and hCG. In contrast, in men in whom gonadotropin deficiency occurs prepubertally, LH or hCG alone usually is insufficient to initiate spermatogenesis; in these subjects, the addition of FSH is necessary for initiating spermatogenesis. Thus, FSH appears to be necessary for programming the spermatogenic machinery at the time of puberty for the initiation of spermatogenesis. Once this programming has occurred and spermatogenesis has been initiated, LH alone can maintain and reinitiate spermatogenesis.

A large number of Y-specific as well as autosomal genes are involved in regulating germ cell development in the testis. Although the number of human genes known to be implicated in the pathophysiology of human infertility is small, a significantly larger database exists in the mouse and *Drosophila*. For instance, 2400 *Drosophila* loci have been implicated in male sterility! Additional autosomal and X- and Y-specific candidate genes that are associated with defects of germ cell replication, meiosis, or spermiogenesis likely will be implicated in infertile men.

The Role of the Y Chromosome in Human Spermatogenesis

The human Y chromosome consists of a small pseudoautosomal region that recombines with homologous regions of the X chromosome; the remaining 95% of Y chromosome (approximately 65 Mb) that does not recombine with the X chromosome is referred to as the *male-specific region of Y* (MSY). In an extraordinary tour de force, Page and colleagues discovered that the MSY contains 156 transcription units that encode 27 proteins.[49] These transcription units are grouped into three classes of euchromatic sequences: X-transposed, X-degenerate, and ampliconic (Fig. 18–7).[49] The ampliconic region is organized into large palindromes that contain several families of multicopy Y-specific genes, all of which are expressed in the testis.[49] The high degree of sequence similarity between the arms of the palindromes is the result of intra-Y gene conversions.[50] Page and colleagues[49] suggest that intra-Y gene conversions not only are possible but that they occur frequently.

The X-transposed sequences have high degree of homology to the X chromosome, and X-degenerate sequences represent what is left of ancient autosomes that were transposed to form X and Y chromosomes.[49] Thus, there is growing recognition that the Y chromosome contains an important collection of testis-specific genes necessary for spermatogenesis,[49,50] and is far from being a garbage dump for former autosomal genes.[49]

Energy Balance and Reproductive Function

Normal reproductive function requires an optimal nutritional intake; caloric deprivation and consequent weight loss as well as excessive food intake and obesity are associated with impairment of reproductive function. Body composition, particularly the amount of body fat, influences the onset of puberty, the length of the reproductive period, the number of offspring, and the age of menopause.[51-53] Weight loss caused by famine, eating disorders, and exercise can impair reproductive function.[54-60] In women, weight loss is associated with delayed pubertal development, cessation of menstruation, and reduced gonadotropin secretion[52,61-69]; the decrease in FSH and LH levels correlates with the degree of weight loss.

Pathways that Link Energy-Sensing Mechanisms and the Reproductive Axis

The turn of the twenty-first century has witnessed substantial advancement in our understanding of the biochemical pathways that link the reproductive system with energy balance (Fig. 18–8). The metabolic signals that regulate hypothalamic GnRH secretion are mediated through leptin and neuropeptide Y.[58,70] Leptin, a hormone secreted by the fat cells, regulates the activity of central nervous system (CNS) effector systems that maintain energy balance.[70-73] Caloric deprivation is associated with reduced circulating levels of leptin as well as LH.[74,75] Leptin administration to calorically deprived humans or mice reverses the inhibition of gonadotropin secretion associated with food restriction.[76,77] Similarly, genetically ob/ob mice with leptin deficiency[78] and humans with congenital leptin deficiency have hypogonadotropic hypogonadism and are infertile[79]; treatment of leptin-deficient patients and mice with leptin restores gonadotropin secretion and fertility.[80] Thus, impaired GnRH secretion associated with energy deficit and weight loss is at least partly a consequence of decreased leptin secretion. Undoubtedly, leptin serves as an important link between energy balance and reproductive axis, although it is unclear whether it is the primary activator of the GnRH pulse generator at the onset of puberty. Emerging evidence suggests that leptin is essential but not sufficient for initiation of puberty.

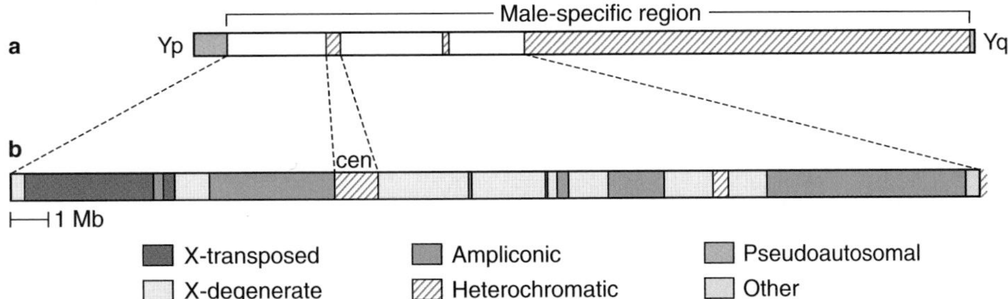

Figure 18–7 ■ Schematic representation of the human Y chromosome. The human Y chromosome consists of a small pseudoautosomal region that recombines with homologous regions of the X chromosome. The remaining 95% of Y chromosome (approximately 65 Mb) that does not recombine with the X chromosome is referred to as the *male-specific region of Y* (MSY). Page and colleagues discovered that the MSY contains many transcription units that are grouped in three classes: X-transposed, X-degenerate, and ampliconic (49). The ampliconic regions contain nine families of multicopy Y-specific genes, all of which are expressed in the testis (35). The X-transposed sequences have high degree of homology to X chromosome, and X-degenerate sequences represent what is left of ancient autosomes that were transposed to form X and Y chromosomes. Yp, short arm of Y chromosome; Yq, long arm of Y chromosome. (Reproduced from Skaletsky H, Kuroda-Kawaguchi T, Minx P, et al. The male-specific region of the Y chromosome is a mosaic of discrete sequence classes. Nature 2003;423:825-837.)

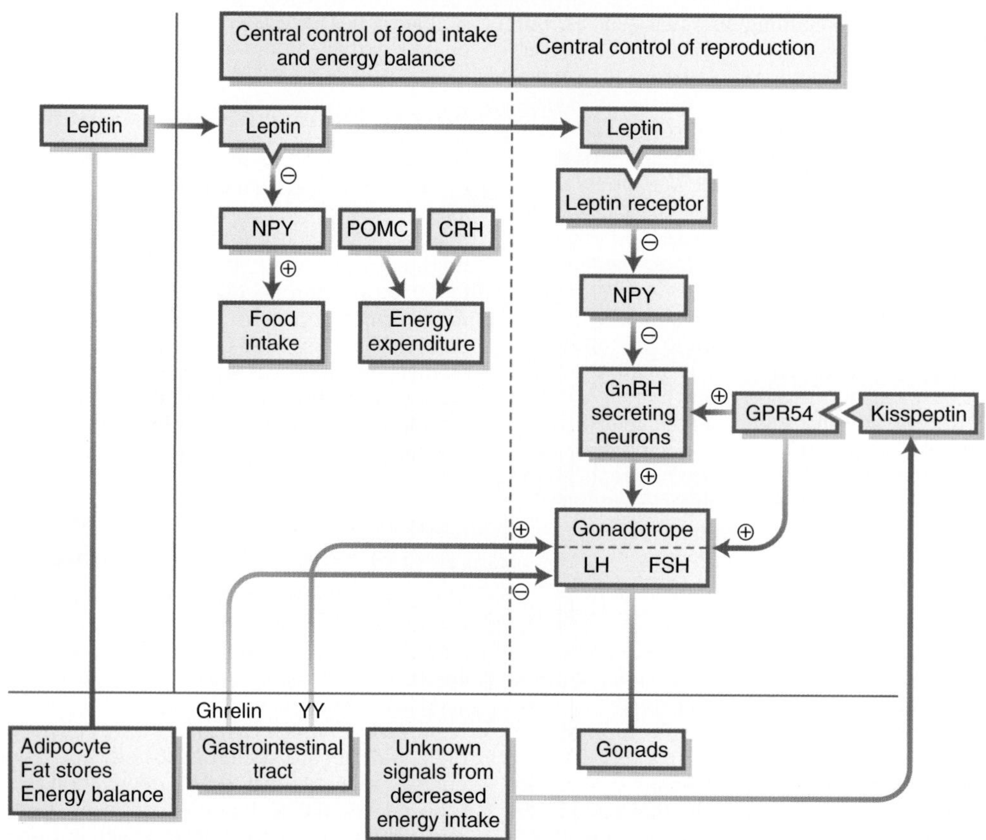

Figure 18–8 ▪ The biochemical pathways that link energy homeostasis and central control of reproduction. The biochemical signals indicating the state of energy stores originate in the adipocytes and are mediated through leptin and neuropeptide Y (NPY). Leptin, the product of the *ob* gene, is secreted by adipocytes and regulates gonadotropin-releasing hormone (GnRH) secretion by down-regulating NPY, which in turn down-regulates GnRH secretion. The net effect of leptin is to stimulate GnRH output. Additionally, leptin also stimulates luteinizing hormone (LH) secretion through a nitric oxide–mediated mechanism. Ghrelin and peptide YY, which originate in the gastrointestinal tract, have also been shown to regulate gonadotropin secretion. Kisspeptin, the natural ligand for the G protein 54 receptor, integrates signals from nutritional intake and energy stores and cross-communicates them to GnRH-secreting neurons and to gonadotropes. Thus, a complex array of signals originating in the energy stores, gastrointestinal tract, and other unknown sites is integrated centrally to regulate gonadotropin secretion and energy intake and expenditure. CRH, corticotropin-releasing hormone; FSH, follicle-stimulating hormone; GPR54, G protein–coupled receptor; POMC, propiomelanocortin.

Leptin stimulates LH secretion by activation of nitric oxide synthase in gonadotropes.[81] Leptin also inhibits neuropeptide Y secretion.[82] Neuropeptide Y has a tonic inhibitory effect on leptin and GnRH secretion.[83,84] Leptin also stimulates nitric oxide production in the mediobasal hypothalamus[81]; NO stimulates GnRH secretion by the hypothalamic GnRH-secreting neurons.[81] Therefore, the net effect of leptin action through stimulation of NO and inhibition of neuropeptide Y is to stimulate hypothalamic GnRH secretion and pituitary LH secretion.

Ghrelin, the natural ligand for growth hormone secretagogue receptor,[85] has been proposed as an additional link between energy deficit and reproductive function.[86-88] Ghrelin, released from the endocrine cells in the gastrointestinal tract,[89,90] inhibits LH secretion, LH response to GnRH, and testosterone response to LH[86,87] in addition to and independent of its effects on appetite and growth hormone secretion.[89-91] Polypeptide YY3-36 is another secreted hormone of gastrointestinal origin that binds to neuropeptide receptor subtypes Y2 and Y5,[92] suppresses food intake, stimulates LH and FSH secretion, and enhances LH responsiveness to GnRH.

The recently cloned G protein–linked receptor 54 (GPR54) plays an important role in integrating signals from energy homeostatic pathways to regulate gonadotropin secretion. Food deprivation is associated with decreased kisspeptin (the ligand for GPR54) and increased GPR54 mRNA expression in rats.[93] In a model of undernutrition, chronic administration of kisspeptin elicits gonadotropin secretion and restores vaginal opening.[93] Collectively, these data suggest that hormones originating in the gastrointestinal tract and energy stores act in concert with the GPR54 receptor signaling to provide important cues for central regulation of reproductive function.

TESTICULAR DISORDERS

Testicular disorders can be classified into disorders of sex-steroid production or action, disorders of germ cell compartment, and testicular neoplasms. Androgen deficiency and gynecomastia are the most prevalent disorders of sex-steroid production. Defects in androgen action encompass mutations in the androgen receptor, steroid 5-α reductase, CYP19 aromatase, or the estrogen receptor alpha genes. Defects of spermatogenesis and sperm function manifest as infertility or subfertility. The clinical consequences of androgenic steroid abuse by athletes and recreational body builders are also described.

Androgen-Deficiency Syndromes in Men

Hypogonadism is a syndrome associated with impaired androgen production or action. Androgen deficiency can result from abnormalities of testicular function (primary hypogonadism), hypothalamic or pituitary regulation of testicular function (secondary hypogonadism),[94] or impairment of androgen action at the target tissue (androgen insensitivity).

Primary testicular failure is characterized by low testosterone levels, impairment of spermatogenesis, and elevated LH and FSH concentrations.[94] Secondary testicular failure results from disorders of hypothalamus or the pituitary and is associated with low testosterone and low or inappropriately normal LH and FSH concentrations.[94] Classifying androgen-deficient men into those with primary or secondary testicular failure is clinically useful because fertility can be induced in men with secondary hypogonadism by administration of gonadotropins or by pulsatile GnRH therapy.[94] In contrast, men with primary testicular failure are unlikely to achieve spontaneous fertility, and therapeutic options include adoption, artificial insemination by using donor sperm, or in rare instances, intracytoplasmic sperm injection (ICSI) using intratesticular sperm.

Causes of Androgen Deficiency in Men

Conditions associated with low testosterone levels are listed in Table 18–1.

Causes of Primary Hypogonadism

The common causes of primary testicular failure include Klinefelter's syndrome, uncorrected cryptorchidism, cancer chemotherapy and radiation, trauma, and orchiectomy.

Klinefelter's Syndrome

Klinefelter's syndrome, the most common chromosomal disorder associated with primary testicular failure and male infertility, is found in 1:500 to 1:1000 live-born boys[95-97] and is the most common recognizable cause of primary testicular failure. The most prevalent karyotype in men with Klinefelter's syndrome is 47,XXY (93%), but 46,XY/47,XXY, 48,XXXY, 48,XXYY, and 49,XXXXY karyotypes have also been reported.[98] The XXY chromosomal constitution has been described in other mammals including mouse, Chinese hamster, cat, dog, sheep, ox, and pig and is associated with sterility.[99] The testes of 47,XXY mammals are devoid of germ cells.[99]

Azoospermia is the rule in men with Klinefelter's syndrome who have the 47,XXY karyotype.[98,100] Men with mosaicism might have germ cells in their testes, especially at a younger age.

Testicular histology in men with Klinefelter's syndrome shows hyalinization of seminiferous tubules and absence of spermatogenesis.[98,100] Patients with mosaicism might have normal size testis and spermatogenesis at puberty. However, progressive degeneration and hyalinization of seminiferous tubules takes place soon after puberty.[100] In some men, the tubular dysgenesis is patchy; degenerating tubules are interspersed with apparently normal tubules. The Leydig cells appear to be increased although their function is impaired.[100]

The 47,XXY karyotype in patients with Klinefelter's syndrome results from nondisjunction during the first meiotic division in one of the parents. Nondisjunction of maternal chromosomes is the cause of 47,XXY karyotype in two thirds of affected men. Advanced maternal age is a risk factor for nondisjunction.[97,101] The mechanism by which an extra X chromosome renders patients infertile is not known. In male germ cells, inactivation of the single X chromosome in primary spermatocytes of heterogametic males is necessary for spermatogenesis to proceed through meiosis. We do not know why X inactivation is essential

TABLE 18–1 CONDITIONS ASSOCIATED WITH LOW TESTOSTERONE LEVELS IN MEN

Common	Less Common	Rare
	PRIMARY GONADAL FAILURE	
Klinefelter's syndrome Uncorrected cryptorchidism	Radiation Chemotherapy Orchitis Trauma Anorchia due to bilateral torsion or vanishing testes syndrome Medications (ketoconazole)	Noonan's syndrome Myotonic dystrophy Mutations in the LH receptor or subunits Type 1 autoimmune polyglandular syndrome
	SECONDARY GONADAL FAILURE	
Chronic disease (HIV infection, COPD, end stage renal disease) Critical illness Hyperprolactinemia Medications (e.g., opiates, anabolic steroids)	Tumors of the hypothalamic-pituitary region Abuse of drugs such as alcohol and marijuana Head injury Surgery Infiltrative disorders (e.g., hemochromatosis, sarcoidosis, histiocytosis) Severe obesity Excessive exercise Eating disorders	Idiopathic hypogonadotropic hypogonadism, Kallmann's syndrome Infections (e.g., TB) Pituitary apoplexy Prader-Willi syndrome
	DUAL	
Aging Alcoholism	Hemochromatosis Sickle cell disease	Congenital adrenal hypoplasia (DAX-1 mutations)

COPD, chronic abstuctive pulmonary disease; LH, luteinizing hormone; TB, tuberculosis.

for male germ cell differentiation in heterogametic species; it is possible that expression of some X-linked genes is detrimental to spermatogenesis. Also, inactivation of the single X may be required for normal sex chromosome pairing.

Most men with Klinefelter's syndrome go though life without a diagnosis.[102] Boys with Klinefelter's syndrome are likely to receive a diagnosis during evaluation for developmental delay and behavioral problems.[102] Men with Klinefelter's syndrome usually come to attention during evaluation for hypogonadism or infertility.[98,102] Children with Klinefelter's syndrome undergo normal pubertal development.[103] Testicular biopsies in boys with Klinefelter's syndrome in various stages of puberty have shown that diploid germ cells are present in the testes in early puberty, but germ cells are lost during pubertal development.[104,105]

Compared with the general population, men with Klinefelter's syndrome have higher overall mortality rates,[106] higher mortality rates from lung cancer, breast cancer, and non-Hodgkin's lymphoma, and lower mortality rates from prostate cancer.[107,108] The relative risk of breast cancer and non-Hodgkin's lymphoma is particularly increased in men with Klinefelter's syndrome.[107,108]

Gonadal Toxicity of Cancer Chemotherapy

Gonadal dysfunction has emerged as an important long-term complication of cancer chemotherapy.[109] This is particularly true of hematological and testicular malignancies in which combination chemotherapy has improved greatly the survival rates. Because these patients are typically young and can expect excellent disease outcome, infertility is a significant issue for many cancer survivors. Also, decreased testosterone levels can contribute to fatigue, sexual dysfunction, altered mood, loss of lean mass, and decreased bone mineral density.[110,111] Although increased frequency of aneuploidy and chromosomal abnormalities have been reported in men who have received cancer chemotherapy,[112,113] no measurable increase in birth defects has been noted to date.[114]

The germ cell compartment displays greater sensitivity to damage by cancer chemotherapeutic agents; however, Leydig cell dysfunction has also been reported.[109,115] The effects of chemotherapy on testicular function depend on the type of chemotherapeutic agent, the cumulative dose, and the nature of the malignancy.[109,116,117] The alkylating agents cyclophosphamide and procarbazine are particularly toxic to the testis. Ninety percent of patients treated with combination chemotherapeutic combinations such as MVPP (mustine, vinblastine, procarbazine, and prednisolone) or MOPP (mustine, vincristine, procarbazine, and prednisolone) that contain procarbazine develop azoospermia.[118,119] A much smaller fraction has low testosterone levels, and approximately 20% to 25% have low normal testosterone levels with elevated LH concentrations suggesting mild Leydig cell dysfunction. Newer chemotherapeutic regimens such as ABVD that do not contain procarbazine are associated with lower frequency of azoospermia than regimens containing procarbazine such as MOPP.[120] High-dose chemotherapy used before and during bone marrow transplantation is also associated with irreversible damage to germinal epithelium, oligospermia or azoospermia, and elevated FSH in a majority of treated men.[121]

The prognosis for fertility and normal gonadal function is better in men with testicular cancers who have received combinations containing platinum; although a large majority of these patients experience a reduction in sperm density after receiving chemotherapy, 80% of men surviving 5 years have normal sperm densities.[122] Similarly, the frequency of low testosterone and elevated LH levels in long-term survivors of testicular cancer is low.[122] Patients treated with high-dose IL-2 for metastatic cancer can experience transient reductions in testosterone levels. The frequency of testicular dysfunction after chemotherapy is not significantly different between prepubertal boys and adults.

Several strategies to prevent germ cell damage during cancer chemotherapy have been explored, but none has been effective in humans. Therefore, cryopreservation of sperm for subsequent use for intrauterine insemination or ICSI has become standard practice for men undergoing cancer chemotherapy and should be offered to patients. Therapeutic approaches based on suppression of testicular function by administration of GnRH analogues or testosterone enanthate have not been consistently effective in preventing germ call damage in men receiving MOPP or MVPP regimens.[123,124] Autologous stem cell implantation into the testes in repopulating the germ cell compartment for restoration of spermatogenesis after completion of chemotherapy has been considered and holds promise.

Testicular Trauma

Because of its location outside the abdomen, testes are particularly vulnerable to trauma. Testicular atrophy can occur in almost 50% of men experiencing blunt trauma to the scrotum.[125]

Infectious Orchitis

Infection of the testes by mumps, echovirus, group B arboviruses, and lymphocytic choriomeningitis can result in testicular atrophy. The incidence of mumps has decreased in recent years. Orchitis complicates the course of mumps infection in about 25% of men infected with the virus, typically 4 to 8 days after the onset of parotitis.[126] In about a third of patients with mumps orchitis, testicular atrophy occurs gradually over a period of several months after the acute illness has subsided.[126] The orchitis might affect only one testis in more 50% of patients; in men with unilateral orchitis, the sperm densities typically return to normal within 1 to 2 years of infection.[126]

Human Immunodeficiency Virus Infection

In early days of the human immunodeficiency virus (HIV) epidemic before the advent of antiretroviral drug therapy, 40% to 50% of HIV-infected men had low testosterone levels.[127] More recent surveys indicate that even among HIV-infected men receiving highly active antiretroviral therapy, 20% to 30% have low total and free testosterone levels.[128,129] SHBG levels are typically increased in HIV-infected men. Eighty percent of HIV-infected men with low testosterone levels have low or normal LH and FSH levels, and 20% have elevated LH and FSH levels.[128] Thus, the pathophysiology of low testosterone levels in HIV-infected men is complex, and defects at all levels of the hypothalamic-pituitary-testicular axis contribute to low testosterone levels. Testicular biopsies from HIV-infected men have revealed loss of architecture of seminiferous tubules, hyalinization, loss of germ cells, and infiltration by mononuclear cells.[130] Low testosterone levels in HIV-infected men are associated with weight loss, accelerated disease progression, decreased lean body mass and decreased exercise capacity, and increased depression scores.[131] Decline in bioavailable testosterone levels precedes the onset of wasting.[132]

Anorchia (Vanishing Testis Syndrome)

Anorchia refers to the absence of testicular tissue in a 46,XY phenotypic male. These patients have normal external male genitalia and normal wolffian duct structures and complete absence of müllerian duct structures,[133,134] indicating that during critical periods of sexual differentiation, the testes must have present and producing testosterone and müllerian inhibiting hormone. The pathogenic factors that cause the testes to atrophy and vanish are not known. Familial occurrence and the association of anorchia with 46,XY gonadal dysgenesis have led to speculation that genetic factors associated with testis determination or descent may be involved.[135,136] However, mutations of SRY, INSL3, and LGR8 (the receptor for INSL3) have not been found in analyses of small samples of patients with anorchia.[137] The prevalence rate of one in 20,000 men for bilateral anorchia and one in 5000 for unilateral anorchia have been reported,[134] but it is possible that the prevalence rates are higher because some cases of anorchia may be mislabeled cryptorchia.

In men with the 46,XY karyotype and nonpalpable testes, a systematic effort to locate the testes is necessary. Measurements of müllerian inhibiting substance, an hCG stimulation test with measurements of testosterone, and magnetic resonance imaging (MRI) scan of the abdomen can help locate an intra-abdominal testis. If the hCG stimulation test and MRI scans do not confirm the presence of an intra-abdominal testes, laparoscopic examination or in some instances exploratory laparotomy may be required to locate the testes and to reposition and anchor them in the scrotum.

Inactivating Mutations of the LH-Receptor Gene

Inactivating mutations of the LH-receptor gene are associated with hypogonadism and Leydig cell hypoplasia. A number of families with resistance to LH action due to inactivating mutations of LH receptor have been reported.[138-148] Men with LH receptor mutations present with a spectrum of phenotypic abnormalities ranging from feminization of external genitalia in 46,XY males to Leydig cell hypoplasia, primary hypogonadism, and delayed sexual development.[138-148] Testicular histology in phenotypic males with LH receptor mutations typically reveals the absence of mature Leydig cells and spermatogenic arrest at the elongated spermatid stage. 46,XX females with LH receptor mutation typically experience normal development of secondary sex characteristics but have increased LH levels and amenorrhea.

Inactivating Mutations of the FSH-Receptor Gene

The loss of function mutation of the gene for the human FSH receptor (2p21) are associated with hypergonadotropic ovarian dysgenesis.[149-153] An extensive investigation of multiple affected Finnish families revealed a C566T transition predicting Ala-189Val substitution in the FSH-receptor gene that was associated with primary amenorrhea, arrest of follicular development, and infertility.[149-153] Expression of the gene in transfected cells showed reduced or no signal transduction. Compared with patients with ovarian dysgenesis who did not have the mutation, patients with the FSH receptor mutation were shorter and had more ovarian follicles. In contrast to female patients, male patients with this mutation were fertile but had reduced sperm counts. Population studies have shown this mutation in about 1% of Finns, with geographic enrichment suggestive of a founder affect.[151]

Other Testicular Disorders Associated with Primary Testicular Failure

Testicular failure can occur as a part of type I, type 2, or type 4 autoimmune polyendocrine syndrome.[154] These patients typically have low testosterone and elevated LH and FSH levels. Antibodies against 17-α hydroxylase and CYP side chain cleavage enzyme have been reported in men with autoimmune polyendocrine syndrome and low testosterone levels.[154]

Men with Down's syndrome (trisomy 21) can have elevated LH and FSH levels and decreased spermatogenesis.

Causes of Secondary Hypogonadism

Hyperprolactinemia, chronic illness, aging, use of opioids and other drugs, eating disorders, and pituitary tumors are the most common causes of secondary hypogonadism.

Hyperprolactinemia can induce androgen deficiency by multiple mechanisms. Most of the studies of the mechanisms of hyperprolactinemia-associated hypogonadism have been conducted in women, and the data have been extrapolated to men. LH pulse frequency is lower in patients with hyperprolactinemia and is restored by bromocriptine therapy[155,156]; prolactin has also been shown to inhibit GnRH release in a neuronal cell line.[157] These data have led to the hypothesis that the primary mechanism of prolactin action is suppression of hypothalamic GnRH secretion.[157] LH pulse amplitude is not decreased in hyperprolactinemic patients,[155] although in oophorectomized rats, high prolactin inhibits LH pulse frequency as well as amplitude. It has been suggested that prolactin might also affect the set point of the gonadostat. There is some evidence, albeit inconclusive, that prolactin might also suppress gonadal response to gonadotropins. In patients with prolactin-secreting pituitary macroadenomas, hypogonadotropic hypogonadism also can occur because of mass effect of the tumor on gonadotropes.

Serum total, free, and bioavailable testosterone and DHEA levels are lower in older men than younger men, even after accounting for potential confounding factors such as time of sampling, concomitant illness, medications, and technical issues related to hormone assays.[158-164] Aging is associated with abnormalities at all levels of the hypothalamic-pituitary-testicular axis; testosterone response to LH and LH response to GnRH are attenuated in older men in comparison to younger men. In addition, the feedback and feed-forward relationships between hypothalamus, pituitary and testis are distorted.[165-168] The increments in LH concentrations in older men are less than those predicted from the decline in serum testosterone concentrations, reflecting both attenuation of pituitary function and resetting of the gonadostat.[169,170] Thus, in many older men with age-related decline in testosterone concentrations, serum LH levels are either normal or only slightly elevated.

Opioid use by patients with cancer-related and noncancer pain or by heroin addicts and patients on methadone maintenance is associated with central hypogonadism characterized by low testosterone levels and low LH and FSH levels.[171-175] The degree of testosterone suppression is related to the opioid dose and the type of opioid used.[171] Thus, buprenorphine has been reported to cause a lesser degree of gonadal suppression than methadone.[176] The mechanisms by which opioids suppress gonadal function are not fully understood, but they involve suppression of GnRH secretion.[177] Veldhuis has suggested that opioids alter the sensitivity of the central GnRH secreting neurons to feedback suppression by endogenous testosterone levels, thus resetting the gonadostat to a lower testosterone level.[178-180] The suppression of testosterone by opioids has clinical consequences, because it is associated with impairment of sexual function, osteoporosis, increased fatigue, anxiety and depression, loss of muscle mass and strength, and reduced quality of life.[171,174]

Genetic Syndromes Associated with Hypogonadotropic Hypogonadism

In men who have hypogonadotropic hypogonadism and in whom detectable causes of gonadotropin deficiency have been excluded, specific hypothalamic syndromes can be recognized by the associated somatic stigmata.[181] A number of hypothalamic syndromes are characterized by the presence of hypogonadotropic hypogonadism in association with a constellation of dysmorphic somatic features such as horseshoe kidney, sensorineural deafness, marked obesity, hyperphagia, polydactyly, retinitis pigmentosa, and mental retardation.[181,182] A diagnosis of these hypothalamic syndromes is made by pattern recognition.

Men who have hypogonadotropic hypogonadism in the absence of a detectable cause have idiopathic hypogonadotropic hypogonadism (IHH), a heterogeneous group of disorders characterized by selective gonadotropin deficiency resulting from an isolated defect in GnRH secretion.[182-184] The primary pathogenic defect in these patients is hypothalamic, and the impaired gonadotropin secretion is secondary to the hypothalamic abnormality in GnRH secretion.

Although anosmia and hyposmia are the best known and the first associations described in this syndrome, a number of other somatic abnormalities have been recorded.[181] The more common associations include color blindness, cleft lip and palate, cranial nerve defects (including eighth nerve deafness), horseshoe-shaped kidneys, cryptorchidism, and optic atrophy.

Heterogeneity of Pulsatile Gonadotropin Secretion in Patients with Idiopathic Hypogonadotropic Hypogonadism

There is considerable heterogeneity in the clinical presentation of IHH.[182,184] Those with the most severe deficiency can present with complete absence of pubertal development, sexual infantilism, and, in some cases, with varying degrees of hypospadias and undescended testes. Male patients can have complete absence of secondary sex characteristics, infantile testes, and azoospermia. Female patients can present with primary amenorrhea. Patients with partial GnRH deficiency can have varying degrees of delay in sexual development in proportion to the severity of gonadotropin deficiency.

Patients with IHH are quite heterogeneous in their LH-secretory profiles.[184] The largest subset comprises patients who display no pulsatile LH secretion at all; these men have the most severe GnRH deficiency. A smaller subset displays low-amplitude pulses. Another subset of patients has LH pulses at a markedly reduced frequency. A fourth subset is characterized by sleep-entrained pulses reminiscent of the pattern seen in early stages of puberty; these patients can be considered to suffer from a "developmental arrest."

Two variants of IHH are particularly interesting. The term *fertile eunuch syndrome* has been used to describe patients who have eunuchoidal proportions and delayed sexual development but normal-sized testes. Such men appear to have sufficient gonadotropins to stimulate high intratesticular testosterone levels and to initiate spermatogenesis but not enough testosterone secretion into the blood to adequately virilize the peripheral tissues; they are, in fact, partially gonadotropin deficient.[185] Another variant with predominantly FSH deficiency has also been described, although these patients are rare.[186]

Genetics of IHH

One third of IHH patients have a positive family history.[183,187] Of those with a positive family history, approximately 20% have an X-linked pattern of inheritance, one third have an autosomal recessive pattern, and one half have an autosomal dominant mode of inheritance.[183,187]

The locus for the X-linked form of Kallmann's syndrome has been assigned to chromosomal region Xp22.3.[188,189] Two groups independently cloned an adhesion-molecule–like protein from this region encoded by the *KALIG-1* (Kallmann's syndrome interval-1) gene.[188,190] The protein product of the *KALIG-1* gene presumably regulates migration of the GnRH and olfactory neurons and their morphogenesis. Mutations in the *KALIG-1* gene have been found in some patients with the X-linked form of IHH, but that can account for only a small fraction of X-linked IHH patients.[191] Additional, as yet unidentified, X-linked genes are likely implicated in other subsets of Kallmann's syndrome.

The GnRH neurons first appear in the epithelium of the olfactory placode in the mouse embryo and then migrate to the forebrain and finally to their ultimate hypothalamic location.[192,193] Such observations suggest that IHH may be a developmental defect resulting from an abnormal migration of the luteinizing hormone–releasing hormone (LHRH) neurons. MRI studies show that the olfactory bulbs and sulci are poorly developed in patients with IHH who have anosmia or hyposmia.[194]

Idiopathic hypogonadotropic hypogonadism and anosmia have also been reported in association with mutations of the fibroblast growth factor receptor 1 *(FGFR1)* gene.[195] Kindreds with *FGFR1* mutations display an autosomal dominant inheritance.[195]

Mutations of the DAX-1 and SF1 Genes are Associated with Hypogonadotropic Hypogonadism and Adrenal Hypoplasia Congenita

Mutations of at least two loci (NROB1 that encodes for the *DAX-1* gene and NR5A1 that encodes for the steroidogenic factor-1 gene) have been associated with congenital adrenal hypoplasia and hypogonadotropic hypogonadism.[196] The product of the *DAX-1* gene is an orphan nuclear receptor.[197,198] The mutations in the C-terminal end of the *DAX-1* gene have been associated with X-linked hypogonadotropic hypogonadism and adrenal insufficiency (congenital adrenal hypoplasia). However, mutations in the *DAX-1* gene are an unusual cause of idiopathic hypogonadotropic hypogonadism, accounting for less than 1% of the cases. These patients typically have normal testosterone response to hCG, indicating normal Leydig cell function, although primary testicular dysfunction has been described in some patients.

Mutations of the steroidogenic factor 1 gene in 46,XY patients also have been associated with congenital adrenal hypoplasia, sex reversal with female phenotype, streak gonads, and hypogonadotropic hypogonadism.[196] Mice with targeted disruption of the murine *SF-1* gene are characterized by gonadal agenesis, female internal genitalia, and primary adrenal failure.[199] The product of the *SF1* gene is an orphan receptor that interacts with *DAX-1* to regulate sexual differentiation and adrenal development.[200]

Mutations of the GnRH Receptor Gene Are Associated with Hypogonadotropic Hypogonadism

Several families with hypogonadotropic hypogonadism due to mutations of the GnRH receptor have been reported.[201] The GnRH receptor is a G-protein–coupled receptor with an extracellular amino-terminus, seven-transmembrane regions and an intracellular carboxy-terminus.[202] Patients with GnRH receptor mutations have a normal sense of smell. In these families, the pattern of inheritance of IHH is autosomal recessive, and consanguinity is often present. The male-to-female distribution among affected persons is equal. GnRH receptor mutations account for almost 40% of cases in families with autosomal recessive pattern of inheritance and 10% of sporadic cases. Mutations in the GnRH receptor gene might alter GnRH binding or ligand-induced signal transduction.[202]

G Protein Receptor 54 Mutations

Mutations of G protein receptor 54 (GPR54) are associated with delayed onset of puberty and hypogonadotropic hypogonadism in men and mice.[203] GPR54 is a member of the rhodopsin family of G protein–coupled receptors, which along with the ligand metastin plays an important role in the regulating pulsatile GnRH secretion and the onset of puberty.[204] Metastins are derived by processing of a single precursor protein, kisspeptin 1[205]; metastin 1-54 and the shorter C-terminal fragment, metastin 45-54 are potent stimulators of GnRH release and less potent stimulators of pituitary LH release. The metastin-induced stimulation of GnRH appears to be independent of leptin. Coincidental with the onset of puberty, Kiss1 and GPR54 mRNA expression is upregulated in the hypothalamus.[206]

Major deletions or rearrangements of the GnRH gene have not been found in patients with IHH by Southern blot analysis or sequencing of polymerase chain reaction (PCR) products.

However, more subtle defects within the GnRH gene have not been completely excluded.

Mutations of Nasal Ectodermal LHRH Factor

Mutations of nasal ectodermal LHRH factor (NELF), whose gene product is involved in neural migration, have been described in a small number of patients with IHH.[207] Similarly, delayed puberty and hypogonadotropic hypogonadism have also been associated with mutations of leptin or its receptor.[208,209]

Known mutations of the *KALIG-1*, GnRH receptor, *GPR54, FGFR1*, and *DAX-1* genes can account for only 30% to 40% of cases of hypogonadotropic hypogonadism.[208] Therefore, additional autosomal and X-linked genes will likely be implicated in other cases of IHH.

Mutations in the Gene Encoding the Follicle Stimulating Hormone β-Subunit Gene

Inherited mutations of the FSHβ genes are uncommon, but they have been reported to produce male hypogonadism and delayed puberty in boys.[210] FSH-deficient male mice are fertile although they have small testes and subnormal spermatogenesis.[211] Female mice deficient in the FSHβ-subunit, produced by embryonic stem cell technology, are infertile, with a block in folliculogenesis prior to antral follicle formation.[211]

A 46,XX patient, homozygous for an FSHβ point mutation, presented with primary amenorrhea, infertility, and low serum FSH levels.[210] Analysis of the FSHβ gene revealed a two-nucleotide deletion that resulted in a frame shift of subsequent codons and premature termination.[210] A relative of the index case was postmenopausal and had subnormal FSH levels. The two point mutations in the FSHβ gene observed in this family were both located in exon 3 at codons 51 and 61.[210]

Hypogonadism Associated with Inactivating Mutations of the LH Beta Gene

A single patient with mutation of the LHβ-subunit gene has been reported[212]; this patient presented with delayed pubertal development. He had increased serum immunoreactive LH levels but decreased bioactive LH concentrations. The mutant LH in this patient had decreased receptor-binding activity due to homozygous substitution of glycine in position 54 with arginine (G54R).[212] The male members of the family who were heterozygous for this mutation had lower testosterone levels.

A polymorphic variant of LH has been reported in Finland and Japan.[213,214] The variant LH has two amino acid substitutions, W8R and I15T, that are associated with increased bioactivity and a reduced serum half-life.[214] The clinical significance of this polymorphism is not known.

Activating Mutations of the LH and FSH Receptor Genes

Activating mutations of the LH receptor gene are associated with gonadotropin-independent sexual precocity. Activating or gain-of-function mutations of the LH receptor are associated with gonadotropin-independent sexual precocity in boys, but they do not produce a discernible phenotype in girls.[215] Analysis of LH receptor in this patient showed a C to T substitution in exon 11 that resulted in an Ala to Val change. When the COS-7 cells were transiently transfected with the wild type or Ala-373Val mutant LH receptor cDNA, the mutant cDNA construct had higher basal and hCG-stimulated cAMP accumulation.

Only a single case of activating mutation of the FSH receptor is on record; this patient was fertile even after surgical hypophysectomy that had lowered his FSH immunoreactivity to undetectable levels[216]

Prader-Willi Syndrome

Patients with Prader-Willi syndrome typically have childhood obesity, neonatal hypotonia, developmental delay, mental retardation, hypogonadism, short stature, and small hands and feet.[217] Hypogonadotropic hypogonadism, cryptorchidism, and micropenis are common.[218,219] The LH response to a single bolus of GnRH is decreased in comparison to obese controls.[218,219] The degree of gonadotropin deficiency in these patients is variable. A few patients with hypergonadotropic hypogonadism have also been described.

Prader-Willi syndrome is a genomic imprinting disorder that commonly results from decreased expression of paternally derived genes in the PWS critical region on chromosome 15q11. Deletions of proximal portion of paternally derived chromosome 15q are the most common cause of decreased expression of paternally derived genes in this region.[220] The maternally derived copies of genes responsible for the Prader-Willi syndrome in proximal 15q are normally silent.[220] Therefore, the deletion of the paternally derived copy of the normally active genes produces the disease. Prader-Willi syndrome can also result if both copies of the gene are derived from the mother because the maternal copies are inactivated presumably by DNA methylation[217]; this condition is known as uniparental disomy. Structural abnormalities of the imprinting center can also produce the Prader-Willi syndrome.

The genes responsible for the Prader-Willi syndrome have not been identified. The genetic diagnosis can be made by using a combination of cytogenetic and molecular approaches, including fluorescent in situ hybridization (FISH) and analysis of allele-specific DNA methylation differences in 15q11-q13.[220]

Developmental Disorders of the Pituitary Due to Mutations of the Homeodomain Transcription Factors

A number of homeodomain transcription factors are involved in the development and differentiation of the different hormone-producing cells within the pituitary gland. Mutations in these transcription factors have been associated with deficiencies of pituitary hormones.[221-226]

Mutations in the *Pit-1* homeodomain transcription factor have been associated with failure of several differentiated cell types to develop within the pituitary gland and deficiencies of GH, prolactin, and TSH.[223,226] These patients have either small or normal-sized pituitary glands. Both autosomal dominant and recessive forms of inheritance have been described, depending on the DNA-binding properties of the mutant protein.

Patients with mutations of *Prop1* have deficiencies of LH and FSH in addition to the deficiencies of GH, prolactin, and TSH.[222,224] ACTH secretion is normal at birth, but corticotrophs can degenerate secondarily. These patients have normal, small, or sometimes large pituitary glands.

Gsx-1, an orphan homeobox gene, is required for normal pituitary development. Homozygous mutations of the *Gsx-1* gene are associated with extreme dwarfism, sexual infantilism, and increased perinatal mortality.[222] The pituitary gland in affected patients is small and hypocellular and has a reduced number of growth hormone– and prolactin-producing cells.

Another homeobox gene, *Hesx1*, encodes a pituitary transcription factor whose mutations are associated with septo-optic dysplasia.[225]

Rieger's Syndrome

A homeodomain gene that is transcribed as two alternately spliced mRNAs that encode for two separate proteins, *Ptx2a* and *Ptx2b*, is a candidate gene for Rieger's syndrome, an autosomal dominant disorder with variable craniofacial, dental, eye, and pituitary anomalies.[227]

Lhx3

Combined pituitary hormone deficiency has been linked to missense mutations in the *Lhx3* gene, which encodes a member of the LIM class of homeodomain proteins.[222,228] Homozygous mutations in *Lhx3* in members of two unrelated consanguineous families were associated with deficiencies of multiple pituitary hormones except ACTH and a rigid cervical spine.[228]

Gonadal Dysfunction in Nutritional Disorders

The Dutch Hunger Winter

Stein and Susser recorded the effects of food scarcity during the German occupation of the Netherlands between October 1944 and May 1945.[54,55] During the German siege, food supplies in certain Dutch cities (famine cities, Fig. 18–9) were curtailed substantially. In some adjacent cities, food supplies were not curtailed by the Germans; Susser and Stein used them as control cities.[54,55] In the famine cities, 50% of women experienced amenorrhea, and the conception rate dropped to about 53% of that observed in control cities.[54,55] The famine cities also witnessed an increase in rates of perinatal mortality, congenital malformations, schizophrenia, and obesity.[54,55]

Weight Change and Fertility in !Kung San of Botswana

The anthropological studies of the !Kung San of Botswana, a tribe of hunter-gatherers until the 1970s, illustrate vividly the relationship of body weight and fertility.[56,57] The body weight of the men and women in the tribe varies substantially throughout the year depending upon the availability of food. In the summer months, the food supply is more abundant and the body weight increases; the number of births in the tribe peaks about 9 months after the peak of body weight (Fig. 18–10),[56,57] illustrating how food availability affects fertility patterns in nature.

Delayed Onset of Menses in Ballet Dancers

The onset and progression of puberty in girls are markedly affected by exercise training and energy drain. Menarche is delayed in ballet dancers compared with normal controls (onset of menarche 15.4 years in ballet dancers vs. 12.6 years in normal controls).[229-231] Periods of rest or reduction in exercise intensity due to injury are associated with rapid sexual development and the resumption of menses.[229-231] Although breast development and menarche are delayed in ballet dancers, the development of pubic hair is not affected, consistent with the proposal that separate mechanisms regulate the onset of adrenarche and menarche. Although ballet dancers have lower body weight and body fat than age-matched controls, we do not know whether the resetting of the hypothalamic GnRH pulse generator in ballet dancers is due to energy drain, low body weight, or low body fat.[231]

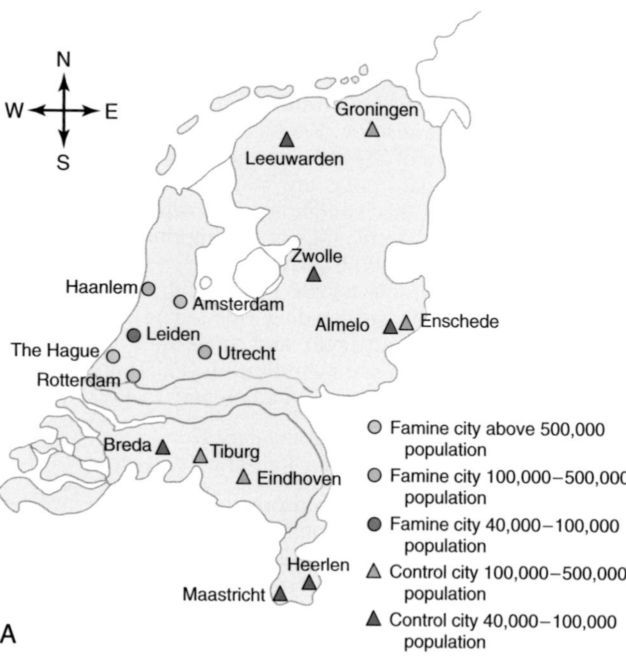

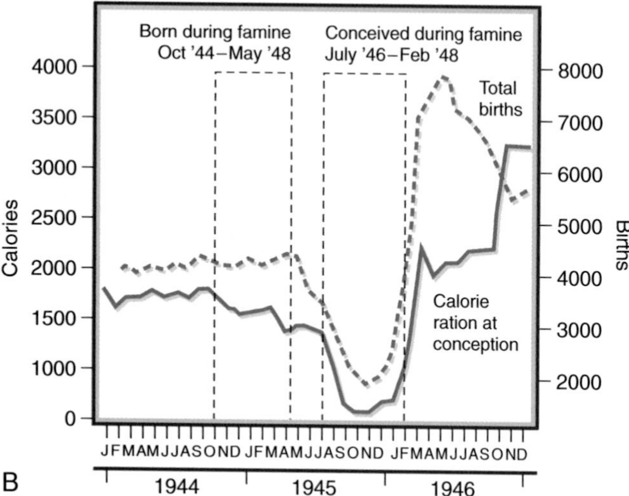

Figure 18–9 ▪ In 1944-1945, the German Army laid siege to the Netherlands and curtailed food supplies to several Dutch cities. Susser and Stein recorded the nutritional intake and health consequences of energy deprivation at a population level in the cities experiencing famine conditions (famine cities, *upper panel*). Several adjacent cities that cooperated with the Germans and did not experience food shortages served as control cities. The *lower panel* shows the average caloric intake and the number of live births. (Reproduced from Stein Z, Susser M. Fertility, fecundity, famine: food rations in the Dutch famine 1944/5 have a causal relation to fertility, and probably to fecundity. Hum Biol 1975;47:131-154; Stein Z, Susser M. The Dutch famine, 1944-1945, and the reproductive process. I. Effects of six indices at birth. Pediatr Res 1975;9:70-76.)

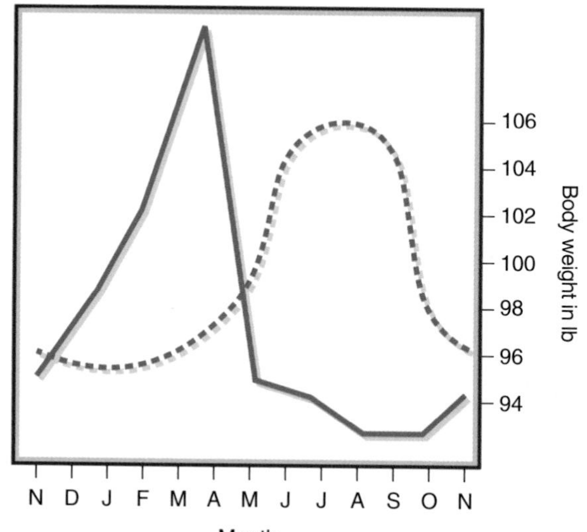

Figure 18–10 ▪ Fertility regulation and body weight in relation to seasonal changes in energy intake in the !Kung San of Botswana. The members of the San tribe were hunter gatherers until 30 years ago, when these studies were conducted. During the spring and summer, food supply was more abundant than in winter. Accordingly, the body weight peaked in late summer. The number of births in the tribe was associated with the body weight after adjustment for the 9-month gestation period. (Adapted from van der Walt LA, Wilmsen EN, Jenkins T. Unusual sex hormone patterns among desert-dwelling hunter-gatherers. J Clin Endocrinol Metab 1978;46:658-663; and van der Walt LA, Wilmsen EN, Levin J, Jenkins T. Endocrine studies on the San ("bushmen") of Botswana. S Afr Med J 1977;52:230-232.)

Frisch[52,62] has proposed that achievement of a minimum fat-to–body mass ratio (approximately 17% fat per body mass) is necessary for triggering the onset of menarche. However, some investigators have questioned whether body fat is the critical determinant of the onset of puberty,[232] because eumenorrheic and amenorrheic athletes do not differ in their body composition.[233]

Reproductive Dysfunction and Hypogonadotropic Hypogonadism in Athletes

There is a high prevalence of amenorrhea, anovulatory cycles, and other menstrual irregularities in adult female athletes, particularly, long-distance runners, dancers, and swimmers.[230] The athletes tend to weigh less and have lower body fat percentage than age-matched healthy controls.[63] In long-distance runners, the number of miles run each week correlates with the degree of menstrual dysfunction. The women athletes typically exhibit hypogonadotropic hypogonadism, presumably due to an acquired hypothalamic GnRH deficiency.[234,235] Some, but not all, female athletes with hypothalamic amenorrhea respond to pulsatile GnRH administration, suggesting that additional pathophysiologic mechanisms may be operative.

Frisch has hypothesized that maintenance of normal reproductive function in women requires a certain minimum fat-to–body mass ratio.[52] Body fat plays an important role in estrogen production and metabolism. Testosterone and androstenedione are converted to estrogens by CYP19 aromatase in adipocytes. Excessively lean women such as marathon runners or those suffering from anorexia nervosa produce a greater amount of catechol estrogens than women with a greater percent of body fat. Catechol estrogens tend to have less estrogenic activity than noncatechol estrogens such as estradiol. Also, there is an inverse relationship between percent body fat and sex hormone–binding globulin concentrations. Therefore, alterations in SHBG concentrations might affect estrogen metabolism and clearance in lean women.

Female athletes have a lower prevalence of breast cancer and other estrogen-dependent reproductive neoplasms than nonathlete controls, presumably due to decreased estrogen exposure.[236-241]

Whereas abnormalities of GnRH secretion and menstrual function are well documented in female athletes, similar reproductive abnormalities have not been widely reported in male athletes. Clinically important hypogonadism is uncommon in male endurance athletes. Serum testosterone and LH concentrations are usually normal or low normal in male endurance athletes.[242] In one study, the frequency and amplitude of LH pulses were significantly lower in runners than in age-matched controls,[243] even though mean plasma LH, FSH, and testosterone concentrations were not significantly different between the two groups. At all doses of GnRH, the response of LH to GnRH was lower in the runners than in the controls.[243] These data indicate that male marathon runners also exhibit perturbations of the hypothalamic GnRH pulse generator, although clinically overt androgen deficiency is less common in male runners than in female runners.[243]

Hypogonadotropic Hypogonadism in Patients with Eating Disorders

Anorexia nervosa, a disorder characterized by distortion of body image and self-induced weight loss, is associated with prepubertal patterns of LH and FSH secretion in which both LH and FSH are low and respond poorly to GnRH stimulation.[60,67,244] Refeeding and restoration of body weight are associated with normalization of pulsatile LH and FSH secretion,[60] illustrating the correlation between energy balance, body weight, and reproductive function. Variants of eating disorders such as bulemia nervosa and mild forms of self-induced dieting are common in young women and may be missed unless the physician maintains a high index of suspicion.

The Effects of Experimental Caloric Deprivation on Reproductive Function in Young Men: The Minnesota Experiment

In the late 1940s, Ancel Keys and coworkers studied human starvation in a historic experiment in which 32 young men volunteered to live on the campus of the University of Minnesota and consume a diet providing approximately 1600 kcal per day, about two thirds of their normal energy requirement (Fig. 18–11).[245,246] The volunteers lost an average of 23% of their initial body weight, more than 70% of body fat and 24% of lean tissue. Keys's group found that a decrease in caloric intake and subsequent weight loss first caused a loss of libido.[246] Continued weight loss resulted in a reduction of prostate fluid and reduced sperm motility. Sperm production was reduced when weight loss approached approximately 25%.[246] Weight gain restored reproductive function in these volunteers.[246]

Reproductive Dysfunction and Endocrine Abnormalities in Obesity

Obesity is associated with a spectrum of endocrine alterations, including changes in the plasma levels, secretion patterns, and clearance rates of circulating sex steroid hormones. In a majority of obese men with mild to moderate obesity, the alterations in total testosterone levels are due to changes in circulating levels of SHBG.[247-250] Because SHBG levels decrease in inverse proportion to the degree of obesity, serum total testosterone levels decrease as body weight increases.[249] Serum free testos-

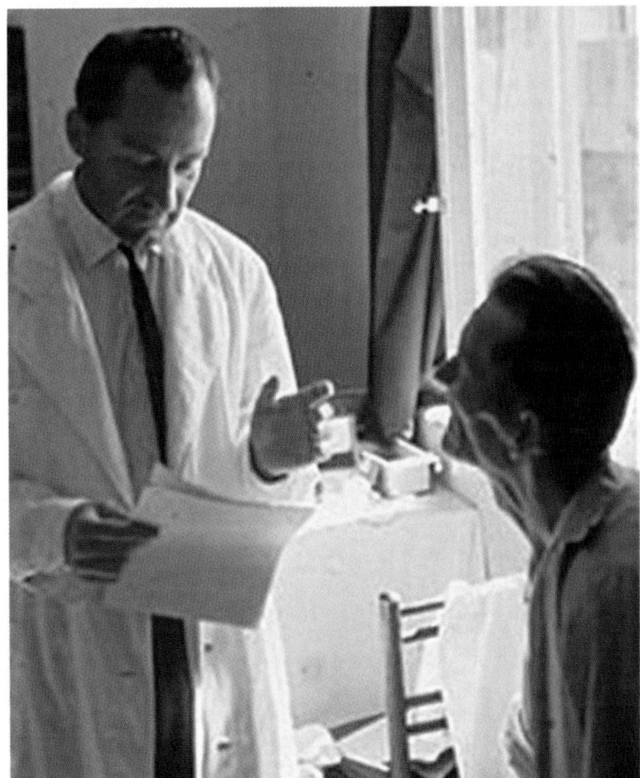

Figure 18–11 ▪ Ancel Keys with one of the volunteers in his study. In the late 1940s, Ancel Keys and coworkers studied the effects of caloric restriction in a historic experiment in which 32 young men volunteered to live on the campus of the University of Minnesota and consume a diet providing approximately two thirds of their normal energy requirement. The volunteers lost an average of 23% of their initial body weight, more than 70% of body fat, and 24% of lean tissue.

terone levels, measured by equilibrium dialysis or as non-SHBG bound testosterone, however, remain within the normal range in a large majority of men with mild to moderate obesity.[249,251]

Lower SHBG levels in obese men have been attributed in part to the hyperinsulinemia associated with obesity.[252-254] Obesity and weight gain are associated with higher insulin levels, which suppress hepatic SHBG production.[255] In contrast, aging and chronic inflammatory conditions are associated with higher SHBG levels.[158,160,256,257] Thus, in obese middle-aged and older men, the effects of adiposity are attenuated by those of age and illness.

A subpopulation of massively obese men may have a defect in the hypothalamic-pituitary axis, as suggested by low free testosterone in the absence of elevated gonadotrophins.[258] Serum estradiol levels may be higher in obese men as compared to healthy, nonobese controls, because of aromatization of testosterone to estradiol in the fat cells.[259,260] Researchers have speculated that very high estrogen levels in massively obese men might suppress GnRH and gonadotropin secretion.[258] Testosterone response to hCG stimulation, an LH-like hormone, is normal in most obese men, indicating normal testicular reserve and function.[261] Weight loss is associated with a reversal of many of these abnormalities including an increase in serum total and free testosterone levels and a decrease in estradiol levels.

A number of congenital hypothalamic syndromes such as the multiple lentigenes syndrome, Laurence-Moon and Bardet-Biedl syndromes, Cohen's syndrome, Borjeson-Forssman-Lehmann syndrome, congenital ichthyosis, Rud's syndrome, cerebellar ataxia, optico-septal dysplasia, and Möbius's syndrome are associated with obesity and hypogonadotropic hypogonadism. The pathophysiology of hypogonadotropic hypogonadism in these disorders is not known, and the diagnosis is made by recognizing the specific somatic abnormalities associated with these syndromes.[181]

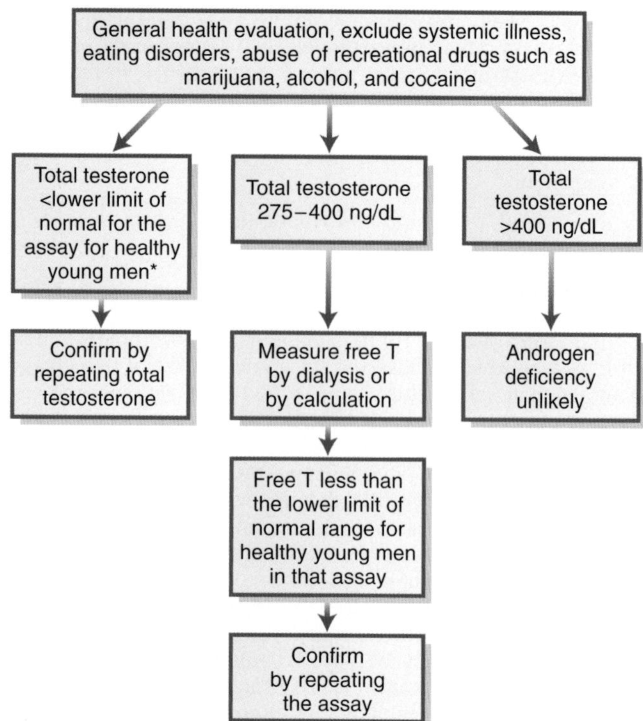

Figure 18–12 ■ Diagnostic work-up of men with suspected androgen deficiency. The reference limits for testosterone assays vary with the type of assay and the laboratory. Therefore, use assay and laboratory-specific reference limits. T, testosterone. (Modified from Bhasin S, Cunningham GR, Hayes FJ, et al. Testosterone therapy in adult men with androgen deficiency syndromes: an endocrine society clinical practice guideline. J Clin Endocrinol Metab 2006;91:1995-2010.)

Diagnosis of Androgen Deficiency

The diagnosis of androgen deficiency proceeds in three steps (Fig. 18–12). The first step includes general health evaluation to ascertain signs and symptoms of androgen deficiency and exclude systemic illness, eating disorders, and lifestyle problems such as excessive exercise or abuse of drugs such as ethanol, marijuana, and opiates. The second step is the measurement of total testosterone level, preferably in an early morning blood sample, using a reliable assay. The third step is measurement of LH level in those deemed androgen deficient to determine whether the defect resides at the testicular level or at the hypothalamic-pituitary site.

Clinical Evaluation of Men Suspected of Androgen Deficiency

An expert panel of the Endocrine Society has advised that the diagnosis of androgen deficiency should only be made in men with characteristic symptoms and signs and unequivocally low testosterone levels.[94] The panel also advised that the diagnosis of androgen deficiency should not be made during an acute or subacute illness.[94]

The symptoms and signs of androgen deficiency are nonspecific and are modified by the age of onset, the severity and duration of androgen deficiency, comorbid illnesses, androgen sensitivity, and previous testosterone therapy.[94] If androgen deficiency has its onset before a patient has completed pubertal development, it often appears as delayed or incomplete sexual development and eunuchoidal proportions (span greater than height by more than 2 cm). Patients with prepubertal onset of androgen deficiency also retain their high-pitched voice and do not experience the temporal recession of hair with advancing age. In men in whom androgen deficiency develops after completion of pubertal maturation, symptoms of androgen deficiency include reduced sexual desire and activity, decreased spontaneous erections, loss of body hair and reduced frequency of shaving, infertility, reduced muscle bulk and strength, hot flushes and sweats, height loss due to atraumatic fracture, small or shrinking testes, and breast enlargement or tenderness. Less-specific symptoms include decreased energy, motivation, and initiative; sad or blue feelings, depressed mood, dysthymia; poor concentration and memory; sleep disturbance and increased sleepiness; increased body fat; and diminished physical or work capacity. In older men, there may be a background of nonspecific aging-associated symptoms.

The threshold testosterone level below which symptoms and signs occur is not known. In the European Male Aging Study, a population-based prospective cohort study of 3369 men recruited from eight European countries, decreased morning erections, decreased sexual desire, erectile dysfunction, and low physical activity had the best association with low testosterone levels.[262] Physical and sexual symptoms are likely to provide greater specificity than psychological symptoms.[262]

Laboratory Evaluation

Measurement of serum total testosterone level, preferably in an early morning specimen, using a reliable assay is crucial to the diagnosis of androgen deficiency (see Fig. 18–12). Total testosterone concentrations, representing the sum of bound and unbound testosterone, are affected by the pulsatile, circadian, and circannual rhythms of testosterone secretion, assay variability, and prevalent SHBG concentrations.[94,263] Testosterone levels are the highest in the morning hours after waking and are lower during the evening hours.[257,264] Therefore, testosterone concentrations should be measured preferably in the morning.

Total testosterone concentrations are affected by changes in SHBG concentrations due to aging, systemic illness, obesity, thyroid hormones, and by many drugs, including testosterone.[18,265] Conditions associated with decreased SHBG concentrations include obesity, the nephrotic syndrome, hypothyroidism, and use of glucocorticoids, progestins, and androgenic steroids.[265] In contrast, aging, hepatic cirrhosis, hyperthyroidism, estrogens, and HIV infection and many systemic illnesses are associated with increased SHBG concentrations.

Measurements of Total and Free Testosterone Concentrations

Total testosterone concentrations usually are measured by radioimmunoassay, immunometric assays, or by liquid chromatography tandem mass spectrometry (LC-MS/MS). Historically, measurements of serum testosterone concentrations involved extraction by organic solvents, separation of testosterone from cross-reacting steroids by chromatography, and then analysis of testosterone concentrations. However, in recent years, to achieve high throughput and automation, most commercial and many research laboratories eliminated the extraction and chromatographic separation steps. These direct, automated radioimmunoassays and immunometric assays have lacked accuracy in the low range of testosterone concentrations that are prevalent in women and some androgen-deficient men.[266] The normative ranges vary across different assays, limiting comparison of data obtained from different laboratories. However, with the use of appropriate assay-specific normative ranges, most assays can distinguish eugonadal and hypogonadal men.[266] LC-MS/MS, widely believed to be the gold standard for measuring sex steroids, is now becoming increasingly available and is poised to become the standard method for measuring sex steroid concentrations in plasma.

Free or unbound testosterone, representing 0.5% to 3% of circulating testosterone, is measured typically by equilibrium dialysis, considered the gold standard. A substantial body of data supports the view that albumin-bound testosterone can dissociate at the tissue level and become bioavailable in some organ systems.[267] Bioavailable testosterone levels are measured by the ammonium sulfate precipitation method, which precipitates SHBG and SHBG-bound testosterone, leaving unbound and albumin-bound testosterone in the supernate (see Fig. 18–2). However, equilibrium dialysis and ammonium sulfate methods are technically challenging and are not widely available in hospital laboratories. Free and bioavailable testosterone concentrations also can be calculated from total testosterone and SHBG concentrations using validated mass action equations.[268]

Algorithms for calculating free and bioavailable testosterone concentrations from total testosterone, albumin, and SHBG concentrations are available on the Internet (www.issam.ch and www.him-link.com). Because SHBG and total testosterone concentrations can be measured more readily in many laboratories than free and bioavailable testosterone concentrations, the use of calculated free testosterone concentrations provides a convenient and reasonable alternative. The tracer analogue displacement assays that are available in many hospital laboratories are inaccurate, and their use is not recommended.[269]

Further Evaluation of Men Deemed Androgen Deficient

In men with androgen deficiency that is diagnosed based on signs and symptoms and low testosterone level, measurements of LH and FSH levels can help determine whether the defect is at the testicular level or the hypothalamic-pituitary level (Fig. 18–13). Men with primary testicular failure, as indicated by elevated LH and FSH and low testosterone levels, should undergo a karyotype analysis to exclude Klinefelter's syndrome, a common cause of primary testicular failure.

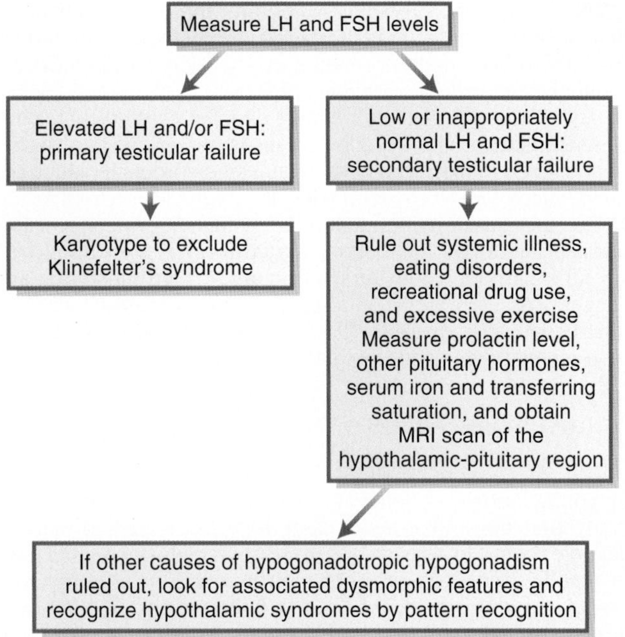
Measure LH and FSH levels
Elevated LH and/or FSH: primary testicular failure
Low or inappropriately normal LH and FSH: secondary testicular failure
Karyotype to exclude Klinefelter's syndrome
Rule out systemic illness, eating disorders, recreational drug use, and excessive exercise Measure prolactin level, other pituitary hormones, serum iron and transferring saturation, and obtain MRI scan of the hypothalamic-pituitary region
If other causes of hypogonadotropic hypogonadism ruled out, look for associated dysmorphic features and recognize hypothalamic syndromes by pattern recognition

Figure 18–13 ▪ Further evaluation of men deemed androgen deficient. FSH, follicle-stimulating hormone; LH, luteinizing hormone.

Men with secondary hypogonadism need further individualized evaluation by measurements of serum prolactin levels, other pituitary hormones, serum iron and transferrin saturation and by MRI scan to exclude hyperprolactinemia, other pituitary hormone deficiencies, hemochromatosis, and space-occupying lesions of the hypothalamus and pituitary. The cost effectiveness of such a diagnostic approach is unknown, because in middle-aged and older men with secondary hypogonadism, the percentage of men who have detectable space-occupying lesions of the hypothalamic-pituitary region is small. The diagnostic yield can be improved by limiting the pituitary workup to men with serum testosterone levels less than 150 ng/dL, panhypopituitarism, hyperprolactinemia, and tumor mass effect, as indicated by headaches or visual field defects.[94] In studies of men presenting with sexual dysfunction and low testosterone levels, the overall prevalence of hypothalamic pituitary space-occupying lesions was low; furthermore, in these studies, men with space-occupying lesions of the hypothalamic-pituitary site had serum testosterone less than 150 ng/dL.[270,271]

Screening and Case Finding

Screening refers to identifying unrecognized disease or defect by using tests or procedures that can be applied rapidly at a population level. In contrast, *case finding* uses procedures to identify existing but previously unsuspected disease that may be unrelated to the chief complaints in a patient seeking medical care. The Endocrine Society expert panel concluded that there was insufficient evidence to justify screening of general population for androgen deficiency.[94] Androgen deficiency does not meet the necessary criteria for population screening because of the lack of data on the public health impact of androgen deficiency. Furthermore, the performance characteristics of the available screening instruments—the Androgen Deficiency in Aging Male (ADAM),[272] the Massachusetts Male Aging Study (MMAS) Scale,[273] and the Aging Males' Symptom Scale

(AMS)[274]—and the predictive value and the cost effectiveness of screening—strategies in the general population are unknown. Also, there is limited information on the long-term health consequences of androgen deficiency.

The Endocrine Society's expert panel suggested that "clinicians consider case detection by measurement of total testosterone levels in men with certain clinical disorders in which the prevalence of low testosterone levels is high or for whom testosterone therapy is recommended".[94] A high prevalence of low testosterone levels has been reported in men presenting with sexual dysfunction, low trauma fracture,[275,276] HIV infection and weight loss,[127-129,132,277-279] end stage renal disease,[280] chronic obstructive lung disease,[281-283] and diabetes mellitus[284] and in men receiving glucocorticoids[285] or opioids.[171,172,176]

Testosterone Therapy in Androgen-Deficient Men

In young androgen-deficient men, testosterone therapy has many benefits and is associated with a low risk of serious adverse events. In a systematic review of mostly open-label trials in healthy androgen-deficient men, testosterone therapy was associated with significant gains in fat-free mass, maximal voluntary strength, and vertebral bone mineral density, as well as a significant decrease in whole body fat mass.[131]

Testosterone therapy improves sexual activity scores and sexual desire.[286-289] Testosterone administration affects many domains of sexual function: it increases the frequency of spontaneous sexual thoughts and fantasies,[288] improves attentiveness to erotic stimuli,[290] and increases the frequency and duration of nocturnal penile erections.[291] Testosterone therapy does not alter the erectile response to visual erotic stimulus[288] or frequency of orgasms in hypogonadal men,[94] although it increases the volume of the ejaculate. In open-label trials, testosterone therapy has been reported to improve positive aspects of mood and reduce negative aspects of mood[292]; randomized clinical trials data on the effects of testosterone therapy on mood are limited and have not shown significantly greater improvements in mood with testosterone therapy than with placebo.[287]

Anecdotally, androgen-deficient men report improvement in sense of well-being and energy after initiation of testosterone therapy. Some studies have reported small and inconsistent effects on visuospatial cognition and verbal memory and verbal fluency.[293,294] Studies of the effects of testosterone therapy on insulin sensitivity have yielded conflicting results.[295-298] Most studies of testosterone therapy in androgen-deficient men have been open-label studies in men selected solely on the basis of low testosterone levels.

Testosterone Preparations and their Clinical Pharmacology

Testosterone replacement can be administered by using one of several available formulations with appropriate attention to its pharmacokinetics (Tables 18–2 and 18–3).

Injectable Testosterone Esters

The esterification of testosterone at the 17-β hydroxyl position makes the molecule hydrophobic and extends its duration of action. The slow release of testosterone ester from its oily depot in the muscle accounts for its extended duration of action. The longer the side chain, the greater the hydrophobicity of the ester and the greater the duration of action. Thus testosterone enanthate and cypionate, with longer side chains, have longer duration of action than testosterone propionate. De-esterification of testosterone esters occurs quickly in plasma, is not rate limiting, and cannot account for the long duration of action.

Within 24 hours after intramuscular administration of 200-mg testosterone enanthate or cypionate, serum testosterone levels rise into the high normal or supraphysiologic range and then gradually decline into the hypogonadal range over the next 2 weeks.[289,299] A bimonthly regimen of testosterone enanthate or cypionate results in highs and lows in serum testosterone levels that may be associated with changes in patient's mood, sexual desire, and activity and energy level.[289,299] The kinetics of testosterone enanthate and cypionate are similar.[300] Although serum estradiol and DHT concentrations increase during testosterone ester administration, serum estradiol to testosterone and dihydrotestosterone to testosterone ratios remain normal.[289,299] With appropriate monitoring, injectable testosterone esters can be adequately dosed and tolerated and are the least expensive of the available testosterone preparations.

Transdermal Testosterone

Testosterone Gel

Two testosterone gels are available commercially.[287,301-306] Pharmacokinetic studies have demonstrated that 5- to 10-g doses applied daily to the skin can raise and maintain serum total and free testosterone concentrations into the mid-normal range in hypogonadal men.[287,303] Average serum total and free testosterone concentrations are uniform throughout the 24-hour period,[287,305] although there may be considerable variation throughout the day in individual patients. The current recommendations are to start with a 5-g dose and adjust the dose based on serum testosterone levels.

The advantages of the testosterone gel are the ease of application, its invisibility after application, and the flexibility of dosing. The major concern about the use of the gel is the potential for transfer to a sexual partner or to children who come in close contact with the patient. Serum dihydrotestosterone to testosterone concentrations are higher in hypogonadal men treated with the testosterone gel than in eugonadal men. Skin tolerability is good, and the frequency of skin irritation is low.

Transdermal Testosterone Patch

One or two 5-mg nongenital testosterone patches can be applied on the nonscrotal skin.[286,307-309] Serum testosterone and estradiol levels are in the mid-normal range 4 to 12 hours after the patch is applied.[308,309] The nongenital patch produces physiologic levels of serum dihydrotestosterone. One 5-mg patch might not be sufficient to increase serum testosterone concentrations into the mid-normal male range in all hypogonadal men; some patients might need daily administration of two 5-mg patches to achieve the target level.[280] The use of nongenital patches is associated with skin irritation in some patients.

Bioadhesive Buccal Testosterone Tablets

Controlled release, bioadhesive 30-mg testosterone tablets applied every 12 hours to buccal mucosa normalize serum testosterone, dihydrotestosterone, and estradiol levels in hypogonadal men.[310-312] Gum problems are associated with the use of buccal tablets in 16% of treated men.

Testosterone Formulations That Are Not Available in the United States

Testosterone undecanoate, when administered orally in oleic acid, is absorbed preferentially through the lymphatics into systemic circulation and is spared the first-pass degradation in the liver. Doses of 40 to 80 mg given two or three times daily are typically used. However, the clinical responses are variable and suboptimal.[313-321] Serum dihydrotestosterone-to-testosterone ratios are higher in hypogonadal men treated with oral testosterone undecanoate as compared to eugonadal men.[313-321]

TABLE 18–2 CLINICAL PHARMACOLOGY OF SOME TESTOSTERONE FORMULATIONS

Formulation	Regimen	Pharmacokinetic Profile	DHT and Estradiol	Advantages	Disadvantages
Testosterone enanthate or cypionate	100 mg IM weekly or 200 mg IM every 2 weeks	After a single IM injection, serum testosterone levels rise into the supraphysiologic range and then decline gradually into the hypogonadal range by the end of the dosing interval	DHT and estradiol levels rise in proportion to the increase in testosterone levels T:DHT and T:E2 ratios do not change	Corrects symptoms of androgen deficiency Relatively inexpensive, if self-administered Flexibility of dosing	Requires IM injection Peaks and valleys in serum testosterone levels
Nongenital transdermal system	One or two patches, designed to nominally deliver 5 to 10 mg testosterone over 24-hr applied daily on nonpressure areas	Restores serum testosterone, DHT, and E2 levels into the physiologic male range	T:DHT and T:E2 levels are in the physiologic male range	Ease of application, corrects symptoms of androgen deficiency, and mimics the normal diurnal rhythm of testosterone secretion Lesser increase in hemoglobin than injectable esters	Serum testosterone levels in some androgen-deficient men maybe in the low normal range; these men may need application of two patches daily Skin irritation at the application site may be a problem for some patients
Testosterone gel	5 to 10 g testosterone gel containing 50 to 100 mg testosterone should be applied daily	Restores serum testosterone and estradiol levels into the physiologic male range	Serum DHT levels are higher and T:DHT ratios are lower in hypogonadal men treated with the testosterone gel than in healthy eugonadal men	Corrects symptoms of androgen deficiency, provides flexibility of dosing, ease of application, good skin tolerability	Potential of transfer to a female partner or child by direct skin-to-skin contact Moderately high DHT levels
17-α-methyl testosterone	This 17-α-alkylated compound should not be used because of potential for liver toxicity	Orally active			Clinical responses variable; potential for liver toxicity Should not be used to treat androgen deficiency
Buccal bioadhesive testosterone tablets	30 mg controlled release, bioadhesive tablets used twice daily	Absorbed from the buccal mucosa	Normalizes serum testosterone and DHT levels in hypogonadal men	Corrects symptoms of androgen deficiency in healthy, hypogonadal men	Gum-related adverse events in 16% of treated men
Oral testosterone undecanoate*	40 to 80 mg orally two or three times daily with meals	When administered in oleic acid, testosterone undecanoate is absorbed through the lympahtics, bypassing the portal system Considerable variability in the same patient on different days and among patients	High DHT:T ratio	Convenience of oral administration	Not approved in the United States Variable clinical responses, variable serum testosterone levels, high DHT:T ratio
Injectable long-acting testosterone undecanoate in oil*	1000 mg injected IM followed by 1000 mg at 6 weeks, then 1000 mg every 12 weeks	When administered at a dose of 1000 mg IM, serum testosterone levels are maintained in the normal range in a majority of treated men	DHT and estradiol levels rise in proportion to the increase in testosterone levels; T:DHT and T:E2 ratios do not change.	Corrects symptoms of androgen deficiency Requires infrequent administration	Requires IM injection of a large volume (4 mL)
Testosterone pellets	Four to six 200-mg pellets implanted SC	Serum testosterone peaks at 1 month and then sustained in normal range for 4 to 6 months	T:DHT and T:E2 ratios do not change	Corrects symptoms of androgen deficiency	Requires surgical incision for insertions; spontaneous extrusion

*This formulation is available outside the United States, but it is not approved currently by the U.S. Food and Drug Administration.
DHT, dihydrotestosterone; E2, estradiol; T, testosterone.
Reproduced from Bhasin S, Cunningham GR, Hayes FJ, et al. Testosterone therapy in adult men with androgen deficiency syndromes: an Endocrine Society clinical practice guideline. J Clin Endocrinol Metab 2006;91:1995-2010.

TABLE 18–3 SOME RECOMMENDED REGIMENS FOR TESTOSTERONE REPLACEMENT THERAPY

Form	Dosing
IN THE UNITED STATES	
Testosterone enanthate or cypionate	75 to 100 mg administered IM weekly, or 150 to 200 mg administered every 2 weeks
Nongenital testosterone patches	One or two 5-mg patches applied nightly over the skin of the back, thigh, or upper arm, away from pressure areas
Testosterone gel	5 to 10 g applied daily over a covered area of skin
Bioadhesive buccal testosterone tablets	30-mg tablet applied to buccal mucosa bid
OUTSIDE THE UNITED STATES*	
Oral testosterone undecanoate	Typically 40 to 80 mg PO bid or tid with meals
Injectable testosterone undecanoate	Typically 1000 mg IM initially and at 6 wk followed by 1000 mg IM every 12 wk
Testosterone pellets	Typically four to six 200-mg pellets implanted every 4-6 mo

Note: These regimens should be viewed as suggestions for initiating testosterone replacement therapy; dose and regimen should be adjusted based on measurement of serum testosterone levels.

*These regimens are available for clinical use in many countries; physicians in those countries who wish to use these formulations should follow the drug regimens approved in those countries.

Adapted from Bhasin S, Cunningham GR, Hayes FJ, et al. Testosterone therapy in adult men with androgen deficiency syndromes: an endocrine society clinical practice guideline. J Clin Endocrinol Metab 2006;91:1995-2010.

Implants of crystalline testosterone are inserted in the subcutaneous tissue by means of a trocar through a small skin incision. Testosterone is released by surface erosion from the implant and absorbed into the systemic circulation. Four to six 200-mg implants can maintain serum testosterone concentrations in the mid- to high-normal range for up to 6 months.[322-326] The need for skin incision for insertion and removal, spontaneous extrusions, and fibrosis at the site of implant insertion are potential drawbacks of this formulation.

Injectable testosterone undecanoate, when administered in oil, can maintain serum testosterone levels in the normal range for 10 to 12 weeks after its IM injection.[327,328] A typical regimen of testosterone undecanoate employs an initial injection of 1000 mg IM, a second injection of 1000 mg at 6 weeks, and IM injections of 1000 mg every 12 weeks thereafter. The relative advantages of this injectable formulation are its long duration of action and lesser degrees of fluctuations in serum testosterone levels than are observed with testosterone enanthate and cypionate. However, testosterone undecanoate is administered in a large volume of oil that causes patient discomfort.

Orally Administered 17-α Alkylated Testosterone Derivatives

Testosterone is well absorbed after its oral administration but undergoes rapid presystemic metabolism after its oral administration. Therefore, it is not possible to achieve sustained blood levels of testosterone after oral administration of crystalline testosterone. 17-α alkylated derivatives of testosterone are relatively resistant to hepatic degradation and can be given orally; however, because of the potential for hepatotoxicity and the availability of alternative and safer formulations, the use of oral 17-α alkylated testosterone derivatives for testosterone replacement is not recommended.[329,330]

Novel Androgen Formulations

A number of novel androgen formulations with better pharmacokinetics or more selective activity profiles are under development. A biodegradable testosterone microsphere formulation provides physiologic testosterone levels for 10 to 11 weeks.[331,332] Long-acting testosterone esters, testosterone buciclate[333,334] and testosterone undecanoate,[335-340] when injected intramuscularly, can maintain circulating testosterone concentrations in the male range for 7 to 12 weeks. Initial clinical trials have demonstrated the feasibility of administering testosterone by the sublingual or buccal routes. 7-α-Methyl-19-nortestosterone is an androgen that cannot be 5-α reduced; therefore, compared to testosterone, it has relatively greater agonist activity on the muscle and gonadotropin suppression but less activity on the prostate.[341-343]

A number of nonsteroidal selective androgen receptor modulators (SARMs) with tissue selectivity are currently under development. These agents can selectively exert androgen activity on muscle, bone, and sexual function, with minimal action on other tissues such as the prostate or the cardiovascular system.[131,344]

Contraindications to Testosterone Therapy

Testosterone therapy should not be administered to men with metastatic prostate cancer or breast cancer because it can promote the growth of these cancers. Testosterone therapy can worsen preexisting erythrocytosis, untreated severe obstructive sleep apnea, and severe congestive heart failure. Because a prostate nodule, induration, or elevated PSA may be an indication of an unrecognized prostate cancer, men with these conditions should undergo a urologic evaluation before being considered for testosterone therapy. Contraindications are listed in Table 18–4.

We do not know whether testosterone therapy can be administered safely to men who have undergone radical prostatectomy for localized prostate cancer and who are deemed disease-free; some have suggested that testosterone therapy may be administered on an individualized basis to such men provided they have undetectable PSA for more than 2 years.[345-347] However, there are no data from randomized, controlled trials to address this issue, and the published studies included very few patients. Therefore, there are insufficient data to recommend such an approach.

Adverse Events Associated with Testosterone Therapy

The frequency of testosterone-related adverse events in open-label trials of healthy young hypogonadal men has been low.[348] The most common testosterone-related adverse events include erythrocytosis, acne, oily skin, and breast tenderness. Although

TABLE 18–4 CONTRAINDICATIONS TO TESTOSTERONE ADMINISTRATION

VERY HIGH RISK OF SERIOUS ADVERSE OUTCOMES
Metastatic prostate cancer Breast cancer
MODERATE TO HIGH RISK OF ADVERSE OUTCOMES
Undiagnosed prostate nodule or induration Unexplained PSA elevation* Erythrocytosis (hematocrit > 50%) Severe BPH symptoms as indicated by an American Urological Association/International Prostate Symptom Score > 19 Unstable severe CHF (class III or IV)

BPH, benign prostatic hyperplasia; CHF, congestive heart failure; PSA, prostate-specific antigen.
*The baseline PSA level above which testosterone therapy should not be given without a urologic evaluation has been the subject of considerable discussion. An expert panel of the Endocrine Society suggested that testosterone therapy should not be administered to men with baseline PSA level > 3 ng/mL without a urologic evaluation to exclude prostate cancer.
From Bhasin S, Cunningham GR, Hayes FJ, et al. Testosterone therapy in adult men with androgen deficiency syndromes: an Endocrine Society clinical practice guideline. J Clin Endocrinol Metab 2006;91:1995-2010.

gynecomastia and induction or worsening of obstructive sleep apnea have been reported, the frequency of these adverse events during testosterone therapy is low. Adverse events are listed in Table 18–5.

Testosterone Effects on the Risk of Atherosclerotic Heart Disease

The widespread perception that testosterone therapy increases the risk of atherosclerotic heart disease is not supported by the available data. The long-term consequences of testosterone supplementation on the risk of heart disease remain unknown. Although supraphysiologic doses of nonaromatizable androgens commonly employed by recreational body builders and athletes decrease plasma high-density lipoprotein (HDL) cholesterol levels,[349,350] physiologic testosterone replacement in older men has been associated with only a modest or no decrease in plasma HDL cholesterol.[94,351,352] Cross-sectional studies of middle-aged men find a direct, rather than an inverse, relationship between serum testosterone levels and plasma HDL cholesterol concentrations[353-355] and an inverse correlation between testosterone levels and visceral fat volume.[356,357] Lower testosterone levels in men are associated with higher levels of dense low-density lipoprotein (LDL) particles and prothrombotic factors.[354,355]

Open-label testosterone trials of testosterone esters in mostly young, hypogonadal men have reported a small decrease in total cholesterol, plasma HDL cholesterol, and LDL cholesterol.[358] Placebo-controlled studies in older men have demonstrated no significant change in plasma HDL cholesterol levels during long-term testosterone administration.[351,352]

Spontaneous[359] and experimentally induced[360] androgen deficiency is associated with increased fat mass. Testosterone therapy decreases fat mass in older men who have low testosterone levels.[131] Testosterone supplementation of middle-aged men with truncal obesity has been reported to reduce visceral fat volume, serum glucose concentration, and blood pressure and to improve insulin sensitivity,[295,296] although improvements in insulin sensitivity by testosterone administration have not been confirmed in other studies. Surgical castration in rats impairs insulin sensitivity; physiologic testosterone replacement reverses this metabolic derangement.[361] However, high doses of testosterone impair insulin sensitivity in castrated rats. Androgens increase insulin-independent glucose uptake[362] and modulate lipoprotein lipase activity in a region-specific manner.[363]

TABLE 18–5 POTENTIAL ADVERSE EFFECTS OF TESTOSTERONE REPLACEMENT

EVIDENCE OF ASSOCIATION
Erythrocytosis Acne and oily skin Detection of subclinical prostate cancer Growth of metastatic prostate cancer Reduced sperm production and fertility
WEAK EVIDENCE OF ASSOCIATION
Gynecomastia Male-pattern baldness (familial) Worsening of BPH symptoms Growth of breast cancer Induction or worsening of obstructive sleep apnea
FORMULATION-SPECIFIC
Oral Tablets Liver function abnormalities (methyltestosterone) Lowering of HDL cholesterol (methyltestosterone)
Pellet Implants Infection and scarring expulsion of pellet
Intramuscular Injections of Testosterone Enanthate or Cypionate Fluctuation in mood or libido Pain at injection site Erythrocytosis (esp. older patients)
Transdermal Patches Skin reactions at application site
Transdermal Gel Potential risk for testosterone transference to partner (need to remind patient to cover application sites with a clothing and to wash skin and hands with soap prior to having skin-to-skin contact with another person)
Buccal Tablets Alterations in taste Irritation of gums

BPH, benign prostatic hyperplasia; HDL, high-density lipoprotein.
From Bhasin S, Cunningham GR, Hayes FJ, et al. Testosterone therapy in adult men with androgen deficiency syndromes: an endocrine society clinical practice guideline. J Clin Endocrinol Metab 2006;91:1995-2010.

Of the 30 cross-sectional studies reviewed by Alexandersen,[364] 18 reported lower testosterone levels in men with coronary heart disease, 11 found similar testosterone levels in controls and men with coronary artery disease and 1 found higher levels of DHEA sulfate. Prospective studies have failed to reveal an association of total testosterone levels and onset of coronary disease.[365,366]

One trial of oral testosterone undecanoate administration reported improvements in angina pectoris in men with coronary heart disease.[367] Testosterone infusion acutely improves coronary blood flow in a canine model.[166-169] The vasodilative effects of testosterone are mediated through L-type calcium channels.[368,369] Androgen-deficient men have impaired vascular reactivity,[370] but the effects of testosterone therapy on vascular reactivity in androgen-deficient men have been inconsistent in clinical trials, some studies showing worsening of vascular reactivity after testosterone therapy.[370-372] In a rodent model of insulin resistance, fructose feeding results in the development of insulin resistance and hypertension.[373] In these fructose-fed rats, gonadectomy prevents worsening of blood pressure; testosterone therapy was necessary for the development of hypertension in fructose-fed rats.[373]

In a mouse model of atherosclerosis that is LDL-receptor deficient,[173] surgical castration accelerates and testosterone therapy retards the progression of atherosclerosis. The magnitude of testosterone effect on atherosclerosis progression is similar to that observed with estrogen administration. Favorable effects of testosterone on atherosclerosis in this mouse model are antagonized by concomitant administration of a CYP19 aromatase inhibitor, suggesting that testosterone effects are mediated through its conversion to estrogen in the vessel wall.[374] Testosterone effects in retarding atherosclerosis progression are independent of plasma lipids.[374] These beneficial effects of testosterone in the LDL receptor null mouse have not been observed consistently in other experimental models.[375]

These data suggest that both supraphysiologic and subphysiologic circulating concentrations of testosterone levels are associated with increased cardiovascular risk, although the evidence is far from conclusive.[366] The effects of testosterone therapy on atherosclerosis progression and cardiovascular event rates have not been examined in men in randomized clinical trials and are important because even small changes in incidence rates of cardiovascular disease could have substantial public health impact.

Testosterone and Prostate Cancer Risk

There is no evidence that testosterone therapy causes prostate cancer.[376] Also, there is no consistent relationship between endogenous serum testosterone levels and the risk of prostate cancer. However, there are a number of areas of concern.

Many older men harbor microscopic foci of cancer in their prostates. We do not know whether testosterone therapy will make these subclinical foci of cancer grow and become clinically overt.

Prostate cancer is a common androgen-dependent tumor, and androgen administration therapy might promote growth of metastatic prostate cancer.[377,378] Therefore, testosterone therapy is contraindicated in men with metastatic prostate cancer.

In addition, Morgentaler and colleagues[379] have reported a high prevalence of biopsy-detectable prostate cancer in men with low total or free testosterone levels despite normal PSA levels and digital rectal examination. However, this study did not have a control group, and we do not know whether sextant biopsies of age-matched controls with normal testosterone levels would yield a similarly high incidence of biopsy-detectable cancer.

Serum PSA levels are lower in testosterone-deficient men and are restored to normal following testosterone therapy.[380,381] However, serum PSA levels do not increase progressively in healthy hypogonadal men with replacement doses of testosterone. In two placebo-controlled trials of testosterone administration in older men, the change in serum PSA levels over 3 years was not significantly different between placebo- and testosterone-treated men.[382,383]

The increase in PSA levels during testosterone therapy might trigger evaluation and biopsy in some patients.[376] More intensive PSA screening and follow-up of men receiving testosterone replacement might lead to increased number of prostate biopsies and detection of subclinical prostate cancers that would have otherwise remained undetected. Testosterone-treated men are at increased risk for prostate biopsy and detection of increased number of prostate events.[348]

Serum PSA levels tend to fluctuate when measured repeatedly in the same patient over time[376] because of interassay variability, age effects, and other biologic factors. Therefore, when serum PSA levels in androgen-deficient men on testosterone replacement therapy show a change from a previously measured value, the clinician has to decide whether the change warrants detailed evaluation of the patient for prostate cancer or whether it is simply due to test-to-test variability in PSA measurement.

Testosterone replacement can be administered safely to men with benign prostatic hypertrophy who have mild to moderate symptom scores. The severity of symptoms associated with benign prostatic hypertrophy can be assessed by using the International Prostate Symptom Score (IPSS)/American Urological Association (AUA) Symptom questionnaire. Androgen deficiency is associated with decreased prostate volume, and androgen replacement increases prostate volumes to those in age-matched controls.[380,381] In patients with preexisting severe symptoms of benign prostatic hypertrophy, even small increases in prostate volume during testosterone administration can exacerbate obstructive symptoms. In these men, testosterone either should not be administered or should be administered with careful monitoring of obstructive symptoms.

Testosterone Therapy and Erythrocytosis

Testosterone therapy increases red cell mass in a dose-dependent manner,[348] presumably through its effects on erythropoietin and stem cell proliferation.[384,385] Therefore, testosterone replacement should not be administered to men with baseline hematocrit of 50% or greater without appropriate evaluation and treatment of erythrocytosis. Administration of testosterone to androgen-deficient young men is typically associated with a small increase in hemoglobin levels. Clinically significant erythrocytosis is uncommon in young hypogonadal men during testosterone replacement therapy, but it can occur in men with sleep apnea, significant smoking history, or chronic obstructive lung disease.

Increase in hemoglobin during testosterone therapy is greater in older men than in young men.[386] Erythrocytosis is the most common drug-related adverse event in published testosterone trials of middle-aged and older men and is the most common cause of discontinuing treatment.[348] Testosterone therapy by means of a transdermal system has been reported to produce a lesser increase in hemoglobin levels than that associated with testosterone esters,[309] presumably because typical regimens of transdermal testosterone systems deliver a smaller dose of testosterone than testosterone esters.

Testosterone therapy should be discontinued when hematocrit is greater than 54%, and therapy should be withheld until hematocrit has fallen to a safe level (<50%), at which time testosterone therapy may be reinitiated at a lower dose.

Testosterone is aromatized to estradiol in many peripheral tissues and can exacerbate breast cancer; therefore, testosterone should not be administered to men with breast cancer.

Testosterone can induce sleep apnea or exacerbate preexisting sleep apnea because of its neuromuscular effects on the upper airway and should not be given to men with severe obstructive sleep apnea without appropriate evaluation and treatment of sleep apnea.[387,388] Men with sleep apnea might have low testosterone levels.[389]

Testosterone administration can transiently induce salt and water retention; therefore, testosterone should not be given or should be given with great caution to patients with severe congestive heart failure and class IV symptoms.

Monitoring of Testosterone Therapy

The Endocrine Society guideline suggests that the men receiving testosterone therapy should be followed at 3 months after starting therapy and then annually thereafter using a standardized monitoring plan to determine whether therapy is effective in correcting symptoms and findings associated with testosterone deficiency and to facilitate early detection of adverse events.[94] Testosterone therapy should aim to raise serum testosterone levels into the mid-normal range. Even in men with primary testicular failure, serum LH levels are not normalized by testosterone doses that restore sexual function and induce clinical improvements. Therefore, serum LH levels have not been used to monitor adequacy of testosterone therapy in androgen-deficient men. Hemoglobin and hematocrit, PSA, and digital prostate examinations should be followed at regular intervals (Table 18–6) in addition to general health evaluation as dictated by community standards.

The most difficult issue in the following hypogonadal men receiving testosterone replacement relates to the criteria that should be used to guide decision to perform prostate biopsy (Table 18– 7). There is considerable variability in PSA measurements from test to test. Some of this variability is due to the inherent assay variability, and some is due to unknown factors.[390-400] Variability can be even greater if measurements are performed in different laboratories that use dissimilar assays.[390-400] The 90% confidence limits for the change in PSA levels between two tests performed 3 to 6 months apart in the placebo-treated men in a study of finasteride in men with benign prostatic hyperplasia was 1.4 ng/mL.[401] Therefore, a change of greater than 1.4 ng/mL in samples drawn 3 to 6 months apart has been used as a criterion for seeking urologic evaluation in some clinical trials of finasteride.[402] As a rough approximation, the interassay coefficient of variation of PSA assays on average has been reported to be 15%.[403,404] The coefficient of variation of the PSA assay should be taken into account when evaluating the change in PSA between samples drawn at different times or when interpreting the PSA velocity.

The administration of replacement doses of testosterone to androgen-deficient men increases serum PSA levels. In a systematic review, the average PSA increase after initiation of testosterone therapy in young, hypogonadal men was 0.3 ng/mL and in older men with low or low normal testosterone levels it was 0.44 ng/mL.[376] The increase in PSA levels after testosterone supplementation in androgen-deficient men generally is less than 0.5 ng/mL, and increments in excess of 1.0 ng/mL over a 3- to 6-month period are unusual. Administration of testosterone to men with baseline PSA levels between 2.5 and 4.0 ng/mL causes PSA levels to exceed 4.0 ng/mL in some men. Increases in PSA levels to greater than 4 ng/mL will trigger a urologic consultation, and many of these men will undergo prostate biopsies, thereby increasing the likelihood of detecting prostatic disease.

In patients in whom sequential PSA measurements are available for more than 2 years, Carter and colleagues[391,397,405,406] have

TABLE 18–6 MONITORING OF MEN RECEIVING TESTOSTERONE THERAPY

Evaluate the patient 3 months after treatment starts and then annually to assess whether symptoms responded to treatment and whether the patient is suffering from any adverse effects.

Monitor testosterone levels 2 or 3 months after initiating testosterone therapy:

- The therapy should aim to raise serum testosterone levels into the mid-normal range.
- Injectable testosterone enanthate or cypionate: Measure serum testosterone levels midway between injections. If testosterone is >700 ng/dL or <350 ng/dL, adjust dose or frequency.
- Transdermal patch: Assess testosterone levels 3 to 12 hr after application of the patch; adjust dose to achieve testosterone levels in the mid-normal range.
- Buccal testosterone bioadhesive tablet: Assess levels immediately before or after application of fresh system.
- Transdermal gel: Assess testosterone level any time after patient has been on treatment for at least 1 week; adjust dose to achieve serum testosterone levels in the mid-normal range.
- Oral testosterone undecanoate*: Monitor serum testosterone levels 3 to 5 hr after ingestion.
- Injectable testosterone undecanoate*: Measure serum testosterone level just prior to each subsequent injection and adjust the dosing interval to maintain serum testosterone in mid-normal range.

Check hematocrit at baseline, at 3 months, and then annually. If hematocrit is > 54%, stop therapy until hematocrit decreases to a safe level; evaluate the patient for hypoxia and sleep apnea; reinitiate therapy with a reduced dose.

Measure bone mineral density of lumbar spine and/or femoral neck after 1 to 2 years of testosterone therapy in hypogonadal men with osteoporosis or low trauma fracture, consistent with regional standard of care.

Perform digital rectal examination and check PSA level before initiating treatment, at 3 months, and then in accordance with guidelines for prostate cancer screening depending on the age and race of the patient.

Evaluate formulation-specific adverse effects at each visit:

- Buccal testosterone tablets: Inquire about alterations in taste and examine the gums and oral mucosa for irritation.
- Injectable testosterone esters: Ask about fluctuations in mood or libido.
- Testosterone patches: Look for skin reaction at the application site.
- Testosterone gels: Advise patients to cover the application site with a shirt and to wash the skin with soap and water before having skin-to-skin contact, because testosterone gels leave a testosterone residue on the skin that can be transferred to a woman or child who might come in close contact. Serum testosterone levels are maintained when the application site is washed 4 to 6 hours after application of the testosterone gel.

*, not approved for clinical use in the United States; PSA, prostate-specific antigen.

Modified from Bhasin S, Cunningham GR, Hayes FJ, et al. Testosterone therapy in adult men with androgen deficiency syndromes: an endocrine society clinical practice guideline. J Clin Endocrinol Metab 2006;91:1995-2010.

TABLE 18–7 INDICATIONS FOR UROLOGIC CONSULTATION IN MEN RECEIVING TESTOSTERONE THERAPY

Verified serum PSA concentration > 4.0 ng/mL

An increase in serum PSA concentration > 1.4 ng/mL within any 12-month period of testosterone treatment

A PSA velocity of > 0.4 ng/mL/year using the PSA level after 6 months of testosterone administration as the reference (only applicable if PSA data are available for a period > 2 years)

Detection of a prostatic abnormality on digital rectal examination

An AUA or IPSS prostate symptom score of > 19

AUA, American Urological Association; IPSS, international prostate symptom score; PSA, prostate-specific antigen.

From Bhasin S, Cunningham GR, Hayes FJ, et al. Testosterone therapy in adult men with androgen deficiency syndromes: an endocrine society clinical practice guideline. J Clin Endocrinol Metab 2006;91:1995-2010.

proposed the use of PSA velocity criterion to identify men at higher risk for prostate cancer. In the Baltimore Longitudinal Study of Aging, when the baseline PSA was between 4 and 10 ng/mL, a rate of change of greater than 0.75 ng/mL per year in PSA was unusual in men with benign prostatic disease.[391,397,405,406] Because most men receiving testosterone therapy have baseline PSA levels lower than 4.0 ng/mL, the criteria established for baseline PSA values between 4 and 10 ng/mL might not be appropriate for use in testosterone trials or during testosterone therapy.

In a recent analysis of data from the Baltimore Longitudinal Aging Study, Fang and colleagues[407] reported the PSA velocity in men who have baseline PSA less than 4 ng/mL. In these men with initial PSA less than 4 ng/mL, using a threshold for PSA velocity of 0.2 ng/mL per year gave a sensitivity of 52.4% and a specificity of 79.4% for detecting prostate cancer; these findings need further confirmation. However, the considerable test-retest variability in PSA levels should be taken into account when evaluating PSA velocity because thresholds for prostate biopsy that are substantially lower than the test-retest variability would likely result in a large number of false triggers for biopsy.

The use of PSA velocity criterion is likely to be more useful in men in whom PSA data are available over many years so that the PSA change over baseline exceeds the expected interassay variability. Carter[391,397,405,406] has emphasized that PSA velocity should not be used for follow-up periods of less than 2 years. Also, estimation of PSA velocity requires multiple PSA measurements over time. PSA velocity is calculated as the total change in PSA from baseline divided by the time in years. A PSA velocity of greater than 0.2 ng/mL per year does not imply that the patient has prostate cancer, nor should it be used to dictate immediate prostate biopsy; rather, it signifies a higher than average risk for developing prostate cancer during the subsequent decades. Therefore, PSA velocity can be useful during long-term follow up of patients over many years. For periods of less than 3 years, we propose that PSA velocity of greater than 0.4 ng/mL per year should warrant a urologic evaluation and more intensive future surveillance for prostate cancer.[376] For follow-up periods exceeding 3 years, a PSA velocity of greater than 0.2 ng/mL per year is likely associated with a greater than average risk of prostate cancer and should warrant a closer follow-up of the patient. The specificity or sensitivity of these PSA velocity criteria has not been tested in prospective testosterone trials.

Testosterone Therapy in Older Men with Age-Related Decline in Testosterone Levels

A number of cross-sectional epidemiologic studies are in agreement that serum total, free, and bioavailable testosterone levels are lower in older men than in younger men, even after accounting for the potential confounding factors such as time of sampling, concomitant illness and medications, and technical issues related to hormone assays.[159,160,162-164,408] Several longitudinal studies[158,160,161] have confirmed a gradual but progressive decline in serum testosterone concentrations from age 20 to 80 years. The diurnal rhythm of testosterone secretion is dampened in older men.[388] Because SHBG levels are higher in older men than younger men,[409] the age-related decline in free and bioavailable testosterone levels is of a greater magnitude than the decline in total testosterone levels. The age-related changes in testosterone levels are affected by comorbid conditions, adiposity, physical activity, and lifestyle factors, including smoking. Men who gain weight and become obese have a greater rate of decline in total testosterone levels[410]; the greater rates of age-related decline in total but not free testosterone levels in men who become overweight is related mostly to a lesser age-related increase in SHBG.[410]

Association of Low Testosterone Levels with Outcomes

Testosterone levels are associated with a number of clinical outcomes in older men in population-based epidemiologic studies, although these associations are weak. For instance, low bioavailable testosterone concentrations are associated with decreased appendicular skeletal muscle mass[276,411-413] and decreased muscle strength.[414] Total and free testosterone levels are also associated with self-reported physical function, as assessed by physical component score and with physical performance.[415] In a survey of healthy older men,[416] bioavailable testosterone levels were positively correlated with muscle strength and bone mineral density and negatively correlated with fat mass. Non–SHBG-bound estradiol was the best predictor of bone mineral density. In other studies, total testosterone levels are inversely correlated with waist-to-hip ratio and visceral fat mass,[357] although the correlation coefficients are not high, suggesting that there are other important determinants of body composition besides testosterone. After adjusting for age and other covariates, testosterone levels are weakly associated with sexual desire and erectile dysfunction in middle-aged and older men.[262,417]

Two[418,419] out of three epidemiologic studies[418-420] that have examined the relationship between testosterone levels and depressive symptoms have reported no significant correlation between these two variables; one study[420] reported an inverse relationship between bioavailable testosterone levels and scores on Beck's Depression Inventory. In a further analysis of the data from the Massachusetts Male Aging Study, Seidman and colleagues[421] found a significant interaction between testosterone levels, the length of the CAG repeats in the androgen receptor gene, and depression scores.

Several epidemiologic studies have also reported an inverse association between serum free testosterone levels and visceral obesity,[356,357] insulin resistance,[422,423] the metabolic syndrome,[424] and the risk of type 2 diabetes mellitus.[355,422,425] In some of these studies, free testosterone concentrations were measured by a tracer analogue method. Measurements of free testosterone by this method are affected by the prevalent SHBG concentrations,[269] leading some experts to question the validity and accuracy of this method. Because of the dependence of the total and free testosterone levels by tracer analogue methods on SHBG concentrations, we cannot exclude the possibility that the relationship between the measured testosterone concentrations and visceral fat and atherosclerosis might reflect the relationship between SHBG and these outcomes. Because insulin is known to inhibit SHBG, obese and insulin-resistant men with higher insulin levels would be expected to have lower SHBG levels and consequently lower testosterone concentrations.

Effects of Testosterone Therapy

Several randomized, placebo-controlled trials of up to 3 years' duration have examined the effects of testosterone supplementation in older men with low-normal to low testosterone concentrations.[382,383,426] In general, testosterone trials in older men were characterized by small sample size, inclusion of healthy older men with low or low-normal testosterone levels who were asymptomatic, and the use of surrogate outcomes. These studies did not have sufficient power to detect either meaningful gains in patient-important outcomes or changes in prostate and cardiovascular event rates. Therefore, the risks and clinical benefits of long-term testosterone therapy in older men with age-related decline in testosterone levels remain unknown.

Body Composition

In a systematic review of placebo-controlled, randomized trials in middle-aged and older men,[44,287,351,383,426-431] testosterone replacement was associated with a significantly greater increase in lean body mass and a greater reduction in fat mass (−2.0 kg; 95% CI −3.1 to −0.8) than placebo. The body weight change did not differ significantly between groups (−0.6 kg; 95% CI −2.0 to +0.8). Testosterone therapy was associated with a greater improvement in grip strength than placebo (3.3 kg; 95% CI 0.7 to 5.8).[351,428,429,432] Changes in performance-based measures of physical function were reported only in a few studies and were inconsistent. One study reported no changes in physical function,[383] and two others reported improvements.[428]

Testosterone therapy did not significantly affect overall quality-of-life scores, as assessed by the Medical Outcomes Study SF-36 questionnaire; however, in comparison with placebo, testosterone therapy was associated with a significantly greater improvement in physical function scores.[94] The systematic review found no significant improvement with testosterone therapy in measures of depression or cognition in older men.

In trials that enrolled men with testosterone levels less than 300 ng/dL, testosterone therapy was associated with significant improvements in libido and inconsistent improvements in erectile function.[94] However, testosterone therapy did not improve either libido or erectile function in men with baseline testosterone greater than 300 ng/dL.

Adverse Events

A recent meta-analysis evaluated the adverse events associated with testosterone therapy in randomized trials in middle-aged and older men.[348] In the 19 studies that met eligibility criteria, 651 men were treated with testosterone and 433 were treated with placebo. The combined rate of all prostate events was significantly greater in testosterone-treated men than in placebo-treated men (OR 1.78; 95% CI 1.07 to 2.95). Rates of prostate cancer, PSA greater than 4 ng/mL, and prostate biopsies were numerically higher in the testosterone group than in the placebo group, although differences between the groups were not individually statistically significant. Testosterone-treated men were nearly four times as likely to have hematocrit greater than 50% as placebo-treated men (OR 3.69; 95% CI 1.82–7.51). Hematocrit increase was the most common adverse event associated with testosterone replacement. The frequency of cardiovascular events, sleep apnea, or death was not significantly different between the two groups.

Thus, there is a significant bias toward detection of more prostate events in testosterone trials. Testosterone treatment increases PSA levels in androgen-deficient men. Because prostate biopsies are triggered usually in response to PSA increases and PSA increases are more likely in testosterone-treated men than in placebo-treated men, the men receiving testosterone therapy are at a greater risk for undergoing prostate biopsy than placebo-treated men. In fact, in the meta-analysis, men in the testosterone group had more than 20 times more biopsies than those in the placebo group. Because of the higher risk of undergoing a prostate biopsy, testosterone-treated men are more likely to receive a diagnosis of a subclinical prostate disorder than placebo-treated men. Strategies to minimize this risk by using a standardized monitoring plan are necessary in clinical trials as well as in clinical practice. These considerations reaffirm the need to monitor hematocrit, PSA, and digital examination of the prostate during testosterone replacement in older men, using a rigorous and standardized monitoring plan.

Risk-to-Benefit Assessment

The available data preclude an assessment of the clinical benefits and the long-term risks of testosterone therapy in older men with age-related decline in testosterone levels. The Endocrine Society's expert panel recommended "against a general policy of offering testosterone therapy to all older men with low testosterone levels." The panel suggested that "clinicians consider offering testosterone therapy on an individualized basis to older men with consistently low testosterone levels on more than one occasion and significant symptoms of androgen deficiency, after appropriate discussion of the uncertainties of the risks and benefits of testosterone therapy in older men." A separate expert panel of the Institute of Medicine also concluded that adequately powered randomized efficacy trials of testosterone therapy are needed in older men who have symptomatic conditions associated with androgen deficiency and unequivocally low testosterone levels. The Institute of Medicine panel, however, suggested that large trials to determine the risks of testosterone therapy should be deferred until efficacy had been established. Therefore, the debate surrounding testosterone therapy of older men is unlikely to be resolved anytime soon.

Gynecomastia

Gynecomastia refers to enlargement of the male breast due to benign proliferation of the glandular tissue.[433,434] Glandular tissue enlargement should be distinguished from excessive accumulation of adipose tissue; glandular tissue is firm and contains fibrous-like cords.[433,434]

Gynecomastia usually is caused by an imbalance between estrogen and androgen action or an increased estrogen-to-androgen ratio due to increased estrogen production, decreased androgen production, or some combination of both.[433,434] Even in men with severe gynecomastia, galactorrhea is uncommon presumably because complete female development of the breast acinar tissue requires the presence of progestagen.[435]

Estrogen Production in Men

Unlike ovulating women, in whom most of the circulating estrogen is derived from the ovaries, 85% of circulating estradiol and more than 95% of circulating estrone in men is derived from extragonadal conversion of testosterone and Δ^4-androstenedione, mostly in the fat and skin.[436,437] Daily production rates of estradiol and estrone have been estimated to be 45 and 65 μg, respectively.[438] Approximately 7 μg of estradiol is secreted directly by the testes, 17 μg is derived from peripheral conversion of testosterone, and 22 μg is derived by 17-keto reduction of estrone by the action of 17-β hydroxysteroid dehydrogenase.[438]

The conversion of testosterone and Δ^4-androstenedione to estradiol and estrone, respectively, requires the coordinate action of the protein product of the aromatase gene, referred to as *CYP19,* and a flavoprotein, NADPH–cytochrome P450 reductase, which transfers reducing equivalents from NADPH to cytochrome P450.[436] The human CYP19 gene is transcribed in the gonads and many extragonadal tissues under the control of tissue-specific promoters that are located within a large 90 kb upstream regulatory region.[436,439] Under the influence of various hormones and growth factors, these promoters regulate the expression of the CYP19 aromatase gene in a tissue-specific manner, directing the transcription of mRNAs that have an identical coding sequence but different 5′ untranslated regions.[439] Estrogen production in the granulosa cells of the ovary in menstruating women is under the control of proximally located promoter II, which is regulated by FSH.[436] In the fat and skin tissues, *CYP19* expression is regulated by 1.3 and 1.4 promoters that are located 0.2 and 73 kb upstream from the coding region.[345,440]

Causes and Pathophysiologic Mechanisms

High prevalence of gynecomastia is observed in the neonatal period, during puberty, and with aging.[433,434,441] Causes of gynecomastia are listed in (Table 18–8).

TABLE 18–8 CAUSES OF GYNECOMASTIA CLASSIFIED BY THE POSTULATED MECHANISMS

INCREASED PRODUCTION OF ESTROGEN PRECURSORS
Adrenal tumors Liver disease 17-β-hydroxysteroid dehydrogenase deficiency
INCREASED AROMATASE ACTIVITY
Increased Activity in Normal Tissue Obesity Aging **Aromatase Dysregulation** Familial aromatase excess syndrome Neoplasms caused by eutopic estrogen production: Sertoli cell tumors (isolated, Peutz-Jeghers syndrome, Carney complex), hCG-producing trophoblastic tumors Neoplasms caused by ectopic estrogen production: feminizing adrenocortical carcinoma, hepatocellular carcinoma
ALTERED TESTOSTERONE-TO-ESTROGEN RATIO DUE TO DECREASED ANDROGEN PRODUCTION OR ACTION
Androgen insensitivity syndrome 5-α reductase deficiency Thyrotoxicosis Klinefelter's syndrome

hCG, human chorionic gonadotropin.
Modified from Braunstein GD. Aromatase and gynecomastia. Endocr Relat Cancer 1999;6:315-324.

Transient breast enlargement in the newborn has been reported in 20% to 30% of newborn babies. It is usually the result of the transplacental transfer of maternal and placental estrogens.

Gynecomastia also is common in pubertal boys[442,443]; breast enlargement appears first in early puberty, presumably reflecting a high estrogen-to-testosterone ratio in the early stages of puberty before testicular testosterone production becomes fully established. Estradiol levels rise more rapidly during early puberty than testosterone levels, resulting in a high estrogen-to-androgen ratio.[444] In most boys, breast enlargement regresses with pubertal progression and rise in testosterone levels so that by age 21, only a small fraction of boys has persistent gynecomastia.

The prevalence of gynecomastia increases with aging and body mass index (BMI)[445] because of increased aromatase activity in adipose tissue. The body mass index correlates with the risk of gynecomastia[445] and the diameter of the breast tissue.[441] Body weight is a good predictor of estrogen production rates in obese men and postmenopausal women.[259] With advancing age, testosterone levels decline, SHBG levels increase, and the peripheral rates of aromatization are higher than in younger men, resulting in an increased estrogen-to-androgen ratio. The higher estrogen production rates in older men are related to an age-related increase in CYP19 activity in the fat tissue[446] and an overall increase in fat mass.

Men with androgen deficiency syndromes often have gynecomastia; continued synthesis of estradiol by aromatization of residual adrenal and gonadal androgens leads to an increased estrogen-to-androgen ratio. Gynecomastia is a characteristic feature of Klinefelter's syndrome. Androgen insensitivity disorders also cause gynecomastia because of unopposed action of estrogens.

Excess estrogen production may be caused by Leydig and Sertoli cell tumors that secrete estrogens or germ cell tumors that secrete hCG.[447] Estrogen-producing Sertoli cell tumors can occur sporadically or in association with Peutz-Jeghers syndrome[448] or Carney complex. hCG also can stimulate Leydig cell estrogen synthesis.

In patients with feminizing adrenal tumors or congenital adrenal hyperplasia, elevated estrogen levels can result from increased production rates of Δ^4-androstenedione, which can be converted to estrone. In patients with liver disease, the catabolism of androstenedione in the liver is reduced; as a result, a greater amount of this precursor becomes available for aromatization in peripheral tissues.[449]

A familial form of prepubertal gynecomastia, inherited as an autosomal dominant or an X-linked disorder, results from increased estrogen production due to excessive aromatase activity in peripheral tissues.[450,451] Male patients with the excessive peripheral aromatase syndrome are characterized by high estradiol levels, prepubertal gynecomastia, accelerated bone age in childhood, and shortened final adult height due to premature epiphyseal fusion.[452] Female patients with this syndrome present with precocious breast development.[451] In some patients with this syndrome, a heterozygous inversion in chromosome 15q21.2-3 has been described; this inversion caused the *CYP19* gene to be excessively transcribed by the constitutively active promoter of other contiguous genes, resulting in increased estrogen production in extragonadal tissues.[450,453]

Administration of some therapeutic agents is associated with gynecomastia. Some of these drugs, such as oral contraceptives, phytoestrogens, and digitalis, have direct estrogenic activity; others such as isoniazid can induce increased estrogen activity. A few drugs inhibit androgen biosynthesis (e.g., ketoconazole) or action (e.g., spironolactone, flutamide, cyproterone acetate, and bicalutamide). Isolated cases of gynecomastia due to inadvertent exposure to estrogenic compounds contained in industrial products or cosmetics have been reported. Thus, gynecomastia has been reported in workers in factories that manufacture diethylstilbestrol or other estrogens and offspring of mothers using estrogen creams. A number of cosmetic creams and lotions contain varying amounts of estrogens. Also, meat, milk, and other dairy products derived from estrogen-treated animals may be inadvertent sources of estrogens.[454]

Diagnosis

Clinical Evaluation

Because some degree of gynecomastia may be observed in up to half of hospitalized men, and because in a vast majority of men gynecomastia is benign, detailed diagnostic evaluation is not indicated in all men presenting with gynecomastia. More extensive evaluation is indicated in lean men and in those with recent onset, rapid growth, tender breast tissue, and very large breast tissue. The diagnostic evaluation should include a careful drug history, examination of the testes, assessment of secondary sex characteristics, and evaluation of liver function.

Laboratory Evaluation

Liver enzymes, serum testosterone, estradiol, androstenedione, LH, and hCG levels should be measured (Fig. 18–14). If testes are small, a karyotype should be obtained to exclude Klinefelter's syndrome. The diagnosis is established in less than half of patients, probably because the alterations of the estrogen-to-androgen ratio are often subtle. Most commercial estrogen assays lack sensitivity in the low male range, making it difficult to detect small changes in estrogen levels and estrogen-to-testosterone ratios.

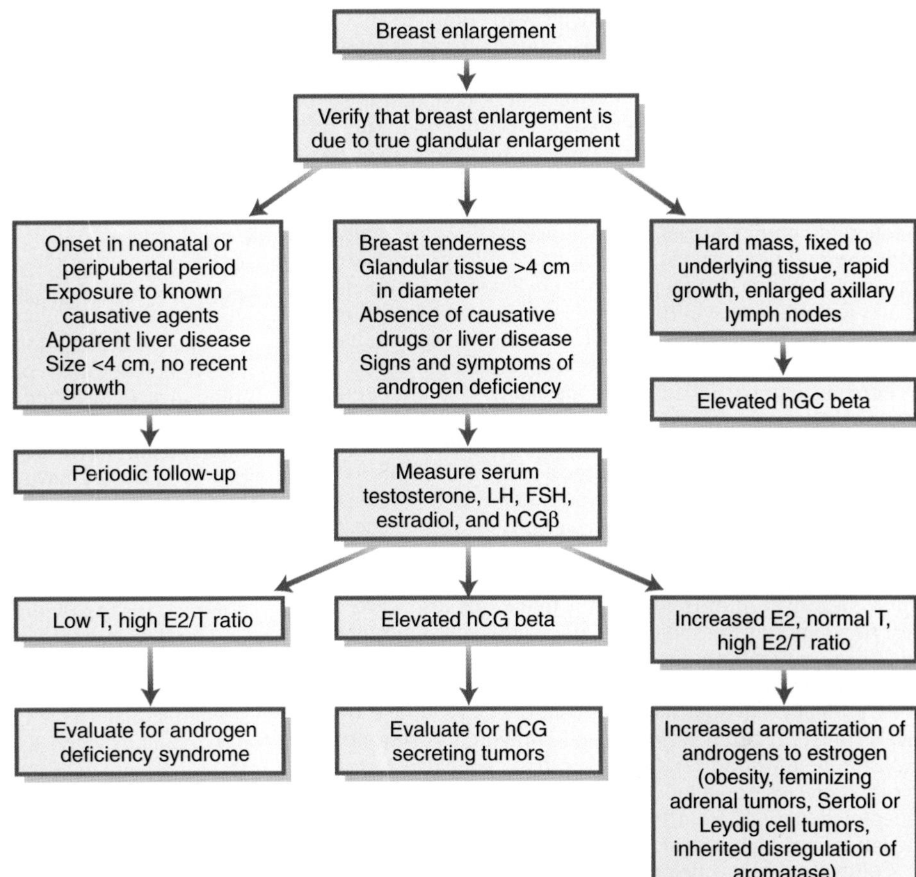

Figure 18–14 ■ Evaluation of a patient with gynecomastia. E2, estradiol 17-β; hCGβ, human chorionic gonadotropin β; T, testosterone.

Gynecomastia and the Risk of Breast Cancer

The risk of breast cancer is increased markedly in men with Klinefelter's syndrome.[107,108,455-461] Although the relative risk of breast cancer is increased in men with primary testicular dysfunction and hyperestrogenism, the absolute increase in risk is small.[462] Obesity also is an important risk factor for breast cancer.[462] It is not clear whether the risk of breast cancer is increased in all men with gynecomastia.[462]

Treatment

When the primary cause can be identified and corrected, breast enlargement usually subsides over several months. However, if gynecomastia is last for more than 1 year, complete reversal of gynecomastia is unusual and surgery is the most effective therapy. Indications for surgery include severe psychological or cosmetic problems, continued growth or tenderness of breast tissue, or suspected malignancy.

Several case reports have documented the beneficial effects of aromatase inhibitors in treating patients with excessive aromatase activity.[463,464] However, the experience with the use of aromatase inhibitors in patients with gynecomastia is largely anecdotal. Although reduction in the breast size has been reported with the use of testolactone in boys with pubertal gynecomastia[465] and in an open-label study of adults with idiopathic gynecomastia,[434] complete disappearance of gynecomastia is unusual with drug therapy. The sample sizes of these open-label studies were small.[434,465] In a randomized clinical trial in boys with pubertal gynecomastia,[466] the percentage of patients with a 50% or greater reduction in total breast volume, measured by ultrasonography, did not differ significantly between the anastrozole and placebo groups.

In patients who have painful gynecomastia and who are not candidates for surgical therapy, treatment with antiestrogens such as tamoxifen reduces pain and breast tissue size in about two thirds of patients.[467-471] Also, tamoxifen has been shown to prevent the development of breast pain and enlargement in patients with prostate cancer who are being treated with antiandrogen therapy.[467] Aromatase inhibitors are likely to be effective in the early proliferative phase of the disorder; in late stages when fibrosis has become established, drug therapy would not be expected to achieve reduction in breast size. Placebo-controlled trials with more potent aromatase inhibitors such as anastrozole, fadrozole, letrozole, or fromestane are needed.

Disorders of Sex-Steroid Action

Testosterone does not only serve as a hormone; it is also converted in many peripheral tissues into two active metabolites, estradiol 17-β and 5-DHT. Testosterone actions in many tissues are mediated through these metabolites. Therefore, androgen action potentially could be impaired as a result of mutations in the androgen receptor, steroid 5-α reductase, the CYP19 aromatase, or the estrogen receptor genes.

Mutations of the Androgen-Receptor Gene

Many androgen actions are mediated through binding of androgen to an intracellular androgen receptor that acts as a ligand-dependent transcription factor. The mutations of the androgen receptor gene have been associated with a wide spectrum of phenotypic abnormalities.[40,472] Patients with complete androgen insensitivity present with male pseudohermaphroditism characterized by a feminine appearance with well-developed breasts, female external genitalia, a blind vaginal pouch, and absence of hair in androgen-sensitive areas.[473] The internal structures that are derived from the müllerian ducts are absent; thus, these patients lack a uterus, cervix, and fallopian tubes. The wolffian structures are also typically absent. These patients often seek medical attention for primary amenorrhea.[473] Occasionally, the undescended testes in the inguinal canal may be mistaken for an inguinal hernia, leading to further evaluation. Complete testicular feminization syndrome is inherited as an X-linked recessive disorder although a third of the patients do not have a family history and likely have a *de novo* mutation.[473]

Persons with partial androgen insensitivity syndrome might have variable phenotype.[474] Some patients with partial androgen insensitivity have a male phenotype and mild abnormalities such as hypospadias, gynecomastia, and infertility; this form of partial androgen insensitivity is also referred to as *Reifenstein's syndrome*.[475,476] Other patients with partial androgen insensitivity present with ambiguous genitalia or with a female appearance and female external genitalia with varying degrees of fusion and clitoromegaly.[476] Androgen receptor mutations also have been described in infertile men who are completely masculinized and have normal hormonal profiles.[475]

Persons with 46,XY karyotype and androgen receptor mutations typically have elevated testosterone, LH, and estradiol levels, but the serum testosterone-to-dihydrotestosterone and testosterone-to-estradiol ratios are normal. Normal testosterone-to-dihydrotestosterone ratios distinguish patients with androgen receptor mutations from those with 5-α reductase mutations; the latter have high testosterone-to-dihydrotestosterone ratios.

Complete or gross deletions of the androgen receptor gene are uncommon in persons with complete androgen insensitivity syndrome; most patients with partial and complete forms of androgen insensitivity have point mutations at several different sites in exons 2 to 8 encoding the DNA-binding and androgen-binding domain of the androgen receptor gene, resulting in amino acid substitutions or a premature stop codon.[40,472,477] Additionally, nucleotide insertions leading to frame shift or premature termination, deletions, and intron mutations in splice site donor or acceptor sites also have been reported.[477]

Mutations in the DNA binding domain result in a mutant androgen receptor protein that has normal hormone binding but that is defective in dimerization or DNA binding, resulting in diminished transcriptional activation.[472] DNA binding domain contains two zinc fingers; the first zinc finger is important for DNA binding, and the second zinc finger is involved in protein-protein interaction and dimerization.[35] Mutations of both zinc fingers have been described and occur with equal frequency.[478,479]

Mutations of the ligand binding domain result in either absent or diminished hormone binding. A relatively high number of mutations have been reported in exons 5 and 7, but mutations in exon 1 and the hinge region of exon 4 are rare.

Adachi and colleagues[480] described a patient with phenotypic findings that were typical of the androgen insensitivity syndrome but in whom no mutation of androgen receptor was found. The activation signal from the AF-1 region of the androgen receptor was disrupted, suggesting a defect in a coactivator protein that interacts with this region.[480]

The lengths of the CAG and GCG trinucleotide repeats that encode polyglutamine and polyglycine tracts in exon 1 of the androgen receptor gene have been inversely correlated to transcriptional activity of androgen receptor protein. An abnormal length of the polyglutamine tract (>40 glutamines) is associated with spinal and bulbar muscular atrophy, also known as *Kennedy's disease*.[481,482] The androgen receptor protein with an expanded polyglutamine tract is cytotoxic to cells, and its proteolytic cleavage causes neuronal cell death.[483] Men with Kennedy's disease often have gynecomastia, increased testosterone and LH concentrations, and evidence of decreased androgen action. Although some studies have reported an association of the lengths of polyglutamine and polyglycine tracts with male infertility (see section on infertility in this chapter) and risk of prostate cancer, others have not confirmed these findings.[484]

Mutations of the Steroid 5-α Reductase Gene

Patients with the autosomal recessive type 2 steroid 5-α reductase deficiency are typically 46,XY males who have normal male internal structures including testes but who exhibit ambiguous or female external genitalia at birth.[10] At puberty, these children undergo partial virilization, and some assume male gender identity, even if they have been brought up as girls in early childhood. Their development suggests that testosterone itself is able to stimulate psychosexual behavior, libido, development of the embryonic wolffian duct, muscle development, voice deepening, spermatogenesis, and axillary and pubic hair growth. In contrast, DHT is required for prostate development and growth and for development of the external genitalia and male patterns of facial and body hair growth or male-pattern baldness.

All the 5-α reductase–deficient kindreds that have been studied to date have been shown to have mutations in steroid 5-α reductase type 2, the predominant form in the prostate. Many patients with congenital deficiency of type 2 5-α reductase have low or low normal DHT levels at puberty, either due to the activity of type 1 isoenzyme or to the residual low activity of type 2 isoenzyme; it is not clear whether the normal muscle development and male psychosexual behavior observed in these patients after puberty is due to the low normal DHT levels or testosterone itself.

Mutations of type 1 steroid 5-α reductase have not been described in humans.

Mutations of the CYP19 Aromatase Gene

The product of the aromatase gene catalyzes the final step in the conversion of C19 sex steroids into C18 estrogens by converting the A ring of the steroid molecule into an aromatic ring. Testosterone effects on trabecular bone resorption, sexual differentiation of the brain, plasma lipids, atherosclerosis progression, epiphyseal fusion, and some types of behavior are mediated through conversion of testosterone to estrogen. Female patients with aromatase gene mutations are masculinized, fail to undergo female pubertal development, have elevated levels of androgens and LH and FSH, and have polycystic ovaries and tall stature.[31] Male patients with CYP19 mutations have delayed epiphyseal fusion, continued linear growth, tall stature, eunuchoidal proportions, osteoporosis and increased bone turnover, and disruption of spermatogenesis and fertility.[30] These men have normal or increased testosterone levels, elevated LH and FSH concentrations, and markedly decreased estradiol levels. Both male and female patients with aromatase gene mutations also have impaired glucose tolerance and hyperinsulinemia.[29,31]

Smith et al[27] reported a single case of estrogen resistance due to an inactivating mutation of the estrogen receptor alpha gene. This male patient had tall stature, continued linear growth beyond pubertal years into adulthood, unfused epiphyses, osteoporosis, normal male external genitalia, normal testosterone concentrations, and elevated estradiol, LH, and FSH concentrations.[27] Treatment with high doses of estrogen that increased serum estradiol levels into the supraphysiologic range was ineffective in inducing bone maturation or epiphyseal fusion.

INFERTILITY AND SUBFERTILITY IN MEN

Definition and Epidemiology

The World Health Organization (WHO) has defined infertility as the inability of a sexually active couple to achieve pregnancy despite unprotected intercourse during the fertile phase of the menstrual cycle for a period of greater than 12 months.[485] The percentage of couples seeking medical treatment for infertility is estimated at 4% to 17%.[486] Three percent to 4% of all couples remain involuntarily childless at the end of their reproductive periods.

The estimates of prevalence rates of infertility and subfertility depend crucially upon the method used to define these conditions.[487,488] The WHO definition was based on studies that used time to pregnancy estimations and found the probability of conception to be 20% per cycle or ~85% to 90% per year.[485,489-492] Even among couples who do not conceive within 12 months, 55% have a live birth within the next 36 months.[493] When the duration of infertility exceeds 4 years, the conception rate per month drops to 1.5%.[494]

Two studies[495,496] suggest that the spontaneous conception rates are higher than had been estimated previously. For instance, in a prospective survey of Chinese female textile workers, 20 to 34 years of age,[495] 50% became pregnant in their first two cycles and 90% in the first six cycles, yielding a monthly fecundity of about 30% to 35%. In a prospective study of German couples,[496] the estimated cumulative probabilities of conception were 38%, 68%, 81%, and 92% at one, three, six, and 12 cycles.

In 20% of infertile couples, the primary problem resides in the male partner; in an additional 26%, problems reside in both the male and the female partner; thus, the male partner contributes to infertility in about half the couples. The occurrence of infertility substantially affects a couple's relationship, quality of life, and health care expenditures.

Causes and Pathophysiology

The frequency of etiologic factors varies among surveys from different centers because of differences in patient referral patterns, the extent of diagnostic investigation, and geography; however, these surveys agree that subfertility and infertility in men are a heterogeneous group of disorders[497] (Table 18–9). Fifteen percent to 20% of infertile men are azoopsermic.[498] An additional 10% have severe oligozoospermia, defined as sperm density less than 1 million/mL. A specific cause of infertility is not determinable in 40% to 60% men.[494] Most infertile men have idiopathic oligozoospermia.[498-500]

Correctable or treatable causes of infertility, such as gonadotropin deficiency and obstruction, are present in only a small number of men, but it is important to recognize them because effective treatment modalities are available.[500] Varicoceles are present in 10% to 30% of men with infertility; their role, if any, in the pathophysiology of male infertility remains unclear. An increasing number of genetic disorders are being implicated in specific abnormalities of germ cell development; in addition, a number of systemic disorders nonspecifically affect spermatogenesis. Of these, Klinefelter's syndrome and Y chromosome microdeletions are the most prevalent disorders, together accounting for 10% to 20% of patients (see Table 18–9). Although the prevalence of antisperm antibodies in infertile men is higher than that in fertile men,[501] the mechanisms by which antisperm antibodies cause infertility are unclear.

Genetic Disorders Associated with Infertility

Genetic Disorders Associated with Impaired Gonadotropin Secretion or Action

Genetic disorders associated with impaired gonadotropin secretion or action were discussed earlier under "Hypogonadism." This section will focus only on the genetic disorders of germ cell development.

Primary Defects of Spermatogenesis

Sex Chromosome Disorders

Five percent of infertile men carries chromosome abnormalities; of these, a majority involves sex chromosomes (4% on average), and 1% involves the autosome.[499,502] The prevalence of sex chromosomal and autosomal abnormalities in infertile men is 15 and 6 times higher than in the general population.[95,502] Klinefelter's syndrome is the most common chromosomal disorder associated with male infertility.

Noonan's Syndrome, the Male Turner's Syndrome

These patients with 46,XY karyotype have male external genitalia but, they exhibit clinical stigmata of Turner's syndrome.[503] The testis size is reduced and testosterone levels are generally low. These men tend to be infertile, and cryptorchidism is common.

TABLE 18–9 COMMON DIAGNOSES IN MEN BEING EVALUATED FOR INFERTILITY

Diagnostic Category	Incidence (%)
Idiopathic infertility	50-60
Primary testicular failure (chromosomal disorders including Klinefelter's syndrome, Y chromosome microdeletions, undescended testis, irradiation, orchitis, drugs)	10-20
Genital tract obstruction (congenital absence of vas, vasectomy, epididymal obstruction)	5
Coital disorders	<1
Hypogonadotropic hypogonadism (pituitary adenomas, panhypopituitarism, idiopathic hypogonadotropic hypogonadism, hyperprolactinemia)	3-4
Varicocele*	15-35
Other (sperm autoimmunity, drugs, toxins, systemic illness)	5

*Although varicoceles are observed with higher frequency in infertile and subfertile men than in fertile men, their role and contribution to infertility remains unclear.
Adapted and modified from Baker et al. (4) with permission.[707]

XYY Syndrome

There is a higher frequency of 47,XYY karyotype in men with tall stature and nodular cystic acne among prisoners and mental hospital patients.[504] 47,XYY men tend to have low intelligence and lower educational levels than healthy controls.

Mixed Gonadal Dysgenesis

Patients with mixed gonadal dysgenesis usually have a 45,X/46,XY karyotype and a testis on one side and a streak gonad on the other.[505,506] External genitalia often show some degree of ambiguity.[505] Phenotypic males with mixed gonadal dysgenesis often have an abdominal testis with normal Leydig cells but diminished or absent germ cells. The dysgenetic gonad is at a high risk for neoplastic degeneration.

XX Males

46,XX males have a masculine appearance and normal-appearing testes, but these patients are typically azoospermic and their LH and FSH levels are elevated.[507] In some XX males, a portion of Y chromosome containing the *Sry* gene may be translocated onto the X chromosome or an autosome, and a few patients may be mosaics and carry some 46,XY cells. These patients are usually sterile because they lack other Y-specific genes required for spermatogenesis.

The Y Chromosome Microdeletion Syndrome

During a meticulous examination of karyotypes, Tiepolo and Zuffardi discovered that men with large interstitial deletions of the long arm of the Y chromosome were infertile and proposed presciently that loci for "azoospermia factor" resided on the long arm of Y chromosome. Large deletions of the long arm of Y chromosome that are visible under the light microscope in late prophase are uncommon in infertile men. However, small deletions of the Y chromosome that are not visible under the microscope in late prophase and, therefore, referred to as microdeletions, are observed in 5% to 10% of infertile men with azoospermia or severe oligozoospermia.[508-519] These microdeletions can be detected by PCR-based sequence-tagged site mapping.[519]

Most infertile men with Y deletions have severe defects of spermatogenesis—they have either azoospermia or severe oligozoospermia.[514,516] A significant fraction of men with Y microdeletions have slightly reduced testicular volumes (<15 mL) and elevated FSH levels, but others have normal testicular volumes and normal FSH levels.[498,508,520] The testicular histologies in men with Y deletions have revealed either Sertoli cell only or germ cell arrest phenotype. There is poor correlation between testicular histology and the location and size of the microdeletion. However, Vogt and colleagues[514] have reported that three loci can be identified in Yq, termed AZFa, AZFb, and AZFc, wherein deletions are associated with specific testicular histopathology.

Several Y-specific gene families, cloned by deletion mapping of infertile men with Yq deletions, have been proposed as candidates for the putative AZF locus; these include the RBM (*R*NA *b*inding *m*otif containing) gene family,[521,522] and the DAZ (*d*eleted in *az*oospermia) gene family.[510,523,524] Both are multiple-copy gene families that contain RNA binding motifs. The RBM gene family has more than 30 copies spread throughout the Y chromosome, and most of the copies are located in deletion intervals 6A and 6B.[525] At least two members of the RBM gene family, RBM-1 and RBM-2, are expressed in the testis.[522] The presence of the RNA-binding motif in the predicted protein sequence suggests that these genes play a role in RNA processing; however, the precise role of the RBM protein(s) in germ cell development remains unclear.

The DAZ gene family is also a multiple-copy gene family.[526] The mouse and *Drosophila* homologues of the DAZ family have been mapped to chromosomes 17 and 3, respectively.[527,528] An autosomal homologue of the DAZ family also has been identified in humans and mapped to chromosome 3.[523,524] The homologues of the autosomal DAZ-like gene, *DAZL1*, are present in all mammalian species; DAZ homologues are present on the Y chromosomes only in great apes, Old World monkeys, and humans. Mutations of the *DAZL1* gene in *Drosophila, boule*, are associated with meiotic arrest and azoospermia.[527] Similarly, mice that are null for *DAZL1* are sterile, providing further evidence that the protein product of *DAZL1* plays an important role in germ cell development.[529] In infertile men with *DAZ* deletions, both meiotic arrest and Sertoli cell–only phenotype have been described; it is possible that germ cell degeneration occurs secondarily.

The precise physiologic function and role of the RBM and DAZ gene families in human spermatogenesis remains unclear. The RNA molecules that are the targets of these RNA binding proteins have not been fully characterized. Using DAZ as bait in a two-hybrid system, Tsui's group[530] identified two novel proteins, DAZ-associated proteins (DAZAP) 1 and 2, that interact with *DAZ* and *DAZL1*. The DAZAP genes have been mapped to chromosomal regions 19p13.3 and 2q33-q34.

Although deletions involving the DAZ genes are the most common in infertile men with Yq deletions, a large portion of Y deletions are outside the DAZ region; some of these involve the *RBM* gene. Additional candidate gene families, including BPY2, CDY1, PRY, and TTY2, have been identified in the AZFc region of the Y chromosome. The role of these additional Y-specific gene families in germ cell development and infertility is not understood. It is also not clear how deletions of one or two copies of the *RBM* or *DAZ* genes could explain infertility when there are multiple copies of these genes elsewhere on the Y chromosome. A significant fraction of infertile men with DAZ deletions is oligozoospermic and not azoospermic. Furthermore, only 5% to 10% of infertile men has Y deletions. These data suggest that additional Y-specific and autosomal genes may be involved in other infertility phenotypes.

Although Y microdeletions have been reported in fertile men, the frequency of Y microdeletions is very low in fertile men and in men with sperm densities greater than 1 million/mL.

Length of the Polyglutamine Tract in the Androgen Receptor Protein and Infertility

Exon 1 of the human androgen receptor contains two polymorphic tracts: the polyglutamine and the polyglycine tracts. The length of the CAG trinucleotide repeat in exon 1 of the androgen receptor gene that encodes for the polyglutamine tract has an inverse correlation with *trans*-activational activity of the androgen receptor protein.[531,532] Some reports indicate that men with idiopathic oligozoospermia have a higher likelihood of having longer polyglutamine tracts than fertile men.[531,532] Dadze and colleagues,[533] on the other hand, found no relationship between the CAG repeat length and impaired spermatogenesis in an sample of infertile men of German origin. Therefore, the validity of this hypothesis remains to be verified.

Cyclic AMP-Response Element Modulator Gene Expression and Spermatogenic Arrest

The cAMP-response element modulator gene encodes a transcription factor that is expressed in postmeiotic germ cells and regulates the balance between germ cell differentiation and apoptosis during spermatogenesis.[534] During spermatogenesis, there is a switch from CREM repressors to CREM activator isoforms in postmeiotic germ cells.[534] Testicular biopsies obtained from infertile men with germ cell arrest have demonstrated the absence of activator isoforms of CREM in postmeiotic germ cells and increased apoptosis.[535,536] These data suggest that germ cell arrest could result from failure of this normal transition from repressor to activator isoforms of CREM in the seminiferous tubule. Null mutations of CREM protein in mice are associated with sterility and spermatogenic arrest characterized by the absence of late spermatids and an increased number of apoptotic germ cells in the seminiferous tubules.[537]

Other Disorders Associated with Infertility

Bilateral Congenital Absence of Vas Deferens and the CFTR Mutations

A majority of patients with the classic pulmonary form of cystic fibrosis suffer from obstructive azoospermia due to congenital absence of the vas deferens. Additionally, mutations in the coding region of the cystic fibrosis conductance regulator gene, *CFTR,* can result in congenital absence of the vas without causing the classical pulmonary disease.[538] Almost 70% of men with congenital absence of the vas deferens harbor mutations of the *CFTR* gene. About 50% are homozygous for the common cystic fibrosis gene abnormality such as F508, and some have compound heterozygosity.

Gonadal Dysfunction Associated with Sickle Cell Disease and β-Thalassemia

A significant fraction of men with sickle cell disease have low testosterone levels. A majority of men with sickle cell disease who have low testosterone levels suffer from primary testicular dysfunction.[539] It is assumed that testicular dysfunction results from microinfarcts in the testis resulting from the vaso-occlusive disease. However, hypogonadotropic hypogonadism due to hypothalamic-pituitary dysfunction has been reported in men with sickle cell disease.

Pituitary and gonadal dysfunction occurs in thalassemia due to iron deposition in these tissues.[540] Hypogonadotropic hypogonadism is the predominant form of androgen deficiency syndrome in men with thalassemia and can be treated effectively with gonadotropin replacement therapy. Pituitary and testicular overload and the resulting hypogonadism can be prevented by prophylactic iron-chelation therapy.

Testicular Dysfunction in Myotonic Dystrophy

An expansion of the CTG repeats in the DMPK gene causes myotonic dystrophy, an autosomal dominant disorder characterized by myotonia, frontal balding, progressive muscle weakness, and testicular atrophy.[541] Among patients with myotonic dystrophy, 75% have testicular atrophy, primarily due to degeneration of the seminiferous tubules. Although Leydig cells are preserved, serum testosterone levels are low in many patients.[542]

Subfertility Associated with Diabetes

Men with diabetes mellitus can experience infertility for many reasons. Men with longstanding diabetes mellitus might have retrograde ejaculation due to autonomic neuropathy. Erectile dysfunction also is highly prevalent in men who have had diabetes for more than 10 years. Men with type 2 diabetes mellitus have a higher prevalence of low testosterone levels than age-matched controls.[284]

Diagnosis

Clinical Evaluation

The evaluation of the infertile couple should include the male and the female partner simultaneously (Fig. 18–15). Initial evaluation should focus on general health; coexisting medical problems such as erectile dysfunction, diabetes mellitus, and autonomic neuropathy that might be associated with retrograde ejaculation; and lifestyle factors such as eating disorders, excessive exercise, and abuse of recreational drugs such as marijuana, cocaine, opiates, and alcohol. The duration of infertility, previous evidence of fertility in the man or the woman, contraceptive use, sexual function, frequency and timing of intercourse in relation to the menstrual cycle, and sexual practices should be ascertained. The timing of pubertal development, shaving frequency, hair loss, and hair distribution should be verified. Additionally, ascertain history of scrotal trauma, genitourinary infection, sexually transmitted disease, and scrotal or inguinal surgery including hernioplasty and vasectomy, cancer, previous treatment with cancer chemotherapeutic agents, and radiation to the inguinal or scrotal area.

Evaluate the patient for signs of androgen deficiency. Body proportions (height to span and upper segment–to–lower segment ratio), voice (high pitched or not), hair distribution including escutcheon, muscle mass and body habitus, and the absence or presence of gynecomastia can point to hypogonadism. Testicular volume should be measured by a Prader orchidometer. Very small testes can point to Klinefelter's syndrome or severe gonadotropin deficiency. Look for cryptorchidism, varicocele, or nodularity of vas deferens. Perform a digital rectal examination to assess prostate size.

Laboratory Evaluation

The laboratory (Figs. 18–15 to 18–17) evaluation should include assessment of general health by obtaining complete blood count, blood chemistries, and urinalysis.[500,543] Three or more semen samples, obtained by masturbation after at least a 48-hour abstinence period, should be assessed for volume, sperm density and count, sperm motility, and sperm morphology. According to WHO, a normal semen specimen has a volume greater than 2 mL, sperm density greater than 20 million/mL, and a total sperm count greater than 40 million per ejaculate. More than 50% of sperm should show forward motility, and

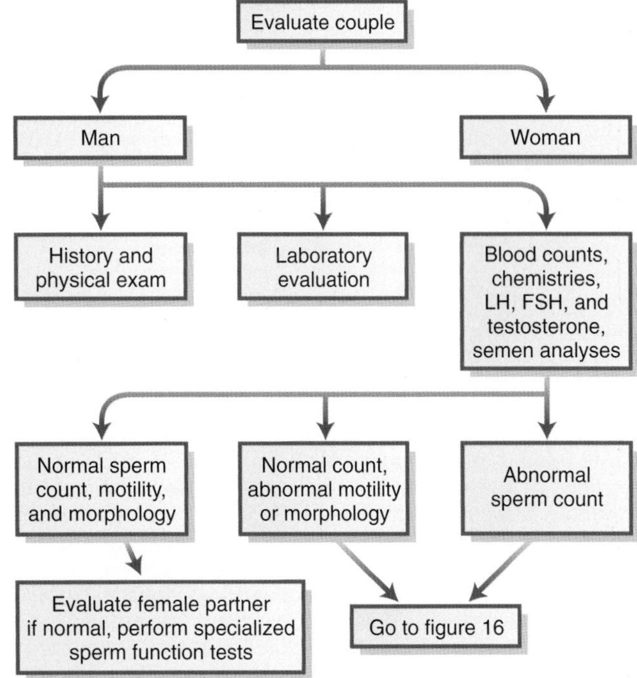

Figure 18–15 ■ Evaluation of an infertile couple. FSH, follicle-stimulating hormone; LH, luteinizing hormone.

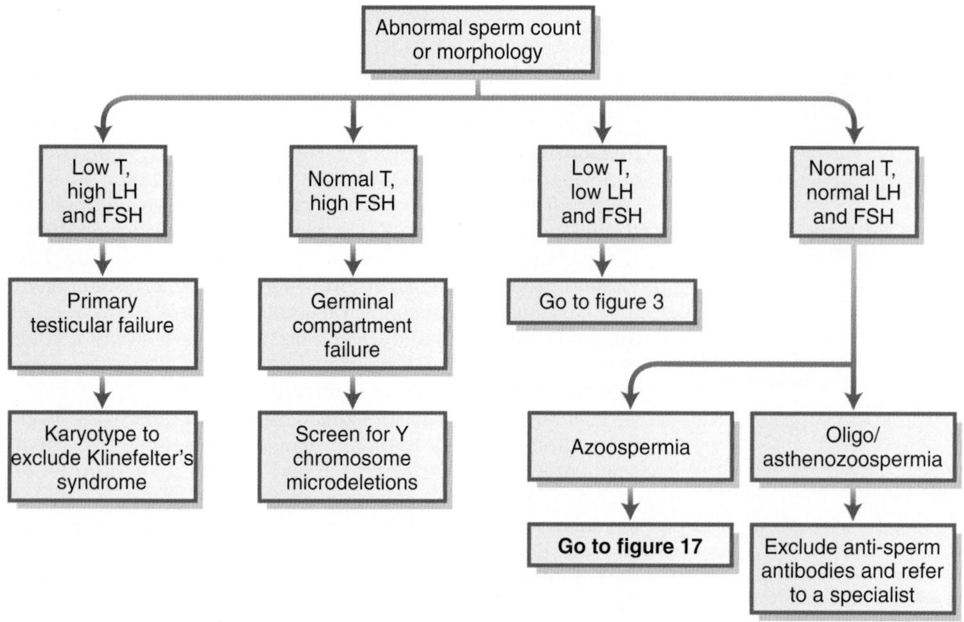

Figure 18–16 ▪ Evaluation of an infertile man with abnormal sperm count and morphology. FSH, follicle-stimulating hormone; LH, luteinizing hormone; T, testosterone.

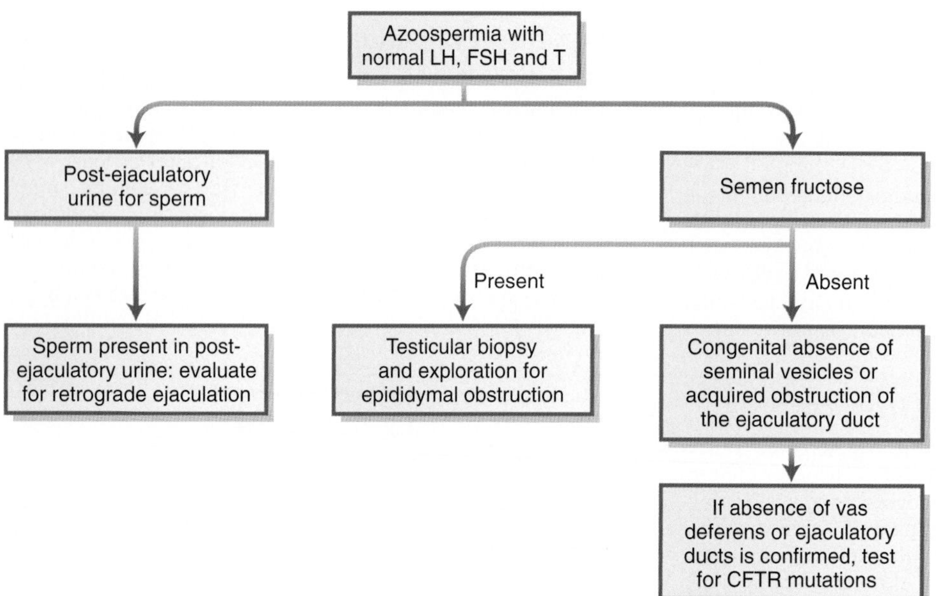

Figure 18–17 ▪ Evaluation of azoospermic men with normal follicle-stimulating hormone (FSH), luteinizing hormone (LH), and testosterone (T) levels. CFTR, cystic fibrosis transmembrane regulator.

more than 30% of cells should have normal morphology.[544,545] The significance of leukocytes in the semen is not clear. The presence of leukocytes in the semen does not necessarily indicate accessory gland infection.

Measurements of total testosterone, LH, and FSH can help diagnose hypogonadism and determine whether hypogonadism is primary or secondary. High LH and FSH levels in the presence of low testosterone concentrations are characteristic of primary testicular failure. Men with primary testicular failure should undergo a karyotype analysis to exclude Klinefelter's syndrome (47,XXY) or its variants. Elevated testosterone and elevated LH levels in a man who appears hypogonadal suggest androgen insensitivity. Men with androgen insensitivity syndrome should undergo analysis of skin fibroblasts for androgen binding or of peripheral lymphocyte DNA for genetic testing for mutations in androgen receptor or 5-α-reductase genes. An isolated increase in serum FSH levels with normal LH and testosterone levels often suggest selective failure of the germ cell compartment. Men who have hypogonadotropic hypogonadism need additional evaluation to determine the cause of gonadotropin deficiency and to rule out hyperprolactinemia, pituitary space-occupying lesions, and hemochromatosis.

In men with azoospermia and normal LH and testosterone levels, obstruction of the urogenital tract due to congenital absence of vas or epididymis or an acquired obstructive lesion should be excluded (see Fig. 18–17). Postejaculatory urine should be checked to exclude retrograde ejaculation. Very low fructose concentrations in the seminal plasma suggest the absence of seminal vesicles or obstruction. In such patients, refer the patient to a urologist for exploration and testicular biopsy to rule out obstruction or germ cell failure. Men with congenital absence of vas deferens or seminal vesicles should be tested for mutations in the cystic fibrosis conductance regulator gene.

Specialized Sperm Function Tests

The utility of specialized sperm tests is limited, and these tests should be performed only in specialized laboratories and only in men who have normal hormone levels and low or normal sperm count.[485,544,545] The sperm function tests include the cervical mucus penetration test, acrosome reaction, zona-free hamster egg penetration test, and human zona pellucida binding test. The clinical utility of the acrosome reaction is not clear. A positive hamster oocyte penetration test indicates that the sperm is able to undergo capacitation and acrosome reaction and can penetrate and fuse with the hamster egg.[544] Although this test has good concordance with fertilization in an in vitro fertilization procedure, it has high frequency of false-negative results.

The computer-aided sperm analysis systems are convenient, but they offer no real advantage over manual methods of assessing sperm morphology, and they are susceptible to error in the estimation of sperm concentration.[544]

Testicular Biopsy

Testicular biopsy may be useful in men with azoospermia and normal testosterone and LH concentrations. In these men, retrograde ejaculation should be excluded by analysis of postejaculatory urine for sperm and of seminal fluid for fructose. If seminal fructose is present, testicular biopsy and exploration should be performed to rule out obstruction and establish the presence of spermatogenesis in the testis.

Testicular biopsy has also been used to retrieve sperm or spermatids for intracytoplasmic sperm injection (ICSI) in men with azoospermia in whom sperm cannot be obtained from the semen. Fertility has been achieved by intracytoplasmic injection of sperm obtained from testicular biopsy in men with azoospermia associated with Klinefelter's syndrome or other causes.

Genetic Testing

Because genetic disorders account for a significant fraction of infertility in men, genetic testing of the infertile man and of the offspring will become increasingly important, especially in couples who are being considered for ICSI. Infertile men who have congenital absence of vas deferens or seminal vesicles should be tested for mutations in the cystic fibrosis transmembrane conductance regulator *(CFTR)* gene.[538]

Screen infertile men with azoospermia or severe oligozoospermia in whom the cause of infertility cannot be ascertained for Y chromosome microdeletions.[520] Consider obtaining a karyotype in infertile men with nonobstructive azoospermia, especially if ICSI is being considered. This is because offspring born after ICSI have a higher frequency of sex chromosome aneuploidy than the general population[546]; in addition, the prevalence of sex chromosome disorders is substantially higher in infertile men, especially among those with azoospermia.[502,547]

Consider mutations in the *CREM* gene in men with postmeiotic germ cell arrest. Many systemic disorders that might be associated with infertility—such as diabetes mellitus, hemoglobinopathies, and myotonic dystrophy—have a genetic basis; these patients also need genetic counseling.

Treatment

The endocrinologist can play a pivotal coordinating role in the treatment of infertile couples by initiating a rational diagnostic evaluation to ascertain a specific treatable cause of infertility and by referring those who require more specialized care. It is particularly important for the endocrinologist to identify and treat gonadotropin deficiency, because hormone replacement therapy in this disorder is highly effective. The endocrinologist should expeditiously ascertain whether the patient has untreatable sterility, in which case the couple should be appropriately counseled about adoption or artificial insemination with donor sperm. In all instances, the endocrinologist should present to the couple a realistic prognosis, the pros and cons of different treatment options, and estimates of costs and should guide the couple away from interventions that have not been shown to be effective.

Induction of Fertility in Men with Hypogonadotropic Hypogonadism

In patients with idiopathic hypogonadotropic hypogonadism, spermatogenesis can be induced by administration of either gonadotropins or pulsatile GnRH infusion. Both pulsatile GnRH therapy and gonadotropin replacement therapy are equally effective in inducing spermatogenesis in men with idiopathic hypogonadotropic hypogonadism.[548-552]

Liu and colleagues[551] compared an hCG/hMG regimen with pulsatile GnRH therapy in its efficacy in inducing spermatogenesis. After 2 years of therapy, 40% of GnRH-treated men and 80% of the hCG/hMG-treated men produced sperm. The sperm concentrations were comparable in the two groups. Buchter and colleagues[553,554] found hCG/hMG and pulsatile GnRH therapy to be equally effective in inducing spermatogenesis. Spermatogenesis was induced in 54 of 57 courses of therapy, and pregnancies occurred in 26 of 36 courses.

The two therapies did not significantly differ either in the time to first appearance of sperm or in pregnancy rates. Successful therapeutic response to GnRH requires the presence of an intact gonadotrope; therefore, this form of therapy is not an option for patients with panhypopituitarism.

Gonadotropin Preparations

Human chorionic gonadotropin (hCG) is purified from the urine of pregnant women and has predominantly LH-like activity; it stimulates Leydig cell testosterone production by interacting with LH/hCG receptors. hMG, derived from the urine of postmenopausal women, contains LH and FSH activities in equal proportions.

Highly purified preparations of hLH and hFSH, derived from human cadaver pituitaries, which had become available for research studies from the National Pituitary Agency of the NIDDK, are no longer recommended. The occurrence of Jakob-Creutzfeldt disease in a few patients treated with earlier preparations of human growth hormone[555] led to the withdrawal and cessation of the use of all human cadaver–derived pituitary hormones for therapeutic purposes. A highly purified hFSH preparation is commercially available for use in gynecologic applications and has been used to treat men with hypogonadotropic hypogonadism.[549]

Recombinant hFSH, expressed in the Chinese hamster ovary cell line and purified to homogeneity, has been approved by FDA for induction of spermatogenesis in men with idiopathic hypogonadotropic hypogonadism.[556,557] The mature β-subunit of rhFSH has seven fewer amino acids than reported in the literature,[60] but it is indistinguishable from purified urinary hFSH in its biologic activity in vitro and in vivo. The pharmacokinetics of urinary hFSH and recombinant hFSH are similar.[556]

Gonadotropin Therapy

Initiate treatment of men with idiopathic hypogonadotropic hypogonadism with 1000 units hCG administered intramuscularly three times a week. Measure serum testosterone levels 6 to 8 weeks after initiation of hCG therapy, 48 to 72 hours after the hCG injection. Adjust the dose to achieve serum testosterone levels in the mid-normal range. Monitor sperm counts on a monthly basis during gonadotropin therapy.

If after 6 months of therapy with hCG alone, serum testosterone levels are in the mid-normal range but the sperm concentrations are low, add FSH. This can be done by using hMG, highly purified FSH, or recombinant FSH. The selection of FSH dose is empirical. Start with 75 IU of FSH three times a week in conjunction with the hCG injections.

If after 3 months of combined treatment, sperm densities are still low, increase the dose of hMG or recombinant FSH to 150 U three times weekly. Forewarn patients at the outset about the potential length and expense of the treatment, and provide conservative estimates of success rates because it can take 18 to 24 months or longer for spermatogenesis to be restored.[548,549,553,557] Couples often tend to get impatient and prematurely disappointed.

Complications

Gonadotropin therapy is usually well tolerated and has low frequency of adverse effects, but it is expensive. Treatment failure due to the development of antibodies to hCG is an uncommon event[558,559] occurring in less than 1% of treated men. Gynecomastia is an uncommon complication of therapy. Allergic reactions are extremely rare.

Outcomes

The two best predictors of success of gonadotropin therapy in hypogonadotropic men are testicular volume at presentation and the time of onset of hypogonadotropism (prepubertally or postpubertally).[548,551] In men with postpubertal onset of hypogonadotropism, spermatogenesis usually can be reinitiated by hCG alone and the success rates are high.[548] On the other hand, men in whom hypogonadotropic hypogonadism developed before pubertal maturation was completed usually do not respond to hCG alone but require combined treatment with hCG and FSH for longer duration, and the overall success rates are lower.

Prior androgen therapy appears not to affect subsequent responsiveness to gonadotropin therapy.[560]

The degree of gonadotropin deficiency, as reflected by the pretreatment testicular volume, is an important determinant of the response to gonadotropin therapy. In general, men with testicular volumes of greater than 8 mL have higher response rates than those with testicular volumes of less than 4 mL.[551] The presence of a coincidental or associated primary testicular abnormality will attenuate the testicular response to gonadotropin therapy. Some patients with IHH also have cryptorchidism; these patients might not respond well to hCG therapy.

Pulsatile GnRH Therapy

Pulsatile administration of GnRH is required to maintain normal LH and FSH output from the pituitary.[561] Continuous infusion of GnRH or administration of a GnRH agonist downregulates LH and FSH secretion.[561,562] The success of GnRH therapy assumes normal pituitary and gonadal function. The pulsatile administration of GnRH should be started with an initial dose of 25 ng/kg per pulse administered subcutaneously every 2 hours by a portable infusion pump.[552,563] Serum testosterone, LH, and FSH levels should be monitored. Adjust the dose of GnRH until the serum testosterone level is in the mid-normal range. There is considerable variability in the GnRH dose requirement among different subjects, and doses ranging from 25 to 200 ng/kg may be required to induce virilization.[563]

After successful induction of secondary sex characteristics, the GnRH dose can be reduced without any adverse effects on serum testosterone, LH, and FSH levels. The gonadotropin secretion and gonadal function can be maintained for extended periods of time (months to years) in a majority of carefully selected patients with IHH by pulsatile GnRH therapy.[552,563]

Complications

Development of anti-GnRH antibodies is an uncommon cause of treatment failure.[552,563] Redness, induration, and subcutaneous infections at the infusion site can occur but are uncommon when proper precautions are taken. Carrying a portable infusion device is cumbersome. Follow-up of these patients often requires considerable physician supervision and laboratory monitoring.

Outcomes

Increases in sperm counts and testicular volume have been reported in more than 70% of treated men, and improvements in sexual function and virilization can be induced in more than 90% of subjects.[552,563] Some patients with IHH have associated cryptorchidism, and these men will likely not respond or will respond suboptimally to pulsatile GnRH treatment. Although induction of virilization by pulsatile GnRH administration in patients with IHH has provided important insights into the mechanisms of puberty and regulation of gonadotropin secretion by GnRH, this approach has no particular advantage over gonadotropin therapy.[551,554]

Treatment Options for Patients with Azoospermia

The prognosis for men with azoospermia, total teratozoospermia, and primary testicular failure with azoospermia is poor.[564] For these men, adoption or artificial insemination using donor sperm are reasonable options. With the advent of ICSI, the prognosis for azoospermic men has improved. There are several case reports of successful pregnancies in partners of men with azoospermia or Klinefelter's syndrome using intracytoplasmic injection of the sperm retrieved from testicular biopsy into the oocyte.[565,566] Palermo and colleagues have reported high success rates with ICSI using spermatozoa surgically retrieved from azoospermic men.[565] Success rates vary considerable among centers depending upon patient selection and experience with the procedure.

The couples who undergo ICSI using testicular spermatozoa should be counseled about the risk of sex chromosome aneuploidy and other genetic disorders being transmitted to the offspring through ICSI.[567] Assisted reproductive technologies, including ICSI, are expensive options. Present a realistic prognosis and dampen expectations at the outset.

Intracytoplasmic Sperm Injection

Intracytoplasmic sperm injection, first used successfully in 1992 for the treatment of infertility, has become a widely used treatment for idiopathic male factor infertility worldwide.[565,568-573] In 2001, more than 114,000 ICSI treatment cycles were performed at 539 centers around the world.[574]

A survey convened by the European Society of Human Reproduction and Embryology reported that the clinical pregnancy rate for each aspiration and transfer for ICSI were 27% and 29%, respectively, in 2002.[575,576] The incidence of multiple gestation is 25% to 35%.[577] The fertilization rates are better for ejaculated and epididymal sperm than for testicular spermatozoa.[570] The pregnancy rates are similar for obstructive and nonobstructive azoospermia. The incidence of oocytes damaged by the procedure remained low (<10%). The pregnancy rates per transfer are higher for fresh sperm than for cryopreserved sperm and are higher for fresh embryos than for frozen-thawed embryos. The results of ICSI are affected by the age of the female partner and the quality of the oocyte. The success rates of ICSI are significantly lower in men in whom sperm has been retrieved from the testis by biopsy and in men with necro- or globozoospermia.

The widespread application of ICSI has raised concern about the safety of this novel technique. The European Society of Human Reproduction and Embryology (ESHRE) has established the ICSI Task Force to annually collect clinical results, the outcome of pregnancy, and the follow-up of children after ICSI to address these important issues.

Multiple gestation with its associated risks of low birth weight and preterm delivery is a frequent complication of ICSI.[569] The risk of obstetric and perinatal complications is higher for pregnancies resulting from ICSI than for naturally conceived pregnancies.[578] The frequency of chromosomal abnormalities is higher in offspring from ICSI than in controls; there is also a small but significant increase in the incidence of chromosome aneuploidy, especially sex chromosome aneuploidy, among offspring from ICSI.[568,570,579-581]

The incidence of major congenital malformations is similar for ICSI and IVF.[580] A small increase in incidence of congenital malformations compared with natural conception has been explained on the basis of the higher prevalence of multiple births. When multiplicity is taken into account, the incidence of major or minor malformations is not increased. However, even among singleton births resulting from assisted reproductive technologies, the risk of low birth weight, preterm delivery, and adverse perinatal outcomes is increased.[569,572,573,578,579]

The developmental outcome of children born after ICSI at 2 and 5 years of age is not significantly different from those born after IVF.[571,582] Also, some reports have suggested increased risk of imprinting disorders, hypospadias, and some types of childhood cancers[583,584]; this issue needs further investigation. Long-term data on the mental and physical well-being of children born through the use of ICSI are not available.

Spontaneous pregnancies in infertile women are associated with a higher risk of obstetric complications and perinatal mortality than spontaneous pregnancies in fertile women.[578] Therefore, it is not apparent whether the complications observed in ICSI pregnancies and births are the consequence of the procedure or of the parental infertility.

ICSI can be effective in many cases of male factor infertility. However, ICSI is an expensive and complicated procedure whose long-term safety is still unclear. Couples should undergo extensive counseling before they are referred for ICSI[578]; adoption or artificial insemination by donor are always reasonable alternatives. Couples should also undergo genetic counseling and testing. Men with idiopathic nonobstructive oligozoospermia or azoospermia should undergo a karyotype and testing for Yq microdeletions before they have ICSI; testing for additional candidate genes may be indicated in some patients. Patients with obstructive azoospermia should be tested for *CFTR* mutations. Additionally, prenatal testing and chorionic villous sampling may be appropriate in many couples undergoing ICSI.

Obstructive Lesions

Microsurgical techniques for treating obstructive lesions have markedly improved. Although the success rates for restoration of patency are high (70% to 90%), the pregnancy rates remain considerably lower (40% to 50%).

Varicoceles in Infertile Men

Varicoceles are present in 10% to 30% of infertile men; however, they are also common in men known to be fertile. Therefore, the role of varicoceles in the pathophysiology of male infertility remains unclear.[585-589]

Although many uncontrolled studies have reported improvements in sperm density and sperm motility after varicocele resection, these data are difficult to interpret because of the lack of an appropriate control group. Many varicocele studies have lacked scientific rigor and are uninterpretable. Only a few controlled clinical trials have been performed, and these trials have failed to show significantly greater improvements in fertility after surgical resection of varicocele than after counseling alone.[585,586] Therefore, there are insufficient data to support a recommendation for surgical resection of varicoceles in most infertile men. However, in the absence of other attractive alternatives, physicians often feel compelled to recommend varicocelectomy or injection of a sclerosing agent.

The expert opinion among urologists favors surgical correction of varicoceles in adolescent boys; the rationale is that there is catch-up growth of the testes after varicocelectomy, which might not occur without the surgical correction. However, prospective data from controlled clinical trials is lacking.

TESTICULAR NEOPLASMS

Epidemiology

Testicular tumors constitute 1% to 2% of malignant tumors in men, although in young and middle-aged men they constitute a greater percentage of all cancers.[590,591] The prevalence rates are higher for whites than for blacks, and the highest prevalence rates of testicular cancers have been reported from Denmark.[590,591] The incidence rates of testicular germ cell tumors have been rising steadily in white men, especially in northern Europe, and have doubled since the 1960s.[592] The risk of testicular neoplasm is increased 50-fold in men with cryptorchidism or previously corrected cryptorchidism.[593] Testicular atrophy, inguinal hernia, and infertility are additional risk factors for testicular germ cell tumors.[594] Among family members of men with testicular germ cell tumors there is higher prevalence of inguinal hernia, cryptorchidism, and hydrocele, suggesting that these conditions may be causally associated with a common defect in urologic development.[595] Adrenal rest tumors occur predominantly in men with poorly controlled congenital adrenal hyperplasia.

Pathophysiology

Testicular germ cell tumors arise during fetal development from cells in the germ cell lineage that are arrested during their maturation.[596] These tumors generally progress through a noninvasive stage called the *intratubular germ cell neoplasia unclassified* (IGCNU) or carcinoma in situ.[596,597] Primordial germ cells undergo considerable imprinting during fetal development; many of these imprinting patterns are erased in testicular germ cell tumors.[598] Thus, hypomethylation of many genes, including the 5′ end of the *XIST* gene, has often been observed in seminomas and nonseminomatous tumors.[599]

Testicular germ cell tumors typically exhibit aneuploidy, and IGCNUs are often triploid.[596,597,600] Gain of function for several genes located on chromosome arm 12p, either because of an isochromosome or as a result of gene amplification, is a common finding in testicular germ cell tumors.[601,602] Other studies have reported altered expression of several genes on 12p, including

CCND2, a regulator of cell cycle; *NANOG* and *STELLAR*, which are involved in maintaining multipotency in germ cells[603,604]; and genes in other chromosomal regions, including *KIT*, *STAT*, and *RAS*, which regulate proliferation and migration of germ cells.[605,606] The molecular basis of the high sensitivity of germ cell tumors to cisplatinum therapy is not fully understood; increased expression of p53 and deficient nucleotide excision repair mechanisms have been suggested as possible means.[607,608]

Classification: Common Types of Testicular Neoplasms

Most testicular neoplasms are of germ cell origin; nongerminal cell tumors of the testis are relatively uncommon.[596] Common types of germ cell tumors include the seminoma, embryonal cell carcinoma, teratoma, choriocarcinoma, and compound tumors that include more than one cell type. Nongerm cell tumors of the testis include Leydig and Sertoli cell neoplasms, adrenal rest tumors, stromal tumors, and mixed cell tumors.

Carcinoma in situ of the testis is characterized by the presence of aneuploid malignant germ cells with clear cytoplasm located within the seminiferous tubules, along the tubular basement membrane, or in the lumen of tubules.[596,597] Approximately 50% of IGCNUs can develop into malignant germ cell tumors in 5 years, and a majority develop into malignant tumors within 7 years. These data point to the malignant nature and invasive potential of IGCNUs and have led to speculation that most germ cell tumors of the testis evolve from this common precursor lesion.

Diagnosis

Testicular neoplasms are detected usually by palpation of a hard testicular mass or metastatic lesion.[596] Five percent to 10% of germ cell tumors arise at extragonadal sites, predominantly retroperitoneum or mediastinum.[609] Intracranial germ cell tumors are rare and are generally located in the pineal gland or suprasellar region.[610]

Many germ cell tumors secrete β-hCG or alpha fetoprotein, and a few secrete carcinoembryonic antigen (CEA), which can serve as useful tumor markers for the diagnosis, treatment, and follow-up of these tumors after chemotherapy.

Leydig cell or Sertoli cell tumors can secrete androgens or estrogens; patients with these tumors might present with isosexual precocity or gynecomastia. hCG-secreting germ cell neoplasms might also manifest with isosexual precocity in boys or gynecomastia in men.

The diagnosis is based on histologic evaluation of testicular biopsy, although the use of fine needle aspiration has been described for the detection of carcinoma in situ. In boys presenting with sexual precocity or gynecomastia, serum testosterone, estradiol, and hCG levels should be measured. Leydig cell tumors secrete both testosterone and estrogens, and Sertoli cell tumors typically secrete only estrogens. In patients with germ cell tumors, hCG, alpha fetoprotein, and CEA should be measured because if they are present, these tumor markers can be useful in following response to therapy and for early detection of recurrences.

Treatment

Testicular germ cell tumors are highly responsive to therapy, even when patients present with advanced disease.[590,591] Orchiectomy or radiotherapy is an effective treatment for patients with unilateral IGCNU, and low-dose radiation is recommended for patients with bilateral IGCNU.[590]

The treatment of testicular germ cell tumors is surgical removal of the primary lesion by orchiectomy followed by adjuvant therapy.[590] The disease-specific survivals in stage I seminoma are 98% or better, whether the adjuvant treatment includes radiotherapy or chemotherapy.[596] Radiotherapy to the paraaortic and paracaval lymph nodes is associated with cure rates of 95% to 98%. Similarly, single-agent carboplatinum treatment has been associated with very low relapse rates.[611] In stage IIA/B seminomas, orchidectomy followed by radiotherapy provides 90% to 95% cure rates.[612] The standard treatment for advanced disease consists of first-line chemotherapy with cisplatin, etoposide, and bleomycin (BEP) followed by surgery in cases with residual tumor.[590,596] In those who do not respond or have residual disease after first-line chemotherapy, second line chemotherapy can salvage a significant proportion. Almost 80% of men with disease in advanced stages can achieve a cure with appropriate treatment.[590,596]

In patients with nonseminomatous germ cell tumors, 5-year survival rates are 94%, 83%, and 71%, respectively, for tumors with good, intermediate, or poor prognosis.[613] Even in patients deemed platinum refractory, response rates of up to 45% have been reported with combination therapies that include gemcitabine and paclitaxel or oxaliplatin-gemcitabine.[613]

The short-term toxicities of systemic chemotherapy of testicular germ cell neoplasms are myelosuppression, nausea and vomiting, pulmonary toxicity, nephropathy, and neuropathy. The long-term toxicities include ototoxicity, impairment of fertility, neuropathy, cardiovascular disease, and secondary malignancies. Because of the young age of these patients and their relatively excellent prognosis for long-term survival, the focus has shifted to minimization of drug toxicity.

ILLICIT USE OF ANDROGENS BY ATHLETES AND RECREATIONAL BODY BUILDERS

Prevalence of Abuse

The exact prevalence of androgenic steroid use by athletes is difficult to determine because the data rely on self-reports, and many users might not admit to the use of these drugs because of fear of self-incrimination. Among professional athletes and Olympians, surveys based on self-report have found high rates of androgenic steroid use.[614,615] From 4 to 6% of high school boys and 1% to 2% of high school girls report using androgenic steroids at least once.[616-619] Similarly high prevalence rates of androgenic steroids have been reported in surveys conducted in other countries.[620,621]

The prevalence of androgenic steroid use among girls has increased since the 1980s.[615,616] In a study published in 1993, Yesalis estimated that approximately one million Americans had used androgenic steroids at some time in their lives.[622] The most egregious example of state-sponsored anabolic steroid doping was uncovered in the former German Democratic Republic after the fall of the communist government.[623]

Pattern of Abuse

Although a large number of androgenic steroids have been known to be abused, the five most commonly abused androgenic steroids include testosterone, nandrolone, stanozolol, methandienone, and methenolol. Surveys of self-reported drug use by athletes and recreational body builders indicate several common patterns[624-626]:

- Intramuscular formulations of androgenic steroids are used far more often than oral formulations[624]; approximately 80% of athletes reporting androgenic steroid use were self-administering intramuscular injections.
- Combinations of androgenic steroids are used more often than single agents.[624,626] Typically, two or more androgenic steroids are used in progressively increasing doses over a period of several weeks in a practice known as *stacking*.
- Athletes and recreational body builders use supraphysiologic doses of testosterone or other androgenic steroids. In one survey,[624] 50% of androgenic steroid users reported using at least 500 mg of testosterone weekly or an equivalent dose of another androgenic steroid; in another survey,[626] almost one fourth of androgenic steroid users used 1000 mg testosterone weekly or an equivalent dose of other androgenic steroids.
- Many androgenic steroid users also abuse other drugs that are perceived in the athletic community to be muscle building, muscle shaping, or performance enhancing.[624] These accessory drugs include stimulants such as amphetamine, clenbuterol, ephedrine, and thyroxine; other anabolic agents such as growth hormone, IGF-1, and insulin; and drugs perceived to reduce adverse effects such as hCG, aromatase inhibitors, or estrogen antagonists.[624] The potential adverse effects of some accessory drugs may be more serious than those of androgenic steroids.

Androgenic Steroids and Athletic Performance

Androgenic steroids increase muscle mass, maximum voluntary strength, and power[350,627,628]; the gains in muscle mass and strength are dose related.[627] Therefore, these drugs might be expected to improve performance in events, such as power lifting, in which performance depends upon muscle strength. It is not surprising that high prevalence rates of androgenic steroid use have been reported among power lifters. Body builders use androgenic steroids to increase skeletal muscle mass and decrease fat mass, which provides greater definition to the muscles.

The use of androgenic steroids by athletes participating in endurance events such as long distance running and bicycling is not easily comprehensible because androgens have not been shown to improve endurance measures such as the lactate threshold and VO_{2max}.[629,630] Androgenic steroids increase hemoglobin levels, which theoretically improves the oxygen-carrying capacity of blood, but even this has not been shown in controlled trials.[631] Researchers speculate that androgenic steroids might allow the athletes to train harder by improving the regenerative response of the skeletal muscle to injury and by their motivational effects; these hypotheses have not been tested rigorously.

The widespread use of androgenic steroids by baseball players and sprint runners also is not easily explained by the available data on the effects of androgenic steroids. The ability to hit a home run against a ball traveling at a speed of 100 mph requires an extraordinary degree of hand-eye coordination—the ability to locate the ball in a specific coordinate of space and to place the bat in that precise coordinate with considerable strength and power. There is some evidence that androgenic steroids decrease reaction time by improving neuromuscular transmission.[632,633] Improved reaction time in conjunction with increased strength and power could potentially explain the perceived improvements in athletic performance by baseball players, although the evidence to support these hypotheses is lacking.

Similarly, in sprint runners who are participating in a 100-m race, the weight gain induced by androgens might be viewed as counterproductive because increased body weight would increase the amount of work done in carrying that body weight against gravity and resistance across the race track. Then why do storied sprinters like Ben Johnson use androgenic steroids? Once again, improved reaction time, the psychological edge gained because of the motivational effects of androgens, and the ability to train harder have been cited as possible explanations without verifiable evidence.

Potential Adverse Effects of Androgenic Steroid Use

Systematic investigations of the adverse effects of androgenic steroids in athletes and recreational body builders have been sparse. These investigations have been hindered by the enormous variability in the types of drugs used; dose, frequency, and duration; age at initiation; and concurrent use of accessory drugs. Furthermore, the veracity of self-reported drug use is always suspect.

It is remarkable that the frequency of serious adverse effects associated with androgenic steroid use has been as low as it has been reported. A number of deaths due to unexpected coronary and cerebrovascular thrombotic events among androgenic steroid users have been reported,[634,635] but these reports are largely anecdotal and do not establish a cause-and-effect relationship. Adverse events associated with androgenic steroid use include deleterious changes in cardiovascular risk factors, including a marked decrease in plasma HDL cholesterol level[636] and changes in clotting factors,[637] suppression of spermatogenesis resulting in infertility, and increase in liver enzymes.[638-640]

The changes in plasma lipids vary depending on the dose, the route of administration (oral or parenteral), and whether the androgen is aromatizable or not. Thus, orally administered 17-α-alkylated nonaromatizable androgens produce greater reductions in plasma HDL cholesterol levels than parenterally administered testosterone. Similarly, elevations of liver enzymes, hepatic neoplasms, and peliosis hepatic have been reported mostly with the use of oral 17-α-alkylated androgenic steroids[638,639] but not with parenterally administered testosterone or its esters.[348]

There are anecdotal reports of the association of androgenic steroid use with "rage reactions." However, placebo-controlled trials of testosterone have not consistently demonstrated a statistically significant increase in anger scores or measures of aggressive behavior.[641-646] There is considerable heterogeneity in the instruments that have been used to measure aggressive behavior, and it is possible that the self-reporting questionnaires were not sufficiently sensitive to detect small but significant changes in aggression. Remarkably, a small number of subjects in the controlled trials have demonstrated marked increases in aggression measures with the use of supraphysiologic doses of testosterone, but a majority of participants show little or no change. It is possible that high doses of androgenic steroids provoke rage reactions in a subset of persons with preexisting psychopathology.

Using a very clever study paradigm, Kouri and colleagues[645] reported that administration of supraphysiologic doses (600 mg weekly) of testosterone enanthate to healthy young men was associated with a significant increase in aggressive responses compared with placebo administration. Testosterone doses that approximated the replacement doses or were slightly higher than the replacement dose did not produce significant changes in aggressive response. In this study, the participants were asked to play a game against a fictitious opponent (the participants were unaware that the opponent was fictitious) in which they had the choice of pressing button A to receive a financial reward or button B that would take money away from a fictitious opponent (aggressive responding). Even though the objective of the game was to achieve the highest monetary gain and the best strategy to achieve that goal was to keep pressing button A, subjects receiving supraphysiologic doses (600 mg weekly) of testosterone enanthate opted to select button B with greater frequency (to punish the fictitious opponent) and thus had higher scores on aggressive responding than those associated with no testosterone or lower doses of testosterone.[645]

Orally administered, 17-α-alkylated androgens also have been associated with insulin resistance and glucose intolerance.[647] There are concerns about potential long-term effects on the risk of prostate and cardiovascular disease; however, the long-term effects of supraphysiologic doses of androgenic steroids are unknown. Increases in left ventricular mass have been reported among users of androgenic steroids[648]; we do not know whether the increase in left ventricular mass is beneficial or deleterious.

Breast tenderness and breast enlargement ("bitch tits" in street parlance) are often associated with the use of aromatizable androgenic steroids. It is not uncommon for athletes to use an aromatase inhibitor or an estrogen antagonist in combination with androgenic steroids to prevent breast enlargement.

Administration of androgenic steroids suppresses endogenous testosterone and sperm production by suppressing the hypothalamic-pituitary-testicular axis.[649,650] Men using androgenic steroids can experience subfertility or infertility.[651] After discontinuing the exogenously administered androgen, recovery of the hypothalamic-pituitary axis can take weeks to months, depending on the dose and duration of prior androgen use.[652-655] During the period immediately after androgens are discontinued, circulating testosterone levels are very low, and the users can experience troublesome symptoms of androgen deficiency, including loss of sexual desire and function, depressed mood, and hot flushes. Some patients who find these withdrawal symptoms difficult to tolerate revert back to using androgenic steroids, thus perpetuating the vicious cycle of abuse, withdrawal symptoms, and dependence.[653-655] Others resort to off-label use of aromatase inhibitors or hCG obtained illicitly based on the folklore widely prevalent in the gymnasia that these agents can accelerate the recovery of the hypothalamic-pituitary-testicular axis, although there is no evidence to support this premise. The long-term suppression of the hypothalamic-pituitary-testicular axis, with its attendant risk of dependence and continued use of androgenic steroids, is a serious complication of androgenic steroid use that has not been widely appreciated.

Self-administration of intramuscular injections increases the risk of infection, muscle abscess, and even sepsis.[625] Transmission of HIV infection has been reported among anabolic steroid users presumably because of needle sharing or the use of improperly sterilized needles and syringes.

Excessive muscle hypertrophy without commensurate adaptations in the associated tendons and connective tissues can predispose athletes using androgenic steroids to the risk of tendon injury and rupture and unusual stress on joints.[656]

Also, 90% of androgenic steroid users abuse additional drugs.[624] Some of these additional drugs of abuse, such as cocaine, amphetamine, and ephedra, may be associated with potentially serious medical complications.

Detection of Illicit Androgenic Steroid

The use of synthetic androgenic steroids was banned in the Olympic games in 1974. Although radioimmunoassay techniques were used initially to detect androgenic steroids in the urine specimens, since 1981, the accredited laboratories have used either gas chromatography–mass spectrometry (GC-MS) or in some instances liquid chromatography mass spectrometry (LC-MS) to detect androgenic steroids that show poor gas chromatographic properties or that are temperature labile.[657] To improve the sensitivity of the gas chromatography, the samples may be derivatized.[658] Thus, silylation is commonly used to derivatize the samples in the analysis of androgenic steroids; this reaction converts the polar groups, such as hydroxyl and keto groups, to less polar trimethylsilyl ethers that improve the signal-to-noise ratio.[658] Also, since the late 1990s, the introduction of high-resolution mass spectrometry (HRMS) and MS/MS has further improved the sensitivity of androgen steroid detection techniques.

For detection of testosterone use, analysis of the testosterone-to-epitestosterone ratio is used in conjunction with isotope ratio combustion mass spectrometry.[659-666] The urinary testosterone-to-epitestosterone ratio typically is less than 6 and is constant in any individual person. There are genetic differences in testosterone-to-epitestosterone ratio. Administration of exogenous testosterone increases the urinary excretion of testosterone glucuronide and increases the testosterone-to-epitestosterone ratio. A testosterone-to-epitestosterone ratio greater than 6:1 is suspicious. Ratios greater than 6 need evaluation of previous urine samples or additional urine samples obtained after a time interval. If the high ratio is due to genetic variation, then all samples obtained from the subject will show the high ratio. A high testosterone-to-epitestosterone ratio that is higher than that observed in previous samples is viewed as a positive test.

If the results of the testosterone-to-epitestosterone ratio test are abnormal and suggest exogenous testosterone use, then additional confirmation by using gas chromatography combustion isotope ratio mass spectrometry is required.[658,661] This method is based on the measurement of the $^{13}C/^{12}C$ isotope ratio in testosterone. In nature, 1.1% of carbon exists as ^{13}C. However, during the chemical synthesis of testosterone, ^{13}C atoms react more slowly than ^{12}C atoms. Therefore, synthetic testosterone, in a manner similar to other organic compounds, has a lower $^{13}C/^{12}C$ ratio than a reference gas standard. During the course of the GC combustion isotope ratio mass spectrometry, the steroids are separated by gas chromatography and oxidized to carbon dioxide in a combustion chamber. The ratio of $^{13}CO_2$ (m/e 45) and $^{12}CO_2$ (m/e 44) is monitored in an isotope ratio mass spectrometer, and the d value is calculated (*d value* refers to the decrease in ^{13}C relative to the reference gas with a standardized $^{13}C/^{12}C$ ratio).[667] A negative d value along with a high testosterone-to-epitestosterone ratio suggests exogenous testosterone administration.

The procedures for collecting and transporting samples for doping tests follow strict rules that have been established by the individual sports organizations.[658] Typically, each urine sample, collected under direct visual oversight of an accredited supervisor, is divided in to two parts (A and B samples) and transported to the testing laboratory using strict chain of custody procedures. If the A sample is deemed positive, then the B sample is analyzed in the presence of the athlete or an authorized representative of the athlete. If the B sample is also positive, then doping with an androgenic steroid is confirmed, and the sports organization can impose punitive sanctions.[658]

Use of Androgen Precursors and Designer Androgens

Δ^4-Androstenedione

Δ^4-Androstenedione, a precursor of testosterone in the testosterone biosynthetic cascade, is converted in the body by 17-hydroxysteroid dehydrogenase to testosterone. Mark Maguire's admission of androstenedione use during an extraordinary season of 53 home runs unleashed a flurry of media stories and heralded a period of rapid growth in over-the-counter sales of dietary supplements such as androstenedione and DHEA.

Androstenedione was sold until recently as a dietary supplement under the Dietary Supplement Health and Education Act.[668,669] Androstenedione's easy availability in nutrition stores made it a popular substance of abuse among recreational body builders.[617,670] Unlike other androgenic steroids, whose sales were regulated within the dictates of the Anabolic Steroid Control Act, androstenedione was sold over the counter, and its sales had not been subject to regulatory oversight of the Food and Drug Administration (FDA) and the Drug Enforcement Agency (DEA). However, the U.S. Congress recently added androstenedione to the list of banned anabolic steroids.

In earlier studies, administration of 100 mg androstenedione orally daily for 7 days produced no significant increases in circulating testosterone concentrations, and administration of a 300-mg dose produced only modest increments in the testosterone area under the curve (AUC) but a much greater increase in circulating estradiol and estrone concentrations.[671-675] In later studies, Jasuja and colleagues[676] demonstrated that 500 mg androstenedione administered thrice daily for 12 weeks to hypogonadal men increased serum testosterone and free testosterone concentrations into the eugonadal range and increased fat-free mass and muscle strength. Also, these studies demonstrated that androstenedione binds androgen receptor, albeit with a substantially lower binding affinity than testosterone, and that it promotes myogenic differentiation in a mesenchymal, multipotent cell line.[676] Similarly, in women, administration of 100 mg androstenedione significantly increased serum testosterone concentrations above the physiologic range for women.[671] As discussed earlier, in female hyenas and several other mammalian species, higher circulating concentrations of androstenedione than those prevalent in humans are associated with virilization.[2] Thus, androstenedione meets all the criteria for an anabolic steroid: it has structural resemblance to testosterone, it binds androgen receptor, it promotes myogenic differentiation in vitro, and it increases muscle mass when administered in sufficiently high doses.[676] Based on these data, the U.S. Congress recently classified androstenedione as an anabolic steroid and banned its over-the-counter sales.

After oral administration of androstenedione, most of the administered dose is inactivated during its presystemic metabolism as indicated by a marked increase in urinary metabolites of androstenedione, including testosterone glucuronide, with only small increases in serum testosterone concentrations.[276] Contamination of dietary supplements with other androgenic steroids because of poor quality control might result in the doping tests becoming positive.[677]

Quality Control Problems in Over-the-Counter Preparations of Androstenedione

Because the manufacture and sale of androstenedione are not regulated by the FDA, there has been a significant quality control problem in over-the-counter preparations of androstenedione.[678,679] In one study, the investigators found considerable variability in androstenedione content of different preparations and even among different batches from the same manufacturer; contamination with other androgens is not uncommon.[677,680]

Potential Adverse Effects of Androstenedione

The long-term side effects of androstenedione use are unknown. Short-term administration of androstenedione is associated with a significant increase in estradiol levels. The long-term consequences of the marked increase in estrogen levels in men taking androstenedione are unknown. In men, the increases in serum estrogen concentrations can affect semen quality, increase inflammation-sensitive markers increasing the risk of cardiovascular events, cause gynecomastia, and induce epigenetic and cytogenetic effects on sperm.

The supplementation of androstenedione decreases HDL levels and increases the LDL/HDL ratio. Other adverse effects of androstenedione stem from the potential increase in testosterone levels. These can include adverse effects on plasma lipids, erythrocytosis, acne, sleep apnea, and increased risk of detecting prostate events.

Given the lack of efficacy data and total absence of long-term safety data, the use of androstenedione is not clinically recommended for any indication, including the treatment of androgen deficiency in men or women.

Dehydroepiandrosterone

DHEA is produced normally in the zona reticularis of the adrenal gland. A weak androgen by itself, it is converted in peripheral tissues to testosterone and estradiol. The circulating levels of DHEA decline markedly with advancing age, so that serum DHEA concentrations in the seventh decade are only about 20% of the peak levels seen in early adult life.[681,682] In addition to its actions as a weak androgen and as an androgen precursor, DHEA might function as a neurosteroid.[683]

DHEA binds androgen receptor with a binding affinity that is substantially lower than that of DHT. A separate G protein–coupled membrane receptor for DHEA has been proposed[684]; however, the existence of such a DHEA-specific membrane receptor needs further confirmation. DHEA also has been shown to modulate the activities of *N*-methyl-*D*-aspartate (NMDA) and γ-aminobutyric acid (GABA) receptors.[685]

Efficacy Trials of DHEA

The literature on DHEA is difficult to interpret for several reasons:

- Many DHEA studies reporting beneficial neurotropic and anticancer effects and immune enhancement were conducted in rodents that have very little endogenous circulating DHEA. Thus, studies in the rodent model have limited applicability to humans.
- The human trials have been characterized by heterogeneity of doses, formulations, and study populations. Doses as high as 1500 mg daily and as low as 25 mg daily have been used.
- Most human studies included small samples and were of relatively short duration.

DHEA studies have been conducted in patients with adrenal insufficiency,[686-690] older men and women,[691-696] peri- and postmenopausal women,[697,698] and patients with autoimmune disease.[699-701] Most intervention trials used 50 mg DHEA daily for 3 to 6 months. A Cochrane review of DHEA trials concluded that there was insufficient evidence of beneficial effect of DHEA on cognition in older men and women.[695] Even higher doses of DHEA administered to older men were found not to produce significant improvements in cognitive function.[696] A randomized, controlled trial has reported greater improvements in bone mineral density in older men and women receiving 50 mg DHEA daily than with placebo.[702]

A number of trials of DHEA supplementation in women with adrenal insufficiency were prompted by the rationale that despite adequate glucocorticoid replacement therapy, patients with adrenal insufficiency report suboptimal quality of life. The results of these studies have been inconsistent. Arlt and colleagues[686] used a double-blind, placebo-controlled crossover study design in women with primary or secondary adrenal insufficiency who received either placebo or 50 mg DHEA daily for 16 weeks each. DHEA administration was associated with improvements in scores for depression and anxiety, sexual function, and circulating osteocalcin levels, but there were no significant changes in body composition.[686] Other trials of DHEA supplementation in women with adrenal insufficiency failed to confirm the beneficial effects of DHEA observed in the Arlt study on mood, well-being, or sexual function.[687-689] Similarly, no consistent effects on body composition, physical function, or insulin sensitivity have been found. Despite unsubstantiated claims in the media and on the Internet, no adequately powered randomized, controlled trials of sufficient duration have been conducted to determine the effects of DHEA administration on cardiovascular event rates or cancer incidence rates.

Pharmacologic doses of DHEA (200 mg daily) have been reported to be associated with modest improvements in systemic lupus erythematosus (SLE) outcomes and a greater reduction in disease flares and disease activity than placebo.[699-701] The effects of DHEA on bone mineral density in patients with SLE have been inconsistent.

Thus, randomized, controlled trials of DHEA have not demonstrated consistent efficacy in any disease state and do not justify DHEA use for any clinical indication at present.

Other Androgen Precursors and Novel Designer Steroids of Abuse

A number of additional steroids that are precursors of testosterone (4-androstenediol and 5-androstenediol in addition to 4-androstenedione and DHEA discussed earlier), dihydrotestosterone (5-α-androstane-3β-17β-diol, 5-α-androstane-3α,17β-diol, 5-α-androstane-3,17-dione, 5-α-androst-1-ene-3,17-dione, 17β-hydroxy-5-α-androst-1-en-3-one, 5-α-androst,1-ene,17 β-diol), or nortestosterone (4-norandrostenedione, 4-norandrostenediol, and 5-norandrostenediol) have been introduced in the underground marketplace[658]; these compounds are weakly androgenic but are converted in the body to potent androgens. Even a precursor (androsta-1,4-diene-3,17-dione) of boldenone (17-β-hydroxyandrosta-1,4-dien-3-one) has been advertised on the internet.[658]

Until recently, the androgenic steroids abused by athletes were typically those that had been synthesized initially for medicinal or veterinary indications. The recent appearance in the market place of designer steroids, such as tetrahydrogestrinone (THG)[703,704] and madol,[705] that were developed solely for abuse and whose synthesis was not driven by any medicinal motivation represents a sinister development.[706] The detection of abuse of novel androgenic steroids for which the detection methods have not been standardized poses considerable challenge to the testing laboratories. Because these designer compounds have never been tested previously in animals or humans, their use by athletes without even the slightest toxicologic or safety data is of enormous health concern. Because there are no published data or prior experience with the use of these novel designer steroids, and because it takes considerable time to generate data of their androgenic and anabolic efficacy that would withstand scientific and legal scrutiny, government agencies have been stymied in their efforts to regulate this underground marketplace.

REFERENCES

1. Kegany GJ, Trombulak SG. Size and function of mammalian testes in relation to body size. J Mammology 1986;67:1-22.
2. Glickman SE, Coscia EM, Frank LG, et al. Androgens and masculinization of genitalia in the spotted hyaena *(Crocuta crocuta)*. 3. Effects of juvenile gonadectomy. J Reprod Fertil 1998;113: 129-135.
3. Glickman SE, Frank LG, Pavgi S, Licht P. Hormonal correlates of "masculinization" in female spotted hyaenas *(Crocuta crocuta)*. 1. Infancy to sexual maturity. J Reprod Fertil 1992;95:451-462.
4. Glickman SE, Frank LG, Davidson JM, et al. Androstenedione may organize or activate sex-reversed traits in female spotted hyenas. Proc Natl Acad Sci U S A 1987;84:3444-3447.
5. Goymann W, East ML, Hofer H. Androgens and the role of female "hyperaggressiveness" in spotted hyenas *(Crocuta crocuta)*. Horm Behav 2001;39:83-92.
6. Wilson JD, Auchus RJ, Leihy MW, et al. 5α-androstane-3α,17β-diol is formed in tammar wallaby pouch young testes by a pathway involving 5α-pregnane-3α,17α-diol-20-one as a key intermediate. Endocrinology 2003;144:575-580.
7. Wilson JD, Shaw G, Renfree MB, et al. Ontogeny and pathway of formation of 5α-androstane-3α,17β-diol in the testes of the immature brushtail possum *Trichosurus vulpecula*. Reprod Fertil Dev 2005;17:603-609.
8. Stechell BP. The testis and tissue transplantation: historical aspects. J Reprod Immunol 1990;18:1-8.
9. George FW, Wilson JD. Sex determination and differentiation. In Knobil E, Wilson JD eds. The Physiology of Reproduction. 2nd edition. New York: Raven Press, 1994:3-26.
10. Wilson JD, Griffin JE, Russel DW. Steroid 5-α reductase-2 deficiency. Endocr Rev 1993;14:557-593.
11. Menderlson CR, Dufau ML, Catt KJ. Gonadotropin stimulation of cyclic adenosine 3′-5′ monophosphate and testosterone production in isolated Leydig cells. J Biol Chem 1975;250:8818-8823.
12. Payne AH, Quinn PG, Rani CS. Regulation of microsome cytochrome P-450 enzymes and testosterone production in Leydig cells. Recent Prog Horm Res 1985;41:153-197.
13. Wahlstrom JT, Huhtaniemi I, Hovatta O, et al. Localization of luteinizing hormone, follicle-stimulating hormone, prolactin, and their receptors in human and rat testis using immunohistochemistry and radioreceptor assays. J Clin Endocrinol Metab 1983;57:825-830.
14. Saez JM. Leydig cells: endocrine, paracrine, and autocrine regulation. Endocr Rev 1994;16:574-626.
15. Carr BR, Parker CR Jr, Ohashi M, et al. Regulation of human fetal testicular secretion of testosterone: low-density lipoprotein-cholesterol and choleterol synthesized de novo as steroid precursor. Am J Obstet Gynecol 1983;146:241-247.
16. Miller WL. Molecular biology of the steroid hormone synthesis. Endocrine Rev 1988;9:295-318.
17. Jasuja R, Ramaraj T, Mac RP, et al. Androstenedione binds androgen receptor, promotes myogenesis in vitro, and increases fat-free mass and muscle strength in hypogonadal men. J Clin Endocrinol Metab 2005;90:855-863.
18. Rosner W. Plasma steroid-binding proteins. Endocrinol Metab Clin North Am 1991;20:697-720.
19. Mendel CM. The free hormone hypothesis: a physiologically based mathematical model. Endocr Rev 1989;10:232-274.
20. Sakiyama R, Pardridge WM, Musto NA. Influx of testosterone-binding globulin (TeBG) and TeBG-bound sex steroid hormones into rat testis and prostate. J Clin Endocrinol Metab 1988;67: 98-103.
21. Nakhla AM, Rosner W. Stimulation of prostate cancer growth by androgens and estrogens through the intermediacy of sex hormone–binding globulin. Endocrinology 1996;137:4126-4129.
22. Hammes A, Andreassen TK, Spoelgen R, et al. Role of endocytosis in cellular uptake of sex steroids. Cell 2005;122:751-762.
23. Andreassen TK. The role of plasma-binding proteins in the cellular uptake of lipophilic vitamins and steroids. Horm Metab Res 2006;38:279-290.
24. Ukkola O, Rankinen T, Gagnon J, et al. A genome-wide linkage scan for steroids and SHBG levels in black and white families: the HERITAGE Family Study. J Clin Endocrinol Metab 2002;87: 3708-3720.

25. Joseph DR. Structure, function, and regulation of androgen-binding protein/sex hormone–binding globulin. Vitam Horm 1994;49:197-280.
26. Besa EC, Bullock LP. The role of the androgen receptor in erythropoiesis. Endocrinology 1981;109:1983-1989.
27. Smith EP, Boyd J, Frank GR, et al. Estrogen resistance caused by a mutation in the estrogen receptor gene in a man. N Engl J Med 1994;331:1056-1061.
28. Carani C, Rochira V, Faustini-Fustini M, et al. Role of oestrogen in male sexual behaviour: insights from the natural model of aromatase deficiency. Clin Endocrinol (Oxf) 1999;51:517-524.
29. Deladoey J, Fluck C, Bex M, et al. Aromatase deficiency caused by a novel P450arom gene mutation: impact of absent estrogen production on serum gonadotropin concentration in a boy. J Clin Endocrinol Metab 1999;84:4050-4054.
30. Morishima A, Grumbach MM, Simpson ER, et al. Aromatase deficiency in male and female siblings caused by a novel mutation and the physiological role of estrogens. J Clin Endocrinol Metab 1995;80:3689-3698.
31. Mullis PE, Yoshimura N, Kuhlmann B, et al. Aromatase deficiency in a female who is compound heterozygote for two new point mutations in the P450arom gene: impact of estrogens on hypergonadotropic hypogonadism, multicystic ovaries, and bone densitometry in childhood. J Clin Endocrinol Metab 1997;82:1739-1745.
32. Russell DW, Wilson JD. Steroid 5-α reductase: two gene/two enzymes. Ann Rev Biochem 1994;63:25-61.
33. Mahendroo MS, Porter A, Russell DW, Word RA. The parturition defect in steroid 5α-reductase type 1 knockout mice is due to impaired cervical ripening. Mol Endocrinol 1999;13:981-992.
34. Bartsch W, Krieg M, Voigt KD. Quantification of endogenous testosterone, 5α-dihydrotestosterone and 5α-androstane-3α,17β-diol in subcellular fractions of the prostate, bulbocavernosus/levator ani muscle, skeletal muscle and heart muscle of the rat. J Steroid Biochem 1980;13:259-264.
35. Simental JA, Sar M, Wilson EM. Domain functions of the androgen receptor. J Steroid Biochem Mol Biol 1992;43:37-41.
36. McPhaul MJ. Molecular defects of the androgen receptor. J Steroid Biochem Mol Biol 1999;69:315-322.
37. McPhaul MJ, Marcelli M, Zoppi S, et al. Genetic basis of endocrine disease. 4. The spectrum of mutations in the androgen receptor gene that causes androgen resistance. J Clin Endocrinol Metab 1993;76:17-23.
38. Lubahn DB, Brown TR, Simental JA, et al. Sequence of the intron/exon junctions of the coding region of the human androgen receptor gene and identification of a point mutation in a family with complete androgen insensitivity. Proc Natl Acad Sci U S A 1989;86:9534-9538.
39. Slagsvold T, Kraus I, Bentzen T, et al. Mutational analysis of the androgen receptor AF-2 (activation function 2) core domain reveals functional and mechanistic differences of conserved residues compared with other nuclear receptors. Mol Endocrinol 2000;14:1603-1617.
40. Quigley CA, De Bellis A, Marschke KB, et al. Androgen receptor defects: historical, clinical, and molecular perspectives. Endocr Rev 1995;16:271-321.
41. Singh R, Artaza JN, Taylor WE, et al. Testosterone inhibits adipogenic differentiation in 3T3-L1 cells: nuclear translocation of androgen receptor complex with β-catenin and T-cell factor 4 may bypass canonical Wnt signaling to down-regulate adipogenic transcription factors. Endocrinology 2006;147:141-154.
42. Singh R, Artaza JN, Taylor WE, et al. Androgens stimulate myogenic differentiation and inhibit adipogenesis in C3H 10T1/2 pluripotent cells through an androgen receptor–mediated pathway. Endocrinology 2003;144:5081-5088.
43. Ferrando AA, Raj D, Wolfe RR. Amino acid control of muscle protein turnover in renal disease. J Ren Nutr 2005;15:34-38.
44. Ferrando AA, Sheffield-Moore M, Paddon-Jones D, et al. Differential anabolic effects of testosterone and amino acid feeding in older men. J Clin Endocrinol Metab 2003;88:358-362.
45. Ferrando AA, Sheffield-Moore M, Wolf SE, et al. Testosterone administration in severe burns ameliorates muscle catabolism. Crit Care Med 2001;29:1936-1942.
46. Ferrando AA, Sheffield-Moore M, Yeckel CW, et al. Testosterone administration to older men improves muscle function: molecular and physiological mechanisms. Am J Physiol Endocrinol Metab 2002;282:E601-E607.
47. Sheffield-Moore M, Urban RJ, Wolf SE, et al. Short-term oxandrolone administration stimulates net muscle protein synthesis in young men. J Clin Endocrinol Metab 1999;84:2705-2711.
48. Wolfe R, Ferrando A, Sheffield-Moore M, Urban R. Testosterone and muscle protein metabolism. Mayo Clin Proc 2000;75(suppl):S55-S59; discussion S59-S60.
49. Skaletsky H, Kuroda-Kawaguchi T, Minx P, et al. The male-specific region of the Y chromosome is a mosaic of discrete sequence classes. Nature 2003;423:825-837.
50. Hawley RS. The human Y chromosome; the rumors of its death have been greatly exaggerated. Cell 2003;113:825-828.
51. Knuth UA, Hull MG, Jacobs HS. Amenorrhoea and loss of weight. Br J Obstet Gynaecol 1977;84:801-807.
52. Frisch RE. Body fat, menarche, fitness and fertility. Hum Reprod 1987;2:521-533.
53. Penny R, Goldstein IP, Frasier SD. Gonadotropin excretion and body composition. Pediatrics 1978;61:294-300.
54. Stein Z, Susser M. Fertility, fecundity, famine: food rations in the Dutch famine 1944/5 have a causal relation to fertility, and probably to fecundity. Hum Biol 1975;47:131-154.
55. Stein Z, Susser M. The Dutch famine, 1944-1945, and the reproductive process. I. Effects of six indices at birth. Pediatr Res 1975;9:70-76.
56. van der Walt LA, Wilmsen EN, Jenkins T. Unusual sex hormone patterns among desert-dwelling hunter-gatherers. J Clin Endocrinol Metab 1978;46:658-663.
57. van der Walt LA, Wilmsen EN, Levin J, Jenkins T. Endocrine studies on the San ("bushmen") of Botswana. S Afr Med J 1977;52:230-232.
58. Foster DL, Nagatani S. Physiological perspectives on leptin as a regulator of reproduction: role in timing puberty. Biol Reprod 1999;60:205-215.
59. Halmi KA, Sherman BM. Gonadotropin response to LH-RH in anorexia nervosa. Arch Gen Psychiatry 1975;32:875-878.
60. Sherman BM, Halmi KA, Zamudio R. LH and FSH response to gonadotropin-releasing hormone in anorexia nervosa: Effect of nutritional rehabilitation. J Clin Endocrinol Metab 1975;41:135-142.
61. Baker ER. Body weight and the initiation of puberty. Clin Obstet Gynecol 1985;28:573-579.
62. Frisch RE. Fatness, menarche, and female fertility. Perspect Biol Med 1985;28:611-633.
63. Frisch RE, Gotz-Welbergen AV, McArthur JW, et al. Delayed menarche and amenorrhea of college athletes in relation to age of onset of training. JAMA 1981;246:1559-1563.
64. Van Der Spuy ZM, Jacobs HS. Weight reduction, fertility and contraception. IPPF Med Bull 1983;17:2-4.
65. Laughlin GA, Dominguez CE, Yen SS. Nutritional and endocrine-metabolic aberrations in women with functional hypothalamic amenorrhea. J Clin Endocrinol Metab 1998;83:25-32.
66. Laughlin GA, Yen SS. Nutritional and endocrine-metabolic aberrations in amenorrheic athletes. J Clin Endocrinol Metab 1996;81:4301-4309.
67. Misra M, Aggarwal A, Miller KK, et al. Effects of anorexia nervosa on clinical, hematologic, biochemical, and bone density parameters in community-dwelling adolescent girls. Pediatrics 2004;114:1574-1583.
68. Bates GW, Bates SR, Whitworth NS. Reproductive failure in women who practice weight control. Fertil Steril 1982;37:373-378.
69. Rock CL, Gorenflo DW, Drewnowski A, Demitrack MA. Nutritional characteristics, eating pathology, and hormonal status in young women. Am J Clin Nutr 1996;64:566-571.
70. Cunningham MJ, Clifton DK, Steiner RA. Leptin's actions on the reproductive axis: perspectives and mechanisms. Biol Reprod 1999;60:216-222.
71. Zhang Y, Proenca R, Maffei M, et al. Positional cloning of the mouse obese gene and its human homologue. Nature 1994;372:425-432.
72. Campfield LA, Smith FJ, Burn P. The OB protein (leptin) pathway—a link between adipose tissue mass and central neural networks. Horm Metab Res 1996;28:619-632.

73. Campfield LA, Smith FJ, Guisez Y, et al. Recombinant mouse OB protein: evidence for a peripheral signal linking adiposity and central neural networks. Science 1995;269:546-549.
74. Weigle DS, Duell PB, Connor WE, et al. Effect of fasting, refeeding, and dietary fat restriction on plasma leptin levels. J Clin Endocrinol Metab 1997;82:561-565.
75. Keim NL, Stern JS, Havel PJ. Relation between circulating leptin concentrations and appetite during a prolonged, moderate energy deficit in women. Am J Clin Nutr 1998;68:794-801.
76. Chan JL, Matarese G, Shetty GK, et al. Differential regulation of metabolic, neuroendocrine, and immune function by leptin in humans. Proc Natl Acad Sci U S A 2006;103:8481-8486.
77. Ahima RS, Prabakaran D, Mantzoros C, et al. Role of leptin in the neuroendocrine response to fasting. Nature 1996;382:250-252.
78. Swerdloff RS, Batt RA, Bray GA. Reproductive hormonal function in the genetically obese (ob/ob) mouse. Endocrinology 1976;98: 1359-1364.
79. Farooqi IS, Matarese G, Lord GM, et al. Beneficial effects of leptin on obesity, T cell hyporesponsiveness, and neuroendocrine/metabolic dysfunction of human congenital leptin deficiency. J Clin Invest 2002;110:1093-1103.
80. Chehab FF, Lim ME, Lu R. Correction of the sterility defect in homozygous obese female mice by treatment with the human recombinant leptin. Nat Genet 1996;12:318-320.
81. Yu WH, Walczewska A, Karanth S, McCann SM. Nitric oxide mediates leptin-induced luteinizing hormone–releasing hormone (LHRH) and LHRH and leptin-induced LH release from the pituitary gland. Endocrinology 1997;138:5055-5058.
82. Barb CR, Kraeling RR, Rampacek GB, Hausman GJ. The role of neuropeptide Y and interaction with leptin in regulating feed intake and luteinizing hormone and growth hormone secretion in the pig. Reproduction 2006;131:1127-1135.
83. Kaynard AH, Pau KY, Hess DL, Spies HG. Third-ventricular infusion of neuropeptide Y suppresses luteinizing hormone secretion in ovariectomized rhesus macaques. Endocrinology 1990;127: 2437-2444.
84. Catzeflis C, Pierroz DD, Rohner-Jeanrenaud F, et al. Neuropeptide Y administered chronically into the lateral ventricle profoundly inhibits both the gonadotropic and the somatotropic axis in intact adult female rats. Endocrinology 1993;132:224-234.
85. Zizzari P, Halem H, Taylor J, et al. Endogenous ghrelin regulates episodic growth hormone (GH) secretion by amplifying GH pulse amplitude: evidence from antagonism of the GH secretagogue-R1a receptor. Endocrinology 2005;146:3836-3842.
86. Fernandez-Fernandez R, Martini AC, Navarro VM, et al. Novel signals for the integration of energy balance and reproduction. Mol Cell Endocrinol 2006;254-255:127-132.
87. Fernandez-Fernandez R, Tena-Sempere M, Navarro VM, et al. Effects of ghrelin upon gonadotropin-releasing hormone and gonadotropin secretion in adult female rats: in vivo and in vitro studies. Neuroendocrinology 2005;82(5-6):245-255. Epub 2006 Apr 20.
88. Fernandez-Fernandez R, Tena-Sempere M, Navarro VM, et al. Effects of ghrelin upon gonadotropin-releasing hormone and gonadotropin secretion in adult female rats: in vivo and in vitro studies. Neuroendocrinology 2006;82(5-6):245-255 [Epub ahead of print].
89. Date Y, Kojima M, Hosoda H, et al. Ghrelin, a novel growth hormone–releasing acylated peptide, is synthesized in a distinct endocrine cell type in the gastrointestinal tracts of rats and humans. Endocrinology 2000;141:4255-4261.
90. Kojima M, Hosoda H, Date Y, et al. Ghrelin is a growth-hormone–releasing acylated peptide from stomach. Nature 1999; 402:656-660.
91. Nakazato M, Murakami N, Date Y, et al. A role for ghrelin in the central regulation of feeding. Nature 2001;409:194-198.
92. Fernandez-Fernandez R, Aguilar E, Tena-Sempere M, Pinilla L. Effects of polypeptide YY(3-36) upon luteinizing hormone–releasing hormone and gonadotropin secretion in prepubertal rats: in vivo and in vitro studies. Endocrinology 2005;146: 1403-1410.
93. Navarro VM, Castellano JM, Fernandez-Fernandez R, et al. Effects of KiSS-1 peptide, the natural ligand of GPR54, on follicle-stimulating hormone secretion in the rat. Endocrinology 2005;146:1689-1697.
94. Bhasin S, Cunningham GR, Hayes FJ, et al. Testosterone therapy in adult men with androgen deficiency syndromes: an endocrine society clinical practice guideline. J Clin Endocrinol Metab 2006;91:1995-2010.
95. Jacobs PA, Melville M, Ratcliffe S, et al. A cytogenetic survey of 11,680 newborn infants. Ann Hum Genet 1974;37:359-376.
96. Hamerton JL, Canning N, Ray M, Smith S. A cytogenetic survey of 14,069 newborn infants. I. Incidence of chromosome abnormalities. Clin Genet 1975;8:223-243.
97. Bojesen A, Juul S, Gravholt CH. Prenatal and postnatal prevalence of Klinefelter syndrome: a national registry study. J Clin Endocrinol Metab 2003;88:622-626.
98. Paulsen CA, Gordon DL, Carpenter RW, et al. Klinefelter's syndrome and its variants: a hormonal and chromosomal study. Recent Prog Horm Res 1968;24:321-363
99. Huckins C, Bullock LP, Long JL. Morphological profiles of cryptorchid XXY mouse testes. Anat Rec 1981;199:507-518.
100. Bandmann HJ, Breit R, Perwein E. Klinefelter's Syndrome. Berlin: Springer-Verlag, 1984.
101. Hook EB. Rates of chromosome abnormalities at different maternal ages. Obstet Gynecol 1981;58:282-285.
102. Abramsky L, Chapple J. 47,XXY (Klinefelter syndrome) and 47,XYY: estimated rates of and indication for postnatal diagnosis with implications for prenatal counselling. Prenat Diagn 1997;17: 363-368.
103. Wikstrom AM, Dunkel L, Wickman S, et al. Are adolescent boys with Klinefelter syndrome androgen deficient? A longitudinal study of Finnish 47,XXY boys. Pediatr Res 2006;59:854-859.
104. Aksglaede L, Wikstrom AM, Rajpert-De Meyts E, et al. Natural history of seminiferous tubule degeneration in Klinefelter syndrome. Hum Reprod Update 2006;12:39-48.
105. Wikstrom AM, Raivio T, Hadziselimovic F, et al. Klinefelter syndrome in adolescence: onset of puberty is associated with accelerated germ cell depletion. J Clin Endocrinol Metab 2004;89: 2263-2270.
106. Bojesen A, Juul S, Birkebaek N, Gravholt CH. Increased mortality in Klinefelter syndrome. J Clin Endocrinol Metab 2004;89: 3830-3834.
107. Swerdlow AJ, Hermon C, Jacobs PA, et al. Mortality and cancer incidence in persons with numerical sex chromosome abnormalities: a cohort study. Ann Hum Genet 2001;65:177-188.
108. Swerdlow AJ, Schoemaker MJ, Higgins CD, et al. Cancer incidence and mortality in men with Klinefelter syndrome: a cohort study. J Natl Cancer Inst 2005;97:1204-1210.
109. Howell SJ, Shalet SM. Spermatogenesis after cancer treatment: damage and recovery. J Natl Cancer Inst Monogr 2005;34:12-17.
110. Howell SJ, Radford JA, Smets EM, Shalet SM. Fatigue, sexual function and mood following treatment for haematological malignancy: the impact of mild Leydig cell dysfunction. Br J Cancer 2000;82:789-793.
111. Holmes SJ, Whitehouse RW, Clark ST, et al. Reduced bone mineral density in men following chemotherapy for Hodgkin's disease. Br J Cancer 1994;70:371-375.
112. Monteil M, Rousseaux S, Chevret E, et al. Increased aneuploid frequency in spermatozoa from a Hodgkin's disease patient after chemotherapy and radiotherapy. Cytogenet Cell Genet 1997;76: 134-138.
113. Robbins WA, Meistrich ML, Moore D, et al. Chemotherapy induces transient sex chromosomal and autosomal aneuploidy in human sperm. Nat Genet 1997;16:74-78.
114. Robbins WA. Cytogenetic damage measured in human sperm following cancer chemotherapy. Mutat Res 1996;355:235-252.
115. Howell SJ, Shalet SM. Effect of cancer therapy on pituitary-testicular axis. Int J Androl 2002;25:269-276.
116. Meistrich ML, Chawla SP, Da Cunha MF, et al. Recovery of sperm production after chemotherapy for osteosarcoma. Cancer 1989;63: 2115-2123.
117. da Cunha MF, Meistrich ML, Fuller LM, et al. Recovery of spermatogenesis after treatment for Hodgkin's disease: limiting dose of MOPP chemotherapy. J Clin Oncol 1984;2:571-577.
118. Whitehead E, Shalet SM, Blackledge G, et al. The effects of Hodgkin's disease and combination chemotherapy on gonadal function in the adult male. Cancer 1982;49:418-422.

119. Whitehead E, Shalet SM, Jones PH, et al. Gonadal function after combination chemotherapy for Hodgkin's disease in childhood. Arch Dis Child 1982;57:287-291.
120. Viviani S, Santoro A, Ragni G, et al. Gonadal toxicity after combination chemotherapy for Hodgkin's disease. Comparative results of MOPP vs ABVD. Eur J Cancer Clin Oncol 1985;21: 601-605.
121. Chatterjee R, Mills W, Katz M, et al. Germ cell failure and Leydig cell insufficiency in post-pubertal males after autologous bone marrow transplantation with BEAM for lymphoma. Bone Marrow Transplant 1994;13:519-522.
122. Hansen SW, Berthelsen JG, von der Maase H. Long-term fertility and Leydig cell function in patients treated for germ cell cancer with cisplatin, vinblastine, and bleomycin versus surveillance. J Clin Oncol 1990;8:1695-1698.
123. Johnson DH, Linde R, Hainsworth JD, et al. Effect of a luteinizing hormone releasing hormone agonist given during combination chemotherapy on posttherapy fertility in male patients with lymphoma: preliminary observations. Blood 1985;65:832-836.
124. Waxman JH, Ahmed R, Smith D, et al. Failure to preserve fertility in patients with Hodgkin's disease. Cancer Chemother Pharmacol 1987;19:159-162.
125. Cross JJ, Berman LH, Elliott PG, Irving S. Scrotal trauma: a cause of testicular atrophy. Clin Radiol 1999;54:317-320.
126. Manson AL. Mumps orchitis. Urology 1990;36:335-338.
127. Dobs AS, Dempsey MA, Ladenson PW, Polk BF. Endocrine disorders in men infected with human immunodeficiency virus. Am J Med 1988;84:611-616.
128. Arver S, Sinha-Hikim I, Beall G, et al. Serum dihydrotestosterone and testosterone concentrations in human immunodeficiency virus–infected men with and without weight loss. J Androl 1999;20:611-618.
129. Rietschel P, Corcoran C, Stanley T, et al. Prevalence of hypogonadism among men with weight loss related to human immunodeficiency virus infection who were receiving highly active antiretroviral therapy. Clin Infect Dis 2000;31:1240-1244.
130. Salehian B, Jacobson D, Swerdloff RS, et al. Testicular pathologic changes and the pituitary-testicular axis during human immunodeficiency virus infection. Endocr Pract 1999;5:1-9.
131. Bhasin S, Calof O, Storer TW, et al. Drug insights: anabolic applications of testosterone and selective androgen receptor modulators in aging and chronic illness. Nature CPEM 2006;2:133-140.
132. Dobs AS, Few WL 3rd, Blackman MR, et al. Serum hormones in men with human immunodeficiency virus–associated wasting. J Clin Endocrinol Metab 1996;81:4108-4112.
133. Edman DC, Winter AJ, Porter JC. Embryonic testicular regression: a clinical spectrum of XY agonadal individuals. Obstet Gynecol 1977;49:208-217.
134. Borrow M, Gough M. Bilateral absence of the testes. Lancet 1970;1:366.
135. Hall J, Morgan A, Blizzard RM. Familial congenital anorchia. Birth Defects Orig Art Ser 1975;11:115-119.
136. Marcantonio SM, Fechner PY, Migeon CJ, et al. Embryonic testicular regression sequence: a part of the clinical spectrum of 46,XY gonadal dysgenesis. Am J Med Genet 1994;49:1-5.
137. Vinci G, Anjot M, Trivin C, et al. An analysis of the genetic factors involved in testicular descent in a cohort of 14 male patients with anorchia. J Clin Endocrinol Metab 2004;89:6282-6285.
138. de Roux N, Milgrom E. Inherited disorders of GnRH and gonadotropin receptors. Mol Cell Endocrinol 2001;179:83-87.
139. Gromoll J, Eiholzer U, Nieschlag E, Simoni M. Male hypogonadism caused by homozygous deletion of exon 10 of the luteinizing hormone (LH) receptor: differential action of human chorionic gonadotropin and LH. J Clin Endocrinol Metab 2000;85: 2281-2286.
140. Latronico AC, Arnhold IJ. Inactivating mutations of LH and FSH receptors—from genotype to phenotype. Pediatr Endocrinol Rev 2006;4:28-31.
141. McDonough PG. Inactivating mutations in the LH receptor—as rare a "a hen with teeth" or as frequent as polycystic ovary syndrome? Fertil Steril 2000;73:655-656.
142. Richter-Unruh A, Martens JW, Verhoef-Post M, et al. Leydig cell hypoplasia: cases with new mutations, new polymorphisms and cases without mutations in the luteinizing hormone receptor gene. Clin Endocrinol (Oxf) 2002;56:103-112.
143. Salameh W, Choucair M, Guo TB, et al. Leydig cell hypoplasia due to inactivation of luteinizing hormone receptor by a novel homozygous nonsense truncation mutation in the seventh transmembrane domain. Mol Cell Endocrinol 2005;229:57-64.
144. Themmen AP, Brunner HG. Luteinizing hormone receptor mutations and sex differentiation. Eur J Endocrinol 1996;134:533-540.
145. Toledo SP, Brunner HG, Kraaij R, et al. An inactivating mutation of the luteinizing hormone receptor causes amenorrhea in a 46,XX female. J Clin Endocrinol Metab 1996;81:3850-3854.
146. Tsigos C, Latronico C, Chrousos GP. Luteinizing hormone resistance syndromes. Ann N Y Acad Sci 1997;816:263-273.
147. Wu SM, Hallermeier KM, Laue L, et al. Inactivation of the luteinizing hormone/chorionic gonadotropin receptor by an insertional mutation in Leydig cell hypoplasia. Mol Endocrinol 1998;12: 1651-1660.
148. Wu SM, Leschek EW, Rennert OM, Chan WY. Luteinizing hormone receptor mutations in disorders of sexual development and cancer. Front Biosci 2000;5:D343-D352.
149. Aittomaki K, Herva R, Stenman UH, et al. Clinical features of primary ovarian failure caused by a point mutation in the follicle-stimulating hormone receptor gene. J Clin Endocrinol Metab 1996;81:3722-3726.
150. Allen LA, Achermann JC, Pakarinen P, et al. A novel loss of function mutation in exon 10 of the FSH receptor gene causing hypergonadotrophic hypogonadism: clinical and molecular characteristics. Hum Reprod 2003;18:251-256.
151. Jiang M, Aittomaki K, Nilsson C, et al. The frequency of an inactivating point mutation (566C→T) of the human follicle-stimulating hormone receptor gene in four populations using allele-specific hybridization and time-resolved fluorometry. J Clin Endocrinol Metab 1998;83:4338-4343.
152. Layman LC, Amde S, Cohen DP, et al. The Finnish follicle-stimulating hormone receptor gene mutation is rare in North American women with 46,XX ovarian failure. Fertil Steril 1998;69:300-302.
153. Loutradis D, Patsoula E, Stefanidis K, et al. Follicle-stimulating hormone receptor gene mutations are not evident in Greek women with premature ovarian failure and poor responders. Gynecol Obstet Invest 2006;61:56-60.
154. Betterle C, Pra CD, Mantero F, Zanchetta R. Autoimmune adrenal insufficiency and autoimmune polyendocrine syndromes: autoantibodies, autoantigens, and their applicability in diagnosis and disease prediction. Endocr Rev 2002;23:327-364.
155. Sauder SE, Frager M, Case GD, et al. Abnormal patterns of pulsatile luteinizing hormone secretion in women with hyperprolactinemia: responses to bromocriptine. J Clin Endocrinol Metab 1984;59: 941-948.
156. Tay CC, Glasier AF, Illingworth PJ, Baird DT. Abnormal 24-hour pattern of pulsatile LH secretion and response to naloxone in women with hyperprolactinemic amenorrhea. Clin Endocrinol (Oxf) 1993;39:599-606.
157. Milenkovic L, D'Angelo G, Kelly PA, Weiner RI. Inhibition of gonadotropin hormone–releasing hormone release by prolactin from GT1 neuronal cell lines through prolactin receptors. Proc Natl Acad Sci U S A 1994;91:1244-1247.
158. Feldman HA, Longcope C, Derby CA, et al. Age trends in the level of serum testosterone and other hormones in middle-aged men: longitudinal results from the Massachusetts Male Aging Study. J Clin Endocrinol Metab 2002;87:589-598.
159. Gray A, Berlin JA, McKinlay JB, Longcope C. An examination of research design effects on the association of testosterone and male aging: results of a meta-analysis. J Clin Epidemiol 1991;44:671-684.
160. Harman SM, Metter EJ, Tobin JD, et al. Longitudinal effects of aging on serum total and free testosterone levels in healthy men. Baltimore Longitudinal Study of Aging. J Clin Endocrinol Metab 2001;86:724-731.
161. Morley JE, Kaiser FE, Perry HM 3rd, et al. Longitudinal changes in testosterone, luteinizing hormone, and follicle-stimulating hormone in healthy older men. Metabolism 1997;46:410-413.
162. Simon D, Preziosi P, Barrett-Connor E, et al. The influence of aging on plasma sex hormones in men: the Telecom Study. Am J Epidemiol 1992;135:783-791.
163. Zmuda JM, Cauley JA, Kriska A, et al. Longitudinal relation between endogenous testosterone and cardiovascular disease risk factors in middle-aged men. A 13-year follow-up of former

Multiple Risk Factor Intervention Trial participants. Am J Epidemiol 1997;146:609-617.

164. Ferrini RL, Barrett-Connor E. Sex hormones and age: a cross-sectional study of testosterone and estradiol and their bioavailable fractions in community-dwelling men. Am J Epidemiol 1998;147:750-754.
165. Harman SM, Tsitouras PD. Reproductive hormones in aging men. I. Measurement of sex steroids, basal luteinizing hormone, and Leydig cell response to human chorionic gonadotropin. J Clin Endocrinol Metab 1980;51:35-40.
166. Veldhuis JD, Veldhuis NJ, Keenan DM, Iranmanesh A. Age diminishes the testicular steroidogenic response to repeated intravenous pulses of recombinant human LH during acute GnRH-receptor blockade in healthy men. Am J Physiol Endocrinol Metab 2005;288: E775-781.
167. Takahashi PY, Liu PY, Roebuck PD, et al. Graded inhibition of pulsatile luteinizing hormone secretion by a selective gonadotropin-releasing hormone (GnRH)-receptor antagonist in healthy men: evidence that age attenuates hypothalamic GnRH outflow. J Clin Endocrinol Metab 2005;90:2768-2774.
168. Keenan DM, Takahashi PY, Liu PY, et al. An ensemble model of the male gonadal axis: illustrative application in aging men. Endocrinology 2006;147:2817-2828.
169. Mulligan T, Iranmanesh A, Johnson ML, et al. Aging alters feed-forward and feedback linkages between LH and testosterone in healthy men. Am J Physiol 1997;273:R1407-1413.
170. Veldhuis JD, Zwart A, Mulligan T, Iranmanesh A. Muting of androgen negative feedback unveils impoverished gonadotropin-releasing hormone/luteinizing hormone secretory reactivity in healthy older men. J Clin Endocrinol Metab 2001;86:529-535.
171. Daniell HW. Hypogonadism in men consuming sustained-action oral opioids. J Pain 2002;3:377-384.
172. Rajagopal A, Vassilopoulou-Sellin R, Palmer JL, et al. Symptomatic hypogonadism in male survivors of cancer with chronic exposure to opioids. Cancer 2004;100:851-858.
173. Abs R, Verhelst J, Maeyaert J, et al. Endocrine consequences of long-term intrathecal administration of opioids. J Clin Endocrinol Metab 2000;85:2215-2222.
174. Daniell HW, Lentz R, Mazer NA. Open-label pilot study of testosterone patch therapy in men with opioid-induced androgen deficiency. J Pain 2006;7:200-210.
175. de la Rosa RE, Hennessey JV. Hypogonadism and methadone: Hypothalamic hypogonadism after long-term use of high-dose methadone. Endocr Pract 1996;2:4-7.
176. Bliesener N, Albrecht S, Schwager A, et al. Plasma testosterone and sexual function in men receiving buprenorphine maintenance for opioid dependence. J Clin Endocrinol Metab 2005;90: 203-206.
177. Rasmussen DD, Liu JH, Wolf PL, Yen SS. Endogenous opioid regulation of gonadotropin-releasing hormone release from the human fetal hypothalamus in vitro. J Clin Endocrinol Metab 1983;57: 881-884.
178. Ellingboe J, Veldhuis JD, Mendelson JH, et al. Effect of endogenous opioid blockade on the amplitude and frequency of pulsatile luteinizing hormone secretion in normal men. J Clin Endocrinol Metab 1982;54:854-857.
179. Evans WS, Weltman JY, Johnson ML, et al. Effects of opioid receptor blockade on luteinizing hormone (LH) pulses and interpulse LH concentrations in normal women during the early phase of the menstrual cycle. J Endocrinol Invest 1992;15:525-531.
180. Veldhuis JD, Rogol AD, Johnson ML. Endogenous opiates modulate the pulsatile secretion of biologically active luteinizing hormone in man. J Clin Invest 1983;72:2031-2040.
181. Rimoin DL, Schimke RN. Mechanisms of gene action in disorders of the endocrine glands. Birth Defects Orig Art Ser 1971;7:5-11.
182. Crowley WF Jr, Whitcomb RW, Jameson JL, et al. Neuroendocrine control of human reproduction in the male. Recent Prog Horm Res 1991;47:27-62.
183. Waldstreicher J, Seminara SB, Jameson JL, et al. The genetic and clinical heterogeneity of gonadotropin-releasing hormone deficiency in the human. J Clin Endocrinol Metab 1996;81: 4388-4395.
184. Spratt DI, Carr DB, Merriam GR, et al. The spectrum of abnormal patterns of gonadotropin-releasing hormone secretion in men with idiopathic hypogonadotropic hypogonadism: clinical and laboratory correlations. J Clin Endocrinol Metab 1987;64:283-291.
185. Smals AG, Kloppenborg PW, van Haelst UJ, et al. Fertile eunuch syndrome versus classic hypogonadotrophic hypogonadism. Acta Endocrinol (Copenh) 1978;87:389-399.
186. Mozaffarian GA, Higley M, Paulsen CA. Clinical studies in an adult male patient with "isolated follicle stimulating hormone (FSH) deficiency." J Androl 1983;4:393-398.
187. Seminara SB, Oliveira LM, Beranova M, et al. Genetics of hypogonadotropic hypogonadism. J Endocrinol Invest 2000;23:560-565.
188. Franco B, Guioli S, Pragliola A, et al. A gene deleted in Kallmann's syndrome shares homology with neural cell adhesion and axonal path-finding molecules. Nature 1991;353:529-536.
189. Ballabio A, Bardoni B, Carrozzo R, et al. Contiguous gene syndromes due to deletions in the distal short arm of the human X chromosome. Proc Natl Acad Sci U S A 1989;86:10001-10005.
190. Legouis R, Hardelin JP, Levilliers J, et al. The candidate gene for the X-linked Kallmann syndrome encodes a protein related to adhesion molecules. Cell 1991;67:423-435.
191. Georgopoulos NA, Pralong FP, Seidman CE, et al. Genetic heterogeneity evidenced by low incidence of KAL-1 gene mutations in sporadic cases of gonadotropin-releasing hormone deficiency. J Clin Endocrinol Metab 1997;82:213-217.
192. Schwanzel-Fukuda M, Pfaff DW. Origin of luteinizing hormone–releasing hormone neurons. Nature 1989;338:161-164.
193. Schwanzel-Fukuda M, Pfaff DW. The migration of luteinizing hormone–releasing hormone (LHRH) neurons from the medial olfactory placode into the medial basal forebrain. Experientia 1990;46:956-962.
194. Klingmuller D, Dewes W, Krahe T, et al. Magnetic resonance imaging of the brain in patients with anosmia and hypothalamic hypogonadism (Kallmann's syndrome). J Clin Endocrinol Metab 1987;65:581-584.
195. Sato N, Katsumata N, Kagami M, et al. Clinical assessment and mutation analysis of Kallmann syndrome 1 (KAL1) and fibroblast growth factor receptor 1 (FGFR1, or KAL2) in five families and 18 sporadic patients. J Clin Endocrinol Metab 2004;89: 1079-1088.
196. Phelan JK, McCabe ERB. Mutations in NROB1 *(DAX1)* and NR5A1 *(SF1)* responsible for adrenal hypoplasia congenita. Human Mutations 2001;18:472-487.
197. Burris TP, Guo W, McCabe ER. The gene responsible for adrenal hypoplasia congenita, *DAX-1,* encodes a nuclear hormone receptor that defines a new class within the superfamily. Recent Prog Horm Res 1996;51:241-259; discussion 259-260.
198. Habiby RL, Boepple P, Nachtigall L, et al. Adrenal hypoplasia congenita with hypogonadotropic hypogonadism: evidence that *DAX-1* mutations lead to combined hypothalmic and pituitary defects in gonadotropin production. J Clin Invest 1996;98: 1055-1062.
199. Luo X, Ikeda Y, Parker KL. A cell-specific receptor is essential for adrenal and gonadal development and sexual differentiation. Cell 1994;77:481-490.
200. Crawford PA, Dorn C, Sadovsky Y, Milbrandt J. Nuclear receptor DAX-1 recruits nuclear receptor corepressor N-CoR to SF-1. Mol Cell Biol 1998;18:2949-2956.
201. de Roux N, Young J, Misrahi M, et al. A family with hypogonadotropic hypogonadism and mutations in the gonadotropin-releasing hormone receptor. N Engl J Med 1997;337:1597-1602.
202. Caron P, Chauvin S, Christin-Maitre S, et al. Resistance of hypogonadic patients with mutated GnRH receptor genes to pulsatile GnRH administration. J Clin Endocrinol Metab 1999;84:990-996.
203. Seminara SB, Messager S, Chatzidaki EE, et al. The GPR54 gene as a regulator of puberty. N Engl J Med 2003;349:1614-1627.
204. Seminara SB. The first kiss—a crucial role for kisspeptin-1 and its receptor, G-protein-coupled receptor 54, in puberty and reproduction. Nature CPEM 2006;2:328-334.
205. Ohtaki T, Shintani Y, Honda S, et al. Metastasis suppressor gene *kiss-1* encodes peptide ligand of a G protein coupled receptor. Nature 2001;411:613-617.
206. Navarro VM, Castellano JM, Fernandez-Fernandez R, et al. Developmental and hormonally regulated mRNA expression of *kiss-1* and its putative receptor, GPR54, in the rat hypothalamus and potent LH releasing activity of KISS-1 peptide. Endocrinology 2004;145:4565-4574.

207. Miura K, Acierno JS, Jr, Seminara SB. Characterization of the human nasal embryonic LHRH factor gene, *NELF*, and a mutation screening among 65 patients with idiopathic hypogonadotropic hypogonadism (IHH). J Hum Genet 2004;49:265-268.
208. Bhagavath B, Podolsky RH, Ozata M, et al. Clinical and molecular characterization of a large sample of patients with hypogonadotropic hypogonadism. Fertil Steril 2006;85:706-713.
209. Layman LC. The molecular basis of human hypogonadotropic hypogonadism. Mol Genet Metab 1999;68:191-199.
210. Layman LC, Lee EJ, Peak DB, et al. Delayed puberty and hypogonadism caused by mutations in the follicle-stimulating hormone β-subunit gene. N Engl J Med 1997;337:607-611.
211. Kumar TR, Wang Y, Lu N, Matzuk MM. Follicle stimulating hormone is required for ovarian follicle maturation but not male fertility. Nat Genet 1997;15:201-204.
212. Weiss J, Axelrod L, Whitcomb RW, et al. Hypogonadism caused by a single amino acid substitution in the β-subunit of luteinizing hormone. N Engl J Med 1992;326:179-183.
213. Nilsson C, Pettersson K, Millar RP, et al. Worldwide frequency of a common genetic variant of luteinizing hormone: an international collaborative research. International Collaborative Research Group. Fertil Steril 1997;67:998-1004.
214. Raivio T, Huhtaniemi I, Anttila R, et al. The role of luteinizing hormone-β gene polymorphism in the onset and progression of puberty in healthy boys. J Clin Endocrinol Metab 1996;81: 3278-3282.
215. Gromoll J, Partsch CJ, Simoni M, Net al. A mutation in the first transmembrane domain of the lutropin receptor causes male precocious puberty. J Clin Endocrinol Metab 1998;83:476-480.
216. Gromoll J, Simoni M, Nordhoff V, et al. Functional and clinical consequences of mutations in the FSH receptor. Mol Cell Endocrinol 1996;125:177-182.
217. Gunay-Aygun M, Schwartz S, Heeger S, et al. The changing purpose of Prader-Willi syndrome clinical diagnostic criteria and proposed revised criteria. Pediatrics 2001;108:E92.
218. Gunay-Aygun M, Cassidy SB, Nicholls RD. Prader-Willi and other syndromes associated with obesity and mental retardation. Behav Genet 1997;27:307-324.
219. Saitoh S, Buiting K, Cassidy SB, et al. Clinical spectrum and molecular diagnosis of Angelman and Prader-Willi syndrome patients with an imprinting mutation. Am J Med Genet 1997;68: 195-206.
220. LaSalle JM, Ritchie RJ, Glatt H, Lalande M. Clonal heterogeneity at allelic methylation sites diagnostic for Prader-Willi and Angelman syndromes. Proc Natl Acad Sci U S A 1998;95:1675-1680.
221. Arnhold IJ, Nery M, Brown MR, et al. Clinical and molecular characterization of a Brazilian patient with Pit-1 deficiency. J Pediatr Endocrinol Metab 1998;11:623-630.
222. Parks JS, Brown MR. Transcription factors regulating pituitary development. Growth Horm IGF Res 1999;9 Suppl B:2-8; discussion 8-11.
223. Pfaffle RW, Parks JS, Brown MR, Heimann G. Pit-1 and pituitary function. J Pediatr Endocrinol 1993;6:229-233.
224. Wu W, Cogan JD, Pfaffle RW, et al. Mutations in PROP1 cause familial combined pituitary hormone deficiency. Nat Genet 1998;18:147-149.
225. Dattani MT, Martinez-Barbera JP, Thomas PQ, et al. Mutations in the homeobox gene *HESX1/Hesx1* associated with septo-optic dysplasia in human and mouse. Nat Genet 1998;19:125-133.
226. Radovick S, Nations M, Du Y, et al. A mutation in the POU-homeodomain of Pit-1 responsible for combined pituitary hormone deficiency. Science 1992;257:1115-1118.
227. Semina EV, Reiter R, Leysens NJ, et al. Cloning and characterization of a novel bicoid-related homeobox transcription factor gene, *RIEG*, involved in Rieger syndrome. Nat Genet 1996;14:392-399.
228. Netchine I, Sobrier ML, Krude H, et al. Mutations in *LHX3* result in a new syndrome revealed by combined pituitary hormone deficiency. Nat Genet 2000;25:182-186.
229. Brooks-Gunn J, Warren MP, Hamilton LH. The relation of eating problems and amenorrhea in ballet dancers. Med Sci Sports Exerc 1987;19:41-44.
230. Warren MP, Perlroth NE. The effects of intense exercise on the female reproductive system. J Endocrinol 2001;170:3-11.
231. Frisch RE, Wyshak G, Vincent L. Delayed menarche and amenorrhea in ballet dancers. N Engl J Med 1980;303:17-19.
232. Glass AR, Harrison R, Swerdloff RS. Effect of undernutrition and amino acid deficiency on the timing of puberty in rats. Pediatr Res 1976;10:951-955.
233. Loucks AB, Horvath SM. Exercise-induced stress responses of amenorrheic and eumenorrheic runners. J Clin Endocrinol Metab 1984;59:1109-1120.
234. Veldhuis JD, Evans WS, Demers LM, et al. Altered neuroendocrine regulation of gonadotropin secretion in women distance runners. J Clin Endocrinol Metab 1985;61:557-563.
235. Loucks AB, Mortola JF, Girton L, Yen SS. Alterations in the hypothalamic-pituitary-ovarian and the hypothalamic-pituitary-adrenal axes in athletic women. J Clin Endocrinol Metab 1989;68: 402-411.
236. Frisch RE, Wyshak G, Albright NL, et al. Lower prevalence of nonreproductive system cancers among female former college athletes. Med Sci Sports Exerc 1989;21:250-253.
237. Frisch RE, Wyshak G, Albright NL, et al. Lower prevalence of breast cancer and cancers of the reproductive system among former college athletes compared to non-athletes. Br J Cancer 1985;52:885-891.
238. Frisch RE, Wyshak G, Albright NL, et al. Lower lifetime occurrence of breast cancer and cancers of the reproductive system among former college athletes. Am J Clin Nutr 1987;45:328-335.
239. Frisch RE, Wyshak G, Witschi J, et al. Lower lifetime occurrence of breast cancer and cancers of the reproductive system among former college athletes. Int J Fertil 1987;32:217-225.
240. Wyshak G, Frisch RE, Albright NL, et al. Lower prevalence of benign diseases of the breast and benign tumours of the reproductive system among former college athletes compared to non-athletes. Br J Cancer 1986;54:841-845.
241. Malin A, Matthews CE, Shu XO, et al. Energy balance and breast cancer risk. Cancer Epidemiol Biomarkers Prev 2005;14: 1496-1501.
242. Rogol AD, Veldhuis JD, Williams FA, Johnson ML. Pulsatile secretion of gonadotropins and prolactin in male marathon runners. Relation to the endogenous opiate system. J Androl 1984;5:21-27.
243. MacConnie SE, Barkan A, Lampman RM, Schork MA, Beitins IZ. Decreased hypothalamic gonadotropin-releasing hormone secretion in male marathon runners. N Engl J Med 1986;315:411-417.
244. Comerci GD. Medical complications of anorexia nervosa and bulimia nervosa. Med Clin North Am 1990;74:1293-1310.
245. Kalm LM, Semba RD. They starved so that others be better fed: remembering Ancel Keys and the Minnesota experiment. J Nutr 2005;135:1347-1352.
246. Keys A, Brazek J, Henschel A, Mickelsen O, Taylor HL. The Biology of Human Starvation. Minneapolis: University of Minnesota Press, 1950.
247. Glass AR, Swerdloff RS, Bray GA, et al. Low serum testosterone and sex-hormone-binding-globulin in massively obese men. J Clin Endocrinol Metab 1977;45:1211-1219.
248. Amatruda JM, Harman SM, Pourmotabbed G, Lockwood DH. Depressed plasma testosterone and fractional binding of testosterone in obese males. J Clin Endocrinol Metab 1978;47:268-271.
249. Vermeulen A. Decreased androgen levels and obesity in men. Ann Med 1996;28:13-15.
250. Vermeulen A, Kaufman JM, Deslypere JP, Thomas G. Attenuated luteinizing hormone (LH) pulse amplitude but normal LH pulse frequency, and its relation to plasma androgens in hypogonadism of obese men. J Clin Endocrinol Metab 1993;76:1140-1146.
251. Zumoff B, Strain GW, Miller LK, et al. Plasma free and non–sex-hormone-binding-globulin-bound testosterone are decreased in obese men in proportion to their degree of obesity. J Clin Endocrinol Metab 1990;71:929-931.
252. Birkeland KI, Hanssen KF, Torjesen PA, Vaaler S. Level of sex hormone-binding globulin is positively correlated with insulin sensitivity in men with type 2 diabetes. J Clin Endocrinol Metab 1993;76:275-278.
253. Laing I, Olukoga AO, Gordon C, Boulton AJ. Serum sex-hormone-binding globulin is related to hepatic and peripheral insulin sensitivity but not to beta-cell function in men and women with type 2 diabetes mellitus. Diabet Med 1998;15:473-479.
254. Giagulli VA, Kaufman JM, Vermeulen A. Pathogenesis of the decreased androgen levels in obese men. J Clin Endocrinol Metab 1994;79:997-1000.

255. Plymate SR, Matej LA, Jones RE, Friedl KE. Inhibition of sex hormone–binding globulin production in the human hepatoma (Hep G2) cell line by insulin and prolactin. J Clin Endocrinol Metab 1988;67:460-464.
256. Crave JC, Lejeune H, Brebant C, et al. Differential effects of insulin and insulin-like growth factor I on the production of plasma steroid–binding globulins by human hepatoblastoma-derived (Hep G2) cells. J Clin Endocrinol Metab 1995;80: 1283-1289.
257. Plymate SR, Tenover JS, Bremner WJ. Circadian variation in testosterone, sex hormone–binding globulin, and calculated non–sex hormone–binding globulin bound testosterone in healthy young and elderly men. J Androl 1989;10:366-371.
258. Strain GW, Zumoff B, Kream J, et al. Mild hypogonadotropic hypogonadism in obese men. Metabolism 1982;31:871-875.
259. Schneider G, Kirschner MA, Berkowitz R, Ertel NH. Increased estrogen production in obese men. J Clin Endocrinol Metab 1979;48:633-638.
260. Zumoff B, Miller LK, Strain GW. Reversal of the hypogonadotropic hypogonadism of obese men by administration of the aromatase inhibitor testolactone. Metabolism 2003;52:1126-1128.
261. Amatruda JM, Hochstein M, Hsu TH, Lockwood DH. Hypothalamic and pituitary dysfunction in obese males. Int J Obes 1982;6:183-189.
262. Arnott JM, Wu FCW, Pye S, et al. A clinically relevant approach to defining the prevalence of late onset hypogonadism in men from the general population. Presented at the 88th Endocrine Society Meeting, Boston, June 20-24, 2006.
263. Diver MJ. Analytical and physiological factors affecting the interpretation of serum testosterone concentration in men. Ann Clin Biochem 2006;43:3-12.
264. Cooke RR, McIntosh JE, McIntosh RP. Circadian variation in serum free and non–SHBG-bound testosterone in normal men: measurements, and simulation using a mass action model. Clin Endocrinol (Oxf) 1993;39:163-171.
265. Rosner W. Sex steroids and the free hormone hypothesis. Cell 2006;124:455-456; author reply 456-457.
266. Wang C, Catlin DH, Demers LM, et al. Measurement of total serum testosterone in adult men: comparison of current laboratory methods versus liquid chromatography-tandem mass spectrometry. J Clin Endocrinol Metab 2004;89:534-543.
267. Manni A, Pardridge WM, Cefalu W, et al. Bioavailability of albumin-bound testosterone. J Clin Endocrinol Metab 1985;61: 705-710.
268. Vermeulen A, Verdonck L, Kaufman JM. A critical evaluation of simple methods for the estimation of free testosterone in serum. J Clin Endocrinol Metab 1999;84:3666-3672.
269. Winters SJ, Kelley DE, Goodpaster B. The analog free testosterone assay: are the results in men clinically useful? Clin Chem 1998;44:2178-2182.
270. Buvat J, Lemaire A. Endocrine screening in 1,022 men with erectile dysfunction: clinical significance and cost-effective strategy. J Urol 1997;158:1764-1767.
271. Citron JT, Ettinger B, Rubinoff H, et al. Prevalence of hypothalamic-pituitary imaging abnormalities in impotent men with secondary hypogonadism. J Urol 1996;155:529-533.
272. Morley JE, Charlton E, Patrick P, et al. Validation of a screening questionnaire for androgen deficiency in aging males. Metabolism 2000;49:1239-1242.
273. Smith KW, Feldman HA, McKinlay JB. Construction and field validation of a self-administered screener for testosterone deficiency (hypogonadism) in ageing men. Clin Endocrinol (Oxf) 2000;53: 703-711.
274. Moore C, Huebler D, Zimmermann T, et al. The Aging Males' Symptoms scale (AMS) as outcome measure for treatment of androgen deficiency. Eur Urol 2004;46:80-87.
275. Stanley HL, Schmitt BP, Poses RM, Deiss WP. Does hypogonadism contribute to the occurrence of a minimal trauma hip fracture in elderly men? J Am Geriatr Soc 1991;39:766-771.
276. Riggs BL, Khosla S, Melton LJ 3rd. Sex steroids and the construction and conservation of the adult skeleton. Endocr Rev 2002; 23:279-302.
277. Wahlstrom JT, Dobs AS. Acute and long-term effects of AIDS and injection drug use on gonadal function. J Acquir Immune Defic Syndr 2000;25(suppl 1):S27-S36.
278. Wahlstrom JT, Tang A, Cofrancesco J, et al. Gonadal hormone levels in injection drug users. Drug Alcohol Depend 2000;60: 311-313.
279. Grinspoon S, Corcoran C, Lee K, et al. Loss of lean body and muscle mass correlates with androgen levels in hypogonadal men with acquired immunodeficiency syndrome and wasting. J Clin Endocrinol Metab 1996;81:4051-4058.
280. Singh AB, Norris K, Modi N, et al. Pharmacokinetics of a transdermal testosterone system in men with end stage renal disease receiving maintenance hemodialysis and healthy hypogonadal men. J Clin Endocrinol Metab 2001;86:2437-2445.
281. Casaburi R. Rationale for anabolic therapy to facilitate rehabilitation in chronic obstructive pulmonary disease. Baillieres Clin Endocrinol Metab 1998;12:407-418.
282. Casaburi R. Skeletal muscle dysfunction in chronic obstructive pulmonary disease. Med Sci Sports Exerc 2001;33:S662-S670.
283. Creutzberg EC, Casaburi R. Endocrinological disturbances in chronic obstructive pulmonary disease. Eur Respir J Suppl 2003;46:76s-80s.
284. Dhindsa S, Prabhakar S, Sethi M, et al. Frequent occurrence of hypogonadotropic hypogonadism in type 2 diabetes. J Clin Endocrinol Metab 2004;89:5462-5468.
285. Reid IR, Ibbertson HK, France JT, Pybus J. Plasma testosterone concentrations in asthmatic men treated with glucocorticoids. Br Med J (Clin Res Ed) 1985;291:574.
286. Arver S, Dobs AS, Meikle AW, et al. Improvement of sexual function in testosterone deficient men treated for 1 year with a permeation enhanced testosterone transdermal system. J Urol 1996;155: 1604-1608.
287. Steidle C, Schwartz S, Jacoby K, et al. AA2500 testosterone gel normalizes androgen levels in aging males with improvements in body composition and sexual function. J Clin Endocrinol Metab 2003;88:2673-2681.
288. Kwan M, Greenleaf WJ, Mann J, et al. The nature of androgen action on male sexuality: a combined laboratory-self-report study on hypogonadal men. J Clin Endocrinol Metab 1983;57:557-562.
289. Snyder PJ, Lawrence DA. Treatment of male hypogonadism with testosterone enanthate. J Clin Endocrinol Metab 1980;51: 1335-1339.
290. Alexander GM, Sherwin BB. The association between testosterone, sexual arousal, and selective attention for erotic stimuli in men. Horm Behav 1991;25:367-381.
291. Cunningham GR, Hirshkowitz M, Korenman SG, Karacan I. Testosterone replacement therapy and sleep-related erections in hypogonadal men. J Clin Endocrinol Metab 1990;70:792-797.
292. Wang C, Alexander G, Berman N, et al. Testosterone replacement therapy improves mood in hypogonadal men—a clinical research center study. J Clin Endocrinol Metab 1996;81:3578-3583.
293. Janowsky JS, Oviatt SK, Orwoll ES. Testosterone influences spatial cognition in older men. Behav Neurosci 1994;108:325-332.
294. Cherrier MM, Asthana S, Plymate S, et al. Testosterone supplementation improves spatial and verbal memory in healthy older men. Neurology 2001;57:80-88.
295. Marin P, Holmang S, Jonsson L, et al. The effects of testosterone treatment on body composition and metabolism in middle-aged obese men. Int J Obes Relat Metab Disord 1992;16:991-997.
296. Marin P, Krotkiewski M, Bjorntorp P. Androgen treatment of middle-aged, obese men: effects on metabolism, muscle and adipose tissues. Eur J Med 1992;1:329-336.
297. Singh AB, Hsia S, Alaupovic P, et al. The effects of varying doses of T on insulin sensitivity, plasma lipids, apolipoproteins, and C-reactive protein in healthy young men. J Clin Endocrinol Metab 2002;87:136-143.
298. Kapoor D, Goodwin E, Channer KS, Jones TH. Testosterone replacement therapy improves insulin resistance, glycaemic control, visceral adiposity and hypercholesterolaemia in hypogonadal men with type 2 diabetes. Eur J Endocrinol 2006;154: 899-906.
299. Sokol RZ, Palacios A, Campfield LA, Saul C, Swerdloff RS. Comparison of the kinetics of injectable testosterone in eugonadal and hypogonadal men. Fertil Steril 1982;37:425-430.
300. Schulte-Beerbuhl M, Nieschlag E. Comparison of testosterone, dihydrotestosterone, luteinizing hormone, and follicle-stimulating hormone in serum after injection of testosterone enanthate of testosterone cypionate. Fertil Steril 1980;33:201-203.

301. Wang ZM, Pierson RN Jr, Heymsfield SB. The five-level model: a new approach to organizing body-composition research. Am J Clin Nutr 1992;56:19-28.
302. Wang C, Swedloff RS, Iranmanesh A, et al. Transdermal testosterone gel improves sexual function, mood, muscle strength, and body composition parameters in hypogonadal men. Testosterone Gel Study Group. J Clin Endocrinol Metab 2000;85:2839-2853.
303. Wang C, Berman N, Longstreth JA, et al. Pharmacokinetics of transdermal testosterone gel in hypogonadal men: application of gel at one site versus four sites: a General Clinical Research Center Study. J Clin Endocrinol Metab 2000;85:964-969.
304. Wang C, Swerdloff RS, Iranmanesh A, et al. Effects of transdermal testosterone gel on bone turnover markers and bone mineral density in hypogonadal men. Clin Endocrinol (Oxf) 2001;54: 739-750.
305. Wang C, Cunningham G, Dobs A, et al. Long-term testosterone gel (AndroGel) treatment maintains beneficial effects on sexual function and mood, lean and fat mass, and bone mineral density in hypogonadal men. J Clin Endocrinol Metab 2004;89: 2085-2098.
306. McNicholas TA, Dean JD, Mulder H, et al. A novel testosterone gel formulation normalizes androgen levels in hypogonadal men, with improvements in body composition and sexual function. BJU Int 2003;91:69-74.
307. Arver S, Dobs AS, Meikle AW, et al. Long-term efficacy and safety of a permeation-enhanced testosterone transdermal system in hypogonadal men. Clin Endocrinol (Oxf) 1997;47:727-737.
308. Dobs AS, Hoover DR, Chen MC, Allen R. Pharmacokinetic characteristics, efficacy, and safety of buccal testosterone in hypogonadal males: a pilot study. J Clin Endocrinol Metab 1998;83: 33-39.
309. Dobs AS, Meikle AW, Arver S, et al. Pharmacokinetics, efficacy, and safety of a permeation-enhanced testosterone transdermal system in comparison with bi-weekly injections of testosterone enanthate for the treatment of hypogonadal men. J Clin Endocrinol Metab 1999;84:3469-3478.
310. Wang C, Swerdloff R, Kipnes M, et al. New testosterone buccal system (Striant) delivers physiological testosterone levels: pharmacokinetics study in hypogonadal men. J Clin Endocrinol Metab 2004;89:3821-3829.
311. Ross RJ, Jabbar A, Jones TH, et al. Pharmacokinetics and tolerability of a bioadhesive buccal testosterone tablet in hypogonadal men. Eur J Endocrinol 2004;150:57-63.
312. Dobs AS, Matsumoto AM, Wang C, Kipnes MS. Short-term pharmacokinetic comparison of a novel testosterone buccal system and a testosterone gel in testosterone deficient men. Curr Med Res Opin 2004;20:729-738.
313. Hirschhauser C, Hopkinson CR, Sturm G, Coert A. Testosterone undecanoate: a new orally active androgen. Acta Endocrinol (Copenh) 1975;80:179-187.
314. Franchimont P, Kicovic PM, Mattei A, Roulier R. Effects of oral testosterone undecanoate in hypogonadal male patients. Clin Endocrinol (Oxf) 1978;9:313-320.
315. Skakkebaek NE, Bancroft J, Davidson DW, Warner P. Androgen replacement with oral testosterone undecanoate in hypogonadal men: a double blind controlled study. Clin Endocrinol (Oxf) 1981;14:49-61.
316. Maisey NM, Bingham J, Marks V, et al. Clinical efficacy of testosterone undecanoate in male hypogonadism. Clin Endocrinol (Oxf) 1981;14:625-629.
317. O'Carroll R, Shapiro C, Bancroft J. Androgens, behaviour and nocturnal erection in hypogonadal men: the effects of varying the replacement dose. Clin Endocrinol (Oxf) 1985;23:527-538.
318. Conway AJ, Boylan LM, Howe C, et al. Randomized clinical trial of testosterone replacement therapy in hypogonadal men. Int J Androl 1988;11:247-264.
319. Gooren LJ. A ten-year safety study of the oral androgen testosterone undecanoate. J Androl 1994;15:212-215.
320. Jockenhovel F, Vogel E, Reinhardt W, Reinwein D. Effects of various modes of androgen substitution therapy on erythropoiesis. Eur J Med Res 1997;2:293-298.
321. Zitzmann M, Nieschlag E. Hormone substitution in male hypogonadism. Mol Cell Endocrinol 2000;161:73-88.
322. Cantrill JA, Dewis P, Large DM, et al. Which testosterone replacement therapy? Clin Endocrinol (Oxf) 1984;21:97-107.
323. Handelsman DJ, Conway AJ, Boylan LM. Pharmacokinetics and pharmacodynamics of testosterone pellets in man. J Clin Endocrinol Metab 1990;71:216-222.
324. Jockenhovel F, Vogel E, Kreutzer M, et al. Pharmacokinetics and pharmacodynamics of subcutaneous testosterone implants in hypogonadal men. Clin Endocrinol (Oxf) 1996;45:61-71.
325. Handelsman DJ, Mackey MA, Howe C, et al. An analysis of testosterone implants for androgen replacement therapy. Clin Endocrinol (Oxf) 1997;47:311-316.
326. Kelleher S, Turner L, Howe C, et al. Extrusion of testosterone pellets: a randomized controlled clinical study. Clin Endocrinol (Oxf) 1999;51:469-471.
327. Kamischke A, Venherm S, Ploger D, et al. Intramuscular testosterone undecanoate and norethisterone enanthate in a clinical trial for male contraception. J Clin Endocrinol Metab 2001;86: 303-309.
328. von Eckardstein S, Nieschlag E. Treatment of male hypogonadism with testosterone undecanoate injected at extended intervals of 12 weeks: a phase II study. J Androl 2002;23:419-425.
329. Loughlin KR, O'Leary MP. Re: Oral androgens in the treatment of hypogonadal impotent men. J Urol 1995;153:1645.
330. Kelleher S, Conway AJ, Handelsman DJ. Blood testosterone threshold for androgen deficiency symptoms. J Clin Endocrinol Metab 2004;89:3813-3817.
331. Bhasin S, Swerdloff RS, Steiner B, et al. A biodegradable testosterone microcapsule formulation provides uniform eugonadal levels of testosterone for 10-11 weeks in hypogonadal men. J Clin Endocrinol Metab 1992;74:75-83.
332. Amory JK, Anawalt BD, Blaskovich PD, et al. Testosterone release from a subcutaneous, biodegradable microcapsule formulation (Viatrel) in hypogonadal men. J Androl 2002;23:84-91.
333. Behre HM, Nieschlag E. Testosterone buciclate (20 Aet-1) in hypogonadal men: pharmacokinetics and pharmacodynamics of the new long-acting androgen ester. J Clin Endocrinol Metab 1992;75: 1204-1210.
334. Kinger S, Pal PC, Rajalakshmi M, et al. Effects of testosterone buciclate on testicular and epididymal sperm functions in bonnet monkeys (Macaca radiata). Contraception 1995;52:121-127.
335. Schubert M, Minnemann T, Hubler D, et al. Intramuscular testosterone undecanoate: pharmacokinetic aspects of a novel testosterone formulation during long-term treatment of men with hypogonadism. J Clin Endocrinol Metab 2004;89:5429-5434.
336. Partsch CJ, Weinbauer GF, Fang R, Nieschlag E. Injectable testosterone undecanoate has more favourable pharmacokinetics and pharmacodynamics than testosterone enanthate. Eur J Endocrinol 1995;132:514-519.
337. Zhang GY, Gu YQ, Wang XH, et al. A pharmacokinetic study of injectable testosterone undecanoate in hypogonadal men. J Androl 1998;19:761-768.
338. Behre HM, Abshagen K, Oettel M, et al. Intramuscular injection of testosterone undecanoate for the treatment of male hypogonadism: phase I studies. Eur J Endocrinol 1999;140:414-419.
339. Zhang GY, Gu YQ, Wang XH, et al. A clinical trial of injectable testosterone undecanoate as a potential male contraceptive in normal Chinese men. J Clin Endocrinol Metab 1999;84: 3642-3647.
340. Nieschlag E, Buchter D, Von Eckardstein S, et al. Repeated intramuscular injections of testosterone undecanoate for substitution therapy in hypogonadal men. Clin Endocrinol (Oxf) 1999;51: 757-763.
341. Anderson RA, Wallace AM, Sattar N, et al. Evidence for tissue selectivity of the synthetic androgen 7α-methyl-19-nortestosterone in hypogonadal men. J Clin Endocrinol Metab 2003;88: 2784-2793.
342. Anderson RA, Martin CW, Kung AW, et al. 7α-Methyl-19-nortestosterone maintains sexual behavior and mood in hypogonadal men. J Clin Endocrinol Metab 1999;84:3556-3562.
343. Suvisaari J, Sundaram K, Noe G, et al. Pharmacokinetics and pharmacodynamics of 7α-methyl-19-nortestosterone after intramuscular administration in healthy men. Hum Reprod 1997;12:967-973.
344. Negro-Vilar A. Selective androgen receptor modulators (SARMs): a novel approach to androgen therapy for the new millennium. J Clin Endocrinol Metab 1999;84:3459-3462.
345. Agarwal PK, Oefelein MG. Testosterone replacement therapy after primary treatment for prostate cancer. J Urol 2005;173:533-536.

346. Kaufman J. A rational approach to androgen therapy for hypogonadal men with prostate cancer. Int J Impot Res 2006;18:26-31.
347. Kaufman JM, Graydon RJ. Androgen replacement after curative radical prostatectomy for prostate cancer in hypogonadal men. J Urol 2004;172:920-922.
348. Calof O, Singh AB, Lee ML, et al. Adverse events associated with testosterone replacement in middle-aged and older men: a meta-analysis of randomized, placebo-controlled trials. J Gerontol A Biol Sci Med Sci 2005;60:1451-1457.
349. Thompson PD, Cullinane EM, Sady SP, et al. Contrasting effects of testosterone and stanozolol on serum lipoprotein levels. JAMA 1989;261:1165-1168.
350. Bhasin S, Storer TW, Berman N, et al. The effects of supraphysiologic doses of testosterone on muscle size and strength in normal men. N Engl J Med 1996;335:1-7.
351. Sih R, Morley JE, Kaiser FE, et al. Testosterone replacement in older hypogonadal men: a 12-month randomized controlled trial. J Clin Endocrinol Metab 1997;82:1661-1667.
352. Snyder PJ, Peachey H, Berlin JA, et al. Effect of transdermal testosterone treatment on serum lipid and apolipoprotein levels in men more than 65 years of age. Am J Med 2001;111:255-260.
353. Barrett-Connor E, Khaw KT. Endogenous sex hormones and cardiovascular disease in men. A prospective population-based study. Circulation 1988;78:539-545.
354. De Pergola G, De Mitrio, V, Sciaraffia, M, et al. Lower androgenicity is associated with higher plasma levels of prothrombotic factors irrespective of age, obesity, body fat distribution, and related metabolic parameters in men. Metabolism 1997;46: 1287-1293.
355. Haffner SM, Laakso M, Miettinen H, et al. Low levels of sex hormone–binding globulin and testosterone are associated with smaller, denser low density lipoprotein in normoglycemic men. J Clin Endocrinol Metab 1996;81:3697-3701.
356. Khaw KT, Barrett-Connor E. Lower endogenous androgens predict central adiposity in men. Ann Epidemiol 1992;2:675-682.
357. Seidell JC, Bjorntorp P, Sjostrom L, et al. Visceral fat accumulation in men is positively associated with insulin, glucose, and C-peptide levels, but negatively with testosterone levels. Metabolism 1990; 39:897-901.
358. Whitsel EA, Boyko EJ, Matsumoto AM, et al. Intramuscular testosterone esters and plasma lipids in hypogonadal men: a meta-analysis. Am J Med 2001;111:261-269.
359. Katznelson L, Rosenthal DI, Rosol MS, et al. Using quantitative CT to assess adipose distribution in adult men with acquired hypogonadism. AJR Am J Roentgenol 1998;170:423-427.
360. Mauras N, Hayes V, Welch S, et al. Testosterone deficiency in young men: marked alterations in whole body protein kinetics, strength, and adiposity. J Clin Endocrinol Metab 1998;83: 1886-1892.
361. Holmang A, Bjorntorp P. The effects of testosterone on insulin sensitivity in male rats. Acta Physiol Scand 1992;146:505-510.
362. Hobbs CJ, Jones RE, Plymate SR. Nandrolone, a 19-nortestosterone, enhances insulin-independent glucose uptake in normal men. J Clin Endocrinol Metab 1996;81:1582-1585.
363. Ramirez ME, McMurry MP, Wiebke GA, et al. Evidence for sex steroid inhibition of lipoprotein lipase in men: comparison of abdominal and femoral adipose tissue. Metabolism 1997;46: 179-185.
364. Alexandersen P, Haarbo J, Christiansen C. The relationship of natural androgens to coronary heart disease in males: a review. Atherosclerosis 1996;125:1-13.
365. Bhasin S, Herbst K. Testosterone and atherosclerosis progression in men. Diabetes Care 2003;26:1929-1931.
366. Liu PY, Death AK, Handelsman DJ. Androgens and cardiovascular disease. Endocr Rev 2003;24:313-340.
367. English KM, Steeds RP, Jones TH, et al. Low-dose transdermal testosterone therapy improves angina threshold in men with chronic stable angina: A randomized, double-blind, placebo-controlled study. Circulation 2000;102:1906-1911.
368. Hall J, Jones RD, Jones TH, et al. Selective inhibition of L-type Ca^{2+} channels in A7r5 cells by physiological levels of testosterone. Endocrinology 2006;147:2675-2680.
369. Scragg JL, Jones RD, Channer KS, et al. Testosterone is a potent inhibitor of L-type Ca^{2+} channels. Biochem Biophys Res Commun 2004;318:503-506.
370. Ong PJ, Patrizi G, Chong WC, et al. Testosterone enhances flow-mediated brachial artery reactivity in men with coronary artery disease. Am J Cardiol 2000;85:269-272.
371. Bernini GP, Sgro M, Moretti A, et al. Endogenous androgens and carotid intimal-medial thickness in women. J Clin Endocrinol Metab 1999;84:2008-2012.
372. Zitzmann M, Brune M, Nieschlag E. Vascular reactivity in hypogonadal men is reduced by androgen substitution. J Clin Endocrinol Metab 2002;87:5030-5037.
373. Vasudevan H, Nagareddy PR, McNeill JH. Gonadectomy prevents endothelial dysfunction in fructose-fed male rats, a factor contributing to the development of hypertension. Am J Physiol Heart Circ Physiol 2006;291(6):H3058-H3064.
374. Nathan L, Shi W, Dinh H, et al. Testosterone inhibits early atherogenesis by conversion to estradiol: critical role of aromatase. Proc Natl Acad Sci U S A 2001;98:3589-3593.
375. Eckardstein A, Wu FC. Testosterone and atherosclerosis. Growth Horm IGF Res 2003;13(Suppl):S72-S84.
376. Bhasin S, Singh AB, Mac RP, et al. Managing the risks of prostate disease during testosterone replacement therapy in older men: recommendations for a standardized monitoring plan. J Androl 2003;24:299-311.
377. Huggins C, Hodges CV. Studies on prostatic cancer: I. The effect of castration, of estrogen and of androgen injection on serum phosphatases in metastatic carcinoma of the prostate. 1941. J Urol 2002;168:9-12.
378. Fowler JE Jr, Whitmore WF Jr. The response of metastatic adenocarcinoma of the prostate to exogenous testosterone. J Urol 1981;126:372-375.
379. Morgentaler A, Bruning CO 3rd, DeWolf WC. Occult prostate cancer in men with low serum testosterone levels. JAMA 1996;276:1904-1906.
380. Behre HM, Bohmeyer J, Nieschlag E. Prostate volume in testosterone-treated and untreated hypogonadal men in comparison to age-matched normal controls. Clin Endocrinol (Oxf) 1994;40: 341-349.
381. Meikle AW, Arver S, Dobs AS, et al. Prostate size in hypogonadal men treated with a nonscrotal permeation-enhanced testosterone transdermal system. Urology 1997;49:191-196.
382. Amory JK, Watts NB, Easley KA, et al. Exogenous testosterone or testosterone with finasteride increases bone mineral density in older men with low serum testosterone. J Clin Endocrinol Metab 2004;89:503-510.
383. Snyder PJ, Peachey H, Hannoush P, et al. Effect of testosterone treatment on body composition and muscle strength in men over 65 years of age. J Clin Endocrinol Metab 1999;84:2647-2653.
384. Mirand EA, Gordon AS, Wenig J. Mechanism of testosterone action in erythropoiesis. Nature 1965;206:270-272.
385. Gordon AS, Zanjani ED, Levere RD, Kappas A. Stimulation of mammalian erythropoiesis by 5β-H steroid metabolites. Proc Natl Acad Sci U S A 1970;65:919-924.
386. Bhasin S, Woodhouse L, Casaburi R, et al. Older men are as responsive as young men to the anabolic effects of graded doses of testosterone on the skeletal muscle. J Clin Endocrinol Metab 2005;90:678-688.
387. Matsumoto AM, Sandblom RE, Schoene RB, et al. Testosterone replacement in hypogonadal men: effects on obstructive sleep apnoea, respiratory drives, and sleep. Clin Endocrinol (Oxf) 1985;22:713-721.
388. Sandblom RE, Matsumoto AM, Schoene RB, et al. Obstructive sleep apnea syndrome induced by testosterone administration. N Engl J Med 1983;308:508-510.
389. Grunstein RR, Handelsman DJ, Lawrence SJ, et al. Neuroendocrine dysfunction in sleep apnea: reversal by continuous positive airways pressure therapy. J Clin Endocrinol Metab 1989;68: 352-358.
390. Riehmann M, Rhodes PR, Cook TD, et al. Analysis of variation in prostate-specific antigen values. Urology 1993;42:390-397.
391. Carter HB, Pearson JD, Waclawiw Z, et al. Prostate-specific antigen variability in men without prostate cancer: effect of sampling interval on prostate-specific antigen velocity. Urology 1995;45: 591-596.
392. Brawer MK, Daum P, Petteway JC, Wener MH. Assay variability in serum prostate-specific antigen determination. Prostate 1995;27: 1-6.

393. Wener MH, Daum PR, Brawer MK. Variation in measurement of prostate-specific antigen: importance of method and lot variability. Clin Chem 1995;41:1730-1737.
394. Roehrborn CG, Pickens GJ, Carmody T 3rd. Variability of repeated serum prostate-specific antigen (PSA) measurements within less than 90 days in a well-defined patient population. Urology 1996;47:59-66.
395. Kadmon D, Weinberg AD, Williams RH, et al. Pitfalls in interpreting prostate specific antigen velocity. J Urol 1996;155:1655-1657.
396. Prestigiacomo AF, Stamey TA. Physiological variation of serum prostate specific antigen in the 4.0 to 10.0 ng/mL range in male volunteers. J Urol 1996;155:1977-1980.
397. Carter HB. PSA variability versus velocity. Urology 1997;49: 305.
398. Oesterling JE, Roy J, Agha A, et al. Biologic variability of prostate-specific antigen and its usefulness as a marker for prostate cancer: effects of finasteride. The Finasteride PSA Study Group. Urology 1997;50:13-18.
399. Oesterling JE, Roy J, Agha A, et al. Biologic variability of prostate-specific antigen and its usefulness as a marker for prostate cancer: effects of finasteride. Finasteride PSA Study Group. Urology 1998;51:58-63.
400. Lujan M, Paez A, Sanchez E, et al. Prostate specific antigen variation in patients without clinically evident prostate cancer. J Urol 1999;162:1311-1313.
401. Gormley GJ, Stoner E, Bruskewitz RC, et al. The effect of finasteride in men with benign prostatic hyperplasia. The Finasteride Study Group. N Engl J Med 1992;327:1185-1191.
402. McConnell JD, Bruskewitz R, Walsh P, et al. The effect of finasteride on the risk of acute urinary retention and the need for surgical treatment among men with benign prostatic hyperplasia. Finasteride Long-Term Efficacy and Safety Study Group. N Engl J Med 1998;338:557-563.
403. Ornstein DK, Smith DS, Rao GS, et al. Biological variation of total, free and percent free serum prostate specific antigen levels in screening volunteers. J Urol 1997;157:2179-2182.
404. Arcangeli CG, Ornstein DK, Keetch DW, Andriole GL. Prostate-specific antigen as a screening test for prostate cancer. The United States experience. Urol Clin North Am 1997;24:299-306.
405. Carter HB, Pearson JD. PSA velocity for the diagnosis of early prostate cancer. A new concept. Urol Clin North Am 1993;20: 665-670.
406. Carter HB, Pearson JD, Metter EJ, et al. Longitudinal evaluation of serum androgen levels in men with and without prostate cancer. Prostate 1995;27:25-31.
407. Fang J, Metter EJ, Landis P, Carter HB. PSA velocity for assessing prostate cancer risk in men with PSA levels between 2.0 and 4.0 ng/mL. Urology 2002;59:889-893; discussion 893-884.
408. Dai WS, Kuller LH, LaPorte RE, et al. The epidemiology of plasma testosterone levels in middle-aged men. Am J Epidemiol 1981;114:804-816.
409. Gray A, Feldman HA, McKinlay JB, Longcope C. Age, disease, and changing sex hormone levels in middle-aged men: results of the Massachusetts Male Aging Study. J Clin Endocrinol Metab 1991;73:1016-1025.
410. Mohr BA, Bhasin S, Link CL, et al. The effect of changes in adiposity on testosterone levels in older men: longitudinal results from the Massachusetts Male Aging Study. Eur J Endocrinol 2006;155: 443-452.
411. Roy TA, Blackman MR, Harman SM, et al. Interrelationships of serum testosterone and free testosterone index with FFM and strength in aging men. Am J Physiol Endocrinol Metab 2002;283: E284-E294.
412. Baumgartner RN, Waters DL, Gallagher D, et al. Predictors of skeletal muscle mass in elderly men and women. Mech Ageing Dev 1999;107:123-136.
413. Lau EM, Lynn HS, Woo JW, et al. Prevalence of and risk factors for sarcopenia in elderly Chinese men and women. J Gerontol A Biol Sci Med Sci 2005;60:213-216.
414. Morley JE, Baumgartner RN, Roubenoff R, et al. Sarcopenia. J Lab Clin Med 2001;137:231-243.
415. O'Donnell AB, Travison TG, Harris SS, et al. Testosterone, dehydroepiandrosterone, and physical performance in older men: results from the Massachusetts Male Aging Study. J Clin Endocrinol Metab 2006;91:425-431.
416. van den Beld AW, Bots ML, Janssen JA, et al. Endogenous hormones and carotid atherosclerosis in elderly men. Am J Epidemiol 2003;157:25-31.
417. Travison TG, Morley JE, Araujo AB, et al. The relationship between libido and testosterone levels in aging men. J Clin Endocrinol Metab 2006;91:2509-2513.
418. Araujo AB, Durante R, Feldman HA, et al. The relationship between depressive symptoms and male erectile dysfunction: cross-sectional results from the Massachusetts Male Aging Study. Psychosom Med 1998;60:458-465.
419. Booth A, Johnson DR, Granger DA. Testosterone and men's health. J Behav Med 1999;22:1-19.
420. Barrett-Connor E, Von Muhlen DG, Kritz-Silverstein D. Bioavailable testosterone and depressed mood in older men: the Rancho Bernardo Study. J Clin Endocrinol Metab 1999;84:573-577.
421. Seidman SN, Araujo AB, Roose SP, McKinlay JB. Testosterone level, androgen receptor polymorphism, and depressive symptoms in middle-aged men. Biol Psychiatry 2001;50:371-376.
422. Haffner SM, Katz MS, Stern MP, Dunn JF. The relationship of sex hormones to hyperinsulinemia and hyperglycemia. Metabolism 1988;37:683-688.
423. Pitteloud N, Mootha VK, Dwyer AA, et al. Relationship between testosterone levels, insulin sensitivity, and mitochondrial function in men. Diabetes Care 2005;28:1636-1642.
424. Blouin K, Despres JP, Couillard C, et al. Contribution of age and declining androgen levels to features of the metabolic syndrome in men. Metabolism 2005;54:1034-1040.
425. Haffner SM. Sex hormones, obesity, fat distribution, type 2 diabetes and insulin resistance: epidemiological and clinical correlation. Int J Obes Relat Metab Disord 2000;24(suppl 2):S56-S58.
426. Kenny AM, Prestwood KM, Gruman CA, et al. Effects of transdermal testosterone on bone and muscle in older men with low bioavailable testosterone levels. J Gerontol A Biol Sci Med Sci 2001;56: M266-M272.
427. Tenover JS. Effects of testosterone supplementation in the aging male. J Clin Endocrinol Metab 1992;75:1092-1098.
428. Page ST, Amory JK, Bowman FD, et al. Exogenous testosterone (T) alone or with finasteride increases physical performance, grip strength, and lean body mass in older men with low serum T. J Clin Endocrinol Metab 2005;90:1502-1510.
429. Wittert GA, Chapman IM, Haren MT, et al. Oral testosterone supplementation increases muscle and decreases fat mass in healthy elderly males with low-normal gonadal status. J Gerontol A Biol Sci Med Sci 2003;58:618-625.
430. Blackman MR, Sorkin JD, Munzer T, et al. Growth hormone and sex steroid administration in healthy aged women and men: a randomized controlled trial. JAMA 2002;288:2282-2292.
431. Harman SM, Blackman MR. The effects of growth hormone and sex steroid on lean body mass, fat mass, muscle strength, cardiovascular endurance and adverse events in healthy elderly women and men. Horm Res 2003;60:121-124.
432. Morley JE, Perry HM 3rd, Kaiser FE, et al. Effects of testosterone replacement therapy in old hypogonadal males: a preliminary study. J Am Geriatr Soc 1993;41:149-152.
433. Braunstein GD. Gynecomastia. N Engl J Med 1993;328:490-495.
434. Braunstein GD. Aromatase and gynecomastia. Endocr Relat Cancer 1999;6:315-324.
435. Kanhai RC, Hage JJ, van Diest PJ, et al. Short-term and long-term histologic effects of castration and estrogen treatment on breast tissue of 14 male-to-female transsexuals in comparison with two chemically castrated men. Am J Surg Pathol 2000;24:74-80.
436. Simpson ER, Mahendroo MS, Means GD, et al. Aromatase cytochrome P450, the enzyme responsible for estrogen biosynthesis. Endocr Rev 1994;15:342-355.
437. Hemsell DL, Grodin JM, Brenner PF, et al. Plasma precursors of estrogen. II. Correlation of the extent of conversion of plasma androstenedione to estrone with age. J Clin Endocrinol Metab 1974;38:476-479.
438. McDonald PC, Maldden JD, Brenner PF, et al. Origin of estrogen in normal men and in women with testicular feminization. J Clin Endocrinol Metab 1979;49:905-916.
439. Sebastian S, Bulun SE. A highly complex organization of the regulatory region of the human *CYP19* (aromatase) gene revealed by the Human Genome Project. J Clin Endocrinol Metab 2001;86: 4600-4602.

440. Mahendroo MS, Mendelson CR, Simpson ER. Tissue-specific and hormonally controlled alternative promoters regulate aromatase cytochrome P450 gene expression in human adipose tissue. J Biol Chem 1993;268:19463-19470.
441. Georgiadis E, Papandreou L, Evangelopoulou C, et al. Incidence of gynaecomastia in 954 young males and its relationship to somatometric parameters. Ann Hum Biol 1994;21:579-587.
442. Ersoz H, Onde ME, Terekeci H, et al. Causes of gynaecomastia in young adult males and factors associated with idiopathic gynaecomastia. Int J Androl 2002;25:312-316.
443. Einav-Bachar R, Phillip M, Aurbach-Klipper Y, Lazar L. Prepubertal gynaecomastia: aetiology, course and outcome. Clin Endocrinol (Oxf) 2004;61:55-60.
444. Lee PA. The relationship of concentrations of serum hormones to pubertal gynecomastia. J Pediatr 1975;86:212-215.
445. Niewoehner CB, Nuttall FQ. Gyneomastia in a hospitalized male population. J Clin Endocrinol Metab 1984;77:633-638.
446. Cleland WH, Menderlson CR, Simpson ER. Effects of aging and obesity on aromatase activity of human adipose cells. J Clin Endocrinol Metab 1985;60:174-177.
447. Young S, Gooneratne S, Straus FH 2nd, et al. Feminizing Sertoli cell tumors in boys with Peutz-Jeghers syndrome. Am J Surg Pathol 1995;19:50-58.
448. Lefevre H, Bouvattier C, Lahlou N, et al. Prepubertal gynecomastia in Peutz-Jeghers syndrome: incomplete penetrance in a familial case and management with an aromatase inhibitor. Eur J Endocrinol 2006;154:221-227.
449. Gordon GG, Olivo J, Rafi F, et al. Conversion of androgens to estrogens in cirrohosis of the liver. J Clin Endocrinol Metab 1975;40:1018-1026.
450. Shozu M, Sebastian S, Takayama K, et al. Estrogen excess associated with novel gain-of-function mutations affecting the aromatase gene. N Engl J Med 2003;348:1855-1865.
451. Stratakis GD, Vottero A, Brodie A, et al. The aromatase excess syndrome is associated with feminization of both sexes and autosomal dominant transmission of aberrant P450 aromatase gene transcription. J Clin Endocrinol Metab 1998;83:1348-1357.
452. Hemsell DL, Edman CD, Marks GG, et al. Massive extraglandular aromatization of plasma androstenedione resulting in feminization of a prepubertal boy. J Clin Invest 1977;60:455-464.
453. Tiulpakov A, Kalintchenko N, Semitcheva T, et al. A potential rearrangement between *CYP19* and *TRPM7* genes on chromosome 15q21.2 as a cause of aromatase excess syndrome. J Clin Endocrinol Metab 2005;90:4184-4190.
454. Hendricks DM, Gray SL, Hoover J. Residue levels of endogenous estrogens in beef tissues. J Anim Sci 1983;57:247-255.
455. Beuers U, Richter WO, Ritter MM, et al. Klinefelter's syndrome and liver adenoma. J Clin Gastroenterol 1991;13:214-216.
456. D'Avanzo B, La Vecchia C. Risk factors for male breast cancer. Br J Cancer 1995;71:1359-1362.
457. Hultborn R, Hanson C, Kopf I, et al. Prevalence of Klinefelter's syndrome in male breast cancer patients. Anticancer Res 1997;17:4293-4297.
458. Meguerditchian AN, Falardeau M, Martin G. Male breast carcinoma. Can J Surg 2002;45:296-302.
459. Sasco AJ, Lowenfels AB, Pasker-de Jong P. Review article: epidemiology of male breast cancer. A meta-analysis of published case-control studies and discussion of selected aetiological factors. Int J Cancer 1993;53:538-549.
460. Wolman SR, Sanford J, Ratner S, Dawson PJ. Breast cancer in males: DNA content and sex chromosome constitution. Mod Pathol 1995;8:239-243.
461. Swerdlow AJ, Higgins CD, Schoemaker MJ, et al. Mortality in patients with Klinefelter syndrome in Britain: a cohort study. J Clin Endocrinol Metab 2005;90:6516-6522.
462. Weiss JR, Moysich KB, Swede H. Epidemiology of male breast cancer. Cancer Epidemiol Biomarkers Prev 2005;14:20-26.
463. Coen P, Kulin H, Ballantine T, et al. An aromatase-producing sex-cord tumor resulting in prepubertal gynecomastia. N Engl J Med 1991;324:317-322.
464. Leiberman E, Zachmann M. Familial adrenal feminization probably due to increased steroid aromatization. Horm Res 1992;37: 96-102.
465. Zachmann M, Eiholzer U, Muritano M, et al. Treatment of pubertal gynaecomastia with testolactone. Acta Endocrinol Suppl (Copenh) 1986;279:218-226.
466. Plourde PV, Reiter EO, Jou HC, et al. Safety and efficacy of anastrozole for the treatment of pubertal gynecomastia: a randomized, double-blind, placebo-controlled trial. J Clin Endocrinol Metab 2004;89:4428-4433.
467. Perdona S, Autorino R, De Placido S, et al. Efficacy of tamoxifen and radiotherapy for prevention and treatment of gynaecomastia and breast pain caused by bicalutamide in prostate cancer: a randomised controlled trial. Lancet Oncol 2005;6:295-300.
468. Derman O, Kanbur NO, Kutluk T. Tamoxifen treatment for pubertal gynecomastia. Int J Adolesc Med Health 2003;15:359-363.
469. Lawrence SE, Faught KA, Vethamuthu J, Lawson ML. Beneficial effects of raloxifene and tamoxifen in the treatment of pubertal gynecomastia. J Pediatr 2004;145:71-76.
470. Hanavadi S, Banerjee D, Monypenny IJ, Mansel RE. The role of tamoxifen in the management of gynaecomastia. Breast 2006;15: 276-280.
471. Khan HN, Rampaul R, Blamey RW. Management of physiological gynaecomastia with tamoxifen. Breast 2004;13:61-65.
472. Brinkmann AO. Molecular basis of androgen insensitivity. Mol Cell Endocrinol 2001;179:105-109.
473. Griffin JE, Leshin M, Wilson JD. Androgen resistance syndromes. Am J Physiol 1982;243:E81-E87.
474. Wilson JD, Harrod MJ, Goldstein JL, et al. Familial incomplete male pseudohermaphroditism, type 1. Evidence for androgen resistance and variable clinical manifestations in a family with the Reifenstein syndrome. N Engl J Med 1974;290:1097-1103.
475. Aiman J, Griffin JE, Gazak JM, et al. Androgen insensitivity as a cause of infertility in otherwise normal men. N Engl J Med 1979;300:223-227.
476. Madden JD, Walsh PC, MacDonald PC, Wilson JD. Clinical and endocrinologic characterization of a patients with the syndrome of incomplete testicular feminization. J Clin Endocrinol Metab 1975;41:751-760.
477. Gottlieb B, Beitel LK, Lumbroso R, et al. Update of the androgen receptor gene mutations database. Human Mutations 1999;14: 103-114.
478. Marcelli M, Zoppi S, Grino PB, et al. A mutation in the DNA-binding domain of the androgen receptor gene causes complete testicular feminization in a patient with receptor-positive androgen resistance. J Clin Invest 1991;87:1123-1126.
479. Zoppi S, Marcelli M, Deslypere JP, et al. Amino acid substitutions in the DNA-binding domain of the human androgen receptor are a frequent cause of receptor-binding positive androgen resistance. Mol Endocrinol 1992;6:409-415.
480. Adachi M, Takayanagi R, Tomura A, et al. Androgen-insensitivity syndrome as a possible coactivator disease. N Engl J Med 2000;343:856-862.
481. La Spada AR, Wilson EM, Lubahn DB, et al. Androgen receptor gene mutations in X-linked spinal and bulbar muscular atrophy. Nature 1991;352:77-79.
482. Nance MA. Clinical aspects of CAG repeat diseases. Brain Pathol 1997;7:881-900.
483. LaFevre-Bernt MA, Ellerby LM. Kennedy's disease. Phosphorylation of the polyglutamine-expanded form of androgen receptor regulates its cleavage by caspase-3 and enhances cell death. J Biol Chem 2003;278:34918-34924.
484. Yong EL, Loy CJ, Sim KS. Androgen receptor gene and male infertility. Hum Reprod Update 2003;9:1-7.
485. World Health Organization. WHO manual for the standardised investigation and diagnosis of infertile couples. Cambridge, UK: Cambridge University Press, 2000.
486. Templeton A. Infertility and the establishment of pregnancy—overview. Br Med Bull 2000;56:577-587.
487. Gnoth C, Godehardt E, Frank-Herrmann P, et al. Definition and prevalence of subfertility and infertility. Hum Reprod 2005;20: 1144-1147.
488. van der Steeg JW, Steures P, Hompes PG, et al. Investigation of the infertile couple: a basic fertility work-up performed within 12 months of trying to conceive generates costs and complications for no particular benefit. Hum Reprod 2005;20:2672-2674.
489. Juul S, Karmaus W, Olsen J. Regional differences in waiting time to pregnancy: pregnancy-based surveys from Denmark, France,

Germany, Italy and Sweden. The European Infertility and Subfecundity Study Group. Hum Reprod 1999;14:1250-1254.
490. Jensen TK, Slama R, Ducot B, et al. Regional differences in waiting time to pregnancy among fertile couples from four European cities. Hum Reprod 2001;16:2697-2704.
491. Hull MG, Glazener CM, Kelly NJ, et al. Population study of causes, treatment, and outcome of infertility. Br Med J (Clin Res Ed) 1985;291:1693-1697.
492. Snick HK, Snick TS, Evers JL, Collins JA. The spontaneous pregnancy prognosis in untreated subfertile couples: the Walcheren primary care study. Hum Reprod 1997;12:1582-1588.
493. Habbema JD, Collins J, Leridon H, et al. Towards less confusing terminology in reproductive medicine: a proposal. Fertil Steril 2004;82:36-40.
494. Dohle GR, Colpi GM, Hargreave TB, et al. EAU guidelines on male infertility. Eur Urol 2005;48:703-711.
495. Wang X, Chen C, Wang L, et al. Conception, early pregnancy loss, and time to clinical pregnancy: a population-based prospective study. Fertil Steril 2003;79:577-584.
496. Gnoth C, Godehardt D, Godehardt E, et al. Time to pregnancy: results of the German prospective study and impact on the management of infertility. Hum Reprod 2003;18:1959-1966.
497. Wong WY, Thomas CM, Merkus JM, et al. Male factor subfertility: possible causes and the impact of nutritional factors. Fertil Steril 2000;73:435-442.
498. Bhasin S, de Kretser DM, Baker HW. Clinical review 64: Pathophysiology and natural history of male infertility. J Clin Endocrinol Metab 1994;79:1525-1529.
499. De Kretser DM, Burger HG, Fortune D, et al. Hormonal, histological and chromosomal studies in adult males with testicular disorders. J Clin Endocrinol Metab 1972;35:392-401.
500. Swerdloff RS, Boyers SP. Evaluation of the male partner of an infertile couple. An algorithmic approach. JAMA 1982;247: 2418-2422.
501. Mazumdar S, Levine AS. Antisperm antibodies: etiology, pathogenesis, diagnosis, and treatment. Fertil Steril 1998;70:799-810.
502. Chandley AC. The chromosomal basis of human infertility. Br Med Bull 1979;35:181-186.
503. Sharland M, Burch M, McKenna WM, Paton MA. A clinical study of Noonan syndrome. Arch Dis Child 1992;67:178-183.
504. Santen RJ, DeKretser DM, Paulsen CA, Vorhees J. Gonadotrophins and testosterone in the XYY syndrome. Lancet 1970;2:371.
505. Davidoff F, Federman DD. Mixed gonadal dysgenesis. Pediatrics 1973;52:725-742.
506. Federman DD, Davidoff FM, Ouellette E. Presumptive Y/D translocation in mixed gonadal dysgenesis. J Med Genet 1967;4: 36-40.
507. Page DC, Brown LG, de la Chapelle A. Exchange of terminal portions of X- and Y-chromosomal short arms in human XX males. Nature 1987;328:437-440.
508. Najmabadi H, Huang V, Yen P, et al. Substantial prevalence of microdeletions of the Y-chromosome in infertile men with idiopathic azoospermia and oligozoospermia detected using a sequence-tagged site-based mapping strategy. J Clin Endocrinol Metab 1996;81:1347-1352.
509. Reijo R, Alagappan RK, Patrizio P, Page DC. Severe oligozoospermia resulting from deletions of azoospermia factor gene on Y chromosome. Lancet 1996;347:1290-1293.
510. Reijo R, Lee TY, Salo P, et al. Diverse spermatogenic defects in humans caused by Y chromosome deletions encompassing a novel RNA-binding protein gene. Nat Genet 1995;10:383-393.
511. Kent-First M, Muallem A, Shultz J, et al. Defining regions of the Y-chromosome responsible for male infertility and identification of a fourth AZF region (AZFd) by Y-chromosome microdeletion detection. Mol Reprod Dev 1999;53:27-41.
512. Pryor JL, Kent-First M, Muallem A, et al. Microdeletions in the Y chromosome of infertile men. N Engl J Med 1997;336:534-539.
513. Ma K, Sharkey A, Kirsch S, et al. Towards the molecular localisation of the AZF locus: mapping of microdeletions in azoospermic men within 14 subintervals of interval 6 of the human Y chromosome. Hum Mol Genet 1992;1:29-33.
514. Vogt P, Chandley AC, Hargreave TB, et al. Microdeletions in interval 6 of the Y chromosome of males with idiopathic sterility point to disruption of AZF, a human spermatogenesis gene. Hum Genet 1992;89:491-496.
515. Ferlin A, Moro E, Garolla A, Foresta C. Human male infertility and Y chromosome deletions: role of the AZF-candidate genes *DAZ, RBM* and *DFFRY.* Hum Reprod 1999;14:1710-1716.
516. Foresta C, Moro E, Ferlin A. Y chromosome microdeletions and alterations of spermatogenesis. Endocr Rev 2001;22:226-239.
517. Maurer B, Gromoll J, Simoni M, Nieschlag E. Prevalence of Y chromosome microdeletions in infertile men who consulted a tertiary care medical centre: the Munster experience. Andrologia 2001;33:27-33.
518. Simoni M, Gromoll J, Dworniczak B, et al. Screening for deletions of the Y chromosome involving the *DAZ* (Deleted in AZoospermia) gene in azoospermia and severe oligozoospermia. Fertil Steril 1997;67:542-547.
519. Simoni M, Kamischke A, Nieschlag E. Current status of the molecular diagnosis of Y-chromosomal microdeletions in the work-up of male infertility. Initiative for international quality control. Hum Reprod 1998;13:1764-1768.
520. Bhasin S, Ma K, de Kretser DM. Y-chromosome microdeletions and male infertility. Ann Med 1997;29:261-263.
521. Ma K, Inglis JD, Sharkey A, et al. A Y chromosome gene family with RNA-binding protein homology: candidates for the azoospermia factor AZF controlling human spermatogenesis. Cell 1993;75: 1287-1295.
522. Najmabadi H, Chai N, Kapali A, et al. Genomic structure of a Y-specific ribonucleic acid binding motif–containing gene: a putative candidate for a subset of male infertility. J Clin Endocrinol Metab 1996;81:2159-2164.
523. Chai NN, Phillips A, Fernandez A, Yen PH. A putative human male infertility gene *DAZLA:* genomic structure and methylation status. Mol Hum Reprod 1997;3:705-708.
524. Yen PH, Chai NN, Salido EC. The human autosomal gene *DAZLA:* testis specificity and a candidate for male infertility. Hum Mol Genet 1996;5:2013-2017.
525. Chai NN, Zhou H, Hernandez J, et al. Structure and organization of the *RBMY* genes on the human Y chromosome: transposition and amplification of an ancestral autosomal *hnRNPG* gene. Genomics 1998;49:283-289.
526. Saxena R, Brown LG, Hawkins T, et al. The *DAZ* gene cluster on the human Y chromosome arose from an autosomal gene that was transposed, repeatedly amplified and pruned. Nat Genet 1996;14:292-299.
527. Eberhart CG, Maines JZ, Wasserman SA. Meiotic cell cycle requirement for a fly homologue of human *DAZ.* Nature 1996;381: 783-785.
528. Cooke H, Lee M, Kerr S, Ruggiu M. A murine homologue of the human *DAZ* gene is autosomal and expressed in male and female gonads. Human Mol Genet 1996;5:513-516.
529. Ruggiu M, Speed R, Taggart M, et al. The mouse *Dazla* gene encodes a cytoplasmic protein essential for gametogenesis. Nature 1997;389:73-77.
530. Tsui S, Dai T, Roettger S, et al. Identification of two novel proteins that interact with germ-cell-specific RNA-binding proteins DAZ and DAZL1. Genomics 2000;65:266-273.
531. Lim HN, Chen H, McBride S, et al. Longer polyglutamine tracts in the androgen receptor are associated with moderate to severe undermasculinized genitalia in XY males. Hum Mol Genet 2000;9:829-834.
532. Tut TG, Ghadessy FJ, Trifiro MA, et al. Long polyglutamine tracts in the androgen receptor are associated with reduced *trans*-activation, impaired sperm production, and male infertility. J Clin Endocrinol Metab 1997;82:3777-3782.
533. Dadze S, Wieland C, Jakubiczka S, et al. The size of the CAG repeat in exon 1 of the androgen receptor gene shows no significant relationship to impaired spermatogenesis in an infertile caucasoid sample of German origin. Mol Hum Reprod 2000;6: 207-214.
534. Tamai KT, Monaco L, Nantel F, et al. Coupling signalling pathways to transcriptional control: nuclear factors responsive to cAMP. Recent Prog Horm Res 1997;52:121-139; discussion 139-140.
535. Weinbauer GF, Behr R, Bergmann M, Nieschlag E. Testicular cAMP responsive element modulator (CREM) protein is expressed in round spermatids but is absent or reduced in men with round spermatid maturation arrest. Mol Hum Reprod 1998;4:9-15.
536. Peri A, Krausz C, Cioppi F, et al. Cyclic adenosine 3′,5′-monophosphate-responsive element modulator gene expression

in germ cells of normo- and oligoazoospermic men. J Clin Endocrinol Metab 1998;83:3722-3726.

537. Blendy JA, Kaestner KH, Weinbauer GF, et al. Severe impairment of spermatogenesis in mice lacking the *CREM* gene. Nature 1996;380:162-165.
538. Anguiano A, Oates RD, Amos JA, et al. Congenital bilateral absence of the vas deferens. A primarily genital form of cystic fibrosis. JAMA 1992;267:1794-1797.
539. Abbasi AA, Prasad AS, Ortega J, et al. Gonadal function abnormalities in sickle cell anemia. Studies in adult male patients. Ann Intern Med 1976;85:601-605.
540. Kletzky OA, Costin G, Marrs RP, et al. Gonadotropin insufficiency in patients with thalassemia major. J Clin Endocrinol Metab 1979;48:901-905.
541. Marchini C, Lonigro R, Verriello L, et al. Correlations between individual clinical manifestations and CTG repeat amplification in myotonic dystrophy. Clin Genet 2000;57:74-82.
542. Takeda R, Ueda M. Pituitary-gonadal function in male patients with myotonic dystrophy—serum luteinizing hormone, follicle stimulating hormone and testosterone levels and histological dmaage of the testis. Acta Endocrinol (Copenh) 1977;84:382-389.
543. Skakkebaek NE, Giwercman A, de Kretser D. Pathogenesis and management of male infertility. Lancet 1994;343:1473-1479.
544. Wang C, Chan SY, Ng M, et al. Diagnostic value of sperm function tests and routine semen analyses in fertile and infertile men. J Androl 1988;9:384-389.
545. World Health Organization. Laboratory Manual for the Examination of Human Semen and Semen-Cervical Mucus Interaction. Cambridge, UK: Cambridge University Press, 1987.
546. Simpson JL, Lamb DJ. Genetic effects of intracytoplasmic sperm injection. Semin Reprod Med 2001;19:239-249.
547. Colombero LT, Hariprashad JJ, Tsai MC, et al. Incidence of sperm aneuploidy in relation to semen characteristics and assisted reproductive outcome. Fertil Steril 1999;72:90-96.
548. Finkel DM, Phillips JL, Snyder PJ. Stimulation of spermatogenesis by gonadotropins in men with hypogonadotropic hypogonadism. N Engl J Med 1985;313:651-655.
549. Burgues S, Calderon MD. Subcutaneous self-administration of highly purified follicle stimulating hormone and human chorionic gonadotrophin for the treatment of male hypogonadotrophic hypogonadism. Spanish Collaborative Group on Male Hypogonadotropic Hypogonadism. Hum Reprod 1997;12:980-986.
550. Santen RJ, Paulsen CA. Hypogonadotropic eunuchoidism. II. Gonadal responsiveness to exogenous gonadotropins. J Clin Endocrinol Metab 1973;36:55-63.
551. Liu L, Banks SM, Barnes KM, Sherins RJ. Two-year comparison of testicular responses to pulsatile gonadotropin-releasing hormone and exogenous gonadotropins from the inception of therapy in men with isolated hypogonadotropic hypogonadism. J Clin Endocrinol Metab 1988;67:1140-1145.
552. Spratt DI, Finkelstein JS, O'Dea LS, et al. Long-term administration of gonadotropin-releasing hormone in men with idiopathic hypogonadotropic hypogonadism. A model for studies of the hormone's physiologic effects. Ann Intern Med 1986;105:848-855.
553. Buchter D, Behre HM, Kliesch S, Nieschlag E. Pulsatile GnRH or human chorionic gonadotropin/human menopausal gonadotropin as effective treatment for men with hypogonadotropic hypogonadism: a review of 42 cases. Eur J Endocrinol 1998;139: 298-303.
554. Kliesch S, Behre HM, Nieschlag E. High efficacy of gonadotropin or pulsatile gonadotropin-releasing hormone treatment in hypogonadotropic hypogonadal men. Eur J Endocrinol 1994;131: 347-354.
555. Fradkin JE, Schonberger LB, Mills JL, et al. Creutzfeldt-Jakob disease in pituitary growth hormone recipients in the United States. JAMA 1991;265:880-884.
556. Recombinant Human FSH Product Development Group. Recombinant follicle stimulating hormone: development of the first biotechnology product for the treatment of infertility. Hum Reprod Update 1998;4:862-881.
557. Liu PY, Turner L, Rushford D, et al. Efficacy and safety of recombinant human follicle stimulating hormone (Gonal-F) with urinary human chorionic gonadotrophin for induction of spermatogenesis and fertility in gonadotrophin-deficient men. Hum Reprod 1999;14:1540-1545.
558. Sokol RZ, McClure RD, Peterson M, Swerdloff RS. Gonadotropin therapy failure secondary to human chorionic gonadotropin-induced antibodies. J Clin Endocrinol Metab 1981;52:929-932.
559. Braunstein GD, Bloch SK, Rasor JL, Winikoff J. Characterization of antihuman chorionic gonadotropin serum antibody appearing after ovulation induction. J Clin Endocrinol Metab 1983;57: 1164-1172.
560. Burger HG, de Kretser DM, Hudson B, Wilson JD. Effects of preceding androgen therapy on testicular response to human pituitary gonadotropin in hypogonadotropic hypogonadism: a study of three patients. Fertil Steril 1981;35:64-68.
561. Belchetz PE, Plant TM, Nakai Y, et al. Hypophysial responses to continuous and intermittent delivery of hypopthalamic gonadotropin-releasing hormone. Science 1978;202:631-633.
562. Knobil E. The neuroendocrine control of the menstrual cycle. Recent Prog Horm Res 1980;36:53-88.
563. Whitcomb RW, Crowley WF Jr. Hypogonadotropic hypogonadism: gonadotropin-releasing hormone therapy. Curr Ther Endocrinol Metab 1997;6:353-355.
564. Burger HG, Baker HW. The treatment of infertility. Annu Rev Med 1987;38:29-40.
565. Palermo GD, Schlegel PN, Hariprashad JJ, et al. Fertilization and pregnancy outcome with intracytoplasmic sperm injection for azoospermic men. Hum Reprod 1999;14:741-748.
566. Bourne H, Stern K, Clarke G, et al. Delivery of normal twins following the intracytoplasmic injection of spermatozoa from a patient with 47,XXY Klinefelter's syndrome. Hum Reprod 1997;12: 2447-2450.
567. Cram DS, Ma K, Bhasin S, et al. Y chromosome analysis of infertile men and their sons conceived through intracytoplasmic sperm injection: vertical transmission of deletions and rarity of de novo deletions. Fertil Steril 2000;74:909-915.
568. Bonduelle M, Camus M, De Vos A, et al. Seven years of intracytoplasmic sperm injection and follow-up of 1987 subsequent children. Hum Reprod 1999;14(suppl 1):243-264.
569. Wright VC, Schieve LA, Reynolds MA, et al. Assisted reproductive technology surveillance—United States, 2001. MMWR Surveill Summ 2004;53:1-20.
570. Tarlatzis BC, Bili H. Intracytoplasmic sperm injection. Survey of world results. Ann N Y Acad Sci 2000;900:336-344.
571. Ponjaert-Kristoffersen I, Bonduelle M, Barnes J, et al. International collaborative study of intracytoplasmic sperm injection–conceived, in vitro fertilization–conceived, and naturally conceived 5-year-old child outcomes: cognitive and motor assessments. Pediatrics 2005;115:e283-289.
572. Schieve LA, Ferre C, Peterson HB, et al. Perinatal outcome among singleton infants conceived through assisted reproductive technology in the United States. Obstet Gynecol 2004;103:1144-1153.
573. Van Steirteghem A, Bonduelle M, Devroey P, Liebaers I. Follow-up of children born after ICSI. Hum Reprod Update 2002;8:111-116.
574. Nyboe Andersen A, Erb K. Register data on assisted reproductive technology (ART) in Europe including a detailed description of ART in Denmark. Int J Androl 2006;29:12-16.
575. Andersen AN, Gianaroli L, Felberbaum R, et al. Assisted reproductive technology in Europe, 2002. Results generated from European registers by ESHRE. Hum Reprod 2006;21:1680-1697.
576. Nygren KG, Andersen AN. Assisted reproductive technology in Europe, 1999. Results generated from European registers by ESHRE. Hum Reprod 2002;17:3260-3274.
577. Feenstra J, van Drie-Pierik RJ, Lacle CF, Stricker BH. Acute myocardial infarction associated with sildenafil. Lancet 1998;352: 957-958.
578. Allen VM, Wilson RD, Cheung A. Pregnancy outcomes after assisted reproductive technology. J Obstet Gynaecol Can 2006;28:220-250.
579. Schieve LA, Rasmussen SA, Buck GM, et al. Are children born after assisted reproductive technology at increased risk for adverse health outcomes? Obstet Gynecol 2004;103:1154-1163.
580. Wennerholm UB, Bergh C, Hamberger L, et al. Incidence of congenital malformations in children born after ICSI. Hum Reprod 2000;15:944-948.
581. Tarlatzis BC, Bili H. Survey on intracytoplasmic sperm injection: report from the ESHRE ICSI Task Force. European Society of Human Reproduction and Embryology. Hum Reprod 1998;13(suppl 1):165-177.

582. Leslie GI, Gibson FL, McMahon C, et al. Children conceived using ICSI do not have an increased risk of delayed mental development at 5 years of age. Hum Reprod 2003;18:2067-2072.
583. Maher ER. Imprinting and assisted reproductive technology. Hum Mol Genet 2005;14(Spec No 1):R133-R138.
584. Maher ER, Afnan M, Barratt CL. Epigenetic risks related to assisted reproductive technologies: epigenetics, imprinting, ART and icebergs? Hum Reprod 2003;18:2508-2511.
585. Nieschlag E, Hertle L, Fischedick A, et al. Update on treatment of varicocele: counselling as effective as occlusion of the vena spermatica. Hum Reprod 1998;13:2147-2150.
586. Nieschlag E, Hertle L, Fischedick A, Behre HM. Treatment of varicocele: counselling as effective as occlusion of the vena spermatica. Hum Reprod 1995;10:347-353.
587. Ismail MT, Sedor J, Hirsch IH. Are sperm motion parameters influenced by varicocele ligation? Fertil Steril 1999;71:886-890.
588. Asci R, Sarikaya S, Buyukalpelli R, et al. The outcome of varicocelectomy in subfertile men with an absent or atrophic right testis. Br J Urol 1998;81:750-752.
589. Segenreich E, Israilov S, Shmuele J, et al. Evaluation of the relationship between semen parameters, pregnancy rate of wives of infertile men with varicocele, and gonadotropin-releasing hormone test before and after varicocelectomy. Urology 1998;52:853-857.
590. Bosl GJ, Motzer RJ. Testicular germ-cell cancer. N Engl J Med 1997;337:242-253.
591. Hartmann JT, Kanz L, Bokemeyer C. Diagnosis and treatment of patients wih testicular germ cell cancer. Drugs 1999;58:257-291.
592. Richiardi L, Bellocco R, Adami HO, et al. Testicular cancer incidence in eight northern European countries: secular and recent trends. Cancer Epidemiol Biomarkers Prev 2004;13:2157-2166.
593. Moller H, Skakkebaek NE. Testicular cancer and cryptorchidism in relation to prenatal factors: case control study in Denmark. Cancer Causes Control 1997;8:904-912.
594. Jacobsen R, Bostofte E, Engholm G, et al. Risk of testicular cancer in men with abnormal semen characteristics: cohort study. BMJ 2000;321:789-792.
595. Tollerud D, Blattner W, Fraser M, et al. Familial testicular cancer and urogenital developmental anomalies. Cancer 1985;55: 1849-1854.
596. Horwich A, Shipley J, Huddart R. Testicular germ-cell cancer. Lancet 2006;367:754-765.
597. Giwercman A, Muller JE, Skakkebaek NE. Prevalence of carcinoma in situ and other histopathological abnormalities in testes from 399 men who died suddenly and unexpectedly. J Urol 1991;145:77-80.
598. Smiraglia DJ, Szymanska J, Kraggerud SM, et al. Distinct epigenetic phenotypes in seminomatous and nonseminomatous testicular germ cell tumors. Oncogene 2002;21:3909-3916.
599. Kawakami T, Okamoto K, Ogawa O, Okada Y. XIST unmethylated DNA fragments in male-derived plasma as a tumor marker for testicular cancer. Lancet 2004;363:40-42.
600. Oosterhuis J, Castedo S, De Jong B. Cytogenetics, ploidy, and differentiation of human testicular, ovarian, and extragonadal germ cell tumors. Cancer Surveys 1990;9:320-332.
601. Ottesen AM, Skakkebaek NE, Lundsteen C, et al. High-resolution comparative genomic hybridization detects extra chromosome arm 12p material in most cases of carcinoma in situ adjacent to overt germ cell tumors, but not before the invasive tumor development. Genes Chromosomes Cancer 2003;38:117-125.
602. Henegariu O, Vance GH, Heiber D, et al. Triple color FISH analysis of 12p amplification in testicular germ-cell tumors using 12p-band specific paiting probes. J Mol Med 1998;76:648-655.
603. Rodriguez S, Jafer O, Goker H, et al. Expression profiling of genes from 12p in testicular germ cell tumors of adolescents and adults associated with i(12p) and amplification of 12p11.2. Oncogene 2003;22:1880-1891.
604. Clark AT, Rodriguez RT, Bodnar MS, et al. Human *STELLAR, NANOG,* and *GDF3* genes are expressed in pluripotent cells and map to chromosome 12p13, a hotspot for teratocarcinoma. Stem Cells 2004;22:169-179.
605. Kemmer K, Corless CL, Fletcher JA, et al. Kit mutations are common in testicular seminoma. Am J Pathol 2004;164:305-313.
606. Li J, Xia F, Li WX. Coactivation of STAT and Ras is required for germ cell proliferation and invasive migration in *Drosophila.* Dev Cell 2003;5:787-798.
607. Kersemaekers AM, Mayer F, Molier M, et al. Role of p53 and MDM2 in treatment response of human germ cell tumors. J Clin Oncol 2002;20:1551-1561.
608. Koberle B, Masters JR, Hartley JA, Wood AD. Defective repair of cisplatin-induced DNA damage caused by reduced XPA protein in testicular germ cell tumors. Curr Biol 1999;9:273-276.
609. Bokemeyer C, Nichols C, Droz J-P, et al. Extragonadal germ cell tumors of the mediastinum and retroperitoneum: results from an international analysis. J Clin Oncol 2002;20:1864-1873.
610. Jennings MT, Gelman R, Hochberg F. Intracranial germ-cell tumors: natural history and pathogenesis. J Neurosurgery 1985;63: 155-167.
611. Oliver RT, Mason MD, Mead GM, et al. Radiotherapy versus single-dose carboplatin in adjuvant treatment of stage I seminomas: a randomised trial. Lancet 2005;366:293-300.
612. Classen J, Schmidberger H, Meisner C, et al. Radiotherapy for stages IIA/B testicular seminomas: final report of a prospective multicenter clinical trial. J Clin Oncol 2003;21:1101-1106.
613. van Dijk MR, Steyerberg J, Habbema DF. Survival of non-seminomatous germ cell cancer patients according to the IGCC classification: an update based on meta-analysis. Eur J Cancer 2005;42:820-826.
614. Yesalis CE 3rd, Bahrke MS, Kopstein AN, Baruskiewicz CK. Incidence anabolic steroid use: a discussion of methodological issues. In Yesalis CE 3rd, ed. Anabolic Steroids in Sports and Exercise, 2nd ed. Champaign, IL: Human Kinetics, 2000:73-115.
615. Bahrke MS, Yesalis CE. Abuse of anabolic androgenic steroids and related substances in sport and exercise. Curr Opin Pharmacol 2004;4:614-620.
616. Bahrke MS, Yesalis CE, Kopstein AN, Stephens JA. Risk factors associated with anabolic-androgenic steroid use among adolescents. Sports Med 2000;29:397-405.
617. Yesalis CE, Barsukiewicz CK, Kopstein AN, Bahrke MS. Trends in anabolic-androgenic steroid use among adolescents. Arch Pediatr Adolesc Med 1997;151:1197-1206.
618. Buckley WE, Yesalis CE 3rd, Friedl KE, et al. Estimated prevalence of anabolic steroid use among male high school seniors. JAMA 1988;260:3441-3445.
619. Irving LM, Wall M, Neumark-Sztainer D, et al. Steroid use among adolescents: findings from project EAT. J Adolescent Health 2002;30:243-252.
620. Melia P, Pipe A, Greenberg L. The use of anabolic-androgenic steroids by Canadian students. Clin J Sport Med 1996;6: 9-14.
621. Handelsman DJ, Gupta L. Prevalence and risk factors for anabolic-androgenic steroid abuse in Australian high school students. Int J Androl 1997;20:159-164.
622. Yesalis CE, Kennedy NJ, Kopstein AN, Bahrke MS. Anabolic-androgenic steroid use in the United States. JAMA 1993;270: 1217-1221.
623. Franke WW, Berendonk B. Hormonal doping and androgenization of athletes: a secret program of the German Democratic Republic government. Clin Chem 1997;43:1262-1279.
624. Evans NA. Gym and tonic: a profile of 100 male steroid users. Br J Sports Med 1997;31:54-58.
625. Evans NA. Local complications of self administered anabolic steroid injections. Br J Sports Med 1997;31:349-350.
626. Pope HG Jr, Katz DL. Psychiatric and medical effects of anabolic-androgenic steroid use. A controlled study of 160 athletes. Arch Gen Psychiatry 1994;51:375-382.
627. Bhasin S, Woodhouse L, Casaburi R, et al. Testosterone dose-response relationships in healthy young men. Am J Physiol Endocrinol Metab 2001;281:E1172-E1181.
628. Storer TW, Magliano L, Woodhouse L, et al. Testosterone dose-dependently increases maximal voluntary strength and leg power, but does not affect fatigability or specific tension. J Clin Endocrinol Metab 2003;88:1478-1485.
629. Baume N, Schumacher YO, Sottas PE, et al. Effect of multiple oral doses of androgenic anabolic steroids on endurance performance and serum indices of physical stress in healthy male subjects. Eur J Appl Physiol 2006;98:329-340.
630. Georgieva KN, Boyadjiev NP. Effects of nandrolone decanoate on VO_{2max}, running economy, and endurance in rats. Med Sci Sports Exerc 2004;36:1336-1341.

631. Hendler ED, Solomon LR. Prospective controlled study of androgen effects on red cell oxygen transport and work capacity in chronic hemodialysis patients. Acta Haematol 1990;83:1-8.
632. Blanco CE, Popper P, Micevych P. Anabolic-androgenic steroid induced alterations in choline acetyltransferase messenger RNA levels of spinal cord motoneurons in the male rat. Neuroscience 1997;78:873-882.
633. Blanco CE, Zhan WZ, Fang YH, Sieck GC. Exogenous testosterone treatment decreases diaphragm neuromuscular transmission failure in male rats. J Appl Physiol 2001;90:850-856.
634. Wight JN Jr, Salem D. Sudden cardiac death and the "athlete's heart." Arch Intern Med 1995;155:1473-1480.
635. Melchert RB, Welder AA. Cardiovascular effects of androgenic-anabolic steroids. Med Sci Sports Exerc 1995;27:1252-1262.
636. Glazer G. Atherogenic effects of anabolic steroids on serum lipid levels. A literature review. Arch Intern Med 1991;151:1925-1933.
637. Ansell JE, Tiarks C, Fairchild VK. Coagulation abnormalities associated with the use of anabolic steroids. Am Heart J 1993; 125:367-371.
638. Soe KL, Soe M, Gluud C. Liver pathology associated with the use of anabolic-androgenic steroids. Liver 1992;12:73-79.
639. Dickerman RD, Pertusi RM, Zachariah NY, et al. Anabolic steroid–induced hepatotoxicity: is it overstated? Clin J Sport Med 1999;9:34-39.
640. Pertusi R, Dickerman RD, McConathy WJ. Evaluation of aminotransferase elevations in a bodybuilder using anabolic steroids: hepatitis or rhabdomyolysis? J Am Osteopath Assoc 2001;101: 391-394.
641. Tricker R, Casaburi R, Storer TW, et al. The effects of supraphysiological doses of testosterone on angry behavior in healthy eugonadal men—a clinical research center study. J Clin Endocrinol Metab 1996;81:3754-3758.
642. Daly RC, Su TP, Schmidt PJ, et al. Neuroendocrine and behavioral effects of high-dose anabolic steroid administration in male normal volunteers. Psychoneuroendocrinology 2003;28:317-331.
643. Su TP, Pagliaro M, Schmidt PJ, et al. Neuropsychiatric effects of anabolic steroids in male normal volunteers. JAMA 1993;269: 2760-2764.
644. Yates WR, Perry PJ, MacIndoe J, et al. Psychosexual effects of three doses of testosterone cycling in normal men. Biol Psychiatry 1999;45:254-260.
645. Kouri EM, Lukas SE, Pope HG Jr, Oliva PS. Increased aggressive responding in male volunteers following the administration of gradually increasing doses of testosterone cypionate. Drug Alcohol Depend 1995;40:73-79.
646. Pope HG Jr, Kouri EM, Hudson JI. Effects of supraphysiologic doses of testosterone on mood and aggression in normal men: a randomized controlled trial. Arch Gen Psychiatry 2000;57:133-140; discussion 155-156.
647. Cohen JC, Hickman R. Insulin resistance and diminished glucose tolerance in powerlifters ingesting anabolic steroids. J Clin Endocrinol Metab 1987;64:960-963.
648. Karila TA, Karjalainen JE, Mantysaari MJ, et al. Anabolic androgenic steroids produce dose-dependant increase in left ventricular mass in power atheletes, and this effect is potentiated by concomitant use of growth hormone. Int J Sports Med 2003;24:337-343.
649. Gill GV. Anabolic steroid induced hypogonadism treated with human chorionic gonadotropin. Postgrad Med J 1998;74:45-46.
650. MacIndoe JH, Perry PJ, Yates WR, et al. Testosterone suppression of the HPT axis. J Investig Med 1997;45:441-447.
651. Lloyd FH, Powell P, Murdoch AP. Anabolic steroid abuse by body builders and male subfertility. BMJ 1996;313:100-101.
652. Jarow JP, Lipshultz LI. Anabolic steroid–induced hypogonadotropic hypogonadism. Am J Sports Med 1990;18:429-431.
653. Brower KJ. Anabolic steroid abuse and dependence. Curr Psychiatry Rep 2002;4:377-387.
654. Brower KJ, Blow FC, Young JP, Hill EM. Symptoms and correlates of anabolic-androgenic steroid dependence. Br J Addict 1991;86: 759-768.
655. Brower KJ, Eliopulos GA, Blow FC, et al. Evidence for physical and psychological dependence on anabolic androgenic steroids in eight weight lifters. Am J Psychiatry 1990;147:510-512.
656. Evans NA, Bowrey DJ, Newman GR. Ultrastructural analysis of ruptured tendon from anabolic steroid users. Injury 1998;29: 769-773.
657. Schanzer W. Metabolism of anabolic androgenic steroids. Clin Chem 1996;42:1001-1020.
658. Schanzer W. Abuse of androgens and detection of illegal use. In Nieschlag E, Behre HM, eds. Testosterone: Action, Deficiency, Substitution, 3rd ed. Cambridge, UK: Cambridge University Press, 2004:715-736.
659. Aguilera R, Becchi M, Grenot C, et al. Detection of testosterone misuse: comparison of two chromatographic sample preparation methods for gas chromatographic-combustion/isotope ratio mass spectrometric analysis. J Chromatogr B Biomed Appl 1996;687: 43-53.
660. Aguilera R, Chapman TE, Starcevic B, et al. Performance characteristics of a carbon isotope ratio method for detecting doping with testosterone based on urine diols: controls and athletes with elevated testosterone/epitestosterone ratios. Clin Chem 2001;47: 292-300.
661. Catlin DH, Hatton CK, Starcevic SH. Issues in detecting abuse of xenobiotic anabolic steroids and testosterone by analysis of athletes' urine. Clin Chem 1997;43:1280-1288.
662. Garle M, Ocka R, Palonek E, Bjorkhem I. Increased urinary testosterone/epitestosterone ratios found in Swedish athletes in connection with a national control program. Evaluation of 28 cases. J Chromatogr B Biomed Appl 1996;687:55-59.
663. Gonzalo-Lumbreras R, Pimentel-Trapero D, Izquierdo-Hornillos R. Development and method validation for testosterone and epitestosterone in human urine samples by liquid chromatography applications. J Chromatogr Sci 2003;41:261-265.
664. Hebestreit M, Flenker U, Buisson C, et al. Application of stable carbon isotope analysis to the detection of testosterone administration to cattle. J Agric Food Chem 2006;54:2850-2858.
665. Saudan C, Baume N, Robinson N, et al. Testosterone and doping control. Br J Sports Med 2006;40(suppl 1):i21-i24.
666. Sottas PE, Baume N, Saudan C, Schweizer C, Kamber M, Saugy M. Bayesian detection of abnormal values in longitudinal biomarkers with an application to T/E ratio. Biostatistics June 19, 2006. Available at http://biostatistics.oxfordjournals.org/cgi/content/abstract/kxl009v1 (accessed January 5, 2007).
667. Shackleton CH, Phillips A, Chang T, Li Y. Confirming testosterone administration by isotope ratio mass spectrometric analysis of urinary androstanediols. Steroids 1997;62:379-387.
668. Kottke MK. Scientific and regulatory aspects of nutraceutical products in the United States. Drug Dev Ind Pharm 1998;24:1177-1195.
669. Stevens K. Dietary Supplement Health and Education Act: quiet but far-reaching consequences. Altern Ther Health Med 1995;1:17-18.
670. Yesalis CE 3rd. Medical, legal, and societal implications of androstenedione use [editorial; comment]. JAMA 1999;281:2043-2044.
671. Leder BZ, Leblanc KM, Longcope C, et al. Effects of oral androstenedione administration on serum testosterone and estradiol levels in postmenopausal women. J Clin Endocrinol Metab 2002;87:5449-5454.
672. Leder BZ, Longcope C, Catlin DH, et al. Oral androstenedione administration and serum testosterone concentrations in young men. JAMA 2000;283:779-782.
673. Brown GA, Vukovich MD, Martini ER, et al. Endocrine responses to chronic androstenedione intake in 30- to 56-year-old men. J Clin Endocrinol Metab 2000;85:4074-4080.
674. Brown GA, Vukovich MD, Martini ER, et al. Effects of androstenedione-herbal supplementation on serum sex hormone concentrations in 30- to 59-year-old men. Int J Vitam Nutr Res 2001;71:293-301.
675. King DS, Sharp RL, Vukovich MD, et al. Effect of oral androstenedione on serum testosterone and adaptations to resistance training in young men: a randomized controlled trial. JAMA 1999; 281:2020-2028.
676. Jasuja R, Ramaraj P, Mac RP, et al. Δ^4-Androstene-3,17-dione binds androgen receptor, promotes myogenesis in vitro, and increases serum testosterone levels, fat-free mass, and muscle strength in hypogonadal men. J Clin Endocrinol Metab 2005;90:855-863.
677. Catlin DH, Leder BZ, Ahrens B, et al. Trace contamination of over-the-counter androstenedione and positive urine test results for a nandrolone metabolite. JAMA 2000;284:2618-2621.
678. Delbeke FT, Van Eenoo P, Van Thuyne W, Desmet N. Prohormones and sport. J Steroid Biochem Mol Biol 2002;83:245-251.

679. van der Merwe PJ, Grobbelaar E. Unintentional doping through the use of contaminated nutritional supplements. S Afr Med J 2005;95:510-511.
680. Geyer H, Parr MK, Mareck U, et al. Analysis of non-hormonal nutritional supplements for anabolic-androgenic steroids—results of an international study. Int J Sports Med 2004;25:124-129.
681. Laughlin GA, Barrett-Connor E. Sexual dimorphism in the influence of advanced aging on adrenal hormone levels: the Rancho Bernardo Study. J Clin Endocrinol Metab 2000;85:3561-3568.
682. Orentreich N, Brind JL, Vogelman JH, et al. Long-term longitudinal measurements of plasma dehydroepiandrosterone sulfate in normal men. J Clin Endocrinol Metab 1992;75:1002-1004.
683. Baulieu EE, Robel P. Dehydroepiandrosterone (DHEA) and dehydroepiandrosterone sulfate (DHEAS) as neuroactive neurosteroids. Proc Natl Acad Sci U S A 1998;95:4089-4091.
684. Liu D, Dillon JS. Dehydroepiandrosterone activates endothelial cell nitric-oxide synthase by a specific plasma membrane receptor coupled to Gα(i2,3). J Biol Chem 2002;277:21379-21388.
685. Demirgoren S, Majewska MD, Spivak CE, London ED. Receptor binding and electrophysiological effects of dehydroepiandrosterone sulfate, an antagonist of the GABAA receptor. Neuroscience 1991;45:127-135.
686. Arlt W, Callies F, van Vlijmen JC, et al. Dehydroepiandrosterone replacement in women with adrenal insufficiency. N Engl J Med 1999;341:1013-1020.
687. Hunt PJ, Gurnell EM, Huppert FA, et al. Improvement in mood and fatigue after dehydroepiandrosterone replacement in Addison's disease in a randomized, double blind trial. J Clin Endocrinol Metab 2000;85:4650-4656.
688. Lovas K, Gebre-Medhin G, Trovik TS, et al. Replacement of dehydroepiandrosterone in adrenal failure: no benefit for subjective health status and sexuality in a 9-month, randomized, parallel group clinical trial. J Clin Endocrinol Metab 2003;88:1112-1118.
689. Johannsson G, Burman P, Wiren L, et al. Low dose dehydroepiandrosterone affects behavior in hypopituitary androgen-deficient women: a placebo-controlled trial. J Clin Endocrinol Metab 2002;87:2046-2052.
690. Gebre-Medhin G, Husebye ES, Mallmin H, et al. Oral dehydroepiandrosterone (DHEA) replacement therapy in women with Addison's disease. Clin Endocrinol (Oxf) 2000;52:775-780.
691. Morales AJ, Haubrich RH, Hwang JY, et al. The effect of six months treatment with a 100 mg daily dose of dehydroepiandrosterone (DHEA) on circulating sex steroids, body composition and muscle strength in age-advanced men and women. Clin Endocrinol (Oxf) 1998;49:421-432.
692. Arlt W, Callies F, Koehler I, et al. Dehydroepiandrosterone supplementation in healthy men with an age-related decline of dehydroepiandrosterone secretion. J Clin Endocrinol Metab 2001;86: 4686-4692.
693. Callies F, Arlt W, Siekmann L, et al. Influence of oral dehydroepiandrosterone (DHEA) on urinary steroid metabolites in males and females. Steroids 2000;65:98-102.
694. Wolkowitz OM, Reus VI, Keebler A, et al. Double-blind treatment of major depression with dehydroepiandrosterone. Am J Psychiatry 1999;156:646-649.
695. Huppert FA, van Niekerk JK. Dehdroepiandrosterone (DHEA) supplementation for cognitive function. Cochrane Database Syst Rev 2001;(2):CD000304.
696. Flynn MA, Weaver-Osterholtz D, Sharpe-Timms KL, et al. Dehydroepiandrosterone replacement in aging humans. J Clin Endocrinol Metab 1999;84:1527-1533.
697. Genazzani AD, Stomati M, Bernardi F, et al. Long-term low-dose dehydroepiandrosterone oral supplementation in early and late postmenopausal women modulates endocrine parameters and synthesis of neuroactive steroids. Fertil Steril 2003;80:1495-1501.
698. Barnhart KT, Freeman E, Grisso JA, et al. The effect of dehydroepiandrosterone supplementation to symptomatic perimenopausal women on serum endocrine profiles, lipid parameters, and health-related quality of life. J Clin Endocrinol Metab 1999;84: 3896-3902.
699. Chang DM, Lan JL, Lin HY, Luo SF. Dehydroepiandrosterone treatment of women with mild-to-moderate systemic lupus erythematosus: a multicenter randomized, double-blind, placebo-controlled trial. Arthritis Rheum 2002;46:2924-2927.
700. Hartkamp A, Geenen R, Godaert GL, et al. The effect of dehydroepiandrosterone on lumbar spine bone mineral density in patients with quiescent systemic lupus erythematosus. Arthritis Rheum 2004;50:3591-3595.
701. van Vollenhoven RF, Park JL, Genovese MC, et al. A double-blind, placebo-controlled, clinical trial of dehydroepiandrosterone in severe systemic lupus erythematosus. Lupus 1999;8:181-187.
702. Jankowski CM, Gozansky WS, Schwartz RS, et al. Effects of dehydroepiandrosterone replacement therapy on bone mineral density in older adults: a randomized, controlled trial. J Clin Endocrinol Metab 2006;91:2986-2993.
703. Catlin DH, Sekera MH, Ahrens BD, et al. Tetrahydrogestrinone: discovery, synthesis, and detection in urine. Rapid Commun Mass Spectrom 2004;18:1245-1049.
704. Jasuja R, Catlin DH, Miller A, et al. Tetrahydrogestrinone is an androgenic steroid that stimulates androgen receptor–mediated, myogenic differentiation in C3H10T1/2 multipotent mesenchymal cells and promotes muscle accretion in orchidectomized male rats. Endocrinology 2005;146:4472-4478.
705. Sekera MH, Ahrens BD, Chang YC, et al. Another designer steroid: discovery, synthesis, and detection of "madol" in urine. Rapid Commun Mass Spectrom 2005;19:781-784.
706. Handelsman DJ. Designer androgens in sport: when too much is never enough. Sci STKE 2004;2004(244):pe41.
707. Baker HWG, Burger HG, de Kretser DM, Hudson B. Relative incidence of etiologic disorders in male infertility. In: Santen RJ, Swerdloff RS, eds. Male Reproducture Dysfunction: diagnosis and management of hypogonadism, infectitity, and improtence. New York: Marcel Dekker 1986:342-372.

CHAPTER 19

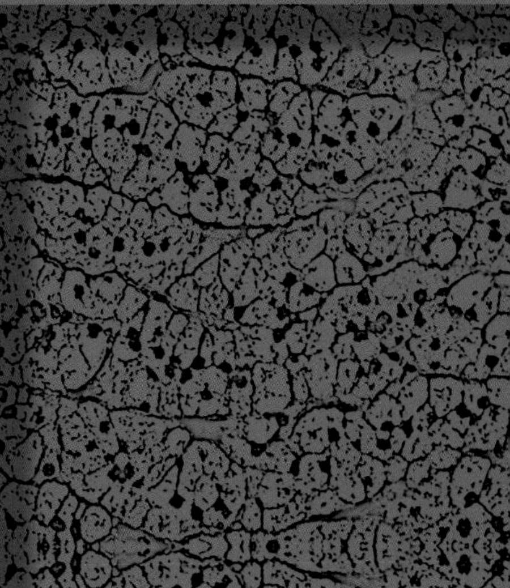

SEXUAL DYSFUNCTION IN MEN AND WOMEN

Shalender Bhasin, Rosemary Basson

Throughout human history, religious dogma and mythology have shaped our views of human sexuality—most of these views were egregiously erroneous. Within this historical context, the creation of the *Kamasutra,* a refreshingly explicit treatise on human sexology, by Vatsayayana Malianaga almost two millennia ago, is a remarkable accomplishment.[1] Human sexuality remained banished from most thoughtful discourse until the middle of the twentieth century, when Michael Kinsey's pioneering epidemiologic investigations provided the first evidence of the considerable variability in sexual practices of American men and women.[2] Subsequent studies by William Masters and Virginia E. Johnson[3] found that both men and women display predictable physiologic responses after sexual stimulation. These landmark descriptions of the human sexual response cycle by Masters and Johnson provided the basis for rational classification of human sexual disorders.[3]

Sigmund Freud ascribed sexual problems in adults to earlier difficulties in maturation of childhood sexuality and development of parent-child relationships. Much acclaimed in an earlier era, Freud's psychoanalytical theories have largely been discredited by recent advances in our understanding of the physiologic and biochemical mechanisms of penile erection and the development of mechanism-specific therapies for erectile dysfunction (ED).

The 1980s and 1990s witnessed steady progress in our understanding of the physicochemical mechanisms that lead to penile tumescence and rigidity. It was recognized that penile erections are a result of cavernosal smooth muscle relaxation and increased penile blood flow.[4] The appreciation of nitric oxide as a key vasodilator in the vascular smooth muscle was a pivotal discovery, recognized later by the award of the Nobel Prize in Physiology or Medicine to Robert F. Furchgott, Louis J. Ignarro, and Ferid Murad. The recognition that nitric oxide caused cavernosal smooth muscle relaxation by simulating guanylyl cyclase provided the theoretical foundation for the discovery of highly effective oral therapies for the treatment of ED.

Excellent epidemiologic surveys, such as the Massachusetts Male Aging Study (MMAS) led by John McKinlay[5] and the National Health and Social Life Survey (NHSLS) led by Laumann and Rosen,[6,7] using modern sampling techniques, revealed high prevalence rates of sexual dysfunction among community dwelling, middle-aged and older men. Recognizing the importance of sexual function as a determinant of quality of life, the World Health Organization declared sexual health a fundamental right of men and women. The confluence of these driving forces in the mid-1990s paved the way for the development of effective oral therapies for ED in men.

Historically, the classification and nomenclature for sexual disorders were based on the *Diagnostic and Statistical Manual of Mental Disorders* (DSM), which is primarily a psychiatric nomenclature, reflecting the belief that sexual disorders in men and women are psychogenic in their origin.[8] In the 1990s, several expert groups updated the clinical definitions of sexual disorders in men.[9,10] The growing recognition that ED is commonly a manifestation of systemic disease and the availability of easy-to-use therapeutic options, including oral and intraurethral drugs, have placed sexual disorders in men within the purview of the primary care provider, where they duly belong. In contrast, the pathophysiology of sexual disorders in women remains poorly understood and no pharmacologic therapies have been approved for this indication, aside from estrogen therapy for dyspareunia associated with vulvovaginal atrophy.

SEXUAL DISORDERS IN MEN

Sexual dysfunction is a more general term that includes libidinal, orgasmic, and ejaculatory dysfunction, in addition to ED.[11] *Erectile dysfunction,* previously referred to as *impotence,* is a more specific term that denotes the inability of the male to attain or maintain an erection sufficient for satisfactory sexual intercourse.[9,10]

Regulation of Sexual Function and the Physiology of Penile Erection

The Human Sexual Response Cycle

William Masters and Virginia E. Johnson[3] found that both men and women display predictable physiologic responses after sexual stimulation that can be categorized in four phases: the excitement phase, the plateau phase, the orgasmic phase, and the resolution phase (Fig. 19–1). During the excitation phase, the heart and breathing rates increase, blood pressure rises, nipples become erect, penis achieves varying degrees of erection, the testes are drawn up, and the skin might undergo a sex flush.[3] The excitation phase is followed by the plateau phase, in which heart rate increases further, sexual pleasure intensifies, bladder sphincter closes, the muscles at the base of the penis contract rhythmically, and men begin to secrete a small amount of seminal fluid.[3]

Achievement of orgasm is associated with contractions of the pelvic muscles and anal sphincter, ejaculation of seminal fluid, a perception of intense pleasure, and release of tension. In the initial emission phase, the seminal fluid collects in the urethral bulb.[12] The subsequent ejaculation of the semen from the penis requires contractions of the periurethral and other pelvic muscles.[12] During the resolution phase, muscles relax, heart rate and blood pressure decrease, and penile erection is lost. Orgasm and ejaculation are followed by a refractory period of varying duration in which men are unable to achieve orgasm again.[3]

Mechanisms of Penile Erection

Penile Anatomy and Blood Flow

The erectile tissue of the penis consists of two dorsally positioned corpora cavernosa and a ventrally placed corpus spongiosum.[13] The erectile tissue of the corpora cavernosa and corpus spongiosum is composed of numerous cavernous spaces separated by trabeculae.[14] These trabeculae are composed mainly of smooth muscle cells that are arranged in a syncytium. Endothelial cells cover the surfaces of the trabeculae.

The penile arterial blood supply is derived from the pudendal arteries, which are branches of the internal iliac arteries (see Fig. 19–1). The pudendal artery, a branch of the hypogastric artery, divides into cavernosal, dorsal penile, and bulbourethral arteries. The cavernosal arteries and their branches, the helicine arteries, provide blood flow to corpora cavernosa.[14] Dilation of the helicine arteries increases the blood flow and pressure in the cavernosal sinuses.[15]

Penile Innervation

The neural input to the penis consists of sympathetic (T11-L2), parasympathetic (S2-S4), and somatic nerves (Table 19–1). Sympathetic and parasympathetic fibers converge in the inferior hypogastric plexus, where the autonomic input to the penis is integrated and communicated to the penis through cavernosal nerves. In humans, the inferior hypogastric ganglionic plexus is located retroperitoneally near the rectum.[13]

Several brain regions, including the amygdala, medial preoptic area, paraventricular nucleus of the hypothalamus, and periaqueductal gray matter act coordinately to effect penile erections. The medial preoptic area of the hypothalamus serves as the integration site for the central nervous system control of erections; it receives sensory input from the amygdala and sends impulses to the paraventricular nuclei of the hypothalamus and the periaqueductal gray matter. Neurons in the paraventricular nuclei project onto the thoracolumbar and sacral nuclei associated with erections.

The parasympathetic input to the penis is proerectile, and sympathetic input is mainly inhibitory. The stimuli from the perineum and lower urinary tract are carried to the penis through the sacral reflex arc.

Hemodynamic Changes During Penile Erection

Penile erection results from a series of biochemical and hemodynamic events that are associated with activation of central nervous system sites involved in regulation of erections, relaxation of cavernosal smooth muscle, increased blood flow into cavernosal sinuses, and venous occlusion resulting in penile engorgement and rigidity.[14] Normal penile erection requires coordinated involvement of intact central and peripheral nervous systems, corpora cavernosa and spongiosa, and normal arterial blood supply and venous drainage.[14]

As cavernosal smooth muscle relaxes and the blood flow to the penis increases, the increased pooling of blood in the cavernosal spaces results in penile engorgement (Fig. 19–2).[4] The expanding corpora cavernosa compress the venules against the rigid tunica albuginea, restricting the venous outflow from the cavernosal spaces.[4] This facilitates entrapment of blood in the cavernosal sinuses, imparting rigidity to the erect penis.

Biochemical Regulation of Cavernosal Smooth Muscle Tone

The tone of the corporal smooth muscle cells determines the erectile state of the penis.[4,15] When the cavernosal smooth muscle cells are relaxed, the penis is engorged with blood and erect. When the cavernosal smooth muscle cells are contracted,

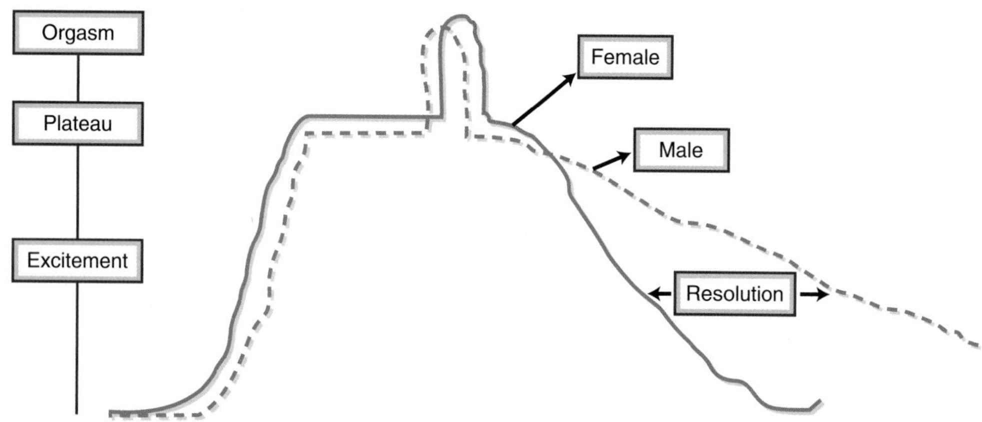

Figure 19–1 ▪ Four phases of the human sexual response cycle as postulated by Masters and Johnson. The resolution phase is prolonged considerably in men, so that men can experience refractoriness to further stimulation for varying lengths of time before they can achieve another orgasm. As discussed in the text, our views of the female response cycle have evolved substantially since then.

TABLE 19–1 INNERVATION OF THE PENIS

Types of Fibers	Location of Neurons in the Spinal Cord	Nerves Carrying the Fibers	General Function
Sympathetic	T10-L2	Prevertebral outflow through the hypogastric and cavernous nerves; additionally, paravertebral outflow through the parasympathetic ganglia and the pudendal or pelvic and cavernous nerves	Generally antierectile; sympathetic innervation plays an important role in regulating seminal emission
Parasympathetic	S2-S4	Cavernosal and pelvic nerves	Proerectile
Somatic	S2-S4	Pudendal nerve	Penile sensation, contraction of the striated muscles during ejaculation

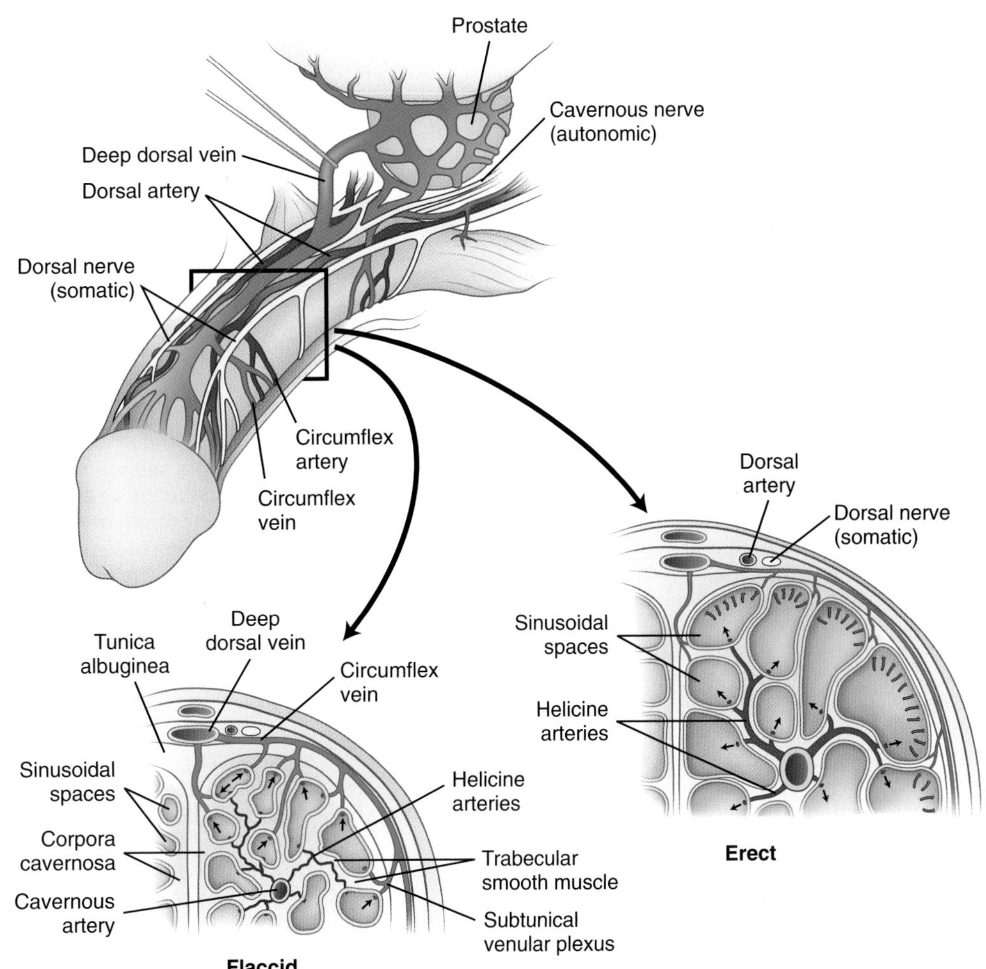

Figure 19–2 ▪ Anatomy and mechanism of penile erection. Corpora cavernosa are made up of trabecular spaces that are surrounded by cavernosal smooth muscle. Helicine arteries provide the arterial supply to the cavernosal spaces. The dorsal nerve provides the sensory innervation to the penis. During erection, the relaxation of the trabecular smooth muscle and increased blood flow result in engorgement of the sinusoidal spaces in the corpora cavernosa. The expansion of the sinusoids compresses the venous return against the tunica albuginea, resulting in entrapment of blood. This imparts rigidity to the tumescent penis. (Adapted from Lue TF. Erectile dysfunction. N Engl J Med 2000; 342:1802-1813.)

there is predominance of sympathetic neural activity, and the penis is flaccid.

The smooth muscle tone in the corpora cavernosa is maintained by the release of stored intracellular calcium into the cytoplasm and influx of calcium through membrane channels.[16] The transmembrane influx of calcium in the cavernosal smooth muscle cells is mediated mostly by L-type voltage-dependent calcium channels,[16] although T-type calcium channels are also expressed in cavernosal smooth muscle cells.[17] An increase in intracellular calcium activates myosin light chain kinase, resulting in phosphorylation of myosin light chain, actin-myosin interactions, and smooth muscle contraction.[14,18]

The transmembrane and intracellular calcium flux in the cavernosal smooth muscle cells is regulated by a number of cellular processes that involve K^+ flux through potassium channels, connexin 43–derived gap junctions, and a number of cholinergic, adrenergic, and noradrenergic noncholinergic mediators (Figs. 19–3 to 19–6).[14,16] The nonadrenergic, noncholinergic mediators include vasoactive intestinal peptide, calcitonin gene-related peptide, and nitric oxide (NO).[14]

Adrenergic pathways, acing through norepinephrine and α_1-adrenergic receptors, activate phospholipase C, which generates diacyl glycerol and inositol triphosphate. Diacyl glycerol activates protein kinase C, which inhibits K^+ channels and

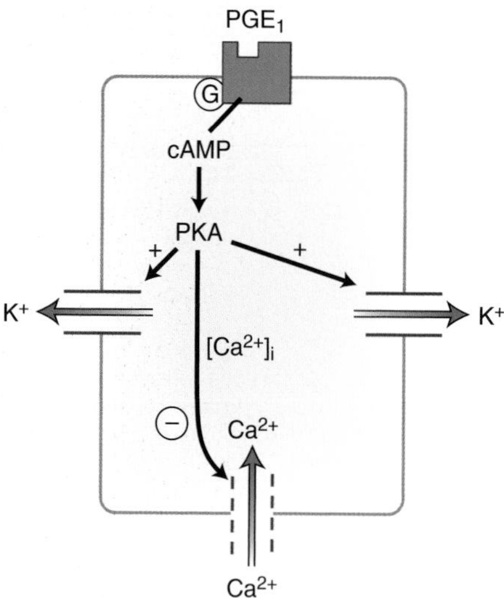

Figure 19–3 ▪ Regulation of cavernosal smooth muscle contractility by PGE_1. The relaxation of the cavernosal smooth muscle is regulated by intracellular cAMP and cGMP. By activation of specific protein kinases, these intracellular second messengers cause sequestration of intracellular calcium, closure of calcium channels, and opening of K^+ channels. This results in a net decrease in intracellular calcium, causing smooth muscle relaxation. PGE_1, by binding to the PGE_1 receptor, increases the intracellular concentrations of cAMP, which activates PKA. PKA promotes the sequestration of intracellular calcium, inhibits cacium influx, and stimulates K^+ channels. The net result is a decrease in intracytoplasmic calcium and smooth muscle relaxation. cAMP, cyclic adnosine monophosphate; cGMP, cyclic guanosine monophosphate; PGE_1, prostaglandin E_1; PKA, protein kinase A. (Adapted from Bhasin S, Benson GS. Male sexual function. In De Kretser D ed. Knobil and Neill's Physiology of Reproduction, 3rd ed. Boston: Academic Press, 2006:1173-1194; and Lue TF. Erectile dysfunction. N Engl J Med 2000;342: 1802-1813.)

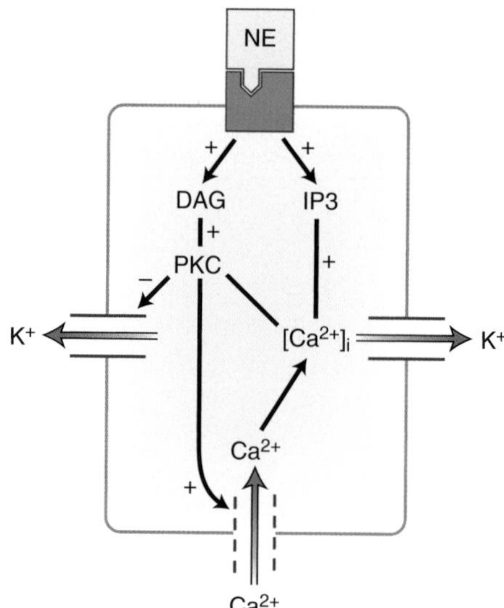

Figure 19–4 ▪ Regulation of cavernosal smooth muscle contractility by norepinephrine. Norepinephrine mediates adrenergic signals, binds to adrenergic receptors, and stimulates diacyl glycerol (DAG) and inositol-3 phosphate (IP3). DAG stimulates protein kinase C (PKC), which, along with IP3, causes an increase in intracytoplasmic calcium and inhibition of K^+ channels. Increased intracellular calcium causes cavernosal smooth muscle contraction and loss of penile erection. (Adapted from Bhasin S, Benson GS. Male sexual function. In De Kretser D ed. Knobil and Neill's Physiology of Reproduction, 3rd ed. Boston: Academic Press, 2006:1173-1194; and Lue TF. Erectile dysfunction. N Engl J Med 2000;342:1802-1813.)

activates transmembrane calcium influx by activating L-type calcium channels (see Fig. 19–4).[19] Inositol 1,4,5-triphosphate (IP_3) increases intracellular calcium by promoting the release of calcium from intracellular calcium stores.[20,21] The net increase in intracellular calcium promotes actin-myosin interactions, resulting in smooth muscle contraction and a flaccid penis.

Prostaglandin E_1 (PGE_1) results in generation of cyclic AMP, which activates protein kinase A. Activated protein kinase A stimulates K^+ channels, resulting in K^+ efflux from the cell (see Fig. 19–3). The protein kinase A–mediated processes also result in a net decrease in intracellular calcium, favoring smooth muscle cell relaxation.

K^+ Channels

At least three types of potassium channels—K_{ATP}, Kv, and the calcium-sensitive K^+ channels, referred to as BK_{Ca} or maxi-K channel, are expressed in the cavernosal smooth muscle cells. Of these, the BK_{Ca} channels are the most important because they account for 90% of K^+ efflux from the cavernosal smooth muscle cells. BK_{Ca} channel openers have been shown to relax cavernosal smooth muscle cells in vitro.[22] Thus, it is not surprising that the strategies that increase BK_{Ca} channel expression in vivo improve erectile capacity in diabetic and older rodents[23] and are being explored as therapy for erectile dysfunction.[24] A phase I human gene therapy trial using this approach is in progress.[24]

Connexin 43 Gap Junctions

The smooth muscle cells in the corpora cavernosa are connected by connexin43 gap junctions that allow the ions and some signaling molecules such as inositol triphosphate to diffuse freely across smooth muscle cells.[25] The ionic changes induced by a stimulus in one smooth muscle cell are communicated rapidly across other smooth muscle cells, resulting in coordinate regulation of the entire corpus cavernosum.[16] Thus, corpora cavernosa can be viewed functionally as a syncytium of interconnected smooth muscle cells (see Fig. 19–5).[16]

Nitric Oxide

Nitric oxide, derived from the nerve terminals innervating the corpora cavernosa, endothelial lining of penile arteries, and cavernosal sinuses, is an important biochemical regulator of cavernosal smooth muscle relaxation. Nitric oxide also induces arterial dilation.[26] The actions of NO on the cavernosal smooth muscle and the arterial blood flow are mediated through the activation of guanylyl cyclase, the production of cyclic guanosine monophosphate (cGMP), and activation of cGMP-dependent protein kinase (PKG) (see Fig. 19–6). cGMP causes smooth muscle relaxation by lowering intracellular calcium. There is some evidence that NO inhibits Rho-kinase–induced cavernosal smooth muscle sensitivity to calcium.[27]

Cyclic Nucleotide Phosphodiesterases

Cyclic nucleotide phosphodiesterases (PDEs) hydrolyze cyclic adenosine monophosphate (cAMP) and cGMP, thus reducing their concentrations within the cavernosal smooth muscle. Of the 13 or more isoforms of cyclic nucleotide phosphodiesterases that have been identified, isoforms 2, 3, 4 and 5 are expressed in the penis.[14,28] Only phosphodiesterase 5 (PDE5) is specific to the NO/cGMP pathway in the corpora cavernosa.[14,28] Hydrolysis of cGMP by this enzyme results in reversal of the smooth muscle relaxation and reversal of penile erection. Sildenafil, vardenafil, and tadalafil are potent and selective inhibitors of the activity of PDE5 that prevent breakdown of cGMP and thereby enhance penile erection.[29]

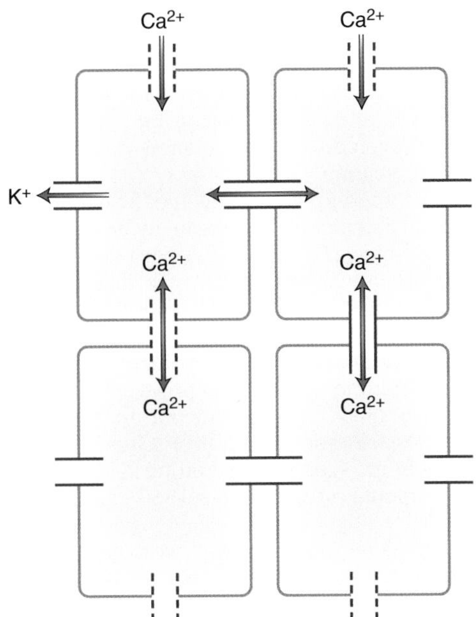

Figure 19–5 ▪ The interconnection of cavernosal smooth muscle cells in the penis. Connexin 43–derived gap junctions connect adjacent corporal smooth muscle cells and allow flow of ions among interconnected smooth muscle cells. Therefore, alterations in action potential and K^+-channel activity in any myocyte affect the adjacent myocytes. (Adapted from Melman A, Christ GJ. Integrative erectile biology. The effects of age and disease on gap junctions and ion channels and their potential value to the treatment of erectile dysfunction. Urol Clin N Am 2001;28:217-230.)

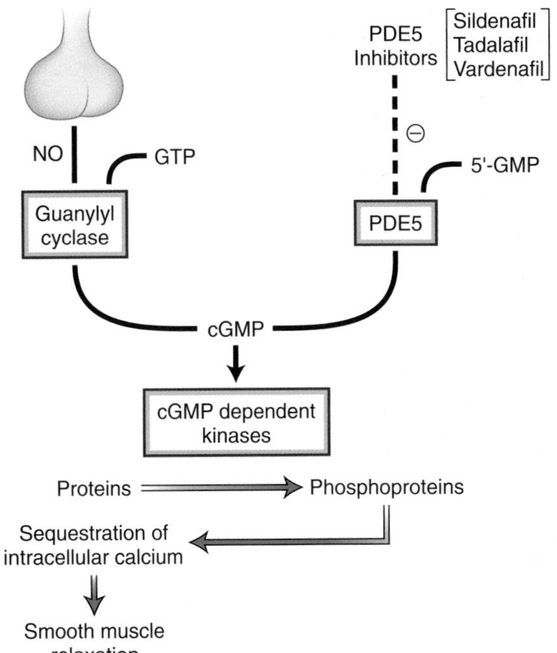

Figure 19–6 ▪ Regulation of cavernosal smooth muscle relaxation by nitric oxide. Cyclic guanosine monophosphate (cGMP) regulates cavernosal smooth muscle relaxation by promoting sequestration of cytoplasmic calcium. Nitric oxide (NO) is released from noradrenergic norcholinergic nerve endings and possibly from the endothelium. NO activates guanylyl cyclase, which generates cGMP, which in turn activates cGMP-dependent kinases, resulting in sequestration of intracellular calcium and smooth muscle relaxation. cGMP is degraded by cyclic nucleotide phosphodiesterases. Sildenafil, vardenafil, and tadalfil are selective inhibitors of PDE isoform 5 that is present in cavernosal smooth muscles. (Adapted from Bhasin S, Benson GS. Male sexual function. In De Kretser D ed. Knobil and Neill's Physiology of Reproduction, 3rd ed. Boston: Academic Press, 2006:1173-1194; and Lue TF. Erectile dysfunction. N Engl J Med 2000;342:1802-1813.)

Regulation of Sensitivity to Intracellular Calcium by Rho A/Rho Kinase Signaling

Considerable attention has focused on the role of Rho kinase in modulating the sensitivity of cavernosal smooth muscle to intracellular calcium (see reference 18). A growing body of evidence suggests that sensitization to intracellular calcium is regulated by the balance between phosphorylation of the regulatory light chain of myosin II by a myosin light chain kinase and its dephosphorylation by a myosin light chain phosphatase (Fig. 19–7).[18] Phosphorylation of regulatory light chain of myosin II is necessary for activation of myosin II adenosine triphosphatases (ATPases) by actin, and its dephosphorylation prevents activation of myosin II ATPases.[18] The ratio of the kinase to phosphatase activities is an important determinant of the contractile sensitivity of the cavernosal smooth muscle cell to intracellular calcium.[18]

Rho A is an approximately 20-kd guanosine triphosphatase (GTPase) that modulates Rho kinase activity, myosin light chain phosphorylation, and calcium sensitivity in smooth muscle cells.[30] The Rho A–GDP (guanosine diphosphate) complex is associated with a GDP dissociation inhibitor (RhoGDI) in its inactive state.[31] A number of intracellular signals can promote an exchange of GDP for GTP on Rho A through the mediation of guanine nucleotide exchange factors.[18] The Rho A–GTP interacts with its downstream effector Rho kinase,[32] increasing the sensitivity of vascular smooth muscle to intracellular calcium by inhibiting the myosin light chain phosphatases.[33] Although the Rho A/Rho kinase expression is not significantly different between young and older rats, the activity of Rho kinase is higher in the cavernosal smooth muscle of older rats than young rats[34]; the age-related increase in Rho kinase activity has been proposed as one possible mechanism to explain the age-related

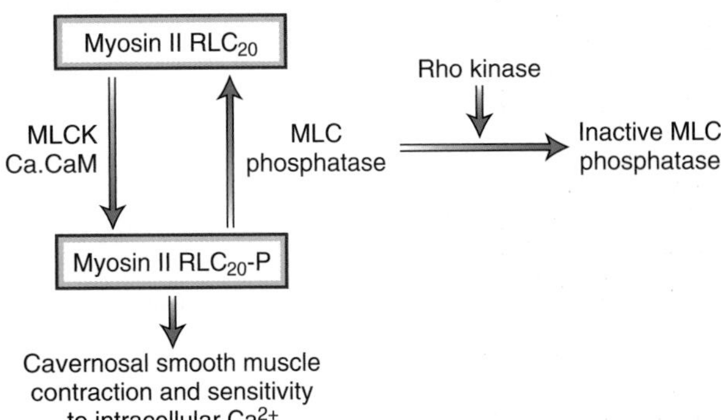

Figure 19–7 ▪ The role of Rho A:Rho kinase in regulation of sensitivity to intracellular Ca^{2+}. Sensitivity to calcium and smooth muscle contractility is regulated by the Rho-A:Rho kinase system. The balance between phsopshorylation of myosin regulatory light chain (myosin II RLC20) kinase and its dephosphorylation by a myosin light chain phosphatase is a major determinant of the smooth muscle sensitization to Ca^{2+}. By inhibiting the activity of myosin light chain (MLC) phosphatase, Rho kinase, the downstream effector of Rho A, can regulate smooth muscle responsiveness to calcium. (Adapted from Somlyo AP, Somlyo AV. Ca^{2+} sensitivity of smooth muscle and nonmuscle myosin II: modulated by G proteins, kinases, and myosin phosphatase. Physiol Rev 2003;83: 1325-1358.)

decrease in erectile capacity in rats.[34] Inhibition of Rho kinase activity in experimental animals increases cavernosal smooth muscle relaxation and improves intracavernosal pressures and penile erections.[34,35] Therefore, inhibitors of Rho A/Rho kinase signaling promise to provide attractive targets for the development of therapies for ED.[18]

The Role of Testosterone in Regulating Sexual Function in Men

Testosterone regulates many domains of sexual function in men and women. Although androgen-deficient men can achieve penile erections, their overall sexual activity is decreased.[5,25] Testosterone promotes sexual thoughts and desire[36] and increases sexual arousal and attentiveness to erotic auditory and other stimuli.[37] Brain imaging studies suggest that processing of sexual stimuli may be altered in androgen-deficient men, with decreased activation in those brain areas that typically are activated in eugonadal men and in androgen-deficient men after testosterone replacement.[38]

Acting on dopaminergic receptors in the medial preoptic area (MPOA) of the hypothalamus, testosterone elicits reward-seeking behavior in male mammals.[39] This may be the basis for testosterone's motivational effects on mammalian sexual behaviour.[39] The roles of the CYP19 aromatase and steroid 5-α reductase systems in mediating androgen effects on sexual function remain unclear. Studies suggest that 5-α reduction of testosterone is not necessary for mediating testosterone's effects on desire, but it is unclear whether aromatization to estradiol is necessary.[40]

Spontaneous, but not stimulus-bound, erections are testosterone responsive (Table 19–2).[36] Androgen-deficient men are able to achieve erection in response to erotic film.[36] Nocturnal erections, temporally related to peaks of nighttime testosterone secretion, are of lower amplitude and duration in androgen-deficient men, and testosterone therapy increases the frequency, fullness, and duration of nocturnal penile tumescence.[41]

TABLE 19–2 DOMAINS OF SEXUAL FUNCTION REGULATED BY TESTOSTERONE

DOMAINS OF SEXUAL FUNCTION THAT ARE IMPROVED BY TESTOSTERONE THERAPY OF ANDROGEN-DEFICIENT MEN
Sexual desire
Spontaneous sexual thoughts
Attentiveness to erotic auditory stimuli
Frequency of nighttime and daytime erections
Duration, magnitude, and frequency of nocturnal penile erections
Overall sexual activity scores
Volume of ejaculate
DOMAINS OF SEXUAL FUNCTION THAT ARE NOT IMPROVED BY TESTOSTERONE THERAPY OR FOR WHICH THERE IS INSUFFICIENT OR INCONCLUSIVE EVIDENCE
Erectile response to visual erotic stimulus
Erectile function in men with erectile dysfunction who have normal testosterone levels
Therapeutic response to selective phosphodiesterase inhibitors
Orgasms

Reproduced with permission from Bhasin S, Enzlin P, Coviello A, Basson R. Sexual dysfunction in men and women with endocerine disorders. Lancet 2007;369:597-611.

Maximum rigidity may require a threshold level of androgen activity[42]: testosterone regulates nitric oxide synthase (NOS) in the cavernosal smooth muscle,[43] exerts trophic effects on cavernosal smooth muscle[44] and ischiocavernosus and bulbospongiosus muscles, and is necessary for the veno-occlusive response. Androgen-deficient men show delayed orgasm and low ejaculatory volume.

Testosterone therapy in androgen-deficient men improves some but not all domains of sexual activity. Testosterone therapy of androgen-deficient men improves sexual desire; spontaneous sexual thoughts; attentiveness to erotic auditory stimuli; frequency of nighttime and daytime erections; duration, magnitude, and frequency of nocturnal penile erections; overall sexual activity scores; and the volume of ejaculate.[36,45,46] However, testosterone does not improve erectile response to visual erotic stimulus,[36] erectile function in men with ED who have normal testosterone levels, or orgasms.[47] There is insufficient evidence to support the proposal that testosterone improves therapeutic response to selective phosphodiesterase inhibitors.[45,48,49]

Androgen deficiency and ED are two independently distributed disorders that coexist in 6% to 10% of middle-aged and older men.[50] Testosterone trials among sildenafil failures have been inconclusive.[48,49]

Classification of Sexual Disorders Based on the Sexual Response Cycle

Sexual disorders have been classified into four categories depending on phase of sexual response cycle in which the abnormality exists:

- Hypoactive sexual desire disorder
- Erectile dysfunction
- Ejaculatory and orgasmic disorders
- Disorders of pain

Classification of the patient's disorder into these categories is important because the etiologic factors, diagnostic tests, and therapeutic strategies vary for each class of sexual disorder.

Hypoactive Sexual Desire Disorder

Hypoactive sexual desire disorder is the persistent or recurrent deficiency (or absence) of sexual fantasies and desire for sexual activity that causes marked distress or interpersonal difficulty and that is not better explained by another disorder, direct physiologic effects of a substance (medication), or general medical condition.[51-53]

A diagnosis of hypoactive sexual desire disorder is appropriate *only* if the person reports distress or interpersonal difficulty due to low sexual desire.[51-53] Low sexual desire is not necessarily pathologic, because low sexual desire may be an appropriate adaptation to relationship and health-related issues.[51-53]

Hypoactive sexual desire disorder is a multifactorial disorder that can result from androgen deficiency, use of medications (SSRIs, antiandrogens, GnRH analogues, antihypertensives, cancer chemotherapeutic agents, anticonvulsants), systemic illness, depression and other psychological problems, other causes of sexual dysfunction, or relationship and differentiation problems. Androgen deficiency is an important, treatable cause of hypoactive sexual desire disorder, and it should be excluded by measuring serum total testosterone levels.

True incidence and prevalence rates of hypoactive sexual desire disorder in the general population are unknown. In studies of referred patient populations, the prevalence rate has been estimated at 5% in men and 22% in women.[7,53] Prevalence rates increase with age.[53,54] Hypoactive sexual desire disorder often coexists with other sexual disorders, such as ED, and can develop as a consequence of other preexisting sexual disorders.[53]

Appropriate evaluation and treatment of hypoactive sexual desire disorder is important because evaluation can lead to detection of treatable androgen deficiency. Also, hypoactive sexual desire in one partner can strain the relationship between sexual partners[55] and lead to ED. Low sexual desire can impede or reduce effectiveness of treatments for other sexual dysfunctions.

There are four important considerations in the evaluation of men with hypoactive sexual desire disorders. An important initial step in evaluation is an interview of the couple to determine whether the patient's primary problem is ED or a sexual desire problem. Second, it is important to ascertain whether the couple has a relationship problem. Establish whether self-stimulation continues despite lack of desire for partnered sex. With availability of Internet sites, sex alone, possibly on a frequent basis, can allow sexual expression in spite of relationship difficulties. Third, a general health evaluation is necessary to exclude systemic illness, depression, and medication use. Testosterone levels should be measured to exclude androgen deficiency, because androgen deficiency is an important treatable cause of hypoactive sexual desire disorder.

Erectile Dysfunction

Erectile dysfunction, previously referred to as *impotence,* is the inability to attain and/or maintain an erection sufficient for satisfactory sexual intercourse.[9,10,14] *Sexual dysfunction* is a more general term that also includes libidinal, orgasmic, and ejaculatory dysfunction in addition to the inability to attain or maintain penile erection. The MMAS[8] and the NHSLS[5,6] revealed a surprisingly high prevalence of erectile dysfunction in men; for instance, in the MMAS,[5] a community-based sample of men in Boston, 52% of men between the ages of 40 and 70 were affected by erectile dysfunction of some degree.

Erectile dysfunction significantly affects quality of life of both the affected man and his partner. In one study, erectile dysfunction had a negative impact on the sexual life of female partners, specifically on their sexual satisfaction and sexual drive.[56]

Prevalence and Incidence

The best data on the prevalence of ED in men have emerged from two cross-sectional studies that have used population-based sampling techniques, the MMAS[5,57] and the NHSLS.[6,7] The MMAS is a cross-sectional as well as longitudinal, community-based epidemiologic survey in which 1,709 men, 40 to 70 years of age, residing in the greater Boston area were surveyed between 1987 and 1989.[5,57] Of these, 847 men were resurveyed between 1995 and 1997.[57] This survey revealed that 52% of men between the ages of 40 and 70 years were affected by erectile dysfunction of some degree; 17.2% of surveyed men reported minimal erectile dysfunction, 25.2% moderate erectile dysfunction, and 9.6% complete erectile dysfunction.[5] The NHSLS was a national probability survey of English-speaking Americans, 18 to 59 years of age, living in the United States.[6,7] This survey also revealed a high prevalence of erectile dysfunction in men; the prevalence of erectile dysfunction increased with increasing age.[6,7]

These two landmark studies and data from several other studies are in agreement that erectile dysfunction is a common problem[6,58,59] affecting 20 to 30 million men in the United States alone. The prevalence of erectile dysfunction increases with age; it affects less than 10% of men younger than 45 years but 75% of men older than 80 years.[5] Men suffering from other medical problems, such as hypertension, diabetes, cardiovascular disease, and end-stage renal disease, have a significantly higher prevalence of erectile dysfunction than healthy men.[5]

There is a paucity of longitudinal data on the incidence rates of ED in men.[57] In the MMAS, the crude incidence rate of ED in white men in the Boston area was found to be 25.9 cases per 1000 man-years.[57] The incidence rates increased from 12.4 cases per 1000 man-years for men 40 to 49 years of age to 29.8 cases per 1000 man-years for men 50 to 59 years of age and 46.4 per 1000 man-years for men 60 to 69 years of age.[60] In another study, incidence rates were derived from a survey of men seen at a preventive medicine clinic. This study found the incidence rates of ED to be less than 3 cases per 1000 man-years among men younger than 45 years and 52 cases per 1000 man-years among men 65 years of age or older. These studies suggest that there were 152 million cases of erectile dysfunction in the world in 1995 and that 600,000 to 700,000 men in the United States develop erectile dysfunction each year.[61]

Risk Factors for Erectile Dysfunction

Epidemiologic studies indicate that the best predictors of the risk of ED are age, history of diabetes mellitus, hypertension, medication use, and cardiovascular disease.[5,58] Advancing age is an important risk factor for ED in men[5,58]: less than 10% of men younger than 40 years and more than 50% of men older than 70 years have ED. In both the MMAS and the NHSLS, the prevalence of ED increased with each decade of life.[5,6]

Among the chronic diseases associated with ED, diabetes mellitus is the most important risk factor. In the MMAS, the age-adjusted risk of complete ED was three times higher in men with a history of treated diabetes mellitus than in those without a history of diabetes mellitus.[5,62] Fifty percent of men with diabetes mellitus will experience ED at some time during the course of their illness.

In the MMAS, treated heart disease, treated hypertension, and hyperlipidemia were associated with significantly increased risk of ED. Among men with treated heart disease and hypertension, the probability of ED was more than two times greater for smokers than for nonsmokers. Smoking also increases the risk of ED in men taking medications for cardiovascular diseases. Cardiovascular disorders, including hypertension, stroke, coronary artery disease, and peripheral vascular disease, are all associated with increased risk of ED. Physical activity is associated with reduced risk of ED.[63]

Several reviews have emphasized the relationship of prescription medications and the occurrence of ED. In the MMAS, the use of antihypertensives, cardiac medication, and oral hypoglycemic drugs was associated with an increased risk of ED. Thiazide diuretics and psychotropic drugs used to treat depression may be the most common drugs associated with ED simply because of the high prevalence of their use. However, a variety of drugs, including almost all antihypertensives, digoxin, H_2-receptor antagonists, anticholinergics, cytotoxic agents, and androgen antagonists, have been implicated in the pathophysiology of ED.

Lower Urinary Tract Symptoms and Erectile Dysfunction

Recent surveys have revealed an association of lower urinary tract symptoms with erectile dysfunction,[64-69] even after adjusting for age and other risk factors. The presence and severity of lower urinary tract symptoms is an independent predictor of ED.[64-70] Because lower urinary tract symptoms and erectile dysfunction are two common conditions in middle-aged and older men, it is possible that this association reflects the coexistence of two highly prevalent conditions.

However, there is growing evidence that the two conditions may be mechanistically linked, because the biochemical mechanisms that regulate bladder detrusor and cavernosal smooth muscle function share many similarities.[68,71] K^+ channels, especially calcium-sensitive K^+ channels (BK_{Ca} channels), Rho A/Rho kinase signaling, L-type calcium channels, and gap junctions are important mediators of detrusor and cavernosal smooth muscle contractility and relaxation. Increased myocyte contractility that characterizes bladder detrusor dysfunction and erectile dysfunction may be mechanistically related to increased Rho kinase activity or impairments of K^+ channel function.[71] Additional proposed hypotheses include increased sympathetic activity and autonomic dysfunction and alterations in nitric oxide generation or PKG activity in the detrusor and cavernosal smooth muscles.[68]

Evaluation

History

The diagnosis of erectile dysfunction is based primarily on patient's self report, and therefore no laboratory test can be a substitute for a good history. The diagnostic workup of the patient with erectile dysfunction should start with an evaluation of general health (Table 19–3).[14,72]

General medical history should be directed at identifying etiologic factors as well as factors that might affect the selection and response to therapy. The presence of diabetes mellitus, coronary artery disease, peripheral vascular disease, and hypertension can suggest a vascular cause. History of stroke, spinal cord or back injury, multiple sclerosis, or dementia can point to a neurologic disorder. Also relevant are history of pelvic trauma, prostate surgery, or priapism. Social history should include ascertainment of recreational drug abuse—particularly tobacco, cocaine, marijuana, opioids, and alcohol. Information about medications, particularly antihypertensives, antiandrogens, antidepressants, and antipsychotic drugs is important because almost a quarter of all cases of ED can be attributed to medications. Psychiatric illnesses, such as depression or psychosis, or drugs used to treat these disorders might be associated with sexual dysfunction.

A detailed sexual history including situational erectile failure, performance anxiety, the nature of relationships, partner expectations, and marital discord needs to be elicited (see Table 19–3).[14,72] It is important to distinguish among inability to achieve erection, changes in sexual desire, failure to achieve orgasm and ejaculation, and dissatisfaction with the sexual relationship. The physician should inquire about the onset, quality, and duration of erections and the presence of nocturnal and early morning erections.

TABLE 19–3 DIAGNOSTIC EVALUATION OF ERECTILE DYSFUNCTION

HISTORY
Ascertain Psychosexual History of:
The strength of marital relationship and marital discord
Depression
Stress
Sexual performance anxiety
Knowledge and beliefs about sexuality
Ascertain Risk Factors:
Diabetes mellitus, hypertension, coronary artery disease, end stage renal disease, and peripheral vascular disease
History of spinal cord injury, stroke, or Alzheimer's disease
Prostate or pelvic surgery
Pelvic injury
Medications such as antihypertensives, antidepressants, antipsychotics, antiandrogens, and inhibitors of androgen production
Use of recreational drugs such as alcohol, cocaine, opiates, and tobacco
Ascertain Factors that Might Affect Choice of Therapy and the Patient's Response to It:
Coexisting coronary artery disease and its symptoms and severity
Exercise tolerance
Use of nitrates or nitrate donors
Use of α-adrenergic blockers
Use of vasodilators for hypertension or congestive heart failure
Use of foods (such as cranberry juice) or drugs (such as erythromycin, protease inhibitors, ketoconazole, and itraconazole) that might affect metabolism of PDE5 inhibitors
PHYSICAL EXAMINATION
Ascertain signs of androgen deficiency, such as loss of secondary sex characteristics, eunuchoid proportions, small testicular volume, or breast enlargement.
Test genital and perineal sensation to evaluate neurologic deficit from spinal cord lesion, previous stroke, or peripheral neuropathy.
Evaluate femoral and pedal pulses and evidence of lower extremity ischemia.
Examine penis to exclude Peyronie's disease.
BASIC LABORATORY EVALUATION THAT SHOULD BE PERFORMED IN ALL MEN WITH ED
Fasting blood glucose
Plasma lipids
Serum testosterone level

ED, erectile dysfunction; PDE, phosophodiesterase.

Self-Reporting Questionnaires

Over the last decade, there has been a general shift away from expensive, time-consuming, and invasive techniques (e.g., penile duplex Doppler ultrasonography, and RigiScan studies) and toward the use of simple, noninvasive self-reporting questionnaires. These questionnaires are valuable because many men with ED do not voluntarily come forward to their physicians and state their sexual complaints. Many men with ED feel embarrassed, and others consider ED to be an inevitable concomitant of the aging process. Some physicians feel uncomfortable discussing issues of such personal nature; this creates an atmosphere that is not conducive to effective communication. The self-reporting questionnaires can help break the ice and facilitate communication. These instruments are widely available and easy to complete, and they can complement or enhance the workup of sexual dysfunction.

The International Index of Erectile Function (IIEF) is a multidimensional scale consisting of 15 questions that address relevant domains of male sexual function.[73] It has been validated in several languages, has been used in many multinational clinical trials, and has been found to have adequate sensitivity and specificity for detecting treatment-related changes, including response to oral erectogenic agents in men with ED. The Male Scale was developed to evaluate a number of sexual function domains and can be used both as an initial screening tool and to evaluate response to therapy.[74]

Considerable effort has been invested in the development of abbreviated questionnaires, such as the Sexual Health Inventory for Men (SHIM), the Brief Male Sexual Function Inventory,[75] and an abridged version of the IIEF.[76] These questionnaires take less time than the IIEF and more concisely address similar aspects of male sexuality.

Physical Examination

A directed physical examination should assess secondary sex characteristics, the presence or absence of breast enlargement, and testicular volume. The examination of the penis evaluates for any unusual curvature, palpable plaques, or superficial lesions. An evaluation of femoral and pedal pulses can provide clues to the presence of peripheral vascular disease. The neurologic examination focuses on the presence of motor weakness, perineal sensation, anal sphincter tone, and bulbocavernosus reflex.

Laboratory Tests Recommended for All Men with ED

The diagnostic evaluation of a man with ED usually includes measurements of hemoglobin, white blood count, blood glucose, blood urea nitrogen (BUN) and creatinine, plasma lipids, and testosterone levels.

Measurement of serum total testosterone concentrations can help detect androgen deficiency. Excluding androgen deficiency in men presenting with ED is important because androgen deficiency may be a manifestation of serious underlying illness such as a pituitary tumor or human immunodeficiency virus (HIV) infection. In addition, testosterone replacement in men with androgen deficiency restores sexual function and can help maintain bone mineral density, muscle mass, and well-being.

If the history, physical exam, and ED questionnaire do not identify any obvious medical concerns needing further workup, then a cost-effective approach is to prescribe a trial of oral PDE5 inhibitor provided there are no contraindications (e.g., nitrate use). See Tables 19–3 and 19–4.

Further Evaluation

Evaluation of Penile Vasculature and Blood Flow

Tests that evaluate the integrity of penile vasculature and blood flow[14,72] are not needed in most patients with ED. They are reserved for patients in whom the results of these tests would alter the management or prognosis and should be performed only by those with considerable experience with their use. The penile brachial blood pressure index is a simple and specific, but it is not a sensitive index of vascular insufficiency.[77,78] It is of historical interest and rarely used today.

Intracavernosal injection of a vasoactive agent such as PGE_1 can be useful as a diagnostic as well as a potential therapeutic modality.[14,72] This procedure can show whether the patient will respond to this therapeutic modality and facilitate patient education about the procedure and its potential side effects. Failure to respond to intracavernosal injection can raise the suspicion of vascular insufficiency or a venous leak that might need further evaluation and treatment.

Most men with erectile dysfunction do not need duplex color sonography, cavernosography, or pelvic angiography.[14,72] For instance, angiography could be useful in a young man with arterial insufficiency associated with pelvic trauma. Similarly, suspicion of congenital or traumatic venous leak in a young man presenting with erectile dysfunction would justify a cavernosography. In each instance, confirmation of the vascular lesion might lead to consideration of surgery. Duplex ultrasonography can provide a noninvasive evaluation of vascular function.[14]

TABLE 19–4 A STEPWISE APPROACH TO TREATMENT OF ERECTILE DYSFUNCTION

All patients and their sexual partners can benefit from and should receive psychosexual counseling.
FIRST-LINE THERAPIES
Oral selective phosphodiesterase inhibitors (sildenafil, vardenafil, or tadalafil)
SECOND-LINE THERAPIES
External vacuum devices Intraurethral alprostadil Intracavernosal injection of alprostadil
THIRD-LINE THERAPIES
Penile prosthesis Vascular surgery

Nocturnal Penile Tumescence

Nocturnal penile tumescence testing is not needed for most patients being evaluated for erectile dysfunction and is recommended only in suspected cases of psychogenic ED, for situational problems, for documented preoperatively poor penile rigidity, or for medico-legal reasons. Although recording of formal nocturnal penile tumescence (NPT) in a sleep laboratory for successive nights can help differentiate organic from psychogenic impotence, this test is expensive and labor intensive. For most cases, a careful history eliciting nighttime or early morning erections provides a reasonable correlation with formal NPT and RigiScan studies.[79]

The introduction of portable RigiScan devices in 1985 has provided clinicians with a reliable means of continuously monitoring penile tumescence and rigidity at home.[79] It is a multicomponent device that the patient wears at bedtime for 2 or 3 nights. It has two wire gauge loops that are placed around the base and tip of the penis that record changes in penile circumference and rigidity. Data are stored and then downloaded via a software program that allows sophisticated interpretation.

Diagnostic Tests to Exclude Androgen Deficiency and Hypothalamic-Pituitary Lesions

There is considerable debate about the usefulness and cost-effectiveness of hormonal evaluation and the extent to which androgen deficiency should be investigated in men presenting with erectile dysfunction. Eight percent to 10% of men with ED have low testosterone levels; the prevalence of androgen deficiency increases with advancing age.[50,80,81] The prevalence of low testosterone levels is not significantly different among men who present with ED and in an age-matched population.[50] These data are consistent with the proposal that ED and androgen deficiency are two common but independently distributed disorders.[50]

However, it is important to exclude androgen deficiency in this patient population. Androgen deficiency is a correctable cause of sexual dysfunction, and some men with ED and low testosterone levels will respond to testosterone replacement. Androgen deficiency might have additional deleterious effects on the patient's health; for instance, androgen deficiency might contribute to osteoporosis and to loss of muscle mass and function.

In large studies,[50,80,81] only a small fraction of men with erectile dysfunction and low testosterone levels have been found to have space-occupying lesions of the hypothalamic-pituitary region. In one large survey, all of the hypothalamic-pituitary lesions were found in men with serum testosterone levels less than 150 ng/dL.[81] Therefore, the cost-effectiveness of the diagnostic workup to rule out an underlying lesion of the hypothalamic-pituitary region can be increased by limiting the workup to men with serum testosterone levels less than 150 ng/dL.

Treatment

The current practice employs a stepwise-approach that first uses minimally invasive therapies that are easy to use and have fewer adverse effects, then progresses to more invasive therapies that might require injections or surgical intervention after the first-line choices have been exhausted (see Table 19–4 and Fig. 19–8). The physician should discuss the risks, benefits, and alternatives of all therapies with the couple. The selection of the therapeutic modality should be based on the underlying etiology, the patient's preference, the nature and strength of the patient's relationship with his sexual partner, and the absence or presence of underlying cardiovascular disease and other comorbid conditions.[14,72] All patients with ED can benefit from psychosexual counseling.[14,72]

In the execution of good medical practice, treatment of all associated medical disorders should be optimized. In men with diabetes mellitus, efforts to optimize glycemic control should be instituted, although improving glycemic control might not improve sexual function. In men with hypertension, control of blood pressure should be optimized and, if possible, the therapeutic regimen may be modified to remove antihypertensive drugs that impair sexual function. This strategy is not always feasible because almost all antihypertensive agents have been associated with sexual dysfunction; the incidence of this adverse event is less with angiotensin converting enzyme inhibitors and angiotensin receptor blockers than with other agents.

First-Line Therapies

Psychosexual Counseling

As Rosen has emphasized, the major goals of psychosexual therapy are to reduce performance anxiety, develop the patient's sexual skills and knowledge, modify negative sexual attitudes, and improve communication between partners.[82] Counseling can be of benefit in both psychogenic and organic causes of sexual dysfunction (Table 19–5).[10]

Masters and Johnson postulated that a person's focus on sexual performance rather than erotic stimulation is a major factor in the pathophysiology of psychogenic ED[82,83]; they referred to this behavior as "spectatoring." Many experts recom-

TABLE 19–5 GOALS OF PSYCHOSEXUAL THERAPY IN MEN WITH SEXUAL DYSFUNCTION
Reduce performance anxiety; train the couple to avoid "spectatoring" and be "sensate focused"
Identify relationship problems and improve partner communication and intimacy
Modify sexual attitudes and beliefs
Improve couple's sexual skills

Adapted from Rosen RC. Psychogenic erectile dysfunction. Classification and management. Urol Clin North Am 2001;28:269-278.

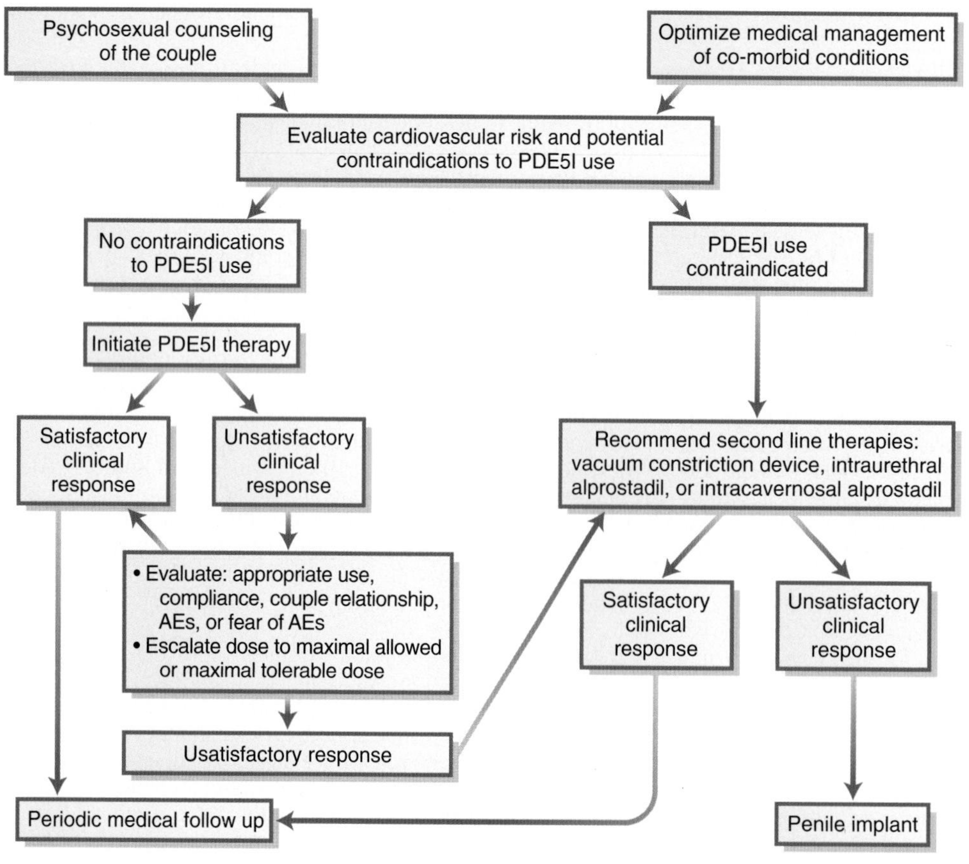

Figure 19–8 ■ An algorithmic approach to the treatment of erectile dysfunction in men. AE, adverse effects; PDE5I, phosphodiesterase 5 inhibitor.

mend a sensate-focus treatment approach in which the couple avoids intercourse and engages in nongenital, nondemanding, pleasure-seeking exercises in order to reduce performance anxiety.[84]

Involving the partner in the counseling process helps dispel misperceptions about the problem, decreases stress, enhances intimacy and ability to talk about sex, and increases the chances of successful outcome.[82,84] Counseling sessions are also helpful in uncovering conflicts in relationships, psychiatric problems, alcohol and drug abuse, and significant misperceptions about sex. Because many men and women harbor misinformation and unrealistic expectations about sexual performance and age-related changes in sexual function, cognitive restructuring techniques are helpful in correcting sexual myths and beliefs.[82] Although psychobehavioral therapy has been claimed to relieve depression and anxiety, there is a paucity of outcome data on the effectiveness of this therapeutic modality.

Selective Phosphodiesterase Inhibitors

Selective PDE5 inhibitors are safe and effective and have become widely accepted as first-line therapy for patients with erectile dysfunction, except in men for whom these drugs are contraindicated.[85]

Mechanisms of Action

Three classes of enzymes—adenylyl cyclase, guanylyl cyclase, and PDEs—play an important role in regulating the intracavernosal concentrations of cAMP and cGMP. Phosphodiesterases hydrolyze cAMP and cGMP, thus reducing their concentrations within the cavernosal smooth muscle.[14,86,87] Although PDE isoforms 2, 3, 4, and 5 are expressed in the penis, only PDE5 is specific to the NO/cGMP pathway in the corpora cavernosa.[88]

Phosphodiesterase inhibitors sildenafil, vardenafil, and tadalafil are relatively selective inhibitors of PDE5 (Table 19–6).[89-94] These drugs block the hydrolysis of cGMP induced by NO,[95,96] thus promoting cavernosal smooth muscle relaxation. The action of these drugs requires an intact NO response as well as constitutive synthesis of cGMP by the smooth muscle cells of the corpora cavernosa. By selectively inhibiting cGMP catabolism in the cavernosal smooth muscle cells, PDE5 inhibitors restore the natural erectile response to sexual stimulation, but they do not produce an erection in the absence of sexual stimulation.

Clinical Pharmacology

Although the three currently available phosphodiesterase inhibitors have some structural similarities, they differ in their selectivity and pharmacokinetics (see Table 19–6). The common adverse effects of the available PDE5 inhibitors—headache, visual problems, and flush—are related to nonselective inhibition of phosphodiesterase isoforms 6 and 11 in other organ systems.[94] The selectivity of PDE5 inhibitor is the ratio of its inhibitory potency for phosphodiesterase isoforms other than type 5 relative to its inhibitory potency for phosphodiesterase isoform.[94] For PDE6, tadalafil is the most selective and sildenafil is the least selective; for PDE11, vardenafil is the most selective and tadalafil is the least selective.[94] The retinal side effects of sildenafil are related to inhibition of PDE6 in the retina. Muscle aches experienced by a small fraction of men using tadalafil may be related to inhibition of PDE11 in the skeletal muscle.[97,98]

Pharmacokinetics

After oral administration of sildenafil, peak plasma concentrations are achieved within 30 to 120 minutes, after which plasma concentrations decline with a half-life of 4 hours (see Table 19–6).[99,100] Vardenafil achieves peak concentrations within 0.7 to 0.9 hours and has a half-life of 4 to 5 hours. In contrast, peak concentrations of tadalafil are achieved at 2 hours, and its half-life of 16.9 hours in young men is significantly longer than the half-lives of sildenafil and vardenafil. The half life of tadalafil is even longer in older men (21.6 hours) in comparison to young men (16.9 hours). Because of the relatively short half-lives of vardenafil and sildenafil, these drugs should be taken 2 to 4 hours before the planned intercourse. In contrast, tadalafil, because of its longer half-life, can be, but does not have to be, taken on demand.

Food, particularly a high-fat meal, and alcohol can delay and decrease the absorption of sildenafil. However, early pharmacokinetic studies have not reported changes in maximum serum concentrations or absorption rates of vardenafil or tadalafil due to food or moderate alcohol ingestion.[101]

TABLE 19–6 CLINICAL PHARMACOLOGY OF SELECTIVE PDE5 INHIBITORS

Characteristic	Sildenafil	Vardenafil	Tadalafil
Commercial name	Viagra	Levitra	Cialis
T_{max}	0.5-2.0 hr	0.7-0.9 hr	2 hr
$T_{1/2}$	3-4 hr	4-5 hr	16.9 hr (young) 21.6 (old)
PDE6 selectivity*	11	25	187
PDE11 selectivity*	780	1160	5
Onset of erection (min)	30 to 60	15 to 45	20 to 30 min
Effect of food and alcohol	C_{max} decreased	Minimal change	No change
Protein binding	96%	94%	94%
Bioavailability	41%	NA	15%

C_{max}, maximum plasma concentration; NA, not available; PDE, phosphodiesterase; $T_{1/2}$, half-life.
*Selectivity refers to the ratio of the IC50 for PDE isoforms other than 5 and IC50 for PDE5. Higher numbers imply greater selectivity. Thus, sildenafil is more selective than tadalafil for PDE5 relative to PDE11, but it is less selective than tadalafil for PDE6 relative to PDE5.
Adapted from Montague DK, Jarow JP, Broderick GA, et al. Chapter 1: The management of erectile dysfunction: an AUA update. J Urol 2005;174:230-239; Yu G, Mason H, Wu X, et al. Substituted pyrazolopyridopyridazines as orally bioavailable potent and selective PDE5 inhibitors: potential agents for treatment of erectile dysfunction. J Med Chem 2003;46:457-460; Grossman EB, Swan SK, Muirhead GJ, et al. The pharmacokinetics and hemodynamics of sildenafil citrate in male hemodialysis patients. Kidney Int 2004;66:367-374; Conti CR, Pepine CJ, Sweeney M. Efficacy and safety of sildenafil citrate in the treatment of erectile dysfunction in patients with ischemic heart disease. Am J Cardiol 1999;83:29C-34C.

Efficacy

All three orally active, selective PDE5 inhibitors—sildenafil, vardenafil, and tadalafil—have been shown to be effective and safe in carefully selected men with ED in randomized clinical trials.[102-106] In men treated with oral selective PDE5 inhibitors, the rates of successful intercourse vary from 50% to 65%, and rates of improved erections vary from 70% to 75%.[102-107] The selective PDE5 inhibitors are effective in men of all ethnic groups and ages[102-106] who have erectile dysfunction due to a multitude of causes, although response rates vary in different patient subgroups.

Introduced to the US market in March 1998, sildenafil (Viagra, Pfizer, New York) was the first effective oral agent for the treatment of ED.[29,96,108,109] The efficacy of sildenafil was demonstrated in a randomized, controlled trial[110] in which 532 men with organic, psychogenic, or mixed erectile dysfunction were randomized to receive placebo or 25, 50, or 100 mg sildenafil for 24 weeks. In this trial, patients on sildenafil experienced greater increments in penile rigidity, frequency of vaginal penetration, and maintenance of erection than those on placebo. Increasing doses of sildenafil were associated with higher mean scores for the questions assessing frequency of penetration and maintenance of erections after sexual penetration.

In a follow-up dose-escalation study,[110] 329 men were randomly assigned to receive placebo or 50 mg sildenafil for 12 weeks. At each follow-up, the dose of sildenafil was increased or decreased by 50% depending upon the therapeutic response or side effects. Sixty-four percent of attempts at intercourse were successful for the men receiving sildenafil, as compared to 22% of men receiving placebo. The mean number of successful attempts per month was 5.9 for men receiving sildenafil and 1.5 for those receiving placebo. The mean scores for orgasms, intercourse satisfaction, and overall satisfaction domain were also significantly higher in the sildenafil group as compared with placebo.[110]

Sildenafil also is an effective treatment for ED in patients with diabetes mellitus.[96] In a randomized trial in 268 men with diabetes mellitus and ED,[96] 56% percent of men receiving sildenafil for 12 weeks reported improved erections compared with 10% of those receiving placebo ($P < 0.001$).

In the vardenafil efficacy trials, 5-, 10-, and 20-mg doses of vardenafil were all superior to placebo in improving erectile function domain scores, and the improvements in erectile function scores were dose related.[111-117] Vardenafil improved rates of vaginal penetration, penile rigidity, intercourse success, and satisfaction with sexual experience in men with ED from diverse causes.[111-117]

Similarly, in randomized, clinical trials, 2.5-, 5-, 10-, and 20-mg doses of tadalafil were each superior to placebo in improving erectile function domain scores.[118-123] The beneficial effects of tadalafil were dose related.[123]

PDE5 inhibitors are effective in men with ED due to a variety of causes including spinal cord injury and radical prostatectomy.[108,124] In general, baseline sexual function correlates positively with response to PDE5 inhibitors, and patients with diabetes mellitus or previous prostate surgery respond less well than patients with psychogenic or vasculogenic ED.[108] Because there is no baseline characteristic that predicts the likelihood of failure to respond to sildenafil therapy, a therapeutic trial of PDE5 inhibitors should be tried in all patients except in those in whom it is contraindicated.[108]

Adverse Effects

In clinical trials, the adverse effects (Table 19–7) that have been reported with greater frequency in men treated with PDE5 inhibitors than in those treated with placebo include headaches, flushing, rhinitis, dyspepsia, and visual disturbances.[125] The occurrence of headache, flushing, and rhinitis, a direct consequence of nonselective PDE5 inhibition in other organ systems, is related to the administered dose. These drugs do not affect semen characteristics.[49] No cases of priapism were noted in the pivotal clinical trials.

TABLE 19–7 COMMON ADVERSE EFFECTS OF SELECTIVE PHOSPHODIESTERASE INHIBITORS

Adverse Event	INCIDENCE (%) Sildenafil	Vardenafil	Tadalafil
Headache	13	16	15
Flushing	10	12	4
Dyspepsia	5	4	12
Nasal congestion	1	10	4
Dizziness	1	2	2
Abnormal vision*	2	<2	—
Back pain*	—	—	7
Myalgia*	—	—	6

*These adverse effects are related to nonselective inhibition of phosphodiesterase isoforms in other tissues.

Adapted from Brock GB, McMahon CG, Chen KK, et al. Efficacy and safety of tadalafil for the treatment of erectile dysfunction: results of integrated analyses. J Urol 2002;168:1332-1336; Morales A, Gingell C, Collins M, et al. Clinical safety of oral sildenafil citrate (Viagra) in the treatment of erectile dysfunction. Int J Impot Res 1998;10:69-73; Wespes E, Amar E, Hatzichristou D, et al. EAU Guidelines on erectile dysfunction: an update. Eur Urol 2006;49:806-815.

Several cases of nonarteritic anterior ischemic optic neuropathy (NAION) have been reported after ingestion of oral PDE5 inhibitor use.[126,127] This condition is characterized sudden onset of monocular visual loss due to acute ischemia of the anterior portion of the optic nerve in the absence of demonstrable arteritis; the ischemia can progress to partial or complete infarction of optic nerve head, resulting in permanent visual loss or visual field cuts.[127] Although a cause-and-effect relationship with PDE5 inhibitor use has not been established,[126] patients with a history of sudden visual loss should not be treated with PDE5 inhibitors without ophthalmologic evaluation.

Cardiovascular and Hemodynamic Effects

In post-marketing surveillance of adverse events associated with sildenafil use, several instances of myocardial infarction and sudden death were reported in men using sildenafil.[128-131] Forty-four of the 130 deaths reported by the US Food and Drug Administration (FDA) from March to November 1998 occurred in temporal relation to the ingestion of sildenafil[128-131]; 16 of these deaths occurred in patients who were taking nitrates. Because most men presenting with ED also have high prevalence of cardiovascular risk factors, it is unclear whether these events were causally related to the ingestion of sildenafil, underlying heart disease, or both.[130]

In a rigorously controlled study,[132] oral administration of 100 mg sildenafil to men with severe coronary artery disease produced only small decreases in systemic blood pressure and no significant changes in cardiac output, heart rate, coronary blood flow, and coronary artery diameter. In a separate analysis of five randomized, placebo-controlled trials of vardenafil, Kloner and colleagues pooled the data on cardiovascular safety profile.[133] The overall frequency of cardiovascular events was similar in vardenafil-treated men and placebo-treated men. However, vardenafil treatment was associated with a mild reduction in blood pressure (4.6 mm Hg decrease in systolic blood pressure) and a small increase in heart rate (2 bpm). This led the American Heart Association to conclude that the preexistence of coronary artery disease by itself does not constitute a contraindication for the use of PDE5 inhibitors.[130]

Drug-Drug Interactions

Sildenafil is metabolized mostly by the P450 2C9 and the P450 3A4 pathways.[130] Cimetidine and erythromycin, inhibitors of P450 3A4, increase the plasma concentrations of sildenafil. HIV protease inhibitors might also alter the activity of the P450 3A4 pathway and affect the clearance of sildenafil.[130] Conversely, sildenafil is an inhibitor of the P450 2C9 metabolic pathway, and its administration could potentially affect the metabolism of drugs metabolized by this system, such as warfarin and tolbutamide.[130] Combined administration of sildenafil and ritonavir results in significantly higher plasma levels of sildenafil than sildenafil given alone.[134] There are similar reactions with other drugs, including saquinavir and itraconazole. Therefore, doses of PDE5 inhibitors should be reduced appropriately in men taking protease inhibitors or erythromycin.

Grapefruit juice can alter oral drug pharmacokinetics by different mechanisms. Grapefruit juice given as a single normal amount (200 to 300 mL) or as whole fresh fruit segments can irreversibly inactivate intestinal P450 3A4, thus reducing presystemic metabolism and increasing oral drug bioavailability of PDE5 inhibitors.[135] Although the magnitude of this problem in clinical practice is unknown, it seems prudent to warn men who are contemplating the use of PDE5 inhibitors not to ingest more than a small amount of grapefruit juice.

The most serious interactions of PDE5 inhibitors are with the nitrates. The vasodilator effects of nitrates are augmented by PDE5 inhibitors; this also applies to inhaled forms of nitrates such as amyl nitrate or nitrites that are sold under the street name "poppers." Concomitant administration of the two drugs can cause a potentially fatal decrease in blood pressure.[130]

Tadalafil and vardenafil are contraindicated in men using α-blockers; the sildenafil label also has a precautionary warning for use with α-blockers. In men with congestive heart failure, those receiving vasodilator drugs, or those who are using complex regimens of antihypertensive drugs, blood pressure should be monitored after initial administration of PDE5 inhibitors.[130,133,136]

Therapeutic Regimens

Excellent therapeutic guidelines have been published by expert panels from several societies.[74,137] To minimize the risk of hypotension and adverse cardiovascular events in association with the use of PDE5 inhibitors, the American Heart Association/American College of Cardiology has published a list of recommendations (Table 19–8), which should be followed rigorously.[130]

In most men with ED, sildenafil is started at an initial dose of 25 or 50 mg. If this dose does not produce any adverse effects, the dose can be titrated to 100 mg.[29,130] Further dose adjustment should be guided by the therapeutic response and occurrence of adverse effects. Typically, unit doses higher than 100 mg are not recommended. Vardenafil should be started at an initial dose of 10 mg; the dose should be increased to 20 mg or decreased to 5 mg depending on the clinical response and the occurrence of adverse effects. Unit doses higher than 20 mg are not recommended. Tadalafil is started at an initial unit dose of 10 mg, with further adjustment of dose based on effectiveness and side effects. Tadalafil need not be taken more frequently than once every 48 hours.

In men taking protease inhibitors (particularly ritonavir and indinavir), erythromycin, ketoconazole, itraconazole, or large amounts of grapefruit, the doses of PDE5 inhibitors should be reduced, and doses greater than 25 mg of sildenafil, 5 mg of vardenafil, or 10 mg of tadalafil are not recommended.

TABLE 19–8 GUIDELINES FOR THE USE OF SELECTIVE PHOSPHODIESTERASE INHIBITORS

Do not administer selective PDE5 inhibitors to men taking long-acting or short-acting nitrate drugs on a regular basis.
If the patient has stable coronary artery disease, is not taking long-acting nitrates, and uses short-acting nitrates only infrequently, the use of a selective PDE5 inhibitor should be guided by careful consideration of risks.
Do not administer selective PDE5 inhibitors within 24 hours of the ingestion of any form of nitrate.
Advise men about the risks of the potential interaction between selective PDE5 inhibitors and nitrates, nitrate donors, and α-adrenergic blockers. Concurrent use of nitrates, nitrate donors, or α-adrenergic blockers could result in hypotension that could be serious or even fatal.
In men with preexisting coronary artery disease, assess the risk of inducing cardiac ischemia during sexual activity before prescribing selective PDE5 inhibitors. This assessment may include a stress test.
In men who are taking vasodilators and diuretics for treatment of hypertension or congestive heart failure, consider the potential risk of inducing hypotension because of potential interaction between PDE5 inhibitors and vasodilators, especially in patients with low blood volume.
In HIV-infected men, consider potential drug-drug interactions between selective PDE5 inhibitors and antiretroviral drugs and antimicrobial agents.

HIV, human immunodeficiency virus; PDE, phosphodiesterase.[4,14,130]

Sildenafil and vardenafil are taken at least 1 hour before sexual intercourse and not more than once in any 24-hour period; because of its longer half-life, tadalafil does not have to be taken immediately before intercourse.

There is insufficient information to determine whether daily administration of selective PDE5 inhibitors is more effective than their on-demand use.[138]

Guidelines for Use of PDE5 Inhibitors in Men with Coronary Artery Disease

Before prescribing PDE5 inhibitors, cardiovascular risk factors should be assessed (see Table 19–8).[130] If the patient has hypertension or symptomatic coronary artery disease, the treatment of those clinical disorders should be addressed first.[14,130] The use of nitrates must be ascertained because PDE5 inhibitors are contraindicated in patients taking any form of nitrates regularly. PDE5 inhibitors should not be used within 24 hours of the use of nitrates or nitrate donors.[130]

Sexual activity can induce coronary ischemia in men with preexisting coronary artery disease[131]; therefore, men contemplating use of ED therapies should undergo assessment of their exercise tolerance. One practical way to assess exercise tolerance is to have the patient climb one or two flight of stairs. If he can safely climb one or two flights of stairs without angina or excessive shortness of breath, he can likely engage in sexual intercourse with a stable partner without similar symptoms. Exercise testing before prescribing PDE5 inhibitors may be indicated in some men with significant heart disease to assess the risk of inducing cardiac ischemia during sexual activity.[130] Selective phosphodiesterase inhibitors have been shown not to impair the ability of patients with stable coronary artery disease to engage in exercise at levels equivalent to that attained during sexual intercourse.[139-142] Similarly, each of the three PDE5 inhibitors has been shown to not to have significant adverse effect on hemodynamics and cardiac events in carefully selected men with erectile dysfunction who did not have any contraindication for the use of PDE5 inhibitors.[139-142] None of the PDE5 inhibitors adversely affects total exercise time or time to ischemia during exercise testing in men with stable angina.

Treatment of Patients Who Do Not Respond to PDE5 Inhibitors

Although oral PDE5 inhibitor therapy has revolutionized the management of ED, not all men respond to this treatment. The cumulative probability of intercourse success with sildenafil citrate increases with the number of attempts, reaching a maximum after eight attempts.[143] Based largely on these data,[143] the failure to respond to phosphodiesterase inhibitor therapy has been defined as the failure to achieve satisfactory response even after eight attempts of either the highest approved dose (e.g., 100 mg sildenafil) or the highest tolerable dose of phosphodiesterase inhibitor, whichever is lower.

Many factors contribute to apparent treatment failure, including failure to take the medication as recommended, suboptimal dose, dose-limiting adverse effects, unaddressed psychological issues, unaddressed partner and relationship issues, incorrect diagnosis, and patient-specific pathophysiologic factors.[144] In clinical trials of PDE5 inhibitors, treatment failures were reported predominantly in men who had diabetes mellitus, non–nerve sparing radical prostatectomy, and high disease severity.[145] In an evaluation of cavernosal smooth muscle biopsies in sildenafil-nonresponders, Wespes and colleagues[146] found severe vascular lesions and cavernosal smooth muscle atrophy and fibrosis to be the underlying pathology.

Patients might not take the medication appropriately due to inadequate instructions, failure to understand the instructions, adverse effects, or fear of adverse effects.[144] Oral PDE5 inhibitors are taken optimally 1 to 2 hours before planned intercourse.[74,137] The medication is unlikely to be effective if it is taken immediately before intercourse; meals and alcohol can further affect the maximal serum concentrations of sildenafil citrate. Similarly, patients might not take the appropriate dose because of side effects or fear of side effects.

Patients whose sexual dysfunction is misdiagnosed erectile dysfunction and whose primary sexual disorder is unresponsive to PDE5 inhibitors may be incorrectly deemed treatment failures. For instance, men with hypoactive sexual desire disorder, Peyronie's disease, or an orgasmic or ejaculatory disorder would not be expected to respond to PDE5 inhibitors. The anxiety associated with resumption of sexual activity, as well as unresolved relationship and partner issues, can attenuate response to treatment. The patient's partner might not be willing or able to engage in sexual activity because of relationship issues, sexual disorder, or real or perceived health issues.

Patients who report lack of satisfactory response to initial administration of PDE5 inhibitors should be asked about the time of drug administration, the dose taken, and adverse effects experienced. Psychological and partner issues should be evaluated. The dose of PDE5 inhibitor should be increased gradually as tolerated. Should the patient not respond to maximal tolerable doses of PDE5 inhibitors, PDE5 inhibitors can be combined with vacuum devices or intraurethral therapy. Second-line therapies such as intracavernosal injections should be pursued. Men who are unresponsive to oral PDE5 inhibitors and second-line therapies might find penile implant an acceptable alternative.[144]

Cost-Effectiveness

A number of studies have evaluated the economic cost of treating ED in men in managed care health plans.[147-150] One computer simulation estimated sildenafil citrate cost to be approximately $11,000 per quality-adjusted life-year (QALY) that it produces.[149] This amount is less than for many other accepted treatments for medical disorders that cost less than $50,000 to $100,000 per QALY; thus, the cost-effectiveness of PDE5 inhibitor therapy compares favorably with other accepted medical therapies. Other analyses have concluded that PDE5 inhibitors and vacuum constriction devices are the most cost-effective of all the available therapeutic options.[147-149]

Several recent analyses of the costs associated with the care of patients with erectile dysfunction have shown that the financial burden imposed by patients with erectile dysfunction on managed care plan is surprisingly small.[149-151] In one such cost utility analysis, the monthly cost of providing erectile dysfunction–related treatment services in a health plan with 100,000 members amounted to less than $0.10 per member.[150] Thus, the failure of many insurance companies to cover the cost of PDE5 inhibitor therapy is not informed by cost utility analyses.

Second-Line Therapies

Vacuum Devices for Inducing Erection

The vacuum device consists of a plastic cylinder, a vacuum pump, and an elastic constriction band.[14,72] The plastic cylinder fits over the penis and is connected to a vacuum pump. The negative pressure created by the vacuum within the cylinder draws blood into the penis, producing an erection. An elastic band slipped around the base of the penis traps the blood in the penis, maintaining an erection as long as the rubber band is retained around the base. The constriction band should not be left in place for more than 30 minutes. Also, only vacuum devices with a pressure-limiting mechanism should be recommended to prevent injury due to high vacuum.[85]

Limited data on the efficacy of vacuum devices from open-label trials indicate that these devices are safe, relatively inexpensive, and moderately effective.[152,153] They can impair ejaculation, resulting in entrapment of semen. Some couples dislike the lack of spontaneity engendered by the use of these devices. Partner cooperation is important for successful use of these devices.[154]

Intraurethral Therapies

An intraurethral system for delivery of alprostadil called MUSE (medicated urethral system for erection; VIVUS, Menlo Park, CA) was released in 1997. Alprostadil is a stable, synthetic form of PGE_1, which increases cAMP levels and decreases intracellular calcium, thereby promoting cavernosal smooth muscle relaxation and penile erection.

Alprostadil, when applied into the urethra, is absorbed through the urethral mucosa and ventral side of the tunica albuginea into the corpus cavernosum. In comparison to intracavernosal injection of PGE_1, intraurethral PGE_1 is easier to administer and has a lower incidence of adverse effects, particularly penile fibrosis.

Alprostadil is available in 125-, 250-, 500-, and 1000-μg strengths. Typically, the initial alprostadil dose of 250 μg is applied in the clinician's office to observe changes in blood pressure or urethral bleeding secondary to misapplication of the device into the urethra.

Initial randomized, placebo-controlled studies reported 40% to 60% success rates, defined as having at least one successful sexual intercourse during a 3-month study period.[155-157] In clinical practice, approximately one third of men using intraurethral alprostadil will respond.[158]

Common side effects of intraurethral alprostadil are penile pain and urethral burning in up to 30% of patients[155-157]; its use also may cause dizziness, hypotension, and syncope in a small fraction of users. Intraurethral alprostadil can cause mild burning or itching in the vagina of the sexual partner. Intraurethral alprostadil should not be used by men whose partners are pregnant or planning to get pregnant.

Intracavernosal Injection of Vasoactive Agents

The use of intracavernosal injections of vasoactive agents has been a cornerstone of the medical management of erectile dysfunction since the early 1980s. Patients can be taught to inject a vasoactive agent into their corpora cavernosa with a 27- or 30-gauge needle prior to planned intercourse. Erections occur typically 15 minutes after intracorporal injection and last 45 to 90 minutes. Although intracavernosal injection therapy is highly effective, it is associated with significantly higher complication rates than oral therapy and should be used only by practitioners who are experienced in the use of this therapy and who can provide emergency medical support to their patients in the event of a serious adverse event, such as priapism. Guidelines are listed in Table 19–9.

Although several different agents—PGE_1, papaverine, and phentolamine—have been used alone or in combination,[155,159-165] only intracavernosal PGE_1 has been approved for clinical use. The long-term data on the efficacy and safety of intracavernosal therapy are sparse.

Several formulations of alprostadil (PGE_1) are commercially available (Caverject, Pharmacia; Prostin VR, Pharmacia; Edex, Schwarz Pharma). PGE_1 binds to PGE_1 receptors on the cavernosal smooth muscle cells, stimulates adenylyl cyclase, increases the concentrations of cAMP, and is a powerful smooth muscle relaxant. The usual dose is 5 to 20 μg, and response to therapy is dose-related and should be titrated.[162]

In one placebo-controlled efficacy trial, the intracavernosal alprostadil injection resulted in satisfactory sexual performance after more than 90% of administrations, and approximately 85% of men and their partners reported satisfactory sexual activity.[162] Intracavernosal alprostadil is more effective than intraurethral alprostadil.[166]

The common adverse effects of intracavernosal therapy include penile pain, hematoma, corporal nodules, penile fibrosis, and the possibility of prolonged erections (priapism, if longer than 4 hours).[162,163,165,167] In an open-label 6-month follow-up of men with erectile dysfunction who were treated with intracavernosal aprostadil,[168] penile pain occurred in 44%, prolonged erection in 8%, priapism in 0.9%, and penile fibrosis in 4%. Despite the effectiveness of this approach in producing rigid erections, many patients do not relish injecting a needle into their penis; therefore, it is not surprising that long-term drop-out rates are high.

Papaverine, derived originally from the poppy seed, is a nonspecific phosphodiesterase inhibitor, which increases both intracellular cAMP and cGMP. It has a greater propensity to induce priapism and fibrosis with long-term use, and efficacy and long-term safety data from randomized, placebo-controlled trials are lacking. Therefore, there is insufficient information to evaluate its efficacy and safety.

Phentolamine is a competitive α_1- and α_2-adrenergic antagonist that contributes to smooth muscle relaxation. As a single agent it is minimally efficacious, but it has been used in combination with other agents to potentiate the effects of papaverine, vasoactive intestinal peptide, or PGE_1.[169] However, randomized clinical trial data on its efficacy and safety are lacking. Therefore, there is insufficient information to evaluate its efficacy and safety.

A serious concern with the use of intracavernosal injection therapy is priapism. In patients who develop a prolonged or painful erection with PGE_1, either brethine, 5 mg, or pseudoephedrine, 60 mg, administered orally may be of benefit. If priapism persists longer than 4 hours, the patient should be instructed to seek medical care in which aspiration alone or with the injection of an α-adrenergic agent is used to induce detumescence. If this fails, surgical therapy may be indicated to reverse a prolonged erection; otherwise, anoxic damage to the cavernosal smooth muscle cells and fibrosis can occur.

TABLE 19–9 GUIDELINES FOR INTRACAVERNOSAL THERAPY

Do not prescribe intracavernosal therapy to men who have psychiatric disorders, hypercoagulable states, or sickle cell disease.
Do not prescribe intracavernosal therapy to men who are receiving anticoagulant therapy or are unable to comprehend the risks or take appropriate action should complications occur.
Designate a physician or a urologist to be available to handle emergencies related to complications of intracavernosal injections, such as prolonged erection and priapism.
Instruct the patient in the injection technique, the risks of intracavernosal therapy, and the steps to be taken in the event of prolonged erection or priapism.
Administer the first injection in the office and observe the blood pressure and heart rate response. This provides an excellent opportunity for educating the patient, observing adverse effects, and determining whether the patient will respond to intracavernosal therapy.
Start with a low dose of alprostadil and titrate the dose based on the erectile response and the duration of erection. Adjust the dose of alprostadil to achieve an erection that is sufficient for sexual intercourse but that does not last more than 30 minutes.
If the erection does not abate in 30 minutes, the patient should be instructed to take a tablet of pseudoephedrine or brethine or an intracavernosal injection of phenylephrine. If this is not effective, the patient should call the designated physician or the urologist and come to the emergency department.

Third-Line Therapies

Penile Prosthesis

The penile prostheses are invasive and costly, but they can be an effective method for restoring erectile function for patients with advanced organic disease who are unresponsive to other medical therapies, have significant structural disorders of the penis (e.g., Peyronie's disease), or have suffered corporal loss from cancer or traumatic injury.[170,171]

Penile implants are paired supports that are placed in each of the two erectile bodies. There are two basic types of penile implants: hydraulic or fluid filled, referred to as inflatable prostheses; and malleable, semirigid, rods which are bendable but always remain firm in the penis.[170,171] Penile prostheses come in a variety of lengths and girths. Implantation surgery usually takes less than an hour and in most cases can be done as an outpatient procedure under general or regional anesthesia.

Infection and mechanical malfunction are the most common problems with penile prostheses. With recent improvements in materials and design, the chance of mechanical malfunction has decreased to 5% to 10% in the first 10 years. Infection occurs in 1% to 3% of cases, but infection rates can be higher in revision surgery, especially in men with diabetes mellitus.

The total cost of penile prosthesis implantation varies from $3000 to $20,000, depending on the type of device used and the community in which the procedure is performed. There are no randomized efficacy trials, but retrospective analyses have reported that more than 80% of patients and 70% of partners are pleased with the prosthesis and the togetherness that it brings to their relationship.[172,173]

A recent industry analysis report projects an increase in the number of penile implant procedures performed through 2010 because of the aging population, a growing awareness of ED, and an increasing number of men with severe forms of ED that will not respond to oral therapies.[172]

Testosterone Replacement

Testosterone treatment does not improve sexual function in impotent men who have normal testosterone levels.[45,47,174] It is not known whether testosterone replacement improves sexual function in impotent men with borderline serum testosterone levels. Many, but not all impotent men with low testosterone levels experience improvements in their libido and overall sexual activity with androgen replacement therapy.[47,175] The response to testosterone supplementation even in this group of men is variable[41,50,80,81] because of the coexistence of other disorders such as diabetes mellitus, hypertension, cardiovascular disease, and psychogenic factors. A meta-analysis[47] of the usefulness of androgen replacement therapy concluded that testosterone administration is associated with greater improvements in sexual function than those associated with placebo in men with erectile dysfunction and low testosterone levels.

ED in middle-aged and older men is often a multifactorial disorder. Common causes of ED include diabetes mellitus, hypertension, medications, peripheral vascular disease, psychogenic factors, and end-stage renal disease. Many of these factors often coexist in the same patient. Therefore, it is not surprising that testosterone treatment alone might not improve sexual function in all men with androgen deficiency. Testosterone induces nitric oxide synthase activity, has trophic effects on cavernosal smooth muscle and ischiocavernosus and bulbospongiosus muscle, and appears essential for achieving optimum venous occlusion in animal models.[44,48,176] Therefore, it is possible that testosterone might improve response to PDE5 inhibitors; this hypothesis has not been rigorously tested.[48]

Therapies with Either Unproven Efficacy or Limited Efficacy Data

There is insufficient efficacy data to support the use of trazodone[177] or yohimbine[178] in men with erectile dysfunction. The literature on the effectiveness of herbal therapies is difficult to interpret because of lack of consistency in product formulations and potencies, contamination of herbal products with PDE5 inhibitors, and paucity of randomized clinical trial data.[85,179] One randomized trial of Korean red ginseng reported this product to be effective in the treatment of ED[180]; these data need further confirmation. Therefore, the use of this or other herbal therapies is not recommended.[85]

Future Therapies

Oral Therapeutic Agents under Development

α-Melanocyte stimulating hormone (α-MSH; Melontan II), a nonselective melanocortin receptor agonist, is a central initiator of erection. It displays dopaminergic agonist activity and beneficial effects on libido. In a double-blind, placebo-controlled crossover study, there was significant improvement in RigiScan events, penile rigidity, and sexual desire in 10 patients with documented ED risk factors. Nausea was the most common adverse event.[181]

PT-141, another synthetic analogue of α-MSH, is an agonist at melanocortin receptors including the MC3R and MC4R.[182-184] Administration of PT-141 to rats and nonhuman primates results in penile erections. Administration of PT-141 to normal men and to patients with erectile dysfunction resulted in a rapid dose-dependent increase in erectile activity. Efficacy trials of PT-141 are in early stages.

Apomorphine, a PDE5 inhibitor, also functions as a dopamine agonist and acts centrally to initiate erection; its main adverse effect is nausea.

Gene Therapy and Erectile Dysfunction

The goal of gene therapy for ED is to introduce novel genetic material into the cavernosal smooth muscle cells in an attempt to restore normal cellular and physiologic function to produce a therapeutic effect.[185] Gene therapy involves administration of a desired gene into the body, delivery of the gene to a targeted cell, and expression of the therapeutic product.

Gene therapy has been proposed as a viable treatment option for diseases that have a vascular origin, such as arteriosclerosis, congestive heart failure, and pulmonary hypertension.[185,186] This suggests that gene therapy may also be employed to treat vascular diseases of the penis, because ED in most cases is a manifestation of vascular disease.

One advantage of applying gene therapy for the treatment of ED is the easily accessible external location of the penis.[187,188] Hence, a tourniquet can be placed around the base of the penis and the desired gene can be administered directly into the corpora cavernosa without entering the systemic circulation. This is a distinct advantage to other gene therapy approaches in which a vector encoding a desired gene is introduced into the systemic circulation. This systemic approach can cause adverse systemic effects, including the gene's being introduced into the incorrect organ or vascular bed. However, this potential adverse effect is minimized when gene therapy vectors are used for treatment of ED, because the penis has its own external circulation, allowing a gene to be transferred and localized in one organ, thus lessening the risk of systemic spillover.

Determination of the number of cells that must be transfected to produce a therapeutic effect is often difficult to determine. However, in the penis, only a small number of cells need to be transfected because the corpus cavernosum smooth muscle cells are interconnected by gap junctions that allow second messenger molecules and ions to be transferred to a number of interconnected smooth muscle cells.[188] Moreover, the low turnover rate of the vascular smooth muscle cells of the penis allows the desired gene to be expressed for long periods of time.

The current strategies of gene therapy for ED treatment have focused on the molecules that regulate corporal smooth muscle relaxation or increase neovascularization (Table 19–10).[189,190] A number of candidate genes have been explored, including the penile-inducible nitric oxide synthase gene, the endothelial nitric oxide synthase (eNOS) gene, *VIP, CGRP,* the maxi-K$^+$ channel gene, *VEGF,* and the brain neurotrophic factor gene.

Garban's group[191] first demonstrated that gene therapy can be performed in the penis by using naked cDNA encoding the penile-inducible nitric oxide synthase gene, leading to physiologic benefit in the aging rat. Christ and colleagues later showed that injection of hSlo cDNA, which encodes the human smooth muscle maxi-K+ channel, into the rat corpora cavernosa can increase gap junction formation and enhance erectile responses to nerve stimulation in the aged rat.[192]

Adenoviral constructs encoding the *eNOS* and *CGRP* genes were shown to reverse age-related erectile dysfunction in rats.[193,194] In these studies, both *eNOS* and *CGRP* expression were sustained for at least 1 month in the corpora cavernosa of the rat penis. Five days after transfection with the AdCMVeNOS or AdRSVeNOS viruses, aged rats had significant increases in erectile function as determined by cavernosal nerve stimulation and pharmacologic injection with the endothelium-dependent vasodilator acetylcholine and the PDE5 inhibitors zaprinast and sildenafil.[193,194]

In one study, intracavernous injection of adeno-associated virus construct carrying the brain derived neurotrophic factor gene improved erectile function after cavernosal nerve injury.[195]

TABLE 19–10 PHYSIOLOGIC TARGETS FOR GENE THERAPY

Gene Target	Vector and Mechanism
Nitric oxide isoforms	Increase eNOS, nNOS, and iNOS activity in the cavernosal smooth muscle
Maxi-K$^+$ channel	Transfer of maxi-K$^+$ channels using a plasmid vector that carries the *hSlo* gene encoding the α-subunit of the maxi-K$^+$ channel
VEGF	Transfer of *VEGF* cDNA into rat corpora cavernosa to promote neovascularization
VEGF with *AAV-BDNF*	Transfer of *VEGF* and brain-derived neurotrophic factor using adeno-associated virus
Neurotrophin 3 gene	Transfer of neurotrophin 3 gene using HSV vector
VIP	Transfection of corpora cavernosa of streptozotocin-treated diabetic rats using pcDNA3 carrying *VIP* cDNA
CGRP	Adenoviral transfer of CGRP in aged rats

CGRP, calcitonin gene-related peptide; eNOS, endothelial nitric oxide synthase; HSV, herpes simplex virus; iNOS, inducible nitric oxide synthase; nNOS, neuronal nitric oxide synthase; VEGF, vascular endothelial growth factor; VIP, vasoactive intestinal polypeptide. Reproduced with permission from Christ GJ, Hodges S. Molecular mechanisms of detrusor and corporal myocyte contraction: identifying targets for pharmacotherapy of bladder and erectile dysfunction. Br J Pharmacol 2006;147(suppl 2):S41-S55.

This neurotrophic factor purportedly restored neuronal NOS in the major pelvic ganglion, thus enhancing the recovery of erectile function after bilateral cavernous nerve injury.[195]

In other studies, intracavernosal vascular endothelial growth factor (VEGF) injection and adeno-associated virus-mediated *VEGF* gene therapy were each shown to reverse venogenic erectile dysfunction in rats.[196] Additional targets for gene therapy include *CGRP*, superoxide dismutase, and Rho A/Rho kinase.[190] These early but innovative studies provide evidence that *in vivo* gene transfer can be accomplished technically and have beneficial physiologic effects on penile erection. A phase I clinical trial of potassium channel gene therapy in patients with ED has been initiated.[24]

The Potential of Stem Cell Therapy

Human mesenchymal stem cells (hMSCs) are bone marrow–derived cells that are endowed with the potential of differentiating into skeletal and smooth muscle cells, as well as adipocytes, osteocytes, and chondrocytes. The hMSCs are attractive gene-delivery vehicles for multiple reasons.[190] These cells can replicate in vitro as well as in vivo, thus providing a large pool of cells. The autologous hMSCs are not immunogenic. Finally, when transplanted into appropriate tissue environment, they have the potential of differentiating into the desired cell type.

Initial studies have demonstrated that rat MSCs, expanded ex vivo and transfected,[190,197,198] when implanted into the corpora cavernosa, are capable of expressing the gene product of interest.[197,198] We do not know whether transplanted hMSCs can differentiate into functional cavernosal smooth muscle cells and thus restore erectile capacity in men with ED.

Ejaculatory Disorders

Ejaculatory disorders include anejaculation, anorgasmia, delayed ejaculation, retrograde ejaculation, premature ejaculation, and painful ejaculation.[11-12] A recent survey has highlighted the high prevalence and clinical importance of ejaculatory disorders.[11] Premature ejaculation is the most prevalent sexual disorder in men 18 to 59 years of age. Retrograde ejaculation due to diabetes-associated autonomic neuropathy is the second most prevalent ejaculatory disorder. Ejaculatory disorders can also lead to infertility.

Mechanisms of Ejaculation

The ejaculatory mechanisms consist of three stages: emission, ejection, and orgasm.[12,199] Although orgasm and seminal fluid ejection often occur contemporaneously, the two processes are regulated by separate mechanisms. *Ejaculation* refers to the ejection of seminal fluid containing sperm and the secretions from seminal vesicles, prostate, and bulbourethral glands; it is regulated primarily by central nervous system activation of the sympathetic nervous system.[200,201] *Emission*, the deposition of seminal fluid into the posterior urethra, depends upon the integrity of the vasa deferentia, seminal vesicles, prostate gland, and bladder neck. This emission is ejaculated out of the urethra by the contractions of the bulbocavernosus and levator ani muscles. The entry of seminal fluid into the bladder is prevented by closure of the bladder sphincter due to sympathetic activation. The sensation associated with the rhythmic contractions of these pelvic floor muscles is referred to as the *orgasm*.[200,201]

The medial preoptic area and the paragigantocellular nucleus integrate seminal fluid emission and ejection with copulatory behavior. The paragigantocellular nucleus though serotonergic pathways inhibits the lumbosacral motor nuclei that are involved in ejaculation.[202,203] When input from the medial preoptic area to paragigantocellular nucleus leads to loss of this inhibition, it results in ejaculation.[199,203] Neural pathways that use serotonin and 5-HT receptors regulate the speed of ejaculation. Thus, administration of serotonin reuptake inhibitors is being explored for the treatment of premature ejaculation.[204,205] A better understanding of the neurochemical mechanisms that regulate ejaculation might provide mechanism-specific targets for treating ejaculatory disorders.

Retrograde ejaculation can be the result of autonomic dysfunction due to autonomic neuropathy associated with diabetes mellitus; sympathectomy; therapy with adrenergic antagonists, some types of antihypertensives, antipsychotics, or antidepressants; bladder neck incompetence; or urethral obstruction.

Following transurethral resection of the prostate, the bladder neck closure mechanism may be damaged. Patients remain continent because of a second, more distal, continence mechanism that is present in the region of the membranous urethra; however, many patients who have undergone transurethral resection of the prostate experience retrograde ejaculation.

WOMEN'S SEXUAL DYSFUNCTION

Assessment of women's sexual dysfunction is often required in the practice of endocrinology. Not only do endocrine disorders lead to sexual symptoms, but also their management can negatively influence sexual function and satisfaction. Moreover, women are often referred to endocrinologists to "rule out a hormonal basis" for their sexual problems. The assumption is that if endocrine disease is excluded (and other medical illness is absent), the problems are psychological.

However, psychological and biologic systems are not separate. Disturbed feelings, emotions, mood, and internal and external stress profoundly alter immunologic, neurologic, and endocrine systems. Sexual function and dysfunction are supreme examples of the mandatory blending of mind and body. The woman with stress-induced hypothalamic amenorrhea affords an example of how emotional stress alters physiology, which in turn reduces sexual response from both the hormonal changes and the psychological reaction to those changes. The lack of menses may be associated with reduced sense of femininity and sexual attractiveness and, hence, sexual desire: the lack of midcycle and premenstrual androgen peaks can further reduce her desire and responsivity. Assessment and treatment of sexual dysfunction in women is therefore biopsychosocial.

Women's Sexual Response Cycle

In women and men there are different phases of sexual response. In men, initial sexual desire (sexual "wanting, hunger, urging"), often precedes deliberate attention to sexual stimuli with subsequent arousal. Women, especially in established relationships, mostly agree to engage sexually or initiate sex with their partners for reasons other than desire.[206,207] Reasons for engaging in sex, identified by qualitative research, include promotion of emotional closeness to the partner, response to romantic environment, and more specifically erotic cues.[208] Empirical, qualitative, and clinical evidence makes it clear that sexual desire, as typified by sexual fantasizing, positively anticipating sexual experiences, and spontaneously thinking about sex in a positive manner has a broad spectrum of frequency among women and that overt desire is infrequent in many sexually functional and satisfied women.[207]

Motivated by one or many reasons (some of them nonsexual), a woman deliberately attends to sexual stimuli, and as a result her subsequent subjective excitement and pleasure triggers feelings of sexual desire.[209,210] Desire and arousal then coexist and augment each other as shown in Figure 19–9. Provided she can stay focused and continue to feel pleasure, and provided the duration of stimulation is sufficiently long and there is no negative outcome (such as pain or partner dysfunction), sexual satisfaction with one, many, or no discreet orgasms fulfills her newly acquired sexual desire. Her original goal or motivation to be sexual will also be achieved. The response is circular, with overlapping phases of variable order. For instance, desire can follow arousal, and high arousal can follow the first orgasm. The figure shows that desire, once triggered, increases the motivation to attend to sexual stimuli and to accept or request more intensely erotic forms of stimulation. Any initial or spontaneous desire will similarly augment the response (see Fig. 19–9).

The model demonstrates the importance of both sexual stimuli and sexual context, and it demonstrates that a response can begin with feelings that are not necessarily sexual. Also contained in the model is the concept of arousability, meaning the ease with which the woman is aroused by sexual stimuli. This concept is important given the evidence that many factors modulate arousal, including feeling desired rather than feeling used, feeling accepted by the partner, finding the partner's behavior attractive, and having a positive body image and positive mood,[208,211] as well as biological factors including testosterone activity.[7,212-215]

Included in evidence-based changes to the conceptualization of woman's sexual response is an emphasis on subjective arousal rather than genital congestion per se.[207] Traditionally, women's arousal has been equated to vaginal lubrication and vulval swelling (as in the DSM-IV-TR [DSM 4th edition, text revision] diagnosis of arousal disorder). However, women view lubrication more as an epiphenomenon.[208] If intravaginal stimulation is part of the couple's interaction, some lubrication is necessary, but neither it nor genital swelling and underlying congestion correlate well with subjective arousal on empirical testing. Unlike penile erection in men, her genital congestion does not robustly reinforce the woman's subjective excitement.[216,217]

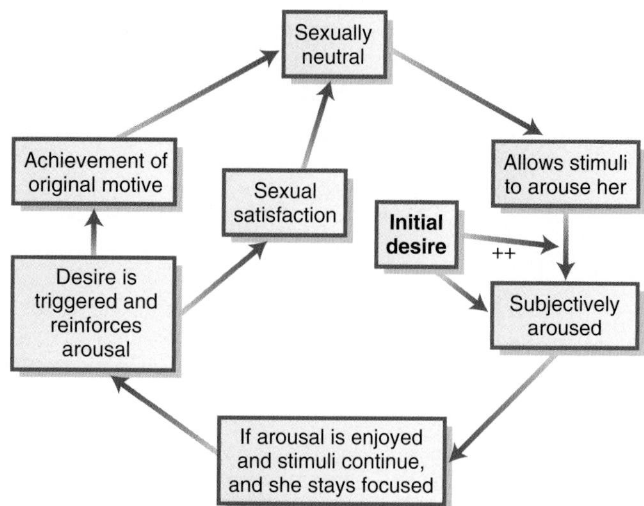

Figure 19–9 ▪ Sexual response cycle reflecting the many reasons women are motivated to be sexual, subjective arousal and excitement in response to stimuli so that (responsive) desire may be triggered. Spontaneous or initial desire can augment the cycle.

This evidence has caused many to question the DSM-IV-TR definitions of sexual disorder. The DSM-IV definitions are commonly employed to guide questions in epidemiologic studies and assessment tools in therapeutic trials. Prevalence rates for women's sexual desire and arousal disorders are therefore in question.

Definitions of Women's Sexual Dysfunction or Disorder

Revisions to the DSM-IV definitions of women's sexual disorders were recently recommended by the International Consensus Committee organized by the American Urological Association Foundation (AUAF), formerly known as the American Foundation of Urologic Disease (AFUD).[207,218] The latest diagnostic entities are shown in Figures 19–10 and 19–11.

Sexual Desire or Interest Disorder

Sexual desire or sexual interest disorder is defined as "absent or diminished feelings of sexual desire or interest, absent sexual thoughts or fantasies and a lack of responsive desire. Motivations (here defined as reasons/incentives), for attempting to become sexually aroused are scarce or absent. The lack of interest is considered to be beyond a normative lessening with life cycle and relationship duration."[218]

This revised definition reflects the fact that lack of any initial or spontaneous desire is within normal experience. It is the additional lack of any triggered or responsive desire that constitutes disorder, usually associated with a lack of subjective arousal and pleasure when engaged in sex and response to other erotic stimuli. The evidence is that initial desire is only a

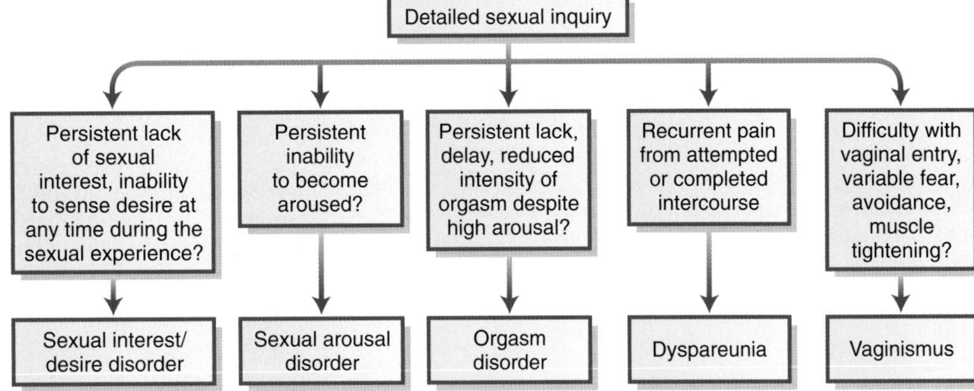

Figure 19–10 ▪ Revised definitions of women's sexual dysfunctions.

reality for some women, most notably when there is a new partner.[219,220]

Combined Arousal Disorder

The diagnostic subtypes of arousal disorders depend on the woman's perception of genital changes and on her recognition of subjective arousal or excitement (see Fig. 19–11). When neither is recognized in response to any kind of sexual stimulation, the diagnosis is "combined arousal disorder."[218] This disorder is defined as "absence of or markedly diminished feelings of sexual arousal (sexual excitement and sexual pleasure), from any type of sexual stimulation as well as complaints of absent or impaired genital sexual arousal, vulvar swelling, lubrication)."[218]

Subjective Arousal Disorder

Women who deny subjective arousal and excitement but recognize some reflex lubrication or genital swelling, or both, are said to have subjective arousal disorder (see Fig. 19–11). This disorder is defined as "absence of or markedly diminished feelings of sexual arousal (sexual excitement and sexual pleasure), from any type of sexual stimulation. Vaginal lubrication or other signs of physical response still occur."[218]

The evidence is that in women with a DSM-IV-TR diagnosis of arousal disorder ("lack of lubrication/swelling response"), the reflex genital response of vasocongestion occurs even when the woman does not report that she finds an erotic stimulus subjectively exciting and is unaware of genital changes.[216] These studies are done by using a tampon-like device called a vaginal photoplethysmograph (VPP), which records increases in congestion of blood around the vagina while simultaneously the woman rates her subjective arousal or excitement. Whereas men when viewing sexual scenes of animals mating report they find the film sexual but not arousing and do not show any erectile response, women viewing the same film similarly report the film is sexual but not arousing and yet, monitoring their vaginal response shows prompt reflexive vasocongestion.[221] Similar increases in clitoral artery blood flow of healthy premenopausal women accompanied both erotic and humorous stimuli.

Genital Sexual Arousal Disorder

A clinical subgroup of women, usually middle aged or older, report "genital deadness," even though nongenital stimuli such as breast stimulation, kissing, stimulating their partner, or reading something erotic are still arousing to them (see Fig. 19–11). This type of dysfunction is termed *genital sexual arousal disorder* and is defined as "complaints of absent or impaired genital sexual arousal. Self-report might include minimal vulval swelling or vaginal lubrication from any type of sexual stimulation and reduced sexual sensations from caressing genitalia. Subjective sexual excitement still occurs from nongenital sexual stimuli."[218]

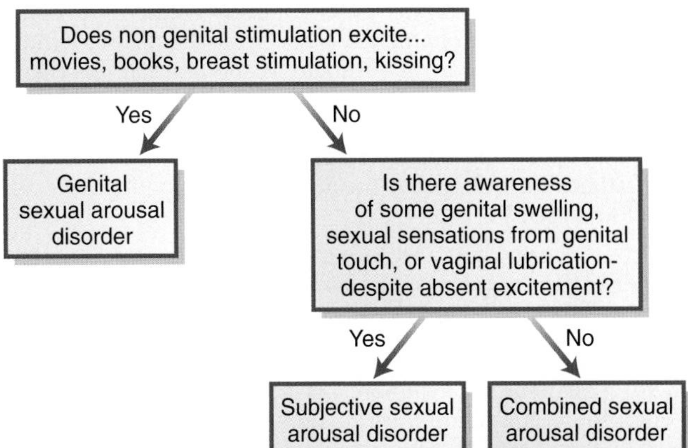

Figure 19–11 ▪ Diagnosis of sexual arousal disorders. Subjective arousal disorder is characterized by absence of or markedly diminished feelings of sexual excitement or sexual pleasure from any type of sexual stimulation. Vaginal lubrication and/or other evidence of physical response is present. Genital sexual arousal disorder is characterized by lack of vulvar swelling, vaginal lubrication, and genital sexual sensation despite subjective feelings of sexual excitement.

It is emphasized again that this is a clinical diagnosis and the small amount of evidence to date suggests that only some of these women have demonstrably reduced reflex vasocongestion in response to mentally sexually arousing erotic stimuli.[222] It would appear that others have lost sexual sensitivity of normally engorged tissues.

Women's Orgasmic Disorder

The patient has women's orgasmic disorder if "despite the self-reported high sexual arousal/excitement, there is either a lack of orgasm, markedly diminished intensity of orgasmic sensations, or marked delay of orgasm from any kind of stimulation."[218] Women with arousal disorders also rarely or never experience orgasm. The revised definition states that disorder is only present when there are difficulties with *any* type of stimulation. The woman who can experience orgasms with self-stimulation does not have an orgasmic disorder.

Vaginismus

Vaginismus is defined as "persistent or recurrent difficulties of the woman to allow vaginal entry of the penis, finger, or any object despite the woman's expressed wish to do so. There is often (phobic) avoidance and anticipation/fear/experience of pain, along with variable and involuntary pelvic muscle contraction. Structural or other physical abnormalities must be ruled out/addressed."[218] Confirmation of this diagnosis is not possible until there has been therapy sufficient to allow a careful introital and vaginal examination. Until then, the diagnosis is presumptive.

Dyspareunia

Dyspareunia is defined as "persistent or recurrent pain with attempted or complete vaginal entry and/or penile vaginal intercourse."[218] There are many causes including, most commonly, vulvar vestibulitis syndrome (VVS, a poorly defined syndrome of unknown etiology characterized by dyspareunia, tenderness localized within the vulvar vestibule, vestibular erythema, and discomfort at the vaginal opening) and vulvar vaginal atrophy. There is often a reflexive muscle tightening consequent to the experiences of pain, but the term "vaginismus" would not be given if there are findings beyond muscle tightening, for example, the allodynia of VVS.

Descriptors as Components of Diagnoses

Women's sexuality is highly contextual. Inappropriate contexts (e.g., insufficient stimuli, lack of attraction to partner, lack of safety) can head to symptoms of sexual dysfunction, even though there is nothing intrinsically wrong with the woman's sex response system.[223]

Alternatively, there may be additional factors in the woman's past experiences or in her personality that are interrupting her sex response cycle. The AUAF International Consensus Committee strongly advocates that the following descriptors be added to any diagnosis of dysfunction:

- Past factors from developmental history affecting psychosexual development
- Present factors—interpersonal, environmental, societal, cultural
- Medical factors

Physiology of Women's Sexual Response

Physiology of Desire and Subjective Arousal

Sexual desire is one of the many motivations to be sexual. Feelings of desire may be triggered by internal cues, such as fantasies or memories, and by external cues, such as an attractive partner, and depend on adequate neuroendocrine function. Multiple neurotransmitters, peptides, and hormones modulate desire and subjective arousal. Stemming mainly from sexually positive and negative effects of pharmacologic agents with known or partially known mechanisms of action, the following factors appear to be prosexual: noradrenalin, dopamine, oxytocin, and serotonin acting on some receptors. Prolactin, serotonin acting on 5-HT_2 and 5-HT_3 receptors and GABA, vasopressin and glutamate inhibit sexual response. These neurotransmitters and peptides are themselves modulated by sex hormones.

Biologic factors do not act independently from environmental factors. Even in animal models it has been shown that either dopamine or progesterone, acting on receptors in the hypothalamus, can cause an increase in sexual behavior in oophorectomized estrogenized female rats. However, the presence of a male animal alongside the cage can cause an identical change in sexual behavior without the administration of either progesterone or dopamine.[224] Similarly in women, arousability and intensity of response can be increased by raising serum testosterone levels in midlife women to those of younger women,[212-215,225] by administering a dopaminergic drug (bupropion),[226] or by a change of partner.[220] Even in rodents, complex networks exist whereby the female assesses the context of potential sexual activity and relates it to past experience and therefore to expectation of reward. In women, factors such as attitudes toward sex, feelings for the partner, past sexual experiences, duration of relationship, and mental and emotional health more strongly modulate desire and arousability than do biologic factors.[223,227-230]

Data supporting these themes stem from nationally representative samples of women. However, in women with chronic disease, the disease itself, its treatment, its psychological effects, and these interpersonal, personal, and contextual issues, all affect sexual response.[231]

Physical Sexual Arousal

A number of physical changes accompany subjective excitement or arousal. Included are genital swelling, increased vaginal lubrication, breast engorgement, nipple erection, and increased skin sensitivity to sexual stimulation; changes in heart rate, blood pressure, muscle tone, breathing, and temperature; and mottling of the skin, a sexual flush of vasodilation over chest and face. These changes result from reflex action of the autonomic nervous system. Within seconds there is increased blood flow to the vagina: vasodilation of the arterioles in the submucosal plexus increases transudation of interstitial fluid from the capillaries, across the epithelium, and into the vaginal lumen. Simultaneously, there is relaxation of smooth muscle cells around the sinusoids in the rami, shaft, and head of the clitoris as well as in the extensions of clitoral tissue known as the vestibular bulbs. The vagina lengthens and dilates, elevating the uterus. The labia become more swollen and darker red, and the lower third of the vagina swells. As the clitoris becomes more swollen, it elevates to lie nearer the symphysis pubis.

When increases in genital congestion in response to visual erotic stimuli are recorded with the VPP, there is highly variable correlation with subjective arousal. This is true for sexually healthy women, as well as women complaining of lack of desire, lack of arousal, and sexual pain.[216,232] Women with a chronic lack of arousal show prompt increases in vaginal congestion, comparable to those of control women. However, they report no subjective sexual excitement in response to the erotic stimulation. Some of these women report negative emotions such as anxiety or embarrassment or sadness. In fact, these latter negative emotions correlate with the increases in congestion. Functional magnetic resonance imaging (MRI) shows activation of a number of areas of the brain during visual erotic stimulation. Unlike these experiments in men, activation of the areas organizing genital vasocongestion does not correlate with the woman's subjective excitement as she views the erotic film while in the MRI tube.[233]

The underlying neurobiology of the genital vasocongestive response is incompletely understood. It does appear to be highly automated and involves release of nitric oxide (NO) from the parasympathetic nerves along with vasoactive intestinal polypeptide (VIP). Acetylcholine (Ach), which blocks noradrenergic vasoconstricting mechanisms and promotes NO release from the endothelium, is also released. Somatic, sympathetic, and parasympathetic nerve pathways are far less separate than was previously believed. There is communication between the NO-containing cavernous nerve to the clitoris and the distal portion of the somatic dorsal nerve of the clitoris from the pudendal nerve. Pelvic sympathetic nerves release primarily vasoconstrictive noradrenalin, adrenalin, and adenosine triphosphate (ATP), but some release ACh, NO, and VIP. In keeping with these findings, it has been repeatedly demonstrated that provoked anxiety in the laboratory situation can, in sexually healthy women, increase vasocongestive response of the genitalia to the erotic stimulation.[234] There has been far less research on the neurotransmission of genital vasocongestion in women than in men, even though NO is thought to be the major neurotransmitter mediating vulval engorgement. Other factors mediating vaginal engorgement include VIP, NO, and another possibly more important unidentified neurotransmitter.[235]

There may be a "cervical motor reflex" such that touch to the cervix reduces pressure in the upper portion of the vagina but increases pressure in the middle and lower portions, accompanied by increased electromyographic activity in the levator ani and puborectalis muscles. It has been hypothesized that during intercourse, penile thrusting on the cervix might cause reflex contraction of the pelvic muscles, thereby facilitating the ballooning of the upper vagina, while the same muscle contraction constricts the lower vagina. Reduced uterine tone can occur in response to mechanical or electrical stimulation of the clitoris. Clitoral stimulation abolishes background tonic uterine muscle contraction such that uterine pressure declines. Possibly, this reflex contributes to the known increase in size and elevation of the uterus with sexual arousal.[236]

The clitoris is a most sexually sensitive area of the body. Clitoral stimulation is usually only enjoyable if nonphysical and nongenital physical stimulation have occurred. Without preceding arousal, direct stimulation can be unpleasant, too intense, and even painful. Little research has occurred into the transmission of sexual sensation, but recent immunohistological studies have identified neurotransmitters thought to be associated with sensation (substance P and calcitonin gene-related peptide [CGRP]), concentrated immediately under the epithelium of the glans clitoris. Recent MRI imaging has confirmed extensive clitoral tissue far beyond the visible portion when the clitoral head is retracted.[237] The clitoris comprises the head, shaft, rami which extend along the pubic arch, periurethral tissue in front of the anterior vaginal wall, as well as bulbar tissue surrounding the anterior distal vagina and contiguous with the periurethral tissue.[237]

There has been minimal research into the underlying physiology of nongenital physical changes and of their correlation with subjective excitement.

Epidemiology

Most epidemiologic studies reflect self-reported symptoms, some using validated questionnaires, rather than carefully diagnosed dysfunctions and disorders on the basis of an in-depth interview. None of the validated assessment questionnaires have yet been modified to reflect the most recent definitions of women's sexual dysfunction modeled on female rather than male sexual response cycles.[218,238] The available questionnaires still reflect the stance that initial desire is necessary for a normal response, and the focus is on genital events more than the subjective experience.[238] Beyond the difficulties arising from changing definitions of desire and arousal disorder, only a few studies report ongoing sexual difficulties as opposed to those present in the past 4 weeks or lasting 2 months, for example. A study of women younger than 44 years in Britain found that although 41% of women reported lack of sexual interest for at least a month in the past year, only 10% reported lack of interest lasting longer than 6 months.[241]

The prevalence of low desire interest disorder in women is unknown. The 30% to 35% of women reporting difficulties or problems with low desire[7,219,239] might in large part reflect women perceiving they have problematic desire because of the standard to which they compare themselves. The standard may be the heightened desire of early relationships or it might be the standard more typical of male sexuality depicted in movies and books as being the norm for women. Understanding that spontaneous or initial desire is only a frequent reality for some women, most notably when there is a new partner,[219,220,228] would reduce the number of women perceiving their experience as abnormal.

Figures for the prevalence of low subjective arousal are also scant; the focus of epidemiology has usually been on just one component of arousal, namely, vaginal lubrication. One study of 979 women in a nationally representative British cohort, aged between 18 and 70 years, found that 17% identified problems with arousal as distinct from vaginal dryness,[240] as did 5% in the SWAN study.[219] Lubrication difficulties have a prevalence of 10% to 30% of women in nationally representative samples.[6,239] These figures are of limited usefulness because it is not known if the low lubrication was accompanied by lack of subjective excitement.

The prevalence of orgasmic disorder is similarly uncertain because some studies report that women with a diagnosed orgasmic disorder have comorbid arousal disorder. Both AUAF and the DSM-IV-TR definitions clarify that a diagnosis of arousal disorder precludes a diagnosis of orgasmic disorder. The range given is from 3.7% to 24%.[6,241] The lower prevalence was from the British study whereby 3.7% were unable to experience orgasm for longer than 6 months and 14.4% reported difficulties for at least 1 month in the previous year.

The prevalence of chronic dyspareunia ranges from 8% to 22%, the prevalence decreasing with age in most studies. The high prevalence of VVS in younger women appears to balance the increased prevalence of dyspareunia from vulvovaginal atrophy in older women. Vestibulitis is thought to affect some 9% of women, with approximately 5% of all women experiencing this condition before age 25 years.[242] Prevalence figures for vaginismus are even less secure. When this condition precludes intercourse completely, it might never be disclosed or it may be disclosed only if conception is planned.

Complexity and Comorbidity of Dysfunction

Consistent with the overlap of phases of sexual response, it is not surprising to find high levels of overlap among various types of sexual dysfunction in women (Fig. 19–12).[243,244] It is becoming increasingly clear that rather than a discrete entity of desire or interest disorder in women, the reality is a more pervasive gradual blunting of sexual response such that women complaining of lack of desire typically have little in the way of intense feelings of arousal and infrequent orgasms.[243] Recent randomized, controlled trials (RCTs) investigating benefit of supplemental transdermal testosterone, although recruiting women with diagnosed "hypoactive sexual desire disorder," show improvements in arousal, pleasure, and orgasm. Indeed the first of these studies showed only improvement in those parameters and not in the "desire" parameter.[212] The problematic response was clearly present despite the diagnostic focus on hypoactive sexual desire disorder.

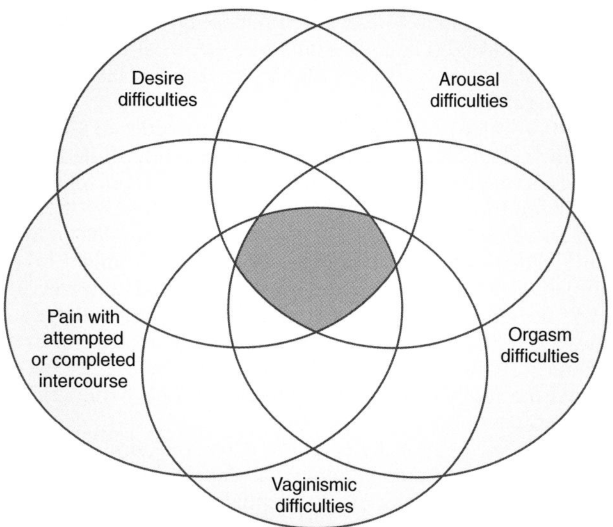

Figure 19–12 ■ Overlap and complexity of women's sexual dysfunctions. Women with sexual dysfunction might have more than one sexual disorder. Also, dysfunction in one sexual function domain can affect other domains secondarily, leading to coexistence of more than one disorder.

Distress About Sexual Dysfunction

Not all women with sexual concerns are distressed about them. A number of larger studies have failed to show an increase of prevalence of desire concerns with age[229,244]; smaller studies have confirmed that sexual desire does decrease with age but distress about that low desire also decreases.[245] The majority of women with dyspareunia report moderate or marked distress.[246] The recent consensus on revised definitions of dysfunction advocates assessing the degree of distress—none, mild, moderate, or severe—when making any diagnosis.

Risk Factors

Both psychological factors and medical conditions alter the biology of sexual response.

Medical Conditions

Depression has been shown to be a major risk factor for women's sexual dysfunction. This is true even before the administration of antidepressants with potentially sexually negative side effects.[247] Of 79 women with major depression prior to medication, 50% reported decreased desire, and similar numbers reported far less sexual arousal when engaging in sex.[247] Of 914 middle-aged women in the SWAN study, those with past history of major depressive illness reported less frequent arousal, less physical pleasure, and less emotional satisfaction in their present relationship.[219] These findings remain significant after controlling for current depressive symptoms, marital status, and psychotropic medication.[248]

Antidepressants, especially those that are more highly serotoninergic, may lessen desire and arousal and delay orgasm. When women are specifically asked about sexual side effects of antidepressants, such side effects are reported by some 70%.[249] Factors predisposing to an antidepressant-associated sexual dysfunction include age, being married as opposed to being single or separated or divorced, being without college or higher education, being without full-time work, having less sexual enjoyment prior to depression, taking concomitant medications of all types, having a comorbid illness that might affect sexual functioning, and having a past history of antidepressant-associated sexual dysfunction.[250]

Reduced Androgen Activity

Although in younger women, ovaries are thought to be responsible for some 50% of androgen production, in midlife and older women the situation is far more variable. When ovaries remain present, their contribution to total androgen activity is highly variable. It is thought that intracellular testosterone production within the brain and other parts of the body including the genitalia, from adrenal prohormones (including DHEA, DHEAS, andro-5-ene-3β, 17β-diol, and Δ^4-androstenedione), account for the majority of testosterone activity in older naturally menopausal women and close to 100% in surgically menopausal women.[251] From the third decade onward, adrenal prohormone production progressively declines such that in the 50- to 60-year-old age group, serum DHEA has already decreased by some 70% compared to peak values in 20- to 30-year-old women.[251]

The cellular androgen deprivation is difficult to measure, given that less than 10% of testosterone produced within cells (other than gonadal and adrenal cells), spills back into the bloodstream.[252] Thus serum levels of testosterone reflect mainly gonadal production. Moreover, the available assays for serum testosterone (free, bioavailable, total) are not designed for the female range and they are very unreliable.[45,253] Liquid chromatography tandem mass spectrometry methods for measuring testosterone levels might soon become widely available. Metabolites resulting from the breakdown of testosterone wherever it was produced—androsterone glucuronide (ADT-G), androstane 3α, 17β-diol glucuronide (3α-diol-G), and androstane 3β,17β-diol glucuronide (3β-diol-G), can be measured.[252] However, assays for these metabolites are currently only available on a research basis, and age-related values in women with and without sexual dysfunction have not yet been established.

It is known that sudden loss of androgen production can result in a sexual syndrome whereby formerly useful sexual stimuli—mental, visual, nongenital touch, genital touch, intercourse—all fail to arouse. Similarly, any former innate or spontaneous desire is lost. Chemotherapy-induced or surgical menopause, especially in younger women, may be associated with this syndrome.[254] However, other women with induced menopause report no sexual changes. A recent prospective nonrandomized study showed that 106 perimenopausal women requiring hysterectomy for benign pathology, choosing hysterectomy with bilateral salpingo-oophorectomy over a hysterectomy alone, showed no deterioration at all in sexual function 1 year after surgery compared with preoperative assessment.[255] The different psychological contexts of unwanted but essential medical intervention versus informed choice may be crucial.

There is minimal evidence correlating sexual function with serum androgen levels in women. Studying 2900 pre- and perimenopausal multiethnic North American women in the SWAN study, total testosterone and free androgen index showed minimal correlation with sexual function.[256] Similarly, measures of free and total testosterone failed to correlate with sexual function in a study of 1021 Australian women aged 18 to 75 years.[257] A low score for sexual response for women older than 45 years was associated with higher odds of having a serum DHEAS level below the 10th percentile for that age group.[257] However, the majority of women with low DHEAS levels did not have any reduced sexual function.[257]

Clearly, there are many unanswered questions, including the variable amounts of remaining adrenal precursors of testosterone, activity of steroidogenic enzymes, changes in number and sensitivity of androgen receptors and coregulators, and interplay between estrogen and androgen. It is assumed but not proven that sexual benefit is afforded by activity at the androgen receptor. However, aromatization to estrogen within the cell may be at least in part responsible. One recent study suggests benefit via the androgen receptor, because the addition of an aromatase inhibitor did not negate the benefit of supplemental testosterone given to postmenopausal women already using transdermal estrogen therapy.[258] Whether testosterone allows benefits simply by reducing SHBG, therefore allowing estrogen to be more bioavailable, is also unclear.

Low Estrogen States

There can be sexual consequences of low estrogen after menopause or childbirth; in association with GnRH agonist treatment, chemotherapy-induced ovarian failure, idiopathic ovarian failure, or surgical menopause; and sometimes in association with low-estrogen combined contraceptives or with depoprogesterone.

With loss of estrogen production from the ovaries, intracellular production of estrogen from testosterone, DHEA, DHEAS, and androstenedione depends on adrenal and ovarian production of these prohormones, numbers of fat cells (an important site of aromatization of testosterone to estradiol), and the presence of the appropriate steroidogenic enzymes to synthesize estrogen or testosterone and DHT from the precursors in the tissue concerned. Recent work clarifies the structure of many tissue-specific genes that encode for the steroidogenic enzymes governing the transformation of the precursors into androgens and/or estrogens.[251,252] There is particular focus on 3β-hydroxysteroid dehydrogenase (3β-HSD), 17β-HSD, 5α-reductase, and aromatase.[252] Thus in the older woman, local biosynthesis of sex hormones applies to estrogens as well as to androgens.

Genital Effects of Low Estrogen

Low estrogen states are typically associated with reduced lubrication in response to sexual stimulation. However, the matter is complex. Visual signs of atrophy and low serum levels of estrogen correlate with basal measures of vaginal congestion, but the percentage increase in congestion in response to erotic stimuli is similar in estrogen-deplete and -replete states.[216] Early results from MRI studies show similar changes in vaginal wall and clitoral volume with sexual stimulation in pre- and postmenopausal women.[259] Estrogen deficiency does not necessarily preclude sufficient lubrication if sexual stimulation is sufficient. Nevertheless, some 30% to 55% of postmenopausal women report sexual symptoms in association with vaginal atrophy.[260]

Low estrogen increases the pH of the vaginal lumen, predisposing to infection, which, in turn, undermines women's sexual self-confidence and contributes to dyspareunia. A review of the mechanism of estrogen acidification of the vagina has changed the traditional view of attributing this to hydrogen peroxide and protons secreted by estrogen-requiring Döderlein's lactobacilli.[261] There is some evidence that vaginal ectocervical cells acidify the vaginal lumen by secreting protons across the apical plasma membrane. It is thought that this active proton secretion occurs throughout life but that it is up-regulated by estrogen.[261]

Symptoms of vaginal dryness, dyspareunia, and vaginal narrowing correlate poorly with visual changes of atrophy, with estrogen levels, and with duration of estrogen lack. Symptoms can occur perimenopausally but sometimes only decades after menopause. Estrogen levels do correlate with ratios between parabasal, intermediate, and superficial vaginal cells. The role of vaginal epithelial cell permeability remains unclear. Nerve endings containing CGRP are present in the vaginal epithelial cells and might modulate their permeability.[262]

Estrogen and Sexual Sensitivity

Reduced sexual sensitivity of the genital and nongenital skin has received little scientific study. A small amount of research using pressure thresholds has demonstrated reduced vulval sensitivity with menopause and increased sensitivity from the use of topical estrogen.[263] Both age and the postmenopausal state have been associated with reduced vibratory sensation in the genital tract, and age by itself affects peripheral nongenital vibration sensation.[264]

The genital "deadness" associated with genital sexual arousal disorder that continues despite estrogen therapy is poorly understood.[218] Reduced genital vasocongestion, despite useful erotic stimulation that does arouse the mind, appears to underlie only a subgroup of women with this disorder. It is therefore suspected, given the large number of vulval androgen receptors, that reduced androgen activity may be involved in this loss of sexual genital sensitivity.[222]

Low Estrogen and Subjective Arousal and Desire

The role of low estrogen in loss of desire and arousability remains unclear. A recent study suggested that sexual responsiveness can be improved by estrogen supplementation to levels between 650 and 759 pM/L, approximately twice the level required to improve local symptoms of vaginal dryness.[265] At least in part, testosterone's benefit may be from increased production of estrogen via aromatization within cells or from increased bioavailability of estrogen due to reduced SHBG.

Breast Cancer

Sexual concerns subsequent to diagnosis and treatment of breast cancer are the most likely areas of distress to persist for more than one year after cancer diagnosis.[254] Chemotherapy plays a major role in causing loss of desire, subjective arousal, vaginal dryness, and dyspareunia.[254] A predictive model for sexual interest and function and satisfaction after breast cancer therapy has evolved from two large independent groups of breast cancer survivors.[254] The most important predictors of sexual satisfaction were absence of vaginal dryness, presence of emotional well-being, a positive body image, a better quality of relationship, and absence of partner sexual problems.[254]

A temporary medical menopause from adjuvant GnRH agonist treatment appears to be associated with reversible sexual dysfunction.[266] Tamoxifen does not consistently alter sexual function.[266] However, aromatase inhibitors by producing a state close to total absence of any estrogen activity can be associated with severe symptoms from vulvovaginal atrophy.[266]

Diabetes

Older studies resulted in conflicting data and were derived from small numbers of subjects without controls, often mixing patients with type 1 and type 2 disease and rarely clarifying estrogen status.

Recent research confirms the biopsychosocial nature of women's sexuality. Five controlled studies confirm links between diabetes-associated sexual dysfunction and depression, as did a previous meta-analysis.[267] Various psychological factors were also linked, including the woman's acceptance of her disease. Sexual difficulties do not appear to correlate with age, duration of disease, BMI, glycemic control, hormonal therapy, complications of disease, or menopausal status.[268-272]

Reduced lubrication is the one sexual dysfunction consistently seen more commonly in women with diabetes than controls.[268-271] Genital vibration sensation has been shown to be reduced in women with diabetes[270]; however, such reduction was not associated with sexual dysfunction. Empirical evidence does not consistantly support the clinical impression that women, especially women with type 1 diabetes, report loss of orgasm function. One study of women with diabetes and renal failure, showed significant impairment of orgasm and clitoral sexual sensation compared with controls.[273]

Psychophysiologic studies are few. In one small study, compared with controls, women with diabetes showed reduced genital congestion but comparable subjective arousal to the erotic stimulus.[274] Data on dyspareunia are scant. A higher prevalence of dyspareunia would be expected, given reduced lubrication and also (despite the evidence of benefit)[275] the reduced prescription of estrogen therapy after menopause if diabetes is present.[275] In addition, the link with chronic candidiasis would be expected to increase prevalence of dyspareunia, perhaps triggering vulvar vestibulitis syndrome in those genetically susceptible. However, prevalence figures for dyspareunia are disconcertingly high in young and middle aged women both with and without diabetes. Prevalence levels of 32% to 62%, 42% to 46% and 26% to 39% for women with type 1, type 2, and no diabetes, respectively[268,272] are reported.

Renal Failure

There has been little research of sexual function in women with renal disease. The associated anovulation (and thus lack of testosterone peak), high prolactin secretion, anemia, comorbid depression and low estrogen state can all impair sexual function. Reduced genital sexual function has been noted in women whose renal failure has been accompanied by hypertriglyceridemia.[273] Subjective arousal can improve after renal transplantation, even though the observed vaginal congestive response to erotica is similar in women receiving hemodialysis, peritoneal dialysis, or transplant.[276]

Cardiovascular Disease

There are very few studies of sexual function in women with cardiovascular disease. In one study, atherosclerotic lesions of the hypogastric and pudendal arteries were associated with reduced lubrication and impaired sexual function. The sexual difficulties became more severe after vascular intervention despite improved overall health.[277] For treated and nontreated premenopausal women with mild hypertension, decreased lubrication has been documented, along with dyspareunia and poor orgasms, compared with age-matched controls.[278]

Medications

A number of commonly prescribed medications can impair sexual function and satisfaction (Table 19–11).

Polycystic Ovarian Syndrome

To date there is no evidence that the higher androgen levels associated with polycystic ovarian syndrome (PCOS) give protection from a complaint of low sexual desire or low sexual arousability. In one sample of 30 women with PCOS presenting for treatment of hirsutism, sexual desire was significantly lower compared with that in a control group.[279]

Hypothalamic-Pituitary Disease

There are few data on sexual dysfunction in women with hypopituitarism. Rarely is testosterone supplemented, the focus usually being on estrogen (and progesterone if the uterus is in place). One recent randomized placebo-controlled study of the effects of testosterone administration in women with hypopituitarism showed improvement in sexual function.[280] Two small RCTs have demonstrated improvement in sexual function from giving 25 to 50 mg DHEA daily to women with secondary adrenal insufficiency and women with hypopituitarism.[281,282]

Adrenal Insufficiency

There are no data on the prevalence of sexual dysfunction. in women with adrenal insufficiency. Results of DHEA supplementation have been inconsistent.[282,283]

Simple Hysterectomy

In women with hysterectomy, studies have not supported a difference in sexual outcome whether hysterectomy is vaginal, subtotal abdominal, or total abdominal.[284-286] Overall, sexual satisfaction has been noted to improve in a majority of women independent of the type of hysterectomy.

Radical Hysterectomy

The autonomic nerves, particularly those in the uterosacral and cardinal ligaments, may be disrupted during radical hysterectomy unless nerve-sparing techniques are used. There are no data on subsequent genital sexual function other than data characterizing the vaginal vasocongestive response to erotica. Photoplethysmographic assessment of congestion during subjectively arousing sexual stimulation in 12 women with past non–nerve-sparing radical hysterectomy revealed reduced maximum response compared with 17 age-matched controls, suggesting that lubrication problems following radical pelvic surgery can result from nerve damage.[287] Nerve-sparing radical hysterectomies for cervical cancer have been introduced, but as yet there are no sexual outcome studies.

Hyperprolactinemia

Women with hyperprolactinemia typically have reduced arousal, reduced orgasm, and increased dyspareunia without demonstrable changes in other hormonal parameters other than the prolactin.[288]

Aging

The degree to which age is a risk factor for sexual dysfunction is unclear. The most common reason women give for discontinuing sexual activity is lack of a partner. Many studies only include women who are "sexually active" (and some only "sexually active with intercourse"), and so available data are limited. Large nationally representative studies have shown little increase in sexual problems with age, but they often do not include those older than 60 years.[229] In other studies, some 40% of older women noted reduced sexual responsivity, along with increased desire for nongenital sexual expression.[220,289] A recent study showed greater prevalence of reduced desire as a function of both menopause status and age, increasing from 22% in the premenopausal group to 32% in the postmenopausal group.[244] As in other studies, low desire was strongly associated with difficulties of arousal and orgasm. One large longitudinal study of women over the 10-year menopausal transition showed a decline in desire and responsivity as a function of both age and menopause[220]: high numbers of menopausal symptoms influenced well-being, which affected sexual responsivity and, in turn, sexual desire and interest. A larger study of 14,000 women from 29 countries found reduced lubrication to be the only age-related factor for women. Unfortunately, the response rate from that study was only 15%, and only women engaging in intercourse in the past year were included.[229]

TABLE 19–11 MEDICATION RISK FACTORS FOR SEXUAL DYSFUNCTION IN WOMEN

Medication	Incidence	Effect	Remedy
Antipsychotics	Sexual dysfunction in up to 73% of patients with schizophrenia	Traditional antipsychotics and risperidone: Reduced dopamine and increased prolactin and cause α-blockade and muscarinic blockade.	Use second-generation antipsychotics, which do not raise prolactin Other mechanisms can still cause dysfunction.
β-blockers	Desire reduction greater than experienced from angiotensin II antagonist	Selective or nonselective blockade can be associated with sexual dysfunction	Use ACE inhibitor, angiotensin receptor antagonist, calcium channel blocker, peripherally acting α-blocker
SSRIs	Sexual side effects in up to 70%	Stimulation of serotonin receptors, including 5-HT_2 receptors	Adding bupropion may be beneficial; benefit shown in one of two RCTs
Antiandrogens: GnRH antagonists, cyproterone acetate, spironolactone in high doses		Suppression of GnRH or LH and/or antagonism of androgen receptor	
Narcotics		Suppression of GnRH	No scientific data on sex hormone supplementation
Antiepileptic drugs		Induction of P450 hepatic enzymes increases SHBG and reduces free testosterone	Some antiepileptic drugs are enzyme neutral, e.g., oxcarbazapine, lamotrigine, levetiraceta, but studies are lacking.
Combined oral contraceptives	Prevalence of associated dysfunction uncertain, but close to 50% of women discontinue OCs within 12 mo, many because of sexual side effects	Increase in SHBG reducing bioavailablility of testosterone; suppression of endogenous testosterone: use of nonandrogenic progestin	No studies are available on testosterone supplementation or comparison of different formulations Consider alternative birth control, e.g., IUD, barrier method, irreversible method

ACE , angiotensin converting enzyme; AED, antiepileptic drug; GnRH, gonadotrophin releasing hormone; 5-HT, serotonin; IUD, intrauterine device; LH, luteinizing hormone; OC, oral contraceptive; RCT, randomized, controlled trial; SHBG, sex hormone–binding globulin; SSRI, selective serotonin reuptake inhibitor.

Adapted with permission from Basson R. Sexual dysfunction in women. New Engl J Med 2006;354(14):1497-1506.

Many studies confirm that older women report less distress about lack of desire compared to younger women.[223] Past studies have shown a shift from genital sex to intimacy as people age such that any activity involving affection, romance, closeness, and companionship may help satisfy the sexual needs of older adults. It is possible that with the advent of effective therapies for erectile dysfunction, these patterns may change. Strong predictors of continued sexual interest are the sexual behavior and enjoyment at an earlier age.

Psychological Factors

Psychosocial factors strongly influence women's sexuality, including partner availability and partner's general and sexual health,[239,290] and the relationship itself.[229] These factors, in turn, determine how well a couple can adapt to changes in sexual life from external factors and their own aging. Personal factors influencing arousability include nonsexual distractions, sexual self-confidence, expectation of reward, feelings for the partner both at that time and generally, and safety issues including adequate birth control, safety from sexually transmitted diseases, unplanned pregnancies, and privacy issues.

Themes from childhood and adolescence can negatively affect a woman's arousability, and these can assume greater importance in later life, perhaps as a result of less-robust sex hormones. A strong need to feel in control, or a need to suppress emotions, might have been the means to survive childhood and adolescence, but those same defenses can preclude healthy sexual response as an adult. Sometimes unresolved anger and resentment toward parental figures is revived by the context of later life—for instance, having to take care of a previously abusive parent. Women can rarely suppress only negative or "unwelcome" emotions; usually all are suppressed, including sexual emotions.

Personality factors can also affect female sexual function. Studies have shown that compared with women with normal sexual function, those complaining of low desire and low arousal have vulnerable self-esteem, higher levels of anxiety and guilt, more negative body image, and more introversion and somatization.[291] Most studies tend not to identify actual psychopathology in women complaining of low desire.[291] For women with orgasmic disorder, the clinical impression is that many are extremely uncomfortable if they are not in control of their circumstances and their bodily functions.

For women with vaginismus, there appears to be a phobic quality to the fear of vaginal penetration. These women usually do not have other phobias other than that of not being able to deliver a baby (believing such an event would cause unimaginable physical trauma). In a substantial subgroup of women with vestibulitis, there is marked fear of negative evaluation by others, marked conscientiousness and self-criticism,[292] and an increase in somatization.[293]

Quality and Age of Partnership

A majority of women complaining of low desire and arousability state that their partnerships are stable and satisfactory—"our only problems are sexual." Lack of conflict, neglect, or abuse and certainty of commitment are, however, by themselves insufficient to nurture women's sexual desire and facilitate arousal. Common themes include unmet need for eroticism and for variety of sexual stimulation and for greater emotional intimacy with the partner. Lack of argument does not equate with feeling close—feeling safe to be vulnerable and to reveal feelings, fears, and hopes to each other.

Being "very good friends" is insufficient sexual context to trigger women's sexual desire. Studies show a normative lessening of innate desire with duration of relationship.[294] The woman's feelings for her partner were identified as one of the two major determinants of freedom from distress about sex in a recent national probability sample.[223] Women's feelings for their partners, or a recent change of partner, were two of the three major determinants of women's desire and responsivity in the longitudinal study of women transitioning to menopause[220] and were major determinants in cross-sectional studies.[228]

Sexual dysfunction in the male partner can also influence a woman's sexual function.[239] Treating a male partner's erectile dysfunction can reverse the woman's sexual complaints, including problematic arousal, lubrication, orgasm, and pain.[290]

Infertility

Both the evaluation of her infertility and the requirement for assisted reproductive techniques can negatively affect a woman's sexual self-image. The goal-oriented intercourse-focused sexual activity while trying to conceive can be sexually unrewarding, and can therefore reduce motivation. Unfortunately, successful pregnancy does not necessarily reverse sexual concerns; unresolved feelings of guilt about the personal responsibility for the infertility and resentment of the multiple procedures for women compared to just semen analysis for men may linger.[295]

Evaluation of the Woman with a Sexual Disorder

Detailed enquiry into the current sexual problems and their context is necessary, preferably seeing both partners together as well as individually. Table 19–12 outlines the information needed to assess and diagnose sexual dysfunction.

Physical examination including pelvic and genital exam is part of routine care (Table 19–13). Unless dyspareunia is involved, it is not often that physical examination identifies the cause of sexual dysfunction. The examination can be therapeutic in confirming normal anatomy and tissue health. For some women with a history of coercive or abusive sexual experiences, such an examination can cause extreme anxiety. The reason the examination is necessary, and an explanation of what will and will not be done, needs to be given before the examination. When the difficulty is vaginismus, examination must be delayed until therapy has allowed an exam to be feasible and a positive therapeutic experience for the woman (see Table 19–13).

Laboratory testing plays a small role in sexual evaluation. Estrogen activity is best detected by examination. Biochemical assessment is limited in the older woman because available assays are for estradiol rather than estrone, the major postmenopausal estrogen. Serum levels of testosterone do not correlate with sexual function, and the available assays currently do not have the required sensitivity at the low levels found in women. Prolactin or thyrotropin can be measured if there are other symptoms that suggest abnormality.

Evidence-Based Treatment Strategies

Evidence-based therapeutic strategies are only just emerging for the treatment of female sexual dysfunction. One of the difficulties is that etiology is usually multifactorial, with the result that management has many components. However, the few RCTs to date usually employ one treatment strategy. Before implementing therapy, an accurate formulation of the problem(s) is necessary. Using the framework of women's sexual response cycle, the following are assessed:

- The various motivations or incentives to be sexual
- The degree of emotional intimacy, trust, respect, and attraction within the relationship
- Sexual context and suitability of stimuli when sex is attempted
- What is going on in the woman's mind as she attempts to become aroused
- Any biologic factors affecting her arousability
- Details of the outcome in terms of both physical and emotional satisfaction and freedom from pain
- Detailed description of any pain, her thoughts and feelings when the pain occurs, her arousal level, and physical findings

Behavioral, Cognitive and Sexual Therapies

Behavioral, cognitive, and sexual therapies continue to be the mainstay of therapy for sexual dysfunction. The kinds of behavior to be addressed are sexual and nonsexual, including the interaction of the partners outside the bedroom. Improving the sexual environment, the stimuli, the timing, and possibly the sexual technique may be involved. The woman's thoughts about herself, her relationship, her sexuality, and her partner, are addressed. Sex therapy focuses more on interpersonal issues as well as sexual details and may include sensate focus techniques.[296-303] These consist of exchanging physical touch, moving from nonsexual to sexual areas of the body similar to systemic desensitization in other behavior therapies that reduce anxiety. When more distant factors are relevant, for instance, when sexual symptoms are thought to result from past (nonsexual) events in childhood and/or from low sexual image, short-term psychotherapy may be necessary.

Unfortunately, outcome data for all these interventions are severely limited (Table 19–14).[304] These data are limited given the different durations of therapy (2 to 20 weeks), differences in follow-up (end of therapy to 3 years), and different ways of evaluating the outcome (clinician-determined, participant-determined, detailed outcome vs. "successful or unsuccessful"). Moreover, diagnosis of dysfunction and therapy has been based on the older model of sexual function. Studies are only just emerging in which change in triggered desire rather than spontaneous desire is measured.[209]

Pharmacologic Interventions

There are no FDA-approved medications for treating sexual dysfunction in women, save for estrogen therapy for dyspareunia related to vulvovaginal atrophy. Table 19–15 shows medications that have been used off label; efficacy data are sparse.[213-215,222,225,226,280-283,305-313] No studies include psychological intervention alongside the prescription of medication. In contrast, in clinical practice, after assessment of both partners,[314,315] typically, combinations of cognitive behavior therapy and sexual

TABLE 19–12 ASSESSMENT OF SEXUAL DYSFUNCTION

Item for Analysis	Method of Analysis
Sexual problem and reason for presenting at this time	Ask patient to describe in her own words. Clarify further with direct questions, giving options rather than leading questions, giving support and encouragement, acknowledgment of embarrassment, and reassurance that sexual problems are common.
Duration, consistency and priority, if more than one problem	Are problems present in all situations? Which problem is most troubling to her?
Context of sexual problems	Emotional intimacy with partner Activity/behavior just prior to sexual activity, privacy, sexual communication, time of day/fatigue level Birth control: adequacy, type, risk of STDs Usefulness of sexual stimulation, sexual knowledge
Rest of each partner's sexual response other than the given problem area	Check this currently and prior to the onset of the sexual problems.
Reaction of each partner	How each has reacted emotionally, sexually, and behaviorally?
Previous help	Compliance with recommendations and effectiveness
QUESTIONS TO ASK EACH PARTNER WHEN SEEN ALONE	
Partner's own assessment of the situation	Sometimes it is easier to disclose symptom severity, e.g., total lack of desire, in the partner's absence.
Sexual response with self-stimulation	Also inquire about sexual thoughts and fantasies.
Past sexual experiences*	Positive, negative aspects
Developmental history*	Relationships to others in the home while growing up Losses, traumas, to whom (if anyone); were they close? Were they shown physical affection, love, respect?
Past or current sexual, emotional, and physical abuse*	Explain that abuse questions are routine and do not necessarily imply causation of the problems. It is helpful to ask if they ever felt hurt or threatened in the relationship and, if so, do they wish to give more information.
Physical health, especially conditions leading to debility and fatigue; difficulty with mobility as in caressing a partner or self-stimulation; difficulties with self-image, e.g., from stomas, disfiguring surgery, continence concerns	Specifically ask about medications with known sexual side effects, including SSRIs, β-blockers, antiandrogens, GnRH agonists, oral contraceptives.
Evaluation of mood	A significant correlation of sexual function and mood (including anxiety and depression) warrants routine screening for mood disorder using either a questionnaire (e.g., Beck Inventory) or semi-structured series of questions.

GnRH, gonadotropin releasing hormone; SSRI, selective serotonin reuptake inhibitor.
*Item may sometimes be omitted (e.g., for a recent problem after decades of healthy sexual function).
Adapted with permission from Basson R. Sexual dysfunction in women. New Engl J Med 2006;354(14):1497-1506.

therapy are given to augment the effect of any investigational drug therapy.

Hormonal Therapies

Estrogen

Local therapy is recommended for dyspareunia associated with vulvovaginal atrophy. Low doses can be supplied by a Silastic vaginal ring or a mucoadhesive vaginal tablet with similar benefit and very low systemic absorption. The available selective estrogen receptor modulators (SERMs) are not estrogen agonists in the vagina. Fortunately, SERMs appear to have many individual and class effects, and lasofoxifene (currently under investigation) has been shown to relieve vaginal atrophy. Tibolone, a synthetic steroid with tissue-specific action, improves vaginal atrophy. Further trials in sexually symptomatic women are awaited and tibolone remains unavailable in North America.

When systemic estrogen is needed it is sometimes necessary to also give additional local estrogen; local estrogen can be continued indefinitely.[316] When estrogen supplementation has ameliorated insomnia or dyspareunia, motivation to be sexual would logically be expected to increase, but this has not been rigorously studied. No significant differences were found between estrogen and placebo groups in reported sexual satisfaction in the Women's Health Initiative trial. However, sexual dysfunction was not a primary focus: specifically, women with marked menopausal symptoms were excluded, and the assessment questionnaire was inadequate.[316]

Testosterone

The role of testosterone therapy to ameliorate women's complaints of low sexual desire, aiming for serum levels that approach those in the normal range of younger women, is currently under investigation. Women are recruited on the basis of symptoms rather than testosterone levels, and five of the six

TABLE 19–13 PHYSICAL EXAMINATION FOR THE WOMAN WITH SEXUAL DYSFUNCTION

Examination	What to Look for
General	Signs of systemic disease leading to low energy, low desire, low arousability: anemia, bradycardia, slow relaxing reflexes of hypothyroidism Signs of connective tissue disease such as scleroderma or Sjögren's, which are associated with vaginal dryness Disabilities that might preclude movements involved in caressing a partner, self-stimulation, intercourse Disfigurements, stomas, catheters that an decrease sexual self-confidence, leading to low desire, low arousability
External genitalia	Sparse pubic hair, suggesting low adrenal androgens Vulvar skin disorders, including lichen sclerosis, which can cause soreness with sexual stimulation Cracks or fissures in the interlabial folds, suggesting chronic candidiasis Labial abnormalities that can cause embarrassment or sexual hesitancy, e.g., particularly long labia or asymmetry
Introitus	Vulvar disease involving introitus, e.g., pallor, friability, loss of elasticity and moisture, vulvar atrophy, lichen sclerosis Recurrent splitting of the posterior fourchette, manifest as just-visible white lines perpendicular to fourchette edge Abnormalities of the hymen Adhesions of the labia minora Swellings in the area of the major vestibular glands Allodynia (pain sensation from touch stimulus) of the crease between the outer hymenal edge and the inner edge of the labia minora, which are typical of vulvar vestibulitis Cystocele, rectocele, or prolapse interfering with the woman's sexual self-image Inability to tighten and relax perivaginal muscles, often associated with hypertonicity of pelvic muscles and mid-vaginal dyspareunia Abnormal vaginal discharge associated with burning dyspareunia
Internal	Pelvic muscle tone Tenderness Trigger points on palpating deep levator ani due to underlying hypertonicity
Full bimanual	Nodules and/or tenderness in the cul-de-sac or vaginal fornix, along uterosacral ligaments Retroverted fixed uterus as cause of deep dyspareunia Tenderness palpating posterior bladder wall from anterior vaginal wall, suggesting bladder pathology

Adapted with permission from Basson R. Sexual dysfunction in women. New Engl J Med 2006;354(14):1497-1506.

recent trials have been in surgically menopausal women.[212-215,225] The women received estrogen therapy: oral in four studies, transdermal in one, and a mixture in one. All studies were industry sponsored, and the (validated) questionnaire used for assessment and change with treatment has not been published. The first study was crossover in design,[212] the remainder were parallel groups.

The first study showed benefit with active drug in sexual response but not in aspects of desire (sexual thoughts, fantasies, initial desire ahead of sexual experiences) and the remainder showed improvements in selected aspects of response and desire. In terms of diary-recorded "sexually satisfying experiences," global outcome differences were small. Pooling the data shows that women receiving testosterone had 1.9 more episodes of satisfying sexual activity per month compared with baseline, whereas those receiving placebo reported 0.9 more than at baseline. Benefit over placebo was observed with patches nominally delivering 300 μg daily but not with either 150 or 450 μg daily.

Studies lasted 24 weeks. The short-term administration has not been associated with significant increases in hirsutism, acne, or virilizing effects. Nor were there changes in lipid parameters.

Despite the documented benefit of transdermal testosterone in estrogen-replete women, there are currently three major factors to preclude any broad recommendation by regulating bodies[314,315] or the American Endocrine Society.[317] The first is that women usually wish to remain sexually active indefinitely, and long-term safety data of testosterone therapy are lacking. Second, there are no data for sexual benefit of testosterone supplementation in estrogen-deficient women; because of the widespread reservations about long-term estrogen therapy, no long-term testosterone therapy can assume concomitant estrogen therapy. The third major reason is lack of clear definition of the target disorder. The recent RCTs are based on the old model of women's sexual response, which assumes women mainly initiate or accept sexual activity for reasons of desire. Studies need to be done in women who are motivated to be sexually active with their partner (for reasons other than desire) but find that their mind and body cannot be aroused by previously useful sexual stimuli. Many such women have been excluded from the recent RCTs given the likelihood that they have infrequent sexual activity, which by itself precluded recruitment.

Management of Vaginismus

Scientific study of management of vaginismus is sparse. That the two partners are involved in the maintenance of the unconsummated nature of the relationship has been repeatedly observed, but details on optimal management of the male partner's sexual caution have not been published.

Standard mechanistic therapy requires a series of visits over a period extending from a few weeks to many months. It involves assisting the woman to be better informed of her own anatomy and to learn to voluntarily open and close the introitus using Kegel and reverse Kegel exercises, preferably observing her ability to change the size of the introitus in a mirror. Changing her concept of "being penetrated" to one of being able to actively surround an object with her vagina is helpful. Daily self-touch as close to the introitus as possible is encouraged, progressing to insertion of the tip of a tampon, a vaginal insert, or her own finger. At this stage, she is encouraged to envisage being able to be examined by opening her labia with her own fingers such

TABLE 19–14 OUTCOME OF PSYCHOLOGICAL THERAPY

Publication	Treatment	Level of Efficacy
Delehanty (O)	DM and assertiveness training vs. waiting list control	82% became orgasmic
Hawton et al (D,A)	Modified sensate focus	57% significant improvement
Heiman and LoPiccolo (O)	CBT, DM, sensate focus vs. waiting list	Increased orgasmic response and initiation of sexual activity
Hurlbert (D,A)	Marital and sex therapy ± orgasm consistency training*	Significant improvements in arousal for sex therapy plus orgasm consistency given vs. sex therapy alone
Hurlbert and Apt (O)	DM and coital alignment	37% receiving coital alignment technique and DM vs. 18% receiving DM alone reported substantial improvements in orgasms experienced during intercourse
McCabe (D,A)	CBT	<50% significant improvement
McMullen and Rosen	DM with bibliotherapy vs. DM and videotape vs. waiting list control	65% and 55% became orgasmic
Sarwer and Durlak (D,A)	Behavioral and sex therapy	64% significant improvement
Trudel et al (D,A)	CBT	74% improved in sexual functioning and quality of marital life

*Orgasm consistency training includes encouragement of self-stimulation, sensate focus therapy with partner, and coital techniques to facilitate clitoral stimulation.

CBT, cognitive behavior therapy; D,A, desire and arousal dysfunction; DM, directed masturbation; O, orgasm dysfunction.

Delehanty R. Changes in assertiveness and changes in orgasmic response occurring in sexual therapy of preorgasmic women. J Sex Marital Ther 1982;8:198-208.

Hawton K, Catalan J, Flagg J. Low sexual desire: sex therapy results and prognostic factors. Behav Res Ther 1991;29:217-224.

Heiman J, LoPiccolo J. Clinical outcome of sex therapy. Effect of daily vs weekly treatment. Arch Gen Psychiatry 1983;40:443-449.

Hurlbert DF. A comparative study using orgasm consistency training in the treatment of women reporting hypoactive sexual desire. J Sex Marital Ther 1993;19:41-55.

Hurlbert DF, Apt C. Coital alignment technique and directed masturbation: a comparative study on female masturbation. J Sex and Marital Therapy 1995;21:21-29.

McCabe MP. Evaluation of a cognitive behavior therapy program for people with sexual dysfunction. J Sex Marital Ther 2001;27:259-271.

McMullen S, Rosen RC. Self-administered masturbation training in the treatment of primary orgasmic dysfunction. J Consult Clin Psychol 1979;47(5):912-918.

Sarwer DB, Durlak JA. A field trial of the effectiveness of behavioral treatment for sexual dysfunctions. J Sex Marital Ther 1997;23:87-97.

Trudel G, Marchand A, Ravart M, et al. The effect of a cognitive behavior treatment program on hypoactive sexual desire disorder in women. Sex Rel Ther 2001;16:145-164.

that her introitus can be viewed both her physician and by herself with the use of a mirror.

To be most informative and therapeutic, the physical exam is done when the woman is ready. The diagnosis is confirmed by excluding any anatomic abnormality or allodynia of vestibulitis or other pathology. Usually the first examination is partial and might involve no touching at all by the physician. Later, more complete examinations can be done. A series of vaginal inserts of increasing diameter is usually recommended. Some women choose to self-stimulate first, allowing physical genital arousal to facilitate the insert placement. Attempts at intercourse are strictly discouraged until larger inserts can be placed. Sharing that placement with her partner allows the woman to learn to share control. Throughout therapy, the couple is encouraged to be sexual in ways that exclude any penetration of the vagina.

Scientific study of the following recommended more holistic approach is also minimal. It consists of

- The mechanistic approach
- Encouragement of nonpenetrative sex with penile vulval (but not vaginal) stimulation
- Addressing the woman's thoughts about something entering her vagina and helping her to change these thoughts
- Addressing the man's general passivity in the relationship if it is felt to be detrimental
- Assisting the couple to cope with the anxiety invoked by the changes they are making; their situation has been tolerable and safe for them, often for very many years before help is sought.

In assisting the couple whose goal is to conceive rather than to have intercourse, once the woman can tolerate replacement of a smaller insert and is able to cooperate with a complete genital exam, she may chose to perform self-insemination of her partner's semen, either at home or with the physician's assistance in the clinic.

Outcome studies of the mechanistic approach are scant but suggest high success rates. The clinical experience is, however, that placement of the larger insert or placement of the partner's penis may well prove possible, but both partners moving on to enjoy intercourse together does not necessarily follow. Better understanding and management of the psychological issues for both partners is advocated.

Dyspareunia

Of the two most common causes of chronic dyspareunia, VVS and vulvovaginal atrophy, evidence-based therapy exists only for the latter. A number of medical, psychological, and surgical approaches to the management of VVS are reviewed in an NIH Consensus Report.[318] Prescription of chronic pain medication and encouragement of nonpenetrative sexual stimulation are the mainstays of conservative therapy. Improved understanding of different etiologic factors, possibly genetically based,[263] might allow scientifically based options of therapy.

TABLE 19–15 OFF LABEL USES OF DRUGS FOR INVESTIGATIONAL TREATMENT OF WOMEN'S SEXUAL DYSFUNCTION

Off-Label Use or Investigational Drug	Comments
SEXUAL INTEREST DESIRE DISORDER, SUBJECTIVE AND COMBINED AROUSAL DISORDERS	
Testosterone (testrogen)	Five multicenter parallel group RCTs of surgically (4 trials[213-215,225]) and naturally (1 trial[306]) menopausal women with diagnosed hypoactive desire disorder (DSM-IV-TR) improved "total satisfying sexual activity" and questionnaire measures of desire and response. No long-term safety data; no data on estrogen deplete women. One RCT of women with hypopituitary states showed improvement in sexual function.[280] Data from trials involving women with adrenal insufficiency are conflicting.[281-283]
DHEA (precursor of estradiol and testosterone)	A study of perimenopausal women with reduced feelings of well-being and low level of desire showed no benefit.[307] Two small studies showed benefit in women with hypopituitarism and in women with secondary hypoadrenal states.[281,282]
Ephedrine (α and β adrenergic agonist)	One RCT crossover study of 20 women.[310] 50 mg ephedrine increased vaginal congestion but not subjective arousal in response to erotic film.
Sildenafil (PDE5 inhibitor)	One level 1 study[305] involving 781 pre- and postmenopausal women with arousal and desire disorders (rather than specifically genital sexual arousal disorder) showed no improved measure of sexual desire, sensation, lubrication, or satisfaction.
Bupropion (doperimen nor adrenalin asonist)	One level 1 study[226] of women with hypoactive desire disorder (DSM-IV-TR) showed improvement in arousability and response but not in desire.
Tibolone (estrogenic, progestogenic, androgenic steroid)	European postmenopausal HT option associated with sexual benefit compared with placebo[308] or menopausal HT involving 17β-estradiol (1 mg) + norethindrone (1 mg). No studies in women with diagnosed sexual dysfunction. Breast safety in question.
Yohimbine (centrally acting noradrenergic) plus arginine (NO precursor)	One RCT crossover study of 24 women: 6 mg yohimbine plus 6 g arginine increased vaginal congestion but not subjective arousal in response to erotic film.[309]
GENITAL SEXUAL AROUSAL DISORDER DESPITE ESTROGEN REPLETE STATUS	
Sildenafil (PDE5 inhibitor)	Laboratory evidence of benefit[222]; clinically difficult to distinguish subgroup with GSAD due to reduced vasocongestion One small study showing benefit[311] No large studies focusing on GSAD
ORGASMIC DISORDER	
Sildenafil (PDE5 inhibitor)	One small RCT showing benefit in orgasmic disorder[312]
Argin Max (herbal supplement)	Small RCT showing benefit at 4 weeks[313]

Note: Only drugs for which at least one randomized trial has been published are listed.
*Only RCTs using testosterone to raise serum levels to values physiologic for younger women are included.
DHEA, dehydroepiandrosterone; GSAD, genital sexual arousal disorder; HT, hormone therapy; NO, nitric oxide; PDE, phosphodiesterase; RCT, randomized, controlled trial.
Adapted with permission from Basson R. Sexual dysfunction in women. New Engl J Med 2006;354(14):1497-1506.

Future Areas of Investigation

The role of intracellular sex hormone production and its intracrine effects needs further clarification. Measures of total androgen activity reflected by the circulating concentrations of androgen metabolites in women with and without dysfunction need further investigation. Development of more selective estrogen and androgen modulators might allow sexual benefits without unwanted adverse effects of either hormone. Randomized trials of combined modalities that include both medical and psychological approaches are much needed.

REFERENCES

1. Bhasin S, Benson GS. Male sexual function. In De Kretser D ed. Knobil and Neill's Physiology of Reproduction, 3rd ed. Boston: Academic Press, 2006:1173-1194.
2. Kinsey AC, Pomeroy WB, Martin CE. Sexual Behavior in the Human Male. Philadelphia: Saunders, 1948.
3. Masters EH, Johnson V. Human Sexual Response. Boston: Little, Brown, 1966.
4. Lue TF, Tanagho EA. Hemodynamics of erection. In Tanagho EA, Lue TF, McClure RD, eds. Contemporary Management of Impotence and Infertility. Baltimore: Williams and Wilkins, 1988:28-38.
5. Feldman HA, Goldstein I, Hatzichristou DG, et al. Impotence and its medical and psychosocial correlates: results of the Massachusetts Male Aging Study. J Urol 1994;151:54-61.
6. Laumann EO, Paik A, Rosen RC. The epidemiology of erectile dysfunction: results from the National Health and Social Life Survey. Int J Impot Res 1999;11(suppl 1):S60-S64.
7. Laumann EO, Paik A, Rosen RC. Sexual dysfunction in the United States: prevalence and predictors. JAMA 1999;281:537-544.
8. Segraves R, Woodards T. Female hypoactive sexual desire disorder: history and current status. J Sex Med 2006;3:408-418.

9. NIH Consensus Development Panel on Impotence. NIH Consensus Conference. Impotence. JAMA 1993;270:83-90.
10. The Process of Care Consensus Panel. The process of care model for evaluation and treatment of erectile dysfunction. Int J Impot Res 1999;11:59-70; discussion 70-74.
11. Benet AE, Melman A. The epidemiology of erectile dysfunction. Urol Clin North Am 1995;22:699-709.
12. Lipshultz LI, McConnell J, Benson GS. Current concepts of the mechanisms of ejaculation. Normal and abnormal states. J Reprod Med 1981;26:499-507.
13. Benson GS, McConnell J, Lipshultz LI, et al. Neuromorphology and neuropharmacology of the human penis: an in vitro study. J Clin Invest 1980;65:506-513.
14. Lue TF. Erectile dysfunction. N Engl J Med 2000;342:1802-1813.
15. Christ GJ. The penis as a vascular organ. The importance of corporal smooth muscle tone in the control of erection. Urol Clin North Am 1995;22:727-745.
16. Christ GJ. Gap junctions and ion channels: relevance to erectile dysfunction. Int J Impot Res 2000;12(suppl 4):S15-S25.
17. Zeng X, Keyser B, Li M, Sikka SC. T-type (α1G) low voltage–activated calcium channel interactions with nitric oxide–cyclic guanosine monophosphate pathway and regulation of calcium homeostasis in human cavernosal cells. J Sex Med 2005;2:620-630; discussion 630-633.
18. Somlyo AP, Somlyo AV. Ca^{2+} sensitivity of smooth muscle and nonmuscle myosin II: modulated by G proteins, kinases, and myosin phosphatase. Physiol Rev 2003;83:1325-1358.
19. O-Uchi J, Komukai K, Kusakari Y, et al. α_1-Adrenoceptor stimulation potentiates L-type Ca^{2+} current through Ca^{2+}/calmodulin-dependent PK II (CaMKII) activation in rat ventricular myocytes. Proc Natl Acad Sci U S A 2005;102:9400-9405.
20. Krall JF, Fittingoff M, Rajfer J. Characterization of cyclic nucleotide and inositol 1,4,5-trisphosphate–sensitive calcium-exchange activity of smooth muscle cells cultured from the human corpora cavernosa. Biol Reprod 1988;39:913-922.
21. Fittingoff M, Krall JF. Changes in inositol polyphosphate-sensitive calcium exchange in aortic smooth muscle cells in vitro. J Cell Physiol 1988;134:297-301.
22. Hewawasam P, Fan W, Ding M, et al. 4-Aryl-3-(hydroxyalkyl)quinolin-2-ones: novel maxi-K channel opening relaxants of corporal smooth muscle targeted for erectile dysfunction. J Med Chem 2003;46:2819-2822.
23. Christ GJ, Day N, Santizo C, et al. Intracorporal injection of hSlo cDNA restores erectile capacity in STZ-diabetic F-344 rats in vivo. Am J Physiol Heart Circ Physiol 2004;287:H1544-H1553.
24. Melman A, Bar-Chama N, McCullough A, et al. The first human trial for gene transfer therapy for the treatment of erectile dysfunction: preliminary results. Eur Urol 2005;48:314-318.
25. Christ GJ, Moreno AP, Melman A, Spray DC. Gap junction–mediated intercellular diffusion of Ca^{2+} in cultured human corporal smooth muscle cells. Am J Physiol 1992;263:C373-C383.
26. Ignarro LJ, Bush PA, Buga GM, et al. Nitric oxide and cyclic GMP formation upon electrical field stimulation cause relaxation of corpus cavernosum smooth muscle. Biochem Biophys Res Commun 1990;170:843-850.
27. Mills TM, Chitaley K, Lewis RW, Webb RC. Nitric oxide inhibits RhoA/Rho-kinase signaling to cause penile erection. Eur J Pharmacol 2002;439:173-174.
28. Naylor AM. Endogenous neurotransmitters mediating penile erection. Br J Urol 1998;81:424-431.
29. Goldstein I, Lue TF, Padma-Nathan H, et al. Oral sildenafil in the treatment of erectile dysfunction. Sildenafil Study Group [see comments] [published erratum appears in N Engl J Med 1998;339(1):59]. N Engl J Med 1998;338:1397-1404.
30. Gong MC, Iizuka K, Nixon G, et al. Role of guanine nucleotide-binding proteins—ras-family or trimeric proteins or both—in Ca^{2+} sensitization of smooth muscle. Proc Natl Acad Sci U S A 1996; 93:1340-1345.
31. Chikumi H, Fukuhara S, Gutkind JS. Regulation of G protein–linked guanine nucleotide exchange factors for Rho, PDZ-RhoGEF, and LARG by tyrosine phosphorylation: evidence of a role for focal adhesion kinase. J Biol Chem 2002;277:12463-12473.
32. Gong MC, Fujihara H, Somlyo AV, Somlyo AP. Translocation of RhoA associated with Ca2+ sensitization of smooth muscle. J Biol Chem 1997;272:10704-10709.
33. Wang H, Eto M, Steers WD, et al. RhoA-mediated Ca^{2+} sensitization in erectile function. J Biol Chem 2002;277:30614-30621.
34. Jin L, Liu T, Lagoda GA, et al. Elevated RhoA/Rho-kinase activity in the aged rat penis: mechanism for age-associated erectile dysfunction. Faseb J 2006;20:536-538.
35. Mills TM, Chitaley K, Wingard CJ, et al. Effect of Rho-kinase inhibition on vasoconstriction in the penile circulation. J Appl Physiol 2001;91:1269-1273.
36. Kwan M, Greenleaf WJ, Mann J, et al. The nature of androgen action on male sexuality: a combined laboratory–self-report study on hypogonadal men. J Clin Endocrinol Metab 1983;57:557-562.
37. Alexander GM, Sherwin BB. The association between testosterone, sexual arousal, and selective attention for erotic stimuli in men. Horm Behav 1991;25:367-381.
38. Redoute J, Stoleru S, Pugeat M, et al. Brain processing of visual sexual stimuli in treated and untreated hypogonadal patients. Psychoneuroendocrinology 2005;30:461-482.
39. King BE, Packard MG, Alexander GM. Affective properties of intra-medial preoptic area injections of testosterone in male rats. Neurosci Lett 1999;269:149-152.
40. Bagatell CJ, Heiman JR, Rivier JE, Bremner WJ. Effects of endogenous testosterone and estradiol on sexual behavior in normal young men [published erratum appears in J Clin Endocrinol Metab 1994;78(6):1520]. J Clin Endocrinol Metab 1994;78:711-716.
41. Carani C, Bancroft J, Granata A, et al. Testosterone and erectile function, nocturnal penile tumescence and rigidity, and erectile response to visual erotic stimuli in hypogonadal and eugonadal men. Psychoneuroendocrinology 1992;17:647-654.
42. Buena F, Swerdloff RS, Steiner BS, et al. Sexual function does not change when serum testosterone levels are pharmacologically varied within the normal male range. Fertil Steril 1993;59: 1118-1123.
43. Lugg JA, Rajfer J, Gonzalez-Cadavid NF. Dihydrotestosterone is the active androgen in the maintenance of nitric oxide-mediated penile erection in the rat. Endocrinology 1995;136:1495-1501.
44. Shabsigh R. The effects of testosterone on the cavernous tissue and erectile function. World J Urol 1997;15:21-26.
45. Bhasin S, Cunningham GR, Hayes FJ, et al. Testosterone therapy in adult men with androgen deficiency syndromes: an endocrine society clinical practice guideline. J Clin Endocrinol Metab 2006;91:1995-2010.
46. Arver S, Dobs AS, Meikle AW, et al. Improvement of sexual function in testosterone deficient men treated for 1 year with a permeation enhanced testosterone transdermal system. J Urol 1996;155: 1604-1608.
47. Jain P, Rademaker AW, McVary KT. Testosterone supplementation for erectile dysfunction: results of a meta-analysis. J Urol 2000;164:371-375.
48. Shabsigh R, Kaufman JM, Steidle C, Padma-Nathan H. Randomized study of testosterone gel as adjunctive therapy to sildenafil in hypogonadal men with erectile dysfunction who do not respond to sildenafil alone. J Urol 2004;172:658-663.
49. Aversa A, Mazzilli F, Rossi T, et al. Effects of sildenafil (Viagra) administration on seminal parameters and post-ejaculatory refractory time in normal males. Hum Reprod 2000;15:131-134.
50. Korenman SG, Morley JE, Mooradian AD, et al. Secondary hypogonadism in older men: its relation to impotence. J Clin Endocrinol Metab 1990;71:963-969.
51. Beck JG. Hypoactive sexual desire disorder: an overview. J Consult Clin Psychol 1995;63:919-927.
52. Rosen RC, Leiblum SR. Hypoactive sexual desire. Psychiatr Clin North Am 1995;18:107-121.
53. Segraves KB, Segraves RT. Hypoactive sexual desire disorder: prevalence and comorbidity in 906 subjects. J Sex Marital Ther 1991;17:55-58.
54. Panser LA, Rhodes T, Girman CJ, et al. Sexual function of men ages 40 to 79 years: the Olmsted County Study of Urinary Symptoms and Health Status Among Men. J Am Geriatr Soc 1995;43:1107-1111.
55. LoPiccolo J. Diagnosis and treatment of male sexual dysfunction. J Sex Marital Ther 1985;11:215-232.
56. Chevret M, Jaudinot E, Sullivan K, et al. Impact of erectile dysfunction (ED) on sexual life of female partners: assessment with the Index of Sexual Life (ISL) questionnaire. J Sex Marital Ther 2004;30:157-172.

57. Johannes CB, Araujo AB, Feldman HA, et al. Incidence of erectile dysfunction in men 40 to 69 years old: longitudinal results from the Massachusetts Male Aging Study. J Urol 2000;163:460-463.
58. Braun M, Wassmer G, Klotz T, et al. Epidemiology of erectile dysfunction: results of the "Cologne Male Survey." Int J Impot Res 2000;12:305-311.
59. McKinlay JB, Digruttolo L, Glasser D, et al. International differences in the epidemiology of male erectile dysfunction. Int J Clin Pract Suppl 1999;102:35.
60. McKinlay JB. The worldwide prevalence and epidemiology of erectile dysfunction. Int J Impot Res 2000;12(suppl 4):S6-S11.
61. Ayta IA, McKinlay JB, Krane RJ. The likely worldwide increase in erectile dysfunction between 1995 and 2025 and some possible policy consequences. BJU Int 1999;84:50-56.
62. Feldman HA, Johannes CB, Derby CA, et al. Erectile dysfunction and coronary risk factors: prospective results from the Massachusetts Male Aging Study. Prev Med 2000;30:328-338.
63. Derby CA, Mohr BA, Goldstein I, et al. Modifiable risk factors and erectile dysfunction: can lifestyle changes modify risk? Urology 2000;56:302-306.
64. Rosen R, Altwein J, Boyle P, et al. Lower urinary tract symptoms and male sexual dysfunction: the multinational survey of the aging male (MSAM-7). Eur Urol 2003;44:637-649.
65. Braun MH, Sommer F, Haupt G, et al. Lower urinary tract symptoms and erectile dysfunction: co-morbidity or typical "Aging Male" symptoms? Results of the "Cologne Male Survey." Eur Urol 2003;44:588-594.
66. Barqawi A, O'Donnell C, Kumar R, et al. Correlation between LUTS (AUA-SS) and erectile dysfunction (SHIM) in an age-matched racially diverse male population: data from the Prostate Cancer Awareness Week (PCAW). Int J Impot Res 2005;17:370-374.
67. Glina S, Santana AW, Azank F, et al. Lower urinary tract symptoms and erectile dysfunction are highly prevalent in ageing men. BJU Int 2006;97:763-765.
68. McVary K. Lower urinary tract symptoms and sexual dysfunction: epidemiology and pathophysiology. BJU Int 2006;97(suppl 2):23-28; discussion 44-45.
69. Paick SH, Meehan A, Lee M, Penson DF, Wessells H. The relationship among lower urinary tract symptoms, prostate specific antigen and erectile dysfunction in men with benign prostatic hyperplasia: results from the proscar long-term efficacy and safety study. J Urol 2005;173:903-907.
70. McVary KT. Interrelation of erectile dysfunction and lower urinary tract symptoms. Drugs Today (Barc) 2005;41:527-536.
71. Christ GJ, Hodges S. Molecular mechanisms of detrusor and corporal myocyte contraction: identifying targets for pharmacotherapy of bladder and erectile dysfunction. Br J Pharmacol 2006;147(suppl 2):S41-S55.
72. NIH Consensus Development Panel on Impotence. HIH Consensus Conference. JAMA 1993;270:83-90.
73. Cappelleri JC, Rosen RC, Smith MD, et al. Diagnostic evaluation of the erectile function domain of the International Index of Erectile Function. Urology 1999;54:346-351.
74. Lue TF, Giuliano F, Montorsi F, et al. Summary of the recommendations on sexual dysfunctions in men. J Sex Med 2004;1:6-23.
75. O'Leary MP, Fowler FJ, Lenderking WR, et al. A brief male sexual function inventory. Urology 1995;46:697-706.
76. Rosen RC, Cappelleri JC, Smith MD, et al. Development and evaluation of an abridged, 5-item version of the International Index of Erectile Function (IIEF-5) as a diagnostic tool for erectile dysfunction. Int J Impot Res 1999;11:319-326.
77. Aitchison M, Aitchison J, Carter R. Is the penile brachial index a reproducible and useful measurement? Br J Urol 1990;66:202-204.
78. Mueller SC, Wallenberg-Pachaly H, Voges GE, Schild HH. Comparison of selective internal iliac pharmaco-angiography, penile brachial index and duplex sonography with pulsed Doppler analysis for the evaluation of vasculogenic (arteriogenic) impotence. J Urol 1990;143:928-932.
79. Brock G. Tumescence monitoring devices: past and present. In Hellstrom, WJG, ed, The Handbook of Sexual Dysfunction. San Francisco: American Society of Andrology, Allen Press, Lawrence, Kamsas 1999:65-69.
80. Buvat J, Lemaire A. Endocrine screening in 1,022 men with erectile dysfunction: clinical significance and cost-effective strategy [see comments]. J Urol 1997;158:1764-1767.
81. Citron JT, Ettinger B, Rubinoff H, et al. Prevalence of hypothalamic-pituitary imaging abnormalities in impotent men with secondary hypogonadism. J Urol 1996;155:529-533.
82. Rosen RC. Psychogenic erectile dysfunction. Classification and management. Urol Clin North Am 2001;28:269-278.
83. Abrahamson DJ, Barlow DH, Beck JG, et al. The effects of attentional focus and partner responsiveness on sexual responding: replication and extension. Arch Sex Behav 1985;14:361-371.
84. Kilmann PR, Boland JP, Norton SP, Davidson E, Caid C. Perspectives of sex therapy outcome: a survey of AASECT providers. J Sex Marital Ther 1986;12:116-138.
85. Montague DK, Jarow JP, Broderick GA, et al. Chapter 1: The management of erectile dysfunction: an AUA update. J Urol 2005;174:230-239.
86. Haning H, Niewohner U, Bischoff E. Phosphodiesterase type 5 (PDE5) inhibitors. Prog Med Chem 2003;41:249-306.
87. Bischoff E. Potency, selectivity, and consequences of nonselectivity of PDE inhibition. Int J Impot Res 2004;16(suppl 1):S11-S14.
88. Boolell M, Allen MJ, Ballard SA, et al. Sildenafil: an orally active type 5 cyclic GMP-specific phosphodiesterase inhibitor for the treatment of penile erectile dysfunction. Int J Impot Res 1996;8:47-52.
89. Taher A, Meyer M, Stief CG, et al. Cyclic nucleotide phosphodiesterase in human cavernous smooth muscle. World J Urol 1997;15:32-35.
90. Jeremy JY, Ballard SA, Naylor AM, et al. Effects of sildenafil, a type-5 cGMP phosphodiesterase inhibitor, and papaverine on cyclic GMP and cyclic AMP levels in the rabbit corpus cavernosum in vitro. Br J Urol 1997;79:958-963.
91. Stief CG, Uckert S, Becker AJ, et al. The effect of the specific phosphodiesterase (PDE) inhibitors on human and rabbit cavernous tissue in vitro and in vivo. J Urol 1998;159:1390-1393.
92. Carter AJ, Ballard SA, Naylor AM. Effect of the selective phosphodiesterase type 5 inhibitor sildenafil on erectile dysfunction in the anesthetized dog. J Urol 1998;160:242-246.
93. Wallis RM, Corbin JD, Francis SH, Ellis P. Tissue distribution of phosphodiesterase families and the effects of sildenafil on tissue cyclic nucleotides, platelet function, and the contractile responses of trabeculae carneae and aortic rings in vitro. Am J Cardiol 1999;83:3C-12C.
94. Saenz de Tejada I, Angulo J, Cuevas P, et al. The phosphodiesterase inhibitory selectivity and the in vitro and in vivo potency of the new PDE5 inhibitor vardenafil. Int J Impot Res 2001;13:282-290.
95. Goldstein I. A 36-week, open label, non-comparative study to assess the long-term safety of sildenafil citrate (Viagra) in patients with erectile dysfunction. Int J Clin Pract Suppl 1999;102:8-9.
96. Rendell MS, Rajfer J, Wicker PA, Smith MD. Sildenafil for treatment of erectile dysfunction in men with diabetes: a randomized controlled trial. Sildenafil Diabetes Study Group [see comments]. JAMA 1999;281:421-426.
97. Yu G, Mason H, Wu X, et al. Substituted pyrazolopyridopyridazines as orally bioavailable potent and selective PDE5 inhibitors: potential agents for treatment of erectile dysfunction. J Med Chem 2003;46:457-460.
98. Seftel AD. Phosphodiesterase type 5 inhibitor differentiation based on selectivity, pharmacokinetic, and efficacy profiles. Clin Cardiol 2004;27:I14-I19.
99. Grossman EB, Swan SK, Muirhead GJ, et al. The pharmacokinetics and hemodynamics of sildenafil citrate in male hemodialysis patients. Kidney Int 2004;66:367-374.
100. Sussman DO. Pharmacokinetics, pharmacodynamics, and efficacy of phosphodiesterase type 5 inhibitors. J Am Osteopath Assoc 2004;104:S11-S15.
101. Rajagopalan P, Mazzu A, Xia C, et al. Effect of high-fat breakfast and moderate-fat evening meal on the pharmacokinetics of vardenafil, an oral phosphodiesterase-5 inhibitor for the treatment of erectile dysfunction. J Clin Pharmacol 2003;43:260-267.
102. Blanker MH, Thomas S, Bohnen AM. Systematic review of Viagra RCTs. Br J Gen Pract 2002;52:329.

103. Burls A, Gold L, Clark W. Systematic review of randomised controlled trials of sildenafil (Viagra) in the treatment of male erectile dysfunction. Br J Gen Pract 2001;51:1004-1012.
104. Fink HA, Mac Donald R, Rutks IR, et al. Sildenafil for male erectile dysfunction: a systematic review and meta-analysis. Arch Intern Med 2002;162:1349-1360.
105. Markou S, Perimenis P, Gyftopoulos K, et al. Vardenafil (Levitra) for erectile dysfunction: a systematic review and meta-analysis of clinical trial reports. Int J Impot Res 2004;16:470-478.
106. Montorsi F, McCullough A. Efficacy of sildenafil citrate in men with erectile dysfunction following radical prostatectomy: a systematic review of clinical data. J Sex Med 2005;2:658-667.
107. Moore RA, Derry S, McQuay HJ. Indirect comparison of interventions using published randomised trials: systematic review of PDE-5 inhibitors for erectile dysfunction. BMC Urol 2005;5:18.
108. Jarow JP, Burnett AL, Geringer AM. Clinical efficacy of sildenafil citrate based on etiology and response to prior treatment [see comments]. J Urol 1999;162:722-725.
109. Dinsmore WW, Hodges M, Hargreaves C, et al. Sildenafil citrate (Viagra) in erectile dysfunction: near normalization in men with broad-spectrum erectile dysfunction compared with age- matched healthy control subjects [published erratum appears in Urology 1999;53(5):1072]. Urology 1999;53:800-805.
110. Goldenberg MM. Safety and efficacy of sildenafil citrate in the treatment of male erectile dysfunction. Clin Ther 1998;20: 1033-1048.
111. Brock G, Nehra A, Lipshultz LI, et al. Safety and efficacy of vardenafil for the treatment of men with erectile dysfunction after radical retropubic prostatectomy. J Urol 2003;170:1278-1283.
112. Donatucci C, Eardley I, Buvat J, et al. Vardenafil improves erectile function in men with erectile dysfunction irrespective of disease severity and disease classification. J Sex Med 2004; 1:301-309.
113. Donatucci C, Taylor T, Thibonnier M, et al. Vardenafil improves patient satisfaction with erection hardness, orgasmic function, and overall sexual experience, while improving quality of life in men with erectile dysfunction. J Sex Med 2004;1:185-192.
114. Hatzichristou D, Montorsi F, Buvat J, et al. The efficacy and safety of flexible-dose vardenafil (Levitra) in a broad population of European men. Eur Urol 2004;45:634-641.
115. Hellstrom WJ, Gittelman M, Karlin G, et al. Vardenafil for treatment of men with erectile dysfunction: efficacy and safety in a randomized, double-blind, placebo-controlled trial. J Androl 2002;23: 763-771.
116. Nehra A, Grantmyre J, Nadel A, et al. Vardenafil improved patient satisfaction with erectile hardness, orgasmic function and sexual experience in men with erectile dysfunction following nerve sparing radical prostatectomy. J Urol 2005;173:2067-2071.
117. Rosen R, Shabsigh R, Berber M, et al. Efficacy and tolerability of vardenafil in men with mild depression and erectile dysfunction: the depression-related improvement with vardenafil for erectile response study. Am J Psychiatry 2006;163:79-87.
118. Brock GB, McMahon CG, Chen KK, et al. Efficacy and safety of tadalafil for the treatment of erectile dysfunction: results of integrated analyses. J Urol 2002;168:1332-1336.
119. Carson C, Shabsigh R, Segal S, et al. Efficacy, safety, and treatment satisfaction of tadalafil versus placebo in patients with erectile dysfunction evaluated at tertiary-care academic centers. Urology 2005;65:353-359.
120. Padma-Nathan H, McMurray JG, Pullman WE, et al. On-demand IC351 (Cialis) enhances erectile function in patients with erectile dysfunction. Int J Impot Res 2001;13:2-9.
121. Porst H, Padma-Nathan H, Giuliano F, et al. Efficacy of tadalafil for the treatment of erectile dysfunction at 24 and 36 hours after dosing: a randomized controlled trial. Urology 2003;62:121-125; discussion 125-126.
122. Saenz de Tejada I, Anglin G, Knight JR, Emmick JT. Effects of tadalafil on erectile dysfunction in men with diabetes. Diabetes Care 2002;25:2159-2164.
123. Staab A, Tillmann C, Forgue ST, et al. Population dose-response model for tadalafil in the treatment of male erectile dysfunction. Pharm Res 2004;21:1463-1470.
124. Giuliano F, Hultling C, el Masry WS, et al. Randomized trial of sildenafil for the treatment of erectile dysfunction in spinal cord injury. Sildenafil Study Group. Ann Neurol 1999;46:15-21.
125. Morales A, Gingell C, Collins M, et al. Clinical safety of oral sildenafil citrate (Viagra) in the treatment of erectile dysfunction. Int J Impot Res 1998;10:69-73.
126. Hatzichristou DG. Phosphodiesterase 5 inhibitors and nonarteritic anterior ischemic optic neuropathy (NAION): coincidence or causality. J Sex Med 2004;2:751-758.
127. Buono L, Foroozan R, Sergott RC, Savino PJ. Nonarteritic anterior ischemic optic neuropathy. Curr Opin Ophthamol 2002;13: 357-361.
128. Feenstra J, Drie-Pierik RJ, Lacle CF, Stricker BH. Acute myocardial infarction associated with sildenafil [letter] [see comments]. Lancet 1998;352:957-958.
129. Zusman RM, Morales A, Glasser DB, Osterloh IH. Overall cardiovascular profile of sildenafil citrate. Am J Cardiol 1999;83: 35C-44C.
130. Cheitlin MD, Hutter AM Jr, Brindis RG, et al. Use of sildenafil (Viagra) in patients with cardiovascular disease. Technology and Practice Executive Committee [published erratum appears in Circulation 1999;100(23):2389] [see comments]. Circulation 1999;99:168-177.
131. Muller JE, Mittleman A, Maclure M, et al. Triggering myocardial infarction by sexual activity. Low absolute risk and prevention by regular physical exertion. Determinants of Myocardial Infarction Onset Study Investigators [see comments]. JAMA 1996;275: 1405-1409.
132. Herrmann HC, Chang G, Klugherz BD, Mahoney PD. Hemodynamic effects of sildenafil in men with severe coronary artery disease. N Engl J Med 2000;342:1622-1626.
133. Kloner RA. Cardiovascular risk and sildenafil. Am J Cardiol 2000;86:57F-61F.
134. Highleyman L. Protease inhibitors and sildenafil (Viagra) should not be combined. BETA 1999;12:3.
135. Bailey DG, Dresser GK. Interactions between grapefruit juice and cardiovascular drugs. Am J Cardiovasc Drugs 2004;4:281-297.
136. Conti CR, Pepine CJ, Sweeney M. Efficacy and safety of sildenafil citrate in the treatment of erectile dysfunction in patients with ischemic heart disease. Am J Cardiol 1999;83:29C-34C.
137. Wespes E, Amar E, Hatzichristou D, et al. EAU Guidelines on erectile dysfunction: an update. Eur Urol 2006;49:806-815.
138. McMahon C. Comparison of efficacy, safety, and tolerability of on-demand tadalafil and daily dosed tadalafil for the treatment of erectile dysfunction. J Sex Med 2005;2:415-425; discussion 425-417.
139. Carson CC 3rd. Cardiac safety in clinical trials of phosphodiesterase 5 inhibitors. Am J Cardiol 2005;96:37M-41M.
140. Jackson G. Hemodynamic and exercise effects of phosphodiesterase 5 inhibitors. Am J Cardiol 2005;96:32M-36M.
141. Kloner RA. Novel phosphodiesterase type 5 inhibitors: assessing hemodynamic effects and safety parameters. Clin Cardiol 2004;27: I20-I25.
142. Thadani U, Smith W, Nash S, et al. The effect of vardenafil, a potent and highly selective phosphodiesterase-5 inhibitor for the treatment of erectile dysfunction, on the cardiovascular response to exercise in patients with coronary artery disease. J Am Coll Cardiol 2002;40:2006-2012.
143. McCullough AR, Barada JH, Fawzy A, et al. Achieving treatment optimization with sildenafil citrate (Viagra) in patients with erectile dysfunction. Urology 2002;60:28-38.
144. Lau DH, Kommu S, Mumtaz FH, et al. The management of phosphodiesterase inhibitor failure. Curr Vasc Pharmacol 2006;4: 89-93.
145. Martinez JM Prognostic factors for response to sildenafil in patients with erectile dysfunction. Eur Urol 40:641-646.
146. Wespes E, Rammal A, Garbar C. Sildenafil no-responders: hemodynamic and morphometric studies. Eur Urol 2005;48:136-139.
147. McGarvey MR. Tough choices: the cost-effectiveness of sildenafil [editorial; comment]. Ann Intern Med 2000;132:994-995.
148. Smith KJ, Roberts MS. The cost-effectiveness of sildenafil [see comments]. Ann Intern Med 2000;132:933-937.
149. Tan HL. Economic cost of male erectile dysfunction using a decision analytic model: for a hypothetical managed-care plan of 100,000 members. Pharmacoeconomics 2000;17:77-107.
150. Sun P, Seftel A, Swindle R, et al. The costs of caring for erectile dysfunction in a managed care setting: evidence from a large national claims database. J Urol 2005;174:1948-1952.

151. Plumb JM, Guest JF. Annual cost of erectile dysfunction to UK society. Pharmacoeconomics 1999;16:699-709.
152. Vrijhof HJ, Delaere KP. Vacuum constriction devices in erectile dysfunction: acceptance and effectiveness in patients with impotence of organic or mixed aetiology. Br J Urol 1994;74:102-105.
153. Cookson MS, Nadig PW. Long-term results with vacuum constriction device. J Urol 1993;149:290-294.
154. Lewis JH, Sidi AA, Reddy PK. A way to help your patients who use vacuum devices. Contemp Urol 1991;3:15-21.
155. Engelhardt PF, Plas E, Hubner WA, Pfluger H. Comparison of intraurethral liposomal and intracavernosal prostaglandin-E_1 in the management of erectile dysfunction. Br J Urol 1998;81: 441-444.
156. Kim ED, McVary KT. Topical prostaglandin-E_1 for the treatment of erectile dysfunction [see comments]. J Urol 1995;153:1828-1830.
157. Peterson CA, Bennett AH, Hellstrom WJ, et al. Erectile response to transurethral alprostadil, prazosin and alprostadil-prazosin combinations. J Urol 1998;159:1523-1527.
158. Fulgham PF, Cochran JS, Denman JL, et al. Disappointing initial results with transurethral alprostadil for erectile dysfunction in a urology practice setting. J Urol 1998;160:2041-2046.
159. Buvat J, Lemaire A, Ratajczyk J. Acceptance, efficacy and preference of sildenafil in patients on long term auto-intracavernosal therapy: a study with follow-up at one year. Int J Impot Res 2002;14:483-486.
160. El-Sakka AI. Intracavernosal prostaglandin E_1 self vs office injection therapy in patients with erectile dysfunction. Int J Impot Res 2006;18:180-185.
161. Heaton JP, Lording D, Liu SN, et al. Intracavernosal alprostadil is effective for the treatment of erectile dysfunction in diabetic men. Int J Impot Res 2001;13:317-321.
162. Linet OI, Ogrinc FG. Efficacy and safety of intracavernosal alprostadil in men with erectile dysfunction. The Alprostadil Study Group. N Engl J Med 1996;334:873-877.
163. Mulhall JP, Daller M, Traish AM, et al. Intracavernosal forskolin: role in management of vasculogenic impotence resistant to standard 3-agent pharmacotherapy. J Urol 1997;158:1752-1758; discussion 1758-1759.
164. Nehra A, Blute ML, Barrett DM, Moreland RB. Rationale for combination therapy of intraurethral prostaglandin E_1 and sildenafil in the salvage of erectile dysfunction patients desiring noninvasive therapy. Int J Impot Res 2002;14(suppl 1):S38-S42.
165. Tsai YS, Lin JS, Lin YM. Safety and efficacy of alprostadil sterile powder (S. Po., CAVERJECT) in diabetic patients with erectile dysfunction. Eur Urol 2000;38:177-183.
166. Shabsigh R, Padma-Nathan H, Gittleman M, et al. Intracavernous alprostadil alfadex is more efficacious, better tolerated, and preferred over intraurethral alprostadil plus optional actis: a comparative, randomized, crossover, multicenter study. Urology 2000;55:109-113.
167. Chew KK. Intracavernosal injection therapy. Does it still have a role in erectile dysfunction? Aust Fam Physician 2001;30:43-46.
168. European Alprostadil Study Group. The long-term safety of alprostadil (prostaglandin-E_1) in patients with erectile dysfunction. Br J Urol 1998;82:538-543.
169. Dinsmore WW, Gingell C, Hackett G, et al. Treating men with predominantly nonpsychogenic erectile dysfunction with intracavernosal vasoactive intestinal polypeptide and phentolamine mesylate in a novel auto-injector system: a multicentre double-blind placebo-controlled study. BJU Int 1999;83:274-279.
170. Hellstrom WJ, Usta MF. Surgical approaches for advanced Peyronie's disease patients. Int J Impot Res 2003;15(suppl 5):S121-S124.
171. Usta MF, Bivalacqua TJ, Sanabria J, et al. Patient and partner satisfaction and long-term results after surgical treatment for Peyronie's disease. Urology 2003;62:105-109.
172. Carson CC, Mulcahy JJ, Govier FE. Efficacy, safety and patient satisfaction outcomes of the AMS 700CX inflatable penile prosthesis: results of a long-term multicenter study. AMS 700CX Study Group. J Urol 2000;164:376-380.
173. Wilson SK, Cleves MA, Delk JR 2nd. Comparison of mechanical reliability of original and enhanced Mentor Alpha I penile prosthesis. J Urol 1999;162:715-718.
174. Carani C, Zini D, Baldini A, et al. Effects of androgen treatment in impotent men with normal and low levels of free testosterone. Arch Sex Behav 1990;19:223-234.
175. Hajjar RR, Kaiser FE, Morley JE. Outcomes of long-term testosterone replacement in older hypogonadal males: a retrospective analysis. J Clin Endocrinol Metab 1997;82:3793-3796.
176. Mills TM, Lewis RW, Stopper VS. Androgenic maintenance of inflow and veno-occlusion during erection in the rat. Biol Reprod 1998;59:1413-1418.
177. Fink HA, MacDonald R, Rutks IR, Wilt TJ. Trazodone for erectile dysfunction: a systematic review and meta-analysis. BJU Int 2003;92:441-446.
178. Lebret T, Herve JM, Gorny P, et al. Efficacy and safety of a novel combination of L-arginine glutamate and yohimbine hydrochloride: a new oral therapy for erectile dysfunction. Eur Urol 2002;41:608-613; discussion 613.
179. Fleshner N, Harvey M, Adomat H, et al. Evidence for pharmacological contamination of herbal erectile function products with type 5 phosphodiesterase inhibitors [abstract]. J Urol 2004;171:314.
180. Hong B, Ji YH, Hong JH, et al. A double-blind crossover study evaluating the efficacy of Korean red ginseng in patients with erectile dysfunction: a preliminary report. J Urol 2002;168: 2070-2073.
181. Wessells H, Gralnek D, Dorr R, et al. Effect of an α-melanocyte stimulating hormone analog on penile erection and sexual desire in men with organic erectile dysfunction. Urology 2000;56: 641-646.
182. Pfaus JG, Shadiack A, Van Soest T, et al. Selective facilitation of sexual solicitation in the female rat by a melanocortin receptor agonist. Proc Natl Acad Sci U S A 2004;101:10201-10204.
183. Rosen RC, Diamond LE, Earle DC, et al. Evaluation of the safety, pharmacokinetics and pharmacodynamic effects of subcutaneously administered PT-141, a melanocortin receptor agonist, in healthy male subjects and in patients with an inadequate response to Viagra. Int J Impot Res 2004;16:135-142.
184. Diamond LE, Earle DC, Rosen RC, et al. Double-blind, placebo-controlled evaluation of the safety, pharmacokinetic properties and pharmacodynamic effects of intranasal PT-141, a melanocortin receptor agonist, in healthy males and patients with mild-to-moderate erectile dysfunction. Int J Impot Res 2004;16:51-59.
185. Nabel EG, Pompil VJ, Plantz GE, Nabel GJ. Gene transfer and vascular disease. Cardiovasc Res 1994;28:445-455.
186. Heistad DD, Faraci FM. Gene therapy for cerebral vascular disease. Stroke 1996;27:1688-1693.
187. Bivalacqua TJ, Hellstrom WJ. Potential application of gene therapy for the treatment of erectile dysfunction. J Androl 2001; 22:183-190.
188. Christ GJ, Melman A. The application of gene therapy to the treatment of erectile dysfunction. Int J Impot Res 1998;10:111-112.
189. Chancellor MB, Yoshimura N, Pruchnic R, Huard J. Gene therapy strategies for urological dysfunction. Trends Mol Med 2001; 7:301-306.
190. Deng W, Bivalacqua TJ, Hellstrom WJ, Kadowitz PJ. Gene and stem cell therapy for erectile dysfunction. Int J Impot Res 2005;17(suppl 1):S57-S63.
191. Garban H, Marquez D, Magee T, et al. Cloning of rat and human inducible penile nitric oxide synthase. Application for gene therapy of erectile dysfunction. Biol Reprod 1997;56: 954-963.
192. Christ GJ, Rehman J, Day N, et al. Intracorporal injection of hSlo cDNA in rats produces physiologically relevant alterations in penile function. Am J Physiol 1998;275:H600-H608.
193. Bivalacqua TJ, Champion HC, Mehta YS, et al. Adenoviral gene transfer of endothelial nitric oxide synthase (eNOS) to the penis improves age-related erectile dysfunction in the rat. Int J Impot Res 2000;12(suppl 3):S8-S17.
194. Champion HC, Bivalacqua TJ, Hyman AL, et al. Gene transfer of endothelial nitric oxide synthase to the penis augments erectile responses in the aged rat. Proc Natl Acad Sci U S A 1999; 96:11648-11652.
195. Burchardt M, Burchardt T, Anastasiadis AG, et al. Application of angiogenic factors for therapy of erectile dysfunction: protein and DNA transfer of VEGF 165 into the rat penis. Urology 2005;66:665-670.
196. Rogers RS, Graziottin TM, Lin CS, et al. Intracavernosal vascular endothelial growth factor (VEGF) injection and adeno-associated virus-mediated VEGF gene therapy prevent and reverse venogenic erectile dysfunction in rats. Int J Impot Res 2003;15:26-37.

197. Deng W, Bivalacqua TJ, Chattergoon NN, et al. Adenoviral gene transfer of eNOS: high-level expression in ex vivo expanded marrow stromal cells. Am J Physiol Cell Physiol 2003;285: C1322-C1329.
198. Deng W, Bivalacqua TJ, Chattergoon NN, et al. Engineering ex vivo–expanded marrow stromal cells to secrete calcitonin gene-related peptide using adenoviral vector. Stem Cells 2004;22: 1279-1291.
199. McMahon CG, Abdo C, Incrocci L, et al. Disorders of orgasm and ejaculation in men. J Sex Med 2004;1:58-65.
200. Yeates WK. Ejaculation and its disorders. Arch Ital Urol Nefrol Androl 1990;62:137-148.
201. Gil-Vernet JM Jr, Alvarez-Vijande R, Gil-Vernet A, Gil-Vernet JM. Ejaculation in men: a dynamic endorectal ultrasonographical study. Br J Urol 1994;73:442-448.
202. Olivier B, Van Oorschot R, Waldinger M. Serotonin, serotonergic receptors, selective serotonin reuptake inhibitors and sexual behavior. Int Clin Psychopharmacol 1998;13(suppl 6):S9-S14.
203. Waldinger M. The neurobiological approach to early ejaculation. J Urol 2002;168:2359-2366.
204. Waldinger MD, Olivier B. Utility of selective serotonin reuptake inhibitors in premature ejaculation. Curr Opin Investig Drugs 2004;5:743-747.
205. Waldinger MD, Zwinderman AH, Olivier B. Antidepressants and ejaculation: a double-blind, randomized, fixed-dose study with mirtazapine and paroxetine. J Clin Psychopharmacol 2003;23: 467-470.
206. Cain VS, Johannes CB, Avis NE, et al. Sexual functioning and practices in a multi-ethnic study of midlife women: baseline results from SWAN. J Sex Res 2003;40:266-276.
207. Basson R. Clinical practice. Sexual desire and arousal disorders in women. N Engl J Med 2006;354:1497-1506.
208. Graham CA, Sanders SA, Milhausen RR, McBride KR. Turning on and turning off: a focus group study of the factors that affect women's sexual arousal. Arch Sex Behav 2004;33:527-538.
209. Basson R. Using a different model for female sexual response to address women's problematic low sexual desire. J Sex Marital Ther 2001;27:395-403.
210. Basson R. Sexual desire and arousal disorders in women. N Engl J Med 2006;354:1497-1506.
211. Galyer KT, Conaglen HM, Hare A, Conaglen JV. The effect of gynecological surgery on sexual desire. J Sex Marital Ther 1999;25:81-88.
212. Shifren JL, Braunstein GD, Simon JA, et al. Transdermal testosterone treatment in women with impaired sexual function after oophorectomy. N Engl J Med 2000;343:682-688.
213. Braunstein GD, Sundwall DA, Katz M, et al. Safety and efficacy of a testosterone patch for the treatment of hypoactive sexual desire disorder in surgically menopausal women: a randomized, placebo-controlled trial. Arch Intern Med 2005;165:1582-1589.
214. Buster JE, Kingsberg SA, Aguirre O, et al. Testosterone patch for low sexual desire in surgically menopausal women: a randomized trial. Obstet Gynecol 2005;105:944-952.
215. Simon J, Braunstein G, Nachtigall L, et al. Testosterone patch increases sexual activity and desire in surgically menopausal women with hypoactive sexual desire disorder. J Clin Endocrinol Metab 2005;90:5226-5233.
216. van Lunsen RH, Laan E. Genital vascular responsiveness and sexual feelings in midlife women: psychophysiologic, brain, and genital imaging studies. Menopause 2004;11:741-748.
217. Cranston-Cuebas MA, Barlow DH. Cognitive and affective contributions to sexual functioning. Ann Rev Sex Res 1990;1: 119-161.
218. Basson R, Leiblum S, Brotto L, et al. Definitions of women's sexual dysfunction reconsidered: advocating expansion and revision. J Psychosom Obstet Gynaecol 2003;24:221-229.
219. Avis N, Zhao X, Johannes CB, et al. Correlates of sexual function among multiethnic middle-aged women: results from the Study of Women's Health Across the Nation (SWAN). Menopause 2005; 12:385-398.
220. Dennerstein L, Lehert P. Modeling mid-aged women's sexual functioning: a prospective, population-based study. J Sex Marital Ther 2004;30:173-183.
221. Chivers ML, Bailey JM. A sex difference in features that elicit genital response. Biol Psychol 2005;70:115-120.
222. Basson R, Brotto LA. Sexual psychophysiology and effects of sildenafil citrate in oestrogenised women with acquired genital arousal disorder and impaired orgasm: a randomised controlled trial. Bjog 2003;110:1014-1024.
223. Bancroft J, Loftus J, Long JS. Distress about sex: a national survey of women in heterosexual relationships. Arch Sex Behav 2003;32:193-208.
224. Blaustein JD. Progestin receptors: neuronal integrators of hormonal and environmental stimulation. Ann N Y Acad Sci 2003;1007:238-250.
225. Davis SR, van der Mooren MJ, van Lunsen RH, et al. The efficacy and safety of a testosterone patch for the treatment of hypoactive sexual desire disorder in surgically menopausal women: A randomized, placebo controlled-trial. Menopause 2006;13:387-396.
226. Segraves RT, Clayton A, Croft H, et al. Bupropion sustained release for the treatment of hypoactive sexual desire disorder in premenopausal women. J Clin Psychopharmacol 2004;24:339-342.
227. Tiefer L, Hall M, Tavris C. Beyond dysfunction: a new view of women's sexual problems. J Sex Marital Ther 2002;28(suppl 1): 225-232.
228. Avis NE, Stellato R, Crawford S, Johannes C, Longcope C. Is there an association between menopause status and sexual functioning? Menopause 2000;7:297-309.
229. Laumann EO, Nicolosi A, Glasser DB, et al. Sexual problems among women and men aged 40-80 y: prevalence and correlates identified in the Global Study of Sexual Attitudes and Behaviors. Int J Impot Res 2005;17:39-57.
230. DeLamater JD, Sill M. Sexual desire in later life. J Sex Res 2005;42:138-149.
231. Barsky JL, Friedman M, Rosen R. Sexual dysfunction and chronic illness: the role of flexibility in coping. J Sex Marital Ther 2006;32:235-253.
232. Meston CM, Gorzalka BB. Differential effects of sympathetic activation on sexual arousal in sexually dysfunctional and functional women. J Abnorm Psychol 1996;105:582-591.
233. Karama S, Lecours AR, Leroux JM, et al. Areas of brain activation in males and females during viewing of erotic film excerpts. Hum Brain Mapp 2002;16:1-13.
234. Palace EM, Gorzalka BB. The enhancing effects of anxiety on arousal in sexually dysfunctional and functional women. J Abnorm Psychol 1990;99:403-411.
235. Creighton SM, Crouch NS, Foxwell NA, Cellek S. Functional evidence for nitrergic neurotransmission in a human clitoral corpus cavernosum: a case study. Int J Impot Res 2004;16:319-324.
236. Shafik A, El-Sibai O, Mostafa R, et al. Response of the internal reproductive organs to clitoral stimulation: the clitorouterine reflex. Int J Impot Res 2005;17:121-126.
237. O'Connell HE, DeLancey JO. Clitoral anatomy in nulliparous, healthy, premenopausal volunteers using unenhanced magnetic resonance imaging. J Urol 2005;173:2060-2063.
238. Althof SE, Dean J, Derogatis LR, et al. Current perspectives on the clinical assessment and diagnosis of female sexual dysfunction and clinical studies of potential therapies: a statement of concern. J Sex Med 2005;2(suppl 3):146-153.
239. Fugl-Meyer K, Fugl-Meyer AR. Sexual disabilities are not singularities. Int J Impot Res 2002;14:487-493.
240. Dunn KM, Croft PR, Hackett GI. Sexual problems: a study of the prevalence and need for health care in the general population. Fam Pract 1998;15:519-524.
241. Mercer CH, Fenton KA, Johnson AM, et al. Sexual function problems and help seeking behaviour in Britain: national probability sample survey. BMJ 2003;327:426-427.
242. Harlow BL, Stewart EG. A population-based assessment of chronic unexplained vulvar pain: have we underestimated the prevalence of vulvodynia? J Am Med Womens Assoc 2003;58:82-88.
243. Hartmann U, Philippsohn S, Heiser K, Ruffer-Hesse C. Low sexual desire in midlife and older women: personality factors, psychosocial development, present sexuality. Menopause 2004;11:726-740.
244. Leiblum SR, Koochaki PE, Rodenberg CA, et al. Hypoactive sexual desire disorder in postmenopausal women: US results from the Women's International Study of Health and Sexuality (WISHeS). Menopause 2006;13:46-56.
245. Hayes R, Dennerstein L. The impact of aging on sexual function and sexual dysfunction in women: a review of population-based studies. J Sex Med 2005;2:317-330.

246. Fugl-Meyer AR, Fugl-Meyer K. Sexual disabilities, problems and satisfaction in 18-74 year old Swedes. Scand J Sexology 1999;2: 79-105.
247. Kennedy SH, Dickens SE, Eisfeld BS, Bagby RM. Sexual dysfunction before antidepressant therapy in major depression. J Affect Disord 1999;56:201-208.
248. Cyranowski JM, Bromberger J, Youk A, et al. Lifetime depression history and sexual function in women at midlife. Arch Sex Behav 2004;33:539-548.
249. Montejo-Gonzalez AL, Llorca G, Izquierdo JA, et al. SSRI-induced sexual dysfunction: fluoxetine, paroxetine, sertraline, and fluvoxamine in a prospective, multicenter, and descriptive clinical study of 344 patients. J Sex Marital Ther 1997;23:176-194.
250. Clayton AH, Pradko JF, Croft HA, et al. Prevalence of sexual dysfunction among newer antidepressants. J Clin Psychiatry 2002;63: 357-366.
251. Labrie F, Belanger A, Cusan L, et al. Marked decline in serum concentrations of adrenal C19 sex steroid precursors and conjugated androgen metabolites during aging. J Clin Endocrinol Metab 1997;82:2396-2402.
252. Labrie F, Luu-The V, Labrie C, et al. Endocrine and intracrine sources of androgens in women: inhibition of breast cancer and other roles of androgens and their precursor dehydroepiandrosterone. Endocr Rev 2003;24:152-182.
253. Padero MC, Bhasin S, Friedman TC. Androgen supplementation in older women: too much hype, not enough data. J Am Geriatr Soc 2002;50:1131-1140.
254. Ganz PA, Desmond KA, Belin TR, et al. Predictors of sexual health in women after a breast cancer diagnosis. J Clin Oncol 1999;17: 2371-2380.
255. Aziz A, Brannstrom M, Bergquist C, Silfverstolpe G. Perimenopausal androgen decline after oophorectomy does not influence sexuality or psychological well-being. Fertil Steril 2005;83: 1021-1028.
256. Santoro N, Torrens J, Crawford S, et al. Correlates of circulating androgens in mid-life women: the study of women's health across the nation. J Clin Endocrinol Metab 2005;90:4836-4845.
257. Davis SR, Davison SL, Donath S, Bell RJ. Circulating androgen levels and self-reported sexual function in women. JAMA 2005;294:91-96.
258. Davis SR, Goldstat R, Papalia MA, et al. Effects of aromatase inhibition on sexual function and well-being in postmenopausal women treated with testosterone: a randomized, placebo-controlled trial. Menopause 2006;13:37-45.
259. Maravilla KR, Cao Y, Heiman JR, et al. Serial MR imaging with MS-325 for evaluating female sexual arousal response: determination of intrasubject reproducibility. J Magn Reson Imaging 2003;18:216-224.
260. van Geelen JM, van de Weijer PH, Arnolds HT. Urogenital symptoms and resulting discomfort in non-institutionalized Dutch women aged 50-75 years. Int Urogynecol J Pelvic Floor Dysfunct 2000;11:9-14.
261. Gorodeski GI, Hopfer U, Liu CC, Margles E. Estrogen acidifies vaginal pH by up-regulation of proton secretion via the apical membrane of vaginal-ectocervical epithelial cells. Endocrinology 2005;146:816-824.
262. Hoyle CH, Stones RW, Robson T, et al. Innervation of vasculature and microvasculature of the human vagina by NOS and neuropeptide-containing nerves. J Anat 1996;188(Pt 3):633-644.
263. Foster DC, Palmer M, Marks J. Effect of vulvovaginal estrogen on sensorimotor response of the lower genital tract: a randomized controlled trial. Obstet Gynecol 1999;94:232-237.
264. Connell K, Guess MK, Bleustein CB, et al. Effects of age, menopause, and comorbidities on neurological function of the female genitalia. Int J Impot Res 2005;17:63-70.
265. Dennerstein L, Lehert P, Burger H. The relative effects of hormones and relationship factors on sexual function of women through the natural menopausal transition. Fertil Steril 2005;84:174-180.
266. Berglund G, Nystedt M, Bolund C, et al. Effect of endocrine treatment on sexuality in premenopausal breast cancer patients: a prospective randomized study. J Clin Oncol 2001;19:2788-2796.
267. de Groot M, Anderson R, Freedland KE, et al. Association of depression and diabetes complications: a meta-analysis. Psychosom Med 2001;63:619-630.
268. Basson RJ, Rucker BM, Laird PG, Conry R. Sexuality of women with diabetes. J Sex Reprod Med 2001;1:11-20.
269. Erol B, Tefekli A, Ozbey I, et al. Sexual dysfunction in type II diabetic females: a comparative study. J Sex Marital Ther 2002; 28(Suppl 1):55-62.
270. Erol B, Tefekli A, Sanli O, et al. Does sexual dysfunction correlate with deterioration of somatic sensory system in diabetic women? Int J Impot Res 2003;15:198-202.
271. Enzlin P, Mathieu C, Van den Bruel A, et al. Sexual dysfunction in women with type 1 diabetes: a controlled study. Diabetes Care 2002;25:672-677.
272. Doruk H, Akbay E, Cayan S, et al. Effect of diabetes mellitus on female sexual function and risk factors. Arch Androl 2005;51:1-6.
273. Peng YS, Chiang CK, Kao TW, et al. Sexual dysfunction in female hemodialysis patients: a multicenter study. Kidney Int 2005; 68:760-765.
274. Wincze JP, Albert A, Bansal S. Sexual arousal in diabetic females: physiological and self-report measures. Arch Sex Behav 1993; 22:587-601.
275. Crespo CJ, Smit E, Snelling A, et al. Hormone replacement therapy and its relationship to lipid and glucose metabolism in diabetic and nondiabetic postmenopausal women: results from the Third National Health and Nutrition Examination Survey (NHANES III). Diabetes Care 2002;25:1675-1680.
276. Toorians AW, Janssen E, Laan E, et al. Chronic renal failure and sexual functioning: clinical status versus objectively assessed sexual response. Nephrol Dial Transplant 1997;12:2654-2663.
277. Hultgren R, Sjogren B, Soderberg M, et al. Sexual function in women suffering from aortoiliac occlusive disease. Eur J Vasc Endovasc Surg 1999;17:306-312.
278. Duncan LE, Lewis C, Jenkins P, Pearson TA. Does hypertension and its pharmacotherapy affect the quality of sexual function in women? Am J Hypertens 2000;13:640-647.
279. Conaglen HM, Conaglen JV. Sexual desire in women presenting for antiandrogen therapy. J Sex Marital Ther 2003;29:255-267.
280. Miller KK, Biller BM, Beauregard C, et al. Effects of testosterone replacement in androgen-deficient women with hypopituitarism: a randomized, double-blind, placebo-controlled study. J Clin Endocrinol Metab 2006;91:1683-1690.
281. Arlt W, Callies F, van Vlijmen JC, et al. Dehydroepiandrosterone replacement in women with adrenal insufficiency. N Engl J Med 1999;341:1013-1020.
282. van Thiel SW, Romijn JA, Pereira AM, et al. Effects of dehydroepiandrostenedione, superimposed on growth hormone substitution, on quality of life and insulin-like growth factor I in patients with secondary adrenal insufficiency: a randomized, placebo-controlled, cross-over trial. J Clin Endocrinol Metab 2005; 90:3295-3303.
283. Lovas K, Gebre-Medhin G, Trovik TS, et al. Replacement of dehydroepiandrosterone in adrenal failure: no benefit for subjective health status and sexuality in a 9-month, randomized, parallel group clinical trial. J Clin Endocrinol Metab 2003;88: 1112-1118.
284. Gimbel H, Zobbe V, Andersen BM, et al. Randomised controlled trial of total compared with subtotal hysterectomy with one-year follow up results. BJOG 2003;110:1088-1098.
285. Kim DH, Lee YS, Lee ES. Alteration of sexual function after classic intrafascial supracervical hysterectomy and total hysterectomy. J Am Assoc Gynecol Laparosc 2003;10:60-64.
286. Roovers JP, van der Bom JG, van der Vaart CH, Heintz AP. Hysterectomy and sexual wellbeing: prospective observational study of vaginal hysterectomy, subtotal abdominal hysterectomy, and total abdominal hysterectomy. BMJ 2003;327:774-778.
287. Maas CP, ter Kuile MM, Laan E, et al. Objective assessment of sexual arousal in women with a history of hysterectomy. BJOG 2004;111:456-462.
288. Kadioglu P, Yalin AS, Tiryakioglu O, et al. Sexual dysfunction in women with hyperprolactinemia: a pilot study report. J Urol 2005;174:1921-1925.
289. Mansfield PK, Koch PB. Qualities midlife women desire in their sexual relationship and their chaning sexual response. Psychol Women Q 1998;22:282-303.
290. Cayan S, Bozlu M, Canpolat B, Akbay E. The assessment of sexual functions in women with male partners complaining of erectile dysfunction: does treatment of male sexual dysfunction improve

female partner's sexual functions? J Sex Marital Ther 2004; 30:333-341.

291. Hartmann U, Heiser K, Ruffer-Hesse C, Kloth G. Female sexual desire disorders: subtypes, classification, personality factors and new directions for treatment. World J Urol 2002;20:79-88.
292. Brotto LA, Basson R, Gehring D. Psychological profiles among women with vulvar vestibulitis syndrome: a chart review. J Psychosom Obstet Gynaecol 2003;24:195-203.
293. Van Lankveld JJ, Weijenborg PT, ter Kuile MM. Psychologic profiles of and sexual function in women with vulvar vestibulitis and their partners. Obstet Gynecol 1996;88:65-70.
294. Klusmann D. Sexual motivation and the duration of partnership. Arch Sex Behav 2002;31:275-287.
295. Verhaak CM, Smeenk JM, van Minnen A, et al. A longitudinal, prospective study on emotional adjustment before, during and after consecutive fertility treatment cycles. Hum Reprod 2005;20:2253-2260.
296. Hawton K, Catalan J, Flagg J. Low sexual desire: sex therapy results and prognostic factors. Behav Res Ther 1991;29:217-224.
297. Hurlbert DF. A comparative study using orgasm consistency training in the treatment of women reporting hypoactive sexual desire. J Sex Marital Ther 1993;19:41-55.
298. Sarwer DB, Durlak JA. A field trial of the effectiveness of behavioral treatment for sexual dysfunctions. J Sex Marital Ther 1997;23:87-97.
299. McCabe MP. Evaluation of a cognitive behavior therapy program for people with sexual dysfunction. J Sex Marital Ther 2001;27: 259-271.
300. Heiman J, LoPiccolo J. Clinical outcome of sex therapy. Effect of daily vs weekly treatment. Arch Gen Psychiatry 1983;40:443-449.
301. Trudel G, Marchand A, Ravart M, et al. The effect of a cognitive behavior treatment program on hypoactive sexual desire disorder in women. Sex Rel Ther 2001;16:145-164.
302. Delehanty R. Changes in assertiveness and changes in orgasmic response occurring in sexual therapy of preorgasmic women. J Sex Marital Ther 1982;8:198-208.
303. Hurlbert DF, Apt C. Coital alignment technique and directed masturbation: a comparative study on female masturbation. J Sex Marital Ther 1995;21:21-29.
304. Heiman JR. Psychologic treatments for female sexual dysfunction: are they effective and do we need them? Arch Sex Behav 2002;31:445-450.
305. Basson BR, McKinnes R, Smith MD, et al. Efficacy and safety of sildenafil citrate in women with sexual dysfunction associated with female sexual arousal. Gend Based Med 2002;11:367-377.
306. Shifren JL, Davis SR, Moreau M, et al. Testosterone patch for the treatment of hypoactive sexual desire disorder in naturally menopausal women: results from the INTIMATE NM1 study. Menopause 2006;13:770-779.
307. Barnhart K, Freeman E, Grisso JA, et al. The effect of dehydroepiandrosterone supplementation to symptomatic perimenopausal women on serum endocrine profiles, lipid parameters and health related quality of life. J Clin Endocrinol Metab 1999;84: 3896-3902.
308. Laan E, van Lunsen RH, Everaerd W. The effects of tibolone on vaginal blood flow, sexual desire and arousability in postmenopausal women. Climacteric 2001;4:28-41.
309. Meston CM, Worcel M. The effects of yohimbine plus l-arginine glutamate on sexual arousal in postmenopausal women with sexual arousal disorder. Arch Sex Behav 2002;31:323-332.
310. Meston CM, Heiman JR. Ephedrine-activated physiological sexual arousal in women. Arch Gen Psychiatry 1998;55:652-656.
311. Caruso S, Intelisano G, Lupo L, et al. Premenopausal women affected by sexual arousal disorder treated with sildenafil: a double-blind cross-over placebo-controlled study. Brit J Obstet Gynecol 2001;108:623-628.
312. Caruso S, Intelisano G, Farina M, et al. The function of seldenafil on female sexual pathways: A double-blind, cross-over placebo controlled study. Euro J Obstet Gynecol 2003;110:201-206.
313. Ito TY, Trant AS, Polan ML. A double-blind placebo-controlled study of Argin Max, a nutritional supplement for enhancement of female sexual function. J Sex Marital Ther 2001;27:541-549.
314. Blake J, Belisle S, Basson R. SOGC Clinical Practice Guideline: Canadian Consensus on Menopause and Osteoporosis. J Obstet Gynecol Can 2006;171:S7-S112.
315. The North American Menopause Society. The role of testosterone therapy in postmenopausal women: position statement of The North American Menopause Society. Menopause 2005;12: 496-511.
316. Hays J, Ockene JK, Brunner RL, et al. Effects of estrogen plus progestin on health-related quality of life. N Engl J Med 2003;348:1839-1854.
317. Wierman M, Basson R, Davis S, et al. Androgen therapy in women: an Endocrine Society Clinical Practice Guideline. J Clin Endocrinol Metab 2006;91:3697-3710.
318. Bachmann G, Rosen R, Pinn V, et al. Vulvodynia: a state-of-the art consensus on definitions, diagnosis and management. J Reprod Med 2006;51:447-456.

SECTION VI

Endocrinology and the Life Span

CHAPTER 20

ENDOCRINE CHANGES IN PREGNANCY

Glenn D. Braunstein

Placental Development

Normal placentation requires a coordinated series of events, beginning with fertilization. The fertilization rate following unprotected regular intercourse during a single menstrual cycle is 25% to 30%. However, in approximately one third of conceptions, there is either failure of implantation or clinical or subclinical spontaneous abortion.[1]

For the first 5 days, preimplantation development takes place within the fallopian tube. During this period, the zygote undergoes cleavage division and, at least through the eight-cell stage, the blastomeres remain totipotential. In the 16-cell stage, differentiation of the innermost cells into the *inner cell mass* and the surrounding cells into the *trophectoderm* occurs. The inner cell mass develops into the fetus, and the trophectoderm gives rise to the placenta and membranes. On approximately day 5 or 6 after fertilization, the blastocyst enters the uterus, but implantation does not occur for another 1 to 2 days. Implantation occurs after the zona pellucida disappears from around the embryo.[2]

Implantation is a complex process that involves apposition of the microvilli present on the trophectoderm cells with pinocytes (fused microvilli) on the endometrial cells, followed by removal of fluid between the cells through pinocytosis by the endometrial cells, a process stimulated by progesterone.[3] Progesterone synthesis by the corpus luteum is stimulated and sustained during this time and for the first 6 to 7 weeks of pregnancy by secretion of human chorionic gonadotropin (hCG) by the trophoblast cells. The hCG is first detected in the maternal serum 6 to 9 days after conception.[4] Attachment of the embryo is enhanced through the expression of a variety of adhesion molecules, including mucins, integrins, and trophinin, a trophoblast-specific cell membrane adhesion protein, as well as cytokines, growth factors, and a variety of transcription factors encoded by Homeobox genes.[3,5]

After the trophoblast attaches to the endometrium during the "window of implantation" 6 to 10 days after ovulation, the embryo invades the endometrium through a complex process involving matrix metalloproteinases and differentiation of the trophectoderm into *cytotrophoblasts* or *syncytiotrophoblasts*. The syncytiotrophoblasts are multinucleated cells formed by the fusion of cytotrophoblasts. The cytotrophoblasts form a column of cells that invade the endometrium, form anchoring villi, and enter the maternal vasculature, eventually replacing the endothelial layer of the endometrial and myometrial spiral arterioles with a layer of cytotrophoblasts (vascular trophoblasts).[6] This process converts the high-resistance, low-capacity uterine vessels into low-resistance, high-volume vessels, essential for growth of the placenta and fetus.[7] At the site of implantation, the endometrial cells undergo decidualization, enlarging and increasing their metabolic activity with enhanced production of tissue inhibitors or metalloproteinase, extracellular matrix proteins, cytokines, and growth factors that modulate the extent of trophoblast invasion and influence trophoblast function.[3,4,8]

The trophoblast cells secrete several angiogenic proteins, including vascular endothelial growth factor, platelet-derived growth factor (PDGF), and basic fibroblast growth factor (bFGF), which stimulate blood vessel development within the villi.[9] The syncytiotrophoblasts form an outer layer of cells in the chorionic villi, between the cytotrophoblast cells and the maternal blood space on the exterior surface. Only three tissues separate the fetal blood from maternal blood: (1) the endothelium of the fetal vessels in the villi, (2) connective tissue, and (3) the trophoblasts; this form of placentation is referred to as *hemochorial.* Thus, in addition to hCG secretion, which is responsible for maintaining early pregnancy, progesterone secretion, required for continuation of pregnancy after the luteal-placental shift, and the synthesis and secretion of other hormones and growth factors (Table 20–1), the syncytiotrophoblasts provide the major site for transportation of oxygen and nutrients to and removal of waste from the fetus.

Substances are transferred across the placenta through transcellular pathways that include carrier-mediated transport (e.g., immunoglobulin G through the Fcγ receptor) and simple extracellular diffusion. The degree of transplacental passage of a

TABLE 20–1 HORMONES, PEPTIDES, AND GROWTH FACTORS PRODUCED BY THE PLACENTA

Hypothalamic analogues
- Gonadotropin-releasing hormone
- Corticotropin-releasing hormone
- Urocortin
- Somatostatin
- Growth hormone-releasing hormone
- Ghrelin
- Thyrotropin-releasing hormone
- Dopamine
- Neuropeptide Y
- Enkephalin

Pituitary analogues
- Chorionic gonadotropin
- Placental lactogen
- Chorionic corticotropin
- β-Endorphin
- α-Melanocyte-stimulating hormone
- Placental variant growth hormone
- Oxytocin

Steroid hormones
- Estrogens
- Progesterone

Other
- Activins
- Inhibins
- Follistatin
- Relaxin
- Calcitonin
- Leptin
- Parathyroid hormone-related protein
- Erythropoietin
- Renin
- Interleukins
- Nitric oxide
- Transforming growth factor-β
- Tumor necrosis factor-α
- Epidermic growth factor
- Insulin-like growth factor I
- Insulin-like growth factor II
- Insulin-like growth factor binding protein-1
- Colony-stimulating factor-1
- Basic fibroblast growth factor
- Corticotropin-releasing hormone binding protein
- Platelet derived growth factor
- Vascular endothelial growth factor
- Endothelin-1
- Anadamide (endocannabinoid)
- Hepatocyte growth factor
- Oncomodulin

hormone from the mother to the fetus through diffusion depends on (1) the rate of placental blood flow, (2) the maternal concentration of the free or readily disassociable from bindius protein(s) hormone, and (3) the molecular mass, lipid solubility, charge, and degree of placental metabolic degradation of the hormone. Maternal-to-fetal transfer occurs for hormones smaller than 700 d, but the placenta is not permeable to hormones larger than 1200 d.[10]

The trophoblast also anchors the placenta and fetus to the uterus and helps protect the fetus, which contains paternal antigens, from rejection by the maternal immune system. This immunologic protection may be mediated by high concentrations of progesterone at the trophoblast-maternal interface and the expression by the trophoblasts of a histocompatibility complex antigen, human leukocyte antigen G (HLA-G), which exhibits reduced polymorphism in comparison with other major HLA antigens.[11] The mass of the trophoblast increases logarithmically during the first trimester, followed by a more gradual increase throughout the remainder of pregnancy. Trophoblastic mass closely correlates with maternal serum concentrations of human placental lactogen (hPL) and pregnancy-specific β_1-glycoprotein throughout pregnancy and with hCG during the first trimester but not during the subsequent trimesters.[12]

Maternal Adaptations to Pregnancy

Myriad physiologic changes take place beginning shortly after implantation. During early pregnancy, these effects are hormonally mediated. In the second and third trimesters, the uteroplacental vascular system and mechanical factors associated with the enlarging gravid uterus combine with the hormonal milieu to alter the function of every system.

General Adaptations

Weight gain averages 12.5 kg, of which the fetus accounts for about 3.4 kg, the placenta 0.65 kg, amniotic fluid 0.8 kg, uterus 1 kg, breasts 0.4 kg, blood 1.5 kg, extravascular fluid 1.5 kg, and maternal fat stores approximately 3.3 kg.[13] The volume of the uterine cavity increases from about 10 mL to an average of 5 L at term, and blood flow through the uteroplacental circulation reaches 450 to 650 mL/minute.[13]

In order to maintain appropriate perfusion of the mother and fetal-placental unit, blood volume increases throughout pregnancy and at term is 40% to 45% higher than in the nonpregnant state. Both the plasma volume and red cell mass increase. The plasma volume increases about 45% to 50% as a result of aldosterone-stimulated sodium and water retention; the red cell mass increases approximately 20% because of increased production resulting from a twofold to threefold increase in erythropoietin secretion. The net effect is a decrease in the hematocrit by about 15% at term.[13]

The renal blood flow and glomerular filtration rate (GFR) increase rapidly and peak during the second trimester, and there is a 50% increase in creatinine clearance, resulting in a reduction in serum creatinine. Atrial natriuretic peptide (ANP) levels increase during pregnancy and may in part be responsible for the increased renal blood flow, GFR, 24-hour urine volume, and natriuresis.[14] An alteration in the osmotic thresholds for the release of vasopressin and activation of the hypothalamic thirst centers, possibly caused by an extragonadal effect of hCG, lead to an approximately 4% reduction in serum osmolality (~10 mOsm/kg).[15]

Several hemodynamic changes are induced by the low-resistance, high-capacity uteroplacental vessels, which in many respects act like an arteriovenous malformation; the increased blood volume; and the large quantities of estrogens, progesterone, and angiotensin present during pregnancy. The changes include an increase in the heart rate by 10 to 15 beats/minute, a 30% to 50% increase in cardiac output resulting from increased stroke volume in early pregnancy and heart rate during the third trimester, a reduction in diastolic blood pressure with little or no change in systolic pressure, and an approximately 20% reduction in peripheral vascular resistance.[13]

The pulmonary vascular resistance is reduced by about one third. Pregnancy is also associated with increases in pulmonary tidal volume by about 30%, which results in a respiratory alkalosis that is compensated by increased bicarbonate excretion by the kidneys; in minute ventilatory volume by 30% to 40%; and in minute oxygen uptake. There are no changes in respiratory rate, maximum breathing capacity, or forced or timed vital capacity. However, there is an approximately 40% reduction in the expiratory reserve because of the elevation of the diaphragm by the enlarged uterus.[13]

Gastrointestinal tract function is altered during pregnancy. Gastric emptying time is decreased by more than 50% at term and the lower esophageal sphincter tone is reduced, which, together with the displacement of the abdominal contents by the pregnant uterus, results in a marked increase in gastroesophageal reflux disease. Motility of the intestine is also reduced, contributing to the constipation that is common during pregnancy. Decreased motility of the gallbladder leads to an increased gallbladder volume and reduced emptying of bile after meals, which results in a more lithogenic bile and an increase in cholelithiasis during pregnancy.[13]

Maternal Endocrine Alterations

Pituitary Gland

The anterior pituitary gland enlarges by an average of 36% during pregnancy, primarily because of a 10-fold increase in lactotroph size and number. This enlargement results in an increase in height and convexity of the pituitary on magnetic resonance imaging. There are reduced numbers of somatotrophs and gonadotrophs and no changes in corticotrophs or thyrotrophs.[16] The posterior pituitary gland diminishes in size during pregnancy.[17]

The marked increase in estrogen levels during pregnancy enhances prolactin synthesis and secretion, and maternal prolactin serum levels increase in parallel with the enlargement of the lactotrophs. At term, the mean serum prolactin concentration is 207 ng/mL (range 35 to 600 ng/mL), in contrast to a mean of 10 ng/mL in nonpregnant premenopausal women. Prolactin is also present in the amniotic fluid and appears to be primarily of decidual origin because the decidua actively synthesizes prolactin. Amniotic fluid prolactin levels are 10 to 100 times higher than in the maternal circulation in early pregnancy, and maternal bromocriptine ingestion does not reduce the amniotic fluid prolactin levels but does reduce the maternal and fetal serum concentrations.[18] Prolactin levels return to the baseline of nonpregnancy approximately 7 days after delivery in the absence of breastfeeding. With breastfeeding, the basal prolactin levels remain elevated for several months but gradually decrease; however, with suckling, there is a brisk rise in prolactin levels within 30 minutes.[16]

Growth hormone (GH) levels in maternal serum throughout pregnancy are unchanged, although the source of immunoreactive GH during gestation does change. Relaxin, secreted by the corpus luteum of pregnancy, and estrogens stimulate GH secretion during early pregnancy.[19] Pituitary GH messenger ribonucleic acid (mRNA) and GH secretion decrease after the 25th week of pregnancy, and beginning in the fourth month of gestation, the placental syncytiotrophoblast secretes a variant of GH in a nonpulsatile pattern.[20,21] In concert with the different sources of GH during the first and second halves of pregnancy, the GH response to provocative stimuli differs in each half. Insulin hypoglycemia or arginine infusion results in an enhanced GH response during the first half of gestation, and there is a decreased response during the second half with respect to the response in nonpregnant women.[16]

Maternal serum concentrations of insulin-like growth factor I (IGF-I) are elevated during the second half of pregnancy, probably through the combined effect of the placental GH variant and hPL, which is evolutionarily related to both GH and prolactin. hPL has somatotropic biologic activity, and its serum concentration increases throughout pregnancy, paralleling that of IGF-I.[20-23] In turn, it is likely that the suppression of pituitary GH synthesis and secretion is due to the high IGF-I concentrations, which in late pregnancy are five times higher than those in nonpregnant women.[21]

Although the placenta synthesizes and secretes biologically active gonadotropin-releasing hormone (GnRH), pituitary gonadotropin production decreases throughout pregnancy, as indicated by a marked reduction in gonadotropin immunoreactivity in the gonadotrophs beginning at 10 weeks of gestation as well as a reduction in serum levels of luteinizing hormone (LH) and follicle-stimulating hormone (FSH).[16] This suppression is probably mediated through the elevated blood levels of ovarian and placental sex steroid hormones along with placental production of inhibin. The suppression is incomplete because administration of exogenous GnRH leads to release of gonadotropins, although the response is blunted in comparison with that of nonpregnant women and does not return to normal until a month after birth.[16]

Mean thyrotropin (hTSH, or thyroid-stimulating hormone) concentrations during the first trimester are significantly lower than in the second and third trimesters or in the nonpregnant state.[24] Much of this early decrease may be accounted for by the intrinsic thyrotropic activity of hCG. The maximal biologic thyrotropic activity in maternal serum corresponds to the peak concentration of hCG at 10 to 12 weeks after the last menstrual period, at a time when there is a reciprocal relationship between the rising hCG levels and falling hTSH concentrations (Fig. 20–1).[24,25] The only time during pregnancy when the free thyroxine concentration in the maternal serum is elevated corresponds

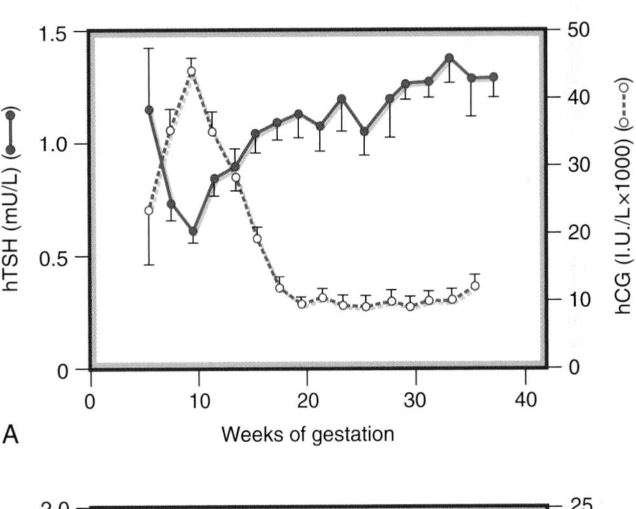

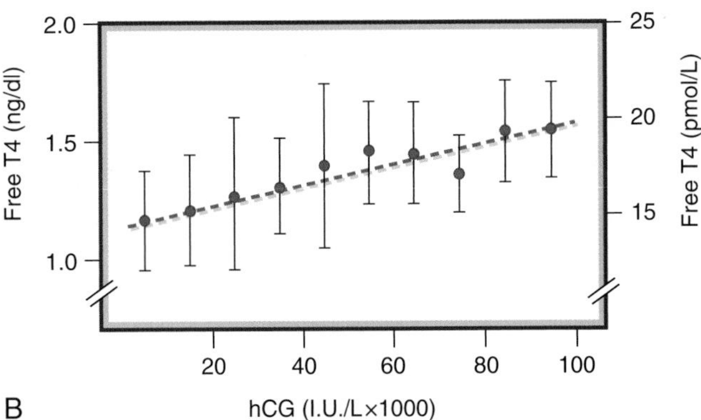

Figure 20–1 ▪ **A,** Serum thyrotropin (hTSH) and human chorionic gonadotropin (hCG) concentrations throughout pregnancy. Between 8 and 14 weeks of gestation, there is a significant negative correlation between the individual hTSH and hCG levels ($P < .001$). Each point represents the mean (±SE). SE, standard error. **B,** Linear regression of maternal serum free thyroxine (T_4) and hCG concentrations during the first half of gestation ($P < .001$). (From Glinoer D, de Nayer P, Bourdoux P, et al. Regulation of maternal thyroid during pregnancy. J Clin Endocrinol Metab 1990;71:276.)

to the time of peak hCG and lowest hTSH, suggesting that the depressed hTSH is the result of feedback suppression by thyroxine. Despite the lower mean hTSH during early pregnancy, the hTSH response to exogenous thyrotropin-releasing hormone (TRH) is normal.[16]

Maternal adrenocorticotropic hormone (ACTH, or corticotropin) levels rise during pregnancy, increasing fourfold over concentrations in the nonpregnant state between 7 and 10 weeks of gestation. There is a further gradual rise to weeks 33 to 37, at which time a mean fivefold increase over prepregnancy values is found, followed by a 50% drop just before parturition and a marked 15-fold increase during the stress of delivery.[26] The ACTH concentration returns to the prepregnancy level within 24 hours of delivery. Both the pituitary gland and the placenta serve as the source of the circulating ACTH during pregnancy, and exogenous corticotropin-releasing hormone (CRH) stimulates the release of ACTH from both tissues in a dose-dependent manner.[26] Biologically active CRH is synthesized and secreted by the placenta and, to a lesser extent, by the decidual and fetal membranes, but in contradistinction to the inhibitory effect on pituitary CRH, glucocorticoids stimulate the expression of placental CRH.[26,27]

Of interest, there appears to be a "disconnect" between CRH and ACTH during pregnancy. One would expect biologically active CRH to stimulate ACTH production. However, the qualitative patterns of CRH production, which shows an exponential rise during the sixth month of gestation, and ACTH secretion, which demonstrates a more gradual rise during pregnancy, are quite different. In addition, the lack of a significant correlation between maternal plasma CRH and ACTH during pregnancy suggests that factors such as the elevated levels of free cortisol in the maternal serum may modulate the response to CRH. Both the circadian rhythm and the ability to respond to stress are maintained throughout pregnancy; however, the ACTH response to exogenous CRH during the third trimester is blunted while the responsiveness to vasopressin is maintained, suggesting that the elevation of CRH in the maternal serum down-regulates the responsiveness to CRH.[26]

Arginine vasopressin (AVP) concentrations in the maternal serum are similar to those in nonpregnant women.[28] During pregnancy, however, there is increased synthesis of AVP, which is offset by the increased metabolic clearance of the hormone through destruction by a trophoblast-derived cysteine aminopeptidase (vasopressinase), whose levels rise throughout pregnancy in parallel with the increase in trophoblastic mass.[28,29] As previously noted, there is a reduced osmolar set-point for thirst and the release of AVP related to the 10 mOsm/kg average decrease in plasma osmolality during pregnancy, possibly reflecting an extragonadotropic effect of hCG.[15] Taking into account the reduced set-point, the AVP response to dehydration and water loading is normal.

Oxytocin levels progressively increase in the maternal blood and parallel the increase in maternal serum estradiol and progesterone.[30] The levels increase further with cervical dilation and vaginal distention during labor and delivery, stimulating contraction of the uterine smooth muscles and enhancing fetal ejection.[30] Uterine oxytocin receptors also increase throughout pregnancy, resulting in a 100-fold increase in oxytocin binding at term in the myometrium.[31]

Thyroid Gland

The thyroid gland enlarges by an average of 18% during pregnancy.[24] The enlargement is associated with an increase in the size of the follicles with increased colloid and enhanced blood volume. This enlargement may be a response to the thyrotropic effect of hCG and asialo-hCG, which may also account for some of the increase in serum thyroglobulin concentrations noted during pregnancy. There is enhanced ^{131}I uptake by the maternal thyroid gland, which undoubtedly reflects the combined effects of hCG stimulation and reduction of the blood levels of iodide by enhanced renal iodide clearance.[24]

The rising estrogen concentrations during pregnancy induce increased hepatic synthesis of thyroxine-binding globulin (TBG) as well as enhanced sialylation of TBG, which decreases its metabolic clearance rate.[25] The results are a twofold increase in TBG and increased total thyroxine (T_4) and triiodothyronine (T_3) levels in maternal serum throughout pregnancy,[24] whereas for most of the gestation, the free T_4 and free T_3 concentrations remain normal. There are no significant changes in the levels of thyroxine-binding prealbumin, but albumin levels are decreased because of the increase in vascular volume.

Parathyroid Glands

During pregnancy, approximately 30 g of calcium is transferred from the maternal compartment to the fetus, with most of the transfer occurring during the last trimester. Maternal total serum calcium levels decrease during pregnancy, with a nadir at 28 to 32 weeks related to the decrease in albumin levels that accompanies the increase in vascular volume. However, the albumin-adjusted total calcium and the ionized calcium concentrations actually rise slightly above the level in the nonpregnant state.[32] The urinary calcium excretion rate increases in parallel with the increased GFR, and intestinal calcium absorption undergoes a twofold increase.[32]

Although some studies have suggested that parathyroid hormone (PTH) levels increase during pregnancy, measurements of intact PTH levels by two-site immunometric assays indicate that they are within the normal, nonpregnancy range throughout pregnancy.[32] In contrast, the circulating concentrations of PTH-related protein (PTHrp) increase throughout pregnancy.[32,33] Many normal tissues produce this protein and the source of the elevated levels during pregnancy is unclear, although the two most likely sites are the mammary tissue and the placenta.[33] This protein is probably involved in placental calcium transport.

The serum levels of 25-hydroxyvitamin D are unchanged during pregnancy, but the estrogen-induced rise in vitamin D–binding globulin results in a twofold increase in 1,25-dihydroxyvitamin D concentrations in maternal serum.[32] There is also a rise in the biologically active free fraction of 1,25-dihydroxyvitamin D, which may reflect both increased maternal renal 1α-hydroxylase activity and the synthesis and secretion of 1,25-dihydroxyvitamin D by the placenta.[32] This increase in the active metabolite of vitamin D may be responsible in part for the enhanced intestinal calcium absorption.

Pancreas

Hyperplasia and hypertrophy of the β cells in the islets of Langerhans are probably the result of stimulation by estrogen and progesterone.[34] During early pregnancy, the glucose requirements of the fetus lead to enhanced transport of glucose across the placenta by facilitated diffusion, and maternal fasting hypoglycemia may be present. Although basal insulin levels may be normal, there is hypersecretion of insulin in response to a meal. Because the half-life of insulin is not altered during pregnancy,[35] this increase represents an increase in synthesis and secretion. The results are enhanced glycogen storage and decreased hepatic glucose production.

As pregnancy progresses, the levels of hPL rise, as do the levels of glucocorticoids, leading to the insulin resistance found during the last half of pregnancy.[36] Thus, in late pregnancy, glucose ingestion results in higher and more sustained levels of glucose and insulin and a greater degree of glucagon suppression than in the nonpregnant state.

Adrenal Glands

As a result of the hyperestrogenemia of pregnancy, hepatic production of cortisol-binding globulin is increased. The increased production results in a doubling of the maternal serum levels cortisol-binding globulin, which in turn results in decreased metabolic clearance of cortisol and a threefold rise in total plasma cortisol by week 26, when the levels reach a plateau until they rise at the onset of labor.[26,37] The rate of cortisol production is increased, and the plasma free cortisol concentrations are also increased.[91] The enhanced cortisol production is due to an increase in the maternal plasma ACTH concentrations and hyperresponsiveness of the adrenal cortex to ACTH stimulation during pregnancy.[26] Cortisol secretion follows that of ACTH, and the diurnal rhythm is maintained during pregnancy.[37] Despite the elevated free cortisol levels, pregnant women do not develop the stigma of glucocorticoid excess, possibly because of the antiglucocorticoid activities of the elevated concentrations of progesterone.

Plasma renin substrate levels are increased as a consequence of the effects of estrogen on the liver. Renin levels are also increased, and increased renin activity results in increased levels of angiotensin II, which lead to an 8- to 10-fold increase in aldosterone production and serum aldosterone levels.[26] The aldosterone levels peak in midpregnancy and are maintained until delivery.

Despite their baseline elevations, the various components of the renin-angiotensin-aldosterone system demonstrate normal responses to positional changes, sodium restriction, and sodium loading. The elevated aldosterone levels do not lead to an increase in serum sodium, a decrease in serum potassium, or an increase in blood pressure, which again may reflect the high progesterone concentrations, which are capable of displacing aldosterone from its renal receptors. Another mineralocorticoid, 11-deoxycorticosterone, shows a 6- to 10-fold increase in concentration at term.[26] Elevated levels of this hormone are due to estrogen-induced extraglandular 21-hydroxylation of progesterone produced by the placenta.[38]

Levels of androstenedione and testosterone, whether they are of adrenal or ovarian origin, are elevated because of the estrogen-induced increase in hepatic synthesis of sex hormone-binding globulin. However, the free androgen levels remain normal or low. The adrenal production rates of dehydroepiandrosterone (DHEA) and dehydroepiandrosterone sulfate (DHEAS) are increased twofold, but the maternal serum concentration of DHEAS is reduced to one third to one half of the nonpregnancy levels because of the enhanced 16-hydroxylation and placental utilization of 16-hydroxydehydroepiandrosterone sulfate in estrogen formation.[38]

Adrenal medullary function remains normal throughout pregnancy. Thus, 24-hour urine catecholamine and plasma epinephrine and norepinephrine levels are similar to concentrations in the nonpregnant state.[39,40]

Placental Hormone Production

Steroid Hormones

Placental steroidogenesis takes place in the syncytiotrophoblast, and synthesis and secretion of estrogens and progesterone increase throughout pregnancy in concert with the increase in the trophoblast mass (Fig. 20–2).[12] The placenta does not express steroidogenic factor-1 (SF-1), a transcription factor that is an important regulator of genes involved in adrenal and gonadal steroid hormone synthesis.[41] As a consequence or in addition, the trophoblast has reduced levels of, or lacks several enzymes important for, the de novo production of estrogens and

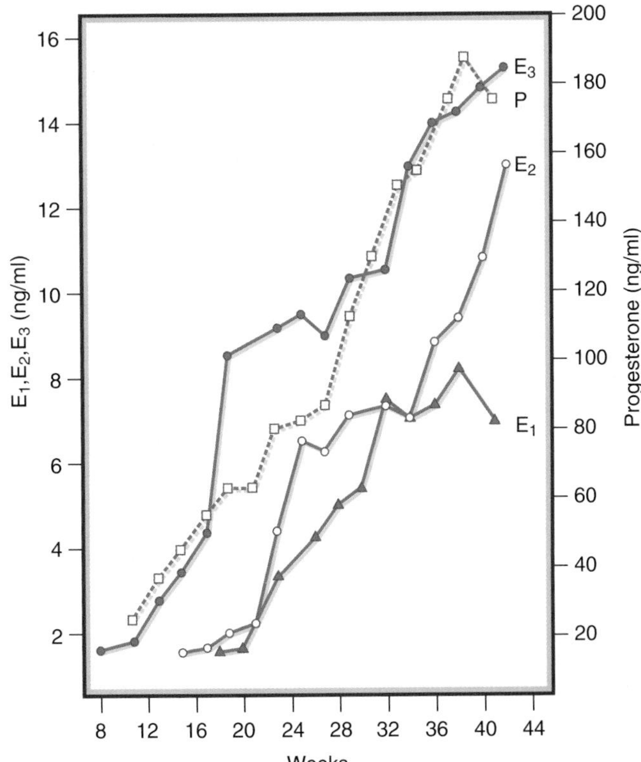

Figure 20–2 ■ Mean plasma concentrations of estrone (E_1), estradiol (E_2), estriol (E_3), and progesterone (P) during pregnancy. (Data from Tulchinsky D, Hobel CJ, Yeager E, et al. Plasma estrone, estradiol, estriol, progesterone, and 17-hydroxyprogesterone in human pregnancy: I. Normal pregnancy. Am J Obstet Gynecol 1972;112:1095; and Levitz M, Young BK. Estrogens and pregnancy. Vitam Horm 1977;35:109.)

progesterone and thus is dependent on precursors of both maternal and fetal origin. This dependence has led to the concept of the *maternal-fetal-placental unit.*[42] These interactions are outlined in Figure 20–3.[43,44]

Progesterone

Although the trophoblast can synthesize cholesterol from acetate, the amount of an essential enzyme needed for cholesterol synthesis, hydroxymethylglutaryl-coenzyme A reductase, in placental microsomes is low because of the inhibitory effects of the high intracellular concentrations of cholesterol that result from progesterone inhibition of cholesterol esterification.[45] Therefore, steroid synthesis by the placenta is dependent on the delivery of low-density lipoproteins (LDLs) and very-low-density lipoproteins (VLDLs) from the maternal circulation. The syncytiotrophoblast contains receptors for LDLs, VLDLs, and high-density lipoproteins (HDLs). Receptor-mediated uptake of LDL cholesterol is stimulated by estrogens, as is the activity of the cholesterol side-chain cleavage/desmolase enzyme (CYP11A1), which converts cholesterol to pregnenolone.[42,46] The placenta lacks the steroidogenic acute regulatory protein (StAR), which mediates the transport of cholesterol from the outer to inner mitochondrial membrane, the site where CYP11A1 acts. Therefore, there must be another mitochondrial transport mechanism present in the placenta. Indeed, altered placental steroid production is not seen in pregnancies with StAR mutations that result in congenital lipoid hyperplasia affecting the adrenals and gonads.[47]

Progesterone is synthesized in the trophoblast from pregnenolone by a placental isoform of 3β-hydroxysteroid dehydro-

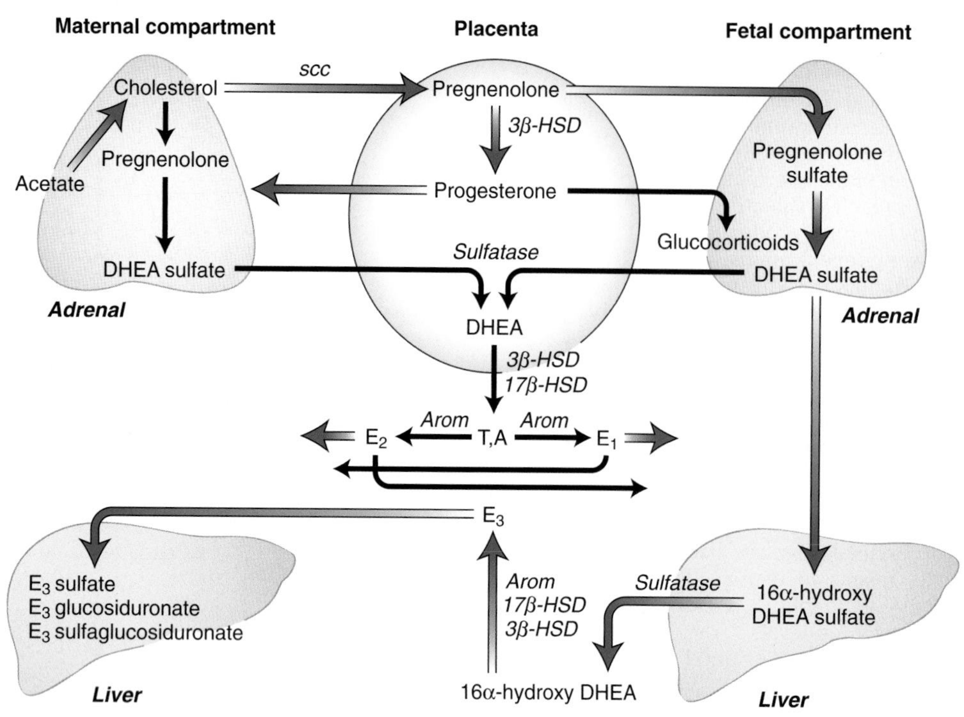

Figure 20–3 ▪ Steroidogenesis in the maternal-fetal-placental unit. *AROM,* Aromatase-enzyme complex; *DHEA,* dehydroepiandrosterone; *HSD,* hydroxysteroid dehydrogenase; *SCC,* cholesterol side-chain cleavage enzyme.

genase (3β-HSD-I).[46] Approximately 90% of the progesterone synthesized is secreted into the maternal compartment, and at term the mean maternal serum concentration is about 150 ng/mL. The fetal adrenals lack 3β-HSD activity, and, therefore, are not essential for progesterone production.[46] Hence, progesterone production continues after fetal death.[48]

Progesterone appears to have multiple functions during pregnancy, the most important being preparation of the uterus for implantation and maintenance of the pregnancy.[42] The corpus luteum is the primary source of progesterone during the first 6 to 8 weeks of pregnancy, after which ovarian progesterone production declines and placental synthesis and secretion become the major source of the hormone (the luteal-placental shift).[48]

Luteectomy, or removal of the ovary containing the corpus luteum, within the first 35 days after conception leads to abortion, but the pregnancy generally continues if these procedures are performed 46 or more days after conception. This indicates that placental progesterone production is sufficient to maintain the pregnancy even before the luteal-placental shift.[48] Administration of the progesterone receptor antagonist mifepristone during the first 49 days after conception results in abortion, again demonstrating that progesterone is essential for the maintenance of early pregnancy.[49]

Progesterone also serves as an important substrate for fetal adrenal glucocorticoid and mineralocorticoid synthesis and maintenance of myometrial quiescence, possibly through inhibition of prostaglandin formation.[42,46] A possible role for the high concentrations of progesterone present at the trophoblast-decidua junction is suppression of cell-mediated rejection of the fetus, which expresses paternal antigens, by maternal T lymphocytes.[42]

Estrogens

The trophoblast lacks 17α-hydroxylase and 17,20-lyase (CYP17) activities and therefore cannot directly convert progesterone to estrogen. Pregnenolone produced in the placenta enters the fetal compartment, where it is taken up by the fetal zone of the adrenal cortex, which also synthesizes pregnenolone from fetal LDL cholesterol. Pregnenolone is conjugated with sulfate by fetal steroid sulfotransferase in the fetal liver and adrenals to form pregnenolone sulfate and is converted in the fetal adrenals to 17α-hydroxy-pregnenolone sulfate and then DHEAS by 17α-hydroxylase and 17,20-lyase (CYP17) activities.[50]

The DHEAS enters the fetal circulation and undergoes hydroxylation in the fetal liver to form 16α-hydroxy-DHEAS, which is converted to 16α-DHEA in the placenta through the action of placental sulfatase. Further metabolism in the trophoblast by 3β-HSD-I, 17β-hydroxysteroid dehydrogenase (17β-HSD), and aromatase (CYP19) leads to the generation of estriol, which is quantitatively the major estrogen in the maternal circulation during pregnancy. The maternal liver actively conjugates estriol with glucosiduronate and sulfate, which are excreted into the urine. Approximately 90% of the estriol present in the maternal serum and urine is derived from fetal precursors, and therefore measurement of estriol levels in serum or urine serves as an index of fetal well-being.[50]

DHEAS from both the fetus and mother is also taken up by the placenta and converted to estradiol by the actions of sulfatase, 3β-HSD-I, 17β-HSD, and aromatase or to estrone by sulfatase, 3β-HSD-I, and aromatase. An estrogen unique to pregnancy, estetrol, is generated by 15α-hydroxylation of 16α-DHEAS in the fetal adrenal followed by enzymatic conversion by placental sulfatase, 3β-HSD-I, 17β-HSD, and aromatase.[51] During pregnancy, estrogens have several actions.[42] They accomplish the following:

1. Enhance receptor-mediated uptake of LDL cholesterol, which is important for normal placental steroid production.
2. Increase uteroplacental blood flow.
3. Increase endometrial prostaglandin synthesis.
4. Prepare the breasts for lactation.

However, estrogen action does not appear to be essential in maintaining pregnancy because a fetus with deletion of the gene encoding placental sulfatase cannot remove the sulfate moiety from 16α-hydroxy-DHEAS and therefore has maternal estrogen levels approaching only about 10% of normal.[52] Similarly, pregnancies complicated by fetal aromatase deficiency may continue to term, again suggesting that the high concentrations of estrogens found in normal pregnancy are not necessary.[53]

Protein Hormones

Human Chorionic Gonadotropin

Chemistry

hCG is a glycoprotein composed of two dissimilar subunits, α and β, which are noncovalently linked through hydrophobic bonding. This molecule shares structural homology with the other glycoprotein hormones, human luteinizing hormone (hLH), hFSH, and hTSH. These hormones have α subunits that contain the same sequence of 92 amino acids and differ only in their carbohydrate composition; the β subunits differ in both amino acid and carbohydrate structure and are responsible for the biologic and immunologic specificity of the heterodimeric (intact) hormones. The 22,200-d β subunit of hCG is composed of 145 amino acids. Approximately 80% of the first 115 amino acids are homologous to those in the β subunit of hLH. hCG has an additional 24 amino acids on its carboxyl-terminal end that enhance its biologic activity.

Both subunits of hCG contain two oligosaccharide chains attached to asparagine residues through N-glycosidic linkages, and the β subunit contains in addition four O-serine–linked oligosaccharide units in the carboxyl-terminal peptide. The carbohydrate composition of hCG contains microheterogeneity and affects hormone clearance and biologic activity. The tertiary structure of hCG is determined by the carbohydrate composition and multiple disulfide bonds within each subunit. The α subunit contains five disulfide bonds; the β subunit has six. In each of the subunits, three of the disulfide bonds form a cystine knot, similar to that found in PDGF-β and transforming growth factor β (TGF-β).[54]

Biosynthesis

The single α subunit gene, located on chromosome 6, is actively expressed in both the cytotrophoblast and syncytiotrophoblast. In contrast, the β subunit is encoded by a cluster of six genes located on chromosome 19 in proximity to the hLH-β gene. Three of the hCG-β genes are actively transcribed during pregnancy, primarily in the syncytiotrophoblast, which thus has the ability to synthesize and secrete free subunits and intact hCG. After synthesis of the protein core, each subunit is glycosylated, undergoes further posttranslational modification through trimming of the carbohydrate, and then combines to form intact hCG.[54]

Secretion of hCG differs from that of many of the other placental proteins, whose secretory pattern parallels that of the trophoblastic mass. hCG is first detected in maternal serum 6 to 9 days after conception.[4] The levels rise in a logarithmic fashion, peaking 8 to 10 weeks after the last menstrual period, followed by a decline to a nadir at 18 weeks, with subsequent levels remaining constant until delivery (Fig. 20–4).[55] The placenta also secretes free subunits. During the first 13 weeks of pregnancy, relatively more β subunit is synthesized than α subunit, and throughout the remainder of pregnancy the opposite occurs.[56] In addition, a hyperglycosylated form of α subunit (*big α*) that is unable to combine with free β subunit is secreted into the maternal serum.

The physiologic factors that regulate hCG secretion in vivo are unknown. Much of the data concerning factors that stimulate or inhibit hCG synthesis and secretion have been derived from in vitro studies and are difficult to extrapolate to the in vivo situation. There is strong circumstantial evidence that GnRH, synthesized in both the cytotrophoblast and syncytiotrophoblast, may be an important factor in hCG secretion. This peptide

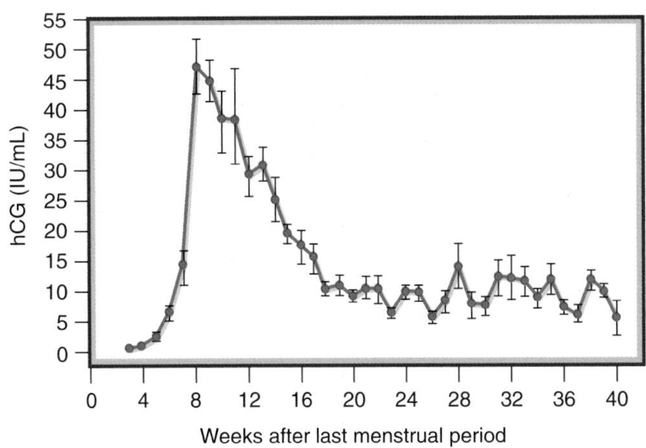

Figure 20-4 ■ Mean (±SE) maternal serum human chorionic gonadotropin (hCG) levels throughout normal pregnancy. (From Braunstein GD, Rasor J, Danzer H, et al. Serum human chorionic gonadotropin levels throughout normal pregnancy. Am J Obstet Gynecol 1976;126:678.)

is identical to hypothalamic GnRH and stimulates placental hCG production both in vitro and in vivo, whereas GnRH antagonists decrease basal hCG secretion.[54,57,58]

Immunohistochemical staining for GnRH in placental tissue is highest at 8 weeks of gestation and lower afterward,[59] roughly paralleling the pattern of hCG production, as do the circulating levels of GnRH measured in maternal serum.[60] In addition, the placenta contains GnRH receptors.[61] Placental GnRH release is stimulated by cyclic adenosine monophosphate (cAMP), prostaglandin E_2, prostaglandin F_2, epinephrine, epidermal growth factor, insulin, and vasoactive intestinal peptide (VIP), factors also noted to increase hCG secretion in vitro.[54,57,62]

Two other peptides synthesized by the cytotrophoblast, activin and inhibin, also modulate GnRH and hCG secretion; activin increases both, and inhibin inhibits the action of GnRH on the syncytiotrophoblast.[57] Increases in hCG production have also been found after trophoblast exposure to FGF, calcium, glucocorticoids, and phorbol esters.[57] Decreased production occurs with TGF-β, follistatin, and progesterone.[57] The decidua may also influence hCG production through paracrine mechanisms.[8] Decidual interleukin-1 stimulates hCG secretion in cultured trophoblasts,[63] while decidual prolactin and an 8- to 10-kd decidual protein inhibit hCG production.[64]

Finally, hCG may autoregulate its own production to some extent. hCG receptors are present on the surface of trophoblastic cells, and the addition of hCG to placental cells in culture stimulates cAMP production as well as proliferation and differentiation of the cytotrophoblasts into syncytiotrophoblasts.[54] Both hCG mRNA and hCG production are stimulated by analogues of cAMP or agents that activate adenylate cyclase, probably through a protein kinase.[54,57] Thus, the net effect of an increase in syncytiotrophoblast mass and cAMP would be enhancement of hCG secretion.

The placenta is not the only site of hCG synthesis. Immunoreactive hCG has been found by immunocytochemistry or by immunoassay of extracts of a wide variety of normal tissues, including spermatozoa, testes, endometrium, kidney, liver, colon, gastric tissue, lung, spleen, heart, fibroblast, brain, and pituitary gland,[65] and the hormone has been shown to be synthesized in some fetal tissues.[54] The pituitary gland appears to be the major source of hCG or an hCG-like material present in nonpregnant individuals. Immunoactive and bioactive hCG has been partially purified from pituitary glands; the material is secreted in vitro by fetal pituitary cells and is shown by immunocytochemistry to be present in gonadotroph-type cells that do not contain hLH or human FSH.[65,66]

Immunoreactive hCG has been measured in sera from normal, nonpregnant individuals, with the highest concentrations found in postmenopausal women.[67,68] In postmenopausal women, this material is secreted in a pulsatile fashion in parallel with hLH pulses, and during the normal menstrual cycle the immunoreactive hCG shows a midcycle peak concomitant with the hLH peak.[67] In both men and postmenopausal women, GnRH stimulates secretion of the hormone, whereas its secretion is inhibited by oral contraceptives in women and by a GnRH agonist in agonadal men.[67,68]

Both gestational and nongestational trophoblastic tumors secrete hCG and its free subunits. The sources of hCG secretion in nongestational trophoblastic neoplasms are the syncytiotrophoblastic cells and in seminomas are the trophoblastic giant cells.[69] In many instances, the tumors produce incomplete forms of hCG or its subunits, and differences in carbohydrate content from the hCG in pregnancy have been especially apparent. A wide variety of nontrophoblastic tumors also secrete hCG, although the predominant moiety appears to be the free β subunit of hCG.[69,70]

Metabolism

After it is secreted, hCG exhibits a biexponential clearance from the circulation with a fast half-life ($T_{1/2}$) of 6 hours and a slow $T_{1/2}$ of close to 36 hours. In contrast, the free β subunit has a 41-minute fast $T_{1/2}$ and a slow $T_{1/2}$ of 4 hours, and the free α subunit has a 13-minute fast $T_{1/2}$ and a 76-minute slow $T_{1/2}$.[71] Approximately 22% of the intact hormone appears in the urine unchanged; the rest undergoes metabolic degradation (Fig. 20–5). One of the early steps is proteolytic cleavage ("nicking")

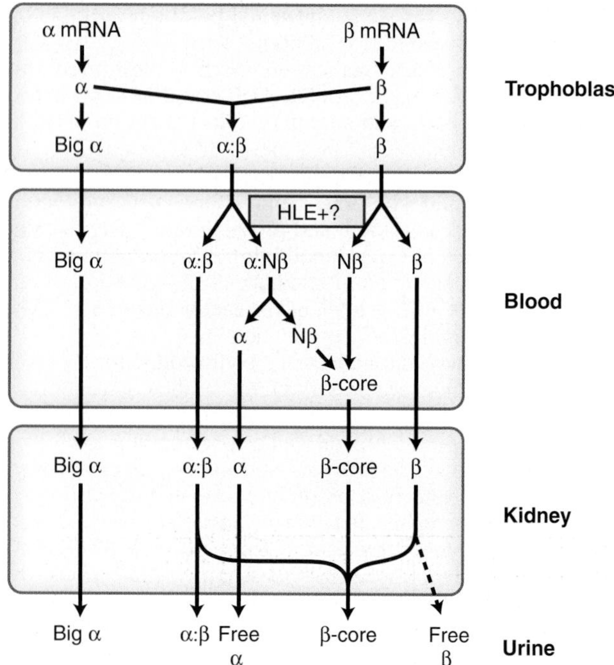

Figure 20-5 ▪ Proposed pathways for metabolism of human chorionic gonadotropin. *α:β,* Intact hCG; *α:Nβ,* hCG with nicked β subunit; *Nβ,* free nicked β subunit; *CTP fragment,* carboxy-terminal fragment; *mRNA,* messenger RNA. (From Braunstein GD. Physiologic functions of human chorionic gonadotropin during pregnancy. In Mochizuki M, Hussa R, eds. Placental Protein Hormones. Amsterdam: Elsevier Science, 1988:33.)

of the β subunit at Val[44]-Leu[45] and Gly[47]-Val[48]. Human leukocyte elastase, present in macrophages and leukocytes, appears to be responsible for some of the nicking of the β subunit.[71]

Nicked hCG is unstable and dissociates into free α subunit and nicked free β subunit. The latter is further metabolized, primarily in the kidney, to produce the β-core fragment, which is composed of the β subunit amino acids 6 to 40 disulfide bridged to amino acids 55 to 92, trimmed of a portion of carbohydrate, and has a molecular mass of 10,479 d.[71] This fragment is the major form of immunoreactive hCG present in the urine in pregnancy. In normal pregnancy, the urine also contains variable quantities of the hyperglycosylated form of α subunit, free α subunit, free β subunit, nicked hCG, nicked free β subunit, carboxyl-terminal fragments of the β subunit, and fragments of the α subunit.[71]

Physiologic Functions

Most, if not all, of the physiologic functions of hCG occur after interaction of the hormone with the hLH-hCG receptor. The receptor gene is located on chromosome 2 and encodes for a G protein–coupled receptor with seven hydrophobic transmembrane domains and a large extracellular amino terminus that binds to hCG (and hLH). The receptor is part of superfamily of receptors, including those for hFSH, hTSH, AVP, VIP, PTH, and receptors for a variety of biogenic amines and neurotransmitters.[54] The hCG-receptor interaction results in increased cAMP production and, in some tissues, increased phosphoinositide turnover.[72]

Because of the close structural homology of the hLH-hCG receptor with the other glycoprotein hormone receptors, hCG may interact with the hTSH and hFSH receptors and thus has weak intrinsic hTSH and hFSH biologic activity. As previously noted, the hTSH-like activity of hCG is clinically manifested during normal pregnancy by the reciprocal decrease in maternal hTSH at the time of the hCG peak between 8 and 12 weeks after the last menstrual period. It is especially important in patients with hydatidiform moles and other forms of trophoblastic disease in which hCG levels may exceed 100,000 IU/L and result in clinical thyrotoxicosis (see Fig. 20–1).[24,25]

One of the major functions of hCG during pregnancy is the "rescue" of the corpus luteum during the conception cycle.[48] During a menstrual cycle without conception, progesterone concentrations in the serum increase for the first 6 to 7 days of the luteal phase, followed by a 3- to 4-day plateau and then a decrease resulting in shedding of the endometrial lining. After conception and implantation, the corpus luteum continues to secrete progesterone and 17-hydroxyprogesterone for another 4 to 6 weeks. The maternal serum progesterone and 17-hydroxyprogesterone concentrations then decrease, indicating a marked diminution in corpus luteum function.[73] The fall in 17-hydroxyprogesterone concentrations continues, but the drop in progesterone levels is only transient. This marks the transition from dependence on ovarian progesterone production to placental progesterone secretion (the luteal-placental shift). As previously noted, luteectomy during the first 50 days after the last menstrual period is associated with a decline in progesterone levels and expulsion of the products of conception. After a therapeutic abortion, progesterone levels also drop rapidly.

Thus, the fetal-placental unit is responsible for the signal to maintain the corpus luteum. The data supporting the idea that hCG is that physiologic signal include the following[48]:

- The presence of hLH-hCG receptors on the corpus luteum
- The early production of hCG by the implanting trophoblast
- The dose-dependent increase in cAMP, progesterone, and estradiol from luteal cells cultured in vitro after exposure to hCG

- The parallel rise of progesterone and hCG in early pregnancy
- The enhanced progesterone secretion and prolongation of the menstrual cycle in nonpregnant women given exogenous hCG during their luteal phase

The inability of hCG to prolong the life of the corpus luteum of pregnancy beyond the sixth to eighth week of pregnancy appears to be due to homologous desensitization of the adenylate cyclase system and the inhibitory effects of the high estrogen levels on progesterone synthesis through inhibition of 3β-hydroxysteroid dehydrogenase and Δ^{5-4}-isomerase in the corpus luteum.

Another physiologic role for hCG is in the differentiation of fetal male genitalia through stimulation of the hLH-hCG receptors on the fetal testicular Leydig cells during the period when differentiation of wolffian duct structures and development of the external genitalia occur. The maximum testosterone production per unit weight of the testes coincides with the maximum binding of ^{125}I-labeled hCG to the fetal testicular receptors at 10 to 12 weeks of development, and fetal Leydig cells produce cAMP and testosterone in vitro after exposure to hCG. The hCG concentrations in fetal serum parallel the fetal testicular testosterone levels at a time when the amount of fetal pituitary hLH is not sufficient to stimulate the testosterone production.[72]

There are several other possible actions of hCG during normal pregnancy. In vitro, hCG stimulates the differentiation of cytotrophoblast to syncytiotrophoblast and hence may play an important paracrine role in regulating syncytiotrophoblast mass and production of trophoblast hormones.[64,74] Additional data supporting this autoregulatory effect of hCG include the in vitro stimulation of placental synthesis of cAMP, activation of glycogen phosphorylase, and incorporation of radiolabeled galactose and leucine into placental proteins upon exposure to hCG.[72] hCG stimulates the secretion of VEGF from the cytotrophoblast, which may be important for placental angiogenesis.[54] Vasodilation of myometrial blood vessels mediated by hCG binding to vascular hCG receptors may enhance uterine blood flow in early pregnancy.[54] The fetal zone of the adrenal releases DHEAS in response to hCG exposure in vitro; therefore, hCG may have adrenocorticotropic activities in concert with fetal pituitary ACTH and placental ACTH.[72]

It has also been suggested that hCG plays a role in the immunosuppression that occurs during pregnancy. Many early studies on this topic were hampered by the use of impure preparations of hCG or the presence of preservatives such as phenol that may alter the end-points of the test systems used to define immunosuppression. In addition, the immunosuppressive effects may be due to gonadal steroid secretion in response to the hCG in the in vivo models used in some of the studies.[75] Relaxin secretion from the corpus luteum is stimulated by hCG both in vivo and in vitro.[54]

Finally, the decrease in osmotic threshold for thirst and AVP release during pregnancy is clearly related to hCG.[28] Whether this decrease is due to a direct effect of hCG or an indirect effect through stimulation of gonadal steroids or interaction with hLH-hCG receptors present in vascular smooth muscle is unclear.

Gestational Trophoblastic Disease

Gestational trophoblastic disease (GTD) includes complete and partial hydatidiform moles, choriocarcinoma, and placental-site trophoblastic tumor.[76] Complete molar pregnancy is the most common variety, occurring in 1 to 2 in 1000 pregnancies. Patients usually present with vaginal bleeding, a uterus that is larger than expected for the duration of pregnancy, anemia, and excessive vomiting. Pathologically, trophoblast hyperplasia, marked edema of the chorionic villi, and absence of fetal tissues are observed. In contrast, partial moles demonstrate focal trophoblast hyperplasia and villous swelling and often have fetal tissues with congenital malformations. Approximately 20% of patients with complete moles develop persistent trophoblastic disease, whereas only 2% to 4% of patients develop persistent disease after partial molar pregnancy. Persistent trophoblastic disease also can occur after a normal term pregnancy as well as in pregnancies that end in spontaneous or induced abortion.

Choriocarcinoma is the most aggressive malignant form of persistent trophoblastic disease and may involve complications from local uterine disease, such as bleeding and rupture of the uterus, or from the effects of metastases, especially those involving the liver, lungs, and brain. The least common form of GTD is placental-site trophoblastic tumor, which is derived from the intermediate trophoblast and is often associated with vaginal bleeding and amenorrhea.[76]

All of these neoplasms secrete hCG, free β subunit, and often additional forms of these molecules. With the exception of placental-site trophoblastic tumor, which secretes relatively low amounts of hCG, the serum and urine concentrations of hCG roughly parallel the tumor burden and provide prognostic information. Thus, hCG measurements in concert with clinical and radiologic findings, especially vaginal ultrasonography findings, are useful for making the diagnosis of GTD. On rare occasions, false-positive, low-level hCG results may be found in some women who have heterophilic antibodies and other interfering substances in their sera.[76] This may lead to a misdiagnosis of GTD. Because these substances are not excreted in the urine, a urine pregnancy test will be negative in the presence of such "phantom hCG."[76]

Hydatidiform moles are initially treated with uterine dilation and evacuation with or without adjunctive single-agent chemotherapy with methotrexate or actinomycin D. Approximately 90% of patients with low-risk, persistent trophoblastic disease are cured by single-agent chemotherapy; 75% of patients with high-risk, metastatic disease are cured by multiagent chemotherapy, including etoposide, methotrexate, actinomycin D, cyclophosphamide, and vincristine. Serial hCG measurements are invaluable for monitoring as they accurately reflect the effect of therapy on the tumor.[76]

Human Placental Lactogen

Also called chorionic somatomammotropin, hPL is a single-chain, nonglycosylated polypeptide composed of 191 amino acid residues and two disulfide bridges, with a molecular mass of 21,600 d.[20,77] It is closely related chemically and biologically to both GH (85% amino acid homology) and prolactin (13% amino acid homology). The hGH-hPL gene cluster is located on the long arm of chromosome 17 and consists of five genes—one coding for pituitary hGH (hGH-N), one for placental hGH (hGH-V), and three for placental hPL (hPL-L, hPL-A, and hPL-B, of which only hPL-A and hPL-B are transcribed).[21,77]

hPL is synthesized and secreted by the syncytiotrophoblast and is detected in maternal serum between 20 and 40 days of gestation.[20] The maternal serum levels rise rapidly and peak at 34 weeks, followed by a plateau (Fig. 20–6).[78] Both the serum concentrations and placental hPL mRNA concentrations are closely correlated with placental weight and syncytiotrophoblastic mass.[78,79] The maternal serum concentrations at term average between 6 and 7 μg/mL; at that time, on the basis of the 9- to 15-minute $T_{1/2}$ of disappearance from the circulation, the placental production rate of hPL is in excess of 1 g/day. The fetal serum levels are 1/50 to 1/100 of the maternal levels.[77]

The physiologic in vivo regulation of hPL synthesis and secretion, other than the constitutive production related to placental mass, is unknown. Several studies have examined the possible role of nutrients in hPL secretion in pregnant women. Neither acute hyperglycemia nor hypoglycemia appeared to alter the hPL concentrations, although prolonged glucose infusions

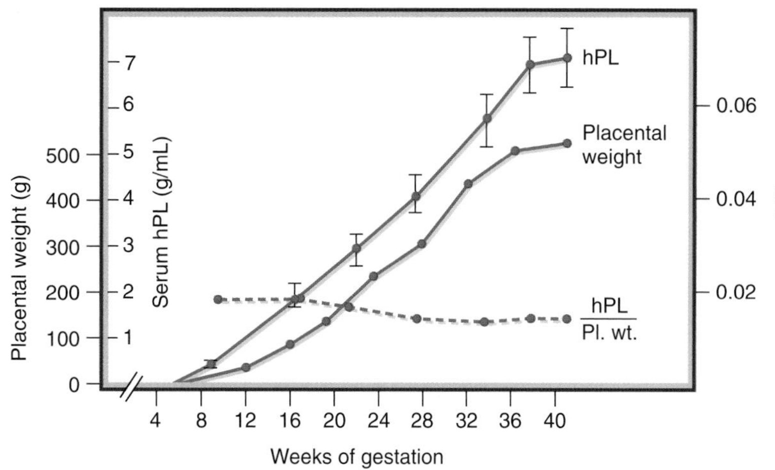

Figure 20–6 ■ Placental weight (Pl. wt.) and maternal serum concentrations of human placental lactogen (hPL) during pregnancy. (From Selenkow HA, Saxena BN, Dana CL. Measurement and pathophysiologic significance of human placental lactogen. In Pecile A, Finzi C, eds. The Feto-Placental Unit. Amsterdam: Excerpta Medica, 1969:340.)

decreased and prolonged fasting increased the concentrations.[20,57,77,80] Arginine infusions, dexamethasone administration, and changes in plasma free fatty acid levels did not affect the maternal hPL concentrations.[81-82] Glucose, estrogens, glucocorticoids, prostaglandins, epinephrine, oxytocin, TRH, GnRH, and l-dopa have been examined in in vitro systems and found to be without consistent effects.[83-86]

Angiotensin II, IGF-I, phospholipase A_2, arachidonic acid, and epidermal growth factor stimulated hPL release in vitro.[57,87] Epidermal growth factor probably enhances production through promotion of cytotrophoblast-to-syncytiotrophoblast differentiation.[87] Apolipoprotein AI also stimulated hPL synthesis and release through cAMP-dependent and arachidonic acid–dependent pathways.[20,88,89] Because changes in the maternal plasma apolipoprotein AI concentrations parallel those of hPL during pregnancy, it is likely that this apoprotein, alone and as part of circulating HDL, is important in the secretion of hPL.[89]

hPL has a number of biologic activities that are qualitatively similar to those of hGH and prolactin and can bind to both the hGH and prolactin receptors.[90] In various bioassay systems, hPL had weak somatotropic and lactogenic effects.[90,91] It appears to be a major regulator of IGF-I production, and during pregnancy, hPL concentrations are correlated with those of IGF-I.[20,91] HPL also affects the metabolism of maternal nutrients. It stimulates pancreatic islet insulin secretion, both directly and after carbohydrate administration,[90,92] and is a diabetogenic factor during pregnancy through its promotion of insulin resistance. It enhances lipolysis, leading to a rise in free fatty acids, which may in part be responsible for the insulin resistance.[90]

The various biologic activities of hPL have led to the hypothesis that the role of hPL during pregnancy is to provide the fetus with a constant supply of glucose and amino acids.[90] The hPL-stimulated lipolysis allows the mother to utilize free fatty acids for energy during fasting, allowing glucose, amino acids, and ketone bodies to cross the placenta for use by the fetus. In addition, hPL has actions in the fetus, promoting amino acid uptake by muscle and stimulating protein production, IGF-I production, and glycogen synthesis.[91]

Despite the proposed importance of hPL in maternal and fetal metabolic homeostasis during pregnancy, its absence does not appear to impair pregnancy. Deficient or absent hPL production related to gene defects has been described in several women who experienced normal pregnancies and delivered normal infants.[93]

Placental Growth Hormone

Placental GH, hGH-V, is synthesized and secreted by the syncytiotrophoblast.[20] Alternate splicing of the hGH-V gene results in two nonglycosylated isoforms with molecular masses of 22 and 26 kd.[21,77] The 22-kd variant may also be glycosylated and circulate as a 26-kd protein.[77] HGH-V is detected in the maternal plasma from 10 weeks of gestation and peaks during the third trimester (Fig. 20–7).[20,21,94,95]

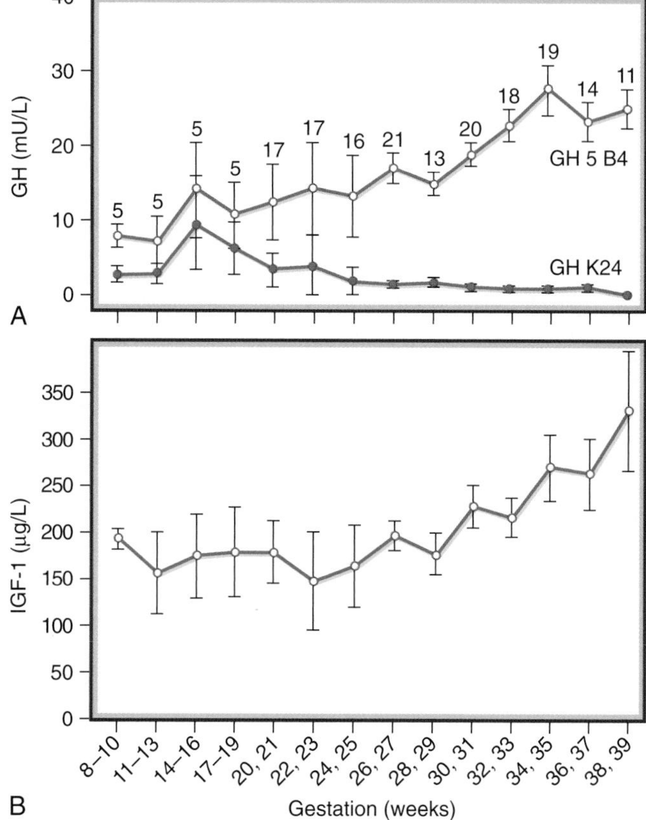

Figure 20–7 ■ Mean (± standard error) of plasma human growth hormone (hGH) **(A)** and insulin-like growth factor I (IGF-I) **(B)** levels throughout pregnancy. The number of individual assays of growth hormone (GH) and IGF-I at each gestational stage is indicated in *A* on top of vertical bars. GH 5 B4 indicates placental GH (hGH-V); GH K24 indicates pituitary GH. (From Mirlesse V, Frankenne F, Alsat E, et al. Placental growth hormone levels in normal pregnancy and in pregnancies with intrauterine growth retardation. Pediatr Res 1993;34:39.)

HGH-V has somatotropic activity and stimulates IGF-I production, and the increase in IGF-I concentrations may in turn be responsible for the suppression of maternal pituitary hGH secretion (see Fig. 20–7).[91,94] Unlike pituitary hGH, hGH-V is not secreted in a pulsatile fashion, nor is it released from the trophoblast by growth hormone–releasing hormone (GHRH), but it is inhibited by glucose. It has been estimated that at term, 85% of the GH biologic activity in maternal serum is due to hGH-V, 12% to hPL, and only 3% to pituitary hGH.[96] Within 48 hours of delivery, pituitary hGH secretion returns to normal.

Human Chorionic Corticotropin

The syncytiotrophoblast synthesizes an ACTH-like peptide, human chorionic corticotropin (hCC), as well as several pro-opiomelanocortin-derived peptides, including β-lipotropin, β-endorphin, and α-melanocyte–stimulating hormone.[26] The maternal serum concentrations of ACTH increase as pregnancy progresses, and the elevation of free cortisol levels during pregnancy may be related in part to both placental hCC and pituitary ACTH production.[26]

HCC secretion is stimulated by CRH, which is probably the most important factor regulating the local production of the peptide through paracrine or autocrine mechanisms, or both, because it is also produced by both the cytotrophoblast and the syncytiotrophoblast. Unlike the situation with the pituitary, glucocorticoids and oxytocin also stimulate hCC release from placental cultures.[27] Indeed, the resistance of maternal plasma ACTH concentrations to suppression after glucocorticoid administration may reflect the placental hCC contribution to the total pool of circulating immunoreactive ACTH.[26]

Hypothalamic Peptides

Gonadotropin-Releasing Hormone

Both the cytotrophoblast and the syncytiotrophoblast synthesize and secrete GnRH, which has the same chemical structure and biologic activity as hypothalamic GnRH.[57,59] Although the GnRH mRNA levels in the placenta are similar throughout gestation, the highest concentrations of the peptide in the placenta and serum are found during the first trimester and correlate with the mass of the cytotrophoblast and peak hCG concentrations.[59,97]

In vitro, GnRH production by placental explants or purified trophoblasts is stimulated by prostaglandins, epinephrine, activin, insulin, epidermal growth factor, VIP, estradiol, and estriol, and secretion is reduced by inhibin, progesterone, and κ-opiate and μ-opiate agonists.[98,99] The syncytiotrophoblast contains low-affinity GnRH receptors, whose concentrations parallel the hCG secretory pattern.[61]

Because GnRH stimulates hCG secretion by placental explants and purified trophoblast cells in vitro, with the response of early to midtrimester placentas being greater than that of term trophoblast, it is reasonable to conclude that GnRH is an important autocrine or paracrine regulator of hCG secretion.[98] The hCG-stimulatory effect of GnRH can be blocked by administration of a GnRH antagonist.[58] Because GnRH stimulates metalloproteinases in cytotrophoblasts, the peptide may be important during implantation.[100]

Corticotropin-Releasing Hormone

Both the cytotrophoblast and the syncytiotrophoblast synthesize and secrete a 41-amino-acid peptide that is identical to hypothalamic CRH.[26,101] CRH mRNA is first detected in trophoblast at 7 weeks of gestation. The levels remaining low during the first 30 weeks of pregnancy but rise 20-fold during the final 5 weeks, a pattern that is parallel to the rise of CRH content in the placenta and concentrations in maternal plasma.[101] In maternal plasma, CRH circulates bound to a 37-kd protein that is synthesized by the placenta, liver, and brain and that reduces the biologic activity of the CRH.[26,101]

In vitro, placental CRF production is stimulated by prostaglandins (E_2 and $F_2\alpha$), norepinephrine, acetylcholine, oxytocin, neuropeptide Y, AVP, angiotensin II, and interleukin-1. Glucocorticoids have been shown to increase both CRH mRNA and peptide, whereas in the hypothalamus suppression is found. CRH secretion is reduced by progesterone and nitric oxide donors. The placenta contains CRH binding sites, and the addition of CRH to cultured placental cells results in a dose-dependent increase in hCC, β-endorphin, and α-melanocyte–stimulating hormone secretion.[26,57,101] Thus, it is likely that CRH has an autocrine or paracrine effect in the placenta.

Whether CRH has a physiologic effect on the maternal pituitary secretion of ACTH is unclear; the circulating CRH may be biologically inactive because of the binding protein. However, just before parturition, the binding protein concentration decreases by approximately 50% and the CRH levels rise.[26,101] At this time, CRH stimulates the synthesis and release of prostaglandins from the decidua, amnion, and chorion, which enhances cervical ripening.[102] The myometrium contains CRH receptors, and CRH may increase myometrial contractility.[101] Thus, CRH may have a role in initiating and promoting parturition. CRH may also stimulate the fetal pituitary production of ACTH, which, in turn, may lead to increased fetal adrenal DHEA production and ultimately estriol synthesis by the fetoplacental unit.[101] In addition to CRH, the syncytiotrophoblast and fetal membranes secrete urocortin 1, which in vitro stimulates placental ACTH, PGE_2, and activin secretion through the CRH receptor.[103]

Other Peptides

A peptide with properties of TRH that is not identical to hypothalamic TRH has been identified in the placenta.[104,105] It is capable of stimulating the release of hTSH in vitro and in vivo.[106,107] It has unknown physiologic significance because there is no convincing evidence that a chorionic thyrotropin exists, and hCG appears to be the major trophoblastic thyrotropin-like substance.

Immunoreactive somatostatin has been identified in the cytotrophoblast in first trimester placentas.[108,109] The levels decrease as pregnancy advances.[108] This pattern has led to the speculation that somatostatin inhibits hPL production and that the loss of inhibition allows the placenta to secrete increasing quantities of hPL.[108] The finding of somatostatin receptors in the placenta adds some indirect support to this hypothesis.[109] However, somatostatin does not inhibit hPL (or hGH-V) production by placental cells exposed to the peptide in vitro.[109]

A substance with GHRH-like activity has been found in the placenta.[110] However, because exposure of placental cells to hypothalamic GHRH does not result in stimulation of hPL or hGH-V secretion, it is unlikely that human placental GHRH is physiologically important.

Several other neuropeptides have been found in the placenta, usually through immunohistochemical techniques. These include methionine enkephalin,[57,111] leucine enkephalin,[111] dynorphin,[111,112] neuropeptide Y,[57,113] and oxytocin.[57,114] The physiologic functions of these placental peptides are unknown. It has been suggested that dynorphin may have a role in the paracrine regulation of hPL release through its binding to placental κ-opiate receptors.[111,112] Neuropeptide Y and oxytocin stimulate the secretion of CRH from placental cells in culture.[62]

Growth Factors

Many growth factors, growth factor-binding proteins, and growth factor receptors have been identified in the placenta. These include IGF-I, IGF-II, relaxin, epidermal growth factor, PDGF, nerve growth factor, FGF, TGF-β, inhibin, activin, and folliculostatin.[57,62] As reviewed earlier, a number of these factors have been implicated in the autocrine or paracrine regulation of placental hormone synthesis and release and placental angiogenesis, and they may have important actions in fetal development. In addition to the placenta, the human endometrium is a rich source of growth factors, cytokines, and vasoactive neuropeptides that are important for uteroplacental function.[8]

REFERENCES

1. Wilcox AJ, Weinberg CR, O'Connor JF, et al. Incidence of early loss of pregnancy. N Engl J Med 1988;319:189.
2. Norwitz ER, Schust DJ, Fisher JJ. Mechanisms of disease: implantation and the survival of early pregnancy. N Engl J Med 2001; 345:1400.
3. Kodaman PH, Taylor HS. Hormonal regulation of implantation. Obstet Gynecol Clin North Am 2004;31:745.
4. Braunstein GD, Grodin JM, Vaitukaitis J, et al. Secretory rates of human chorionic gonadotropin by normal trophoblast. Am J Obstet Gynecol 1973;115:447.
5. Dey S, Lim H, Das SK, et al. Molecular cues to implantation. Endocrin Rev 2004;117:53.
6. Cross JC, Werb Z, Fisher SJ. Implantation and the placenta: key pieces of the development puzzle. Science 1994;266:1508.
7. Greiss FC Jr, Anderson SG, Still JG. Uterine pressure-flow relationships during early gestation. Am J Obstet Gynecol 1976;126:799.
8. Tabibzadeh S. Human endometrium: an active site of cytokine production and action. Endocr Rev 1991;2:272.
9. Gordon JD, Shifren JL, Foulk RA, et al. Angiogenesis in the human female reproductive tract. Obstet Gynecol Surv 1995;50:688.
10. Fisher DA. Endocrinology of fetal development. In Larsen PR Kronenberg HM, Melmed S, Polansky KS, eds. Williams Textbook of Endocrinology. Philadelphia: WB Saunders, 2003:811.
11. Szekerese-Bartho J. Immunological relationship between the mother and the fetus. Int Rev Immunol 2002;24:471.
12. Braunstein GD, Rasor JL, Engvall E, et al. Interrelationships of human chorionic gonadotropin, human placental lactogen, and pregnancy-specific beta 1-glycoprotein throughout normal human gestation. Am J Obstet Gynecol 1980;138:1205.
13. Cunningham EG, Leveno KJ, Bloom SL, et al. (eds) Maternal physiology. In Williams Obstetrics, New York: McGraw-Hill, 2005:121.
14. Castro LC, Hobel CJ, Gornbein J. Plasma levels of atrial natriuretic peptide in normal and hypertensive pregnancies: a meta-analysis. Am J Obstet Gynecol 1994;171:1642.
15. Lindheimer MD, Davison JM. Osmoregulation, the secretion of arginine vasopressin and its metabolism during pregnancy. Eur J Endocrinol 1995;132:133.
16. Foyouzi N, Yr Frisbaek BA, Norwitz ER. Pituitary gland and pregnancy. Obstet Gynecol Clin North Am 2004;31:873.
17. Elster AD, Sanders TG, Vines FS, et al. Size and shape of the pituitary gland during pregnancy and post partum: measurement with MR imaging. Radiology 1991;181:531.
18. Lehtovirta P, Ranta T. Effect of short-term bromocriptine treatment on amniotic fluid prolactin concentration in the first half of pregnancy. Acta Endocrinol 1981;97:559.
19. Emmi AM, Skurnick J, Goldsmith LT, et al. Ovarian control of pituitary hormone secretion in early human pregnancy. J Clin Endocrinol Metab 1991;72:1359.
20. Handwerger S, Brar A. Placental lactogen, placental growth hormone, and decidual prolactin. Semin Reprod Endocrinol 1992;10:106.
21. Alsat E, Guibourdenche J, Luton D, et al. Human placental growth hormone. Am J Obstet Gynecol 1997;177:1526.
22. Walker WH, Fitzpatrick SL, Barrera-Saldana HA, et al. The human placental lactogen genes: structure, function, evolution and transcriptional regulation. Endocr Rev 1991;12:316.
23. Zimkeller W. Current topic: the role of growth hormone and insulin-like growth factors for placental growth and development. Placenta 2000;21:451.
24. Glinoer D. The regulation of thyroid function in pregnancy: pathways of endocrine adaptation from physiology to pathology. Endocr Rev 1997;18:404.
25. Glinoer D, de Nayer P, Bourdoux P, et al. Regulation of maternal thyroid during pregnancy. J Clin Endocrinol Metab 1990;71:276.
26. Lindsay JR, Nieman LK. The hypothalamic-pituitary-adrenal axis in pregnancy: challenges in disease detection and treatment. Endocrin Rev 2005;26:775.
27. Jones SA, Brooks AN, Challis JR. Steroids modulate corticotropin-releasing hormone production in human fetal membranes and placenta. J Clin Endocrinol Metab 1989;68:825.
28. Davison JM, Shiells EA, Philips PR, et al. Serial evaluation of vasopressin release and thirst in human pregnancy. Role of human chorionic gonadotrophin in the osmoregulatory changes of gestation. J Clin Invest 1988;81:798.
29. Davison JM, Sheills EA, Barron WM, et al. Changes in the metabolic clearance of vasopressin and in plasma vasopressinase throughout human pregnancy. J Clin Invest 1989;83:1313.
30. Leake RD, Weitzman RE, Glatz TH, et al. Plasma oxytocin concentrations in men, nonpregnant women, and pregnant women before and during spontaneous labor. J Clin Endocrinol Metab 1981; 53:730.
31. Zeeman GG, Khan-Dawood FS, Dawood MY. Oxytocin and its receptor in pregnancy and parturition: current concepts and clinical implications. Obstet Gynecol 1997;89:873.
32. Kovacs CS. Calcium and bone metabolism in pregnancy and lactation. J Clin Endocrinol Metab 2001;86:2344.
33. Strewler GJ. Mechanisms of disease: the physiology of parathyroid hormone-related protein. N Engl J Med 2000;342:177
34. Costrini NV, Kalkhoff RK. Relative effects of pregnancy, estradiol, and progesterone on plasma insulin and pancreatic islet insulin secretion. J Clin Invest 1971;50:992.
35. Lind T, Bell S, Gilmore E, et al. Insulin disappearance rate in pregnant and non-pregnant women, and in non-pregnant women given GHRIH. Eur J Clin Invest 1977;7:47.
36. Galerneau F, Inzucchi SE. Diabetes mellitus in pregnancy. Obstet Gynecol Clin North Am 2004;31:907.
37. Carr BR, Parker CR Jr, Madden JD, et al. Maternal plasma adrenocorticotropin and cortisol relationships throughout human pregnancy. Am J Obstet Gynecol 1981;139:416.
38. Rainey WE, Rehman KS, Carr BR. Fetal and maternal adrenals in human pregnancy. Obstet Gynecol Clin North Am 2004;31: 817.
39. Zuspan FP. Urinary excretion of epinephrine and norepinephrine during pregnancy. J Clin Endocrinol Metab 1970;30:357.
40. Tunbridge RD, Donnai P. Plasma noradrenaline in normal pregnancy and in hypertension of late pregnancy. Br J Obstet Gynaecol 1981;88:105.
41. Ramayya MS, Zhou J, Kino T, et al. Steroidogenic factor 1 messenger ribonucleic acid expression in steroidogenic and nonsteroidogenic human tissues: Northern blot and in situ hybridization studies. J Clin Endocrinol Metab 1997;82:1799.
42. Pepe GJ, Albrecht ED. Actions of placental and fetal adrenal steroid hormones in primate pregnancy. Endocr Rev 1995;16:608.
43. Tulchinsky D, Hobel CJ, Yeager E, et al. Plasma estrone, estradiol, estriol, progesterone, and 17-hydroxyprogesterone in human pregnancy. I. Normal pregnancy. Am J Obstet Gynecol 1972;112:1095.
44. Levitz M, Young BK. Estrogens in pregnancy. Vitam Horm 1977;35:109.
45. Simpson ER, Burkhart MF. Regulation of cholesterol metabolism by human choriocarcinoma cells in culture: effect of lipoproteins and progesterone on cholesteryl ester synthesis. Arch Biochem Biophys 1980;200:86.
46. Kallen CB. Steroid hormone synthesis in pregnancy. Obstet Gynecol Clin North Am 2004;31:795.
47. Bose HS, Sugawara T, Strauss JF III, et al. The pathophysiology and genetics of congenital lipoid adrenal hyperplasia. International Congenital Lipoid Adrenal Hyperplasia Consortium. N Engl J Med 1996;335:1870.
48. Braunstein GD. Evidence favoring human chorionic gonadotropin as the physiological "rescuer" of the corpus luteum during early pregnancy. Early Pregnancy 1996;2:183.
49. Spitz IM, Bardin CW. Drug therapy: mifepristone (RU486)—a modulator of progestin and glucocorticoid action. N Engl J Med 1993;329:404.
50. Miller WL. Steroid hormone biosynthesis and actions in the materno-feto-placental unit. Clin Perinatol 1998;25:799.
51. Heikkila J, Luukkainen T. Urinary excretion of estriol and 15 alpha-hydroxyestriol in complicated pregnancies. Am J Obstet Gynecol 1971;110:509.

52. Ryan KJ. Placental synthesis of steroid hormones. In Tulchinsky D, Ryan KJ, eds. Maternal-Fetal Endocrinology. Philadelphia: WB Saunders, 1980:3.
53. Shozu M, Akasofu K, Harada T, et al. A new cause of female pseudohermaphroditism: placental aromatase deficiency. J Clin Endocrinol Metab 1991;72:560.
54. Keay SD, Vatish M, Karteris E, et al. The role of hCG in reproductive medicine. Br J Obstet Gynaecol 2004;111:1218.
55. Braunstein GD, Rasor J, Danzer H, et al. Serum human chorionic gonadotropin levels throughout normal pregnancy. Am J Obstet Gynecol 1976;126:678.
56. Ozturk M, Bellet D, Manil L, et al. Physiological studies of human chorionic gonadotropin (hCG), alpha hCG, and beta hCG as measured by specific monoclonal immunoradiometric assays. Endocrinology 1987;120:549.
57. Sullivan MHF. Endocrine cell lines from the placenta. Mol Cell Endocrinol 2004;228:103.
58. Siler-Khodr TM, Khodr GS, Vickery BH, et al. Inhibition of hCG, alpha hCG and progesterone release from human placental tissue in vitro by a GnRH antagonist. Life Sci 1983;32:2741.
59. Miyake A, Sakumoto T, Aono T, et al. Changes in luteinizing hormone-releasing hormone in human placenta throughout pregnancy. Obstet Gynecol 1982;60:444.
60. Siler-Khodr TM, Khodr GS, Valenzuela G. Immunoreactive gonadotropin-releasing hormone level in maternal circulation throughout pregnancy. Am J Obstet Gynecol 1984;150:376.
61. Currie AJ, Fraser HM, Sharpe RM. Human placental receptors for luteinizing hormone releasing hormone. Biochem Biophys Res Commun 1981;99:332.
62. Petraglia F, Santuz M, Florio P, et al. Paracrine regulation of human placenta: control of hormonogenesis. J Reprod Immunol 1998;39: 221.
63. Masuhiro K, Matsuzaki N, Nishino E, et al. Trophoblast-derived interleukin-1 (IL-1) stimulates the release of human chorionic gonadotropin by activating IL-6 and IL-6-receptor system in first trimester human trophoblasts. J Clin Endocrinol Metab 1991; 72:594.
64. Ren SG, Braunstein GD. Decidua produces a protein that inhibits choriogonadotrophin release from human trophoblasts. J Clin Invest 1991;87:326.
65. Braunstein GD, Kamdar V, Rasor J, et al. Widespread distribution of a chorionic gonadotropin-like substance in normal human tissues. J Clin Endocrinol Metab 1979;49:917.
66. Odell WD, Griffin J, Bashey HM, et al. Secretion of chorionic gonadotropin by cultured human pituitary cells. J Clin Endocrinol Metab 1990;71:1318.
67. Odell WD, Griffin J. Pulsatile secretion of human chorionic gonadotropin in normal adults. N Engl J Med 1987;317:1688.
68. Stenman UH, Alfthan H, Ranta T, et al. Serum levels of human chorionic gonadotropin in nonpregnant women and men are modulated by gonadotropin-releasing hormone and sex steroids. J Clin Endocrinol Metab 1987;64:730.
69. Braunstein GD. Placental proteins as tumor markers. In Herberman RB, Mercer DW, eds. Immunodiagnosis of Cancer. New York: Marcel Dekker, 1991:673.
70. Stenman U-H, Alfthan H, Hotakainen K. Human chorionic gonadotropin in cancer. Clin Biochem 2004;37:549.
71. Braunstein GD. Beta core fragment: structure, production, metabolism, and clinical utility. In Lustbader JW, Puett D, Ruddon RW, eds. Glycoprotein Hormones. New York: Springer-Verlag, 1994: 293.
72. Braunstein GD. Physiologic functions of human chorionic gonadotropin during pregnancy. In Mochizuki M, Hussa R, eds. Placental Protein Hormones. Amsterdam: Elsevier Science Publishers, 1988:33.
73. Yoshimi T, Strott CA, Marshall JR, et al. Corpus luteum function in early pregnancy. J Clin Endocrinol Metab 1969;29:225
74. North RA, Whitehead R, Larkins RG. Stimulation by human chorionic gonadotropin of prostaglandin synthesis by early human placental tissue. J Clin Endocrinol Metab 1991;73:60.
75. Nisula B, Bartocci A. Choriogonadotropin and immunity: a reevaluation. Ann Endocrinol 1984;45:315.
76. Soper Jt, Mutch DG, Schink JC. Diagnosis and treatment of gestational trophoblastic disease: ACOG Practice Bulletin No. 53. Gynecol Oncol 2004;93:575.
77. Barrera-Saldana HA. Growth hormone and placental lactogen: biology, medicine and biotechnology. Gene 1998;211:11.
78. Selenkow HA, Saxena BN, Dana CL. Measurement and pathophysiologic significance of human placental lactogen. In Pecile A, Finzi C, eds. The Feto-Placental Unit. Amsterdam: Excerpta Medica, 1969:340.
79. Hoshina M, Boothby M, Boime I. Cytological localization of chorionic gonadotropin alpha and placental lactogen mRNAs during development of the human placenta. J Cell Biol 1982;93:190.
80. Gaspard U, Sandront H, Luyckx A. Glucose-insulin interaction and the modulation of human placental lactogen (HPL) secretion during pregnancy. J Obstet Gynaecol Br Commonw 1974;81:201.
81. Morris HH, Vinik AI, Mulvihal M. Effects of acute alterations in maternal free fatty acid concentration on human chorionic somatomammotropin secretion. Am J Obstet Gynecol 1974; 119:224.
82. Ylikorkala O, Kauppila A. Effect of dexamethasone on serum levels of human placental lactogen during the last trimester of pregnancy. J Obstet Gynaecol Br Commonw 1974;81:368.
83. Niven PA, Buhi WC, Spellacy WN. The effect of intravenous oestrogen injections on plasma human placental lactogen levels. J Obstet Gynaecol Br Commonw 1974;81:466.
84. Belleville F, Lasbennes A, Nabet P, et al. Study of compounds capable of intervening in the in vitro regulation of the secretion of chorionic somatomammotropin by placenta in culture. C R Seances Soc Biol Fil 1974;168:1057.
85. Handwerger S, Barrett J, Tyrey L, et al. Differential effect of cyclic adenosine monophosphate on the secretion of human placental lactogen and human chorionic gonadotropin. J Clin Endocrinol Metab 1973;36:1268.
86. Hershman JM, Kojima A, Friesen HG. Effect of thyrotropin-releasing hormone on human pituitary thyrotropin, prolactin, placental lactogen, and chorionic thyrotropin. J Clin Endocrinol Metab 1973;36:497.
87. Wilson EA, Jawad MJ, Vernon MW. Effect of epidermal growth factor on hormone secretion by term placenta in organ culture. Am J Obstet Gynecol 1984;149:579.
88. Handwerger S, Quarfordt S, Barrett J, et al. Apolipoproteins AI, AII, and CI stimulate placental lactogen release from human placental tissue. A novel action of high density lipoprotein apolipoproteins. J Clin Invest 1987;79:625.
89. Desoye G, Schweditsch MO, Pfeiffer KP, et al. Correlation of hormones with lipid and lipoprotein levels during normal pregnancy and postpartum. J Clin Endocrinol Metab 1987;64:704.
90. Eberhardt NL, Jiang SW, Shepard AR, et al. Hormonal and cell-specific regulation of the human growth hormone and chorionic somatomammotropin genes. Prog Nucleic Acid Res Mol Biol 1996;54:127.
91. Handwerger S, Freemark M. The roles of placental growth hormone and placental lactogen in the regulation of human fetal growth and development. J Pediatr Endocrinol Metab 2000;13:343.
92. Sorenson RL, Brelje TC. Adaptation of islets of Langerhans to pregnancy: beta-cell growth, enhanced insulin secretion and the role of lactogenic hormones. Horm Metab Res 1997;29:301.
93. Sideri M, De Virgiliis G, Guidobono F, et al. Immunologically undetectable human placental lactogen in a normal pregnancy. Br J Obstet Gynaecol 1983;90:771.
94. Mirlesse V, Frankenne F, Alsat E, et al. Placental growth hormone levels in normal pregnancy and in pregnancies with intrauterine growth retardation. Pediatr Res 1993;34:39.
95. Lonberg U, Damm P, Andersson AM, et al. Increase in maternal placental growth hormone during pregnancy and disappearance during parturition in normal and growth hormone-deficient pregnancies. Am J Obstet Gynecol 2003;188:247.
96. Petraglia F, Florio P, Nappi C, et al. Peptide signaling in human placenta and membranes: autocrine, paracrine, and endocrine mechanisms. Endocr Rev 1996;17:156.
97. Kelly AC, Rodgers A, Dong KW, et al. Gonadotropin-releasing hormone and chorionic gonadotropin gene expression in human placental development. DNA Cell Biol 1991;10:411.
98. Petraglia F, Lim AT, Vale W. Adenosine 3′,5′-monophosphate, prostaglandins, and epinephrine stimulate the secretion of immunoreactive gonadotropin-releasing hormone from cultured human placental cells. J Clin Endocrinol Metab 1987;65:1020.

99. Petraglia F, Vaughan J, Vale W. Steroid hormones modulate the release of immunoreactive gonadotropin-releasing hormone from cultured human placental cells. J Clin Endocrinol Metab 1990; 70:1173.
100. Chou CS, Zhu H, MacCalman CD, et al. Regulatory effects of gonadotropin-releasing hormone (GnRH) I and GnRH II on the levels of matrix metalloproteinase (MMP)-2, MMP-9, and tissue inhibitor of metalloproteinase-1 in primary cultures of human extravillous cytotrophoblasts. J Clin Endocrinol Metab 2003;88:4781
101. Fadalti M, Pezzani I, Cobellis L, et al. Placental corticotrophin-releasing factor. An update. Ann N Y Acad Sci 2000;900:89.
102. Jones SA, Challis JR. Local stimulation of prostaglandin production by corticotropin-releasing hormone in human fetal membranes and placenta. Biochem Biophys Res Commun 1989;159: 192.
103. Florio P, Vale W, Petraglia F. Urocortins in human reproduction. Peptides 2004;25:1751.
104. Youngblood WW, Humm J, Lipton MA, et al. Thyrotropin-releasing hormone-like bioactivity in placenta: evidence for the existence of substances other than Pyroglu-His-Pro-NH2 (TRH) capable of stimulating pituitary thyrotropin release. Endocrinology 1980;106:541.
105. Bajoria R, Babawale M. Ontogeny of endogenous secretion of immunoreactive-thyrotropin releasing hormone by the human placenta. J Clin Endocrinol Metab 1998;83:4148.
106. Gibbons JM Jr, Mitnick M, Chieffo V. In vitro biosynthesis of TSH- and LH-releasing factors by the human placenta. Am J Obstet Gynecol 1975;121:127.
107. Shambaugh G III, Kubek M, Wilber JF. Thyrotropin-releasing hormone activity in the human placenta. J Clin Endocrinol Metab 1979;48:483.
108. Watkins WB, Yen SS. Somatostatin in cytotrophoblast of the immature human placenta: localization by immunoperoxidase cytochemistry. J Clin Endocrinol Metab 1980;50:969.
109. Caron P, Buscail L, Beckers A, et al. Expression of somatostatin receptor SST4 in human placenta and absence of octreotide effect on human placental growth hormone concentration during pregnancy. J Clin Endocrinol Metab 1997;82:3771.
110. Berry SA, Srivastava CH, Rubin LR, et al. Growth hormone-releasing hormone-like messenger ribonucleic acid and immunoreactive peptide are present in human testis and placenta. J Clin Endocrinol Metab 1992;75:281.
111. Ahmed MS, Cemerikie B, Agbas A. Properties and functions of human placental opioid system. Life Sci 1992;50:83.
112. Lemaire S, Valette A, Chouinard L. Purification and identification of multiple forms of dynorphin in human placenta. Neuropeptides 1983;3:181.
113. Petraglia F, Calza L, Giardino L, et al. Identification of immunoreactive neuropeptide-gamma in human placenta: localization, secretion, and binding sites. Endocrinology 1989;124:2016.
114. Fields PA, Eldridge RK, Fuchs AR, et al. Human placental and bovine corpora luteal oxytocin. Endocrinology 1983;112:1544.

CHAPTER 21

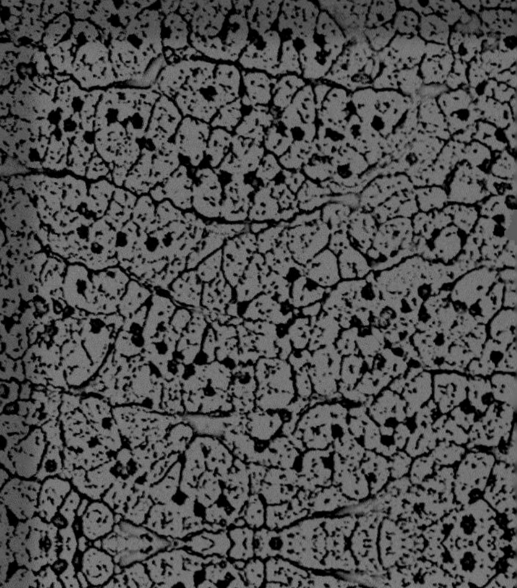

ENDOCRINOLOGY OF FETAL DEVELOPMENT

Delbert A. Fisher

Introduction

The unfolding of our understanding of mammalian pregnancy and fetal development represents one of the dramatic chapters of scientific progress during the past half-century. Successful pregnancy involves complex genetic, cellular, and hormonal interactions facilitating implantation, placentation, embryonic and fetal development, parturition, and fetal adaptation to extrauterine life. An array of transcription factors and epigenetic events program embryogenesis and fetal development in concert with autocrine, paracrine, and endocrine networks of hormones and growth factors that provide the cellular communication coordinating maternal-placental-fetal interactions and fetal maturation. Unique features of the placental-fetal endocrine environment include the growing spectrum of placental hormones and growth factors and a variety of fetal endocrine adaptations to the intrauterine environment (Table 21–1) The fetal adrenal cortex, the paraaortic chromaffin system including the paired organs of Zuckerkandl, and the intermediate lobe of the pituitary are prominent among these. Vasotocin, the parent neurohypophyseal hormone in submammalian species, is expressed transiently during fetal life, and calcitonin, a largely vestigial hormone in adult mammals, plays a significant role in fetal calcium and bone metabolism.

In addition, the active adrenal glucocorticoid, cortisol, and the thyroid hormones are largely inactive during much of fetal life because of the production of inactive analogues. Hormones and growth factors that play prominent roles in the fetus include catecholamines, parathyroid hormone–related protein (PTHrP), antimüllerian hormone, insulin-like growth factor II (IGF-II), transforming growth factor α (TGF-α), and the neuroregulins. In the perinatal period, cortisol serves to modulate the functional adaptations requisite for extrauterine survival. In addition, hormonal programming during the fetal-perinatal period conditions the adult functional characteristics of selected endocrine systems. This chapter reviews the current status of our understanding of the maternal-placental-fetal endocrine and growth factor milieu, maturation of the fetal endocrine systems, and adaptations of the fetal endocrine system to extrauterine life.

PLACENTAL HORMONE TRANSFER

The fetal endocrine milieu is largely independent of maternal hormones because the placenta is impermeable to most peptide hormones. Hormones larger than 0.7 to 1.2 kd have little or no access to the fetal compartment.[1] The exception is immunoglobulin G, which is actively transported from mother to fetus during the latter half of gestation.[2] Steroid and thyroid hormones and catecholamines do cross the placenta but several of these are metabolized en route, including cortisol, estradiol, thyroxine, triiodothyronine, and catecholamines.[3-7] The placental cells contain an active 11β-hydroxysteroid dehydrogenase (11βHSD) that catalyzes the conversion of most of the cortisol to inactive cortisone.[4-5] Placental 17βHSD is considered to prevent passage of excessive estrogens to the fetus by catalyzing inactivation of estradiol to estrone.[6] Placental tissue also contains an iodothyronine inner ring monodeiodinase, which deiodinates most of the T_4 to inactive reverse triiodothyronine (rT_3) and converts active 3,5,3′-triiodothyronine (T_3) to inactive diiodothyronine.[7,8]

TABLE 21–1 FEATURES OF THE FETAL ENDOCRINE ENVIRONMENT

PLACENTAL HORMONE PRODUCTION
Estrogens Progesterone Neuropeptides Growth factors
NEUTRALIZATION OF HORMONE ACTIONS
Growth hormone Cortisol Thyroxine Catecholamines
UNIQUE FETAL ENDOCRINE SYSTEMS
Fetal adrenal cortex Paraaortic chromaffin system Intermediate lobe of the pituitary
PROMINENT FETAL HORMONES OR METABOLITES
Vasotocin Calcitonin Cortisone Reverse triiodothyronine (rT_3) Sulfated iodothyronines Ectopic neuropeptides
FETAL ENDOCRINE SYSTEM ADAPTATIONS
Adrenal-placental interactions Testicular control of male phenotypic differentiation Developmentally regulated growth factor control of fetal growth Neuropeptides and fetal water metabolism Parathyroid glands and placental calcium transport Catecholamine and vasopressin responses to hypoxia Cortisol programming for extrauterine exposure Catecholamine and cortisol control of extrauterine adaptation Perinatal hormonal programming

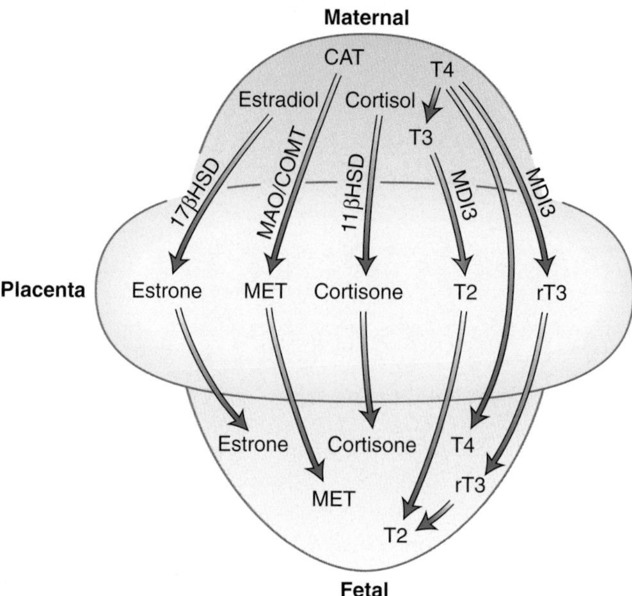

Figure 21–1 ▪ Placental neutralization of biologic activity of several potent hormones during maternal-fetal transfer. *CAT,* Catecholamines; *MET,* metanephrines; *T4,* thyroxine; *T3,* 3,5,3′ triiodothyronine; *rT3,* 3,3′5′ (reverse) triiodothyronine; *T2,* diiodothyronine. The neutralizing enzymes, 17βHSD and 11βHSD, are shown. *MAO,* Monoamine oxidase; *COMT,* catechol *O*-methyltransferase; *MDI3,* iodothyronine monodeiodinase, type 3. See text for details.

Catecholamine-degrading enzymes in placental tissue include both monoamine oxidase and catechol *O*-methyltransferase,[3,9] and both metanephrine and dihydroxymandelic acid metabolites of catecholamines are present in placental homogenates (Fig. 21–1).

ECTOPIC FETAL HORMONE PRODUCTION

Kidney, liver, and testes from 16- to 20-week-old human fetuses produce immunoreactive and bioactive human chorionic gonadotropin (hCG) in vitro.[10,11] Kidney tissue produces nearly half as much hCG per milligram of protein as placenta; liver activity is lower. Adrenocorticotropic hormone (ACTH)-like immunoreactivity is present in relatively high concentrations in neonatal rat pancreas and kidney.[12] This material is presumably derived from a pro-opiomelanocortin (POMC) parent molecule. Hypothalamic neuropeptides are present in a variety of adult tissues, particularly in the pancreas and gut.[13-17] In the fetus, hypothalamic neuropeptides are also present in the gut and tissues derived from it. High concentrations of thyrotropin-releasing hormone (TRH) and somatostatin immunoreactivity have been reported in neonatal rat pancreas and gastrointestinal tract tissues, whereas hypothalamic concentrations of these immunoreactive substances are low.[18,19] These neuropeptides have immunoreactive and chromatographic properties similar to those of the synthetic hypothalamic peptides. Encephalectomy does not alter the circulating TRH levels in the neonatal rat, whereas significant reductions are produced by pancreatectomy. In the sheep fetus, thyroid hormones modulate pancreatic and gut TRH concentrations, which suggests thyroid hormone control of extrahypothalamic *TRH* gene transcription or translation in the fetus.[20] TRH and somatostatin also are present in the human neonatal pancreas and in blood of the human newborn where both hormones are derived mostly from extrahypothalamic sources.[21-24] The presence of TRH at high concentrations in fetal ovine blood and the modulation of fetal pancreatic, placental, and blood TRH levels by thyroid hormones suggest a role for extrahypothalamic TRH in the control of fetal pituitary thyrotropin secretion before the near-term maturation of hypothalamic TRH.[20] The role of extraneural somatostatin in the fetus is undefined.

FETAL ENDOCRINE SYSTEMS

Anterior Pituitary and Target Organs

The human fetal forebrain is identifiable by 3 weeks of gestation, the diencephalon and telencephalon by 5 weeks. Rathke's pouch, the buccal precursor of the anterior pituitary gland, separates from the primitive pharyngeal stomodeum by 5 weeks of gestation.[20,25] The neural components of the transducer system (the hypothalamus, the pituitary stalk, and the posterior pituitary) are largely developed by 7 weeks of gestation, and the bony floor of the sella turcica is present by this time, separating the adenohypophysis from the primitive gut. Capillaries develop within the proliferating anterior pituitary mesenchymal tissue around Rathke's pouch and the diencephalon by 8 weeks of gestation, and intact hypothalamic-pituitary portal vessels are present by 12 to 17 weeks. Maturation of the pituitary portal vascular system continues, and the system becomes functionally intact during the period of histologic differentiation of the hypothalamus and development of the portal vascular extension into hypothalamic tissue; this maturation process extends to 30 to 35 weeks of gestation.

The hypothalamic cell condensations, which represent the hypothalamic nuclei, and the interconnecting fiber tracts are demonstrable histologically by 15 to 18 weeks of gestation.[20,25] Hypothalamic cells and diencephalic fiber tracts for the hypothalamic neuropeptides somatostatin, corticotropin-releasing hormone (CRH), growth hormone–releasing hormone (GHRH), and gonadotropin-releasing hormone (GnRH) are also visible by this time. Concentrations of dopamine, TRH, GnRH, and somatostatin are significant in hypothalamic tissue by 10 to 14 weeks of gestation. Specialized anterior pituitary cell types, including lactotropes, somatotropes, corticotropes, thyrotropes, and gonadotropes, can be recognized in the anterior pituitary between 7 and 16 weeks of gestation. Anterior pituitary hormones—including growth hormone (GH), prolactin (PRL), thyroid-stimulating hormone (TSH), luteinizing hormone (LH), follicle-stimulating hormone (FSH), and ACTH—are detectable by radioimmunoassay between 10 and 17 weeks of gestation. Thus, the anatomy and biosynthetic mechanisms that make up the hypothalamic-pituitary neuroendocrine transducer appear to be functional by 12 to 17 weeks of gestation in humans.

This embryogenic process is regulated by a series of homeodomain proteins or transcription factors that have been characterized by mutation analysis and gene transfection, and gene knockout studies in mice. Mutations of the homeobox genes sonic hedgehog *(SHH), ZIC1,* and *SIX3* have been identified in patients with holoprosencephaly.[26,27] *HESX1* homeobox gene mutations have been shown in siblings with septo-optic dysplasia in association with midline brain defects and pituitary hypoplasia.[28] *GL13* mutations result in the Pallister-Hall syndrome associated with hypothalamic disorganization and hypopituitarism.[29] Other genes involved in hypothalamic development include *PAX6, SIX3, SIX6, SIM1, SIM2, SF1,* and *BRN2.*[1,30-32] Early pituitary transcription factors include the Rathke pouch homeobox gene *(RPX), LHX3,* and *LHX4.* Later factors *PROP1* and *PIT1* program development and function of the pituitary cells producing GH, TSH, and PRL.[29-36] *TPIT* gene mutation is associated with ACTH deficiency.[35] Mutations in *PROP1* and *PIT1* have been described in patients with familial hypopituitarism (Fig. 21–2).[33,36]

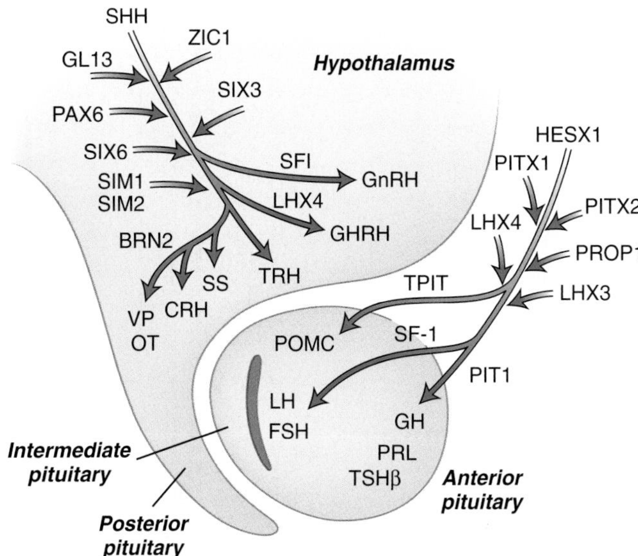

Figure 21–2 ▪ Illustration of the homeobox genes programming hypothalamic and pituitary embryogenesis and function. *SHH* and *ZIC1* are the sonic hedgehog and *Drosophila* odd-paired homologues, mutations of which have been shown to cause human holoprosencephaly. *SIX3* and *SIX6* are mammalian homologues of Drosphila sine oculis homeobox genes. *SIX3* mutations have been associated with holoprosencephaly. *GL1-3* transription factor mutations cause hypothalamic dysfunction (Pallister-Hall syndrome). *HESX1* is the Rathke pouch homeobox gene (also referred to as *RPX*) involved in anterior pituitary gland embryogenesis. *PITX1* and *PITX2* are bicoid-related homeodomain transcription factors involved with both hypothalamic and pituitary development. *LHX3* and *LHX4* are LIM class homeodomain transcription factors that are also essential for normal pituitary embryogenesis. *PROP1* and *PIT1* defects in mice and humans lead to growth hormone (GH), prolactin (PRL), and thyroid-stimulating hormone (TSH) deficiency. TPIT mutation is associated with isolated ACTH deficiency. LH-FSH deficiency is associated with *LHX3* mutation. *FSH,* Follicle-stimulating hormone; *LH,* luteinizing hormone; *POMC,* pro-opiomelanocortin; *TRH,* thyrotropin-releasing hormone; *SS,* somatostatin; *CRH,* corticotropin-releasing hormone; *VP,* vasopressin; *OT,* oxytocin. See text for details and see references 29-36.

Growth Hormone and Prolactin

The human fetal pituitary gland can synthesize and secrete GH by 8 to 10 weeks of gestation.[1,25] Pituitary GH content increases from about 1 nmol (20 ng) at 10 weeks to 45 nmol (1000 ng) at 16 weeks of gestation. Fetal plasma GH levels in cord blood samples are in the range 1 to 4 nmol/L during the first trimester and increase to a mean peak of approximately 6 nmol/L at midgestation. Plasma GH levels fall progressively during the second half of gestation to a mean value of 1.5 nmol/L at term.[25] Pituitary GH mRNA and GH content generally parallel the increase in plasma GH concentration between 16 and 24 weeks of gestation.[37] This pattern of ontogenesis of plasma GH reflects a progressive maturation of hypothalamic-pituitary and forebrain function. The responses of plasma GH to somatostatin and GHRH and to insulin and arginine are mature at term in human infants.[25,38]

The high plasma GH concentrations at midgestation after the development of the pituitary portal vascular system may reflect unrestrained secretion.[25] Studies of 9 to 16-week-old human fetal pituitary cells in culture have shown a predominant response to GHRH and a limited effect of somatostatin, which suggests that the inhibitory action of somatostatin develops later in gestation.[39] This interpretation has been substantiated by in vivo studies in the sheep fetus, which have shown a failure of somatostatin to inhibit GHRH-stimulated GH release early in the third trimester and maturation of the inhibitory effect of somatostatin near term.[25] Thus, a predominant GHRH enhancement and limited somatostatin inhibition of GH secretion at midgestation presumably relate to a limited capacity for inhibition of GH release by somatomedin feedback. In addition, there may be unrestrained GH secretion at the pituitary cell level or immaturity of limbic and forebrain inhibitory circuitry that modulates hypothalamic function, or both.[25] Whatever the mechanisms, control of GH secretion matures progressively during the last half of gestation and the early weeks of postnatal life so that mature responses to sleep, glucose, and L-dopa are present by 3 months of age.

The ontogenesis of fetal plasma PRL differs significantly from that of GH; levels are low until 25 to 30 weeks of gestation and

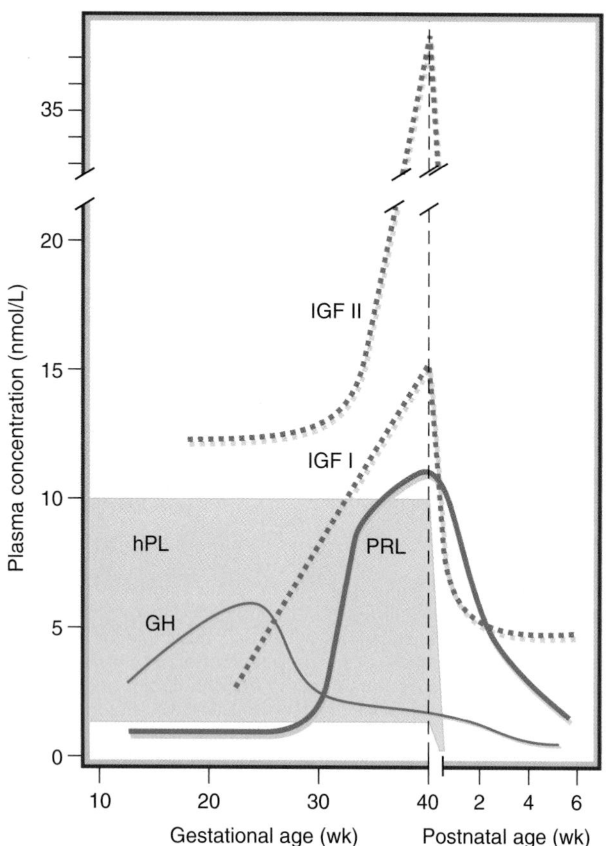

Figure 21–3 ▪ Patterns of change of fetal plasma human placental lactogen (hPL), growth hormone (GH), prolactin (PRL), insulin-like growth factor I (IGF-I), and insulin-like growth factor II (IGF-II) during gestation and in the neonatal period. The range of fetal plasma HPL concentrations is shown in the *pink area*. (Data from Bennett A, Wilson DM, Liu R, et al. J Clin Endocrinol Metab 1983;57:609-612; Kaplan SL, Grumbach MM, Aubert ML. Recent Prog Horm Res 1976;32:161-243; Bala RM, Lopatka J, Leung A, et al. Clin Endocrinol Metab 1981;52: 508-512.)

increase to a mean peak value of approximately 11 nmol/L at term[25] (Fig. 21–3). Pituitary PRL content increases progressively from 12 to 15 weeks, and in vitro fetal pituitary cells from midgestation fetuses show limited autonomous PRL secretion, although PRL release increases in response to TRH and decreases in response to dopamine. Brain and hypothalamic control of PRL matures late in gestation and during the first months of extrauterine life.[25,38] Estrogen stimulates PRL synthesis and release by pituitary cells, and the marked increase in fetal plasma PRL concentration in the last trimester parallels the increase in fetal plasma estrogen levels, although lagging by several weeks.[25,38] Anencephalic fetuses have plasma PRL concentrations in the normal or low-normal range. These data support a role for estrogen in stimulating fetal PRL release. The fetal sheep exhibits a similar pattern of fetal plasma PRL levels, indicating that maturation and integration of brain and hypothalamic mechanisms modulating PRL release develop late in gestation and in the postnatal period, accounting for the delayed postnatal fall in plasma PRL level in the neonate of this species.[25]

There is a general tendency toward hypersecretion of fetal pituitary hormones during the last half of gestation, and pituitary hormones found at high levels in cord blood from aborted human fetuses and premature human infants include GH, TSH, ACTH, β-endorphin, β-lipotropin, LH, and FSH.[25,38] Development of hypothalamic-pituitary control is complex, involving maturational events in the cortex and midbrain, the hypothalamus and hypothalamic-pituitary portal vascular system, peripheral endocrine systems, and the placenta itself, including hormone, growth factor, and neuropeptide production. The fetal pituitary hyperfunction appears to be related more to relatively delayed maturation of the central nervous system and hypothalamic control with unrestrained secretion of stimulating hypothalamic hormones than to the action of placental neuropeptides.[25]

Postnatally, GH acts through receptors in liver and other tissues to stimulate production of IGF-I and, to a lesser degree, IGF-II. Prenatally, in contrast, GH receptor mRNA levels and receptor binding are low in fetal liver, although receptor mRNA is present in other fetal tissues.[25] The growth of anencephalic fetuses is nearly normal, however, suggesting that factors other than GH stimulate fetal IGF production. Nutritional factors are known to play a role.[40,41] PRL receptors are present in most fetal tissues during the first trimester of gestation, and it is likely that lactogenic hormones have a significant role in organ and tissue development early in gestation.[40,42] The coordinate increase in fetal adipose tissue and adipose tissue PRL receptors PRLR1 and PRLR2 suggests that PRL may play a role in growth and maturation of fetal adipose tissue later in gestation.[43] PRL also may play a role in fetal skeletal maturation.[43] Ovine placental lactogen stimulates glycogen synthesis in fetal ovine liver, and HPL stimulates amino acid transport, DNA synthesis, and IGF-I production in human fetal fibroblasts and muscle cells. GH and PRL have little activity in these tissues.[42] (See Fetal Growth.)

Adrenal System

The primordia of the adrenal glands can be recognized just cephalad of the bilaterally developing mesonephros by 3 to 4 weeks of gestation.[44,45] The fetal adrenal is composed of three functional zones, a fetal zone capable of production of C_{19} androgens, a transitional zone with enzymes for cortisol production, and an outer definitive zone producing mineralocorticoids. The large eosinophilic cells of the fetal zone are well differentiated by 9 to 12 weeks of gestation and are capable of active steroidogenesis. The fetal adrenal gland grows rapidly and progressively in mass; the combined glandular weight is approximately 8 g at term, when the fetal zone makes up about 80% of the mass of the gland with a relative size 10- to 20-fold that of the adult adrenal.[10,44,45]

Fetal adrenal cortical development is under control of several genes and growth factors. The genes include those coding for the orphan nuclear receptors SF-1 (steroidogenic factor-1) and DAX-1 (dosage-sensitive sex reversal, adrenal hypoplasia congenita, X-chromosome factor)[46-48] (Fig. 21–4). These genes show coordinate expression in adrenal cortex, testis, ovary, hypothalamus, and pituitary tissues. *SF-1* gene knockout mice manifest adrenal and gonadal agenesis, gonadotropin deficiency, and absence of the hypothalamic ventromedial nucleus.[47] Inactivating *DAX-1* gene mutations are associated with adrenal hypoplasia and gonadotropin deficiency.[47] Several other transcription factors including *WT1, LIM1* and *PBX1* are involved earlier in the complex genetic cascade programming adrenal gland organogenesis from the coelomic epithelium and urogenital ridge.[47,48] The steroidogenic acute regulatory protein (StAR) is a rate-limiting factor in adrenal steroidogenesis. *StAR* knockout mice manifest glucocorticoid and mineralocorticoid deficiency and female genitalia in XY animals.[49] In humans, inactivating *StAR* mutations cause adrenal hypoplasia and adrenal hormone insufficiency.[49]

Adrenal gland development is mediated by a variety of growth factors. Proliferation of both the fetal and definitive zones is stimulated by fibroblast growth factor and EGF, and the

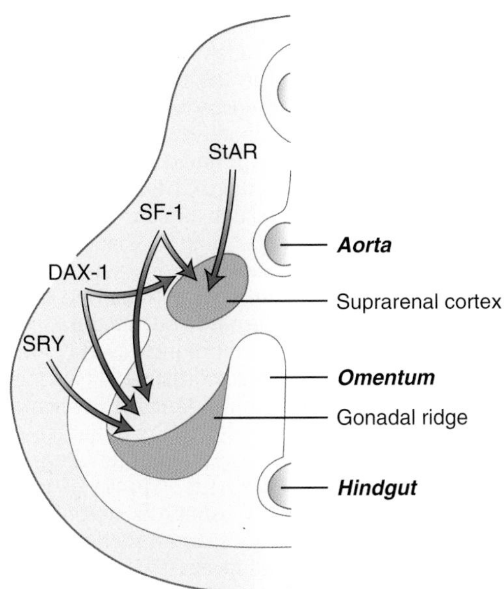

Figure 21–4 ■ Hemi-cross-section of a 5-week human embryo with location of the adrenal primordia (suprarenal cortices) and gonadal ridges. The homeobox genes programming adrenal and gonadal embryogenesis are indicated. *SF-1* (steroidogenic factor 1) is involved in testicular and ovarian development, whereas *SRY* is the single critical regulator of testicular embryogenesis. Inactivation of the *DAX1* gene leads to adrenal hypoplasia. The steroidogenic acute regulatory protein (StAR) is the rate-limiting factor for adrenal steroidogenesis. See text for details.

fetal adrenal expresses high levels of IGF-II mRNA and protein, which are responsive to ACTH.[10] Moreover, IGF-II augments ACTH-stimulated expression of steroidogenic enzymes and stimulates steroid hormone production in fetal adrenal cortical cells, suggesting a role in adrenal regulation during fetal and postnatal life.[10] The pattern of enzyme maturation in the fetal adrenal suggests that cortisol production by the definitive zone does not occur de novo from cholesterol until 30 weeks of gestation but some production using progesterone as precursor probably occurs earlier.[10]

The fetal adrenal expresses the same five steroidogenic apoenzymes as the adult gland: two microsomal enzymes with 17-hydroxylase and 17,20-desmolase (CYP17 or P450c17) and 21-hydroxylase (CYP21A2 or P450c21) activities, respectively, plus two mitochondrial cytochrome P450 enzymes providing cholesterol side-chain cleavage (CYP11A1 or P450scc) and C_{11}/C_{18} hydroxylation of the parent steroid structure (CYP11B1/CYP11B2 or P450c11/aldosterone synthase). A fifth enzyme, expressed by the smooth endoplasmic reticulum, exhibits both 3β-hydroxysteroid dehydrogenase (3βHSD) and Δ^4, Δ^5-isomerase activities.[44,45] Quantitative differences in the relative activities of these enzymes are found, however, between cells derived from the fetal versus the definitive zones and these differences are largely due to regulated steroidogenic gene transcription.[44] The fetal zone has relatively high steroid sulfotransferase activity, and because of the low 3βHSD and high sulfotransferase activities, the major steroid products of the fetal adrenal are dehydroepiandrosterone (DHEA), dehydroepiandrosterone sulfate (DHEAS), pregnenolone sulfate, several $\Delta^5$3β-hydroxysteroids, and limited amounts of $\Delta^5$3-ketosteroids, including cortisol and aldosterone.[44,45] The definitive zone contributes only a small fraction of total fetal adrenal steroid output. Cholesterol, the major substrate for fetal adrenal steroidogenesis, is derived from circulating low-density lipoprotein (LDL) and from de novo adrenal synthesis. LDL cholesterol, largely of fetal liver and testicular origin, contributes 70% of the total. The fetal zone contains more LDL binding sites and manifests a greater rate of de novo cholesterol synthesis than does the definitive zone, in keeping with its greater steroidogenic activity. Both ACTH and angiotensin II receptors (AT_1 and AT_2) are present on fetal adrenal cells early in gestation. ACTH stimulates steroid production by activating StAR and increasing delivery of substrate cholesterol to P450 scc; angiotensin II inhibits 3βHSD activity and promotes DHEA production in the fetal zone.[44] Both fetal adrenal cortisol and placental estradiol regulate hepatic synthesis of cholesterol in the fetus.

The major stimulus to fetal adrenal function is fetal pituitary ACTH.[10,44,50] Although placental hCG may support early adrenal growth, the involution of the adrenal gland that occurs after 15 weeks in the anencephalic fetus suggests a crucial role for pituitary-derived factors. CRH protein has been demonstrated in fetal baboon pituitary, adrenal, liver, kidney, and lung tissues during the last third of gestation. Levels in pituitary are highest (300 to 500 pg/mg protein); levels in adrenal and lung and liver and kidney tissues average 20 to 30 and 5 to 10 pg/mg protein, respectively.[51] *CRH* gene knockout in mice leads to neonatal death due to pulmonary hypoplasia, suggesting that CRH-stimulated glucocorticoid production is essential for adrenergic chromaffin and normal lung development.[52] Circulating CRH levels are elevated in the fetus largely from extrahypothalamic and placental sources.[10,51,53] Maternal levels of CRH are elevated during the last trimester of gestation and reach values of 0.5 to 1 nmol/L at term; normal values in nonpregnant women are less than 0.01 nmol/L.[54] This placental CRH is bioactive and levels correlate with maternal cortisol concentrations, suggesting that this circulating placental CRH plays a role in stimulating maternal corticotropin release. Fetal plasma CRH levels at term, however, are approximately 0.03 nmol/L and, relative to the presumably high levels in pituitary portal blood, probably have little role in modulating fetal corticotropin release. Midgestation fetal plasma corticotropin concentrations average about 55 pmol/L (250 pg/mL), levels that maximally stimulate fetal adrenal steroidogenesis, and concentrations are higher throughout gestation than in postnatal life, although they fall near term[10,44] (Fig. 21–5). Arginine vasopressin (AVP) and catecholamines also are significant stimuli for fetal ACTH secretion.[55]

The paradox of human fetal adrenal function is that steroidogenesis is programmed largely to production of inactive products.[44] The gland is maximally stimulated to maintain fetal cortisol levels and ACTH feedback homeostasis but is programmed by the steroidogenic enzyme expression pattern (e.g., relative 3βHSD deficiency) to produce inactive DHEA and pregnenolone and their sulfate conjugates. Much of the DHEA is converted to 16-hydroxy-DHEAS by the fetal adrenal and fetal liver. As already discussed, this programming is designed to provide DHEA substrate for placental estrone and estradiol production; 16-hydroxy-DHEA undergoes metabolism to estriol in the placenta. Fetal DHEAS production and maternal estriol concentrations increase progressively to term; DHEAS production approximates 200 mg/day near term.[10] In the anencephalic fetus, placental estrogen production is reduced to about 10% of normal.[10,44] In pregnant baboons in which placental estrogen production was suppressed by administration of an aromatase inhibitor, the volume of the fetal zone of the fetal adrenal increased markedly.[56] This effect was reversed by administration of inhibitor plus estrogen, suggesting that estrogen selectively suppresses fetal zone growth and development during the second half of primate pregnancy. It is proposed that this represents a feedback system to regulate secretion of fetal adrenal DHEA to maintain normal fetal-placental function and development.[56] Near term the fetal cortisol production rate in blood, per unit body weight, is similar to that in the adult.[44] About two thirds of fetal cortisol is derived from the fetal adrenal glands, and one

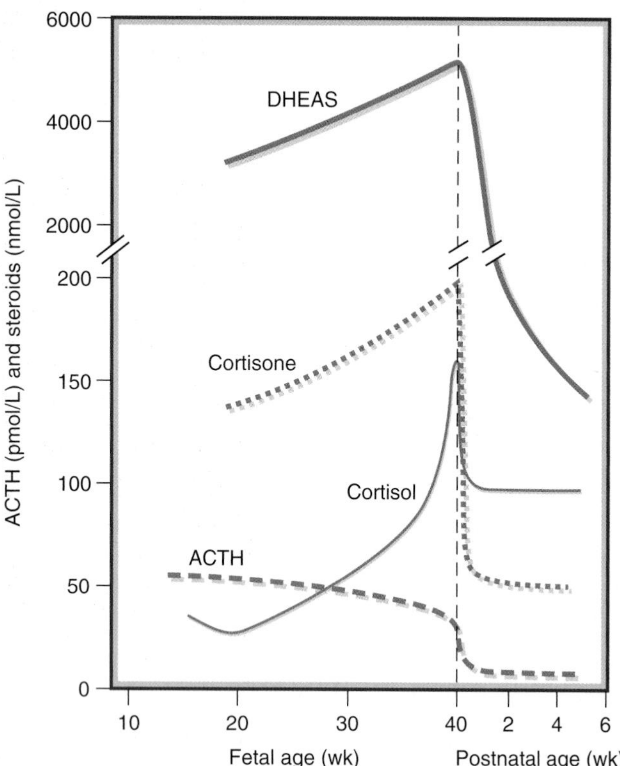

Figure 21–5 ▪ Patterns of change of fetal plasma adrenocorticotropic hormone (ACTH), cortisol, cortisone, and dehydroepiandrosterone sulfate (DHEAS) during gestation and in the neonatal period. The trend of average values is shown for each hormone in nanomoles per liter. Note the broken scale for DHEAS. (Data from Winters AJ, Oliver C, Colston C, et al. J Clin Endocrinol Metab 1974;39:269-273; Murphy BEP. Am J Obstet Gynecol 1982;144:276-282; Beitins IZ, Bayard F, Ances FIG, et al. Pediatr Res 1973;7:509-513; Winter JSD. In Polin RA, Fox WW, Abman SH, eds. Fetal and Neonatal Physiology. Philadelphia: WB Saunders, 2004:115-1925.)

third is derived from placental transfer.[44] The metabolic clearance of cortisol in the fetus is rapid; 80% is oxidized in fetal tissues or placenta to cortisone or further metabolites.[44]

The corticotropin feedback control system matures progressively during the second half of gestation and the early neonatal period. Dexamethasone can suppress the human fetal pituitary-adrenal axis at term but not at 18 to 20 weeks of gestation.[44] In the fetal sheep, hypothalamic and pituitary glucocorticoid receptors are present at midgestation and corticotropin suppressibility can be demonstrated by the midpoint of the third trimester of gestation.[57] The number of glucocorticoid receptors in the sheep fetal hypothalamus increases at term at the time of increasing glucocorticoid levels, suggesting that some process in the fetus allows the normal autoregulation of glucocorticoid receptors to be overridden at term.[58]

Adrenal hormone receptors, including glucocorticoid receptors (GRs) and mineralocorticoid receptors (MRs), are members of the nuclear receptor superfamily of steroid hormone, thyroid hormone, vitamin D, and retinoid receptors.[59] GRs are present in most body tissues by the second trimester and play an important role in fetal development. Mice lacking GR receptor function manifest enlarged and disorganized adrenal cortices, adrenal medullary atrophy, lung hypoplasia, and defective gluconeogenesis.[52,59] They appear normal at birth but are not viable.

GRs are present at birth and are probably present at midgestation in most tissues, including placenta, lung, brain, liver, and gut.[44,58,60] Fetal cortisol is converted to cortisone through an 11β hydroxysteroid dehydrogenase (11βHSD) in fetal tissues, and levels of circulating cortisone in the fetus at midgestation are fourfold to fivefold higher than cortisol concentrations (see Fig. 21–5). Cortisone is a relatively inactive glucocorticoid, and this metabolism protects the anabolic milieu of the fetus because cortisol can retard both placental and fetal growth.[61] As term approaches, selected fetal tissues including liver and lung express 11-ketosteroid reductase activity that promotes local conversion of cortisone to cortisol.[44] Cortisol serves as an important stimulus to prepare the fetus for extrauterine survival. An increase in fetal cortisol concentration occurs during the last 10 weeks of gestation and is the result of increased cortisol secretion and decreased conversion to cortisone.[44] This increase in fetal cortisol production has an important role in the maturation of several fetal systems or functions that are critical to extrauterine survival.[44,62] (See Transition to Extrauterine Life.)

The human fetal adrenal gland is capable of aldosterone secretion near term, and fetal plasma aldosterone concentrations in infants who are born by cesarean section are threefold to fourfold higher than maternal levels.[44,63] Vaginal delivery and maternal salt restriction increase levels in both mother and infant. The increased aldosterone levels in the fetus are due to increased fetal adrenal secretion and persist during the first year of extrauterine life.[63] However, there is a poor correlation between plasma renin activity (PRA) and aldosterone levels in cord blood.[64] Aldosterone secretion is low in the midgestation human fetal adrenal and is unresponsive to the secretagogues that are known to modulate aldosterone production in the adult. In sheep, fetal aldosterone becomes responsive to PRA and angiotensin II in the neonatal period.[65] In this species, in which late fetal aldosterone levels are also high compared with adult levels, furosemide stimulates PRA but not aldosterone during the third trimester; the aldosterone response to furosemide (and PRA) is delayed until the neonatal period.[65,66] This situation also appears to be the case in the human fetus and neonate.

MRs are present in fetal tissues from 12 to 16 weeks of gestation.[67] MR immunoreactivity is detectable in fetal kidney, skin, hair follicles, trachea and bronchioles, esophagus, stomach, small intestine, colon, and pancreatic exocrine ducts. The role of MRs in these fetal tissues remains unclear. MR knockout mice appear normal at birth but demonstrate defects in mineralocorticoid and renin-angiotensin system functions in the postnatal period.[68]

Angiotensin II levels in the sheep fetus are similar to maternal values, and blockade of fetal production with angiotensin-converting enzyme inhibitors decreases the fetal glomerular filtration rate.[66] Both subtypes of angiotensin receptors, AT_1 and AT_2, are detectable in various tissues early in fetal development.[69] AT_1 receptor mRNA expression in the fetal sheep kidney is low early in gestation, increases in the latter third of pregnancy, and decreases postnatally; AT_2 mRNA levels, in contrast, are high at midgestation and decrease during the third trimester.[69] These changes are believed to reflect growth factor mediated changes in cells that contain AT in various tissues. Hormonal factors modulate fetal renal AT gene expression in sheep; angiotensin II suppresses both AT_1 and AT_2, and cortisol increases AT_1 gene expression in kidney and lungs.[69,70]

The role of the fetal renin-angiotensin system is not clear; rather than modulating renal sodium excretion through aldosterone, it may maintain renal excretion of salt and water into amniotic fluid to prevent oligohydramnios.[66] This renal effect is presumably mediated by modulation of arterial pressure. The mechanism for the high aldosterone levels in the fetal and neonatal periods remains unclear. Atrial natriuretic peptide (ANP), a cardiac hormone, is known to inhibit aldosterone secretion. Because plasma atrial natriuretic factor concentrations (ANP, BNP and CNP) are high in the fetus, the increased PRA and aldosterone levels are not due to relative atrial natriuretic factor deficiency.[71]

Aldosterone affects renal sodium excretion in the fetal sheep and in premature infants.[44,65] Manifestations of mineralocorticoid deficiency in the newborn term infant can occur as a result of aldosterone deficiency or competition for binding to renal MRs by other steroids such as 17-hydroxyprogesterone.[44] Relatively reduced glomerular filtration in the newborn limits sodium loss initially, but by 1 week of age aldosterone deficiency produces the characteristic manifestations of hyponatremia, hyperkalemia, and volume depletion.

Thyroid System

The thyroid gland is a derivative of the primitive buccopharyngeal cavity and develops from contributions of two anlagen, a midline thickening of the pharyngeal floor (median anlage) and paired caudal extensions of the fourth pharyngobranchial pouches (lateral anlagen).[72,73] These structures are discernible by 16 to 17 days of gestation, and by 24 days the median anlage develops a thin, flasklike diverticulum extending from the floor of the buccal cavity to the fourth branchial arch. By 50 days of gestation, the median and lateral anlagen have fused and the buccal stalk has ruptured. During this period, the thyroid gland migrates caudally to its definitive location in the anterior neck. By 70 days of gestation, colloid is visible histologically and thyroglobulin synthesis and iodide accumulation can be demonstrated within the gland. During the final follicular phase of development, colloid spaces increase in size and there is progressive cell growth and accumulation of thyroid hormones. At 12 weeks of gestation, the fetal thyroid gland weighs about 80 mg, and at term it weighs 1 to 1.5 g. The parathyroid glands develop between 5 and 12 weeks of gestation from the third and fourth pharyngeal pouches.

Four or more homeobox genes are involved in thyroid and parathyroid gland embryogenesis. These include the genes for thyroid transcription factors *HEX (Hhex), TTF1 (Titf1/Nkx2.1), TTF2 (Titf2/Foxe1)*, and *PAX8*[73-75] (Fig. 21–6). *HEX* gene knockout in mice is associated with thyroid agenesis or severe hypoplasia. *TTF2* knockout results in thyroid dysgenesis and cleft palate. *TTF1* knockout produces pulmonary hypoplasia and thyroid agenesis. Inactivating *PAX8* mutations produce thyroid hypoplasia and renal anomalies. *TTF1* knockout also produces parafollicular C-cell aplasia. The *HOX* genes appear to be important in the expression of *TTF1* and *PAX8*. *HOX15* gene disruption in mice results in parathyroid gland aplasia.[75] *TTF1, TTF2, PAX8*, and TSH receptor gene mutations account for less than 10% of patients with familial thyroid dysgenesis and congenital hypothyroidism.[76] Most cases of congenital hypothyroidism occur sporadically, and the pathogenesis in these cases remains unclear.

Pituitary and plasma thyrotropin (TSH) concentrations begin to increase during the second trimester in the human fetus, about the time that pituitary portal vascular continuity develops[73,77] (Fig. 21–7). Plasma thyrotropin levels increase progressively during the last half of gestation. Plasma T_4-binding globulin and total T_4 concentrations increase progressively from low levels at 16 to 18 weeks of gestation to maximal levels at 35 to 40 weeks. Free T_4 levels also increase as a consequence of the increase in T_4 production. The increases in plasma TSH and T_4 levels during the third trimester reflect a progressive maturation of hypothalamic pituitary control and of thyroid gland responsiveness to TSH. Pituitary TSH secretion is responsive to hypothyroxinemia and to TRH early in the third trimester.[73] Premature infants born at 26 to 28 weeks of gestation respond to exogenous TRH with an increase in plasma TSH concentration comparable to that in adults.[78] However, their TSH response to extrauterine

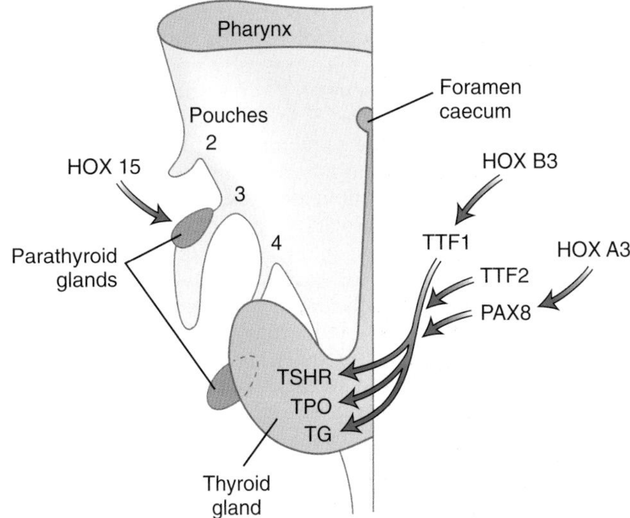

Figure 21–6 ▪ Illustration of the homeobox genes programming development of the thyroid and parathyroid glands. *HEX* is involved early in the integrated cascade programming thyroid gland embryogenesis. *HOXB3* and *HOXA3* may be responsible for activation of thyroid transcription factors TTF1 and TTF2, respectively, during early embryogenesis. *PAX8* is essential in the cascade. These factors are also involved in thyroid follicular cell function, promoting thyroglobulin (TG), thyroid peroxidase (TPO), and thyroid-stimulating hormone receptor (TSHR) gene transcription. *HOX15* gene knockout in mice causes parathyroid gland aplasia. See text for details.

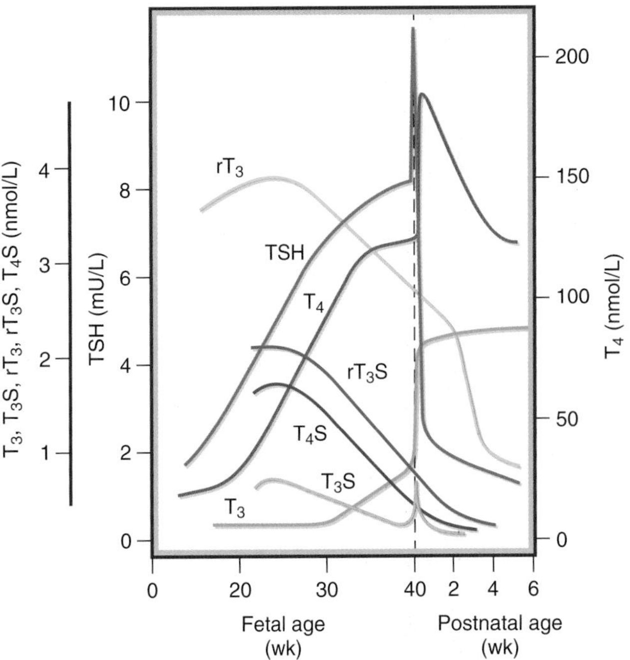

Figure 21–7 ▪ Patterns of change of fetal plasma thyroid-stimulating hormone (TSH), thyroxine (T_4), triiodothyronine (T_3), reverse T_3 (rT_3), and iodothyronine sulfates (T_4S, rT_3S, and T_3S) during gestation and in the neonatal period. The patterns for T_4S and rT_3S are based on limited 30-week data. (Data from Fisher DA, Klein AH. N Engl J Med 1981;304:702-712; Santini F, Chiovato L, Ghirri P, et al. J Clin Endocrinol Metab 1999;84:493-498; Burrow GN, Fisher DA, Larsen PR. N Engl J Med 1994;331:1072-1078.)

exposure is reduced indicating hypothalamic immaturity. Hypothalamic-pituitary-thyroid control matures during an interval corresponding to the late third trimester and early neonatal period of human development.[77,79] The period of parallel increases in fetal TSH and free T_4 levels during the latter half of gestation is followed by the sequential TSH and free T_4 surges in the early neonatal period and a final slow equilibration of the TSH/free T_4 ratio to adult values during infancy and childhood.[79-81] This maturation includes coordinate maturation of hypothalamic TRH secretion, pituitary TRH sensitivity, thyrotropin negative-feedback control, and thyroid follicular cell responsiveness to TSH. Functionally, the fetus progresses from a state of both primary (thyroidal) and tertiary (hypothalamic) hypothyroidism at midgestation through a state of mild tertiary hypothyroidism during the final weeks in utero to a fully mature hypothalamic-pituitary-thyroid axis by 2 months postnatally. In premature infants, the neonatal free T_4 increments also are reduced relative to term infants at 31 to 34 weeks, attenuated at 28 to 30 weeks, and absent in 23- to 27-week infants.[81]

The adult thyroid follicular cell can modify iodine transport or uptake with changes in dietary iodine intake, independent of variations in serum thyrotropin levels.[82,83] Before 36 to 40 weeks of gestation, the thyroid gland lacks this autoregulatory mechanism and is susceptible to iodine-induced inhibition of thyroid hormone synthesis.[78,83] The fetal thyroid follicular cell, when exposed to high circulating levels of iodide, is unable to reduce iodide trapping and prevent the high intracellular iodide concentrations that produce the blockade of hormone synthesis referred to as the *Wolff-Chaikoff effect.* Failure of the immature thyroid to exhibit autoregulation is probably due to failure of downregulation of thyroid cell membrane sodium-iodide symporter units, which may be related to the absence or reduced iodination of an 8- to 10-kd protein in the thyroid follicular cell.[82,83] In addition to maturation of autoregulation, thyroidal responsiveness to thyrotropin increases during the last trimester.[73]

The metabolism of thyroid hormones occurs through a progressive series of monodeiodinations.[77,84] Three deiodinase enzymes act to remove an iodine atom from the outer (phenolic) ring or the inner (tyrosyl) ring of the tetraiodothyronine (T_4) molecule, thus activating or inactivating, respectively, the hormone. The deiodinases are encoded by separate genes and share sequence homology. Most of the circulating, biologically active T_3 in adults is derived by outer-ring monodeiodination of T_4 in liver and other nonthyroidal tissues; biologically inactive rT_3 derives from inner-ring deiodination of T_4 in peripheral tissues. The type I enzyme (D1), an outer-ring monodeiodinase, is a high-Michaelis-constant (K_m) enzyme inhibited by propylthiouracil and stimulated by thyroid hormone. It deiodinates T_4 to T_3 and rT_3 to T2. 3,3′ diiodothyronine (T_2). D1 also has inner ring deiodinase activity converting T_3 to T_2. The type II outer-ring monodeiodinase (D2) is a low-K_m enzyme insensitive to propylthiouracil and inhibited by thyroid hormone. It deiodinates T_4 to T_3 and rT_3 to T_2. Type III monodeiodinase (D3) inactivates T_4 and T_3 via inner-ring deiodination of T_4 to rT_3 and of T_3 to T_2. D1 is largely responsible for production of T_3 that escapes from the cells, especially liver and kidney, into the circulation, whereas D2 is responsible for production of local tissue T_3. Inactive rT_3 also diffuses out of most tissues to appear in plasma.

The distribution of the deiodinases has been characterized in rodent and human tissues as shown in Table 21–2.[84] D2 plays an important role in supplying T_3 to developing brain tissue, regulating thermogenesis in brown adipose tissue in the neonatal period, and in regulation of pituitary TSH secretion. D3 activity is present in placenta, liver, and perhaps fetal skin, accounting for the higher levels of rT_3 in the fetus and limiting the metabolic effects of thyroid hormones during much of fetal life. There is little conversion of T_4 to circulating T_3 via D1 deiodination until midgestation in the human fetus; plasma T_3 levels are low (<0.2 nmol/L [<15 ng/dL]) until 30 weeks of gestation, after which the mean value increases to 0.7 nmol/L (50 ng/dL) at term[85] (see Fig. 21–7). Sulfation is active in fetal tissues, and the predominant thyroid hormone metabolites in the fetus are iodothyronine sulfates.[77,86,87] High levels of phenolsulfotransferases (SULT) have been characterized in fetal liver, lung, and brain by midgestation. SULT activities decrease rapidly in the neonatal period.[87] In the last third of gestation in fetal sheep, the mean plasma production rates for T_4 and metabolites in µg/kg body weight per day are T_4, 40; T_4 sulfate (T_4S), 10; rT_3, 5; rT_3S, 12; T_3, 2; and T_3S, 2. All metabolites are biologically inactive except for T_3 and perhaps T_3S, so that 90% of the T_4 metabolites in the fetus are biologically inactive.[86] The sulfated metabolites accumulate in fetal serum as a result of the low D1 activity in fetal tissues and because the sulfated iodothyronines are not substrates for D3.[82,86] The production rate of T_3 increases progressively between 30 weeks of gestation and term because of maturation of D1 activity in the liver and other tissues and because of decreasing D3 activity in placenta.[73,88] In the fetal sheep, hepatic D1 activity increases progressively during the last trimester.[89]

It has long been assumed that thyroid hormones passively diffuse into cells. However, several classes of cell membrane iodothyronine transporters have been recently described questioning this hypothesis.[90-92] These transporters belong to different families of organic anion, amino acid, and monocarboxylate solute carriers including the anion transporting polypeptide (OATP) family and the solute carrier family 21 (SLC21).[90-92] The significance of these transporters is not yet clear, but mutation of the human monocarboxylate transporter 8 (MCT8), a member of the SLC21 family, shown to be a specific thyroid hormone transporter present in developing brain, leads to a syndrome of combined thyroid dysfunction and psychomotor retardation.[91,92] MCT8 expression in neonatal mice has been localized to neurons in the olfactory bulb, cerebral cortex, hippocampus, and amygdala. Presumably all thyroid hormone–sensitive cell populations express iodothyronine membrane transporters. A cell surface T_4 receptor also has been characterized as αVβ3 integrin that serves as the initiation site for T_4-induced activation of the MAPK pathway mediating T_4-induced activation of the MAPK pathway for angiogenesis and perhaps actin polymerization and neuronal migration.[93] The ontogenesis and significance of these cell surface receptors and membrane transporters in fetal development remain to be further defined.

TABLE 21–2 DEIODINASE EXPRESSION IN HUMAN AND RODENT TISSUES

	DEIODINASE EXPRESSION		
Tissue	**D1**	**D2**	**D3**
Brain	X	X	X
Pituitary	X	X	
Thyroid	X	X*	
Liver	X		X†
Kidney	X		
Ovary	X		X
Ear		X*	
Heart		X*	
Muscle		X†	
Skin		X	X
Testes		X	X
Uterus		X	X
Brown fat		X	

*Expressed in human only.
†Expressed only in fetus.
See reference 84.

Classical thyroid hormone actions are mediated via functional thyroid hormone nuclear receptors, members of the steroid, retinoid, vitamin D family of nuclear transcription factors. Two genes code for the receptors, TRα on chromosome 17 and TRβ on chromosome 3.[94] The genes code for four classical receptor isoforms—TRα1, TRα2, TRβ1, and TRβ2. TRα1, TRβ1, and TRβ2 bind thyroid hormones (T_3/T_4 affinity, 10/1) and bind to DNA to effect gene transcription. TRα2 does not bind thyroid hormone but binds to DNA and can inhibit binding of other TRs. The TRs exist as monomers, homodimers, and heterodimers with other nuclear receptor family members such as retinoid X (RXR). Other TR transcripts, including TRΔα1 and TRΔα2, have been characterized. These do not bind DNA or T_3 but can inhibit TR and retinoid receptor activities.[95] The TRs are expressed developmentally and differentially in various fetal and adult tissues. TRα proteins are present in most tissues. TRβ1 is expressed in liver, kidney, and lung, and in developing brain, cochlea, and pituitary. TRβ2 expression is restricted largely to the pituitary gland, retina, and cochlea.[73,94] The receptors function redundantly, as indicated by knockout studies in mice, but predominant effects of one or another TR have been characterized (Table 21–3). Knockout of both the TRα and TRβ genes in mice is not lethal but results in elevated TSH levels, deafness, bradycardia, and decreased postnatal growth with delayed bone maturation.[73,94,95] Lethality occurs in association with improper intestinal development associated with persistent TRΔα isoforms in TRα or combined TRα and TRβ knockout mice.[95] In the fetal rat brain, TRα1 mRNA and receptor binding are detectable by 12 to 14 days of gestation (term is 21 days), increasing to maximal levels at birth. The TRβ1 isoform is detected at birth and increases approximately 40-fold in the early postnatal period.[73,96] In human fetal brain, TRα1 and TRβ1 isoforms and receptor binding are present by 8 to 10 weeks of gestation; TRα1 transcripts and receptor occupancy increase 8- to 10-fold by 16 to 18 weeks.[73,97,98] Liver, heart, and lung receptor binding can be identified by 13 to 18 weeks.[73,98,99]

Despite the limited maternal-fetal placental transfer of thyroxine and the predominant production of inactive thyroid hormone metabolites in the human fetus, significant levels of free T_4 via placental transfer are present in fetal fluids early in gestation and from fetal thyroid production during later gestation.[73,96] Early in gestation placental transfer is the only source of T_4 in fetal fluids and is essential for normal fetal neurodevelopment. T_4 is detectable in human coelomic fluid at levels of 0.5 to 2 nmol/L between 6 and 11 weeks of gestation, before the onset of fetal thyroid function.[100] Significant placental transfer continues to term when serum T_4 levels in the athyroid fetus range from 30 to 70 nmol/L (2.3 to 5.4 μg/dL).[101] Isotopic equilibrium studies with pregnant rats at term suggest that 15% to 20% of the T_4 in fetal tissues is of maternal origin.[102] As indicated, thyroid hormones cross the placenta early in gestation supplying the low levels of free T_4 essential for brain development between 12 and 20 weeks, before the onset of fetal thyroid hormone production.[96] Most thyroid hormone in the fetal compartment is inactivated to sulfated and deiodinated analogues until the perinatal period.[77,86,87] This neutralization of active circulating thyroid hormone maintains the low T_3 metabolic state, facilitating fetal growth and programmed tissue maturation. Thyroid hormone–programmed development of selective fetal tissues requires the interaction of local tissue D1, D2, thyroid receptors, receptor coactivators, and thyroid responsive genes. In most responsive tissues the timing of maturation events is controlled by the state of the thyroid receptors acting as a molecular switch.[95,103] In the absence of T_3, the unliganded receptor (aporeceptor) recruits corepressors, repressing gene transcription. Non–T_3-binding receptors also can repress transcription by inhibiting receptor DNA binding. Local tissue maturation events are initiated by the coincident availability of T_3, liganded T_3 receptor, T_3-mediated receptor exchange of corepressor with coactivators for creation of an active holoreceptor, and activation of responsive gene transcription.

In several of these tissues, programming events have been studied in transgenic mice, including brain, liver, heart, intestine, and bone tissues, thermogenesis, and spleen erythropoiesis.[103-109] The timing of these events in the mouse range from early midbrain neuronal development at gestational day 15 through perinatal activation of hepatic enzymes, cardiac ion channels, and spleen erythropoiesis to postnatal brain, intestinal, and bone maturation and thermogenesis. In this species, parturition occurs at a gestation age equivalent to human midgestation. In hypothyroid mice, repressive effects of aporeceptors have been shown to delay tissue maturation in brain, bone, intestine, spleen, and heart.[106] The increase in circulating T_3 levels associated with parturition in mice and humans normally triggers development of tissue functions essential to postnatal metabolism and homeostatis (e.g., hepatic, intestinal, and cardiac functions and brown fat thermogenesis); thyroid hormone–stimulated maturation of vision and hearing appear to be triggered by the local expression of D2 mediating local T_3 production, postnatally in the mouse and probably toward the end of the second midtrimester in the human fetus.[84]

In humans, T_3-mediated maturation of fetal tissues, including liver, heart, brown adipose tissue, and bone, become thyroid hormone–responsive during late gestation and during the perinatal period. Classical signs of congenital hypothyroidism (jaundice, lethargy, feeding difficulties, macroglossia, myxedema, hypothermia, growth retardation, and progressive developmental delay and IQ deterioration) accrue during the early weeks and months of extrauterine life as maternal T_4 becomes unavailable and the non–central nervous system (CNS) tissues become thyroid hormone–responsive.[73,77] Maternal hypothyroxinemia has been associated with attention deficit disorder and/or 5 to 10 points of IQ deficit in the offspring of such pregnancies.[73,96] The period of brain dependency for thyroid hormone extends postnatally to 2 to 3 years of age, but the early weeks and months of life are most critical. Untreated thyroid agenesis is associated with a loss of 5 to 7 IQ points monthly during the first months of postnatal life, and over 6 to 8 months can amount to a 30- to 40-point IQ deficit.[99]

TABLE 21–3 PREDOMINANT THYROID HORMONE RECEPTOR SUBTYPE FUNCTIONS IN DEVELOPING MICE

Brain TRα1, TRβ1	Thermogenesis TRα1, TRβ1, TRβ2
Pituitary TSH secretion TRβ2, TRα1	Inner ear TRα1, TRβ2
Pituitary GH secretion TRα1	Retina TRβ2
Bone maturation TRα1	Intestine TRα1
Liver TRβ1	Heart TRα1

See references 94 and 95.

Pituitary-Gonadal Axis

The mammalian gonad is derived from two tissue anlagen, the primordial germ cells of the yolk sac wall and somatic, stromal cells that migrate from the primitive mesonephros.[110,111] By 4 to

5 weeks of gestation, the germ cells have begun their migration from the yolk sac and the gonadal ridge has appeared as a derivative of the mesonephros. The germ cells are incorporated into the developing gonadal ridge during the sixth week, when the primitive gonad is composed of a surface epithelium, primitive gonadal cords continuous with the epithelium, and a dense cellular mass referred to as the gonadal blastema including the steroidogenic cell precursors.[110] Embryogenesis of the gonads is programmed by genes coding for the male sexual determinant SRY as well as SF-1 and DAX-1.[112,113] SRY is the single critical regulator of male gonadal differentiation. SF-1 is also required for testicular and perhaps ovarian development and mediates müllerian-inhibiting hormone gene expression and gonadotropin production. SF-1 and DAX-1 are orphan receptors of the steroid-thyroid hormone family of nuclear receptors and appear to interact as heterodimers coordinately involved in the regulation of target genes in the adrenal glands and in hypothalamic gonadotroph cells and the ventromedial hypothalamic nucleus.[112,113] A current view of the pathways for genes programming gonadal differentiation is shown (Fig. 21–8). The full menu of downstream gene targets remains to be defined, but the net result is the highly organized pattern of gonadal development and phenotypic sexual differentiation. Fetal pituitary gonadotropins are not required for gonadal development or sexual differentiation; LH or FSH receptor knockout mice are born phenotypically normal.[114] Human mutations in several of the genes programming gonadal differentiation have been described.[111] Loss of function mutations of *SRY* or *SOX1* produce XY sex reversal while gain of function mutations produce XX sex reversal. *SF1* mutations have been associated with XY sex reversal with gonadal agenesis. *WT1* mutations produce several syndromes associated with abnormal testicular embryogenesis (WAGR, Denys-Drash and Frasier syndromes). *WNT4* gain of function mutations result in XX sex reversal, and *DAX1* mutations produce XY sex reversal.[111]

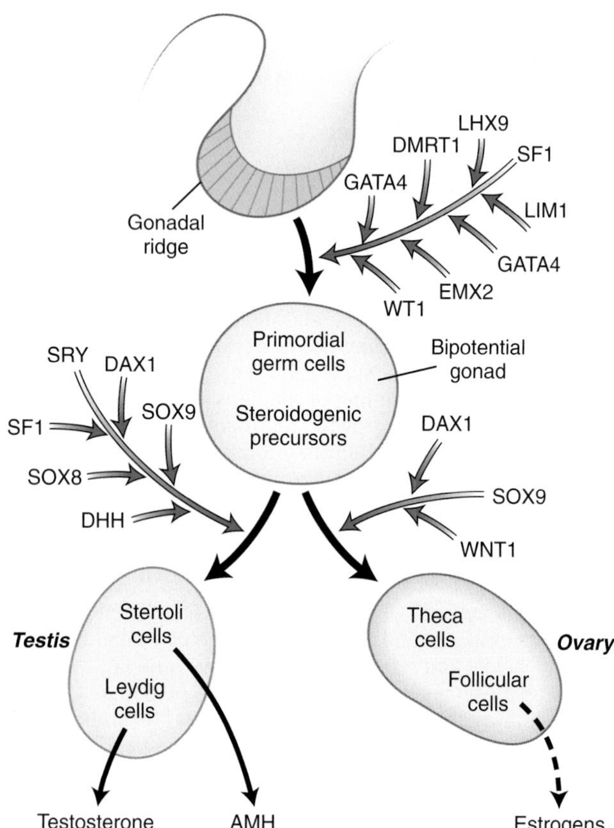

Figure 21–8 ▪ Summary of the molecular and cellular events of gonadal differentiation. *AMH*, Antimüllerian hormone or müllerian inhibiting substance. (The molecular cascades were developed from references 112 and 113. See text for details.)

Male gonadal differentiation begins at 7 weeks of gestation with organization of the gonadal blastema into interstitium and germ cell-containing testicular cords. The primitive cords lose their connections with the epithelium, primitive Sertoli cells and spermatogonia become visible within the cords, and the epithelium differentiates to form the tunica albuginea.[115] Leydig cells derived from the undifferentiated interstitium are visible by the end of the eighth week of gestation and are capable of androgen synthesis at this time. By 14 weeks of gestation, these cells make up as much as 50% of the cell mass, but as the tubules develop, they account for a smaller percentage of the tissue. The fetal testes grow from approximately 20 mg at 14 weeks of gestation to 800 mg at birth; at 5 to 6 months they descend into the inguinal canal in association with the epididymis and the ductus deferens.[115]

In females, differentiation of ovaries begins during the seventh week of gestation. The gonadal blastema differentiates into interstitium and medullary cords containing the primitive germ cells now referred to as *oogonia*. The cords degenerate and cortical layers of surface epithelium, containing individual small oogonia, appear. By 11 to 12 weeks of gestation, clusters of dividing oogonia are surrounded by cord cells within the cortex; the medulla at this time consists largely of connective tissue.[116] At 12 weeks of gestation, primitive granulosa cells begin to replicate and many of the large oogonia in the deepest layers of the cortex enter their first meiotic division. Primordial follicles are first observed at about 18 weeks of gestation and the number increases rapidly thereafter.[117] However, the number of oocytes progressively declines from a peak of 3 to 6 million at 5 months gestation to approximately 2 million at term.[10,117] Germ cell proliferation and apoptosis are ongoing simultaneously. Proliferating oocytes cluster and the clusters break down with the development of follicles because only those oocytes enfolded by developing granulosa cells (as primordial follicles) survive.[10,117] By 5 months of gestation and during the 7th month stroma-derived thecal cells develop around the primordial follicles as they mature to primary follicles. This process continues after birth, again progressing toward the superficial layers. Each fetal ovary weighs about 15 mg at 14 weeks of gestation and 300 to 350 mg at birth.[116] The number of surviving primary follicles at birth correlates with the duration of postpubertal ovulation. Interstitial cells with characteristics of steroid-producing cells are present after 12 weeks, and during the third trimester theca cells with steroidogenic capacity surround the developing follicles.[10] Significant aromatase activity also is present, but few if any steroids are produced by the ovary during development.[10,116]

In the male, the development of Leydig cells leads to an increase in fetal testosterone production between gestational weeks 10 and 20[115] (Fig. 21–9). In vitro studies in the rat have shown that hCG binding to fetal testis cells does not downregulate LH receptors. If this is true in vivo, continuous exposure of the Leydig cell to hCG would not desensitize the fetal testis and would allow the maintenance of augmented testosterone production during development. Fetal LH may contribute to fetal Leydig cell function, but quantitatively hCG is the predominant gonadotropin. Testosterone itself, acting through the androgen receptor, stimulates differentiation of the primitive mesonephric ducts into bilateral ductus deferens, epididymides, seminal vesicles, and ejaculatory ducts. Androgen receptors appear in the mesenchyme of urogenital structures at 8 weeks of gestation, followed by appearance of the receptors in the epithelium during development at 9 to 12 weeks.[118] There was no difference in receptor expression in male and female

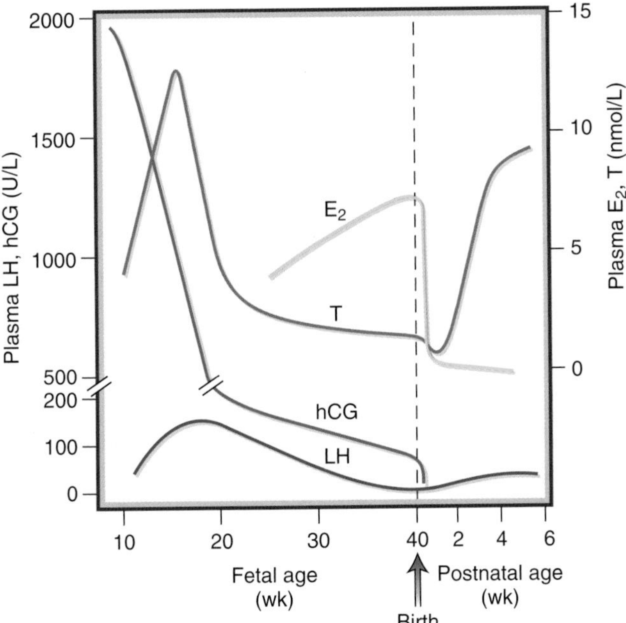

Figure 21–9 ▪ Patterns of change of plasma levels of human chorionic gonadotropin (hCG), luteinizing hormone (LH), testosterone (T), and estradiol (E_2) in a male fetus during gestation and in the neonatal period. (Data from Reyes FI, Boroditsky RS, Winter JS, et al. J Clin Endocrinol Metab 1974;38:612-617; Kaplan SL, Grumbach MM, Aubert ML. Recent Prog Horm Res 1975;32:161-243; Winter JS, Faiman C, Hobson WC, et al. J Clin Endocrinol Metab 1975;40:545-551; Forest MG, Cathiard AM. J Clin Endocrinol Metab 1975;41:977-980; Penny R, Parlow AF, Frasier SD. Pediatrics 1979;64:604-608).

fetuses. Dihydrotestosterone stimulates male differentiation of the urogenital sinus and external genitalia, including differentiation of the prostate, growth of the genital tubercle to form a phallus, and fusion of the urogenital folds to form the penile urethra. Dihydrotestosterone is formed from testosterone by the 5α-reductase enzyme within the urogenital sinus and urogenital tubercle and acts through the same androgen receptor that mediates the action of testosterone in the wolffian ducts.

The fetal testis also produces antimüllerian hormone (AMH), which causes dedifferentiation of the müllerian duct system in the male fetus.[119,120] AMH is a glycoprotein with a monomer molecular size of approximately 72 kd and multimer sizes ranging from 145 to 235 kd. It is produced by testicular Sertoli cells and reaches the müllerian ducts largely by diffusion; duct regression in vitro requires a 24- to 36-hour exposure to AMH, which is synthesized early in gestation, with production peaking at the time of müllerian duct regression. Biosynthesis continues throughout gestation and decreases after birth. *AMH* gene expression is activated by the *SRY* gene.[119] AMH also has autocrine and paracrine effects on testicular steroidogenic function during fetal life.[120] Male phenotypic differentiation is mediated by testicular testosterone and AMH, and occurs between 8 and 14 weeks of gestation. In the female fetus, the müllerian duct system differentiates in the absence of AMH, the mesonephric ducts fail to develop in the absence of testosterone, and the undifferentiated urogenital sinus and external genitalia mature into female structures. Mutation of the AMH gene results in a persistent müllerian duct syndrome in the XY fetus.[119]

Estrogen effects are mediated by cognate receptors, members of the large family of steroid and thyroid hormone, vitamin D, and retinoid receptors.[121,122] Two receptors, ERα and ERβ, have been identified with 96% and 58% homology in the DNA-binding and ligand-binding domains, respectively. Expression profiles of mRNAs of both receptors, products of separate genes, have been characterized in the 16- to 23-week human fetus. One or both receptor mRNAs are present in most tissues. ERβ message is predominant, particularly in testis, ovary, spleen, thymus, adrenal, brain, kidney, and skin. ERα message is prominent in uterus with relatively low levels in most other tissues.[121,122] The significance of estrogen receptors in fetal development remains unclear. Knockout of the ERα gene in mice does not impair fetal development of any tissue, but adult females are infertile with hypoplastic uteri and polycystic ovaries and adult males manifest decreased fertility.[122] ERβ knockout mice develop normally and female adults are fertile with normal sexual behavior; adult males reproduce normally but have prostate and bladder hyperplasia.[121] It is known that estrogens regulate DHEA production in the baboon and human fetal adrenal.[121] Knockout of both ERα and ERβ genes also has little impact on fetal development, but after birth the uterus, fallopian tubes, vagina, and cervix in females are hypoplastic and unresponsive to estrogen.[122]

Both androgens and estrogens are involved in the structural development of the rat brain.[123] Gonadal hormones also control gonadotropin production in the brain that results in cyclic ovarian function and normal function of the testes.[124,125] Testosterone administration to neonatal female rats produces permanent inhibition of cyclic hypothalamic control through local aromatization to estradiol and estrogen receptor binding. In primates and humans, estrogens seem to be more effective in this regard. However, there is no evidence for permanent programming in the primate, and there appear to be no major tissue biochemical differences between the sexes in utero to account for sexual dimorphic behavioral or gonadotropic programming.[125] Thus, the mechanisms for these effects are not yet clear in the primate and human fetus.

Intermediate Lobe of the Pituitary

The intermediate lobe of the pituitary gland is prominent in both the human and the sheep fetus. Intermediate lobe cells begin to disappear near term and are virtually absent in the adult human pituitary, although the intermediate lobe in the adult of some lower species is anatomically and functionally distinct.[126] The major secretory products of the intermediate lobe are α-MSH and β-endorphin derived from cleavage of the POMC molecule.[127] Cleavage of POMC in the anterior lobe results predominantly in corticotropin and β-lipotropin formation. In rhesus monkeys and humans, the fetal pituitary contains high concentrations of compounds resembling α-MSH and corticotropin-like intermediate lobe peptide.[128] In the human fetus, α-MSH levels decrease with increasing fetal age.[34] The circulating levels of both β-endorphin and β-lipotropin are high in the fetal lamb, and the ratio of β-endorphin to β-lipotropin increases during hypoxic stimulation of the anterior pituitary.[34] Because hypoxia provokes corticotropin release and β-lipotropin production from the anterior pituitary, these data have been interpreted to suggest that basal β-endorphin levels in the fetus originate in the intermediate lobe.[29] α-MSH and corticotropin-like intermediate lobe peptide may play a role in fetal adrenal activation, and α-MSH may play a role in fetal growth.[129,130] However, these effects are probably minor. The processing of pituitary POMC in the human fetus by the end of the second trimester is similar to that in the adult, but the role of these intermediate lobe peptides in the fetus remains obscure.[131]

Posterior Pituitary

The fetal neurohypophysis is well developed by 10 to 12 weeks of gestation and contains both AVP (also called *antidiuretic hormone*) and oxytocin (OT).[132,133] In addition, arginine vasotocin (AVT), the parent neurohypophyseal hormone in submammalian vertebrates, is present in the fetal pituitary and pineal glands and in adult pineal glands from several mammalian species, including humans.[134] AVT is present in the pituitary during fetal life and disappears in the neonatal period. In adult mammals, instillation of AVT into cerebrospinal fluid inhibits gonadotropin and corticotropin release, stimulates PRL release by the anterior pituitary, and induces sleep; however, its physiologic importance in these regards remains unclear. The role of AVT in the fetal pineal gland is unknown (see Fig. 21–2).

In the fetal sheep, the baseline fetal plasma AVP concentrations are similar to maternal levels after midgestation. During the last trimester of gestation, fetal hypothalamic and pituitary responsiveness to both volume and osmolar stimuli for AVP secretion are well developed and AVP exerts antidiuretic effects on the fetal kidney.[132,133] Baseline plasma levels of AVT in fetal sheep during the last trimester approximate values for AVP and OT.[134] Presumably this AVT is derived from the posterior pituitary, but the stimuli for AVT secretion in the fetus are not defined. The neurohypophyseal peptides are synthesized as large precursor molecules (neurophysins) and processed to bioactive amidated peptides.[135] Enzymatic processing involves progressive cleavage of carboxyl terminal–extended peptides producing sequentially (for OT) OT-glycine-lysine-arginine (OTGKR), OTGK, OTG, and OT. Similar progressive processing yields AVPG and AVP from the AVP neurophysin. Enzymatic processing of neurophysins matures progressively in the fetus so that early in gestation fetal plasma contains relatively large concentrations of the extended peptides. For OT, the ratio of OT-extended peptides to OT in fetal sheep serum is approximately 35 : 1 early in gestation and 3 : 1 late in gestation.[135]

In the fetus, AVP appears to function as a stress-responsive hormone. Perhaps the major potential stress for the fetus is hypoxia, and the response of AVP to hypoxia is increased compared with the maternal response and with the fetal AVP responses to osmolar stimuli.[133,136-138] Plasma AVP concentrations in human cord blood are elevated in association with intrauterine bradycardia and meconium passage.[137] The vasopressor action of AVP may be important in the maintenance of fetal circulatory homeostasis during hemorrhage and hypoxia; AVP has a limited effect on fetoplacental blood flow.[132,138] Fetal hypoxia is also a major stimulus for catecholamine release. There is little information on interaction between AVP and catecholamines during fetal hypoxia, but both fetal hypoxia and AVP stimulate anterior pituitary function.[138] A role for AVP as a CRH is established in the adult, and the ovine fetal pituitary responds separately and synergistically to AVP and CRH early in the third trimester.[139] The role of AVP in controlling fetal corticotropin release seems to decrease with gestational age. It is not known whether AVT functions as a fetal CRH.

OT receptors have been demonstrated in human fetal membranes at term, and AVP receptors have been found in renal medullary membranes of newborn sheep.[140-142] Both AVP and AVT evoke antidiuretic actions in the sheep fetus during the last third of gestation, and both hormones act to conserve water for the fetus by inhibiting fluid loss into amniotic fluid through the lungs and kidneys.[132,133] Aquaporin-1, aquaporin-2, and aquaporin-3 water channel receptors are present in the human fetal and newborn kidney, and the ability of the newborn infant to regulate free water clearance in response to volume and osmolar stimuli has been demonstrated.[143,144] Whether AVT exerts its effects through AVP receptors or separate fetal AVT receptors is not clear. Maximal concentrating capacity by the fetal kidney is limited to about 600 mmol/L. This limitation is due not to inadequate AVP stimulation, but rather to inherent immaturity of the renal tubules.

Fetal Autonomic Nervous System

The primordia of the sympathetic trunk ganglia are visible in the human fetus by 6 to 7 weeks of gestation. The preaortic sympathetic primordia at this time are composed of primitive sympathetic neurons and chromaffin cells, which condense into chains of cell masses along the abdominal aorta. By 10 to 12 weeks of gestation the paired adrenal masses are well developed. In addition, numerous extramedullary paraganglia (derived from preaortic condensations of sympathetic neurons and chromaffin cells) are scattered throughout the abdominal and pelvic sympathetic plexuses.[145] Each of these extramedullary paraganglia may reach a maximal diameter of 2 to 3 mm by 28 to 30 weeks of gestation. The largest of the paraganglia, the organs of Zuckerkandl near the origin of the inferior mesenteric arteries, enlarge to 10 to 15 mm in length at term. After birth, the paraganglia gradually atrophy and disappear by 2 to 3 years of age. With increasing gestational age, there is progressive growth of the adrenal medullae, increasing catecholamine content of the adrenal medullae, and progressive maturation of medullary functional capacity. Histologically, the adrenal medullae are somewhat immature at birth, but by the age of 1 they resemble the adult glands.

Both chromaffin and sympathetic nerve cells are derived from common neuroectodermal stem cells. In mice, the sympathoadrenal progenitor cells first aggregate at the dorsal aorta where they migrate in a dorsolateral direction to form sympathetic ganglia or ventrally to colonize the adrenal glands.[146] In the adrenal glands they differentiate into neuroendocrine cells, expressing tyrosine hydroxylase and dopamine β hydroxylase in response to a series of transcription factors including *PHOX2B, MASH1, PHOX2A,* and *dHAND*.[146] The *PHOX2B* gene is pivotal in development of most relays of the autonomic nervous system, and mutation of this gene has been associated with the congenital hypoventilation syndrome, with Hirschsprung disease and with a predisposition to neuroblastoma.[147] Sympathetic nervous system development is NGF-dependent, and injections of NGF antiserum into neonatal rats lead to degeneration of immature chromaffin cells, sympathetic cells, and pheochromoblasts.[148] Whether NGF and other growth factors are involved in the transient life span and function of the paraganglia in the human fetus and neonate is not clear. The role of placental NGF in maturation of the fetal autonomic nervous system is also unclear.

Catecholamines are present in the paraaortic chromaffin tissue by 10 to 15 weeks of gestation, and concentrations increase until term. The predominant catecholamine is norepinephrine (NE), presumably because of low activity of phenylethanolamine *N*-methyltransferase in paraaortic chromaffin tissue. This enzyme, which catalyzes the methylation of NE to epinephrine, appears to be activated by the high levels of cortisol that diffuse into the adrenal medulla from the adrenal cortex; in contrast, cortisol levels in extramedullary chromaffin tissue are low.[145,149,150] In fetal mammals, the chromaffin cells of the adrenal medulla can respond directly to asphyxia, long before splanchnic innervation develops, by secreting NE; the noninnervated paraaortic tissue responds similarly. In the fetal sheep, a similar developmental transition occurs between days 120 and 135 of the 150-day gestation.[145,149,150] The CNS responds to stimuli that evoke sympathetic nervous system responses before the adrenomedullary splanchnic innervation, but the adrenal medulla is relatively unresponsive to such stimuli. The transition is heralded by an adrenomedullary response to hypoglycemia mediated by the CNS.[149] This response is present in developing sheep, monkeys, and human fetuses during the third trimester of gestation.[151-153] Central and adrenal enkephalins are also involved in fetal autonomic nervous system function, and pretreatment with naloxone potentiates and methadone inhibits the catecholamine response to hypoxia.[145,150]

Basal plasma epinephrine, NE, and dopamine levels during the last third of gestation in sheep decrease as term approaches.[153,154] The metabolic clearance rate of epinephrine increases with gestational age, whereas the production rate remains unchanged, indicating that the decreasing basal catecholamine levels that occur with fetal age are due to maturation of clearance mechanisms.[154] The fetal sheep responds to maternal exercise or hypoxia with increased catecholamine levels.[155] The human neonate responds to parturition with an increase in plasma epinephrine and NE concentrations, and these responses are augmented by hypoxia and acidosis.[145,149] In the newborn infant catecholamine secretion also increases after cold exposure and hypoglycemia.[149,152]

Catecholamines are critical for fetal cardiovascular function and fetal survival. Gene knockout studies in mice, targeting either tyrosine hydroxylase or dopamine β-hydroxylase, produced fetal catecholamine deficiency and midgestation fetal death in 90% of the mutant embryos.[156,157] In addition, fetal catecholamines are the major stress hormones in the fetus.[149-152] The fetal adrenal and the paraaortic chromaffin masses discharge large amounts of catecholamines directly into the circulation in response to fetal hypoxia.[149] Moreover, the defense against fetal hypoxia involves catecholamine actions mediated through cardiac α-receptors that are unique to immature animals. α-Adrenergic receptors predominate in immature cardiac tissue and gradually decline in number as β-adrenergic receptors increase with maturation. Chromaffin tissue in the fetus is also innervated by opiate receptors and contains relatively large amounts of opiate peptides that appear to be co-secreted with the catecholamines.[149] The extent to which these peptides or pituitary endorphins are involved in modulating fetal catecholamine secretion remains unclear.

Parathyroid Hormone/ Calcitonin System

Parathyroid gland development from the third and fourth pharyngeal pouches proceeds in synchrony with thyroid embryogenesis.[72,73] The third pouches encounter the migrating thyroid anlage, and the parathyroid anlagen are carried caudally with the thyroid gland, finally coming to rest at the lower poles of the thyroid lobes as the inferior parathyroid glands. The fourth pouches encounter the thyroid anlage later and come to rest at the upper poles of the thyroid lobes as the superior parathyroid glands. The individual parathyroid glands increase in diameter from less than 0.1 mm at 14 weeks of gestation to 1 to 2 mm at birth. The fifth pouches contribute paired ultimobranchial bodies that are incorporated into the developing thyroid gland as the parafollicular or C cells that secrete calcitonin. Both endocrine systems are functional during the second and third trimesters (see Fig. 21–6). Disruption of the *HOX15* gene in mice results in parathyroid gland aplasia, indicating that this gene functions as part of the gene cascade programming normal thyroid-parathyroid gland development. Additional genes involved in parathyroid gland embryogenesis include *GCMB, GATA3, CRKL*, and *TBX1*.[158,159] *CRKL* and *TBX1* mutations have been associated with the DiGeorge syndrome and *GATA3* mutation with a DiGeorge-like syndrome; *GCMB* mutation leads to isolated hypoparathyroidism.[158]

Studies in fetal sheep and monkey and measurements in human preterm and term infants indicate that high concentrations of fetal calcium (averaging 2.75 to 3 mmol/L in the last trimester) are maintained by active placental transport from maternal blood.[160,161] The transport of calcium occurs across the syncytiotrophoblast, which contains a calcium-binding protein that buffers intracellular calcium ions as they are transported across the syncytial cell to the basement membrane. An adenosine triphosphate (ATP)-dependent calcium pump transports the calcium across the cell membrane to the fetal circulation.[161] The placental calcium pump is stimulated by a midmolecule portion of PTHrP secreted by the fetal parathyroid gland and by the placenta, where it may exert a paracrine effect.[161-163] The placenta is impermeable to PTH, PTHrP, and calcitonin, but 25-hydroxyvitamin D and 1,25-dihydroxyvitamin D are transported across the placenta and free vitamin D levels in fetal blood are similar to or higher than maternal values.[160,161]

Thyroparathyroidectomy in the fetal sheep causes a rapid decrease in fetal plasma calcium concentration and a loss of the placental calcium gradient.[160] In mice, knockout of the gene for PTHrP abolished the maternal-fetal calcium gradient and placental transport of calcium was reduced.[161,164] Placental calcium transport in these models was restored by the midmolecule fragment of PTHrP (amino acids 67 to 86) but not by PTH or PTHrP fragments 1 to 34, which activate the PTH/PTHrP receptor.[163,164] Thus, a second as yet unidentified PTHrP receptor recognizing the PTHrP 38 to 94 ligand appears to be involved in placental calcium pump activation.[161]

Other factors are also involved in maintenance of fetal serum calcium levels because knockout of the mouse gene for PTH-PTHrP also results in hypocalcemia in the presence of normal or increased placental calcium transport.[160,162] PTH and PTHrP, through the PTH-PTHrP receptor, presumably modulate fetal skeletal calcium flux, calcium excretion through the fetal kidney, and perhaps reabsorption of calcium from amniotic fluid. PTHrP has a major role in fetal bone development and metabolism as well as fetal calcium homeostasis. PTHrP knockout mice display increased ossification of the basal portion of the skull, long bones, vertebral bodies, and pelvic bones and mineralization of the normally cartilaginous portions of the ribs and sternum; as a result of the cartilaginous mineralization, the animals die of asphyxiation in the early neonatal period.[161,164]

Fetal nephrectomy also reduces fetal calcium concentrations, and the hypocalcemia can be prevented by administration of 1,25-dihydroxyvitamin D ($1,25[OH]_2D$).[160] Moreover, infusion into the sheep fetus of antibody to $1,25(OH)_2D$ reduced the placental calcium gradient.[160] Thus, fetal PTHrP and PTH appear to stimulate fetal renal $1,25(OH)_2D$ production, which acts to enhance maternal-fetal transport of calcium by the placenta. The fetal kidney can synthesize $1,25(OH)_2D$ via 1-hydroxylation of 25-hydroxycholecalciferol, and the placenta contains both $1,25(OH)_2D$ receptors and a vitamin D–dependent calcium-binding protein. In the sheep fetus, the endogenous production rate of $1,25(OH)_2D$ during the last third of gestation was six times greater than that in the mother.[164] The metabolic clearance of $1,25(OH)_2D$ was also higher in the fetus than in the mother.

The fetal parathyroid-placental axis promotes maternal-fetal transfer of bone mineral and accretion of fetal bone mineral. The high blood levels of calcitonin in the fetus, probably resulting from the chronic stimulation by fetal hypercalcemia, are thought to contribute to the fetal bone mineral accretion.[159,160] A prominent effect of calcitonin is to inhibit bone resorption, and the high fetal serum calcium concentrations coupled with high circulating calcitonin promote bone mineral anabolism.[159] Placental calcitonin production may contribute to the calcitonin in fetal plasma, but the persistence of high plasma levels in neonatal plasma argues for predominant fetal production. Also, $1,25(OH)_2D$ or $24,25(OH)_2D$ may play a role in fetal cartilage growth and bone mineral accretion.[165] These concepts are summarized in Figure 21–10.

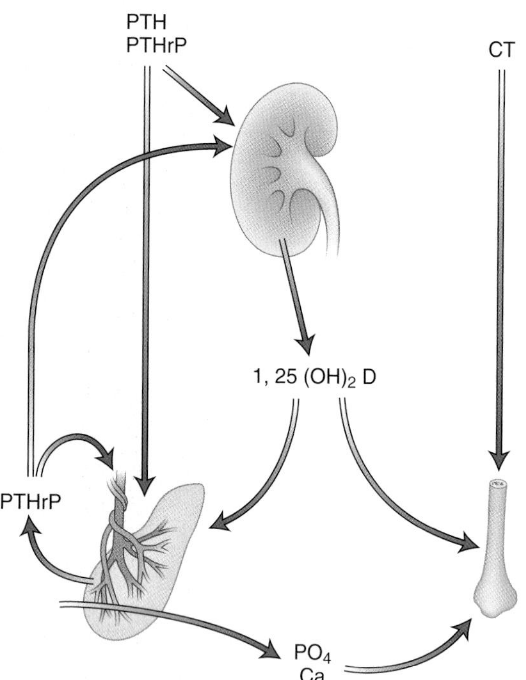

Figure 21–10 ▪ Proposed actions of parathyroid hormone (PTH), PTH-related protein (PTHrP), and calcitonin (CT) in the fetus. PTHrP and perhaps PTH from the parathyroid glands and PTHrP from the placenta act on the placenta to promote calcium (Ca) and phosphate (PO_4) transport from the maternal to the fetal circulation to maintain the relative fetal hypercalcemia and the high rate of fetal bone formation during the last half of gestation. PTHrP also acts on the kidney to promote 1-hydroxylation of 25-hydroxycholecalciferol to 1,25-dihydroxyvitamin D, 1,25(OH)2D, which augments placental calcium transport and promotes fetal bone growth. High fetal CT levels tend to promote bone accretion. See text for details.

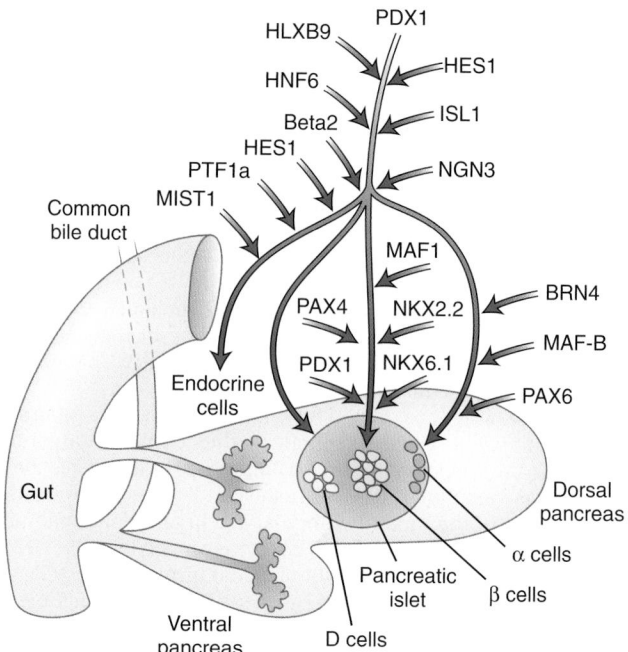

Figure 21–11 ▪ Expression of transcription factors during pancreatic embryogenesis. Knockout of *PDX1, HLXB9,* or *ISL-1* is associated with early arrest of pancreatic development. *HLXB9* knockout leads to failure of the pancreatic dorsal bud to develop with decreased β cell number in the remnant pancreas. *HES-1* or neurogenin 3 *(NGN3)* disruption leads to aplasia or hypoplasia of the islets of Langerhans. Disruption of the downstream transcription factors impairs formation of the β cells or alpha cells. *SOX9* and *HNF3*β (not shown) are required for early foregut formation and pancreas specification. (From Habener JF, Kemp DM, Thomas MJ. Mini review: transcriptional regulation in pancreatic development. Endocrinology 2005;146:1025-1034.)

Endocrine Pancreas: Insulin and Glucagon

Embryogenesis of the pancreas is mediated by a series of homeobox genes and transcription factors in the mouse programming pancreatic budding from the gut tube, development of branching ducts and undifferentiated epithelium, differentiation of exocrine and endocrine cell lineages, and organization of the endocrine cells into islets of Langerhans. The process in mice begins at day 8 of the 21-day gestation and extends 2 to 3 weeks after birth[166] (Fig. 21–11). Studies in mice have shown that *PDX-1, HLXB9, ISL-1,* or *HES1* gene knockout results in pancreatic agenesis or dysgenesis. *NGN3* or *Beta2* knockout leads to complete absence of endocrine cells while knockout of the lower pathway genes shown in Figure 21–11 impair specific islet cell differentiation.[166] Members of the EGF family of growth factors, laminin, and perhaps other growth factors including the IGFs contribute to pancreatic growth and differentiation.[167,168]

The human fetal pancreas is identifiable by 4 weeks of gestation, and α and β cells can be recognized by 8 to 9 weeks. Insulin, glucagon, somatostatin, and pancreatic polypeptide are measurable by 8 to 10 weeks of gestation.[169] α Cells are more numerous than β cells in the early fetal pancreas and reach a relative peak at midgestation; β cells increase throughout the second half of gestation so that by term the ratio of α cells to β cells is approximately 1 : 1. The insulin content of the pancreas increases from less than 3.6 pmol/g (0.5 U/g) at 7 to 10 weeks to 30 pmol/g (4 U/g) at 16 to 25 weeks of gestation and 93 pmol/g (13 U/g) near term; the concentration in the adult pancreas is approximately 14 pmol/g (2 U/g).[170]

Although the fetal β cell is functional by 14 to 24 weeks of gestation, secretion of insulin by the fetal pancreas is low. Insulin release from the fetal rat pancreas in vitro in response to glucose or pyruvate is minimal but can be stimulated by leucine, arginine, tolbutamide, or potassium chloride, indicating that parts of the secretory mechanism are functional in the fetus.[170-172] Insulin secretion in adult islets is mediated by two or more mechanisms, including stimulation of the adenylate cyclase system with production of cAMP and inhibition of potassium efflux, which leads to depolarization of the cell membrane and opening of voltage-dependent calcium channels. The former mechanism, although suppressed in the fetal islets, can be augmented by theophylline, but calcium channel activation does not occur in fetal islets in response to initiators of insulin release that cause depolarization of adult islet cells.[172] The infusion of glucose or arginine in pregnant women before hysterotomy fails to provoke fetal insulin secretion at midgestation or near term, and plasma insulin levels in the late human fetus are relatively unresponsive to high glucose concentrations before the onset of labor.[170]

Similar observations have been made in the monkey. In this species, neither glucose nor arginine stimulated fetal insulin release near term but glucagon evoked prompt insulin secretion.[170] Late in gestation in the ovine fetus, epinephrine inhibits insulin release through a receptor pathway.[170] In the anencephalic human fetus, the endocrine pancreas develops normally if maternal carbohydrate metabolism is not impaired, but β cell hypertrophy and hyperplasia do not occur in the anencephalic fetus or in decapitated fetal rabbits exposed to chronic hyperglycemia. This lack of β cell response to hyperglycemia may be the result of GH deficiency because GH stimulates insulin gene expression and may play a permissive role in β cell hyperplasia and hypertrophy.[168]

Pancreatic glucagon concentrations are relatively high in fetal plasma and increase progressively with fetal age.[170,171] The fetal pancreatic glucagon content at midgestation is approximately 6 μg/g, compared with an adult level of 2 μg/g. As is true for insulin, the capacity for glucagon secretion is blunted in the fetus. Hyperglycemia does not suppress fetal plasma glucagon levels in rats, monkeys, or sheep, and acute hypoglycemia does not evoke glucagon secretion in the rat fetus. Amino acids, which are important secretagogues for insulin and glucagon in the adult, probably have little role in modulating insulin and glucagon secretion in the preterm fetus. However, infusion of alanine into women at term increases both maternal and cord blood glucagon levels, indicating a fetal glucagon response to amino acids in the term fetus. Catecholamines also evoke glucagon release in the near-term ovine fetus.[170]

Thus, the fetal pancreatic islet cells, although histologically mature and capable of hormone synthesis and hyperplasia, are relatively immature functionally at birth with regard to the capacity to secrete both insulin and glucagon. The rapid maturation of responsiveness to glucose in the neonatal period in both premature and mature infants suggests that this blunted state may be a secondary result of the relatively stable fetal serum glucose levels maintained by placental transfer of maternal glucose rather than a primary, temporally fixed maturation process. The blunted capacity for insulin and glucagon secretion has been related to a deficient capacity of the fetal pancreatic islet cells to generate cAMP or a rapid destruction of cAMP by phosphodiesterase, or both.[170]

Insulin and glucagon are normally not necessary for substrate metabolism in the fetus.[171] Glucose is obtained by placental transfer through facilitated diffusion The fetal respiratory quotient is approximately 1, which suggests that glucose is the primary energy substrate for the fetus. Other substrates such as amino acids and lactate may also be utilized in the human as in the sheep fetus. However, at least early in gestation, hepatic metabolism and substrate utilization appear to be independent of insulin and to be modulated in an autoregulatory fashion by glucose.[170] In addition, the constant supply of glucose normally precludes the necessity for endogenous gluconeogenesis, and gluconeogenic enzyme activities are low in the fetal liver.

Glycogen storage in the fetus is modulated by fetal glucocorticoids and probably by placental lactogen (HPL). Fetal insulin plays a role near term, when insulin also has the capacity to increase fetal glucose uptake and lipogenesis.[170,171] Insulin receptors are present on most fetal cells in higher numbers than on adult cells; moreover, hyperinsulinemia fails to down-regulate fetal insulin receptors.[170] Fetal hepatic glucagon receptors, in contrast, are reduced in number, and fetal liver is relatively resistant to the glycemic effect of glucagon. These conditions tend to potentiate the fetal anabolic milieu during the period of rapid growth in the last trimester of gestation.

NEUTRALIZATION OF HORMONE ACTIONS IN THE FETUS

After the period of embryogenesis, the fetal milieu is programmed to optimize body growth and organ development through an array of generalized and specialized growth factors. (See Fetal Growth.) These function in a stable metabolic environment with substrate supply maintained by the placenta. The endocrine-metabolic systems characterizing the extrauterine environment are programmed to maintain metabolic stability in a changing external environment with intermittent substrate provision. Hormonal systems in the fetus are programmed to maintain anabolism with minimal hormonal perturbation. Thus, production of catabolic and thermogenic hormones is limited and the effects of the hormones altering metabolic substrate supply and distribution pathways are muted (Table 21–4).

TABLE 21–4 NEUTRALIZATION OF HORMONE ACTIONS IN THE FETUS*

PRODUCTION OF INACTIVE METABOLITES	
Active Hormone	**Inactive Metabolites**
Cortisol	Cortisone
Thyroxine (T_4)	rT_3, T_4S, rT_3S
Triiodothyronine (T_3)	T_3S, T_2
DELAYED EXPRESSION OR NEUTRALIZATION OF RECEPTORS	
Active Hormone	**Receptor**
Growth hormone (GH)	GHR
Thyroid hormone	Trα, TRβ
Catecholamines	βAR
Estrogens	ER
Glucagon	GR
LIMITED HORMONE SECRETION	
Active Hormone	**Secretory Cell**
Insulin	Islet cell β
Glucagon	Islet cell α

*See text for details.
rT_3, Reverse T_3; *T_4S*, T_4 sulfate.

Limitation of Hormone Secretion

The human fetal pancreas is functional during the second trimester, but secretion of insulin in response to glucose or pyruvate is minimal until the neonatal period.[170,171] Glucagon secretion is also blunted, although fetal blood glucagon levels are relatively high. Fetal islet hyperplasia and increased insulin secretion occur in response to chronic hyperglycemia as in the infant of the diabetic mother, and insulin release can be stimulated by acute fetal infusions of leucine, arginine, or tolbutamide.[170,172] Moreover, responsiveness of both insulin and glucagon secretion to glucose develops rapidly in the neonatal period.[170] It is not clear whether the limited fetal islet cell responsiveness is due to the relatively stable fetal serum glucose levels or a temporally fixed maturation process. (See Endocrine Pancreas: Insulin and Glucagon.)

Production of Inactive Metabolites

Throughout the latter part of gestation, cortisol is metabolized in fetal tissues to inactive cortisone through an 11βHSD. The placenta is permeable to steroid hormones including cortisol. During midgestation, placental 11βHSD activity is low and some cortisol is transferred to the fetus. Placental 11βHSD activity increases during the second half of pregnancy under the control of placental estrogens, and enzyme activity near term is high.[10,173] Thus, maternal-fetal cortisol transfer decreases progressively. In addition, although many adult tissues can convert cortisone to cortisol, conversion is limited during most of fetal life. Consequently, most of the cortisol that crosses the placenta or is produced by the fetus is inactivated to cortisone by the placenta or by fetal tissues.

Levels of cortisone in fetal plasma exceed those of cortisol by threefold to fourfold until after 30 weeks of gestation (see Fig. 21–5). Teleologically, this would help preserve the anabolic and growth-promoting milieu of the fetus and minimize premature maturational and parturitional effects of cortisol. After 30 weeks, the ratio of cortisol to cortisone in fetal tissues and plasma increases as a result of increased fetal secretion and decreased conversion of cortisol to cortisone within the placenta and fetal tissues.[173] Cortisol has important maturational action on several fetal tissues near term. (See Transition to Extrauterine Life.)

Fetal thyroid hormone metabolism is characterized by conversion of active thyroid hormones to inactive rT_3 and inactive sulfated iodothyronines and by limited receptor and postreceptor responsiveness to thyroid hormone in selected tissues.[77,86] The placenta contains an iodothyronine inner-ring monodeiodinase that catalyzes conversion of maternal T_4 to rT_3. In addition, the fetal sheep liver and kidney, in contrast to the adult liver and kidney, manifest low levels of iodothyronine type I outer-ring monodeiodinase activity so that conversion of T_4 to active T_3 is limited and large amounts of inactive iodothyronine sulfoconjugates accumulate.[77,88] As a consequence, plasma T_3 levels in the fetus remain low until the last few weeks of gestation (see Fig. 21–7). Selected fetal tissues (brain, brown adipose tissue) have active iodothyronine, type II, outer-ring monodeiodinase activities that contribute to local tissue T_3 concentrations; local T_3 is important in development, particularly in the hypothyroid fetus.[77,174] Near term and in the neonatal period in the human fetus, the dramatic increase in plasma T_3 levels, and presumably T_3 production, heralds the onset of thyroid hormone actions on growth and development and on metabolism (see Fig. 21–7).

Neutralization of Receptor Response

Selected ovine fetal tissues seem relatively unresponsive to thyroid hormones. Fetal ovine liver and kidney thermogenesis (as evidenced by oxygen consumption, Na^+,K^+-ATPase activity, and mitochondrial α-glycerophosphate activity) is unresponsive to exogenous T_3 during the third trimester, and thyroid hormone responsiveness in a number of tissues (cardiac, hepatic, renal, and skin) develops only during the perinatal period.[175] β-Adrenergic receptor binding in heart and lung of the ovine fetus is unresponsive to T_3 late in the third trimester but increases in response to T_3 in the neonatal period.[73,175] In rodent species, in which development at birth is comparable to human fetal development at midgestation, pituitary GH concentrations become responsive to thyroid hormone only during the first weeks of extrauterine life.[176] Mouse submandibular gland EGF and NGF levels become responsive to thyroid hormone during the second week of life, as do urine and kidney EGF concentrations and hepatic EGF receptor levels.[177,178] Mouse skin EGF levels and EGF receptors are responsive during the first neonatal week.[179,180] Thus, despite the presence of nuclear T_3 receptors in significant concentrations in developing rat and sheep, many thyroid hormone actions in these species are delayed.[181] The mechanism of this delayed thyroid hormone responsiveness is not clear; developmental programming of iodothyronine monodeiodinase expression and gene expression programming via unliganded thyroid receptors (TR) or TR interacting corepressors probably all play a role.

The effect of the high circulating concentrations of GH in the fetus is also limited. Fetal somatic growth is only partially GH-dependent; indeed, the GH-deficient fetus has little or no growth retardation.[33,42] The paucity of fetal GH effects is due to delayed maturation of GH receptors or postreceptor mechanisms. In animals such as sheep, hepatic GH receptor binding appears only during the neonatal period.[33,42] Receptor deficiency may also be a factor in the limited PRL bioactivity in the fetus near term.[42]

There is less information on fetal hormone responsiveness in other systems. β-Adrenergic receptor binding in heart and lung of the sheep fetus is relatively low near term and increases in the neonatal period in response to thyroid hormones.[175] Moreover, premature lambs have an augmented plasma catecholamine surge at birth but have a relatively mild increase in plasma free fatty acid levels, which suggests reduced catecholamine responsiveness.[182] The high levels of progesterone and estrogens in fetal blood also seem to have limited effects in the fetus. Progesterone receptors are present in low concentration in fetal guinea pig kidney, lung, and uterus at midgestation and increase progressively until term.[183] Estrogen receptors appear in neonatal rat uterus, oviduct, cervix, and vagina during the first 10 days of extrauterine life, and both ERα and ERβ mRNAs are present in human fetal tissues during the second trimester.[121,184] The human neonate often manifests mild breast enlargement at birth, and vaginal estrogenation may be evident in female infants at birth. Estrogen effects otherwise appear limited (see Table 21–4).

FETAL GROWTH

Insulin-Like Growth Factors

The IGFs are involved in regulation of uterine and placental growth during pregnancy and in early embryonic and fetal development IGF-I, EGF, and estrogens are mitogens for endometrial stromal cells, and the endometrial contents of IGF-I and IGF-I mRNA are high at implantation and during early embryogenesis in the sow.[185] Uterine IGF-I and IGF-I mRNA levels decrease progressively with advancing gestation.[185] Placental tissue also contains IGF-I and IGF-II mRNAs, significant concentrations of the respective proteins, and IGF-I receptors.[10] Autocrine and paracrine roles for the IGFs in uterine and placental tissues are postulated. IGF-I and insulin are produced by embryonic tissues during the prepancreatic stage of mouse development, and both factors stimulate growth of embryonic mouse cells.[186] Studies of transgenic mice with null mutations of the genes encoding *IGF-I, IGF-II*, or the IGF-I receptor have defined the role of the somatomedins; the birth weight of the embryos lacking IGF-I or IGF-II was 60% of that of the control mice. When both genes were inactive, birth weight was reduced another 30%, and mice lacking IGF-I receptor had birth weights averaging 45% of control values.[40] IGF-II deficient mice also manifest intrauterine growth retardation in association with a small placenta. They have near normal postnatal growth but delayed bone development.[40] IGF-II receptor knockout fetal mice are 30% overweight, suggesting a negative growth modulating effect of this receptor. The normal growth in fetuses with both IGF-I and IGF-II receptor knockout is due to IGF-I signaling via the insulin receptor; combined IGF-I, IGF-II, and insulin receptor knockout results in severe intrauterine growth retardation and fetal death. Knockout of individual IGF binding proteins has little effect on fetal or placental growth.[40]

IGF binding proteins are present as early as 5 weeks of gestation, and prenatally as postnatally, the IGF's circulate associated with binding proteins.[40] Thus, during fetal and postnatal life, plasma concentrations of IGFs are relatively high compared with tissue concentrations. In the fetus, IGF-II levels are five to six times higher than those of IGF-I, in contrast to these levels in children and adults, and levels of both increase progressively throughout gestation.[187] Fetal levels of both peptides at term are 30% to 50% of adult levels. In most studies, cord blood IGF-I concentrations correlate with birth size.[40] Despite the fetal growth-enhancing effects of IGF-II, blood levels are only weakly related to size at birth, largely because of the inhibiting effect of soluble IGF-II receptor (IGFIIR).[188] Soluble IGFIIR is derived through proteolytic cleavage of the transmembrane region of the receptor in many tissues. IGF receptors have been identified as early as 5 weeks of gestation and are widespread in fetal tissues.[40] IGF-I stimulates glycogenesis in cultured fetal rat hepatocytes and induces formation of myotubes in cultured myoblasts. IGF-II is active in cultured muscle and neonatal rat astroglial cells. Insulin receptors are increased in fetal cells and are resistant to down-regulation; no similar data are available for the IGF-I receptor.

As discussed earlier, the control of IGF production differs in fetal and postnatal life. GH receptors are relatively deficient and receptors for placental lactogen (HPL) predominate in fetal tissues.[42,43] GH does play a minor role in the fetus as reflected in the low IGF levels and slight reduction in birth weight and length in infants with GH resistance (Laron dwarfism). HPL stimulates IGF-I production and augments amino acid transport and DNA synthesis in human fetal fibroblasts and muscle cells.[42] IGF-I and IGF-II levels are reduced in fetuses of protein-starved pregnant rats and the low IGF-II levels are reversed by HPL.[189] Thyroidectomy of the third trimester sheep fetus impairs skeletal muscle growth in association with a decrease in muscle GH receptor mRNA and IGF-I mRNA without an effect on IGF-II levels.[190] This period is equivalent to the postnatal period in the human and there is no evidence that thyroid hormones modulate GH receptor or IGF-I levels in the human fetus. Glucocorticoids can inhibit fetal growth, presumably by inhibiting IGF gene transcription.[190] Nutrition is the major factor modulating IGF production in the fetus. IGF levels fall in suckling rats deprived of milk, and IGF-I and IGF-II levels are reduced in fetuses of protein-starved pregnant rats and placentally restricted sheep.[40,41] These data support the view that the IGFs are important in embryonic and fetal growth and that in the fetus they are regulated, at least in part, by HPL and by nutritional substrate derived transplacentally. The high levels of IGF-II in fetal rat serum, the high levels of IGF-II mRNA in fetal tissues, and the presence of a truncated form of IGF-I in human fetal brain tissue suggest unique developmental actions of these peptides (Table 21–5).

Insulin

Insulin has been proposed to act as a fetal growth factor. Infants born to women with diabetes mellitus may have hyperinsulinemia associated with increased birth weight.[191] Most of this increased weight is accounted for by body fat; there is little increase in body length, but some organomegaly may occur. Infants with hyperinsulinemia caused by nesidioblastosis or the Beckwith-Wiedemann syndrome may also have increased somatic growth in utero. Conversely, the human fetus with pancreatic agenesis is small and has decreased muscle bulk and little or no adipose tissue.[191] Mice with insulin or insulin receptor gene mutations have a 10% decrease in birth weight and early neonatal death with hyperglycemia and ketonemia.[40] Insulin receptor mutations in humans lead to severe intrauterine growth retardation and limited postnatal weight gain.[40] In contrast to mice, the human fetus during the latter half of gestation has a significant increase in adipose mass, and adipose tissue is highly sensitive to insulin. In clinical conditions associated with fetal hyperinsulinemia, the human neonate is born large for gestation age, largely due to increased lipogenesis mediated by insulin or IGF-I receptors.

TABLE 21–5 GROWTH FACTORS AND FETAL GROWTH*

Tissues Affected	Growth Factors
Neural tissue	BNF, NT3, NGF Neuregulin, TGF-α, EGF IGF-I, IGF-II
Ectodermal derivatives	TGF-α, EGF, PDGF IGF-II, IGF-I
Mesodermal derivatives	IGF-II, IGF-I TGF-α, EGF, FGF family, insulin, PDGF
Endodermal derivatives	IGF-II, IGF-I TGF-α, EGF, FGF
Hematopoietic tissues	HGF, EGF, PDGF Colony-stimulating factors
Specialized tissues	
Adipose tissue	Insulin
Skeletal tissue	PTHrP, IGF-I, IGF-II Calcitonin

*This listing will be expanded and more detailed as knockout and other information develops.

BNF, Brain-derived neurotropic factor; *EGF,* epidermal growth factor; *FGF,* fibroblast growth factor; *HGF,* hematopoietic growth factor; *IGF-II,* insulin-like growth factor; *NGF,* nerve growth factor; *NT3,* neurotropin 3; *PDGF,* platelet-derived growth factor; *PTHrP,* parathyroid hormone–related protein; *TGF-α,* transforming growth factor α.

Epidermal Growth Factor-Transforming Growth Factor System

The EGF/TGF-α system has been characterized in considerable detail.[192,193] EGF is a 6-kd peptide product of a large 1207–amino-acid precursor molecule and acts through a 170-kd membrane receptor glycoprotein. This receptor, like the IGF receptor, has intrinsic tyrosine kinase activity, and tyrosine kinase-mediated autophosphorylation is a critical event in EGF signal transduction. TGF-α, which has 35% amino acid homology with murine EGF and 44% homology with human EGF, also acts through the EGF receptor system.[192,193] Several additional family members have been characterized, including amphiregulin, heparin-binding EGF, betacellulin, and neuregulins.[193] Three additional receptors are referred to as ErbB2, ErbB3, and ErbB4 in animals; the human receptors are referred to as human EGF receptor (HER) 2, 3, and 4.[193]

EGF, pre-pro-EGF mRNA, and EGF receptors are present in most tissues in the postnatal rodent, but mRNA levels are highest in salivary glands and kidneys. EGF and pre-pro-EGF mRNA levels are absent or low in the fetal mouse and remain low in mouse tissues during the early neonatal period.[192] Nonetheless, the EGF receptor knockout mouse exhibits epithelial immaturity and multiorgan failure with early death.[194] Tissue concentrations of both EGF and EGF mRNA increase in the mouse during the first 2 months of postnatal life; indeed, levels of EGF in the salivary glands increase several thousand-fold between 3 weeks and 3 months of age. Mouse urinary levels increase 200-fold, and kidney concentrations increase 10-fold between

1 week and 2 months of age. EGF concentrations in mouse ocular tissues increase 100-fold during the first week of life.[192] Liver EGF concentrations increase more slowly, as do serum levels, and there is a high degree of correlation between serum and liver EGF levels in the developing mouse.[192] Thus, the production of EGF in the rodent is accelerated during the early neonatal period, and it is during this time that most hormone-stimulated growth and development occur.

Fetal mouse and human tissues have high levels of TGF-α.[192,195,196] Immunoreactive TGF-α concentrations in mice are measurable at relatively high levels in lung, brain, liver, and kidney tissues in the fetal neonatal/rat, and the ontogenic pattern of TGF-α is tissue specific; most late fetal tissues studied contained TGF-α, and levels persisted or increased in most tissues through the period of growth and development.[195] In rodents and sheep, EGF provokes precocious eyelid opening and tooth eruption in neonatal animals; stimulates lung maturation; promotes palatal development in organ culture; stimulates gastrointestinal maturation; evokes secretion of pituitary hormones including GH, PRL, and corticotropin; and stimulates secretion of chorionic gonadotropin and placental lactogen by the placenta.[192,194] Both EGF and TGF-α compete for binding to the EGF receptor, and both factors accelerate eye opening and tooth eruption in the neonatal rodent, presumably through interaction with the same EGF receptor.[192]

Considerable evidence suggests a role for the EGF family of growth factors in mammalian CNS development.[197] EGF, TGF-α, neuregulins, and the EGF receptors are widely distributed in the nervous system.[192,197-200] EGF promotes proliferation of astroglial cells, acts as an astroglial differentiation factor, and enhances survival and outgrowth of selected neuronal cells.[197,198] Transgenic mice with a deficiency of neuregulin, ErbB2, ErbB3, or ErbB4 die in utero with cardiac anomalies and developmental anomalies of the hindbrain, midbrain, and ventral forebrain[199,200] (see Table 21–5).

EGF also plays an important role in rodent pregnancy. Maternal salivary gland and plasma EGF concentrations in the mouse increase fourfold to fivefold during pregnancy.[201] Removal of the salivary glands prevents the increase in plasma EGF; moreover, salivary gland removal reduces the number of mice completing term pregnancy (by 50%), decreases the percentage of live pups, and decreases the crown-rump length of fetuses delivered.[201] Administration of EGF antiserum to pregnant mice without salivary glands further increases the abortion rate, whereas administration of EGF improves pregnancy outcome.[201] Because maternal EGF is too large a molecule to traverse the placental barrier, an effect on maternal metabolism and/or the placenta are likely.[201] The placenta is richly endowed with EGF receptors, and placental tissue binds and degrades EGF to constituent amino acids.[192] TGF-α also is produced by the maternal deciduus in rodents, and stimulates proliferation of decidual tissue and decidual prolactin production.

Nerve Growth Factor

NGF is a 13-kd protein that is present at high concentrations in mouse salivary gland and at low concentrations in many adult tissues.[193] It is also produced by human placental tissue. It is the original member of an expanding family of neurotropic growth factors that now include brain-derived neurotropic factor, neurotropin 3, and two less well characterized factors; these ligands act via two receptors, NGF and NGF2 (or Trk).[193,202] NGF binds to high-affinity plasma membrane receptors and is internalized and transported to subcellular organelles, including the nucleus, in neurons of the peripheral nervous system. It promotes neurite outgrowth and enhances tyrosine hydroxylase and dopamine β-hydroxylase activities in developing sympathetic neurons. NGF acts on undifferentiated sympathetic cell precursors to evoke both hyperplastic and hypertrophic effects and plays a permissive role in stimulating the development of immature autonomic neurons along either a sympathetic or a cholinergic pathway.[193,203]

The injection of NGF in neonatal mice causes a marked increase in the volume of the superior cervical ganglia and increases the nerve supply of body organs. Likewise, injection of NGF antiserum during early neonatal life results in a decrease in the size of the superior cervical ganglia, reduction in tyrosine hydroxylase activity, and permanent sympathectomy.[203] Maternal NGF autoantibodies in rats and rabbits impair autonomic nervous system development in utero.[204] This impairment affects sympathetic and dorsal root ganglia and autonomic innervation of peripheral organs. NGF is produced by neonatal mouse astroglial cells in tissue culture, is present in developing mouse brain tissue, and with brain-derived neurotropic factor and neurotropin 3 plays an important role in brain development.[201,202,205] Thyroid hormones and testosterone modulate postnatal NGF levels in the submandibular gland of the mouse. Thyroid hormones increase NGF, neurotropin 3, and brain-derived neurotropic factor mRNA levels in adult rat brain.[192,206]

Other Factors

Additional growth factors are involved in fetal growth and development, including hematopoietic growth factors, platelet-derived growth factors (PDGFs), fibroblast growth factors, vascular endothelial growth factor, and members of the TGF-β family.[40,193] Hematopoietic growth factors are also active in the fetus during development; erythropoietin in the fetal sheep is produced by the liver rather than the kidney and erythropoietin gene expression in fetal sheep is regulated by glucocorticoids.[207] A switch to kidney production occurs after parturition.[208] Postnatally, thyroid hormones, testosterone, and hypoxia modulate erythropoietin production. PDGF represents a family of homodimers and heterodimers of PDGF-A and PDGF-B chains derived from two gene loci.[209] Two PDGF receptors have been characterized, PDGFα and PDGFβ. The genes for PDGF and its receptors are expressed in many tissues. *PDGF-A* gene inactivation in mice leads to defects in lung, skin, intestine, testes, and brain resulting in early postnatal death.[209] *PDGF-B* gene inactivation leads to microvessel disruption and leakage with hemorrhage and edema and intrauterine death.

The fibroblast growth factor (FGF) family of heparin-binding growth factors now includes 17 members with diverse effects on development, angiogenesis, wound healing, and other biologic systems.[210-211] These effects are mediated by ligand-activated tyrosine protein kinase receptors (FGFRs) transcribed from four related genes. Several receptor isoforms are products of alternative RNA splicing.[40,193] Targeted disruptions of *FGF* and *FGFR* genes in mice have defined critical roles in development.[193,210] FGF3-deficient mice show tail and inner ear defects. Knockout of the *FGF4* gene is lethal, leading to early death. Knockout of the *FGFR1* gene also leads to early fetal death. *FGF10* knockout mice die at birth because of pulmonary agenesis. FGF4, FGF8, FGF9, FGF10, or FGF17 deficiency is associated with limb deformities. FGF8 deficiency leads to abnormal left-right axis patterning. In mice, *FGFR3* knockout results in chondrocyte hypertrophy and increased bone length.[193] In humans, a variety of gain-of-function FGFR mutations are associated with chondrodysplasias and craniosynostosis syndromes.[193] FGF, like EGF, stimulates the production of hCG from a choriocarcinoma cell line.[211] These observations and the fact that the placenta contains FGF, NGF, TGF-α, TGF-β, IGF-I, and IGF-II suggest that the placenta plays an important role in modulating fetal growth (see Table 21–5).

TRANSITION TO EXTRAUTERINE LIFE

The transition to extrauterine life involves abrupt delivery from the protected intrauterine environment and succor by the placenta to the relatively hostile extrauterine environment. The neonate must initiate air breathing and defend against hypothermia, hypoglycemia, and hypocalcemia as the placental supply of energy and nutritional substrate is removed. Both the adrenal cortex and the autonomic nervous system, including the paraaortic chromaffin system, are essential for extrauterine adaptation. Longer-term transition requires adaptation to an environment of intermittent nutrient supply and transient substrate deficiency and requires maturation of the secretory control mechanisms for the PTH-calcitonin system and the endocrine pancreas.

Cortisol Surge

In most mammals, a cortisol surge occurs near term and is mediated by increased cortisol production by the fetal adrenal and a decreased rate of conversion of cortisol to cortisone. Pepe and Albrecht have proposed that the preterm fetal cortisol surge is due to the progressive stimulation by estrogens of placental 11βHSD activity and the subsequent increase in placental conversion of cortisol to cortisone.[173] The resulting decrease in maternal-to-fetal cortisol transfer results in stimulation of fetal CRH and corticotropin secretion through the negative-feedback control loop. The concomitant estrogen-stimulated increase in 11βHSD activity in fetal tissues potentiates the relative fetal cortisol deficiency and the CRH-corticotropin response.[173] Placental CRH may also potentiate fetal adrenal activation.

The cortisol surge augments surfactant synthesis in lung tissue; increases lung liquid reabsorption; increases adrenomedullary phenylethanolamine *N*-methyltransferase activity, which in turn increases methylation of NE to epinephrine; increases hepatic iodothyronine outer-ring monodeiodinase activity and hence increases conversion of T_4 to T_3; decreases sensitivity of the ductus arteriosus to prostaglandins, which facilitates ductus closure; induces maturation of several enzymes and transport processes of the small intestine; and stimulates maturation of hepatic enzymes[62,212] (Fig. 21–12). In some cases, these events involve increased synthesis of specific proteins or enzymes. In other instances, such as the action on the ductus arteriosus, the mechanism remains obscure.

Secondary effects of cortisol also promote extrauterine adaptations. The increased T_3 levels stimulate β-adrenergic receptor binding, potentiate surfactant synthesis in lung tissue, and increase the sensitivity of brown adipose tissue to NE. The sig-

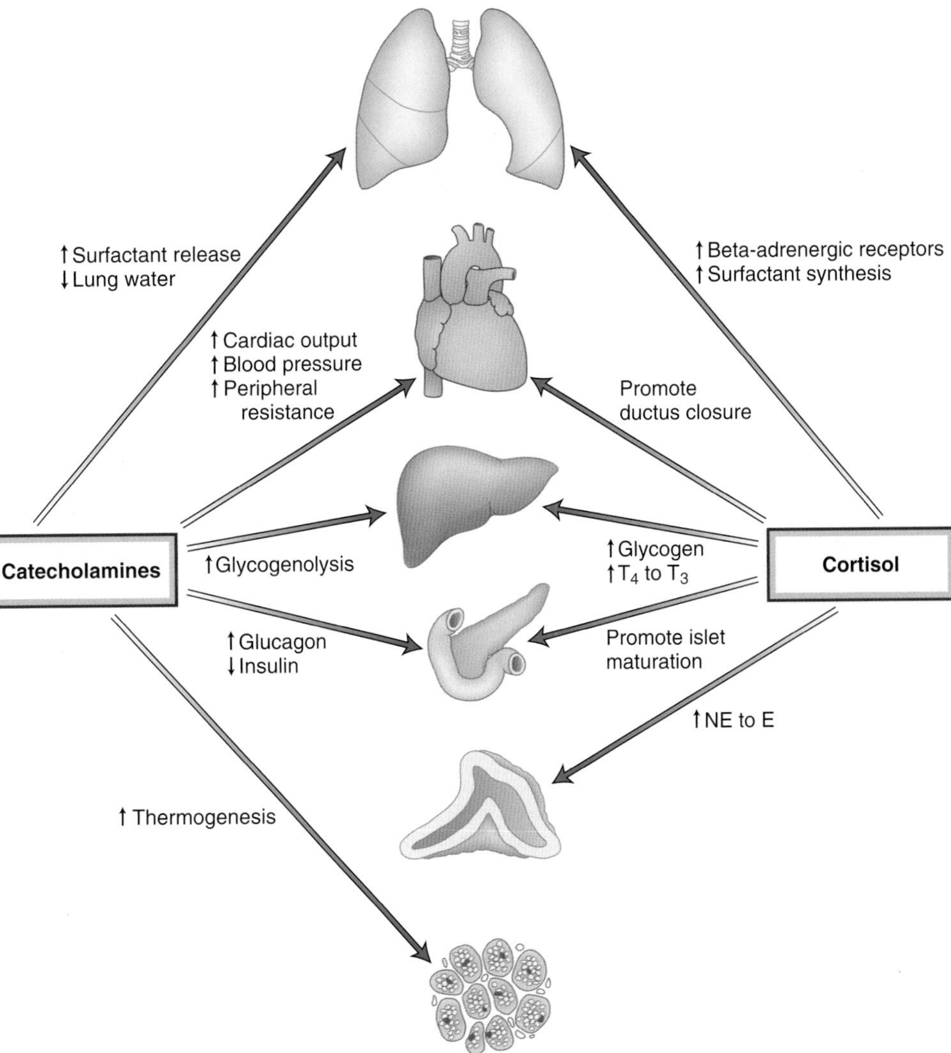

Figure 21–12 ■ Actions of cortisol and catecholamines during fetal adaptation to the extrauterine environment. The prenatal cortisol surge acts to promote functional maturation of several organ systems as indicated. The neonatal catecholamine surge triggers or potentiates a number of the extrauterine cardiopulmonary and metabolic functional adaptations that are critical to extrauterine survival. See text for details. *BAT*, Brown adipose tissue; *E*, epinephrine; *NE*, norepinephrine; *T_3*, triiodothyronine; *T_4*, thyroxine.

nificance of prenatal cortisol is demonstrated by the effects of gene-targeted CRH or glucocorticoid receptor deficiency in mice; the progeny of homozygous CRH-deficient or glucocorticoid receptor-deficient animals die in the first 12 hours with lung dysplasia and surfactant deficiency.[213,214]

Catecholamine Surge

Parturition also evokes a dramatic catecholamine surge in the newborn, resulting in extraordinarily high levels of NE, epinephrine, and dopamine in cord blood.[145] As indicated earlier, plasma NE concentrations exceed epinephrine levels because of peripheral and adrenomedullary and paraaortic catecholamine release. Cord blood NE levels of 15 nmol/L (2500 pg/mL) and epinephrine levels of 2 nmol/L (370 pg/mL) are common after spontaneous delivery of term infants.[145] Levels of 25 nmol/L (4200 pg/mL) of NE and 35 nmol/L (640 pg/mL) of epinephrine are common in cord blood of premature infants. These changes evoke critical cardiovascular adaptations, including increased blood pressure and increased cardiac inotropic effects; increased glucagon secretion; decreased insulin secretion; increased thermogenesis in brown adipose tissue and increased plasma free fatty acid levels; and pulmonary adaptation, including mobilization of pulmonary fluid and increased surfactant release.[145,149,212]

Thermogenesis in Neonatal Brown Adipose Tissue

Brown adipose tissue is the major site of thermogenesis in the newborn and is especially prominent in the mammalian fetus. The largest accumulations of brown adipose tissue envelop the kidneys and adrenal glands, and smaller amounts surround the blood vessels of the mediastinum and neck.[215] The mass of brown adipose tissue peaks at the time of birth and gradually decreases during the early weeks of life. Surgical removal of this tissue leads to neonatal hypothermia. NE, through β-adrenergic receptors, stimulates thermogenesis by brown adipose tissue, and optimal responsiveness of this tissue to NE is dependent on thyroid hormone.[215,216] Brown adipose tissue is rich in mitochondria containing a unique 32-kd protein (thermogenin) that uncouples oxidation and phosphorylation of adenosine diphosphate, reduces ATP production, and consequently enhances thermogenesis.[215,217] Thermogenin is T_3-dependent, and brown adipose tissue contains a 5′-monoiodothyronine deiodinase that deiodinates T4 locally to T3.[215,217] Full maturation of catecholamine-stimulated cellular respiration in brown adipose tissue occurs before delivery in the ovine fetus and requires thyroid hormone.[215,218] Fetal thyroidectomy in this species leads to marked hypothermia, with low plasma free fatty acid levels and increased plasma epinephrine concentrations.[218] In vitro, basal brown adipose tissue thermogenesis and NE-stimulated and dibutyryl cAMP-stimulated thermogenesis are decreased by fetal thyroidectomy.

The rapid onset of thermogenesis in brown adipose tissue is essential for survival in newborn infants. Catecholamine release is the stimulus for brown adipose tissue thermogenesis in the early neonatal period, and responsiveness to catecholamines is markedly increased by cutting of the umbilical cord.[216] Fetal hypoxia and placental inhibitors, including prostaglandin E_2 and adenosine, appear to inhibit brown adipose tissue thermogenesis in utero.[216] Cord cutting, neonatal cooling, catecholamine stimulation, and augmented conversion of T_4 to T_3 in brown adipose tissue in the neonatal period are the essential features that mediate and condition newborn thermogenesis.

Calcium Homeostasis

The neonate must adjust rapidly from a *high-calcium* environment regulated by PTHrP and calcitonin to a *low-calcium* environment that requires regulation by PTH and vitamin D. With removal of the placenta in term infants, plasma total calcium concentration falls and reaches a nadir of approximately 2.3 mmol/L (9 mg/dL),[161] and the ionized calcium concentration reaches a low level of about 1.2 mmol/L (4.8 mg/dL) by 24 hours of life.[219] Plasma PTH levels are relatively low in the neonatal period and are minimally responsive to hypocalcemia during the first 2 to 3 days of life. Calcitonin concentrations are high in cord blood (~2000 ng/L), increase further during the early neonatal period, and remain high for several days after birth.[161,220] The relatively obtunded PTH response and the high calcitonin levels lead to a 2- to 3-day period of transient neonatal hypocalcemia.[220,221] Inhibition of calcitonin secretion and stimulation of PTH secretion gradually result in increased serum calcium levels in the neonate. The disappearance of PTHrP in the neonatal lamb is approximately coincident with the time of restoration of calcium levels to the adult range.[161] The mechanism of transition from PTHrP to PTH secretion by the neonatal parathyroid glands is not clear.

Calcium homeostasis is also affected in the human newborn period by the low level of glomerular filtration that persists for several days.[220,221] In addition, renal responsiveness to PTH is reduced in the first few days of life. These factors limit phosphate excretion and predispose the neonate to hyperphosphatemia, particularly if the diet includes high-phosphate milk such as unmodified cow's milk. Premature infants, relative to term infants, tend to have lower PTH and higher calcitonin levels and more immature kidney function; in these infants, neonatal hypocalcemia may be more marked and prolonged and the incidence of symptomatic hypocalcemia is higher. Birth asphyxia also predisposes the neonate to hypocalcemia.[221] Infants born to mothers with hypercalcemia related to hyperparathyroidism have a high incidence of symptomatic hypocalcemia. These infants have a more marked suppression of parathyroid function and a longer period of transient hypoparathyroidism in the neonatal period. PTH secretion and calcium homeostasis usually return to normal in 1 to 2 weeks in full-term infants and within 2 to 3 weeks in the small premature infant.

Glucose Homeostasis

The abrupt withdrawal of the placental glucose supply leads to a prompt fall in plasma glucose in the term neonate.[170,171] The low glucose and high catecholamine levels stimulate glucagon secretion, and the plasma glucagon level peaks within 2 hours after birth.[170,171] Plasma insulin levels are low at birth and tend to fall further with hypoglycemia. The early glucagon response is short-lived; however, levels remain at about 100 ng/L for the first 12 to 24 hours, and the glucagon/insulin ratio is high enough to stabilize glucose levels in the range 2.8 to 4 mmol/L (50 to 70 mg/dL) during this period. The early glucagon and catecholamine surges deplete hepatic glycogen stores so that the return of plasma glucose levels to normal after 12 to 18 hours requires maturation of hepatic gluconeogenesis under the stimulus of a high plasma glucagon/insulin ratio.[171] Glucagon secretion gradually increases during the early hours after birth, especially with protein feeding, which stimulates gut glucagon release and pancreatic glucagon secretion.[170,171] Premature infants have more severe and prolonged hypoglycemia because of reduced glycogen stores and impaired hepatic gluconeogenesis. Infants born to diabetic mothers have more severe neonatal hypoglycemia because of relative hyperinsulinism. In the healthy term infant, glucose homeostasis is achieved within 5 to 7 days of life; in premature infants, 1 to 2 weeks may be required.

Other Hormonal Adaptations

Delivery of the placenta results in decreases in fetal blood levels of estrogens, progesterone, hCG, and HPL. The fall in estrogen levels presumably removes the major stimulus to fetal pituitary PRL release, and PRL levels decrease within several weeks. The relatively delayed fall may be due to lactotrope hyperplasia in the fetal pituitary or to delayed maturation of hypothalamic dopamine secretion. The gradual fall of GH levels during the early weeks of life is due to delayed maturation of hypothalamic-pituitary feedback control of GH release.[25] In the neonatal primate there are concomitant decreases in plasma GH levels and GH responsiveness to exogenous GHRH.[222] The mechanisms remain unclear; changes in secretion or in pituitary sensitivity to GHRH or somatostatin, or both, may be involved. IGF-I and IGF-II levels fall to infantile values within a few days, presumably because of the removal of placental HPL and placental IGF production (see Fig. 21–3).

In male infants (see Fig. 21–9), after a transient fall in testosterone levels as the hCG stimulus abates, pituitary LH secretion rebounds modestly and there is a secondary surge of plasma testosterone that persists at significant levels for several weeks.[25,223] This surge is mediated by hypothalamic GnRH; blockade of neonatal activation of the pituitary-testicular axis with a GnRH agonist in neonatal monkeys ablates the neonatal increments in LH and testosterone.[224] Such a blockade also results in subnormal increments in plasma LH and testosterone levels and subnormal testicular enlargement at puberty in these animals, suggesting that neonatal GnRH release with pituitary-testicular activation may be critical for normal sexual maturation of male primates.[224] In females, a transient, secondary surge in FSH may transiently elevate estrogen levels.

Delivery results in a reversal of the high fetal cortisone/cortisol ratio, and plasma cortisol concentrations are higher in the neonate despite relatively lower plasma corticotropin concentrations (see Fig. 21–5). Presumably, this increase is due to decreased inhibition of adrenal 3βHSD by estrogen and perhaps to removal of a placental CRH action on fetal pituitary corticotropin release. Plasma DHEAS and DHEA levels fall as the fetal adrenal atrophies.

The increase in serum thyrotropin levels during the early minutes after birth is due to cooling of the neonate in the extrauterine environment.[73,77] In term infants, the thyrotropin surge peaks at 30 minutes at a concentration of about 70 mU/L (see Fig. 21–7). This peak evokes increased secretion of T_4 and T_3 by the thyroid gland. In addition, increased conversion of T_4 to T_3 by liver and other tissues maintains the T_3 level in the extrauterine range of 1.6 to 3.4 nmol/L (105 to 220 ng/dL). The reequilibration of thyrotropin levels to the normal extrauterine range is probably due to the readjustment of prevailing serum T_3 levels and to maturation of feedback control of thyrotropin by thyroid hormones during the early weeks of life.[73,79] Production of rT_3 by fetal and neonatal tissues abates by 3 to 4 weeks of age, at which time serum rT_3 reaches adult levels.

PROGRAMMING OF DEVELOPING ENDOCRINE SYSTEMS

During the past several decades, the concept of fetal endocrine systems plasticity has evolved from experiments in several mammalian species indicating that hormonal programming occurs during a critical fetal or perinatal period of development. There is a growing list of examples. In the female rodent, transient neonatal androgen administration masculinizes the pattern of hypothalamic control of GnRH secretion and pituitary gonadotropin secretion, masculinizes adult behavior and adult sexual activity, permanently alters the pattern of GH secretion, increases longitudinal bone growth and body weight, and masculinizes the pattern of hepatic steroid metabolism.[225,226] Prenatal androgens program the timing of neuroendocrine puberty in sheep; the higher the dose of prenatal testosterone, the earlier the initiation of the pubertal LH rise.[227] Estrogen administration to pregnant rats during the last third of gestation produces cryptorchid male offspring and may permanently suppress spermatogenesis in adult males.[228] Transient levothyroxine administration to neonatal rodents leads to growth retardation, delayed puberty, decreased adult pituitary weight, decreased pituitary TRH concentrations, low serum thyrotropin levels, and decreased thyrotropin responsiveness to propylthiouracil challenge.[229,230] Administration of insulin or alloxan to neonatal rats produces permanent alteration of glucose tolerance.[231] A single dose of vasopressin to the neonatal rat permanently enhances the adult response to vasopressin.[232] Fetal exposure to high maternal glucocorticoid levels in the rat inhibits fetal growth and leads to subsequent hypertension in the offspring.[233] Moreover it has been observed that the permanent programming can be transmitted to later generations, leading to the concept of epigenetic effects.[231,234]

The concept of fetal programming has been extended more recently with the observation of ecologic associations of fetal and early life health indicators (e.g., birth size, infant mortality) and adult diseases. The concept, advanced in the 1980s, that adult diseases have fetal and perinatal genesis has been referred to as the *Barker hypothesis*.[235] There is now extensive documentation of the association of intrauterine growth retardation (IUGR, low birth weight for gestational age) with an increased risk of later hypertension, insulin resistance, diabetes, and cardiovascular and coronary heart disease.[236-243] The programming involves epigenetic, neuroendocrine, hormonal receptor, and metabolic alterations involving the placenta and fetus.[244-252]

Epigenetic effects include genetic imprinting. Imprinted genes are a class of genes in placental mammals and marsupials whose expression depends on the placental origin.[244-250] Imprinting is controlled epigenetically (by such factors as nutrition) via DNA methylation and chromatin modifications. In mice, imprinted genes in the placenta regulate the supply of nutrients; in the fetus, they control nutrient metabolism.[244] In mice, approximately 60 imprinted genes have been identified, and for most the imprinting status is conserved in humans; many of these are involved in the control of fetal growth.[250] Paternally expressed imprinted genes tend to enhance while the maternally expressed genes suppress fetal growth. Knockout of paternally expressed genes for IGF-II, PEG1, PEG2, and insulin result in IUGR, whereas knockout of the maternal genes *H19, IGF-IIr,* or overexpression of *IGF-II* result in fetal overgrowth.[244] Other genetic alterations including modification of tandem repeats in the insulin gene have been described.[245]

Hormones in the fetus are derived from the placenta, from the mother, from fetal endocrine glands, and from circulating precursor in fetal or placental tissues (Fig. 21–13). These extensive networks linking maternal-placental-fetal endocrine interactions, and the apparent plasticity of developing endocrine and metabolic systems, facilitates endocrine system programming. As indicated, the programming may be relatively system limited.[225-233] Other examples include the observation many years ago that diethylstilbestrol administration to pregnant women increased the prevalence of vaginal adenocarcinoma in

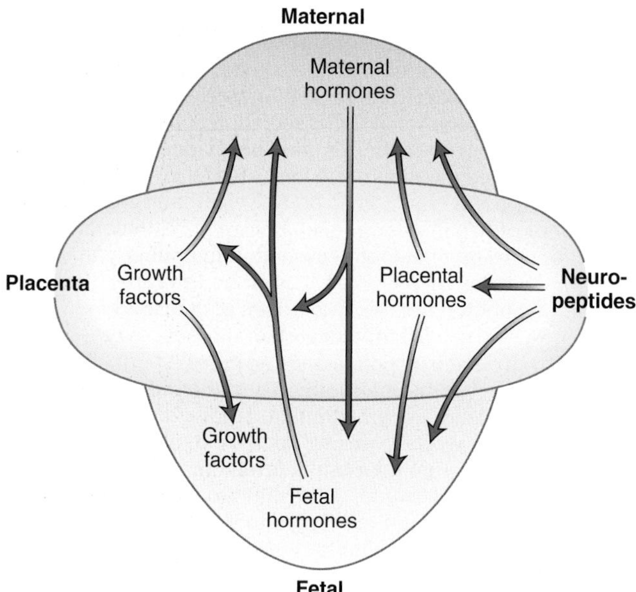

Figure 21–13 ▪ The extensive networks linking maternal-placental-fetal endocrine interactions facilitating fetal endocrine programming during the critical periods of fetal development. Developing endocrine system's plasticity extends into the perinatal period. The extent of placental growth factor transfer to the maternal and fetal compartments remains unclear. See text for details.

female offspring during the second and third decades of life.[241] More recently it was shown that prenatal or neonatal diethylstilbestrol exposure in hamsters and mice perturbs normal uterine development by affecting the genetic pathways programming uterine differentiation and resulting in hyperplastic and neoplastic uterine lesions with increased levels of cJun, cFos, Myc, Bax, and Bcl-x.[253,254] Excessive androgen exposure during fetal life has been associated with later polycystic ovarian syndrome (PCOS).[241] Hormonal programming also is demonstrable in cell lines and in unicellular organisms, in which a single exposure to a hormone can produce persistent alteration of the hormonal response characteristics or prohormone processing.[255,256] Undernutrition during pregnancy in the rat results in the offspring developing obesity, hyperinsulinemia, and hyperleptinemia during adult life; this phenotype is potentiated when the offspring are fed a high-fat diet.[257] Neonatal leptin treatment normalized the programmed phenotype indicating that metabolic programming may be reversible during the period of developmental plasticity.[257]

The effects of maternal undernutrition and fetal IUGR extend to several systems, and it is hypothesized that excessive maternal-fetal glucocorticoids play a significant programming role. Glucocorticoids have wide ranging effects in the fetus, altering receptors, enzymes, ion channels, and transporters in a variety of cells and tissues in the late gestation fetus and can induce programming of other endocrine systems. Throughout gestation, they modify *GLUT* gene expression in placenta and fetus, influence IGF and glucocorticoid receptor gene expression in various tissues, affect expression of several transcription factors, and affect a wide variety of enzymes in placenta, liver, kidney, intestine, and lung.[247] Maternal undernutrition, stress, and placental dysfunction are associated with increased maternal and fetal glucocorticoid levels, which contribute importantly to IUGR and programmed alterations in adult endocrine systems and metabolism.[239,247,248]

MATERNAL AND FETAL MEDICINE

The foregoing review summarizes current understanding of the intrauterine endocrine milieu and highlights progress in this challenging frontier of medicine. This progress has set the stage for fetal endocrine disease diagnosis, therapy of fetal endocrine and metabolic disorders, management of disorders of fetal growth, and diagnosis and management of perinatal or neonatal endocrine dysfunction. In addition, understanding of developmental endocrinology is increasingly relevant to management strategies for premature infants and infants and children with fetal growth retardation and for our understanding of the pathogenesis of adult endocrine and metabolic diseases.

We are now entering the era of direct access to and management of the intrauterine environment with provision of medical and surgical fetal therapy, entailing both potential advantages and risks.[258] With expansion of the application and scope of amniotic fluid fetal cell sampling, maternal plasma DNA analysis, and the advent of fetal visualization and intrauterine fetal blood sampling, direct access for fetal diagnosis is now possible.[259-262] Intrauterine diagnosis and treatment of fetal adrenal and thyroid disorders have become the standard of care.[263,264] Intravenous nutritional supplementation of fetal sheep can prevent some forms of growth retardation, and chronic fetal therapy through indwelling pumps is feasible in animal fetuses.[265] These approaches, coupled with increasing availability of synthetic hormones and growth factor agonists and antagonists, facilitate direct fetal endocrine therapy. In addition, intrauterine stem cell transplantation has been successful in the correction of congenital hematologic disease. The fetus in early gestation is a favorable recipient of cellular therapy, and fetal cell transplantation may be applicable to therapy for selected endocrine and metabolic disease.[266,267] Finally, there is a growing experience with fetal and neonatal gene therapy in animals.[268]

REFERENCES

1. Fisher DA. Fetal and neonatal endocrinology. In DeGroot LJ, Jameson JL, eds. Endocrinology, 5th ed. Philadelphia: Elsevier Saunders 2006, pp 3369-3386.
2. Palfi M, Selbing A. Placental transport of maternal immunoglobulin G. Am J Reprod Immunol 1998;39:24-26.
3. Sodha RJ, Proegler M, Schneider H. Transfer and metabolism of norepinephrine studied from maternal to fetal and fetal to maternal sides in the in vitro perfused human placental life. Am J Obstet Gynecol 1984;148:474-481.
4. Benediktsson R, Calder A, Edwards CRW, et al. Placental 11β-hydroxysteroid dehydrogenase: a key regulator of fetal glucocorticoid exposure. Clin Endocrinol (Oxf) 1997;46:161-166.
5. Murphy BEP. Cortisol and cortisone in human fetal development. J Steroid Biochem 1979;11:509-513.
6. Takeyama J, Sasano H, Suzuki T, et al. 17β-Hydroxysteroid dehydrogenase types 1 and 2 in human placenta: an immunohistochemical study with correlation to placental development. J Clin Endocrinol Metab 1998;83:3710-3715.
7. Krysin E, Brzezinska-Slebodzinska E, Slebodzinski AB. Divergent deiodination of thyroid hormones in the separated parts of the fetal and maternal placenta in pigs. J Endocrinol 1997;155: 295-303.
8. Roti E, Gnudi A, Braverman LE. The placental transport, synthesis and metabolism of hormones and drugs which affect thyroid function. Endocr Rev 1983;4:131-149.
9. Iisalo E, Castren O. The enzymatic inactivation of noradrenaline in human placental tissue. Ann Med Exp Biol Fenn 1967;45: 253-257.
10. Mesiano S, Jaffe RB. Neuroendocrine-metabolic regulation of pregnancy. In Strauss JF III, Barbieri RL, eds. Reproductive Endocrinology, 5th ed. Philadelphia: WB Saunders, 2004:327-366.

11. Goldsmith PC, McGregor WG, Raymoure WJ, et al. Cellular localization of chorionic gonadotropin in human fetal liver and kidney. J Clin Endocrinol Metab 1983;57:654-661.
12. Kapcala LP. Immunoassayable adrenocorticotropin in peripheral organs: concentrations during early development. Life Sci 1985; 37:2283-2290.
13. Martino E, Lernmark A, Seo H, et al. High concentration of thyrotropin releasing hormone in pancreatic islets. Proc Natl Acad Sci U S A 1978;75:4265-4267.
14. Pekary AE, Meyer NV, Vaillant C, et al. Thyrotropin releasing hormone and a homologous peptide in the male rat reproductive system. Biochem Biophys Res Commun 1980;95:993-1000.
15. Suda T, Tomori N, Tozawa F, et al. Distribution and characterization of immunoreactive corticotropin-releasing factor in human tissues. J Clin Endocrinol Metab 1984;59:861-866.
16. Thompson RC, Seasholtz AF, Herbert E. Rat corticotropin releasing hormone gene: sequence and tissue specific expression. Mol Endocrinol 1987;1:363-370.
17. Shibaski T, Kiyosawa Y, Masuda A, et al. Distribution of growth hormone releasing hormone-like immunoreactivity in human tissue extracts. J Clin Endocrinol Metab 1984;59:263-268.
18. Wu P, Jackson IMD. Identification, characterization and localization of thyrotropin releasing hormone precursor peptides in perinatal rat pancreas. Regul Pept 1988;22:347-360.
19. Koshimizu T. The development of pancreatic and gastrointestinal somatostatin-like immunoreactivity and its relationship to feeding in neonatal rats. Endocrinology 1983;112:911-916.
20. Polk DH, Reviczky AL, Lam RW, et al. Thyrotropin releasing hormone in the ovine fetus: ontogeny and effect of thyroid hormone. Am J Physiol 1991;23:E53-E58.
21. Rahier J, Wallon J, Henquin JC. Abundance of somatostatin cells in the human neonatal pancreas. Diabetologia 1980;18:251-254.
22. Leduque P, Aratan-Spire S, Czernichow P, et al. Ontogenesis of thyrotropin-releasing hormone in the human fetal pancreas. J Clin Invest 1986;78:1028-1034.
23. Saito H, Saito S, Sano T, et al. Fetal and maternal plasma levels of immunoreactive somatostatin at delivery: evidence for its increase in the umbilical artery and its arteriovenous gradient in the fetoplacental circulation. J Clin Endocrinol Metab 1983;56:567-571.
24. Koshimizu T, Ohyama Y, Yokota Y, et al. Peripheral plasma concentrations of somatostatin-like immunoreactivity in newborns and infants. J Clin Endocrinol Metab 1985;61:78-82.
25. Grumbach MM, Gluckman PD. The human fetal hypothalamus and pituitary gland: the maturation of neuroendocrine mechanisms controlling secretion of fetal pituitary growth hormone, prolactin, gonadotropins, adrenocorticotropin-related peptides, and thyrotropin. In Tulchinsky D, Little AB, eds. Maternal Fetal Endocrinology, 2nd ed. Philadelphia: WB Saunders, 1994:193-261.
26. Roessler E, Belloni E, Gaudenz K, et al. Mutations in the human Sonic Hedgehog gene cause holoprosencephaly. Nat Genet 1996;14:357-360.
27. Brown SA, Warburton D, Brown LY, et al. Holoprosencephaly due to mutation in ZIC1, a homologue of *Drosophila* odd-paired. Nat Genet 1998;20:180-183.
28. Dattani MT, Martinez-Barbera JP, Thomas PQ, et al. *HESX1* a novel homeobox gene implicated in septo-optic dysplasia (Abstract 06). Horm Res 1998;8(suppl 3).
29. Parks JS, Brown MR. Consequences of mutations in pituitary transcription factor genes. In Pescovitz OH, Eugster EA, eds. Pediatric Endocrinology. Philadelphia: Lippincott Williams and Wilkins, 2004:80-89.
30. Tran PV, Savage JJ, Ingraham HA, et al. Molecular genetics of hypothalamic-pituitary development. In Pescovitz OH, Eugster EA, eds. Pediatric Endocrinology. Philadelphia: Lippincott Williams and Wilkins, 2004:63-79.
31. Millis PE. Transcription factors in pituitary gland development and their clinical impact on phenotype. Horm Res 2000;54:107-119.
32. Goshu E, Jin H, Lovejoy J, et al. SIM2 contributes to neuroendocrine hormone gene expression in the anterior pituitary. Molec Endocrinol 2004;18:1251-1262.
33. Cohen LE, Radovik S. Molecular basis of combined pituitary hormone deficiencies. Endocrine Rev 2002;23:431-442.
34. Charles MA, Suh H, Hjalt TA, et al. PITX genes are required for cell survival and Lhx3 activation. Mol Endocrinol 2005;19:1893-1903.
35. Vallette-Kasic S, Brue T, Pulichino AM, et al. Congenital isolated adrenocorticotropin deficiency: an underestimated cause of neonatal death, explained by TPIT gene mutations. J Clin Endocrinol Metab 2005;90:1323-1331.
36. Wu W, Cogan JD, Pfaffle RM, et al. Mutations in PROP-1 cause familial combined pituitary hormone deficiency. Nat Genet 1998;18:147-149.
37. Mulchahey JJ, DiBlasio AM, Martin MC, et al. Hormone production and peptide regulation of the human fetal pituitary gland. Endocr Rev 1987;8:406-425.
38. Suganuma N, Seo H, Yamamoto N, et al. The ontogeny of growth hormone in the human fetal pituitary. Am J Obstet Gynecol 1989;160:729-733.
39. Goodyear CG, Sellen JM, Fuks M, et al. Regulation of growth hormone secretion from human fetal pituitaries, interactions between growth hormone releasing factor and somatostatin. Reprod Nutr Dev 1987;27:461-470.
40. DeLeon DD, Cohen P, Katz LEL. Growth factor regulation of fetal growth. In Polin RA, Fox WW, Abman SH, eds. Fetal and Neonatal Physiology, 3rd ed. Philadelphia: WB Saunders, 2004:1880-1890.
41. Kind KL, Owens JA, Robinson JS, et al. Effect of restriction of placental growth on expression of IGFs in fetal sheep: relationship to fetal growth, circulating IGFs and binding proteins. J Endocrinol 1995;146:23-34.
42. Gluckman PD, Pinal CS. Growth hormone and prolactin. In Polin RA, Fox WW, Abman SH, eds. Fetal and Neonatal Physiology, 3rd ed. Philadelphia: WB Saunders, 2004:1891-1895.
43. Clement-Lacroix P, Ormandy C, Lepescheux L, et al. Osteoblasts are a new target for prolactin analysis of bone formation in prolactin receptor knockout mice. Endocrinology 1999;140: 3404-3410.
44. Winter JSD. Fetal and neonatal adrenocortical physiology. In Polin RA, Fox WW, Abman SH, eds. Fetal and Neonatal Physiology. Philadelphia: WB Saunders, 2004:1915-1925.
45. Geller DH, Miller WL. Molecular development of the adrenal gland. In Pescovitz OH, Eugster EA, eds. Pediatric Endocrinology. Philadelphia, Lippincott Williams and Wilkins, 2004:548-567.
46. Ikeda Y, Swain A, Weber TH, et al. Steroidogenic factor 1 and DAX-1 localize in multiple cell lineages: potential links in endocrine development. Mol Endocrinol 1996;10:1261-1272.
47. Hammer GD, Parker KL, Schimmer BP. Minireview: transcriptional regulation of adrenocortical development. Endocrinology 2005; 146:1018-1024.
48. Fujieda K, Tajima T. Molecular basis of adrenal insufficiency. Pediatric Res 2005;57:62R-69R.
49. Miller WL. Steroid hormone biosynthesis and actions in the materno-feto-placental unit. Clin Perinatal 1998;25:799-817.
50. Leavitt MG, Albrecht EO, Pepe GJ. Development of the baboon fetal adrenal gland: regulation of the ontogenesis of the definitive and transitional zones by adrenocorticotropin. J Clin Endocrinol Metab 1999;84:3831-3835.
51. Dotzler DA, Digeronimo JJ, Yoder BA, et al. Distribution of corticotrophin releasing hormone in the fetus, newborn, juvenile and adult baboon. Pediatr Res 2004;55:120-125.
52. Cole TJ, Blendy JA, Monaghan AD, et al. Targeted disruption of the glucocorticoid receptor gene blocks adrenergic chromaffin development and severely retards lung maturation. Genes Dev 1995; 9:1608-1625.
53. Thompson M, Smith R. The action of hypothalamic and placental corticotrophin releasing factor on the corticotrope. Mol Cell Endocrinol 1989;62:1-12.
54. Goland RS, Wardlow SL, Blum M, et al. Biologically active corticotropin-releasing hormone in maternal and fetal plasma during pregnancy. Am J Obstet Gynecol 1988;159:884-890.
55. Rivier C, Vale W. Neuroendocrine interactions between corticotrophin releasing factor and vasopressin on adrenocorticotropic hormone secretion in the rat. In Schrier WW, ed. Vasopressin. New York: Raven, 1985:181-188.
56. Albrecht ED, Aberdeen GW, Pepe GJ. Estrogen elicits cortical zone specific effects on development of the primate fetal adrenal gland. Endocrinology 2005;146:1737-1744.
57. Rose JC, Turner CS, Ray DeW, et al. Evidence that cortisol inhibits basal adrenocorticotropin secretion in the sheep fetus by 0.70 gestation. Endocrinology 1988;123:1307-1313.

58. Yang K, Jones SA, Challis JRG. Changes in glucocorticoid receptor number in the hypothalamus of the sheep fetus with gestational age and after adrenocorticotropin treatment. Endocrinology 1990;126:11-17.
59. McKenna NT, Moore DD. Nuclear receptors: structure, function and cofactors. In DeGroot LJ, tameson JL, eds. Endocrinology 5th ed. Philadelphia: Elsevier Saunders, 2006:277-287.
60. Pavlik A, Buresova M. The neonatal cerebellum: the highest level of glucocorticoid receptors in the brain. Dev Brain Res 1984; 12:13-20.
61. Johnson JW, Mitzner W, Beck JC, et al. Long term effects of betamethasone in fetal development. Am J Obstet Gynecol 1981;141: 1053-1064.
62. Liggins GC. The role of cortisol in preparing the fetus for birth. Reprod Fertil Dev 1994;6:141-150.
63. Beitins IZ, Graham GG, Kowarski A, et al. Adrenal function in normal infants and in marasmus and kwashiorkor: plasma aldosterone concentration and aldosterone secretion rate. J Pediatr 1974;84:444-451.
64. Katz FH, Beck P, Makowski EL. The renin-aldosterone system in mother and fetus at term. Am J Obstet Gynecol 1974;118:51-55.
65. Siegel SR, Fisher DA. Ontogeny of the renin-angiotensin-aldosterone system in the fetal and newborn lamb. Pediatr Res 1980;14:99-102.
66. Lumbers ER. Functions of the renin-angiotensin system during development. Clin Exp Pharmacol Physiol 1995;22:499-505.
67. Berger S, Bleich M, Schmid N, et al. Mineralocorticoid receptor knockout mice: pathophysiology of Na+ metabolism. Proc Natl Acad Sci U S A 1998;95:9424-9429.
68. Hirasawa G, Sasano H, Suzuki T, et al. 11β-Hydroxysteroid dehydrogenase type 2 and mineralocorticoid receptor in human fetal development. J Clin Endocrinol Metab 1999;84:1453-1458.
69. Robillard JE, Page WV, Matthews MS, et al. Differential gene expression and regulation of renal angiotensin II receptor subtypes (AT1 and AT2) during fetal life in sheep. Pediatr Res 1995;38:896-904.
70. Chen K, Carey LC, Liu J, et al. The effect of hypothalamo-pituitary disconnection on the renin-angiotensin system in the late gestation sheep. Am J Physiol Regul Integr Comp Physiol 2005;288: R1279-R1287.
71. Walther T, Schultheiss HP, Tschope C, et al. Natriuretic peptide system in fetal heart and circulation. J Hypertens 2002;20: 785-791.
72. Santisteban P. Development and anatomy of the hypothalamic-pituitary axis. In Braverman LE, Utiger RD, eds. The Thyroid, 9th ed. Philadelphia: JB Lippincott, 2005:8-25.
73. Brown RS, Huang SA, Fisher DA. The maturation of thyroid function in the perinatal period and during childhood. In Braverman LE, Utiger RD, eds. The Thyroid, 9th ed. Philadelphia: JB Lippincott, 2005:1013-1028.
74. Parlato R, Rosica A, Rodriguez-Mallon A, et al. An integrated regulatory network controlling survival and migration in thyroid organogenesis. Dev Biol 2004;276:464-475.
75. Trueba SS, Auge J, Mattei G, et al. PAX8, TITF1 and FOXE1 gene expression patterns during human development: new insights into human thyroid development and thyroid dysgenesis-associated malformations. J Clin Endocrinol Metab 2005;90:455-462.
76. Chisaka O, Capecchi MR. Regionally restricted developmental defects resulting from targeted disruption of the mouse homeobox gene hox-1.5. Nature 1991;350:473-479.
77. Burrow GN, Fisher DA, Larsen PR. Maternal and fetal thyroid function. N Engl J Med 1994;331:1072-1078.
78. Roti E. Regulation of thyroid stimulating hormone (TSH) secretion in the fetus and neonate. J Endocrinol Invest 1988;11:145-158.
79. Fisher DA, Nelson JC, Carlton EI, et al. Maturation of human hypothalamic-pituitary-thyroid function and control. Thyroid 2000;10: 229-234.
80. Murphy N, Home R, vanToor, et al. The hypothalamic-pituitary-thyroid axis in preterm infants: changes in the first 24 hours of postnatal life. J Clin Endocrinol Metab 2004;89:2824-2831.
81. Williams FLR, Simpson J, Delahunty C, et al. Developmental trends in cord and postpartum serum thyroid hormones in preterm infants. J Clin Endocr Metab 2004;89:5314-5320.
82. Eng PHK, Cardona GR, Fang SL, et al. Escape from the acute Wolff-Chaikoff effect is associated with a decrease in thyroid sodium/iodide symporter messenger ribonucleic acid and protein. Endocrinology 1999;140:3404-3410.
83. Sherwin JR. Development of regulatory mechanisms in the thyroid: failure of iodide to suppress iodide transport activity. Proc Soc Exp Biol Med 1982;169:458-462.
84. St. Germain DL, Hernandez A, Schneider MJ, et al. Insights into the role of deiodinases from studies of genetically modified animals. Thyroid 2005;15:905-916.
85. Hume R, Simpson J, Delahunty C, et al. Human fetal and cord serum thyroid hormones: developmental trends and interrelationships. J Clin Endocrinol Metab 2004;89:4097-4103.
86. Polk DH, Reviczky A, Wu SY, et al. Metabolism of sulfoconjugated thyroid hormone derivatives in developing sheep. Am J Physiol 1994;266:E892-E896.
87. Kerry R, Hume R, Kaptein E, et al. Sulfation of thyroid hormone and dopamine during human development: ontogeny of phenol sulfotransferases and arylsulfatase in liver, lung, and brain. J Clin Endocrinol Metab 2001;86:2734-2742.
88. Richard K, Hume R, Kaptein E, et al. Ontogeny of iodothyronine deiodinases in human liver. J Clin Endocrinol Metab 1998;83: 2868-2874.
89. Polk DH, Wu WY, Wright C, et al. Ontogeny of thyroid hormone effect on tissue 5′-monodeiodinase activity in fetal sheep. Am J Physiol 1988;254:E337-E341.
90. Jansen J, Friesema ECH, Milici C, et al. Thyroid hormone transporters in health and disease. Thyroid 2005;15:757-768.
91. Heuer H, Maier ML, Iden S, et al. The monocarboxylate transporter 8 linked to human psychomotor retardation is highly expressed in thyroid hormone-sensitive neuron populations. Endocrinology 2005;146:1701-1706.
92. Dumitrescu AM, Liao XH, Best TB, et al. A novel syndrome combining thyroid and neurological abnormalities is associated with mutations in a monocarboxylate transporter gene. Am J Hum Genet 2004;74:168-175.
93. Bergh JJ, Lin HY, Lansing L, et al. Integrin αVβ3 contains a cell surface receptor site for thyroid hormone that is linked to activation of mitogen-activated protein kinase and induction of angiogenesis. Endocrinology 2005;146:2864-2871.
94. Yen P. Genomic and nongenomic actions of thyroid hormones. In Braverman LE, Utiger RD, eds. The Thyroid, 9th ed. Philadelphia: Lippincott Williams and Wilkins, 2005:135-150.
95. Flamant F, Samarut J: Thyroid hormone receptors: lessons from knockout and knockin mutant mice. Trends Endocrinol Metab 2005;14:85-90.
96. Morreale de Escobar G, Obregon MJ, Escobar del Rey F. Role of thyroid hormone during early brain development. Eur J Endocrinol 2004;151:U25-U37.
97. Kilby MD, Giltoes N, McCabe C, et al. Expression of thyroid receptor isoforms in the human fetal central nervous system and the effects of intrauterine growth retardation. Clin Endocrinol (Oxf) 2000;53:469-477.
98. Iskaros J, Pickard M, Evans I, et al. Thyroid hormone receptor gene expression in first trimester human fetal brain. J Clin Endocrinol Metab 2000;85:2620-2623.
99. Rajatapiti P, Kester MHA, de Krijger RR, et al. Expression of glucocorticoid, retinoid, and thyroid hormone receptors during human lung development. J Clin Endocrinol Metab 2005;90: 4309-4314.
100. Contempre B, Jauniaux E, Calvo R, et al. Detection of thyroid hormones in human embryonic cavities during the first trimester of pregnancy. J Clin Endocrinol Metab 1993;77:1719-1722.
101. Vulsma T, Gons MH, de Vijlder JJ. Maternal-fetal transfer of thyroxine in congenital hypothyroidism due to a total organification defect or thyroid agenesis. N Engl J Med 1989;321:13-16.
102. Morreale De Escobar G, Calvo R, Obregon MJ, et al. Contribution of maternal thyroxine to fetal thyroxine pools in normal rats near term. Endocrinology 1990;126:2765-2767.
103. Sadow PM, Chassande O, Koo EK, et al. Regulation of expression of thyroid hormone receptor isoforms and coactivators in liver and heart by thyroid hormone. Mol Cell Endocrinol 2003;203:65-75.
104. Quignodon L, Legrand C, Allioli N, et al. Thyroid hormone signaling is highly heterogeneous during pre- and postnatal brain development. J Molec Endocrinol 2004;33:467-476.
105. Plateroti M, Gauthier K, Domon-Dell C, et al. Functional interference between thyroid hormone receptor α (TRα) and natural

truncated TRΔα isoforms in the control of intestinal development. Mol Cell Biol 2001;21:4761-4772.
106. Mai W, Janier MF, Allioli N, et al. Thyroid hormone receptor α is a molecular switch of cardiac function between fetal and postnatal life. Proc Natl Acad Sci U S A 2004;101:10332-10337.
107. Harvey CB, O'Shea PJ, Scott AJ, et al. Molecular mechanisms of thyroid hormone effects on bone growth and function. Mol Gen Metab 2002;75:17-30.
108. Marrit H, Schifman A, Stepanyan Z, et al. Temperature homeostasis in transgenic mice lacking thyroid receptor α gene products. Endocrinology 2004;146:2872-2884.
109. Angelin-Duclos C, Domenget C, Kolbus A, et al. Thyroid hormone T3 acting through the thyroid hormone α receptor is necessary for implementation of erythropoiesis in the neonatal spleen environment in the mouse. Development 2005;132:325-934.
110. Erickson RP, Blecher SR. Genetics of sex determination and differentiation. In Polin RA, Fox WW, Abman SH, eds. Fetal and Neonatal Physiology, 3rd ed. Philadelphia: WB Saunders, 2004: 1935-1941.
111. Lee MM. Molecular genetic control of sex differentiation. In Pescovitz OH, Eugster EA, eds. Pediatric Endocrinology. Philadelphia, Lippincott Williams and Wilkins, 2004:231-242.
112. Harley VR, Clarkson MJ, Argentaro A. The molecular action and regulation of the testis-determining factors, SRY (sex determining region of the Y chromosome) and SOX9 [SRY-related high-mobility group (HMG) Box 9]. Endocr Rev 2003;24:466-487.
113. Park SY, Jameson JL. Minireview: transcriptional regulation of gonadal development and differentiation. Endocrinology 2005; 146:1035-1042.
114. Zang FP, Poutanen M, Wilbertz J, et al. Normal prenatal but arrested postnatal sexual development of luteinizing hormone receptor knockout (LURKO) mice. Mol Endocrinol 2001;15: 172-183.
115. Aslan AR, Kogan BA, Gondos B. Testicular development. In Polin RA, Fox WW, Abmans SH, eds. Fetal and Neonatal Physiology, 3rd ed. Philadelphia: WB Saunders, 2004:1950-1955.
116. Byskov AG, Westergaard LG. Differentiation of the ovary. In Polin RA, Fox WW, Abman SH, eds. Fetal and Neonatal Physiology, 3rd ed. Philadelphila: WB Saunders, 2004:1941-1949.
117. Fulton N, da Silva SJM, Bayne RAL, et al.. Germ cell proliferation and apoptosis in the developing human ovary. J Clin Endocrinol Metab 2005;90:4664-4670.
118. Sajjad Y, Quenby S, Nickson P, et al. Immunohistochemical localization of androgen receptors in the urogenital tracts of human embryos. Reproduction 2004;128:331-339.
119. Josso N, Belville C, Dicard JY. Mutations in AMH and its receptors. Endocrinology 2003;13:247-251.
120. Roviller Fabre V, Carmona S, Abou Merhi A, et al. Effect of antimüllerian hormone on Sertoli and Leydig cell functions in fetal and immature rats. Endocrinology 1998;139:1213-1220.
121. Brandenberger AW, Tee MK, Lee JY, et al. Tissue distribution of estrogen receptors alpha (ERα) and beta (ERβ) mRNA in the midgestation human fetus. J Clin Endocrinol Metab 1997;82: 3509-3512.
122. Couse JF, Korach KS. Estrogen receptor null mice: what have we learned and where will they lead us? Endocrine Rev 1999;20: 358-417.
123. Falgueras AG, Pinos H, Collado P, et al. The role of the androgen receptor in CNS masculinization. Brain Res 2005;1035:13-23.
124. Naftolin F, Brawer JB. The effect of estrogens on hypothalamic structure and function. Am J Obstet Gynecol 1978;132:758-765.
125. Sholl SA, Goy RW, Kim KL. 5α-reductase, aromatase, and androgen receptor levels in the monkey brain during fetal development. Endocrinology 1989;124:627-634.
126. Visser M, Swaab DF. Life span changes in the presence of alpha-melanocyte-stimulating-hormone-containing cells in the human pituitary. J Dev Physiol 1979;1:161-178.
127. Perry RA, Mulvogue HM, McMillen IC, et al. Immunohistochemical localization of ACTH in the adult and fetal sheep pituitary. J Dev Physiol 1985;7:397-404.
128. Silman RE, Holland T, Chard T, et al. The ACTH family tree of the rhesus monkey changes with development. Nature 1978;276: 526-528.
129. Glickman JA, Carson GD, Challis JRG. Differential effects of synthetic adrenocorticotropin and melanocyte stimulating hormone on adrenal formation in human and sheep fetus. Endocrinology 1979;104:34-39.
130. Swaab DF, Martin JT. Functions of alpha melanotropin and other opiomelanocortin peptides in labour, intrauterine growth and brain development. Ciba Found Symp 1981;81:196-217.
131. Facchinetti F, Storchi AR, Petraglia F, et al. Ontogeny of pituitary β-endorphin and related peptides in the human embryo and fetus. Am J Obstet Gynecol 1987;156:735-739.
132. Leake RD, Fisher DA. Ontogeny of vasopressin in man. In Czernichow P, Robinson AG, eds. Diabetes Insipidus in Man, Frontiers in Hormone Research, vol 13. Basel: S Karger, 1985:42-51.
133. Leake RD. The fetal-maternal neurohypophysial system. In Polin RA, Fox WW, eds. Fetal and Neonatal Physiology, 2nd ed. Philadelphia: WB Saunders, 1998:2442-2446.
134. Ervin MG, Leake RD, Ross MG, et al. Arginine vasotocin in ovine maternal and fetal blood, fetal urine, and amniotic fluid. J Clin Invest 1985;75:1696-1701.
135. Morris M, Castro M, Rose JC. Alterations in prohormone processing during early development in the fetal sheep. Am J Physiol 1992;263:R738-R740.
136. Zhao X, Nijland MJM, Ervin G, et al. Regulation of hypothalamic arginine vasopressin content in fetal sheep: effect of acute tonicity alterations and fetal maturation. Am J Obstet Gynecol 1998;179: 899-905.
137. DeVane GW, Porter JC. An apparent stress-induced release of arginine vasopressin by human neonates. J Clin Endocrinol Metab 1980;51:1412-1416.
138. Matthews SG, Challis JRG. Regulation of CRH and AVP mRNA in the developing ovine hypothalamus: effects of stress and glucocorticoids. Am J Physiol 1995;268:E1096-E1107.
139. Brooks AN, White A. Activation of pituitary adrenal function in fetal sheep by corticotrophin-releasing factor and arginine vasopressin. J Endocrinol 1990;124:27-35.
140. Benedetto MT, DeCicco F, Rossiello F, et al. Oxytocin receptor in human fetal membranes at term and during labor. J Steroid Biochem 1990;35:205-208.
141. Tribollet E, Charpak S, Schmidt A, et al. Appearance and transient expression of oxytocin receptors in fetal, infant and peripubertal rat brain studied by autoradiography and electrophysiology. J Neurosci 1989;9:1764-1773.
142. Ervin MG, Miller SJ, Ramseyer LJ, et al. Renal arginine vasopressin receptors in newborn and adult sheep. Clin Res 1990;38:170A.
143. Devuyst O, Burrow CR, Smithe BL, et al. Expression of aquaporins 1 and 2 during nephrogenesis and in autosomal dominant polycystic kidney disease. Am J Physiol 1996;271:F169-F183.
144. Baum MA, Ruddy MK, Hosselet CA, et al. The perinatal expression of aquaporin-2 and aquaporin-3 in developing kidney. Pediatr Res 1998;43:783-790.
145. Padbury JF. Functional maturation of the adrenal medulla and peripheral sympathetic nervous system. Baillieres Clin Endocrinol Metab 1989;33:689-705.
146. Huber K, Karch N, Ernsberger U, et al. The role of PHOX2B in chromaffin cell development. Dev Biol 2005;279:501-508.
147. Gaultier C, Trang H, Dauger S, et al. Pediatric disorders with autoimmune dysfunction: What role for PHOX2B? Pediatr Res 2005;58:1-6.
148. Aloe L, Levi-Montalcini R. Nerve growth factor-induced transformation of immature chromaffin cells in vivo into sympathetic neurons: effect of antiserum to nerve growth factor. Proc Natl Acad Sci U S A 1979;76:1246-1250.
149. Slotkin TA, Seidler FJ. Adrenomedullary catecholamine release in the fetus and newborn: secretory mechanisms and their role in stress and survival. J Dev Physiol 1988;10:1-16.
150. Stonestreet BS, Piasecki GJ, Susa JB, et al. Effects of insulin infusion on catecholamine concentration in fetal sheep. Am J Obstet Gynecol 1989;160:740-745.
151. Cohen WR, Piasecki GJ, Cohn HE, et al. Plasma catecholamines in the hypoxaemic fetal rhesus monkey. J Dev Physiol 1987;9:507-515.
152. Pryds O, Christensen NJ, Friis-Hansen B. Increased cerebral blood flow and plasma epinephrine in hypoglycemic, preterm neonates. Pediatrics 1990;85:172-176.
153. Palmer SM, Oakes GK, Lam RW, et al. Catecholamine physiology in the ovine fetus. I: Gestational age variation in basal plasma concentrations. Am J Obstet Gynecol 1984;149:420-425.

154. Palmer SM, Oakes GK, Lam RW, et al. Catecholamine physiology in the ovine fetus. II: Metabolic clearance rate of epinephrine. Am J Physiol 1984;246:E350-E355.
155. Palmer SM, Oakes GK, Champion JA, et al. Catecholamine physiology in the ovine fetus. III: Maternal and fetal response to acute maternal exercise. Am J Obstet Gynecol 1984;149:426-434.
156. Zhou QY, Ouaife CJ, Palmiter RD. Targeted disruption of the tyrosine hydroxylase gene reveals that catecholamines are required for mouse fetal development. Nature 1995;374:640-643.
157. Thomas SA, Matsumoto AM, Palmiter RD. Noradrenaline is essential for mouse fetal development. Nature 1995;374:643-646.
158. Hochberg Ze'ev, Tiosano D. Disorders of mineral metabolism. In Pescovitz OH, Eugster EA, eds. Pediatric Endocrinology. Philadelphia: Lippincott Williams and Wilkins, 2004:614-640.
159. Miao D, He B, Karaplis C, et al. Parathyroid hormone is essential for normal fetal bone formation. J Clin Invest 2002;109:1173-1182.
160. Prada JA. Calcium-regulating hormones. In Polin RA, Fox WW, eds. Fetal and Neonatal Physiology, 2nd ed. Philadelphia: WB Saunders, 1998:2287-2296.
161. Kovaks CS, Kronenberg HM: Maternal-fetal calcium and bone metabolism during pregnancy, puerperium and lactation. Endocr Rev 1997;18:832-872.
162. Care AD, Abbas SK, Pickard DW, et al. Stimulation of ovine placental transport of calcium and magnesium by mid-molecule fragments of human parathyroid hormone-related protein. J Exp Physiol 1990;75:605-608.
163. Kovacs CS, Lanske B, Hunzelman JL, et al. Parathyroid hormone-related peptide (PTHrP) regulates fetal-placental calcium transport through a receptor distinct from the PTH/PTHrP receptor. Proc Natl Acad Sci U S A 1996;93:15233-15238.
164. Karaplis AC, Luz A, Glowacki J, et al. Lethal skeletal dysplasia from targeted disruption of the parathyroid hormone-related protein gene. Genes Dev 1994;8:277-289.
165. Ross R, Halbert K, Tsang RC. Determination of the production and metabolic clearance rates of 1,25-dihydroxyvitamin D_3 in the pregnant sheep and its chronically catheterized fetus by primed infusion technique. Pediatr Res 1989;26:633-638.
166. Habener JF, Kemp DM, Thomas MJ. Mini review: transcriptional regulation in pancreatic development. Endocrinology 2005;146:1025-1034.
167. Jiang FX, Harrison LC. Laminin-1 and epidermal growth factor family members co-stimulate fetal pancreas cell proliferation and colony formation. Differentiation 2005;73:45-49.
168. Formby B, Ullrich A, Coussens L, et al. Growth hormone stimulates insulin gene expression in cultured human fetal pancreatic islets. J Clin Endocrinol Metab 1988;66:1075-1079.
169. Edlund H. Pancreatic organogenesis: developmental mechanisms and implications for therapy. Nat Rev Genet 2002;3:524-532.
170. Sperling MA. Carbohydrate metabolism: insulin and glucagons. In Tulchinsky D, Little AB, eds. Maternal-Fetal Endocrinology, 2nd ed. Philadelphia: WB Saunders, 1994:380-400.
171. Girard J. Control of fetal and neonatal glucose metabolism by pancreatic hormones. Baillieres Clin Endocrinol Metab 1989;3:817-836.
172. Ammon HP, Glocker C, Waldner RG, et al. Insulin release from pancreatic islets of fetal rats mediated by leucine, b-BCH, tolbutamide, glibenclamide, arginine, potassium chloride, and theophylline does not require stimulation of Ca^2+ net uptake. Cell Calcium 1989;10:441-450.
173. Pepe GJ, Albrecht ED. Actions of placental and fetal adrenal steroid hormones in primate pregnancy. Endocr Rev 1995;16:608-648.
174. Ruiz de Ona C, Obregon MJ, Escobar del Rey F, et al. Developmental changes in rat brain 5′-deiodinase and thyroid hormones during the fetal period: the effects of fetal hypothyroidism and maternal thyroid hormones. Pediatr Res 1988;24:588-594.
175. Polk DH, Cheromcha D, Reviczky A, et al. Nuclear thyroid hormone receptors: ontogeny and thyroid hormone effects in sheep. Am J Physiol 1989;256:E543-E549.
176. Coulombe P, Ruel J, Dussault JH. Effects of neonatal hypo- and hyperthyroidism on pituitary growth hormone content in the rat. Endocrinology 1980;107:2027-2033.
177. Lakshmanan J, Perheentupa J, Macaso T, et al. Acquisition of urine, kidney and submandibular gland epidermal growth factor responsiveness to thyroxine administration in neonatal mice. Acta Endocrinol 1985;109:511-516.
178. Alm J, Scott SM, Fisher DA. Epidermal growth factor receptor ontogeny in mice with congenital hypothyroidism. J Dev Physiol 1986;8:377-385.
179. Hoath SB, Lakshmanan J, Fisher DA. Thyroid hormone effects on skin and hepatic epidermal growth factor concentrations in neonatal and adult mice. Biol Neonate 1984;45:49-52.
180. Hoath SB, Lakshmanan J, Fisher DA. Epidermal growth factor binding to neonatal mouse skin explants and membrane preparations: effect of triiodothyronine. Pediatr Res 1985;19:277-280.
181. Perez Castillo A, Bernal J, Ferriero B, et al. The early ontogenesis of thyroid hormone receptor in the rat fetus. Endocrinology 1985;117:2457-2461.
182. Padbury JF, Lam RW, Newnham JP, et al. Neonatal adaptation: greater neurosympathetic system activity in preterm than full term sheep at birth. Am J Physiol 1985;248:E443-E449.
183. Pasqualini JR, Sumida C, Gelly C, et al. Progesterone receptors in the fetal uterus and ovary of the guinea pig: evolution during fetal development and induction and stimulation in estradiol-primed animals. J Steroid Biochem 1976;7:1031-1038.
184. Yamashita S, Newbold RR, McLachlan JA, et al. Developmental pattern of estrogen receptor expression in female mouse genital tracts. Endocrinology 1989;125:2888-2896.
185. Simmen FA, Simmon RCM, Letcher LR, et al. IGFs in pregnancy: developmental expression in uterus and mammary gland and paracrine actions during embryonic and neonatal growth. In LeRoith D, Raizada MK, eds. Molecular and Cellular Biology of Insulin-Like Growth Factors and Their Receptors. New York: Plenum, 1989:195-208.
186. Spaventi R, Antica M, Pavelic K. Insulin and insulin-like growth factor I (IGF I) in early mouse embryogenesis. Development 1990;108:491-495.
187. Forhead AJ, Li J, Gilmour RS, et al. Thyroid hormone and the mRNA of the GH receptor and IGFs in skeletal muscle of fetal sheep. Am J Physiol Endocrinol Metab 2002;282:E80-E86.
188. Ong K, Kratzsch J, Kiess W, et al. Size at birth and cord blood levels of insulin, insulin-like growth factor (IGF-I), IGF-II, IGF binding protein-1 (IGFBP-1), IGFBP-3 and the soluble IGF-II/mannose-6-phosphate receptor in term human infants. J Clin Endocrinol Metab 2000;85:4266-4269.
189. Pilistine SJ, Moses AC, Munro HN. Placental lactogen administration reverses the effect of low protein diet on maternal and fetal somatomedin levels in the pregnant rat. Proc Natl Acad Sci U S A 1984;81:5853-5857.
190. Gohlke BC, Fahnenstich H, Dame C, et al. Longitudinal data for intrauterine levels of fetal IGF-I and IGF-II. Horm Res 2004;61:200-204.
191. Accili D, Drago J, Lee EJ, et al. Early neonatal death in mice homozygous for a null allele of the insulin receptor gene. Nat Genet 1996;12:106-109.
192. Fisher DA, Lakshmanan J. Metabolism and effects of EGF and related growth factors in mammals. Endocr Rev 1990;11:418-442.
193. Rotwein P. Peptide growth factors other than insulin-like growth factors or cytokines. In DeGroot LJ, Jameson JL, eds. Endocrinology, 5th ed. Philadelphia: Elsevier Saunders, 2006:675-695.
194. Meittinen PJ, Berger JE, Menesses J, et al. Epithelial immaturity and multiorgan failure in mice lacking epidermal growth factor receptor. Nature 1995;376:337-341.
195. Brown PI, Lam R, Lakshmanan J, et al. Transforming growth factor alpha in developing rats. Am J Physiol 1990;259:E256-E260.
196. Hemmings R, Langlais J, Falcone T, et al. Human embryos produce transforming growth factor α activity and insulin-like growth factor II. Fertil Steril 1992;58:101-104.
197. Mazzoni IE, Kenigsberg RL. Effects of epidermal growth factor in the mammalian central nervous system. Drug Dev Res 1992;26:111-128.
198. Kitchens DL, Snyder EY, Gottlieb DI. FGF and EGF are mitogens for immortalized neural progenitors. J Neurobiol 1990;21:356-375.
199. Santa-Olalla J, Covarrubias L. Epidermal growth factor, transforming growth factor-α, and fibroblast growth factor differentially influence neural precursor cells of mouse embryonic mesencephalon. J Neurosci Res 1995;42:172-183.

200. Lee KF, Simon H, Chen C, et al. Requirement for neuregulin receptor erbB2 in neural and cardiac development. Nature 1995;378:394-398.
201. Kamei Y, Tsutsumi O, Kuwabara Y, et al. Intrauterine growth retardation and fetal losses are caused by epidermal growth factor deficiency in mice. Am J Physiol 1993;264:R597-R600.
202. Yan Q, Elliott J, Snider WD. Brain derived neurotrophic factor rescues spinal motor neurons from axotomy-induced cell death. Nature 1992;360:753-755.
203. Gospodarowicz D. Epidermal and nerve growth factors in mammalian development. Annu Rev Physiol 1981;43:251-263.
204. Padbury JF, Lam RW, Polk DH, et al. Autoimmune sympathectomy in fetal rabbits. J Dev Physiol 1986;8:369-376.
205. Tarris RH, Weichsel ME Jr, Fisher DA. Synthesis and secretion of a nerve growth stimulating factor by neonatal mouse astrocyte cells in vitro. Pediatr Res 1986;20:367-372.
206. Giordano T, Pan JB, Casuto D, et al. Thyroid hormone regulation of NGF, NT3 and BDNF RNA in the adult rat brain. Mol Brain Res 1992;16:239-245.
207. Lim GB, Dodic M, Earnest L, et al. Regulation of erythropoietin gene expression in fetal sheep by glucocorticoids. Endocrinology 1996;137:1658-1663.
208. Moritz KM, Lim GB, Wintour EM. Developmental regulation of erythropoietin and erythropoiesis. Am J Physiol 1997;273:R1829-R1844.
209. Betsholtz C. Functions of platelet-derived growth factor and its receptors deduced from gene inactivation in mice. J Clin Ligand Assay 2000;23:206-213.
210. Lewandoski M, Sun X, Martin GR. Fgf8 signalling from the AER is essential for normal limb development. Nat Genet 2000;26:460-463.
211. Oberbauer AM, Linkhart TA, Mohan S, et al. Fibroblast growth factor enhances human chorionic gonadotropin synthesis independent of mitogenic stimulation in Jar choriocarcinoma cells. Endocrinology 1988;123:2696-2700.
212. Wallace MJ, Hooper SB, Harding R. Effects of elevated fetal cortisol concentrations on the volume, secretion, and reabsorption of lung liquid. Am J Physiol 1995;269:R881-R887.
213. Muglia L, Jacobson L, Dikkes P, et al. Corticotropin-releasing hormone deficiency reveals major fetal but not adult glucocorticoid need. Nature 1995;373:427-432.
214. Cole TJ, Blendy JA, Monaghan P, et al. Targeted disruption of the glucocorticoid receptor gene blocks adrenergic chromaffin cell development and severely retards lung maturation. Genes Dev 1995;9:1608-1621.
215. Polk DH. Thyroid hormone effects on neonatal thermogenesis. Semin Perinatol 1988;12:151-156.
216. Gunn TR, Gluckman PD. Perinatal thermogenesis. Early Hum Dev 1995;42:169-183.
217. Obregon MJ, Pitamber R, Jacobsson A, et al. Euthyroid status is essential for the perinatal increase in thermogenin mRNA in brown adipose tissue of rat pups. Biochem Biophys Res Commun 1987;148:9-14.
218. Polk DH, Padbury JF, Callegari CC, et al. Effect of fetal thyroidectomy on newborn thermogenesis in lambs. Pediatr Res 1987;21:453-457.
219. Longhead JL, Minouni F, Tsang RC. Serum ionized calcium concentrations in normal neonates. Am J Dis Child 1988;142:516-518.
220. Venkataraman PS, Tsang RC, Chen IW, et al. Pathogenesis of early neonatal hypocalcemia: studies of serum calcitonin, gastrin and plasma glucagon. J Pediatr 1987;110:599-603.
221. Mimoumi F, Tsang RC. Perinatal mineral metabolism. In Tulchinsky D, Little AB, eds. Maternal-Fetal Endocrinology, 2nd ed. Philadelphia: WB Saunders, 1994:402-417.
222. Wheeler MD, Styne DM. Longitudinal changes in growth hormone response to growth hormone-releasing hormone in neonatal rhesus monkeys. Pediatr Res 1990;28:15-18.
223. Penny R, Parlow AF, Frasier O. Testosterone and estradiol concentrations in paired maternal and cord sera and their correlation with the concentration of chorionic gonadotropin. Pediatrics 1979;64:604-608.
224. Mann DR, Gould KG, Collins DC, et al. Blockade of neonatal activation of the pituitary-testicular axis: effect on peripubertal luteinizing hormone and testosterone secretion and on testicular development in male monkeys. J Clin Endocrinol Metab 1989;68:600-607.
225. Dohler KD. The special case of hormonal imprinting: the neonatal influence on sex. Experientia 1986;42:759-769.
226. Resko JA, Roselli CE. Prenatal hormones organize sex differences in the neuroendocrine reproductive system: observations on guinea pigs and nonhuman primates. Cell Mol Neurobiol 1997;17:627-648.
227. Kosut SS, Wood RI, Herbosa-Encaracion C, et al. Prenatal androgens time neuroendocrine puberty in the sheep: effect of testosterone dose. Endocrinology 1997;138:1072-1077.
228. Grocock CA, Charlton HM, Pike MC. Role of fetal pituitary in cryptorchidism induced by exogenous maternal oestrogen during pregnancy in mice. J Reprod Fertil 1988;83:295-300.
229. Martin SM, Moberg GP. Effects of early neonatal thyroxine treatment on development of the thyroid and adrenal axes in rats. Life Sci 1981;29:1683-1688.
230. Walker P, Courtin F. Transient neonatal hyperthyroidism results in hypothyroidism in the adult rat. Endocrinology 1985;116:2246-2250.
231. Csaba G, Inczefi Gonda A, Dobozy O. Hereditary transmission in the F_1 generation of hormonal imprinting (receptor memory) induced in rats by neonatal exposure to insulin. Acta Physiol Hung 1984;63:93-99.
232. Csaba G, Ronai A, Laszlo V, et al. Amplification of hormone receptors by neonatal oxytocin and vasopressin treatment. Horm Metab Res 1980;12:28-31.
233. Benediktsson R, Lindsay RD, Noble J, et al. Glucocorticoid exposure in utero: new model for adult hypertension. Lancet 1993;341:339-341.
234. Drake AJ, Walker BR, Seckl JR. Intergenerational consequences of fetal programming by in utero exposure to glucocorticoids in rats. Am J Physiol Regul Integr Comp Physiol 2005;288:R34-R38.
235. Lackland DR. Fetal and early life determinants of hypertension in adults: implications for study. Hypertension 2004;44:811-812.
236. Barker DJP. Fetal programming of coronary heart disease. Trends Endocrinol Metab 2002;13:364-368.
237. Barker DJP. The developmental origins of chronic adult disease. Acta Paediatr Suppl 2004;336:26-33.
238. Ozanne SE, Hales CN. Early programming of glucose-insulin metabolism. Trends Endocrinol Metab 2002;13:368-373.
239. Matthews SG. Early programming of the hypothalamo-pituitary-adrenal axis. Trends Endocrinol Metab 2002;13:373-380.
240. Young BS. Programming of sympatho adrenal function. Trends Endocrinol Metab 2002;13:381-385.
241. Davies MJ, Norman RJ. Programming and reproductive function. Trends Endocrinol Metab 2002;13:386-392.
242. Holt RIG. Fetal programming of the growth hormone-insulin-like growth factor axis. Trends Endocrinol Metab 2002;13:392-402.
243. Dodic M, Moritz K, Koukoulas I, et al. Programmed hypertension: kidney, brain or both. Trends Endocrinol Metab 2002;13:403-408.
244. Reik W, Constancia M, Fowdey A, et al. Regulation of supply and demand for maternal nutrients in mammals by imprinted genes. J Physiol 2003;547:35-44.
245. Ibanez L, Ong K, Potau N, et al. Insulin gene variable number of tandem repeat genotype and the low birth weight, precocious pubarche, and hyperinsulinism sequence. J Clin Endocrinol Metab 2001;86:5788-5793.
246. Ijzerman RG, Stehouwer CDA, de Geus EJ, et al. Low birth weight is associated with increased sympathetic activity: dependence on genetic factors. Circulation 2003;108:566-571.
247. Fowden AL, Forhead AJ. Endocrine mechanisms of intrauterine programming. Reproduction 2004;127:515-526.
248. Slone-Wilcoxon J, Redei EE. Maternal-fetal glucocorticoid milieu programs hypothalamic-pituitary-thyroid function of adult offspring. Endocrinology 2004;145:4068-4072.
249. Lavcola L, Perrini S, Belsanti G, et al. Intrauterine growth restriction in humans is associated with abnormalities in placental insulin-like growth factor signaling. Endocrinology 2005;146:1498-1505.
250. Waterland RA, Jirtle RL. Early nutrition, epigenetic changes at transposons and imprinted genes, and enhanced susceptibility to adult chronic diseases. Nutrition 2004;20:63-68.

251. McMullen S, Langley-Evans SC. Maternal low-protein diet in rat pregnancy programs blood pressure through sex-specific mechanisms. Am J Physiol regul Integr Physiol 2005;288:R85-R90.
252. Bunt JC, Tataranni PA, Salbe AD. Intrauterine exposure to diabetes is a determinant of hemoglobin A(1)c and systolic blood pressure in Pima Indian children. J Clin Endocrinol Metab 2005;90: 3225-3229.
253. Zheng X, Hendry WJ III. Neonatal stilbestrol treatment alters the estrogen-related expression of both cell proliferation and apoptosis-related proto-oncogene (c-jun, dfos, cmyc, bax, bcl-2 and bcl-x) in the hamster uterus. Cell Growth Diff 1997;8:425-434.
254. Huang WW, Yin Y, Bi Q, et al. Developmental diethylstilbestrol exposure alters genetic pathways of uterine cytodifferentiation. Mol Endocrinol 2005;19:669-682.
255. Csaba G. Receptor ontogeny and hormonal imprinting. Experientia 1986;42:750-759.
256. Sato SM, Mains MI, Adzick MS, et al. Plasticity in the adrenocorticotropin-related peptides produced by primary cultures of neonatal rat pituitary. Endocrinology 1988;122:68-77.
257. Vickers MH, Gluckman PD, Coveny HH, et al. Neonatal leptin treatment reverses developmental programming. Endocrinology 2005;146:4211-4216.
258. Flake AW. Fetal therapy: medical and surgical approaches. In Creasy RK, Resnik R, eds. Maternal-Fetal Medicine, 4th ed. Philadelphia: WB Saunders, 1999:365-377.
259. Harman CR. Assessment of fetal health. In Creasy RK, Resnik R, eds. Maternal-Fetal Medicine, 5th ed.. Philadelphia: WB Saunders, 2004:357-401.
260. Resnick R, Creasy RK. Intrauterine growth restriction, In Creasy RK, Resnick R, eds. Maternal Fetal Medicine, 5th ed. Philadelphia: WB Saunders, 2004:495-512.
261. Bianchi DW. Prenatal exclusion of recessively inherited disorders: should maternal plasma analysis precede invasive techniques. Clin Chem 2002;48:689-690.
262. Manning FA. General principles and applications of ultrasonography. In Creasy RK, Resnik R, eds. Maternal-Fetal Medicine, 5th ed. Philadelphia: WB Saunders, 2004:315-355.
263. Fisher DA. Fetal thyroid function: diagnosis and management of fetal thyroid disorders. Clin Obstet Gynecol 1997;40:16-31.
264. New MI, Carlton A, Obeid J, et al. Update: prenatal diagnosis for congenital adrenal hyperplasia in 595 pregnancies. Endocrinologist 2003;13:233-239.
265. Charlton V, Johengen M. Fetal intravenous nutritional supplementation ameliorates the development of embolization-induced growth retardation in sheep. Pediatr Res 1987;22:55-61.
266. Flake AW, Zanjani ED. In utero hematopoietic stem cell transplantation. JAMA 1997;278:932-937.
267. Lin RY, Kubo A, Keller GM, et al. Committing embryonic stem cells to differentiate into thyrocyte-like cells in vitro. Endocrinology 2003;144:2644-2649.
268. Waddington SN, Kennea NL, Buckley SMK, et al. Fetal and neonatal gene therapy: benefits and pitfalls. Gene Therapy 2004;11: 592-597.

CHAPTER 22

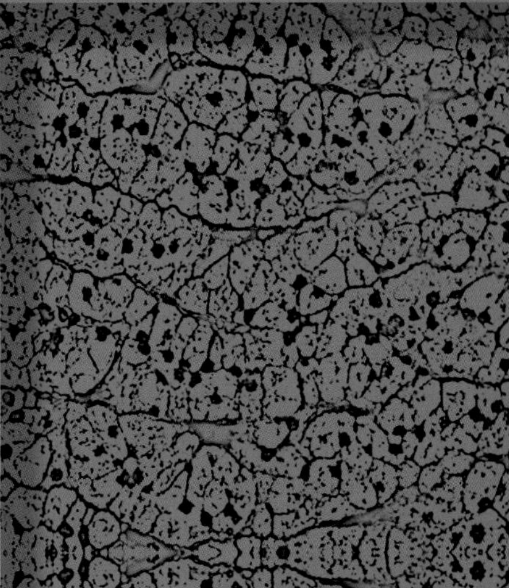

DISORDERS OF SEX DEVELOPMENT

John C. Achermann and Ieuan A. Hughes

INTRODUCTION

Under most circumstances, the distinction between male and female is considered absolute so that sex assignment at birth is instantaneous. Allied to this analysis of the somatotype is the assignation of gender, which is confined to either male or female in the vast majority of human societies. Ambiguity of the external genitalia sufficient to prevent instantaneous sex assignment at birth is rare but it is estimated that abnormalities of the external genitalia that need formal investigation occur in 1 in 4000 births.[1]

The investigation and management of infants and young people with disorders of sex development requires an understanding of the embryology of the urogenital system and the mechanism of normal hormone production and action. Previous editions of the textbook have emphasized the advances that have taken place in the cognate sciences that have now allowed many of the causes of abnormal genital development to be better characterized.[2] Many of the advances in identifying key genes involved in normal sex determination and sex differentiation have emanated from detailed clinicopathologic assessment of prismatic cases. Nevertheless, much remains to be explained in causation, particularly for the underandrogenized male who has some form of gonadal dysgenesis or indeed the male who has normal testes determination, androgen production, and action, but has abnormal external genital development. Application of techniques such as tissue-specific microarrays and whole genome scans will provide further inroads to the understanding of those disorders that currently remain unexplained.

Clarity in terminology is fundamental to the understanding of disorders of sex development and their management. This applies not only to health professionals but also to patients and their families. The importance of this element of management was a key component of a consensus statement published by a faculty of world experts involved in the management of intersex disorders.[3,4] It was agreed that the term *intersex* should be abandoned in view of pejorative elements and be replaced by the generic term *disorders of sex development (DSD),* which now entitles the latest edition of this chapter. Linked to this change is the recommendation to abandon nomenclature such as *male pseudohermaphroditism, female pseudohermaphroditism,* and *true hermaphroditism.* The alternative nomenclature is shown in Table 22–1. How this can be used for classification of the causes of DSD is discussed in the section on abnormal sex development. There has been a major change in how the problem of DSD is managed, with families and the affected individual at an appropriate age being fully engaged in decision making borne out of a process that involves disclosure commensurate with changing cognitive and psychological development. The need to understand the embryology and genetic and hormonal control of normal sex development underpins the investigation and management of an individual with DSD.

DEVELOPMENT OF THE REPRODUCTIVE SYSTEMS

Development of the reproductive systems begins at around 4 to 5 weeks' gestation in humans and might be considered complete following the development of secondary sexual characteristics and fertility (the production of viable gametes) after puberty. Sex development is a dynamic process requiring the appropriate and timely interaction of a multitude of genes, proteins, signaling molecules, paracrine factors, and endocrine stimuli.[5-8] Marked differences in the basic mechanisms of sex determination, differentiation, and reproductive strategy have evolved between different species, with fascinating variability in sex chromosome complement, gonad development, and gametogenesis throughout the animal kingdom.[9-11] Here we focus on the basic mechanisms of reproductive development in humans. We also review important insight that is being obtained from studies in normal and transgenic mice, and the relevance of these findings to individuals with DSD.

The basic processes of normal development are divided into (1) sex determination and sex differentiation, (2) development of the hypothalamic-gonadotrope axis in the fetus, and (3) the hypothalamic-pituitary-gonadal axis in infancy and childhood. A more detailed overview of normal and disordered puberty is provided in Chapter 24.

Sex Determination and Sex Differentiation

Sex determination is the process whereby the bipotential gonad develops into either a testis or an ovary.

Sex differentiation requires the developing gonad to function appropriately to produce peptide hormones and steroids.

In the male, the process of sex differentiation involves regression of müllerian structures (uterus, fallopian tubes, and upper one third of the vagina), stabilization of wolffian structures (which develop into the seminal vesicles, vasa deferentia, and epididymides), androgenization of the external genitalia (penis and scrotum), and descent of the testes from their origin in the urogenital ridge to their final position in the scrotum (Fig. 22–1).

In the female, the ovary is generally steroidogenically quiescent until the time of puberty, when estrogen synthesis stimulates breast and uterine development, and follicular development results in regular menstrual cycles. Thus, defects in ovarian development usually first manifest in adolescence. Indeed, ovarian development and differentiation has been viewed in the past as a "default" process, which occurs in the absence of the chromosomal, genetic, and endocrine signals deemed actively necessary to "make a male." Whilst male sex differentiation is undoubtedly a more active developmental process—as defined in the classic experiments of Alfred Jost—recent studies of gene expression are showing that a specific complement of genes are implicated in ovarian development and integrity, some of which (e.g., *RSPO1*) may actively antagonize testis differentiation.[12-15] Even the concept of a fixed and quiescent population of ovarian germ cells at birth has now been challenged.[16] Thus, ovarian development likely involves many active processes rather than being simply the "default mechanism" proposed previously.

Classically, sex determination and sex differentiation can be divided into three major components: chromosomal sex (i.e., the presence of a Y or X chromosome); gonadal sex (the presence of a testis or ovary); and phenotypic or anatomic sex (the presence of "male" or "female" external and internal genitalia) (Fig. 22–2). None of these processes absolutely defines one's "sex," and psychosexual development ("brain sex") may be an unpredictable outcome of several factors. Furthermore, the presence or absence of a Y chromosome or well-formed testis should not be the focus of how a physician views an individual with a disorder of sex development once a diagnosis or management plan has been established. However, considering sex development in terms of chromosomal sex, gonadal sex, and phenotypic (or anatomic) sex can be a very useful way of understanding the processes involved in reproductive development, and can be a helpful construct for the investigation and diagnosis of patients with these conditions, especially because the (somatic) karyotype is usually readily available as one of the first and potentially guiding investigations. Thus, the chromosomal/gonadal/phenotypic model is the one presented here.

TABLE 22–1 PROPOSED REVISED NOMENCLATURE FOLLOWING THE CONSENSUS MEETING

Previous	Proposed
INTERSEX	**DISORDERS OF SEX DEVELOPMENT (DSD)**
Male pseudohermaphrodite Undervirilization of an XY male Undermasculinization of an XY male	46,XY DSD
Female pseudohermaphrodite Overvirilization of an XX female Masculinization of an XX female	46,XX DSD
True hermaphrodite	Ovotesticular DSD
XX male or XX sex reversal	46,XX testicular DSD
XY sex reversal	46,XY complete gonadal dysgenesis

Reproduced with permission from Hughes IA, Houk C, Ahmed SF, et al. Consensus statement on management of intersex disorders. Arch Dis Child 2006;91:554-562.

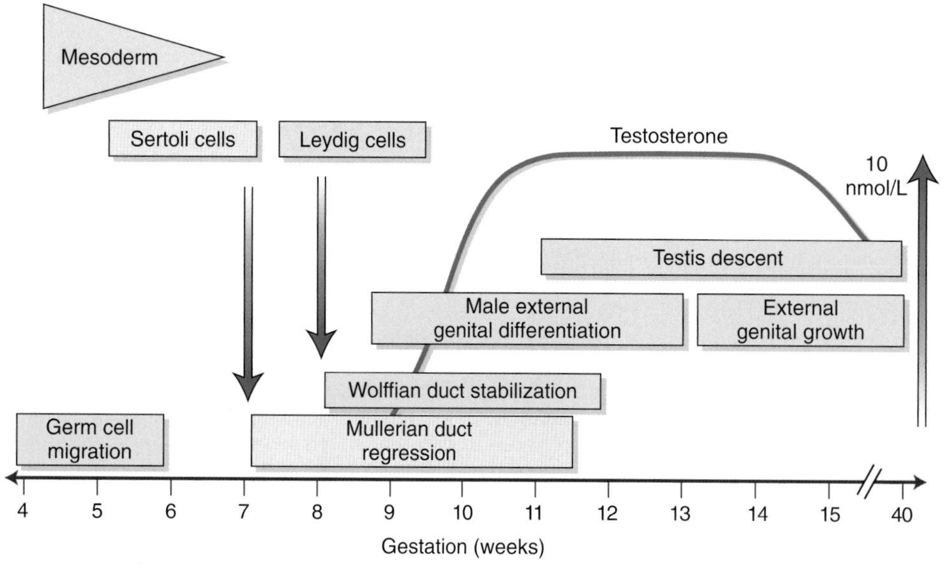

Figure 22–1 ■ Events temporally related to sex differentiation in the male fetus. Mesoderm refers to the tissue source for Sertoli and Leydig cell formation. The continuous line depicts the rise in fetal serum testosterone, the peak concentration being around 10 nmol/L (300 ng/dL).

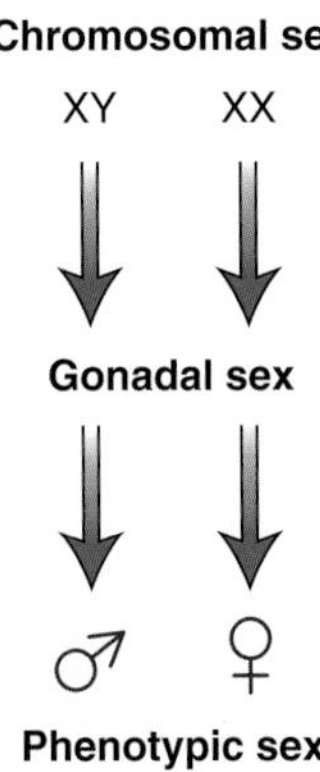

Figure 22–2 ▪ Dividing sex development into three major components can provide a useful framework for diagnosis and classification. Chromosomal sex refers to the karyotype (46,XX, 46,XY, or variants). Gonadal sex refers to the presence of a testis or ovary following the process of *sex determination.* Phenotypic (anatomic) sex refers to the appearance of the external genitalia and internal structures following the process of *sex differentiation.*

Chromosomal Sex

Chromosomal sex describes the complement of sex chromosomes present in an individual (e.g., 46,XY; 46,XX). In humans, the usual complement of 46 chromosomes consists of 22 pairs of autosomes (identified numerically from 1 to 22 based on decreasing size) as well as a pair of sex chromosomes, XX or XY (Fig. 22–3). Other species have different numbers of chromosomes, or may have sexually dimorphic autosomes.[9-11]

In humans, chromosomal sex is generally determined at the time of fertilization when two haploid gametes (ova and sperm, 23 chromosomes each) fuse to generate a diploid zygote (46 chromosomes). Gametes are ultimately derived from germ cells, which initially replicate their chromosome complement, then undergo a series of two meiotic divisions (meiosis I [reduction division], meiosis II) to produce haploid ova or sperm (Fig. 22–4). Normal ova have a single X chromosome. Normal sperm contain either a single Y chromosome or a single X chromosome, resulting in 46,XY or 46,XX zygotes, respectively, following fertilization.

Nondisjunction is the failure of either of a pair of sister chromatids to separate during anaphase (see Fig. 22–4).[17,18] *Meiotic* nondisjunction during gametogenesis can result in ova or sperm with gain or loss of sex chromosomal material. Fertilization by such gametes can give rise to a zygote with an imbalance in sex chromosome number, termed *sex chromosome aneuploidy.* For example, zygotes with a single X (45,X) have Turner's syndrome and presence of an extra X causes Klinefelter's syndrome (47,XXY) or triple X syndrome (47,XXX).[18] Zygotes with no X chromosomal material (45,Y) are nonviable.

In contrast, *mitotic* nondisjunction can occur in the zygote, resulting in an imbalance in sex chromosome number in a proportion or subset of cells, and termed *sex chromosome mosaicism* (e.g., 45,X/46,XY) (see Fig. 22–4). In such cases, the two (or more) cell lines originate from a single zygote. This situation differs from *chimerism,* which is the existence of two or more cell lines with different genetic origins in one individual. Chimerism can occur by (1) double fertilization (dispermy) of a binucleate ovum, (2) fusion of two complete zygotes or morulae before implantation, or (3) fertilization by separate sperm of an ovum and its polar body. Chimerism is difficult to detect if the separate cell lines have the same sex chromosomes. However, if the different cell lines are of different sexes, a 46,XX/46,XY karyotype occurs. This form of true *sex chromosome chimerism* is very rare in humans, but is seen more frequently in cattle in a condition called *freemartinism,* which results from admixture of hematopoietic and primordial germ cells between biovular twins of opposite sex through anastomotic placental channels. The consequences of some of these events in humans are discussed in the section on Sex Chromosome DSD.

The Y Chromosome

Although the Y chromosome was initially thought to be inert, the detection of a 46,XY karyotype in males and a 47,XXY karyotype in men with Klinefelter's syndrome provided evidence that the Y chromosome carries a gene (or genes) responsible for male sex-determination. In fact, the presence of a single Y chromosome is generally sufficient to drive testis development even in the presence of multiple copies of chromosome X.

The human Y chromosome is approximately 60 Mb in length and represents only 2% of the human genome DNA (Fig. 22–5).[19,20] The Y chromosome consists of the highly variable and largely genetically inactive heterochromatic region on the long arm; the remnants of a conserved region; and autosomal-derived regions that are estimated to have been added approximately 80-130 million years ago. It is thought that Y-chromosomal genes encode only 60 proteins. Whilst some of these genes have putative roles in growth, cognition, and tooth development, a number of genes are involved in reproductive development and function. For example, a cluster of genes at Yq11.22 (e.g., AZFc region) is essential for spermatogenesis, whereas genes within the gonadoblastoma locus (e.g., TSPY) increase the risk of malignancy when present in dysgenetic gonads. Deletions of other genetic loci (*gr/gr*) result in susceptibility to germ cell tumors.[21-24]

The euchromatic (conserved) portion of the Y chromosome consists of a Y-specific segment, and regions at the distal ends of both the short and long arms called the *pseudoautosomal regions* (PARs) (see Fig. 22–5).[19] These PARs are homologous to the distal ends of the short and long arms of the X chromosome, and are the only regions involved in pairing and recombination during meiosis. This process is essential for proper distribution of recombined sex chromosomal material to daughter cells. PAR1 (distal short arm, Yp and Xp) contains at least 10 genes, including the homeobox gene SHOX (PHOG). SHOX haploinsufficiency contributes to the short stature associated with Turner's syndrome, Xp- or Yp- deletions, and Leri-Weill syndrome (dyschondrosteosis). These regions are not subject to dosage compensation (i.e., gene inactivation) (see below). PAR2 (distal long arm) contains a number of genes that are mostly growth factors and signaling molecules.

The quest for a testis-determining factor (TDF) on the Y chromosome began over 50 years ago. The discovery by Eichwald and Silmser in 1955 of a male cell membrane-specific antigen that causes rejection of skin grafts by female mice led to the H-Y antigen being pursued as a candidate TDF.[25] Subsequently, Page and associates proposed in 1987 that the sex-determining function of the Y chromosome is located within a 140-kb segment of the short arm, within the Y-specific euchromatic portion.[26] A zinc-finger transcription factor, ZFY, was the initial candidate in this region. However, it was the description by Palmer and colleagues in 1989 of several 46,XX *males* who harbored Y-to-X translocations of Y chromosomal material that was distal (telomeric) to the ZFY locus that finally refuted the role of ZFY as the putative testis determing gene and helped to focus on a 35 kilobase region of the Y chromosome close to the pseudoautosomal boundary.[27] This region was shown to contain a putative transcription factor (termed *sex-determining region, Y* or SRY) expressed in appropriate tissues (see Fig. 22–5).

Before long, a series of elegant reports in mice and humans established SRY as the likely primary Y-chromosomal testis-determining gene.[28-30] However, it was the generation of trans-

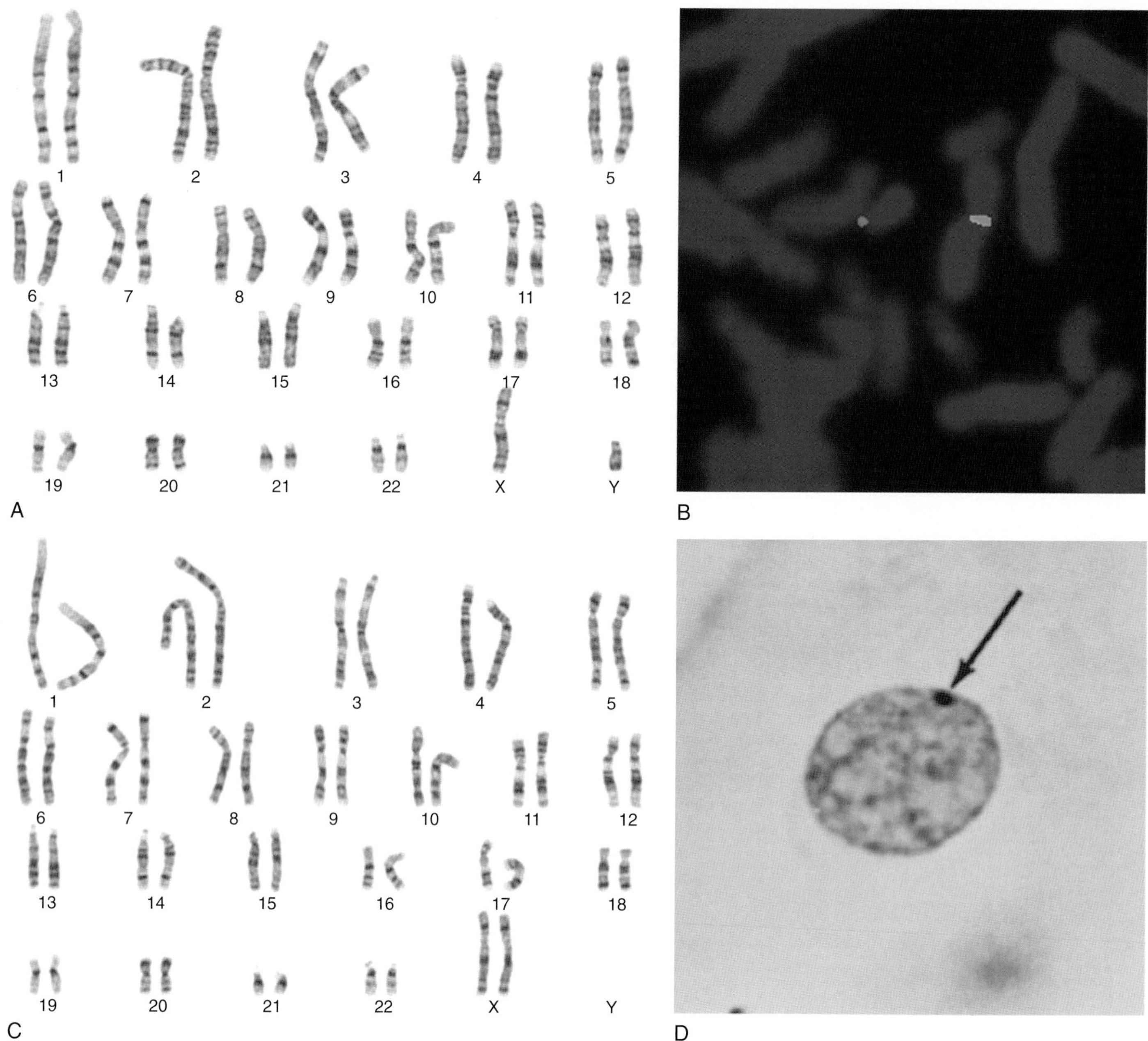

Figure 22–3 ▪ Cytogenetic and fluorescent in-situ hybridization (FISH) studies. **A,** Male (46,XY) G-banded karyotype. **B,** FISH analysis in a male (46,XY) using fluorescent probes directed against SRY (spectrum red) and against the X centromere (spectrum green). **C,** Female (46,XX) G-banded karyotype. **D,** Photomicrograph showing the X chromatin body (Barr body, *arrow*) in the nucleus of buccal mucosa cells from a 46,XX female (thionine stain, ×2000). (Images **A** to **C** courtesy of Mr Lee Grimsley and Dr Jonathan Waters, North East London Regional Cytogenetics Laboratory, Great Ormond Street Hospital NHS Trust, London, UK.)

genic XX mice specifically expressing the Sry locus (14 kb) that provided the first definitive proof that Sry is a testis-determining gene; some of these mice had a male phenotype, developed testes (with absent spermatogenesis) and showed male sexual mating behavior (Fig. 22–6).[31] This work was supported soon afterward by reports of deletions and loss of function mutations in SRY in humans with 46,XY complete gonadal dysgenesis (Swyer syndrome) (see below and *46,XY DSD*).[29,32,33]

The X Chromosome

The X chromosome is a relatively large and gene rich chromosome compared to the Y chromosome, consisting of about 160 Mb of genomic DNA (see Fig. 22–5).[19,34,35] This DNA contains 5% of the haploid genome, and more than 1000 expressed genes of which about 800 encode proteins. X-chromosomal genes play an important role in sex development in both the male and female, both at the level of the gonad and gametogenesis as well as in hypothalamic-pituitary (gonadotrope) function (e.g., androgen receptor, KAL1, DAX1, SOX3). More than 100 X chromosome genes are expressed in the testis.[34] However, most X linked genes are unrelated to sex development and have a diverse range of cellular functions.

The X chromosome contains pseudoautosomal regions (PARs) at the distal end of each arm, similar to the PARs of the Y chromosome (see Fig. 22–5).[19] These regions, as well as

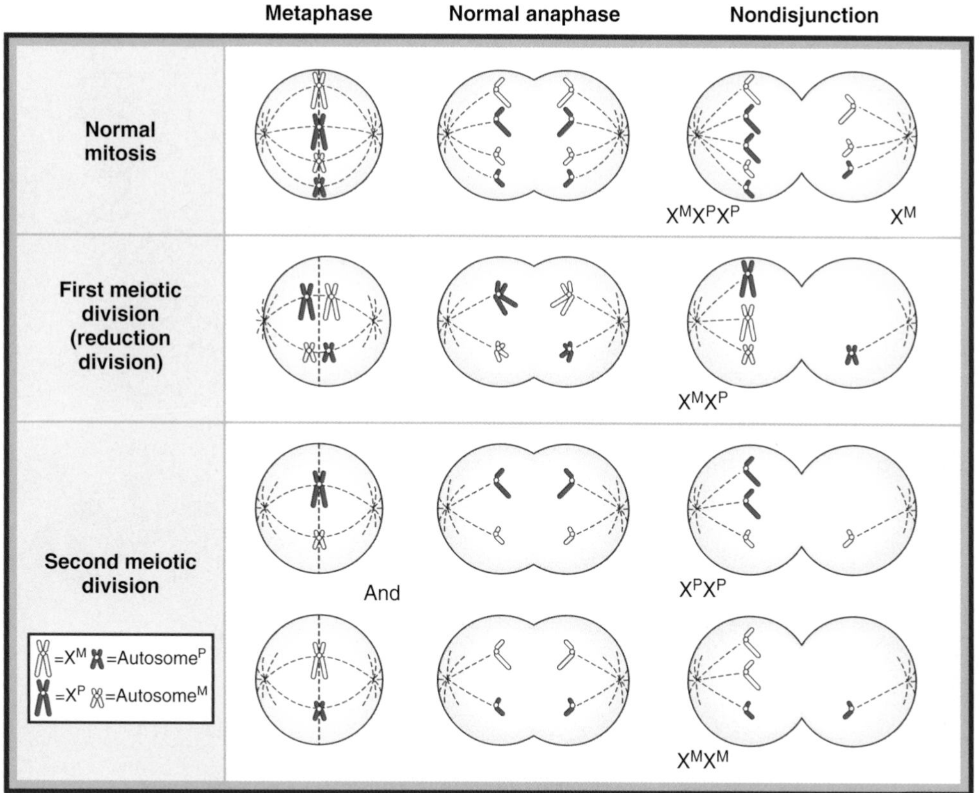

Figure 22–4 ▪ Types of cell division. A female somatic cell is represented. At the metaphase plate are two X chromosomes and two homologous autosomes of group 21 to 22. Division occurs through the centromere, giving rise to two daughter cells of identical chromosomal composition. Replication of each arm into two chromatids takes place while the chromosomes are extended and before the next metaphase. The first meiotic division involves pairing of homologous chromosomes. The centromere does not divide in this cell division. It is by chance whether the maternal (X^M) or paternal (X^P) member of each pair goes to the respective daughter cells. During the complex prophase of first meiotic division *(not shown)*, multiple chiasmata are formed between the chromosomes of each pair, facilitating exchanges of chromosomal segments (crossing over) between them. During the second meiotic division, the centromere again divides, giving rise to daughter cells identical to the parent cell. This division more nearly resembles mitosis than the first meiotic division. Nondisjunction can take place in mitosis or in the first or second meiotic division; representative examples are illustrated.

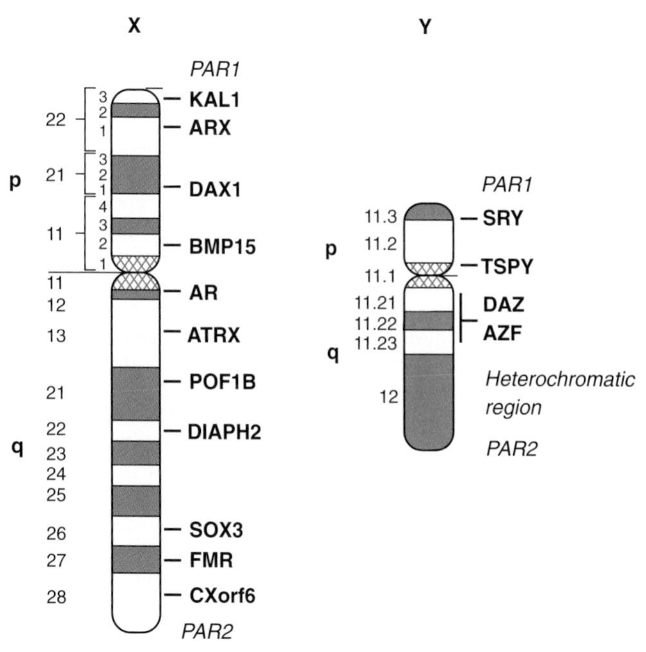

Figure 22–5 ▪ Schematic diagrams of the X chromosome *(left panel)* and Y chromosome *(right panel)* showing key regions and genes involved in sex development and reproduction. *p,* Short arm; *q,* long arm; *PAR,* pseudoautosomal region; *KAL1,* Kallman syndrome, 1; *ARX,* aristaless-related homeobox, X-linked; *DAX1,* dosage-sensitive sex reversal congenital adrenal hypoplasia critical region on the X chromosome, 1; *BMP15,* bone morphogenetic protein, 15; *AR,* androgen receptor; *ATRX,* α-thalassemia, X-linked mental retardation; *POF1B,* actin-binding protein, 34 kd; *DIAP2,* human homologue of the *Drosophila* diaphanous gene; *SOX3,* SRY-related HMG-box, 3; *FMR,* fragile X, mental retardation; *SRY,* sex-determining region Y; *TSPY,* testes-specific protein Y; *DAZ,* deleted in azoospermia; *AZF,* azoospermia factor.

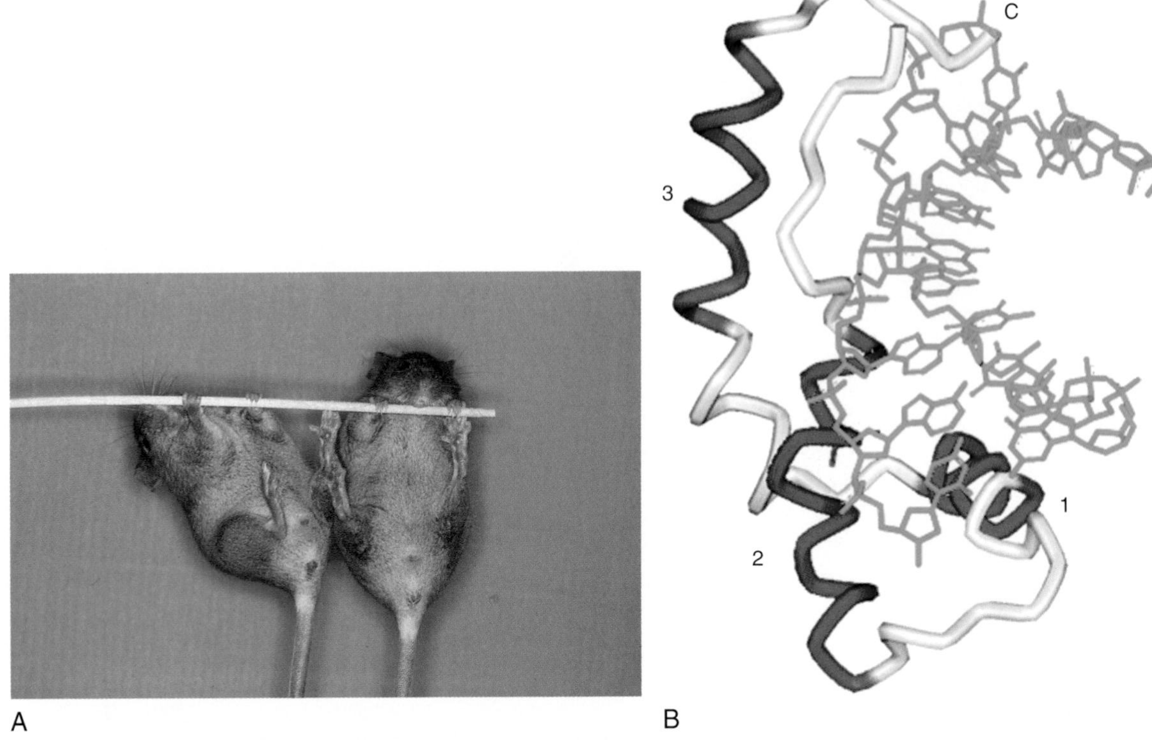

Figure 22–6 ▪ **A,** The XX*Sry*+ mouse *(right)* has testis development and a male phenotype providing convincing evidence that *Sry* is a testis-determining gene. A normal XY male littermate is shown for comparison *(left)*. **B,** A model of the structure of the SRY HMG box bound to DNA. The HMG domain contains three α-helices (red), which adopt an L-shaped conformation. Binding of this region of SRY to the minor groove of DNA (green) causes it to bend and unwind. (**A** Courtesy of Professor Robin Lovell-Badge, National Institute of Medical Research, London, UK; **B** Reproduced with permission from Harley VR, Clarkson MJ, Argentaro A. The molecular action and regulation of the testis-determing factors, SRY [sex-determining region on the Y chromosome] and SOX9 [SRY-related high-mobility group {HMG} box 9]. Endocr Rev 2003;24:466-487. Copyright 2003, The Endocrine Society.)

several genes in their boundaries, do not undergo X-inactivation and function in an autosomal fashion with their homologues on the Y-chromosomal PARs. A large number of genes on the X chromosome are located outside the PARs and do not have homologues on the Y chromosome. As many of these genes are involved in a wide range of cellular processes unrelated to sex development or sex-specific function, a process must exist to maintain the balance in expressed copy number (gene dosage) of these genes in males (with a single X chromosome) and females (with two X chromosomes).

The first insight into a mechanism that could explain correction of this potential imbalance came following the identification in 1949 of the X chromatin body (Barr body) in a proportion of cells in females (see Fig. 22–3). Subsequent studies showed that this X chromatin is derived from only one of the two X chromosomes in interphase nuclei of these somatic cells.[36] Grumbach and colleagues showed that the X chromosome giving rise to X chromatin completes DNA synthesis later than any other chromosome. These findings led to the concept that only one X chromosome is genetically active during interphase, whereas the other X chromosome is heterochromatinized and relatively inactive. This change in activation state occurs in early gestation in humans (12 to 18 days, late blastocyte stage) and is a multistep process leading to stable and epigenetic silencing of genes on all X chromosomes in excess of one ("the Lyon hypothesis").[37] However, female germ cells beyond the stage of oogonia are exempt from X inactivation, in keeping with the need for a second X chromosome for germ cell and ovarian development.

The process of X inactivation involves a number of important steps including (1) chromosome counting, (2) *random* selection of which X chromosome to inactivate (maternal or paternal), and (3) silencing—the initiation, establishment, and maintenance of X-inactivation. These complex molecular and cellular silencing processes involve DNA methylation, histone acetylation, and maintainence of inactivation by a noncoding RNA gene *XIST* located in the X-inactivating center and its antisense transcript Tsix (XIC, Xq13).[38,39] Once inactivation has occurred, the inactive state of that particular X chromosome is transmitted to all descendants of that cell, so that normal females effectively function as genetic mosaics insofar as X-linked traits are concerned. If the initial population of cells is small, "skewed" X-inactivation can occur as a chance event despite random inactivation. In such situations, heterozygous female carriers of an X-linked disorder may manifest symptoms of the condition. Indeed, recent evidence suggests that X-inactivation profiles exhibit extensive variability.[40] Furthermore, recent studies have proposed that some genes on the X chromosome in males and the active chromosome in females actually undergo a further process of up-regulation so that the ratio of sex chromosome/autosome expression is maintained.[39,41] In addition, a subset of genes on the X chromosome may be imprinted. The implications of these concepts for sex development are as yet unclear, although it is established that several X-chromosomal (e.g.,

DAX1) and autosomal (e.g. WNT4) genes have dose-dependent effects on gonad development.

It was hoped that studying families with ovarian failure or women with Turner's syndrome who have chromosomal variations, such as partial loss of X material, would lead to the loci for key genes involved in ovarian development and function.[42-44] Although several X-chromosomal loci and genes for premature ovarian failure (POF) have been identified (e.g., POF1, Xq26-q28, *FMR* premutations; POF2A, Xq22, *DIAPH2;* POF2B, Xq21, *POF1B [actin binding protein];* POF4, Xp11.2, *BMP15;* N.B. POF3, *FOXL2* is on 3q23),[45-51] and certain variants of Turner's syndrome are more likely to have ovarian dysfunction (e.g., isochromosome for Xq), it is likely that the accelerated oocyte atresia in Turner's syndrome is the result of impaired meiosis and subsequent germ cell apoptosis secondary to the sex chromosome imbalance, rather than simply loss of certain genetic loci containing ovarian development genes.[42]

Gonadal Sex

Gonadal sex refers to the development of the gonadal tissue as testis or ovary. The principle embryologic and morphologic changes involved in gonad development are shown in Figure 22–7 and in excellent reviews by Brennan[5] and by Wilhelm.[8]

The Bipotential Gonad

The primitive gonad arises from a condensation of the medioventral region of the urogenital ridge at approximately 4 to 5 weeks' gestation in humans (see Fig. 22–7). The primitive gonad separates from the adrenal primordium at around 5 weeks' gestation but remains bipotential ("indifferent") until about 40 days' gestation in humans. Thus, testes and ovaries are morphologically indistinguishable from each other until approximately 42 days (12-mm stage).

Several important genes are expressed in the developing urogenital ridge, which facilitate formation of the bipotential gonad (e.g., *Emx2, Lim1, Lhx9, M33, Pod1, Gata4*) (Fig. 22–8). Deletion of these genes causes gonadal dysgenesis in mice, but human mutations associated with DSD phenotypes have not yet been described.

Emx2 is a mouse homologue of the *Drosophila* empty spiracles (*Ems*) gene involved in head morphogenesis. It is expressed early in the development of the urogenital system, so *Emx2* null mice have absent kidneys, ureters, gonads, and genital tracts as well as developmental abnormalities of the brain.[52] Although heterozygous mutations in *EMX2* have been found in patients with schizencephaly (without gonadal dysgenesis), mutations causing a gonadal phenotype in humans have not yet been reported.[53]

The homeobox gene *Lhx1* (*Lim1*) is expressed in the intermediate mesoderm and nephrogenic cords. Targeted deletion of this gene in mice results in a failure to develop kidneys, gonads, and anterior brain structures.[54] Human *LIM1* mutations have not yet been described although the expected phenotype would be quite severe. The related homeobox gene *Lhx9* is also expressed in the brain, limb buds, and urogenital ridge, but deletion of this gene in mice leads to gonadal dysgenesis alone.[55] No human *LHX9* mutations have been identified to date, despite a study of 41 patients with 46,XY gonadal dysgenesis.[56]

Other genes implicated in early gonad development are *M33, Pod1* and *GATA4.*[57-59] *M33* is the mouse homologue of the *Drosophila* polycomb genes, which may play a role in chromatin modification and gene silencing. Deletion of this gene in mice causes impaired 46,XY sex development through effects early in the sex development pathway.[57] *Pod1* encodes a basic helix-loop-helix transcription factor that appears to be essential for gonad development in both sexes.[58] *Gata4* (and its co-factor, *Fog2*) encodes a transcriptional regulator involved in early gonadal and cardiac development. Mice with deletion of these genes have cardiac defects and variable gonadal phenotypes.[59]

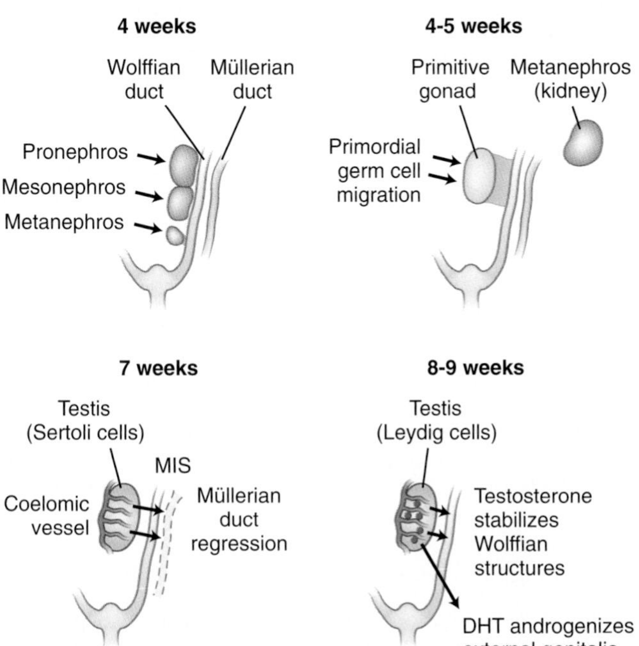

Figure 22–7 ▪ Schematic representation of the principal morphologic and functional events during early gonad/testis development in humans. *DHT,* dihydrotestosterone. (Modified with permission from Achermann JC, Jameson JL. Testis determination. Top Endocrinol 2003;22:10-14. © Chapterhouse Codex.)

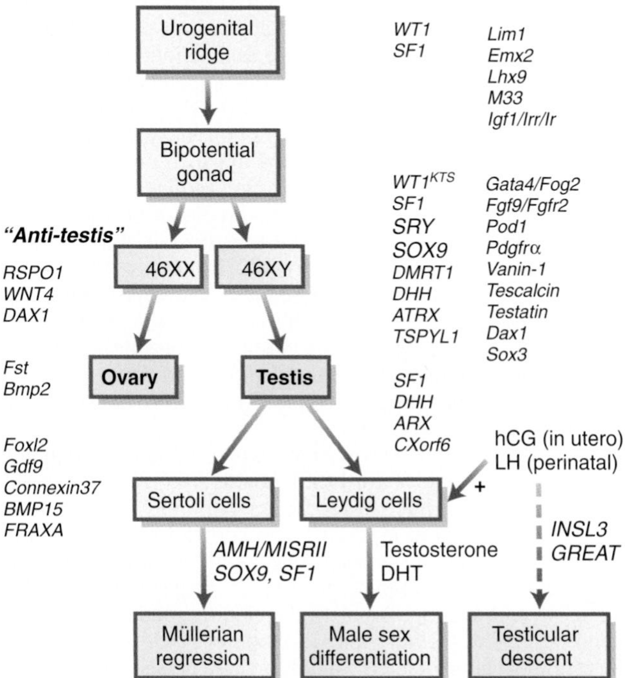

Figure 22–8 ▪ Overview of the major events involved in sex determination and sex differentiation. Mutations or deletions in the genes shown in upper case letters have been reported or proposed as causes of DSD or gonadal failure in humans. The genes and factors shown in lower case letters have been proposed to play an important role in sex development, largely from studies of mice.

Haploinsufficiency and point mutations in *GATA4* have been identified in patients with cardiac defects but no human mutations associated with gonadal dysgenesis have been reported to date. Finally, deletion of multiple components of the insulin signaling pathway (insulin receptor, insulin-related receptor and insulin-like growth factor 1 receptor) has recently been shown to have marked effects on the early stages of testis development and downstream *Sry* expression.[60] This work adds to the body of literature showing the importance of signaling factors in endocrine development, and highlights the concept of functional redundancy, in that the phenotype was only apparent when all three receptor types were deleted simultaneously.

The role of transcription factors such as Wilms' tumor–related gene-1 (WT1) and steroidogenic factor-1 (SF1) in early gonad development is better understood as mice models are well characterized and human mutations in these genes have been found in patients with impaired gonad development (see *46,XY DSD*) (see Fig. 22–8).

WT1 (11p13) is a four-zinc finger transcription factor expressed in the developing genital ridge, kidney, gonads, and mesothelium.[61-62] Homozygous deletion of the gene encoding *Wt1* in mice prevents gonad and kidney development.[63] The WT1 protein is subject to complex posttranslational modification and splicing processes, and it is believed that at least 24 WT1 isoforms exist.[64,65] The most common variants include (1) an isoform with alternative splicing of exon 5 and insertion of an additional 17 amino acids in the middle of the protein and (2) the use of an alternative splice donor site for exon 9 resulting in addition of three amino acids (lysine-threonine-serine, "+KTS") between zinc finger 3 and 4. It is believed that the +KTS and −KTS isoforms have different cellular function and differential effects on gonad and renal development.[66-67] Thus, the ratio of +KTS:−KTS isoforms may be important. Whilst some insight into the roles of different isoforms of WT1 is being obtained from transgenic mice,[67] the overall role of WT1 in cellular biology is complex and incompletely understood.

In humans, WT1 transcripts can be detected in the indifferent gonadal ridge when it first forms at 32 days postovulation.[68] Deletions or mutations of WT1 cause well-defined syndromes in humans. Haploinsufficiency of WT1 due to deletion of the chromosomal locus containing *WT1* and *PAX6* (11p13) causes WAGR syndrome (*W*ilms tumor, *a*niridia, *g*enitourinary abnormalities, and mental *r*etardation).[69] Dominant negative point mutations in WT1 cause Denys-Drash syndrome (gonadal dysgenesis, genital ambiguity, nephropathy, and predisposition to Wilms' tumor),[70] whereas mutations in the exon 9 splice site of *WT1,* causing an altered ratio of +KTS to −KTS isoforms of WT1, result in Frasier syndrome (gonadal dysgenesis, late-onset nephropathy, and predisposition to gonadoblastoma) (see *46,XY DSD* and Fig. 22–20).[71,72] Although these isoforms may play different roles in regulating various stages of renal and gonad development, it is likely that significant phenotypic overlap in these latter two conditions exists.[73]

Another key transcription factor expressed in the urogenital ridge is steroidogenic factor-1 (SF1/Ad4BP, *NR5A1*) (9q33).[74] SF1 is a member of the nuclear receptor superfamily that regulates the transcription of at least 30 genes known to be involved in gonadal development, adrenal development, steroidogenesis, and reproduction. Complete deletion of the gene encoding Sf1 in mice results in apoptosis of the developing gonad and adrenal gland during early embryonic development.[75] Other features of these homozygous-deleted animals include persistent müllerian structures and impaired androgenization in XY animals, hypogonadotropic hypogonadism, abnormalities of the ventromedial hypothalamus, and late-onset obesity in adult animals rescued by adrenal transplantation.[76,77] Heterozygous animals have reduced gonadal size and impaired adrenal stress responses.[78,79]

SF1 is expressed during the early stages of urogenital ridge formation in humans (32 days postovulation) where it is involved in maintaining gonadal integrity and permitting testicular differentiation.[68] Consistent with the mouse phenotype, heterozygous or homozygous loss of function mutations has been described in two patients with primary adrenal failure, severe 46,XY gonadal dysgenesis, and persistent müllerian structures (see *46,XY DSD*).[80,81] Furthermore, haploinsufficiency of SF1 is emerging as a relatively frequent cause of 46,XY DSD. Data in mice suggest that SF1 plays a critical role in testis development, and SF1 may regulate downstream targets such as *SRY* and *SOX9.*[82] In contrast, SF1 may play a less significant role in the ovary compared to the testis. Data to support this hypothesis include the relatively mild ovarian phenotype following targeted deletion of Sf1 in the ovary of mice,[83] the report of apparently normal ovarian development in a girl with adrenal failure due to a heterozygous SF1 mutation,[84] and the transmission of heterozygous Sf1 mutations from normal mothers to 46,XY children with impaired androgenization in a sex-limited dominant fashion (see 46,XY DSD).[85]

In addition to the single gene defects outlined above, a number of chromosomal duplications or deletions have been reported in association with impaired gonad development in patients. Thus, dosage-sensitive overexpression or underexpression of key factors in these regions may interfere with normal sex development. For example, duplication of a region of the X chromosome (Xp21, *dosage-sensitive sex-reversal*) containing the gene *DAX1* (*NR0B1*) has been reported in a small number of 46,XY patients with impaired testicular development or ovotestes.[86] These reports suggested that the orphan nuclear receptor DAX1 could act to antagonize testis development as an "anti-testis" gene. This concept has been supported by in vitro studies showing that DAX1 can repress SF1 transactivation and from studies in mice where overexpression of *Dax1* causes impaired male development in the presence of a "weakened" *Sry* locus (*Poshiavinus*).[87] However, targeted deletion of *Dax1* in a similar mouse strain also causes impaired testis development or ovotestis, and patients with X-linked adrenal hypoplasia congenita (due to mutations in *DAX1*) have abnormal testis architecture and infertility, suggesting that critical doses of these factors have important roles; both underactivity or overactivity could have deleterious effects at different stages of gonadal development.[88]

Impaired gonadal development has also been described in a 46,XY individual with duplication of 1p35, which resulted in overexpression of the signaling molecule WNT4.[89] This observation is consistent with the results of DAX1 overexpression, and DAX1 may be a functional target of the WNT4 signaling pathway. However, the duplicated locus in this patient likely contained other important genes, such as *RSPO1,* so the phenotype may have been influenced by altered expression dosages of several factors.

In addition to these regions of genomic duplication, more than 30 chromosomal rearrangements and deletions have been described in individuals with reproductive disorders. The most frequent ones associated with abnormalities of testis development (9p24, 10q25-qter, Xq13 or 16p13.3-pter) are considered below.

Primordial Germ Cell (PGC) Migration

Primordial germ cells are the embryonic precursors of gametes (spermatocytes or ova). Surprisingly, in all species, primordial germ cells arise some distance from the developing gonad, and undergo a process of migration during the early stages of embryogenesis.[90,91] In humans, PGCs arise from pluripotent epiblast cells and are initially located in the 24-day embryo in a region of the dorsal endoderm of the yolk sac close to the allantoic evagination (see Fig. 22–7). Following mitotic division, PGCs migrate into the primitive gonad between 4 and 5 weeks' gestation, under the influence of signaling molecules, receptors, and extracellular matrix proteins, such as c-KIT, Steel, β1-integrin, E-cadherin, and IFITM1/3.[91,92] Gonadal colonization is mediated by SDF1 and its receptor CXCR4.[93]

In the first few months of gestation, PGCs undergo multiple cycles of mitotic division. In the testis, a "self-renewable" population of germ cells exists. These undifferentiated PGCs are maintained by factors such as OCT4, whereas Plzf is required in adult male germ cells for stem cell self-renewal.[94] Most PGCs commit to differentiation, following the expression of signaling molecules and transcription factors such as Pog. After several cycles of mitotic division, these cells enter mitotic arrest.[95] Subsequent testicular development can occur in the absence of this germ cell population.[96] Meiosis only occurs during the progress of spermatogenesis during puberty (see Chapter 18).

In the developing ovary, primordial ova (oogonia) undergo mitotic expansion in the first few months of gestation (5 to 24 weeks) followed by meiotic division (8 to 36 weeks) and a process of meiotic arrest (ooctyes).[95] Although it was originally thought that entry into meiosis occurred autonomously, recent data suggest that retinoic acid signaling from the mesonephros may stimulate this process.[97,98] Male germ cells may be protected from this signal by virtue of their location within the testis cord and by Sertoli cell expression of CYP26B1, which breaks down retinoic acid. Meiotic arrest occurs in the first prophase when the chromatids of homologous pairs have begun to separate but are fixed by chiasmata (diplotene stage) and is maintained by Gpr3 (see also Chapter 16).[99] The presence of these primordial germ cells and subsequent meiotic oocytes is critical for differentiation of prefollicular cells into follicular cells, and for the maintaining ovarian development.

More than 6 million oogonia and prophase oocytes exist in the developing ovary around 16 weeks of gestation, and formation of oogonia from primordial germ cells ceases by 7 months' gestation. At this stage, some oocytes remain in undifferentiated nests whereas others associate with somatic pregranulosa cells to form primitive or primordial follicles. However, approximately 80% of oogonia fail to form follicles and undergo apoptosis, so that only 1 million germ cells are present in the ovary at the time of birth. These "resting" primordial follicles can remain in this stage of development throughout the woman's reproductive life, and meiosis only progresses in response to ovulation of the graafian follicle (approximately 400 in a woman's reproductive lifetime). It was widely held that the population of germ cells present at birth represents a "fixed pool" that gradually reduces with time through apoptosis (and ovulation). However, this view has been challenged recently by reports of a potential self-renewable population of germline stem cells in the mouse ovary that are active into adult life or by potential repopulation of the ovary by germ cells from bone marrow.[16] Whether such mechanisms exist in primates is currently the subject of much debate.[100]

Testis Determination

Testis determination is an active process that begins around 6 weeks' gestation in humans and consists of several distinct genetic and morphologic events.[5,8] One of the first and most significant events in testis determination is a transient wave of SRY expression through the undifferentiated gonad. Data from several species indicate that Sry expression must reach a certain threshold within a definite time window for testis development to occur.[8,101,102] Initially, this expression occurs centrally, then in cells located at the cranial and caudal poles.

In humans, *SRY* is a single exon gene (Yp11.3) that encodes a 204 amino acid high mobility group (HMG)-box transcription factor.[28,82] Mutations and deletions in *SRY* tend to cluster within the region encoding the HMG box and have been reported in approximately 10% to 15% of patients with sporadic or familial 46,XY gonadal dysgenesis (see *46,XY DSD* and Fig. 22–21).[29,32,82] As described above, translocation or transgenic expression of Sry is sufficient to induce testis development in XX patients and mice (see Y chromosome) (see Fig. 22–6).[31]

In humans, SRY is first detected in the XY gonad at approximately 41 days' gestation, just before differentiation of the bipotential gonad into a testis.[103] Expression levels peak at day 44 when testicular cords are first visible but, unlike in the mouse, SRY expression does not switch off completely in humans. Rather, low-level SRY expression is confined to Sertoli cells (day 52) where it persists into adulthood.

The HMG box of human SRY is a 79 amino acid structure that has moderate homology with Sry in other species (approximately 70%) as well as with the HMG box of related SOX (*S*RY-like HMG b*ox*) proteins (60%) (see *46,XY DSD* and Fig. 22–21).[82] The HMG box consists of three α-helices, which are able to adopt an "L" or boomerang-shaped configuration (see Fig. 22–6). The HMG box binds to variations on specific response elements (AACAAT/A) in the minor groove of DNA and induces a 40- to 85-degree structural bend in its target, depending on the sequence. The precise function of protein-directed DNA bending is not known, although this interaction results in minor groove expansion, DNA unwinding, and altered base stacking.[82,104-106] These effects likely alter DNA architecture in chromatin and may permit the interaction of other protein complexes with the DNA, resulting in activation or repression. Other important domains in SRY are two nuclear localization signals that can interact with calmodulin and importin β to regulate cellular localization[107]; several serine residues in the amino-terminus of SRY that can undergo phosphorylation and influence DNA binding[108]; and a carboxyl terminal seven amino acid motif that interacts with PDZ domains of SiP1 (SRY-interacting protein 1).[109] This interacting protein is thought to be important for SRY function in humans, as it may replace the function of the long carboxyl terminal glutamate-rich repeat domain (285 amino acid) of *Sry* found in mice. Human SRY lacks a classic transactivation domain; most human mutations in SRY interfere with DNA-binding or nuclear localization.[82,105,110-112]

SRY expression is believed to "switch" the fate of the progenitor cells into pre-Sertoli cells; elegant studies of chimeric XX-XY gonads have shown that most Sertoli cells are XY derived.[113] These SRY-positive cells can signal to other cell lineages to induce male-specific differentiation.[8,114-116] The onset of SRY expression is followed by marked cellular proliferation and the migration of mesonephric cells into developing testis (Fig. 22–9).[117-119] These mesonephric cells are thought to differentiate into Leydig, endothelial and peritubular myoid cells, depending on their interactions with somatic cells in the gonad. However, although SRY was shown convincingly to be the primary Y-testis determining gene more than 15 years ago, relatively little is known about the regulation of SRY expression. Some studies have shown that SF1, WT1 and Sp1 can all regulate SRY promoter activity *in vitro,* but the exact mechanisms that turn on SRY in vivo are unclear.[120] Furthermore, most of the downstream targets of SRY remain elusive. Indeed, it is still unclear whether SRY acts primarily as an activator of gene transcription, a repressor, or both.[82] Various hypotheses have proposed that Sry might disrupt binding and function of a repressor, resulting in downstream up-regulation of key genes such as SOX9, FGF9 or DHH.[121]

SOX9 is an SRY-related HMG box factor (3 exons, 509 amino acids) that shows up-regulation and nuclear localization in the developing male gonad shortly after the initial wave of SRY expression.[103,122-125] In humans, SOX9 becomes strongly localized to the developing sex cords (44 to 52 days postovulation) and is expressed in Sertoli cells thereafter.[103] SOX9 is also expressed in the developing cartilage under the regulation of PTHRP/Indian

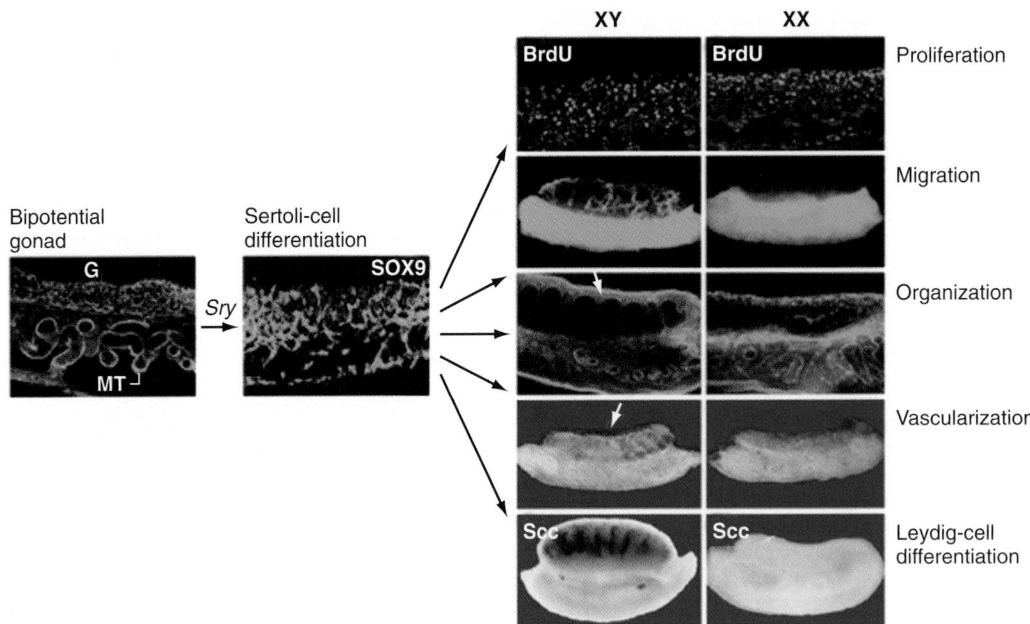

Figure 22–9 ▪ Key morphologic changes in the developing testis in mice. No morphologic differences between the XY and XX gonad are seen during the bipotential gonad stage (10.5 to 11.5 days postcoitum [dpc]) *(far left panel)*. In XY gonads, Sry expression is followed by expression and nuclear localization of Sox9 (blue) in pre-Sertoli cells *(second panel)*, resulting in Sertoli-cell differentiation by 11.5 dpc (vasculature and germ cells are labeled with platelet endothelial cell adhesion molecule (PECAM) and appear green). Between 11.5 and 12.5 dpc, distinct changes occur in the XY gonad *(left column)*, which are not seen in the XX gonad *(right column)*. These changes include proliferation of coelomic epithelial cells (measured by BrdU incorporation; *red, arrow*); migration of cells from the mesonephros (shown by recombinant culture of a wild-type gonad and a mesonephros in which the cells express green fluorescent protein); structural organization of testis cords (detected by laminin deposition, green); male-specific vascularization (by light microscopy with blood cells indicated by an arrow); and Leydig cell differentiation (detected by mRNA in situhybdridization for the steroidogenic enzyme, P450scc). (Reproduced by permission from Macmillan Publishers Ltd: Brennan J, Capel B. One tissue, two fates: molecular genetic events that underlie testis versus ovary development. Nat Rev Genet 2004;5:509-521.)

hedgehog signaling pathways. Heterozygous mutations or deletions in SOX9 cause camptomelic dysplasia, a form of severe skeletal dysplasia associated with variable gonadal dysgenesis in approximately 75% of patients.[82,122,123] Mutations have been found in the HMG box of SOX9, but also in the carboxyl terminal transactivation domain and in a region that interacts with heat-shock proteins (HSP70) (see 46,XY DSD and Fig. 22–21).[82,126,127]

Although SOX9 expression is a potential target of SRY, an important body of evidence has emerged to show that SOX9 is a "testis-determining factor" in its own right. In addition to the loss-of-function mutations in SOX9 causing gonadal dysgenesis, overexpression of SOX9 due to mosaic duplication of the locus containing *SOX9* (17q24.3-q25.1) has been reported in a 46,XX individual with ambiguous genitalia.[128] Furthermore, transgenic expression of Sox9 in mice results in testis development in XX animals, and the XX *odsex* (*ods*) mouse develops as a male due to disruption of a regulatory element 1 MB upstream of Sox9 that causes testis-specific overexpression of the Sox9 during development.[129-131] Thus, the regulatory region of the SOX9 promoter is very large. In fact, breakpoints have been reported up to 350 kb from the start of the SOX9 gene in patients with camptomelic dysplasia and gonadal dysgenesis.

Around the time of SRY and SOX9 expression (and nuclear localization), the developing testis undergoes a series of distinct cellular and morphologic changes (see Fig. 22–9). Our current understanding of these processes has resulted largely from studies in mice.[5]

As outlined above, the first stage of testis development involves a proliferation of Sf1 positive somatic cells, resulting in an increase in Sertoli cell precursors and Sertoli cell differentiation. This process is influenced by growth factors, such as Fgf9 and the receptor Fgfr2.[132] These primitive Sertoli cells coalesce with peritubular myoid cells to form primary sex cords, which then condense to form primitive seminiferous cords at around 7 weeks' gestation in humans. Sex cord development is supported by a striking reorganization of the gonadal vasculature in the developing testis, but not the ovary (see Fig. 22–9).[5,133] These changes include the development of a discrete coelomic vessel, restriction of endothelial cells to the interstitial space between the sex cords, and increased branching of blood vessels. The development of these vascular systems is influenced by growth factor signaling systems, such as Pdgfrα, and can be repressed by the Wnt4/follistatin system.[134-136] These changes in vascular architectural play an important role in determining cellular patterning and organization in the developing testis, in supporting paracrine interactions, and in the export of androgens from the developing Leydig cells to the perineal and systemic circulation.

Although the expression of SRY plays a crucial role as a "testis-determining factor," it is becoming clear that many other factors are necessary for normal early testis development (see Fig. 22–8). Some of these factors may be expressed exclusively within the developing testis, whereas others may play a facilitative role in supporting gonad development and are expressed in other developing tissues too (e.g., brain).

Desert hedgehog (*DHH*) is a member of the hedgehog signaling pathway that is expressed in mouse embryonic Sertoli cells and interstitium, and plays a key role in the differentiation of peritubular myoid cells through its action on the *Patched* receptor.[137] The peritubular myoid cells are flat smooth-muscle–like cells that ensheath the testis cords and are necessary for cord development and structural integrity. Deletion of *Dhh* in the mouse leads to impaired differentiation of peritubular myoid cells and Leydig cells, and to impaired androgenization in males.[138,139] In humans, *DHH* mutations have been reported in patients with impaired testicular development, with or without minifascicular neuropathy.[140]

DMRT1 (*double sex, mab3, related transcription factor 1*) (9p24.3) encodes a 373 amino acid protein, which is homologous to the sex-development *double sex* gene of *Drosophila* and *mab3* gene of *Caenorhabitus elegans*. *DMRT1* shows a male-specific pattern expression in the developing genital ridge and is expressed in the developing Sertoli cells by 7 weeks' gestation.[141,142] Deletion of *dmrt1* in the mouse results in normal androgenization but regression of testes later in embryonic development.[143] No specific point mutations in *DMRT1* have been described in humans, but impaired gonadal development and 46,XY DSD are well established features of the 9p deletion syndrome, suggesting that haploinsufficiency of the *DMRT* locus may be a cause of testicular dysgenesis in humans.[144]

ARX (*aristaless-related homeobox, X-linked*) encodes a transcription factor that regulates neuronal migration and brain development as well as Leydig cell development. Deletion of *Arx* in the mouse causes abnormal neuronal development and a block in Leydig cell differentiation.[145] Mutations in *ARX* in humans cause X-linked lissencephaly and ambiguous genitalia (XLAG).[145] In addition, signaling through PDGF and the PDGFRA has been shown to be important in fetal and adult Leydig cell differentiation following deletion of these genes in mice.[146,147]

Other genes proposed to play a role in early testis development have been identified following chromosome deletions or differential expression studies. For example, *tescalcin* encodes a calcium-binding protein that is expressed in the early mouse fetal testes and *testatin* encodes a cystatin-related gene expressed in the fetal gonads and adult testes.[148,149] *ATRX* (Xq13.3, also known as *XH2* and *XNP*) is a transcription factor deleted in the α-thalassemia mental retardation syndrome.[150,151] This syndrome includes a range of genital phenotypes from partial gonadal dysgenesis to micropenis. The locus containing *SOX8* is deleted in the ATR-16 (α-thalassemia mental retardation) syndrome affecting the tip of chromosome 16p,[152] and terminal deletions of chromosome 10 (10q25-qter) are frequently associated with urogenital abnormalities and sometimes complete gonadal dysgenesis.[153] Indeed, more than 50 syndromic conditions or human chromosomal rearrangements have now been reported in association with a range of urogenital phenotypes.[154] Furthermore, gene expression profiling in the embryonic mouse gonad is starting to reveal a host of expressed and differentially expressed genes involved in testicular and ovarian development (see below).

Ovarian Development

Ovarian development was believed to be a constitutive ("default") process for many years, as an external female phenotype occurs in the absence of gonadal tissue and müllerian structures persist in the absence of anti müllerian hormone (AMH; also known as müllerian inhibiting substance, MIS). Although the presence of primordial germ cells was known to be necessary to maintain ovarian integrity, it is emerging that ovarian development is an active process that requires expression of a set of specific genes, as well as factors necessary to actively prevent testis development.

A number of genes have now been implicated in ovarian and follicular development (FIGα, Dazla, Bmp8b, Smad5, connexin 37, Foxl2, and POF genes listed previously).[45-51,155,156] Furthermore, recent studies comparing gene expression profiles in the testes and ovaries of mice at critical stages of fetal development (e10.5 to e13.5) have shown that a specific subset of ovarian genes are "turned-on" soon after the onset of testis determination (e.g., follistatin, cyclin kinases inhibitors) (Fig. 22–10).[13,14] It is unclear whether any ovarian *determining* genes exist or whether these factors play a role in maintaining ovarian development in the absence of testis-determining gene expression. However, it seems likely that certain active processes are involved, as many of the genes (e.g., Wnt4, RSPO1) may actually function, as do meiotic germ cells, to antagonize testis development.[15,157,158,159]

Phenotypic (or Anatomic) Sex

The developing gonad produces several steroid and peptide hormones that mediate sexual differentiation and result in the phenotypic sex seen at birth. Alfred Jost first showed the importance of fetal testicular androgens in this process in 1947.[12] In his classic experiments, Jost demonstrated that surgical removal of the gonads during embryonic development of the rabbit resulted in development of female reproductive characteristics, regardless of chromosomal sex of the embryo.

Male Sexual Differentiation

Sertoli Cells and Müllerian Regression

Sertoli cells play a key role in supporting germ cell survival and produce two important peptide hormones, anti müllerian hormone (AMH; also known as müllerian inhibiting substance, MIS), and inhibin B. AMH/MIS is a member of the TGF-β superfamily and is first secreted in humans from around 7 weeks' gestation under the regulation of key transcription factors such as SOX9, SF1, WT1, and GATA4 (see Figs. 22–1 and 22–7).[160,161] AMH/MIS, a glycoprotein homodimer, causes regression of müllerian structures (fallopian tubes, uterus, upper two thirds of the vagina) by its paracrine action on the AMH type II receptor (AMH2R; MIS type II receptor, MISIIR). The AMH type II receptor forms a serine/threonine kinase heterodimeric receptor complex with ALK2 to induce apoptosis through secondary paracrine signals, such as matrix metalloproteinase 2 (MMP2).[161,162] Müllerian structures appear to be maximally sensitive to AMH/MIS between 9 and 12 weeks' gestation, a time when the developing testis produces peak concentrations of AMH/MIS but before the onset of significant AMH/MIS production by the developing ovary. Consequently, boys with mutations in either AMH/MIS or the AMH type II receptor gene can present with persistent müllerian duct syndrome (PMDS) and undescended testes, but otherwise normal external genitalia. In contrast, severe forms of 46,XY gonadal dysgenesis can result in persistent müllerian structures due to impaired Sertoli cell development and AMH/MIS release. In some cases, a hemiuterus will be present if testicular development is more severely affected on that side, but it is likely that androgenization of the external genitalia will also be impaired. Notably, defects confined to Leydig cell steroidogenesis in 46,XY DSD will not be associated with persistent müllerian structures in that Sertoli cell production of AMH/MIS is unaffected. In normal boys, a small müllerian remnant can sometimes persist as a testicular appendage. Inhibin B suppresses pituitary FSH activity, but its local role during testis development is less clear. Furthermore, it is emerging that both AMH/MIS and inhibin B may have important functions throughout life at multiple levels of the HPG axis (see later).[163]

Fetal Leydig Cells and Steroidogenesis

Fetal Leydig cells develop within the interstitium of the developing testis and secrete androgens by 8 to 9 weeks' gestation (see Fig. 22–1).[164] Human chorionic gonadotropin/luteinizing hormone (hCG/LH) receptors are only present on the Leydig

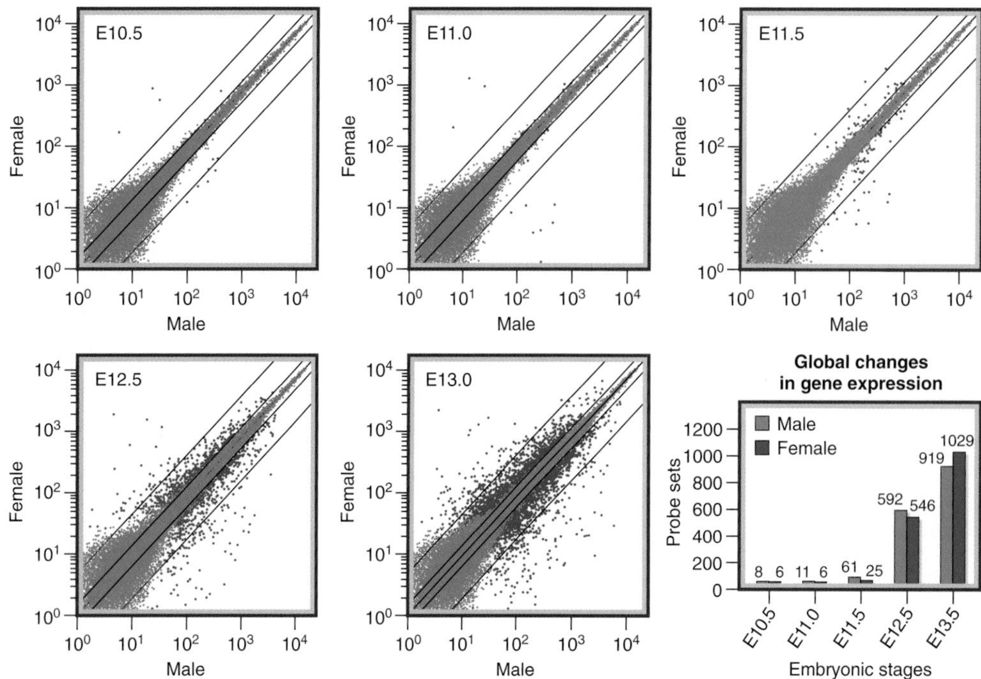

Figure 22–10 ▪ Scatterplot of global differences in gene expression during gonad development in the male and female mouse between e10.5 and e13.5 (log2-scaled expression signals). Blue dots represent genes with statistically similar expression levels. Red dots represent genes whose expression profiles were found to be sexually dimorphic (>1.5-fold, black diagonal lines). These data reveal a distinct complement of gene expression in the ovary as well as the testis during these critical periods of organogenesis. (Reproduced from Nef S, Schaad O, Stallings NR, et al. Gene expression during sex determination reveals a robust female genetic program at the onset of ovarian development. Dev Biol 2005;287:361-377.)

cells from around 10 to 12 weeks' gestation, suggesting that the initial secretion of testosterone is independent of hCG and fetal LH. A massive expansion in fetal Leydig cells occurs between 14 and 18 weeks' gestation, resulting in marked increase in testosterone secretion around 16 weeks.[165,166] Fetal Leydig cell steroidogenesis is stimulated by placental hCG during the first two trimesters of pregnancy, but the developing hypothalamic-gonadotrope system produces significant amounts of luteinizing hormone from around 20 weeks' gestation.[167]

The pathways of testicular steroidogenesis are shown in Figure 22–11. The role of individual enzymes is discussed in detail in relation to individual steroidogenic defects (see Disorders of Sex Development) and in several excellent reviews.[168] In brief, cholesterol is taken up into Leydig cells via LDL or HDL receptors, or is generated de novo by cholesterol synthesis pathways or from cholesterol ester. Stimulation of the hCG/LH receptor by the appropriate glycoprotein hormone increases the ability of steroidogenic acute regulatory protein (StAR) to facili-ate movement of cholesterol from the outer to inner mitochondrial membrane. The first and rate-limiting step in steroid hormone synthesis involves three distinct reactions: 20α-hydroxylation, 22-hydroxylation, and cleavage of the cholesterol side-chain to generate pregnenolone and isocaproic acid. These steps are catalyzed by a single enzyme, P450scc (*CYP11A1*). Pregnenolone can either be converted to progesterone by the microsomal enzyme 3β-hydroxysteroid dehydrogenase type 2 (Δ5→Δ4 isomerase) (*HSD3B2*), or undergoes 17α-hydroxylation by P450c17 (*CYP17*) to yield 17-hydroxypregnenolone. P450c17 also has 17,20-lyase activity, which can cleave the C17,20 carbon bond of 17-hydroxypregnenolone to generate dehydroepiandrosterone (DHEA). This 17,20-lyase activity is favored by the presence of Δ5 substrates, redox partners such as P450 oxidoreductase and cytochrome b5, and serine phosphorylation. These reactions are facilitated by the relative abundance of these factors in the Leydig cell in humans, so that the main pathway to androgen production is through conversion of 17-hydroxypregnenolone to DHEA rather than through conversion of 17-hydroxyprogesterone to androstenedione.[169] Subsequent testosterone production can occur through conversion of DHEA to androstenedione (by 3β-hydroxysteroid dehydrogenase type 2), followed by the actions of 17β-hydroxysteroid dehydrogenase type 3 (*HSD17B3*) to generate testosterone, or via the intermediate metabolite androstenediol (see Fig. 22–11). During male sex development, testosterone undergoes local conversion to dihydrotestosterone (DHT) by 5α-reductase type 2. Dihydrotestosterone has high-affinity action on the androgen receptor to result in androgenization of the external genitalia. Recent studies based on the phenotype of patients with P450 oxidoreductase deficiency and the fetal Tamar Wallaby have proposed that an alternative pathway to DHT production might also exist in the human fetal testis (see 46,XYDSD, P450 oxidoreductase).[170,171]

Local production of testosterone is believed to be necessary for stabilization of wolffian structures such as the epididymides, vasa deferentia, and seminal vesicles, whereas the potent metabolite dihydrotestosterone induces androgenization of the external genitalia and urogenital sinus (Fig. 22–12). In the male, the urogenital sinus develops into the prostate and prostatic urethra, the genital tubercle develops into the glans penis, the urogenital (urethral) folds fuse to form the shaft of the penis, and the urogenital (labioscrotal) swellings form the scrotum (Figs. 22–13 and 22–14). The distinction between a clitoris and a penis at this stage is based primarily on size and whether the labis minora fuse to form a corpus spongiosum. The effects of androgenization on the genital tubercle between 8 and 10 weeks' gestation has been shown recently by Goto et al (see Fig. 22–14).[172]

Both testosterone and DHT mediate their effects via the androgen receptor (AR) (Xq11-q12), which is a transcription

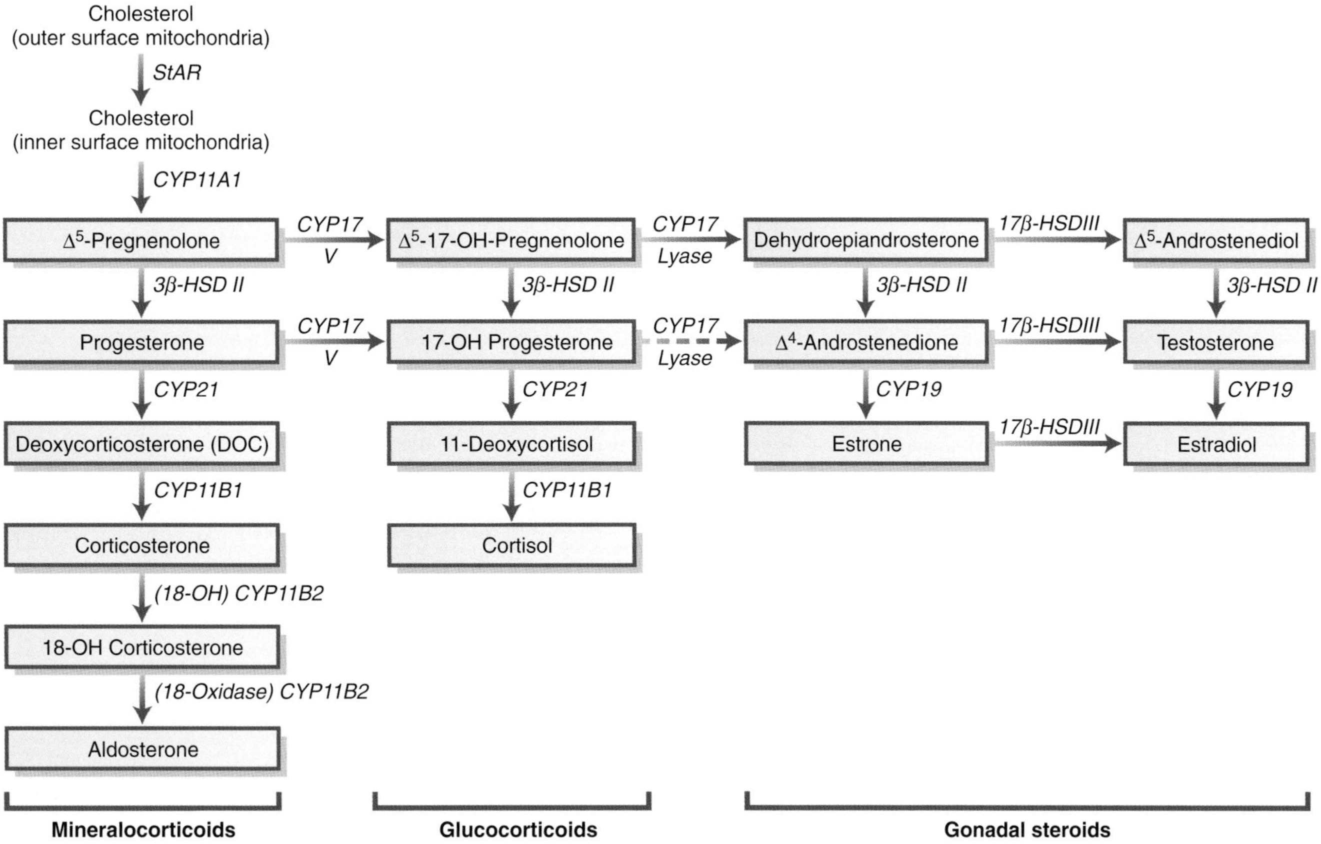

Cholesterol
(outer surface mitochondria)
↓ *StAR*
Cholesterol
(inner surface mitochondria)
↓ *CYP11A1*

Mineralocorticoids		Glucocorticoids		Gonadal steroids		
Δ^5-Pregnenolone	→ *CYP17 V* →	Δ^5-17-OH-Pregnenolone	→ *CYP17 Lyase* →	Dehydroepiandrosterone	→ *17β-HSDIII* →	Δ^5-Androstenediol
↓ *3β-HSD II*		↓ *3β-HSD II*		↓ *3β-HSD II*		↓ *3β-HSD II*
Progesterone	→ *CYP17 V* →	17-OH Progesterone	- - → *CYP17 Lyase* - - →	Δ^4-Androstenedione	→ *17β-HSDIII* →	Testosterone
↓ *CYP21*		↓ *CYP21*		↓ *CYP19*		↓ *CYP19*
Deoxycorticosterone (DOC)		11-Deoxycortisol		Estrone	→ *17β-HSDIII* →	Estradiol
↓ *CYP11B1*		↓ *CYP11B1*				
Corticosterone		Cortisol				
↓ *(18-OH) CYP11B2*						
18-OH Corticosterone						
↓ *(18-Oxidase) CYP11B2*						
Aldosterone						

Figure 22–11 ▪ Schematic diagram of the steroid biosynthetic pathways leading to androgen production in the testis. In humans, the main pathway to androgen production is through conversion of 17-hydroxypregnenolone to dehydroepiandrosterone (DHEA) rather than through conversion of 17-hydroxyprogesterone to androstenedione. Subsequent testosterone biosynthesis can occur through conversion of DHEA to androstenedione (by 3β-hydroxysteroid dehydrogenase type 2), followed by the actions of 17β-hydroxysteroid dehydrogenase type 3 to generate testosterone, or via the intermediate metabolite androstenediol. During male sex development, testosterone undergoes local conversion to dihydrotestosterone (DHT) by 5α-reductase type 2 (not shown). Dihydrotestosterone has high-affinity action on the androgen receptor to result in androgenization of the external genitalia. Recent studies based on the phenotype of patients with P450 oxidoreductase deficiency and the Tamer Wallaby have proposed that an alternative pathway to DHT production might also exist in the human fetal testis. The pathways responsible for mineralocorticoid and glucocorticoid synthesis are present in the adrenal gland.

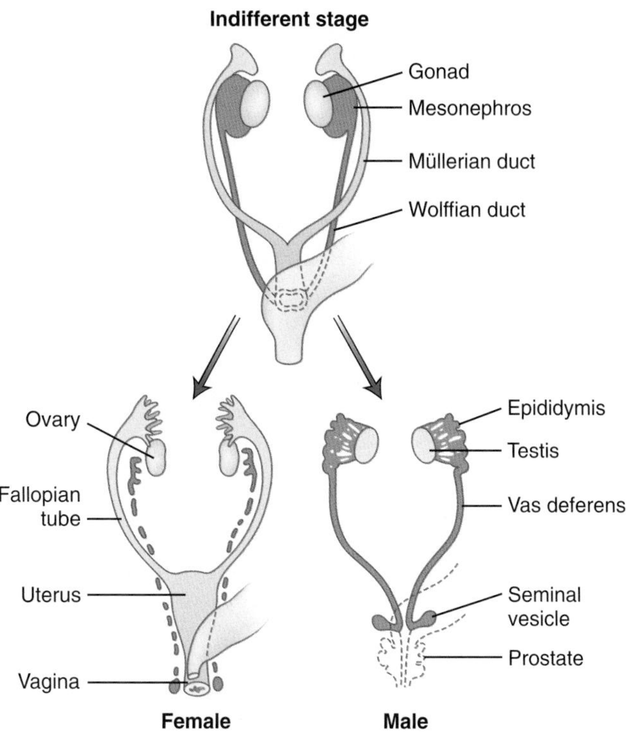

Figure 22–12 ▪ Embryonic differentiation of female and male genital ducts from wolffian and müllerian primordial, prior to descent of the testes into the scrotum. In females, müllerian structures persist to form the fallopian tubes, uterus, and upper portion of the vagina. The lower portion of the vagina and urethra are derived from the urogenital sinus. In males, wolffian structures develop into the epididymes, vasa deferentia, and seminal vesicles, whereas the prostate and prostatic urethra are derived from the urogenital sinus. In some cases, a small müllerian remnant can persist in males as a testicular appendage.

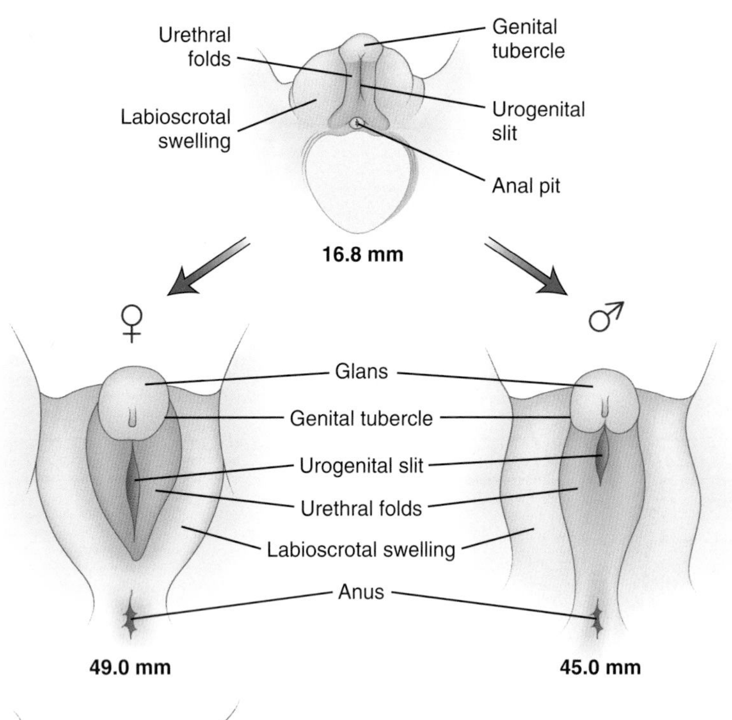

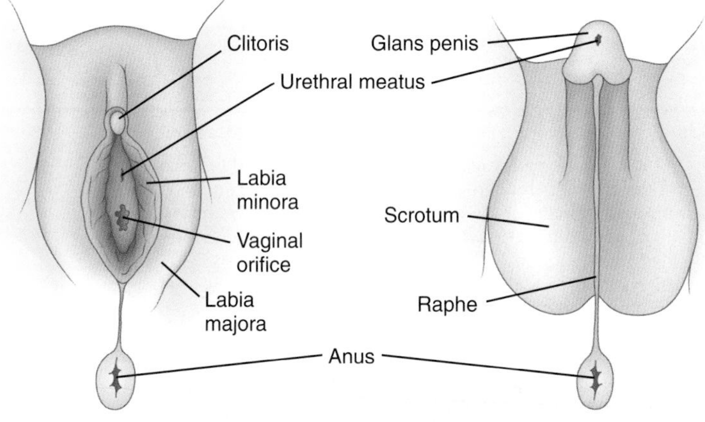

Figure 22–13 ▪ Differentiation of male and female external genitalia. (Adapted from Spaulding MH. The development of the external genitalia in the human embryo. Contrib Embryol Carnegie Inst 1921;13: 69-88.)

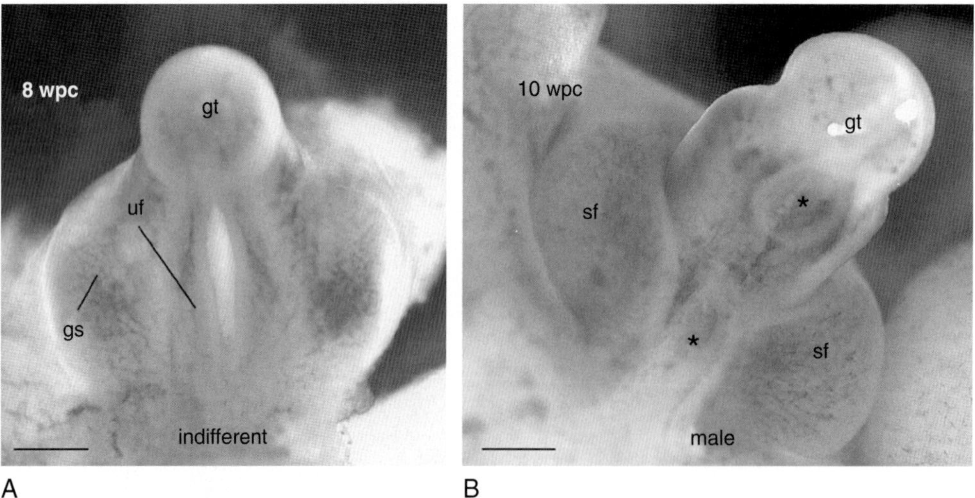

Figure 22–14 ▪ Differentiation of male external genitalia in humans between 8 and 10 weeks postconception (wpc). **A,** Undifferentiated human external genitalia at 8 wpc. **B,** Differentiation of scrotal folds and fusion of the urethral folds (asterisks mark patent regions, either side) at 10 wpc. *gs,* Genital swelling; *gt,* genital tubercle; *sf,* scrotal folds; *uf,* urethral folds. Scale bars: 500 μm. (Reproduced with permission of the American Society for Clinical Investigation from Goto M, Piper Hanley K, Marcos J, et al. In humans, early cortisol biosynthesis provides a mechanism to safeguard female sexual development. J Clin Invest 2006;116:872-874. Copyright 2006 by American Society for Clinical Investigation.)

factor (see 46,XY DSD, Androgen Action). Surprisingly little is known about AR targets, both in the developing wolffian structures (testosterone-responsive) as well as in the key target tissues (DHT-responsive). However, varying degrees of impaired androgen action are seen in a range of syndromic conditions, which may reflect defects in genes that mediate target-tissue responsiveness and genital tubercle growth (e.g., HOXA 10, HOXA13).[8] Indeed, recent studies in mice have revealed a number of factors necessary for development of the wolffian ducts (e.g., Gdf7, Bmps [4, 7, 8a, 8b], Hoxa10, Hoxa11), as well as for growth of the genital tubercle (Fgfs, Shh, Wnts, Hoxa13, Hoxd13, Bmp/noggin, ephrin signalling).[8]

Testis Descent

Testicular descent is a two-stage process that starts at around 12 weeks' gestation and is usually complete by the middle of the third trimester.[173] The initial *transabdominal* stage of testicular descent involves contraction and thickening of the gubernacular ligament. This stage is mediated by the testis itself, following secretion of factors such as insulin-like 3 (*INSL3,* relaxin-like factor) and its G-protein coupled receptor, GREAT (LGR8).[174] Other testicular factors are likely to be involved in testicular descent, in that most dysgenetic testes are intraabdominal. The subsequent *transinguinal* phase of testicular descent involves stimulation by androgens and LH.

Subsequent Testicular Development

During the second and third trimesters, the testes show several distinct morphologic changes, including a reduction in fetal Leydig cell mass, and elongation and coiling of seminiferous cords. There is no further significant development of germ cells during this time, and seminiferous cords do not canalize until later in childhood. Nevertheless, certain developmental insults can affect the testis at this stage. For example, "vanishing (absent) testis syndrome" likely represents a late fetal event in that boys with this condition have adequate virilization and no müllerian structures.

Female Sexual Differentiation

The processes of female sexual differentiation are less obvious than in the male and do not involve significant changes in the external genitalia. Müllerian structures persist to form the fallopian tubes, uterus and upper portion of the vagina (see Fig. 22–12). Normal uterine development occurs in the absence of the ovary, but is not a "passive" process as a host of factors are required for uterine development (e.g., Pax2, Lim1, Emx2, Wnt4/Lp, Hoxa13) and differentiation (e.g., Wnt7a, Hoxa10, Hoxa11, Hoxa13, progesterone and estrogen receptors).[175] The lack of local testosterone production leads to degeneration of wolffian structures. The urogenital sinus develops into the urethra and lower portion of the vagina, the genital tubercle develops into the clitoris, the urogenital (urethral) folds form the labia minora, and the urogenital (labioscrotal) swellings form the labia majora (see Figs. 22–12 and 22–13).

In contrast to the testis, the developing ovary does not express FSH and hCG/LH receptors until after 16 weeks' gestation. At around 20 weeks' gestation, plasma concentrations of FSH reach a peak and the first primary follicles are formed.[167] By 25 weeks' gestation, the ovary has developed definitive morphologic characteristics. Folliculogenesis can proceed and a few graafian follicles will have developed by the third trimester. However, the amount of estrogen secreted by the developing ovary is likely to be insignificant compared to placenta estrogen synthesis, and the ovary is believed to remain generally quiescent until activation at the time of puberty. Abnormalities in several factors (e.g., connexin 37, GDF9, FSH receptors, estrogen receptor β, progesterone receptor) can interfere with this early folliculogenesis.

Several conditions can affect female sexual development in utero. Exposure of the fetus to androgens results in androgenization of the external genitalia.[172] A uterus will be present, but usually the local testosterone concentration is not sufficient to stabilize wolffian structures as the androgens are usually adrenal in origin. Most frequently, androgenization of the 46,XX fetus is due to disorders of adrenal steroidogenesis (21-hydroxylase deficiency, 11β-hydroxylase deficiency, oxidoreductase deficiency) or due to the mild androgenic effects following conversion of excess DHEA in 3β-hydroxysteroid dehydrogenase deficiency type II (see 46,XX DSD). Rare causes of androgenization include aromatase deficiency, glucocorticoid resistance, and maternal virilizing tumors (e.g., luteoma of pregnancy). Exposure to certain chemical agents in pregnancy has also been proposed as a cause of fetal androgenization. Other developmental abnormalities of the female genital tract (e.g., Mayer-Rokitansky-Kuster-Hauser syndrome) are discussed in the section on 46,XX DSD.

Psychosexual Development

Psychosexual development is traditionally viewed as having a number of distinct components (Table 22–2). *Gender identity* refers to a person's self-representation or identification as male or female (with the caveat that some individuals may not identify exclusively with either). *Gender role* (sex-typical behaviors) describes the expression or portrayal of psychological characteristics that are sexually dimorphic within the general population, such as toy preferences and physical aggression. *Sexual orientation* refers to choice of sexual partner and erotic interest (heterosexual, bisexual, homosexual) and includes behavior, fantasies, and attractions.

The past 50 years has seen a number of opposing theories about the origins of psychosexual development, and debate about the relative contributions of chromosomes, hormones, brain structure, and societal and family influences on the various components outlined above. Much of this work has focused on the study of rodents as well as nonhuman primate species. For example, Young and colleagues first showed in 1959 that exposure of guinea pigs to testosterone during pregnancy resulted in altered mating behavior of female offspring.[176] Such effects may be most pronounced during a critical window of exposure and, in rodents, may be dependent in part on aromatization of these androgens to estrogens, as well as receptor availability and social environment.[177,178] More recently, interest has focussed on the role of genes and chromosomes on sex behavior. For example, studies of differential gene expression patterns in the developing mouse brain have shown upregulation of different X and Y chromosomal genes in early embryonic life, even before the onset of significant androgen secretion by the developing testis in males.[179] Furthermore, studies of mice where *Sry* had been deleted (XYSry-) or trans-

TABLE 22–2 OVERVIEW OF TERMINOLOGY IN GENDER-RELATED BEHAVIOR

Gender identity	Identification of sex as male or female
Gender role	Expression of sexually dimorphic behavior
	Aggression
	Parenting rehearsal
	Peer and group interactions
	Labeling (e.g., "tomboy")
	Grooming behavior
Sexual orientation	Choice of sexual partner

genically expressed (XXSry+) showed certain neuroanatomic differences between XY and XX mice independent of gonad development and endocrine status.[180,181] Taken together, these findings suggest that factors related to chromosome complement have at least the potential to affect psychosexual development independent of sex hormone action.

Understanding the complex issues related to human psychosexual development is much more challenging, especially as gender identity is a component of psychosexual development that cannot readily be assessed in nonhuman species. For many years, it was believed that gender identity would be concordant with assigned sex, provided that the child was raised unambiguously and appropriate surgical "correction" and hormone therapy were instituted concordant with the gender chosen. This theory assumed psychosexual neutrality at birth, but has been challenged in the past decade by a refocusing on the potential importance of prenatal (e.g., endocrine) and innate (e.g., chromosomal) influences on psychosexual development. Direct data to assess such effects in humans are limited but, for example, studies in women with complete androgen insensitivity syndrome (CAIS) would argue against a strong behavioral role for Y chromosome genes in human psychosexual development, as the karyotype is 46,XY but psychosexual development is female.[182,183]

In contrast, prenatal exposure to androgens does influence certain aspects of psychosexual development in humans.[184,185] Girls with congenital adrenal hyperplasia (CAH) who harbor more severe mutations and have more marked genital androgenization, are more likely to play more with boys' toys, with long-term effects evident into adulthood.[186,187] Prenatal androgen exposure can also be associated with other psychological characteristics such as sexual orientation. However, evidence for a strong association between prenatal androgens and *gender identity* does not exist.[188] Although gender dissatisfaction (unhappiness with assigned sex) is more common in individuals with DSD, more than 90% of 46,XX individuals with CAH who are assigned female gender in infancy actually identify as female.[189] Furthermore, the causes of gender dissatisfaction in general are poorly understood and are hard to predict from karyotype, prenatal androgen exposure, degree of genital virilization, or assigned gender.[190-192] Because gender identity, sex-typical behavior, and sexual orientation are separate components of psychosexual development, it is important to appreciate that homosexual orientation (relative to sex of rearing) or strong cross-sex interest in an individual with DSD is not necessarily an indication of incorrect gender assignment.[3]

Challenges in assessing gender identity in young children make it difficult to know when this is generally established, although this is thought to be between 18 and 36 months, and possibly younger.[193] Many of the reported sexually dimorphic differences in brain structures reported at puberty or in adulthood are not seen in early childhood, so are not useful at present for guiding gender assignment. [194,195] Potential plasticity in psychosexual development may exist, as evident from studies in some patients with conditions such as 5α-reductase deficiency who may change their gender role in adolescence. Thus, a better understanding of the processes of human psychosexual development, as well as the influences of different forms of DSD, is needed to help make early gender assignment decisions and to guide psychological support in the future.

Development of the Hypothalamic-Gonadotrope Axis in the Fetus

Fetal hypothalamic-gonadotrope development occurs from 6 weeks' gestation, in parallel with the processes of sex determination and sexual differentiation in humans. Pituitary gonadotropin release probably does not influence the gonad until around 20 weeks' gestation.[167] Detailed descriptions of the development of the neuroendocrine system and congenital disorders of the hypothalamic-pituitary axis are provided in Chapters 7 and 8, respectively. However, development of the hypothalamic-gonadotrope axis has some unique features, and abnormalities in this process can cause congenital forms of hypogonadotropic hypogonadism (HH).

Development and Migration of GnRH-Synthesizing Neurons

Embryonic development of the hypothalamic GnRH neurosecretory system is intimately related to development of the extracranial and intracranial olfactory apparatus and, in all species studied, the GnRH-synthesizing neurons originate *extracranially* before migrating to their final position in the fetal hypothalamus (Fig. 22–15).[196]

In humans, GnRH-synthesizing neurons first appear in the embryonic medial olfactory placode at around 6 weeks' gestation and begin to migrate along axons of the terminal vomeronasal nerve complex on an N-CAM–rich scaffold. At around 6.5 weeks' gestation, these migrating neurons pass through the primitive cribriform plate and penetrate the forebrain, medial and caudal to the developing olfactory bulbs. GnRH neurons then migrate posteriorly in the submeningeal space by the interhemispheric fissure, before proceeding laterally to reach their final position in the fetal mediobasal hypothalamus from around 14 weeks' gestation.[196] Fetal GnRH neuron migration is complete by around 19 weeks' gestation, by which stage pulsatile GnRH release is established.

A number of cell adhesion molecules and signaling factors have been implicated in this migratory process (e.g., anosmin-1/*KAL1*, FGFR1, NELF, AXL/GAS6), and GnRH neurons express different transcription factors at different stages of maturation. Furthermore, other neuroendocrine cells comigrate with GnRH-synthesizing neurons. Some of these cells synthesis neurotransmitters and hormones such as neuropeptide Y, leptin, corticotropin-releasing factor (CRF), and glutamate, factors that may interact with GnRH neurons along the migratory path or in their final position in the hypothalamus. The association of GnRH neuronal migration with development of the olfactory system explains the association of some forms of HH with anosmia (lack of a sense of smell) in Kallmann syndrome. This condition can be due to mutations in a number of different X-linked and autosomal genes (*KAL1,* FGFR1, NELF, PROK2, PROKR2), which are discussed in more detail in Chapter 24.[196-199]

GnRH Synthesis and Action

GnRH-synthesizing neurons are localized throughout the hypothalamus, with a concentration in the arcuate nucleus. GnRH is synthesized as a precursor polypeptide, which undergoes cleavage and enzymatic processing to form a mature ten amino-acid hormone that is stored in secretory granules. GnRH is released from neuronal projections at the medial eminence into the portal blood system in a pulsatile manner to stimulate GnRH receptors on the anterior pituitary gonadotropes. GnRH pulsatility is thought to be established in the second trimester and may be modulated at various stages of development by the G-protein–coupled receptor, GPR54, and its ligand kisspeptin, as well as a host of other neuroendocrine factors and regulators. No mutations in GnRH have been identified in humans, but congenital HH has been reported in patients with GnRH receptor mutations and in defects of GPR54.[200-201] HH can also occur in humans due to abnormalities in GnRH processing

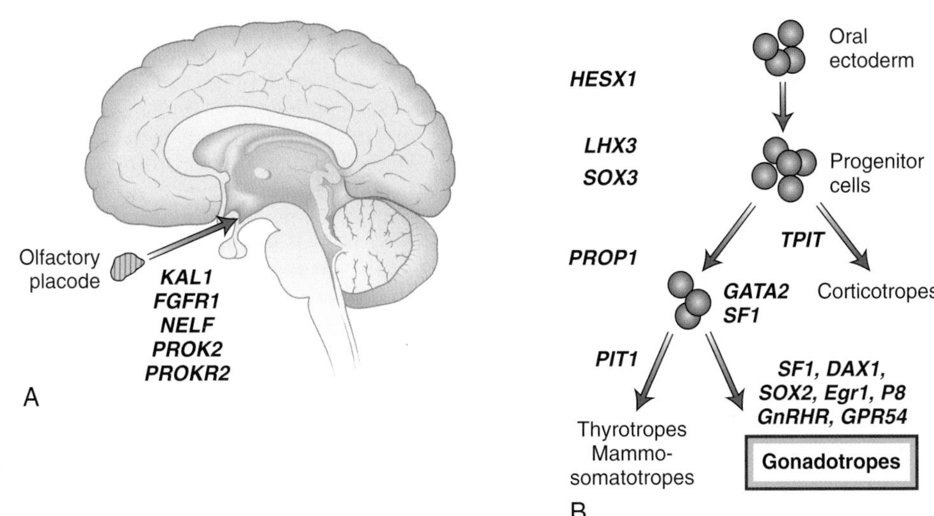

Figure 22–15 ■ Development of the hypothalamic-gonadotrope axis in humans. **A,** Migration of GnRH neurons from the olfactory placode to the fetal hypothalamus is facilitated by proteins such as anosmin-1 *(KAL1),* FGFR1, NELF, PROK2 and PROKR2. Defects in these factors have been reported in association with Kallmann syndrome (hypogonadotropic hypogonadism and anosmia). **B,** Differentiation of the anterior pituitary gland. The gradient of factors such as GATA2/SF1 and TPIT may provide a "switch" for gonadotrope differentiation. Variations in several transcription factors are associated with multiple pituitary hormone deficiency in humans (HESX1, LHX3, SOX3, PROP1). Mutations affecting isolated gonadotrope factors have not yet been described, except as part of complex phenotypes associated with mutations in SF1, DAX1, and SOX2. Defects in the GnRH receptor and GPR54 have also been reported in individuals with congenital hypogonadotropic hypogonadism.

(prohormone convertase-1, *PCSK1*) and leptin/leptin receptor signaling.

Pituitary Gonadotrope Development and Function

During development, cells destined to form the anterior pituitary arise within the oral ectoderm and Rathke's pouch, and undergo a process of differentiation into corticotropes, thyrotropes, mammosomatotropes, and gonadotropes (see Fig. 22–15). The mechanisms underlying these processes are discussed in Chapter 8. Developmental events that affect differentiation of early progenitor cells can cause congenital gonadotropin insufficiency as part of a multiple pituitary hormone deficiency. For example, mutations or variations in transcription factors such as HESX1, LHX3, SOX3, and PROP1 have all been associated with HH, although in some cases the onset of this is often delayed until adolescence (e.g., PROP1).

Differentiation of the gonadotropin cell line from other pituitary lineages may be controlled by gradient-dependent "switches" such as GATA2 and Tpit (TBX19).[202-203] A limited number of factors that appear to affect gonadotrope function have been identified, including SF1, DAX1, and SOX2. Patients with mutations in SF1 may have partial deficits in gonadotropin synthesis, but the phenotype is more complex because it involves gonadal dysgenesis too. Mutations in DAX1 cause X-linked adrenal hypoplasia congenita. HH is an established part of this condition, but only approximately 10% of boys with this condition have evidence of congenital gonadotropin insufficiency, and the HPG axis is usually intact in early postnatal life.[204] SOX2 mutations can cause congenital HH with developmental delay and microphthalmia.[205]

Gonadotropins

Fetal pituitary gonadotropin synthesis and release begins from around 14 weeks' gestation and peaks around 20 to 22 weeks' gestation.[167] Synthesis of these hormones is regulated by hypothalamic GnRH, downstream signaling mechanisms such as PACAP, and transcription factors such as SF-1, DAX-1, Pitx1, Egr-1 (LHβ), and p8 (LHβ).[206] The β subunits of these hormones undergo posttranslational modification and heterodimerize with a common α-subunit to form the mature glycoprotein hormones, FSH and LH.

The gonadotropin hormones are also influenced by inhibin, activin, and follistatin. Inhibin is a heterodimeric hormone consisting of a α-subunit bound to one of two distinct β-subunits, βA or βB. Inhibin A and inhibin B are produced by the gonads (predominantly ovarian granulosa cells and testicular Sertoli cells, respectively) and placenta, and suppress FSH. Activins stimulate FSH, and consist of homodimers or heterodimers of inhibin β-subunits (activin A, activin B, or activin AB). Follistatin binds activin to attenuate its action and reduce FSH release. These hormones are likely to function at a local (paracrine) level in the pituitary as well as having a systemic influence on gonadotropin release, and signal through TGFβ/Smad pathways.

Mutations in genes encoding the gonadotropin hormones, LH and FSH, have been described in a small number of patients with abnormalities of puberty or spermatogenesis, but severe congenital abnormalities associated with these conditions have not yet been described.[207] Of particular note, the two males with inactivating mutations of the LHβ subunit had descended testes and no evidence of hypospadias. These findings confirm the important role of placental hCG signaling through the LH/hCG receptor as the primary mediator of fetal Leydig cell androgen production.[208,209]

The Hypothalamic-Pituitary (Gonadotrope)-Gonadal Axis in Infancy and Childhood

At birth, the infant is removed from the influence of maternal and placental hormones and undergoes a series of distinct endocrine changes.

Postnatal Endocrine Changes in Boys

In the male, low concentrations of testosterone can be detected by standard assays at birth, but these fall in the first few days of life. Thereafter, a reactivation of the HPG axis occurs from around 6 weeks of age, which results in peaks of testosterone nearing mid-pubertal levels at between 2 and 3 months after birth (Fig. 22–16).[210,211] This peak of testosterone is associated with an acceleration in penile growth.[211] The HPG axis then becomes relatively quiescent by 4 to 6 months of age, until the onset of puberty in late childhood.

Inhibin B concentrations are high at birth and fall in the first 2 years of life before once again rising with the onset of puberty between 11 and 15 years (see Fig. 22–16).[212,213] In contrast, AMH/MIS concentrations remain high from birth through childhood, and decline to low concentrations with the onset of puberty (see Fig. 22–16).[160,214] Thus, AMH and inhibin B can be useful markers of active testicular tissue in boys with cryptorchidism, anorchia, and 46,XY DSD. Inls3 assays may provide a useful additional marker of testicular integrity in the future.

Postnatal Endocrine Changes in Girls

The early postnatal endocrine events in girls are less well understood. Placental estrogen exposure can result in breast development before birth, and a small episode of menstrual bleeding can occur several days after birth following withdrawal of estrogen and progesterone. It remains unclear whether girls have a discrete activation of the HPG axis in infancy. However, detectable concentrations of estradiol (5 to 20 pg/mL; 20 to 80 pmol/L), and inhibin B (50 to 200 pg/mL) can be measured in the first few months of life, and surprisingly high concentrations of FSH with marked interindividual variability can be found during infancy and early childhood (median 3.8 IU/L [1.2 to 18.8 IU/L, 2.5% to 97.5%] at 3 months of age in healthy, term girls).[215] Inhibin A has been proposed as a test of ovarian tissue in the newborn period in children with possible true hermaphroditism, but this hormone is below the limits of detection in many normal term newborn girls.

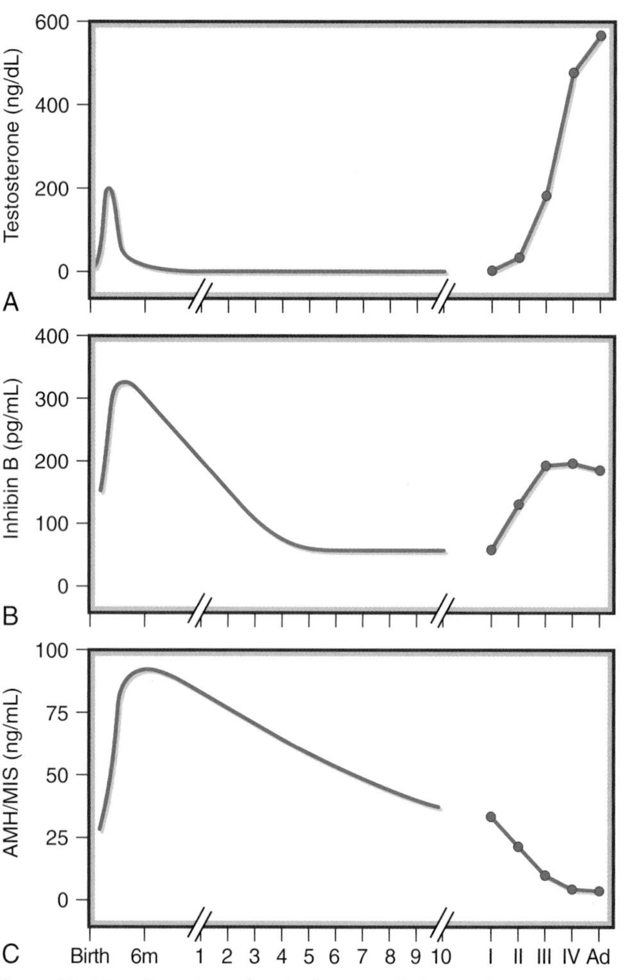

Figure 22–16 ▪ Overview of typical postnatal changes in testosterone, AMH, and inhibin B in normal males from birth to adulthood. Pubertal stages (I-IV) are indicated. (Conversions: testosterone, ng/dL ×0.0347 for nmol/L; AMH/MIS, ng/mL ×7.14 for pmol/L.)

DISORDERS OF SEX DEVELOPMENT

Introduction

Disorders of sex development (DSD) can have a wide range of presenting phenotypes depending on the underlying condition as well as its severity. Thus, individuals with these conditions can present to many different health care professions, including neonatologists, geneticists, urologists, gynecologists, or internists. For example, when an infant is born with ambiguous genitalia, the need for further investigation is usually clear. However, 46,XY individuals with complete 17α-hydroxylase/17,20-lyase deficiency may first present in early adolescence on account of hypertension and delayed puberty, or a young woman with complete androgen insensitivity syndrome (46,XY) may first present to a gynecologist with amenorrhea.

Significant progress in our understanding of the molecular basis of gonad development has also occurred within the past 20 years. Although several single gene disorders causing gonadal dysgenesis in humans have now been described, and many more candidate genes are emerging following studies in mice, the percentage of patients with disorders of gonad development who can be diagnosed at the molecular level remains disappointingly low (approximately 15% to 20%). Defining the exact basis of DSDs can have important implications for gender assignment, predicting response to treatment (e.g., androgen supplementation), assessing associated features (e.g., adrenal dysfunction) or the risk of tumorigenesis, and determining likely fertility options as well as long-term counseling for the individuals and their family. However, long-term outcome studies are often inadequate, and an evidence-based approach to management is not possible in many cases at present.

Nomenclature and Classification of Disorders of Sex Development

The proposal to change terminology by replacing *intersex* with the DSD acronym has led to a new classification for disorders of sex development.[3,4] DSD has been defined as "*congenital conditions in which development of chromosomal, gonadal, or anatomic sex is atypical.*" Such a definition is wide-ranging to cover conditions such as cloacal extrophy but sufficiently specific not to embrace, for example, disorders of puberty. The most common cause of ambiguous genitalia of the newborn, congenital adrenal hyperplasia, is classified as 46,XX DSD while the next most commont cause, partial androgen insensitivity syndrome, is classified as 46,XY DSD. Table 22–3 illustrates how such a classification system can be applied to DSD. The list is not exhaustive but provides a framework for the following discussion of the more common causes of DSD.

TABLE 22–3 AN EXAMPLE OF A DSD CLASSIFICATION

Sex Chromosome DSD	46,XY DSD	46,XX DSD
A: 47,XXY (Klinefelter's syndrome and variants) B: 45,X (Turner's syndrome and variants) C: 45,X/46,XY (mixed gonadal dysgenesis) D: 46,XX/46,XY (chimerism)	A: Disorders of gonadal (testis) development 1. Complete or partial gonadal dysgenesis (e.g., *SRY, SOX9, SF1, WT1, DHH, etc.*) 2. Ovotesticular DSD 3. Testis regression	A: Disorders of gonadal (ovary) development 1. Gonadal dysgenesis 2. Ovotesticular DSD 3. Testicular DSD (e.g., *SRY+, dup SOX9, RSPO1*)
	B: Disorders in androgen synthesis or action 1. Disorders of androgen synthesis LH receptor mutations Smith-Lemli-Opitz syndrome Steroidogenic acute regulatory protein mutations Cholesterol side chain cleavage (*CYP11A1*) 3β-hydroxysteroid dehydrogenase 2 (*HSD3B2*) 17α-hydroxylase/17,20-lyase (*CYP17*) P450 oxidoreductase (*POR*) 17β-hydroxysteroid dehydrogenase (*HSD17B3*) 5α-reductase 2 (*SRD5A2*) 2. Disorders of androgen action Androgen insensitivity syndrome Drugs and environmental modulators	B: Androgen excess 1. Fetal 3β-hydroxysteroid dehydrogenase 2 (*HSD3B2*) 21-hydroxylase (*CYP21A2*) P450 oxidoreductase (*POR*) 11β-hydroxylase (*CYP11B1*) Glucocorticoid receptor mutations 2. Fetoplacental Aromatase (*CYP19*) deficiency Oxidoreductase (*POR*) deficiency 3. Maternal Maternal virilizing tumors (e.g., luteomas) Androgenic drugs
	C: Other 1. Syndromic associations of male genital development (e.g. cloacal anomalies, Robinow, Aarskog, hand-foot-genital, popliteal pterygium) 2. Persistent müllerian duct syndrome 3. Vanishing testis syndrome 4. Isolated hypospadias (*CXorf6*) 5. Congenital hypogonadotropic hypogonadism 6. Cryptorchidism (*INSL3, GREAT*) 7. Environmental influences	C: Other 1. Syndromic associations (e.g. cloacal anomalies) 2. Müllerian agenesis/hypoplasia (e.g., MURCS) 3. Uterine abnormalities (e.g., MODY5) 4. Vaginal atresias (e.g., McKusick-Kaufman) 5. Labial adhesions

Here, we divide disorders of sex development into (1) sex chromosome disorders (sex chromosome DSD); (2) disorders of testis development and androgenization (46,XY DSD, including male pseudohermaphroditism); and (3) disorders of ovary development and androgen excess (46,XX DSD, including female pseudohermaphroditism) (see Fig. 22–2).

Sex Chromosome Disorders (Sex Chromosome DSD)

Disorders in the number of sex chromomes (sex chromosome aneuploidy) can be termed *sex chromosome DSD.* These conditions include Klinefelter's syndrome (47,XXY and its variants); Turner's syndrome (45,X and its variants); mixed gonadal dysgenesis (45,X/46,XY mosaicism and its variants); and true sex chromosome chimerism (46,XY/46,XX) (Table 22–4). A 45,Y cell line is nonviable. In many cases the diagnosis of these conditions will only be made in adolescence or adult life, due to associated features, impaired pubertal development, or infertility. Thus, a more detailed description of the long-term management of some of these conditions is provided in the relevant chapters (e.g., Turner's syndrome and Klinefelter's syndrome, Chapter 24).

Klinefelter's Syndrome (47,XXY) and Its Variants

Klinefelter's syndrome (KS) is the most frequent form of sex chromosome aneuploidy with a reported incidence of between 1:500 and 1:1000 live births.[216] The classic form of KS is associated with a 47,XXY karyotype and results following meiotic nondisjunction of the sex chromosomes during gametogenesis (Fig. 22–17; see Fig. 22–4).[18,216] In approximately 40% of cases this represents an abnormality during spermatogenesis, whereas approximately 60% of cases occur during oogenesis. Mosaic forms of KS (46,XY/47,XXY) represent mitotic nondisjunction within the developing zygote and are thought to occur in approximately 10% of individuals with this condition (see Fig. 22–4). Other chromosomal variants associated with KS (e.g., 48,XXXY) have been reported.

An overview of the clinical features of KS and its variants is presented in Table 22–4.[216,217] In the most severe situations, a young man might be diagnosed on account of small testes, gynecomastia, poor androgenization at puberty, eunuchoid proportions, or infertility. Other features, such as learning difficulties, may occur. However, it is likely that the clinical detection of KS based on postnatal karyotyping is biased to detecting those individuals with a more severe phenotype, and that a significant proportion of men with mosaic forms of KS or with milder phenotypes may not be diagnosed.

The development of testes and a male phenotype in individuals with KS provides important evidence for the key role of the Y chromosome in testis determination and subsequent prenatal androgen production. However, micropenis and hypospadias may be a presenting feature in some cases (personal observation) and early postnatal gonadotropin concentrations are reported to be elevated in some studies.[218,219]

A more predictable elevation in gonadotropin concentrations (FSH, LH) occurs in the preadolescence and periadolescence

TABLE 22–4 CLINICAL FEATURES OF SEX CHROMOSOME DSD

Condition	Karyotype	Gonad	Internal Genitalia	Features
Klinefelter's syndrome	47,XXY and variants	Hyalinized testes	No uterus	Small testis, azoospermia, hypoandrogenemia; tall stature and increased leg-length; increased incidence of learning difficulties, obesity, breast tumors, varicose veins, impaired glucose tolerance
Turner's syndrome	45,X and variants	Streak gonad or immature ovary	Uterus	Childhood: lymphedema, shield chest, web neck, low hair line; cardiac defects and coarctation of the aorta; renal and urinary abnormalities; short stature, cubitus valgus, hypoplastic nails, scoliosis; otitis media and hearing loss; ptosis and amblyopia; nevi; autoimmune thyroid disease; visuospatial learning difficulties Adulthood: pubertal failure, primary amenorrhea; hypertension; aortic root dilatation and dissection; sensorineural hearing loss; increased risk of cardiovascular disease, inflammatory bowel disease, colon cancer, thyroid disease, glucose intolerance and diabetes mellitus, osteoporosis (NB some of these may be related to estrogen deficiency).
Mixed gonadal dysgenesis	45,X/46, XY and variants	Testis or dysgenetic gonad	Variable	Increased risk of gonadal tumors; short stature; some features of Turner's syndrome may be present.
Ovotesticular DSD	46,XX/46,XY chimerism	Testis, ovary or ovotestis	Variable	Possible increased risk of gonadal tumors.

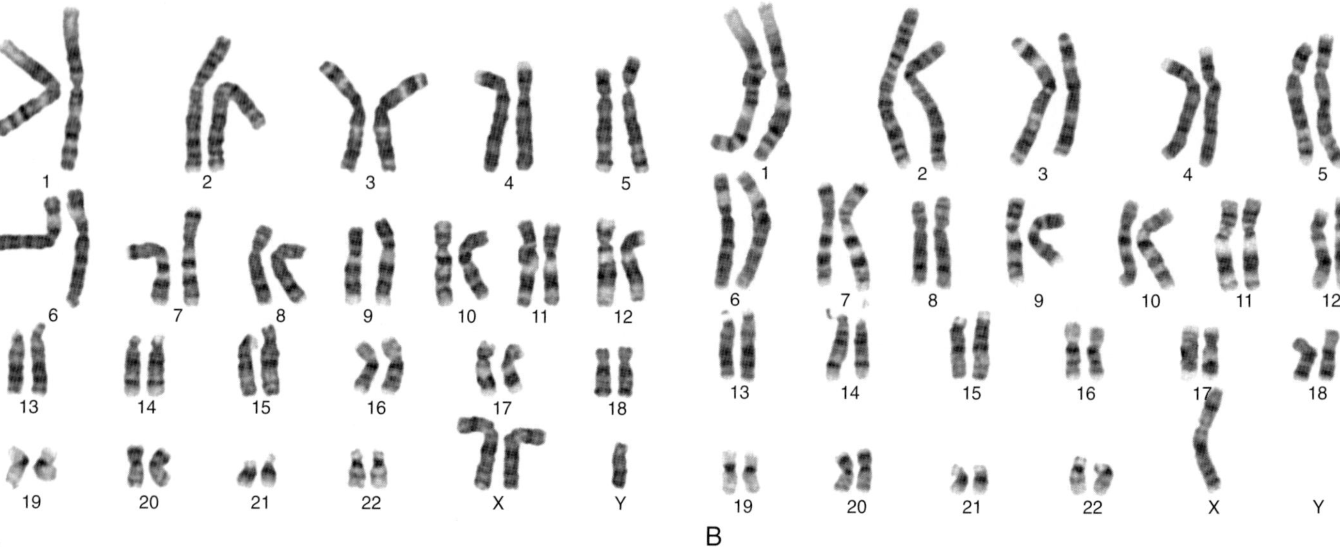

Figure 22–17 ▪ G-banded karyotypes of Klinefelter's syndrome (47,XXY) **(A)** and Turner's syndrome (45,X) **(B)**. **C,** Structural changes of the X chromosome seen in variants of Turner's syndrome (*from left to right,* normal X; ring chromosome [r(X)(p22.3q22)]; short-arm deletion [del(X)(p21)]; long-arm deletion [del(X)(q21.31)]; isochromosome [I(X)(q10)]). (Images courtesy of Mr Lee Grimsley and Dr Jonathan Waters, North East London Regional Cytogenetics Laboratory, Great Ormond Street Hospital NHS Trust, London, UK.)

period in patients with KS following activation of the hypothalamic-pituitary-gonadal axis.[216] By the time of adolescence, plasma concentrations of FSH are increased in 90% of patients with KS, and plasma concentrations of LH in 80% of cases. Other serum markers of testicular function (prepubertal AMH, peripubertal inhibin B, midpubertal Insl3) are often below normal ranges.[220-221] Although some androgenization usually occurs during puberty in classic KS, plasma testosterone is decreased in 50% to 75% of cases.[216] Testes usually remain small and firm (median length 2.5 cm [4 ml]; almost always less than 3.5 cm [12 mls], and typically appear inappropriately small for the degree of androgenization.[217] Serum estradiol is often raised, which contributes to the gynecomastia often observed during the adolescent period.

Testicular biopsy is not warranted clinically because the diagnosis can usually be made on karyotyping from peripheral blood cells. However, studies where testicular histology has been obtained report germ cell depletion, progressive hyalinization of seminiferous tubules and Leydig cell hyperplasia following chronic LH stimulation. A significant proportion of men with KS receive testosterone supplementation to fully induce puberty and to support sexual characteristics, libido, and bone mineralization into adult life. An overview of the management of KS in adolescence and adulthood is provided in Chapters 18 and 24. Whilst some cases of spontaneous fertility have been reported for mosaic forms of KS (46,XY/47,XXY), the prospects for fertility in classic KS were thought to be poor. However, recent studies of combining testicular sperm extraction (TESE) with intracytoplasmic sperm injection (ISCI) have reported successful pregnancies in approximately 50% of men with classic KS (47,XXY) in specialist centers.[222] The potential risk of the transmission of sex-chromosome aneuploidy must be considered, and the benefits of this approach may decrease with age, suggesting that progressive deterioration in testicular function is a feature of KS.

Turner's Syndrome (45,X) and Its Variants

Turner's syndrome (TS) is the second most frequent form of sex-chromosome aneuploidy with an incidence of approximately 1 : 2500.[42] The classic form of TS is associated with a 45,X karyotype and occurs in approximately one half of individuals with this condition (see Fig. 22–17). Mosaic forms of TS (45,X/46,XX) account for approximately one fourth of individuals with this condition, whereas the remainder have structural abnormalities of the X chromosome such as long- or short-arm deletions, isochromosomes or ring chromosomes (see Fig. 22–17).[42,223]

A 45,X chromosome constitution may be the consequence of nondisjunction or chromosome loss during gametogenesis in either parent that results in a sperm or ovum lacking a sex chromosome (see Fig. 22–4). Although errors in mitosis in a normal zygote often lead to mosaicism, a purely 45,X constitution may arise at the first cleavage division from anaphase lag with loss of a sex chromosome or, less likely, from mitotic nondisjunction with failure of the complementary 47,XXX or 47,XYY cell line to survive.[17] Indeed, it has been estimated that around 2% of all zygotes have a 45,X karyotype, and around 7% of spontaneous abortuses have a 45,X karyotype, making this the most frequent chromosomal anomaly in humans.

The clinical features of TS are highly variable and may differ depending on the age of the child and time of diagnosis. For example, a prenatal diagnosis of TS may be made incidentally following amniocentesis or chorionic villous sampling for an incidental reason, such as advanced maternal age, or following the detection of increased nuchal translucency on fetal ultrasound scan.[223,224] In early infancy, the diagnosis should be considered in females with lymphedema, nuchal folds, low hair line, or left-sided cardiac defects. Unexplained growth failure or somatic features (e.g., abnormal nails, shield chest, abnormal carrying angle, recurrent ear infections) might point to the diagnosis during childhood, whereas TS should certainly be considered in all girls with pubertal delay or pubertal failure. An overview of clinical features associated with TS is provided in Table 22–4 and more detailed analysis of investigation and management of individuals with this condition is provided in Chapter 24. Timely and appropriate introduction of estrogens is necessary in adolescence to ensure adequate breast and uterine development, thereby optimizing the opportunity to carry a pregnancy by ovum donation in the future.[224,225] Turner women benefit from dedicated long-term follow-up with a focus on issues such as cardiovascular, bone and reproductive health, and hearing.[82,224,225]

Girls with classic TS show ovarian dysgenesis, which highlights the importance of two copies of the X chromosome for ovarian development and integrity. Indeed, studies of TS embryos have shown normal germ cell migration and normal ovarian development until around the third month of gestation.[226] However, accelerated germ cell apoptosis and subsequent oocyte atresia occur, which results in progressive degeneration of the ovary in the prenatal or postnatal period. With these gonadal changes, LH and FSH tend to rise in late childhood following activation of the hypothalamic pulse generator. Nevertheless, sufficient estrogen synthesis for puberty to commence in adolescence occurs in approximately 25% of Turner girls (10% in 45,X; 30% to 40% in 45,X/46,XX mosaicism) and menstruation occurs in around 2% of cases.[42,227] Gonadectomy is not usually required except when a Y fragment containing the TSPY locus is present; in these cases the risk of gonadoblastoma is increased.[23,228] It is currently unclear whether any follicular tissue could be usefully cryopreserved in girls in whom spontaneous puberty has occurred.[229,230]

45,X/46,XY Mosaicism (Mixed Gonadal Dysgenesis) and Variants

A mosaic 45,X/46,XY karyotype (sometimes referred to as "mixed gonadal dysgenesis") probably arises through anaphase lag during mitosis in the zygote, although Y chromosomal abnormalities are sometimes seen and interchromosomal rearrangements with loss of structural abnormal Y material may be a common mechanism for variants of this condition. Although the classic form of this condition is associated with 45,X/46,XY mosaicism, 45,X/47,XYY or 45,X/46,XY/47,XYY mosaic karyotypes have also been reported.

The clinical phenotype associated with a 45,X/46,XY mosaicism is highly variable and the true prevalence of this condition is not known (see Table 22–4). Historically, those individuals with the most severe forms of 45,X/46,XY mosaicism have been referred for further assessment, and most series of patients reported in the literature have likely reflected this bias.[231,232]

Reported genital phenotypes associated with 45,X/46,XY mosaicism range from normal female external genitalia or mild clitoromegaly through all stages of ambiguous genitalia to hypospadias or a normal penis.[231,232] Gonadal phenotypes range from streak gonads, through dysgenetic testes to testes with normal histological architecture. In rare cases, ovarian-like stroma and sparse primordial follicles may be present. The gonads may be positioned anywhere along the pathway of testicular descent, with streaklike gonads more likely to be intraabdominal and well-formed testes to be in the inguinoscrotal region. Müllerian structures may be present in the most severe cases, due to impaired AMH production by Sertoli cells. Marked differences in gonadal development and histology can be seen between the right and the left, or even within a single gonad, which gave rise to the term *mixed gonadal dysgenesis.*[2] Indeed, the presence of a hemiuterus and fallopian tube on the side of the most severely affected gonad in some cases provides important supportive evidence for the paracrine actions of AMH on developing müllerian structures.

Somatic features associated with a 45,X/46,XY karyotype are also highly variable, and are not always correlated well with the gonadal phenotype.[232] At the most severe end of the spectrum, clinical features reminiscent of Turner's syndrome may be seen, such as short stature, nuchal folds, low-set hairline, and cardiac and renal abnormalities. Detailed evaluation and long-term follow-up of these patients may be warranted, as for Turner's syndrome (see Chapter 24). In other cases, a slight reduction in predicted height might be the only somatic manifestation. It is unclear whether detailed, ongoing monitoring for Turner's syndrome–associated features is required for this group of individuals, but a low threshold should be maintained for monitoring associated features (e.g., thyroid function, hearing, cardiac anomalies) if there are any concerns.

Gender assignment can be difficult in individuals with 45,X/46,XY and a number of factors need to be taken into consideration, including genital appearance and urogenital anatomy, risk of gonadal malignancy, fertility and reproductive options and likely gender identity, sex role behavior, and psychosexual functioning.

Most infants with female or minimally androgenized genitalia are raised as female and the presence of a uterus or hemiuterus allows the potential for pregnancy by ovum donation in the future. Intraabdominal streak and dysgenetic gonads are thought to be at significant risk of malignancy and should be removed.[233,234] Estrogen replacement will be required to induce breast and uterine development in adolescence, and the addition of progestins will allow menstruation when a uterus is present. Growth-promoting agents have been used on an individual basis when short stature or Turner's syndrome–like features are present, but no proper trials have been performed in this group of patients. Similarly, no long-term outcome data on gender identity or psychosexual functioning are currently available.

Infants with hypospadias and reasonable phallic development are usually raised as male. Testosterone can be given to promote phallic growth in infancy and hypospadias repair is usually undertaken as a two-stage procedure. Attempts should be made to perform orchidopexy as a one- or two-stage procedure, because there is believed to be a significant risk of malignancy in these gonads so careful monitoring is necessary.[23] Gonads that cannot be placed within the scrotum are usually removed.[234] Gonads that can be secured within the scrotum need careful monitoring and biopsy in early adolescence to assess for carcinoma in situ.[23] Puberty needs to be carefully monitored in this group of patients to ensure adequate endogenous testosterone production, and in some cases testosterone supplementation is needed. Loss of height potential is generally unpredictable, but needs careful monitoring.

Assignment of gender and management of a 45,X/46,XY child with *highly ambiguous genitalia* can be a very difficult situation for parents and physicians, and long-term outcome data in this group are not available. Limited data suggest that approximately 60% of infants with this phenotype will be raised female, but will be infertile, will have no uterus, will require gonadectomy, and are likely to undergo urogenital surgery.[2] In contrast, those raised as male will require multiple hypospadias surgeries, may have poor corporal tissue, will be infertile if dysgenetic gonads are present that need to be removed, and may have a significantly reduced height potential. Such situations highlight the need for a multidisciplinary approach in the assessment and management of such patients, and long-term monitoring and support. Long-term outcome data from larger studies may provide better guidance on the management of this group of individuals in the future.

In addition to the most severe cases described above, it is also emerging that a 45,X/46,XY mosaic karyotype is compatible with a normal male phenotype and apparently normal testis development. Initial cases of normal males with a 45,X/46,XY karyotype were described following screening of family members as potential bone marrow transplant donors,[2] but more recent studies of amniocentesis have shown that 90% of fetuses diagnosed as 45,X/46,XY by amniocentesis and confirmed as having this karyotype postnatally have normal male genitalia and apparently normal testes.[235,236] Moreover, there seems to be limited correlation between the degree of mosaicism on peripheral blood sampling and gonadal or somatic phenotype. Follow-up data on this cohort are currently limited, hypothalamic-pituitary gonadal function has not been reported in detail, and fertility outcome and tumor risk is not known. Although a 45,X/46,XY karyotype is a relatively rare finding in men presenting with testicular tumors or in the infertility clinic, more detailed long-term studies of the 45,X/46,XY male cohort are required to know whether detailed follow-up is necessary. It might seem prudent to monitor gonadal function in this cohort and to assess for evidence of testicular carcinoma in situ in adolescence, its but endenic is currently lacking.

Ovotesticular DSD (True Hermaphroditism), 46,XX/46,XY Chimerism, and Variants

The diagnosis of ovotesticular DSD (also known as "true hermaphroditism") requires the presence of both ovarian tissue (containing follicles) and testicular tissue in either the same or opposite gonads (Fig. 22–18; see Table 22–4). Gonadal stroma arranged in whorls, similar to those found in the ovary but lacking oocytes, should not be considered sufficient evidence to designate the rudimentary gonad as an ovary.[2]

Ovotesticular DSD is a relatively rare condition but has been reported in around 500 individuals worldwide. Although 46,XX/46,XY chimerism (due to double fertilization or ovum fusion, see Normal Development) does occur in a proportion of these patients, especially in North America and Europe, most individuals with 46,XX/46,XY chimerism do not have this condi-

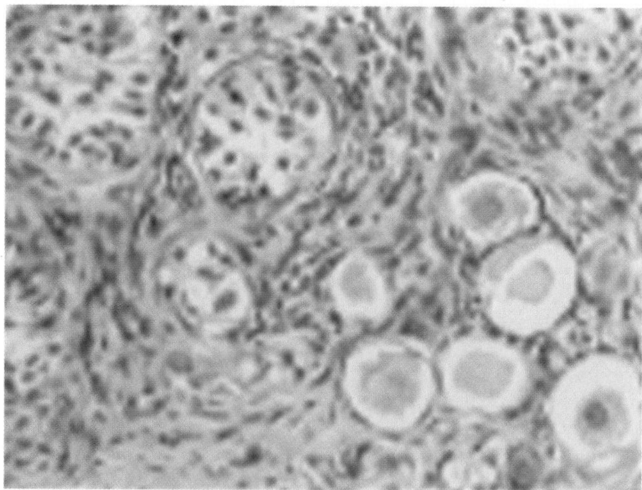

Figure 22–18 ■ Ovotestis showing immature seminiferous tubules lined with Sertoli cells and germ cells *(upper left)* and ovarian tissue with follicles *(lower right)* (H & E stain, 400× magnification). (Courtesy of Dr. Neil Sebire, Great Ormond Street Hospital NHS Trust, London, UK.)

tion (Table 22–5).[237] Indeed, the majority of patients with ovotesticular DSD have a 46,XX karyotype, especially in South and Western Africa.[237-239] The molecular basis of this disorder is not currently know, but familial cases have been reported, and both autosomal recessive and sex-limited autosomal dominant transmission have been proposed. Sry translocations are rare.[240] Ovotesticular DSD associated with a 46,XY karyotype is rare, and may represent cryptic gonadal mosaicism for a Y chromosome deletion or early sex-determining gene mutation. Thus, ovotesticular DSD likely represents a number of different etiologies.

Patients with ovotesticular DSD may be subclassified according to the type and location of the gonads.[2] *Lateral* cases (20%) have a testis on one side and an ovary on the other. *Bilateral* cases (30%) have testicular and ovarian tissue present bilaterally, usually as ovotestes. *Unilateral* cases (50%) have an ovotestis present on one side and an ovary or testis on the other. In most cases of ovotesticular DSD, the ovary (or ovotestis) is more frequently found on the left hand side of the body, whereas the testis (or ovotestis) is found more often on the right.[241] An ovary is likely to be in its normal anatomic position, whereas the testis or ovotestis can be anywhere along the pathway of testicular descent, and is often found in the right inguinal region.

The differentiation of the genital tract and development of secondary sex characteristics are very variable in ovotesticular DSD.[242] Most patients who present early have ambiguous genitalia or significant hypospadias. Cryptorchidism is common, but at least one gonad is palpable usually in the labioscrotal fold or inguinal region, more often on the right, and often associated with an inguinal hernia. The differentiation of the genital ducts usually follows that of the gonad, and a hemiuterus or rudimentary uterus is often present on the side of the ovary/ovotestis.

Breast development at the time of puberty is common in ovotesticular DSD. Menses occurs in a significant proportion of cases and ovulation and pregnancy has been reported in a number of patients with a 46,XX karyotype, especially when an ovary is present. However, progressive androgenization can occur in girls with significant testicular tissue, which can result in voice changes and clitoral enlargement during adolescence if left untreated. Individuals raised as male often present with hypospadias and undescended testes, although bilateral scrotal ovotestes have been reported. These individuals can experience significant estrogenization around the time of puberty and may have cyclical hematuria if a uterus is present. Spermatogenesis is reportedly rare and interstitial fibrosis of the testis is common.

Although rare, the diagnosis of ovotesticular DSD should be considered in all patients with ambiguous genitalia, especially when there is more pronounced scrotalization or detection of a gonad on the right. A 46,XX/46,XY karyotype strongly supports the diagnosis, but the detection of a 46,XX or 46,XY karyotype does not exclude the diagnosis. Pelvic imaging, for example, with ultrasound or magnetic resonance imaging (MRI) is useful for visualizing internal genitalia. The presence of testicular tissue may be detected by the measurement of basal testosterone, AMH and inhibin B in the first months of life, as well as testosterone increase following hCG stimulation. Ovarian tissue is more difficult to detect in early childhood, although estradiol response to repeated injection of recombinant human FSH has been used and inhibin A may be useful for detection of ovarian follicles before 4 months of age or after 10 years of age. Examination under anesthesia and laparoscopy may provide the most detailed information about internal structures and allows biopsy to confirm the diagnosis of ovotesticular DSD when all other forms of DSD have been excluded.

The management of ovotesticular DSD varies depending upon the age at diagnosis, genital development, internal structures, and reproductive capacity. Either a male or female assignment may be appropriate in the young infant in whom a strong gender identity has not yet been established. Those individuals with a 46,XX karyotype and a uterus are likely to have functional ovarian tissue and female assignment is likely to be appropriate. Potentially functional testicular tissue should be removed and monitored postoperatively by serum AMH levels and by showing a lack of testosterone response to hCG stimulation. The risk of malignant transformation in the ovarian tissue of 46,XX patients is not known.

A male gender assignment may be more appropriate if there is reasonable phallic development and müllerian structures are absent or very poorly formed. Ovarian tissue is usually removed to prevent estrogenization at puberty and remnant müllerian structures can be removed by an experienced surgeon. The prevalence of gonadoblastoma and/or germinoma arising in the testicular tissue of patients with 46,XX ovotesticular DSD has been estimated at 3% to 4 % and the ovotesticular tissue is usually dysgenetic, so removal of this testicular tissue has been advocated.[23] However, the management of a histologically normal scrotally positioned testis is more difficult, and careful monitoring and biopsy for carcinoma in situ in adolescence may be an appropriate strategy.

Gender identity is an important consideration in patients with ovotesticular DSD who first present in late childhood or adolescence, due to androgenization in girls or estrogenization in boys. In most cases, gender identity is consistent with sex of rearing. The discordant gonad and dysgenetic tissue should be removed to prevent further androgenization in girls and estrogenization in boys, following appropriate counseling. Sex hormone supplementation may be required for complete pubertal development.

TABLE 22–5 Relative Frequency of Different Karyotypes in Individuals with Ovotesticular DSD (True Hermaphroditism)

Location	46,XX/46,XY	46,XX	46,XY
North America	21%	72%	7%
Europe	41%	52%	7%
Africa	—	97%	—

Adapted from Krob G, Braun A, Kuhnle U. True hermphroditism: geographical distribution, clinical findings, chromosomes and gonadal histology. Eur J Pediatr 1994;153:2-10.

Disorders of Testis Development and Androgenization (46,XY DSD, Including Male Pseudohermaphroditism)

46,XY DSD can be divided into (1) disorders of testis development, (2) disorders of androgen synthesis, (3) disorders of androgen action, and (4) other conditions affecting sex development (Table 22–6; see also Fig. 22–8).

Disorders of Testis Development

Disorders of testis development can have a spectrum of phenotypes and presentations. In the most extreme cases, *complete testicular dysgenesis* is associated with a complete lack of androgenization of the external genitalia, and persistent müllerian structures due to insufficient MIS/AMH production (sometimes called *Swyer syndrome*). In contrast, *partial gonadal dysgenesis* may be associated with clitoromegaly or ambiguous genitalia. A uterus and vagina may or may not be present. It is also possible that a subset of less severe forms of male

TABLE 22–6 OVERVIEW OF SOME OF THE MOST IMPORTANT GENES CURRENTLY KNOWN TO BE INVOLVED IN DSD

Gene	Protein	OMIM	Locus	Inheritance	Gonad	Müllerian Structures	External Genitalia	Associated Features/Variant Phenotypes
A. CAUSES OF 46,XY DSD								
Disorders of Gonadal (Testicular) Development: Single Gene Disorders								
WT1	TF	607102	11p13	AD	Dysgenetic testis	±	Female or ambiguous	Wilms' tumor, renal abnormalities, gonadal tumors (WAGR, Denys-Drash and Frasier syndromes)
SF1 (NR5A1)	Nuclear receptor TF	184757	9q33	AD/AR	Dysgenetic testis (variable)	±	Female, ambiguous or hypospadias	More severe phenotypes include primary adrenal failure; milder phenotypes have isolated partial gonadal dysgenesis and/or impaired androgenization
SRY	TF	480000	Yp11.3	Y	Dysgenetic testis or ovotestis	±	Female or ambiguous	
SOX9	TF	608160	17q24-q25	AD	Dysgenetic testis or ovotestis	±	Female or ambiguous	Camptomelic dysplasia (17q24 rearrangements have a milder phenotype than point mutations)
DHH	Signaling molecule	605423	12q13.1	AR	Dysgenetic testis, testis	+	Female	The severe phenotype of one patient included minifascicular neuropathy, other patients have isolated gonadal dysgenesis
ARX	TF	300382	Xp22.13	X	Dysgenetic testis (Leydig)	–	Ambiguous	X-linked lissencephaly, epilepsy, temperature instability
TSPYL1	? chromatin remodeling	604714	6q22-23	AR	Dysgenetic testis	–	Female or ambiguous	Sudden infant death
Cxorf6	Unknown	300120	Xq28	X	Normal (Leydig cell dysfunction)	–	Hypospadias	
Disorders of Gonadal (Testicular) Development: Chromosomal Changes Involving Key Candidate Genes								
DMRT1	TF	602424	9p24.3	Monosomic deletion	Dysgenetic testis	±	Female or ambiguous	Mental retardation
ATRX	Helicase (?chromatin remodeling)	300032	Xq13.3	X	Dysgenetic testis	–	Female, ambiguous or male	α-Thalassemia, mental retardation
DAX1 (NR0B1)	Nuclear receptor TF	300018	Xp21.3	dupXp21	Dysgenetic testis or ovary	±	Female or ambiguous	
WNT4	Signaling molecule	603490	1p35	dup1p35	Dysgenetic testis	+	Ambiguous	Mental retardation
Disorders in Hormone Synthesis or Action								
DHCR7	Enzyme	602858	11q12-q13	AR	Testis	–	Variable	Smith-Lemli-Opitz syndrome: coarse facies, second-third toe syndactyly, failure to thrive, developmental delay, cardiac and visceral abnormalities

Table continued on following page 807

TABLE 22–6 OVERVIEW OF SOME OF THE MOST IMPORTANT GENES CURRENTLY KNOWN TO BE INVOLVED IN DSD (Continued)

Gene	Protein	OMIM	Locus	Inheritance	Gonad	Müllerian Structures	External Genitalia	Associated Features/Variant Phenotypes
LHGCR	G-protein receptor	152790	2p21	AR	Testis	–	Female, ambiguous or micropenis	Leydig cell hypoplasia
STAR	Mitochondrial associated protein	600617	8p11.2	AR	Testis	–	Female	Congenital lipoid adrenal hyperplasia (primary adrenal failure), pubertal failure
CYP11A1	Enzyme	118485	15q23-q24	AR	Testis	–	Female or ambiguous	Congenital adrenal hyperplasia (primary adrenal failure), pubertal failure
HSD3B2	Enzyme	201810	1p13.1	AR	Testis	–	Ambiguous	CAH, primary adrenal failure, ↑ Δ5:Δ4 ratio
CYP17	Enzyme	202110	10q24.3	AR	Testis	–	Female, ambiguous or micropenis	CAH, hypertension due to ↑ 11-deoxycorticosterone (except in isolated 17,20-lyase deficiency)
POR (P450 oxido reductase)	CYP enzyme electron donor	124015	7q11.2	AR	Testis	–	Male or ambiguous	Mixed features of 21-hydroxylase deficiency, 17α-hydroxylase/17,20-lyase deficiency and aromatase deficiency; sometimes associated with Antley Bixler craniosynostosis
HSD17B3	Enzyme	605573	9q22	AR	Testis	–	Female or ambiguous	Partial androgenization at puberty, ↑ androstenedione: testosterone ratio
SRD5A2	Enzyme	607306	2p23	AR	Testis	–	Ambiguous or micropenis	Partial androgenization at puberty, ↑ testosterone:DHT ratio
Androgen receptor	Nuclear receptor TF	313700	Xq11-q12	X	Testis	–	Female, ambiguous, micropenis or normal male	Phenotypic spectrum from complete androgen insensitivity syndrome (female external genitalia) and partial androgen insensitivity (ambiguous) to normal male genitalia/infertility
AMH	Signaling molecule	600957	19p13.3-p13.2	AR	Testis	+	Normal male	Persistent müllerian duct syndrome (PMDS). Male external genitalia, bilateral cryptorchidism.
AMH-Receptor	Serine-threonine kinase transmembrane receptor	600956	12q13	AR	Testis	+	Normal male	

Table continued on following page 808

TABLE 22–6 OVERVIEW OF SOME OF THE MOST IMPORTANT GENES CURRENTLY KNOWN TO BE INVOLVED IN DSD (Continued)

Gene	Protein	OMIM	Locus	Inheritance	Gonad	Müllerian Structures	External Genitalia	Associated Features/Variant Phenotypes
B. CAUSES OF 46,XX DSD								
Disorders of Gonadal (Ovarian) Development								
SRY	TF	480000	Yp11.3	translocation	Testis or ovotestis	–	Male or ambiguous	
SOX9	TF	608160	17q24	dup17q24	ND	–	Male or ambiguous	
RSPO1	Thrombospondin (Wnt signaling)	609595	1p34.3	AR	Testis	–	Male	Palmar-plantar hyperkeratosis, squamous cell carcinoma
Androgen Excess								
HSD3B2	Enzyme	201810	1p13	AR	Ovary	+	Clitoromegaly (mild)	CAH, primary adrenal failure, partial androgenization due to ↑ conversion of DHEA
CYP21A2	Enzyme	201910	6p21-p23	AR	Ovary	+	Ambiguous; rarely Prader V	CAH, phenotypic spectrum from severe salt-losing forms associated with adrenal failure to simple virilizing forms with compensated adrenal function, ↑ 17-hydroxy-progesterone
CYP11B1	Enzyme	202010	8q21-q22	AR	Ovary	+	Ambiguous; rarely Prader V	CAH, hypertension due to ↑ 11-deoxycortico-sterone
POR (P450 oxidoreductase)	CYP enzyme electron donor	124015	7q11.2	AR	Ovary	+	Normal or ambiguous	Mixed features of 21-hydroxylase deficiency, 17α-hydroxylase/17,20-lyase deficiency and aromatase deficiency; associated with Antley Bixler craniosynostosis
CYP19	Enzyme	107910	15q21	AR	Ovary	+	Ambiguous	Maternal androgenization during pregnancy, absent breast development at puberty, except in partial cases
Glucocorticoid receptor	Nuclear receptor TF	138040	5q31	AR	Ovary	+	Normal or ambiguous	↑ ACTH, 17-hydroxy-progesterone, cortisol, mineralocorticoids and androgens; failure of dexamethasone suppression (NB patient heterozygous for a mutation in CYP21)

AR, Autosomal recessive; *AD,* autosomal dominant (often de novo mutation); *Y,* Y chromosomal; *X,* X-chromosomal; *TF,* transcription factor; *ND,* not determined; *CAH,* congenital adrenal hyperplasia; *ACTH,* adrenocorticotropin. +, present; –, absent.

Chromosomal rearrangements likely to include key genes are included.

Adapted with permission from Achermann JC, Ozisik G, Meeks JJ, et al. Genetic causes of human reproductive disease. J Clin Endocrinol Metab 2002;87:2447-2454. © 2002 The Endocrine Society.

reproductive development, such as isolated hypospadias, testicular regression, micropenis, or male infertility may represent milder variants of these more severe phenotypes.

Several single gene disorders have now been described in patients with varying degrees of testicular dysgenesis. An overview of these factors is provided in Table 22–6, and a description of the role of these factors in normal development has been discussed previously (see Normal Development). These factors have largely been discovered as candidate genes based on mouse phenotypes, or when gonadal dysgenesis is part of a more complex syndrome. In such cases, the presence of any associated features can help to direct genetic analysis appropriately. It is important to remember that a genetic diagnosis is reached in only around 20% to 30% of cases of 46,XY testicular dysgenesis at present.

Steroidogenic Factor 1 (SF1)

Steroidogenic factor 1 (SF1/Ad4BP, *NR5A1*) (9q33) is a member of the nuclear receptor superfamily that regulates the transcription of at least 30 genes known to be involved in gonadal development, adrenal development, steroidogenesis, and reproduction.[74] Complete deletion of the gene encoding Sf1 in mice results in apoptosis of the developing gonad and adrenal gland during early embryonic development.[75] XY animals are phenotypically female and have persistent müllerian structures. Abnormalities of the ventromedial hypothalamus and variable hypogonadotropic hypogonadism are also described.

Given the phenotypic findings in the mouse, SF1 mutations were first reported in two 46,XY individuals with female external genitalia, persistent müllerian structures and primary adrenal failure.[80,81] These changes both resulted in impaired DNA binding; the first mutation was a de novo heterozygous Gly35Glu change in the P-box primary DNA-binding region of SF1, whereas the second mutation was a recessively inherited homozygous Arg92Gln mutation in the A-box secondary DNA-binding region (Fig. 22–19).

More recently a number of heterozygous nonsense, frameshift, and missense mutations have been reported in SF1 in association with 46,XY DSD.[85,243-246] These mutations are likely to cause haploinsufficiency of SF1, resulting in a phenotype of mild gonadal dysgenesis, significantly impaired androgenization, and normal adrenal function, and can be inherited from the mother in a sex-limited dominant fashion (i.e., the mother carries the mutation but is unaffected). Milder cases of SF1 mutation are found with severe hypospadias, and polymorphic variants of SF1 with partial loss of function have been reported in association with micropenis or cryptorchidism.[247,248] Thus, it it emerging that variable loss of SF1 activity is associated primarily with testicular dysfunction in humans.

Wilms' Tumor-Related Gene-1 (WT1)

Wilms' tumor-related gene-1 (WT1) (11p13) is a four-zinc finger transcription factor expressed in the developing genital ridge, kidney, gonads, and mesothelium.[61-62] Homozygous deletion of the gene encoding *Wt1* in mice prevents gonad and kidney development.[62] The WT1 protein has several different isoforms that have complex roles in sex development, as outlined previously (Normal Sex Development, Bipotential Gonad) and shown in Figure 22–20. The important role of WT1 in human testis development has been confirmed through the description of various WT1 mutations in patients with WAGR syndrome, Denys-Drash syndrome, and Frasier syndrome.

WAGR syndrome (*W*ilms' tumor, *a*niridia, *g*enitourinary abnormalities, and mental *r*etardation) is a distinct syndrome caused by deletion of a region of chromosome 11p13.[249] The resultant phenotype is likely to be the consequence of haploinsufiiciency of WT1, together with loss of developmental genes such as *PAX6*, which is involved in eye development. Renal abnormalities also include renal agenesis and horseshoe kidney. Genitourinary abnormalities are usually relatively mild and include hypospadias, cryptorchidism, and ureteral atresia.

Denys-Drash syndrome (DDS) is characterized by gonadal dysgenesis, severe congenital or early-onset nephropathy

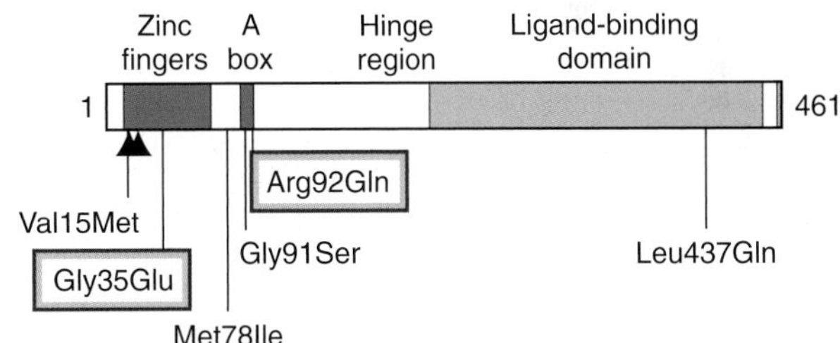

Figure 22–19 ▪ Structure of SF1 showing key domains and mutations associated with a 46,XY gonadal phenotype described to date. The Gly35Glu (heterozygous) and Arg92Gln (homozygous) changes (boxed) affect DNA-binding regions of the protein (P-box and A-box, respectively) and are associated with marked underandrogenization, dysgenetic gonads, müllerian structures and primary adrenal failure. More recently, a number of heterozygous frameshift and nonsense mutations (▲) as well as missense mutations (indicated) have been described in 46,XY individuals with milder forms of gonadal dysgenesis and severe underandrogenization but normal adrenal function. (Modified with permission from Lin L, Philibert P, Ferraz-de-Souza B, et al. Heterozygous missense mutations in steroidogenic factor-1 [SF1/Ad4BP, NR5A1] are associated with 46,XY disorders of sex development with normal adrenal function. J Clin Endocrinol Metab 2007;92:991-999. Copyright 2007, The Endocrine Society.)

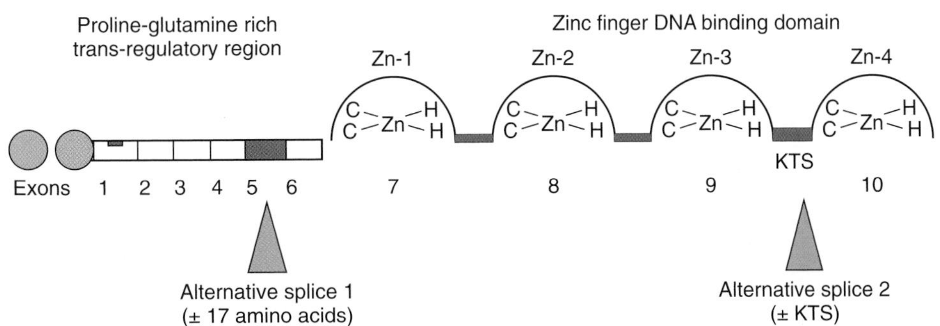

Figure 22–20 ▪ Schematic diagram showing the structure of WT1 and the changes associated with exon 5 and exon 9 (+KTS) isoforms. Many point mutations associated with Denys-Drash syndrome are located within zinc fingers 2 and 3 (especially Arg394), whereas mutations affecting the exon 9 splice site are associated with Frasier syndrome. (Modified with permission from Koziell A, Grundy R. Frasier and Denys-Drash syndromes: different disorders or part of a spectrum? Arch Dis Child 1999;81:365-369. © BMJ Publishing Group 1999.)

(diffuse mesangial sclerosis), and predisposition to Wilms' tumor.[70] Most 46,XY patients with DDS present with genital ambiguity in the newborn period, although normal male or female phenotypes have been described. The presence or absence of müllerian structures depends on the degree of Sertoli cell dysfunction. DDS usually results from heterozygous de novo point mutations in WT1 that have a dominant negative effect on the function of the wild-type protein. These point mutations usually affect the DNA binding region (zinc-fingers) of WT1. The risk of early-onset end-stage renal failure is high, and Wilms' tumor usually develops in the first decade of life. Gonadoblastoma occurs in less than 10% of cases.

Frasier syndrome (FS) usually results from heterozygous mutations in the donor splice site of exon 9 of WT1.[71,72] These changes are predicted to result in an imbalance in the ratio of +KTS to −KTS isoforms of WT1. FS is characterized by streak gonads, a 46,XY female phenotype with müllerian structures and later-onset nephropathy (focal segmental glomerulosclerosis) that usually causes renal failure in the second decade of life. There is a high risk of gonadal tumors such as gonadoblastoma in FS patients.[23] In practice, DDS and FS may represent a continuum of phenotypes rather than distinct conditions.[73] Milder variants of these conditions may also occur; a man with hypospadias was found to have late-onset nephropathy due to a WT1 mutation.[250] Taken together, these cases highlight the importance of considering this diagnosis in 46,XY DSD and performing urinalysis for proteinuria in cases of 46,XY DSD. Management of patients with WT1 mutations includes monitoring and treatment of renal function, assessment for the development of Wilms' tumor, and gonadectomy in DDS patients with a Y chromosome and in individuals with FS (see Table 22–22).[23]

Sex-Determining Region, Y (SRY)

The sequence of events leading to the identification of SRY as the primary "testis-determining gene" is described in the first section of this chapter, as is an overview of the actions of SRY in testis development. SRY is a 204 amino-acid HMG-box transcription factor that is encoded by a single exon on the Y chromosome (Yp11.3) (see Fig. 22–5).[28,29,82] The description of inactivating mutations in SRY in patients with 46,XY gonadal dysgenesis confirmed the key role this factor plays in testis determination in humans.[29,32,33,110-112] Approximately 15% of individuals with the complete form of 46,XY gonadal dysgenesis have inactivating mutations in *SRY*.[82] Most of the mutations occur in the HMG-box DNA-binding domain of the SRY protein (Fig. 22–21), a region involved in binding to and bending DNA.[82,104] Rare mutations in the 5′ and 3′ flanking regions in patients have led to complete and partial gonadal dysgenesis, respectively.[251-255] The HMG box contains two nuclear localization signals [NLS]) that bind calmodulin and importin B.[82] Mutations in these nuclear localization signal domains in the HMG box of SRY result in failure to transport the SRY protein into the nucleus and result in consequent XY gonadal dysgenesis.[107]

SRY-Box 9 (SOX9)

Heterozygous mutations of the autosomal *SOX9* gene (17q24-q25) cause camptomelic dysplasia.[82,122,123] Features of this condition include bowed long bones, hypoplastic scapula, a deformed pelvis, 11 pairs of ribs, a small thoracic cage, cleft palate, macrocephaly, micrognathia, hypertelorism, and a variety of cardiac and renal defects. Death from respiratory distress often occurs in the neonatal period, but long-term survival has been reported.

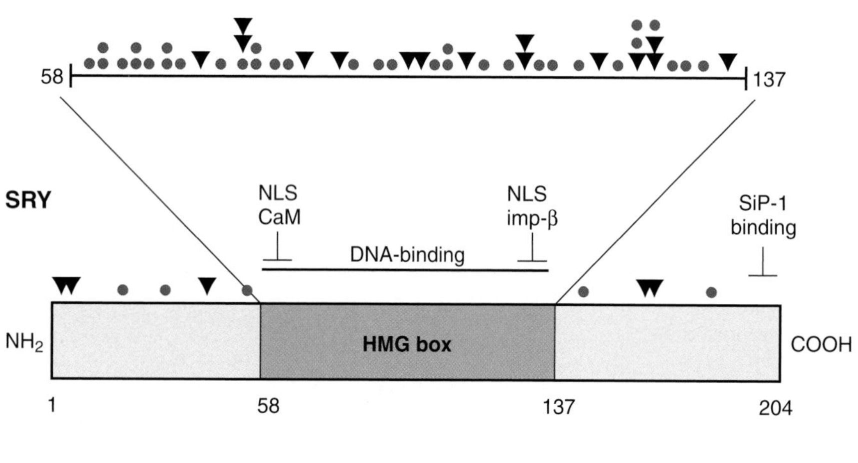

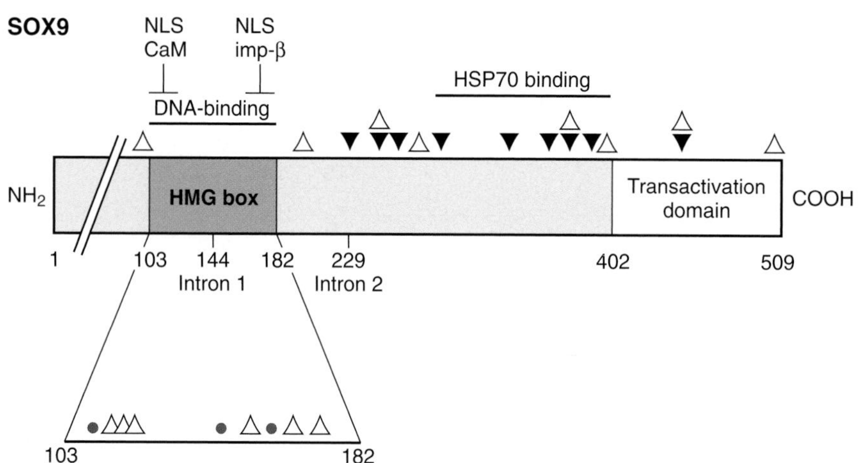

Figure 22–21 ▪ Human SRY and SOX9 protein and reported mutations. **A,** Diagram of SRY. The HMG box is an 80 amino acid DNA-binding domain with two nuclear localization signals (NLS) at either end: CaM, calmodulin, and imp β, importin β. The last seven amino acids of SRY can bind to either of the PDZ domains found in SRY-interacting protein 1 (SIP-1). The *solid circles* indicate missense mutations reported in the SRY protein affecting testicular development, which cluster within the HMG-box. Nonsense and frameshift mutations in SRY are shown by *solid arrowheads.* **B,** Diagram of SOX9. SOX9 has an HMG box with two nuclear localization signals similar to the structure of SRY. However, SOX9 is encoded by three exons, binds to heat shock protein 70 (HSP70), and has a *trans*-activation domain at the carboxyl-terminal end, unlike SRY. Selected mutations causing 46,XY DSD and camptomelic dysplasia are indicated by the *solid circles* (missense) and *solid arrowheads* (nonsense and frameshift). Those mutations causing only camptomelia in 46,XY males or affecting 46,XX females are indicated by the *open triangles.*

SOX9 is now emerging as an important testis-determining gene in its own right and may be one of the key regulators of testis determination downstream of SRY (see Normal Sex Development). Consistent with this, three fourths of affected 46,XY patients have dysgenetic gonads, but a complete spectrum of genital phenotypes can be seen from completely male to completely female appearances.[82] Histologic examination of the gonads from 46,XY patients with ambiguous or female external genitalia shows varying degrees of testicular dysgenesis extending to streak gonads with primordial follicles or even "ovaries."[256] Müllerian structures may or may not be present depending on the degree of gonadal dysgenesis. Affected 46,XX females have normal external genitalia and apparently normal ovaries.

The locus for camptomelic dysplasia with 46,XY DSD was mapped to 17q24.3-q25.1 following studies of three patients with balanced de novo reciprocal translocations, and the proposal of *Sox9* as a candidate gene based on expression studies in the mouse.[124,125] Subsequently, missense, nonsense, frameshift, and splice junction mutations have been detected in the *SOX9* gene in patients with camptomelic dysplasia with or without gonadal dysgenesis.[82] These mutations are usually heterozygous de novo changes, although in rare cases multiple siblings have been affected due to germline mosaicism for a *SOX9* mutation in a parent.[256] Of note, the gonadal phenotype in this kindred varied in the two affected 46,XY siblings; one of them had dysgenetic gonads and the other was reported to have "normal" ovaries.

The *SOX9* gene has three exons and two introns and encodes a 509-residue protein that contains an HMG box with 71% homology to that of the SRY protein and a carboxyl terminal *trans*-activation domain (see Fig. 22–21). Unlike SRY, where most mutations are located within the HMG-box, SOX9 mutations are located throughout the protein with little relation between functional domains and phenotype. Chromosomal translocations that disrupt regulatory elements upstream of the SOX9 promoter can be associated with a less severe phenotype, or camptomelic dysplasia without gonadal abnormalities.

Desert Hedgehog (DHH)

The hedgehog signaling pathways play an important role in many aspects of neuronal, skeletal, and endocrine development, and a homozygous mutation in *desert hedgehog* (*DHH*) was reported in a patient with partial gonadal dysgenesis and minifascicular neuropathy.[140] Subsequently, a number of *DHH* changes were reported in association with complete 46,XY gonadal dysgenesis, but with no apparent neurologic features.[257]

ARX

ARX (aristaless-related homeobox, X-linked) is a transcription factor that plays a central role in neuronal migration and the *Arx* knockout mouse has a profound myelination defect. *ARX* was considered a candidate gene for the X-linked lissencephaly ambiguous genitalia (XLAG) syndrome and mutations in *ARX* have been described in several patients with this condition.[145] This unusual form of lissencephaly is associated with severe epilepsy and thermal instability. The genital abnormality most likely represents a defect in Leydig cell function. A number of additional *ARX* mutations have now been described in patients with neurologic defects (e.g., infantile spasms) without significant disorders of sex development.

TSPYL1

An association between 46,XY gonadal dysgenesis and sudden infant death syndrome has been characterized in a large Amish kindred and termed SIDDT (sudden infant death, dysgenetic testes).[258] An autosomal recessive gene responsible for this condition has been identified, *TSPYL1* (testis-specific protein-like-1), which encodes a protein of unknown function, but which may be involved in chromatin remodeling.

CXorf6

CXorf6 is a gene on the X chromosome that encodes a hypothetical protein expressed in the developing testes. Hemizygous mutations in CXorf6 have been described in cases of isolated severe hypospadias, which may represent a defect in testicular Leydig cell development as well as an impaired end-organ (genital tubercle) response to androgen.[259]

Chromosomal Rearrangements Associated with Gonadal (Testicular) Dysgenesis

Abnormalities of genital development are reported with a number of chromosomal deletions, duplications, and rearrangements.[154] Some of the most frequent changes are seen with deletions of 9p24-pter, 10q25-qter, and Xq13, and with duplications of Xp21.

Deletions of 9p24-pter likely disrupt *DMRT1* (*double sex, mab3, related transcription factor 1*) (9p24.3), a gene with sex-specific homologues in *Drosophila* (*double sex*) and *Caenorhabitus elegans* (*mab3*), and which is expressed in early gonad development (see Normal Sex Development).[141,143] No specific point mutations in DMRT1 have been described in humans, but impaired gonadal development and 46,XY DSD are well established features of the 9p deletion syndrome, suggesting that haploinsufficiency of the *DMRT* locus may be a cause of testicular dysgenesis in humans.[142,144]

Terminal deletions of chromosome 10 (10q25-qter) are frequently associated with urogenital abnormalities and sometimes complete gonadal dysgenesis.[153] The gene in this locus has not yet been identified.

Deletions of Xq13.3 and of the tip of chromosome 16p cause α-thalassemia mental retardation (ATR) syndromes that may have gonadal dysgenesis as part of the phenotype.[150,152] The Xq13.3 locus contains the transcription factor *ATRX* (also known as *XH2* and *XNP*), whereas the *SOX8* gene is located on 16p.[151,152]

Duplications of the Xp21.3 region that contains the *DAX1* gene can cause abnormal testis development in rare cases.[86] The role of *DAX1* and the *WNT4* pathway (duplication 1p35) in "opposing" testis development is discussed previously (Normal Sex Development).[89]

Syndromic Causes of 46,XY DSD

In addition to those specific syndromes outlined above, variable degrees of testicular dysgenesis and/or impaired genital development (e.g., hypospadias, cryptorchism, scrotal transposition) are seen in a large number of discrete syndromes.[154] In some situations a genetic basis has been identified, but in many cases the etiology is currently unknown.

46,XY DSD is also often associated with intrauterine growth restriction (IUGR). Of note, monozygotic twins have shown disparate genital development, with the growth-restricted one having ambiguous genitalia and the larger one appearing as a normal male.[260] The mechanism of this association is unclear. However, more common genetic causes of 46,XY DSD (e.g., SRY mutations, SF1 mutations, androgen receptor mutations) are rarely found in this group of IUGR patients.

Disorders of Androgen Synthesis

Defects anywhere along the pathway of androgen synthesis and target organ action can result in impaired androgenization and 46,XY DSD (male pseudohermaphroditism) (see Normal Development, Table 22–6, and Fig. 22–11).

Cholesterol Synthesis Defects: Smith-Lemli-Opitz Syndrome (7-Dehydrocholesterol Reductase Deficiency)

Smith-Lemli-Opitz (SLO) syndrome has a broad phenotypic spectrum but typically includes microcephaly, mental retardation, cardiac defects, ptosis, upturned nose, micrognathia, cleft palate, polydactyly, syndactyly of toes (especially second and third toes), severe hypospadias, micropenis, and growth failure.[261] The abnormalities of the external genitalia in approximately 65% of 46,XY patients vary from micropenis and hypospadias to complete failure of androgenization, resulting in a female phenotype. SLO syndrome is caused by a deficiency of 7-dehydrocholesterol reductase (sterol Δ7-reductase, DHCR7), the phylogenetically conserved sterol-sensing domain-containing enzyme required for the last step in the biosynthetic pathway from acetate to cholesterol. Cholesterol is necessary not only as a substrate for steroid synthesis, but also intermediates of cholesterol synthesis may have important interactions with hedgehog signaling pathways. SLO syndrome is diagnosed by finding elevated plasma levels of 7-dehydrocholesterol and low cholesterol. The gene encoding this enzyme *(DHCR7)* maps to 11q12-q13 and more than 70 different mutations have now been described.[262] Thus, measurement of serum 7-DHC should be considered in all underandrogenized males with relevant phenotypic features, however mild. Testis development is apparently normal, and normal, elevated, or low concentrations of plasma testosterone have been described in affected male infants with intact hypothalamic-pituitary-gonadotropin function. Compromised adrenal function can occur in rare cases.

LH Receptor Mutations (LH/hCG Resistance, Leydig Cell Hypoplasia)

Mutations in the LH/hCG receptor *(LHCGR)* cause impaired responsiveness to hCG and/or LH with Leydig cell agenesis or hypoplasia.[207,263] Phenotypically, the external genitalia vary from a normal-appearing female appearance to males with micropenis (Table 22–7). Müllerian derivatives are absent in all patients and rudimentary wolffian derivatives have been present, even in some patients with severely underandrogenized external genitalia. This finding may reflect some early hCG-independent mechanisms of testosterone synthesis between 8 and 10 weeks' gestation.[2] Small, undescended testes are usually found in the inguinal region in the most severe forms of this Leydig cell hypoplasia. Patients with milder phenotypes may have appropriately descended testes of relatively normal size, as the Leydig cell population contributes only about 10% to testicular volume. On histologic examination, the testes lack distinct Leydig cells in prepubertal patients. Postpubertal patients have absent or decreased numbers of Leydig cells without Reinke's crystalloids, normal-appearing Sertoli cells, and discrete seminiferous tubules with spermatogenic arrest. This observation highlights the important role of intratesticular androgen in the final stages of sperm maturation.

TABLE 22–7 CLINICAL FEATURES OF LEYDIG CELL HYPOPLASIA IN 46,XY INDIVIDUALS

Karyotype:	46, XY
Inheritance:	Autosomal recessive; mutations in *LHCGR* gene
Genitalia:	Female, hypospadias or micropenis
Wolffian duct derivatives:	Hypoplastic
Müllerian duct derivatives:	Absent
Gonads:	Testes
Habitus:	Underandrogenization with variable failure of sex hormone production at puberty
Hormone profile:	Low T and DHT; elevated LH (and FSH); exaggerated LH response to LHRH stimulation; poor T and DHT response to hCG stimulation

DHT, Dihydrotestosterone; *FSH,* follicle-stimulating hormone; *hCG,* human chorionic gonadotropin; *LH,* luteinizing hormone; *T,* testosterone.

The typical biochemical profile of Leydig cell hypoplasia is elevated basal and LHRH-stimulated LH (and FSH) levels in early infancy or at puberty.[207] In childhood, when the GnRH pulse generator is quiescent, basal LH levels may sometimes still be detected above the normal range. Plasma levels of 17-OHP, androstenedione, and testosterone are low, with little or no response to prolonged hCG stimulation. Plasma LH falls following testosterone administration. Less marked biochemical changes can occur with milder forms of this condition.

To date, approximately 30 different homozygous or compound heterozygous mutations have been reported in the LH/hCG receptor gene (*LHCGR*) in individuals with various forms of this condition (Fig. 22–22).[207,264-266] The original reports of Kremer and colleagues[264] and Latronico and associates[265] described homozygous Ala593Pro and Arg554Stop mutations, respectively, in 46,XY phenotypic females with Leydig cell hypoplasia, hypergonadotropic hypogonadism, and no testosterone response to hCG stimulation. Of note, an affected 46,XX sister showed normal sexual maturation at puberty, but had elevated LH and amenorrhea, demonstrating that the LH receptor is not necessary for estrogen synthesis but is necessary for normal ovulation in females.[207] These mutations impair hCG stimulation of intracellular cyclic AMP in in vitro studies through disturbances in hCG binding, intracellular signaling, or receptor stability and trafficking, depending on the nature of the change. Partial loss of function mutations in the LH/hCG receptor causing milder phenotypes such as micropenis have, to date, tended to localize within the seventh transmembrane domain (Ser616Tyr, Ile625Lys) (see Fig. 22–22).[265,267] Individuals with complete Leydig cell hypoplasia are raised female and require estrogens at puberty. Gonadectomy is usually performed. If a male gender assignment is decided, then testosterone supplements may be given in early infancy and to support puberty. The risk of gonadal malignancy is unknown.[23]

Steroidogenic Acute Regulatory Protein Defects (StAR, Lipoid CAH)

Steroidogenic acute regulatory protein (StAR) is a 30-kd mitochondrial protein present in the adrenal gland and gonads that plays a key role in facilitating the rapid movement of cholesterol from the outer to the inner mitochondrial membrane.[268,269] This process is necessary to allow de novo steroid biosynthesis in response to an increase in ACTH or angiotensin II (in the adrenal gland), or an LH pulse (in the gonad). The exact mechanism by which StAR facilitates this movement is still unclear, but it is likely that the protein remains on the mitochondrial surface in a molten globule structure.[269] Although it is well established that a limited amount of cholesterol transfer is StAR-independent (14%), this protein certainly plays a central role in the acute regulation of adrenal and gonadal steroidogenesis.

Consistent with these actions, patients with recessively inherited defects in StAR develop a severe form of primary adrenal failure termed *lipoid congenital adrenal hyperplasia* (lipoid CAH).[270] Patients with this condition tend to present with severe glucocorticoid deficiency early in life (e.g., hypoglycemia, hyperpigmentation) and progressive mineralocorticoid insufficiency resulting in hyponatremia, hyperkalemia, dehydration, acidosis, and collapse (Table 22–8). Little or no C_{18}-, C_{19}-, and C_{21}-steroids are detectable in plasma or urine, even after corticotropin or hCG stimulation. Females (46,XX) with lipoid CAH

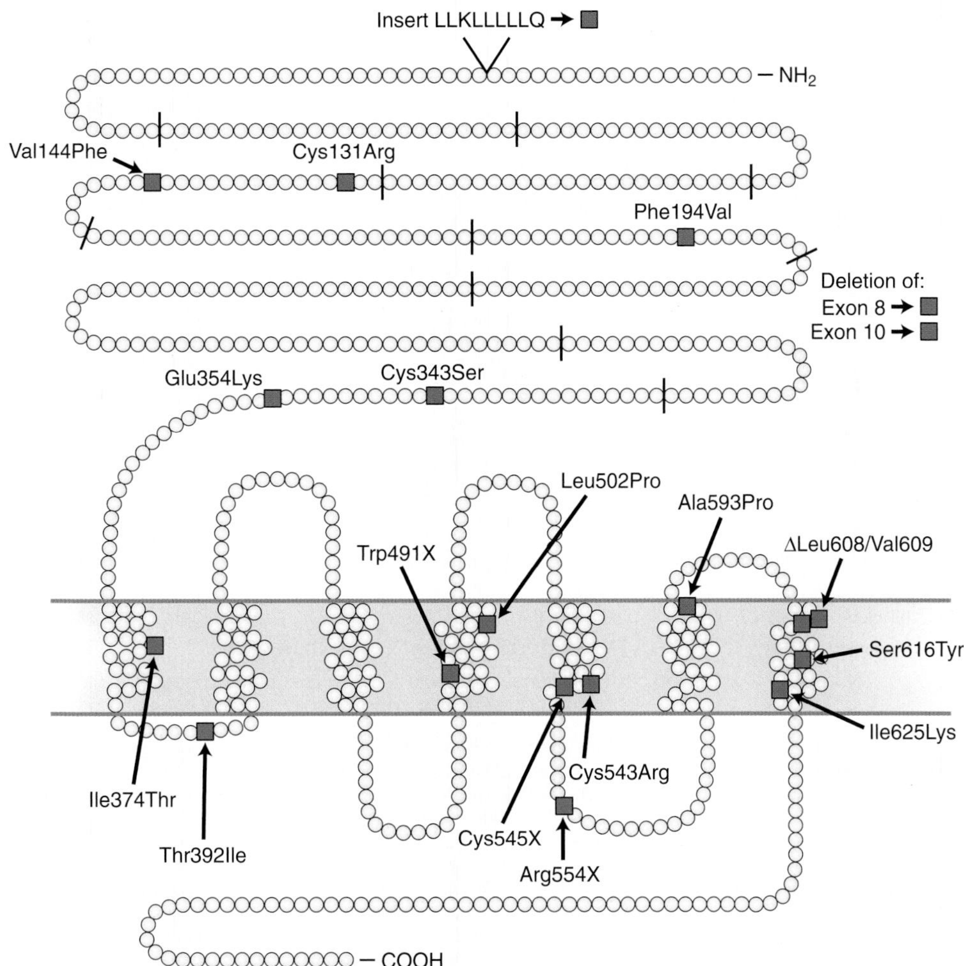

Figure 22–22 ▪ Diagram of the seven transmembrane domain LH/hCG receptor with selected inactivating mutations shown by *filled squares*. Most of these changes are associated with marked underandrogenization. However, the mutations at residues 616 and 625 in the seventh transmembrane domain are associated with a milder phenotype of micropenis.

TABLE 22–8 CLINICAL FEATURES OF LIPOID CAH IN 46,XY INDIVIDUALS

Karyotype	46, XY
Inheritance	Autosomal recessive; mutations in *StAR* gene
Genitalia	Female; rarely ambiguous or male
Wolffian duct derivatives	Hypoplastic or normal
Müllerian duct derivatives	Absent
Gonads	Testes
Habitus	Severe adrenal insufficiency in infancy with salt loss; failure of pubertal development; rare "nonclassic" cases associated with isolated glucocorticoid deficiency
Hormone profile	Usually deficiency of glucocorticoids, mineralocorticoids and sex steroids except rare "nonclassic" cases

have normal genitalia and a uterus. In 46,XY individuals, mutations in StAR typically cause a marked deficiency in testosterone synthesis by fetal Leydig cells so that completely female genitalia are seen. Testes may be abdominal, inguinal, or in the labia. A blind vaginal pouch is present and müllerian structures will have regressed. Thus, a karyotype should be performed in all "girls" presenting with early-onset adrenal failure.

The typical finding in lipoid CAH—as the name suggests—is lipid accumulation within steroidogenic cells. In the steroid-deficient state, the tropic drive by ACTH, angiotensin II, and LH causes increased cholesterol uptake and synthesis by steroidogenic cells. Coupled with the inability of StAR to facilitate cholesterol movement into mitochondria, this leads to marked accumulation of cholesterol in cells and results in the appearance of enlarged lipid-laden adrenal glands seen on MRI or computed tomograph (CT) scan. Eventually this cholesterol accumulation causes engorgement and results in disruption of the structural and functional integrity of the cell: the "two-hit" hypothesis (Fig. 22–23).[271] The StAR knockout mouse has a similar phenotype to patients with congenital lipoid adrenal hyperplasia, consistent with the two-hit hypothesis model.[272] StAR is *not* necessary for placental progesterone production, unlike P450scc (see below).

The two-hit hypothesis also explains why 46,XX girls with lipoid CAH show evidence of estrogenization and breast development at puberty, but have progressive hypergonadotropic hypogonadism.[271] Follicular cells are relatively quiescent in utero and before puberty; hence, they are undamaged. At the beginning of each cycle, they are recruited, and a small amount of estradiol can be produced as a result of StAR-independent mechanisms. This can occur until the follicular cells are

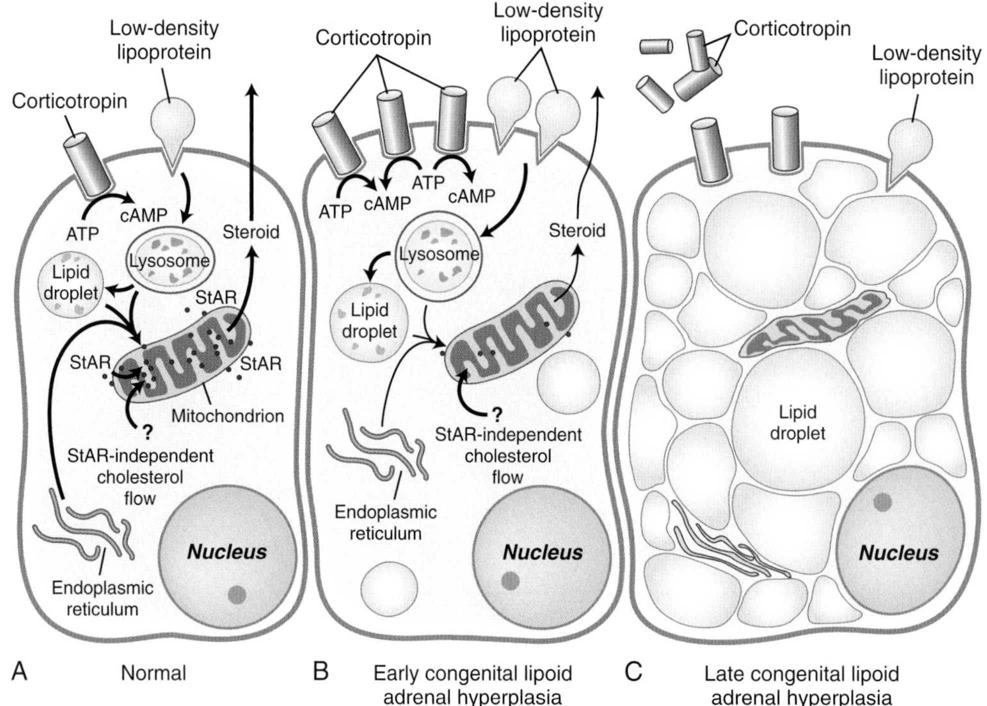

Figure 22–23 ▪ Model of the steroid-synthesizing cell (adrenal/gonadal) showing conversion of cholesterol to steroids. **A,** Cholesterol from low-density lipoprotein, from cholesterol esters stored in lipid droplets, and from endogenous synthesis in the endoplasmic reticulum is transported from the outer mitochondrial membrane to the inner membrane. This transport is facilitated by StAR (steroidogenic acute regulatory protein) as well as by other, StAR-independent mechanisms. In the mitochondria, steroid synthesis then ensues as a result of the conversion of cholesterol to Δ^5-pregnenolone by the enzyme CYP11A1 (P450scc). **B,** In patients with lipoid congenital adrenal hyperplasia, a mutation in the gene encoding StAR results in little or no activity of the mutant StAR, causing greatly diminished cholesterol transport into the mitochondria. Low levels of steroidogenesis via mechanisms independent of StAR can occur; however, increased corticotropin (or LH/FSH) secretion results in cholesterol accumulation in the cells as lipid droplets. **C,** Continued stimulation and resultant accumulation of cholesterol causes engorgement of these cells, with both mechanical and chemical perturbation of the cell function. This results in primary adrenal insufficiency and impaired androgen biosynthesis by fetal Leydig cells. Females with lipoid congenital adrenal hyperplasia feminize at puberty and menstruate but have progressive hypergonadotropic hypogonadism. It has been hypothesized by Bose and colleagues that this occurs because the follicular cells are relatively quiescent in utero and before puberty; hence, they are undamaged. At the beginning of each cycle, follicles are recruited, and a small amount of estradiol can be produced as a result of StAR-independent mechanisms. This can occur until the follicular cells are engorged and rendered nonfunctional. (From Bose HS, Sujiwara T, Strauss JF III, et al. The pathophysiology and genetics of congenital lipoid adrenal hyperplasia. N Engl J Med 1996;335:1870-1878. Copyright 1996, Massachusetts Medical Society.)

engorged and rendered nonfunctional. Thus, puberty can occur but any cycles are anovulatory as progesterone synthesis in the latter half of the cycle is disturbed. Polycystic ovaries and progressive ovarian failure usually ensue if left untreated.

Although more than 20 different StAR mutations have now been described in patients from around the world, lipoid CAH is especially prevalent in Japan and Korea where it is the second most common steroidogenic disorder after CYP21 deficiency (Fig. 22–24).[271,273-275] Most Japanese patients and virtually all Korean patients harbor the Gln258Stop mutation, which is estimated to be carried by 1 in 300 of the population.[274] Other geographic clusters include the Leu260Pro mutation in patients of Swiss ancestry, Arg188Cys in Eastern Saudi Arabia, and Arg182Leu in Palestinians. Most of these mutations show complete loss of function, although in rare cases presentation with salt-loss may not occur until about 1 year of age. Furthermore, a "nonclassic" form of lipoid CAH has recently been described due to point mutations in StAR that retain approximately 20% function.[276] These children presented with progressive glucocorticoid deficiency between 2 and 4 years of age; affected males had normal androgenization of the external genitalia. Treatment of "classic" lipoid CAH includes glucocorticoid and mineralocorticoid replacement and salt supplementation in early life. Gonadectomy is usually performed in individuals with a 46,XY karyotype. Estrogen treatment is given to induce puberty, and to 46,XX females when gonadal failure occurs.

P450 Side-Chain Cleavage (P450scc, CYP11A1) Deficiency

P450scc is the mitochondrial enzyme that converts cholesterol to pregnenolone by three distinct enzymatic reactions: 20α-hydroxylation, 22-hydroxylation, and cleavage of the cholesterol side-chain. P450scc is therefore responsible for the first and rate-limiting step in steroid synthesis, which is necessary for pregnenolone production by the placenta as well as for mineralocorticoid, glucorticoid, and androgen production by the adrenal glands and gonads.

Although a natural model of lipoid CAH due to P450scc deficiency exists in the rabbit,[277] it was believed that severe loss of P450scc activity in humans would be incompatible with survival; placental progesterone production is necessary to support pregnancy after the second trimester in higher primates (luteoplacental shift) but not in rodents. However, a small number of mutations in P450scc have now been described (Table 22–9).

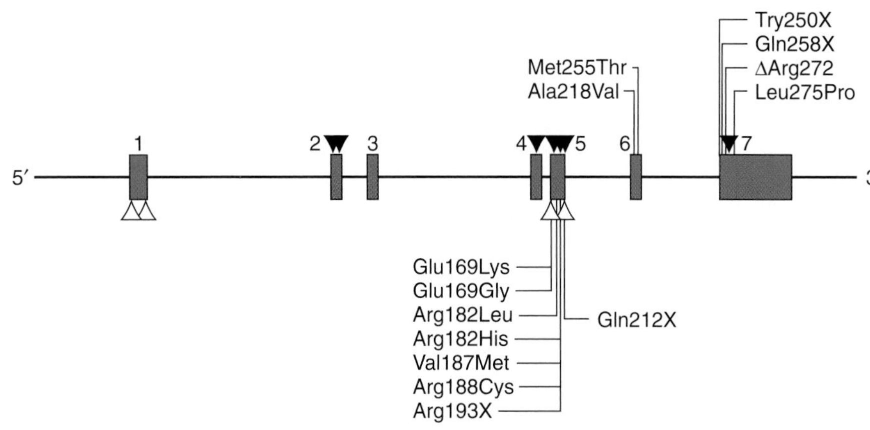

Figure 22–24 ▪ Diagram of selected mutations identified in the StAR gene associated with lipoid congenital adrenal hyperplasia. The numbered solid boxes depict the exons. The three letter abbreviation for amino acids is used to indicate the position of missense mutations; X, indicates a nonsense (stop) mutation; insertions and deletions resulting in frameshift *(filled arrowheads)* and splice site mutations *(open arrowheads)* are shown. Although StAR mutations are especially frequent in Japan, Korea, and regions in the Middle East, an increasing number of sporadic changes in StAR are being detected in other countries. Furthermore, two missense mutations at residues 187 and 188 have been described with a nonclassic late-onset phenotype of glucocorticoid insufficiency.

TABLE 22–9 CLINICAL FEATURES OF P450SCC DEFICIENCY IN 46,XY INDIVIDUALS

Karyotype	46, XY
Inheritance	Autosomal recessive; mutations in *CYP11A1* gene
Genitalia	Female; rarely ambiguous
Wolffian duct derivatives	Hypoplastic or normal
Müllerian duct derivatives	Absent
Gonads	Testes (or absent)
Habitus	Severe adrenal insufficiency in infancy with salt loss ranging to milder adrenal insufficiency with onset in childhood; prematurity associated in one case
Hormone profile	Usually deficiency of glucocorticoids, mineralocorticoids, and sex steroids

At the mildest end of the spectrum, a heterozygous mutation in P450scc has been reported in a 46,XY child with clitoromegaly and delayed onset of primary adrenal failure at 4 years of age.[278] In contrast, complete disruption of P450 activity due to a frameshift mutation in *CYP11A1* has been reported in a 46,XY infant with a female phenotype and severe early-onset salt-losing adrenal failure.[279] Of note, this child was born prematurely at 31 weeks' gestation, suggesting possible disruption of placental steroidogenesis.

3β-Hydroxysteroid Dehydrogenase/$\Delta^{4,5}$-Isomerase Type 2 (HSD3B2) Deficiency

3β-hydroxysteroid dehydrogenase deficiency (3β-HSD) is a rare cause of CAH and is one of the steroidogenic deficiencies that affects both adrenal and gonadal steroid production. The autosomal recessive disorder is a consequence of mutations in *HSD3B2*, the gene encoding the 3β-HSD/$\Delta^{4,5}$-isomerase type 2 isozyme, which is expressed mainly in the adrenals and gonads. This enzyme catalyses a crucial step in the biosynthesis of all steroid hormones, the conversion of Δ^5- to Δ^4-steroids (see Fig. 22–11). There are two isoenzymes isolated in humans. The type 1 isozyme is expressed in the placenta and in peripheral tissues such as the skin (mainly sebaceous glands), breast, and prostate. Types 1 and 2 isoenzymes are 93.5% homologous in protein structure with their genes located on chromosome lp13.1.[280] The type 1 isozyme is not associated with CAH. Human pregnancy is maintained by high levels of progesterone produced by placental 3β-HSD type 1 activity; thus, a homozygous type 1 gene defect would not be compatible with survival of an affected fetus.

TABLE 22–10 CLINICAL FEATURES OF 3β-HYDROXYSTEROID DEHYDROGENASE II DEFICIENCY IN 46,XY INDIVIDUALS

Karyotype	46, XY
Inheritance	Autosomal recessive; mutations in *HSD3B2* gene
Genitalia	Ambiguous; hypospadiac male
Wolffian duct derivatives	Normal
Müllerian duct derivatives	Absent
Gonads	Testes
Habitus	Severe adrenal insufficiency in infancy; poor virilization at puberty with gynecomastia. Mild form: no mineralocorticoid deficiency, premature adrenarche→mild virilization
Hormone profile	Increased concentrations of Δ^5 C_{21}- and C_{19}-steroids (e.g., 17-hydroxypregnenolone/cortisol ratio response to corticotropin; 17-hydroxypregnenolone and DHEA suppressible by dexamethasone

Classical 3β-HSD type 2 deficiency is subdivided into salt-losing and non–salt-losing forms. Males with 3β-HSD type 2 deficiency have clinical features as summarized in Table 22–10. The external genitalia are usually ambiguous, with a small penis, severe hypospadias, partial labioscrotal fusion, a urogenital sinus, and a blind vaginal pouch.

Newborns with severe 3β-HSD 2 deficiency develop adrenal insufficiency soon after birth. 46,XY males with partial deficiency of 3β-HSD 2 are not salt losers in that they have mutant enzymes that retain 2% to 10% of 3β-HSD 2 enzymatic activity, as assessed by transiently expressing the mutant in intact cells.[281] Gynecomastia can occur at puberty in both affected males and affected females. This is presumably the result of 3β-HSD 1–mediated peripheral conversion of Δ^5-C_{19}-steroids to Δ^4-C_{19}-steroids and aromatization to estrogens.[282] Indeed normal puberty and fertility has been reported in males with a null mutation in the *HSD3B2* gene.[283,284]

The biochemical profile indicative of classic 3β-HSD 2 deficiency is straightforward based on an elevated ratio of $\Delta^5 : \Delta^4$ steroids, determined either in plasma or urine. The most specific analyte to confirm the diagnosis is 17-hydroxypregnenolone which is greater than 100 nmol/L either basally or after ACTH stimulation.[281] However, this steroid is only measured in specialist laboratories. The concentrations of Δ^4-steroids such as 17-hydroxyprogesterone and androstenedione may also be elevated in 3β-HSD 2 deficiency, again as a result of peripheral type I 3β-HSD activity. In a neonatal screening program, elevated 17-hydroxyprogesterone in a salt-loser with 3β-HSD 2 deficiency may invoke a diagnosis of 21-hydroxylase deficiency.[285]

HSD3B2 is a four exon gene encoding for 371 amino acids. About 36 different mutations are now reported with many affected individuals being compound heterozygotes (Fig. 22–25). The concordance between genotype and phenotype is close so that the salt-losing versus the non–salt-losing form of 3β-HSD 2 deficiency is quite predictable. Examples of mutants that retain no enzyme activity and cause the severe, salt-losing form include Gly15Asp, Leu108Trp, Glu142Lys, Pro186Leu, Leu205Pro, Pro222Gln, Tyr253Asn, and Thr259Arg. In contrast, mutations such as Ala10Val and Ala245Pro retain considerable enzyme activity and were found in males with perineoscrotal hypospadias and no salt loss. A late-onset form of 3β-HSD 2 deficiency is also described, manifest generally as premature pubarche and idiopathic hirsutism in females. Clearer biochemical markers consistent with mutation-proven 3β-HSD 2 deficiency have now been derived for this late-onset group.[286,287] These include ACTH-stimulated 17-hydroxypregnenolone and 17-hydroxypregnenolone : cortisol ratios 54 and 38 SD above the control means, respectively. However, biochemical phenotyping is not possible for carrier detection in families with known *HSD3B2* mutations.[288] Targeting analysis of this gene in patients with idiopathic hypospadias yields, at best, only subtle changes in a small minority of cases.[289]

17α-Hydroxylase/17,20-Lyase (CYP17) Deficiency

P450c17 (*CYP17*) is a microsomal enzyme with both 17α-hydroxylase and 17,20-lyase activity that is expressed in the adrenals and gonads, but not in the placenta or in ovarian granulosa cells.[290-292] The 17α-hydroxylase action of P450c17 catalyzes the conversion of pregnenolone (Δ^5) to 17-hydroxypregnenolone, and progesterone (Δ^4) to 17-hydroxyprogesterone (17-OHP) (see Fig. 22–11). The 17,20-lyase action of P450c17 can covert 17-hydroxypregnenolone (Δ^5) to DHEA, and 17-OHP (Δ^4) to androstenedione (see Fig. 22–11). P450c17 is bound to the smooth endoplasmic reticulum where it accepts electrons from a specific flavoprotein, NADPH-P450 oxidoreductase. The 17,20-lyase activity of P450c17 is favored by the presence of Δ5 substrates, redox partners such as P450 oxidoreductase and cytochrome b5, and serine phosphorylation. Furthermore, unlike in rodents, the Δ^5-17,20-lyase activity of human P450c17 is about 50 times more efficient than its Δ^4-17,20-lyase activity, so very little androstenedione is formed directly from 17-OHP and the principal pathway to androgen production is via DHEA.[169] P450c17 also has 16α-hydroxylase activity.

Defects in P450c17 action can result in two different forms of CAH: most frequently, *combined 17α-hydroxylase/17,20-lyase deficiency* is seen, but rare cases of *isolated 17,20-lyase deficiency* have been reported (Tables 22–11 and 22–12).[292]

Combined 17α-hydroxylase/17,20-lyase deficiency is a relatively rare form of CAH, although an increasing number of cases are being reported worldwide.[293] A prevalence of approximately 1 : 50,000 individuals is reported. The classic phenotype of complete combined 17α-hydroxylase/17,20-lyase deficiency is of a phenotypic female (46,XX, or underandrogenized 46,XY) who presents with an absence of secondary sexual characteristics

TABLE 22–11 CLINICAL FEATURES OF COMBINED 17α-HYDROXYLASE/17,20-LYASE DEFICIENCY IN 46,XY INDIVIDUALS

Karyotype	46, XY
Inheritance	Autosomal recessive; mutations in *CYP17* gene
Genitalia	Female, ambiguous or hypospadiac male
Wolffian duct derivatives	Absent or hypoplastic
Müllerian duct derivatives	Absent
Gonads	Testes
Habitus	Absent or poor virilization at puberty; gynecomastia; hypertension
Hormone profile	Decreased T; increased LH and FSH; increased plasma deoxycorticosterone, corticosterone and progesterone; decreased plasma renin activity
	Low renin hypertension with hypokalemic alkalosis

FSH, follicle-stimulating hormone; LH, luteinizing hormone; T, testosterone.

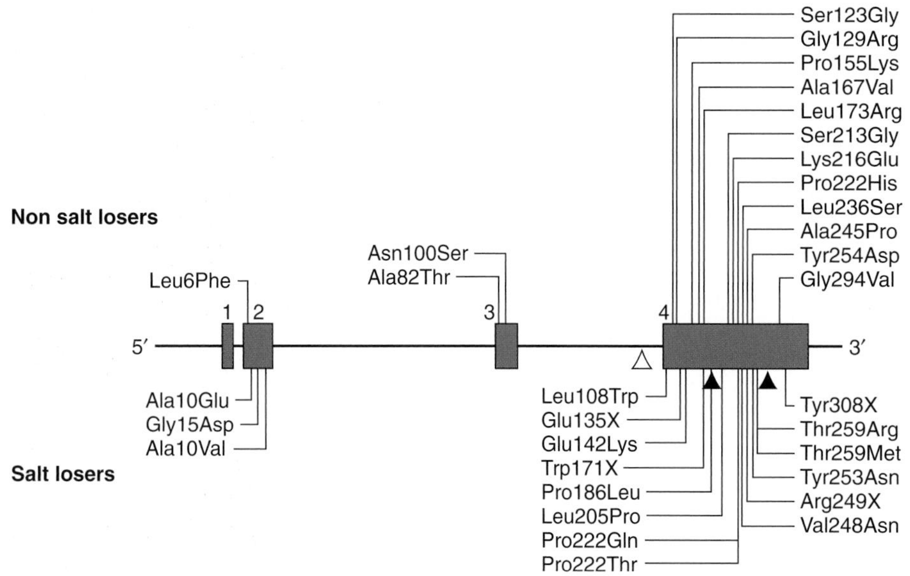

Figure 22–25 ▪ Diagram of the 3β-hydroxysteroid dehydrogenase type 2 *(HSD3B2)* gene depicting the mutations that result in 3β-HSD deficiency. The numbered *solid boxes* depict the exons. Mutations are subdivided according to association with salt-losing and non–salt-losing states. The three-letter abbreviation for amino acids is used to indicate the position of missense mutations; X, indicates a nonsense (stop) mutation; insertions and deletions resulting in frameshift *(filled arrowheads)* and splice site mutations *(open arrowheads)* are shown.

(hypergonadotropic hypogonadism) at puberty and is found to have low renin hypertension and hypokalemic alkalosis (see Table 22–11).

This classic phenotype and underlying biochemistry can be explained by the enzyme deficiency (see Fig. 22–11).[262] A defect in 17α-hydroxylation in both the adrenal cortex and gonads results in impaired synthesis of 17-hydroxyprogesterone and 17-hydroxypregnenolone and thus of cortisol, androgens, and estrogens. Decreased cortisol synthesis causes increased corticotropin secretion, which results in excessive secretion of 17-deoxysteroids by the adrenal cortex, including the mineralocorticoids DOC, corticosterone, and 18-hydroxycorticosterone. Excess DOC secretion leads to hypertension, hypokalemic alkalosis, and suppression of the renin-angiotensin system. Diminished aldosterone synthesis and secretion is sometimes reported. Corticosterone is a weak glucocorticoid; the high plasma concentrations in this disorder prevent the signs and symptoms of cortisol deficiency (e.g., hypoglycemia) and modulate the secretion of corticotropin.

Affected 46,XX females have normal female internal and external genital tracts, but the ovaries cannot secrete estrogens at puberty, resulting in absent breast development and hypogonadism with elevated plasma FSH and LH levels. In addition, the lack of adrenal and ovarian androgens can result in little or no growth of pubic and axillary hair. In affected 46,XX individuals, the ovaries have a high proportion of atretic follicles and some ovaries contain an increased number of enlarged follicular cysts.

Affected 46,XY individuals with complete combined 17α-hydroxylase/17,20-lyase deficiency who are diagnosed in adolescence usually have female external genitalia and a blind vaginal pouch (see Table 22–11). Testes may be intraabdominal, in the inguinal canal, or in the labioscrotal folds. Inguinal herniae are common, müllerian structures are absent, and wolffian derivatives are hypoplastic. Bone age is frequently delayed and prolonged linear growth can lead to tall stature. Pubic and axillary hair is absent or sparse, and hypergonadotropic hypogonadism is associated with a failure to develop secondary sexual characteristic at puberty. Excessive secretion of DOC and corticosterone usually leads to low renin hypertension and hypokalemic alkalosis, as in 46,XX girls with this condition.

Complete 17α-hydroxylase/17,20-lyase deficiency is associated with a variety of mutations in the *CYP17* gene, which cause complete loss of function in assays of enzyme activity. These changes include a range of missense, frameshift, and nonsense mutations (Fig. 22–26). The most common mutation is the four base-pair duplication in exon 8, shared by Mennonites and individuals in the Friesland region of the Netherlands, which is attributed to a founder effect originating in Friesland. Other geographic clusters include an in-frame deletion of residues 487-489 in Southeast Asia, and the Arg362Cys and Trp406Arg missense mutations found among Brazilians of Portuguese and Spanish ancestry, respectively.[292,294,295]

Partial forms of combined 17α-hydroxylase/17,20-lyase deficiency have also been described. This condition most frequently presents as a 46,XY infant with ambiguous genitalia or severe hypospadias, in whom the steroid profile is consistent with this diagnosis of P450c17 deficiency. Hypertension may or may not be present in partial forms of combined 17α-hydroxylase/17,20-

TABLE 22–12 CLINICAL FEATURES OF ISOLATED 17,20-LYASE DEFICIENCY IN 46,XY INDIVIDUALS

Karyotype	46, XY
Inheritance	Autosomal recessive; mutations in *CYP17* gene, usually affecting key redox domains
Genitalia	Female, ambiguous or hypospadiac male
Wolffian duct derivatives	Absent or hypoplastic
Müllerian duct derivatives	Absent
Gonads	Testes
Habitus	Absent or poor virilization at puberty; gynecomastia
Hormone profile	Decreased plasma T, DHEA, androstenedione, and estradiol; abnormal increase in plasma 17-hydroxyprogesterone and 17-hydroxypregnenolone; increased LH and FSH; increased ratio of C_{21}-deoxysteroids to C_{19}-steroids (DHEA, androstenedione) after hCG stimulation

DHEA, Dehydroepiandrosterone; FSH, follicle-stimulating hormone; LH, luteinizing hormone; T, testosterone.

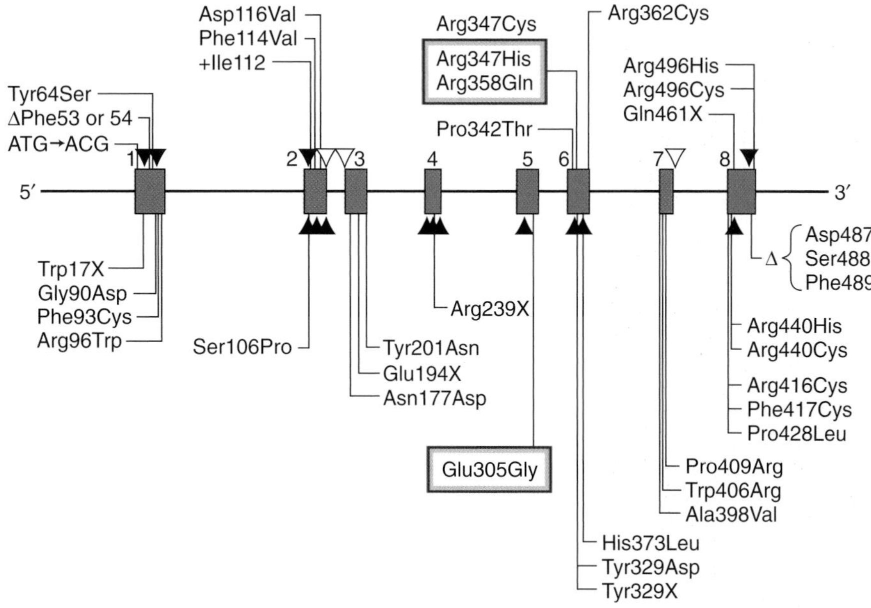

Figure 22–26 ▪ Diagram of selected mutations in the *CYP17* gene (17α-hydroxylase/17,20-lyase deficiency). The numbered *solid boxes* depict the exons. The three-letter abbreviation for amino acids is used to indicate the position of missense mutations; X, indicates a nonsense (stop) mutation; insertions and deletions resulting in frameshift and splice site mutations are shown by *filled arrowheads* and *open arrowheads,* respectively. All of these mutations cause 17α-hydroxylase deficiency. Several missense mutations such as those at codons 305, 347, and 358 *(boxed)* have been associated with "isolated" 17,20-lyase deficiency.

lyase deficiency and aldosterone secretion may be normal or even elevated. Corticosterone levels, which are usually 50- to 100-fold higher than normal, provide adequate glucocorticoid effects and prevent symptoms of cortisol deficiency. The development of male secondary sexual characteristics at puberty may be incomplete and gynecomastia is often seen. This rare condition has been reported due to a phenylalanine deletion at codon 53 or 54,[296] in a patient compound heterozygous for a null mutation in P450c17 together with a Pro342Thr mutation with 20% of normal 17α-hydroxylase activity;[297] and in a small number of additional cases in which some residual enzyme function is seen. Analysis of these patients suggests that 5% of normal activity in a 46,XX female is sufficient to allow estrogen production with normal secondary sexual characteristics and irregular menses, whereas more than 25% of normal activity appears to be necessary to achieve normal androgenization of the external genitalia of affected 46,XY males.

Isolated 17,20-lyase activity has been reported in a small number of cases.[298] These 46,XY patients usually have genital ambiguity, normal secretion of glucocorticoids and mineralocorticoids, and marked reduction in sex steroid synthesis (see Table 22–12). The first two patients shown to have a molecular defect in P450c17 harbored homozygous point mutations in the enzyme (Arg347His, Arg358Gln), which specifically interfered with 17,20-lyase activity by changing the distribution of surface charges in the redox-partner binding site.[299,300] Other patients have been reported with similar mutations, or where a point mutation (Glu305Gly) specifically alters the conformation of the substrate binding site.[301] Of note, a splice site mutation in the redox partner cytochrome b5 has been reported in a 46,XY child with ambiguous genitalia and methemoglobinemia, although extensive endocrinologic data are not reported.[302] Defects in the other key redox partner—P450 oxidoreductase—are described below.

The diagnosis of 17α-hydroxylase deficiency should be suspected in all cases of 46,XY DSD and is strongly supported by the discovery of hyporeninemic hypertension and hypokalemic alkalosis, as well as a lack of secondary sex characteristics at puberty.[262] Plasma concentrations of corticotropin, DOC, corticosterone, and progesterone are high, and those of 17α-hydroxyprogesterone, cortisol, and gonadal steroids are low. Replacement therapy with physiologic doses of glucocorticoids suppresses DOC and corticosterone secretion and normalizes serum potassium levels, blood pressure, and plasma renin and aldosterone levels. Gonadectomy is performed in 46,XY patients who have a female gender assignment. Appropriate gonadal steroid replacement therapy is indicated at puberty.

P450 Oxidoreductase (POR) Deficiency

P450 oxidoreductase (*POR*) is a membrane-bound flavoprotein that plays a central role in electron transfer from NADPH to P450 enzymes (Fig. 22–27).[303] The crucial role of P450 oxidoreductase in the 17,20-lyase reaction of P450c17 has been outlined above, but it is also clear that P450 oxidoreductase interacts with all 57 microsomal P450 enzymes, including P450c21 (21-hydroxylase) and P450c19 (aromatase), as well as many cytochrome P450 enzymes system involved in hepatic drug metabolism.

A potential role for P450 oxidoreductase in human steroidogenesis emerged following the description of several patients with apparent combined deficiencies of P450c17 and P450c21.[304] Furthermore, ambiguous genitalia and unusual patterns of combined steroidogenic defects have been described in a subset of patients with Antley-Bixler syndrome (ABS), a form of skeletal dysplasia that is characterized by craniosynostosis, brachycephaly, midface hypoplasia, proptosis, choanal stenosis, radioulnar or radiohumeral synostosis, bowed femora, and arachnodactyly.[305]

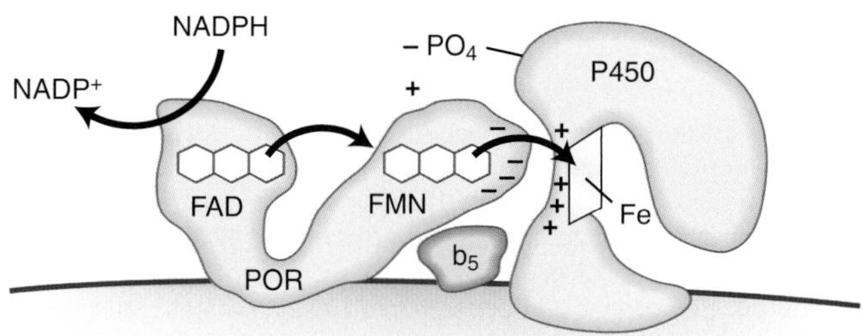

Figure 22–27 ▪ Cartoon of the role of P450 oxidoreductase (POR) in electron transfer to microsomal (type II) P450 enzymes. NADPH interacts with POR, bound to the endoplasmic reticulum, and transfers a pair of electrons to the FAD moiety. This change in charge results in altered conformation, which allows the electrons to pass from the FAD to the FMN moiety. Following further realignment, the FMN domain can interact with the redox partner binding site of the P450 enzyme (e.g., P450c17, P450c21, P450c19), permitting electron transfer to the active heme group of the enzyme, which results in substrate catalysis. The interaction of POR and the P450 is coordinated by negatively charged acidic residues on the surface of the FMN domain of POR and positively charged basic residues in the redox partner binding site of the P450. In the case of human P450c17, this interaction is facilitated by the allosteric action of cytochrome b_5 and by serine phosphorylation of P450c17. (Reproduced with permission from Miller WL. Minireview: regulation of steroidogenesis by electron transfer. Endocrinology 2005;146:2544-2550. © 2005 The Endocrine Society.)

TABLE 22–13 CLINICAL FEATURES OF P450 OXIDOREDUCTASE DEFICIENCY IN 46,XY INDIVIDUALS

Karyotype	46, XY
Inheritance	Autosomal recessive; mutations in *POR* gene
Genitalia	Ambiguous; hypospadias or normal male
Wolffian duct derivatives	Absent or hypoplastic
Müllerian duct derivatives	Absent
Gonads	Testes
Habitus	Variable androgenization at birth; variable virilization at puberty; glucocorticoid deficiency; no severe mineralocorticoid deficiency; features of Antley-Bixler syndrome (craniosynostosis, skeletal dysplasia) in some cases
Hormone profile	Evidence of combined P450c17 and P450c21 insufficiency; normal or low cortisol with poor response to ACTH stimulation; elevated 17-hydroxyprogesterone; T low

ACTH, Adrenocorticotropin.

The first recessively inherited human mutations in P450 oxidoreductase were described in 2004 and a significant number of *POR* changes have already been described in patients with marked phenotypic variability (Table 22–13).[306,170] At the most severe end of the spectrum is ABS with ambiguous genitalia, or patients with apparent combined P450c17 and P450c21 deficiency but no skeletal phenotype. However, milder defects in P450 oxidoreductase have also been seen in women with a form of polycystic ovary syndrome or in men with mild gonadal insufficiency. A range of P450 oxidoreductase activity is associated with this spectrum of phenotypes. Although experience is limited at present, two mutations are emerging as being especially common: Arg287Pro is the most prevalent mutation in patients of European ancestry whereas the Arg457His mutation is common in Japan.[170,306-308] Furthermore, activating mutations in fibroblast growth factor receptor 2 have also been reported in association with ABS; in these cases, ambiguous genitalia or steroidogenic defects are not present.

Most patients with P450 oxidoreductase deficiency have normal electrolytes and mineralocorticoid function (see Table 22–13).[308] Cortisol insufficiency can be present or, if basal levels are adequate, the response to ACTH stimulation is reduced. Serum 17-hydroxyprogesterone is usually elevated, with a variable response to ACTH stimulation, and sex steroids tend to be low, especially outside the early neonatal period. Of particular importance is the fact that P450 oxidoreductase deficiency can be associated with ambiguous genitalia in both sexes (46,XY and 46,XX). Underandrogenization of 46,XY males most likely results from disturbed 17,20-lyase activity during fetal Leydig cell steroidogenesis. The partial androgenization of 46,XX infants may be the result of a disturbance in aromatase activity, as P450 oxidoreductase is an electron donor for this enzyme and aromatase deficiency causes prenatal androgenization of the developing 46,XX fetus (see Aromatase Deficiency in 46,XX DSD). Alternatively, a "backdoor" pathway of androgen biosynthesis has been described in certain species such as the fetal Tamar Wallaby.[170,171] In this model system, 17-OHP can be converted to DHT without using androstenedione or testosterone as an intermediate. Data are emerging that this pathway may also be functional during human development.

17β-Hydroxysteroid Dehydrogenase Type 3 (HSD17B3) Deficiency (Fig. 22–28)

The 17β-HSD reaction in the human is mediated by six known isozymes that catalyze the reduction of androstenedione, DHEA, and estrone to testosterone, Δ^5-androstenediol, and estradiol, respectively, as well as the reverse reaction (see Fig. 22–11).[309] The 17β-HSD 3 enzyme utilizes NADPH as a cofactor; its gene, designated *HSD17B3,* contain 11 exons and is located on chromosome 9q22. The type 3 isoenzyme is expressed primarily in the testes, where it favors the conversion of the weak androgen substrate, androstenedione, to the more biologically active testosterone (see Fig. 22–11).

17β-HSD 3 deficiency (also called 17β-hydroxysteroid oxidoreductase or 17-ketosteroid reductase) as one of the causes of 46,XY DSD was first reported by Saez and colleagues.[310,311] Many cases have now been reported and the phenotype well characterized (Table 22–14).[312-314] Most affected males have female external genitalia at birth, although a few infants may present with ambiguous genitalia. The testes are usually located in the inguinal canal, the wolffian ducts are stabilized to form epididymides, vas deferens, seminal vesicles, and ejaculatory ducts, and there is a blind vaginal pouch. Affected infants are invariably assigned a female sex and may mistakenly be assumed to have complete androgen insensitivity syndrome (see later). Profound virilization occurs at puberty in the form of deepening of the voice, hirsutism, muscle development, and clitoromegaly. This is often how the condition must be distinguished from other causes of virilization arising at puberty in subjects raised female. The pubertal increase in testosterone is mostly from extraglandular conversion from androstenedione. We have speculated that this is mediated by genetic and/or environmental induction of enzyme activities of the aldoketoreductase family IC (AKRIC) such as the 17β-HSD type 5 isoenzyme, also known as AKRIC3.[315,316] There is also increased androstenedione substrate at puberty and partial 17β-HSD 3 activity in the testes in some cases. In a large cohort of patients from a consanguineous population in the Gaza Strip, the phallus was described as reaching lengths of 4 to 8 cm.[317] The *HSD17B3* mutation reported in this population (Arg80Gln) is associated with 15% to 20% retention of normal 17β-HSD3 activity (see Fig. 22–26). The development of gynecomastia at puberty occurs from estrogens derived from the conversion of androstenedione by aromatase in extraglandular tissue and the action of the 17β-HSD 1 or 17β-HSD 2 isoenzymes. The striking virilization at puberty, similar to patients with 5α-reductase-2 deficiency, has resulted in gender role reassignment from female to male in some cases. In general, patients presenting as androgenized females at puberty undergo urgent gonadectomy and reduction clitoroplasty and maintenance of female gender. The typical biochemical profile in 17β-HSD3 deficiency is an elevated androstenedione level relative to testosterone (see Table 22–14). Expressed as a ratio of testosterone:androstenedione (and following an hCG

TABLE 22–14 CLINICAL FEATURES OF 17β-HYDROXYSTEROID DEHYDROGENASE TYPE 3 DEFICIENCY IN 46,XY INDIVIDUALS

Karyotype	46, XY
Inheritance	Autosomal recessive; mutations in *HSD17B3* gene
Genitalia	Female→ambiguous; blind vaginal pouch
Wolffian duct derivatives	Present
Müllerian duct derivatives	Absent
Gonads	Testes (usually undescended)
Habitus	Virilization at puberty (phallus enlargement, deepening of voice, and development of facial and body hair); gynecomastia variable
Hormone profile	Increased plasma estrone and androstenedione; decreased ratio of plasma testosterone/androstenedione and estradiol after hCG stimulation test; increased plasma FSH and LH levels

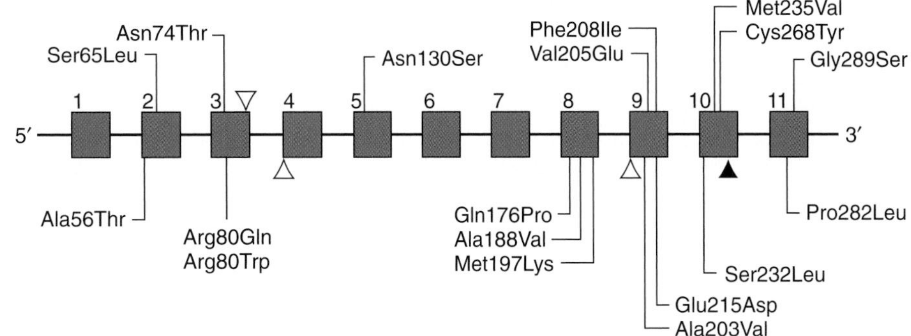

Figure 22–28 ▪ Diagram of the 17β-hydroxysteroid dehydrogenase type 3 *(HSD17B3)* gene depicting the mutations that result in 17β-HSD deficiency. The numbered *solid boxes* depict the exons. The three-letter abbreviation for amino acids is used to indicate the position of missense mutations; X, indicates a nonsense (stop) mutation; insertions and deletions resulting in frameshift *(filled arrowheads)* and splice site mutations *(open arrowheads)* are shown.

stimulation test before puberty), values less than 0.8 are generally found in these patients.[318] Testicular vein sampling at the time of gonadectomy shows a markedly increased androstenedione gradient relative to testosterone.

Only mutations in the *HSD17B3* gene that encodes the testis-specific enzyme are a cause of this form of 46,XY DSD. A total of 21 mutations in patients with 17β-HSD3 deficiency are now described (see Fig. 22–28). The majority are missense mutations and some patients are compound heterozygotes. Expression studies of the mutant enzymes in heterologous cells generally show complete absence of activity in the conversion of androstenedione to testosterone compared with the normal enzyme. A single nucleotide polymorphism in exon 11 resulting in Gly289Ser confers a significant increase in risk for prostate cancer.[319] A similar study undertaken in women with polycystic ovary syndrome showed no association between the polymorphism and this condition.[320] Women homozygous or compound heterozygous for *HSD17B3* mutations are asymptomatic. The presence of wolffian duct derivatives in the form of a normal vas deferens and epididymis in patients with homozygous mutations that result in complete absence of enzymatic activity is intriguing. A similar finding occurs in a significant number of patients with CAIS due to a missense mutation in the *AR* gene.[321] Androgens can diffuse directly into the adjacent wolffian ducts to elicit a paracrine effect. Fetal androstenedione levels are expected to be increased. Although this is a weak androgen, its potency using a reporter gene assay indicated it was almost as potent as testosterone and DHT when tested at concentrations greater than 10 nM.[322]

Establishing the diagnosis of 17β-HSD3 deficiency soon after birth, either because of finding inguinal testes in a phenotypic female infant, or ambiguity of the external genitalia, raises the question of sex assigment. Because of the experience of gender role change at puberty in affected families as reported in Gaza, it has been proposed that these patients could be given male gender assignment at diagnosis.[323] This study reported 46,XY males with female external genitalia treated early with testosterone, followed later by first-stage genitoplasty. The majority achieved a reasonable cosmetic result with a penile length within the normal range. There are no more recent studies that report on outcome in infants assigned a male sex of rearing. Phenotypic variability within affected families can also influence gender assignment.[315] That gender role changes at puberty has been reported in 39% to 64% of cases raised as girls should be discussed with families when providing evidence for gender assignment after birth.[190]

Steroid 5α-Reductase Type 2 Deficiency

This defect in androgen biosynthesis, as with 17β-HSD deficiency, is characterized by a 46,XY karyotype, normally differentiated testes, male internal ducts, but external genitalia that may be more ambiguous at birth. Again 5α-RD deficiency shares the striking degree of virilization, which occurs at puberty. The classic features of this enzyme deficiency are summarized in Table 22–15. The description of a genetic isolate from villages in the southwestern part of the Dominican Republic and a subsequent review of the biochemical and molecular features underlines the importance of DHT in the development of the male phenotype.[324-327] At birth, there is a clitoris-like, hypospadiac phallus, a bifid scrotum, a urogenital sinus, and a blind vaginal pouch. Testes differentiate normally and are located either in the inguinal canal or the labioscrotal folds. No müllerian structures are present. The wolffian ducts are stabilized so that the epididymis, vas deferens, and seminal vesicle are well differentiated; the ejaculatory ducts usually terminate in the blind vaginal pouch. The prostate is hypoplastic. Affected males virilize to a variable degree at puberty. The voice deepens, muscle mass increases, the phallus enlarges to 4 to 8 cm in length, the bifid scrotum becomes rugated and pigmented, and the testes enlarge and descend into the labioscrotal folds. None of the postpubertal affected males have acne, temporal hair recession, or enlargement of the prostate, and they do not develop gynecomastia. There is normal libido with penile erections. Histology of the testes shows Leydig cell hyperplasia and decreased spermatogenesis, the latter probably secondary to the cryptorchidism.[328] Nevertheless, some of the Dominican cohort had normal sperm counts. One man fathered a child following intrauterine insemination and two affected brothers in a Swedish family were spontaneously fertile having previously had hypospadias repair in childhood.[329,330] Gender role changes occur frequently in 5α-RD deficiency, particularly where clusters of cases occur in geographic regions such as the Dominican Republic, New Guinea,[331] South Lebanon, and Turkey. Overall, gender role changes in 56% to 63% of cases.[332] Females homozygous for 5α-RD deficiency undergo normal puberty but delayed menarche, and fertility is normal.[333]

Table 22–15 CLINICAL FEATURES OF 5α-REDUCTASE-2 DEFICIENCY IN 46,XY INDIVIDUALS

Karyotype	46, XY
Inheritance	Autosomal recessive; mutations in *SRD5A2* gene
Genitalia	Usually ambiguous with small, hypospadiac phallus; blind vaginal pouch
Wolffian duct derivatives	Normal
Müllerian duct derivatives	Absent
Gonads	Normal testes
Habitus	Decreased facial and body hair, no temporal hair recession, prostate not palpable
Hormone profile	Decreased ratio of 5α/5β C_{21}- and C_{19}-steroids in urine; increased T/DHT ratio before and after hCG stimulation; modest increase in plasma LH; decreased conversion of T to DHT in vitro

DHT, dihydrotestosterone; hCG, human chorionic gonadotropin; LH, luteinizing hormone; T, testosterone.

The biochemical profile in 5α-RD deficiency typically shows elevated testosterone : DHT ratios, which need to be determined after hCG stimulation when investigations are undertaken before puberty (see Table 22–15). The ratio generally exceeds 30 : 1. Serum LH and FSH levels may be normal or elevated after puberty. An additional and useful diagnostic feature is a diminished ratio of urinary 5α to 5β-reduced C_{19}- and C_{21}-steroids. The diagnosis can still be confirmed biochemically after gonadectomy because of persistent effect on C_{21} 5α/5β-reduced steroids such as allo-tetrahydrocortisol and tetrahydrocortisol, but this is more accurate after 6 months of age.

Early diagnosis of 5α-RD2 deficiency is important because of its bearing on sex assignment. The natural history of this condition whereby there is a propensity in some patients for change to a male gender role with virilization at puberty mandates a male gender assignment when there is ambiguous or underandrogenized genitalia at birth.[334] DHT, which can be applied topically as a cream, increases penile length and facilitates repair of the hypospadias.[335,336] Much higher doses of DHT given systemically are needed to promote phallic growth in adulthood.

5α-RD2 deficiency is transmitted as an autosomal recessive trait. There are two microsomal 5α-RD enzymes that catalyze the NADPH-dependent conversion of testosterone to DHT. 5α-RD2 is a 254 amino acid protein encoded by the *SRD5A2* gene on chromosome 2p23.[326] The type 2 isozyme is expressed predominantly in the primordial of the prostate and external genitalia but not in the wolffian ducts until after their differentiation in to the male internal genital ducts.[337] The type 1 isoenzyme is expressed in skin, including human genital skin fibroblasts. It has been suggested that this isoenzyme may contribute to the virilization that occurs in 5α-RD–deficient patients at puberty.[338]

5α-RD2 deficiency is genetically heterogeneous and more than 40 mutations have been detected in the *SRD5A2* gene (Fig. 22–29). Mutations are distributed in all five exons; the majority are missense mutations and a complete gene deletion is found in the New Guinea population. The resulting enzymatic dysfunction ranges from complete loss of activity to impaired substrate and cofactor binding, and enzyme instability. There is little correlation between the severity of the clinical phenotype and the nature of the mutation. A significant number of cases are compound heterozygotes, while consanguinity is also common. Male heterozygotes are normal.

Disorders of Androgen Action

The key role of androgens in male sex differentiation cannot be better illustrated than the consequence of total lack of response to androgens in target tissues—a complete female phenotype in a 46,XY individual with normally formed testes producing age-appropriate testosterone levels. This is *the* paradigm of a hormone resistance syndrome. To understand the pathophysiology of the various clinical syndromes associated with complete or partial resistance to androgens, it is necessary to briefly review the mechanism of normal androgen action.

Male sex differentiation and the subsequent acquisition of secondary sex characteristics at puberty, and the onset of spermatogenesis, are all mediated by androgens binding to a single intracellular androgen receptor (AR) ubiquitously expressed in target tissue. The AR is one of a quartet of nuclear receptors (glucocorticoid, mineralocorticoid, progesterone and androgen) that are closely related within a large superfamily and can activate gene transcription via a common hormone response element. The single copy gene encoding the AR is located on Xq11-q12 and is made up of eight exons, which encode a protein of 919 amino acid residues. The major functional domains comprise an N-terminal transactivation domain (NTD) encoded by exon 1, a central highly conserved DNA binding domain (DBD) encoded by exons 2 and 3, a hinge region, which connects the DBD to the ligand binding domain and the C-terminal ligand binding domain (LBD) encoded by exons 4 to 8 (Fig. 22–30). The DBD is highly conserved amongst nuclear receptors and contains cysteine residues that coordinate zinc atoms to form the zinc fingers characteristic of all nuclear receptors and many other transcription factors. The first zinc finger contains a P-box,

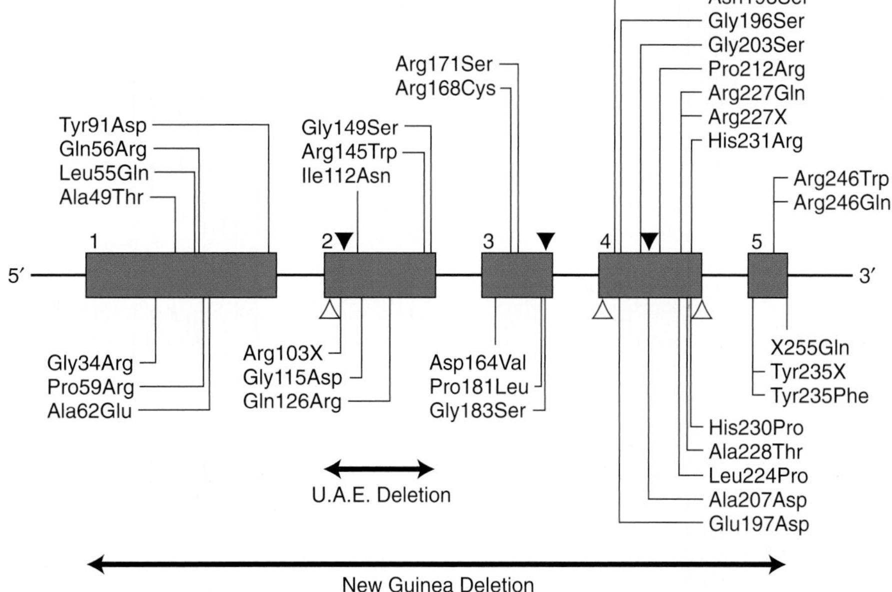

Figure 22–29 ▪ Diagram of the 5α-reductase type 2 *(SRD5A2)* gene depicting the mutations that result in 5α-reductase deficiency. The numbered *solid boxes* depict the exons. The three-letter abbreviation for amino acids is used to indicate the position of missense mutations; X, indicates a nonsense (stop) mutation; insertions and deletions resulting in frameshift and splice site mutations are shown by *filled arrowheads* and *open arrowheads,* respectively. Large deletions found in affected UAE (United Arab Emirates) and New Guinea populations are shown. (Adapted from Grumbach MM, Hughes IA, Conte FA. Disorders of sex differentiation. In Larsen PR, et al, eds. Williams Textbook of Endocrinology, 10th ed. Philadelphia: Saunders, 2003, with additional data provided courtesy of Dr. Julianne Imperato-McGinley, Department of Medicine, Weill Medical College of Cornell University, NY.)

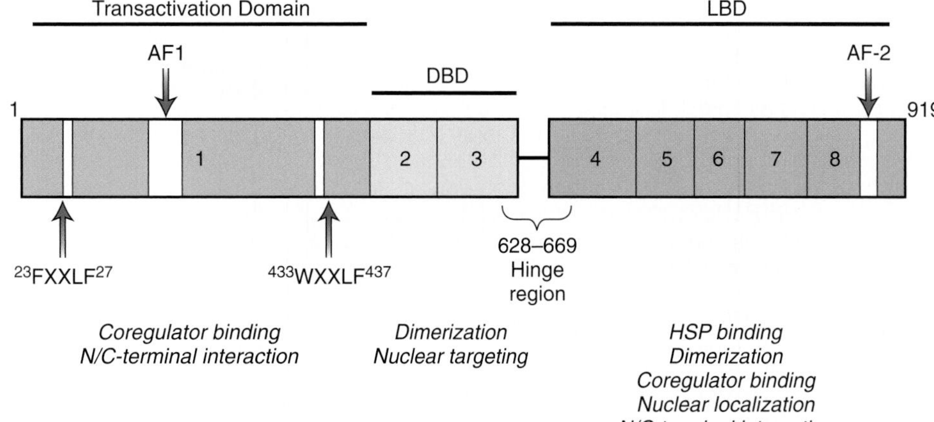

Figure 22–30 ▪ Schematic diagram of the androgen receptor showing the major functional domains and subsidiary functions. Single amino acid codes are used; X is any amino acid. *AF,* Activation function; *DBD,* DNA binding domain; *LBD,* ligand binding domain; *HSP,* heat-shock protein. Numbers outside the structure refer to amino acids (AR is 919 amino acid residues); numbers 1-8 inside the structure refer to AR exons.

which recognizes the androgen response element for direct DNA binding. The second zinc finger containing the D-box is involved in protein:protein interactions and also stabilizes the unit for receptor dimerization. The subsidiary functions operated by these domains are shown in Figure 22-30 and include dimerization, binding to coregulator proteins, interaction with heat-shock proteins, and transcriptional regulation. The two subdomains most involved in activation of transcription are the motif activation function-1 (AF1) in the NTD and the motif activation function-2 (AF2) in the LBD. AF1 is ligand independent whereas AF2 is ligand dependent and also interacts with the p160 steroid receptor coactivators such as SRC1, SRC2/TIF2, and SRC3.[339] For most nuclear receptors, there is a strong interaction between the AF2 subdomain and LXXLL (where L is a leucine and X is any amino acid) motifs in the coactivators. In the case of the AR, however, this interaction is weaker and the AF2 subdomain interacts in an intramolecular manner with its cognate AF1 subdomain in the NTD.[340] This N/C interaction is a relatively unique feature of the AR and is mediated by interaction with the FXXLF (F, phenylalamine) motif in AF1 comprising amino acid residues 23-27. N/C interaction stabilizes the AR and slows down the dissociation of the ligand from its receptor. Further modulation of AR function occurs posttranslationally via processes such as phosphorylation and SUMOylation.

A unique feature of the AR is homopolymeric stretches of amino acids within the NTD. A sequence of CAG repeats in exon 1 encodes for a stretch of glutamines, which ranges from 11-31 repeats in the general population with a mean of 21 repeats. Another repeat of glycines ranges from 10 to 25 in the general population with an average of 23 glycines. In vitro studies show that the length of the CAG repeat is inversely proportional to the activity of the AR as a transcription factor.[341]

Figure 22–31 illustrates androgens interacting with the AR on entering target cells and subsequent activation of target genes. A single receptor binds all androgens, with testosterone being converted to DHT, biologically more potent by virtue of dissociating from the AR at a slower rate. The AR in the unliganded state is located in the cytoplasm complexed to heat-shock proteins (HSPs) such as HSP70 and HSP90. These in turn are also complexed to cochaperone proteins such as FKBP52.[342] Binding of ligand to its receptor initiates dissociation from these complexes to allow translocation of the AR into the nucleus where it binds as a homodimer to a DNA hormone response element, comprising the consensus inverted repeat, GGTACAnnnTGTTCT. The action of the AR is further modulated by interaction with coregulatory proteins, which function either as coactivators or corepressors.[339] These proteins are postulated to function as a physical bridge connecting the receptor to the basal transcription machinery and thereby interacts the ligand-bound AR with chromatin. There are many coactivators that act in a generic fashion (e.g., the SRC and CBP/p300 family of proteins) but there are also others—such as ARA24, ARA54, ARA55 and ARA70—that are relatively specific to the AR.

The crystal structure of the DBD and LBD, complexed with ligand, is shown in Figure 22–32. The three-dimensional structure of a nuclear receptor LBD comprises 12α helices associated with antiparallel β sheets arranged in the form of a tripartite sandwich. A hydrophobic pocket is formed by helices 3, 4, 5, 7, 11, and 12, to which the ligand is bound on contact with its cognate receptor. Helix 12 is the outermost α-helix, which folds back on top of the ligand hydrophobic pocket like a lid closing on a box. This has been referred to as the "mousetrap" effect to capture the ligand and retain it by slowing the rate of ligand-receptor dissociation. This trapping effect by helix 12 also permits interaction between the LBD and AF2 subdomain and the LXXLL motif in associated coregulator proteins. Information about the structural and functional aspects of the AR has been gleaned not only from studying the effects of amino acid residue manipulations using site-directed mutagenesis, but also from analysis of the functional consequences of AR mutations that lead to various degrees of androgen resistance. The role of the AR in mediating androgen action indicates the pleiotropic effects, which occur when the function of the AR is disrupted. These are clinically manifest as syndromes of androgen insensitivity, classified as complete, partial, and minimal according to severity of hormone resistance.[343]

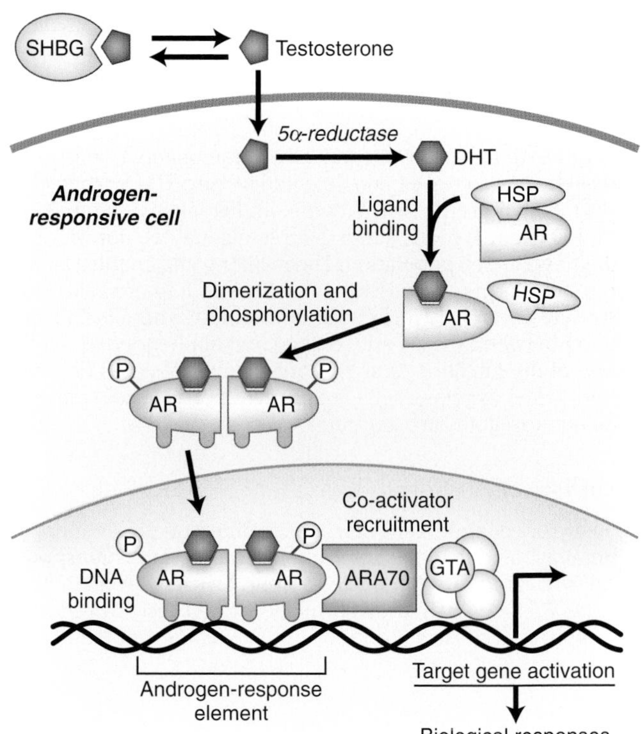

Figure 22–31 ■ A schematic diagram of androgen action in a target cell. Circulating testosterone bound predominantly to sex hormone–binding globulin (SHBG) enters the cell in free form where it is converted to DHT, a more potent androgen. Both androgens bind to a single cytoplasmic androgen receptor (AR) complexed to heat-shock proteins (HSPs) and other cochaperones such as FKBP52. Androgen binding dissociates the AR from HSPs where AR-bound androgen translocates to the nucleus, binding to DNA response elements as a homodimer. Coactivators, such as ARA70, bind to the AR complex to mediate interaction with the general transcription apparatus (GTA). This results in transcription of androgen-responsive genes and pleiotropic biologic responses; examples of such responses would include male sex differentiation, growth, muscle and bone development, spermatogenesis, and prostate growth. *P*, Phosphorylation. (Adapted from Feldman BJ, Feldman D. The development of androgen-independent prostate cancer. Nature Ref Cancer 2001;1:34-45.© 2001 Nature Publishing Group.)

Complete Androgen Insensitivity Syndrome (CAIS)
(Table 22–16)

The phenotype of CAIS is that of a normal female. Estimates on the prevalence of this X-linked recessive disorder range from 1 in 20,400 genetic males to 1 in 99,000 genetic males.[344,345] The typical mode of presentation is an adolescent female who has breast development with a pubertal growth spurt but has not had her menarche. Clinical assessment also confirms the absence or scanty growth of pubic and axillary hair. The uterus is absent as a result of normal AMH action, although there may be müllerian remnants. Surprisingly, the wolffian ducts are stabilized in many patients with well developed vas deferens and epididymis observed when gonadectomy is performed.[321] The main differential at this age is XY complete gonadal dysgen-

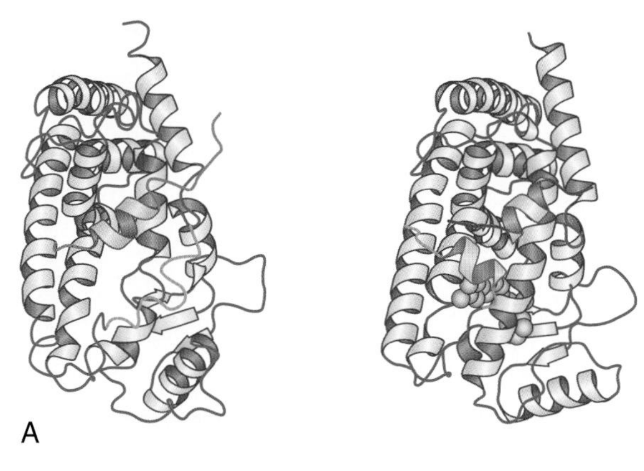

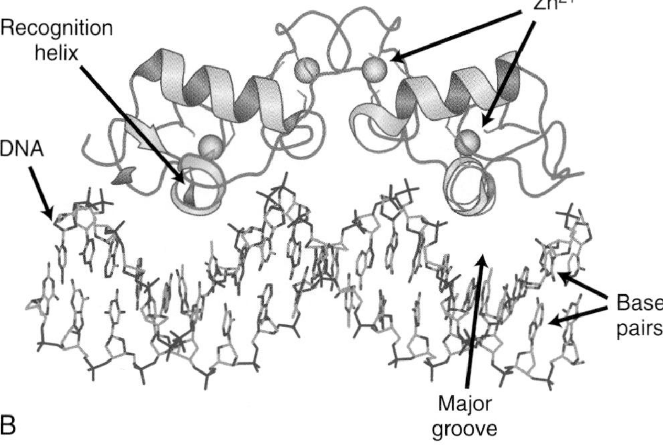

Figure 22–32 ▪ Diagram of the representative crystal structure of the ligand-binding domain (LBD) and DNA-binding domain (DBD) of a nuclear receptor. **A,** LBD structure of PPARa bound to a corepressor peptide, which displaces helix12 from an "active" conformation *(left)* and the LBD structure of PPARα bound to a coactivator peptide which renders helix 12 in an "active" conformation. **B,** DBD structure of the AR binding via its two zinc fingers to DNA response elements. (Courtesy of Professor John Schwabe, Department of Biochemistry, University of Leicester, Leicester, UK.)

esis (Swyer syndrome), which is distinguished by poor breast development and a shorter stature. CAIS may also present in early infancy with bilateral inguinal or labial swellings. 17β-HSD deficiency may also present in this manner. Bilateral inguinal herniae are rare in girls and it has been estimated that 1% to 2% of such cases have CAIS. Consequently, it is now generally recommended that a CAIS diagnosis be considered in all girls with this type of hernia and the presence of a Y chromosome be checked either by FISH analysis or on full karyotype. If the contents of the hernial sac contain gonads, a biopsy should be taken in concert with the cytogenetic studies.[346] It is not unusual to obtain the history of an older female sibling having had an inguinal hernia repair in infancy and when the karyotype is subsequently checked, the sibling is also found to have CAIS.

It is increasingly common for the sex of the infant to be determined before birth by analysis of the fetal karyotype because of maternal risk factors for congenital malformation. Fetal sexing is possible by three-dimensional ultrasound as early as the first trimester. Consequently, presentation can be via a mismatch between the result of fetal sexing and the subsequent birth phenotype.

TABLE 22–16 CLINICAL FEATURES OF COMPLETE ANDROGEN INSENSITIVITY SYNDROME

Karyotype	46, XY
Inheritance	X-linked recessive; mutations in *AR* gene
Genitalia	Female with blind vaginal pouch
Wolffian duct derivatives	Often present, depending on mutation type
Müllerian duct derivatives	Absent or vestigial
Gonads	Testes
Habitus	Scant or absent pubic and axillary hair; breast development and female habitus at puberty; primary amenorrhea
Hormone and metabolic profile	Increased LH and testosterone levels; increased estradiol (for male reference range); FSH levels often normal or slightly increased. Resistance to androgenic and metabolic effects of testosterone

FSH, follicle-stimulating hormone; LH, luteinizing hormone.

TABLE 22–17 CLINICAL FEATURES OF PARTIAL ANDROGEN INSENSITIVITY SYNDROME

Karyotype	46, XY
Inheritance	X-linked recessive; mutations in *AR* gene
External genitalia	Ambiguous with blind vaginal pouch→ undermasculinized→isolated hypospadias →normal male with infertility (mild AIS)
Wolffian duct derivatives	Often normal
Müllerian duct derivatives	Absent
Gonads	Testes (usually undescended)
Habitus	Decreased to normal axillary and pubic hair, beard growth, and body hair; gynecomastia common at puberty
Hormone and metabolic profile	Increased LH and testosterone concentrations; increased estradiol (for men); FSH levels may be normal or slightly increased Partial resistance to androgenic and metabolic effects of testosterone

FSH, follicle-stimulating hormone; LH, luteinizing hormone.

Partial Androgen Insensitivity Syndrome (PAIS)
(Table 22–17)

This terminology implies some biological response to androgens leading to male undermasculinization. The external genitalia may be ambiguous at birth, but the prototypic phenotype for PAIS is characterized by perineoscrotal hypospadias, micropenis, and a bifid scrotum. The testes may also be undescended. The more severe form of PAIS, presenting as isolated clitoromegaly, is only marginally different from CAIS. The milder end of the spectrum of PAIS includes isolated hypospadias, while isolated micropenis does not appear to be a manifestation of PAIS.

The list of differentials to consider within the 46,XY DSD category is much larger with the PAIS phenotype. They can be broadly classified as partial gonadal dysgenesis, a defect in androgen biosynthesis (LH receptor, SF1, 17β-HSD and 5α-RD deficiencies) and mixed gonadal dysgenesis in association with 45,X/46,XY mosaicism.

Minimal or Mild Androgen Insensitivity Syndrome (MAIS)

This category of AIS was realized following investigations for male factor infertility, which suggested a defect in androgen action.[347] Several large surveys of males with oligospermia and normal testosterone levels with increased LH concentrations have shown that a small percentage have AIS as based on finding a mutation in the *AR* gene. High doses of androgens may overcome the spermatogenic defect.[348] MAIS may also manifest just with gynecomastia in young adulthood and perhaps a history of having a minor hypospadias repair in childhood. Cancer of the breast is rare in males but the risk is increased in MAIS and PAIS.[349] There is an association between longer glutamine repeats in the AR and male breast cancer, generally.[350]

Hormone Profile

The typical hormone profile in a postpubertal patient with CAIS and intact gonads comprises a testosterone level within or above the adult male range, increased LH, and normal or slightly elevated FSH. Serum estradiol is also increased, both directly from the testis and as a result of peripheral aromatization. A similar gonadotrophin and sex steroid profile occurs in PAIS.[351] Concentrations of sex hormone–binding globulin (SHBG) are sexually dimorphic with levels in CAIS similar to those found in normal females. This hepatic resistance to the action of androgens has been proposed as a simple marker of androgen responsiveness in XY cases of DSD.[352] A short course of stanazolol (0.2 mg/kg/day), a synthetic non-aromatizable androgen is administered orally for 3 days and the decrement in serum SHBG levels measured up to 8 days thereafter. This is of the order of 45% to 55% in normals, whereas in CAIS there is an insignificant change in SHBG concentration. There is a moderate response in PAIS, but overlapping with normals. The test has use in diagnosis and in predicting androgen responsiveness in 46,XY DSD infants with ambiguous genitalia. In addition, AMH/MIS is normal or raised in AIS, but low in gonadal dysgenesis.[353]

Male infants have an LH-induced surge in serum testosterone concentrations during the first few months of life, which is manifest as some growth of the penis.[211] Isolated case reports have suggested the surge does not occur in CAIS; this was confirmed in a study of 10 infants with CAIS proven to have an AR mutation.[354] Testosterone levels did increase following hCG stimulation. In contrast, infants with PAIS have a spontaneous neonatal testosterone surge. Such observations provide some insight into the control mechanisms of hypothalamic-pituitary-gonadal cyclicity.[355] It is generally believed that a female infant with bilateral inguinal swellings and a 46,XY karyotype is sufficient to make a diagnosis of CAIS. As in cases of 46,XY DSD where there is ambiguity of the external genitalia, baseline gonadotropins with sex steroids before and after hCG stimulation should be measured.

A further biochemical test that is helpful in the investigation of androgen resistance, but is only available in research laboratories, is measurement of androgen binding in genital skin fibroblasts.[356] The AR is ubiquitously expressed and in greater quantities in genital versus nongenital skin. It is possible to obtain a small punch biopsy of foreskin at the time of hypospadias repair or from labial skin in the case of patients with CAIS having an examination under anesthetic or undergoing gonadectomy. Binding assays using radiolabeled DHT or synthetic androgens such as mibolerone provide a quantitative and qualitative analysis of the AR. Figure 22–33 shows a Scatchard plot derived from a saturation binding assay indicating that androgens bind to the AR with high affinity. The assay can be used to define the nature of AR dysfunction, which gives rise to either a CAIS or PAIS phenotype. The former is typically associated with absent or markedly reduced binding, whereas a reduced binding affinity (indicated by a high Kd) is the usual abnormality seen in PAIS. Further information on the qualitative aspects of AR function can be determined from experiments to assess whether binding is thermolabile and the rate at which the androgen dissociates from its receptor.[357] The cells are also a source of RNA for the study of mutations which reside in noncoding regions. Furthermore, receptor expression can be studied by Western blot analysis as illustrated in Figure 22–33.

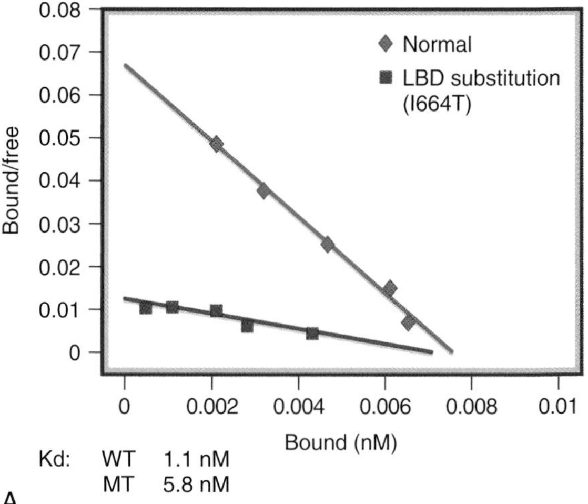

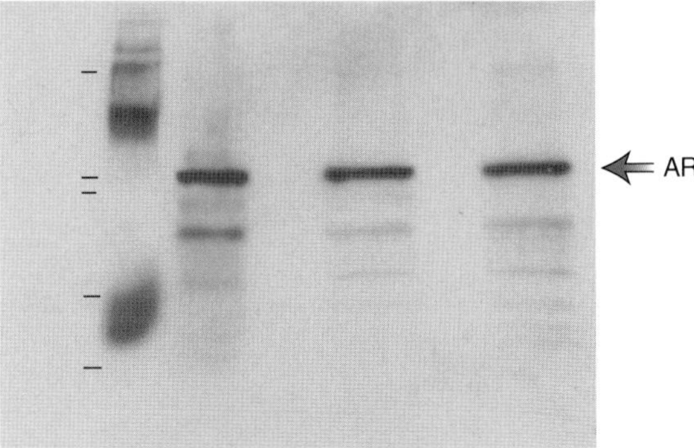

Figure 22–33 ■ **A,** Scatchard plot of specific androgen binding in genital skin fibroblasts (GSF). The intercept on the X axis is the Bmax, the receptor concentration, and the slope of the line calculates the Kd, a measure of binding affinity. A mutant AR due to a missense mutation (Ile664Thr) in the LBD has a six fold higher kd and reduced binding affinity compared with the wild-type AR. **B,** Western blot analysis of GSF proteins showing expression of the AR protein; size markers are illustrated. (Data are courtesy of Trevor Bunch, Department of Paediatrics, University of Cambridge, Cambridge, UK.)

Molecular Pathogenesis of Androgen Insensitivity Syndromes

Information about the various mutations that affect the AR and give rise to clinical disease is recorded on an International Mutation Database at McGill University (*http://www.androgendb.mcgill.ca*). A map of most of the reported mutations is shown in Figure 22–34. The majority of mutations relate to syndromes of androgen insensitivity but in addition, somatic mutations identified in prostate carcinoma are listed. The database comprises more than 750 entries, which encompass more than 300 different mutations that can cause AIS. There is no specific "hot spot" of mutations, but certain locations, such as exon 5, are affected more frequently. About two thirds of reported mutations are located in the LBD, approximately 20% in the DBD and a small minority in the NTD, despite this region of the AR being encoded by the largest of the eight exons. This region of the gene is GC

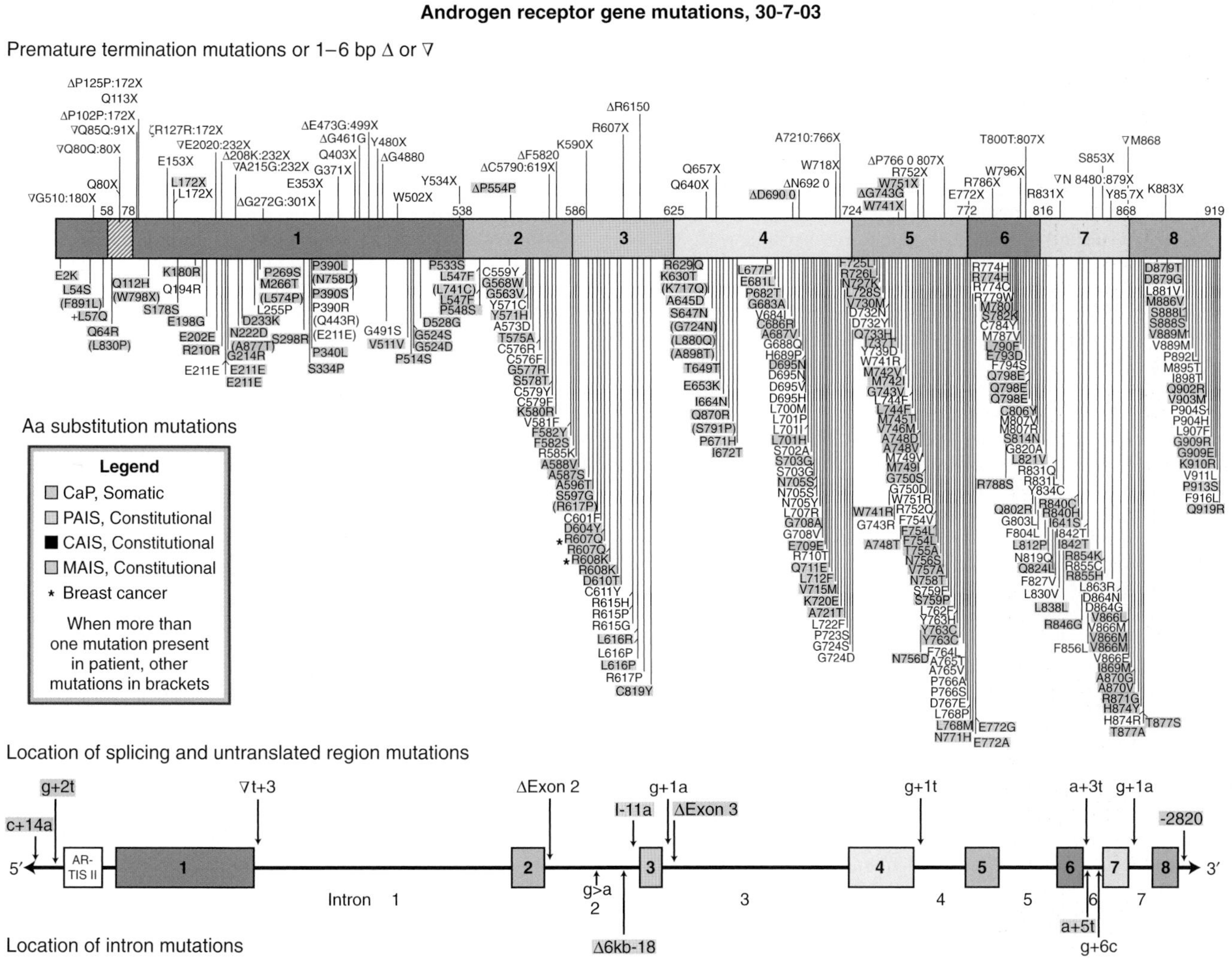

Androgen receptor gene mutations, 30-7-03

Premature termination mutations or 1–6 bp Δ or ∇

Aa substitution mutations

Legend
- CaP, Somatic
- PAIS, Constitutional
- CAIS, Constitutional
- MAIS, Constitutional
- * Breast cancer

When more than one mutation present in patient, other mutations in brackets

Location of splicing and untranslated region mutations

Location of intron mutations

Figure 22–34 ▪ Overview of androgen receptor (AR) mutations that cause different forms of androgen insensitivity syndrome (AIS). (From the McGill Androgen Receptor Gene Mutation Database *http://www.androgen.mcgill.ca*).

rich and difficult to sequence, so it is possible that the distribution of mutations in the NTD is underrepresented.

The range of mutation types affecting the *AR* gene is similar to that found in most single gene disorders. Complete or partial gene deletions are uncommon and the most frequent type of mutation is single base substitutions resulting in amino acid substitutions or premature stop codons. Nucleotide insertions, exon duplications, and intronic mutations affecting splice donor and acceptor sites are also reported. Figure 22–35 illustrates the spread of mutations identified in the authors' laboratory, which is also consistent with the pattern documented on the McGill Database. Finding a mutation, particularly if missense, does not necessarily imply pathogenicity. It is generally necessary to recreate the mutant AR for functional studies using a reporter gene assay. This is particularly the case where the mutation is novel and is associated with a PAIS phenotype. It is also possible to undertake structure-guided modeling of the mutant protein to provide insight into AR dysfunction.[358] Having a large database of mutations with some phenotype details is also of clinical use as reference. A detailed analysis of mutations is not appropriate here, but some examples serve to highlight information that is of relevance to clinical management and to explain the mode of action of the AR as a transcription factor. Thus, the presence of *increased* androgen binding in two sisters with CAIS was

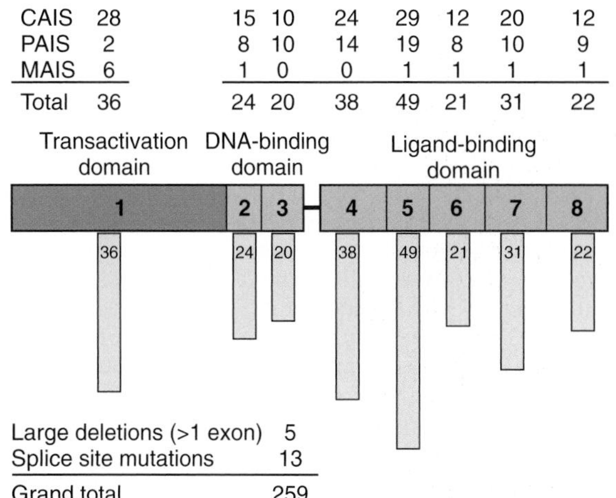

CAIS 28 15 10 24 29 12 20 12
PAIS 2 8 10 14 19 8 10 9
MAIS 6 1 0 0 1 1 1 1
Total 36 24 20 38 49 21 31 22
Transactivation domain
DNA-binding domain
Ligand-binding domain
1 2 3 4 5 6 7 8
36 24 20 38 49 21 31 22
Large deletions (>1 exon) 5
Splice site mutations 13
Grand total 259

Figure 22–35 ▪ Frequency of androgen receptor (AR) gene mutation recorded on the Cambridge DSD Database, related to phenotype. *MAIS,* Minimal/mild androgen insensitivity syndrome.

explained by deletion of exon 3 (encoding the first zinc finger in the DBD), which ablated binding to DNA but left androgen binding intact.[359]

There is considerable heterogeneity in the phenotypic expression of a particular mutation, sometimes even within families. For example, a missense mutation at codon 703 in exon 4 of the LBD, which changes a serine to a glycine, is reported in four separate individuals on the McGill Database. One patient had a normal female phenotype consistent with CAIS. The other three cases all had ambiguous genitalia consistent with PAIS, but the degree of androgenization of the external genitalia was sufficiently variable that two were raised male, whereas the remaining case of PAIS was raised female.[360,361] Rarely, two affected members in the same family can be phenotypically CAIS and PAIS, respectively. X-linked disorders are associated with a high rate of mutations that are *de novo*; the rate in AIS is about 30%. Such mutations arise either as a single mutational event in a parental germ cell (in the case of AIS, this would be the mother) or as a germ cell mosaicism in the maternal gonad. When the mutation arises at the postzygotic stage, the index case is a somatic mosaic. This gives rise to expression of both mutant and wild-type AR in different target tissues, including the external genitalia. Perhaps one third of *de novo* mutations in AIS arise at the postzygotic stage and would explain some of the variable phenotype in PAIS.[362] Other modulatory factors include differences in 5α-RD2 expression and reduced AR transcription and translation.[363,364] The intramolecular interaction between the N-terminal and C-terminal domains is a key component of nuclear receptor function. A supplementary feature of N/C interaction unique to the AR is the weaker affinity of binding between the AR AF2 subdomain and the LXXLL motifs of SRC/p160 coactivator as compared with a much stronger binding of AF2 to cognate motifs FXXLF and WXXLF in the N-terminal domain.[365] It is by studying mutations in the AR AF2 subdomain causing AIS that it has been possible to clarify the important role of N/C interaction in stabilizing androgen binding to the hydrophobic pocket in the LBD.[366-368]

AIS without an AR Mutation

Reference has been made to the role of coactivators that serve to provide a physical bridge between the liganded AR homodimer bound to hormone response elements and the recruitment of RNA polymerase II to initiate transcription.[339] It is possible that patients with CAIS or PAIS in whom no mutation has been found in the *AR* gene may have a mutant coactivator protein to explain the androgen resistance. The coregulator family of proteins number in excess of 150, of which approximately 45 proteins have been identified as being relatively specific for AR function. In a study of the two AR-related coactivators, ARA24 and ARA 70, no substantive variations were found in amino acid residues in a series of patients with PAIS and a normal AR.[369,370] Disruption of the steroid receptor coactivator-3 (SRC3) in mice results in a phenotype of general hormone resistance, including features consistent with PAIS.[371] The *SRC3* gene contains a variable tract of CAG/CAA triplets that encode a polyglutamine repeat. The lengths of glutamine repeats were found to be shorter in PAIS subjects compared to controls.[372] Such variation in the SRC-3 protein may modulate or destabilize receptor-coactivator interactions. The large number of coregulator proteins, their array of mechanisms to modulate transcription, and promiscuous binding to nuclear receptors in general makes it unlikely that a single mutant protein in this family would explain the mechanism of androgen resistance in CAIS or PAIS patients who have a normal AR. One patient with CAIS has been reported in whom it was proposed that the molecular abnormality was a coactivator protein dysfunction based on evidence from AR-GR chimeric experiments in genital skin fibroblasts of a defect in transmission of the transactivating signal from the AF1 region to the basal transcriptional machinery.[373,374] Glutathione-S-transferase studies identified that a 90-kd protein, normally present in fibroblasts, was absent. However, the nature of this coactivator protein has not been characterized. Targeted disruption of *FKBP52*, a cochaperone protein for HSPs, causes a phenotype in the mouse consistent with PAIS.[342] It is possible that variations in the protein are evident in some patients with severe hypospadias.

The polymorphic regions in the N-terminal domain of the AR have biologic relevance to disease as summarized in Table 22–18. The most compelling evidence is the toxic gain-of-function from polyglutamine hyperexpansion (more than 40 repeats) found in Kennedy's disease or spinal and bulbar muscular atrophy, SBMA.[375] Affected males have testicular atrophy, decreased spermatogenesis, and gynecomastia despite elevated androgen levels in keeping with a degree of androgen resistance. An abnormally expanded CAG repeat to 44 residues has been reported in one case of hypospadias.[376] Generally, variations in the length of the polyglutamine tract are merely in association with disorders such as hypospadias,[377] reduced spermatogenesis,[378] and the phenotype of Klinefelter's syndrome.[379] An association between shorter CAG repeats and relative hyperandrogenic states is found in prostate cancer,[380] androgenetic alopecia and acne,[381] and ovarian hyperandrogenism.[382] The latter study was conducted in a group of girls with precocious pubarche drawn from a Catalan population with shorter CAG repeat alleles than a comparable UK population, indicating that the genetic background may influence the prevalence of androgenic effects. The number of glycines was also significantly longer in patients with cryptorchidism and in a separate group with hypospadias compared with controls.[383] When CAG (glutamine) and GGN (glycine) lengths are analyzed together in the context of a missense mutation in the *AR* gene causing AIS, the combined effects appear to modulate the phenotypic expression of a given AR mutant in different affected individuals.[384]

Management

Gender assignment and sex of rearing is uniformly female in CAIS. Inguinal hernias need repair when presentation is in infancy with an option at this stage to perform gonadectomy. There is no uniformity in practice for early versus late gonadectomy. Relevant points of discussion are the merits of spontaneous puberty from gonads in situ versus induction of puberty with estrogen replacement, and the risk of a gonadal tumor if gonad-

TABLE 22–18 DISEASE ASSOCIATIONS WITH VARIATIONS IN THE AR GLUTAMINE REPEAT

Shortened (CAG)n	Increased (CAG)n
Prostate cancer	*Above normal range*
Ovarian hyperandrogenism	SBMA (Kennedy's disease)
Androgenetic alopecia	Hypospadias (one reported case)
Aspects of Klinefelter phenotype	
Response to androgen treatment	*Within normal range*
Central obesity	Male infertility
Mental retardation	Gynecomastia
Endometrial cancer	Hypospadias
Coronary artery disease severity	Aspects of Klinefelter phenotype
	Bone density
	Breast cancer

ectomy is delayed until adulthood. If gonadectomy is undertaken early, estrogen replacement using a gradual increase in doses of ethinyl oestradiol (initially 2 μg daily) is started at 10 to 11 years of age. Replacement doses up to 20 μg daily are reached by around 15 years of age; thereafter, adult estrogen replacement may continue orally or be changed to transdermal preparations. Adjunctive replacement with progestins is seldom used in view of the absence of a uterus. Adults with CAIS report an improved well-being with androgen replacement, particularly when introduced after gonadectomy. The mechanism of this androgenic effect is not understood. The onset of puberty occurs at the same age as in normal girls when the gonads are intact.[385] Pubic hair occurred slightly later (median 14 yr) while axillary hair was generally absent. Adult height in CAIS is close to target male height. Bone mineral density is decreased in CAIS compared to 5α-RD deficiency, illustrating the direct role of androgens in bone mineralization. Adult bone mineral density in CAIS is similar whether gonadectomy occurs before or after puberty.

There is an increased risk of gonadal tumors in DSD, particularly in the presence of a Y chromosome.[23,386,387] Seminoma, an invasive type II germ cell tumor, can develop in later adulthood in AIS. This is preceded by an in situ neoplastic change termed *intratubular germ cell neoplasia unclassified* (ITGNU). A more commonly recognized histologic term for this lesion is carcinoma in situ (CIS). The tumor outcome of CIS is more likely to be a gonadoblastoma when the gonad is not well differentiated. The abundance of primordial germ cells in the tubules (the ITGNU lesion) represents a delay in germ cell maturation into spermatogonia.[388] CIS cells originate from primordial germ cells (also referred to as gonocytes) and express immunohistochemical markers such as placental-like alkaline phosphatase (PLAP), c-KIT (a receptor for stem cell factor), AP-2γ, Oct-3/4, and NANOG.[389] The initiating events for neoplastic transformation from the CIS state are not known. Normal androgen production and action are a requirement for germ cell maturation. Environmental chemicals, which act as endocrine disruptors during fetal life, may disturb the prevailing androgen:estrogen balance.[390] This proposal aims to explain the increased incidence in testis tumors, which is often associated with abnormal spermatogenesis, undescended testes, and hypospadias. The prevalence of germ cell tumors in CAIS has previously been reported as 25% to 30% in adulthood.[391,392] Recent estimates from larger numbers are as low as 0.8% for CAIS and 5.5% for AIS overall.[23,393] The timing of gonadectomy is now generally in early adulthood and some adults with CAIS are opting for no gonadectomy.

Surgery in CAIS is confined to gonadectomy and perhaps vaginoplasty procedures. Laparoscopic procedures are routine for removal of intraabdominal testes. Those sited in the inguinal region can be removed during herniorrhaphy or by a laparoscopy-assisted transinguinal approach. The vagina in CAIS is blind-ending and shortened. The regular use of graded vaginal dilators during adolescence is generally successful with only a minority of women requiring a vaginoplasty. The prepubertal girl with CAIS requires an examination under anesthetic around the age of puberty to evaluate the vaginal anatomy.

The early management of PAIS centers on the decision about gender assignment and the subsequent plan and timing for surgery consequent upon that decision. The phenotypic heterogeneity seen in PAIS has been emphasized. The majority of PAIS infants are raised male. Surgical procedures required include orchidopexy, chordee correction, and urethral reconstruction for the hypospadias. In some cases, several procedures implemented into adult life are required before full reconstruction has taken place. Large doses of androgen may be required to promote phallic growth; the results of functional studies of any mutant AR that has been identified can be a useful predictor of the likely response. In practice, a course of androgen injections in early infancy is often used to assess androgen responsiveness, which can be a contributory factor in sex assignment. A monthly course of three 25-mg intramuscular injections of Sustanon (a mixture of testosterone esters) is a common protocol. It is important to quantify the response and an androgenization score, which takes account of penis size, testis position, and site of urethral orifice, is reliable and simple to apply.[394]

The risk of germ cell tumor of the testis is higher in PAIS with the prevalence as high as 50% if the gonad is nonscrotal in position.[395] A patient with PAIS raised male should have careful monitoring of scrotal testes. It is recommended that a biopsy be performed at puberty. If CIS is present, there is debate about whether the contralateral testis should be biopsied. Unilateral CIS is treated by gonadectomy; bilateral CIS (rare) is managed with local low-dose radiotherapy, which effectively eradicates CIS.[396] Regular self-examination and testicular ultrasonography to screen for microliths is also recommended screening.

The management of PAIS is complicated by the low incidence of proven *AR* mutations in cases that meet the phenotypic criteria consistent with incomplete resistance to androgens. In most reported series, which have included molecular analysis of the *AR* gene in a large number of cases, only about one fourth of patients have a mutation in the coding region of the gene.[397,398] Yet, the features of PAIS cases with and without a mutant AR are indistinguishable other than a family history of AIS being more common when a PAIS case has an identified *AR* gene mutation.[361] What causes the phenotype in the majority of PAIS cases with a normal AR is not known. Hypospadias is a common birth defect and is associated with fetal growth restraint as based on reduced birth weight for gestational age.[399,400] That androgenization of the external genitalia takes place during the first and early part of the second trimester suggests a possible link with either placental dysfunction or early fetal growth-related genes. Information on outcome in adult life for parameters such as physical health, sexual function, fertility, quality of life, and social participation is particularly scanty in males with PAIS. In a group of 14 individuals with PAIS, 23% were dissatisfied with the gender assigned to them as infants regardless of now being male or female.[401] Another study of 15 adult males with PAIS reported major impairment of sexual function.[402] This is in contrast to data in women with CAIS who report satisfaction with gender assignment, sexual function, and psychological outcome.[182,403] Sex assignment in MAIS is male and clinical presentation is not until adolescence because of gynecomastia or for investigation of male factor infertility in adulthood.[404] Reduction mammoplasty is required for the gynecomastia.

Counseling

AIS is an X-linked recessive condition; in 30% of cases the mutation arises spontaneously. Knowledge of the causative mutation in the index case can be applied for carrier detection, which may extend through a number of generations (Fig. 22–36). Analysis of the CAG repeats provides information on the pattern of inheritance of the maternal X chromosome and thus carrier status. It is particularly useful in cases of a phenotype consistent with PAIS but a mutant AR is excluded by the pattern of allele transmission. Other causes such as an androgen biosynthetic defect, may then need to be considered.

An important component of counseling in AIS is disclosure of the diagnosis at an age and cognitive appropriate stage. Historically, the principles of beneficence (the commitment by health care professionals to deliver care that provides the maximum benefit to the patient) and nonmaleficence (the duty to avoid causing harm) were applied to AIS in the mistaken belief that nondisclosure of the diagnosis was the appropriate management.[405] Now, most clinicians ensure that adults with AIS and the parents of affected children are fully informed about

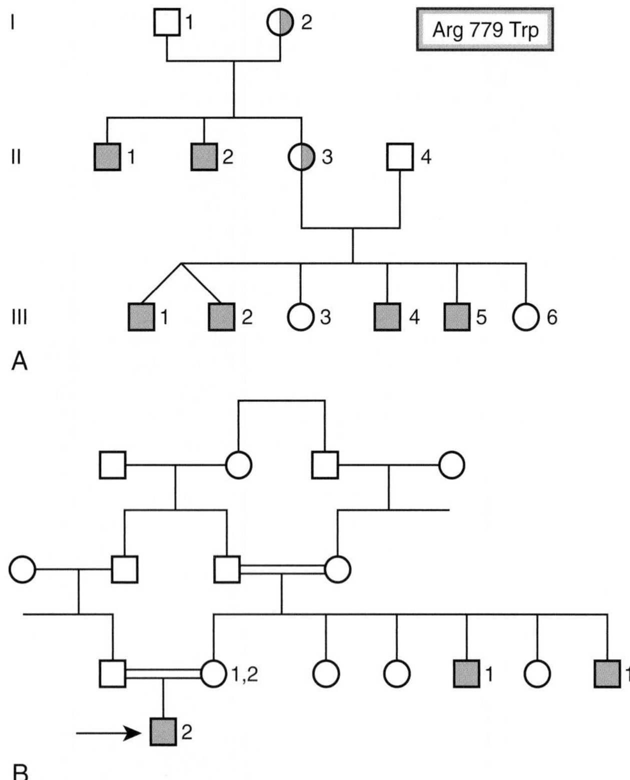

Figure 22–36 ■ **A,** X-linked inheritance pattern in a family with CAIS due to a missense mutation in the ligand-binding domain of the androgen receptor (AR). Subjects I.2 and II.3 are the female carriers. **B,** Inheritance of androgen receptor CAG repeats. Affected members in this consanguineous family are indicated by the closed symbols. The index case, denoted by the arrow, has inherited a different (CAG)n allele from his mother compared with his two affected uncles. This excludes a mutation in the *AR* gene as the cause of a PAIS phenotype.

the condition and are appraised of the management options. A comprehensive, regularly updated review is available on the Internet.[406] Much of the enlightened change in practice has arisen from improved team networking with advocacy groups such as the Androgen Insensitivity Syndrome Support Group (AISSG) and its allied groups established in several countries (*http://www.medhelp.org/www/ais*), including Australia.[407] Parents of children with AIS need considerable support in planning and implementing disclosure for their child once the diagnosis has been established. In common with the principles of disclosure in other childhood chronic medical conditions, relaying facts about chromosomes, gonads, genital anatomy, and fertility is a collaborative process, which requires an individualized approach commensurate with the child's changing cognitive and psychological development.[3,4] Such a partnership approach mandates a psychologist experienced in DSD counseling as a member of the multidisciplinary team.

Other Conditions Affecting 46,XY Sex Development

Persistent Müllerian Duct Syndrome

Antimüllerian hormone (AMH; also known as *müllerian inhibiting substance,* MIS) is a glycoprotein homodimer that is secreted by the Sertoli cells of the developing testes from around 7 weeks' gestation and acts via the AMH type II receptor (AMH2R, MIS II receptor) between 8 and 12 weeks' gestation to cause regression of the müllerian duct (see Normal Sex Development).[160,161]

AMH/MIS is encoded by a 2.75-kb gene containing five exons in the region of chromosome 19p13.3. The AMH/MIS II receptor is a serine/threonine kinase with a single transmembrane domain that is encoded by an 11 exon gene on 12q13.[162] Exons 1 to 3 code for the signal sequence and the extracellular domain of the AMH II receptor, exon 4 codes for the transmembrane domain, and exons 5 through 11 code for the intracellular serine/threonine domain.

Persistent müllerian duct syndrome (PMDS, herniae uteri inguinale) is a condition in which 46,XY males have well-developed testes and normal male ducts and external genitalia, but have müllerian duct derivatives. The diagnosis is often not made until a fallopian tube and uterus are encountered in patients undergoing inguinal hernia repair, orchiopexy, or abdominal surgery. Because of the trend for early surgical repair of an inguinal hernia or undescended testis, more cases are detected in infancy or early childhood. There are two anatomic forms. In the more prevalent form, there is a hernia containing a partially descended or scrotal testis and the ipsilateral tube and uterus are in the hernia. In some instances, the contralateral testis and tube are present in the hernial sac as well. The presence of transverse testicular ectopia should suggest PMDS. In the second form, the uterus, tubes, and testes are in the pelvis.

PMDS in normally differentiated males can result from failure of the testes to synthesize or secrete bioactive AMH/MIS or from a defect in the response of the duct to AMH/MIS because of an AMH II receptor defect. To date, approximately half of all genetically proven cases of PMDS are due to defects in AMH/MIS and half are due to mutations in its receptor (Fig. 22–37).[408] *AMH* gene mutations are most common in Mediterranean and Northern African/Middle Eastern countries.[409] Most familial mutations are homozygous. In contrast, mutations in the gene encoding the AMH/MIS II receptor are more common in France and Northern Europe and are often compound heterozygous mutations.[410] In an extensive study of 69 families with PMDS, 28 different mutations in the *AMH* gene were detected in 31 families (see Fig. 22–37).[408,409] Both homozygous and compound heterozygous mutations were found in affected families, including splicing, missense, nonsense, and deletion mutations affecting the whole gene but mainly exon 1 and the 3′ region of exon 5. Deleterious mutations in the AMH/MIS type II receptor gene (*AMH2R*) were detected in 27 families, including deletion, missense, and nonsense mutations (see Fig. 22–37). The most common mutation was a 27-base pair deletion in exon 10.[411] No abnormality in *AMH* or *AMH2R* genes was detected in 11 families (16% of the total number). Measurement of serum AMH/MIS can provide a useful means for guiding genetic analysis; patients with PMDS caused by mutations of the *AMH* gene have low or undetectable levels of serum AMH/MIS, whereas AMH/MIS concentrations are often high normal or elevated in patients with mutations of the AMH/MIS II receptor.

Treatment of PMDS is directed toward an attempt to ensure fertility in males, a difficult issue because of the anatomic findings. Testicular differentiation and function are normal in these patients, but an increased prevalence of testicular degeneration has been described, which is probably secondary to torsion of the testes. Anatomic abnormalities of the epididymis and the vas deferens are common. Infertility may result from late orchiopexy or from mechanical problems associated with entrapment of the vas deferens in the müllerian derivatives. Early orchiopexy, proximal salpingectomy (leaving the epididymis attached to the fimbriae of the fallopian tube), dissection of the vas deferens from the lateral walls of the uterus, and a complete hysterectomy are recommended as a useful surgical approach. These structures can be left in place if there is risk of damaging the genital ducts. Men with high pelvic testes rarely have successful orchiopexy, and many of these individuals are androgen deficient.

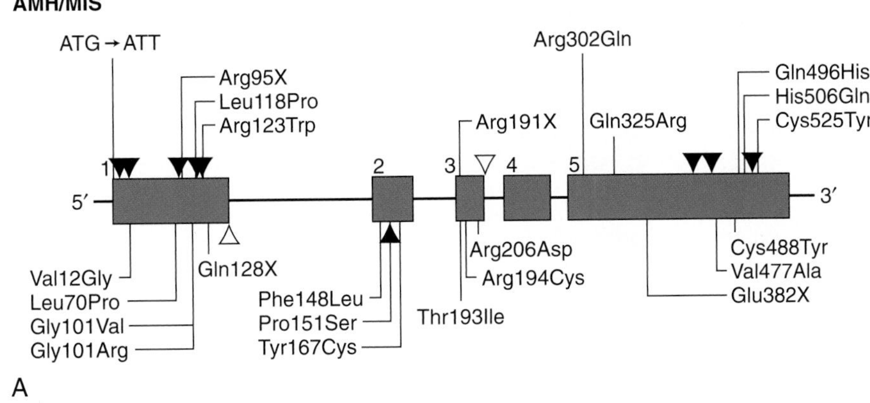

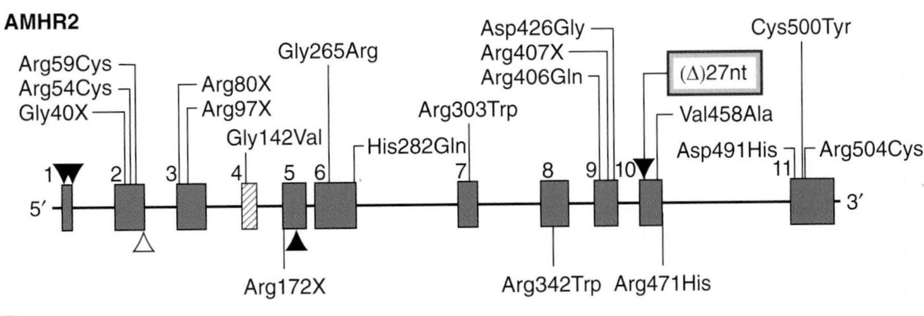

Figure 22–37 ■ **A,** Diagram of the mutations in the antimüllerian hormone (AMH/MIS) gene that cause persistent müllerian duct syndrome. The numbered *solid boxes* depict the exons. The three-letter abbreviation for amino acids is used to indicate the position of missense mutations; X, indicates a nonsense (stop) mutation; insertions and deletions resulting in frameshift and splice site mutations are shown by *filled arrowheads* and *open arrowheads,* respectively. **B,** Diagram of selected mutations in the gene for the AMH receptor type II *(AMHR2).* The numbered *solid boxes* depict the exons. Exons 1 to 3 encode the extracellular domain of the receptor. Exon 4 *(diagonal lines)* encodes the transmembrane domain, and exons 5 through 11 encode the intracytoplasmic domain. Different forms of mutation are depicted as outlined above. Δ27nt *(open box)* is a 27-nucleotide deletion, the most common *AMHR2* mutation causing the persistent müllerian duct syndrome. (**A** Redrawn from Imbeaud S, Carré Eusebe D, Rey R, et al. Molecular genetics of the persistent müllerian duct syndrome: a study of 19 families. Hum Mol Genet 1994;3:125-131. By permission of Oxford University Press. **B** Redrawn from Imbeaud S, Belville C, Messike-Zeitoun L, et al. A 27 base-pair deletion of the antimüllerian type II receptor gene is the most common cause of the persistent müllerian duct syndrome. Hum Mol Genet 1996;5:1269-1277. By permission of Oxford University Press.)

Hypospadias

Hypospadias is incomplete fusion of the penile urethra defined by an arrest in development of the urethral spongiosum and ventral prepuce.[412] The normal embryologic correction of penile curvature is also interrupted. It is a common congenital anomaly, with birth prevalence estimated around 3 to 4 per 1000 live births. There has been a suggestion of an increase in incidence worldwide[413,414] but also evidence that trends have not changed in recent decades.[415,416] Despite extensive effort at investigation, the cause is unknown in the majority of cases.[412,417,418] The occasional case of isolated hypospadias has been identified with a mutation in *WT1, SF1, LHR, CYP17,* or the *AR* gene. The *CXorf6* gene on chromosome Xq28 has been found to be mutated in some cases of hypospadias.[259] A mutation screen of *BMP4, BMP7, HOXA4, and HOXB6* identified mutations in 14 of 90 cases of hypospadias in a Chinese population, but all in the heterozygous state.[419] Mutations in *HOXA13* are found in the hand-foot-genital syndrome, which includes hypospadias.[420] There is a familial clustering of cases in hypospadias with a 7% incidence of one or more additional affected family members.[421] Furthermore, the twinning rate is higher than in the general population, of which two thirds are monozygotic.

Associations observed in hypospadias include increased maternal age, mother exposed to diethylstilbestrol in utero, paternal subfertility, maternal vegetarian diet, maternal smoking, assisted reproductive techniques, paternal exposure to pesticides, and fetal growth restriction.[422] The association with low birth weight is consistent across all studies of idiopathic hypospadias and suggests a link between early fetal growth factors and the completion of fusion of the urethra by the early second trimester. Gene expression profiles during urethral development in the mouse indicate a number of signaling pathways are involved.[423]

Management is surgical, the aim being to relocate the urethral meatus on to the glans and straighten the penis by correcting any chordee in order to give a normal forward-directed urinary stream and the ability to have satisfactory sexual intercourse. Numerous techniques are described; repairs may require more than one stage, usually starting at 6 to 12 months of age. Complications include fistula formation, meatal stenosis, urethral stricture, and residual chordee. Outcome data in large series are lacking, but there is some evidence of satisfactory function but less so for cosmetic appearance.[424,425]

Anorchia and Cryptorchidism

The term, *vanishing testis syndrome,* was coined for the phenotype of bilateral anorchia in an otherwise normally developed male infant.[2] It recognizes the presence of normal testes in early gestation operating to induce müllerian duct regression, stabilize wolffian duct development, and differentiate male external genitalia. Any ambiguity of the external genitalia suggests a variant of the syndrome related to some form of XY gonadal dysgenesis. Bilateral anorchia with normal differentiated but small phallus (micropenis) is also a recognized variant of the syndrome.[426] The cause is unknown other than invoking an interruption to the testis blood supply from a torsion or vascular occlusion event in utero. Surgical exploration and histologic findings typically show testicular nubbins as remnants of gonads, which are associated with a vas deferens in the majority and some epididymal tissue.[427,428] The presence of hemosiderin-laden macrophages and dystrophic calcification is in keeping with the vascular accident hypothesis.

Establishing complete anorchia is based on a combination of biochemical tests, imaging studies, and surgical exploration.[429] An undetectable serum AMH level is a reliable marker when evaluating infants with nonpalpable gonads.[430] This, coupled with elevated serum gonadotropins and an absent testosterone response to hCG stimulation, is predictive of the absence of testes. A low inhibin B level is also confirmatory. Imaging with CT or MRI may be useful before laparoscopy. Most centers would still undertake surgical exploration to remove testicular remnants even though there is usually no evidence of malignancy found. Such a procedure could be deferred until the time of insertion of prostheses.

Testes that have not descended at birth (cryptorchidism) is the most common congenital abnormality in boys, affecting 2% to 9% male live births.[431] The strong association with low birth weight is well recognized, as are disorders of the pituitary-gonadal axis such as hypogonadotrophic hypogonadism and the androgen insensitivity syndrome. The latter observations are in keeping with the role of androgens in the inguinoscrotal phase of testis descent. The first phase of transabdominal migration is under the control of insulin-like factor 3 (Insl3) produced by Leydig cells.[174] Mutations in *INSL3* and the gene for its receptor, *LGR8/GREAT,* are only rarely found in boys with cryptorchidism.[432-434] Higher exposure to pesticides has been reported in cryptorchid boys based on analyses of breast milk samples as a proxy to fetal exposure.[435]

Environmental Chemicals

This apparent increase in male reproductive tract disorders such as testis cancer, abnormal spermatogenesis, cryptorchidism, and hypospadias has led to the concept that testicular dysgenesis syndrome (TDS) of fetal origin may be triggered by environmental chemicals disrupting an androgen/estrogen balance critical for normal sex development.[436] The clearest evidence that certain chemicals such as herbicides, fungicides, bisphenol A, and phthalates can act as endocrine disruptors is derived from observations of wildlife and laboratory animal experiments. It remains uncertain whether there is also a new and emerging public health problem.[437] The possible role of environmental factors in an apparent increase in hypospadias and cryptorchidism has already been mentioned. Direct evidence of toxic effects in humans has yet to be established. Increased estrogenic bioactivity has been found in the newborn serum of some infants with idiopathic 46,XY DSD whose mothers were exposed to endocrine disruptors during pregnancy.[438] The anogenital distance in newborn rodents is a sensitive index following maternal exposure to androgens and antiandrogens. Data on this anthropometric measure in normal male infants are not yet available, but a preliminary study has reported reduced anogenital distance in male infants related to prenatal phthalate exposure.[439]

The relevance of these epidemiologic and experimental findings to the assessment of an individual case of DSD remains uncertain. Major programs of research such as CREDO (Cluster of Research into Endocrine Disruption in Europe) supported by the European Commission and projects undertaken by the National Institute of Environmental Health Sciences and the National Toxicology Program are underway to determine the risks posed to human health by environmental chemicals. In the meantime, it would seem sensible to reduce levels of chemicals to as low as is reasonably practicable.

Disorders of Ovary Development and Androgen Excess (46,XX DSD, Including Female Pseudohermaphroditism)

46,XX DSD can be divided into (1) disorders of ovarian development, (2) disorders of androgen synthesis, and (3) other conditions affecting sex development (see Table 22–6).

Disorders of Ovary Development

Disorders of ovarian development (ovarian dysgenesis or resistance) do not usually manifest until puberty, when a failure of estrogenization becomes apparent. In contrast, several well-defined but poorly understood disorders of gonadal development can result in a 46,XX individual having an ovary containing testicular tissue ("46,XX ovotesticular DSD/true hermaphrodite"), or even the development of a testis capable of producing enough androgen for a male phenotype and sufficient AMH/MIS to regress the uterus ("46,XX testicular DSD/XX males").

Ovarian Dysgenesis

Ovarian dysgenesis is most frequently seen in association with sex chromosome aneuploidy (Turner syndrome; 45,X and variants) where progressive ovarian apoptosis is evident (see sections on Ovarian Development and Sex Chromosome DSD). Ovarian resistance occurs due to mutations in the FSH receptor and presents at puberty.[207] Ovarian dysfunction can also occur with a wide range of multisystem syndromes, often involving DNA-repair mechanisms (e.g., Perrault, Maximilian, Quayle and Copeland, Pober, Malouf, Nijmegen, Cockayne, Rothmund-Thompson, Werner syndromes; also ataxia telangiectasia).[154,155] A number of nonmetabolic causes of premature ovarian failure have now been described[45-51] (e.g., POF1, Xq26-q28, *FMR* premutations; POF2A, Xq22, *DIAPH2;* POF2B, Xq21, *POF1B [actin binding protein];* POF3, 3q22, *FOXL2;* POF4, Xp11.2, *BMP15*), as well as mitochondrial disorders such as POLG.[440] Although these conditions usually present with early menopause, it is possible that more severe forms of some of these disorders might interfere with earlier aspects of ovarian development.

46,XX Ovotesticular DSD ("True Hermaphrodites") and 46,XX Testicular DSD ("46,XX Males")

In rare conditions, the developing ovary may contain an element of testicular tissue (46,XX ovotesticular DSD, "true hermaphrodite") or may even develop as a functioning testis (46,XX testicular DSD, "46,XX male"). In 46,XX ovotesticular DSD, the infant usually presents with ambiguous genitalia at birth and progressive virilization at puberty if the gonad is not removed. In contrast, 46,XX testicular DSD is usually associated with a normal male phenotype and absence of müllerian structures. However, the testis is not capable of supporting spermatogenesis because crucial genes on the Y chromosome are absent.

A detailed review of the presentation, endocrinology, and management of 46,XX ovotesticular DSD is included in the section on Sex Chromosome DSD, because many of the issues faced are similar to those with 46,XX/46,XY chimerism. It is important to note, though, that a 46,XX karyotype is the most frequent finding in ovotesticular DSD, especially in patients from Sub-Saharan Africa.[238] As familial cases have been described, it is likely that a genetic basis exists in some cases, although the exact etiology is unknown. Translocation of a testis-determining gene has been found in rare cases (e.g., SRY, SOX9).[128] Whether 46,XX DSD can result from milder changes in ovarian testis repressor genes (e.g., *RSPO1*, see below) remains to be seen.

Patients with 46,XX testicular DSD ("XX males") often present first with male factor infertility. In some cases, a family history may be present. Because different family members can have different phenotypes, it is possible that 46,XX testicular DSD represents the most severe end of the spectrum of ovarian transdifferentiation phenotypes. Most reported 46,XX males (up to 80%) harbor translocations of Y-chromosomal material containing the testis-determining factor, SRY.[82,27] This finding helped considerably in mapping the SRY gene in the first instance (see Normal Sex Development) and in some situations residual ovarian tissue (ovotestis) develops. Individuals with SRY-translocations can be diagnosed by FISH analysis using a probe directed to this gene (see Fig. 22–3). A number of SRY-negative cases have been reported. Recently, loss-of-function mutations in an ovarian gene *RSPO1* (encoding respondin-1) have been reported in 46,XX testicular DSD with palmar-plantar hyperkeratosis and squamous cell carcinoma.[15] This factor, which mediates the WNT4 signaling pathway, is the first ovarian-specific repressor of testis development described. Loss of function in respondin-1 in the developing gonad of 46,XX individuals results in testis development and an infertile male phenotype. It is likely that additional factors, which may act as repressors of SRY and testis determination, will be found in other individuals who are SRY negative.

Disorders of Androgen Excess

An overview of the steroid biosynthetic disorders causing androgen excess and 46,XX DSD is shown in Table 22–6. Although 21-hydroxylase deficiency is by far the most common form of this condition, it is important that alternative diagnoses are considered as approaches to counseling and management may vary.

3β-Hydroxysteroid Dehydrogenase (HSD3B2) Deficiency

3β-Hydroxysteroid dehydrogenase/$\Delta^{4,5}$-isomerase (3β-HSD) catalyzes the conversion of Δ^5 steroids to Δ^4 steroids and is required for the generation of mineralocorticoids, glucocorticoids, and more potent androgens (testosterone, DHT) by the adrenal glands and gonads (see Fig. 22–11). A detailed description of 3β-HSD actions and the consequences of deficiency of the type 2 enzyme is provided in the section on 46,XY DSD, in that this defect results in adrenal insufficiency with variable defects in androgenization of the developing male fetus.

Defects in 3β-HSD type 2 (*HSD3B2*) can also present in 46,XX females. Severe recessively inherited defects in enzyme function can cause mild clitoral enlargement at birth in girls with glucocorticoid deficiency (with or without salt loss). This mild androgenization occurs not as a direct androgenic effect of the excess DHEA but as a result of its conversion, as well as that of other Δ^5-3β-hydroxy C19-steroids, to testosterone by the 3β-HSD type 1 isozyme in the placenta and in the peripheral tissues of the fetus. This conversion, coupled with the limited capacity of the placenta to aromatize androgens to estrogens early in gestation, can lead to an increase in circulating androgens in the female fetus and in a minority of patients to modest clitoromegaly. Milder (nonclassic) forms of 3β-HSD type 2 deficiency have been reported to be a cause of premature pubarche in girls. Furthermore, breast development can occur at puberty in affected females, presumably by peripheral conversions of Δ^5-C_{19}-steroids to Δ^4-C_{19}-steroids by the 3β-HSD type 1 isozyme expressed principally in peripheral tissues, and by the subsequent aromatization of androgens to estrogens. Menses has been reported in treated females with this condition.

The diagnosis of 3β-HSD type 2 deficiency can be challenging in nonclassic forms of this condition.[288] In general, Δ^5 steroids are raised (e.g., 17-hydroxypregnenolone, DHEA and its sulfate) and the ratio of Δ^5 steroids to Δ^4 steroids (e.g., 17-hydroxyprogesterone : cortisol ratio) is markedly increased, especially following stimulation with intravenous ACTH. The urinary steroid profile can also be informative as 17-ketosteroids and especially DHEAS and 16-hydrox DHEAS are elevated. Of note, basal plasma concentrations of *17-hydroxyprogesterone* can be increased as a result of peripheral conversion of Δ^5-17-hydroxypregnenolone to 17-hydroxyprogesterone by the type I enzyme. This finding may lead to potential confusion with alternative forms of CAH, such as 21-hydroxylase deficiency or oxidoreductase deficiency. Furthermore, mild forms of 3β-HSD type 2 may present in a similar fashion to virilizing adrenal tumors. Suppression of the increased plasma and urinary levels of C19- and C21-3β-hydroxysteroids by glucocorticoids distinguishes 3β-HSD deficiency in such cases. Treatment for 3β-HSD is with glucocorticoid, mineralocorticoid,and salt supplementation, as appropriate, and estrogen replacement to induce puberty.

21-Hydroxylase (CYP21) Deficiency

In the context of DSD, 21-hydroxylase deficiency (see Fig. 22–11) is the most common cause of ambiguous genitalia of the newborn. It is primarily a disorder of adrenal steroidogenesis and is discussed in Chapter 14. A number of additional components are included of relevance to this chapter.

A female fetus with 21-hydroxylase deficiency can become androgenized to varying degrees as illustrated by the Prader classification (Fig. 22–38). The fact that CYP21 deficiency may androgenize a female sufficiently to result in a male phenotype at birth (with nonpalpable testes) is indicative of exposure to extremely high circulating concentrations of androgens. Indeed, serum concentrations of testosterone are invariably within the adult male range (and sometimes higher) in CAH due to CYP21 deficiency. That androgenization can be prevented if dexamethasone is administered to the mother early enough in gestation indicates an intact fetal pituitary-adrenal axis that is responsive to negative feedback regulation. This is indeed the case based on studies of human fetal adrenal explants that synthesize cortisol, androstenedione, and testosterone under ACTH regulation, which, in turn, is subject to negative feedback by glucocorticoids.[172] The precise route to increased adrenal production is possibly via the "backdoor" pathway to androgen synthesis.[170,441] Nevertheless, high fetal concentrations of 17OH-progesterone, androstenedione, and testosterone is the hall-

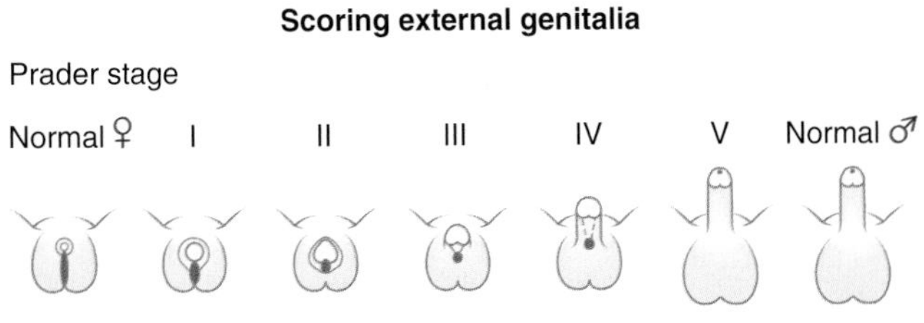

Figure 22–38 ▪ Prader classification of the degree of androgenization in a female with CAH.

mark of androgenization in CAH due to CYP21 deficiency. More than 75% of cases are also salt-losers due to the inability to synthesize sufficient mineralocorticoids. The two forms are readily explained by the nature of the mutation, which affects the *CYP21* gene on chromosome 6p21.3. The concordance between genotype and phenotype for the single gene disorder is remarkably precise (Fig. 22–39). In patients who are compound heterozygotes, the phenotype is generally concordant with the milder allele. More than 90% of cases are the result of *CYP21* deletion or one of nine mutations derived from the nonfunctional pseudogene *CYP21P* (see Fig. 22–39). Rarer mutations arise spontaneously, accounting for only 5% of *CYP21* mutations. Worldwide, more than 80 non-pseudogene-derived mutations are reported on the CYP21A2 database *http://www.imm.ki.se/CYPalleles/cyp21.htm.*

The diagnosis of CYP21 deficiency in a newborn with ambiguous genitalia is really confirmed by markedly elevated serum 17-hydroxyprogesterone concentrations (>300 nmol/L) after the first 48 hours. Sick, preterm infants can have moderately raised steroid levels so that an ACTH stimulation may be needed to resolve any diagnostic confusion. The affected male generally has no alerting clinical signs at birth and if a salt-loser, does not decompensate with hypokalemia, hyperkalemia, and weight loss until 1 to 2 weeks after birth. Hence the introduction of newborn screening programs to measure blood spot 17OH-progesterone concentrations soon after birth in a number of countries. The practice has not been universally adopted in developed countries, which suggests that an evidence-base for beneficial versus harmful effects of screening remains to be established.[443,444] Of major relevance to DSD is the potential to prevent ambiguous genitalia of the newborn through prenatal treatment with dexamethasone.[445,446] The treatment is effective if dexamethasone is started by 6 to 7 weeks of gestation according to the protocol outlined in Figure 22–40. Also shown are those mutations associated with the more severe form of CAH for which prenatal dexamethasone treatment would be beneficial. There is concern that exposure of the fetus to dexamethasone may cause adverse effects in the growing child, especially males and unaffected females (seven out of eight cases) receive treatment for about 4 to 5 weeks until the karyotype and *CYP21* analysis is known. Analysis of free fetal DNA in maternal blood as early as 7 weeks of gestation for Y chromosome markers using real-time quantitative PCR can be used to avoid dexamethasone exposure for the male fetus.[447] A further option is preimplantation genetic diagnosis to avoid the need for prenatal dexamethasone treatment altogether.[448]

An increase in morbidity or mortality has not been observed in fetuses treated with dexamethasone to term and monitored through infancy and early childhood.[449,445] Furthermore, cognitive and motor development based on questionnaires appeared not to be adversely affected by exposure to dexamethasone.[450] However, direct examination of 26 children who had been exposed to dexamethasone (maternal dose 20 μg/kg/day) from gestational age 6 to 7 weeks did show adverse effects on verbal working memory compared with controls.[451] It is recommended that continuation of prenatal treatment for CAH be conducted in prospective studies using agreed protocols for long-term monitoring.[452]

P450 Oxidoreductase (POR) Deficiency

P450 oxidoreductase (*POR*) is a membrane-bound flavoprotein that plays a central role in electron transfer from NADPH to all microsomal P450 enzymes, including P450c17, P450c21 (21-hydroxylase), and P450c19 (aromatase) (see Fig. 22–27). Defects in P450 oxidoreductase can cause apparent combined P450c17 and P450c21 deficiency, with or without Antley-Bixler syndrome, a form of craniosynostosis. These conditions are described in detail in the section on 46,XY DSD (Disorders of Androgen Synthesis).[303-308] However, it is important to note that P450 oxidoreductase deficiency can be associated with ambiguous genitalia in both 46,XX and 46,XY infants. The androgenization of 46,XX fetuses may result from a defect in aromatase activity, or via a proposed "backdoor" pathway of DHT production that does not involve androstenedione or testosterone as intermediates.[170,171] Children with this condition usually have cortisol deficiency but mineralocorticoid function is relatively preserved.

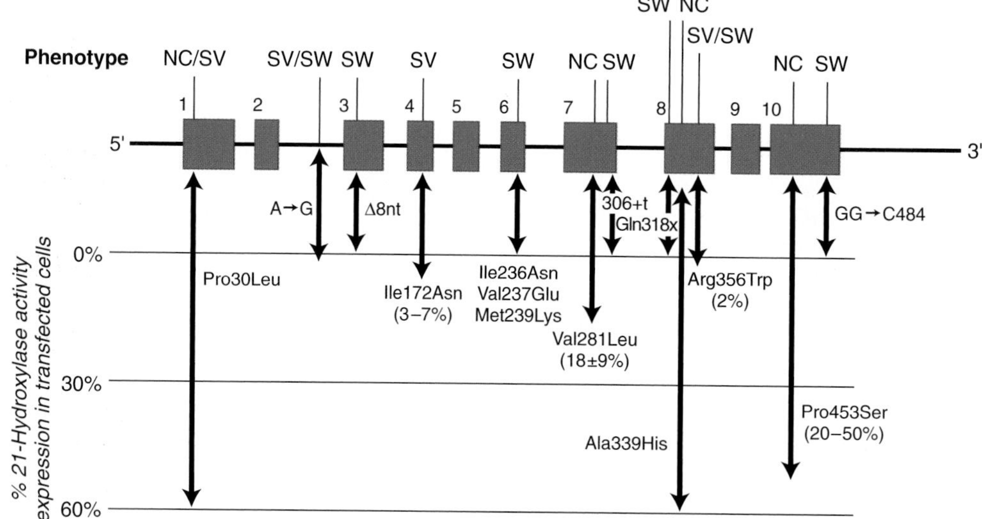

Figure 22–39 ▪ Diagram of the *CYP21* gene and locations of the mutations that cause more than 90% of cases of 21-hydroxylase deficiency. The numbered boxes are the exons. The three-letter abbreviation for amino acids is used; X indicates a nonsense (stop) mutation. An adenine (A) to guanine (G) transition in intron 2 causes a common splice site mutation. Other mutations include an 8-nucleotide deletion ((αnt) in exon 3, a thymidine insertion at codon 306 (306+T), and a guanine (G) to cytosine (C) transition at codon 484. The activity of the mutant enzymes, expressed as a percentage of wild-type, is indicated on the vertical axis and in parentheses for some missense mutations. *NC,* Nonclassic form; *SV,* simple virilizing; *SW,* salt wasting.

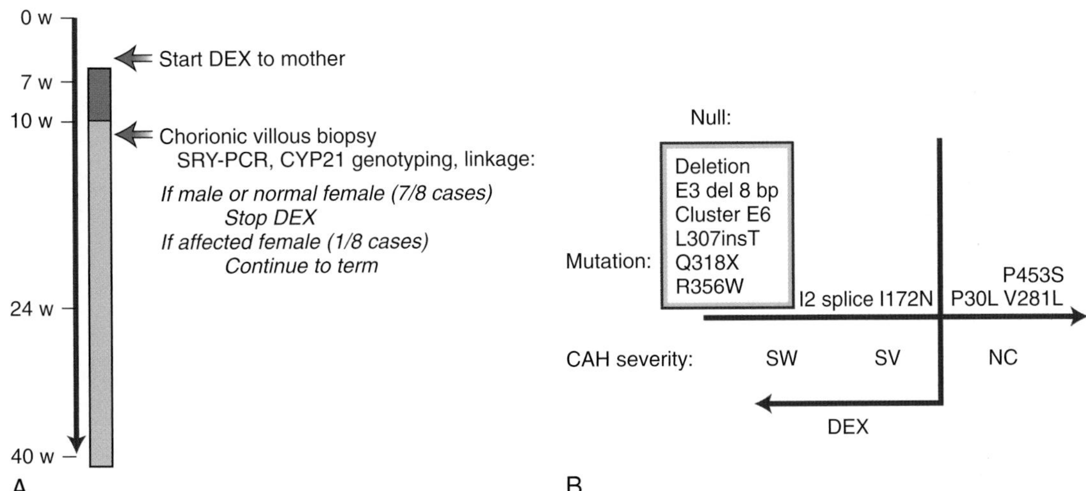

Figure 22–40 ■ Prenatal management of 21-hydroxylase deficiency. **A,** Protocol for dexamethasone (DEX) treatment; the standard dose is 20 µg/kg maternal body weight per day administered orally in three divided doses. The vertical bar indicates critical periods of androgen action, the solid bar represents the period during the first trimester when fusion of the labia and displacement of the vaginal opening into a male-like urethra occurs. The clitoris is sensitive to androgens throughout gestation. **B,** Genotype and phenotype associations in 21-hydroxylase deficiency according to the most common *CYP21* mutations (see also Fig. 22–39). The single letter code for amino acids is shown. The severity of CAH is classified according to SW, SV, NC categories; prenatal treatment is restricted to families segregating mutations associated with the SW and SV phenotypes. (Adapted with permission from Lajic S, Nordenström A, Ritzen EM, et al. Prenatal treatment of congenital adrenal hyperplasia. Eur J Endocrinol 2004;2151(suppl):U63-U69.)

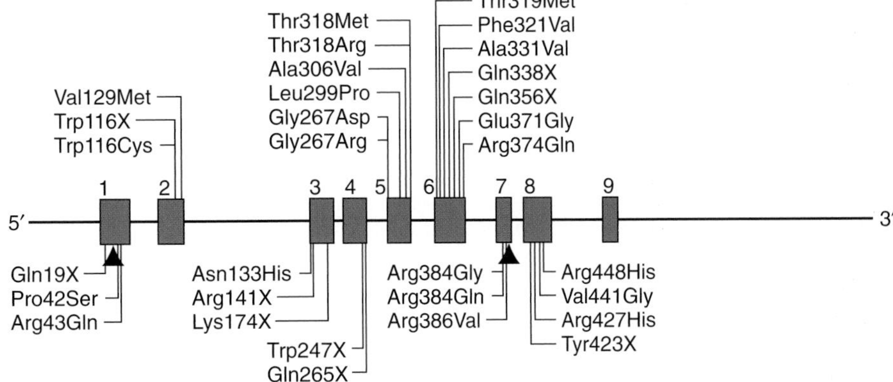

Figure 22–41 ■ Diagram of the *CYP11B1* gene and locations of the mutations causing 11β-hydroxylase deficiency. The numbered solid boxes depict the exons. The three letter abbreviation for amino acids is used; X, indicates a nonsense (stop) mutation. A deletion of cytosine (C) at codon 32 and the addition of two nucleotides at codon 394 cause frameshift mutations (▲).

11β-Hydroxylase (CYP11B1) Deficiency

This disorder in adrenal steroidogenesis can also profoundly androgenize an affected female fetus and accounts for 5% to 8% of patients with CAH; there is a clustering of cases in Moroccan Jews. Apart from causing ambiguous genitalia in the newborn, 11β-hydroxylase deficiency presents later with hypertension. This is the result of accumulation of 11-deoxycorticosterone leading to salt and fluid retention. Plasma renin is suppressed. 11β-hydroxylase is encoded by the *CYP11B1* gene, which is located on chromosome 8q21-22 in tandem with *CYP11B2,* which encodes aldosterone synthase, the enzyme catalyzing the conversion of deoxycorticosterone to corticosterone and thence to aldosterone.[453] A selection of the *CYP11B1* mutations that cause 11β-hydroxylase deficiency are shown in Figure 22–41. A total 53 mutations are now listed on the Human Gene Mutation Database (HGMD), the majority of which are missense mutations. Arg448 appears to be a relative "hotspot" for mutations, with Arg448His possibly a founder mutation in the Moroccan Jewish population. However, screening a healthy representative group from this population did not reveal a high carrier rate for mutations at codon 448.[454] It is possible to establish a prenatal diagnosis of 11β-hydroxylase deficiency and, as with 21-hydroxylase deficiency, virilization of an affected female fetus can be prevented with maternal dexamethasone administration.[453]

Familial Glucocorticoid Resistance

Glucocorticoid resistance is a rare disorder, usually caused by sporadic heterozygous mutations in the glucocorticoid receptor (α isoform).[455] Partial end-organ insensitivity to glucocorticoid action coupled with impaired feedback mechanisms result in excess ACTH secretion and elevated circulating cortisol levels, without the clinical features of Cushing's syndrome. Elevated mineralocorticoids (causing hypertension and hypokalemia) and elevated adrenal androgens (causing hirsutism and acne) are frequently seen.

Most GRα mutations are heterozygous changes that cause a partial loss of function through altering ligand-binding, nuclear localization, co-activator interactions, and target gene transcription, often with some degree of dominant negative activity. Complete loss of the GRα gene in mice is lethal, so it is unclear whether complete glucocorticoid resistance could occur in

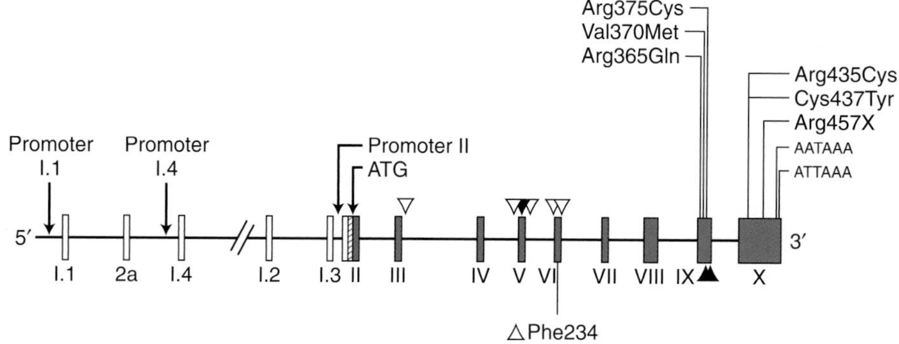

Figure 22–42 ▪ Diagram of the *CYP19* ($P450_{arom}$) gene and selected mutations causing aromatase deficiency. The numbered *solid boxes* represent translated exons. The septum in the open box in exon II represents the 3′ acceptor splice junction for the untranslated exons. The multiple alternate promoters and the untranslated exons *(open boxes)* are indicated. The three-letter abbreviation for amino acids is used to indicate the position of missense mutations; X, indicates a nonsense (stop) mutation; insertions and deletions resulting in frameshift and splice site mutations are shown by *filled arrowheads* and *open arrowheads,* respectively. In addition to the mutations causing classic aromatase deficiency, a homozygous Arg435Cys mutation and deletion of a phenylalanine residue at position 234 are both associated with a partial aromatase insufficiency phenotype. (Modified from Morishima A, Grumbach MM, Simpson ER, et al. Aromatase deficiency in male and female siblings caused by a novel mutation and the physiological role of estrogens. J Clin Endocrinol Metab 1995; 80:3689-3698. © 1995, The Endocrine Society.)

humans and, if it did, whether any excess androgens generated prenatally would cause genital ambiguity at birth. One homozygous GRα mutation (Val571Ala) has been reported in a Brazilian girl who had a large clitoris, posterior labioscrotal fusion, and a urogenital sinus at birth.[456] This mutation caused marked reduction in GRα function, without complete loss of receptor activity. She also harbored a heterozygous mutation in *CYP21.* At 9 years of age, studies showed low renin hypertension and hypokalemia with increased plasma DOC and corticosterone, high concentrations of plasma ACTH and cortisol, and impaired suppression of plasma cortisol during a dexamethasone test. Consistent with her advanced bone age and progressive virilization, the concentrations of plasma testosterone, androstenedione, and 17-hydroxyprogesterone were elevated. Thus, more severe GRα mutations may present mild 46,XX DSD, although the phenotype may have been modified in this case by the coexistence of a heterozygous P450c21 change.

Aromatase (CYP19) Deficiency

Aromatase (*CYP19A1,* cytochrome $P450_{arom}$, or P450c19, formerly estrogen synthetase) is the only cytochrome P450 enzyme known to catalyze the conversion of androgens (C_{19} steroids) to estrogens (C_{18} steroids) in vertebrate species.[457] Aromatase is expressed in many tissues, including the placenta, ovary, brain, bone, vascular endothelium, breast, and adipose tissue, where it is regulated by a number of tissue-specific promoters to convert testosterone to estradiol and androstenedione to estrone (Fig. 22–42). Thus, aromatase plays a crucial role in the local production of estrogens as well as in the synthesis of circulating estrogens from the ovary at the time of puberty.

Aromatase deficiency due to recessively inherited mutations in *CYP19* has now been described in approximately 10 girls with 46,XX DSD (female pseudohermaphroditism). The clinical and biochemical features of this condition underscore the key role aromatase plays in the fetoplacental unit, and this condition is sometimes referred to as *placental aromatase deficiency.* Aromatase plays a critical role in protecting the fetus from excessive androgen exposure in utero (Fig. 22–43 and described in detail in the figure legend). In the absence of aromatase, estrogen cannot be synthesized by the placenta, and large quantities of placental testosterone and androstenedione are transferred to the fetal and maternal circulation, resulting in androgenization of the female fetus and virilization of the mother during pregnancy.[458] Putative CYP19 deficiency has been described in

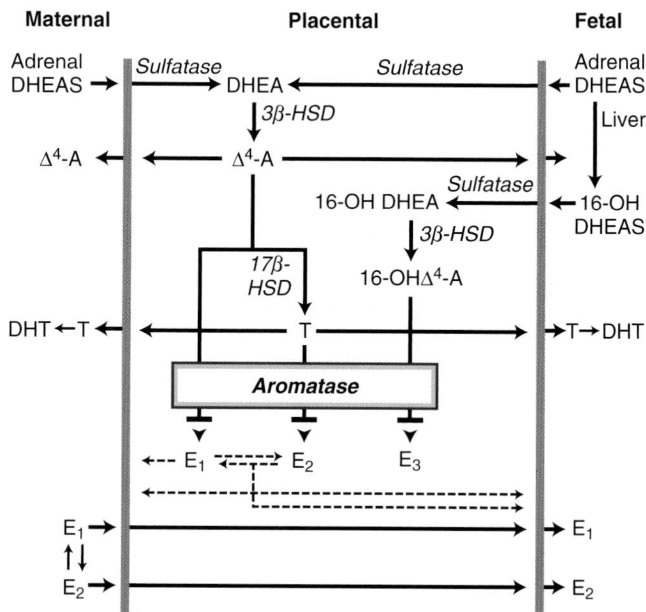

Figure 22–43 ▪ Aromatase plays a crucial role in protecting the fetus from excessive androgen exposure in utero. The placenta lacks CYP17 enzymatic activity and thus cannot convert C21-steroids such as progesterone to C19-steroids and thereafter to estrogens. During gestation, large quantities of DHEAS are produced in the fetal adrenal gland and by the maternal adrenal. DHEAS is 16α-hydroxylated in the fetal adrenal and liver. 16α-Hydroxy-DHEAS from the fetus and DHEAS from the fetus and mother are transferred to the placental unit, where the sulfate moiety is cleaved by placental sulfatase. These steroids can then be converted to androstenedione and 16α-hydroxyandrostenedione by 3β-HSD type I $\Delta^{4,5}$-isomerase; to testosterone and 16α-hydroxytestosterone by 17β-HSD; and to estrogens (mainly estriol from 16α-hydroxy-DHEA) by placental aromatase. Androstenedione and 16α-hydroxyandrostenedione may be aromatized directly to estrogens. *3β-HSD,* 3β-hydroxysteroid dehydrogenase/$\Delta^{4,5}$-isomerase; *17β-HSD,* 17β-hydroxysteroid dehydrogenase; *DHEA,* dehydroepiandrosterone; *DHEAS,* DHEA sulfate; *DHT,* dihydrotestosterone; *T,* testosterone; *Δ^4-A,* androstenedione; *E_1,* estrone; *E_2,* estradiol; *E_3,* estriol. (Modified and redrawn from Conte FA, Grumbach MM, Ito Y, et al. A syndrome of female pseudohermaphrodism, hypergonadotropic hypogonadism, and multicystic ovaries associated with missense mutations in the gene encoding aromatase ($P450_{arom}$). J Clin Endocrinol Metab 1994;78:1287-1292. © 1994, The Endocrine Society.)

the spotted hyena, which provides, in part, an explanation for the strikingly masculinized external genitalia and aggressive behavior of the female spotted hyena, especially during pregancy.[459]

Affected females (46,XX) with aromatase insufficiency are born with clitoromegaly, varying degrees of posterior fusion, scrotalization of the labioscrotal folds, and, in some infants with a urogenital sinus, a single perineal orifice.[460,461] There is often a striking history of maternal virilization after the second trimester of pregnancy (e.g., acne, hair growth, voice changes) coupled with elevated maternal androgen levels, which generally resolve after the infant is born. As expected for a steroidogenic defect, affected girls (46,XX) have normal müllerian structures. The histology of the ovaries in infancy is normal, but under increased FSH stimulation in the absence of ovarian aromatase, multiple enlarged follicular cysts develop. At puberty affected females have hypergonadotropic hypogonadism, typically fail to develop female secondary sexual characteristics, and exhibit progressive virilization. Plasma androstenedione and testosterone are elevated, and estrone and estradiol levels are low or unmeasurable. The ovaries enlarge and develop multiple cysts at puberty; in one affected female, polycystic ovaries were detected in infancy. The hypergonadotropism and the multiple ovarian cysts respond to estrogen replacement therapy, but in some cases temporary treatment with an antiandrogen is necessary.[462]

In addition to a role in the reproductive axis, aromatase deficiency has implications for bone development, metabolism, and immune function, as determined by the long-term follow-up of the small numbers of women (46,XX) and men (46,XY) with aromatase deficiency, as well as from studies of aromatase knockout mice. Males only present after puberty and have tall stature, delayed bone maturation and epiphyseal fusion, and osteopenia, suggesting that estrogens are essential for the prevention of osteoporosis in males and females and for normal skeletal maturation and proportions.[463] This phenotype is similar to that of a man with an inactivating estrogen receptor-α mutation.[464] Hyperinsulinemia and abnormal plasma lipids have also been reported in aromatase deficiency, which may in part reflect estrogen insufficiency but may also reflect specific actions of aromatase itself. The finding of apparently normal psychosexual development in the three aromatase-deficient adolescent or adult patients and in the man with an estrogen receptor defect suggests that estrogen does not play a critical role in sex differentiation of the human brain, as has been reported in nonprimate mammals.

Approximately 15 different aromatase (*CYP19A1*) mutations have been described to date in males and females with this condition (see Fig. 22–42). These changes are inherited in a recessive fashion and are present in a homozygous or compound heterozygous state. Functional assays of aromatase activity have shown severe loss of enzyme function (<0.3%) in all cases associated with classic aromatase deficiency, other than approximately 1% activity for the Arg435Cys change found in a compound heterozygous state together with the null Cys437Tyr mutation.[460] Although this patient had a classic presentation at birth, maternal virilization during pregnancy was reportedly absent. Furthermore, the Arg435Cys change has now been reported in a homozygous state in a girl who presented with androgenized genitalia at birth but who showed limited breast development in puberty.[465] In addition, deletion of a single phenylalanine residue (Phe234del) causing partial loss of aromatase activity has been described in an androgenized 46,XX individual who showed significant breast development in puberty (Tanner stage 4).[465] Thus, a spectrum of phenotypes may be seen with aromatase insufficiency in humans. This important diagnosis should be considered in all androgenized 46,XX infants when more common forms of CAH (e.g., 21-hydroxylase) have been excluded. A history of maternal virilization in pregnancy should always be sought, and increased levels of Δ^4-androstenedione, testosterone, and DHT and low levels of plasma estriol, urinary estriol and amniotic fluid estrone, estradiol, and estriol may be detected.

Maternal Androgen Excess

Maternal sources of androgens that may virilize a female fetus are either endogenous from adrenal and ovarian tumors, or exogenous from maternal ingestion of androgenic compounds. Danazol, a synthetic derivative of ethisterone with androgenic, antiestrogenic, and antiprogestogenic activities, is used in diverse conditions such as endometriosis, benign fibrocystic breast disease, and hereditary angioedema and in women with unexplained subfertility. It crosses the placenta and is contraindicated in pregnancy in view of reports that a female fetus may become androgenized.[466] Evidence that danazol competitively inhibits aromatase activity in endometriosis-derived stromal cells may partly explain its androgenic effects on the fetus.[467] Ovarian causes of virilization include primary malignancy, benign lesions such as luteoma and hyperreactio luteinalis, and polycystic ovary syndrome. Recurrence in subsequent pregnancies and maternal virilization can occur with luteomas, most commonly in multiparous women of Afro-Caribbean descent.[468] As in fetal aromatase deficiency previously discussed, a similar pattern of recurrent hyperandrogenization without evidence of placental aromatase deficiency has been reported.[468]

Other Conditions Affecting 46,XX Sex Development

A number of syndromic associations can cause developmental genital abnormalities in 46,XX girls, although these are less frequent than the syndromic associations resulting in underandrogenization in 46,XY males. Complex urogenital anomalies such as cloacal extrophy can affect both sexes and require major reconstructive surgery for bladder and bowel function, as well as for the lower genital system.

Abnormalities in uterine development can result in bicornate uterus (Fryns syndrome), uterine hemiagenesis or hypoplasia, or uterine agenesis. These conditions can be associated with renal, cardiac and cervical spinal abnormalities as part of Mayer-Rokitansky-Kuster-Hauser syndrome or MURCS (*mü*llerian, *r*enal, *c*ervical *s*pine).[470] The etiology of these conditions is not known in most women, although some familial cases have been described, and a mutation in *WNT4* has been reported in a patient with absent müllerian structures (uterus, upper vagina), unilateral renal agenesis, and mild hyperandrogenemia.[471] Uterine abnormalities have also been associated with maturity-onset diabetes of the young type 5 (MODY5, *HNF1β*) and with vaginal abnormalities with hand-foot-genital syndrome (*HOXA13*) and McKusick-Kaufman syndrome (*BBS6*). A prominent clitoris can be associated with conditions such as Fraser syndrome or neurofibromatosis, so careful evaluation is necessary before a hyperandrogenic cause is diagnosed.

Other common conditions that might be mistaken for a more serious underlying disorder include apparent clitoromegaly seen in premature or ex-premature babies or when little labial adipose tissue is present. Thus, assessment by a surgeon of physician with experience of normal variability in clitoral size is important. Labial adhesions are also a common finding in the newborn girl. Often they will dissolve spontaneously, although estrogen cream can be used to accelerate the process. Transient menstrual bleeding in the first week of life can be seen frequently in female infants, following the withdrawal of large amounts of estrogens and progesterones following birth. This finding can be alarming for parents, but it rapidly resolves and no treatment is needed.

INVESTIGATION AND MANAGEMENT OF DISORDERS OF SEX DEVELOPMENT

The majority of cases of DSD present at birth, the prototypical example being ambiguous genitalia of the newborn. In these circumstances, health professionals should be open in acknowledging that it is not possible to make an instant gender assignment until a number of investigations are completed. Gender assignment must be avoided until the appropriate assessment has been undertaken by an expert multidisciplinary team. Subsequently, all individuals should receive a gender assignment, while any surgical procedure needed to make the genitalia concordant with that assignment can, if necessary, be deferred until later. It is mandatory to communicate openly with patients and families, with their concerns respected and addressed in confidence.

The composition of a multidisciplinary team is self-evident, including specialists in endocrinology, surgery, gynecology, genetics, psychology plus where necessary, a medical ethicist, legal adviser, and social worker. Discussion at this early stage should be conducted by a team member with appropriate communication skills. Support groups can play an important role to ensure the delivery of care is of appropriate standard.

Table 22–19 lists the problems in a newborn infant that merit investigation as a possible DSD. Deviation from the genital anatomy of the "ideal" male or female based on one literature search is estimated to be as high as 2% live births. Table 22–20 provides some reference anthropometric data gathered from the literature that is included in the consensus statement on DSD.[3,4] The Prader scoring system is useful to assess the degree of external virilization in 46,XX DSD due, for example, to CAH (see Fig. 22–38) while in a case of 46,XY DSD, the external androgenization/masculinization score is a useful assessment both basally and after androgen treatment (Fig. 22–44).[394] An exhaustive list of investigations that may be needed to establish a diagnosis is not included in this chapter because the choice of test is center-specific and no single evaluation protocol can be recommended in all circumstances. Hormone measurements need to be interpreted in relation to the specific assay characteristics and to normal values for gestational and chronologic age gathered by laboratories that comply with criteria stipulated by appropriate external quality control schemes. Table 22–21 lists those tests that may be needed to investigate a newborn with ambiguous genitalia. Molecular studies now play a major part in attempting a definitive diagnosis in DSD, although this still remains unsatisfactory in 46,XY DSD.[398] Whilst DSD is not a medical emergency, the detection and treatment of any associated *adrenal disorder* can be. Thus, close clinical and biochemical vigilance for salt-loss or glucocorticoid deficiency is needed in the assessment of all children presenting with a DSD phenotype until a specific diagnosis is reached.

Factors that influence gender assignment include the underlying diagnosis, appearance of the genitalia, surgical options in relation to technical advances, potential for fertility, the views of the family as well as social and cultural aspects. More than 90% of CAH females and all CAIS females identify as females; the Prader V CAH that may be instantly assigned male at birth by mistake should be raised female if a correct diagnosis is made early. The generalization that the age of 18 months is the upper limit of imposed gender reassignment should be treated with caution and viewed conservatively. The difficult choices that may need to be considered in XY DSD conditions such as

TABLE 22–19 NEWBORN PROBLEMS THAT MERIT DSD INVESTIGATION

Ambiguous genitalia
Apparent female genitalia with:
- *Enlarged clitoris*
- *Posterior labial fusion*
- *Inguinal/labial mass*

Apparent male genitalia with:
- *Nonpalpable testes*
- *Isolated perineoscrotal hypospadias*
- *Severe hypospadias, undescended testes, micropenis*

Family history of DSD, such as CAIS
Discordance between genital appearance and prenatal karyotype

TABLE 22–20 ANTHROPOMETRIC MEASUREMENTS OF THE EXTERNAL GENITALIA

Sex	Population	Age	Stretched Penile Length (PL) Mean (cm)±SD	Penile Width Mean (cm)±SD	Mean Testicular Volume (cc)
M	USA	30 wk GA	2.5±0.4		
M	USA	Full term	3.5±0.4	1.1±0.1	0.52 (median)
M	Japan	Term -14 yr	2.9±0.4 – 8.3±0.8		
M	Australia	24-36 wk GA	PL=2.27+(0.16 GA)		
M	Chinese	Term	3.1±0.3	1.07±0.09	
M	India	Term	3.6±0.4	1.14±0.07	
M	N America	Term	3.4±0.3	1.13±0.08	
M	Europe	10 years	6.4±0.4		0.95-1.20
M	Europe	Adult	13.3±1.6		16.5-18.2
Sex	**Population**	**Age**	**Clitoral length Mean (mm)±SD**	**Clitoral width Mean (mm)±SD**	**Perineum length Mean (mm)+SD**
F	USA	Full term	4.0±1.24	3.32±0.78	
F	USA	Adult Nulliparous	15.4±4.3		
F	USA	Adult	19.1±8.7	5.5±1.7	31.3±8.5

Reproduced with permission from Hughes IA, Houk C, Ahmed SF, Lee PA. Consensus statement on management of intersex disorders. Arch Dis Child 2006;91:554-562.

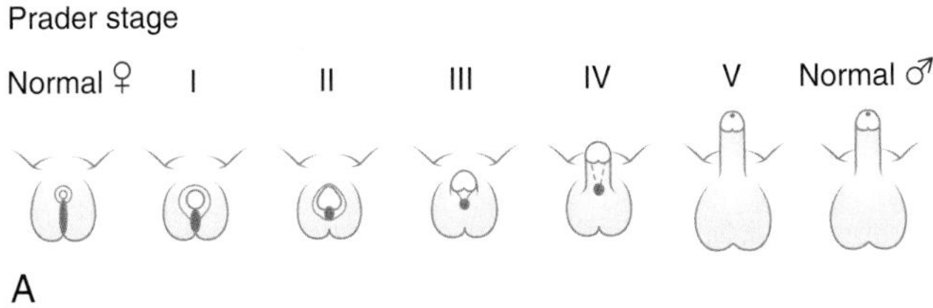

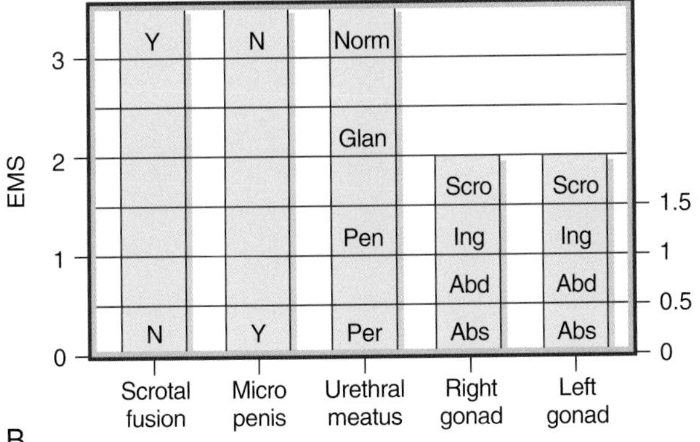

Figure 22–44 ■ **A,** Prader staging for scoring the degree of androgenization of the external genitalia in a female infant with CAH. **B,** External masculinization score (EMS) to assess degree of underandrogenization in an individual with 46,XY DSD. The score is based on the presence or absence of a micropenis and bifid scrotum, the location of the urethral meatus, and the position of the testes.[394]

mixed gonadal dysgenesis (45,X/46,XY mosaicism), 17β-HSD, and 5α-RD deficiencies have been mentioned.

Surgical management is clearly dictated by the gender assignation and, increasingly, a desire to involve the patient in decision making. In the case of CAH, for example, clitoroplasty should only be considered for Prader stage III or more, with an emphasis on functional outcome rather than the cosmetic appearance. This practice recognizes that damage may occur to the clitoral neurovascular bundles with subsequent adverse effects on sexual function.[472]

There remains debate about the timing of vaginoplasty, recognizing that if there are complications arising from a persistent urogenital sinus such as urinary infection or incontinence, then early surgery is necessary. A vaginoplasty undertaken in infancy generally needs to be refined at the time of puberty. Vaginal dilatation should not be undertaken in childhood. The use of vaginal dilators in young adulthood is often successful in avoiding the need for bowel vaginoplasty, especially in women with CAH and CAIS. The mainstay of surgical treatment in patients raised male is hypospadias repair, with correction of chordee and orchidopexy for undescended testes. The magnitude and complexity of phalloplasty in adulthood should be taken into account during the initial counseling period if successful gender assignment is dependent on this procedure. The risk of gonadal tumors in various categories of DSD has already been mentioned in the relevant sections and is summarized in Table 22–22.[32] Gonadectomy needs to be performed before puberty in PAIS, 17β-HSD, and 5α-RD deficiencies and in 45,X/46,XY mixed gonadal dysgenesis raised female. Preservation of the component of ovotestis concordant with the sex of rearing should be a long-term goal in ovotesticular DSD in view of some

TABLE 22–21 INVESTIGATING A NEWBORN WITH AMBIGUOUS GENITALIA

Genetics	FISH* (X and Y specific probes) Karyotype* Save DNA with consent
Endocrine	17OH-progesterone,* 11-deoxycortisol, 17OH-pregnenolone Routine serum biochemistry*; urinalysis* Renin, ACTH Testosterone,* androstenedione, DHT Gonadotropins, AMH, inhibin B Urinary steroids by GC-MS Dynamic tests: ACTH stimulation hCG stimulation Save serum
Imaging	Abdominopelvic and renal ultrasound* CT, MRI Cystourethroscopy, sinogram
Surgical	Laparoscopy Gonadal biopsies

*Indicates first-line investigations where results are available within days (see Table 22–19). For images of G-banded karyotypes and FISH analysis, see Fig. 22–3.

potential for fertility. In specialized centers for DSD management, cryopreservation of gonadal material is increasingly undertaken in view of the possibilities to preserve fertility in cancer patients by this means.[473] However, there is no evidence currently that this is successful in DSD.

While the main focus of this chapter has been on presentation and management of DSD in infancy and childhood, a DSD condition may present for the first time in adolescence. Table 22–23 lists some of the disorders that may present at puberty with signs of virilization or feminization at variance with the sex of rearing. In the case of a girl who develops signs of virilization at puberty because of 17β-HSD deficiency, for example, there is urgency in reducing the effects of androgens, which may not be completely reversible, such as deepening of the voice. Treatment with a GnRH analogue and an antiandrogen is helpful, pending arranging gonadectomy. It is not uncommon that investigating an adolescent for primary amenorrhea reveals a 46,XY DSD associated with CAIS, gonadal dysgenesis, or CYP17 deficiency. Establishing a 46,XX karyotype at adolescence in a male is less common and may be a serendipitous finding during investigations for infertility.

Transfer of care for adolescents with DSD to the cognate adult services is essential to ensure hormone replacement treatment is provided with appropriate preparations and doses. It is important to monitor bone density to ensure optimal bone mineral accumulation. Psychological support is equally important to provide through adolescence and young adulthood. Some adolescents may report significant gender dysphoria and if gender reassignment is sought, they should be supported and managed by specialists skilled in gender identity disorders. There is unanimity amongst all specialists working in DSD that outcome data are needed if decisions taken in infancy that have life-long consequences are to be reached from an evidence base. This mandates DSD management to be undertaken by a multidisciplinary team working from specialized centers committed to collaborating nationally and internationally in prospective, multicenter studies.

TABLE 22–22 RISK OF GERM CELL MALIGNANCY ACCORDING TO DIAGNOSIS

Risk Group	Disorder	Malignancy Risk (%)	Recommended Action	NUMBERS:	
				Studies (n)	Patients (n)
High	GD[a] (+Y)[b] intra-abd.	15-35	Gonadectomy[c]	12	350
	PAIS nonscrotal	50	Gonadectomy[c]	2	24
	Frasier	60	Gonadectomy[c]	1	15
	Denys-Drash (+Y)	40	Gonadectomy[c]	1	5
Intermediate	Turner (+Y)	12	Gonadectomy[c]	11	43
	17β-HSD	28	Watchful waiting	2	7
	GD (+Y)[b] scrotal	Unknown	Biopsy[d] and irrad.?	0	0
	PAIS scrotal gonad	Unknown	Biopsy[d] and irrad.?	0	0
Low	CAIS	2	Biopsy[d] and ???	2	55
	Ovotesticular DSD	3	Testis. tissue removal ?	3	426
	Turner (−Y)	1	None	11	557
No (?)	5α-reductase	0	Unresolved	1	3
	Leydig cell hypoplasia	0	Unresolved	1	2

[a]Gonadal dysgenesis (including not further specified, 46XY, 45X/46XY, mixed, partial, complete).
[b]GBY region positive, including the *TSPY* gene.
[c]At time of diagnosis.
[d]At puberty, allowing investigation of at least 30 seminiferous tubules, preferentially diagnosis based on OCT3/4 immunohistochemistry.

Reproduced with permission from Hughes IA, Houk C, Ahmed SF, Lee PA. Consensus statement on management of intersex disorders. Arch Dis Child 2006;91:554-562.

TABLE 22–23 DSD PRESENTING IN ADOLESCENCE

Prepubertal Sex of Rearing	Karyotype	DSD
Female	46,XY	17β-HSD deficiency 5α-RD deficiency PAIS CAIS* Swyer syndrome (complete gonadal dysgenesis)* CYP17 deficiency*
Male	46,XX	Ovotesticular DSD (feminization from ovarian tissue) (infertility) XX male CAH (usually present earlier with precocious puberty)

*Presentation is primary amenorrhea±lack of puberty.

ACKNOWLEDGMENTS

We recognize the major contributions made to this chapter in previous editors by Dr. Melvin Grumbach and Dr. Felix Conte. JCA holds a Wellcome Trust Senior Research Fellowship in Clinical Science (079666).

REFERENCES

1. Sax L. How common is intersex? A response to Anne Fausto-Sterling. J Sex Res 2002;39:174-178.
2. Grumbach MM, Hughes IA, Conte FA. Disorders of sex differentiation. In Larsen PR, Kronenberg HM, Melmed S, et al, eds. Williams Textbook of Endocrinology, 10th ed. Philadelphia: WB Saunders, 2003:842-1002.
3. Hughes IA, Houk C, Ahmed SF, et al. Consensus statement on management of intersex disorders. Arch Dis Child 2006;91: 554-563.
4. Lee PA, Houk CP, Ahmed SF, et al. Consensus statement on management of intersex disorders. International Consensus Conference on Intersex. Pediatrics 2006;118:753-757.
5. Brennan J, Capel B. One tissue, two fates: molecular genetic events that underlie testis versus ovary development. Nat Rev Genet 2004;5:509-521.
6. Park SY, Jameson JL. Minireview: transcriptional regulation of gonadal development and differentiation. Endocrinology 2005; 146:1035-1042.
7. Nikolova G, Vilain E. Mechanisms of disease: Transcription factors in sex determination—relevance to human disorders of sex development. Nat Clin Pract Endocrinol Metab 2006;2:231-238.
8. Wilhelm D, Koopman P. The making of maleness: towards an integrated view of male sexual development. Nat Rev Genet 2006;7:620-631.
9. Ezaz T, Stiglec R, Veyrunes F, et al. Relationships between vertebrate ZW and XY sex chromosome systems. Curr Biol 2006; 16:736-743.
10. Matsubara K, Tarui H, Toriba M, et al. Evidence for different origin of sex chromosomes in snakes, birds, and mammals and step-wise differentiation of snake chromosomes. Proc Natl Acad Sci U S A 2006;103:18031-18032.
11. Sarre SD, Georges A, Quinn A. The ends of a continuum: genetic and temperature-dependent sex determination in reptiles. Bioessays 2004;26:639-645.
12. Jost A. Recherches sur la differentiation sexualle de l'embryo de lapin. Arch Anat Microsc Morph Exp 1947;36:271-315.
13. Nef S, Schaad O, Stallings NR, et al. Gene expression during sex determination reveals a robust female genetic program at the onset of ovarian development. Dev Biol 2005;287:361-367.
14. Beverdam A, Koopman P. Expression profiling of purified mouse gonadal somatic cells during the critical time window of sex determination reveals novel candidate genes for human sexual dysgenesis syndromes. Hum Mol Genet 2006;15:417-431.
15. Parma P, Radi O, Vidal V, et al. R-spondin1 is essential in sex determination, skin differentiation and malignancy. Nat Genet 2006;38:1304-1309.
16. Johnson J, Canning J, Kaneko T, et al. Germline stem cells and follicular renewal in the postnatal mammalian ovary. Nature 2004;428:145-150.

17. Hall H, Hunt P, Hassold T. Meiosis and sex chromosome aneuploidy: how meiotic errors cause aneuploidy; how aneuploidy causes meiotic errors. Curr Opin Genet Dev 2006;16:323-329.
18. Thomas NS, Hassold TJ. Aberrant recombination and the origin of Klinefelter syndrome. Hum Reprod Update 2003;9:309-317.
19. Ross MT, Bentley DR, Tyler-Smith C. The sequences of the human sex chromosomes. Curr Opin Genet Dev 2006;16:213-218.
20. Tilford CA, Kuroda-Kawaguchi T, Skaletsky H, et al. A physical map of the human Y chromosome. Nature 2001;409:943-945.
21. Kuroda-Kawaguchi T, Skaletsky H, Brown LG, et al. The AZFc region of the Y chromosome features massive palindromes and uniform recurrent deletions in infertile men. Nat Genet 2001; 29:279-286.
22. McElreavey K, Ravel C, Chantot-Bastaraud S, et al. Y chromosome variants and male reproductive function. Int J Androl 2006;29: 298-303.
23. Cools M, Drop SL, Wolffenbuttel KP, et al. Germ cell tumors in the intersex gonad: old paths, new directions, moving frontiers. Endocr Rev 2006;27:468-484.
24. Nathanson KL, Kanetsky PA, Hawes R, et al. The Y deletion gr/gr and susceptibility to testicular germ cell tumor. Am J Hum Genet 2005;77:1034-1043.
25. Goldberg E. HY antigen and sex determination. Philos Trans R Soc Lond B Biol Sci 1988;322:72-81.
26. Mardon G, Page DC. The sex determining region of the mouse Y chromosome encodes a protein with a highly acidic domain and 13 zinc fingers. Cell 1989;56:765-770.
27. Palmer MS, Sinclair AH, Berta P, et al. Genetic evidence that ZFY is not the testis-determining factor. Nature 1989;342:937-939.
28. Sinclair AH, Berta P, Palmer MS, et al. A gene from the human sex determining region encodes a protein with homology to a conserved DNA-binding motif. Nature 1990;346:240-244.
29. Berta P, Ross Hawkins J, Sinclair AH, et al. Genetic evidence equating SRY and the testis determining factor. Nature 1990;348: 448-450.
30. Koopman P, Munsterberg A, Capel B, et al. Expression of a candidate sex determining gene during mouse testis differentiation. Nature 1990;348:450-452.
31. Koopman P, Gubbay J, Vivian N, et al. Male development of chromosomally female mice transgenic for Sry. Nature 1991;351: 117-121.
32. Jager RJ, Anvret M, Hall K, et al. A human XY female with a frame shift mutation in the candidate testis-determining gene SRY. Nature 1990;348:452-454.
33. Goodfellow PN, Lovell-Badge R. SRY and sex determination in mammals. Annu Rev Genet 1993;27:271-292.
34. Ross MT, Grafham DV, Coffey AJ, et al. The DNA sequence of the human X chromosome. Nature 2005;434:325-337.
35. Harsha HC, Suresh S, Amanchy R, et al. A manually curated functional annotation of the human X chromosome. Nat Genet 2005; 37:331-332.
36. Grumbach MM, Morishima A, Taylor JH. Human sex chromosome abnormalities in relation to DNA replication and heterochromatinization. Proc Natl Acad Sci U S A 1963;49:581-589.
37. Lyon MF. The X inactivation centre and X chromosome imprinting. Eur J Hum Genet 1994;2:255-261.
38. Whitelaw E. Unravelling the X in sex. Dev Cell 2006;11:759-762.
39. Heard E, Disteche CM. Dosage compensation in mammals: fine-tuning the expression of the X-chromosome. Genes Dev 2006;20: 1848-1867.
40. Carrel L, Willard HF. X-inactivation profile reveals extensive variability in X-linked gene expression in females. Nature 2005;434: 400-404.
41. Nguyen DK, Disteche CM. Dosage compensation of the active X chromosome in mammals. Nat Genet 2006;38:47-53.
42. Elsheikh M, Dunger DB, Conway GS, et al. Turner's syndrome in adulthood. Endocr Rev 2002;23:120-140.
43. Schlessinger D, Herrera L, Crisponi L, et al. Genes and translocations involved in POF. Am J Med Genet 2002;222:328-333.
44. Davison RM, Davis CJ, Conway GS. The X chromosome and ovarian failure. Clin Endocrinol 1999;51:673-679.
45. Murray A, Webb J, Grimley S, et al. Studies of FRAXA and FRAXE in women with premature ovarian failure. J Med Genet 1998;35: 637-640.
46. Sala C, Arrigo G, Torri G, et al. Eleven X chromosome breakpoints associated with premature ovarian failure (POF) map to a 15-Mb YAC contig spanning Xq21. Genomics 1997;40:123-131.
47. Lacombe A, Lee H, Zahed L, et al. Disruption of POF1B binding to nonmuscle actin filaments is associated with premature ovarian failure. Am J Hum Genet 2006;79:113-119.
48. Di Pasquale E, Beck-Peccoz P, Persan L. Hypergonadotropic ovarian failure associated with an inherited mutation of human bone morphogenetic protein-15 (BMP15) gene. Am J Hum Genet 2004;75:106-111.
49. Dixit H, Rao LK, Padmalatha VV, et al. Missense mutations in the BMP15 gene are associated with ovarian failure. Hum Genet 2006;119:408-415.
50. Crisponi L, Deiana M, Loi A, et al. The putative forkhead transcription factor FOXL2 is mutated in blepharophimosis/ptosis/epicanthus inversus syndrome. Nat Genet 2001;27:159-166.
51. Harris SE, Chand AL, Winship IM, et al. Identification of novel mutations in FOXL2 associated with premature ovarian failure. Mol Hum Reprod 2002;8:729-733.
52. Miyamoto N, Yoshida M, Kuratani S, et al. Defects of urogenital development in mice lacking *Emx2*. Development 1997;124: 1653-1664.
53. Brunelli S, Faiella A, Capra V, et al. Germline mutation in the homeobox gene EMX2 in patients with severe schizencephaly. Nat Genet 1996;12:94-96.
54. Shawlot W, Behringer RR. Requirement for Lim1 in head-organizer function. Nature 1995;374:425-430.
55. Birk OS, Casiano DE, Wassif CA, et al. The LIM homeobox gene *Lhx9* is essential for mouse gonad formation. Nature 2000; 403:909-913.
56. Ottolenghi C, Moreira-Filho C, Mendonca BB, et al. Absence of mutations involving the LIM homeobox domain gene LHX9 in 46,XY gonadal agenesis and dysgenesis. J Clin Endocrinol Metab 2001;86:2465-2469.
57. Katoh-Fukui Y, Tsuchiya R, Shiroishi T, et al. Male-to-female sex reversal in M33 mutant mice. Nature 1998;393:688-692.
58. Cui S, Ross A, Stallings N, et al. Disrupted gonadogenesis and male-to-female sex reversal in Pod1 knockout mice. Development 2004;131:4095-5105.
59. Tevosian SG, Albrecht KH, Crispino JD, et al. Gonadal differentiation, sex determination and normal *Sry* expression in mice require direct interaction between transcription partners GATA4 and FOG2. Development 2002;129:4627-4634.
60. Nef S, Verma-Kurvari S, Merenmies J, et al. Testis determination requires insulin receptor family function in mice. Nature 2003; 426:291-295.
61. Call KM, Glaser T, Ito CY, et al. Isolation and characterization of a zinc finger polypeptide gene at the human chromosome 11 Wilms tumor locus. Cell 1990;60:509-520.
62. Pritchard-Jones K, Fleming S, Davidson D, et al. The candidate Wilms' tumor gene is involved in genitourinary development. Nature 1990;346:194-197.
63. Kreidberg JA, Sariola H, Loring JM, et al. WT1 is required for early kidney development. Cell 1993;74:679-691.
64. Hastie ND. Life, sex, and WT1 isoforms-three amino acids can make all the difference. Cell 2001;106:391-394.
65. Hohenstein P, Hastie ND. The many facets of the Wilms' tumour gene, WT1. Hum Mol Genet 2006;15:R196-R201.
66. Nachtigal MW, Hirokawa Y, Enyeart-VanHouten DL, et al. Wilms' tumor 1 and Dax-1 modulate the orphan nuclear receptor SF-1 in sex-specific gene expression. Cell 1998;93:445-454.
67. Hammes A, Guo JK, Lutsch G, et al. Two splice variants of the Wilms' tumor 1 gene have distinct functions during sex determination and nephron formation. Cell 2001;106:319-329.
68. Hanley NA, Ball SG, Clement-Jones M, et al. Expression of steroidogenic factor 1 and Wilms' tumour 1 during early human gonadal development and sex determination. Mech Dev 1999; 87:175-180.
69. Francke U, Holmes LB, Atkins L, et al. Aniridia-Wilms' tumor association: evidence for specific deletion of 11p13. Cytogenetics Cell Genet 1979;24:185-192.
70. Pelletier J, Bruening W, Kashtan CE, et al. Germline mutations in the Wilms tumor suppressor gene are associated with abnormal urogenital development in Denys-Drash syndrome. Cell 1991;67: 437-447.

71. Barbaux X, Niandet P, Gubler M-C, et al. Donor splice-site mutations in WTI are responsible for Frasier syndrome. Nat Genet 1997;17:467-470.
72. Klamt B, Koziell A, Poulat F, et al. Frasier syndrome is caused by defective alternative splicing of WT1 leading to an altered ratio of WT1 +/-KTS splice isoforms. Hum Mol Genet 1998;7:709-714.
73. Koziell A, Charmandari E, Hindmarsh PC, et al. Frasier syndrome, part of the Denys Drash continuum or simply a WT1 gene associated disorder of intersex and nephropathy? Clin Endocrinol 2000;52:519-524.
74. Parker Kl, Rice DA, Lala DS, et al. Steroidogenic factor 1: an essential mediator of endocrine development. Recent Prog Horm Res 2002;57:19-36.
75. Luo X, Ikeda Y, Parker KL. A cell-specific nuclear receptor is essential for adrenal and gonadal development and sexual differentiation. Cell 1994;77:481-490.
76. Tran PV, Lee MB, Marin O, et al. Requirement of the orphan nuclear receptor SF-1 in terminal differentiation of ventromedial hypothalamic neurons. Mol Cell Neurosci. 2003;22:441-453.
77. Majdic G, Young M, Gomez-Sanches E, et al. Knockout mice lacking steroidogenic factor 1 are a novel genetic model of hypothalamic obesity. Endocrinology 2002;143:607-614.
78. Park SY, Meeks JJ, Raverot G, et al. Nuclear receptors Sf1 and Dax1 function cooperatively to mediate somatic cell differentiation during testis development. Development 2005;132:2415-2423.
79. Bland ML, Jamieson CA, Akana SF, et al. Haploinsufficiency of steroidogenic factor-1 in mice disrupts adrenal development leading to an impaired stress response. Proc Natl Acad Sci U S A 2001;97:14488-14493.
80. Achermann JC, Ito M, Ito M, et al. A mutation in the gene encoding steroidogenic factor-1 causes XY sex reversal and adrenal failure in humans. Nat Genet 1999;22:125-126.
81. Achermann JC, Ozisik G, Ito M, et al. Gonadal determination and adrenal development are regulated by the orphan nuclear receptor, steroidogenic factor-1 in a dose dependent manner. J Clin Endocrinol Metab 2002;87:1829-1833.
82. Harley VR, Clarkson MJ, Argentaro A. The molecular action and regulation of the testis-determing factors, SRY (sex-determining region on the Y chromosome) and SOX9 [SRY-related high-mobility group (HMG) box 9]. Endocr Rev 2003;24:466-487.
83. Jeyasuria P, Ikeda Y, Jamin SP, et al. Cell-specific knockout of steroidogenic factor 1 reveals its essential roles in gonadal function. Mol Endocrinol 2004;18:1610-1619.
84. Biason-Lauber A, Schoenle EJ. Apparently normal ovarian differentiation in a prepubertal girl with transcriptionally inactive steroidogenic factor 1 (NR5A1/SF-1) and adrenocortical insufficiency. Am J Hum Genet 2000;67:1563-1568.
85. Lin L, Pascal P, Ferraz-de-Souza B, et al. Heterozygous missense mutations in steroidogenic factor 1 (SF1/Ad4BP, NR5A1) are associated with 46,XY disorders of sex development with normal adrenal function. J Clin Endocrinol Metab 2007;92:991-999.
86. Bardoni B, Zanaria E, Guioli S, et al. A dosage sensitive locus at chromosome Xp21 is involved in male to female sex reversal. Nat Genet 1994;7:497-501.
87. Swain A, Narvaez V, Burgoyne P, et al. Dax1 antagonizes Sry action in mammalian sex determination. Nature 1998;391:761-767.
88. Meeks JJ, Weiss J, Jameson JL. Dax1 is required for testis determination. Nat Genet 2003;34:32-33.
89. Jordan BK, Mohammed M, Ching ST, et al. Up-regulation of WNT-4 signaling and dosage-sensitive sex reversal in humans. Am J Hum Genet 2001;68:1102-1109.
90. Molyneaux KA, Stallock J, Schaible K, et al. Time-lapse analysis of living mouse germ cell migration. Dev Biol 2001;240:488-498.
91. Kunwar PS, Siekhaus DE, Lehmann R. In vivo migration: a germ cell perspective. Annu Rev Cell Dev Biol 2006;22:237-265.
92. Tanaka SS, Yamaguchi YL, Tsoi B, et al. IFITM/Mil/fragilis family proteins IFITM1 and IFITM3 play distinct roles in mouse primordial germ cell homing and repulsion. Dev Cell 2005;9:745-756.
93. Molyneaux KA, Zinszner H, Kunwar, PS, et al. The chemokine SDF1/CXCL12 and its receptor CXCR4 regulate mouse germ cell migration and survival. Development 2003;130:4279-4286.
94. Buaas FW, Kirsh AL, Sharma M, et al. Plzf is required in adult male germ cells for stem cell self-renewal. Nat Genet 2004;36:647-652.
95. McLaren A. Germ and somatic cell lineages in the developing gonad. Mol Cell Endocrinol 2000;163:3-9.
96. Kurohmaru M, Kanai Y, Hayashi Y. A cytological and cytoskeletal comparison of Sertoli cells without germ cell and those with germ cells using the W/WV mutant mouse. Tissue Cell 1992;24: 895-903.
97. Bowles J, Knight D, Smith C, et al. Retinoid signaling determines germ cell fate in mice. Science 2006;312:596-600.
98. Koubova J, Menke DB, Zhou Q, et al. Retinoic acid regulates sex-specific timing of meiotic initiation in mice. Proc Natl Acad Sci U S A 2006;103:2474-2479.
99. Mehlmann LM. Stops and starts in mammalian oocytes: recent advances in understanding the regulation of meiotic arrest and oocyte maturation. Reproduction 2005;130:791-799.
100. Telfer EE, Gosden RG, Byskov AG, et al. Editorial: on regenerating the ovary and generating controversy. Cell 2005;122:821-822.
101. Bullejos M, Koopman P. Delayed *Sry* and *Sox9* expression in developing mouse gonads underlies B6-Y^{DOM} sex reversal. Dev Biol 2005;278:473-481.
102. Polanco JC, Koopman P. Sry and the hesitant beginnings of male development. Dev Biol 2007;302:13-24.
103. Hanley NA, Hagan DM, Clement-Jones M, et al. SRY, SOX9, and DAX1 expression patterns during human sex determination and gonadal development. Mech Dev 2000;91:403-407.
104. Harley VR, Jackson DI, Hextall PJ, et al. DNA binding activity of recombinant SRY from normal males and XY females. Science 1992;255:453-456.
105. Pontiggia A, Rimini R, Harvey VR, et al. Sex-reversing mutations affect the architecture of SRY-DNA complexes. EMBO J 1994;13: 6115-6124.
106. Werner MH, Huth JR, Gronenborn AM, et al. Molecular basis of human 46,XY sex reversal revealed from the three-dimensional solution structure of the human SRY DNA complex. Cell 1995;81: 705-714.
107. Sim H, Rimmer K, Kelly S, et al. Defective calmodulin-mediated nuclear transport of the sex-determining region of the Y chromosome (SRY) in XY sex reversal. Mol Endocrinol 2005;7:1884-1892.
108. Desclozeaux M, Poulat F, de Santa Barbara P, et al. Phosphorylation of an N-terminal motif enhances DNA-binding activity of the human SRY protein. J Biol Chem 1998;273:7988-7995.
109. Poulat F, Barbara PS, Desclozeaux M, et al. The human testis determining factor SRY binds a nuclear factor containing PDZ protein interaction domains. J Biol Chem 1997;272:7167-7172.
110. Schmitt-Ney M, Thiele H, Kaltwasser P, et al. Two novel SRY missense mutations reducing DNA binding identified in XY females and their mosaic fathers. Am J Hum Genet 1995;56: 862-869.
111. Jäger R, Harley V, Pfeiffer R, et al. A familial mutation in the testis-determining gene *SRY* shared by both sexes. Hum Genet 1992;90: 350-355.
112. Li B, Zhang W, Chan G, et al. Human sex reversal due to impaired nuclear localization of SRY. A clinical correlation. J Biol Chem 2001;276:46480-46484.
113. Burgoyne PS, Buehr M, Koopman P. Cell-autonomous action of the testis-determining gene: Sertoli cells are exclusively XY in XX-XY chimaeric mouse testes. Development 1988;102:443-450.
114. Albrecht KH, Eicher EM. Evidence that Sry is expressed in pre-Sertoli cells and Sertoli and granulosa cells have a common precursor. Dev Biol 2001;240:92-107.
115. Wilhelm D, Martinson F, Bradford S, et al. Sertoli cell differentiation is induced both cell-autonomously and through prostaglandin signaling during mammalian sex determination. Dev Biol 2005; 287:111-124.
116. Malki S, Nef S, Notarnicola C, et al. Prostaglandin D2 induces nuclear import of the sex-determining factor SOX9 via its cAMP-PKA phosphorylation. EMBO J 2005;24:1798-1809.
117. Schmahl J, Eicher EM, Washburn LL, et al. Sry induces cell proliferation in the mouse gonad. Development 2000;127:65-73.
118. Martineau J, Nordqvist K, Tilmann C, et al. Male-specific cell migration into the developing gonad. Curr Biol 1997;7:958-968.
119. Capel B, Albrecht KH, Washburn LL, et al. Migration of mesonephric cells into the mammalian gonad depends on Sry. Mech Dev 1999;84:127-131.
120. de Santa Barbara P, Mejean C, Moniot B, et al. Steroidogenic factor-1 contributes to the cyclic-adenosine monophosphate down-regulation of human SRY gene expression. Biol Reprod 2001;64: 775-783.

121. McElreavey K, Vilain E, Abbas N, et al. A regulatory cascade hypothesis for mammalian sex determination: SRY represses a negative regulator of male development. Proc Natl Acad Sci U S A 1993;90:3368-3372.
122. Foster JW, Dominguez-Steglich MA, Guioli S, et al. Campomelic dysplasia and autosomal sex reversal caused by mutations in an SRY-related gene. Nature 1994;372:525-530.
123. Wagner T, Wirth J, Meyer J, et al. Autosomal sex reversal and campomelic dysplasia are caused by mutations in and around the *SRY*-related gene *SOX9*. Cell 1994;79:1111-1120.
124. Morais da Silva S, Hacker A, Harley V, et al. Sox 9 expression during gonadal development implies a conserved role for the gene in testis differentiation in mammals and birds. Nat Genet 1996;14:62-68.
125. Kent J, Wheatley SC, Andrews JE, et al. A male-specific role for SOX9 in vertebrate sex determination. Development 1996;122: 2813-2822.
126. Südbeck P, Schmitz ML, Baeuerle PA, et al. Sex reversal by loss of the C-terminal transactivation domain of human SOX9. Nat Genet 1996;13:230-232.
127. Preiss S, Argentaro A, Clayton A, et al. Compound effects of point mutations causing campomelic dysplasia/autosomal sex reversal upon SOX9 structure, nuclear transport, DNA binding, and transcriptional activation. J Biol Chem 2001;276:27864-27872.
128. Huang B, Wang S, Ning Y, et al. Autosomal XX sex reversal caused by duplication of SOX9. Am J Med Genet 1999;87:349-353.
129. Vidal VP, Chaboissier MC, de Rooij DG, et al. Sox9 induces testis development in XX transgenic mice. Nat Genet 2001;28: 216-217.
130. Qin Y, Bishop CE. Sox9 is sufficient for functional testis development producing fertile male mice in the absence of Sry. Hum Mol Genet 2005;14:1221-1229.
131. Bishop CE, Whitworth DJ, Qin Y, et al. A transgenic insertion upstream of Sox9 is associated with dominant XX sex reversal in the mouse. Nat Genet 2000;26:490-494.
132. Colvin JS, Green RP, Schmahl J, et al. Male-to-female sex reversal in mice lacking fibroblast growth factor 9. Cell 2001;104:875-889.
133. Brennan J, Karl J, Capel B. Divergent vascular mechanisms downstream of Sry establish the arterial system in the XY gonad. Dev Biol 2002;244:418-428.
134. Jeays-Ward K, Hoyle C, Brennan J, et al. Endothelial and steroidogenic cell migration are regulated by WNT4 in the developing mammalian gonad. Development 2003;130:3663-3670.
135. Yao HH, Matsuk MM, Jorgez CJ, et al. Follistatin operates downstream of Wnt4 in mammalian ovary organogenesis. Dev Dyn 2004;230:210-215.
136. Kim Y, Kobayashi A, Sekido R et al. Fgf9 and Wnt4 act as antagonistic signals to regulate mammalian sex determination. PloS Biol 2006;4:e187.
137. Clark AM, Garland KK, Russell LD. *Desert hedgehog* (*Dhh*) gene is required in the mouse testis for formation of adult-type Leydig cells and normal development of peritubular cells and seminiferous tubules. Biol Reprod 2000;63:1825-1838.
138. Pierucci-Alves F, Clark A, and Russell L. A developmental study of the *Desert hedgehog*-null mouse testis. Biol Reprod 2001;65: 1392-1402.
139. Yao HH, Whoriskey W, Capel B. Desert Hedgehog/Patched 1 signaling specifies fetal Leydig cell fate in testis organogenesis. Genes Dev 2002;16:1433-1440.
140. Umehara F, Tate G, Itoh K, et al. A novel mutation of desert hedgehog in a patient with 46,XY partial gonadal dysgenesis accompanied by minifascicular neuropathy. Am J Hum Genet 2000;67: 1302-1305.
141. Moniot B, Berta P, Scherer G, et al. Male specific expression suggests role of DMRT1 in human sex determination. Mech Dev 2000;91:323-325.
142. Ottolenghi C, Veitia R, Quintana-Murci L, et al. The region on 9p associated with 46,XY sex reversal contains several transcripts expressed in the urogenital system and a novel double sex-related domain. Genomics 2000;64:170-178.
143. Raymond CS, Murphy MW, O'Sullivan MG, et al. Dmrt1, a gene related to worm and fly sexual regulators, is required for mammalian testis differentiation. Genes Dev 2000;14:2587-2595.
144. Huret JL, Leonard C, Forestier B, et al. Eleven new cases of del(9p) and features from 80 cases. J Med Genet 1988;25:741-749.
145. Kitamura K, Yanazawa M, Sugiyama N, et al. Mutation of ARX causes abnormal development of forebrain and testes in mice and X-linked lissencephaly with abnormal genitalia in humans. Nat Genet 2002;32:359-369.
146. Brennan J, Tilmann C, Capel B. Pdgfr- mediates testis cord organization and fetal Leydig cell development in the XY gonad. Genes Dev 2003;17:800-810.
147. Gnessi L, Basciani S, Mariani S, et al. Leydig cell loss and spermatogenic arrest in platelet-derived growth factor (PDGF)-A-deficient mice. J Cell Biol 2000;149:1019-1026.
148. Perera EM, Martin H, Seeherunvong T, et al. Tescalcin, a novel gene encoding a putative EF-hand Ca(2+)-binding protein, Col9a3, and renin are expressed in the mouse testis during the early stages of gonadal differentiation. Endocrinology 2001;142: 455-463.
149. Töhönen V, Österlund C, Nordqvist K. Testatin: a cystatin-related gene expressed during early testis development. Proc Natl Acad Sci U S A 1998;95:14208-14213.
150. Gibbons RJ, Higgs DR. Molecular-clinical spectrum of the ATR-X syndrome. Am J Med Genet 2000;97:204-212.
151. Ion A, Telvi L, Chaussain JL, et al. A novel mutation in the putative DNA helicase XH2 is responsible for male to female sex reversal associated with an atypical form of ATRX syndrome. Am J Hum Genet 1996;58:1185-1191.
152. Pfeifer D, Poulat F, Holinski-Feder E, et al. The SOX8 gene is located within 700 kb of the tip of chromosome 16p and is deleted in a patient with ATR-16 syndrome. Genomics 2000;63:108-116.
153. Waggoner DJ, Chow CK, Dowton SB, et al. Partial monosomy of distal 10q: three new cases and a review. Am J Med Genet 1999;86:1-5.
154. Pinsky L, Erickson RP, Schimke RN, eds. Genetic Disorders of Human Sexual Development. New York: Oxford University Press, 1999.
155. Simpson JL, Rajkovic A. Ovarian differentiation and gonadal failure. Am J Med Genet 1999;89:186-200.
156. Matzuk MM, Burns KH, Viveiros MM, et al. Intercellular communication in the mammalian ovary: oocytes carry the conversation. Science 2002;296:2178-2180.
157. Yao HH, et al. Meiotic germ cells antagonize mesonephric cell migration and testis cord formation in mouse gonads. Development 2003;130:5895-5902.
158. Vainio S, Heikkila M, Kispert A, et al. Female development in mammals is regulated by Wnt-4 signalling. Nature 1999;397: 405-409.
159. Couse JF, Hewitt SC, Bunch DO, et al. Postnatal sex reversal of the ovaries in mice lacking estrogen receptors alpha and beta. Science 1999;286:2328-2331.
160. Teixeira J, Maheswaran S, Donahoe PK. Mullerian inhibiting substance: an instructive developmental hormone with diagnostic and possible therapeutic applications. Endocr Rev 2001;22: 657-674.
161. Josso N, Clemente N. Transduction pathway of anti-Mullerian hormone, a sex-specific member of the TGF-beta family. Trends Endocrinol Metab 2003;14:91-97.
162. Visser JA. AMH signaling: from receptor to target gene. Mol Cell Endocrinol 2003;211:65-73.
163. Bedecarrats GY, O'Neill FH, Norwitz ER, et al. Regulation of gonadotropin gene expression by Mullerian inhibiting substance. Proc Natl Acad Sci U S A 2003;100:9348-9353.
164. Siiteri PK, Wilson JD. Testosterone formation and metabolism during male sexual differentiation in the human embryo. J Clin Endocrinol Metab 1974;38:113-125.
165. Murray TJ, Fowler PA, Abramovich DR, et al. Human fetal testis: second trimester proliferative and steroidogenic capacities. J Clin Endocrinol Metab 2000;85:4812-4817.
166. Tapanainen JS, Kellokumpu-Lehtinen P, Pelliniemi L, et al. Age-related changes in endogenous steroids of human fetal testis during early and midpregnancy. J Clin Endocrinol Metab 1981; 52:98-102.
167. Kaplan SL, Grumbach MM. Pituitary and placental gonadotrophins and sex steroids in the human and sub-human primate fetus. Clin Endocrinol Metab 1978;7:487-511.
168. Payne AH, Hales DB. Overview of steroidogenic enzymes in the pathway from cholesterol to active steroid hormones. Endocr Rev 2004;25:947-970.

169. Fluck CE, Miller WL, Auchus RJ. The 17, 20-lyase activity of cytochrome p450c17 from human fetal testis favors the delta5 steroidogenic pathway.J Clin Endocrinol Metab 2003;88:3762-3766.
170. Arlt W, Walker EA, Draper N, et al. Congenital adrenal hyperplasia caused by mutant P450 oxidoreductase and human androgen synthesis: analytical study. Lancet 2004;363:2128-2135.
171. Auchus RJ. The backdoor pathway to dihydrotestosterone. Trends Endocrinol Metab 2004;15:432-438.
172. Goto M, Piper Hanley K, Marcos J, et al. In humans, early cortisol biosynthesis provides a mechanism to safeguard female sexual development. J Clin Invest 2006;116:953-960.
173. Hutson JM, Hasthorpe S. Testicular descent and cryptorchidism: the state of the art in 2004. J Pediatr Surg 2005;40:297-302.
174. Zimmermann S, Steig G, Emmen JM, et al. Targeted disruption of the Insl3 gene causes bilateral cryptorchidism. Mol Endocrinol 1999;13:681-691.
175. Kobayashi A, Behringer RR. Developmental genetics of the female reproductive tract in mammals. Nat Rev Genet 2003;4: 751-766.
176. Phoenix CH, Goy RW, Gerall AA, et al. Organizing action of prenatally administered testosterone proprionate on the tissues mediating mating behaviour in the female guinea pig. Endocrinology 1959;65:369-382.
177. Wallen K. Hormonal influences on sexually differentiated behavior in nonhuman primates. Front Neuroendocrinol 2005;26:7-26.
178. Wallen K. Nature needs nurture: the interaction of hormonal and social influences on the development of behavioral sex differences in rhesus monkeys. Horm Behav 1996;30:364-378.
179. Dewing P, Shi T, Horvath S, et al. Sexually dimorphic gene expression in mouse brain precedes gonadal differentiation. Brain Res Mol Brain Res 2003;118:82-90.
180. De Vries GJ, Rissman EF, Simerly RB, et al. A model system for study of sex chromosome effects on sexually dimorphic neural and behavioral traits. J Neurosci 2002;22:9005-9014.
181. Arnold AP, Xu J, Grisham W, et al. Minireview: Sex chromosomes and brain sexual differentiation. Endocrinology 2004;145: 1057-1062.
182. Hines M, Ahmed F, Hughes IA. Psychological outcomes and gender-related development in complete androgen insensitivity syndrome. Arch Sex Behav 2003;32:93-101.
183. Mazur T. Gender dysphoria and gender change in androgen insensitivity or micropenis. Arch. Sex Behav 2005;34:411-421.
184. Cohen-Bendahan CCC, van de Beek C, Berenbaum SA. Prenatal sex hormone effects on child and adult sex-typed behavior: methods and findings. Neurosci Biobehav Rev 2005;29:353-384.
185. Meyer-Bahlburg HF. Gender and sexuality in congenital adrenal hyperplasia. Endocrinol Metab Clin North Am 2001;30:155-171.
186. Nordenström A, Servin A, Bohlin G, et al. Sex-typed toy play behavior correlates with the degree of prenatal androgen exposure assessed by CYP21 genotype in girls with congenital adrenal hyperplasia. J Clin Endocrinol Metab 2002;87:5119-5124.
187. Meyer-Bahlburg HF, Dolezal C, Baker SW, et al. Gender development in women with congenital adrenal hyperplasic as a function of disorder severity. Arch Sex Behav 2006;35:667-684.
188. Meyer-Bahlburg HF, Dolezal C, Baker SW, et al. Prenatal androgenization affects gender-related behavior but not gender identity in 5-12-year-old girls with congenital adrenal hyperplasia. Arch Sex Behav 2004;33:97-104.
189. Dessens AB, Slijper FM, Drop SL. Gender dysphoria and gender change in chromosomal females with congenital adrenal hyperplasia. Arch Sex Behav 2005;32:389-397.
190. Cohen-Kettenis PT. Gender change in 46,XY persons with 5-alpha-reductase-2 deficiency and 17-beta-hydroxysteroid dehydrogenase-3 deficiency. Arch Sex Behav 2005;34:399-410.
191. Meyer-Bahlburg HF. Gender identity outcome in female-raised 46,XY persons with penile agenesis, cloacal exstrophy of the bladder, or penile ablation. Arch Sex Behav 2005;34:423-438.
192. Zucker KJ. Intersexuality and gender identity differentiation. Ann Rev Sex Res 1999;10:1-69.
193. Martin CL, Ruble DN, Szkrybalo J. Cognitive theories of early gender development. Psychol Bull 2002;128:903-933.
194. Luders E, Narr K, Thompson PM, et al. Gender differences in cortical complexity. Nat Neurosci 2004;7:799-800.
195. Paus T. Mapping brain maturation and cognitive development during adolescence. Trends Cogn Sci 2005;9:60-68.
196. MacColl G, Quinton R, Bouloux PMG. GnRH neuronal development: insights into hypogonadotropic hypogonadism. Trends Endocrinol Metab 2002;13:112-118.
197. Dode C, Levilliers J, Dupont J-M, et al. Loss-of-function mutations in FGFR1 cause autosomal dominant Kallmann syndrome. Nat Genet 2003;33:463-465.
198. Miura K, Acierno JS Jr, Seminara SB. Characterization of the human nasal embryonic LHRH factor gene, NELF, and a mutation screening among 65 patients with idiopathic hypogonadotropic hypogonadism (IHH). J Hum Genet 2004;49:265-268.
199. Dode C, Teixeira L, Levilliers J, et al. Kallmann syndrome: mutations in the genes encoding prokineticin-2 and prokineticin receptor-2. PloS Genet 2006;2:e175.
200. Millar RP, Lu ZL, Pawson AJ, et al. Gonadotropin-releasing hormone receptors. Endocr Rev 2004;25:235-275.
201. Seminara SB, Messager S, Chatzidaki EE, et al. The GPR54 gene as a regulator of puberty. N Engl J Med 2003;23:1614-1627.
202. Dasen JS, O'Connell SM, Flynn SE, et al. Reciprocal interactions of Pit1 and GATA2 mediate signaling gradient-induced determination of pituitary cell types. Cell 1999;97:587-598.
203. Pulichino AM, Vallette-Kasic S, Tsai JP, et al. Tpit determines alternate fates during pituitary cell differentiation. Genes Dev 2003;17:738-747.
204. Lin L, Gu WX, Ozisik G, et al. Analysis of DAX1 (NR0B1) and steroidogenic factor-1 (NR5A1) in children and adults with primary adrenal failure: ten years' experience. J Clin Endocrinol Metab 2006;91:3048-3054.
205. Kelberman D, et al. Mutations within Sox2/SOX2 are associated with abnormalities in the hypothalamo-pituitary-gonadal axis in mice and humans. J Clin Invest 2006;116:2442-2455.
206. Quirk CC, Seachrist DD, Nilson JH. Embryonic expression of the luteinizing hormone beta gene appears to be coupled to the transient appearance of p8, a high mobility group-related transcription factor. J Biol Chem 2003;278:1680-1685.
207. Themmen APN, Huhtaniemi IT. Mutations of gonadotropins and gonadotropin receptors: elucidating the physiology and pathophysiology of pituitary-gonadal function. Endocr Rev 2000;21: 551-583.
208. Weiss J, Axelrod L, Whitcomb RW, et al. Hypogonadism caused by a single amino acid substitution in the beta subunit of luteinizing hormone.N Engl J Med 1992;16:326:179-183.
209. Valdes-Socin H, Salvi R, Daly AF, et al. Hypogonadism in a patient with a mutation in the luteinizing hormone beta-subunit gene. N Engl J Med 2004;351:2619-2625.
210. Forest MG, Sizonenko PC, Cathiard AM, et al. Hypophyso-gonadal function in humans during the first year of life. 1. Evidence for testicular activity in early infancy. J Clin Invest 1974;53:819-828.
211. Boas M, Boisen KA, Virtanen HE, et al. Postnatal penile length and growth rate correlate to serum testosterone levels: a longitudinal study of 1962 normal boys. Eur J Endocrinol 2006;154: 125-129.
212. Crofton PM, Illingworth PJ, Groome NP, et al. Changes in dimeric inhibin A and B during normal early puberty in boys and girls. Clin Endocrinol 1997;46:109-114.
213. Kubini K, Zachmann M, Albers N, et al. Basal inhibin B and the testosterone response to human chorionic gonadotropin correlate in prepubertal boys. J Clin Endocrinol Metab 2000;85: 134-138.
214. Lee MM, Misra M, Donahoe PK, et al. MIS/AMH in the assessment of cryptorchidism and intersex conditions. Mol Cell Endocrinol 2003;211:91-98.
215. Chellakooty M, Schmidt IM, Haavisto AM, et al. Inhibin A, inhibin B, follicle-stimulating hormone, luteinizing hormone, estradiol, and sex hormone-binding globulin levels in 473 healthy infant girls. J Clin Endocrinol Metab 2003;88:3515-1520.
216. Lanfranco F, Kamischke A, Zitzmann M, et al. Klinefelter's syndrome. Lancet 2004;364:273-283.
217. Amory JK, Anawalt BD, Paulsen CA, et al. Klinefelter's syndrome. Lancet 2000;356:333-335.
218. Salbenblatt JA, Bender BG, Puck MH, et al. Pituitary-gonadal function in Klinefelter syndrome before and during puberty. Pediatr Res 1985;19:82-86.
219. Wang C, Baker HWG, Burger HG, et al. Hormonal studies in Klinefelter syndrome. Clin Endocrinol 1975;4:399-411.

220. Wikstrom AM, Hoei-Hansen CE, Dunkel L, et al. Immunoexpression of androgen receptor and nine markers of maturation in the testes of adolescent boys with Klinefelter syndrome: Evidence for degeneration of germ cells at the onset of meiosis. J Clin Endocrinol Metab 2007;92:714-719.
221. Wikstrom AM, Bay K, Hero M, et al. Serum insulin-like factor 3 levels during puberty in healthy boys and boys with Klinefelter syndrome. J Clin Endocrinol Metab 2006;91:4705-4708.
222. Schiff JD, Palermo GD, Veeck LL, et al. Success of testicular sperm extraction and intracytoplasmic sperm injection in men with Klinefelter syndrome. J Clin Endocrinol Metab 2005;90: 6263-6267.
223. Sybert VP, McCauley E. Turner's syndrome. N Engl J Med 2004;351: 12227-1238.
224. Bondy CA. Turner Syndrome Study Group. Care of girls and women with Turner syndrome: a guideline of the Turner Syndrome Study Group. J Clin Endocrinol Metab 2007;92:10-25.
225. Ranke MB, Saenger P. Turner's syndrome. Lancet 2001;358: 309-314.
226. Singh RF, Carr DH. The anatomy and histology of XO human embryos and fetuses. Anat Rec 1966;155:369-384.
227. Pasquino AM, Passeri F, Pucarelli I, et al. Spontaneous pubertal development in Turner's syndrome. Italian Study Group for Turner's syndrome. J Clin Endocrinol Metab 1997;82:1810-1813.
228. Gravholt CH, Fedder J, Naeraa RW, et al. Occurrence of gonadoblastoma in females with Turner syndrome and Y chromosome material-a population study. J Clin Endocrinol Metab 2000;85: 3199-3202.
229. Hreinsson JG, Otala M, Fridstrom M, et al. Follicles are found in the ovaries of adolescent girls with Turner's syndrome. J Clin Endocrinol Metab 2002;87:3618-3623.
230. Reynaud K, Cortvrindt R, Verlinde F, et al. Number of ovarian follicles in human fetuses with the 45,X karyotype. Fertil Steril 2004;81:1112-1119.
231. Knudtzon J, Aarskog D. 45,X/46,XY mosaicism. A clinical review and report of ten cases. Eur J Pediatr 1987;146:266-271.
232. Telvi L, Lebbar A, Del Pino O, et al. 45,X/46,XY mosaicism: report of 27 cases. Pediatrics 1999;104:304-308.
233. Müller J, Skakkebaek NE, Ritzen M, et al. Carcinoma in situ of the testis in children with 45,X/46,XY gonadal dysgenesis. J Pediatr 1985;106:431-436.
234. Müller J, Ritzen EM, Ivarsson SA, et al. Management of males with 45,X/46,XY gonadal dysgenesis. Horm Res 1999;52:11-14.
235. Hsu LY. Prenatal diagnosis of 45,X/46,XY mosaicism—a review and update. Prenat Diagn 1989;9:31-48.
236. Chang HJ, Clark RD, Bachman H. The phenotype of 45,X/46,XY mosaicism: an analysis of 92 prenatally diagnosed cases. Am J Hum Genet 1990;46:156-167.
237. Krob G, Braun A, Kuhnle U: True hermaphroditism: geographical distribution, clinical findings, chromosomes and gonadal histology. Eur J Pediatr 1994;153:2-10.
238. Spurdle AB, Shankman S, Ramsay M. XX true hermaphroditism in Southern African blacks: exclusion of SRY sequences had uniparental disomy of the X chromosome. Am J Med Genet 1995;55: 53-56.
239. Wiersma R. Management of the African child with true hermaphroditism. J Pediatr Surg 2001;36:397-399.
240. McElreavey K, Rappaport R, Vilain E, et al. A minority of 46,XX true hermaphrodites are positive for the Y DNA sequence including SRY. Hum Genet 1992;90:121-125.
241. Aaronson IA. True hermaphroditism. A review of 41 cases with observations on testicular histology and function. Br J Urol 1985;57:775-779.
242. Damiani D, Fellous M, McElreavey K, et al. True hermaphroditism: clinical aspects and molecular studies in 16 cases. Eur J Endocrinol 1997;136:201-204.
243. Correa RV, Domenice S, Bingham NC, et al. A microdeletion in the ligand binding domain of human steroidogenic factor 1 causes XY sex reversal without adrenal insufficiency. J Clin Endocrinol Metab 2004;89:1767-1772.
244. Hasegawa T, Fukami M, Sato N, et al. Testicular dysgenesis without adrenal insufficiency in a 46,XY patient with a heterozygous inactive mutation of steroidogenic factor-1. J Clin Endocrinol Metab 2004;89:5930-5931.
245. Mallet D, Bretones P, Michel-Calemard L, et al. Gonadal dysgenesis without adrenal insufficiency in a 46, XY patient heterozygous for the nonsense C16X mutation: a case of SF1 haploinsufficiency. J Clin Endocrinol Metab 2004;89:4829-4832.
246. Jameson JL. Of mice and men: the tale of steroidogenic factor-1. J Clin Endocrinol Metab 2004;89:5927-5929.
247. Wada Y, Okada M, Hasegawa T, et al. Association of severe micropenis with Gly146Ala polymorphism in the gene for steroidogenic factor-1. Endocr J 2005;52:445-448.
248. Wada Y, Okada M, Fukami M, et al. Association of cryptorchidism with Gly146Ala polymorphism in the gene for steroidogenic factor-1. Fertil Steril 2006;85:787-790.
249. Fischbach BV, Trout KL, Lewis J, et al. WAGR syndrome: a clinical review of 54 cases. Pediatrics 2005;116:984-988.
250. Kohler B, Schumacher V, l'Allemand D, et al. Germline Wilms tumor suppressor gene (WT1) mutation leading to isolated genital malformation without Wilms tumor or nephropathy. J Pediatr 2001;138:421-424.
251. Brown S, Yu C, Lanzano P, et al. A de novo mutation (Gln2Stop) at the 5′ end of the SRY gene leads to sex reversal with partial ovarian function. Am J Hum Genet 1998;62:189-192.
252. Tajima T, Nakae J, Shinohara N, et al. A novel mutation localized in the 3′ non-HMG box region of the SRY gene in 46,XY gonadal dysgenesis. Hum Mol Genet 1994;3:1187-1189.
253. Hawkins JR, Taylor A, Goodfellow PN, et al. Evidence for increased prevalence of SRY mutations in XY females with complete rather than partial gonadal dysgenesis. Am J Hum Genet 1992;51: 979-984.
254. McElreavey K, Vilain E, Abbas N, et al. XY sex reversal associated with a deletion 5′ to the SRY "HMG box" in the testis-determining region. Proc Natl Acad Sci U S A 1992;89:11016-11020.
255. Vilain E, McElreavey K, Jaubert F, et al. Familial case with sequence variant in the testis-determining region associated with two sex phenotypes. Am J Hum Genet 1992;50:1008-1011.
256. Cameron FJ, Hageman RM, Cooke-Yarborough C, et al. A novel germ line mutation in SOX9 causes familial campomelic dysplasia and sex reversal. Hum Mol Genet 1996;5:1625-1630.
257. Canto P, Soderlund D, Reyes E, et al. Mutations in the desert hedgehog (DHH) gene in patients with 46,XY complete pure gonadal dysgenesis. J Clin Endocrinol Metab 2004;89:4480-4483.
258. Puffenberger EG, Hu-Lince D, Parod JM, et al. Mapping of sudden infant death with dysgenesis of the testes syndrome (SIDDT) by a SNP genome scan and identification of TSPYL loss of function. Proc Natl Acad Sci U S A 2004;101:11689-11694.
259. Fukami M, Wada Y, Miyabayashi K, et al. CXorf6 is a causative gene for hypospadias. Nat Genet 2006;38:1369-1371.
260. Mendonca BB, Billerbeck AE, de Zegher F. Nongenetic male pseudohermaphroditism and reduced prenatal growth. N Engl J Med 2001;345:1135.
261. Kelly RI, Heenekam RC. The Smith-Lemli-Opitz syndrome. J Med Gent 2000;37:321-335.
262. Fitzky BU, Witsch-Baumgartner M, Erdel M, et al. Mutations in the Δ7-sterol reductase gene in patients with the Smith-Lemli-Opitz syndrome. Proc Natl Acad Sci U S A 1998;95:8181-8186.
263. Berthezene F, Forest MG, Grimaud JA, et al. Leydig cell agenesis: a cause of male pseudohermaphroditism. N Engl J Med 1976; 295:969-972.
264. Kremer H, Kraaij R, Toledo S, et al. Male pseudohermaphroditism due to a homozygous missense mutation of the luteinizing hormone receptor gene. Nat Genet 1995;9:160-164.
265. Latronico AC, Anasti J, Arnhold IJP, et al. Brief report: testicular and ovarian resistance to luteinizing hormone caused by homozygous inactivating mutations of the luteinizing hormone receptor gene. N Engl J Med 1996;334:507-512.
266. Wu SM, Hallermeier KM, Laue L, et al. Inactivation of the luteinizing hormone/chorionic gonadotropin receptor by an insertional mutation in Leydig cell hypoplasia. Mol Endocrinol 1998;12: 1651-1660.
267. Martens JWM, Verhoef-Post M, Abelin N, et al. A homozygous mutation in the luteinizing hormone receptor causes partial Leydig cell hypoplasia: correlation between receptor activity and phenotype. Mol Endocrinol 1998;12:775-784.
268. Lin D, Sugawara T, Strauss JF III, et al. Role of steroidogenic acute regulatory protein in adrenal and gonadal steroidogenesis. Science 1995;267:1828-1831.

269. Miller WL. StAR search—What we know about how the steroidogenic acute regulatory protein mediates mitochondrial cholesterol import. Mol Endocrinol 2007;21:589-601.
270. Prader A, Gurtner HP. Das Syndrom des Pseudohermaphroditismus masculinus bei kongenitaler NebennierenrindenHyperplasie ohne Androgenuberproduktion (adrenaler Pseudohermaphrotidismus masculinus). Helv Paediatr Acta 1955;10:397-412.
271. Bose HS, Sugawara T, Strauss JF III, et al. The pathophysiology and genetics of congenital lipoid adrenal hyperplasia. N Engl J Med 1996;335:1870-1878.
272. Caron K, Soo S-C, Wetsel W, et al. Targeted disruption of the mouse gene encoding steroidogenic acute regulatory protein provides insights into congenital lipoid adrenal hyperplasia. Proc Natl Acad Sci U S A 1997;94:11540-11545.
273. Bose HS, Pescouitz OH, Miller WL. Spontaneous feminization in a 46,XX female patient with adrenal hyperplasia due to a homozygous frame shift mutation in the steroidogenic reactive protein. J Clin Endocrinol Metab 1997;82:1511-1515.
274. Nakae J, Tajima T, Sugawara T, et al. Analysis of the steroidogenic acute regulatory protein (StAR) gene in Japanese patients with congenital lipoid adrenal hyperplasia. Hum Mol Genet 1997;6: 571-576.
275. Bose HS, Sato S, Aisenberg J, et al. Mutations in the steroidogenic acute regulatory protein (StAR) in six patients with congenital lipoid adrenal hyperplasia. J Clin Endocrinol Metab 2000;85: 3636-3639.
276. Baker BY, Lin L, Kim CJ, et al. Nonclassic congenital lipoid adrenal hyperplasia: a new disorder of the steroidogenic acute regulatory protein with very late presentation and normal male genitalia. J Clin Endocrinol Metab 2006;91:4781-4785.
277. Yang X, Iwamoto K, Wang M, et al. Inherited congenital adrenal hyperplasia in the rabbit is caused by a deletion in the gene encoding cytochrome P450 cholesterol sidechain cleavage enzyme. Endocrinology 1993;132:1977-1982.
278. Tajima T, Fujieda K, Kouda N, et al. Heterozygous mutation in the cholesterol side chain cleavage enzyme (p450scc) gene in a patient with 46,XY sex reversal and adrenal insufficiency. J Clin Endocrinol Metab 2001;86:3820-3825.
279. Hiort O, Holterhus PM, Werner R, et al. Homozygous disruption of P450 side-chain cleavage (CYP11A1) is associated with prematurity, complete 46,XY sex reversal, and severe adrenal failure. J Clin Endocrinol Metab 2005;90:538-541.
280. Simard J, Ricketts M-L, Gingras S, et al. Molecular biology of the 3β-hydroxysteroid dehydrogenase/Δ^5-Δ^4 isomerase gene family. Endocr Rev 2005;26:525-582.
281. Moisan AM, Ricketts ML, Tardy V, et al. New insight into the molecular basis of 3β-hydroxysteroid dehydrogenase deficiency: identification of eight mutations in the HSD3B2 gene eleven patients from seven new families and comparison of the functional properties of twenty-five mutant enzymes. J Clin Endocrinol Metab 1999;84:4410-4425.
282. Alos N, Moisan AM, Ward L, et al. A novel A10E homozygous mutation in the HSD3B2 gene causing severe salt-wasting 3β-hydroxysteroid dehydrogenase deficiency in 46,XX and 46,XY French-Canadians: evaluation of gonadal function after puberty. J Clin Endocrinol Metab 2000;85:1968-1974.
283. Parks GA, Bermudez JA, Anast CS, et al. Pubertal boy with the 3β-hydroxysteroid dehydrogenase defect. J Clin Endocrinol Metab 1971;33:269-278.
284. Rheaume E, Simard J, Morel Y, et al. Congenital adrenal hyperplasia due to point mutations in the type II 3 beta-hydroxysteroid dehydrogenase gene. Nat Genet 1992;1:239-245.
285. Johannsen TH, Mallet D, Dige-Petersen H, et al. Delayed diagnosis of congenital adrenal hyperplasia with salt wasting due to type II 3β-hydroxysteroid dehydrogenase deficiency. J Clin Endocrinol Metab 2005;90:2076-2080.
286. Lutfallah C, Wang W, Mason JI, et al. Newly proposed hormonal criteria via genotypic proof for type II 3beta-hydroxysteroid dehydrogenase deficiency. J Clin Endocrinol Metab 2002;87: 2611-2622.
287. Mermejo LM, Elias LL, Marui S, et al. Refining hormonal diagnosis of type II 3 beta-hydroxysteroid dehydrogenase deficiency in patients with premature pubarche and hirsutism based on HSD3B2 genotyping. J Clin Endocrinol Metab 2005;90: 1287-1293.
288. Pang S, Carbunaru G, Haider A, et al. Carriers for type II 3beta-hydroxysteroid dehydrogenase (HSD3B2) deficiency can only be identified by HSD3B2 genotype study and not by hormone test. Clin Endocrinol 2003;58:323-331.
289. Codner E, Okuma C, Iniguez G, et al. Molecular study of the 3 beta-hydroxysteroid dehydrogenase gene type II in patients with hypospadias. J Clin Endocrinol Metab 2004;89:957-964.
290. New MI. Male pseudohermaphrodism due to a 17-alpha-hydroxylase deficiency. J Clin Invest 1970;49:1930-1941.
291. Winter JSD, Couch RM, Muller J, et al. Combined 17-hydroxylase and 17/20 desmolase deficiencies: evidence for synthesis of a defective cytochrome P450c17. J Clin Endocrinol Metab 1989; 68:309-316.
292. Auchus RJ. The genetics, pathophysiology, and management of human deficiencies of P450c17. Endocrinol Metab Clin North Am 2001;30:101-119.
293. Miller WL. Steroid 17alpha-hydroxylase deficiency—not rare everywhere. J Clin Endocrinol Metab 2004;89:40-42.
294. Martin RM, Lin CJ, Costa EM, et al. P450c17 deficiency in Brazilian patients: biochemical diagnosis through progesterone levels confirmed by CYP17 genotyping. J Clin Endocrinol Metab 2003;88: 5739-5746.
295. Costa-Santos M, Kater CE, Auchus RJ, Brazilian Congenital Adrenal Hyperplasia Multicenter Study Group. Two prevalent CYP17 mutations and genotype-phenotype correlations in 24 Brazilian patients with 17-hydroxylase deficiency. J Clin Endocrinol Metab 2004; 89:49-60.
296. Yanase T, Kagimoto M, Suzuki B, et al. Deletion of a phenylalanine in the N-terminal region of human cytochrome P-450(17α) results in combined 17α-hydroxylase/17,20-lyase deficiency. J Biol Chem 1989;264:18076-18082.
297. Ahlgren R, Yanase T, Simpson ER, et al. Compound heterozygous mutations (Arg239stop, Pro342Thr) in the CYP17 (P450 17-alpha) gene lead to ambiguous external genitalia in a male with partial combined 17 alpha-hydroxylase/17,20 lyase deficiency. J Clin Endocrinol Metab 1992;74:667-672.
298. Geller DH, Auchus RJ, Mendonca BB, et al. The genetic and functional basis of isolated 17,20 lyase deficiency. Nat Genet 1997;17: 201-205.
299. Geller DH, Auchus RJ, Miller WL. P450c17 mutations R347H and R358Q selectively disrupt 17,20-lyase activity by disrupting interactions with P450 oxidoreductase and cytochrome b5. Mol Endocrinol 1999;13:167-175.
300. Auchus RJ, Miller WL. Molecular modeling of human P450c17 (17-alpha-hydroxylase/17,20-lyase): insights into reaction mechanisms and effects of mutations. Mol Endocrinol 1999;13:1169-1182.
301. Sherbert DP, Tosiano D, Kwist KM, et al. CYP17 mutation E305G causes isolated 17,20-lyase deficiency by selectively altering substrate binding. J Biol Chem 2003;278:48563-48569.
302. Giordano SJ, Kaftory A, Steggles AW. A splicing mutation in the cytchrome b_5 gene from a patient with congenital methemoglobinemia and pseudohermaphrodism. Hum Genet 1994;93:568-570.
303. Miller WL. Minireview: regulation of steroidogenesis by electron transfer. Endocrinology 2005;146:2544-2550.
304. Peterson RE, Imperato-McGinley J, Gautier T, Shackleton, C. Male pseudohermaphroditism due to multiple defects in steroid-biosynthetic microsomal mixed-function oxidases: a new variant of congenital adrenal hyperplasia. N Engl J Med 1985;313: 1182-1191.
305. Reardon W, Smith A, Honour JW, et al. Evidence for digenic inheritance in some cases of Antley-Bixler syndrome? J Med Genet 2000;37:26-32.
306. Fluck CE, Tajima T, Pandey AV, et al. Mutant P450 oxidoreductase causes disordered steroidogenesis with and without Antley-Bixler syndrome. Nat Genet 2004;36:228-230.
307. Huang N, Pandey AV, Agrawal V, et al. Diversity and function of mutations in P450 oxidoreductase in patients with Antley-Bixler syndrome and disordered steroidogenesis. Am J Hum Genet 2005;76:729-749.
308. Miller WL, Huang N, Pandey AV, et al. P450 oxidoreductase deficiency: a new disorder of steroidogenesis. Ann N Y Acad Sci 2005;1061:100-108.
309. Labrie F, Luu-The V, Lin SX, et al. Role of 17 beta-hydroxysteroid dehydrogenases in sex steroid formation in peripheral intracrine tissues. Trends Endocrinol Metab 2000;11:421-427.

310. Saez JM, de Perett E, Morera AM, et al. Familial male pseudohermaphroditism with gynaecomastia due to a testicular 17-ketosteroid reductase defect. I. In vivo studies. J Clin Endocrinol Metab 1971;32:604-610.
311. Saez JM, Morera AM, de Peretti E, et al. Further in vivo studies in male pseudohermaphroditism with gynaecomastia due to a testicular 17-ketosteroid reductase defect (compared to a case of testicular feminization). J Clin Endocrinol Metab 1972;34: 598-600.
312. Andersson S, Geissler WM, Wu L, et al. Molecular genetics and pathophysiology of 17 beta-hydroxysteroid dehydrogenase 3 deficiency. J Clin Endocrinol Metab 1996;81:130-136.
313. Boehmer AL, Brinkmann AO, Sandkuijl LA, et al. 17 beta-hydroxysteroid dehydrogenase-3 deficiency: diagnosis, phenotypic variability, population genetics, and worldwide distribution of ancient and de novo mutations. J Clin Endocrinol Metab 1999;84: 4713-4721.
314. Twesten W, Holterhus P, Sippell WG, et al. Clinical, endocrine and molecular genetic findings in patients with 17beta-hydroxysteroid dehydrogenase deficiency. Horm Res 2002;53:26-31.
315. Lee YS, Kirk JM, Stanhope RG, et al. Phenotypic variability in 17β-hydroxysteroid dehydrogenase-3 deficiency and diagnostic pitfalls. Clin Endocrinol (Oxf.) 2007;67:20-28.
316. Qiu W, Zhou M, Labrie F, et al. Crystal structures of the multispecific 17beta-hydroxysteroid dehydrogenase type 5: critical androgen regulation in human peripheral tissues. Mol Endocrinol 2004;18:1798-17807.
317. Rösler A. Steroid 17 beta-hydroxysteroid dehydrogenase deficiency in man: an inherited form of male pseudohermaphroditism. J Steroid Biochem Mol Biol 1992;43:989-1002.
318. Faisal SF, Iqbal A, Hughes IA. The testosterone : androstenedione ratio in male undermasculinization. Clin Endocrinol 2000;53: 697-702.
319. Margiotti K, Kim E, Pearce CL, et al. Association of the G289S single nucleotide polymorphism in the HSD17B3 gene with prostate cancer in Italian men. Prostate 2002;53:65-68.
320. Moghrabi N, Hughes IA, Dunaif A, et al. Deleterious missense mutations and silent polymorphism in the human 17beta-hydroxysteroid dehydrogenase 3 gene (HSD17B3). J Clin Endocrinol Metab 1998:83;2855-2860.
321. Hannema SE, Scott IS, Hodapp J, et al. Residual activity of mutant androgen receptors explains wolffian duct development in the complete androgen insensitivity syndrome. J Clin Endocrinol Metab 2004;89:5815-5822.
322. Khan N, Sharma KK, Andersson S, et al. Human 17beta-hydroxysteroid dehydrogenases types 1, 2 and 3 catalyse bi-directional equilibrium reactions, rather than unidirectional metabolism, in HEK-293 cells. Arch Biochem Biophys 2004;429:50-59.
323. Gross DJ, Landau H, Kohn G, et al. Male pseudohermaphroditism due to 17 beta-hydroxysteroid dehydrogenase deficiency: gender assignment in early infancy. Acta Endocrinol 1986;112:238-246.
324. Imperato-McGinley J, Guerrero L, Gautier T, et al. Steroid 5a-reductase deficiency in man: an inherited form of male pseudohermaphroditism. Science 1974;186:1213-1215.
325. Andersson S, Berman DM, Jenkins EP, et al. Deletion of steroid 5-alpha-reductase 2 gene in male pseudohermaphroditism. Nature 1991;354:159-161.
326. Wilson JD, Griffin JE, Russell DW. Steroid 5a-reductase 2 deficiency. Endocr Rev 2003;14:577-593.
327. Imperato-McGinley J, Zhu Y-S. Androgens and male physiology the syndrome of 5a-reductase-2 deficiency. Mol Cell Endocrinol 2002;198:51-59.
328. Cai LQ, Fratianni CM, Gautier T, et al. Dihydrotestosterone regulation of semen in male pseudohermaphrodites with 5 alpha-reductase-2 deficiency. J Clin Endocrinol Metab 1994;79:409-414.
329. Katz MD, Kligman I, Cai L-Q, et al. Paternity by intrauterine insemination with sperm from a man with 5a-reductase-2 deficiency. N Engl J Med 1997;336:994-997.
330. Nordenskjold A, Ivarsson SA. Molecular characterization of 5 alpha-reductase type 2 deficiency and fertility in a Swedish family. J Clin Endocrinol Metab 1998;83:3236-3238.
331. Herdt GH, Davidson J. The Sambia "Turnim-Man": sociocultural and clinical aspects of gender formation in male pseudohermaphrodites with 5-alpha-reductase deficiency in Papua, New Guinea. Arch Sex Behav 1988;17:33-56.
332. Cohen-Kettenis PT. Gender change in 46,XY persons with 5alpha-reductase-2 deficiency and 17beta-hydroxysteroid dehydrogenase-3 deficiency. Arch Sex Behav 2005;34:399-410.
333. Katz MD, Cai LQ, Zhu YS, et al. The biochemical and phenotypic characterization of females homozygous for 5 alpha-reductase 2 deficiency. J Clin Endocrinol Metab 1995;80:3160-3167.
334. Forti G, Falchetti A, Santoro S, et al. Steroid 5 alpha-reductase 2 deficiency: virilization in early infancy may be due to partial function of mutant enzyme. Clin Endocrinol 1996;44:477-482.
335. Odame I, Donaldson MCD, Wallace AM, et al. Early diagnosis and management of 5 alpha-reductase deficiency. Arch Dis Child 1992;67:720-723.
336. Charmandari E, Dattani MT, Perry LA, et al. Kinetics and effect of percutaneous administration of dihydrotestosterone in children. Horm Res 2001;56:177-181.
337. Levine AC, Wang JP, Ren M, et al. Immunohistochemical localization of steroid 5 alpha-reductase 2 in the human male fetal reproductive tract and adult prostate. J Clin Endocrinol Metab 1996;81:384-389.
338. Thiele S, Hoppe U, Holterhus P-M, et al. Isoenzyme type 1 of 5alpha-reductase is abundantly transcribed in normal human genital skin fibroblasts and may play an important role in masculinisation of 5alpha-reductase type 2 deficient males. Eur J Endocrinol 2005;152:875-880.
339. Heinlein CA, Chang C. Androgen receptor (AR) coregulators: an overview. Endocr Rev 2002;23:175-200.
340. Bevan CL, Hoare S, Claessens F, et al. The AF1 and AF2 domains of the androgen receptor interact with distinct regions of SRC1. Mol Cell Biol 1999;19:8383-8392.
341. Tut TG, Ghadessy FJ, Trifiro MA, et al. Long polyglutamine tracts in the androgen receptor are associated with reduced trans-activation, impaired sperm production, and male infertility. J Clin Endocrinol Metab 1997;82:3777-2782.
342. Cheung-Flynn J, Prapapanich V, Cox MB, et al. Physiological role for the cochaperone FKBP52 in androgen receptor signalling. Mol Endocrinol 2005;19:1654-1666.
343. Quigley C, De Bellis A, Marschke KB, et al. Androgen receptor defects: historical, clinical, and molecular perspectives. Endocr Rev 1995;16:271-321.
344. Banksboll S, Qvist I, Lebech PE, et al. Testicular feminization syndrome and associated gonadal tumours in Denmark. Acta Obstet Gynecol Scand 1992;71:63-66.
345. Boehmer AL Brinkmann AO, Bruggenwirth H, et al. Genotype versus phenotype in families with androgen insensitivity syndrome. J Clin Endocrinol Metab 2001;86:4151-4160.
346. Deeb A, Hughes IA. Inguinal hernia in female infants: a cue to check the sex chromosomes? BJU Int 2005;96:401-403.
347. Yong EL, Loy CJ, Sim KS. Androgen receptor gene and male infertility. Hum Reprod Update 2003;9:1-7.
348. Ong YC, Wong HB, Adaikan G, et al. Directed pharmacological therapy of ambiguous genitalia due to an androgen receptor gene mutation. Lancet 1999;354:1444-1445.
349. Poujol N, Lobaccaro JM, Chiche L, et al. Functional and structural analysis of R607Q and R608K androgen receptor substitutions associated with male breast cancer. Mol Cell Endocrinol 1997; 130:43-51.
350. MacLean HE, Brown RW, Beilin J, et al. Increased frequency of long androgen receptor CAG repeats in male breast cancers. Breast Cancer Res Treat 2004;88:239-246.
351. Ahmed SF, Cheng A, Hughes IA. Assessment of the gonadotropin-gonadal axis in androgen insensitivity syndrome. Arch Dis Child 1999;80:324-329.
352. Sinnecker GH, Hiort O, Nitsche EM, et al. Functional assessment and clinical classification of androgen sensitivity in patients with mutations of the androgen receptor gene. German Collaborative Intersex Study Group. Eur J Pediatr 1997;1:7-14.
353. Rey RA, Belville C, Nihoul-Fekete C, et al. Evaluation of gonadal function in 107 intersex patients by means of serum antimullerian hormone. J Clin Endocrinol Metab 1999;84:627-631.
354. Bouvattier C, Carel JC, Lecointre C, et al. Postnatal changes of T, LH, and FSH in 46,XY infants with mutations in the AR gene. J Clin Endocrinol Metab 2002;87:29-32.
355. Quigley CA. Editorial: the postnatal gonadotropin and sex steroid surge—insights from the androgen insensitivity syndrome. J Clin Endocrinol Metab 2002;87:24-28.

356. Hughes IA, Evans BAJ. The fibroblast as a model for androgen resistant stages. Clin Endocrinol 1988;28:565-579.
357. Shkolny DL, Beitel LK, Ginsberg J, et al. Discordant measures of androgen-binding kinetics in two mutant androgen receptors causing mild or partial androgen insensitivity, respectively. J Clin Endocrinol Metab 1999;84:805-810.
358. Nagy L, Schwabe JW. Mechanism of the nuclear receptor molecular switch. Trends Biochem Sci 2004;29:317-324.
359. Quigley CA, Evans BAJ, Simental JA, et al. Complete androgen insensitivity due to deletion of exon c of the androgen receptor gene highlights the functional importance of the second zinc finger of the androgen receptor in vivo. Mol Endocrinol 1992;6:1103-1112.
360. Radmayr C, Culig Z, Glatzl J, et al. Androgen receptor point mutations as the underlying molecular defect in 2 patients with androgen insensitivity syndrome. J Urol 1997;158:1553-1556.
361. Deeb A, Mason C, Lee YS, et al. Correlation between genotype, phenotype and sex of rearing in 111 patients with partial androgen insensitivity syndrome. Clin Endocrinol 2005;63:56-62.
362. Kohler B, Lumbroso S, Leger J, et al. Androgen insensitivity syndrome: somatic mosaicism of the androgen receptor in seven families and consequences for sex assignment and genetic counselling. J Clin Endocrinol Metab 2005;90:106-111.
363. Boehmer AL, Brinkmann AO, Nijman RM, et al. Phenotypic variation in a family with partial androgen insensitivity syndrome explained by differences in 5alpha dihydrotestosterone availability. J Clin Endocrinol Metab 2001;86:1240-1246.
364. Holterhus PM, Werner R, Hoppe U, et al. Molecular features and clinical phenotypes in androgen insensitivity syndrome in the absence and presence of androgen receptor gene mutations. J Mol Med 2005;83:1005-1113.
365. He B, Kemppainen JA, Wilson EM. FXXLF and WXXLF sequences mediate the NH2-terminal interaction with the ligand binding domain of the androgen receptor. J Biol Chem 2000;275: 22986-22994.
366. Quigley CA, Tan JA, He B, et al. Partial androgen insensitivity with phenotypic variation caused by androgen receptor mutations that disrupt activation function 2 and the NH(2)- and carboxyl-terminal interaction. Mech Ageing Dev 2004;125:683-695.
367. He B, Gampe RT Jr, Hnat AT, et al. Probing the functional link between androgen receptor coactivator and ligand-binding sites in prostate cancer and androgen insensitivity. J Biol Chem 2006;281:6648-6663.
368. Jääskeläinen J, Deeb A, Schwabe JW, et al. Human androgen receptor gene ligand-binding domain mutations leading to disrupted interaction between the N- and C-terminal domains. J Mol Endocrinol 2006;36:361-368.
369. Mongan NP, Lim HN, Hughes IA. Genetic evidence to exclude the androgen receptor-polyglutamine associated coactivator, ARA-24, as a cause of male undermasculinisation. Eur J Endocrinol 2001;145:809-811.
370. Lim HN, Hawkins JR, Hughes IA. Genetic evidence to exclude the androgen receptor co-factor, ARA70 (NCOA4) as a candidate gene for the causation of undermasculinised genitalia. Clin Genet 2001;59:284-286.
371. Xu J, Liao L, Ning G, et al. The steroid receptor coactivator SRC-3 (p/CIP/RAC3/AIB1/ACTR/TRAM-1) is required for normal growth, puberty, female reproductive function, and mammary gland development. Proc Natl Acad Sci USA 2000;97:6379-6384.
372. Mongan NP, Jääskeläinen J, Bhattacharyya S, et al. Steroid receptor coactivator-3 glutamine repeat polymorphism and the androgen insensitivity syndrome. Eur J Endocrinol 2003;148:277-279.
373. Adachi M, Takayanagi R, Tomura A, et al. Androgen-insensitivity syndrome as a possible coactivator disease. N Engl J Med 2000; 343:856-862.
374. Hughes IA. A novel explanation for resistance to androgens. N Engl J Med 2000;343:881-882.
375. La Spada AR, Wilson EM, Lubahn DB, et al. Androgen receptor gene mutations in X-linked spinal and bulbar muscular atrophy. Nature 1991;352:77-79.
376. Ogata T, Muroya K, Ishii T, et al. Undermasculinized genitalia in a boy with an abnormally expanded CAG repeat length in the androgen receptor gene. Clin Endocrinol 2001;54:835-838.
377. Lim HN, Chen H, McBride S, et al. Longer polyglutamine tracts in the androgen receptor are associated with moderate to severe undermasculinized genitalia in XY males. Hum Mol Genet 2000; 9:829-834.
378. Mengual L, Oriola J, Ascaso C, et al. An increased CAG repeat length in the androgen receptor gene in azoospermic ICSI candidates. J Androl 2003;24:279-284.
379. Zinn AR, Ramos P, Elder FF, et al. Androgen receptor CAGn repeat length influences phenotype of 47,XXY (Klinefelter) syndrome. J Clin Endocrinol Metab 2005;90:5041-5046.
380. Tsujimoto Y, Takakuwa T, Takayama H, et al. In situ shortening of CAG repeat length within the androgen receptor gene in prostatic cancer and its possible precursors. Prostate 2004;58:283-290.
381. Zitzmann M, Nieschlag E. The CAG repeat polymorphism within the androgen receptor gene and maleness. Int J Androl 2003;26: 76-83.
382. Ibanez L, Ong KK, Mongan N, et al. Androgen receptor gene CAG repeat polymorphism in the development of ovarian hyperndrogenism. J Clin Endocrinol Metab 2003;88:3333-3338.
383. Aschim EL, Nordenskjold A, Giwercman A, et al. Linkage between cryptorchidism, hypospadias, and GGN repeat length in the androgen receptor gene. J Clin Endocrinol Metab 2004;89:5105-5109.
384. Werner R, Holterhus PM, Binder G, et al. The A645D mutation in the hinge region of the human androgen receptor (AR) gene modulates AR activity, depending on the context of the polymorphic glutamine and glycine repeats. J Clin Endocrinol Metab 2006;91: 3515-3520.
385. Papadimitriou DT, Linglart A, Morel Y, et al. Puberty in subjects with complete androgen insensitivity syndrome. Horm Res 2006; 65:126-131.
386. Savage MO, Lowe DG. Gonadal neoplasia and abnormal sexual differentiation. Clin Endocrinol 1990;32:519-533.
387. Levin HS. Tumors of the testis in intersex conditions. Urol Clin North Am 2000;27:543-551.
388. Rajpert-De Meyts E, Jorgensen N, Brondum-Nielsen K, et al. Developmental arrest of germ cells in the pathogenesis of germ cell neoplasia. APMIS 1998;106:198-204.
389. Almstrup K, Sonne SB, Hoei-Hansen CE, et al. From embryonic stem cells to testicular germ cell cancer—should we be concerned? Int J Androl 2006;29:211-218.
390. Rajpert-De Meyts E. Developmental model for the pathogenesis of testicular carcinoma in situ: genetic and environmental aspects. Hum Reprod Update 2006;12:303-323.
391. Rutgers JL, Scully RE. The androgen insensitivity syndrome (testicular feminization): a clinicopathologic study of 43 cases. Int J Gynecol Pathol 1991;10:126-144.
392. Cassio A, Cacciari E, D'Errico A, et al. Incidence of intratubular germ cell neoplasia in androgen insensitivity syndrome. Acta Endocrinol (Copenh) 1990;123:416-422.
393. Hannema SE, Scott IS, Rajpert-De Meyts E, et al. Testicular development in the complete androgen insensitivity syndrome. J Pathol 2006;208:518-527.
394. Ahmed SF, Khwaja O, Hughes IA. The role of a clinical score in the assessment of ambiguous genitalia. BJU Int 2000;85:120-124.
395. Cools M, van Aerde K, Kersemaekers AM, et al. Morphological and immunohistochemical differences between gonadal maturation delay and early germ cell neoplasia in patients with undervirilization syndromes. J Clin Endocrinol Metab 2005;90:5295-5303.
396. Hoei-Hansen CE, Rajpert-De Meyts E, Daugaard G, et al. Carcinoma in situ testis, the progenitor of testicular germ cell tumours: a clinical review. Ann Oncol 2005;16:863-868.
397. Ahmed SF, Cheng A, Dovey L, et al. Phenotypic features, androgen receptor binding, and mutational analysis in 278 clinical cases reported as androgen insensitivity syndrome. J Clin Endocrinol Metab 2000;85:658-665.
398. Morel Y, Rey R, Teinturier C, et al. Aetiological diagnosis of male sex ambiguity: a collaborative study. Eur J Pediatr 2002;161: 49-59.
399. Hughes IA, Northstone K, Golding J, ALSPAC Study Team. Reduced birth weight in boys with hypospadias: an index of androgen dysfunction? Arch Dis Child Fetal Neonatal Ed 2002;87:F150-F151.
400. Main KM, Jensen RB, Asklund C, et al. Low birth weight and male reproductive function. Horm Res 2006;65:116-122.
401. Migeon CJ, Wisniewski AB, Gearhart JP, et al. Ambiguous genitalia with perineoscrotal hypospadias in 46,XY individuals: long-term medical, surgical, and psychosexual outcome. Pediatrics 110:e31, 2002.

402. Bouvattier C, Mignot B, Lefevre H, et al. Impaired sexual activity in male adults with partial androgen insensitivity. J Clin Endocrinol Metab 2006;91:3310-3315.
403. Wisniewski AB, Migeon CJ, Meyer-Bahlburg HF, et al. Complete androgen insensitivity syndrome: long-term medical, surgical and psychosexual outcome. J Clin Endocrinol Metab 2000;85: 2664-2669.
404. Gottlieb B, Lombroso R, Beitel LK, et al. Molecular pathology of the androgen receptor in male (in)fertility. Reprod Biomed Online 2005;10:42-48.
405. Conn J, Gillam L, Conway GS. Revealing the diagnosis of androgen insensitivity syndrome in adulthood. BMJ 2005;331:628-630.
406. Gottlieb B, Beitel LK, Trifiro MA. Androgen Insensitivity Syndrome. Gene Reviews 2006. http://www.geneclinics.org. Last updated 19 Sept 2006.
407. Warne G. Support groups for CAH and AIS. Endocrinologist 2003; 13:175-178.
408. Josso N, Belville C, de Clemente N, et al. AMH and AMH receptor defects in persistent müllerian duct syndrome. Hum Reprod Update 2005;11:351-356.
409. Imbeaud S, Carre-Eusebe D, Rey R, et al. Molecular genetics of the persistent müllerian duct syndrome: a study of 19 families. Hum Mol Genet 1994;13:25-131.
410. Imbeaud S, Faure E, Lamarre I, et al. Insensitivity to anti müllerian hormone due to a mutation in the human antimüllerian hormone receptor. Nat Genet 1995;11:382-388.
411. Imbeaud S, Belville C, Messika-Zeitoun L, et al. A 27 base pair deletion of the antimüllerian type II receptor gene is the most common cause of the persistent müllerian duct syndrome. Hum Mol Genet 1996;5:1269-1277.
412. Baskin LS, Ebbers MB. Hypospadias: anatomy, etiology, and technique. J Ped Surg 2006;41:463-472.
413. Paulozzi LJ. International trends in rates of hypospadias and cryptorchidism. Environ Health Perspect 1999;107:297-302.
414. Nelson CP, Park JM, Wan J, et al. The increasing incidence of congenital penile anomalies in the United States J Urol 2005; 174:1573-1576.
415. Ahmed SF, Dobbie R, Finlayson AR, et al. Prevalence of hypospadias and other genital anomalies among singleton births, 1988-1997, in Scotland. Arch Dis Child Fetal Neonatal Ed 2004;89: F149-F151.
416. Abdullah N, Pearce M, Parker L, et al. Birth prevalence of cryptorchidism and hypospadias in northern England, 1993-2000. Arch Dis Child Dec 7 Epub ahead of print, 2006.
417. Rey RA, Codner E, Iniguez G, et al. Low risk of impaired testicular Sertoli and Leydig cell functions in boys with isolated hypospadias. J Clin Endocrinol Metab 2005;90:6035-6040.
418. Holmes NM, Miller WL, Baskin LS, Lack of defects in androgen production in children with hypospadias. J Clin Endocrinol Metab 2004;89:2811-2816.
419. Chen T, Li Q, Xu J, et al. Mutation screening of BMP4, BMP7, HOXA4 and HOXB6 genes in Chinese patients with hypospadias. Eur J Hum Genet 2007;15:23-28.
420. Goodman FR, Bacchelli C, Brady AF, et al. Novel *HOXA13* mutations and the phenotypic spectrum of hand-foot-genital syndrome. Am J Hum Genet 2000;67:197-202.
421. Fredell L, Kockum I, Hansson E, et al. Heredity of hypospadias and the significance of low birth weight. J Urol 2002;167: 1423-1427.
422. Brouwers MM, Feitz WFJ, Roelofs LA, et al. Risk factors for hypospadias. Eur J Pediatr 2007;166:671-678.
423. Li J, Willingham E, Baskin LS. Gene expression profiles in mouse urethral development. BJU Int 2006;98:880-885.
424. Mureau MA, Slijper FM, Slob AK, et al. Satisfaction with penile appearance after hypospadias surgery: the patient and surgeon view. J Urol 1996;155:703-706.
425. Aho MO, Tammela OK, Somppi EM, et al. Sexual and social life of men operated in childhood for hypospadias and phimosis. A comparative study. Eur Urol 2000;37:95-100.
426. Zenaty D, Dijoud F, Morel Y, et al. Bilateral anorchia in infancy: occurrence of micropenis and the effect of testosterone treatment. J Pediatr 2006;149:687-691.
427. Law H, Mushtaq I, Wingrove K, et al. Histopathological features of testicular regression syndrome: relation to patient age and implications for management. Fet Pediatr Pathol 2006;25:119-129.
428. Emir H, Ayik B, Eliçevik M, et al. Histological evaluation of the testicular nubbins in patients with nonpalpable testis: assessment of etiology and surgical approach. Pediatr Surg Int 2007;23: 41-44.
429. McEachern R, Houle AM, Garel L, et al. Lost and found testes: the importance of the hCG stimulation test and other testicular markers to confirm a surgical declaration of anorchia. Horm Res 2004; 62:124-128.
430. Lee MM, Donahoe PK, Silverman BL, et al. Measurements of serum müllerian inhibiting substance in the evaluation of children with nonpalpable gonads. N Engl J Med 1997;336:1480-1486.
431. Boisen KA, Chellakooty M, Schmidt IM, et al. Hypospadias in a cohort of 1072 Danish newborn boys: prevalence and relationship to placental weight, anthropometrical measurements at birth, and reproductive hormone levels at three months of age. J Clin Endocrinol Metab 2005;90:4041-4046.
432. Gorlov IP, Kamat A, Bogatcheva NV, et al. Mutations of the GREAT gene cause cryptorchidism. Hum Molec Genet 2002;11: 2309-2318.
433. Ferlin A, Simonato M, Bartoloni L, et al. The INSL3-LGR8/GREAT ligand-receptor pair in human cryptorchidism. J Clin Endocrinol Metab 2003;88:4273-4279.
434. Yamazawa K, Wada Y, Sasagawa I, et al. Mutation and polymorphism analyses of INSL3 and LGR8/GREAT in 62 Japanese patients with cryptorchidism. Horm Res 2006;67:73-76.
435. Damgaard IN, Skakkebaek NE, Toppari J, et al. Persistent pesticides in human breast milk and cryptorchidism. Environ Health Perspect 2006;114:1133-1138.
436. Bay K, Asklund C, Skakkebaek NE, et al. Testicular dysgenesis syndrome: possible role of endocrine disruptors. Best Pract Res Clin Endocrinol Metab 2006;20:77-90.
437. Acerini CL, Hughes IA. Endocrine disrupting chemicals: a new and emerging public health problem? Arch Dis Child 2006;91: 633-641.
438. Paris F, Jeandel C, Servant N, et al. Increased serum estrogenic bioactivity in three male newborns with ambiguous genitalia: a potential consequence of prenatal exposure to environmental endocrine disruptors. Environ Res 2006;100:39-43.
439. Swan SH, Main KM, Liu F, et al. Decrease in anogenital distance among male infants with prenatal phthalate exposure. Environ Health Perspect 2005;113:1056-1061.
440. Pagnamenta AT, Taanman JW, Wilson CJ, et al. Dominant inheritance of premature ovarian failure associated with mutant mitochondrial DNA polymerase gamma. Hum Reprod 2006;21: 2467-2473.
441. Hanley NA, Arlt W. The human fetal adrenal cortex and the window of sexual differentiation. Trends Endocrinol Metab 2006;17: 391-397.
442. Robins T, Bellanne-Chantelot C, Barbaro M, et al. Characterization of novel missense mutations in *CYP21* causing congenital adrenal hyperplasia. J Mol Med 2007;85:243-251.
443. Hughes IA. Prenatal treatment of congenital adrenal hyperplasia: do we have enough evidence? Treat Endocrinol 2006;5:1-6.
444. Grosse SD, Van Vliet G. How many deaths can be prevented by newborn screening for congenital adrenal hyperplasia? Horm Res 2007;67:284-291.
445. New MI, Carlson A, Obeid J, et al. Prenatal diagnosis for congenital adrenal hyperplasia in 532 pregnancies. J Clin Endocrinol Metab 2001;86:5651-5657.
446. Joint LWPES/ESPE CAH Working Group. Consensus statement on 21-hydroxylase deficiency. J Clin Endocrinol Metab 2002;87: 4048-4053.
447. Rijnders RJP, Christiaens GCML, Bossers B, et al. Clinical applications of cell-free fetal DNA from maternal plasma. Obstet Gynecol 2004;103:157-164.
448. Van de Velde H, Sermon K, De Vos A, et al. Fluorescent PCR and automated fragment analysis in preimplantation genetic diagnosis for 21-hydroxylase deficiency in congenital adrenal hyperplasia. Mol Hum Reprod 1999;5:691-696.
449. Forest MG, Morel Y, David M. Prenatal treatment of congenital adrenal hyperplasia. Trends Endocrinol Metab 1998;9:284-289.
450. Meyer-Bahlburg HF, Dolezal C, Baker SW, et al. Cognitive and motor development of children with and without congenital adrenal hyperplasia after early-prenatal dexamethasone. J Clin Endocrinol Metab 2004;89:610-614.

451. Hirvikoski T, Nordenström A, Lindholm T, et al. Cognitive functions in children at risk for congenital adrenal hyperplasia treated prenatally with dexamethasone. J Clin Endocrinol Metab 2007;92:542-548.
452. Lajic S, Nordenström A, Ritzén EM, Wedell A. Prenatal treatment of congenital adrenal hyperplasia. Eur J Endocrinol 2004; 2151(suppl):U63-U69.
453. White PC. Steroid 11 beta-hydroxylase deficiency and related disorders. Endocrinol Metab Clin North Am 2001;20:61-79.
454. Paperna T, Gershoni-Baruch R, Badarneh K, et al. Mutations in CYP11B1 and congenital adrenal hyperplasia in Moroccan Jews. J Clin Endocrinol Metab 2005;90:5463-5465.
455. Charmandari E, Kino T, Chrousos GP. Familial/sporadic glucocorticoid resistance: clinical phenotype and molecular mechanisms. Ann N Y Acad Sci 2004;1024:168-181.
456. Mendonca BB, Leite MV, de Castro M, et al. Female pseudohermaphroditism caused by a novel homozygous missense mutation of the GR gene. J Clin Endocrinol Metab 2002;87:1805-1809.
457. Simpson ER, Clyne C, Rubin G, et al. Aromatase—a brief overview. Annu Rev Physiol 2002;64:93-127.
458. Shozu M, Akasofu K, Harada T, et al. A new cause of female pseudohermaphroditism: placental aromatase deficiency. J Clin Endocrinol Metab 1991;72:560-566.
459. Yalcinkaya TM, Siiteri PK, Vigne JL, et al. A mechanism for virilization of female spotted hyenas in utero. Science 1993;260: 1929-1931.
460. Ito Y, Fisher CR, Conte FA, et al. Molecular basis of aromatase deficiency in an adult female with sexual infantilism and polycystic ovaries. Proc Natl Acad Sci U S A 1993;90:11673-11677.
461. Conte FA, Grumbach MM, Ito Y, et al. A syndrome of female pseudohermaphrodism, hypergonadotropic hypogonadism, and multicystic ovaries associated with missense mutations in the gene encoding aromatase (P450arom). J Clin Endocrinol Metab 1994;78: 1287-1292.
462. Mullis PE, Yoshimura N, Kuhlmann B, et al. Aromatase deficiency in a female who is compound heterozygote for two new point mutations in the P450arom gene: impact of estrogens on hypergonadotropic hypogonadism, multicystic ovaries, and bone densitometry in childhood. J Clin Endocrinol Metab 1997;82:1739-1745.
463. Carani C, Qin K, Simoni M, et al. Effect of testosterone and estradiol in a man with aromatase deficiency. N Engl J Med 1997;337:91-95.
464. Smith EP, Boyd J, Frank GR, et al. Estrogen resistance caused by a mutation in the estrogen receptor gene in a man. N Engl J Med 1994;331:1056-1061.
465. Lin L, Ercan O, Raza J, et al. Variable phenotypes associated with aromatase (CYP19) insufficiency in humans. J Clin Endocrinol Metab Dec 12 2007;92:982-990.
466. Brunskill J. The effects of fetal exposure to Danazol. Br J Obstet Gynaecol 1992;99:212-214.
467. Murakami K, Nomura K, Shinohara K, et al. Danazol inhibits aromatase activity of endometriosis-derived stromal cells by a competitive mechanism. Fertil Steril 2006;86:291-297.
468. Holt HB, Medbak S, Kirk D, et al. Recurrent severe hyperandrogenism during pregnancy: a case report. J Clin Pathol 2005;58: 439-442.
469. Lo JC, Grumbach MM. Pregnancy outcomes in women with congenital virilizing adrenal hyperplasia. Endocrinol Metab Clin North Am 2001;30:207-229.
470. Oppelt P, Renner SP, Kellermann A, et al. Clinical aspects of Mayer-Rokitansky-Kuester-Hauser syndrome: recommendations for clinical diagnosis and staging. Hum Reprod 2006;21:792-797.
471. Biason-Lauber A, Konrad D, Navratil F, et al. A WNT4 mutation associated with Mullerian-duct regression and virilization in a 46,XX woman. N Engl J Med 2004;351:792-798.
472. Crouch NS, Minto CL, Laio LM, et al. Genital sensation after feminizing genitoplasty for congenital adrenal hyperplasia: a pilot study. BJU Int 2004;93:135-138.
473. Whitworth A. New options expand possibilities for fertility preservation in cancer patients. J Natl Cancer Inst 2006;98:1358-1360.

CHAPTER 23

NORMAL AND ABERRANT GROWTH

Edward O. Reiter and Ron G. Rosenfeld

NORMAL GROWTH

Childhood is a time of growth, a process that is complex and involves the interaction of multiple, diverse factors, the "cumulative sum of millions of unsynchronized cell replications."[1-3] Growth is common to all multicellular organisms and occurs by cell replication and enlargement along with the nonhomogeneous processes of cell and organ differentiation. The overall morphologic development, the rates of cellular division in different organ systems at different times, and the ultimate outcome are determined by the genetic composition of the individual interacting with external phenomena, including the quality and quantity of nutrition, as well as psychosocial and economic factors. Human growth is a relatively tightly regulated phenotype in that 1 standard deviation of adult height represents about only 4% of the mean adult height. In exploring abnormalities of growth in this chapter, the complex interrelationships among hormones and growth factors with subtle variabilities in structure, their membrane receptors, and seemingly redundant intracellular signaling factors cannot be ignored and presumably depict a story whose depth is just now being appreciated.

The very nature of linear height growth, whether occurring as a continuous process or with periodic bursts of growth and arrest,[3-5] has been hard to characterize definitively. During 1 year of growth monitoring, there may be marked seasonal variations of height and weight gain with several monthly bursts of weight and then height growth.[6] Some normal children may have a broad growth channel with many showing diverse, but characteristic, growth tracks.[7] Nonetheless, even though the process of growth is multifactorial and complex, children usually grow in a remarkably predictable manner. Deviation from such a normal pattern of growth can be the first manifestation of a wide variety of disease processes, including both endocrine and nonendocrine disorders and involving virtually any organ system of the body. Frequent and accurate assessment of growth is, therefore, of primary importance in the care of children.

Phases of Normal Growth

Growth occurs at differing rates during intrauterine life, early and mid-childhood, and adolescence, before its cessation after fusion of long bone and vertebral epiphyseal growth plates. Prenatal growth averages 1.2 to 1.5 cm per week but varies dramatically (Fig. 23–1); mid-gestational length growth velocity of 2.5 cm per week falls to almost 0.5 cm per week immediately before birth. Growth velocity (Figs. 23–2 and 23–3) during the first 2 years of life averages about 15 cm per year, and slows to approximately 6 cm per year during middle childhood. Pubertal growth begins earlier in girls than in boys, but is 3 to 5 cm greater in magnitude in boys than in girls. The actual assessment of total pubertal growth does, of course, depend upon the time of initiation. This is defined by the standard Tanner stages to determine pubertal onset or by more complex assessments of the actual "take-off" of growth by modeling techniques. The latter would suggest that the pubertal growth spurt starts earlier and accounts for a greater percentage of total growth.[8] About 40% of total pubertal growth occurs before Tanner 2 breast development in girls and 23% before testicular volume exceeds 3 mL in boys. The amount of pubertal growth, using this methodology, is greater than 30 cm and has less gender difference. The peak height velocity during the pubertal growth spurt is comparable to the rate of growth during the second year of life. The time of onset of the pubertal growth spurt varies in normal children, reflecting the concept of a "tempo of growth" or rate of maturation, as emphasized by Tanner.[9] In most normal children, the final height is not influenced by the chronologic time of the onset of the pubertal growth spurt, though the sex-related differences in adult height of approximately 13 cm are due, in part, to an earlier cessation of growth in females.[9] Growth ceases when the skeleton achieves adult maturity. This occurs when chondrocyte proliferation in the growth plate slows and senescent changes occur in a process seemingly intrinsic to the biology of the growth plate.[10] Some data suggest that the cessation of the growth process may precede epiphyseal fusion.[11]

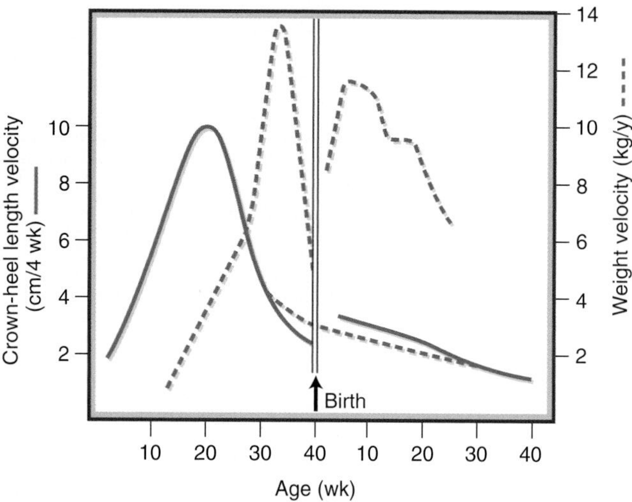

Figure 23–1 ■ Rate of linear growth and weight gain in utero and during first 40 weeks after birth. Note that length velocity is expressed in centimeters per week. The solid line depicts actual linear growth rate; the dashed line connecting the prenatal and postnatal length velocity lines depicts the theoretical curve for no uterine restriction late in gestation. The lighter dashed line depicts weight velocity. (From data in Tanner JM. Fetus into Man. Cambridge, MA: Harvard University Press, 1978.)

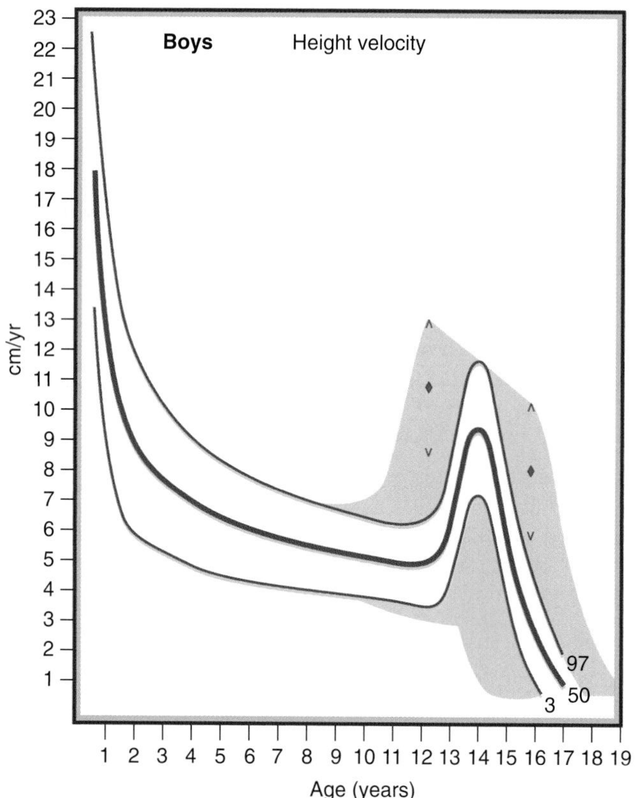

Figure 23–2 ■ Height velocity chart for boys constructed from longitudinal observations of British children. The 97th, 50th, and 3rd percentile curves define the general pattern of growth during puberty. Shaded areas define velocities of children who have peak velocities at ages up to 2 standard deviations before or after the average age depicted by the percentile lines. *Arrows* and *diamonds* mark the 97th, 50th, and 3rd percentiles of peak velocity when the peak occurs at these early or late limits. (Modified from charts prepared by Tanner JM and Whitehouse RH from data published in references 129, 1680, and 1699. Reproduced with permission of Tanner JM and Castlemead Publications, Ward's Publishing Services, Herts, UK.)

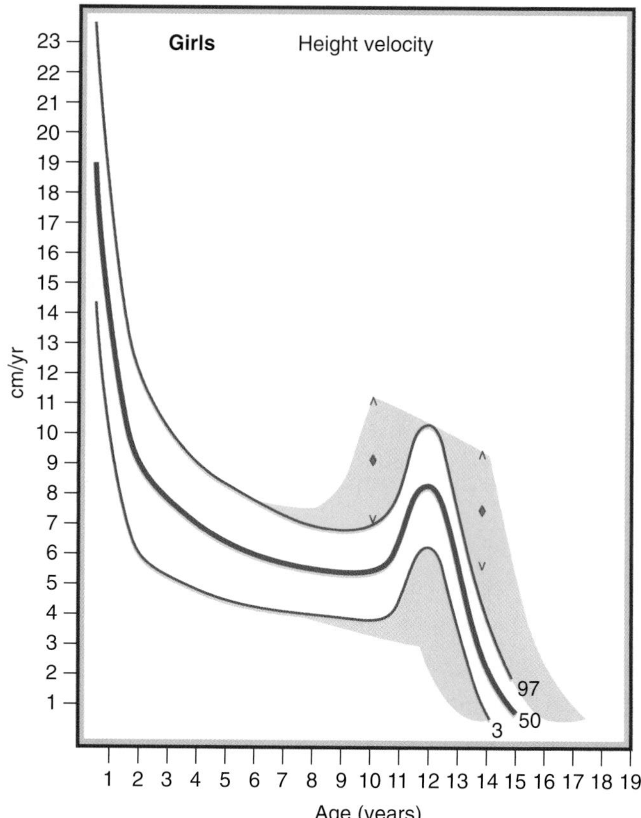

Figure 23–3 ■ Height velocity chart for girls See legend for Figure 23–2. (Modified and reproduced with permission of Tanner JM and Castlemead Publications, Ward's Publishing Services, Herts, UK.)

Karlberg and associates have resolved the normal linear growth curve into three additive, partially superimposible phases.[12,13] The components of this model include an "infancy" phase, starting in midgestation and then rapidly decelerating until about 3 to 4 years of age; a "childhood" phase, slowly decelerating during early adolescence; and a sigmoid-shaped "puberty" phase that involves the adolescent growth spurt. Hormonal concomitants of these phases have been suggested, but as seen in this chapter, the interplay of the growth hormone (GH)/insulin-like growth factor (IGF) axis, gonadal steroids, and thyroxine is complex, and attempts to define individual predominance of one hormone at any time of life as likely an oversimplification. The recognition of nonhormonal regulation of growth plate biology is an important concept.

Measurement

Assessment of growth requires accurate and reproducible determinations of height. Supine length is routinely measured in children younger than 2 years of age, and erect height is assessed in older children. The inherent inaccuracies involved in measuring length in infants are often obscured by the rapid skeletal growth during this period. For measurement of supine length (Fig. 23–4), it is best to use a firm box with an inflexible board against which the head lies, together with a movable footboard on which the feet are placed perpendicular to the plane of the supine length of the infant. Optimally, the child should be relaxed, the legs should be fully extended, and the head should be positioned in the "Frankfurt plane," with the line connecting the outer canthus of the eyes and the external auditory meatus perpendicular to the long axis of the trunk.

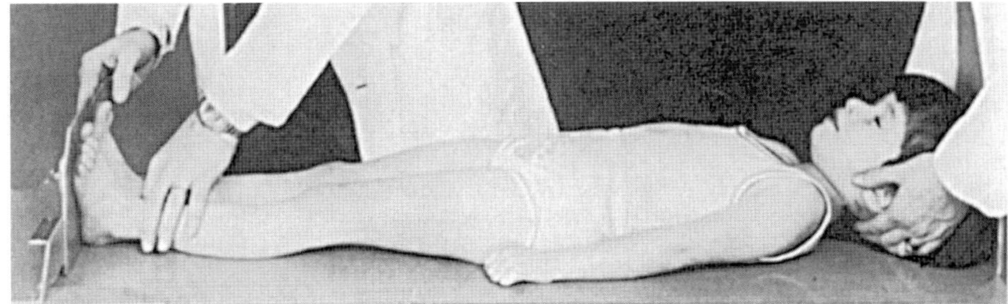

Figure 23–4 ▪ Technique for measuring recumbent length. (A device suitable for measurement of length of infants can be purchased from Raven Equipment Limited, Essex, UK.) (Photograph courtesy of Noel Cameron.)

When children are old enough (and physically capable) to stand erect, it is best to employ a wall-mounted "Harpenden" stadiometer, similar to that designed by Tanner and Whitehouse for the British Harpenden Growth Study. The traditional measuring device of a flexible arm mounted to a weight balance is notoriously unreliable and does not provide accurate serial measurements.

As with length measurements in infants, positioning of the child in the stadiometer is critical (Fig. 23–5); the child should be fully erect, with the head in the Frankfurt plane; the back of the head, thoracic spine, buttocks, and heels should touch the vertical axis of the stadiometer, and the heels should be together. Every effort should be made to correct discrepancies related to lordosis or scoliosis; and, ideally, serial measurements should be made at the same time of day, since standing height may undergo diurnal variation.

Height determinations should be performed by a trained individual, rather than by an inexperienced member of the staff. We recommend that lengths and heights be measured in triplicate, that variation should be no more than 0.3 cm, and that the mean height should be recorded. For determination of height velocity when several measurements are being made within a short period, the same individual should perform the determinations to eliminate inter-observer variability. Even when every effort is made to obtain accurate height measurements, a minimum interval of 6 months is necessary for meaningful height velocity computation. Nine to 12 months' data are preferable so that errors of measurement are minimized and the seasonal variation in height velocity is assimilated into the data.

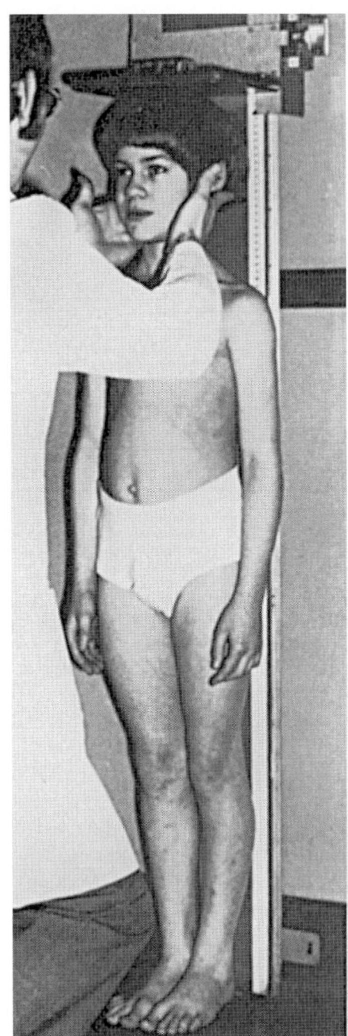

Figure 23–5 ▪ Technique for measuring erect height using the Harpenden stadiometer with direct digital display of height. (Devices of this type are available from Holtain Ltd, Wales, UK, and Seritex Inc, Carlstadt, NM.)

Growth Charts

Evaluation of a child's height must be done in the context of normal standards with the international data that are available. Such standards can be either cross-sectional or longitudinal. Most American pediatric endocrine clinics continue to use the cross-sectional data provided by the National Center for Health Statistics (NCHS), which were originally introduced in 1977. Epidemiologic limitations exist in these growth charts. The original infant charts, for example, were derived from a private study of a group of subjects who were primarily Caucasian, formula-fed, middle-class infants from southwestern Ohio. Data employed for older children came from national health examination surveys conducted from 1963 to 1974. The NCHS (now part of the Centers for Disease Control and Prevention [CDC]) has recently provided a set of 16 new growth charts (8 each for males and females), representing revisions of 14 existing charts, as well as the introduction of new charts for body mass index ($BMI=wt/ht^2$) (www.cdc.gov/growthcharts) (Figs. 23–6 to 23–13).[14] These latter charts more clearly define the presence of the obesity epidemic. The height charts show little change in average height over the last 25 years, despite the perception that today's children are taller than those from 3 decades ago.

These charts compare individual children with the 5th, 10th, 25th, 50th, 75th, 90th, and 95th percentiles of normal American children. There are, however, two major limitations of these charts when applied to the individual child. First, they do not satisfactorily define children below the 5th or above the 95th percentiles, the very children in whom it is most critical to define the degree to which they deviate from the normal growth centiles. The NCHS data are useful in computing standard devia-

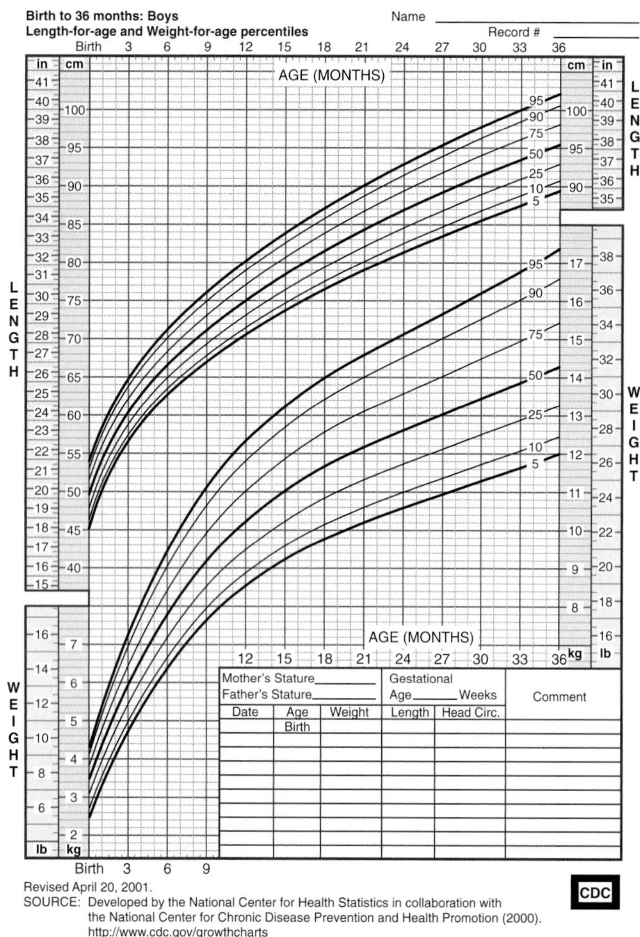

Figure 23–6 ▪ Length-for-age and weight-for-age percentiles for boys (birth to 36 months) developed by the National Center for Health Statistics in collaboration with the National Center for Chronic Disease Prevention and Health Promotion (2000). Available at http://www.cdc.gov/growthcharts.

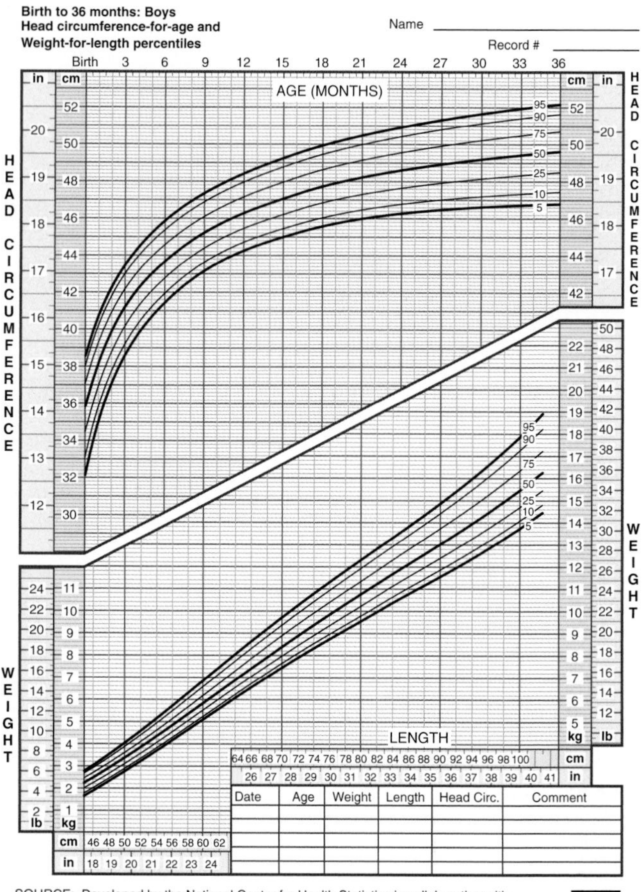

Figure 23–7 ▪ Head circumference-for-age and weight-for-length percentiles for boys (birth to 36 months) developed by the National Center for Health Statistics in collaboration with the National Center for Chronic Disease Prevention and Health Promotion (2000). Available at http://www.cdc.gov/growthcharts.

tion scores (SDS), which are more helpful, because a short child can be described as, for example, −4.2 or −2.5 SDS from normal. A height SDS for age is calculated as follows: SDS equals height minus mean height for normal children at this age and sex divided by the SD of height for normal children at this age and sex. As these are defined by cross-sectional data, however, childhood SDS are not directly comparable with SDS during adolescence, when variation in growth rate and maturational tempo can be large. Second, cross-sectional data are of greater value during infancy and childhood than in adolescence, because differences in the timing of pubertal onset can considerably influence normal growth rates. To address this issue, Tanner and colleagues[15] developed longitudinal growth charts, in an effort to construct the curve shapes with centile widths obtained from a large cross-sectional survey, thus accounting for variability in the timing of puberty. Such charts are of particular value in assessing growth during adolescence and puberty and for plotting sequential growth data on any given child.

The data from cross-sectional and longitudinal growth studies have been employed to develop *height velocity* standards (see Figs. 23–2 and 23–3). It is important to emphasize that carefully documented height velocity data are invaluable in assessing the child with abnormalities of growth. Although there is considerable variability in the normal height velocity in children of different ages, between the age of 2 years and the onset of puberty, children normally grow with remarkable fidelity relative to the normal growth curves. Any "crossing" of height percentiles during this age period should always be considered abnormal and always warrants further evaluation.

Syndrome-specific growth curves have been developed for a number of clinical conditions associated with growth failure, such as Turner's syndrome,[16] achondroplasia,[17] and Down's syndrome.[18] Such growth profiles are invaluable for tracking the growth of children with these clinical conditions. Deviation of growth from the appropriate disease-related growth curve suggests the possibility of a second underlying cause such as acquired autoimmune hypothyroidism in Down's or Turner's syndromes.

Body Proportions

Many abnormal growth states, including both short stature and excessive stature, are characterized by *disproportionate* growth. The following determinations should be made as part of the evaluation of short stature: (1) occipitofrontal head circumference; (2) lower body segment: distance from top of pubic sym-

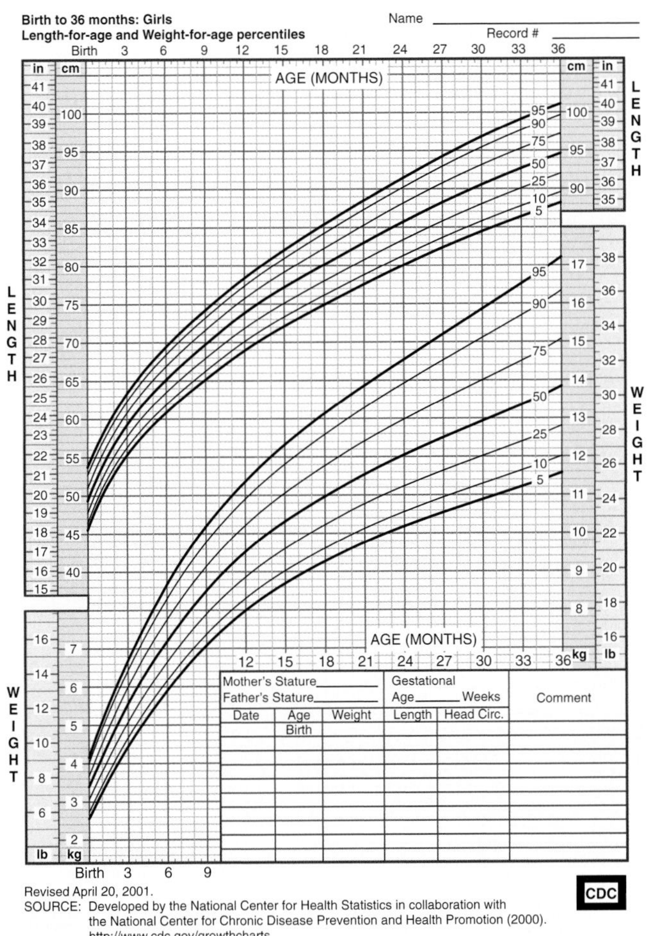

Figure 23–8 ▪ Length-for-age and weight-for-age percentiles for girls (birth to 36 months) developed by the National Center for Health Statistics in collaboration with the National Center for Chronic Disease Prevention and Health Promotion (2000). Available at http://www.cdc.gov/growthcharts.

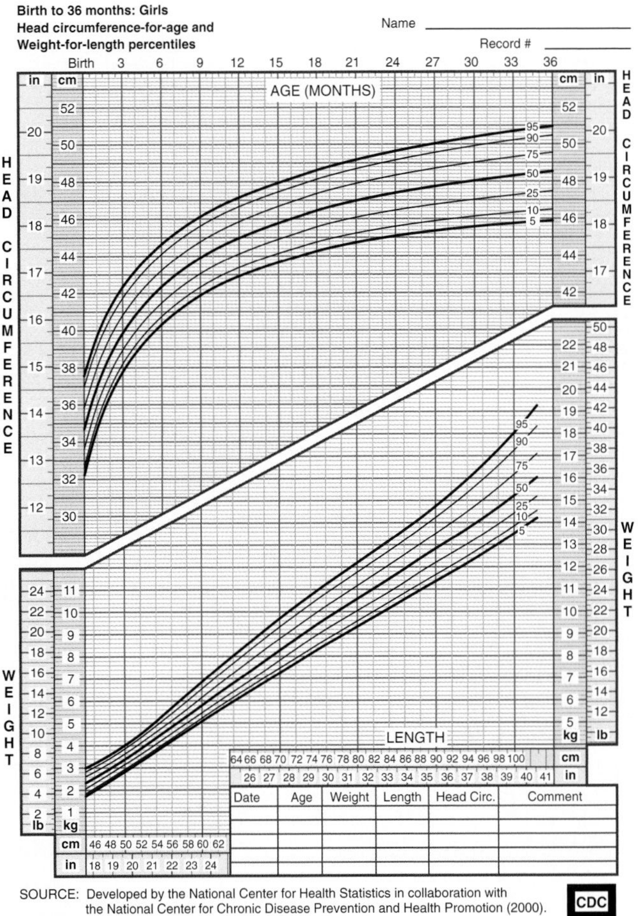

Figure 23–9 ▪ Head circumference-for-age and weight-for-length percentiles for girls (birth to 36 months) developed by the National Center for Health Statistics in collaboration with the National Center for Chronic Disease Prevention and Health Promotion (2000). Available at http://www.cdc.gov/growthcharts.

physis to the floor; (3) upper body segment: the sitting height (height of stool should be subtracted from standing height); (4) arm span. Published standards exist for these body proportion measurements, which must be evaluated relative to the patient's age.[19] The upper segment to lower segment ratio, for example, ranges from 1.7 in the neonate to slightly less than 1.0 in the adult.

Skeletal Maturation ("Bone Age")

The growth potential in the tubular bones can be assessed by evaluation of the progression of ossification within the epiphyses. The ossification centers of the skeleton appear and progress in a predictable sequence in normal children, and skeletal maturation can be compared with normal age-related standards. This forms the basis of "bone age" or "skeletal age," the only readily available quantitative determination of net somatic maturation and, thus, a mirror of the tempo of growth and maturation. It is not clear what factors determine this normal maturational pattern, but it is certain that genetic factors and multiple hormones, including thyroxine, GH, and gonadal steroids, are involved.[20] Studies in patients with mutations of the gene for the estrogen receptor[21] or for the aromatase enzyme[22-24] demonstrated that estrogen is primarily responsible for epiphyseal fusion,[25] although it seems unlikely that estrogen is solely responsible for all aspects of skeletal maturation.

After the neonatal period, a radiograph of the left hand and wrist is commonly used for comparison with the published standards of Greulich and Pyle.[26] An alternative method for assessing bone age from radiographs of the left hand involves a scoring system for developmentally identified stages of each of 20 individual bones,[27] a technique that has been adapted for computerized assessment.[28,29] The left hand is used because radiographs of the entire skeleton would be tedious and expensive and would involve additional radiation exposure. However, the hand does not contribute to height, and accurate evaluation of growth potential might require radiographs of the legs and spine.

A number of important caveats concerning bone age must be considered. Experience in determination of bone age is essential to minimize intraobserver variance, and clinical studies involving bone age generally benefit from having a single reader perform all interpretations. The normal rate of skeletal maturation differs between boys and girls, and among different ethnic groups. The standards of Greulich and Pyle are separable by sex, but were developed in American white children between 1931 and 1942. Finally, both the Greulich and

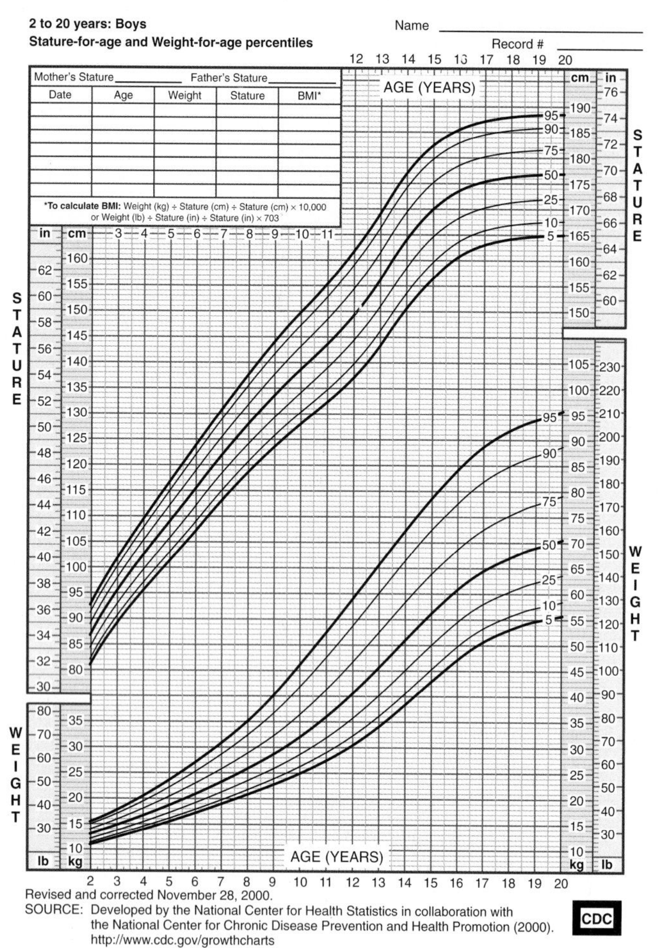

Figure 23–10 ▪ Stature-for-age and weight-for-age percentiles for boys (2 to 20 years) developed by the National Center for Health Statistics in collaboration with the National Center for Chronic Disease Prevention and Health Promotion (2000). Available at http://www.cdc.gov/growthcharts.

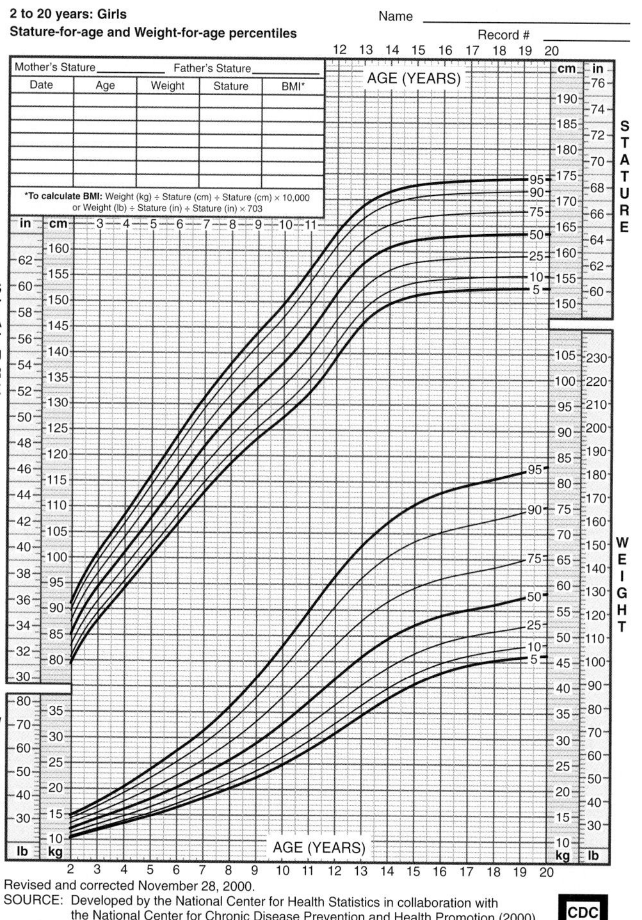

Figure 23–11 ▪ Stature-for-age and weight-for-age percentiles for girls (2 to 20 years) developed by the National Center for Health Statistics in collaboration with the National Center for Chronic Disease Prevention and Health Promotion (2000). Available at http://www.cdc.gov/growthcharts.

Pyle and the Tanner and Whitehouse standards involved *normal* children[30] and may not be applicable to children with skeletal dysplasias, endocrine abnormalities, or other forms of growth retardation or acceleration.

As the biology of the growth plate is studied, it becomes apparent that the hormonal milieu, as well as the intrinsic (and finite) capacity of chondrocytes to proliferate, ultimately lead to growth cessation.[31] The bone age is a reflection of the degree of growth plate senescence and, thus, is a useful adjunct in estimating growth opportunity.

Prediction of Adult Height

The extent of skeletal maturation observed in an individual can be employed to predict the ultimate height potential. Such predictions are based upon the observation that the more delayed the bone age (relative to the chronologic age), the longer the time before epiphyseal fusion prevents further growth. The most commonly used method for height prediction, based upon Greulich and Pyle's "Radiographic Atlas of Skeletal Development,"[26] was developed by Bayley and Pinneau,[32] and relies upon bone age, height, and a semiquantitative allowance for chronologic age (Table 23–1). The system of Tanner and colleagues[27] employs height, bone age, chronologic age, and, during puberty, height and bone age increments during the previous year, as well as menarchal status. Roche and associates[33] have employed the combination of height, bone age, chronologic age, midparental height, and weight. Attempts have been made to calculate final height predictions without requiring the use of skeletal age[34] by utilizing multiple regression analyses with available data such as height, weight, birth measurements, and midparental stature. All of these systems are, by nature, empiric, and are not absolute predictors. The more advanced the bone age, the greater the accuracy of the adult height prediction, because a more advanced bone age places a patient closer to final height.

All methods of predicting adult height are based upon data from normal children, and none has been documented to be accurate in children with growth abnormalities. For this kind of precision, it would be necessary to develop disease-specific (e.g., achondroplasia, Turner's syndrome) atlases of skeletal maturation. The height prediction tables must also be used with care in assessing height outcomes, for example, in patients with precocious puberty treated with gonadotropin-releasing hormone agonists to avoid data misinterpretation. It is fair to say that the clinical endocrinologist must not give height predictions a value that is greater than a reasonable estimate.

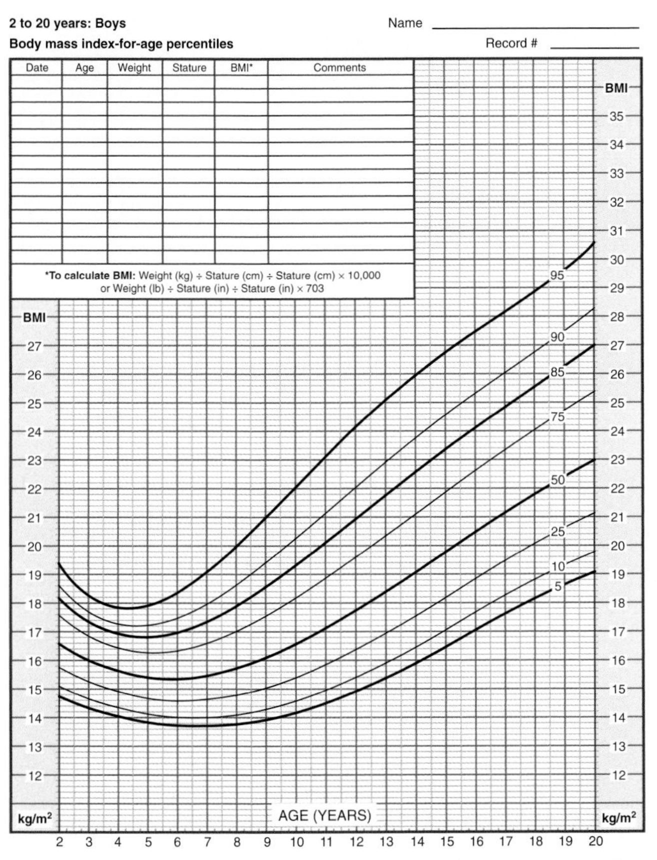

Figure 23–12 ■ Body mass index-for-age percentiles for boys (2 to 20 years) developed by the National Center for Health Statistics in collaboration with the National Center for Chronic Disease Prevention and Health Promotion (2000). Available at http://www.cdc.gov/growthcharts.

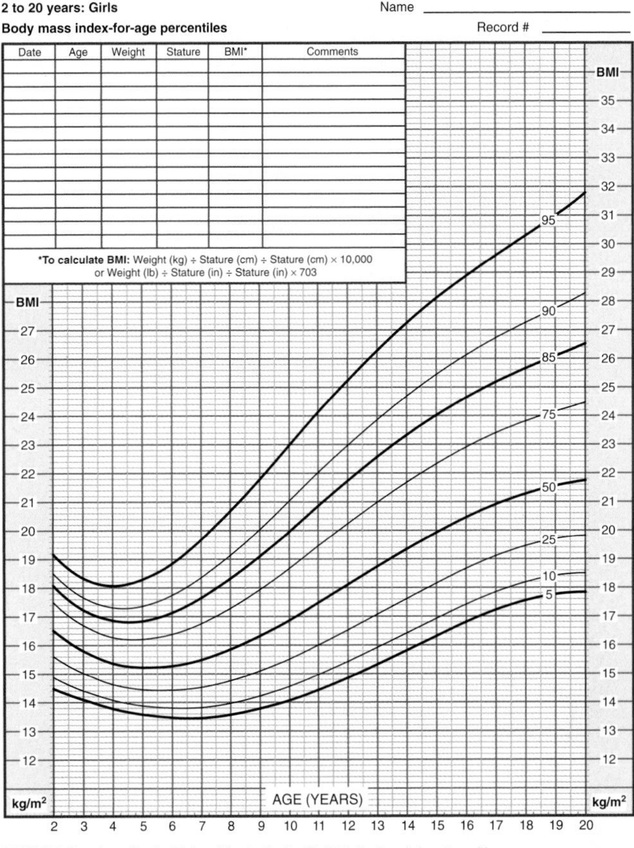

Figure 23–13 ■ Body mass index-for-age percentiles for girls (2 to 20 years) developed by the National Center for Health Statistics in collaboration with the National Center for Chronic Disease Prevention and Health Promotion (2000). Available at http://www.cdc.gov/growthcharts.

Parental Target Height

Because genetic factors are important determinants of growth and height potential, it is useful to assess a patient's stature relative to that of siblings and parents. Tanner and associates developed a growth chart modifying the heights of children, ages 2 to 9 years, by the midparental height.[35] A child's predicted adult height (see above) may also be related to a "parental target height," namely the mean parental height with the addition or subtraction of 6.5 cm for boys and girls, respectively. The 2 standard deviation range (2 SD) for this calculated parental target height is about ± 10 cm, so that calculated target heights, like predicted adult heights, are approximations. In children with extremely short stature (>–3 SD), the father's height may more strongly correlate with the patient's height, while the mother's height may more greatly influence birth length.[36] Recent statistical reassessment shows a tendency for regression to the mean of the children's height as related to the midparental target height.[37] Failure to realize this may lead to inappropriately using short parental height as an explanation for marked short stature in a child. Nevertheless, when a child's growth pattern clearly deviates from that of parents or siblings, the possibility of underlying pathology should be considered. Although it is certainly important to measure the heights of parents and siblings, rather than accepting their statural claims, one must recall as well that it is not always possible to conveniently and definitively identify the true biologic parents.

Secular Changes in Height

There are surprisingly few data concerning the stature of "modern man" until the measurement of military recruits became customary in the eighteenth century. Skeletal remains from the last ice age would appear to indicate that adult stature 10,000 to 20,000 years ago was not substantially different from that of contemporary humanity, although this record is obviously fragmentary.[38] It has been suggested that a reduction in stature was observed with the introduction of agriculture approximately 5000 years ago, with growth attenuation resulting from the combined effects of nutrient deficiency, population growth, and the spread of infectious diseases. Military recruits in the eighteenth and nineteenth century were clearly shorter than those today, although it must be recognized that such data are impacted by the fact that soldiers were commonly recruited from the lower socioeconomic classes, and that poor health and nutrition contributed not only to poor growth but also to late maturity.[39] Whereas men in the twentieth century averaged 5 to 10 cm greater height than those in the eighteenth century, much of this height gain has occurred over the last 100 years, and

TABLE 23–1 PREDICTION OF ADULT STATURE

Bone Age (yr-mo)	Fraction of Adult Height Attained at Each Bone Age					
	Girls			Boys		
	Retarded	Average*	Advanced	Retarded	Average*	Advanced
6-0	0.733	0.720		0.680		
6-3	0.742	0.729		0.690		
6-6	0.751	0.738		0.700		
6-9	0.763	0.751		0.709		
7-0	0.770	0.757	0.712	0.718	0.695	0.670
7-3	0.779	0.765	0.722	0.728	0.702	0.676
7-6	0.788	0.772	0.732	0.738	0.709	0.683
7-9	0.797	0.782	0.742	0.747	0.716	0.689
8-0	0.804	0.790	0.750	0.756	0.723	0.696
8-3	0.813	0.801	0.760	0.765	0.731	0.703
8-6	0.823	0.810	0.771	0.773	0.739	0.709
8-9	0.836	0.821	0.784	0.779	0.746	0.715
9-0	0.841	0.827	0.790	0.786	0.752	0.720
9-3	0.851	0.836	0.800	0.794	0.761	0.728
9-6	0.858	0.844	0.809	0.800	0.769	0.734
9-9	0.866	0.853	0.819	0.807	0.777	0.741
10-0	0.874	0.862	0.828	0.812	0.784	0.747
10-3	0.884	0.874	0.841	0.816	0.791	0.753
10-6	0.896	0.884	0.856	0.819	0.795	0.758
10-9	0.907	0.896	0.870	0.821	0.800	0.763
11-0	0.918	0.906	0.883	0.823	0.804	0.767
11-3	0.922	0.910	0.887	0.827	0.812	0.776
11-6	0.926	0.914	0.891	0.832	0.818	0.786
11-9	0.929	0.918	0.897	0.839	0.827	0.800
12-0	0.932	0.922	0.901	0.845	0.834	0.809
12-3	0.942	0.932	0.913	0.852	0.843	0.818
12-6	0.949	0.941	0.924	0.860	0.853	0.828
12-9	0.957	0.950	0.935	0.869	0.863	0.839
13-0	0.964	0.958	0.945	0.880	0.876	0.850
13-3	0.971	0.967	0.955		0.890	0.863
13-6	0.977	0.974	0.963		0.902	0.875
13-9	0.981	0.978	0.968		0.914	0.890
14-0	0.983	0.980	0.972		0.927	0.905
14-3	0.986	0.983	0.977		0.938	0.918
14-6	0.989	0.986	0.980		0.948	0.930
14-9	0.992	0.988	0.983		0.958	0.943
15-0	0.994	0.990	0.986		0.968	0.958
15-3	0.995	0.991	0.988		0.973	0.967
15-6	0.996	0.993	0.990		0.976	0.971
15-9	0.997	0.994	0.992		0.980	0.976
16-0	0.998	0.996	0.993		0.982	0.980
16-3	0.999	0.996	0.994		0.985	0.983
16-6	0.999	0.997	0.995		0.987	0.985
16-9	0.9995	0.998	0.997		0.989	0.988
17-0	1.00	0.999	0.998		0.991	0.990
17-3					0.993	
17-6		0.9995	0.9995		0.994	
17-9					0.995	
18-0		1.00			0.996	
18-3					0.998	
18-6					1.00	

Table derived from Post EM, Richman RA (reference 1682) based upon the data of Bayley and Pinneau (reference 32). These tables have been organized in an easy-to-use slide-rule format ("Adult Height Predictor," copyright 1987 Ron G. Rosenfeld.)

probably reflects the dramatic improvement in overall nutrition and health seen in the Western world. Thus, secular changes in height appear to reflect fundamental alterations in the standard of living, rather than major genomic differences among populations; economic advances in developing countries would be predicted to lead to improvement in adult stature and a reduction in international differences in growth.

ENDOCRINE REGULATION OF GROWTH

The Pituitary

The concept of the pituitary as a "master gland," controlling the endocrine activities of the body, has been replaced by recognition of the importance of the brain and, particularly, the hypothalamus in regulating hormonal production and secretion. Nevertheless, the pituitary gland is central to understanding the regulation of growth.

Embryologically, the pituitary gland is formed from two distinct sources:[40] Rathke's pouch, a diverticulum of the primitive oral cavity (stomodeal ectoderm), gives rise to the adenohypophysis. The neurohypophysis (posterior pituitary) originates in the neural ectoderm of the floor of the forebrain, which also develops into the third ventricle. The adenohypophysis normally constitutes 80% of the weight of the pituitary and consists of anterior, intermediate, and infundibular lobes. In humans, the anterior lobe is the largest component and houses the most hormone producing cells.

Rathke's pouch, the origin of the adenohypophysis, can be identified in the 3-mm embryo during the third week of pregnancy. GH-producing cells can be found in the adenohypophysis by 9 weeks of gestation[41] and vascular connections between the anterior lobe of the pituitary and the hypothalamus develop at about this time,[42,43] although hormone production can occur in the pituitary in the absence of connections with the hypothalamus. Somatotropes frequently can be demonstrated in the pituitary in anencephalic newborns.[44] Nevertheless, it appears likely that the initiation of development of the anterior pituitary is dependent upon responsiveness of the oral ectoderm to inducing factors from the ventral diencephalon (Fig. 23–14).[45-53] A complex orchestration of temporally sequenced and geographically restricted expression of multiple extracellular signaling peptides and intracellular transcription factors regulates this developmental process.[51,52] The developing pituitary and hypothalamus are in close anatomic juxtaposition and their embryonic development is likely to be codependent. Some of the diencephalic factors that have been identified as critical in formation and patterning of Rathke's pouch, which, in the mouse, is initiated on embryonic day 8 (e8) are bone morphogenetic proteins 4 and 2 (BMP4/2), Wnt5a, and fibroblast growth factor 8 (FGF8).[45,51,54] The dorsal neuroepithelial signal, BMP4, is needed for "organ commitment" of the pituitary, whereas a BMP2 (ventral) and FGF8 (dorsal) gradient determines pituitary cell phenotypes (i.e., gonadotropes and the Pit-1 dependent lines, somatotropes, lactotropes and thyrotropes [ventral], and melanotropes and corticotropes [dorsal]).[45,46,48,51] It seems that reciprocal interaction of at least two transcription factors, Pit-1 and GATA-2, is important in implementing the cell-determination signals of BMP2 and FGF8.[45,55] Explant studies in the mouse have demonstrated that if Rathke's pouch is removed from the oral ectoderm on e10.5 and incubated in appropriate culture medium, differentiation of each of the pituitary cell types continues, indicating that by that point, organogenesis of the anterior pituitary is no longer dependent upon hypothalamic signals,[51] although such signals may remain critically involved in pituitary hormone production.

As described, a number of pituitary-specific transcription factors are involved in the determination of pituitary cell lineages and cell-specific expression of anterior pituitary hormones. To date, defects in multiple homeodomain transcription factors shown to be involved in human anterior pituitary development and differentiation have now been associated with various combinations of pituitary hormone deficiencies (see Fig. 23–14 and Table 23–5).[20,52,53,56]

In the adult, the mean pituitary size is 13×9×6 mm.[57] The mean weight of 600 mg, with a range of 400 to 900 mg, is slightly greater in women than in men and increases during pregnancy.[58] In the newborn, pituitary weight averages about 100 mg. Normally the pituitary resides in the sella turcica, immediately above and partially surrounded by the sphenoid bone. The volume of the sella turcica is a good index of pituitary size and may be reduced in the child with pituitary hypoplasia or increased in some with *PROP-1* defects (see Table 23–5). The anatomic proximity between the optic chiasm and the pituitary is important, because hypoplasia of the optic chiasm may occur together with hypothalamic/pituitary dysfunction in the syndrome of septo-optic dysplasia.[59] Children with congenital blindness or nystagmus should be monitored carefully for hypopituitarism. Similarly, suprasellar growth of a pituitary tumor may initially manifest with visual complaints or evidence of decreases in peripheral vision.

The existence of a portal circulatory system within the pituitary is critical for normal pituitary function. The blood supply of the pituitary is shown in Figure 23–15.[42,43] Hypothalamic peptides, produced in neurons that terminate in the infundibulum, enter the primary plexus of the hypophyseal portal circulation and are transported via the hypophyseal portal veins to the capillaries of the anterior pituitary. This portal system thus provides a means of communication between the neurons of the hypothalamus and the anterior pituitary.

Growth Hormone

Chemistry

Human GH is produced as a single chain, 191 amino acid, 22-kd protein (Fig. 23–16).[60] It is not glycosylated, but contains two intramolecular disulfide bonds. GH shares sequence homology with prolactin, chorionic somatomammotropin (CS) (placental lactogen), and a 22-kd GH variant (GH-V) secreted only by the placenta[61] that differs from pituitary GH by 13 amino acids. The genes for these proteins have probably evolved from a common ancestral gene, even though the genes are located on different chromosomes (chromosome 6 for prolactin and chromosome 17 for GH).[62] The genes for GH, prolactin, and placental lactogen share a common structural organization, with four introns separating five exons. In fact, the GH subfamily contains five members, whose genes are located on a 78-kb section of chromosome 17; the 5′ to 3′ order of the genes are GH, a CS pseudogene, CS-A, GH-V, and CS-B.[63]

Normally, about 75% of GH produced by the pituitary is of the mature, 22-kd form. Alternative splicing of the second codon results in deletion of amino acids 32-46, yielding a 20-kd form, which normally accounts for 5% to 10% of pituitary GH.[62] The remainder of pituitary GH includes desamidated and *N*-acetylated forms and various GH oligomers.

Secretion

The pulsatile pattern characteristic of GH secretion largely reflects the interplay of two hypothalamic regulatory peptides,

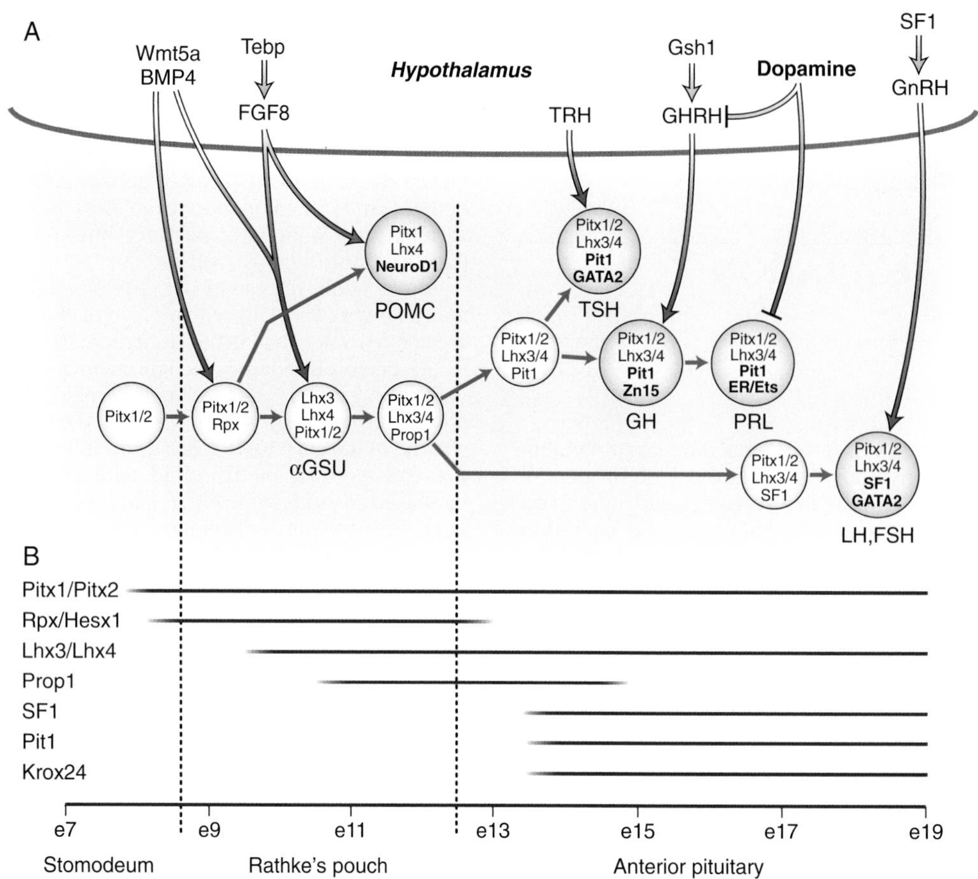

Figure 23–14 ▪ Development of pituitary cell lineages. **A,** Schematic representation of pituitary cell precursors showing the expression of prevalent transcription factors at each stage of development. Terminally differentiated cells are shown as larger and shaded circles together with the hormones produced (lineage-specific transcription factors are highlighted in bold in these cells). The interaction with transcription factors and signaling molecules in the hypothalamus is also noted. Transcription factors are represented in lower case (except for SF1 and GATA2), whereas signaling molecules appear in upper case. **B,** Schema showing the timing of appearance and disappearance of pituitary transcription factors during mouse embryogenesis. *BMP4,* Bone morphogenic protein 4; e, embryonic day; *ER,* estrogen receptor; *FGF8,* fibroblast growth factor 8; *FSH,* follicle-stimulating hormone; *GHRH,* growth hormone–releasing hormone; *GnRH,* gonadotropin-releasing hormone; *αGSU,* α-glycoprotein subunit; *LH,* luteinizing hormone; *POMC,* pro-opiomelanocortin; *PRL,* prolactin; *SF1,* steroidogenic factor 1; *TRH,* thyrotropin-releasing hormone; *TSH,* thyroid-stimulating hormone; *Wmt5a,* wingless type MMTV integration site family, member 5A; *Hesx1,* homeobox expressed in ES1 cells (Rathke's pouch homeobox, Rpx). (Reprinted with permission from Lopez-Bermejo A, Buckway CK, Rosenfeld RG. Genetic defects of the growth hormone-insulin-like growth factor axis. Trends Endocrinol 2000;11:43, 2000.)

growth hormone–releasing hormone (GHRH) and somatostatin (somatotropin release–inhibiting factor [SRIF]), with presumed modulation by other putative GH-releasing factors.[64] GHRH activity is species-specific, presumably reflecting the specificity of binding to a G protein–related receptor on the pituitary somatotropes. Regulation of GH production by GHRH is mediated largely at the level of transcription and is enhanced by increases in intracellular cyclic adenosine monophosphate (cAMP) levels. The GHRH receptor is a member of the G protein–coupled receptor family B-III, also called the secretin family, and has partial sequence identity with receptors for VIP, secretin, calcitonin and parathyroid hormone.[65,66] In the dwarf transgenic mouse model with diminished GHRH production, pituitary somatotrope proliferation is markedly decreased.[67] Mutations of the GHRH gene itself have not yet been reported, but anatomic and functional abnormalities of the connection between the hypothalamus and the anterior pituitary, which prevent interaction of GHRH with its receptor on the somatotrope, are considered to be the most important causes of clinical GH deficiency in children. The Gsh-1 homeobox gene, which is expressed in the developing central nervous system[68] but not in the pituitary, plays an important role, nonetheless, in mouse pituitary development. Mice with mutations in this gene do not produce GHRH and presumably also do not produce gonadotropin-releasing hormone (GnRH), because there are anterior pituitary hypoplasia and deficiencies of GH, prolactin, and luteinizing hormone (LH).[69] The effects of this gene on hypothalamic releasing factors are analogous to those of the Pit-1 or *PROP1* genes (see below) at the pituitary level.

Somatostatin appears to affect the timing and amplitude of pulsatile GH secretion rather than to regulate GH synthesis. The pulsatile secretion of GH in vivo is believed to result from a simultaneous reduction in hypothalamic somatostatin release and increase in GHRH release.[70] Conversely, a trough of GH secretion occurs when somatostatin is released in the face of diminished GHRH activity.

The regulation of the reciprocal secretion of GHRH and somatostatin is imperfectly understood. Multiple neurotransmitters and neuropeptides are involved in regulation of release of these hypothalamic factors.[71] These factors influence GH secretion with stress, sleep, hemorrhage, fasting, hypoglycemia, and exercise and form the basis for a number of GH-stimulatory tests employed in the evaluation of GH secretory capacity/reserve. GH secretion is also influenced by a variety of nonpeptide hormones, including androgens,[72,73] estrogens,[74] thyroxine,[75] and glucocorticoids.[76,77] The mechanisms by which these hormones regulate GH secretion may involve actions at both the hypothalamic and pituitary levels. Practically speaking, hypothyroidism and glucocorticoid excess may each blunt spontaneous and provocative GH secretion. Gonadal steroids appear to be responsible for the rise in GH secretion characteristic of puberty.

Synthetic hexapeptides capable of stimulating GH secretion are termed *GH-secretagogues* (GHSs).[78,79] These peptides stimulate GH release and enhance the GH response to GHRH, although they work at receptors distinct from those for GHRH, at hypothalamic and pituitary sites.[78,79] Finding 40% to 60% homology to the G-protein–coupled GHS receptor in the pufferfish indicates that the structure and function of this receptor has been highly conserved for around 400 million years, certainly suggesting a fundamental role for the natural ligand of this receptor.[79] Kojima and colleagues[80] identified a putative endogenous ligand, a 28 amino acid with the serine 3 residue n-octanoylated, referred to as *ghrelin*. It is found primarily in the stomach (and throughout the gastrointestinal tract[81]) but also in the hypothalamus, heart, lung, and adipose tissue. Administration of ghrelin stimulates food intake and obesity[82] and raises plasma GH concentrations[80,83-85] and, to a lesser extent, adrenocorticotropic hormone (ACTH).[85] These data suggest that ghrelin is an important stimulus for nutrient allocation for growth and metabolism and a central component of the GH regulatory system. PACAP (pituitary adenylate cyclase–activating peptide), a hypothalamic peptide possibly involved in the regulation of GH secretion, is a member of the PACAP/glucagon superfamily.[86,87] The developmental abnormality holoprosencephaly, which can be associated with GH deficiency, may be caused by gene defects affecting PACAP and PACAP-R expression.[87,88]

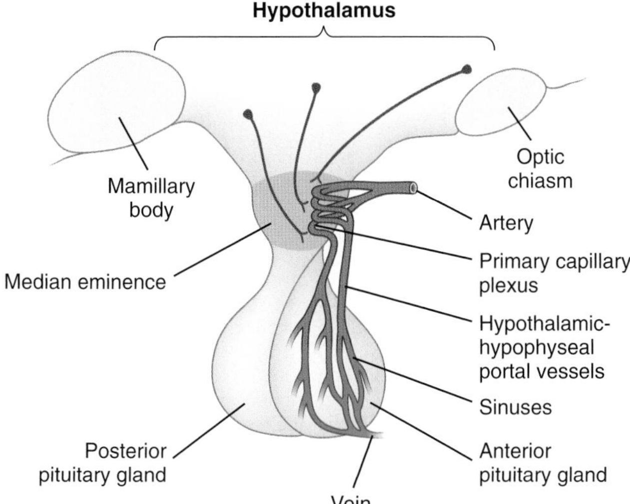

Figure 23–15 ■ The main components of the hypothalamic-pituitary portal system. (From Guyton AC, Hall JC. Human physiology and mechanisms of disease, 6th ed. WB Saunders, Philadelphia: 1997:600, with permission.)

The synthesis and secretion of GH are also regulated by the IGF peptides. Receptors specific for IGF-I and IGF-II have been identified in varied pituitary cell systems.[89,90] Inhibition of GH secretion by IGF-I and/or IGF-II in rat anterior pituitary cells has been demonstrated in a perifusion system[91] and spontaneous GH secretion is diminished in humans treated with synthetic IGF-I.[92]

Studies of GH Secretion in Humans

The episodic release of GH from the pituitary somatotropes results in intermittent increases in serum levels of GH separated by periods of low or undetectable levels, during which time GH secretion is minimal.[93,94] The pulsatile nature of GH secretion has been demonstrated by frequent serum sampling, coupled with the use of sensitive immunofluorometric or chemoluminescent assays of GH.[94] Under normal circumstances serum GH levels are less than 0.04 μg/L between secretory bursts. It is, consequently, impractical to assess GH secretion by random serum sampling. Extensive sampling studies at different ages, in

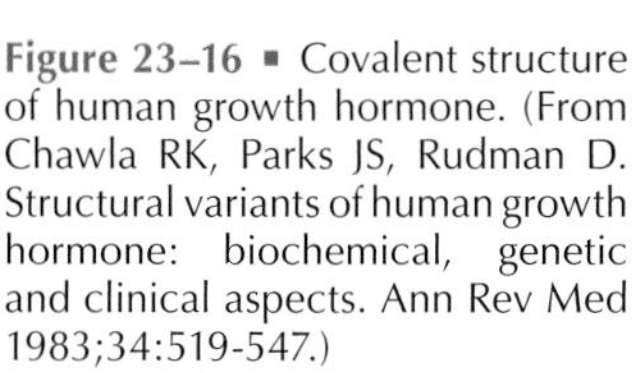
Figure 23–16 ■ Covalent structure of human growth hormone. (From Chawla RK, Parks JS, Rudman D. Structural variants of human growth hormone: biochemical, genetic and clinical aspects. Ann Rev Med 1983;34:519-547.)

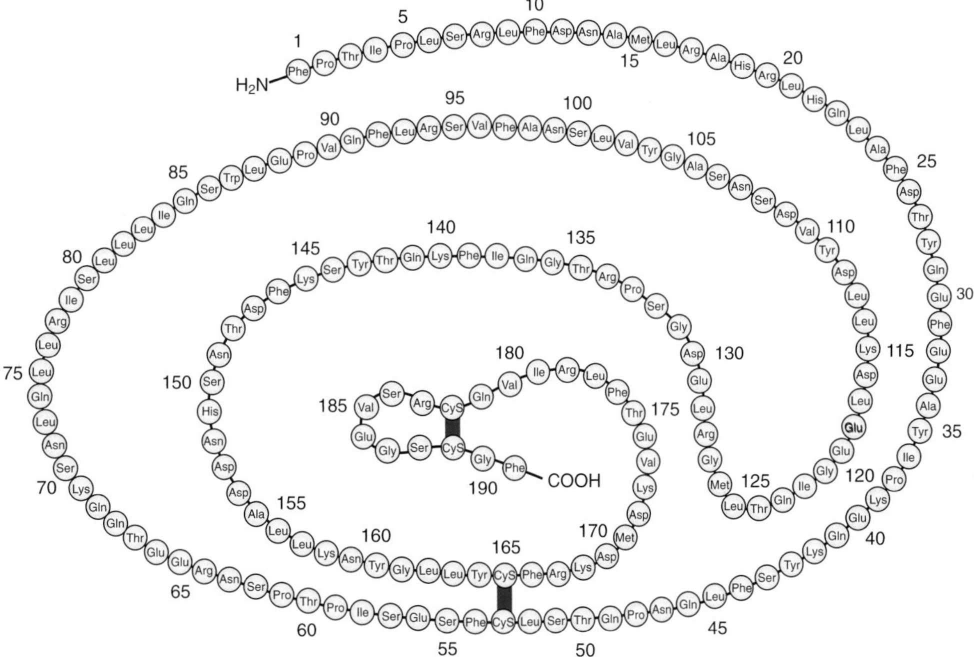

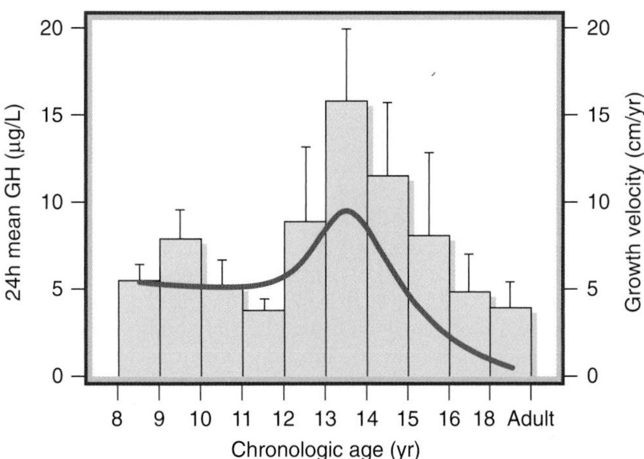

Figure 23–17 ▪ Relation between 24-hour mean growth hormone (GH) levels and age in boys and men. The bars represent values for the 24-hour mean (+SE) levels of GH (left axis) from 60 24-hour GH profiles of healthy boys and men subdivided according to chronologic age. An idealized growth velocity curve reproduced from the 50th percentile values for whole year height velocity of North American boys[15] is superimposed. (From Martha PM Jr, Rogol AD, Veldhuis JD, et al. Alterations in the pulsatile properties of circulating growth hormone concentrations during puberty in boys. J Clin Endocrinol Metab 1989;69:563-570.)

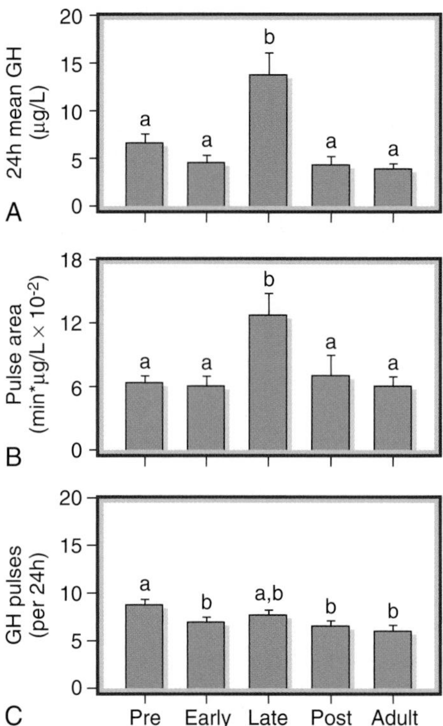

Figure 23–18 ▪ **A,** The mean (+SE) 24-hour levels of growth hormone (GH) for groups of normal boys at varied stages of pubertal maturation. **B,** The mean (+SE) area under the GH concentration versus time curve for individual GH pulses, as identified by the cluster pulse detection algorithm. **C,** The number of GH pulses (+SE) as detected by the cluster algorithm, in the 24-hour GH concentration profiles for boys in each of the pubertal study groups. Note that the mean 24-hour GH concentration changes are largely mediated by changes in amount of GH secreted per pulse, rather than frequency of pulses. In each panel, bars bearing the same letter are statistically indistinguishable. (From Martha PM Jr, Rogol AD, Veldhuis JD, et al. Alterations in the pulsatile properties of circulating growth hormone concentrations during puberty in boys. J Clin Endocrinol Metab 69:563-570.)

normal persons and in many abnormal conditions have defined GH pulses, basal secretion, and diurnal variability. Computer programs have been developed to indicate whether changes in GH levels in various life periods and under diverse clinical circumstances occur because of a change of secretory mass or of pulse frequency, of altered clearance, or of a combination of these processes.[93-96] Deconvolution techniques allow accurate estimates of the quantity of GH secreted per burst, GH clearance kinetics, pulse amplitudes and frequencies, and an overall calculation of endogenous GH production. Approximate entropy, a model-free measure, is applied to quantify the degree of orderliness of GH release patterns.[97,98] The impact of the specific nature of pulsatile GH secretion upon its biologic actions is under study.[93,94] For example, it appears that better statural growth is associated with large swings of GH output but of relatively uniform magnitude in an irregular sequence (high approximate entropy).[99,100]

GH-secreting cells have been identified by 9 to 12 weeks of gestation, and immunoreactive pituitary GH is present by 7 to 9 weeks of gestation.[101,102] Fetal pituicytes secrete GH in vitro by 5 weeks,[103] before the hypothalamic-portal vascular system is differentiated.[104] Pit-1 mRNA and pit-1 protein are expressed by at least 6 weeks of gestation; their abundant presence early in gestation suggests an important role in cytodifferentiation and cell proliferation.[105] GH can be identified in fetal serum by the end of the first trimester, with peak levels of around 150 μg/L in midgestation.[101,102] Serum levels fall throughout the latter part of pregnancy and are lower in term than in premature infants, perhaps reflecting feedback by the higher serum levels of IGF peptides characteristic of the later stages of gestation.[106,107] Mean levels of GH decrease from values of 25 to 35 μg/L in the neonatal period to approximately 5-7 μg/L through childhood and early puberty.[102,108,109] Twenty-four GH secretion peaks during adolescence, undoubtedly contributing to the high serum levels of IGF-I characteristic of puberty. The increase in GH production during mid to late puberty is due both to enhanced pulse amplitude and increased mass of GH per secretory burst, rather than to a change in pulse frequency[93,97,108] (Figs. 23–17 and 23–18).[109] Greater irregularity in GH secretion corresponds to greater linear growth.[110] In the face of stable levels of the growth hormone–binding protein (GHBP),[111,112] the enhanced pubertal GH production appears to be associated with higher levels of "free" GH (Fig. 23–19), potentially facilitating the delivery of IGF-I to target tissues. This enhanced activity of the GH-IGF axis contributes to the insulin resistance occurring during puberty.[113] GH and IGF production begins to decline by late adolescence[95] and continues to fall throughout adult life. Normal young adult men generally experience 6 to 10 GH secretory bursts per 24 hours, a value similar to that in younger children and in adolescents.[94,108] On the other hand, 24-hour GH production rates for normal men range from 0.25 to 0.52 mg/m^2 surface area,[77,114] about 20% to 30% of pubertal levels; this is largely due to decreased GH pulse amplitude with age.[108] Indeed, puberty may be considered, with some justification, a period of "physiological acromegaly," while aging, with its decrease in GH secretion, has been termed "the somatopause."[74,115]

Physiologic states that impact GH secretion, in addition to maturation and aging, include sleep,[116] nutritional status,[117] fasting, exercise,[118] stress,[118] and gonadal steroids.[72,73] Maximal GH secretion occurs during the night, especially at the onset of the first slow wave sleep (stages III and IV). Rapid eye movement sleep is, on the other hand, associated with low GH secretion.[116,119] A circadian rhythm of somatostatin secretion, upon which is superimposed episodic bursts of GHRH release, may help explain the nocturnal augmentation of GH produc-

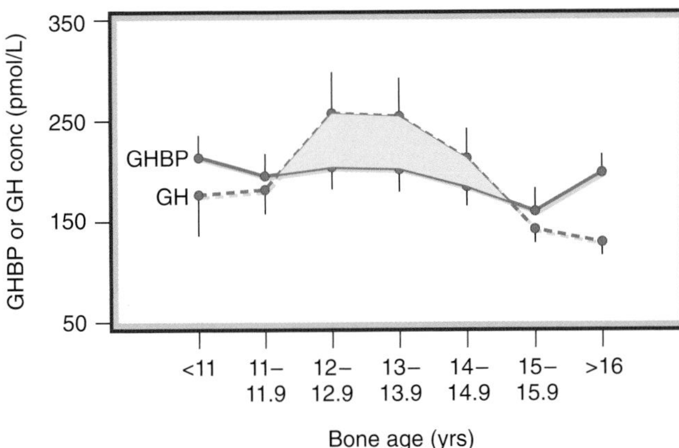

Figure 23–19 ■ Levels of growth hormone (GH) and growth hormone–binding protein (GHBP) measured in normal pubertal boys throughout adolescence. The GHBP levels do not significantly change during puberty, but there is a significant increment of GH production and, therefore, of GH levels during this same time. These data suggest that there may be greater amounts of "free GH" during this period, leading to greater production of IGF-I. (Based on data from references 109 and 111.)

tion.[120] When testosterone was administered to boys with delayed puberty, spontaneous GH release was enhanced, but such a change was not duplicated by administration of nonaromatizable androgens, emphasizing the possible unique importance of estrogen upon GH secretion.[95,121-123] The effects of testosterone on serum IGF-I levels may in part be independent of GH in that individuals with mutations of the GH receptor still experience a modest rise in serum IGF-I during puberty.[124] With a combination of deconvolution analysis, approximate entropy, and cosine regression analysis, Veldhuis and associates[97,123] carefully evaluated intensive GH sampling data, derived from measurements in sensitive GH assays, in prepubertal and pubertal children of both genders. In addition to the amplified secretory burst mass due to jointly increased GH pulse amplitude and duration, they found that sex steroids selectively affected facets of GH neurosecretory control: estrogen increases basal GH secretion rate and irregularity of GH release patterns, while testosterone stimulates greater GH secretory burst mass and IGF-I concentrations.

Obesity is characterized by lowered GH production, reflected by a diminished number of GH secretory bursts and shorter half-life duration.[117,125] Obesity in childhood and adolescence, similarly, is characterized by decreased GH production, but normal IGF and increased GHBP levels and often-increased linear growth.[125] The hyperinsulinism associated with obesity causes lowered IGFBP-1 and, perhaps, higher "free" IGF-I levels.[126] Endogenous GH secretion and levels achieved during provocative tests in these obese subjects[127] approximate the diagnostic range of GH deficiency. Fasting increases both the number and amplitude of GH secretory bursts, presumably reflecting decreased somatostatin secretion and enhanced GHRH release, while lowering GHBP concentrations. Rapid changes in levels of IGFBPs in response to altered nutrition and changes of insulin levels may modify the effect of IGF-I upon its negative feed-back and effector sites.[94,125] Body mass also influences GH production in normal prepubertal and pubertal children and adults.[108,128,129]

GH Receptor (GH-R)/GH Binding Protein (GHBP)

Leung and colleagues[130] cloned both the rabbit and human cDNAs for the GH receptor. Each contains an open reading frame of 638 amino acids and encodes a mature receptor of 620 amino acids and a predicted molecular weight of 70 kd before glycosylation. There are three domains—an extracellular, hormone-binding domain, a single membrane-spanning domain, and a cytoplasmic domain. In humans, the most important circulating GH binding protein appears to be derived from proteolytic cleavage of the extracellular domain of the receptor.[131] In the mouse[132] and rat,[133] on the other hand, there are multiple transcripts for the GH receptor; the larger 3.4- to 4.8-kb transcript codes for the intact receptor and the 1.2- to 1.9-kb transcript codes for the soluble GHBP.

The coding and 3′-untranslated regions of the human GH-R are encoded by nine exons, numbered 2 to 10.[134] The gene for the human GH-R is located on chromosome 5p13.1-p12, where it spans more than 87 kb.[135] Exons 3 to 7 encode the extracellular, GH-binding domain. Two isoforms of the GH-R have been found in humans, a full-length form and one that had a deletion of exon 3 (d3-GH-R) with loss of a 22 amino acid segment.[136] Several recent studies[137-139] have suggested that short children with d3-GH-R (approximately 50% of Europeans are either homozygous or heterozygous for the allele encoding d3-GH-R) are more responsive to GH treatment, a potentially important observation that requires prospective study and mechanistic explanation.[140] The GH-R shows sequence homology with the prolactin receptor and with receptors for interleukin (IL)-2, -3, -4, -6, and -7, as well as receptors for erythropoietin, granulocyte-macrophage colony stimulating factor, and interferon.[134] The GH-R is a member of the class 1 hematopoietic cytokine family.[141] Examination of the crystal structure of the GH–GH-R complex revealed that the complex consisted of one molecule of GH bound to two GH-R molecules, initially suggesting that GH induced receptor dimerization as a necessary step in its action.[142] Later studies, however, indicate that the receptor may be constitutively dimerized and that receptor activation involves a GH-induced conformational change.[143,144]

After binding to its receptor, GH stimulates phosphorylation of a protein with an apparent molecular weight of 120 kd.[145] Although it was originally suspected that the GH receptor might be capable of autophosphorylation, it is now apparent that the major tyrosine-phosphorylated protein is associated with the receptor, rather than being the receptor itself, which has been proven to lack intrinsic kinase activity. JAK2 (Janus kinase 2) has been identified as the critical GH receptor–associated tyrosine kinase.[146] This has been supported by studies showing that the loss of ability of the GH-R to bind JAK2 results in loss of GH-induced GH-R signaling, and by the observation that conditional knockout of the *JAK2* gene in mice decoupled the GH-R from downstream signaling.[147,148] Recruitment and/or activation of JAK2 molecules by the GH-R promotes their enzymatic activity via cross-phosphorylation, and the active kinases then phosphorylate critical tyrosines on the intracellular portion of the GH-R itself, thereby providing docking sites for critical intermediary proteins, such as the STATs (signal transducers and activators of transcription).[149] There are seven known mammalian STATs; of these, STAT5b appears to be most critically involved in mediating the growth-promoting actions of the GH-R, as indicated by several gene disruption studies in rodent models.[150-152] The report of two cases of homozygous human STAT5b mutations, presenting with severe growth failure and GH resistance, has further substantiated the critical intermediary role of STAT5b in GH regulation of *IGF-I* gene transcription and growth.[153,154] STAT proteins dock, via their src-homology-2 (SH2) domain to phosphotyrosines on ligand-activated receptors, such as the GH-R, and are subsequently phosphorylated on single tyrosines at the C-terminus of the protein, dimerize, translocate to the nucleus, bind to DNA through their DNA-binding domain, and regulate gene transcription. The identification of STAT5b response elements in intron 2 of the rat IGF-I gene further sup-

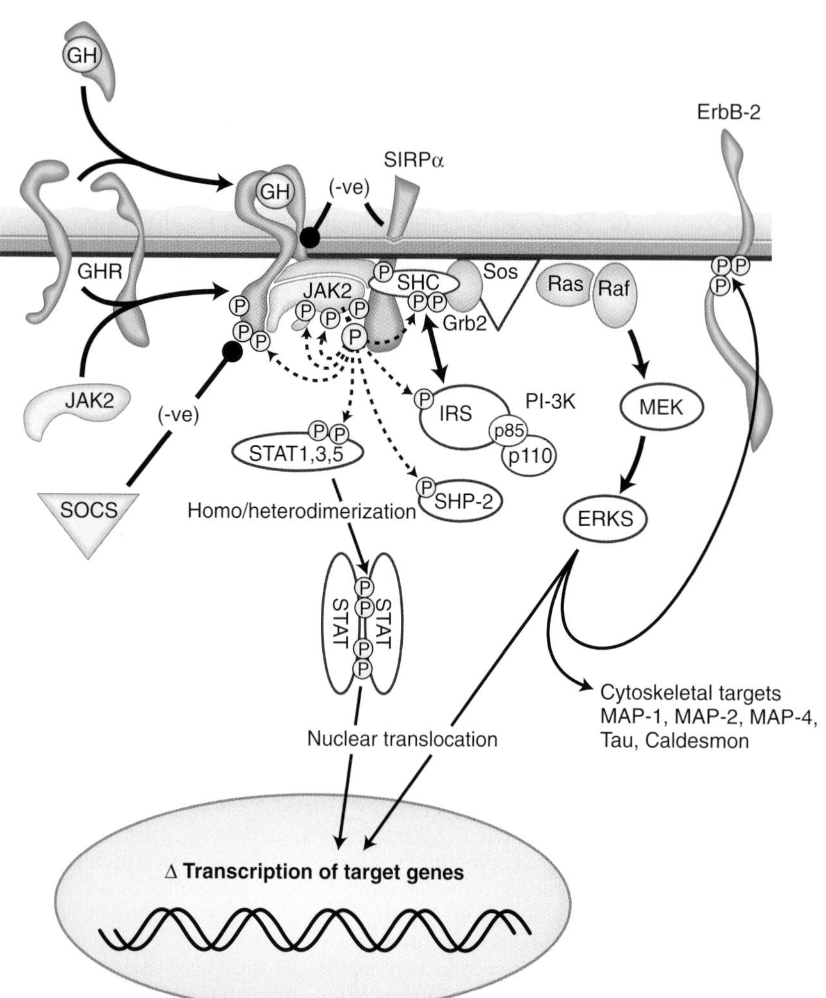

Figure 23–20 ▪ A model depicting intracellular signaling intermediates induced by binding of growth hormone (GH) with the GH receptor (GHR). *ERK,* Extracellular signal-regulated kinase; *GRB,* growth factor receptor–binding protein; *JAK,* Janus kinase; *IRS,* insulin receptor substrate; *MAP,* mitogen-activated protein kinase; *MEK,* MAPK-ERK kinase; *PKC,* protein kinase C; *PLC,* phospholipase C; *SHP2,* protein tyrosine phosphatase; *SOCS,* suppressors of cytokine signaling; *STAT,* signal transducer and activator of transcription. (From Le Roith DC, Bondy S, Yakar J-L, et al. The somatomedin hypothesis: 2001. Endocrine Rev 2001;22:53-74.)

ports the key role of STAT5b in GH regulation of skeletal growth.[155]

The presumed sequence of steps in GH action is shown in Figure 23–20.

1. Binding of a molecule of GH, through each of two specific sites, to the membrane-associated, dimerized GH-R.
2. Interaction of the GH-R with JAK2. Tyrosine phosphorylation of both JAK2 and key residues on the intracellular portion of the GH-R, thereby providing docking sites for other signal mediators.
3. Recruitment of STAT5b (it is unclear whether any of the other STATs, including STAT5a, play a role in IGF-I gene transcription in humans) to phosphorylated tyrosine residues on activated receptors.
4. Phosphorylation of STAT5b.
5. Dissociation of phosphorylated STAT5b from the GH-R.
6. Dimerization of STAT5b and entry into nucleus.
7. Binding to DNA and initiation of gene transcription.

GH- and JAK2-dependent phosphorylation and activation have been demonstrated for many cytoplasmic signaling molecules which, after forming homodimers or heterodimers, translocate into the nucleus, bind DNA, and activate transcription.[156-158] How all of these seemingly redundant pathways interact to mediate the various anabolic and metabolic actions of GH remains to be elucidated. The role of the MAPK/ERK signaling pathway in mediating GH actions on skeletal growth remains unclear, despite the report of a dysfunctional GH variant (Ile179Met GH), which reportedly induced phosphorylation of STAT5, but only poorly activated ERK.[159] Similarly, the PI3K/AKT pathway, which is capable of activation by multiple growth factors and cytokines, plays an unclear role in GH stimulation of growth. The potential negative modulation of these pathways by intracellular phosphatases and the actions of SOCS2 and CIS will likely further affect growth responses.

The major GHBP in human plasma binds GH with high specificity and affinity but with relatively low capacity, as only about 45% of circulating GH is bound.[112,160,161] The GHBP is, in essence, the extracellular domain of the GH receptor and has an apparent molecular weight of approximately 55 kd. An additional GHBP, not related to the GH receptor, binds approximately 5% to 10% of circulating GH with lower affinity.[112] GHBP prolongs the half-life of GH, presumably by impairing its glomerular filtration, and modulates its binding to the GH receptor. In general, GHBP levels reflect GH receptor levels and activity; that is, low levels are associated with states of GH insensitivity.[112]

Levels of GHBP are low in early life, rise through childhood, and plateau during the pubertal years and adulthood.[111,162,163] Levels are usually constant for a given individual once puberty is reached.[111] Impaired nutrition, diabetes mellitus, hypothyroidism, chronic liver disease, and a spectrum of inherited abnormalities of the GH receptor are associated with low levels of GHBP, while obesity, refeeding, early pregnancy, and estrogen treatment can cause elevated levels of GHBP.[112] A direct correlation exists between GHBP levels and body mass index.[164] Serum GHBP levels correlate inversely with 24-hour GH production[111]; this reciprocal relationship between GH production and GHBP in normal subjects may result from adjustments of GH secretion to accommodate GH receptor levels, which may be genetically determined or modulated by environmental factors such as nutritional status.[164,165] Assays of serum levels of GHBP are useful in identifying subjects with GH insensitivity due to genetic abnormalities of the GH-R.[166,167] Patients with GH insensitivity due to nonreceptor abnormalities, defects of the intracellular domain of the GH-R, or inability of the receptor to dimerize may, however, have normal serum levels of GHBP.[124,168-170]

Inhibition of GH signaling by several members of the GH-inducible suppressors of cytokine signaling (SOCS) family has been reported.[171] The importance of SOCS proteins in controlling growth is demonstrated by the finding of gigantism in SOCS-2 knockout mice, an effect which appears to require the presence of GH and the activation of STAT5b.[172,173] Endotoxin and proinflammatory cytokines, such as IL-1β and tumor necrosis factor α (TNF-α), which can also induce SOCS proteins,[174] can produce GH insensitivity. SOCS-3, induced by IL-1β and TNF-α, or by endotoxin in vivo may play a role in the GH insensitivity induced by sepsis.[175] Critically ill patients with septic shock treated with GH had increased mortality,[176] possibly related to induction of GH insensitivity in specific tissues as a consequence of endotoxin- and cytokinemia.

GH Actions

According to the somatomedin hypothesis, the anabolic actions of GH are mediated through the IGF peptides.[177,178] Although this theory is largely true, GH is also capable of inducing effects that are independent of IGF activity. Indeed, the actions of GH and IGF are, on occasion, contradictory, as evident in the "diabetogenic" actions of GH[179,180] and the glucose-lowering activity of IGFs. Green and colleagues[181] have attempted to resolve some of these differences in a "dual effector" model, in which GH stimulates precursor cells, such as prechondrocytes, to differentiate. When differentiated cells or neighboring cells then secrete IGFs, these peptides act as mitogens and stimulate clonal expansion. This hypothesis is based upon the ability of IGF peptides to work, not only as hormones that are transported through the blood, but also as paracrine or autocrine growth factors.

GH has a variety of metabolic actions, some of which appear to be independent of IGF production, such as enhancement of lipolysis,[182] stimulation of amino acid transport in diaphragm[183] and heart,[184] and enhancement of hepatic protein synthesis. Thus, there are multiple sites of GH action and, frequently, it is not entirely clear which of these actions are mediated through the IGF system and which might represent IGF-independent effects of GH.[185] Potential IGF-independent sites of action for GH include (1) *epiphysis:* stimulation of epiphyseal growth; (2) *bone:* stimulation of osteoclast differentiation and activity, stimulation of osteoblast activity, and increase of bone mass by endochondral bone formation; (3) *adipose tissue:* acute insulin-like effects, followed by increased lipolysis, inhibition of lipoprotein lipase, stimulation of hormone-sensitive lipase, decreased glucose transport, and decreased lipogenesis; and (4) *muscle:* increased amino acid transport, increased nitrogen retention, increased lean tissue, and increased energy expenditure. The concept of IGF-independent actions of GH is supported by in vivo studies, in which IGF-I cannot duplicate all of the effects of GH, such as nitrogen retention and insulin resistance.[186] The administration of GH for 1 to 3 weeks to calorically restricted normal or obese men results in significant nitrogen retention, although this effect does not persist with prolonged therapy.[187]

The question of whether GH has an effect upon growth that is not IGF-mediated was addressed by studies involving simultaneous targeted disruption of the genes for both IGF-I and the GH-R in mice, which resulted in a more severe attenuation of postnatal growth than was observed with knockout of either gene alone, indicating that GH and IGF-I promote growth by both common and independent functions.[188] However, experience, at least in humans, would suggest that the contribution of GH beyond its ability to stimulate the IGF axis (including IGF-I, IGFBP-3, and the acid-labile subunit) is modest, at most, and that the IGF system should be viewed as the major mediator of GH's actions on skeletal growth.[154] The observation that the variations in growth associated with the exon 3 deletion of GH-R were not reflected in changes in IGF-I levels suggests the possibility that an IGF-independent action of GH upon growing cartilage could occur.[137,138]

Insulin-like Growth Factors

Historical Background

The insulin-like growth factors (or somatomedins) are a family of peptides that are, in part, GH-dependent and that mediate many of the anabolic and mitogenic actions of GH. They were originally identified in 1957 by their ability to stimulate [^{35}S] sulfate incorporation into rat cartilage and were termed *sulfation factor.*[177] Concurrent investigations indicated that only a component of the insulin-like activity of normal serum could be blocked by the addition of antiinsulin antibodies. The remaining activity, termed *nonsuppressible insulin-like activity* (NSILA), was subsequently demonstrated to contain two soluble, low-molecular-weight (7 kd) forms, named NSILA-I and -II.[189,190] A third line of investigation arose from studies by Dulak and Temin[191] on the mitogenic nature of bovine serum; the mitogenic factor was termed *multiplication stimulating activity* (MSA) and shares metabolic and mitogenic activities with both sulfation factor and NSILA. It soon became apparent that each of these independent approaches was identifying the same, or greatly similar, proteins.

In 1972, the restrictive labels of *sulfation factor* and *NSILA* were replaced by the term *somatomedin* (SM).[192] The following criteria for a somatomedin were established: (1) the concentration in serum must be GH-dependent; (2) the factor must possess insulin-like activity in extraskeletal tissues; (3) the factor must promote the incorporation of sulfate into cartilage; and (4) the factor must stimulate DNA synthesis and cell multiplication. Purification yielded two somatomedin peptides, a basic peptide (SM-C), and a neutral peptide (SM-A).[193,194] In 1978, Rinderknecht and Humbel[195,196] isolated two active somatomedins from human plasma and after demonstrating a striking structural resemblance to proinsulin, renamed them *insulin-like growth factors* (IGFs).

IGF Structure and Molecular Biology

IGF-I, a basic peptide of 70 amino acids, correlates with SM-C, and IGF-II is a slightly acidic peptide of 67 amino acids. The two peptides share 45 of 73 possible amino acid positions and have approximately 50% amino acid homology to insulin.[178,195,196] Like insulin, both IGFs have A and B chains connected by disulfide bonds. The connecting C-peptide region is 12 amino acids long for IGF-I and 8 amino acids for IGF-II, bearing no homology with the C-peptide region of proinsulin. IGF-I and -II also differ from proinsulin in possessing carboxyl-terminal extensions, or D-peptides, of 8 and 6 amino acids, respectively. This structural similarity explains the ability of both IGFs to bind to the insulin receptor and of insulin to bind to the type I IGF receptor (see below). On the other hand, structural differences probably also explain the failure of insulin to bind with high affinity to the IGF-binding proteins (see later).

IGF Variants

There are several variants of the two IGF peptides. Rinderknecht and Humbel[196] reported that up to one fourth of the IGF-II isolated from human plasma lacked the *N*-terminal alanine. Jansen and colleagues[197] demonstrated that an IGF-II cDNA isolated from a human liver library predicted an IGF-II variant in which Ser^{29} was replaced by Arg-Leu-Pro-Gly, and Zumstein and colleagues[198] identified this variant peptide subsequently in human plasma. Zumstein and colleagues isolated a 10-kd IGF-II variant from human plasma that contains a 21-residue carboxyl-terminal extension, representing a portion of the E domain of proIGF-II (see below). In one peptide fragment isolated, Ser^{33} was replaced by Cys-Gly-Asp. A 25-kd IGF-II variant was isolated by Gowan and associates,[199] presumably representing a carboxyl-terminal extension.

The significance of "big" IGF-II forms is still uncertain. In general, these variants appear capable of binding to IGF and insulin receptors and to IGFBPs, and can participate in formation of the 150-kd (IGF)-(IGFBP-3)-(acid-labile subunit) ternary complex. Big IGF-II can be produced by mesenchymal tumors and can cause non–islet-cell tumor hypoglycemia (NICTH). Daughaday and associates[200] described a patient with a leiomyosarcoma and recurrent hypoglycemia, in whom 70% of serum IGF-II was in higher molecular weight forms. Removal of the tumor eliminated big IGF-II from the serum and corrected the hypoglycemia. The presence of big IGF-II in NICTH has been confirmed in multiple laboratories, but it is unclear why hypoglycemia occurs in the face of normal *total* serum IGF-II levels. Zapf[201] has proposed that NICTH occurs when secretion of big IGF-II results in suppression of GH, insulin, and 7-kd IGF-II, leading to decreased production of IGF-I, IGFBP-3, and the acid-labile subunit and increased production of IGFBP-2. This leads to a shift in the distribution of IGF-II from the 150-kd ternary complex to the 40- to 50-kd molecular weight complex, comprising IGFBP-3, IGFBP-2, and a number of other low-molecular-weight IGFBPs. It is presumed that this results in increased bioavailability of IGF-II to target tissues, enhanced glucose consumption, and decreased hepatic glucose production.

Big forms of IGF-I have not been as thoroughly documented as were IGF-II. Powell and colleagues,[202] however, have reported that IGF-I forms with an apparent molecular weight as high as 19 kd may be found in uremic serum. Large molecular forms of IGF-I have also been identified in conditioned media of human fibroblast cell lines.

Two IGF-I precursor molecules have been identified.[178] The first 134 amino acids of each are identical, comprising the signal peptide (48 amino acids), the mature IGF-I molecule (70 amino acids), and the first 16 amino acids of the E domain of the precursor. IGF-IA has additional 19 amino acids and IGF-IB has additional 61 amino acids (total 195 residues). Alternative splicing of the IGF-I gene presumably generates the two mRNAs. The primary IGF-II translation product in human, rat, and mouse contains 180 amino acids, including a 24-residue signal peptide, the 67 amino acid mature IGF-II sequence, and a carboxyl-terminal E-peptide of 89 amino acids.

The IGF-I Gene (Fig. 23–21)

The IGF genes are expressed differently in the embryo, fetus, child and adult.[178,203-205] Single large genes encode both IGF-I and -II. The human IGF-I gene is located on the long arm of chromosome 12[206,207] and contains at least six exons. Exons 1 and 2 encode alternative signal peptides, probably each containing several transcription start sites. Exons 3 and 4 encode the remaining signal peptide, the remainder of the mature IGF-I molecule and part of the trailer peptide (E-peptide). Exons 5 and 6 encode alternatively used segments of the trailer peptide (resulting in the IGF-IA and IGF-IB forms) and 3′ untranslated sequences with multiple different polyadenylation sites. The wide diversity of IGF-I mRNAs thus reflects (1) multiple leader exons and transcription start sites; (2) alternative splicing of exons 5 or 6; and (3) multiple polyadenylation sites in exon 6.

The IGF-II Gene (Fig. 23–22)

The human IGF-II gene is located on the short arm of chromosome 11[206-208] adjacent to the insulin gene and spans 35 kb of genomic DNA, containing 9 exons. Exons 1-6 encode 5′ untranslated RNA; exon 7 encodes the signal peptide and most of the mature protein, while exon 8 encodes the carboxyl-terminal portion of the protein and part of the trailer peptide, whose coding is completed in exon 9.

Thus, multiple mRNA species exist for both IGF-I and IGF-II allowing for tissue-specific expression of specific transcripts and for developmental and hormonal regulation. The mechanisms involved in the regulation of IGF gene expression include the existence of multiple promoters, heterogeneous transcription initiation within each of the promoters, alternative splicing of various exons, differential RNA polyadenylation, and variable mRNA stability. Translation of IGF-I genes may also be under complex control.

Regulation of IGF Gene Expression

Growth hormone appears to be the primary regulator of IGF-I gene transcription, which begins as early as 30 minutes after intraperitoneal injection of GH into hypophysectomized rats.[209] Transcriptional activation by GH affects both IGF-I promoters equivalently, resulting in a 20-fold rise in IGF-I mRNA. This coordinated, rapid induction of all IGF-I mRNA species coincides with induction of Spi 2.1 gene by GH, although the relationship between these two processes is still not clear.[209] Furthermore there may be tissue to tissue variability in GH-induced expression of IGF-I mRNA.[210] Other factors that influence IGF-I gene expression include estrogen, which stimulates IGF-I mRNA expression in the uterus but inhibits GH-stimulated IGF-I transcription in the liver.[211] The pubertal rise in serum IGF-I levels reflects the effect of gonadal steroids on IGF-I transcription, some of which results from the pubertal rise in GH secretion and some of which is due to a direct effect of gonadal steroids on IGF synthesis or secretion, because a modest pubertal rise in serum IGF levels is also observed in patients with GH insensitivity. Estradiol administration to a GHR-KO mouse stimulates growth and hepatic IGF-I synthesis.[212]

It now appears, as described above, that STAT5b is the most critical mediator of GH-induced activation of IGF-I gene transcription, an observation underscored by studies involving target disruption of the STAT5b gene in mouse models[150-152] and by the reports of two patients with severe GH insensitivity associated with homozygosity for mutations of the STAT5b gene.[153,154] Two adjacent STAT5 binding sites have been identified in the second intron of the rat IGF-I gene, within a region previously identified as undergoing acute changes in chromatin structure after GH treatment.[155]

The factors involved in the regulation of IGF-II gene expression are less clear.[213] In humans and rats, IGF-II gene expression is high in fetal life and has been detected as early as the blastocyst stage in mice.[214] Serum levels of IGF-II are high in midgestation in pregnant rabbits.[215] Fetal tissues generally have high IGF-II mRNA levels that decline postnatally, although brain IGF-II mRNA remains high in the adult rat.[216] IGF-II mRNA is expressed constitutively in a number of mesenchymal and embryonic tumors, including Wilms',[217,218] rhabdomyosarcoma, neuroblastoma, pheochromocytoma, hepatoblastoma, leiomyoma, leiomyosarcoma, liposarcoma, and colon carcinoma.[219-223] Production of "big" IGF-II by these tumors may cause non–islet-cell tumor hypoglycemia (NICTH, see above).[200] A tumor

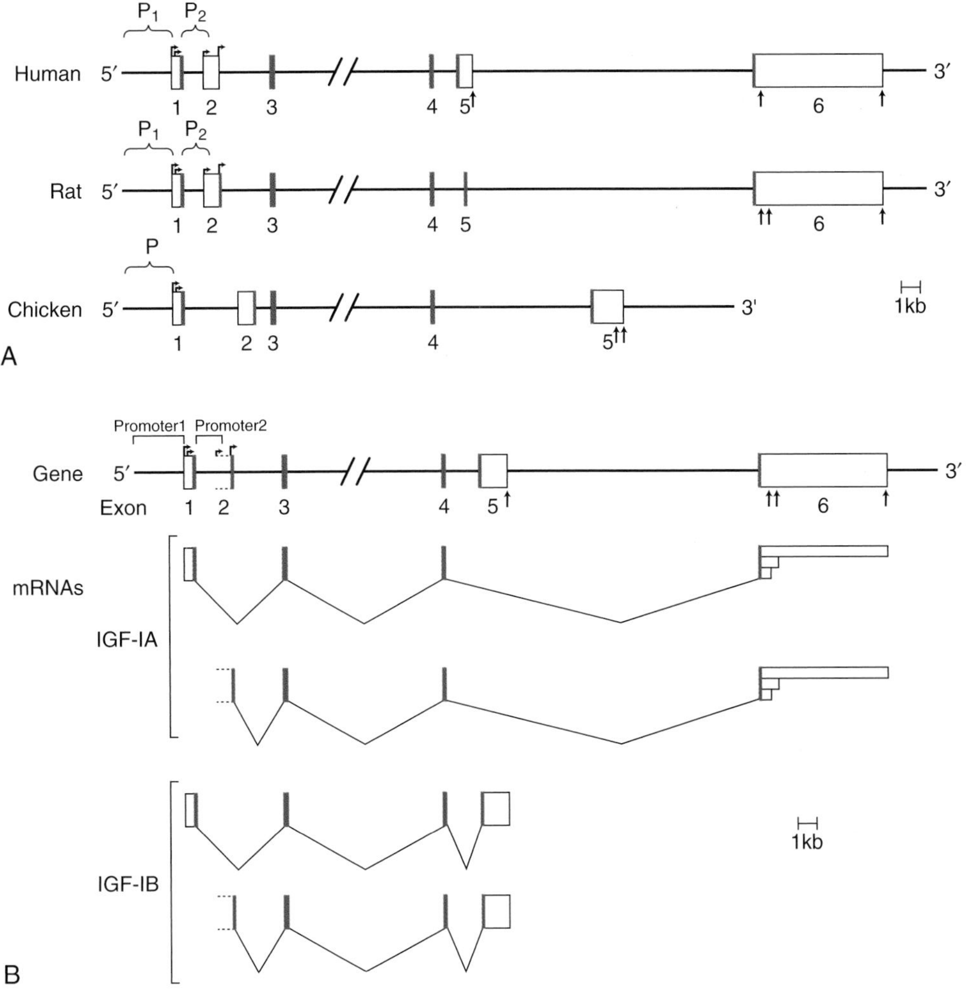

Figure 23–21 ■ Structure of the IGF-I gene. **A,** The organization of the genes encoding human, rat, and chicken IGF-I is depicted. Exons are represented by *boxes* (coding regions are in *black*, noncoding in *white*), polyadenylation sites by arrows, and promoter regions by a bracket and the letter P. The full extent of the second and last human exons and the second rat exon has not been determined, as indicated by the *dotted lines*. **B,** Structure and expression of the human IGF-I gene. The structure of the different human IGF-I mRNAs is displayed below the map of the gene. Sites of pre-mRNA processing are indicated by the *thin lines*. Sites of differential polyadenylation are marked at the 3′ end of the gene by *vertical arrows* and in the mRNAs by *horizontal boxes* of varying length. (From Rotwein P. Structure, evolution, expression and regulation of insulin-like growth factors I and II. Growth Factors 1991;5:3-18.)

suppressor gene associated with Wilms' tumor (WT1) has been mapped to 11p13, close to the IGF-II locus (11p15.5), consistent with the possibility of a direct effect of WT1 on IGF-II gene transcription and suggesting an autocrine role for IGF-II in some tumors.[224,225] This may be relevant in the embryonal tumors of Beckwith-Wiedemann syndrome, in which there may be loss of heterozygosity in the 11p15 maternally derived chromosome and paternal isodisomy, consistent with parental imprinting and a twofold increase in gene dosage of the active IGF-II allele.[226]

IGF Imprinting

Gene regulation for the IGF system may also be subject to genomic imprinting, a process that influences the expression of specific genes. Certain autosomal genes are only expressed from one of the two theoretically available alleles, in a manner that is specific for the parent of origin. The result is a heritable difference in gene expression depending on whether a specific allele is inherited from the mother or the father. Allele-specific imprinting is exemplified by abnormalities of chromosome 15q11-13, where deletions of the paternal chromosome result in the Prader-Willi syndrome (PWS), and deletions of the maternal locus are associated with Angelman syndrome, two phenotypically distinct conditions. The molecular mechanisms responsible for genomic imprinting involve variable DNA methylation.

The first evidence for imprinting in the IGF axis emerged from studies of targeted gene disruption of Igf2 in the mouse[227] that caused fetal growth retardation only when the disrupted allele was inherited from the father (i.e., maternally imprinted).[228] The human IGF-II gene is similarly imprinted.[226,229,230] In tissues where only maternal chromosomes are present, such as ovarian teratomas, no IGF-II expression is observed, whereas gene expression is observed in tissues in which only paternal chromosomes are present (complete hydatidiform mole).[231] Loss of imprinting (or "relaxation" of imprinting) of the IGF-II gene has been observed in rhabdomyosarcomas, lung cancers, Wilms' tumors, and choriocarcinoma.[218,219,222] In such situations, IGF-II may act as an autocrine or paracrine growth factor for neoplastic tissue. Furthermore, in Wilms' tumor, loss of imprinting of the IGF-II gene is associated with reduced expression of the putative tumor suppressor gene H19.[225,232] The H19 gene appears to be imprinted in a reciprocal manner to igf2/IGF2, and the two genes may be coordinately regulated, in that the genes are located near each other on the same chromosome.

The genes for the type II IGF receptor, which is the same as the cation-independent mannose-6-phosphate receptor, are also imprinted, although in a different manner.[233] Thus, the mouse Igf2 receptor gene and the human IGF-2 receptor gene are both expressed by the maternal allele (i.e., paternally imprinted). If IGF-II functions as a fetal growth factor, there is, thus, potential for both maternal and paternal regulation of fetal size.

Targeted Disruption of IGF Genes

The role of the IGF axis in fetal growth has been firmly established by a series of studies involving IGF and IGF receptor null mutations.[234] Unlike GH and GH receptor knockouts,[235,236] which

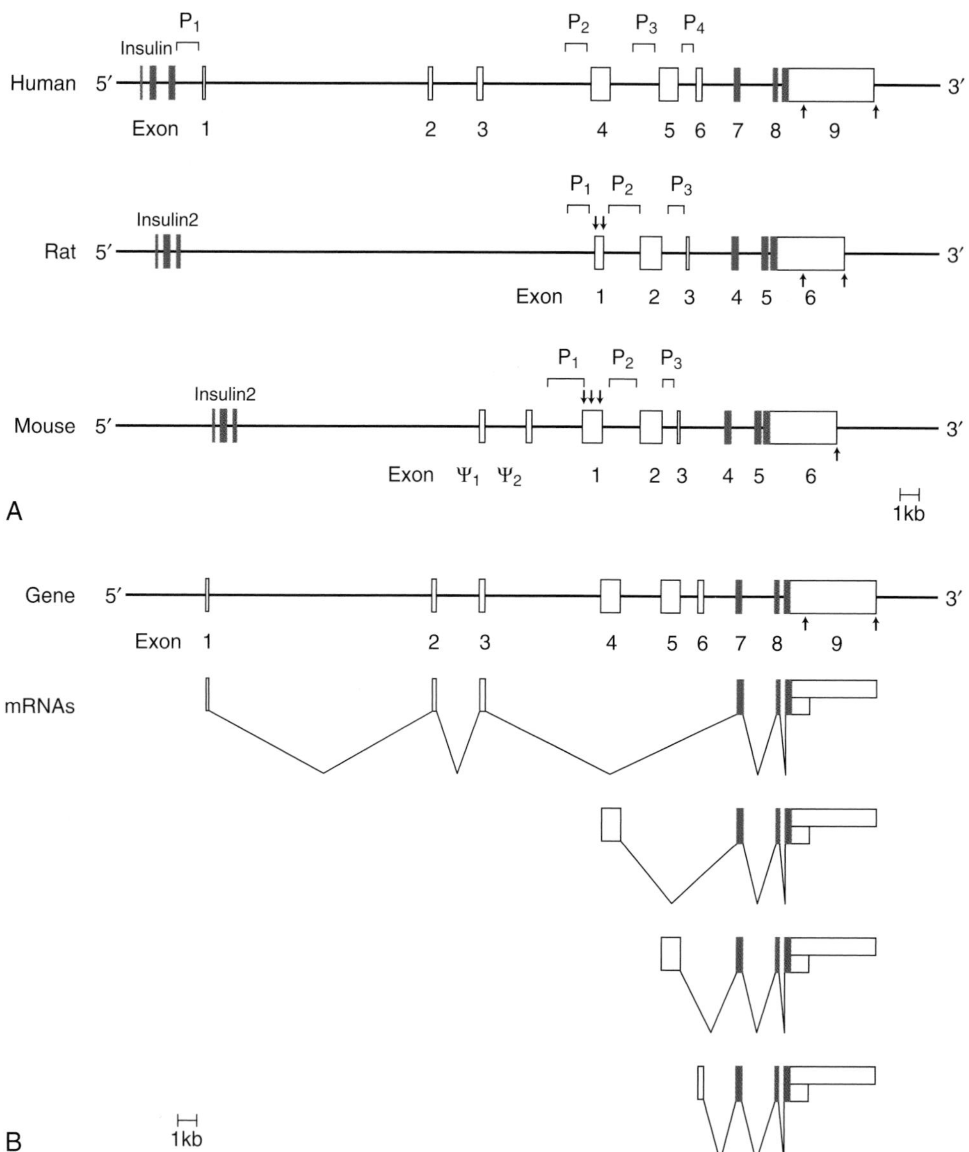

Figure 23–22 ▪ Structure of the IGF-II gene. **A,** The organization of human, rat, and mouse IGF-II genes is shown. Exons are represented by boxes (coding regions are in black and noncoding in white), polyadenylation sites by thick vertical arrows, and promoter regions by a bracket and the letter P. The multiple transcription initiation sites for mouse and rat exon 1 are marked by the thin vertical arrows. The locations of mouse pseudo-exons 1 and 2 are indicated. **B,** Structure and expression of the human IGF-II gene. The structure of different human IGF-II mRNAs is displayed below the map of the gene. The patterns of mRNA processing are indicated by the thin lines. Sites of differential polyadenylation are marked at the 3′ end of the gene by vertical arrows and in the mRNAs by horizontal boxes of varying length. (From Rotwein P. Structure, evolution, expression and regulation of insulin-like growth factors I and II. Growth Factors 1991;5:3-18.)

are near normal size at birth, mice with knockouts of the gene for either IGF-I *or* IGF-II have birthweights approximately 60% of normal.[227,228,237] Mouse mutants lacking both IGF-I and the GH receptor are only 17% of normal size.[188] These observations indicate that both IGF-I and IGF-II are important embryonic and fetal growth factors, but that GH itself does have some modest apparent IGF-independent roles as well. Although fetal size was proportionately reduced in both situations and although morphogenesis was grossly normal, a higher neonatal death rate was observed following disruption of the gene for IGF-I. Growth delay began on day e11 for IGF-II knockouts and on day e13.5 for IGF-I knockouts. Those mice with IGF-I gene disruptions who survived the immediate neonatal period continued to have growth failure postnatally, with weights 30% of normal by 2 months of age. Indeed, postnatal growth was poorer than that observed in mice with GH-R, GHRH receptor mutations, or pit-1 mutations, indicating that both GH-dependent and GH-independent factors are necessary for normal growth. A similar prenatal and postnatal growth phenotype has been observed in the one reported case of an IGF-I gene deletion,[238] as well as a more recent report of a bioinactive IGF-I molecule, resulting from a missense mutation,[239] thereby supporting the critical role of IGF-I in both prenatal and postnatal growth. When the genes for both IGF-I and IGF-II were disrupted, weight at birth was only 30% of normal, and all animals died shortly after birth, apparently from respiratory insufficiency secondary to muscular hypoplasia. Specific ablation of hepatic IGF-I production through the Cre/loxP recombination system confirmed that the liver is the principal source of circulating IGF-I, but demonstrated that an 80% lowering of serum IGF-I levels had no apparent effect on postnatal growth[240-243] suggesting that postnatal growth was relatively independent of hepatic IGF-I production. Presumably, either local (paracrine) chondrocyte production of IGF-I or other tissues (perhaps adipose) maintain adequate endocrine sources of IGF-I to account for growth preservation, or, alternatively, free IGF-I levels remained within the normal range as a result of the reciprocal increase in GH production, as well as the lowering of serum IGFBPs. Supportive data for the predominant role in growth of locally produced IGF-I is the only modest decrement of postnatal growth seen in ALS null mice.[244] These murine models are complex, as IGFBP-3 levels are reduced despite increased GH and, in contrast to the human, rise after treatment with exogenous IGF-I. Furthermore, the "free" IGF-I levels are normal in these animals but do not prevent an increment of GH production.[242,245]

By crossing the liver-derived IGF-I gene-deleted mice (LID) with acid labile subunit (ALS) gene-deleted mice (ALSKO), an 85% to 90% reduction in serum IGF-I was achieved, and, in this case, early postnatal growth retardation was observed.[246] These findings suggest that postnatal growth is dependent upon both endocrine (i.e., hepatic) and tissue IGF-I, although definite conclusions are problematic in the face of the elevated GH production and perturbations of the IGFBP system observed in these studies.

Knockout of the gene for the type 1 IGF receptor resulted in birthweights 45% of normal and 100% neonatal lethality.[247] Abuzzahab and colleagues[248] have reported two patients with intrauterine growth retardation and postnatal growth failure, despite elevated serum IGF-I concentrations. One patient was a compound heterozygote for point mutations in exon 2 of the IGF-1R gene, leading to decreased receptor affinity for IGF-I, while the second had a nonsense mutation of one allele, resulting in reduced numbers of IGF-1 receptors. In mice, concurrent knockout of genes for IGF-I and the type 1 IGF receptor resulted in no further reduction in birth size (45% of normal), consistent with the concept that all IGF-I actions in fetal life are mediated through this receptor. On the other hand, simultaneous knockout of the genes for IGF-II and the type 1 IGF receptor resulted in further reduction of birth size to 30% of normal (as with simultaneous knockouts of IGF-I and IGF-II), suggesting that some of the fetal anabolic actions of IGF-II are mediated by a secondary mechanism (perhaps, placental growth or IGF-II interactions with the insulin receptor). This pathway does not appear to involve the type 2 IGF receptor, because knockout of this paternally imprinted gene results in an *increased* birthweight but death in late gestation or at birth.[249] Because this receptor normally degrades IGF-II, increased growth reflects excess IGF-II acting through the IGF-I receptor; there is, however, variable accumulation of IGF-II in such mouse tissues.[250] Knockout of the type 2 IGF receptor plus IGF-II causes a birthweight 60% of normal (as is the case with knockout of IGF-II alone), but allows fetal survival.[251]

Several conclusions can be drawn from these studies: (1) IGF-I is important for both fetal and postnatal growth; (2) IGF-II is a major fetal growth factor, but has little, if any, role in postnatal growth; (3) the type 1 IGF receptor mediates anabolic actions of both IGF-I and IGF-II; (4) the type 2 IGF receptor is bifunctional, serving to both target lysosomal enzymes and to enhance IGF-II turnover; (5) IGF-I production is involved in normal fertility; (6) placental growth is only impaired with IGF-II knockouts; (7) GH and the GHR play little role in prenatal growth; (8) IGF-I is the major mediator of GH's effects on postnatal growth, although GH and the GHR may have a small IGF-independent effect. Whether these studies in mice are fully applicable to humans is yet unknown.

IGF Peptide Assays

Bioassay methods for IGF activity have included stimulation of [^{35}S] sulfate incorporation, using various modifications of the original method described by Salmon and Daughaday.[177,252,253] A wide variety of other bioassays have utilized stimulation of the synthesis of DNA,[254] RNA,[255] or protein[256] or of glucose uptake.[256] Such assays are cumbersome, subject to interference by IGFBPs, and incapable of distinguishing between IGF-I and IGF-II. When SM-C (and later, IGF-I and IGF-II) was purified, it became possible to develop radioreceptor (RRA)[257,258] and competitive protein binding assays[259,260]; development of specific antibodies permitted the development of accurate and specific measurement of IGF I and IGF II.[261-265]

The issue of IGFBPs must be dealt with in any IGF assay.[266] For example, the discrepant results found in uremic sera assayed for IGF by bioassay, RRA, and immunoassay are due to the interference of IGFBPs[267]; such interference is a particular problem in conditions with a relatively high IGFBP/IGF peptide ratio and at the extremes of the assay (i.e., GH deficiency or acromegaly). The most effective way to deal with IGFBPs is to separate them from IGF peptides by chromatography under acidic conditions.[268] This is, however, a labor-intensive procedure, and has been occasionally replaced by an acid ethanol extraction procedure.[269] While this latter method may be reasonably effective for most serum samples, it is problematic in conditions of high IGFBP/IGF peptide ratios, such as conditioned media from cell lines and sera from newborns and from subjects with GH deficiency or uremia.

Alternative methodologies include the use of antibodies generated against synthetic peptides, such as the C-peptide region of IGF-I or -II, which does not bind to IGFBPs. In general, such antibodies have high specificity, but relatively low affinity. An alternative approach, developed by Blum and colleagues,[270] involves use of an antibody with high specificity for IGF-II, which permits the addition of excess unlabeled IGF-I to saturate endogenous IGFBPs. Bang and associates[271] have bypassed the interference of IGFBPs by employing a truncated IGF-I radioligand, which has decreased affinity for IGFBPs. At the current time, the most practical and effective way to perform accurate IGF assays with minimal interference by IGFBPs is to utilize the "sandwich" assay method.[272] These assays, which can be performed in either ELISA or IRMA, do not employ a radiolabeled IGF molecule, which can bind to IGFBPs, as in conventional RIAs, and lead to erroneous readings if IGFBPs are elevated.[273] The absolute IGF values obtained in many of the assays may be falsely high because of low purity and inconsistent amino acid analyses of local standards, but this can be avoided by the use of the WHO IRR 87/518 calibration standard, although questions have been raised concerning the purity of even this preparation.[274] Most importantly, to date no valid interlaboratory comparative studies of serum IGF-I concentrations have been published. Thus, although there appear to be any number of clinically useful IGF-I assays, each laboratory must develop its own population-specific reference ranges. Even here, care must be taken to assure that the "normative data" derive from a properly analyzed subject sample that matches the clinical samples to be tested, as ethnic variations, as well as nutritional and environmental factors may impact "normal" serum IGF-I concentrations.

In recent years, a number of assays have been developed that purport to measure "free" or "free dissociable" IGF-I as a means of assessing concentrations of IGF-I peptides that circulate unbound to IGFBPs.[275] Both the accuracy and the physiologic relevance of these determinations remain open to debate, in that liver-derived IGF-I appears to enter the circulation already complexed with high-affinity IGFBPs. The relative contributions of nonhepatic IGF-I production and IGFBP proteolysis to the generation of free IGF-I remain to be resolved.

Serum Levels of IGF Peptides

In human fetal serum, IGF-I levels are relatively low and are positively correlated with gestational age.[276,277] Some,[276-278] but not all, groups[279] have reported a correlation between fetal cord serum IGF-I levels and birthweight. IGF-I levels in human newborn serum are generally 30% to 50% of adult levels. Serum levels rise during childhood and attain adult levels at the onset of sexual maturation[280] (Fig. 23–23). During puberty, IGF-I levels rise to 2 to 3 times the adult range, reflecting a phase of "physiological acromegaly" characteristic of adolescence.[281] Thus, levels during adolescence correlate better with Tanner stage (or

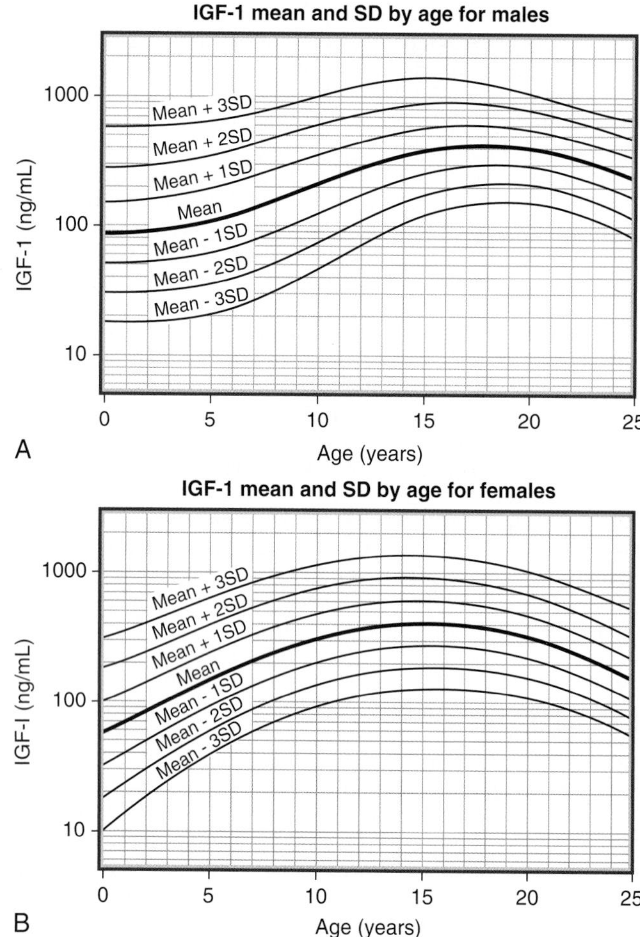

Figure 23–23 ▪ Normal serum levels of IGF-I (μg/L) for males **(A)** and females **(B)**. Lines represent the mean±3 SD. (Data courtesy of Diagnostic Systems Laboratories, Inc., Webster, TX.)

bone age) than with chronologic age. Girls with gonadal dysgenesis show no adolescent increase in serum IGF-I, clearly establishing the association of the pubertal rise in IGF-I with the production of gonadal steroids.[282-284] The pubertal rise in gonadal steroids may stimulate IGF-I production indirectly, by first leading to a rise in GH secretion, but patients with GH insensitivity due to GH receptor mutations show a modest pubertal rise in serum IGF-I despite a *decline* in GH levels, thereby suggesting a direct effect of gonadal steroids upon IGF-I.[92]

After adolescence, or at least after 20 to 30 years of age, serum IGF-I levels demonstrate a gradual and progressive age-associated fall,[285,286] a decline that is possibly responsible for the negative nitrogen balance, decrease in muscle mass, and osteoporosis characteristic of aging.[285] This provocative hypothesis is unproven but has generated interest in the potential use of GH and/or IGF-I therapy in normal aging.

Human newborn levels of IGF-II are generally 50% of adult levels. By 1 year of age, however, adult levels are attained, with little, if any subsequent decline, even up to the seventh or eighth decade. This pattern of IGF-II levels in humans is different than that in the rat or mouse, in which serum IGF-II levels are also high in the fetus but rapidly decline postnatally to undetectable levels in the adult.[287,288]

Measurement of IGF Levels in Growth Disorders

The GH dependency of the IGFs was established in the initial report from Salmon and Daughaday[177] and further clarified with the development of sensitive and specific immunoassays that distinguish between IGF-I and IGF-II.[264] IGF-I levels are more GH-dependent than are IGF-II levels and are more likely to reflect subtle differences in GH secretory patterns. However, serum IGF-I levels, as stated above, are influenced by age, degree of sexual maturation, and nutritional status, as well. As a result, construction of age-defined normative values is important, but problematic. IGF-I levels in normal children younger than 5 years of age are low and there is overlap between the normal range and values in GH-deficient children. Assessment of serum IGF-II levels is less age-dependent, especially after 1 year of age, but IGF-II is less GH-dependent than is IGF-I.

Moore and colleagues[289] performed GH stimulation tests in 78 children with heights below the 5th percentile and serum IGF-I levels <0.5 U/mL. While 19 of these children were subsequently diagnosed as GH deficient on the basis of standard provocative tests, there was overlap of serum IGF-I levels between GH-deficient children and children with other forms of short stature and normal provocative GH levels. It was only in children with bone ages >12 years that serum IGF-I levels permitted discrimination between GH deficiency and normal short children. Similarly, Reiter and Lovinger[290] found that 4 of 16 children with low provocative GH levels had normal serum IGF-I levels, whereas 7 of 25 children with normal provocative GH levels had low serum IGF-I levels.

Rosenfeld and colleagues[265] evaluated the efficacy of IGF-I and IGF-II measurements in 68 GH-deficient patients, 197 children with normal stature, and 44 normal children with short stature (Figs. 23–24 and 23–25). Eighteen percent of the putative GH-deficient children had serum IGF-I levels within the normal range for age, and 32% of normal short children had low IGF-I levels. Low IGF-II levels were found in 52% of GH-deficient children and in 35% of normal short children. However, the use of combined IGF-I/IGF-II assays provided better discrimination. Only 4% of GH-deficient children had normal plasma levels of both IGF-I and IGF-II. Furthermore, only 0.5% of normal children and 11% of normal short children had low serum levels of both IGF-I and IGF-II.

The observation that many "normal short" children have low serum levels of IGF-I, IGF-II, or both, calls into question the criteria by which the diagnosis of GH deficiency is made. Given that provocative GH testing is both arbitrary and nonphysiologic and given the inherent variability in GH assays, it is not surprising that the correlation between IGF-I levels and provocative GH levels is imperfect. These points are further supported by recent observations with immunoassays for IGFBP-3 (see below).

Given the critical role of the IGF system in mammalian growth and, in particular, the influence of IGF-I on postnatal growth, Rosenfeld proposed in 1996 that the term *IGF deficiency* (IGFD) be employed for diagnostic categorization.[291] This concept has been expanded by subcategorizing IGFD into secondary (i.e., resulting from defects of GH production) and primary states (i.e., resulting from defects of GH sensitivity or IGF-I gene deletions/mutations).[292,293] The concept of IGFD is expanded below.

IGF Receptors

The binding of IGFs to the insulin receptor provides an explanation for their insulin-like activity.[294] Shortly thereafter, Megyesi and coworkers[295] identified distinct receptors for insulin and IGF in rat hepatic membranes. At least two classes of IGF receptors exist; insulin, at high levels, competes for occupancy of one form of IGF receptor, but has essentially no affinity for the second form of receptor.

Structural characterization of these receptors documented the differences in the two forms of receptor (Fig. 23–26).[296,297] The type 1 IGF receptor is closely related to the insulin receptor;

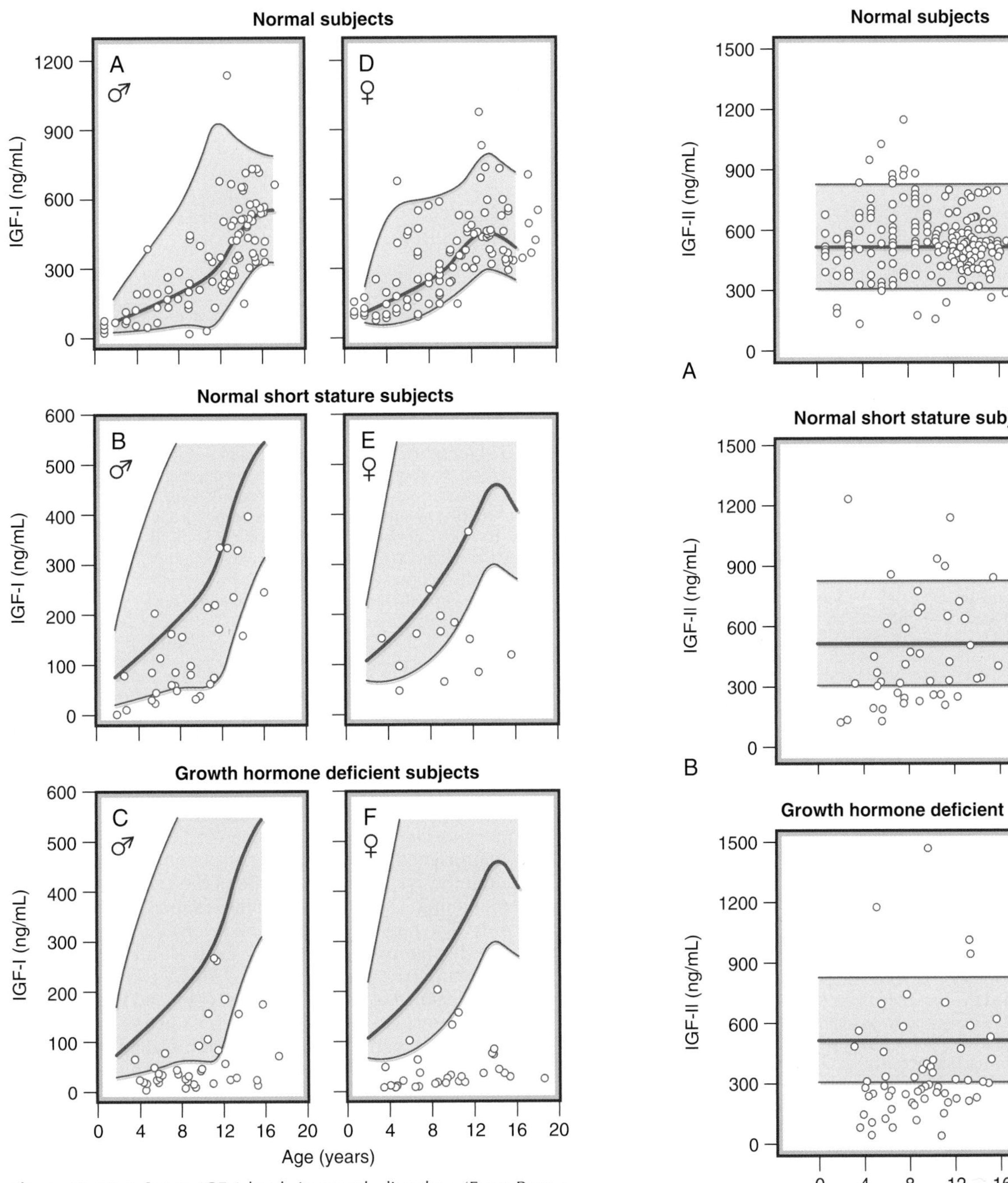

Figure 23–24 ■ Serum IGF-1 levels in growth disorders. (From Rosenfeld RG, Wilson DM, Lee PD, et al. Insulin-like growth factors I and II in the evaluation of growth retardation. J Pediatr 1986;109:428-433.)

Figure 23–25 ■ Serum IGF-II levels in growth disorders. (From Rosenfeld RG, Wilson DM, Lee PD, et al. Insulin-like growth factors I and II in the evaluation of growth retardation. J Pediatr 1986;109:428-433.)

both are heterotetramers comprising two membrane-spanning α subunits and two intracellular β subunits. The α subunits contain the binding sites for IGF-I and are linked by disulfide bonds. The β subunits contain a transmembrane domain and an adenosine triphosphate (ATP)-binding site and a tyrosine kinase domain that constitute the presumed signal transduction mechanism for the receptor. One mole of the full heterotetrameric receptor appears to bind 1 mole of ligand.

Although the type 1 IGF receptor has been commonly termed the "IGF-I receptor," the receptor binds both IGF-I and IGF-II with high affinity, and both IGF peptides appear capable of activating tyrosine kinase by binding to this receptor. In studies involving transfection and overexpression of the type 1 IGF receptor cDNA, the K_DD for IGF-I is typically in the 0.2- to 1-nM range; affinity for IGF-II is usually slightly less, but varies from study to study. The affinity of the type 1 receptor for insulin is generally 100-fold less, thereby explaining the relatively weak mitogenic effect of insulin.

Ullrich and coworkers[298] deduced the structure of the human type 1 IGF receptor from cDNA; the mature peptide constitutes 1337 amino acids with a predicted molecular mass of 151,869 (Fig. 23–27). The translated α-β heterodimer is subsequently

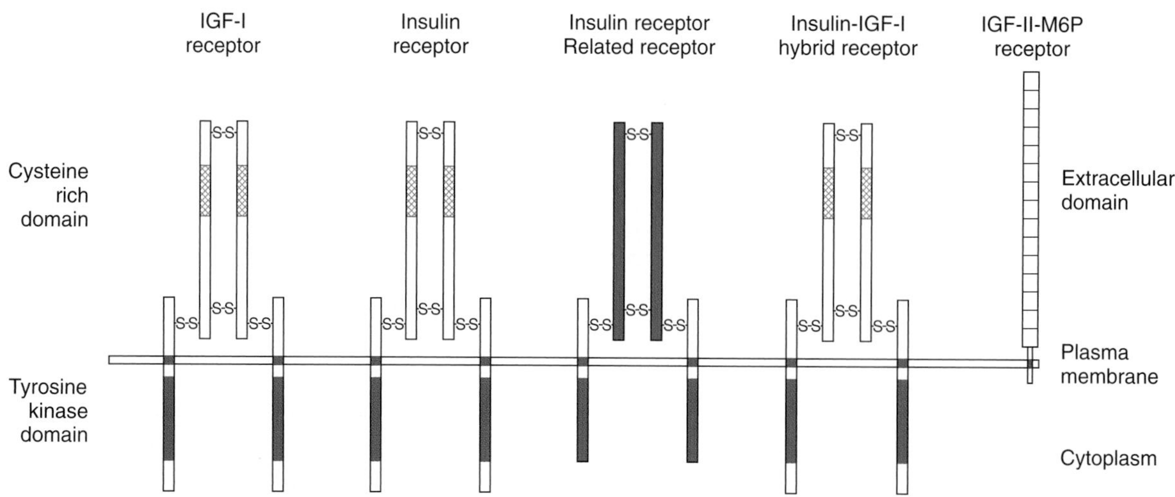

Figure 23–26 ▪ Structure of the IGF receptors. The insulin and IGF-I receptors are both heterotetrameric complexes composed of extracellular α-subunits that bind the ligands and β-subunits that anchor the receptor in the membrane and that contain tyrosine kinase activity in their cytoplasmic domains. The tyrosine kinase domain of the insulin receptor related receptor (IRR) is homologous to the tyrosine kinase domains of the insulin and IGF-I receptors. The C-terminal domain is deleted in the IRR. Hybrids consist of a hemireceptor from both insulin and IGF-I receptors. The IGF-II/M6P receptor is not structurally related to the IGF-I and insulin receptors or the IRR, having a short cytoplasmic tail and no tyrosine kinase activity. (From LeRoith D, Werner H, Geitner-Johnson D, et al. Molecular and cellular aspects of the insulin-like growth factor I receptor. Endocr Rev 1995;16:143-163).

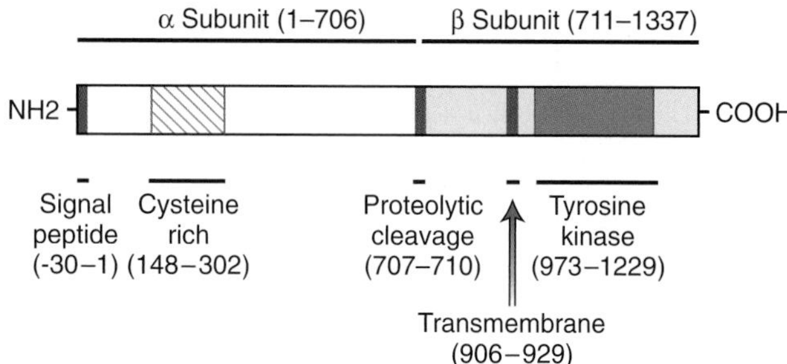

Figure 23–27 ▪ Structure of the human IGF-I receptor precursor. Molecular cloning of human IGF-I receptor cDNAs isolated from a placental library revealed the presence of an open reading frame of 4101 nucleotides. The 1367 amino acid polypeptide contains, at its N-terminus, a 30 amino acid hydrophobic signal peptide, which is responsible for the transfer of the nascent protein chain into the endoplasmic reticulum. After digestion by endopeptidases at a proteolytic cleavage site (Arg-Lys-Arg-Arg) located at residues 707-710, α and β subunits are released and linked by disulfide bonds to give the configuration of the mature heterotetrameric receptor. Shown in this diagrammatic representation are, in addition, the cysteine-rich domain of the α subunit and the transmembrane and tyrosine kinase domains of the β subunit. (From LeRoith D, Werner H, Beitner-Johnson D, et al. Molecular and cellular aspects of the insulin-like growth factor I receptor. Endocr Rev 1995;16:143-163.)

cleaved at an Arg-Lys-Arg-Arg sequence at positions 707-710, and the released α and β subunits are linked by disulfide bonds to form the mature $(\alpha\beta)_2$-receptor in which two α chains are joined by secondary disulfide bonds. The α subunits are extracellular and contain a cysteine-rich domain, which is critical for IGF binding. As is the case with the insulin receptor, the β subunit has a short extracellular domain, a hydrophobic transmembrane domain, and the intracellular tyrosine kinase domain and ATP binding site. Like the insulin receptor, the type 1 IGF receptor undergoes ligand-induced autophosphorylation, principally on tyrosines 1131, 1135, and 1136.[299-302] Both the insulin and type 1 IGF receptors are believed to have evolved from a common ancestor protein but are encoded by genes on separate chromosomes (chromosome 15 for the type 1 IGF receptor[303] and chromosome 19 for the insulin receptor).

The type 1 IGF receptor gene spans greater than 100 kb of genomic DNA, with 21 exons; the genomic organization resembles that of the insulin receptor gene.[298,304] Exons 1-3 code for the 5′ untranslated region, the signal peptide, the N-terminal region, and the cysteine-rich domain of the α subunit involved in ligand binding. The remainder of the α subunit is encoded by exons 4–10. The peptide cleavage site involved in generation of the α and β subunits is encoded by exon 11, and the tyrosine kinase domain of the β subunit is encoded by exons 16–20. It is in the latter region that the type 1 IGF receptor and insulin receptor share the greatest sequence homology, ranging from 80% to 95%; interspecies homology in this region of the receptors is also high. Exon 21 encodes 3′-untranslated sequences.

Type 1 IGF receptor mRNA has been identified in virtually every tissue except liver.[305,306] By Northern blot hybridization, human mRNA reveals two bands of 11 and 7 kb; in rat tissues, only the 11 kb band is observed.[307] Type 1 IGF receptor mRNA is most abundant in embryonic tissues, and appears to decrease with age. The type 1 IGF receptor is present at the embryonic 8-cell stage (the type 2 IGF receptor is first demonstrable at the 2-cell stage) and becomes widely expressed postimplantation, consistent with the observation that this receptor is essential for normal fetal growth.

As with other growth factor receptor tyrosine kinases, binding of ligand (IGF-I or IGF-II) induces receptor autophosphorylation of critical tyrosine residues in the type 1 receptor.[299-302] Mutations of the ATP-binding site or of critical tyrosine residues in the β subunit result in loss of IGF-stimulated thymidine incorporation and glucose uptake. Autophosphorylation appears to occur by transphosphorylation of sites on the opposite β subunit.[308,309] The activated type 1 IGF receptor is capable of phosphorylating other tyrosine-containing substrates, such as IRS-1 (insulin receptor substrate 1), a 185-kd protein that is the predominant substrate of the insulin receptor kinase and IRS-2 (Fig. 23–28).[310] IRS-1 contains specific phosphotyrosine

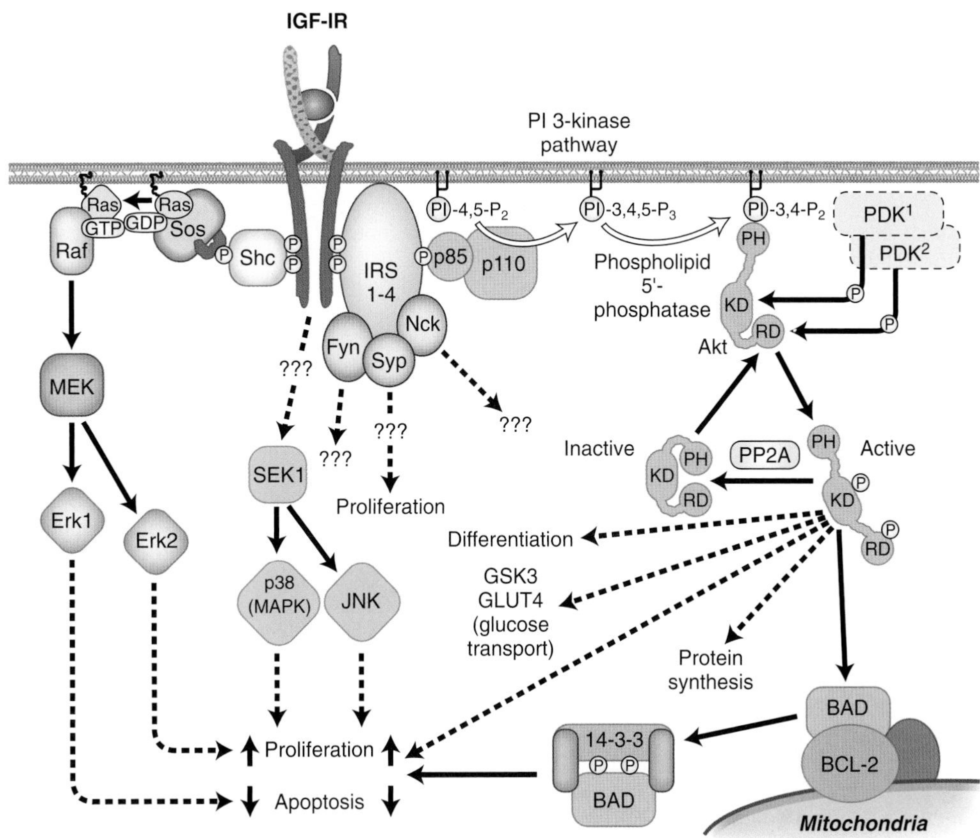

Figure 23–28 ▪ Schematic representation of intracellular signaling pathways of the IGF-I receptor. Upon binding IGF-I, the IGF-receptor undergoes autophosphorylation at multiple tyrosine residues. The intrinsic kinase activity of the receptor also phosphorylates IRS-1 at multiple tyrosine residues. Various SH domain–containing proteins, including PI 3-kinase, Syp, Fyn, and Nck, associate with specific phosphotyrosine-containing motifs within IRS-1. These docking proteins recruit diverse other intracellular substrates, which then activate a cascade of protein kinases including Raf-1 and one or more related kinases, MAP kinases (or MEKs), the MAP kinases, and others. These protein kinases, in turn, activate various other elements, including nuclear transcription factors. Alterations in expression of various IGF-I–responsive genes result in longer-term effects of IGF-I, including growth and differentiation. This model of signal transduction cascades also shows a potential mechanism for inhibition of apoptosis. (From Le Roith D, Bondy C, Yakar S, et al. The somatomedin hypothesis: 2001. Endocrine Rev 2001;22:53-74.)

motifs that can associate with proteins containing SH2 (src homology 2) domains, such as PI3-kinase (phosphatidylinositol-3 kinase),[311] Grb2 (growth factor receptor-bound protein 2),[312] Syp (a phosphotyrosine phosphatase),[311] and Nck (an oncogenic protein).[313] The substrates, which are phosphorylated by the IGF receptor, include the members of the IRS family, particularly IRS-1 and IRS-2, and both of the knockout mice models for these genes result in poor growth (as well as insulin resistance).[314] Other IRS molecules may have a negative feedback role in regulating IGF action.[315] Activation of the type 1 IGF receptor also leads to tyrosine phosphorylation of Shc (src homology domain-containing protein),[316] which then associates with Grb2 and activates Ras, leading to a cascade of protein kinases, including Raf, MAP kinase kinases, MAP kinases, and S6 kinase.[317-319] Thus, phosphorylation of IRS-1 by either the type 1 IGF or insulin receptor activates multiple signaling cascades that ultimately influence nuclear transcription and gene expression. It is, presumably, at this level that the IGF peptides exert their mitogenic and anabolic actions. Given that insulin and IGF peptides activate similar, if not identical, signaling pathways through their own specific receptors, it is unclear how the cell distinguishes between these overlapping ligands. Whether this merely reflects the relative levels of receptors or whether divergent downstream pathways exist for insulin and IGF action remain questions for future investigation.[320]

While targeted disruption of the gene for the type 1 IGF receptor causes fetal growth retardation, a clear role for this receptor in the cell cycle has not been established. Fibroblast cell lines derived from mouse embryos homozygous for the knockout gene still undergo cell cycle–dependent division, although at a slower rate.[321-323] On the other hand, the transformed phenotype of some cells may be critically dependent upon expression of the type 1 IGF receptor. The SV40TAg is capable of inducing a transformed phenotype in a cell only in the presence of intact type 1 IGF receptors.[323] NIH 3T3 cells and Rat-1 fibroblasts that are made to overexpress the type 1 IGF receptor develop IGF-I–dependent neoplastic transformation, with colony formation in soft agar and tumor formation in nude rats.[324] Prager and associates[325] have shown that truncation of the type 1 IGF receptor at the amino terminus increases transforming potential, suggesting that the α subunit normally restricts this function and that the binding of IGF to the receptor releases constraints on mitogenic stimulation.

Variants of both the α and β subunits are present in placenta,[326] muscle,[326,327] and brain.[328] These variants may explain seemingly anomalous competitive binding studies.[329-331] The molecular mechanisms for the formation of such receptor variants have not been identified, nor is it clear if they differentially bind IGF-I, IGF-II, or insulin. The formation of IGF-insulin receptor hybrids that contain an α-IGF hemireceptor disulfide-linked to an α-insulin hemireceptor (see Fig. 23–26)[332-334] appears to be ligand-dependent,[335] and studies with monoclonal antibodies specific for the insulin or type 1 IGF receptor suggest that such receptors develop in cells with abundant native receptors, such as muscle and placenta.[336,337] Such hybrids have near-normal affinity for IGF-I but decreased affinity for insulin. The physiologic significance of such hybrid receptors is unknown.

The type 2 IGF receptor bears no structural homology with either the insulin or type 1 IGF receptors. It has an apparent M_r=220,000 under nonreducing conditions and 250,000 after reduction, indicating that it is a monomeric protein. The cloned human type 2 receptor cDNA predicts a molecular mass of 270,294 and a lengthy extracellular domain containing 15 repeat sequences of 147 residues each, a 23-residue transmembrane domain, and a small cytoplasmic domain consisting of only 164 residues.[338] The receptor does not contain an intrinsic tyrosine kinase domain or any other recognized signal transduction mechanism. The type 2 IGF receptor is identical to the cation-independent mannose-6-phosphate (CIM6P) receptor, a protein involved in the intracellular lysosomal targeting of acid hydrolases and other mannosylated proteins.[339,340] Most of these receptors are located on intracellular membranes, in equilibrium with receptors on the plasma membrane.[341]

Why this receptor binds both IGF-II and M6P-containing lysosomal enzymes is unknown. Unlike the type 1 IGF receptor, which binds both IGF peptides with high affinity and insulin with 100-fold lower affinity, the type 2 receptor only binds IGF-II with high affinity, the K_D ranging from 0.017 to 0.7 nM; IGF-I binds with lower affinity, and insulin does not bind at all.[341] One mole of IGF-II binds per mole of receptor. IGF-II and M6P bind to different portions of the receptor, but the two ligands do show some reciprocal inhibitory effects upon receptor binding, suggesting that IGF-II may affect the sorting of lysosomal enzymes. Alternatively, this receptor may be important to the degradation of IGF-II. Knockout of the gene for the type 2 IGF receptor in mice causes macrosomia and fetal death, consistent with a potential role in IGF-II degradation.

The mitogenic and metabolic actions of both IGF-I and IGF-II appear to be mediated through the type 1 IGF receptor because monoclonal antibodies directed against the IGF-I binding site on the type 1 IGF receptor inhibit the ability of both IGF-I and IGF-II to stimulate thymidine incorporation and cell replication.[342,343] Similarly, polyclonal antibodies that block IGF-II binding to the type 2 IGF/M6P receptor do not block IGF-II actions.[344-346] In addition, IGF-II analogues with decreased affinity for the type 1 receptor but preserved affinity for the type II receptor are less potent than IGF-II in stimulating DNA synthesis.[195] Interestingly, the M6P receptor in hepatic tissues from chicken[347] or frog[348] does not bind IGF-II. Presumably, the mitogenic actions of IGF-II in these species are mediated solely through the type 1 IGF receptor.

Nevertheless, some IGF-II actions may be mediated via the type 2 IGF receptor. Rogers and Hammerman[349] have suggested that the type 2 receptor is involved in production of inositol triphosphate and diacylglycerol in proximal tubules and canine kidney membranes. Tally and coworkers[329] have reported that IGF-II stimulates the growth of a K562 human erythroleukemia cell line, an action not duplicated by either IGF-I or insulin. Minniti and colleagues[330] reported that IGF-II appears capable of acting as an autocrine growth factor and cell motility factor for human rhabdomyosarcoma cells, actions apparently mediated through the type 2 receptor, and IGF-II may activate a calcium-permeable cation channel via the type 2 IGF receptor, perhaps through coupling to a pertussis toxin–sensitive guanine nucleotide binding protein (G_i protein).[331,335,350-353] In cells transfected with the human type 2 IGF receptor cDNA, IGF-II decreased cAMP accumulation promoted by cholera toxin or forskolin. Mutations or truncation of the small cytoplasmic domain of the receptor prevented these IGF-II actions. The type 2 IGF receptor also binds other molecules such as M6P-containing enzymes (e.g., cathepsin and urokinase), which may be important in the removal of these enzymes from the cellular environment, thus modulating tissue remodeling.[354] In addition, the type 2 IGF receptor binds retinoic acid and may mediate some of the growth inhibitory effects of retinoids.[355] As discussed earlier, knockout of the type 2 IGF receptor results in excessive growth so this receptor may act as a growth inhibitory component of the IGF system responding to and mediating multiple antimitogenic systems.[356]

IGF Binding Proteins (Fig. 23–29)

In contrast to insulin the IGFs circulate in plasma complexed to a family of binding proteins that extend the serum half-life of the IGF peptides, transport the IGFs to target cells, and modulate the interaction of the IGFs with surface membrane receptors.[357,358] The identification and characterization of IGFBPs in body fluids[359] and in conditioned media from cultured cells has been facilitated by the development of a number of biochemical and assay techniques, including gel chromatography, radioreceptor assays, affinity cross-linking, Western ligand blotting,[360] immunoblotting, and specific radioimmunoassays. However, study of

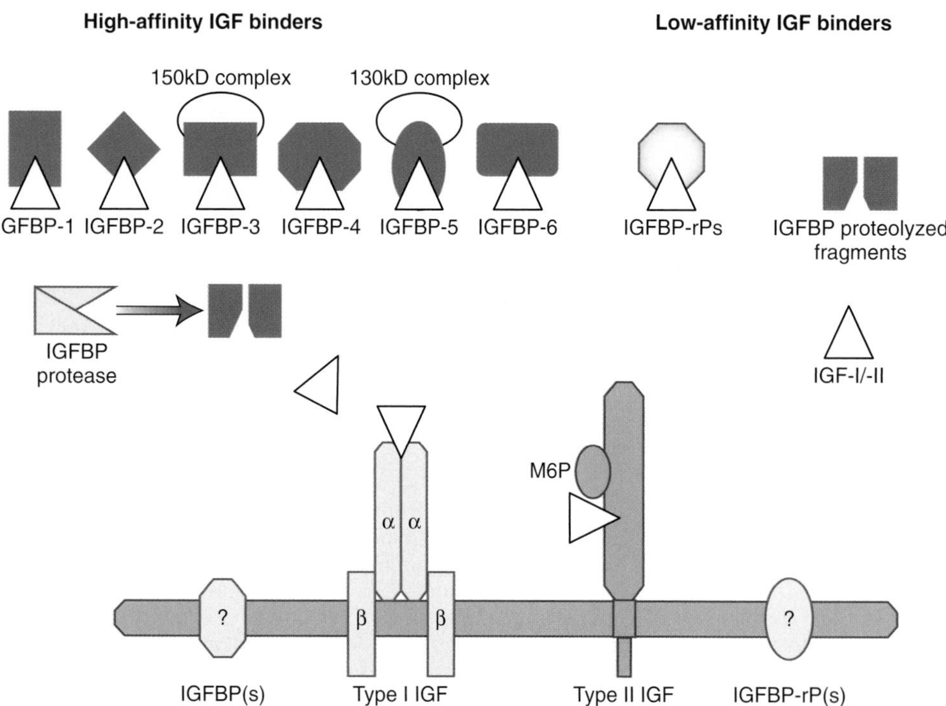

Figure 23–29 ▪ Schematic representation of the IGF system, including IGF ligands (IGF-I and II), binding proteins (both high- and low-affinity binders), IGFBP proteases, type I and type II IGF receptors, and potential IGFBP(s) and IGFBP-rP(s) receptors. *MCP,* Mannose-6-phosphate. (From Hwa V, Oh Y, Rosenfeld RG. The insulin-like growth factor-binding protein [IGFBP] superfamily. Endocr Rev 1999;20:761-787, copyright Endocrine Society.)

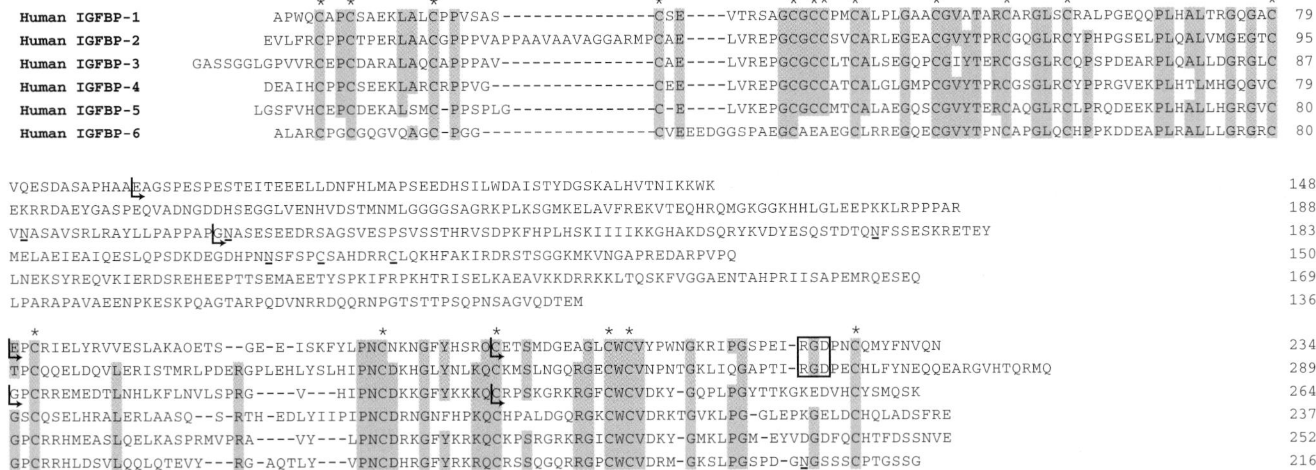

Figure 23–30 ■ Amino acid sequences of human IGFBP 1-6, deduced from nucleotide sequences. Sequences in the amino terminal and carboxy terminal residues are aligned to show maximal homologies. Dashes indicate gaps. Residues that are identical in five or six of the six IGFBPs are shaded. (From Rechler MM. Insulin-like growth factor binding proteins. Vit Horm 1993;47:114.)

the molecular biology of the IGFBPs has provided the most information concerning their structural interrelationship.

IGFBP Structure

To date, the cDNAs for six distinct human and rat IGFBPs have been cloned and sequenced.[357] Their structural characteristics are summarized in Figure 23–30. The amino acid sequences of the six cloned mammalian IGFBPs are highly conserved. Within a species, the IGFBPs share an overall amino acid sequence homology on the order of 50%, and between species there is more than 80% sequence homology for individual IGFBPs. Perhaps the most impressive similarity in structure is the conservation of the number and placement of the cysteine residues. The total number of cysteines varies from 16 to 20 (18 cysteines are conserved in human IGFBPs 1-5; IGFBP-6 conserves 16 of the 18, and IGFBP-4 has 2 additional cysteines in the middle region of the protein), and each of the IGFBPs has cysteine-rich regions at the amino and carboxyl termini. Conservation of the spatial order of the cysteines presumably indicates that the secondary structure of the IGFBPs, which is dependent upon disulfide bonding, must also be conserved. This hypothesis is supported by the observation that the combination of isolated N- and C-domains of the IGFBPs does not restore IGF binding affinity to that of the full-length IGFBPs.[361]

Disulfide bonding is essential for formation of the IGF binding site of each IGFBP; reduction of the disulfide proteins results in loss of IGF binding. On the other hand, the middle region of the IGFBPs is not well conserved, containing N-glycosylation sites for IGFBP-3 and -4, and two additional cysteine residues in IGFBP-4. Some of the more specialized properties of the IGFBPs, such as cell-association, IGF enhancement, and IGF-independent actions (see later) may be dependent upon specific sequences in these midregions.

An RGD (arginine-glycine-aspartic acid) sequence near the carboxy-terminus of IGFBP-1 and -2[362] is the minimum sequence required for the binding of many extracellular matrix proteins to membrane receptors of the integrin protein family, and IGFBPs may associate with the cell surface through such amino acid sequences.[363] However, IGFBP-3, which lacks an RGD sequence, also binds to cell membranes,[364,365] possibly to specific receptors[366] (see below).

Under most conditions, the IGFBPs appear to inhibit IGF action, presumably by competing with IGF receptors for binding IGF peptides.[367] For example, IGF analogues with decreased affinity for IGFBPs have increased biologic potency.[368-370] In studies involving transfection of the hIGFBP-3 gene into fibroblasts, increased expression of IGFBP-3 inhibited cell growth, even in the absence of added IGF, suggesting a direct inhibitory role of the binding protein.[371] Under some conditions, however, the IGFBPs appear to enhance IGF action, perhaps by facilitating the delivery of IGF to target receptors.[372]

The discovery of several groups of cysteine-rich proteins that contain domains similar to the amino-terminus of the IGFBPs has led to the proposal of an IGFBP superfamily,[373] which includes the family of six high-affinity IGFBPs, as well as a number of IGFBP-related proteins (IGFBP-rPs). Three of the IGFBP-rPs (Mac25/IGFBP-rP1; connective tissue growth factor, CTGF/IGFBP-rP2; NovH/IGFBP-rP3) have been shown to bind IGFs, although with considerably lower affinity than the IGFBPs. Like the IGFBPs, the IGFBP-rPs are modular proteins and the highly preserved amino-terminal domain appears to represent the consequence of exon shuffling of an ancestral gene. The role, if any, of the IGFBP-rPs in normal IGF physiology is unclear, but it seems likely that they influence cell growth by both IGF-independent and IGF-dependent mechanisms.

Analysis of IGFBPs is further complicated by the presence of IGFBP proteases, which degrade IGFBP.[374,375] Initially reported in the serum of pregnant women,[374,375] proteases for IGFBP-2, -3, -4, and -5 are present in serum, seminal plasma,[376] cerebrospinal fluid,[377] and urine,[378] consistent with a potential role in IGF-II degradation. It is likely that multiple IGFBP proteases exist, including calcium-dependent serine proteases, kallikreins, cathepsins,[379] and matrix metalloproteases.[380] Proteolysis of IGFBPs complicates their assay and must be taken into consideration when measuring the various IGFBPs in biologic fluids.[381] The physiologic significance of limited proteolysis of IGFBPs remains to be determined, although protease activity usually decreases the affinity of the IGFBP for IGF peptides (Fig. 23–31) and may enhance the mitogenic and anabolic effects of IGF peptides in this way. In prostate epithelial cells,[382-384] prostate-specific antigen acts as a potent IGFBP-3 protease (Figs. 23–32 and 23–33), and in rat granulosa cells,[385] follicle-stimulating hormone (FSH) induces an IGFBP-5 protease.

IGFBPs as Carrier Proteins

Given the high affinity of the IGFBPs for IGF-I and IGF-II (Kd 10^{-10} to 10^{-11} M), virtually all IGF-I and IGF-II in serum is complexed to IGFBPs.[386] In normal adult serum, 75% to 80% of the IGF peptides is carried in a ternary complex consisting of one molecule of IGF plus one molecule of IGFBP-3 plus one molecule of an 88-kd protein termed the *acid-labile subunit* (ALS).[387,388] Binding of ALS to form the full ternary complex occurs after the binding of IGF by IGFBP-3 or IGFBP-5, although ALS may bind to IGFBP-3 even in the absence of IGF.[389] The 150-kd ternary complex is too large to leave the vascular compartment and extends the half-life of IGF peptides from approximately 10 minutes for IGF alone to 1 to 2 hours for IGF in the IGF-IGFBP-3 binary complex to 12 to 15 hours for IGF in the ternary complex.[390] The fact that both IGFBP-3 and ALS are GH-dependent provides an additional mechanism for GH regulation of the IGF axis. Although IGF-I administration to hypophysectomized rats increases serum levels of IGFBP-3,[391-393] no sustained increase in serum levels of IGFBP-3 occurs in humans following administration of IGF-I.[92,394] ALS levels may even decline after IGF-I administration, presumably reflecting IGF feedback inhibition of pituitary GH secretion.[394,395] Thus, in serum of patients with GH deficiency or GH insensitivity, little IGF is present in the 150-kd ternary complex, most being found in the lower molecular weight IGF–GFBP-3 complex or bound by other IGFBPs. While GH administration to GH-deficient patients shifts IGF from the 40- to 50-kd low-molecular-weight peak to the 150-kd high-molecular-weight peak,[396,397] a similar phenomenon is not observed following IGF-I treatment.[396]

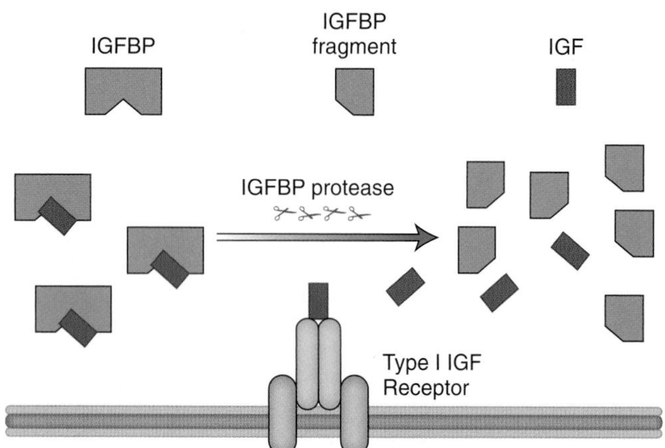

Figure 23–31 ▪ Schematic representation of the effect of IGFBP proteases on IGF action. In this model, proteolysis of IGFBPs results in a reduction in their affinity for IGF ligands, resulting in enhanced binding of IGF peptides by IGF receptor. (From Cohen P, Rosenfeld RG. The IGF axis. In Rosenbloom AL, ed. Human Growth Hormone, Basic and Scientific Aspects. Boca Raton, FL: CRC Press, 1995:43-58.)

IGF peptides in the 40- to 50-kd molecular-weight peak may not be restricted to the vascular compartment. IGFBP-1, -2, and -4, at least, can probably cross endothelial barriers.[398] In the fetus and neonate, where IGFBP-3 levels are relatively low, and in GH deficiency and GH insensitivity, binding of IGFs by IGFBP-1, -2, -4, and -5 may predominate over binding to IGFBP-3.[287,396,399] Similarly, in tumor-induced hypoglycemia associated with increased serum levels of IGF-II, ternary complex formation may be decreased, and most IGF peptides are found in the low-molecular-weight peak.

IGFBPs as Modulators of IGF Action

In general, the binding affinity of IGFBPs for IGF peptides is higher than that of IGF receptors, implying that IGFBPs can modulate IGF binding to its receptors, thereby regulating IGF biologic actions (Fig. 23–34).[386] Co-incubation of cells with IGF-I and a molar excess of IGFBP-3 results in an inhibition of IGF-I–stimulated thymidine incorporation in human fibroblasts, lipogenesis in rat epididymal adipocytes,[400] and glucose consumption in mouse fibroblasts.[401] Termination of inhibition apparently requires dissociation of IGFs from the IGF-IGFBP complex by mass action, proteolysis, or other mechanisms. IGFBP proteases have been identified in a wide variety of body fluids and cell

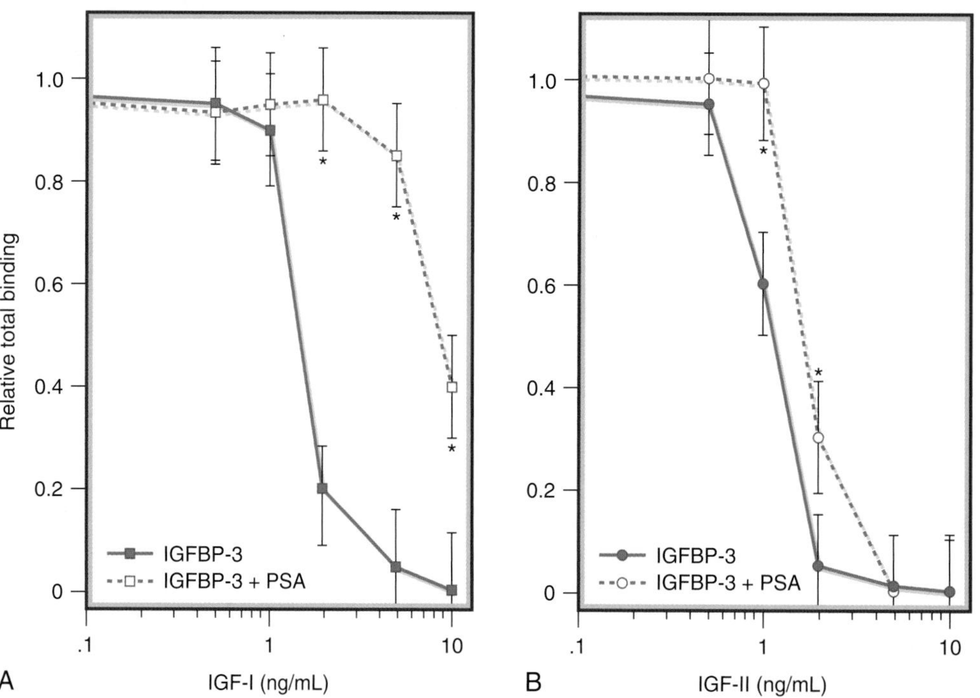

Figure 23–32 ▪ The effect of IGFBP-3 proteolysis by prostate-specific antigen on IGFBP-3 affinity for IGF-I **(A)** and IGF-II **(B)**. (From Cohen P, Peehl DM, Graves HC, et al. Biological effects of prostate specific antigen as an insulin-like growth factor binding protein-3 protease. J Endocrinol 1994;142:407-415.)

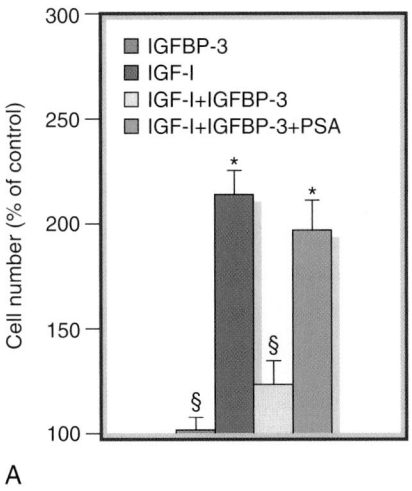

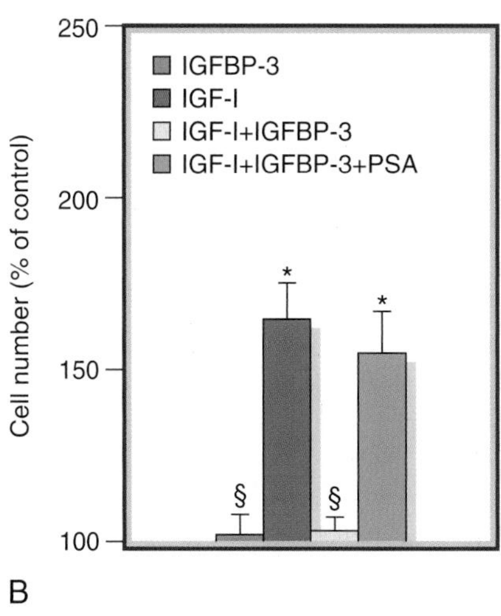

Figure 23–33 ▪ The effect of IGFBP-3 proteolysis by prostate-specific antigen (PSA) on the ability of IGFBP-3 to inhibit IGF-I **(A)** and IGF-II action **(B).** (From Cohen P, Peehl DM, Graves HC, et al. Biological effects of prostate specific antigen as an insulin-like growth factor binding protein-3 protease. J Endocrinol 1994;142: 407-415.)

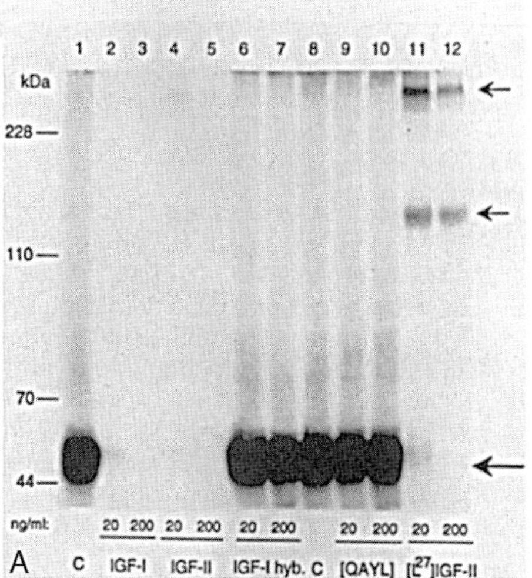

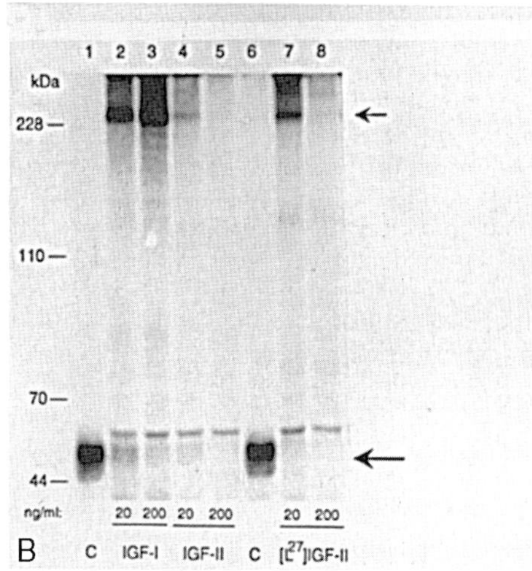

Figure 23–34 ▪ Affinity cross-linking of [^{125}I]IGF-I **(A)** and [^{125}I]IGF-II **(B)** to membranes from Hs578T breast cancer cells. In the absence of unlabeled IGF peptide (lane 1), IGF predominantly bound to 40- to 45-kd IGFBP-3; no type 1 or type 2 IGF receptors were observed. Iodinated IGF was readily displaceable by unlabeled IGF-I or IGF-II (lanes 2 to 5), but not by unlabeled IGF-I/insulin hybrid molecule (lanes 6 and 7) or by an IGF analogue with decreased affinity for IGFBPs (QAYL, lanes 9 and 10 in A). However, addition of [Leu^{27}] IGF-II, which decreased affinity for the type I IGF receptor (lanes 11 to 12 in A and lanes 7 to 8 in **B**, resulted in "unmasking" of the 130-kd α subunit of the type I IGF receptor **(A)** and the 250-kd type II IGF receptor in **B**. (From Oh Y, Muller HL, Lamson G, et al. Insulin-like growth factor (IGF)-independent action of IGF-binding protein-3 in Hs578T human breast cancer cells. Cell surface binding and growth inhibition. J Biol Chem 1993;268:14964-14971.)

culture media,[379,380,382,383,385] and are postulated to play a role in altering IGF availability by lowering the affinities of IGFBPs for their ligand, thereby increasing the availability of IGFs to cell membrane receptors[384,402] (see earlier).

Under certain conditions, the IGFBPs potentiate IGF action. In human and bovine fibroblasts, DNA synthesis and α-aminoisobutyric acid transport are augmented when cells are preincubated with IGFBP-3, whereas IGFBP-3 is inhibitory if added at the same time as IGF-I.[403,404] These observations have suggested that cell association of IGFBP-3 during preincubation is essential for its IGF-potentiating effect, perhaps allowing IGFBP-3 to serve as a reservoir for IGFs and bringing the ligand into closer proximity to the type 1 IGF receptors. This cell-surface association of IGFBP-3 may involve interaction with

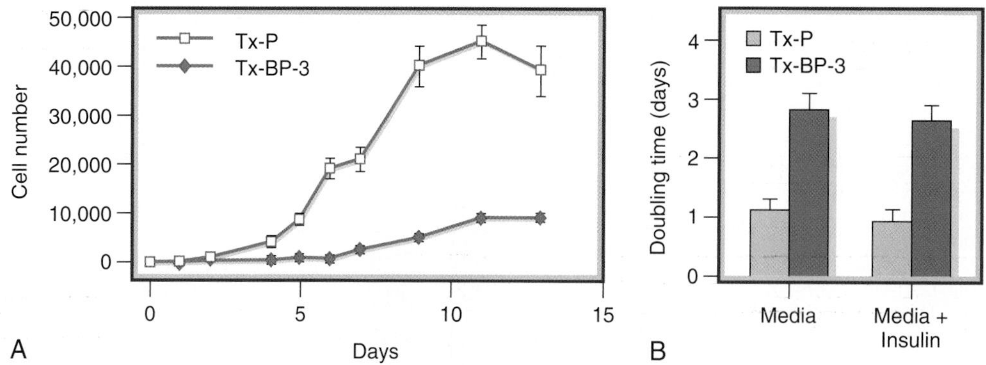

Figure 23–35 ▪ Effect of transfection of Balb/c fibroblasts with a human IGFBP-3 cDNA (Tx-BP-3) or with the control plasmid (Tx-P) on cell growth. Transfection with the IGFBP-3 cDNA resulted in a decreased cell proliferation **(A)** and increased cell doubling time **(B)**. The latter effect could not be overcome with insulin, supporting the concept that the inhibitory effects of IGFBP-3 are IGF-independent. (From Cohen P, Lamson G, Okajima T, et al. Transfection of the human insulin-like growth factor binding protein-3 gene into Balb/c fibroblasts inhibits cellular growth. Mol Endocrinol 1993;7:380-386.)

heparin and heparin sulfate proteoglycans on the cell membrane or specific IGFBP-3 receptors.[366]

IGF-Independent Actions of IGFBPs

The IGFBPs are bioactive molecules that, in addition to binding IGF, have a variety of IGF- independent functions. These include growth inhibition in some cell types,[405] growth stimulation in other tissues,[406] direct induction of apoptosis,[407] and modulation of the effects of other non-IGF growth factors. These effects of IGFBPs may be mediated by binding of IGFBPs to their own receptors. The IGFBP-signaling pathways are currently being unraveled and involve interaction of IGFBPs with nuclear retinoid receptors as well as with other molecules on the cell surface and in the cytoplasm.[408]

IGFBP-3 itself appears to have intrinsic inhibitory effects on cells, independent of its interaction with IGF. Villaudy and colleagues[409] found that the stimulation of DNA synthesis by basic FGF is inhibited by simultaneous treatment with IGFBP-3, even in the presence of levels of insulin, suggesting that sequestration of IGF peptides from type 1 IGF receptors is not the only means whereby IGFBP-3 inhibits cell growth. IGFBP-3 is also more effective than immunoneutralization of IGF-I in inhibiting serum-stimulated DNA synthesis, and IGFBP-3 inhibits FSH-stimulated DNA synthesis in cultured ovarian granulosa cells, with or without added IGF.[410] Under the same conditions, IGFBP-2 is less inhibitory, despite its higher affinity for IGF peptides. Expression of a transfected human IGFBP-3 cDNA in mouse fibroblasts inhibits both IGF-stimulated and insulin-stimulated cell proliferation (Fig. 23–35).[371] Similar studies in fibroblasts derived from mouse embryos homozygous for a targeted disruption of the type 1 IGF receptor again demonstrated inhibition with overexpression of IGFBP-3.[411] These studies strongly support an IGF-independent action for IGFBP-3 (Fig. 23–36).

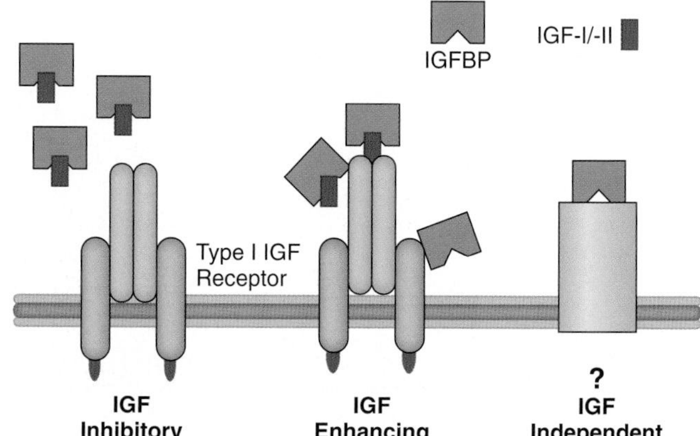

Figure 23–36 ▪ Theoretical mechanisms of cellular IGFBP actions.

IGFBP-3 binds with high affinity to the surface of various cell types, including human breast cancer cells and rat chondrocytes, and inhibits monolayer growth of these cells in an IGF-independent manner (Fig. 23–37).[366,412,413] Furthermore, transcriptional regulation of IGFBP-3 expression may be the mechanism for the inhibition of breast cancer cell growth by both TGF-2 and retinoic acid (Fig. 23–38).[414-417] Reduction of IGFBP-3 production through the use of IGFBP-3 antisense oligodeoxynucleotides decreases the inhibitory effects of both TGF-2 and retinoic acid, suggesting that IGFBP-3 production may be a common pathway for multiple hormones and growth factors involved in the modulation of cell growth.[414] For example, estrogen inhibits expression and secretion of IGFBP-3, whereas antiestrogens stimulate production of IGFBP-3 in estrogen receptor–positive human breast cancer cells.[418] Similarly, the mitogenic action of EGF in human cervical epithelial cells is associated with inhibition of IGFBP-3 expression, and the inhibitory effect of retinoic acid is accompanied by increased IGFBP-3 expression.[419] Regulation of IGFBP-3 gene expression plays a role in signaling by p53, a potent tumor-suppressor protein.[420]

The presence of cell membrane proteins or receptors that specifically bind IGFBP-3 provides a potential mechanism for IGF-independent growth inhibitory actions of IGFBP-3 (Fig. 23–39).[366] IGFBP-3 may inhibit cell growth both by sequestering IGF ligands (IGF-dependent action of IGFBP-3) and by binding to the cell surface (IGF-independent action of IGFBP-3). IGFBP-3 proteases may not only degrade intact IGFBP-3 to forms with lower affinities for IGFs, but also generate IGFBP-3 fragments with enhanced affinity for cell surface IGFBP-3–interacting proteins or receptors. A proteolytic fragment of IGFBP-3 that fails to bind IGFs still retains its ability to inhibit cell proliferation.[421]

Characteristics of Insulin-Like Growth Factor Binding Proteins 1 to 6

IGFBP-1

IGFBP-1 was the first of the IGFBPs to be purified and to have its cDNA cloned.[422] The protein was actually identified and purified

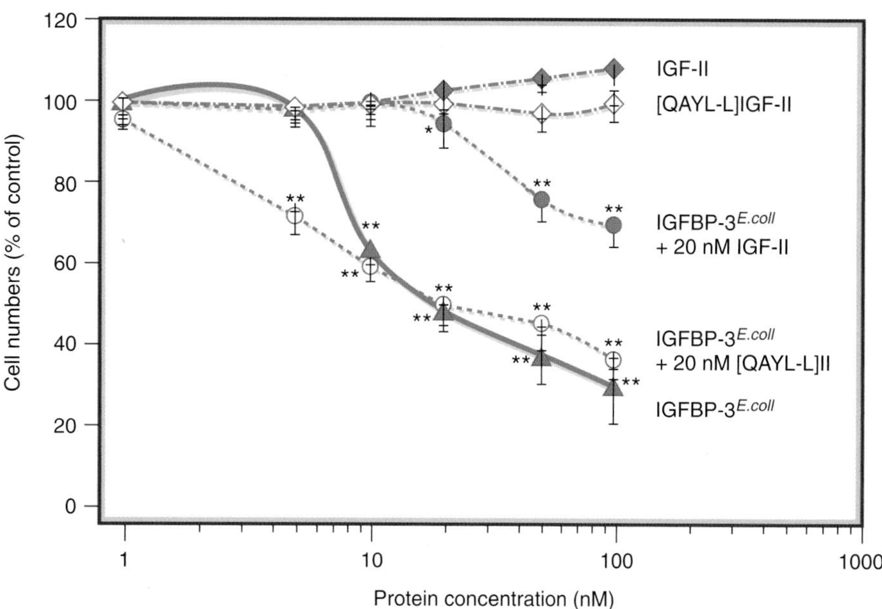

Figure 23–37 ▪ Inhibition of Hs578T breast cancer cell growth by IGFBP-3 is IGF-independent. Recombinant IGFBP-3 from *Escherichia coli* results in decreased cell number and cannot be overcome by the addition of an IGF analogue with normal affinity for IGF receptors, but decreased affinity for IGFPB-3 (QUAYL-Leu-IGF-II). On the other hand, IGF-II, which itself does not stimulate cell proliferation in Hs578T cells, partially releases cells from the growth-inhibitory effects of IGFBP-3, presumably by causing dissociation of IGFBP-3 from the cell membrane. (From Oh Y, Muller HL, Lamson G, et al. Insulin-like growth factor (IGF)-independent action of IGF binding protein-3 in Hs578T human breast cancer cells. J Biol Chem 1993;268:14964-14971.)

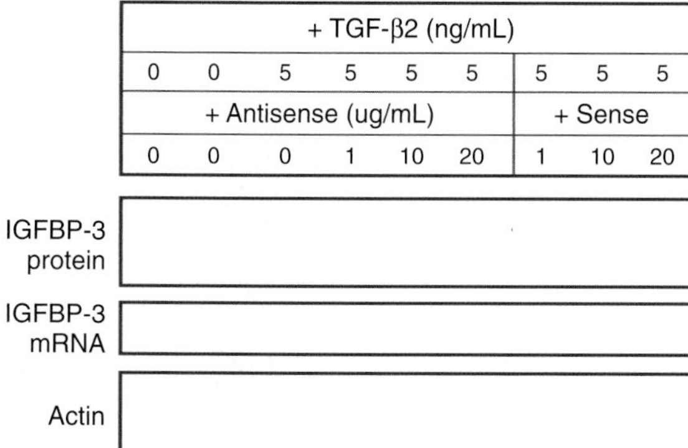

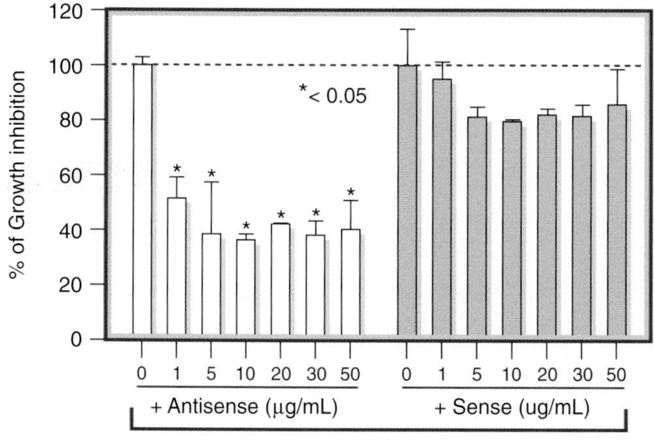

Figure 23–38 ▪ TGF-β2 inhibits Hs578T cell growth by transcriptional regulation of IGFBP-3. Reduction in IGFBP-3 mRNA and protein levels through the use of an IGFBP-3 antisense oligodeoxynucleotide resulted in significant reduction in the growth inhibitory actions of TGF-β2. (From Oh Y, Muller HL, Ng L, et al. TGF-β2-induced cell growth inhibition in human breast cancer cells is mediated through IGFBP-3 action. J Biol Chem 1995;270:13589-13592.)

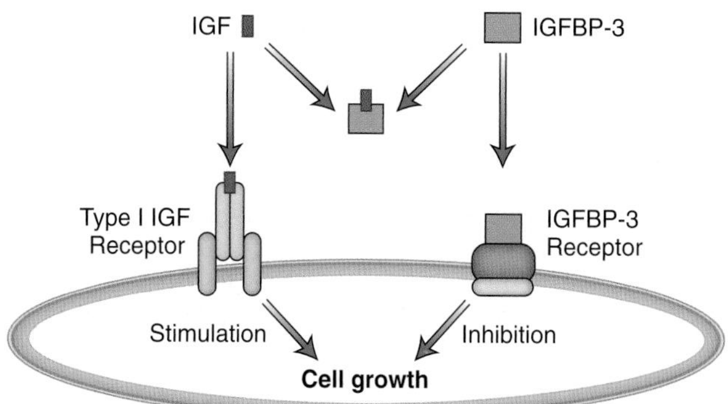

Figure 23–39 ▪ Schematic diagram of IGF-dependent and IGF-independent actions of IGFBP-3, the latter being mediated through a putative membrane-associated IGFBP-3 receptor.

from several different tissues, including amniotic fluid[423] and HepG2 conditioned media,[424] placental membranes (placental protein 12),[425] and endometrium (pregnancy-associated α1-globulin).[426] Its gene is 5.2 kb long, located on the short arm of chromosome 7, and comprising four exons.[427] The mature protein is 30 kd and is nonglycosylated. Messenger RNA for IGFBP-1 is strongly expressed in decidua (although not in placental trophoblasts), liver, and kidney.

IGFBP-1 may be involved in reproductive functions, including endometrial cycling,[428] oocyte maturation,[429] and fetal growth.[399,430] It is the major IGFBP in fetal serum in early gestation, reaching levels as high as 3000 μg/L by the second trimester. Levels of IGFBP-1 in newborn serum are inversely correlated with birthweight, consistent with an inhibitory role on fetal IGF action.

IGFBP-1 also appears to have an important metabolic role, in that its gene expression is enhanced in catabolic states,[287,431,432] and serum levels undergo diurnal variation.[433] Insulin suppresses and glucocorticoids enhance IGFBP-1 mRNA levels.[431,434] The acute modulation of serum IGFBP-1 levels may regulate the free fraction of circulating IGF peptides.[431,433] For example, administration of IGFBP-1 transiently reduces the glucose-lowering capability of IGF-I in rats.[435]

While most in vitro studies are consistent with an inhibitory effect of IGFBP-1 on IGF actions, presumably reflecting interference with IGF ligand-receptor interactions,[358] IGFBP-1 potentiates IGF effects in certain cell systems,[436] possibly as the result of the binding of IGFBP-1 to cell membranes through its Arg-Gly-Asp (RGD) sequence; RGD is an integrin receptor recognition sequence that presumably allows IGFBP-1 to associate with the $\alpha_5\beta_1$ integrin (fibronectin) receptor.[363] The ability of IGFBP-1 to inhibit or potentiate IGF action may depend upon posttranslational modifications of IGFBP-1, such as phosphorylation, which appears to enhance IGFBP-1 affinity for IGF-I and thereby inhibit IGF action.[437]

IGFBP-2

The IGFBP-2 gene is located on the long arm of chromosome 2.[438,439] A single 1.6-kb mRNA yields a mature protein of approximately 34 kd. Like IGFBP-1, IGFBP-2 is highly expressed in fetal tissues, particularly in the central nervous system.[440] IGFBP-2 is also similar to IGFBP-1 in its lack of N-glycosylation and in the presence of an RGD sequence, perhaps allowing cell association and potentiation of IGF action.[441] Nevertheless, knockout of the IGFBP-2 gene[442] or overexpression of IGFBP-1 in transgenic mice[443] appears to have little effect on phenotype, possibly reflecting "redundancy" in the IGFBP system, in which one IGFBP can compensate for loss of another.

The existence of a low-molecular-weight IGFBP in cerebrospinal fluid was inferred from studies demonstrating a 34-kd IGFBP that did not react with antibodies to IGFBP-1 (or IGFBP-3).[444] This IGFBP appeared to be consistent with a previous observation of CSF IGFBPs with preferential affinity for IGF-II.[445] IGFBP-2 is expressed in secretory endometrium and endometrial tumors[428] and is the major IGFBP in seminal fluid and in the conditioned media of prostatic epithelial cells.[446] Interestingly, IGFBP-2 gene expression is markedly reduced in prostatic stromal cells from patients with benign prostatic hyperplasia, suggesting that IGFBP-2 may inhibit stromal growth.[447] Serum levels of IGFBP-2 are frequently elevated in patients with prostatic carcinoma.[448]

IGFBP-3

The IGFBP-3 gene is located on chromosome 7 in proximity to the gene for IGFBP-1.[449] It contains four exons homologous to those of IGFBP-1 and -2 and a fifth exon, consisting of 3′ untranslated sequences. In all human tissues studied to date, a single 2.6-kb mRNA has been observed, while an additional 1.7-kb mRNA species suggests alternative splicing in baboons.[450] Messenger RNA levels are high in liver, but IGFBP-3 appears to be synthesized in hepatic endothelia (portal venous and sinusoidal) and Kupffer cells, whereas ALS is synthesized in hepatocytes.[451,452]

IGFBP-3 is GH-dependent, either due to a direct GH effect or to regulation by IGF. IGF-I administration to hypophysectomized rats increases serum levels of IGFBP-3.[391-393] On the other hand, IGF-I treatment of patients with GH insensitivity does not greatly alter serum IGFBP-3 levels,[92,363,379] while GH treatment of GH-deficient patients does increase serum levels. Whether these observations mean that GH has a direct effect on IGFBP-3 or reflects GH regulation of ALS and ternary complex formation is unclear, although it appears likely that both factors are contributory.

The mature IGFBP-3 protein has a molecular weight of approximately 29 kd, but, because it is N-glycosylated, normally migrates as a doublet-triplet of 40 to 46 kd. Glycosylation does not appear to alter its affinity for IGF-I or -II.[453] IGFBP-3 also undergoes serine phosphorylation of IGFBP-3, although its physiologic significance is uncertain.[454] Perhaps the most significant posttranslational modification of IGFBP-3 is proteolysis (see above). Discrepancies between immunoblot analyses and radioimmunoassays for IGFBP-3 reflect the altered affinity of IGFBP-3 fragments for IGF ligands, although some proteolytic fragments of IGFBP-3 are capable of ternary complex formation.[381] In pregnancy serum, the predominant form of IGFBP-3 is a glycosylated 29-kd fragment. A similar size IGFBP-3 fragment is present in serum from patients who are postsurgical or catabolic[455] and from patients with non–insulin-dependent diabetes mellitus.[456]

IGFBP-3 is the predominant IGFBP in adult serum, where it carries approximately 75% of the total IGF, primarily as part of the 150-kd ternary complex. IGFBP-3 and IGFBP-5 are the only IGFBPs to form this complex, which involves the binding of the binary IGF-IGFBP complex to the 85-kd ALS. It is believed that formation of this ternary complex limits IGF access to target cells, while at the same time prolonging serum half-lives of both the IGF peptide and its binding protein.[457] Serum levels of both IGFBP-3 and ALS are reduced in patients with GH deficiency or GH insensitivity, conditions in which assays for serum IGFBP-3 have important diagnostic value (see below).

IGFBP-3 associates with cell membranes. Affinity cross-linking studies employing [^{125}I] IGF-I and a human breast cancer cell line have demonstrated no binding to the type 1 IGF receptor but rather to membrane-associated 45-kd IGFBP-3 (see Fig. 23–34). When IGF analogues with selective affinity for IGFBPs were added, a typical 135-kd α subunit of the type 1 IGF receptor was uncovered, demonstrating that membrane-associated IGFBP-3, with its high affinity for IGF peptides, normally "masks" the IGF receptors. Oh and colleagues[414] demonstrated that the binding of IGFBP-3 to cell membrane proteins was specific, cation-dependent, and of high affinity. Whether these proteins constitute genuine "IGFBP-3 receptors" remains to be demonstrated, although they may mediate IGF-independent actions of IGFBP-3. Alternatively, IGFBP-3 may associate with heparin-containing proteoglycans both in the extracellular matrix and in the cell membrane, in that both IGFBP-3 and IGFBP-5 contain heparin-binding consensus sequences in their COOH-termini.[458] However, treatment of cell monolayers with heparinase or chondroitinase has only minor effect on IGFBP-3 binding. IGFBP-3 and, probably, IGFBP-5 appear to localize to the nucleus of target cells, although the role of nuclear transport in the IGF-independent actions of IGFBP-3 is still uncertain. Additionally, IGFBP-3, perhaps the most promiscuous of the IGFBPs, can bind to multiple other molecular partners, although the relationship between these binding actions and IGFBP function remain unclear.

Like other IGFBPs, IGFBP-3 inhibits IGF action, especially when the binding protein is present in excess. Presumably, inhibition of IGF action by IGFBP-3 reflects a sequestering of IGF peptides away from the type 1 receptor. Proteolysis of IGFBP-3, resulting in a decrease in affinity for IGF ligands, decreases the inhibitory effects of the binding protein.

IGFBP-4

The IGFBP-4 gene, located on chromosome 17, contains four exons.[459] A single 2.6 kd mRNA has been identified with high expression in liver. The protein is the smallest of the IGFBPs with 237 amino acids in humans including 20 cysteines and one N-linked glycosylation site. In immunoblots of most biologic fluids, IGFBP-4 is a 24/28-kd doublet; deglycosylation eliminates the 28-kd band.[460] IGFBP-4 appears to interact with connective tissues,[461] but there is no evidence of membrane association, consistent with a primary role for IGFBP-4 as a soluble, extracellular IGFBP.

IGFBP-4 was initially isolated on the basis of its ability to inhibit IGF-stimulated cell proliferation in bone,[462] and there is no evidence for any IGF-potentiating effects. The inhibitory effects of IGFBP-4 are reduced by proteolysis of the protein, much as has been observed with IGFBP-3 degradation. IGFBP-4 proteases are produced by a wide variety of cells, including neuroblastoma,[463] smooth muscle,[464] fibroblasts,[465] osteoblasts,[466] and prostatic epithelium.[467] Activation of IGFBP-4 proteolysis occurs in the presence of IGF-I or IGF-II, presumably reflecting a conformational change in IGFBP-4 resulting from IGF occupancy.[468,469] The clinical use of IGFBP-4 measurements is as yet minor.[470]

IGFBP-5

cDNAs for IGFBP-5 have been isolated and sequenced from rat ovary and human placenta and from a human osteosarcoma.[471,472] The gene is located on chromosome 5 and contains 4 exons. A single 6.0-kb mRNA is expressed in a wide variety of tissues, particularly in kidney. Mature IGFBP-5 is produced as a 252 amino acid protein with no N-linked glycosylation sites but with one O-linked glycosylation site.[473]

The addition of excess IGFBP-5 to human osteosarcoma cells inhibits IGF-I-stimulated DNA and glycogen synthesis.[474] However, when IGFBP-5 adheres to fibroblast extracellular matrix, it potentiates the growth stimulatory effects of IGF on DNA synthesis.[475] The affinity of IGFBP-5 for IGF-I is reduced approximately sevenfold when the binding protein is associated with extracellular matrix, providing a potential mechanism for release of IGFs to cell surface receptors. Association of IGFBP-5 with extracellular matrix also appears to protect it from proteolysis.[476] Addition of IGFBP-5 to conditioned medium from fibroblasts results in proteolysis to a 21-kd fragment that does not potentiate IGF action, while the deposition of IGFBP-5 in extracellular matrix of fibroblasts makes it relatively resistant to degradation. Andress and Birnbaum[477] have purified a 23-kd IGFBP-5 fragment from U-2 osteosarcoma cells that has reduced affinity for IGFs but enhances IGF-I–stimulated mitogenesis. The 23-kd IGFBP-5 fragment stimulates mitogenesis in an IGF-independent manner, presumably by binding to a specific "receptor" on the cell membrane.

Unlike proteolysis of IGFBP-4, which is enhanced by addition of IGFs, degradation of IGFBP-5 is inhibited by the binding of IGF peptides.[34,385,473] Proteolysis of IGFBP-5 results in the formation of 16- to 23-kd fragments demonstrated on immunoblots. Degradation of IGFBP-5 may have particular importance in the regulation of granulosa cell activity. In healthy ovarian follicles, neither IGFBP-4 nor -5 is expressed, whereas both binding proteins are expressed in atretic follicles, thereby providing a mechanism for intrafollicular regulation of IGF action.[478,479] Furthermore, FSH enhances IGF action in the ovary and stimulates IGFBP-5 proteolysis.[385]

IGFBP-5 and IGFBP-4 also appear to be major IGFBPs in bone, where, in addition to inhibiting IGF actions, IGFBP-5 may promote IGF-receptor interactions. Thus, depending on the conditions, IGFBP-5 can either inhibit or potentiate IGF actions.

IGFBP-6

The human IGFBP-6 gene is located on chromosome 12 and contains 4 exons. IGFBP-6 transcripts include a major 1.3-kb mRNA and a minor 2.2-kb transcript.[480] The mature peptide contains 216 amino acids and has a molecular mass of approximately 23 kd, although it may migrate at a higher molecular weight on SDS gels, presumably reflecting O-glycosylation.[481] Although IGFBP-6 binds both IGF-I and -II, it has a significantly greater affinity for IGF-II.[482] IGFBP-6 is found in relatively high levels in cerebrospinal fluid, as is also the case for IGFBP-2, which also binds IGF-II with selectively high affinity. IGFBP-6 may also have a role in regulating ovarian activity, perhaps by functioning as an antigonadotropin.[483]

Radioimmunoassays for the IGFBPs

Specific radioimmunoassays have been developed for IGFBP-1,[484-486] -2,[448] -3,[381,487,488] -4,[489] -5, and -6. Measurement of IGFBP-3 appears to have the greatest clinical value because it is GH-dependent (Fig. 23–40). Blum and colleagues[488] have suggested that immunoassay of serum levels of IGFBP-3 may be superior to IGF-I assays in the diagnosis of GH deficiency, since normal levels of IGF-I are so low in young children and since many "normal" short children have low levels of IGF-I. Because IGFBP-3 determinations reflect the levels of both IGF-I and IGF-II, their age-dependency is not nearly as striking as that of IGF-I; even in young children normal levels are above 500 μg/L. The use of IGFBP assays in the evaluation of IGF deficiency and GH deficiency is discussed below. Measurement of IGFBP levels in biologic fluids may be useful for evaluation of malignancies or other pathologic states in which the IGFBP levels may be altered.

Radioassays for ALS are also available.[490] Low serum concentrations of ALS are consistent with both GH deficiency and GH insensitivity and may be of use in identifying patients with mutations of the ALS gene.

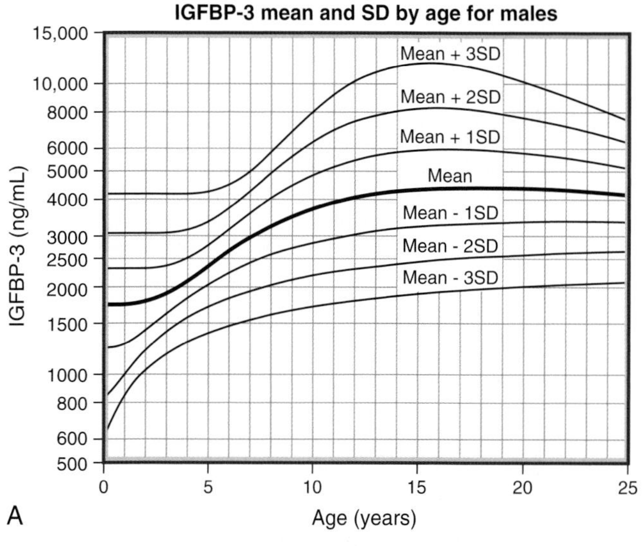

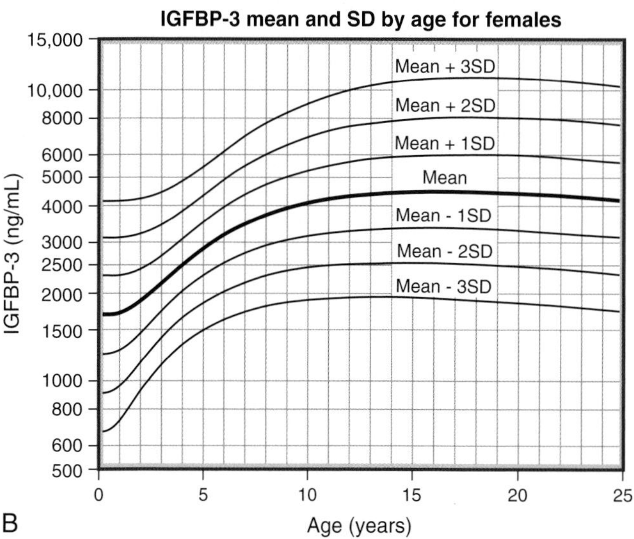

Figure 23–40 ▪ Normal serum levels of IGFBP-3 (μg/mL) for males **(A)** and females **(B)**. Lines represent the mean±3 SD. (Data courtesy of Diagnostic Systems Laboratories, Inc., Webster, TX.)

Gonadal Steroids

While androgens and estrogens do not contribute substantially to normal growth before puberty, the adolescent rise in serum gonadal steroid levels is an important part of the pubertal growth spurt. States of androgen or estrogen excess before epiphyseal fusion cause rapid linear growth and skeletal maturation. Thus, just as growth deceleration requires evaluation, growth acceleration can be as abnormal and may be a sign of precocious puberty or virilizing congenital adrenal hyperplasia.

A GH-replete state is obligatory for a normal growth response to gonadal steroids and children with GH deficiency do not have a normal growth response to either endogenous or exogenous androgens. Gonadal steroids work, in part, by enhancing GH secretion and by stimulating IGF-I production directly, as evidenced by the rise in serum IGF-I levels and pubertal growth spurt in children with mutations of the GH receptor.[124]

Both androgens and estrogens increase skeletal maturation. It is likely that androgens primarily act in this regard after conversion to estrogens by aromatase in extraglandular tissues, but presumably may also have independent actions. Indeed, mutation of the estrogen receptor in a man was associated with tall stature and open epiphyses,[21] and similar findings occur in patients with mutations of the gene encoding the aromatase enzyme.[22,23] In addition, women with an estrogen receptor variant have increased height,[491] while estrogen receptor polymorphisms, but not serum estradiol levels, are related to bone density and height in males.[492]

Skeletal development, in terms of bone mass accretion, is an important pubertal phenomenon and is largely mediated by estrogen action.[493-495] A longitudinal analysis of pubertal calcium accretion found that approximately 26% of adult calcium is laid down during the two adolescent years of maximal growth.[496] A small, but significant, contributor to calcium absorption is the positive association with taller stature in growing adolescents.[497] More than 90% of skeletal mass is present by 18 years of age[498] and estrogens appear to regulate the timing of the growth spurt, stabilization of bone modeling, and endosteal mineral apposition.[493,499] Rubin has described a schema by which early and midpuberty are times of linear growth and increased bone mineral content and areal density (a reflection of bone growth, perhaps largely mediated by the GH-IGF-estrogen synergism.[500] It appears that pubertal males have stronger bones than females, perhaps due to greater bone deposition on the periosteal surface in contrast to increased bone on the endocortical surface in females.[501] Late puberty is characterized by bone maturation (epiphyseal closure) and increased volumetric density (true bone mineral density that is not size-based), which are apparently mediated more clearly by estrogen. Late menarche and delayed puberty appear to be risk factors for later osteopenia,[502] but some data exist to suggest that low bone mass may already be present prepubertally in these individuals.[503] Independent and synergistic effects of gonadal steroids, GH, and IGF-I also contribute to the attainment of peak bone mass in adults.

Thyroid Hormone

Thyroid hormone is a major contributor to postnatal growth, although, like GH, it is of relatively little importance to growth of the fetus. Hypothyroidism postnatally can cause profound growth failure and virtual arrest of skeletal maturation. In addition to a direct effect on epiphyseal cartilage, thyroid hormones appear to have a permissive effect on GH secretion. Patients with hypothyroidism have decreased spontaneous GH secretion and blunted responses to GH provocative tests. Treatment with thyroid hormone results in rapid "catch-up" growth, which is typically accompanied by marked skeletal maturation, potentially causing overly rapid epiphyseal fusion and compromise of adult height.

GROWTH RETARDATION

A classification of growth retardation is listed in Table 23–2. Growth disorders are subdivided into (1) primary growth abnormalities, (2) secondary growth disorders, and (3) idiopathic short stature (ISS). In primary growth abnormalities, the defects appear to be intrinsic to the growth plate. These are best exemplified by osteochondrodysplasias and many chromosomal disorders, but also include conditions of resistance to IGF and SHOX gene mutations. In secondary growth disorders, growth failure results from chronic disease or endocrine disorders. The category of "IGF deficiency" can result secondarily from GHRH, GHRH-R, or GH deficiencies or, primarily, from GH-R, GH signaling, or IGF gene dysfunction. ISS includes variants of normal, such as constitutional delay of growth and maturation and genetic short stature. It is important to note that terms such as ISS in large part reflect our ignorance concerning the multigenic regulation of growth. It is certain that many cases of ISS and genetic short stature (not to mention "normal" variations in stature) reflect subtle genetic variability, including, but clearly not limited to, heterozygosity for mutations of the genes for the GHR, IGF-1R, IGF-I, and other growth factors.[504]

Primary Growth Abnormalities

Osteochondrodysplasias

The osteochondrodysplasias encompass a heterogeneous group of disorders characterized by intrinsic abnormalities of cartilage and/or bone.[505,506] These conditions share the following features: (1) genetic transmission; (2) abnormalities in the size and/or shape of bones of the limbs, spine, and/or skull; and (3) radiologic abnormalities of the bones (generally). More than 100 osteochondrodysplastic conditions have been identified to date on the basis of physical features and radiologic characteristics, and biochemical, molecular, and genetic studies of these condi-

TABLE 23–2 CLASSIFICATION OF GROWTH RETARDATION

I. Primary Growth Abnormalities
   A. Osteochondrodysplasias
   B. Chromosomal abnormalities
   C. Intrauterine growth retardation
II. Secondary Growth Disorders
   A. Malnutrition
   B. Chronic disease
   C. Endocrine disorders
      1. Hypothyroidism
      2. Cushing syndrome
      3. Pseudohypoparathyroidism
      4. Rickets
         a. Hypophosphatemic rickets
      5. IGF deficiency (see Table 23–7)
III. Idiopathic Short Stature
   1. Genetic short stature
   2. Constitutional delay of growth and maturation
   3. Heterozygous defects of the GH receptor

TABLE 23–3 CLASSIFICATION OF OSTEOCHONDRODYSPLASIAS

I. Defects of the Tubular (and Flat) Bones and/or Axial Skeleton
  A. Achondroplasia group
  B. Achondrogenesis
  C. Spondylodysplastic group (perinatally lethal)
  D. Metatropic dysplasia group
  E. Short rib dysplasia group (with/without polydactyly)
  F. Atelosteogenesis/diastrophic dysplasia group
  G. Kniest-Stickler dysplasia group
  H. Spondyloepiphyseal dysplasia congenita group
  I. Other spondylo epi-(meta)-physeal dysplasias
  J. Dysostosis multiplex group
  K. Spondylometaphyseal dysplasias
  L. Epiphyseal dysplasias
  M. Chondrodysplasia punctata (stippled epiphyses) group
  N. Metaphyseal dysplasias
  O. Brachyrachia (short spine dysplasia)
  P. Mesomelic dysplasias
  Q. Acro/acro-mesomelic dysplasias
  R. Dysplasias with significant (but not exclusive) membranous bone involvement
  S. Bent bone dysplasia group
  T. Multiple dislocations with dysplasias
  U. Osteodysplastic primordial dwarfism group
  V. Dysplasias with increased bone density
  W. Dysplasias with defective mineralization
  X. Dysplasias with increased bone density
II. Disorganized Development of Cartilaginous and Fibrous Components of the Skeleton
III. Idiopathic Osteolyses

tions will undoubtedly lead to the recognition of additional types. An international classification for the osteochondrodysplasias developed in 1970[507] and revised in 1978[508] and 1992[505] is summarized in Table 23–3. Of note, the category of dysostoses has been dropped from the classification, which focuses on developmental disorders of bone and cartilage.

Diagnosis of osteochondrodysplasias can be difficult. Although the underlying molecular and biochemical defects have been identified in many of these conditions, clinical and radiologic evaluation remains central to the diagnosis. Frequently, the clinical features are characteristic, and the diagnosis can be made at birth or even prenatally by ultrasound. The family history is critical, although many cases are due to fresh mutations, as is generally the case in the classic autosomal dominant achondroplasia and hypochondroplasia. Measurement of body proportions should include arm span, sitting height, upper/lower body segments, and head circumference. Clinical and radiologic evaluation should be used to determine whether involvement is of the long bones, skull, and/or vertebrae and whether abnormalities are primarily at the epiphyses, metaphyses, or diaphyses.

Achondroplasia

This is the most common of the osteochondrodysplasias, with a frequency of approximately 1 : 26,000. Although transmitted as an autosomal dominant disorder, 80% to 90% of cases appear to be due to new mutations. Achondroplasia is due to a mutation in a transmembranous domain of the gene for fibroblast growth factor receptor 3 (FGFR3)[509,510] located on the short arm of chromosome 4 (4p16.3) (reviewed in references 511 through 513). The vast majority of cases identified to date are due to activating mutations at a "hot spot" at nucleotide 1138 (codon 380, gly380arg) of the FGFR3 gene and because these mutations create new recognition sites for restriction enzymes, they can be easily diagnosed. To date, the mutation rate reported at this site indicates that it may be the most mutable gene in the human genome. The homogeneity of mutation in achondroplasia probably explains the minimal heterogeneity in its phenotype. Infants homozygous for this condition have severe disease, typically dying in infancy from respiratory insufficiency due to the small thorax. Diminished growth velocity is present from infancy, although short stature may not be evident until after 2 years of age. Mean adult heights in males and females are 130 and 120 cm, respectively.[514] Growth curves for achondroplasia have been developed and are of value in following up patients.[17]

With increasing age, the diagnosis of achondroplasia becomes easier in that these patients develop characteristic abnormalities of the skeleton, including megalocephaly, low nasal bridge, lumbar lordosis, short trident hand, and rhizomelia (shortness of the proximal legs and arms) with skin redundancy. Radiologic findings include small, cuboid-shaped vertebral bodies with short pedicles and progressive narrowing of the lumbar interpedicular distance. The iliac wings are small, with narrow sciatic notches. The small foramen magnum may lead to hydrocephalus, and spinal cord and/or root compression may result from kyphosis, stenosis of the spinal canal, or disc lesions.[515,516] GH secretion in these children is comparable to that in normal children.[517] In a mouse with an equivalent FGFR3 mutation showing many features of human achondroplasia, there is ligand-independent dimerization and phosphorylation of FGFR3 with activation of STAT proteins and up-regulation of cell-cycle inhibition.[518] Additionally, such mutant mice also exhibit down-regulation of expression of the Indian hedgehog and PTHrP receptor genes, which are also involved in bone formation.[519] As a result of the overexpression of this receptor activity, there is abnormal chondrogenesis and osteogenesis during endochondral ossification.

Hypochondroplasia

Hypochondroplasia is an autosomal dominant disorder, previously described as a "mild form" of achondroplasia, that frequently results from a mutation (Asn540Lys) in the FGFR3 gene.[513,520,521] Although achondroplasia and hypochondroplasia are, thus, the results of mutations of the same genes, the specific mutations differ and the two disorders do not occur in the same family.[522] About 70% of affected individuals are heterozygous for a mutation in FGFR3 gene, but locus heterogeneity exists as other unidentified mutations cause a very similar phenotype.[513] Mullis and colleagues,[523] using restriction enzyme analysis, suggested that the IGF-I gene may be a candidate gene for hypochondroplasia, but other molecular abnormalities are likely to be found. The facial features of achondroplasia are absent, and both the short stature and rhizomelia are less pronounced. Adult heights typically are in the 120- to 150-cm range. In contrast to achondroplasia, poor growth may not be evident until after 2 years of age, but stature then deviates progressively from normal. Occasionally, the disproportionate short stature is not apparent until adulthood. Outward bowing of the legs may be accompanied by genu varum. Lumbar interpedicular distances diminish between L1 and L5, and, as with achondroplasia, there may be flaring of the pelvis and narrow sciatic notches. The diagnosis is exceedingly difficult to make in young children. Mild variants of the syndrome may not be clinically distinguishable from normal and radiologic studies should be performed if a question arises.

SHOX Deficiency Syndromes

The pseudoautosomal region of distal Xp and Yp (region escaping inactivation) includes a gene known as SHOX (short stature homeobox-containing gene), mutations of which are associated with syndromes of poor growth and skeletal dysplasia, including Leri-Weil dyschondrosteosis (LWD), Turner Syndrome, and Langer's mesomelic dwarfism.[524] The latter entity is caused by homozygous gene defects, the others being due to haploinsufficiency. The majority of patients (73%) share a distinct region (5-kb) for breakpoints, suggesting a "hot spot" for mutations.[525] The skeletal manifestations of these disorders have been associated with those areas in which there is intrauterine expression of SHOX.[526,527] The SHOX protein may affect cellular proliferation and apoptosis of chondrocytes in the growth plate.[527] The auxologic finding of relatively short limbs suggests this gene defect,[528] which has been found in about 2% of children with so-called idiopathic short stature. This finding eliminates the "idiopathic" and stresses the need for careful physical assessment. The more profound findings in LWD, compared with Turner's syndrome, may reflect the impact of pubertal estrogen exposure in LWD,[526] but the presence of some findings in prepubertal children and boys does not entirely support this notion.

Mutations in the Natriuretic Peptide Receptor (NPR-B)

Endochondral growth is regulated by multiple endocrine, paracrine, and autocrine factors, with many inborn errors having been identified.[529] Of great interest, albeit extremely rare, is the syndrome of acromesomelic dysplasia in which growth is remarkably impaired leading to adult heights that may be more than 5 SD below the mean. A homozygous mutation in the homodimeric transmembrane natriuretic receptor B in which binding of the ligand C-type natriuretic peptide is impaired has been implicated. Olney and associates[530] have identified a family in which obligatory heterozygotes have been found to be significantly shorter than [E1]normal, suggesting that heterozygosity for this condition may, on occasion, be mistaken for idiopathic short stature. In this sense, heterozygous mutations of NPR-B, like heterozygosity for SHOX defects, demonstrate that a subset of children with unexplained short stature may, in fact, have mild forms of classic osteochondrodysplasias.

Chromosomal Abnormalities

Abnormalities of autosomes or sex chromosomes may cause growth retardation, frequently associated with somatic abnormalities and mental retardation, as in deletion of chromosome 5 or trisomy 18 or 13. Such abnormalities, however, may be subtle, and, for example, the diagnosis of Turner's syndrome (TS) must be considered in any girl with unexplained short stature. In many cases, the precise cause of growth failure is not clear because the genetic defects do not affect known components of the GH-IGF system. The chromosomal lesion may directly influence normal tissue growth and development, or, indirectly, modulate local responsivity to IGF or other growth factors at the growth plate.

Down's Syndrome

Trisomy 21, or Down's syndrome, is probably the most common chromosomal disorder associated with growth retardation, affecting approximately 1 in 600 live births. On average, newborns with Down's syndrome have birthweights 500 g below normal and are 2 to 3 cm shorter. Growth failure continues postnatally and is typically associated with delayed skeletal maturation and a delayed and incomplete pubertal growth spurt. Adult heights range from 135 to 170 cm in men and 127 to 158 cm in women.[18] The etiology of growth failure in Down's syndrome and in other autosomal defects is unknown. Attempts to find underlying hormonal explanations for growth retardation have been unsuccessful, even though hypothyroidism due to Hashimoto's thyroiditis is more common than normal in Down's syndrome and should be sought. Marginal levels of GH secretion and low serum levels of IGF-I have been reported in Down's syndrome and exogenous GH may be efficacious in the short term (references found in reference 20). It is more likely, however, that the growth failure reflects a generalized biochemical abnormality of the epiphyseal growth plate. Although GH treatment in children with Down's syndrome and growth hormone deficiency (GHD) will augment growth velocity, there is no improvement of mental or gross motor development. Some improvement in fine motor development has been noted.[531] We do not believe GH treatment is indicated outside of study protocols, because there has been a persistent concern regarding development of leukemia in such children without exposure to exogenous GH.

Turner's Syndrome

In girls with Turner's syndrome (gonadal dysgenesis), short stature is the single most common feature, occurring more frequently than delayed puberty, cubitus valgus, or webbing of the neck.[532-534] In large series of such individuals, short stature occurs in 95% to 100% of girls with a 45,X karyotype.[535-537] Several distinct phases of growth have been identified in girls with Turner's syndrome[538-540]: (1) mild intrauterine growth retardation (IUGR), with mean birthweights and lengths of 2800 g and 48.3 cm, respectively; (2) slow growth recognized during early infancy and falling to −3 SD by 3 years of age[541]; (3) delayed onset of the "childhood phase" of growth[12,13,540] and progressive decline in height velocity from age 3 years until approximately 14 years of age, resulting in further deviation from normal height percentiles; and (4) a prolonged adolescent growth phase, characterized by a partial return toward normal height, followed by delayed epiphyseal fusion. Mean adult heights in the United States and Europe range from 142.0 to 146.8 cm (lower in Asia). There are important genetic and ethnic influences upon growth in these girls. Parental height correlates well with final patient height,[542,543] and a cross-cultural study in 15 countries demonstrated a very strong correlation ($r = 0.91$) between final height in Turner's syndrome and in the normal population with an approximate 20-cm deficit.[535]

The cause of growth failure in Turner's syndrome remains unclear. These girls have many features of a skeletal dysplasia and are haploinsufficient for the SHOX gene (short stature homeobox-containing gene) located in the pseudoautosomal region of the short arm of the X chromosome.[544] When contrasting heights in Turner's syndrome to that of Leri-Weil dyschondrosteosis, which has a SHOX deletion, it seems that the SHOX defect may account for about two thirds of the height deficit in Turner's syndrome.[545] Mutations and deletions of this gene are associated with poor height growth and several syndromes of skeletal dysplasia, including Madelung's deformity, which is also seen in Turner's syndrome.[544,546,547] The incidence of intrauterine growth retardation is much greater in those girls lacking two copies of the SHOX gene (46% vs. 7%).[548] Most patients have normal GH and IGF levels during childhood; reports of low GH or IGF levels in adolescents with Turner's syndrome are likely due to low serum levels of gonadal steroids.[549] Growth impairment is clinically evident before the period when activity of the GH-IGF axis is decreased. Nevertheless, GH therapy is capable of both accelerating short-term growth and increasing adult height.[537,550,551] This diagnosis must be considered in all girls with unexplained growth failure and especially in girls who are short for family but are growing between the 5th and 10th percentiles in the first decade of life. Nonetheless, the mean age at diagnosis lagged 5.3 years behind the age at which Turner's syndrome patients fell below the 5th percentile,[552] at which point its frequency is approximately 1/100. Such data affirm the need for vigorous assessment of all girls who are either absolutely short or relatively small for family heights.

18q Deletions

Deletion of the long arm of chromosome 18 has an estimated prevalence of 1 in 40,000 live births. In a review of 50 cases, 64% of children (mean age 5.8±4.5 years) had heights greater than 2 SD below the mean, only 6% being greater than 0 SDS.[553] Fifteen percent had serum IGF-I concentrations and 9% IGFBP-3 concentrations below −2 SD. Seventy-two percent of children had reduced GH responses to provocative testing, although such testing was not always rigorous. In a group of 13 children GH-treated for an average of 37 months, net height increase compared to 10 untreated was approximately+2 SD, but more intriguing was a "clinically significant" increment in cognitive measures.[554] These latter data are strengthened by a longer GH treatment trial in small for gestational age (SGA) children (see later).

Intrauterine Growth Retardation

Infants with IUGR comprise a heterogeneous group with birthweight and/or length below the 3rd or 10th percentile for gestational age depending on the study.[555] They may also be referred to as small for gestational age (SGA) infants, in contrast to those who are appropriate for gestational age (AGA). The importance of this distinction, in addition to a number of issues influencing neonatal morbidity, is in the prediction of later growth: most AGA low-birthweight infants experience catch-up growth during the first 2 years of life, in contrast to the slower, attenuated growth of SGA infants who may have persistent height deficits throughout childhood and adolescence. First trimester growth failure has been closely associated with low birthweight and low birthweight percentile.[556] The earlier in gestation that fetal growth is impaired, the less likely that complete recapture of lost growth will occur.

IUGR can arise from abnormalities in the fetus, the placenta, or the mother (Table 23–4). Factors affecting fetal growth include nutrition provided by the maternal-placental system, alterations of fetal IGF production, and as yet unclarified genes. Although it is understandable why uterine constraint or twin pregnancies might result in limited fetal growth, the reason for abnormal fetal growth in most cases of IUGR is unclear.

The implications of IUGR may extend beyond fetal life. Although most SGA infants exhibit catch-up growth by 2 years of age, a large subgroup remains small. In a retrospective study of 47 individuals who had IUGR, 23 men had a mean adult height of 162 cm, and 24 women had a mean adult height of 148 cm.[557] Larger studies[555] demonstrate that SGA children had a fivefold to sevenfold greater chance of short stature than AGA children did. Ten percent to 15% of SGA infants will have short stature, and this group makes up as much as 20% of all short children. In a study of a more severely affected neonatal intensive care unit (ICU) SGA population, 27% had not yet achieved catch-up by 6 years of age.[558] Final adult height is −0.8 to −0.9 SD, which is a mean deficit of 3.6 to 4 cm when adjusted for family stature.[559] The endocrinologic mechanisms of the poor growth are varied but may include abnormalities of GH production and secretory patterns and insensitivity to GH and IGF-I action. Alterations of levels of the GH-dependent peptides do not seem to predict subsequent growth patterns,[555,560,561] although ghrelin levels have been correlated with postnatal catch-up growth.[561]

The childhood and adolescent endocrine disorders associated with the subset of the SGA children, who show a striking increment of weight gain during the first several years of life, include premature adrenarche, insulin resistance, functional ovarian hyperandrogenism, and an attenuated pubertal growth spurt.[562] Furthermore, such SGA infants have an increased risk of hypertension, maturity-onset diabetes, and cardiovascular disease later in life.[563-565] These data support the Barker hypothesis, which states that the fetal metabolic responses to a nutritionally hostile intrauterine environment may lead, most strikingly in the setting of childhood and adolescent obesity, to inappropriate extrauterine consequences that result in ovarian dysfunction and the metabolic syndrome.[566-569] These problems do not appear to occur in SGA babies without "catch-up" growth, although insulin resistance has been described.[570] Whether IUGR is *causally* related to these disorders or is a symptom of an underlying inborn metabolic disorder is not yet known.

TABLE 23–4 CAUSES OF INTRAUTERINE GROWTH RETARDATION

I. Intrinsic Fetal Abnormalities
   A. Chromosomal disorders
   B. Syndromes associated with primary growth failure
      1. Russell-Silver syndrome
      2. Seckel's syndrome
      3. Noonan's syndrome
      4. Progeria
      5. Cockayne's syndrome
      6. Bloom's syndrome
      7. Prader-Willi syndrome
      8. Rubenstein-Taybi syndrome
   C. Congenital infections
   D. Congenital anomalies
II. Placental Abnormalities
   A. Abnormal implantation of the placenta
   B. Placental vascular insufficiency; infarction
   C. Vascular malformations
III. Maternal Disorders
   A. Malnutrition
   B. Constraints on uterine growth
   C. Vascular disorders
      1. Hypertension
      2. Toxemia
      3. Severe diabetes mellitus
   D. Uterine malformations
   E. Drug ingestion
      1. Tobacco
      2. Alcohol
      3. Narcotics

Derived from Underwood LE, Van Wyk JJ. Normal and aberrant growth. In Wilson JD, Foster DW, eds. Williams Textbook of Endocrinology Philadelphia: WB Saunders, 1991:1079-1138.

Intrinsic Fetal Factors

In contrast to the role of the endocrine system in postnatal growth, intrauterine growth is less dependent upon fetal pituitary hormones.[571,572] Athyreotic and agonadal infants are of normal length and weight at birth. Pituitary GH is synthesized and secreted by the latter half of the first trimester, with midgestational levels peaking at 150 μg/L and then falling to around 30 μg/L at term.[101] Because the anencephalic fetus is normal in size, the pituitary was thought to be unnecessary for fetal growth.[573,574] However, documentation of birth size of rats and humans with congenital GHD[575-578] and of human newborns with mutations of the GH or GH receptor genes[124] indicates that GH from the fetal pituitary makes a small contribution to birth size. Infants with neonatal GHD are around −0.5 to −1.5 SD below the mean in length and are heavy for this length.[576-578]

These observations should not be interpreted to mean that the IGF axis is unimportant in fetal growth. Gene knockout studies causing elimination of paracrine/autocrine production of IGF-I, IGF-II, as well as of the type 1 IGF receptor, impair fetal growth although placenta size is normal.[227,228,247,579] Circulating IGF-I levels in fetal and cord blood correlate with fetal size and are reduced in IUGR, especially in situations associated with decreased growth velocity.[107,580-582] Similar data suggestive of marked GH insensitivity are found in the first week of life following severe fetal malnutrition.[583] The molar ratio of IGF-II to the IGF-II receptor was also related to birthweight and placenta weight.[584] The initial case of a deletion of the IGF-I gene had profound intrauterine growth failure.[238,585] The implication of that report is that local tissue production of IGF-I is critical for intrauterine growth and that its regulation is largely GH-independent. Human umbilical cord lymphocytes have increased numbers of IGF receptors[586] and mRNAs for both IGF-I and -II are abundant in fetal tissues.[587,588] Exogenous IGF-I administration increases neonatal growth rate and protein and fat accretion in pigs with IUGR.[589] Hepatic levels of GH receptor mRNA and of GH receptor are low in the fetus,[101,590,591] perhaps explaining the modest impact of GH upon IGF production and linear growth. In neonates with IUGR GH levels are elevated,[592] and exogenous GH treatment has little or no effect upon growth, body composition, or energy expenditure,[593,594] further supporting a state of relative insensitivity to GH at this developmental stage. With defects of the GH receptor, neonatal IGF levels are low,[101] suggesting a role for GH in regulating IGF production at the very late stages of gestation. Similarly, the IGFBPs are identifiable in serum and other biological fluids in the fetus and newborn.[399] However, serum levels of IGFBP-3 and ALS, the major serum carriers of IGF peptides in the adult, are low in the fetus and newborn. Thus, the components of the IGF system are apparently regulated directly by glucose levels or indirectly by fetal insulin secretion, with less impact of GH levels.[595-597] The role of insulin production in fetal growth is demonstrated by somatic overgrowth of the hyperinsulinemic infants of diabetic mothers and of infants with the syndrome of persistent neonatal hyperinsulinemic hypoglycemia (nesidioblastosis).[598-600] In contrast, infants with pancreatic agenesis or with abnormalities of the insulin receptor in the "leprechaun" syndrome are small for gestational age.[598] Furthermore, the inverse relationship of insulin and IGFBP-1 levels and the finding that fetal IGFBP-1 levels are elevated in IUGR[597] support an important role for insulin in fetal growth regulation. In addition to these well-characterized endocrine profiles, cord blood cortisol levels are inversely related to IGF-I and directly to IGFBP-3 concentrations.[582] In infants with IUGR, a close correlation (r=−0.54) was observed between cord blood cortisol levels and skeletal growth during the first 3 months of life. This is the period during which substantial catch-up growth occurs in some, but clearly not all, IUGR infants.[601] In those with the greatest catch-up growth, evidence for many of the components of the metabolic syndrome becomes apparent by adolescent years or earlier. There are further data that suggest that a hostile intrauterine environment leading to premature delivery and then the adverse circumstances (nutritionally and otherwise) may also result in insulin resistance, increased abdominal adiposity, and later-life obesity in AGA-infants.[602-604] This suggests that the immediate postnatal period, as well as intrauterine life, may strongly influence long-term outcomes.

Infants with IUGR exhibiting poor postnatal growth, particularly when the abnormalities are intrinsic to the fetus, have frequently been categorized as having "primordial growth failure." These children also have resistance to the action of the GH-IGF axis, which also may lead to insulin resistance.[605] The use of GH treatment in such infants is discussed later. The complex role of GH treatment of these children in influencing the propensity to insulin resistance is not clear, but has not yet resulted in the appearance of clinical diabetes. Several syndromes are briefly discussed in the following paragraphs.

Russell-Silver Syndrome (RSS)

This condition was independently described by Russell[606] and by Silver and associates.[607] Although this syndrome is probably due to a heterogeneous group of disorders, the common findings include IUGR, postnatal growth failure, congenital hemihypertrophy, and small, triangular facies.[608-611] Nonspecific findings include clinodactyly, precocious puberty, delayed closure of the fontanels, and delayed bone age.[608-610] Adults are short with final heights around −4 SD below the mean.[609,611] Endogenous GH secretion in prepubertal RSS children is similar to that in other short IUGR children and less than in AGA short children.[601,612] Because no genetic or biochemical basis for this disorder has been identified, RSS is often used incorrectly as a designation for IUGR of unknown etiology. Maternal uniparental disomy of chromosome 7 exists in 7% to 10% of cases.[54,613-615] Candidate genes in chromosome region 7p11-13, such as those for IGFBP-1, IGFBP-3, and EGF-R, all show bi-allelic expression, but a growth suppression gene, GRB10, which binds to the insulin and IGF-I receptors and replicates asynchronously, remains a candidate gene for overexpression.[615,616] Paternally expressed imprinted genes at 7q32, PEG/MEST, and g2-COP are other candidates.[614,617,618]

Seckel's Syndrome

Although originally described by Mann and Russell in 1959,[619] this condition is most commonly termed *Seckel's syndrome* or *Seckel's birdheaded dwarfism.*[620] Seckel's syndrome is an autosomal recessive disorder characterized by IUGR and severe postnatal growth failure, combined with microcephaly, prominent nose, and micrognathia. Final height is typically 90 to 110 cm, with moderate to severe mental retardation. The nature of the underlying defect is unknown, although the gene defect may be at 3q22.1-q24.[621]

Noonan's Syndrome

Although this condition shares certain phenotypic features with Turner's syndrome, the two disorders are clearly distinct.[622,623] In Noonan's syndrome, the sex chromosomes are normal, and transmission is apparently autosomal dominant, although about 50% of cases are sporadic. Approximately half of the patients have been found to have heterozygous missense mutations of PTNP11, leading to a gain-of-function mutation of a nonreceptor type II tyrosine phosphatase SHP-2 (enhancing intracellular dephosphorylation).[624-626] Both males and females may be affected, explaining the misleading terms "Turner-like syndrome" and "male Turner syndrome." Affected individuals typically have webbing of the neck, a low posterior hairline, ptosis, cubitus valgus, and malformed ears. Cardiac abnormalities are primarily right-sided (pulmonary valve, more frequently in the mutation positive patients), rather than the left-sided lesions (aorta, aortic valve) characteristic of Turner's syndrome. Although birthweight is generally within the normal range, mean growth in length and weight is below the third percentile through much of childhood, with a falling height velocity not dissimilar to that seen in Turner's syndrome, except for the late and attenuated pubertal increment characteristic of the latter condition.[627,628] GH secretory abnormalities do not account for the short stature, although endogenous GH production may be reduced somewhat.[629,630] Presumably, the increase of function mutation leading to enhanced intracellular phosphatase activity would diminish the effectiveness of GH-induced IGF production.[631-633] Microphallus and cryptorchidism are common, and puberty may be delayed or incomplete. Mental retardation of variable degrees is present in approximately 25% to 50% of patients.

Progeria

The senile appearance characteristic of progeria (Hutchinson-Gilford syndrome) is typically apparent by 2 years of age.[634] There is a progressive loss of subcutaneous fat, accompanied by alopecia, hypoplasia of the nails, joint limitation, early onset of atherosclerosis, typically followed by angina, myocardial infarction, hypertension, and congestive heart failure. Skeletal hypoplasia results in severe growth retardation, which typically becomes evident by 6 to 18 months of age.

Cockayne's Syndrome

Cockayne's syndrome, like progeria, is characterized by a premature senile appearance.[635] Retinal degeneration, photosensitivity of the skin, and impaired hearing may also be present. Growth failure typically appears at 2 to 4 years of age. Transmission is as an autosomal recessive disorder.

Prader-Willi Syndrome

In Prader-Willi syndrome (PWS),[636] growth failure may be evident at birth and is more impressive postnatally. It is considered at length in the section on IGF deficiency syndrome due to hypothalamic dysfunction.

Other syndromes associated with moderate to profound growth failure include Bloom's syndrome, de Lange's syndrome, leprechaunism (mutations of the insulin receptor gene), Ellis-van Creveld syndrome, Aarskog's syndrome, Rubenstein-Taybi syndrome, mulibrey nanism (Perheentupa's syndrome), Dubowitz's syndrome, and Johanson-Blizzard syndrome.[637] It is perhaps of interest that the gene for the ghrelin receptor is close to the mapped location of the de Lange syndrome.[638]

Maternal and Placental Factors

Maternal factors and placental insufficiency can impair fetal growth. While such affected infants have better growth potential than do infants with "primordial growth failure," postnatal growth is not always normal. Maternal nutrition is an important contributor to fetal growth and to growth during the first year of life.[639] Fetal growth retardation may also result from alcohol consumption during pregnancy[640-642] and from use of cocaine,[643] marijuana,[643] or tobacco.[644] The mechanisms for such drug-induced fetal growth retardation are unclear but probably include uterine vasoconstriction and vascular insufficiency, placental abruption, and premature rupture of membranes. Although maternal tobacco use is, statistically, a major contributor to reduced fetal size, it is unlikely, by itself, to result in severe IUGR. The maternal hormonal milieu is affected by placental steroids and peptides, especially placental GH and human placental lactogen (HPL), also termed *human chorionic somatomammotropin* (HCS), which influence the production of maternal IGF-I.[595] Maternal IGF affects placental function and may facilitate transport of nutrients to the fetus, and maternal IGF-I levels have been found to correlate with fetal growth.[645,646] Hasegawa and colleagues[647] have found increased levels of free (non–IGFBP-bound) IGF-I levels during normal human pregnancy, possibly due to accelerated proteolysis of IGFBP-3.

The placenta has multiple functions, including the transporting of nutrients, oxygen, and waste, as well as the production of hormones, and it consumes oxygen and glucose brought to it by the uterine circulation. Placental GH affects maternal IGF production that in turn affects placental function. The finding of normal levels of placental GH and IGF-I in a woman with Pit-1 deficiency supports the importance of placental GH action.[648] Additionally, ghrelin message and peptide are present in human placentae during the first trimester.[638] HPL is a major regulator of glucose, amino acid and lipid metabolism in the mother, aiding in the mobilization of nutrients for transport into the fetus. Damage to the placenta by vascular disease, infection, or intrinsic abnormalities of the syncytiotrophoblasts can impair these important functions. Sometimes, examination of the placenta will yield diagnostic information as to the cause of IUGR. An X-linked homeobox gene, Esx1, detected only in extraembryonic tissues and human testis, is a chromosomally imprinted regulator of placental morphogenesis.[649-651] Heterozygous and homozygous mutant mice were born 20% smaller than normal and had large edematous placentae.[650] Vasculature was abnormal at the maternal-fetal interface, presumably causing the growth retardation.

Secondary Growth Disorders

Malnutrition

Given the worldwide presence of undernutrition, it is not surprising that inadequate caloric and/or protein intake is the most common cause of growth failure.[652] *Marasmus* refers to cases with an overall deficiency of calories including protein malnutrition. Subcutaneous fat is minimal, and protein wasting is marked. *Kwashiorkor*, on the other hand, refers specifically to inadequate protein intake, although it may also be characterized by some caloric undernutrition. In both conditions, multiple deficiencies of vitamins and minerals are apparent.[653] Frequently, the two conditions overlap. Decreased weight growth generally precedes the failure of linear growth by a very short time in the neonatal period and by several years at older ages. Stunting of growth due to caloric and/or protein malnutrition in early life will often have lifelong consequences, with diminished skeletal growth.[654]

Both acute and chronic malnutrition affects the GH-IGF system. The impaired growth is usually associated with elevated basal and/or stimulated serum GH levels,[655] but in generalized malnutrition (marasmus), GH levels may be normal or low.[656] In both conditions, serum IGF-I levels are reduced.[657,658] Malnutrition may, consequently, be considered a form of GH insensitivity, with serum IGF-I levels reduced despite normal or elevated GH levels. GHBP levels, as a reflection of GH receptor content, are decreased.[432,659] GH insensitivity may be an adaptive response, whereby protein is spared by the lipolytic and antiinsulin actions of GH.[660,661] Reduced serum IGF-I levels would serve to shift calories from anabolic to survival requirements. These adaptive mechanisms are accompanied by changes in serum IGFBPs to further limit IGF action during periods of malnutrition.[659,662]

Neonatal nutrition of normal babies may play an important subsequent role in intellectual development and statural growth. In a normal population of 8- to 9-year old children, IGF-I levels correlated with intelligence quotient, with each increase of 100 ng/mL associated with an increase of 3.2 IQ points.[663] Babies who are breastfed are taller in later childhood and in adulthood.[664] IGF-I levels during middle childhood years are positively related to the amount of breastfeeding and correlate with the taller stature.[665] Formula-fed (higher protein intake) babies grow more rapidly and gain more weight in infancy.[432] They have higher IGF-I levels in early life, but lower IGF-I in adulthood along with shorter stature.[666] In population studies, mean mid-childhood height differences of 1 cm are associated with as little as 2 to 3 ng/mL differences in IGF-I concentrations.[665,667] Whether these findings are related to an early, nutrition-related setting of the hypothalamic-pituitary-IGF axis that ultimately results in greater IGF production in the initially lower protein-fed group is an interesting and testable hypothesis.

Inadequate calorie/protein intake complicates many chronic diseases that are characterized by growth failure. Anorexia is a common feature of renal failure and inflammatory bowel disease, and occurs with cyanotic heart disease, congestive heart failure, central nervous system disease, and other illnesses. Some of these conditions may, furthermore, be characterized by deficiencies of specific dietary components, such as zinc, iron, and vitamins necessary for normal growth and development.

Undernutrition may also be voluntary, as with dieting and food fads (Fig. 23–41).[668] Caloric restriction is especially common in girls during adolescence, in whom it may be associated with anxiety concerning obesity, and in gymnasts and ballet dancers. Anorexia nervosa and bulimia are extremes of "voluntary" caloric deprivation and are commonly associated with impaired growth prior to epiphyseal fusion that may result in diminished final adult height.[669-671] Adolescent bone mineral accretion is impaired and significant osteopenia may persist into adulthood.[672,673] Later in adolescence, malnutrition may cause delayed puberty and/or menarche and a variety of metabolic alterations. In anorexia nervosa, hormonal profiles are similar to those in protein-energy malnutrition,[669-671,674] with high basal levels of GH but low levels of IGF-I, IGFBP-3, and GHBP. GHBP and IGFBP-3 levels correlate with body mass index as in normal children.[111,669,675] The hormones of the GH-IGF axis return to normal levels with refeeding.[659,669,675]

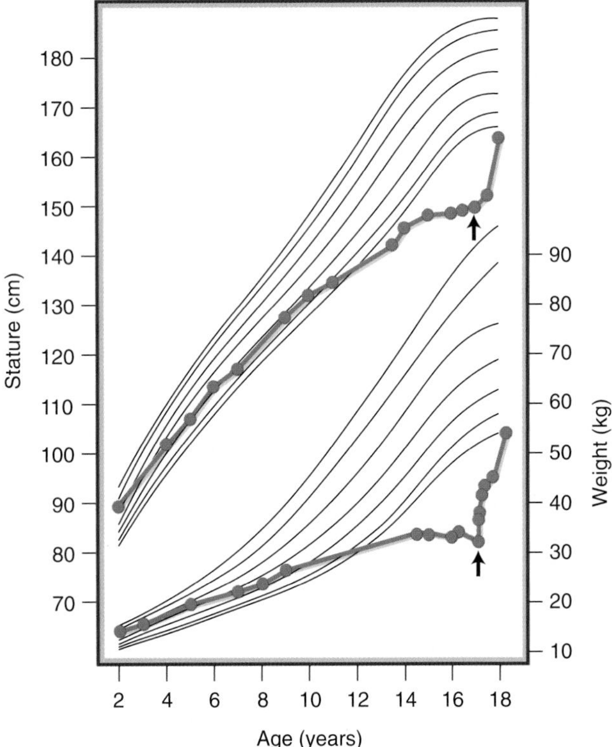

Figure 23–41 ▪ Curves of weight and height of a child who had growth failure resulting from prolonged self-imposed caloric restriction because of a fear of becoming obese. Note that crossing of percentiles on the weight curve preceded that for the height curve, and when the caloric intake was normalized (*arrow*), the gain in weight occurred before the improvement in linear growth. Also note that at the end of the prolonged period of caloric restriction, weight age (10.2 years) was less than height age (12 years). (Pugliese MT, Lifshitz F, Grad G, et al. Fear of obesity: a cause of short stature and delayed puberty. N Engl J Med 1983;309:513-518. Reprinted by permission of the New England Journal of Medicine.)

A complex clinical state of emaciation with high levels of GH, but at least initially normal linear growth and IGF concentrations, is the diencephalic syndrome.[676] Hypothalamic tumors cause this failure to thrive, with the later appearance of classic central nervous system (CNS) signs and symptoms; this condition differs from anorexia nervosa in that the IGF levels do not reflect the state of severe GH resistance seen in the latter state.

Chronic Diseases[677]

Malabsorption/Gastrointestinal Diseases

Intestinal disorders that impair absorption of calories or protein cause growth failure, for many of the reasons cited above.[660,678,679] Growth retardation may predate other manifestations of malabsorption and/or chronic inflammatory bowel disease. Accordingly, celiac disease (gluten-induced enteropathy) and regional enteritis (Crohn's disease) should be considered in the differential diagnosis of unexplained growth failure. Serum levels of IGF-I may be reduced,[660,680] reflecting the malnutrition, and it is critical to discriminate between these conditions and GHD or related disorders causing IGF-I deficiency. Documentation of malabsorption requires demonstration of fecal wasting of calories, especially fecal fat, along with other measures of gut dysfunction such as the d-xylose or breath hydrogen studies.

In celiac disease, an immune-mediated disorder in which the intestinal mucosa is damaged by dietary gluten (Fig. 23–42), impaired linear growth may be the first manifestation of

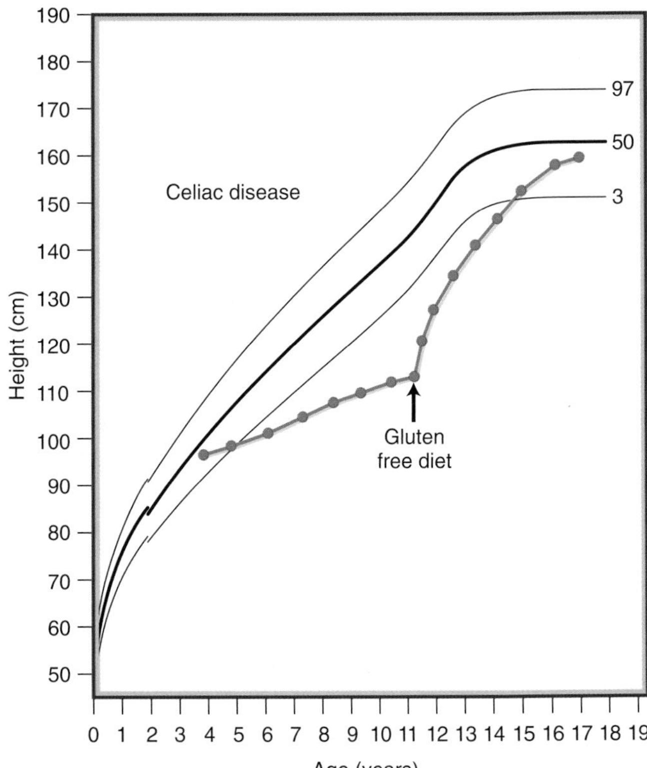

Figure 23–42 ▪ Catch-up growth in a girl with gluten-induced enteropathy (celiac disease). After 8 years of growth impairment, the patient was placed on a gluten-free diet and demonstrated substantial catch-up growth. Note the return to the previous growth percentiles. (Courtesy of J. M. Tanner.)

disease.[660,681-684] The degree of growth impairment may be similar in patients with or without gastrointestinal symptoms.[660] It is associated, as well, with Turner's syndrome, type 1 diabetes mellitus, Down's syndrome, and Williams syndrome. In European studies, celiac disease is the cause of unexplained growth impairment in 5% to 20% of unselected patients, although this high frequency does not hold true in many centers, and may reflect varying stringency in the diagnostic criteria employed.[682-684] The onset and progression of puberty may be delayed and menarche may be late.[681] Measurement of an IgA tissue transglutaminase antibody[685] is the currently recommended screening test. One must remember that IgA deficiency is the most common imunodeficiency when assessing the antibody data. Nonetheless, the diagnosis of celiac disease ultimately requires demonstration of the characteristic mucosal flattening in small bowel biopsy. The incidence of childhood celiac disease in the United States is around 0.9%.[686] Changes in the serologic profiles mirror the clinical status, obviating the need for subsequent biopsies. Gluten withdrawal is a highly effective treatment for celiac disease and results in rapid catch-up growth and decreased clinical symptoms during the first 6 to 12 months of treatment.[660,681] Low IGF-I and IGFBP-3 levels return to normal during this period.[680,687] Most children who receive appropriate dietary management ultimately achieve a normal final height.[688,689]

Growth failure in Crohn's disease, which correlates with disease severity,[690] is probably due to a combination of malnutrition from malabsorption and anorexia, chronic inflammation,[678,679] inadequacy of trace minerals in the diet, and use of glucocorticoids.[691] IGF-I levels are low, especially with impaired growth.[660,679] One third to two thirds or more of children with Crohn's disease have impaired growth at diagnosis and occasional patients have significant growth failure as the first evidence of Crohn's disease.[660,679,692,693] Osteopenia is common.[673,694] An elevated erythrocyte sedimentation rate, anemia, and low serum albumin are useful clues, but diagnosis ultimately requires colonoscopy and biopsy, along with gastrointestinal imaging studies. Long-term treatment includes enteral and parenteral nutrition, antiinflammatory agents, alternate day steroid therapy, and judicious operative intervention. Newer therapeutic alternatives may include GH.[695,696] Permanent impairment of linear growth and deficits of final height may occur in 30% of patients.[691] Around 20% of patients at adult height are more than 8 cm below the midparental target height.[697]

Chronic Liver Disease

Impaired linear growth and short stature with chronic liver disease in childhood[698-701] are caused by decreased food intake, fat and fat-soluble vitamin malabsorption, trace element deficiencies, and abnormalities of the GH-IGF system.[701,702] Decreased levels of IGF-I, IGF-II, and IGFBP-3 and increased GH secretion define the acquired GH insensitivity syndrome.[703-706] A close correlation between GH-dependent peptides and liver function indicates the dominant regulatory role of damaged hepatocytes in the growth retardation characteristic of end-stage liver failure.[703] Low levels of full-length and truncated GH receptors in the cirrhotic liver and consequent diminished release of GHBP substantiate the GH insensitivity.[707] Despite provision of adequate calories, insensitivity to the action of GH persists.[701,704] Liver transplantation prolongs life expectancy, but linear growth is variably improved in the early posttransplantation years.[700,705,708,709] Exogenous glucocorticoid administration presumably plays a major role in the continued growth retardation[700,709]; GH and IGF-I production are normal, but the amount of "free IGF" may be decreased as IGFBP-3 levels are relatively high.[705,708] Posttransplantation growth is inversely correlated with age and directly correlated with degree of growth impairment at transplantation.[699,700] Exogenous GH treatment, for a period of 18 months, enhances growth rates and increases median height SDS by 0.7 units.[710,711]

Cardiovascular Disease

Congenital heart disease with cyanosis or chronic congestive heart failure can cause growth failure.[712-714] As many as 27% of children with varied cardiac lesions were below the 3rd percentile for height and weight in one survey,[715] and 70% were lower than the 50th percentile in another.[716] Because cardiac defects are usually congenital, many infants have dysmorphic features and IUGR. Inadequate caloric intake is the most common cause of growth impairment in children with congenital heart disease[714,716,717] frequently associated with anorexia and vomiting. Chronic congestive heart failure is associated with malabsorption that includes protein-losing enteropathy, intestinal lymphangiectasia, and steatorrhea. Greater cardiac and respiratory work and the relatively higher ratio of metabolically active, energy-utilizing brain and heart to the growth-retarded body mass (cardiac cachexia[718]) cause an increased basal metabolic rate in these children.[719-721] Food intake that appears adequate for the child's weight, thus, is often inadequate for normal growth. The degree of cyanosis or hypoxia does correlate with the degree of growth impairment.[714,716,722] Decreased levels of IGF-I and IGFBP-3,[723,724] normal levels of GH, and hepatic GH receptors in chronically hypoxemic newborn sheep[724] suggest GH insensitivity distal to the GH receptor. Linear growth and pubertal maturation depend upon left ventricular function in children and adolescents with complicated rheumatic heart disease.[725]

Corrective surgery may restore normal growth, frequently after a phase of "catch-up" growth with normalization of energy expenditure.[720,726] Surgery must, on occasion, be delayed until the infant reaches an appropriate size, resulting in the conundrum that surgery corrects growth failure but cannot be performed because the infant is too small. In these situations, meticulous attention to caloric support and alleviation of hypoxia and heart failure are necessary to promote growth before surgery. Fortunately, this problem has diminished because of operative successes in the neonatal period. The nutritional management of these infants includes calorie-dense feedings because of the need to restrict fluids, calcium supplementation because of the use of diuretics that may cause calcium loss in the urine, and iron to maintain an enhanced rate of erythropoiesis.

Renal Disease

All conditions that impair renal function can impair growth.[727-731] Uremia and renal tubular acidosis can cause growth failure before other clinical manifestations become evident. The growth impairment results from multiple mechanisms, including inadequate formation of 1,25-dihydroxycholecalciferol (1,25 $[OH]_2D$), with resultant osteopenia, decreased caloric intake, loss of electrolytes necessary for normal growth, metabolic acidosis, protein wasting, insulin resistance, chronic anemia, and compromised cardiac function, as well as from impairment of GH and IGF production and action. In nephropathic cystinosis, acquired hypothyroidism contributes to the inadequate growth.[732] Sixty percent to 75% of patients with chronic renal failure treated before the GH therapeutic era had final adult heights more than −2 SD below the mean.[733]

Children and adolescents have normal or elevated circulating levels of GH, depending upon the degree of renal failure.[728,729,734-738] In children with end-stage renal disease on dialysis (ESRD) or preterminal chronic renal failure (CRF), the half-life of GH is prolonged twofold.[703] The number of secretory bursts was increased in ESRD by twofold to threefold over CRF and controls, and the mean levels of GH were 2.5-fold higher in ESRD than in CRF or controls. Overall, children with ESRD had a substantially higher GH production than either CRF patients or controls. Early reports of decreased serum IGF levels in uremia were an artifact due to inadequate separation of IGF from IGFBPs prior to assay.[267] Decreased hepatic IGF production[739] is possibly due to low hepatic GH receptor gene expression.[740] Additionally, the uremic state may cause a postreceptor defect in GH signal transduction by diminishing phosphorylation and nuclear translocation of GH-activated STAT proteins.[741,742] Serum IGF-I and -II levels are, however, usually normal,[728,734,735,743] but increases in serum IGFBPs, especially IGFBP-1 and IGFBP-6,[728,729,734,743,744] may inhibit IGF action.[745-748] In nephrotic syndrome, serum levels of IGF-I and IGFBP-3 are low because of urinary loss of IGF-IGFBP complexes.[730] Chronic glucocorticoid therapy for a variety of renal disorders can exacerbate growth retardation by diminishing GH release and blunting IGF-I action at growth plates.[747,749-751] Chronic renal disease, especially ESRD, with increased GH levels and production, low levels of IGF-I, and poor growth is, thus, a state of relative resistance to GH and, in some instances, to IGF-I, as well.[733,745-748,752]

Even after successful renal transplantation, growth may not be normal.[753-757] In the large cohort of patients in the North American Pediatric Renal Transplant Cooperative Study,[755,757,758] mean height increased after transplantation by only 0.11 SD in the first 4.5 years. The youngest age group (younger than 2 years) had the largest deficit and the most catch-up (0.94 SD); children between 6 and 17 years had no improvement in height SD score. Although their younger age group had a 16% mortality,[755] more recent studies[759,760] suggest that transplantation may have an acceptable high risk in such patients. Growth-retarded posttransplantation children, whether receiving daily or alternate-day glucocorticoid treatment, have decreased GH secretion, normal levels of IGF-I and IGFBP-1, and elevated levels of IGFBP-3. They differ from ESRD patients in that IGFBP-1 levels are not strikingly elevated, perhaps because of altered glucose tolerance and hyperinsulinism due to chronic glucocorticoid therapy.[747] Overall, height SDS at the time of transplantation and use of alternate-day glucocorticoid therapy posttransplant correlate positively with final height, and longer duration of reduced GFR and higher cumulative dose of prednisone have a negative impact; other factors such as gender, age at transplantation, diagnosis, and number of transplants do not seem to have significant impact on adult height.[753] The importance of height at the time of transplantation in determining final adult height, despite the complex posttransplantation health issues, confirms the value of improving growth velocity and absolute height before transplantation. Children who receive tacrolimus (FK-506)-based immunosuppression, allowing discontinuation of glucocorticoids, have normal growth and absence of obesity.[761]

Although the growth failure of renal disease in the pretransplantation period is not specifically due to either GH or IGF deficiency, GH therapy accelerates skeletal growth and is approved by the Food and Drug Administration (FDA) for use. Such treatment probably increases the molar ratio of IGF peptides to IGFBPs and may override the inhibitory actions of IGFBPs. GH administration may also be useful for treatment of posttransplantation growth failure.[762-765]

Hematologic Disorders

Chronic anemias, such as sickle cell disease, are characterized by growth failure.[766,767] In general, the decrease in height and weight is greater in adolescent years than earlier, as the onset of the adolescent growth spurt is delayed and menarche is late.[766-768] The adolescent growth and final adult height in sickle cell disease, however, may be normal.[768] The causes of growth retardation probably include impaired oxygen delivery to tissues, increased work of the cardiovascular system, energy demands of increased hematopoiesis, and impaired nutrition. Long-term chronic transfusion therapy as part of stroke prevention treatment is associated with enhanced growth.[769] The GH-IGF system probably does not have an important role in the growth impairment of sickle cell anemia.

In thalassemia, in addition to the consequences of chronic anemia, endocrine deficiencies can result from chronic transfusions and accompanying hemosiderosis.[770] Despite vigorous efforts to maintain hemoglobin levels near normal and to avoid iron overload, growth failure is still a common feature of thalassemia, especially in male adolescents.[771] The patients tend to show body disproportion with truncal shortening but normal leg length. It is likely that anemia, impaired IGF-I synthesis, hypothyroidism, gonadal failure, and hypogonadotropic hypogonadism all contribute to growth failure in this disorder. GH insensitivity in some cases is suggested by generally adequate GH production with low IGF-I levels.[772,773] Several groups have reported data on treatment of thalassemia patients in whom GH production seemed diminished. In most patients, GH treatment increases growth at least initially.[772,774] In a longer term study (average duration 59 months) starting with young (7.2 years) patients, an increased growth velocity was maintained throughout the treatment period[775]; when treatment was initiated at an older age (13.6 years), final height was not improved.[776] A small number of adults with thalassemia are found to have continued GHD so that GH treatment for cardiac and bone health reasons may be important in this disease.[777] About half of the patients in the International Fanconi Anemia Registry have short stature. GH deficiency was demonstrated by provocative testing (22 of 48) or with assessment of endogenous secretion (13 of 13) in a group with mean height of −2.23 SDS.[778]

In pure red cell aplasia,[779] approximately 30% of patients demonstrate growth retardation. The frequency increases with age (42% in individuals older than 16 years) and with treatment programs such as chronic transfusions or glucocorticoids.

Diabetes Mellitus

Although weight loss may occur immediately before the onset of clinically apparent insulin-dependent diabetes mellitus (IDDM), children with new-onset diabetes are frequently taller than their peer group, possibly because GH and insulin levels are increased during the preclinical evolution of the disease.[780-782] Most children with IDDM grow quite normally, even those with marginal control,[783] especially in prepubertal years, although growth velocity may decrease during puberty.[784] Growth failure, however, can occur in diabetic children with longstanding poor glycemic control.[785,786] The Mauriac syndrome[787] describes children with poorly regulated IDDM, severe growth failure, and hepatosplenomegaly due to excess hepatic glycogen deposition. This type of growth retardation has become increasingly rare with modern diabetes care.

Many pathophysiologic processes, including malnutrition, chronic intermittent acidosis, increased glucocorticoid production, hypothyroidism, impaired calcium balance, and "end organ unresponsiveness" to either GH or IGF, may contribute to growth failure in IDDM.[780,788-790] IGF-I and IGFBP-3 levels are diminished in the face of enhanced GH production,[791-795] reflecting acquired GH insensitivity; GHBP levels are decreased,[788,794] supporting the concept of impaired GH receptor number or function. Furthermore, IGFBP-1 is normally suppressed by insulin and hypoinsulinemia results in elevated serum IGFBP-1 levels, which may inhibit IGF action.[794,796-799] In contrast to the situation in adolescents and adults, IGFBP-1 levels are not elevated in well-growing prepubertal children.[798] On the contrary, increased IGFBP-3 proteolysis may enhance the bioactivity of the available IGF-I.[795,800] Most children with IDDM, however, attain normal cellular nutrition and growth factor action despite intermittent hypoinsulinemia and derangements of peripheral indices of the GH-IGF system.

Even though glycemic control is inversely correlated with IGF I levels,[789,791,794,796,801] the correlation between glycemic control and growth is weak. With conflicting reports as to the influence of glycemic regulation on growth,[780,781,802,803] a longitudinal study[803] of 46 children whose diabetes began before age 10 indicated that initial heights at diagnosis were normal and that the final height SDS was minimally reduced from that at onset. In boys, despite a delay of about 2.5 years in onset of puberty, total pubertal height gain was normal. In girls with diabetes, however, total pubertal height gain was diminished and the age of menarche was delayed; the effects of altered insulin and IGF-I levels upon ovarian function have not been assessed in such patients. Chronic metabolic control did not correlate with the pubertal height gain or with the normal final heights. Nevertheless, good glycemic control at certain maturational periods, such as puberty, may improve growth during those intervals.[780,793,804]

Inborn Errors of Metabolism

Inborn errors of metabolism are often accompanied by growth failure that may be pronounced. Glycogen storage disease, the mucopolysaccharidoses, glycoproteinoses, and mucolipidoses are characterized by poor growth. Many inborn metabolic disorders are also associated with significant skeletal dysplasia. In a small number of patients with organic acidoses, such as methylmalonic and propionic acidurias, IGF-I levels are low and GH levels are normal, suggesting a possible state of GH insensitivity related to nutritional status.[805] Preliminary data suggest that exogenous GH treatment may improve the metabolic status of such children.[805,806]

Pulmonary Disease

Growth can be retarded in children with asthma who have not received glucocorticoid therapy.[807,808] Mean height and growth velocity and degree of growth failure are related to the severity of the asthma.[807,808] Delayed pubertal maturation in such patients is also associated with growth deceleration in early teenage years.[807,809] Impaired nutrition and increased energy requirements, along with chronic stress, especially with nocturnal asthma and enhanced endogenous glucocorticoid production, cause poor linear growth. The lowered growth in asthmatic children does not appear to be associated with abnormalities of the GH-IGF axis.[810] Glucocorticoid therapy, generally given to more severely affected patients, further impairs growth throughout childhood.[811-813] Synthetic glucocorticoids, such as prednisone or dexamethasone, may have a greater growth-suppressive effect than equivalent therapeutic doses of cortisol, presumably because the biopotency of the synthetic agents may be underestimated. Alternate-day or aerosolized glucocorticoid therapy often ameliorates growth retardation and can be associated with an accelerated catch-up phase.[807,812] The use of spacer devices and effective nebulizer solutions may permit use of inhaled glucocorticoids in young children without growth impairment.[814-816] Clearly, however, sufficient glucocorticoid delivered by any route can diminish growth and impede the function of the adrenal gland.[817] Nonetheless, judicious utilization of inhaled glucocorticoid results in normal adult height despite long-term exposure and an initial decrement of linear growth velocity.[818] Indeed, examination of near adult heights of Swedish men with asthma demonstrated an improvement in the mean difference between "severe" asthmatics and normal controls in the era of inhaled corticosteroid use.[819] Overall, normal adult height is usually achieved.[820,821]

Bronchopulmonary dysplasia (BPD), a sequela of hyaline membrane disease and prematurity, has an incidence as high as 35% in very low birthweight infants (<1500 g).[822] The use of dexamethasone in the neonatal treatment of BPD causes a transient cessation of growth[823] and has engendered long-term concern for neurodevelopment and somatic growth.[824] Growth in surviving infants is poor through early childhood,[825-827] but the defect generally disappears by 8 years of age.[828-830] Long-term hypoxemia, poor nutrition, chronic pulmonary infections, and reactive airway disease are responsible for the poor early growth.

In patients with cystic fibrosis (CF), chronic pulmonary infection with bronchiectasis, pancreatic insufficiency with exocrine and endocrine inadequacy, malabsorption, and malnutrition all contribute to decreased growth and late sexual maturation. In 17,857 patients with CF, mean height was at the 21st percentile and mean weight was at the 9th percentile.[831] Early impairment of height and weight growth and retardation of skeletal maturation may progress or plateau during midchildhood years but become most marked in the preadolescent period when growth and maturational changes are frequently delayed.[831-833] The degree of growth retardation is related most closely to the severity and variability of the pulmonary disease rather than to pancreatic dysfunction.[834,835] The degree of steatorrhea does not correlate well with growth impairment, though improved nutrition programs enhance the overall clinical picture.[836,837] Adult heights in surviving patients with CF approach the normal range.[677] Endocrine abnormalities, such as failure of both α and β islet cells with decreased glucagon and insulin production do not seem to influence prepubertal growth patterns in children with CF. The incidence of diabetes mellitus increases as patients live past the second decade.[831] Alterations of vitamin D metabolism, while potentially affecting skeletal mineralization, do not diminish growth.[838] Delayed sexual maturation in which GnRH administration evokes a prepubertal pattern of pituitary gonadotropin secretion in adolescent patients is similar to that in constitutional delay of growth and maturation (CDGM).[839,840] The GH-IGF axis shows evidence for some degree of acquired GH insensitivity with lowered mean IGF-I and elevated GH levels.[841] Treatment of prepubertal children with CF with GH for 1 year resulted in an anabolic effect, with greater growth velocity and nitrogen retention and increased protein and decreased fat stores.[842,843] In a 2-year GH treatment program of CF patients who received enteral nutrition before and during GH therapy, auxologic parameters continued to improve.[844] Pulmonary function improved in most patients. A 4-year longitudinal study utilizing the National CF Foundation registry found that improved nutrition status and growth were associated with a slower age-related decrement of pulmonary function.[845] Current perspective would suggest that GH treatment should be adjunctive to an aggressive nutritional program, appropriate pulmonary care without glucocorticoid administration, and careful assessment of carbohydrate metabolism.[846]

Chronic Inflammation/Infection

Poor growth is a characteristic feature of chronic inflammatory disease and recurrent serious infection. We have discussed impaired growth associated with such disorders as Crohn's disease, CF, and asthma in which inflammatory processes may be significant. De Benedetti and colleagues,[847] studying juvenile rheumatoid arthritis in humans and a transgenic murine model expressing excessive IL-6, demonstrated an IL-6–mediated decrease in IGF-I production to be a credible mechanism by which chronic inflammatory disease could lead to poor growth. The close relationship of the GH receptor to that of multiple cytokines[141] makes this an interesting hypothesis. A complex cascade of cytokines, as part of the inflammatory response to acute and chronic infection, can impact the endocrine system at many levels,[848,849] impairing mineral and nutrient metabolism and the growth and remodeling of bone,[850] along with impairing IGF-I production by diminishing the JAK2/STAT5 signal transduction pathway efficiency.[851]

Exposure to human immunodeficiency virus (HIV) in children and adolescents occurs through perinatal transmission, blood transfusions, drug usage, and sexual contact. Growth failure is a cardinal feature of childhood acquired immunodeficiency syndrome (AIDS).[852-857] Mean length and weight measurements during early childhood years are at or below −1 SD below the mean, but weight-for-height data may be normal[855,857] in contrast to the "wasting" syndrome described in adult patients with AIDS.[858,859] In a drug treatment study of 88 HIV-infected children with a mean age of 3.1 years, more than 90% were below the 50th percentile for both height and weight; only 44% of this group survived 4 years after initiation of the study. Height or growth velocity are not useful predictive indicators for survival.[855] Impaired bone quality is found in perinatally affected prepubertal children, seemingly related to low IGF-I levels.[860] In hemophiliac boys with HIV, growth impairment, delayed pubertal onset, and progression and lower skeletal age were common.[856] Despite the delayed pubertal maturation, serum testosterone levels were not significantly decreased. In a short-term treatment trial with standard doses of GH, height and weight growth increased, while protein catabolism diminished, without any adverse effect upon viral burden.[861] In many developing countries, chronic infestation with parasites, such as schistosomiasis, hookworm, and roundworm, contribute to nutritional debilitation and growth failure.[862]

Endocrine Disorders

Hypothyroidism

Growth may be retarded in children with hypothyroidism, but the development of newborn screening programs for congenital hypothyroidism (CH) has resulted in more prompt diagnosis and treatment of such newborns (approximately 1/4100 live births). Growth and bone mineral density in appropriately treated infants and children with CH is normal for age,[863-865] so that skeletal maturation approximates chronologic age.[864] These data do demonstrate the essential role of thyroxine in linear growth during the first year of life.[866] Pubertal growth and maturation and final adult height are normal in well-treated CH.[867] Many features of adult myxedema are present in children with hypothyroidism, but this is not always the case. The most prominent manifestation of acquired hypothyroidism is growth failure, which may be profound.[868] In acquired hypothyroidism, growth retardation may take several years to become clinically evident, but, once present, is typically severe and progressive. The poor growth is more apparent in height than in weight gain, so those children tend to be overweight for height. Rivkees and coworkers[868] have reported a mean 4.2-year delay between slowing of growth and the diagnosis of hypothyroidism. At diagnosis, girls were 4.04 SD below and boys 3.15 SD below mean heights for age. (This is one of many situations in which the diagnosis of short stature is later in girls than in boys.) Body proportion is immature with an increased upper to lower body segment ratio. Skeletal age is usually markedly delayed. Although chronic hypothyroidism is usually associated with delayed puberty, precocious puberty and premature menarche can occur in hypothyroid children (see Chapter 24).

The diagnosis of primary hypothyroidism is usually straightforward. Serum levels of T_4 are reduced, and TSH levels are elevated. The presence of antithyroid antibodies (usually thyroperoxidase antibodies) is consistent with a diagnosis of Hashimoto's thyroiditis, the most common cause of acquired childhood hypothyroidism in the United States. Isolated secondary or tertiary hypothyroidism, due to thyroid-stimulating hormone (TSH) or thyrotropin-releasing hormone (TRH) deficiency, respectively, is a rare cause of hypothyroidism.

Replacement therapy results in rapid catch-up growth. Nevertheless, accelerated growth may not restore full growth potential, because skeletal maturation is rapid during the first 18 months of treatment. In one study of profoundly hypothyroid children, those treated at a mean chronologic age of 11 years had adult heights approximately −2 SD below the mean, final heights that were lower than midparental and predicted adult heights.[868] The deficit in adult stature correlated with the duration of hypothyroidism before initiation of treatment. In a study of hypothyroid children treated at a mean age of 9 years and with a 3-year delay of bone age,[869] mean height SDS for bone age fell from +0.59 to −0.55 in girls and from +1.6 to −0.87 in boys. Catch-up growth may be particularly compromised when therapy is initiated near puberty.[870] Based on these studies it may be appropriate to use lower than usual replacement dosages of levothyroxine and/or to consider a pharmacologic delay of puberty and epiphyseal fusion.

Cushing's Syndrome

Glucocorticoid excess impairs skeletal growth, interferes with normal bone metabolism by inhibiting osteoblastic activity, and enhances bone resorption,[871-873] effects related to the duration of steroid excess,[874] regardless of whether Cushing's syndrome is due to ACTH hypersecretion, adrenal tumor, or glucocorticoid administration. The effects of glucocorticoids are probably at the level of the epiphysis,[747,749,750,875] because GH secretion and serum concentrations of IGF peptides and IGFBPs are usually normal.[873,876] GH treatment cannot completely overcome the growth-inhibiting effects of excess glucocorticoids, although short-term GH or IGF-I administration can diminish many of the catabolic effects.[872,877,878] Linear growth in children receiving glucocorticoids falls during GH therapy if the exogenous prednisone dose is greater than 0.35 mg/kg/day.[873,879] The "toxic" effects of glucocorticoids upon the epiphysis may persist, in part, after correction of chronic glucocorticoid excess, and patients frequently do not attain target heights.[880,881] The longer the duration and the greater the intensity of glucocorticoid excess, the less likely is catch-up growth to be completed. Therefore, exposure to excess glucocorticoids should be limited as much as the underlying condition allows, frequently by the use of alternate-day therapy or inhalants.

Adrenal tumors secreting large amounts of glucocorticoids can produce excess androgens, which may mask growth-inhibitory effects of glucocorticoids. In addition, Cushing's syndrome in children may not cause all the clinical signs and symptoms associated with the disorder in adults and may present with growth arrest. However, Cushing's syndrome is an unlikely diagnosis in children with obesity, because exogenous obesity is associated with normal or even accelerated skeletal growth, and because growth deceleration is generally evident by the time other signs of Cushing's syndrome appear (Fig. 23–43). In a series of 10 children and adolescents treated for Cushing's disease with surgery and cranial irradiation, mean final height was −1.36 SDS. Post-therapy GHD was common and GH replacement contributed to a positive change of the difference between height and target height from the height at diagnosis until final height (−1.72 to −0.93 SDS).[882,883]

Pseudohypoparathyroidism

This condition is discussed in detail in Chapter 27, but is included here because growth failure is a common feature.[884] This condition typically combines growth failure, characteristic dysmor-

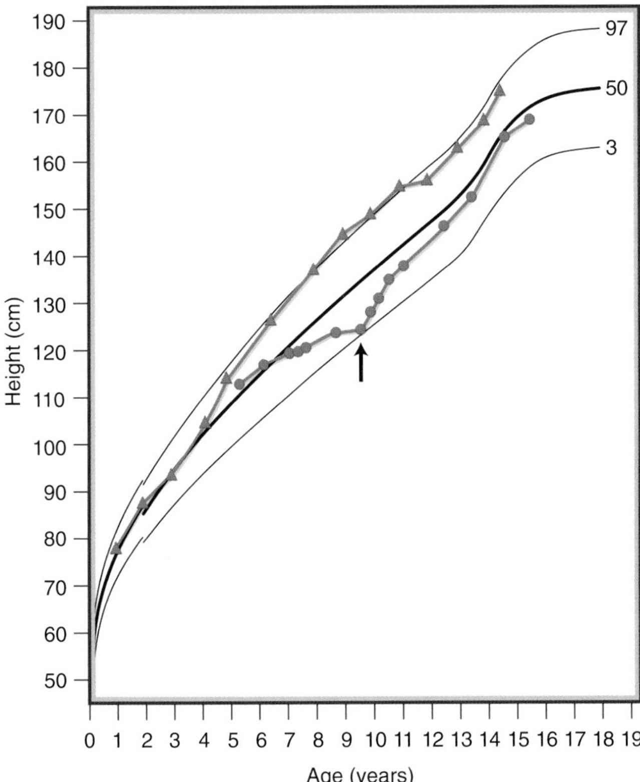

Figure 23–43 ■ Growth curves of two boys with obesity. The boy depicted by the circles had cortisol excess related to Cushing's disease. He had onset of rapid weight gain associated with a decrease in linear growth velocity at age 7. Diagnosis was made and an adrenalectomy (*arrow*) was performed at $9^1/_2$ years with an almost immediate increase in growth rate and striking catch-up. The boy whose growth is depicted by triangles had exogenous obesity. At age $9^1/_2$, his weight was approximately the same as that of the patient with Cushing's disease, but his height was at the 97th percentile, reflecting the enhancement of linear growth in individual was exogenous obesity.

phic features, and hypocalcemia and hyperphosphatemia secondary to end-organ resistance to parathyroid hormone. Children with pseudohypoparathyroidism are characterized by short and truncal obesity, short metacarpals, subcutaneous calcifications, round facies, and mental retardation. Resistance to GHRH-induced GH release has been reported,[885] but studies to demonstrate beneficial effects of exogenous GH remain to be done.

Rickets

In the past, hypovitaminosis D was a major cause of short stature often associated with other causes of growth failure, such as malnutrition, prematurity, malabsorption, hepatic disease, or chronic renal failure (see Chapter 28). In isolated vitamin D deficiency, breastfed infants typically have poor exposure to sunlight and are not nutritionally supplemented with vitamin D. Characteristic skeletal manifestations of rickets include frontal bossing, craniotabes, rachitic rosary, and bowing of the legs. Such children usually begin to synthesize $1,25(OH)_2D$ as they become older, broaden their diet, and have increased exposure to sunlight, with amelioration of the transient early decrease of linear growth velocity. The association of vitamin D receptor gene polymorphism with birth length, growth rate, adult stature, and bone mineral density[886-890] further emphasizes the importance of vitamin D in normal growth. Additionally, vitamin D- and estrogen receptor genotypes appear to interactively affect infant growth, especially in males.[888,891] The presence of high-affinity binding sites for the vitamin D receptor DNA binding domain in the GH promoter suggests that the vitamin D receptor may actually modulate GH expression.[892]

Hypophosphatemic Rickets

This X-linked dominant disorder is due to decreased renal tubular reabsorption of phosphate related to mutations in the phosphate regulating endopeptidase gene (PHEX, Xp22.1). Other hypophosphatemic syndromes include autosomal dominant hypophosphatemic rickets, hereditary hypophosphatemic rickets with hypercalciuria, and tumor-induced osteomalacia (See Chapter 28).[893] In all of these conditions, there are increased levels of FGF23, perhaps a major phosphaturic agent.[894] The features are usually more severe in boys and include short stature,[779,895] prominent bowing of the legs, and (sometimes) rachitic signs.[896] The metabolic and skeletal abnormalities cannot be overcome by vitamin D therapy alone, hence the older name *vitamin D–resistant rickets*. Treatment of hypophosphatemic rickets requires oral phosphate replacement, but such therapy may result in poor calcium absorption from the intestine. The addition of calcitriol to oral phosphate increases intestinal phosphate absorption and prevents hypocalcemia and secondary hyperparathyroidism. Such combined therapy does improve the rickets but does not necessarily correct growth.[893,897-899] Potential growth-related benefits of this regimen appear dependent on the initiation of therapy in early infancy, with achievement of greater childhood and adult height.[895] There is no clear association between endogenous GH secretion, IGF-I, or phosphate levels and height in this disorder.[900-902] Nevertheless, GH therapy in eight trials including 83 patients has resulted in an enhancement of skeletal growth and improvement in bone mineral density.[903-905] In 14 of these patients, treatment for 4 to 5 years resulted in a height gain of up to 1.2 SDS.

IGF-I Deficiency

The growing appreciation of the central role of the IGF system in mammalian growth, paralleled by the recognition of limitations to the clinical and biochemical diagnosis of GH deficiency, has led to the proposal that the concept of IGF deficiency (IGFD) may provide a more meaningful way to evaluate and categorize patients with some forms of growth failure.[293,906,907] As useful as this categorization may prove, it is important to recognize that, at least currently, it is somewhat limited by issues concerning IGF assays: (1) marked age- and pubertal-dependence of serum IGF-I concentrations; (2) effect of nutrition and chronic inflammation on serum IGF-I concentrations; (3) the often slow decline in serum IGF-I concentrations in patients with evolving GHD, especially following cranial irradiation; and (4) lack of standardized normative data. Nevertheless, this classification serves to recognize the important diagnostic value of IGF assays in the evaluation of children with growth failure, and further serves to emphasize the critical role of IGF-I in both prenatal and postnatal growth.

IGFD can be divided into primary and secondary causes (see Table 23–7). Secondary IGFD includes those disorders in which IGF deficiency results from defects of GH production, on either a hypothalamic or pituitary basis. Secondary IGFD can be the consequence of damage to the hypothalamus and/or pituitary resulting from trauma, infection, tumors, radiation, inflammation, and so on, as well as an increasingly recognized group of molecular defects in pituitary development. Primary IGFD represents a constellation of disorders characterized by decreased IGF-I production in the presence of normal or even elevated GH secretion (states of insensitivity to GH action

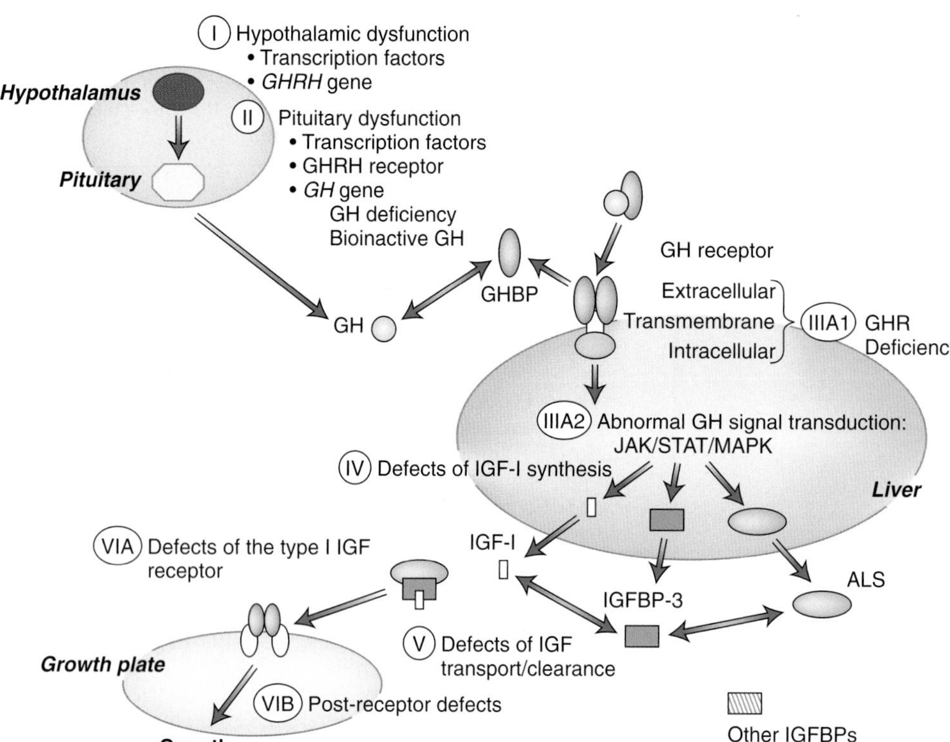

Figure 23–44 ■ The hypothalamic-pituitary-IGF axis: sites of established and hypothetical defects (established defects: black Roman numerals; hypothetical defects: white Roman numerals). *ALS,* Acid-labile subunit; *GH,* growth hormone; *GHBP,* GH-binding protein; *GHRH,* GH-releasing hormone; *IGF,* insulin-like growth factor; *IGF-BP,* IGF-binding protein; *JAK,* Janus kinase; *MAPK,* mitogen-activated protein kinase; *STAT,* signal transducer and activator of transcription. (Reprinted with permission from Lopez-Bermejo A, Buckway CK, Rosenfeld RG. Genetic defects of the growth hormone-insulin-like growth factor axis. Trends Endocrinol Metab 2000;11:43.)

[GHI]). To date, eight different molecular defects have been identified as causes of primary IGFD (Fig. 23–44). A potential system for analysis of known and potential genetic errors in patients with IGF deficiency syndrome is shown in Figure 23–45.

Clinical Features of IGF Deficiency

The clinical features of IGFD are dictated, to a large extent, by whether the deficiency of IGF-I occurred throughout gestation, or only late in pregnancy and postnatally. As demonstrated by murine knockout studies (see above) and many specific human mutations (see below), IGF-I is critically involved in both prenatal and postnatal growth. In utero, however, IGF-I production, at least until the very late stages of gestation, is essentially GH-independent, while in postnatal life, it is profoundly GH-dependent. Thus, IGFD due to hypothalamic dysfunction with abnormalities of GHRH, endogenous GHS or SRIF synthesis or secretion, primary or secondary decreased pituitary GH production, or GHI resulting from abnormalities of the GHR or its signaling cascade all share a common phenotype. The similarity among these patients emphasizes the role of IGF-I in mediating most of the anabolic and growth-promoting actions of GH, as well as the pivotal role of the GH-IGF axis in postnatal growth. This point is further supported by the capability of IGF-I therapy to correct growth in children with mutations of the GHR gene. Accordingly, the typical clinical features of severe IGF deficiency are shared by all of these conditions. If GH or IGF deficiency is acquired, clinical signs and symptoms appear at a later age.

The presence or absence of IUGR is determined, to a large extent, by when the IGF deficient state commenced. Thus, patients with secondary IGFD, or with primary IGFD resulting from defects of GH action, such as abnormalities of the GHR or its signaling cascade, tend to have near-normal birth size, reflecting the largely GH-independent nature of IGF production in utero. Typically, birth length and weight are within 10% of normal in such situations, and growth failure may not become obvious until several months of postnatal age.[576-578,908] When IGFD results from defects of the IGF-I gene,[238] however, IGFD is evident early in gestation and results in significant fetal growth retardation.

Although at least 50% of infants diagnosed with IGFD before 2 years of age have birth lengths more than 2 SD below the mean (both in isolated GHD and in multiple pituitary hormone deficiencies), mean birthweight is around −1 SD, lending an appearance of relative adiposity, even in the neonatal period.[577] These data further support some degree of an intrauterine role of the GH-IGF system in growth regulation, although much of IGF production in utero is GH-independent. Abnormalities of the hypothalamic-pituitary area defined by magnetic resonance imaging (MRI) include dysgenesis of the pituitary stalk, ectopic placement of the posterior pituitary inferior to the median eminence, and diminished volume of the anterior pituitary (Fig. 23–46).[101,909-913] There is a high frequency of breech deliveries and perinatal asphyxia reported to be associated with congenital GHD, although it is not entirely clear as to which is cause and which is effect (see below). Neonatal morbidity can include hypoglycemia and prolonged jaundice with direct hyperbilirubinemia due to cholestasis and giant cell hepatitis.[914,915] When GHD is combined with deficiency of ACTH and TSH, hypoglycemia may be severe. The combination of GHD with gonadotropin deficiency can cause microphallus, cryptorchidism, and hypoplasia of the scrotum.[916] GHD (or GHI) should, therefore, be considered in the differential diagnosis of neonatal hypoglycemia and of microphallus/cryptorchidism.

Postnatal growth is abnormal in severe congenital IGF deficiency (Fig. 23–47). Most surveys of GHD and GHI indicate that growth failure can occur during the first months of life.[576-578,917,918] By 6 to 12 months of age, the growth rate is definitely slow and deviates from the normal growth curve, with lengths 3 to 4 SD below the mean. This stresses the importance of normal IGF-I production and action in the neonatal period and early child-

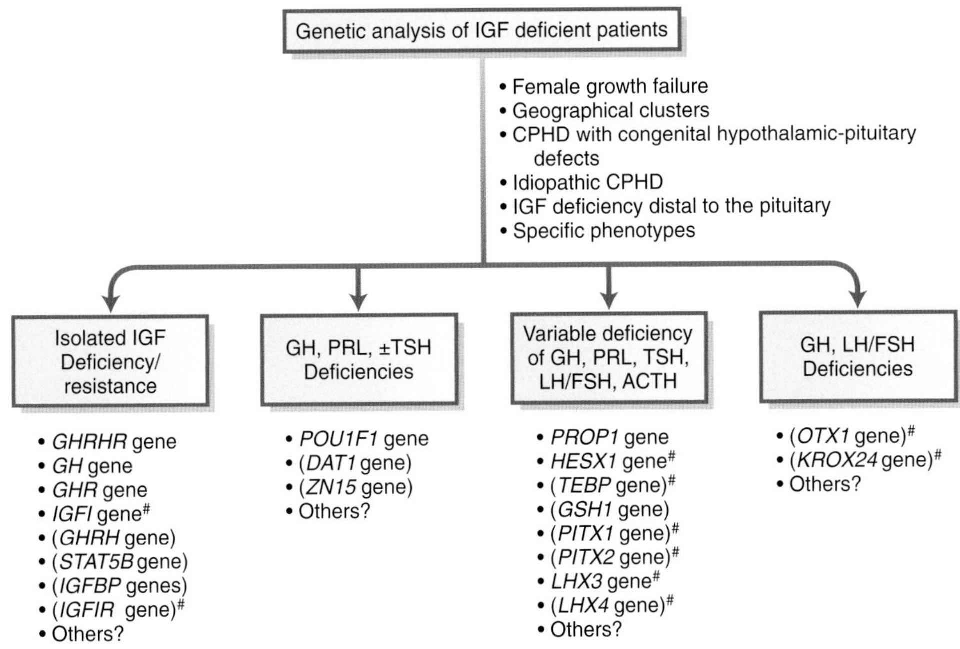

Figure 23–45 ▪ Decision tree for investigation of genetic defects in patients with insulin-like growth factor deficiency. Hypothetical genetic defects are presented in parentheses. #, Abnormalities in other organs and structures beside the hypothalamus-pituitary-IGF axis are expected to occur as a result of these genetic defects. *ACTH,* Adrenocorticotropic hormone; *CPHD,* combined pituitary hormone deficiencies; *FSH,* follicle-stimulating hormone; *GH,* growth hormone; *GHR,* GH receptor; *GHRHR,* GH-releasing hormone receptor; *IGF,* insulin-like growth factor; *IGFIR,* IGF-I receptor; *LH,* luteinizing hormone; *PRL,* prolactin; *STAT5,* signal transducer and activator of transcription 5; *TSH,* thyroid-stimulating hormone. (Reprinted with permission from Lopez-Bermejo A, Buckway CK, Rosenfeld RG. Genetic defects of the growth hormone-insulin-like growth factor axis. Trends Endocrinol Metab 2000;11:43.)

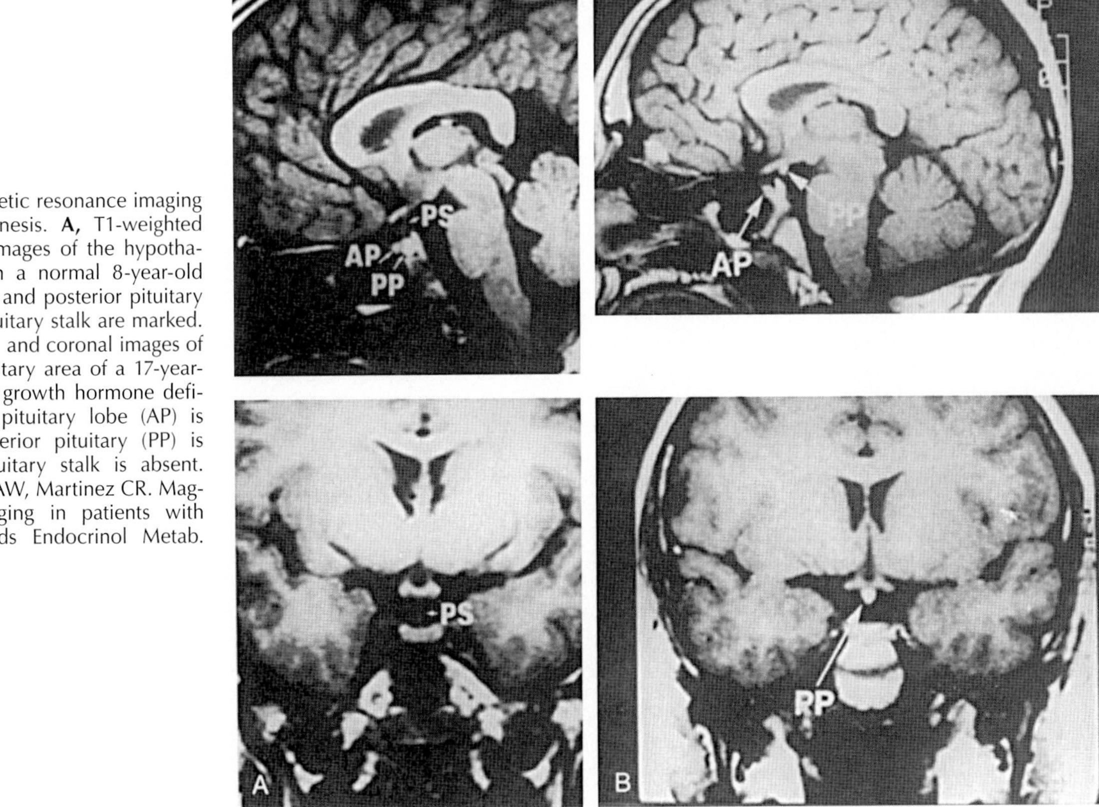

Figure 23–46 ▪ Magnetic resonance imaging of infundibular dysgenesis. **A,** T1-weighted sagittal and coronal images of the hypothalamic-pituitary area in a normal 8-year-old girl. The anterior (AP) and posterior pituitary (PP) lobes and the pituitary stalk are marked. **B,** T1-weighted sagittal and coronal images of the hypothalamic-pituitary area of a 17-year-old boy with isolated growth hormone deficiency. The anterior pituitary lobe (AP) is hypoplastic, the posterior pituitary (PP) is ectopic, and the pituitary stalk is absent. (Reprinted from Root AW, Martinez CR. Magnetic resonance imaging in patients with hypopituitarism. Trends Endocrinol Metab. 1992;3:283-287.)

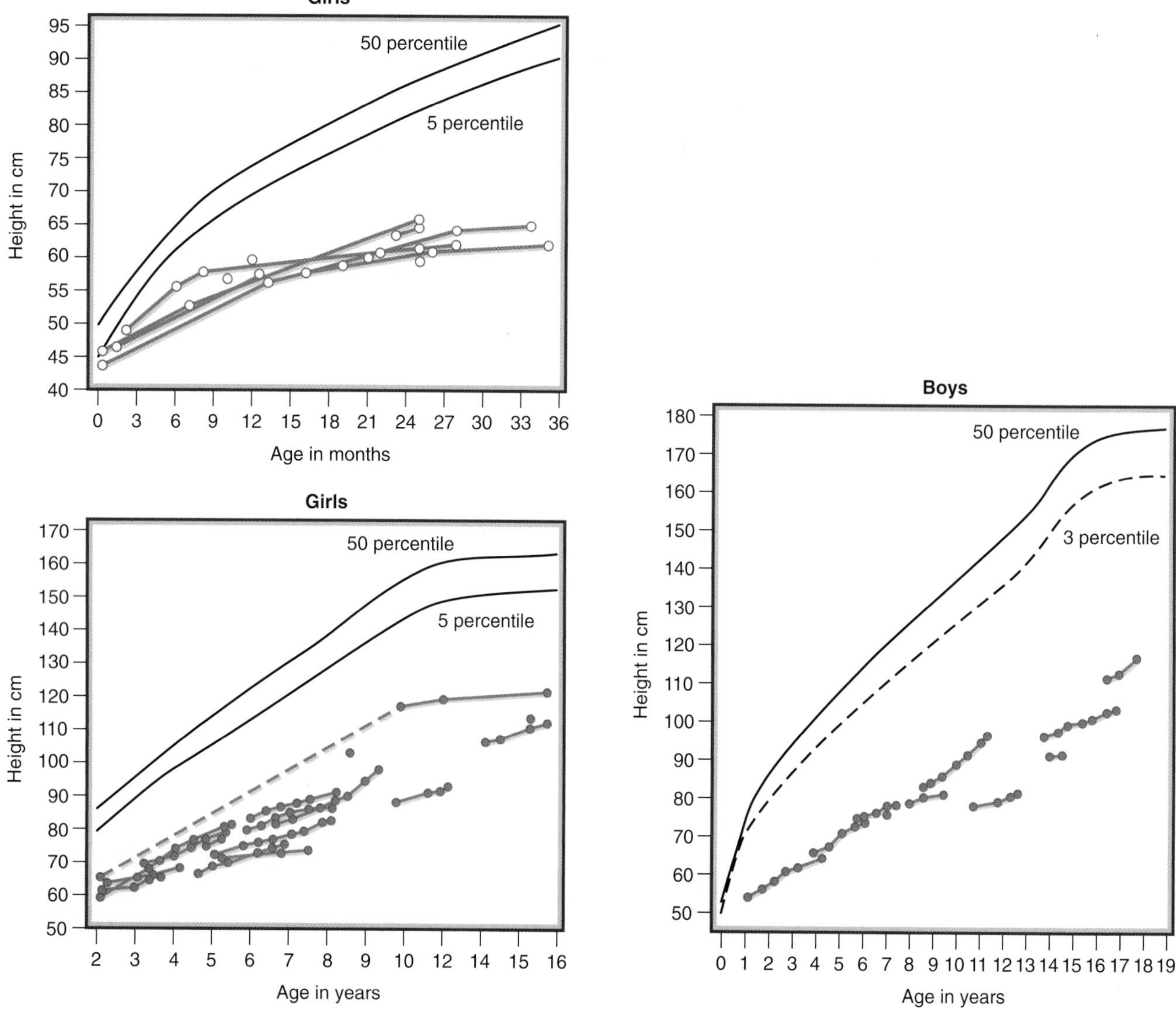

Figure 23–47 ▪ Height measurements for Ecuadorian children with IGF deficiency resulting from GH insensitivity. (From Rosenfeld RG, Rosenbloom AL, Guevara-Aguirre J. Growth hormone [GH] resistance due to primary GH receptor deficiency. Endocr Rev 1994;15:369-390.)

hood. We emphasize that the single most important clinical manifestation of IGF deficiency of all etiologies is growth failure, and careful documentation of growth rates is critical to making the correct diagnosis. Deviation from the normal growth curve should always be a cause of concern; between 2 years of age and the onset of puberty, growth deceleration (or acceleration) must *always* be considered pathologic.

Skeletal proportions tend to be relatively normal but correlate better with bone age than with chronologic age. Skeletal age may be delayed to less than 60% of the chronologic age, but, in the absence of hypothyroidism, is similar to the height age.[917] In acquired GHD, as from a CNS tumor that causes increased intracranial pressure, bone age may approximate the chronologic age; delayed skeletal maturation should not, therefore, be required for the diagnosis of GHD. Assessment of volumetric bone mineral density reveals decreased mineralization beyond that dependent upon small size.[919] Weight/height ratios tend to be increased, and fat distribution is often "infantile" or "doll-like" in pattern. Musculature is poor, especially in infancy, and can cause delay in gross motor development and lead to the erroneous impression of mental retardation in an immature-appearing child. Facial bone growth may be particularly retarded with an underdeveloped nasal bridge and frontal bossing (Fig. 23–48). Fontanel closure is often delayed, but the overall growth of the skull is normal, leading to cephalic/facial disproportion and the appearance of hydrocephalus. The voice is infantile because of hypoplasia of the larynx. Hair growth is sparse and thin, especially during early life; nail growth is also slow. Even with normal gonadotropin production, the penis is small, and puberty is usually delayed.

Final height data in patients with untreated GH deficiency are not plentiful.[920-923] Wit and colleagues summarized data from 22 untreated men and 14 women with severe isolated GH deficiency who had a mean final height SDS of −4.7. In 19 patients with multiple pituitary hormone deficiencies, thus lacking in gonadal steroids, mean final height was −3.1 SDS.[923]

Causes of IGF-I Deficiency

Two surveys of nearly 108,000 GH-treated patients, corresponding to nearly 400,000 patient-years, in databases managed by

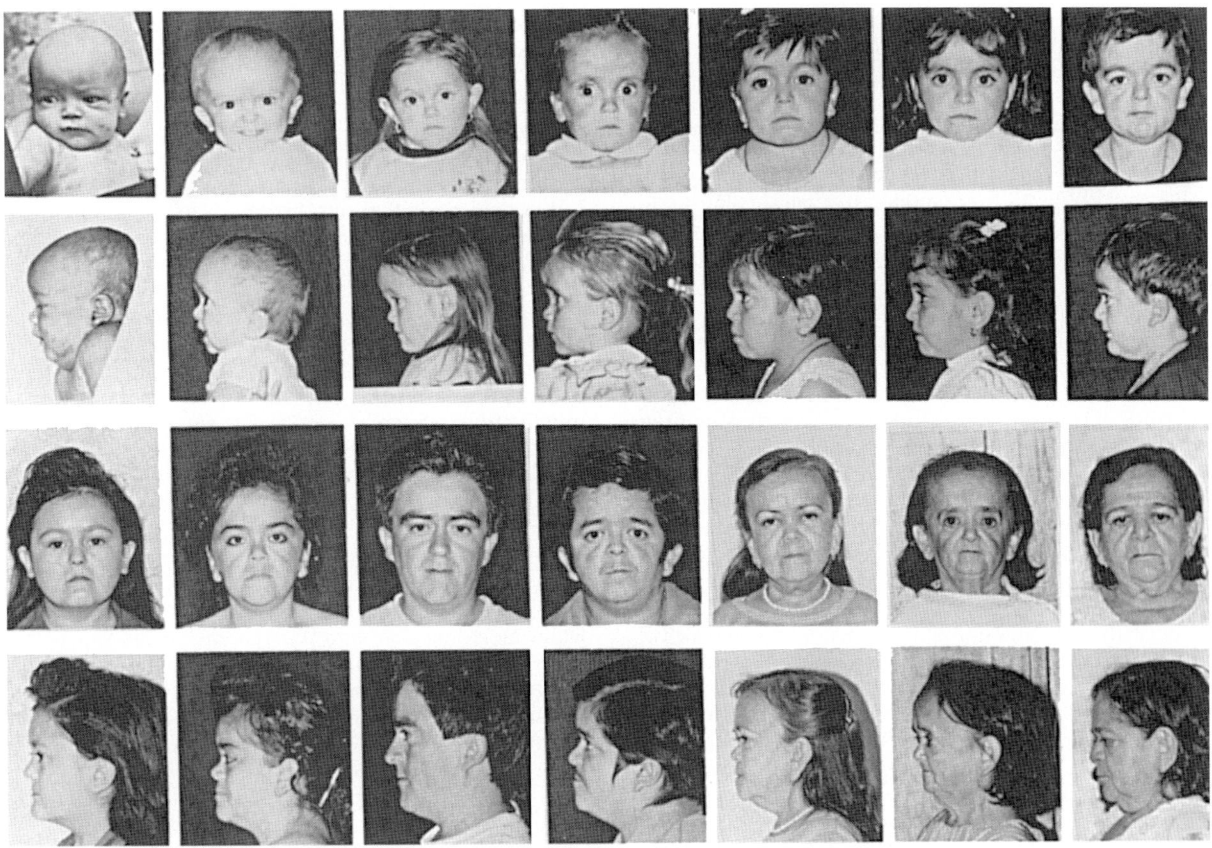

Figure 23–48 ▪ Facial appearance of Ecuadorian patients with IGF deficiency due to GH insensitivity. (From Rosenfeld RG, Rosenbloom AL, Guevara-Aguirre J. Growth hormone [GH] resistance due to primary GH receptor deficiency. Endocr Rev 1994;15:369-390; photography by A.L. Rosenbloom, M.D.)

Pfizer (KIGS) and Genentech (NCGS), cared for by pediatric endocrinologists throughout the world include a substantial proportion of the internationally treated patients.[924-926] The patients are diverse and include subjects with GHD and with Turner's syndrome and miscellaneous other disorders. About 59% of the total group, or approximately 65,000 patients, had GHD (as defined by a stimulated GH level of <10 μg/L) of whom 78% had "idiopathic" GHD and 22% had "acquired" or "organic" (neoplasms, trauma, inflammation, miscellaneous) causes of GHD. The latter group includes patients with congenital (developmental) GHD-associated syndromes. The organic/acquired group is probably underestimated because many of the patients classified as idiopathic had not had definitive imaging assessments of the hypothalamic-pituitary region and possibly have congenital structural abnormalities.

With the availability of synthetic IGF-I for treatment of patients with inherited abnormalities of the GH receptor, around 300 patients with primary IGFD resulting from primary GHI have been identified. This is an exceedingly small number of subjects, even with the addition of the potentially larger group of individuals with heterozygous abnormalities of the GH receptor.[927,928] To this must be added patients with even rarer forms of primary IGFD, such as defects of GH receptor signaling (JAK-STAT) and defects of the IGF-I gene. In contrast, patients with secondary GHI, including those with malnutrition or chronic systemic disease, must be considered as potentially a huge number, on a worldwide basis.

An incidence of GHD of 1 : 60,000 live births has been reported from the United Kingdom[929] and a survey of Scottish schoolchildren indicated prevalence as high as 1 : 4000.[930] The best estimate in the United States population is approximately 1 : 3480.[931] It is likely, however, that childhood GHD is an *overdiagnosed condition.* In particular, the diagnosis of acquired, idiopathic, isolated GHD should always be suspect. Although one may argue that (1) destructive or inflammatory lesions of the hypothalamus or pituitary may only affect GH secretion, or (2) isolated GHD due to a mild mutation/deletion of the GHRH receptor gene or GH gene may appear late, or (3) CPHD (combined pituitary hormone deficiencies) may first present with what appears to be isolated GHD, such circumstances appear to be rare. In the absence of anatomic abnormalities evident on imaging studies, and/or biochemical evidence of CPHD, the diagnosis of acquired, isolated, idiopathic GHD demands careful and thorough documentation, with greater skepticism as children approach teenage. The entity of partial, transient GH insufficiency related to sex steroid deficiency in delayed puberty is particularly confounding and most likely represents a temporary physiologic variant.

Secondary IGF Deficiency–Hypothalamic-Pituitary Abnormalities

Many of the disorders that affect hypothalamic regulation of GH synthesis and secretion also impact directly upon pituitary function. Consequently, it is not always possible to establish definitively the primacy of hypothalamic or pituitary dysfunction, hence the term *idiopathic.* Nevertheless, congenital (developmental) or functional abnormalities of the hypothalamus account for most "idiopathic" cases of hypopituitarism, and many such cases of GHD will prove to have a molecular basis. Acquired structural damage to this area (e.g., neoplastic, traumatic) causes one fourth of GHD cases.

Hypothalamic Dysfunction: Genetic Abnormalities. Hypothalamic factors involved in regulating GH synthesis and secretion include, but may not be limited to, GHRH, GHS, endogenous GH-releasing peptides such as ghrelin, PACAP, galanin,[932] and somatostatin. Mutations of the genes encoding these or other hypothalamic peptides may explain some cases of IGF deficiency due to hypothalamic dysfunction. To date, however, mutations of the genes encoding GHRH have not been identified,[933-935] although murine models have been described.[936,937] The importance of the GHRH presence is further accentuated by the finding that long-term treatment of GHRO-KO mice with a GHS (GHRP-2) is unsuccessful.[895] Normal growth is reported in the ghrelin-/- mouse.[938,939] Targeted disruption of the murine homeobox gene T/ebp, expressed in the ventral diencephalon but not in Rathke's pouch or in the pituitary during embryogenesis, results in early ablation of the pituitary primordium.[50] A Gsh-1 homeobox gene, expressed in varied parts of the developing murine central nervous system,[68] plays an important role in pituitary development, in that mutant strains have impaired production of GHRH with anterior pituitary hypoplasia and GHD.[69] The broad impact of defects of this gene upon hypothalamic-releasing factors may be similar to mutations of the Pit-1 gene, because deficiencies of prolactin and LH also occur.[69] Deletions of the murine dopamine transporter (DAT) results in increased dopaminergic tone, anterior pituitary hypoplasia, and dwarfism.[940] This suggests an important role for hypothalamic dopamine in pituitary development.

Congenital Malformations Involving the Hypothalamus. Hypothalamic dysfunction from congenital malformations of the brain or hypothalamus is a common cause of hypopituitarism. As noted above, patients with early diagnosed congenital GHD frequently have an abnormal pituitary stalk, ectopia of the posterior pituitary, and hypoplasia of the anterior pituitary. Anencephaly results in a pituitary gland that is small or abnormally formed and is frequently ectopic.[101,941,942] Despite the loss of hypothalamic regulation, somatotropes differentiate and proliferate, although in diminished overall mass.[44] During intrauterine life, serum GH and IGF-I levels are 30% to 50% of the normal range,[107] and pituitary GH content at birth about 15% to 20% of normal,[101,107] with similarly low neonatal plasma GH levels.[102,943,944] Holoprosencephaly, due to abnormal midline development of the embryonic forebrain, usually has hypothalamic insufficiency[945,946] and has been associated with two separate heterozygous mutations.[88,947] These are associated with diminished signalling by sonic hedgehog (shh), a critical factor in forebrain development and influenced by loss of function mutations of the GL12 gene.[948] Chromosomal-mediated abnormalities of PACAP and PACAP-R expression may be associated with some cases.[87] Facial dysmorphism of holoprosencephaly ranges from cyclopia to hypertelorism, accompanied by absence of the nasal septum, midline clefts of the palate or lip, and sometimes a single central incisor. GH deficiency may be accompanied by other pituitary hormone insufficiencies. The incidence of GH deficiency is increased in cases of simple clefts of the lip and/or palate alone,[949,950] and children with cleft palates who grow abnormally require further evaluation.

In its complete form, the rare syndrome of *septo-optic dysplasia* combines hypoplasia or absence of the optic chiasm and/or optic nerves, agenesis or hypoplasia of the septum pellucidum and/or corpus callosum, and hypothalamic insufficiency.[951-953] The extent of the anatomic and functional abnormalities can vary but generally in parallel to each other.[951,952] GH deficiency can occur by itself, or in combination with deficiencies of TSH, ACTH, and/or gonadotropins. About 50% to 70% of children with severe anatomic defects have hypopituitarism or, at least, identifiable abnormalities of the GH-IGF axis,[101,954,955] and the diagnosis should be considered in any child with growth failure associated with pendular or rotatory nystagmus or impaired vision and a small optic nerve disc. In some patients, hypoplastic or interrupted pituitary stalks and ectopic posterior pituitary placement have been identified by MRI.[101,953,956] It is not clear whether this disorder is inherited, but there is an increased incidence in offspring of young mothers, in first-born children, in areas of high unemployment, and in babies exposed to intrauterine medications, smoking, alcohol, and diabetes.[957,958] Mutations of HESX1, a paired-like homeodomain gene, expressed early in pituitary and forebrain development, are associated with familial forms of septo-optic dysplasia.[959-961] Three of 228 patients with a broad spectrum of congenital pituitary defects ranging from pituitary hypoplasia to septo-optic dysplasia were found to have heterozygous mutations of the HESX1 gene.[962] A very short girl (−4.6 SDS) with consanguineous parents was found to have a homozygous missense mutation with MRI findings of an attenuated infundibular stalk, pituitary hypoplasia, and ectopic posterior pituitary lobe *without* optic nerve abnormalities.[963] This patient had a mutation that demonstrated an impairment of HESX1 function as a transcriptional repressor, while including TSH and ACTH deficiencies similar to those seen in PROP1 deficiencies. Transgenic mice lacking this gene exhibit a variety of anterior midline CNS defects (e.g., abnormalities of corpus callosum, septum pellucidum, and anophthalmia or microphthalmia) and pituitary dysplasia.[56,959,964]

In most patients, so-called idiopathic hypopituitarism or GHD is presumed to be due to abnormalities of synthesis or secretion of hypothalamic hypophysiotropic factors.[78,965,966] In a number of reports, "idiopathic" GHD is associated with MRI findings of an ectopic neurohypophysis, pituitary stalk dysgenesis, and hypoplasia or aplasia of the anterior pituitary. In series involving 397 children with isolated GHD or with combined pituitary hormone deficiencies (CPHD), 54% had the characteristic MRI findings; 93% of CPHD patients were abnormal in contrast to 32% of patients with isolated GHD.[911-913,967-970] Abrahams and colleagues[909] studied 35 patients with idiopathic GHD and found that those with MRI abnormalities could be divided into two groups: (1) 43% had an ectopic neurohypophysis (neurohypophysis located near the median eminence), absent infundibulum, and absence of the normal posterior pituitary bright spot; (2) 43% had a small anterior pituitary, either as an isolated finding or combined with an ectopic neurohypophysis. Overall, those patients with the most striking abnormalities of the hypothalamic-pituitary region, largely those with CPHD, had the smallest anterior pituitary glands.[912,970] Patients with more severe deficiencies of GH have greater frequency of significant morphologic abnormalities.[971,972]

Although the increased incidence of breech presentation and birth trauma with neonatal asphyxia in congenital idiopathic hypopituitarism has led some to suggest an etiologic role for these occurrences,[968,973] the syndrome of pituitary stalk dysgenesis with congenital hypopituitarism is probably due to abnormal development, and the perinatal difficulties are likely the consequence, rather than the cause of the abnormalities. Findings of a similar MRI appearance in patients with septo-optic dysplasia,[101,953] in association with type I Arnold Chiari syndrome and syringomyelia,[101,917,970] as well as possibly in holoprosencephaly[101] and the occurrence of micropenis with this syndrome[101,576-578,916] all support the concept that congenital hypopituitarism is a genetic or developmental malformation, not a birth injury. A single report of an apparent autosomal dominant mutation of early brain development with infundibular dysgenesis associated with GHD supports the primary nature of the anomaly.[974] Further indirect evidence in studies[975] of isolated, complete anterior pituitary aplasia indicates that hypothalamic hypopituitarism and breech delivery are consequences of congenital midline brain defects, although perinatal residua of breech delivery may exacerbate ischemic damage to the hypothalamic-pituitary unit.

The MRI findings described above for early diagnosed patients with hypopituitarism are also found in children diagnosed at a later age. Most of these children have hypothalamic dysfunction as the cause of diminished pituitary hormone secretion. In the older group, as in the infants, structural, acquired hypothalamic, stalk, or pituitary abnormalities must be considered.

Patients with myelomeningocele with long-term survival have growth failure, decreased bone mineral density, and pubertal abnormalities.[976-978] Diminished growth is due to maldevelopment of the vertebral-skeletal system and to diverse midline CNS developmental anomalies such as hydrocephalus and Arnold-Chiari malformation. Many have hypothalamic-pituitary dysfunction including GHD and precocious puberty.[976,977] GH treatment does improve growth in these patients, although most of the growth is in the trunk and arms.[976,979,980] In children with shunted hydrocephalus, nearly two thirds have endocrine abnormalities.[981,982] As a group, heights of prepubertal patients were about 1 SD below control populations and they had a higher BMI. Sixteen of 54 (30%) had inadequate GH production associated with lower pituitary heights found on MRI.[981,983] Early and accelerated pubertal maturation contributes to reduced final height.[983]

Trauma of the Brain and/or Hypothalamus. Head trauma, resulting from boxing and varied injuries, may cause isolated GHD or multiple anterior pituitary deficiencies,[984-988] and some series of patients with GHD indicate an increased incidence of birth trauma, such as breech deliveries, extensive use of forceps, prolonged labor, or abrupt delivery. Although GHD *may* be a consequence of a difficult delivery or hypoxemic perinatal period, it is more commonly associated with developmental abnormality deficiencies (as discussed above), or due to head trauma later in life. In a series of 22 head-injured adolescents and adults, nearly 40% had some degree of hypopituitarism.[985]

Inflammation of the Brain and/or Hypothalamus. Bacterial, viral, or fungal infections may result in hypothalamic/pituitary insufficiency,[989,990] and the hypothalamus and/or pituitary may also be involved in sarcoidosis.[991]

Tumors of the Brain and/or Hypothalamus. Brain tumors are a major cause of hypothalamic insufficiency,[992] especially midline brain tumors, such as germinomas, meningiomas, gliomas, ependymomas, and gliomas of the optic nerve. Although short stature and GHD are most often associated with suprasellar lesions in neurofibromatosis, they may also exist without such lesions; whether growth impairment antedates the pathologic findings is not yet clear.[993,994] Metastases from extracranial carcinomas are rare in children, but hypothalamic insufficiency can result from local extension of craniopharyngeal carcinoma or Hodgkin's disease of the nasopharynx. The laboratory diagnosis of GHD in children with brain tumors may be difficult because levels of both IGF-I and IGFBP-3 are poor predictors especially in pubertal patients.[995] Craniopharyngiomas and histiocytosis can cause hypothalamic dysfunction but are discussed under "Pituitary GH Deficiency".

Radiation of the Brain and/or Hypothalamus. Cranial radiation appears to be an increasing cause of hypothalamic-pituitary dysfunction.[996-1001] Taken in aggregate there may be as many as 4000 pediatric cancer survivors who have GHD resulting from the broad range of cancer treatments.[1002] Radiation may impair both hypothalamic and pituitary function, and it is often not easy to discriminate between damage at the two levels. The hypothalamus is more radiosensitive than the pituitary and is more often the site of damage, especially in the dose range usually given to children with malignancy.[998] Thyroidal and gonadal function also may be directly impaired by certain radiation therapies. The degree of pituitary dysfunction is relative to the dose of radiation received. Low doses typically cause isolated GHD and higher doses may cause multiple pituitary deficiencies. The majority of long-term survivors develop GHD with the adverse effect of radiotherapy directly related to the biologically effective dose to the hypothalamus.[1001] Within 5 years of radiation, nearly 100% of children receiving more than 30 Gy over 3 weeks to the hypothalamic-pituitary axis had subnormal GH responses to provocative tests,[999,1003] while GHD may not become apparent for a decade or more after lower doses (18 to 24 Gy).[1002] The degree of pituitary deficiency is also a function of the length of time after radiation[1004]; children who test normally at 1 year post-therapy may develop pituitary deficiencies later. Additionally, hyperleptinemia, decreased insulin sensitivity, and increased fat mass may occur.[1005] Before development of GH secretory deficiency, GH insensitivity with low levels of IGF-I, IGFBP-3, and GHBP (presumably caused by the malignancy and the intensive chemotherapy and radiotherapy regimens) may decrease growth velocity.[1006-1008] Chemotherapy regimens by themselves may impair final adult height, although not nearly to the extent seen after radiation.[1007,1009] When such therapy is stopped, prepubertal children will have some degree of catch-up growth, but they may also have persistent abnormalities of the IGF/IGFBP system.[1008] Even when serum GH responses to provocative testing are normal, spontaneous GH secretion may be blunted at X-ray doses as low as 18 to 24 Gy.[1010] The marked reduction in GH secretion seen in these patients is largely dependent upon a decrease in pulse amplitude rather than frequency, with several studies suggesting that radiation affects GH secretion in a quantitative not qualitative fashion.[1011,1012] Although acquired GHD impairs final height,[1009,1013,1014] the relation of diminished GH production to levels of the GH-dependent peptides, IGF-I and IGFBP-3, is variable[1015,1016] and relates to the severity of the GHD.[1017] With long-term follow-up, however, correlations were found between nocturnal GH secretion, levels of IGF-I and IGFBP-3, and pituitary size.[1015]

Poor linear growth from decreased GH secretion may be exacerbated by the impact of radiation itself with inadequate pubertal acceleration of spinal growth.[998,1018-1021] Surprisingly, cranial radiation can result in precocious puberty, especially in children irradiated at young ages,[1022-1025] causing early epiphyseal fusion. Sexual precocity appears to occur more frequently with low doses of radiation,[1022,1026] and gonadotropin deficiency is likely at high doses.[1027] The rate of pubertal progression, however, does not appear to be accelerated.[1023] Treatment with GnRH analogues may be necessary to suppress the hypothalamic-pituitary gonadal axis in an attempt to attain normal final height.[1028] Three possibilities must be considered in following up children after craniospinal radiation: evolving hypopituitarism, decreased spinal growth potential, and early puberty with premature epiphyseal fusion. Children with documented GHD and growth failure are candidates for exogenous GH treatment[998,1023,1029-1031]; there is no evidence for enhanced relapses of the primary neoplasm in patients treated with GH,[1032-1036] but there appears to be a variable growth response to GH;[1021,1023,1031,1037,1038] spinal growth impairment, inadequate or delayed treatment, and sexual precocity may limit linear growth. Girls treated with GH after spinal radiation seem less adversely affected than boys, having typically completed a greater component of total spinal growth by the time GH treatment is used.[1031]

Bone marrow transplantation (BMT) for patients with inborn errors of metabolism, aplastic anemias, and malignancies requires preparative regimens that include total lymphoid or total body radiation, often with chemotherapy, and sometimes including cranial radiation.[1029,1039] Children in whom the clinical condition requires modest treatment programs before BMT have minimal loss of growth after BMT.[1029,1039-1041] In children who have cranial radiation followed by high-dose chemotherapy and total body radiation, especially in a single dose as preparative regimens, growth failure is almost inevitable 2 to 5 years after BMT.[1041-1046] Pubertal growth is most affected.[1041] If the total body radiation is fractionated and if cranial radiation was not previously needed, growth velocity and height 3 years after BMT are not compromised.[1039,1045-1047] In the absence of cranial radiation, there is a poor correlation between GH production and levels of IGF-1 or IGFBP-3 and growth in children after BMT,[1029,1046,1048] suggesting the importance of such factors as nutrition and radiation-induced vertebral dysplasia or hypothyroidism.[1049] Mean final heights in 28 long-term survivors of BMT were about 1 SD lower than at the time of the transplantation but still within the normal range in all but one patient[1050]; such data suggest a conservative approach with regard to exogenous hormonal treatment.

Psychosocial Dwarfism. An extreme form of failure to thrive is termed *psychosocial dwarfism* or *emotional deprivation dwarfism.*[1051-1053] Most cases of failure to thrive can be traced back to a poor home environment and inadequate parenting, with improved weight gain and growth upon removal of the infant from the dysfunctional home. Some children have been reported, however, to show dramatic behavioral manifestations beyond those in the typical failure-to-thrive infant, namely bizarre eating and drinking habits, such as drinking from toilets, social withdrawal, and primitive speech.[1052] Hyperphagia and abnormalities of GH production may be associated.[1054] GH secretion is low in response to pharmacologic stimuli but returns to normal upon removal from the home. Concomitantly, eating and behavioral habits returned to normal and a period of catch-up growth ensued. Careful assessment of endogenous GH secretion showed reversal of the GH insufficiency within 3 weeks, including enhancement of GH pulse amplitude and a variable increase of pulse frequency.[1054-1056] The reversibility of GH secretory defects and the later growth increment in the context of the clinical findings described above confirm the diagnosis of psychosocial dwarfism.[1053,1056-1058]

The neuroendocrinologic mechanisms involved in psychosocial dwarfism remain to be elucidated. GH secretion is abnormal and ACTH and TSH levels may also be low, although some patients have high plasma cortisol levels.[1053] Even when GH secretion is reduced, treatment with GH is not usually of benefit until the psychosocial situation is improved.[1053] Management of the environmental causes of the growth failure is imperative and often associated with substantial growth. In our experience, although psychosocial dysfunction is a common cause of failure to thrive in infancy, the constellation of bizarre behaviors described in psychosocial dwarfism is rare.

The fact that GH production is impaired in adults with varied psychiatric disorders[1059,1060] and given the growth aberrations of functional GHD with psychosocial dwarfism together suggest that children with emotional problems may have impaired GH secretion and growth.[1061] Indeed, depression in children, as adults, can lower GH production,[1062] and in girls, anxiety disorders predict a modest height loss in adults.[1061]

GH Neurosecretory Dysfunction. Because tests of GH secretion following pharmacologic provocation may not accurately reflect normal GH secretion, it has been argued that a subset of children with "GH neurosecretory dysfunction" may be identified by frequent or continuous serum sampling over a 12- to 24-hour period.[1063,1064] This condition is characterized by short stature and poor growth, normal serum GH response to provocative testing, and reduced IGF-I and 24-hour serum GH levels. Prior cranial radiation may be the most common cause of these findings. Patients with *idiopathic short stature* (see below) do not appear to have diminished 24-hour GH production rates, especially when the very broad range of data in normal and short normal children is considered.[108,109,1065-1067] There appears to be little doubt that some children with "GH neurosecretory dysfunction" secrete insufficient amounts of GH, even if they pass provocative GH testing; whether they should be identified by 24-hour GH sampling or by determination of the GH-dependent peptides is unclear.

Prader-Willi Syndrome. PWS is a genetically determined syndrome complex, with a frequency of 1 in 10,000 to 25,000 live births, that includes profound neonatal hypotonia and subsequent diminished muscle mass and strength.[636,1068] Growth failure may be evident at birth, is more impressive postnatally, with mean adult heights more than 2 SD below the mean and almost always below the midparental height target range.[1068,1069] Cryptorchidism and microphallus are present neonatally and hypogonadotropic hypogonadism may persist into adult life. With advancing age, hyperphagia and obesity become prominent. The genetic defect in PWS is a functional deletion of the paternal allele within chromosome 15q11-13[1070-1072] in an area that includes many genes whose relationship to the clinical findings remain unclear. Most patients with PWS have deletions of the long arm of the paternally derived chromosome 15; in some, both copies of 15q may be maternally derived, (uniparental disomy), while rarely there may be mutations of the imprinting center of chromosome 15q.[1068]

The probable cause of the short stature in PWS is deficient GH production due to as yet undefined hypothalamic dysfunction.[1069] MRI assessment of the hypothalamic-pituitary area does not yield evidence for congenital structural abnormalities. The body habitus and composition are similar to classic GHD, including small hands and feet, increased fat mass, and low muscle mass and bone mineral density.[1073,1074] Low mean serum GH levels or inadequate responses after provocative testing may reflect the impact of obesity, but serum levels of GH-dependent peptides are low in PWS, in contrast to the findings in exogenous obesity where these factors are produced normally despite diminished GH production.[1068,1075-1080] Thus, PWS is an IGF deficiency condition due to inadequate GH production, although the possibility of failure of upregulation of GH action, as seen in obesity, may yet be found to play a role. GH treatment of growth failure in PWS is now an FDA-approved indication. Treatment results in improved growth velocity, normalization of final height potential, increased muscle mass and strength, and decreased fat mass.[1068,1081,1082] In view of the risk for developing obesity-related insulin resistance and diabetes mellitus, glycemic status must be monitored closely during GH therapy. The increased occurrence of death by apnea in PWS is a great concern and has led to close scrutiny of GH-treated patients, although there is no absolute demonstration of a relationship.[1083,1084]

"Acquired, Idiopathic, Isolated GHD". In most pediatric endocrine centers, many children receiving GH are diagnosed with acquired, idiopathic, isolated GHD. As noted earlier, this diagnosis should always be considered somewhat suspect, especially peripubertally, although some patients may actually have undiagnosed gene defects in GH production or secretion, or they may be showing the first manifestation of combined pituitary hormone deficiency. Multiple studies have reported data on retesting patients with GH-treated GHD during or after cessation of therapy. All of the vagaries of different GH assays and GH provocative tests, varied "cutoff" levels of GH normalcy, diagnostic categorization of patients, and radiologic interpretation of MRI findings certainly affect these evaluations. Nonetheless, several clear conclusions emerge. In 464 patients with isolated GHD, 207 (44%) had normal GH levels during provocative retesting.[1085-1092] More than 70% of subjects initially diagnosed as having "partial" GHD had normalization on retesting.[1089] In contrast, approximately 96% of 148 patients with combined pituitary hormone deficiency, with or without structural abnormalities of the hypothalamic-pituitary area, had sustained

GHD.[1086,1087,1089-1093] The presence of multiple anterior pituitary hormone deficiencies or structural disease would seem to obviate the need for subsequent retesting in the majority of cases. Whether these results simply cast doubt upon the validity of the initial GH tests (or GH provocative testing in general) or whether children with earlier GHD may truly normalize is not clear. The entity of partial, transient GHD associated with delayed puberty certainly may be an example of this latter situation.[95,1094]

Pituitary GH Deficiency. As discussed above, many of the disease processes that impair hypothalamic regulation of GH secretion also impair pituitary function. Another group of abnormalities specifically affects pituitary somatotrope development and function.

Genetic Abnormalities of GH Production, Secretion, or Bioactivity. As many as 3% to 30% of patients with GHD have an affected parent, sibling, or child,[933,934,1095] and multiple genetic causes of GHD have been recently described.[56,1096] This text discusses inborn errors of genes for nuclear transcription factors affecting hypothalamic-pituitary development, the GHRH receptor, and the GH gene, each of which can cause GHD and IGF deficiency.

Genetic Abnormalities Resulting in Combined Pituitary Hormone Deficiency (CPHD; Table 23–5*).* Septo-optic dysplasia with pituitary abnormalities as profound as aplasia[961] and its relationship to *HESX1* are discussed above. The gene *PROP1* (denoting prophet of Pit1) encodes a paired-like 226 amino acid homeodomain protein, which is involved in the early determination and differentiation of multiple anterior pituitary cell forms

TABLE 23–5 GENETIC DEFECTS OF THE GH-IGF AXIS RESULTING IN IGF DEFICIENCY[52,56,1684]

Mutant gene	Inheritance	Phenotype	Refs	Murine Homolog	Refs
GHD due to hypothalamic-pituitary dysfunction					
Developmental abnormalities					
HESX1	AR	Septo-optic dysplasia Variable involvement of pituitary hormones	959-961	*Hesx1/Rpx*	56, 959, 964
PROP1	AR	GH, PRL, TSH, LH, FSH deficiencies Variable degree of ACTH deficiency	1097, 1685	Prop1 (Ames mouse)	1097, 1685
POU1F1 (Pit1)	AR, AD	GH, PRL deficiency Variable degree of TSH deficiency	935, 1120, 1124, 1130, 1132	*Pit1/Ghf1* (Snell and Jackson mouse)	1123
RIEG	AD	Rieger syndrome IGHD	1135, 1136	*Rieg* Pitx2	1137-1139
LHX3	AR	GH, TSH, LH, FSH, prolactin deficiencies	1145, 1686	Lhx3	1687
LHX4	AD	GH, TSH, ACTH deficiencies	1688	Lhx4	1689, 1690
SOX3	XL	GH deficiency, mental retardation	1144, 1688, 1691	Sox3	1692
GLI2	AD	Holoprosencephaly, hypopituitarism	948	Gli1+Gli2	1693
GLI3	AD	Pallister-Hall syndrome Hypopituitarism	1694, 1695	Gli3	1696
IGHD					
GHRH	?	None yet		GHRHKO mouse	936
GHRHR	AR	IGHD, type IB form of IGHD	1153-1156	*Ghrhr* (little mouse)	1119, 1121, 1159-1161
GHS-R	AD	GHD ISS	1148-1150	ghsr mouse, *antisense GHSR mRNA*	1151, 1152
GH1	AR	Type IA form of IGHD	935, 1162	*Gh* (spontaneous dwarf rat)	1697
	AR	Type IB form IGHD	935, 1096, 1125		
	AD	Type II form of IGHD	935, 1096, 1125		
	X-linked	Type III form of IGHD Hypogamma-globulinemia	1173		
	AD	Bioinactive GH molecule	1177, 1178		
GHI					
GHR				Ghr	235
Extracellular domain	AR, AD	IGF- I deficiency Decreased or normal GHBP	124, 1208, 1209		
Transmembrane domain	AR	IGF-I deficiency Normal or increased GHBP	170, 1210		
Intracellular domain	AD	IGF-I deficiency Normal or increased GHBP	1212, 1213		
Primary defects of IGF synthesis					
IGFI	AR	IGF-I deficiency IUGR and postnatal growth failure	238	Igfl	247

ACTH, Adrenocorticotropic hormone; AD, autosomal dominant; AR, autosomal recessive; FSH, follicle-stimulating hormone; GH, growth hormone; GHBP, GH-binding protein; GHD, GH deficiency; GHI, GH insensitivity; GHR, GH receptor; GHRH, GH-releasing hormone; GHRHR, GHRH receptor; IGF, insulin-like growth factor; IGHD, isolated GHD; LH, luteinizing hormone; PRL, prolactin; TSH, thyroid-stimulating hormone.

and is necessary for POUI1F1 (Pit1) expression.[1097,1098] Mutation of this gene is responsible for a form of murine pituitary-dependent dwarfism, the Ames mouse.[56,1097,1098] Abnormalities of human PROP1 result in CPHD, characterized by variable and often age-dependent degrees of deficiency of GH, prolactin, TSH, FSH, LH, and, occasionally, ACTH.[1097,1099,1100] Gonadotropin abnormalities are particularly diverse in that approximately 30% of patients have spontaneous pubertal development including menarche before ultimately developing hypogonadotropic hypogonadism.[1099,1101] A case of apparently normal growth without GH has also been found in a child with PROP1 deficiency.[1102,1103] Striking variability has been described in pituitary size with very large glands, possibly arising from the intermediate lobe,[1104] having a hyperintense T1 signal occasionally demonstrated by MRI.[1097,1100,1105,1106] These may then undergo involution leaving a large empty sella in patients with complete anterior hypopituitarism including ACTH deficiency.[1107-1109] The ACTH deficiency may develop in the fourth or fifth decades.[1110] Multiple *PROP1* (chromosome 5q35, OMIM601538) abnormalities have been identified and include missense, frameshift, and splicing mutations. A GA repeat in exon 2 (295-CGA-GAG-AGT-303) has been reported to be a "hot spot" in *PROP1;* any combination of a GA or AG deletion in this repeat region results in a frameshift in the coding sequence and premature termination at codon 109.[1101,1111] Similar abnormalities result from homozygous lesions at other sites on exon 2 affecting codons 73, 88, and 149.[1100,1112,1113] Furthermore, compound heterozygosity for two mutations was detected in 36% of children from four families, as two different common deletions both led to a stop codon at position 109.[1113] These mutations all result in loss of the DNA-binding and C-terminal trans-activating domains of *PROP1.* There does not appear to be strong correlation between phenotype and genotype.[1101] Large-scale screening of patients with CPHD has found 54% with *PROP1* mutations.[1097,1101] In two series of families with multiple affected individuals, however, *PROP1* mutations accounted for all of the 25 siblings. Such frequencies far exceed those reported for *POU1F1* mutations[1114] and emphasize a central role for *PROP1* in pituitary cellular differentiation. A contrasting assessment, nonetheless, is reported from England where 27 children with CPHD had no evidence of *PROP1* mutations, thus demonstrating geographic variability in causes of CPHD.[1115]

The *POU1F1* (*Pit-1,GHF-1*) gene (chromosome 3p11, OMIM173110) encodes Pit1, a member of a large family of transcription factors, referred to as POU-domain proteins, and is responsible for pituitary-specific transcription of genes for GH, prolactin, TSH, and the GHRH receptor.[1096,1116-1119] Additionally, the 290 amino acid Pit-1 protein activates transcription of genes that regulate differentiation, proliferation, and survival of somatotropes, lactotropes, and thyrotropes.[934,1119-1121] Both Snell (dw/dwS) and Jackson (dw/dwJ) dwarf mice have GH, prolactin, and TSH deficiency associated with mutations or rearrangements of the murine *pit1* gene.[1122,1123] Many different mutations of the *POU1F1* gene have been found internationally in families with GHD and prolactin deficiency and variable defects in TSH secretion.[56,935,1096,1120,1124-1129] These mutations are transmitted as autosomal recessive or dominant traits and cause variable peptide hormone deficiencies with or without anterior pituitary hypoplasia.[935,1096,1120,1125-1128,1130-1132] The most common mutation is an R271W substitution affecting the POU homeodomain, encoding a mutant protein that binds with increased affinity to DNA and acts as a dominant inhibitor of transcription.[880,1133] The mutations involve sites affecting *Pit-1* DNA-binding, dimerization, or target gene transactivation. Phenotypic variability occurs among patients with apparently similar genotypes.[1131] It does not appear that ACTH or gonadotropin deficiencies occur, as is frequently the case with *PROP1* defects,[1132] but adrenarche appears absent or delayed in patients with this mutation.[1134]

Haploinsufficiency of the homeobox gene, *RIEG*(Ptx2), results in Rieger's syndrome, an autosomal dominant disorder that involves abnormal development of the anterior chamber of the eye, teeth, and umbilicus, with an occasional association with GHD.[1135,1136] The *rieg/pitx2* null mouse is characterized by multiple pituitary hormone deficiencies.[1137-1139] Mutations of another homeobox gene, *Optx2,*[1140] and that for BMP-4, a member of the TGF-β superfamily,[1141] are also associated with eye maldevelopment and pituitary hypoplasia. Multiple other genes (and thus, likely genetic defects) in the regulation of pituitary development with varied CNS anomalies are being discovered in murine models.[51,56] At least three other transcription factors (Lhx3, Lhx4, and SOX3) have been associated with anterior pituitary deficiencies, along with varied neural and neurodevelopmental abnormalities.[52,1142-1144] Lhx3 mutation has multiple pituitary hormone deficiency, associated with neck rigidity, and in at least one case, the presence of a hypodense pituitary mass lesion suggesting a microadenoma.[1145] Lhx4 appears to activate transcription from POUIF1, thus demonstrating how a mutant Lhx4 protein could alter GH expression.[1146] Overall, however, mutations of the genes studied to date have been very unusual in cases of sporadic CPHD, especially in those with hypothalamic-pituitary area structural abnormalities noted on MRI.[1115,1147]

Molecular Defects of GHRH. Despite extensive assessment, mutations of the gene encoding GHRH, which would be predicted to cause an IGF deficiency phenotype, have not been identified,[56,933] although expression of GHRH is suppressed in mutations of murine neural genes *Gsh1*[68,69] and *DAT1* (dopamine transporter).[940] The failure to demonstrate a GHRH mutation remains a surprise because this would appear to be a likely candidate for familial GHD. A murine model for ablation of the GHRH gene (GHRHKO) demonstrates a similar phenotype to that described for GHD due to molecular defects of the GHRH-R.[936] Abnormalities of the endogenous "GHSs" remain to be identified as causes of IGF deficiency, but mutations of GHS-R[79] have been reported in three families.[1148-1150] It is transmitted as an autosomal dominant trait, causing loss of the constitutive activity of the receptor. Responsivity to ghrelin, however, is maintained and obesity has appeared in teenage years. The mechanisms by which GHS-R mutations cause short stature are not clear; one child had GHD, but another had an idiopathic short stature laboratory phenotype. Two different murine models for this entity have been described with varying degrees of growth impairment.[1151,1152] Mutations causing constitutive or enhanced ligand-mediated activation of the G-protein–related somatostatin receptor to yield chronic inhibition of GH also have not yet been reported.

Molecular Defects of the GHRH Receptor (GHRH-R). Although no defects of the GHRH gene have yet been reported, multiple kindreds have been found with homozygous mutations of the GHRH-R gene.[1153-1156] Wajnrajch and colleagues reported the first human cases of a mutation in the GHRH-R gene (chromosome 7) in two cousins with IGF deficiency and profound growth failure. The gene defect resulted in a markedly truncated GHRH receptor protein that lacked the membrane-spanning regions and the G-protein–binding site. The affected children had undetectable GH release during standard provocative tests and after exogenous GHRH administration, but responded to GH treatment. Another series of 18 patients with the same point mutation was found in Pakistan ("dwarfism of Sindh")[1154] and in two members of a Tamoulean family from Sri Lanka.[1155] The largest kindred with a mutation of GHRH-R has been identified in Brazil[1156]; a donor splice mutation in position 1 of exon 1 also results in a severely truncated GHRH protein. The patients in all of the groups have striking short stature (often more than −5 SD) and a lack of other features of GHD, such as microphallus, truncal obesity, and hypoglycemia, but they have profound abnormalities of the GH-IGF axis.[1154,1157] The absence of the GHRH-R in the testis does not preclude fertility.[1154] The patients respond well to exogenous GH without antibody formation. Heterozygotes may have minimal height deficits and may show moderate biochemical deficiencies of the GH-IGF axis.[1154] Despite extensive study, the geographic separation and ethnic differences do not suggest recent (more than 200 years) contact among the families from the Indian subcontinent. The present likely explanation for all four families is that of a "founder effect" or one-time mutations in each group with propagation within geographically isolated gene pools.[1156] In an analysis of 30 families with IGHD type IB, Salvatori and colleagues[1158] found new missense mutations in transmembrane and intracellular domains of GHRH-R in three families (10%) with two affected members in each. Transfection experiments indicated normal cellular expression of these mutant receptors. Mutation of the gene for GHRH-R in its ligand-binding domain has also been identified in the *little* mouse (lit/lit),[1159] leading to dwarfism and decreased numbers of somatotropes.[1119,1160,1161] In this model, the fetal somatotrope mass is normal and hypoplasia, but not absence, of the somatotropes is only evident postnatally.[1119,1121,1160,1161] Such data suggest that GHRH is not an essential factor for fetal differentiation of the somatotropes and that GHRH-independent cells persist or that mutation does not cause total loss of GHRH function.

Genetic Abnormalities of GH Production and/or Secretion Resulting in Isolated GHD (IGHD). Four forms of isolated GHD due to errors of the GH gene have been reported (see Table 23–5).[52,934,1096] The gene encoding GH (*GH1*) is located on chromosome 17q23 in a cluster that includes two genes for placental lactogen (HPL), a pseudogene for HPL, and the *GH2* gene that encodes placental GH.[933,1095] *GH1* and *GH2* differ in mRNA splicing pattern: GH1 generates 20- and 22-kd proteins (of approximately equal bioactivity), while *GH2* yields a protein differing from GH1 in 13 amino acid residues. Isolated GHD type IA (GHD IA) results primarily from large deletions, with rare microdeletions and single base pair substitutions of the *GH1* gene that prevent synthesis or secretion of the hormone.[1162] GHD IA is inherited as an autosomal recessive trait and affected individuals have profound congenital GHD. Because GH is not produced even in fetal life, patients are immunologically intolerant of GH and, typically, develop anti-GH antibodies when treated with either pituitary-derived or recombinant DNA-derived GH. When antibodies prevent patients from responding to GH, GHD IA can be viewed as a form of GH insensitivity, and such patients are candidates for IGF-I therapy. The less severe form of autosomal recessive GHD (IGHD IB) also may result from mutations or rearrangements of the GH1 gene that cause production of an aberrant GH molecule that retains some function or at least generates immune tolerance. The phenotypic variability is greater than in IGHD 1A.[52] These patients usually respond to exogenous GH therapy without antibody production. The very low frequency (1.7%) of GH1 gene mutations in familial type 1B IGHD suggests the importance of studying the *GH1* gene promoter region in patients with unexplained GHD.[1096,1163] In a group of 65 children with IGHD IB, the GHRH receptor gene was normal in domains coding for the extracellular region,[1164] but mutations in transmembrane and intracellular gene domains were found in 10% of families with IGHD IB.[1158]

IGHDII is inherited as an autosomal dominant trait. Such patients may have splice site, intronic, or missense mutations of the *GH1* gene. The most common cause appears to be those mutations that inactivate the 5′ splice donor site of intron 3, resulting in skipping of exon 3[56,1096] and producing a molecule that cannot fold normally. It is likely that the 17.5-kd GH isoform mutant functions in a dominant-negative manner suppressing intracellular accumulation and secretion of wild-type GH.[1165-1168] In patients with missense mutations in exon 4 or 5, clinical presentation is quite variable with some evidence for reversibility of the impairment of intracellular GH storage and secretion by GH treatment.[1169] Mullis and coworkers[1170] studied 57 subjects from 19 families and found that patients with IGHDII not only have a variable phenotype in terms of onset, severity, and progression of GHD, but also may demonstrate later onset of ACTH or TSH deficiencies and pituitary hypoplasia. An extensive assessment of *GH1* gene mutations in short children with and without GHD did reveal a substantial number of heterozygous mutations.[1171] Even though these are not primary explanations for the growth impairment, these findings may contribute to the variation of the growth process. Finally, as many as 16% of families with autosomal dominant GHD do not have a definable GH-1 mutation, suggesting that mutations in other gene(s) may play a role in this condition.[1172]

Type III GHD, transmitted as an X-linked trait with associated hypogammaglobulinemia,[1173] has not yet been related to a mutation of the *GH1* gene. A large Australian kindred demonstrated GHD with a variable spectrum of pituitary hormonal deficiencies that may be caused by duplication of the Xq25-Xq28 region.[1174]

Bioinactive GH. Serum GH exists in multiple molecular forms, reflecting the consequences of alternative posttranscriptional or posttranslational processing of the mRNA or protein respectively. Some of these forms are presumed to have defects in the amino acid sequences required for binding of GH to its receptor and different molecular forms of GH may have varying potencies for stimulating skeletal growth, although this remains to be rigorously proved. Short stature with normal GH immunoreactivity but reduced biopotency has been suggested,[1175,1176] but the molecular abnormalities have only been characterized in a very few such situations, and many cases of alleged bioinactive GH have not been rigorously proven.[1177,1178] In one child with extreme short stature (−6.1 SDS), a mutant GH caused by a single missense heterozygous mutation (cys to arg, codon 77 of *GH-1* gene) bound with greater affinity than normal to GHBP and the GH-receptor and inhibited the action of normal GH. The child grew more (6 vs. 3.9 cm/yr) during a period of exogenous GH in moderate dosage. Strangely, the father had the same genetic abnormality but did not express the mutant hormone. In the second patient[1178] with marked short stature (−3.6 SDS), a heterozygous A to G substitution on exon 4 of GH led to a glycine to arginine substitution. This mutation is located in site 2 of GH molecular binding with its receptor and apparently led to failure of appropriate molecular rotation of the dimerized receptor and subsequent diminished tyrosine phosphorylation and the GH-mediated intracellular cascade of events. Bioactivity determined in a mouse B-cell lymphoma line was about 33% of immunoreactivity.[1179] Exogenous GH substantially increased growth velocity (4.5 to 11.0 cm/yr). An Ile179Met substitution found in a short child was characterized by normal STAT5 activation, but a 50% decrement of ERK activation.[159] This novel finding demonstrated the complexity of GH's functional interaction with its receptor, but since STAT5b is clearly the major (if not sole) GH-dependent mediator of IGF-I gene transcription, the role of this mutation is not clear. Six GH heterozygous variants with evidence of impairment of JAK/STAT activation found on screening of short children suggest the need for continuing to examine the GH molecule for variations in success at receptor activation.[1171] These reports are all of heterozygotes and have unclear genotype-phenotype correlation. In one of the more convincing cases of bioinactive GH reported to date, Besson and associates[1180] found a homozygous missense mutation (G705C) leading to absence of two disulfide bridges in a short (−3.6 SDS) Serbian boy. Both GHR binding and JAK2/STAT5 signaling activity were markedly reduced.

There remain other patients, however, in whom diminished bioactivity by sensitive in vitro assays is not reflected by comparable alteration in immunoreactivity. The absence of *GH1* mutations suggests the importance of abnormal posttranslational modifications of GH or other peripheral mechanisms.[368,1181] The complex net relationships of subtle differences in structure, both of GH and GHR, occurring through populations of polymorphism variations is likely to account for a portion of the range of human height.

Trauma (See Above)

Inflammation (See Above)

Tumors Involving the Pituitary. Many tumors that impair hypothalamic function also impact pituitary secretion of GH. In addition, *craniopharyngiomas* are a major cause of pituitary insufficiency.[1182-1184] These tumors arise from remnants of Rathke's pouch, the diverticulum of the roof of the embryonic oral cavity that normally gives rise to the anterior pituitary. Genetic defects in this condition, although certainly reasonable to suspect, have not yet been identified. This tumor is a congenital malformation present at birth and gradually grows over the ensuing years. The tumor arises from rests of squamous cells at the junction of the adenohypophysis and neurohypophysis and forms a cyst as it enlarges, which contains degenerated cells and may calcify but does not undergo malignant degeneration. The cyst fluid ranges from a "machinery oil" to a shimmering cholesterol-laden liquid, and the calcifications may be microscopic or gross.[1185] About 75% of craniopharyngiomas arise in the suprasellar region, the remainder resembling pituitary adenomas.[1185-1190]

Craniopharyngiomas can cause manifestations at any age from infancy to adulthood but usually present in mid-childhood. The most common presentation is due to increased intracranial pressure, including headaches, vomiting, and oculomotor abnormalities. Visual field defects result from compression of the optic chiasm and papilledema or optic atrophy may be present. Visual and olfactory hallucinations have been reported, as have seizures and dementia. Most children with craniopharyngiomas have evidence of growth failure at the time of presentation, and, retrospectively, often have had reduced growth since infancy.[1191] GH and the gonadotropins are the most commonly affected pituitary hormones in children and adults, but deficiency of TSH and/or ACTH may also occur; diabetes insipidus is present in 25% to 50%.[1185-1187,1192] Fifty percent to 80% of patients have abnormalities of at least one anterior pituitary hormone at diagnosis.[1186,1192] Although lateral skull films may demonstrate enlargement or distortion of the sella turcica, frequently accompanied by suprasellar calcifications, some children have normal results on plain films. MRI is the most sensitive diagnostic technique, allowing identification of cystic and solid components and delineation of anatomic relationships necessary for a rational operative approach. Operative intervention either via craniotomy or transphenoidal resection may result in partial or almost complete removal of the lesion. Postoperative irradiation, especially when tumor resection is incomplete, is commonly used. In some patients, especially those who become obese, a syndrome of normal linear growth without GH may occur. The metabolic syndrome with evidence of insulin insensitivity and increased BMI is common and a predictor of potential major long-term morbidity.[1191,1193,1194] The long-term childhood and adolescent consequences of craniopharyngioma are substantial with many quality-of-life issues exacerbating the hypopituitarism.

Pituitary adenomas (see Chapter 8) are infrequent during childhood and adolescence, accounting for less than 5% of patients undergoing surgery at large centers.[1189,1190,1195] Nearly two thirds of tumors immunochemically stain for prolactin, and a small number stain for GH. GH-secreting pituitary adenomas are exceedingly unusual in youth. There is a variable experience as to the invasive nature of pituitary adenomas, although the prevailing opinion is that they are less aggressive in children than in adults.[1189,1195] In 56 patients at the Mayo Clinic with non-ACTH secreting adenomas removed transphenoidally, macroadenomas were about one third more frequent than microadenomas, with cases in girls outnumbering those in boys 3.3 to 1.[1189] The macroadenoma patients had an approximately 50% incidence of hypopituitarism, compared with none in patients with microadenomas; long-term cure rates were 55% to 65% for both tumor sizes.

The localized or generalized proliferation of mononuclear macrophages (histiocytes) characterizes Langerhans cell histiocytosis, a diverse disorder occurring at all ages, with peak incidence at ages 1 to 4 years.[1196] Endocrinologists are more familiar with the term *histiocytosis X,* which includes three related disorders: solitary bony disease (eosinophilic granuloma), Hand-Schüller-Christian disease (chronic disease with diabetes insipidus, exophthalmos, and multiple calvarial lesions), and disseminated histiocytosis X (Letterer-Siwe, with widespread visceral involvement). These syndromes are characterized by an infiltration and accumulation of Langerhans cells in the involved areas, such as skull, hypothalamic-pituitary stalk, CNS, and viscera. Although these disorders, especially Hand-Schüller-Christian, are classically associated with diabetes insipidus, approximately 50% to 75% of patients in selected series have growth failure and GHD at the time of presentation.[1197-1199] In contrast, a French national registry (n=589) found GHD in 61 subjects, with overall endocrine dysfunction in 148. In this latter group, an evolving neurodegenerative syndrome (in 10% of patients with 15-year follow-up) seemed associated with pituitary involvement.[1200] Only 1% of unselected children with Langerhans cell histiocytosis living in Canada during a 15-year period had GHD.[1201]

Primary IGF Deficiency: Inherited and Acquired Syndromes of Insensitivity to GH Action (Table 23–6)

The term *primary IGFD* encompasses a variety of genetic and acquired conditions (Table 23–7), which share the characteristics of decreased serum IGF-I concentrations (typically, less than –2 SD), growth failure, and normal-increased serum GH (Fig. 23–49).[124,1202] Although the category of primary IGFD includes patients with GH insensitivity (GHI), the term *IGFD* is preferred, because (1) no suitable biochemical criteria for GHI (other than in its most severe form) have been developed to date and (2) patients with IGF gene defects are more properly labeled as IGF deficient, rather than categorizing them by their resistance to GH action. Furthermore, the phenotypes of various conditions characterized by IGFD are dependent upon the molecular basis for the deficiency, and whether decreased IGF production begins in utero or in late pregnancy, or postnatally (see below).

Abnormalities of the GH Receptor. The initial report, by Laron and colleagues[1203] of primary GH insensitivity (GHI) described "three siblings with hypoglycemia and other clinical and laboratory signs of growth hormone deficiency, but with abnormally high levels of immunoreactive serum growth hormone." To date, approximately 250 cases have been identified worldwide,[56,124,1167] most from the Mediterranean region or from Ecuador.[1204] These individuals do not respond to exogenous GH, in terms of growth, metabolic changes, or of increases in serum levels of IGF-I and IGFBP-3.[92] Cellular unresponsiveness to GH was demonstrated in vitro by the failure of GH to stimulate erythroid progenitor cells from the peripheral blood of patients,[1205] and direct evidence of receptor dysfunction was provided by the demonstration that microsomes obtained by liver biopsy do not bind radiolabeled GH.[1206] GHBP activity is usually (75% to 80%) undetectable in the sera of patients with this disorder.[166,167]

TABLE 23–6 CLINICAL FEATURES OF CLASSIC GROWTH HORMONE INSENSITIVITY

GROWTH AND DEVELOPMENT
Birthweight: near-normal Birth length: may be slightly decreased Postnatal growth: severe growth failure Bone age: delayed, but may be advanced relative to height age Genitalia: micropenis in childhood; normal for body size in adults Puberty: delayed 3 to 7 years Sexual function and fertility: normal
CRANIOFACIES
Hair: sparse before age 7 years Forehead: prominent; frontal bossing Skull: normal head circumference; craniofacial disproportion due to small facies Facies: small Nasal bridge: hypoplastic Orbits: shallow Dentition: delayed eruption Sclerae: blue Voice: high-pitched
MUSCULOSKELETAL/METABOLIC/MISCELLANEOUS
Hypoglycemia: in infants and children; fasting symptoms in some adults Walking and motor milestones: delayed Hips: dysplasia; avascular necrosis of femoral head Elbow: limited extensibility Skin: thin, prematurely aged Osteopenia

Studies of the GHR gene in several Israeli patients indicated that some, but not most, contained gene deletions,[1207] and a wide variety of homozygous point mutations in this gene (missense, nonsense, and abnormal splicing) have been identified subsequently.[124,1167,1208,1209] The initially described gene deletion involved exons 3, 5, and 6 (although later studies have shown that the loss of exon 3, itself, may be a normal variant of the GHR gene). The deletion of exons 5 and 6, however, resulted in a frameshift and a premature translational stop signal, with the consequent encoding of a receptor lacking most of the extracellular GH-binding domain. More than 60 distinct mutations of the *GHR* gene, resulting in GHI, have been reported to date.[907] Most of the mutations are in the extracellular (GH-binding) domain of the GHR. As a result, the ability of the receptor to bind GH is impaired, which is reflected in a deficiency of circulating GH-binding protein (GHBP) when assayed by methodologies that measure either intact protein or GH-binding ability. At least one mutation of the extracellular domain does not affect GH binding but prevents dimerization of the receptor.[169]

Normal GH binding (either to the receptor or to the circulating GHBP) may also be observed in the case of mutations affecting the transmembrane or intracellular domains of the GHR. Woods and colleagues[170] described two cousins with severe GHR and homozygous mutations at the 5′ splice donor site of intron 8, resulting in a mutant GH receptor without functional transmembrane or intracellular domains. A similar defect was found in a Druse girl with a mutation of the 3′ acceptor site of intron 7.[1210] Serum levels of GHBP were elevated as the mutant receptor protein apparently becomes detached from the cell receptor surface.

TABLE 23–7 IGF DEFICIENCY SYNDROMES

SECONDARY
GH deficiency resulting from hypothalamic dysfunction GH deficiency resulting from pituitary dysfunction GH deficiency resulting from GH gene deletion Inactivating mutations of the GH gene (bioinactive GH)
PRIMARY
Molecular Defects Abnormalities of the GH receptor affecting GH binding Abnormalities of the GHR affecting receptor dimerization Abnormalities of the GH receptor affecting receptor anchoring Abnormalities of the GH receptor affecting GH signal transduction GHR signaling defects ALS mutations IGF-I gene deletions Inactivating mutations of the IGF-I gene (bioinactive IGF-I) **Acquired Defects** Circulating antibodies to GH that inhibit GH action Circulating antibodies to the GH receptor Malnutrition/catabolic states Liver disease Inflammatory disease

ALS, Acid-labile subunit; GH, growth hormone; IGF, insulin-like growth factor.

Several mutations/deletions affecting the intracellular domain of the GHR have been reported.[1210-1216] Two defects directly involving the intracellular domain have been reported to result in dominantly inherited GHI. In one, a girl and her mother, both with short stature and biochemical evidence of GHI, were found to be heterozygous for a single G to C transversion in the 3′-splice acceptor site of intron 8, resulting in a truncated GH receptor 1-277 lacking most of the intracellular domain.[1212] A second report described high serum GHBP concentrations in two Japanese siblings and their mother who were characterized by partial GH insensitivity.[1213] The patients and their mother had a heterozygous point mutation that disrupted the 5′-splice donor site of intron 9, causing skipping of exon 9 and the appearance of a premature stop codon in exon 10, and resulting in the same GH 1-277 receptor molecule as described by Ayling and coworkers.[1212] Under in vitro conditions, the Japanese mutation has been shown to result in a GH receptor molecule that behaves in a dominant negative manner, presumably by retaining an ability to dimerize with the normal GHR and thereby inhibiting GH-induced tyrosine phosphorylation of STAT5.[1217] Mutations resulting in C-terminal deletions of the intracellular domain of the GHR have been shown to exhibit normal GH binding and JAK2 phosphorylation, but impaired phosphorylation of STAT5b, again underscoring the critical role of this transcription factor in GH action.[1047,1218]

As described above, a dominant negative effect has been described for mutations, resulting in the loss of the intracellular domain of the GHR, but the question of whether heterozygosity for defects of the extracellular domain can result in short stature remains open to debate. Heterozygosity for defects of the GH receptor has been reported to cause some degree of relative GHI with modest growth improvement only occurring in response to high doses of GH.[927,928,1219,1220] Such observations raise the important question of whether heterozygosity for GHI can result in a clinically important phenotype and whether some children

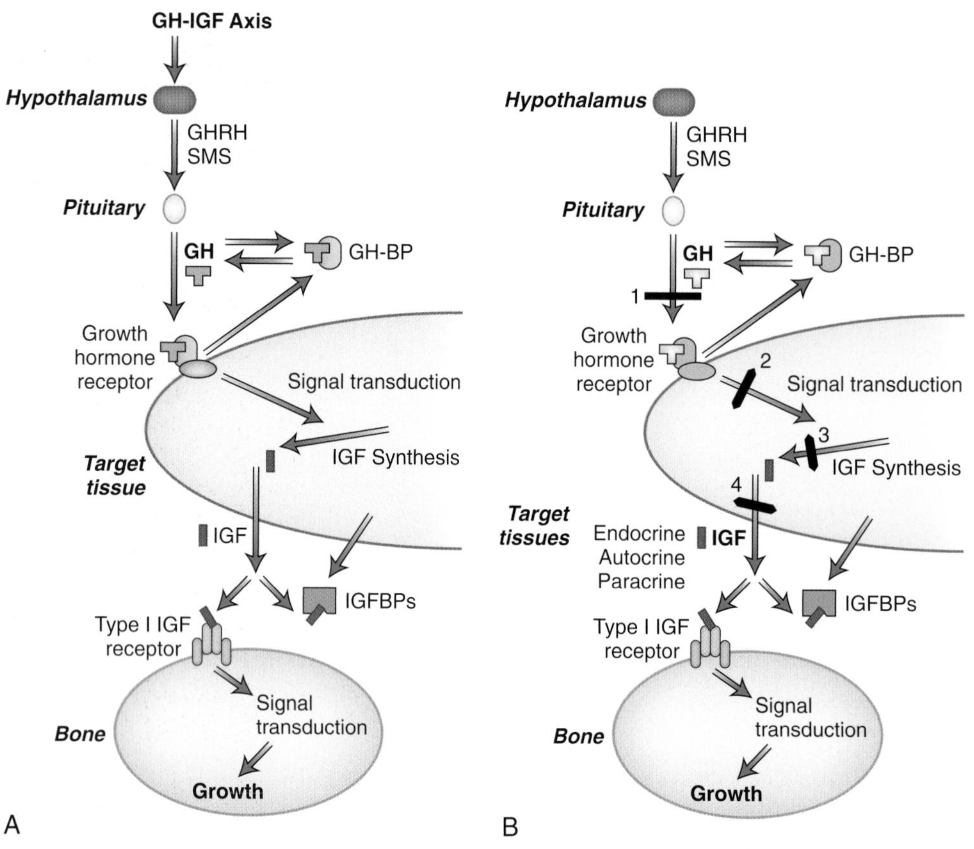

Figure 23–49 ▪ The normal GH-IGF axis **(A)** and the GH-IGF axis showing four potential biochemical defects capable of causing GH insensitivity **(B):** (1) abnormalities of the GH receptor and/or binding protein; (2) abnormal signal transduction, resulting from a defect in the intracellular domain of the GH receptor or postreceptor; (3) defect of IGF synthesis; (4) defect of IGF secretion. (From Rosenfeld RG, Rosenbloom AL, Guevara-Aguirre J. Growth hormone [GH] resistance due to primary GH receptor deficiency. Endocr Rev 1994;15: 369-390.)

labeled as "idiopathic short stature" may harbor such mutations. Given the requirement for dimerization of the GH receptor, there is the potential for an abnormal protein to have varying degrees of dominant negative effect. Ross and colleagues[1221] described a truncated (1–279) GH receptor splice variant whose differential production could act to regulate GHBP production and, more importantly, to modulate GH receptor signaling in a negative fashion.

In summary, the clinical features of GHI due to GH receptor deficiency are identical to those of other forms of severe IGF deficiency, such as congenital GHD, but as with GHD there is a wide range of clinical phenotypes. Basal serum GH levels are typically elevated in children, but may be normal in adults (Fig. 23–50). Most patients have decreased serum GHBP levels but normal or even elevated serum GHBP concentrations do not exclude the diagnosis of GHRD, in that mutations of the GH receptor dimerization domain and in the intracellular domain have been described. Those with measurable GHBP tend to be taller.[1167] Serum IGF-I, IGF-II, and IGFBP-3 levels are profoundly reduced (Fig. 23–51), but partial clinical and biochemical phenotypes have been described, typically but not always related to milder mutations of the GH receptor gene, resulting in only a modest reduction in binding activity and/or receptor action.[56,1167,1210]

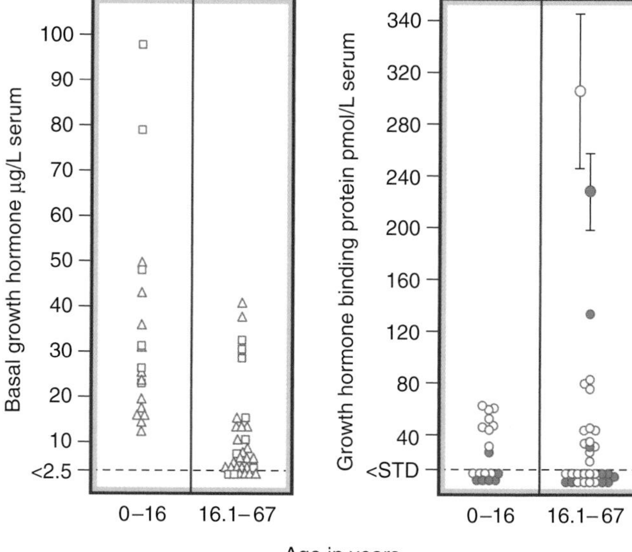

Figure 23–50 ▪ Serum GH and GHBP levels in sera of patients from Ecuador with GH receptor deficiency. (From Rosenfeld RG, Rosenbloom AL, Guevara-Acquirre J. Growth hormone [GH] resistance due to primary GH receptor deficiency. Endocr Rev 1994;15:369-390.)

GHR Signaling Defects. While some cases of primary IGFD with normal serum GHBP have proved to have defects of the transmembrane or intracellular domain of the GH receptor, patients have been reported with similar clinical and biochemical phenotypes, but with normal sequencing of the GH receptor gene.[1222,1223] Until recently, such cases, even when characterized by apparently abnormal activation of the STAT or MAPK pathways, have had no demonstrable molecular basis. Kofoed and colleagues,[153] however, reported a 16-year-old girl with a height of −7.5 SD and markedly low serum concentrations of IGF-I, IGFBP-3, and ALS, despite normal serum concentrations of GHBP and a normal GHR gene sequence. The patient, born to consanguineous parents, proved to be homozygous for a point mutation, resulting in a substitution of proline for alanine at position 630 of the STAT5b gene, with resulting marked decrease

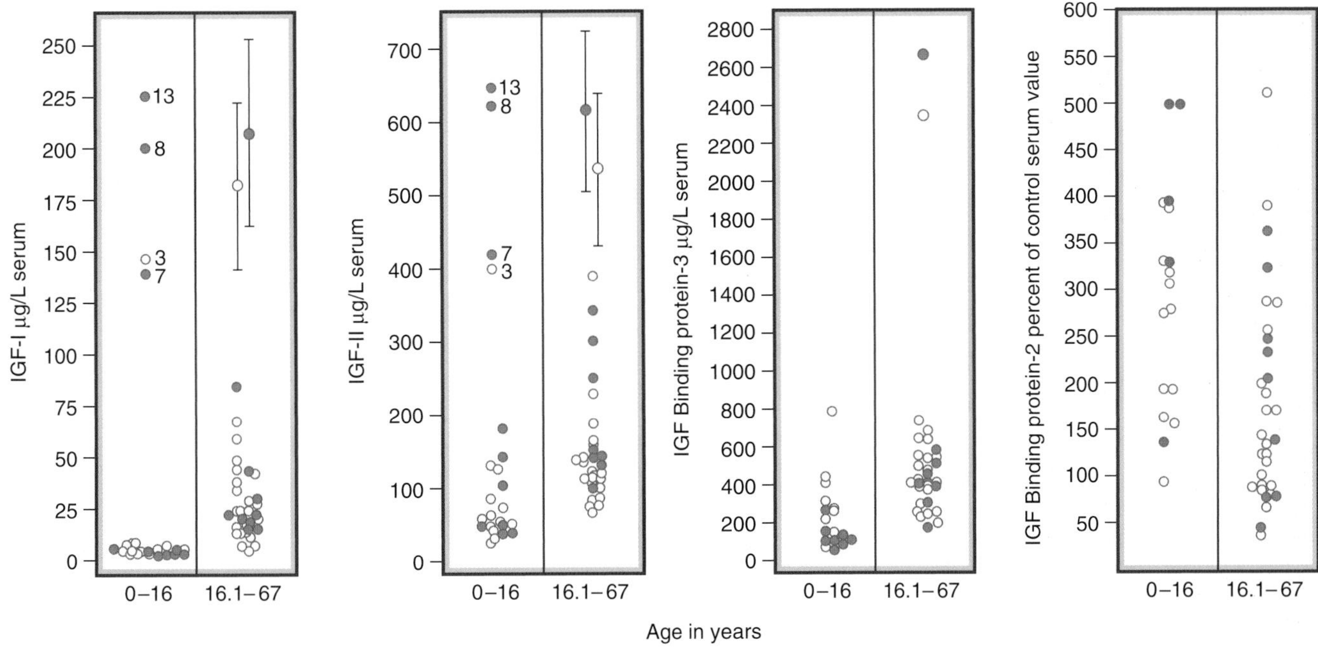

Figure 23–51 ■ Serum levels of IGF-I, IGF-II, IGFBP-2, and IGFBP-3 in patients from Ecuador with GH receptor deficiency. (From Rosenfeld RG, Rosenbloom AL, Guevara-Acquirre J. Growth hormone [GH] resistance due to primary GH receptor deficiency. Endocr Rev 1994;15:369-390.)

in phosphorylation of tyrosine,[699] a critical step in the pathway to STAT activation of IGF-I gene transcription. Subsequent investigations indicated that the mutant STAT5b could not function as a signal transducer or transcription factor, presumably because of an inability to dock with phosphophotyrosines on GH-activated receptors, as well as an inability to form a stable interaction with DNA.[1224] The A630P STAT5b was shown to be characterized by aberrant folding and diminished solubility, resulting in aggregation and formation of cytoplasmic inclusion bodies.[1225] A second case of severe primary IGFD and GH insensitivity, resulting from a novel mutation of STAT5b has been reported.[154] The patient was shown to be homozygous for a single nucleotide insertion in exon 10 of the STAT5b gene, leading to early protein termination. Because STAT5b is involved in the signaling pathway for multiple cytokines, it is of note that both patients had evidence of immune dysfunction and recurrent pulmonary infections. The growth and clinical characteristics of these two patients strongly support the hypothesis that STAT5b mediates the overwhelming majority, if not all, of GH's effects on IGF-I gene transcription. To date, no convincing mutations of the genes for JAK2 or MAPK have been implicated in primary IGFD and GH insensitivity. It is quite possible that severe mutations of JAK2 (which is involved in signaling for multiple growth factors and cytokines) are incompatible with life.

ALS Mutations. Markedly reduced serum concentrations of IGF-I and IGFBP-3 have also been observed in two cases involving mutations of the ALS gene.[1226,1227] Of note is that in both cases, even though serum concentrations of IGF-I and IGFBP-3 were as low as in patients with mutations of the GHR or STAT5b genes, growth was only modestly affected; indeed, the index case[1226] actually attained an adult height within the normal range. Whether the relatively normal growth reflects the greater importance of locally produced IGF-I or whether it reflects altered kinetics of serum IGF-I in the face of reduced concentrations of binding proteins remains uncertain.

IGF-I Gene Deletion. Woods and coworkers[238] described a 15-year-old boy with a partial deletion of the IGF-I gene yielding a truncated IGF-I molecule. Severe prenatal and postnatal (−6.7 SDS) growth retardation and insensitivity to exogenous GH were consistent with the expectations of the phenotype of IGF-I deficiency commencing in utero. Sensorineural deafness, mental retardation, and microcephaly suggest a role for prenatal IGF-I in CNS development. Hyperinsulinism and insulin resistance were presumably due to overproduction of GH. IGF-I levels were exceedingly low, but IGFBP-3 and GHBP levels were normal. The patient is homozygous for deletions of exons 4 and 5 of the IGF-I gene, with both parents being heterozygous carriers and, perhaps, mildly affected, themselves. While unresponsive to GH therapy, the patient was able to accelerate growth velocity, improve body composition, although with greater fat, increase bone mineralization, and decrease insulin resistance upon treatment with IGF-I.[1228,1229]

Inactivating Mutations of the IGF-I Gene. An adult patient with a phenotype virtually identical to that of the patient with the IGF-I gene deletion (i.e., IUGR, severe postnatal growth failure, microcephaly, developmental delay, and sensorineural deafness) has been identified and found to have markedly elevated serum concentrations of IGF-I.[239] The patient was found to be homozygous for a point mutation resulting in a substitution of methionine for valine at position 44. The resulting abnormal IGF-I molecule was shown to have markedly reduced affinity for the IGF-I receptor and only poorly stimulated autophosphorylation of the IGF1 receptor or to activate PKB/Akt or Erk in skin fibroblasts.[1230] This report constitutes the first convincing case of "bioinactive" IGF-I, with the phenotype of severe primary IGFD, commencing in utero, despite elevated serum levels of abnormal IGF-I. Family members who were heterozygous for this mutation were found to have significantly lower birthweight, final height, and head circumference than was the case for wild-type family members, suggesting an effect of heterozygosity for this mutation on IGF-I function.

Genetic Insensitivity to IGF Action. Conditions of insensitivity to IGF-I action include abnormalities of (1) IGF transport and clearance, which would alter presentation of IGF to its receptor; (2) the IGF receptor itself; and (3) postreceptor signaling activation. Such patients would be expected to be exceedingly small, both during prenatal and postnatal life, have elevated GH and normal to high IGF-I levels, and poor growth responses to GH and (presumably) IGF-I administration.

Primary Defects of IGF Transport and Clearance. In fibroblasts from a single short child of 127 studied, Tollefsen and colleagues[1231] found a marked resistance to IGF-I stimulated α-aminoisobutyric acid uptake and thymidine incorporation. An IGF-variant with 600-fold lower binding affinity for IGFBPs stimulated the fibroblasts of this child and normal children, thus eliminating a primary IGF-I receptor defect. This patient's fibroblasts secreted more IGFBPs than normal and had a 10-fold increase in a cell-surface protein similar in size though no immunoreactivity to IGFBP-1.

Barreca and coworkers[1232] studied a short boy (−6 SDS) with increased GH, normal IGF-I, and 20- to 30-fold elevated IGFBP-1 levels. Growth failure seemed due to inhibition of IGF-I action by IGFBP-1. Short-term treatment with GH led to suppression of IGFBP-1, increased ternary complexed-IGF-I, and a marked increase of growth rate.

Interestingly, no convincing cases of defects of IGFBP-3 production or action as causes of short stature have been reported to date.

Primary Defects of IGF-I Receptor Production or Responsivity. In mouse knockout models, homozygous mutations of the IGF-I receptor result in profound growth failure and neonatal mortality. Heterozygous mutations are phenotypically similar to wild-type mice. In the African Efe pygmies, a series of studies[1233] demonstrated extreme insensitivity to the in vitro growth-enhancing effects of IGF-I. Reduced IGF-I receptor transcripts and sites with resultant diminished tyrosine phosphorylation and postreceptor signaling, although no definable receptor mutation, are suggested explanations.[1234]

Patients with IUGR and postnatal growth failure associated with defects of the IGF1R[248,1235] have been reported. Clinical findings have included microcephaly and mild mental retardation, as well. Serum IGF-I concentrations were normal to elevated, but binding of IGF-I was shown to be reduced. Whether such mutations will prove to be a common cause of combined IUGR and postnatal growth failure remains to be determined.

In leprechaunism, a syndrome of growth failure and insulin receptor dysfunction, there is variable IGF-I insensitivity.[1233,1236] The profound abnormality of the insulin receptor suggests that heterodimeric insulin and IGF-I receptor combinations could possibly lead to failed activation of the IGF-I signaling cascade. Because the IGF-I receptor gene resides at 15q26.3, deletions of the distal long arm of chromosome 15 or ring chromosome 15 may lead to hemizygosity for the IGF-I receptor.[1233,1237] Although such patients may have IUGR and striking postnatal growth failure, lack of a biologic response to IGF-I has not been conclusively demonstrated.[1237] Whether growth failure in such patients is due to altered levels of IGF-I receptor or represents the net effect of the loss of other genes located on 15q remains to be determined.

Diagnosis of IGF Deficiency Syndrome: GH Deficiency

Because the proper means of diagnosing GHD is controversial,[1238] the concept of the *IGF deficiency syndrome* becomes even more relevant. With availability of highly specific assays for the IGF peptides and binding proteins and with increasing understanding of the GH-IGF axis, evaluation of patients with growth failure should include a combination of careful auxologic assessment and appropriate measures of the GH-IGF system. Documenting a deficiency of IGF levels and concomitant alterations in serum concentrations of IGFBPs suggests an abnormality of GH secretion or activity and makes necessary a thorough evaluation of hypothalamic-pituitary-IGF function. At the same time, it must be noted that serum concentrations of IGFs may only be surrogates for more physiologically relevant tissue concentrations of these growth factors.

The foundation for the diagnosis of IGF deficiency is the careful documentation of serial heights and determination of height velocity. In the absence of other evidence of pituitary GH secretory dysfunction, it is usually unnecessary to perform tests of GH secretion. Thus, even in children below the 5th percentile in height (which, obviously, applies to 5% of the normal population), documentation of a normal height velocity (above the 25th percentile for several years) makes the diagnosis of IGF deficiency and GHD highly unlikely.

Assessment of pituitary GH production is difficult because GH secretion is pulsatile with the most consistent surges occurring at times of slow-wave electroencephalographic rhythms during stages 3 and 4 of sleep. The regulation of GH secretion involves at least two hypothalamic factors, GHRH and somatostatin, as well as multiple other peptides and neurotransmitters. Spontaneous GH secretion varies with gender, age, pubertal stage, and nutritional status, all of which must be factored into the evaluation of GH production.

Between normal pulses of GH secretion, serum GH levels are low (often <0.1 μg/L), below the limits of sensitivity of most conventional assays (usually <0.2μg/L). Accordingly, measurement of random serum GH concentrations is virtually useless in diagnosing GHD, but may be useful in the diagnosis of GHI and GH excess. Measurement of GH "secretory reserve," therefore, relies on the use of physiologic or pharmacologic stimuli, and such "provocative tests" have been the basis for the diagnosis of GHD for more than 30 years.[1238,1239] Physiologic stimuli include fasting, sleep, and exercise, and pharmacologic stimuli include levodopa, clonidine, glucagon, propranolol, arginine, and insulin (references found in reference 20). Stimulation tests have often been divided into "screening tests" (exercise, fasting, levodopa, clonidine), which are characterized by ease of administration, low toxicity, low risk, and low specificity) and "definitive tests" (arginine, insulin, glucagon). To improve specificity, provocative tests are customarily combined or given sequentially. We have, for example, often used fasting plus oral clonidine as a "screening test," to be followed by fasting plus intravenous sequential arginine, oral clonidine, levodopa, or insulin as a "definitive test." It is generally accepted that a child must "fail" provocative tests with at least two separate stimuli to be considered as having GHD. Standard provocative GH tests are summarized in Table 23–8.

Although provocative GH testing has been the foundation for the diagnosis of GHD since GH assays first became available, they have come under criticism for a number of reasons[1238,1240]:

1. *Nonphysiologic provocative GH testing.* None of the standard pharmacologic provocative tests satisfactorily mimic the normal secretory pattern of pituitary GH. Even when naturally occurring regulatory peptides are used for stimulation, their dosage, route of administration, and interactions with other regulatory factors in a testing situation are artificial. Furthermore, because most endocrine centers use several different stimulation tests, there are no validated means of resolving conflicting data from two or more provocative tests.[1241] To emphasize this point, Guyda[1242] reported on 6373 GH stimulation tests performed on 3233 short French children; 11 different pharmacologic tests were employed with 62 of the possible 66 pairs employed at least once and the most frequent combination of tests used only in 12.7% of patients.

TABLE 23–8 TESTS TO PROVOKE GROWTH HORMONE SECRETION

Stimulus	Dosage	Times Samples Are Taken (min)	Comments
Exercise	Step climbing; exercise cycle for 10 minutes	0, 10, 20	Observe child closely when on the steps
Levodopa	<15 kg: 125 mg 10-30 kg: 250 mg >30 kg: 500 mg	0, 60, 90	Nausea, rarely emesis
Clonidine	0.15 mg/m^2	0, 30, 60, 90	Tiredness, postural hypotension
Arginine HCl (IV)	0.5 g/kg (max 30 g) 10% arginine HCl in 0.9% NaCl over 30 min	0, 15, 30, 45, 60	
Insulin (IV)*	0.05 to 0.1 unit/kg	0, 15, 30, 60, 75, 90, 120	Hypoglycemia, requires close supervision
Glucagon (IM)	0.03 mg/kg (max 1 mg)	0, 30, 60, 90, 120, 150, 180	Nausea, occasional emesis
GHRH (IV)	1 μg/kg	0, 15, 30, 45, 60, 90, 120	Flushing, metallic taste

Tests should be performed after an overnight fast. Many investigators suggest that prepubertal children should be "primed" with gonadal steroids, e.g., 5 mg Premarin orally the night before and the morning of the test or with 50 to 100 μg/day ethinyl estradiol for 3 consecutive days before testing or 100 ng depot testosterone 3 days before testing. This, of course, alters the patient's steady-state and performs the provocative test in a steroid-rich environment. Patients must be euthyroid at the time of testing.
*Insulin-induced hypoglycemia is a potential risk of this procedure, which is designed to lower the blood glucose by at least 50%. Documentation of appropriate lowering of blood glucose is recommended. If GHD is suspected, the lower dosage of insulin is usually administered, especially in infants. $D_{10}W$ and glucagon should be available.

2. *Arbitrary definitions of "subnormal" response to provocative tests.* Different centers vary in the definition of a "normal" response to stimulation tests. Whereas early reports generally employed a cutoff level of 2.5 μg/L, this cutoff was gradually increased to 7 μg/L and with the availability of recombinant DNA-derived GH, increased to 10 μg/L, although there are no data for validating higher arbitrary cutoff values.[1240,1243] The initial levels of GH that were used to define GHD were based on the study of patients with profound "classical" findings or organic destruction of the adenohypophysis.[1244] The lack of documentation of defined normal responses can be seen in the use of vague terminology such as "lack of adequate endogenous growth hormone secretion"[1245] and "inadequate secretion of normal endogenous growth hormone".[1246] Many new GH assays measure GH immunopotency at 33% to 50% of earlier assays, but there has not been a systematic reassessment of "new normal" GH cutoff levels nor of critical evaluation by many endocrinologists of which assay their center might be using.[1242,1247]
3. *Age dependency and use of gonadal steroids.* Serum GH levels rise during puberty, typically because of an increase in pulse-amplitude rather than an increase in pulse frequency.[108,121] Before puberty and during the early phases of puberty, GH secretion may normally be so low as to blur the discrimination between GHD and constitutional delay of growth and maturation.[1248] Many children who "fail" provocative testing before the onset of puberty prove to have "normal" GH secretion after puberty or after administration of exogenous gonadal steroids.[1094,1249-1251] In a placebo-controlled comparison of estrogen priming in children with GHD and ISS, the GH provocative tests performed after priming (using 9 μg/L as a cutoff with a polyclonal GH assay) had a diagnostic efficiency of 98%.[1252] A well-controlled study of provocative GH testing in children of normal stature documented the inherent problems of such testing and the need for standardization of gonadal steroid administration during stimulation tests in peripubertal children.[1253] When exercise and arginine-insulin stimulation tests were administered to these normal children, the lower limit of normal (−2 SD) for peak serum GH concentration in prepubertal children was only 1.9 μg/L, while in children of Tanner stage 5 puberty, this level was 9.3 μg/L. When estrogen was administered before provocative testing, the lower 95% confidence limit for the normal serum GH range rose to 7.2 μg/L. When estrogen was not administered, the serum GH level did not rise above 7 μg/L during three provocative tests. These normally growing children could, potentially, have been erroneously labeled as having GHD in 61% of normal prepubertal children. Furthermore, the finding of similar GH values in slow-growing, short children emphasizes the difficulty of basing this important diagnosis on provocative test data that use a "magic" number as an arbitrary cutoff for normal.
4. *Variability of GH assays limiting discriminatory power.* Many studies have demonstrated as much as threefold variability in the measurement of serum GH levels among established laboratories.[1254,1255] This is explained, at least in part, by the presence of several molecular forms of GH in serum and by the use of different monoclonal antibodies in contrast to older polyclonal antibodies; variations in the choice of standards, labeling techniques, and assay buffers (matrix) are also contributory. The consequence is that children labeled as GHD by one assay are considered normal by another. This is an unacceptable situation for clinicians, who may be unaware of the type and source of GH assay being used by a given laboratory.[1256] A highly sensitive immunofunctional GH assay has been developed recently, which measures concentrations of GH capable of binding to GHBP. It is not clear, however, that such assays necessarily have any advantages over standard radioimmunoassays for routine GH measurements.[1257] Using arginine/L-dopa or arginine/insulin stimulation tests, approximately 50% of normal children had peak GH concentrations less than 7 ng/mL, and 30% of less than 5 ng/mL, whether GH was measured by immunofunctional assay or ELISA.
5. *Expense, discomfort, and risks of provocative GH testing.* Provocative testing typically requires multiple timed blood samples and the parenteral administration of drugs. The resulting discomfort to the patient and expense are self-evident. In addition, tests involving insulin administration carry the risk of hypoglycemia and seizures, and should be performed only by experienced medical personnel and under appropriate patient supervision. Deaths have been reported from insulin-induced hypoglycemia and from its overly vigorous correction with parenteral glucose.[1258]
6. *Poor reproducibility of provocative tests.* The reproducibility of provocative GH tests has never been adequately docu-

mented, even when GH levels are measured with the same assay.[1259]

Another diagnostic approach involves measurement of spontaneous GH secretion. This can be done either by multiple sampling (every 5 to 30 minutes) over a 12- to 24-hour period or by continuous blood withdrawal over 12 to 24 hours.[1063,1064,1260-1262] The former method allows one to evaluate and characterize GH pulsatility, while the latter only permits determination of mean GH concentration. Both approaches are subject to many of the same limitations as provocative GH testing. The expense and discomfort of such testing are obvious, and, although it was thought that this approach might be more reproducible than provocative GH tests, variability remains a problem.[1263-1265] The ability of such tests to discriminate between children with GHD and those with "normal" short stature. Rose and coworkers[1065] reported that measurement of spontaneous GH secretion identified only 57% of children with GHD as defined by provocative testing. Similarly, Lanes[1066] reported that one fourth of normally growing children have low overnight GH levels, and a longitudinal study of normal boys through puberty demonstrated a wide intersubject variance, including many "low" 24-hour GH production rates, despite fully normal growth.[108,109]

Given the problems with GH testing, it is not surprising that provocative tests and 24-hour GH profiles do not always correlate. It is likely that 12- to 24-hour GH profiles can identify most children with GHD and is superior, both in sensitivity and specificity, to provocative GH testing. Urinary GH assessment has not yet evolved into a useful integrative methodology. "Neurosecretory dysfunction" probably does exist in children after cranial radiation and likely does characterize a subgroup of children with GHD and IGF deficiency. The expense and discomfort of such GH profiles and the problems in GH determinations preclude it, however, from being the test of choice in establishing the diagnosis of GHD in most cases.

Despite the many problems with GH measurements described above, there continues to be a value in determination of GH secretory capacity in the diagnostic evaluation of a child with IGF deficiency. Documentation of normal (or increased) GH levels is necessary in discriminating between primary and secondary IGF deficiency. The documented presence of GH deficiency should alert the clinician to the possibility of other pituitary deficiencies. Additionally, the presence of pituitary dysfunction mandates clinical and radiologic evaluation for evidence of congenital or acquired structural defects of the hypothalamus and/or pituitary, including the possibility of intracranial tumors. Finally, documentation of GHD, either alone or combined with other pituitary deficiencies, may warrant evaluation for molecular defects of GH production.

An alternative means of diagnosing GHD is the assessment of IGF-I and -II and their binding proteins.[261,262,264,290] GHD then becomes part of the differential diagnosis of IGF deficiency, which includes hypothalamic dysfunction, pituitary insufficiency, and GHI. With the development of sensitive and specific assays for IGF-I, IGF-II, and the IGFBPs, it has become clear that these peptides accurately reflect integrated GH status of pediatric patients. Furthermore, IGF-I and -II normally circulate in serum in sufficiently high levels that assay sensitivity is not an issue. Serum levels of both peptides are relatively constant during the day so that provocative testing or multiple sampling is not necessary. However, IGF-I assays do have potential limitations:

1. IGFBPs potentially interfere with radioimmunoassays, radioreceptor assays, and bioassays.[267-269] These binding proteins must either be removed by acid gel chromatography (which is labor-intensive)[267-269] or blocked by the addition of excess IGF-II (which requires a high-affinity, high-specificity antibody for IGF-I).[277] An alternative approach is to employ a radiolabeled IGF-I analogue with reduced affinity for IGFBPs.[271]
2. Serum IGF-I levels are age-dependent,[263,280,281] being lowest in young children (younger than 5 years of age), a period during which one most wishes to have an accurate diagnostic test.
3. Serum IGF-I levels may be low in conditions other than GHD such as primary GHI (Laron syndrome) and secondary GHI (e.g., malnutrition, liver disease).
4. Serum concentrations of IGF-I (and IGFBP-3) are frequently normal in adult-onset GHD and in children with GHD resulting from brain tumors and/or cranial irradiation.
5. Interlaboratory differences of absolute IGF values, although not as striking as with GH, may be substantial.

Even when these caveats are considered, the correlation between serum IGF-I levels and provocative or spontaneous GH measurements is imperfect. In a group of children younger than 10 years of age, IGF-I levels were below −2 SD in only 8/15 children with a diagnosis of GHD based upon provocative testing (53.3% sensitivity), and normal in 47/48 children with a normal GH response (97.9% specificity).[1266] We believe, however, that this imperfect correlation more likely reflects limitations of GH testing rather than inadequacies of IGF measurements. However, when serum levels of both IGF-I and -II are determined, the correlation with GH testing improves, because serum IGF-II levels are low in GHD and normally do not increase with age after 1 year.[264] In one study, 18% of patients with low provocative GH levels had IGF-I concentrations in the normal range, but only 4% of "GHD" patients had normal serum levels of both IGF-I and -II.[264] Serum levels of IGF-I and -II were both reduced in only 0.5% of normal children and in 11% of normal short children.

The assay of GH-dependent IGFBP-3, normally the major serum carrier of IGF peptides, is an additional means of diagnosing IGF deficiency due to GHD[381,487,488] because the concentrations of IGFBP-3 correlate with the sum of the levels of IGF-I and -II:

1. The immunoassay of IGFBP-3 is technically simple and does not require separation of the binding protein from IGF peptides.
2. Normal serum levels of IGFBP-3 are high, typically in the 1 to 5 mg/L range, so that assay sensitivity is not an issue.
3. Serum IGFBP-3 levels vary with age to a lesser degree than is the case for IGF-I. Even in infants, serum IGFBP-3 levels are sufficiently high to allow discrimination of low values from the normal range.
4. Serum IGFBP-3 levels are less dependent on nutrition than IGF-I, reflecting the "stabilizing" effect of IGF-II levels.
5. IGFBP-3 levels are GH-dependent.

The utility of IGFBP-3 assays in the diagnosis of GHD was evaluated by Blum and colleagues,[488] who found that serum IGFBP-3 levels were below the 5th percentile for age in 128/132 of children (97%) diagnosed with GHD by conventional criteria (height less than 3rd percentile, height velocity less than 10th percentile, and peak serum GH less than 10 μg/L). At the same time, 124/130 (95%) of non-GHD, short children had normal IGFBP-3 levels; it is likely that this group of GHD patients consisted largely of children with severe GHD, because such a clear correlation between provocative GH testing and serum IGFBP-3 levels has not been consistently observed. For example, in one study the sensitivity of the IGFBP-3 assay in complete GHD (peak GH less than 5 μg/L) was 93%, but only 43% in partial GHD (peak GH 5 to 10 μg/L).[1267] In another study, 100% of children with severe GHD (peak GH less than 1 μg/L) and low serum IGF-I also had decreased serum IGFBP-3; four of eight children with GHD and normal serum IGF-I levels had reduced IGFBP-3 levels; and 10 of 23 normal short children (43%) had decreased serum IGFBP-3.[1268] In the latter study, 18% of patients had discordance between IGFBP-3 levels and provocative GH testing. Juul and Skakkebaek found that 47/48 prepubertal, but only 74/94 pubertal children, with normal GH provocative test results had normal IGFBP-3 levels.[1269] There is the additional concern that IGFBP-3 levels may be "falsely" normal in patients with GHD due to intracranial lesions.[1270] The addition of a radioimmunoassay for IGFBP-2 further enhanced the ability of IGF axis measures to identify children who were GHD by conventional criteria.[1268]

The correlation between IGF-I and IGFBP-3 levels and assessments of spontaneous GH secretion is also imperfect. Even in normal children the correlation between 24-hour GH secretion and serum IGF-I and IGFBP-3 levels is modest (r=0.78 and r=0.62, respectively).[1271]

It is not possible to resolve fully conflicts between assays of the IGF axis and measurements of GH secretion, as there is no definitive way to diagnose GHD, but studies of patients with GH receptor deficiency support the utility of IGF-related determinations.[124,1272,1273] Although such patients may have normal or elevated serum GH levels, mutations or deletions of the GH receptor gene render them unresponsive to GH, making them "functionally GH deficient." In approximately 70 instances of GH receptor gene mutations, all had markedly reduced serum levels of both IGF-I and IGFBP-3.[1272] Even so, both IGF-I and IGFBP-3 correlated significantly with height. Measurements of IGF-I and IGFBP-3 levels have been used in other studies to establish the diagnosis of GHI.[1274,1275]

Assessment of the Child with Poor Growth

The most important parameter in assessing children with growth failure is careful clinical evaluation, including accurate serial measurements of height and height velocity. Figure 23–52 provides an algorithm for the evaluation of the child with growth failure. The many illness-related causes of diminished growth are discussed in prior sections. The possibility of hypothalamic/pituitary dysfunction should always be considered in children with documented growth deceleration, particularly in the face of known or suspected CNS pathology (e.g., tumors, radiation, malformations, infection, trauma, blindness, nystagmus). Similarly, the neonate with hypoglycemia and/or microphallus warrants evaluation of pituitary function (including MRI), and children with documented TSH, ACTH, ADH, or gonadotropin deficiency are candidates for GHD. For children with proportional short stature and documented growth deceleration, assessment of serum IGF-I and IGFBP-3 is warranted, and, based upon the results, the possibilities of hypothalamic dysfunction, pituitary insufficiency, and GHI can be investigated.

Recommendations by the GH Research Society (GRS)[1276] for defining GHD recognize no "gold standard" for that diagnosis and propose that in a child with slow growth, whose history and auxology suggest GHD (Table 23–9), testing for GH/IGF-I deficiency requires the measurement of IGF-I and IGFBP-3 levels as well as GH provocation tests (after hypothyroidism has been excluded). In suspected isolated GHD, two GH provocation tests (sequential or on separate days) are required, but in those with defined CNS pathology, history of irradiation, CPHD, or a genetic defect, one GH test will suffice. In patients who have had cranial irradiation or malformations of the hypothalamic-pituitary unit, GHD may evolve over years and its diagnosis requires serial testing. Some patients with auxology suggestive of GHD, however, may have IGF-I and/or IGFBP-3 levels below the normal range on repeated tests but GH responses in provocation tests above the "cutoff" level. Such children do not have classical GHD but nonetheless may have an abnormality of the GH-IGF axis and, after the exclusion of systemic disorders affecting the synthesis or action of IGF-I, could be considered for GH treatment. A cranial MRI scan with particular attention to the hypothalamic-pituitary region should be carried out in any child diagnosed as having GHD. These recommendations stress the importance of rational clinical judgment rather than specific tests in characterization of childhood GHD.

TABLE 23–9 KEY HISTORY AND PHYSICAL EXAMINATION FINDINGS THAT MAY INDICATE THAT GROWTH HORMONE DEFICIENCY COULD BE PRESENT (THE GRS 2000 CRITERIA[1276])

- In the neonate, hypoglycemia, prolonged jaundice, microphallus, or traumatic delivery
- Cranial irradiation
- Head trauma or central nervous system infection
- Consanguinity and/or an affected family member
- Craniofacial midline abnormalities
- Severe short stature (<–3 SD)
- Height less than –2 SD and a height velocity over 1 year less than –1 SD
- A decrease in height SD of more than 0.5 over 1 year in children older than 2 years of age
- A height velocity below –2 SD over 1 year
- A height velocity more than 1.5 SD below the mean sustained over 2 years
- Signs indicative of an intracranial lesion
- Signs of multiple pituitary hormone deficiency (MPHD)
- Neonatal symptoms and signs of growth hormone deficiency

Ultimately, the diagnosis of GHD (or IGF deficiency) should be made on the basis of combined clinical and laboratory criteria. Short children who have well-documented normal height velocities do not, generally, require evaluation of GH secretion, and the finding of normal serum levels of IGF-I and/or IGFBP-3 is confirmatory for the absence of defects of the GH-IGF axis. Children with Turner's syndrome and short stature should not be required to undergo GH testing to qualify for GH therapy, because such treatment is not predicated on abnormal GH secretion. On the other hand, the child with documented growth deceleration requires further evaluation, even if tests of GH secretion appear normal. Documentation of decreased serum IGF-I and IGFBP-3 levels would then substantiate the diagnosis of IGF deficiency, and the differential diagnoses of GHD and GHI would need to be considered. The child with a history of cranial irradiation, decreased height velocity, and reduced serum levels of IGF-I and IGFBP-3 should be considered to have GHD (or GHR), even in the face of normal provocative tests.[1010] Alternatively, such patients may have normal IGFBP-3 levels with low GH levels in pharmacologic tests.[1269,1270] This approach still leaves a place for measurements of GH secretion. Such determinations are critical for distinguishing between GHD and GHI as causes of IGF deficiency. Documentation of abnormal pituitary GH secretion raises the possibility of intracranial tumors and the potential for deficiency of other pituitary hormones. Evaluation for GHD permits concomitant assessment of ACTH/cortisol secretion during insulin-induced hypoglycemia.

The diagnosis of GHD in a newborn is especially challenging. The presence of micropenis in a male newborn should always lead to an evaluation of the GH-IGF axis. A GH level must be measured in the presence of neonatal hypoglycemia occurring in the absence of a metabolic disorder such as hyperammonemia or carnitine deficiency syndromes. A level of less than 20 ng/mL in a polyclonal radioimmunoassay suggests GHD. The use of standard GH stimulation tests is not recommended in neonates with the exception of the glucagon test; it is often of value to measure serum GH during an episode of documented

Step 1—Defining the risk of IGF deficiency syndrome

Auxologic abnormalities
- Severe short stature (height SDS <-3 SD)
- Severe growth deceleration (height velocity SDS <-2 SD over 12 months)
- Height <-2 SD and height velocity <-1.0 SD over 12 months
- Height <-1.5 SD and height velocity <-1.5 SD over 2 years

Risk factors
- History of a brain tumor, cranial irradiation, or other documented organic or congenital hypothalamic-pituitary abnormality
- Incidental finding of hypothalamic-pituitary abnormality on MRI
- If any of the above exists, proceed with Step 2; if not, follow clinically and return to Step 1 in 6 months

Step 2—Screening for IGF deficiency and other diseases

A. Order a laboratory panel including a bone age, free T_4, and TSH, chromosomes (in females), and nonendocrine tests; if indicated, refer back to primary care physician or treat diagnosed conditions as appropriate.

and

B. Order an IGF-I and an IGFBP-3 level.
- If IGF-I/IGFBP-3 are both above the -1 SD, follow clinically and return to Step 1 in 6 months.
- If IGF-I/IGFBP-3 are both below -2 SD, proceed to Step 4. If MRI is abnormal, GH provocative testing is optional (Table 23–8)
- Otherwise, proceed to Step 3. If this is a patient with delayed adolescence, consider sex steroid treatment prior to Step 3.

Step 3—Testing GH secretion

This step can be bypassed if a clear GHD risk factor and a severe IGF deficiency are identified.

- Perform two of the following GH stimulation tests (if appropriate, estrogen prime) (see Table 23–8):
  - Clonidine
  - Arginine
  - Insulin
  - Glucagon
  - L-Dopa
  - Propranolol
- If all GH levels are below 10, go to Step 4.
- If peak GH >15 ng/mL, obtain GHBP; if GHBP <-2 SD, consider an IGF-generation test and, if abnormal, IGF treatment.
- If peak GH >15 ng/mL and GHBP is normal, follow clinically and return to Step 1 in 6 months.
- If peak GH is between 10 and 15 ng/mL, go back to Step 2 in 6 months.

Step 4—Evaluating the pituitary

- Perform MRI, with particular emphasis on hypothalamic-pituitary anatomy
- Test HPA axis, if not already done (CRH stimulation or ITT), and teach cortisol supplementation as needed (must do this if the MRI is abnormal).
- Consider molecular evaluation of GH, GHR, or GHRHR and other potential genetic defects (Fig. 23–14)

Step 5—Treating for growth promotion

- Initiate GH treatment at appropriate dose levels.
- If GHIS is suspected, consider IGF therapy, if available.
- Regularly evaluate growth parameters, IGF-I, and IGFBP-3, as well as compliance and safety (see Table 23-13).
- GH secretion should be retested, according to adult GH assessment protocols, at the end of growth.

Figure 23–52 ▪ Clinical and biochemical evaluation of growth failure: seeking the diagnosis of IGF deficiency syndrome. The goal of step 1 is to define the patient to be assessed. Step 2 seeks a wide array of "diseases" associated with poor growth. Step 3 relates to the possibility of GH provocative testing. Step 4 defines assessment of the hypothalamic-pituitary morphology and the consideration of ACTH deficiency. Nonetheless, the primary evaluation is for "IGF deficiency," with studies designed to delineate hypothalamic or pituitary abnormalities or growth hormone insensitivity.

hypoglycemia. Normative data are not available for stimulated serum GH levels, but a cutoff of 25 ng/mL is probably appropriate and stimulated values under 20 certainly should raise suspicion. MRI is es-sential when the diagnosis is suspected and useful clinical information defining developmental abnormalities of the hypothalamic-pituitary area may be available sooner than GH assay data. An IGFBP-3 level is of value for the diagnosis of neonatal GHD, but IGF-I levels are rarely helpful.[1277] In fact, serum IGFBP-3 should be performed as the test of choice in suspected neonatal GHD.

In summary, a child should be considered a candidate for GH therapy, if he or she meets one of these auxologic criteria, supported by biochemical evidence of GH deficiency based on sex-steroid-primed provocative tests, and/or evidence of IGF deficiency based on measurement of IGF-I and IGFBP-3 concentrations. Such cases need also to have MR imaging of the hypothalamus-pituitary and assessment of other pituitary hormone deficiencies. It is understood that this approach will result in GH treatment of some children with "idiopathic, isolated" GH deficiency or IGF deficiency, and that such cases require careful monitoring of both pituitary status and responsiveness to GH treatment. The latter can be assessed relative to recently developed predictive models[1278,1279] and the diagnosis of GHD reconsidered in the child with idiopathic, isolated GHD, a normal MRI, and a subnormal clinical response to GH.

Diagnosis of Primary IGF Deficiency

Primary IGFD is characterized by low serum IGF-I concentrations in the presence of normal (or increased) production of GH. While previously classified as GH insensitivity (GHI), it is now apparent that primary IGFD has multiple molecular etiologies, including defects of the GHR, defects of the GH signaling cascade, defects of IGF binding proteins, and defects of IGF-I, itself. While the hallmark of all of these conditions is low serum IGF-I, complete biochemical assessment of the GH-IGF axis can help point to the correct molecular etiology (see Table 23–5). It is, consequently, important to assess multiple biochemical parameters in such cases, including serum IGF-I, IGF-II, IGFBP-3, ALS, and GHBP. Basal and stimulated GH levels are, typically, normal or increased in such cases. IGF generation studies are of value in demonstrating GH insensitivity, but, by themselves, cannot completely discriminate among the various causes of primary IGFD, and, accordingly, molecular studies may be required.

Savage and colleagues[1273,1280] devised a scoring system for evaluating short children for the diagnosis of GH receptor deficiency, based upon five parameters: (1) basal serum GH greater than 10 mU/L (approximately 5 μg/L); (2) serum IGF-I less than 50 μg/L; (3) height SDS less than −3; (4) serum GHBP less than 10% (based upon binding of [^{125}I] GH); and (5) a rise in serum IGF-I levels after GH administration of less than twofold the intra-assay variation (approximately 10%). Blum and associates[1281] proposed that these criteria could be strengthened by (1) evaluating GH secretory profiles rather than isolated basal levels; (2) employing an age-dependent range and the 0.1 percentile as the cutoff level for evaluation of serum IGF-I concentrations; (3) employing highly sensitive IGF-I immunoassays and defining a failed GH response as the inability to increase serum IGF-I levels by at least 15 μg/L; and (4) measuring both basal and GH-stimulated IGFBP-3 levels. These criteria fit well with the population of GHRD patients in Ecuador, but that is a homogeneous population with severe GHI.[124,1272] The applicability of these criteria elsewhere remains to be evaluated. An important biochemical marker is the response of IGF-I (and possibly, IGFBP-3) to GH stimulation.[1282-1284]

Several diagnostic points may be elicited from Table 23–10:

1. The presence of IUGR (in addition to postnatal growth failure) suggests intrauterine IGFD or resistance, and points to a diagnosis of IGF-I gene deletions, bioinactive IGF-I, or IGF receptor abnormalities.
2. Low GHBP suggests a defect in the extracellular domain of the GHR, but normal (or increased) GHBP may be seen in some defects of the GHR or GH signaling cascade.
3. A markedly elevated IGF-I is consistent with bioinactive IGF.
4. IGFBP-3 and ALS concentrations may be increased in cases of molecular defects of IGF-I.

The diagnosis of primary IGFD mandates, additionally, that the possibilities of malnutrition or GHD be eliminated.

TABLE 23–10 POTENTIAL MOLECULAR REASONS FOR THE SYNDROME OF IDIOPATHIC SHORT STATURE

LOW SERUM CONCENTRATIONS OF IGF-I: IGF DEFICIENCY
Diminished total 24-hour growth hormone (GH) synthesis and secretion
"Mild" abnormalities of the GH receptor
Heterozygosity for mutations or deletions of the GH receptor gene
"Mild" defects of post GH receptor signaling (JAK/STAT system)
Polymorphisms of the IGF gene resulting in altered transcription and/or translational efficiency
Abnormalities of IGF binding proteins
NORMAL OR ELEVATED SERUM CONCENTRATIONS OF IGF-I: IGF RESISTANCE
Bioinactive IGF-I, resulting from inactivating mutations of the IGF-I gene
Abnormalities of IGF binding proteins
"Mild" abnormalities of the IGF receptor
"Mild" defects of post IGF receptor signaling
End-organ resistance to IGF action at the epiphyseal growth plate

Modified from Rosenfeld RG. The molecular basis of idiopathic short stature. Growth Horm IGF Res 2005;15S:3-5.

Idiopathic Short Stature

There remains a large cadre of short children in whom the cause of their diminished stature is unknown or "idiopathic." Many children and early adolescents are short (<3rd percentile), have slowed linear growth velocity (<25th percentile), may have delayed skeletal maturation and an impaired or attenuated pubertal growth spurt, with or without a family history manifesting some or all of these clinical features, and have no chronic illnesses or apparent endocrinopathies. Such children usually have normal GH secretory dynamics, although provocative tests may be blunted under some circumstances. GH-dependent peptides are frequently (but not invariably) lower than expected on a chronologic though often not skeletal age basis. Treatment with exogenous GH usually augments linear growth. These children have often been considered variants of normal growth and, if untreated, may achieve a final adult height within the range considered acceptable for the family. It should be noted, however, that many of these children are as short as those with GHD and so cannot simply be considered "normal, short children." The etiology of the slowed childhood growth and frequently delayed pubertal spurt has not been established in most of these children. As this is the largest group of short children, continuing efforts are underway to develop a rational categorization and to develop the means of defining these children within the possible abnormalities of the GH-IGF axis. Multiple groups of patients are included in this broad category, including those with constitutional delay of growth and maturation and so-called genetic or familial short stature. The genetic characterization of the former syndrome, with an emphasis upon the timing and tempo of pubertal onset and progression, is beyond the scope of this chapter. Familial short stature, while not usually in the range of the dramatic genetic syndromes resulting in extremely poor growth described above, generally results in an adult whose height is close to or below the bottom of the normal range, but appropriate for family. It must be noted that this should not be considered totally reassuring, because there is growing recognition of subtle genetic defects contributing to growth failure and masquerading as "benign" familial short stature. ISS is the remaining large but uncharacterized group of children. These children presumably have more subtle disorders of the hypothalamic-pituitary-IGF axis[907,928] than those described in the discussion of primary IGFD (see Table 23–10). Heterozygous mutations throughout the growth system, a relatively greater preponderance of blockers of the GH-signaling cascade, such as enhanced intracellular phosphatase activity and production of such signaling factors as SOC2 and CIS, and gene-mediated alterations in patterns of GH or IGF production await to be described.

TABLE 23–11 CRITERIA FOR PRESUMPTIVE DIAGNOSIS OF CONSTITUTIONAL DELAY OF GROWTH AND MATURATION

1. No history of systemic illness
2. Normal nutrition
3. Normal physical examination, including body proportions
4. Normal thyroid and GH levels
5. Normal complete blood count, sedimentation rate, electrolytes, blood urea nitrogen
6. Height at or below the 3rd percentile, but with annual growth rate greater than 5th percentile for age
7. Delayed puberty
   Males: failure to achieve Tanner G2 stage by age 13.8 years or P2 by 15.6 years
   Females: failure to achieve Tanner B2 stage by age 13.3 years
8. Delayed bone age
9. Normal predicted adult height:
   Males: >163 cm (64″)
   Females: >150 cm (59″)

Constitutional Delay of Growth and Maturation

The term *constitutional delay*[1285,1286] describes children with a normal variant of maturational tempo characterized by short stature but relatively normal growth rates during childhood, delayed puberty with a late and attenuated pubertal growth spurt, and attainment of normal adult height. Most children with constitutional delay begin to deviate from the normal growth curve during the early years of life and by age 2 years are at or slightly below the 5th percentile for height.[1287] During mid-childhood years, height SDS may gradually drift lower, but this does not appear to affect adult height outcome.[1288] Final height, though usually within the normal population range, is often in the lower part of the parental height target zone,[1289-1291] with few patients exceeding that target height. The predicted final height, especially when the skeletal age is extremely delayed, is greater than that usually achieved, but is difficult to reliably anticipate.[1292-1294] The delayed growth spurt may adversely affect growth of the spine and mineralization of the vertebrae, which is not overcome when the pubertal growth acceleration finally occurs, thus limiting the final height.[1293,1295] The osteopenia reported in men with a history of delayed puberty[1295] may be due to a profound alteration of normal pubertal bone mineral accretion or to a prepubertal and continuing deficit in bone mass that is an intrinsic part of CDGM.[502,503] These children do also tend to be thin (though certainly not uniformly) and data suggesting the presence of a hypermetabolic state, possibly contributing to impaired anabolism, have been reported.[1296]

GH secretion may be decreased with transient partial GH deficiency at the time of the delayed pubertal growth spurt, apparently the consequence of inadequate production of gonadal steroids.[95,1094,1297,1298] Such children would be expected to have delayed skeletal ages, normal or slightly low serum IGF-I but usually normal IGFBP-3 levels for skeletal age, and normal GH provocative tests (if pretreated with gonadal steroids). Overnight GH secretion is generally normal in these children when control groups are carefully matched.[1067] By definition, children with pure CDGM should have bone ages sufficiently delayed to result in normal predicted adult heights (greater than 163 cm in males and greater than 150 cm in females) (Table 23–11), although the correlation between predicted and final height is imperfect and must be viewed with caution.[1292,1293,1299] When CDGM occurs in the context of familial short stature (see below), however, children may experience both a delayed adolescent growth spurt *and* a short final height.

As stated above, some have attributed the diminished growth in the peripubertal period in CDGM to a transient GH deficiency or to a "lazy" pituitary, a concept that probably reflects the inadequacies of GH testing, especially the failure to pretreat patients with a brief course of gonadal steroids.[95,1253] Low serum levels of IGF-I and IGFBP-3 and/or a poor GH response to provocative testing (after priming with gonadal steroids) should mandate an investigation for underlying pathology, such as intracranial tumors. While CDGM has, historically, been viewed as a benign condition, an alternative perspective is that it is the product of subtle defects of the GH-IGF axis, which is then, in part, compensated for by delayed epiphyseal fusion.

Genetic (Familial) Short Stature

The control of growth in childhood and the final height attained are polygenic in nature. For this reason, familial height impacts upon the growth of an individual, and evaluation of a specific growth pattern must be placed in the context of familial growth and stature. Formulas have been developed for determination of parental target height, and growth curves that relate a child's height to parental height are available.[35] As a general rule, a child who is growing at a rate that is inconsistent with that of siblings or parents warrants further evaluation.

Furthermore, many organic diseases characterized by growth retardation are genetically transmitted. This list includes multiple etiologies, such as GH insensitivity due to mutations of the GH receptor gene, GH gene deletions, mutations of the *PROP-1* or *POUF-1* gene, pseudohypoparathyroidism, diabetes mellitus, and some forms of hypothyroidism. Inherited nonendocrine diseases characterized by short stature include osteochondrodysplasias (see above), dysmorphic syndromes associated with IUGR (see above), inborn errors of metabolism, renal disease, and thalassemia (see below). Identifying short stature as inherited thus does not, by itself, relieve the clinician of responsibility for determining the underlying cause of growth failure.

Nonetheless, a constellation of clinical findings describes a normal variant referred to as *genetic short stature* (GSS) (or familial short stature) that differs from the syndrome of constitutional delay of growth and maturation discussed above. In GSS, childhood growth is at or below the 5th percentile, but the velocity is generally normal. The onset and progression of puberty are normal or even slightly early and more rapid than normal so that skeletal age is concordant with chronologic age. Parental height is short (both parents are often below the 10th percentile) and pubertal maturation is normal. Final heights in these individuals are short and in the target zone for the family.[1291] The GH-IGF system is normal, but exogenous GH therapy during middle childhood years may increase linear growth velocity substantially without disproportionate augmentation of skeletal maturation. Whether long-term GH treatment enhances final height outcome, however, is not clear.

Subtle, Less Well Characterized Defects within the GH-IGF Axis

Gene-mediated defects throughout the GH-IGF axis have been described above as dramatic causes of IGFD. More intriguing in the consideration of the causes of the short stature syndrome currently labeled as idiopathic are subtle defects reflecting all of the steps from the brain to the effector steps of IGF action. The range of insufficiency of GH production is well known and has been largely described by GH provocative testing and measurement of the GH-dependent peptides. Another universe of potential abnormalities of GH action was defined as *primary IGFD;* a similar broad range of causes of insufficiency of the transduction of GH or IGF action (as for GH production) seems reasonable to expect. The cascade of seemingly redundant and overlapping intracellular pathways (both stimulatory and inhibitory, as noted above) provides nearly endless combinations of up- and down-regulatory outcomes that result in statural variations. Table 23–11 depicts a potential categorization of ISS with distinction based on IGF-I levels.[504]

The functional level of the GH receptor may be genetically determined, although modulated by such factors as nutritional status; GH production appears to be inversely related to GH-receptor/GHBP levels.[164,165] Accordingly, GHBP levels have been assessed in subjects with ISS.[1300-1302] Serum levels of GHBP in 90% of children with ISS are lower than the normal mean, 20% being below the normal range, especially a subgroup with low IGF-I and higher mean 12-hour levels of GH.[1300,1301] Such data raise the possibility that an abnormality of GH receptor content or structure could impair GH action. The inverse relationship of GHBP levels to GH production is consistent with this hypothesis.[111] In a small group of patients with growth failure, low levels of IGF-I, and poor response to exogenous GH, heterozygous GH-receptor mutations were present in 28%.[927] In contrast to the rarity of homozygous GH-receptor mutations in GHR, heterozygosity is more common and may be a frequent cause of short stature.[212,928,1219] In heterozygotes, protein from the mutant allele may disrupt the normal dimerization and rotation that is needed for normal GH-receptor activation, leading to diminished GH action and growth impairment.[144] Even when individuals heterozygous for GHR mutations have normal stature, it is possible that this reflects compensatory oversecretion of GH or an adjustment from the receptor. Thus, subtle defects of GH action, when coupled with other relatively minor genetic perturbations of the GH-IGF axis, may result in short stature.

The IGF-I/IGFBP-3 generation test following 4 days of GH administration reveals many patients with findings of low basal and provoked peptides and occasional modestly elevated GH levels that might represent lesser degrees of IGFD.[1282-1284,1303] It seems reasonable to speculate that the severe forms of IGFD represent the "tip of the iceberg" and that the range of molecular defects, probably best assessed by studies of polymorphism (e.g., the exon 3 deletion of GH-R), will be broad. As noted above, large numbers of children with ISS do have lowered serum concentrations of IGF-I, which in the face of normal or elevated GH levels, will need to be examined with genomic and proteomic studies to identify more subtle defects of the GHR, GH signaling cascade, and IGF gene expression.[504]

TREATMENT OF GROWTH DISORDERS

When growth failure is the result of a chronic underlying disease, such as renal failure, cystic fibrosis, or malabsorption, therapy first must be directed at treatment of the underlying condition. Although growth acceleration may occur in such children with GH or IGF-I therapy, complete catch-up requires correction of the primary medical problem. If treatment of the underlying condition involves glucocorticoids, growth failure may be profound and is unlikely to be correctable until steroids are reduced or discontinued.

Correction of growth failure associated with chronic hypothyroidism requires appropriate thyroid replacement. As discussed earlier, thyroid therapy causes dramatic catch-up growth but also markedly accelerates skeletal maturation, potentially limiting adult height. More gradual thyroid replacement and/or the use of gonadotropin inhibitors to delay puberty may be necessary to obtain maximal final height.

Treatment of Constitutional Delay

Constitutional delay of growth and maturation (CDGM) is a normal variant, with (by definition) potential for a normal (although delayed) pubertal maturation and a normal (albeit diminished for target zone) adult height. Most subjects can be managed by careful evaluation to rule out other causes of abnormal growth and/or delayed puberty combined with appropriate explanation and counseling. The skeletal age and Bayley-Pinneau table are often helpful in explaining the potential for normal growth to the patient and parents. A family history of constitutional delay is also, frequently, a source of reassurance. On occasion, however, the stigmata of short stature and delayed maturation may be psychologically disabling for the preadolescent or teenager. Some adolescents with delayed puberty have poor self-images and limited social involvement.[1304] In such patients and in some in whom pubertal delay is predicted based on the overall clinical picture, there is a role for the judicious use of short-term gonadal steroids.

Two aspects of this syndrome are addressed by androgen treatment: *short stature,* especially in boys between ages 10 and 14, and *delayed puberty* after age 14. In the younger group, in whom CDGM is apparent, the orally administered synthetic androgen oxandrolone has been used extensively.[1305] In several controlled studies,[1306-1311] oxandrolone therapy for 3 months to 4 years increased linear growth velocity by 3 to 5 cm per year without adverse effects or decreasing either actual[1311-1313] or predicted[1308,1312,1314] final height. The growth-promoting effects of oxandrolone appear related to its androgenic and anabolic effects rather than to augmentation of the GH-IGF axis.[1315,1316] Currently recommended treatment is 0.1 mg/kg orally per day. In older boys, in whom delayed pubertal maturation is highly stressful and anxiety-provoking, testosterone enanthate has been administered intramuscularly with success.[1305,1306,1317] Criteria for therapy of such adolescents should include (1) a minimal age of 14 years; (2) height below the 3rd percentile; (3) prepubertal or early Tanner G2 stage with an early morning serum testosterone less than 3.5 nmol/L (<1 ng/mL); and (4) a poor self-image that does not respond to reassurance alone. Therapy consists of intramuscular testosterone enanthate, 50 to 200 mg every 3 to 4 weeks for a total of four to six injections.[1304,1318] Patients typically show early secondary sex characteristics by the fourth injection and grow an average of 10 cm in the ensuing year. Despite attempts to choose subjects carefully for treatment programs in CDGM, a spectrum of activation of the reproductive system is inevitable; growth responses to short courses of therapy are best in the boys who have early pubertal gonadotropin secretory patterns.[1319] Testosterone enhances growth velocity by direct actions and also increases GH production, and may have a direct effect on IGF-I secretion, as well.[95,121,122,127,1320,1321] Brief testosterone regimens do not cause overly rapid skeletal maturation, compromise adult height, or suppress pubertal maturation.[1322] It is important to emphasize to the patient that he is normal, that therapy is short-term and designed to provide some pubertal development earlier than he would on his own, and that treatment will not necessarily increase adult height. In such situations, the combination of short-term androgen therapy, reassurance, and counseling help the boys with constitutional delay to cope with a difficult adolescence.

The availability of several new forms of testosterone, which are approved for adults with hypogonadism, provides adolescents with an opportunity for a choice among different androgen replacement therapies. Although effectiveness of these preparations has not been demonstrated in children with constitutional delay, the authors have personal experience with their successful use, finding an equivalent response to that obtained with testosterone injections. Testosterone gel is painless and easy to apply and has proved popular since its release.[1323] Testosterone patches also avoid the need for injections, but work best when applied to the scrotum and are often accompanied by complaints of itching.[1324] The dosing of these alternative forms of therapy in children and adolescents is not yet established. In view of the important role of estrogen in the process of skeletal maturation, aromatase inhibitors could be used in conjunction with androgen therapy to prevent an acceleration of bone age and further enhance final adult height.[1325] Near final height data on the combined use of an aromatase inhibitor (letrozole) and testosterone show an increase of 5 to 6 cm over prediction.[1325] Pubertal maturation and growth are enhanced by the androgen activity, while the skeletal maturation is attenuated enough to achieve good height outcome.

Patients must be reevaluated to ensure that they enter "true" puberty. One year after testosterone treatment, boys should have testicular enlargement and a serum testosterone in the pubertal range. If this is not the case, the diagnosis of hypothalamic-pituitary insufficiency or hypogonadotropic hypogonadism should be considered. Although the diagnosis of constitutional growth delay remains most likely in such patients, some eventually prove to be gonadotropin deficient, especially if still prepubertal late in adolescence.

Referrals for constitutional delay are more common in boys than girls, undoubtedly reflecting our cultural values. When constitutional delay is a problem in girls, short-term estrogen therapy can be employed, but the advancement of bone is a greater hazard at doses that enhance growth velocity and sexual maturation. The use of GH in patients with constitutional delay is discussed below.

Treatment of Growth Hormone Deficiency

Nomenclature and Potency Estimation

The nomenclature for the various biosynthetic GH preparations reflects the source and the chemical composition of the product. Somatropin refers to GH of the same amino acid sequence as that in naturally occurring human GH. Somatropin from human pituitary glands is abbreviated *GH* or *pit-GH;* recombinant origin somatropin is termed *recombinant GH* or *rGH.* Somatrem refers to the methionine derivative of recombinant GH and is abbreviated *met-rGH.* Although the latter preparation is a more antigenic preparation, that propensity is not clinically relevant; despite the presence of anti-GH antibodies, growth responses to met-rGH were similar to those seen in patients treated with rGH.[1326,1327] This derivative of GH is no longer available for use. We refer to the biosynthetic preparations as GH in subsequent discussions.

The biopotency of commercially available biosynthetic GH preparations, expressed as international units per milligram of the new World Health Organization (WHO) rGH reference reagent for somatropin,[88/624] is 3 IU/mg.[1328] It was necessary to standardize the early GH preparations by bioassay because of variable production techniques (e.g., extraction, column purification). The most common bioassays have been the hypophysectomized rat weight-gain assay, the tibial width assay, and the more sensitive Nb2 rat lymphoma proliferation assay.[1328-1331] With the availability of purified and essentially equivalent recombinant GH products, the requirement for bioassays has become an FDA requisite to substantiate biologic activity rather than to assess potential differences between preparations. The bioassays are likely to be replaced by in vitro binding assays using GH receptors or GHBP derived from molecular techniques.[1328]

Historical Perspective

Because untreated patients with IGF deficiency syndrome have profound short stature (averaging nearly −5 SDS[920-923]), the clinical urgency to use GH therapy as soon as it was available is apparent.[1243] The action of GH is highly species-specific and humans do not respond to animal-derived GH.[1332] Unlike most other hormones, the only GH that is biologically active in humans is primate GH. Human cadaver pituitary glands were for many years the only practical source of primate GH for treatment of GHD, and more than 27,000 children with GHD worldwide were treated with pit-GH.[1333] The limited supplies of pit-GH, low doses, and interrupted treatment regimens resulted in incomplete growth increments; usually therapy was discontinued in boys who reached 5′5″ and in girls who reached 5′. Nonetheless, this treatment did increase linear growth and in many patients enhanced final adult height. The dose-response relationship and the relation of age to GH response were recognized during this period.[1334]

Distribution of pit-GH was halted in the United States and most of Europe in 1985 because of concern about a causal relationship with Creutzfeldt-Jakob disease (CJD), a rare and fatal spongiform encephalopathy that had been previously reported to be capable of iatrogenic transmission through human tissue.[1335,1336] In North America and Europe, this disorder has an incidence of approximately 1 case per million in the general population; it is exceedingly rare before the age of 50 years. To date, more than 160 young adults who had received human cadaver pituitary products have been identified with cases of CJD, with the sad likelihood that all affected patients will die of the disease.[1337-1339] In patients in the United States, the onset of CJD was 14 to 33 years after starting treatment, while the large cohort of French patients had a median incubation period approximately 5 years shorter.[1339] There is still no CJD in Americans who began treatment after new methods of purifying hormone began in the United States in 1977. Vigilant surveillance for this dreadful complication continues (www.niddk.nih.gov/health/endo/pubs/creutz/updatecomp.htm),[1340,1341] although the incubation period is now more than 30 years.

Fortunately, by the time the risks of pituitary-derived GH were discovered, biosynthetic GH was being tested for safety and efficacy.[1326,1342,1343] The original recombinant GH mimicked pit-GH in regard to both anabolic and metabolic actions and was scrupulously scrutinized for monoisomerism, antigenic bacterial products, and toxins of any sort. GH has universally replaced pit-GH as the treatment for children with GHD.

Treatment Regimens

The recommended therapy starting dose of GH in GHD is 0.18 to 0.35 mg/kg body weight per week, administered in seven daily doses, with the mean American dose being 0.3 mg/kg/wk.[1344] Alternative regimens include a 6 day/week or 3 day/week schedule, with the same weekly dosage, but are not as successful. In general, the growth response to GH is a function of the log-dose given, so that increasing dosages further enhance growth velocities,[1278,1333,1334] but daily dosing may be the most important treatment parameter.[1345] Either subcutaneous or intramuscular administration has equivalent growth-promoting activity[1346]; the former is now used exclusively. GH is available in several vehicles and multiple systems are used for administration (Table 23–12). The standard preparations include lyophilized GH, which is highly water-soluble and may be brought into solution with a small volume of diluent and a "ready-to-use" aqueous solution with 28-day stability. A sustained-release preparation of GH with protein integrity in a poly(lactide-coglycolide) polymer that is biocompatible and biodegradable permitted once- or twice monthly treatments.[1347] This vehicle for GH is no longer available, but several others are undergoing clinical trials.[1348,1349] Either reconstituted or liquid GH is most frequently administered with pen devices that are characterized by ease of use, accuracy, and "hidden needles." At this time, all of the commercially available GH preparations yield comparable growth outcomes. GH treatment should be continued after growth ceases, because GH has other important metabolic effects, including support of normal gonadal function[1350] and attainment of normal adult bone mineral density and body composition (see discussion under "Treatment during tronsition to adulthood and in adulthood"). A report from the Drug and Therapeutics committee of the Lawson Wilkins Pediatric Endocrine Society summarized the society's views on the use of GH in children with diverse syndromes of short stature.[1351]

Growth responses to exogenous GH vary, depending on the frequency of administration, dosage, age (greater absolute gain in a younger child, though not necessarily of growth velocity SDS), weight, GH receptor type and amount, as assessed by serum GHBP levels, and, perhaps, seasonality.[139,164,165,1352,1353] On the general regimen of daily GH at the recommended doses, nonetheless, the typical GHD child accelerates growth from a pretreatment rate of 3 to 4 cm/yr to 10 to 12 cm/yr in year 1 of therapy and 7 to 9 cm/yr in years 2 and 3. Progressive waning of GH efficacy occurs and is poorly understood. The importance of dosage frequency is illustrated (Figs. 23–53 and 23–54) by data from a carefully done assessment of growth responses of prepubertal naive GHD children randomly assigned to receive thrice-weekly or daily GH at the same total weekly dose (0.30 mg/kg/wk).[1345] The mean total height gain during this period was 9.7 cm greater in the daily-treated patients (38.4 vs. 28.7 cm, $P<.0002$) with similar increments in skeletal maturation and no acceleration of the onset of puberty. Mean height SDS at the end of 4 years was +0.2, or at the midpoint of normal for age. Studies utilizing varying dosing of GH based on gender, growth responsivity, and growth factor concentrations suggest the need for greater sophistication and individualization of the current treatment regimens.[1354,1355] At a dosage of 0.30 mg/kg/wk, the approximate current cost of GH therapy for a 20-kg child is $12,000 to $15,000 per year.

Sophisticated mathematical models[1278,1279] have examined many laboratory and auxologic parameters that influence response to GH therapy. Because age at onset of treatment is inversely correlated with growth responses, and because the smaller, lighter child requires less GH (with marked economic benefit), growth data in early treated children are important to assess. In short-term studies of 134 patients[908,1356,1357] treated before age 3, marked early catch-up growth occurred with a mean height gain of around 3 SDS by 4 years of therapy, allowing most children to reach the normal height range by midchildhood. Mean height in one study[908] reached −0.4 SDS after 8 years of treatment. Near-adult height data in 13 patients treated before 5 years[1358] did not differ from the midparental target height (−0.9 vs. −0.7 SDS). In a group of 25 children treated before 12 months of age,[1359] adult height also matched the target height despite low dosage and less frequent administration. In an analysis of postmarketing data for development of a growth prediction model, a greater height gain per GH amount occurred in the very young children, but a seemingly lowered sensitivity to endogenous GH in early infancy adds complexity to interpretation of these data.[1360] If long-term outcome studies continue to show excellent growth responses with achievement of genetic target height *and* adherence to treatment regimens in very young children, recommendations for early treatment would be appropriate.[1361]

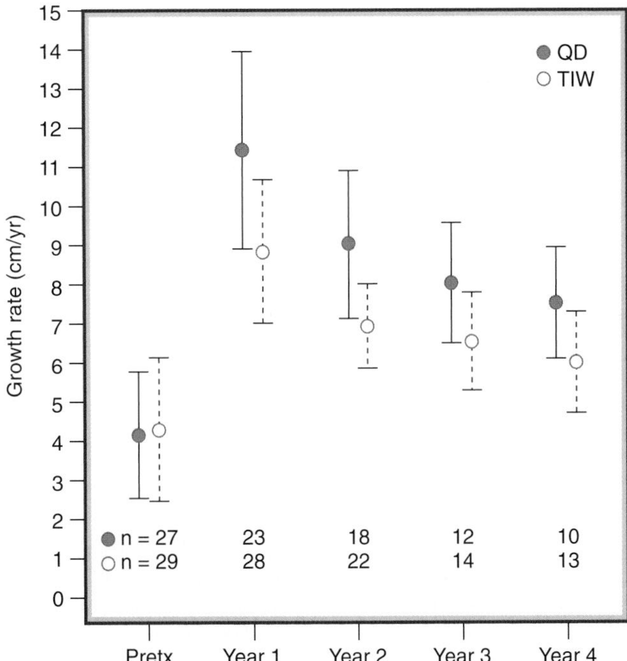

Figure 23–53 ▪ Annual growth velocity (mean±SD) for prepubertal GHD patients before and during 4 years of growth hormone (GH) treatment, contrasting results with daily (QD) and thrice-weekly injections (TIW). The mean annual growth velocity in the QD group was significantly greater than that of the TIW group during each year, although significance diminished from year 1 to year 4. (From MacGillivray MH, Baptista J, Johanson A, et al. Outcome of a four-year randomized study of daily versus three times weekly somatropin treatment in prepubertal naive growth hormone deficient children. J Clin Endocrinol Metab 1996;81:1806-1809. Reproduced by permission of MacGillivray, MH.)

TABLE 23–12 NEW MODALITIES FOR TREATMENT OF GROWTH HORMONE DEFICIENCY

Liquid formulations
Pen-type delivery devices
Oral secretagogues
Long-acting growth hormone (GH) formulations
GH-releasing hormone, both short- and long-acting
Inhaled GH delivery systems

Longer Term/Adult Height Results

Much information on growth has been reported about pit-GH-treated children, generally thrice-weekly and intramuscularly administered. Five-year data are available from Bundak and colleagues[1362] on a group of 58 prepubertal and 20 pubertal children with GHD. The younger group increased its height from −3.6 SDS to −2 SDS, while the pubertal children grew to −2.3 SDS. The height SDS for bone age, however, did not increase; thus, further loss of adult height was prevented, but there was no increase in the adult height prediction. The importance of early initiation of treatment is stressed by such data. Similarly, Libber and coworkers[1363] found that GH therapy increased mean height from about −4.2 SDS to −2.3 SDS. Bierich[1364] reviewed nine trials of pit-GH to determine effect on final height. Overall, a dose-response relationship was noted between doses of 0.11 and 0.25 mg/kg/week. The greatest SDS increment of 2.7 occurred with the highest dosage of pit-GH. The pretreatment heights ranged from −5.6 to −3.6 SDS, with adult heights achieving −3.6 to −1.6 SDS. Final height data from the same large U.S. center permit a contrast of pit-GH and rGH therapeutic results. The mean final height was −2.0 SDS in the former group, which received only 0.1 mg/kg/wk, in contrast to −1.5 SDS in the rGH group treated with 0.3 mg/kg/wk.[1344]

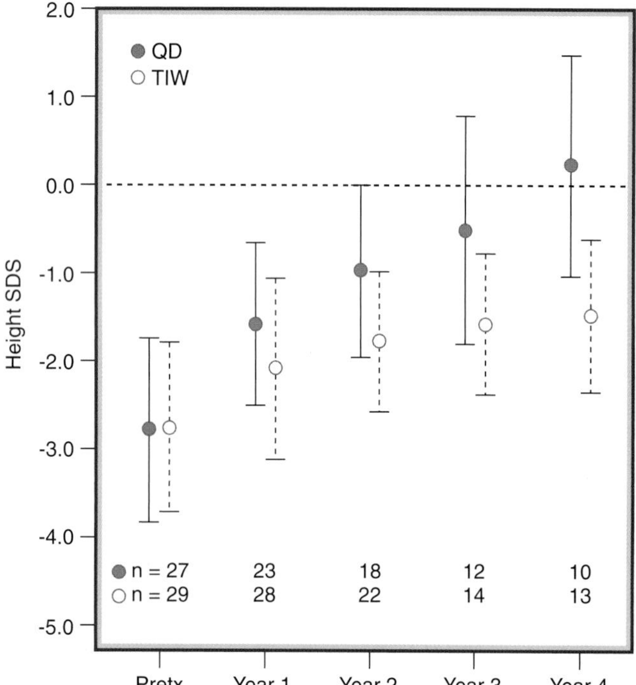

Figure 23–54 ▪ Height SDS (mean±SD) for prepubertal GHD patients before and during 4 years of GH treatment, contrasting results with daily (QD) and thrice-weekly injections (TIW). The mean SDS in the QD group was significantly greater throughout the treatment period. Younger patients had the greatest increase in height SDS and the effect of age was more marked in the QD group. (From MacGillivray MH, Baptista J, Johanson A, et al. Outcome of a four-year randomized study of daily versus three times weekly somatropin treatment in prepubertal naive growth hormone deficient children. J Clin Endocrinol Metab 1996;81:1806-1809. Reproduced by permission of MacGillivray, MH.)

Patients treated largely with biosynthetic GH[82,1243,1266,1344,1358,1365-1371] have improved actual or near-final adult height SDS, with average final height in more than 1400 patients approximating −1.3 SD. Data from the two largest databases,[1266,1369-1371] representing the North American and European experiences, as reported by pediatric endocrinologists, are shown in Table 23–13.

Despite this availability of GH therapy, long-term studies still show that most patients fail to reach their genetic target heights. Evaluation of adult heights in 121 patients with childhood GHD treated in the Genentech GH research trials indicated a mean adult height in both male and female patients of −0.7 SDS, with 106 being within 2 SDS for normal adult Americans.[1367] Even in these closely followed patients, however, a −0.4 to −0.6 SDS difference from midparental target height still occurred. The achievement of the genetic target *is* possible, however, as a Swedish subgroup (in the KIGS database) of consistently treated patients reached a median final height SDS of −0.32, which was equivalent to the midparental target height.[1370] By multiple regression analysis, factors found to correlate with enhanced adult height were baseline height, younger age at onset of treatment, longer treatment duration especially during prepubertal years, and a greater growth velocity during the first year of treatment[1371] (Figs. 23–55 and 23–56). Increased height velocity and subsequent superior adult height outcome, although with considerable overlap, were demonstrated in children with GHD who carried one or both GHR alleles with an exon 3 deletion.[139,140] Whereas the development of recombinant GH has solved the problem of supply experienced in the pituitary GH era, delays in diagnosis and initiation of therapy have still compromised adult height.

In an effort to increase final height of GHD patients, the use of high-dose GH during puberty has been studied, based on the rationale that GH secretion normally rises twofold to fourfold during the pubertal growth spurt with dramatic concomitant increases in serum IGF-I levels and that the pubertal growth spurt normally accounts for approximately 17% of adult male height and 12% of adult female height. Earlier studies by Stanhope and associates[1372,1373] indicated that little difference in height gain could be observed when adolescent patients were

TABLE 23–13 ADULT HEIGHT IN CHILDREN WITH GROWTH HORMONE DEFICIENCY TREATED WITH BIOSYNTHETIC GROWTH HORMONE

Study	Sex	"n"	Dose*	Duration (yr)	Age (yr)	Ht SDS	Δ Ht SDS	Ht vs MPH
KIGS[1371]								
	M	351	.22	7.5	18.2	−0.8	+1.6	−0.2
	F	200	.20	6.9	16.6	−1.0	+1.6	−0.5
NCGS[1369,1698]								
	M	2095	0.28	5.2	18.2	−1.1	+1.4	−0.7
	F	1116	0.29	5.0	16.7	−1.3	+1.6	−0.9

*Growth hormone dose is mg/kg/week.
KIGS, Pharmacia International growth database; MPH, midparental target height; NCGS, Genentech National Cooperative Growth Study.

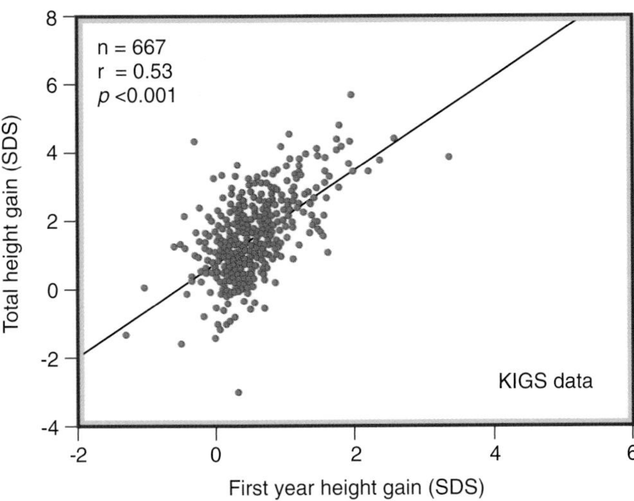

Figure 23–55 ▪ Relationship between first-year change in height SD score (SDS) and total change in height SDS between start of growth hormone (GH) treatment and near-final height in children with idiopathic isolated GH deficiency. (Modified with permission from Reiter EO, Price DA, Wilton P, et al. Effect of growth hormone [GH] treatment on the final height of 1258 patients with idiopathic GH deficiency: analysis of a large international database. J Clin Endocrinol Metab 2006;91.)

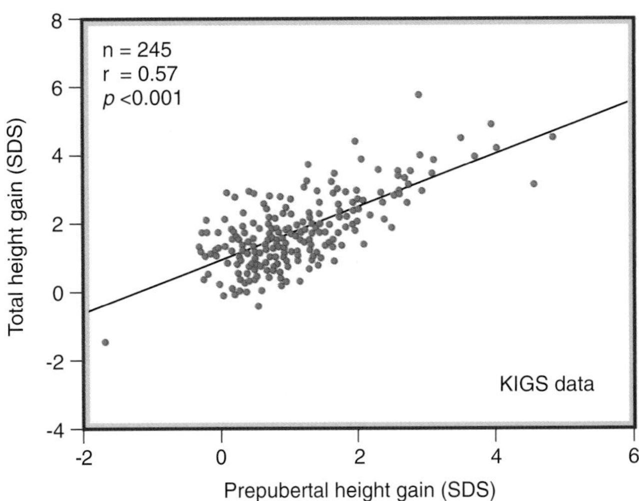

Figure 23–56 ▪ Relationship between prepubertal change in height SD score (SDS) and total change in height SDS between start of growth hormone (GH) treatment and near-final height in children with idiopathic, isolated GH deficiency. (Modified with permission from Reiter EO, Price DA, Wilton P, et al. Effect of growth hormone [GH] treatment on the final height of 1258 patients with idiopathic GH deficiency: analysis of a large international database. J Clin Endocrinol Metab 2006;91;2047-2054.)

treated with 30 vs. 15 IU/m^2/wk of GH (approximately 0.04 vs. 0.02 mg/kg/day). Mauras and colleagues,[1374] however, evaluated higher pubertal GH doses (0.1 vs. 0.043 mg/kg/day) and found that the higher dosage resulted in a 4.6-cm increase in near-final height. Mean height SDS achieved in the 0.043 mg/kg/day group (as in the earlier report[1367]) was −0.7±0.9, but was 0.0±1.2 in the 0.1 mg/kg/day group. The higher GH dosage did not result in more rapid acceleration of skeletal maturation.

The use of higher doses of GH, the ability to treat until growth cessation, early initiation of treatment, progressive weight-related dose increments, attention to compliance with daily administration, and appropriate thyroid hormone and glucocorticoid replacement therapy are important factors in these improved adult height outcomes. As final height correlates with height at the onset of puberty in the GHD patients,[1352,1366,1375-1377] every effort must be made to enhance growth velocity during prepuberty. In data from NCGS and KIGS, the height gained during puberty in patients with GHD was generally comparable to that in healthy children with delayed bone ages.[1369,1378] The pubertal height gain is negatively correlated with the age of pubertal onset in normal and GH-treated children.[1379,1380]

The earlier the age of pubertal onset, the lower the final height outcome,[1369,1378] and GHD patients with delayed puberty or hypogonadotropic hypogonadism have a taller adult height.[920,1352,1381] When normal or precocious puberty limits the response to GH, it may be appropriate to delay puberty by the use of a GnRH agonist[1382-1384] or with an aromatase inhibitor to attenuate the rate of skeletal maturation.[1325,1385] Use of these strategies in pubertal GHD patient groups, however suggestive, is not yet clearly documented to enhance final height.[1386-1392] Data from both KIGS[1393] and NCGS[1369,1394,1395] have not demonstrated value to the addition of GnRH agonists to GH treatment regimens. Utilization of aromatase inhibition[1385,1396-1399] may be a more effective regimen in boys in that they would get growth benefit from continued androgen presence while the elimination of estrogen would slow bone age advancement. Short-term treatment has not impaired skeletal mineralization[1400] nor altered spermatogenesis.[1401] Attempts at altering aromatase activity in girls have not been reported. The long-term safety of the plan to alter aromatase activity remains to be demonstrated. In an uncontrolled study, the selective estrogen receptor modulator, tamoxifen, slowed skeletal maturation and increased height prediction when used in conjunction with GH in pubertal males.[1402] The current recommendation regarding attempts to enhance growth outcomes must center upon initiation of GH treatment in an early, aggressive, and closely optimized manner, rather than at attempts at solely gaining substantial SDS increments by altering the pubertal process.

Treatment of Prader-Willi Syndrome

GH treatment of growth failure in PWS is an FDA-approved indication with the recommended dose being approximately 1 mg/m^2/day or 0.24 mg/kg/wk. Numerous clinical trials document efficacy and confirm that the characteristic IGF deficiency state is due to GH deficiency. After 5 years of GH therapy, Lindgren and Ritzen[1082] (at a dose of 0.23 mg/kg/wk) showed that mean height SDS approached 0.5 with a gain of nearly 2 SDS. Other shorter term (6 to 24 months) treatment programs have found increased growth rates, but also provide important information on the changes in abnormal metabolic parameters during GH treatment. Such data demonstrate reduction in body fat mass, an increase in the percentage of fat-free mass, improved muscle strength and agility, increased fat oxidation, and, perhaps, behavioral improvement.[1078,1079,1081,1142,1403] Respiratory muscle weakness, which is found in PWS, was improved after GH treatment.[1079] GH treatment of infants and toddlers beginning before 18 months of age increased mobility and improved body composition, certainly a provocative finding if these benefits would persist throughout childhood.[1080,1404] In view of the association of insulin resistance and type 2 diabetes mellitus with obesity, glycemic status should be monitored in GH-treated patients with PWS,[1068] although it seems that they are more insulin sensitive than one might predict from their obesity.

Although death from presumed obesity-induced hypoventilation or apneic events in PWS without GH treatment is well described, the occurrence of such deaths during GH administration raises the question of an exacerbation of this condition by

GH.[1083,1405] Tonsillar hypertrophy and fluid retention associated with GH therapy are potential risk factors. Nonetheless, as respiratory and overall muscle strength improve, with early evidence of beneficial effects upon respiratory function, it does not seem that GH is a proven causal factor. There is also the suggestion that GH may actually lower the risk of such deaths.[1084] The obesity-hypoventilation syndrome is more likely the etiologic factor, suggesting that ventilatory and pulmonary function, with polysomnography studies, should be undertaken before and, possibly, during GH treatment.[1083,1406]

A final issue with PWS patients relates to GH treatment through the life cycle. In view of the childhood findings of low lean body mass and high fat content, osteopenia, and some degree of glucose intolerance ameliorated by GH, the issue of long-term therapy through adulthood must be considered and studied.[1407,1408]

TABLE 23–14 ELEMENTS OF MONITORING GROWTH HORMONE THERAPY

Close follow-up with a pediatric endocrinologist every 3 to 4 months
Determination of growth response (change in height SD-score)
Interval measurements of serum IGF-I and IGFBP-3 levels (every 3 to 6 months) and annual assessment of fasting glucose/insulin ratio and thyroid function tests
Screening for potential adverse effects
Evaluation of compliance
Consideration of dose adjustment based on IGF values, growth response, and comparison to growth prediction models

IGF, Insulin-like growth factor.

Combined Pituitary Hormone Deficiencies

If GHD is part of a multiple pituitary insufficiency, it is necessary to address each endocrine deficiency both for general medical reasons and to ensure maximal effect of GH therapy. TSH deficiency is often "unmasked" during the initial phase of therapy, and thyroid function should be assessed both before the onset of therapy and during the first 3 months of GH treatment,[1409] and at least on an annual basis thereafter. The pituitary-adrenal axis is customarily evaluated during the insulin stimulation test in the workup for GHD. If ACTH secretion is impaired, patients should be placed on the lowest safe maintenance dose of glucocorticoids, certainly no more than 10 mg/m^2/day of hydrocortisone and less, if possible. Higher doses impair the growth response to GH therapy, but may be necessary during times of stress. Long-term evolution of glucocorticoid deficiency is critical to monitor, especially in adults with PROP1 mutations (discussed earlier).

Gonadotropin deficiency may be evident in the infant with microphallus. This can usually be treated with 3 or 4 monthly injections of 25 mg of testosterone enanthate.[1410] Management at puberty can be more complicated, in that the physical and psychological benefits of promoting sexual maturation must be balanced against the effects of epiphyseal fusion. When GH therapy is initiated in childhood and growth is normal before adolescence, it is appropriate to begin gonadal steroid replacement at a normal age (e.g., 11 to 12 years of age in girls and 12 to 13 years of age in boys). In boys, this can be done by beginning with monthly injections of 50 to 100 mg of testosterone enanthate, gradually increasing to 200 mg per month, and eventually moving to the appropriate adult replacement regimen as determined by the monitoring of plasma testosterone levels. In girls, therapy involves use of conjugated estrogens or ethinyl estradiol, and eventual cycling with estrogen and progesterone.

Monitoring Growth Hormone Therapy

(Table 20–14)

While most pediatric endocrinologists simply document changes in growth velocity as the single parameter of therapeutic efficacy, this may not be sufficient. Treatment models that predict growth rate[1278,1279] with quite narrow confidence limits provide quantitative estimates of whether the individual patient is responding appropriately to GH. A model[1278] explaining 61% of growth response variability for the first year of therapy includes inverse relationships with maximum GH response during provocative testing, age, and height SDS minus midparental height SDS and positive correlation with body weight SDS, GH dose, and birthweight SDS.[1411,1412] The single most important predictive factor for years 2 through 4 is the first-year–height velocity. Models that further enhance individual patient predictions continue to be developed.[1413] Clearly, after age at diagnosis, GH dose management is the variable most affected by the clinician. Changes in levels of the GH-dependent peptides, IGF-I and IGFBP-3, ALS, and the aggregate ternary complex, as well as of leptin, correlate with growth responses.[1414-1416] Measurement of these may give added information on the growth-promoting and fat-mobilizing actions of GH, as well as of the spectrum of childhood responsivity to exogenous GH. Specifically, modifying the GH dose based upon frequent monitoring of IGF-I levels, combined with documentation of the growth response, seems reasonable and may enhance growth outcomes by greater individualization of the treatment program. Safety monitoring should include 6 to 12 monthly assessments of IGF-I, IGFBP-3, and perhaps annual measurement of fasting glucose/insulin ratios.[1417]

Poor Growth Responses

The growth response to GH typically attenuates after several years, but should continue to be equal to or greater than the normal height velocity for age throughout treatment. Using the statistical growth treatment models may prove valuable in judging therapeutic efficacy.[1278,1279] A suboptimal response to GH can be due to several causes: (1) poor compliance, (2) improper preparation of GH for administration or incorrect injection techniques, (3) subclinical hypothyroidism, (4) coexisting systemic disease, (5) excessive glucocorticoid therapy, (6) prior irradiation of the spine, (7) epiphyseal fusion, (8) anti-GH antibodies, or (9) incorrect diagnosis of GHD as the explanation for growth retardation. Although 10% to 20% of recipients of recombinant GH develop anti-GH antibodies, growth failure is rarely due to such antibodies.[1326,1327,1418] Maximal growth response to GH usually can be obtained by early diagnosis and initiation of therapy and by careful attention to compliance and psychological support. Although in many earlier studies large numbers of boys and especially girls with idiopathic GHD did not achieve normal adult heights, it is our belief that normal height (i.e., reaching the family-specific target height) can be reached in most cases. It should be emphasized that the referral of short girls and their ultimate treatment with GH remains less frequent than that of boys.[1419] When molecular studies describing the IGF deficiency syndromes and complex intracellular signaling events following GH and GHR interaction are considered, the wide spectrum of growth outcomes becomes understandable and expected.

Despite the efficacy of GH in accelerating growth in GHD children and bringing adult height into the normal range if treatment is begun sufficiently early, several studies have indicated that the long-term prognosis for such patients is guarded, even though there is much more follow-up assessment needed in the modern era.[1243,1420,1421] The educational, vocational, and social outlook for adults who had childhood GHD is frequently suboptimal. Whether this reflects subtle intellectual deficits or the consequences of lower expectations of patients, families, or teachers remains to be determined. In any case, patients with GHD should be followed up carefully throughout life.

Treatment During the Transition to Adulthood and in Adulthood

A growing challenge to the management of patients with GHD has been the issues surrounding their care after the growth process has ceased.[1422] This period from mid- to late teenage years until the mid-20s is a normal physiologic phase during which peak bone and muscle mass are achieved and the independence and self-sufficiency characteristic of adulthood are achieved. It is also a time during which care of pediatric patients is transferred to endocrinologists who treat adults.

Clinical consequences of GHD in adults and potential benefits of GH therapy in such patients have been described.[1423-1426] Signs and symptoms of adult GHD have included reduced lean body mass and musculature, increased body fat, reduced bone mineral density, reduced exercise performance, and increased plasma cholesterol. Adults with GHD have had significantly increased risk of death from cardiovascular causes, a finding potentially linked to increased visceral adiposity and other cardiovascular risk factors.[1427,1428] GHD adults have been found to have "impaired psychological well-being and quality of life," characterized by depression, anxiety, reduced energy and vitality, and social isolation.[1429] Several placebo-controlled studies have demonstrated that GH therapy of adult GHD patients results in marked alterations in body composition, fat distribution, bone density, and sense of well-being.[1421,1424,1425,1430]

Based on the adult data, which suggest profound metabolic derangements associated with untreated GHD, continuation of GH treatment in the late adolescent patient who shows persistent GHD is an important issue. Documentation of persistent GHD, however, is important. In nearly 500 patients with isolated GHD, 207 (44%) had normal GH levels during provocative retesting.[1085-1092] In contrast, approximately 96% of patients with combined pituitary hormone deficiency, with or without structural abnormalities of the hypothalamic-pituitary area, had sustained GHD.[1086,1087,1089-1093] The presence of multiple anterior pituitary hormone deficiencies or structural disease would seem to obviate the need for subsequent retesting. The data are not absolute so clinical judgment is of paramount importance.[1636,1971,2214] The strict pharmacologic definition of GHD in that age group is difficult as shown by Maghnie and colleagues,[1431] who demonstrated that one should not use the much lower GH responses to testing which characterize older adults. This issue of testing validity may have influenced the dichotomy noted between the patient populations in testing "positive" on the provocative tests. As in the childhood population, it does not necessarily seem reasonable to rely on artificial cutoffs in pharmacologic provocative tests, but to include broader clinical and laboratory data.

Many patients do not wish to continue the daily GH regimen, but data do support strong consideration for sustained treatment. After 1 to 2 years off GH therapy, IGF-I and IGFBP-3 levels decrease substantially below baseline levels.[1432-1436] Resumption of GH normalizes these levels, although there is a strong suggestion that there is a gender-based difference in GH requirements, with females needing higher GH doses.[1434-1436] Loss of energy and strength is frequent,[1073] while some quality-of-life data suggest age-specific psychological issues in untreated severe GHD transition patients.[1437,1438] Quality-of-life data with rigorous study designs are lacking in GH-treated childhood GHD.[1439,1440] Total body and abdominal fat in untreated patients increases significantly, while lean body mass is lost relative to controls or comparable GH-treated patients or those after reinstitution of therapy.[1432,1433,1435,1441,1442]

As bone mass accrual is not completed until the third decade, late adolescence is an important time for GH sufficiency, in order to prevent later osteopenia.[673,1422] There have been numerous GH treatment studies carried out in the transition age group to assess the impact of bone mineralization.[1434-1436,1443,1444] Differences in age of onset of retreatment, duration of therapy, GH dosage, and gender distribution have led to variations in results. In general, however, the data affirm the concept that reinstitution of treatment with GH enables progression of bone mineralization to appropriate adult levels. Bone density assessment in patients with childhood-onset isolated GHD, who "tested" negative for GHD in adulthood, showed lower bone mineralization than controls and a correlation with IGF-I levels.[1445] Such bone findings challenge the simplistic view of diagnosing GHD simply on the basis of pharmacologic provocative testing.

The cardiovascular risk of stopping GH treatment has also been examined. Colao and associates showed modest left ventricular ejection fraction decrements that paralleled IGF levels when stopping and re-starting GH in a group of adolescents with GHD.[1446] The overall IGF levels were rather low, so cardiac changes were relatively modest. It should be recalled that GH treatment during childhood, while altering cardiac size, does not seem to change cardiac function.[1447] Mauras and associates did not show cardiac changes with a wide array of functional studies in a similar transition-age group,[1436] but it is of interest that their patients had relatively high IGF-I levels (mean=427 ng/mL) at GH discontinuation, suggesting a degree of "protectiveness" in the subsequent period off GH treatment. Nonetheless, abnormal cardiovascular risk factors, such as elevated concentrations of lipids, fibrinogen, inflammatory markers, and homocysteine, along with platelet hyperactivation, in untreated GHD adolescents may occur.[1448-1450] In prepubertal children with GHD, normalization of homocysteine levels and of markers of oxidative stress is achieved with GH treatment,[1451,1452] buttressing the notion of important effects of GH upon cardiovascular health. Cardiac function and those factors affecting vascular biology are targets, therefore, in the spectrum of GH-mediated body compositional changes.

These studies affirm the necessity of continuing GH treatment in late adolescence, albeit at lower doses than in childhood, to prevent development of adverse cardiovascular risk, diminished bone mineralization and an overall lowering of energy level. Whether the diversity of treatment and response data discussed above relates to the efficacy of the childhood GH therapeutic process is not clear, but the period of time off GH and the degree of persistent GHD would seem likely predictors of the clinical status at the time of reinitiation of GH treatment.

Our current method of assessing the late adolescent patient is based on the retesting data discussed earlier and several workshop recommendations.[1276,1422] An algorithm to guide this transition is shown in Figure 23–57. Upon completion of skeletal growth, GH therapy should be halted for approximately 2 to 3 months and the patient then thoroughly reevaluated. In places where an insulin tolerance test is mandatory for the patient to qualify for further GH therapy, this test should be performed; other pituitary hormones, especially glucocorticoids, and serum IGF-I and IGFBP-3 levels are also measured. The opportunity should be taken to assess body composition, bone mineral density, fasting lipids, insulin, and quality of life, before and after discontinuation of GH therapy. These studies establish baseline

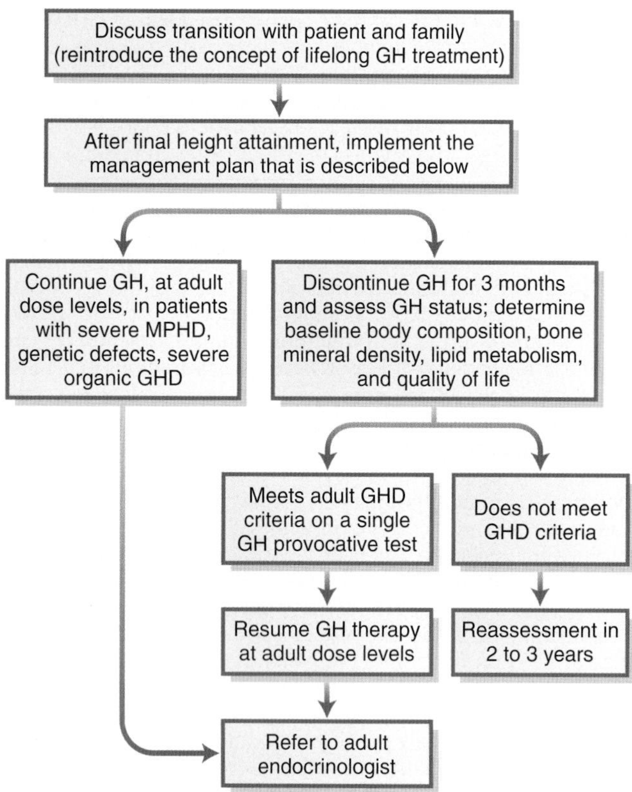

Figure 23–57 ▪ Algorithm for transition to adult treatment of growth hormone deficiency. *GH,* Growth hormore; *GHD,* Growth hormore deficiency; *MPHD,* multiple pituitary hormone deficiencies.

data prior to long-term GH treatment and also are used for longitudinal assessment of untreated patients. The likelihood of GHD persisting into adult life in patients with CPHD, structural abnormalities of the hypothalamus-pituitary, or documented hypothalamic-pituitary molecular defects far exceeds that in patients with idiopathic, isolated GHD. In patients with documented molecular defects of GH production, or CPHD, or with structural abnormalities or histories of cranial irradiation, an argument can be made that a low serum IGF-I concentration may obviate the need for repeat provocative GH testing. This would generally describe the clinically useful designation as a high- or low-risk patient for continuation of GHD requiring GH treatment.

In summary, a conservative approach would suggest that all children diagnosed with GHD should be retested by insulin-provocative tests upon completion of skeletal growth, and before a commitment is made for long-term adult treatment. A strong argument can be made, however, that patients with the very high likelihood of persistent GHD do not necessarily require retesting, or, at most, should have IGF-I and IGFBP-3 concentrations determined. On the other hand, the child who has carried a diagnosis of idiopathic, isolated GHD should *always* be retested. When the diagnosis of adult GHD is established, continuation of GH therapy is strongly recommended. Caution should be exercised when considering the decision of continuing GH therapy in conditions where there is a known risk of diabetes or malignancy. This is an opportunity for a thorough clinical reassessment, with a determination of the need for other hormonal replacement. The transition to adult GH replacement should be arranged as a close collaboration between the endocrinologists who treat pediatric patients and those who treat adult patients, and they should discuss the reinitiation of treatment with the patient. A discussion of many transition issues was reported by Clayton and associates following a European consensus meeting.[1422]

Growth Hormone Treatment of Other Forms of Short Stature

The availability of GH has made it possible to use the hormone for treatment of other forms of short stature. Theoretically, it should be possible to accelerate growth in any child so as to achieve a height greater than indicated by genetic potential. A survey of 251 pediatric endocrinologists suggested that 30% to 50% would consider treating short children with a wide array of diagnoses, including Russell-Silver and Noonan syndromes, IUGR, and steroid-induced growth suppression.[1256] Indeed, children with growth failure due to multiple different disorders have received GH and have grown substantially.[924,925]

Although these data arise from large, uncontrolled NCGS and KIGS databases, certain trends do emerge. On purely auxologic grounds, it is difficult to discriminate between responses to GH, over at least 4 years, in children diagnosed with GHD by current clinical and laboratory criteria versus children with a wide variety of other clinical conditions associated with growth failure; although mean growth rates between patient groups may differ, overlap is substantial.[925] If such data are taken in the context that responsiveness to GH, rather than an arbitrary diagnosis of GHD, should determine appropriateness of GH therapy,[1085] prospective evaluations of such treatment in many clinical states of poor growth should ensue. Whether such therapy is safe and whether it justifies the cost and potential risks are more complicated. Additionally, questions have been raised about the appropriateness of "cosmetic" hormonal therapy. These are not issues that are presently answered. Guidelines have been developed by the Lawson Wilkins Pediatric Endocrine Society and the Growth Hormone Research Society to provide a rational framework in this area.[1276,1351] The 2006 FDA-approved indications for GH treatment in childhood and adolescence are GHD, PWS, chronic renal failure, Turner's syndrome, and growth failure due to either prior IUGR or ISS. GH insufficiency need not be documented except in GHD.

Chronic Renal Failure (Figs. 23–58 and 23–59)

GH accelerates growth in children with chronic renal failure at least over 5 years of therapy.[1453-1456] Using a GH dosage of 0.05 mg/kg/day, Fine and colleagues[1457] reported a mean first-year growth rate of 10.7 cm in GH recipients and 6.5 cm in the placebo group; in the second year, GH-treated patients had a mean growth rate of 7.8 cm/yr versus 5.5 cm/yr in placebo recipients, resulting in an improvement of height SDS from −2.9 to −1.5. Twenty patients who were treated for 5 years reached a normal height SDS of −0.7, having had a mean height increase of 40 cm.[1456] The youngest patients (younger than 2.5 years of age) had the most impressive growth response to GH therapy (14.1 cm/yr). Deleterious effects on renal function or progression of osteodystrophy were not observed.[1458,1459] This treatment regimen does not adversely affect renal graft function after transplantation, nor is there significant "catch-down" growth following the transplantation.[1460] The final height in 38 German children treated with GH for an average of 5.3 years was −1.6 ± 1.2 SDS, an increment of 1.4 SDS over the pretreatment baseline. The final height of an untreated control group was −2.1 ± 1.2 or 0.6 SDS below baseline.[1461] Long-term GH treatment has also been shown to be safe and effective for extremely short (−4.0 SDS) children with nephropathic cystinosis and should be considered if nutrition and cysteamine treatment do not prevent growth failure.[1462] As children are often short at the time of renal transplantation, have hormone findings of relative GH insensitivity, and receive chronic prednisone

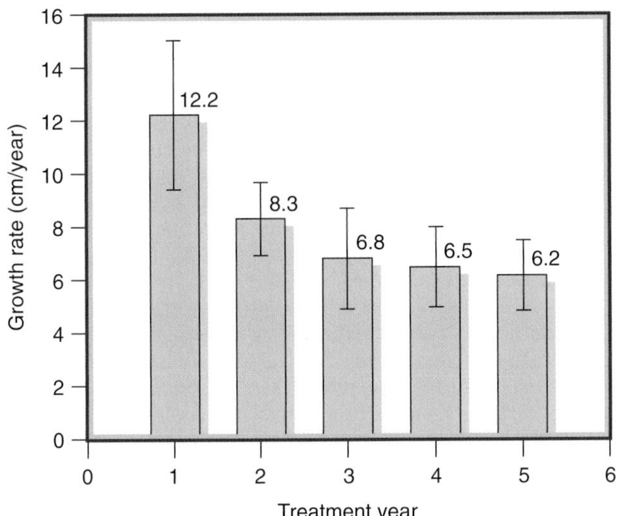

Figure 23–58 ▪ Annual growth velocity in 20 growth-retarded prepubertal patients with chronic renal insufficiency who were treated with growth hormone. (From Fine RN, Kohaut E, Brown D, et al. Long-term treatment of growth retarded children with chronic renal insufficiency with recombinant human growth hormone. Kidney Int 1996;49:781-785. Reproduced with permission of Fine, RN.)

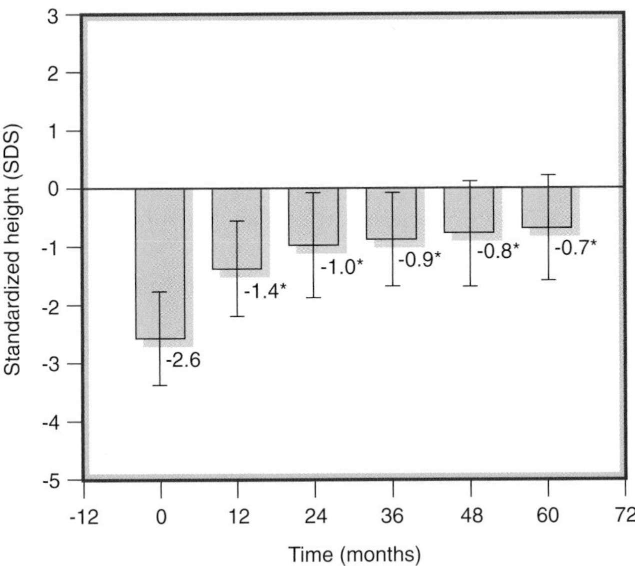

Figure 23–59 ▪ Height SDS (mean±SD) in 20 growth-retarded prepubertal patients with chronic renal insufficiency. Note that the basal height is outside the normal range (at −2.6 SD), enters the normal range within 1 year of treatment, and is not different from the mean by the 5th year of growth hormone therapy. (From Fine RN, Kohaut E, Brown D, et al. Long-term treatment of growth retarded children with chronic renal insufficiency with recombinant human growth hormone. Kidney Int 1996;49:781-785. Reproduced with permission of Fine, RN.)

therapy, GH is sometimes administered in the posttransplantation period. Data for 1 to 2 years of treatment of such children and adolescents[762-764,1463] indicate a large increment of growth velocity at year 1 and a smaller benefit at year 2. As with GH treatment of chronic renal failure, the pharmacologic regimen overcomes the relative GH insensitivity. Considerable assessment must yet be undertaken to demonstrate whether there is increased growth over a longer term, that renal function does not deteriorate during therapy, and that the risk of rejection is not enhanced. GH treatment does not appear to cause an accelerated decline of allograft function[1464-1466] nor changes in histopathologic findings,[1467] but the exacerbation of chronic rejection by GH therapy remains a possibility.[1468] Use of nonsteroid-based immunosuppressive regimens may obviate the need for posttransplantation GH treatment.

Turner's Syndrome

Patients with Turner's syndrome have a final height, averaging 143 cm in the United States,[16,537] that is about 20 cm lower than the mean final height of normal women.[535] Extensive trials of therapy have involved androgens, estrogens, and GH. Androgens have either no effect or cause modest gains in final adult height, despite frequent reports of short-term improvement in growth velocity (references listed in reference 20). Although estrogen deficiency is probably not involved in the growth failure of Turner's syndrome, especially that in infancy and childhood years, low-dose therapy has been unsuccessfully used in an attempt to enhance growth.[1469-1480] These studies consistently show modest, transient increments of growth velocity, invariably accompanied by advancement of skeletal maturation. Final height outcome is not improved and often is impaired. Planning for the needed estrogen replacement for ovarian failure should take into account its effects on growth outcome and different regimens sought to achieve the desired normalization of pubertal maturation.

Before the availability of recombinant GH, there were conflicting data concerning the efficacy of pit-GH in this disorder,[1481,1482] but the ability of GH to accelerate growth has now been demonstrated in multiple reports.[535-537,549,1483-1487] Growth responses are not affected by the karyotype. In 1983, a randomized, controlled North American study of GH (at a dose of 0.375 mg/kg/wk) with or without added oxandrolone was initiated, with mean age of onset of treatment approximately 9 years.[1483] Analysis of all 62 girls enrolled in the study at near final height showed a mean stature of 152.1 cm in the GH plus oxandrolone group (a gain of 10.3 cm compared to the height predictions derived from Lyon and colleagues,[16] whereas girls receiving GH alone averaged 150.4 cm (a gain of 8.4 cm) (Fig. 23–60).[537] In another arm of this study, addition of estrogen to the GH regimen before age 15 years lowered the final height gain from 8.4 cm to 5.1 cm.[1488] In a reassessment of North American data in NCGS, early initiation of GH treatment was shown to allow estrogen administration at a physiologic age without loss of adult height.[1489,1490] Several other recent studies[550,1491] using higher doses of GH have shown even greater gains in adult height outcomes. Sas and coworkers, in a multicenter trial, using a maximum GH dose of approximately 0.63 mg/kg/wk for 4.8 estrogen-free GH treatment years beginning at mean age 8.1 years, had a gain of 16 cm over the modified Lyon and colleagues' projection.[16,550] In their group receiving a similar GH dose to the American studies, a height gain of 12.5 cm was achieved by age 16 with 4.8 estrogen-free GH treatment years starting at 7.9 years. In these girls, induction of puberty at a normal (not delayed) age was associated with these excellent height outcomes.[1492] Carel and colleagues,[1491] using 0.7 mg/kg/wk in a group that received 5.1 estrogen-free GH treatment years beginning at 10.2 years, gained 10.6 cm over the projections of Lyon and colleagues.[16] Their conventional dose group (0.3 mg/kg/wk) gained only 5.2 cm with 3.0 estrogen-free GH treatment years starting at 11 years. The substantial variations in the GH-induced growth increments in these studies are presumably related to GH dose, duration of estrogen-free GH treatment years, the age of initiation of GH and estrogen administration, as well as the population and parental adult heights. Additionally, a protein polymorphism of GH-R based on a genomic

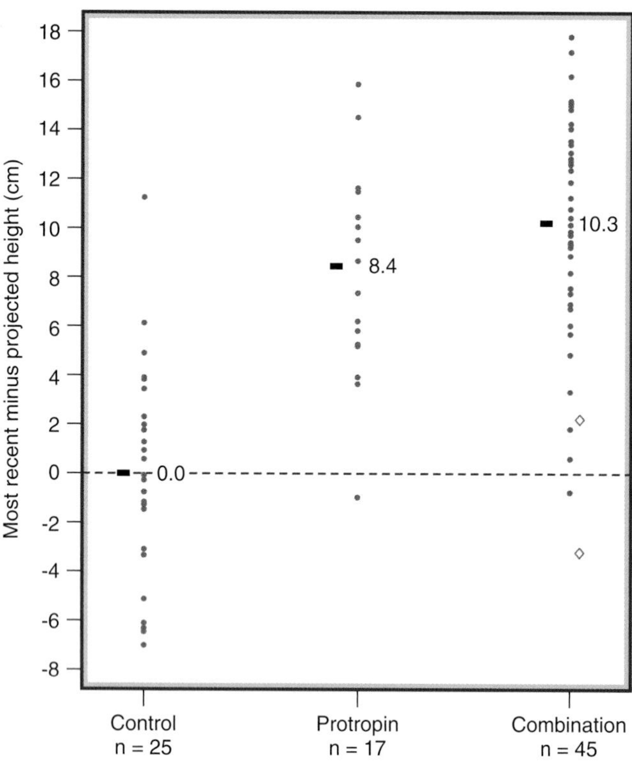

Figure 23–60 ▪ Adult heights of Turner's patients treated with growth hormone (n=17) or combination GH=oxandrolone (n=45), or of historical Turner's controls (n=25), relative to each subject's projected adult height (indicated by the dotted zero line). The mean increments in adult height relative to the projected adult height are indicated. The diamond symbols in the combination group indicate two subjects with poor compliance who terminated treatment early. (From Rosenfeld RG, Attie KM, Frane J, et al. Growth hormone treatment of Turner syndrome: beneficial effect on adult height. J Pediatr 1998;132:319-324.)

deletion of exon 3 has been reported to be associated with increased responsivity to GH in girls with Turner syndrome.[138] Transdermal or depot estrogen administration, as opposed to oral estrogen, may also contribute positively to growth outcomes.[1493,1494] In these higher dose treatment studies, hyperinsulinism with presumed insulin resistance was evident though reversible.[1491,1495] Other data suggest that impaired insulin secretion may ultimately be the significant issue in the Turner's syndrome patients,[1496,1497] although to date long-term GH therapy has been well tolerated.

Some uncertainty existed, however, because none of these studies were placebo-controlled to adult height, and some studies have yielded much poorer height outcomes.[551] Finally, in a randomized, controlled, multicentered Canadian study, the mean height gain ascribed to GH treatment was 7.3 cm at 1 year after cessation of the treatment protocol. Estrogen was initiated at 13 years of age.[1498] Another temporally matched control study from Italy showed a gain of 8.1 cm.[1499] These studies corroborate and support the information that had accumulated from historic data on natural growth in Turner's syndrome juxtaposed to the available GH treatment results. Such data, in aggregate, provide convincing support that GH can both accelerate growth velocity and increase adult height.

We recommend seeking the diagnosis vigorously at any age in every girl with otherwise unexplained short stature and initiating therapy at that young age (i.e., at diagnosis or in early childhood). One must bear in mind that growth velocity in untreated Turner's syndrome girls can be slowed as early as the 1- to 3-year-old period.[539,540] We generally treat with the FDA-approved GH dosage of 0.375 mg/kg/wk and closely monitor adherence to the regimen with auxologic and IGF-I measurements, along with assuring continued normal thyroid status. Oxandrolone may be added to the regimen in the late-diagnosed girl. We initiate estrogen therapy at an appropriate physiologic age in those girls in whom GH had been started at a young age, but delay estrogen as long as clinically reasonable in those in whom GH therapy was initiated at a late age. Often, growth-promoting and pubertal needs must be balanced and the therapeutic approach should be individualized. The diminished areal bone density in Turner's syndrome is enhanced by GH, but estrogen therapy is needed to normalize volumetric density (i.e., not simply size-related).[1500] Absence of an adverse impact of GH upon aortic diameters is reassuring, given the predisposition of such patients for dissecting aneurysms.[1134] Utilization of statistical prediction models for long-term growth in Turner's syndrome may permit a more quantitative assessment of individual therapeutic efficacy.[1501]

Despite our enthusiasm for aggressive GH treatment of girls with Turner's syndrome and the generally excellent quality-of-life assessments in adulthood,[986,1502] an array of health-related issues in these individuals may persist, despite achievement of adequate adult height. Carel and colleagues[1503] reviewed health outcomes of 568 French GH-treated Turner's syndrome adult women (in their mid-20s) with mean height of 150.9 cm (having gained about 9 cm over prediction) and found that neither height nor height gain were associated with quality-of-life scores. Rather, issues surrounding cardiologic and otologic health concerns, along with a delay in pubertal initiation beyond 15 years, were of greater concern. In contrast, a long-term follow-up assessment of 49 women from The Netherlands, who had reached a mean adult height of 160.7 cm (a gain of more than 15 cm), suggested that the high quality-of-life scores were, indeed, related to height gain and adequate estrogenization. These studies are not controlled, but emphasize the broad range of health concerns in Turner's syndrome women and affirm the need for multidisciplinary follow-up care.

Down's Syndrome

The encouraging results of GH trials in Turner's syndrome led to studies of GH in Down's syndrome. In several preliminary studies, GH accelerated growth in such patients, although ethical issues were raised concerning the appropriateness of such therapy.[1504-1507] In the uncontrolled NCGS experience, 23 children experienced a 1.3 SDS height gain over the first 4 years of GH therapy.[925] No convincing data exist that GH improves neurologic or intellectual function in such patients. The increased risk of diabetes mellitus and leukemia in children with Down's syndrome might be augmented by GH therapy.[1508]

Intrauterine Growth Retardation (Born Small for Gestational Age)

The studies employing GH in short children with IUGR are hampered by the heterogeneity of this group of patients, whose poor growth may reflect maternal factors, chromosomal disorders, dysmorphic syndromes, toxins, and so on. Indeed, the low levels of IGF-I and IGFBP-3 in many infants with IUGR, apparently related to fetal malnutrition, do not seem to predict the degree of subsequent growth impairment,[1509] although continuing low levels are associated with poor catch-up growth.[560] Short post-SGA children make up a substantial portion of growth-retarded patients seen in pediatric endocrine practices.[559,601,1510]

Because these children may have heights in the range seen in IGF deficiency syndrome, therapeutic attempts certainly are appropriate, assuming that the insulin resistance noted in these thin, small post-SGA children[570] does not become a clinical issue. Encouraging growth responses have been obtained with GH treatment. A randomized, placebo-controlled, double-blind, two-dose (0.13 and 0.4 mg/kg/week) study of 95 children on GH therapy was serially reported during 3 years of treatment and then after 1 year off GH.[1511,1512] After this period, mean height was within the normal range in the high-dose GH group (−1.76±0.17 SDS) and higher than in the low dose group (−2.46±0.39 SDS); skeletal maturation in the two groups advanced 5.3±0.4 and 4.6±0.7 years, respectively, over the 4-year study, but remained 1 to 2 years below chronologic age. Several other 2-year multicenter trials utilizing doses ranging from 0.23 to 0.7 mg/kg/wk also showed enhanced growth velocity (gaining 5 to 10 cm more than control groups), but bone age advanced 2.7 years.[1513,1514] These data clearly show acceleration of growth in IUGR children who are very short during middle childhood years. While an approximation to the growth velocity of their peers may be enough benefit to justify GH treatment, many questions regarding long-term efficacy of GH therapy upon final height have been answered. Sas and colleagues[1515] contrasted prepubertal SGA children receiving 0.23 (n=23) to 0.47 mg/kg/wk (n=16) over a 5-year period. Mean height SDS increment of 3.3±0.7 in the higher dose group exceeded that in the lower (2.4±0.5). Despite a mean skeletal age increase of 7 years during the study, predicted adult height increased 9.1±2.8 and 14.0±5.5 cm in the two groups. De Zegher and his colleagues[1516,1517] used several different regimens, including continuous treatment with 0.23 to 0.45 mg/kg/wk for 6 years and a discontinuous program of 0.23 to 0.7 mg/kg/wk for 2 years followed by no therapy or one additional 2-year course at these varied doses. The mean dose in the discontinuous treated children was 0.22 mg/kg/wk over the 6 years, but they received 46% fewer injections. Mean height SDS gains were approximately 2.0 in these regimens, with mean parent adjusted height SDS at about −0.5. Bone age advanced 7.3±0.1 years over the 6-year period and remained slightly delayed. At 8 years of therapy,[1517] the children were still growing and had reached approximately 12 cm over predicted adult height. Onset of puberty was not accelerated in these studies.[1515-1517] In reviewing data for the first 28 children reaching adult height, shorter children benefit initially from a higher GH dose (greater than 50 μg/kg/day or greater than 0.35 mg/kg/wk) while long-term achievement of quite acceptable height could be attained with a lower mean dose (~33 μg/kg/day or 0.23 mg/kg/wk).[1518] In 77 Swedish children who received long-term GH treatment, mean final height was −1.2 SDS, with 86% within the target range for families.[1519] The younger, smaller, and lighter children grew best, with the greatest catch-up growth occurring during the prepubertal years. In a prediction model derived from KIGS SGA data, Ranke and coworkers[1520] found that youth and GH dose were strong predictors of initial growth, but that the growth achieved during the first year was a powerful predictor of later growth. Furthermore, the polymorphism of GH-R based on the exon 3 genomic deletion has been reported to be associated with somewhat greater responsivity to GH than predicted in SGA children.[137,138]

In a report from the long-term Dutch SGA treatment trial (mean duration of therapy being 8 years), mean height had reached the parental target, with 91% of children within the normal range.[1521] Additionally, and most provocatively, intelligence quotient, behavior, and self-perception scores increased significantly and approximated those of normal Dutch children. A positive association of IGF-I levels and intelligence quotient in a normal 8- to 9-year-old childhood population supports such findings.[663] The importance of the IGF/IGFBP system in neurodevelopment gives credence to these observations,[1522] although corroborative studies are necessary and the potential implications of such intriguing data remain to be explored.[1523]

GH therapy for this group of patients, which accounts for about 20% of short children, has received FDA approval. No systematic evidence of meaningful increases in insulin resistance was found in these study patients, in contrast to its high prevalence in IUGR children who are growing well (or excessively) and potentially evolving into the adult "syndrome X."[555,562] A small group of GH-treated SGA children who did develop insulin resistance still had evidence of it 3 months after cessation of GH treatment.[1524] The complexity of the metabolic derangements in the SGA population demands that long-term follow-up of treated children be undertaken to determine whether cardiovascular risk factors also will appear despite their earlier thin habitus.[1525,1526]

Osteochondrodysplasias

GH therapy has been studied in several skeletal dysplasias. The largest published study in achondroplasia involved 40 children; during the first year of treatment, the height velocity increased from 3.8 to 6.6 cm/yr and in year 2, the height velocity decreased to approximately 5 cm/yr.[1527] A modest improvement was seen in the ratio of lower limb length to height. Although GH was well-tolerated, atlantoaxial dislocation during GH therapy has been reported in one patient. In another study, normal growth velocity was achieved for up to 6 years in 35 subjects with a significant increment in height SDS for at least 4 years[1528]; in this study, vertebral growth was disproportionately greater than limb growth. Bridges and Brook[1529] reported on the effects of GH therapy in 27 patients with hypochondroplasia; response was maximal during the first year of treatment, but substantial benefit was seen through 4 years of treatment in pubertal subjects. Much of the growth response represents an increase of spinal length; with leg-lengthening procedures some patients may achieve adult height within the normal range.[1530] Experience with GH treatment is limited in other skeletal disorders, such as dyschondrosteosis, hereditary multiple exostoses, osteogenesis imperfecta, and Ellis-van Creveld syndrome. On the other hand, the experience with GH in patients heterozygous for abnormalities of the SHOX gene (both Turner's syndrome and Leri-Weil syndrome) has indicated that GH therapy may be of benefit in some relatively mild skeletal dysplasias.

Noonan's Syndrome

Most experience with GH therapy of short stature in Noonan's syndrome has been limited to small uncontrolled studies in which few patients have reached final height.[623,925,1531] The clinical diagnosis of a dysmorphic syndrome potentially makes the treatment groups heterogeneous, although identification of a mutant gene PTNN11[624] will help with characterization. Overall, treatment results for 3 to 4 years are generally similar to those attained in Turner's syndrome, with mean growth velocities improving by 2 to 4 cm/yr over baseline rates of approximately 4 cm/yr over the first 4 years of therapy, gaining from about −3.5 to −1.7 SDS of stature without inordinate advancement of bone age.[623,631-633,925,1531] Those children with identifiable PTPN II mutations are reported to have a poorer response to GH treatment in terms of growth and IGF production suggesting impaired efficiency of phosphorylation-dependent GH signaling pathways[631-633] Although initial anecdotal experience suggested progression of ventricular hypertrophic cardiomyopathy, this has not been found in larger, carefully monitored studies.[623,1532]

Juvenile Chronic (Idiopathic) Arthritis

Growth retardation has been a common finding in chronic juvenile arthritis, presumably related to the widespread inflammatory process, glucocorticoid therapy, and variable resistance to the actions of GH. Multiple short- and long-term studies have been reported,[1533-1536] with the best data found in a 4-year study[1536] in which height SDS improved by 1.0 in the treated group, but fell by 0.7 in untreated children. Lean mass and bone mineral density improvements have been found.[1535]

Idiopathic Short Stature (Subtle Errors throughout the Growth Axis)

Although the term *idiopathic short stature* (ISS), by definition, involves children without identifiable causes of growth retardation, it clearly encompasses a *heterogeneous* group that includes children with constitutional growth delay, genetic short stature, and subtle defects of the GH-IGF axis, such as heterozygous mutations of the GH receptor gene. Even though they are often grouped in one category, children with ISS have been shown to have a broad range of provocative GH responses, including marginally normal to elevated, but have a wide range of serum IGF concentrations, ranging from normal to unequivocally IGF deficient. This group also includes children with unidentified syndromes and as yet unidentified chronic illnesses or endocrine disorders. For example, children with heterozygous mutations of the GH receptor may have subnormal growth, diminished IGF and GHBP levels, and impaired responsiveness to exogenous GH administration, although this may be true for some GHR mutations, but not others. ISS children may experience stressful behavioral circumstances, but studies suggest variable relationships of psychosocial problems to the short stature.[1061,1537-1540] Nonetheless, hormonal intervention to enhance growth, hoping to diminish such difficulties, has been used. As noted above, specific etiologies are often unknown, but GH treatment has been utilized widely.[925] Important questions have been raised about the financial, ethical, and psychosocial impact of GH therapy of "normal" short children.[1539,1541-1544] Given the cost of GH, the financial implications of treating such children (whether at the bottom 5%, 3%, 1%, or 0.1%) is considerable. The point is well taken that 5% of the population will always be below the 5th percentile, whether we treat with GH or not, and focusing upon short stature potentially handicaps an otherwise normal child, psychologically or socially. No convincing data have yet been presented to show that GH treatment of short children definitively improves psychological, social, or educational function.[1544-1546] A possible exception is the improved intellectual function in SGA childen treated with GH.[1521] Furthermore, final adult height in the subset of children with constitutional delay of growth and maturation (probably a common inclusion, though not ISS as defined in the FDA approval) may be adequate without any treatment, in at least some children.[1289-1291] Finally, the treatment risks (however minimal) of GH therapy, both known and unknown, must be considered when treatment of otherwise apparently normal children, even if exceedingly small, is a legitimate concern.[1547] The failure to report levels of IGF-I, IGFBP-3, and GHBP in many studies, and differing interpretations of endogenous GH secretion studies (e.g., assay variance, control group size), in addition to the heterogeneity of the patient groups, confounds assessment of response data. Nevertheless, it is clear that many children who do not meet conventional criteria for the diagnosis of GHD and who fall under the heading of ISS are as growth-retarded as children with bona-fide GHD and might be considered suitable candidates for growth-promoting therapy.

Uncontrolled Growth Hormone Treatment Trials in Idiopathic Short Stature

Published clinical trials have often not contained long-term control groups and have reported variable growth responses.[1548-1552] Most short children treated with GH have growth acceleration ("catch-up"), which generally is sustained over the first several years of therapy[925] (although attenuation of the response occurs as in all other instances of GH treatment). It appears that slower pretreatment growth velocity and higher weight/height ratio, factors suggesting GHD, and lesser degrees of bone age retardation are associated with better early growth responses.[1553] Longer-term data are now available to begin to determine the impact of therapy on adult height. Nearly 3000 children, with 153 having reached final height, were classified as ISS in KIGS[1554] in 1999. GH treatment (0.2 to 0.25 mg/kg/wk) resulted in achievement of target height in familial (FSS) short stature patients, although at a relatively short stature (−1.7 SDS in males and −2.2 SDS in females) with a mean gain during therapy of 0.6 to 0.9 SDS. In non-FSS children, the mean final height was greater in males (−1.4 SDS), but not in females (−2.3 SDS), with mean gains having been 1.3 and 0.9 SDS, respectively. These latter heights are, nonetheless, distant from the midparental target heights that were near 0 SDS. Hintz and colleagues[1555] assessed adult height in 80 North American children with ISS treated for up to 10 years at a GH dose of 0.3 mg/kg/wk. Mean height SDS at conclusion was −1.4, with a gain of 1.3 SDS, quite similar to the broader KIGS experience. Although this study was not placebo-controlled, the data were compared to predicted and actual final heights of two groups of short children followed up for similar periods. Treated boys achieved 9.2 cm and girls 5.7 cm greater gain in final over predicted heights, compared to the untreated children.

Controlled Growth Hormone Treatment Trials in Idiopathic Short Stature

Controlled studies also have demonstrated clear gains of height among ISS children. A meta-analysis looking at an aggregate group of 1089 children suggested efficacy of treatment.[1556] Four controlled trials with adult height data showed treatment benefits of 0.54 to 0.84 SDS, corresponding to a mean effect of 5 to 6 cm. We focus on several specific studies. McCaughey and coworkers[1557] showed that GH treatment (about 0.34 mg/kg/wk) of eight prepubertal girls led to a mean height SDS of −1.14 after 6.2 years of treatment. This was a 7.6 cm greater gain than in the control groups whose mean height SDS (−2.55) did not change during the study. The studies that ultimately led to approval of GH treatment in the United States included the long-term, randomized, double-blind, placebo-controlled trial at the National Institutes of Health by Leschek and her associates[1558] and the randomized dosing trial of the European Idiopathic Short Stature Study Group.[1559] In the former trial, utilizing a less optimal regimen of 0.22 mg/kg/wk given thrice-weekly, for subjects with a mean starting height of nearly −3 SDS, the treated children had mean final height gain of 3.7 cm over the control group. In the latter randomized study, employing GH doses of 0.24 and 0.37 mg/kg/wk, given as a six-dose per week regimen in children with mean starting heights of −3.0 to −3.4 SDS, the higher dose group exceeded the lower by 3.6 cm, achieving a final height of −1.12 SDS. Combining the data from the two trials showed a cumulative gain of 7.3 cm in the group treated with 0.37 mg/kg/wk over the placebo-treated children. Concerns had been raised that GH treatment might accelerate pubertal onset and progression, resulting in failure to improve height SDS for bone age,[1560,1561] thereby offsetting the positive responses observed during early years of GH treatment of ISS.[1562] In the higher dose-treated group just described,[1563] there was no evidence of accelerated pubertal or skeletal maturation in contrast to data reported by Kamp and colleagues[1564] at a 30% greater GH dose. This matter of advancing maturation has not been substantiated by additional studies.[1554,1557,1565-1567] Taken together these data show that GH treatment of prepubertal children with ISS does increase growth velocity and final height.

Safety, along with efficacy, is of paramount importance in the GH treatment of children with ISS. In the earlier study of Hintz and colleagues,[1555] careful monitoring did not reveal any discernible metabolic side effects.[1566] In two recent studies of GH-treated ISS children, no evidence of increased adverse events relative to other GH-treated groups was noted.[1568,1569] Nonetheless, the long-term safety profile of GH usage in this indication deserves special monitoring in view of the heterogeneity of the patient population and the inclusion of children whose heights are only modestly below the normal range.[1547]

In summary, in view of (1) the current limitations in the definitive discrimination between GHD and the less classic syndromes of primary IGFD; (2) the inadequate understanding of neurosecretory defects of GH secretion; (3) the inadequate recognition of "partial" GHD or GHI; and (4) the need to move to a more global concept of "IGF deficiency," it seems unfair to prevent GH therapy of short children who do not meet a narrow definition of GHD (i.e., provocative testing), which we recognize as inadequate. As noted above, many of these children are comparable clinically and in responsivity to GH to classic GHD patients. Accordingly, we recommend the following approach:

1. Continue therapeutic trials of ISS to adult height.
2. Appropriate evaluation should include thorough analysis of the GH-IGF axis (with GHBP levels, serum IGF-I and IGFBP-3 concentrations, and, where appropriate, IGF responses to GH treatment, before labeling a short child as "normal."
3. Proper assessment of pretreatment growth velocity should be over a minimum of a 6-month period and preferably for 12 months.
4. Decisions concerning therapy should be individualized, with careful attention to the needs and expectations of the child and family. In the otherwise normal child with severe short stature (at least 2.25 SD below the mean for age) and a failure to show convincing evidence for spontaneous catch-up growth, a *trial* of GH therapy should be discussed with the patient and family. This discussion should include an assessment of normal growth patterns, familial growth patterns, and the predicted pubertal and statural development. The inconveniences, discomforts, and potential risks of GH treatment should be fully described. It is the clinician's responsibility to ensure that expectations of the child and the parents are realistic in regard to short-term growth and ultimate height. Where appropriate, counseling and psychological support should be provided.
5. If a trial of GH therapy is desired, treatment should be for a minimum of 6 months. We recommend the FDA-approved dosage of 0.37 mg/kg/wk.
6. Therapy with GH should be continued beyond 6 months only if growth is accelerated (defined as an increase in the height velocity of at least 2 cm/yr). Efficacy of treatment requires continuous monitoring, both in terms of growth and in measurement of the GH-dependent peptides. Delineation of patients with resistance to GH treatment with IGF insufficiency should lead to consideration of IGF-I therapy as an alternative. The use of complex, nonlinear multivariate models to assess growth response is recommended, but requires further refinement.
7. Growth acceleration with GH treatment does not relieve the clinician of seeking an underlying etiology for the child's growth failure. Appropriate studies should be repeated, when indicated.
8. Treatment must be carefully monitored for side effects of GH treatment.
9. Continued psychological support should be provided for the child and family. This includes guiding the patient through puberty and providing posttreatment follow-up.

Miscellaneous Causes of Growth Failure

In addition to the clinical conditions described above, GH has been employed in treatment of short stature associated with a variety of other conditions associated with postnatal growth failure. In general, such trials have been uncontrolled and have not included sufficient numbers of subjects for efficacy to be evaluated. Examination of such treatments should be continued in the large international databases.

Normal Aging and Other Catabolic States

Detailed consideration of the potential use of GH in normal aging is beyond the scope of this chapter. The rationale for such therapy is based upon the concept of the "somatopause," referring to the fact that GH secretion normally declines progressively after 30 years of age, as reflected in decreasing IGF-I levels. Aging can be viewed as a catabolic state, with the potential that GH therapy might reverse or retard the loss of muscle mass and strength and the decrease in bone density with aging. Clinical studies are in progress.

Growth failure, often with impaired final adult height, is a characteristic clinical finding in endogenous or exogenous Cushing's syndrome. Excess glucocorticoids cause a catabolic state characterized by increased proteolysis, decreased protein synthesis, lowered osteoblastic and increased osteolytic activity, and insulin resistance.[1570] GH treatment blunts some of these catabolic actions, but increases the insulin resistance.[1571] Mauras[878] showed that IGF-I therapy similarly induces an anabolic response, despite excess glucocorticoids, but does not cause insulin resistance. GH treatment in the posttransplantation period[1464-1466] and in other glucocorticoid-treated children[873] causes some height increments, but not as good a response as in individuals not on glucocorticoids. GH does enhance bone formation and increases osteoblastic activity in such children.[1572] The marked increase in IGF-I levels during GH treatment may be sufficient to overcome the local insensitivity to IGF action.[749,750,875]

GH therapy is also being investigated in catabolic states, such as burns, tumor cachexia, major abdominal surgery, AIDS, sepsis, metabolic acidosis, and situations requiring total parenteral alimentation.

Side Effects of Growth Hormone

Pituitary-derived human GH had an enviable safety record for a quarter of a century, but proved to be the agent for transmission of the fatal spongiform encephalopathy, Creutzfeldt-Jakob disease (CJD).[1335,1336] Although pit-GH was removed from use in the United States in 1985 and, later, throughout the world, more than 160 patients with GH-derived CJD have been identified and cases are likely to continue to be found over the next several decades.[1337-1339] Although this risk does not exist with recombinant DNA-derived GH, the experience with pituitary GH serves as a grim reminder of the potential toxicity that can reside in "normal" products and "physiological replacement."

Extensive experience with recombinant GH over more than 20 years has been encouraging.[1034,1035,1243,1573,1574] Concerns have been raised about a number of potential complications, which clearly require continued follow-up and assessment. This evaluation has been greatly facilitated by the extensive databases established by GH manufacturers, in particular Genentech (National Collaborative Growth Study, NCGS)[1034,1573,1575] and Pharmacia (Pharmacia International Growth Database, KIGS).[924,1035,1576]

Development of Leukemia

The development of leukemia as a complication of GH therapy was first reported in five cases from Japan in 1988,[1577] and to date more than 50 cases of leukemia have been reported in GH-treated cases. Many of the cases are from Japan,[1578] but some are from the United States.[1573,1579] One difficulty in assessing the role of GH treatment in this disorder is that many GHD children have conditions that may predispose to the development of leukemia, such as histories of prior malignancies, irradiation, or syndromes which themselves are associated with the development of leukemia, even in the absence of GH therapy (e.g., Bloom's syndrome, Down's syndrome, Fanconi's anemia). GH-treated patients who develop leukemia do so at a later age than the normal population. Patients have included recipients of both pit-GH and rGH, and leukemia has occurred both during treatment and following termination of therapy. Calculations of relative risk are imprecise but vary from sevenfold in Japan to twofold to fourfold in the United States. Leukemia has been reported in GHD individuals *without any history of GH therapy*, raising the possibility that the GHD state, by itself, might be a predisposing factor.[1576,1580]

It is not possible to be certain whether GH is a causative agent in the development of leukemia. If it is, the increase in risk appears modest and may arise from the underlying state rather than from GH therapy. The number of cases worldwide of new leukemia in children treated with GH, but in whom there are no known risk factors, is approximately what would be expected on a patient-year basis.[1034,1581,1582] This issue should be discussed with all potential recipients of GH, but it appears that the risk is limited to those children with high risk factors. Particular care should be used in prescribing GH therapy for children with past histories of leukemia or lymphoma or other disorders conveying an increased risk of leukemia. In a study of more than 600 children with prior leukemia and who were treated with GH, the relapse rate was within the expected range, consistent with no effect of GH replacement therapy on recurrence of leukemia.[1035,1573,1583] In addition, data from 59,158 GH-treated patients with more than 193,000 patient-years at risk did not reveal an increased risk for nonleukemic extracranial neoplasms.[1034,1035]

Recurrence of Central Nervous System Tumors

Because many recipients of GH have acquired GHD because of CNS tumors or their treatment, the possibility of tumor recurrence with therapy is of obvious importance. Estimates of CNS tumor recurrence rates in non–GH-treated children and adolescents are difficult to obtain, bearing in mind the vast array of treatment programs utilized in the past 3 decades. In a total of 1083 patients compiled in 11 reports who were not treated with GH, 209 (19.3%) had recurrences.[1583-1593] Such data in a heterogeneous group, including craniopharyngiomas, gliomas, ependymomas, medulloblastomas, and germ cell tumors, provide a background for assessing recurrence rates in GH-treated youth. Reports from nine centers, encompassing 390 patients, indicate recurrence in 64 patients, or 16.4%, at the time of publication,[1583,1584,1593-1598] not much different than the recurrence rate observed in a much larger number of untreated patients. In a particularly well-done comparative study at three pediatric neurooncology centers having data on 1071 brain tumor patients (180 treated with GH for a mean treatment period of 6.4 years, with 31 followed for more than 10 years), relative risk of recurrence or death was similar in both groups.[1597] In a study of 361 cancer survivors (including 172 brain tumor patients), disease recurrence of all cancers in GH-treated children did not differ from those not treated. There was, however, an overall increased risk (3.21[1.88-5.46 95% CI]) of second neoplasms, mostly meningiomas.[1036] A similar increased risk for second neoplasms, largely meningiomas, was found in GH-treated adult patients.[1599] Cranial irradiation seems to be a most important predisposing factor, but the role of GH remains uncertain. Extensive analysis of 4410 patients with brain tumor or craniopharyngioma histories before GH therapy in the NCGS and KIGS databases[1034,1035] showed a similar lack of increased tumor recurrence. In the NCGS series, recurrence rates of the most common CNS neoplasms, craniopharyngioma (6.4%), primary neuroectodermal tumors (medulloblastoma, ependymoma) (7.2%), and low-grade glioma (18.1%) were lower or similar to those reported in non–GH-treated children.[1583,1600,1601] Despite these comforting data, the relatively short median follow-up times, even in the huge international databases, must temper the willingness to eliminate any relationship of GH therapy to recurrence of intracranial neoplasia.

Pseudotumor Cerebri

Pseudotumor cerebri (idiopathic intracranial hypertension; IIH) has been reported in GH-treated patients.[1034,1035,1602] The disorder may develop within months of starting treatment or as long as 5 years into the course; it appears to be more frequent in patients with renal failure than in those with GHD.[1034] The mechanism for the effect is unclear, but may reflect changes in fluid dynamics within the CNS. Pseudotumor has also been described following thyroid hormone replacement in hypothyroidism. In any case, clinicians should be alert to complaints of headache, nausea, dizziness, ataxia, or visual changes. Significant fluid retention with edema or hypertension is rare.[1603] Because of the possible association of pseudopapilledema with GHD, perhaps representing a variant of optic nerve hypoplasia,[1604] careful ophthalmologic evaluation should be undertaken in patients with suspected GH therapy–associated pseudotumor cerebri to avoid overdiagnosis and invasive treatments.

Slipped Capital Femoral Epiphysis

Slipped capital femoral epiphysis (SCFE) is associated with both hypothyroidism and GHD. Whether GH therapy plays a role in SCFE has been difficult to determine, in part because the incidence of SCFE varies with age, sex, race, and geographic locale, being reported between 2 and 142 cases per 100,000. The data in the KIGS and NCGS studies are in this range.[1034,1035] Accordingly, while SCFE cannot be attributed to GH therapy per se, complaints of hip and knee pain and/or limp should be evaluated carefully. The situation of such pain in the setting of a child having an exceedingly rapid growth rate should make one consider this diagnosis.

Diabetes Mellitus

The association of GH treatment with insulin resistance is well documented.[1605] A retrospective analysis of the KIGS database found 43/23,333 children with abnormalities of glucose regulation, including 11 with type 1 and 18 with type 2 diabetes mellitus.[1133] The heterogeneity of this patient group and the failure to corroborate these findings with a similar retrospective analysis of NCGS data (type 2, 6.2/100,000) put the report into question. Nonetheless, the reduction of insulin sensitivity by GH is a concern that demands close assessment of high-risk patients such as those with PWS or Turner's syndromes, or with a history of IUGR. At present it would seem most likely that the relationship of the development of diabetes mellitus in childhood/adolescent GH recipients is due to a common genetic linkage rather than a GH side effect,[1606] but studies of the impact of decades of GH therapy on insulin sensitivity are warranted.

Miscellaneous Side Effects[1034,1035]

Other potential side effects of GH therapy include prepubertal gynecomastia,[1607] pancreatitis,[1608] growth of nevi,[1609,1610] although typically without evidence of malignant degeneration,[1573] behavioral changes, scoliosis and kyphosis, worsening of neurofibromatosis, hypertrophy of tonsils and adenoids, and sleep apnea. A report[1611] of reduced testicular volume and elevated gonadotropin levels in four young adult males previously treated with GH for ISS has not been confirmed by a double-blind, placebo-controlled study[1612] nor by the international databases.[1613] This list is, obviously, only partial. It is best for the clinician to remember that GH and the peptide growth factors it regulates are potent mitogens with diverse metabolic and anabolic actions. All patients receiving GH treatment, even as replacement therapy, must be carefully monitored for side effects.

For the most part, the side effects of GH are minimal and rare. When they occur, careful history and physical examination are adequate to identify their presence. Management of these side effects may include either transient reduction of dosage or temporary discontinuation of GH.[1276] In the absence of other risk factors, there is no evidence that the risk of leukemia, brain tumor recurrence, slipped capital femoral epiphysis, or diabetes mellitus is increased in recipients of long-term GH treatment. Any patient receiving GH, who has a second major medical condition, such as being a tumor survivor, should be followed up in conjunction with an appropriate specialist such as an oncologist or a neurosurgeon. While GH has been shown to increase the mortality of critically ill patients in the ICU,[176] there is no evidence that GH replacement therapy needs to be discontinued during intercurrent illness in GHD children.

The Question of Long-Term Cancer Risk

Several epidemiologic studies suggest an association between high serum IGF-I levels and an increased incidence of malignancies.[1614,1615] The calculated risk of cancer in those studies was also increased for patients with low IGFBP-3 levels. While additional studies are being conducted to verify or disprove these associations, GH's role also should be carefully examined. Although IGF-I levels were not statistically associated with cancer risk, the combination of high IGF-I and low IGFBP-3 was related to a heightened risk.[1616] As GH positively influences production of both peptides, this casts doubt on its role as a driving force in the IGF-cancer relationship. A potential confounder in these studies is the variability of serum IGF-I levels that may be observed normally and the consequent substantial movement of a given individual's risk designation in differing quartiles when multiple samples are obtained.[1617] Additionally, the effects of high IGFBP-3 levels on the incidence of premenopausal breast cancer further underscore the complexity of these relationships.[1618] The necessity of long-term, well-designed studies with sufficient patients is apparent, in order to prevent potentially incorrect and inappropriately ominous conclusions.[1619] Epidemiologic studies assessing the risk of malignancy in patients with acromegaly found differing results, with some[1620-1622] but not others[1623,1624] identifying significant associations between acromegaly and colon cancer risk. Small size, uncontrolled retrospective nature, and multiple possible sources of bias make these reports difficult to interpret. The largest study to date, reviewing more than 1000 patients, indicated no overall increased cancer incidence in acromegaly.[1625] Although colon cancer risk was also not increased in that study, mortality was higher in this population, suggesting an effect of GH or IGF-I on established tumors.[1626] A recent prospective analysis of colon cancer and colonic polyps in acromegalics did not observe an association between these two diseases when using either autopsy series or prospective colonoscopy screening series for the control population.[1627] Acromegaly is associated with a marked increase in the incidence of benign hyperplasia of several organs, including colonic polyps.[1628] Such findings suggest that the GH-IGF axis may lead to symptomatic benign proliferative disease, which could be associated with symptoms, such as rectal bleeding, that would then lead to a potential detection (or ascertainment) bias.

Children receiving GH do not appear to have a greater risk of de novo or recurrent tumors.[1034,1035,1243] A cohort of 1848 patients treated with GH in the United Kingdom was assessed after as long as 40 years and found to have increased rates of colorectal cancer and Hodgkin's disease, but the tumor-associated deaths were such a low number that a single patient death would markedly alter the risk ratios.[1629,1630] No increased incidence of cancer was found in GH recipients among adults who were treated for GH deficiency.[1423,1631] These reports represent imperfect, uncontrolled studies, but the experience gained through them strongly suggests that GH therapy is not associated with future development of neoplasms in the absence of other risk factors. The use of IGF-I and IGFBP-3 in the monitoring of GH recipients, both adult and pediatric, has been recommended and endorsed by international bodies such as the GH Research Society,[1276] and the Drug and Therapeutics Committees of Lawson Wilkins Pediatric Endocrine Society and European Society of Pediatric Endocrinology.[1629,1632] Until the issue of cancer risk in GH therapy is fully resolved, the prudent approach appears to be regular monitoring of both IGF-I and IGFBP-3 and altering the GH dose to ensure that the theoretical risk profile induced by GH therapy is favorable. This can be done by avoiding the unlikely situation of a GH-treated patient having an IGF-I level at the upper end and IGFBP-3 at the lower end of the normal ranges. In the twenty-first century, many GH-deficient patients will receive lifelong GH replacement, emphasizing the importance of long-term, regular monitoring of IGF-I and IGFBP-3.[1417] Although many issues still remain in fully discerning the relationship, if any, between the GH-IGF axis and the risk of cancer, current data strongly suggest the safety of present indications for use of GH in children and adults.[1633]

Treatment of Primary IGF Deficiency: Use of IGF-I

The production of IGF peptides by recombinant DNA technology has permitted clinical trials of IGF therapy. IGF-I administration to normal adult male volunteers as a single intravenous injection of 100 μg/kg caused hypoglycemia within 15 minutes.[1634] On a molar basis, IGF-I has approximately 6% of the hypoglycemic potency of insulin. In contrast, intravenous infusions of IGF-I to normal men at a rate of 20 μg/kg/hr resulted in serum IGF-I levels within the normal range and did not produce hypoglycemia, but did suppress GH levels, increase creatinine clearance, and decrease plasma urea nitrogen.[1635]

The most obvious clinical use of IGF-I therapy is in patients with GHI. In patients with GH receptor deficiency (GHRD), intravenous bolus administration of IGF-I caused acute symptomatic hypoglycemia, presumably reflecting the insulin-like actions of IGF-I coupled to the low serum levels of IGFBP-3.[1636] The subcutaneous administration of IGF-I to eight GHRD patients, at a dosage of 150 μg/kg/day for 7 days, did not cause symptomatic hypoglycemia.[1637] Vaccarello and colleagues[92] treated six adults with GHRD for 7 days with subcutaneous IGF-I at a dosage of

40 μg/kg every 12 hours. Normal serum IGF-I levels were maintained for 2 to 6 hours postinjection, followed by a rapid decline, because of low serum levels of IGFBP-3. Hypoglycemia did not occur, mean 24-hour GH levels were suppressed, and urinary calcium was increased.

A number of short-term growth-related studies with IGF-I treatment at varied doses have been reported. Laron and associates[1638] reported growth acceleration to rates of 8.8 to 13.6 cm/yr in five children treated with a single daily dose of 150 μg IGF-I/kg for 3 to 10 months. Similarly, Walker and colleagues[1639] found an increase in growth rate from 6.5 to 11.4 cm/yr in a GHRD patient treated with twice-daily subcutaneous injections of 120 μg IGF-I/kg. Wilton and coworkers[1640] reported collaborative data on the treatment of 30 patients, ages 3 to 23 years, with GHI from GHRD or GHD-IA with anti-GH antibodies; the dosage of IGF-I varied from 40 to 120 μg/kg given twice daily. With the exception of the two oldest individuals, growth rates increased in all subjects by at least 2 cm/yr. A mean increment of more than 4 cm/yr in growth velocity was found in 11 prepubertal children treated with 80 μg/kg twice a day.[1641] This latter study also demonstrated a significant inverse relationship between growth response to exogenous IGF-I and the severity of the GHI phenotype.

Longer term studies of IGF-I treatment of GHI have demonstrated a persistent, but progressively waning effect.[1642] Data from 17 patients in a European collaborative trial, treated for at least 4 years, showed an increase in mean height SDS from −6.5 to −4.9, with two adolescents reaching the 3rd percentile, and emphasize the importance of early diagnosis and initiation of therapy (Fig. 23–61). Side effects included hypoglycemia, headache, convulsions, urolithiasis, and papilledema; the latter, which suggests the possibility of pseudotumor cerebri, resolved spontaneously while receiving IGF-I. In the longest treatment study, Backeljauw and Underwood[1643,1644] showed data similar to the European study, with an initial burst of growth followed by slowing to just above baseline by the sixth year of therapy. Height SDS improved from −5.6 to −4.2 by the end of the sixth year.

A randomized, double-blind, placebo-controlled trial of IGF-I therapy in GHRD has been performed in Ecuador, probably the only place where the patient population is sufficiently large and homogeneous to permit such investigation.[1645] Growth rates in subjects receiving IGF-I increased from 2.9 to 8.6 cm/yr over the first year of therapy. The placebo group grew 4.4 cm/yr during the same time, and then their growth rate increased to 8.4 cm/yr during IGF-I treatment. Incidence of hypoglycemia was equal in the two groups. One recipient of IGF-I developed papilledema, which resolved spontaneously while on treatment.

Although these early studies are promising, little is known about the long-term effects of IGF-I or about the optimal dose or frequency of administration. When all clinical studies are combined, the total number of children treated to date is still only several hundred, and relatively few have been treated for longer than 5 years. Taken together, the IGF-I treatment studies show that the growth response, while significant, is neither as successful nor as long-lived as that of GHD children treated with exogenous GH. The failure of serum levels of IGFBP-3 to increase with IGF-I administration underscores the relevance of the IGFBPs to IGF pharmacokinetics.[92,1646] The possibility that local production of IGF-I at the growth plate may be critical for optimal growth also requires consideration. Nevertheless, these data indicate that the IGF peptides, long considered to function as autocrine or paracrine growth factors, can act as classic endocrine hormones.

Two IGF-I preparations have received FDA approval recently: one is IGF-I alone, while the other is a combination of IGF-I:IGFBP-3. While both drugs show promise in treatment of severe primary IGFD, no comparative studies have been performed to date. The use of IGF-I in milder forms of primary IGFD is also the subject of current investigations.

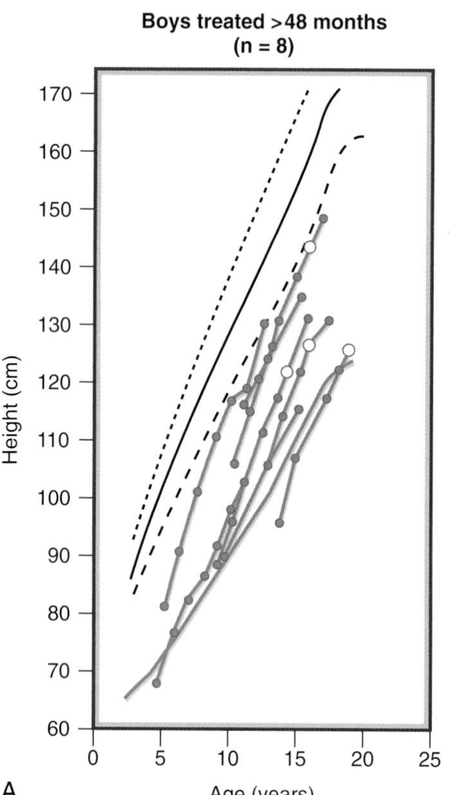

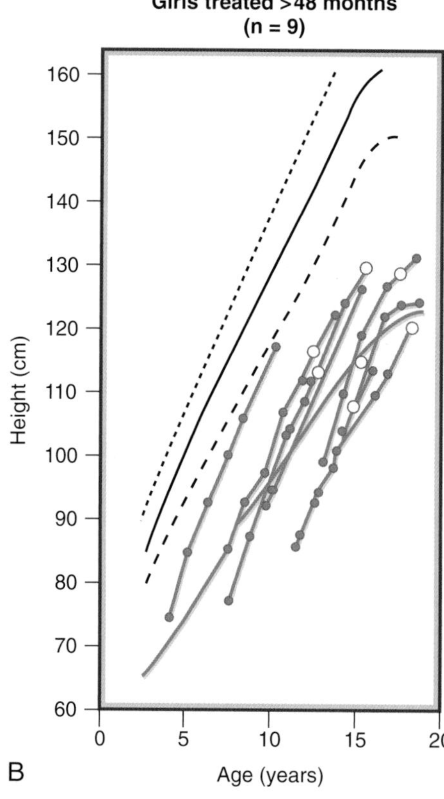

Figure 23–61 ▪ Growth during IGF-I treatment of GH insensitivity, relative to normal standards (Tanner) and median for untreated patients (Laron). Open circles indicate the onset of puberty. (From Ranke MB, Savage MO, Chatelain PG, et al. Long-term growth of patients with growth hormone insensitivity syndrome with IGF-I. Results of the European Multicentre Study. The Working Group on Growth Hormone Insensitivity Syndromes. Horm Res 1999;51:128-134.)

EXCESS GROWTH AND TALL STATURE (Table 20–15)

Although as many children have heights greater than 2 SD above the mean as have heights greater than 2 SD below the mean, referral for tall stature is less common than for short stature. This pattern speaks eloquently to the psychosocial pressures to which children with "growth disorders" are subjected. Nevertheless, it is critical to identify those situations wherein tall stature or an accelerated growth rate provides a clue for the diagnosis of an underlying disorder.

Statural Overgrowth in the Fetus

Maternal diabetes mellitus is the most common cause of large-for-gestational age infants (height or weight greater than the 90th percentile for gestational age). Even in the absence of clinical symptoms or a family history, the birth of an excessively large infant should lead to evaluation for maternal (or gestational) diabetes.

Two relatively rare syndromes can also cause large-for-gestational age infants. Children with cerebral gigantism (also known as Sotos syndrome)[1646-1648] are typically above the 90th percentile for both length and weight at birth. Additional clinical features include a prominent forehead; dolichocephaly; macrocephaly; high arched palate; hypertelorism with an unusual slant to the eyes; prominent ears, jaw, and chin; large hands and feet with thickened subcutaneous tissue; mental retardation; and motor incoordination. Although such children continue to grow rapidly during the early years of childhood, puberty is usually early and causes premature epiphyseal fusion. Most patients have a final height within the normal population range.[1648] GH secretion and serum IGF levels are normal, and no specific cause of the overgrowth in cerebral gigantism has been identified. Most patients (~80%) with Sotos syndrome possess a loss of function mutation in the NSD1 gene whose product is a nucleus-localized, basic transcriptional factor.[1649]

Beckwith-Wiedemann syndrome (BWS) is the most common (1/13,700) of a group of disorders associated with excessive somatic and specific organ growth, collectively referred to as overgrowth syndromes, apparently caused by excess availability of the growth factor insulin-like growth factor-II (IGF-II) encoded by the gene *Igf2.*[681] BWS is characterized by fetal macrosomia with omphalocele[1650] with its clinical features due to selective organomegaly, including macroglossia, renal medullary hyperplasia, and neonatal hypoglycemia due to islet cell hyperplasia.[1651] As with cerebral gigantism, excessive fetal, neonatal, and childhood growth ultimately leads to early epiphyseal fusion, without an increase in adult height.[1652] Although an association between BWS and disordered regulation of IGF-II gene transcription exists, no consistent postnatal abnormality of the GH-IGF axis has been identified to date.[1653,1654] Under normal conditions, the IGF-II gene is imprinted (i.e., the paternally derived gene for IGF-II is expressed and the maternally transmitted gene is not active).[1655] Four children with somatic overgrowth but not the diagnostic features of BWS had IGF-II gene overexpression.[1656] Various lines of investigation have localized "imprinted" genes involved in BWS and associated childhood tumors to chromosome 11p15.5. These include, in addition to *Igf2,* the gene H19, which is involved in *Igf2* suppression, as well as the gene WT-1 (the Wilms' tumor gene).[225] Mutations in GPC3, a glypican gene that codes for an IGF-II neutralizing membrane receptor, cause the related Simpson-Golabi-Behmel overgrowth syndrome.[1657,1658]

TABLE 23–15 DIFFERENTIAL DIAGNOSIS OF STATURAL OVERGROWTH

FETAL OVERGROWTH
Maternal diabetes mellitus Cerebral gigantism (Sotos syndrome) Weaver's syndrome Beckwith-Wiedemann syndrome Other IGF-II excess syndromes
POSTNATAL OVERGROWTH LEADING TO CHILDHOOD TALL STATURE
Familial (constitutional) tall stature Cerebral gigantism Beckwith-Wiedemann syndrome Exogenous obesity Excess growth hormone (GH) secretion (pituitary gigantism) McCune-Albright syndrome or multiple endocrine neoplasia (MEN) associated with excess GH secretion Precocious puberty Marfan's syndrome Klinefelter's syndrome (XXY) Weaver's syndrome Fragile X syndrome Homocystinuria XYY Hyperthyroidism
POSTNATAL OVERGROWTH LEADING TO ADULT TALL STATURE
Familial (constitutional) tall stature Androgen or estrogen deficiency/estrogen resistance (in males) Testicular feminization Excess GH secretion Marfan's syndrome Klinefelter's syndrome (XXY) XYY

Postnatal Statural Overgrowth

As stated above, both cerebral gigantism and BWS are associated with rapid perinatal growth, but rapid growth usually ends by early to mid-childhood. Nevertheless, these conditions should be considered when tall stature in childhood is accompanied by the characteristic phenotypic features or with a history of unexplained fetal overgrowth. As in the case of the child with growth failure, crossing height percentiles between infancy and the onset of puberty is an indication for further evaluation. Although such growth patterns are frequently not of concern to parents, overly rapid statural growth can indicate serious underlying pathology and warrants evaluation. Furthermore, as with short stature, children with tall stature must be evaluated in the context of familial growth and pubertal patterns.

Familial (Constitutional) Tall Stature

GH secretion and levels of IGF-I and IGFBP-3 in familial tall stature (FTS) are often in the upper normal range.[1271] Tauber and colleagues[1659] divided 65 children with FTS into a subset with high GH secretion rates (5.4±2.3 mg/L/mm) and frequent secretory bursts (5.1±1.6/day) and another subset with lower GH secretion (2.1±.5 mg/L/mm) and fewer episodic spikes (3.3±1.3/day). IGF-I levels were higher in the group producing more GH and were normal in the low GH group. They postulated that both enhanced secretion of GH and greater efficiency of GH-mediated IGF-I production might be potential causes of FTS.

As with short stature, children with tall stature must be evaluated relative to familial growth patterns and parental target height.[1660] When a family history of tall stature is available, support and reassurance are frequently all that is required. A careful assessment of pubertal status and bone age facilitates prediction of adult height and usually obviates the need for hormonal therapy. Standard height prediction, using Bailey-Pinneau tables, especially in children younger than age 12, tend to overestimate final height and confidence limits are large,[1661-1663] particularly in boys. We discourage therapy for boys with predicted adult heights less than 198 cm (6′6″) and girls with predicted adult heights less than 183 cm (6′). Indeed, societal changes in attitudes toward tall individuals appear to discourage treatment, except in extreme circumstances. The majority of patients treated for tall stature in the past were female, but heights well above the mean for girls have become increasingly acceptable socially and psychologically. The number of patients treated in the United States has fallen markedly over the last 3 decades. Therapy when necessary is aimed at the acceleration of puberty in order to cause premature epiphyseal fusion.[1664,1665] Accordingly, the optimal time for treatment is before the onset of puberty. The earlier the intervention, the more likely that adult height can be decreased, although patients are not usually referred until late childhood or early puberty. Although some success with lower dosages had been reported, administration of ethinyl estradiol to tall girls at a dose of 0.15 to 0.30 mg/day is a reasonable starting level in girls and can be increased, if necessary, and if well-tolerated, to 0.50 mg/day. Conjugated estrogens, 7.5 to 10 mg/day have also been successful. If breakthrough bleeding occurs, cyclic progestogens may be added to the estrogen therapy. Treatment should be continued until epiphyses fuse, because posttreatment growth may be substantial if treatment is stopped early.[1663]

The mechanism of estrogen action is probably complex, in that estrogen can affect both GH secretion and serum IGF levels and, more importantly, act directly on the epiphysis. Estrogen mediates epiphyseal fusion in both girls and boys.[21-23] In prepubertal girls, estrogen therapy reduces adult height by as much as 5 to 6 cm relative to predictions. When therapy is initiated after the onset of puberty, the decrement in adult height is not likely to be as large.

The use of high-dose estrogen in otherwise normal children must be weighed against the known (and unknown) toxicity of such therapy,[1666] including nausea, weight gain, edema, and hypertension. During the initial phases of therapy, growth is paradoxically accelerated as the child rapidly progresses through puberty. Other potential problems, such as thromboembolism, cystic hyperplasia of the breast, endometrial hyperplasia, and cancer have not been definitively related to estrogen therapy in children, but should be discussed with the patient and family.

Therapy in boys with tall stature is even more problematic. For the reasons discussed above, estrogen is likely to be most efficacious in accelerating epiphyseal fusion, but is obviously undesirable in males. Androgens will also accelerate skeletal maturation, presumably via aromatization to estrogen but at the price of rapid virilization. Benefits and potential side effects must, therefore, be balanced and therapy should be individualized.

Obesity

Obesity is frequently associated with rapid skeletal growth and early onset of puberty.[1667] Patients with obesity tend to have diminished overall GH production, but normal to high GHBP, and IGF-I levels appear to be capable of maintaining adequate or enhanced linear growth velocity. Early activation of adrenal androgenesis and premature pubarche are common. Bone age is usually modestly accelerated so that both puberty and epiphyseal fusion occur early and adult height is normal. This association between obesity and rapid growth is so characteristic that the child with obesity and *short stature* should always be evaluated for underlying pathology, such as hypothyroidism, GH deficiency, Cushing's syndrome, or PWS.

Excess GH Secretion

Pituitary gigantism is a rare condition, analogous to acromegaly in the adult (see Chapter 8).[1668-1670] GH-secreting tumors of the pituitary are, typically, eosinophilic or chromophobe adenomas. Their etiology is uncertain, although many result from somatic mutations that generate constitutively activated G-proteins with reduced GTPase activity (see Chapter 8).[1671] The resulting increase in intracellular cAMP in the pituitary leads to increased GH secretion. McCune-Albright syndrome, which is also caused by mutations resulting in constitutive activation of G-proteins, may also be characterized by somatotropic tumors and excess GH secretion.[1672,1673] GH-secreting tumors have also been reported in multiple endocrine neoplasia and in association with neurofibromatosis and tuberous sclerosis (see Chapter 8).[1674] GH excess that occurs before epiphyseal fusion results in rapid growth and attainment of adult heights above the expected genetic potential. When GH hypersecretion is accompanied by gonadotropin deficiency, accelerated linear growth may persist for decades, as in the case of the Alton giant, who reached a height of 280 cm by the time of his death in his 20s.[1675] Manifestations typical of acromegaly may also appear, such as soft tissue swelling, enlargement of the nose, ears, and jaw with coarsening of the facial features, pronounced increases in hand and foot size, diaphoresis, galactorrhea, and menstrual irregularity.

Serum IGF-I levels are elevated, although high IGF-I levels may also be a normal manifestation of puberty. Basal serum GH levels may be normal or increased, but serum GH is not suppressed by administration of glucose (1.75 g/kg body weight, up to a maximum of 100 g).

Although abnormalities of the sella turcica are often evident on lateral skull films, the demonstration of increased GH-IGF secretion should lead to radiologic evaluation of the hypothalamus and pituitary by MRI or CT. Definitive therapy requires surgical ablation of the tumor. Fortunately, this can usually be accomplished by transphenoidal pituitary surgery, although macroadenomas may require a more aggressive surgical approach. As described in Chapter 8, the use of somatostatin analogues, dopamine agonists, and GH-receptor antagonists are important components of treatment programs for GH-excess.

Precocious Puberty

Precocious puberty, whether centrally mediated (increased gonadotropin secretion, GnRH-dependent) or peripherally mediated (increased androgen and/or estrogen secretion, GnRH-independent) results in accelerated linear growth in childhood, mimicking the pubertal growth spurt. Because skeletal maturation is also accelerated, adult height is frequently compromised. The diagnostic evaluation and management of precocious puberty are discussed in Chapter 24.

Miscellaneous Causes of Tall Stature

Marfan's syndrome, an autosomal dominant disorder of collagen metabolism, is characterized by hyperextensible joints, dislocation of the lens, kyphoscoliosis, and dissecting aortic aneurysm and often leads to long, thin bones, that result in arachnodactyly and moderately tall stature. Marfan's syndrome is caused by mutations in the fibrillin-1 (*FBN1*) gene. The abnormal fibrillin-1 monomers from the mutated gene disrupt the normal aggregation of fibrillin-1, impairing microfibril formation. Homocystinuria, an autosomal recessive disorder, phenotypically resembles Marfan's syndrome, although patients are usually mentally retarded. The rate of linear growth may increase modestly in hyperthyroidism. Tall stature has been found in patients with familial ACTH resistance due to a defective ACTH receptor.[1676]

Dosage effects of the SHOX gene may result in tall stature.[1677] In females with three copies of the SHOX gene and gonadal dysgenesis, adult stature was +2 to +2.9 SDS.[1678,1679] In women with 47,XXX karyotype, mean final heights are around 5 to 10 cm taller, and in men with 47,XXY karyotype (Klinefelter's syndrome), around 3.5 cm taller than population means.[1678,1680,1681] Males with an XYY karyotype may also have moderate tall stature. In addition to the SHOX effects, however, the variable degree of estrogen production in some of these syndromes must influence skeletal maturation and final height.[25]

It is worth commenting that while delayed puberty may be associated with short stature in childhood, as with constitutional delay, failure to enter puberty and complete sexual maturation may result in sustained growth during adult life with ultimate tall stature and a characteristic eunuchoid habitus. The description of tall stature with open epiphyses resulting from mutation of the estrogen receptor or from aromatase deficiency underscores the fundamental role of estrogen in promoting epiphyseal fusion and termination of normal skeletal growth.[21-23]

REFERENCES

1. Kaplan SL. Normal and abnormal growth. In Rudolph AM, ed. Pediatrics. New York: Appleton-Century Crofts, 1977.
2. Reiter EO, Witt MF. Physical growth and development. In Braham RL, Morris ME, eds. Textbook of Pediatric Dentistry. Baltimore: Williams & Wilkins, 1985:2-23.
3. Heinrichs C, Munson PJ, Counts DR, et al. Patterns of human growth. Science 1995;268:442-444.
4. Lampl M, Velhuis JD, Johnson ML. Saltation and stasis: a model of human growth. Science 1992;258:801-803.
5. Lampl M, Cameron N, Veldhuis JD, et al. Patterns of human growth: response. Science 1995;268:445-447.
6. Tillmann V, Thalange NKS, Foster PJ, et al. The relationship between stature, growth, and short-term changes in height and weight in normal prepubertal children. Pediatr Res 1998;44: 882-886.
7. Hermanussen M, Lange S, Grasedyck L. Growth tracks in early childhood. Acta Paediatr 2001;90:381-386.
8. Martin DD, Hauspie RC, Ranke MB. Total pubertal growth and markers of puberty onset in adolescents with GHD: comparison between mathematical growth analysis and pubertal staging methods. Horm Res 2005;63:95-101.
9. Tanner JM. Auxology. In Kappy MS, Blizzard RM, Migeon CJ, eds. The Diagnosis and Treatment of Endocrine Disorders. Springfield, IL: Charles C. Thomas, 1994:137-192.
10. Nilsson O, Baron J. Fundamental limits on longitudinal bone growth: growth plate senescence and epiphyseal fusion. Trends Endocrinol Metab 2004;15:370-374.
11. Parfitt AM. Misconceptions (1): epiphyseal fusion causes cessation of growth. Bone 2002;30:337-339.
12. Karlberg J, Engstrom I, Karlberg P, et al. Analysis of linear growth using a mathematical model. 1. From birth to three years. Acta Paediatr Scand 1987;76:478-488.
13. Karlberg J, Fryer JG, Engstrom I, et al. Analysis of linear growth using a mathematical model. II. From 3 to 21 years. Acta Paediatr Scand (Suppl) 1987;337:12-29.
14. Ogden CL, Kuczmarski RJ, Flegal KM, et al. Centers for Disease Control and Prevention 2000 growth charts for the United States: improvements to the 1977 National Center for Health Statistics version. Pediatrics 2002;109:45-60.
15. Tanner JM, Davies SW. Clinical longitudinal standards for height and height velocity for North American children. J Pediatr 1985;107:317.
16. Lyon AL, Preece MA, Grant DB. Growth curve for girls with Turner syndrome. Arch Dis Child 1985;60:932-935.
17. Horton WA, Rotter JI, Rimoin DL, et al. Standard growth curves for achondroplasia. J Pediatr 1978;93:435-438.
18. Cronk C, Crocker AC, Pueschel SM, et al. Growth charts for children with Down syndrome: 1 month to 18 years of age. Pediatrics 1988;81:102-110.
19. Bayer LM, Bayley L. Growth Diagnosis. Chicago: University of Chicago Press, 1959:226-231.
20. Reiter EO, Rosenfeld RG. Normal and aberrant growth. In Larsen PR, Kronenberg HM, Melmed S, et al, eds. Williams Textbook of Endocrinology. Philadelphia: Saunders, 2002:1003-1114.
21. Smith EP, Boyd J, Frank GR, et al. Estrogen resistance caused by a mutation in the estrogen-receptor gene in a man. N Engl J Med 1994;331:1056-1061.
22. Conte FA, Grumbach MM, Ito Y, et al. A syndrome of female pseudohermaphroditism, hypergonadotropic hypogonadism, and multicystic ovaries associated with missense mutations in the gene encoding aromatase (P450arom). J Clin Endocrinol Metab 1994;78:1287-1292.
23. Morishima A, Grumbach MM, Simpson ER, et al. Aromatase deficiency in male and female siblings caused by a novel mutation and the physiological role of estrogens. J Clin Endocrinol Metab 1995;80:3689-3698.
24. Bilezikian J, Morishima A, Bell J, et al. Increased bone mass as a result of estrogen therapy in a man with aromatase deficiency. N Engl J Med 1998;339:599-603.
25. Grumbach MM, Auchus RJ. Estrogen: consequences and implications of human mutations in synthesis and action. J Clin Endocrinol Metab 1999;84:4677-4694.
26. Greulich WW, Pyle SI. Radiographic Atlas of Skeletal Development of the Hand and Wrist. Stanford, CA: Stanford University Press, 1959.
27. Tanner JM, Whitehouse RH, Cameron N, et al. Assessment of Skeletal Maturity and Prediction of Adult Height (TW2 Method). New York: Academic Press, 1983.
28. Tanner JM, Oshman D, Lindgren G, et al. Reliability of computer-assisted estimates of Tanner-Whitehouse skeletal maturity [CASAS]: comparison with manual method. Horm Res 1994; 42:288-294.
29. Van Teunenbroek A, De Waal W, Roks A, et al. Computer-aided skeletal age scores in healthy children, girls with Turner syndrome, and in children with constitutionally tall stature. Pediatr Res 1996;39:360-367.
30. Roche AF, Davila GH, Eyman SL. A comparison between Greulich-Pyle and Tanner-Whitehouse assessments of skeletal maturity. Radiology 1971;98:273-280.
31. Emons JA, Boersma B, Baron J, et al. Catch-up growth: testing the hypothesis of delayed growth plate senescence in humans. J Pediatr 2005;147:843-846.
32. Bayley N, Pinneau SR. Tables for predicting adult height from skeletal age: revised for use with the Greulich-Pyle hand standards. J Pediatr 1952;40:423-441.
33. Roche AF, Wainer H, Thissen D. The RWT method for the prediction of adult stature. Pediatrics 1975;56:1026-1033.
34. Khamis HJ, Roche AF. Predicting adult stature without using skeletal age: the Khamis-Roche method. Pediatrics 1994;94:504-507.
35. Tanner JM, Goldstein H, Whitehouse RH. Standards for children's height at ages 2-9 years allowing for height of parents. Arch Dis Child 1970;45:755-762.
36. Giacobbi V, Trivin C, Lawson-Body E, et al. Extremely short stature: influence of each parent's height on clinical-biological features. Horm Res 2003;60:272-276.
37. Wright CM, Cheetham TD. The strengths and limitations of parental heights as a predictor of attained height. Arch Dis Child 1999;81:257-260.
38. Ruff C. Variation in human size and shape. Annu Rev Anthropol 2002;31:211-232.
39. Tanner JM. A History of the Study of Human Growth. Cambridge: Cambridge University Press, 1981.

40. Ikeda H, Suzuki J, Sasano N, et al. The development and morphogenesis of the human pituitary gland. Anat Embryol (Berl) 1988; 178:327-336.
41. Goodyer CG. Ontogeny of pituitary hormone secretion. In Collu R, Ducharme JR, Guyda HJ, eds. Pediatric Endocrinology. New York: Raven, 1989:125-169.
42. Stanfield JP. The blood supply of the human pituitary gland. J Anat 1960;94:257-273.
43. Gorcyzca W, Hardy J. Arterial supply of the human anterior pituitary gland. Neurosurgery 1987;20:369-378.
44. Pilavdzic D, Kovacs K, Asa SL. Pituitary morphology in anencephalic human fetuses. Neuroendocrinology 1997;65:164-172.
45. Rosenfeld MG, Briata P, Dasen J, et al. Multistep signaling and transcriptional requirements for pituitary organogenesis. Recent Prog Horm Res 2000;55:1-13.
46. Ericson J, Norlin S, Jessell TM, et al. Integrated FGF and BMP signaling controls the progression of progenitor cell differentiation and the emergence of pattern in the embryonic anterior pituitary. Development 1999;125:1005-1015.
47. Kioussi C, Carriere C, Rosenfeld MG. A model for the development of the hypothalamic-pituitary axis: transcribing the hypophysis. Mech Dev 1999;81:23-35.
48. Sheng HZ, Westphal H. Early steps in pituitary organogenesis. Trends Genet 1999;15:236-240.
49. Burrows HL, Douglas KR, Seasholtz AF, et al. Genealogy of the anterior pituitary gland: Tracing a family tree. Trends Endocrinol Metab 1999;10:343-353.
50. Takuma N, Sheng HZ, Furuta Y, et al. Formation of Rathke's pouch requires dual induction from the diencephalon. Development 1998;125:4835-4840.
51. Treier M, Gleiberman AS, O'Connell SM, et al. Multistep signaling requirements for pituitary organogenesis in vivo. Genes Dev 2000;12:1691-1704.
52. Mullis PE. Genetic control of growth. Eur J Endocrinol 2005; 152:11-31.
53. Dattani MT. Growth hormone deficiency and combined pituitary hormone deficiency: does the genotype matter? Clin Endocrinol (Oxf) 2005;63:121-130.
54. Moore GE, Abu-Amero S, Wakeling E, et al. The search for the gene for Silver-Russell syndrome. Acta Paediatr Suppl 1999; 433:42-48.
55. Dasen JS, O'Connell SM, Flynn SE, et al. Reciprocal interactions of Pit1 and GATA2 mediate signaling gradient-induced determination of pituitary cell types. Cell 1999;97:587-598.
56. Lopez-Bermejo A, Buckway CK, Rosenfeld RG. Genetic defects of the growth-hormone insulin-like growth factor axis. Trends Endocrinol Metab 2000;11:39-49.
57. Thorner MO, Vance ML, Horvath E, et al. The anterior pituitary. In Wilson JD, Foster DW, eds. Williams Textbook of Endocrinology. Philadelphia: WB Saunders, 1991:210-221.
58. Scheithauer BW, Sano T, Kovacs K, et al. The pituitary gland in pregnancy: a clinicopathologic and immunohistochemical study of 69 cases. Mayo Clin Proc 1990;65:461-474.
59. Hoyt WF, Kaplan SL, Grumbach MM, et al. Septo-optic dysplasia and pituitary dwarfism. Lancet 1970;1:893-894.
60. Baumann G. Heterogeneity of growth hormone. In Bercu B, ed. Basic and Clinical Aspects of Growth Hormone. New York: Plenum, 1988:13-31.
61. Frankenne F, Closset J, Gomez F, et al. The physiology of growth hormones (GHs) in pregnant women and partial characterization of the placental GH variant. J Clin Endocrinol Metab 1988;66: 1171-1180.
62. Cooke NE, Ray J, Watson MA, et al. Human growth hormone gene and the highly homologous growth hormone variant gene display different splicing patterns. J Clin Invest 1988;82:270-275.
63. Miller WL, Eberhardt NL. Structure and evaluation of the growth hormone gene family. Annu Rev Med 1983;34:519.
64. Frohman LA, Kineman RD, Kamegi J, et al. Secretagogues and the somatotrope: signaling and proliferation. Recent Prog Horm Res 2000;55:269-290.
65. Miller TL, Godfrey PA, Dealmeida VI, et al. The rat growth hormone-releasing hormone receptor gene structure, regulation, and generation of receptor isoforms with different signaling properties. Endocrinology 1999;140:4152-4165.
66. Mayo KE, Miller T, DeAlmeida V, et al. Regulation of the pituitary somatotroph cell by GHRH and its receptor. Recent Prog Horm Res 2000;55:237-266.
67. Kineman RD, Aleppo G, Frohman LA. The tyrosine hydroxylase-human growth hormone (GH) transgenic mouse as a model of hypothalamic GH deficiency: growth retardation is the result of a selective reduction in somatotrope numbers despite normal somatotrope function. Endocrinology 1996;137:4630-4636.
68. Valerius MT, Li H, Stock JL, Weinstein M, et al. Gsh-1: a novel murine homeobox gene expressed in the central nervous system. Dev Dynamics 1995;203:337-351.
69. Li H, Zeitler PS, Valerius MT, et al. Gsh-1, an orphan Hox gene, is required for normal pituitary development. EMBO J 1996;15: 714-724.
70. Hartman ML, Faria AC, Vance ML, et al. Temporal sequence of in vivo growth hormone secretory events in man. Am J Physiol 1991;260:E101-E110.
71. Frohman LA. Neurotransmitters as regulators of endocrine function. In Krieger DT, Hughes JC, eds. Neuroendocrinology. Sunderland, MA: Sinauer Associates, 1980.
72. Deller JJ, Plunket DC, Forsham PH. Growth hormone studies in growth retardation: therapeutic response to administration of androgen. Calif Med 1996;104:359.
73. Zeitler P, Argente J, Chowen-Breede JA, et al. Growth hormone releasing hormone messenger ribonucleic acid in the hypothalamus of the adult male rat is increased by testosterone. Endocrinology 1990;127:362-368.
74. Ho KY, Evans WS, Bilzzard RM, et al. Effects of sex and age on the 24-hour profile of growth hormone secretion in man: importance of endogenous estradiol concentrations. J Clin Endocrinol Metab 1987;64:51-58.
75. Katz HP, Youlton R, Kaplan SL, et al. Growth and growth hormone. III. Growth hormone release in children with primary hypothyroidism and thyrotoxicosis. J Clin Endocrinol Metab 1969;29: 346.
76. Frantz AG, Rabkin MT. Human growth hormone. Clinical measurement, response to hypoglycemia and suppression by corticosteroids. N Engl J Med 1964;271:1375-1381.
77. Thompson RG, Rodriguez A, Kowarski A, et al. Growth hormone: metabolic clearance rates in normal adults and effect of prednisone. J Clin Invest 1972;51:3193-3199.
78. Korbonits M, Grossman AB. Growth hormone-releasing peptide and its analogues. Trends Endocrinol Metab 1995;6:43-49.
79. Smith RG, Palyha OC, Feighner SD, et al. Growth hormone releasing substances: types and their receptors. Horm Res 1999;51: 1-8.
80. Kojima M, Hosoda H, Date Y, et al. Ghrelin is a growth-hormone-releasing acylated peptide from the stomach. Nature 1999;402: 656-660.
81. Date Y, Kojima M, Hosoda H, et al. Ghrelin, a novel growth hormone-releasing acylated peptide, is synthesized in a distinct endocrine cell type in the gastrointestinal tract of rats and humans. Endocrinology 2000;141:4255-4261.
82. Birnbacher R, Riedl S, Frisch H. Long-term treatment in children with hypopituitarism: pubertal development and final height. Horm Res 1998;49:80-85.
83. Takaya K, Ariyasu H, Kanamoto N, et al. Ghrelin strongly stimulates growth hormone (GH) release in humans. J Clin Endocrinol Metab 2000;85:4908-4911.
84. Hosada H, Kojima M, Matsuo H, et al. Purification and characterization of rat des-Gln14-Ghrelin, a second endogenous ligand for the growth hormone secretagogue receptor. J Biol Chem 2000;275:1995-2000.
85. Wren AM, Small CJ, Ward HL, et al. The novel peptide ghrelin stimulates food intake and growth hormone secretion. Endocrinology 2000;141:4325-4328.
86. Goth MI, Lyons CE, Canny BJ, et al. Pituitary adenylate cyclase activating polypeptides, growth hormone (GH) releasing peptide and GH releasing hormone stimulate GH release through distinct pituitary receptors. Endocrinology 1992;130:939-944.
87. Sherwood NM, Krueckl SL, McRory JE. The origin and function of the pituitary adenylate cyclase-activating polypeptide (PACAP)/glucagon superfamily. Endocrine Rev 2000;21:619-670.

88. Roessler E, Muenke M. Holoprosencephaly: a paradigm for the complex genetics of brain development. J Inher Metab Dis 1998;481-497.
89. Rosenfeld RG, Ceda G, Wilson DM, et al. Characterization of high-affinity receptors for insulin-like growth factors-I and -II on rat anterior pituitary cells. Endocrinology 1984;114:1571-1575.
90. Ceda GP, Hoffman AR, Silverberg GD, et al. Regulation of growth hormone release from cultured human pituitary adenomas of somatomedins and insulin. J Clin Endocrinol Metab 1985;60: 1204-1209.
91. Ceda GP, Davis RG, Rosenfeld RG, et al. The growth hormone (GH) releasing hormone (GHRH)-GH-somatomedin axis: evidence for rapid inhibition of GHRH-elicited GH release by insulin-like growth factors I and II. Endocrinology 1987;120:1658-1662.
92. Vaccarello MA, Diamond FB Jr, Guevara-Aguirre J, et al. Hormonal and metabolic affects and pharmacokinetics of recombinant insulin-like growth factor-I in growth hormone receptor deficiency (GHRD)/Laron syndrome. J Clin Endocrinol Metab 1993;77:273-280.
93. Hartman ML, Veldhuis JD, Thorner MO. Normal control of growth hormone secretion. Horm Res 1993;40:37-47.
94. Veldhuis JD, Liem AY, South S, et al. Differential impact of age, sex steroid hormones, and obesity on basal versus pulsatile growth hormone secretion in men as assessed in an ultrasensitive chemiluminescence assay. J Clin Endocrinol Metab 1995;80:3209-3222.
95. Martha PM Jr, Reiter EO. Pubertal growth and growth hormone secretion. Endocrinol Metab Clin North Am 1991;20:165-182.
96. Veldhuis JD, Johnson ML. Deconvolution analysis of hormone data. Methods Enzymol 1992;210:539-575.
97. Veldhuis JD, Roemmich JN, Rogol AD. Gender and sexual maturation-dependent contrasts in the neuroregulation of growth hormone secretion in prepubertal and late adolescent males and females—a general clinical research center-based study. J Clin Endocrinol Metab 2000;85:2385-2394.
98. Hartman ML, Pincus SM, Johnson ML, et al. Enhanced basal and disorderly growth hormone secretion distinguish acromegalic from normal pulsatile growth hormone release. J Clin Invest 1994;94:1277-1288.
99. Gill MS, Thalange NK, Foster PJ, et al. Regular fluctuations in growth hormone (GH) release determine normal human growth. Growth Horm IGF Res 1999;9:114-122.
100. Tillmann V, Gill MS, Thalange NK, et al. Short-term changes in growth and urinary growth hormone, insulin-like growth factor-I and markers of bone turnover excretion in healthy prepubertal children. Growth Horm IGF Res 2000;10:28-36.
101. Grumbach MM, Gluckman PD. The human fetal hypothalamic and pituitary gland: the maturation of neuroendocrine mechanisms controlling secretion of fetal pituitary growth hormone, prolactin, gonadotropin, adrenocorticotropin-related peptides and thyrotropin. In Tulchinsky D, Little AB, eds. Maternal and Fetal Endocrinology. Philadelphia: WB Saunders, 1994:193-261.
102. Kaplan SL, Grumbach MM, Aubert ML. The ontogenesis of pituitary hormones and hypothalamic factors in the human fetus: maturation of central nervous system regulation of anterior pituitary function. Recent Prog Horm Res 1976;32:161-243.
103. Siler-Khodr TM, Morgenstern IL, Greenwood FC. Hormone synthesis and release from human fetal adenohypophysis in vitro. J Clin Endocrinol Metab 1974;39:891-905.
104. Thliveris JA, Currie RW. Observations of the hypothalamophyseal portal vasculature in the developing human fetus. Am J Anat 1980;157:441-444.
105. Puy LA, Asa SL. The ontogeny of Pit-1 expression in the human fetal pituitary gland. Neuroendocrinology 1996;63:349-355.
106. Gluckman PD, Grumbach MM, Kaplan SL. The neuroendocrine regulation and function of growth hormone and prolactin in the mammalian fetus. Endocr Rev 1981;2:363-395.
107. Arosio M, Cortelazzi D, Persani L, et al. Circulating levels of growth hormone, insulin-like growth factor-I and prolactin in normal, growth-retarded and anencephalic human fetuses. J Endocrinol Invest 1995;18:346-353.
108. Martha PM Jr, Gorman KM, Blizzard RM, et al. Endogenous growth hormone secretion and clearance rates in normal boys, as determined by deconvolution analysis: relationship to age, pubertal status and body mass. J Clin Endocrinol Metab 1992;74:336-344.
109. Martha PM, Rogol AD, Veldhuis JD, et al. Alterations in the pulsatile properties of circulating growth hormone concentrations during puberty in boys. J Clin Endocrinol Metab 1989;69: 563-570.
110. Pincus SM, Veldhuis JD, Rogol AD. Longitudinal changes in growth hormone secretory process irregularity assessed transpubertally in healthy boys. Am J Physiol Endocrinol Metab 2000;279: E417-E424.
111. Martha PM Jr, Rogol AD, Blizzard RM, et al. Growth hormone-binding protein activity is inversely related to 24-hour growth hormone release in normal boys. J Clin Endocrinol Metab 1991;73:175-181.
112. Baumann G, Shaw MA, Amburn K. Circulating growth hormone binding proteins. J Endocrinol Invest 1994;17:67-81.
113. Moran A, Jacobs DR Jr, Steinberger J, et al. Association between the insulin resistance of puberty and the insulin-like growth factor-I/growth hormone axis. J Clin Endocrinol Metab 2002;87:4817-4820.
114. MacGillivray MH, Frohman LA, Doe J. Metabolic clearance and production rates of human growth hormone in subjects with normal and abnormal growth. J Clin Endocrinol Metab 1970;30: 632-638.
115. Rudman D, Kutner MH, Rogers CM, et al. Impaired growth hormone secretion in the adult population: relation to age and adiposity. J Clin Invest 1981;67:1361-1369.
116. Van Cauter E, Caufriez A, Kerkhofs M, et al. Sleep, awakenings, and insulin-like growth factor-I modulate the growth hormone (GH) secretory response to GH-releasing hormone. J Clin Endocrinol Metab 1992;74:1451-1459.
117. Veldhuis JD, Iranmanesh A, Ho KK, et al. Dual defects in pulsatile growth hormone secretion and clearance subserve the hyposomatotropism of obesity in man. J Clin Endocrinol Metab 1991; 72:51-59.
118. Schalch DS. The influence of physical stress and exercise on growth hormone and insulin secretion in man. J Lab Clin Med 1967;69:256.
119. Holl RW, Hartman ML, Veldhuis JD, et al. Thirty second sampling of plasma growth hormone in man: correlation with sleep stages. J Clin Endocrinol Metab 1991;72:854-861.
120. Jaffe CA, Turgeon DK, Friberg RD, et al. Nocturnal augmentation of growth hormone (GH) secretion is preserved during repetitive bolus administration of GH-releasing hormone: potential involvement of endogenous somatostatin—a clinical research center study. J Clin Endocrinol Metab 1995;80: 3321-3326.
121. Mauras N, Blizzard RM, Link K, et al. Augmentation of growth hormone secretion during puberty: evidence for a pulse amplitude-modulated phenomenon. J Clin Endocrinol Metab 1987; 64:596-601.
122. Keenan BS, Richards GE, Ponder SW, et al. Androgen-stimulated pubertal growth: the effects of testosterone and dihydrotestosterone on growth hormone and insulin-like growth factor-I in the treatment of short stature and delayed puberty. J Clin Endocrinol Metab 1993;76:996-1001.
123. Veldhuis JD, Metzger DL, Martha PM Jr, et al. Estrogen and testosterone, but not a nonaromatizable androgen, direct network integration of the hypothalamo-somatotrope (growth hormone)-insulin-like growth factor I axis in the human: evidence from pubertal pathophysiology and sex steroid hormone replacement. J Clin Endocrinol Metab 1997;82:3414-3420.
124. Rosenfeld RG, Rosenbloom AL, Guevara-Aguirre J. Growth hormone (GH) insensitivity due to primary GH receptor deficiency. Endocr Rev 1994;15:369-390.
125. Argente J, Caballo N, Barrios V, et al. Multiple endocrine abnormalities of the growth hormone and insulin-like growth factor axis in prepubertal children with exogenous obesity: effect of short- and long-term weight reduction. J Clin Endocrinol Metab 1997;82:2076-2083.
126. Attia N, Tamborlane WV, Heptulla R, et al. The metabolic syndrome and insulin-like growth factor I regulation in adolescent obesity. J Clin Endocrinol Metab 1998;83:1467-1471.
127. Metzger DL, Kerrigan JR. Estrogen blockade with tamoxifen diminishes growth hormone secretion in boys: evidence for a stimulatory role of endogenous estrogens during male adolescence. J Clin Endocrinol Metab 1994;79:513-518.

128. Martin-Hernandez T, Diaz-Galvez M, Torres-Cuadro A, et al. Growth hormone secretion in normal prepubertal children: importance of relations between endogenous secretion, pulsatility and body mass. Clin Endocrinol 1996;44:327-334.
129. Iranmanesh A, Lizarralde G, Veldhuis JD. Age and relative adiposity are specific negative determinants of the frequency and amplitude of growth hormone (GH) secretory bursts and the half-life of endogenous GH in healthy men. J Clin Endocrinol Metab 1991;73:1081-1088.
130. Leung DW, Spencer SA, Cachianes G, et al. Growth hormone receptor and serum binding protein: purification, cloning and expression. Nature 1987;330:537-543.
131. Trivedi B, Daughaday WH. Release of growth hormone binding protein from IM-9 lymphocytes by endopeptidase is dependent on sulfhydryl group inactivation. Endocrinology 1988;123: 2201-2206.
132. Smith WC, Kuniyoshi J, Talamantes F. Mouse serum growth hormone (GH) binding protein has GH receptor extracellular and substituted transmembrane domains. Mol Endocrinol 1989;3: 984-990.
133. Sadeghi H, Wang BS, Lumunglas AL, et al. Identification of the origin of the growth hormone-binding protein in rat serum. Mol Endocrinol 1990;4:1799-1805.
134. Kelly PA, Djiane J, Postel-Vinay M-C, et al. The prolactin/growth hormone receptor family. Endocr Rev 1991;12:235-251.
135. Barton DE, Foellmer BE, Wood WI, et al. Chromosome mapping of the growth hormone receptor gene in man and mouse. Cytogenet Cell Genet 1989;50:137-141.
136. Pantel J, Machinis K, Sobrier ML, et al. Species-specific alternative splice mimicry at the growth hormone receptor locus revealed by the lineage of retroelements during primate evolution. J Biol Chem 2000;275:18664-18669.
137. Dos SC, Essioux L, Teinturier C, et al. A common polymorphism of the growth hormone receptor is associated with increased responsiveness to growth hormone. Nat Genet 2004;36:720-724.
138. Binder G, Baur F, Schweizer R, et al. The d3-Growth Hormone (GH) receptor polymorphism is associated with increased responsiveness to GH in Turner syndrome and short small-for-gestational-age children. J Clin Endocrinol Metab 2006;91: 659-664.
139. Jorge AA, Marchisotti FG, Montenegro LR, et al. Growth hormone (GH) pharmacogenetics: influence of GH receptor exon 3 retention or deletion on first-year growth response and final height in patients with severe GH deficiency. J Clin Endocrinol Metab 2006;91:1076-1080.
140. Rosenfeld RG. Editorial: the pharmacogenomics of human growth. J Clin Endocrinol Metab 2006;91:795-796.
141. Bazan JF. Hemopoietic receptors and helical cytokines. Immunol Today 1990;11:350-354.
142. deVos AM, Ultsch M, Kossiakoff AA. Human growth hormone and extracellular domain of its receptor: crystal structure of the complex. Science 1992;255:306-312.
143. Wan Y, McDevitt A, Shen B, et al. Increased site 1 affinity improves biopotency of porcine growth hormone. Evidence against diffusion dependent receptor dimerization. J Biol Chem 2004;279: 44775-44784.
144. Brown RJ, Adams JJ, Pelekanos RA, et al. Model for growth hormone receptor activation based on subunit rotation within a receptor dimer. Nat Struct Mol Biol 2005;12:814-821.
145. Carter-Su C, Stubbart JR, Wang XY, et al. Phosphorylation of highly purified growth hormone receptors by a growth hormone receptor-associated tyrosine kinase. J Biol Chem 1989;264: 18654-18661.
146. Argetsinger LS, Campbell GS, Yang X, et al. Identification of JAK2 as a growth hormone receptor-associated tyrosine kinase. Cell 1993;74:237-244.
147. Yi W, Kim SO, Jiang J, et al. Growth hormone receptor cytoplasmic domain differentially promotes tyrosine phosphorylation of signal transducers and activators of transcription 5b and 3 by activated JAK2 kinase. Mol Endocrinol 1996;10:1425-1443.
148. Krempler A, Qi Y, Triplett AA, et al. Generation of a conditional knockout allele for the Janus kinase 2 (Jak2) gene in mice. Genesis 2004;40:52-57.
149. Hwa V, Rosenfeld RG. Downstream mechanisms of growth hormone action. In Deciphering Growth: Research and Perspectives in Endocrine Interactions. Berlin: Springer-Verlag, 2005.
150. Udy GB, Towers RP, Snell RG, et al. Requirement of STAT5b for sexual dimorphism of body growth rates and liver gene expression. Proc Natl Acad Sci U S A 1997;94:7239-7244.
151. Teglund S, McKay C, Schuetz E, et al. Stat5a and Stat5b proteins have essential and nonessential, or redundant, roles in cytokine responses. Cell 1998;93:841-850.
152. Rowland JE, Lichanska AM, Kerr LM, et al. In vivo analysis of growth hormone receptor signaling domains and their associated transcripts. Mol Cell Biol 2005;25:66-77.
153. Kofoed EM, Hwa V, Little B, et al. Growth hormone insensitivity associated with a STAT5b mutation. N Engl J Med 2003;349: 1139-1147.
154. Hwa V, Little B, Adiyaman P, et al. Severe growth hormone insensitivity resulting from total absence of signal transducer and activator of transcription 5b. J Clin Endocrinol Metab 2005;90: 4260-4266.
155. Woelfle J, Chia DJ, Rotwein P. Mechanisms of growth hormone (GH) action. Identification of conserved Stat5 binding sites that mediate GH-induced insulin-like growth factor-I gene activation. J Biol Chem 2003;278:51261-51266.
156. Schindler C, Darnell JE Jr. Transcriptional responses to polypeptide ligands: the JAK-STAT pathway. Ann Rev Biochem 1995;64: 621-651.
157. Ihle JN, Kerr IM. Jaks and Stats in signaling by the cytokine receptor family. Trends Genet 1995;11:69-74.
158. Dinerstein-Cali H, Ferrag F, Kayser C, et al. Growth hormone (GH) induces formation of protein complexes involving Stat5, Erk2, Shc and serine phosphorylated proteins. Mol Cell Endocrinol 2000;166:89-99.
159. Lewis MD, Horan M, Millar DS, et al. A novel dysfunctional growth hormone variant (Ile179Met) exhibits a decreased ability to activate the extracellular signal-regulated kinase pathway. J Clin Endocrinol Metab 2004;89:1068-1075.
160. Baumann G, Stolar MW, Amburn K, et al. A specific growth hormone-binding protein in human plasma: initial characterization. J Clin Endocrinol Metab 1986;62:134-141.
161. Herington AC, Ymer S, Stevenson J. Identification and characterization of specific binding proteins for growth hormone in normal human sera. J Clin Invest 1986;77:1817-1823.
162. Holl RW, Snehotta R, Siegler B, et al. Binding protein for human growth hormone: effects of weight and age. Horm Res 1991;35: 190-197.
163. Massa G, deZegher F, Vanderschueren-Lodeweyckz M. Serum growth hormone binding proteins in the human fetus and infant. Pediatr Res 1992;32:69-72.
164. Martha PM, Reiter EO, Davila N, et al. The role of body mass in the response to growth hormone therapy. J Clin Endocrinol Metab 1992;75:1470-1473.
165. Martha PM, Reiter EO, Davila N, et al. Serum growth hormone (GH)-binding protein/receptor: an important determinant of GH responsiveness. J Clin Endocrinol Metab 1992;75:1464-1469.
166. Daughaday WH, Trivedi B. Absence of serum growth hormone binding protein in patients with growth hormone receptor (Laron dwarfism). Proc Natl Acad Sci U S A 1987;84:4636-4640.
167. Baumann G, Shaw MA, Winter RJ. Absence of plasma growth hormone-binding protein in Laron-type dwarfism. J Clin Endocrinol Metab 1987;65:814-816.
168. Buchanan CR, Maheshwari HG, Norman MR, et al. Laron-type dwarfism with apparently normal high affinity serum growth hormone-binding protein. Clin Endocrinol (Oxf) 1991;35: 179-185.
169. Douquesnoy P, Sobrier ML, Duriez B. A single amino acid substitution in the exoplasmic domain of the human growth hormone (GH) receptor confers familial GH resistance (Laron syndrome) with positive GH-binding activity by abolishing receptor homodimerization. EMBO J 1994;13:1386-1395.
170. Woods KA, Fraser NC, Postel-Vinay MC, et al. A homozygous splice site mutation affecting the intracellular domain of the growth hormone (GH) receptor resulting in Laron syndrome with elevated GH-binding protein. J Clin Endocrinol Metab 1996;81: 1686-1690.
171. Hansen JA, Londberg K, Hilton DJ, et al. Mechanism of inhibition of growth hormone receptor signaling by suppressor of

cytokine signaling proteins. Mol Endocrinol 1999;13:1832-1843.
172. Metcalf D, Greenhalgh CJ, Viney E, et al. Gigantism in mice lacking suppressor cytokine signaling-2. Nature 2000;405:1069-1073.
173. Greenhalgh CJ, Bertolino P, Asa SL, et al. Growth enhancement in suppressor of cytokine signaling 2 (SOCS-2)-deficient mice is dependent on signal transducer and activator of transcription 5b (STAT5b). Mol Endocrinol 2002;16:1394-1406.
174. Colson A, Le Cam A, Maiter D, et al. Potentiation of growth hormone-induced liver suppressors of cytokine signaling messenger ribonucleic acid by cytokines. Endocrinology 2000;141:3687-3695.
175. Mao Y, Ling PR, Fitzgibbons TP, et al. Endotoxin-induced inhibition of growth hormone signaling in rat liver in vivo. Endocrinology 1999;140:5505-5515.
176. Takala J, Ruokonen E, Webster NR, et al. Increased mortality associated with growth hormone treatment in critically ill adults. N Engl J Med 1999;341:785-792.
177. Salmon WD Jr, Daughaday WH. A hormonally controlled serum factor which stimulates sulfate incorporation by cartilage in vitro. J Lab Clin Med 1957;49:825-836.
178. Daughaday WH, Rotwein P. Insulin-like growth factors I and II. Peptide, messenger ribonucleic acid and gene structures, serum and tissue concentrations. Endocr Rev 1989;10:68-91.
179. Sherwin RS, Schulman GA, Hendler R, et al. Effect of growth hormone on oral glucose tolerance and circulating metabolic rules in man. Diabetologia 1983;24:155-161.
180. Rosenfeld RG, Wilson DM, Dollar LA, et al. Both human pituitary growth hormone and recombinant DNA-derived human growth hormone cause insulin resistance at a postreceptor level. J Clin Endocrinol Metab 1982;54:1033-1038.
181. Green H, Morikawa M, Nixon T. A dual effector theory of growth hormone action. Differentiation 1985;29:195-198.
182. Gerich JE, Lorenzi M, Bier DM, et al. Effects of physiologic levels of glucagon and growth hormone on human carbohydrate and lipid metabolism. Studies involving administration of exogenous hormone during suppression of endogenous hormone secretion with somatostatin. J Clin Invest 1976;57:875-884.
183. Kostyo JL, Hotchkiss J, Knobil E. Stimulation of amino acid transport in isolated diaphragm by growth hormone added in vitro. Science 1959;130:1653-1656.
184. Hjalmarson A, Isaksson O, Ahmen K. Effects of growth hormone and insulin on amino acid transport in perfused rat heart. Am J Physiol 1969;217:1795-1802.
185. Carrel AL, Allen DB. Effects of growth hormone on body composition and bone metabolism. Endocrine 2000;12:163-172.
186. Griffin EE, Miller LL. Effects of hypophysectomy of liver donor on net synthesis of specific plasma proteins by the isolated perfused rat liver: modulation of synthesis of albumin, fibrinogen, alpha 1-acid glycoprotein, alpha 2-(acute phase)-globulin, and haptoglobin by insulin, cortisol, triiodothyronine, and growth hormone. J Biol Chem 1974;249:5062-5069.
187. Snyder DK, Clemmons DR, Underwood LE. Treatment of obese, diet-restricted subjects with growth hormone for 11 weeks: effects on anabolism, lipolysis, and body composition. J Clin Endocrinol Metab 1988;67:54-61.
188. Lupu F, Terwilliger JD, Lee K, et al. Roles of growth hormone and insulin-like growth factor I in mouse postnatal growth. Dev Biol 2001;229:141-162.
189. Burgi H, Muller WA, Humbel RE, et al. Non-suppressible insulin-like activity of human serum. I. Physicochemical properties, extraction and partial purification. Biochem Biophys Acta 1966;121:349-359.
190. Froesch ER, Zapf J, Meuli C, et al. Biological properties of NSILA-S. Adv Metab Disord 1975;8:211-235.
191. Dulak NC, Temin HM. A partially purified polypeptide fraction from rat liver cell conditioned medium with multiplication-stimulating activity for embryo fibroblasts. J Cell Physiol 1973;81:153-160.
192. Daughaday WH, Hall K, Raben MS, et al. Somatomedin: proposed designation for sulphation factor. Nature 1972;235:107.
193. Hall K, Takano K, Fryklund L, et al. Somatomedins. Adv Metab Disord 1975;8:19-46.
194. Van Wyk JJ, Underwood LE, Hintz RL, et al. The somatomedins: a family of insulin-like hormones under growth hormone control. Recent Prog Horm Res 1974;30:259-318.
195. Rinderknecht E, Humbel RE. The amino acid sequence of human insulin-like growth factor I and its structural homology with pro-insulin. J Biol Chem 1978;253:2769-2776.
196. Rinderknecht E, Humbel RE. Primary structure of human insulin-like growth factor II. FEBS Lett 1978;89:283-286.
197. Jansen M, Van Schaik SM, Van Tol H, et al. Nucleotide sequence of cDNAs encoding precursors of human insulin-like growth factor II (IGF-II) and an IGF-II variant. FEBS Lett 1985;179:243.
198. Zumstein PP, Luthi C, Humbel RE. Amino acid sequence of a variant pro-form of insulin-like growth factor II. Proc Natl Acad Sci U S A 1985;82:3169.
199. Gowan LK, Hampton B, Hill DJ, et al. Purification and characterization of a unique high molecular weight form of insulin-like growth factor II. Endocrinology 1987;121:449-458.
200. Daughaday WH, Emaneule MA, Brooks MH, et al. Insulin-like growth factor II synthesis and secretion by a leiomyosarcoma with associated hypoglycemia. N Engl J Med 1988;319:1434-1440.
201. Zapf J. Insulin-like growth factor binding proteins and tumor hypoglycemia. Trends Endocrinol Metab 1995;6:37-42.
202. Powell DR, Lee PD, Chang D, et al. Antiserum developed for the E-peptide region of insulin-like growth factor IA prohormone recognizes a serum protein by both immunoblot and radioimmunoassay. J Clin Endocrinol Metab 1987;65:868.
203. Sussenbach JS. The gene structure of the insulin-like growth factor family. Prog Growth Factor Res 1989;1:33-48.
204. Lund PK, Moats-Staats BM, Hynes MA, et al. Somatomedin-C/insulin-like growth factor-I and insulin-like growth factor-II mRNAs in rat fetal and adult tissues. J Biol Chem 1986;261:14539-14544.
205. Brown AL, Graham DE, Nissley SP, et al. Developmental regulation of insulin-like growth factor II mRNA in different rat tissues. J Biol Chem 1986;261:13144-13150.
206. Brissenden JE, Ullrich A, Francke U. Human chromosomal mapping of genes for insulin-like growth factors I and II and epidermal growth factor. Nature 1984;310:781-784.
207. Tricoli JV, Rall LB, Scott J, et al. Localization of insulin-like growth factor genes to human chromosomes 11 and 12. Nature 1984;310:784-785.
208. Bell GI, Gerhard DS, Fong NM, et al. Isolation of the human insulin-like growth factor genes. Insulin-like growth factor II and insulin genes are contiguous. Proc Natl Acad Sci U S A 1985;82:6450-6454.
209. Yoon JB, Berry SA, Seelig S, et al. An inducible nuclear factor binds to a growth hormone-regulated gene. J Biol Chem 1990;265:19947-19954.
210. Lowe WL Jr, Roberts CT Jr, Lasky SR, et al. Differential expression of alternative 5′ untranslated regions in mRNAs encoding rat insulin-like growth factor I. Proc Natl Acad Sci U S A 1987;84:8946-8950.
211. Murphy LJ, Friesen HG. Differential effects of estrogen and growth hormone on uterine and hepatic insulin-like growth factor I gene expression in the ovariectomized hypophysectomized rat. Endocrinology 1988;122:325-332.
212. Bonioli E, Taro M, Rosa CL, et al. Heterozygous mutations of growth hormone receptor gene in children with idiopathic short stature. Growth Horm IGF Res 2005;15:405-410.
213. Holthuizen PE, Rodenburg RJT, Scheper W, et al. Regulation of IGF-II gene expression and posttranscriptional processing of IGF-II mRNAs. In Baxter RC, Gluckman PD, Rosenfeld RG, eds. The Insulin-Like Growth Factors and Their Regulatory Proteins. Amsterdam: Elsevier Science, 1994:43-53.
214. Rappolee DA, Sturm KS, Behrendtsen O, et al. Insulin-like growth factor II acts through an endogenous growth pathway regulated by imprinting in early mouse embryos. Genes Dev 1992;6:939-952.
215. Nason KS, Binder ND, Labarta JI, et al. IGF-II and IGF-binding proteins increase dramatically during rabbit pregnancy. J Endocrinol 1996;148:121-130.
216. Stylianopoulou F, Herbert J, Soares MB, et al. Expression of the insulin-like growth factor II gene in the choroid plexus and the leptomeninges of the adult rat central nervous system. Cell Biol 1988;85:141-145.

217. Reeve AE, Eccles MR, Wilkins RJ, et al. Expression of insulin-like growth factor-II transcripts in Wilms tumour. Nature 1985;317: 258-260.
218. Ogawa O, Eccles MR, Szeto J, et al. Relaxation of insulin-like growth factor II gene imprinting implicated in Wilms' tumor. Nature 1993;362:749-751.
219. Zhan S, Shapiro D, Zhang L, et al. Concordant loss of imprinting of the human insulin-like growth factor II gene promoters in cancer. J Biol Chem 1995;270:27983-27986.
220. El-Badry OM, Helman LJ, Chatten J, et al. Insulin-like growth factor II-mediated proliferation of human neuroblastoma. J Clin Invest 1991;87:648-657.
221. Haselbacher GK, Irminger JC, Zapf J, et al. Insulin-like growth factor in human adrenal pheochromocytomas and Wilms tumors: expression of the mRNA and protein level. Proc Natl Acad Sci U S A 1987;84:1104-1106.
222. Rainier S, Johnson LA, Dobry CJ, et al. Relaxation of imprinted genes in human cancer. Nature 1993;362:747-749.
223. Tricoli JV, Rall LB, Karakousis CP, et al. Enhanced levels of insulin-like growth factor messenger RNA in human colon carcinomas and liposarcomas. Cancer Res 1986;46:6169-6173.
224. Werner H, Roberts CT Jr, LeRoith D. Transcriptional repression of the IGF-II and IGF-I receptor genes by tumor suppressor WT1: implications for normal kidney development and Wilms' tumor. In Baxter RC, Gluckman PD, Rosenfeld RG, eds. The Insulin-Like Growth Factors and Their Regulatory Proteins. Amsterdam: Elsevier Science, 1994:107-115.
225. Mahar ER, Reik W. Beckwith-Wiedemann syndrome: imprinting in clusters revisited. J Clin Invest 2000;105:247-252.
226. Ohlsson R, Nystrom A, Pfeifer-Ohlsson S, et al. IGF2 is parentally imprinted during human embryogenesis and in the Beckwith-Wiedemann syndrome. Nat Genet 1993;4:94-97.
227. DeChiara TM, Efstratiadis A, Robertson EJ. A growth-deficiency phenotype in heterozygous mice carrying an insulin-like growth factor II gene disrupted by targeting. Nature 1990;345:78-80.
228. Baker J, Liu JP, Robertson EJ, et al. Role of insulin-like growth factors in embryonic and postnatal growth. Cell 1993;75:73-82.
229. Giannoukakis N, Deal C, Paquette J, et al. Parental genomic imprinting of the human IGF2 gene. Nat Genet 1993;4:98-100.
230. Deal CL. Parental genomic imprinting. Curr Opin Pediatr 1995;7:445-458.
231. Mutter GL, Stewart CL, Chaponot ML, et al. Oppositely imprinted genes H19 and insulin-like growth factor 2 are coexpressed in human androgenetic trophoblast. Am J Hum Genet 1993;53: 1096-1102.
232. Steenman MJ, Rainier S, Dobry CJ, et al. Loss of imprinting of IGF2 is linked to reduced expression and abnormal methylation of H19 in Wilm's tumor patients. Nat Genet 1994;7:433-438.
233. Barlow DP, Stoger R, Hermann BG, et al. The mouse insulin-like growth factor type-2 receptor is imprinted and closely linked to the Tme locus. Nature 1991;349:84-87.
234. Efstratiadis A. Genetics of mouse growth. Int J Dev Biol 1998;42: 955-976.
235. Zhou Y, Xu BC, Maheshawari HG, He L, et al. A mammalian model for Laron syndrome produced by targeted disruption of the mouse growth hormone receptor/binding protein gene (the Laron mouse). Proc Nat Acad Sci U S A 1997;94:13215-13220.
236. Sims NA, Clement-Lacroix P, Da Ponte F, et al. Bone homeostasis in growth hormone receptor-null mice is restored by IGF-I but independent of Stat5. J Clin Invest 2000;1006:1095-1103.
237. Liu JP, Baker J, Perkins AS, et al. Mice carrying null mutations of the genes encoding insulin-like growth factor I (Igf-1) and type 1 IGF receptor (Igf1r). Cell 1993;75:73-82.
238. Woods KA, Camacho-Hubner C, Savage MO, et al. Intrauterine growth retardation and postnatal growth failure associated with deletion of the insulin-like growth factor I gene. N Engl J Med 1996;335:1342-1349.
239. Walenkamp MJ, Karperien M, Pereira AM, et al. Homozygous and heterozygous expression of a novel insulin-like growth factor-I mutation. J Clin Endocrinol Metab 2005;90:2855-2864.
240. Sjogren K, Liu JL, Blad K, et al. Liver-derived insulin-like growth factor I (IGF-I) is the principal source of IGF-I in blood but is not required for postnatal body growth in mice. Proc Nat Acad Sci U S A 1999;96:7088-7092.
241. Yakar S, Liu J-L, Stannard B, et al. Normal growth and development in the absence of hepatic insulin-like growth factor I. Proc Natl Acad Sci U S A 1999;96:7324-7329.
242. Le Roith D, Bondy C, Yakar S, et al. The somatomedin hypothesis: 2001. Endocrine Rev 2001;22:53-74.
243. Butler AA, LeRoith D. Minireview: tissue-specific versus generalized gene targeting of the igf1 and igf1r genes and their roles in insulin-like growth factor physiology. J Clin Endocrinol Metab 2001;142:1685-1688.
244. Ueki I, Ooi GT, Tremblay ML, et al. Inactivation of the acid labile subunit gene in mice results in mild retardation of postnatal growth despite profound disruptions in the circulating insulin-like growth factor system. Proc Natl Acad Sci U S A 2000;97: 6868-6873.
245. Le Roith D, Scavo L, Butler A. What is the role of circulating IGF-I? Trend Endocrinol Metab 2001;12:48-52.
246. Yakar S, Rosen CJ, Beamer WG, et al. Circulating levels of IGF-1 directly regulate bone growth and density. J Clin Invest 2002;110: 771-781.
247. Liu JP, Baker J, Perkins AS, et al. Mice carrying null mutations of the genes encoding insulin-like growth factor I (Igf-1) and type 1 IGF receptor (Igf1r). Cell 1993;75:73-82.
248. Abuzzahab MJ, Schneider A, Goddard A, et al. IGF-I receptor mutations resulting in intrauterine and postnatal growth retardation. N Engl J Med 2003;349:2211-2222.
249. Lau MM, Stewart CE, Liu Z, et al. Loss of the imprinted IGF2/cation-independent mannose 6-phosphate receptor results in fetal overgrowth and perinatal lethality. Genes Dev 1994;8: 2953-2963.
250. Nolan CM, Lawlor MA. Variable accumulation of insulin-like growth factor II in mouse tissues deficient in insulin-like growth factor II receptor. Int J Biochem Cell Biol 1999;31:1421-1433.
251. Filson AJ, Louvi A, Efstratiadis A, et al. Rescue of the T-associated maternal effect in mice carrying null mutations in Igf-2 and Igf2r, two reciprocally imprinted genes. Development 1993;118: 731-736.
252. Hall K. Quantitative determination of the sulphation factor activity in human serum. Acta Endocrinol (Kbh) 1970;63:338-350.
253. Phillips LS, Herington AC, Daughaday WH. Somatomedin stimulation of sulfate incorporation in porcine costal cartilage discs. Endocrinology 1974;94:856-863.
254. Garland JT, Lottes ME, Kozak S, et al. Stimulation of DNA synthesis in isolated chondrocytes by sulfation factor. Endocrinology 1972;90:1086-1090.
255. Garland JT, Buchanan F. Stimulation of RNA and protein synthesis in isolated chondrocytes by human serum. J Clin Endocrinol Metab 1976;43:842-846.
256. Meuli C, Froesch ER. Effects of insulin and of NSILA-S on the perfused rat heart: glucose uptake, lactate production and efflux of 3-O-methyl glucose. Eur J Clin Invest 1975;5:93-99.
257. Hall K, Takano K, Fryklund L. Radioreceptor assay for somatomedin A. J Clin Endocrinol Metab 1974;39:973-976.
258. Van Wyk JJ, Underwood LE, Baseman JB, et al. Explorations of the insulin-like and growth-promoting properties of somatomedin C by membrane receptor assays. Adv Metab Disord 1974;8: 128-150.
259. Zapf J, Kaufmann U, Eigenmann EJ, et al. Determination of non-suppressible insulin-like activity in human serum by a sensitive protein-binding assay. Clin Chem 1977;23:677-682.
260. Schalch DS, Heinrich UE, Koch JG, et al. Nonsuppressible insulin-like activity (NSILA). Development of a new sensitive competitive protein-binding assay for determination of serum levels. J Clin Endocrinol Metab 1978;46:664-671.
261. Furlanetto RW, Underwood LE, Van Wyk JJ, et al. Estimation of somatomedin-C levels in normals and patients with pituitary disease by radioimmunoassay. J Clin Invest 1977;60:646-756.
262. Zapf J, Walter H, Froesch ER. Radioimmunological determination of insulin-like growth factors I and II in normal subjects and in patients with growth disorders and extrapancreatic tumor hypoglycemia. J Clin Invest 1981;68:1321-1330.
263. Bala RM, Bhaumick B. Radioimmunoassay of a basic somatomedin: comparison of various assay techniques and somatomedin levels in various sera. J Clin Endocrinol Metab 1979;49:770-777.

264. Baxter RC, Axiak S, Raison RL. Monoclonal antibody against human somatomedin-C/insulin-like growth factor I. J Clin Endocrinol Metab 1982;54:474-476.
265. Rosenfeld RG, Wilson DM, Lee PD, et al. Insulin-like growth factors I and II in the evaluation of growth retardation. J Pediatr 1986;109:428-433.
266. Daughaday WH, Kapadia M, Mariz I. Serum somatomedin binding proteins: physiologic significance and interference in radioligand assay. J Lab Clin Med 1986;109:355-363.
267. Powell DR, Rosenfeld RG, Baker BK, et al. Serum somatomedin levels in adults with chronic renal failure: the importance of measuring insulin-like growth factor (IGF)-1 and -2 in acid chromatographed uremic serum. J Clin Endocrinol Metab 1986;63:1186-1192.
268. Horner JM, Liu F, Hintz RL. Comparison of [125I] somatomedin-A and [125I] somatomedin C radioreceptor assays for somatomedin peptide content in whole and acid-chromatographed plasma. J Clin Endocrinol Metab 1978;47:1287-1295.
269. Daughaday WH, Mariz IK, Blethen SL. Inhibition of access of bound somatomedin to membrane receptor and immunobinding sites: a comparison of radioreceptor and radioimmunoassay of somatomedin in native and acid-ethanol-extracted serum. J Clin Endocrinol Metab 1980;51:781-788.
270. Blum WF, Ranke MB, Bierich JR. A specific radioimmunoassay for IGF-II: the interference of IGF binding proteins can be blocked by excess IGF-I. Acta Endocrinol 1988;118:374-380.
271. Bang P, Ericksson U, Sara V, et al. Comparison of acid ethanol extraction and acid gel filtration prior to IGF-I and IGF-II radioimmunoassays: improvement of determinations in acid ethanol extracts by the use of a truncated IGF-I as radioligand. Acta Endocrinol (Copenh) 1991;124:620-629.
272. Khosravi MJ, Diamondi A, Mistry J, et al. Noncompetitive ELISA for human serum insulin-like growth factor-I. Clin Chem 1996;42:1147-1154.
273. Cohen P. Implications of IGF-I elevations in prostate cancer sera. J Nat Cancer Inst 1998;12:876-879.
274. Quarmby V, Quan C, Ling V, et al. How much insulin-like growth factor I (IGF-I) circulates? Impact of standardization on IGF-I assay accuracy. J Clin Endocrinol Metab 2000;83:1211-1216.
275. Bang P, Ahlsen M, Berg U, et al. Free insulin-like growth factor I: are we hunting a ghost? Horm Res 2001;55(suppl 2):84-93.
276. Bennett A, Wilson DM, Liu F, et al. Levels of insulin-like growth factor-I and -II in human cord blood. J Clin Endocrinol Metab 1983;57:609-612.
277. Gluckman PD, Barrett-Johnson JJ, Butler JH, et al. Studies of insulin-like growth factor I and II by specific radioligand assays in umbilical cord blood. Clin Endocrinol 1983;19:405-413.
278. Lassare C, Hardouin S, Daffos F, et al. Serum insulin-like growth factors and their binding proteins in the human fetus. Relationships with growth in normal subjects and in subjects with intrauterine growth retardation. Pediatr Res 1991;29:219-225.
279. Hall K, Hansson U, Lundin G, et al. Serum levels of somatomedins and somatomedin-binding protein in pregnant women with type I or gestational diabetes and their infants. J Clin Endocrinol Metab 1986;63:1300-1305.
280. Luna AM, Wilson DM, Wibbelsman CJ, et al. Somatomedins in adolescence: a cross-sectional study of the effect of puberty on plasma insulin-like growth factor I and II levels. J Clin Endocrinol Metab 1983;57:258-271.
281. Cara JF, Rosenfield RL, Furlanetto RW. A longitudinal study of the relationship of plasma somatomedin-C concentration to the pubertal growth spurt. Am J Dis Child 1987;141:562-564.
282. Cuttler L, Van Vliet G, Conte FA, et al. Somatomedin-C levels in children and adolescents with gonadal dysgenesis: differences from age-matched normal females and effect of chronic estrogen replacement therapy. J Clin Endocrinol Metab 1985;60:1087-1091.
283. Rosenfeld RG, Hintz RL, Johanson AJ, et al. Methionyl human growth hormone and oxandrolone in Turner syndrome: preliminary results of a prospective randomized trial. J Pediatr 1986;109:936-940.
284. Copeland KC. Effects of acute high dose and chronic low dose estrogen on plasma somatomedin-C and growth in patients with Turner's syndrome. J Clin Endocrinol Metab 1988;66:1278-1282.
285. Rudman D, Feller AG, Nagraj HS, et al. Effects of human growth hormone in men over 60 years old. N Engl J Med 1990;323:1-6.
286. Johanson AJ, Blizzard RM. Low somatomedin-C levels in older men rise in response to growth hormone administration. Johns Hopkins Med J 1981;149:115-117.
287. Donovan SM, Oh Y, Pham H, et al. Ontogeny of serum insulin-like growth factor binding proteins in the rat. Endocrinology 1989;125:2621-2627.
288. Glasscock GF, Gelber SE, Lamson G, et al. Pituitary control of growth in the neonatal rat: effects of neonatal hypophysectomy on somatic and organ growth, serum insulin-like growth factors (IGF)-I and -II levels, and expression of IGF binding proteins. Endocrinology 1990;127:1792-1803.
289. Moore DC, Ruvalcaba RH, Smith EK, et al. Plasma somatomedin-C as a screening test for growth hormone deficiency in children and adolescents. Horm Res 1982;16:49-55.
290. Reiter EO, Lovinger RD. The use of a commercially available somatomedin-C radioimmunoassay in patients with disorders of growth. J Pediatr 1981;99:720-724.
291. Rosenfeld RG. Biochemical diagnostic strategies in the evaluation of short stature: the diagnosis of insulin-like growth factor deficiency. Horm Res 1996;46:170-173.
292. Laron Z. The essential role of IGF-I: lessons from the long-term study and treatment of children and adults with Laron syndrome. J Clin Endocrinol Metab 1999;84:4397-4404.
293. Rosenfeld RG. The IGF system: new developments relevant to pediatric practice. In IGF-I and IGF Binding Proteins. Basic Research and Clinical Management. Basal: Karger, 2005:1-10.
294. Hintz RL, Clemmons DR, Underwood LE, et al. Competitive binding of somatomedin to the insulin receptors of adipocytes, chondrocytes and liver membranes. Proc Natl Acad Sci U S A 1972;69:2351-2353.
295. Megyesi K, Kahn CR, Roth J, et al. Insulin and non-suppressible insulin-like activity (NSILA-s): evidence for separate plasma membrane receptor sites. Biochem Biophys Res Commun 1974;57:307-315.
296. Oh Y, Muller H, Neely EK, et al. New concepts in insulin-like growth factor receptor physiology. Growth Reg 1993;3:113-123.
297. LeRoith D, Werner H, Beitner-Johnson D, et al. Molecular and cellular aspects of the insulin-like growth factor I receptor. Endocr Rev 1995;16:143-163.
298. Ullrich A, Gray A, Tam AW, et al. Insulin-like growth factor I receptor primary structure: comparison with insulin receptor suggests structural determinants that define functional specificity. EMBO J 1986;5:2503-2512.
299. Kato H, Faria TN, Stannard B, et al. Role of tyrosine kinase activity in signal transduction by the insulin-like growth factor-I (IGF-I) receptor. J Biol Chem 1993;265:2655-2661.
300. Kato H, Faria TN, Stannard B, et al. Essential role of tyrosine residues 1131, 1135, and 1136 of the insulin-like growth factor-I (IGF-I) receptor in IGF-I action. Mol Endocrinol 1994;8:40-50.
301. Yamaski H, Prager D, Gebremedhin S, et al. Human insulin-like growth factor I receptor 950 tyrosine is required for somatotroph growth factor signal transduction. J Biol Chem 1992;267:20953-20958.
302. Gronborg M, Wulff BS, Rasmussen JS, et al. Structure-function relationship of the insulin-like growth factor-I receptor tyrosine kinase. J Biol Chem 1993;258:23435-23440.
303. Abbott AM, Bueno R, Pedrini MT, et al. Insulin-like growth factor I receptor gene structure. J Biol Chem 1992;267:10759-10763.
304. Ullrich A, Bell JR, Chen EY, et al. Human insulin receptor and its relationship to the tyrosine kinase family of oncogenes. Nature 1985;313:756-761.
305. Bondy CA, Werner H, Roberts CT Jr, et al. Cellular pattern of insulin-like growth factor-I (IGF-I) and type I IGF receptor gene expression in early organogenesis: comparison with IGF-II gene expression. Mol Endocrinol 1990;4:1386-1398.
306. Werner H, Woloschak M, Adamo M, et al. Developmental regulation of the rat insulin-like growth factor I receptor gene. Proc Natl Acad Sci U S A 1989;86:7451-7455.
307. Lowe WL Jr, Adamo M, Werner H, et al. Regulation by fasting of rat insulin-like growth factor I and its receptor. Effects on gene expression and binding. J Clin Invest 1989;84:619-626.
308. Frattali AL, Pessin JE. Relationship between alpha subunit ligand occupancy and beta subunit autophosphorylation in insulin/

insulin-like growth factor-1 hybrid receptors. J Biol Chem 1993; 268:7393-7400.
309. Treadway JL, Morrison BD, Soos MA, et al. Transdominant inhibition of tyrosine kinase activity in mutant insulin/insulin-like growth factor I hybrid receptors. Proc Natl Acad Sci U S A 1991;88:214-218.
310. Shemer J, Adamo M, Wilson GL, et al. Insulin and insulin-like growth factor-I stimulate a common endogenous phosphoprotein substrate (pp185) in intact neuroblastoma cells. J Biol Chem 1987;262:15476-15482.
311. Kuhne MR, Pawson T, Lienhard GE, et al. The insulin receptor substrate-1 associates with the SH2-containing phosphotyrosine phosphatase Syp. J Biol Chem 1993;268:11479-11481.
312. Skolnik EY, Batzer A, Li N, et al. The function of GRB2 in linking the insulin receptor to ras signaling pathways. Science 1993;260:1953-1955.
313. Lee CH, Li W, Nishimura R, et al. Nck associates with the SH2 domain-docking protein IRS-1 in insulin-stimulated cells. Proc Natl Acad Sci U S A 1993;90:11713-11717.
314. Kadowaki T, Tanemoto H, Tobe K, et al. Insulin resistance and growth retardation in mice lacking insulin receptor substrate-1 and identification of insulin receptor substrate-2. Diabet Med 1996;13:103-108.
315. Tsuruzoe K, Emkey R, Kriauciunas KM, et al. Insulin receptor substrate 3 (IRS-3) and IRS-4 impair IRS-1- and IRS-2 mediated signaling. Mol Cell Biol 2001;21:26-38.
316. Sasaoka T, Rose DW, Juhn BH, et al. Evidence for a functional role of Shc proteins in mitogenic signaling induced by insulin, insulin-like growth factor-I, and epidermal growth factor. J Biol Chem 1994;269:13689-13694.
317. Lamphere L, Leinhard GE. Components of signaling pathways for insulin and insulin-like growth factor-I in muscle myoblasts and myotubes. Endocrinology 1992;131:2196-2202.
318. Oemar BS, Law NM, Rosenzweig SA. Insulin-like growth factor-I induces tyrosyl phosphorylation of nuclear proteins. J Biol Chem 1991;266:27241-27244.
319. Werner H, LeRoith D. The insulin-like growth factor-I receptor signaling pathways are important for tumorigenesis and inhibition of apoptosis. Crit Rev Oncol 1997;8:71-92.
320. Chao MV. Growth factor signaling: where is the specificity? Cell 1992;68:995-997.
321. Porcu P, Ferber A, Pietrzkowski Z, et al. The growth-stimulatory effect of Simian virus 40 T antigen requires the interaction of insulin-like growth factor I with its receptor. Mol Cell Biol 1992;12:5069-5077.
322. Baserga R. The double life of the IGF-I receptor. Receptor 1992;2: 261-266.
323. Sell C, Rubini M, Rubin R, et al. Simian virus 40 large tumor antigen is unable to transform mouse embryonic fibroblasts lacking type I insulin-like growth factor receptor. Proc Natl Acad Sci U S A 1993;90:11217-11221.
324. Kaleko M, Rutter WJ, Miller AD. Overexpression of the human insulin-like growth factor I receptor promotes ligand-dependent neoplastic transformation. Mol Cell Biol 1990;10:464-473.
325. Prager D, Li HL, Asa S, et al. Dominant negative inhibition of tumorigenesis in vivo by human insulin-like growth factor I receptor mutant. Proc Natl Acad Sci U S A 1994;91:2181-2185.
326. Alexandrides TK, Chen JH, Bueno R, et al. Evidence for two insulin-like growth factor I receptors with distinct primary structure that are differentially expressed during development. Regul Pept 1993;48:279-290.
327. Alexandrides TK, Smith RJ. A novel fetal insulin-like growth factor (IGF) I receptor. Mechanism for increased IGF-I and insulin-stimulated tyrosine kinase activity in fetal muscle. J Biol Chem 1989;264:12922-12930.
328. Garofalo RS, Rosen OM. Insulin and insulin-like growth factor I (IGF-I) receptors during central nervous system development: expression of two immunologically distinct IGF-I receptor b subunits. Mol Cell Biol 1989;9:2806-2817.
329. Tally M, Li CH, Hall K. IGF-2 stimulated growth mediated by the somatomedin type 2 receptor. Biochem Biophys Res Commun 1987;148:811-816.
330. Minniti CP, Kohn EC, Grubb JH, et al. The insulin-like growth factor II (IGF-II)/mannose 6-phosphate receptor mediates IGF-II-induced motility in human rhabdomyosarcoma cells. J Biol Chem 1992;267:9000-9004.
331. Nishimoto I, Murayama Y, Katada T, et al. Possible direct linkage of insulin-like growth factor-II receptor with guanine nucleotide-binding proteins. J Biol Chem 1989;264:14029-14038.
332. Moxham CP, Duronio V, Jacobs S. Insulin-like growth factor I receptor beta subunit heterogeneity. Evidence for hybrid tetramers composed of insulin-like growth factor I and insulin receptor heterodimers. J Biol Chem 1989;264:13238-13244.
333. Soos MA, Siddle K. Immunological relationships between receptors for insulin and insulin-like growth factor I. Evidence for structural heterogeneity of insulin-like growth factor I receptors involving hybrids with insulin receptors. Biochem J 1989;263: 553-563.
334. Moxham CP, Jacobs S. Insulin/IGF-I receptor hybrids: a mechanism for increasing receptor diversity. J Cell Biochem 1992;48: 136-140.
335. Misra P, Hintz RL, Rosenfeld RG. Structural and immunological characterization of insulin-like growth factor II binding to IM-9 cells. J Clin Endocrinol Metab 1986;63:1400-1405.
336. Soos MA, Field CE, Siddle K. Purified hybrid insulin/insulin-like growth factor-I, but not insulin, with high affinity. Biochem J 1993;290:419-425.
337. Kasuya J, Paz B, Madduz BA, et al. Characterization of human placental insulin-like growth factor-I/insulin hybrid receptors by protein microsequencing and purification. Biochemistry 1993;32:13531-13536.
338. Morgan DO, Edman JC, Strandring DN, et al. Insulin-like growth factor II receptor as a multifunctional binding protein. Nature 1987;329:301-307.
339. MacDonald RG, Pfeffer SR, Coussens L, et al. A single receptor binds both insulin-like growth factor II and mannose-6-phosphate. Science 1988;239:1134-1137.
340. Kornfeld S. Trafficking of lysosomal enzymes. FASEB J 1987;1: 462-468.
341. Rosenfeld RG, Conover CA, Hodges D, et al. Heterogeneity of insulin-like growth factor-I affinity for the insulin-like growth factor-II receptor: comparison of natural, synthetic and recombinant DNA-derived insulin-like growth factor-I. Biochem Biophys Res Commun 1987;143:195-205.
342. Beukers M, Oh Y, Zhang H, et al. [Leu27] insulin-like growth factor II is highly selective for the type II IGF receptor in binding, cross-linking and thymidine incorporation. Endocrinology 1991;128:1201-1203.
343. Furlanetto RW, DiCarlo JN, Wisehart C. The type II insulin-like growth factor receptor does not mediate deoxyribonucleic acid synthesis in human fibroblasts. J Clin Endocrinol Metab 1987;64:1142-1149.
344. Mottola C, Czech MP. The type II insulin-like growth factor receptor does not mediate DNA synthesis in H-35 hepatoma cells. J Biol Chem 1984;259:12705-12713.
345. Kiess W, Haskell JF, Lee L, et al. An antibody that blocks insulin-like growth factor (IGF) binding to the type II IGF receptor is neither an agonist nor an inhibitor of IGF-stimulated biologic response in L6 myoblasts. J Biol Chem 1987;162:12756-12761.
346. Adashi EY, Resnick CE, Rosenfeld RG. Insulin-like growth factor-I (IGF-I) hormonal action in cultured rat granulosa cells: mediation via type I but not type II IGF receptors. Endocrinology 1989;126:216-222.
347. Canfield WM, Kornfeld S. The chicken liver cation-independent mannose-6-phosphate receptor lacks the high affinity binding site for insulin-like growth factor II. J Biol Chem 1989;264:7100-7103.
348. Clairmont KB, Czech MP. Chicken and Xenopus mannose 6-phosphate receptors fail to bind insulin-like growth factor II. J Biol Chem 1989;264:16390-16392.
349. Rogers SA, Hammerman MR. Insulin-like growth factor II stimulates production of inositol triphosphate in proximal tubular basolateral membranes from canine kidney. Proc Natl Acad Sci U S A 1988;85:4037-4041.
350. Jonas HA, Cox AJ. Insulin-like growth factor binding to the atypical insulin receptors of a human lymphoid-derived cell line (IM-9). Biochem J 1990;266:737-742.
351. Feltz SM, Swanson SM, Wemmie JA, et al. Functional properties of an isolated heterodimeric human placenta insulin-like growth factor I complex. Biochemistry 1988;27:3234-3242.
352. Treadway JL, Morrison BD, Goldfine ID, et al. Assembly of insulin/insulin-like growth factor-1 hybrid receptors in vitro. J Biol Chem 1989;264:21450-21453.

353. Soos MA, Siddle K. Immunological relationships between receptors for insulin and insulin-like growth factor I. Biochemistry 1989;263:553-563.
354. Braulke T. Type -2 IGF receptor: a multi-ligand binding protein. Horm Metab Res 1999;31:242-246.
355. Kang JX, Bell J, Beard RL, et al. Mannose 6-phosphate/insulin-like growth factor II receptor mediates the growth -inhibitory effects of retinoids. Cell Growth Differ 1999;10:591-600.
356. Melnick M, Chen H, Buckley S, et al. Insulin-like growth factor II receptor, transforming growth factor-beta, and Cdk4 expression and the developmental epigenetics of mouse palate morphogenesis and dysmorphogenesis. Dev Dyn 1998;211:11-25.
357. Rechler MM. Insulin-like growth factor binding proteins. Vitam Horm 1993;47:1-114.
358. Jones JI, Clemmons DR. Insulin-like growth factors and their binding proteins: biological actions. Endocr Rev 1995;16:3-34.
359. Hintz RL, Liu F. Demonstration of specific plasma protein binding sites for somatomedin. J Clin Endocrinol Metab 1977;45:988-995.
360. Hossenlopp P, Surin D, Segovia-Quinson B, et al. Analysis of serum insulin-like growth factor binding proteins using western blotting: use of the method for titration of the binding proteins and competitive binding studies. Anal Biochem 1986;154: 138-143.
361. Bach LA, Headey SJ, Norton RS. IGF-binding proteins—the pieces are falling into place. Trends Endocrinol Metab 2005;16:228-234.
362. Brewer MT, Stetler GL, Squires CH, et al. Cloning, characterization, and expression of a human insulin-like growth factor binding protein. Biochem Biophys Res Commun 1988;152:1289-1297.
363. Jones JI, Gockerman A, Busby WH, et al. Insulin-like growth factor binding protein 1 stimulates cell migration and binds to the a5b1 integrin by means of its Arg-Gly-Asp sequence. Proc Natl Acad Sci U S A 1993;90:10553-10557.
364. Oh Y, Muller H, Pham H, et al. Non-receptor mediated, post-transcriptional regulation of insulin-like growth factor binding protein (IGFBP)-3 in Hs578T human breast cancer cells. Endocrinology 1992;131:3123-3125.
365. Oh Y, Muller H, Lamson G, et al. Insulin-like growth factor (IGF)-independent action of IGF binding protein (BP)-3 in Hs578T human breast cancer cells. Cell surface binding and growth inhibition. J Biol Chem 1993;268:14964-14971.
366. Oh Y, Muller HL, Pham H, et al. Demonstration of receptors for insulin-like growth factor binding protein-3 (IGFBP-3) on Hs578T human breast cancer cells. J Biol Chem 1993;268:26045-26048.
367. Ritvos O, Ranta T, Julkanen J, et al. Insulin-like growth factor (IGF) binding protein from human decidua inhibits the binding and biological action of IGF-I in cultured choriocarcinoma cells. Endocrinology 1988;122:2150-2157.
368. Ross M, Francis GL, Szabo L, et al. Insulin-like growth factor (IGF)-binding proteins inhibit the biological activities of IGF-I and IGF-II but not des-(1-3)-IGF-I. Biochem J 1989;258:267-272.
369. Clemmons DR, Cascieri MA, Camacho-Hubner C, et al. Discrete alterations of the insulin-like growth factor I molecule which alter its affinity for insulin-like growth factor-binding proteins result in changes in bioactivity. J Biol Chem 1990;265:12210-12216.
370. Okajima T, Nakamura K, Zhang H, et al. Sensitive colorimetric bioassays for insulin-like growth factor (IGF) stimulation of cell proliferation and glucose consumption: use in studies of IGF analogs. Endocrinology 1992;130:2201-2212.
371. Cohen P, Lamson G, Okajima T, et al. Transfection of the human insulin-like growth factor binding protein-3 gene into Balb/c fibroblasts inhibits cellular growth. Mol Endocrinol 1993;7:380-386.
372. Elgin RC, Busby WH, Clemmons DR. An insulin-like growth factor (IGF) binding protein enhances the biologic response to IGF-I. Proc Natl Acad Sci U S A 1987;84:3254-3258.
373. Hwa V, Oh Y, Rosenfeld RG. The insulin-like growth factor-binding protein (IGFBP) superfamily. Endocrine Rev 1999;20:761-787.
374. Giudice LC, Farrell EM, Pham H, et al. Insulin-like growth factor binding proteins in the maternal serum throughout gestation and in the puerperium: effects of a pregnancy-associated protease activity. J Clin Endocrinol Meta 1990;71:1330-1338.
375. Hossenlopp P, Segovia B, Lassaree C, et al. Evidence of enzymatic degradation of insulin-like growth factor binding proteins in the 150K complex during pregnancy. J Clin Endocrinol Metab 1990;71:797-805.
376. Cohen P, Graves HC, Peehl DM, et al. Prostate-specific antigen (PSA) is an insulin-like growth factor binding protein-3 protease found in seminal plasma. J Clin Endocrinol 1992;75:1046-1053.
377. Muller H, Oh Y, Gargosky SE, et al. Concentrations of insulin-like growth factor binding protein-3, insulin-like growth factors and IGFBP-3 protease activity in cerebrospinal fluid (CSF) of children with leukemia, brain tumors, or meningitis. J Clin Endocrinol Metab 1993;77:1113-1119.
378. Lee D-Y, Park S-K, Yorgin P, et al. Alteration in insulin-like growth factor binding proteins (IGFBPs) and IGFBP-3 protease activity in serum and urine from acute and chronic renal failure. J Clin Endocrinol Metab 1994;79:1376-1382.
379. Conover CA, De Leon DD. Acid-activated insulin-like growth factor-binding protein-3 proteolysis in normal and transformed cells. Role of cathepsin. J Biol Chem 1994;269:7076-7080.
380. Fowlkes JL, Enghild JJ, Suzuki K, et al. Matrix metalloproteinases degrade insulin-like growth factor-binding protein-3 in dermal fibroblast cultures. J Biol Chem 1994;269:16766-16773.
381. Gargosky SE, Pham H, Wilson KF, et al. Measurement and characterization of insulin-like growth factor binding protein-3 in human biological fluids: discrepancies between radioimmunoassay and ligand blotting. Endocrinology 1992;131:3051-3060.
382. Cohen P, Graves HC, Peehl DM, et al. Prostate-specific antigen (PSA) is an insulin-like growth factor binding protein-3 protease found in seminal plasma. J Clin Endocrinol Metab 1992;75: 1046-1053.
383. Angelloz-Nicoud P, Binoux M. Autocrine regulation of cell proliferation by the insulin-like growth factor (IGF) and IGF binding protein-3 protease system in a human prostate carcinoma cell line (PC-3). Endocrinology 1995;136:5485-5492.
384. Cohen P, Peehl DM, Graves HC, et al. Biological effects of prostate specific antigen as an insulin-like growth factor binding protein-3 protease. J Endocrinol 1994;142:407-415.
385. Fielder PJ, Pham H, Adashi EY, et al. Insulin-like growth factors (IGFs) block FSH-induced proteolysis of IGF-binding protein-5 (BP-5) in cultured rat granulosa cells. Endocrinology 1993;133: 415-418.
386. Oh Y, Muller HL, Lee DY, et al. Characterization of the affinities of insulin-like growth factor (IGF)-binding proteins 1-4 for IGF-I, IGF-II, IGF-I/insulin hybrid, and IGF-I analogs. Endocrinology 1993;132:1337-1344.
387. Leong SR, Baxter RC, Camerato T, et al. Structure and functional expression of acid labile subunit of the insulin-like growth factor binding protein complex. Mol Endocrinol 1992;6:870-876.
388. Baxter RC, Martin JL. Structure of the Mr 140,000 growth hormone-dependent insulin-like growth factor binding protein complex: demonstration by reconstitution and affinity labeling. Proc Natl Acad Sci U S A 1989;86:6898-6902.
389. Barreca A, Ponzani P, Arvigo M, et al. Effect of the acid-labile subunit on the binding of insulin-like growth factor (IGF)-binding protein-3 to $[^{125}I]$IGF-I. Endocrinol Metab 1995;80: 1318-1324.
390. Guler HP, Zapf J, Schmid C, et al. Insulin-like growth factors I and II in a healthy man. Estimations of half-lives and production rates. Acta Endocrinol 1989;121:753-758.
391. Zapf J, Hauri C, Waldvogel M, et al. Recombinant human insulin-like growth factor I induces its own specific carrier protein in hypophysectomized and diabetic rats. Proc Natl Acad Sci U S A 1989;86:3813-3817.
392. Clemmons DR, Thissen JP, Maes M, et al. Insulin-like growth factor-I (IGF-I) infusion into hypophysectomized or protein-deprived rats induces specific IGF binding proteins in serum. Endocrinology 1989;25:2967-2972.
393. Glasscock GF, Hein AN, Miller JA, et al. Effects of continuous infusion of insulin-like growth factor I and II, alone and in combination with thyroxine or growth hormone, on the neonatal hypophysectomized rat. Endocrinology 1992;130:203-210.
394. Wilson KF, Fielder PJ, Guevara-Aguirre J, et al. Long-term effects of insulin-like growth factor (IGF)-I treatment on serum IGFs and IGF binding proteins in adolescent patients with growth hormone receptor deficiency. Clin Endocrinol 1995;42:399-407.
395. Walker JL, Baxter RC, Young S, et al. Effects of recombinant insulin-like growth factor I on IGF binding proteins and the acid-labile subunit in growth hormone insensitivity syndrome. Growth Regulat 1993;3:109-112.
396. Gargosky SE, Wilson KF, Fielder PJ, et al. The composition and distribution of insulin-like growth factors (IGFs) and IGF-binding

proteins (IGFBPs) in the serum of growth hormone receptor-deficient patients: effects of IGF-I therapy on IGFBP-3. J Clin Endocrinol Metab 1993;77:1683-1689.
397. Gargosky SE, Tapanainen P, Rosenfeld RG. Administration of growth hormone (GH), but not insulin-like growth factor-I (IGF-I), by continuous infusion can induce the formation of the 150-kilodalton IGF-binding protein-3 complex in GH-deficient rats. Endocrinology 1994;134:2267-2276.
398. Bar RS, Boes M, Clemmons DR, et al. Insulin differentially alters transcapillary movement of intravascular IGFBP-1, IGFBP-2 and endothelial cell IGF binding proteins in rat heart. Endocrinology 1990;127:497-499.
399. Giudice LC, de Zegher F, Gargosky SE, et al. Insulin-like growth factors and their binding proteins in the term and preterm human fetus with normal and extremes of intrauterine growth and in the neonatal period. J Clin Endocrinol Metab 1995;80:1548-1555.
400. Rechler MM, Nissley SP. Insulin-like growth factors. In Sporn MB, Roberts AB, eds. Peptide Growth Factors and Their Receptors. Berlin: Springer-Verlag, 1990:263-367.
401. Okajima T, Iwashita M, Takeda Y, et al. Inhibitory effects of insulin-like growth factor (IGF)-binding proteins-1 and -3 on IGF-activated glucose consumption in mouse Balb/c 3T3 fibroblasts. J Endocrinol 1993;136:457-470.
402. Lamson G, Giudice LC, Cohen P, et al. Proteolysis of IGFBP-3 may be a common regulatory mechanism of IGF action in vivo. Growth Regulat 1993;3:91-95.
403. De Mellow JS, Baxter RC. Growth hormone-dependent insulin-like growth factor (IGF) binding protein both inhibits and potentiates IGF-I-stimulated DNA synthesis in human skin fibroblasts. Biochem Biophys Res Commun 1988;156:199-204.
404. Conover CA, Ronk M, Lombana F, et al. Structural and biological characterization of bovine insulin-like growth factor binding protein-3. Endocrinology 1990;127:2795-2803.
405. Oh Y, Muller HL, Ng L, et al. Transforming growth factor-beta-induced cell growth inhibition in human breast cancer cells is mediated through insulin-like growth factor binding protein-3 action. J Biol Chem 1995;270:13589-13592.
406. Conover CA, Bale LK, Durham SK, et al. Insulin-like growth factor (IGF) binding protein-3 potentiation of IGF action is mediated through the phosphotidylinositol-3-kinase pathway and is associated with alteration in protein kinase B/AKT sensitivity. Endocrinology 2000;141:3098-3103.
407. Rajah R, Valentinis B, Cohen P. Insulin-like growth factor (IGF) binding protein-3 induces apoptosis and mediates the effects of transforming growth factor-beta on programmed cell death through a p53- and IGF-independent mechanism. J Biol Chem 2000;275:33607-33613.
408. Liu B, Lee HY, Weinzimer SA, et al. Direct functional interactions between insulin-like growth factor-binding protein-3 and retinoid X receptor-alpha regulate transcriptional signaling and apoptosis. J Biol Chem 2000;275:33607-33613.
409. Villaudy J, Delbe J, Blat C, et al. An IGF binding protein is an inhibitor of FGF stimulation. J Cell Physiol 1991;149:492-496.
410. Bicsak TA, Simonaka M, Malkowski M, et al. Insulin-like growth factor binding protein (IGFBP) inhibition of granulosa cell function: effect of cyclic adenosine 3′, 5′-monophosphate, deoxyribonucleic acid synthesis, and comparison with the effect of an IGF-I antibody. Endocrinology 1990;126:2184-2189.
411. Valentis B, Bhala A, DeAngelis T, et al. The human insulin-like growth factor (IGF) binding protein-3 inhibits the growth of fibroblasts with a targeted disruption of the IGF-I receptor gene. Mol Endocrinol 1995;9:361-367.
412. Oh Y, Muller HL, Lamson G, et al. Insulin-like growth factor (IGF)-independent action of IGF binding protein-3 in Hs578T human breast cancer cells. J Biol Chem 1993;268:14964-14971.
413. Spagnoli A, Hwa V, Horton WA, et al. Antiproliferative effects of insulin-like growth factor binding protein-3 (IGFBP-3) in mesenchymal chondrogenic cell line RCJ3.1C5.18. J Biol Chem 2001; 276:5533-5540.
414. Oh Y, Muller HL, Ng L, et al. TGF-B2-induced cell growth inhibition in human breast cancer cells is mediated through IGFBP-3 action. J Biol Chem 1995;270:13589-13592.
415. Martin JL, Coverley JA, Pathson ST, et al. Insulin-like growth factor binding protein-3 production by MCF-7 breast cancer cells: stimulation by retinoic acid and cyclic adenosine monophosphate and differential effects of estradiol. Endocrinology 1995;136: 1219-1226.
416. Fontana JA, Burrows-Meszu A, Clemmons DR, et al. Retinoid modulation of insulin-like growth factor binding proteins and inhibition of breast carcinoma proliferation. Endocrinology 1991;128:1115-1122.
417. Sheikh MS, Shao ZM, Hussain A, et al. Regulation of insulin-like growth factor binding protein-1, 2, 3, 4, 5, and 6: synthesis, secretion, and gene expression in estrogen receptor-negative human breast cancer cells. J Cell Physiol 1993;155:556-567.
418. Huynh H, Yang X, Pollak M. Estradiol and antiestrogens regulate a growth inhibitory insulin-like growth factor binding protein-3 autocrine loop in human breast cancer cells. J Biol Chem 1996;271:1016-1021.
419. Leyen SA, Hembree JR, Eckert RL. Regulation of insulin-like growth factor-I binding protein-3 levels by epidermal growth factor and retinoic acid in cervical epithelial cells. J Cell Physiology 1994;160:265-274.
420. Buckbinder L, Talbott R, Velasco-Miguel S, et al. Induction of the growth inhibitor IGF-binding protein-3 by p53. Nature 1995;377: 646-649.
421. Lalou C, Lassarre C, Binoux M. A proteolytic fragment of insulin-like growth factor (IGF) binding protein-3 that fails to bind IGFs inhibits the mitogenic effects of IGF-I and insulin. Endocrinology 1996;137:3206-3212.
422. Lee YL, Hintz RL, James PM, et al. Insulin-like growth factor (IGF) bind protein complementary deoxyribonucleic acid from human HEP G2 hepatoma cells: predicted protein sequence suggests an IGF binding domain different from those of the IGF-I and IGF-II receptors. Molec Endocrinol 1988;2:404-411.
423. Drop SL, Valiquette G, Guyda HJ, et al. Partial purification and characterization of a binding protein for insulin-like activity (ILAs) in human amniotic fluid: a possible inhibitor of insulin-like activity. Acta Endocrinol (Copenh) 1979;90:505-518.
424. Moses AC, Freinkel AJ, Knowles BB, et al. Demonstration that a human hepatoma cell line produces a specific insulin-like growth factor carrier protein. J Clin Endocrinol Metab 1983;56: 1003-1008.
425. Rutanen EM, Koistinen R, Wahlstrom T, et al. Synthesis of placental protein 12 by human decidua. Endocrinology 1985;116: 1304-1309.
426. Koistinen R, Kalkkinen N, Huhtala M-L, et al. Placental protein 12 is a decidual protein that binds somatomedin and has an identical N-terminal amino acid sequence with somatomedin-binding protein from human amniotic fluid. Endocrinology 1986;118: 1375-1378.
427. Brinkman A, Groffen CA, Kortleve DJ, et al. Organization of the gene encoding the insulin-like growth factor binding protein IBP-1. Biochem Biophys Res Commun 1988;157:898-907.
428. Giudice LC, Irwin JC, Dsupin BA, et al. Insulin-like growth factors (IGFs), IGF binding proteins (IGFBPs) and IGFBP protease in human uterine endometrium. Their potential relevance to endometrial cyclic function and maternal-embryonic interactions. In Baxter RC, Gluckman PD, Rosenfeld RG, eds. The Insulin-Like Growth Factors and Their Regulatory Proteins. Amsterdam: Elsevier, 1994:351-361.
429. Adashi EY. Regulation of intrafollicular IGFBPs: possible relevance to ovarian follicular selection. In Baxter RC, Gluckman PD, Rosenfeld RG, eds. The Insulin-Like Growth Factors and Their Regulatory Proteins. Amsterdam: Elsevier, 1994:341-350.
430. Unterman TG, Simmons RA, Glick RP, et al. Circulating levels of insulin, insulin-like growth factor-I (IGF-I), IGF-II, and IGF-binding proteins in the small for gestational age fetal rat. Endocrinology 1993;132:327-336.
431. Lee PD, Conover CA, Powell DA. Regulation and function of insulin-like growth factor binding protein-1. Proc Soc Expl Biol Med 1993;204:4-29.
432. Thissen J-P, Ketelslegers J-M, Underwood LE. Nutritional regulation of the insulin-like growth factors. Endocr Rev 1994;15: 80-101.
433. Cotterill AM, Cowell CT, Baxter RC, et al. Regulation of the growth hormone-independent growth factor-binding protein in children. J Clin Endocrinol Metab 1988;67:882-887.

434. Powell DR, Suwanichkul A, Cubbage ML, et al. Insulin inhibits transcription of the human gene for insulin-like growth factor binding protein-1. J Biol Chem 1991;266:18868-18876.
435. Lewitt MS, Saunders H, Cooney GJ, et al. Effect of human insulin-like growth factor-binding protein-1 on the half-life and action of administered insulin-like growth factor-I in rats. J Endocrinol 1993;136:253-260.
436. Koistinen R, Itkonen O, Selenius P, et al. Insulin-like growth factor binding protein-1 inhibits binding of IGF-I on fetal skin fibroblasts but stimulates their DNA synthesis. Biochem Biophys Res Commun 1990;173:408-415.
437. Jones JI, D'Ercole AJ, Camacho-Hubner C, et al. Phosphorylation of insulin-like growth factor binding protein in cell culture and in vivo. Effects on affinity for IGF-I. Proc Natl Acad Sci USA 1991;88:7481-7485.
438. Binkert C, Margot JB, Landwehr J, et al. Structure of the human insulin-like growth factor binding protein-2 gene. Mol Endocrinol 1992;6:826-836.
439. Agarwal N, Hsieh CL, Sills D, et al. Sequence analysis, expression and chromosomal localization of a gene, isolated from a subtracted human retina cDNA library, that encodes an insulin-like growth factor binding protein (IGFBP2). Exp Eye Res 1991;52:549-561.
440. Lamson G, Pham H, Oh Y, et al. Expression of the BRL-3A insulin-like growth factor binding protein (rBP-30) in the rat central nervous system. Endocrinology 1989;123:1100-1102.
441. Bourner MJ, Busby WH, Seigel NR, et al. Cloning and sequence determination of bovine insulin-like growth factor binding protein-2 (IGFBP-2). Comparison of its structural and functional properties with IGFBP-1. J Cell Biochem 1992;48:215-226.
442. Wood TL, Rogler L, Streck RD, et al. Targeted disruption of IGFBP-2 gene. Growth Regul 1993;3:5-8.
443. Dai Z, Xing Y, Borney CM, et al. Human insulin-like growth factor binding protein-1 (hIGFBP-1) in transgenic mice. Characterization and insights into the regulation of IGFBP-1 expression. Endocrinology 1994;135:1316-1327.
444. Rosenfeld RG, Pham H, Conover CA, et al. Structural and immunological comparison of insulin-like growth factor (IGF) binding proteins of cerebrospinal and amniotic fluids. J Clin Endocrinol Metab 1989;68:636-646.
445. Binoux M, Hardouin S, Lassarre C, et al. Evidence for production by the liver of two IGF binding proteins with similar molecular weights but different affinities for IGF-I and IGF-II. Their relationship with serum and cerebrospinal fluid IGF binding proteins. J Clin Endocrinol Metab 1982;55:600-602.
446. Rosenfeld RG, Pham H, Oh Y, et al. Identification of insulin-like growth factor binding protein-2 (IGF-BP-2) and a low molecular weight IGF-BP in human seminal plasma. J Clin Endocrinol Metab 1989;69:963-965.
447. Cohen P, Peehl DM, Baker B, et al. Insulin-like growth factor axis abnormalities in prostatic stromal cells from patients with benign prostatic hyperplasia. J Clin Endocrinol Metab 1994;79:1410-1415.
448. Cohen P, Peehl DM, Stamey TA, et al. Elevated levels of insulin-like growth factor binding protein-2 in the serum of prostate cancer patients. J Clin Endocrinol Metab 1993;76:1031-1035.
449. Cubbage ML, Suwanichkal A, Powell DR. Insulin-like growth factor binding protein-3. Organization of the human chromosomal gene and demonstration of promoter activity. J Biol Chem 1990;265:12642-12649.
450. Gargosky SE, Giudice LC, Rosenfeld RG, et al. Different molecular and messenger ribonucleic acid forms of insulin-like growth factor binding protein-3 in the pregnant baboon. J Endocrinol 1995;147:449-461.
451. Arany E, Afford S, Strain AJ, et al. Different cellular synthesis of insulin-like growth factor binding protein-1 (IGFBP-1) and IGFBP-3 within human liver. J Clin Endocrinol Metab 1994;79:1871-1976.
452. Chin E, Zhou J, Dai J, et al. Cellular localization and regulation of gene expression for components of the insulin-like growth factor ternary binding complex. Endocrinology 1994;134:2498-2504.
453. Baxter RC. Insulin-like growth factor binding proteins in the human circulation. A review. Horm Res 1994;42:140-144.
454. Hoech WG, Mukku VR. Identification of the major sites of phosphorylation in IGF binding protein-3. J Cell Biochem 1994;56:262-273.
455. Holly J, Claffey DC, Cwyfan-Hughes SC, et al. Proteases acting on IGFBPs. Their occurrence and physiological significance. Growth Regul 1992;3:88-91.
456. Bang P, Brismar K, Rosenfeld RG. Increased proteolysis of insulin-like growth factor-binding protein-3 (IGFBP-3) in noninsulin-dependent diabetes mellitus serum, with elevation of a 29-kilodalton (kDa) glycosylated IGFBP-3 fragment contained in the approximately 130- to 150-kDa ternary complex. J Clin Endocrinol Metab 1994;78:1119-1127.
457. Janosi JB, Ramsland PA, Mott MR, et al. The acid-labile subunit of the serum insulin-like growth factor-binding protein complexes. Structural determination by molecular modeling and electron microscopy. J Biol Chem 1999;274:23328-23332.
458. Booth BA, Boes M, Andress DL, et al. IGFBP-3 and IGFBP-5 association with endothelial cells: role of C-terminal heparin binding domain. Growth Regul 1995;5:1-17.
459. Gao L, Ling N, Shimasaki S. Structure of the rat insulin-like growth factor binding protein-4 gene. Biochem Biophys Res Commun 1993;190:1053-1059.
460. Ceda GP, Fielder PJ, Henzel WJ, et al. Differential effects of insulin-like growth factor (IGF)-I and IGF-II on the expression of IGF binding proteins (IGFBPs) in a rat neuroblastoma cell line. Isolation and characterization of two forms of IGFBP-4. Endocrinology 1991;128:2815-2824.
461. Boes M, Booth BA, Sandra A, et al. Insulin-like growth factor binding protein (IGFBP)-4 accounts for the connective tissue distribution of endothelial cell IGFBPs perfused through the isolated heart. Endocrinology 1992;133:327-330.
462. Mohan S, Bautista CM, Wergedal J, et al. Isolation of an inhibitory insulin-like growth factor (IGF) binding protein from bone cell-conditioned medium. A potential local regulator of IGF action. Proc Natl Acad Sci U S A 1989;88:8338-8342.
463. Cheung PT, Wu J, Banach W, et al. Glucocorticoid regulation of an insulin-like growth factor binding protein-4 protease produced by a rat neuronal cell line. Endocrinology 1994;135:1328-1335.
464. Cohick WS, Gockerman A, Clemmons DR. Vascular smooth muscle cells synthesize two forms of insulin-like growth factor binding proteins which are regulated differently by the insulin-like growth factors. J Cell Physiol 1993;157:52-60.
465. Conover CA, Kiefer MC, Zapf J. Postranslational regulation of insulin-like growth factor binding protein-4 in normal and transformed human fibroblasts. J Clin Invest 1993;91:1129-1137.
466. Durham SK, Kiefer MC, Roggs BL, et al. Regulation of insulin-like growth factor binding protein-4 by a specific insulin-like growth factor binding protein-4 proteinase in normal osteoblast-like cells. Implications in bone cell physiology. J Bone Miner Res 1994;9:111-117.
467. Lee KO, Oh Y, Giudice LC, et al. Identification of insulin-like growth factor binding protein-3 (IGFBP-3) fragments and IGFBP-5 proteolytic activity in human seminal plasma. A comparison of normal and vasectomized men. J Clin Endocrinol Metab 1994;79:1367-1372.
468. Neely EK, Rosenfeld RG. Insulin-like growth factors (IGFs) reduce IGF-binding protein-4 (IGFBP-4) concentration and stimulate IGFBP-3 independently of IGF receptors in human fibroblasts and epidermal cells. Endocrinology 1992;130:985-993.
469. Fowlkes J, Freemark M. Evidence for a novel insulin-like growth factor (IGF)-dependent protease regulating IGF binding protein-4 in dermal fibroblasts. Endocrinology 1992;131:2071-2076.
470. Van Doorn J, Cornelissen AJ, van Buul-Offers SC. Plasma levels of insulin-like growth factor binding protein-4 (IGFBP-4) under normal and pathological conditions. Clin Endocrinol 2001;54:655-664.
471. Shimasaki S, Shimonaka J, Zhang HP, et al. Identification of five different insulin-like growth factor binding proteins (IGFBPs) from adult rat serum and molecular cloning of a novel IGFBP-5 in rat and human. J Biol Chem 1991;266:10646-10653.
472. Kiefer MC, Ioh RS, Bauer DM, et al. Molecular cloning of a new human insulin-like growth factor binding protein. Biochem Biophys Res Commun 1991;176:219-225.

473. Conover CA, Kiefer MC. Regulation and biological effect of endogenous insulin-like growth factor binding protein-5 in human osteoblast cells. J Clin Endocrinol Metab 1993;76:1153-1159.
474. Kiefer MC, Schmid C, Waldvogel M, et al. Characterization of recombinant human insulin-like growth factor binding proteins 4, 5 and 6 produced in yeast. J Biol Chem 1992;267:12692-12699.
475. Jones JL, Gockerman A, Busby WH Jr, et al. Extracellular matrix contains insulin-like growth factor binding protein-5: potentiation of the effects of IGF-I. J Cell Biol 1993;121:679-687.
476. Clemmons DR, Nam TJ, Busby WH, et al. Modification of IGF action by insulin-like growth factor binding protein-5. In Baxter RC, Gluckman PD, Rosenfeld RG, eds. The Insulin-Like Growth Factors and Their Regulatory Proteins. Amsterdam: Elsevier, 1994:183-191.
477. Andress DL, Birnbaum RS. Human osteoblast-derived insulin-like growth factor (IGF) binding protein-5 stimulates osteoblast mitogenesis and potentiates IGF action. J Biol Chem 1992;267: 22467-22472.
478. Adashi EY, Resnick CE, Hurwitz A, et al. The intra-ovarian IGF system. Growth Reg 1992;2:10-15.
479. Shimasaki S, Tanahashi H, Onoda N, et al. Transcriptional and posttranscriptional regulation of IGFBP-4 and -5 in cultured rat granulosa cells. In Baxter RC, Gluckman PD, Rosenfeld RG, eds. The Insulin-Like Growth Factors and Their Regulatory Proteins. Amsterdam: Elsevier, 1994:193-204.
480. Kiefer MC, Masiarz FR, Bauer DM, et al. Identification and molecular cloning of two new 30 kDa insulin-like growth factor binding proteins isolated from adult human serum. J Biol Chem 1991; 266:9043-9049.
481. Bach LA, Thotakura NR, Rechler MM. Human insulin-like growth factor binding protein-6 is O-glycosylated. Growth Reg 1993;3: 59-62.
482. Roghani M, Lassarre C, Zapf J, et al. Two insulin-like growth factor (IGF) binding proteins are responsible for the selective affinity for IGF-II of cerebrospinal fluid binding proteins. J Clin Endocrinol Metab 1991;73:658-666.
483. Rohan RM, Ricciarelli E, Kiefer MC, et al. Rat ovarian insulin-like growth factor binding protein-6, a hormonally regulated theca-interstitial-selective species with limited antigonadotropic activity. Endocrinology 1993;132:2507-2512.
484. Drop SL, Valiquette G, Guyda HJ, et al. Partial purification and characterization of a binding protein for insulin-like activity (ILAs) in human amniotic fluid: a possible inhibitor of insulin-like activity. Acta Endocrinol 1979;90:505-518.
485. Povoa G, Roovete A, Hall K. Cross-reaction of a serum somatomedin-binding protein in a radioimmunoassay developed for somatomedin-binding protein isolated from human amniotic fluid. Acta Endocrinol 1984;107:563-570.
486. Baxter RC, Cowell CT. Diurnal variation of growth hormone-independent binding protein for insulin-like growth factors in humans. Clin Endocrinol Metab 1987;65:432-440.
487. Baxter RC, Martin JL. Radioimmunoassay of growth hormone dependent insulin-like growth factor binding protein in human plasma. J Clin Invest 1986;78:1504-1512.
488. Blum WF, Ranke MB, Kietzmann K, et al. A specific radioimmunoassay for the growth hormone-dependent somatomedin-binding protein: its use for diagnosis of GH deficiency. J Clin Endocrinol Metab 1990;70:1292-1298.
489. Honda Y, Landale EC, Strong DD, et al. Recombinant synthesis of insulin-like growth factor-binding protein-4 (IGFBP-4): development, validation and application of a radioimmunoassay for IGFBP-4 in human serum and other biological fluids. J Clin Endocrinol Metab 1996;81:1389-1396.
490. Khosravi MJ, Diamandi A, Mistry J, et al. Acid-labile subunit of human insulin-like growth factor-binding protein complex: measurement, molecular, and clinical evaluation. J Clin Endocrinol Metab 1997;82:3944-3951.
491. Lehrer S, Rabin J, Stone J, et al. Association of an estrogen receptor variant with increased height in women. Horm Metab Res 1994;26:486-488.
492. Lorentzon M, Lorentzon R, Backstrom T, et al. Estrogen receptor gene polymorphism, but not estradiol levels, is related to bone density in healthy adolescent boys: a cross-sectional and longitudinal study. J Clin Endocrinol Metab 1990;84:4597-4601.
493. Matkovic V. Editorial: skeletal development and bone turnover revisited. J Clin Endocrinol Metab 1996;81:2013-2016.
494. Abrams SA, O'Brien KO, Stuff JE. Changes in calcium kinetics associated with menarche. J Clin Endocrinol Metab 1996; 81:2017-2020.
495. Slemenda CW, Reister TK, Hui SL, et al. Influences on skeletal mineralization in children and adolescents: evidence for varying effects of sexual maturation and physical activity. J Pediatr 1996;125:201-207.
496. Bailey DA, Martin AD, McKay HA, et al. Calcium accretion in girls and boys during puberty: a longitudinal analysis. J Bone Miner Res 2000;15:2245-2250.
497. Abrams SA, Griffin IJ, Hawthorne KM, et al. Height and height Z-score are related to calcium absorption in five- to fifteen-year-old girls. J Clin Endocrinol Metab 2005;90:5077-5081.
498. Theintz G, Buchs B, Rizzoli R, et al. Longitudinal monitoring of bone mass accumulation in healthy adolescents: evidence for a marked reduction after 16 years of age at the levels of lumbar spine and femoral neck in female subjects. J Clin Endocrinol Metab 1992;75:1060-1065.
499. Libanti C, Baylink DJ, Lois-Wenzel E, et al. Studies on the potential mediators of skeletal changes occurring during puberty in girls. J Clin Endocrinol Metab 1999;84:2807-2814.
500. Rubin K. Pubertal development and bone. Curr Opin Endocrinol Diab 7:65-70.
501. Schoenau E, Neu CM, Rauch F, et al. The development of bone strength at the proximal radius during childhood and adolescence. J Clin Endocrinol Metab 2001;86:613-618.
502. Bonjour J-P. Delayed puberty and peak bone mass. Eur J Endocrinol 1998;139:257-259.
503. Moreira-Andres MN, Canizo FJ, de la Cruz FJ, et al. Bone mineral status in prepubertal children with constitutional delay of growth and pubertal maturation. Eur J Endocrinol 1998;139:271-275.
504. Rosenfeld RG. The molecular basis of idiopathic short stature. Growth Horm IGF Res 2005;15 Suppl A:3-5.
505. Spranger J. International classification of osteochondrodysplasias. Eur J Pediatr 1992;151:407-415.
506. Pauli RM. Osteochondrodysplasia with mild clinical manifestations: a guide for endocrinologists and others. Growth Genet Horm 1995;11(1):1-5.
507. Maroteaux P. Nomenclature internationale des maladies osseuses constitutionnelles. Ann Radiol 1970;13:455-464.
508. Rimoin DL. International nomenclature of constitutional diseases of bone: revision—May 1977. J Pediatr 1978;93:614-616.
509. Shiang R, Thompson LM, Zhu Y-Z, et al. Mutations in the transmembrane domain of FGFR3 cause the most common genetic form of dwarfism, achondroplasia. Cell 1994;78:335-342.
510. Rousseau F, Bonaventure J, Legeai-Mallet L, et al. Mutations in the gene encoding fibroblast growth factor receptor-3 in achondroplasia. Nature 1994;371:252-254.
511. Francomano CA. The genetic basis of dwarfism. N Engl J Med 1995;332:58-59.
512. Bellus GA, Hefferon TW, Ortiz de Luna RI, et al. Achondroplasia is defined by recurrent G380R mutations of FGFR3. Am J Human Genet 1995;56:368-373.
513. Vajo Z, Francomano CA, Wilkin DJ. The molecular and genetic basis of fibroblast growth factor receptor 3 disorders: the achondroplasia family of skeletal dysplasia, Muenke craniosynostosis, and Crouzon syndrome with acanthosis nigricans. Endocr Rev 2000;21:23-39.
514. Yamate T, Kanzaki S, Tanaka H, et al. Growth hormone (GH) treatment in achondroplasia. J Pediatr Endocrinol 1993;6:45-52.
515. Hecht JT, Butler IJ. Neurologic morbidity associated with achondroplasia. J Child Neurol 1990;5:84-97.
516. Hahn YS, Engelhard HH, Naidish T, et al. Paraplegia resulting from thoracolumbar stenosis in a seven-month-old achondroplastic dwarf. Pediatr Neurosci 1989;15:39-43.
517. Waters KA, Kirjavainen T, Jimenez M, et al. Overnight growth hormone secretion in achondroplasia: deconvolution analysis, correlation with sleep state, and changes after treatment of obstructive sleep apnea. Pediatr Res 1996;39:547-553.
518. Chen L, Adar R, Yang X, et al. Gly369Cys mutation in mouse FGFR3 causes achondroplasia by affecting both chondrogenesis and osteogenesis. J Clin Invest 1999;104:1517-1525.

519. Chen L, Li C, Qiao W, et al. A Ser (365)→Cys mutation of fibroblast growth factor receptor 3 in mouse downregulates Ihh/PTHrP signals and causes severe achondroplasia. Hum Mol Genet 2001;10:457-465.
520. Ramaswami U, Hindmarsh PC, Brook CG. Geneotype and phenotype in hypochondroplasia. J Pediatr 1998;133:99-102.
521. Prinster C, Carrera P, Del Maschio M, et al. Comparison of clinical-radiological and molecular findings in hypochondroplasia. Am J Med Genet 1998;75:109-112.
522. Stollov I, Kilpatrick M, Tsipouras P. A common FGFR3 gene mutation is present in achondroplasia but not in hypochondroplasia. Am J Med Genet 1995;55:127-133.
523. Mullis PE, Patel MS, Brickell PM, et al. Growth characteristics and response to growth hormone therapy in patients with hypochondroplasia: genetic linkage of the insulin-like growth factor I gene at chromosome 12q23 to the disease in a subgroup of these patients. Clin Endocrinol 1991;34:265-274.
524. Ross JL, Kowal K, Quigley CA, et al. The phenotype of short stature homeobox gene (SHOX) deficiency in childhood: contrasting children with Leri-Weill dyschondrosteosis and Turner syndrome. J Pediatr 2005;147:499-507.
525. Schneider KU, Sabherwal N, Jantz K, et al. Identification of a major recombination hotspot in patients with short stature and SHOX deficiency. Am J Hum Genet 2005;77:89-96.
526. Ogata T, Fukami, M. Clinical features in SHOX haploinsufficiency: diagnostic and therapeutic implications. Growth Genet Horm 2004;20:17-23.
527. Marchini A, Marttila T, Winter A, et al. The short stature homeodomain protein SHOX induces cellular growth arrest and apoptosis and is expressed in human growth plate chondrocytes. J Biol Chem 2004;279:37103-37114.
528. Binder G, Ranke MB, Martin DD. Auxology is a valuable instrument for the clinical diagnosis of SHOX haploinsufficiency in school-age children with unexplained short stature. J Clin Endocrinol Metab 2003;88:4891-4896.
529. Bartels CF, Bukulmez H, Padayatti P, et al. Mutations in the transmembrane natriuretic peptide receptor NPR-B impair skeletal growth and cause acromesomelic dysplasia, type Maroteaux. Am J Hum Genet 2004;75:27-34.
530. Olney RC, Bukulmez H, Bartels CF, et al. Heterozygous mutations in natriuretic peptide receptor-B (NPR2) are associated with short stature. J Clin Endocrinol Metab 2006;91:1229-1232.
531. Anneren G, Tuvemo T, Gustafsson J. Growth hormone therapy in young children with Down syndrome and a clinical comparison of Down and Prader-Willi syndromes. Growth Horm IGF Res 2000;10(suppl B):87-91.
532. Turner Syndrome. Rosinfeld RG, Grumbach, MM (eds) New York: Marcel Dekker, 1990.
533. Turner Syndrome: Growth Promoting Therapies: Proceedings of a Workshop on Turner Syndrome. Amsterdam: Excerpta Medica, 1991.
534. Basic and Clinical Approach to Turner Syndrome: Proceedings of the 3rd International Symposium on Turner Syndrome. Amsterdam: Excerpta Medica, 1993.
535. Rochiccioli P, David M, Malpuech G, et al. Study of final height in Turner's syndrome: ethnic and genetic influences. Acta Paediatr 1994;83:305-308.
536. Nilsson KO, Wikland KA, Alm J, et al. Improved final height in girls with Turner's syndrome treated with growth hormone and oxandrolone. J Clin Endocrinol Metab 1996;81:635-640.
537. Rosenfeld RG, Attie KM, Frane J, et al. Growth hormone treatment of Turner syndrome: beneficial effect on adult height. J Pediatr 1998;132:319-324.
538. Ranke MB, Pfluger H, Rosendahl W, et al. Turner syndrome: spontaneous growth in 150 cases and review of the literature. Eur J Pediatr 1983;141:81-88.
539. Davenport ML, Punyasavatsut N, Gunther D, et al. Turner syndrome: a pattern of early growth failure. Acta Paediatr Suppl 1999;443:118-121.
540. Even L, Cohen A, Marbach N, et al. Longitudinal analysis of growth over the first 3 years of life in Turner's syndrome. J Pediatr 2000;137:460-464.
541. Davenport ML, Punyasavatsut N, Stewart PW, et al. Growth failure in early life: an important manifestation of Turner syndrome. Horm Res 2002;57:157-164.
542. Brook CG, Gasser T, Werder EA, et al. Height correlations between parents and mature offspring in normal subjects and in subjects with Turner's and Klinefelter's and other syndromes. Ann Hum Biol 1977;4:17-22.
543. Massa G, Vanderschueren-Lodeweyckx M, Malvaux P. Linear growth in patients with Turner syndrome: influence of spontaneous puberty and parental height. Eur J Pediatr 1990;149:246-250.
544. Blaschke RJ, Rappold GA. SHOX: growth, Leri-Weill and Turner syndromes. Trends Endocrinol Metab 2000;11:227-230.
545. Ross JL, Scott C Jr, Marttila P, et al. Phenotypes associated with SHOX deficiency. J Clin Endocrinol Metab 2001;86:5674-5680.
546. Kosho T, Muroya K, Nagai T, et al. Skeletal features and growth patterns in 14 patients with haploinsufficiency of SHOX: implications for the development of Turner syndrome. J Clin Endocrinol Metab 1999;84:4613-4621.
547. Clement-Jones M, Schiller S, Rao E, et al. The short stature homeobox gene SHOX is involved in skeletal abnormalities in Turner syndrome. Hum Mol Genet 2000;9:695-702.
548. Yaegashi N, Uehara S, Ogawa H, et al. Association of intrauterine growth retardation with monosomy of the terminal segment of the short arm of the X chromosome in patients with Turner's syndrome. Gynecol Obstet Invest 2000;50:237-241.
549. Ross JL, Long LM, Loriaux DL, et al. Growth hormone secretory dynamics in Turner syndrome. J Pediatr 1985;106:202-206.
550. Sas TC, De Muinck Keizer-Schrama SM, Stijnen T, et al. Normalization of height in girls with Turner syndrome after long-term growth hormone treatment: results of a randomized dose-response trial. J Clin Endocrinol Metab 1999;84:4607-4612.
551. Saenger P. Growth-promoting strategies in Turner's syndrome. J Clin Endocrinol Metab 1999;84:4345-4348.
552. Savendahl L, Davenport ML. Delayed diagnosis of Turner's syndrome: proposed guidelines for change. J Pediatr 2000;137: 455-459.
553. Hale DE, Cody JD, Baillargeon J, et al. The spectrum of growth abnormalities in children with 18q deletions. J Clin Endocrinol Metab 2000;85:4450-4454.
554. Cody JD, Semrud-Clikeman M, Hardies LJ, et al. Growth hormone benefits children with 18q deletions. Am J Med Genet A 2005; 137:9-15.
555. Lee PA, Kendig JW, Kerrigan JR. Persistent short stature, other potential outcomes, and the effect of growth hormone treatment in children who are born small for gestational age. Pediatrics 2003;112:150-162.
556. Smith GC, Smith MF, McNay MB, et al. First-trimester growth and the risk of low birth weight. N Engl J Med 1999;339:1817-1822.
557. Chaussain JL, Colle M, Ducret JP. Adult height in children with prepubertal short stature secondary to intrauterine growth retardation. Acta Paediatr Suppl 1994;399:72-73.
558. Seminara S, Rapisardi G, La Cauza F, et al. Catch-up growth in short-at-birth NICU graduates. Horm Res 2000;53:139-143.
559. Leger J, Limoni C, Collin D, et al. Prediction factors in the determination of final height in subjects born small for gestational age. Pediatr Res 1998;43:808-812.
560. Ali O, Cohen P. Insulin-like growth factors and their binding proteins in children born small for gestational age: implication for growth hormone therapy. Horm Res 2003;60(suppl 3): 115-123.
561. Gohlke BC, Huber A, Hecher K, et al. Fetal insulin-like growth factor (IGF)-I, IGF-II, and ghrelin in association with birth weight and postnatal growth in monozygotic twins with discordant growth. J Clin Endocrinol Metab 2005;90:2270-2274.
562. Ibanez L, DiMartino-Nardi J, Potau N, et al. Premature adrenarche-normal variant of forerunner of adult disease. Endocrine Rev 2000;21:671-696.
563. Barker DJ, Gluckman PD, Dodrey KM, et al. Fetal nutrition and cardiovascular disease in adult life. Lancet 1993;341:938-941.
564. Barker DJ. Growth in utero and coronary heart disease. Nutr Rev 1996;54:S1-S7.
565. Osmond C, Barker DJ. Fetal, infant, and childhood growth are predictors of coronary heart disease, diabetes, and hypertension in adult men and women. Environ Health Perspect 2000;108: 545-553.
566. Barker DJ. Fetal and infant origins of adult disease. London, Br Med J 1992.

567. Gluckman PD, Hanson MA. Living with the past: evolution, development, and patterns of disease. Science 2004;305:1733-1736.
568. Gluckman PD, Hanson MA, Morton SM, et al. Life-long echoes—a critical analysis of the developmental origins of adult disease model. Biol Neonate 2005;87:127-139.
569. Barker DJ, Bagby SP. Developmental antecedents of cardiovascular disease: a historical perspective. J Am Soc Nephrol 2005; 16:2537-2544.
570. Hofman PL, Cutfield WS, Robinson EM, et al. Insulin resistance in short children with intrauterine growth retardation. J Clin Endocrinol Metab 1997;82:402-406.
571. D'Ercole AJ, Underwood LE. Regulation of fetal growth by hormones and growth factors. In Falkner F, Tanner JM, eds. Human Growth: A Comprehensive Treatise, Vol I. Developmental Biology, Prenatal Growth. New York: Plenum, 1986:327-338.
572. Sizonenko PC, Aubert ML. Pre- and perinatal endocrinology. In Falkner F, Tanner JM, eds. Human Growth: A Comprehensive Treatise, Vol I. Developmental Biology, Prenatal Growth. New York: Plenum, 1986:339-376.
573. Gluckman P, Harding J. The regulation of fetal growth. In Hernandez M, Argente J, eds. Human Growth: Basic and Clinical Aspects. Amsterdam, Elsevier, 1992:253-276.
574. Cooke PS, Nicoll CS. Hormonal control of fetal growth. Physiologist 1983;26:317-323.
575. Kim JD, Nanto-Salonen K, Szczepankiewicz JR, et al. Evidence of pituitary regulation of somatic growth, insulin-like growth factors-I and -II and their binding proteins in the fetal rat. Pediatr Res 1993;33:144-151.
576. Wit JM, van Unen H. Growth of infants with neonatal growth hormone deficiency. Arch Dis Child 1992;67:920-924.
577. Gluckman PD, Gunn AJ, Wray A, et al. Congenital idiopathic growth hormone deficiency associated with prenatal and early postnatal growth failure. J Pediatr 1992;121:920-923.
578. DeLuca F, Bernasconi S, Blandino A, et al. Auxological, clinical, and neuroradiological findings in infants with early onset growth hormone deficiency. Acta Paediatr Scand 1995;84:561-565.
579. Jones JI, Clemmons DR. Insulin-like growth factors and their binding proteins: biological actions. Endocrine Rev 1995;16: 3-34.
580. Spencer JA, Chang TC, Jones J, et al. Third trimester fetal growth and umbilical venous blood concentrations of IGF-I, IGFBP-1, and growth hormone at term. Arch Dis Child 1995;73:F87-F90.
581. Leger J, Oury JF, Noel M, et al. Growth factors and intrauterine growth retardation. I. Serum growth hormone, insulin-like growth factor (IGF)-I, IGF-II, and IGF binding protein 3 levels in normally grown and growth-retarded human fetuses during the second half of gestation. Pediatr Res 1996;40:94-100.
582. Cianfarani S, Germani D, Rossi L, et al. IGF-I and IGF-binding protein-1 are related to cortisol in human cord blood. Eur J Endocrinol 1998;138:524-529.
583. Cance-Rouzaud A, Laborie S, Bieth E, et al. Growth hormone, insulin-like growth factor-I and insulin-like growth factor binding protein-3 are regulated differently in small-for-gestational-age and appropriate-for-gestational-age neonates. Biol Neonate 1998;73:347-355.
584. Ong K, Kratzsch J, Kiess W, et al. Size at birth and cord blood levels of insulin, insulin-like growth factor I (IGF-I), IGF-II, IGF-binding protein-1 (IGFBP-1), IGFBP-3, and soluble IGF-II/mannose-6-phosphate receptor in term human infants. J Clin Endocrinol Metab 2000;85:4266-4269.
585. Woods KA, Camacho-Hubner C, Barter D, et al. Insulin-like growth factor I gene deletion causing intrauterine growth retardation and severe short stature. Acta Paediatr Suppl 1997;423: 39-45.
586. Rosenfeld RG, Thorsson AV, Hintz RL. Increased somatomedin receptor sites in newborn circulating mononuclear cells. J Clin Endocrinol Metab 1979;48:456-461.
587. D'Ercole AJ. Somatomedins/insulin-like growth factors and fetal development. J Dev Physiol 1987;9:481-495.
588. Han VK, D'Ercole AJ, Lund PK. Cellular localization of somatomedin (insulin-like growth factor) messenger RNA in the human fetus. Science 1987;236:193-197.
589. Schoknecht PA, Ebner S, Skottner A, et al. Exogenous insulin-like growth factor-I increases weight gain in intrauterine growth-retarded neonatal pigs. Pediatr Res 1997;42:201-207.
590. Klempt M, Bingham B, Breier BH, et al. Tissue distribution and ontogeny of growth hormone receptor mRNA and ligand binding to hepatic tissue in the midgestation sheep fetus. Endocrinology 1993;132:1071-1077.
591. Gluckman PD, Butler JH, Elliott TB. The ontogeny of somatotropic binding sites in ovine hepatic membranes. Endocrinology 1983;112:1607-1612.
592. de Zegher F, Kimpen J, Raus J, et al. Hypersomatotropism in the dysmature infant at term and preterm birth. Biol Neonate 1990;58:188-191.
593. Wollmann HA, Ranke MB. GH treatment in neonates. Acta Paediatr 1996;85:398-400.
594. van Toledo-Eppinga L, Houdijk EC, Cranendonk A, et al. Effects of recombinant human growth hormone treatment in intrauterine growth-retarded preterm newborn infants on growth, body composition and energy expenditure. Acta Paediatr 1996;85:476-481.
595. Evain-Brion D. Hormonal regulation of fetal growth. Horm Res 1994;42:207-214.
596. Oliver MH, Harding JE, Breier BH, et al. Glucose but not a mixed amino acid infusion regulates insulin-like growth factor I concentrations in fetal sheep. Pediatr Res 1993;34:62-65.
597. Chard T. Insulin-like growth factors and their binding proteins in normal and abnormal fetal growth. Growth Regulation 1994;4:91-100.
598. Warshaw JB. Intrauterine growth restriction revisited. Growth Genet Horm 1992;8:5-8.
599. Milner RD. Nesidioblastosis unravelled. Arch Dis Child 1996;74: 369-372.
600. Soliman AT, Alsalmi I, Darwish A, et al. Growth and endocrine function after near total pancreatectomy for hyperinsulinemic hypoglycemia. Arch Dis Child 1996;74:379-385.
601. Albertsson-Wikland K, Boguszewski M, Karlberg J. Children born small for gestational age: postnatal growth and hormonal status. Horm Res 1998;49:7-13.
602. Hofman PL, Regan F, Cutfield WS. Prematurity—another example of perinatal metabolic programming? Horm Res 2006;66:33-39.
603. Euser AM, Finken MJ, Keijzer-Veen MG, et al. Associations between prenatal and infancy weight gain and BMI, fat mass, and fat distribution in young adulthood: a prospective cohort study in males and females born very preterm. Am J Clin Nutr 2005;81:480-487.
604. Atkinson SA, Randall-Simpson J. Factors influencing body composition of premature infants at term-adjusted age. Ann N Y Acad Sci 2000;904:393-399.
605. Woods KA, van Helvoirt M, Ong KK, et al. The somatotropic axis in short children born small for gestational age: relation to insulin resistance. Pediatr Res 2002;51:76-80.
606. Russell AA. A syndrome of "intrauterine" dwarfism recognizable at birth with craniofacial dysostosis, disproportionately short arms and other anomalies (5 examples). Proc R Soc Med 1954;47:1040-1044.
607. Silver HK. Asymmetry, short stature and variations in sexual development: syndrome of congenital malformations. Am J Dis Child 1964;107:495-515.
608. Angehrn V, Zachmann M, Prader A. Silver-Russell syndrome. Observations in 20 patients. Helv Paediatr Acta 1979;34:297-308.
609. Davies PS, Valley R, Preece MA. Adolescent growth and pubertal progression in the Silver-Russell syndrome. Arch Dis Child 1988;63:130-135.
610. Saal HM, Pagon RA, Pepin MG. Re-evaluation of Russell-Silver syndrome. J Pediatr 1985;107:733-737.
611. Wollman HA, Kirchner T, Enders H, et al. Growth and symptoms in Silver-Russell syndrome: review on the basis of 386 patients. Eur J Pediatr 1995;154:958-968.
612. Boguszewski M, Rosberg S, Albertsson-Wikland K. Spontaneous 24-hour growth hormone profiles in prepubertal small for gestational age children. J Clin Endocrinol Metab 1995;80:2599-2602.
613. Eggermann T, Wollmann HA, Kuner R, et al. Molecular studies in 37 Silver-Russell syndrome patients: frequency and etiology of uniparental disomy. Hum Genet 1998;100:415-419.
614. Hall JG. Russell-Silver syndrome begins to be unraveled. Growth Genet Horm 2000;16:35.
615. Monk D, Wakeling EL, Proud V, et al. Duplication of 7p11.2-p13, including GRB10, in Silver-Russell syndrome. Am J Hum Genet 2000;66:36-46.

616. Miyoshi N, Kuroiwa Y, Kohda T, et al. Identification of the Megl/Grb10 imprinted gene on mouse proximal chromosome 11, a candidate for the Silver-Russell syndrome gene. Proc Natl Acad Sci U S A 1998;95:1102-1107.
617. Lefebvre L, Viville S, Barton SC, et al. Abnormal maternal behavior and growth retardation associated with loss of the imprinted gene Mest. Nature Genetics 1998;20:163-169.
618. Blagitko N, Schulz U, Schinzel AA, et al. gamma2-COP, a novel imprinted gene on chromosome 7q32, defines a new imprinting cluster in the human genome. Hum Mol Genet 1999;8: 2387-2396.
619. Mann TP, Russell A. Study of a microcephalic midget of extreme type. Proc R Soc Med 1959;52:1024-1027.
620. Harper RG, Orti E, Baker RK. Birdheaded dwarfs (Seckel's syndrome). A familial pattern of developmental, dental, skeletal, genital, and central nervous system anomalies. J Pediatr 1967;70: 799-804.
621. Goodship J, Gill H, Carter J, et al. Autozygosity mapping of a Seckel syndrome locus to chromosome 3q22.1-q24. Am J Hum Genet 2000;67:498-503.
622. Collins E, Turner G. The Noonan syndrome—a review of the clinical and genetic features of 27 cases. J Pediatr 1973;83:941-950.
623. Kelnar CJ. Growth hormone therapy in Noonan syndrome. Horm Res 2000;53:77-81.
624. Tartaglia M, Mehler EL, Goldberg R, et al. Mutations in PTPN11, encoding the protein tyrosine phosphatase SHP-2, cause Noonan syndrome. Nat Genet 2001;29:465-468.
625. Kosaki K, Suzuki T, Muroya K, et al. PTPN11 (protein-tyrosine phosphatase, nonreceptor-type 11) mutations in seven Japanese patients with Noonan syndrome. J Clin Endocrinol Metab 2002;87:3529-3533.
626. Jongmans M, Otten B, Noordam K, et al. Genetics and variation in phenotype in Noonan syndrome. Horm Res 2004;62(suppl 3):56-59.
627. Patton MA. Noonan syndrome: a review. Growth Genet Horm 1994;10:1-3.
628. Ranke MB, Heidemann P, Knupfer C, et al. Noonan syndrome: growth and clinical manifestations in 144 cases. Eur J Pediatr 1988;148:22-27.
629. Witt DR, Keena BA, Hall JG, et al. Growth curves for height in Noonan syndrome. Clin Genet 1986;30:150-153.
630. Bernardini S, Spadoni GL, Cianfarani S, et al. Growth hormone secretion in Noonan's syndrome. J Pediatr Endocrinol 1991;4: 217-221.
631. Ferreira LV, Souza SA, Arnhold IJ, et al. PTPN11 (protein tyrosine phosphatase, nonreceptor type 11) mutations and response to growth hormone therapy in children with Noonan syndrome. J Clin Endocrinol Metab 2005;90:5156-5160.
632. Binder G, Neuer K, Ranke MB, et al. PTPN11 mutations are associated with mild growth hormone resistance in individuals with Noonan syndrome. J Clin Endocrinol Metab 2005;90:5377-5381.
633. Limal JM, Parfait B, Cabrol S, et al. Noonan syndrome: relationships between genotype, growth, and growth factors. J Clin Endocrinol Metab 2006;91:300-306.
634. Rosenbloom AL, DeBusk FL. Progeria of Hutchinson-Gilford: a caricature of aging. Am Heart J 1971;82:287-289.
635. MacDonald WB, Fitch KD, Lewis IC. Cockayne's syndrome. An heredo-familial disorder of growth and development. Pediatrics 1960;25:997-1007.
636. Bray GA, Dahms WT, Swerdloff RS, et al. The Prader-Willi syndrome. A study of 40 patients and review of the literature. Medicine 1983;62:59-80.
637. Jones KL. Smith's Recognizable Patterns of Human Malformation. Philadelphia: WB Saunders, 1988.
638. Gualillo O, Caminmos JE, Blanco M, et al. Ghrelin, a novel placental-derived hormone. Endocrinology 2001;142:788-794.
639. Edwards LE, Alton IR, Barrada MI, et al. Pregnancy in the underweight woman: course, outcome and growth patterns of the infant. Am J Obstet Gynecol 1979;135:297-302.
640. Ouellette EM, Rosett HL, Rosman NP, et al. Adverse effects on offspring of maternal alcohol abuse during pregnancy. N Engl J Med 1977;297:528-530.
641. Jones KL, Smith DW, Streissguth AP. Outcome in offspring of chronic alcoholic women. Lancet 1974;1:1076-1078.
642. Abel EL. Consumption of alcohol during pregnancy: a review of effects on growth and development of offspring. Hum Biol 1982;54:421-453.
643. Zuckerman B, Frank DA, Hingson R, et al. Effects of maternal marijuana and cocaine use on fetal growth. N Engl J Med 1989; 320:762-768.
644. Abel EL. Smoking during pregnancy: a review of effects on growth and development of offspring. Hum Biol 1980;52:593-625.
645. Hall K, Enberg G, Hellem D, et al. Somatomedin levels in pregnancy: longitudinal study in healthy subjects and in pregnancies with intrauterine growth retardation. J Clin Endocrinol Metab 1984;59:587-594.
646. Mirlesse V, Frankenne F, Alsat E, et al. Placental growth hormone levels in normal pregnancy and in pregnancies with intrauterine growth retardation. Pediatr Res 1993;34:439-442.
647. Hasegawa T, Hasegawa Y, Takada M, et al. The free form of insulin-like growth factor I increases in circulation during normal human pregnancy. J Clin Endocrinol Metab 1995;80:3284-3286.
648. Verhaeghe J, Bougoussa M, Van Herck E, et al. Placental growth hormone and IGF-I in a pregnant woman with Pit-1 deficiency. Clin Endocrinol 2000;53:656-647.
649. Li Y, Lemaire P, Behringer RR. Esx1, a novel X chromosome-linked homeobox gene expressed in mouse extraembryonic tissues and male germ cells. Dev Biol 1997;188:85-95.
650. Li Y, Behringer RR. Esx1 is an X-chromosome-imprinted regulator of placental development and fetal growth. Nat Genet 1998;20: 309-311.
651. Fohn LE, Behringer RR. ESX1L, a novel X chromosome-linked human homeobox gene expressed in the placenta and testis. Genomics 2001;74:105-108.
652. Graham GC, Adrianzen T, Rabold J, et al. Later growth of malnourished children. Am J Dis Child 1982;136:348-352.
653. Allen LH. Nutritional influences on linear growth: a general review. Eur J Clin Nutrition 1994;48(suppl 1):75-89.
654. Liu Y, Albertsson-Wikland K, Karlberg J. Long-term consequences of early linear growth retardation (stunting) in Swedish children. Pediatr Res 2000;47:475-480.
655. Pimstone B, Berbezat G, Hansen JD, et al. Growth hormone and protein-calorie malnutrition. Impaired suppression during induced hyperglycemia. Lancet 1967;2:1333-1334.
656. Beas F, Contreras I, Maccioni A, et al. Growth hormone in infant malnutrition: the arginine test in marasmus and kwashiorkor. Br J Nutr 1971;26:169-175.
657. Grant DB, Hambley J, Becker D, et al. Reduced sulphation factor in undernourished children. Arch Dis Child 1973;48:596-600.
658. Soliman AT, Hassan AE, Aref MK, et al. Serum insulin-like growth factors I and II concentrations and growth hormone and insulin responses to arginine infusion in children with protein-energy malnutrition before and after nutritional rehabilitation. Pediatr Res 1986;20:1122-1130.
659. Zamboni G, Dufillot D, Antoniazzi F, et al. Growth hormone-binding proteins and insulin-like growth factor-binding proteins in protein-energy malnutrition, before and after nutritional rehabilitation. Pediatr Res 1996;39:410-414.
660. Mayer E, Stern M. Growth failure in gastrointestinal diseases. Bailliere's Clin Endocrinol Metab 1992;6:645-663.
661. Phillips LS. Nutrition, somatomedins, and the brain. Metabolism 1986;35:78-87.
662. Donovan SM, Atilano LC, Hintz RL, et al. Differential regulation of the insulin-like growth factors (IGF-I and IGF-II) and IGF binding proteins during malnutrition in the neonatal rat. Endocrinology 1991;129:149-157.
663. Gunnell D, Miller LL, Rogers I, et al. Association of insulin-like growth factor I and insulin-like growth factor-binding protein-3 with intelligence quotient among 8- to 9-year-old children in the Avon Longitudinal Study of Parents and Children. Pediatrics 2005;116:e681-e686.
664. Martin RM, Smith GD, Mangtani P, et al. Association between breast feeding and growth: the Boyd-Orr cohort study. Arch Dis Child Fetal Neonatal Ed 2002;87:F193-F201.
665. Martin RM, Holly JM, Smith GD, et al. Could associations between breastfeeding and insulin-like growth factors underlie associations of breastfeeding with adult chronic disease? The Avon Longitudinal Study of Parents and Children. Clin Endocrinol (Oxf) 2005;62:728-737.

666. Ben Shlomo Y, Holly J, McCarthy A, et al. Prenatal and postnatal milk supplementation and adult insulin-like growth factor I: long-term follow-up of a randomized controlled trial. Cancer Epidemiol Biomarkers Prev 2005;14:1336-1339.
667. Fall CH, Pandit AN, Law CM, et al. Size at birth and plasma insulin-like growth factor-1 concentrations. Arch Dis Child 1995;73:287-293.
668. Pugliese MT, Lifshitz F, Grad G, et al. Fear of obesity: a cause of short stature and delayed puberty. N Engl J Med 1983;309:513-518.
669. Golden NH, Kreitzer P, Jacobson MS, et al. Disturbances in growth hormone secretion and action in adolescents with anorexia nervosa. J Pediatr 1994;125:655-660.
670. Root AW, Powers PS. Anorexia nervosa presenting as growth retardation in adolescents. J Adolesc Health Care 1983;4:25-30.
671. Russell GF. Premenarchal anorexia nervosa and its sequelae. J Psychiatr Res 1985;19:363-369.
672. Miller KK, Klibanski A. Amenorrheic bone loss. J Clin Endocrinol Metab 1999;84:1775-1783.
673. Soyka L, Fairfield WP, Klibanski A. Hormonal determinants and disorders of peak bone mass in children. J Clin Endocrinol Metab 2000;85:3951-3963.
674. Postel-Vinay M-C, Saab C, Gourmelen M. Nutritional status and growth hormone-binding protein. Horm Res 1995;44:177-181.
675. Counts DR, Gwirtsman H, Carlsson LM, et al. The effects of anorexia nervosa and refeeding on growth hormone-binding protein, the insulin-like growth factors (IGFs), and the IGF-binding proteins. J Clin Endocrinol Metab 1992;75:762-766.
676. Fleischman A, Brue C, Poussaint TY, et al. Diencephalic syndrome: a cause of failure to thrive and a model of partial growth hormone resistance. Pediatrics 2005;115:e742-e748.
677. Preece MA, Law CM, Davies PS. The growth of children with chronic paediatric disease. Clin Endocrinol Metab 1986;15:453-477.
678. Sentongo TA, Semeao EJ, Piccoli DA, et al. Growth, body composition, and nutritional status in children and adolescents with Crohn's disease. J Pediatr Gastroenterol Nutr 2000;31:33-40.
679. Savage MO, Beattie RM, Camacho-Hubner C, et al. Growth in Crohn's disease. Acta Paediatr Suppl 1999;88:89-92.
680. Lucuratolo N, Pugliese G, Pricci F, et al. The circulating insulin-like growth factor system in children with coeliac disease: an additional marker for disease activity. Diabetes Metab Res Rev 1999;15:254-260.
681. Auricchio S, Greco L, Troncone R. Gluten-sensitive enteropathy in childhood. Pediatr Clin North Am 1988;35:157-187.
682. DeLuca F, Astori M, Pandullo E, et al. Effects of a gluten-free diet on catch-up growth and height prognosis in coeliac children with growth retardation recognized after the age of 5 years. Eur J Pediatr 1988;47:188-191.
683. Stenhammer L, Fallstrom SP, Jansson G, et al. Coeliac disease in children of short stature without gastrointestinal symptoms. Eur J Pediatr 1986;145:185-186.
684. Radzikowski T, Zalewski TK, Kapuscinska A, et al. Short stature due to unrecognized coeliac disease. Eur J Pediatr 1988;147:334-335.
685. Hill ID, Dirks MH, Liptak GS, et al. Guideline for the diagnosis and treatment of celiac disease in children: recommendations of the North American Society for Pediatric Gastroenterology, Hepatology and Nutrition. J Pediatr Gastroenterol Nutr 2005;40:1-19.
686. Hoffenberg EJ, MacKenzie T, Barriga KJ, et al. A prospective study of the incidence of childhood celiac disease. J Pediatr 2003;143:308-314.
687. Hernandez M, Argente J, Navarro A, et al. Growth in malnutrition related to gastrointestinal diseases: coeliac disease. Horm Res 1992;38(suppl 1):79-84.
688. Bode SH, Bachmann EH, Gudmand-Hoyer E, et al. Stature of adult coeliac patients: no evidence for decreased attained height. Eur J Clin Nutr 1991;45:145-149.
689. Cacciari E, Corazza GR, Salardi S, et al. What will be the adult height of coeliac patients? Eur J Pediatr 1991;150:407-409.
690. Wine E, Reif SS, Leshinsky-Silver E, et al. Pediatric Crohn's disease and growth retardation: the role of genotype, phenotype, and disease severity. Pediatrics 2004;114:1281-1286.
691. Kirschner BS. Growth and development in chronic inflammatory bowel disease. Acta Paediar Scand Suppl 1990;366:98-104.
692. Gryboski JD, Spiro HM. Prognosis in children with Crohn's disease. Gastroenterology 1978;74:807-817.
693. Kanof ME, Lake AM, Bayless TM. Decreased height velocity in children and adolescents before the diagnosis of Crohn's disease. Gastroenterology 1988;95:1523-1527.
694. Cowan FJ, Warner JT, Dunstan J, et al. Inflammatory bowel disease and predisposition to osteopenia. Arch Dis Child 1997;76:325-329.
695. Slonim AE, Bulone L, Damore MB, et al. A preliminary study of growth hormone therapy for Crohn's disease. N Engl J Med 2000;342:1633-1637.
696. Mauras N, George D, Evans J, et al. Growth hormone has anabolic effects in glucocorticosteroid-dependent children with inflammatory bowel disease: a pilot study. Metabolism 2002;51:127-135.
697. Sawczenko A, Ballinger AB, Savage MO, et al. Clinical features affecting final adult height in patients with pediatric-onset Crohn's disease. Pediatrics 2006;118:124-129.
698. Wasserman D, Zemel BS, Mulberg AE, et al. Growth, nutritional status, body composition, and energy expenditure in prepubertal children with Alagille syndrome. J Pediatr 1999;134:172-177.
699. Viner RM, Forton JT, Cole TJ, et al. Growth of long term survivors of liver transplantation. Arch Dis Child 1999;80:235-240.
700. Bartosh SM, Thomas SE, Sutton MM, et al. Linear growth after pediatric liver transplantation. J Pediatr 1999;135:624-631.
701. Bucuvalas JC, Cutfield W, Horn J, et al. Resistance to the growth promoting and metabolic effects of growth hormone in children with chronic liver disease. J Pediatr 1990;117:397-402.
702. Russell WE. Growth hormone, somatomedins, and the liver. Semin Liver Dis 1985;5:46-58.
703. Donaghy A, Ross R, Gimson A, et al. Growth hormone, insulin-like growth factor binding proteins 1 and 3 in chronic liver disease. Hepatology 1995;21:680-688.
704. Quirk P, Owens P, Moyse K, et al. Insulin-like growth factors I and II are reduced in plasma from growth-retarded children with chronic liver disease. Growth Reg 1994;4:35-38.
705. Holt RI, Jones JS, Stone NM, et al. Sequential changes in insulin-like growth factor I (IGF-I) and IGF-binding proteins in children with endstage liver disease before and after successful orthotopic liver transplantation. J Clin Endocrinol Metab 1996;81:160-168.
706. Maghnie M, Barreca A, Ventura M, et al. Failure to increase insulin-like growth factor-I synthesis is involved in the mechanisms of growth retardation of children with inherited liver disorders. Clin Endocrinol 1998;48:747-755.
707. Shen XY, Holt RI, Miell JP, et al. Cirrhotic liver expresses low levels of the full-length and truncated growth hormone receptors. J Clin Endocrinol Metab 1998;83:2532-2538.
708. Sarna S, Sipila I, Vihervuori E, et al. Growth delay after liver transplantation in childhood: studies of underlying mechanisms. Pediatr Res 1995;38:366-372.
709. Codoner-French P, Bernard O, Alvarez F. Long-term follow-up of growth in height after successful liver transplantation. J Pediatr 1994;124:368-373.
710. Sarna S, Sipila I, Ronnholm K, et al. Recombinant human growth hormone improves growth in children receiving glucocorticoid treatment after liver transplantation. J Clin Endocrinol Metab 1996;81:1476-1482.
711. Rodeck B, Kardorff R, Melter M, et al. Improvement of growth after growth hormone treatment in children who undergo liver transplantation. J Pediatr Gastroenterol Nutr 2000;31:286-290.
712. Bayer LM, Robinson SJ. Growth history of children with congenital heart defects. Am J Dis Child 1969;117:564-572.
713. Feldt RH, Strickler GB, Weidman WH. Growth of children with congenital heart disease. Am J Dis Child 1969;117:573-579.
714. Gilger M, Mensen C, Kessler B, et al. Nutrition, growth and the gastrointestinal system: basic knowledge for the pediatric cardiologist. In Garson A Jr, Bricker JT, McNamara DG, eds. The Science and Practice of Pediatric Cardiology. Philadelphia: Lea & Febiger, 1990:2354-2370.
715. Mehrizi A, Drash A. Growth disturbances in congenital heart disease. J Pediatr 1962;61:418-429.
716. Nadas AS, Rosenthal A, Crigler JF. Nutritional considerations in the prognosis and treatment of children with congenital heart disease. In Suskind RM, ed. Textbook of Pediatric Nutrition. New York: Raven Press, 1987:537-544.

717. McLean WC. Protein energy malnutrition. In Grand RJ, Sutphen JL, Dietz WH, eds. Pediatric Nutrition: Theory and Practice. Stoneham, MA: Butterworth's, 1987:421-431.
718. Naeye RL. Anatomic features of growth failure in congenital heart disease. Pediatrics 1967;39:433-440.
719. Wahlig TM, Georgieff MK. The effects of illness on neonatal metabolism and nutritional management. Clin Prenatal 1995; 22:77-79.
720. Leitch CA, Karn CA, Ensing GJ, et al. Energy expenditure after surgical repair in children with cyanotic congenital heart disease. J Pediatr 2000;137:381-385.
721. Leitch CA, Karn CA, Peppard RJ, et al. Increased energy expenditure in infants with cyanotic congenital heart disease. J Pediatr 1998;133:755-760.
722. Linde LM, Dunn OJ, Schireson R, et al. Growth in children with congenital heart disease. J Pediatr 1967;70:413-419.
723. Barton JS, Hindmarsh PC, Preece MA. Serum insulin-like growth factor I in congenital heart disease. Arch Dis Child 1996; 75:162-163.
724. Bernstein D, Jasper JR, Rosenfeld RG, et al. Decreased serum insulin-like growth factor-I associated with growth failure in newborn lambs with experimental cyanotic heart disease. J Clin Invest 1992;89:1128-1132.
725. Soliman AT, El Naway A, El Azzoni O, et al. Growth parameters and endocrine function in relation to echocardiographic parameters in children and adolescents with compensated rheumatic heart disease. J Trop Pediatr 1997;43:4-9.
726. Schuurmans FM, Pulles-Heintzberger CF, Gerver WJ, et al. Long-term growth of children with congenital heart disease: a retrospective study. Acta Paediatr 1998;87:1250-1255.
727. Holliday MA. Symposium on metabolism and growth in children with kidney disease. Kidney Int 1978;14:299-382.
728. Kohaut EC. Chronic renal disease and growth in childhood. Curr Opin Pediatr 1995;7:171-175.
729. Mehls O, Blum WF, Schaefer F, et al. Growth failure in renal disease. Bailliere's Clin Endocrinol Metab 1992;6:665-685.
730. Lee D-Y, Park SK, Kim J-S. Insulin-like growth factor-I (IGF-I) and IGF-binding proteins in children with nephrotic syndrome. J Clin Endocrinol Metab 1996;81:1856-1860.
731. Kuizon BD, Salusky IB. Growth retardation in children with chronic renal failure. J Bone Miner Res 1999;14:1680-1690.
732. Kimonis VE, Troendle J, Rose SR, et al. Effects of early cysteamine therapy on thyroid function and growth in nephropathic cystinosis. J Clin Endocrinol Metab 1995;80:3257-3261.
733. Warady BA, Jabs K. New hormones in the therapeutic arsenal of chronic renal failure. Pediatr Clin North Am 1995;42:1551-1577.
734. Tonshoff B, Mehls O. Growth retardation in children with chronic renal insufficiency: current aspects of pathophysiology and treatment. J Nephrol 1955;8:133-142.
735. Tonshoff B, Veldhuis JD, Heinrich U, et al. Deconvolutuion analysis of spontaneous nocturnal growth hormone secretion in prepubertal children with preterminal chronic renal failure and with end-stage renal disease. Pediatr Res 1995;37:86-93.
736. Ramirez G, O'Neill WM Jr, Bloomer A, et al. Abnormalities in the regulation of growth hormone in chronic renal failure. Arch Intern Med 1978;138:267-271.
737. Hokken-Koelega AC, Hackeng WH, Stijen T, et al. Twenty-four-hour plasma growth hormone (GH) profiles, urinary GH excretion, and plasma insulin-like growth factor-I and -II levels in prepubertal children with chronic renal insufficiency and severe growth retardation. J Clin Endocrinol Metab 1990;71:688-695.
738. Schaefer F, Hamill G, Stanhope R, et al. Cooperative Study Group on Pubertal Development in Chronic Renal Failure 1991. Pulsatile growth hormone secretion in peri-pubertal patients with chronic renal failure. J Pediatr 1991;119:568-577.
739. Blum WF. Insulin-like growth factors (IGFs) and IGF binding proteins in chronic renal failure: evidence for reduced secretion of IGFs. Acta Paediatr Scand Suppl 1991;379:24-31.
740. Tonshoff B, Eden S, Weiser E, et al. Reduced hepatic growth hormone (GH) receptor gene expression and increased plasma GH binding protein in experimental uremia. Kidney Int 1994;45:1085-1092.
741. Schaefer F, Chen Y, Tsao T, et al. Impaired JAK-STAT signal transduction contributes to growth hormone resistance in chronic uremia. J Clin Invest 2001;108:467-475.
742. Rabkin R, Sun DF, Chen Y, et al. Growth hormone resistance in uremia, a role for impaired JAK/STAT signaling. Pediatr Nephrol 2005;20:313-318.
743. Hokken-Koelega AC, Stijnen T, De Muinck Keizer-Schrama SM, et al. Placebo-controlled, double-blind, cross-over trial of growth hormone treatment in prepubertal children with chronic renal failure. Lancet 1991;338:585-590.
744. Rees L, Maxwell H. The hypothalamo-pituitary-growth hormone insulin-like growth factor 1 axis in children with chronic renal failure. Kidney Int 1996;47(Suppl 53):S109-S114.
745. Blum WF, Ranke MB, Kietzmann K, et al. Growth hormone resistance and inhibition of somatomedin activity by excess of insulin-like growth factor binding protein in uremia. Pediatr Nephrol 1991;5:539-545.
746. Saenger P, Wiedemann E, Schwartz E, et al. Somatomedin and growth after renal transplantation. Pediatr Res 1974;8:162-169.
747. Hokken-Koelega AC, Stijnen T, De Muinck Keizer-Schrama SM, et al. Levels of growth hormone, insulin-like growth factor-I (IGF-I) and -II, IGF-binding protein-1 and -3, and cortisol in prednisone-treated children with growth retardation after renal transplantation. J Clin Endocrinol Metab 1993;77:932-938.
748. Hanna JD, Santos F, Foreman JW. Insulin-like growth factor-I gene expression in the tibial epiphyseal growth plate of growth hormone-treated uremic rats. Kidney Int 1995;17:1374-1382.
749. Unterman TG, Phillips LS. Glucocorticoid effects on somatomedins and somatomedin inhibitors. J Clin Endocrinol Metab 1985;61:618-626.
750. Allen DB. Growth suppression by glucocorticoid therapy. Pediatr Rounds 1995;4:1-5.
751. Fine RN, Tejani A. Renal transplantation in children. Nephron 1987;47:81-86.
752. Ding H, Gao X-L, Hirschberg R, et al. Impaired actions of insulin-like growth factor I on protein synthesis and degradation in skeletal muscle of rats with chronic renal failure: evidence for a postreceptor defect. J Clin Invest 1996;97:1064-1075.
753. Hokken-Koelega AC, Van Zaal MA, de Ridder MA, et al. Growth after renal transplantation in prepubertal children: impact of various treatment modalities. Pediatr Res 1994;35:367-371.
754. Hokken-Koelega AC, Van Zaal MA, Van Bergen W, et al. Final height and its predictive factors after renal transplantation in childhood. Pediatr Res 1994;36:323-328.
755. Tejani A, Fine R, Alexander S, et al. Factors predictive of sustained growth in children after renal transplantation. J Pediatr 1993; 122:397-402.
756. Schaefer F, Haffner D, Wuhl E, et al. Long-term experience with growth hormone treatment in children with chronic renal failure. Perit Dial Int 1999;19(suppl 2):467-472.
757. Fine RN. Growth post renal-transplantation in children: lessons from the North American Pediatric Renal Transplant Cooperative Study (NAPRTCS). Pediatr Transplant 1997;1:85-89.
758. Tejani A, Stablein DM, Donaldson L, et al. Steady improvement in short-term graft survival of pediatric renal transplants: the NAPRTCS experience. Clin Transpl 1999;95-110.
759. Millam MT, Sarwal MM, Lemley KV, et al. A 100% 2-year graft survival can be attained in high-risk 158 kg or smaller infant recipients of kidney allografts. Arch Surg 2000;135:1063-1068.
760. Kari JA, Romagnoli J, Duffy P, et al. Renal transplantation in children under 5 years of age. Pediatr Nephrol 2000;13:730-736.
761. Ellis D. Growth and renal function after steroid-free tacrolimus-based immunosuppression in children with renal transplants. Pediatr Nephrol 2000;14:689-694.
762. Hokken-Koelega AC, de Ridder MA, De Muinck Keizer-Schrama SM, et al. Growth hormone treatment in growth-retarded adolescents after renal transplant. Lancet 1994;343:1313-1317.
763. Van Dop C, Jabs KL, Donohoue PA, et al. Accelerated growth rates in children treated with growth hormone after renal transplantation. J Pediatr 1992;120:244-250.
764. Ingulli E, Tejani A. An analytical review of growth hormone studies in children after renal transplantation. Pediatr Nephrol 1995;9:S61-S65.
765. Riedl S, Lebl J, Kluge M, et al. Treatment of peripubertal children after renal transplantation (RTX) with recombinant human growth hormone: auxological and effects on insulin-like growth factor-I (IGF-I) and IGF-binding protein-3 (IGFBP-3) during 24 months. J Pediatr Endocrinol Metab 1998;11:713-718.

766. Henderson RA, Saavedra JM, Dover GJ. Prevalence of impaired growth in children with homozygous sickle cell anemia. Am J Med Sci 1994;307:405-407.
767. Modebe O, Ifenu SA. Growth retardation in homozygous sickle cell disease: role of calorie intake and possible gender-related differences. Am J Hematol 1994;44:149-154.
768. Singhal A, Thomas P, Cook R, et al. Delayed adolescent growth in homozygous sickle cell disease. Arch Dis Child 1994;71: 404-408.
769. Wang WC, Morales KH, Scher CD, et al. Effect of long-term transfusion on growth in children with sickle cell anemia: results of the STOP trial. J Pediatr 2005;147:244-247.
770. Saka N, Sukur M, Bundak R, et al. Growth and puberty in thalassemia major. J Pediatr Endocrinol Metab 1995;8:181-186.
771. Filosa A, Di Maio S, Baron I, et al. Final height and body disproportion in thalassemic boys and girls with spontaneous or induced puberty. Acta Paediatr 2000;89:1295-1301.
772. Low LC, Kwan EY, Lim YJ, et al. Growth hormone treatment of short Chinese children with β-thalassemia major without GH deficiency. Clin Endocrinol 1995;42:359-363.
773. DeLuca G, Maggioline M, Bria M, et al. GH secretion in thalassemic patients with short stature. Horm Res 1995;44:158-163.
774. Scacchi M, Danesi L, DeMartin M, et al. Treatment with biosynthetic growth hormone of short thalassemic patients with impaired growth hormone secretion. Clin Endocrinol 1991;35: 335-339.
775. Masala A, Atzeni MM, Alagna S, et al. Growth hormone secretion in polytransfused prepubertal patients with homozygous beta-thalassemia. Effect of long-term recombinant GH (recGH) therapy. J Endocrinol Invest 2003;26:623-628.
776. Cavallo L, De Sanctis V, Cisternino M, et al. Final height in short polytransfused thalassemia major patients treated with recombinant growth hormone. J Endocrinol Invest 2005;28:363-366.
777. La Rosa C, De Sanctis V, Mangiagli A, et al. Growth hormone secretion in adult patients with thalassaemia. Clin Endocrinol (Oxf) 2005;62:667-671.
778. Wajnrajch MP, Gertner J, Huma Z, et al. Evaluation of growth and hormonal status in patients referred to the international Fanconi anemia registry. Pediatrics 2001;107:744-754.
779. McNair SL, Stickler GB. Growth in familial hypophosphatemic vitamin-D-resistant rickets. N Engl J Med 1969;281:512-516.
780. Malone JI. Growth and sexual maturation in children with insulin-dependent diabetes mellitus. Curr Opin Ped 1993;5:494-498.
781. Thon A, Heinze E, Feilen KD, et al. Development of height and weight in children with diabetes mellitus: report on two prospective multicentre studies, one cross-sectional, one longitudinal. Eur J Pediatr 1992;151:258-262.
782. Bognetti E, Cristina M, Bonfanti R, et al. Growth changes in children and adolescents with short-term diabetes. Diabetes Care 1998;21:1226-1229.
783. Hjelt K, Braendholt V, Kamper J, et al. Growth in children with diabetes mellitus. Dan Med Bull 1983;30:28-33.
784. Jackson RL, Holland E, Chatman ID, et al. Growth and maturation of children with insulin-dependent diabetes mellitus. Diabetes Care 1978;1:96-107.
785. Vanelli M, DeFanti J, Adinolfi B, et al. Clinical data regarding the growth of diabetic children. Horm Res 1992;37:65-69.
786. Rogers DG, Sherman LD, Gabbay KH. Effect of puberty on insulin-like growth factor and HbA1 in Type I diabetes. Diabetes Care 1991;141031-141035.
787. Mandell F, Berenberg W. The Mauriac syndrome. Am J Dis Child 1974;127:900-902.
788. Menon RK, Arslaninan S, May B, et al. Diminished growth hormone binding protein in children with insulin-dependent diabetes mellitus. J Clin Endocrinol Metab 1992;74:934-938.
789. Froesch ER, Hussain M. Metabolic effects of insulin-like growth factor I with special reference to diabetes. Acta Paediatr Scand 1994;399:165-170.
790. Malone JI, Lowitt S, Duncan JA, et al. Hypercalciuria, hyperphosphaturia and growth retardation in children with diabetes mellitus. Pediatrics 1986;78:298-304.
791. Clayton KL, Holly JM, Carlsson LM. Loss of the normal relationship between growth hormone, growth hormone binding protein and insulin like growth factor in adolescents with insulin dependent diabetes mellitus. Clin Endocrinol 1994;41:517-524.
792. Bereket A, Lang CH, Blethen SL, et al. Effect of insulin on IGF system in children with new onset insulin dependent diabetes mellitus. J Clin Endocrinol Metab 1995;80:1312-1317.
793. Rudolf MC, Sherwin RS, Markowitz R, et al. Effect of intensive insulin treatment on linear growth in the young diabetic patient. J Pediatr 1982;101:333-339.
794. Munoz MT, Barrios V, Pozo J, et al. Insulin-like growth factor I, its binding proteins 1 and 3, and growth hormone-binding protein in children and adolescents with insulin-dependent diabetes mellitus: clinical implications. Pediatr Res 1996;39:992-998.
795. Bereket A, Lang CH, Wilson TA. Alterations in the growth hormone-insulin-like growth factor axis in insulin dependent diabetes mellitus. Horm Metab Res 1999;31:172-181.
796. Dunger DB. Insulin and insulin-like growth factors in diabetes mellitus. Arch Dis Child 1995;72:469-471.
797. Suikkari AM, Koivisto VA, Rutanen EM, et al. Insulin regulates the serum levels of low molecular weight insulin-like growth factor binding protein. J Clin Endocrinol Metab 1988;66:266-272.
798. Batch JA, Baxter RC, Werther G. Abnormal regulation of insulin-like growth factor binding proteins in adolescents with insulin-dependent diabetes mellitus. J Clin Endocrinol Metab 1991;73: 964-968.
799. Taylor AM, Dunger DB, Preece MA, et al. The growth hormone independent insulin-like growth factor-I binding protein BP-28 is associated with serum insulin-like growth factor I inhibitory bioactivity in adolescent insulin-dependent diabetes mellitus. Clin Endocrinol 1990;32:229-239.
800. Bereket A, Lang CH, Blethen SL, et al. Insulin-like growth factor binding protein-3 proteolysis in children with insulin dependent diabetes mellitus: a possible role for insulin in the regulation of IGFBP-3 protease activity. J Clin Endocrinol Metab 1995;80: 2282-2288.
801. Winter RJ, Phillips LS, Klein MN, et al. Somatomedin activity and diabetic control in children with insulin-dependent diabetes. Diabetes 1979;28:952-954.
802. Clarson D, Daneman D, Ehrlich RM. The relation of metabolic control to growth and pubertal development in children with insulin-dependent diabetes. Diabetes Res 1985;2:237-241.
803. Du Caju MV, Rooman RP, Op De Beeck L. Longitudinal data on growth and final height in diabetic children. Pediatr Res 1995;38:607-611.
804. Tamborlane WV, Hintz RL, Bergman M, et al. Insulin-infusion-pump treatment of diabetes: influence of improved metabolic control on plasma somatomedin levels. N Engl J Med 1981;305: 303-307.
805. Marsden D, Barshop BA, Capistrano-Estrada S, et al. Anabolic effect of human growth hormone: management of inherited disorders of catabolic pathways. Biochem Med Metab Biol 1994;52:145-154.
806. Bain MD, Nussey SS, Jones M, et al. Use of human somatotropin in the treatment of a patient with methylmalonic aciduria. Eur J Pediatr 1995;154:850-852.
807. Russell G. Asthma and growth. Arch Dis Child 1993;69:695-698.
808. Cohen MB, Abram LE. Growth patterns of allergic children. J Allergy 1948;19:165-171.
809. Balfour-Lynn L. Growth and childhood asthma. Arch Dis Child 1986;61:1049-1055.
810. Crowley S, Hindmarsh PC, Matthews DR, et al. Growth and the growth hormone axis in prepubertal children with asthma. J Pediatr 1995;126:297-303.
811. Ninan TK, Russell G. Asthma, inhaled corticosteroid treatment and growth. Arch Dis Child 1992;67:703-705.
812. Nassif E, Weinberger M, Sherman, et al. Extrapulmonary effects of maintenance corticosteroid therapy with alternate-day prednisolone and inhaled beclomethasone in children with chronic asthma. J Allergy Clin Immunol 1987;80:518-528.
813. Falliers CJ, Tan LS, Szentivanyi J, et al. Childhood asthma and steroid therapy as influences on growth. Am J Dis Child 1963;105: 127-137.
814. Reid A, Murphy C, Steen HJ, et al. Linear growth of very young asthmatic children treated with high-dose nebulized budesonide. Acta Paediatr 1996;85:421-424.
815. Versano I, Volovitz B, Malik H, et al. Safety of 1 year of treatment with budesonide in young children with asthma. J Allergy Clin Immunol 1990;85:914-920.

816. Volovitz B, Amir J, Malik H, et al. Growth and pituitary-adrenal function in children with severe asthma treated with inhaled budesonide. N Engl J Med 1996;329:1703-1708.
817. Todd G, Dunlop K, McNaboe J, et al. Growth and adrenal suppression in asthmatic children treated with high-dose fluticasone propionate. Lancet 1996;348:27-29.
818. Agertoft L, Pedersen S. Effect of long-term treatment with inhaled budesonide on adult height in children with asthma. N Engl J Med 2000;343:1064-1069.
819. Norjavaara E, de Verdier MG, Lindmark B. Reduced height in Swedish men with asthma at the age of conscription for military service. J Pediatr 2000;137:25-29.
820. Martin AJ, McLennan LA, Landau LI, et al. The natural history of childhood asthma to adult life. BMJ 1980;280:1397-1400.
821. Shohat M, Shohat T, Kedem R, et al. Childhood asthma and growth outcome. Arch Dis Child 1987;62:63-65.
822. Avery ME, Tooley W, Keller J, et al. Is chronic lung disease in low birth weight infants preventable. A survey of eight centers. Pediatrics 1987;79:26-30.
823. Gibson AT, Pearse RG, Wales JK. Growth retardation after dexamethasone administration: assessment by knemometry. Arch Dis Child 1993;69:505-509.
824. Finer NN, Craft A, Vaucher YE, et al. Postnatal steroids: short-term gain, long-term pain? J Pediatr 2000;137:9-13.
825. Kurzner SI, Garg M, Bautista D, et al. Growth failure in infants with bronchopulmonary dysplasia: nutrition and elevated resting metabolic expenditure. Pediatrics 1988;81:379-384.
826. Yu V, Orgill A, Lim S, et al. Growth and development of very low-birth-weight infants recovering from bronchopulmonary dysplasia. Arch Dis Child 1983;58:791-794.
827. Meisels S, Plunkett J, Roloff D, et al. Growth and development of preterm infants with respiratory distress syndrome and bronchopulmonary dysplasia. Pediatrics 1986;77:345-352.
828. Vrlenich LA, Bozynski ME, Shyr Y, et al. The effect of bronchopulmonary dysplasia on growth at school age. Pediatrics 1995;95:855-859.
829. Ross G, Lipper E, Auld P. Growth achievement of very low-birth-weight premature children at school age. J Pediatr 1990;117: 307-309.
830. Robertson M, Etches P, Goldson E, et al. Eight year school performance, neurodevelopmental, and growth outcome of neonates with bronchopulmonary dysplasia: a comparative study. Pediatrics 1992;89:365-372.
831. FitzSimmons SC. The changing epidemiology of cystic fibrosis. J Pediatr 1993;122:1-9.
832. Landon C, Rosenfeld RG. Short stature and pubertal delay in male adolescents with cystic fibrosis. Am J Dis Child 1984;138: 388-391.
833. Karlberg J, Kjellmer I, Kristiansson B. Linear growth in children with cystic fibrosis. I. Birth to 8 years of age. Acta Paediatr Scand 1991;80:508-514.
834. Lapey A, Kattwinkel J, DiSant'Agnese PA, et al. Steatorrhea and azotorrhea and their relation to growth and nutrition in adolescents and young adults with cystic fibrosis. J Pediatr 1974;84: 328-334.
835. Mearns M. Growth and development. In Hodson E, Norman A, Batten J, eds. Cystic Fibrosis. London: Bailliere Tindall, 1983: 183-196.
836. Shepherd RW, Holt TL, Thomas BJ, et al. Nutritional rehabilitation in cystic fibrosis: controlled studies of effects on nutritional growth retardation, body protein turnover, and course of pulmonary disease. J Pediatr 1986;109:788-794.
837. Reiter EO, Gerstle RS. Cystic fibrosis in puberty and adolescence. In Lerner RM, Petersen AC, Brooks-Gunn J, eds. Encyclopedia of Adolescence. New York: Garland Publishing, 1991:187-195.
838. Reiter EO, Brugman SM, Pike JW, et al. Vitamin D metabolites in adolescents and young adults with cystic fibrosis: effects of sun and season. J Pediatr 1985;106:21-26.
839. Reiter EO, Stern RC, Root AW. The reproductive system in cystic fibrosis. II. Changes in gonadotrophins and sex steroids following LHRH. Clin Endocrinol 1982;16:127-137.
840. Aswani N, Taylor CJ, McGaw J, et al. Pubertal growth and development in cystic fibrosis: a retrospective review. Acta Paediatr 2003;92:1029-1032.
841. Laursen EM, Juul A, Lanng S, et al. Diminished concentrations of insulin-like growth factor I in cystic fibrosis. Arch Dis Child 1995;72:494-497.
842. Huseman CA, Columbo JL, Brooks MA, et al. Anabolic effect of biosynthetic growth hormone in cystic fibrosis. Pediatr Pulmonol 1996;22:90-95.
843. Hardin DS, Stratton R, Kramer JC, et al. Growth hormone improves weight velocity and height velocity in prepubertal children with cystic fibrosis. Horm Metab Res 1998;30:636-641.
844. Hardin DS, Rice J, Ahn C, et al. Growth hormone treatment enhances nutrition and growth in children with cystic fibrosis receiving enteral nutrition. J Pediatr 2005;146:324-328.
845. Zemel BS, Jawad AF, FitzSimmons S, et al. Longitudinal relationship among growth, nutritional status, and pulmonary function in children with cystic fibrosis: analysis of the Cystic Fibrosis Foundation National CF Patient Registry. J Pediatr 2000;137: 374-380.
846. Colombo C, Battezzati A. Growth failure in cystic fibrosis: a true need for anabolic agents? J Pediatr 2005;146:303-305.
847. De Benedetti F, Alonzi T, Moretta A, et al. Interleukin 6 causes growth impairment in transgenic mice through a decrease in insulin-like growth factor-I. J Clin Invest 1997;99: 643-650.
848. McCann SM, Lyson K, Karanth S, et al. Role of cytokines in the endocrine system. Ann N Y Acad Sci 1994;740:50-63.
849. Vassilopoulou-Sellin R. Endocrine effects of cytokines. Oncology 1994;8:43-50.
850. Skerry TM. The effects of the inflammatory response on bone growth. Eur J Clin Nutr 1994;48(suppl 1):190-198.
851. Lang CH, Hong-Brown L, Frost RA. Cytokine inhibition of JAK-STAT signaling: a new mechanism of growth hormone resistance. Pediatr Nephrol 2005;20:306-312.
852. Abrams EJ, Rogers MF. Pediatric HIV infection. Baillieres Clin Haematol 1991;4:333-339.
853. McKinney RE, Robertson JW, Duke Pediatric AIDS Clinical Trials Unit. Effect of human immunodeficiency virus infection on the growth of young children. J Pediatr 1993;123:579-582.
854. Saavedra JM, Henderson RA, Perman JA, et al. Longitudinal assessment of growth in children born to mothers with human immunodeficiency virus infection. Arch Pediatr Adolesc Med 1995;149:497-502.
855. McKinney RE, Wilfert C, AIDS Clinical Trials Group Protocol 043 Study Group. Growth as a prognostic indicator in children with immunodeficiency virus infection treated with zidovudine. J Pediatr 1994;125:728-733.
856. Gertner JM, Kaufman FR, Donfield SM, et al. Delayed somatic growth and pubertal development in human immunodeficiency virus-infected hemophiliac boys: Hemophilia Growth and Development Study. J Pediatr 1994;124:896-902.
857. Moye J, Rich KC, Kalish LA, et al. Natural history of somatic growth in infants born to women infected by human immunodeficiency virus. J Pediatr 1996;128:58-69.
858. Grunfeld C. What causes wasting in AIDS? N Engl J Med 1996; 333:123-124.
859. Grunfeld C, Feingold KR. Metabolic disturbances and wasting in the acquired immunodeficiency syndrome. N Engl J Med 1992; 327:329-337.
860. Stagi S, Bindi G, Galluzzi F, et al. Changed bone status in human immunodeficiency virus type 1 (HIV-1) perinatally infected children is related to low serum free IGF-I. Clin Endocrinol (Oxf) 2004;61:692-699.
861. Hardin DS, Rice J, Doyle ME, et al. Growth hormone improves protein catabolism and growth in prepubertal children with HIV infection. Clin Endocrinol (Oxf) 2005;63:259-262.
862. Infections as deterrents of growth. Nutr Rev 1981;39:328.
863. Chiesa A, de Papendieck G, Keselman A, et al. Growth follow-up in 100 children with congenital hypothyroidism before and during treatment. J Pediatr Endocrinol 1994;7:211-217.
864. Grant DB. Growth in early treated congenital hypothyroidism. Arch Dis Child 1994;70:464-468.
865. Salerno M, Lettiero T, Esposito-del Puente A, et al. Effect of long-term L-thyroxine treatment on bone mineral density in young adults with congenital hypothyroidism. Eur J Endocrinol 2004; 151:689-694.

866. Heyerdahl S, Ilicki A, Karlbarg J, et al. Linear growth in early-treated children with congenital hypothyroidism. Acta Paediatr 1997;86:479-483.
867. Dickerman Z, De Vries L. Prepubertal and pubertal growth, timing and duration of puberty, and attained adult height in patients with congenital hypothyroidism(CH) detected by the neonatal screening programmed for CH—a longitudinal study. Clin Endocrinol 1997;47:649-654.
868. Rivkees SA, Bode HH, Crawford JD. Long-term growth in juvenile acquired hypothyroidism. N Engl J Med 1988;318:599-602.
869. Pantsiouou S, Stanhope R, Urena M, et al. Growth prognosis and growth after menarche in primary hypothyroidism. Arch Dis Child 1991;66:838-840.
870. Boersma B, Otten BJ, Stoelings GB, et al. Catch-up growth after prolonged hypothyroidism. Eur J Pediatr 1996;155:362-367.
871. Reid IR. Pathogenesis and treatment of steroid osteoporosis. Clin Endocrinol 1989;30:83-103.
872. Giustina A, Bussi AR, Jacobello C, et al. Effects of recombinant human growth hormone (GH) on bone and intermediary metabolism in patients receiving chronic glucocorticoid treatment with suppressed endogenous GH response to GH-releasing hormone. J Clin Endocrinol Metab 1995;80:122-129.
873. Allen DB, Goldberg BD. Stimulation of a collagen synthesis and linear growth by growth hormone in glucocorticoid-treated children. Pediatrics 1992;89:416-421.
874. Schatz M, Dudl J, Zeiger RS, et al. Osteoporosis in corticosteroid-treated asthmatic patients: clinical correlates. Allerg Proc 1993; 14:341-345.
875. Luo J, Murphy LJ. Dexamethasone inhibits growth hormone induction of insulin-like growth factor-I (IGF-I) messenger ribonucleic acid (mRNA) in hypophysectomized rats and reduces IGF-I mRNA abundance in the intact rat. Endocrinology 1989;125:165-171.
876. Magiakou MA, Mastorakos G, Gomez MT, et al. Suppressed spontaneous and stimulated growth hormone secretion in patients with Cushing's disease before and after surgical cure. J Clin Endocrinol Metab 1994;78:131-137.
877. Horber FF, Haymond MV. Human growth hormone prevents the protein catabolic side effects of prednisone in humans. J Clin Invest 1990;86:265-272.
878. Mauras N, Beaufrere B. rhIGF-I enhances whole body protein anabolism and significantly diminishes the protein-catabolic effects of prednisone in humans without a diabetogenic effect. J Clin Endocrinol Metab 1995;80:869-874.
879. Rivkees SA, Danon M, Herrin J. Prednisone dose limitation of growth hormone treatment of steroid-induced growth failure. J Pediatr 1994;125:322-325.
880. Mosier HD, Smith FG, Schultz MA. Failure of catch-up growth after Cushing's syndrome in childhood. Am J Dis Child 1972;124: 251-253.
881. Leong GM, Mercado-Asis LB, Reynolds JC, et al. The effect of Cushing's disease on bone mineral density, body composition, growth and puberty; a report of identical adolescent twin pair. J Clin Endorinol Metab 1996;81:1905-1911.
882. Lebrethon M-C, Grossman AB, Afshar F, et al. Linear growth and final height after treatment for Cushing's disease in childhood. J Clin Endocrinol Metab 2000;85:3262-3265.
883. Savage MO, Lienhardt A, Lebrethon M-C, et al. Cushing's disease in childhood: presentation, investigation, treatment and long-term outcome. Horm Res 2001;55:24-30.
884. Schwindinger WF, Levine MA. Albright hereditary osteodystrophy. Endocrinologist 1994;4:17-27.
885. Mantovani G, Maghnie M, Weber G, et al. Growth hormone-releasing hormone resistance in pseudohypoparathyroidism type ia: new evidence for imprinting of the Gs alpha gene. J Clin Endocrinol Metab 2003;88:4070-4074.
886. Minamitani K, Takahashi Y, Minagawa M, et al. Difference in height associated with a translation start site polymorphism in the vitamin D receptor gene. Pediatr Res 1998;44:628-632.
887. Lorentzon M, Lorentzon R, Nordstrom P. Vitamin D receptor gene polymorphism is associated with birth weight, growth to adolescence, and adult stature in healthy Caucasian men: a cross-sectional and longitudinal study. J Clin Endocrinol Metab 2000;85:1666-1671.
888. Suarez F, Zeghoud F, Rossignol C, et al. Association between vitamin D receptor gene polymorphism and sex-dependent growth during the first two years of life. J Clin Endocrinol Metab 1997;82:2966-2970.
889. Kanan RM, Varanasi SS, Francis RM, et al. Vitamin D receptor gene start codon polymorphism (FokI) and bone mineral density in healthy male subjects. Clin Endocrinol 2000;53:93-98.
890. Arai H, Miyamoto KI, Taketani Y, et al. A vitamin D receptor gene polymorphism translation initiation codon: effect on protein activity and relation to bone mineral density in Japanese women. J Bone Min Res 1997;12:915-921.
891. Suarez F, Rossignol C, Garabedian M. Interactive effect of estradiol and vitamin D receptor gene polymorphisms as a possible determinant of growth in male and female infants. J Clin Endocrinol Metab 1998;83:3563-3568.
892. Alonso M, Segura C, Dieguez C, et al. High-affinity binding sites to the vitamin D receptor DNA binding domain in the human growth hormone promoter. Biochem Biophys Res Commun 2000;247:882-887.
893. Cho HY, Lee BH, Kang JH, et al. A clinical and molecular genetic study of hypophosphatemic rickets in children. Pediatr Res 2005;58:329-333.
894. Shimada T, Hasegawa H, Yamazaki Y, et al. FGF-23 is a potent regulator of vitamin D metabolism and phosphate homeostasis. J Bone Min Res 2004;19:429-435.
895. Makitie O, Doria A, Kooh SW, et al. Early treatment improves growth and biochemical and radiographic outcome in X-linked hypophosphatemic rickets. J Clin Endocrinol Metab 2003;88: 3591-3597.
896. Chan JC. Renal hypophosphatemic rickets—a review. Int J Pediatr Nephrol 1982;3:305-310.
897. Glorieux FH, Marie PJ, Pettifor JM, et al. Bone response to phosphate salts, ergocalciferol and calcitriol in hypophosphatemic vitamin D resistant rickets. N Engl J Med 1980;303: 1023-1031.
898. Petersen DJ, Boniface AM, Schranck FW, et al. X-linked hypophosphatemic rickets: a study (with literature review) of linear growth response to calcitriol and phosphate therapy. J Bone Min Res 1992;7:583-597.
899. Balsan S, Tieder M. Linear growth in patients with hypophosphatemic vitamin D-resistant rickets: influence of treatment regimen and parental height. J Pediatr 1990;116:365-371.
900. Bistritzer T, Chalew SA, Hanukoglu A, et al. Does growth hormone influence the severity of phosphopenic rickets? Eur J Pediatr 1990;150:26-29.
901. Jasper H, Cassinelli H. Growth hormone and insulin-like growth factor I plasma levels in patients with hypophosphatemic rickets. J Pediatr Endocrinol 1993;6:179-184.
902. Saggese G, Barancelli GI, Vertelloni S, et al. Growth hormone secretion in poorly growing children with renal hypophosphatemic rickets. Eur J Pediatr 1994;153:548-555.
903. Wilson DM, Lee PD, Morris AH, et al. Growth hormone therapy in hypophosphatemic rickets. Am J Dis Child 1991;145:1165-1170.
904. Wilson DM. Growth hormone and hypophosphatemic rickets. J Pediatr Endocrinol Metab 2000;13:993-998.
905. Baroncelli GI, Bertelloni S, Ceccarelli C, et al. Effect of growth hormone treatment on final height, phosphate metabolism, and bone mineral density in children with X-linked hypophosphatemic rickets. J Pediatr 2001;138:236-243.
906. Rosenfeld RG, Hwa V. Toward a molecular basis for idiopathic short stature. J Clin Endocrinol Metab 2004;89:1066-1067.
907. Rosenfeld RG. Molecular mechanisms of IGF-I deficiency. Horm Res 2006;65(suppl 1):15-20.
908. Huet F, Carel JC, Nivelon JL, et al. Long-term results of GH therapy in GH-deficient children treated before 1 year of age. Eur J Endocrinol 1999;140:29-34.
909. Abrahams JJ, Trefelner E, Boulware SD. Idiopathic growth hormone deficiency: MR findings in 35 patients. Am J Neuroradiol 1991;12:155-160.
910. Maghnie M, Genovese E, Villa A, et al. Dynamic MRI in the congenital agenesis of the neural pituitary stalk syndrome: the role of the vascular pituitary stalk in predicting residual anterior pituitary function. Clin Endocrinol 1996;45:281-290.
911. Root AW, Martinez CR. Magnetic resonance imaging in patients with hypopituitarism. Trends Endocrinol Metab 1992;3:283-287.

912. Triulzi F, Scotti G, diNatale B, et al. Evidence of a congenital midline brain anomaly in pituitary dwarfs: a magnetic resonance imaging study in 101 patients. Pediatrics 1994;93:409-416.
913. Nagel BH, Palmbach M, Peterson D, et al. Magnetic resonance image of 91 children with different causes of short stature: pituitary size reflects growth hormone secretion. Eur J Pediatr 1997;156:758-763.
914. Copeland KC, Franks RC, Ramamurthy R. Neonatal hyperbilirubinemia and hypoglycemia in congenital hypopituitarism. Clin Pediatr 1981;20:523-526.
915. Choo-Kang LR, Sun C-CJ, Counts DR. Cholestasis and hypoglycemia: manifestations of congenital anterior hypopituitarism. J Clin Endocrinol Metab 1996;81:2786-2789.
916. Lovinger RD, Kaplan SL, Grumbach MM. Congenital hypopituitarism associated with neonatal hypoglycemia and microphallus: four cases secondary to hypothalamic hormone deficiencies. J Pediatr 1975;87:1171-1181.
917. Goodman HG, Grumbach MM, Kaplan SL. Growth and growth hormone. II. A comparison of isolated growth hormone deficiency and multiple pituitary hormone deficiency in 35 patients with idiopathic hypopituitary disease. N Engl J Med 1968; 278:57-68.
918. Mehta A, Hindmarsh PC, Stanhope RG, et al. The role of growth hormone in determining birth size and early postnatal growth, using congenital growth hormone deficiency (GHD) as a model. Clin Endocrinol (Oxf) 2005;63:223-231.
919. Baroncelli GI, Bertelloni S, Ceccarelli C, et al. Measurement of volumetric bone mineral density accurately determines degree of lumbar undermineralization in children with growth hormone deficiency. J Clin Endocrinol Metab 1998;83:3150.
920. Wit JM, Kamp G, Rikken B. Spontaneous growth and response to growth hormone treatment in children with growth hormone deficiency and idiopathic short stature. Pediatr Res 1996; 39:295-302.
921. Rimoin DL, Merimee TJ, Rabinowitz D, et al. Genetic aspects of clinical endocrinology. Rec Prog Horm Res 1968;24:365-437.
922. Ranke MB. A note on adults with growth hormone deficiency. Acta Paediatr Scand Suppl 1987;331:80-82.
923. van der Werff ten Bosch JJ, Bot A. Growth of males with idiopathic hypopituitarism without growth hormone treatment. Clin Endocrinol 1990;32:707-717.
924. Ranke MB, Wilton PM. Growth Hormone therapy in KIGS—10 years' experience. Heidelberg-Leipzig: Johann Ambrosius Barth Verlag, 1999.
925. Rosenfeld RG, Buckway CK. Should we treat genetic syndromes? J Pediatr Endocrinol Metab 2000;13:971-981.
926. Bell J, Bolar K, Swinford RD, et al. Long-term safety of recombinant human growth hormone (rhGH): The National Cooperative Growth Study (NCGS) experience. 87th Annual Meeting of the Endocrine Society, San Diego, 2005.
927. Goddard AD, Covello R, Shiuh ML, et al. Mutation of the growth hormone receptor in children with idiopathic short stature. N Engl J Med 1995;333:1093-1098.
928. Rosenfeld RG. Broadening the growth hormone insensitivity syndrome. N Engl J Med 1995;333:1145-1146.
929. Parkin JM. Incidence of growth hormone deficiency. Arch Dis Child 1974;49:904-905.
930. Vimpani GV, Vimpani AF, Lidgard GP, et al. Prevalence of severe growth hormone deficiency. Br Med J 1977;2:427-430.
931. Lindsay R, Feldkamp M, Harris D, et al. Utah Growth Study: growth standards and the prevalence of growth hormone deficiency. J Pediatr 1994;125:29-35.
932. Melander T, Hokfelt T, Rokaeus A. Distribution of galaninlike immunoreactivity in the rat central nervous system. J Comp Neurol 1986;218:175-217.
933. Perez Juarado LA, Argente J. Molecular basis of familial growth hormone deficiency. Horm Res 1994;42:189-197.
934. Parks JS, Pfaffle RW, Brown MR, et al. Growth hormone deficiency. In Weintraub BD, ed. Molecular Endocrinology: Basic Concepts and Clinical Correlations. New York: Raven Press, 1995:473-490.
935. Cogan JD, Phillips JA, Sakati N, et al. Heterogeneous growth hormone (GH) gene mutations in familial GH deficiency. J Clin Endocrinol Metab 1993;76:1224-1228.
936. Alba M, Salvatori R. A mouse with targeted ablation of the growth hormone-releasing hormone gene: a new model of isolated growth hormone deficiency. Endocrinology 2004;145:4134-4143.
937. Le Tissier PR, Carmignac DF, Lilley S, et al. Hypothalamic growth hormone-releasing hormone (GHRH) deficiency: targeted ablation of GHRH neurons in mice using a viral ion channel transgene. Mol Endocrinol 2005;19:1251-1262.
938. Sun Y, Ahmed S, Smith RG. Deletion of ghrelin impairs neither growth nor appetite. Mol Cell Biol 2003;23:7973-7981.
939. Wortley KE, Anderson KD, Garcia K, et al. Genetic deletion of ghrelin does not decrease food intake but influences metabolic fuel preference. Proc Natl Acad Sci U S A 2004;101:8227-8232.
940. Bosse R, Fumagalli F, Jaber M, et al. Anterior pituitary hypoplasia and dwarfism in mice lacking the dopamine transporter. Neuron 1997;19:127-138.
941. Ch'in KY. The endocrine glands of anencephalic foetuses. Chinese Med J 1938;2(suppl):63-90.
942. Lemire RJ, Beckwith JB, Warkany J. Anencephaly. New York: Raven Press: 1978.
943. Grumbach MM, Kaplan SL. Ontogenesis of growth hormone, insulin, prolactin and gonadotropin secretion in the human foetus. In Cross DW, Nathanielsz P, eds. Foetal and Neonatal Physiology: Proceedings of Sir Joseph Barcroft Centenary Symposium. Cambridge: Cambridge University Press, 1973:462.
944. Grumbach MM, Kaplan SL. Fetal pituitary hormones and the maturation of central nervous system regulation of anterior pituitary function. In Gluck L, ed. Modern Perinatal Medicine. Chicago: Year Book Medical Publishers, 1974:247.
945. Hintz RL, Menking M, Sotos JF. Familial holoprosencephaly with endocrine dysgenesis. J Pediatr 1968;72:81-87.
946. Lieblich JM, Rosen SW, Guyda H, et al. The syndrome of basal encephalocele and hypothalamic pituitary dysfunction. Ann Intern Med 1978;89:910-916.
947. Brown SA, Warburton D, Brown LY, et al. Holoprosencephaly due to mutations in ZIC2, a homologue of Drosophila odd-paired. Nat Genet 1998;20:180-183.
948. Roessler E, Du YZ, Mullor JL, et al. Loss-of-function mutations in the human GLI2 gene are associated with pituitary anomalies and holoprosencephaly-like features. Proc Natl Acad Sci U S A 2003; 100:13424-13429.
949. Rudman D, Davis GT, Priest JH, et al. Prevalence of growth hormone deficiency in children with cleft lip or palate. J Pediatr 1978;93:378-382.
950. Izenberg N, Rosenblum M, Parks JS. The endocrine spectrum of septo-optic dysplasia. Clin Pediatr 1984;23:632-636.
951. Wilson DM, Enzmann DR, Hintz RL, et al. Cranial computed tomography in septo-optic dysplasia: discordance of clinical and radiological features. Neuroradiology 1984;26:279-283.
952. Willnow S, Kiess W, Butenandt O, et al. Endocrine disorders in septo-optic dysplasia (De Morsier syndrome)—evaluation and follow-up of 18 patients. Eur J Pediatr 1998;155:179-184.
953. Hellstrom A, Wiklund L-M, Svensson E, et al. Midline brain lesions in children with hormone insufficiency indicate early prenatal damage. Acta Paediatr Scand 1998;87:528-536.
954. Kaplan SL, Grumbach MM. Pathophysiology of GH deficiency and other disorders of GH metabolism. In LaCauza C, Root AW, eds. Problems in Pediatric Endocrinology. Serono Symposia, Vol 32. London: Academic Press, 1980:45.
955. Ahmad T, Garcia-Filion P, Borchert M, et al. Endocrinological and auxological abnormalities in young children with optic nerve hypoplasia: a prospective study. J Pediatr 2006;148:78-84.
956. Stickler GB, Morgenstern BZ. Hypophosphatemic rickets: final height and clinical symptoms in adults. Lancet 1989;2:902-905.
957. Patel L, McNally RJ, Harrison E, et al. Geographical distribution of optic nerve hypoplasia and septo-optic dysplasia in Northwest England. J Pediatr 2006;148:85-88.
958. Tornqvist K, Ericsson A, Kallen B. Optic nerve hypoplasia: risk factors and epidemiology. Acta Ophthalmol Scand 2002;80: 300-304.
959. Dattani MT, Martinez-Barbera JP, Thomas PQ, et al. HESX1: a novel gene implicated in a familial form of septo-optic dysplasia. Acta Paediatr Suppl 1999;433:49-54.

960. Hermesz E, Mackem S, Mahon KA. Rpx: a novel anterior-restricted homeobox gene progressively activated in the prechordal plate, anterior neural plate, and Rathke's pouch of the mouse embryo. Development 1996;122:41-52.
961. Sobrier ML, Netchine I, Heinrichs C, et al. Alu-element insertion in the homeodomain of HESX1 and aplasia of the anterior pituitary. Hum Mutat 2005;25:503.
962. Thomas PQ, Dattani MT, Brickman JM, et al. Heterozygous HESX1 mutations associated with isolated congenital pituitary hypoplasia and septo-optic dysplasia. Hum Mol Genet 2001;10: 39-45.
963. Carvalho LR, Woods KS, Mendonca BB, et al. A homozygous mutation in HESX1 is associated with evolving hypopituitarism due to impaired repressor-corepressor interaction. J Clin Invest 2003;112:1192-1201.
964. Dattani MT, Martinez-Barbera J-P, Thomas PQ, et al. Mutations in the homeobox gene HESX1/Hesx1 associated with septo-optic dysplasia in human and mouse. Nat Genet 1998;19:125-133.
965. Tuilipakov AN, Bulatov AA, Peterkova AV, et al. Growth hormone (GH)-releasing effects of synthetic peptide GH-releasing peptide-2 and GH-releasing hormone (1-29NH2) in children with GH insufficiency and idiopathic short stature. Metabolism 1995;44:1199-1204.
966. Pombo M, Barreiro J, Penalva A, et al. Absence of growth hormone (GH) secretion after administration of GH-releasing hormone (GHRH). GH-releasing peptide (GHRP-6), or GHRH plus GHRP-6 in children with neonatal pituitary stalk transection. J Clin Endocrinol Metab 1995;80:3180-3184.
967. Cacciari E, Zucchini S, Carla G, et al. Endocrine function and morphological findings in patients with disorders of the hypothalamo-pituitary area: a study with magnetic resonance. Arch Dis Child 1990;65:1199-1202.
968. Maghnie M, Larizza D, Triulzi F, et al. Hypopituitarism and stalk agenesis: a congenital syndrome worsened by breech delivery? Horm Res 1991;35:104-108.
969. Brown RS, Bhatia V, Hayes E. An apparent cluster of congenital hypopituitarism in central Massachusetts: magnetic resonance imaging and hormonal studies. J Clin Endocrinol Metab 1991;72:12-18.
970. Argyopoulou M, Perignon F, Brauner R, et al. Magnetic resonance imaging in the diagnosis of growth hormone deficiency. J Pediatr 1992;120:886-891.
971. Hamilton J, Blaser S, Daneman D. MR imaging in idiopathic growth hormone deficiency. AJNR Am J Neuroradiol 1998;19: 1609-1615.
972. Kornreich L, Horev G, Lazar L, et al. MR findings in growth hormone deficiency: correlation with severity of hypopituitarism. AJNR Am J Neuroradiol 1998;19:1495-1499.
973. Kuroiwa T, Okabe Y, Hasuo K, et al. MR imaging of pituitary dwarfism. AJNR Am J Neuroradiol 1991;12:161-164.
974. Hamilton J, Chitayat D, Blaser S, et al. Familial growth hormone deficiency associated with MRI abnormalities. Am J Med Genet 1998;80:128-132.
975. de Zegher F, Kaplan SL, Grumbach MM, et al. The foetal pituitary, postmaturity and breech presentation. Acta Paediatr 1995;83: 1100-1102.
976. Trollmann R, Strehl E, Wenzel D, et al. Does growth hormone (GH) enhance growth in GH-deficient children with myelomeningocele? J Clin Endocrinol Metab 2000;85:2740-2743.
977. Trollmann R, Dorr HG, Strehl E, et al. Growth and pubertal development in patients with meningomyelocele: a retrospective analysis. Acta Paediatr 1996;85:76-80.
978. Quan A, Adams R, Ekmark E, et al. Bone mineral density in children with myelomeningocele. Pediatrics 1998;102:E34-1-E34-6.
979. Rotenstein D, Reigel DH. Growth hormone treatment of children with neural tube defects: results from 6 months to 6 years. J Pediatr 1996;128:184-187.
980. Satin-Smith MS, Katz LL, et al. Arm span as measurement of response to growth hormone (GH) treatment in a group of children with meningomyelocele and GH deficiency. J Clin Endocrinol Metab 1996;81:1654-1656.
981. Lopponen T, Paakko E, Laitien J, et al. Pituitary size and function in children and adolescents with shunted hydrocephalus. Clin Endocrinol 1997;46:691-699.
982. Lopponen T, Saukkonen AL, Serlo W, et al. Reduced levels of growth hormone, insulin-like growth factor-I and binding protein-3 in patients with shunted hydrocephalus. Arch Dis Child 1997; 77:32-37.
983. Lopponen T, Saukkonen AL, Serlo W, et al. Slow prepubertal linear growth but early pubertal growth spurt in patients with shunted hydrocephalus. Pediatrics 1995;95:917-923.
984. Miller WL, Kaplan SL, Grumbach MM. Child abuse as a cause of post-traumatic hypopituitarism. N Engl J Med 1980;302:724-728.
985. Kelly DF, Gonzalo IT, Cohan P, et al. Hypopituitarism following traumatic brain injury and aneurysmal subarachnoid hemorrhage: a preliminary report. J Neurosurg 2000;93:743-752.
986. Carel JC. Growth hormone in Turner syndrome: twenty years after, what can we tell our patients? J Clin Endocrinol Metab 2005;90:3793-3794.
987. Leal-Cerro A, Flores JM, Rincon M, et al. Prevalence of hypopituitarism and growth hormone deficiency in adults long-term after severe traumatic brain injury. Clin Endocrinol (Oxf) 2005; 62:525-532.
988. Bondanelli M, Ambrosio MR, Zatelli MC, et al. Hypopituitarism after traumatic brain injury. Eur J Endocrinol 2005;152:679-691.
989. Mayfield RK, Levine JH, Gordon L, et al. Lymphadenoid hypophysitis presenting as a pituitary tumor. Am J Med 1980;69:619-623.
990. Bartsocas CS, Pantelakis SN. Human growth hormone therapy in hypopituitarism due to tuberculous meningitis. Acta Paediatr Scand 1973;62:304-306.
991. Stuart CA, Neelon FA, Lebovitz HE. Hypothalamic insufficiency: the cause of hypopituitarism in sarcoidosis. Ann Intern Med 1978;88:589-594.
992. Costin G. Endocrine disorders associated with tumors of the pituitary and hypothalamus. Pediatr Clin North Am 1979;26:15-31.
993. Vassilopoulou-Sellin R, Klein MJ, Slopis JK. Growth hormone deficiency in children with neurofibromatosis type I without suprasellar lesions. Pediatr Neurology 2000;22:355-358.
994. Carmi D, Shohat M, Metzker A, et al. Growth, puberty, and endocrine function in patients with sporadic or familial neurofibromatosis type I. Pediatrics 1999;103:1257-1262.
995. Weinzimer SA, Homan SA, Ferry RJ, et al. Serum IGF-I and IGFBP-3 concentrations do not accurately predict growth hormone deficiency in children with brain tumours. Clin Endocrinol 1999;51:339-345.
996. Brauner R, Rappaport R, Prevot C, et al. A prospective study of the development of growth hormone deficiency in children given cranial irradiation, and its relation to statural growth. J Clin Endocrinol Metab 1989;68:346-351.
997. Albertsson-Wikland K, Lannering B, Marky I, et al. A longitudinal study on growth and spontaneous growth hormone (GH) secretion in children with irradiated brain tumors. Acta Paediatr Scand 1987;76:966-973.
998. Sklar CA, Constine LS. Chronic neuroendocrinological sequelae of radiation therapy. Int J Radiat Oncol Biol Phys 1995;31: 1113-1121.
999. Clayton PE, Shalet SM. Dose dependency of time of onset of radiation-induced growth hormone deficiency. J Pediatr 1991;118: 226-228.
1000. Brennan BM, Rahim A, Mackie EM, et al. Growth hormone status in adults treated for acute lymphoblastic leukaemia in childhood. Clin Endocrinol 1998;48:777-783.
1001. Schmiegelow M, Lassen S, Poulsen HS, et al. Cranial irradiation of childhood brain tumours: Growth hormone deficiency and its relation to the biological effective dose of irradiation in a large population based study. Clin Endocrinol 2000;53:191-197.
1002. Sklar C. Editorial: paying the price for cure—treating cancer survivors with growth hormone. J Clin Endocrinol Metab 2000;85: 4441-4443.
1003. Rappaport R, Brauner R. Growth and endocrine disorders secondary to cranial irradiation. Pediatr Res 1989;25:561-567.
1004. Littley MD, Shalet SM, Beardwell CG, et al. Radiation-induced hypopituitarism is dose-dependent. Clin Endocrinol 1989;31: 361-373.
1005. Bulow B, Link K, Ahren B, et al. Survivors of childhood acute lymphoblastic leukaemia, with radiation-induced GH deficiency, exhibit hyperleptinaemia and impaired insulin sensitivity, unaf-

fected by 12 months of GH treatment. Clin Endocrinol (Oxf) 2004;61:683-691.
1006. Nivot S, Benelli C, Clot JP, et al. Nonparallel changes of growth hormone (GH) and insulin-like growth factor-I, insulin-like growth factor binding protein-3, and GH-binding protein, after craniospinal irradiation and chemotherapy. J Clin Endocrinol Metab 1995;78:597-601.
1007. Ogilvy-Stuart AL, Shalet SM. Effect of chemotherapy on growth. Acta Paediatr Suppl 1995;411:52-56.
1008. Arguelles B, Barrios V, Pozo J, et al. Modifications of growth velocity and the insulin-like growth factor system in children with acute lymphoblastic leukemia: a longitudinal study. J Clin Endocrinol Metab 2000;85:4087-4092.
1009. Sklar C, Mertens A, Walter A, et al. Final height after treatment for childhood acute lymphoblastic leukemia: comparison of no cranial irradiation with 1800 and 2400 centigrays of cranial irradiation. J Pediatr 1993;123:56-64.
1010. Stubberfield TG, Byrne GC, Jones TW. Growth and growth hormone secretion after treatment for acute lymphoblastic leukemia in childhood. J Pediatr Heme Oncol 1995;17:167-171.
1011. Darzy KH, Murray RD, Gleeson HK, et al. The impact of short-term fasting on the dynamics of 24-hour growth hormone (GH) secretion in patients with severe radiation-induced GH deficiency. J Clin Endocrinol Metab 2006;91:987-994.
1012. Darzy KH, Pezzoli SS, Thorner MO, et al. The dynamics of growth hormone (GH) secretion in adult cancer survivors with severe GH deficiency acquired after brain irradiation in childhood for nonpituitary brain tumors: evidence for preserved pulsatility and diurnal variation with increased secretory disorderliness. J Clin Endocrinol Metab 2005;90:2794-2803.
1013. Katz JA, Pollack BH, Jacaruso D, et al. Finally attained height in patients successfully treated for childhood acute lymphoblastic leukemia. J Pediatr 1993;123:546-552.
1014. Achermann JC, Hindmarsh PC, Brook CG. The relationship between growth hormone and insulin-like growth factor axis in long-term survivors of childhood brain tumors. Clin Endocrinol 1998;49:639-645.
1015. Talvensaari KK, Lanning M, Paako E, et al. Pituitary size assessed with magnetic resonance imaging as a measure of growth hormone in long term survivors of childhood cancer. J Clin Endocrinol Metab 1994;79:1122-1127.
1016. Sklar CA, Sarafoglou K, Whittam E. Effects of insulin-like growth factor binding protein 3 in predicting the growth hormone response to provocative testing in children treated with cranial irradiation. Acta Endocrinol 1993;129:511-515.
1017. Adan L, Trivin C, Sainte-Rose C, et al. GH deficiency caused by cranial irradiation during childhood: factors and markers in young adults. J Clin Endocrinol Metab 2001;86:5245-5251.
1018. Donaldson SS, Kaplan HS. Complications of treatment of Hodgkin's disease in children. Cancer Treat Rep 1982;66:977-989.
1019. Wallace WHB, Shalet SM, Morris-Jones PH, et al. Effect of abdominal irradiation on growth in boys treated for a Wilms' tumor. Med Pediatr Oncol 1990;18:441-446.
1020. Davies HA, Didcock E, Didi A, et al. Growth, puberty obesity after treatment for leukemia. Acta Paediatr 1995;411:45-50.
1021. Brownstein CM, Mertens AC, Mitby PA, et al. Factors that affect final height and change in height standard deviation scores in survivors of childhood cancer treated with growth hormone: a report from the childhood cancer survivor study. J Clin Endocrinol Metab 2004;89:4422-4427.
1022. Leiper AD, Stanhope R, Kitching P, et al. Precocious and premature puberty associated with treatment of acute lymphoblastic leukemia. Arch Dis Child 1987;62:1107-1112.
1023. Ogilvy-Stuart AL, Shalet SM. Growth and puberty after growth hormone treatment after irradiation for brain tumors. Arch Dis Child 1995;73:141-146.
1024. Ogilvy-Stuart AL, Clayton PE, Shalet SM. Cranial irradiation and early puberty. J Clin Endocrinol Metab 1994;78:1282-1286.
1025. Oberfield SE, Soranno D, Nirenberg A, et al. Age at onset of puberty following high dose central nervous system radiation. Arch Pediatr Adolesc Med 1996;150:589-592.
1026. Quigley C, Cowell C, Jimenez M, et al. Normal or early development of puberty despite gonadal damage in children treated for acute lymphoblastic leukemia. N Engl J Med 1989;321:143-151.
1027. Constine LS, Woolf PD, Cann D, et al. Hypothalamic-pituitary dysfunction after radiation for brain tumors. N Engl J Med 1993;328:87-94.
1028. Cara JF, Kreiter ML, Rosenfield RL. Height prognosis of children with true precocious puberty and growth hormone deficiency: effect of combination therapy with gonadotropin releasing hormone agonist and growth hormone. J Pediatr 1992;120: 709-715.
1029. Sklar CA. Growth following therapy for childhood cancer. Cancer Invest 1995;13:511-516.
1030. Kim RJ, Janss A, Shanis D, et al. Adult heights attained by children with hypothalamic/chiasmatic glioma treated with growth hormone. J Clin Endocrinol Metab 2004;89:4999-5002.
1031. Lerner SE, Huang GJ, McMahon D, et al. Growth hormone therapy in children after cranial/craniospinal radiation therapy: sexually dimorphic outcomes. J Clin Endocrinol Metab 2004;89: 6100-6104.
1032. Ogilvy-Stuart AL, Ryder WD, Gattamanemi HR, et al. Growth hormone and tumor recurrence. Br Med J 1992;304:1601-1605.
1033. Moshang T. Is brain tumor recurrence increased following growth hormone treatment? Trends Endocrinol Metab 1995;6:205-209.
1034. Maneatis T, Baptista J, Connelly K, et al. Growth hormone safety update from the National Cooperative Growth Study. J Pediatr Endocrinol Metab 2000;13:1035-1044.
1035. Wilton P. Adverse events during GH treatment: 10 years' experience in KIGS, a pharmacoepidemiological survey. In Ranke MB, Wilton P, eds. Growth Hormone Therapy in KIGS—10 Years' Experience. Heidelberg-Leipzig: Johann Ambrosius Barth Verlag, 1999:349-364.
1036. Sklar CA, Mertens AC, Mitby P, et al. Risk of disease recurrence and second neoplasms in survivors of childhood cancer treated with growth hormone: a report from the Childhood Cancer Survivor Study. J Clin Endocrinol Metab 2002;87:3136-3141.
1037. Sulmont V, Brauner R, Fontoura M, et al. Response to growth hormone treatment and final height after cranial or craniospinal irradiation. Acta Paediatr Scand 1990;79:542-549.
1038. Lannering B, Marky I, Mellander L, et al. Growth hormone secretion and response to growth hormone therapy after treatment for brain tumor. Acta Pediatr Scand 1988;343:146-151.
1039. Sklar C. Growth and endocrine disturbances after bone marrow transplantation in childhood. Acta Paediatr Suppl 1995;411: 57-61.
1040. Bushhouse S, Ramsay NK, Pescovitz OH, et al. Growth in children following irradiation for bone marrow transplantation. Am J Pediatr Hematol Oncol 1989;11:134-140.
1041. Clement-De Boers A, Oostdijk W, Van Weel-Sipman MH, et al. Final height and hormonal function after bone marrow transplantation in children. J Pediatr 1996;129:544-550.
1042. Giri N, Davis EA, Vowels MR. Long-term complications following BMT in children. J Pediatr Child Health 1993;29:201-205.
1043. Sanders JE. Endocrine problems in children after bone marrow transplant for hematologic malignancies. Bone Marrow Transplant 1991;8(suppl 1):2-4.
1044. Bozzola M, Giorgiani G, Locatelli F, et al. Growth in children after bone marrow transplantation. Horm Res 1993;39:122-126.
1045. Brauner R, Fontoura M, Zucker JM, et al. Growth and growth hormone secretion after bone marrow transplantation. Arch Dis Child 1993;68:458-463.
1046. Thomas BC, Stanhope R, Plowman PN, et al. Endocrine function following single fraction and frationated total body irradiation for bone marrow transplantation in childhood. Acta Endocrinol 1993;128:508-512.
1047. Horikawa R, Hellmann P, Cella SG, et al. Growth hormone-releasing factor (GRF) regulates expression of its own receptor. Endocrinology 1996;137:2642-2645.
1048. Ogilvy-Stuart AL, Clark DJ, Wallace WH, et al. Endocrine deficit after fractionated total body irradiation. Arch Dis Child 1992;67:1107-1110.
1049. Sklar CA, Kim TH, Ramsay NK. Thyroid function among long-term survivors of bone marrow transplantation. Am J Med 1982;73: 688-694.
1050. Cohen A, Rovelli A, Van-Lint MT, et al. Final height of patients who underwent bone marrow transplantation during childhood. Arch Dis Child 1996;74:437-440.

1051. Blizzard RM. Psychosocial short stature. In Lifshitz F, ed. Pediatric Endocrinology. New York: Marcel Dekker, 1985:87-107.
1052. Powell GF, Brasel JA, Blizzard RM. Emotional deprivation and growth retardation simulating idiopathic hypopituitarism. I. Clinical evaluation of the syndrome. N Engl J Med 1967;276: 1271-1278.
1053. Blizzard RM, Bulatovic A. Psychosocial short stature: a syndrome with many variables. Clin Endocrinol Metab 1992;6:687-712.
1054. Skuse D, Albanese A, Stanhope R, et al. A new stress-related syndrome of growth failure and hyperphagia in children, associated with reversibility of growth-hormone insufficiency. Lancet 1996;348:353-358.
1055. Stanhope R, Adlard P, Hamill G, et al. Physiological growth hormone (GH) secretion during the recovery from psychosocial dwarfism; a case report. Clin Endocrinol 1988;28:335-339.
1056. Albanese A, Hamill G, Jones J, et al. Reversibility of physiological growth hormone secretion in children with psychosocial dwarfism. Clin Endocrinol 1994;40:687-692.
1057. Skuse D. Emotional abuse and delay in growth. Br Med J 1989;299:113-115.
1058. Miller JD, Tannenbaum GS, Colle E, et al. Daytime pulsatile growth hormone secretion in short prepubertal children. Clin Endocrinol 1982;27:581-591.
1059. Brambilla F, Perna G, Garberi A, et al. Alpha-2 adrenergic receptor sensitivity in panic disorder. I. GH response to GHRH and clonidine stimulation in panic disorder. Psychoneuroendocrinology 1995;20:1-9.
1060. Charney DS, Heninger GR, Sternberg DE, et al. Adrenergic receptor sensitivity in depression. Effects of clonidine in depressed patients and healthy subjects. Arch Gen Psychiatry 1982;39: 290-294.
1061. Pine DS, Cohen P, Brook J. Emotional problems during youth as predictors of stature during early adulthood: Results from a prospective epidemiologic study. Pediatrics 1996;97:856-863.
1062. Jensen JB, Garfinkel BD. Growth hormone dysregulation in children with major depressive disorder. J Am Acad Child Adolesc Psychiatry 1990;29:295-301.
1063. Spiliotis BE, August GP, Hung W, et al. Growth hormone neurosecretory dysfunction: a treatable cause of short stature. JAMA 1984;252:2223-2230.
1064. Bercu BB, Shulman D, Root AW, et al. Growth hormone (GH) provocative testing frequently does not reflect endogenous GH secretion. J Clin Endocrinol Metab 1986;63:709-716.
1065. Rose SR, Ross JL, Uriarte M, et al. The advantage of measuring stimulated as compared with spontaneous growth hormone levels in the diagnosis of growth hormone deficiency. N Engl J Med 1988;319:201-207.
1066. Lanes R. Diagnostic limitations of spontaneous growth hormone measurements in normally growing prepubertal children. Am J Dis Child 1989;143:1284-1286.
1067. Rose SR, Municchi G, Barnes K, et al. Overnight growth hormone concentrations are usually normal in pubertal children with idiopathic short stature—a clinical research center study. J Clin Endocrinol Metab 1996;81:1063-1068.
1068. Lee PD, Allen DB, Angulo MA, et al. Consensus statement—Prader-Willi syndrome: growth hormone (GH)/insulin-like growth factor deficiency and GH treatment. Endocrinologist 2000;10: 71S-73S.
1069. Eiholzer U, Bachmann S, l'Allemand D. Is there growth hormone deficiency in Prader-Willi syndrome? Horm Res 2000;53:44-42.
1070. Francke U. Prader-Willi syndrome: chromosomal and gene aberrations. Growth Genet Horm 1994;10:4-7.
1071. Gladstone AP. Prader-Willi syndrome: advances in genetics, pathophysiology and treatment. Trend Endocrinol Metab 2004;15: 12-20.
1072. Carrel AL, Allen DB. Growth hormone and Prader-Willi syndrome: what we know and have yet to learn. Endocrinologist 2003;13: 106-111.
1073. Hulthen L, Bengtsson BA, Sunnerhagen KS, et al. GH is needed for the maturation of muscle mass and strength in adolescents. J Clin Endocrinol Metab 2001;86:4765-4770.
1074. Vestergaard P, Kristensen K, Bruun JM, et al. Reduced bone mineral density and increased bone turnover in Prader-Willi syndrome compared with controls matched for sex and body mass index—a cross-sectional study. J Pediatr 2004;144:614-619.
1075. Costeff H, Holm VA, Ruvalcaba R, et al. Growth hormone secretion in Prader Willi syndrome. Acta Paediatr Scand 1990;79: 1059-1062.
1076. Cappa M, Grossi A, Borrelli P, et al. Growth hormone (GH) response to combined pyridostigmine and GH-releasing hormone administration in patients with Prader-Labhard-Willi syndrome. Horm Res 1993;39:51-55.
1077. Angulo M, Castro-Magana M, Uy J. Pituitary evaluation and growth hormone treatment in Prader-Willi syndrome. J Pediatr Endocrinol 1991;4:167-173.
1078. Lindgren AC, Hagenas L, Muller J, et al. Growth hormone treatment of children with Prader-Willi syndrome affects linear growth and body composition favourably. Acta Paediatr 1998;87:28-31.
1079. Carrel AL, Myers SE, Whitman BY, et al. Growth hormone improves body composition, fat utilization, physical strength and agility, and growth in Prader-Willi syndrome: a controlled study. J Pediatr 1999;134:215-221.
1080. Carrel AL, Moerchen V, Myers SE, et al. Growth hormone improves mobility and body composition in infants and toddlers with Prader-Willi syndrome. J Pediatr 2004;145:744-749.
1081. Myers SE, Carrel AL, Whitman BY, et al. Sustained benefit after 2 years of growth hormone on body composition, fat utilization, physical strength and agility, and growth in Prader-Willi syndrome. J Pediatr 2000;137:42-49.
1082. Lindgren AC, Ritzen EM. Five years of growth hormone treatment in children with Prader-Willi syndrome. Acta Paediatr Suppl 1999;433:109-111.
1083. Eiholzer U. Deaths in children with Prader-Willi syndrome. Horm Res 2005;63:33-39.
1084. Lee PD. Growth hormone and mortality in Prader-Willi Syndrome. Growth Genet Horm 2006;22:1-8.
1085. Allen DB, Fost NC. Growth hormone therapy for short stature: panacea or Pandora's box? J Pediatr 1990;117(1 Pt 1):16-21.
1086. Maghnie M, Strigazzi C, Tinelli C, et al. Growth hormone (GH) deficiency (GHD) of childhood onset: reassessment of GH status and evaluation of the predictive criteria for permanent GHD in young adults. J Clin Endocrinol Metab 1999;84(12): 1324-1328.
1087. Longobardi S, Merola B, Pivonello R, et al. Reevaluation of growth hormone (GH) secretion in 69 adults diagnosed as GH-deficient patients during childhood. J Clin Endocrinol Metab 1996;81: 1244-1247.
1088. Cacciari E, Tassoni P, Cicognani A, et al. Value and limits of pharmacological and physiological tests to diagnose growth hormone (GH) deficiency and predict therapy response: First and second retesting during replacement therapy of patients defined as GH deficient. J Clin Endocrinol Metab 1994;79: 1663-1669.
1089. Tauber M, Moulin P, Pienkowski C, et al. Growth hormone (GH) retesting and auxological data in 131 GH-deficient patients after completion of treatment. J Clin Endocrinol Metab 1997;82: 352-356.
1090. Nicolson A, Toogood AA, Rahim A, et al. The prevalence of severe growth hormone deficiency in adults who received growth hormone. Clin Endocrinol (Oxf) 1996;44:311-316.
1091. Rutherford OM, Jones DA, Round JM, et al. Changes in skeletal muscle and body composition after discontinuation of growth hormone treatment in growth hormone deficient young adults. Clin Endocrinol (Oxf) 1991;34:469-475.
1092. Clayton PE, Price DA, Shalet SM. Growth hormone state after completion of treatment with growth hormone. Arch Dis Child 1987;62:222-226.
1093. Juul A, Kastrup KW, Pedersen SA, et al. Growth hormone (GH) provocative retesting of 108 young adults with childhood-onset GH deficiency and the diagnostic value of insulin-like growth factor I (IGF-I) and IGF-binding protein-3. J Clin Endocrinol Metab 1997;82:1195-1291.
1094. Gourmelen M, Pham-Huu-Trung MT, Girard F. Transient partial GH deficiency in prepubertal children with delay of growth. Pediatr Res 1979;13:221-224.
1095. Phillips JA, Cogan JD. Molecular basis of familial human growth hormone deficiency. J Clin Endocrinol Metab 1994;76:11-16.
1096. Procter AM, Phillips JA III, Cooper DN. The molecular genetics of growth hormone deficiency. Hum Genet 1998;103:255-272.

1097. Parks JS, Brown MR, Hurley DL, et al. Heritable disorders of pituitary development. J Clin Endocrinol Metab 1999;84:4362-4370.
1098. Sornson MW, Wu W, Dasen JS, et al. Pituitary lineage determination by the Prophet of Pit-1 homeodomain factor defective in Ames dwarfism. Nature 1996;384:327-333.
1099. Fluck C, Deladoey J, Rutishauser K, et al. Phenotypic variability in familial combined pituitary hormone deficiency caused by a PROP1 gene mutation resulting in the substitution of Arg → Cys at codon 120 (R120C). J Clin Endocrinol Metab 1998;83:3727-3734.
1100. Osorio MG, Kopp P, Marui S, et al. Combined pituitary hormone deficiency caused by a novel mutation of a highly conserved residue (F88S) in the homeodomain of PROP-1. J Clin Endocrinol Metab 2000;85:2779-2785.
1101. Deladoey J, Fluck C, Buyukgebiz A, et al. "Hot spot" in the PROP1 gene responsible for combined pituitary hormone deficiency. J Clin Endocrinol Metab 1999;84:1645-1650.
1102. Dattani MT. GH deficiency might be associated with normal height in PROP1 deficiency. Clin Endocrinol (Oxf) 2002;57:157-158.
1103. Arroyo A, Pernasetti F, Vasilyev VV, et al. A unique case of combined pituitary hormone deficiency caused by a PROP1 gene mutation (R120C) associated with normal height and absent puberty. Clin Endocrinol (Oxf) 2002;57:283-291.
1104. Voutetakis A, Argyropoulou M, Sertedaki A, et al. Pituitary magnetic resonance imaging in 15 patients with PROP1 gene mutations: pituitary enlargement may originate from the intermediate lobe. J Clin Endocrinol Metab 2004;89:2200-2206.
1105. Rosenbloom AL, Almonte AS, Brown MR, et al. Clinical and biochemical phenotype of familial anterior hypopituitarism from mutation of the PROP1 gene. J Clin Endocrinol Metab 1999;84:50-57.
1106. Mendonca BB, Osorio MG, Latronica AC, et al. Longitudinal hormonal and pituitary imaging changes in two families with combined pituitary hormone deficiency due to deletion of A301,G302 in the PROP1 gene. J Clin Endocrinol Metab 1999;84:942-945.
1107. Agarwal G, Bhatia V, Cook S, et al. Adrenocorticotropin deficiency in combined pituitary hormone deficiency patients homozygous for a novel PROP1 mutation. J Clin Endocrinol Metab 2000;85:4556-4561.
1108. Asteria C, Oliveira JH, Abucham J, et al. Central hypocortisolism as part of combined pituitary hormone deficiency due to mutations of PROP-1 gene. Eur J Endocrinol 2000;143:347-352.
1109. Bottner A, Keller E, Kratzsch J, et al. PROP1 mutations cause progressive deterioration of anterior pituitary function including adrenal insufficiency: a longitudinal analysis. J Clin Endocrinol Metab 2004;89:5256-5265.
1110. Pavel ME, Hensen J, Pfaffle R, et al. Long-term follow-up of childhood-onset hypopituitarism in patients with the PROP-1 gene mutation. Horm Res 2003;60:168-173.
1111. Vallette-Kasic S, Barlier A, Teinturier C, et al. PROP1 gene screening in patients with multiple pituitary hormone deficiency reveals two sites of hypermutability and a high incidence of corticotroph deficiency. J Clin Endocrinol Metab 2001;86:4529-4535.
1112. Duquesnoy P, Roy A, Dastot F, et al. Human Prop-1: cloning, mapping, genomic structure. Mutations in familial combined pituitary hormone deficiency. FEBS Lett 1998;437:216-220.
1113. Fofanova O, Takamura N, Kinoshita E, et al. Compound heterozygous deletion of the PROP-1 gene in children with combined pituitary hormone deficiency. J Clin Endocrinol Metab 1998;83:2601-2604.
1114. Fofanova OV, Takamura N, Kinoshita E, et al. Rarity of PIT1 involvement in children from Russia with combined pituitary hormone deficiency. Am J Med Genet 1998;77:360-365.
1115. Rainbow LA, Rees SA, Shaikh MG, et al. Mutation analysis of POUF-1, PROP-1 and HESX-1 show low frequency of mutations in children with sporadic forms of combined pituitary hormone deficiency and septo-optic dysplasia. Clin Endocrinol (Oxf) 2005;62:163-168.
1116. Nelson C, Albert VR, Elsholtz HP, et al. Activation of cell-specific expression of rat growth hormone and prolactin genes by a common transcription factor. Science 1988;239:1400-1405.
1117. Mangalam HJ, Albert VR, Ingraham HA, et al. A pituitary POU domain protein, pit-1, activates both growth hormone and prolactin promoters transcriptionally. Genes Dev 1989;3:946-958.
1118. Li S, Crenshaw EB III, Rawson EJ, et al. Dwarf locus mutants lacking three pituitary cell types result from mutations in the POU-domain gene pit-1. Nature 1990;347:528-532.
1119. Lin S-C, Lin CR, Gukovsky I, et al. Molecular basis of the little mouse phenotype and implications for cell type-specific growth. Nature 1993;364:208-213.
1120. Parks JS, Kinoshita EI, Pfaffle RW. Pit-1 and hypopituitarism. Trends Endocrinol Metab 1993;4:81-85.
1121. Montminy M. The road not taken. Nature 1993;364:190-191.
1122. Pfaffle RW, DiMattia GE, Parks JS, et al. Mutation of the POU-specific domain of Pit-1 and hypopituitarism without pituitary hypoplasia. Science 1992;257:1118-1121.
1123. Buckwalter MS, Katz RW, Camper SA. Localization of the panhypopituitary dwarf mutation (df) on mouse chromosome 11 in an intersubspecific backcross. Genomics 1991;10:515-526.
1124. Wit JM, Drayer NM, Jansen M, et al. Total deficiency of growth hormone and prolactin and partial deficiency of thyroid stimulating hormone in two Dutch families: a new variant of hereditary pituitary deficiency. Horm Res 1989;32:170-177.
1125. Cogan JD, Phillips JA, Schenkman SS, et al. Familial growth hormone deficiency: a model of dominant and recessive mutations affecting a monomeric protein. J Clin Endocrinol Metab 1994;79:1261-1265.
1126. Cohen LE, Wondisford PE, Salvatoni A, et al. A "hot spot" in the Pit-1 gene responsible for combined pituitary hormone deficiency: clinical and molecular correlates. J Clin Endocrinol Metab 1995;80:679-684.
1127. Tatsumi KI, Miyai K, Notomi T, et al. Cretinism with combined hormone deficiency caused by a mutation in the Pit-1 gene. Nature Genet 1992;1:56-58.
1128. Pellegrini-Bouiller I, Belicar P, Barlier A, et al. A new mutation of the gene encoding the transcription factor Pit-1 is responsible for combined pituitary hormone deficiency. J Clin Endocrinol Metab 1996;81:2790-2796.
1129. Haqq AM, Stadler DD, Jackson RH, et al. Effects of growth hormone on pulmonary function, sleep quality, behavior, cognition, growth velocity, body composition, and resting energy expenditure in Prader-Willi syndrome. J Clin Endocrinol Metab 2003;88:2206-2212.
1130. Radovick S, Nations M, Du Y, et al. A mutation in the POU-homeodomain of pit-1 responsible for combined pituitary hormone deficiency. Science 1992;257:1115-1118.
1131. Pfaffle R, Kim C, Otten B, et al. Pit 1: Clinical aspects. Horm Res 1996;45(suppl 1):25-28.
1132. Turton JP, Reynaud R, Mehta A, et al. Novel mutations within the POU1F1 gene associated with variable combined pituitary hormone deficiency. J Clin Endocrinol Metab 2005;90:4762-4770.
1133. Cutfield WS, Wilton P, Bennmarker H, et al. Incidence of diabetes mellitus and impaired glucose tolerance in children and adolescents receiving growth-hormone treatment. Lancet 2000;355:610-613.
1134. Bondy CA, Van PL, Bakalov VK, et al. Growth hormone treatment and aortic dimensions in Turner syndrome. J Clin Endocrinol Metab 2006;91:1785-1788.
1135. Russell-Aulet M, Shairo B, Jaffe CA, et al. Peak bone mass in young healthy men is correlated with the magnitude of endogenous growth hormone secretion. J Clin Endocrinol Metab 1998;83:3463-3468.
1136. Amendt BA, Sutherland LB, Semina E, et al. The molecular basis of Rieger syndrome. J Biol Chem 1998;273:20066-20072.
1137. Gage PJ, Camper SA. Pituitary homeobox 2, a novel member of the bicoid-related family of homeobox genes, is a potential regulator of anterior structure formation. Hum Mol Genet 1997;6:457-464.
1138. Semina EV, Reiter R, Leysens NJ, et al. Cloning and characterization of a novel bicoid-related homeobox transcription factor gene, RIEG, involved in Rieger syndrome. Nat Genet 1996;14:392-399.
1139. Charles MA, Suh H, Hjalt TA, et al. PITX genes are required for cell survival and Lhx3 activation. Mol Endocrinol 2005;19:1893-1903.
1140. Toy J, Yang J-M, Leppert GS, et al. The Optx2 homeobox gene is expressed in early precursors of the eye and activates retina-specific genes. Proc Nat Acad Sci U S A 1998;95:10643-10648.

1141. Lemyre E, Lemieux N, Decarie JC, et al. Del (14)(q22.1q23.2) in a patient with anophthalmia and pituitary hypoplasia. Am J Med Genet 1998;77:162-165.
1142. Whitman BY, Myers MG, Carrel AL, et al. The behavioral impact of growth hormone treatment for children and adolescents with Prader-Willi syndrome: a 2-year controlled study. Pediatrics 2005;109(e35):308-309.
1143. Bona G, Paracchini R, Giordano M, et al. Genetic defects in GH synthesis and secretion. Eur J Endocrinol 2004;151(suppl 1): S3-S9.
1144. Woods KS, Cundall M, Turton J, et al. Over- and underdosage of SOX3 is associated with infundibular hypoplasia and hypopituitarism. Am J Hum Genet 2005;76:833-849.
1145. Bhangoo AP, Hunter CS, Savage JJ, et al. Clinical case seminar: a novel LHX3 mutation presenting as combined pituitary hormonal deficiency. J Clin Endocrinol Metab 2006;91:747-753.
1146. Machinis K, Amselem S. Functional relationship between LHX4 and POU1F1 in light of the LHX4 mutation identified in patients with pituitary defects. J Clin Endocrinol Metab 2005;90: 5456-5462.
1147. Kim SS, Kim Y, Shin YL, et al. Clinical characteristics and molecular analysis of PIT1, PROP1,LHX3, and HESX1 in combined pituitary hormone deficiency patients with abnormal pituitary MR imaging. Horm Res 2003;60:277-283.
1148. Pantel J, Legendre M, Cabrol S, et al. Loss of constitutive activity of the growth hormone secretagogue receptor in familial short stature. J Clin Invest 2006;116:760-768.
1149. Holst B, Schwartz TW. Ghrelin receptor mutations—too little height and too much hunger. J Clin Invest 2006;116:637-641.
1150. Wang HJ, Geller F, Dempfle A, et al. Ghrelin receptor gene: identification of several sequence variants in extremely obese children and adolescents, healthy normal-weight and underweight students, and children with short normal stature. J Clin Endocrinol Metab 2004;89:157-162.
1151. Shuto Y, Shibasaki T, Otagiri A, et al. Hypothalamic growth hormone secretagogue receptor regulates growth hormone secretion, feeding, and adiposity. J Clin Invest 2002;109: 1429-1436.
1152. Sun Y, Wang P, Zheng H, et al. Ghrelin stimulation of growth hormone release and appetite is mediated through the growth hormone secretagogue receptor. Proc Natl Acad Sci U S A 2004;101:4679-4684.
1153. Wajnrajch MP, Gertner JM, Harbison MD, et al. Nonsense mutations of the human growth hormone releasing hormone receptor (GHRHR) causes growth failure analogous to that of the little (lit) mouse. Nat Genet 1996;12:88-90.
1154. Maheshwari HG, Silverman BL, Dupuis J, et al. Phenotype and genetic analysis of a syndrome caused by an inactivating mutation in the growth hormone-releasing hormone receptor: dwarfism of Sindh. J Clin Endocrinol Metab 1998;83:4065-4074.
1155. Netchine I, Talon P, Dastot F, et al. Extensive phenotypic analysis of a family with growth hormone (GH) deficiency caused by a mutation in the GH-releasing hormone receptor gene. J Clin Endocrinol Metab 1998;83:432-436.
1156. Salvatori R, Hayashida CY, Aguiar-Oliveira MH, et al. Familial dwarfism due to a novel mutation of the growth hormone-releasing hormone receptor gene. J Clin Endocrinol Metab 1999; 84:917-923.
1157. Aguiar-Oliveira MH, Gill MS, de A'Barretto ES, et al. Effect of severe growth hormone (GH) deficiency due to a mutation in the GH-releasing hormone receptor on insulin-like growth factors (IGFs), IGF-binding proteins, and ternary complex formation throughout life. J Clin Endocrinol Metab 1999;84:4118-4126.
1158. Salvatori R, Fan X, Phillips JA III, et al. Three new mutations in the gene for the growth hormone (GH)-releasing hormone receptor in familial isolated GH deficiency type IB. J Clin Endocrinol Metab 2001;86:273-279.
1159. Gaylinn BD, Dealmeida VI, Lyons CE Jr, et al. The mutant growth hormone-releasing hormone (GHRH) receptor of the Little mouse does not bind GHRH. Endocrinology 1999;140: 5066-5074.
1160. Godfrey P, Rahal JO, Beamer WG, et al. GHRH receptor of little mouse contains missense mutation in the extracellular domain that disrupts receptor function. Nat Genet 1993;4:227-232.
1161. Mayo KE, Godfrey PA, Suhr ST, et al. Growth hormone-releasing hormone: synthesis and signaling. Rec Prog Horm Res 1995;50:35-73.
1162. Illig R, Prader A, Ferrandez A, et al. Hereditary prenatal growth hormone deficiency with increased tendency to growth hormone antibody formation ("A-type" of isolated growth hormone deficiency). Acta Paediatr Scand 1971;60:607.
1163. Wagner JK, Eble A, Hindmarsh PC, et al. Prevalence of human GH-1 gene alterations in patients with isolated growth hormone deficiency. Pediatr Res 1998;43:105-110.
1164. Cao Y, Wagner JK, Hindmarsh PC, et al. Isolated growth hormone deficiency: testing the little mouse hypothesis in man and exclusion of mutations within the extracellular domain of the growth hormone releasing hormone receptor. Pediatr Res 1995;38: 962-966.
1165. Hayashi Y, Yamamoto M, Ohmori S, et al. Inhibition of growth hormone (GH) secretion by a mutant GH-I gene product in neuroendocrine cells containing secretory granules: an implication for isolated GH deficiency inherited in an autosomal dominant manner. J Clin Endocrinol Metab 1999;84:2134-2139.
1166. Lee MS, Wajnrajch MP, Kim SS, et al. Autosomal dominant growth hormone (GH) deficiency type II: the del32-71-GH deletion mutant suppresses secretion of wild-type GH. J Clin Endocrinol Metab 2000;141:883-890.
1167. Woods KA, Dastot F, Preece MA, et al. Phenotype: genotype relationships in growth hormone insensitivity syndrome. J Clin Endocrinol Metab 1997;82:3529-3535.
1168. Binder G, Keller E, Mix M, et al. Isolated GH deficiency with dominant inheritance: new mutations, new insights. J Clin Endocrinol Metab 2001;86:3877-3881.
1169. Deladoey J, Stocker P, Mullis PE. Autosomal dominant GH deficiency due to Arg183His GH-1 gene mutation: clinical and molecular evidence of impaired regulated GH secretion. J Clin Endocrinol Metab 2001;86:3941-3947.
1170. Mullis PE, Robinson IC, Salemi S, et al. Isolated autosomal dominant growth hormone deficiency: an evolving pituitary deficit? A multicenter follow-up study. J Clin Endocrinol Metab 2005;90:2089-2096.
1171. Millar DS, Lewis MD, Horan M, et al. Novel mutations of the growth hormone 1 (GH1) gene disclosed by modulation of the clinical selection criteria for individuals with short stature. Hum Mutat 2003;21:424-440.
1172. Fintini D, Salvatori R, Salemi S, et al. Autosomal-dominant isolated growth hormone deficiency (IGHD type II) with normal GH-1 gene. Horm Res 2006;65:76-82.
1173. Fleisher TA, White RM, Broder S, et al. X-linked hypogammaglobulinemia and isolated growth hormone deficiency. N Engl J Med 1980;302:1429-1434.
1174. Solomon NM, Nouri S, Warne GL, et al. Increased gene dosage at Xq26-q27 is associated with X-linked hypopituitarism. Genomics 2002;79:553-559.
1175. Valenta LJ, Sigel MB, Lesniak MA, et al. Pituitary dwarfism in a patient with circulating abnormal growth hormone polymers. N Engl J Med 1985;312:214-217.
1176. Kowarski AA, Schneider J, Ben-Galim E, et al. Growth failure with normal serum RIA-GH and low somatomedin activity: somatomedin restoration and growth acceleration after exogenous GH. J Clin Endocrinol Metab 1978;47:461-464.
1177. Takahashi Y, Kaji H, Okimura Y, et al. Short stature caused by a mutant growth hormone. N Engl J Med 1996;334:432-436.
1178. Takahashi Y, Shirono H, Arisaka O, et al. Biologically inactive growth hormone caused by an amino acid substitution. J Clin Invest 1997;100:1159-1165.
1179. Ishikawa M, Nimura A, Horikawa R, et al. A novel specific bioassay for serum human growth hormone. J Clin Endocrinol Metab 2000;85:4274-4279.
1180. Besson A, Salemi S, Deladoey J, et al. Short stature caused by a biologically inactive mutant growth hormone (GH-C53S). J Clin Endocrinol Metab 2005;90:2493-2499.
1181. Radetti G, Bossola M, Pagani S, et al. Growth hormone immunoreactivity does not reflect bioactivity. Pediatr Res 2000;48: 619-622.
1182. Jenkins JS, Gilberg CJ, Ang V. Hypothalamic-pituitary function in patients with craniopharyngiomas. J Clin Endocrinol Metab 1976;43:394-399.

1183. Thomsett MJ, Conte FA, Kaplan SL, et al. Endocrine and neurologic outcome in childhood craniopharyngioma. Review of effect of treatment in 42 patients. J Pediatr 1980;97:728-735.
1184. Lafferty AR, Chrousos GP. Pituitary tumors in children and adolescents. J Clin Endocrinol Metab 1999;84:4317-4323.
1185. Laws ER, Thapar K. The diagnosis and management of craniopharyngioma. Growth Genet Hormones 1994;10:6-10.
1186. Paja M, Lucas T, Garcia-Uria J, et al. Hypothalamic-pituitary dysfunction in patients with craniopharyngioma. Clin Endocrinol 1995;42:467-473.
1187. Rivarola M, Mendilaharzu H, Warman M, et al. Endocrine disorders in 66 suprasellar and pineal tumors of patients with prepubertal and pubertal ages. Horm Res 1992;37:1-6.
1188. Kane LA, Leinung MC, Scheithauer BW, et al. Pituitary adenomas in childhood and adolescence. J Clin Endocrinol Metab 1994;79:1135-1140.
1189. Frailioli B, Ferrante L, Celli P. Pituitary adenomas with onset during puberty: features and treatment. J Neurosurg 1983;59: 590-595.
1190. Maira G, Anile C. Pituitary tumors in childhood and adolescence. Can J Neurol Sci 1990;65:733-744.
1191. Muller HL, Emser A, Faldum A, et al. Longitudinal study on growth and body mass index before and after diagnosis of childhood craniopharyngioma. J Clin Endocrinol Metab 2004;89: 3298-3305.
1192. DeVile CJ, Grant DB, Hayward RD, et al. Growth and endocrine sequelae of craniopharyngioma. Arch Dis Child 1996;75:108-114.
1193. Geffner M, Lundberg M, Koltowska-Haggstrom M, et al. Changes in height, weight, and body mass index in children with craniopharyngioma after three years of growth hormone therapy: analysis of KIGS (Pfizer International Growth Database). J Clin Endocrinol Metab 2004;89:5435-5440.
1194. Srinivasan S, Ogle GD, Garnett SP, et al. Features of the metabolic syndrome after childhood craniopharyngioma. J Clin Endocrinol Metab 2004;89:81-86.
1195. Richmond IL, Wilson CB. Pituitary adenomas in childhood and adolescence. J Neurosurg 1978;49:163-168.
1196. Egeler RM, D'Angio GJ. Langerhans cell histiocytosis. J Pediatr 1996;127:1-11.
1197. Braunstein GD, Kohler PO. Pituitary function in Hand-Schuller-Christian disease. Evidence for deficient growth hormone release in patients with short stature. N Engl J Med 1972;286:1225-1229.
1198. Broadbent V, Dunger DN, Yeomans E, et al. Anterior pituitary function and computed tomography/magnetic resonance imaging in patients with Langerhans cell histiocytosis and diabetes insipidus. Med Pediatr Oncol 1993;21:649-654.
1199. Maghnie M, Cosi G, Genovese E, et al. Central diabetes insipidus in children and young adults. N Engl J Med 2000;343:998-1007.
1200. Donadieu J, Rolon MA, Thomas C, et al. Endocrine involvement in pediatric-onset Langerhans' cell histiocytosis: a population-based study. J Pediatr 2004;144:344-350.
1201. Dean HJ, Bishop A, Winter JS. Growth hormone deficiency in patients with histiocytosis X. J Pediatr 1996;109:615-618.
1202. Laron Z, Blum W, Chatelain P, et al. Classification of growth hormone insensitivity syndrome. J Pediatr 1993;122:241.
1203. Laron Z, Pertzelan A, Mannheimer S. Genetic pituitary dwarfism with high serum concentration of growth hormone—a new inborn error of metabolism? Isr J Med Sci 1966;2:152-155.
1204. Rosenbloom AL, Guevara-Aguirre J, Rosenfeld RG, et al. The little men of Loja: growth hormone receptor deficiency in an inbred population of southern Ecuador. N Engl J Med 1990;323: 1367-1374.
1205. Golde DW, Bersch N, Kaplan SA, et al. Peripheral unresponsiveness to human growth hormone in Laron dwarfism. N Engl J Med 1980;303:1156-1159.
1206. Eshet R, Laron Z, Pertzelan A, et al. Defect of human growth hormone receptors in the liver of two patients with Laron-type dwarfism. Isr J Med Sci 1984;20:8-11.
1207. Godowski PJ, Leung DW, Meacham LR, et al. Characterization of the human growth hormone receptor gene and demonstration of a partial gene deletion in two patients with Laron-type dwarfism. Proc Natl Acad Sci U S A 1989;86:8083-8087.
1208. Amselem S, Duquesnoy P, Attree O, et al. Laron dwarfism and mutations of the growth hormone-receptor gene. N Engl J Med 1989;321:989-995.
1209. Berg MA, Guevara-Aguirre J, Rosenbloom AL, et al. Mutation creating a new splice site in the growth hormone receptor genes of 37 Ecuadorian patients with Laron syndrome. Hum Mutation 1992;1:24-34.
1210. Silbergeld A, Dastot F, Klinger B, et al. Intronic mutation in the growth hormone (GH) receptor gene from a girl with Laron syndrome and extremely high GH binding protein: extended phenotypic study in a very large pedigree. J Pediatr Endocrinol Metab 1997;10:265-274.
1211. Kaji H, Nose O, Tajiri H, et al. Novel compound heterozygous mutations of growth hormone (GH) receptor gene in a patient with GH insensitivity syndrome. J Clin Endocrinol Metab 1997;82:3705-3709.
1212. Ayling RM, Ross R, Towner P, et al. A dominant-negative mutation of the growth hormone receptor causes familial short stature. Nat Genet 1997;16:13-14.
1213. Iida K, Takahashi Y, Kaji H, et al. Growth hormone (GH) insensitivity syndrome with high serum GH-binding protein levels caused by a heterozygous splice site mutation of the GH receptor gene producing a lack of intracellular domain. J Clin Endocrinol Metab 1998;83:531-537.
1214. Gastier JM, Berg MA, Vesterhus P, et al. Diverse deletions in the growth hormone receptor gene cause growth hormone insensitivity syndrome. Hum Mutat 2000;16:323-333.
1215. Milward A, Metherell L, Maamra M, et al. Growth hormone (GH) insensitivity syndrome due to a GH receptor truncated after box1, resulting in isolated failure of STAT 5 signal transduction. J Clin Endocrinol Metab 2004;89:1259-1266.
1216. Tiulpakov A, Rubtsov P, Dedov I, et al. A novel C-terminal growth hormone receptor (GHR) mutation results in impaired GHR-STAT5 but normal STAT-3 signaling. J Clin Endocrinol Metab 2005;90:542-547.
1217. Iida K, Takahashi Y, Kaji H, et al. Functional characterization of truncated growth hormone (GH) receptor-(1-277) causing partial GH insensitivity syndrome with high GH-binding protein. J Clin Endocrinol Metab 1999;84:1011-1016.
1218. Szabo M, Butz MR, Banerjee SA, et al. Autofeedback suppression of growth hormone (GH) secretion in transgenic mice expressing a human GH reported targeted by tyrosine hydroxylase 5′-flanking sequences to the hypothalamus. Endocrinology 1995; 136:4044-4048.
1219. Attie KM. Editorial: Mutations of the growth hormone receptor—widening the search. J Clin Endocrinol Metab 1996;81: 1683-1685.
1220. Sanchez JE, Perera E, Baumbach L, et al. Growth hormone receptor mutations in children with idiopathic short stature. J Clin Endocrinol Metab 1998;83:4079-4083.
1221. Ross RJ, Esposito N, Shen XY, et al. A short isoform of the human growth hormone receptor functions as a dominant negative inhibitor of the full-length receptor and generates large amounts of binding protein. Mol Endocrinol 1997;11:265-273.
1222. Johnston LB, Woods KA, Rose SJ, et al. The broad spectrum of inherited growth hormone insensitivity syndrome. Trends Endocrinol Metab 1998;9:228-232.
1223. Freeth JS, Silva CM, Whatmore AJ, et al. Activation of the signal transducers and activators of transcription signaling pathway by growth hormone (GH) in skin fibroblasts from normal and GH-binding positive Laron syndrome children. Endocrinology 1998;139:20-28.
1224. Fang P, Kofoed EM, Little BM, et al. A mutant STAT5b, associated with growth hormone insensitivity and IGF-I deficiency, cannot function as a signal transducer or transcription factor. J Clin Endocrinol Metab 2006;91:1526-1534.
1225. Chia DJ, Subbian E, Buck TM, et al. Aberrant folding of a mutant Stat5b causes growth hormone insensitivity and proteasomal dysfunction. J Biol Chem 2005;281:6522-6558.
1226. Domene HM, Bengolea SV, Martinez AS, et al. Deficiency of the circulating insulin-like growth factor system associated with inactivation of the acid-labile subunit gene. N Engl J Med 2004; 350:570-577.
1227. Hwa V, Haeusler G, Pratt KL, et al. Total absence of acid labile subunit (ALS) resulting in severe IGF deficiency and moderate growth failure. J Clin Endocrinol Metab 2006;91;1826-1831.
1228. Woods KA, Camacho-Hubner C, Bergman RN, et al. Effects of insulin-like growth factor I (IGF-I) therapy on body composition

and insulin resistance in IGF-I gene deletion. J Clin Endocrinol Metab 2000;85:1407-1411.

1229. Camacho-Hubner C, Woods KA, Miraki-Moud F, et al. Effects of recombinant human insulin-like growth factor I (IGF-I) therapy on the growth hormone-IGF system of a patient with a partial IGF-I gene deletion. J Clin Endocrinol Metab 1999;84:1611-1616.
1230. Denley A, Wang CC, McNeil KA, et al. Structural and functional characteristics of the Val44Met insulin-like growth factor I missense mutation: correlation with effects on growth and development. Mol Endocrinol 2005;19:711-721.
1231. Tollefsen SE, Heath-Monnig E, Cascieri MA, et al. Endogenous insulin-like growth factor (IGF) binding proteins cause IF+GF-I resistance in cultured fibroblasts from a patient with short stature. J Clin Invest 1991;87:1241-1250.
1232. Barreca A, Bozzola M, Cesarone A, et al. Short stature associated with high circulating insulin-like growth factor (IGF)-binding protein-1 and low circulating IGF-II: Effect of growth hormone therapy. J Clin Endocrinol Metab 1998;83:3534-3541.
1233. Jain S, Golde DW, Bailey R, et al. Insulin-like growth factor-I resistance. Endocr Rev 1998;19:625-646.
1234. Hattori Y, Vera JC, Rivas CI, et al. Decreased insulin-like growth factor I receptor expression and function in immortalized African pygmy T cells. J Clin Endocrinol Metab 1996;81:2257-2263.
1235. Raile K, Klammt J, Schneider A, et al. Clinical and functional characteristics of the human Arg59Ter insulin-like growth factor I receptor (IGF1R) mutation: implications for a gene dosage effect of the human IGF1R. J Clin Endocrinol Metab 2006;91: 2264-2271.
1236. Wertheimer E, Lu SP, Backeljauw PF, et al. Homozygous deletion of the human insulin receptor gene results in leprechaunism. Nat Genet 1993;5:71-73.
1237. Siebler T, Lopaczynski W, Terry EL, et al. Insulin-like growth factor I receptor expression and function in fibroblasts from two patients with deletion of the distal long arm of chromosome 15. J Clin Endocrinol Metab 1995;80:3447-3457.
1238. Rosenfeld RG, Albertsson-Wikland K, Cassorla F, et al. The diagnosis of childhood growth hormone deficiency revisited. J Clin Endocrinol Metab 1995;80:1532-1540.
1239. Frasier SD. A review of growth hormone stimulation tests in children. Pediatrics 1974;53:929-937.
1240. Reiter EO, Martha PM Jr. Pharmacological testing of growth hormone secretion. Horm Res 1990;33:121-127.
1241. Raiti S, Davis WT, Blizzard RM. A comparison of the effects of insulin hypoglycemia and arginine infusion on release of human growth hormone. Lancet 1967;2:1182-1183.
1242. Guyda HJ. Growth hormone testing and the short child. Pediatr Res 2000;48:579-580.
1243. Grumbach MM, Bin-Abbas BS, Kaplan SL. The growth hormone cascade: progress and long-term results of growth hormone treatment in growth hormone deficiency. Horm Res 1998;49 (suppl 2):41-57.
1244. Kaplan SL, Abrams CA, Bell JJ. Growth and growth hormone. I. Changes in serum levels of growth hormone following hypoglycemia in 134 children with growth retardation. Pediatr Res 1968;2:43-63.
1245. Physicians' Desk Reference. Montvale, NJ: Medical Economics Data Production Company, 1994:1004.
1246. Physicians' Desk Reference. Montvale, NJ: Medical Economics Data Production Company, 1994:1228.
1247. Guyda HJ. Four decades of growth hormone therapy for short children: what have we achieved? J Clin Endocrinol Metab 1999;84:4307-4316.
1248. Rosenfeld RG. Evaluation of growth and maturation in adolescence. Pediatr Rev 1982;4:175-183.
1249. Lippe B, Wong S-L, Kaplan SA. Simultaneous assessment of growth hormone and ACTH reserve in children pretreated with diethylstilbestrol. J Clin Endocr 1971;33:949-956.
1250. Chernausek SD. Laboratory diagnosis of growth disorders. In Hintz RL, Rosenfeld RG, eds. Growth Abnormalities. Contemporary Issues in Endocrinology and Metabolism. New York: Churchill Livingstone, 1987:231-254.
1251. Cacciari E, Tassoni P, Parisi G, et al. Pitfalls in diagnosing impaired growth hormone (GH) secretion: retesting after replacement therapy of 63 children defined as GH deficient. J Clin Endocrinol Metab 1992;74:1284-1289.
1252. Martinez AS, Domene HM, Ropelato MG, et al. Estrogen priming effect on growth hormone (GH) provocative testing: a useful tool for the diagnosis of GH deficiency. J Clin Endocrinol Metab 2000;85:4168-4172.
1253. Marin G, Domene HM, Barnes KM, et al. The effects of estrogen priming and puberty on the growth hormone response to standardized treadmill exercise and arginine-insulin in normal girls and boys. J Clin Endocrinol Metab 1994;79:537-541.
1254. Reiter EO, Morris AH, MacGillivray MH, et al. Variable estimates of serum growth hormone concentrations by difference radioassay systems. J Clin Endocrinol Metab 1988;66:68-71.
1255. Celniker AC, Chem AB, Wert RM Jr, et al. Variability in the quantitation of circulating growth hormone using commercial immunoassays. J Clin Endocrinol Metab 1989;68:469-476.
1256. Wyatt DT, Mark D, Slyper A. Survey of growth hormone treatment practices by 251 pediatric endocrinologists. J Clin Endocrinol Metab 1995;80:3292-3297.
1257. Mauras N, Walton P, Nicar M, et al. Growth hormone stimulation testing in both short and normal statured children: use of an immunofunctional assay. Pediatr Res 2000;48:614-618.
1258. Shah A, Stanhope R, Matthews D. Hazards of pharmacological tests of growth hormone secretion in childhood. Br Med J 1992;304:173-174.
1259. Eddy RL, Gilliland PF, Ibarra JD Jr, et al. Human growth hormone release. Comparison of provocative test procedures. Am J Med 1974;56:179-185.
1260. Zadik Z, Chalew SA, Raiti S, et al. Do short children secrete insufficient growth hormone? Pediatrics 1985;76:355-360.
1261. Thompson RG, Rodriguez A, Kowarski AA, et al. Growth hormone: metabolic clearance rates, integrated concentrations and production rates in normal adults and the effects of prednisone. J Clin Invest 1972;51:3193-3199.
1262. Zadik Z, Chalew SA, McCarter RJ, et al. The influence of age on the 24-hour integrated concentrations of growth hormone in normal individuals. J Clin Endocrinol Metab 1985;60:153.
1263. Zadik Z, Chalew SA, Gilula Z, et al. Reproducibility growth hormone testing procedures: a comparison between 24-hour integrated concentration and pharmacological stimulation. J Clin Endocrinol Metab 1990;71:1127-1130.
1264. Tassoni P, Cacciari E, Cau M, et al. Variability of growth hormone response to pharmacological and sleep tests performed twice in short children. J Clin Endocrinol Metab 1990;71:230-234.
1265. Donaldson DL, Hollowell JG, Pan F, et al. Growth hormone secretory profiles: variation on consecutive nights. J Pediatr 1989; 115:51-56.
1266. Cutfield WS, Lindberg A, Chatelain P, et al. Final height following growth hormone treatment of idiopathic growth hormone deficiency in KIGS. In Ranke MB, Wilton P, eds. Growth Hormone Therapy in KIGS—10 Years' Experience. Heidelberg-Leipzig: Johann Ambrosius Barth Verlag, 1999:93-110.
1267. Hasegawa Y, Hasegawa T, Aso T, et al. Usefulness and limitation of measurement of insulin-like growth factor binding protein-3 (IGFBP-3) for diagnosis of growth hormone deficiency. Endocrinol Japan 1992;39:585-591.
1268. Smith WJ, Nam TJ, Underwood LE, et al. Use of insulin-like growth factor binding protein-2 (IGFBP-2), IGFBP-3, and IGF-I for assessing growth hormone status in short children. J Clin Endocrinol Metab 1993;77:1294-1299.
1269. Juul A, Skakkebaek NE. Prediction of the outcome of growth hormone provocative testing in short children by measurement of serum levels of insulin-like growth factor I and insulin-like growth factor binding protein 3. J Pediatr 1997;130: 197-204.
1270. Tillmann V, Shalet SM, Price DA, et al. Serum insulin-like growth factor-I, IGF binding protein -3 and IGFBP-3 protease activity after cranial irradiation. Horm Res 1998;50:71-77.
1271. Blum WF, Albertsson-Wikland K, Rosberg S, et al. Serum levels of insulin-like growth factor I (IGF-I) and IGF binding protein 3 reflect spontaneous growth hormone secretion. J Clin Endocrinol Metab 1993;76:1610-1616.
1272. Guevara-Aguirre J, Rosenbloom AL, Fielder PJ, et al. Growth hormone receptor deficiency in Ecuador: clinical and biochemical phenotype in two populations. J Clin Endocrinol Metab 1993;76:417-423.

1273. Savage MO, Blu WF, Ranke MB, et al. Clinical features and endocrine status in patients with growth hormone insensitivity (Laron syndrome). J Clin Endocrinol Metab 1993;77:1465-1471.
1274. Thalange NK, Price DA, Gill MS, et al. Insulin-like growth factor binding protein-3 generation: an index of growth hormone insensitivity. Pediatr Res 1996;39:849-855.
1275. Blum WF, Cotterill AM, Postel-Vinay MC, et al. Improvement in the diagnostic criteria in growth hormone insensitivity syndrome: solutions and pitfalls. Acta Paediatr Scand Suppl 1994;399: 117-124.
1276. GH Research Society. Consensus guidelines for the diagnosis and treatment of growth hormone (GH) deficiency in childhood and adolescence: summary statement of the GH Research Society. J Clin Endocrinol Metab 2000;85:3990-3993.
1277. Bhala A, Harris M, Cohen P. Insulin-like growth factors and their binding proteins in critically ill infants. J Pediatr Endocrinol 1998;11:451-459.
1278. Ranke MB, Lindberg A, Chatelain P, et al, on behalf of the KIGS International Board. Derivation and validation of a mathematical model for predicting the response to exogenous recombinant human growth hormone (GH) in prepubertal children with idiopathic GH deficiency. J Clin Endocrinol Metab 1999;84: 1174-1183.
1279. Albertsson-Wikland K, Kristrom B, Rosber S, et al. Validated multivariate models predicting the growth response to GH treatment in individual short children with a broad range in GH secretion capacities. Pediatr Res 2000;48:475-484.
1280. Savage MO, Rosenfeld RG. Growth hormone insensitivity: a proposed revised classification. Acta Paediatr Suppl 1999;428:147.
1281. Blum WF, Ranke MB, Savage MO. Insulin-like growth factors and their binding proteins in patients with growth hormone receptor deficiency: suggestions for new diagnostic criteria. Acta Paediatr Scand Suppl 1992;383:125-126.
1282. Buckway CK, Guevara-Aguirre J, Pratt KL, et al. The insulin-like growth factor-I (IGF-I) generation test revisited: a marker of growth hormone sensitivity. J Clin Endocrinol Metab 2001; 86:5176-5183.
1283. Buckway CK, Selva KA, Pratt KL, et al. Insulin-like growth factor binding protein-3 generation as a measure of GH sensitivity. J Clin Endocrinol Metab 2002;87:4754-4765.
1284. Selva KA, Buckway CK, Sexton G, et al. Reproducibility in patterns of IGF generation with special reference to idiopathic short stature. Horm Res 2003;60:237-246.
1285. Clayton PE, Shalet SM, Price DA. Endocrine manipulation of constitutional delay in growth and puberty. J Endocrinol 1988;116: 321-323.
1286. Burstein S, Rosenfield RL. Constitutional delay in growth and development. In Hintz RL, Rosenfeld RG, eds. Growth Abnormalities. New York: Churchill Livingstone, 1987:167-186.
1287. Horner JM, Thorsson AV, Hintz RL. Growth deceleration pattern in children with constitutional short stature: an aid to diagnosis. Pediatrics 1978;62:529-534.
1288. Du Caju MV, Op De Beeck L, Sys SU, et al. Progressive deceleration in growth as an early sign of delayed puberty in boys. Horm Res 2000;54:126-130.
1289. Crowne EC, Shalet SM, Wallace WH, et al. Final height in boys with untreated constitutional delay in growth and puberty. Arch Dis Child 1990;65:1109-1112.
1290. LaFranchi S, Hanna CE, Mandel SH. Constitutional delay of growth: expected versus final adult height. Pediatrics 1991;87: 82-87.
1291. Ranke MB, Grauer ML, Kistner K, et al. Spontaneous adult height in idiopathic short stature. Horm Res 1995;44:152-157.
1292. Blethen SL, Gaines S, Weldon V. Comparison of predicted and adult heights in short boys: effect of androgen therapy. Pediatr Res 1984;18:467-469.
1293. Albanese A, Stanhope R. Predictive factors in the determination of final height in boys with constitutional delay of growth and puberty. J Pediatr 1995;126:545-550.
1294. Krajewska-Siuda E, Malecka-Tendera E, Krajewski-Siuda K. Are short boys with constitutional delay of growth and puberty candidates for rGH therapy according to FDA recommendations? Horm Res 2006;65:192-196.
1295. Finkelstein JS, Neer RM, Biller BM, et al. Osteopenia in men with a history of delayed puberty. N Engl J Med 1992;326:600-604.
1296. Han JC, Balagopal P, Sweeten S, et al. Evidence for hypermetabolism in boys with constitutional delay of growth and maturation. J Clin Endocrinol Metab 2006;91:2081-2086.
1297. Eastman CJ, Lazarus L, Stuart MC, et al. The effect of puberty on growth hormone secretion in boys with short stature and delayed adolescence. Aust N Z J Med 1971;1:154-159.
1298. Deller JJ Jr, Boulis MW, Harriss WE, et al. Growth hormone response patterns to sex hormone administration in growth retardation. Am J Med Sci 1970;259:292-297.
1299. Volta C, Ghizzoni L, Buono T, et al. Final height in a group of untreated children with constitutional growth delay. Helv Paediat Acta 1988;43:171-176.
1300. Attie KM, Carlsson LM, Rundle AC, et al. Evidence for partial growth hormone insensitivity among patients with idiopathic short stature. J Pediatr 1995;127:244-250.
1301. Carlsson LM, Attie KM, Compton PG, et al. Reduced concentration of serum growth hormone-binding protein in children with idiopathic short stature. J Clin Endocrinol Metab 1994;78: 1325-1330.
1302. Davila N, Moreira-Andres M, Alcanez J, et al. Serum growth hormone-binding protein is decreased in prepubertal children with idiopathic short stature. J Endocrinol Invest 1996;19: 348-352.
1303. Cotterill AM, Camacho-Hubner C, Duquesnoy P, et al. Changes in serum IGF-I and IGFBP-3 concentrations during IGF-I generation test performed prospectively in children with short stature. Clin Endocrinol 1998;48:719-724.
1304. Rosenfeld RG, Northcraft GB, Hintz RL. A prospective, randomized trial of testosterone treatment of constitutional short stature in adolescent males. Pediatrics 1982;69:681-687.
1305. Blizzard RM, Hindmarsh PC, Stanhope R. Oxandrolone therapy: 25 years experience. Growth Genet Horm 1991;7:1-6.
1306. Buyukgebiz A, Hindmarsh C, Brook CD. Treatment of constitutional delay of growth and puberty with oxandrolone compared with growth hormone. Arch Dis Child 1990;65:448-449.
1307. Clayton PE, Shalet SM, Price DA, et al. Growth and growth hormone responses to oxandrolone in boys with constitutional delay of growth and puberty (CDGP). Clin Endocrinol 1988;23: 123-130.
1308. Joss EE, Schmidt JA, Zuppinger KA. Oxandrolone in constitutionally delayed growth, a longitudinal study up to final height. J Clin Endocrinol Metab 1989;69:1109-1115.
1309. Marti-Henneberg C, Niirianen A, Rappaport MD. Oxandrolone treatment of constitutional short stature in boys during adolescence: effect on linear growth, bone age, pubic hair and testicular development. J Pediatrics 1975;86:783-788.
1310. Stanhope R, Buchanan CR, Fenn GC, et al. Double-blinded placebo controlled trial of low dose oxandrolone in the treatment of boys with constitutional delay of growth and puberty. Arch Dis Child 1988;63:501-505.
1311. Wilson DM, McCauley E, Brown DR, et al, and Bio-Technology General Corporation Cooperative Study Group. Oxandrolone treatment in constitutionally delayed growth and puberty. Pediatrics 1995;96:1095-1100.
1312. Tse WY, Buyukgebiz A, Hindmarsh PC, et al. Long-term outcome of oxandrolone treatment in boys with constitutional delay of growth and puberty. J Pediatr 1990;117:588-591.
1313. Papadimitriou S, Wacharasindhu S, Preece MA, et al. Treatment of constitutional growth delay in prepubertal boys with a prolonged course of low dose oxandrolone. Arch Dis Child 1991; 66:841-843.
1314. Hochberg Z, Korman S. Oxandrolone therapy for short stature. J Pediatr Endocrinol (Israel) 1987;2:115-120.
1315. Link K, Blizzard RM, Evans WS, et al. The effect of androgens on growth hormone response in children with constitutional growth delay. J Clin Endocrinol Metab 1986;52:159-164.
1316. Malhotra A, Poon E, Tse WY, et al. The effects of oxandrolone on the growth hormone and gonadal axes in boys with constitutional delay of growth and puberty. Clin Endocrinol 1993; 38:393-398.
1317. Kulin HE, Reiter EO. Managing the patient with delay in puberty development. Endocrinologist 1992;2:231-239.
1318. Richman RA, Kirsch LR. Testosterone treatment in adolescent boys with constitutional delay in growth and development. N Engl J Med 1988;319:1563-1567.

1319. Crowne EC, Wallace WH, Moore C, et al. Degree of activation of the pituitary-testicular axis in early pubertal boys with constitutional delay of growth and puberty determines the growth response to treatment with testosterone or oxandrolone. J Clin Endocrinol Metab 1995;80:1869-1875.
1320. Link K, Blizzard RM, Evans WS, et al. The effect of androgens on the pulsatile release and twenty-four-hour mean concentration of growth hormone in peripubertal males. J Clin Endocrinol Metab 1986;62:159-164.
1321. Metzger DL, Kerrigan JR. Androgen receptor blockade with flutamide enhances growth hormone secretion in late pubertal males: evidence for independent actions of estrogen and androgen. J Clin Endocrinol Metab 1993;76:1147-1152.
1322. Wilson DM, Kei J, Hintz RL, et al. Effects of testosterone enanthate therapy for pubertal delay. Am J Dis Child 1988;142:96-99.
1323. Wang C, Swerdloff RS, Iranmanesh A. Transdermal testosterone gel improves sexual function, mood, muscle strength and body composition parameters in hypogonadal men. Testosterone Gel Study Group. J Clin Endocrinol Metab 2000;85:2839-2853.
1324. Ahmed SR, Boucher AE, Manni A, et al. Transdermal testosterone therapy in the treatment of male hypogonadism. J Clin Endocrinol Metab 1988;66:546-551.
1325. Wickman S, Sipila I, Ankarberg-Lindgren C, et al. A specific aromatase inhibitor and potential increase in adult height in boys with delayed puberty: a radomised controlled trial. Lancet 2001;357:1743-1748.
1326. Kaplan SL, Underwood LE, August GP, et al. Clinical studies with recombinant-DNA-derived methionyl human growth hormone in growth hormone deficient children. Lancet 1986;i:697-700.
1327. Underwood LE, Moore WV. Antibodies to growth hormone: measurement and meaning. Growth Genet Horm 1987;3:1-3.
1328. MacGillivray MH, Blizzard RM. Rationale for dosing recombinant human growth hormone by weight rather than units. Growth Genet Horm 1994;10:7-9.
1329. Marx W, Simpson ME, Evans HM. Bioassay of growth hormone at anterior pituitary. Endocrinology 1942;30:1-10.
1330. Wilhelmi AE. Measurement: bioassay. In Berson SA, Yalow RS, eds. Peptide Hormones: Methods in Investigative and Diagnostic Endocrinology. New York: North-Holland Publishing, 1973: 296-302.
1331. Binder G, Benz MR, Elmlinger M, et al. Reduced human growth hormone (hGH) bioactivity with a defect of the GH-1 gene in three patients with rhGH responsive growth failure. Clin Endocrinol (Oxf) 1999;51:89-95.
1332. Blizzard RM. Growth hormone as a therapeutic agent. Growth Genet Horm 2005;21:49-54.
1333. Frasier SD. Human pituitary growth hormone (hGH) therapy in growth hormone deficiency. Endocr Rev 1983;4:155-170.
1334. Frasier SD, Costin G, Lippe BM, et al. A dose-response curve for human growth hormone. J Clin Endocrinol Metab 1981;53: 1213-1217.
1335. Fradkin JE. Creutzfeldt-Jakob disease in pituitary growth hormone recipients. Endocrinologist 1993;3:108-114.
1336. Buchanan CR, Preece MA, Milner RD. Mortality, neoplasia, and Creutzfeldt-Jakob disease in patients treated with human pituitary growth hormone in the United States. Br Med J 1991;302: 824-828.
1337. Tintner R, Brown P, Hedley-Whyte ET, et al. Neuropathologic verification of Creutzfeldt-Jakob disease in the exhumed American recipient of human growth hormone: epidemiologic and pathogenetic implications. Neurology 1986;36:932-936.
1338. Hintz RL. The prismatic case of Creutzfeldt-Jakob disease associated with pituitary growth hormone treatment. J Clin Endocrinol Metab 1995;80:2298-2301.
1339. d'Aignaux JH, Costagliola D, Maccario J, et al. Incubation period of Creutzfeldt-Jakob disease in human growth hormone recipients in France. Neurology 1999;53:1197-1201.
1340. Swerdlow AJ, Higgins CD, Adlard P, et al. Creutzfeldt-Jakob disease in United Kingdom patients treated with human pituitary growth hormone. Neurology 2003;61:783-791.
1341. Mills JL, Schonberger LB, Wysowski DK, et al. Long-term mortality in the United States cohort of pituitary-derived growth hormone recipients. J Pediatr 2004;144:430-436.
1342. Rosenfeld RG, Aggarwal BB, Hintz RL, et al. Recombinant DNA-derived methionyl growth hormone is similar in membrane binding properties to human pituitary growth hormone. Biochem Biophys Res Commun 1982;106:202-209.
1343. Hintz RL, Rosenfeld RG, Wilson DM, et al. Biosynthetic methionyl-human growth hormone is biologically active in adult humans. Lancet 1982;1:1276-1279.
1344. MacGillivray MH, Blethen SL, Buchlis JG, et al. Current dosing of growth hormone in children with growth hormone deficiency: how physiologic? Pediatrics 1998;102:527-530.
1345. MacGillivray MH, Baptista J, Johanson A, et al. Outcome of a four year randomized study of daily versus three times weekly somatropin treatment in prepubertal naive growth hormone deficient children. J Clin Endocrinol Metab 1996;81:1806-1809.
1346. Wilson DM, Baker B, Hintz RL, et al. Subcutaneous versus intramuscular growth hormone therapy: growth and acute somatomedin response. Pediatrics 1985;76:361-364.
1347. Reiter EO, Attie KM, Moshang T, et al. A multicenter study of the efficacy and safety of sustained-release growth hormone in the treatment of naive pediatric patients with growth hormone deficiency. J Clin Endocrinol Metab 2001;86:4700-4706.
1348. Murray F, Basu S, Kipnes M, et al. Pharmacokinetics and pharmacodynamics of a novel long-acting crystalline growth hormone formulation (ALTU-238) in normal healthy men and women. Horm Res 2005;64(suppl 1):312 (abstr).
1349. Kim DH, Lee BC, Shin JH, et al. Efficacy and safety following six-month treatment with a sustained release human growth hormone (LB03002) in children with growth hormone deficiency (GHD). Horm Res 2005;64(suppl 1):49 (abstr).
1350. Ranke MB. Growth hormone therapy in children: when to stop? Horm Res 1995;43:122-125.
1351. Willson TA, Rose SJ, Cohen P, et al. Update of guidelines for the use of growth hormone in children: the Lawson Wilkins Pediatric Endocrinology Society Drug and Therapeutics Committee. J Pediatr 2003;143:415-421.
1352. Price DA, Ranke MB. Final height following growth hormone treatment. In Ranke MB, Gunnarsson R, eds. Progress in Growth Hormone Therapy—5 Years of KIGS. Mannheim: J&J Verlag, 1994:129-144.
1353. Land C, Blum WF, Stabrey A, et al. Seasonality of growth response to GH therapy in prepubertal children with idiopathic growth hormone deficiency. Eur J Endocrinol 2005;152:727-733.
1354. Cohen P, Bright GM, Rogol AD, et al. Effects of dose and gender on the growth and growth factor response to GH in GH-deficient children: implications for efficacy and safety. J Clin Endocrinol Metab 2002;87:90-98.
1355. Cohen P, Rogol AD, Howard C, et al. IGF-based dosing of growth hormone accelerates the growth velocity of children with growth hormone deficiency (GHD) and idiopathic short stature. Horm Res 2005;64(suppl 1):48.
1356. Boersma B, Rikken B, Wit JM. Catch-up growth in early treated patients with growth hormone deficiency. Arch Dis Child 1995;72:427-431.
1357. Rappaport R, Mugnier E, Limoni C, et al. A 5-year prospective study of growth hormone (GH) deficient children treated with GH before the age of 3 years. J Clin Endocrinol Metab 1997; 82:452-456.
1358. de Luca F, Maghnie M, Arrigo T, et al. Final height outcome of growth hormone-deficient patients treated since less than five years of age. Acta Paediatr 1996;85:1167-1171.
1359. Carel JC, Huet F, Chaussain JL. Treatment of growth hormone deficiency in very young children. Horm Res 2003;60:10-17.
1360. Ranke MB, Lindberg A, Albertsson-Wikland K, et al. Increased response, but lower responsiveness, to growth hormone (GH) in very young children (aged 0-3 years) with idiopathic GH deficiency: analysis of data from KIGS. J Clin Endocrinol Metab 2005;90:1966-1971.
1361. Saenger P. Growth hormone in growth hormone deficiency. BMJ 2002;325:58-59.
1362. Bundak R, Hindmarsh PC, Brook CG. Long-term auxologic effects of human growth hormone. J Pediatr 1988;112:875-879.
1363. Libber SM, Plotnick LP, Johanson AJ, et al. Long-term follow-up of hypopituitary patients treated with human growth hormone. Medicine 1990;69:46-55.
1364. Bierich JR. Final height in hypopituitary patients after treatment with HGH. In Bierch JR, Cacciari E, Raiti S, eds. Growth abnormalities. New York: Raven, 1989:161-174.

1365. Bramswig JH, Schlosser H, Kiese K. Final height in children with growth hormone deficiency. Horm Res 1995;43:126-128.
1366. Severi F. Final height in children with growth hormone deficiency. Horm Res 1995;43:138-140.
1367. Blethen SL, Baptista J, Kuntze J, et al. Adult height in growth hormone (GH)-deficient children treated with biosynthetic GH. J Clin Endocrinol Metab 1997;82:418-420.
1368. Bernasconi S, Arrigo T, Wasniewski M, et al. Long-term results with growth hormone therapy in idiopathic hypopituitarism. Horm Res 2000;53:55-59.
1369. August GP, Julius JR, Blethen SL. Adult height in children with growth hormone deficiency who are treated with biosynthetic growth hormone: The National Cooperative Growth Study experience. Pediatrics 1998;102:512-516.
1370. Cutfield W, Lindberg A, Albertsson-Wikland K, et al. Final height in idiopathic growth hormone deficiency: the KIGS experience. Acta Paediatr Suppl 1999;428:72-75.
1371. Reiter EO, Price DA, Wilton P, et al. Effect of growth hormone (GH) treatment on the final height of 1258 patients with idiopathic GH deficiency: analysis of a large international dtabase. J Clin Endocrinol Metab 2006;91:2047-2054.
1372. Stanhope R, Urena M, Hindmarsh P, et al. Management of growth hormone deficiency through puberty. Acta Paediatr Scand Suppl 1991;372:47-52.
1373. Stanhope R, Albanese A, Hindmarsh P, et al. The effects of growth hormone therapy on spontaneous sexual development. Horm Res 1992;38:9-13.
1374. Mauras N, Attie KM, Reiter EO, et al. High dose recombinant human growth hormone (GH) treatment of GH-deficient patients in puberty increases near-final height: a randomized, multicenter trial. J Clin Endocrinol Metab 2000;85:3653-3660.
1375. Frisch H, Birnbacher R. Final height and pubertal development in children with growth hormone deficiency after long-term treatment. Horm Res 1995;43:132-134.
1376. Burns EC, Tanner JM, Preece MA, et al. Final height and pubertal development in 55 children with idiopathic growth hormone deficiency, treated for between 2 and 15 years with human growth hormone. Eur J Pediatr 1981;137:155-164.
1377. Bourguignon JP, Vandeweghe M, Vanderschuren-Lodeweyckx M, et al. Pubertal growth and final height in hypopituitary boys: a minor role of bone age at onset of puberty. J Clin Endocrinol Metab 1986;63:376-382.
1378. Ranke MB, Price DA, Albertsson-Wikland K, et al. Factors determining pubertal growth and final height in growth hormone treatment of idiopathic growth hormone deficiency. Horm Res 1997;48:62-71.
1379. Ranke MB, Martin DD, Lindberg A. Prediction model of total pubertal growth in idiopathic growth hormone deficiency: analysis of data from KIGS. Horm Res 2003;60:58-59.
1380. Carel JC. Can we increase adolescent growth? Eur J Endocrinol 2004;151(suppl 3):U101-U108.
1381. Hibi I, Tanaka T, Tanae A, et al. The influence of gonadal function and the effect of gonadal suppression treatment on final height in growth hormone (GH)-treated GH-deficient children. J Clin Endocrinol Metab 1989;69:221-226.
1382. Saggese G, Cesaretti G, Andreani G, et al. Combined treatment with growth hormone and gonadotropin-releasing hormone analogues in children with isolated growth hormone deficiency. Acta Endocrinol 1992;127:307-312.
1383. Toublanc JE, Couptrie C, Garnier P, et al. The effects of treatment combining an agonist of gonadotropin-releasing hormone with growth hormone in pubertal patients with isolated growth hormone deficiency. Acta Endocrinol 1989;120:795-799.
1384. Adan L, Souberbielle JC, Zucker JM, et al. Adult height in 24 patients treated for growth hormone deficiency and early puberty. J Clin Endocrinol Metab 1997;82:229-233.
1385. Dunkel L, Wickman S. Novel treatment of short stature with aromatase inhibitors. J Steroid Biochem Mol Biol 2003;86:345-356.
1386. Balducci R, Toscano V, Mangiantini A, et al. Adult height in short normal adolescent girls treated with gonadotropin-releasing hormone analog and growth hormone. J Clin Endocrinol Metab 1995;80:3596-3600.
1387. Saggese G, Pasquino AM, Bertelloni S, et al. Effect of combined treatment with gonadotropin releasing hormone analogue and growth hormone in patients with central precocious puberty who had subnormal growth velocity and impaired height prognosis. Acta Paediatr 1995;84:299-304.
1388. Pasquino AM, Municchi G, Pucarelli I, et al. Combined treatment with gonadotropin-releasing hormone analog and growth hormone in central precocious puberty. J Clin Endocrinol Metab 1996;81:948-951.
1389. Job JC, Toublanc JE, Landier F. Growth of short normal children in puberty treated for three years with growth hormone alone or in association with gonadotropin-releasing hormone agonist. Horm Res 1994;41:177-184.
1390. Mericq MV, Eggers M, Avila A, et al. Near final height in pubertal growth hormone (GH)–deficient patients treated with GH alone or in combination with luteinizing hormone–releasing hormone analog: results of a prospective, randomized trial. J Clin Endocrinol Metab 2000;85:569-573.
1391. Walvoord EC, Pescovitz OH. Combined use of growth hormone and gonadotropin-releasing hormone analogues in precocious puberty: theoretic and practical considerations. Pediatrics 1999;104:1010-1014.
1392. Codner E, Mericq V, Cassorla F. Optimizing growth hormone therapy during puberty. Horm Res 1997;48:16-20.
1393. Ranke MB, Lindberg A. Early-onset idiopathic growth hormone deficiency within KIGS. Horm Res 2003;60:18-21.
1394. Kohn B, Julius JR, Blethen SL. Combined use of growth hormone and gonadotropin-releasing hormone analogues: the National Cooperative Growth Study Experience. Pediatrics 1999;104:1014-1017.
1395. Reiter EO. A brief review of the addition of gonadotropin-releasing hormone agonists (GnRH-Ag) to growth hormone (GH) treatment of children with idiopathic growth hormone deficiency: previously published studies from America. Mol Cell Endocrinol 2006;254-255:221-225.
1396. Grumbach MM. Estrogen, bone, growth and sex: a sea change in conventional wisdom. J Pediatr Endocrinol Metab 2000;13:1439-1455.
1397. Zhou P, Shah B, Prasad K, et al. Letrozole significantly improves growth potential in a pubertal boy with growth hormone deficiency. Pediatrics 2005;115:e245-e248.
1398. Eugster EA. Aromatase inhibitors in precocious puberty: rationale and experience to date. Treat Endocrinol 2004;3:141-151.
1399. Mauras N, Welch S, Rini A, et al. An open label 12-month pilot trial on the effects of the aromatase inhibitor anastrozole in growth hormone (GH)-treated GH deficient adolescent boys. J Pediatr Endocrinol Metab 2004;17:1597-1606.
1400. Wickman S, Kajantie E, Dunkel L. Effects of suppression of estrogen action by the p450 aromatase inhibitor letrozole on bone mineral density and bone turnover in pubertal boys. J Clin Endocrinol Metab 2003;88:3785-3793.
1401. Mauras N, Bell J, Snow BG, et al. Sperm analysis in growth hormone-deficient adolescents previously treated with an aromatase inhibitor: comparison with normal controls. Fertil Steril 2005;84:239-242.
1402. Kreher NC, Eugster EA, Shankar RR. The use of tamoxifen to improve height potential in short pubertal boys. Pediatrics 2005;116:1513-1515.
1403. Davies PS, Evans S, Broomhead S, et al. Effect of growth hormone on height, weight, and body composition in Prader-Willi syndrome. Arch Dis Child 1998;78:474-476.
1404. Eiholzer U, l'Allemand D, Schlumpf M, et al. Growth hormone and body composition in children younger than 2 years with Prader-Willi syndrome. J Pediatr 2004;144:753-758.
1405. VanVliet G, Deal C, Crock P, et al. Sudden death in growth hormone-treated children with Prader-Willi syndrome. J Pediatr 2004;144:129-131.
1406. Nagai T, Obata K, Tonoki H, et al. Cause of sudden, unexpected death of Prader-Willi syndrome patients with or without growth hormone treatment. Am J Med Genet A 2005;136:45-48.
1407. Hoybye C, Thoren M. Somatropin therapy in adults with Prader-Willi syndrome. Treat Endocrinol 2004;3:153-160.
1408. Hoybye C, Frystyk J, Thoren M. The growth hormone-insulin-like growth factor axis in adult patients with Prader Willi syndrome. Growth Horm IGF Res 2003;13:269-274.
1409. Lippe BM, Van Herle AJ, Lafranchi SH, et al. Reversible hypothyroidism in growth-hormone deficient children treated with

human growth hormone. J Clin Endocrinol Metab 1975;40: 612-618.
1410. Guthrie RD, Smith SW, Graham CB. Testosterone treatment for micropenis during early childhood. J Pediatr 1973;83:247-252.
1411. Achermann JC, Hamdani K, Hindmarsh PC, et al. Birth weight influences the initial response to growth hormone treatment in growth hormone-insufficient children. Pediatrics 1998;102: 342-345.
1412. Cacciari E, Zucchini S, Cicognani A, et al. Birth weight affects final height in patients treated for growth hormone deficiency. Clin Endocrinol 1999;51:733-739.
1413. de Ridder MA, Stijnen T, Drop SL, et al. Validation of a calibrated prediction model for response to growth hormone treatment in an independent cohort. Horm Res 2006;66:13-16.
1414. Mandel SH, Moreland E, Rosenfeld RG, et al. The effect of GH therapy on the immunoreactive forms and distribution of IGFBP-3, IGF-I, the acid-labile subunit, and growth rate in GH-deficient children. Endocrine 1997;7:351-360.
1415. Tillmann V, Patel L, Gill MS, et al. Monitoring serum insulin-like growth factor-1 (IGF-I), IGF-binding protein-3 (IGFBP-3), IGF-I/IGFBP-3 molar ratio and leptin during growth hormone treatment for disordered growth. Clin Endocrinol 2000;53:329-336.
1416. Kristrom B, Carlsson B, Rosber S, et al. Short-term changes in serum leptin levels provide a strong metabolic marker for the growth response to growth hormone treatment in children. J Clin Endocrinol Metab 1998;83:2735-2541.
1417. Wetterau L, Cohen P. Role of insulin-like growth factor monitoring in optimizing growth hormone therapy. J Pediatr Endocrinol Metab 2000;13:1371-1376.
1418. Pirazzoli P, Cacciari E, Mandini M, et al. Follow-up of antibodies to growth hormone in 210 growth hormone-deficient children treated with different commercial preparations. Acta Paediatr 1995;84:1223-1226.
1419. Grimberg A, Kutikov JK, Cucchiara AJ. Sex differences in patients referred for evaluation of poor growth. J Pediatr 2005;146: 212-216.
1420. Dean HJ, McTaggart TL, Fish DG, et al. The educational vocational, and marital status of growth hormone-deficient adults treated with growth hormone during childhood. Am J Dis Child 1985;139:1105-1110.
1421. Salomon F, Cuneo RC, Hesp R, et al. The effects of treatment with recombinant human growth hormone on body composition and metabolism in adults with growth hormone deficiency. N Engl J Med 1989;321:1797-1803.
1422. Clayton PE, Cuneo RC, Juul A, et al. Consensus statement on the management of the GH-treated adolescent in the transition to adult care. Eur J Endocrinol 2005;152:165-170.
1423. Abs R, Bengtsson BA, Hernberg-Stahl E, et al. GH replacement in 1034 growth hormone deficient hypopituitary adults: demographic and clinical characteristics, dosing and safety. Clin Endocrinol (Oxf) 1999;50:703-713.
1424. Bengtsson BA, Johannsson G, Shalet SM, et al. Therapeutic controversy: treatment of growth hormone deficiency in adults. J Clin Endocrinol Metab 2000;85:933-942.
1425. Carroll PV, Christ ER, Members of GRS Scientific Committee. Growth hormone deficiency in adulthood and the effects of growth hormone replacement: a review. J Clin Endocrinol Metab 1998;83:382-395.
1426. Attanasio AF, Bates PC, Ho KK, et al. Human growth hormone replacement in adult hypopituitary patients: long-term effects on body composition and lipid status—3-year results from the HypoCCS Database. J Clin Endocrinol Metab 2002;87:1600-1606.
1427. Rosen T, Bengtsson B-A. Premature mortality due to cardiovascular disease in hypopituitarism. Lancet 1990;336:285-288.
1428. Maison P, Griffin S, Nicoue-Beglah M, et al. Impact of growth hormone (GH) treatment on cardiovascular risk factors in GH-deficient adults: a metaanalysis of blinded, randomized, placebo-controlled trials. J Clin Endocrinol Metab 2004;89:2192-2199.
1429. Hull KL, Harvey S. Growth hormone therapy and quality of life: possibilities, pitfalls and mechanisms. J Endocrinol 2003;179: 311-333.
1430. Bengtsson B-A, Eden S, Lonn L, et al. Treatment of adults with growth hormone deficiency with recombinant human growth hormone. J Clin Endocrinol Metab 1993;76:309-317.
1431. Maghnie M, Aimaretti G, Bellone S, et al. Diagnosis of GH deficiency in the transition period: accuracy of insulin tolerance test and insulin-like growth factor-I measurement. Eur J Endocrinol 2005;152:589-596.
1432. Vahl N, Juul A, Jorgensen JO, et al. Continuation of growth hormone (GH) replacement in GH-deficient patients during transition from childhood to adulthood: a two year placebo-controlled study. J Clin Endocrinol Metab 2000;85:1874-1881.
1433. Johannsson G, Albertsson-Wikland K, Bengtsson B-A. Discontinuation of growth hormone (GH) treatment: metabolic effects in GH-deficient and GH-sufficient adolescent patients compared with control subjects. J Clin Endocrinol Metab 1999;84: 4516-4524.
1434. Shalet SM, Shavrikova E, Cromer M, et al. Effect of growth hormone (GH) treatment on bone in postpubertal GH-deficient patients: a 2-year randomized, controlled, dose-ranging study. J Clin Endocrinol Metab 2003;88:4124-4129.
1435. Attanasio AF, Shavrikova E, Blum WF, et al. Continued growth hormone (GH) treatment after final height is necessary to complete somatic development in childhood-onset GH-deficient patients. J Clin Endocrinol Metab 2004;89:4857-4862.
1436. Mauras N, Pescovitz OH, Allada V, et al. Limited efficacy of growth hormone (GH) during transition of GH-deficient patients from adolescence to adulthood: a phase III multicenter, double-blind, randomized two-year trial. J Clin Endocrinol Metab 2005;90: 3946-3955.
1437. Attanasio AF, Shavrikova EP, Blum WF, et al. Quality of life in childhood onset growth hormone-deficient patients in the transition phase from childhood to adulthood. J Clin Endocrinol Metab 2005;90:4525-4529.
1438. Stouthart PJ, Deijen JB, Roffel M, et al. Quality of life of growth hormone (GH) deficient young adults during discontinuation and restart of GH therapy. Psychoneuroendocrinology 2003;28: 612-626.
1439. Sheppard L, Eiser C, Davies HA, et al. The effects of growth hormone treatment on health-related quality of life in children. Horm Res 2006;65:243-249.
1440. Sandberg DE. Health-related quality of life as a primary endpoint for growth hormone therapy. Horm Res 2006;65:250-252.
1441. Cowan FJ, Evans WD, Gregory JW. Metabolic effects of discontinuing growth hormone treatment. Arch Dis Child 1999;80: 517-523.
1442. Tauber M, Jouret B, Cartault A, et al. Adolescents with partial growth hormone (GH) deficiency develop alterations of body composition after GH discontinuation and require follow-up. J Clin Endocrinol Metab 2003;88:5101-5106.
1443. Drake WM, Carroll PV, Maher KT, et al. The effect of cessation of growth hormone (GH) therapy on bone mineral accretion in GH-deficient adolescents at the completion of linear growth. J Clin Endocrinol Metab 2003;88:1658-1663.
1444. Underwood LE, Attie KM, Baptista J. Growth hormone (GH) dose-response in young adults with childhood-onset GH deficiency: a two-year, multicenter, multiple-dose, placebo-controlled study. J Clin Endocrinol Metab 2003;88:5273-5280.
1445. Lange M, Muller J, Svendsen OL, et al. The impact of idiopathic childhood-onset growth hormone deficiency (GHD) on bone mass in subjects without adult GHD. Clin Endocrinol (Oxf) 2005;62:18-23.
1446. Colao A, Di Somma C, Salerno M, et al. The cardiovascular risk of GH-deficient adolescents. J Clin Endocrinol Metab 2002; 87:3650-3655.
1447. Salerno M, Esposito V, Spinelli L, et al. Left ventricular mass and function in children with GH deficiency before and during 12 months GH replacement therapy. Clin Endocrinol (Oxf) 2004; 60:630-636.
1448. Lanes R, Paoli M, Carrillo E, et al. Cardiovascular risk of young growth-hormone-deficient adolescents. Differences in growth-hormone-treated and untreated patients. Horm Res 2003;60: 291-296.
1449. Lanes R, Paoli M, Carrillo E, et al. Peripheral inflammatory and fibrinolytic markers in adolescents with growth hormone deficiency: relation to postprandial dyslipidemia. J Pediatr 2004;145: 657-661.
1450. Reis F, Campos MV, Bastos M, et al. Platelet hyperactivation in maintained growth hormone-deficient childhood patients after

therapy withdrawal as a putative earlier marker of increased cardiovascular risk. J Clin Endocrinol Metab 2005;90:98-105.
1451. Mohn A, Marzio D, Giannini C, et al. Alterations in the oxidant-antioxidant status in prepubertal children with growth hormone deficiency: effect of growth hormone replacement therapy. Clin Endocrinol (Oxf) 2005;63:537-542.
1452. Esposito V, Di Biase S, Lettiero T, et al. Serum homocysteine concentrations in children with growth hormone (GH) deficiency before and after 12 months GH replacement. Clin Endocrinol (Oxf) 2004;61:607-611.
1453. Mardh G, Lundin K, Borg B, et al. Growth hormone replacement therapy in adult hypopituitary patients with growth hormone deficiency: combined data from 12 European placebo-controlled clinical trials. Endocrinol Metab 1994;1(suppl A):43-49.
1454. Hokken-Koelega AC, Stijnen T, de John MC, et al. Double blind trial comparing the effects of two doses of growth hormone in prepubertal patients with chronic renal insufficiency. J Clin Endocrinol Metab 1994;79:1185-1190.
1455. Mehls O, Broyer M, European/Australian Study Group. Growth response to recombinant human growth hormone in short prepubertal children with chronic renal failure with or without dialysis. Acta Paediatr Suppl 1994;399:1-7.
1456. Fine RN, Kohaut E, Brown D, et al. Long-term treatment of growth retarded children with chronic renal insufficiency with recombinant human growth. Kidney Int 1996;49:781-785.
1457. Fine RN, Kohaut EC, Brown D, et al. Growth after recombinant human growth hormone treatment in children with chronic renal failure: report of a multicenter randomized double-blind placebo-controlled study. J Pediatr 1994;124:374-382.
1458. Fine RN. Recombinant human growth hormone in children with chronic renal insufficiency—clinical update: 1995. Kidney Int 1996;49(suppl 53):S115-S116.
1459. Watkins SL. Bone disease in patients receiving growth hormone. Kidney Int 1996;49(suppl 53):S126-S127.
1460. Fine RN, Sullivan EK, Kuntze J, et al. The impact of recombinant human growth hormone treatment during chronic renal insufficiency on renal transplant patients. J Pediatr 2000;136:372-382.
1461. Haffner D, Schaefer F, Nissel R, et al. Effect of growth hormone treatment on the adult height of children with chronic renal failure. N Engl J Med 2000;343:923-930.
1462. Wuhl E, Haffner D, Broyer M, et al. Long-term treatment with growth hormone in short children with nephropathic cystinosis. J Pediatr 2001;138:880-887.
1463. Van Es A. Growth hormone treatment in short children with chronic renal failure and after renal transplantation: combined data from European clinical trials. Acta Paediatr Scand Suppl 1991;379:42-48.
1464. Fine RN. Allograft rejection in growth hormone and non-growth hormone treated children. J Pediatr Endocrinol 1994;7:127-133.
1465. Chavers BM, Doherty L, Nevins TE, et al. Effects of growth hormone on kidney function in pediatric transplant recipients. Pediatr Nephrol 1995;9:176-181.
1466. Benfield MR, Parker KL, Waldo FB, et al. Growth hormone in the treatment of growth failure in children after renal transplantation. Kidney Int 1993;44(suppl 43):S62-S64.
1467. Laine J, Krogerus L, Sarna S, et al. Recombinant human growth hormone treatment; its effect on renal allograft function and histology. Transplantation 1996;61:898-903.
1468. Fine RN. Growth hormone in children with chronic renal insufficiency and end-stage renal disease. Endocrinologist 1998;8:160-169.
1469. Bohnet HG. New aspects of oestrogen/gestation-induced growth and endocrine changes in individuals with Turner syndrome. Eur J Pediatr 1986;145:275-279.
1470. Demetriou E, Emans SJ, Crigler JF Jr. Final height in estrogen-treated patients with Turner syndrome. J Obstet Gynecol 1984;64:459-464.
1471. Job JC. How sex steroids can modify the effect of growth hormone on growth in Turner syndrome. In Hibi I, Takano K, eds. Basic and Clinical Approach to Turner Syndrome. Amsterdam Elsevier Science, 1993:279-286.
1472. Kastrup KW. Oestrogen therapy in Turner syndrome. Acta Paediatr Scand Suppl 1988;343:43-46.
1473. Kastrup KW. Growth and development in girls with Turner's syndrome during early therapy with low doses of estradiol. Acta Endocrinol Copenh Suppl 1986;279:157-163.
1474. Knudtzon J, Aarskog D. Results of two years of growth hormone treatment followed by combined growth hormone and oestradiol in Turner syndrome. The Norwegian Turner Study Group. Horm Res 1993;39(suppl 2):7-17.
1475. Martinez A, Heinrich JJ, Domene H, et al. Growth in Turner's syndrome: long-term treatment with low dose ethinyl estradiol. J Clin Endocrinol Metab 1987;65:253-257.
1476. Naeraa RW, Nielsen J, Kastrup KW. Growth hormone and 17B-oestradiol treatment of Turner girls—2 year results. Eur J Pediatr 1994;153:72-77.
1477. Pasquino AM, Boscherini B. Effect of low-dose estrogen on growth in Turner syndrome. In Ranke MB, Rosenfeld RG, eds. Turner Syndrome: Growth Promoting Therapies. Amsterdam: Elsevier Science, 1991:181-185.
1478. Ranke MB, Haug F, Blum WF, et al. Effect on growth of patients with Turner's syndrome treated with low estrogen doses. Acta Endocrinol Copenh Suppl 1986;279:153-156.
1479. Ross JL, Cassorla FG, Skerda MC, et al. A preliminary study of the effect of estrogen dose on growth in Turner's syndrome. N Engl J Med 1983;309:1104-1106.
1480. Schwartzberg M, Senior B, Sadeghi-Nejad AB. Final height in girls with Turner syndrome treated with low-dose ethinyl estradiol (EE2). Pediatr Res 1992;31:84A.
1481. Rudman D, Goldsmith M, Kutner M, et al. Effect of growth hormone and oxandrolone singly and together on growth rate in girls with X chromosome abnormalities. J Pediatr 1980;96:132-135.
1482. Forbes AP, Jacobsen JG, Carroll EL, et al. Studies of growth arrest in gonadal dysgenesis: response to exogenous human growth hormone. Metabolism 1962;11:56-75.
1483. Rosenfeld RG, Hintz RL, Johanson AJ, et al. Three-year results of a randomized prospective trial of methionyl human growth hormone and oxandrolone in Turner syndrome. J Pediatr 1988;113:393-400.
1484. Takano K, Hizuka N, Shizume K. Treatment of Turner's syndrome with methionyl human growth hormone for six months. Acta Endocrinol (Copenh) 1986;112:130-137.
1485. Rongen-Westerlaken C, Wit JM, Drop SL, et al. Methionyl human growth hormone in Turner's syndrome. Arch Dis Child 1988;63:1211-1217.
1486. Massa G, Otten BJ, De Muinck Keizer-Schrama SM, et al. Treatment with two growth hormone regimens in girls with Turner syndrome: final height results. Horm Res 1995;43:144-146.
1487. Rocchiccioli P, Battin J, Bertrand AM, et al. [Final stature in cases of Turner's syndrome treated with growth hormone]. Arch Pediatr 1994;1:359-362.
1488. Chernausek SD, Attie KM, Cara JF, et al. Growth hormone therapy of Turner syndrome: the impact of estrogen replacement on final height. J Clin Endocrinol Metab 2000;85:2439-2445.
1489. Reiter EO, Baptista J, Price L, et al. Effect of the age at initiation of GH treatment on estrogen use and near adult height in Turner Syndrome. In Saenger PH, Pasquino AM, eds. Amsterdam 5th International Turner Symposium—Optimizing Health Care for Turner Patients in the 21st Century. 2000:199-209.
1490. Reiter EO, Blethen SL, Baptista J, et al. Early initiation of growth hormone treatment allows age-appropriate estrogen use in Turner syndrome. J Clin Endocrinol Metab 2001;86:1936-1941.
1491. Carel JC, Mathivon L, Gendrel C, et al. Near normalization of final height with adapted doses of growth hormone in Turner's syndrome. J Clin Endocrinol Metab 1998;83:1462-1466.
1492. van Pareren YK, de Muinck Keizer-Schrama SM, Stijnen T, et al. Final height in girls with Turner syndrome after long-term growth hormone treatment in three dosages and low dose estrogens. J Clin Endocrinol Metab 2003;88:1119-1125.
1493. Soriano-Guillen L, Coste J, Ecosse E, et al. Adult height and pubertal growth in Turner syndrome after treatment with recombinant growth hormone. J Clin Endocrinol Metab 2005;90:5197-5204.
1494. Rosenfield RL, Devine N, Hunold JJ, et al. Salutary effects of combining early very low-dose systemic estradiol with growth hormone therapy in girls with Turner syndrome. J Clin Endocrinol Metab 2005;90:6424-6430.
1495. van Pareren YK, de Muinck Keizer-Schrama SM, Stijnen T, et al. Effect of discontinuation of long-term growth hormone treatment

on carbohydrate metabolism and risk factors for cardiovascular disease in girls with Turner syndrome. J Clin Endocrinol Metab 2002;87:5442-5448.
1496. Radetti G, Pasquino B, Gottardi E, et al. Insulin sensitivity in Turner's syndrome: influence of GH treatment. Eur J Endocrinol 2004;151:351-354.
1497. Bakalov VK, Cooley MM, Quon MJ, et al. Impaired insulin secretion in the Turner metabolic syndrome. J Clin Endocrinol Metab 2004;89:3516-3520.
1498. The Canadian Growth Hormone Advisory Committee. Impact of growth hormone supplementation on adult height in Turner syndrome: results of the Canadian randomized controlled trial. J Clin Endocrinol Metab 2005;90:3360-3398.
1499. Pasquino AM, Pucarelli I, Segni M, et al. Adult height in sixty girls with Turner syndrome treated with growth hormone matched with an untreated group. J Endocrinol Invest 2005;28:350-356.
1500. Bertelloni S, Cinquanta L, Baroncelli GI, et al. Volumetric bone mineral density in young women with Turner's syndrome treated with estrogens or estrogens plus growth hormone. Horm Res 2000;53:72-76.
1501. Ranke MB, Lindberg A, Chatelain P, et al. Prediction of long-term response to recombinant human growth hormone in Turner syndrome: development and validation of mathematical models. J Clin Endocrinol Metab 2000;85:4212-4218.
1502. Bannink EM, Raat H, Mulder PG, et al. Quality of life after growth hormone therapy and induced puberty in women with Turner syndrome. J Pediatr 2006;148:95-101.
1503. Carel JC, Ecosse E, Bastie-Sigeac I, et al. Quality of life determinants in young women with Turner's syndrome after growth hormone treatment: results of the StaTur Population-Based Cohort Study. J Clin Endocrinol Metab 2005;90:1992-1997.
1504. Anneren G, Sara VR, Hall K, et al. Growth and somatomedin responses to growth hormone in Down's syndrome. Arch Dis Child 1986;61:48-52.
1505. Anneren G, Gustavson KH, Sara VR, et al. Normalized growth velocity in children with Down's syndrome during growth hormone therapy. J Intell Disabil Res 1993;37:381-387.
1506. Neyzi O, Darendelilier F. Growth hormone treatment in syndromes with short stature including Down syndrome, Prader-Labhardt-Willi syndrome, von Recklinghausen syndrome, Williams syndrome and others. In Ranke MB, Gunnarsson R, eds. Progress in Growth Hormone Therapy—5 Years of KIGS. Mannheim: J&J Verlag, 1994:240-245.
1507. Torrado C, Bastian W, Wisniewski KE, et al. Treatment of children with Down syndrome and growth retardation with recombinant human growth hormone. J Pediatr 1991;119:478-483.
1508. Allen DB, Frasier SD, Foley TP, et al. Growth hormone for children with Down syndrome. J Pediatr 1993;123:742-743.
1509. Leger J, Noel M, Limal JM, et al. Growth factors and intrauterine growth retardation. II. Growth hormone, insulin-like growth factor (IGF) I, and IGF-binding protein 3 levels in children with intrauterine growth retardation compared with normal control subjects: prospective study from birth to two years of age. Pediatr Res 1996;40:101-107.
1510. Strauss RS, Dietz WH. Growth and development of term children born with low birth weight: effects of genetic and environmental factors. J Pediatr 1998;133:67-72.
1511. Chatelain P, Job JC, Blanchard J, et al. Dose-dependent catch-up growth after 2 years of growth hormone treatment in intrauterine growth retarded children. J Clin Endocrinol Metab 1994;78: 1454-1460.
1512. Job JC, Chaussain JL, Job B, et al. Follow-up of three years of treatment with growth hormone and of one post-treatment year, in children with severe growth retardation of intrauterine onset. Pediatr Res 1996;39:354-359.
1513. Chaussain JL, Colle M, Landier F. Effects of growth hormone therapy in prepubertal children with short stature secondary to intrauterine growth retardation. Acta Paediatr 1994;399:74-75.
1514. de Zegher F, Maes M, Gargosky SE, et al. High-dose growth hormone treatment of short children born small for gestational age. J Clin Endocrinol Metab 1996;81:1887-1892.
1515. Sas T, De Waal W, Mulder P, et al. Growth hormone treatment in children with short stature born small for gestational age: 5 year results in a randomized, double-blind, dose-response trial. J Clin Endocrinol Metab 1999;84:3064-3070.
1516. de Zegher F, De Caju MV, Heinrichs C, et al. Early, discontinuous, high dose growth hormone treatment to normalize height and weight of short children born small for gestational age: results over 6 years. J Clin Endocrinol Metab 1999;84:1558-1561.
1517. de Zegher F, Albertsson-Wikland K, Wollmann HA, et al. Growth hormone treatment of short children born small for gestational age: growth responses with continuous and discontinuous regimens. J Clin Endocrinol Metab 2000;85:2816-2821.
1518. de Zegher F, Hokken-Koelega A. Growth hormone therapy for children born small for gestational age: height gain is less dose dependent over the long term than over the short term. Pediatrics 2005;115:e458-e462.
1519. Dahlgren J, Wikland KA. Final height in short children born small for gestational age treated with growth hormone. Pediatr Res 2005;57:216-222.
1520. Ranke MB, Lindberg A, Cowell CT, et al. Prediction of response to growth hormone treatment in short children born small for gestational age: analysis of data from KIGS (Pharmacia International Growth Database). J Clin Endocrinol Metab 2003;88: 125-131.
1521. van Pareren YK, Duivenvoorden HJ, Slijper FS, et al. Intelligence and psychosocial functioning during long-term growth hormone therapy in children born small for gestational age. J Clin Endocrinol Metab 2004;89:5295-5302.
1522. Russo VC, Gluckman PD, Feldman EL, et al. The insulin-like growth factor system and its pleiotropic functions in brain. Endocr Rev 2005;26:916-943.
1523. Sands SA. Intelligence and psychosocial functioning during long-term growth hormone therapy in children born small for gestational age. J Clin Endocrinol Metab 2004;89:5292-5294.
1524. Cutfield WS, Jackson WE, Jefferies C, et al. Reduced insulin sensitivity during growth hormone therapy for short children born small for gestational age. J Pediatr 2003;142:113-116.
1525. Arends NJ, Boonstra VH, Duivenvoorden HJ, et al. Reduced insulin sensitivity and the presence of cardiovascular risk factors in short prepubertal children born small for gestational age (SGA). Clin Endocrinol (Oxf) 2005;62:44-50.
1526. Dunger DB, Ong KK. Babies born small for gestational age: insulin sensitivity and growth hormone treatment. Horm Res 2005;64(suppl 3):58-65.
1527. Seino Y, Yamate T, Kanzaki S, et al. Achondroplasia: effect of growth hormone in 40 patients. Clin Pediatr Endocrinol 1994; 3(suppl 4):41-45.
1528. Ramaswami U, Rumsby G, Spoudeas HA, et al. Treatment of achondroplasia with growth hormone: six years of experience. Pediatr Res 1999;46:435-439.
1529. Bridges NA, Brook CG. Progress report: growth hormone in skeletal dysplasia. Horm Res 1994;42:231-234.
1530. Ramaswami U, Hindmarsh PC, Brook CG. Growth hormone therapy in hypochondroplasia. Acta Paediatr Suppl 1999;428: 116-117.
1531. Romano AA, Blethen SL, Dana K, et al. Growth hormone treatment in Noonan syndrome: The National Cooperative Growth Study experience. J Pediatr 1996;128:S18-S21.
1532. Cotterill AM, McKenna WJ, Brady AF, et al. The short-term effects of growth hormone therapy on height velocity and cardiac ventricular wall thickness in children with Noonan's Syndrome. J Clin Endocrinol Metab 1996;81:2291-2297.
1533. Saha MT, Haapasaari J, Hannula S, et al. Growth hormone is effective in the treatment of severe growth retardation in children with juvenile chronic arthritis. Double blind placebo-controlled followup study. J Rheumatol 2004;31:1413-1417.
1534. Bechtold S, Ripperger P, Muhlbayer D, et al. GH therapy in juvenile chronic arthritis: results of a two year controlled study on growth and bone. J Clin Endocrinol Metab 2001;86:5737-5744.
1535. Simon D, Lucidarme N, Prieur AM, et al. Effects on growth and body composition of growth hormone treatment in children with juvenile idiopathic arthritis requiring steroid therapy. J Rheumatol 2003;30:2492-2499.
1536. Bechtold S, Ripperger P, Hafner R, et al. Growth hormone improves height in patients with juvenile idiopathic arthritis: 4-year data of a controlled study. J Pediatr 2003;143:512-519.
1537. Stabler B, Siegel PT, Clopper RR, et al. Behavior changes after growth hormone treatment of children with short stature. J Pediatr 1998;133:366-373.

1538. Voss LD, Mulligan J. Bullying in school: are short pupils at risk? Questionnaire study in a cohort. BMJ 2000;320:612-613.
1539. Voss LD. Growth hormone therapy for the short normal child: who needs it and who wants it? The case against growth hormone therapy. J Pediatr 2000;136:103-106, 109-110.
1540. Saenger P. Growth hormone therapy for the short normal child: who needs it and who wants it ? The case in support of growth hormone therapy. J Pediatr 2000;136:106-108.
1541. Underwood LE, Rieser PA. Is it ethical to treat healthy short children with growth hormone? Acta Paediatr Scand Suppl 1989; 362:18-23.
1542. Allen DB, Brook CGD, Bridges NA, et al. Therapeutic controversies: growth hormone (GH) treatment of non-GH deficient subjects. J Clin Endocrinol 1994;79:1239-1248.
1543. Allen DB, Fost N. hGH for short stature: ethical issues raised by expanded access. J Pediatr 2004;144:648-652.
1544. Sandberg DE, Colsman M. Growth hormone treatment of short stature: status of the quality of life rationale. Horm Res 2005;63:275-283.
1545. Ross JL, Sandberg DE, Rose SR, et al. Psychological adaptation in children with idiopathic short stature treated with growth hormone or placebo. J Clin Endocrinol Metab 2004;89: 4873-4878.
1546. Voss LD, Sandberg DE. The psychological burden of short stature: evidence against. Eur J Endocrinol 2004;151(suppl 1):29-33.
1547. Cuttler L. Editorial: safety and efficacy of growth hormone treatment for idiopathic short stature. J Clin Endocrinol Metab 2005;90:5502-5504.
1548. Van Vliet G, Styne DM, Kaplan SL, et al. Growth hormone treatment for short stature. N Engl J Med 1983;309:1016-1022.
1549. Gertner JM, Genel M, Gianfredi SP, et al. Prospective clinical trial of human growth hormone in short children without growth hormone deficiency. J Pediatr 1984;104:172-176.
1550. Hopwood NJ, Hintz RL, Gertner JM, et al. Growth response of children with non-growth hormone deficiency and marked short stature during three years of growth hormone therapy. J Pediatr 1993;123:215-222.
1551. Zadik Z, Chalew S, Zung A, et al. Effect of long-term growth hormone therapy on bone age and pubertal maturation in boys with and without classical growth hormone deficiency. J Pediatr 1994;125:189-195.
1552. Weise KL, Nahata MC. Growth hormone use in children with idiopathic short stature. Ann Pharmacother 2004;38:1460-1468.
1553. Spagnoli A, Spadoni GL, Cianfarani S, et al. Prediction of the outcome of growth hormone therapy in children with idiopathic short stature. J Pediatr 1995;126:905-909.
1554. Wit J-M. Growth hormone treatment of idiopathic short stature. In Ranke MB, Wilton P, eds. Growth Hormone Therapy in KIGS—10 Years' Experience. Heidelberg-Leipzig: Johann Ambrosius Verlag, 1999:225-244.
1555. Hintz RL, Attie KM, Baptista J, et al. Effect of growth hormone treatment on adult height of children with idiopathic short stature. N Engl J Med 1999;340:502-507.
1556. Finkelstein BS, Imperiale TF, Speroff T, et al. Effect of growth hormone therapy on height in children with idiopathic short stature. Arch Pediatr Adolesc Med 2002;156:230-240.
1557. McCaughey ES, Mulligan J, Voss LD, et al. Randomised trial of growth hormone in short normal girls. Lancet 1998;351:940-944.
1558. Leschek EW, Rose SR, Yanovski JA, et al. Effect of growth hormone treatment on adult height in peripubertal children with idiopathic short stature: a randomized, double-blind, placebo-controlled trial. J Clin Endocrinol Metab 2004;89:3140-3148.
1559. Wit JM, Rekers-Mombarg LT, Cutler GB, et al. Growth hormone (GH) treatment to final height in children with idiopathic short stature: evidence for a dose effect. J Pediatr 2005;146:45-53.
1560. de Zegher F, Maes M, Heinrichs C, et al. High-dose growth hormone therapy for short children born small for gestational age. Acta Paediatr Scand Suppl 1994;399:77-78.
1561. Loche S, Cambiaso P, Setzu S, et al. Final height after growth hormone therapy in non-growth-hormone-deficient children with short stature. J Pediatr 1994;125:196-200.
1562. Cowell CT. Growth hormone therapy in idiopathic short stature in the Kabi International Growth Study. In Ranke MB, Gunnarsson R, eds. Progress in Growth Hormone Therapy—5 Years of KIGS. Mannheim: J&J Verlag, 1994;216-229.
1563. Crowe BJ, Rekers-Mombarg LT, Robling K, et al. Effect of growth hormone dose on bone maturation and puberty in children with idiopathic short stature. J Clin Endocrinol Metab 2006;91: 169-175.
1564. Kamp GA, Waelkens JJ, De Muinck Keizer-Schrama SM, et al. High dose growth hormone treatment induces acceleration of skeletal maturation and an earlier onset of puberty in children with idiopathic short stature. Arch Dis Child 2002;87:215-220.
1565. Buchlis JG, Irizarry L, Crotzer BC, et al. Comparison of final heights of growth hormone-treated vs. untreated children with idiopathic growth failure. J Clin Endocrinol Metab 1998; 83:1075-1079.
1566. Saenger P, Attie KM, DiMartino-Nardi J, et al. Metabolic consequences of 5-year growth hormone (GH) therapy in children treated with GH for idiopathic short stature. J Clin Endocrinol Metab 1998;83:3115-3120.
1567. Kelnar CJ, Albertsson-Wikland K, Hintz RL, et al. Should we treat children with idiopathic short stature? Horm Res 1999;52: 150-157.
1568. Kemp SF, Kuntze J, Attie KM, et al. Efficacy and safety results of long-term growth hormone treatment of idiopathic short stature. J Clin Endocrinol Metab 2005;90:5247-5253.
1569. Quigley CA, Gill AM, Crowe BJ, et al. Safety of growth hormone treatment in pediatric patients with idiopathic short stature. J Clin Endocrinol Metab 2005;90:5188-5196.
1570. Robinson IC, Gabrielsson B, Klaus G, et al. Glucocorticoids and growth problems. Acta Paediatr Suppl 1995;411:81-86.
1571. Reusz GS, Hoyer PF, Lucas M, et al. X linked hypophosphatemia: treatment, height gain, and nephrocalcinosis. Arch Dis Child 1990;65:1125-1128.
1572. Sanchez CP, Goodman WG, Brandli D, et al. Skeletal response to recombinant human growth hormone (rhGH) in children treated with long-term glucocorticoids. J Bone Min Res 1995;10:2-6.
1573. Blethen SL, Allen DB, Graves D, et al. Safety of recombinant DNA-derived growth hormone (rhGH): the National Cooperative Growth Study experience. J Clin Endocrinol Metab 1996;81: 1704-1710.
1574. Cowell CT, Dietsch S. Adverse events during growth hormone therapy. J Pediatr Endocrinol Metab 1995;8:243-252.
1575. Wyatt D. Lessons from the national cooperative growth study. Eur J Endocrinol 2004;151(suppl 1):55-59.
1576. Blethen SL. Complications of growth hormone therapy in children. Curr Opinion Pediatr 1995;7:466-471.
1577. Watanabe S, Yamaguchi N, Tsunematsu Y, et al. Risk factors for leukemia occurrence among growth hormone users. Jpn J Cancer 1989;80:822-825.
1578. Fisher DA, Job J-C, Preece M, et al. Leukemia in patients treated with growth hormone. Lancet 1988;1:1159-1160.
1579. Fradkin JE, Mills JL, Schonberger LB, et al. Risk of leukemia after treatment with pituitary growth hormone. JAMA 1993;270: 2829-2832.
1580. Wilton P. Adverse events during growth hormone treatment: 5 years' experience. In Ranke MB, Gunnarsson R, eds. Progress in Growth Hormone Therapy—5 Years of KIGS. Mannheim: J&J Verlag, 1994;291-307.
1581. Blethen SL. Leukemia in children treated with growth hormone. Trends Endocrinol Metab 1999;9:367-370.
1582. Nishi Y, Tanaka T, Takano K, et al. Recent status in the occurrence of leukemia in growth hormone-treated patients in Japan. J Clin Endocrinol Metab 1999;84:1961-1965.
1583. Oglivy-Stuart AL, Ryder WD, Gattamaneni HR, et al. Growth hormone and tumor recurrence. Br Med J 1992;304:1601-1605.
1584. Arslanian SA, Becker DJ, Lee PA, et al. Growth hormone therapy and tumor recurrence: findings in children with brain neoplasms and hypopituitarism. Am J Dis Child 1985;139:347-350.
1585. Bloom HJ, Glees J, Bell J. The treatment and long-term prognosis of children with intracranial tumors: a study of 610 cases, 1950-81. Int J Radiat Oncol Biol Phys 1990;18:723-745.
1586. Davis CH, Joglekar VM. Cerebellar astrocytomas in children and young adults. J Neurol Neurosurg Psychiatry 1981;44:820-828.

1587. Halperin EC. Pediatric brain stem tumors: patterns of treatment failure and their implications for radiotherapy. Int J Radiat Oncol Biol Phys 1985;11:1293-1298.
1588. Hoffman HJ, De Silva M, Humphreys RP, et al. Aggressive surgical management of craniopharyngiomas in children. J Neurosurg 1992;76:47-52.
1589. Lapras C, Patet JD, Mottolese C, et al. Craniopharyngiomas in childhood: analysis of 42 cases. Prog Exp Tumor Res 1987;30: 350-358.
1590. Nishio S, Fukui M, Takeshita I, et al. Recurrent medulloblastoma in children. Neurol Med Chir 1986;26:19-25.
1591. Schuler D, Somolo P, Borsi J, et al. New drug combination for the treatment of relapsed brain tumors in children. Pediatr Hematol Oncol 1988;5:153-156.
1592. Torres CF, Rebsamen S, Silber JH, et al. Surveillance scanning of children with medulloblastoma. N Engl J Med 1994;330:892-895.
1593. Uematsu Y, Tsuura Y, Miyamoto K, et al. The recurrence of primary intracranial germinomas. J Neuro Oncol 1992;13:247-256.
1594. Clayton PE, Shalet SM, Gattamaneni HR, et al. Does growth hormone cause relapse of brain tumors? Lancet 1987;1:711-713.
1595. Rodens KP, Kaplan SL, Grumbach MM, et al. Does growth hormone therapy increase the frequency of tumor recurrence in children with brain tumors? Acta Endocrinol 1987;28(suppl): 188-189.
1596. Moshang T Jr. Is brain tumor recurrence increased following growth hormone treatment? Trends Endocrinol Metab 1995; 6:205-209.
1597. Swerdlow AJ, Reddingius RE, Higgins CD, et al. Growth hormone treatment of children with brain tumors and risk of tumor recurrence. J Clin Endocrinol Metab 2000;85:4444-4449.
1598. Karavitaki N, Warner JT, Marland A, et al. GH replacement does not increase the risk of recurrence in patients with craniopharyngioma. Clin Endocrinol (Oxf) 2006;64:556-560.
1599. Jostel A, Mukherjee A, Hulse PA, et al. Adult growth hormone replacement therapy and neuroimaging surveillance in brain tumour survivors. Clin Endocrinol (Oxf) 2005;62:698-705.
1600. Weiss M, Sutton L, Marcial V, et al. The role of radiation therapy in the management of childhood craniopharyngioma. J Rad Oncol Biol Physics 1989;17:1313-1321.
1601. Packer RJ, Sutton LN, Elterman R, et al. Outcome for children with medulloblastoma treated with radiation and cisplatin, CCNU, and vincristine chemotherapy. J Neurosurg 1994;81:690-698.
1602. Malozowski S, Tanner LA, Wysoluski D, et al. Growth hormone, insulin-like growth factor-I, and benign intracranial hypertension. N Engl J Med 1993;329:665-666.
1603. Ranke MB. Effects of growth hormone on the metabolism of lipids and water and their potential causing adverse events during growth hormone treatment. Horm Res 1993;39:104-106.
1604. Collett-Solberg P, Liu GT, Satin-Smith M, et al. Pseudopapilledema and congenital disc anomalies in growth hormone deficiency (GHD). J Pediatr Endocrinol Metab 1998;11:261-265.
1605. Alford FP, Hew FP, Christopher MC, et al. Insulin sensitivity in growth hormone (GH) deficient adults and effects of GH replacement therapy. J Endocrinol Invest 1999;22:28-32.
1606. Wetterau L, Cohen P. New paradigms for growth hormone therapy in children. Horm Res 2000;53:31-36.
1607. Malozowski S, Stadel BV. Prepubertal gynecomastia during growth hormone therapy. J Pediatr 1995;126:659-661.
1608. Malozowski S, Hung W, Scott DC. Acute pancreatitis associated with growth hormone therapy for short stature. N Engl J Med 1995;332:401-402.
1609. Bourguignon JP, Pierard GE, Ernould C, et al. Effects of human growth hormone therapy on melanocytic naevi. Lancet 1993;341: 1505-1506.
1610. Pierard GE, Pierard-Franchimont C. Morphometric evaluation of the growth of nevi. Ann Dermatol Venereol 1993;120:605-609.
1611. Bertelloni S, Baroncelli GI, Viacava P, et al. Can growth hormone treatment in boys without growth hormone deficiency impair testicular function? J Pediatr 1999;135:367-370.
1612. Leschek EW, Troendle JF, Yanovski JA, et al. Effect of growth hormone treatment on testicular function, puberty, and adrenarche in boys with non-growth hormone-deficient short stature: a randomized, double-blind, placebo-controlled trial. J Pediatr 2001;138:406-410.
1613. Frasier SD. A red flag unfurled? Growth hormone treatment and testicular function. J Pediatr 1999;135:278-279.
1614. Chan JM, Stampfer MJ, Giovannucci E, et al. Plasma insulin-like growth factor-I and prostate cancer risk: a prospective study. Science 1998;279:563-566.
1615. Hankinson SE, Willett WC, Colditz GA, et al. Circulating concentrations of insulin-like growth factor-I and risk of breast cancer. Lancet 1998;351:1393-1396.
1616. Ma J, Pollak MN, Giovannucci E, et al. Prospective study of colorectal cancer risk in men and plasma levels of insulin-like growth factor (IGF)-I and IGF-binding protein-3. J Natl Cancer Inst 1999;91:620-625.
1617. Milani D, Carmichael JD, Welkowitz J, et al. Variability and reliability of single serum IGF-I measurements: impact on determining predictability of risk ratios in disease development. J Clin Endocrinol Metab 2004;89:2271-2274.
1618. Renehan AG, Zwahlen M, Minder C, et al. Insulin-like growth factor (IGF)-I, IGF binding protein-3, and cancer risk: systematic review and meta-regression analysis. Lancet 2004;363: 1346-1353.
1619. Wolk A. The growth hormone and insulin-like growth factor I axis, and cancer. Lancet 2004;363:1336-1337.
1620. Ron E, Gridley G, Hrubec Z, et al. Acromegaly and gastrointestinal cancer. Cancer 1991;68:1673-1677.
1621. Popovic V, Damjanovic S, Micic D, et al. Increased incidence of neoplasia in patients with pituitary adenomas. Clin Endocrinol (Oxf) 1998;49:441-445.
1622. Bengtsson BA, Eden S, Ernest I, et al. Epidemiology and long-term survival in acromegaly. Acta Med Scand 1998;223:327-335.
1623. Delhougne B, Deneux C, Abs R, et al. The prevalence of colonic polyps in acromegaly: a colonoscopic and pathological study in 103 patients. J Clin Endocrinol Metab 1995;80:3223-3226.
1624. Ladas SD, Thalassinos NC, Loannides G, et al. Does acromegaly really predispose to an increased prevalence of gastrointestinal tumours? Clin Endocrinol (Oxf) 1994;41:597-601.
1625. Orme SM, McNally RJ, Cartwright RA, et al. Mortality and cancer incidence in acromegaly. J Clin Endocrinol Metab 1998;83: 2730-2734.
1626. Sonksen PH, Jacobs H, Orme S, et al. Acromegaly and colonic cancer. Clin Endocrinol 1997;47:647-648.
1627. Renehan AG, O'Dwyer ST, Shalet SM. Colorectal neoplasia in acromegaly: the reported increase prevalence is overestimated. Gut 2000;46:440-441.
1628. Colao A, Balzano A, Ferone D, et al. Increase prevalence of colonic polyps and altered lymphocyte subset pattern in the colonic lamina propria in acromegaly. Clin Endocrinol (Oxf) 1997;47:23-28.
1629. Sperling MA, Saenger PH, Ray H, et al. Growth hormone treatment and neoplasia—coincidence or consequence? J Clin Endocrinol Metab 2002;87:5351-5352.
1630. Swerdlow AJ, Higgins CD, Adlard P, et al. Risk of cancer in patients treated with human pituitary growth hormone in the UK, 1959-85: a cohort study. Lancet 2002;360:273-277.
1631. Tuffli GA, Johanson A, Rundle AC, et al. Lack of increased risk for extracranial, nonleukemic neoplasms in recipients of recombinant deoxyribonucleic acid growth hormone. J Clin Endocrinol Metab 1995;80:1416-1422.
1632. Juul A, Bernasconi S, Carel JC, et al. Growth hormone treatment and risk of solid tumours. A statement from the Drugs and Therapeutics Committee of the European Society for Paediatric Endocrinology (ESPE). Horm Res 2003;60:103-104.
1633. Cohen P, Clemmons DR, Rosenfeld RG. Does the GH-IGF axis play a role in cancer pathogenesis? Growth Horm IGF Res 2000; 10:1-9.
1634. Guler HP, Zapf J, Froesch ER. Short-term metabolic effects and half-lives of intravenously administered insulin-like growth factor I in healthy adults. N Engl J Med 1987;317:137-140.
1635. Guler HP, Schmid C, Zapf J, et al. Effects of recombinant insulin-like growth factor-I on insulin secretion and renal function in normal human subjects. Proc Natl Acad Sci U S A 1989; 86:2868-2872.
1636. Laron Z, Klinger B, Erster B, et al. Effects of acute administration of insulin-like growth factor-I in patients with Laron-type dwarfism. Lancet 1988;2:1170-1172.

1637. Laron Z, Klinger B, Jensen JT, et al. Biochemical and hormonal changes induced by one week of administration of rIGF-I to patients with Laron type dwarfism. Clin Endocrinol (Oxf) 1991;35:145-150.
1638. Laron Z, Anin S, Klipper-Auerbach Y, et al. Effects of insulin-like growth factor-I on linear growth, head circumference, and body fat in patients with Laron-type dwarfism. Lancet 1992;339: 1258-1261.
1639. Walker J, Van Wyk JJ, Underwood LE. Stimulation of statural growth by recombinant insulin-like growth factor-I in a child with growth hormone insensitivity syndrome (Laron type). J Pediatr 1992;121:641-646.
1640. Wilton P. Treatment with recombinant insulin-like growth factor-I of children with growth hormone receptor deficiency (Laron syndrome). Kabi Pharmacia Study Group on Insulin-like Growth Factor 1 Treatment in Growth Hormone Insensitivity Syndromes. Acta Paediatr Suppl 1992;282:137-141.
1641. Azcona C, Preece MA, Rose SJ, et al. Growth response to rhIGF-I 80 μg/kg twice daily in children with growth hormone insensitivity syndrome: relationship to severity of clinical phenotype. Clin Endocrinol 1999;51:787-792.
1642. Ranke MB, Savage MO, Chatelain PG, et al. Long-term growth of patients with growth hormone insensitivity syndrome with IGF-I. Results of the European Multicentre Study. The Working Group on Growth Hormone Insensitivity Syndromes. Horm Res 1999;51:128-134.
1643. Backeljauw PF, Underwood LE, GHIS Collaborative Group. Therapy for 6.5-7.5 years with recombinant insulin-like growth factor I in children with growth hormone insensitivity syndrome: a clinical research center study. J Clin Endocrinol Metab 2001;86:1504-1510.
1644. Backeljauw PF, Chernausek SD. Treatment of insulin-like growth factor deficiency with IGF-I: studies in humans. Horm Res 2006;65(suppl 1):21-27.
1645. Guevara-Aguirre J, Vasconez O, Martinez V, et al. A randomized, double-blind, placebo-controlled trial on safety and efficacy of recombinant human insulin-like growth factor-I in children with growth hormone receptor deficiency. J Clin Endocrinol Metab 1995;80:1393-1398.
1646. Sotos JF, Cutler EA, Dodge P. Cerebral gigantism. Am J Dis Child 1977;131:625-627.
1647. Wit JM, Beemer FA, Barth PG, et al. Cerebral gigantism (Sotos syndrome). Compiled data of 22 cases. Eur J Pediatr 1985;144: 131-140.
1648. Agwu JC, Shaw NJ, Kirk J, et al. Growth in Sotos syndrome. Arch Dis Child 1999;80:339-342.
1649. Waggoner DJ, Raca G, Welch K, et al. NSD1 analysis for Sotos syndrome: insights and perspectives from the clinical laboratory. Genet Med 2005;7:524-533.
1650. Sotelo-Avila C, Gonzalez-Crussi F, Fowler JW. Complete and incomplete forms of Beckwith-Wiedemann syndrome: their oncogenic potential. J Pediatr 1980;96:47-50.
1651. Elliott M, Bayly R, Cole T, et al. Clinical features and natural history of Beckwith-Wiedemann syndrome: presentation of 74 new cases. Clin Genetics 1994;46:168-174.
1652. Weng EY, Moeschler JB, Graham JM Jr. Longitudinal observations on 15 children with Wiedemann-Beckwith syndrome. Am J Med Genet 1995;56:366-373.
1653. Drummond IA, Madden SL, Rohwer-Nutter, et al. Repression of the insulin-like growth factor II gene by the Wilms' tumor suppressor WT1. Science 1992;257:674-678.
1654. Schofield PN, Nystrom A, Smith J, et al. Expression of a high molecular weight form of insulin-like growth factor II in a Beckwith-Wiedemann syndrome associated adrenocortical adenoma. Cancer Lett 1995;94:71-77.
1655. Kubota T, Saitoh S, Matsumoto T, et al. Excess functional copy of allele at chromosomal region 11p15 may cause Wiedemann-Beckwith syndrome. Am J Med Genet 1994;49:378-383.
1656. Morison IM, Becroft DM, Taniguchi T, et al. Somatic overgrowth associated with overexpression of insulin-like growth factor II. Nature Med 1996;2:311-316.
1657. Cano-Gauci DF, Song HH, Yang H, et al. Glypican-3-deficient mice exhibit developmental overgrowth and some of the abnormalities typical of Simpson-Golabi-Behmel syndrome. J Cell Biol 1999;146:255-264.
1658. Veugelers M, Cat BD, Muyldermans SY, et al. Mutational analysis of the GPC3/GPC4 glypican gene cluster on Xq26 in patients with Simpson-Golabi-Behmel syndrome: identification of loss-of-function mutations in the GPC3 gene. Hum Mol Genet 2000;22: 1321-1328.
1659. Tauber M, Pienkowski C, Rochiccioli P. Growth hormone secretion in children and adolescents with familial tall stature. Eur J Pediatr 1994;153:311-316.
1660. Dickerman Z, Loewinger J, Laron Z. The pattern of growth in children with constitutional tall stature from birth to age 9 years: a longitudinal study. Acta Paediatr Scand 1984;73:530-536.
1661. Josse EE, Temperli R, Mullis PE. Adult height in constitutionally tall stature: accuracy of five different height prediction methods. Arch Dis Child 1992;67:1357-1362.
1662. Ignatius A, Lenko HL, Perheentupa J. Oestrogen treatment of tall girls: effect decreases with age. Acta Paediatr Scand 1991;80: 712-717.
1663. De Waal WJ, Greyn-Fokker MH, Stijnen TH, et al. Accuracy of final height prediction and effect of growth reductive therapy in 362 constitutionally tall children. J Clin Endocrinol Metab 1996;81:1206-1216.
1664. Bierich JR. Estrogen treatment of girls with constitutional tall stature. Pediatrics 1978;62(December suppl):1196-1201.
1665. Sorgo W, Scholler K, Heinze F, et al. Critical analysis of height reduction in oestrogen-treated tall girls. Eur J Pediatr 1984; 142:260-265.
1666. Trygstad O. Oestrogen treatment of adolescent tall girls; short term side effects. Acta Endocrinol 1986;113(suppl 279):170-173.
1667. Forbes GB. Nutrition and growth. J Pediatr 1977;91:40.
1668. Spence HJ, Trias EP, Raiti S. Acromegaly in a 9 1/2-year-old boy. Am J Dis Child 1972;123:504-506.
1669. AvRuskin TW, Sau K, Tang S, et al. Childhood acromegaly: successful therapy with conventional radiation and effects of chlorpromazine on growth hormone and prolactin secretion. J Clin Endocrinol Metab 1973;37:380.
1670. DeMajo SF, Onativia A. Acromegaly and gigantism in a boy: comparison with three overgrown non-acromegalic children. Pediatr 1960;57:382.
1671. Lefkowitz RJ. G proteins in medicine. N Engl J Med 1995;332: 186-187.
1672. Lightner ES, Winter JS. Treatment of juvenile acromegaly with bromocriptine. J Pediatr 1981;98:494-496.
1673. Geffner ME, Nagel RA, Dietrich RB, et al. Treatment of acromegaly with a somatostatin analog in a patient with McCune-Albright syndrome. J Pediatr 1987;3:740-743.
1674. Hoffman WH, Perrin JS, Halac E, et al. Acromegalic gigantism and tuberous sclerosis. J Pediatr 1978;93:478.
1675. Daughaday WH. Extreme gigantism. Analysis of growth velocity and occurrence of severe peripheral neuropathy and neuropathic arthropathy (Charcot joints). N Engl J Med 1977;297:1267-1269.
1676. Elis LL, Huebner A, Metherell LA, et al. Tall stature in familial glucocorticoid deficiency. Clin Endocrinol 2000;53:423-430.
1677. Ogata T, Kosho T, Wakui K, et al. Short stature homeobox-containing gene duplication on the der(X) chromosome in a female with 45X/46,Xder(X), gonadal dysgenesis, and tall stature. J Clin Endocrinol Metab 2000;85:2927-2930.
1678. Ogata T, Matsuo N. Sex chromosome aberrations and stature: deduction of the principal factors involved in the determination of adult height. Hum Genet 1993;91:551-562.
1679. Nakamura Y, Suehiro Y, Sugino N, et al. A case of 46,X, der(X)(pter →q21::q21→pter) with gonadal dysgenesis, tall stature and endometriosis. Fertil Steril 2001;75:1224-1225.
1680. Tanner JM, Whitehouse RH, Takaishi M. Standards from birth to maturity for height, weight, height velocity, and weight velocity: British children, 1965 part II. Arch Dis Child 1966;41:613-635.
1681. Tanner JM, Whitehouse RH, Takaishi M. Standards from birth to maturity for height, weight, height velocity and weight velocity, British children, 1965. Arch Dis Child 1966;41:454-471.
1682. Post EM, Richman RA. A condensed table for predicting adult stature. J Pediatr 1981;98:440-442.
1683. Underwood LE, Van Wyk JJ. Normal and aberrant growth. In Wilson JD, Foster DW, eds. Williams Textbook of Endocrinology. Philadelphia: WB Saunders, 1991:1079-1138.
1684. Dattani MT. Novel insights into the aetiology and pathogenesis of hypopituitarism. Horm Res 2004;62(suppl 3):1-13.

1685. Wu W, Cogan JD, Pfaffle RW, et al. Mutations in PROP1 cause familial combined pituitary hormone deficiency. Nature Genet 1998;18:147-149.
1686. Netchine I, Sobrier ML, Krude H, et al. Mutations in LHX3 result in a new syndrome revealed by combined pituitary hormone deficiency. Nat Genet 2000;25:182-186.
1687. Sheng HZ, Zhadanov AB, Mosinger B Jr, et al. Specification of pituitary cell lineages by the LIM homeobox gene Lhx3. Science 1996;272:1004-1007.
1688. Laumonnier F, Ronce N, Hamel BC, et al. Transcription factor SOX3 is involved in X-linked mental retardation with growth hormone deficiency. Am J Hum Genet 2002;71:1450-1455.
1689. Sheng HZ, Moriyama K, Yamashita T, et al. Multistep control of pituitary organogenesis. Science 1997;278:1809-1812.
1690. Li H, Witte DP, Branford WW, et al. Gsh-4 encodes a LIM-type homeodomain, is expressed in the developing central nervous system and is required for early postnatal survival. EMBO J 1994;13:2876-2885.
1691. Laumonnier F, Ronce N, Hamel BC, et al. Transcription factor SOX3 is involved in X-linked mental retardation with growth hormone deficiency. Am J Hum Genet 2002;71:1450-1455.
1692. Rizzoti K, Brunelli S, Carmignac D, et al. SOX3 is required during the formation of the hypothalamo-pituitary axis. Nat Genet 2004;36:247-255.
1693. Park HL, Bai C, Platt KA, et al. Mouse Gli1 mutants are viable but have defects in SHH signaling in combination with a Gli2 mutation. Development 2000;127:1593-1605.
1694. Shin SH, Kogerman P, Lindstrom E, et al. GLI3 mutations in human disorders mimic Drosophila cubitus interruptus protein functions and localization. Proc Natl Acad Sci U S A 1999;96: 2880-2884.
1695. Radhakrishna U, Bornholdt D, Scott HS, et al. The phenotypic spectrum of GLI3 morphopathies includes autosomal dominant preaxial polydactyly type-IV and postaxial polydactyly type-A/B; No phenotype prediction from the position of GLI3 mutations. Am J Hum Genet 1999;65:645-655.
1696. Bose J, Grotewold L, Ruther U. Pallister-Hall syndrome phenotype in mice mutant for Gli3. Hum Mol Genet 2002;11:1129-1135.
1697. Takeuchi T, Suzuki H, Sakurai S, et al. Molecular mechanism of growth hormone (GH) deficiency in the spontaneous dwarf rat: detection of abnormal splicing of GH messenger ribonucleic acid by the polymerase chain reaction. Endocrinology 1990;126: 31-38.
1698. Dana K, Baptista J, Blethen SL. Updated NCGS data. Personal communication, 2001.
1699. Tanner JM, Whitehouse RH. Clinical longitudinal standards for height, weight, height velocity, weight velocity and the stages of puberty. Arch Dis Child 1976;51:170-179.
1700. Rotwein P. Structure, evolution, expression and regulation of insulin-like growth factors I and II. Growth Factors 1991;5:3-18.
1701. Cohen P, Rosenfeld RG. The IGF axis. In Rosenbloom AL, ed. Human Growth Hormone, Basic and Scientific Aspects. Boca Raton, FL: CRC Press, 1995:279-285.

CHAPTER 24

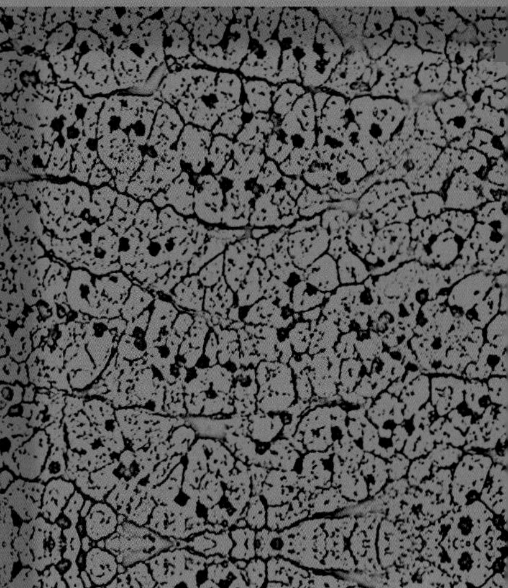

PUBERTY: ONTOGENY, NEUROENDOCRINOLOGY, PHYSIOLOGY, AND DISORDERS

Dennis M. Styne and Melvin M. Grumbach

INTRODUCTION

Puberty is not a de novo event but rather a phase in the continuum in the development of gonadal function and the ontogeny of the hypothalamic-pituitary-gonadal system from the fetus to full sexual maturation and fertility. During puberty secondary sexual characteristics appear and the adolescent growth spurt occurs, resulting in the striking sex dimorphism of mature individuals, fertility is achieved, and profound psychological effects ensue.[1] These changes arise by stimulation of the gonads by pituitary gonadotropins and a subsequent increase in gonadal steroid output; puberty is a consequence of CNS maturation entraining physical maturation. Adolescence usually relates to psychosocial aspects of the teenage years and is accompanied by the onset of adult patterns of sociosexual and economic behavior.[2] Humans are the most reproductively successful of mammals, and many anthropologists have attributed this success to the prolonged pattern of human growth and development[3,4] and to the delay in attaining full sexual maturity.[2,5] The human scheme of growth involves the development of two stages: a childhood stage and an adolescent stage that includes an adolescent or pubertal growth spurt (Fig. 24–1). Not even our closest biologic relative, the chimpanzee (estimated divergence of the chimpanzee and human lineages is 4 million to 5 million years ago), which matures twice as rapidly as the human, unequivocally exhibits these two stages including the unique human pubertal growth spurt. Evolution theorists proposed that a critical part of human success and of many biosocial characteristics emanate from the learning and practice of adult behaviors related to sex and childrearing, particularly provisioning children (not just infants) with food,[2] which is unique to humans.[6] These include learning skills related to production of food, cooperative hunting, division of labor according to sex, sharing food, tool making, and adjustment to the social organization and cultural environment. Bogin, on the other hand, noting that tool making preceded the evolutionary development of adolescence, suggested that, in addition, the evolution and value of human childhood and adolescence and this unique pattern of growth and development has had a significant role in the comparatively striking reproductive advantage and success of humans.[2,5,7,8] Mayr has called this process of selection "selection

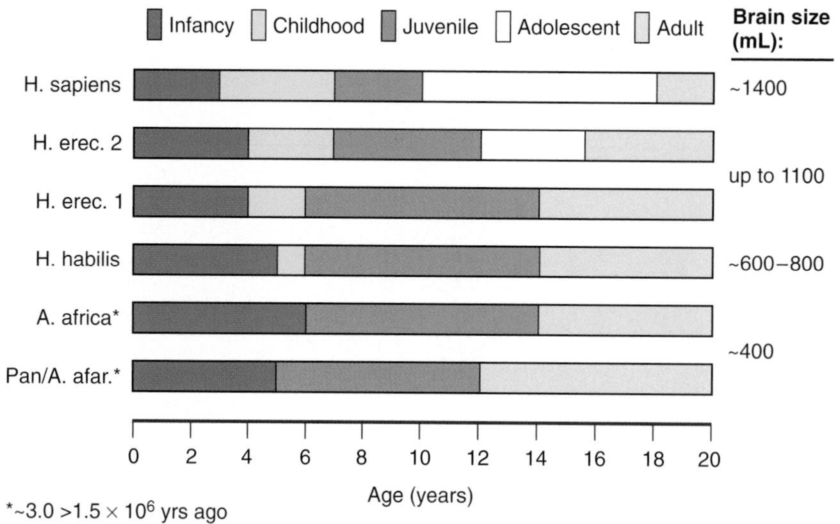

Figure 24–1 ▪ A summary and proposed scheme of the evolution of the human pattern of postnatal growth and development during the first 20 years of life. A. afar, *Australopithecus afarensis,* a "bipedal chimpanzee"; A. africa, *Australopithecus africanus;* H. habilis, *Homo habilis* (the toolmaker); H. erec 1, early *Homo erectus;* H. erec 2, late *Homo erectus;* H. sapiens, *Homo sapiens.* The early hominid australopithecine specimens from South Africa date to about 3.0 to 1.5 million years ago. *H. afarensis,* while a hominid (the family of all human species), retained many anatomic features of nonhominid species, for example, an adult brain size of about 400 mL compared with *H. habilis* (650 to 800 mL), early *H. erectus* (850 to 900 mL), late *H. erectus* (up to 1100 mL), and modern *H. sapiens* (about 1400 mL). Infancy is defined as the period when the mother's breast milk is the sole or most important source of nutrition and in preindustrialized societies ends at about 36 months. Childhood is the period after weaning, when the child is dependent on others for food and protection; this period ends when the growth of the brain in weight is almost complete, at about age 7 years. The juvenile stage is defined as prepubertal individuals who are no longer dependent on their parents for survival. The adolescent stage that begins with the onset of puberty, ends when adult height is attained.[2,5] The pattern in *A. afarensis* is no different from that in the chimpanzee *(Pan troglodytes).* Note the first appearance of the childhood stage, *H. habilis* (arising about 2 million years ago) and the first appearance of the adolescent stage in *H. erectus* 2 (about 500,000 years ago); *H. sapiens* arose about 120,000 to 150,000 years ago. (Modified from Bogin B. Growth and development: recent evolutionary and biocultural research. In Boaz NT, Wolfe LD, eds. Biological Anthropology: The State of the Science. Bend, OR: International Institute for Human Evolutionary Research, 1995:49-70.)

for reproductive success."[9] The transition from the range of age normally considered adolescence to adult life presents important implications for a change in the manner that medical care is presented in modern times due to changes in the individual's autonomy and implications of legal distinctions: some have suggested that this "transition period" be considered another stage of the life span.[10]

In the developed world, as detailed below, reproductive maturity, using menarche as a proxy marker, occurs years earlier than psychosocial maturation occurs, causing a mismatch between biologic stages and psychosocial expectations and transitions (Fig. 24–2).[11] In past eras, such as Neolithic times or the Greek or Roman eras, there was not apparently such a mismatch, as menarche occured at an age similar to what it does today (9 to 14 years) and psychosocial maturation in a simpler world occurred at an age close to that of reproductive maturity.[12,13] With increased population, the advent of agriculture and the growth of cities and later urban centers, menarche occurred later and the complexity of life led to a delay in the attainment of an adult role in society. Now, with improved nutritional status and improved health, the age of menarche has decreased but the age of social adulthood remains later, causing a discrepancy that may never have occurred before in human history.

Influences are posited to exert effects in the reported decrease in the age of menarche in children from the developing world who suffer poor prenatal nutrition who are adopted into families of the developed world.[14-20] There is evidence that poor prenatal nutrition tends to advance the age of menarche[21-24] and adrenarche[25] and to cause an earlier age of

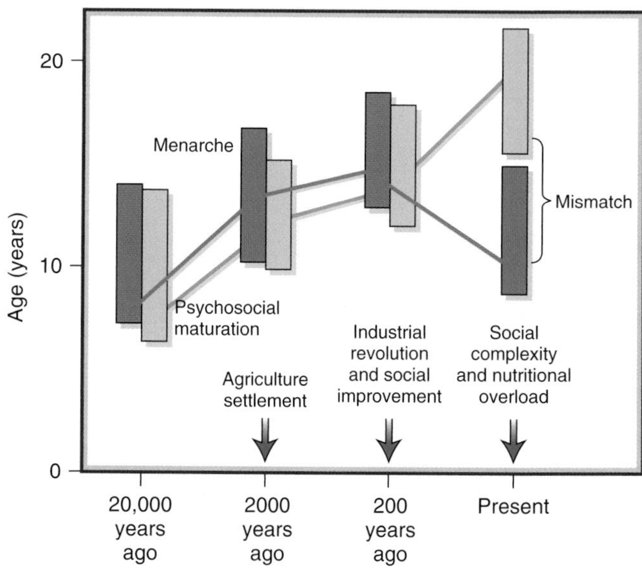

Figure 24–2 ▪ The relationship between the likely range of ages of menarche (green) and achievement of psychosocial maturity (pink) from 20 000 years ago to the present day. The mismatch in timing between these two processes is a novel phenomenon. (From Gluckman PD, Hanson MA. Evolution, development, and timing of puberty. Trends Endocrinol Metab 2006;17[1]:7-12)

puberty. Then a secondary effect of increased nutrition leading to overweight or obesity in girls, lowers the age of puberty further. Thus, children adopted from the developing world into an environment of affluence experience precocious puberty. Longitudinal studies show that low birth weight followed by the rapid weight gain in infancy of catch-up growth may lead to tall childhood stature and early pubertal development (Fig. 24–3).[26] Girls who are longer and lighter at birth and subsequently have greater body mass index (BMI) values at 8 years tend to have earlier menarche.[27] Puberty viewed in a life history approach allows an evolutionary perspective of the process. Theories aiminig to explain influcences on the age of puberty address energetics, stress-suppression, psychosocial acceleration, paternal investment, and child development, all of which may have various effects on the timing and progression of pubertal development (the influence of stress is discussed below).[28]

Influences on the Secular Trend in the Age of Menarche

While historical records show that puberty occurs at an earlier age today than in the past, most evidence derives from the age of menarche, which is removed by several years from the first sign of secondary development in girls.[29-33] Furthermore, historical evidence reflects changes in health and socioeconomic status in regions where it was collected. This leads to complexity in the interpretation of modern national data.

The method of ascertainment of the age of menarche affects the results of surveys. Contemporaneous recordings are performed with the probit method of asking for "yes" or "no" answers to the question "are you menstruating," but the results may be incorrect due to social pressures of the culture and socioeconomic group considered.[34] Recalled age of menarche are used in other studies and considered to be accurate within 1 year of accuracy (in 90% of cases) during the teenage years[35,36] and in older women, to 30 years after the event,[37] but these also may be altered due to social pressures of the culture and socioeconomic group considered.[34]

The "Developed World"

The average age of menarche in industrialized European countries has decreased 2 to 3 months per decade over the past 150 years, and in the United States the decrease has been approximately 2 to 3 months per decade in the last century (Fig. 24–4).[30-32,38] However, this secular trend has slowed or ceased in "developed" countries such as the United States, Australia, and Western Europe (e.g., Britain and Holland among others) since approximately 1940 presumably due to improved socioeconomic status, health, and benefits of urbanization, and because there is a relatively small range of ages of menarche in the "well-off" developed world.[30-32,39-41] Not only has the age of menarche decreased but the standard deviation of the mean has also decreased, suggesting a diminished number of those maturing very late as might be found in disadvantaged subjects.[42] Teasing out the various factors involved in any remaining, more subtle secular trends will require further long-term study and new methodologic approaches in areas where nutrition and health are optimal or nearly optimal.[43] The socioeconomic status differences in menarcheal age has narrowed or disappeared in most of these Western countries where the lower socioeconomic classes do not have an increased burden of disease or malnutrition (for an example in the United States, see reference 44).[45-47] but that does not necessarily hold elsewhere in the world (see below). In Denmark, Spain, and Brazil, there remains evidence for a continued decline in the age of menarche, at least in certain local regions of these countries.[48-51] Remarkably, a reverse secular trend is reported in Northern Italy (in women born between 1950 and 1959) and certain other areas of Europe leading to a later age of menarche; this has been attributed putatively to a resurgence of physical and psychological stress such as was seen in previous eras, such as World War II.[43,52,53]

According to the most recent survey by the U.S. National Center for Health Statistics (although it is more than 30 years old), the age of menarche in the United States is 12.8 years,[54,55] and recent data published in 1997[56] (the Pediatric Research in Office Settings [PROS] study described later) indicate that this age remains similar for Caucasians but not for African-American

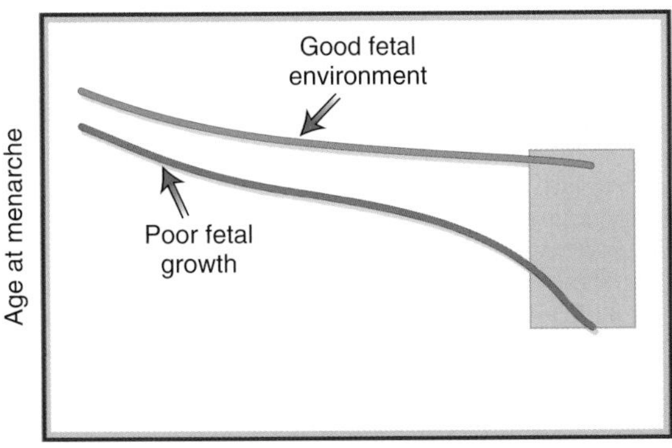

Figure 24–3 ▪ The relationship between childhood nutrition and the age of menarche is shown for children of different birth sizes as a series of contour lines. There is an inverse relationship between the age of menarche and childhood nutritional status but being born smaller also advances menarche. The prenatal influence is more marked at higher postnatal nutritional levels. (From Gluckman PD, Hanson MA. Changing times: the evolution of puberty. Mol Cell Endocrinol 2006; 254-255:26-31)

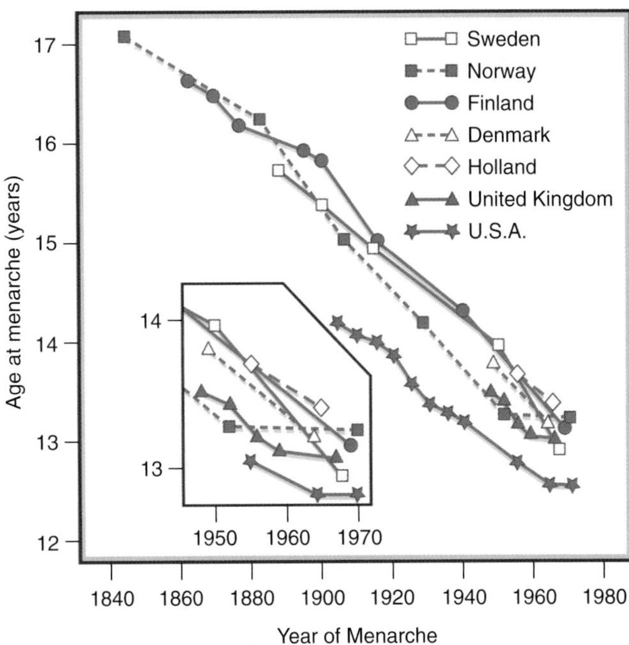

Figure 24–4 ▪ Changes in age at menarche, 1840 to 1978, illustrating the advance in the age at menarche in Western Europe and the United States since 1840 and the slowing of this trend since about 1965. (Modified from Tanner M, Eveleth PB. Variability between populations in growth and development at puberty. In Berenberg SR, ed. Puberty, Biologic and Psychosocial Components. Leiden: HE Stenfert Kroese, 1975:256-273.)

girls in whom the mean age of menarche is 6 months earlier.[57] Data from the Bogalusa Heart Study in the 1970s demonstrated menarche 0.14 year later in African-Americans compared to white girls,[58] and a similar pattern was found in South Africa in the 1980s.[59] This suggest a genetic difference in the age of menarche in addition to environmental factors. However, during the the 20-year study period in Bogalusa, the median menarcheal age decreased by approximately 9.5 months among African-American girls versus approximately 2 months among white girls,[60] leading to a 4-month difference. In addition, between 5 and 9 years of age, black girls were taller and weighed more than white girls, and these characteristics were predictive of a relatively early (before age 11.0 years) menarche. Longitudinal and cross-sectional study of age of menarche in most available studies demonstrate a decrease of 3 months in white girls and 5.5 months in U.S. black girls between 1960 and 1990.[61] African-American girls are advanced in secondary sexual development compared with Caucasian American girls of the same age during the first three stages of puberty; this may be related, in part, to differences in nutrition that have increased over time, leading to the higher prevalence of obesity in African-American girls, although, as stated above, there appears to be a genetic influence in ethnic differences as well.[57,62,63] Furthermore, an advancement in bone age in African-American girls versus white girls was reported in several studies[64-66] and was attributed to increased adiposity found in African-American girls.[67]

There is a disturbing, well-known trend in the United States and elsewhere of an increasing prevalence in childhood overweight (defined by the Centers for Disease Control and Prevention [CDC] as a BMI (calculated as weight in [kg/(height in meters)^2]) >95th percentile for age) and at risk for overweight (defined by the CDC as BMI>85th percentile for age).[68,69] Many[38,70-75] but not all[76,77] studies, cross-sectional and longitudinal, found an inverse relationship between menarcheal age and BMI or other reflections of adiposity (Table 24–1). An increase in subjects' BMI between National Health Evaluation Survey (NHES) and National Health and Nutrition Evaluation Survey (NHANES III) was associated with a decrease in the age of menarche from 12.75 to 12.54 years. If the population in the 1970s (the time of the NHES) had the same range of BMI values as found in the 1990s (the time of NHANES III), the projected age of menarche would have been 12.54 years in NHES, as it was in NHANES III according to one estimation.[78]

Longitudinal study of 180 girls from 5 to 9 years of age demonstrated that higher percent body fat at 5 years; higher percent body fat, higher BMI percentile, or larger waist circumference at 7 years; larger increases in percent body fat from 5 to 9 years of age; and larger increases in waist circumference from 7 to 9 years of age were more likely to exhibit earlier pubertal development at 9 years.[79] A more recent longitudinal study of 354 girls from the National Institute of Child Health and Human Development Study of Early Child Care and Youth Development demonstrated that higher BMI z score in girls as young as 36 months of age and higher rate of change of BMI between 36 months old and grade 1 are associated with earlier puberty, which suggests that increasing rates of obesity in the United States may result in an earlier average age of onset of puberty for US girls.

The longitudinal National Heart, Lung and Blood Institute Growth and Health Study followed 1266 white and 1313 African-American girls from 9 or 10 years of age for 10 or more years. The mean age of menarche in whites was 12.7 years and in African-Americans was 12.1 years with a direct relationship between weight and BMI and age of menarche.[71] A total of 51.6% of these girls started puberty with only one manifestation: those with breast development first (thelarche pattern) rather than the appearance of pubic hair (adrenarche pattern) had an earlier menarche (12. 6 versus 13.1 years respectively), which was associated with a greater BMI and body weight, which was not true for those starting puberty with the initial appearance of pubic hair.[80] Participants in the Girls Health Enrichment Multisite Studies demonstrated a greater prevalence for risk of overweight or overweight between ages 8 and 10 years if they were in puberty or had advanced breast development.[81] A recent reanalysis of the PROS study data[56] yielded a relationship between BMI corrected for age with an earlier onset of puberty and of reaching various stages of puberty, including menarche, for Caucasian girls. This relationship of age of onset of puberty to BMI was less evident in African-American girls in this study, pointing to other factors including genetics.[74] Furthermore, the recent study of boys in the United States of various ethnic groups, while controversial, if accurate, indicates a direct relationship of BMI to age of onset of puberty in boys.[82]

The national longitudinal study of adolescent health is a representative cross-sectional survey of ethnic groups with extra samples from certain minority groups. The mean menarcheal age[63] in wave 2 (14,738 girls) found that African-American girls were 1.55 times more likely than white girls to have menarche before 11 years, considered as early menarche, and Mexican-Americans were 1.76 times more likely to do so than whites. Asians were 1.65 more likely than whites to mature later than 14 years. Overweight was twice as likely to be found in those with early menarche, whereas African-American girls had 2.57-fold greater likelihood of being at risk for overweight if they had menarche before 11 years. In fact, 57.5% of early menarcheal African-Americans had BMI greater than the 85th percentile and 32.5% had BMI greater than the 95th percentile.

Large national studies of pubertal development in the United States are often reanalyzed with different statistical techniques applied to subgroups of the population chosen for particular characteristics or ethnicity; this may explain why the reported age of any stage of pubertal development may differ between publications studying the same sample.[54,55,57,83,84]

Each gain of BMI unit decreased the age of onset of puberty 0.6 year in Swedish boys and 0.7 year in girls; it also reduced the height gain in adolescence 0.88 cm for boys and 0.51 cm for girls, although there was no effect of BMI on final height.[85] Children in Denmark showed no secular trend to earlier pubertal development but increased BMI was associated with earlier pubertal development.[86]

TABLE 24–1 NIPPLE DIAMETER COMPARED WITH BREAST AND PUBIC HAIR STAGES: COMPARISON OF LONGITUDINAL AND CROSS-SECTIONAL DATA

Stage	NIPPLE SIZE (MM)*	
	Cross-Sectional Data	Longitudinal Data
Breast		
1	2.89 (0.81)	3.0 (0.77)
2	3.28 (0.89)	3.37 (0.96)
3	4.07 (1.32)	4.72 (1.40)†
4	7.74 (1.64)†	7.25 (1.46)†
5	9.94 (1.38)†	9.41 (1.45)†
Pubic hair		
1	2.95 (1.02)	3.14 (1.31)
2	3.32 (0.91)	3.69 (1.34)
3	4.11 (1.54)	4.44 (1.17)†
4	7.15 (1.81)†	6.54 (1.47)†
5	9.66 (1.59)†	8.98 (1.56)†

*Results are means ± standard deviation (SD; in parentheses).
†Significantly different from previous stage, $P < .05$.

However, over the past 40 years, menarcheal age in the Caucasian subjects of the Fels Longitudinal Study has remained stable, even as BMI has increased with no relationship between the two. Those subjects with early menarche have a tendency to increase BMI after menarche so that the early menarche occurred first, with increased BMI following.[87] Furthermore, women of the Fels Study who were born in previous decades back to the 1930s, compared to those born in more recent decades and followed longitudinally revealed a decrease in the age of menarche but no concomitant increase in BMI during childhood, although adult BMI values did increase later. Thus, the longitudinal Fels study demonstrates that increased weight appears to be a consequence, rather than a determinant, of the age at menarche and that secular changes in BMI and in the mean age at menarche could be independent phenomena.[89] Early menarche may be a marker for a later increase in BMI. Indeed, there is a rise in BMI, waist circumference, hip circumference, serum luteinizing hormone (LH), androstenedione, testosterone, and dehydroepiandrosterone sulfate (DHEAS) in the few years following menarche.[90] This may be a reflection of polycystic ovarian syndrome.

While moderate obesity is associated with earlier menarche,[62,63,91] pathologic obesity is reportedly associated with delayed age of menarche.[92] The prevelance of polyovarian cystic syndrome in the population however makes it more difficult to determine whether it is primarily weight that exerts the effect.

We conclude from these data, if the effects from BMI are removed, the trend to earlier menarche in the entire population of United States has either ceased or slowed considerably in our era in that most, but not all, large cohorts show no statistically significant change in the age of menarche in the overall population. The decrease in the age of menarche in the African-American population reported in some studies may be an effect of nutritional factors. However, there is increasing evidence that future studies will demonstrate an unequivocal decrease in the age of puberty due to the effects of overweight and obesity.

Leptin, acting as a metabolic messenger between the fat cell and the hypothalamus, was once thought to stimulate the onset of puberty, but more recent studies support the role of leptin as permissive rather than the trigger of the process (reviewed below).

The composition of diet as well as the number of calories in the diet may also relate to menarche. The longitudinal Harvard Longitudinal Studies of Childhood Health and Development found that girls had earlier menarche if they were taller and consumed more animal protein and less vegetable protein as early as 3 to 5 years of age; earlier peak growth velocity occurred if they had higher dietary fat intake at 1 to 2 years of age and higher animal protein intake at 6 to 8 years. Peak velocity increased if, controlling for body size, more calories and animal protein was consumed 2 years before peak growth.[94] However, in contrast,[95] otherwise healthy, prepubertal, 8- to 10-year-olds with elevated low-density lipoprotein (LDL) cholesterol who were given a low-fat diet for a median of 7 years follow-up had no difference between these groups in age of menarche or pubertal progression but they did have lower estradiol, lower non–sex hormone–binding globulin-bound estradiol, lower estrone, and lower estrone sulfate levels during the follicular phase of the menstrual cycle while testosterone concentrations were 27.2% higher during the luteal phase of the menstrual cycle and luteal phase progesterone level was 52.9% lower compared to control girls on a standard diet. A study of Quebecois girls confirmed no effect of fat intake on menarche but also found that no aspect of dietary composition affected menarche, although increase in calories alone was associated with a decrease in the age of menarche[96,97] (see below for a discussion of obesity and puberty). The effect of fat in the diet may be compounded by the effect of estrogen added to commercial beef production cows, which is concentrated in fatty tissue. While safety standards are in place, new ultrasensative estrogen assays may demonstrate that the amount of estrogen consumed has biological effect on children, although no such data exist as yet. There is a positive relationship between high fiber intake and age of menarche,[98-101] which holds true in a comparison of 46 countries. Because diets low in protein are often high in fiber, this might be a compensatory mechanism to ensure adequate nutritional status before reproduction is possible. Lifelong vegetarian dietary intake does not, however, affect the age of menarche.[102]

One reason for the secular trend in the decrease of age of menarche is the modern treatment of chronic diseases that previously increased the age of menarche. Still, delay can occur in any serious chronic condition that is not adequately treated. For example, celiac disease can delay menarche and decrease growth in childhood, as can asthma or even infection with *Helicobacter pylori*.[103-105] Blindness may advance the age of menarche.[106-109]

The "Developing World"

The interaction of socioeconomic conditions, nutrition, energy expenditure, and states of health and puberty is presently of particular importance in areas of the world where nutrition is suboptimal.[110-112] Stunting is common in sub-Saharan Africa, more in younger children than older children, and menarche is about 1.2 years delayed in this area compared to that in African-American girls.[113] Mozambique is one of the poorest countries in Africa with a mean age of menarche of 13.9 years, which has not changed in the last 40 years; the lowest socioeconomic groups and the least educated families have the latest menarche.[114] A lower age of menarche in Brazil is related to the initial social class of the family (reflected by parental education) in that daughters of less educated fathers demonstrate a stronger secular trend toward earlier menarche than those living in better conditions for at least a generation beforehand.[115] In Oaxaca, Mexico, the age at menarche has declined by 1.8 years over about 23 years, 0.78 year/decade, a greater velocity of decrease compared to that of Europe and the United States, noted above,[116] indicating the extent that more severe social changes exert upon the rate of decrease in the age of menarche in some locations. There is no trend toward earlier menarche in the nomadic Lapp culture, in which the standard of living changed little between 1870 and 1930.[112] Greenlandic girls presently have menarche 3 years earlier (12.63 yr) compared to 100 years ago, with the present age of menarche of girls in Greenland being 3 months earlier than in Denmark. The height of children in Greenland has also increased but adult heights remain several centimeters below those in Denmark.[117] In South Korea, a decrease of 4.12 years in the age of menarche has occurred in the last 67 years (0.62 yr/decade decrease) in concert with a gain in adult height of 22.5 cm.[118]

Certain areas of South America and Africa exhibit a pattern in which rural children fare better and have earlier puberty and taller stature than urban children, demonstrating a disturbing trend of adverse health and nutritional conditions in crowded urban centers.[119,120] On the contrary, urban boys in Zambia entered puberty on the average 1.2 years earlier than rural boys, apparently due to inadequate nutrition in that rural region.[121] Zambian rural girls progress through puberty and finish developing at an age similar to urban girls; this is attributed to culturally determined preferential feeding during puberty.[122]

Historical records support the effects of improving standards of living. There was a closer inverse relationship between the gross national product at the time of birth than at the time of menarche in Norway between 1860 and 1950, showing that improved socioeconomic factors operate more strongly early in life than later ages near menarche.[123]

The onset of secondary sexual development in girls of the Kikuyu in Kenya is 13.0 years with menarche at 15.9 years,[124] in contrast to the age of onset of puberty in African-American girls of 8.9 years with menarche at 12.2 years.[56] The Kikuyu start later and have a shorter time of transition to menarche than the American girls. Kikuyu boys enter puberty before or at the same age as Kikuyu girls.[124] Furthermore, boys of the Hadza of Tanzania enter puberty 2 years earlier than girls.[124] This contrasts the pattern of earlier onset of puberty in girls than boys by about 6 months in the developed world.

Thus, malnourished individuals have later age of menarche across the world.[28c] The sum of these reports indicates that those populations existing in the most difficult conditions who experience improvement in socioeconomic status demonstrate a greater decrease in the age of menarche: once a minimum of nutritional status or state of health is reached, the effects of socioeconomic status upon the age of menarche is minimized or eliminated.

Stress and Puberty

Stress may add to the disparity between the age of menarche in the developed and developing world in addition to nutritional effect. Several psychological theories address this relationship.[28] A life history approach suggests that the stress-suppression theory explains some influences on the age of puberty as do the theories of energetics, psychosocial acceleration, paternal investment, and child development.[28] The presence of a father increases the level of paternal investment in the family and the absence of a father at an early age, a factor likely to increase stress, increases the likelihood of early menarche (older than 12 years) by threefold[125] and of acceleration of puberty in boys as well.[126,127] The age of voice breaking in Bach's choir in Leipzig increased during the war of Austrian Succession in 1727-1749,[111] which in effect could be due to nutritional changes or to stress. During World War II and the hostilities in the former Yugoslavia, the age of menarche increased; again, nutritional changes may be a factor in these times although the effect of stress was here invoked as a cause for delaying menarche.[28,128-130] In Poland lower socioeconomic conditions did not delay menarche as did family dysfunction.[131] On the other hand, study of 523 girls who lived in families free of strong traumatic events compared to 1817 girls whose family dysfunction exposed them to prolonged distress demonstrated a lower mean age of menarche in the dysfunctional families (13.0 years, significantly lower that 13.11 years for the girls in average families).[132]

Sexual abuse is associated with earlier onset of puberty as well as earlier menarche compared to a control population.[133-136] The data do not analyze how early sexual development might itself influence the occurrence of sexual abuse.

While maternal age at menarche tends to predict daughters' age at menarche, breast development, weight, and depressive affect were also predictive of age at menarche, with family relations (including the absence of a father at least in some studies) more strongly predicting age at menarche than breast development or weight. Thus the question arises of whether psychological stress decreases the age of menarche or whether stress arises from earlier menarche.[137]

An alternative biologic hypothesis is suggested to explain lower age of menarche in stressful family environment. Short alleles of the GGC repeat polymorphism of the androgen receptor (AR) gene are associated with aggression and impulsivity, increased number of sexual partners, sexual compulsivity, lifetime number of sex partners in males and paternal divorce, father absence as well as early age of menarche in females. This implies a genetic basis to the relationship between absence of father and early puberty in girls in that this allele can be transferred from the father (who later in her life is absent) to the daughter who develops early menarche.[138] However, others find no relationship between the GGC-repeat polymorphism and aberrant fathering behavior, but adverse early experiences, early menarche, and early sexual activity were related in the cohort.[135]

Puberty begins at a later age and pubertal development lasts longer at high altitudes than at low altitudes even when nutritional status is similar.[139-144] The number of offspring born at high altitudes does not decrease even though reproduction is complicated by late menarche and a shortened period of fertility; a secular trend toward earlier menarche in the Andean population suggests improvement in living conditions.[145]

A convergence of the onset of menses in women or girls living together was noted[146] and subsequent studies supported synchrony of the timing of the spontaneous onset of menses in women living together or when axillary odor scent (presumably containing pheromones) was administered to women. Sensitivity to odor relates to development and gender in that 17-year-old males were less able to detect androstadienone or androstenone than 13 year old males while females demonstrated no such trend; this may be due to the increased presence of these odoriferous substances in older males compared to younger males and compared to females of both ages.[147] Others found in college women and older subjects that closeness of sleeping conditions was not a prerequisite to synchronizing menstrual cycles but being close friends was of significance.[148,149] The methodology of studies of menstrual synchrony was heavily criticized based upon the variable cycle length found among women.[150-153]

In a study of 3000 U.S. and Norwegian women, menarche peaked in December-January and in July.[154] U.S. women born before 1970 had more frequent winter menarche and an older age of menarche while those born after 1970 tended towards summer menarche at a younger age. In rural Brazil, birth month correlated to month of menarche, with a peak in December (in the southern hemisphere a period of spring-summer transition); this may be related to release from a pattern of stress because this time of year is the end of the school year, the start of vacation, and the time when rural workers receive a major portion of harvest pay.[155]

There is a North to South decrease in the age of menarche in Europe,[42] either due to environmental factors or genetic influences. Reduction or elimination of the secular trend toward earlier puberty in the present era supports the effects of environment on the age of puberty or menarche in that improvements in the environmental state may be responsible for the diminution of the secular trend.

The important role played by genetic factors in the onset of puberty, is illustrated by the similar age of menarche in members of an ethnic population and in mother-daughter and sibling pairs.[156-158] The age of menarche from the California Childhood Health and Development Study confirms the influence of the age of menarche in a mother upon the age of menarche of her daughter, but found no influence of early life family stress upon early menarche such as discussed above.[159] The correlation between mother and daughter should theoretically be equal to sister-sister ages of menarche if only genetic factors are operative, but because sistler-sister correlations are higher than mother daughter correlations, environmental influences must add to genetic factors.[160]

Evidence for the influence of genetics upon the age of menarche is found in study of twins: the concordance of the ages of pubertal developmental stages and menarche are closer between monozygotic than dizygotic twins.[161-165] Because monozygotic twins reared together have more similar ages of menarche than those reared apart and because dizygotic twins reared together were less similar than either points to environmental influences upon genetic factors. Some twin research suggests that additive genetic factors account for 96% of variance in the age of puberty in girls and 88% of the variance in boys (although other sources from the United States, Australia, Great Britain, Finland, and Norway find genetic effects accounting for between 50% and 80%) with the rest due to shared and nonshared environmental influences.[28,166-172]

Presently there remains a difference in the age of attainment of stages of puberty in different countries even if stability in socioeconomic factors are reached. For example, Japanese boys undergo changes in testicular size about 1 year earlier than Swiss boys reach the same stages.[173] Thus, when socioeconomic and environmental factors lead to good nutrition, general health, and infant care, the age of onset of puberty in normal children appears determined largely by genetic factors.[157]

Menarche occurs later in left-handed girls and menopause occurs earlier in left-handed women, suggesting a relationship between functional brain asymmetry and hypothalamic pituitary ovarian function.[174] Males with left handedness and early maturation appeared to associate with increased mathematical scores while, females with left handedness and late maturation were associated with significantly decreased mathematical scores.[175]

Certain genes are related to pubertal development. The CYP3A4 gene, which metabolizes testosterone, was associated with the age of puberty in girls,[176] the LEP gene (1875) leptin gene variant and maternal age at birth (age of mother >or <30 yrs) was additively associated with menarche,[177] and XbaI and PvuII polymorphisms of the estrogen receptor α gene are related to the age of menarche.[178] Homozygosity for the 5′-UTR variant of the cytochrome P450c17α (CYP17) gene, located on chromosome 10q24.3, which encodes the enzyme cytochrome P450c17α, is modestly correlated to the recalled age of menarche in adult women.[179]Girls with longer (>8) TAAAA repeats in their SHBG gene have later age of menarche than those with fewer repeats.[180,181] These and other factors are studied with animal models to determine influence of genes upon pubertal development.[182,183]

Health Effects of the Age of Menarche

Many but not all international studies show that earlier age at menarche is associated with a greater risk of development of breast cancer[184-186]: menarche at younger than 12 years increases the risk by about 50% compared with girls of menarche at 16 years,[187-189] and the risk of breast cancer decreases 9% while the risk for postmenopausal breast cancer decreases 4%.[190] Adolescents with higher BMI have a lower risk of premenopausal breast cancer although, in contrast, decreased BMI during early adulthood is more preventive of this condition.[191] In disease discordant monozygotic twins, the one with cancer recalled puberty to be earlier and in disease concordant twins, the one with earlier menarche had the earlier diagnosis of breast cancer.[192] Women with breast cancer were taller and leaner in childhood and increased height velocity at age 4 to 7 years and at age 11 to 15 years and higher BMI increased this risk. These variables were particularly significant in women with early menarche (menarche at age younger than 12.5 years).[193]

On the other hand, women who developed breast cancer did not reveal a relationship with recalled menarcheal age, although the women did recall body shape silhouette increases (more adipose tissue) at age 8, and increased body shape at menarche was related to breast cancer.[194] In a study of 117,415 Danish women, an increased risk of breast cancer occurred in those with high birth weight, increased height at 14 years of age, high BMI at 14 years of age, and early age at peak growth but no relationship to age of menarche.[195] Large size in childhood only minimally modified the increased risk of premenopausal breast cancer in women in study.[196]

Of 200 nine-year-old girls, those with increased CYP3A4 activity, which primarily metabolizes testosterone, showed a striking association with the onset of puberty, as noted above.[176] However, high-activity CYP17 alleles involved in estrogen formation and high-activity CYP1A2 and CYP1B1 alleles, whose gene products metabolize estradiol, were not associated with pubertal stage. Furthermore, CYP1B1, CYP3A4, and CYP3A5 variants were more common in African-American girls than in Hispanic or Caucasian girls, a distribution that reflects the more common occurrence of breast cancer in African-American women.

There is indirect evidence relating earlier menarche to increasing likelihood of hepatocellular carcinoma.[197] On the contrary, later age of menarche (after 14 years) is associated with an increased risk of glioma or non-Hodgkin's lymphoma.[198,199]

Evidence from the Fels longitudinal growth study of Caucasian girls revealed that girls with self-reported menarcheal age younger than 11.9 years (23% of the sample. This age may be classified as early) had adverse cardiovascular risk factors such as elevated blood pressure and glucose intolerance unrelated to body composition.[200]

Surveys of Army recruits, schoolchildren, and workers in Europe and America, as well as historical records of slaves in the United States, show that large portions of the population in the past 2 centuries continued to grow a considerable amount into their early 20s, whereas modern adolescents cease to grow and reach stable heights by about 17 years of age.[30,31] The adult heights attained during the eighteenth and nineteenth centuries were often at modern 25th percentiles or less. Comparison between the growth charts developed by the CDC in 1978 and 2001 shows no continued increase in height in children of all ages during this period (available at *http://www.cdc.gov/nchs/about/major/nhanes/growthcharts/clinical_charts.htm*). In Europe, however, a secular trend toward increasing adult height continues, although there is a dampening if not cessation of the secular trend in menarche in many areas showing how these phenomena are independent.[53] While ethnic-specific growth charts are available for some groups, usually all ethnic groups are plotted on the standard CDC growth chart CDC charts are found at http://www.cdc.gov/growthcharts/.[201]

PHYSICAL CHANGES OF PUBERTY

Secondary Sexual Characteristics

Tanner[32] developed objective standard description of the most useful signs of sexual maturation (Figs. 24–5 through 24–7) derived from photographs of 192 girls and 228 boys in a residential home in England. Of note is that they are not based upon direct physical examination and the lower socioeconomic status of the subjects may have implications for the generalization of the age of onset of puberty to children in optimal social situations.

Female

Two distinct phenomena occur in the female. The development of the breast and its modified apocrine glands[202,203] is primarily under the control of estrogens secreted by the ovaries (see Fig. 24–5); the growth of pubic and axillary hair (see Fig. 24–6) are mainly under the influence of androgens secreted by the adrenal

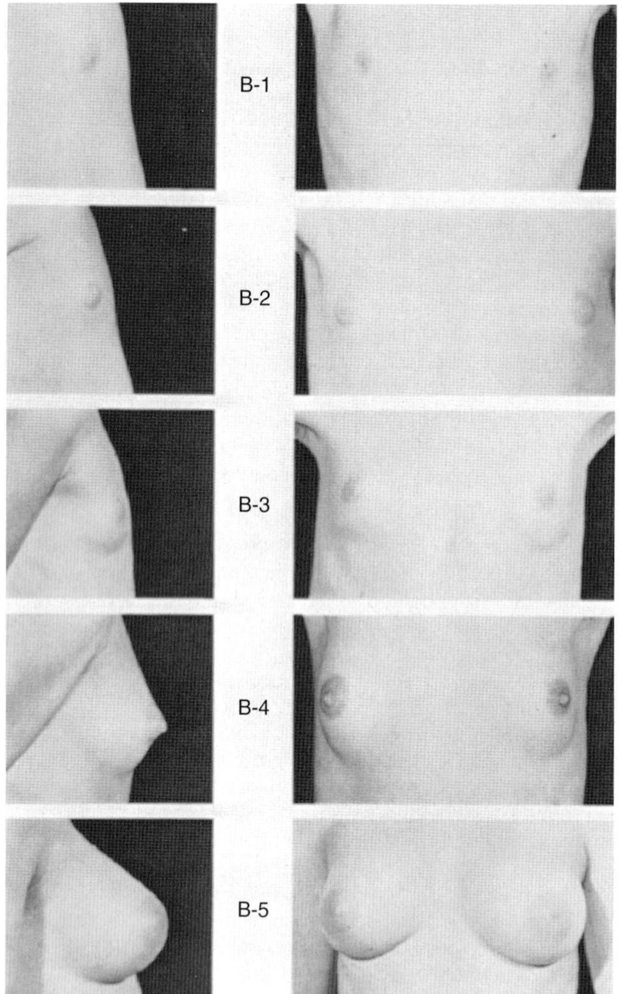

Figure 24–5 ▪ Stages of breast development according to Marshall and Tanner[2689] and Reynolds and Wines.[210] Stage 1: preadolescent; elevation of papilla only. Stage 2: breast bud stage; elevation of breast and papilla as a small mound, enlargement of areolar diameter. Stage 3: further enlargement of breast and areola with no separation of their contours. Stage 4: projection of areola and papilla to form a secondary mound above the level of the breast. Stage 5: mature stage; projection of papilla only, resulting from recession of the areola to the general contour of the breast. (Photographs from Van Wieringen JD, Wafelbakker F, Verbrugge HP, et al. Growth Diagrams 1965 Netherlands: Second National Survey on 0-24 Year Olds. Netherlands Institute for Preventative Medicine TNO. Groningen, Wolters-Noordhoff, 1971.)

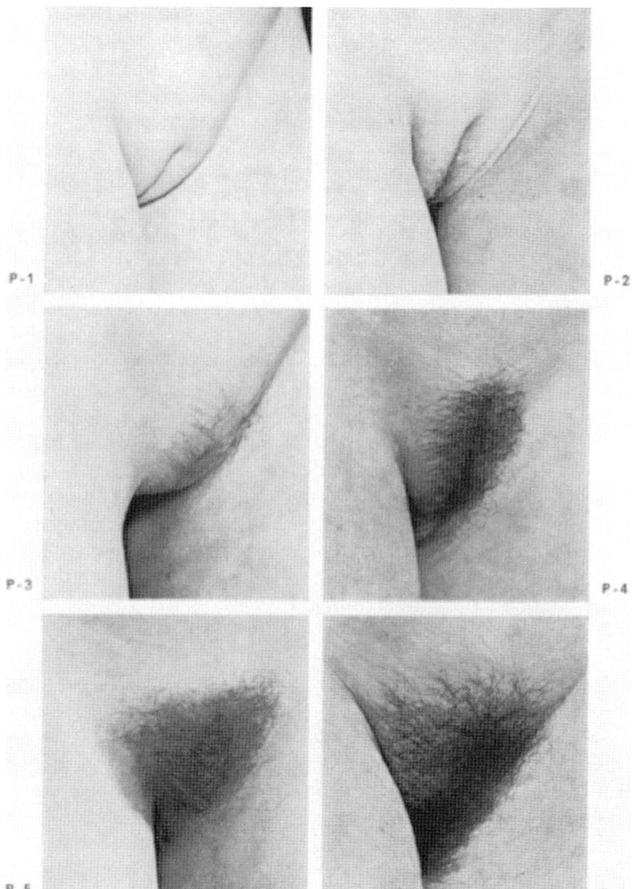

Figure 24–6 ▪ Stages of female pubic hair development, according to Marshall and Tanner,[2689] Reynolds and Wines,[210] and Dupertuis and colleagues.[2690] Stage 1: preadolescent; the vellus over the pubes is not further developed than that over the anterior abdominal wall; that is, there is no pubic hair. Stage 2: sparse growth of long, slightly pigmented, downy hair, straight or only slightly curled, appearing chiefly along the labia. This stage is difficult to see on photographs. Stage 3: hair is considerably darker, coarser, and curlier. The hair spreads sparsely over the junction of the pubic region. Stage 4: hair is now adult in type, but the area covered by it is still considerably smaller than in most adults. There is no spread to the medial surface of the thighs. Stage 5: hair is adult in quantity and type, distributed as an inverse triangle of the classical feminine pattern. The spread is to the medial surface of the thighs but not up the linea alba or elsewhere above the base of the inverse triangle. (Photographs from Van Wieringen JD, Wafelbakker F, Verbrugge HP, et al. Growth Diagrams 1965 Netherlands: Second National Survey on 0-24 Year Olds. Netherlands Institute for Preventative Medicine TNO. Groningen, Wolters-Noordhoff, 1971.)

cortex and the ovary. The glandular and connective tissue of the mammary gland begins to develop at the onset of pubertal maturation. Thus, lobules composed of small ductules and cellular connective tissue develop to a more pronounced degree in the female at puberty. Proliferation of fatty and connective tissue accounts for 80% of the volume of the adult, nonlactating female breast.[202] Breast cancer develops in rodents exposed to environmental estrogenic toxins (endocrine disruptors) that alter normal mammary development, and this same relationship is postulated to occur in girls exposed to endocrine-disrupting chemicals.[204-207] Aromatase is present in adipose tissue,[208] and it is theoretically possible that estrogen produced in chest adipose tissue might stimulate breast development at an earlier age, as seen in the aromatase excess syndrome.

The classification of the stages of breast development[209] depends on specific characteristics common to the female breast but does not include size or inherent shape of the breasts, which are determined by genetic and nutritional factors (see Fig. 24–5). Four stages were described by Stratz,[209] a fifth was added by Reynolds and Wines,[210] and modifications were made to the schema by Tanner,[32] who produced the most widely utilized staging. The initial breast development may be unilateral for several months and may be cause for unfounded concern by girls or parents; needless surgical biopsies are carried out for this normal variation. If concern about the exceptionally unlikely risk case of breast cancer during puberty arises, ultrasound evaluation is suggested due to the dense nature of the tissue at this stage.[211] Agenesis of the breast, inherited or sporadic, allows no glandular or fat enlargement regardless of the level of estrogen stimulation.[212] Virginal breast hypertrophy, extreme and rapid increase in breast size at the onset of puberty, is rare[213] but it is attributed, at least in part, to increased sensitivity to estrogen action,[214] or to increased local estrogen synthesis and growth factors. One family had this condition associated with anonychia.[215]

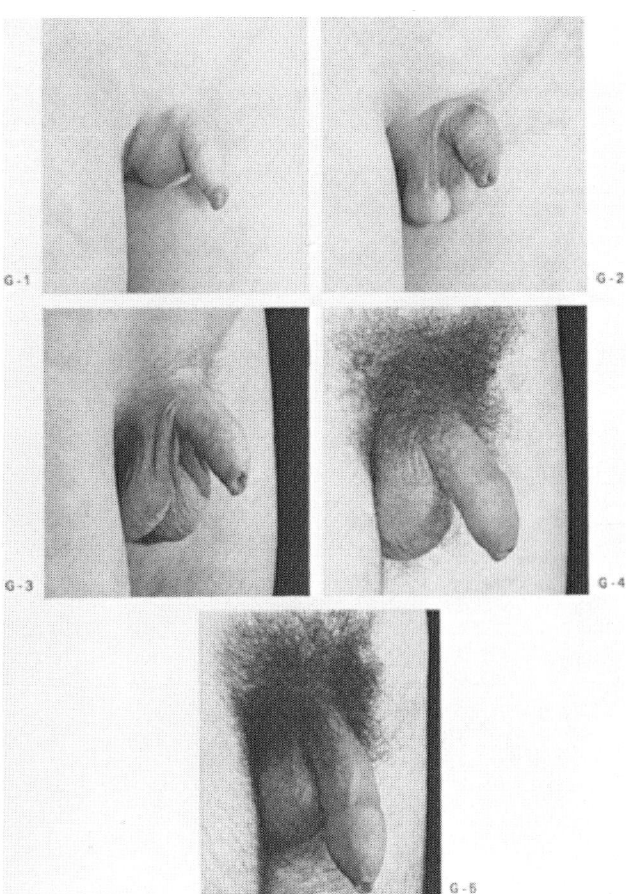

Figure 24–7 ▪ Stages of male genital development and pubic hair development, according to Marshall and Tanner,[2691] Reynolds and Wines,[236] and Dupertuis and colleagues.[2690] *Genital development:* Stage 1: preadolescent. Testes, scrotum, and penis are about the same size and proportion as in early childhood. Stage 2: the scrotum and testes have enlarged; the scrotal skin shows a change in texture and also some reddening. Stage 3: growth of the penis has occurred, at first mainly in length but with some increase in breadth; there is further growth of the testes and scrotum. Stage 4: the penis is further enlarged in length and breadth with development of the glans. The testes and scrotum are further enlarged. The scrotal skin has further darkened. Stage 5: genitalia are adult in size and shape. No further enlargement takes place after stage 5 is reached. *Pubic hair development:* Stage 1: preadolescent; the vellus over the pubic region is not further developed than that over the abdominal wall; that is, there is no pubic hair. Stage 2: sparse growth of long, slightly pigmented, downy hair, straight or slightly curled, appearing chiefly at the base of the penis. Stage 3: hair is considerably darker, coarser, and curlier and spreads sparsely over the junction of the pubes. Stage 4: hair is now adult in type, but the area it covers is still considerably smaller than in most adults. There is no spread to the medial surface of the thighs. Stage 5: hair is adult in quantity and type, distributed as an inverse triangle. The spread is to the medial surface of the thighs but not up the linea alba or elsewhere above the base of the inverse triangle. Most men will have further spread of the pubic hair. (Photographs from Van Wieringen JD, Wafelbakker F, Verbrugge HP, et al. Growth Diagrams 1965 Netherlands: Second National Survey on 0-24 Year Olds. Netherlands Institute for Preventative Medicine TNO. Groningen, Wolters-Noordhoff, 1971.)

TABLE 24–2 REPORTED MEAN AGES (YEARS) AT ONSET OF SEXUAL MATURITY STAGES IN FEMALES

Study	Longitudinal or Cross-sectional	No. of Subjects	Age Range	BREAST STAGES				PUBIC HAIR STAGES					
				B2	B3	B4	B5	PH2	PH3	PH4	PH5	PHV	Menarche
Marshall and Tanner (1969),[2689] United Kingdom	L	192	8-18	11.1	12.1	13.1	15.3	—	12.4	12.9	14.4	12.1	13.5
Billewicz et al. (1981),[2692] United Kingdom	L	753	9-17	10.8	12.0	13.1	14.0	—	—	—	—		
Roy et al. (1972),[2693] France	L	80	7-15	11.4	12.5	13.4	—	11.3	12.4	13.2	—	12	13
Taranger (1976),[2694] Sweden	L	90	8-17	11.0	11.8	13.1	15.6	11.5	12.0	12.9	15.2		
Largo and Prader (1983),[321] Switzerland	L	142	8-18	10.9	12.2	13.2	14.0	10.4	12.2	13.0	14.0	12.2	13.4
Van Wieringen et al. (1971),[2695] Holland				11.0	12.1	13.4	15.2	11.3	12.2	13.3	14.9		
Neyzi et al. (1975),[2696] Turkey	C	1,468	9-17	10.0	11.6	12.8	15.2	10.8	11.6	12.3	13.6		
Villarreal et al. (1989),[2697] Mexican-American	C	699	10-17	10.9	12.2	13.9	15.1	11.2	12.4	14.1	15.5		
Roche et al. (1995),[237] United States (Ohio)	L	67	9.5-16	11.2	12.0	12.4	—	11	11.8	12.4	13.1		
Herman-Giddens (1997),[56] United States	C	17,077	3-12										
African-American		1,638		8.9	10.2	—	—	8.8	10.4				
White		15,439		10.0	11.3	—	—	10.5	11.5				

Changes in the diameter of the papilla of the nipple are sequential and linked to stages of pubertal development. Nipple papilla diameter does not increase much during pubic hair stage 1 to 3 or breast stage 1 to 3 (diameter is 3 to 4 mm) but does increase after breast stage 3, providing an objective method of differentiating stage 4 from 5 (final diameter is approximately 9 mm) (Table 24–2).[216,217]

The stage of breast development usually progresses along with the stage of pubic hair development in normal girls, but as different endocrine organs control these two processes and these organs mature at different ages, and discordance can occur in disease states, their stages should be classified separately for greatest accuracy (Tables 24–3 and 24–4 and Fig. 24–8). Where thelarche occurs first the age of menarche

TABLE 24–3 DESCRIPTIVE STATISTICS FOR THE TIMING OF SEXUAL MATURITY STAGES IN FEMALES

BREAST STAGES				
	ONSET OF STAGE		MEAN AGE FOR STAGE	
Stage	**Mean**	**SD**	**Mean**	**SD**
Stage 2				
Roche et al. (Ohio)[237]	11.2	0.7	11.3	1.1
Herman-Giddens et al. (USA)[56]				
African-American	8.9	1.9		
White	10.0	1.8		
Stage 3				
Roche et al. (Ohio)[237]	12.0	1.0	12.5	1.5
Herman-Giddens et al. (USA)[56]				
African-American	10.2	1.4		
White	11.3	1.4		
Stage 4				
Roche et al. (Ohio)[237]	12.4	0.9		
TANNER PUBIC HAIR				
Tanner Stage 2				
Roche et al. (Ohio)[237]	11.0	0.5		
Herman-Giddens et al. (USA)[56]				
African-American	8.8	2.0		
White	10.5	1.7		
Tanner Stage 3				
Roche et al. (Ohio)[237]	11.8	1.0		
Herman-Giddens et al. (USA)[56]				
African-American	10.4	1.6		
White	11.5	1.2		
Tanner Stage 4				
Roche et al. (Ohio)[237]	12.4	0.8		
MENARCHE				
Herman-Giddens et al. (USA)				
African-American	12.2	1.2		
White	12.9	1.2		
Percent Menstruating	*At Age 11*		*At Age 12*	
African-American	27.9%*		62.1%	
White	13.4%*		35.2%	
Onset Axillary Hair (Stage 2)				
African-American	10.1 ± 2.0			
White	11.8 ± 1.9			

*African-American girls enter puberty approximately 1 to 1½ years earlier than white girls and begin menses 8½ months earlier.

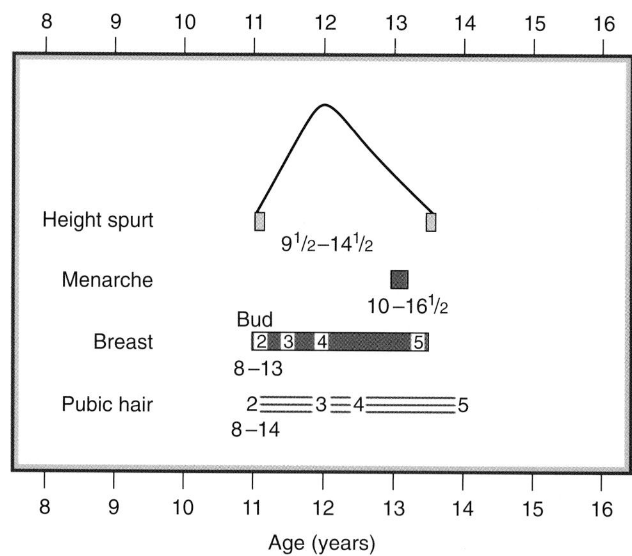

Figure 24–8 ▪ The sequence of events at puberty in females. The design of the figure is described in the legend of Figure 24–9. (From Marshall WA, Tanner JM. Variations in pattern of pubertal changes in girls. Arch Dis Child 1969;44:291-303.)

reportedly is earlier while if adrenarche occurs first, menarche is later. Pubertal maturation in girls and the relationship to anthropometric changes: pathways through puberty. HYPERLINK "http://www.ncbi.nlm.nih.gov/sites/entrez?Db=pubmed&Cmd=ShowDetailView&TermToSearch=12838192&ordinalpos=1&itool=EntrezSystem2.PEntrez.Pubmed.Pubmed_ResultsPanel.Pubmed_RVDocSum"Biro FM, Lucky AW, Simbartl LA, Barton BA, Daniels SR, Striegel-Moore R, Kronsberg SS, Morrison JA. J Pediatr. 2003 Jun;142(6):643-6.

Increase in height velocity (rather than breast development) is the first sign of puberty in girls, although breast budding is what is first noted by most lay or medical observers.

Dulling and thickening of the vaginal mucosa from the prepubertal reddish glistening appearance occur due to the cornification of the lining cells and the secretion of clear or whitish discharge increases in the months before menarche as a result of estrogen action.[218] Girls may notice yellowish or whitish discharge on their underwear at this stage. The vaginal pH decreases as menarche approaches due to the increase of lactic acid produced by lactobacilli in the vaginal flora. The length of the vagina increases from about 8 cm at onset of puberty to 11 cm at menarche. Thickening, protrusion, and rugation of the labia majora and minora occur. Fat is deposited in the area of the mons pubis, and the labia majora becomes wrinkled in appearance. Occasionally, the labia minora may enlarge on one or both sides enough to suggest a tumor. This childhood asymmetric labium majus enlargement has recently been characterized and suggested to be a disorder of prepuberty or early puberty.[219] The clitoris enlarges slightly, and the urethral opening becomes more prominent. Photographic atlases of normal female prepubertal genitalia are available and include standards for the variation in appearance of the hymenal opening; this information is invaluable in the examination of a victim of suspected child abuse.[220]

Male

The growth and maturation of the penis usually correlates closely with pubic hair development, because both features are under androgen control, but for the most accurate assessment, the stages of pubic hair development and genital development should be determined independently and recorded separately; in this way, discordant stages are a clue to potential disease states of the adrenal gland or testes (Fig. 24–9 and see Fig. 24–7) (Tables 24–5, 24–6 and 24–7).

Growth of the testes is usually the first sign of puberty in the male, and it begins approximately 6 months after the average age of initiation of breast development in girls. Pubertal testicular enlargement is indicated when the longitudinal measurement of a testis is greater than 2.5 cm (excluding the epididymis), or the volume is greater than 4 mL. The testicular volume index ([length×width of right testis+length×width of left testis]/2) and testicular volume, measured by comparing the testes with ellipsoids of known volume, correlate with the stages of puberty (Table 24–7).[221,222] A longitudinal study supports the utility of adding a stage 2a when testicular volume is 3 mL; further pubertal progression occurred within 6 months in 82% of boys who

TABLE 24–4 COMPARISON OF MENARCHEAL AGES REPORTED BY VARIOUS STUDIES

AGE OR MENARCHE (yr)					Ages (yr):				
Sample	**Year Studied**	**Plan**	**Evaluation**	**n**	**Overall**	**White**	**A-A**	**M-A**	**Comments**
Britain	1969	Long	Probit	192 a		13.5			
NHANES III	1963-1970	Cross	Recalled	3272	born 1940-1960	12.8			
					born 1890-1910	13.5			
							12.52		
NHANES III	1988-1994	Cross	Yes/No	330 a		12.7			Menarcheal age black<white
			Probit	419 b			12.3		
				419 c				12.5	
NHANES III	1988-1994	Cross	Yes/No	2510	12.43				Menarcheal age black<white
			Probit	710 a		12.6			
				917 b			12.06		
				883 c				12.3	
PROS	1992-1993	Cross	Status Quo-Probit	17077 a		12.9			Menarcheal age black<white
				1638 b			12.16		
NHLB Growth	1987-1997	Long	Recalled	1092 a		12.7			Menarcheal age black<white
				1164 b			12.1		BMI inversely proportional to menarcheal age
Bogalusa	1973-1974	Cross		5552		12.7			
							12.9		
	1992-1994	Cross				12.5			
							12.1		
	1973-1994	Long		2508					Menarcheal age black<white
						12.6			BMI inversely proportional to menarcheal age
							12.3		
NHES	1963-1970	Status Quo	Yes/No-Status Quo	3272	12.75				
						12.8			
							12.48		
	1988-1994	Status Quo	Median Yes/No	1414	12.54				Age of menarche NHANES III< NHES
						12.6			Growing difference in menarcheal age white-black
							12.14		BMI inversely proportional to age of menarche

Where the *n* of individual populations is stated, *a* represents white, *b* African American, and *c* Mexican American.
A-A, African American; *M-A,* Mexican American; *Cross,* cross sectional; *Long,* longitudinal.
From Styne DM. Puberty, obesity and ethnicity. Trends Endocrinol Metab 2004;15(10):472-478.

had reached this 3-mL phase (Table 24–8).[223] The most significant changes in serum testosterone and calculated free testosterone occur at the transition of testicular volume between 1 to 2, 2 to 3, 6 to 8, and 10 to 15 mL, suggesting the denotation of stages pre1 (testis, 1 mL), pre2 (testis, 2 mL), early (testis, 3 to 6 mL), mid (testis, 8 to 12 mL), late1 (testis, 15 to 25 mL, the boy has not reached final height), and late2 (testis, 15 to 25 mL, the boy has reached final height).[224] The right testis is normally larger than the left, and the left testis is located lower in the scrotum than the right testis.

The phallus should be measured stretched while in the flaccid state, because there is much variation between individuals in the length of the unstretched penis. The length of the erectile tissue (excluding the foreskin) increases from an average of 6.2 cm in the prepubertal state to 12.4±2.7 cm in the Caucasian adult. Ethnic differences have been noted; the mean value in African-American men is 14.6 cm and in Asians, 10.6 cm.[225]

As in girls, the areolar diameter increases in boys during puberty with a distinct separation between the sexes occurring

TABLE 24–5 REPORTED MEAN AGES (YEARS) AT ONSET OF SEXUAL MATURITY STAGES IN MALES

Study	Longitudinal or Cross-sectional	No. of Subjects	Age Range	GENITAL STAGES				PUBIC HAIR STAGES			
				G2	G3	G4	G5	PH2	PH3	PH4	PH5
Marshall and Tanner (1970),[2691] United Kingdom	L/C			11.6	12.9	13.8	14.19	—	13.9	14.4	15.2
Roy (1972), France[2693]	L			12.0	13.1	14.3	—	12.4	13.4	14.3	—
Taranger (1976),[2694] Sweden	L	122	9-17	12.2	13.1	13.9	15.1	12.5	13.4	14.1	15.5
Largo and Prader (1983),[2698] Switzerland	L	142	8-18	11.2	12.9	13.8	14.7	12.2	13.5	14.2	14.9
Van Wieringen et al. (1971),[2695] Holland				11.3	13.1	14.0	15.3	11.7	13.1	14	15.0
Neyzi et al. (1975),[2699] Turkey	C	1530	9-17	—	—	—	—	12.3	13.8	16.1	—
Villarreal et al. (1989), Mexican-American	C	704	10-17	12.4	13.5	14.6	16.3	12.8	13.6	14.6	16.1
Roche et al. (1995),[237] United States (Ohio)	L	78	9.5-16	11.2	12.1	13.5	14.3	11.2	12.1	13.4	14.3

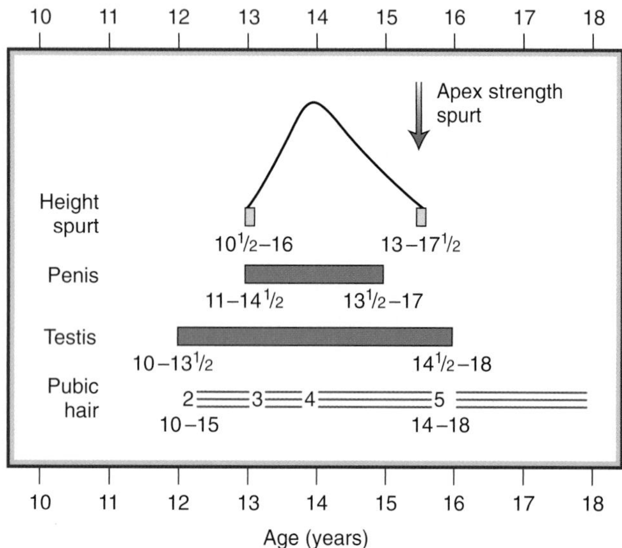

Figure 24–9 ▪ Diagram of the sequence of events at puberty in males. An average is represented in relation to the scale of ages; the range of ages within which some of the changes occur is indicated by the numbers below. (From Marshall WA, Tanner JM. Variations in the pattern of pubertal changes in boys. Arch Dis Child 1970;45:13-23.)

in stage 4 when female areolar diameter increases much more than male values.[226] In gynecomastia, the areolar diameter increases above normal.

Limits of Normal Pubertal Development in the United States

Guidelines for the normal variation in pubertal development in the United States are controversial in girls. Physical examination with palpation of testes in boys or breasts in girls by trained observers is the most accurate method of assessment of pubertal development, but limited numbers of trained personnel and subjects' refusal of embarrassing examinations lead to the use of proxy measures. Detection of the onset of stage 2 breast development in an overweight girl may be difficult even for a trained observer (although assessment of stage 3 is generally obvious). This may lead to a specious decrease of the reported age of onset of thelarche.

Visual observation of the stage of development in person (not by photographs) is one step removed from physical examination and palpation; errors in the evaluation of breast tissue in obese girls or the stage of testicular enlargement in boys may occur. Visual observation by multiple rather than limited numbers of observers is utilized in the NHANES III (National Health and Nutrition Examination Survey III 1988-1994) and the NHES (National Health Examination Survey) that occurred more than 20 years earlier. A study from PROS (Pediatric Research in Office Setting), a network fostered by the American Academy of Pediatrics, utilized specially trained pediatricians, nurse practitioners, or physician assistants who used visual inspection in all and palpation in 30% of the study population. To improve accuracy, all observers had to pass a practical test to verify competency in pubertal assessment.[56]

Photographs or drawings of pubertal development allow self-reporting or parental reporting of pubertal progress to avoid the embarrassment of a secondary sexual examination in normal children and adolescents[227,228]; correlations of self ratings with physical examiners range widely from 0.48 to 0.91,[28,229] compared with physicians' examinations or visual observation of the subject. Unfortunately, the answers to self-assessment may be influenced by the subject's views of what is considered normal or by wishes to confirm with normal development.[230-232] Answers may be less accurate in some ethnic groups than others,[233] and obese girls may overestimate breast developmental stage while boys may overestimate pubic hair development.[234] Physical examination by a trained observer remains the "gold standard" for staging pubertal development.

The U.S. Health Examination Survey began with subjects of 12 years of age and, although useful in defining the upper limits of normal pubertal development, the survey is uninformative about the lower limits of the age of onset of puberty.[55,57,235] The results of this study, with extrapolation, added to earlier studies set the lower range of normal puberty to 8 years in girls and in boys to 9 years.[210,236] A more recent longitudinal study (see Table 24–6) of Caucasian boys and girls started at 9.5 years of age and adds much to the determination of the mean age of attainment of stages of puberty[237]; however, it starts too late to include those normal children entering puberty at an earlier age (Table 24–6). Two studies utilized data from the NHANES III: one[83] found mean onset of stage 2 breast development for African-Americans, Mexican-Americans, and whites was 9.5 years, 9.8 years, and 10.3 years, respectively, and for stage 2 pubic hair was 9.5 years, 10.3 years, and 10.5 years, respectively, using a sample of 1623 girls, whereas the other study[238] found the ages for onset of stage 2 breast development was 9.5 years for African-

TABLE 24–6 DESCRIPTIVE STATISTICS FOR THE TIMING OF SEXUAL MATURITY STAGES IN WHITE MALES (OHIO)[97]

GENITAL STAGES				
	ONSET OF STAGE		MEAN AGE FOR STAGE	
Stage	Mean	SD	Mean	SD
2	11.2	0.7	11.3	1.0
3	12.1	0.8	12.6	1.0
4	13.5	0.7	14.5	1.1
5	14.3	1.1	—	—
PUBIC HAIR STAGES				
	ONSET OF STAGE		MEAN AGE FOR STAGE	
Stage	Mean	SD	Mean	SD
2	11.2	0.8	11.3	0.9
3	12.1	1.0	12.4	1.0
4	13.4	0.9	13.7	0.9
5	14.3	0.8	14.8	1.0
6	15.3	0.8	—	—

TABLE 24–7 CORRELATION OF TESTICULAR VOLUME WITH STAGE OF PUBERTAL DEVELOPMENT

Parameter	PUBERTAL STAGE				
	1	2	3	4	5
TV*	1.8	4.5	8.2	10.5	—
Volume (cm^3)†	2.5	3.4	9.1	11.8	14
Volume (cm^3)‡	1.8	4.2	10	11	15
Volume (cm^3)§	1.8	5.0	9.5	12.5	17

*Testicular volume index calculatd by (length × width of right testis + length × width of left testis) ÷ 2. Data from Burr et al. and August et al.

†Volume estimated by comparison with ellipsoid of known volume (orchidometer) that is equal to or smaller than the testes. Data from Zachmann et al.

‡Volume by comparison with orchidometer. Data from Waaler et al.

§Measurement with calipers and average volume of both testes calculated by 0.52 × longitudinal axis × transverse axis. Data from Waaler et al.

TABLE 24–8 MEAN VALUES OF AGE, HEIGHT, WEIGHT, BODY MASS INDEX, AND SERUM HORMONE LEVELS BY PUBERTAL STAGE IN 515 (OHIO) BOYS (237 AFRICAN-AMERICAN, 278 WHITE; AGE 10-15 YR AT INTAKE) FOLLOWED EVERY 6 MONTHS FOR 3 YEARS

Variable	PUBERTAL STAGE					
	PS1†	PS2a	PS2b	PS3	PS4	PS5
Age (yr)	11.44*	12.18*	12.79*	13.74*	14.63*	15.19*
Height (cm)	144.2*	149.8*	154.6*	162.3*	169.9*	173.3*
Weight (kg)	38.18*	41.65*	47.27*	54.67*	61.11*	66.88*
Body mass index (kg/m^2)	18.1*	18.4*	19.5*	20.6*	21.0*	22.2*
Testosterone: nmol/L (ng/dL)						
Black subjects	0.8 (23)*	3.0 (86)*	4.9 (141)*	11.5 (331)*	13.4 (338)*	15.5 (449)*
White subjects	0.6 (16)*	2.9 (83)*	4.6 (132)*	9.7 (281)*	13.3 (383)*	14.6 (422)*
Free testosterone: pmol/L (ng/dL)	11 (0.33)*	60 (1.74)*	114 (3.28)*	294 (8.49)*	413 (11.9)*	504 (14.5)*
DHEAS: μmol/L (μg/dL)	2.71 (99.7)*	3.31 (121.8)*	4.04 (148.7)*	4.75 (175.0)*	5.08 (187.0)*	5.89 (217.0)*
TeBG (nmol/L)	34.6	33.3	28.4*	21.5*	14.4*	10.7*

*Duncan post-hoc analysis significant at $P < .01$.

†PS1, absence of pubic hair, testicular volume <3 mL; PS2a, absence of pubic hair, testicular volume ≥3 mL; PS2b, Tanner stage 2 pubic hair; PS3-5, Tanner pubic hair stages.

DHEAS, Dehydroepiandrosterone sulfate; *TeBG*, testosterone-binding globulin.

Modified from Biro FM, Lucky AW, Hoster GA, et al. Pubertal staging in boys. J Pediatr 1995;127:40-46.

American, 9.8 years for Mexican-American, and 10.4 years for white girls, while the onset of stage 2 pubic hair was 10.4 years for white, 9.4 years for African-American, and 10.6 years for Mexican-American girls in a sample of 2145 girls (see Tables 24–1 through 4).

The PROS cross-sectional study sponsored by the American Academy of Pediatrics of a convenience sample of 17,070 girls visiting the office of 225 specially trained pediatricians across the United States started at 3 years of age but ended at 12 years of age and so excludes a proportion of normal children who enter puberty at a later age.[56] However, the authors point out that the probit statistical method can be used to estimate events from which only a portion of the population has achieved the event.[239] The standard deviation of the longitudinal study[237] was low, 1.0 years or less in most cases, while the cross-sectional study had a larger standard deviation of approximately 2 years.[56] This may be due to the difference in the study design, but it may reflect a limit in the spread of the upper end of the normal pubertal curve (rarely does even the subject with the most severe constitutional delay spontaneously enter puberty after 18 years of age) where there may be a skewing of the normal age of onset of puberty to an earlier spread of ages.

The latest and largest multiracial and ethnic study of the age of onset of puberty in 2114 American boys ages 8 through 19 years suggests a decrease has occurred over the last decades, but the observations are controversial,[82] as is the report of the data in girls presented above. Using the NHANES (National Health and Nutrition Examination) III database, the authors determined that the onset of pubic hair occurs earlier in African-American boys than in Caucasian boys with a tendency to later onset in Mexican-American boys. Between the ages of 8 and 9 years, no Caucasian boys had pubic hair, whereas 5.3% of African-American boys were at least at Tanner stage 2.[82] The age of genital development was based upon the visual change in scrotal skin and enlargement of the testes (an unsatisfactory method of assessing the size of the testes compared to direct examination); by the beginning of age 8, the earliest age studied, 29.35% of Caucasian boys, 37.8% of African-American boys, and 27.3% of Mexican-American boys purportedly had genital development. Furthermore, the height and weight of boys reaching the earlier stages of puberty was greater than reported in the past, although the adult heights and weight were equivalent to past data. However, a number of aspects of this study have been questioned.[240] For example, the observers for NHANES III did not measure testicular volume, an important factor in the assessment of pubertal development, and a one-stage variance was allowed between the observers' findings and the quality control, a variance that is quite significant between stage 1 and 2 of pubertal development in boys as this defines the very onset of puberty. Thus, just as there is difficulty in determining the difference between stage 1 and 2 of breast development, there is substantial difficulty in determining the difference between stage 1 and 2 of genital development without a direct assessment of testicular size. These observations are being further investigated by a new PROS project studying pubertal development in boys. If confirmed that there is an earlier onset of puberty in a substantial number of boys below the previously accepted lower age limit of 9 years, the guidelines for normal pubertal development in boys will have to be revised downward from 9 years.

Obesity is found in hypogonadal boys and in those who carry the diagnosis of Froelich's syndrome (adiposodysgenesis, originally described in a patient with tuberculosis involving the hypothalamic pituitary axis), a term, now rarely used, which combines findings of obesity and hypogonadism due to a hypothalamic-pituitary disorder. Characteristically it is considered that obese boys enter puberty early but there are reports that obesity is associated with delayed puberty rather than early puberty.[241]

The PROS study led to the conclusion that puberty in girls begins earlier in the United States than was the case 3 to 4 decades ago but there is no comparably large study starting early enough upon which to base this conclusion in past decades. Thus, a secular trend toward earlier puberty in girls cannot be supported from this data set alone.[242,243] The most recent comprehensive evaluation compared data available from US HES (3042 white boys, 478 African-American boys, 2065 white girls, and 505 African-American girls studied from 1966 to 1970), from Hispanic Health and Nutrition Examination Survey (HHANES: 717 Mexican-American boys, 512 Mexican-American girls from 1982 to 1984), and from NHANES III (259 white boys, 411 African-American boys, 291 white girls, 415 African-American girls, 576 Mexican-American boys, and 512 Mexican-American girls from 1988 to 1994).[244] The analysis showed no strong evidence of a secular trend toward earlier puberty between 1966 and 1994 in non-Hispanic black boys and non-Hispanic black and white girls, although there is some evidence of earlier puberty in non-Hispanic white boys between 1966 and 1994 and in Mexican-American boys and girls between 1982 and 1994.[238,242] There remains controversy in the literature as to whether puberty is starting earlier in the present era based upon various large studies, but if puberty can not definitely be proved to start earlier as yet, if the obesity epidemic continues, puberty will be earlier in the future.

The length of pubertal development relates to the age of onset of puberty in some studies. Spanish investigators demonstrated that the earlier normal girls entered puberty, the longer the duration of puberty before menarche.[245-247] Thus, girls who started puberty at 9, 10, 11, 12, and 13 years of age, experienced menarche 2.77, 2.27, 1.78, 1.44, and 0.65 years later, respectively, demonstrating a normalizing trend that keeps the age of menarche relatively stable in the group as a whole in one of these studies.[245] This is in contrast to a suggestion of a decrease in the time to transit puberty from start to end in Dutch and Swedish boys and girls (reported in reference 42).

In summary, there appears to be no consistently supported significant change in the age of puberty in the United States based upon limited data, which are so often collected in differing ways such that comparison is flawed. It is clear that the African-American girls develop before white girls regardless of socioeconomic issues. There is evidence, but not proof, that rising BMI in childhood is associated with earlier pubertal maturation, which may partly account for the increasing difference in ages between these ethnic groups (it is proven that early puberty is associated with elevated BMI in later life) if it is true that increasing BMI leads to early puberty rather than the other way around. Thus, if the population continues to progress to ever increasing BMI values and if obesity does indeed lead to earlier puberty rather than vice versa, an irrefutable decrease in the age of puberty in the overall population of girls may be realized in the future. Clearly the United States is lacking a comprehensive, large, longitudinal study based on direct physical examination rather than observation that would start early enough to include the youngest normal pubertal subjects and last long enough to include the oldest. Such a study must be balanced as to ethnic groups and the planners must use the predicted increase of certain ethnic populations in the United States so that in a few decades we do not conclude that we did not study enough of one or another ethnic group in the early 2000s. In fact, we are in just that unfortunate position as we look back from the present and try to draw conclusions about a secular trend.[242]

International data are available for the age of pubertal stages collected in cross-sectional and longitudinal studies (see Tables 24–3 and 24–5). The results show similarities to United States data in boys, but the data differ for girls.

We can combine the studies above to establish reasonable clinical guidelines for the limits of normal puberty. The mean age for a Caucasian boy to reach genital stage 2 or pubic hair stage 2 in the longitudinal study is 11.2 years with a standard deviation of 0.7 years: (±2.5 standard deviations ranges from 8.9 to 13.3 and may be simplified by saying the mean age of onset of puberty in boys is 11 years with the limits of ±2.5 SD at 9 to 14 years of age using the longitudinal data and some of the cross sectioal data.[237] For the rest of this chapter we will use the ages of 9 and 14 years as the lower and upper bounds of puberty in boys, although it is quite possible that some normal boys, especially African-American boys, enter puberty or adrenarche between 8 and 9 years of age.

In the evaluation of girls, it may be difficult for the physician to detect the onset of stage 2 breast development during an office visit while assessment of stage 3 is generally obvious. Using the longitudinal data of a mean age of 11.2 and a standard deviation of 0.7 year, the normal range is defined as 8.9 to 13.3 years. This correlates well with the U.S. Health Examination Survey of 1977.[57] Using the large number of Caucasian and African-American girls in the cross-sectional PROS study[56] and using the average ages of stage 2 and stage 3 from that study, the mean age of breast development for Caucasian girls is 10.6 years with 2.5 standard deviations encompassing 6.7 to 14.5

years. However, in the cross-sectional study, 3.0% of Caucasian girls had stage 2 breast development by 6 years and 5.0% by 7 years, whereas 6.4% of African-Americans had stage 2 breast development by 6 years and 15.4% by 7 years. African-American girls have an earlier onset of pubertal development of about 1 year, even though their average age of menarche in the cross-sectional study was only 8½ months different (12.2 years for African-Americans and 12.9 for Caucasians). We may combine these findings and set the mean at 10.6 years for Caucasian girls and the range between 7 and 13 years and accept 8.9 years as the mean age for African-American girls with the range of normal from 6 to 13 years.

These data provide guidelines for choosing which candidates with early onset of puberty are candidates for expensive diagnostic tests and for consideration of long-term therapy, because many of the children who appeared to have mild sexual precocity in years past may now may be considered to represent normal variation. It would be inappropriate to extensively study all normal girls found just below these lower limits of normal. We emphasize that family history, the rapidity of development of secondary sex characteristics, the rate of growth, and the presence or absence of central nervous system (CNS) or other types of disease must enter into the decision of whether to evaluate a child. As we have recommended in the previous editions, the Drug and Therapeutics and Executive Committees of the Lawson Wilkins Pediatric Endocrine Society supports such a revision of the lower limits of the normal age of onset of puberty to age 7 in white girls and age 6 in African-American girls with no changes in the current guidelines for evaluating boys, as before, as evaluation is still suggested for those with signs of puberty younger than 9 years for evalulation.[248]

Several studies present the likelihood of missing serious endocrine disorders if these new guidelines are followed. One study of 223 girls between 6 and 8 years of age at one center referred for diagnoses associated with precocious puberty found 12.3% having diagnosable endocrine disease such as congenital adrenal hyperplasia or neurofibromatosis rather than simply a normal variation of pubertal development that would have been missed by the age criteria alone. (Midyett, 2003; 111(1):47-51.) However, the age criteria are meant for subjects that have a normal pattern of pubertal development without any sign of chronic disease or other manifestations. Those patients who veer from these basic rules would have been evaluated because they violate the prime criteria of normal clinical presentation. Another center reported that out of 107 patients referred for evaluation of precocious puberty, only 9% could be classified as truly having precious puberty and some of those were only mildly affected and did not need intervention; thus, only 4% of the entire group required therapy.[249] Another study found that of 453 children referred for precocious puberty, 34% had idiopathic central precocious puberty with some between the ages of 7 and 8 years (and most presumably being Caucasian although these details were not presented).[250] These authors cautioned continued surveillance of those with early puberty, advice that we fully support. With all of these studies it may be inferred that if the examining physician looks for signs and symptoms of disease rather than just relying on the age criteria, somewhat less than 10% of true precious puberty will be missed and of those, some cases, and probably many, will be so mild as to not need intervention and may represent variations of normal.

A multinational study from Europe suggests that valid indications for a CNS magnetic resonance imaging (MRI) scan in the diagnosis of precocious puberty are (1) an age of onset of puberty in girls before 6 years (certainly in agreement with our recommendations) or (2) an estradiol value over the 45th percentile for girls with central precocious puberty according to the standards of the laboratory performing the study, which is an additional new criteria.[251] Even though estradiol values vary over a 24-hour period, those girls with a substantial increase most likely would have substantial pubertal progression and would awaken clinical concern of a diagnosis other than normal variation. Further problems with specificity and sensitivity of methods predating LC/MS-MS (liquid chromatography tandem mass spectrometry) techniques (read below) raise further concern about interpretation of estrogen values in children. This guideline may best be retested after invoking LC/MS-MS techniques.

Other Dimorphic Physical Changes of Puberty

The larynx and vocal folds are targets of endocrine changes in boys and girls.[252] In boys, both the membranous and cartilaginous components of the vocal cords lengthen during puberty. In the peripubertal period, the length of the vocal cords in both boys and girls is about 12 to 15 mm, of which the membranous portion is 7 to 8 mm. In adult men, the vocal cords attain a length of 18 to 23 mm (membranous portion 12 to 16 mm), whereas in women the cords enlarge only slightly (13 to 18 mm). In the castrati whose vocal brilliance had a great influence on the lyrical Italian operas of past centuries, the membranous component of the vocal cords was the same length as in prepubertal boys and even shorter than in women.[253] During puberty, the male larynx, cricothyroid cartilage, and laryngeal muscles enlarge. The relatively largest change in singing and speaking frequencies occur between Tanner genital stage 3 and 4,[254,255] breaking of the voice occurs at approximately 13 years, and the adult voice is achieved by about 15 years.[256] The singing voice changes after the deepening of the speaking voice by one octave.[257]

Facial hair in boys is first apparent on the corners of the upper lip and the upper cheeks; it then spreads to the midline of the lower lip and finally to the sides and the lower border of the chin. The first stage of facial hair development usually occurs during pubic hair stage 3 (average age of 14.9 in the United States), and the last stage occurs after pubic hair stage 5 and genital stage 5.

Axillary hair appears at approximately 14 years in boys. Ninety-three percent of African-American girls have axillary hair by age 12, in contrast to 68% of white girls.[56] Axillary sweat glands begin to function as the hair appears. The appearance of circumanal hair slightly precedes that of axillary hair in boys.

Comedones, acne, and seborrhea of the scalp appear as a result of the increased secretion of gonadal and adrenal sex steroids.[258-260] Early onset acne correlates with the development of severe acne later in puberty. The most serious variety, acne fulminans, occurs mainly in pubertal males.[261] Acne vulgaris, the most prevalent skin disorder in adolescence, appears at a mean age of 12.2 years ± 1.4 years SD (range 9 to 15 years) in boys and progresses with advancement through puberty. However, acne vulgaris can be the first notable signs of puberty in a girl, preceding pubic hair and breast development.[258] Analysis of the Nurses Study indicates intake of milk and skim milk is related to the development of acne, an association suggested, but not proven, to be due to the hormone content of milk.[262] At late prepuberty, comedones are present in many boys and 100% of boys have comedones by genital stage 5.

Dental hygiene is often worse in boys than girls after the onset of puberty; this is also the age when gingivitis begins to appear along with the formation of pockets at the gum line.[263] There is a positive correlation between sex steroid concentrations and the presence of the bacteria most responsible for the inflammation of gingivitis in boys and girls.[264,265]

Facial morphology changes with pubertal development, leading to the mature appearance. Thus, the mandible and nose enlarge more in boys, but they and the maxilla, brow, frontal sinuses, and middle and posterior fossae enlarge in both sexes, mainly during the pubertal growth spurt. Children with isosexual precocity have the facial appearance of older children, and individuals with delayed puberty have the facies of younger children. There is a greater change in various measurements of the face compared to measurements of the skull with the jaw showing the most increase.[266]

The size of the thyroid gland evaluated by ultrasonography increases roughly 40% to 50% with growth in height, weight, surface area, and fat-free mass during puberty but not with BMI.[267] Lymphoid tissue growth reaches a maximum at about age 12 and thereafter decreases with pubertal progression. The mean heart rate and maximal oxygen uptake do not change in boys with the passage of peak height velocity, but respiratory quotient increases at the time of peak height velocity.[268]

The pituitary gland enlarges more in the female. In an MRI study, the height of the pituitary gland was no greater than 6 mm before puberty, was 8 to 10 mm in teenage females and had a spherical appearance in some, was no more than 7 mm in teenage males, and decreased in young adults of both sexes.[269]

Other Biochemical Changes of Puberty

A host of other physiologic and biochemical measurements change with the onset of puberty and must be interpreted in terms of the stage of pubertal development; age-related standards should be used in all laboratories but often are not, leaving the interpreting clinician to need to turn to a textbook of pediatrics or the *Harriet Lane Handbook*. Serum inorganic phosphate, alkaline phosphatase, serum osteocalcin (Gla-protein level) and urinary pyridinoline, deoxypyridinoline, and galactosyl-hydroxylysine excretion reflect the increased osteoblastic activity and growth rate at that time in both sexes.[270-275] Tartrate-resistant acid phosphatase isoform 5b also rises with pubertal growth and is proposed as another index of bone turnover at this age.[276] Serum urate rises at the end of pubertal development in average boys but obese boys experience a rise earlier in puberty.[277] Hemoglobin increases at puberty in boys; the effect appears mediated by androgen rather than growth hormone or IGF-1 as treatment of constitutionally delayed boys with testosterone and letrozole, the later to block aromatization to estrogen, resulted in increased hemoglobin even in the absence of a rise in IGF-I.[278]

Gonadal Development and Function

Female Ovarian and Uterine Development in Puberty (Also See Chapter 16)[279-282]

The peak number of germ cells in the fetal ovary is attained at 16 to 20 weeks' gestation. Primordial follicles appear beginning at 20 weeks of fetal life and soon thereafter primary follicles appear; they constitute the lifelong store of follicles for the individual as no more arise. Follicle-stimulating hormone (FSH) receptors have not been detected in midtrimester human fetal ovaries; fetal pituitary FSH is not required for proliferation of oogonia, oocyte differentiation, or formation of primordial follicles.[279] During fetal life and childhood, follicular growth to the large antral stage occurs, but before menarche, all developing follicles are destined to undergo atresia (Fig. 24–10).[281,283] Large preovulatory follicles are rarely present before puberty. Other aspects of follicular growth are found in Chapter 21.

The ultrasound appearance of the prepubertal ovary changes after pulsatile gonadotropin secretion increases and a multicystic appearance appears with more than six follicles of at least 4 mm in diameter; this appearance differs from that found in the polycystic ovarian syndrome.[284-286] During prepuberty, the ovarian volume is 0.2 to 1.6 mL on ultrasound scans, and after the onset of puberty, the volume increases to 2.8 to 15 mL.[287,288] Tall girls have greater ovarian volume than average size girls. Ultrasonographic studies (Fig. 24–11) show that the corpus of the uterus increases during pubertal progression from an initial tubular shape to a bulbous structure and that the length of the uterus increases from 2 to 3 cm to 5 to 8 cm[229] and the volume from 0.4 to 1.6 mL to 3 to 15 mL.[288] The addition of color Doppler studies is proposed to improve accuracy of diagnosis of precocious puberty and to differentiate the condition from premature thelarche; Doppler study showed the lowest impedance of the uterine artery to be in girls with established central precocious puberty.[290]

Endometriosis is considered to be an estrogen-dependent process but there is a remarkable report of 5 premenarcheal girls, of whom at least one was reported to be in breast stage 1, with proven endometriosis diagnosed after investigation for chronic abdominal pain; it was suggested that this etiology for abdominal pain is more common than was ever considered.[291] One proposed explanation for early onset of endometriosis is the possibility that the condition results from müllerian rests.[289-291]

Menarche (See Chapter 16)

Although there is significant variation, Menarche usually occurs in the 6-month period preceding or following the fusion of the second and first distal phalanges and the appearance of the sesamoid bone[293]; this corresponds to Tanner stage 4 in most cases. The 95th percentile for menarche is 14.5 years, although many textbooks define primary amenorrhea as absence of menses at 16 years of age: the reconsideration of the age of onset of female puberty may lead to a reconsideration of the age of definition of primary amenorrhea.[294] Anovulatory cycles are common in the first years after menarche.[295,296] There is a reported prevalence of 55% anovulation in the first 2 years after menarche that decreases to 20% anovulatory cycles by the fifth year; others have observed a lower number of ovulatory events shortly after menarche as well as 5 years after the event.[297,298] With the prevalence of polycystic ovarian syndrome (PCOS), it is unclear how often delayed regularity is an early sign of PCOS or is just normal variation. While the majority of early pubertal females are infertile in terms of risk of pregnancy, a substantial number are fertile, as evidenced by the prevalence of early teenage pregnancy. While the number of early teenage pregnancies is decreasing, in 2000 there were 8519 births to girls 10 to 14 years of age.[299] The latest final birth rate data available for the youngest teenagers declined to 0.6 births per 1000 females age 10 to 14 years in 2003, compared with 0.7 in 2002; the 2003 rate was less than one-half the rate reported during 1989 to 1994 (1.4 per 1000).[300]

Male Testicular Development in Puberty (Also See Chapters 13 and 29)[279]

The testes are active during the prepubertal period, albeit at a lower level of activity than during pubertal development.[301] During pubertal development the testes increase in size, principally because of the growth of the seminiferous tubules associated with the onset of spermatogenetic activity, and mitosis of Sertoli cells,[302] and testosterone production increases (Fig. 24–12 and Table 24–9).[303] The Sertoli cells are the major cell type in the seminiferous cords in prepuberty and early puberty, but in the adult, germ cells predominate. During progression through

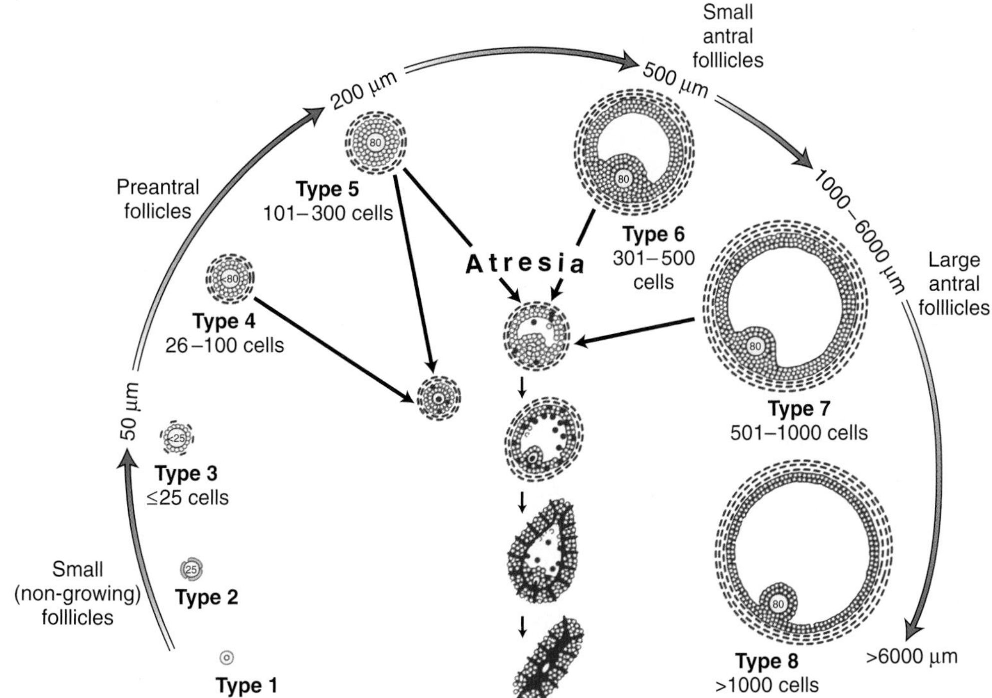

Figure 24–10 ▪ Schematic representation of the growth of ovarian follicles during infancy and childhood. Type 1 (primordial follicle) and type 2 (primary follicle) are composed of a small oocyte and a few to a ring of flat granulosa cells. In the diplotene (nesting) stage of prophase, primary follicles are the predominant form of oocyte and constitute the reservoir of cells from which follicular growth occurs. Types 3 to 5 (preantral follicles) are follicles that have entered the growth phase; the oocyte is enlarging and is surrounded by a zona pellucida, and granulosa cells increase in number and differentiate. The growth of the oocyte is complete by the end of the preantral stage, and the increased follicular size is due to follicular growth and fluid accumulation. Types 6 to 8 represent antral follicles (graafian follicles) and contain a fully grown oocyte, a large number of granulosa cells, a fluid-filled cavity, and a well-developed theca external to the basement membrane. Large preovulatory follicles are absent (10,000 to 15,000 μm). Follicular growth and atresia take place throughout childhood; all follicles that enter the growth phase become atretic, and this can occur at any stage in their development but mainly involves large antral follicles. (From Peters H, Byskov AG, Grinsted J. Follicular growth in fetal and prepubertal ovaries of humans and other primates. Clin Endocrinol Metab 1978;7:469-485.)

TABLE 24–9 CELLULAR ACTIVITY IN HUMAN TESTIS AT DIFFERENT STAGES OF DEVELOPMENT

Stage	Germ Cells	Sertoli Cells	Leydig Cells
Prepubertal	Prespermatogenic cells present	Predominant cells in seminiferous cords	Scattered, partially differentiated cells present
Pubertal	Initiation of spermatogenesis	Increased complexity, formation of occlusive junctions	Fully differentiated cells appear
Adult	Active spermatogenesis, predominant cells	Individual cells associated with groups of germ cells	Groups of fully differentiated cells present

From Gondos B, Kogan S. Testicular development during puberty. In Grumbach MM, Sizonenko PC, Aubert ML, eds. Control of the Onset of Puberty. Baltimore: Williams & Wilkins, 1990:387-398. © 1990, the Williams & Wilkins Co., Baltimore.

puberty, the Sertoli cells cease to undergo mitosis, differentiate into adult-type Sertoli cells, and form occlusive junctions with the development of the blood-testicular barrier. Although Leydig cells can be detected in early gestation and again during the neonatal period of testosterone secretion, during childhood the interstitial tissue is composed principally of undifferentiated mesenchyme-type cells. With pubertal development and rising serum luteinizing hormone (LH) levels, adult-type Leydig cells appear. It is suggested that three phases of Leydig cell maturation be recognized associated with ages of increased testosterone production; 14 to 18 weeks of fetal life, 2 to 3 months after birth, and from puberty through adulthood.[304,305] The seminal vesicle enlarges through childhood to puberty to hold 3.4 to 4.5 mL, or 70%, of the seminal fluid.[306] The mean blood flow in the testes increases to adult values, as measured by Doppler sonography, in boys with greater than 4 cm^3 testicular volume.[307]

Absent or very poor detection of estrogen receptor (ER) α by histochemistry and by RNA expression was observed in three age groups of prepubertal testes: GR1, newborns (1- to 21-day-old neonates); GR2, postnatal activation stage (1- to 7-month-old infants); GR3, childhood (12- to 60-month-old boys). Leydig cells of newborns and 1- to 7-month-olds showed strong immunostaining of aromatase and P450 side chain cleavage (scc) but

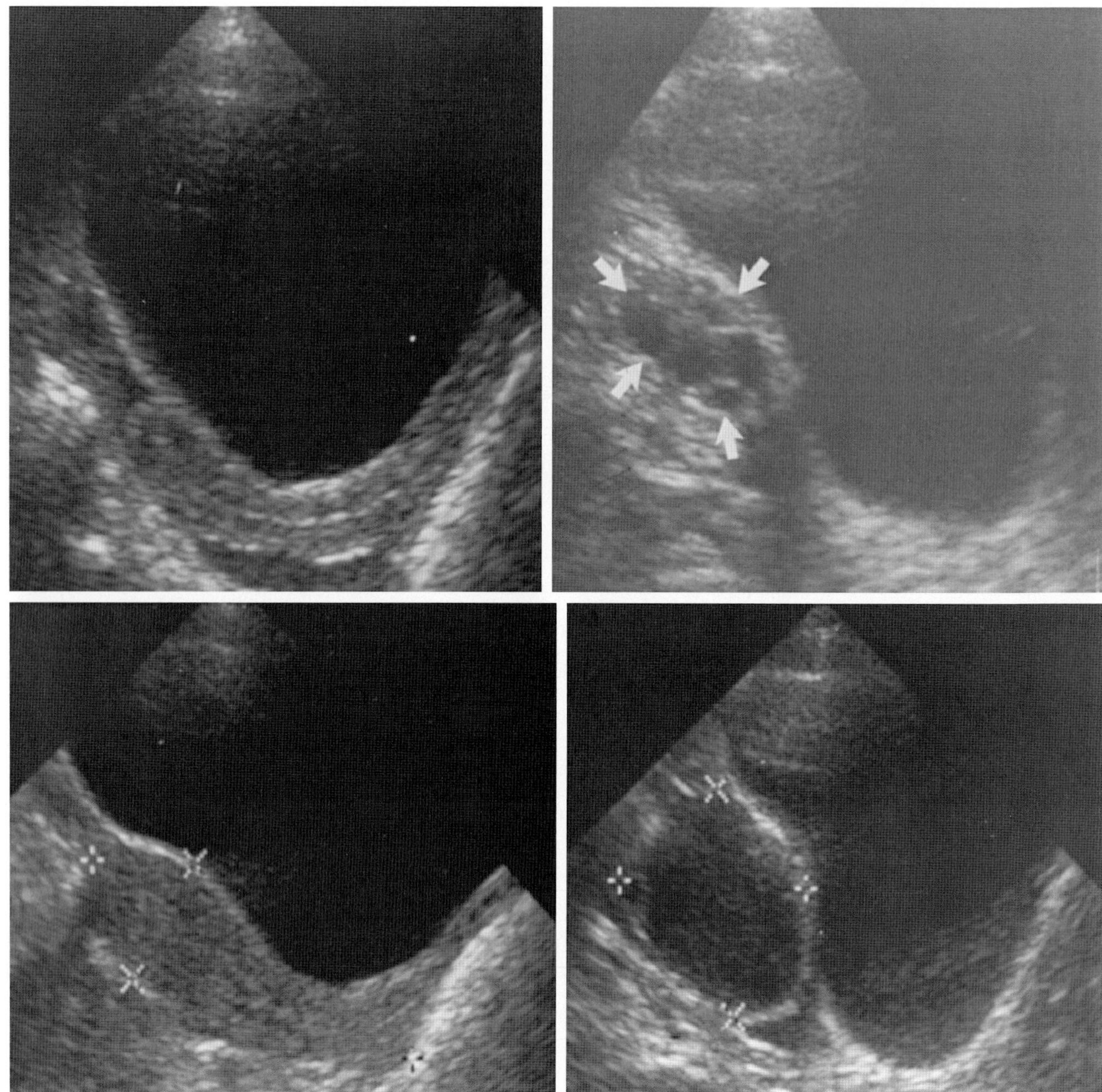

Figure 24–11 ▪ High-resolution pelvic ultrasonography. *Top left,* Prepubertal uterus. *Top right,* Prepubertal ovary demonstrating four small follicular cysts *(arrows)*. *Bottom left,* Pubertal postmenarchal uterus. *Bottom right,* Ovarian cyst in a girl with true precocious puberty.

weak staining of ERβ and androgen receptor (AR). Interstitial cells (ICs) and Sertoli cells (SCs) expressed ERβ, particularly in the newborn and 1- to 7-month-olds. Strong expression of AR was found in peritubular cells (PCs). Expression of all of these markers was weakest in prepuberty. In gonocytes and spermatogonia, aromatase and ERβ were immunoexpressed strongly whereas no expression of ERα, AR, or P450scc was detected. The authors proposed that in newborn and infantile testis, testosterone acting on PCs might modulate infant Leydig cell differentiation, whereas the absence of AR in Sertoli cells prevents development of spermatogenesis.[308]

Spermatogenesis

The first histologic evidence of spermatogenesis appears between ages 11 and 15 years. Spermaturia in the first morning urine specimen, probably reflecting the maturation of spermatogenesis,[309-311] occurs at a mean chronologic age of 13.3 (other studies found 16 years) at a mean pubic hair stage of 2.5. However, spermaturia was detected in 2 of 28 normal boys with bilateral testicular volumes of 3 mL and no other signs of puberty.[312] Spermaturia is more prevalent in early puberty than in late puberty, suggesting that there may be a continuous flow of sperm through the urethra in early puberty but that ejaculation is necessary for sperm to appear in the urine in late puberty.[313] Normospermia (sperm concentration, morphology, motility) is not present until a bone age of 17 years.[314,315] The first conscious ejaculation occurs at a mean chronologic age of $13^1/_2$ in normal boys and at a mean bone age of $13^1/_2$ in boys with delayed puberty.[316] The potential for fertility is reached before an adult phenotype is attained, before the attainment of adult

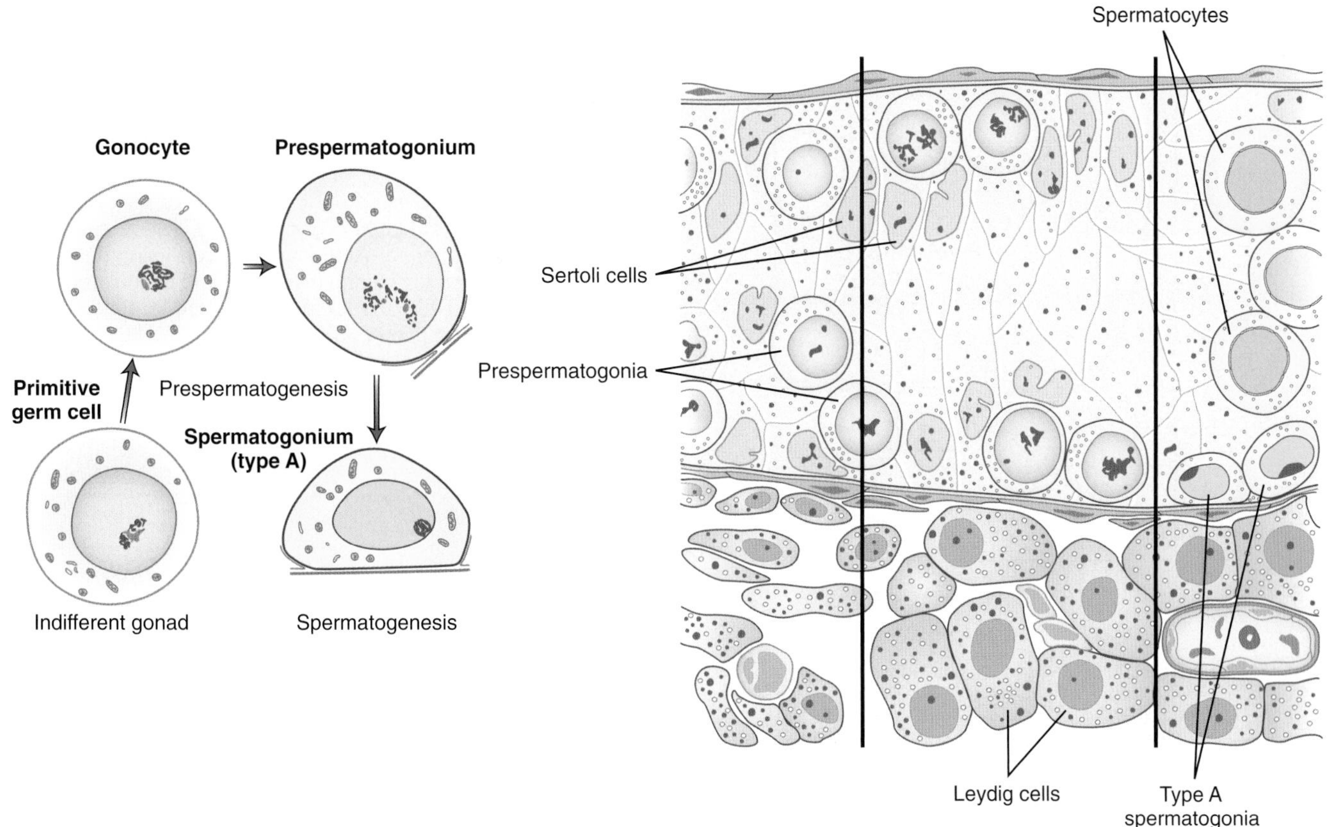

Figure 24–12 ■ *Left,* Diagram illustrating developmental stages of testicular germ cells based on electron microscopic findings in the rabbit. Note differences between prespermatogonium and spermatogonium. *Right,* Diagram showing maturation of testicular cell types in the rabbit from prepubertal appearance at left to onset of spermatogenesis at right. Interstitial cells undergo changes in shape, size, and arrangement in the process of Leydig cell differentiation. (From Gondos B. Testicular development. In Johnson AD, Gomes WR, eds. The Testis, vol 4. New York, Academic Press, 1977:1-37.)

plasma testosterone concentrations and before peak height velocity is reached.[309]

Adolescent Growth

Pubertal Growth Spurt

Prepubertal height and growth velocity are similar in boys and girls. The greatest postnatal growth occurs in infancy and decreases to the nadir known as the minimal prespurt velocity just before the pubertal growth spurt. The minimal prespurt growth velocity of prepuberty is the slowest period of growth in childhood, with boys averaging 0.46 cm/yr and girls averaging 0.48 cm/yr of deceleration before the pubertal growth spurt.[317] During puberty, boys and girls experience a growth velocity greater than at any postnatal age since infancy. The pubertal growth spurt may be divided for purposes of comparison into three stages: the time of prespurt minimal growth velocity in peripuberty just before the spurt (takeoff velocity); the time of most rapid growth, or peak height velocity (PHV); and the stage of decreased velocity and cessation of growth at epiphyseal fusion. Boys reach peak height velocity approximately 2 years later than girls and are taller at takeoff (Fig. 24–13 and Table 24–10); peak height velocity occurs during stage 3 to 4 of puberty in most boys (see Tables 24–4, 24–5, and 24–7; see Figure 24–8) and is completed by stage 5 in more than 95% of boys,[318] in English studies while a Canadian longitudinal study found PHV usually occurring in pubic hair stage 4.[319] Boys achieve a peak height velocity of 9.5 cm/yr at about a mean of 13.5 years with a greater PHV in those who mature earlier than those who mature later.[320] The pubertal growth spurt in girls (PHV in girls reaches a mean of 8.3 cm/yr at a mean chronologic age of 11.5 years) occurs between stages 2 and 3 (see Table 24–3 and Fig. 24–9)[209,321] in European studies while a Canadian longitudinal study found PHV occurring in pubic hair stage 3 or 4.[319] Boys grew a mean of 28 cm and girls grew 25 cm between takeoff and cessation of growth in a study in the United Kingdom.[322] The mean height difference of 12.5 cm between adult men and women in the Zurich growth study resulted partly from the greater prespurt growth of boys (+1.5 cm); partly from the height difference at age of takeoff, with boys being taller at their later age of takeoff than girls (+6.5 cm); partly from the greater gain in height of boys during the pubertal growth spurt (+6 cm); and partly from the greater postspurt growth in girls (−1.5 cm).[323] However, more recent analysis of U.S. children suggest that 8 to 11 cm of increased height gained during the pubertal growth spurt in boys is mainly responsible for the difference in adult height between the sexes.[320,323]

There are several mathematical models that attempt to define the various stages of the pubertal growth curve. Takeoff in children with growth hormone deficiency, determined by mathematical analysis via the Preece-Baines model 1,[324] occurred at a mean of 1.4 years before testicular enlargement in boys and was a mean of 2 years before breast stage 2 in girls.[325] Another model based on longitudinal data, separates the infancy, childhood, and pubertal phases of growth and allows evaluation of growth despite the variation in the age of the onset of puberty. A slowly decelerating childhood component is the base, with a sigmoidal pubertal component added during secondary sexual development (Fig. 24–14). This model provides a new means of predict-

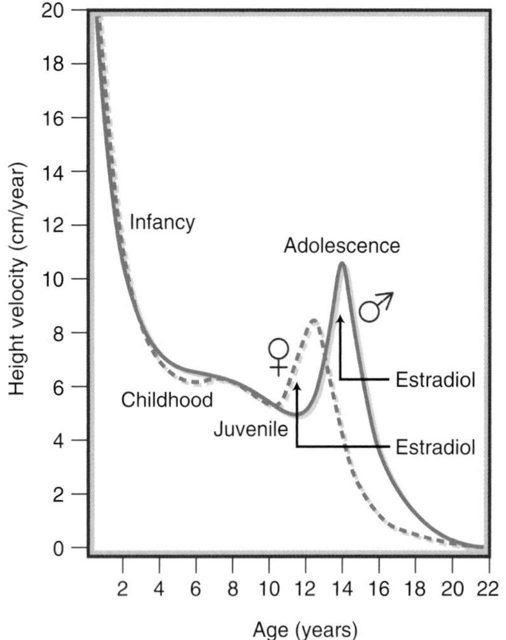

Figure 24–13 ▪ The adolescent growth spurt in girls and boys (growth velocity curves). Note the later onset of the pubertal growth spurt in boys and the approximately 2-year difference in peak height velocity and the greater magnitude of peak height velocity compared with girls. The timing of the effects of estradiol is indicated. Progressive epiphyseal fusion terminates the growth spurt and leads to final or adult height. (From Grumbach MM. Estrogen, bone, growth, and sex: a sea change in conventional wisdom. J Pediatr Endocrinol Metab 2000;13[Suppl 6]:1439-1455.)

ing adult height, the height adjusted for pubertal onset (HAPO).[326] Variations on this technique of height prediction use the ICP (infancy-childhood-puberty) growth curve either (1) without bone age (IPP) or (2) without bone age but with the use of parental height information (ICPN) when available.[327] The ICP model detected the onset of the pubertal growth spurt, predicted the actual magnitude of the pubertal growth spurt, and predicted adult height using only the age of onset of puberty and a measurement of height.[328] Tanner and Davies[329] have constructed growth curves for American children using data from the National Center for Health Statistics and calculated data from theoretical growth curves can be adjusted for time of peak height velocity (see Chapter 23).

TABLE 24–10 DIFFERENCE IN THE RELATIONSHIP OF ONSET OF PUBERTAL GROWTH TO SEXUAL MATURATION IN BOYS AND GIRLS

GIRLS
The onset of the pubertal growth spurt precedes or is associated with the earliest signs of female secondary sexual maturation (e.g., sexual hair, breast development).
BOYS
The onset of sexual maturation, including testicular enlargement and male secondary sexual characteristics, precedes the onset of the pubertal growth spurt. Peak height velocity is not achieved until a late stage of sexual maturation (stage III-IV).

From Grumbach MM. Estrogen, bone, growth, and sex: a sea change in conventional wisdom. J Pediatr Endocrinol Metab 2000;13(suppl 6):1439-1455.

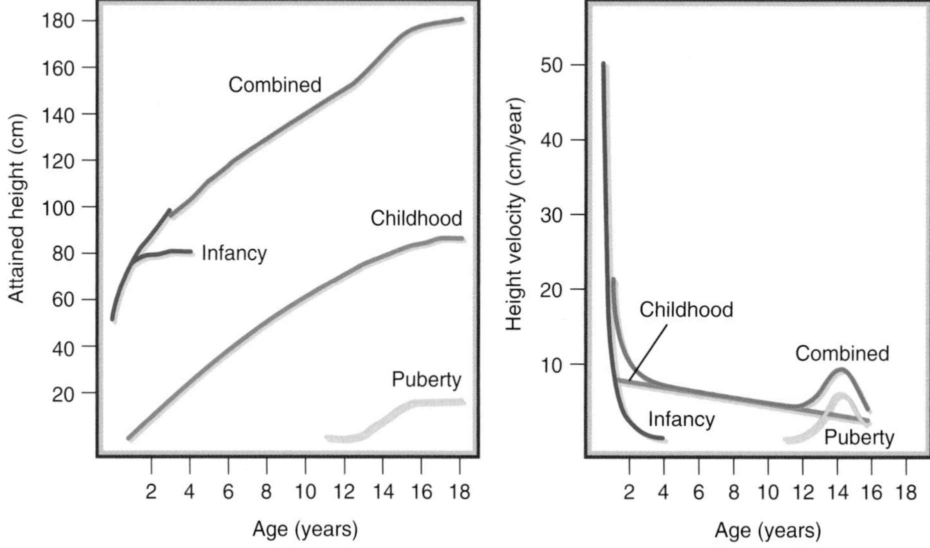

Figure 24–14 ▪ The infancy, childhood, and puberty (ICP) model of Karlberg for mean attained height *(left)* and height velocity *(right)* for boys. The mean value for each component (infancy, childhood, puberty) and their sums (combined growth, *right;* combined velocity, *left*) are plotted. The growth curve for an individual represents the additive effect of the three biologic phases of the growth process (ICP). Karlberg has provided mathematical functions for each component of his model. *Infancy:* This component starts before birth and falls off by age 3 to 4 years. It can be described by the exponential function $y=a+b[1-\exp(-ct)]$. Average total gain in height for Swedish boys is 79.0 cm (44.0% of final height) and for girls is 76.8 cm (46.2%). *Childhood:* This phase begins at the end of the first year of life and continues to mature height. A second-degree polynomial function describes this component: $y=a+bt+ct^2$. Average total gain in height for boys is 85.2 cm (47.4%) and for girls is 78.4 cm (47.3%). *Puberty:* The model for the pubertal growth spurt is a logistic function: $y=a/[1+\exp(-b(t-t_v))]$. Average total gain in height for boys is 15.4 cm (8.6%) and for girls is 10.9 cm (6.5%); y designates attained height at time t in years from birth; a, b, and c are constants; t_v is the age at peak height velocity. (Adapted from Karlberg J. On the construction of the infancy-childhood-puberty growth standard. Acta Paediatr Scand Suppl 1989;356:26-37.)

Daily, meticulous observations of girls during puberty over 120 to 150 days show stasis periods in each girl (3 to 7 events lasting between 7 and 22 consecutive days) as well as steep changes in each girl (1 to 4 episodes with the sum of these steep changes calculated as a percentage of total growth during the study period ranging from 15.3% to 42.9%) and continuous growth the remainder of time with no rhythms or cycles found.[330] Thus, clinicians observe an integrated growth rate during puberty, rather than these varying complex patterns that occur during shorter periods of observation.

In a large Swedish registry, faster linear growth during infancy and childhood was associated with earlier peak height velocity during adolescence but less height gain between 8 and 18 years, whereas greater height and BMI at birth were associated with later peak height velocity in adolescence and more height gain between ages 8 and 18.[331]

Because girls reach peak height velocity about 1.3 years before menarche, there is limited growth potential after menarche; most girls grow only about 2.5 cm in height after menarche,[209] although there is a variation from 1 to as much as 7 cm. The ages at menarche, takeoff, and peak height velocity are not good predictors of adult height because the duration of pubertal growth is the more important determinant of final height; later onset of puberty and consequent increase in height at takeoff of the pubertal growth spurt can be balanced by a decrease in actual height achieved during peak height velocity and result in no net change in adult height. However, early onset of puberty can diminish ultimate adult stature,[332] prolonged delay of puberty[333] can increase stature and an older age of menarche leads to taller adult height in women.[190] The age at peak height velocity and the age at initiation of puberty correlate well with the rate of passage through the stages of pubertal development in normal children.[317] All that can be deduced by physical examination of a boy is that if he is in early puberty, he is likely to have significant growth left, whereas in late puberty limited growth is likely.

Both stature and the upper/lower segment ratio, defined as the length from the top of the pubic ramus to the top of the head divided by the distance from the top of the pubic ramus to the sole of the foot, change markedly during the peripubertal and early pubertal periods because of the elongation of the extremities.[334] At birth the U/L ration is about 1.7, at 1 year is 1.4, and at 10 years is 1.0 in a normal healthy individual. The legs begin to grow before the trunk, although late in puberty, during the growth spurt, growth of the legs is similar to growth of the upper torso.[335] The mean upper/lower segment ratio of Caucasian adults is 0.92, and that of African-American adults is 0.85. There are no differences in upper/lower segment ratio between the sexes; however, the ratio of sitting height to standing height is higher in pubertal and adult females than in males.[30,32] In general, hypogonadal patients have delayed epiphyseal fusion and lack a pubertal growth spurt; therefore, their extremities grow for a prolonged period, leading to a decreased upper/lower segment ratio and an increased span for height, a condition known as eunuchoid proportions. Eunuchoid proportions are found in subjects with defects in estrogen synthesis and estrogen receptor deficiency but normal proportions occur in complete androgen insensitivity syndrome demonstrating the primary role of estrogen in mitigating or establishing these proportions.[336-338] The distal parts of the extremities, the hands and feet, grow before the proximal parts; a rapid increase in shoe size is a harbinger of the pubertal growth spurt. Boys with Klinefelter's syndrome have long legs, but not long arms, as a physical feature apparent before the onset of puberty. The shoulders become wider in boys, whereas the hips enlarge more in girls; the ratio of biacromial (shoulder) breadth to bicrystal (hip) breadth remains constant in boys at about 1.37 but decreases in girls from 1.35 to 1.27.[32] The female pelvic inlet widens, mainly because of the growth of the os acetabuli. The size of the head approaches the adult size by age 10 years and the brain reaches 95% of adult size by the onset of puberty (see more about brain development below).[32]

Hormonal Control of the Pubertal Growth Spurt

Postnatal growth follows a pattern of (1) a very high growth rate just after birth but (2) a decleration following and (3) continuing until 3 years of age, (4) a slower phase of deceleration up to puberty followed by (5) the pubertal growth spurt, the second greatest period of postnatal growth, which is followed by (6) maturation of the spine and long bones until adult height is reached.[320] Many factors influence the growth plate.[172] The adolescent growth spurt in normal girls and boys depends on both estradiol and growth hormone (GH)[336,337,339-341] among other factors.

Hormonal control of the pubertal growth spurt is complex (Figs. 24–15 and 24–16). Growth hormone (GH) clearly is involved in increasing growth at puberty through the stimulation of insulin-like growth factor I (IGF-I, previously called somatomedin-C) production. Gonadal steroids have two effects

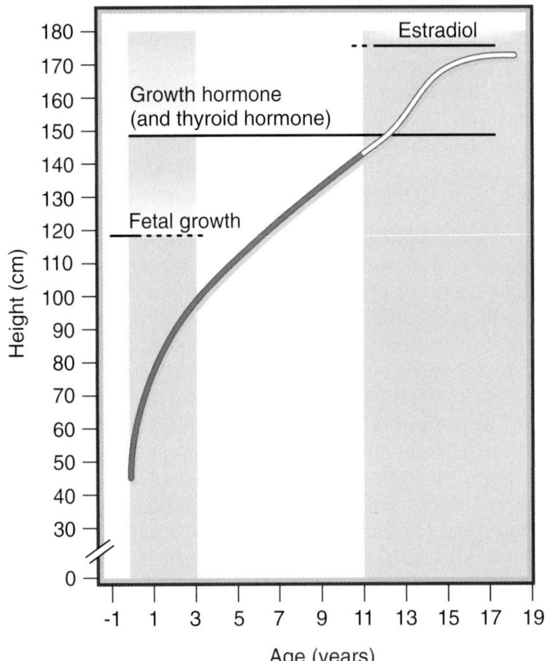

Figure 24–15 ▪ A schematic male growth chart with the features of the ICP (infancy, childhood, puberty) pattern overlaid and illustrating the predominant endocrine mechanisms controlling each phase of growth. The first shaded area emphasizes the decreasing velocity of infantile growth as the individual leaves the rapid growth phase of fetal life. The clear area is the childhood phase, which continues and magnifies the decreased velocity of growth into a plateau of rather constant growth during childhood. These two phases depend, in large part, on the effects of growth hormone (GH) and thyroid hormone with no or little effect derived from gonadal steroids. Finally, there is the period of the pubertal growth spurt in which gonadal steroids exert their direct and indirect effects. Gonadal steroids exert direct effects on the bone by stimulating the generation of insulin-like growth factor I (IGF-I) and other growth factors locally, and exert indirect effects by stimulating increased GH secretion which, in turn, exerts its own effects on bone and stimulates the production of IGF-I. In the female, the major gonadal steroid involved in the pubertal growth spurt is estradiol, whereas in the male, testosterone and estradiol (arising mainly from the aromatization of testosterone) are the major gonadal steroids. From Grumbach MM. Estrogen, bone, growth, and sex: A sea change in conventional wisdom. J Pediatr Endocrinol Metab 2000; 13 (suppl 6):1439-1455.

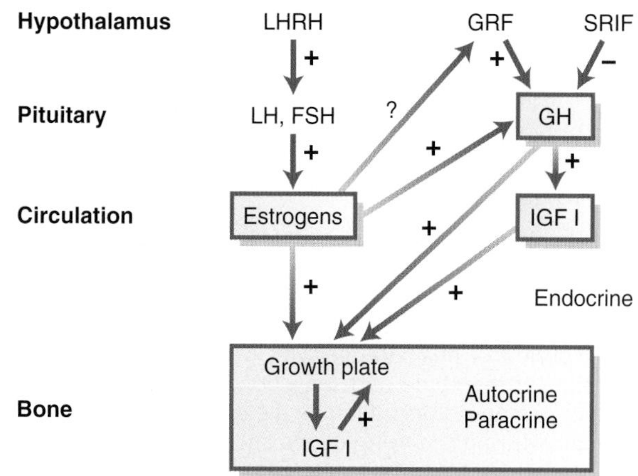

Figure 24–16 ▪ Interactions of the major growth-promoting hormones during puberty. Plus (+) indicates stimulatory action, minus (–) inhibitory action. Circulating insulin-like growth factor I (IGF-I) arises mainly from liver, but other tissues also contribute (endocrine action). Growth hormone and gonadal steroids have a direct stimulatory effect on the generation of IGF-I (paracrine action) locally in bone and cartilage cells. For simplification, the feedback loops for IGF-I and gonadal steroids on the hypothalamic pituitary unit are omitted.

on pubertal growth: (1) induction of an increase in GH secretion and thus the consequent increase in IGF-I production, thereby indirectly stimulating pubertal growth, and (2) a direct effect on cartilage and bone by stimulating local production of IGF-I, among other local factors.[342-344,337]

Gonadal Steroids

In the developing human skeleton, gonadal steroids have growth-promoting and maturational actions on chondrocytes and osteoblasts among other bone constituents.[336,337,345] The latter action, which eventually leads to epiphyseal fusion and the cessation of longitudinal growth in both boys and girls, is mediated mainly by estrogen either directly secreted (in girls) or arising from the conversion of testosterone and androstenedione to estrogen in peripheral tissues by aromatase. The detection of estrogen resistance due to a null mutation in the gene encoding the estrogen receptor and of derangements in the CYP19 gene leading to severe cytochrome P450 aromatase deficiency have highlighted the cardinal role of estradiol but not testosterone in both boys and girls in the pubertal growth spurt, complete epiphyseal maturation, and normal skeletal proportions and mineralization.[336,337] Individuals with a mutation in the estrogen receptor α gene or the CYP19 gene encoding aromatase continue to grow, lack a pubertal growth spurt, and have open epiphyses and osteopenia.[336,337,339-341] Furthermore, estrogen treatment of men with aromatase deficiency leads to epiphyseal closure and cessation of growth, and a striking increase in bone mass.[346-348] On the other hand, patients with aromatase excess, who produce excess estrogen, have advanced skeletal maturation, rapid growth, and may ultimately reach short adult stature.[349] (See below.)

Although estradiol secreted by the ovary has been recognized for more than 2 decades as the major sex steroid responsible for the pubertal growth spurt, skeletal maturation, and bone mineral accrual in the female, until the detection of the rare human genetic defects in estrogen synthesis or action, conventional wisdom dictated that in the male, testosterone mediated these maturational changes during puberty. In the male as well as the female, estrogen (not androgen) is the critical sex hormone in the pubertal growth spurt, skeletal maturation, accrual of peak bone mass, and maintenance of bone mass in the adult. Estrogen stimulates chondrogenesis in the epiphyseal

TABLE 24–11 EARLIER CLINICAL CLUES TO THE EFFECT OF ESTROGEN ON GROWTH AND SKELETAL MATURATION IN THE MALE

Complete androgen insensitivity (resistance) syndrome (Zachmann M, Prader A, Sobel EH, et al. Pubertal growth in patients with androgen insensitivity: indirect evidence for the importance of estrogen in pubertal growth of girls. J Pediatr 1986;108:694-697)

Short-term estradiol administration increased rate of ulnar growth in prepubertal boys (Caruso-Nicoletti M, Cassorla FG, Skerda MC, et al. Short term, low dose estradiol accelerates ulnar growth in boys. J Clin Endocrinol Metab 1985;61:896-898)

Aromatase inhibitor decreased rapid growth and skeletal maturation in testotoxicosis whereas antiandrogen had no effect on skeletal maturation (Laue L, Jones J, Barnes K, et al. Treatment of familial male precocious puberty with spironolactone and deslorelin. J Clin Endocrinol Metab 1993;76:151-155)

Aromatase excess syndrome in boys associated with increased rate of growth and skeletal maturation, elevated plasma estrogen concentrations, but prepubertal testosterone values (Stratakis CA, Vottero A, Brodie A, et al. The aromatase excess syndrome is associated with feminization of both sexes and autosomal dominant transmission of aberrant P450 aromatase gene transcription. J Clin Endocrinol Metab 1998;83:1349-1357)

Estrogen-secreting tumors: adrenal and testicular neoplasms (especially Peutz-Jeghers syndrome) (Bulun SE, Rosenthal IM, Brodie AM, et al. Use of tissue-specific promoters in the regulation of aromatase cytochrome P450 gene expression in human testicular and ovarian sex cord tumors, as well as in normal fetal and adult gonads. J Clin Endocrinol Metab 1993;77:1616-1621)

From Grumbach MM. Estrogen, bone, growth, and sex: a sea change in conventional wisdom. J Pediatr Endocrinol Metab 2000;13(suppl 6):1439-1455.

growth plate,[350] increasing pubertal linear growth. At puberty, estrogen promotes skeletal maturation and the gradual progressive closure of the epiphyseal growth plate.[336] The use of a supersensitive assay for plasma estradiol[351,352] in prepubertal and pubertal boys revealed a high positive correlation between estradiol concentrations and peak growth velocity (but not serum growth hormone), which was greatest about 3 years after the onset of puberty,[353] further implicating estrogen in the pubertal growth spurt and skeletal maturation of boys as well as girls.

Surprisingly little is known about the mechanism of action of estrogen on the skeletal growth plates[337,350,350a] (Table 24–11) although information is accruing. There are estrogen receptors, both ERα and ERβ and the membranous estrogen receptor GPR30 in the growth plate chondrocytes.[172] Histologic study of the bone and cartilage of rodents treated with corticosteroids or estrogen and clinical evaluation of children with precocious puberty supports the theory that senescence of the growth plate occurs due estrogen exposure in precocious puberty, causing decreased growth during treatment with gonadotropin-releasing hormone (GnRH) agonists.[354]

The high rate of bone turnover in early puberty followed by a decrease in periosteal apposition and endosteal resorption within cortical bone, and in bone remodeling within cortical and cancellous bone is mediated by apoptosis of chondrocytes in the growth plate and osteoclasts within cortical and cancellous bone effected at least in part by estrogen. This leads to a reduction in bone turnover markers at menarche reflecting the closure of the epiphyseal growth plates.[355] Girls with Turner's syndrome without estrogen exposure retain elevated markers of bone turnover.[356] Prepubertal girls with Turner's syndrome tend to lose bone but that ceases when estrogen therapy begins; thus, administration of estrogen might best be started earliler.[357] During puberty and into the third decade, estrogen has an anabolic effect on the osteoblast and an apoptotic effect on the osteoclast, increasing bone mineral acquisition in the axial and appendicular skeleton. Furthermore, in the adult, estrogen is important in maintaining the constancy of bone mass through its effect on bone remodeling and bone turnover (Table 24–12).[337,358]

Testosterone also has a direct action on bone in the human male; androgen receptors are found in human tibiae growth plates[359,360] in osteoblasts[361] and chondrocytes, osteocytes, mononuclear cells, and endothelial cells of blood vessels in the bone marrow.[362] Androgens that cannot be aromatized to estrogen still cause an increase in growth rate, presumably due to interaction with these receptors.[363] The greater increase in periosteal bone deposition, and the resultant thickening of cortical bone and greater bone strength, which seems to be determined by relatively higher periosteal bone formation and, therefore, greater bone dimensions[364] in boys, is probably related to a direct effect of testosterone.[365] Thus, androgens may protect men against osteoporosis via maintenance of cancellous bone mass and expansion of cortical bone.[364] Experiments in mice suggest that ERβ may mediate growth-limiting effects of estrogens in the female but does not seem to be involved in the regulation of bone size in males.

A pubertal growth spurt leading to adult height close to that of genotypic men occurs in individuals with the complete form of androgen resistance,[366] demonstrating the critical role of estrogen rather than androgen in the adolescent growth spurt in boys. In a study of 18 adult XY women with the complete androgen insensitivity syndrome, with appropriate estrogen replacement therapy, six (30%) exceeded 5'11" in height. In addition, a modest decrease in Bone Mineral Density (BMD) Z-scores were noted at the spine but not hip using age-specific female standard values, but the reductions were greater against male standards and when apparent BMD (a measure of volumetric BMD) was used. There was also a disturbing increase in prevalence of fractures in the affected women even with estrogen replacement. This suggests that lack of a direct effect of testosterone on the skeleton, especially the spine, has a part in the defects in bone mineralization in women with complete androgen insensitivity (see Table 24–11).[367]

Growth Hormone

GH release is stimulated by hypothalamic GH-releasing hormone (GHRH), but another class of 6 and 7 amino acid peptides (GH-releasing peptide, or GHRP) also stimulate GH release independently and in a manner additive to GHRH. GHRP stimulates the release of GH in the absence of GHRH as well as in its presence.

GH secretion approximately doubles during puberty in both boys and girls,[368-375] but decreases after pubertal development; the greater rise in girls starts at an earlier age and pubertal stage than in boys due to the earlier onset of puberty in girls.[30,31] GH secretion increases coincident with the onset of breast development (Tanner stage 2) and is maximal at Tanner stage 3 to 4 breast development; in boys, in contrast, GH rises later and peaks at stage 4 genital development. GH secretion and IGF-I levels decrease after late puberty in both sexes. Adolescents of normal height have an inverse relationship between weight and GH levels.[376] Increased GH pulse amplitude and content of GH secreted per pulse (not frequency or metabolic clearance rate or intersecratory burst interval and half-life of GH) in the basal state are mainly responsible for the augmented GH levels.[373,377,378]

Stimulated GH secretion also increases at puberty; of 88 subjects of normal height, 61% of prepubertal children did not raise their GH peak above 7 ng/mL after exercise, arginine, or L-Dopa, but by stage two puberty, 44% met the 7-ng/mL level, by stage three, 11% met the level, and at stage four and five, 100% did so.[379,380] GH secretion increases in puberty in the basal state as well as after GHRH or GHRP stimulation.[381,382] However, hexarelin, a 6 amino acid GHRP stimulates as much growth hormone secretion in prepuberty as in puberty.[383] Circulating ghrelin is mostly of gastrointestinal (GI) origin and may not reflect hypothalamic function, but serum values decrease from infancy through puberty.[384]

The increase in estradiol at puberty, in boys from testicular secretion and especially extraglandular synthesis from testosterone and androstenedione, and in girls from secretion by the ovaries, is the principal mediator of the increased pulse amplitude and the amount of GH secreted per pulse.[385] Administration of exogenous androgens in delayed puberty raises GH secretion. Transdermal application of testosterone increases spontaneous GH secretion overnight independent of GHRH because infusion of GnRH antagonist does not affect this phenomenon.[386] The effect of testosterone, however, is mediated mainly through its conversion to estradiol[387] in that treatment of late pubertal boys with tamoxifen (estrogen receptor blocker) causes smaller GH secretory peaks and fewer GH secretory episodes.[388] Exogenous estrogen increases the peak GH reached after insulin-induced hypoglycemia, exercise, and arginine.[379] This priming effect of estrogen on GH secretion is used in clinical practice because estrogen administered before a provocative test in prepubertal subjects increases the GH response.[389] Androgens that cannot be aromatized to estrogen (e.g., oxandrolone and dihydrotestosterone) have less effect upon GH secretion; contrariwise, androgen receptor blockade with flutamide increases GH secretion.[388,390,391] Dihydrotestosterone, which is not aromatized to estrogen, does not increase GH secretion or the plasma concentration of IGF-I and may decrease the integrated GH secretion, but still stimulates increased growth rate, suggesting a possible direct effect of androgen on pubertal growth independent of GH[342] or estradiol. Increased GH secretion also occurs in sexual precocity. GH secretion decreases with the fall in gonadal steroid levels after treatment of children with true precocious puberty with potent luteinizing hormone–releasing hormone (GnRH) agonists.[369,392,393]

In a series of 26 GH-deficient women who had spontaneous puberty, 39% had menarche after 16 years of age and almost 50% continued to have menstrual disorders.[394]

GH deficiency[395] or GH resistance[396] causes an attenuated pubertal growth spurt, indicating the importance of GH and IGF-I. Severe primary or secondary hypogonadism leads to a

TABLE 24–12 SOME SITES OF ESTROGEN ACTION ON BONE

Linear growth: chondrogenesis—proliferation and differentiation of growth plate chondrocytes—and its link to osteogenesis
Skeletal maturation: the gradual, progressive ossification of the epiphyseal growth plate during puberty, possibly as a consequence of both estrogen-induced vascular and osteoblastic invasion and the termination of chondrogenesis
Accrual of bone mass during puberty and into the third decade
Estrogen and the constancy of bone mass in the adult: remodeling, maintenance, and repair—the osteoclast and the osteoblast and osteocyte

From Grumbach MM. Estrogen, bone, growth, and sex: a sea change in conventional wisdom. J Pediatr Endocrinol Metab 2000;13(suppl 6):1439-1455.

minimal or absent growth spurt, demonstrating the primary role of gonadal steroids in pubertal growth. Hypopituitary patients deficient in both GH and gonadotropins do not have an adolescent growth spurt when GH alone is replaced; gonadal steroids must also be given, substantiating the interaction of GH and gonadal steroids in the pubertal growth spurt.[335,397] In normal puberty, neither the magnitude of the increase in GH secretion nor the concentration of plasma IGF-I correlate with peak height velocity of the pubertal growth spurt. While a threshold level of GH secretion is necessary, the extent of the growth spurt correlates with gonadal sex steroid secretion. Individuals with both true precocious puberty and GH deficiency (usually a consequence of cranial irradiation for a brain tumor) have a growth spurt clinically indistinguishable from that of true precocious puberty and normal GH secretion.[342] After treatment with a GnRH agonist for sexual precocity, patients with GH deficiency and true precocious puberty decrease their growth velocity along with the suppression of their pubertal progression,[342] illustrating the direct effect of gonadal steroids, principally estradiol, on the pubertal growth spurt.

The concentration of plasma IGF-I increases during puberty, induced by increased GH secretion, to reach an earlier peak in girls than in boys[392,398-400] and then decreases to adult levels (Fig. 24–17). Plasma IGF-I concentrations are high for chronologic age in sexual precocity and low in delayed puberty. Estrogen mediates the pubertal increase in IGF-I concentration through increased secretion of GH,[392] with an additional effect through the gonadal steroid-induced local generation of IGF-I in cartilage and bone.[342] Treatment with GnRH agonist of a 16-year-old male with a homozygous mutation in the WSXWS-like motif of the human GH receptor (GHR) causing Laron syndrome led to a further decrease in the already low serum IGF-I and IGF binding protein 3 (IGFBP-3), which did not reverse with dihydrotestosterone treatment, suggesting a direct effect of estradiol on IGF-I production.[401] Children with true precocious puberty treated with a GnRH agonist show suppression of the untreated elevated serum GH concentrations and a decrease of plasma IGF-I concentration, although not to prepubertal values, supporting the concept that GH is the major, but not only, factor that raises circulating IGF-I levels in puberty.[392,393] A confounding factor is the relative role of hepatic-generated circulating IGF-I (endocrine role) and of locally produced IGF-I (paracrine/autocrine role) in linear growth. For example, mice with a selectively and totally deleted hepatic IGF-I gene have strikingly reduced circulating levels of IGF-I but normal postnatal body and bone growth.[402,403]

GH stimulates local IGF-I production in resting zone chondrocytes, located at the epiphyseal end of the growth plate in the area known as the reserve zone or stem cell zone,[404] and in the perichondrium through GH receptors in the chondrocytes.[405] This IGF-I production stimulates via autocrine/paracrine effects the clonal expansion of proliferating chondrocytes derived from the resting chondrocyte/germ cells; either GH or IGF-I can reduce the stem cell cycle time, proliferating cell cycle time, and duration of the hypertrophic phase, a phase that leads to apoptosis, leaving the cells serving as a scaffold for the mineralization and production of new bone.[406,407]

Urinary GH excretion reflects serum levels and changes with pubertal development[408,409] with a peak reached at pubertal stage 3 to 4, higher in boys than in girls.[410,411]

Growth Hormone Binding Protein (GHBP)

GHBP has the same amino acid sequence as the extracellular component of the GH receptor and serum concentrations are directly related to the amount of cellular GH receptors; in normal

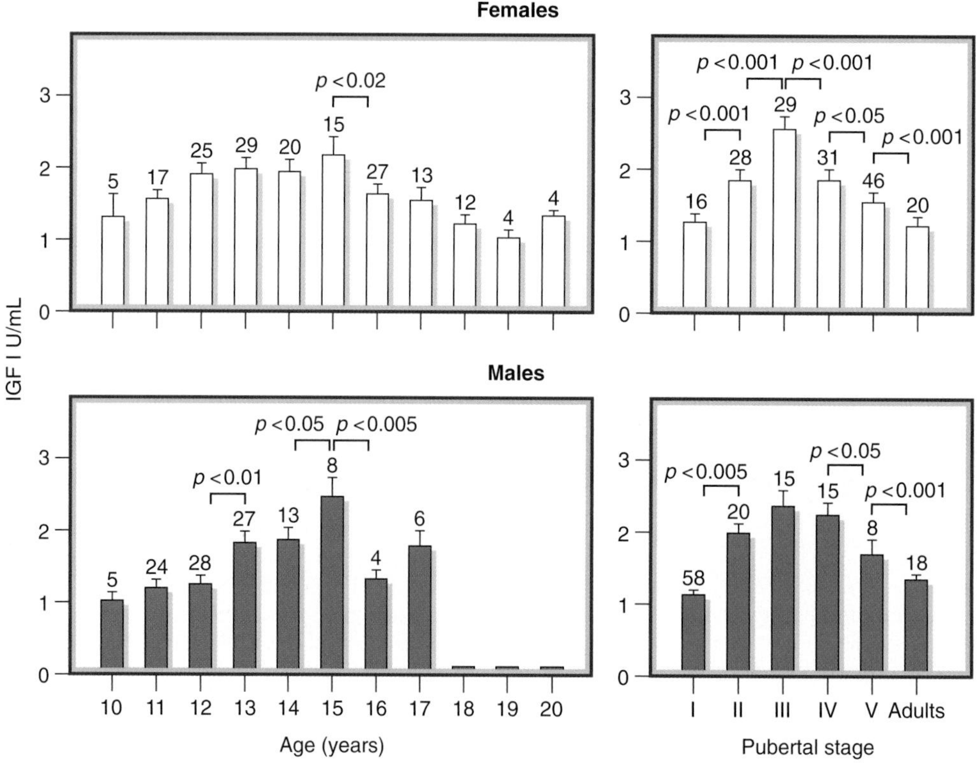

Figure 24–17 ▪ Serum insulin-like growth factor I (IGF-I; also called somatomedin C, SMC) in females and males stratified by age *(left)* and by pubertal stage *(right)*. Males attain peak IGF-I levels at 15 years (2.5±0.2 U/mL) at pubertal (genital) stage 3 (2.3±0.2 U/mL). IGF-I concentrations reach a plateau between ages 12 and 15 in females (about 2 U/mL) and peak at pubertal (breast) stage 3 (2.5±0.2 U/mL). The mean concentrations during puberty are higher than both adult and prepubertal values.

children, plasma GHBP is inversely related to 24-hour GH secretion.[412] Serum GHBP rises early in childhood and through puberty in some cross-sectional studies,[413,414] but not in others.[415] In a longitudinal study[416] in which plasma GHBP did not change appreciably with the onset of puberty, it was suggested that at the time of the pubertal growth spurt there is a relative increase in unbound (free) growth hormone in relation to GH bound to GHBP. GHBP is related to adiposity, and it may be this factor that accounts for the increased levels of GHBP in girls compared to boys, for the rise in GHBP in girls with precocious puberty, and for the negative influence of testosterone on GHBP levels.[417]

Insulin-Like Growth Factor I

Concentrations of IGF-I rise during puberty to levels higher than those of prepubertal or adult subjects, remain elevated past the time of peak height velocity with a peak attained 1 or 2 years after the pubertal growth spurt, thus later in boys than in girls, and then fall to normal adult levels (see Fig. 24–17).[392,398,413,418-420] The pattern of the GH-dependent serum IGFBP-3 in pubertal development is similar to that of serum IGF-I. However, serum IGFBP-3 concentrations correlate with BMI even though IGF-I does not.[421] Measurement of free IGF-I shows the same pattern of change with development as the measurement of total IGF-I, a slow rise in serum free IGF-I in prepuberty followed by a steeper rise during puberty.[422] A decrease of free IGF-I is described with age in the later stages of puberty.[400,423] The increase in the serum ratio of IGF-I to IGFBP-3 at the time of the pubertal growth spurt appears to be due to production proteolysis of IGFBP-3 does not change in puberty in normal children.[421,424,425] The testosterone level in boys and the estradiol level in girls correlate with the rise in IGF-I concentration, but gonadal steroids are not the direct cause of the increase in circulating IGF-I levels; rather, GH secretion approximately doubles during puberty due to the effect of estrogen causing augmented release of GH (see earlier).

Serum IGF-II shows no pubertal peak and falls during adulthood in boys.

Other Hormones

Children with chronic adrenal insufficiency with appropriate replacement therapy have a normal pubertal growth spurt despite deficient adrenal androgen secretion, indicating a minimal impact of these adrenal androgens on normal growth at puberty.[426] There are glucocorticoid receptors in human growth plates, mostly in hypertrophic chondrocytes.[427]

Hypothyroid subjects lack a pubertal growth spurt even when the disorder is accompanied by sexual precocity.[428] Thyroid hormone has a permissive role in the pubertal growth spurt but is a requisite for normal growth. Hypothyroidism decreases GH secretion, affecting growth indirectly. However, thyroid hormone also interacts with the thyroid hormone receptors (TF) α1 and TFβ, whose proteins are found in early proliferating chondrocytes of the human growth plate and the mRNA found in other developing stages of chondrocytes and osteoblasts.[429,430] However, thyroid hormones also interact with the local effects of IGF-I and GH at the growth plate.[172]

Bone Age

Skeletal maturation is assessed by comparing radiographs of the hand, the knee, or the elbow with standards of maturation in a normal population.[431-434] Ossification centers appear in early life, the bones mature in shape and size and develop articulation of surfaces, and ultimately the epiphyses or growth plates fuse with their shafts. Bone age, an index of physiologic maturation, does not have a well-defined relationship in normal children to the onset of puberty as it appears to be more variable than chronologic age.[435] However, bone age is useful for predicting the age of menarche and in boys the onset of normal, premature, and delayed puberty correlates better with the onset of secondary sexual development than does chronologic age. Bone age advancement has no relationship to the passage through puberty in normal boys.[435] Some studies suggest a strong relationship between the timing of the pubertal growth spurt and rate of skeletal maturation.[436] The timing and rate of growth in stature and rate of skeletal maturation are highly integrated genetic processes.[163] Another view is that while peak height velocity occurs at limited range of bone ages, the takeoff of the pubertal spurt occurs at a wider range of bone ages.[437]

Bone age, height, and chronologic age can be used for the prediction of final adult height from the Bayley-Pinneau tables[438] or by the use of the RWT,[439] Tanner-Whitehouse,[432] or Walker[440] techniques. Skeletal maturation is more advanced in girls than in boys of the same chronologic age as the early pubertal bone ages of 11 years in girls and 13 in boys are equivalent stages of bone maturation by the hand-wrist method. African-American children have slightly more advanced bone ages than do Caucasian children of the same chronologic ages.[441] difference between bone age and chronologic age must exceed 2 SD to be of biologic significance. Standard deviations of bone age in normal children may range from a few months in infancy compared to 1 year in later adolescence; thus, a 2-year variation of bone age from chronologic age is within normal limits in middle teenage years. As commonly estimated, bone age is imprecise and a qualitative measure rather than a quantitative measure.[433] The development of techniques for scanning radiographs coupled with computer analysis may increase the precision of the procedure.[442-445]

Patients with hemiplegia due to cerebral palsy have a less advanced bone age on the affected side than the normal side.[446] This difference (mean of 7.3 months) is greater than the difference noted between left and right side in normal children (less than 6 months). In cerebral palsy, diminished linear growth (height), low lumbar-spine bone density, and low body fat as measured by triceps skinfolds were all independently associated with delays in skeletal maturation.[447]

Skeletal Density

Osteoporosis and osteopenia are important conditions of the adult which have origins in youth; increasing interest focuses upon bone health in children and adolescents, including the effects of nutrition, exercise, and genetics on normal skeletal development.[448-450]

Areal bone mineral density represents a two-dimensional image and is a function of the size of bone; this is the measurement most often available clinically with commercial DXA devices. The mineral content of the bone attenuates the radiation beam; this is what is classically considered when measuring bone density using commercial DXA devices. Smaller bones attenuate the radiation beam used for detection less than do larger bones, and this factor must be considered in interpretation. Bone mineral density of the total body, lumbar spine, and femoral neck measured by dual energy X-ray absorptiometry increases at a mean annualized rate of 0.047 g/cm^2 for boys and 0.039 g/cm^2 for girls. Recent data from longitudinal total body DXA study suggest that boys accumulate 407 g/yr and girls 322 g/yr of mineral or 359 mg/day for boys and 284 mg/day for girls; thus, 26% of adult calcium is laid down during the 2 adolescent years of peak calcium accretion of 14 years (mean) for boys and 12.5 years for girls.[451] Bone mineral density approaches a peak in girls by the age of 16 years, and in boys by about 17 years, the difference in the timings related to the disparity in peak height velocity; the rate then decreases reaching a plateau in the third decade of life.[452,259] While quantitative computed tomography (CT) scanning demonstrates an increase in the cortical bone density of the lumbar spine with age, less increase in cancellous bone density with age occurs until the later stages of puberty.[453] Increased bone mineral density correlates well with height, weight (a main determinant of bone density in adolescent and postpubertal females),[454,455] age, pubertal development, and BMI, but has less relationship with serum IGF-I.[456,457] Some consider the concept of age of peak bone density attainment too simplistic and prefer to consider the strength of the bone and its geometry.[458]

Volumetric bone density Apparent Volumentric Bone Mineral Density (BMAD) represents the amount of bone within the periosteal envelope and is of more physiologic importance as it does not rely upon the size of the bone that is changing during growth (Fig. 24–18). Volumetric bone density grows in a region-specific pattern, and conditions in childhood and adolescence that affect the accrual of bone mineral have a differing effect based upon the length of time the affected bone has remaining to achieve its maximum mineral content; thus, deficits may occur in limb dimensions (prepuberty), spine dimensions (early puberty), or vBMD by interference with mineral accrual (late puberty).[459]

A calculation for BMAD is:

Spine BMAD = spine BMC divided by (spine area)$^{1.5}$ or spine BMC/square root of (spine area) (spine area) (spine area).

Femoral neck BMAD = femoral neck BMC divided by (femoral neck area)^2

Whole body = BMC divided by height (in cm) was used as an means of correcting for bone size

The patterns of areal or volumetric bone density differ during development.[460,461,462]

DXA manufacturer devices provide standards for BMD for young adult but until recently not for children or adolescents. Children are often referred for evaluation of osteoporosis as their DXA results are compared to young adult values when in fact they have not yet reached maximal bone density. Bone size reaches its adult value and peak height velocity occurs before maximal bone mineral content is reached[463,464]; these factors may result in a period of increased fragility and susceptibility to trauma characteristic of adolescence. Lean body mass is related to skeletal density (stronger in boys than girls) and fat mass and skeletal density (stronger in girls than boys).[465] Standards are available to interpret bone mineral content in terms of lean body mass, which appears better related to normal bone growth than chronologic age.[466]

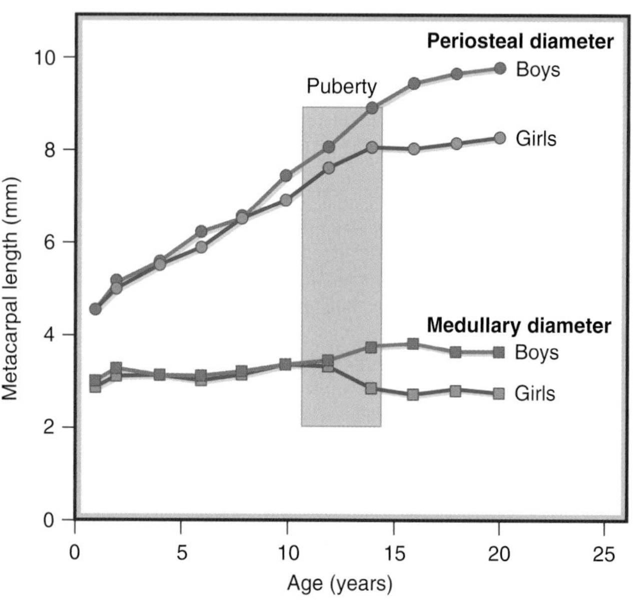

Figure 24–18 ▪ Periosteal diameter of the metacarpal bones does not differ before puberty in boys and girls. During puberty the periosteal diameter expands in boys and ceases to expand in girls whereas medullary diameter remains fairly constant in boys throughout growth but contracts in girls. [Reproduced with permission from S. Garn: Nutritional Perspectives, Charles C. Thomas, Springfield, IL, 1970 (From Seeman E. Pathogenesis of bone fragility in women and men. Lancet 2002;359[9320]:841-1850).]

There are normative data for pediatric DXA studies available from various centers, sometimes including various ethnic groups.[452,462,466-480]

An applet available on the Stanford University website (*http://www-stat-class.Stanford.EDU/pediatric-bones*) generates a Z-score for BMD or BMAD measurements at the lumbar spine (L2-4), hip, or whole body using the Hologic 1000W with respect to the age, gender, and ethnicity of the subject.

In sum, bone densitometry is useful in assessing the attainment of bone mass and the risk of osteoporosis and fracture but appropriate standards must be used in the evaluation. Quantitative ultrasound standards are in development which may simplify the process in teenagers.[481,482]

However, Seeman describes certain fallacies in interpretation of densitometry: (1) "volumetric bone mineral density (BMD) increases during growth. It does not. Growth builds a bigger, not more dense, skeleton"; (2) peak volumetric BMD is higher in men than women. It is not. Bone size is greater but is underestimated in patients with larger bones than controls. The misconceptions occur since the result of areal bone density is the BMC per unit projected bone area of the bone in the coronal plane, or an areal BMC (g/cm^2). 'Areal' is often deleted, and 'content' is replaced by density, so BMC per unit projected area is too often called 'bone mineral density' or 'BMD' while in fact volumetric bone 'density' is the desired measurement.[461] Thus, while bone mineral content may normally be higher in boys than girls and rise with development, volumetric bone density is identical in boys and girls.[483]

The increase in bone mineral density during the prepubertal and pubertal years is owing to the increase in the size of the long bones.[462] Legs grow more rapidly than the trunk in prepubertal girls, but during puberty there is more truncal growth.[484] Periosteal apposition is demonstrated by pQCT scanning of the midshaft tibia in a longitudinal study of pubertal subjects throughout puberty with no appreciable endosteal apposition.[485] Boys develop greater bone size due to increased periosteal apposition (increasing bone strength) and endosteal resorption than girls, who add bone on the endocortical surface, which may serve as a reservoir for calcium for later lactation and pregnancy.[486] Longitudinal study showed that cortical and volumetric bone mineral density increased in the radius and tibia, periosteal apposition increased before menarche, and periosteal and endomysial apposition occurred after menarche.[487] The growth rates of cross-sectional area (CSA) and BMC of the distal radius peaked at 16 and 9 months before menarche, respectively, rather than simultaniosuly.[487]

Birth weight, weight gain during infancy, and the years 9 through 12 influence bone mass achieved at 21 years.[488] The bone mineral density at the beginning of puberty predicted the peak bone mass at sexual maturity and appeared to predict the likelihood of osteoporosis as an adult in longitudinal studies suggesting a method of identification of those most in need of intervention.[489] Limb dimensions may suffer with disease in prepuberty while spine dimensions may be affected in early puberty and volumetric bone mineral content may change in late pubertal pathologic conditions (Fig. 24–19).[459,464,468,490-492]

In contrast to the long bones, volumetric bone density increases at the spine in both sexes.[459,461,468,472,490-498]

The mechanostat concept posits that developmental changes in bone strength are secondary to the increasing loads imposed

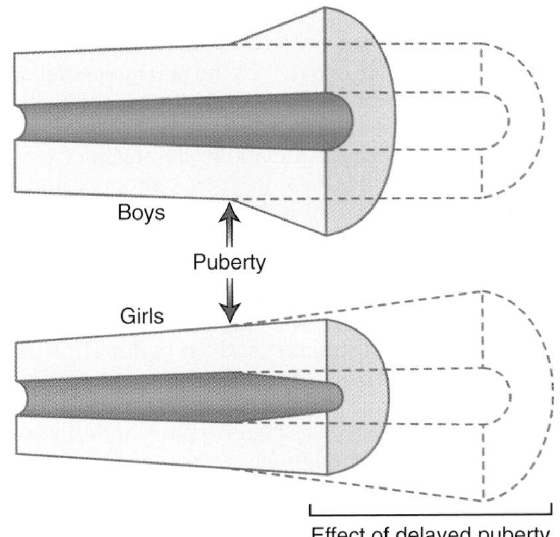

Figure 24–19 ▪ In boys, delayed puberty may reduce periosteal apposition, leaving a smaller bone with a thinner cortex but normal medullary diameter (*top*). In girls, delayed puberty may result in reduced endocortical apposition, leaving a normal or larger bone (if periosteal apposition continues in absence of the inhibitory effect of estrogen) with a thinner cortex and larger medullary diameter (*bottom*). (From Seeman E. Pathogenesis of bone fragility in women and men. Lancet 2002; 359[9320]:1841-1850).

by larger muscle forces that, in turn, stimulate bone mineral acquisition: a rise in lean body mass occurs before peak bone mineral content in longitudinal study.[499] Fat mass later exerts more influence on this process.[500,501] Increased physical activity is generally beneficial for bone health but excessive running, gymnastics, and cheerleading, for example, is progressively more likely to lead to stress fractures.[502] Femoral head strength increases markedly during puberty and femoral neck increases in density more with impact-loading sports such as running (compared to active load sports such as swimming).[503-506] Only 3 to 12 minutes of daily exercise increases femoral bone density in early pubertal children[507,508] with greater increases during puberty.[504,506,509-512]

Prepubertal girls engaged in gymnastics demonstrate increased bone density in the limbs more used and in a dose-response manner,[513,514] and longitudinal study of gymnasts and their mothers demonstrate that these effects are not mainly due to genetic influences.[515] Female adolescent middle distance runners and soccer players have increased bone density,[516] although the effects only lasts as long as activity continues.[517] However, the acquisition of mineral content in pubertal artistic gymnasts is normal when compared to bone age but delayed if compared to chronologic age.[518]

Calcium intake during puberty strongly affects bone density later in life in most, but not all, studies.[519-524] But pubertal girls are estimated to get well below recommended intake levels and even recommended levels may be too low for optimal mineralization.[495,520,525] Children avoiding dairy products without calcium supplementation have an increased prevalence of fractures in the prepubertal period, even with minor trauma.[526] Early pubertal girls cannot increase GI calcium absorption enough to compensate for a poor diet as older individuals may.[527] African-American children retain more calcium than Caucasians and the bone structure is thicker in African-American children[528]; the difference in vertebral bone density appears to develop by late puberty.[529]

Extra calcium administration may increase bone accretion and may safely be accomplished by increased dairy product intake in many sudies,[530-534] but the effect of increased ingestion of calcium may only last as long as the calcium is actually administered.[535-537] Calcium supplementation can still increase bone mineral density and lower parathyroid hormone (PTH) values if given after menarche.[538] One longitudinal study showed increased bone density in girls with calcium and exercise combined but no effect with only calcium administration,[539] whereas another showed no relationship of physical activity and calcium intake to bone density and geometry.[519] Girls with the lowest calcium intake in one study had relatively delayed bone age, delayed pubertal development, and no effect on bone density, but PTH was higher.[540] Calcium supplementation of 850 mg/day in prepuberty led to earlier menarche in longitudinal study and increased areal bone mineral density in those who had earlier menarche.[541] Increased sodium intake at the expense of calcium intake adversely affects bone accretion. Increased calcium intake does not disturb the magnesium balance of the individual. Zinc is another factor related to bone mineral density in puberty.[543]

Randomized placebo-controlled clinical trials between 1985 and 2005 in normal children extending for at least 3 months revealed a small effect of calcium supplementation in the upper limb, but the increase in BMD was not thought to influence the likelihood of a fracture later in life.[544] However, such lack of effects apply only to normal children and studies of subjects with disorders of puberty that affect bone development may reveal other findings.

There is a complex mix of genetic and environmental influences on bone mineral density.[545] Co-twin studies are designed to decrease the influence of genetics in the study of calcium-supplemented diets and bone density. A co-twin study of pubertal girls demonstrated increased bone mineral density in the spine.[546,547] Study of prepubertal twin girls determined that 9 months of high impact exercise increased BMD in the proximal femur if the children were not already active.[548] There is a correlation between the bone density of children and their parents with osteoporosis demonstrating the importance of the pubertal period of bone accretion; indeed, there is a relationship of bone density between generations: if the effects of age and puberty are eliminated,[520,549,550] 60% to 80% of variance in peak bone mass is attributed to genetic factors.[520]

Vitamin D status is also of concern in that 32% of girls with low calcium intake were also vitamin D–deficient and had elevated serum PTH and Tartrate-resistant acid phosphatase 5b (TRAP) 5b, as well as significantly lower cortical volumetric BMD of the distal radius and tibia shaft[551]; another 46% had low normal concentrations of vitamin D. Thus, deficient calcium and vitamin D can lead to secondary hyperparathyroidism in adolescence. The Fokl polymorphism of the vitamin D receptor is related to calcium absorption and total body calcium for those adolescents taking in more than 800 mg/day compared to those taking in less.[552] The Fokl F allele is related to total body BMD and spine BMD but not femoral neck BMD more than the ff alleles.[553]

Girls with heterozygote ER-α genotype (Pp) and high physical activity (PA) had significantly higher bone mass and BMD as well as thicker cortex at loaded bone sites (as compared to the distal radius, which is not a weight-bearing bone) than their low counterparts.[554] The results suggest that high physical activity benefits those with heterozygous ER genotypes and one may compensate one's less favorable Pp genotype by increasing leisure PA at early puberty.

Studies of male athletes are less common than those of girls, but 16- to 19-year-old athletic boys can still gain more bone mass in the spine and femora than nonathletic controls.[555] In the prepubertal stage, boys actively engaged in soccer have greater BMD in lumbar and femoral areas.[556]

Abnormalities of puberty impair bone accretion in both sexes and is mainly a consequence of estrogen deficiency, either due to decreased secretion or peripheral aromatization of androgens. Urinary adrenal C19 hormone metabolites are related to achievement of increased proximal radial diaphyseal bone strength.[557] Prepubertal boys with constitutional delay in puberty have decreased bone density for age[558] and decreased areal bone density as adults in early studies[559-561]; however, normal volumetric bone density was more recently found in adults previously affected by constitutional delay, or primary hypogonadism,[562-565] demonstrating catch-up to normal values of bone density with maturation, but reduced total-body bone mass caused by by reduced limb bone mass and size.[566] Cross-sectional study of boys with constitutional delay suggested normal bone turnover during this period.[567]

Testosterone administration in normal prepubertal boys increases calcium retention and bone growth,[568] increases bone density in adolescents with constitutional delay,[563] raises serum osteocalcin, and increases bone density in male hypogonadotropic hypogonadism.[569] Bone density is increased in females with excess androgens.[570-572] Decreased bone density occurs in Klinefelter's syndrome; testosterone replacement is recommended in those with low serum testosterone.[573] Girls with anorexia nervosa, hypothalamic amenorrhea, or ovarian failure have decreased bone density.[574-576] Children with true precocious puberty have increased bone density but successful treatment with GnRH agonist decreases bone density again.[577-581]

Bone turnover is reflected by changes in biochemical markers. The most significant indicators of bone turnover are bone-specific alkaline phosphatase, osteocalcin, and urinary deoxpyridinoline, which reach a peak at midpuberty and decrease thereafter. Lesser changes are reflected in concentrations of carboxyterminal pyridinoline cross-linked telopepetide, immunoreactive urinary pyridinolines, and urinary galactosyl hydroxylysine.[270] Estrogen appears responsible for the decrease in bone turnover in late puberty.[582] Evolutionary theory suggests that positive effects of estrogen on bone density added to mechanical loading allow women to carry increased weight for pregnancy and lactation; this process is unnecessary after reproduction so osteoporosis becomes more common at menopause.[583]

Body Composition

Lean body mass, skeletal mass, and body fat are equal in prepubertal boys and girls, but by maturity, men have 1.5 times the lean body mass and almost 1.5 times the skeletal mass of women, whereas women have twice as much body fat as men. Lean body mass increases by 6 years in girls and 9.5 years in boys. Boys aquire fat-free mass more quickly and for a longer period than girls during puberty; stability is attained by 15 to 16 years in girls and 2 to 3 years later in boys.[320] Fat mass increases in girls at an average rate of 1.14 kg/yr while boys do not change fat mass during the pubertal years, leading to a greater value in girls than boys with age.[320] Graphs of percent change per year in lean mass, bone mineral composition, and fat mass demonstrate characteristic patterns with development.[584]

Weight is not necessarily a reflection of body fat: the BMI (calculated as weight/height^2) is often invoked in describing the shape of the body in age-adjusted terms and is used as a better, if imperfect, reflection of body fat.[585-587] BMI changes with age and there is no specific number indicating normal or abnormal BMI at all stages of development as there is for adults. Thus, reference to charts of BMI versus age and sex between the 3rd and 97th percentiles are available at *www.CDC.gov* for interpretation of BMI values.

Increased visceral fat (or the intraabdominal adipose tissue [IAAT]) in obese teenagers is associated with hypertriglyceridemia, decreased high-density lipoprotein (HDL) cholesterol and small denser, cholesterol-laden very-low-density lipoprotein (VLDL) particles; subcutaneous fat is associated with large, lipid-laden VLDL particles, which are removed directly from the circulation and pose less risk.[588,589] The subcutaneous adipose tissue that leads to visibly different body forms is only an imperfect reflection of this internal distribution of fat cells,[590] as increased IAAT may cause metabolic derangements without increased total body fat. Recent studies support the role of increased intraabdominal fat in children as a cause of insulin resistance and dyslipidemia.[591] Waist/hip ratios may not reflect intraabdominal adipose tissue in children and adolescents,[592] but there is renewed interest in the waist circumference in children as a reflection of IAAT; standards are available.[593,594]

The generalized distribution of fat in males (central fat or apple-shaped; android), which is different from females (lower body fat predominance or pear-shaped; gynoid) develops largely during puberty as males become more android than they were in prepuberty although girls start and remain gynecoid.[595,596] There are ethnic differences in the pattern of change; Asians have the most significant changes.[597]

Dual-energy X-ray absorptiometry (DXA) is used to determine the percentage of body fat, water, and bone mineral with great accuracy,[598] but it cannot differentiate visceral from subcutaneous adipose tissue. CT scanning was used until the validation of MRI to determine intraabdominal (IAAT) subcutaneous (SAAT) fat distribution without the use of radiation.[246,599,600] In addition, equations utilize anthropomorphic data to determine IAAT and SAAT.[601]

A "strength spurt" occurs during puberty after the pubertal growth spurt.[32,602] Muscle mass is 54% of body weight in adolescent boys and 42% of body weight in adolescent girls with the difference partly due to men having more muscle cells and a greater size of individual muscle cells. There is little gender difference before 8 years of age, but by 14 years boys develop greater lean leg mass and greater power than girls.[603]

Obesity, Puberty, and the Metabolic Syndrome

Between the last two National Health and Nutrition Examination Studies (NHANES II to III), roughly in the last 20 years, there was more than a quadrupling of the prevalence of individuals over the 95th percentile for BMI for gender and age in childhood and adolescence (denoted by the CDC as "overweight") to a prevalence of 17.1% and a 50% increase in those above the 85th percentile (denoted as "at risk for overweight").[604]

Excessive body fat during childhood and adolescence has significant medical effects early and later in life.[605] Indeed, many[606-612] but not all,[613] follow-up studies extending over 4 to 6 decades show increased mortality and morbidity in adults who had increased BMI in early life.

Serum Lipids in Normal Puberty and in Obesity

Testosterone increases serum LDL cholesterol and decreases HDL cholesterol concentrations, accounting for the adverse LDL/HDL ratio in adult males compared with adult females.[614,615] Post-heparin hepatic lipase activity is increased by exogenous androgens (and decreased by estrogens), accounting for the decrease in HDL after androgen treatment or after a rise in endogenous androgen secretion.[616]

The epidemic of obesity has led to the advent of the metabolic syndrome in youth.[617-619,620-622] While familial hypercholesterolemia leads to carotid intimal plaques by puberty,[623] random autopsies demonstrate macro or micro evidence of arteriosclerosis in "normal" youth and the tendency is increased by obesity.[624] By 15 to 19 years of age, 2% of autopsied males in a recent study had advanced (American Heart Association grade 4 or 5) atherosclerotic coronary artery lesions associated with increased serum cholesterol, obesity, and hypertension.[625]

Elevated cholesterol in children and adolescents track to adult values in longitudinal studies.[617,626-629] The clustering of components of syndrome X (dyslipidemia, hyperinsulinemia) intensified as BMI increased in children studied longitudinally in the Bogalusa Heart Study.[630]

On the other hand, girls are already expressing dissatisfaction with their weight in the third to the fifth grade,[631,632] and restrictive dieting begins.[632] Depending upon the study, although there is evidence that African-American girls more often try to gain weight, apparently due to parental suggestion that they are too thin.[62,633] Nutrition suffers with dieting because the content of fruits and vegetables as well as calcium and vitamins is decreased.[632,634]

Insulin and Insulin Resistance

Insulin resistance is a hallmark of obesity and is thought to be the etiology or an associated factor in the metabolic syndrome associated with cardiac disease.[635,636] However, fasting insulin concentration increases twofold to threefold with peak height velocity, insulin secretion after a glucose load increases over prepubertal levels, insulin-mediated glucose disposal in peripheral tissues decreases in the hyperinsulinemic euglycemic clamp or the minimal model frequently sampled intravenous glucose tolerance test or IVGTT[637] showing increased insulin resistance during normal puberty[638]: insulin sensitivity is inversely related to pubertal stage and BMI.[639] The best indicators of insulin sensitivity are dynamic tests using euglycemic clamp techniques or variations of glucose tolerance tests.[618] The response of insulin to an oral glucose tolerance test is greater in African-American subjects than white subjects at all stages of pubertal development; this ethnic difference in insulin resistance is suggested as a cause for the increased incidence of non–insulin-dependent diabetes mellitus (NIDDM) in African-American adults compared to white adults[640] and appears to offer a similar explanation in the ethnic disparity in youth with Caucasians teenagers having more insulin sensitivity than African-American or Hispanic youth.[641,642] Insulin resistance is present early in the course of Turner's syndrome and thalassemia major.[643] In Turner's syndrome, there is an underlying increase in insulin resistance, but there seems to be low or absent risk of these conditions developing with GH treatment.[644]

With the recent increased prevalence in type 2 diabetes, screening criteria are proposed but remain under evaluation. At present screening is recommended for a child with BMI>85th percentile who has one of the following two criteria: (1) a family history of type 2 DM, (2) signs of insulin resistance (acanthosis nigricans, PCOS, hypertension, or dyslipidemia), or (3) is a member of certain ethnic groups (African-American, Native American, Hispanic American, and more recently, Asian American). If a fasting plasma glucose is greater than 126 mg/dL or a 2-hour postprandial value is more than 200 mg/dL, or if there are symptoms such as weight loss, polyuria, or polydipsia and a casual plasma glucose is more than 200 mg/dL, the diagnosis of DM is likely and determination of the type of DM is appropriate.[645]

Obesity is hypothesized to act as an accelerator that causes DM type 1 to appear at an earlier age but not to change the risk of the condition when a whole life is considered.[646] Girls who have the IL6-174G>C SNP, a gene influenced by estrogen, have an earlier onset of diabetes but boys do not.[647]

Patients with type 1 (insulin-dependent) diabetes mellitus usually require an increase in the dose of insulin for euglycemic control at puberty, as noted above.[648-650] The cause of insulin resistance has been attributed, at least in part, to increased fat oxidation at puberty, which correlates with rising serum IGF-I and may be linked to increased growth hormone secretion.[651] However, there is no evidence that GH treatment alone increases the likelihood of development of type 2 diabetes or impaired glucose tolerance.[652] Weight gain increases in children with type 1 DM during puberty, leading to a higher incidence of obesity in children with IDDM than expected from family patterns.[653] Some adolescents with IDDM, predominantly girls, reduce their insulin use in order to lose weight, with dire consequences.

Retinopathy due to IDDM characteristically appears in the teenage years or later, but duration and control of diabetes in the prepubertal years are contributing factors; there is an increased appreciation of the prevalence of retinopathy in the prepubertal years.[654-660] The vitreous fluorophotometry penetration ratio increases at the time of puberty, indicating a decrease in the blood-retinal barrier during this period.[661] The American Diabetes Association recommends screening for microalbuminuria, an indicator of the development of diabetic nephropathy; microalbuminuria may develop quite early in puberty rather than at the later stages as previously suggested.[662]

A normal individual adapts to the changes in pubertal insulin physiology, but an individual at risk for type 2 diabetes may not adapt to the insulin resistance and, with the accompanying defect in pancreatic β cell function,[663] characteristic of type 2 diabetes will often develop clinical type 2 diabetes during the pubertal years (or earlier). Type 2 DM in children or adolescents should not be confused with the six variations of maturity onset diabetes of the young (MODY),[664] all inherited as an autosomal dominant trait with slowly progressive loss of pancreatic β cell function in individuals who need not be obese.

Several syndromes of insulin resistance combine hyperglycemia and virilization[665,666] (also see PCOS). The Kahn type A syndrome features include a lean, muscular adolescent female phenotype with acanthosis nigricans, hirsutism, oligomenorrhea or amenorrhea, and ovarian hyperthecosis with stromal hyperplasia associated with abnormalities of the insulin receptor gene. Hyperandrogenism, insulin resistance, acanthosis nigricans (HAIR-AN) syndrome and polycystic ovary syndrome (PCOS) are less severe than Kahn type A and usually manifest in adolescent females. Robson-Mendenhall is a syndrome of severe insulin resistance (possibly leading to diabetic ketoacidosis), dysmorphic facies, acanthosis nigricans, thickened nails, hirsutism, dental dysplasia, abdominal distention, and phallic or clitoral enlargement. The Robson-Mendenhall syndrome, similar to the Donahue Leprechaunism syndrome, which shares some features, is due to homozygous or compound heterozygote defects in the insulin receptor gene. Kahn type B syndrome is due to inhibitory or stimulatory antibodies to the insulin receptor, sometimes with acanthosis nigricans and ovarian hyperandrogenism; this syndrome can occur in ataxia-telangiectasia syndrome of otherwise normal adolescents. Individuals with the Seip-Berardinelli syndrome combine lipodystrophy and severe insulin resistance and complete or partial absence of subcutaneous fat with increased growth and skeletal maturation, muscle hypertrophy, acanthosis nigricans, hypertrichosis, organomegaly, and mild hypertrophy of the external genitalia. Most of these NIDDM syndromes can be treated with oral hypoglycemic agents initially; progression of the disorder may require the use of insulin. Several girls with these syndromes of insulin resistance are described with low serum gonadotropin values but the expected hyperinsulinism; none even if in stage 4 of pubertal development responded to GnRH and all but one had at least one enlarged ovary, suggesting a direct role for insulin in stimulating the growth of the ovary.[667] The hypoleptinemic state of various degrees of lipodystrophy does not appear to affect pubertal progression but administration of leptin to such individuals has led to resumption of menstrual periods in some women and adjustment of testosterone production toward normal in males.[668]

Insulin resistance is characteristic of the state of functional ovarian hyperandrogenism seen after a history of premature pubarche[669]; these two conditions are more frequent in children with a history of low birth weight.[669-672] Obese teenage girls with predominant abdominal adiposity have insulin resistance and are at higher risk for the development of breast cancer; abdominal adiposity may be recognized in the prepubertal state and is associated with early puberty, early menarche, and a longer exposure to an endocrine profile predisposing to breast cancer.[186,673-676]

Blood Pressure

Blood pressure (BP) is related to the height of the child using appropriate standards (the latest standards are available at *http://pediatrics.aappublications.org/cgi/content/full/114/2/S2/555*). BP increases with pubertal maturation, related to increased stature, but now hypertension is becoming common in puberty as a comorbid condition of obesity.[677] Increased BP at puberty is dependent upon BMI[678] as well as height, factors that are interrelated.[620,679-691] BP in childhood and adolescence is predictive of adult BP (tracking across development).[618,687,692,693] BP rises in African-American children at lower BMIs than in Caucasian children, making the problem worse in the African-American population. In sexual precocity, BP rises above prepubertal levels to values commensurate with body size and BMI.[694]

CENTRAL NERVOUS SYSTEM ANATOMY, FUNCTION, AND EEG RHYTHM

Brain anatomy and function changes substantially during late childhood and adolescence. Behavior and psychopathology that becomes evident at this time has its orgins in these changes as well as exposures dating from early life and the prenatal period, all interacting with a genetic basis. Puberty is the time of appearance of the ability to solve complex problems in a mature manner. There is an increase in cortical metabolic rate in infancy followed by a late childhood decline to adult levels; this decline ceases by the end of the second decade. The prefrontal association cortex, an area of the brain concerned with forward planning and regulatory control of emotional behavior, continues to develop until the age of 20.[6] Stress at various stages of development may cause psychological manifestation during puberty long after the occurrence in early childhood.[695]

The anatomic changes revealed by functional MRI studies of the prefrontal cortex, an area involved with emotional regulation and planning, which occur during a time of physical maturation are likely to relate to many of the characteristic behavior changes of puberty.[6] The volume of white matter increases linearly between 4 and 22 years due to an increase in myelination during development while there are more complex changes in gray matter.[696-699] A reduction in cortical synaptic density and neuronal density,[700] analogous to programmed cell death, occurs between 2 and16 years, and this "pruning" of synapses appears linked to improved memory.[701] This change in gray matter follows a U-shaped curve of increase from age 6 years. Recent longitudinal studies utilizing dynamic mapping of human cortical development demonstrate that higher order association cortices (e.g., those involved in executive function, attention, and motor coordination) mature after lower order somatosensory, motor, and visual cortices mature, and those areas phylogenetically older mature before new ones.[702,703] However, it is not yet possible to determine the effects of endocrine changes of puberty on brain remodeling or vice versa in humans, although studies on the subject are underway.[704]

Brian plasticity decreases during puberty; the inability to learn to speak a foreign language without an accent after puberty[705] or recovery of a child from the effects of a CNS injury that in an adult might lead to aphasia are examples. Such loss of plasticity may be maladaptive to our rapidly changing world and extended life span compared to prehistoric times.[706] Plasticity allowed developmental learning before puberty, but lack of plasticity and a standard response to conditions in the adult allowed success in that static environment.

Mania, depression, obsessive-compulsive disorders and schizophrenia are more common after puberty, postulated to be related to alterations in the normal changes in brain architecture and function that occur during puberty.[707,708]

Sleep Patterns In Puberty

Increased sleep is characteristic of the period of growth and development across species.[709] Because sleep is a time of vulnerability, threats leading to stress is antithetical to normal sleep and a feeling of safety is thought to be necessary to allow sleep to proceed normally as the adolescent is preparing for independence and increased self-care in a possibly hostile world.[709] A rising complexity of brain function during puberty is reflected in increases in the amplitude and frequency of delta waves (0- to 3-Hz EEG waves) is found during deep sleep.[710] The function of deep sleep (slow-wave or non-REM sleep) is thought to be restorative[711] to learning, and other activities of the waking state and the most restorative portion is during high-amplitude delta-wave sleep. During adolescence, the time spent in deep (stage 4) sleep declines by 40% to 50% and increased (19.7%) stage 2 sleep occurs with pubertal development.[712] The decline of slow-wave sleep during adolescence may reflect developmental changes of the brain.

When an individual is allowed to "run free," the period is entrained (synchronized) to the earth's 24-hour light-dark cycle,[713] as humans had little to do after dark and evolution favored an early bedtime, but within this schedule developmental changes occur. One-year-old infants sleep an average of 11 hours per day while by age 18 the mean, if circumstances permit, is 8 hours.[709] Older people have earlier waking times and rate themselves as more morning-like than adolescents or young adults; as children are also morning-like, there is a U-shaped curve of preferred times of awakening with development. This change to "eveningness" from "morningness" during puberty appears related to biologic, in contrast to social, factors (in the past social factors were previously thought to be more important).[714,715] Thus, without the pressure of work, school, and the like, adolescents would stay up longer and awaken hours later than a normal weekday schedule would dictate—a schedule far different than they followed at a younger age.[716] Those adolescents with early school starts awaken earlier than those with later school starts, but do not change the time they go to sleep, leading to great variation in the amount of sleep attained.[717] Data from the National Longitudinal Study of Adolescent Health showed decreased self-reported sleep duration during self-reported pubertal development with females reporting more problems with sleep (e.g., insomnia, insufficient sleep, awakening tired) as puberty progressed, with no such relationship in males.[718] Futhermore, there is an increase in daytime sleepiness during adolescence, particularly during midpuberty up to stage 3-4, even if total sleep time is held constant during longitudinal multiyear studies.[709] With voluntary sleep deprivation, such as is found with late night homework habits, sleepiness can reach levels seen in narcolepsy and sleep apnea. Adolescents adapt more poorly to changes in sleep patterns, such as is seen in the difference in hours awake between the school week and the weekend, than other age groups, and are able to shift to a later schedule more easily than shifting to an earlier schedule.[719] When self-selected bedtimes are late during summer but have to be changed to allow school attendance, the adjustment is particularly lengthy and difficult in adolescents returning to school.

It was recently proposed, after study of 27,000 individuals, that the point of inflection from eveningness during adolescence (following morningness in childhood) to morningness in adulthood might be a useful marker to the end of adolescence, a sign that the developmental remodeling of brain pathways is completed.[720,721] The age of this inflection point is about 20.9 years in males and 19.5 years in females having an earlier change than males (Fig. 24–20).

Normal Pubertal Behavior and Pathology in Puberty

While the attainment of an adult role in society occurs within a few years of achievement of reproductive maturity in non-Westernized societies,[722] the more technologically advanced the society, the more protracted the length of time society allows for adolescent psychosocial development.[723] The prolonged current period of the "adolescence role" in society, ranging from the ages of 11 years to 20 years in America, arose recently in human history, dating to no more than the last 100 years in Western society (Fig. 24–2).

"The most important psychological and psychosocial changes in adolescence are the emergence of abstract thinking, the growing ability of absorbing the perspectives or viewpoints of others, an increased ability of introspection, the development of personal and sexual identity, the establishment of a system of values, increasing autonomy from family and personal independence, greater importance of peer relationships of sometimes subcultural quality, and the emergence of skills and coping strategies to overcome problems and crises."[724]

Adolescence may be divided into three periods by chronologic age: early, middle, and late adolescence. However, these periods may be reached at different "maturational" ages since rates of physiologic maturation differ in individuals within these age groups.[725-727]

Early adolescence, during ages 11 to 15 years, encompasses most of the physical changes of puberty and includes a profound social change from the sheltered, single classroom environment of elementary school to the multiple classroom and multiple teacher experience of junior high school. The individual develops a maturing, but not mature, abstract thought and decision-making processes in contrast to the concrete reasoning of childhood.

Middle adolescence, ages 15 to 17 years, the period of the high school years, is a calmer period than early adolescence; the school experience is not a striking change and many of the most prominent biologic and physical changes of puberty are past. There is acceptance of some increased autonomy (drivers' permits and licenses are allowed), but the individual still lives

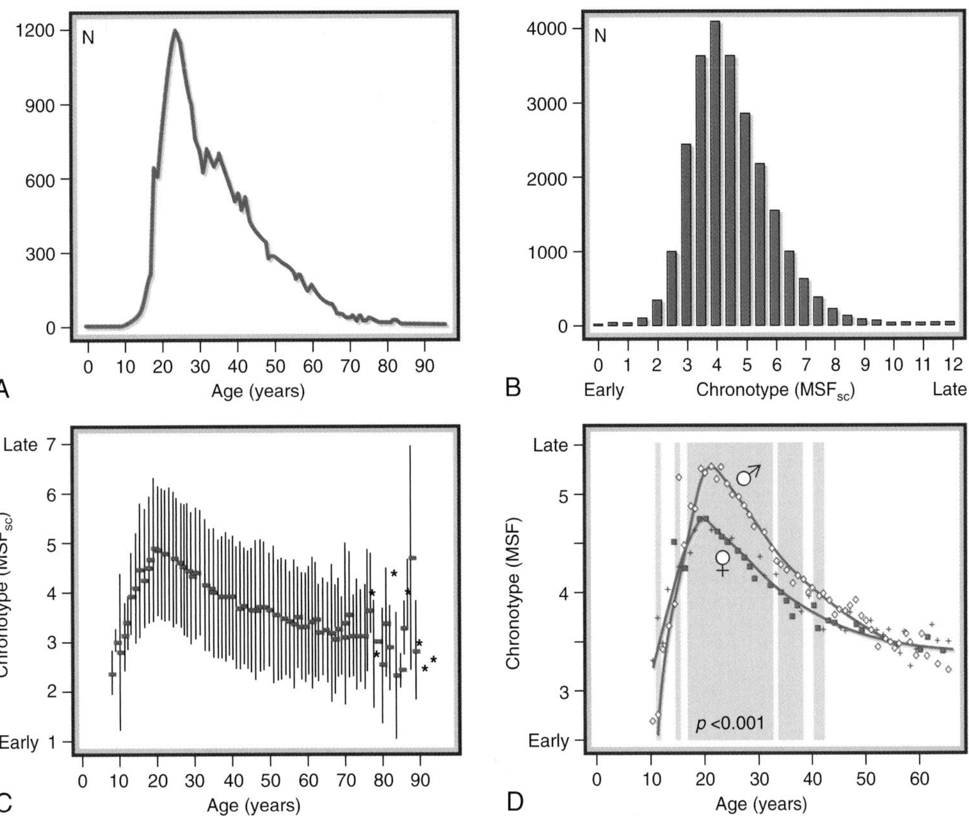

Figure 24–20 ▪ Assessment of chronotype using the MCTQ database (N≈25,000). (A) Age distribution within the database. (B) Distribution of chronotypes. (C) Age-dependent changes in average chronotype (± SD) are highly systematic (except for the age groups of 19, 21, 22, and 23, all other age-dependent averages ± SD are significantly different from that of age group 20; t-test, $p < 0.001$). (D) Age-dependent changes of chronotype are different for males and females (filled circles and black line: females; open circles and gray line: males). Gray areas indicate significant male–female differences (t-test, $p < 0.001$). (From Roenneberg T, Kuehnle T, Pramstaller PP, et al. A marker for the end of adolescence. Curr Biol 2004;14[24]:R1038-R1039).

at home. The individual emotionally moves away from the family and is less influenced by his or her peer group than are early adolescent individuals; friendships take an increasingly important role.

Late adolescence starts at the senior year of high school and is the age of acceptance of adult roles in work, family, and community. If the individual attends college, this stage is prolonged.

Behavior and Normal Puberty

Almost 100 years ago, Hall,[728] without using what would be considered contemporary research techniques, characterized the maturing child as experiencing "Sturm und Drang" (storm and stress), which is normally restrained by cultural influences. Contrary to this view, most recent empirical studies describe adolescent development as a continuous, adaptive phase of emotional growth more characterized by stability than disorder and by harmonious relationships between generations rather than conflict.[723,729] While mood changes are normally more rapid and marked in the teenage years than in adults (occurring over hours or days), these shifts must be differentiated from longstanding mood and behavior changes of serious psychopathology. Thus, "turmoil" or truly tumultuous behavior in adolescence is not a normal phase but may reflect actual psychopathology that will require diagnosis and treatment.[722]

A 4-year longitudinal study of normal first-year U.S. high school students showed that 25% experienced "continuous growth" characterized by smooth, well-adjusted functioning despite stressful situations; 34% experienced "surgent growth," demonstrating good adaptation in general and short periods of difficulty and distress after some stressful situations; and 21% were judged to be in "turmoil," characterized by mood swings, anxiety, and depression and mainly came from homes characterized by conflict, familial mental illness, and socioeconomic distress.[730] Many with adolescent turmoil "did not grow out of it" when studied 5 years later and had eventual diagnoses of unipolar and bipolar depressive disorders.[731] It may be concluded that 80% to 90% of adolescents do well psychologically during puberty and are happy individuals, but 10% to 20% have significant difficulties.[732]

Mood and Self-Image in Puberty

Young girls at the beginning of puberty frequently exhibit a negative self-image but positive body image, positive peer relationships, and superior adjustment improvement are noted with continued breast development.[733] Mood in adolescence is not closely related to stage of puberty but a significant curvilinear trend for depressive affect (increase, then decrease), impulse control (decrease, then increase), and according to level of serum estradiol.[734] Such data suggest that hormonal changes may be more important than physical changes as determinants of certain mood and behavior patterns at adolescence.

Behavior in Variations of the Normal Age of Onset of Puberty

Within the normal limits of pubertal development, early maturing girls and late maturing boys have the greatest prevalence of adjustment reactions in puberty and thereafter.[735] Both boys and girls who mature earlier have an increased risk of sexual abuse.[736]

While early developing boys are perceived to be more mature, attractive, and smart, and are given more leadership roles, late developing boys are more insecure, more susceptible to lower levels of self-esteem and body image,[737] and more vulnerable to peer pressure, especially in working class and minority groups. Much of the problem of late maturation is said to focus upon the decreased height of the individual rather than the lack of sexual development.[738] Social maturation lags even after androgen treatment in severe constitutional delay in puberty.[739] Delayed social maturation may put boys at risk for missing educational opportunities.[740]

In contrast to boys, early maturing girls tend to experience more difficulty, especially in the junior high school setting where they may attract the attention of older, more mature boys and have a higher prevalence of internalizing symptoms and disorders.[741] Early puberty may lead to negative body image in girls, compared to boys in whom the effect is positive. Early maturation may increase a propensity to violent behavior, which is fostered by living in a disadvantaged neighborhood.[742] Early pubertal maturation in girls may be related to a small IQ advantage over late maturing girls.[743] Late maturing girls are often more comfortable, remaining with the support of their families longer and are less often brought to medical attention than late maturing boys.[722] Both early and late maturing girls have a tendency to engage in health risking behaviors involving strategies to lose weight, strategies to increase muscle, disordered eating, use of food supplements and steroids, and exercise dependence, tendencies not found in boys at the same developmental stages.[744]

Menarche is delayed in lean ballet dancers compared to a control group of non-ballerina girls of the same age and compared to their own mothers.[745] The dancers studied were less likely to date than age-matched peers and while menarcheal status had no effect on dating behavior in non-dance controls, the dancers who did achieve menarche were more likely to date.[746]

Psychological Problems and Puberty

The age of onset of many psychological conditions appears to have decreased.[6] When the conditions extend from adolescence to the adult stage, they are more severe. Longstanding psychopathology may first appear and be misdiagnosed as a temporary problem of adjustment reactions of adolescence.[747]

Depression in Puberty

Reports of attempted suicide increase sharply during puberty, and suicide now ranks fourth as a cause of death among 15- to 19-year-olds.[723,748,749]

Depression becomes more frequent in girls than girls by midpuberty.[750,751] The frequency of depression correlated better to serum sex steroid concentrations than to LH or FSH values or the physical changes of puberty.[752] Because late menarche is related to increased likelihood of depression in adult women, production of estrogen may be a factor.[753]

Changes in the stress response with pubertal development, in girls more than in boys, is implicated in the development of various psychopathological diagnoses in childhood depression.[754,755] It is postulated that periods of biologic transition, such as puberty, are times of increased psychological vulnerability, which allows depression to manifest due to a malfunction of the stress response.[756]

An estimated 1.7% to 5.5% of adolescents have seasonal affective disorders[757] with dysregulated circadian activity rhythms.[758]

Panic attacks usually first appear during puberty.[759]

Schizophrenia in Puberty

Childhood onset of schizophrenia is rare but the prevalence rises with the onset of puberty and boys are more often affected than girls. Because adult onset of schizophrenia is more common in women than men, estrogen may raise the threshold for schizophrenia in women until the age of menopause when more severe cases occur in women than in men.[760]

The increase in schizophrenia at puberty may be due to anatomic changes in the prefrontal cortex that have been studied in monkeys.[761] Remodeling of this area may be particularly vulnerable to adverse influence at the time of puberty.

Risk-Taking Behavior

Adolescents who function at lower levels of cognitive complexity or concrete thinking and have an early onset of puberty demonstrate an increase in risk-taking behavior.[762,763] The age of onset of cigarette smoking and alcohol use is proportional to the age of onset of puberty in girls; earlier maturing girls partake earlier; boys may follow the same pattern.[764,765]

Sexuality in Puberty

Early and middle adolescence is the period of introduction to sexuality for many, but not for a majority of teenagers.[766-768] There was an increase in sexual intercourse in urban teenage girls between 1971 and 1981.[768] In the last decade, the mean age of first intercourse was 17.5 years for Caucasian males, 15.5 years for African-American males, 17 years for Hispanic males, 18.5 years for Caucasian females, 17.5 years for African-American females, and 18.5 years for Hispanic females.[766,768] By age 15, only 13% of teenage girls have ever had sex, but by 17 years, the totals rise above 50% with 52% of girls and 59% of boys reporting intercourse. By the time they reach age 19 years, 7 in 10 teenagers have engaged in sexual intercourse (*http://www.guttmacher.org/pubs/fb_sex_ed02.html*). Factors such as the onset of puberty, weak self-concept, having tried smoking or drinking, and not being overweight were significantly associated with early sexual activity in girls. For boys, older age, a poor relationship with parents, low household income, and having tried smoking were factors significantly associated with sexual activity.[769]

Fertility is reached well before adult phenotype is acquired. Although there has been a 27% decrease in pregnancies in African-American girls 15 to 17 years old (99.5 to 72.9 per 1000), and a 6% decrease in Caucasians (25.7 to 24.1 per 1000) over the last 20 years, the problem is still substantial. In 2000, there were 8519 births to mothers 10 to 14 years of age, the lowest value since 1966, a rate of 0.6 per 1000 in the US.[299]

Sexuality appears correlated with testosterone production in boys in some studies, but in others it appears modified by the social effects of pubertal maturation.[770-772] Correlation of salivary testosterone determinations (pitfalls of these assays are below) every month over 3 years with sexual activity in boys revealed that rising testosterone is associated with sexual activity. When pubertal status was controlled, rising testosterone was related to sexuality and falling levels to decreased sexual activity[773]; a similar pattern occurred in girls. Follicular phase levels of testosterone in girls in the eighth to tenth grades were associated with increased frequency of thinking about sex and masturbation.[774] Peer influences exerted a strong effect on masturbation activity, the progression of sexuality, and the transition to first coitus. But the relationship with testosterone became nonsignificant when Caucasian girls who attended religious services regularly were considered, while the relationship remained significant if girls who did not regularly attend religious services were considered.[775]

The social pressures are more mixed in their messages to girls, both encouraging sexuality and restricting it in a way more disparate than encountered by boys.[776] Surely, the earlier onset of puberty today compared to previous centuries has had a profound effect on societal norms of sexual behavior.[13,767-778]

A randomized, double blind, placebo-controlled, crossover clinical trial of boys and girls with delayed puberty evaluated the effects of administration of oral conjugated estrogen to girls and testosterone enanthate to boys at three dose levels, which were intended to simulate early, middle, and late pubertal levels.[779] Boys had increased nocturnal emission and touching behaviors at the mid- and high doses but no other effects. Girls demonstrated a significant increase in "necking" related to the administration of estrogen only at the late pubertal dose and no other effects. Thus, administration of physiologic (rather than higher) doses of sex steroids to boys or girls with delayed puberty had few effects on sexual behaviors and responses. However, the data included patients with various conditions, so the results cannot be directed to a single clinical disorder. Furthermore, a 3-month period may be considered too short to allow the study of the evolution of sexuality. Nonetheless, it may be concluded at present that exogenous testosterone or estrogen administered to reflect physiologic levels has modest or no significant effects on boys and girls respectively.

Analysis of data from the National Longitudinal Study of Adolescent Health (Add Health) (including approximately 12,000 adolescents enrolled in the seventh to twelfth grades) revealed adolescents at the upper and lower ends of the intelligence distribution were less likely to have sex. Higher intelligence was also associated with postponement of the initiation of the full range of partnered sexual activities.[780]

Epilepsy and Headaches in Puberty

Primary reading epilepsy, juvenile absence epilepsy, juvenile myoclonic epilepsy, and epilepsy with grand mal on awakening increases in prevalence during puberty[781,782] although, benign epilepsy with centrotemporal (rolandic) spikes, the most common idiopathic epilepsy, often goes into remission at puberty. While GABA is an inhibitory neurotransmitter thought to restrict the onset of puberty by decreasing GnRH secretion, the use of GABAergic drugs in clinical treatment of epilepsy in children does not appear to delay of the onset or progression of puberty.[783]

Migraine headaches also increase in prevalence during puberty until there is a twofold excess in girls over boys by the late teens.[784] Indeed headache complaints were found in seventh to twelfth grade girls in contrast to the higher prevalence of musculoskeletal complaints in boys; those whose pubertal development differed from the average tended to voice more complaints.[785]

HORMONAL AND METABOLIC CHANGES IN PUBERTY (Table 24–13)

Puberty is a stage in a continuum extending from sexual differentiation and the ontogeny of the hypothalamic-pituitary gonadotropin-gonadal apparatus in the fetus to the completion of sexual maturation.[786,787] Increased amplitude and alterations of the patterns of GnRH secretion at puberty initiates and regulates the sequential increases in the secretion of pituitary gonadotropins and gonadal steroids that culminate in fertility.

Gonadotropins

Because of the pulsatile secretion of GnRH, gonadotropin secretion is also episodic. The measurement of gonadotropins has

TABLE 24–13 CARDINAL HORMONAL CHARACTERISTICS OF PUBERTY

Increased amplitude of LH pulses (initially at night)
Increased LH response to intravenous GnRH
Increased estradiol secretion in girls and testosterone secretion in boys
Increased GH secretion
Increased serum IGF-I concentration
Increased prolactin secretion in girls

GH, Growth hormone; *IGF-I*, insulin-like growth factor I; *LH*, luteinizing hormone; *GnRH*, gonadotropin-releasing hormone.

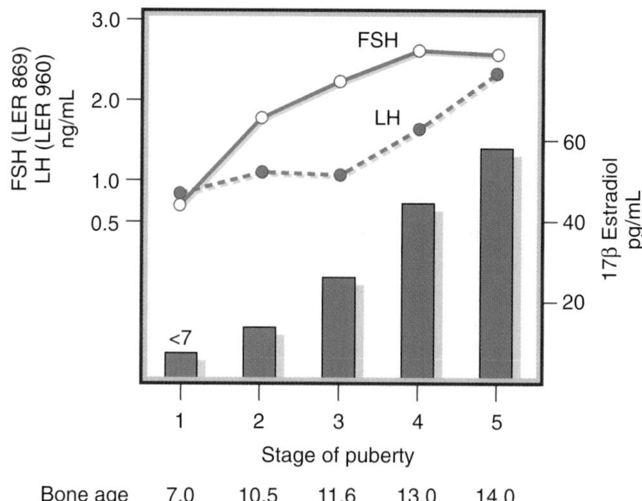

Figure 24–21 ■ Mean plasma estradiol, follicle-stimulating hormone (FSH), and luteinizing hormone (LH) concentrations in prepubertal and pubertal females by pubertal stage of maturation (1=prepubertal; 5=menstruating adolescents) and the mean bone age for each stage. Single daytime values of gonadotropins have limited usefulness because of pulsatility of gonadotropin release and the increased amplitude of LH pulses during sleep through puberty. The gonadal steroid values, however, are useful in determining the stage of pubertal development. To convert FSH values (LER-869) to international units per liter, multiply by 8.4. To convert LH values (LER-960) to international units per liter, multiply by 3.8. To convert estradiol values to picomoles per liter, multiply by 3.671. (From Grumbach MM. Onset of puberty. In Berenberg SR, ed. Puberty, Biologic and Social Components. Leiden: HE Stenfert Kroese, 1975:1-21. Reprinted by permission of Kluwer Academic Publishers.)

increased from relatively insensitive and nonspecific assays to the newer immunometric supersensitive assays that allow accurate measurement in small pediatric samples that may be obtained in sequence without harm due to excessive volume. The results of measurements using these ultrasensitive assays allow the accurate determination of basal levels of serum LH and FSH, and the results are lower than previously reported by the older assays.

During the first 2 years after birth in girls and the first 6-8 months in boys, plasma levels of LH and FSH rise intermittently to adult values and occasionally higher but then remain low until puberty. Ultrasensitive assays and third generation assays for LH and FSH[788-794] confirm earlier evidence of pulsatile secretion of the gonadotropins in prepuberty[795-798] and indicate that the basal immunoreactive levels of LH are much lower than previously reported.[788-790,793,794] The serum FSH level is higher than the LH level in prepubertal boys and girls.[799] There is a more striking rise in serum LH amplitude by at least 1 year before the onset of puberty (the peripubertal period or the time that immediately precedes the signs of sexual maturation),[791,793,794] while FSH rises more consistently through male puberty rather than before with increased pulse amplitude.[790,793,800,801] An increase in LH pulse frequency at puberty onset was not found in cross-sectional or longitudinal studies[802] in boys[803] or girls,[794] despite the striking increase in LH pulse amplitude. An increased amplitude of LH and FSH secretion occurs at night in prepubertal boys and girls by 5 years of age,[793,794] the amplitude of such peaks increase, and daytime secretion increases with the progression of pubertal development.[788,789,796,798,804-807] The augmented release of pulsatile LH during sleep is prominent during puberty.[804,805,808] Although it has been difficult to characterize a diurnal variation of immunoreactive FSH secretion, secretion of bioactive FSH was reported to increase at night during sleep and is more resistant to testosterone-induced suppression than is immunoreactive LH.[801,809]

In girls, FSH levels rise during the early stages of puberty, and LH levels tend to rise in the later stages; from beginning to late puberty, the LH concentration rises over 100-fold. In boys, FSH levels rise progressively through puberty, and LH levels rise and reach an early plateau (Figs. 24–21 and 24–22).[790,810-816]

There is a temporal concordance of LH pulses with FSH pulses of 43%. Primary testicular failure is associated with enhanced amplitude and frequency of both FSH and LH pulses.[786,796]

Disorderly patterns of secretion of LH but not FSH were noted just before the onset of puberty followed by, first, increased orderliness in early puberty and, then, increased disorderliness again in later puberty. This suggests a more integrated feedback system operates in early puberty, which is followed by less stability.[817] Ultrasensitive LH assays provide indirect evidence of a diurnal variation of GnRH secretion with a preponderance at night; the frequency is similar to that of the early pubertal period although the amplitude of LH does not increase until the peripubertal period.[790,792,805,807,818]

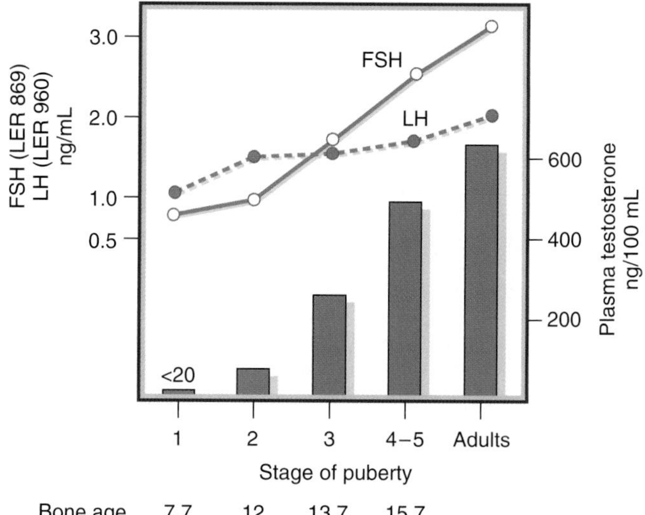

Figure 24–22 ■ Mean plasma testosterone (after solvent extraction and chromatography)[813] and gonadotropin levels in normal boys by stage of maturation (1=prepubertal) and mean bone age for each stage. (See legend for Fig. 24–21.) To convert testosterone values to nanomoles per liter, multiply by 0.03467. (From Grumbach MM. Onset of puberty. In Berenberg SR, ed. Puberty, Biologic and Social Components. Leiden: HE Stenfert Kroese, 1975:1-21. Reprinted by permission of Kluwer Academic Publishers.)

Doses of exogenous GnRH that are relatively ineffective in stimulating gonadotropin or gonadal steroid secretion before puberty become effective with the onset of puberty[786]; thus an amplification occurs in the hypothalamic-pituitary-gonadal axis with progression of puberty.[786,800,819] While the GnRH test usually requires multiple sampling after the administration of GnRH, a single determination at 30, 45, or 60 minutes may suffice with the new sensitive assays.[820] Furthermore, the use of a GnRH agonist (e.g., nafarelin leuprolide) in a single dose with determination of serum gonadotropins, and sex steroids can help differentiate the pubertal from the prepubertal state.[821,822] The basal values of serum LH and FSH measured in modern supersensitive assays are reported to predict the onset of pubertal development as well as GnRH testing; a value of serum LH greater than 0.4 mIU/mL, measured by immunochemiluminometric assay is consistent with the onset of puberty (but the cutoff will be laboratory specific).[810,815,823] Moreover, the use of these ultrasensitive assays to determine concentration of LH and FSH in urine reveals a pattern of a fivefold increase in urinary FSH in boys and girls and a 50-fold increase in urinary LH in boys and a 100-fold rise in girls during puberty.[824]

Qualitative[825] as well as the well-defined quantitative changes occur in the pattern of FSH and LH in the pituitary gland, serum, and urine during development. The pattern of glycosylation of the α and β subunits of the gonadotropins is influenced by maturation, GnRH secretion, and the action of gonadal steroids on the pituitary gonadotropes. Variation in glycosylation, which affects the size and charge of the hormone, is the principal cause of the heterogeneity of FSH and LH and the large number of isoforms that vary according to the more acidic or more basic charge.[826,827] This pleomorphism has an important effect on the biologic half-life and biologic activity, and provides an additional mechanism of regulating the biologic activity of the gonadotropins.[801,826-832] Discrepancies between serum bioactivity and immunoactivity of LH during pubertal development are reported by some,[801,809,831,833-836] but not all.[836] However, a change in the isoforms of FSH released during puberty favors the secretion of increased bioactive FSH, which may favor reproductive development.[837]

Gonadal Steroids (Table 24–14)

Only recently has it been appreciated that many actions on linear skeletal growth, skeletal maturation, and accretion of bone mass thought to be due to testosterone in the male are mainly attributable to its peripheral aromatization to estrogen.

Testosterone

The Leydig cells of the testes produce testosterone and, in lesser amounts, androstenedione, α 5-androstenediol, dihydrotestosterone, and estradiol, although a small amount of testosterone is derived from extraglandular conversion of androstenedione secreted by the testes and the adrenal.[838] In the female, extraglandular conversion of ovarian and adrenal[826] androstenedione accounts for almost all of the circulating testosterone.

Previous methods of determination of low levels of sex steroids in children have been heavily criticized as inaccurate.[839,840] In fact, the measurement of testosterone in women, where levels are similar to those of children, are suggested to be "no better than a guess."[841] This insensitivity is mainly due to the presence of interfering substances and relative insensitivity of antibodies used in assays. Now, larger national laboratories are beginning to utilize liquid chromatography tandem mass spectrometry (LC/MS-MS), which allows the accurate measurement of extremely low values present in pediatric samples.[842] This is especially critical for the determination of the concentration of plasma estradiol. Virtually all of the commercial immunoassay platforms which use unextracted plasma give spurious, high estradiol values in children.[842] These newer techniques may lead to revision of some of the results reported below.

Prepubertal boys and girls have plasma testosterone concentrations of less than 0.3 nmol/L (0.1 ng/mL)[790,793,794,813,843] (except during the first 3 to 5 months of infancy in the male, when pubertal levels are found).[279,844-846] Nighttime elevations of serum testosterone levels are detectable in the male by 5 years of age, before the onset of physical signs of puberty, and increase during early puberty after the appearance of sleep-entrained secretion of LH[790,804,847] and increased pituitary sensitivity to GnRH; the 60 minutes of lag between the peak of LH and the increase in testosterone is presumably due to synthesis and secretion of the steroid.[790,848] In the daytime, increases in testosterone levels are detectable at approximately 11 years in boys after the testis volume is greater than 4 mL, with a consistent increase throughout puberty.[813,843] The steepest increment in testosterone occurs between pubertal stages 2 and 3 in males (see Fig. 24–22 and Table 24–15).[843] The ratio of testosterone to epitestosterone in the urine, which has been used to evaluate "doping" of athletes, may be elevated normally during puberty.

Free testosterone measurements may be determined by dialysis or by calculation using testosterone values and available protein binding sites; the accuracy of the testosterone assay affects the result and can be problematic.[842] Free testosterone values are low or nondetectable until the age of normal pubertal development, at which time they rise in boys and girls.[849]

A sensitive mammalian cell recombinant bioassay for androgen bioactivity strongly correlates with serum immunoreactive testosterone concentration but not with 5α-dihydrotestosterone, dehydroepiandrosterone, or androstenedione.[850] Bioactive testosterone measured in this assay increased with pubertal development in concert with progression of pubic hair and penile development in constitutional delay in puberty.[851] Another bioassay was used to detect pesticide androgenic effects.[852] In contrast to this specific bioassay, a novel highly sensitive transcriptional androgen receptor–mediated bioassay system demonstrated higher circulating values of bioactive androgen in menopausal women than revealed by immunoassays; this assay has not yet been used in children.[853]

The values of sex steroids measured in saliva are much lower than found in the serum, but trauma (even brushing teeth) leading to blood in the specimen can influence the results and all is based upon the accuracy of the basic assay as noted above.[842] Furthermore, the steroid in saliva is not a direct representation of free steroid in the serum as is often claimed. Testosterone in saliva is said in some reports to correlate well with serum levels of testosterone in normal subjects and in patients with chronic disease such as cystic fibrosis.[854,855] Salivary progesterone is said to rise with the progression of puberty.[856] Salivary DHEA is higher after the onset of puberty than before.[857] Salivary steroid measurements, if accurate, can increase the ability of investigators to address the relationship between development and behavior in a noninvasive manner,[858] but it may take the use of LC/MS-MS in salivary assays to achieve such accuracy.

Estrogens

In the female, estradiol is secreted principally (90%) by the ovary; a small fraction of circulating estradiol arises from the extraglandular conversion of testosterone and androstenedione. In the male, approximately 75% of estradiol is derived from extraglandular aromatization of testosterone and (indirectly) androstenedione and 25% is from testicular secretion.[838] Aromatase is absent or present in barely detectable amounts in prepubertal testes but maximal amounts appear in late puberty; in normal testes, aromatase is predominantly present in the Leydig cells but in testicular tumors of either Sertoli or Leydig cells, for example, associated with the Peutz-Jeghers syndrome, the Sertoli cells of the tumor express aromatase.[859,860]

TABLE 24–14 STEROID VOLUMES IN PUBERTAL DEVELOPMENT: DIFFERING METHODS OF VARIOUS NATIONAL LABORATORIES

Gonadal Steroid	Reference Intervals								Volume Requirements (Pediatric Minimums)
Testosterone, by LC-MS/MS	Males				Females				0.18 mL serum (Quest) 0.5 mL serum (Esoterix) 0.15 mL serum (ARUP)
		Quest, in ng/dL	Esoterix, in ng/dL	ARUP, in ng/dL		Quest, in ng/dL	Esoterix, in ng/dL	ARUP, in ng/dL	
	1-10 days	<187	75-400 at term Levels decrease during first week to 20-50. Levels increase from 20-60 days to 60-400, then levels decrease to prepubertal range.	Level decreases rapidly in first week to 20-50, then increases to 60-400 between 20 and 60 days. Levels then decline to prepubertal ranges by 7 mo.	1-10 days	<24	20-64 at term Levels decrease to <10 during first month.	Levels decrease during the first month to less than 10 and remain at this level until puberty.	
	1-3 months	72-344			1-3 months	<17			
	3-5 mo	<201			3-5 mo	<12			
	5-7 mo	<59			5-7 mo	<13			
	7-12 mo	<16			7-12 mo	<11			
	Tanner stage I	<5	<3-10	<16	Tanner stage I	<8	<3-10	1-16	
	Tanner stage II	<167	18-150	2-156	Tanner stage II	<24	7-28	4-40	
	Tanner stage III	21-719	100-320	7-762	Tanner stage III	<28	15-35	10-60	
	Tanner stage IV	25-912	200-650	164-854	Tanner stage IV	<31	13-32	8-62	
	Tanner stage V	110-975	350-970	233-940	Tanner stage V	<33	20-38	12-68	
Testosterone, extraction, chromatography, RIA									0.5 mL serum (Quest)
Testosterone, chemiluminescence									1 mL serum (Quest)
Testosterone, electrochemiluminescent IA									0.3 mL serum (ARUP)

DHT, RIA	Males				Females				0.6 mL serum (ARUP)
				ARUP, in pg/mL				ARUP, in pg/mL	
			Term Newborn	50-600			Term Newborn	20-150	
			1 wk-6 mo	120-850			1 wk-9 yr	0-49.9	
			7 mo-9 yr	0-49.9			10-49 yr	50-170	
			10-19 yr	0-553					
DHT, extraction, chromatography, RIA	Males				Females				0.5 mL serum (Esoterix) 1.1 mL serum (Quest)
		Quest, in ng/dL				Quest, in ng/dL			
	1-6 mo	12-85			1-6 mo	<5			
	Prepubertal	<5			Prepubertal	<5			
	Tanner II-III	3-33			Tanner II-III	5-19			
	Tanner IV-V	22-75			Tanner IV-V	3-30			
Androstenedione, RIA	Males				Females				0.1 mL serum (ARUP)
				ARUP, in ng/mL				ARUP, in ng/mL	
	Male children			0.1-0.5	Female children			0.1-0.5	
Androstenedione, extraction, chromatography, RIA									0.25 mL serum (Esoterix) 0.5 mL serum (Quest)
Estradiol, LC-MS/MS									1.2 mL serum (Esoterix)
Estradiol, chemiluminescent immunoassay	Males				Females				0.2 mL serum (ARUP)
				ARUP, in pg/mL				ARUP, in pg/mL	
			0-8 yr	7-8			0-8 yr	7-14	
			9-10 yr	7-11			9-10 yr	7-32	
			11-12 yr	7-22			11-12 yr	7-38	
			13-14 yr	7-24			13-14 yr	10-91	
			15-16 yr	11-33			15-16 yr	17-181	
			17-50 yr	18-67			17-40 yr	23-170	

Table continued on following page 1006

TABLE 24–14 STEROID VOLUMES IN PUBERTAL DEVELOPMENT: DIFFERING METHODS OF VARIOUS NATIONAL LABORATORIES (Continued)

Gonadal Steroid	Reference Intervals						Volume Requirements (Pediatric Minimums)
Estradiol, extraction chromatography, RIA	Males			Females			0.6 mL (Quest)
		Quest, in pg/mL			Quest, in pg/mL		
	Tanner stage I	3-15		Tanner stage I	5-10		
	Tanner stage II	3-10		Tanner stage II	5-115		
	Tanner stage III	5-15		Tanner stage III	5-180		
	Tanner stage IV	3-40		Tanner stage IV	25-345		
	Tanner stage V	15-45		Tanner stage V	25-410		
Estrone, LC-MS/MS							1.2 mL serum (Esoterix)
Estrone, RIA	Males			Females			0.15 mL serum (ARUP)
			ARUP, in pg/mL			ARUP, in pg/mL	
	Prepubertal		<25	Prepubertal		<25	
	Adult		<65	Early follicular phase		<150	
				Luteal phase		100-250	
				Late follicular phase		<200	
Estrone, extraction, chromatography, RIA	Males			Females			1.1 mL serum (Quest)
		Quest, in pg/mL			Quest, in pg/mL		
	Prepubertal	5-15		Prepubertal	5-15		
	Tanner II	10-22		Tanner II	10-33		
	Tanner III	17-25		Tanner III	15-43		
	Tanner IV	21-35		Tanner IV	16-77		
	Tanner V	18-45		Tanner V	29-77		

From Albrecht and Styne, in press 2007

In the fetus and at term, estrogen is high due to conversion of fetal and maternal adrenal C19 steroids to estrogen by the placenta but drops precipitously in the first few days of life. Plasma estradiol levels are so low in prepuberty that detection by standard immunoassays was difficult, but a rise through puberty[814] and a diurnal rhythm were described (see Fig. 24–21 and Table 24–15).[861] Estrone levels rise early and reach a plateau by midpuberty.[814] A highly sensitive bioassay demonstrated higher estradiol concentrations in girls than in boys before puberty[351] with a rise through puberty until the pubertal growth spurt (there is a significant correlation between peak growth velocity and the rise in estradiol concentration (Fig. 24–13); the rise is earlier in girls than boys but bioactive estradiol levels are equivalent at peak growth velocity) and a decrease thereafter.[337,352,353] The higher estrogen levels in prepubertal girls may be an important factor in the more advanced levels of skeletal maturation in girls and play a part in the earlier onset of sexual maturation in girls than in boys.[337] Furthermore, a new human cell bioassay measuring total estrogenic bioactivity, rather than solely estradiol, in children was reported[862] with an extremely sensitive detection limit of less than 1 pg/mL.

The daily peak of estradiol in early pubertal girls occurs about 6 to 9 hours after the peak of serum LH detected during the night,[863] apparently related to time for synthesis. In all stages of puberty, boys have higher concentrations of estrone than estradiol, and levels of both estrogens are lower than those in girls at comparable stages.[790,864]

TABLE 24–15 DIFFERENCES IN THE TIMING OF THE ONSET OF ESTROGEN SYNTHESIS IN GIRLS AND BOYS

GIRLS
Follicle-stimulating hormone (FSH) from late fetal life through puberty stimulates aromatase and estrogen synthesis by the ovary.
BOYS
FSH leads to enlargement of the testes, the earliest sign of puberty in the male; spermarche occurs early in puberty and spermaturia at a mean age of 13.3 years before the sharp rise in testosterone levels and peak height velocity.
Estrogen synthesis is not detectable in fetal or prepubertal Leydig cells and is at a very low level, until luteinizing hormone stimulates
Leydig cell aromatase at late stage II to stage III of male secondary sexual maturation. Estradiol does not reach the level found in girls in early puberty who exhibit a pubertal growth spurt until at least midpuberty.

Adrenal Androgens

There is a progressive increase in plasma levels of Δ5-steroids, dehydroepiandrosterone (DHEA) and dehydroepiandrosterone sulfate (DHEAS), in both boys and girls beginning before age 8 (skeletal age of 6 to 8) and continuing through early adulthood (Table 24–16); the increase in the secretion of adrenal androgen and its precursors is known as *adrenarche* while the appearance of pubic hair caused by adrenarche is known as *pubarche*. Plasma DHEA has a diurnal rhythm similar to that of cortisol, but plasma DHEAS shows less variation and is a useful biochemical marker of adrenarche.

Sex Steroid–Binding Globulin (Testosterone-Binding Globulin)

Between 97% and 99% of circulating testosterone and estradiol is reversibly bound to SSBG; prepubertal levels of SSBG are approximately equal in boys and girls, but a decrease in TeBG level occurs with advancing prepubertal age and the concomitant increase in the plasma gonadal steroid levels. At puberty there is a small decrease in SSBG levels in girls and as a consequence of testosterone, a greater decrease in boys.[865-867] The drop noted increased activity of normal boys is attenuated in boys treated with tamoxifen even with advancing pubertal development.[868] The rise in adrenal androgen levels at adrenarche may explain the early drop in SSBG levels, which allows more circulating free hormone at a given concentration of testosterone.[869] Although the plasma concentration of testosterone is 20 times greater in men than in women, the concentration of free testosterone is 40 times greater.[870-873] Boys with hypogonadotropic hypogonadism and patients with the androgen resistance syndrome show the same characteristic fall in SSBG levels at puberty, but values are intermediate between those of normal adult males and females.[874,875] SSBG production is downregulated by GH administration in prepubertal children, perhaps

TABLE 24–16 MEAN SERUM CONCENTRATIONS OF DEHYDROEPIANDROSTERONE SULFATE DURING CHILDHOOD

	CONCENTRATION, μmol/L (ng/mL), AT CHRONOLOGIC AGE					
	6-8 yr	**8-10 yr**	**10-12 yr**	**12-14 yr**	**14-16 yr**	**16-20 yr**
Boys	0.5 (188)	1.6 (586)	3.4 (1260)	3.6 (1330)	7.2 (2640)	7.2 (2640)
Girls	0.8 (306)	3.2 (1170)	3.1 (1130)	4.6 (1690)	6.9 (2540)	6.3 (2320)

	CONCENTRATION, μmol/L (ng/mL), AT BONE AGE				
	6-8 yr	**8-10 yr**	**10-12 yr**	**12-14 yr**	**14-16 yr**
Boys	0.98 (360)	1.6 (574)	3.4 (1250)	5.8 (2150)	10.9 (4030)
Girls	0.73 (276)	3.1 (1130)	4.33 (1560)	7.1 (2610)	3.9 (1450)

Modified from Reiter EO, Fuldauer VG, Root AW. Secretion of the adrenal androgen, dehydroepiandrosterone sulfate, during normal infancy, childhood, and adolescence, in sick infants, and in children with endocrinologic abnormalities. J Pediatr 1977;90:766-770.

by the action of IGF-I.[876] SSBG is decreased in prepubertal children with diabetes mellitus.[877]

Prolactin

Prolactin levels rise in girls during puberty. Prepubertal mean (± standard error) plasma prolactin concentrations are 4.0±0.5 μg/L in boys and 4.5±0.6 μg/L in girls. Late pubertal girls and adult women have higher concentrations of prolactin (7.5±0.7 and 8.3±0.7 μg/L), whereas the mean concentration in adult men is 5.2±0.4 μg/L.[878] This sex difference quite likely is a consequence of the higher estradiol levels during puberty in girls and in women.

Inhibin, Activin, Follistatin

Originally, inhibin, activin, and follistatin were revealed by their effect on FSH secretion: inhibin and follistatin inhibit and activin stimulates FSH β subunit expression and hence FSH biosynthesis and secretion. It is now recognized that they are synthesized in a variety of tissues in addition to the gonads and have diverse activities apart from those on the reproductive apparatus.[879] Two distinct binding proteins for inhibin and activin have been described and are present in the circulation, the gonads, and other tissues: α2-macroglobulin, a high-capacity, low-affinity binding protein; and follistatin, a glycosylated single peptide chain that functions not only as a high-affinity binding protein but also as a regulator of activin bioactivity (e.g., in the pituitary gland, a site of synthesis of both activin and follistatin).[879,880] Inhibin, a heterodimeric glycoprotein product of the Sertoli cell of the testes and the ovarian granulosa cell (as well as the placenta and other tissues), exerts a direct negative feedback action on the secretion of FSH from the pituitary. Inhibin is composed of an α subunit and one of two β subunits, βA or βB, which form inhibin A or inhibin B, respectively, dimers with apparently identical function. Inhibin is a member of the transforming growth factor-β superfamily that includes antimüllerian hormone (AMH, also called müllerian-inhibiting factor) and the dimers of two inhibin subunits, activin A and activin B, which stimulate the release of FSH from pituitary cells.[879] Synthesis and secretion of gonadal inhibin is induced by FSH. Inhibin plays a role in the feedback regulation of FSH secretion during puberty in males and females.[879-881] In men, inhibin B is a major feedback regulator of FSH release.[882] (Inhibin B and inhibin A exhibit specific patterns of secretion during the menstrual cycle.[883])

The assay for plasma "inhibin" is confounded by the fact that the dimeric inhibins occur in a wide range of molecular weights, including combinations of precursor forms of each of the subunits as well as a precursor of the α-subunit of inhibin, pro-α-C. The "Monash" radioimmunoassay detects the dimeric inhibins, inhibin A and B as well as pro-α-C and related peptides, and is essentially a nondiscriminatory total inhibin assay.[884] With the development of highly specific enzyme-linked immunoabsorbent assays for the mature 31-kd inhibin A and inhibin B dimers and for inhibin pro-α-C,[879,885] the detection of sex-specific differences in the pattern of inhibin secretion has advanced our knowledge of the biologic action of inhibin and the clinical usefulness of inhibin determinations.[885-887]

During pregnancy, the placenta secretes inhibin A and the fetal membranes secrete both inhibin A and B,[888] whereas, at least for the first 20 weeks of gestation, only inhibin A was detected in maternal serum.[889] In umbilical cord serum from term female newborn infants, no inhibin dimer was detected, whereas cord serum from male newborns contained inhibin B, the only inhibin detected in adult males; the median value was 167 pg/mL.[888] In the human fetal testis α- and βB (but not βA) subunits are present in both Sertoli and Leydig cells at 16 weeks' gestation; by 24 weeks' gestation, immunoexpression of both subunits was greater in the Sertoli cells. Postnatally, the expression of both subunits was decreased by 4 months of age. Inhibin subunits were not detected in the fetal ovary, nor was immunoreactive follistatin present in fetal or neonatal gonads.[890] These findings are consistent with inhibin A and inhibin B values in midgestation and term fetuses.[891]

Immunoreactive "inhibin-like" activity measured by the Monash assay increases in both boys and girls during puberty, with mean plasma levels increasing in boys from 161 to 442 U/L and in girls from 97 to 231 U/L between stage 1 and stage 5.[892] In boys, the rise in serum immunoreactive "inhibin" was relatively constant during puberty, increasing 1.5-fold between a testis volume of 1 mL and 10 mL[893] However, as discussed above, the early "inhibin" immunoassays cross-react with inactive monomeric inhibin precursors. There is a striking sex dimorphism in the pattern of circulating inhibin B and A from fetal life through full sexual maturation.[894] In large cross-sectional studies[895,896] using highly specific inhibin B and inhibin A immunoassays, which correlate with the bioactivity of inhibin and distinguish inhibin B from inhibin A,[897] the mean concentration of serum inhibin B increased between prepuberty (a stage when it is higher than the undetectable levels in castrate men)[898,899] and the first stage of puberty; when the strong correlation with chronologic age was taken into account, a correlation with LH and testosterone values remained. From genital stage 2 puberty on, inhibin B levels were relatively constant, despite a rise in the mean concentration of serum FSH between stage II and III after which the FSH value was relatively unchanged. By genital stage III, a negative partial correlation between inhibin B and FSH was found, which persisted as puberty advanced,[895] and by genital stage IV, there was a clear negative correlation of inhibin with serum FSH.[900,901] Crofton and colleagues found dimeric inhibin B rose twice in development, reflecting the two periods of Sertoli cell proliferation during infancy and early puberty while an inverse relationship between inhibin and FSH is seen at midpuberty and thereafter indicating the development of the negative feedback inhibition.[902] In the early stages of puberty, inhibin B values closely relate to LH and testosterone but by stage 3, when inhibin B values peak, this relation is lost and inhibin B becomes more closely related to FSH.[903]

Serum inhibin A and B increase early in puberty in girls although there are individual increases in the prepubertal period directly related to FSH levels demonstrating sporadic follicular development in the infant and child due to FSH stimulation.[904] Inhibin B is predominant in the follicular phase and inhibin A during the luteal phase.[885,886,896,894] More specifically, inhibin A and inhibin B peak in mid puberty and inhibin B thereafter decreases.[905] During the early stages of puberty, inhibin B values are related to estradiol and FSH values but these relationships diminish with the progression of puberty.[906] While there is no significant change in activin during female puberty, follistatin decreases from a midpuberty peak to later values that fall below prepubertal values.

Serum values of FSH regulating proteins follow circadian patterns. In seven pubertal girls, LH and FSH were higher from 2200 to 0800 than the rest of the day, inhibin B reached a nadir between 17:00 and 22:45 hours just prior to the nighttime increase in FSH, and follistatin concentrations reached the greatest concentrations between 05:00 and 11:00 hours while activin-A concentrations declined coincident with the nighttime increase in FSH in pubertal girls.[907] Diurnal variations of inhibin B in boys in the peripubertal or early pubertal period demonstrate a fall in inhibin during the night as LH and subsequently testosterone rise, demonstrating a negative feedback effect of testosterone on inhibin B secretion.[908] FSH treatment, which raises testosterone secretion, suppresses inhibin B, demonstrating the ability of testosterone to negatively influence inhibin B secretion.[909] A study to determine the relationship between FSH and its regulatory factors at different stages of puberty invoked administration of GnRH agonist, which led to an increase in FSH by 30 minutes and an increase in inhibin B in girls older than 5 years of age by 8 hours and in boys by 20 hours.[910] Baseline inhibin B was greater in boys than girls, while baseline activin A concentrations were greater in girls and activin did not change with GnRH agonist. The administration of testosterone to boys in Tanner stage 2 led to decreased FSH and LH, increased activin, and decreased inhibin B, but no change in follistatin. Estradiol administered to girls in Tanner stage 1 or 2 led to decreased LH and FSH and increased activin A but no change in inhibin B or follistatin, while administering estradiol to girls with Turner's syndrome led to decreased serum FSH but the effectively nondetectable levels of activin and inhibin did not change.[911]

Serum inhibins and FSH are markedly elevated in chronic renal failure but are reduced after renal transplantation.[912]

A low concentration of inhibin B in men and pubertal boys is an indicator of impaired seminiferous tubule function.[913] Early pubertal boys with testicular defects have higher FSH concentrations and low inhibin levels.[914] Inhibin B is the form most closely related to testicular function and is absent in orchidectomized men.[898] Inhibin B is related to Sertoli cell function in prepuberty, but a developmental change occurs during puberty so that later in life, inhibin B is related to spermatogenesis. Prepubertal boys with the Sertoli cell only syndrome had normal inhibin B levels, whereas in postpubertal affected boys and men with Sertoli cell only syndrome and early stage spermatogenic arrest have undetectable or low levels of inhibin B while those with late stage spermatogenic arrest or obstructive azoospermia have normal or near normal levels of serum inhibin B.[899,915] It is suggested that in prepuberty both the α inhibin and β B subunits are expressed in Sertoli cells, but during puberty and in men, fully differentiated Sertoli cells express only the α-subunit and the β-subunit is expressed in germ cells; inhibin B in the adult appears to be a product of both germ and Sertoli cells. In prepubertal boys, basal plasma inhibin B concentrations have a high correlation with the incremental testosterone response to the administration of hCG and provides a useful assessment of both the presence of testes and its function. In true precocious puberty, inhibin B values are in the pubertal range and decrease with GnRH agonist therapy. [916]

Antimüllerian Hormone

AMH a 14-kd glycoprotein dimer structurally related to the subunit of inhibin and transforming growth factor (TGF)-β, is produced by the Sertoli cell of the fetal testis and later in gestation by granulosa cells of the fetal ovary. Immunoassayable concentrations of AMH (or MIS, müllerian inhibitory substance)[917] rise from birth to relatively high levels in the first year in newborn males, decrease by age 10 yrs, and decrease further during puberty.[918] Newborn females have low or nondetectable serum levels of AMH, which rise only slightly thereafter; serum AMH concentrations are virtually undetectable in most girls just before puberty.[917,919,920]

Serum AMH and inhibin B are inversely related to androgen concentrations in pubertal boys and values in boys with true precocious puberty are appropriate for pubertal stage rather than chronologic age; elevated serum AMH concentrations occur in the newborn period, (decreasing at puberty), and in older individuals with androgen resistance.[921-923] Treatment with rFSH and hCG in hypogonadotropic hypogonadism increases testosterone and decreases the elevated levels of serum AMH (due to immature Sertoli cells) as well as inhibin B, further demonstrating this relationship.[909,924] AMH is slightly higher in delayed puberty than in pubertal age-matched controls and lower in those with testicular dysgenesis associated with impaired virilization than in normal boys. Serum AMH is a useful index of intratesticular testosterone concentrations. Boys with isolated cryptorchidism have normal values of AMH while AMH is absent in anorchia, allowing differential diagnosis.[923,925] Dysgenetic testes secrete only low serum AMH levels; the testosterone response to hCG will indicate the presence of testicular tissue.[925] Histologic study of five cases of testicular dysgenesis demonstrated carcinoma in situ and retention of normal AMH staining in the immature Sertoli cells but absence of germ cell–specific RNA-binding motif (RBM) protein (encoded by the Y chromosome) in all but normal germs cells.[926] This suggests distortion of the development of germ cells in carcinoma in situ and that the germinal component is the origin of the cancer in testicular dysgenesis. AMH is a useful gonadal tumor marker as values are elevated in males with primitive Sertoli-like tumors and in girls and women with a granulosa cell tumor.[918]

Insulin Like-3 or INSL3

During puberty, serum INSL3, a protein produced by the Leydig cell, rises in normal boys under LH stimulation and its secretion is increased in boys given letrozole. Values do not increase in Klinefelter's syndrome, in which the initial rise levels off during midpuberty.[927] INSL3 may serve as another indication of Leydig cell function.

Prostate-Specific Antigen

Prostate-specific antigen (PSA) is detectable in male and female cord blood and in the serum of infants, but PSA concentrations decrease to undetectable levels during childhood. PSA concentrations rise to the measurable range with the onset of puberty in the male and correlate with the progression of pubertal stage, the size of the testes, and serum LH and testosterone concentrations and presumably the prostate.[928,929] PSA values are increased to the pubertal range in boys with idiopathic true precocious puberty, and decrease with GnRH agonist treatment.[930]

Study of cadaveric prostatic tissue from teenage subjects reveals the gene expression of this tissue, including but not limited to Nkx3.1, TMEPAI, TGFBR3, FASN, ANKH, TGFBR2, FAAH, S100P, HoxB13, fibronectin, and TSC2. Some of these are androgen responsive and may provide information on the precursors to prostate disorders later in life.[931]

Cortisol

Although no change occurs in the secretory rate of cortisol, salivary cortisol values increase slightly and correlate with pubertal stage without a sex difference.[932]

CENTRAL NERVOUS SYSTEM AND PUBERTY

The onset of puberty is a consequence of maturational changes, including the development of secondary sexual characteristics, the adolescent growth spurt, the attainment of fertility, and the psychosocial changes entrain from the maturation of the gonads and the increase in gonadal steroid secretion.[786,787,933] The events characterizing the development of gonadal function can be viewed as a continuum extending from sexual differentiation and the ontogenesis of the hypothalamic-pituitary-gonadotropin-gonadal system[279,799,934] through a juvenile pause (in which the system is largely quiescent)[787,935] to the attainment of full sexual maturation and fertility during puberty. These developmental and maturational events have as their end-point procreation. Two independent but associated processes (controlled by different mechanisms but closely linked temporally) are involved in the increased secretion of gonadal steroids in the peripubertal and pubertal period. The first, adrenarche, the increase in adrenal androgen secretion,[426,936] precedes by 2 years or so the second, gonadarche, the consequence of the pubertal reactivation of the hypothalamic-pituitary-gonadotropin-gonadal apparatus.[787,935]

Puberty is a developmental milestone that involves the disinhibition or reaugmentation of the hypothalamic GnRH pulse generator and gonadotropin secretion. The hypothalamic GnRH pulse generator-pituitary system in the human functions during fetal life and early infancy,[279,787,799,935,937] is suppressed to a low level of activity during childhood (the juvenile pause), and is derepressed or reactivated during puberty.[787,799,935] In this light, puberty does not represent the initiation or first occurrence of pulsatile secretion of GnRH or pituitary gonadotropins but the reactivation or disinhibition of GnRH neurosecretory neurons in the medial basal hypothalamus and the endogenous, apparently self-sustaining oscillatory secretion of GnRH after the period of quiescent activity during childhood. An increase in the pulsatile release of GnRH heralds the onset of puberty in the primate as well as other mammals.[279,934,935,937,938] The CNS, and not the hypothalamic GnRH pulse generator, pituitary gland, gonads, or gonadal steroid target tissues, restrains activation of the hypothalamic-pituitary-gonadal system during the prepubertal years according to a large body of evidence.[786,787,938-943] This inhibitory effect of the CNS appears to be mediated through the hypothalamus on the neurosecretory neurons that synthesize and secrete GnRH in a pulsatile manner.

Certain CNS lesions involving the hypothalamus and nearby structures can advance as well as delay the onset of human puberty (Table 24–17).[786,787,944,945] True or central precocious puberty (CPP) including cyclic ovulation in girls and spermatogenesis in boys can occur secondary to a variety of CNS disorders. Several regulatory systems that control puberty are (Fig. 24–23):

1. In humans and nonhuman primates, the *neural component* controlling gonadotropin secretion resides in the medial basal hypothalamus including the arcuate region.[946] Incredibly there are only about 1500 to 2000 transducer GnRH neurosecretory neurons, which are not segregated into a specific nucleus but are functionally interconnected. These GnRH neurons (the GnRH pulse generator),[947,948] which drive and control the pituitary gonadal components, translate neural signals into a periodic, oscillatory chemical signal, GnRH, in a coordinated manner. These pulses appear to be generated by a propagated depolarization, the firing of action potentials in individual cells, and the resulting influx of calcium through L-type calcium channels.[949-952] GnRH, a decapeptide, is synthesized as part of a larger precursor protein; the gene, which contains four exons and three introns,[953] is located on the short arm of chromosome 8.
2. The *pituitary gonadotropes,* which contain the seven-transmembrane domain Gs coupled LH/hCG receptors,[954] in response to the GnRH rhythmic signal, release LH and FSH in a pulsatile manner. Each LH (and FSH) pulse is induced by a pulse of GnRH.
3. The *gonads,* which are modulated primarily by the amplitude of the gonadotropin pulse, transmit the episodic gonadotropin signal into pulsatile secretion of gonadal steroids.[955]

This control mechanism, with its three principal components (medial basal hypothalamic GnRH neurosecretory neurons, pituitary gonadotropes, and gonadotropin-responsive elements of the gonad), is common to all mammalian species. At the last two levels—the pituitary gland and the gonad—the target cells contain receptors for the peptide hormones that mediate the cellular response to the signal.[954-958] Although the fundamental properties of the hypothalamic GnRH pulse generator-pituitary-gonadal complex are common to all mammalian species, diverse adaptive mechanisms and strategies have evolved among species and between the sexes that influence the biology and timing of puberty.[959,960] Photoperiodicity and seasonal breeding, biologic clocks, and pheromones are integral parts of the pubertal process in some species but not in the control of human puberty. Other environmental factors and cues that play a role in the human are less critical than in most mammals. Many well-established CNS regulatory mechanisms that affect the GnRH pulse generator and puberty onset in nonprimates may be of minor or of no documented significance in primates. The most enlightening studies on the neuroendocrinology of human puberty have emerged from studies in the human and the nonhuman primate.

TABLE 24–17 HYPOTHESIS OF THE CONTROL OF THE ONSET OF HUMAN PUBERTY

1. *Central Dogma:* The CNS exercises the only major restraint on the onset of puberty. The neuroendocrine control of puberty is mediated by the hypothalamic GnRH-secreting neruosecretory neurons in the medial basal hypothalamus, which act as an endogenous pulse generator (oscillator).
2. The development of reproductive function is a continuum extending from sexual differentiation and the ontogeny of the hypothalamic-pituitary-gonadal system in the fetus to the attainment of full sexual maturation and fertility.
3. In the prepubertal child the GnRH pulse generator, operative in the fetus and infant, functions at a low level of activity (the juvenile pause) because of steroid-independent and steroid-dependent inhibitory mechanisms.
4. Puberty represents the *reactivation* (disinhibition) of the CNS suppressed GnRH pulse generator characteristic of late infancy and childhood, leading to increased amplitude and frequency of GnRH pulsatile discharges, to increased stimulation of the pituitary gonadotropes, and finally to gonadal maturation. Hormonally, puberty is initiated by the recrudescence of augmented pulsatile GnRH and gonadotropin secretion, mainly at night.

CNS, Central nervous system; *GnRH,* luteinizing hormone–releasing hormone.

From Grumbach MM, Kaplan SL. The neuroendocrinology of human puberty: an ontogenetic perspective. In Grumbach MM, Sizonenko PC, Aubert ML, eds. Control of the Onset of Puberty. Baltimore: Williams & Wilkins, 1990:1-68.

Pattern of Gonadotropin Secretion

Tonic Secretion

Tonic, or basal, secretion is regulated by a negative, or inhibitory, feedback mechanism in which changes in the concentration of circulating gonadal steroids and inhibin result in reciprocal changes in the secretion of pituitary gonadotropins. This is the pattern of secretion in the male and one of the control mechanisms in the female.

Cyclic secretion involves a positive, or stimulatory, feedback mechanism in which an increase in circulating estrogens, to a critical level and of sufficient duration, initiates the synchronous release of LH and FSH (the preovulatory LH surge) that is characteristic of the normal adult woman before menopause.

Pulsatile Secretion

In vitro studies suggest that the generation of the GnRH pulse is an intrinsic property of the GnRH neurosecretory neuronal network and that other factors modulate the fundamental autorhythmicity of the GnRH neuron including the downstream

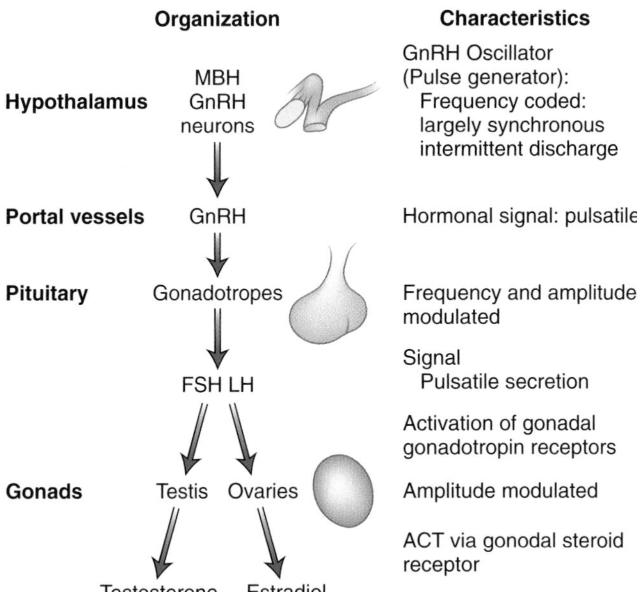

Figure 24–23 ▪ Organization and characteristics of the hypothalamic-pituitary gonadotroph-gonadal system. The medial basal hypothalamus (MBH) contains the transducer luteinizing hormone–releasing hormone (GnRH) neurosecretory neurons. These neurons translate neural signals into a periodic, oscillatory chemical signal, GnRH. This MBH complex functions as an GnRH pulse generator (oscillator), which is frequency coded and releases GnRH from its axon terminals at the median eminence as a largely synchronous intermittent discharge into the primary capillary plexus of the hypothalamicohypophysial portal circulation. The GnRH pulse generator is influenced by biogenic amine neurotransmitters, peptidergic neuromodulators, neuroexcitatory amino acids, and neural pathways. During the follicular phase in the adult female and the adult male, an GnRH pulse (estimated indirectly by monitoring LH pulses in peripheral blood) occurs approximately every 90 to 120 minutes throughout the day. Changes in the frequency and probably in the amplitude of the GnRH secretory episodes modulate the pattern of LH and follicle-stimulating hormone (FSH). The major site of action of testosterone and progesterone is on the GnRH pulse generator, as these two classes of steroids decrease LH pulse frequency, but a pituitary site of action has also been described. Estrogens have major direct inhibitory and stimulatory effects on the GnRH-primed pituitary gonadotroph; the inhibitory, or negative, feedback action is associated with a decrease in both the frequency and the amplitude of pituitary LH secretion. On the other hand, evidence also supports a negative and positive feedback action of estrogen on the GnRH pulse generator. Inhibin has a direct inhibitory effect on the pituitary gland and the secretion of FSH. The secretion of gonadal steroids by the gonads is controlled mainly by the amplitude of the gonadotropin signal. (Adapted from Grumbach MM, Kaplan SL. The neuroendocrinology of human puberty: an ontogenetic perspective. In Grumbach MM, Sizonenko PC, Aubert ML, eds. Control of the Onset of Puberty. Baltimore: Williams & Wilkins, 1990:1-68.)

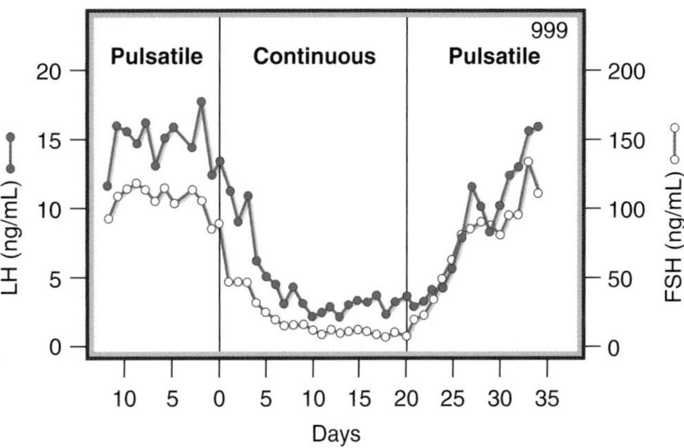

Figure 24–24 ▪ The Knobil Paradigim. Effect of pulsatile administration of luteinizing hormone-releasing hormone (GnRH) in contrast to continuous infusion of GnRH in adult oophorectomized rhesus monkeys in which gonadotropin secretion has been abolished by lesions that ablated the medial basal hypothalamic GnRH pulse generator. Note the high concentrations of plasma LH and follicle-stimulating hormone (FSH) in monkeys given one GnRH pulse per hour, the suppression of gonadotropin secretion by continuous infusion of GnRH even though the total dose of GnRH was the same, and the restoration of FSH and LH secretion when the pulsatile mode of GnRH administration was reinitiated. (From Belchetz PE, Plant TM, Nakai Y, et al. Hypophysial responses to continuous and intermittent delivery of hypothalamic gonadotropin releasing hormone. Science 1978;202:631-633.)

effects of cAMP-gated cation channels on the regulation of pulsatility by cAMP.[961] The immortalized GnRH neurosecretory neuronal cell line exhibits spontaneous, synchronized autorhythmicity in the release of GnRH.[950,952,962] Cultured monkey GnRH-1 neurons exhibit spontaneous pulsatile release of GnRH at a frequency similar to that observed in vivo while patch clamped primary GnRH neurons show disordered patterns of release that are sensitive to increased extracellular potassium; firing activity can be stimulated by exposure to estrogen in a manner that appears to function through the estrogen receptor.[963] Taken together, these observations suggest that a stimulatory input is not required for pulsatile GnRH secretion.

The secretion of FSH and LH is always pulsatile or episodic, regardless of developmental stage, due to the pulsatility of the GnRH pulse generator. GnRH stimulates the release of both FSH and LH, but the pulsatile secretion of immunoreactive FSH in normal adults is less prominent; this is attributed in part to the longer half-life of FSH than LH, to differences in the factors that modulate the action of GnRH on FSH and LH release by the gonadotropes (especially gonadal steroids, inhibin, and possibly activin and follistatin), and to intrinsic differences in the secretory pattern of the two gonadotropins. For example, a change in the frequency of GnRH pulses can modify the ratio of FSH to LH released; midfollicular phase concentrations of estradiol and adult male concentrations of plasma testosterone have a greater inhibitory effect on the response of FSH than on that of LH to pulsatile injections of GnRH.[964-966]

Knobil and associates[947,951,967] first revealed the essential nature of a periodic, oscillatory GnRH signal for the regulation of gonadotropin secretion. Inhibition of gonadotropin secretion results from the continuous infusion of GnRH because of desensitization of GnRH receptors on the gonadotrope.[956,957,968] Intermittent, or pulsatile, administration (e.g., GnRH 1 μg/min for 6 min every hour) restored pulsatile release of LH and FSH in adult monkeys in which hypothalamic lesions obliterated the arcuate nucleus region and thus eliminated endogenous GnRH secretion.[947,967] Furthermore, pulsatile GnRH administration reestablished gonadotropin secretion in animals in which gonadotropin secretion had been suppressed by the continuous infusion of GnRH (Fig. 24–24). Thus, the GnRH signal to the pituitary gonadotropes of the adult is frequency coded.

The GnRH neurosecretory neurons of the hypothalamic GnRH pulse generator that arise in the olfactory placode (see below) exhibit spontaneous autorhythmicity[951,952,962,969-972] and function intrinsically as a neuronal oscillator for the entrainment of the repetitive release of GnRH (Fig. 24–25). Current evidence[973] suggests that the autorhythmicity in the GnRH neurosecretory neurons[950,974-980] involve cAMP and cyclic nucleotide-gated cation channels associated with oscillatory increases in intracellular Ca^{2+}, a hallmark of neurosecretion and gap junctional communication.[981] Cycles of transcription and translation are not integral components of the oscillator but are

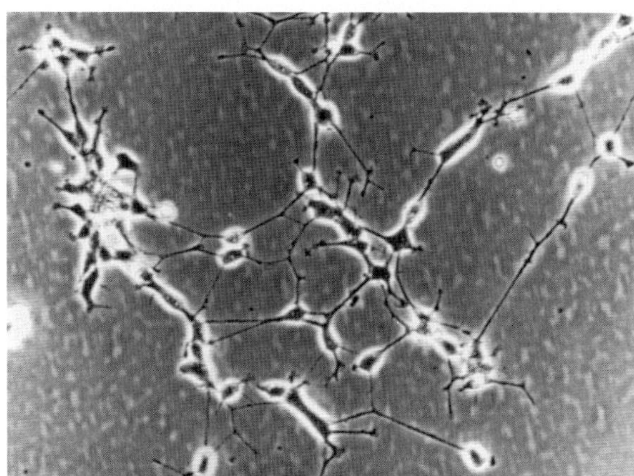

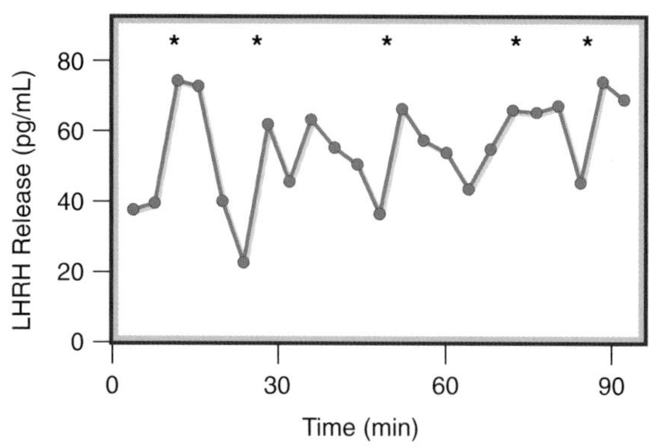

Figure 24–25 ▪ The immortalized hypothalamic luteinizing hormone–releasing hormone (GnRH) neuronal cell line. *Left,* Phase-contrast micrograph illustrating the neuronal phenotype (GT1-3 cell line) including the extension of multiple long neurites, cell-cell contacts, and growth cones. The neuroendocrine function of GT cells is limited to expression of GnRH and GAP. Magnification×175. *Right,* Demonstration of autonomous GnRH (gonadotropin-releasing hormone, GnRH) pulses at about 20-minute intervals by the GnRH neurons in culture. This is the same frequency as that for LH pulses in vivo, in castrated adult mice and rats. To convert GnRH values to picomoles per liter, multiply by 0.8460. (Micrograph from Mellon PL, Windle II, Goldsmith PC, et al. Immortalization of hypothalamic GnRH neurons by genetically targeted tumorigenesis. Neuron 1990;5:1-10. Copyright by Cell Press. Graph courtesy of G. Martinez de la Escalera and R.I. Weiner.)

necessary for replenishment of constituents.[982] Moreover, the immortalized GnRH neuronal cell line contains neuronal nitric oxide (NO) synthase,[983] so NO generated by GnRH neurons may act as a an intercellular as well as intracellular messenger.[983,984] Furthermore, GnRH acting as an autocrine factor may play a role in the synchronization mechanism.[946] GnRH is synthesized in these neurons and released episodically from axon terminals at the median eminence into the primary plexus of the hypothalamic-hypophyseal portal circulation. The hormone is then transported by the portal vessels to the anterior pituitary gland to produce the pulsatile LH and FSH secretion.

Ontogeny

Studies in the mouse,[985-988] rhesus monkey,[989,990] human,[991,992] and all vertebrates examined[993a] indicate that GnRH neurons arise in the embryo from the epithelium of the olfactory placode and migrate in a rostrocaudal direction by an ordered spatiotemporal course along the pathway of the nervous terminalis-vermonasal complex to the forebrain; the latter also originates in the olfactory placode and forms a connection between the nasal septum and the forebrain (Figs. 24–26 and 24–27). This contrasts to the pattern of Growth Hormone Releasin Factor (GRF), TRF, or CRF neurosecretory neurons that originate from ventricular zones within the embryonic forebrain.[994,995]

In the mouse, in vitro and in vivo studies using the GnRH green fluorescent protein model demonstrate an increase in dendritic and somal spines in adult mice compared to juveniles, suggesting an increase in direct excitatory inputs to GnRH neurons and increased glutametergic stimulation of GnRH neurons across the time of puberty.[996,997] Embryonic GnRH neurons of the olfactory placode and the hypothalamus coexpress mRNAs for GnRH and the type 1 GnRH receptor. These neurons demonstrate spontaneous electrical pulsatile activity, which can be stimulated by GnRH agonist and abolished by GnRH antagonist in the same pattern as GnRH pulses themselves, all in a calcium-dependent manner in that the intracellular calcium responses themselves are stimulated by the agonist and inhibited by the antagonist.

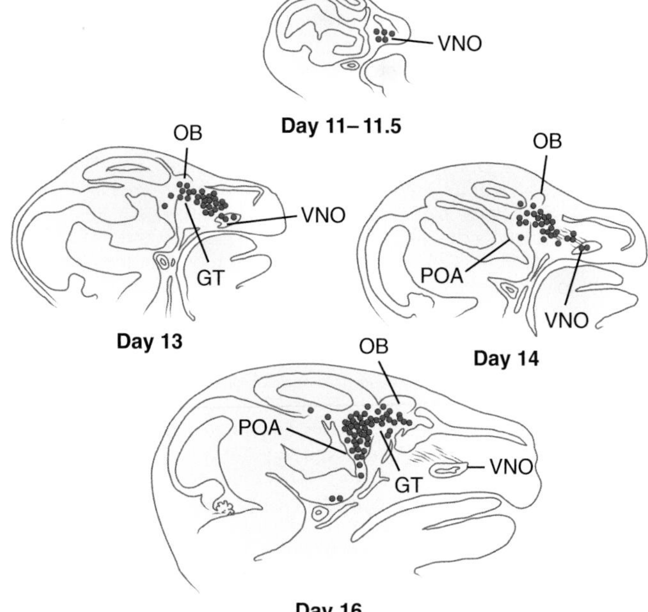

Figure 24–26 ▪ Ontogeny of luteinizing hormone–releasing hormone (GnRH) neurons in the mouse. The route of migration of the GnRH neurosecretory neurons *(black dots)* in the mouse embryo is shown from their origin in the medial olfactory placode (a platelike thickening of embryonic ectoderm) in the nasal region through the forebrain into the hypothalamus and preoptic areas. At embryonic (E) day 11 to 11.5, GnRH cells are in the anlage of the vomeronasal organ and medial wall of the olfactory placode. By E day 13, the number of GnRH neurons has increased, and most are in the nasal septum with the nervus terminalis and the vomeronasal nerves; only a few cells are in the brain. By E day 14, the majority of GnRH cells are in the ganglion terminale and the central root of the nervus terminalis and arch through the forebrain to the hypothalamus. By E day 16, most of the GnRH neurons are in the hypothalamus and preoptic areas, and the migration is almost complete. *GT,* Ganglion terminale; *OB,* olfactory bulb; *POA,* preoptic area, *VNO,* vomeronasal organ. (Adapted from Schwanzel-Fukuda M, Pfaff DW. Origin of luteinizing hormone-releasing hormone neurons. Nature 1989;338:161-164. Reprinted by permission from Nature, Vol. 338, pp. 161-164. Copyright 1989 Macmillan Magazines Ltd.)

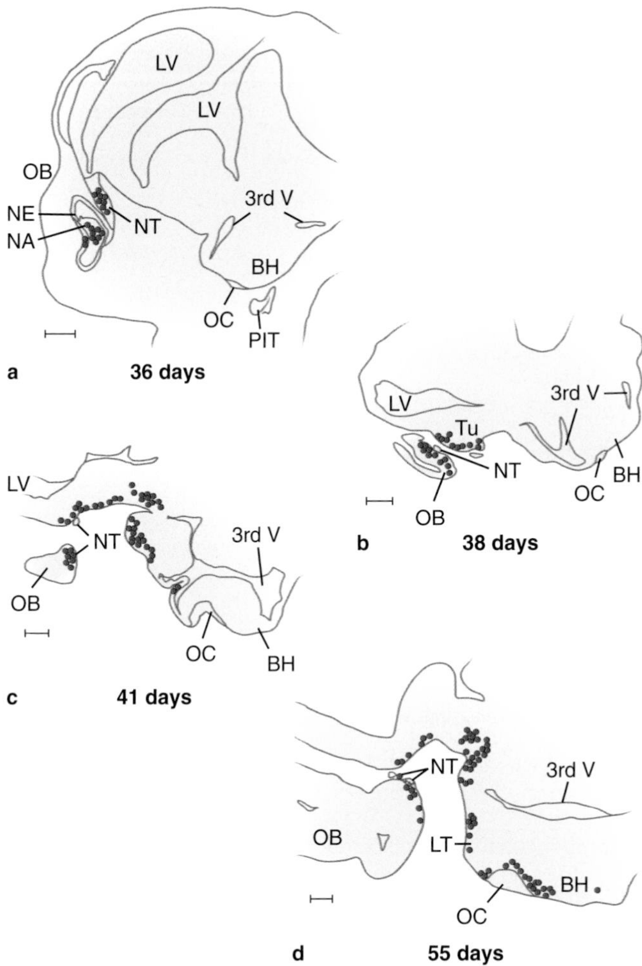

Figure 24–27 ▪ Ontogeny of the luteinizing hormone–releasing hormone (GnRH) neurons in the rhesus monkey. In the 36-day embryo, the GnRH cells *(black dots)* are located deep in the nasal septum along the path of the nervus terminals but not within the brain. By day 38, GnRH cells are clustered along the dorsal region of the olfactory bulbs and nervus terminalis with a few cells arching back along the ventral surface of the forebrain. By 55 days, the GnRH neurons are in the process of migration, but clusters of GnRH cells have entered the central nervous system and reached the basal hypothalamus. *BH,* Basal hypothalamus; *LT,* lamina terminalis; *LV,* lateral ventricle; *NA,* nasal area; *NE,* nasal epithelium; *NT,* nervus terminalis; *OB,* olfactory bulb; *OC,* optic chiasm; *Tu,* olfactory tubercle. (Adapted from Ronnekleiv OK, Resko JA. Ontogeny of gonadotropin-releasing hormone-containing neurons in early fetal development of rhesus macaques. Endocrinology 1990;126:498-511. Copyright by The Endocrine Society.)

The Human Fetus

Schwanzel-Fukuda and colleagues[991] found no GnRH neurosecretory neurons in the brain, including the hypothalamus, in a 19-wk gestational male human fetus with Kallmann's syndrome (see later). However, dense clusters of GnRH cells and fibers were present in the nose, including the nasal septum and cribriform plate, and within the dural layers of the meninges under the forebrain. The olfactory bulbs were absent. In subsequent studies, GnRH immunoreactivity was observed in the epithelium of the medial aspect of the olfactory placode by 42 days of gestation but not at 28 to 32 days.[992] Thus, the GnRH neurosecretory neurons migrate from the olfactory placode to the hypothalamus in humans as well as in other mammals.[994]

Aberrant migration of the GnRH neurons leads to delayed or absent pubertal development. Hypogonadotropic hypogonadism and anosmia or hyposmia are cardinal features of Kallmann's syndrome and the CHARGE syndrome described below.

In the mouse, the number of GnRH neurons in the adult is similar to that in late fetal life and the numbers of the GnRH neurons as well as the GnRH mRNA levels in the nonhuman primate do not appear to change during pubertal development. Furthermore, the ability of the GnRH neuron to respond to electrical or neurochemical (e.g., glutaminergic, kisspeptinergic) stimuli does not change with pubertal development.[999]

GnRH has been detected in human embryonic brain extracts by 4.5 weeks gestation and in the fetal hypothalamus by 6 weeks (Table 24–18); furthermore, the fetal pituitary gonadotropes are responsive to GnRH.[799] The hypothalamic-hypophyseal portal system is functional by 11.5 weeks of gestation,[1000,1001] and by 16 weeks axon fibers that contain GnRH are present in the median eminence and terminate in contact with capillaries of the portal system.[279,787,799,937]

In fetal sheep, the hypothalamus secretes GnRH in a pulsatile manner.[1002,1003] thus the available data are consistent with the development of a human fetal hypothalamic GnRH pulse generator by at least the end of the first trimester.

The human fetal gonad is affected by placental gonadotropins and by fetal pituitary FSH and LH.[279,937] The placental gonadotropin hCG may play an important role in the secretion of testosterone by the Leydig cells of the fetal testes during the masculinization of the wolffian ducts and the external genitalia at 8 to 13 week's gestation. However, it is uncertain whether functional hCG/LH and FSH receptors are present in the fetal testis by 12 weeks of gestation[1004-1006] and whether the early fetal testis responds to hCG. Fetal Leydig cells are a unique population of Leydig cells limited to the fetus and infant, which regress to be followed by the differentiation of adult type Leydig cells in the peripubertal period.[279,937,1007-1010]

In comparison with the adult-type, fetal Leydig cells form tightly opposed clusters joined by gap junctions and lack Reinke crystals; are resistant to hcG/LH-induced desensitization—indeed, hCG/LH produce up-regulation of LH/hCG receptors; and contain little aromatase activity and few estradiol receptors. In contrast to the fetal testis, FSH receptors in the fetal ovary appear[1006] only late in the second trimester, a stage well after completion of male phenotypic differentiation, demonstrating a sex difference in the stage of gestation at which fetal pituitary gonadotropins have an important effect on the development of the fetal gonad. In the anencephalic fetus (which is deficient in hypothalamic GRH, resulting in deficiency of pituitary gonadotropins), the testes appear hypoplastic by early in the third trimester; however, the ovaries in this disorder are normal until at least 32 weeks of gestation.[279,937,944,1011]

The human fetal pituitary gland contains FSH and LH by 10 weeks of gestation, secretion begins by 11 to 12 weeks, and the gonadotropin content increases until approximately 25 to 29 weeks of gestation (Figs. 24–28 and 24–29).[279,799,934,937,944] Fetal serum LH and FSH concentrations rise to peak levels by midgestation and then decrease to low values in umbilical venous blood at term (see Figs. 24–28 and 24–29). The serum concentration of FSH and LH and of bioactive FSH at 17 to 24 weeks' gestation are strikingly higher in female than male fetuses, and in both sexes decreased remarkably between 25 and 40 weeks' gestation.[1012] Mean FSH and LH concentrations are elevated at the beginning of the third trimester and decreased with advancing gestational age to undetectable values in term fetuses.[1012] Mean FSH value are higher in female fetuses between 26 and 36 weeks, whereas the mean LH level is higher in males.[1013] In the ovine fetus, LH and FSH are secreted in a pulsatile manner in response to the episodic secretion of fetal hypothalamic GnRH (Fig. 24–30); human fetal pituitary gonadotropins are probably released in the same mode. The mean FSH and LH

TABLE 24–18 THE EARLY DEVELOPMENT OF THE HUMAN FETAL PITUITARY AND HYPOTHALAMUS

Gestational Age (wk)	Hypothalamus	Pituitary	Portal Circulation
3	Forebrain appears		
4		Rathke's pouch in contact with stomodeum	
5	Diencephalon differentiated	Rathke's pouch separated from stomodeum and in contact with infundibulum; pituitary in culture can secrete corticotropin, prolactin, GH, FSH	
6	Premammillary preoptic nucleus; GnRH detected	Intermediate-lobe primordia; cell cords penetrate mesenchyme around Rathke's pouch.	
7	Arcuate, supraoptic nucleus	Sphenoidal plate forms	
8	Median eminence differentiated: TRH detected*	Basophils appear	Capillaries in mesenchyme
9	Paraventricular nucleus; dorsal medial nucleus	Pars tuberalis formed: β-endorphin detected*	
10	Serotonin and norepinephrine detected*	Acidophils appear	
11	Mammillary nucleus; primary (hypothalamic) portal plexus present; β-endorphin and opioidergic neurons detected*	Secondary (pituitary) portal plexus present catecholamines (IF)†	Functional hypothalamic-hypophyseal portal system
12	Dopamine present		
13	Corticotropin-releasing hormone detected*	α-Melanocyte-stimulating hormone detected	
14	Fully differentiated hypothalamus	Adult form of hypophysis developed	

*Hormone detected at this gestational age but may be present earlier.
†IF, detected by immunofluorescer.
FSH, Follicle-stimulating hormone; *GH,* growth hormone; *GnRH,* luteinizing hormone–releasing hormone; *TRH,* thyrotropin-releasing hormone.
Modified from Gluckman P, Grumbach MM, Kaplan SL. The human fetal hypothalamus and pituitary gland. In Tulchinsky D, Ryan KJ, eds. Maternal-Fetal Endocrinology. Philadelphia: WB Saunders, 1980:196-232.

content of fetal pituitary glands are greater in female than in male fetuses at midgestation. This difference has been ascribed to the higher concentration of plasma testosterone between 11 and 24 weeks in the male fetus (the only major difference in gonadal steroids between the male and female fetus) and fetal testicular inhibin.[279,937] The decrease in both serum FSH and LH concentrations toward term during late gestation is attributed to the maturation of the negative feedback mechanism, the development of gonadal steroid receptors in the hypothalamic-pituitary unit,[799,934,1014] and the effect of inhibin.[279,937]

Consistent with this sequence of events, in vitro studies indicate that the human fetal pituitary gland is responsive to GnRH as early as 10 weeks of gestation[1015]; the GnRH-stimulated release of LH is greater in second-trimester fetal pituitary cells cultured from females than males and is augmented by estradiol in both sexes.[1016] In vivo studies[1017] during middle and late gestation demonstrate the stimulating action of exogenous GnRH on fetal FSH and LH release by 16 weeks of gestation with a striking sex difference in the FSH response and a fall in responsivity to GnRH in late gestation (see Figs. 24–21 and 24–22). The anencephalic infant and some infants with neonatal hypothalamic hypopituitarism[279,937] have an absent or diminished gonadotropin response to GnRH,[279,799] in contrast to the brisk increase demonstrated in the normal infant.

Thus, a pattern of increasing synthesis and secretion of FSH and LH leading to peak serum concentrations at castrate levels, probably the result of relatively autonomous, unrestrained activity of the fetal hypothalamic GnRH pulse generator and subsequent stimulation of the fetal gonadotropes by GnRH, is followed by a decline after midgestation persisting to term, probably due to maturation of the negative feedback mechanism[1014] and increasing sensitivity of the GnRH pulse generator to the inhibitory effects of the high concentration of sex steroids (estrogens and progesterone from the placenta and in the male, testosterone from the fetal testes) in the fetal circulation[787,799] and in the male fetus to a contributory effect on the decrease in FSH by testicular inhibin in late gestation.[279,937] The increasing CNS control of gonadotropin secretion seems to require the maturation of gonadal steroid receptors (intracellular or on the cell surface or both) in the fetal hypothalamus and in the pituitary gonadotropes (see Figs. 24–21 and 24–23).[799,1018]

The Sheep Fetus

The fetal sheep model in which indwelling vascular catheters are placed in the fetus and pregnant ewe afford an opportunity for mechanistic studies as the ontogeny of fetal gonadotropins, hypothalamic GnRH, and gonadal steroids is similar to that in the human fetus.[279,787,799,937,1000] The length of gestation in the sheep is about 145 days (see Fig. 24–23).

By gestation 60% of the secretion of fetal LH and FSH is pulsatile[1002] and mediated by the hypothalamic GnRH pulse generator.[787,1003,1014] Sex difference in gonadotropin secretion occurs in both the ovine and the human fetus,[787] as orchiectomy (but not oophorectomy) in the ovine fetus leads to an increase in pulsatile secretion of LH (and to a lesser degree FSH).[1019] Opiodergic neurons have a tonic suppressive effect on the pulsatile release of GnRH in the ovine fetus,[787,1020] while the excitatory amino acid analogue N-methyl-D-aspartate (NMDA) evokes an LH pulse mediated by GnRH. The excitatory amino acids, glutamate and aspartate, can stimulate the GnRH pulse generator,[1021] directly as well as indirectly (Fig. 24–31).[962,1022] Glutamate is present in abundance in the hypothalamus and is released from glutaminergic neurons by exocytosis in an ATP- and calcium-dependent process.[1023] Furthermore, FSH stimulates inhibin synthesis by the ovine fetal testis and ovary, and administration of an inhibin-rich extract inhibits fetal FSH but not LH secretion, evidence of the functional capacity of the FSH-fetal gonadal inhibin feedback system.[1024,1025] These observations provide support for an operative hypothalamic GnRH-pituitary gonadotropin unit by at least 30% of gestation in the human fetus and 40% of gestation in the ovine fetus and for the central role of the CNS in this process.

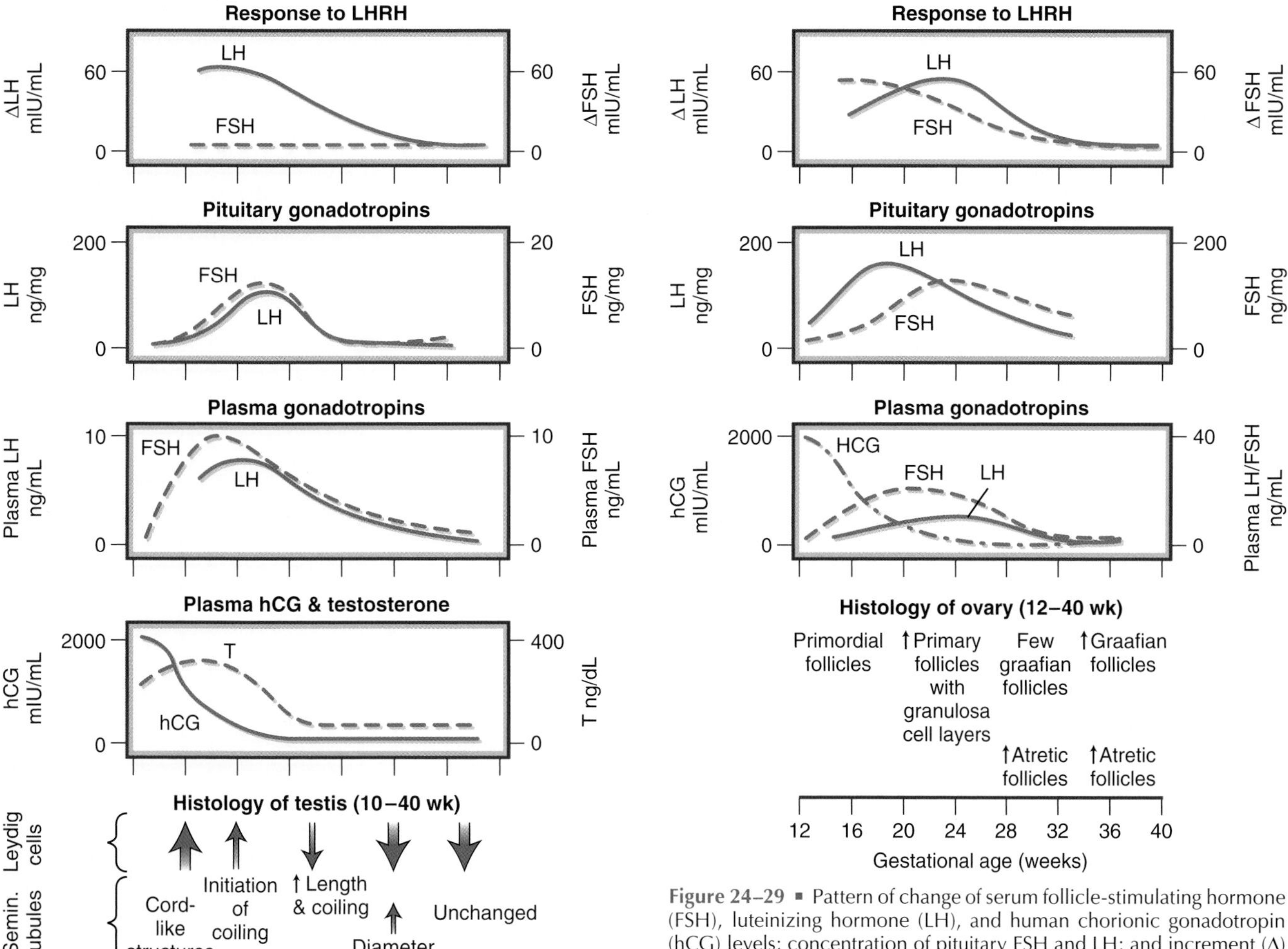

Figure 24–28 ▪ Comparison of the pattern of change of serum testosterone, human chorionic gonadotropin (hCG), and serum and pituitary luteinizing hormone (LH) (LER-960) and follicle-stimulating hormone (FSH) (LER-869) levels in the human male fetus during gestation in relation to the morphologic changes in fetal testis. The top graph illustrates the regression curve for the increment (Δ) between a baseline plasma LH and FSH level and the 15-minute response to administration of GnRH to the male fetus plotted as a function of gestational age. The scale masks the slight increase in plasma FSH. Data were recalculated from Takagi and colleagues. Takagi S, Yoshida T. [Feto-placental relation in fetal endocrine function]. Horumon To Rinsho 1973; 21(2):173-179. The evidence supports the hypothesis that the hypothalamic GnRH pulse generator is functional early in gestation and mediates the rise in serum concentration of fetal pituitary gonadotrophs. To convert plasma hCG values to international units per liter, multiply by 1.0. Other conversions are in the legends of Figures 24–21 and 24–22. (Modified from Kaplan SL, Grumbach MM. Pituitary and placental gonadotropins and sex steroids in the human and subhuman primate fetus. Clin Endocrinol Metab 1978;7:487-511; and Gluckman PD, Grumbach MM, Kaplan SL. The human fetal hypothalamus and pituitary gland. In Tulchinsky D, Ryan KJ, eds. Maternal-Fetal Endocrinology. Philadelphia, WB Saunders, 1980:196-232.)

Figure 24–29 ▪ Pattern of change of serum follicle-stimulating hormone (FSH), luteinizing hormone (LH), and human chorionic gonadotropin (hCG) levels; concentration of pituitary FSH and LH; and increment (Δ) between baseline FSH and LH and the 15-minute response to administration of GnRH in the human female fetus during gestation with the development of the fetal ovary. See legends of Figures 24–21, 24–22, and 24–28 for conversions to SI units. (Modified from Kaplan SL, Grumbach MM. Pituitary and placental gonadotropins and sex steroids in the human and subhuman primate fetus. Clin Endocrinol Metab 1978;7:487-511.)

The Human Neonate and Infant

The hypothalamic regulatory mechanisms for pituitary gonadotropins, as for other pituitary hormones, are not fully developed at birth.[787] In both sexes, the concentration of plasma FSH and LH is low in cord blood as a consequence of the inhibitory effect of the high levels of placental derived estrogens but within a few minutes after birth in the male neonate, but not the female, the concentration of LH increases abruptly in peripheral blood (about 10-fold) followed by an increase in serum testosterone concentration during the first 3 hours that persists for 12 hours or more.[1026] After the fall in circulating levels of steroids of placental origin (especially estrogens) during the first few days after birth, the concentration of serum FSH and LH increases and exhibits a pulsatile pattern with wide perturbations during the first few months. FSH pulse amplitude is much greater in the female infant and is associated with a larger FSH response to GnRH throughout childhood; LH pulses are of greater magnitude in the male (Fig. 24–32). This striking sex difference also is present in agonadal male and female infants[787,1027] and in the infant rhesus monkey.[1028,1029] This sex difference (see Fig. 24–32) may in part be related to the effect of testosterone in the male fetus on the development and function of the hypothalamic-pituitary apparatus.[279,937]

The high gonadotropin concentrations are associated with a proliferation of Sertoli cells and gonocytes (and their transformation into spermatogonia)[1030] a transient second wave of differentiation of fetal-type Leydig cells and increased serum testosterone levels in male infants during the first few postnatal months[1010] there also are increased estradiol levels intermittently during the first year of life and part of the second year in females.[1031,1032] The mean FSH concentration is higher in females than in males during the first few years of life. By approximately 6 months of age in the male and 2 to 3 years of age in the female, the concentration of plasma gonadotropins decreases to the low levels that are present until the onset of puberty. Thus, the restraint of the hypothalamic GnRH pulse generator and the suppression of pulsatile GnRH secretion (and thus LH release) do not attain the prepubertal level of quiescence until late infancy or early childhood and earlier in boys than girls.[787,1033]

The rise in circulating gonadotropins, sex hormones, and inhibin in both sexes during infancy, the so-called postnatal surge (or "minipuberty") is well documented.[937] In sum, the neonatal-midinfancy surge in pulsatile gonadotropin secretion is attributable to an increase in GnRH pulse amplitude and is associated in the male infant with the following:[937]

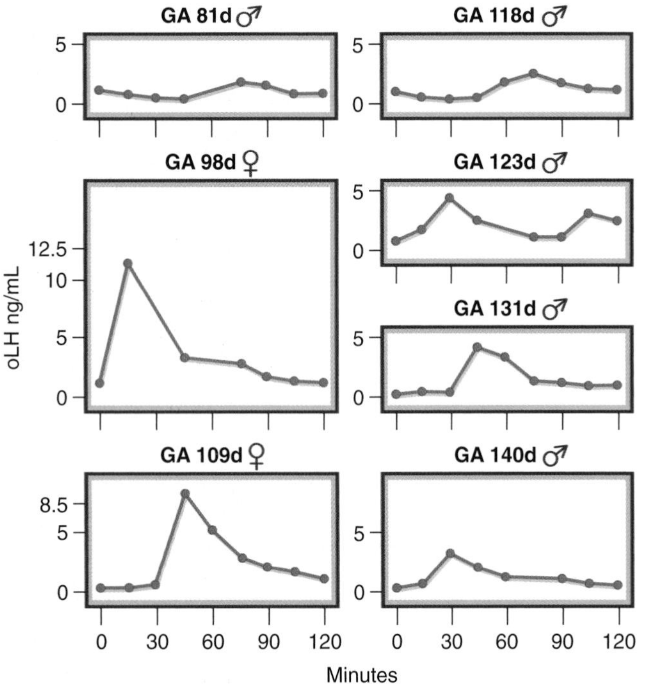

Figure 24–30 ▪ Pulsatile luteinizing hormone (LH) secretion in the ovine fetus. *GA,* Gestational age. The length of gestation is 145 days in the sheep. (From Clark SJ, Ellis N, Styne DM, et al. Hormone ontogeny in the ovine fetus. XVII. Demonstration of pulsatile luteinizing hormone secretion by the fetal pituitary gland. Endocrinology 1984;115:1774-1779. Copyright by The Endocrine Society.)

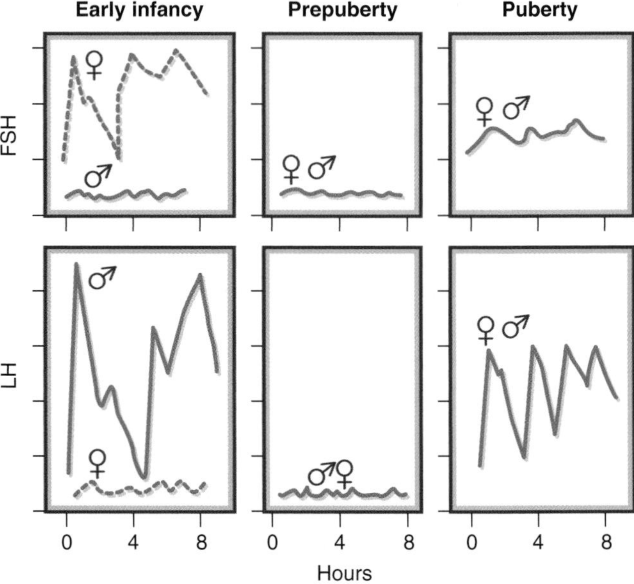

Figure 24–32 ▪ Change in the pattern of pulsatile follicle-stimulating hormone (FSH) and luteinizing hormone (LH) secretion in early infancy, childhood, and puberty. The data for early infancy are derived from Waldhauser and colleagues. Waldhauser F, Weissenbacher G, Frisch H, Pollak A. Pulsatile secretion of gonadotropins in early infancy. Eur J Pediatr 1981; 137:71-74. Note the pulsatile secretion in the infant and the striking difference in the amplitude of FSH and LH pulses between male and female infants. After infancy, the amplitude and frequency of gonadotropin pulses decrease greatly for almost a decade (juvenile pause) until the onset of puberty. (From Grumbach MM, Kaplan SL. The neuroendocrinology of human puberty: an ontogenetic perspective. In Grumbach MM, Sizonenko PC, Aubert ML, eds. Control of the Onset of Puberty. Baltimore: Williams & Wilkins, 1990:1-68.)

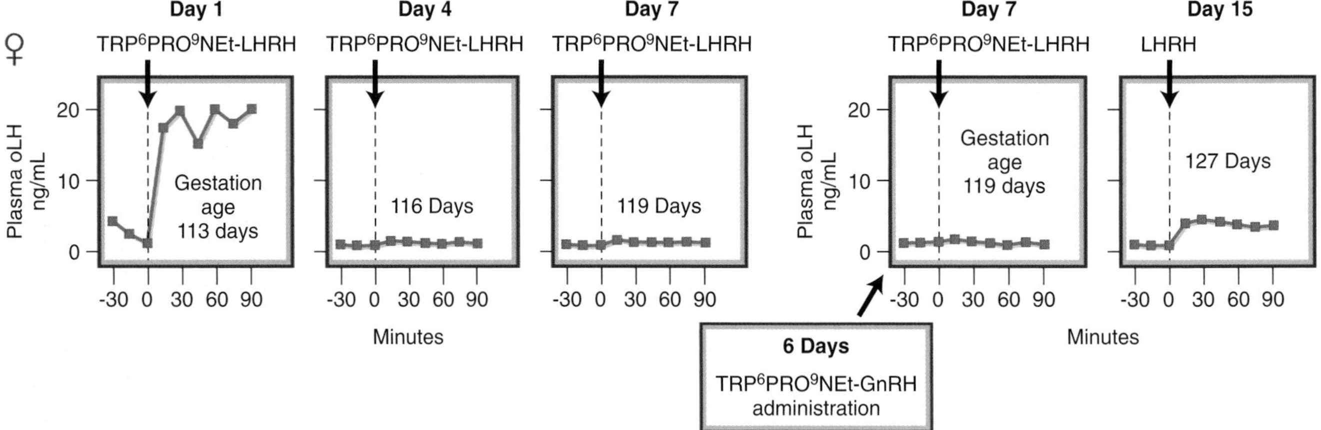

Figure 24–31 ▪ *Left,* The effect in the ovine fetus of administration for 7 days of luteinizing hormone–releasing hormone (GnRH) agonist (10 μg intravenously daily) on the acute LH response to GnRH agonist. *Right,* Recovery of the LH response was impaired 8 days after discontinuing GnRH agonist administration to the ovine fetus. (From Grumbach MM, Kaplan SL. The neuroendocrinology of human puberty: an ontogenetic perspective. In Grumbach MM, Sizonenko PC, Aubert ML, eds. Control of the Onset of Puberty. Baltimore: Williams & Wilkins, 1990:1-68.)

- Increase in testicular volume (by direct measurement) due to increase in seminiferous tubule length (approximately sixfold increase in year 1).
- Rapid expansion of Sertoli cell population (makes up approximately 85% to 95% of seminiferous tubular cell mass).
- High concentration of circulating inhibin B (low in hypogonadotropic hypogonadism).

Sertoli cell number, including postnatal proliferation, is a determinant of spermatogenic function.The postnatal surge apparently is not essential for masculine-typical psychosexual development; the brain in congenital hypogonadotropic hypogonadism including Kallmann's syndrome is masculinized by testosterone therapy at puberty despite the lack of an infantile surge in gonadotropins and testosterone. Of interest, an LH and testosterone surge is absent in the complete androgen insensitivity syndrome. Parenthetically, in the McCune-Albright syndrome, an activating mutation in the Gsα gene primarily expressed in the Sertoli cell can cause macroorchidism due to Sertoli cell proliferation and hyperfunction with increased concentration of serum inhibin B and AMH but without increased testosterone levels due to Leydig cell hyperplasia, elevated gonadotropins, or signs of puberty.[937] The increase in circulating testosterone in the normal male infant may lead to facial comedones and even acneiform lesions, and the increase in gonadotropins may lead to a transient increase in testicular size, but there may be more subtle changes.

The transient postnatal to midinfancy function of the GnRH pulse generator in the male infant may be related to future spermatogenic function and fertility.[1034-1036] Sertoli cells and germ cells proliferate for about 100 days after birth, indicating mitotic activity including the transformation of gonocytes into Ad (dark) spermatogonia (the stem cell for spermatogenesis) and subsequently a decrease after about 6 months, mainly by apoptosis[1030] at an age coincident with the waning of gonadotropins and testosterone.

Neural Control

The timing of puberty has been linked to the vague, but generally accepted, concept of "maturation" of the CNS. The maturation is the outcome or consequence of the totality of environmental and genetic factors that retard or accelerate the onset of puberty. It is a provocative but unproven hypothesis that a metabolic signal related to body composition is an important factor in the maturation or activation of the hypothalamic GnRH pulse generator and not a result of the early hormonal and body composition changes in human puberty. In either event, clinical and experimental data support the contention that the factors influencing the timing of puberty are expressed finally through CNS regulation of the onset of puberty.[786,787,939,940,973,1037-1039] In the human, the pineal gland and melatonin do not appear to have a major effect on this control system.[787,1040-1050]

Timing and Onset of Puberty

Genetic Neural Control

Many levels control the onset of pubertal development so a systems biology approach holds promise in characterizing the complex components of this neural and neuroendocrine network. It appears that normal and some types of abnormal puberty are under polygenic control.[1051] Whereas the increased pulsatile release of GnRH is most frequently considered, this change is caused by a balance in the inhibitory and excitatory factors via coordinated changes in transsynaptic and glial-neuronal communication, increase in stimulatory factors, most prominently glutamate and kisspeptin, and decrease in inhibitory tone, mostly via gamma aminobutyric acid (GABA)ergic and opioidergic neurons, all ultimately controlled by gene expression. Glial cells affect GnRH secretion though growth factor dependent cell-cell signaling coordinated by numerous unrelated genes. A second level of genes is postulated to control cell-cell interaction. Lastly, a third highest level of control occurs via transcriptional regulation of the subordinate genes by other of the higher-level genes that maintain the function and integration of the network. New genomic and metabolomic methods and a systems biology approach should illuminate these complex processes.

Although the action of multiple genes (quantitative or polygenic inheritance) on the time of onset of puberty (or, for example, on stature[1052,1053]) has long been recognized, little is known about the gene loci involved in this complex quantitative trait or the effect of gene interactions (epistaxis) on this paradigm of complex traits.[1054-1059] Genetic factors are estimated to account for 50% to 80% of the variation in the onset of normal puberty. These complex traits are now analyzed by study of linkage analysis (e.g., quantitative trait loci are shown to relate to the age of menarche)[1060] and large-scale haplotype-based association studies (e.g., variation in GnRH1 and GnRH receptor proteins do not seem to be related to pubertal onset in a significant manner).[1061] Pedigree analyses have revealed relative risks of delay in puberty in kindreds with histories of constitutional delay compared to those without; for example, for first-degree relatives, the risk for 2 SD delay in the onset of puberty is 4.8.[1062] There are clear genetic influences on the time of onset of puberty in monogenetic disorders, such as Kal 1 or GRP54 mutations (see below) that can prevent pubertal development.

Nutrition and Metabolic Control

The genetic influences on the time of onset of puberty and its course are influenced by environmental factors operating through the CNS. The latter include socioeconomic factors, nutrition, general health, geography, and altitude discussed above. It has long been postulated that some alteration of body metabolism linked to energy metabolism may affect the CNS restraints on pubertal onset and progression.[960,1063,1064]

The role of nutritional factors and body composition in the onset of menarche[1064-1066] is supported by the earlier age of menarche in moderately obese girls[92]; delayed menarche in states of malnutrition and chronic disease, in twins, and after early rigorous athletic or ballet training; and the relationship of weight and diminished body fat to changes in gonadotropin secretion and amenorrhea in girls with anorexia nervosa,[1067] voluntary weight loss, and strenuous physical conditioning.[1068-1071] An "invariant mean weight" (48 kg) for the initiation of the pubertal spurt in weight, the maximal rate of weight gain, and menarche in healthy girls regardless of chronologic age was proposed[1066,1072-1074] but the concept generated controversy and criticism[1057,1076-1080] in part because the empirical estimations and the equations used to determine fat mass were challenged and because no direct measurements supported the theory.[1081-1083] A recent 5-year longitudinal study of 469 girls revealed that puberty began at different chronologic ages but there was a similar percentage of body fat associated with the onset.[1084] On the other hand, other studies report no change in body fat or body composition at the time of menarche that accompany the change in hormone production although substantial changes occur in early puberty and in premenarcheal in girls.[77,1085]

The relationship of adipose tissue mass, fat metabolism, and energy balance to reproduction was illuminated by the discovery of the genes encoding leptin, an adipocyte satiety factor,[1086-1091] and its receptor.[1092] In rodents it stimulates energy expenditure among a variety of other actions. Leptin is a highly conserved 167 amino acid cytokine-like protein produced mainly but not exclusively by adipose tissue; a mutant gene was first isolated from the very obese ob/ob mouse by positional cloning.[1086] Soon thereafter the leptin receptor was cloned,[1092] which is a member of the gp family of cytokine receptors, and the mutation identified in the obese db/db mouse.[1093]

Both ob/ob and db/db mice[1094] are not only obese but also exhibit hypogonadotropic hypogonadism providing evidence for an important role of leptin in reproduction. Correction of the infertility in ob/ob mice is achieved by administration of recombinant leptin.[1095-1098] The pubertal delay associated with food restriction in the rat was partially reversed by the administration of leptin and suggested that a fall in circulating leptin below a critical level would occur with 30% to 75% food restriction.[1099,1100] However, leptin administration to normal prepubertal rats did not advance the time of onset of puberty.[1099] The sum of studies in rodents indicates a critical threshold level of leptin was necessary for puberty to begin and advance, but leptin alone (as in administration to normal rodents) was insufficient to promote puberty[1101] but was one, among several, permissive factors (Fig. 24–33).[1102]

Among the various sites of action of leptin in the hypothalamus, one site seems to be a direct action on hypothalamic GnRH neurons; in the rodent, these neurosecretory neurons contain leptin receptors (including the Ob-Rb isoform) and release GnRH in response to leptin.[1103-1105] Leptin may act also indirectly on the GnRH pulse generator (Fig. 24–34).[1106,1107]

In the male rhesus monkey, leptin levels were similar during the advancement of prepuberty to puberty.[1108,1109] In the peripubertal rhesus monkey 3 to 5 years old, fasted for 2 days, the administration of leptin prevented the decrease in plasma gonadotropins detected in the untreated animals.[1110] Continuous infusion of leptin into the lateral ventricle of agonadal male monkeys failed to evoke an increase in GnRH on gonadotropin secretion.

Leptin is a well-established afferent satiety factor acting on the hypothalamus, including nuclei controlling appetite, to suppress appetite.[279,937,1111-1113] Leptin reflects body fat and hence energy stores and has an important role in the control of body weight and the regulation of metabolism.[1089,1091,1111,1112] Leptin is secreted in a pulsatile manner[1114] and exhibits a diurnal rhythm with a peak at night and a nadir in the morning.[1111,1112,1115] Considerable interest has focused on the potential role of leptin in the control of the onset of puberty—from a proposal that it was an essential, if not a key, factor in triggering the onset of puberty to one in which it had a more subsidiary role.

Is leptin the peripheral somatic trigger for the onset of puberty to the CNS, or does it have a permissive role, signaling the hypothalamus and the GnRH pulse generator that a critical energy store[77,1064,1065] has been attained? While the first longitudinal study of plasma leptin in normal boys before and during puberty suggested that there was a brief rise in circulating leptin at the onset of puberty,[2709] two large cross-sectional studies[1116,1117] and a longitudinal study[1118] of serum leptin levels in prepubertal and pubertal boys and girls later showed leptin to increase gradually during the prepubertal years with similar levels in both sexes.[1118] During puberty, leptin continued to rise in girls, whereas in boys the leptin mean levels peaked at Tanner stage 2.[1116,1117,2710] and decreased to prepubertal concentrations by genital stage 5 (see Fig. 24–33). The decrease is attributed to the effect of testosterone on leptin secretion.[1119,1120] Adipose tissue mass, percentage body fat, and age were correlated with leptin levels among other variables,[1116-1118,1121] but there was no correlation between 24-hour serum estradiol and leptin concentrations in nonobese and obese prepubertal and early pubertal girls.[1115] Serum leptin rises after administration of pulsatile GnRH administration for 36 hours to children with delayed puberty but not after a single dose of buserelin, suggesting that rather than leptin triggering puberty, pubertal increase in GnRH pulsatility increases leptin.[1122]

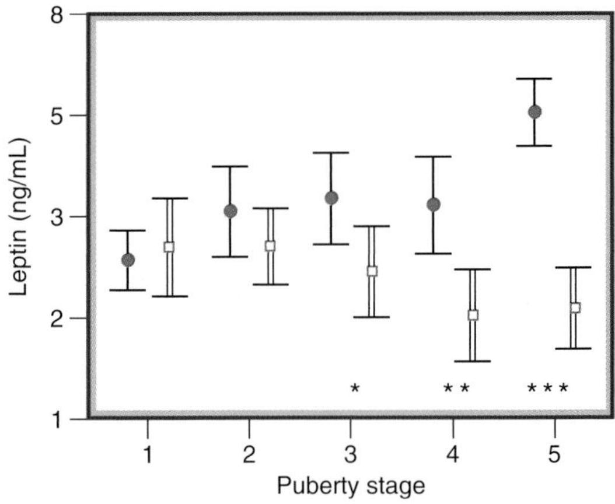

Figure 24–33 ▪ Mean leptin ±95% CI (log scale) by puberty stage in boys and girls, with significant sex differences marked. (*$P<.05$; **$P<.005$; ***$P<.0005$). (From Ahmed ML, Ong KK, Morrell NJ, et al. Longitudinal study of leptin concentrations during puberty. J Clin Endocrinol Metab 1999;84:902.)

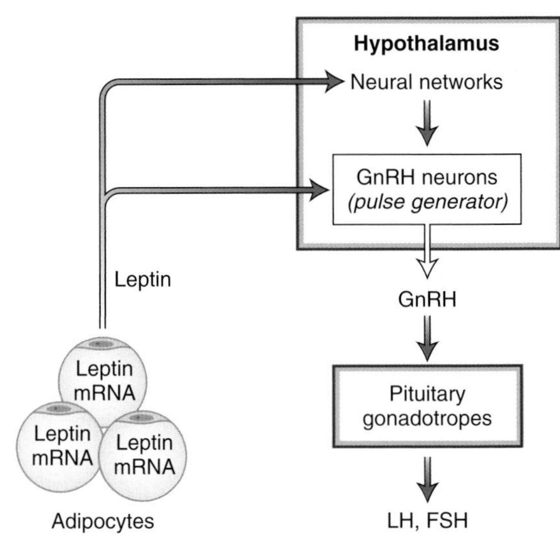

Figure 24–34 ▪ The postulated action of leptin secreted by adipocytes on the hypothalamic luteinizing hormone–releasing hormone (GnRH) pulse generator. Its indirect action through hypothalamic neural networks is illustrated as well as direct action. Leptin appears to function as a permissive factor, not a trigger, in the onset of human puberty. Although leptin is reported to advance puberty in rodents, its role in "triggering" puberty in humans has not been established and is speculative. *FSH,* Follicle-stimulating hormone; *mRNA,* messenger ribonucleic acid. *(See text.)*

In the human, leptin circulates in both a free and a high molecular weight bound form.[1123] Leptin-binding activity in serum is highest in childhood and decreases to relatively low levels during puberty.[1124] Free leptin is postulated to have more relevance than total leptin measured in the circulation to reproductive development.[1125] The soluble leptin receptor appears higher in males than females and is inversely related to leptin levels later in development in females,[1125] as a study of a 132 monozygotic female twin pairs and 48 dizygotic female twin pairs demonstrated a rise in leptin throughout puberty and a decrease in the soluble leptin receptor between stages 1 and 2, leading to a rise in the free leptin index between stage 1 and 2. There was a greater heritability of the soluble leptin receptor than of leptin,[1126] and there was also a high heritability of free IGF-I values. There is no known relationship between leptin and leptin receptor gene polymorphism and constitutional delay in puberty (CDP); however the presence of a short allele of leptin was associated with heavier weight while those who were thin and had significant bone age delay and increased frequency of parental pubertal delay were less likely to have this leptin short allele.[1127]

As in the Ob/Ob mouse, humans with a homozygous mutation in the leptin gene[1128] or the leptin receptor[1129] not only have morbid obesity but also a striking delay in puberty owing to hypogonadotropic hypogonadism.

In a pedigree affected by a stop codon mutation in the gene encoding leptin, a 23-year-old man had failed to attain puberty due to hypogonadotropic hypogonadism[1128] and two affected women were prepubertal and amenorrheic until at 29 years, one began to have irregular scanty periods and at 36 years another began to menstruate monthly. A 9-year-old girl with a bone age of 13 years affected with congenital leptin deficiency lost weight and had an early pubertal pattern of LH release to the administration of GnRH following treatment with recombinant leptin.[1130] A 4-year-old affected relative of this 9-year-old girl benefited from the metabolic improvement with leptin administration but did not under go early pubertal development, indicating the permissive nature of leptin on puberty.[943]

Boys with CDP have lower mean levels of leptin than expected and can enter puberty without an increase in circulating leptin. In two women with congenital lipoatrophic diabetes (Berardinelli-Seip syndrome), which is associated with absence of both subcutaneous and visceral adipose tissue, the severe hypoleptinemia did not lead to a delay in menarche and one of the women had three unaffected children.[1120] These observations suggest that severe leptin deficiency causes hypogonadotropic hypogonadism, and that a critical level of leptin and a leptin signal are required to achieve puberty but a *rise* in leptin is *not* required to trigger puberty.[1118,1121]

In sum, accumulating evidence supports the function of leptin as a permissive factor (tonic mediator) and not a trigger (phasic mediator) in the onset of human puberty (Table 24–19).[973,1131] Recently, studies in the mouse have shown that leptin binds to kisspeptin containing neurons. This finding supports an interaction between leptin and the kisspeptin GPR54 signaling.

To relate metabolism to the onset of puberty, a longitudinal study of boys followed up for the 18 months leading up to an increase in morning salivary testosterone concentrations, the boys had a relatively constant basal metabolic rate (BMR)/lean body mass (LBM) ratio but an increase in the ratio of BMR/total daily energy expenditure. The suggestion is that a subtle energy-dependent process is in play, possibly related to an increase in brain BMR as a secondary phenomenon at the initiation of puberty or that a central rise in BMR is a signal for the onset of puberty.[1132,1133]

Ghrelin is the natural ligand for the growth hormone secretagoge receptor but also serves as a orexogenic signal that is increased after food deprivation; ghrelin is usually negatively correlated with body mass index.[1134] Ghrelin administration delays pubertal development in rats due to gonadal and central effects suggesting a link between malnutrition and the decrease in reproductive development or function.[1135]

Adiponectin is an adipocytokine produced in fat cells, producing antidiabetic and antiatherogenic effects and exerting antiinflammatory effects. Adiponectin decreases in the face of excess fat mass in obesity and is suppressed by rising testosterone and DHEAS, falling during pubertal development in males and remaining rather stable in females with advancing Tanner srage.[1136,1137]

Restin is an adipocytokine belonging to the restin-like molecule family of cysteine-rich molecules (RELM). Values increase with pubertal development in boys and, although the evidence is weaker, appears to be true of girls as well. Because resistin serum levels were elevated in mouse models of obesity, resistin was considered to be a potential link between insulin resistance and obesity, but serum resistin appears to relate more to pubertal development than insulin resistance.[1138]

TABLE 24–19 LEPTIN AND PUBERTY: A PERMISSIVE FACTOR, NOT A TRIGGER FOR THE ONSET OF PUBERTY

PRO TRIGGER
Congenital leptin deficiency or congenital leptin resistance related to mutations is associated with delayed puberty and hypogonadotropin deficiency, evidence that the virtual absence of leptin or the leptin signal leads to severe hypogonadotropic hypogonadism.
In congenital leptin deficiency, administration of leptin led to a reduction in weight and an early pubertal pattern of luteinizing hormone release in an affected prepubertal girl.
However:
PRO PERMISSIVE
A sharp rise in circulating leptin does not occur at the onset of puberty.
In prepubertal and early pubertal girls, the rise in serum leptin did not correlate with the increase in serum estradiol.
In constitutional delay in growth and adolescence, an increase in prepubertal leptin levels is not essential for the onset of puberty.
In congenital lipoatrophic diabetes, despite the absence of subcutaneous and visceral adipose tissue and, as a consequence, severe hypoleptinemia, puberty can occur at the usual age and fertility is reported.
Supportive experimental data in the rodent, sheep, and nonhuman primate.

(From Grumbach MM. The neuroendocrinology of human puberty revisited. Horm Res 2002; 57(suppl 2):2-14.)

Mechanisms of Control

In rodents, exteroceptive factors and cues, including light, olfaction, and pheromones, have an important influence, by way of the CNS, on gonadotropin secretion.[959,960] In seasonal breeding species, such as sheep, the length of the light-dark cycle is critical and the pattern of gonadotropin secretion is different.[1139] In contrast, male and female primates exhibit an estrogen-provoked LH surge. In brief, diverse strategies and adaptive mechanisms have evolved to control puberty in different species.[935,938,943,941,1139-1142]

In humans and subhuman primates, after development and function in the fetus, infantile surge of increased LH and FSH secretion occurs, followed by a decade of suppression (but not absence of activity of the hypothalamic GnRH pulse generator and resulting quiescence of the pituitary gonadotropin-gonadal axis, the prepubertal period or juvenile pause (Table 24–20),[279,787,935,938,942,1143] until the gradual disinhibition and reactivation mainly at night during late childhood[787,1144,1145,935,938,942,943] and finally, the increased amplitude of the GnRH pulses, which are reflected in the progressively increased and changing pattern of circulating LH pulses, with the approach of and during puberty (Fig. 24–31).

Two interacting mechanisms have been proposed to explain the juvenile pause (Fig. 24–35)[787,1144] the negative feedback mechanism (gonadal steroid dependent) and "intrinsic" CNS inhibitory mechanism (gonadal steroid independent).

TABLE 24–20 POTENTIAL COMPONENTS OF THE INTRINSIC CENTRAL NERVOUS SYSTEM INHIBITORY MECHANISM ("JUVENILE PAUSE")

I. Inhibitory
   A. Inhibitory central neurotransmitter-neuromodulatory pathways
      1. γ-Aminobutyric acid (the main inhibitory factor)
      2. Endogenous opioid peptides
II. Stimulatory
   A. Stimulatory central neurotransmitter-neuromodulatory pathways
      1. Excitatory amino acids
      2. Calcium-mobilizing agonists
      3. Noradrenergic
      4. Dopaminergic
      5. Neuropeptide Y (NPY)
      6. Nitric oxide
      7. Prostaglandins, PGE_2
   B. Other brain peptides
      1. Neurotrophic and growth peptides
      2. Activin A
      3. Endothelin −1, −2, −3

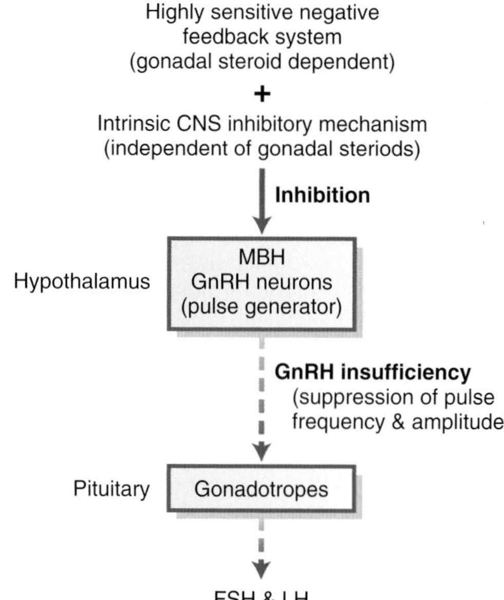

Figure 24–35 ▪ Postulated dual mechanism of restraint of puberty involves both gonadal steroid-dependent and gonadal steroid-independent (intrinsic central nervous system inhibitory mechanism) processes. *MBH,* Medial basal hypothalamus. (Modified from Grumbach MM, Kaplan SL. The neuroendocrinology of human puberty: an ontogenetic perspective. In Grumbach MM, Sizonenko PC, Aubert ML, eds. Control of the Onset of Puberty. Baltimore: Williams & Wilkins, 1990:1-68.)

The principal evidence for an operative negative feedback mechanism in prepubertal children[786,787] is as follows:

1. The pituitary of the prepubertal child secretes small amounts of FSH and LH, showing a low level of activity of the hypothalamic-pituitary-gonadal complex.
2. In agonadal infants and prepubertal children (e.g., Turner's syndrome), secretion of FSH and, to a lesser degree, LH is increased, suggesting that even low levels of hormones secreted by the normal prepubertal gonad inhibit gonadotropin secretion by a sensitive, functional, tonic, negative feedback mechanism (Fig. 24–36).[786,787,1032,1144,1145]
3. The low level of gonadotropin secretion in childhood is shut off by administration of small amounts of gonadal steroids, showing that the hypothalamic-pituitary gonadotropin unit is highly sensitive (approximately 6 to 15 times more sensitive than in the adult) to the feedback effect of gonadal steroids (Fig. 24–37).[786,787,1146] The ontogeny of the negative feedback mechanism beginning in the fetus is described above (see Figs. 24–28 and 24–29).[786,787]

In "intrinsic" CNS inhibitory mechanism (gonadal steroid independent), the diphasic pattern of basal and GnRH-induced FSH and LH secretion from infancy to adulthood is similar in normal individuals and in agonadal patients, but in the latter gonadotropin concentrations are higher, except during the middle childhood nadir.[1144,1145] The high concentration of plasma FSH and LH in agonadal children between infancy and about age 4 years and the increased gonadotropin reserve reflect the absence of gonadal steroid inhibition (Fig. 24–38) of the hypothalamic-pituitary unit by the low levels of plasma gonadal steroids.[787] However, the striking fall in gonadotropin secretion between ages 4 and 11 suggests the presence of a CNS inhibitory mechanism restraining the hypothalamic GnRH pulse generator, independent of gonadal steroid secretion. The resulting fall in gonadotropin secretion in agonadal children is not due to gonadal steroid feedback (because functional gonads are lacking) or to increased secretion of adrenal steroids (because concentrations are low and glucocorticoid suppression of the adrenal does not augment the concentration of circulating gonadotropins).[787] Thus, a CNS steroid-independent inhibitory mechanism for suppression of the hypothalamic GnRH pulse generator seems to be the dominant factor in restraint of puberty between ages 4 and 11[787,1147] and a gradual loss of this intrinsic

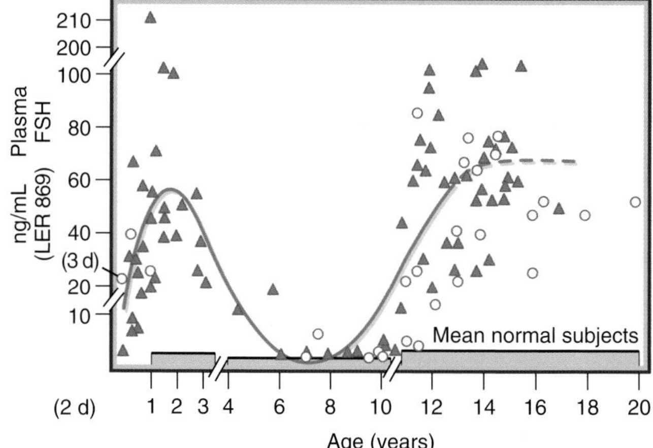

Figure 24–36 ▪ Change in pattern of the plasma concentration of follicle-stimulating hormone (FSH) with age in 58 patients with the syndrome of gonadal dysgenesis. Mixed longitudinal ($n=23$) and cross-sectional ($n=35$) data. Triangles designate patients with 45,X karyotype. Circles indicate Turner's syndrome patients with X chromosome mosaicism or structural abnormalities of the X chromosome, or both. Note the values in the 2- and 3-day-old infants. The solid line represents a regression line of best fit. The hatched area indicates the mean plasma values in normal females. To convert FSH values to international units per liter, multiply by 8.4. (From Conte FA, Grumbach MM, Kaplan SL. A diphasic pattern of gonadotropin secretion in patients with the syndrome of gonadal dysgenesis. J Clin Endocrinol Metab 1975;40:670-674. Copyright by The Endocrine Society.)

CNS inhibitory mechanism would lead to disinhibition or reactivation of the GnRH pulse generator at puberty.

Interaction of negative feedback mechanism and intrinsic CNS inhibitory mechanism both appear to interact to restrain puberty (see Fig. 24–38). During the first 2 to 3 years of life, the gonadal steroid negative feedback mechanism seems dominant,

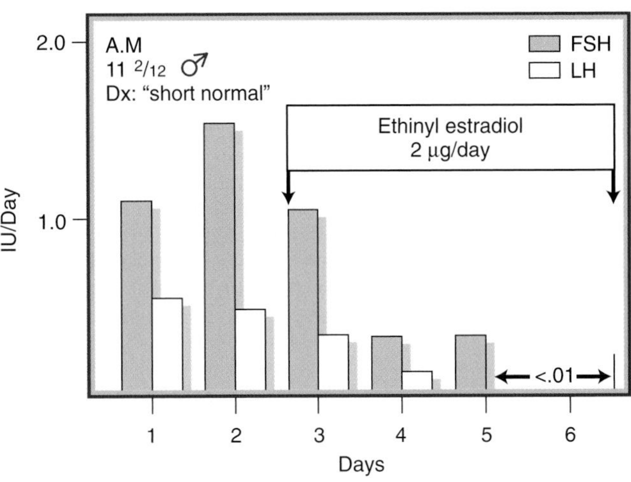

Figure 24–37 ▪ Effect of administration of ethinyl estradiol (2 µg/day) on the urinary excretion of luteinizing hormone (LH) and follicle-stimulating hormone (FSH) in a prepubertal normal male age 11 years, 2 months. Note the rapid and significant decrease in LH and FSH levels by day 3 after treatment with estradiol; by day 4 the excretion of FSH and LH is less than 0.01 IU. (From Kelch RP, Kaplan SL, Grumbach MM. Suppression of urinary and plasma follicle-stimulating hormone by exogenous estrogens in prepubertal and pubertal children. J Clin Invest 1973;52:1122-1128. Copyright of the American Society for Clinical Investigation.)

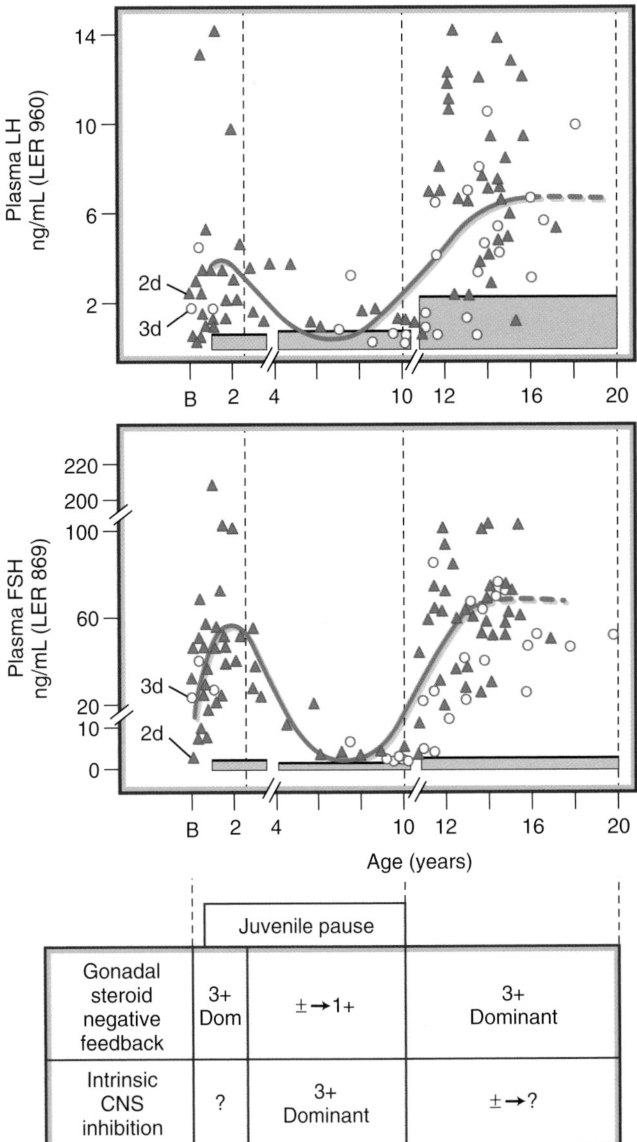

Figure 24–38 ▪ Interaction of the negative feedback mechanism and the putative intrinsic central nervous system (CNS) inhibitory mechanism in restraining puberty as extrapolated from the pattern of change in the concentrations of follicle-stimulating hormone (FSH) and luteinizing hormone (LH) in agonadal infants, children, and adolescents. (See Fig. 24–37 for key to symbols; the solid line is the regression curve of best fit; the solid bars connote the mean normal concentrations +1 SD of FSH and LH.) For about the first 3 years of life, the sensitive gonadal steroid, negative feedback mechanism has a dominant role in restraining gonadotropin secretion, as exemplified by the high gonadotropin concentrations in this age group in the absence of gonads (and gonadal steroid feedback). A major role of the intrinsic CNS inhibitory mechanism in this age group is unlikely in light of the rise in gonadotropins to castrate levels in the absence of functional gonads. From 4 to 6 years of age, the postulated intrinsic CNS inhibitory mechanism is dominant, as indicated by the fall in FSH and LH concentrations in the absence of gonads. Even in this age group, the augmented gonadotropin response evoked by GnRH and the slightly higher mean basal gonadotropin concentrations in agonadal individuals support a role, although a subsidiary one, for gonadal steroid negative feedback in the suppression of gonadotropin secretion during this period of the juvenile pause. The authors suggest that the intrinsic CNS inhibitory mechanism suppresses the functional GnRH pulse generator. Finally, after about 10 years of age, the CNS inhibition gradually wanes, resulting in disinhibition of the GnRH pulse generator. The gonadal steroid negative feedback mechanism with an adult-type set-point and inhibin play a dominant role in regulating the GnRH pulse generator-pituitary gonadotropin system. For conversion to SI units, see the legend of Figure 24–21. (Modified from Grumbach MM, Kaplan SL. The neuroendocrinology of human puberty: an ontogenetic perspective. In Grumbach MM, Sizonenko PC, Aubert ML, eds. Control of the Onset of Puberty. Baltimore: Williams & Wilkins, 1990:1-68.)

but beginning at about 3 years of age, the intrinsic CNS inhibitory mechanism becomes dominant and remains so during the rest of the juvenile pause, as evidenced by the fall in FSH and LH levels between ages 3 and 10 despite the lack of functional gonads. However, during this segment of the juvenile pause, the negative feedback mechanism remains operative: agonadal patients in this age group have higher mean plasma FSH levels than normal prepubertal children and a greater FSH and LH response to the acute administration of GnRH.[1144,1145] As puberty approaches, the CNS inhibitory mechanism gradually wanes, initially during nighttime sleep, and the hypothalamic GnRH pulse generator becomes less sensitive to gonadal steroid negative feedback (Fig. 24–39).[787] After the onset of puberty, gonadal steroid negative feedback attains the set-point characteristic of the adult and is again the dominant mechanism in restraining gonadotropin secretion (along with inhibin), as reflected in the increased gonadotropin concentrations characteristic of the adolescent with severe primary hypogonadism (see Fig. 24–38). A similar pattern has been described in the infant monkey.[1028] The postulated ontogeny of this dual mechanism of restraint of puberty is illustrated in Figure 24–39. Many neural, neurotransmitter/neuromodulator, hormonal, growth factors, and metabolic factors[1148-1154] as well as exteroceptive influences and cues can influence the activity of the GnRH pulse generator, but the nature of the intrinsic CNS inhibitory mechanism remains elusive.[938] In the rhesus monkey, despite the damping of the GnRH pulse generator during the juvenile pause,[1155] the content of hypothalamic GnRH and the GnRH messenger RNA during this phase is similar to that in the infant and adult monkey. Low-amplitude LH and FSH pulses are detectable by sensitive and specific immunoradiometric assays in the juvenile pause demonstrates a low level of activity of the GnRH pulse genera-

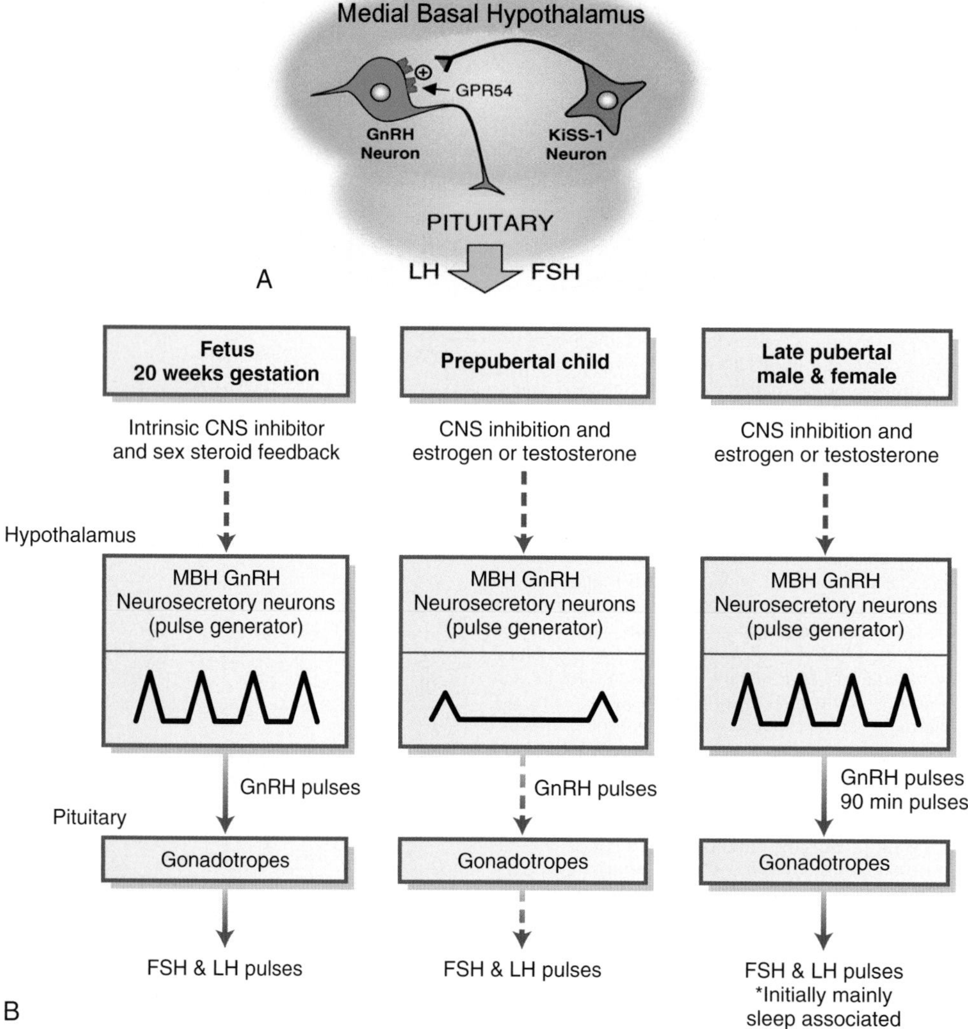

Figure 24–39 ▪ **A,** Kisspeptin–GPR54 and the GnRH neuron. KiSS-1 mRNA expressing neurons in the medial basal hypothalamus synapse with GnRH neurons. Activation of the kisspeptin receptor GPR54 on the GnRH neuron entrains the release of GnRH into the portal circulation which induces the gonadotropes to release LH and FSH. Diagram modified from Smith JT, Clifton DK, Steiner RA. Regulation of the neuroendocrine reproductive axis by kisspeptin-GPR54 signaling. Reproduction 2006; 131:623-630. **B,** Postulated ontogeny of the dual mechanism for the inhibition of puberty. Interrupted arrows indicate inhibition. Note the action of both components during the juvenile pause (prepuberty). See Figure 24–38 for the relative role of these two mechanisms during development. GnRH, MBH, medial basal hypothalamus. (Modified from Grumbach MM, Kaplan SL. The neuroendocrinology of human puberty: an ontogenetic perspective. In Grumbach MM, Sizonenko PC, Aubert ML, eds. Control of the Onset of Puberty. Baltimore: Williams & Wilkins, 1990:1-68.)

tor.[1156,1157,790-792,818] The end of the juvenile pause is marked by an increase in LH pulse amplitude most evident during the early hours of sleep.[1156,1157]

Potential Components of the Intrinsic CNS Inhibitory Mechanism

Children with true precocious puberty associated with posterior hypothalamic neoplasms (usually a pilocytic astrocytoma), radiation of the CNS, midline CNS developmental abnormalities such as septo-optic dysplasia with deficiency of one or more pituitary hormones, or other CNS lesions provide indirect evidence for an inhibitory neural component located in or projecting through the posterior hypothalamus. These lesions compromise the neural pathway inhibiting the hypothalamic GnRH pulse generator, resulting in its disinhibition and activation leading to true (or central) precocious puberty.[787] For example, a suprasellar arachnoid cyst can cause true precocious puberty by compressing and distorting the hypothalamus[787] but the puberty is reversed with regression of the hormonal and physical features of puberty after decompression of the cyst due to reversal of the disinhibition of the CNS inhibitory mechanism of the posterior pituitary (Fig. 24–40). In addition, precocious sexual maturation can be induced in the juvenile female rhesus monkey by posterior hypothalamic lesions[1158]; such lesions advance the age at onset of a pubertal increase in LH secretion and the time of the first positive feedback effects of estrogen.[1159]

The GnRH-secreting hypothalamic hamartoma, a heterotypic mass of nervous tissue that contains GnRH neurosecretory neurons[1160,1161] attached to the tuber cinereum or the floor of the third ventricle, can cause true precocious puberty.[1162] The GnRH neurons within the hamartoma with their axon fibers projecting to the median eminence secrete GnRH in pulsatile fashion. We consider the hypothalamic hamartoma an "ectopic GnRH pulse generator" that functions independently of the CNS inhibitory mechanism that normally restrains the hypothalamic GnRH pulse generator (Fig. 24–41).[787,1162] An analogy can be drawn between the GnRH-secreting hypothalamic hamartoma and the rescue of fertility in the GnRH-deficient hypogonadal mouse (hyp/hyg) by transplantation of fetal or neonatal hypothalamic tissue into the third ventricle.[1163,1164] Some rare, large hypothalamic hamartomas that cause true precocious puberty contain TGF-α, an astroglial-derived growth factor, with few or no GnRH neurosecretory neurons, raising the possibility that the secretion of TGF-α may interact directly or indirectly to stimulate GnRH release.

Noradrenergic, dopaminergic, serotoninergic, and opioidergic pathways; inhibitory neurotransmitters (e.g., γ-aminobutyric acid), excitatory amino acids (e.g., glutamic and aspartic acids), nitrinergic transmitters, other brain peptides, including neurotrophic and growth factors, and corticotropin-releasing hormone affect the hypothalamic GnRH pulse generator (see Table 24–21).[941,1140,1148-1154,1021,1165-1172] The studies of Plant[942] in the monkey and of others in the human exclude melatonin as a critical restraining factor in primates.[787,1041-1043,1173] Likewise, endogenous opioid peptides do not appear to play an important role in the juvenile pause.[1174-1178]

A critical and landmark advance in our understanding of the nature of the juvenile phase and central inhibition of the GnRH pulse generator was provided by Terasawa and her colleagues when the GnRH pulse generator was demonstrated to be inhibited by GABA (the most important inhibitory neurotransmitter in the primate brain) and GABAergic neurons during prepuberty but that exogenous administration of GABA in prepuberty is ineffective because of the high local endogenous GABA levels (Fig. 24–42).[938,1156,1157,1179-1182] Both GAD 65 and GAD 67 forms of glutamic acid decarboxylase (GAD), the enzyme that catalyzes the conversion of glutamate to GABA. are present in in the mediobasal hypothalamus, the site of the GnRH pulse generator. Antisense oligodeoxynucleotides for GAD 67 and GAD 65 mRNAs infused into the stalk median eminence of prepubertal monkeys induced a striking increase in GnRH release whereas nonsense D-oligos did not.[1179] These latter studies provide additional support for GABA, arising from interneurons, as the the intrinsic CNS inhibitor during the juvenile pause of prepuberty.[1180] GABA acting through both $GABA_A$ and $GABA_B$ receptors affects GnRH secretion in the perifused mouse GT1 GnRH-releasing neuronal cell line.[1183-1185] Conversely, the administration of chronic repetitive administration of bicuculline, GABA inhibitor, into the base of the third ventricle of a prepubertal monkey causes premature menarche and the onset of the first ovulation.[1182] While GABA is inhibitory in the juvenile and adult brain, early in brain development through the postnatal period, GABAergic synaptic transmission is excitatory and increases intracellular Ca^{2+} concentration.[1186,1187] It seems possible that the transition from the dominance of the gonadal steroid-dependent negative-feedback mechanism in infancy and early childhood to the dominance of the intrinsic CNS inhibitory mechanism is associated with the developmental switch of GABAergic synaptic transmission from excitatory to inhibitory.

Thus, the onset of puberty in the rhesus monkey is characterized by the decrease in GABAergic (and possibly neuropeptide Y [NPY]) inhibition of the hypothalamic GnRH pulse generator and the increased release of glutamate,[938,1188] the major excitatory amino acid neurotransmitter in the hypothalamus.[1189,1170,1190] The sensitivity to the stimulatory glutaminergic input into the GnRH pulse generator increases strikingly after the onset of puberty,[1191] but it is the reduction in GABAergic inhibition that is the critical factor in disinhibition of the GnRH pulse generator.[938]

A persistent question has been how a single central signal can activate GnRH neurons to cause LH release and bring about ovulation by simultaneous suppression of GABA and stimulation of glutamate release, both of which each converge in the anteroventral periventricular nucleus (AVPV). Recently is was reported that nearly all neurons in the AVPV of female rats express both vesicular glutamate transporter 2 (VGLUT2), a marker of hypothalamic glutamatergic neurons, as well as glutamic acid decarboxylase and vesicular GABA transporter (VGAT), markers of GABAergic neurons. These dual-phenotype neurons are twice as prevalent in females than males and are the main targets of E2 in the region.[1192] Moreover, dual-phenotype synaptic terminals contact GnRH neurons, and at the time of the surge, VGAT-containing vesicles decrease and VGLUT2-containing vesicles increase in these terminals. Dual-phenotype GABA/glutamate neurons may act as central transducers of hormonal and neural signals to GnRH neurons.

Excitatory N-methyl-d-aspartate (NMDA) amino acid neurotransmitter receptors are widely distributed throughout the CNS including the hypothalamus.[1022] NMDA stimulates LH release in neonatal[1193] and adult[1194] rats, fetal sheep,[1021,1166] and prepubertal[1190] and adult[1195] rhesus monkeys. NMDA evokes GnRH secretion from rat hypothalamic explants[1196] from a GnRH neuronal cell line[1197] but does not have a direct effect on pituitary gonadotropes.[1166] Parenthetically, NMDA administration acutely stimulates the GnRH pulse generator in the ovine fetus, providing additional evidence of NMDA receptors on fetal GnRH neurons and the functional capacity of the fetal pulse generator.[1021] Immortalized GnRH neurons contain ionotropic NMDA receptors that mediate the release of GnRH by NMDA.[1198] The prepubertal male rhesus monkey may be forced to enter puberty by repetitive intravenous administration of NMDA; in both the prepubertal and pubertal female rhesus, NMDA administered centrally and peripherally induced the release of GnRH.[938,1188,1199]

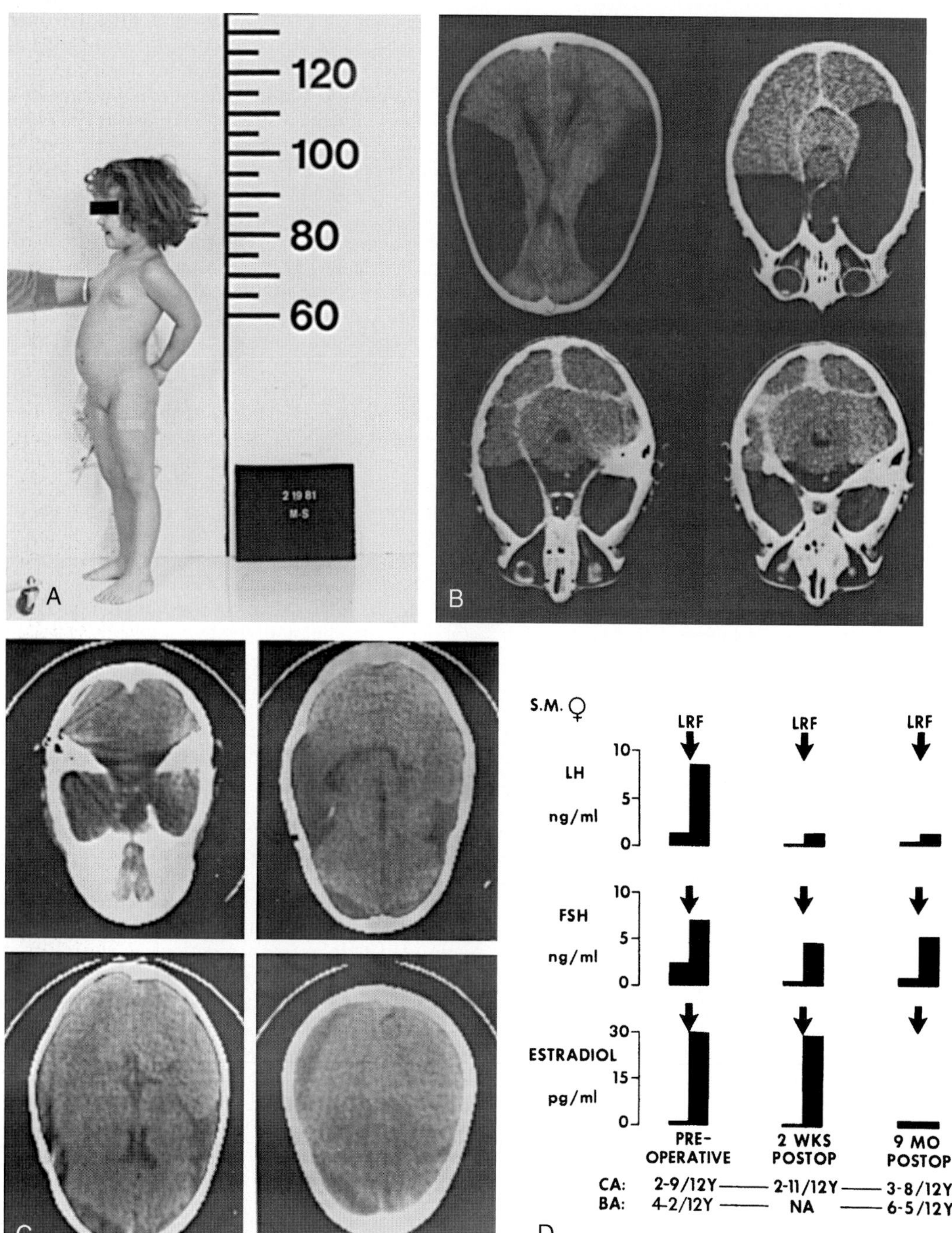

Figure 24–40 ▪ **A,** True precocious puberty in a 2 9/12-year-old girl secondary to a large bilateral congenital suprasellar arachnoid cyst. Signs of sexual precocity were noted during the preceding year. The head circumference was +5 SD above the mean value for age, and frontal bossing was present. Breasts were Tanner stage 3. Serum estradiol, 26 pg/mL; estrone, 38 pg/mL; dehydroepiandrosterone sulfate (DHEAS), less than 3 μg/dL. The serum luteinizing hormone (LH) concentration rose from 1.4 to 8.7 ng/mL (LER-960) after IV administration of gonadotropin-releasing hormone GnRH, which constitutes a pubertal response. Bone age, 3 6/12 years. Pelvic ultrasonography showed pubertal-size uterus and ovaries. To convert estrone values to picomoles per liter, multiply by 3.699. To convert DHEAS values to micromoles per liter, multiply by 0.02714. For other conversions, see legend for Figure 24–21. **B,** Cranial computed tomography (CT) scans for SM showing low-density fluid collection in the middle cranial fossa, thinning of the cortex, and striking compression of the lateral and third ventricles. **C,** Cranial CT scans 8 months later, after decompression of the arachnoid cyst and creation of a communication between the cyst and the basal cerebrospinal fluid cisterns and a cystoperitoneal shunt. Note the striking decrease in size of the fluid collections and expansion of the cerebral cortex. **D,** Basal and peak LH and follicle-stimulating hormone (FSH) concentrations after GnRH administration in SM and serum estradiol values before surgical decompression and 2 weeks and 9 months after surgical decompression of the arachnoid cyst. Note prepubertal LH response to GnRH and fall in serum estradiol level by 9 months after surgery. The bone age had increased by 3 years over an 11-month period, but the velocity returned to normal. The patient remained prepubertal during follow-up. (From Grumbach MM, Kaplan SL. The neuroendocrinology of human puberty: an ontogenetic perspective. In Grumbach MM, Sizonenko PC, Aubert ML, eds. Control of the Onset of Puberty. Baltimore: Williams & Wilkins, 1990:1-68.)

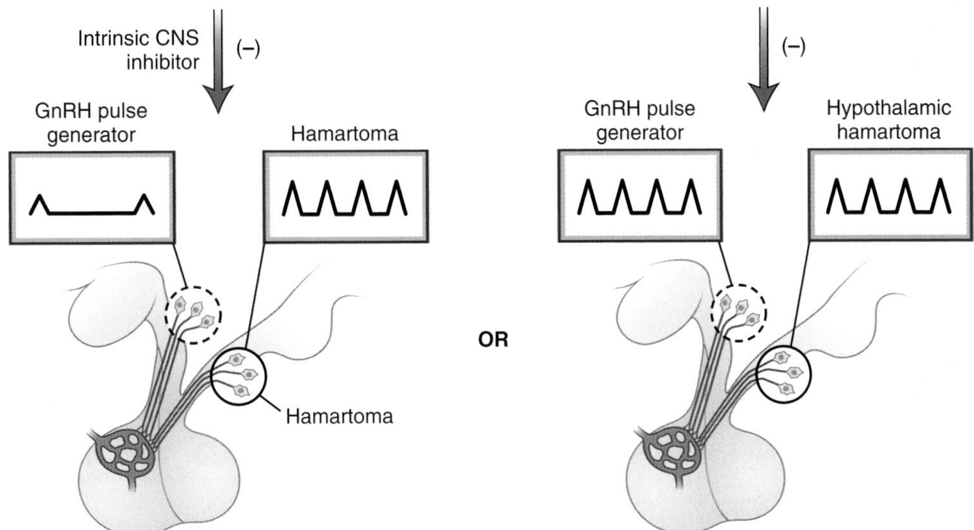

Figure 24–41 ■ Hypothalamic hamartoma as an ectopic luteinizing hormone–releasing hormone (GnRH) pulse generator that escapes the intrinsic central nervous system inhibitory mechanism and results in true precocious puberty. Two possible mechanisms are proposed. *Left,* The GnRH neurosecretory neurons in the hamartoma functioning as an GnRH pulse generator without activation of the suppressed normally located GnRH pulse generator. *Right,* The hamartoma acting as an ectopic GnRH pulse generator but communicating with and activating (possibly through axonic connections or by GnRH itself) the normally located hypothalamic GnRH pulse generator, which then functions synchronously with the hamartoma.

Recent description of the role of kisspeptins and their receptors, GRP54, in the CNS hypothalamic-pituitary-gonadal axis has led to a flurry of investigation (Figs. 24–43 and 24–44).[1200-1203] KISS-1 is a human metastasis suppressor gene at gene map locus 19p13.3 and KiSS-1 mRNA is found in placenta, testes, pancreas, liver, small intestine, and brain, mainly in the hypothalamus and basal ganglion.[1204,1205] The product of the KiSS-1 gene is a 145 amino acid peptide but the secreted product of the KISS-1 gene is a 54 amino acid known as metastin or kisspeptin, which binds to an endogenous receptor; a variety of shorter forms also are proteolytically cleaved, including kisspeptin 10, whose activity is comparable to the 54 amino acid product. GPR54 (metastin 54 receptor, a G protein–coupled receptor of the rhodopsin family). This receptor protein is found in the brain, mainly in the hypothalamus and basal ganglia, and in the placenta from where it was first isolated and sequenced. KiSS-1 mRNA is present in the primate in the medial arcuate nucleus and in the mouse in the arcuate, periventricular and anteroventral periventricular nuclei and in the regions important in reproductive function.[1206,1207]

GPR54 is coupled to the Gq subclass of G proteins and is expressed with in GnRH neurons in the rat, in the medial and lateral sections of the arcuate nucleus and the ventral aspect of the ventromedial hypothalamus in mice[1208] and in primates.[1206] As GPR54 is also located in areas not involved in reproduction, it quite likely has other functions. While the expression of GRP54 mRNA does not increase with development in the mouse, kisspeptin mRNA increases dramatically in the forebrain and the number of receptors responsive to kisspeptin increase with development[1209]; the activation of GnRH neurons by kisspeptin at puberty in both adult and prepubertal animals, including non-human primates, reflects an increase in kisspeptin input and a posttranscriptional change in GPR54 signaling within the GnRH neuron. Increases in kisspeptin lead to increased GnRH release.

Mice transfected with GPR54 genes exhibited hypogonadotropic hypogonadism, as is the case with inactivating mutations in the GPR54 gene in the human.[1211] The null GPR54 mice had normal content of GnRH in their hypothalamus[1211] and were responsive to GnRH or gonadotropin administration, suggesting normal function of the GnRH and LH and FSH receptors despite the mutation. The intact mouse also releases significant LH boluses after kisspeptin administration, an effect that is abolished in the GRP 54 -/- mouse, which lacks the receptor.[1208] Underfed prepubertal mice have decreased hypothalamic Kiss-1, but kisspeptin administration led to increases in GRP-54 mRNA which in turn led to increased GnRH and LH secretion.[998] Chronic kisspeptin administration to these underfed mice restored vaginal opening and enhanced gonadtoropin and enstrogen responses.

Administration of kisspeptin-54 into the RPOA, MPOA, PVN, and arcuate nuclei of the hypothalamus of male adult rats increased plasma luteinizing hormone and testosterone substantially[1212] and intracerebral kisspeptin administration stimulated the release of FSH.[1213,1214] Since the release of FSH is abolished with blockade of GnRH, GnRH modulates the central actions of kisspeptin in the rodent. In the rat, the mRNA for kisspeptin and its receptor increase at puberty and administration of intracerebral injection of kisspeptin in prepubertal female rats caused large peaks of LH and advanced vaginal opening as a sign of pubertal development as well as premature ovulation.[1215,1216] The ovulation elicited by peripheral kisspeptin in the prepubertal female rat is abolished by blocking GnRH.[1217]

KiSS-1 and GPR54 mRNA expression is found in the region of the arcuate nucleus of the monkey and while KISS-1 increases with puberty in intact male and female monkeys, GPR54 mRNA levels increase in intact females but not in agonadal male monkeys. Administration of Kiss-1 via intracerebral catheters to GnRH primed juvenile female rhesus monkeys stimulates GnRH release; this release is abolished by infusion of GnRH antagonist. These findings led to a postulate that KISS-1 signaling through the GPR54 receptor of primate hypothalamus may be activated at the end of the juvenile pause and contribute to the pubertal resurgence of pulsatile GnRH release of puberty.[1206] Remarkably, just as continuous infusion of GnRH suppresses GnRH release, continuous infusion of kisspeptin decreases the response of gonadotropes in the agonadal male monkey to boluses of kisspeptin. However, the release of FSH and LH after a bolus of NMDA or GnRH was maintained, demonstrating that

TABLE 24–21 POSTULATED ONTOGENY OF THE HYPOTHALAMIC-PITUITARY-GONADAL CIRCUIT

FETUS
Medial basal hypothalamic GnRH neurosecretory neurons (pulse generator) operative by 80 days of gestation Pulsatile secretion of FSH and LH by 80 days of gestation Initially unrestrained secretion of GnRH (100 to 150 days of gestation) Maturation of negative gonadal steroid feedback mechanism by 150 days of gestation—sex difference Low level of GnRH secretion at term
EARLY INFANCY
Hypothalamic GnRH pulse generator highly functional after 12 days of age Prominent FSH and LH episodic discharges until approximately 6 months of age in males and 18 months of age in females, with transient increase in plasma levels of testosterone and estradiol in males and females, respectively
LATE INFANCY AND CHILDHOOD
Intrinsic CNS inhibition of hypothalamic GnRH pulse generator operative; predominant mechanism in childhood; maximal sensitivity by approximately 4 years of age Negative feedback control of FSH and LH secretion highly sensitive to gonadal steroids (low set-point) GnRH pulse generator inhibited; low amplitude and frequency of GnRH discharges Low secretion of FSH, LH, and gonadal steroids
LATE PREPUBERTAL PERIOD
Decreasing effectiveness of intrinsic CNS inhibitory influences and decreasing sensitivity of hypothalamic-pituitary unit to gonadal steroids (increased set-point) Increased amplitude and frequency of GnRH pulses, initially most prominent with sleep (nocturnal) Increased sensitivity of gonadotrophs to GnRH Increased secretion of FSH and LH Increased responsiveness of gonad to FSH and LH Increased secretion of gonadal hormones
PUBERTY
Further decrease in CNS restraint of hypothalamic GnRH pulse generator and of the sensitivity of negative feedback mechanism to gonadal steroids Prominent sleep-associated increase in episodic secretion of GnRH gradually changes to adult pattern of pulses about every 90 minutes Pulsatile secretion of LH follows pattern of GnRH pulses Progressive development of secondary sexual characteristics Spermatogenesis in males Middle to late puberty—operative positive feedback mechanism and capacity to exhibit an estrogen-induced LH surge Ovulation in females

CNS, Central nervous system; *FSH,* follicle-stimulating hormone; *LH,* luteinizing hormone; *GnRH,* LH-releasing hormone.

Modified from Grumbach MM, Roth JC, Kaplan SL, et al. Hypothalamic-pituitary regulation of puberty in man: evidence and concepts derived from clinical research. In Grumbach MM, Grave GD, Mayer FE, eds. Control of the Onset of Puberty. New York: John Wiley & Sons, 1974:115-166.

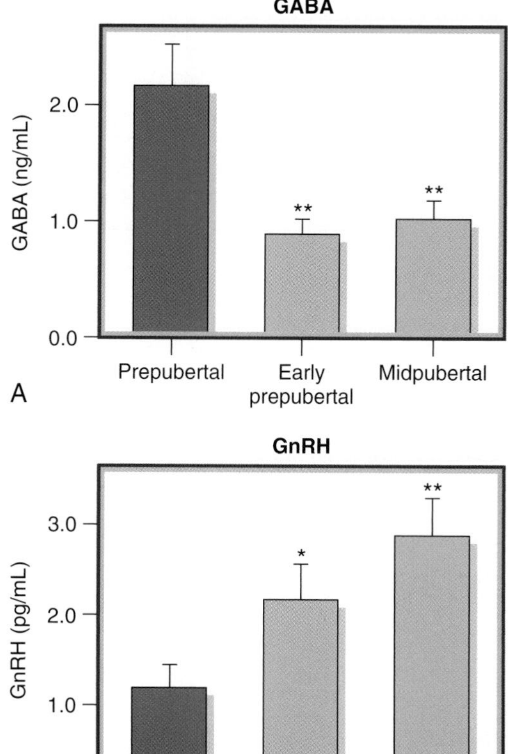

Figure 24–42 ▪ The striking developmental changes in γ-aminobutyric acid (GABA) and gonadotropin-releasing hormone (GnRH; luteinizing hormone–releasing hormone) release between the prepubertal and the pubertal rhesus monkey as measured in 10-minute perfusate samples from the stalk median eminence. In each animal, multiple samples were obtained. Mean±SEM; ***P*<.01; **P*<.05 versus prepubertal monkeys. (From Mitsushima D, Hei DL, Terasawa E. γ-Aminobutyric acid is an inhibitory neurotransmitter restricting the release of luteinizing hormone-releasing hormone before the onset of puberty. Proc Natl Acad Sci U S A 1994;91:395-399.)

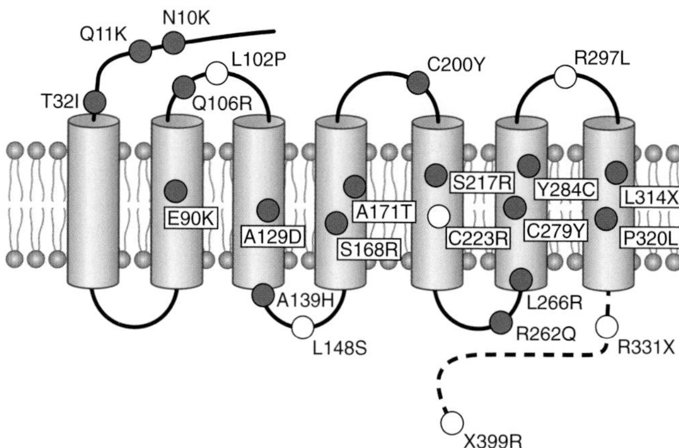

Figure 24–43 ▪ Inactivating mutations of the GnRHR *(closed circle)* and GPR54 *(open circle)* identified in patients with isolated hypogonadotropic hypogonadism. Dashed line indicates the intracellular domain of GPR54. (From de Roux N. GnRH receptor and GPR54 inactivation in isolated gonadotropic deficiency. The seven transmembrane G-protein-coupled receptor model is used for illustration. Best Pract Res Clin Endocrinol Metab 2006;20(4):515-528).

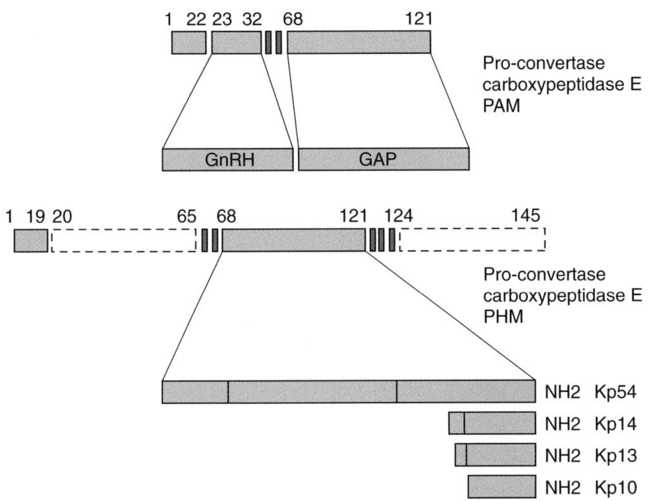

Figure 24–44 ▪ Posttranslational maturation of gonadotropin-releasing hormone (GnRH) (upper figure) and kisspeptins (Kp). Doublets of basic residues and glycine are indicated by black vertical bars. Enzymes involved in the normal maturation are indicated. *PAM,* Peptidyl glycine α-amidating mono-oxygenase; *PHM,* peptidyl α-hydroxylating mono-oxygenase. (From de Roux N. GnRH receptor and GPR54 inactivation in isolated gonadotropic deficiency. Best Pract Res Clin Endocrinol Metab 2006;20[4]:515-528).

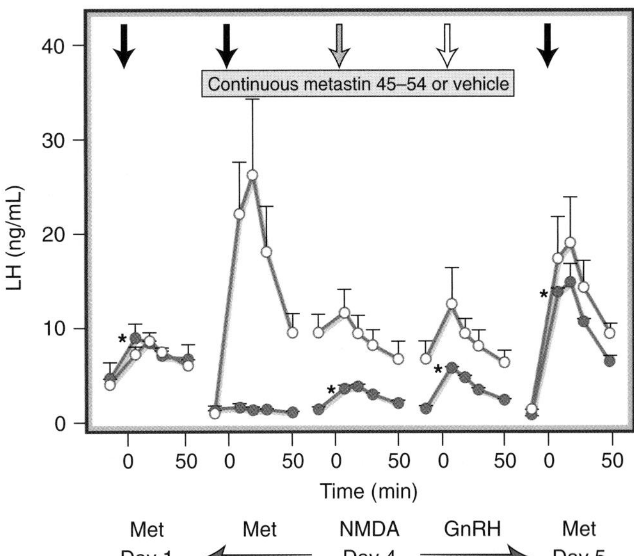

Figure 24–45 ▪ Effect of single sequential boluses of hu metastin 45-54 (Met Kisspeptin 10) *(black arrow)*, NMDA *(gray arrow)*, and GnRH *(white arrow)* on plasma LH concentrations (mean±SEM) during the last 3 hours of the 98-hour intravenous infusion (*shaded horizontal box*) of hu metastin 45-54 at a dose of 100 μg/hr (•) or vehicle (Veh) (○) compared with the LH response to the same bolus of hu metastin 45-54 1 hour before (day 1) and 21 hours after (day 5) the termination of continuous hu metastin 45-54 or vehicle infusion. *, Infusion of hu metastin 45-54 (•) significantly different ($P<.05$) from preinjection mean; n=3. (From Seminara SB, Dipietro MJ, Ramaswamy S, et al. Continuous human metastin 45-54 infusion desensitizes G protein-coupled receptor 54-induced gonadotropin-releasing hormone release monitored indirectly in the juvenile male rhesus monkey (*Macaca mulatta*): a finding with therapeutic implications. Endocrinology 2006;147[5]:2122-2126.)

the desensitization of the GRP54 receptors was selective to kisspeptin administration (Fig. 24–45).[1218] This down-sensitization of the GRP54 receptors after continuous kisspeptin infusion may have a therapeutic function in central precocious puberty in the future, just as GnRH agonists are used.

GPR54 mRNA is expressed in the pituitary gland, is evidence that kisspeptin act directly on the gonadotrope[1219] in vivo to cause LH secretion is unproven.[1213] In the sheep, kisspeptin colocalizes to a high proportion of GnRH-receptor cells in the preoptic area, as well as various neuronal fibers within the external, neurosecretory zone of the median eminence.

Kisspeptin 54 administered intravenously to men and subcutaneously to women causes a dose dependent increase in plasma LH and FSH; in women the greatest increment in gonadotropins occurred in the preovulatory phase of the menstrual cycle.[1219a,1219b] These observations are an indication of the potential use of kisspeptins as an additional approach to the manipulation of the hypothalamic-pituitary gonadotropin-gonadal apparatus independent of GnRH agonists and antagonists.

Estrogen has a dual effect on kisspeptin neurons in the basal hypothalamus of mice. It suppresses Kiss mRNA in some neurons whereas it increases it in others.[1210a,1221b]

Leptin indirectly influences the regulation of the GnRH neuronal network by its direct action on hypothalamic kisspeptinergic neurons. Kisspeptin appears to act as a central effector for the effect of leptin on GnRH neurons.[1214,1217a]

The generation of mice with a targeted deletion of the Kissl gene has further clarified the role of kisspeptin and its G-protein-coupled receptor GPR54, especially its specificity.[1220] The male and female Kissl null mice had absent puberty and hypogonadotropic hypogonadism; the phenotype did not differ from that of the mice bearing a loss of function mutation in the GPR54 gene. The Kiss-1 knockout mice provided proof in vivo that kisspeptins are the physiologic ligands of the GPR54 receptor. The remarkable specificity of hypothalamic kisspeptin-GPR54 signaling is supported by the apparent absence of disruption of other physiological systems in the Kiss-1 null mouse. Spontaneous mutations in the GPR54 gene in humans are rare but instructive in elucidating the role of the kisspeptin/GPR54 signaling in pubertal development.

Mounting evidence in rodents, sheep and primates provides strong support to the critical role of kisspeptin-GPR54 signaling in the initiation and maintenance of puberty.[1210a,1221,1221a,1221b] A default in this pathway prevents passage through puberty. It is necessary to be mindful of other neurotransmitter systems that have been implicated in the control of the onset of puberty, e.g., GABA and glutamate,[938] transforming growth factors alpha[1222], EAP1 (enhanced at puberty 1 gene).[1222a,1223] There are large gaps in our knowledge of the interaction of these neurotransmitters on the disinhibition and reawakening of the GnRH neuronal network. Developmentally what increases Kiss mRNA and kisspeptin release and GPR54 receptors at puberty onset, and, for example, what mechanism decreases GABA inhibition and promotes glutamate stimulation at the onset of puberty. Even though the kisspeptin-GPR54 is a "gatekeeper of puberty", nothing is known about its activation on ontogeny. These observations provide additional evidence that the hypothalamic GnRH neurosecretory neuron is not a limiting factor in puberty because the GnRH pulse generator, the anterior pituitary gland, gonads, and gonadal steroid end organs are functionally intact in the fetus and prepubertally, and can be fully activated by the appropriate stimulus. Hence, the CNS restraint of puberty lies above the level of the autorhythmic GnRH neurosecretory neurons in the hypothalamus. Figure 24–46 contrasts the direct and/or indirect effects of the GABA inhibitory and the excitatory amino acid (as represented by NMDA and other glutamate receptors) stimulatory neurotransmitters such as kisspeptin on GnRH release. In the primate, the GABA hypo-

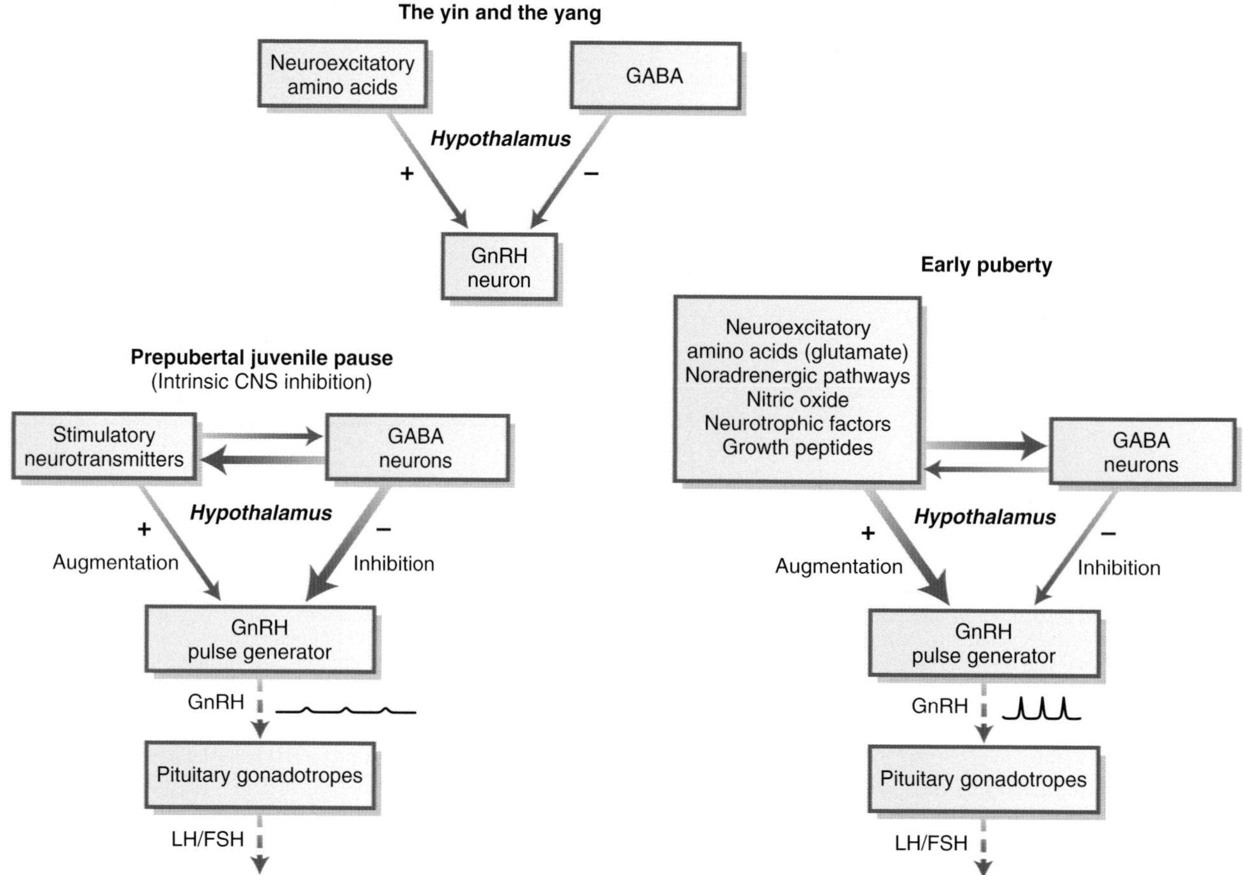

Figure 24–46 ▪ The yin and the yang of the neuroendocrinology of the prepubertal juvenile pause and its intrinsic central inhibition of the luteinizing hormone–releasing hormone (GnRH) pulse generator and the reversal of this inhibition and termination of the juvenile pause, which leads to the onset of puberty. The GABAergic neuronal network and its neurotransmitter γ-aminobutyric acid (GABA) constitute the most ubiquitous inhibitory transmitter in the hypothalamus as well as the brain. During the prepubertal juvenile pause, this neurotransmitter system appears to play the major neural role in inhibiting the GnRH pulse generator. (Suppression of GABA inhibition during this period promptly results in reactivation of the suppressed GnRH pulse generator in the rhesus monkey.) With the approach of puberty, GABA inhibition of the GnRH pulse generator wanes, and its reactivation gradually occurs. This reactivation is quite likely augmented by stimulatory neurotransmitters (e.g., kisspeptin excitatory amino acids), some of which are dependent on increased gonadal steroids for their activation, and by neurotrophic factors and growth peptides. A critical component of the reawakening of the GnRH neuronal network is the increase, independently of sex steroids, in KiSS-1 mRNA expression in kisspeptinergic neurons in the medial basal hypothalamus, the secretion of kisspeptins, the cognate ligands for the GPR54 receptor on the surface of the GnRH neuron.[1206] As a consequence, the amplitude and, to a lesser extent, the frequency of GnRH pulses increase, which, in turn, leads to increased pulsatile secretion of follicle-stimulating hormone (FSH) and LH and the activation of the ovary and testis. As shown experimentally in the monkey, the GnRH pulse generator can function in the absence of hypothalamic stimulatory factors. The nature of and factor or factors responsible for this transition from central inhibition and the postulated dominance of GABA to the release of inhibition and reactivation of the GnRH pulse generator are unknown.

thalamic neural network seems to be the major component of the intrinsic CNS inhibitory mechanism during the juvenile pause.

Sleep-Associated LH Release and Onset of Puberty

In sensitive radioimmunoassays, a diurnal rhythm of serum LH, FSH, and testosterone is already demonstrable in 5- to 6-year-old short but otherwise normal girls, demonstrating that the preparation for the changes of puberty starts long before the physical features appear and the classic endocrine markers of puberty occur (see Fig. 24–32).[787,793,1044,1156,1157,1225,1226] While adult men as well as women during most phases of the menstrual cycle have little difference in the amplitude or frequency of LH pulses during a 24-hour period, in pubertal children sleep-associated pulsatile release of LH is prominent in early and midpuberty[1227]; only in late puberty were prominent LH-secretory episodes detected during the day, but they were still less than during sleep until the adult pattern was finally achieved. Augmented LH release during sleep leads to a rise in the plasma concentration of testosterone at night in boys, in children with true (or central) precocious puberty, in glucocorticoid-treated children with congenital adrenal hyperplasia who have an advanced bone age and an early onset of true puberty (Fig. 24–47), and in agonadal patients during the pubertal age period, suggesting that it is not dependent on gonadal function.[804,1227,1228] There is significantly increased excretion of urinary LH in prepubertal

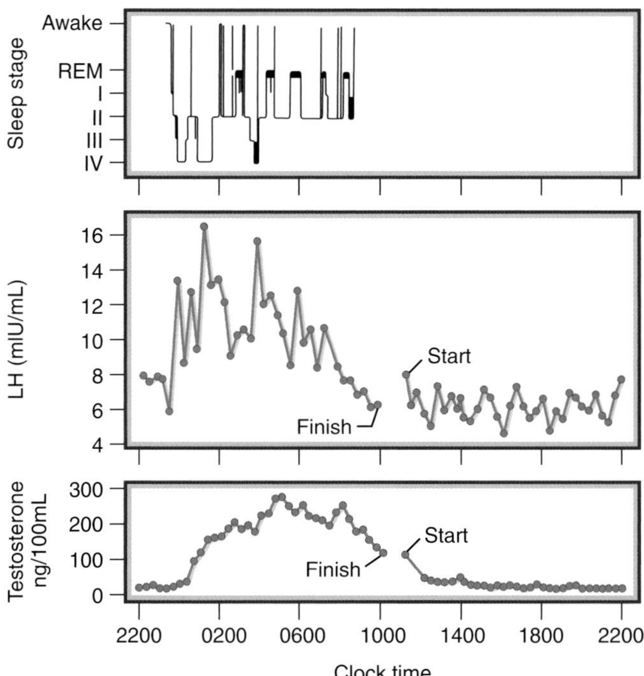

Figure 24–47 ▪ Plasma luteinizing hormone (LH) and testosterone sampled every 20 minutes in a 14-year-old boy in pubertal stage 2. The histogram displaying sleep stage sequence is depicted above the period of nocturnal sleep. Sleep stages are rapid eye movement (REM) with stages I to IV shown by depth of line graph. Plasma LH is expressed as mIU/mL. Plasma testosterone is expressed as nanograms per 100 mL. To convert LH values to international units per liter, multiply by 1.0. To convert testosterone values to nanomoles per liter, multiply by 0.03467. (From Boyar RM, Rosenfeld RS, Kapen S, et al. Human puberty: simultaneous augmented secretion of luteinizing hormone and testosterone during sleep. J Clin Invest 1974;54:609-618. Copyright of the American Society for Clinical Investigation.)

children at night compared to during the day (see Fig. 24–47).[1229]

Sleep-enhanced LH secretion can be viewed as a maturational phenomenon related to changes in the CNS and in the hypothalamic restraint of GnRH release. Episodic release of gonadotropins is suppressed by anti-GnRH antibodies and by the administration of gonadal steroids or of certain catecholaminergic agonists and antagonists, and is augmented by the opioid antagonist naloxone. Naloxone does not alter the testosterone-mediated suppression of LH nor does it alter the testosterone effects upon LH pulsatility in early to midpubertal boys.[1230] We have suggested that an increase in endogenous GnRH secretion at puberty has a priming effect on the gonadotrope[786] and leads to increased sensitivity of the pituitary to GnRH (either endogenous or exogenous). In the monkey, a striking increase in the pulse amplitude and putatively an increase in pulse frequency occurs between prepuberty and puberty.[942,1232] Sleep-associated LH release in the peripubertal period correlates with the increased sensitivity of the pituitary gonadotropes to administration of GnRH in the peripubertal period and in puberty, and is an indication that the hypothalamic GnRH pulse generator initially is less inhibited during sleep, even in prepubertal children.

Pituitary and Gonadal Sensitivity to Tropic Stimuli

If the increased secretion of gonadotropins at the beginning of puberty is a consequence of changes in both neural and hormonal restraints on the synthesis and pulsatile secretion of GnRH, disinhibition and reaugmentation of the GnRH pulse generator should lead to priming of the gonadotropes, increased pulsatile gonadotropin secretion from the pituitary, and finally augmented output of steroids by the gonad. Endogenous GnRH secretion is estimated indirectly and qualitatively by determining the pulsatile pattern of LH and by the gonadotropin response to exogenous GnRH at different stages[1233,1234] and in disorders of the hypothalamic-pituitary-gonadal system. The release of LH after administration of GnRH is minimal in prepubertal children beyond infancy, increases during the peripubertal period and puberty (Fig. 24–48),[786,787] and is still greater in adults (depending on the phase of the menstrual cycle in women).[1235,1236] The results support the concept that the prepubertal state is characterized by functional GnRH deficiency.[786,787,933,935,1232] FSH release after the administration of GnRH is comparable in prepubertal, pubertal, and adult males, indicating similar pituitary sensitivity to GnRH, but females release more FSH than males at all stages of sexual maturation.[786,1233] There is a striking reversal of the FSH/LH ratio after the administration of GnRH to both males and females between prepuberty and puberty (see Fig. 24–48).[786]

These observations suggest a striking change in pituitary sensitivity to GnRH in prepubertal and pubertal individuals as well as a sex difference in the "dynamic reserve" of pituitary FSH,[786] in that the pituitary gonadotropes of prepubertal females are more sensitive to GnRH than those of prepubertal males, even though the concentration of circulating gonadal steroids is very low in both sexes at this stage of maturation. Prepubertal girls have a larger readily releasable pool of pituitary FSH than prepubertal or pubertal males, possibly related in part to the higher concentration of inhibin B in prepubertal boys (see Fig. 24–48); these may be factors in the higher frequency of idiopathic true precocious puberty in girls and in the occurrence of premature thelarche.[1237] The available data are consistent with the hypothesis that less GnRH is required for FSH than for LH release.

This change in responsiveness of the gonadotropes is apparently mediated by increased pulsatile secretion of GnRH.[786,787] The increased LH response to synthetic GnRH is one of the earliest hormonal markers of puberty onset. The degree of previous exposure of gonadotropes to endogenous GnRH appears to affect both the magnitude and the quality of LH responses to a single intravenous dose of GnRH. Studies of the effects of acute and long-term administration of synthetic GnRH in hypergonadotropic hypogonadism, hypogonadotropic hypogonadism, constitutional delayed growth and adolescence, and idiopathic precocious puberty support this concept of "self-pri ming."[786,800,819,1228,1234,1238-1243] With the approach of puberty, the derepression of the hypothalamic GnRH pulse generator and the increased pulsatile secretion of GnRH augment pituitary sensitivity to GnRH and enlarge the reserve of LH.[941,947,964,965,1244] Reduction in the frequency of exogenous GnRH pulses from one per hour to one every 3 hours in the adult rhesus monkey with ablative hypothalamic lesions that eliminate endogenous GnRH secretion increased the FSH/LH ratio,[964] suggesting that GnRH pulse frequency is one factor affecting relative secretion of FSH and LH. Furthermore, inhibin and endogenous gonadal steroids may also affect this ratio through action on the hypothalamus, the pituitary gland, or both.

Pulsatile administration of GnRH to prepubertal monkeys promptly initiates puberty (and, in females, ovulatory menstrual cycles) and restores complete gonadal function in adult monkeys with hypothalamic lesions.[941,942,1244-1246] Similar studies in the human yielded comparable results in prepubertal children and in adults with hypothalamic hypogonadotropic hypogonadism.[965,1174,1225,1239-1243,1247] These results provide further support for reactivation of the hypothalamic GnRH pulse generator as the first hormonal change in the onset of puberty.

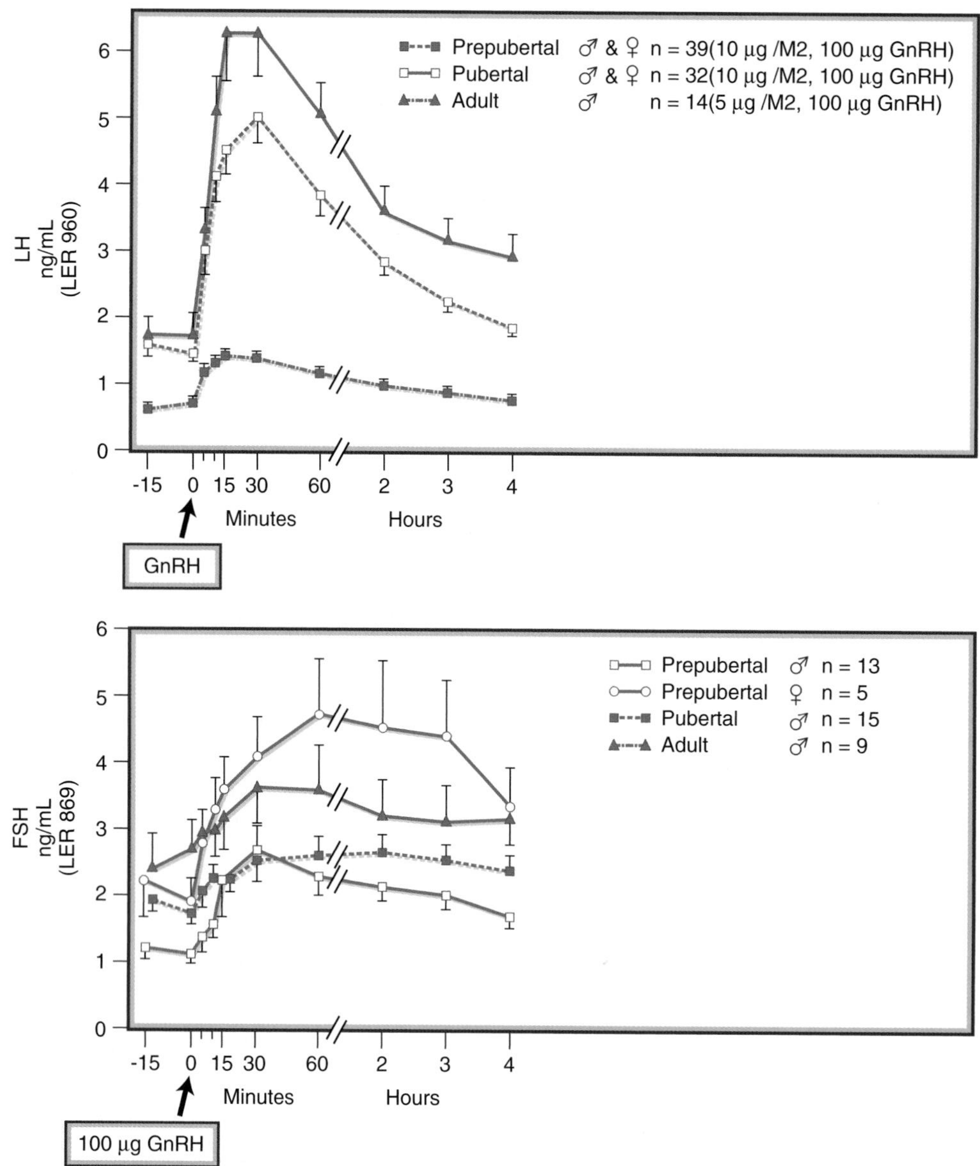

Figure 24–48 ▪ Changes in plasma luteinizing hormone (LH) *(top)* and follicle-stimulating hormone (FSH) *(bottom)* levels in prepubertal, pubertal, and adult individuals. Note the limited LH response in prepubertal children compared with that of pubertal and adult subjects. The FSH response to LH-releasing hormone (GnRH) is similar in prepubertal, pubertal, or adult males. In females, the FSH response is significantly greater than that of prepubertal, pubertal, or adult males. For conversion to SI units, see the legend for Figure 24–21. (Modified from Grumbach MM, Roth JC, Kaplan SL, et al. Hypothalamic pituitary regulation of puberty in man: evidence and concepts derived from clinical research. In Grumbach MM, Grave GD, Mayer FE, eds. Control of the Onset of Puberty. New York: John Wiley & Sons, 1974:115-166.)

Responsiveness of the gonads to gonadotropins also increases during puberty. For example, the augmented testosterone secretion in response to administration of hCG at puberty in boys[1248] is probably a consequence of the priming effect of the increase in endogenous secretion of LH (in the presence of FSH)[1249] in the Leydig cell.

Maturation of Positive Feedback Mechanism

Estrogen exerts suppressive effects from late fetal life to peripuberty when the positive action of endogenous (or exogenous) estradiol on gonadotropin release is not demonstrated.[786,787,1250] Hence, acquisition of positive feedback, a requisite for ovulation, is a late maturational event in puberty and, from the present evidence, probably does not occur before midpuberty in normal girls.[786,787,1250,1251] The positive feedback effect requires an increased concentration of plasma estradiol for a sufficient length of time during the latter part of the follicular phase in later pubertal or adult women.[947,1235,1252]

Among the requirements for a positive feedback action of estradiol on gonadotropin release at puberty[786] are (1) ovarian follicles primed by FSH to secrete sufficient estradiol to reach and maintain a critical level in the circulation, (2) a pituitary gland that is sensitized to GnRH and contains a large enough pool of releasable LH to support an LH surge, and (3) controversial in the human but not in lower animals, sufficient GnRH stores for the GnRH neurosecretory neurons to respond with an acute increase in GnRH release in addition to the usual adult pattern of pulsatile GnRH secretion.

An important site of action of estradiol is at the level of the anterior pituitary but estrogen has dual sites of action,[1253] including a negative as well as positive feedback action on the hypothalamus.[1253a] Knobil and Plant[1254] have shown in the rhesus monkey that positive as well as negative feedback can occur in adult ovariectomized females in whom the medial basal hypothalamus is surgically disconnected from the remainder of the CNS. Estradiol has a positive feedback effect directly on the pituitary gland in normal women, and prolonged administration of estradiol is accompanied by an augmented LH response to GnRH administration in women.[1236] In monkeys with hypothalamic lesions, unvarying, intermittent GnRH administration leads to sufficient estradiol release from the ovary to induce an ovulatory LH surge in the absence of an increase in the dose of the GnRH pulses.[947,1246] The fact that the major positive feedback action on the pituitary gland is demonstrable in the absence of an increase in pulsatile GnRH secretion suggests that the failure to elicit a positive feedback action with administration of estradiol into prepubertal girls could be related to the inadequate GnRH pulses or insufficient LH reserve, respectively, or by both components.

Gonadotropin cyclicity[1255,1256] and estradiol-induced positive feedback can be demonstrated by midpuberty and before menarche but may be insufficient to induce an ovulatory LH surge even when there is an adequate pituitary store of readily releasable LH and FSH.[1,7861033,1250,1251] The ovary does not secrete estradiol at a high level or long enough to induce an ovulatory LH surge. We visualize the process leading to ovulation as a gradual one in which the ovary (the Zeitgeber for ovulation[947]) and the hypothalamic-pituitary gonadotropin complex become progressively more integrated and synchronous until, finally, an ovary primed for ovulation secretes sufficient estradiol to induce an ovulatory LH surge.[1033]

As many as 55% to 90% of cycles are anovulatory during the first 2 years after menarche but the proportion decreases to less than 20% of cycles by 5 years after menarche.[295,1255,1257] The mechanism of ovulation seems unstable and immature and does not appear to have attained the fine tuning and synchronization requisite for maintenance of regular ovulatory cycles. However, the high prevelance of PCOS adds to the irregularity of menses and anovulation in puberty as well.

Summary of Present Concept

Puberty is not an immutable process; it can be arrested or even reversed. Environmental factors and certain disorders that affect the onset or progression of puberty mediate their effects by direct or indirect suppression of the hypothalamic GnRH pulse generator and its periodic oscillatory signal, GnRH. Table 24–21 lists some of these factors.

ADRENAL ANDROGENS AND ADRENARCHE

Speculation has focused on the mechanism of adrenarche (the adrenal component of pubertal maturation), the fact that adrenarche occurs earlier than gonadarche (the maturation of the hypothalamic-pituitary-gonadal system), and the interaction between adrenal and gonadal hormones at puberty.[426,1258,1259]

Nature and Regulation of Adrenal Androgens

The major adrenal androgen precursors secreted by the adrenal cortex are DHEA, DHEAS, and androstenedione, which can undergo extraglandular metabolism to lead to physiologically active testosterone and estradiol[336]; however, none of the adrenal androgens themselves directly activate the androgen receptor. DHEA and especially DHEAS (which binds avidly to serum proteins, particularly albumin) are useful biochemical markers of adrenal androgen secretion and the onset of adrenarche. Androstenedione is the major androgen secreted by the ovary during and after puberty and is more readily converted to potent androgens than DHEA or DHEAS.

Cross-sectional and longitudinal studies have demonstrated a progressive increase in the plasma concentration of DHEA and DHEAS in boys and girls by about the age of 6 (6 to 8 years' skeletal age, approximately 2 years before the increase in gonadotropin and gonadal steroid secretion) that continues through puberty (age 13 to 15),[426,1260-1263] reaches a peak at age 20 to 30, and then gradually decreases (Fig. 24–49).[1259,1264] The increase is not associated with increased sensitivity of the pituitary gonadotropes to GnRH[1237] or with sleep-associated LH secretion and occurs at an age when the hypothalamic-pituitary-gonadal complex is functioning at a low level.[426]

Associated with the increase in the adrenal secretion of DHEA and DHEAS (and independent of a change in the secretion of cortisol or aldosterone) is the appearance and growth of the zona reticularis (the principal source of DHEA and DHEAS) coincident with adrenarche (see Fig. 24–49).[1264]

In contrast to the zona glomerulosa and fasciculata, four main features distinguish the zona reticularis:

1. A low level of expression of 3β-hydroxysteroid/4,5-isomerase type 2 and cytochrome P450c21 mRNAs and enzyme activities.[1265-1267]
2. Abundant dehydroepiandrosterone (hydroxysteroid) sulfotransferase activity.[1265,1266]
3. Relative increase in 17,20 lyase to 17α-hydroxylase activity of P450c17, the enzyme which catalyzes both activities.[1265,1266] The above characteristics are shared by the fetal zone of the fetal adrenal cortex.[1265,1268,1269]
4. Expression of major histocompatibility complex (MHC) class II (HLA-DR) antigens,[1270,1271] which are not expressed in the fetal zone of the fetal adrenal cortex.[1271]

In contrast to the zona fasciculata, the zona reticularis has an increased ratio of 17,20 lyase/17α-hydroxylase. Mutation in human P450c17 (arginine 347 to alanine) resulted in strikingly decreased 17,20 lyase activity but retention of 17α-hydroxylase activity.[1272,1273] Two XY phenotypic females with hypergonadotropic hypogonadism and normal mineralocorticoid and glucocorticoid function had isolated 17,20 lyase deficiency due to homozygous mutations at either the arginine 347 residue or arginine 358 in P450c17.[a]

In contrast to these observations of loss of 17,20 lyase activity with retention of 17α-hydroxylase activity, Miller and colleagues showed that the ratio of human 17,20 lyase/17α-hydroxylase activities was increased by increased phosphorylation of serine and threonine residues on the P450c17 enzyme,[1274] by the increased abundance of redox partners such as cytochrome P450 oxidoreductase, and by b5, which preferentially promotes 17,20-lyase activity by allosterically affecting the interaction between P450c17 and P450 oxidoreductase.[1272,1275] These latter studies provide a provisional hypothesis of the mechanisms that appear to be involved in the relatively increased 17,20 lyase activity of the zona reticularis, but not its regulation (Fig. 24–50).

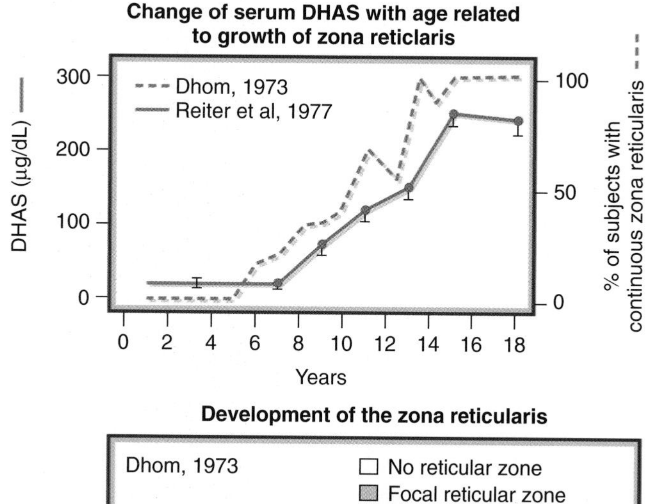

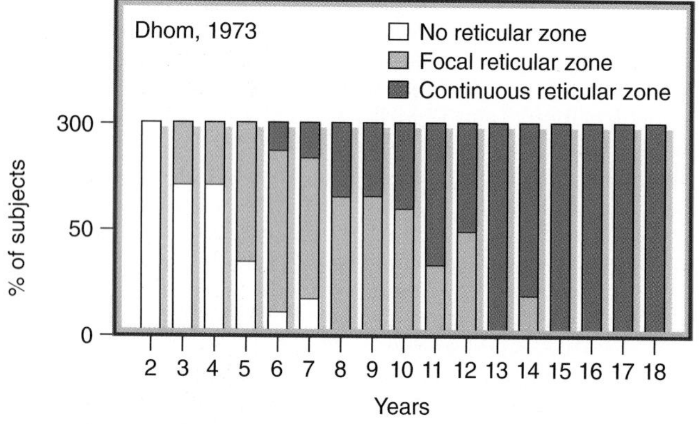

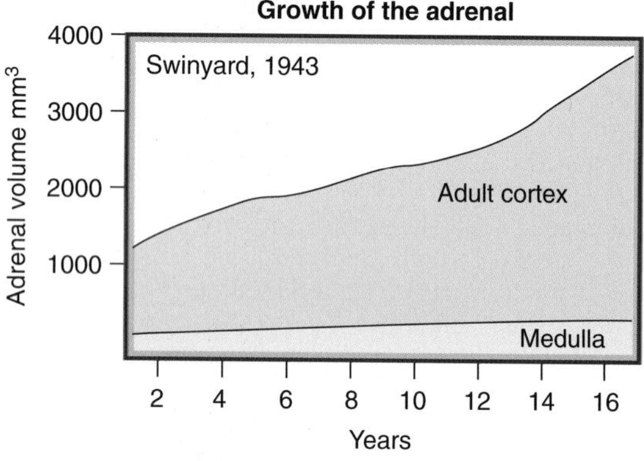

Figure 24–49 ▪ Relation of plasma dehydroepiandrosterone sulfate (DHEAS [DHAS]) to growth of the zona reticularis and increase in adrenal volume with age. *Top,* The close correlation between the development of the zona reticularis and the increase in plasma DHEAS level. *Middle,* The age at which either focal islands of reticular tissue or a continuous reticular zone was found in a series of patients with sudden death who had not had an antecedent illness. *Bottom,* The increase in adrenal volume at the time of puberty. For conversion to SI units, see the legend of Figure 24–41. (From Grumbach MM, Richards HE, Conte FA, et al. Clinical disorders of adrenal function and puberty: assessment of the role of the adrenal cortex and abnormal puberty in man and evidence for an ACTH-like pituitary adrenal androgen stimulating hormone. In James VHT, Serio M, Giusti G, et al, eds. The Endocrine Function of the Human Adrenal Cortex. New York: Academic Press, 1978:583-612.)

There are several hypotheses about the control of adrenal androgen secretion[426,936,1258,1272,1276] Regulation of adrenal androgen secretion in the zona reticularis is postulated to be based on a dual control mechanism: (1) corticotropin (ACTH, adrenocorticotropin) is obligatory, as evidenced, for example, by the findings in ACTH deficiency or resistance,[1277] for (2) the action of an unidentified adrenal androgen-stimulating factor, possibly pituitary in origin or from a nonadrenal source, or an intraadrenal event.[426] This concept is illustrated in Figure 24–51.[1045] Corticotropin-releasing hormone (CRH) has been advanced as an adrenal androgen secretagogue through its stimulatory action on the zona reticularis. The intravenous infusion of hCRH into dexamethasone-suppressed young men induced within 3 hours of DHEA, DHEAS, and androstenedione.[1278] Similar results were obtained in adolescent girls with hyperandrogenism and a history of premature adrenarche.[1278,1279] CRH directly stimulates DHEAS secretion and the expression of P450c17 by the fetal adrenal cortical cells.[1280,1281] Leptin in vitro vigorously stimulates 17,20-lyase activity and transiently stimulates 17α-hydroxylase activity of the microsomal enzyme CYP17, implying a role in adrenarche,[1282] but no clinical evidence suggests a pivotal role of leptin in adrenarche. Despite much effort, a distinct hormone or factor that in addition to ACTH stimulates the zona reticularis and adrenal androgen secretion has not been isolated, and the mechanism regulating adrenarche remains unknown.[1283]

A distinct adrenal androgen-stimulating factor, whether of pituitary, intra-adrenal, or other origin, could explain the following observations[426]:

1. The spurt in adrenal growth and the differentiation and growth of the zona reticularis at adrenarche occur independently of an increase in ACTH or cortisol secretion but correlate with the increase in plasma DHEAS (see Fig. 24–49).
2. Cortisol and adrenal androgen secretions vary independently with age, during normal as well as premature adrenarche, and in Cushing's disease, starvation, malnutrition, anorexia nervosa, and chronic disease.
3. Unlike cortisol secretion, the secretion of DHEA and DHEAS in response to ACTH administration varies with age.
4. Dissociation of adrenarche and gonadarche occurs in a variety of disorders of sexual maturation,[24-51] including premature adrenarche (onset of pubic or axillary hair before age 8), chronic adrenal insufficiency, true precocious puberty (when the onset is before age 6), primary hypogonadism, isolated gonadotropin deficiency, and anorexia nervosa.[1259]

A longitudinal study of 42 children demonstrated that an increase in BMI (not the value itself at any age) is related to the rise in the urinary excretion of DHEAS, suggesting that a change in nutritional status is one physiologic regulator of adrenarche.[1284]

Adrenal Androgens and Puberty

The earlier onset of adrenarche than gonadarche and the contribution of adrenal androgens to the growth of pubic and axillary hair have led some to suggest that in normal children adrenal androgens are an important factor in the onset of puberty and the maturation of the hypothalamic-pituitary-gonadal complex.

Although true precocious puberty may occur in circumstances in which the prepubertal child has previously been exposed to excessive levels of androgens from an endogenous or an exogenous source (e.g., after the initiation of glucocorticoid therapy in congenital virilizing adrenal hyperplasia or after removal of a sex steroid–secreting adrenal or gonadal neoplasm),[426,1285] there is little evidence that adrenal androgens play an important qualitative or rate-limiting role in the onset of puberty in normal children.[426] Most patients with premature adrenarche who secrete excessive amounts of adrenal androgens for their age enter puberty and experience menarche within the normal age range.[426] Moreover, prepubertal children who have congenital or acquired chronic adrenal insufficiency (Addison's disease) and, consequently, have deficient or absent adrenal androgen secretion usually have a normal onset of and

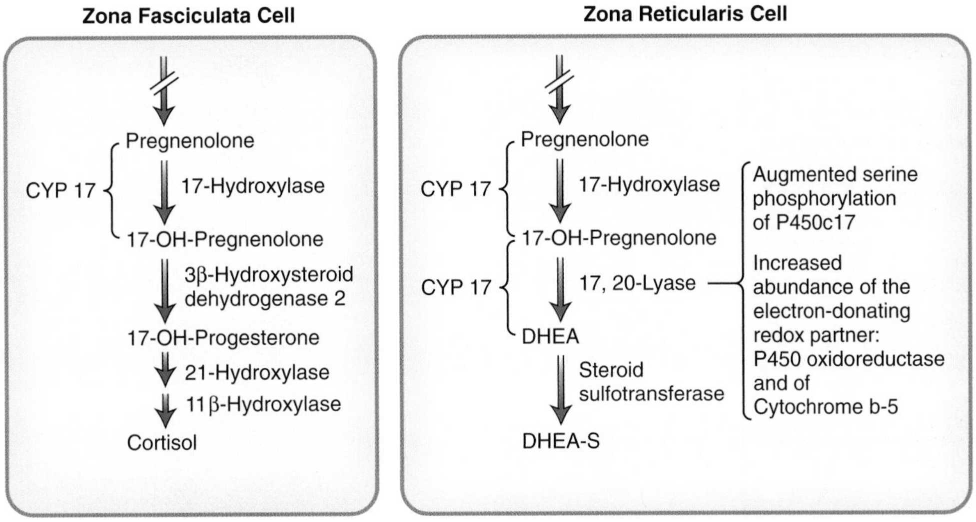

Zona Fasciculata Cell

Pregnenolone → (CYP 17: 17-Hydroxylase) → 17-OH-Pregnenolone → (3β-Hydroxysteroid dehydrogenase 2) → 17-OH-Progesterone → (21-Hydroxylase) → (11β-Hydroxylase) → Cortisol

Zona Reticularis Cell

Pregnenolone → (CYP 17: 17-Hydroxylase) → 17-OH-Pregnenolone → (CYP 17: 17, 20-Lyase) → DHEA → (Steroid sulfotransferase) → DHEA-S

Augmented serine phosphorylation of P450c17

Increased abundance of the electron-donating redox partner: P450 oxidoreductase and of Cytochrome b-5

Figure 24–50 ▪ Adrenarche and the zona reticularis. The rise in circulating dehydroepiandrosterone sulfate (DHEAS) is the biochemical hallmark of adrenarche. The diagram compares and contrasts the major steroidogenic pathway in the zona fasciculata with that in the zona reticularis. In contrast to the zona fasciculata, the expression of 3β-hydroxysteroid, $\Delta^{4,5}$ isomerase type 2 messenger ribonucleic acid (mRNA) and its activity (the enzyme that irreversibly traps Δ^5 precursors into Δ^4 steroids) is very low in the zona reticularis, whereas the expression of and activity of steroid sulfotransferase is high. A single gene, *CYP17,* encodes a single enzyme that has both 17α-hydroxylase and 17,20-lyase activity, but the ratio of 17,20-lyase to 17α-hydroxylase activity is relatively high in the zona reticularis compared with that in the zona fasciculata. Some of the factors that seem to augment the increased 17,20-lyase activity of *CYP17* are the augmented serine phosphorylation of the enzyme and the apparent increased abundance of the electron-donating redox partner, including P450 reductase and of cytochrome b_5. *(See text.)*

progression through puberty when given appropriate glucocorticoid and mineralocorticoid replacement therapy.[426] Studies in children with chronic adrenal insufficiency, isolated gonadotropin deficiency, hypergonadotropic hypogonadism, and androgen resistance suggest that in girls and boys adrenal androgens are not essential for the adolescent growth spurt, whereas gonadal steroids secreted by the testis and ovary are and act in concert with GH.[426] The transient increase in height velocity (about 1.5 cm/year in both sexes) that occurs in middle childhood (6 to 7 years) and lasts about 2 years terminates while serum DHEAS continues to increase, and is related to the cyclic pattern of prepubertal growth and to genetic regulation of growth rather than an increase in either adrenal androgen or GH secretion.[1274,1286,1287]

DISORDERS OF PUBERTY

Delayed Puberty and Sexual Infantilism (Table 24–22)

As stated earlier, reasonable upper limits of the normal age of onset of puberty is 14 years of age in boys and 13 years in girls. Patients who will undergo spontaneous but delayed puberty must be differentiated from those with disorders associated with permanent sexual infantilism that require treatment. Diagnosis could be constitutional (idiopathic) delay, hypogonadotropic hypogonadism, or primary gonadal failure with hypergonadotropic hypogonadism. Functionally, delayed puberty can be divided into disorders that affect the operation of the GnRH pulse generator, the pituitary gland, or the gonad.

Idiopathic (Constitutional) Delay in Growth and Puberty[1288]

Otherwise healthy girls who spontaneously enter puberty after the age of 13 and boys who begin after 14 years have constitutional delay in growth and adolescence. Affected individuals usually are short (2 SD below the mean value for height for age) at evaluation and have been shorter than their classmates for years, although growth velocity and height are usually appropriate for bone age (Fig. 24–52 and Table 24–23). Family history in as many as 77% of cases reveals a mother who had delayed menarche or a father (or sibling) who did not enter puberty until late (age 14 to 18 years), and the pattern in some cases suggests dominant inheritance with incomplete penetrance.[1062,1289] Constitutional delay in development may be considered physiologic immaturity with a slow tempo of maturation; as a result of the delay in the reactivation of the GnRH pulse generator, affected children have a functional deficiency of GnRH for chronologic age but not for the stage of physiologic development. Adrenarche and gonadarche occur later in individuals with constitutional (idiopathic) delay in growth and adolescence,[1289] whereas adrenarche usually occurs at a normal age in patients with isolated gonadotropin deficiency.[1259,1290] These patients have a retarded bone age at presentation but, on achieving a bone age of approximately 12 to 14 years for boys and 11 to 13 years for girls, they can be expected to show the earliest stages of sexual maturation, although bone age is certainly not a fully reliable indicator. The U.S. Health Examination Survey showed that 5.7% of boys with a bone age of 14 years lacked pubic hair (stage 1) and 4% were in genital stage 1, whereas at bone age of 15 years, only 0.2% were still in pubic hair stage 1 and 0.8% were still in genital stage 1. This study started at an age at which the same descriptive information could not be determined for girls.[235]

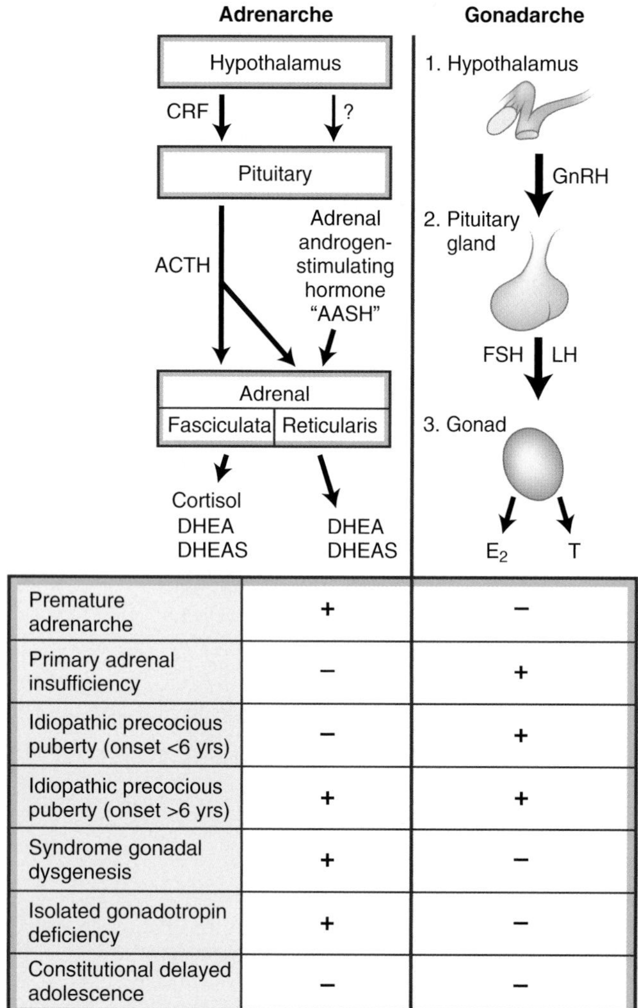

	Adrenarche	Gonadarche
Premature adrenarche	+	−
Primary adrenal insufficiency	−	+
Idiopathic precocious puberty (onset <6 yrs)	−	+
Idiopathic precocious puberty (onset >6 yrs)	+	+
Syndrome gonadal dysgenesis	+	−
Isolated gonadotropin deficiency	+	−
Constitutional delayed adolescence	−	−

Figure 24–51 ▪ Hypothesis of the control of pituitary adrenal androgen secretion by a putative separate adrenal androgen-stimulating hormone acting on a corticotropin (ACTH)-primed adrenal cortex. Although this diagram suggests that "AASH" arises from the pituitary gland, a distinct pituitary factor with AASH activity has not been isolated; an extrapituitary factor is not excluded. The lower part of the diagram shows the relationship of adrenarche to gonadarche, including dissociation in various clinical disorders of sexual development (+, present; –, absent). (Modified from Sklar CA, Kaplan SL, Grumbach MM. Evidence for dissociation between adrenarche and gonadarche: studies in patients with idiopathic precocious puberty, gonadal dysgenesis, isolated gonadotropin deficiency, and constitutionally delayed puberty. J Clin Endocrinol Metab 1980;51:548-556. Copyright by The Endocrine Society.)

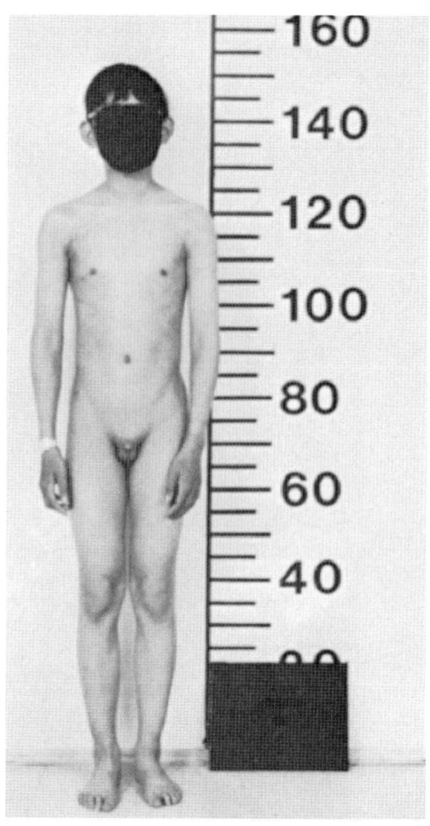

Figure 24–52 ▪ A boy 16 years, 2 months of age, with constitutional delay in growth and puberty. Height, 149.5 cm (4 SD below the mean value for age); upper/lower body ratio, 1.1 (retarded for age); phallus, 6.0×1.6 cm; testes, 2.5×1.4 cm; the scrotum showed early thinning. At a chronologic age of 15 years and 4 months, the bone age was 11 years and the sella turcica was normal. The plasma concentration of luteinizing hormone (LH) was 0.7 ng/mL (LER-960); follicle-stimulating hormone (FSH), 0.5 ng/mL (LER-869). On LH-releasing hormone (GnRH) testing, the plasma concentration of LH increased to 2.2 ng/mL (an increment of 1.5 ng/mL), and the testosterone level rose from 52 to 77 ng/dL. The testes subsequently spontaneously enlarged, and the patient progressed through puberty. For conversion to SI units, see the legends of Figures 24–21 and 24–22. (From Styne DM, Grumbach MM. Puberty in the male and female: its physiology and disorders. In Yen SCC, Jaffe RB, eds. Reproductive Endocrinology, 2nd ed. Philadelphia: WB Saunders, 1986:313-384.)

In one large series, 25% of patients with constitutional delay were over the 85th percentile BMI for age and the bone age of these subjects was less delayed than the more classic thin patients.[1289] Furthermore, there is evidence that the heavier boys with constitutional delay end up taller than the thinner ones related to their midparental height and suggests the possibility of differing etiologies between the boys with classic thin constitutional delay and those who have constitutional delay and are heavier.[1291] There is no impairment of olfaction as in Kallmann's syndrome and undescended testes are uncommon in boys constitutionally delayed in puberty. Plasma gonadal steroid levels may be low at the time of presentation, but as bone age advances, serum gonadotropin concentration and the amplitude of LH pulses increase (initially at night), and both the basal serum gonadotropin concentrations measured by third generation assays and the LH response to GnRH or GnRH agonists all reflect maturation of the hypothalamic-pituitary system.

In most cases, the first signs of secondary sexual development occur within 1 year after LH rises to pubertal levels after administration of 100 µg of intravenous synthetic GnRH or subcutaneous GnRH agonist or within 1 y after gonadotropin and testosterone or estradiol concentrations begin to increase spontaneously above prepubertal values.[786,787] An 8 AM serum testosterone value of 0.7 nmol/L (20 ng/dL) heralds the development of phenotypic puberty in boys within 12 to 15 months.[1292] Constitutional delay in growth and puberty is more common in boys and may be a counterpart of constitutional true precocious puberty, a condition many times more common in girls. Full sexual maturity will be reached, but the process takes longer than usual. On the other hand, familial short stature is a physiologic variant of growth in which the velocity of development and bone age are normal but stature is decreased, whereas constitutional delay in growth and adolescence is a disorder of tempo that secondarily impairs growth distance. The combination of both constitutional delay in puberty and familial short stature,

TABLE 24–22 CLASSIFICATION OF DELAYED PUBERTY AND SEXUAL INFANTILISM

IDIOPATHIC (CONSTITUTIONAL) DELAY IN GROWTH AND PUBERTY (DELAYED ACTIVATION OF HYPOTHALAMIC LRF PULSE GENERATOR)

HYPOGONADOTROPIC HYPOGONADISM: SEXUAL INFANTILISM RELATED TO GONADOTROPIN DEFICIENCY

Central nervous system (CNS) disorders
- Tumors
  - Graniopharyngiomas
  - Germinomas
  - Other germ cell tumors
  - Hypothalamic and optic gliomas
  - Astrocytomas
  - Pituitary tumors (including MEN-1, prolactinoma)
- Other causes
  - Langerhans' histiocytosis
  - Postinfectious lesions of the CNS
  - Vascular abnormalities of the CNS
  - Radiation therapy
  - Congenital malformations especially associated with craniofacial anomalies
  - Head trauma
  - Lymphocytic hypophysitis

Isolated Gonadotropin Deficiency
- Kallmann's syndrome
  - With hyposmia or anosmia
  - Without anosmia
- LHRH receptor mutation
- Congenital adrenal hypoplasia (*DAX1* mutation)
- Isolated LH deficiency
- Isolated FSH deficiency
- Prohormone convertase 1 deficiency (PCI)

Idiopathic and Genetic Forms of Multiple Pituitary Hormone Deficiencies Including PROP-1 Mutation

Miscellaneous Disorders
- Prader-Willi syndrome
- Laurence-Moon and Bardet-Biedl syndromes
- Functional gonadotropin deficiency
  - Chronic systemic disease and malnutrition
    - Sickle cell disease
    - Cystic fibrosis
    - Acquired immunodeficiency syndrome (AIDS)
    - Chronic gastroenteric disease
    - Chronic renal disease
  - Malnutrition
  - Anorexia nervosa
  - Bulimia
  - Psychogenic amenorrhea
  - Impaired puberty and delayed menarche in female athletes and ballet dancers (exercise amenorrhea)
  - Hypothyroidism
  - Diabetes mellitus
  - Cushing's disease
  - Hyperprolactinemia
  - Marijuana use
  - Gaucher's disease

HYPERGONADOTROPIC HYPOGONADISM

Males
- The syndrome of seminiferous tubular dysgenesis and its variants (Klinefelter's syndrome)
- Other forms of primary testicular failure
  - Chemotherapy
  - Radiation therapy
  - Testicular steroid biosynthetic defects
  - Sertoli-only syndrome
  - LH receptor mutation
  - Anorchia and cryptorchidism
- Trauma/surgery

Females
- The syndrome of gonadal dysgenesis (Turner's syndrome) and its variants
- XX and XY gonadal dysgenesis
  - Familial and sporadic XX gonadal dysgenesis and its variants
  - Familial and sporadic XY gonadal dysgenesis and its variants
- Aromatase deficiency
- Other forms of primary ovarian failure
  - Premature menopause
  - Radiation therapy
  - Chemotherapy
  - Autoimmune oophoritis
  - Galactosemia
  - Glycoprotein syndrome type 1
  - Resistant ovary
  - FSH receptor mutation
  - LH/hCG resistance
  - Polycystic ovarian disease
  - Trauma/surgery
  - Noonan's or pseudo-Turner's syndrome
  - Ovarian steroid biosynthetic defects

TABLE 24–23 CONSTITUTIONAL DELAY IN GROWTH AND ADOLESCENCE

- A variation of normal
- Males more often seek assistance
- Family history of delayed menarche or delayed secondary sexual characteristics
- Height is often below the fifth percentile, but growth rate is normal for skeletal age
- Onset of adrenarche is delayed
- The combination of genetic short stature and constitutional delay leads to more profound short stature
- Final height is less than predicted

leads to conspicuous shortness during adolescence, especially when other children increase their growth velocity, and referrals occur more often with this combination than with either condition alone. Not one test yet reliably distinguishes between constitutional delay in growth and puberty and isolated hypogonadotropic hypogonadism, so that watchful waiting is usually in order.

Growth rate before the actual onset of puberty in constitutional delay is often suboptimal for chronologic age but growth velocity usually increases to normal levels after puberty begins.[1293] Affected boys seem to be more distressed by short stature than by delay in sexual development.[1294-1297] A theoretical model of growth in delayed puberty is proposed based upon the ICP growth chart presented earlier in this text and prepubertal growth rates over a range of ages is available.[1298]

GH release in the basal state, as well as in response to GH secretagogues, including the administration of GH-releasing hormone, may be decreased in children with constitutional delay in puberty.[1299,1300] The amplitude of GH secretion and the GH response to GH-releasing hormone is greater after the administration of exogenous (aromatizable) androgens or estrogens.[372,1301-1304] Thus, constitutional delay in puberty may constitute a state of functional temporary GH insufficiency for chronologic age but not for bone age. IGF-I interacts with gonadotropins in the ovary and testis, and the relatively low secretion of GH (and presumably intragonadal IGF-I) in constitutional delayed puberty may impair the gonadal response to gonadotropins.[1305]

Patients with constitutional delay in adolescence and growth do not reach their predicted height in some[1297,1306-1308] but not all reports.[1309] Lack of growth of the spine in relation to leg length leads to eunuchoid proportions (decreased upper to lower segment ratio) when the subject reaches adulthood; the greater this segmental disproportion is, the closer the patient is to reaching target height.[1310,1311] An alternative explanation for reduced adult stature is that the patients most likely to be referred are those that combine genetic short stature with constitutional delay in growth and puberty.[1308] The magnitude of the catch-up linear growth during puberty in boys is a major determinant of adult height.[1312] Heavier individuals with constitutional delay reach greater height than those who are thinner.[1289] When the genetic tendency for growth is greater, subjects with constitutional delay in puberty reach normal stature.

Prepubertal children with constitutional delay are reported to have decreased bone mineral density.[1313] The bone mineral status in men with a previous history of constitutional delay in pubertry is still controversial, partlydue to the techniques of the study. Originally, low axial bone mineral density was reported[559,1314,1315]; however, later, reports of normal volumetric bone density measured by pQCT techniques[564,336] in contrast to the decreased peak bone mass due to hypergonadotropic or hypogonadotropic hypogonadism appeared. Recent longitudinal studies find impaired periosteal expansion during delayed puberty.[1316] Cross-sectional studies in delayed puberty found normal mean alkaline phosphatase, osteocalcin, and deoxypyridinoline for pubertal stage.[1317] Longitudinal studies determining the best methods of evaluation may ultimately resolve this question.

Girls with constitutional delay in growth and puberty[1307] have a mean deficit in adult height of 2.4 cm below the mean predicted height, although the range of adult height varies about ±10 cm from predictions.

Because 15% to 20% of adult height is gained during puberty, many approaches were tried to increase stature in otherwise normal short children.[1318] Delaying the onset or progression of puberty by the use of GnRH agonist in a placebo-controlled randomized study in boys and girls with idiopathic short stature led to a mean gain in height of 4.2 cm; the effect is greater in boys than girls. However, a decrease in bone density 1 year after cessation led to warnings that routine administration of this treatment carries substantial risk and is not recommended.[1319] The additional psychological risk of delaying puberty in otherwise normal children should also be considered.[1320]

Growth hormone would seem like a therapy likely to increase adult height in constitutional delay. Earlier, the use of growth hormone therapy was not shown to increase the final height in constitutional delay even if growth velocity does transiently increase with growth hormone therapy.[1321] The gain in height from the use of growth hormone in children diagnosed with idiopathic short stature (along with others diagnosed with growth hormone deficiency) in a multicenter study was small with many appearing to reach the same height with or without treatment.[1322] Even though the Food and Drug Administration (FDA) approved GH treatment for children predicted to reach an adult height less than the 1st percentile (160 cm), which would include some with constitutional delay, starting growth hormone in the pubertal age range is late for significant effect in that length of therapy is related to increase in stature. GH rises during pubertal development and GH therapy in larger doses is approved by the FDA for subjects with GH deficiency during puberty in an attempt to mimic the normal pubertal GH physiology. However, analysis of thousands of GH-deficient subjects treated in post marketing surveys demonstrates only moderate effects of increased GH doses during puberty upon adult height. Male gender had a positive effect and age of onset of puberty had a negative effect, and both overshadowed the effects of the change in dose on adult hieght.[1323]

Some have combined GnRH agonist therapy with GH treatment to increase final height in children who are normal except for genetic short stature or in children with small for gestational age (SGA) but the preliminary results are either inconclusive[1324] or show increased predicted or near final height (which does not necessarily translate into increased adult height)[1325-1327]; this approach to treatment remains experimental.[1328-1333,1327] Recent review of a large database from post marketing survey does not support efficacy of this approach,[1334] and there is no good follow-up evaluation to adult height.[1318] Thus, this combination cannot be supported by substantial evidence.

The cost of GH is exceptionally high in non–GH-deficient short stature, $14,000 per centimeter or $35,000 per inch gained.[1335,1336] In addition, payors are reluctant in many cases to cover the cost of the GH therapy in those without confirmed GH deficiency.[1337] There are few controlled studies to adult height but strong recommendations for more to determine the efficacy of this treatment in short normal children.[1338]

Since the critical role of estradiol in skeletal maturation was appreciated, it was postulated that treatment with a potent aromatase inhibitor would improve adult height by inhibiting skeletal maturation.[336,337,341] A double-blind, randomized, placebo-controlled study, in which boys with constitutional delay in puberty were treated with either a 6-month course of monthly testosterone or testosterone with an added 12-month trial of daily oral letrazole (a potent fourth generation aromatase inhibitor), gave preliminary evidence of efficacy. In the letrazole plus testosterone group, the mean increase in predicted adult height was 5.1 cm, although the boys were not followed to adult height.[1339] The boys in the group treated with testosterone and letrazole had increased bioactive testosterone, analyzed by a new cellular assay, compared to control boys.[851] These early observations suggest that adult height can be increased by inhibition of estradiol synthesis and by the dampening of the rate of skeletal maturation without affecting the development of male secondary sex characteristics and other publications have supported this.[1339-1341] These short-term studies reveal no significant effect upon bone metabolism or structure.[1340,1342] A 1-year study of the aromatase inhibitor, anastrazole, in combination with GH compared to GH treatment alone demonstrated no ill effects of anastrazole on body composition, plasma lipids, bone metabolism, or the tempo of puberty (although estrogen decreased as expected in the use of anastrozole),[1343] but there was no effect of this therapy upon predicted height in this study. This treatment is not supported in long-term studies up to adult height and concerns about possible effects on bone density must be addressed in long-term studies, before this therapy can be recommended.[1342]

Hypogonadotropic Hypogonadism: Sexual Infantilism Related to Gonadotropin Deficiency

Insufficient pulsatile secretion of GnRH and the resulting FSH and LH deficiency lead to delayed sexual maturation. The phenotype in hypogonadotropic hypogonadism (HH) can vary from severe sexual infantilism to apparent constitutional delay of puberty (indeed both conditions are found in the same family).[1344] The deficiency of pulsatile GnRH may be quantitative—either absolute or relative—or qualitative, as, especially in females, it may involve abnormalities in the amplitude or frequency of GnRH pulses or in both components (Fig. 24–53).[1238,1345,1346]

Patients with isolated HH usually are of normal height in early or middle adolescent years, whereas patients with CDP usually have a normal growth rate for bone age but are short for chronologic age. In contrast to subjects with CDP, subjects with HH usually do not have a normal response to GnRH stimulation, nor do they have a pulsatile LH profile commensurate with bone age. While serum concentrations of plasma FSH and LH and urinary gonadotropins are low, the differences are relative rather than absolute and are not diagnostic in the individual.

HH may be secondary to a genetic or developmental defect present at birth but undetected until the age of expected puberty, or it may be due to a tumor, inflammatory process, vascular lesion, radiation, or trauma to the hypothalamus. Similarly, HH may arise from lesions or defects that involve the pituitary gland directly. When GH is affected as well as gonadotropins, impaired growth is manifested by decreased growth velocity, especially during the expected pubertal growth spurt, and short stature.

CNS Disorders: Tumors

Extrasellar masses may interfere with GnRH synthesis, secretion, or stimulation of pituitary gonadotropes. Most patients with hypothalamic-pituitary tumors causing gonadotropin deficiency also have one or more additional pituitary hormone deficiencies (or, an increased serum prolactin with prolactinomas). Those with GH deficiency due to a neoplasm have late onset of growth failure compared with those who have idiopathic and familial hypopituitarism, who have growth failure early in life. The presence of both anterior and posterior (i.e. central diabetes insipidus) pituitary deficiencies in infancy suggests a midline developmental defect but it is this combination developing after infancy that ominously suggests an expanding CNS lesion.

Craniopharyngioma

This common CNS neoplasm of nonglial origin and the most common brain tumor associated with hypothalamic-pituitary dysfunction and sexual infantilism is craniopharyngioma. Usually suprasellar, this tumor of Rathke pouch originates from epithelial rests along the pituitary stalk that extend superiorly to the hypothalamus; craniopharyngiomas may reside within the sella turcica or, more rarely, craniopharyngiomas may be found in the nasopharynx[1347] or the third ventricle.[1348] Craniopharyngiomas are usually symptomatic before age 20.[1349] The peak incidence occurs between ages 6 and 14.[1350-1352] CNS signs develop as the tumor encroaches on surrounding structures.

Symptoms of craniopharyngioma include headache, visual disturbances, short stature, symptoms of diabetes insipidus (DI), vomiting, and weakness of one or more limbs.[1351-1353] Visual

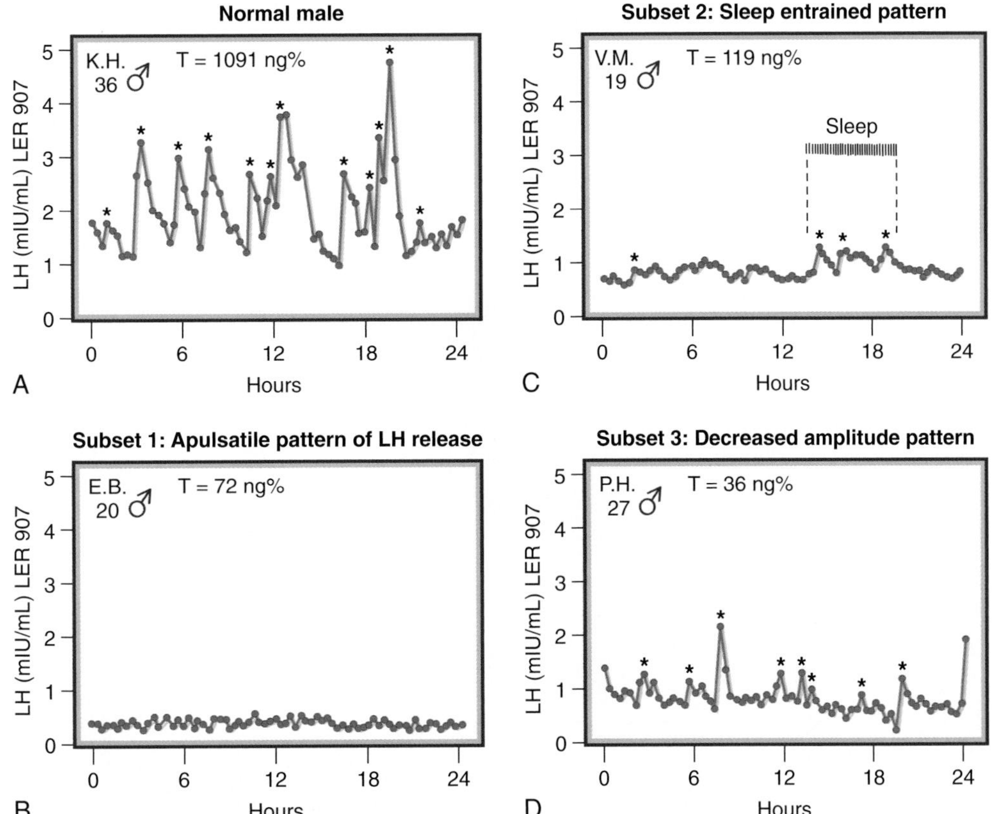

Figure 24–53 ■ The various patterns of pulsatile luteinizing hormone (LH) secretion that can occur in isolated hypogonadotropic hypogonadism (**B** to **D**) compared with LH secretion in a normal man **(A)**. **A,** The discrete LH pulses occurring about every 2 hours in a normal 36-year-old man. **B,** Typical apulsatile LH pattern associated with a low testosterone concentration usually found in isolated hypogonadotropic hypogonadism. **C,** Pattern of developmental arrest with low-amplitude nocturnal LH pulses apparent only during sleep. **D,** Low-amplitude LH pulse pattern during sleep and wake periods. To convert LH values to international units per liter, multiply by 1.0. (From Spratt DI, Crowley WF. Hypogonadotropic hypogonadism: GnRH therapy. In Krieger DT, Bardin CW, eds. Current Therapy in Endocrinology and Metabolism, 1985-1986. Toronto: BC Decker, 1985:155-159.)

defects (including bilateral temporal field deficits), optic atrophy or papilledema, and signs of GH deficiency, delayed puberty, and hypothyroidism are the signs of craniopharyngioma.[1351,1352] Most patients are below the mean in height and height velocity at the time of diagnosis; a long indolent course is possible.[1352] Deficiencies of gonadotropins, GH, thyrotropin (TSH), ACTH, and vasopressin (AVP) are common. The serum concentration of prolactin may be normal, low, or increased, depending upon size and location of the tumor. Delayed bone age is common and may point to the onset of tumor growth.

About 70% of patients with craniopharyngioma have suprasellar or intrasellar calcification (found in less than 1% of normals) and an abnormal sella turcica.[1352] Coincidental finding of calcification or abnormalities of the sella on skull X-ray films obtained for other indications including orthodontic reasons may lead to diagnosis in asymptomatic patients.[1350,1352,1354] CT scans (but not MRI scans) reveal fine calcifications that are not apparent on lateral skull X-ray films, and CT or MRI scans with contrast (the diagnostic procedure of choice) can determine whether the tumor is cystic or solid and indicate the presence of hydrocephalus (Fig. 24–54).[1355]

Smaller craniopharyngiomas, usually intrasellar, can be treated by transsphenoidal microsurgery, but larger or suprasellar masses usually require craniotomy, so the approach must be individualized.[1356] A survey of 40 patients with attempted complete removal without radiation therapy revealed a recurrence rate of 42%.[1357] The combination of limited tumor removal and radiation therapy leads to at least as satisfactory a neurologic prognosis, better cognitive outcome, and better endocrine outcome as attempts at complete surgical extirpation.[1352,1358-1361] Radical removal of craniopharyngioma leads to the need for gonadal steroids and growth hormone replacement; 91% requiring glucocorticoids and 50% becoming severely obese postoperatively in one series.[1357] Postoperative hyperphagia and obesity can be striking (BMI>5 SD) and correlate with the magnitude of hypothalamic damage on cranial MRI.[1362] Injury to the hypothalamic ventromedial nuclei (associated with increased parasympathetic activity and hyperinsulinemia) and/or the paraventricular nuclei may cause these findings.[1363] Hypersecretion of insulin is implicated in the growth and obesity, and suppression of insulin may be helpful.[1364,1365] Aberrant sleep patterns and even narcolepsy and daytime somnolence may follow surgical treatment of craniophayngiomas.[1366-1372] Melatonin may improve sleep patterns.[1369,1373] While the endocrine complications are manageable, combination of ADH insufficiency (DI) and impaired sense of thirst remain one of the most complex management problems.[1349]

Rathke-cleft cysts are often discovered as incidental findings on MRI, but can produce symptoms and signs indistinguishable from those of a craniopharyngioma. Precocious or delayed puberty may be a feature of the cysts.[1374,1375] Surgical drainage and excision of the cyst wall is customary.[1376]

Other Extrasellar Tumors

Germinomas (pinealomas, ectopic pinealomas, atypical teratomas, or dysgerminomas)[1377] or other germ cell tumors of the CNS are the most common extrasellar tumors that arise in suprasellar hypothalamic region, in the pineal region and encroach on the hypothalamus to cause sexual infantilism. Out of all primary CNS tumors, germinomas are rare. The second decade is one of the two peak age ranges for all germ cell tumors (the other is infancy). They are more often found in males.[1378] Polydipsia and polyuria are among the most common symptoms,[1379] followed by visual difficulties and abnormalities of growth and puberty.[1380] Deficiencies of vasopressin and GH are most common, but other anterior pituitary hormone deficiencies (including gonadotropin deficiency) and elevated serum prolactin levels are frequent. Determinations of the concentration of hCG in spinal fluid and in serum, as well as of α-fetoprotein, are useful tumor markers in children and adolescents with germ cell tumors. Germ cell tumors in boys cause isosexual GnRH-independent

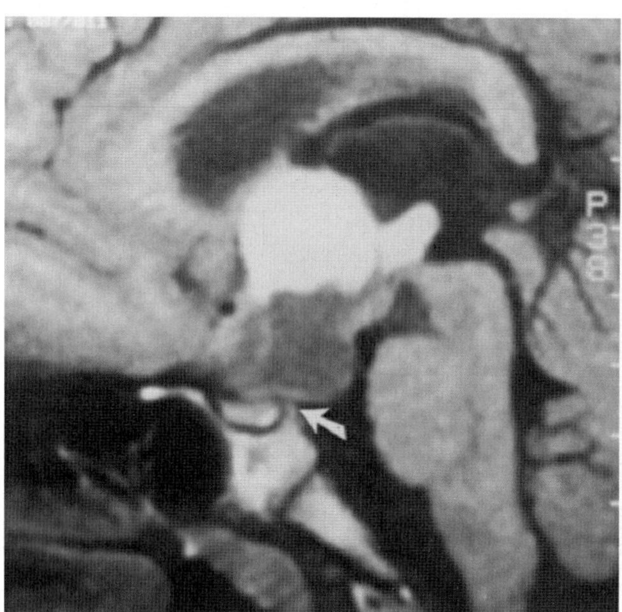

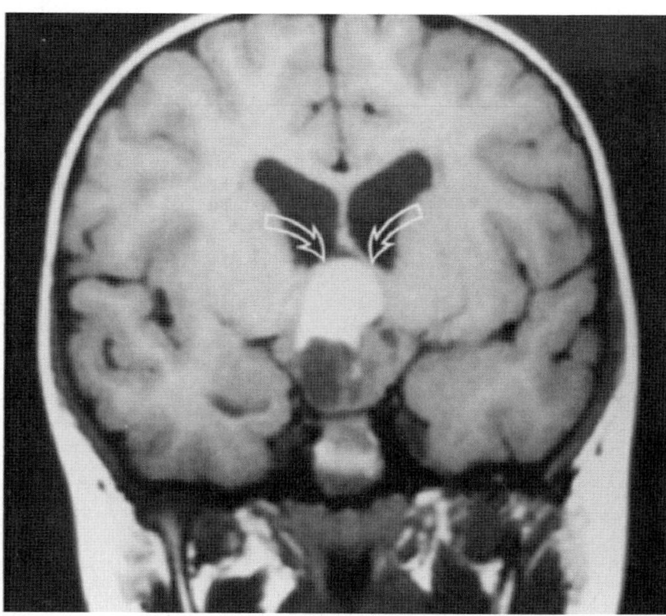

Figure 24–54 ▪ Craniopharyngioma in a short 5-year-old girl with a history of frontal headaches, impaired vision, and poor growth. *Left,* Midline sagittal T1-weighted image that shows a hyperintense region superiorly and an inferior hypointense region. The combination of hyperintense and hypointense areas in a non–contrast-enhanced examination is the most characteristic finding in craniopharyngioma. Note erosion of dorsum sellae *(solid white arrow)* and posterior pituitary bright spot. *Right,* Coronal-weighted T1 image shows tumor extending upward to the inferior frontal horns, narrowing the foramen of Monro and causing mild hydrocephalus. The open white arrows indicate the upper border of the hyperintense area of the tumor.

sexual precocity by secretion of hCG (see section on sexual precocity, page 99) as well. A single hCG-secreting suprasellar teratoma produced mild sexual precocity in a 6-year-old girl who had nondetectable serum concentrations of LH and FSH. Pubertal development was possibly due to aromatase activity of the teratoma; with regression of the tumor, the breast budding disappeared.[1381]

Subependymal spread along the lining of the third ventricle is common in germ cell tumors, and seeding may involve the lower spinal cord and corda equina. MRI scans with contrast enhancement are useful in the diagnosis of tumors more than 0.5 cm in diameter and in the detection of isolated enlargement of the pituitary stalk, an early finding.[1379] Hypothalamic-pituitary abnormalities on MRI relate to functional defects such as DI.[1379,1380] Periodic MRI monitoring is indicated whenever thickening of the pituitary stalk occurs, especially with DI. The pituitary gland increases in size 100% between year 1 and 15, but the pineal gland does not normally change in size after 1 year; any later enlargement should awaken suspicion of a mass lesion.[1382] Pineal cysts are a rare cause of central precocious puberty.[1383] Radiation is the preferred treatment for pur germ cell tumors such as germinomas; surgery is rarely indicated except for biopsy to establish a tissue diagnosis.[1379,1384] However, both radiation therapy and chemotherapy are recommended for a mixed germ cell tumor.

Hypothalamic and optic gliomas or astrocytomas, as part of neurofibromatosis (Von Recklinghausen disease) or independently, can also cause sexual infantilism (see page 107).[1385-1387]

Pituitary Tumors

Only 2% to 6% of all pituitary adenomas occur in childhood and adolescence. Most pituitary tumors in this age group are prolacitnomas with GH, ACTH secreting or nonfunctioning adenomas less commonly[1388] although one report states that the corticotrope adenoma is the most common prepubertal adenoma.[1389]

A recent survey of 44 cases reported that 61% were macroadenomas (more often in boys, hypopituitarism and growth failure are common) and 39% were microadenomas (more often in girls, delayed puberty is common).[1390-1394] In our patients, only 2 of 29 had delayed onset of puberty,[1394] although primary amenorrhea was the presenting symptom in 13 of 20 pubertal females. Presenting symptoms include oligoamenorrhea and galactorrhea in the girls, and headache in the boys. Galactorrhea may only be demonstrable by manual manipulation of the nipples (blood samples for prolactin should be obtained before examination or many hours later because manipulation of the nipples raises prolactin). Transsphenoidal resection of microprolactinomas in children and adolescents is an effective treatment.[1394] The dopamine agonist bromergocryptine may decrease serum prolactin concentrations and decrease the tumor size[1395]; we use this approach before surgery to reduce the size of the tumor in large macroprolactinomas and when resection of the adenoma is incomplete. Pubertal progression and normal menstrual function in girls usually follows reduction in serum prolactin levels. However, pituitary apoplexy followed cabergoline treatment of a macroprolactinoma in a 16-year-old, a complication known in adults treated with bromocriptine.[1396] High serum levels of macroprolactin, a complex of immunoglobulin G and monomeric prolactin with little biologic activity in vivo, cross-reacts in commercial prolactin assays leading to pseudohyperprolactinemia.[1397] Clinical evaluation should help decrease misdiagnosis of prolactinomas in such casese.

Other CNS Disorders Leading to Delayed Puberty

Langerhans' cell histiocytosis (Hans-Schuller-Christian disease, or histiocytosis X). This clonal proliferative disorder of Langerhans' histiocytes or their precursors,[1398,1399] is characterized by the infiltration of lipid-laden histiocytic cells or foam cells in the skin, viscera, and bone.[1400-1402] DI, due to infiltration of the hypothalamus and/or the pituitary stalk, is the most common endocrine manifestation,[1403] with GH deficiency and delayed puberty possible.[1404,1405] Involvement of the lung, liver, and spleen, as well as cystlike areas in flat and long bones and in the dorsolumbar spine occurs. "Floating teeth" within rarefied bone of the mandible and absent or loose teeth, as well as exophthalmos due to infiltration of the orbit are seen. Mastoid or temporal bone involvement may lead to chronic otitis media.[1406] Treatment with glucocorticoids, antineoplastic agents, and radiation is promising in terms of survival but more than 50% of patients have late sequelae or progression.[1402,1405-1407] The natural waxing and waning course of this disease makes evaluation of therapy difficult.[1408,1409]

Postinfectious Inflammatory Lesions of the CNS, Vascular Abnormalities, and Head Trauma

Tuberculous or sarcoid granulomas of the CNS are associated with delayed puberty[1410]; indeed the original case of "adiposogenital dystrophy" or Frohlich's syndrome is thought to be due to tuberculosis rather than neoplasm. Hydrocephalus may cause delayed puberty that can be reversed with decompression[1411,1412] as can pressure from a subarachnoid cyst as noted above (see page 75).

Radiation of the CNS

Radiation of the CNS for treatment of tumors, leukemia, or neoplasms of the head and the face may result in the gradual onset of hypothalamic-pituitary failure.[1413] Although GH deficiency is the most common hormone disorder resulting from radiation, gonadotropin deficiency also occurs,[1172,1414] as does hypothyroidism and decreased bone density.[1415] Decreased growth due to GH deficiency with early onset of puberty can lead to a decrease in the adult height of children with acute lymphocytic leukemia treated with CNS radiation.[1416] The advance in the age of the onset of puberty is reported to be positively correlated with the age of diagnosis of the condition for which the radiation was given (earlier age of onset of puberty with earlier age of diagnosis) and positively correlated with BMI at diagnosis.[1417] However, girls receiving 25 gy of CNS irradiation after 7 years of age were reportedly more likely to have delayed puberty while those treated earlier were not affected in the onset of puberty, although they had diminished ultimate height.[1418] Newer radiation treatment regimens using 18 gy instead of 24 gy for various malignancies may have less influence on advancing the age of menarche and may lead to less long-term morbidity.[1419-1421] Self reported fertility is lower in women who received CNS radiotherapy for acute lymphocytic leukemia (ALL) about the time of menarche,[1422] although this long-term study included women on the average in their ealy 20s and longer follow-up of fertility may change the results. Other reports confirm the possibility of hypogonadotropic hypogonadism in those treated with CNS irradiation.[1423] It is clear that any child treated with CNS irradiation must be monitored for development of these complications over time. It is further recommended that those treated with chemotherapy alone for childhood malignancies be monitored annually for the development of endocrine complications.[1424,1425]

Isolated Hypogonadal Hypogonadism

A developmental defect of the hypothalamus involving the GnRH pulse generator and/or the gonadotropes without an anatomic lesion causes the selective deficiency of gonadotropins, isolated hypogonadal hypogonadism (IHH) (Table 24–24).[1243,1247,1346,1391,1426-1430] Puberty fails to begin by 14 years in boys and 13 years in girls or the pubertal maturation is incomplete or transient. In boys, micropenis or undescended testes, or both, are evidence of a fetal testosterone deficiency. Prepubertal concentration of gonadal sex steroid values (testosterone in boys; estradiol in girls) and low serum gonadotropin levels or values within the normal range (normal in the basal state but not in the secretory state) are characteristic. Concentrations of gonadal sex steroids and gonadotropins are low, pulsatile LH secretion is virtually absent, and the LH response to GnRH or of GnRH agonist is deficient in the severe form. The testes are small and may be hard to detect; serum inhibin B, an estimate of seminiferous tubule function, is low.[1431,1432]

IHH may occur in families (about 20% to 30% of patients) or sporadically. In contrast to CNS tumors (patients usually have GH deficiency and growth failure) and CDP (patients are short for chronologic age), height is appropriate for age in IHH (Fig. 24–55). Because gonadal steroids, particularly estradiol, are too low to cause epiphyseal fusion at the normal age, increased arm span for height and decreased upper/lower ratios (eunuchoid body proportions) occur and, if untreated, growth continues and adult height is tall.[1433,1434]

Kallmann's Syndrome (Table 24–25)

Anosmia or hyposmia resulting from agenesis or hypoplasia of the olfactory lobes and/or sulci is associated with GnRH deficiency in this most common form of IHH.[1426,1435] First noted in the autopsy of a 40-year-old man with micropenis, small cryptorchid testes and absence of the olfactory bulbs in 1856,[1436] Franz Kallmann later described a familial pattern in 1944.[1435] The (Fig. 24–56) is about 1/10,000 in males and 40,000 in females. Even though the loss of olfaction usually correlates with the

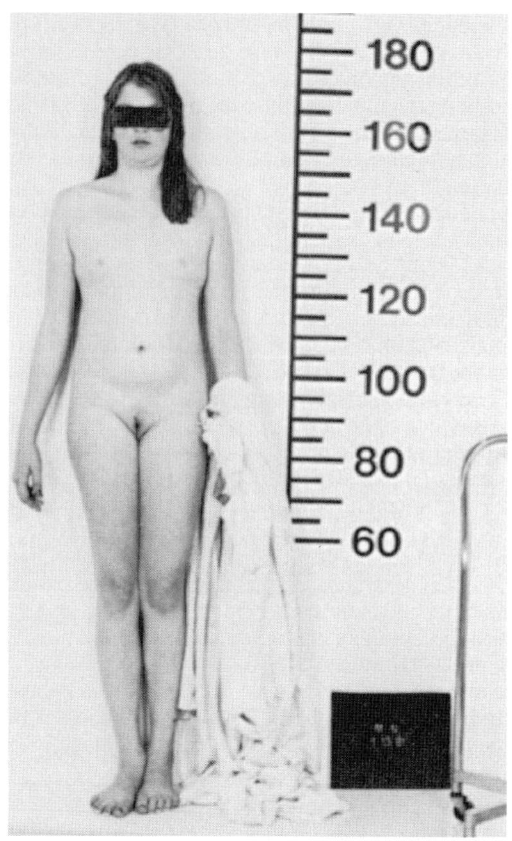

Figure 24–55 ▪ A girl 18 years and 8 months of age with isolated gonadotropin deficiency (sexual infantilism and primary amenorrhea). Height was 173 cm (+1 SD), weight was 66.5 kg (+1 SD), and skeletal age was 13 years. Adrenarche with pubic hair development occurred at age 13½ years. At the time of the photograph, pubic hair was in stage 3 and there was slight breast and nipple development resulting from a previous short course of estrogen therapy. Immature labia minora and majora were noted, and no estrogen effect was present on the vaginal mucosa. Olfactory testing was normal. The plasma luteinizing hormone (LH) (LER-960) level after LH-releasing hormone (GnRH) administration rose from 0.5 to 1.8 ng/mL (a prepubertal response). Serum estradiol was undetectable. The dehydroepiandrosterone sulfate (DHEAS) level was 92 µg/dL (appropriate for pubic hair stage 2). Note the discrepancy between adrenarche and gonadarche. For conversion to SI units, see the legends of Figures 24–21 and 24–40. (From Styne DM, Grumbach MM. Puberty in the male and female: its physiology and disorders. In Yen SCC, Jaffe RB, eds. Reproductive Endocrinology, 2nd ed. Philadelphia: WB Saunders, 1986:313-384.)

TABLE 24–24 ISOLATED GONADOTROPIN DEFICIENCY

- Males more commonly affected
- Familial (more common in females) or sporadic (more common in males)
- Height normal for age; tall adult height if untreated
- Eunuchoid skeletal proportions
- Delayed bone age
- Small, often cryptorchid testes: diameter <2.5 cm prepubertal size; phallus may be small
- Normal adrenarche
- Examine for anosmia or hyposmia (Kallmann's syndrome)
- Look for associated malformations (facial, central nervous system, skeletal, renal)

TABLE 24–25 ISOLATED GONADOTROPIN DEFICIENCY: CLINICAL FEATURES IN 20 ADOLESCENT BOYS

Classification	Age and Range* (yr)	Testicular Enlargement	Undescended Testes	Gynecomastia	Ocular Anomalies	Other Anomalies
Euosmic	$3^{5}/_{12}$-$20^{6}/_{12}$	3/10	3/10	2/10	3/10	6/10†
Anosmic or hyposmic	7-8	2/10	8/10	6/10	7/10	7/10‡
Total		5/20	11/20	8/20	10/20	13/20

*First evaluated at University of California, San Francisco, Pediatric Endocrine Clinic. All of the patients had delayed puberty; mean height was normal for age.
†Cohen syndrome (1); congenital adrenal hypoplasia (1).
‡Absent kidney (1); talipes, camptodactyly (1).

degree of GnRH deficiency, even in complete anosmia the GnRH deficiency may be partial (see discussion of the fertile eunuch syndrome page 76).[1432,1437] Because affected individuals often do not notice impaired olfaction, testing with graded dilutions of pure scents is necessary.[1438] Rarely, affected males who are severely delayed in puberty may spontaneously increase their testicular size and enter full puberty.[1439,1440] Kallmann patients lack or have diminished nocturnal pulses of gonadotropins found in normal prepubertal boys although daytime valules are equal.[1441] Undescended testes and gynecomastia are common in this and all types of hypogonadotropic hypogonadism in boys.[1431] The magnitude of the GnRH deficiency correlates with the size of the testes. Micropenis occurs in about one half of males with Kallman's syndrome (KS).[1442]

Associated defects inconstantly present are cleft lip, cleft palate, imperfect facial fusion, seizure disorders, short metacarpals, pes cavus, neurosensory hearing loss (rarely found in the X-linked form),[1443] cerebellar ataxia and nystagmus, ocular motor abnormalities,[1444] unilateral or rarely bilateral renal aplasia or dysplasia,[1445] and, limited to the X-linked form, mirror movements of the upper extremities (bimanual synkinesia) (see Table 24–26).[1197,1435,1446,1447]

One of the striking features of isolated hypogonadotropic hypogonadism is the clinical heterogeneity in gonadal function and phenotype within and between families with the same genetic mutation. This variability in clinical manifestations within and across families with a shared apparent monogenic defect confounds prediction of the phenotype within a pedigree. Because of this clinical heterogeneity, IHH is clinically classified as Kallmann syndrome (with anosmia or hyposmia) or normosmic IHH. As discussed below, the clinical phenotype including olfactory abnormalities is variable even within affected families. Recent genetic analyses provide novel insight into both the intrafamilial and interfamilial heterogeneity by detecting oligogeneity in genetic mutations causing IHH[1447a].

This syndrome is genetically heterogeneous and can be transmitted as an X-linked, autosomal dominant or autosomal recessive trait. Initial reports of infertile males suggested an X-linked mode of inheritance[1435] now denoted as KAL 1. The Xp22.3 locus is the site of the KAL-1 gene, an X-linked gene that

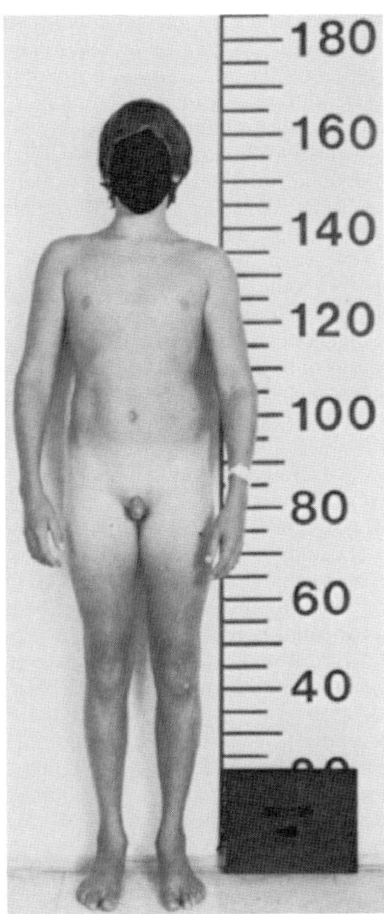

Figure 24–56 ▪ A boy of 15 years and 10 months with isolated gonadotropin deficiency and anosmia (Kallmann's syndrome). He had undescended testes, but after administration of 10,000 U of human chorionic gonadotropin (hCG) the testes descended and were palpable in the scrotum. Height, 163.9 cm (−1.5 SD); the upper/lower body ratio was 0.86, which is eunuchoid. The phallus measured 6.3×1.8 cm, and the testes were 1.2×0.8 cm. The concentration of plasma luteinizing hormone (LH) was less than 0.3 ng/mL; of follicle-stimulating hormone (FSH), 1.2 ng/mL; of testosterone, 16 ng/dL. After 100 μg of LH-releasing hormone (GnRH), the plasma LH (LER-960) was 0.7 ng/mL and FSH (LER-869) 2.4 ng/mL. For conversion to SI units, see the legends of Figures 24–21 and 24–22. (From Styne DM, Grumbach MM. Puberty in the male and female: its physiology and disorders. In Yen SCC, Jaffe RB, eds. Reproductive Endocrinology, 2nd ed. Philadelphia: WB Saunders, 1986:313-384.)

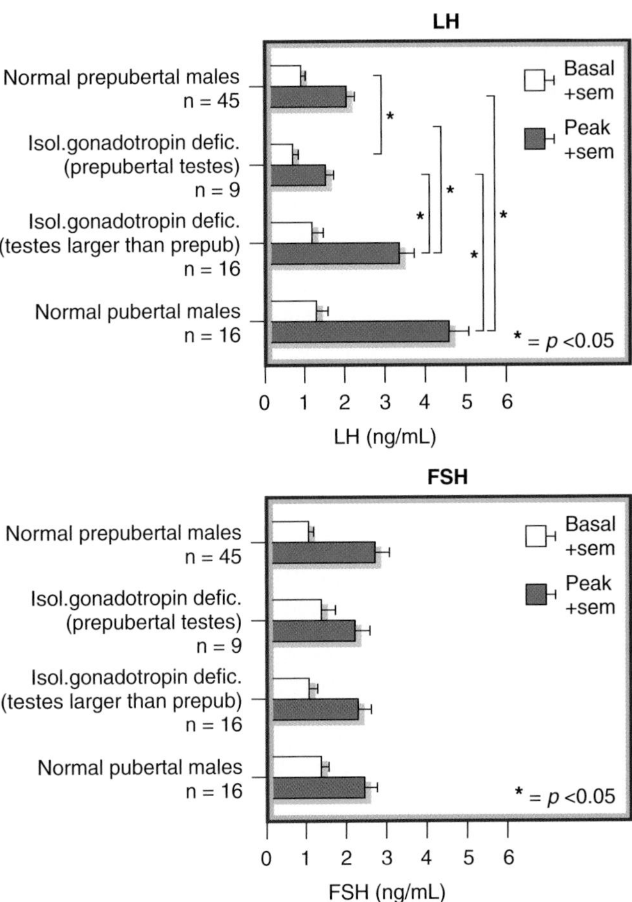

Figure 24–57 ▪ Serum luteinizing hormone (LH) and follicle-stimulating hormone (FSH) responses to the administration of LH-releasing hormone (GnRH) in 25 males with an isolated gonadotropin deficiency with or without anosmia, segregated according to whether the volume of the testes was prepubertal or greater than 2.5 cm^3; testicular volume in those with testes greater than 2.5 cm^3 were as large as 4 cm^3. Basal and GnRH-stimulated gonadotropin levels after the intravenous injection of 100 μg GnRH (peak value) are shown. $P<.05$. For conversion to SI units, see the legend of Figure 24–21. (From Van Dop C, Burstein S, Conte FA, et al. Isolated gonadotropin deficiency in boys: clinical characteristics and growth. J Pediatr 1987;111:684-692.)

TABLE 24–26 FEATURES OF KALLMANN'S SYNDROME

Clinical
- GnRH deficiency: absent or arrested puberty
- Anosmia or hyposmia
- In infancy: microphallus; cryptorchidism
- Normal stature and growth in childhood
- Normal adrenarche
- Eunuchoid proportions
- Associated midline defects (e.g., cleft lip, cleft palate, midline cranial anomalies)
- MRI: aplasia or hypoplasia of olfactory bulbs and/or sulci

Prevalence: approximately 1 in 7500 males, 1 in 50,000 females; one-tenth prevalence of Klinefelter's syndrome

Inheritance: sporadic and familial cases; genetic heterogeneity
- X linked
  - X-lined recessive (Kallmann et al.[1114])
  - X chromosome deletion: Xp22.3 (Ballabio et al.[1129])
- Autosomal
  - Dominant (sex limitation) (Santen and Paulsen[1132]; Merriam et al.[1133])
  - Recessive (White et al.[1134])

Anatomy: developmental field defect
- Aplasia or hypoplasia of olfactory bulb and sulcus
- Arrested migration of GnRH neurosecretory neurons from olfactory placode to medial basal hypothalamus

GnRH, Luteinizing hormone-releasing hormone.

escapes X-inactivation and maps 1.5 megabases proximal to the steroid sulfatase gene at the same locus. The KAL-1 gene encodes a 680 amino acid glycoprotein, anosmin-1, with characteristics of an extracellular neural adhesion molecule that could function as a pathfinder in the guidance of GnRH neurons in their migration to the medial basal hypothalamus (see page 43). The developmental distribution of immunoreactive anosmin-1 in the human embryo and fetus demonstrates its widespread distribution including the olfactory placode and forebrain by week 5 to 6 as well as the mesonephros and metanephros, precartilaginous skeleton, inner ear, and cerebellum. All of the structures and organs affected by the symptoms are sites of expression of the KAL gene in the human fetus (see Table 24–25).[1448,1449]

A variety of deletions and mutations of the KAL 1 gene have been described including large and small (exon) deletions,[1197,1447,1450] point mutations, and a variety of non-sense mutations leading to frameshift and premature stop codons.[1197,1451,1452] The KAL1 mutations are more prevalent in Japanese than Caucasian patients and can be associated with normal olfactory function.[1453] The defect in some rare patients with no KAL 1 mutation but X-linked inheritance may be located in the promoter region of the KAL gene.[1454] KS associated with X-linked ichthyosis caused by steroid sulfatase deficiency, mental retardation, and chondroplasia punctata occurs in a contiguous gene syndrome.[1455] Only 14% of familial cases and 11% of sporadic cases have mutations in the KAL gene on the X chromosome, but it is these that are more likely to have complete absence of gonadotropin secretory pulses and absence of migration of GnRH neurons to the hypothalamus.[1456] Hypogonadotropic hypogonadism is rarely due to a mutation in the KAL 1 gene in female subjects.[1457]

The autosomal dominant form is known as Kallmann's syndrome 2 (KAL 2) and the associated gene is KAL2 or the fibroblast growth factor receptor 1 gene (FGFR1) with a gene map locus 8p11.2-p11.1.[1442,1458] A report of an affected male who fathered an affected son after treatment with hCG further supports autosomal dominant inheritance.[1459]

KAL 2 occurs with or without anosmia/hyposmia; it is associated with mental retardation, choanal atresia, short stature, congenital heart defects, and sensorineural hearing loss and has more variation in presentation than those with KAL 1. The loss of function mutation of the FGFR1 gene interferes with the migration of the olfactory cells to the olfactory bulb.[1460] Anosmin-1 may act through the FGFR1 to bring about FGF signaling. KAL 1 partially escapes inactivation in females, and it is postulated that enough KAL 1 is produced despite FGF1 haploinsufficiency in affected females to maintain adequate FGF signaling to allow olfactory function and GnRH neuron migration. One kindred of Kallmann's syndrome contained four women with FGFR1 mutations that were transmitted to affected male offspring, although the mother had normal reproduction and olfaction.[1460] While gain of function mutations of the FGFR1 gene is associated with craniosynostosis, a loss of function mutation is not associated with lack of fusion of the cranial sutures. One kindred is reported with FGFR1 mutation (Arg(622)X) in the tyrosine kinase domain in which some of the manifestations were temporary; the mother of the proband had delayed puberty and the maternal grandmother had anosmia, while the proband with KAL 2 exhibited normal LH, testosterone production and spermatogenesis after earlier testosterone therapy.[1461] An unusual kindred with a proband demonstrating severe ear anomalies, mandibular hypoplasia, thoracic dystrophia, and other usual findings was associated with an Arg622 mutation in the FGFR1 gene: investigation for hypogonadism is indicated when such facial abnormalities occur.[1462] Prevalence of the FGFR1 mutations in Japan is equal to the prevalence in Caucasians.[1453]

Apparent autosomal recessive inheritance characterizes other kindreds[1463] in Kallmann's syndrome 3 or KAL 3. Unilateral renal agenesis, hypotelorism, cleft lip and palate, and midline cranial fusion defect occur. While renal aplasia is characteristic of KAL1 mutations and KAL 3 and cleft palate and dental agenesis are characteristic of FGFR1 mutations in KAL 2, these findings can occur in Kallmann's patients without KAL1 and FGFR1 mutations.[1453]

Thus, the various forms of Kallmann's syndrome are due to heterogeneous mutations[1426,1442,1456,1458,1463] in which the phenotype can vary. For example, a 20-year-old man with the complete picture of Kallmann's syndrome had an identical twin brother (proved by genetic fingerprinting) with anosmia but a normal adult phenotype and normal plasma testosterone and gonadotropin concentrations.[1464]

In Kallmann's syndrome, fetal GnRH neurosecretory neurons do not migrate from the olfactory placode to the medial basal hypothalamus, where they should constitute the GnRH pulse generator (see earlier) but instead end in a tangle around the cribriform plate and in the dural layers adjacent to the meninges beneath the forebrain.[991] Abnormal or absent olfactory bulbs or folds on MRI scans result in some (Fig. 24–58).[1465,1466] Other postulated defects that might interfere with GnRH neuron migration are caused by mutations in the genes for neural cell adhesion molecules (NCAM) and related proteins, such as tenascin, laminin, and phosphacan, as well as various glycoconjugates.

Coronal and axial cranial MRI scans of the olfactory bulbs and sulci reflect this defect in about 90% of cases and can point to the diagnosis,[1467,1465] especially in affected infants and prepubertal-age children.[1465] Of 64 individuals with Kallmann's syndrome, 56% had bilateral agenesis of the olfactory bulbs (2% unilateral); 56% had absent or abnormal olfactory sulci bilaterally (17% unilateral).[1451] By fetal MRI, olfactory sulci are detectable from 30 weeks gestational age and olfactory bulbs from 30 to 34 weeks gestational age.[1468a]

The CHARGE syndrome includes a host of congenital anomalies including hypogonadotropic hypogonadism, abnormal olfactory bulbs, and defective olfaction.[1468] This syndrome has been associated with a mutation in the CHD7 gene, a member

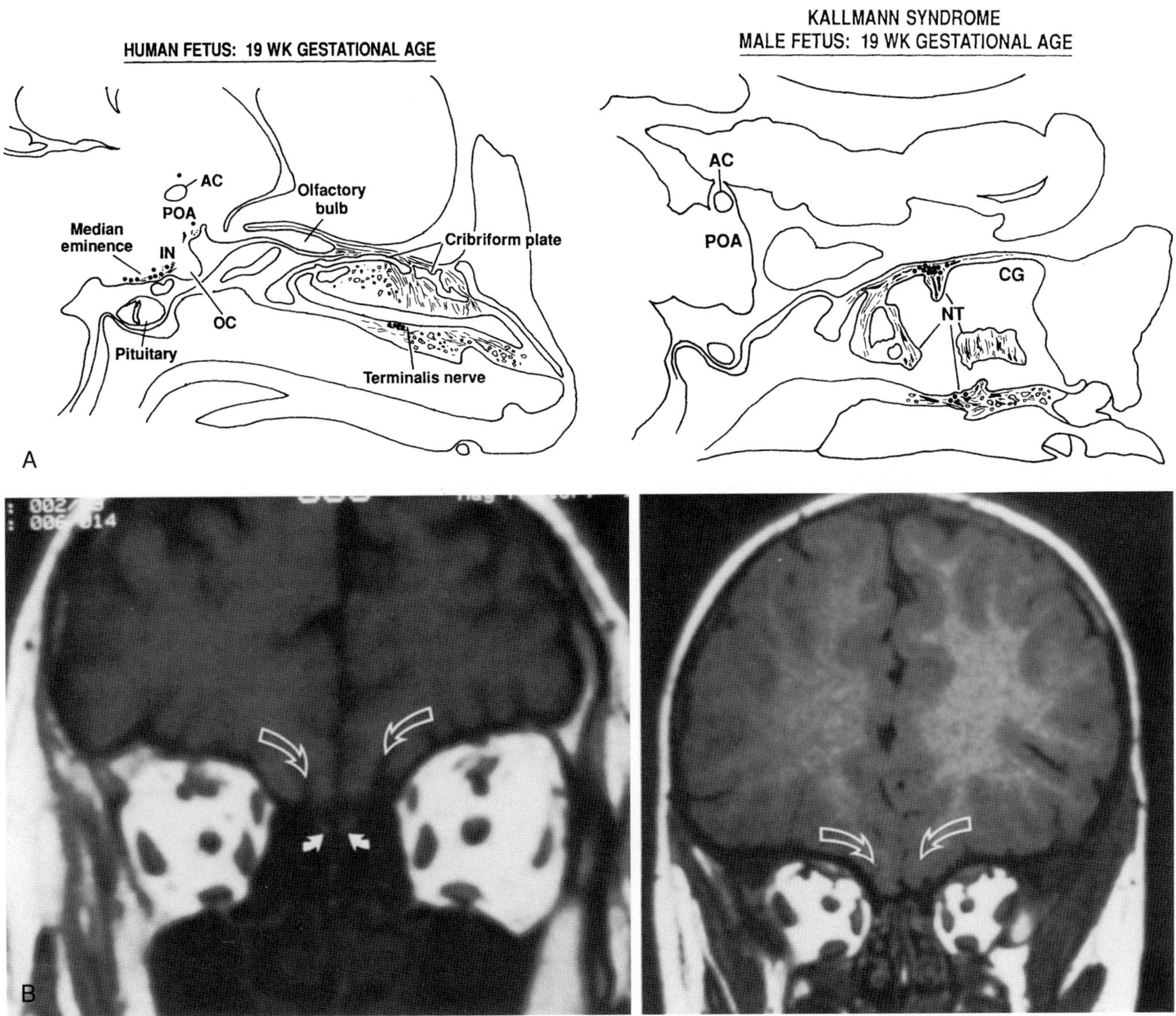

Figure 24–58 ▪ Comparison of the brain and nasal cavities of a normal 19-week-old male fetus *(upper left)* and those of a male fetus of similar age with Kallmann's syndrome caused by an X chromosome deletion at Xp22.3 *(upper right)*. In the normal fetal brain the luteinizing hormone–releasing hormone (GnRH) neurosecretory neurons *(black dots)* are located in the hypothalamic area including the medial basal hypothalamus; the anterior hypothalamic area; and, of interest regarding hypothalamic hamartoma as an ectopic GnRH pulse generator, the premammillary and retromammillary areas. A small cluster of GnRH neurons is present among the fibers of the terminalis nerve on the floor of the nasal septum. In the male fetus with Kallmann's syndrome, no GnRH neurons were detected in the hypothalamic region including the basal hypothalamus, median eminence, and preoptic area. The GnRH cells fail to migrate to and enter the brain from their origin in the nose; these cells end in a tangle beneath the forebrain on the dorsal surface of the cribriform plate and in the nasal cavity. *AC,* Anterior commissure; *CG,* crista galli; *IN,* infundibular nucleus; *NT,* terminalis nerve; *OC,* optic chiasm; *POA,* preoptic area. Lower panels show magnetic resonance imaging scans of brain (coronal section, TI-weighted image). *Lower left,* Normal olfactory sulci *(open white arrows)* and bulbs *(small solid white arrows)* in a 15-year-old boy. *Lower right,* Absent olfactory sulci *(open white arrows)* and bulbs in a 17-year-old anosmic, sexually infantile boy with Kallmann's syndrome.

of the chromodomain helicase DNA-binding family and the SEMA3E gene (semaphorin 3E).

Other Forms of Isolated Hypogonadotropic Hypogonadism

Inheritance of HH (Table 24–26) with none of the other features of Kallmann's syndrome may be found in autosomal dominant (gene map locus 19p13.3, 9q34.3), autosomal recessive (gene map locus 8p21-p11.2), or X-linked recessive (gene map locus Xp21) locations.[1469-1471] Males with cerebellar ataxia and deficient gonadotropin production are reported in kindreds with X-linked inheritance (possibly a variant form of Kallmann's syndrome), and hypogonadotropic hypogonadism may be associated with the multiple lentigines and basal cell nevus syndromes.

The combination of human genetic studies and mouse models has led to the discovery of many genes involved in gonadotropin regulation (Table 24–27).[924] An autosomal

TABLE 24–27 MOLECULAR BASIS FOR DEVELOPMENT DISORDERS ASSOCIATED WITH HYPOGONADOTROPIC HYPOGONADISM

ISOLATED HYPOGONADOTROPIC HYPOGONADISM	
Gene	**Phenotype**
Kallmann syndrome or normosmic IHH (with the same mutant gene)	
KAL1	X-linked Kallmann syndrome, anosmia/hyposmia, renal agenesis
FGFR1 (fibroblast growth factor) (KAL2)	Autosomal dominant Kallmann syndrome (± recessive) Anosmia/Hyposmia, cleft lip/palate
FGF8 (fibroblast growth factor 8) (ligand for FGFR1)	
NELF (nasal embryonic LHRH factor)	
PROK2 (prokineticin 2)	
PROKR2 (G-protein-coupled receptor)	
Normosmic Isolated Hypogonadotropic Hypogonadism	
GNRHR (GnRH receptor; G-protein-coupled receptor)	Autosomal recessive (± dominant)
GPR54 (kisspeptin G-protein-coupled receptor 54	Autosomal recessive
SNRPN (small nuclear ribonucleoprotein polypeptide SmN)	Prader Willi Syndrome
Lack of function of paternal 15q11-q13 region or maternal uniparental disomy	Obesity
LEP (leptin)	Autosomal recessive Obesity
LEPR (leptin receptor)	Autosomal recessive Obesity
DAX1	X-linked recessive Adrenal Hypoplasia

MULTIPLE PITUITARY HORMONE DEFICIENCIES		
Gene	**Hormone Deficiencies**	**Complex Phenotype**
PROP1 (POU1F1)	Autosomal recessive GH, PRL, TSH, and LH/FSH (less commonly later onset ACTH deficiency)	
HESX1 (RPX)	Autosomal recessive; and heterozygous mutations Multiple pituitary including diabetes insipidus but LH/FSH uncommon	Septo-optic dysplasia
LHX3	Autosomal recessive GH, PRL, TSH, FSH/LH	Rigid cervical spine
PHF6	X-linked; GH, TSH, ACTH, LH/FSH	Borjeson-Lehmann syndrome: mental retardation; facies

*HESX1, Homeobox gene expressed in ES cells; PHF6, plant homeo domain-like finger gene; FGFR1, fibroblast growth factor receptor 1; GNRHR, GnRH receptor; SNRPN, small nuclear ribonucleoprotein polypeptide SmN; LEP, leptin; LEPR, leptin receptor; DAX1, dosage-sensitive sex reversal-adrenal hyperplasia congenita critical region on the X chromosome, gene 1; PROP1, prophet of Pit-1; LHX3, lim homeobox gene 3.

recessive form has been described in the mouse (hyg/hyg) in which there is a deletion of a part of the GnRH gene, although there has been no case of GnRH deletion identified in a human as yet. The mutant RNA is incapable of generating functional GnRH.[1472]

KISS-GRP54 Axis

KISS1 is a human metastasis suppressor gene, which is the ligand for the GRP 54 receptor as described earlier; this axis in the resurgena of GnRH signaling at the onset of puberty as demonstrated in cases of HH with defects in the axis. A consanguineous kindred with IHH had homozygous deletions of 155 nucleotides in the GPR54 gene encompassing the splicing acceptor site of intron 4-exon 5 junction and part of exon 5 in all affected family members,[1473] while unaffected family members had no deletion or only one mutant allele. Another kindred had an L148S mutation in GPR54, while another had two separate mutations, R331X and X399R, in the gene.[1211] The later patient had decreased secretion of GnRH and decreased response to GnRH administration. A line of mice transfected with the affected gene exhibited hypogonadotropic hypogonadism with decreased GnRH in the hypothalamus but were responsive to GnRH or gonadotropin administration. KISS-GRP 54 axis mutations are rare[1474], less than 5% in patients with IHH. An affected male infant with micropenis and undescended testes first studied at 2 months of age had low concentrations of plasma FSH and LH[1474a] and no evidence of infantile surge in gonadotropins ("minipuberty" of infancy) (937). The micropenis is evidence that kisspeptin-GPR54 signaling is functional in the late fetus and infant.

The human equivalent of the mouse nasal embryonic GnRH factor gene (Nelf) is NELF; a mutation of this gene was found in one of 65 patients with IHH but in none of 100 controls, suggesting a role for this mutation in the etiology of IHH.[1475]

GnRH Receptor Mutations

No mutation in the human GnRH gene (GnRH 1 at gene map locus 8p21-p11.2) is reported,[1476] in contrast to the mutation described in the hyg/hyg mouse.[1472] On the other hand, mutations in the gene encoding the GnRH receptor (gene map locus Gene map locus 4q21.2), the G protein–coupled seven-transmembrane segments, lead to familial and sporadic patterns of various degrees of hypogonadotropic hypogonadism with normosmia.[1469,1471,1477-1482] Mutations in HH with amino acid substitutions in the extracellular N-terminal domain (Thr32Ile), second extracellular loop (Cys200Tyr), third intracellular loop

(Leu266Arg), and sixth transmembrane helix (Cys279Tyr) affected specific GnRH binding.[1483,1484] Except for Thr32Ile, there was no significant inositol phosphate accumulation after GnRH stimulation, thus demonstrating loss of function even if binding was accomplished; however, an increased dose of GnRH allowed stimulation of gonadotropin subunit and gonadotropin releasing hormone receptor (GnRHR) promoters as well as the ability to partially activate extracellular signal-regulated kinase 1 and stimulate CRE-luciferase activity. A higher dose of GnRH caused the Cys200Tyr mutant to stimulate gonadotropin subunit and GnRHR promoter activity as this mutant reduces cell-surface receptor expression. Another human GnRH receptor (hGnRHR) gene mutation of a highly conserved sequence located in the second transmembrane helix impairs hGnRHR-effector coupling due to loss of surface expression of the receptor leading to a severe manifestation of IHH.[1485] Four families with autosomal recessive IHH had no defects within the coding sequence of the GnRHR or of the GnRH gene itself, GnRH1: the authors postulated the presence of a novel, as-yet-undiscovered gene for this condition.[1476] Classically IHH owing to a mutation in the GnRH receptor is inherited as an autosomal recessive trait. However, recent studies suggest the rare occurrence of autosomal dominant transmission.

Certain GnRH receptor defects may be "rescued" by pharmacologic agents that can act as a folding template can correct the structural defects caused by the mutations, allowing function to occur. A small, membrane-permeant molecule demonstrated pharmacologic rescue (ligand binding and restoration of receptor coupling to effector) of five naturally occurring GnRH receptor (GnRHR) missense mutations of the GnRH receptor in families with IHH.[1486] These molecules also allowed rescue of intentionally manufactured defective receptors with internal or terminal deletions or substitutions at sites expected to be involved in establishment of tertiary receptor structure.[1484] This approach may allow a therapeutic approach to other conditions due to mutations causing protein misfolding.

The clinical presentation of patients with mutations in the GnRH receptor is heterogeneous as impairment of signal transmission is highly variable (ranging from severe features of isolated hypogonadotropic hypogonadism, to sexual infantilism, to long delayed puberty with reversal in adulthood, to relatively mild hypogonadism and infertility) even within the same pedigree and especially in patients with compound heterozygous mutations.[1487] In one woman with impaired GnRH receptor function, the use of pulsatile GnRH treatment induced ovulation and allowed a successful pregnancy.[1488] In all types of congenital gonadotropin deficiency, male patients are likely to manifest micropenis (penile length less than 2.0 cm at birth [and in infancy]) due to lack of fetal gonadotropin stimulation of fetal testes during the last half of gestation. Rarely, boys with congenital growth hormone deficiency have micropenis even if gonadotropin function is normal.[1489] Testosterone therapy is effective (see treatment on page 94); sex reversal is contraindicated in these cases of microphallus.

X-Linked Congenital Adrenal Hypoplasia and Hypogonadotropic Hypogonadism

A rare deletion or mutation in the dax1 gene (*d*osage-sensitive sex reversal-*a*drenal hypoplasia congenita gene on the *X* chromosome gene *1*, gene map locus Xp21.3-p21.2)[1490-1494] leads to an X-linked recessive disorder of adrenocortical organogenesis. The dax1 gene encodes an orphan receptor, a member of the nuclear receptor superfamily, which is a putative transcriptional repressor. dax1 locus undergoes X inactivation. It maps to the DSS (*d*osage *s*ensitive *s*ex reversal) locus (Xp21); a double dose of the dax1 is associated with a female phenotype or ambiguous genitalia in 46XY males. dax1 protein has a novel domain in the amino terminus, which contains two putative unique zinc finger motifs, and the carboxy terminus contains a conserved ligand binding domain,[1491,1493] which binds DNA and localizes in the nucleus and contains a transcriptional silencing domain that antagonizes SF1 transactivation function.[1495,1496] DAX1 has a steroidogenic factor-1 (sf1) response element in the 5 promoter region.[1497,1498] sf1 is another orphan member of the nuclear hormone receptor superfamily; both dax1 and sf1 are expressed in the adrenals, gonads, pituitary, and hypothalamus,[1499] which raises the possibility of an important interaction between these two genes and their products.

Rare abnormalities of the dax1 gene are characterized by severe glucocorticoid, mineralocorticoid, and, at puberty, androgen deficiency.[1500-1505] The abnormal structure of the adrenal cortex resembles that of the fetal zone made up of disorganized vacuolated cytomegalic cells with normal mature cortex.[1502,1504,1506,1507] The severe primary adrenal insufficiency with hyponatremia, hyperkalemia, acidosis, and hypoglycemia (failure to thrive, vomiting, poor feeding, dehydration, circulatory collapse, increased pigmentation) is lethal if untreated early in life of affected boys.[1502,1504] Adrenoleukodystrophy may present with adrenal failure long before neurologic symptoms develop and some cases of X-linked Addison's disease may represent this diagnosis. This condition is in the differential diagnosis for adrenal hypoplasia. Plasma renin activity; plasma cortisol, and aldosterone levels are low. Symptomatic adrenal insufficiency may first present in later childhood. In the infant male, signs of salt-wasting are usually the most prominent feature but cortisol deficiency is present and detectable, and the adrenal insufficiency includes deficient secretion of the zona reticularis steroids, dehydroepiandrosterone and its sulfoconjugate. An early sign of elevated ACTH is increased skin pigmentation. The testes are undescended in less than one half of the patients; micropenis is rare, but occasionally urogenital abnormalities and hearing loss are present. Boys who do not present with clinical evidence of adrenal insufficiency in infancy often have a more insidious onset during childhood or as adults.[1508-1511] In a pedigree in which two affected boys had a hemizygous DAX1 nonsense mutation and neonatal onset of adrenal insufficiency, a maternal aunt who was homozygous for the mutation had sexual infantilism and primary amenorrhea, but even after decades of follow-up maintained normal adrenal function. A maternal grandfather who carried the same mutation was asymptomatic.[1512] This pedigree again highlights the limitations and complexities of genotype and phenotype correlations.[1513] Most commonly, due to hypogonadotropic hypogonadism, signs of sexual maturation at the age of puberty are lacking including the absence of pubic and axillary hair and testicular enlargement; the concentrations of serum FSH, LH, and testosterone are low.[1500-1504] Delayed puberty is a manifestation in some female carriers of a DAX1 mutation.[1514]

For many years, the nature of the hypogonadotropic hypogonadism in this condition has been uncertain.[1501-1504] Intragenic mutations in the dax1 gene[1491,1492,1515,1516] (frameshift mutations; nonsense mutations, and missense mutations[1490,1491,1493,1515-1518]) indicate that the hypogonadotropic hypogonadism is an intrinsic characteristic of the disorder, a manifestation of the single gene mutation and not due to the involvement of a contiguous gene. Second, the dax1 gene is not only expressed in the adrenal cortex and testes (and weakly in the ovary),[1490,1515] but also in the hypothalamus and pituitary.[1493,1519] Thus, there is evidence of both GnRH deficiency and an abnormality in the gonadotropes, giving a mixed picture of both hypothalamic and intrinsic gonadotrope defects[1504] with absent or erratic pulsatile secretion of LH. Even if basal immunoreactive LH and FSH levels are normal, gonadotropins seem to lack bioactivity.[1518] In some affected boys, the GnRH pulse generator-pituitary gonadotropin apparatus is intact and functional in infancy and early childhood as the GnRH-gonadotrope defects are not manifest until later in childhood or the peripubertal period.[1509,1520-1522]

Azoospermia unresponsive to gonadotropin treatment was detected in a few affected men.[1511,1514]

Two cases of dax1 frameshift mutations demonstrate adrenal failure and GnRH-independent sexual precocity that is suppressible by glucocorticoid therapy but not by GnRH agonist. The exceedingly high ACTH levels, possibly acting through the human melanocortin 1 receptor present in human Leydig cells, may be the underlying cause of the increased steroidogenesis and testosterone secretion that was reversed by glucocorticoid treatment. In addition, because DAX1 inhibits the SF1 transactivation, a regulator of steroidogenic genes, the loss of DAX1 inhibition of SF1 transcriptional activity also may have a role.[1523,1524]

A deletion of the adrenal hypoplasia congenita locus (at Xp21) can include the glycerol kinase (GK) and Duchenne's muscular dystrophy (DMD) genes if it extends centromerically, or mental retardation if there is extension toward the telomere leading to a contiguous gene syndrome.[1525]

Other mutations of the X chromosome may be associated with IHH. Two brothers are reported with hypogonadotropic hypogonadism, obesity, and short stature associated with a maternally inherited pericentric inversion (X)(p11.4q11.2): because the break point is not related to other genes associated with pubertal disorders, it is not clear if this is a functional relationship or a coincidence.[1526]

Other Presentations of Hypogonadotropic Hypogonadism

Mutation in the prohormone convertase 1 (PC1) gene led to extreme childhood obesity, hypocortisolemia, defects in conversion of proinsulin to insulin leading to hypoglycemia and isolated partial hypogonadotropic hypogonadism allowing spontaneous pubertal development but primary ammenorrhea.[1527,1528] The HH postulated to relate to impaired processing of GnRH or neuropeptides involved in its secretion. The findings in another subject extended to gastrointestinal disturbance and small intestinal malabsorption related to monosaccharide and fats, and elevation in progastrin and proglucagon, showing that prohormone processing in enteroendocrine cells was abnormal.[1529]

Isolated LH Deficiency

Isolated LH deficiency (the fertile eunuch syndrome) is associated with deficient testosterone production (which responds to administration of hCG) in the presence of variable spermatogenesis[1530]; the disorder may be idiopathic or secondary to a hypothalamic pituitary neoplasm. A homozygous gln106-to-arg mutation in the first extracellular loop of the GnRH receptor at gene map locus 4q21.2. was found with normal testicular volume (17 mL) in one subject, but with apulsatile, low gonadotropin values and low testosterone values.[1487] After hCG stimulation, the subject developed adequate spermatogenesis to father a child and after cessation of hCG treatment, he demonstrated adult testosterone values and pulsatile gonadotropin secretion, an example of reversibility of the syndrome.

Isolated Bioinactive LH

The only known patient had a striking discrepancy between elevated immunoactive and absent bioactive LH due to a mutation in the gene encoding the βLH subunit[1470] in a 17-year-old male with a history of delayed puberty. The subject had a homozygous mutation in exon 3 of the βLH subunit gene (glutamine 54 arginine). Apparently, absent Leydig cells and arrested spermatogenesis improved with hCG treatment. The heterozygote mother exhibited only 50% of normal binding of serum LH to the LH receptor.[1531] The patients normal male sex differentiation was likely due to the action of hCG during the second third trimester. The absence of a micropenis, found in male infants with congenital GnRH deficiency, suggests possible initially bioactive LH in utrero.[1532]

Isolated FSH Deficiency

Mutations in FSH β-subunit, either homozygous or compound heterozygous, are reported in three females and two males[955,1470,1533-1536] with delayed puberty or poorly developed secondary sex characteristics, and primary amenorrhea but normal adrenarche in the women. The LH concentration was elevated, serum estradiol was low, and immunoactive FSH was absent. Two of three women had a homozygous nonsense mutation in the FSH β-subunit gene (Val 61 X) at gene map locus 11p13 and the other was a compound heterozygote (Cys 51 Gly/Val 61 X). The two men had azoospermia, small, soft testes, and absence of serum FSH: one had normal puberty and LH and testosterone values with a missense mutation Cys 82 Arg substitution,[1537] and the other man had slightly delayed puberty, low testosterone and inhibin B, and high LH with a nonsense mutation (Val 61 X).[1537,1538]

Midline Developmental Defects

Septo-optic or optic dysplasia is caused by abnormal development of the prosencephalon, leading to small, dysplastic, pale optic discs, with a double outline and pendular (evenly moving side to side) nystagmus; blindness may occur. Midline hypothalamic defect may cause GH deficiency, DI and ACTH, TSH, and gonadotropin deficiency. Short stature and delayed puberty may result, although true precocious puberty is an alternative (see later).[1539] The septum pellucidum is often absent in association with optic hypoplasia or dysplasia, which is readily demonstrable by imaging techniques.[279,1540] In our series, the syndrome is associated with decreased maternal age. The pituitary gland may be hypoplastic, due to the lack of hypothalamic stimulatory factors and the neurohypophysis may have an ectopic location noted by the location of the posterior pituitary hot spot on MRI.[1541] The condition is usually sporadic but one brother and sister were affected from a consanguineous union[1542] and a mutation in the HESX1 gene map locus 3p21.2-p21.1 is found rarely.[1543,1544] Abnormalities of the corpus callosum and cerebellum are common MRI imaging. Four groups are described: (1) normal MRI results, (2) abnormalities of the septum pellucidum with a normal hypothalamic pituitary area, (3) abnormalities of the hypothalamic pituitary area and a normal septum pellucidum, and (4) abnormalities in both areas.[1545] No endocrine abnormalities were described in group 1, but the others had progressively more endocrine abnormalities, with precocious puberty most common in group 2. Early diagnosis is important due to the risk of sudden death associated with adrenal insufficiency.[1546]

The solitary median maxillary incisor syndrome is associated with the eponymous midline defect as well as prominent midpalatal ridge (torus palatinus) and hypopituitarism.[1547] The defect in this autosomal dominant condition is in the sonic hedgehog gene at gene map locus 7q3.[1548,1549]

Other congenital midline defects ranging from complete dysraphism and holoprosencephaly to cleft palate or lip are also associated with hypothalamic-pituitary dysfunction.[1411] Delayed puberty is rarely described in duplication of the hypophysis.[1550] Myelomeningocele (myelodysplasia) is associated with endocrine abnormalities, including hypothalamic hypothyroidism, hyperprolactinemia, and elevated gonadotropin concentrations as well as true precocious puberty.[1551,1552]

Hypopituitary Dwarfism (Fig. 24–59)

Autosomal recessive mutations in homeobox genes encoding transcription factors involved in the early aspects of pituitary development lead to hypogonadotropic hypogonadism and other pituitary hormone deficiencies[1553] in addition to HESX1 mentioned above. Prop1 mutations[1554,1555] at gene map locus 5q cause GH and TSH deficiency as well as delayed puberty or the late onset of secondary hypogonadism in adulthood.[1555] In one study of 73 patients with "idiopathic" multiple pituitary hormone deficiencies, 35 had a mutation in Prop1.[1556] Homozygous R73C mutation of PROP1 allowed spontaneous puberty in 2 of 10 affected family members.[1557] ACTH deficiency is more rarely a feature of Prop1 deficiency.[1558] Homozygous mutations in the *LHX3* gene[1559] at gene map locus 9q34.3, which encodes a member of the LIM class of homeodomain proteins, are associated with multiple pituitary hormone deficiencies including LH and FSH and severe restriction of head rotation.[1559]

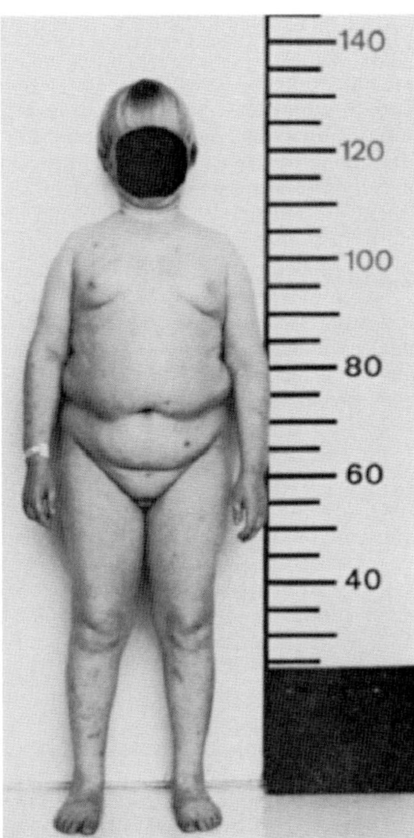

Figure 24–59 ▪ A 20-year-old male with idiopathic hypopituitary dwarfism and deficiencies of gonadotropins, thyrotropin, corticotropin, and growth hormone, who had a history of arrested hydrocephalus. Height, 129 cm (−8 SD); the phallus was 2 cm in length, and the testes measured 1.5×1 cm. He had received thyroid and glucocorticoid replacement. Basal luteinizing hormone (LH) was less than 0.2 ng/mL (LER-960), follicle-stimulating hormone (FSH) was 0.5 ng/mL (LER-869), and testosterone was less than 0.1 ng/mL. In response to 100 µg of LH-releasing hormone (GnRH), the plasma LH concentration increased slightly to 0.6 ng/mL, and there was no increase in plasma testosterone. The excretion of urinary 17-ketosteroids was 1.1 mg/24 hr. The bone age was 10 years, and the volume of the sella turcica was small on skull radiographs. For conversion to SI units, see the legends for Figures 24–21 and 24–22. (From Styne DM, Grumbach MM. Puberty in the male and female: its physiology and disorders. In Yen SCC, Jaffe RB, eds. Reproductive Endocrinology, 2nd ed. Philadelphia: WB Saunders, 1986:313-384.)

The familial forms of multiple pituitary hormone deficiencies with either autosomal recessive or X-linked inheritance are less common.[395,1554-1556,1558,1560-1562] The degree of hormone deficit and the age of onset of pituitary hormone deficiencies may vary within a single kindred with the same genetic defect.

The X-linked form of hypopituitarism can be associated with duplication of the SOX3 gene.[1563]

There is an association between breech delivery, especially in males, perinatal distress, and idiopathic hypopituitarism.[279,1564] Malformations of the pituitary stalk demonstrable by MRI are common in such patients.[279] Common to many patients with idiopathic hypopituitary dwarfism is early onset of growth failure; late onset of diminished growth is an ominous finding suggesting the presence of a CNS tumor.

Isolated GH deficiency allows spontaneous pubertal development when the bone age reaches the pubertal stage of 11 to 13 years,[395,1564,1565] usually after the corresponding chronologic age is reached, while associated gonadotropin deficiency does not allow spontaneous puberty, even when the bone age advances to the pubertal stage during GH therapy.

While normal boys have greater variation of bone age with the onset of puberty than chronologic age (bone age determination adds little over chronologic age to the prediction of the onset of puberty in normal subjects),[435] greater synchrony occurs in boys with early puberty due to congenital adrenal hyperplasia or testotoxicosis as well as those with delayed puberty due to constitutional delay.

The absence of GH and gonadotropins allows long-term but slow growth to increased adult height; the height at the onset of puberty and the height in relation to bone age determines the final height that is possible.[1566] GH treatment can increase the rate of pubertal development that was delayed by the GH deficiency so that GH treatment begun in pubertal children who have a limited height potential, limits adult stature. GnRH agonists to suppress pubertal development in addition to GH has been suggested to increase final height,[1567] but concerns about decreased bone density with the use of GnRH agonist in the absence of precocious puberty causes worry about this combination[1319] (see earlier). The judicious use of low-dose testosterone in GH-deficient boys of pubertal age with associated gonadotropin deficiency does not seem to impair growth achieved by GH replacement.[1568]

Miscellaneous Conditions

Prader-Willi Syndrome

This autosomal dominant syndrome of a tendency for intrauterine growth retardation, delayed onset of and ultimately poor fetal activity, infantile central hypotonia, and lethargy followed by early onset childhood hyperphagia, pathologic obesity and carbohydrate intolerance, short stature, small hands and feet, mild to moderate mental retardation, emotional instability including perseveration, obsessions and compulsions, and characteristic facies with almond-shaped eyes, triangular mouth, and narrow bifrontal diameter is associated with delayed puberty and hypogonadotropic hypogonadism caused by hypothalamic dysfunction. Despite the late or absent puberty, there is a tendency to early adrenarche[1569-1574] or even precocious puberty in a minority of cases.[1575]

Affected boys usually have micropenis and cryptorchidism with underdeveloped scrotum being common.[1575] Female subjects have underdevelopment of the labia majora or labia minora or clitoris. Amenorrhea may occur in about half of cases with irregular menses being common in others.[1575] Weight reduction may lead to menarche in some females because severe obesity may play a role in the impaired puberty in some patients.

The role of relative GH deficiency in this disorder is uncertain and controversial (see reference 1576 for a contrary view). In June 2000, the FDA approved Prader-Willi syndrome as an indication for GH treatment in affected children without a requirement for assessing growth hormone secretion; genetic testing is used to confirm the clinical diagnosis of the syndrome. The decision to approve rhGH treatment was strongly influenced by long-term randomized control trials in Prader-Willi syndrome.[1577-1579] GH treatment decreases body fat but increases fat utilization, lean body mass, linear growth, energy expenditure, and possible improvement in physical strength, and motor development. The recommended dose is 1.0 to 1.5 mg/m^2/day (0.03 to 0.05 mg/kg/day). Children with Prader-Willi syndrome were previously known to have a risk for sudden death due to GI, respiratory, or cardiac complications.[1580-1585] However, the report of sudden deaths due to respiratory complications during GH treatment led to recommendation for evaluation for sleep apnea or respiratory difficulties before instituting GH therapy.[1586-1588]

This distinct genetic disorder with a frequency of about 1 in 20,000, is very rarely familial (the recurrence risk depends on the type of the genetic defect) and is caused by abnormalities involving the long arm of chromosome 15 in the region q11-q13. Approximately 70% of Prader-Willi cases are caused by a paternal deletion of 15q11-q13 (commonly about 3 to 5 mega-base pairs in size); 20% to 25% of cases have maternal uniparental disomy (either isodisomy or heterodisomy) where both chromosomes 15 are derived from the mother, possibly by non-disjunction during maternal meiosis, and represent a striking example of genomic imprinting. In 2% to 5%, an imprinting center defect has been detected.[1573,1589-1593] This lack of a functional paternal 15q11-q13 region, caused by any of a variety of genetic mechanisms,[1574] can result in the syndrome. One imprinted gene, SNRPN (small nuclear ribonucleoprotein associated polypeptide SmN) implicated in splicing pre-mRNA, is expressed in the brain including the hypothalamus, and has been advanced as one etiology of the syndrome.[1594,1595] A study of the hypothalamic paraventricular nucleus describes a decrease in the number of immunoreactive oxytocin-containing cells—"putative satiety" neurosecretory neurons.[1596]

Elevated serum concentrations of the growth hormone secretagogue and orexigenic GI hormone ghrelin are found in the basal state in Prader-Willi syndrome as well as after meals, when values should be suppressed,[1597,1598] and are suggested as a possible cause of the insatiable appetite. Administration of the somatostatin analogue, octreotide, leads to a decrease in basal ghrelin values and some decrease in values after meals,[1599] but no change in appetite was demonstrated in preliminary study.

Laurence-Moon and Bardet-Biedl Syndromes

The Laurence-Moon syndrome[1600-1602] is frequently combined with the Bardet-Biedl syndrome; both are rare autosomal recessive traits and both combine retinitis pigmentosum and hypogonadism of various etiologies. Many Bardet-Biedl patients have developmental delay, as do all Laurence-Moon patients. The Laurence-Moon syndrome, however, was considered to be associated with spastic paraplegia, whereas the Bardet-Biedl syndrome had postaxial polydactyly, onset of obesity usually in early infancy, renal dysplasia, and a relatively high prevalence among the Bedouin of the Middle East. The genetically and phenotypically heterogenous Bardet-Biedl syndrome is linked to 6 loci which map to gene map locus 20p12, 16q21, 15q22.3-q23, 14q32.1, 11q13, 4q27, 3p12-q13, and 2q31. In most cases, three mutant genes are required for a phenotype.[1603-1605] However, a 22-year study of 26 families in Newfoundland revealed such lack of correlation of phenotype with genotype that the authors state that there is no justification for now separating Bardet-Biedl syndrome from Laurence-Moon syndrome.[1606] Similar findings are present in the Biemond syndrome II with iris coloboma, hypogenitalism, obesity, polydactyly, and developmental delay, but it is a distinct entity.[1607]

Functional Gonadotropin Deficiencies

The effects of malnutrition, which can lead to functional hypogonadotropic hypogonadism, should be separated from the primary effects of chronic systemic disease, because some have direct effects upon the function of the hypothalamic-pituitary unit or the gonads. Thus, even if nutrition is adequate, puberty may be affected. In general, weight loss of any cause to less than 80% of ideal weight for height can lead to gonadotropin deficiency[1065,1608] and low serum leptin levels; weight regain usually restores hypothalamic-pituitary gonadal function over a variable period,[1609] although the weight needed to restart menstrual periods is variable between individuals and is related to the weight at which menstruation first ceased.[1610] If adequate nutrition and body weight are maintained in patients with regional enteritis, chronic gastrointestinal[1605] or pulmonary disease,[1611] gonadotropin secretion is usually adequate. Cystic fibrosis also delays puberty and age of peak height velocity, in large part through malnutrition.[259,1612-1614] The age of menarche in girls with cystic fibrosis is related to maternal age, as expected, but is delayed approximately 1 year compared to their mothers, mainly related to nutritional status.[1615] However, even with normal pubertal progression, boys with cystic fibrosis almost universally have oligospermia caused by obstruction of the spermatic ducts unrelated to their nutritional status.[1616] The greater prevalence of reproductive difficulties in male patients with cystic fibrosis compared with female patients may be due to the greater prevalence of the cystic fibrosis transmembrane regulator (CFTR) in male reproductive tissues such as the epididymis and vas deferens and as a consequence more viscid luminal contents, which ultimately damage the testes and even lead to absence of the epididymides and the vas differentia.[1617,1618] Normal ovaries do not express the CFTR, while endometrial tissue only expresses it after puberty with variable levels in cervical epithelium and fallopian tubes. Even though the CFTR gene and its protein is expressed in the human hypothalamus, in an immortizalized mouse, hypothalamic GnRH-secreting cell line mutations in the CFTR gene did not appear to affect LH and FSH secretion.

Jamaican boys and girls with sickle-cell disease have delay in the pubertal growth spurt and in peak height velocity, although final height is comparable to normal adults; girls were said to have a marginally to significantly delayed onset of menstruation.[1619] Boys with sickle cell anemia often exhibit impaired Leydig cell function caused by ischemia of the testes, gonadotropin deficiency, or both factors.[1620]

Thalassemia carries the risk of hemochromatosis due to transfusional iron deposition in the pituitary and hypothalamus and as a consequence, hypogonadotropic hypogonadism[1621-1624] as well as impairment of testicular function.[1625] Primary hypothyroidism is prevalent in this condition, but is only part of the problem of sexual maturation and growth failure due to GH deficiency.[1626-1628] Before the advent of subcutaneous chelation therapy (with monitoring of serum ferritin), complete absence of pubertal development occurred in over 40% of patients with thalassemia.[1629,1630] The gonads can be stimulated by exogenous gonadotropins, and satisfactory sexual development including fertility can be promoted by the use of hCG and hFSH in many patients without gonadal damage,[1621,1622,1631-1633] but in children with poor control, pituitary, adrenal, and gonadal damage may be severe.[1634] Of note, desferrioxamine therapy may cause skeletal dysplasia and compromise pubertal growth.[1635] Decreased bone mineral density in thalassemia makes early recognition and treatment of the problem all the more important.[1636,1637]

Cytotoxic effects of the alkylating agents used to prepare patients for bone marrow transplant in this condition add to the problem.[1638] Treatment after the onset of puberty is safer for gonadal function in boys but not necessarily for girls.[1639] Girls with early bone marrow transplantation and apparently normal pubertal development have elevated serum FSH and menstrual abnormalities ranging in severity to amenorrhea,[1640] suggesting that gonadal impairment is universal in girls with thalassemia major after bone marrow transplantation.[1641]

Growth in stature was delayed in boys affected with acquired immunodeficiency syndrome (AIDS) even if weight for height was equal to that of normal boys. Remarkably, serum testosterone concentrations were not affected by AIDS, but bone age was delayed, as was the progression through the stages of puberty. Because GH secretion is rarely affected by AIDS, the poor growth appeared more related to the delay in pubertal development.[1642] These concerns apply to children with prenatally acquired human immunodeficiency virus (HIV) infection as well.[1643,1644] Prepubertal children with HIV infection have lower IGFBP3 values than case controls and the DHEAS/cortisol ratio was higher in infected children as well.[1645]

Chronic GI disease (e.g., Crohn's disease) is often accompanied by delayed puberty; therapy to restore nutrition, if successful, enables puberty to progress. There is compromise of the pubertal growth spurt from active inflammatory bowel disease, especially if glucocorticoid therapy is necessary.[1646] Coeliac disease decreases the growth rate in childhood and adolescence but with appropriate dietary restrictions final adult height appears normal.[1647]

Chronic renal disease has been associated with delayed pubertal development[1648,1649] and decreased pulsatile gonadotropin secretion due to a decrease in the mass of bioactive and immunoactive LH secreted rather than an alteration of the frequency; successful renal transplantation usually restores gonadotropin secretion and improves growth.[1649-1652] Immunoreactive gonadotropin concentrations may be elevated, presumably because of impaired renal clearance, but the response to GnRH is blunted in severe renal impairment.[1653,1654] TeBG is elevated in chronic renal failure and free testosterone is low.[1655] Survivors of renal transplantation who are having immune suppression and alternate-day steroid treatment often have delayed onset of puberty and decreased pulsatility of GH and gonadotropins at night.[1656,1657]

Patients with nephrotic syndrome have poor pubertal growth, poor secondary sexual development, and deficient gonadotropin secretion in a pattern resembling constitutional delay in puberty.[1656] Glomerulonephritis treated with alternate-day glucocorticoid therapy leads to a late, diminished but prolonged pubertal growth spurt, which can lead to a normal final height.[1658]

Children with early onset of leukemia and long-term remission experience puberty at an appropriate age or with only slight delay, whereas patients with initial symptoms of leukemia in late childhood may have considerable delay of pubertal development.[1659] Radiation treatment to the CNS may cause hypogonadotropic hypogonadism and/or growth hormone deficiency, and radiation to the abdomen or pelvis and certain types of chemotherapy, especially if administered during puberty, may impair gonadal function and cause primary hypogonadism,[1660] although ovarian function may return even in the face of elevation of serum gonadotropins.[1661] Total body irradiation for bone marrow transplant may lead to decrease in growth in spite of normal growth hormone secretion. Children with leukemia treated with CNS irradiation demonstrated a diminished pubertal growth spurt and diminished final height.[1662-1664] Long-term follow-up studies point out the rising incidence of the metabolic syndrome in childhood cancer survivors.[1415,1665-1667]

Hypothyroidism may delay the onset of puberty or menarche (except in extreme cases described below in which puberty starts early); treatment with levothyroxine will reverse this pattern but there is likely to be a permanent loss of height if diagnosis is delayed. Poorly controlled diabetes mellitus can lead to poor growth, fatty infiltration of the liver, and sexual infantilism (Mauriac syndrome),[1668,1669] probably related to poor nutritional status; prepubertal children are most vulnerable to poor glycemic control while pubertal subjects exhibit normal growth unless severe hyperglycemia occurs.[1670] The degree of control necessary to avoid these complications cannot be exactly quantified, but adolescents with even moderately poor control frequently manifest some degree of growth impairment and delayed puberty or irregular menses.[1671] Cushing's disease can be associated with delayed onset or arrest of gonadarche, which usually is corrected by transsphenoidal removal of an ACTH-secreting pituitary adenoma.[1672,1673]

Anorexia Nervosa and Variants

Anorexia nervosa, a common cause of gonadotropin deficiency in adolescence, is a functional disorder which can cause lifelong endocrine abnormalities, increasing in prevalence in girls (the third most common chronic disease of adolescent girls), starting at ever younger ages, but rare in boys, characterized by a distorted body image, obsessive fear of obesity, and food avoidance that can cause severe self-induced weight loss (to less than 85% of normal weight for age and height or BMI less than 17.5 kg/m^2 after cessation of growth), primary or secondary amenorrhea in affected females as well as widespread endocrine disorders, and even death (specific diagnostic details are in the DSM-IV criteria of the American Psychiatric Association[1674]) (also see Chapter 16).[1675] Other common features include onset in middle adolescence,[1676] hyperactivity, defective thermoregulation with hypothermia and sensitivity to cold, constipation, bradycardia and hypotension, decreased basal metabolic rate, dry skin, fine downy hypertrichosis, peripheral edema, and parotid enlargement.[1677-1679] The pathogenesis is multifactorial and includes a genetic factor and a well-characterized psychological component.[1680,1681] Before the diagnosis of anorexia nervosa is made, organic disease must be eliminated; a girl with macroprolactinoma presented with signs consistent with anorexia nervosa.[1392] The prevalence of anorexia nervosa is increased in Turner's syndrome. The HH in many patients with anorexia nervosa is related only in part to weight loss.[1677,1679] The onset of amenorrhea precedes the onset of severe weight loss.

This condition must be considered in the differential diagnosis of growth failure.[1682] In anorexia nervosa the concentrations of plasma FSH, LH, leptin, and estradiol and the excretion of urinary gonadotropins are characteristically low. In adult women, there may be a reversion to a circadian rhythm of LH secretion and to the sleep-associated increase in episodic LH secretion characteristic of early puberty; in severe cases, the amplitude of the pulsatile episodes is diminished and resembles the pattern in prepubertal children.[1683] Similarly, the LH response to GnRH correlates with the severity of the weight loss.[1684,1685] With weight less than 75% of the appropriate weight and a strikingly reduced BMI, there is either a blunted or an absent LH response to the administration of synthetic GnRH and undetectable or small LH pulses. Pulsatile administration of intravenous GnRH at 90- to 120-minute intervals can produce LH pulses that are indistinguishable from the normal pubertal pattern,[1683] demonstrating functional GnRH deficiency in the amenorrhea of anorexia nervosa. Serum leptin levels are low, remarkably so with severe malnutrition consistent with the strikingly decreased mass of adipose tissue and increase with regaining weight.[1686-1688] Other hormonal changes include an increased mean concentration of plasma GH and plasma cortisol; low levels of plasma IGF-I, DHEAS, and plasma triiodothyronine with normal levels of thyroxine (unless associated with the "low thyroxine syndrome") and TSH; a decreased rise in serum prolactin after the administration of thyrotropin-releasing hormone

(TRH) or insulin-induced hypoglycemia,[1689,1690] and a diminished capacity to concentrate urine.

A study of 60 adolescents with anorexia nervosa in a free living condition compared to 60 average age-matched girls demonstrated significantly lower heart rates, lower systolic blood pressure, and lower body temperature compared with control subjects; 22% were anemic and 22% leukopenic.[1691] The ratio of bone age to chronologic age was significantly lower in girls with anorexia nervosa versus control subjects and correlated positively with duration of illness and markers of nutritional status. All measures of bone mineral density were lower in anorexia nervosa, with the most significant predictors of bone density being lean body mass, BMI, and age at menarche. Although the mean age at menarche did not differ between the groups, the proportion of those who were premenarcheal with anorexia nervosa was significantly higher despite comparable maturity of the groups reflected by bone age. Free leptin was an important determinant of menstrual recovery in longitudinal study.[1692]

Normal endocrine and metabolic function may follow weight gain, but the amenorrhea may persist for months, suggesting persistent hypothalamic dysfunction[1693] (also see Chapter 25). Treatment of this disorder requires skillful management, understanding, patience, and psychiatric consultation.[1681] In view of the mortality risk, parenteral alimentation may be indicated in resistant patients with severe weight loss, especially in the presence of infection or an electrolyte imbalance.

Functional amenorrhea can also occur in women of normal weight but decreased percent body fat and is characterized by normal basal levels of gonadotropin and normal gonadotropin response to GnRH stimulation but lack of or an inadequate midcycle LH surge and a decrease in normal pulsatile secretion (amplitude and/or frequency) of gonadotropins.[1694,1695] In addition, these patients have higher average cortisol values, decreased free T_4, free T_3, and total T_4 with normal TSH levels, decreased leptin concentrations, quite likely due to subtle dysfunction of eating patterns and altered energy expenditure.[1696] The consequences range in severity from severe estrogen deficiency to anovulation to a short luteal phase. Reduced bone density is of concern.

Bulimia nervosa is thought to be a variant of anorexia nervosa,[1681,1697] occurring in about 1.5% of young women. In this disorder the individual consumes large amounts of food, but food gorging is followed by induced vomiting.[1693] A hand lesion from the induced vomiting (Russell's sign) and an abnormal level of serum electrolytes are useful clinical markers. Abuse of laxatives, diet pills, and diuretics is frequent. Although weight loss is not frequent, amenorrhea is common.[1698] Bulimia is especially prevalent in high school and college women students. A history of childhood sexual abuse is more frequent than in unaffected adolescents.

Cessation of growth can occur in infants and young children with psychosocial dwarfism. Stressful social situations can also inhibit growth and physical pubertal development at adolescence[1699] (reviewed in the earlier section of this chapter).

Exercise, Hypo-ovarianism, and Amenorrhea (The Female Athlete Triad)

In 1992, the American College of Sports Medicine defined the female athletic triad of primary or secondary amenorrhea, disordered eating, and osteoporosis (see references 1700 and 1701). The bone density of female long distance runners is greater in those with regular menses compared to those with menstrual irregularities.[1702] Athletes who began strenuous training before menarche have a delay in menarcheal age.[1079,1703] Osteopenia in later life may result from amenorrhea in ballet dancers even with estrogen replacement.[1704] (see below). While there are substantial endocrine effects of excessive athletic training in girls described above, elite prepubertal and pubertal female athletes suffer relatively few physical injuries.[1705] Because there is no demonstrable effect on pubertal development from moderate exercise in subelite female runners, moderate exercise should not be discouraged during adolescence.[1706]

Bulemia, anorexia nervosa, or anorexia athletica is most often found in girls engaged in sports emphasizing weight.[1707,1708] Teenage ballet dancers are lighter, have less body fat, and have a high incidence of delayed puberty and of primary and secondary amenorrhea than less physically active girls. Factors other than decreased body weight can impair pubertal progression and delay menarche through inhibition of the hypothalamic GnRH pulse generator in healthy ballet dancers and female athletes.[1068-1071,1079,1693,1709,1710]

Genetic influences overlie changes due to weight or activity because there is a positive correlation between the delayed menarche found in athletic girls and the age of menarche of their mothers.[1711] However, there is a relationship between the choice of sport and constitutional factors, with no indication that the sport causes changes in growth rate or height.[1712,1713] Artistic and rhythmic gymnasts have delay in menarche when compared with their mothers and sisters,[518,1714,1715] artistic gymnasts having a more significant delay.[1716,1717] Higher bone density is reported in the femurs of gymnasts compared to ballet dancers and controls, but lower radial bone density is reported in the gymnasts and ballet dancers; a positive relation between serum leptin and tibial bone density is fouind.[1718]

Both thinness and strenuous physical activity appear to act synergistically, but strenuous exercise training by itself may inhibit the GnRH pulse generator possibly mediated in part by endogenous opioidergic pathways involving β-endorphin. When the strenuous physical activity is interrupted (e.g., by injury), puberty advances, and menarche often occurs within a few months in those with amenorrhea, in some cases before significant change in body composition or weight.[1693] Even though gonadarche is retarded, adrenarche is not delayed.[1068,1719]

Thus, female athletes of normal weight who have less fat and more muscle than nonathletic girls (e.g., ice skaters or swimmers) are also at risk for delayed puberty and for primary and secondary amenorrhea.[1068,1719] However, the mechanism apparently is different from the hypothalamic amenorrhea in runners and ballet dancers. In swimmers, menstrual cycles frequently were irregular and anovulatory rather than absent; the plasma concentration of dehydroepiandrosterone sulfate and LH were higher than normal, and plasma estrogen levels were normal.[1720,1700]

Prospective study of gymnasts contrasted with swimmers demonstrated decreased growth velocity, stunting in leg length growth, and decreased height prediction in the gymnasts; extensive gymnastics training starting before puberty and continuing through puberty leads to a decrease in adult height.[1721-1723] These studies suggest that extensive training (10 to 12 hr/wk) may be excessive for prepubertal girls. However, a longitudinal study of rhythmic female gymnasts exercising 10 hours per week showed a delay in the tempo of pubertal development and delayed menarche but no deficit in adult stature.[1724] Thus, the biology of pubertal delay in female athletes is controversial still.

Prolactin levels may be elevated in women athletes and could contribute to the delayed menarche found in this group.[1394,1725] Indeed, osteopenia can result from the resulting chronic hypoestrogenism.[1726]

Scoliosis in girls usually develops during the pubertal growth spurt and more often occurs in girls with a more rapid pubertal

Undescended testes remain at a higher temperature than descended testes and undescended testes have a maturation arrest at the conversion of the gonocyte to the spermatogonia; this appears to direct the testes toward malignant degeneration.[1814] In a Copenhagen study, the risk of neoplasia was 5% in patients with an intraabdominal testis, abnormalities of the external genitalia, or an abnormal sex chromosome karyotype compared to 0% (0 out of 1185) in patients with cryptorchidism who lacked these characteristics.[1840] A study of testicular cancer in England reported that the increasing performance of orchiopexy before 10 years of age appears to have reduced the increased risk of testicular carcinoma associated with undescended testes.[1841] There is a very small risk of carcinoma of the testes in prepuberty, but the absence of carcinoma in situ in prepuberty is not an assurance that carcinoma will not develop in adult life. Periodic sonography of the testis of affected patients is recommended after the onset of puberty.[1842,1843] One year is a useful age to consider orchiopexy for undescended testes as it is an age at which the likelihood of spontaneous descent lessens but the benefits to the testes of orchiopexy remain.[1829] The prevalence of antisperm antibodies are reportedly as high as 38% in men with cryptorchidism undergoing operation before puberty,[1844] although a recent study found no antibodies in the sera of men who had dartos pouch orchiopexy or other means of testicular fixation, suggesting this phenomenon may be technique specific.[1845]

Retractile testes are considered a normal variation but the risk of ascent of one significantly retractile testis to a location below the inguinal canal may be as high as 50%.[289] Ascended testes are typically unilateral and located distal to the inguinal canal. About 40% of ascended testes redescend.[1846] The finding of one case of testicular carcinoma in a boy with spontaneous descent led to suggestion of the need to follow such cases in the long term.[1847] Thus, because ascended and significantly retractile testes may be theoretically prone to germ cell maldevelopment and one case of carcinoma is documented, it is reasonable to consider orchiopexy in retractile testes as is recommended for congenital cryptorchidism.

The risk of breast cancer is increased in men with a history of undescended testes, orchiopexy, orchitis, testicular injury, infertility, or any cause of delayed puberty. This risk is associated with the gynecomastia, which occurs in these conditions.[1848]

Girls

Syndrome of Gonadal Dysgenesis and Its Variants (Turner's Syndrome) (See Chapter 22)[1143,1849-1854]

The most common form of hypergonadotropic hypogonadism in the female is the syndrome of gonadal dysgenesis, or Turner's syndrome, and its variants, a sporadic disorder with an incidence of 1 per 2500 liveborn girls,[1849,1855,1856] in which all (X chromosome monosomy with haploinsufficiency) or part of the second sex chromosome (partial sex chromosome monosomy) is absent. About 99% of 45,X concepti abort spontaneously and 1 in 15 spontaneous abortions has a 45,X karyotype.[1857,1858] The 45,X karyotype is associated with female phenotype, short stature, sexual infantilism, and various somatic abnormalities.

Sex chromosome mosaicism or structural abnormalities of an X or Y chromosome may modify the features of this syndrome, although about 40% of the individuals with the features noted above have mosaicism or structural abnormalities of the X chromosome. The syndrome of gonadal dysgenesis and its variants is a continuum ranging from the typical 45,X phenotype to a normal male or female phenotype.[1143] Recently, comprehensive recommendations for the diagnosis and management of Turner's syndrome were presented by an international committee.[1859]

45,X Turner's Syndrome (Fig. 24–61)

Short stature and sexual infantilism are invariable features of sex chromatin-negative 45,X gonadal dysgenesis, or Turner's syndrome. This karyotype is found in approximately 60% of cases of Turner's syndrome.[1143,1858] The short stature is due to loss of a homeobox-containing gene located on the pseudoautosomal region (PAR 1) of the short arms of the X (Xp22) and Yp11.3 chromosomes,[1860,1861] which encodes an osteogenic factor.[1861] The gene is called SHOX (*s*hort stature *h*omeob*ox*-containing gene[1860] or, previously, PHOG (*p*seudoautosomal *h*omeobox *o*steogenic *g*ene).[1861] It is located on the pseudoautosomal region of the short arm of the X and Y chromosome and hence escapes X inactivation. SHOX haploinsufficiency is responsible for, in addition to abnormal growth, mesomelic growth retardation and Madelung deformity of the wrist (bilateral bowing of the radius with a dorsal subluxation of the distal ulna)[1862,1863] in Leri-Weill dyschondrosteosis (SHOX haploinsufficiency). Langer mesomelic dysplasia, which includes severe dwarfism with striking hypoplasia or aplasia of the ulnar and fibula, is due to SHOX nullizygosity. SHOX haploinsufficiency appears to be responsible for −2.0 SD of the approximately −3.0 SD deficit in stature and the skeletal abnormalities in Turner's syndrome.[1864-1867] On the contrary, patient with complete gonadal dysgenesis and tall stature had a 45,X/46X,der(X) and three doses of the SHOX gene due to the SHOX duplication on the der(X) chromosome.[1868] A method of relating Shox genotype to phenotypic manifestations has been developed.[1869]

Turner's syndrome may be recognized in the newborn period or before. Abortuses with 45,X have edema and large hygromas of the neck, which may be seen on prenatal ultrasound studies; this lymphatic defect is the basis for the loose skin folds that ultimately form the webbed neck (pterygium colli). Affected newborn infants may also have lymphedema of the extremities; the term *Bonnevie-Ullrich syndrome* has been applied to newborn infants with these features of Turner's syndrome. (See Chapter 22.)

Frequent features are distinct facies with micrognathia, "fishmouth" appearance, high-arched palate with dental abnormalities, epicanthal folds, ptosis, low-set or deformed ears, short neck with low hairline, webbing (pterygium colli), and recurrent otitis media, often leading to impaired hearing (25% affected adults require hearing aids).[1143,1870] A broad shield-like chest leads to the appearance of wide-spaced nipples; the areolae are often hypoplastic. Skeletal defects include short fourth metacarpals and cubitus valgus (which may develop after birth), Madelung deformity of the wrist (in about 7%), genu valgum, and scoliosis. There are extensive pigmented nevi, tendency to keloid formation, and hypoplastic nails.[1143,1871] Lymphatic obstruction leads not only to the infantile puffiness of extremities and pterygium colli but also to a distinctive shape of the ears. Cardiovascular anomalies affect the left side of the heart and include coarctation of the aorta in about 10% (40% have associated webbing of the neck), aortic stenosis, and bicuspid aortic valves; the latter individuals are at risk for a dissecting aortic aneurysm.[1872] An echocardiogram of the cardiovascular system must be performed and prophylactic antibiotics are indicated if an anatomic abnormality is demonstrated. Abnormal pelvocaliceal collecting systems, abnormal position or alignment of the kidneys, and abnormal vascular supply to the kidney are encountered in 30% to 60% of patients, and recurrent urinary tract infections are common.[1873] Defects of the gastrointestinal

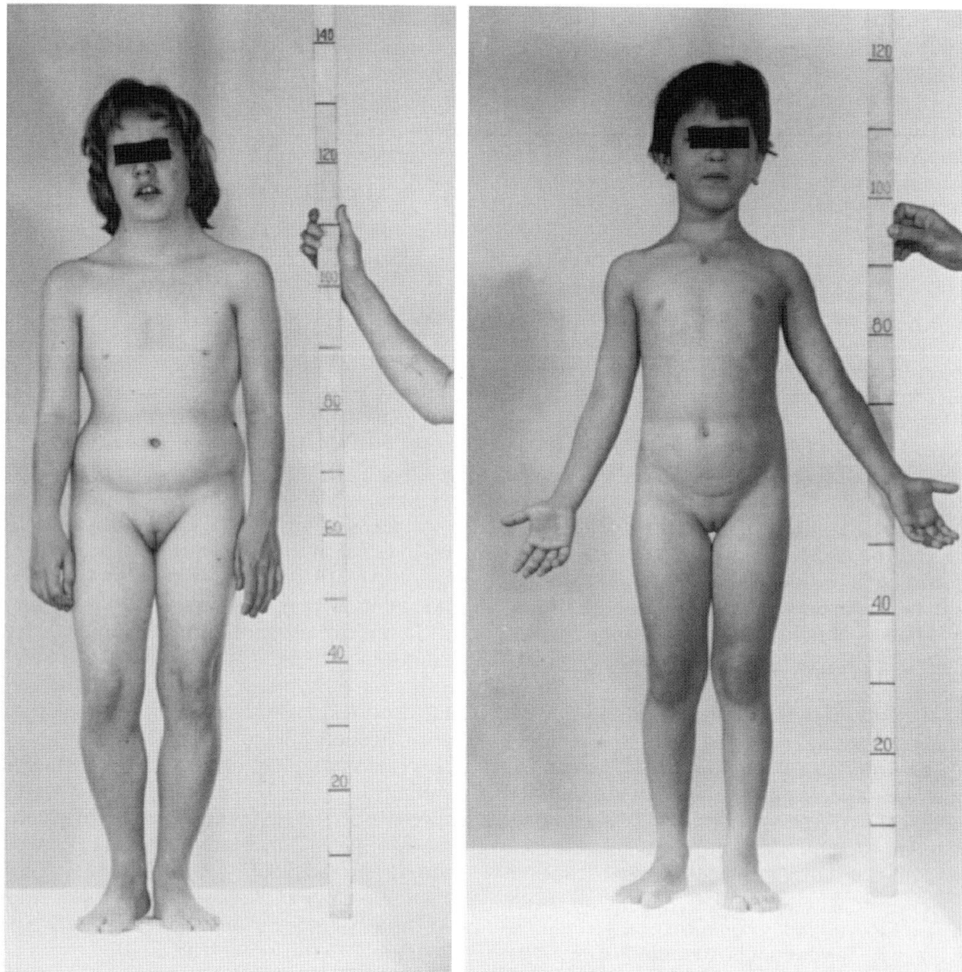

Figure 24–61 ▪ *Left,* A 14 10/12-year-old patient with the typical form of the syndrome of gonadal dysgenesis (Turner's syndrome). The X chromatin pattern was negative, and the karyotype was 45,X. She was short (height 134.5 cm; height age 9 5/12 years) and sexually infantile except for the appearance of sparse pubic hair, and exhibited characteristic stigmata of the syndrome: a short webbed neck, shield-like chest with widely separated nipples, bilateral metacarpal signs, puffiness over the dorsum of the fingers, cubitus valgus, increased number of pigmented nevi, characteristic facies, and low-set ears. The bone age was 13 6/12 years; urinary 17-ketosteroids 5.1 mg/day; urinary gonadotropin greater than 100 mU/day. Vaginal smears and the urocytogram showed an immature pattern in which cornified squamous cells were absent. With estrogen therapy, female secondary sexual characteristics were induced; the cyclic administration resulted in periodic estrogen withdrawal bleeding. *Right,* A 45,X, 9 11/12-year-old patient with Turner's syndrome. Apart from short stature (height 118 cm; age 6 10/12 years), increased pigmented nevi, and subtle changes in the fingers and toes, she had few somatic anomalies. In contrast to the patient at the left, the main clinical feature was short stature.

system include intestinal telangiectasias and hemangiomatoses that rarely can lead to massive gastrointestinal bleeding. Furthermore, the prevalence of inflammatory bowel disease, chronic liver disease, and colon cancer is increased.[1853,1874] Autoimmune diseases, such as Hashimoto's thyroiditis (16-fold relative risk) and Graves' disease, are common,[1875] and an association with juvenile rheumatoid arthritis and psoriatic arthritis is described.

The age of diagnosis of Turner's syndrome continues to be delayed with the exception of newborns with the striking phenotype of the Bonnevie-Ullrich syndrome. It is recommended that all prepubertal age girls below –2.0 SD who have at least two somatic stigmata of the syndrome have a karyotype analysis; early diagnosis is of key importance for optimal management of the growth failure and the detection of occult features of the syndrome.[1876]

Pelvic ultrasonography or MRI usually permits the detection of even a small, infantile uterus and reveal streak gonads. Ultrasensitive estrogen bioassays now confirm decreased ovarian function in girls with Turner's syndrome as estradiol values are significantly lower than found in average girls.[1877] Long-term follow-up of affected women previously treated with growth hormone and estrogen demonstrated normal adult uterine length only in those with 45X/46XX karyotypes while those with pure 45X karyotypes had smaller uterus length and volume.[1878] The streak gonads result in sexual infantilism; rarely, probably in about 10% of cases, puberty, menarche, and, even more rarely, pregnancy may occur.[1143] Others with some of the variants described later have been able to achieve fertility and deliver normal infants.[1879] One woman with 45X karyotype in skin, blood, and ovary is reported to have had spontaneous puberty, became pregnant three times, and gave birth to a child with 45X karyotype as well as another with normal karyotype. The third pregnancy ended in spontaneous abortion.[1880] Affected adults can undergo hormone replacement to prepare the uterus to receive a donated embryo and proceed to delivery. Unfortunately, deaths are reported in patients receiving donated ovum associated with dissection or rupture of the aorta, leading to caution in recommending this technique.[1881,1882]

Intrauterine growth retardation with a mean deficit in birth length of 2.6 cm (−1.24 SD) and a slow childhood growth rate results in a loss of about 8 to 9 cm (−3.0 SD) by age 3 years.[1883] A major portion of the height deficit occurs during the first 3 years of life. There is a decrease in growth rate at the time of expected puberty and absent pubertal growth spurt in those without pubertal development.[1884,1885] Those subjects who undergo spontaneous puberty have decreased growth in the first year after birth with another decrease at 7 to 8 years. This may reflect a suppressive effect of estrogen on growth in those retaining some ovarian function.[1886] Untreated individuals with Turner's syndrome in the United Kingdom and United States have a mean final height of approximately 142 to 143 cm,[1884] about 20 cm less than the average height of normal women; the adult stature of these patients correlates with midparental height and with the height of unaffected women of the same ethnic group.[1887,1888] Haploinsufficiency of the SHOX gene is estimated to contribute two thirds of the height deficit. It is postulated that a second gene on the short arm of the X, which does not undergo X inactivation, contributes the other one third of the deficit (see above). In Turner's syndrome with spontaneous puberty, pubertal height velocity was transiently higher than in girls with amenorrhea, but final adult height was not different.[1143]

Specific growth curves are available for plotting the growth of affected children.[1884,1885]

Growth hormone treatment is approved by the FDA for Turner's syndrome to increase height. The average height gain has varied from 4 to 16 cm,[1889-1891] with a systematic review of the literature showing a 5-cm gain to be most likely.[1892] This variability in gain in height is incompletely understood, but many factors have been implicated, including the age of initiation of therapy, dose duration, age (and especially number of years from beginning hGH treatment) of beginning estrogen replacement, number of injections per week, compliance, and whether the last measured height represented an adult height.[1893-1896] The weekly dose of hGH is 0.375 mg/kg divided into seven daily doses but it is important to individualize the dose. A treatment regimen that gradually increased the dose 0.63 mg/kg/wk elicited a 16.0±4.1 cm increase in height. Early initiation of hGH therapy (e.g., 2 to 8 years of age) and a mean duration of treatment of about 7 years can lead the majority of treated Turner's patients to achieve a final height greater than 150 cm; a Dutch study reported the mean final height was 162.3±6.1 cm.[1897] Turner's syndrome treated with GH who have spontaneous onset of puberty reportedly reach a shorter adult height[1898] or no difference in adult height[1899] compared to those in whom puberty is induced. With an early age of initiation of GH therapy, low-dose estrogen can be introduced at an appropriate age (about age 13) without compromising adult height.[1900] Percutaneous estrogen may be more beneficial than oral estrogen therapy.[1901] Adult height of 149 to 155 cm[1902] is reported compared to an untreated control group that reached a height of 142 cm even if estrogen administration starts at the normal age of puberty or GH administration starts at a later age.[1903]

Evaluation of bone density is technique specific,[1904-1906] but GH treatment of Turner's syndrome for at least 1 year showed no difference in volumetric bone mineral density, although lean body mass was higher and fat mass was lower than in the controls.[1907,1908] GH treatment of Turner's patients has been safe, and untoward events are infrequent.[1889-1893,1909,1910] There is some degree of improvement of the abnormal body proportions of Turner's syndrome with hGH treatment but the disproportionate growth of the foot may dissuade some girls from continuing treatment to maximal benefit on height.[1897] The addition of estrogen therapy at low doses has been reported either to exert no effect on adult height or to actually reduce the adult height obtained with growth hormone therapy administered alone.[1909-1917] Indeed, the length of time exposed to GH before estrogen treatment is said to be the major determinant of whether GH and estrogen treatment increased final height[1900] (see Chapter 22). However, it is postulated that if growth hormone is started early enough (e.g., 2 to 8 years of age), estrogen therapy may be added at an age (approximately 13 years) appropriate for the institution of puberty (see discussion for Turner's syndrome).[1918] Counseling and a peer support group are exceedingly important components of the long-term management.[1919]

A recent nationwide survey of 632 Danish girls with Turner's syndrome demonstrated an increased prevalence of fractures, mainly in the forearm, compared to controls: the prevalence was higher still in the absence of ovarian function and in girls with family history of fractures and presumed familial disorders of bone density.[1920] Thus it appears that estrogen therapy is critical for the prevention and repair of osteoporosis but in adolescents and adults, the optimal dose preparation and site of delivery for the prevention of osteoporosis is not known.

Girls younger than 6 years with Turner's syndrome did not perceive that they had a problem with height but by 7 to 12 and especially by 13 to 15 years, affected Turner's girls have a strong desire for growth hormone therapy and even unrealistic expectations of what growth hormone therapy might accomplish in terms of adult height.[1921] However, growth hormone therapy improved self-esteem even if there remained a significant difference in height between Turner's girls and the normal range. With the increased growth rate, girls felt better about their attractiveness, intelligence, and popularity; and they perceived that they experienced less teasing; there was no effect on school performance with growth hormone therapy.[1922] Growth hormone did not affect the nonverbal neurocognitive defects in Turner's syndrome,[1923] IQ, or achievement scores.[1924] Height gained with growth hormone therapy in Turner's syndrome did not affect quality of life, although cardiac defects and otologic complications did affect quality of life.[1925] Girls who have discontinued GH therapy after reaching adult height showed no evidence of depression but still had remaining problems with self-perception and bodily attitude despite significant height gains.[1926] Thus, psychological problems in Turner's syndrome are not necessarily diminished with GH treatment and an increase in adult height.

About 50% of patients with Turner's syndrome have a tendency toward impaired glucose tolerance without GH treatment.[1927] In some this may be due to associated obesity, and risk of type 2 diabetes mellitus is increased.[1928] Although glucose values do not change with GH therapy, insulin levels reversibly rise during treatment, indicating an additional degree of insulin resistance caused by the growth hormone.[1929] Turner's syndrome patients as young as 11 years can have elevated serum cholesterol concentrations (before treatment with growth hormone or estrogen).[1930]

The biphasic pattern of gonadotropin secretion in normal infancy and childhood (see Fig. 24-36) is exaggerated in Turner's syndrome. Thus, baseline gonadotropin concentrations and peak LH and FSH values after GnRH administration are above normal between birth and 4 years of age and again after age 10. Baseline values of FSH are 3 to 10 times higher than LH values. However, between ages 4 and 10, mean gonadotropin concentrations in this syndrome are similar to the mean values in normal girls (see Figs. 24–40 and 24–42) and are lower than those before age 4 and after age 10.[1144,1145]

The appearance of pubic hair, pubarche, is often delayed in the syndrome of gonadal dysgenesis, even though adrenarche, as assessed by the increase in concentration of plasma DHEAS, occurs at the normal age.[1259] Girls with ovarian failure demonstrate early adrenarche, and therefore higher serum values of DHEAS, but later pubarche, whereas those who demonstrate at least beginning breast development follow a course of adrenarche similar to unaffected girls.[1931] This suggests that ovarian function is necessary to convert DHEA to active androgens responsible for the appearance of pubic hair in normal girls. Because the pubic hair of affected individuals is sparse, but estrogen therapy increases the growth of pubic hair despite a lack of increase in adrenal androgen secretion, estrogen also affects pubic hair appearance.[1932]

Turner's syndrome girls resemble normal girls in verbal and language skills, but there are frequently difficulties with memory and attention, and with arithmetic skills, due to mistakes on operation and alignment processes.[1933] Girls with 45X mosaicism associated with a 46XX cell line 45,X/46,XX scored closer to normal than those with other types of mosaicisms. However, girls with Turner's syndrome can score higher on reading achievement tests than predicted by IQ or age; this hyperliteracy is a strength in many girls with this disorder. Only 3.3% of girls with Turner's syndrome have mental retardation in the absence of a variant of Turner's syndrome caused by a ring X chromosome.[1934]

Whereas IQ is normal in Turner's syndrome when verbal ability, including comprehension and vocabulary, is considered, visuoconstructional or visual-perceptual spatiotemporal processing, visuomotor coordination,[1935,1936] and mathematical ability (particularly in geometry) may be impaired, leading to a decrease in the performance of IQ.[1928,1937] However, one study found no specific deficits in visuospatial or tactile-spatial tasks in these children.[1938] A recent study found no difference in lateralization and performance of motor tasks in Turner's syndrome versus controls; there was superior performance of the dominant or right hand in contrast to the nondominant or left hand.[1939] Impaired abilities in association with executive dysfunction and decreased attention span can lead to learning difficulties.[1940,1939] Hyperactive behavior in these patients usually improves after the age of puberty.[1936] It is useful to monitor the patient's progress in high school mathematics.

There are consistent MRI abnormalities in the right parietal lobe and the occipital lobes in Turner's syndrome, which show decreased volumes in these areas, which are implicated in visuospatial processing. Using positron-emission tomography, decreased glucose metabolism is found in the right parietal band occipital lobes.[1941-1943] These anatomic data relate to the difficulties in visual spatial skills found in most studies of girls with Turner's syndrome, because these problems are most closely inked to the right parietal region.[1944]

There is an increased risk of impaired social adjustment in Turner's syndrome.[1945,1946] 45,X demonstrated a significant decrease in social competence score and an increase in total behavior problems, social, and attention problems. Girls had difficulty in schooling, in peer relationships, and in concentration, and had problems with immaturity, hyperactivity, nervousness, and withdrawn behaviors. The origin of the X chromosome was not determined in this study.[1947,1948] In other studies, structural abnormalities of the X chromosome were associated with more behavior problems than a missing X chromosome or mosaicism of the X chromosomes.[1949] Mental retardation and a "severe" phenotype is associated with small ring X chromosomes that undergo X inactivation resulting in X chromosome disomy for genes that undergo X inactivation.[1950]

The neurocognitive phenotype associated with Turner's syndrome maps to distal Xp.[1951] 45,X individuals in whom the X is of paternal origin (X^p) show better adjustment and "social cognition" as a group than X^m individuals.[1947,1952] This difference has been attributed to the imprinting of a gene inherited from the mother located on X^m (but which is not imprinted on X^p).[1947] The first example of an imprinted gene on the X chromosome, the locus resides in the pericentric region of the short arm or on the long arm of the X chromosome. Skuse and colleagues[1947] postulate that this imprinted gene may play a role in male-female differences in social behavior and developmental disorders. The risk is higher if the single X chromosome comes from the mother rather than the father. Individuals with Turner's syndrome have difficulty in inferring affective intention from facial appearance. As an explanation for these phenomena, there appears to be a locus on the X chromosome on Xq or close to the centromere on Xp which escapes X inactivation and affects social cognition.[1921,1953,1954] This locus is apparently imprinted and not expressed from the maternally derived X chromosome. If the locus was inherited from the father, the 45,X individuals were significantly better adjusted, with superior verbal and higher-order executive function skills, which mediate social interactions. If expressed only on the paternally derived X chromosome, the existence of this putative locus may explain, in part, why 46,XY males (whose single X chromosome is maternal) are more vulnerable to developmental disorders of language and social cognition, such as autism, than are 46,XX females. The origin of the single X chromosome affects memory performance as well in that those with a maternal derived X have increased verbal forgetting but normal nonverbal forgetting while those with a paternal derived X chromosome have the opposite pattern of problems.[1955]

The increase in mental health problems documented in Turner's syndrome may also be rooted in the increased peer ridicule experienced by girls with Turner's syndrome as opposed to a biologic abnormality.[1956]

The results of a double-blind study of estrogen vs. placebo treatment for 1 to 3 years in 7- to 9-year-old girls with Turner's syndrome show placebo-treated Turner's girls performed less well than either control girls or estrogen-treated Turner's syndrome girls in memory tests, suggesting that estrogen replacement therapy improves verbal and nonverbal memory. This raises the possibility that a prepubertal deficit in estrogen may affect performance of these tasks as well as a potential role for low dose estrogen replacement therapy in late prepubertal girls with Turner's syndrome.[1957] These results are similar to the improvement in short- and long-term verbal memory found in postmenopausal or surgically castrated women treated with estrogen replacement therapy.[1958,1959] Treatment with estrogen for a period of over 4 years appeared to move the self-esteem scores for girls with Turner's syndrome and psychological well-being toward normal control values as they reached 16 years of age compared to a significant difference in these scores that was documented at 12 years of age. No such change occurred in the non–estrogen-treated group, suggesting that it was the estrogen effects that caused the change rather than the passage of years.

Several mechanisms are proposed to explain these estrogen effects: (1) estrogen acts as a neuromodulator in a transient time frame, (2) estrogen alters synapse formation and remodeling in a permanent time frame, or (3) both mechanisms. Thus, estrogen may function as an organizational agent in the brain of the young but as a stabilizing agent in older individuals.

Because of the multiplicity of complications affected individuals might encounter, transition of girls with Turner's syndrome to adult care is best carried out by an experienced team ideally composed of endocrinologist; cardiologist; nephrologist; reproductive endocrinologist; audiologic physician; ear, nose, and throat surgeon; plastic surgeon; dentist; and psychologist.[1960]

Sex Chromatin–Positive Variants of the Syndrome of Gonadal Dysgenesis

Mosaicism of 45,X/46,XX, 45,X/47,XXX, or 45,X/46,XX/47,XXX chromosomes is associated with a chromatin-positive buccal smear and usually fewer manifestations of the syndrome of gonadal dysgenesis. Likewise, structural abnormalities of the X chromosome can be associated with fewer phenotypic features of the syndrome. Lack of genetic material on the long or the short arm of the second X chromosome can cause decreased gonadal function; loss of all or part of the short arm of the X leads to the physical findings of Turner's syndrome (see Chapter 22).[1143] Depending on the location and extent of the deletion on the short arm of the X chromosome, these patients are more likely to have modest pubertal growth and some spontaneous pubertal development.[1961]

Sex Chromatin–Negative Variants of Gonadal Dysgenesis

These variants include 45,X/46,XY mosaicism and structural abnormalities of the Y chromosome. Affected individuals vary in phenotype from that of classic gonadal dysgenesis to that of ambiguous genitalia to phenotypic males.[1143] Patients may present with short stature, delayed puberty, and a history of hypospadias repair.[1962] There is variable testicular differentiation, ranging from a streak gonad to functioning testes. Patients with mosaicism involving a Y cell line or abnormalities of the Y chromosome are at risk for neoplastic transformation of the dysgenetic testes. Gonadoblastomas, benign nonmetastasizing tumors, may arise within the gonad and produce either testosterone or estrogens; the neoplasm may become calcified sufficiently to be detected on an abdominal radiograph. Thus, the appearance of feminization or virilization in a patient with dysgenetic gonads and a Y cell line may indicate gonadoblastoma formation. Of greater significance is the increased prevalence of malignant germ cell tumors, arising within the dysgenetic gonad or gonadoblastoma.[1963] Examples are dysgerminomas, mature teratomas, and testicular intraepithelial neoplasia.[1964] Such tumors occur more often in postpubertal subjects and rarely in children.[1965] The management of gonads in patients with a Y cell line is discussed in Chapter 22 and in reference 1143.

46,XX and 46,XY Gonadal Dysgenesis

Pure gonadal dysgenesis refers to phenotypic females with sexual infantilism and a 46,XX or 46,XY karyotype without chromosomal abnormalities.[1143]

Familial and Sporadic 46,XX Gonadal Dysgenesis and Its Variants

The usual phenotype of 46,XX gonadal dysgenesis includes normal stature, sexual infantilism, bilateral streak gonad, normal female internal and external genitalia, and primary amenorrhea. The streak gonad occasionally produces estrogens or androgens, but malignant transformation is rare. Incomplete forms of this condition may result in hypoplastic ovaries that produce enough estrogen to cause some breast development and a few menstrual periods followed by secondary amenorrhea. This heterogeneous syndrome[1966] occurs sporadically or with autosomal recessive inheritance and in some instances is associated with other congenital malformations; some familial cases have been associated with sensorineural deafness (Perrault's syndrome)[1143] (see below).

Familial and Sporadic 46,XY Gonadal Dysgenesis and Its Variants

A phenotype that includes female genitalia with or without clitoral enlargement, normal or tall stature, bilateral streak gonads, normal müllerian structures, sexual infantilism, and a eunuchoid habitus is typical of 46,XY gonadal dysgenesis. About 15% of the patients have a deletion or mutation in the SRY gene. If the dysgenetic testes produce significant amounts of testosterone, slight clitoral enlargement may occur at birth and virilization may ensue at puberty. The incomplete form of 46,XY gonadal dysgenesis may involve any degree of ambiguity of the external genitalia and internal ducts. The risk of neoplastic transformation of the streak gonads or dysgenetic testes is increased, and gonadectomy is indicated.[1143] The disorder is usually transmitted as an X-linked or sex-limited autosomal dominant trait, less commonly as an autosomal recessive trait[1143] (see Chapter 22). A novel homozygous missense mutation in exon 1 of the desert hedgehog gene is reported in a patient with polyneuropathy associated with partial XY gonadal dysgenesis.[1967]

Other Causes of Primary Ovarian Failure

Primary ovarian failure is increasing in prevalence as a consequence of the long-term effects of cytotoxic chemotherapy and radiation is increasing in prevalence as these agents prolong life in children and adolescents with cancer just as occurs in the testes of males so treated.[1780]

Radiation therapy that includes the ovaries within the field can cause primary ovarian failure.[1792] A dose of 4 Gy to the ovaries will lead to sterility in 30% of young women and 100% of older women.[1793] It is useful to surgically move the ovaries out of the radiation field if they are not the actual target of the therapy, thereby greatly decreasing the dose of radiation to the ovaries. Ovarian transposition before radiation therapy is compatible with normal menses, pubertal development, and pregnancy in most cases.[1968] The uterus may also be affected by radiation and may not expand normally during pregnancy.

Chemotherapy

Successful treatment of childhood acute lymphoblastic leukemia is now commonplace. In a large study by Quigley and colleagues,[1969] after cytotoxic chemotherapy, boys and girls had extensive germ cell damage as evidenced by increased FSH secretion and boys had decreased testicular size for the stage of puberty. The concentration of plasma inhibin B is usually decreased, a sensitive indicator of damage to the germinal epithelium.[1970] Many of the girls at puberty had evidence of a compensated decrease in ovarian follicular function. Quite likely as a result of cranial irradiation, the mean age of menarche was advanced about 12 months despite the ovarian damage; puberty was not advanced in the boys. The type of chemotherapy relates to the effects upon the gonads. The ovary is less vulnerable to the effects of radiation and chemotherapy than the testis. The prevalence of ovarian damage does not appear to be high in that fertility and regular menses are reported in a majority of females who were treated as children.[1971] Nevertheless, age at treatment has a significant role: treatment between 13 and 19 years of age was associated with a more than twofold increase in premature ovarian failure during the third decade.[1972] Adjuvant chemotherapy for localized osteosarcoma in the prepubertal period is compatible with ovarian function and fertility.[1973] Parenthetically, early pubertal growth spurt and tall stature are increased in subjects with Ewing's sarcoma and osteosarcoma. Attempts to protect the gonads by suppressing the pituitary-gonadal axis with gonadal steroids or GnRH agonists are ineffective. Careful endocrine follow-up of children and adolescents treated with chemotherapy or radiotherapy is essential.

Premature menopause may occur at any age before the normal climacteric and has been reported in adolescent girls. Cessation of ovarian function usually presents as secondary amenorrhea. Autoimmune oophoritis can cause ovarian failure leading to primary amenorrhea, oligomenorrhea, arrest of puberty, and occasionally cystic enlargement of the ovaries.[1974-1978] Most often it is associated with other autoimmune endocrinopathies, especially autoimmune Addison's disease wherein it may precede the onset of adrenal insufficiency but it rarely, if ever, occurs in isolated premature ovarian failure[1974,1978,1979] (see Chapter 16). Glucocorticoid therapy may improve ovarian function, at least temporarily.

Thirty-six percent of women with type I autoimmune polyglandular insufficiency, also known as APECED, a rare systemic autoimmune disorder (hypoparathyroidism, adrenal insufficiency, gonadal failure, diabetes mellitus, pernicious anemia, hypothyroidism, chronic hepatitis, mucocutaneous candidiasis, dystrophic nail hypoplasia, vitiligo, alopecia, keratinopathy, and intestinal malabsorption), exhibited ovarian failure before age 20, whereas only 4% of affected men had testicular failure by this age.[1976] This autosomal recessive disorder is due to more than 42 mutations in AIRE-1 gene at gene map locus 21q22.3.[1980] study of genotype and phenotype correlations only demonstrated a higher prevalence of candidiasis in the patients with the most common mutation, arg257 to ter, although HLA class II is a significant determinant.[1981] This is in contrast to earlier studies suggesting a phenotype-genotype correlation in other features.

Autoimmune oophoritis is present in more than 20% of patients with autoimmune adrenal insufficiency. Various autoantibodies have been detected in autoimmune oophoritis including autoantibodies to cytochrome P450 steroidogenic en zymes[1982,1974,1978,1979,1983] some are organ specific, whereas others react with antigens in more than one tissue and more than one cell type.[1975]

Resistant ovary is a heterogeneous cause of primary hypogonadism, a syndrome associated with elevated concentrations of plasma FSH and LH and ovaries that contain primordial follicles.[1984,1985] The syndrome is usually idiopathic but an increasing number of genetic abnormalities are described in addition to the more common X-chromosomal defects.[1986]

Homozygous galactosemia due to mutation in the galactose-1-phosphate uridylyltransferase gene (GALT) is commonly associated with primary ovarian failure (from failure to develop puberty to primary or secondary amenorrhea and premature menopause), but puberty is usually normal in males and the risk of testicular dysfunction is low[1987]; compound heterozygotes have normal onset of puberty.[1987,1988] Dietary restriction programs have not prevented the ovarian failure nor are other means of avoiding ovarian failure effective. The pathogenesis of galactose-induced ovarian toxicity remains unclear but probably involves galactose itself and its metabolites such as galactitol and UDP-galactose. The pathophysiology of ovarian failure may be due to direct toxicity of galactose of its such as UDP-galactose, deficient galactosylation of glycoproteins and glycolipids, oxidative stress, and activation of apoptosis.[1989] Most cases are detected by newborn screening programs.[1990]

A rare autosomal dominant disorder involving eyelid dysplasia and premature ovarian failure is due to haploinsufficiency of the FOXL2 gene, a member of the winged helix/forkhead family of transcription factors.[1991] The eyelid abnormalities include small palpebral fissures, ptosis, and a small skinfold extending inward and upward from the lower lid (epicanthus inversus). The gene is expressed in the follicular cells, and the mutations that lead to haploinsufficiency are associated with an increased rate of follicular atresia. The degree of ovarian failure is variable from primary amenorrhea to irregular menses and premature ovarian failure, varying from normal-appearing ovaries on ultrasonography to streak gonads, and on ovarian biopsy a variable number of primordial follicles.[1992] The infertility component of the syndrome is limited to the female.

The congential disorders of glycosylation-1 (carbohydrate-deficient glycoprotein syndrome type Ia), an autosomal recessive disorder associated with circulating glycoproteins deficient in their terminal carbohydrate moieties, include a wide range of glycoproteins, enzymes, binding proteins, and coagulation factors.[1993] A typical isoform pattern of serum transferrin by isoelectric focusing is used as a diagnostic test. The dominant clinical feature is the neurologic manifestations of involvement of the central and peripheral nervous system among the other organ systems affected is the pituitary-gonadal system.

The hypergonadotropic-hypogonadism is more severe in females because males virilize at puberty. There are two interesting aspects: both the ovary and the pituitary gland are affected. The affected girls have sexual infantilism; the ovaries are hypoplastic or atrophic. High serum FSH and LH levels exhibited normal electrophoretic isoform patterns, but appear to have decreased but not absent FSH bioactivity in an FSH bioassay, and yet in the only three girls tested, a response to the administration of human menopausal gonadotropin was indicated by an increase in serum estradiol and in one patient, ovarian follicular growth. These observations suggest an abnormality in both the FSH molecule and the ovary, in the latter case a defect in the configuration and activation of the FSH receptor itself and the binding of ligand or a post receptor defect.[1994,1995]

FSH Receptor Gene Mutations and Hypergonadotropic Hypogonadism: FSH Receptor Resistance[955]

The FSH receptor is a member of the G protein–linked receptor seven-transmembrane superfamily; it has a large, extended extracellular ligand binding domain.[1996,1997] The gene for the FSH receptor is at gene map locus 2p21-p16. An autosomal recessive disorder due to a mutation in the extracellular ligand-binding domain of the FSH receptor in affected females in six Finnish families mainly from the north central region[1806,1998] resulted in delayed (40%) or normal puberty but primary amenorrhea, elevated gonadotropins, and hypergonadotropic ovarian dysgenesis with arrest of ovarian follicular development at the primary follicle stage and continued atresia.[1998,1999] The clinical features are very similar to the findings in FSH-deficient mice generated by targeted disruption of the gene encoding the FSH β-subunit.[2000] Quite likely this disorder is responsible for most cases of the "resistant" ovary syndrome. The FSH receptor gene contains nine small exons (1-9), which encode the extracellular ligand-binding domain, and one large exon (10), which designates the remainder of the receptor including the seven-transmembrane and the intracellular domains.[1996] The Finnish mutation, an alanine 1989 valine substitution, is in the extracellular domain.[2001] Expression of the mutation in transfected cells indicated a small FSH effect on cAMP production, a striking reduction of FSH-binding capacity, but apparently normal binding affinity.[2001]

The FSH receptor mutation in the Finnish patients is not a null mutation. It remains to be determined if the loss or complete inactivation of the FSH receptor will lead to failure of puberty and sexual infantilism or to estrogen synthesis by the immature ovarian follicles described in the FSH-β subunit knockout mouse.[2000] Affected males in these families are normally masculinized at puberty but tend to have small testes. They have a variable degree of spermatogenic insufficiency, but not azoospermia, increased plasma concentrations of FSH and LH, decreased inhibin B levels, and normal plasma testosterone values.[2002]

LH/hCG resistance due to mutations in the gene encoding the seven-transmembrane LH/hCG receptor is discussed in Chapter 22. In the affected XY individual, this autosomal recessive disorder leads to varying degrees of male pseudohermaphrodism as would be predicted, with the mildest case represented by isolated micropenis.[1809,1810] Less severe mutations of the LH/hCG receptor could be associated with delayed puberty. In the affected female, on the other hand, LH/hCG resistance does not affect pubertal maturation but leads to amenorrhea with high serum LH levels but normal FSH and estradiol concentrations.[2003]

Polycystic ovary syndrome or functional ovarian hyperandrogenism does not delay the onset of puberty but often delays menarche or causes menstrual abnormalities (see Chapter 22 for complete discussion).[2004-2007] Polycystic ovarian syndrome is more common in girls with type 1 diabetes mellitus.[2008] It is important to realize the serious long-term metabolic consequences such as dyslipidemia and insulin resistance over and above androgen excess and reproductive difficulties.[2009]

Noonan's Syndrome (Pseudo-Turner's Syndrome, Ullrich Syndrome) (See Chapter 23)

Individuals with Noonan's syndrome have webbed neck, ptosis, down-slanting palpebral fissures, low-set ears, short stature, cubitus valgus, and lymphedema, and hence this phenotype has been called *pseudo-Turner's syndrome.*[1143] Features that differentiate these individuals from those with Turner's syndrome include triangular facies, pectus excavatum, right-sided heart disease (e.g., pulmonic stenosis, often with valve dysplasia, or atrial septal defect) compared to the left-sided heart disease in Turner's syndrome, hypertrophic cardiomyopathy, varied blood clotting defects, and an increased incidence of mental retardation. Females with Noonan's syndrome have normal ovarian function. Males have normal differentiation of external genitalia but may have undescended testes; germinal aplasia or hypoplasia and impaired Leydig cell function may be present.[2010] Puberty may be delayed, with an average of 2 years.[2011] Stature is decreased, usually following the −2 SD curve; the pubertal growth spurt is often delayed or attenuated but final height usually is at the low limits of normal.[2012] hGH administration increased the growth rate but long-term reports are not yet available although there does not appear to be adverse effects on cardiac function from GH treatment.[2013,2014] Adult males with Noonan's syndrome are reported to have osteopenia, which has been attributed to estrogen deficiency because estrogen administration improves the decreased bone mineral content.[2015] Patients who have sufficient ovarian function to undergo spontaneous pubertal development and menarche have adequate bone mineral density compared to those in whom puberty was induced by estrogen and who exhibited osteopenia despite hormone replacement.[2016] Noonan's syndrome is inherited as an autosomal dominant trait.[1143] A gene implicated in Noonan's syndrome has been localized to the long arm of chromosome 12 (12q 24.1). The incidence is estimated at 1/1000 to 1/5000. One parent may have features of the syndrome in 40% to 60% of cases. About 50% of patients are thought to be the result of new mutations.

Chronic renal failure is combined with gonadal dysgenesis in the *Frasier syndrome.*[2017] While most cases present with ambiguous genitalia, this diagnosis should be considered in any phenotypic female with end-stage renal disease (due to focal segmental glomerulosclerosis) and sexual infantilism; the karyotype may be 46,XY or 46,XX.[2018]

Diagnosis of Delayed Puberty and Sexual Infantilism (Figs. 24–62 and 24–63; Table 24–28)

When girls remain prepubertal at 13 years or boys remain prepubertal at 14, the physician must make a clinical judgment as to which are variants of the norm and which require extensive evaluation and treatment. A boy who has not completed secondary sexual maturation within 4.5 years after onset of puberty or a girl who does not menstruate within 5 years after onset may have a hypothalamic, pituitary, or gonadal disorder. The diagnosis of hypergonadotropic hypogonadism is readily established by elevation of random plasma LH and FSH concentrations. However, the differential diagnosis of hypogonadotropic hypogonadism versus constitutional delay in growth and adolescence is more difficult because of the overlap in physical and laboratory findings in the two conditions, including inability to differentiate between normal and low concentrations of serum gonadotropins (Table 24–29). The majority of boys with pubertal delay have a self-limited variant in the tempo of growth and pubertal onset, CDP. The task of the physician is, on the one hand, to avoid a costly investigation of an essentially healthy boy while on the other, identifying those who have an underlying disorder compromising the hypothalamic-pituitary gonadotropin-gonadal system.

History taking must elicit all symptoms of chronic or intermittent illnesses and all details pertaining to growth and development as well as questioning about the patient's sense of smell. Has puberty failed to occur or did it begin but failed to progress or even regressed? Disorders of pregnancy, abnormalities of labor and delivery, and birth trauma, if present in the patient's history, suggest that a congenital or neonatal event may be related to the delay in puberty. Poor linear growth and poor nutritional status during the neonatal period and childhood may reflect longstanding abnormalities of development. Family history may reveal disorders of puberty or infertility, anosmia, or hyposmia in relatives as well as delay in the age at onset of puberty in parents or siblings. Recalled age of pubertal onset is relatively reliable in women[2019] but less often accurate in men. A history of consanguinity is important in the detection of autosomal recessive disorders.

The physical examination starts with determination of height and weight, the upper/lower segment ratio or sitting height is calculated and the arm span is measured and compared with the height. A growth chart is plotted to represent graphically the increase in stature and to assess growth velocity from birth (see Chapter 23). Late onset of growth failure usually indicates a serious condition requiring evaluation as soon as it is noted. Weight is plotted to determine states of malnutrition. BMI should be calculated and plotted by age and gender in this era of epidemic obesity or to further determine nutritional status. The height velocity should be documented over a period of at least 6 months, preferably 12 months. The signs of puberty are noted, and the stage of secondary sexual development is determined by physical examination according to the standards presented earlier (see Figs. 24–5 to 24–7). Questionnaires utilizing pictures are used to allow children to determine their own stage of

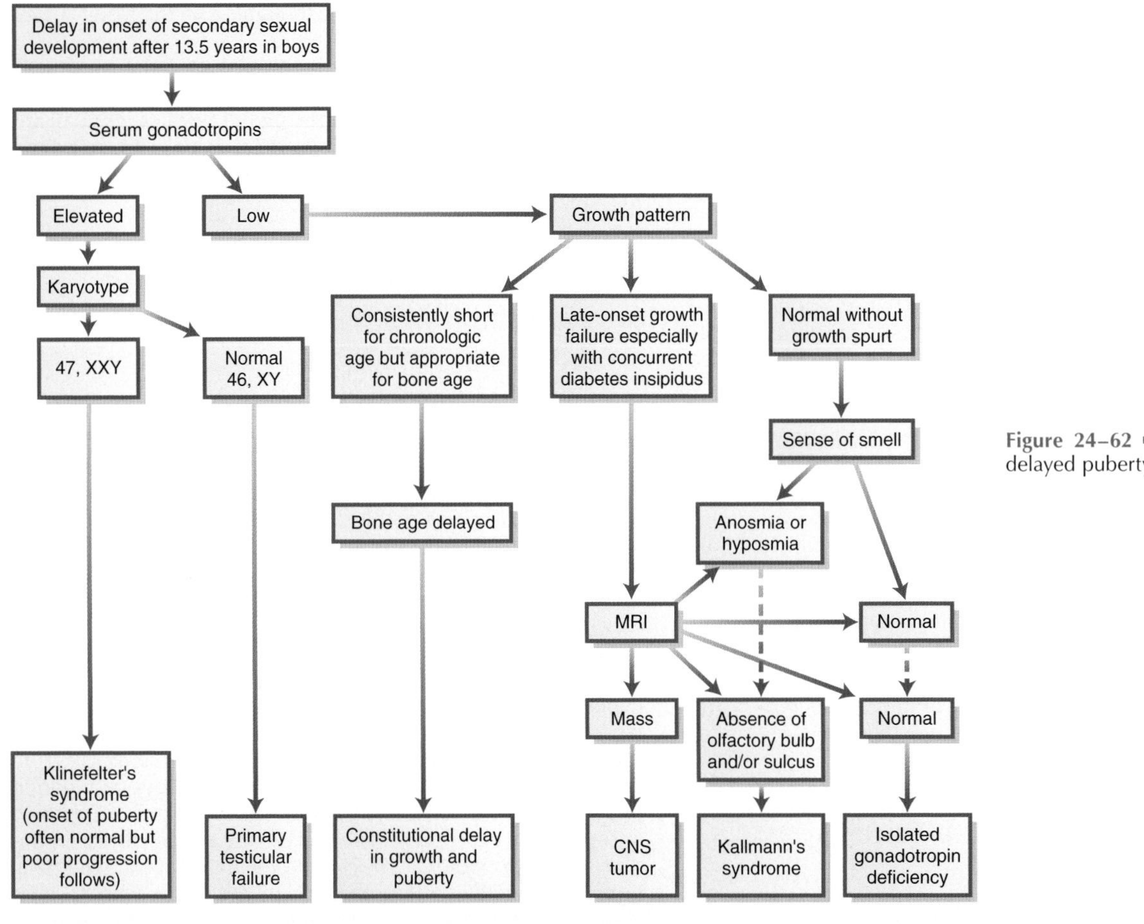

Figure 24–62 ▪ The evaluation of delayed puberty in boys.

TABLE 24–28 DIFFERENTIAL DIAGNOSTIC FEATURES OF DELAYED PUBERTY AND SEXUAL INFANTILISM

Condition	Stature	Plasma Gonadotropins	GnRH Test LH Response	Plasma Gonadal Steroids	Plasma DHEAS	Karyotype	Olfaction
Constitutional delay in growth and adolescence	Short for chronologic age, usually appropriate for bone age	Prepubertal, later pubertal	Prepubertal, later pubertal	Low, later normal	Low for chronologic age, appropriate for bone age	Normal	Normal
Hypogonadotropic hypogonadism							
Isolated gonadotropin deficiency	Normal, absent pubertal growth spurt	Low	Prepubertal or no response	Low	Appropriate for chronologic age	Normal	Normal
Kallmann's syndrome	Normal, absent pubertal growth spurt	Low	Prepubertal or no response	Low	Appropriate for chronologic age	Normal	Anosmia or hyposmia
Idiopathic multiple pituitary hormone deficiencies	Short stature and poor growth since early childhood	Low	Prepubertal or no response	Low	Usually low	Normal	Normal
Hypothalamic-pituitary tumors	Late onset decrease in growth velocity	Low	Prepubertal or no response	Low	Normal or low for chronologic age	Normal	Normal
Primary gonadal failure							
Syndrome of gonadal dysgenesis (Turner's syndrome) and variants	Short stature since childhood	High	Hyperresponse for age	Low	Normal for chronologic age	45,X or variant	Normal
Klinefelter's syndrome and variants	Normal to tall	High	Hyperresponse at puberty	Low or normal	Normal for chronologic age	47,XXY or variant	Normal
Familial XX or XY gonadal dysgenesis	Normal	High	Hyperresponse for age	Low	Normal for chronologic age	46,XX or 46,XY	Normal

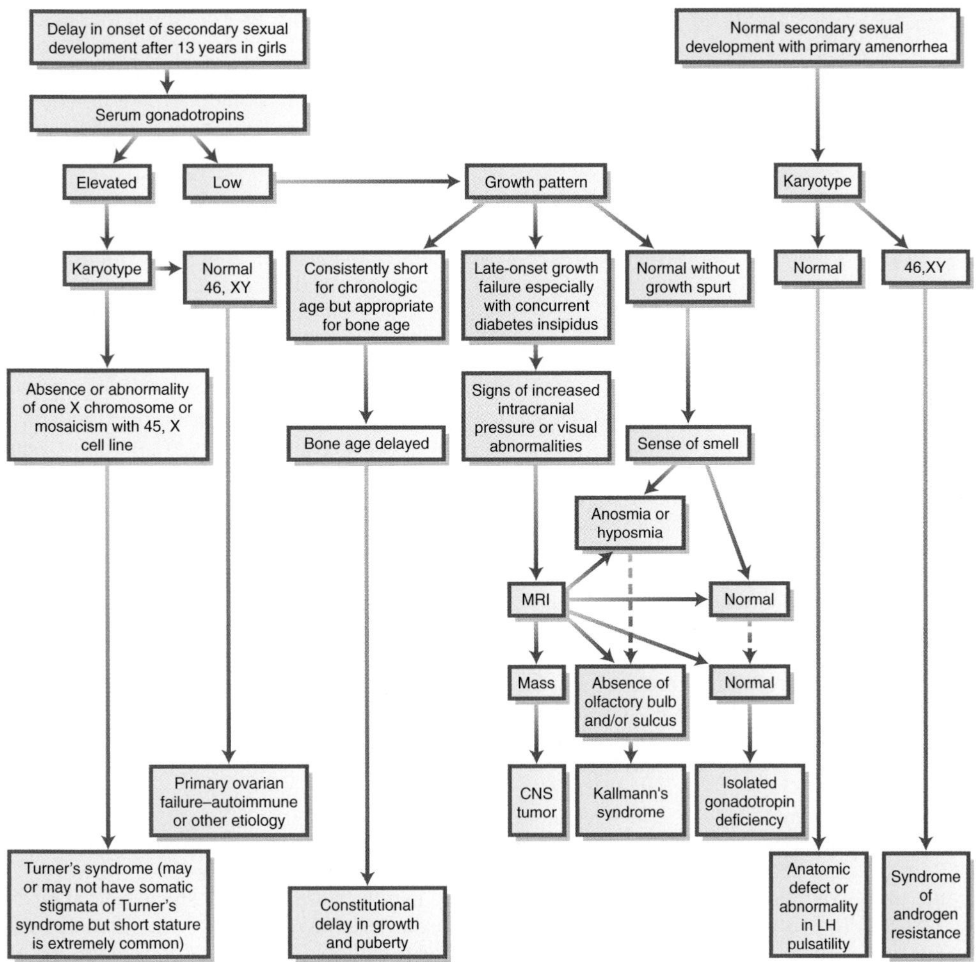

Figure 24–63 ▪ The evaluation of delayed puberty in girls.

TABLE 24–29 ENDOCRINE DIAGNOSIS OF CONSTITUTIONAL DELAYED ADOLESCENCE AND HYPOGONADOTROPIC HYPOGONADISM

No single test reliably discriminates between the two diagnoses.
Onset of puberty in boys is indicated by
- Testes >2.5 cm in diameter
- Serum testosterone concentration >50 ng/dL
- Pubertal LH response to GnRH bolus
- Pubertal pattern of LH pulsatility

LH, Luteinizing hormone; *GnRH,* LH-releasing hormone.

puberty in some studies, but they do not replace the physical examination and there is a tendency to overestimate development early in puberty and underestimate late in puberty.[230,2020] The length and width of the testes is measured in boys or the volume is assessed using an orchidometer. The length and diameter of the stretched and penis is determined in boys, and the diameter of glandular breast tissue and areolar size are noted in girls. The presence or absence of galactorrhea is noted. Obese boys often appear to have a small penis because of excessive adipose tissue surrounding the phallus; only when the fat is retracted can the full extent of phallic development be assessed. (This is among the most common causes of inappropriate referral for hypogonadism.) The extent of pubic and axillary hair is noted, as is the degree of acne or comedones. The possibility of cryptorchidism or retractile testes should be differentiated if no testes are palpated in the scrotum. Neurologic examination, including examination of the optic discs and visual fields by frontal confrontation perimetry, may reveal findings suggesting the presence of a CNS neoplasm or a developmental defect. Determination of olfaction is important in that many patients with Kallmann's syndrome wait years for the correct diagnosis to be made even in the presence of classic findings.[2021] A high index of suspicion by the physician is important. The stigmata of gonadal dysgenesis (Turner's syndrome) or the small testes and gynecomastia of Klinefelter's syndrome may suggest one of these diagnoses. Complete physical examination including the lungs, heart, kidney, and the gastrointestinal tract is also important in the search for a chronic disorder that may delay puberty.

Laboratory studies (Table 24–30) include determination of plasma LH and FSH concentrations in sensitive third-generation assays in pediatric endocrine laboratories, measurement of the rise in LH level after GnRH or GnRH agonist administration, determination of testosterone concentrations in boys and estradiol levels in girls in pediatric endocrine laboratories, and measurements of thyroxine and prolactin concentrations in boys and girls if the clinical features warrant. It is important to use one of the few national endocrine laboratories for the determinations of the hormones of puberty as most local laboratories are only interested in differentiating the normal, higher adult values from inappropriately low levels and cannot determine

TABLE 24–30 ENDOCRINE AND IMAGING STUDIES IN DELAYED ADOLESCENCE

Initial assessment
- Plasma testosterone or estradiol
- Plasma FSH and LH
- Plasma thyroxine (and prolactin)
- Bone age and lateral skull roentgenograph
- Test of olfaction

Follow-up studies
- Karyotype (short, phenotypic females)
- MRI with contrast enhancement
- Pelvic ultrasonography (females)
- GnRH test
- hCG test (males)
- Pattern of pulsatile LH secretion
- Visual acuity and visual fields

FSH, Follicle-stimulating hormone; *hCG,* human chorionic gonadotropin; *LH,* luteinizing hormone; *MRI,* magnetic resonance imaging.

the gradations of the low levels found in puberty. Recently, several national laboratories are using liquid chromatography tandem mass spectrometry methods for improved sensitivity and specificity and determinations in children (and women) for increased accuracy.[842] New ultrasensitive bioassays may also be made available commercially for determination of low values of testosterone and estradiol[352,1877,851] or total androgen or estrogen.[853,862]

Radiographic examination may include bone age determination and, if the diagnosis is at all consistent with a CNS lesion, an MRI scan of the brain with specific attention to the pituitary and hypothalamic area using contrast. CT scanning can detect calcification in contrast to MRI scans (or plain X-ray films in most cases). Ultrasound evaluation of the uterus and ovaries provides useful information about the state of development of these structures[2022] if the ultrasonographer has experience with children and young adolescents.

Assessment of chromosomal karyotype should be considered in all short girls, even in the absence of somatic signs of Turner's syndrome and especially if puberty is delayed, and in boys with suspected Klinefelter's stigmata or behavior.

A presumptive diagnosis of constitutional delay in growth and adolescence is made if the history and growth chart reveal a history of short stature but consistent growth rate for skeletal age (and no signs or symptoms of hypothalamic lesions), if the family history includes parents or siblings with delayed puberty, if the physical examination (including assessment of the olfactory threshold) is normal, if optic discs and visual fields are normal, and if the bone age is significantly delayed. In classic cases, an MRI scan of the hypothalamic-pituitary region may not be necessary. The rate of growth in these patients is usually appropriate for bone age; a decrease in growth velocity occurs in some normal children just before the appearance of secondary sexual characteristics and may awaken concerns if such a pattern occurs in these subjects. Furthermore, in these individuals the onset at puberty correlates better with bone age than with chronologic age (although bone age is not any better at estimating the onset of puberty in normal boys than is chronologic age[435]). Elevated concentrations of gonadotropins and gonadal steroids to early pubertal levels precede secondary sexual development by several months; thus, measurements of serum LH, FSH, estradiol, or testosterone levels in appropriate assays may help in predicting future development. The third-generation LH assays are reported sufficiently sensitive to allow in most boys the determination of the onset of endocrine puberty on a single blood sample but a dynamic GnRH test may be performed. The use of 10 micrograms of GnRH instead of 100 mcg is stated to differentiate constitutional delay from hypogonadotropic hypogonadism, but the virtual absence of GnRH supplies makes this contention not practical for clinical use.[2023] The measurement of gonadotropins 40 minutes to one hour after an subcutaneous injection of GnRH agonist is proposed as another test of dynamic secretion of gonadotropins in the absence of native GnRH supplies.[2024-2026]

Measurement of 8 AM serum testosterone is said to be an accurate indication of impending pubertal development; a value of greater than 0.7 nmol/L (20 ng/dL) predicts enlargement of testes to greater than 4 mL by 12 months in 77% of cases and in 15 months in 100% of cases, while in those with a value less than 0.7 nmol/L only 12% entered puberty in 12 months and only 25% entered puberty in 15 months. This technique may help predict spontaneous pubertal development but still requires considerable watching and waiting.[1292] A 5-year longitudinal study of boys with delay of pubertal onset aimed to determine indicators of CDP versus HH.[2027] An initial basal morning testosterone level greater than 1.7 nmol/L was observed in 55% of patients with constitutional delay exclusively (predictive positive value [PPV] = 100%; predictive negative value [PNV] = 59%). For those with basal morning testosterone level less than 1.7 nmol/L CDP, a measurement of the LH peak 3 hours after the GnRH agonist Triptorelin had a PPV of 100% if the upper threshold was set at 14 IU/L and the PNV was 72%. Because no lower threshold could discriminate hypogonadotropic hypogonadism from constitutional delay if the LH peak 3 hours after Triptorelin less than 14 IU/L, hCG stimulation was invoked. In constitutional delay, the PPV of a serum testosterone increment greater than 9 nmol/L (PNV=72%) after hCG stimulation was 100% and in IHH patients, the PPV of a rise in testosterone of less than 3 nmol/L (PNV=82%) after hCG was 100%. However, 29% of the studied population had a rise in testosterone after hCG between these thresholds and could not be classified by testing alone, limiting these techniques. Another study suggests that a ratio of peak to basal free α gonadotropin subunit after GnRH greater than 3.7 to 4.8 will differentiate constitutional delay from hypogonadotropic hypogonadism.[2028] These methods require continued evaluation before they become standard clinically and at present there does not appear to be a practical and reliable endocrine test for indisputably differentiating between constitutional delay in growth and adolescence from hypogonadotropic hypogonadism. Watchful waiting remains the procedure of choice if a patient does not fulfill the above criteria and fall into a diagnosable grouping.

A typical patient with isolated gonadotropin deficiency is of average height for age and has eunuchoid proportions; low plasma concentrations of gonadal steroids, LH, and FSH; and no increase or a blunted response of LH after GnRH or GnRH agonist administration. The amplitude and usually the frequency of LH pulses are decreased when serial blood samples are studied over a 24-hour period. In some but not all forms of Kallmann's syndrome, the sense of smell is absent or impaired. However, as stated, differentiation of isolated gonadotropin deficiency in the absence of hyposmia or anosmia from constitutional delay in puberty may be difficult at initial study. Gonadotropin-deficient patients may be as short as those with constitutional delay in growth and adolescence, and concentrations of LH and FSH in hypogonadotropic hypogonadism may be indistinguishable from those of normal prepubertal children or children with constitutional delay. Sometimes years of observation are necessary to detect the appearance of spontaneous and progressive signs of secondary sexual development or to document rising concentrations of gonadotropins or gonadal steroids before the diagnosis is clear. There is a tendency for hypogonadotropic patients to undergo adrenarche at a normal age and to have a higher DHEAS concentration than those with constitutional delay in growth. This pattern is helpful in the differential diagnosis.[1259,2029,2030] In general, but not in all cases, absence of the first signs of sexual maturation or failure of a rise in gonadotropins or gonadal steroid levels by age 18 in the presence of a normal concentration of serum DHEAS for chronologic age supports the diagnosis of isolated gonadotropin deficiency.

Patients with deficiency of gonadotropins combined with deficiency of other pituitary hormones require careful evaluation for a CNS neoplasm. Visual field or optic disc abnormalities support the diagnosis of CNS tumor. Even if these tests are normal, a cranial MRI scan should be done to evaluate the pituitary gland and stalk and the hypothalamic region. MRI appears superior to CT scanning to detect mass lesions and developmental abnormalities of the hypothalamic-pituitary region.[2031,2032]

Treatment of Delayed Puberty and Sexual Infantilism (Table 24–31)

Patients with constitutional delay in growth and adolescence ultimately have spontaneous onset and progression through puberty. Often, reassurance and continued observation to ensure that the expected sexual maturation occurs are sufficient. However, the stigma of appearing less mature than one's peers can cause psychological stress; such individuals may be unable to participate in the dating activities their friends are starting, smaller size may lead them to avoid participation in athletics, immature appearance may lead to ridicule, especially in the locker room, and school work may suffer with their poor self-image.[2033,2034] Some children feel such intense peer pressure and low self-esteem that only the appearance of signs of puberty will reassure them and enable them to participate in sports and social activities with their peers. Poor self-image in late-maturing boys may carry into adulthood even after normal puberty ensues.[2033,2034] The growth retardation appears more often responsible for most of the stress rather than the delay in pubertal development itself.[2035]

TABLE 24–31 MANAGEMENT AND TREATMENT OF DELAYED PUBERTY

OBJECTIVE
Determine site and etiology of abnormality Induce and maintain secondary sexual characteristics Induce pubertal growth spurt Prevent the potential short-term and long-term psychological, personality, and social handicaps of delayed puberty Ensure normal libido and potency Attain fertility
THERAPY
Concerned but not anxious or socially handicapped adolescent: Reassurance and follow-up (tincture of time) Repeat evaluation (including serum testosterone or estradiol) in 6 mo Psychosocial handicaps, anxiety, highly concerned: Therapy for 4 mo with Boys: testosterone enanthate 100 mg intramuscularyly every 4 wk at 14-14.5 yr of age, or overnight transdermal testosterone patch Girls: ethinyl estradiol 5-10 μg daily by mouth or conjugated estrogens 0.3 mg daily by mouth or overnight ethinyl estradiol patch at 13 yr of age No therapy for 4-6 mo; reevaluate status including serum testosterone or estradiol; if indicated repeat treatment regimen

For psychological reasons, in boys of age 14 or older who show no signs of puberty, a 3- to 6-month course of testosterone enanthate, cypionate or cycloproprionate (50 mg sometimes up to 100 mg intramuscularly every 4 weeks) may be helpful.[2036-2038] Decades of experience confirm no effect on final height of such low dosage for short term.[2039,2040] The low dose of testosterone enanthate is generally considered to be safe but can raise apoB and decrease HDL-C and apoAI (estradiol increases HDL-C and decreased triglycerides, LDL cholesterol, and apoB) as an expected effect.[2041] Furthermore, starting with the higher dose of 100 mg could lead to priapism in treatment of naïve boys, so care, lower dosage, and short-acting preparation are advisable.

Alkylated testosterone preparations are to be avoided because of the risk of peliosis hepatitis (hemorrhagic liver cysts), which are not related to dose or duration of treatment; whereas regression is possible with discontinuation of testosterone treatment, and progression to liver failure can occur.[2042,2043]

A course of low-dose oxandrolone (0.05 mg/kg/day, maximum dose 2.5 mg/day)[2044] is sometimes used as an oral alternative to intramuscular testosterone enanthate; this agent increases growth through androgenic effects reflected by suppression of LH and FSH but does not stimulate GH secretion as it is not aromatized to estrogen.[2045] The temporary increase in growth velocity found with oxandrolone does not affect final height in most studies,[2046-2048] although predicted height is said to increase with an oral dose of 0.7 mg/kg per week.[2040] Oral treatment with 2.5 mg of fluoxymesterone (Halotestin) for 6 to 60 months will allow increased pubertal development without adverse effect upon final height, although the necessity to take a daily dose may decrease compliance.[714] Testosterone undecenoate at 40 mg/day is likewise an effective but expensive treatment for those opting for an oral therapy.[2049-2051] This treatment can increase growth rate but does not result in a change in LH pulsatility, mean overnight LH, testosterone, SHBG, free androgen index, PSA, or testicular volume values. Transdermal testosterone may be applied as a daily patch or a gel, although experience with these forms of androgen is more limited than with the other forms. Preliminary experience suggests that overnight (approximately 8 to 9 hours) or every other night use of a 2.5 mg (Androderm patch) can achieve physiologic testosterone levels, lower SHBG levels, promote growth and virilization, and increase bone mineral density in hypogonadal teenagers without significant side effects.[2052] An overnight study of transdermal testosterone (Virormone [5 mg]) applied overnight (8 or 12 hours) for 4-week periods in boys with delayed puberty and short stature raised salivary testosterone, stimulated leg growth measured by knemometry (sensitive short-term measurements of leg growth) and stimulated bone turnover reflected by increased serum alkaline phosphatase.[2053] Testosterone cream is approved for adults and is now undergoing clinical trials for use in teenagers with delayed puberty. It may replace the use of parenteral testosterone.

While the use of exogenous androgens may improve self-image and start the secondary sexual changes of puberty, low-dose androgens neither improve final height nor change the eunuchoid proportions.[2054] One recent study from Israel reports that 6000 units of vitamin A (and 12 mg of iron) per day promotes pubertal development in affected boys as effectively as androgen administration; this implies that vitamin A deficiency was an etiologic factor in the constitutional delay[2055] but this contention has not been proven as yet.

For girls of age 13 or older, a 3- to 4-month course of ethinyl estradiol (5 μg/day orally) or conjugated estrogens (0.3 mg/day orally) may be used to initiate maturation of the secondary sexual characteristics without unduly advancing bone age or limiting final height.[2056,2057] Transdermal estrogen has been used in clinical trials for decades in the treatment of delayed puberty or hypogonadism with beneficial results on physical development and bone density.[2058-2061] However, there is new support for such therapy due to the understanding of the adverse effects of oral estrogen that enters the portal circulation initially at high dosage (first pass) and stimulates the production of proteins such as C reactive protein, angiotensin precursor, and activated protein C, which are involved in cardiac complications. This is in contrast to dermal estrogen that is administered in lower dosage and reaches its therapeutic targets relatively unchanged and in lower, more physiologic concentrations: there is no change in these listed proteins with dermal estrogen administration.[2062] Estrogen patches are undergoing clinical testing for use in initiating or promoting pubertal development in hypogonadal or delayed pubertal girls and promise to replace parenteral therapy.

As described above, the long-term safety and effects on bone density of aromatase inhibitor therapy is unknown.

If during the 3 to 6 months after discontinuing gonadal steroid therapy spontaneous puberty does not ensue or the concentrations of plasma gonadotropins and plasma testosterone in boys or plasma estradiol in girls do not increase, the treatment may be repeated. Usually, only one or two courses of therapy are necessary. When treatment is discontinued after bone age has advanced, for example, to 12 to 13 years in girls or 13 or 14 years in boys, patients with constitutional delay usually continue pubertal development on their own, whereas those with gonadotropin deficiency do not progress and may, in fact, regress.

Functional hypogonadotropic hypogonadism associated with chronic disease is treated by alleviating the underlying problem. Delayed puberty in this situation is usually a result of inadequate nutrition and low weight or excessive energy expenditure; when weight returns to normal values, puberty usually occurs spontaneously. Treatment with thyroxine will allow normal pubertal development in hypothyroid patients with delayed puberty.

Congenital or acquired gonadotropin deficiency as a result of a lesion or surgery requires replacement therapy with gonadal steroids at an age approximating the normal age of onset of puberty (Tables 24–32 and 24–33). An exception may occur when GH deficiency coexists with gonadotropin deficiency; if bone age advancement and epiphyseal fusion are brought about by testosterone or estradiol replacement before therapy with GH causes adequate linear growth, adult height will be compromised. However, if puberty is not initiated early enough, the patient may suffer psychological damage. It is generally advisable to initiate puberty in such patients with low-dose gonadal steroids by age 14 in boys and age 13 in girls regardless of the definitive diagnosis of gonadotropin deficiency; thus these children with GH deficiency would be treated similarly to those with isolated delayed puberty. Isolated GH-deficient patients may have a delayed onset of puberty; with growth hormone administration usually puberty occurs at an appropriate age but may progress faster than in normal individuals.[1919,2063] A study of children with GH deficiency showed a correlation between the age of onset of induced puberty and final height in patients who were also gonadotropin deficient, whereas those who underwent spontaneous puberty, which occurred earlier than the age of hormone-induced puberty in the gonadotropin-deficient children, had a decreased final height; this supports the advisability of waiting to initiate puberty in GH- and gonadotropin-deficient subjects.[2064] Height at the onset of puberty is also correlated with final height in GH-deficient children.[2065] However, artificially delaying puberty with a GnRH analogue to attempt to achieve a greater final height in patients has been attempted in isolated GH deficiency[2066] or with normal variant short stature, but concern over decreased bone density seen in subjects treated with GnRH analogues leads to warnings about the use of this agent in GH-deficient patients as well.[1319]

TABLE 24–32 HORMONAL SUBSTITUTION THERAPY IN BOYS WITH HYPOGONADISM

Goal: to approximate normal adolescent development *when diagnosis is established*

Initial therapy: at 13 yr of age, testosterone enanthate (or other long-acting testosterone ester) 50 mg intramuscularly every month for about 9 mo (6-12 mo)

Over the next 3 to 4 yr: gradually increase dose to adult replacement dose of 200 mg every 2-3 wk

Begin *replacement therapy in boys with suspected hypogonadotropic hypogonadism* by bone age ≤14 yr

To induce fertility at appropriate time in hypogonadetropic hypogonadism: pulsatile GnRH or FSH and hCG therapy

TABLE 24–33 HORMONAL SUBSTITUTION THERAPY IN GIRLS WITH HYPOGONADISM

When diagnosis of hypogonadism is firmly established (e.g., girls with 45,X gonadal dysgenesis), begin hormonal substitution therapy at 12-13 yr of age

Goal: to approximate normal adolescent development

Initial therapy: ethinyl estradiol 5 μg by mouth or conjugated estrogen 0.3 mg (or less) by mouth daily for 4-6 mo or preferably estradiol transdermally

After 6 mo of therapy (or sooner if "breakthrough" bleeding occurs) begin cyclic therapy:
- Estrogen: first 21 days of month
- Progestagen: (e.g., medroxyprogesterone acetate 5 mg by mouth) 12th to 21st day of month
- Gradually increase dose of estrogen over next 2-3 yr to conjugated estrogen 0.6-1.25 mg or ethinyl estradiol 10-20 μg daily for first 21 days of month or estradiol patch

In hypogonadotropic hypogonadism: to induce ovulation at appropriate time: pulsatile GnRH or FSH and hCG therapy

Microphallus due to hypothalamic deficiencies[937] may be treated with one or two 3-month courses of testosterone enanthate, 25 mg per month given IM, to enlarge the size of the penis.[2067,2068] While concern was raised that early testosterone therapy might not allow the attainment of a normal adult penile size, experience has proven otherwise. Furthermore, the concern that the penis might not respond to androgens later in life if exposed to testosterone in childhood, a pattern noted in the rat, proved incorrect.[225] Positive psychological outcome as well as attainment of normal stretched penile length are reported.[1489,2069] Thus it is appropriate to treat male infants and children with micropenis due to gonadotropin or growth hormone deficiency with short courses of androgens to enlarge the penis into the normal childhood range.[1489] Patients with isolated congenital GH deficiency occasionally have micropenis, which may be successfully treated with growth hormone replacement alone.[2070] It is not appropriate to sex reverse a male infant because of microphallus owing to fetal testosterone or GH deficiency.

Episodic administration of GnRH elicits pulsatile LH and FSH release and gonadal stimulation in prepubertal children or hypogonadotropic patients.[1239,1242,1243] Portable pumps are used to administer episodic GnRH over prolonged periods (see Chapter 23).[1241] Pulsatile GnRH therapy can induce puberty and promote the development of secondary sexual characteristics and spermatogenesis in men[2071-2076] and ovulation in women[2077,2078] but is not practical for the routine induction of puberty in adolescent boys and girls with gonadotropin deficiency. Pregnancy can be achieved with this regimen in women and spermatogenesis in men with hypogonadotropic hypogonadism. A lower frequency of GnRH administration favors FSH secretion while a faster frequency favors LH secretion and, ultimately, has been associated with a PCOS-like picture,[2079] although, in general, the hypothalamic-pituitary-gonadal axis is sufficiently robust to accommodate various frequencies of GnRH secretion.[2080]

HCG and human menopausal gonadotropin can be used as effective substitutes for recombinant human pituitary LH and FSH to produce full gonadal maturation, but again, this regimen is cumbersome and expensive.[2081] Thus long-term gonadal steroid replacement therapy is the treatment of choice for hypothalamic or pituitary gonadotropin deficiency until fertility is desired.[2082]

Hypergonadotropic hypogonadism is treated by replacement of testosterone in boys and estradiol in girls. For treatment of gonadal dysgenesis, estrogen therapy should be initiated when the patient is age 13 (bone age more than 11 years) to allow secondary sexual development at an appropriate chronologic age. The Klinefelter's syndrome is compatible with varying degrees of masculinization at puberty; some but not all patients require testosterone replacement. The concentration of plasma testosterone and LH should be monitored every 6 months during puberty and yearly thereafter. If the LH level rises more than 2.5 SD above the mean value or the testosterone level decreases below the normal range for age, testosterone replacement therapy is indicated. FSH will be increased due to lack of inhibin from affected testes.

Patients receiving gonadal steroid replacement follow the same treatment regimen whether the diagnosis is hypogonadotropic hypogonadism or hypergonadotropic hypogonadism (see Tables 24–32 and 24–33). Various testosterone preparations are available with several routes of administration as noted under the treatment of CDP above (reviewed in reference 2083). Alkylated testosterone preparations are to be avoided because of the risk of peliosis hepatitis (hemorrhagic liver cysts), which are not related to dose or duration of treatment; while regression is possible with discontinuation of testosterone treatment, progression to liver failure can occur.[2042,2043] Males may receive testosterone enanthate, propionate, or cypionate, 50-100 mg every 4 weeks IM at the start although priapism is reported with the higher starting dose in a testosterone naïve boy; later the dosage is gradually increased to 200 to 300 mg every 2 to 3 weeks. Low-dose replacement therapy is appropriate until well into the pubertal growth spurt[332] (also see Chapters 13 and 14). Testosterone may be administered by cutaneous patch on scrotal skin or nonsexual skin to cause secondary sexual development in hypogonadal adolescents; patches may be given at night to recreate the diurnal variation of testosterone seen in early puberty. Physiologic values of serum testosterone may be reached with these patches along with secondary sexual development.[2052,2084] A teenage boy may be less likely to apply a patch daily and biweekly or monthly injections may allow better compliance; nonetheless, we and others find 2.5-mg and 5-mg dermal testosterone patches may be useful in motivated teenagers. New testosterone gel preparations, usually rubbed onto the forearms, are approved for adults but not for adolescents as yet. Testosterone ointment may be used as therapy for microphallus to enlarge the size of the phallus intentionally[2085] but an infant contacting the skin of an individual with testosterone gel (before it is absorbed into the intended subject's skin) runs the risk of unplanned testosterone effects.[2086,2087]

Initially, girls age 12 to 13 are given ethinyl estradiol, 5 μg/day orally, or conjugated estrogens, 0.3 mg/day by mouth, on the first 21 days of the month for about 6 months. The dose is gradually increased over the next 2 to 3 years to 10 μg of ethinyl estradiol or 0.6 to 1.25 mg of conjugated estrogen for the first 21 days of the month. The maintenance dose should be the minimal amount to maintain secondary sexual characteristics, sustain withdrawal bleeding, and prevent osteoporosis. After breakthrough bleeding occurs, or no later than 6 months after the start of cyclic therapy, a progestogen (e.g., medroxyprogesterone acetate, 5 mg/day) is added on days 12 through 21 of the month. Undesirable effects are uncommon but may include weight gain, headache, nausea, peripheral edema, and mild hypertension. The benefits of transdermal estrogen treatment is discussed above. Recently, application of portions of transdermal 17β estradiol patches at night were shown to mimic levels of estrogen produced in early puberty and to slowly bring about breast development.[2058] Other therapeutic schedules are possible.[2059,2061,2088,2089] Estradiol gel in increasing dose from 0.1 to 1.5 mg over a 5-year period is reported to be safe and effective as replacement therapy in girls with Turner's syndrome.[2090] As with testosterone, there must be care that the preparation is not placed in contact with young children or else untoward estrogen effects may occur. Patches and gels are not approved for use in adolescents as yet.

There is a concern about the increased risk of endometrial and breast carcinoma in patients receiving long-term estrogen replacement therapy including patients with Turner's syndrome (see Chapter 23). The use of progestational agents to antagonize the effect of estrogens reduces the risk of endometrial cancer, but the best answer as to the optimal dose of estrogen and progesterone to enhance development without unduly increasing the risk of cancer must come from future studies (see Chapter 23). Estrogen replacement is important for its antiosteoporosis action on bone. Bone density is decreased in Turner's syndrome, at least in part, because of hypogonadism at puberty, and this tendency becomes more severe with age in patients who discontinue or do not receive estrogen replacement therapy.[2091,2092]

Transdermal estrogen is shown to increase bone density in subjects with Turner's syndrome who have finished statural growth.[2060] Surprisingly, we lack adequate controlled studies on optional sex steroid replacement regimens in young adolescent women.

Biosynthetic hGH therapy in Turner's syndrome causes an increase in growth rate with an increase in final height approaching or reaching the lower range of the normal growth curves possible, especially with a dose higher than used in GH deficiency [see more detailed earlier discussion in the Turner's syndrome section]. Patients with hypopituitarism may complain of sparse pubic hair growth or, in girls, total absence of pubic hair. Pubic hair will thicken further in affected males with hCG treatment which adds the testicular contribution of testosterone to the exogenous testosterone therapy. GH therapy in GH- and gonadotropin-deficient males enhances the steroidogenic response of the testes to hCG administration.[2093] Furthermore, adolescent or young adult women have been given low dose (25 mg) of long-acting intramuscular testosterone every 4 weeks to stimulate the growth of pubic hair without virilization.[2094] Oral DHEAS treatment is suggested to improve pubic hair growth in hypopitutiary girls.[2095]

The result of treatment with testosterone in boys with radiation induced primary testicular failure is normal final height although in patients with concomitant spinal irradiation, the upper to lower segment ratio was very much reduced, indicating impaired spinal growth.[2096]

SEXUAL PRECOCITY

Sexual precocity (Table 24–34) may be considered as the appearance of any sign of secondary sexual maturation below the lower limits of the normal onset of puberty: 9 years for boys, 7 years for Caucasian girls, and 6 years for African-American

TABLE 24–34 CLASSIFICATION OF SEXUAL PRECOCITY

TRUE PRECODIOUS PUBERTY OR COMPLETE ISOSEXUAL PRECOCITY (GnRH-DEPENDENT SEXUAL PRECOCITY OR PREMATURE ACTIVATION OF THE HYPOTHALAMIC GnRH PULSE GENERATOR)

Idiopathic true precocious puberty
CNS tumors
  Optic glioma associated with neurofibromatosis type 1
  Hypothalamic astrocytoma Gain-of-function mutation of GPR54 gene
Other CNS disorders
  Developmental abnormalities including hypothalamic hamartoma of the tuber cinereum
  Encephalitis
  Static encephalopathy
  Brain abscess
  Sarcoid or tubercular granuloma
  Head trauma
  Hydrocephalus
  Arachnoid cyst
  Myelomeningocele
  Vascular lesion
  Cranial irradiation
True precocious puberty after late treatment of congenital virilizing adrenal hyperplasia or other previous chronic exposure to sex steroids

INCOMPLETE ISOSEXUAL PRECOCITY (HYPOTHALAMIC GnRH-INDEPENDENT)

Males
Gonadotropin-secreting tumors
  hCG-secreting CNS tumors (e.g., chorioepitheliomas, germinoma, teratoma)
  hCG-secreting tumors located outside the CNS (hepatoma, teratoma, choriocarcinoma)
Increased androgen secretion by adrenal or testis
  Congenital adrenal hyperplasia (CYP21 and CYP11B1 deficiencies)
  Virilizing adrenal neoplasm
  Leydig cell adenoma
  Familial testotoxicosis (sex-limited autosomal dominant pituitary gonadotropin-independent precocious Leydig cell and germ cell maturation)
  Cortisol resistance syndrome

Females
  Ovarian cyst
  Estrogen-secreting ovarian or adrenal neoplasm
  Peutz-Jeghers syndrome
In Both Sexes
  McCune-Albright syndrome
  Hypothyroidism
  Iatrogenic or exogenous sexual precocity (including inadvertent exposure to estrogens in food, drugs, or cosmetics)

VARIATIONS OF PUBERTAL DEVELOPMENT
Premature thelarche Premature isolated menarche Premature adrenarche Adolescent gynecomastia in boys Macro-orchidism
CONTRASEXUAL PRECOCITY

Feminization in Males
  Adrenal neoplasm
  Chorioepithelioma
  CYP11B1 deficiency
  Late-onset adrenal hyperplasia
  Testicular neoplasm (Peutz-Jeghers syndrome)
  Increased extraglandular conversion of circulating adrenal androgens to estrogen
  Iatrogenic (exposure to estrogens)
Virilization in Females
  Congenital adrenal hyperplasia
    CYP21 deficiency
    CYP11B1 deficiency
    3β-HSD deficiency
  Virilizing adrenal neoplasm (Cushing's syndrome)
  Virilizing ovarian neoplasm (e.g., arrhenoblastoma)
  Iatrogenic (exposure to androgens)
  Cortisol resistance syndrome
  Aromatase deficiency

GnRH, Luteinizing hormone-releasing factor (GnRH); *CNS,* central nervous system; *CYP21,* 21-hydroxylase; *CYP11B1,* 11-hydroxylase; 3β-*HSD,* 3β-hydroxysteroid dehydrogenase 4,5-isomerase.

Modified from Grumbach MM. True or central precocious puberty. In Kreiger DT, Bardin CW, eds. Current Therapy in Endocrinology and Metabolism, 1985-1986. Toronto: BC Decker, 1985:4-8.

girls (detailed on page 12). These cutoffs assume that there is no sign or symptoms of CNS disorders or other serious disease that might cause sexual precocity puberty. These guidelines, presented in a previous version of this chapter, are similar to those proposed by the Drug and Therapeutics and Executive Committees of the Lawson Wilkins Pediatric Endocrine Society.[248] Careful evaluation is essential at these lower age ranges in evaluating girls with only minimal, relatively nonprogressive signs of sexual precocity. As stated on page 13 there is controversy about these newer limits but if the cautions described are heeded, the limits are appropriate.

If sexual precocity results from premature reactivation of the hypothalamic GnRH pulse generator-pituitary gonadotropin-gonadal axis, the condition is complete isosexual precocity, or true or central precocious puberty (CPP), and is GnRH dependent. Pulsatile LH release has a pubertal pattern and the rise in the concentration of LH after GnRH administration is indistinguishable from the normal pubertal pattern of serum LH. If extrapituitary secretion of gonadotropins or secretion of gonadal steroids independent of pulsatile GnRH stimulation leads to virilization in boys or feminization in girls, the condition is termed *incomplete isosexual precocity* (ICP), *pseudoprecocious puberty,* or *GnRH-independent sexual precocity.* The production of excessive estrogens in males leads to inappropriate feminization, and the production of increased androgen levels in females leads to inappropriate virilization; these conditions are termed *contrasexual precocity* (or heterosexual precocity). Disorders causing sexual precocity are thus separated into those in which the increased secretion of gonadal steroids depends on GnRH stimulation of pituitary gonadotropins and those in which it is unrelated to activation of the hypothalamic GnRH pulse generator.

In all forms of sexual precocity, increased gonadal steroid secretion increases height velocity, somatic development, and the rate of skeletal maturation and, because of premature epiphyseal fusion, can lead to the paradox of tall stature in childhood but short adult height. Data on the final height in true precocious puberty are scarce (see Table 24–34), but several studies of untreated females with idiopathic central precocious puberty demonstrated a mean final height of 151 to 155 cm.[2097-2105] There are few reports of final height in boys with untreated precocious puberty (Table 24–35).[2098] In the boys followed to adult stature by Thamdrup,[2099] the mean height was 155.4 cm±8.3 SD and all were well below midparent height and far below the father's height.

Serum alkaline phosphatase reflects growth and IGF-I concentrations reflect the degree of sexual development rather than chronologic age as do most chemistry and hematology values.[2106] The serum concentrations of the propeptide of type III procollagen (P-III-NP) in normal puberty and in true precocious puberty parallel the normal pubertal growth curve and also parallel the changes in growth rate in children treated with GnRH agonists.[2107-2109] Blood pressure matches that of height- and weight-related normal subjects rather than age-matched normals according to the latest standards for blood pressure.[2110]

True or Central Precocious Puberty: Complete Isosexual Precocity (GnRH-Dependent Sexual Precocity)

In our series of over 200 patients with CPP,[2097] girls had true precocious puberty five times more commonly than boys, and the idiopathic form was eight times more common in girls than in boys (Table 24–36). Others report a 10-fold increased prevalence of precocious puberty in girls than boys.[2111] CNS abnormalities occurred at least as often as idiopathic true precocious puberty in boys, whereas in girls neurologic lesions were a fifth as common as idiopathic disorders. Thus it is essential to search for a CNS etiology for true precocious puberty, especially in boys as sexual precocity may be the only manifestation of a CNS tumor (Table 24–37).[1147,2097,2112,2113] However, most children referred for evaluation have the benign variants premature thelarche or premature adrenarche.[249]

TABLE 24–35 HISTORICAL CONTROLS OF UNTREATED CHILDREN WITH TRUE PRECOCIOUS PUBERTY

Reference	No. of Patients (Women/Men)	FINAL Ht (cm)*	
		Women	Men
Thamdrup[2099]	26/8	151.3 ± 8.8	155.4 ± 8.3
Sigurjonsdottir and Hayles[2102]	40/11	152.7 ± 8.0	156.0 ± 7.3
Werder et al[2105]	4/0	150.9 ± 5.0	
Lee[2103]	15/0	155.3 ± 9.6	
UCSF	8/4	153.8 ± 6.8	159.6 ± 8.7
Total	93/23	152.7 ± 8.6	155.6 ± 7.7

*Mean ± 1 SD.

From Paul D, Conte FA, Grumbach MM, et al. Long-term effect of gonadotropin-releasing hormone agonist therapy on final and near-final height in 26 children with true precocious puberty treated at a median age of less than 5 years. J Clin Endocrinol Metab 1995;80:546-551.

Long-Term Follow-up of True Precocious Puberty

Pregnancy has occurred in patients with true or central precocious puberty as early as 5 years of age[2114] (an unfortunate result of childhood sexual abuse). In our experience as well as others', normal pregnancies have occurred in women who had idiopathic true precocious puberty,[2115] a CNS abnormality triggering true precocious puberty,[2097,2102] or premature menarche. In the isosexual precocity of the McCune-Albright syndrome, there are also reports of adult fertility.[945,2116,2117] Recent report of 46 women studied 12.5 years after cessation of treatment with GnRH agonist revealed an adult height 1.6 cm or 0.3 SD below target height. There is no evidence as yet of reproductive impairment nor apparent PCOS or hirsutism.[2118]

Idiopathic True or Central Precocious Puberty

Girls of age 6 to 8 with the onset of puberty represent one end of the range of ages of the onset of normal puberty,[56] and are

TABLE 24–36 DISTRIBUTION BY SEX OF CHILDREN WITH IDIOPATHIC AND NEUROGENIC PRECOCIOUS PUBERTY

Series	IDIOPATHIC		NEUROGENIC	
	Male	Female	Male	Female
Thamdrup (1961)[2099]	4	34	7	11
Wilkins (1965)[945]	13	67	10	5
Sigurjonsdottir and Hayles (1968)[2102]	8	54	16	16
University of California, San Francisco (1981)*	13	121	26	45

*Unpublished.

TABLE 24–37 ETIOLOGY OF TRUE PRECOCIOUS PUBERTY*

Etiology	Number and Sex
Idiopathic	121F, 13M
Others causes	
CNS-hypothalamic tumors including hamartomas	11F, 15M
Arachnoid cyst	2F, 1M
Hydrocephalus	6F, 1M
Head trauma (child abuse)	1F
Perinatal asphyxia, cerebral palsy	3F, 1M
Encephalitis or meningitis	3F, 1M
Sex chromosome abnormalities (47,XXY; 48,XXXY)	2M
Nonspecific seizure disorder or mental retardation	26F, 16M
Degenerative CNS disease	3M
Congenital virilizing adrenal hyperplasia with secondary true precocious puberty	3M

*Data from University of California, San Francisco, Pediatric Endocrine Clinic.

From Kaplan SL, Grumbach MM. Pathogenesis of sexual precocity. In Grumbach MM, Sizonenko PC, et al, eds. Control of the Onset of Puberty. Baltimore: Williams & Wilkins, 1990:620-660. © 1990, the Williams & Wilkins Co., Baltimore.

examples the early example of normal variation just as those with constitutional delay in growth and adolescence fall in the older age segment of the distribution. The nature of the striking sex difference in the prevalence of idiopathic true precocious puberty (females>>males) in contrast to constitutional delay in growth and puberty (males>>females) is poorly understood. There may be a history of early maturation in families of the affected subjects.[1289,2119] Rarely, true precocious puberty is transmitted as an autosomal recessive trait in boys and girls.[2097,2120] A familial pattern was far more likely to occur in girls than boys.[180] However, most children develop CPP with no familial tendency and no signs of organic disease; these children have idiopathic CPP. This condition, which may be manifest in infancy (see Table 24–37), is commonly associated with electroencephalographic abnormalities.[2121] The age at onset in girls in about 50% of cases is 6 to 7 years, in about 25% it is 2 to 6 years, and in 18% in infancy (Fig. 24–64).[2097] Organic forms of true precocious puberty, especially if associated with hypothalamic hamartoma, has an earlier mean age of onset than the idiopathic form.[1162,2097]

In boys (Fig. 24–65), the testes usually enlarge under gonadotropin stimulation before any other signs of puberty are seen; in girls (see Fig. 24–64), an increase in the rate of growth, the appearance of breast development, enlargement of the labia minora, and maturational changes in the vaginal mucosa are the usual presenting signs, with variable manifestations of pubic hair depending on the age at onset. Progression of secondary sexual maturation may be more rapid than normal, but a waxing and waning course of development may occur.[2122] Spermatogenesis in males and ovulation in females often occur, and fertility is possible. The rapid growth is associated with the increased GH secretion and elevation of serum IGF-I levels due to stimulation by estradiol.[336,337,369,392] The ratio of bone age to chronologic age and the rise of IGF-I above normal values for age are predictive of outcome: more mildly affected children progress less rapidly and tend to maintain their target height, and may be a benign entity.[2123] Patients with slowly progressive or unsustained puberty have little or no loss of predicted final height[2122] and are characterized by the presence of normal or only slightly elevated estrogen and IGF-I concentrations.[2123] If height prediction is normal at the time of diagnosis rather than reduced, the patient does not require therapy.[2124-2126]

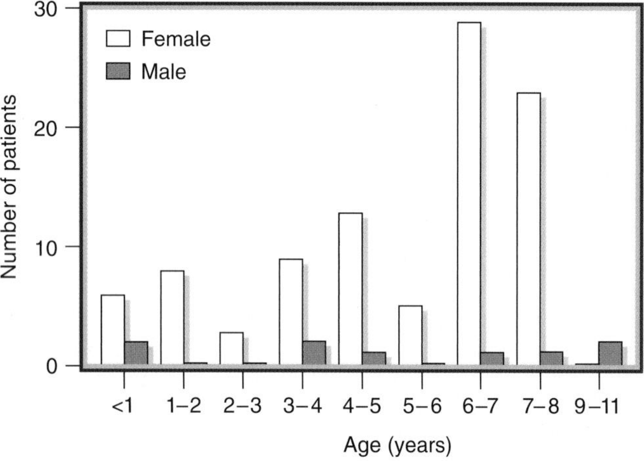

Figure 24–64 ■ Age at onset of idiopathic true precocious puberty in 106 children. Open bars, female; hatched bars, male. At all ages, the frequency is greater in females than in males. The peak prevalence in girls is between ages 6 and 8 years. (From Kaplan SL, Grumbach MM. The neuroendocrinology of human puberty: an ontogenetic perspective. In Grumbach MM, Sizonenko PC, Aubert ML, eds. Control of the Onset of Puberty. Baltimore: Williams & Wilkins, 1990:1-68.)

The uterus and ovaries increase in size in CPP. The ovaries also may develop a multicystic appearance (but not a polycystic appearance) that may remain even after successful treatment with a GnRH agonist.[2127] True precocious puberty in females does not lead to premature menopause. However, in girls there is increased risk for the development of carcinoma of the breast[184-187,189] in adulthood. Psychosexual development[2128,2129] is advanced only modestly in patients with sexual precocity (about one and a half years in girls with idiopathic true precocious puberty).[2130] The pituitary gland undergoes hypertrophy in early infancy, puberty, and pregnancy and also increases in size on MRI in patients with central precocious puberty.[269,2131,2132] T1-weighted images indicate a convex upper border of the pituitary gland in patients in normal or central precocious puberty indicating the similarity in the physiologic changes of both conditions. Pituitary gland hyperplasia (height greater than 1 cm) is a rare finding reported in central precocious puberty.[2133] The empty sella syndrome is less frequently observed in patients with central precocious puberty than in patients with pituitary hypofunction. While empty sella was found in 10% of children imaged for suspected hypothalamic-pituitary disorders including hypogonadotropic hypogonadism, the incidence in the general population is not known.[2134-2136]

The gonadotropin and gonadal steroid concentrations in plasma, the LH response to GnRH administration, and the amplitude and frequency of LH pulses are in the normal pubertal range (Figs. 24–66 and 24–67 and see Fig. 24–48).[814,1228,1237] The new third-generation gonadotropin assays allow the diagnosis of true precocious puberty by single serum sample determination for LH in the basal state or 40 minutes after a single subcutaneous dose of GnRH[2024,2137-2139] with high specificity and sensitivity. Adrenarche usually does not accompany gonadarche in girls with true precocious puberty younger than age 5 or 6.[1259] Pubic hair is sparse or absent initially in girls of this age. When the onset of true precocious puberty occurs after age 6, it is usually associated with early adrenarche for chronologic age but not for bone age.

A small proportion of patients with CPP, proven by a pubertal response of LH to GnRH and increased pulsatile LH secretion at night, may either revert spontaneously to a more immature pubertal state, persist without further progression, or fluctuate between progression and regression.[2097,2122,2123,2140-2142] There is a continuum in girls from premature thelarche through unsustained or slowly progressive precocious puberty to the relatively rapid progression of sexual maturation, once begun, in true precocious puberty.[2111]

CNS Tumors Causing True Precocious Puberty

Sexual precocity may be the first manifestation of a hypothalamic tumor of any cell type when it arises in or impinges on the posterior hypothalamus. However, neurologic symptoms such as headaches and visual disturbances may develop, and children may have DI, hydrocephalus, or optic atrophy caused by an enlarging tumor in addition to precocious puberty.[2097,2102]

CPP resulting from CNS tumors (Tables 24–35 through 24–38) has about the same prevalence in boys and girls; however, in boys, who have a lower overall prevalence of precocious puberty, neurologic abnormalities account for two thirds of those with true precocious puberty, and in our experience a CNS tumor was present in at least half of this group.[2097] A CNS neoplasm must be considered in the differential diagnosis of any patient with true precocious puberty.[945,1147,1386,2102,2143] The location of CNS tumors causing true precocious puberty makes surgical removal difficult. A conservative approach calls for

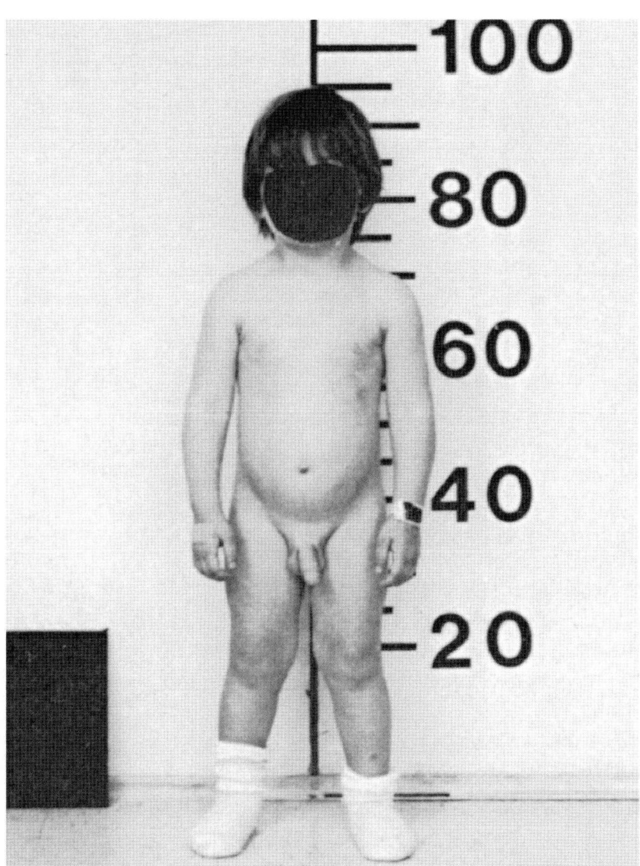

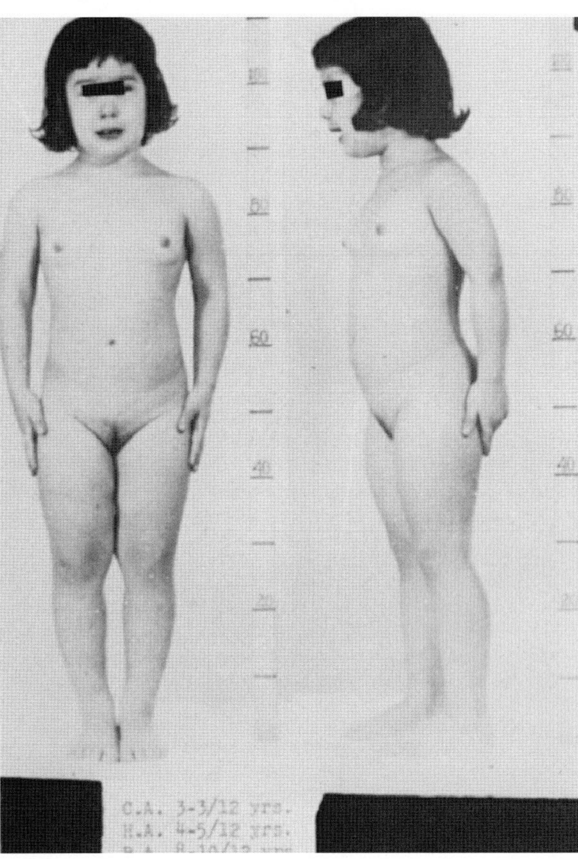

Figure 24–65 ▪ *Left,* A boy 2 years and 5 months of age with idiopathic precocious puberty. He had pubic hair and phallic and testicular enlargement by 10 months of age. At 1 year of age, his height was 86 cm (+4 SD); the phallus measured 10×3.5 cm, and the testes measured 2.5×1.5 cm. Plasma luteinizing hormone (LH) was 1.9 ng/mL (LER-960); follicle-stimulating hormone (FSH) 1.2 ng/mL (LER-869); and testosterone 416 ng/dL. After 100 µg of LH-releasing hormone (GnRH), the plasma LH increased to 8.4 ng/mL and FSH to 1.8 ng/mL, a pubertal response. When photographed, the patient had been treated with medroxyprogesterone acetate for 1.5 years. His height was 95.2 cm (+1 SD), the phallus was 6×3 cm, and the testes were 2.4×1.3 cm. Basal concentrations of LH (LER-960) were 0.9 ng/mL; FSH (LER-869) 0.8 ng/mL; and testosterone 7 ng/dL. After 100 µg of GnRH, LH concentrations rose to 2.3 ng/mL, whereas FSH concentrations did not change when he was on treatment with medroxyprogesterone acetate. For conversion to SI units, see the legends of Figures 24–21 and 24–22. *Right,* A 3 3/12-year-old girl with idiopathic true precocious puberty who had recurrent vaginal bleeding since 9 months of age. Height age, 4 5/12 years; bone age, 8 10/12 years. (*Left,* From Styne DM, Grumbach MM. Puberty in the male and female: its physiology and disorders. In Yen SCC, Jaffe RB, eds. Reproductive Endocrinology, 2nd ed. Philadelphia: WB Saunders, 1986:313-384.)

TABLE 24–38 CLASSIFICATION OF CENTRAL NERVOUS SYSTEM TUMORS ASSOCIATED WITH ISOSEXUAL PRECOCITY AT UNIVERSITY OF CALIFORNIA, SAN FRANCISCO

10% of all true precocious puberty patients: CNS tumors, hypothalamic (*n* = 26)
Males—IPP/organic precocious puberty = 13/15 =0.9/1
Females—IPP/organic precocious puberty = 121/11 = 12/1
GnRH-dependent true precocious puberty
Astrocytoma 3M, 5F
Hamartomas 3M, 3F
Neurofibromatosis 5M, 1F
Craniopharyngioma 2F
GnRH-independent incomplete sexual precocity
hCG-secreting tumor* 4M

*CNS and extra-CNS neoplasms.
IPP, Idiopathic true or central precocious puberty.

biopsy of the neoplasm and radiation or chemotherapy or both depending on the pathologic findings. Optic and hypothalamic glioma (often associated with neurofibromatosis),[2144] astrocytoma, ependymoma, and, rarely, craniopharyngioma may cause true precocious puberty, either by impinging on the neural pathways that inhibit the GnRH pulse generator in childhood or as a consequence of cranial radiation for therapy of a brain tumor.

The prevalence of CPP is increased after cranial radiation for local tumors or leukemia[342,1417,2145,2146] even if radiotherapy targets the pituitary gland.[2147] The combination of GH deficiency and central precocious puberty can occur in children previously subjected to therapeutic radiation of the CNS in association with a CNS neoplasm or, in those with a variety of CNS abnormalities, including developmental malformations and head trauma.[342] The lack of GH may not be apparent because of the increased growth resulting from the elevated gonadal steroid levels; GH-deficient children with CPP grow slower than GH-sufficient children with CPP but faster than GH-deficient children without

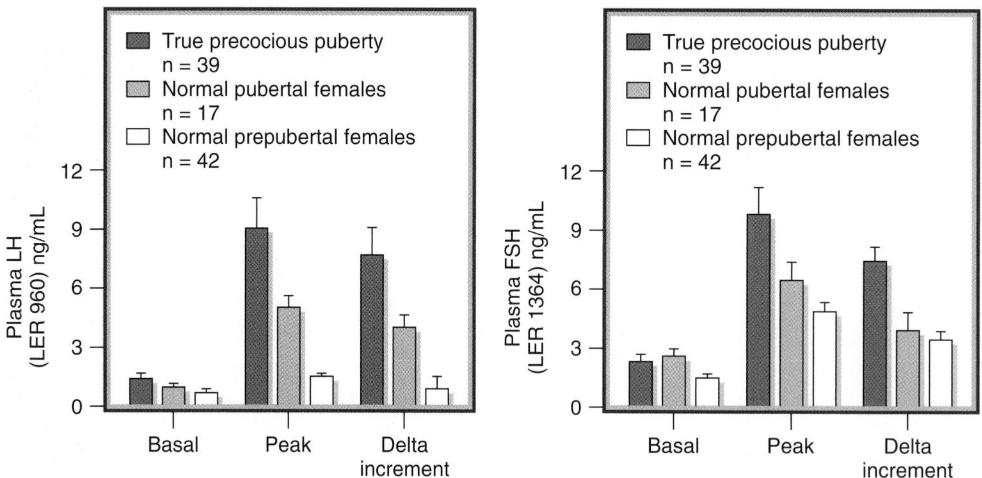

Figure 24–66 ▪ *Left,* Mean basal plasma luteinizing hormone (LH) level (LER-960) and mean peak and increment after intravenous LH-releasing hormone (GnRH) (100 μg) in normal prepubertal and pubertal females and in females with idiopathic true precocious puberty. The mean peak and increments of plasma LH are higher in true precocious puberty than in normal puberty. *Right,* Basal follicle-stimulating hormone (FSH) level (LER-1364) and mean peak and increment after intravenous GnRH (100 μg) in normal prepubertal and pubertal females with true precocious puberty. The concentration of FSH and the response to GnRH were greater in females with true precocious puberty and normal puberty than in prepubertal females. (From Kaplan SL, Grumbach MM. Pathogenesis of sexual precocity. In Grumbach MM, Sizonenko PC, Aubert ML, eds. Control of the Onset of Puberty. Baltimore: Williams & Wilkins, 1990:620-660.)

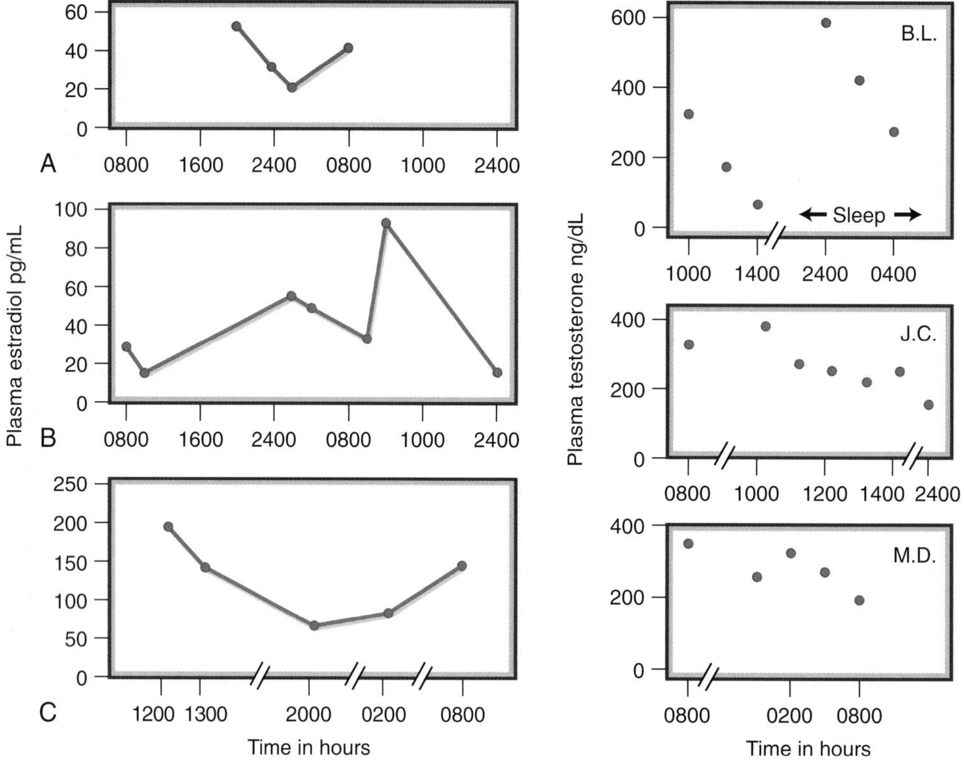

Figure 24–67 ▪ *Left,* Serial determinations of plasma estradiol in three girls with idiopathic true precocious puberty. Note the striking fluctuations in values. *Right,* Serial determinations of plasma testosterone in three boys with true precocious puberty (B.L. and J.C. have a hypothalamic hamartoma; M.D. has the idiopathic form). For conversion to SI units, see the legends for Figures 24–21 and 24–22. (From Kaplan SL, Grumbach MM. Pathogenesis of sexual precocity. In Grumbach MM, Sizonenko PC, Aubert ML, eds. Control of the Onset of Puberty. Baltimore: Williams & Wilkins, 1990:620-660.)

sexual precocity. GH-deficient children with CPP have IGF-I concentrations intermediate between the higher levels found in GH-sufficient children with sexual precocity and the lower levels found in the prepubertal GH-deficient children.[342] GH deficiency and true precocious puberty can occur with CNS radiation doses of only 18 to 47 Gy while gonadotropin deficiency, thyrotropin deficiency, and adrenocorticotropin deficiency usually occur with doses greater than 40 Gy, as does hypoprolactinemia.[342,2148] Treatment with a combination of GH and GnRH agonist is indicated in these patients with CDP and GH deficiency and results in better growth and improved height prognosis over the use of GnRH agonist alone.[1913,2149] Because GH secretion is related to BMI, it is important to rule out a decrease in GH secretion due to increased BMI in true precocious puberty before interpreting the decrease as evidence of GH deficiency.[2150]

Hamartomas of the Tuber Cinereum

These congenital malformations are composed of a heterotopic mass of nervous tissue containing GnRH neurosecretory neurons, fiber bundles, and glial cells—frequently associated with true precocious puberty (Fig. 24–68), usually before the patient is 3 years of age (Table 24–39).[1160,1677,2097,2151] Hypothalamic hamartomas may be sessile or pedunculated and are usually attached to the posterior hypothalamus between the tuber cinereum and the mamillary bodies. These masses project into the suprasellar cistern, and the pedunculated hamartoma has a distinct stalk; hamartomas present a characteristic appearance tat does not change with time as hamartomas of the tuber cinereum are not true neoplasms[1160-1162,2152-2154] in that long-term follow-up demonstrates lack of growth on monitoring by periodic CT or MRI scans.[1162,2155-2157] They appear on a CT scan or MRI as an isodense, abnormal fullness of the interpeduncular, prepontine, and posterior suprasellar cisterns, occasionally with distortion of the anterior third ventricle[2158,2159] although one case of pedunculated hamartoma was associated with a large craniopharyngeal canal and sellar spine leading to the appearance of a duplicated pituitary gland.[2160] The appearance and location have relationships to the clinical manifestation with distortion of the third ventricle more closely related to the occurrence of seizures.[2161] There is no enhancement with contrast material.[2162]

MRI using T2-weighted imaging gives the best visualization of the lesion (Fig. 24–69).[1162,2163,2164] However, the solid component of hamartomas may be missed when associated with a subarachnoid cyst if lower resolution MRI studies are invoked.[2165]

The etiology of the development of the hypothalamic hamartoma may be the converse of the lack of migration of GnRH

TABLE 24–39 CLINICAL AND LABORATORY CHARACTERISTICS OF CHILDREN WITH TRUE PRECOCIOUS PUBERTY CAUSED BY HYPOTHALAMIC HAMARTOMA

Characteristic	University of California, San Francisco (n = 12: 6M, 6F)	Hochman et al,* (n = 27: 18M, 9F)
Age at onset of pubertal signs		
Birth to 1 yr	4	6
1 to 2 yr	4	17
2 to 4 yr	3	6
7 yr	1	1
Neurologic signs		
Seizures including gelastic type	3/12	11/24
Headache and visual symptoms	1/12	5/24
None	7/12	7/24

*Literature review.

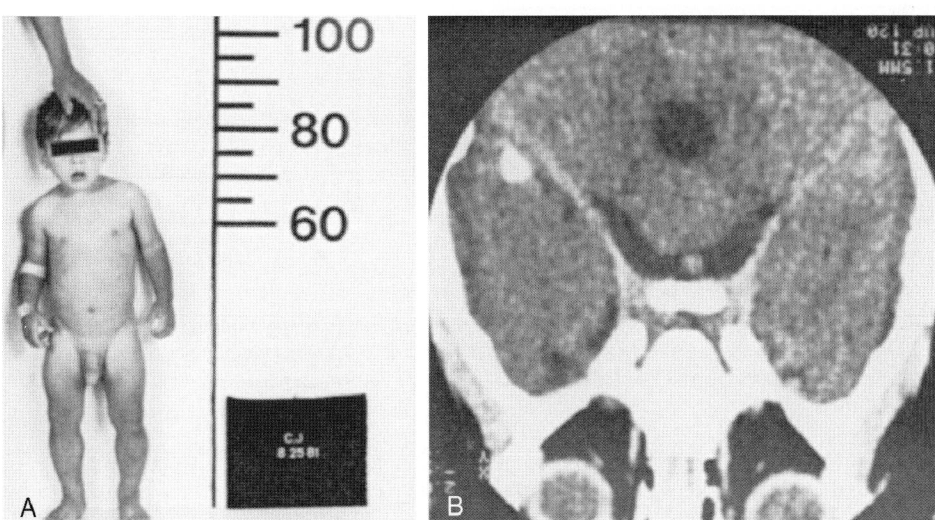

Figure 24–68 ■ **A,** A 17-month-old male infant with hamartoma of the tuber cinereum and true precocious puberty. At 8 months of age, secondary sexual development was noted, and the patient was misdiagnosed as having congenital virilizing adrenal hyperplasia. He was treated with glucocorticoids, which slowed his growth but did not affect his sexual development and bone age advancement. When he was first seen at 17 months, height was 84.2 cm; weight was 14.8 kg; the pubic hair stage was stage II; the penis was 10.4×2.2 cm; the testes were 1.5×2.8 cm; and the scrotum was thinned and rugated. The bone age was 4 3/12 years. After gonadotropin–releasing hormone (GnRH) administration, the LH level rose from 0.5 to 3.1 ng/dL (LER-960), the follicle-stimulating hormone (FSH) level from 0.5 to 1.2 ng/mL (LER-869), and the testosterone level from 409 to 450 ng/dL. Dehydroepiandrosterone sulfate (DHEAS) was 17 μg/dL (preadrenarchal value). The patient was treated with a potent long-acting LHRH agonist deslorelin (D-Trp^{6}Pro^{9}NEt-GnRH), which resulted in arrest of his pubertal advancement and a striking decrease in the plasma concentration of testosterone, LH pulses, and the response to exogenous GnRH. **B,** Computed tomographic scan of the patient, demonstrating a 1.5-cm mass posterior and rostral to the dorsum sella, which depresses the flow of the third ventricle. For conversion to SI units, see the legends for Figures 24–21, 24–22, and 24–40. (From Styne DM, Grumbach MM. Puberty in the male and female: its physiology and disorders. In Yen SCC, Jaffe RB, eds. Reproductive Endocrinology, 2nd ed. Philadelphia: WB Saunders, 1986:313-384.)

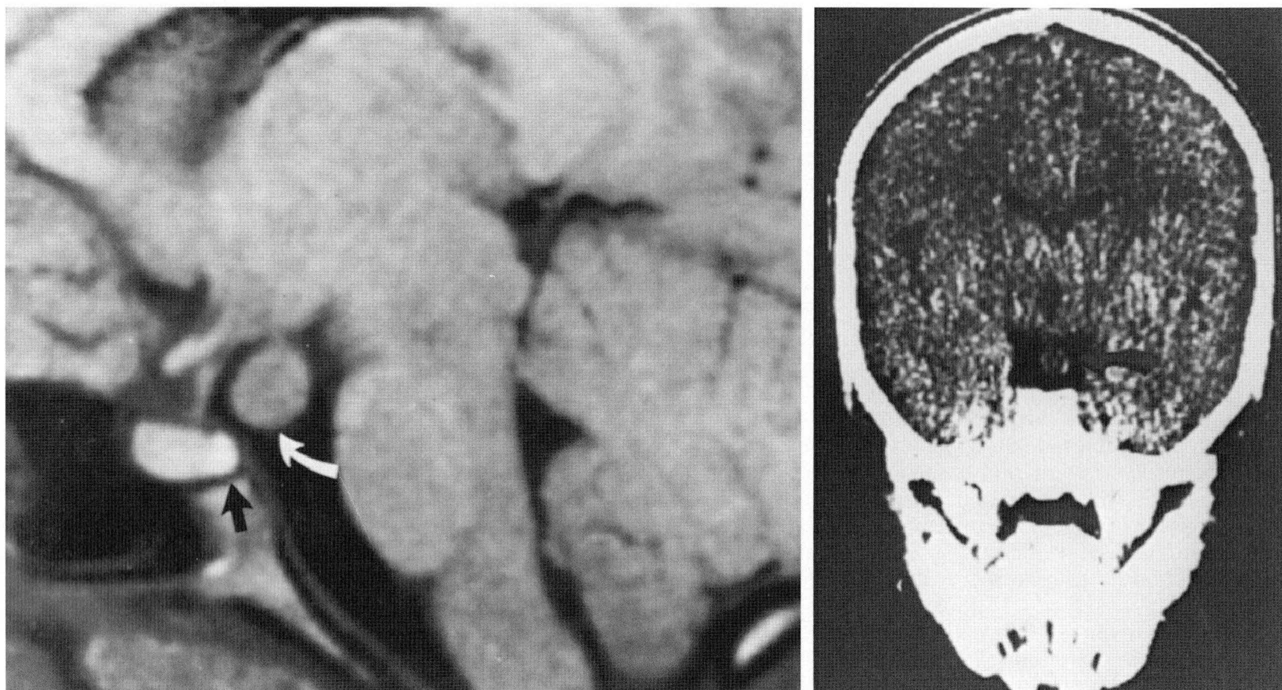

Figure 24–69 ▪ *Left,* Magnetic resonance imaging scan demonstrating a hypothalamic hamartoma *(solid white arrow)* in a 4-year-old boy with true precocious puberty; sagittal T1-weighted image. The posterior pituitary hot spot is designated by the solid black arrow. *Right,* Computed tomographic brain scan (coronal section) showing an isodense, pedunculated, collar button-shaped hypothalamic hamartoma *(arrow)* in a 2-year-old girl with true precocious puberty.

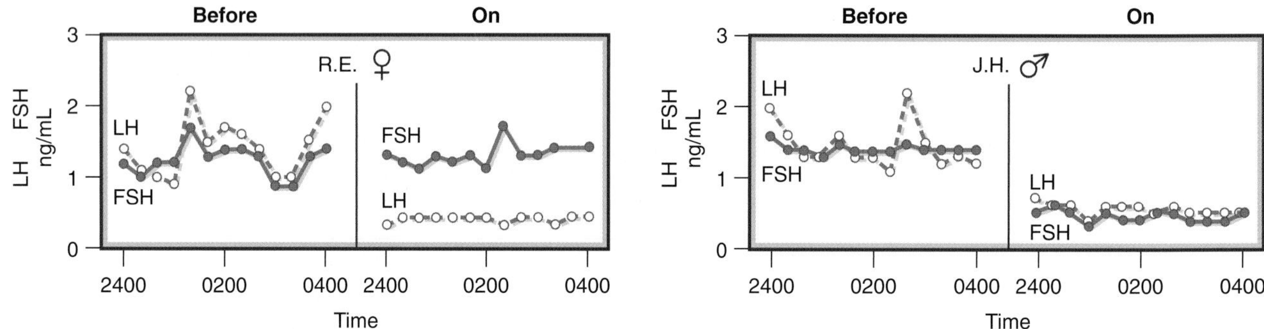

Figure 24–70 ▪ Pulsatile luteinizing hormone (LH) secretion before and during GnRH agonist therapy in a boy *(right)* and a girl *(left)* with true precocious puberty secondary to a hypothalamic hamartoma. For conversion to SI units, see the legend for Figure 24–21.

neurons in Kallmann's syndrome due to the lack of production of adhesion molecules coded by the KAL gene. We may postulate that in the hypothalamic hamartoma, the KAL gene protein among other axon-guiding factors may cause the majority of the total complement of 1500 or so GnRH neurons to migrate to the hamartoma or alternatively there may be a stimulus to progenitor cells capable of synthesizing GnRH to do so while located in the hamartoma.

Hamartomas associated with CPP contain ectopic GnRH neurosecretory cells similar to the GnRH-containing neurons in the medial basal hypothalamus. This developmental abnormality exerts its endocrine effects by the elaboration and pulsatile release of GnRH.[1147,2097] Indeed, GnRH-containing fibers have been identified passing from the hamartoma toward the median eminence.[2097,2152] We have suggested that the GnRH-containing neurosecretory neurons in the tumor are unrestrained by the intrinsic CNS mechanism that inhibits the normal GnRH pulse generator and act as an ectopic GnRH pulse generator,[787,939] either independently or in synchrony with the GnRH neurosecretory neurons in the medial basal hypothalamus to produce intermittent secretory bursts of GnRH[787] (see Fig. 24–42). The GnRH is transported to the pituitary by way of the portal circulation and elicits pulsatile release of LH (Fig. 24–70). If the hamartoma were to secrete GnRH in a continuous fashion, true precocious puberty should not occur as the GnRH receptors would be desensitized. (About 10% of hypothalamic hamartomas are not associated with true precocious puberty.)

The hypothalamic hamartoma of two young girls with rapidly progressive true precocious puberty did not contain immunoreactive GnRH neurons but the mass showed a network of TGF-α-containing astroglial cells.[2166] As discussed earlier (see page 54) this suggests that some hypothalamic hamartomas by virtue of the increased production of TGF-α, a member of the epidermal growth factor family and neuregulins synthesized by hypothalamic and astroglial cells through paracrine mechanisms, effect the release of bioactive factors including prostaglandin E2, which act on GnRH neurons to increase GnRH secretion. However, these hamartomas were much larger than the typical hypothalamic hamartoma associated with true precocious puberty,[1160,1162] as the mass bulged into the third ventricle in one girl, and in the other the pituitary gland was hypertrophic and bulged through the diaphragm sellae.[2166] Activation of the GnRH pulse generator through a mass effect and the compromise of restraint mechanisms may be the mechanism of CPP rather than TGF-α signaling. Thus, hypothalamic hamartomas are postulated to elict their effects by neurons able to produce GnRH within the HH, by the ability to control neurons synaptically connected to GnRH neurons or to neuronal networks including GnRH neurons in the HH itself or signaling-competent astrocytic and ependymoglial cells,[2167] although more studies are needed to clarify this hypothesis in humans. The precocious sexual development can be controlled by treatment with GnRH agonist therapy.[2156,2168,2169] Although some have advocated neurosurgical removal of these hamartomas for the occurrence of precocious puberty alone,[2170,2171] we do not recommend neurosurgical extirpation in the absence of strong evidence of growth of the mass or of an associated complication such as intractable seizures or hydrocephalus.[1147,1162,2097,2171-2173]

Before 1980 there were 37 patients in the literature with hamartomas of the tuber cinereum but since 1980 many more have been reported with the advent of CT and MRI brain scans[2151,2153,2174] (see Fig. 24–69 and Table 24–39).[2175,2176] Of girls with CPP at the NIH, 16% had a hypothalamic hamartoma, 40% had other CNS abnormalities, and 60% had idiopathic CPP. Of boys with CPP, 10% had idiopathic CPP, 50% had a hypothalamic hamartoma, and the rest had other CNS abnormalities including hypothalamic neoplasms.

Hypothalamic hamartomas that cause true precocious puberty can be associated with laughing (gelastic),[2177] petit mal, or generalized tonic-clonic seizures; mental retardation; behavioral disturbances; and dysmorphic syndromes beginning as early as the neonatal period.[1162,2151,2178-2180] Males are more likely to have seizures with these lesions. Seizures can be caused by a hamartoma in the absence of precocious puberty.[2161,2181] The occurrence of seizure is uncommon when the mass diameter of the hamartoma is less than 10 mm whereas a larger mass is associated with a high risk.[1162] Larger hamartomas are also associated with precocious puberty.[2157] Gelastic seizure are less amenable to antiepileptic therapy than other hamartoma related seizures and may require surgical treatment; endoscopic technique is increasingly employed.[259,2182-2185]

Refractory seizures have replaced precocious puberty as the main reason to perform surgery in cases of hamartomas of the tuber cinereum. In cases of intractable seizures, gamma knife procedures are another approach with reported success especially in small lesions.[2186,2187] The endocrine result of surgery on these lesion is rarely reported but one series of 29 subjects states that hypernatremia, low thyroxine, low growth hormone, and weight gain are encountered.[2188] Prior unsuccessful surgery may increase the risk for endocrinopathy in these patients. The postoperative endocrine disturbances appear to be transient, mild or asymptomatic, but increased appetite and weight gain appeared in 25% and may present an enduring problem. Although there are cases in which removal of a hypothalamic hamartoma has led to reversal of the pubertal process,[1160,2154,2174] deaths have been reported after attempted operative removal.[1160] We strongly recommend medical therapy with GnRH agonist in lieu of surgery for the treatment of precocious puberty associated with these hamartomas if seizures are absent or under control.

The Pallister Hall syndrome (PHS) is associated with polydactyly, imperfect anus, bifid epiglottis, and hypopituitarism with seizures.[2189] This syndrome is not usually associated with precocious puberty but one apparent case is reported as well as one with hypoparathyroidism.[2190]

Other CNS Conditions

CPP may occur secondary to encephalitis, static cerebral encephalopathy, brain abscess, or sarcoid granulomas or tuberculous granulomas of the hypothalamus, with or without tuberculous meningitis.[1413,2191,2192] CPP can occur after severe head trauma[2193] (usually in girls), and it has been associated with the cerebral atrophy or focal encephalomalacia, following cerebral edema complicating the treatment of severe diabetic ketoacidosis.[2194] Children with nontumor hydrocephalus, even if shunted, experience earlier pubertal development and those who have not been adequately treated may develop true precocious pub erty.[2191,2097,2195,710] Delayed puberty is an alternative outcome in a minority of affected children.[1412] The growth pattern of children with severe hydrocephalus often includes poor prepubertal growth and an early pubertal growth spurt leading to decreased final height.[2196]

Arachnoid cysts arising de novo, after infection, or after surgery can cause premature sexual development, possibly with associated GH deficiency.[787,2097,2197,2198] Head nodding, abnormal gait, and abnormalities of visual fields are reported in 30% to 40% of cases. Erosion or enlargement of the sella turcica into a J shape may occur. Decompression and extirpation of a suprasellar arachnoid cyst can reverse the sexual precocity (see Fig. 24–40).[787,2199,2200]

Neurofibromatosis type 1 (von Recklinghausen's disease) is associated with a propensity to develop the optic chiasmal tumors that are the most common,[2201] but not the only[2202] cause for a child with neurofibromatosis to develop CPP. Most optic gliomas appear in the first decade, but only about 20% to 30% become symptomatic; these tumors rarely progress in the years after diagnosis.[1079,2201,2203,2204] The tumor suppressor NF1 gene located on the long arm of chromosome 17 (q11.2), which has a high mutation rate, encodes a 327-kd protein, neurofibromin, which is widely expressed, even though neurofibromatosis 1 involves mainly tissues derived from the neural crest.[2205-2207] A wide variety of mutations of the gene have been reported, especially deletions, nonsense mutations, and truncating mutations distributed over the coding region of the NF1 gene.[2204] In sporadic cases, the new mutation originates in the paternally derived NF1 allele in the vast majority of instances, which suggests a role for genomic imprinting.[2208] Concentrations of midkine (MK) and stem cell factor, but not epidermal growth factor, were found to be substantially increased in serum of NF1 patients compared with healthy controls and serve as a diagnostic feature.[2209] Serum MK levels increase dramatically in patients older than 18 years of age, apparently as a feature of pubertal development. Because serum from NF1 patients enhance proliferation of human neurofibroma-derived primary Schwann cells and endothelial cells, enhanced circulating growth factor levels contribute to diffuse tumorigenesis in NF1.

Neurofibromatosis type 1 is characterized by multiple pigmented areas and overgrowth of nerve sheaths and fibrous tissue elements (Fig. 24–71).[1385,1386,2210,2211] Multiple café au lait spots are frequent and are smoother in outline (coast of California appearance) than those of the McCune-Albright syndrome (coast of Maine appearance). The diagnosis is made if two or more of the following are observed: (1) six or more café au lait macules, the greatest diameter of which is more than 5 mm in prepubertal and more than 12.5 mm in postpubertal subjects; (2) two or more neurofibromas of any type or one plexiform neurofibroma; (3) freckling in the axilla or inguinal region; (4) optic glioma; (5) two or more iris Lisch nodules (ophthalmic hamartomas that occur more frequently after the onset of

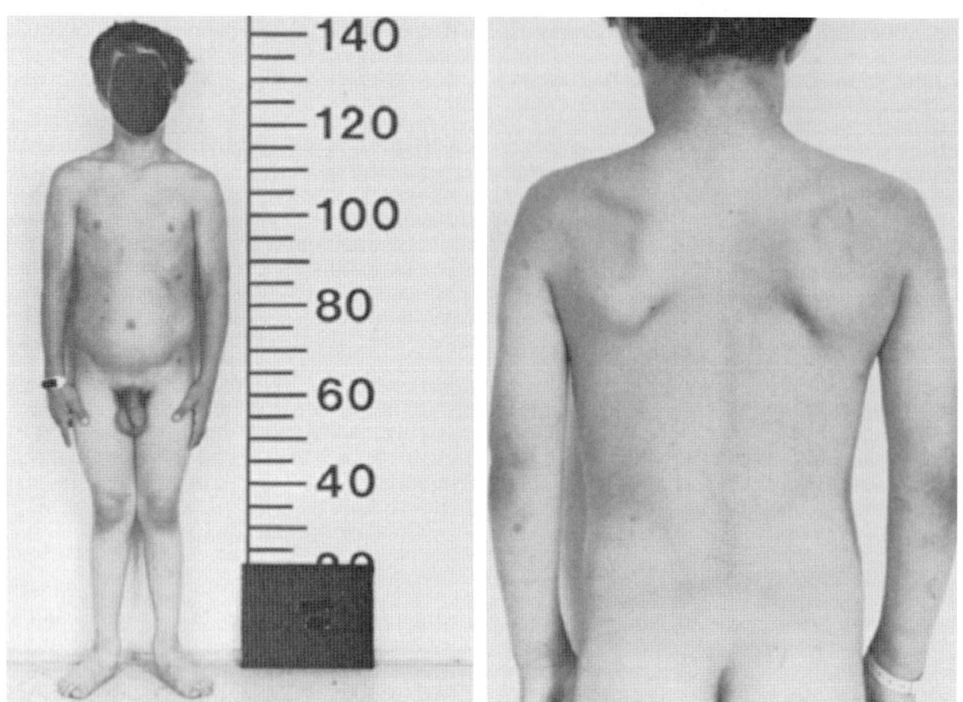

Figure 24–71 ▪ A boy of 8 years and 8 months with neurofibromatosis and precocious puberty, secondary to a hypothalamic glioma. He had tonic-clonic seizures at $2^1/_2$ years and rapid growth starting at 4 years; an enlarged penis and testes and the presence of pubic hair were first noted at $7^1/_2$ years. At this time, his height was 139.9 cm (+1.4 SD); the phallus was 9×3 cm; the right testis measured 5.5×3.2 cm and the left measured 5.4×2.9 cm. He had stage 3 pubic hair and 24 large café-au-lait spots. Computed tomographic scans and pneumoencephalography revealed a 1.5×2.5 cm hypothalamic mass, which was treated with radiation. The plasma concentration of luteinizing hormone (LH) was 0.5 ng/mL (LER-960); follicle-stimulating hormone (FSH) 0.4 ng/mL (LER-869); testosterone 221 ng/dL. After 100 μg of intravenous LH-releasing hormone (LHRH), the peak concentration of LH was 4.9 ng/mL, and that of FSH 1.4 ng/mL, a pubertal response. For conversion to SI units, see the legends for Figures 24–21 and 24–22. (From Styne DM, Grumbach MM. Puberty in the male and female: its physiology and disorders. In Yen SCC, Jaffe RB, eds. Reproductive Endocrinology, 2nd ed. Philadelphia: WB Saunders, 1986:313-384.)

puberty)[2212]; (6) a distinctive osseous lesion such as sphenboid dysplasia or pseudoarthrosis; (7) a first-degree relative with neurofibromatosis type 1 according to the preceding criteria.[2204,2211,2213]

Neurofibromas of the skin in neurofibromatosis may be subcutaneous sessile or deep plexiform masses in children; pedunculated lesions develop in later childhood. Internal neurofibromas cause most of the complications. Bone abnormalities such as cysts and pseudoarthrosis, hemihypertrophy, bowing, scoliosis, and skull and facial defects are common (20%); dumbbell-shaped tumors of spinal nerve roots may cause pain, sensory and motor dysfunction, and bone erosions; gliomas or neurofibromas of any part of the CNS, including the optic nerves and hypothalamus, may calcify. Lisch nodules of the iris are frequent, particularly in adults.[2204,2213] Sarcomatous degeneration occurs in 5% to 15% of patients. Other neoplasms include CNS astrocytomas often involving the visual pathways, ependymomas, meningiomas, neurofibrosarcomas, rhabdomyosarcomas, and nonlymphocytic leukemias.[2214] Pheochromocytoma may develop in affected adults.

The clinical manifestations of neurofibromatosis include seizures, visual defects, and either delayed or true precocious puberty.[2210] While some manifestations of NF-1 are quite common such as café au lait spots, found in 99% of a series of 297 subjects, precocious puberty is rarer, found in 3.2% of that series.[2215] Growth hormone deficiency is possible at presentation, but after radiation therapy for associated optic glioma, growth hormone, TSH, ACTH, and gonadotropin deficiency may develop.[2216] Developmental delay occurs more often in this population but usually is not severe.[2217] There is also an increased incidence of psychiatric disease.[2218] Most affected children have some manifestations of the disease by 1 year of age.[1385,1386,2207,2210,2211] Screening MRI scans are recommended for early detection of CNS tumors.

Other CNS abnormalities associated with true precocious puberty but without demonstrable lesions on imaging study include epilepsy,[2121] laughing seizures,[2219] mental retardation, and the posttraumatic state.[2220] Septo-optic dysplasia (described earlier) may be associated not only with multiple pituitary hormone deficiencies and delayed puberty but also rarely with true precocious puberty.[1539,2146,2221] Thus there may be coexisting deficiencies of some pituitary hormones and excessive secretion of others, including prolactin.[2222] Myelomeningocele (myelodysplasia) patients have an increased prevalence of endocrine abnormalities, including hypothalamic hypothyroidism, hyperprolactinemia, and elevated gonadotropin concentrations, which in some patients is associated with true precocious puberty.[1175,1552]

CPP in Children Adopted from Developing Countries[2223]

An increased prevalence of CPP occurred in children (with established birth dates) from developing countries adopted after 3 years of age into families in Sweden, Netherlands, France, and Italy[1725] and in children referred after suffereing kwashiorkor before to 3 years of age.[2224] As well as in the In Sweden, the adopted Indian children had pubertal growth spurts similar to those of Swedish children, but the loss of height in childhood and the early puberty appeared to be responsible for a decrease in adult height.[2225] As noted on page 3, one explanation for the CPP links the tendency to early puberty after SGA with a secondary influence of overweight or obesity decreasing the age of pubertal development.[12,13] A confounding factor in the study of adopted children is the finding that children of immigrant groups who have been born in their new country may have earlier puberty than the children of the predominant ethic group of that country; influences might be genetic or might be due to cultural and dietary differences but could complicate the analysis.[2227] Foreign children who immigrated to Belgium with their biologic families from developing countries had greatly elevated concentration of the organochlorine pesticide DDT derivative P,P'-DOE raising the possibility of a role for endocrine disrupters in their CPP, although this is unproven as yet.[2226]

The use of GnRH agonist in addition to GH treatment increased final height in at least two groups of affected children[17,1326] although this combination therapy may have drawbacks discussed above. One group of adopted children with early puberty benefited more from the GnRHa therapy than the added GH therapy but adult height was increased.[2228] The combination of adoption, living in a culture foreign to the background at birth, and precocious puberty makes these children vulnerable to psychic trauma, which must always be considered.[18]

True Precocious Puberty after Virilizing Disorders

Correction of longstanding virilization may be followed by development of true precocious puberty with activation of the hypothalamic-pituitary gonadotropin-gonadal system. This secondary true precocious puberty occurs in congenital virilizing adrenal hyperplasia with advanced bone age when glucocorticoid replacement therapy starts after 4 to 8 years.[426,945,1237,2229] CPP is also been documented in children who received or were exposed to androgens or estrogens for long periods during early childhood for a variety of conditions.

Marfan's Syndrome

Marfan's syndrome may be associated with tall stature and early peak height velocity and menarche[2230] compared to North American averages.

Management of True Precocious Puberty

Table 24–40, which addresses the major psychosocial and clinical goals of therapy for CPP.[2172] (See also reference 2231 for important psychosocial issues.) Three principal agents have been used in the medical treatment of true precocious puberty whether idiopathic or neurologic: medroxyprogesterone acetate, cyproterone acetate, and superactive GnRH agonists.

Medroxyprogesterone Acetate and Cyproterone Acetate

Medroxyprogesterone and cyproterone reversed or arrested the progression of secondary sexual characteristics but had no apparent or a small effect on final height, especially in affected girls,[2103-2105,1143] although more encouraging results from long-term treatment with medroxyprogesterone acetate on final height are reported more recently.[2232] Medroxyprogesterone acetate inhibits gonadotropin secretion by its action on the hypothalamic GnRH pulse generator-pituitary gonadotropin unit and has a direct suppressive effect on gonadal steroidogenesis through 3 beta-hydroxysteroid dehydrogenase 3β HSDII.[2233] Medroxyprogesterone acetate has glucocorticoid action and can suppress ACTH and cortisol secretion, increase appetite and lead to excessive weight gain, and induce hypertension and a cushingoid facies and appearance.[1147,2097,2234]

Cyproterone acetate has been used outside the United States for the treatment of true precocious puberty[2104,2105,2235] with advantages and disadvantages similar to those of medroxyprogesterone acetate.[1147] Cyproterone acetate has antiandrogenic, antigonadotropic, and progestational properties. Cyproterone acetate suppresses the secretion of ACTH and the plasma concentration of cortisol. Fatigue and weakness are common side effects, probably as a consequence of secondary adrenal insufficiency. This agent lacks gluconeogenic activity and does not appear to produce cushingoid features.

The long-term effects of either of these agents on fertility is not known. For the treatment of true precocious puberty, medroxyprogesterone, and cyproterone acetate have been replaced by the much more effective GnRH agonists; however, they may be backup agents for the occasional patients who develop untoward effects from GnRH agonist therapy.

Superactive GnRH Agonists

The GnRH agonists, synthetic analogues of the amino acid sequence of the natural GnRH decapeptide, are the treatment of choice for CPP of any cause (Tables 24–41 and 24–42).[2236,2237]

TABLE 24–40 OBJECTIVES FOR THE MANAGEMENT AND TREATMENT OF TRUE PRECOCIOUS PUBERTY

- Detection and treatment of an expanding intracranial lesion
- Arrest of premature sexual maturation until the normal age at onset of puberty
- Regression of secondary sexual characteristics already present
- Attainment of normal mature height; suppression of the rapid rate of skeletal maturation
- Prevention of emotional disorders and handicaps and alleviation of parental anxiety; promotion of understanding by counseling, early sex education, and acceleration of social age
- Reduction of risk of sexual abuse and early sexual debut
- Prevention of pregnancy in girls
- Preservation of future fertility
- Diminish the increased risk of breast cancer associated with early menarche

From Grumbach MM. True or central precocious puberty. In Krieger DT, Bardin CW, eds. Current Therapy in Endocrinology and Metabolism, 1985-1986. Toronto: BC Decker, 1989:4-8.

TABLE 24–41 ACTION OF GONADOTROPIN-RELEASING HORMONE AGONISTS IN TRUE PRECOCIOUS PUBERTY

- A selective, highly specific pharmacologic clamp on the secretion of gonadotropin that produces a "medical gonadectomy"
  - Chronic administration induces desensitization of the pituitary gonadotrope to the action of endogenous GnRH
- As a consequence
  - Inhibition of pulsatile secretion of LH and FSH
  - Inhibition of gonadotropin secretion results in a striking decrease in gonadal steroid output by testes or ovaries and reduction in gonadal size

TABLE 24–42 GONADOTROPIN–RELEASING HORMONE AGONISTS: PHARMACOLOGIC TREATMENT OF TRUE PRECOCIOUS PUBERTY

Structure of Natural GnRH and Substitutions in GnRH Agonist Analogues			Relative Potency	Formula	Dosage Form	Dose	References
<Glu-His-Pro-Ser-Trp-Gly-Leu-Arg-Pro-Gly-NH_2> 1 2 3 4 5 6 7 8 9 10			1	GnRH			
Deslorelin	D-Trp^6	–NEt	150	[D-Trp^{6}Pro^{9}NEt]GnRH	Subcutaneous Depot-intramuscular	4-8 μg/kg/day	1147, 2176, 2168, 2242, 2243, 2246, 2248, & 2700
Nafarelin	D-Nal(2)^6		150	[D-Nal(2)^{6}Pro^{9}NEt]GnRH	Subcutaneous	4 μg/kg/day	1147, 2248
					Intranasal	800-1600 μg/day	1147, 2248, 2243
Leuprolide	D-Leu^6	-NEt	20	[D-Leu^6-Pro^{9}NEt]GnRH	Subcutaneous	20-50 μg/kg/day	2701
					Depot-intramuscular	140-300 μg/kg/mo	2284, Kaplan and Grumbach 1991*
Buserelin	D-Ser(tBu)^6	-NEt	20	[D-Ser(tBu)^{6}Pro^{9}NEt]GnRH	Subcutaneous	20-40 μg/kg/day	2244, 2252, 2702 & 2703
					Intranasal	1200-1800 μg/day	2244, 2247, 2703, 2704, 2705, 2706
Tryptorelin	D-Trp^6		35	[D-Trp^6]GnRH	Subcutaneous	20-40 μg/kg/day	2708
					Depot-instramuscular	60 μg/kg/mo	2287
Histerelin long-acting (12 month) pellet	D-His(Bzt)^6	-NEt	150	[D-His(Bzt)^{6}NEt]GnRH	Subcutaneous	8-10 μg/kg/d	Boepple and Crowley 1991*

*Not published.

GnRH, Luteinizing hormone–releasing hormone.

Modified from Grumbach MM, Kaplan SL. Recent advances in the diagnosis and management of sexual precocity. Acta Paediatr Jpn 1988;30(suppl):155-175.

After initial stimulation, these pharmacologic agents suppress pulsatile LH and FSH release, gonadal steroid output, and gametogenesis similar to the effects of continuous administration of natural GnRH, which suppresses gonadotropin secretion[947,967,1254] after an initial, brief stimulation of gonadotropin release. The agonist binds to the GnRH receptor on gonadotropes, and desensitization of the gonadotrope to GnRH, downregulation, and loss of receptors follow. When receptor levels return to normal, desensitization persists as a result of uncoupling of the receptors from the intracellular signaling effector pathway.[956,957,2238] This regimen functions as a selective, highly specific pharmacologic clamp on the secretion of gonadotropins without interfering directly with release of the other pituitary hormones. In essence, the regimen produces a reversible medical gonadectomy (see Table 24–41). The superactive agonist analogues of GnRH have about 15 to 200 times the potency of the natural GnRH decapeptide, prolonged action, and low toxicity (see Table 24–42). Replacing the glycine-amide terminus of GnRH with alkyl amines, as in [Pro9-ethylamide(NEt)]GnRH, substituting certain D-amino acids at position 6, as in [D-Trp6]GnRH, and making bulky hydrophobic alterations at position 6, as in [D-Nal^2]GnRH, increase the potency and duration of action.[2239] These changes make the molecule more resistant to enzymatic degradation, increase the binding affinity of the analogue for the receptor on the pituitary gonadotrope, increase hydrophobicity, and, with some analogues, increase binding to plasma proteins.[956,957,1147,2239-2241]

The suppressive effects of the agonists on gonadotropin secretion make them useful in the treatment of true precocious puberty,[1147,2236,2242-2248] although they are also used in endometriosis and prostatic carcinoma. Various agonists are available (see Table 24–42). Presently, the depot formulation of leuprorelin (leuprolide acetate) is the only depot preparation that may be given every 4 weeks (there is a preparation that is given every 12 weeks approved by FDA for adults but not for children); long-term studies have established its efficacy and safety.[2236,2249-2251] The bioavailability of agonists given intranasally is much reduced,[1147,2252] as reflected in the need to use a high dose at more frequent intervals. The effectiveness of GnRH agonists in the treatment of true precocious puberty varies with the potency of the analogue, dose, route of administration, and compliance.[1147,2236,2248,2253-2257]

Treatment of CPP with a potent GnRH agonist results in 1 to 3 days of increased FSH and LH release and a rise in circulating gonadal steroid levels followed after 7 to 14 days of treatment by suppression of pulsatile secretion of LH and FSH and of the pubertal LH response to the administration of native GnRH (Figs. 24–72 and 24–73). The isoforms of gonadotropins tend toward a more basic charge (see Figs. 24–72 and 24–73). A plasma estradiol concentration of less than 18 pmol/L

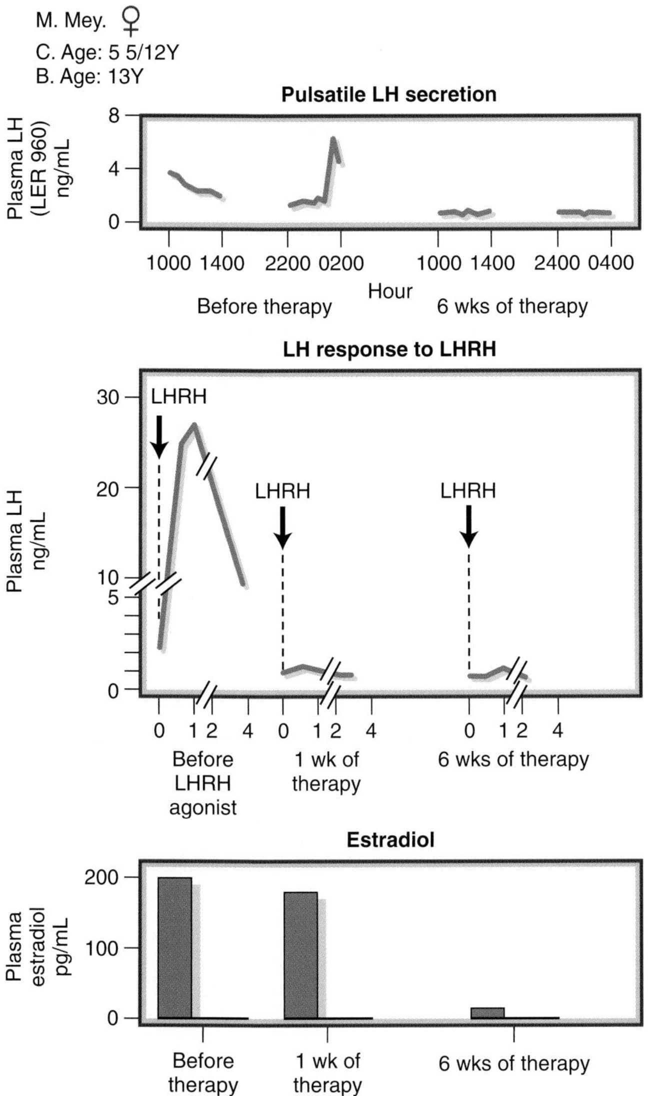

Figure 24–72 ▪ Effect of administration of the luteinizing hormone–releasing hormone (GnRH) agonist deslorelin (4 µg/kg/day subcutaneously) on pulsatile secretion of LH *(top)*, LH response to GnRH *(middle)*, and plasma concentration of estradiol *(bottom)* in a 5 1/12-year-old girl with idiopathic true precocious puberty. This patient, who had a bone age of 13 years when treatment was begun, has been administered deslorelin for 7 years. During this period, the estimated predicted final height increased by 15 cm. Surprisingly, the bone age advanced by only about 6 months on serial examinations for several years. For conversion to SI units, see the legend for Figure 24–17. (Modified from Grumbach MM, Kaplan SL. Recent advances in the diagnosis and management of sexual precocity. Acta Paediatr Jpn 1988;30[suppl]:155-175.)

(5 pg/mL) in girls and a plasma testosterone level of less than 0.7 nmol/L (20 ng/dL) in boys indicate adequate gonadal suppression in about within 2 to 4 weeks in girls and 6 weeks in boys. GnRH agonist therapy does not affect the secretion of adrenal androgens.[1147,2168,2242]

Changes in secondary sexual characteristics within the first 6 mo of therapy (Fig. 24–74) include reduction in breast size and decrease in pubic hair, cessation of menses if present before treatment, and decreased size of the uterus and ovaries as assessed by pelvic sonography in girls. Some girls have recurrent episodes of hot flushes and moodiness. In boys, pubic hair thins, the testes decrease in size, acne and seborrhea regress, penile erections and masturbation become much less frequent, the high energy level and aggressive behavior diminishes, and self-esteem improves.

Height velocity decreases about 60% during the first year of therapy. Skeletal maturation slows dramatically during the first 3 years, to a rate often less than the progression in chronologic age. From the second year on, height velocity for bone age is usually appropriate (Fig. 24–75). Bone age is suggested to represent a surrogate for growth plate senescence due to prior exposure to estrogens. Those with the longest courses before treatment, with the most advanced physical findings, and with the most rapid bone age advancement before therapy have the lowest growth velocities on treatment. Thus, the rate of growth on treatment with GnRH agonists is inversely related to the bone age at start of therapy[354] and best results occur when treatment is begun soon after the onset of precocity and when the bone age is advanced only a few years.[2236,2258,2259] There is a striking benefit to those children treated before 5 years of age (girls height 164.3±7.7 cm) compared to those treated after age 5 years (157.6±6.6 cm) and compared to untreated patients (152.7±8.6 cm).[2098] Adult height in children treated with GnRH agonists are increased especially with therapy starting before 6 years of age than after 8 years of age (Table 24–43).[2098,2236,2260-2269] An adult height within target height occurs in about 90% of girls and boys.[2270] We recommend the treatment of all affected children in whom puberty began before 6 years of age to ensure an optimal prognosis for adult height. The age which is optimal to discontinue therapy is still open to question in that the posttreatment growth spurt is important in determining adult height.[2271,2272]

The addition of hGH treatment to the GnRH regimen is a consideration when growth velocity is reduced sufficiently over a 6-month period to compromised predicted final height.[2273] This is in contrast to the concern raised over therapy with GnRH agonist and GH in normal variant short stature of CDP.

A preliminary study of GnRH antagonist (cetrorelix) appeared to bring about more rapid suppression of gonadotropin secretion and the elimination of the "flare-up" of gonadotropin secretion after administration of GnRH agonist.[2274] There are no publications at present concerning the use of cetrorelix as a sole treatment of precocious puberty but one unsual case of a girl with purported gonadotropin-independent precocious puberty who responded to this treatment brings up a possible direct effect of the agent on ovarian function.[2275]

Girls with CPP have a tendency toward obesity (a mean BMI greater than that of normal girls of the same chronologic age), unrelated to treatment with GnRH agonist.[2156,2276,2277] as there is no substantial evidence that GnRHa treatment fosters the development of obesity. The BMI before therapy predicts the BMI value after cessation.[2277-2279] However, a recent longitudinal study suggests that with adequate gonadotropin suppression, BMI for age may improve over at least 2 years of therapy.[2280] Serum leptin in precocious puberty remains in line with average children of similar BMI and pubertal development.[2281]

The IGF-I concentration in CPP correlates best with the stage of puberty and the plasma concentration of testosterone or estradiol.[392] Treatment with GnRH agonists reduces the level of IGF-I to the normal range for bone age but not for chronologic age.[392] Gonadal steroids increase plasma IGF-I concentrations in true precocious puberty as well as in normal puberty. Secretion of GH is increased in true precocious puberty to a level comparable to that in normal puberty.[369,2282] Treatment with GnRH agonists usually results in a decrease in GH secretion, most strikingly during sleep, and in a decrease in GH response to provocative stimuli. It is suggested that the serum concentration of GH and GHBP activity is a better reflection of the suppression of growth velocity with GnRH agonist than is serum IGF-I and IGFBP-3.[2283,2284]

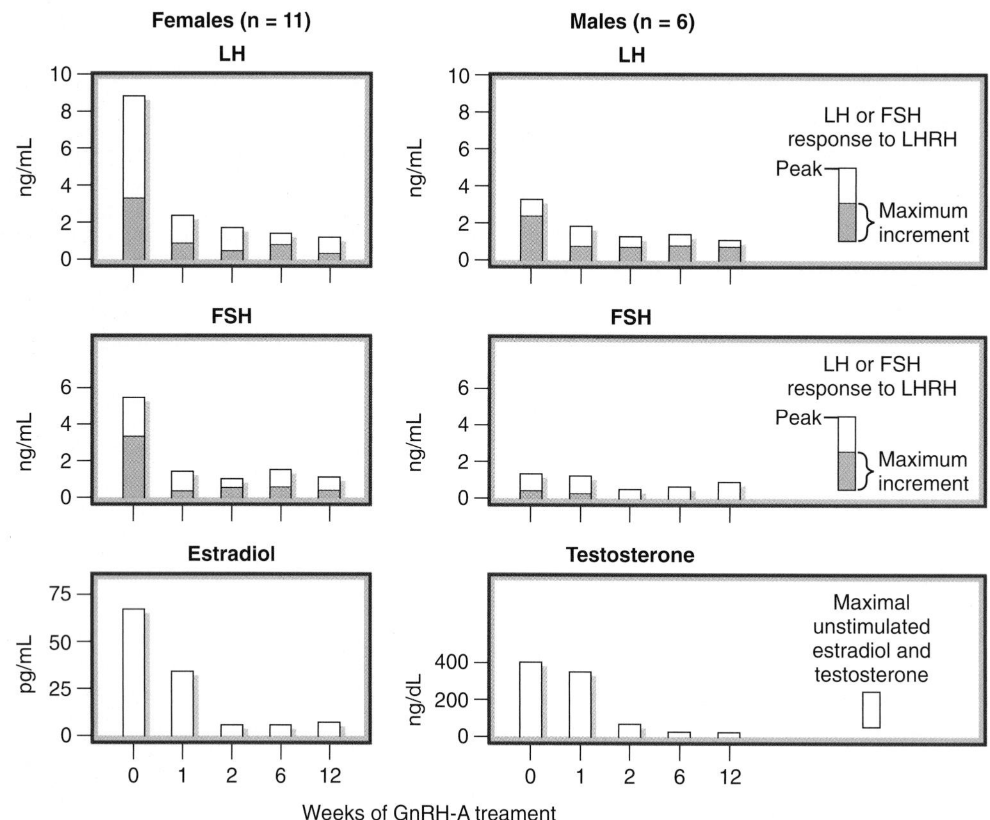

Figure 24–73 ▪ Deslorelin treatment (4 μg/kg/day subcutaneously) of girls and boys with true precocious puberty: effect during the first 12 weeks of treatment on the luteinizing hormone (LH) and follicle-stimulating hormone (FSH) response to a challenge with LH-releasing hormone (GnRH) (mean peak response and maximum increment) and on the maximal unstimulated concentration of plasma estradiol in the girls and of plasma testosterone in the boys. Note the relatively rapid change from pubertal values to prepubertal values. For conversion to SI units, see the legends of Figures 24–21 and 24–22. (From Styne DM, Harris DA, Egli CA, et al. Treatment of true precocious puberty with a potent luteinizing hormone releasing factor agonist: effect on growth, sexual maturation, pelvic sonography, and the hypothalamic pituitary gonadal axis. J Clin Endocrinol Metab 1985;61:142-181. Copyright by The Endocrine Society.)

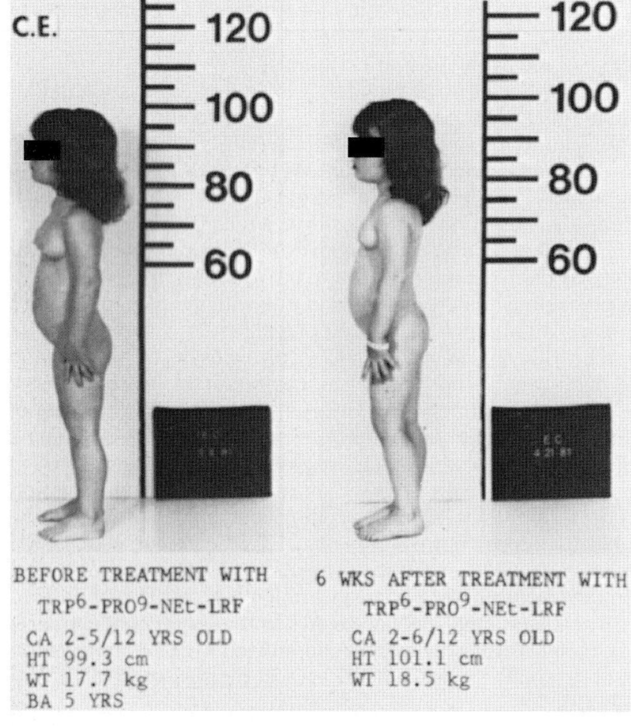

Figure 24–74 ▪ A 2 5/12-year-old girl with true precocious puberty after 6 weeks of deslorelin therapy (4 μg/day subcutaneously). Note the regression in the size of the breasts; however, the rapid rate of growth had not decreased. At the end of 1 year of therapy, growth rate was suppressed to 4 cm/year, and bone age advanced only 1 year. *CA,* Chronologic age; *HT,* height; *WT,* weight; *BA,* bone age. (From Styne DM, Grumbach MM. Puberty in the male and female: its physiology and disorders. In Yen SCC, Jaffe RB, eds. Reproductive Endocrinology, 2nd ed. Philadelphia: WB Saunders, 1986:313-384.)

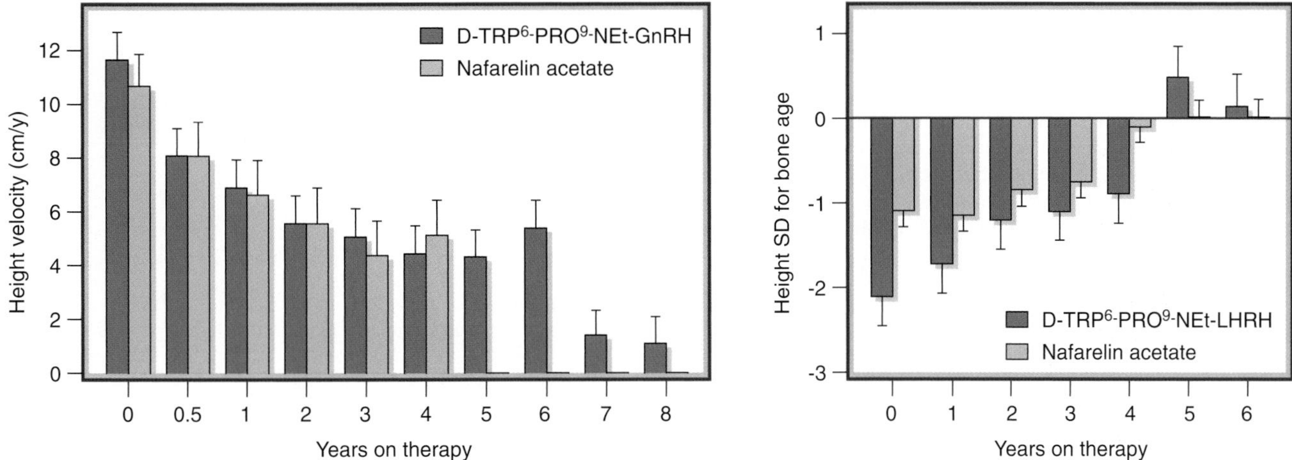

Figure 24–75 ▪ Effect of Gonadotropin–releasing hormone (GnRH) agonist therapy in true precocious puberty on growth. *Left,* Changes in mean height velocity (cm/year±1 SE) after the initiation of GnRH agonist therapy with DTrp[6]Pro[9]Net (GnRH) (deslorelin) *(filled bars)* or with nafarelin *(hatched bars)*. A sharp decrease in height velocity occurred within 1 year. *Right,* Mean (±1 SE) height for bone age before and during GnRH agonist treatment. The discrepancy between height and the more advanced bone age decreases (reverts to normal) with chronic GnRH agonist treatment. (From Kaplan SL, Grumbach MM. True precocious puberty: treatment with GnRH agonists. In Delemarre-Van de Waal H, Plant TM, van Rees GP, et al, eds. Control of the Onset of Puberty III. Amsterdam: Elsevier, 1989:357-373.)

TABLE 24–43 COMPARISON OF CURRENT HEIGHT (ADULT OR NEAR ADULT) AND HEIGHT GAIN OF GONADOTROPIN–RELEASING HORMONE AGONIST–TREATED PATIENTS

	No. of Patients	MEAN CURRENT HT (CM) Female	Male	Mean Ht Gain (cm)[a]
Untreated[b]				
Total	116	152.7 ± 8.6	155.6 ± 7.7	
<5 yr	41	150.2 ± 7.6	153.3 ± 7.1	
>5 yr	75	153.4 ± 8.4	161.3 ± 6.0	
GnRH-treated[d]				
UCSF	26	160.5 ± 6.6	166.3 ± 12.2	
<5 yr[c]	11	164.3 ± 7.7	172.1	10.0 (female); 11.1 (male)
>5 yr[c]	15	157.6 ± 6.6	163.3 ± 13.0	4.0 (female); 6.0 (male)
Ref.				
Oerter	40	157.8 ± 5.9	168.8 ± 8.3	5.2 (female), 6.7 (male)
Kaull	8	151.2 ± 5.9		5.8 (female)
Boepple	26	154.4		4.1 (female)

[a]Final predicted height—intitial predicted height (Bayley-Pinneau method).
[b]Final height.
[c]CA at start of therapy.
[d]Final or nearly final height.
From Paul D, Conte FA, Grumbach MM, Kaplan SL. Long-term effect of gonadotropin-releasing hormone agonist therapy on final and near-final height in 26 children with true precocious puberty treated at a median age of less than 5 years. J Clin Endocrinal Metab 1995;80:546-551.

The use of depot formulations of GnRH agonists provides continuous exposure to the agonist with a single IM injection every 4 weeks (or 12 weeks in a formulation not yet approved for children and a new preparation of subcutaneous annual administration of GnRH agonist in a pellet type formulation) and minimizes the problem of poor compliance.[1966,2098,2285-2287] However, irregular or inadequate treatment or poor compliance results in persistent or intermittent increase in the concentration of plasma gonadal steroids. Regular assessment is essential, initially at intervals of 1 to 3 months, including periodic determinations of plasma testosterone levels in boys and estradiol levels in girls; the change in basal concentrations of LH and FSH in third-generation assays or the LH and FSH response to exogenous GnRH or GnRH agonists; measurement of growth, bone age, and secondary sexual characteristics; and in girls serial evaluations of ovarian morphology and uterine size by pelvic sonography. A decrease in the size of ovaries and uterus on pelvic sonography occurs with successful treatment with GnRH agonist.[2168,2288] Recently as GnRH became more difficult to obtain, evaluating the rise in serum LH and FSH 30 to 120 minutes after the administration of GnRH agonist was invoked.[2289,2290] LH and FSH responses to GnRH agonist suppress with effective therapy, but because standards for pubertal responses differ between laboratories, actual cutoff values may differ in clinical practice.

Whereas the urinary excretion of LH correlates with the stage of pubertal development in normals, urinary gonadotropin determinations are not sufficiently sensitive to be used for monitoring purposes.[1807] Regularly scheduled visits also provide the opportunity for continued counseling.

When treatment is discontinued, even after 8 years, gonadal suppression is reversed within a few weeks to months with a rise in the concentration of plasma gonadal steroids, progression of sexual maturation, and return of menses.[2262,2291,2156] Menarche occurred at an average of 1.2 to 1.5 years after discontinuing therapy (with a range of 0 to 60 months). Ovulation occurred in 50% of girls 1 year after menarche and in 90% of those studied, 2 or more years after menarche.[2292] Mean ovarian volume was found to be and to remain greater than in normals, and LH response to GnRH was below normal response.[2156,2270,2293] Results in boys with true precocious puberty after GnRH therapy was discontinued also confirm the reversible nature of the therapy in that gonadotropins in the basal or GnRH stimulated state return to normal pubertal values by 1 year after cessation of therapy.[2169] However, testicular size may take longer to reach normal values. In a long-term study, young adult women who had been treated for CPP with a long-acting GnRH agonist had normal adult pituitary gonadotropin-ovarian function.[2293a]

Before beginning treatment, it is essential to establish the rapidly progressive nature of the sexual precocity.[2126,2265] In a subset of girls, the tempo is relatively slow and the sexual precocity may not be sustained.[2097,2122,2248] The growth rate slows to normal for age, skeletal maturation progresses in accordance with chronologic age, and there is little to no risk of impairment of final height. In some girls we have observed within a 1- to 2-month period the return of a pubertal pattern of LH pulsatility during sleep, of a pubertal LH response to GnRH, and of the concentration of plasma estradiol to a pubertal state; unlike the typical patient, such girls do not exhibit the initial hyperresponse of plasma estradiol and LH to the GnRH agonist or the physical changes of estrogen effect and tend to have lower serum IGF-I.[2294,2295] Many girls in this subset have clinical and hormonal features that fall between those of premature thelarche and true precocious puberty and are typical of neither condition,[2296] so-called exaggerated thelarche. About 10% of girls with apparently classic premature thelarche will progress to definite true precocious puberty with no signs at the time of first presentation to differentiate them from girls who continued with the pattern of premature thelarche; the majority in this situation have the onset of breast development noted after 2 years of age.[2297] Therapy is not indicated if a pubertal pattern of pulsatile LH secretion during sleep is not present or if the basal LH measured in the ultrasensative assay or the LH response to exogenous GnRH of GnRH agonist is prepubertal (Table 24–44). The most severely affected girls are the ones who respond best to GnRH agonist therapy.[2265,2298]

Psychosocial factors and parental anxiety that adversely affect the well-being of the child need to be assessed in the decision to initiate GnRH agonist treatment.

Adverse Effects

Rare reactions to GnRH agonists include local and systemic allergic reactions, including asthmatic episodes when the agent is given intranasally. However, the prevalence of a sterile abscess at the site of intramuscular injection of long-acting repository preparations, including leuprorelin and triptorelin, is clearly increased (5% to 10%), unpredictable, and intermittent, and in most instances is related to the polylactic and polyglycotic polymer and not to the GnRH agonist itself.[2250,2299] Switching to daily subcutaneous injections of nondepot preparations or to intranasal preparations is rarely associated with a recurrence. A small increase in serum prolactin above normal limits is described in girls following treatment with GnRH agonist but not galactorrhea.[2300] Volumetric BMD and peak bone mass are normal during and after discontinuation of GnRH the rapy.[580,259,2262,2301,2302] Calcium and vitamin D intake must be ensured during treatment to achieve optimal skeletal health, and this must be routinely evaluated.[2303] However, high fruit and vegetable intake (defined in this study as more than 3 servings per day, lower than the U.S. government recommends) is desirable in all children and may serve in early puberty as a factor to increase bone density, possibly due to decreasing calcium excretion in the urine.[2304]

Four patients developed slipped capital femoral epiphyses during or just after treatment of CPP with GnRH agonist.[2305,2306] Slipped capital epiphyses (SCFE) occurs mostly during the earliest phase of puberty when growth is beginning to increase and does not occur after fusion of the triradiate cartilage,[2307] so these cases may have a different etiology (SCFE) than found in average pubertal children.

TABLE 24–44 INDICATIONS FOR THERAPY WITH GONADOTROPIN-RELEASING HORMONE AGONISTS IN TRUE OR CENTRAL PRECOCIOUS PUBERTY

In children with clinical and unequivocal endocrine features of idiopathic true precocious puberty:
- Rapid advancement over a period of 6 mo to 1 yr of secondary sex characteristics, height, height velocity, and bone age (increased >2.5 SD for chronologic age) in affected boys and girls
- A plasma testosterone concentration sustained >2.5 nmol/L (>75 ng/dL) in boys younger than 8 yr of age determined by sensitive, specific immunoassay
- A plasma estradiol, recurrently ≥36 pmol/L (≥10 pg/mL) determined by a sensitive, specific assay capable of quantifying low concentrations of estradiol
- Onset of menarche (and recurrent menses) in girls younger than 9 yr of age
- Psychosocial factors and parental anxiety, including evidence that the child's psychosocial well-being is adversely affected

In children with neurogenic or organic true precocious puberty, especially those with associated GH deficiency, the course is almost invariable progressive and LHRH treatment should not be delayed

Psychosocial Aspects

Psychological management is a critical aspect of the care of children with true precocious puberty.[1147,2034,2172,2308] With the advanced physical maturation for chronologic age, these children tend to seek friends closer to their size, strength, and physical development. Difficulties may arise because they lack the social skills of older children. Sex education of the child and the family is essential and must be given in a skillful, sensitive, and explicit manner; the risks of sexual abuse in both sexes and of pregnancy in girls need to be discussed. The parents need to be informed about the management of menses. The onset of sexual activity may be earlier than average, but generally remains within the normal range.[2128] It is imperative to provide support in handling the increased height, the advanced sexual maturation, and the effects of gonadal steroids on behavior, activity, and emotional stability. The unrealistic demands and expectations that arise from the discrepancy between the physique and the chronologic, mental, and psychosexual age require wise counseling, as do the reaction to ridicule by peers and the concern about being different from age mates. Some of these problems have been mitigated by school acceleration, advancing the child one or two grades, if this is consistent with the mental and emotional development. These comments are applicable to children with all forms of sexual precocity. The effectiveness of GnRH agonists has reduced but not eliminated many of these issues in true precocious puberty.[2172]

The GnRH agonists are useful in conjunction with GH in the management of patients with organic or neurogenic true precocious puberty, especially those with associated GH deficiency (usually as a result of radiation of the brain) and has been advocated even in the absence of precocious puberty[2309] to allow a longer period of GH treatment before epiphyseal fusion.[2310,2066] A few, usually short-term, studies utilized the combination with variable results. This regimen is experimental; its cost effectiveness needs to be considered (see above in the section considering the hormone control of the pubertal growth spurt).[1327,1330,1331,1336,2311-2314] However, concern over the use of GnRH agonsts in children with short stature but not precocious puberty raises concern about decreasing adult bone density so this combination cannot recommended.[1319] On the other hand, the combination of GnRH agonist and GH is useful to increase adult height in GH-deficient patients of pubertal age,[1325] although the effects on bone density must be considered.

GnRH agonists are effective in both boys and girls with idiopathic true precocious puberty, the androgen-induced form of secondary true precocious puberty following therapy of virilizing congenital adrenal hyperplasia with glucocorticoids, and organic or neurogenic forms of true precocious puberty associated with hamartomas of the tuber cinereum, hypothalamic neoplasms, and other CNS lesions.[2168,2242,2315] Although there are reports in the literature of surgical removal of hamartomas of the tuber cinereum,[1161,2154,2174,2316-2319] the ease of medical treatment of the sexual precocity associated with this congenital malformation, the finding that the mass does not enlarge on MRI or CT brain scans, and the risks of an adverse outcome of surgical intervention in this region of the CNS[1161] support the choice of GnRH agonists over surgical intervention (see above).

An aromatase inhibitor, such as letrozole, will decrease or eliminate the effect of estrogen on bone age advancement. This effect may be useful to improve height prognosis in sexual precocity in boys.[336,337,1339,1341,2320-2322] Controlled studies are necessary to establish safety and efficacy and, especially, effects on adult bone density (Table 24–45).

TABLE 24–45 POTENTIAL USE OF AROMATASE INHIBITORS OR ESTROGEN RECEPTOR ANTAGONISTS TO RESTRAIN SKELETAL MATURATION IN DISORDERS OF GROWTH AND SEXUAL MATURATION

Growth disorders or variants of normal growth (to restrain epiphyseal maturation)
Isolated growth hormone deficiency
Genetic short stature/constitutional delay in growth
Sexual precocity
Congenital virilizing adrenal hyperplasia in male and female
To reduce dose of glucocorticoid
To inhibit conversion of C19 steroids to estrogens (or estrogen action)
With/without use of C17/20 lyase inhibitor of anti-androgen
Testotoxicosis
To inhibit conversion of C19 steroids to estrogens
McCune-Albright syndrome
To inhibit conversion of C19 steroids to estrogens (or estrogen action)
Adolescent gynecomastia
To inhibit estrogen synthesis (or estrogen action)

From Grumbach MM. Estrogen, bone, growth, and sex: a sea change in conventional wisdom. J Pediatr Endocrinol Metab 2000;13(suppl 6):1439-1455.

Incomplete form of Isosexual Precocity: GnRH-Independent Sexual Precocity

In this group of disorders, the secretion of testosterone in boys and estrogen in girls is independent of the hypothalamic GnRH pulse generator (see Table 24–34): there is no pubertal LH response to GnRH or GnRH agonist and there is no pubertal pattern of pulsatile LH secretion. Patients do not respond to chronic GnRH agonist with suppression of gonadal steroid output. Incomplete form of isosexual precocity (ISP) is a consequence of gonadal or adrenal steroid secretion independent of GnRH, of iatrogenic exposure to gonadal steroids, or, in boys, of rare hCG- or LH-secreting tumors.

Boys

Chorionic Gonadotropin-Secreting Tumors

Several types of germ cell tumors secrete hCG, which may cross react in some older polyclonal LH assays. Boys with hCG-secreting neoplasms have slightly enlarged testes (not to a size consistent with the size of the phallus and other male secondary sex characteristics) and may be difficult to differentiate from boys in the early stages of CPP on the basis of physical examination alone.[2097,2323] However, plasma hCG levels are elevated without an increase in the concentration of FSH or LH measured in specific assays. Hepatomas and hepatoblastomas present with hepatomegaly or firm, irregular liver nodules, anemia, and precocious puberty; these malignant liver tumors cause or smooth hepatic enlargement (Fig. 24–76).[2324] hCG is localized to multinucleated tumor giant cells; α-fetoprotein was found in the embryonal-type tumor cells of the hepatoblastoma in one case.[2325] The mean age at onset is 2 years and 8 months, but average survival is only 10.7 months after diagnosis.[2326-2328] Infantile choriocarcinoma is also associated with elevated hCG and is thought to originate in the placenta; infants may be diagnosed at 1 month with survival of only 3 months.[2329] About 20% of mediastinal germ cell tumors occur in boys with 47,XXY or mosaic Klinefelter's syndrome, a prevalence 30 to 50 times more common than in unaffected boys.[1776,2330,2331] Plasma α-fetoprotein is a useful additional marker for yolk sac (endodermal sinus) or mixed germ cell tumors.[2332] The cells in the tumor that secrete α-fetoprotein appear to differ from those that secrete hCG. Rarely, the germ cells contain sufficient aromatase activity to convert circulating C19 precursors (of adrenal origin after adrenarche) to estradiol, which in some instances is sufficient to induce breast development.[1381,2333,2334]

Some teratomas, chorioepitheliomas, or mixed germ cell tumors in the hypothalamic region (or in the mediastinum, the lungs, the gonads, or the retroperitoneum) and certain pineal tumors (usually a germ cell tumor or mixed germ cell tumor),[2323,2335,2336] less commonly a chorioepithelioma or its variants, cause sexual precocity in boys by secreting hCG rather than by activating the pituitary gonadotropin-gonadal axis by the hypothalamic GnRH pulse generator. Calcification of the pineal is found in 8% to 11% of 8- to 11-year-old children and by itself is not indicative of a tumor. Intracranial germ cell tumors account for 3% to 11% of malignant CNS tumors in children and adolescents with a predominance in the Far East.[2337,2338] Germ cell tumors of the hypothalamus or pineal region constitute less than 1% of primary CNS tumors in Western countries but account for 4.5% of such tumors in Japan. The prevalence of intracranial

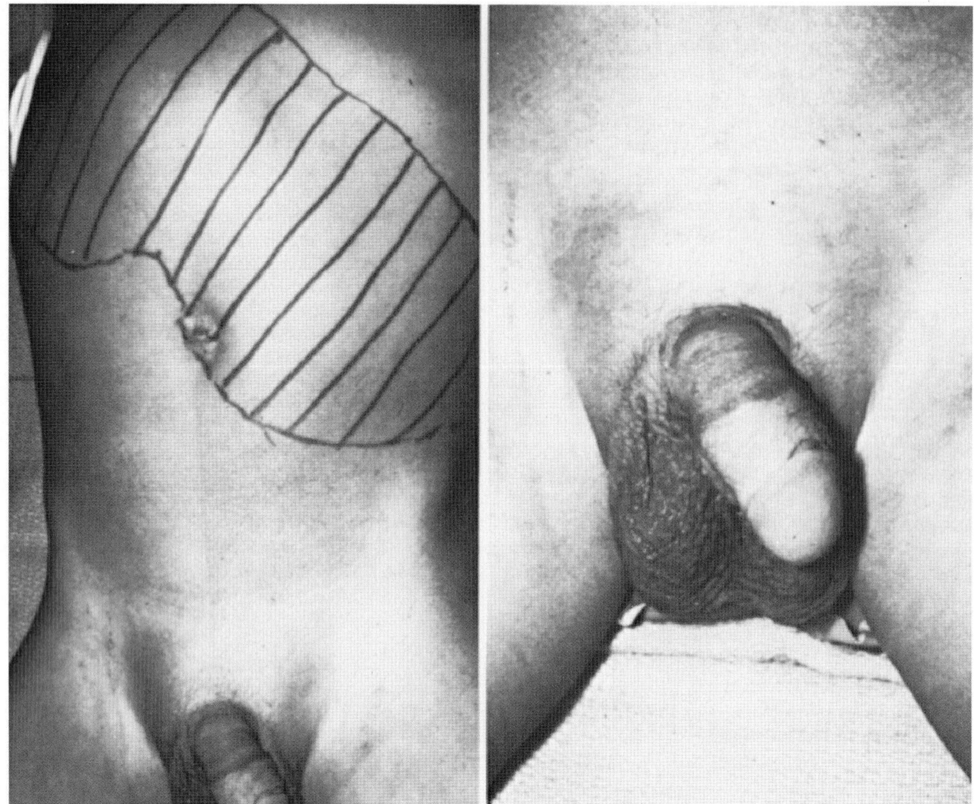

Figure 24–76 ▪ A 1 5/12-year-old boy with a human chorionic gonadotropin (hCG)-secreting hepatoblastoma. Note the outline of the large liver *(left)* and the penile enlargement *(right)*. The testes were 2×1 cm, and pubic hair was stage 2. The plasma hCG level was 50 mIU/mL; plasma testosterone 168 ng/dL; and plasma α-fetoprotein 160,000 ng/mL. Metastatic lesions in both lungs were seen on the radiograph of the chest. To convert testosterone values to SI units, see the legend of Figure 24–21. To convert hCG values to international units per liter, multiply by 1.0. To convert α-fetoprotein values to micrograms per liter, multiply by 1.0. (From Kaplan SL, Grumbach MM. Pathogenesis of sexual precocity. In Grumbach MM, Sizonenko PC, Aubert ML, eds. Control of the Onset of Puberty. Baltimore: Williams & Wilkins, 1990:620-660.)

germ cell tumors are 2.6 times more common in males than females[2339] but germ cell tumors in the suprasellar-hypothalamic region do not exhibit a sex predominance and are generally associated with pituitary hormone deficiencies including DI.[1379] Germ cell tumors do not cause gonadotropin-induced isosexual precocity in females because of the paucity of effects of hCG in prepubertal females. However, CPP may occur through disinhibition of the hypothalamic GnRH pulse generator by local effects mass effects. Germ cell tumors that secrete hCG are rarely located in the thalamus and basal ganglia. In "true" pure CNS germ cell tumors (germinomas), hCG cannot be readily detectable in the circulation, but may be detected in the cerebrospinal fluid.[1379] In mixed germ cell tumors, on the other hand, hCG is commonly present in the blood as well as in cerebrospinal fluid. Extreme elevation of hCG in a CNS tumor is so suggestive of a primary intracranial choriocarcinoma (PICCC)/germ-cell tumor (GCT)), with high risk for tumor hemorrhage during biopsy, that surgical removal or debulking rather than diagnostic biopsy could be the initial operative approach.[2340]

Mixed germ cell tumors and especially "pure" germinomas are radiosensitive, and regression of sexual precocity may occur if the bone age is less than 11 years, only to progress later into normal puberty.[2323] Long-term survival is reported as 88% after appropriate therapy.[2341]

Pineal cysts are a rare cause of central precocious puberty.[1383]

All pituitary adenomas, including gonadotropin-secreting pituitary adenomas, are exceedingly rare in children. One series found 61% were macroadenomas and 39% were microadenomas.[1390] An LH- (basal serum LH of 900 IU/L with no rise after GnRH) and prolactin-secreting (215 μg/L) pituitary adenoma caused sexual precocity in two boys (serum testosterone 7 nmol/L [200 ng/dL]).[2342,2343] Prepubertal values returned after removal of these "chromophobe" adenomas with suprasellar extension.

Precocious Androgen Secretion Caused by Congenital Adrenal Hyperplasia, Virilizing Adrenal Tumor, or Leydig Cell Tumor

Virilizing congenital adrenal hyperplasia caused by a defect in 21-hydroxylation (CYP21, cytochrome P-450c21 deficiency) leads to elevated androgen concentrations and masculinization and is a common cause of GnRH-independent sexual precocity in boys (see Chapter 22 and review in reference 2344).[1143] Approximately 75% of patients with P-450c21 deficiency have salt loss resulting from impaired aldosterone secretion and have low serum sodium and high serum potassium concentrations. Increased plasma concentrations of 17-hydroxyprogesterone, increased levels of urinary 17-ketosteroids and pregnanetriol, and advanced bone age and rapid growth are characteristic. Treatment with glucocorticoids suppresses the abnormal androgen secretion and arrests virilization; treatment with mineralocorticoids, when necessary, corrects the electrolyte imbalance. A rarer form of virilizing adrenal hyperplasia is usually accompanied by hypertension and is caused by 11β-hydroxylase deficiency; the progressive virilization ceases and the blood pressure falls to normal with glucocorticoid therapy. All forms of congenital adrenal hyperplasia are inherited as autosomal recessive traits.[1143] Untreated virilizing congenital adrenal hyperplasia causes anovulatory amenorrhea in females and oligospermia in males, reversible with treatment (see Chapter 22). Treatment of virilizing CAH may reveal GnRH-dependent CPP (secondary CPP) as a consequence of the advanced somatic and hypothalamic maturation due to long exposure to adrenal androgen. Further difficulty is presented in the treatment of congenital adrenal hyperplasia during the pubertal years when androgen secretion normally increases and increased clearance of glucocorticoids at puberty in girls may alter dosing requirements.[2345]

Virilizing adrenal carcinomas or adenomas secrete large amounts of DHEA and DHEAS and on occasion testosterone. Glucocorticoids do not suppress the increased secretion of adrenal androgens to the normal range for age in carcinoma as occurs in CAH. Cushing's syndrome resulting from adrenal carcinoma may cause isosexual precocity and growth failure in boys. Rarely, an adrenal adenoma may produce both testosterone and aldosterone leading to sexual precocity and hypertension with hypokalemia.[2346,2347]

Adrenal rests, or heterotopic adrenal tissue in the testes, testicular adrenal rest tumors (TART) may enlarge (sometimes to massive size) with endogenous ACTH stimulation in boys with untreated or inadequately treated CAH and may mimic bilateral or unilateral interstitial cell tumors (see Chapter 22). MRI sonography including Doppler flow studies of the testes are useful to define the extent and nature of the testicular masses. In boys in whom the testicular tumors are autonomous and unresponsive to glucocorticoid therapy or improved compliance, surgical management including enucleation of the tumor has been useful in preventing further damage to the testes and improving the potential for fertility.[2348] In 8 men, "testis-sparing" surgery did not improve testicular function even though the removal of the adrenal rests was successful. LH receptors have been detected on adrenal/cortical cells,[2349-2352] and LH may stimulate the testes in some patients.

Leydig cell tumor is a rare cause of sexual precocity in boys; unilateral enlargement (often nodular) of the testis usually occurs in this neoplasm (although 5% to 10% are bilateral), in contrast to the usually normal size (small)of both testes for chronologic age in boys with congenital adrenal hyperplasia or a virilizing adrenal tumor.[945,2353] An LH receptor activating mutation was detected in three boys with a sporadic Leydig cell adenoma.[2354]

Women with a previous history of congenital adrenal hyperplasia or a virilizing tumor may exhibit ovarian hyperandrogenism associated with persistent elevation of LH despite successful treatment of their initial virilizing condition in childhood: this is not usually the case in women who have late onset congenital adrenal hyperplasia.[2355]

Familial or Sporadic Testotoxicosis (Familial Male-Limited Gonadotropin-Independent Sexual Precocity with Premature Leydig Cell and Germ Cell Maturation)

A unique form of sexual precocity in males is pituitary gonadotropin-independent familial premature Leydig cell and germ cell maturation, or testotoxicosis.[2356-2362] Andrew Shenker brought to our attention a report of this condition by R.K. Stone in 1852.[2363] Affected boys have secondary sexual development with penile enlargement, which may be present at birth,[2357] and bilateral enlargement of testes to the early or midpubertal range, although the testes often are smaller than expected in relation to penile growth and pubertal maturation (Fig. 24–77). Premature Leydig and Sertoli cell maturation and spermatogenesis is found in the testes; Leydig cell hyperplasia may occur.[2356,2357,2359] The Leydig cells in affected boys produce dimeric inhibin B as well as testosterone,[2364] and Leydig cells and spermatogonia stain positively for the α and beta B segments of inhibin. The rate of linear growth is rapid, skeletal maturation is advanced, and muscular development is prominent. Prepubertal basal and GnRH-stimulated gonadotropin concentrations and lack of a pubertal pattern of LH pulsatility (measured by immunologic or bioassay techniques) normal pubertal or adult levels and clearance of testosterone are characteristic (Table 24–46).[2357] The onset of adrenarche and its biochemical marker, serum DHEAS, correlate with bone age rather than chronologic age. Treatment with a GnRH agonist does not suppress the testicular function or maturation.[2357,2361] In late childhood or early adolescence, fertility is achieved and an adult pattern of LH secretion and response to GnRH is demonstrable[2358]; secondary GnRH-dependent true precocious puberty may be superimposed on the substrate of testotoxicosis.[2358,2359,2365] In some adults, impaired spermatogenic function is associated with elevated concentrations of plasma FSH.[2021,2358] Testotoxicosis may occur sporadically, quite likely as a consequence of a germ-line mutation or even a postzygotic one, but is usually inherited as a sex-limited autosomal dominant trait[2358] and probably accounts for the earlier descriptions of "true" precocious puberty in families in which only males were affected. A kindred with nine generations of affected males has been reported.[2358] Obligatory female carriers of the trait were unaffected because constitutional activation of the LH receptor on the ovary causes no ill effects.[2358,2365]

In 1993, Shenker and colleagues[2366] and Kremer and associates[2367] independently described heterozygous activating mutations of the heterotrimeric Gs protein-coupled LH/CG receptor, which in concert transduce the LH/CG signal to the main effector, adenyl cyclase (Fig. 24–78). The LH receptor, cloned from the human,[2368,2369] is a glycoprotein of 80 to 90 kd belonging to a subfamily of the seven-transmembrane–spanning, G protein–coupled receptors. The gene is localized to chromosome 2p21 (the same as the FSH receptor), which spans at least 70 kb, and contains 11 exons separated by 10 introns. The large glycosylated amino terminal extracellular hormone binding domain of the 701 amino acid LH/hCG receptor[2369] is encoded by exon 1 to 10. A single exon, the large exon 11, encodes the entire G-linked transmembrane domain with its 7α-helical segments connected by alternating extracellular and intracellular loops, the intracellular domain and the three untranslated region—almost two thirds of the receptor (see Fig. 24–78).[1805,2370-2372] Thirteen constitutively activating heterozygous missense mutations (in more than 60 reported patients) all residing within exon 11 have

TABLE 24–46 TESTOTOXICOSIS: CLINICAL AND LABORATORY CHARACTERISTICS

Sex-limited autosomal dominant inheritance; activating mutation in the gene encoding the LH receptor
Early onset of sexual precocity in boys with bilateral testicular enlargement
Prepubertal immunologic and biologic LH response to GnRH, prepubertal LH pulse secretory pattern
Concentration of plasma testosterone in pubertal range
Premature Leydig cell and seminiferous tubule maturation
No CNS, adrenal, or testicular abnormalities demonstrable by radiologic or hormonal studies
Lack of suppression of plasma testosterone or physical signs of puberty by GnRH agonist

CNS, Central nervous system; *LH*, luteinizing hormone; *GnRH*, gonadotropin-releasing hormone.

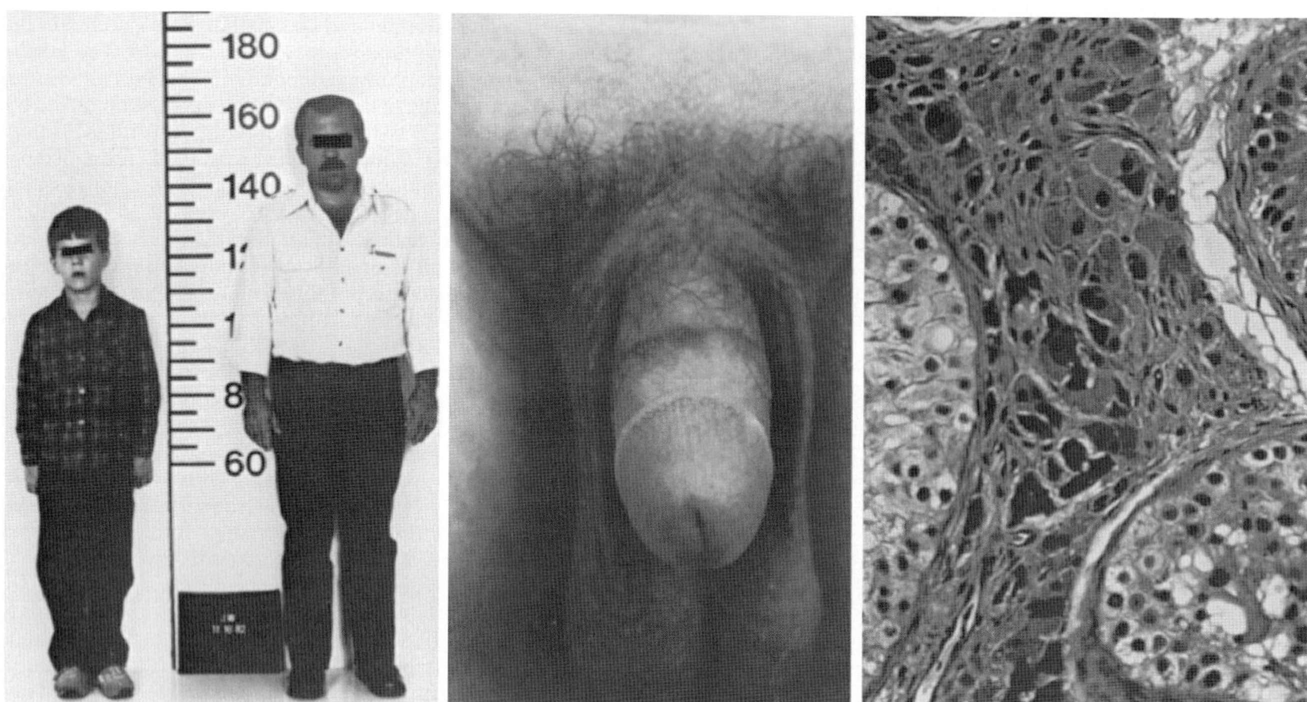

Figure 24–77 ▪ Familial testotoxicosis. *Left,* A 5½-year-old boy and his 28-year-old father with the disorder. The boy exhibited signs of sexual precocity by 3 years of age. Height was 130.6 cm (+4.8 SD); bone age 12½ years. The plasma testosterone level was 267 ng/dL; dihydrotestosterone 46 ng/dL; dehydroepiandrosterone sulfate (DHEAS) 23 µg/dL. The plasma luteinizing hormone (LH) and follicle-stimulating hormone (FSH) levels were low, and neither rose after treatment. Pulsatile LH secretion was not demonstrable. Treatment with deslorelin, an LHRH agonist, was without effect. The father had begun sexual maturation by 3 years of age and had reached a final height of 162.6 cm in his early teens. The plasma testosterone level was 294 ng/dL; LH 0.5 ng/mL (LER-960); and FSH 0.5 ng/mL (LER-869). The father had an adult-type LH and FSH response to LHRH; the LH level increased to 7.5 ng/mL, and the FSH level to 2 ng/mL. At least 28 male family members over nine generations are affected. To convert dihydrotestosterone values to nanomoles per liter, multiply by 0.03467. For other conversions to SI units, see the legends of Figures 24–21 and 24–22. *Center,* External genitalia of the 5½-year-old boy. The penis measured 12×2.8 cm; the right testis was 4×2 cm, and the left testis 3.5×2.5 cm. *Right,* Testis of the boy showed Leydig cell maturation without Reinke crystalloids and spermatogenesis (Mallory trichome).

been reported (see Fig. 24–78); six involve the transmembrane helix VI, two the flanking third cytoplasmic loop, and one each in helix V and helix II and less commonly mutations in the first transmembrane helix.[2366,2367,2373-2377] Thus, nine mutations are between amino acid residues 542 and 581, suggesting a "hotspot." There appears to be a limited repertoire of mutations in American boys consistent with a founder effect; European pedigrees are more diverse.[2378,2379] A model of the transmembrane domain of the receptor provides novel suggestions on the structural and functional effects of these activating mutations.[2380] Transfected cultured cells with these mutations exhibited increased basal cAMP production in the absence of agonist, observations consistent with a constitutive activating mutation.[2378] Various possibilities for the conformational changes in the LH receptor that lead to its constitutive activation have been considered.[2381] Inactivating mutations of the LH/CG receptor and their clinical consequences are discussed in Chapter 22.

In one Polish family, the disorder, a mutation of M298T in the second transmembrane domain of the LH receptor, led to sexual precocity in one boy but not in the mother, who carried the same mutation, nor in her father, the maternal grandfather or his son, the maternal uncle, suggesting the involvement of epigenetic factors.[2382] Three boys with sexual precocity due to a sporadic Leydig cell adenoma had an Asp578His mutation in the tumor (Fig 24–79).[2354,955]

Boys with GnRH-independent, pituitary gonadotropin-independent maturation of the testes do not respond to chronic administration of a GnRH agonist with suppression of testosterone secretion, in contrast to the characteristic response in patients with true precocious puberty.[2357] However, testosterone secretion, height velocity and rate of bone maturation, and aggressive and hyperactive behavior have been decreased by treatment with oral medroxyprogesterone acetate.[1147,2357]

Two other therapies have been used (Table 24–47). Ketoconazole, an orally active substituted imidazole derivative, suppresses gonadal and adrenal biosynthesis at several steps.[2383] In the dosage used in testotoxicosis (200 mg every 8 to 12 hours orally),[2360,2384] ketoconazole mainly inhibits the enzyme cytochrome P450c17, which regulates both 17-hydroxylation and the scission (17,20 lyase) of 17α-hydroxypregnenolone to dehydroepiandrosterone (see page 62). However, even at the recommended dose, the agent produces a mild transient decrease in cortisol secretion and interferes with binding of testosterone to TeBG. Secondary true precocious puberty often occurs when the bone age advances to or has already reached the pubertal range (usually more than 11.5 years), at which time addition of a GnRH agonist is appropriate.[2360] Ketoconazole can cause hepatic injury, which is usually mild and reversible, but rarely hepatotoxicity is severe.[2383] Furthermore, reversible renal injury, rash, and interstitial pneumonia are reported in a patient who tolerated lower doses suggesting a dose response effect.[2385] Even so, five patients treated with ketoconazole experienced no side effects other than one mild and transient elevation of lilver enzymes, had appropriate age of onset of true puberty, and

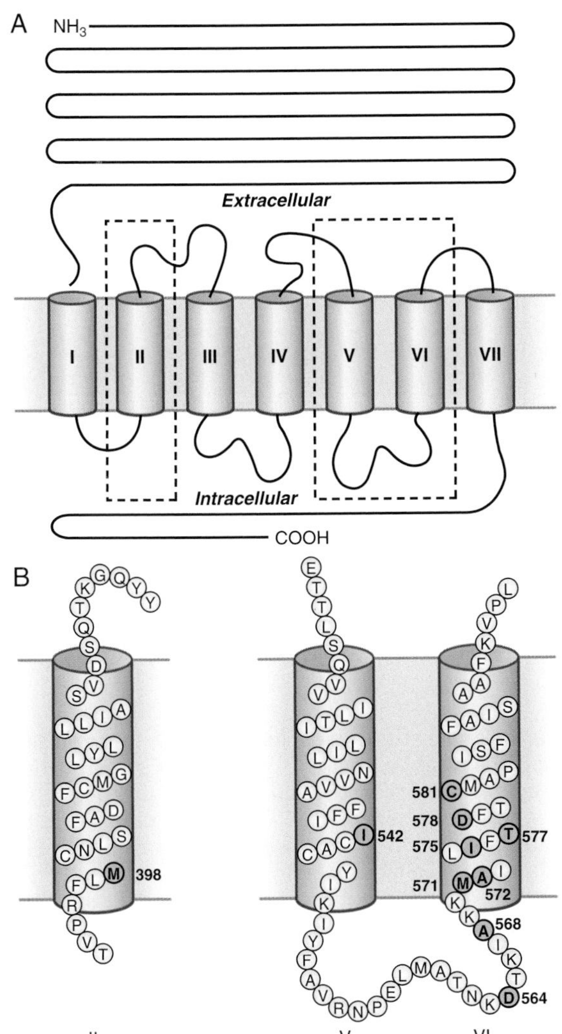

Figure 24–78 ■ **A,** The serpentine seven transmembrane G_s protein coupled hLH/hCG receptor with its large extracellular domain and the intracellular domain. The seven helical transmembrane domains are indicated by Roman numerals. **B,** The two-dimensional seven-transmembrane topology of the hLH/hCG receptor with positions of constitutively activating mutations causing testotoxicosis (male-limited autosomal dominant sexual precocity). The mutations are indicated by solid circles and the residue number. Note the cluster of mutations in the VI transmembrane helix and third cytoplasmic loop. The aspartine 578-glycine mutation is the most common. (Redrawn from Yano K, Kohn LD, Saji M, et al. A case of male limited precocious puberty caused by a point mutation in the second transmembrane domain of the luteinizing hormone choriogonadotropin receptor gene. Biochem Biophys Res Commun 1996;220:1036-1042.)

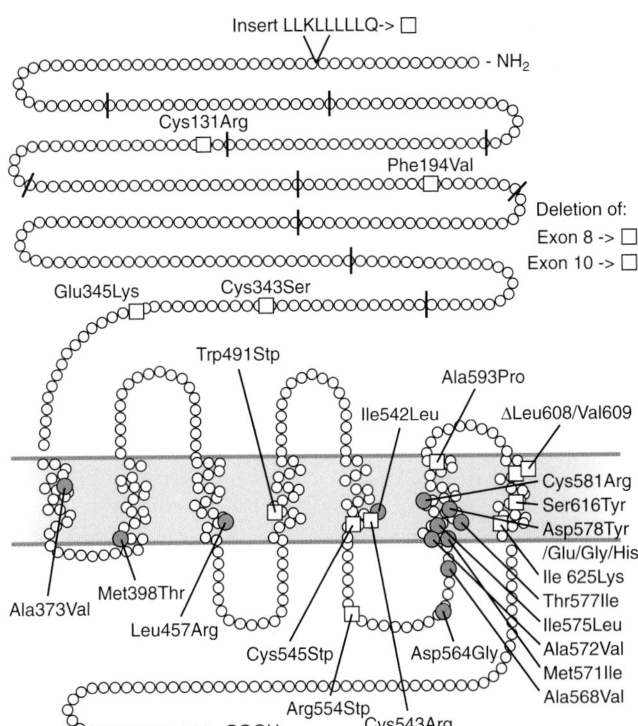

Figure 24–79 ■ Mutations in the luteinizing hormone (LH) receptor protein. Schematic structure of the LH receptor protein and localization of the inactivating *(open squares)* and activating *(filled circles)* mutations currently known in the human LH receptor. The short lines across the amino acid chain separate the 11 exons. (From Themmen APN, Huhtaniemi IT. Mutations of gonadotropins and gonadotropin receptors. Endocr Rev 2000;21[5]:551-583.)

reached adult height almost identical to target height, a mean increase of 8 cm over initially predicted height, suggesting great benefit to this therapy in this condition.[2386]

Another therapeutic approach has been the use of the antiandrogen (and antimineralocorticoid) spironolactone combined with testolactone, an inhibitor of cytochrome P-450 aromatase (CYP19), the key enzyme in the conversion of androgens to estrogens.[2387] Because these boys often develop secondary central precocious puberty after control with spironolactone and testolactone, the addition of GnRH agonist is a useful step to suppress pituitary gonadotropin secretion.[2388] More potent and specific nonsteroidal antiandrogens such as flutamide and nilutamide[2389] and aromatase inhibitors, such as letrozole[2390,2391] to inhibit the rate of skeletal maturation and linear growth by suppressing estradiol synthesis, potentially have greater therapeutic efficacy.[336,337] Striking clinical improvements occurred in two patients treated with anastrozole (1 mg/day) and bicalutamide, a potent third generation nonsteroidal antiandrogen.[2387a] Table 24–47 lists the various agents used in the treatment of testotoxicosis. Which of these agents or combination of agents will be effective for long term treatment and safe remains to be determined.

A single case study of an untreated affected boy revealed no true precocious puberty but the expected pattern of rapid growth and early cessation but adult height of (174 cm) was within target height range (171.5 to 188.5 cm), indicating the importance of individual approaches to affected boys when considering treatment to maximize height.[2392]

Gonadotropin-Independent Sexual Precocity and Pseudohypoparathyroidism Type Ia due to a Gsα Mutation

Mutations in Gsα, can either constitutively activate or inactivate adenyl cyclase.[2393] Two boys who presented in infancy with classic pseudohypoparathyroidism type Ia (PHPIa), a disorder characterized by resistance to hormones whose action is mediated by cAMP, developed signs of sexual precocity with the hormonal characteristics of testotoxicosis (gonadotropin-independent sexual precocity) at about 24 months of age.[2394] They both had a unique alanine 366 to serine mutation[2394] in one allele of the Gsα gene; the alanine residue is absolutely conserved in all heterotrimeric G proteins. PHPIa is due to a wide variety of inactivating mutations in Gsα, which lead to about a 50% reduction in Gsα activity in functional assays.[2395]

The paradox of a Gsα mutation causing both inactivation and pseudohypoparathyroidism and constitutive activation and

TABLE 24–47 PHARMACOLOGIC THERAPY FOR SEXUAL PRECOCITY

Disorder	Treatment	Action and Rationale
GnRH dependent		
True or central precocious puberty	GnRH agonists	Desensitization of gonadotropes; blocks action of endogenous GnRH
GnRH independent		
Incomplete sexual precocity		
Girls		
Autonomous ovarian cysts	Medroxyprogesterone acetate	Inhibition of ovarian steroidogenesis; regression of cyst (inhibition of FSH release)
McCune-Albright syndrome	Medroxyprogesterone acetate*	Inhibition of ovarian steroidogenesis; regression of cyst (inhibition of FSH release)
	Third-generation aromatase inhibitor, e.g., letrozole	Inhibition of P-450 aromatase; blocks estrogen synthesis
Boys		
Familial testotoxicosis	Ketoconazole*	Inhibition of P-450-c17 (CYP17) (mainly 17,20-lyase activity)
	Flutamide orbicalatamide and	Antiandrogen
	letrozole or anactrozole	Inhibition of aromatase; blocks estrogen synthesis
	Medroxyprogesterone acetate*	Inhibition of testicular steroidogenesis

*If true precocious puberty develops, an LHRH agonist can be added.

GnRH, Luterinizing hormone–releasing hormone.

Modified from Grumbach MM, Kaplan SL. Recent advances in the diagnosis and management of sexual precocity. Acta Paediatr Jpn 1988:30(suppl):155-175.

testotoxicosis was resolved by in vitro studies.[2396] In cultured cells, the Gsα Ala 366 Ser mutant protein was rapidly degraded at 37° C but constitutively activated adenyl cyclase at 33° C.[2396] Unlike other activating mutations of Gsα that involve mutations inhibiting its intrinsic GTPase activity and decreasing the rate of hydrolysis of GTP to GDP, the mutation in the two boys caused accelerated dissociation of GDP at 33° C in transfected Leydig cells but was rapidly degraded at 37° C in a lymphoma cell line[2396] and in skin fibroblasts at both 33° C and 37° C[2394] transfected with the mutation. These observations explain the clinical consequences of increased Gsα activity in the testis, which are 3° to 5° C cooler than the body and the tissue specificity and temperature dependency of the mutation.[2396] The mother of one patient appeared to be a mosaic for the Gsα mutation whereas a germ line mutation is likely in the other boy.[2394]

Girls

ISP in girls (see Table 24–34) is caused by autonomous estrogen secretion by an ovarian cyst or tumor or by an adrenal neoplasm or by inadvertent exposure to estrogen. Girls harboring a teratoma or teratocarcinoma (or a CNS germ cell tumor) that secretes hCG have had sexual precocity caused by concurrent estrogen secretion by the tumor but no effect from the effects of hCG alone; these girls also may have galactorrhea, especially if chorionic somatomammotropin (hCS, hPL) is also secreted.

Autonomous Ovarian Follicular Cysts

The most common childhood estrogen-secreting ovarian mass and ovarian cause of sexual precocity is the follicular cyst.[2397] Antral follicles up to about 8 mm in diameter are common in the ovaries of normal prepubertal girls[283,2398,2399] and may be seen in third-trimester fetuses and newborn infants.[2400-2404] They may appear and regress spontaneously. Large follicular cysts may be discovered because of the presence of an abdominal mass or abdominal pain, especially after torsion or as an unexpected finding on pelvic sonography performed for other reasons. Occasionally, the antral follicles secrete estrogen and may enlarge to form large masses, or the follicular cysts may recur and cause recurrent signs of sexual precocity and acyclic vaginal bleeding. Enlarged antral follicles or cysts occur in premature thelarche, true precocious puberty, and transient or incomplete sexual precocity.[2097,2405-2407,2141] In some ovarian follicular cysts, the transient or recurrent sexual precocity is GnRH-independent (Fig. 24–80). The concentration of estradiol fluctuates, usually correlating with changes in the size of the follicular cyst when monitored by pelvic sonography,[2408,2409] and may increase to levels found in a granulosa cell tumor although values may also be in the pubertal range but they do not have increased plasma granulosa cell tumor markers such as antimüllerian hormone and inhibin.[814,2097,2407] The concentration of LH is suppressed, a pubertal pattern of pulsatile LH secretion is absent, and the LH rise induced by GnRH is prepubertal.[2097,2406,2141,2407] It is curious that a constitutive activating mutation of the FSH receptor is undescribed in a female, especially because a heterozygous mutation, Asp 567 Gly has been detected in the third intracellular loop of the FSH receptor in a hypophysectomized man who, despite the gonadotropin deficiency, was fertile and had normal sized testes.[2410] This is a site of activating mutations in the LH receptor. Accordingly, the possibility that some girls with recurrent ovarian cysts harbor an activating mutation of the FSH receptor seems worthy of study. The McCune-Albright syndrome needs to be considered in any girl with recurrent ovarian cysts even in the apparent initial absence of other features of this disorder due to somatic activating mutations in the gene encoding the α-subunit of the heterotrimeric Gs protein (see below). The luteinization of follicular cysts may be related to subtle elevations and increased pulses of plasma FSH. Ovarian cysts and sexual precocity have been associated with the fragile X syndrome in girls.[2411]

An unusual syndrome of estradiol-secreting ovarian cysts in preterm infants born before 30 weeks' gestation is associated with edema of the labia majora and, in some instances, of the lower abdominal wall.[2402] The LH and FSH response to GnRH suggested GnRH-dependence. Treatment with medroxyprogesterone acetate was associated with regression of the cysts. A case of massive ovarian edema associated with ovarian cysts found in a 6-month-old with breast and pubic hair development is reported.[2412]

GnRH agonists are useful in the treatment of ovarian follicular cysts associated with CPP (GnRH-dependent) but not so-called autonomous cysts. However, girls with "autonomously" functioning ovarian follicular cysts, whether recurrent or an

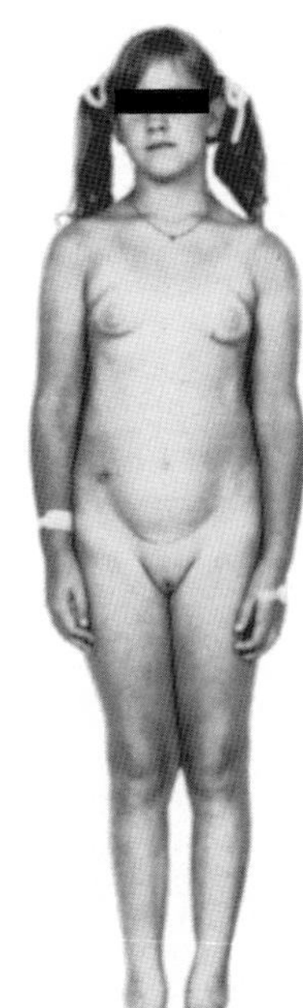

FOLLICULAR CYST OF OVARY
(Pt. G.B.)
AGE OF ONSET: 2 10/12 Y
P.E. AT AGE 4 10/12 Y
HT: 122.8 cm (+3.2 SD)
BREASTS: III, PH: 2
LAB: LRF: LH: 0.4 to 0.7 ng/ml, FSH: 0.4 to 0.8 ng/ml
E_2: 180 pg/ml
BA: 6 Y, CA: 4 10/12
Rx: 5 3/12: REMOVAL OF OVARIAN CYST
CYST FLUID: 25,000 pg/ml E_1
>34,000 pg/ml E_2
MPA: AGE 5 5/12 to 9 0/12 Y
LRF: PREPUBERTAL LH RESPONSE
E_2: <10 pg/ml
REMISSION WITH NO PROGRESSION OF PUBERTAL SIGNS
6 11/12 Y, ON MPA

Figure 24–80 ■ A 4 10/12-year-old girl with recurrent "autonomous" follicular cysts of the ovary. *MPA*, Medroxyprogesterone acetate (oral). For conversion to SI units, see the legend for Figure 24–21. (From Kaplan SL, Grumbach MM. Pathogenesis of sexual precocity. In Grumbach MM, Sizonenko PC, Aubert ML, eds. Control of the Onset of Puberty. Baltimore: Williams & Wilkins, 1990:620-660.)

isolated episode, often respond to treatment with oral medroxyprogesterone acetate but not to GnRH agonists. Medroxyprogesterone acetate also seems to prevent recurrence and accelerate involution of the follicular cysts[2097,2407] and reduce the risk of torsion. The use of one of the new, potent aromatase inhibitors such as letrozole to reduce estradiol secretion is another potential approach to treatment.[2413] Surgical intervention is rarely indicated; a large or persistent cyst can be reduced by puncture at laparoscopy. The size of the cyst can be monitored readily by pelvic sonography.

Ovarian Tumors

Ovarian tumors are the most common genitourinary tumors of girls[2414] but are rare in the prepubertal period, accounting for about 1% of all tumors in girls younger than 17 years and most are benign according to some,[2415-2417] but not all studies.[2418] Discrepancy between studies may be due to method of classification of cysts and potentially malignant lesions. The majority of ovarian tumors arise from germ cells or sex cord stromal cells in childhood with less than 20% being of epithelial origin in contrast to adults where the majority of tumors are of epithelial origin.[2419,2420] Early diagnosis of most childhood tumors of the ovary allow successful cure unlike ovarian cancer in women.[2421] Most of these tumors present with pain or an abdominal mass. Tumors less than 5 cm at diagnosis are more likely nonneoplastic, whereas those over 10 cm are more likely to be neoplastic.[2397] Ultrasonography is helpful in evaluation but will not usually lead to the correct histologic diagnosis. The successful use of tumor markers for diagnosis varies by etiology: for example in one series, cystic teratomas may have LDH and ESR elevation; immature teratomas have LDH, AFT, and CA 125 elevated; granulose cell tumors have sex steroids (estradiol and/or testosterone) elevated.[2418]

Granulosa Cell Tumor of the Ovary

This tumor is rare in childhood, although theca cell tumors are even less common.[2422,2423] Characteristic histologic features of juvenile granulosa cell tumors include nodular architecture, follicle formation, abundant interstitial and intrafollicular acid mucopolysaccharide-rich fluid, irregular microcysts, individual cell necrosis, and high mitotic activity (mean activity, 11 mitotic figures per 10 high-power fields). Size can vary from 2.5 to 25 cm with a mean diameter of 12 cm. The interstitial mucinous fluid consists predominantly of hyaluronic acid.[2424] Prognosis is good, in that only about 3% of patients die of the disease. However, the age of diagnosis is related to the prognosis and delay leads to substantial complications. Girls presenting with isosexual precocity who were correctly diagnosed had no intraabdominal spread and had stage FIGO (Federation of Gynecology and Obstetrics) stage 1 A in one series while those presenting with acute abdominal symptoms had 50% prevalence of intraabdominal spread and two recurrences after surgery. When the diagnosis was made after normal puberty had begun, some girls had virilization and abdominal symptoms, 80% had intraabdominal spread, and 30% had recurrence FIGO stage 1c or 11c. Delay of diagnosis for 3 to 11 months was associated with significant morbidity.[2425]

Approximately 80% of granulosa cell tumors can be palpated on bimanual examination while less than 5% are bilateral or clinically malignant. The concentration of plasma estradiol may increase to high levels[2426] while serum FSH and LH concentrations are usually suppressed. Antimüllerian hormone and inhibin are sensitive tumor markers[2427-2431] and are used to screen for metastases. An elevated estradiol in a patient younger than age 9, or an abnormal rise in concentration of plasma antimüllerian hormone, or inhibin at any age suggests recurrence or metastasis.

Occasionally, gonadoblastomas in streak gonads, rare lipoid tumors, cystadenomas, and ovarian carcinomas secrete estrogens, androgens, or both hormones. Even with successful resection of a gonadal sex steroid–secreting neoplasm, the child is at risk for secondary CPP in the future. Gonadal tumors composed of a mixture of germ cells and sex cord stromal cells that are distinct from gonadoblastoma are usually benign when discovered in female infants or children with 46,XX karyotypes,[2432,2433] although neoplastic transformation is a risk,[2434,2435] as two cases of metastasizing malignant mixed germ cell-sex cord-stromal tumors are described in prepubertal girls with isosexual precocity. α-Fetoprotein and other tumor markers aid in diagnosis.

Peutz-Jeghers Syndrome

This autosomal dominant syndrome of mucocutaneous pigmentation of the lips, buccal mucosa, fingers, and toes, gastrointestinal hamartomatous polyposis, and a predisposition to malignancy is associated with a rare, distinctive sex cord tumor with annular tubules in both boys and girls.[2436-2438] Estrogen secretion by the tumor may lead to feminization and incomplete sexual precocity in boys as well as girls. Less frequently, an epithelial tumor of the ovary, dysgerminoma, or a feminizing Sertoli-Leydig cell tumor has been found in patients with Peutz-Jeghers syndrome.[2439,2440] Children with this disorder should be examined at regular intervals for the presence of gonadal tumors by pelvic sonography. The syndrome is due to mutations in the gene on 9p13.3 encoding a serine/threonine protein kinase STK11 leading to haploinsufficiency of this novel tumor-suppressing gene.[2441-2444]

Sex cord stromal tumors derive from the coelomic epithelium or mesenchymal cells of the embryonic gonads and are composed of granulosa, theca, Leydig, and Sertoli cells. Estrogen secretion from these tumors can cause pseudoprecocious puberty, whereas androgen secretion can cause virilization. Both inhibin A and B activin are produced as is antimüllerian factor; all serve as useful tumor markers.[2429,2445,2446] Sex cord-stromal tumors not associated with Peutz-Jeghers syndrome are malignant in 25% of patients; these tumors may grow quite large while those associated with Peutz-Jeghers syndrome are often small and multiple, and contain calcifications.[2447]

Adrenal Adenomas

Adrenocortical tumors are rare in childhood (0.6% of all childhood tumors and 0.3% of all malignant childhood tumors) but most produce steroid hormones in childhood while those in adults usually do not. The median age of diagnosis is 4 years but 41 % appear before 2 years and 71% before 5 years of age. Most cause virilization or Cushing's syndrome but adrenal tumors may produce estrogen as well as androgens and cause sexual precocity in a girl or gynecomastia in a boy. One adrenal adenoma found in a 7-year-old girl expressed the gene for aromatase demonstrating that the tumor could directly produce estrogen[2448] to a level of 145 pg/mL, in the range found in adrenal carcinomas.

Incomplete Sexual Precocity: Boys and Girls

McCune-Albright Syndrome

This sporadic syndrome[2449,2450] occurs about twice as often in girls as in boys and is due to somatic activating mutations in the gene (GNAS 1) encoding the α-subunit of the trimeric guanosine triphosphate(GTP)-binding protein (Gαs) that stimulates adenyl cyclase. It is characterized by the triad of irregularly edged hyperpigmented macules (café au lait spots); a slowly progressive bone disorder, and polyostotic fibrous dysplasia that can involve any bone; it is frequently associated with facial asymmetry and hyperostosis of the base of the skull; and, it is more commonly associated with GnRH-independent sexual precocity in girls (Fig. 24–81 and Table 24–48).[2117,2395,2451] At least two of the features must be present to consider the diagnosis. Autonomous hyperfunction most commonly involves the ovary, but other endocrine involvement includes thyroid (nodular hyperplasia with thyrotoxicosis or, remarkably, with euthyroid status)[1783] adrenal (multiple hyperplastic nodules with Cushing's syndrome),[2451] pituitary (adenoma or mammosomatotroph hyperplasia with gigantism and acromegaly and hyperprolactinemia),[2452] and parathyroids (adenoma or hyperplasia with hyperparathyroidism).[2117] In addition, hypophosphatemic vitamin D–resistant rickets or osteomalacia occurs, either because of overproduction of a phosphaturic factor, phospha-

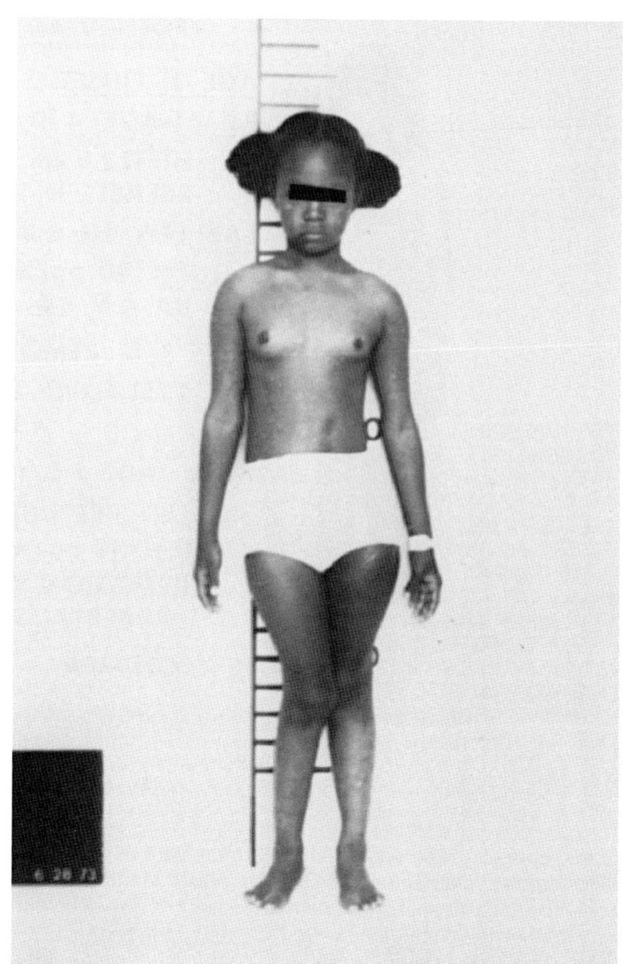

Figure 24–81 ▪ A 7 4/12-year-old girl with luteinizing hormone–releasing hormone (GnRH)-independent sexual precocity associated with McCune-Albright syndrome. She had breast development since infancy, which increased noticeably at about 3 years of age; 6 months later episodes of recurrent vaginal bleeding began. Growth of pubic hair was noted at about 4 to 5 years of age. At age 5 1/12 years the bone age was 6 11/12 years; height was +1 SD above the mean value for age. By 6½ years of age, when she was seen at the University of California, San Francisco, the bone age had advanced to 9 years, and height was at +1 SD. Breasts were at Tanner stage 4; pubic hair at stage 3. Extensive irregular café-au-lait macules cover the right side of the face, left lower abdomen and thigh, and both buttocks. A bone survey showed widespread involvement of the long bones with typical polyostotic fibrous dysplasia, and the floor of the anterior fossa of the skull was sclerotic and the diploetic space widened. She has had two pathologic fractures through bone cysts in the right upper femur. Note the osseous deformities. Plasma estradiol concentrations were consistently in the pubertal range; LH response to GnRH was prepubertal. Results of thyroid function studies were normal, including the thyrotropin response to thyrotropin-releasing hormone administration and antithyroid antibodies were not detected. Treatment with oral medroxyprogesterone acetate suppressed menses and arrested pubertal development but did not slow skeletal maturation. Her final height is 142 cm (−2.5 SD). Menstrual cycles are regular.

TABLE 24–48 CLINICAL MANIFESTATIONS OF MCCUNE-ALBRIGHT SYNDROME IN 158 REPORTED PATIENTS*

Manifestation	Patiens (%) (n = 158)	Male (n = 53)	Female (n = 105)	AGE AT DIAGNOSIS		Comments
				yr	(range)	
Fibrous dysplasia	97	51	103	7.7	(0-52)	Polystotic more common than monostotic
Café-au-lait lesion	85	49	86	7.7	(0-52)	Variable size and number of lesions, irregular border ("coast of Maine")
Sexual precocity	52	8	74	4.9	(0.3-9)	Common initial manifestation
Acromegaly/gigantism	27	20	22	14.8	(0.2-42)	17/26 with adenoma on MRI/CT
Hyperprolactinemia	15	9	14	16.0	(0.2-42)	23/42 of acromegalic with ↑ PRL
Hyperthyroidism	19	7	23	14.4	(0.5-37)	Enthyroid goiter is common
Hypercortisolism	5	4	5	4.4	(0.2-17)	All primary adrenal
Myxomas	5	3	5	34	(17-50)	Extremity myxomas
Osteosarcoma	2	1	2	36	(34-37)	At site of fibrous dysplasia, not related to prior radiation therapy
Rickets/osteomalacia	3	1	3	27.3	(8-52)	Responsive to phosphorus plus calcitriol
Cardiac abnormalities	11	8	9		(0.1-66)	Arrhythmias and CHF reported
Hepatic abnormalities	10	6	10	1.9	(0.3-4)	Neonatal icterus is most common

*Evaluations include clinical and biochemical data; other rarely described manifestations include metabolic acidosis, nephrocalcinosis, developmental delay, thymic and splenic hyperplasia, and colonic polyps.

CHF, Congestive heart failure; *CT*, computed tomography; *MRI*, Magnetic resonance imaging; *PRL*, prolactin.

Modified from Ringel MD, Schwindinger WF, Levine MA. Clinical implication of genetic defects in G proteins: the molecular basis of McCune-Albright syndrome and Albright hereditary osteodystrophy. Medicine (Baltimore) 1996;75:171-184.

tonin[2453] secreted by the bone lesions, or an intrinsic renal abnormality leading to the excess generation of nephrogenous cAMP in the proximal tubule and resulting in decreased reabsorption of phosphate.[2454] Hepatocellular dysfunction may occur due to expression of the mutant-activating gene in liver cells[2455] leading to jaundice associated with hepatobiliary disease and pancreatitis.[2455] Another nonendocrine manifestation is cardiac disease, which carries the risk of cardiac arrhythmia and sudden death. This is a sporadic condition that can be concordant or discordant in monoygotic twins.[2456]

Considering children with at least one of the signs of McCune-Albright syndrome, 24% had the classic triad, 33% had two signs, and 40% had only one classic sign. The mutation was identified in 43% of the patients when no affected tissue could be tested but if an affected tissue was available, the mutation was found in more than 90% of the patients no matter what the number of signs. The mutation was detected in 46% of blood samples in patients presenting the classic triad, but only 21% and 8% in patients with two and one sign, respectively, were found. The mutation was found in 33% of the 39 cases of isolated peripheral precocious puberty. Patients with monostotic fibrous dysplasia, isolated GnRH-independent sexual precocity, neonatal liver cholestasis, and the classic McCune-Albright syndrome all had the same molecular defect.[2457] While most endocrine organs involved in McCune-Albright syndrome patients were not associated with parent specificity,[2458] pituitary adenomas secreting GH expressed NESP55 transcripts, which are mono-allelically expressed from the maternal alleles rather than exon 1A paternal allele. Mutation of the GNAS1 involving replacement of arginine by histidine in codon 201 (R201H [+] is associated with apparent premature or exaggerated thelarche and early menarche.)[2459]

The majority of patients have pigmented skin lesions in infancy, which usually increase in size along with body growth.[2460] The irregular border café -au-lait macules usually do not cross the midline, but they may, and often are located on the same side as the main bone lesions and have a segmented distribution.[2449]

The skeletal lesions in the cortex are dysplastic and are filled with spindle cells with poorly organized collagen support; they take the form of scattered cystic areas of rarefaction on radiography and often result in pathologic fractures and progressive deformities (Fig. 24–82).[2461] Technetium bone scintography has been the most sensitive approach to the detection of bone lesions before they are visible radiographically. Fractures are most common during the 6th to 10th year but decline thereafter and are more frequent if phosphaturia is present.[2462] Patients referred for fibrous dysplsia of the bone in one or more locations are often found to have endocrine or dermatologic manifestations of McCune-Albright syndrome as well as GNAS1 mutations so suspicion should be kept high in fibrous lesions.[2463] If the skull is involved, there may be entrapment and compression of optic or auditory nerve foramina, which can lead to blindness, deafness, facial asymmetry, and ptosis. Asymmetry of the jaw is another manifestation of McCune-Albright syndrome.[2462,2464] Fifty percent of affected children in one series manifested bone abnormalities by 8 years of age.[2460] Increased serum GH levels have an adverse effect on the skull deformities; depending upon age of onset: somatostatin analogues have variable efficacy. Radiation therapy of the hypothalamic-pituitary area may be invoked but carries a risk of later occurrence of sarcoma. Rapid control of elevated GH can be achieved by the use of pegvisomant.[2465]

The sexual precocity often begins in the first 2 years and is frequently heralded by menstrual bleeding all due to an autonomously functioning luteinized follicular cysts of the ovary in girls (Table 24–49).[2097,2117] The ovaries contain no corpora lutea and commonly exhibit asymmetrical enlargement as a result of a large solitary follicular cyst, which characteristically enlarges and spontaneously regresses, only to recur (Fig. 24–83).[2097,2117,2361,2451,2466,2467] Serum estradiol is elevated (at times to extraordinarily high levels); in contrast, the LH response to GnRH is prepubertal and the pubertal pattern of nighttime LH pulses is absent at the onset and during the initial years.[2097,2468,2469] Later in the course of the sexual precocity, when the bone age approaches 12 years, the GnRH pulse generator becomes opera-

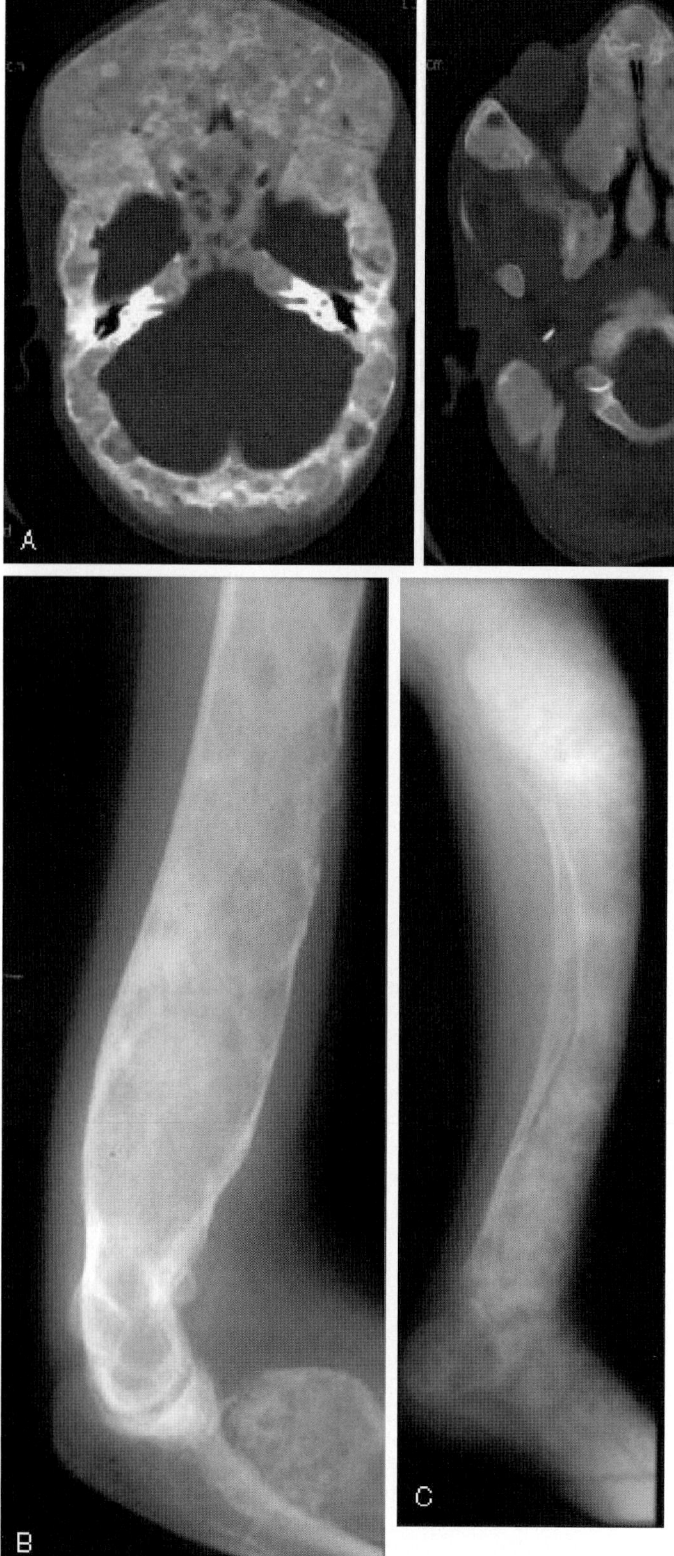

Figure 24–82 ▪ Bone lesions in McCune-Albright syndrome. **A,** The skull with severe thickening primarily at the base due to fibrous dysplasia. The auditory and optic nerves could be caught in narrowed foramina but that is not the case in these patients. **B** and **C,** Distortions of the long bones, which can develop into a "shepherd's crock" appearance; note the multiple bone cysts.

tive and ovulatory cycles ensue. Thus, an affected girl may progress from GnRH-independent puberty to GnRH-dependent puberty (see Table 24–47).[2097,2468,2470] GnRH agonists are not effective for treatment in the GnRH-independent stage. Testolactone (40 mg/kg/day orally),[2471] a relatively weak aromatase inhibitor, has been of equivocal usefulness,[2472] and some patients become resistant to the drug.[2473] The use of the new, highly potent, specific, third-generation aromatase inhibitors, such as letrozole, may be more effective,[336,337] but experience with fadrozole has not yet demonstrated clinical efficacy in girls with McCune-Albright syndrome.[2474] After a single case report of treatment with tamoxifen, an antiestrogen, showed decrease in

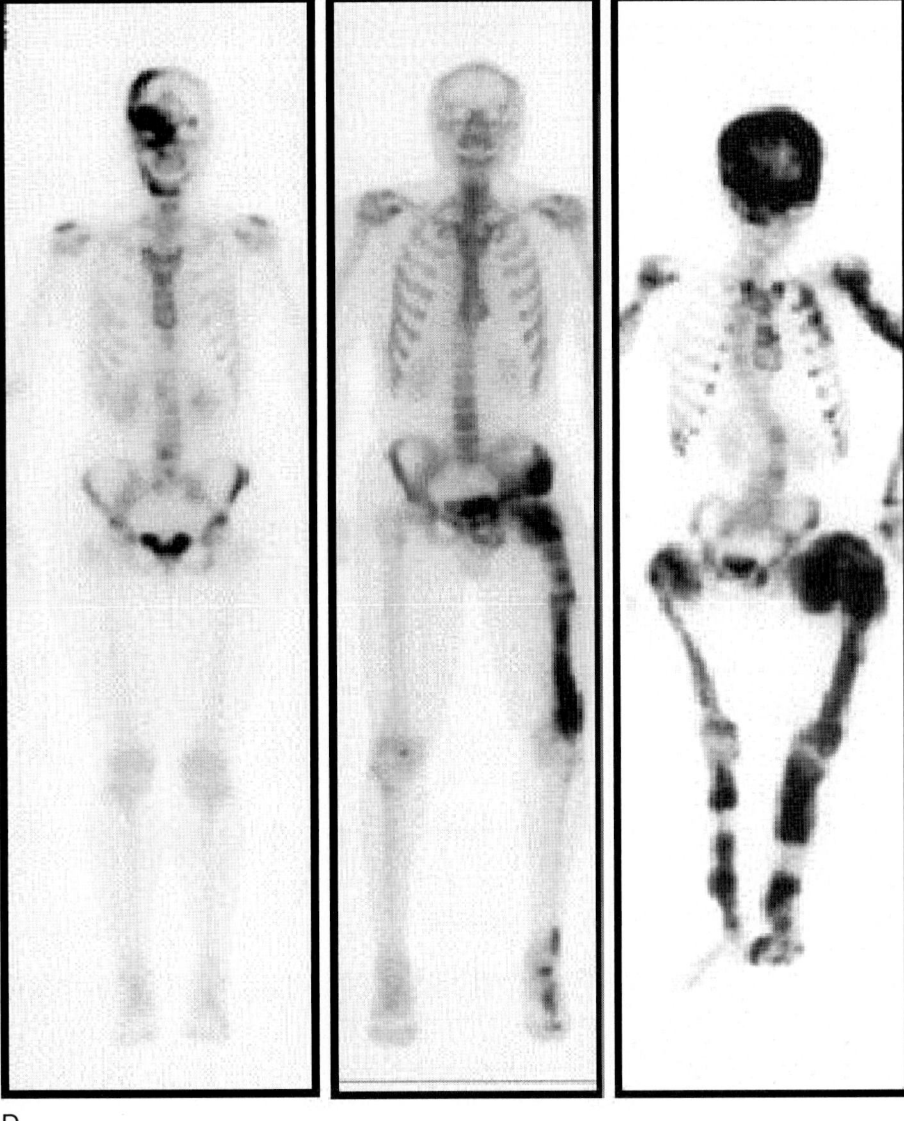

Figure 24–82, cont'd ▪ **D,** Bone scan showing the areas of remodeling that "light up" depending upon the area affected in individual patients. There are examples of patients primarily affected in the craniofacial area, in the appendicular area, and in both areas as well as the axial skeleton. (Courtesy of Michael T. Collins, M.D., National Institutes of Health, Bethesda, MD, and Sandra Gorges, M.D., University of California, Davis.)

bone age advancement, growth rate, menses, and pubertal development,[2475] a multicenter trial demonstrated the utility of this agent in decreasing vaginal bleeding and decreasing the rate of bone age advancement and growth rate in affected girls.[2476] However, ovarian and uterine volumes remained elevated.

Sexual precocity is rare in boys with McCune-Albright syndrome.[2117,2477,2395] Affected boys may have asymmetric enlargement of the testes in addition to signs of sexual precocity. The histologic changes and hormonal findings are reminiscent of those in testotoxicosis: the seminiferous tubules are enlarged and exhibit spermatogenesis; Leydig cells may be hyperplastic.[2117,2477] A 3.8-year-old boy with the McCune-Albright syndrome (several café -au-lait lesions on the back and polyostotic fibrous dysplasia) had an Arg201His mutation detected in bone and testis tissue and the unusual feature of macroorchidism (right testis 9 mL, left testis 7 mL) and the absence of sexual precocity. While basal and GnRH stimulated gonadotropins and sex steroid levels were prepubertal, serum inhibin B and antimüllerian hormone concentrations were strikingly elevated. The testes on histology showed that most seminiferous tubules were "slightly" increased in diameter and filled with Sertoli cells but lacked a lumen. The tubules stained intensively for inhibin B_B subunit; mature Leydig cells were absent.[2478] An increased incidence of the rare condition, testicular microlithiasis, was described in boys with McCune-Albright syndrome evaluated by ultrasonography.[2479]

McCune-Albright syndrome may occur concordantly or discordantly in monozygotic twins; familial cases have not been described. In 1986, Happle[2480] posited that the disorder is caused by an autosomal "dominant" lethal gene that results in loss of the zygote in utero and that cells bearing this mutation survive only in embryos mosaic for the lethal gene. The early somatic mutation would lead to a mosaic cell pattern of the distribution of cells containing the mutation. The severity of the disorder would depend on the proportion of mutant cells in various embryonic tissues. The description of somatic mutations in human endocrine tumors that convert the peptide chain of the Gs protein into a putative oncogene (referred to as a *gsp* mutation)[2481] raised the possibility of a similar defect in the McCune-Albright syndrome that both affect a differentiated function such as a signaling pathway and mediate the regulation of proliferation. These hypotheses are established in that mutations in the gene encoding the α-subunit of the stimulatory G protein for adenyl cyclase were identified in the tissues of children with the McCune-Albright syndrome.

TABLE 24–49 A PATIENT WITH MCCUNE-ALBRIGHT SYNDROME AND RECURRENT OVARIAN CYSTS

Chronologic Age (yr)	Bone Age (yr)	Height (cm)	Physical Signs*	Basal and Post-LHRH[‡]	Plasma Estradiol, pmol/L (pg/mL)	Radiograph, Long Bones
$1\frac{4}{12}$	$1\frac{3}{12}$	81.1	Café au lait pigmentation, B2, PH1 Vaginal bleeding (× 2 mo)	LH 0.6-1.3[†] (LER-960) FSH 1.9-3.2[†] (LER-869) (DHEAS <0.14 μmol/L [<50 ng/nL])	40 (11)	Normal
$1\frac{8}{12}$			B1, PH1			
$2\frac{6}{12}$	$2\frac{6}{12}$	92.4	B2, PH2 Vaginal bleeding	LH 0.6-1.1 FSH 1.9-3.2 (DHEAS <0.14 μmol/L [<50 ng/mL])	55-66 (15-18)	Normal
$3\frac{3}{12}$		98.3	B1, PH1			
$3\frac{10}{12}$	$3\frac{10}{12}$		B2, PH1	LH 1.1-2.0 FSH 1-1.7	51-95 (14-26)	Normal
$4\frac{3}{12}$			B1, PH1		7.3-7.3 (20-20)	Polyostotic fibrous dysplasia of fermurs
$5\frac{11}{12}$	6	123.4	B3, PH2 Vaginal bleeding (× 2 mo)	LH 1.1-4.3 FSH 1.0-2.0		
$6\frac{6}{12}$	$7\frac{10}{12}$	128.5	B3, PH2 Oral medroxyprogesterone acetate, 10 mg bid stated		<5	
$7\frac{10}{12}$	$8\frac{10}{12}$	136.8				
$8\frac{7}{12}$		142.2				

*B2, breast stage 2; PH1, public hair stage 1.
[†]ng/mL To conver ng/mL to IU/L, multiply LH value by 3.8 and FSH value by 8.4.
[‡]Note the prepubertal LH response to GnRH consistent with GnRH-independent sexual precocity until age 5 11/12 yr, and the pubertal LH response at 5 11/12 yr consistent with the development of secondary true precocious puberty (GnRH-dependent). Note discrepancy between gonadarche and adrenarche as evidenced by preadrenarchal concentration of DHEAS.

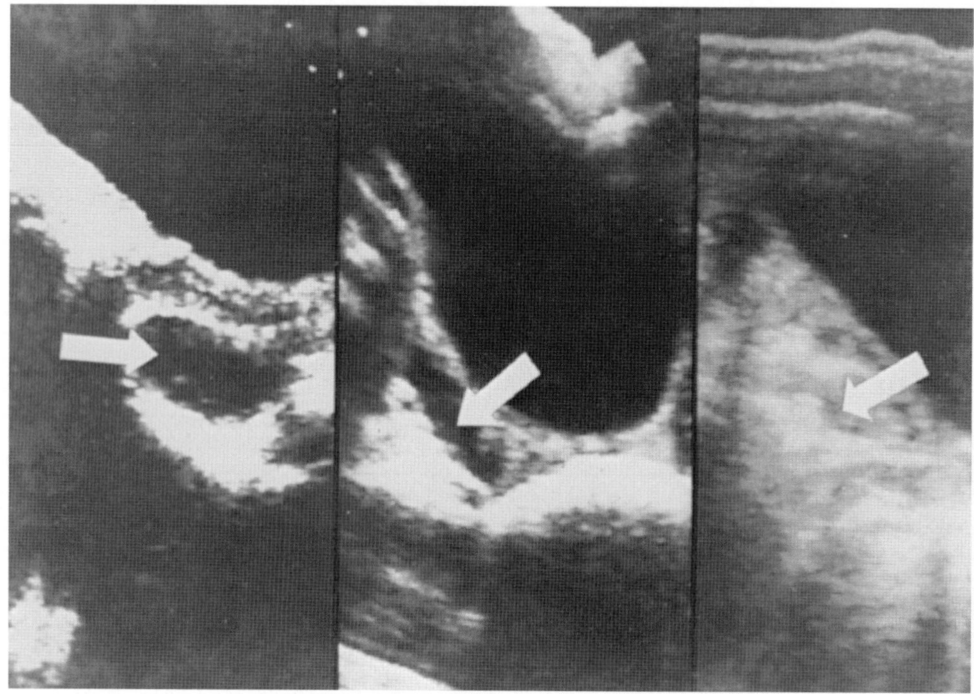

Figure 24–83 ▪ Serial pelvic ultrasonograms at 2-week intervals in a 6-year-old girl with McCune-Albright syndrome. Breast development and vaginal bleeding coincided with the enlargement of the ovarian cyst. With the spontaneous regression of the large ovarian cyst, the breasts regressed in size and vaginal bleeding ceased. (From Kaplan SL, Grumbach MM. Pathogenesis of sexual precocity. In Grumbach MM, Sizonenko PC, Aubert ML, eds. Control of the Onset of Puberty. Baltimore: Williams & Wilkins, 1990:620-660.)

The heterotrimeric guanine nucleotide binding proteins (G proteins) are a subfamily within the large superfamily of GTP-binding proteins and serve to transduce signals from a large number of cell-surface receptors with a common structural motif of seven-membrane–spanning domains to their intracellular effector molecules, including enzymes and ion channels; in essence, they couple serpentine cell-surface receptors to effectors (Fig. 24–84). For Gs, the stimulatory G-protein, the effector is adenyl cyclase, which is controlled by Gs and an inhibitory (Gi) G protein (reviewed in references 2393, 2482, and 2483). The heterotrimer is composed of (1) an α-subunit (39 to 45 kd) that binds GTP and has intrinsic GTPase activity, which converts GTP to GDP; (2) a β-subunit (35 to 36 kd) and a smaller β-subunit (7 to 8 kd) that are tightly but noncovalently associated with each other. Each of the subunits is encoded by a distinct gene. The G proteins function as "conformational switches." The GDP-liganded α-subunit is bound to the βγ subunits and is in an inactivated state. When the cell-surface receptor is activated by its ligand or agonists, the GDP is catalytically released from the α-subunit and enables GTP to bind. This leads to dissociation of the GTP-activated α-subunit, its dissociation from the bound βγ subunits, and activation of the effector, adenyl cyclase. When GTP is hydrolyzed by the intrinsic GTPase activity of Gsα, the α and βγ subunits reassociate and the α-subunit is now in the off or inactive conformation. The three-dimensional structure of the heterotrimeric G proteins has been determined.[2484-2488]

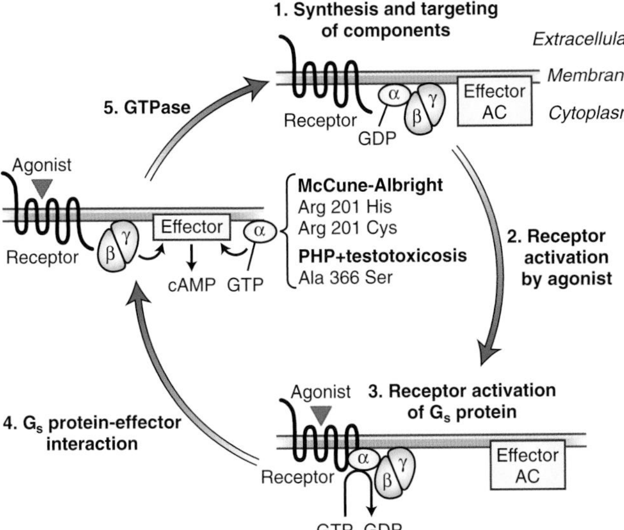

Figure 24–84 ▪ The G protein guanosine triphosphatase (GTPase) cycle. The heterotrimeric guanine nucleotide-binding proteins (G proteins) composed of three subunits (α, β, γ) couple cell-surface receptors consisting of a single serpentine polypeptide having seven helical membrane-spanning domains with an effector, in this instance, adenylate cyclase (AC) that catalyzes the transformation of adenosine triphosphate (ATP) to cyclic adenosine monophosphate (cAMP). The G protein stimulation subunit α, $G_{s\alpha}$, mediates the stimulation of cAMP generation. In the inactive, unstimulated state, the G protein is a heterotrimer and GDP is tightly bound to the α subunit. When the cell-surface receptor is activated by its cognate agonist, the receptor catalyzes the release of the tightly bound GDP, which enables GTP to bind to the α subunit. The GTP-bound α subunit (α-GTP) dissociates from the tightly bound βγ dimer, and both play a role in the G protein activation of the effector, adenylate cyclase. The intrinsic GTPase activity of the α subunit ends the stimulation of the effector by converting the bound α-GTP to α-GDP; as a consequence, the α subunit again returns to its inactive state and reassociates with high affinity with the βγ subunit, yielding the α, β, γ heterotrimer. Disorders of signal transduction can arise from germ cell or somatic mutations at any of the five stages of the cycle. The gain-of-function, activating somatic mutations in the *GNAS1* gene that encodes the G $G_{s\alpha}$ subunit and leads to McCune-Albright syndrome (shown in the bracket), involves the highly conserved arginine 201 residue. These mutations inhibit the intrinsic GTPase activity of the α subunit and hence the conversion of the bound GTP to GDP. *(See text.)* Alanine 366-to-serine mutation (shown in the bracket) was detected in two boys, both of whom had pseudohypothyroidism Ia (PHP) and testotoxicosis. The mutant protein was constitutively activated in the Leydig cells at the scrotal temperature (32° to 33° C), leading to testotoxicosis, but was rapidly degraded at body temperature, 37° C, which led to PHP1a. *(See text.)* (Modified from Spiegel AM. Mutations in G proteins and G protein-coupled receptors in endocrine disease. J Clin Endocrinol Metab 1996;81:2434-2442.)

Activating heterozygous mutations in the Gs α-subunit that occurred as an early postzygotic event are described in the McCune-Albright syndrome. The somatic constitutive activating mutation, which leads to excess cAMP production and in some tissues cAMP-induced hyperplasia,[2487] has a mosaic pattern and the proportion of the hyperactive mutant to normal cells varies in different tissues, contributing, at least in part, to the varied clinical findings, severity, its sporadic nature, and the discordant occurrence in monozygotic twins. A germ line mutation is presumed to be lethal to the embryo. Two gain of function somatic missense mutations have been described in this order, both of which involve the arginine 201 residue of the α-subunit,[2393] the site of covalent modification by cholera toxin: arginine 201 with either a cysteine or histidine substitution (see Fig. 24–84).[2395,2489-2492] The arginine 201 residue is critical for α-subunit GTPase activity, and each of the two mutations decreases the GTPase activity of the Gsα-subunit and leads to constitutive activation. These activating mutations have been found in all tissues affected in the syndrome,[2493,2494] including bone lesions.

Juvenile Hypothyroidism

Longstanding untreated primary hypothyroidism, usually a consequence of Hashimoto's thyroiditis, is an uncommon cause of incomplete isosexual precocity[428,2495,2496] in both girls and boys and occurs in association with impaired growth and delayed skeletal maturation. If the concentration of plasma prolactin is elevated, galactorrhea may be demonstrable, more commonly in affected girls than boys (Figs. 24–85 and 24–86). Girls have breast development, enlarged labia minora, and estrogenic changes in the vaginal smear, usually without the appearance of pubic hair.[428,2497-2499] Some girls have irregular vaginal bleeding,[428,2500] which could proceed to metrorrhagia,[2501,2502] and solitary or multiple ovarian cysts may be demonstrable by pelvic sonography or by physical examination.[428,2503,2504] It is important to recognize the condition to avoid unnecessary surgery, which would be a tragic mistake in lieu of the success of medical management.[2505] In about 80% of boys with juvenile hypothyroidism, the testes are enlarged because of an increase in the size of the seminiferous tubules, but signs of virilization and Leydig cell maturation are absent[2506,2507] and the plasma concentration of testosterone is prepubertal. Enlargement of the sella turcica and the pituitary gland (see Fig. 24–86) has led to the misdiagnosis of a pituitary neoplasm. The hypothyroidism, incomplete sexual maturation, galactorrhea, and pituitary enlargement are reversed or corrected by levothyroxine therapy within a few months.[428]

In 1960, Van Wyk and Grumbach[428] suggested that the syndrome resulted from hormonal "overlap" in negative feedback regulation with increased secretion of gonadotropins, prolactin, and TSH as a consequence of the chronic hypothyroidism. With the advent of radioimmunoassays for pituitary hormones, increased prolactin secretion was documented in children[2496] and adults with primary hypothyroidism and in affected girls with the syndrome.[2497] GH release is usually decreased as in uncomplicated primary hypothyroidism.[2508,2509]

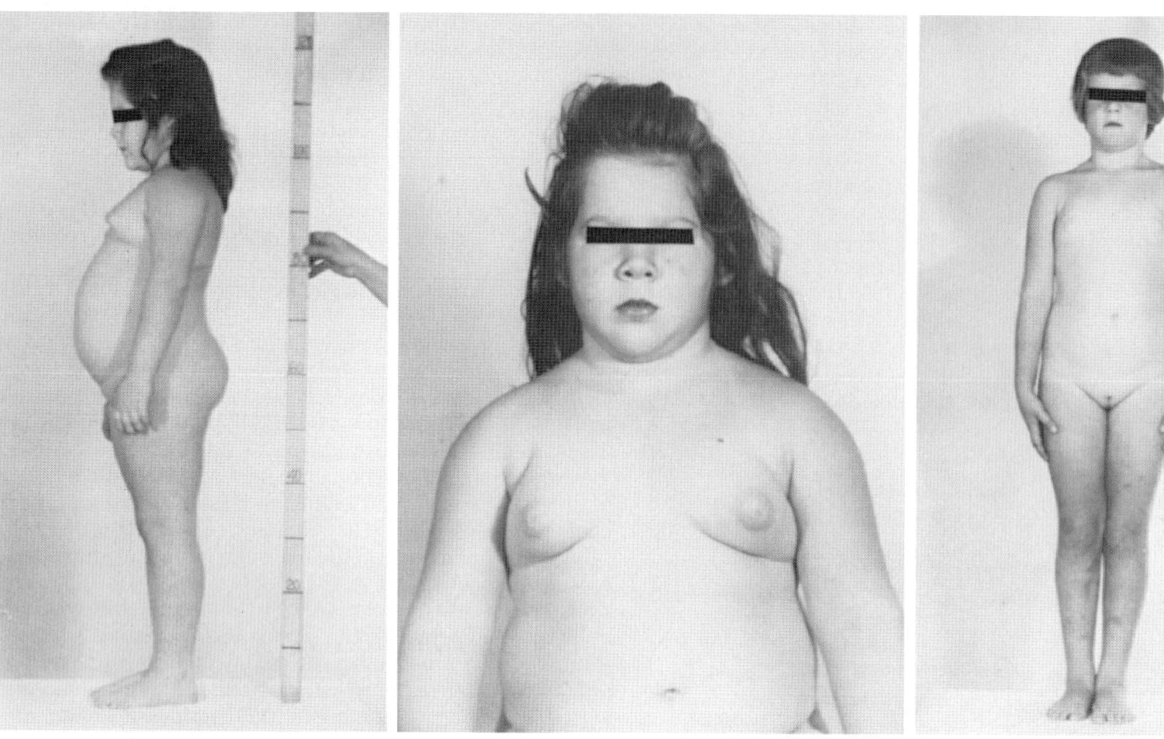

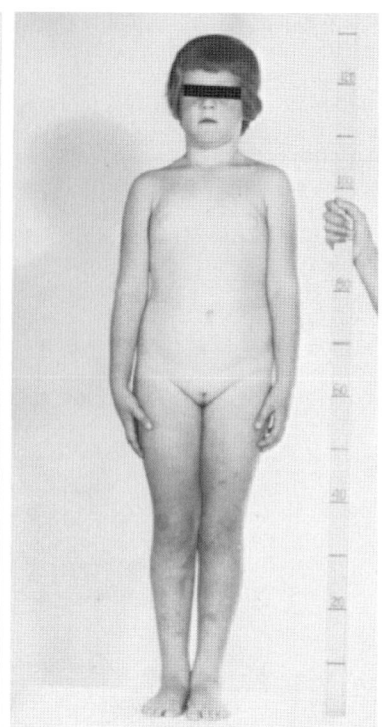

Figure 24–85 ▪ *Left* and *center,* Severe, chronic hypothyroidism of Hashimoto's thyroiditis in a 7 1/12-year-old girl with sexual precocity (without pubic or axillary hair), episodic vaginal bleeding, and galactorrhea. She had symptoms of hypothyroidism and a sharply decreased rate of growth over the previous 2 years (height, −1 SD; bone age, 5 3/12 years). Breast development was Tanner stage 3; the labia minora were enlarged, and the vaginal mucosa was dull pink, thickened, and rugated with evidence of an estrogenic effect. No acne, seborrhea, or hirsutism was present. The uterus was of adolescent size, and the endometrial mucosa was in a proliferative phase. Urinary gonadotropins were barely detectable by bioassay. *Right,* Striking change in appearance after 8 months of thyroid hormone treatment. She had grown 7 cm in height and lost 8.1 kg in weight; the breasts had decreased in size, galactorrhea was no longer demonstrable, the labia minora had regressed, and the vaginal mucosa was pink and glistening (no estrogen effect). Ten weeks after the initiation of thyroid hormone replacement therapy, she developed a right slipped capital femoral epiphysis that was repaired surgically; recovery was uneventful.

However, the explanation for the sexual maturation remains uncertain. Pubertal development in primary hypothyroidism is usually delayed and is only rarely advanced for chronologic age. By using radioimmunoassays for FSH and LH in which the cross-reaction with TSH is negligible, an increased (pubertal) concentration of plasma immunoreactive and bioactive FSH but not LH has been detected.[2508-2510] Bioactive LH activity is also low. In addition, increased FSH pulsatility, mainly at night, but not LH release was demonstrated in patients with the syndrome and in some children with primary hypothyroidism who did not exhibit premature sexual maturation.[2508-2510] The increased FSH release and the high FSH/LH ratio (in contrast to that in normal puberty) seem to account for the increased ovarian estrogen secretion in girls and for the enlarged testes without signs of virilization in affected boys; the suggestion here is that FSH-induced Sertoli cell proliferation is an important determinant of mature testis size.[302,2511,2512] A GnRH-independent mechanism is quite likely in that GnRH did not suppress the pubertal LH levels.[2510] Pulsatile TSH release is increased at night and administration of TRH appears to increase FSH release in normal children (but not adults). Moreover, the FSH response to TRH, but not GnRH, is augmented in primary hypothyroidism[2509] and this FSH response to TRH can occur in gonadotropin-secreting pituitary adenomas. If the latter observations are confirmed, it is likely that the incomplete sexual precocity and the increased prolactin secretion and galactorrhea are a consequence of the increased release of TRH, the increased sensitivity of the mammotropes and gonadotropes to TRH, or both. This mechanism,[428] which has gained recent support,[2510] would explain the relatively rapid and complete reversal of the syndrome by levothyroxine treatment. Human recombinant TSH at a dose about 1000-fold greater than hFSH evoked a dose-dependent cAMP response in COS-7 cells transfected with the human FSH receptor, which suggests another possible mechanism for the FSH- (or FSH-like) dependent but GnRH-independent sexual precocity.[2513] In 7 girls and 1 boy with the syndrome, no mutations in the hFSHR were detected. In transfected cultured cells containing the hFSHR, LFSHR polymorphisms had no effect on the cAMP response to hTSH. The hFSHR transfected cells responded to high doses of hTSH.[2513a] A direct effect of severe hypothyroidism on the prepubertal testis, which leads to overproliferation of Sertoli cells, also has been advanced as an explication of the macroorchidism.[2507]

Diagnosis of Sexual Precocity (Table 24–50 and Figs. 24–87 to 24–89)

The separation of patients with self-limited benign disorders, such as premature adrenarche or premature thelarche, or normal but early puberty, from those with serious or even potentially fatal disorders is the first step in evaluation. The history may reveal symptoms suggesting perinatal abnormalities or injuries, previous infections, adventitious ingestion of or exposure to gonadal steroids, or the presence of similar conditions in

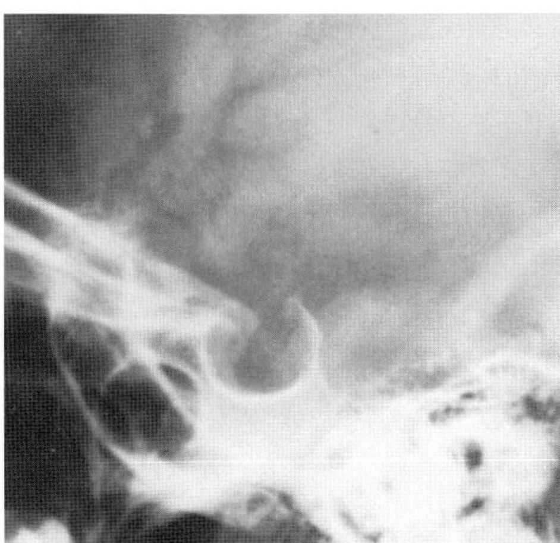

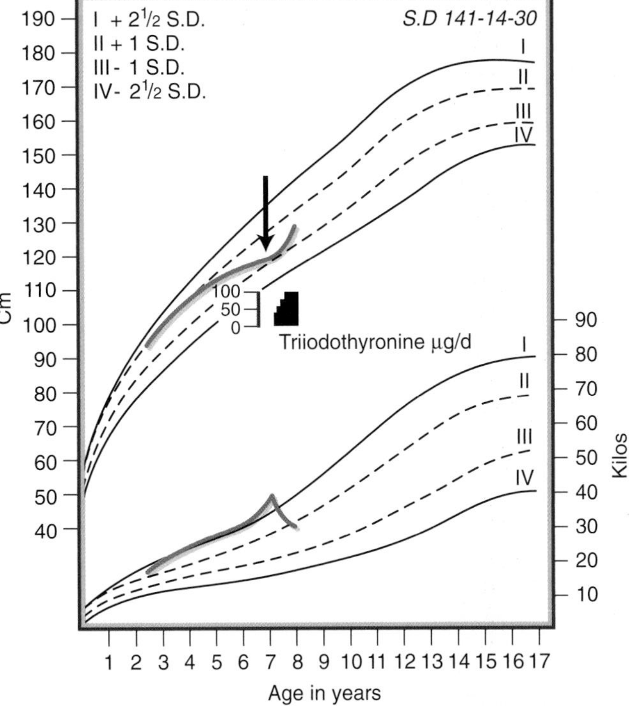

Figure 24–86 ▪ *Left,* Radiograph of the skull of a patient with hypothyroidism illustrating an enlarged pituitary fossa in the lateral view. The dorsum sellae was thin and demineralized, and the floor had a double contour line. The area of the sella turcica was 150 mm². Pneumoencephalography showed a suprasellar mass impinging on the cisterna chiasmatica. After thyroid hormone treatment for 8 months, the area of the sella had decreased 30% in volume to 100 mm², the dorsum sellae had remineralized, and the double floor was no longer evident. *Right,* Growth curve illustrating the decrease in growth rate despite the sexual precocity and the catch-up growth induced by thyroid hormone therapy. (From Van Wyk JJ, Grumbach MM. Syndrome of precocious menstruation and galactorrhea in juvenile hypothyroidism: an example of hormonal overlap in pituitary feedback. J Pediatr 1960;57:416-435.)

family members. In addition, previous measurements should be plotted on a growth chart to determine height velocity and the age of onset of any increase in the rate of growth.

Important aspects of the physical examination include description of the secondary sexual development according to Tanner stages; measurement of the penis and the testes in boys and breast tissue in girls; and examination for acne, oily skin, facial and body hair, pubic and axillary hair development, apocrine gland odor, muscular development, and galactorrhea. A careful examination of the external genitalia should be done with a nonrelated chaperone present, as the performance of such an examination has been interpreted by patients as sexual abuse in some cases.[2514] A thorough neurologic examination is indicated, with emphasis on assessment of the visual fields and optic discs, and search for signs of increased intracranial pressure; evaluation for skin lesions of the McCune-Albright syndrome or neurofibromatosis; and examination for abdominal, gonadal, or adnexal masses and for coexisting endocrine disease. Bone age is determined in all cases.

Ultrasonography of the ovary and uterus is exceedingly useful in evaluation of affected girls[2409] because standards are available for the shape and volume of the uterus and the ovaries.[2515-2518] The largest measurement of uterine size by sonograph in infants and children on ultrasound is found at puberty and in the neonatal period.[2517] The upper limit of uterine length in the prepubertal state is 3.5 cm.[2515] Furthermore, a uterine volume of greater than 1.8 mL is quite specific for the onset of puberty while increased ovarian volume is less specific. Patients with premature thelarche were indistinguishable from age-matched controls when this sonographic standard was used.[288] The presence of microcysts and macrocysts of the ovary can be detected on ultrasound as well.[2409] Cysts may be found in the ovaries in true precocious puberty or GnRH-independent isosexual precocity, but the cysts usually are less than 9 mm in the former and greater than 9 mm in the latter.[2017]

Measurements of basal plasma gonadotropin concentrations and the LH response to administration of GnRH or GnRH agonist or the amplitude and frequency of LH pulses, especially at night, using third-generation assays, and the plasma concentration of testosterone in boys and of estradiol in girls using LCMSMS assays are of primary importance in diagnosis. Girls early in the course of true precocious puberty have elevation of estradiol associated with increasing LH levels but not necessarily an increase in the concentration of FSH.[2519] Determination of thyroxine concentration is indicated when hypothyroidism is suspected. CPP in males usually begins with enlargement of the testes, followed by other signs of secondary sexual maturation. A Leydig cell tumor usually causes asymmetric enlargement of the testes, whereas an extragonadal hCG-secreting tumor is associated with less marked testicular enlargement than occurs at the same stage of masculinization in true precocious puberty. Adrenal rests in the testes may enlarge under chronic stimulation from ACTH in inadequately treated congenital adrenal hyperplasia or noncompliant boys and may be bilateral, although they are unlikely to closely mimic normal pubertal testicular development.[2520] An elevated hCG level with a prepubertal, or supressed, GnRH test indicates an ectopic, autonomous, gonadotropin-secreting tumor. If this tumor is in the CNS, abnormalities are likely present on MRI or CT brain scans. Enlargement of the liver or a mediastinal, retroperitoneal mass

TABLE 24–50 DIFFERENTIAL DIAGNOSIS OF SEXUAL PRECOCITY

	Plasma Gonadotropins	LH Response to GnRH	Serum Sex Sterold Concentration	Gonadal Size	Miscellaneous
True Precocious Puberty (premature reactivation of GnRH pulse generator)	Prominent LH pulses, initially during sleep	Pubertal LH response	Pubertal values of testosterone or estradiol	Normal pubertal testicular enlargement or ovarian and uterine enlargement (by ultrasonography)	MRI of brain to rule out CNS tumor or other abnormality; skeletal survey for McCune-Albright syndrome
Incomplete Sexual Precocity (pituitary gonadotropin-independent)					
Males					
Chorionic gonado-tropin-secreting tumor in males	High hCG, low LH	Prepubertal LH response	Pubertal value of testosterone	Slight to moderate uniform enlargement of testes	Hepatomegaly suggests hepatoblas-toma; CT scan of brain if chorionic gonadotropin-secreting CNS tumor suspected
Leydig cell tumor in males	Suppressed	No LH response	Very high testosterone	Irregular asymmetrical enlargement of testes	
Familial testotoxicosis	Suppressed	No LH response	Pubertal values of testosterone	Testes symmetrical and larger than 2.5 cm but smaller than expected for pubertal development; spermatogenesis occurs	Familial; probably sex-limited, autosomal dominant trait
Virilizing congenital adrenal hyperplasia	Prepubertal	Prepubertal LH response	Elevated 17-OHP in CYP21 deficiency or elevated 11-deoxycortisol in CYP11B1 deficiency	Testes prepubertal	Autosomal recessive, may be congenital or late-onset form, may have salt loss in CYP21 deficiency or hypertension in CYP11B1 deficiency
Virilizing adrenal tumor	Prepubertal	Prepubertal LH response	High DHEAS and androstenedione values	Testes prepubertal	CT, MRI, or ultrasonography of abdomen
Premature adrenarche arche	Prepubertal	Prepubertal LH response	Prepubertal testosterone, DHEAS, or urinary 17-ketosteriod values appropriate for public hair stage 2	Textes prepubertal	Onset usually after 6 years of age; more frequent in CNS-injured children

Females					
Granulosa cell tumor (follicular cysts may present similarly)	Suppressed	Prepubertal LH response	Very high estradiol	Ovarian enlargement on physical examination, CT, or ultrasonography	Tumor often palpable on abdominal examination
Follicular cyst	Suppressed	Prepubertal LH response	Prepubertal to very high estradiol	Ovarian enlargement on physical examination, CT, or ultrasonography	Single or recurrent epiodes of menses and/or breast development; exclude McCune-Albright syndrome
Feminizing adrenal tumor	Suppressed	Prepubertal LH response	High estradiol and DHEAS values	Ovaries prepubertal	Unilateral adrenal mass
Premature thelarche	Prepubertal	Prepubertal LH, pubertal estradiol response	Prepubertal or early	Ovaries prepubertal	Onset usually before 3 years of age
Premature adrenarche	Prepubertal	Prepubertal LH response	Prepubertal estradiol; DHEAS or urinary 17-ketosteriod values appropriate for public hair stage 2	Ovaries prepubertal	Onset usually after 6 years of age; more frequent in brain-injured children
Late-onset virilizing congenital adrenal hyperplasia	Prepubertal	Prepubertal LH response	Elevated 17-OHP in basal or corticotropin-stimulated state	Ovaries prepubertal	Autosomal recessive
In Both Sexes					
McCune-Albright syndrome	Suppressed	Suppressed	Sex steroid pubertal or higher	Ovarian (on ultrasound); slight testicular enlargement	Skeletal survey for polyostotic fibrous dysplasia and skin examination for café au lait spots
Primary hypothyroidism	LH prepubertal; FSH may be slightly elevated	Prepubertal FSH may be increased	Estradiol may be pubertal	Testicular enlargement; ovaries cystic	TSH and prolactin elevated; T_4 low

CNS, Central nervous system; *CT*, computed tomography; *DHEAS*, dehydroepiandrosterone sulfate; *hCG*, human chorionic gonadotropin; *LH*, luteinizing hormone; MRI, magnetic resonance imaging; *17-OHP*, 17-hydroxyprogesterone; *T_4*, thyroxine; *TSH*, thyrotropin.

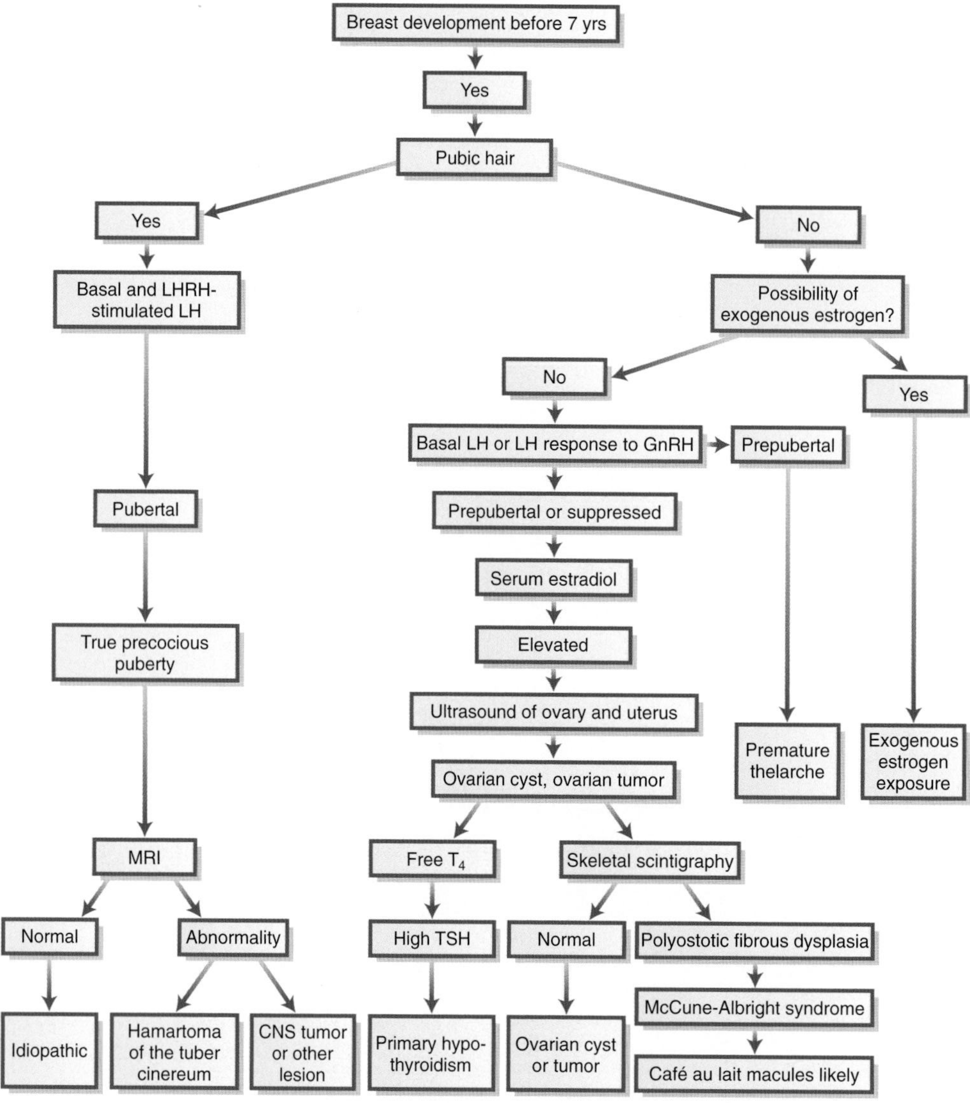

Figure 24–87 ▪ The diagnosis of sexual precocity in girls.

in boys with sexual precocity suggests an hCG-producing hepatic or germ cell tumor; the possibility of Klinefelter's syndrome needs to be considered with the latter.

Pubertal concentrations of LH and FSH, a pubertal mode of pulsatile LH secretion (initially during sleep), and/or pubertal LH response in the GnRH or GnRH agonist confirms the diagnosis of CPP (and in boys differentiates true precocity from familial testotoxicosis). A CNS tumor must be considered as a potential cause of this premature activation of the hypothalamic GnRH pulse generator. The evaluation for a CNS tumor as a cause of true precocious puberty is similar to the investigation of an hCG-secreting tumor of the CNS. Although CT scanning is now a well-established procedure for determining the presence of a CNS abnormality,[2521] MRI with contrast is more sensitive for the detection of small tumors in the hypothalamus, such as a hamartoma of the tuber cinereum (see Fig. 24–70).[1459,2164,2522] The use of contrast adds to diagnostic certainty and is recommended for MRI of the CNS.[2523] All boys with CPP should have CNS MRI evaluation but girls do not always receive the same recommendation as a CNS tumor is less likely in girls than in boys to be the cause of CPP. However, studies using MRI or CT brain scans indicate that the hypothalamic hamartoma is more prevalent in both boys and girls with so-called idiopathic true precocious puberty than was previously suspected. An unselected group of girls with precocious puberty and no other symptoms underwent CNS MRI; 15% had intracranial pathology and the authors found no clinical difference between them and the 85% who did not,[2524] suggesting CNS MRI is indicated in girls with precocious puberty as well.

The height of the pituitary gland on MRI correlates with advancing age and with pubertal development.[2525] Patients with true precocious puberty and higher peak LH/FSH ratios had pituitary heights exceeding 6 mm on the average while those with a lower LH/FSH ratio or precocious thelarche had lower heights of approximately 5 mm.[2526] The shape of the pituitary gland is also of importance; a convex appearance rather than a flat top is associated with true precocious puberty of all etiologies.[2132] The size and shape of the pituitary gland does not decrease with successful GnRH therapy.[2527]

The premature appearance of pubic hair, phallic enlargement, and other signs of virilization in a male without enlargement of the testes or the liver suggests the diagnosis of congenital virilizing CAH, virilizing adrenal tumor, or, rarely, Cushing's syndrome. Measurement of plasma 17-hydroxyprogesterone and DHEAS concentrations and their suppressibility with glucocorticoids will distinguish adrenal hyperplasia from a virilizing adrenal tumor. If growth rate is suppressed, the possibility of primary hypothyroidism or of Cushing syndrome is raised; ele-

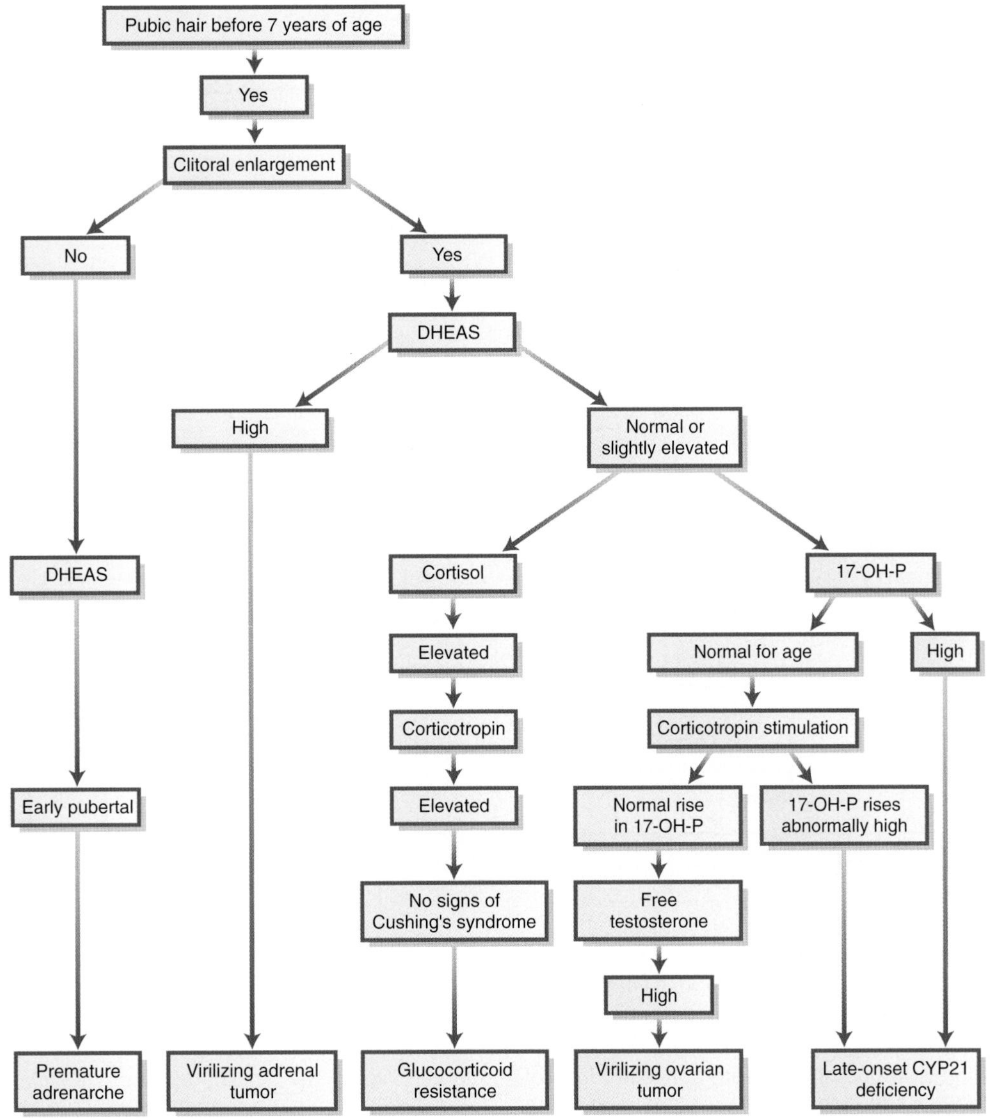

Figure 24–88 ▪ The evaluation of pubic hair in normal phenotypic girls before 7 years.

vated plasma concentrations of cortisol, urinary free cortisol, 17-hydroxycorticosteroid, or salivary cortisol after suppression with dexamethasone confirm the latter diagnosis. The appearance in a girl of pubic hair and other signs of virilization, such as clitoral enlargement, acne, deepening voice, muscular development, or growth spurt, is caused by CAH, virilizing adrenal tumor, or virilizing ovarian tumor. Cushing's syndrome caused by an adrenocortical carcinoma can cause virilization associated with growth failure and a virilizing adrenocortical carcinoma can present with so much androgen effect that the Cushing's syndrome is not apparent but rapid growth and virilization is noted; estradiol may be secreted by these tumors as well as androgens.[2528] Virilizing ovarian tumors can be detected by pelvic ultrasound.

The appearance of pubic hair without other signs of puberty in boys or girls, increased growth, or bone age advancement is usually a result of premature adrenarche but may be the first sign of sexual precocity or of adrenal virilism from other causes.

In a girl, breast development associated with dulling and thickening of the vaginal mucosa and enlargement of the labia minora indicates significant estrogen secretion or iatrogenic exposure to estrogen. The differential diagnosis includes true precocious puberty, an estrogen-secreting neoplasm, and a cyst of the ovary. If the plasma concentrations of gonadotropins are in the pubertal range, if LH pulses of pubertal amplitude are detected, or if a pubertal LH response to GnRH or GnRH agonist is elicited, true precocious puberty is present. Unfortunately one child is described with pubertal level serum LH due to heterophile antibodies interfering with the LH assay and fallaciously elevating the values in the basal and stimulated state; after addition of antimouse antibody, LH values decreased. As always, clinical observation should be congruent with laboratory findings.[2529] Estrogen concentrations in girls early in normal or true precocious puberty are in the prepubertal range much of the day, and a single determination may be inadequate to reflect ovarian function (see Fig. 24–67).[337,2097]

If the concentration of plasma estradiol is elevated but gonadotropin levels are low, an estrogen-secreting cyst or neoplasm is present or exogenous estrogens are exerting effects. Ovarian tumors of moderate size can be palpated by bimanual examination. Advances in pelvic sonography allow the delineation of ovarian cysts or tumors and the determination of uterine size. This procedure has become an essential component of the diagnostic evaluation.[2022] An estrogen-secreting neoplasm of the ovary is usually accompanied by high estradiol concentrations

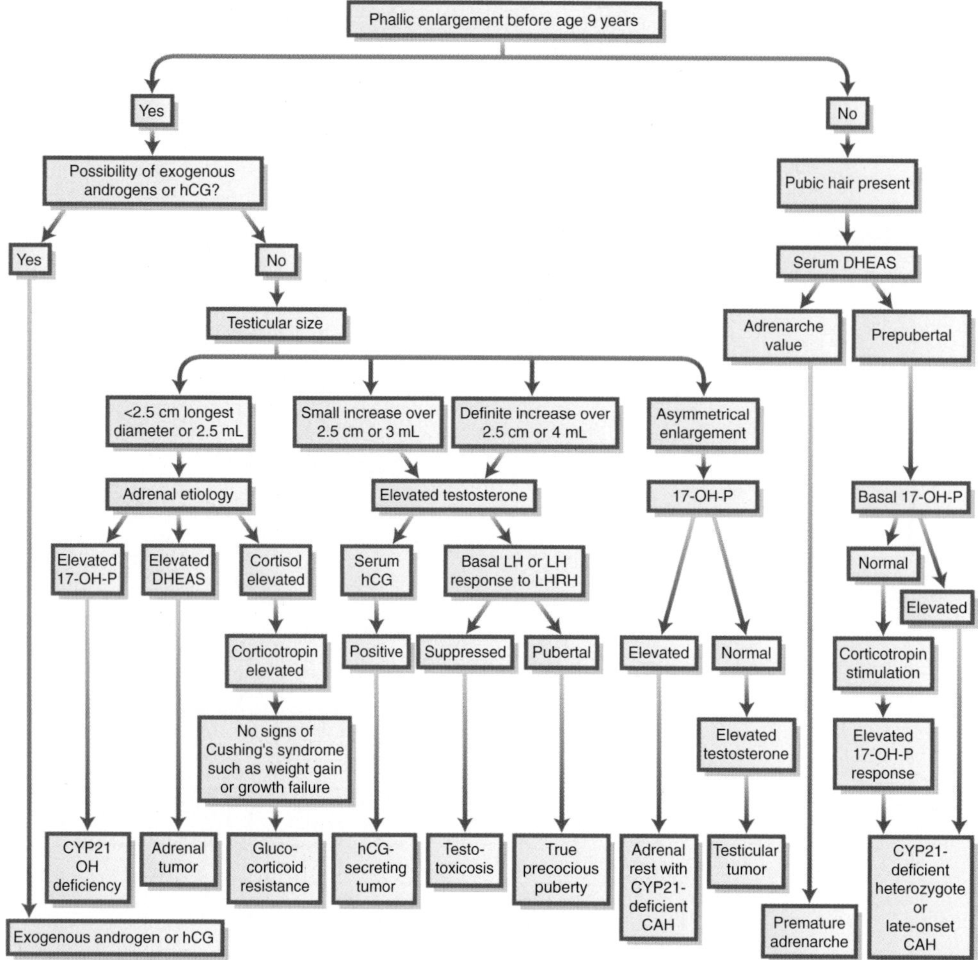

Figure 24–89 ▪ The diagnosis of sexual precocity in a phenotypic male.

but some ovarian cysts are associated with concentrations of estradiol as high as those in granulosa cell tumors. The differential diagnosis between these cysts and ovarian neoplasms rarely requires exploratory laparotomy or laparoscopy and usually can be resolved by pelvic sonography and by the use of tumor markers. Breast development in the absence of other estrogen effects is almost always a result of premature thelarche.

Iatrogenic Sexual Precocity and Endocrine Disruptors

Prepubertal children are remarkably sensitive to exogenous gonadal steroids and may show signs of sexual maturation resulting from overlooked sources of androgens or estrogens, such as ingested or absorbed tonics, lotions, or creams that contain or are inadvertently contaminated with an estrogen.[2530-2532] Hair creams and straighteners may contain estrogenic substances; this source of exogenous estrogens is more frequently encountered in an African-American population.[2533] The amount of estrogen available from these sources is unclear, but it is estimated that a dermal exposure to estrogen might add up to more than 300 mcg, far in excess of a therapeutic dose[2534] and possibly greater in infants and children exposed to estrogen dermal gel. Children who inhaled estrogen dust have developed sexual precocity. A short course of application of estrogen cream is used to treat labial adhesions, but long courses may lead to breast development or even withdrawal bleeding. In addition to breast development, pigmentation of the areolae and the linea alba and the appearance of pubic hair may be seen in children exposed to estrogen. One 21-month-old boy developed enlarged penis, pubic hair appearance, and rapid growth without testicular enlargement when the child was exposed to testosterone contaminating hydrocortisone cream used to treat eczema.[2535] The administration of hCG to boys with undescended testes may induce secretion of testosterone sufficient to cause incomplete sexual precocity.

Food is another potential source of estrogen or endocrine disruptors.[2536] Epidemics of gynecomastia in boys and thelarche in girls have occurred in schoolchildren in Italy;[2537,2538] meat contaminated by estrogens was suspected in some cases.[2539] However, no etiology was uncovered in Milan and environs where 21.1% of 1- to 2-year-old girls and 36.6% of 1- to 2-year-old boys were reported with premature thelarche or gyncecomastia.[2540] During a 10-year period, more than 600 cases of gynecomastia in boys and premature thelarche or incomplete sexual precocity in girls were discovered in Puerto Rico, the highest prevalence noted in the world, a prevalence about 10 to 15 times higher than a survey in Olmsted, MN.[2541-2543] Maternal ovarian cysts were demonstrated in two thirds of affected Puerto Rican girls.[2541,2544] The wide publicity given these observations and the questions raised about contamination of the food supply by the clandestine use of estrogens as growth-promoting agents for meat production caused anxiety among parents, cattle raisers, and farmers. It was suggested that the use of estrogen preparations in animals to stimulate weight gain led to ingestion of estrogen-contaminated meat. While this idea has not been confirmed by selected analyses of meat, poultry, and milk in Puerto Rico by the U.S. Department of Agriculture, it has not been excluded.[2544] Guidelines by the FDA define a limit of not more that 1% of normal daily estrogen production of prepubertal children as a safe intake of estrogen,[2545] which translates into 0.43 ng/day for boys and 3.24 ng/day for girls using the most recent data from extremely sensitive estrogen assays.[2532] While an increased prevalence of soy formula intake was described in affected girls, other studies do not link soy formula and premature thelarche or other auxologic effects, suggesting no result of phytoestrogen in this exposure.[2546] A possible association has been advanced between plasticizers with documented estrogenic and antiandrogenic activity and premature thelarche in Puerto Rico. Significantly elevated concentrations of phthalate and its major metabolites were found in 28 girls (68%) of a cohort with premature breast development in Puerto Rico.[2547] Criticisms of this finding arise because phthalates do not have estrogenic in vivo activity and have a short half-life, suggesting that because these girls were brought to evaluation due to premature thelarche, they must have been exposed, most likely from food, just before sampling and the values in their blood was so high and the level of metabolites of phthalates so low that the possibility of contamination by laboratory apparatus must arise.[2548]

Girls breastfed or exposed during intrauterine life to polybrominated biphenyls (PBBs) following an accidental exposure of their mothers in Michigan experienced early menarche (by about 1 year) and early appearance of pubic hair but not breast development compared to girls who were not exposed and to girls who were not breastfed.[2549]

Endocrine disruptors must be studied in more detail before cause and effect is established but there is some evidence that environmental agents are affecting pubertal development.[2550,2551] Environmental polychlorinated biphenyls (PCBs) are still present in many locations years after being banned. In some cases epidemiologic evidence is used to implicate such substances affecting puberty; in a circumscribed area of 2 villages in Tuscany, there was a 9.56 increase in relative risk for precocious puberty treated by GnRH agonist, compared to surrounding areas, suggesting an endocrine disruptor present in the area.[2552] Increased lead levels in Mohawk girls on the border of New York State and Canada delayed the age of menarche, while increased PCB levels promoted it.[2553] Variations in BMI exerted no effect, which is interesting as these toxic substances are concentrated in adipose tissue at all ages.[2554] In the NHANES III survey, a lead level of 3 mcg/dL delayed all measures of pubertal development including menarche and breast development in African-American girls for several months compared to those with lead levels less than 1 mcg/dL. No such delay was found in Caucasian girls.[2555] Another analysis of data from NHANES III using cutoffs of lead levels starting at 0.7 to 2.0 mcg/dL found delay in menarche and pubic hair appearance with increasing exposure but no effect on breast development; apparently this occurred in all included ethnic groups.[2556] Follow-up of adolescents exposed to DEHP (Di(2-ethylhexyl) phthalate, a component of polyvinylchloride (PVC) that is used in plastic tubing and medical devices) in the neonatal period through extra corporeal membrane oxygenation of (ECHMO) demonstrated no effects on pubertal development despite the findings of disruption of development in animals exposed to this substance.[2557] A preliminary report of boys exposed to aerial spraying of endosulfan in almond orchards in India suggests a delay in pubertal development.[2558]

A widespread exposure to 2,3,7,8-Tetrachlorodibenzo-*p*-dioxin (TCDD), an extremely potent antiestrogenic xenobiotic, due to a chemical exposure in Italy, was not associated with a change in the age of menarche, even though experimental exposure in rodents actually causes a delay in vaginal opening and other reproductive effects.[2559] However, a reanalysis of these data looking at the girls who were younger than 8 years at exposure, who presumably had the highest dose per BMI compared to older girls, showed a tendency for a decrease in the age of menarche, suggesting that age of exposure to environmental endocrine disruptors modulates their effects.[2560]

There is a high frequency of reproductive problems in adult Danish men such as impaired semen quality and testicular cancer in Denmark, but there is an increase in infantile testicular cancer as well.[2561] Furthermore, a 4.6% total rate of hypospadius was discovered in Danish newborns, some not noted until the foreskin was retracted.[2562] When compared to data from Finland, where there was a prevelance of 2.4%, the prevalence of 9.0% in a prospective study suggested environmental agents rather than genetic influences were responsible.[2563] Testes are larger in infant boys from Finland and inhibin B concentrations higher in comparison to measurements in Denmark, supporting the theory that environmental agents are a factor.[2563,2564] Phthalates were found in the breast milk of mothers from both countries and, although there was no relationship to the finding of hypospadias, there was indication of alteration of reproductive hormones in the boys in a pattern suggesting effects of these substances on the Leydig cells.[2563,2565]

Boys exposed to PCBs and polychlorinated dibenzofurans (PCDFs) in utero due to contamination of rice ingested by the mothers had decreased testosterone and increased estrogen compared to controls, although there was no difference on physical examination or in age of onset of puberty.[2566] This preliminary study suggests disruption of endocrine function after intrauterine exposure but must be confirmed by further observations. Boys exposed to DDT in utero did not demonstrate any abnormalities in puberty in a study from Philadelphia.[2567] However, a Chinese study of in utero exposure to the heat-degradation products of PCBs, mainly PCDFs, demonstrated defects in sperm production after puberty.[2568]

The sudy of endocrine disruptors is active, but the ultimate effects of environmental agents on reproductive development is not yet clear.

Feminization in Boys and Virilization in Girls (Contrasexual Precocity)

Boys

Feminization in a boy before the age of puberty is rare. Rarely, an estrogen-secreting adrenal adenoma[2569] or a chorionepithelioma may cause gynecomastia. Gynecomastia has been reported in a 1-year-old boy with 11-hydroxylase deficiency[2570] and in boys with late-onset congenital adrenal hyperplasia.

Aromatase Excess Syndrome

Gynecomastia in prepubertal boys can also be caused by increased extraglandular aromatization of C19 steroids of adrenal origin such as androstenedione and hence increased extraglandular estrogen production in sporadic or familial cases.[2571-2573] This autosomal dominant disorder leading to excess estrogen synthesis from C19 precursors due to aromatase overexpression, especially in fat and skin, is a consequence of gain-of-function mutations of CYP19, the gene encoding aromatase due to a chromosome arrangement, which gave rise to a cryptic promoter.[2574] Kindreds are reported with an autosomal dominant pattern of prepubertal gynecomastia and adult hypogonadism but not short stature in the presence of elevated serum estrone but less or no elevation of estradiol. The mutations in the CYP19 gene in these patients appeared different from those in the families above with gain of function mutations due to gene inversions.[2575] Turkish kindred found a potential rearrangement between CYP19 and TRPM7 genes on chromosome 15q21.2 as a cause of aromatase excess syndrome.[2576]

Feminizing testicular tumors may cause gynecomastia in boys younger than age 6 with the Peutz-Jeghers syndrome.[2436-2438] Both testes may be enlarged, and the histology indicates sex cord or Sertoli cell tumors that form annular tubules and often have areas of calcification; increased estradiol secretion is noted in the basal state, and a further rise occurs after hCG administration. Otherwise, feminizing Sertoli cell tumors are very rare in boys.[2440] Sonography or MRI scans of the testes may be useful in the diagnosis.[2440,2577]

In one series 5% of 581 boys referred for evaluation of gynecomastia were prepubertal at diagnosis (mean age of 9 years) and in 93.2% no underlying cause was identified.[2578] Spontaneous resolution was recorded in 6 boys, no change in 15, and further breast enlargement in 6. Pubertal onset of gynecomastia was documented in 13 boys at 12 years.[2579]

Girls

Virilization in a girl indicates organic disease except for premature adrenarche. CAH resulting from 21-hydroxylase or 11β-hydroxylase deficiency and androgen-producing tumors of the adrenal can cause virilization and are discussed earlier as occurring in males. 3β-Hydroxydehydrogenase/Δ4,5-isomerase deficiency is a rare type of congenital adrenal hyperplasia characterized by elevated 5-17-hydroxypregnenolone, DHEA, and DHEAS levels and, in the severe form, decreased secretion of aldosterone and cortisol. Severely affected patients have mineralocorticoid and glucocorticoid deficiency and may die in infancy. Excess adrenal androgens lead to virilization in utero and to ambiguous external genitalia, including clitoral enlargement in females with continued virilization after birth[1143] (see Chapter 22). Milder forms of this disorder can cause hirsutism in women. 46,XY Phenotypic women with incomplete forms of androgen resistance syndrome or with 17β-hydroxysteroid dehydrogenase type 3 deficiency may have virilization as well as breast development at the time of expected puberty. Mutations in the CYP19 gene, which encodes aromatase, are not only associated with intrauterine masculinization of the external genitalia in affected XX individuals but also with progressive virilization, lack of female secondary sex characteristics, multicystic ovaries at the age of puberty, tall stature, and osteopenia.[339,341] Polycystic ovarian syndrome in pubertal girls is frequently associated with varying degrees of virilization (see below: polycystic ovarian disease).

Cushing's syndrome resulting from adrenal carcinoma usually manifests as growth failure with or without virilization, obesity, and moon facies; striae may not appear for months to years later.

The syndrome of glucocorticoid resistance manifests in various degrees. Some patients demonstrate hyperandrogenic signs such as acne, hirsutism, male type baldness, menstrual irregularities, and oligoanovulation and infertility.[2580] Dexamethasone decreased the excessive adrenal androgen secretion, virilization, and advancing bone age found in a prepubertal boy with general glucocorticiod resistance.[2581]

Arrhenoblastoma, the most common virilizing ovarian tumor, is rare in children. Lipoid cell tumor of the ovary and gonadoblastoma are even more unusual sources of androgens.[2582,2583]

VARIATIONS OF PUBERTAL DEVELOPMENT

Premature Thelarche

Unilateral or bilateral breast enlargement without other signs of sexual maturation (e.g., sexual hair and growth of the labia minora and the uterus) is not uncommon in infancy and childhood as premature thelarche. The disorder usually occurs by age 2 (in over 80%) and rarely after age 4.[2584,2585] In a retrospective study in Minnesota, the incidence of premature thelarche was 21.2 per 100,000 patient-years, 60% of cases were noted between 6 months and 2 years of age, and most regressed in 6 months to 6 years after diagnosis, although a few persisted until puberty. When 10- to 35-year follow-up was available, no untoward effects on later health, growth, or fertility were evident.[2586] The breast enlargement usually regresses after a few months,[2587,2585] but occasionally persists for years or lasts until the onset of normal puberty; in about half of affected girls, the breast development, which is characteristically cyclic, lasts 3 to 5 years. Usually, significant nipple and areolae development is absent and estrogen-induced thickening and dulling of the vaginal mucosa is uncommon. Enlargement of the uterus on ultrasonography (greater than 1.8 mL volume and length greater than 36 mm) is rare. Measurement of the ellipsoid volume of the uterus (V=longitudinal diameter×anteroposteri or diameter×transverse diameter×0.523) is the most sensitive and specific discriminator between premature thelarche and early true precocious puberty[288] and provides better early discrimination than the LH response to GnRH or GnRH agonist. Growth in stature is normal.[945,2584,2588-2590]

This is a benign self-limited disorder compatible with normal pubertal development at an appropriate age; only reassurance and follow-up are usually necessary. The appearance of premature thelarche can, however, be the harbinger of further sexual maturation in a minority of cases as discussed e arlier.[945,2588,2591,2585,2297,2409] Because the development may be unilateral, it is important to consider the condition in girls with unilateral breast development so that needless worry about a breast neoplasm is not stimulated in the parents and no unnecessary surgical procedure is carried out. Indeed, the removal of tissue in premature thealrche may leave the child with no possibility of future breast development.[2020] In selected instances, sonography of the breast is useful in distinguishing unilateral premature thelarche from less benign conditions.[2592] The most common cause of breast mass in the pubertal girl is fibroadenoma; whereas metastatic disease may locate in the pubertal breast, breast carcinoma is exceedingly rare.[2592]

Plasma estradiol levels are slightly higher for age in premature thelarche when determined by a highly sensitive estrogen assay.[2593] However, there is usually no significant increase in plasma levels of TeBG or in thyroxin-binding globulin, indicators of estrogen action on circulating plasma proteins,[2594] although a modest increase of TeBG for age has been reported.[2050] The urocytogram often reveals an estrogen effect on squamous epithelial cells in the urine.[814,2595]

The concentration of serum FSH may be in the pubertal range, nocturnal FSH pulsatility has been detected, and the rise in FSH elicited by the administration of GnRH may be augmented for chronologic age, with an FSH/LH ratio higher in precocious thelarche than in normal individuals or girls with true precocious puberty.[1237,2584,2142,2596] However, these results overlap those in normal prepubertal girls.

As postulated for some recurrent ovarian cysts, premature thelarche appears to result from the ovarian response to transient increases in FSH levels and possible variations in ovarian sensitivity to FSH.[1237,2595] The LH response to GnRH is prepubertal in all cases.[1237,2597] Plasma inhibin B and FSH are higher in girls with precocious thelarche than in controls, in a range similar to that of precocious puberty.[2598] Activin concentrations have not been reported; the possible role of a paracrine-acting pituitary factor in stimulating FSH independent of GnRH is not known.

Sonograms of the ovary often show one or several cysts larger than 0.5 cm that disappear and reappear, usually correlating with changes in the size of the breasts[2409,2596] but the volume of the ovary and uterus is prepubertal.[2599,288] Unfortunately, in clinical practice, it is rare to find the cyst at the time of presentation and or at ultrasound study.

"Exaggerated thelarche" is described as premature thelarche with the added findings of advanced bone age and increased growth rate, estrogen effects in addition to thelarche. The endocrine measurements in the basal state are in the normal prepubertal range whereas after GnRH agonist stimulation, the FSH but not LH rose higher than in controls or true precocious puberty.[2600] Mutation of the GNAS1 involving replacement of arginine by histidine in codon 201 (R201H [+]) is associated with apparent premature or exaggerated thelarche and early menarche.[2459]

Premature Isolated Menarche

Rarely, girls begin periodic vaginal bleeding at age 1 to 9 years without any other signs of secondary sexual development.[2601-2603] The bleeding can recur for 1 to 6 years and then cease. At the normal age of puberty (3 to 11 years later), secondary sexual development and menses ensue and follow a normal pattern, as does stature. Fertility was later demonstrated after a normal onset of puberty in women with this variant of pubertal development. The etiology is uncertain, but it may be a counterpart of premature thelarche. There is a predominance of FSH secretion but the gonadotropin secretion is not characteristic of true premature puberty.[2604]

Isolated menarche may appear before other manifestations of sexual precocity in the McCune-Albright syndrome and in the premature sexual maturation that can occur in juvenile hypothyroidism.

Before the diagnosis of premature menarche is accepted, all other causes of vaginal bleeding and precocious estrogen secretion and of exposure to exogenous estrogens should be excluded, including neoplasms, granulomas, infection of the vagina or cervix, or a foreign body.[2605] In a series of 50 girls who had vaginal bleeding before age 10 years, a local lesion was found in about 50%; half of the latter had a malignant neoplasm (usually a rhabdomyosarcoma) and the other half had no discernible cause.[2606] In another report, a foreign body was responsible for 25% of vaginal bleeding in prepubertal girls.[2607] A careful examination for trauma, such as that caused by sexual abuse, is indicated. Urethral prolapse may be misdiagnosed as vaginal bleeding.

Premature Adrenarche (Pubarche)

Premature adrenarche[2608-2610] is the precocious appearance of pubic hair and/or axillary hair and less commonly an apocrine odor, comedones, and acne, without other signs of puberty or virilization; it is characterized by premature and mild adrenal hyperandrogenism.[936] Premature adrenarche refers to the rise in serum concentrations of adrenal androgens that cause the appearance of the pubic hair. In the past, this designation was assigned to the appearance of these clinical features before age 8 years in girls or age 9 years in boys. While in boys the age of 9 years still seems appropriate, the age of 8 years can no longer be used for American girls. At 6 years of age, 9.5% (range 5.7% to 16.4%) and at 8 years of age, 34.3% of African-American girls had Tanner stage 2 or greater pubic hair, whereas 1.4% (range 0.9% to 2.2%) and 7.7% of white girls, at these ages, respectively, had pubic hair (mean ages are shown in Table 24–3) in the PROS study. Accordingly, we recommend the diagnosis of premature pubarche be limited to African-American girls younger than 5 years of age and Caucasian-American girls younger than age 7 years, which should affect the age at which laboratory studies are initiated unless there are other signs of virilization such as clitoromegaly or rapid growth.

Premature adrenarche is about 10 times more common in girls than boys. The prevalence is increased in children with CNS abnormalities without a clear sex difference; the electroencephalogram may be abnormal[2121,2611] in the absence of other neurologic findings. Familial transmission is uncommon.[2612] Premature adrenarche is commonly slowly progressive and does not have an untoward effect on either the onset or normal progression of gonadarche or final adult height.[426] Nonetheless, there is a relationship between reduced fetal growth leading to intrauterine growth retardation, the increased prevalence of premature adrenarche and hyperinsulinism, and ovarian hyperandrogenism in life[2613] (see below).

Plasma concentrations of DHEA, DHEAS, androstenedione, testosterone, 17-hydroxyprogesterone and 17-hydroxypregnenolone are comparable to values normally found in pubic hair stage 2.[1261,2608,2614-2616] ACTH stimulation increases serum DHEA and DHEAS concentrations and the excretion of urinary 17-ketosteroids, but the concentrations of plasma 17-hydroxyprogesterone and 17-hydroxypregnenolone do not increase to the levels found in individuals with virilizing forms of congenital adrenal hyperplasia.[2615,2617,2618] Shorter androgen receptor gene CAG number, indicative of increased androgen sensitivity is found, in girls with precocious adrenarche in affected girls.[2619] As in CAH, dexamethasone suppresses adrenal androgen and androgen precursor secretion.[2615,2616] Serum gonadotropin levels in the basal state and after GnRH are in the prepubertal range in premature adrenarche.[1237,2620] Premature adrenarche occurs independently of gonadarche and is due to some factor other than increased secretion of GnRH or ACTH[1259] (see adrenarche, page 62). Bone age and height are slightly advanced for chronologic age but normal adult height is commonly achieved,[2621-2623] with the rare exception of some individuals with unusually high values of adrenal androgens, hirsutism, acne, and a bone age greater than 2.5 SD above the mean value for chronologic age. In a follow-up study of 20 girls, the functional adrenal hyperandrogenism in premature adrenarche was limited to childhood.[2622]

In our view, premature adrenarche is a developmentally regulated, normal variation in the differentiation, growth, and function of the zona reticularis of the adrenal cortex, marked biochemically by the precocious increase in the concentration of plasma DHEAS to more than 40 mcg/dL.[426] The latter is quite likely related to the independent increase of 17,20 lyase activity in the developing zona reticularis mediated by the increased phosphorylation of serine and threonine residues on the P450c17 enzyme, and the increased abundance of cytochrome b5 and of electron-donating redox partners such as cytochrome P450 oxidoreductase and cytochrome b5, essential for the 17,20 lyase activity of this functional microsomal enzyme (see Fig. 24–50).[2617] Nonetheless, the factor stimulating the development and function of the zona reticularis, independent of ACTH, remains elusive (see adrenarche, p. 62). In the past, the failure to recognize the earlier onset of normal adrenarche, particularly the striking ethnic differences in African-American, Hispanic, and Latin populations, has contributed to the overdiagnosis of premature adrenarche (e.g., see references 2621, 2624, and 2625), and, in some instances, needless laboratory studies.

The appearance of premature pubarche can be a manifestation of nonclassic congenital adrenal hyperplasia caused by homozygous or compound heterozygous missense mutations in the CYP21 gene encoding cytochrome P450c21.[2626] This condition can readily be detected by a plasma 17-hydroxyprogesterone response to ACTH that is at least 6 SD above the mean value. The prevalence of 21-hydroxylase deficiency in children with premature adrenarche is low,[2622,2627,2628] except in some ethnic groups[2629-2631] (e.g., Hispanic, Italians, and Ashkenazi Jews) in whom the prevalence may be as high as 20% to 30%.[2630,2631] The phenotype of premature pubarche is also associated with the rarer nonclassical 11β-hydroxylase deficiency.

There has been controversy about the prevalence and significance of 3β-hydroxysteroid dehydrogenase deficiency, and the pervasive belief that a mutation in the gene encoding this enzyme was a common cause of premature adrenarche and nonclassic 3β-HSD deficiency.[2630] The possibility of a mutation in the open receding frame of 3β-HSD of the type 2 or type 1 gene 1 has been excluded as all but an uncommon cause of this condition.[2632-2634] Mutations in the 3β-HSD type 2 gene have been associated with a 17-hydroxypregnenolone response to ACTH that exceeds or equals the mean normal value by 6 SD. Of 26 families studied, only one family with a mutation, alanine 82 threonine, had affected females who exhibited preature pubarche; in this family, the affected male was a male pseudohermaphrodite.[2635] Thus, a mutation in the 3β-HSD type 2 or type 1 gene is an uncommon cause of premature pubarche, exaggerated adrenarche, and of hirsute adolescent girls and women. The cause of the "mild deficiency" in 3β-HSD2 activity is unknown, but it may be multifactorial and lead to a wide range in the secretory capacity of the zona reticularis. A family constellation is described with a dominant pattern of inheritance[2612] of elevated adrenal androgens and androgen precursors that presented as premature pubarche; later affected individuals developed hirsutism and anovulation. Several investigators joined to propose hormonal standards for the diagnosis of 3β-HSD deficiency in cases of apparent premature pubarche and state that: ACTH stimulated Δ5 17P values must exceed 294 nmol/L or 54 SD above the mean for Tanner stage 2 (17±5 nmol/L) or a ratio of 17-hydroxypregnenolone (Δ5-17P) to cortisol (F) of 363, which is 3.0 SD above the mean ratio of 20±5. Recent studies relating genotype and hormonal analyses in the basal and ACTH- stimulated case confirmed that significant elevations of 17-hydroxypregnenolone (Δ5-17P) to cortisol (F) ratios are necessary to prove true 3β-HSD in genetically proven disease[2636] and that this is a rare disorder in patients presenting with putative premature adrenarche.[2637] However, patients with a constellation of findings of PCOS may have more subtle elevations of these values and present a picture of adrenal impairment of 3β-HSD activity in the absence of mutations in the gene coding for the enzyme; these children presenting with premature pubarche are postualateed to later develop clinical PCOS.[2636]

DHEA is a stimulus to sebaceous gland activity,[2638] and prepubertal acne or comedones may appear in association with elevated serum DHEAS concentrations in some children without the appearance of pubic hair, suggesting a variant of premature adrenarche may manifest in this manner.[2639-2641]

More significant androgen effects such as clitoral or penile enlargement, rapid growth, hirsutism, deepening of the voice, for example, excludes premature adrenarche and indicates a more severe form of hyperandrogenism.

The concept of "exaggerated adrenarche"[2627] was first advanced[2642] in relation to a postulated childhood antecedent of the polycystic ovary syndrome, the hallmarks of which are hyperandrogenism, hirsutism, anovulation, amenorrhea or oligomenorrhea, and insulin resistance and compensatory hyperinsulinemia, with its attendant risk of major metabolic sequelae including type 2 diabetes mellitus, dyslipidemia, and an increased propensity to coronary heart disease, and in about 50% of affected women, obesity.[2624,2643-2648] It has been extended to include rare instances of premature adrenarche associated with excessive responses of 17-hydroxypregnenolone, DHEAS, and androstenedione to ACTH found in women with functional adrenal hyperandrogenism.

While premature adrenarche was usually considered a benign condition with no substantial long-term risk, accumulating observations indicate that girls with premature adrenarche are at increased risk of developing functional ovarian hyperandrogenism and the polycystic ovarian syndrome, hyperinsulinism, acanthosis nigricans, and dyslipidemia in adolescence and adult life, especially if fetal growth was reduced and birth weight was low.[936] Affected girls have BMI values similar to controls but differing distribution of fat with an increased likelihood of increased waist circumference along with increased measure of insulin resistance.[2649]

Polycystic Ovarian Disease

Polycystic ovarian syndrome is the most common endocrine disease, estimated to affect 10% of women.[2650,2651] This condition is considered equivalent to the metabolic syndrome in its many manifestations in females. Recent review of diagnostic criteria support most of the original 1990 recommendations.[2007] A discussion of this condition is found in chapter 16. Premature adrenarche is a risk factor for the later development of the polycystic ovary syndrome and functional ovarian hyperandrogenism in adolescent and adult women. The magnitude of this risk is unknown but appears to be rare, except in girls with a history of decreased fetal growth.[2613,2652-2654,936,2622,2627] However, catch-up growth in children who were SGA may be an important factor in the development of PCOS. Serum androstenedione and DHEAS were related to weight gain between 1 and 3 years of age as well as to current weight and were inversely related to birth weight in an 880-member cohort of 8-year-olds.[25] However, not all researchers find a relationship between increase in premature adrenarche and small for gestational age birth weight; a Dutch study could not confirm such a relationship in 181 subjects born SGA compared to 170 subjects born appropriate for gestational age.[2655] In the absence of premature adrenarche, the age of onset of puberty in SGA children is in the normal range[2656] and is not affected by GH therapy.[2657] Recently, an association of premature adrenarche with prematurity as well as SGA birth was reported.[2658]

Plasma plasminogen activator inhibitor-1, a marker of risk for cardiovascular disease including in women with PCOS, was increased in girls with premature adrenarche, especially those with low birth weights, and may be useful in the identification of those with a greater risk of developing PCOS.[2659] Certain ethnic groups, especially African-American and Hispanic girls, carry a higher risk of the association of premature adrenarche with the metabolic syndrome (obesity, hyperinsulinism, dyslipidemia, and other factors increasing the risk of later coronary heart disease) and the development of the polycystic ovary syndrome in late adolescence and early adulthood,[936,2660-2662] especially if decreased insulin sensitivity and acanthosis nigricans accompany the premature adrenarche.[2661] Of interest, the adrenal steroid pattern in the black and Hispanic patients in the latter study[2662] did not differ from children with uncomplicated premature adrenarche.

As discussed above, hyperinsulinism is associated with many metabolic and endocrine conditions and functional ovarian hyperandrogenism, which in some cases is heralded by premature adrenarche.[2663] When the role of insulin resistance and hyperinsulinism was recognized in the pathogenesis of the polycystic ovary syndrome, therapeutic approaches to reduce insulin resistance were introduced, especially the use of insulin sensitizers. Among the latter, the most widely used drug is metformin because of its low prevalence of adverse effects and therapeutic efficacy. Its major effect is in decreasing gluconeogenesis from the liver rather than insulin sensitizing. In early studies in the treatment of PCOS, this agent, has decreased insulin resistance, ovarian hyperandrogenism, and hirsutism in both obese and nonobese patients;[2006,2664,2665] The safety and efficacy of metformin in 82 children and adolescents with type 2 diabetes mellitus (10 to 16 years of age) is supported by a short-term randomized control trial,[2666] Useful preliminary data support the safety of its use in adolescents with insulin resistance and functional ovarian hyperandrogenism although metformin is not approved for such use.

A trial of metformin in girls just past menarche with a history of low birth weight and premature adrenarche who are therefore at risk for development of PCOS prevented this predicted course.[2667,2668] Treatment of 8-year-old girls with similar risk factors appeared to diminish the risk factor during short-term studies.[2667,2668] These beneficial effects on body composition, dyslipidemia, insulin resistance, etc., are present only during therapy in that they revert to increased risk factors after discontinuation of metformin.

Troglitazone is another potent insulin sensitizer, which in a well-controlled study improved hirsutism and ovulation in PCOS (but is not yet approved for use in children).[2669] In an in vitro study, troglitazone but not metformin directly inhibited the steroidogenic enzymes P450c17 and 3β-hydroxydehydrogenase.[2670] Again the potential toxicity of these agents in children and adolescents remains to be determined. These are promising approaches to a still poorly understood syndrome that often becomes manifest during adolescence. Many aspects need to be addressed in the management of this heterogeneous disorder, and include, apart from pharmacologic agents, concern about nutrition and physical activity, which are also shown to improve the findings of PCOS (see Chapter 16).

Girls with reduced fetal growth are at risk for a reduced number of ovarian primordial follicles at birth and for small ovaries and – uterus at puberty. They may have and an increased serum FSH and decreased estradiol concentrations, suggesting relative ovarian resistance to FSH.

Adolescent Gynecomastia (see Chapter 18)

Normal pubertal boys, usually in the early stages of puberty, may have either unilateral breast enlargement (approximately 25% of boys)[2671] or bilateral breast enlargement (approximately 50% to 65% of boys),[2672] of varying degrees, commonly between chronologic ages 14 to 14½ years or pubic hair stages 3 and 4. In these boys the plasma concentrations of testosterone and estrogen are normal for the stage of puberty. Pubertal gynecomastia is usually associated with an elevated ratio of the concentration of serum estradiol to testosterone.[2673-2676] In a prospective study, adolescent boys with gynecomastia had a lower mean free testosterone concentration, lower weight, higher plasma TeBG levels, and a tendency toward earlier onset of puberty and more rapid progression through puberty.[2671] In one study a significant decrease in the concentration ratio of plasma androstenedione to estrone and estradiol and a similarly low ratio of DHEAS to estrone and estradiol were described in boys with pubertal gynecomastia who had normal ratios of plasma testosterone to estrone and estradiol. It was postulated that either decreased adrenal production of androgens or more likely increased peripheral conversion of adrenal androgens to estrogens was a factor in the development of pubertal gynecomastia.[2677] An elevated ratio of testosterone to dihydrotestosterone, presumably due to a decrease in 5α reductase activity, is suggested in the etiology of gynecomastia as well.[2678] Immunoreactive estrogen, androgen, and progesterone receptors localized to the nucleus of ductal cells was detected in all of 30 patients with gynecomastia but aromatase immunoreactivity, limited to stromal cells, was detected in only 37% of cases.[2679]

Trials of therapy with aromatase inhibitors, antiestrogens or exogenous androgens have generally been disappointing but may be able to decrease tenderness associated with gynecomastia if not the size of the tissue itself.[2680] Tamoxifen or raloxifene are reported to decrease the gynecomastia compared to watchful waiting but larger studies are recommended to prove the utility of the approach.[2681,2682]

Pubertal gynecomastia usually resolves spontaneously within 1 to 2 years of onset, and reassurance and continued observation are often adequate treatment. Nevertheless, some boys have conspicuous gynecomastia and sufficient psychological distress to warrant a reduction mammoplasty.[2683] Liposuction is an alternative approach, but its efficacy in adolescent gynecomastia remains to be established. Rarely, untreated gynecomastia persists into adulthood, as illustrated by a patient who had persistent unilateral gynecomastia that began during puberty and contralateral Poland syndrome of hypoplasia of the chest, breast tissue, and nipple.[2684]

Gynecomastia is a component of the Klinefelter's syndrome, of anorchia, primary and secondary hypogonadism, biosynthetic defects in testosterone synthesis, increased aromatase activity in adipose and other tissues (aromatase excess syndrome), Sertoli cell tumors, adventitious exposure to estrogens in meat or cosmetics, and variants of the androgen resistance syndromes, including Rosewater's syndrome (familial hypogonadism and gynecomastia) and Reifenstein's syndrome (hypospadias, hypogonadism, and gynecomastia). These disorders usually have characteristic findings or environmental circumstances that allow ready differentiation from the normal gynecomastia of puberty.[1143] Gynecomastia has been described in association with the administration of drugs such as cimetidine, spironolactone, digitalis, phenothiazines, and GH therapy,[2685] as well as in the use of marijuana.

Macro-Orchidism

Macro-orchidism, without androgenization, is a rare manifestation of the McCune-Albright syndrome[2478] and is an occasional finding in prepubertal boys with longstanding primary hypothyroidism. The latter form of testicular enlargement appears to result from increased FSH secretion independent of a pubertal increase in LH secretion or a pubertal LH response to GnRH. Testicular adrenal rests in congenital adrenal hyperplasia and a lymphoma can cause bilateral macro-orchidism. It was a feature of severe aromatase deficiency in a young male adult[341] and in men with an FSH-secreting pituitary macroadenoma. Bilateral megalotestes (26 mL testicular volume) in adults can occur as a normal variant.[2686] One may speculate that some instances of bilateral macro-orchidism are due to a heterozygous constitutive activating mutation of the FSH receptor. As noted above, prepubertal enlargement of the testes was reported with a single base deletion at codon 434 (1301delT) of the DAX1 gene with prepubertal testosterone and gonadotropin values.[1524]

The fragile X syndrome is associated with mental retardation, a long face, large prominent ears, and macro-orchidism in 80% of affected pubertal boys. Macro-orchidism may be evident only after careful measurements. The enlarged testes are due to increased interstitial volume and excessive connective tissue, including increased peritubular collagen fibers,[2687] rather than to increase in the seminiferous tubules. Enlargement of the testes is demonstrable in the prepubertal period in most patients with fragile X syndrome, but the onset of true macro-orchidism (>4 cm) only occurs in the later prepubertal period.[2688]

REFERENCES

1. Grumbach MM. Onset of puberty. In: Berenberg SR, ed. Puberty, Biologic and Social Components. Leiden: H. E. Stenfert Kroese, 1975:1-21.

2. Bogin B. Growth and development: recent evolutionary and biocultural research. In: Boaz NT, Wolfe DL, eds. Bend, OR: International Institute for Human Evolutionary Research, 1995: 49-70.
3. Dean C, Leakey MG, Reid D, et al. Growth processes in teeth distinguish modern humans from Homo erectus and earlier hominins. Nature 2001;414(6864):628-631.
4. Moggi-Cecchi J. Questions of growth. Nature 2001;414(6864): 595-597.
5. Bogin B. Adolescence in evolutionary perspective. Acta Paediatr Suppl 1994;406:29-35; discussion 36.
6. Keverne EB. Understanding well-being in the evolutionary context of brain development. Philos Trans R Soc Lond B Biol Sci 2004;359(1449):1349-1358.
7. Conroy GC, Kuykendall K. Paleopediatrics: or when did human infants really become human? Am J Phys Anthropol 1995;98: 121-131.
8. Tattersall I. Out of Africa again . . . and again? Sc American 1997;276(4):60-67.
9. Mayr E. The objects of selection. Proc Natl Acad Sci USA 1997;94:2091-2094.
10. Rosenfeld RG, Nicodemus BC. The transition from adolescence to adult life: physiology of the "transition" phase and its evolutionary basis. Horm Res 2003;60(Suppl 1):74-77.
11. Gluckman PD, Hanson MA. Mismatch : why our world no longer fits our bodies. New York: Oxford University Press, 2006.
12. Gluckman PD, Hanson MA. Changing times: the evolution of puberty. Mol Cell Endocrinol 2006;254-255:26-31.
13. Gluckman PD, Hanson MA. Evolution, development and timing of puberty. Trends Endocrinol Metab 2006;17(1):7-12.
14. Bourguignon JP, Gerard A, Alvarez Gonzalez ML, et al. Effects of changes in nutritional conditions on timing of puberty: clinical evidence from adopted children and experimental studies in the male rat. Horm Res 1992;38(Suppl 1):97-105.
15. Kempers MJ, Otten BJ. Idiopathic precocious puberty versus puberty in adopted children;auxological response to gonadotrophin-releasing hormone agonist treatment and final height. Eur J Endocrinol 2002;147(5):609-616.
16. Mul D, Oostdijk W, Drop SL. Early puberty in adopted children. Horm Res 2002;57(1-2):1-9.
17. Mul D, Oostdijk W, Waelkens JJ, et al. Gonadotrophin releasing hormone agonist treatment with or without recombinant human GH in adopted children with early puberty. Clin Endocrinol (Oxf) 2001;55(1):121-129.
18. Officioso A, Ferri P, Esposito V, et al. Adopted girls with idiopathic central precocious puberty: observations about character. J Pediatr Endocrinol Metab 2004;17(10):1385-1392.
19. Proos LA, Karlberg J, Hofvander Y, et al. Pubertal linear growth of Indian girls adopted in Sweden. Acta Paediatr 1993;82: 641-644.
20. Tuvemo T, Gustafsson J, Proos LA. Growth hormone treatment during suppression of early puberty in adopted girls. Swedish Growth Hormone Advisory Group. Acta Paediatr 1999;88(9): 928-932.
21. Ibanez L, Ferrer A, Marcos MV, et al. Early puberty: rapid progression and reduced final height in girls with low birth weight. Pediatrics 2000;106(5):E72.
22. Koziel S, Jankowska, et al. Effect of low versus normal birthweight on menarche in 14-year-old Polish girls. J Paediatr Child Health 2002;38(3):268-271.
23. Adair LS. Size at birth predicts age at menarche. Pediatrics 2001;107(4):E59.
24. Voordouw JJ, van Weissenbruch MM, Delemarre-van de Waal HA. Intrauterine growth retardation and puberty in girls. Twin Res 2001;4(5):299-306.
25. Ong KK, Potau N, Petry CJ, et al. Opposing influences of prenatal and postnatal weight gain on adrenarche in normal boys and girls. J Clin Endocrinol Metab 2004;89(6):2647-2651.
26. Dunger DB, Ahmed ML, Ong KK. Early and late weight gain and the timing of puberty. Mol Cell Endocrinol 2006;254-255:140-145.
27. Tam CS, de Zegher F, Garnett SP, et al. Opposing influences of prenatal and postnatal growth on the timing of menarche. J Clin Endocrinol Metab 2006;91(11):4369-4373.
28. Ellis BJ. Timing of pubertal maturation in girls: an integrated life history approach. Psychol Bull 2004;130(6):920-958.
29. Tanner JM. Aristotle: De generatione animalium. In: Tanner JM, ed. A History of the Study of Human Growth. Cambridge: Cambridge University Press, 1981:7.
30. Marshall WA, Tanner JM. Puberty. In Falkner F, Tanner JM, eds. Human Growth. New York: Plenum CY, 1986:171-209.
31. Tanner JM. A History of the Study of Human Growth. Cambridge: Cambridge University Press, 1981.
32. Tanner JM. Growth at Adolescence. Springfield, IL: Charles C Thomas, 1962.
33. Wyshak G, Frisch RE. Evidence for a secular trend in age of menarche. N Engl J Med 1982;306:1033-1035.
34. Artaria MD, Henneberg M. Why did they lie? Socio-economic bias in reporting menarcheal age. Ann Hum Biol 2000;27(6):561-569.
35. Koo MM, Rohan TE. Accuracy of short-term recall of age at menarche. Ann Hum Biol 1997;24(1):61-64.
36. Williams RL, Cheyne KL, Houtkooper LK, et al. Adolescent self-assessment of sexual maturation. Effects of fatness classification and actual sexual maturation stage. J Adolesc Health Care 1988;9(6):480-482.
37. Tryggvadottir L, Tulinius H, Larusdottir M. A decline and a halt in mean age at menarche in Iceland. Ann Hum Biol 1994;21(2): 179-186.
38. Okasha M, McCarron P, McEwen J, et al. Age at menarche: secular trends and association with adult anthropometric measures. Ann Hum Biol 2001;28(1):68-78.
39. Damon A. Larger body size and earlier menarche: the end may be in sight. Soc Biol 1974;21:8-11.
40. Nicholson AB, Hanley C. Indices of physiological maturity: derivation and interrelationships. Child Dev 1953;24(1):3-38.
41. Zacharias L, Wurtman RJ, Schatzoff M. Sexual maturation in contemporary American girls. Am J Obstet Gynecol 1970;108: 833-846.
42. Parent AS, Teilmann G, Juul A, et al. The timing of normal puberty and the age limits of sexual precocity: variations around the world, secular trends, and changes after migration. Endocr Rev 2003;24(5):668-693.
43. Ong KK, Ahmed ML, Dunger DB. Lessons from large population studies on timing and tempo of puberty (secular trends and relation to body size): the European trend. Mol Cell Endocrinol 2006;254-255:8-12.
44. Ellis BJ, McFadyen-Ketchum S, Dodge KA, et al. Quality of early family relationships and individual differences in the timing of pubertal maturation in girls: a longitudinal test of an evolutionary model. J Pers Soc Psychol 1999;77(2):387-401.
45. Gerver WJ, De Bruin R, Drayer NM. A persisting secular trend for body measurements in Dutch children. The Oosterwolde II Study. Acta Paediatr 1994;83:812-814.
46. Whincup PH, Gilg JA, Odoki K, et al. Age of menarche in contemporary British teenagers: survey of girls born between 1982 and 1986. BMJ 2001;322(7294):1095-1096.
47. Loesch DZ, Stokes K, Huggins RM. Secular trend in body height and weight of Australian children and adolescents. Am J Phys Anthropol 2000;111(4):545-556.
48. Olesen AW, Jeune B, Boldsen JL. A continuous decline in menarcheal age in Denmark. Ann Hum Biol 2000;27(4):377-386.
49. Marrodan MD, Mesa MS, Arechiga J, et al. Trend in menarcheal age in Spain: rural and urban comparison during a recent period. Ann Hum Biol 2000;27(3):313-319.
50. Kac G, Auxiliadora de Santa Cruz Coel, et al. Secular trend in age at menarche for women born between 1920 and 1979 in Rio de Janeiro, Brazil. Ann Hum Biol 2000;27(4):423-428.
51. Danubio ME, De Simone M, Vecchi F, et al. Age at menarche and age of onset of pubertal characteristics in 6-14-year-old girls from the Province of L'Aquila (Abruzzo, Italy). Am J Hum Biol 2004; 16(4):470-478.
52. Veronesi FM, Gueresi P. Trend in menarcheal age and socioeconomic influence in Bologna (northern Italy). Ann Hum Biol 1994;21:187-196.
53. Cole TJ. Secular trends in growth. Proc Nutr Soc 2000;59(2): 317-324.
54. Zacharias L, Rand M, Wurtman R. A prospective study of sexual development in American girls: the statistics of menarche. Obstet Gynecol Surv 1976;31:325-337.
55. MacMahon B. Age at menarche. National Health Survey. DHEW Publication No. (HRA) 74-1615, Series 11, No. 133. Washington, DC: 1973.

56. Herman-Giddens ME, Slora EJ, Wasserman RC, et al. Secondary sexual characteristics and menses in young girls seen in office practice: a study from the Pediatric Research in Office Settings network. Pediatrics 1997;99:505-512.
57. Harlan WR, Harlan EA, Grillo GP. Secondary sex characteristics of girls 12 to 17 years of age: the U.S. Health Examination Survey. J Pediatr 1980;96:1074-1078.
58. Foster TA, Voors AW, Webber LS, et al. Anthropometric and maturation measurements of children, ages 5 to 14 years, in a biracial community—the Bogalusa Heart Study. Am J Clin Nutr 1977; 30(4):582-591.
59. Chaning-Pearce SM, Solomon L. Pubertal development in black and white Johannesburg girls. S Afr Med J 1987;71:22-24.
60. Freedman DS, Khan LK, Serdula MK, et al. Relation of age at menarche to race, time period, and anthropometric dimensions: the Bogalusa Heart Study. Pediatrics 2002;110(4):e43.
61. Himes JH. Examining the evidence for recent secular changes in the timing of puberty in US children in light of increases in the prevalence of obesity. Mol Cell Endocrinol 2006;254-255: 13-21.
62. Morrison JA, Barton B, Biro FM, et al. Sexual maturation and obesity in 9- and 10-year-old black and white girls: the National Heart, Lung, and Blood Institute Growth and Health Study. J Pediatr 1994;124:889-895.
63. Adair LS, Gordon-Larsen P. Maturational timing and overweight prevalence in US adolescent girls. Am J Public Health 2001;91(4): 642-644.
64. Ontell FK, Ivanovic M, Ablin DS, et al. Bone age in children of diverse ethnicity. AJR Am J Roentgenol 1996;167(6):1395-1398.
65. Loder RT, Estle DT, Morrison K, et al. Applicability of the Greulich and Pyle skeletal age standards to black and white children of today. Am J Dis Child 1993;147(12):1329-1333.
66. Malina RM. Skeletal maturation studied longitudinally over one year in American Whites and Negroes six though thirteen years of age. Hum Biol 1970;42(3):377-390.
67. Russell DL, Keil MF, Bonat SH, et al. The relation between skeletal maturation and adiposity in African American and Caucasian children. J Pediatr 2001;139(6):844-848.
68. Troiano RP, Flegal KM, Kuczmarski RJ, et al. Overweight prevalence and trends for children and adolescents. The National Health and Nutrition Examination Surveys, 1963 to 1991. Arch Pediatr Adolesc Med 1995;149(10):1085-1091.
69. Styne DM. Childhood obesity. Prevalence and significance. Pediatr Clin North Am 2001;48(4):823-854.
70. Power C, Lake JK, Cole TJ. Measurement and long-term health risks of child and adolescent fatness. Int J Obes Relat Metab Disord 1997;21(7):507-526.
71. Biro FM, McMahon RP, Striegel-Moore R, et al. Impact of timing of pubertal maturation on growth in black and white female adolescents: The National Heart, Lung, and Blood Institute Growth and Health Study. J Pediatr 2001;138(5):636-643.
72. Freedman DS, Srinivasan SR, Harsha DW, et al. Relation of body fat patterning to lipid and lipoprotein concentrations in children and adolescents: the Bogalusa Heart Study. Am J Clin Nutr 1989;50(5):930-939.
73. Freedman DS, Khan LK, Serdula MK, et al. Relation of age at menarche to race, time period, and anthropometric dimensions: the Bogalusa Heart Study. Pediatrics 2002;110(4):e43.
74. Kaplowitz PB, Slora EJ, Wasserman RC, et al. Earlier onset of puberty in girls: relation to increased body mass index and race. Pediatrics 2001;108(2):347-353.
75. Wattigney WA, Srinivasan SR, Chen W, et al. Secular trend of earlier onset of menarche with increasing obesity in black and white girls: the Bogalusa Heart Study. Ethn Dis 1999;9(2): 181-189.
76. Frisancho AR, Housh CH. The relationship of maturity rate to body size and body proportions in children and adults. Hum Biol 1988;60(5):759-770.
77. de Ridder CM, Thijssen JH, Bruning PF, et al. Body fat mass, body fat distribution, and pubertal development: a longitudinal study of physical and hormonal sexual maturation of girls. J Clin Endocrinol Metab 1992;75:442-446.
78. Anderson SE, Dallal GE, Must A. Relative weight and race influence average age at menarche: results from two nationally representative surveys of US girls studied 25 years apart. Pediatrics 2003;111(4 Pt 1):844-850.
79. Davison KK, Susman EJ, Birch LL. Percent body fat at age 5 predicts earlier pubertal development among girls at age 9. Pediatrics 2003;111(4 Pt 1):815-821.
80. Biro FM, Lucky AW, Simbartl LA, et al. Pubertal maturation in girls and the relationship to anthropometric changes: pathways through puberty. J Pediatr 2003;142(6):643-646.
81. Himes JH, Obarzanek E, Baranowski T, et al. Early sexual maturation, body composition, and obesity in African-American girls. Obes Res 2004;12 Suppl:64S-72S.
82. Herman-Giddens ME, Wang L, Koch G. Secondary sexual characteristics in boys. Arch Pediatr Adolesc Med 2001;155: 1022-1028.
83. Wu T, Mendola P, Buck GM. Ethnic differences in the presence of secondary sex characteristics and menarche among US girls: the Third National Health and Nutrition Examination Survey, 1988-1994. Pediatrics 2002;110(4):752-757.
84. Chumlea WC, Schubert CM, Roche AF, et al. Age at menarche and racial comparisons in US girls. Pediatrics 2003;111(1): 110-113.
85. He Q, Karlberg J. BMI in childhood and its association with height gain, timing of puberty, and final height. Pediatr Res 2001;49(2): 244-251.
86. Juul A, Teilmann G, Scheike T, et al. Pubertal development in Danish children: comparison of recent European and US data. Int J Androl 2006;29(1):247-255.
87. Demerath EW, Li J, Sun SS, et al. Fifty-year trends in serial body mass index during adolescence in girls: the Fels Longitudinal Study. Am J Clin Nutr 2004;80(2):441-446.
88. Demerath EW, Towne B, Chumlea WC, et al. Recent decline in age at menarche: the Fels Longitudinal Study. Am J Hum Biol 2004;16(4):453-457.
89. Broekmans FJ, Fauser BC. Diagnostic criteria for polycystic ovarian syndrome. Endocrine 2006;30(1):3-11.
90. van Hooff MH, Voorhorst FJ, Kaptein MB, et al. Insulin, androgen, and gonadotropin concentrations, body mass index, and waist to hip ratio in the first years after menarche in girls with regular menstrual cycles, irregular menstrual cycles, or oligomenorrhea. J Clin Endocrinol Metab 2000;85(4):1394-1400.
91. Garn SM, LaVelle M, Rosenberg KR, et al. Maturational timing as a factor in female fatness and obesity. Am J Clin Nutr 1986; 43(6):879-883.
92. Hartz AJ, Barboriak PN, Wong A. The association of obesity with infertility and related menstrual abnormalities in women. Int J Obes 1979;3:57-73.
93. Kelesidis T, Mantzoros CS. The emerging role of leptin in humans. Pediatr Endocrinol Rev 2006;3(3):239-248.
94. Berkey CS, Gardner JD, Frazier AL, et al. Relation of childhood diet and body size to menarche and adolescent growth in girls. Am J Epidemiol 2000;152(5):446-452.
95. Dorgan JF, Hunsberger SA, McMahon RP, et al. Diet and sex hormones in girls: findings from a randomized controlled clinical trial. J Natl Cancer Inst 2003;95(2):132-141.
96. Meyer F, Moisan J, Marcoux D, et al. Dietary and physical determinants of menarche. Epidemiology 1990;1(5):377-381.
97. Moisan J, Meyer F, Gingras S. Diet and age at menarche. Cancer Causes Control 1990;1(2):149-154.
98. de Ridder CM, Thijssen JH, Van 't Veer P, et al. Dietary habits, sexual maturation, and plasma hormones in pubertal girls: a longitudinal study [see comments]. Am J Clin Nutr 1991;54: 805-813.
99. Koo MM, Rohan TE, Jain M, et al. A cohort study of dietary fibre intake and menarche. Public Health Nutr 2002;5(2): 353-360.
100. Soriguer FJ, Gonzalez-Romero S, Esteva I, et al. Does the intake of nuts and seeds alter the appearance of menarche? Acta Obstet Gynecol Scand 1995;74:455-461.
101. Hughes RE, Jones E. Intake of dietary fibre and the age of menarche. Ann Hum Biol 1985;12(4):325-332.
102. Rosell M, Appleby P, Key T. Height, age at menarche, body weight and body mass index in life-long vegetarians. Public Health Nutr 2005;8(7):870-875.
103. Treem WR. Emerging concepts in celiac disease. Curr Opin Pediatr 2004 Oct;16(5):552-559.
104. Patel P, Mendall MA, Khulusi S, et al. *Helicobacter pylori* infection in childhood: risk factors and effect on growth. BMJ 1994; 309(6962):1119-1123.

105. Moudiou T, Theophilatou D, Priftis K, et al. Growth of asthmatic children before long-term treatment with inhaled corticosteroids. J Asthma 2003;40(6):667-671.
106. Zacharias L, Wurtman RJ. Blindness: its relation to age of menarche. Science 1964;144:1154-1155.
107. Magee K, Basinska J, Quarrington B, et al. Blindness and menarche. Life Sci 1970;9:7-12.
108. Thomas JB, Pizzarello DJ. Blindness, biologic rhythms, and menarche. Obstet Gynecol 1967;30(4):507-509.
109. Zacharias L, Wurtman RJ. Blindness and menarche. Obstet Gynecol 1969;33(5):603-608.
110. Buffon H. Histoire Naturelle. In: Tanner JM, ed. A History of the Study of Human Growth. Cambridge: Cambridge University Press, 1981:83.
111. Daw SF. Age of boys' puberty in Leipzig, 1727-49, as indicated by voice breaking in J.S. Bach's choir members. Hum Biol 1970;42: 87-89.
112. Kill V. Stature and growth of Norwegian men during past 200 years. Skr Nor Vidensk Akad 1939;2(6):1-175.
113. Leenstra T, Petersen LT, Kariuki SK, et al. Prevalence and severity of malnutrition and age at menarche; cross-sectional studies in adolescent schoolgirls in western Kenya. Eur J Clin Nutr 2005;59(1):41-48.
114. Padez C. Age at menarche of schoolgirls in Maputo, Mozambique. Ann Hum Biol 2003;30(4):487-495.
115. Junqueira Do LM, Faerstein E, De Souza LC, et al. Family socioeconomic background modified secular trends in age at menarche: evidence from the Pro-Saude Study (Rio de Janeiro, Brazil). Ann Hum Biol 2003;30(3):347-352.
116. Malina RM, Pena Reyes ME, Tan SK, et al. Secular change in age at menarche in rural Oaxaca, southern Mexico: 1968-2000. Ann Hum Biol 2004;31(6):634-646.
117. Becker-Christensen FG. Growth in Greenland: development of body proportions and menarcheal age in Greenlandic children. Int J Circumpolar Health 2003;62(3):284-295.
118. Hwang JY, Shin C, Frongillo EA, et al. Secular trend in age at menarche for South Korean women born between 1920 and 1986: the Ansan Study. Ann Hum Biol 2003;30(4):434-442.
119. Delemarre-Van de Waal HA. Environmental factors influencing growth and pubertal development. Environ Health Perspect 1993;101 Suppl 2:39-44.
120. Morabia A, Costanza MC. International variability in ages at menarche, first livebirth, and menopause. World Health Organization Collaborative Study of Neoplasia and Steroid Contraceptives. Am J Epidemiol 1998;148(12):1195-1205.
121. Campbell BC, Gillett-Netting R, Meloy M. Timing of reproductive maturation in rural versus urban Tonga boys, Zambia. Ann Hum Biol 2004;31(2):213-227.
122. Gillett-Netting R, Meloy M, Campbell BC. Catch-up reproductive maturation in rural Tonga girls, Zambia? Am J Hum Biol 2004;16(6):658-669.
123. Liestol K. Social conditions and menarcheal age: the importance of early years of life. Ann Hum Biol 1982;9(6): 521-537.
124. Worthman C. Bio-cutural interactions in human development. In: Pereira M, Fairbanks L, eds. Juvenile primates: life history, development and behavior. Oxford: Oxford University Press, 1993: 339-358.
125. Jones B, Leeton J, McLeod I, et al. Factors influencing the age of menarche in a lower socio-economic group in Melbourne. Med J Aust 1972;2(10):533-535.
126. Maestripieri D, Roney JR, DeBias N, et al. Father absence, menarche and interest in infants among adolescent girls. Dev Sci 2004;7(5):560-566.
127. Mustanski BS, Viken RJ, Kaprio J, et al. Genetic and environmental influences on pubertal development: longitudinal data from Finnish twins at ages 11 and 14. Dev Psychol 2004;40(6): 1188-1198.
128. Wellens R, Malina RM, Beunen G, et al. Age at menarche in Flemish girls: current status and secular change in the 20th century. Ann Hum Biol 1990;17(2):145-152.
129. Hoel DG, Wakabayashi T, Pike MC. Secular trends in the distributions of the breast cancer risk factors—menarche, first birth, menopause, and weight—in Hiroshima and Nagasaki, Japan. Am J Epidemiol 1983;118(1):78-89.
130. Prebeg Z, Bralic I. Changes in menarcheal age in girls exposed to war conditions. Am J Human Biol 2000;12(4):503-508.
131. Hulanicka B, Gronkiewicz L, Koniarek J. Effect of familial distress on growth and maturation of girls: a longitudinal study. Am J Human Biol 2001;13(6):771-776.
132. Toromanovic A, Tahirovic H. Menarcheal age of girls from dysfunctional families. Bosn J Basic Med Sci 2004;4(3):5-6.
133. Brown J, Cohen P, Chen H, et al. Sexual trajectories of abused and neglected youths. J Dev Behav Pediatr 2004;25(2):77-82.
134. Herman-Giddens ME, Sandler AD, Friedman NE. Sexual precocity in girls. An association with sexual abuse? Am J Dis Child 1988;142:431-433.
135. Jorm AF, Christensen H, Rodgers B, et al. Association of adverse childhood experiences, age of menarche, and adult reproductive behavior: does the androgen receptor gene play a role? Am J Med Genet B Neuropsychiatr Genet 2004;125(1):105-111.
136. Romans SE, Martin JM, Gendall K, et al. Age of menarche: the role of some psychosocial factors. Psychol Med 2003;33(5): 933-939.
137. Graber JA, Brooks-Gunn J, Warren MP. The antecedents of menarcheal age: heredity, family environment, and stressful life events. Child Dev 1995;66(2):346-359.
138. Comings DE, Muhleman D, Johnson JP, et al. Parent-daughter transmission of the androgen receptor gene as an explanation of the effect of father absence on age of menarche. Child Dev 2002;73(4):1046-1051.
139. Freyre EA, Ortiz MV. The effect of altitude on adolescent growth and development. J Adolesc Health Care 1988;9:144-149.
140. Beall CM. Ages at menopause and menarche in a high-altitude Himalayan population. Ann Hum Biol 1983;10(4):365-370.
141. Vitzthum VJ, Wiley AS. The proximate determinants of fertility in populations exposed to chronic hypoxia. High Alt Med Biol 2003;4(2):125-39.
142. Gonzales GF, Villena A. Body mass index and age at menarche in Peruvian children living at high altitude and at sea level. Hum Biol 1996;68(2):265-275.
143. Greksa LP. Age of menarche in Bolivian girls of European and Aymara ancestry. Ann Hum Biol 1990;17(1):49-53.
144. Singh L, Thapar M. Age at menarche among the Bhotias of Mana Valley. Anthropol Anz 1983;41(4):259-262.
145. Crognier E, Villena M, Vargas E. Reproduction in high altitude Aymara: physiological stress and fertility planning? J Biosoc Sci 2002;34(4):463-473.
146. McClintock MK. Menstrual synchrony and suppression. Nature 1971;229(5282):244-245.
147. Hummel T, Krone F, Lundstrom JN, et al. Androstadienone odor thresholds in adolescents. Horm Behav 2005;47(3):306-310.
148. Casper RC. Women's Health: Hormones, Emotions, and Behavior. Cambridge: Cambridge University Press, 1998.
149. Persky H. Psychoendocrinology of Human Sexual Behavior. New York: Praeger, 1987.
150. Wilson HC. A critical review of menstrual synchrony research. Psychoneuroendocrinology 1992;17(6):565-591.
151. Schank JC. A multitude of errors in menstrual-synchrony research: replies to Weller and Weller (2002) and Graham (2002). J Comp Psychol 2002;116(3):319-322.
152. Schank JC. Avoiding synchrony as a strategy of female mate choice. Nonlinear Dynamics Psychol Life Sci 2004;8(2):147-176.
153. Schank JC. Menstrual-cycle variability and measurement: further cause for doubt. Psychoneuroendocrinology 2000;25(8): 837-847.
154. Brundtland GH, Liestol K. Seasonal variations in menarche in Oslo. Ann Hum Biol 1982;9(1):35-43.
155. Tavares CH, Barbieri MA, Bettiol H, et al. Monthly distribution of menarche among schoolgirls from a municipality in Southeastern Brazil. Am J Hum Biol 2004;16(1):17-23.
156. Moisan J, Meyer F, Gingras S. A nested case-control study of the correlates of early menarche. Am J Epidemiol 1990;132(5): 953-961.
157. Zacharias L, Wurtman RJ. Age at menarche. N Engl J Med 1969;280:868-875.
158. Palmert MR, Hirschhorn JN. Genetic approaches to stature, pubertal timing, and other complex traits. Mol Genet Metab 2003;80(1-2):1-10.

159. Campbell BC, Udry JR. Stress and age at menarche of mothers and daughters. J Biosoc Sci 1995;27(2):127-134.
160. Malina RM, Ryan RC, Bonci CM. Age at menarche in athletes and their mothers and sisters. Ann Hum Biol 1994;21(5):417-422.
161. Meyer JM, Eaves LJ, Heath AC, Martin NG. Estimating genetic influences on the age-at-menarche: a survival analysis approach. Am J Med Genet 1991;39(2):148-154.
162. Loesch DZ, Huggins R, Rogucka E, Hoang NH, Hopper JL. Genetic correlates of menarcheal age: a multivariate twin study. Ann Hum Biol 1995;22(6):470-490.
163. Loesch DZ, Hopper JL, Rogucka E, Huggins RM. Timing and genetic rapport between growth in skeletal maturity and height around puberty: similarities and differences between girls and boys. Am J Hum Genet 1995;56:753-759.
164. Fischbein S. Onset of puberty in MX and DZ twins. Acta Genet Med Gemellol (Roma) 1977;26(2):151-158.
165. Fischbein S. Intra-pair similarity in physical growth of opposite-sex twin pairs during puberty. Ann Hum Biol 1983;10:135-145.
166. Eaves L, Silberg J, Foley D, et al. Genetic and environmental influences on the relative timing of pubertal change. Twin Res 2004;7(5):471-481.
167. Golden WL. Reproductive histories in a Norwegian twin population: evaluation of the maternal effect in early spontaneous abortion. Acta Genet Med Gemellol (Roma) 1981;30(2):91-165.
168. Kaprio J, Rimpela A, Winter T, et al. Common genetic influences on BMI and age at menarche. Hum Biol 1995;67(5):739-753.
169. Treloar SA, Martin NG. Age at menarche as a fitness trait: nonadditive genetic variance detected in a large twin sample. Am J Hum Genet 1990;47(1):137-148.
170. van den Akker OB, Stein GS, Neale MC, et al. Genetic and environmental variation in menstrual cycle: histories of two British twin samples. Acta Genet Med Gemellol (Roma) 1987;36(4): 541-548.
171. Towne B, Czerwinski SA, Demerath EW, et al. Heritability of age at menarche in girls from the Fels Longitudinal Study. Am J Phys Anthropol 2005;128(1):210-219.
172. van der Eerden BC, Karperien M, Wit JM. Systemic and local regulation of the growth plate. Endocr Rev 2003;24(6):782-801.
173. Matsuo N, Anzo M, Sato S, et al. Testicular volume in Japanese boys up to the age of 15 years. Eur J Pediatr 2000;159(11): 843-845.
174. Orbak Z. Does handedness and altitude affect age at menarche? J Trop Pediatr 2005;51(4):216-218.
175. Sappington J, Topolski R. Maths performance as a function of sex, laterality, and age of pubertal onset. Laterality 2005;10(4): 369-379.
176. Kadlubar FF, Berkowitz GS, Delongchamp RR, et al. The CYP3A4*1B variant is related to the onset of puberty, a known risk factor for the development of breast cancer. Cancer Epidemiol Biomarkers Prev 2003;12(4):327-331.
177. Comings DE, Gade R, Muhleman D, et al. The LEP gene and age of menarche: maternal age as a potential cause of hidden stratification in association studies. Mol Genet Metab 2001;73(3): 204-210.
178. Stavrou I, Zois C, Ioannidis JP, et al. Association of polymorphisms of the oestrogen receptor alpha gene with the age of menarche. Hum Reprod 2002;17(4):1101-1105.
179. Sharp L, Cardy AH, Cotton SC, et al. CYP17 gene polymorphisms: prevalence and associations with hormone levels and related factors. A HuGE review. Am J Epidemiol 2004;160(8):729-740.
180. De Vries L, Kauschansky A, Shohat M, et al. Familial central precocious puberty suggests autosomal dominant inheritance. J Clin Endocrinol Metab 2004;89(4):1794-1800.
181. Xita N, Tsatsoulis A, Stavrou I, et al. Association of SHBG gene polymorphism with menarche. Mol Hum Reprod 2005;11(6): 459-462.
182. Nathan BM, Hodges CA, Supelak PJ, et al. A quantitative trait locus on chromosome 6 regulates the onset of puberty in mice. Endocrinology 2006;147(11):5132-5138.
183. Nathan BM, Hodges CA, Palmert MR. The use of mouse chromosome substitution strains to investigate the genetic regulation of pubertal timing. Mol Cell Endocrinol 2006;254-255:103-108.
184. Morabia A, Costanza MC. Reproductive factors and incidence of breast cancer: an international ecological study. Soz Praventivmed 2000;45(6):247-257.
185. Gao YT, Shu XO, Dai Q, et al. Association of menstrual and reproductive factors with breast cancer risk: results from the Shanghai Breast Cancer Study. Int J Cancer 2000;87(2):295-300.
186. Stoll BA, Vatten LJ, Kvinnsland S. Does early physical maturity influence breast cancer risk? Acta Oncol 1994;33:171-176.
187. MacMahon B, Trichopoulos D, Brown J, et al. Age at menarche, urine estrogens and breast cancer risk. Int J Cancer 1982; 30(4):427-431.
188. Apter D, Vihko R. Early menarche, a risk factor for breast cancer, indicates early onset of ovulatory cycles. J Clin Endocrinol Metab 1983;57:82-86.
189. Persson I. Estrogens in the causation of breast, endometrial and ovarian cancers—evidence and hypotheses from epidemiological findings. J Steroid Biochem Mol Biol 2000;74(5):357-364.
190. Clavel-Chapelon F, Gerber M. Reproductive factors and breast cancer risk. Do they differ according to age at diagnosis? Breast Cancer Res Treat 2002;72(2):107-115.
191. Michels KB, Willett WC. Breast cancer—early life matters. N Engl J Med 2004;351(16):1679-1681.
192. Hamilton AS, Mack TM. Puberty and genetic susceptibility to breast cancer in a case-control study in twins. N Engl J Med 2003;348(23):2313-2322.
193. De Stavola BL, dos Santos Silva I, McCormack V, et al. Childhood growth and breast cancer. Am J Epidemiol 2004;159(7):671-682.
194. Tehard B, Kaaks R, Clavel-Chapelon F. Body silhouette, menstrual function at adolescence and breast cancer risk in the E3N cohort study. Br J Cancer 2005;92(11):2042-2048.
195. Ahlgren M, Melbye M, Wohlfahrt J, et al. Growth patterns and the risk of breast cancer in women. N Engl J Med 2004;351(16): 1619-1626.
196. dos Santos Silva I, De Stavola BL, Hardy RJ, et al. Is the association of birth weight with premenopausal breast cancer risk mediated through childhood growth? Br J Cancer 2004;91(3): 519-524.
197. Mucci LA, Kuper HE, Tamimi R, et al. Age at menarche and age at menopause in relation to hepatocellular carcinoma in women. Br J Obstet Gynaecol 2001;108(3):291-294.
198. Hatch EE, Linet MS, Zhang J, et al. Reproductive and hormonal factors and risk of brain tumors in adult females. Int J Cancer 2005;114(5):797-805.
199. Zhang Y, Holford TR, Leaderer B, et al. Menstrual and reproductive factors and risk of non-Hodgkin's lymphoma among Connecticut women. Am J Epidemiol 2004;160(8):766-773.
200. Remsberg KE, Demerath EW, Schubert CM, et al. Early menarche and the development of cardiovascular disease risk factors in adolescent girls: the Fels Longitudinal Study. J Clin Endocrinol Metab 2005;90(5):2718-2724.
201. Berkey CS, Dockery DW, Wang X, et al. Longitudinal height velocity standards for U.S. adolescents. Stat Med 1993;12: 403-414.
202. Rillema JA. Development of the mammary gland and lactation. Trends Endocrinol Metab 1994;5:149-154.
203. Drife JO. Breast development in puberty. Ann N Y Acad Sci 1986;464:58-65.
204. Fenton SE. Endocrine-disrupting compounds and mammary gland development: early exposure and later life consequences. Endocrinology 2006;147(6 Suppl):S18-S24.
205. Rayner JL, Enoch RR, Fenton SE. Adverse effects of prenatal exposure to atrazine during a critical period of mammary gland growth. Toxicol Sci 2005;87(1):255-266.
206. Rayner JL, Wood C, Fenton SE. Exposure parameters necessary for delayed puberty and mammary gland development in Long-Evans rats exposed in utero to atrazine. Toxicol Appl Pharmacol 2004;195(1):23-34.
207. Wang XJ, Bartolucci-Page E, Fenton SE, et al. Altered mammary gland development in male rats exposed to genistein and methoxychlor. Toxicol Sci 2006;91(1):93-103.
208. Bulun SE, Noble LS, Takayama K, et al. Endocrine disorders associated with inappropriately high aromatase expression. J Steroid Biochem Mol Biol 1997;61(3-6):133-139.
209. Stratz CH. Der Korper des Kindes und Seine Pflege. Stuttgart: Ferdinand Enke, 1909.
210. Reynolds EL, Wines JV. Individualized differences in physical changes associated with adolescence in girls. Am J Dis Child 1948;75:329-350.

211. Templeman C, Hertweck SP. Breast disorders in the pediatric and adolescent patient. Obstet Gynecol Clin North Am 2000;27(1):19-34.
212. Lin KY, Nguyen DB, Williams RM. Complete breast absence revisited. Plast Reconstr Surg 2000;106(1):98-101.
213. Griffith JR. Virginal breast hypertrophy. J Adolesc Health Care 1989;10(5):423-432.
214. O'Hare PM, Frieden IJ. Virginal breast hypertrophy. Pediatr Dermatol 2000;17(4):277-281.
215. Govrin-Yehudain J, Kogan L, Cohen HI, et al. Familial juvenile hypertrophy of the breast. J Adolesc Health 2004;35(2):151-155.
216. Rohn RD. Papilla (nipple) development during female puberty. Adolesc Health Care 1982;2:217.
217. Rohn RD. Nipple (papilla) development in puberty: longitudinal observations in girls. Pediatrics 1987;79:745-747.
218. Paavonen J. Physiology and ecology of the vagina. Scand J Infect Dis Suppl 1983;40:31-35.
219. Vargas SO, Kozakewich HP, Boyd TK, et al. Childhood asymmetric labium majus enlargement: mimicking a neoplasm. Am J Surg Pathol 2005;29(8):1007-1016.
220. McCann J. Color Atlas of Child Sexual Abuse. Chicago: Year Book Medical, 1989.
221. Taskinen S, Taavitsainen M, Wikstrom S. Measurement of testicular volume: comparison of 3 different methods. J Urol 1996; 155:930-933.
222. Zachmann M, Prader A, Kind HP, et al. Testicular volume during adolescence. Cross-sectional and longitudinal studies. Helv Paediatr Acta 1974;29:61-72.
223. Biro FM, Lucky AW, Huster GA, et al. Pubertal staging in boys. J Pediatr 1995;127:40-46.
224. Ankarberg-Lindgren C, Norjavaara E. Changes of diurnal rhythm and levels of total and free testosterone secretion from pre to late puberty in boys: testis size of 3 mL is a transition stage to puberty. Eur J Endocrinol 2004;151(6):747-757.
225. Sutherland RS, Kogan BA, Baskin LS, et al. The effect of prepubertal androgen exposure on adult penile length. J Urol 1996;156:783-787.
226. Rohn RD. Papilla (nipple) development in puberty. The adolescent male. J Adolesc Health Care 1985;6:429-432.
227. Duke PM, Litt IF, Gross RT. Adolescents self-assessment of sexual maturation. Pediatrics 1980;66:918-920.
228. Dorn LD, Susman EJ, Nottelmann ED, et al. Perceptions of puberty: adolescent, parent, and health care personnel. Dev Psychol 1990;26:322-329.
229. Coleman L, Coleman J. The measurement of puberty: a review. J Adolesc 2002;25(5):535-550.
230. Schlossberger NM, Turner RA, Irwin CEJ. Validity of self-report of pubertal maturation in early adolescents [see comments]. J Adolesc Health 1992;13:109-113.
231. Taylor SJ, Whincup PH, Hindmarsh PC, et al. Performance of a new pubertal self-assessment questionnaire: a preliminary study. Paediatr Perinat Epidemiol 2001;15(1):88-94.
232. Finkelstein JW, D'Arcangelo MR, Susman EJ, et al. Self-assessment of physical sexual maturation in boys and girls with delayed puberty. J Adolesc Health 1999;25(6):379-381.
233. Wu Y, Schreiber GB, Klementowicz V, et al. Racial differences in accuracy of self-assessment of sexual maturation among young black and white girls. J Adolesc Health 2001;28(3):197-203.
234. Bonat S, Pathomvanich A, Keil MF, et al. Self-assessment of pubertal stage in overweight children. Pediatrics 2002;110(4):743-747.
235. Harlan WR, Grillo GP, Cornoni-Huntley J, et al. Secondary sex characteristics of boys 12 to 17 years of age: the U.S. Health Examination Survey. J Pediatr 1979;95:293-297.
236. Reynolds EL, Wines JV. Physical changes associated with adolescence in boys. Am J Dis Child 1951;82:529-547.
237. Roche AF, Wellens R, Attie KM, et al. The timing of sexual maturation in a group of U.S. white youths. J Pediatr Endocrinol 1995;8:11-18.
238. Sun SS, Schubert CM, Chumlea WC, et al. National estimates of the timing of sexual maturation and racial differences among US children. Pediatrics 2002;110(5):911-919.
239. Herman-Giddens ME, Kaplowitz PB, Wasserman R. Navigating the recent articles on girls' puberty in Pediatrics: what do we know and where do we go from here? Pediatrics 2004;113(4):911-917.
240. Reiter EO, Lee PA. Have the onset and tempo of puberty changed? Arch Pediatr Adolesc Med 2001;155:988-989.
241. Kaplowitz P. Delayed puberty in obese boys: comparison with constitutional delayed puberty and response to testosterone therapy. J Pediatr 1998;133(6):745-749.
242. Styne DM. Puberty, obesity and ethnicity. Trends Endocrinol Metab 2004;15(10):472-478.
243. Lee PA, Guo SS, Kulin HE. Age of puberty: data from the United States of America. APMIS 2001;109(2):81-88.
244. Sun SS, Schubert CM, Liang R et al. Is sexual maturity occurring earlier among U.S. children? J Adolesc Health 2005;37(5):345-355.
245. Marti-Henneberg C, Vizmanos B. The duration of puberty in girls is related to the timing of its onset. J Pediatr 1997;131(4):618-621.
246. de Ridder CM, de Boer RW, Seidell JC, et al. Body fat distribution in pubertal girls quantified by magnetic resonance imaging. Int J Obes Relat Metab Disord 1992;16:443-449.
247. Bourguignon JP. Variations in duration of pubertal growth: a mechanism compensating for differences in timing of puberty and minimizing their effects on final height. Belgian Study Group for Paediatric Endocrinology. Acta Paediatr Scand Suppl 1988;347:16-24.
248. Kaplowitz PB, Oberfield SE. Reexamination of the age limit for defining when puberty is precocious in girls in the United States: implications for evaluation and treatment. Drug and Therapeutics and Executive Committees of the Lawson Wilkins Pediatric Endocrine Society. Pediatrics 1999;104(4 Pt 1):936-941.
249. Kaplowitz P. Clinical characteristics of 104 children referred for evaluation of precocious puberty. J Clin Endocrinol Metab 2004;89(8):3644-3650.
250. De Vries L, Phillip M. Children referred for signs of early puberty warrant endocrine evaluation and follow-up. J Clin Endocrinol Metab 2005;90(1):593-594.
251. Chalumeau M, Hadjiathanasiou CG, Ng SM, et al. Selecting girls with precocious puberty for brain imaging: validation of European evidence-based diagnosis rule. J Pediatr 2003;143(4):445-450.
252. Amir O, Biron-Shental T. The impact of hormonal fluctuations on female vocal folds. Curr Opin Otolaryngol Head Neck Surg 2004;12(3):180-184.
253. Peschel ER, Peschel RE. Medical insights into the castrati in opera. Am Sci 1987;75:578-583.
254. Harries M, Hawkins S, Hacking J, et al. Changes in the male voice at puberty: vocal fold length and its relationship to the fundamental frequency of the voice. J Laryngol Otol 1998; 112(5):451-454.
255. Harries ML, Walker JM, Williams DM, et al. Changes in the male voice at puberty. Arch Dis Child 1997;77(5):445-447.
256. Karlberg P, Taranger J. The somatic development of children in a Swedish urban community. Acta Paediatr Scand Suppl 1976;258:1-148.
257. Amy dlB, Sanchez S. [A comparative acoustic study of the speaking and singing voice during the adolescent's break of the voice]. Rev Laryngol Otol Rhinol (Bord) 2000;121(5):325-328.
258. Lucky AW, Biro FM, Simbartl LA, et al. Predictors of severity of acne vulgaris in young adolescent girls: results of a five-year longitudinal study. J Pediatr 1997;130:30-39.
259. Barth JH, Clark S. Acne and hirsuties in teenagers. Best Pract Res Clin Obstet Gynaecol 2003;17(1):131-148.
260. Barth JH, Clark S. Acne and hirsuties in teenagers. Best Pract Res Clin Obstet Gynaecol 2003;17(1):131-148.
261. Traupe H, Von Muhlendahl KE, Bramswig J, et al. Acne of the fulminans type following testosterone therapy in three excessively tall boys. Arch Dermatol 1988;124:414-417.
262. Adebamowo CA, Spiegelman D, Danby FW, et al. High school dietary dairy intake and teenage acne. J Am Acad Dermatol 2005;52(2):207-214.
263. Addy M, Hunter ML, Kingdon A, et al. An 8-year study of changes in oral hygiene and periodontal health during adolescence. Int J Paediatr Dent 1994;4:75-80.
264. Nakagawa S, Fujii H, Machida Y, et al. A longitudinal study from prepuberty to puberty of gingivitis. Correlation between the

occurrence of *Prevotella intermedia* and sex hormones. J Clin Periodontol 1994;21:658-665.
265. Gusberti FA, Mombelli A, Lang NP, et al. Changes in subgingival microbiota during puberty. A 4-year longitudinal study. J Clin Periodontol 1990;17:685-692.
266. Cozza P, Stirpe G, Condo R, et al. Craniofacial and body growth: a cross-sectional anthropometric pilot study on children during prepubertal period. Eur J Paediatr Dent 2005;6(2):90-96.
267. Boyanov MA, Temelkova NL, Popivanov PP. Determinants of thyroid volume in schoolchildren: fat-free mass versus body fat mass—a cross-sectional study. Endocr Pract 2004;10(5):409-416.
268. Vanden Eynde B, Vienne D, Vuylsteke-Wauters M, et al. Aerobic power and pubertal peak height velocity in Belgian boys. Eur J Appl Physiol 1988;57:430-434.
269. Elster AD, Chen MY, Williams DW 3rd, et al. Pituitary gland: MR imaging of physiologic hypertrophy in adolescence. Radiology 1990;174:681-685.
270. Calvo MS, Eyre DR, Gundberg CM. Molecular basis and clinical application of biologic markers of bone turnover. Endocr Rev 1996;17:333-368.
271. Johansen JS, Giwercman A, Hartwell D, et al. Serum bone Gla-protein as a marker of bone growth in children and adolescents: correlation with age, height, serum insulin-like growth factor I, and serum testosterone. J Clin Endocrinol Metab 1988;67: 273-278.
272. Crofton PM, Stirling HF, Schonau E, et al. Bone alkaline phosphatase and collagen markers as early predictors of height velocity response to growth-promoting treatments in short normal children. Clin Endocrinol (Oxf) 1996;44:385-394.
273. Fujimoto S, Kubo T, Tanaka H, et al. Urinary pyridinoline and deoxypyridinoline in healthy children and in children with growth hormone deficiency. J Clin Endocrinol Metab 1995;80: 1922-1928.
274. Rauch F, Schnabel D ASM, Remer T, et al. Urinary excretion of galactosyl-hydroxylysine is a marker of growth in children. J Clin Endocrinol Metab 1995;80:1295-1300.
275. Sen AT, Derman O, Kinik E. The relationship between osteocalcin levels and sexual stages of puberty in male children. Turk J Pediatr 2000;42(4):281-285.
276. Chen CJ, Chao TY, Janckila AJ, et al. Evaluation of the activity of tartrate-resistant acid phosphatase isoform 5b in normal Chinese children—a novel marker for bone growth. J Pediatr Endocrinol Metab 2005;18(1):55-62.
277. Garbagnati E. Urate changes in lean and obese boys during pubertal development. Metabolism 1996;45:203-205.
278. Hero M, Wickman S, Hanhijarvi R, et al. Pubertal upregulation of erythropoiesis in boys is determined primarily by androgen. J Pediatr 2005;146(2):245-252.
279. Grumbach MM, Gluckman PD. The human fetal hypothalamus and pituitary gland; the maturation of neuroendocrine mechanisms controlling the secretion of fetal pituitary growth hormone, prolactin, gonadotropin, and adrenocorticotropin-related peptides and thyrotropin. In Tulchinsky D, Little AB, eds. Maternal-Fetal Endocrinology. Philadelphia: WB Saunders, 1994: 193-261.
280. Rabinovici J, Jaffe RB. Development and regulation of growth and differentiated function in human and subhuman primate fetal gonads. Endocr Rev 1990;11:532-551.
281. Ross GT. Follicular development: the life cycle of the follicle and puberty. In Grumbach MM, Sizonenko PC, Aubert MI, eds. Control of the Onset of Puberty. Baltimore: Williams & Wilkins, 1990:376-386.
282. Gougeon A. Regulation of ovarian follicular development in primates: facts and hypotheses. Endocr Rev 1996;17:121-155.
283. Peters H, Byskov AG, Grinsted J. Follicular growth in fetal and prepubertal ovaries of humans and other primates. Clin Endocrinol Metab 1978;7:469-485.
284. Stanhope R, Adams J, Jacobs HS, et al. Ovarian ultrasound assessment in normal children, idiopathic precocious puberty, and during low dose pulsatile gonadotrophin releasing hormone treatment of hypogonadotrophic hypogonadism. Arch Dis Child 1985;60(2):116-119.
285. Adams J, Franks S, Polson DW, et al. Multifollicular ovaries: clinical and endocrine features and response to pulsatile gonadotropin releasing hormone. Lancet 1985;2(8469-70):1375-1379.
286. Bridges NA, Cooke A, Healy MJ, et al. Standards for ovarian volume in childhood and puberty. Fertil Steril 1993;60:456-460.
287. Salardi S, Orsini LF, Cacciari E, et al. Pelvic ultrasonography in premenarcheal girls: relation to puberty and sex hormone concentrations. Arch Dis Child 1985;60:120-125.
288. Haber HP, Wollmann HA, Ranke MB. Pelvic ultrasonography: early differentiation between isolated premature thelarche and central precocious puberty. Eur J Pediatr 1995;154:182-186.
289. Garel L, Dubois J, Grignon A, et al. US of the pediatric female pelvis: a clinical perspective. Radiographics 2001;21(6):1393-1407.
290. Battaglia C, Mancini F, Regnani G, et al. Pelvic ultrasound and color Doppler findings in different isosexual precocities. Ultrasound Obstet Gynecol 2003;22(3):277-283.
291. Marsh EE, Laufer MR. Endometriosis in premenarcheal girls who do not have an associated obstructive anomaly. Fertil Steril 2005;83(3):758-760.
292. Batt RE, Mitwally MF. Endometriosis from thelarche to midteens: pathogenesis and prognosis, prevention and pedagogy. J Pediatr Adolesc Gynecol 2003;16(6):337-347.
293. Onat J, Ertem B. Age at menarche: relationship to socioeconomic status, growth rate in stature and weight, and skeletal and sexual maturation. Am J Hum Biol 1995;7:741-750.
294. Mitan LA, Slap GB. Adolescent menstrual disorders. Update. Med Clin North Am 2000;84(4):851-868.
295. Apter D, Vihko R. Serum pregnenolone, progesterone, 17-hydroxyprogesterone, testosterone and 5 alpha-dihydrotestosterone during female puberty. J Clin Endocrinol Metab 1977;45: 1039-1048.
296. Pakarinen A, Hammond GL, Vihko R. Serum pregnenolone, progesterone, 17alpha-hydroxyprogesterone, androstenedione, testosterone, 5alpha-dihydrotestosterone and androsterone during puberty in boys. Clin Endocrinol (Oxf) 1979;11:465-474.
297. Metcalf MG, MacKenzie JA. Incidence of ovulation in young women. J Biosoc Sci 1980;12:345-352.
298. Lemarchand-Beraud T, Zufferey MM, Reymond M. Maturation of the hypothalamo-pituitary ovarian axis in adolescent girls. J Clin Endocrinol Metab 1982;54:241-246.
299. BIrths: Final data for 2000. National Vital Statistics Reports: CDC 2002;50(5).
300. Martin JA, Brady E, Hamilton P, et al. Births: final data for 2003. National Vital Statistics Reports: CDC 2005;54(2):1-116.
301. Chemes HE. Infancy is not a quiescent period of testicular development. Int J Androl 2001;24(1):2-7.
302. Cortes D, Muller J, Skakkebaek NE. Proliferation of Sertoli cells during development of the human testis assessed by stereological methods. Int J Androl 1987;10:589-596.
303. Gondos B, Kogan SJ. Testicular development during puberty. In Grumbach MM., Sizonenko PC, Aubert ML, et al, eds. Control of the Onset of Puberty. 1990:387-402.
304. Saez JM. Leydig cells: endocrine, paracrine, and autocrine regulation. Endocr Rev 1994;15(5):574-626.
305. Prince FP. The triphasic nature of Leydig cell development in humans, and comments on nomenclature. J Endocrinol 2001; 168(2):213-216.
306. Aumuller G, Riva A. Morphology and functions of the human seminal vesicle. Andrologia 1992;24:183-196.
307. Paltiel HJ, Rupich RC, Babcock DS. Maturational changes in arterial impedance of the normal testis in boys: Doppler sonographic study. AJR Am J Roentgenol 1994;163:1189-1193.
308. Berensztein EB, Baquedano MS, Gonzalez CR, et al. Expression of aromatase, estrogen receptor alpha and beta, androgen receptor, and cytochrome P-450scc in the human early prepubertal testis. Pediatr Res 2006;60(6):740-744.
309. Nielsen CT, Skakkebaek NE, Darling JA, et al. Longitudinal study of testosterone and luteinizing hormone (LH) in relation to spermarche, pubic hair, height and sitting height in normal boys. Acta Endocrinol [Suppl] 1986;279:98-106.
310. Richardson DW, Short RV. Time of onset of sperm production in boys. J Biosoc Sci Suppl 1978;15-25.

311. Weissenberg R, Hirsch M, Shemesh J, et al. Evaluation of the morphology of sperm in urine of adolescent boys. Int J Androl 1984;7(4):348-351.
312. Nysom K, Pedersen JL, Jorgensen M, et al. Spermaturia in two normal boys without other signs of puberty. Acta Paediatr 1994; 83:520-521.
313. Pedersen JL, Nysom K, Jorgensen M, et al. Spermaturia and puberty. Arch Dis Child 1993;69:384-387.
314. Janczewski Z, Bablok L. Semen characteristics in pubertal boys. II. Semen quality in relation to bone age. Arch Androl 1985;15:207-211.
315. Janczewski Z, Bablok L. Semen characteristics in pubertal boys. III. Semen quality and somatosexual development. Arch Androl 1985;15:213-218.
316. Laron Z, Arad J, Gurewitz R, et al. Age at first conscious ejaculation: a milestone in male puberty. Helv Paediatr Acta 1980;35: 13-20.
317. Largo RH, Gasser T, Prader A, et al. Analysis of the adolescent growth spurt using smoothing spline functions. Ann Hum Biol 1978;5(5):421-434.
318. Ilyes I, Mahunka I, Sari B. [Insulin resistance in childhood obesity]. Orv Hetil 1992;133(35):2221-2224.
319. Sherar LB, Baxter-Jones AD, Mirwald RL. Limitations to the use of secondary sex characteristics for gender comparisons. Ann Hum Biol 2004;31(5):586-593.
320. Veldhuis JD, Roemmich JN, Richmond EJ, et al. Endocrine control of body composition in infancy, childhood, and puberty. Endocr Rev 2005;26(1):114-146.
321. Largo RH, Prader A. Pubertal development in Swiss girls. Helv Paediatr Acta 1983;38:229-243.
322. Tanner JM, Whitehouse RH, Marubini E, et al. The adolescent growth spurt of boys and girls of the Harpenden growth study. Ann Hum Biol 1976;3:109-126.
323. Gasser T, Sheehy A, Molinari L, et al. Sex dimorphism in growth. Annals of Human Biology 2000;27(2):187-197.
324. Preece MA, Baines MJ. A new family of mathematical models describing the human growth curve. Ann Hum Biol 1978;5(1): 1-24.
325. Martin DD, Hauspie RC, Ranke MB. Total pubertal growth and markers of puberty onset in adolescents with GHD: comparison between mathematical growth analysis and pubertal staging methods. Horm Res 2005;63(2):95-101.
326. Karlberg J, Fryer JG, Engstrom I, et al. Analysis of linear growth using a mathematical model. II. From 3 to 21 years of age. Acta Paediatr Scand Suppl 1987;337:12-29.
327. Limony Y, Zadik Z, Pic AK, et al. Improved method for predicting adult height of pubertal boys using a mathematical model. Horm Res 1993;40:117-122.
328. Karlberg J, Kwan CW, Gelander L, Albertsson-Wikland K. Pubertal growth assessment. Horm Res 2003;60(Suppl 1): 27-35.
329. Tanner JM, Davies PSW. Clinical longitudinal standards for height and height velocity for North American children. J Pediatr 1985;107:317-329.
330. Caino S, Kelmansky D, Lejarraga H, et al. Short-term growth at adolescence in healthy girls. Ann Hum Biol 2004;31(2): 182-195.
331. Luo ZC, Cheung YB, He Q, et al. Growth in early life and its relation to pubertal growth. Epidemiology 2003;14(1):65-73.
332. Bourguignon JP. Linear growth as a function of age at onset of puberty and sex steroid dosage: therapeutic implications. Endocr Rev 1988;9:467-488.
333. Hugg U, Juranger J. Height and height velocity in early, average and late maturers followed to the age of 25: a prospective longitudinal study of Swedish urban children from birth to adulthood. Ann Hum Biol 1991;18:47-56.
334. McKusick VA. Heritable Disorders of Connective Tissue. St Louis: CV Mosby, 1972.
335. Tanner JM, Whitehouse RH, Hughes PCR, et al. Relative importance of growth hormone and sex steroids for the growth at puberty of trunk length, limb length, and muscle width in growth hormone-deficient children. J Pediatr 1976;89:1000-1008.
336. Grumbach MM, Auchus RJ. Estrogen: consequences and implication of human mutations in synthesis and action. J Clin Endocrinol Metab 1999;84:4677-4694.
337. Grumbach MM. Estrogen, bone, growth, and sex: a sea change in conventional wisdom. J Pediatr Endocrinol Metab 2000;13(suppl 6):1439-1455.
338. Rochira V, Balestrieri A, Faustini-Fustini M, et al. Role of estrogen on bone in the human male: insights from the natural models of congenital estrogen deficiency. Mol Cell Endocrinol 2001; 178(1-2):215-220.
339. Conte FA, Grumbach MM, Ito Y, et al. A syndrome of female pseudohermaphrodism, hypergonadotropic hypogonadism and multicystic ovaries associated with missense mutations in the gene encoding aromatase (P450 arom). J Clin Endocrinol Metab 1994;78:1287-1292.
340. Smith EP, Boyd J, Frank GR, et al. Estrogen resistance caused by a mutation by the estrogen-receptor in a man. N Engl J Med 1994;331:1056-1061.
341. Morishima A, Grumbach MM, Simpson ER, et al. Aromatase deficiency in male and female siblings caused by a novel mutation and the physiological role of estrogens. J Clin Endocrinol Metab 1995;80:3689-3698.
342. Attie KM, Ramirez NR, Conte FA, et al. The pubertal growth spurt in eight patients with true precocious puberty and growth hormone deficiency: evidence for a direct role of sex steroids. J Clin Endocrinol Metab 1990;71:975-983.
343. Van Wyk JJ, Smith EP. Insulin-like growth factors and skeletal growth: possibilities for therapeutic interventions. J Clin Endocrinol Metab 1999;84(12):4349-4354.
344. Rogol AD. Growth at puberty: interaction of androgens and growth hormone. Med Sci Sports Exerc 1994;26:767-770.
345. Riggs BL, Khosla S, Melton LJ. The contribution of sex steroids to the construction and conservation of the adult skeleton. Endocr Rev 2002;23(3):279-302.
346. Bilezikian JP, Morishima A, Bell J, et al. Increased bone mass as a result of estrogen therapy in a man with aromatase deficiency. N Engl J Med 1998;339(9):599-603.
347. Carani C, Qin K, Simoni M, et al. Effect of testosterone and estradiol in a man with aromatase deficiency. N Engl J Med 1997;337(2):91-95.
348. Rochira V, Faustini-Fustini M, Balestrieri A, et al. Estrogen replacement therapy in a man with congenital aromatase deficiency: effects of different doses of transdermal estradiol on bone mineral density and hormonal parameters. J Clin Endocrinol Metab 2000;85(5):1841-1845.
349. Stratakis CA, Vottero A, Brodie A, et al. The aromatase excess syndrome is associated with feminization of both sexes and autosomal dominant transmission of aberrant P450 aromatase gene transcription. J Clin Endocrinol Metab 1998;83(4): 1348-1357.
350. Weise M, De Levi S, Barnes KM, et al. Effects of estrogen on growth plate senescence and epiphyseal fusion. Proc Natl Acad Sci U S A 2001;98(12):6871-6876.
350a. Chagin AS, Chrysis D, Takigawa M, et al. Locally produced estrogen promotes fetal rat metatarsal bone growth; an effect mediated through increased chondrocyte proliferation and decreased apoptosis. J Endocrinol 2006;188(2):193-203.
351. Klein KO, Baron J, Colli MJ, et al. Estrogen levels in childhood determined by an ultrasensitive recombinant cell bioassay. J Clin Invest 1994;94:2475-2480.
352. Ikegami S, Moriwake T, Tanaka H, et al. An ultrasensitive assay revealed age-related changes in serum oestradiol at low concentrations in both sexes from infancy to puberty. Clin Endocrinol 2001;55:789-795.
353. Klein KO, Martha PMJ, Blizzard RM, et al. A longitudinal assessment of hormonal and physical alterations during normal puberty in boys. II. Estrogen levels as determined by an ultrasensitive bioassay. J Clin Endocrinol Metab 1996;81:3203-3207.
354. Weise M, Flor A, Barnes KM, et al. Determinants of growth during gonadotropin-releasing hormone analog therapy for precocious puberty. J Clin Endocrinol Metab 2004;89(1):103-107.
355. Eastell R. Role of oestrogen in the regulation of bone turnover at the menarche. J Endocrinol 2005;185(2):223-234.
356. Garnett SP, Hogler W, Blades B, et al. Relation between hormones and body composition, including bone, in prepubertal children. Am J Clin Nutr 2004;80(4):966-972.
357. Hogler W, Briody J, Moore B, et al. Importance of estrogen on bone health in Turner syndrome: a cross-sectional and longitu-

dinal study using dual-energy X-ray absorptiometry. J Clin Endocrinol Metab 2004;89(1):193-199.
358. Manolagas SC. Birth and death of bone cells: basic regulatory mechanisms and implications for the pathogenesis and treatment of osteoporosis. Endocr Rev 2000;21(2):115-137.
359. Abu EO, Horner A, Kusec V, et al. The localization of androgen receptors in human bone. J Clin Endocrinol Metab 1997; 82(10):3493-3497.
360. Noble B, Routledge J, Stevens H, et al. Androgen receptors in bone-forming tissue. Horm Res 1999;51(1):31-36.
361. Vanderschueren D, Bouillon R. Androgens and bone. Calcif Tissue Int 1995;56:341-346.
362. Compston JE. Sex steroids and bone. Physiol Rev 2001;81(1): 419-447.
363. Cassorla FG, Skerda MC, Valk IM, et al. The effects of sex steroids on ulnar growth during adolescence. J Clin Endocrinol Metab 1984;58:717-720.
364. Vanderschueren D, Vandenput L, Boonen S, et al. Androgens and bone. Endocr Rev 2004;25(3):389-425.
365. Schoenau E, Neu CM, Rauch F, et al. The development of bone strength at the proximal radius during childhood and adolescence. J Clin Endocrinol Metab 2001;86(2):613-618.
366. Zachman M, Prader A, Sobel E, et al. Pubertal growth in patients with androgen insensitivity: indirect evidence for the importance of estrogens in pubertal growth of girls. J Pediatr 1986;108: 694-697.
367. Marcus R, Leary D, Schneider DL, et al. The contribution of testosterone to skeletal development and maintenance: lessons from the androgen insensitivity syndrome. J Clin Endocrinol Metab 2000;85(3):1032-1037.
368. Martha PM Jr, Rogol AD, Veldhuis JD, et al. Alterations in the pulsatile properties of circulating growth hormone concentrations during puberty in boys. J Clin Endocrinol Metab 1989; 69:563-570.
369. Ross JL, Pescovitz OH, Barnes K, et al. Growth hormone secretory dynamics in children with precocious puberty. Ann Hum Biol 1989;16:397-406.
370. Costin G, Kaufman FR, Brasel JA. Growth hormone secretory dynamics in subjects with normal stature. J Pediatr 1989;115: 537-544.
371. Garnier P, Raynaud F, Job JC. Growth hormone secretion during sleep. I. Comparison with GH responses to conventional pharmacologic stimuli in pubertal and early pubertal short subjects. Effects of treatment with human GH in patients with discrepant measurements of GH secretion. Horm Res 1988;29:133-139.
372. Link K, Blizzard RM, Evans WS, et al. The effect of androgens on the pulsatile release and the twenty-four-hour mean concentration of growth hormone in peripubertal males. J Clin Endocrinol Metab 1986;62:159-164.
373. Martha PM Jr, Rogol AD, Veldhuis JD. Alterations in the pulsatile properties of circulating growth hormone concentrations during puberty in boys. J Clin Endocrinol Metab 1989;69:563-570.
374. Mauras N, Blizzard RM, Link K, et al. Augmentation of growth hormone secretion during puberty: evidence for a pulse amplitude-modulated phenomenon. J Clin Endocrinol Metab 1987;64:596-601.
375. Wennink JM, Delemarre-van de Waal HA, Schoemaker R, et al. Growth hormone secretion patterns in relation to LH and estradiol secretion throughout normal female puberty. Acta Endocrinol (Copenh) 1991;124:129-135.
376. Albertsson-Wikland K, Rosberg S, Karlberg J, et al. Analysis of 24-hour growth hormone profiles in healthy boys and girls of normal stature: relation to puberty. J Clin Endocrinol Metab 1994;78:1195-1201.
377. Martha PMJ, Gorman KM, Blizzard RM, et al. Endogenous growth hormone secretion and clearance rates in normal boys, as determined by deconvolution analysis: relationship to age, pubertal status, and body mass. J Clin Endocrinol Metab 1992;74: 336-344.
378. Veldhuis JD, Roemmich JN, Rogol AD. Gender and sexual maturation-dependent contrasts in the neuroregulation of growth hormone secretion in prepubertal and late adolescent males and females—a general clinical research center-based study. J Clin Endocrinol Metab 2000;85(7):2385-2394.
379. Marin G, Domene HM, Barnes KM, et al. The effects of estrogen priming and puberty on the growth hormone response to standardized treadmill exercise and arginine-insulin in normal girls and boys. J Clin Endocrinol Metab 1994;79:537-541.
380. Bouix O, Brun JF, Fedou C, et al. Plasma beta-endorphin, corticotrophin and growth hormone responses to exercise in pubertal and prepubertal children. Horm Metab Res 1994;26:195-199.
381. Mericq V, Cassorla F, Garcia H, et al. Growth hormone (GH) responses to GH-releasing peptide and to GH-releasing hormone in GH-deficient children. J Clin Endocrinol Metab 1995;80: 1681-1684.
382. Laron Z, Bowers CY, Hirsch D, et al. Growth hormone-releasing activity of growth hormone-releasing peptide-1 (a synthetic heptapeptide) in children and adolescents. Acta Endocrinol (Copenh) 1993;129:424-426.
383. Loche S, Cambiaso P, Carta D, et al. The growth hormone-releasing activity of hexarelin, a new synthetic hexapeptide, in short normal and obese children and in hypopituitary subjects. J Clin Endocrinol Metab 1995;80:674-678.
384. Soriano-Guillen L, Barrios V, Chowen JA, et al. Ghrelin levels from fetal life through early adulthood: relationship with endocrine and metabolic and anthropometric measures. J Pediatr 2004; 144(1):30-35.
385. Whatmore AJ, Hall CM, Jones J, et al. Ghrelin concentrations in healthy children and adolescents. Clin Endocrinol (Oxf) 2003;59(5):649-654.
386. Racine MS, Symons KV, Foster CM, et al. Augmentation of growth hormone secretion after testosterone treatment in boys with constitutional delay of growth and adolescence: evidence against an increase in hypothalamic secretion of growth hormone-releasing hormone. J Clin Endocrinol Metab 2004;89(7):3326-3331.
387. Eakman GD, Dallas JS, Ponder SW, Keenan BS. The effects of testosterone and dihydrotestosterone on hypothalamic regulation of growth hormone secretion. J Clin Endocrinol Metab 1996;81:1217-1223.
388. Metzger DL, Kerrigan JR. Estrogen receptor blockade with tamoxifen diminishes growth hormone secretion in boys: evidence for a stimulatory role of endogenous estrogens during male adolescence. J Clin Endocrinol Metab 1994;79:513-518.
389. Muller G, Keller A, Reich A, et al. Priming with testosterone enhances stimulated growth hormone secretion in boys with delayed puberty. J Pediatr Endocrinol Metab 2004;17(1):77-83.
390. Kerrigan JR, Veldhuis JD, Rogol AD. Androgen-receptor blockade enhances pulsatile luteinizing hormone production in late pubertal males: evidence for a hypothalamic site of physiologic androgen feedback action. Pediatr Res 1994;35:102-106.
391. Keenan BS, Richards GE, Ponder SW, et al. Androgen-stimulated pubertal growth: the effects of testosterone and dihydrotestosterone on growth hormone and insulin-like growth factor-I in the treatment of short stature and delayed puberty. J Clin Endocrinol Metab 1993;76:996-1001.
392. Harris DA, Van Vliet G, Egli CA, et al. Somatomedin-C in normal puberty and in true precocious puberty before and after treatment with a potent luteinizing hormone-releasing hormone agonist. J Clin Endocrinol Metab 1985;61:152-159.
393. Mansfield MJ, Rudlin CR, Crigler Jr, et al. Changes in growth and serum growth hormone and plasma somatomedin-C levels during suppression of gonadal sex steroid secretion in girls with central precocious puberty. J Clin Endocrinol Metab 1988;66:3-9.
394. de Boer JA, Schoemaker J, van der Veen, et al. Impaired reproductive function in women treated for growth hormone deficiency during childhood. Clin Endocrinol (Oxf) 1997;46(6): 681-689.
395. Rimoin DL, Merimee TJ, Rabinowitz D, et al. Genetic aspects of clinical endocrinology. Recent Prog Horm Res 1968;24:365-437.
396. Phillips JA III. Inherited defects in growth hormone synthesis and action. In Scriver CR, Beaudet AI, Sly WS, et al, eds. The metabolic and molecular bases of inherited disease. New York: McGraw-Hill/Medical Publishing Division, 2001.
397. Aynsley-Green A, Zachmann M, Prader A. Interrelation of the therapeutic effects of growth hormone and testosterone on growth in hypopituitarism. J Pediatr 1976;89:992-999.
398. Bala RM, Lopatka J, Leung A. Serum immunoreactive somatomedin levels in normal adults, pregnant women at term, children at

various ages, and children with constitutionally delayed growth. J Clin Endocrinol Metab 1981;52:508-512.
399. Lofqvist C, Andersson E, Gelander L, et al. Reference values for IGF-I throughout childhood and adolescence: a model that accounts simultaneously for the effect of gender, age, and puberty. J Clin Endocrinol Metab 2001;86(12):5870-5876.
400. Juul A, Bang P, Hertel NT, et al. Serum insulin-like growth factor-I in 1030 healthy children, adolescents, and adults: relation to age, sex, stage of puberty, testicular size, and body mass index. J Clin Endocrinol Metab 1994;78:744-752.
401. Jorge AA, Souza SC, Arnhold IJ, et al. The first homozygous mutation (S226I) in the highly-conserved WSXWS-like motif of the GH receptor causing Laron syndrome: suppression of GH secretion by GnRH analogue therapy not restored by dihydrotestosterone administration. Clin Endocrinol (Oxf) 2004;60(1):36-40.
402. Sjogren K, Liu JL, Blad K, et al. Liver-derived insulin-like growth factor I (IGF-I) is the principal source of IGF-I in blood but is not required for postnatal body growth in mice. Proc Natl Acad Sci U S A 1999;96(12):7088-7092.
403. Yakar S, Liu JL, Stannard B, et al. Normal growth and development in the absence of hepatic insulin-like growth factor I. Proc Natl Acad Sci U S A 1999;96(13):7324-7329.
404. Isaksson OG, Lindahl A, Nilsson A, et al. Mechanism of the stimulatory effect of growth hormone on longitudinal bone growth. Endocr Rev 1987;8(4):426-438.
405. Werther GA, Haynes KM, Barnard R, et al. Visual demonstration of growth hormone receptors on human growth plate chondrocytes. J Clin Endocrinol Metab 1990;70:1725-1731.
406. Hunziker EB, Wagner J, Zapf J. Differential effects of insulin-like growth factor I and growth hormone on developmental stages of rat growth plate chondrocytes in vivo. J Clin Invest 1994;93(3):1078-1086.
407. Ohlsson C, Nilsson A, Isaksson O, et al. Growth hormone induces multiplication of the slowly cycling germinal cells of the rat tibial growth plate. Proc Natl Acad Sci U S A 1992;89(20):9826-9830.
408. Skinner AM, Price DA, Addison GM, et al. The influence of age, size, pubertal status and renal factors on urinary growth hormone excretion in normal children and adolescents. Growth Regul 1992;2:156-160.
409. Crowne EC, Wallace WH, Shalet SM, et al. Relationship between urinary and serum growth hormone and pubertal status. Arch Dis Child 1992;67:91-95.
410. Main KM, Jarden M, Angelo L, et al. The impact of gender and puberty on reference values for urinary growth hormone excretion: a study of 3 morning urine samples in 517 healthy children and adults. J Clin Endocrinol Metab 1994;79:865-871.
411. Patel L, Skinner AM, Price DA, et al. The influence of body mass index on growth hormone secretion in normal and short statured children. Growth Regul 1994;4:29-34.
412. Martha PMJ, Rogol AD, Blizzard RM, et al. Growth hormone-binding protein activity is inversely related to 24-hour growth hormone release in normal boys. J Clin Endocrinol Metab 1991;73:175-181.
413. Argente J, Barrios V, Pozo J, et al. Normative data for insulin-like growth factors (IGFs), IGF-binding proteins, and growth hormone-binding protein in a healthy Spanish pediatric population: age- and sex-related changes. J Clin Endocrinol Metab 1993;77: 1522-1528.
414. Merimee TJ, Russell B, Quinn S. Growth hormone-binding proteins of human serum: developmental patterns in normal man. J Clin Endocrinol Metab 1992;75:852-854.
415. Massa G, Bouillon R, Vanderschueren-Lodeweyckx M. Serum levels of growth hormone-binding protein and insulin-like growth factor-I during puberty. Clin Endocrinol (Oxf) 1992;37:175-180.
416. Martha PMJ, Rogol AD, Carlsson LM, Gesundheit N, Blizzard RM. A longitudinal assessment of hormonal and physical alterations during normal puberty in boys. I. Serum growth hormone-binding protein. J Clin Endocrinol Metab 1993;77:452-457.
417. Juul A, Fisker S, Scheike T, et al. Serum levels of growth hormone binding protein in children with normal and precocious puberty: relation to age, gender, body composition and gonadal steroids. Clin Endocrinol 2000;52(2):165-172.
418. Rosenfield RL, Furlanetto R, Bock D. Relationship of somatomedin-C concentrations to pubertal changes. J Pediatr 1983; 103:723-728.
419. Luna AM, Wilson DM, Wibbelsman CJ, et al. Somatomedins in adolescence: a cross-sectional study of the effect of puberty on plasma insulin-like growth factor I and II levels. J Clin Endocrinol Metab 1983;57:268-271.
420. Hesse V, Jahreis G, Schambach H, et al. Insulin-like growth factor I correlations to changes of the hormonal status in puberty and age. Exp Clin Endocrinol 1994;102:289-298.
421. Juul A, Dalgaard P, Blum WF, et al. Serum levels of insulin-like growth factor (IGF)-binding protein-3 (IGFBP-3) in healthy infants, children, and adolescents: the relation to IGF-I, IGF-II, IGFBP-1, IGFBP-2, age, sex, body mass index, and pubertal maturation. J Clin Endocrinol Metab 1995;80:2534-2542.
422. Hasegawa Y, Hasegawa T, Takada M, et al. Plasma free insulin-like growth factor I concentrations in growth hormone deficiency in children and adolescents. Eur J Endocrinol 1996;134:184-189.
423. Lofqvist C, Andersson E, Gelander L, et al. Reference values for insulin-like growth factor-binding protein-3 (IGFBP-3) and the ratio of insulin-like growth factor-I to IGFBP-3 throughout childhood and adolescence. J Clin Endocrinol Metab 2005;90(3): 1420-1427.
424. Juul A, Flyvbjerg A, Frystyk J, et al. Serum concentrations of free and total insulin-like growth factor-I, IGF binding proteins -1 and -3 and IGFBP-3 protease activity in boys with normal or precocious puberty. Clin Endocrinol (Oxf) 1996;44:515-523.
425. Wilson DM, Stene MA, Killen JD, et al. Insulin-like growth factor binding protein-3 in normal pubertal girls. Acta Endocrinol (Copenh) 1992;126:381-386.
426. Grumbach MM, Richards GE, Conte FA, et al. Clinical disorders of adrenal function and puberty: an assessment of the role of the adrenal cortex in normal and abnormal puberty in man and evidence for an ACTH-like pituitary adrenal androgen stimulating hormone. In James VHT, Serio M, Giusti G, et al, eds. The Endocrine Function of the Human Adrenal Cortex, Serono Symposium. New York: Academic Press, 1977:583-612.
427. Abu EO, Horner A, Kusec V, et al. The localization of the functional glucocorticoid receptor alpha in human bone. J Clin Endocrinol Metab 2000;85(2):883-889.
428. Van Wyk JJ, Grumbach MM. Syndrome of precocious menstruation and galactorrhea in juvenile hypothyroidism: an example of hormonal overlap in pituitary feedback. J Pediatr 1960;57: 416-435.
429. Abu EO, Bord S, Horner A, et al. The expression of thyroid hormone receptors in human bone. Bone 1997;21(2):137-142.
430. Abu EO, Horner A, Teti A, et al. The localization of thyroid hormone receptor mRNAs in human bone. Thyroid 2000;10(4): 287-293.
431. Greulich WS, Pyle SI. Radiographic Atlas of Skeletal Development of the Hand and Wrist. Stanford, CA: PB-Stanford University Press, 1959.
432. Tanner JM, Whitehouse RH, Marshall WA, et al. Assessment of Skeletal Maturity and Prediction of Adult Height: TW 2 Method. New York: Academic, 1975.
433. Aicardi G, Vignolo M, Milani S, et al. Assessment of skeletal maturity of the hand-wrist and knee: a comparison among methods. Am J Human Biol 2000;12(5):610-615.
434. Sauvegrain J, Nahum H, Carle F. [Bone maturation. Importance of the determination of the bone age. Methods of evaluation (general review)]. Ann Radiol (Paris) 1962;5:535-541.
435. Flor-Cisneros A, Roemmich JN, Rogol AD, et al. Bone age and onset of puberty in normal boys. Mol Cell Endocrinol 2006; 254-255:202-206.
436. Marshall WA. Inter-relationships of skeletal maturation, sexual development and somatic growth in man. Ann. Hum Biol 1974;1:29-40.
437. Hauspie R, Bielicki T, Koniarek J. Skeletal maturity at onset of the adolescent growth spurt and at peak height velocity for growth in height: a threshold effect? Ann Hum Biol 1995;18:23-29.
438. Bayley N, Pinneau SR. Tables for predicting adult height from skeletal age: revised for use with the Greulich-Pyle standards. J Pediatr 1952;40:441-423.
439. Roche AF, Wainer H, Thissen D. The RWT method for the prediction of adult stature. Pediatrics 1975;56:1026-1033.
440. Walker RN. Standards for somatotyping children. I. Prediction of young adult height from children's growth data. Ann Hum Biol 1974;1:149-158.

441. Roche AF. Skeletal maturity of children 6-11 years: racial, geographic area of residence, socioeconomic differentials. National Health Survey. DHEW Vital and Health Statistics Series 11, No. 149. Washington, DC: Government Printing Office, 1975.
442. Pietka E, Gertych A, Pospiecha Euro KS, et al. Computer-assisted bone age assessment: graphical user interface for image processing and comparison. J Digit Imaging 2004;17(3):175-188.
443. Tanner JM, Gibbons RD. Automatic bone age measurement using computerized image analysis. J Pediatr Endocrinol 1994;7: 141-145.
444. Gross GW, Boone JM, Bishop DM. Pediatric skeletal age: determination with neural networks. Radiology 1995;195:689-695.
445. Van Teunenbroek A, De Waal W, Roks A, et al. Computer-aided skeletal age scores in healthy children, girls with Turner syndrome, and in children with constitutionally tall stature. Pediatr Res 1996;39:360-367.
446. Roberts CD, Vogtle L, Stevenson RD. Effect of hemiplegia on skeletal maturation. J Pediatr 1994;125:824-828.
447. Henderson RC, Gilbert SR, Clement ME, et al. Altered skeletal maturation in moderate to severe cerebral palsy. Dev Med Child Neurol 2005;47(4):229-236.
448. Seeman E. Pathogenesis of bone fragility in women and men. Lancet 2002;359(9320):1841-1850.
449. Seeman E. Periosteal bone formation—a neglected determinant of bone strength. N Engl J Med 2003;349(4):320-323.
450. Mora S, Gilsanz V. Establishment of peak bone mass. Endocrinol Metab Clin North Am 2003;32(1):39-63.
451. Bailey DA, Martin AD, McKay HA, et al. Calcium accretion in girls and boys during puberty: a longitudinal analysis. J Bone Miner Res 2000;15(11):2245-2250.
452. Bachrach LK, Hastie T, Wang M, et.al. Bone mineral acquisition in healthy Asian, Hispanic, black and Caucasian youth: a longitudinal study. J Clin Endocrinol Metab 1999;84:4702-4712.
453. Mora S, Goodman WG, Loro ML, et al. Age-related changes in cortical and cancellous vertebral bone density in girls: assessment with quantitative CT. AJR Am J Roentgenol 1994;162: 405-409.
454. Rico H, Revilla M, Villa LF, et al. Determinants of total-body and regional bone mineral content and density in postpubertal normal women. Metabolism 1994;43:263-266.
455. Du X, Greenfield H, Fraser DR, et al. Low body weight and its association with bone health and pubertal maturation in Chinese girls. Eur J Clin Nutr 2003;57(5):693-700.
456. Lloyd T, Rollings N, Andon MB, et al. Determinants of bone density in young women. I. Relationships among pubertal development, total body bone mass, and total body bone density in premenarchal females. J Clin Endocrinol Metab 1992;75: 383-387.
457. Moreira-Andres MN, Papapietro K, Canizo FJ, et al. Correlations between bone mineral density, insulin-like growth factor I and auxological variables. Eur J Endocrinol 1995;132:573-579.
458. Schonau E. The peak bone mass concept: is it still relevant? Pediatr Nephrol 2004;19(8):825-831.
459. Bass S, Delmas PD, Pearce G, et al. The differing tempo of growth in bone size, mass, and density in girls is region-specific. J Clin Invest 1999;104(6):795-804.
460. Seeman E. From density to structure: growing up and growing old on the surfaces of bone. J Bone Miner Res 1997;12(4): 509-521.
461. Seeman E. Clinical review 137: Sexual dimorphism in skeletal size, density, and strength. J Clin Endocrinol Metab 2001;86(10): 4576-4584.
462. Lu PW, Cowell CT, LLoyd-Jones SA, et al. Volumetric bone mineral density in normal subjects, aged 5-27 years. J Clin Endocrinol Metab 1996;81(4):1586-1590.
463. Bradney M, Karlsson MK, Duan Y, et al. Heterogeneity in the growth of the axial and appendicular skeleton in boys: implications for the pathogenesis of bone fragility in men. J Bone Miner Res 2000;15(10):1871-1878.
464. Bonjour JP, Theintz G, Law F, et al. Peak bone mass. Osteoporos Int 1994;4(Suppl 1):7-13.
465. Arabi A, Tamim H, Nabulsi M, et al. Sex differences in the effect of body-composition variables on bone mass in healthy children and adolescents. Am J Clin Nutr 2004;80(5):1428-1435.
466. Crabtree NJ, Kibirige MS, Fordham JN, et al. The relationship between lean body mass and bone mineral content in paediatric health and disease. Bone 2004;35(4):965-972.
467. Southard RN, Morris JD, Mahan JD, et al. Bone mass in healthy children: measurement with quantitative DXA. Radiology 1991; 179(3):735-738.
468. Bonjour JP, Theintz G, Buchs B, et al. Critical years and stages of puberty for spinal and femoral bone mass accumulation during adolescence. J Clin Endocrinol Metab 1991;73:555-563.
469. Faulkner RA, Bailey DA, Drinkwater DT, et al. Bone densitometry in Canadian children 8-17 years of Age. Calcif Tissue Int 1996;59(5):344-351.
470. Sabatier JP, Guaydier-Souquieres G, Laroche D, et al. Bone mineral acquisition during adolescence and early adulthood: a study in 574 healthy females 10-24 years of age. Osteoporos Int 1996;6(2):141-148.
471. van der Sluis I, de Ridder MA, Boot AM, et al. Reference data for bone density and body composition measured with dual energy x ray absorptiometry in white children and young adults. Arch Dis Child 2002;87(4):341-347.
472. del Rio L, Carrascosa A, Pons F, et al. Bone mineral density of the lumbar spine in white Mediterranean Spanish children and adolescents: changes related to age, sex, and puberty. Pediatr Res 1994;35:362-366.
473. Ellis KJ, Shypailo RJ, Hardin DS, et al. Z score prediction model for assessment of bone mineral content in pediatric diseases. J Bone Miner Res 2001;16(9):1658-1664.
474. Taylor A, Konrad PT, Norman ME, et al. Total body bone mineral density in young children: influence of head bone mineral density. J Bone Miner Res 1997;12(4):652-655.
475. Van Coeverden SC, de Ridder CM, Roos JC, et al. Pubertal maturation characteristics and the rate of bone mass development longitudinally toward menarche. J Bone Min Res 2001;16(4): 774-781.
476. Hogler W, Briody J, Woodhead HJ, et al. Importance of lean mass in the interpretation of total body densitometry in children and adolescents. J Pediatr 2003;143(1):81-88.
477. Binkley TL, Specker BL, Wittig TA. Centile curves for bone densitometry measurements in healthy males and females ages 5-22 yr. J Clin Densitom 2002;5(4):343-353.
478. Kelly TL, Crane G, Baran DT. Single X-ray absorptiometry of the forearm: precision, correlation, and reference data. Calcif Tissue Int 1994;54(3):212-218.
479. Genanat HK, Engelke K, Fuerst T, et al. Noninvasive assessment of bone mineral and structure:state of the art. J Bone Miner Res 1992;7:137-145.
480. Lu PW, Briody JN, Ogle GD, et al. Bone mineral density of total body, spine, and femoral neck in children and young adults: a cross-sectional and longitudinal study. J Bone Miner Res 1994;9:1451-1458.
481. Lappe JM, Stegman M, Davies KM, et al. A prospective study of quantitative ultrasound in children and adolescents. J Clin Densitom 2000;3(2):167-175.
482. Lum CK, Wang MC, Moore E, et al. A comparison of calcaneus ultrasound and dual X-ray absorptiometry in healthy North American youths and young adults. J Clin Densitom 1999;2(4): 403-411.
483. Zamberlan N, Radetti G, Paganini C, et al. Evaluation of cortical thickness and bone density by roentgen microdensitometry in growing males and females. Eur J Pediatr 1996;155:377-382.
484. Baxter-Jones AD, Mirwald RL, McKay HA, et al. A longitudinal analysis of sex differences in bone mineral accrual in healthy 8-19-year-old boys and girls. Ann Hum Biol 2003;30(2):160-175.
485. Kontulainen SA, Macdonald HM, Khan KM, et al. Examining bone surfaces across puberty: a 20-month pQCT trial. J Bone Miner Res 2005;20(7):1202-1207.
486. Schoenau E, Neu CM, Rauch F, et al. The development of bone strength at the proximal radius during childhood and adolescence. J Clin Endocrinol Metab 2001;86(2):613-618.
487. Wang Q, Alen M, Nicholson P, et al. Growth patterns at distal radius and tibial shaft in pubertal girls: a 2-year longitudinal study. J Bone Miner Res 2005;20(6):954-961.
488. Saito T, Nakamura K, Okuda Y, et al. Weight gain in childhood and bone mass in female college students. J Bone Miner Metab 2005;23(1):69-75.

489. Loro ML, Sayre J, Roe TF, et al. Early identification of children predisposed to low peak bone mass and osteoporosis later in life. J Clin Endocrinol Metab 2000;85(10):3908-3918.
490. Bachrach LK. Bone mineralization in childhood and adolescence. Curr Opin Pediatr 1993;5:467-473.
491. Grimston SK, Morrison K, Harder JA, et al. Bone mineral density during puberty in western Canadian children. Bone Miner 1992;19:85-96.
492. Theintz G, Buchs B, Rizzoli R, et al. Longitudinal monitoring of bone mass accumulation in healthy adolescents: evidence for a marked reduction after 16 years of age at the levels of lumbar spine and femoral neck in female subjects. J Clin Endocrinol Metab 1992;75:1060-1065.
493. Weaver CM, Peacock M, Martin BR, et al. Calcium retention estimated from indicators of skeletal status in adolescent girls and young women. Am J Clin Nutr 1996;64:67-70.
494. Carrie Fassler AL, Bonjour JP. Osteoporosis as a pediatric problem. Pediatr Clin North Am 1995;42:811-824.
495. Matkovic V, Jelic T, Wardlaw GM, et al. Timing of peak bone mass in Caucasian females and its implication for the prevention of osteoporosis. Inference from a cross-sectional model. J Clin Invest 1994;93:799-808.
496. Proesmans W, Goos G, Emma F, et al. Total body mineral mass measured with dual photon absorptiometry in healthy children. Eur J Pediatr 1994;153:807-812.
497. Kroger H, Kotaniemi A, Kroger L, et al. Development of bone mass and bone density of the spine and femoral neck—a prospective study of 65 children and adolescents. Bone Miner 1993;23:171-182.
498. Bachrach LK, Hastie T, Wang MC, et al. Bone mineral acquisition in healthy Asian, Hispanic, black, and Caucasian youth: a longitudinal study. J Clin Endocrinol Metab 1999;84(12):4702-4712.
499. Rauch F, Bailey DA, Baxter-Jones A, et al. The "muscle-bone unit" during the pubertal growth spurt. Bone 2004;34(5):771-775.
500. Young D, Hopper JL, MacInnis RJ, et al. Changes in body composition as determinants of longitudinal changes in bone mineral measures in 8 to 26-year-old female twins. Osteoporos Int 2001;12(6):506-515.
501. Van Langendonck L, Claessens AL, Lysens R, Koninckx PR, Beunen G. Association between bone, body composition and strength in premenarcheal girls and postmenopausal women. Ann Hum Biol 2004;31(2):228-244.
502. Loud KJ, Gordon CM, Micheli LJ, et al. Correlates of stress fractures among preadolescent and adolescent girls. Pediatrics 2005;115(4):e399-e406.
503. van der Meulen MC, Ashford MWJ, Kiratli BJ, et al. Determinants of femoral geometry and structure during adolescent growth. J Orthop Res 1996;14:22-29.
504. Lehtonen-Veromaa M, Mottonen T, Irjala K, et al. A 1-year prospective study on the relationship between physical activity, markers of bone metabolism, and bone acquisition in peripubertal girls. J Clin Endocrinol Metab 2000;85(10):3726-3732.
505. Lehtonen-Veromaa M, Mottonen T, Nuotio I, et al. Influence of physical activity on ultrasound and dual-energy X-ray absorptiometry bone measurements in peripubertal girls: a cross-sectional study. Calcif Tissue Int 2000;66(4):248-254.
506. Lehtonen-Veromaa M, Mottonen T, Svedstrom E, et al. Physical activity and bone mineral acquisition in peripubertal girls. Scand J Med Sci Sports 2000;10(4):236-243.
507. McKay HA, MacLean L, Petit M, et al. "Bounce at the Bell": a novel program of short bouts of exercise improves proximal femur bone mass in early pubertal children. Br J Sports Med 2005; 39(8):521-526.
508. Mackelvie KJ, Petit MA, Khan KM, et al. Bone mass and structure are enhanced following a 2-year randomized controlled trial of exercise in prepubertal boys. Bone 2004;34(4):755-764.
509. Johannsen N, Binkley T, Englert V, et al. Bone response to jumping is site-specific in children: a randomized trial. Bone 2003; 33(4):533-539.
510. Wang QJ, Suominen H, Nicholson PH, et al. Influence of physical activity and maturation status on bone mass and geometry in early pubertal girls. Scand J Med Sci Sports 2005;15(2):100-106.
511. Nickols-Richardson SM, Modlesky CM, O'Connor PJ, et al. Premenarcheal gymnasts possess higher bone mineral density than controls. Med Sci Sports Exerc 2000;32(1):63-69.
512. Lloyd T, Chinchilli VM, Johnson-Rollings N, et al. Adult female hip bone density reflects teenage sports-exercise patterns but not teenage calcium intake. Pediatrics 2000;106(1 Pt 1): 40-44.
513. Laing EM, Wilson AR, Modlesky CM, et al. Initial years of recreational artistic gymnastics training improves lumbar spine bone mineral accrual in 4- to 8-year-old females. J Bone Miner Res 2005;20(3):509-519.
514. Scerpella TA, Davenport M, Morganti CM, et al. Dose related association of impact activity and bone mineral density in prepubertal girls. Calcif Tissue Int 2003;72(1):24-31.
515. Nurmi-Lawton JA, Baxter-Jones AD, Mirwald RL, et al. Evidence of sustained skeletal benefits from impact-loading exercise in young females: a 3-year longitudinal study. J Bone Miner Res 2004;19(2):314-322.
516. Greene DA, Naughton GA, Briody JN, et al. Bone strength index in adolescent girls: does physical activity make a difference? Br J Sports Med 2005;39(9):622-627.
517. Valdimarsson O, Alborg HG, Duppe H, et al. Reduced training is associated with increased loss of BMD. J Bone Miner Res 2005;20(6):906-912.
518. Markou KB, Mylonas P, Theodoropoulou A, et al. The influence of intensive physical exercise on bone acquisition in adolescent elite female and male artistic gymnasts. J Clin Endocrinol Metab 2004;89(9):4383-4387.
519. Kardinaal AF, Hoorneman G, Vaananen K, et al. Determinants of bone mass and bone geometry in adolescent and young adult women. Calcif Tissue Int 2000;66(2):81-89.
520. Bachrach LK. Acquisition of optimal bone mass in childhood and adolescence. Trends Endocrinol Metab 2001;12(1):22-28.
521. Weaver CM, Peacock M, Johnston CC Jr. Adolescent nutrition in the prevention of postmenopausal osteoporosis. J Clin Endocrinol Metab 1999;84(6):1839-1843.
522. Rubin K, Schirduan V, Gendreau P, et al. Predictors of axial and peripheral bone mineral density in healthy children and adolescents, with special attention to the role of puberty. J Pediatr 1993;123:863-870.
523. Sentipal JM, Wardlaw GM, Mahan J, et al. Influence of calcium intake and growth indexes on vertebral bone mineral density in young females. Am J Clin Nutr 1991;54:425-428.
524. Dibba B, Prentice A, Ceesay M, et al. Effect of calcium supplementation on bone mineral accretion in Gambian children accustomed to a low-calcium diet. Am J Clin Nutr 2000;71(2):544-549.
525. Abrams SA, Stuff JE. Calcium metabolism in girls: current dietary intakes lead to low rates of calcium absorption and retention during puberty. Am J Clin Nutr 1994;60:739-743.
526. Goulding A, Rockell JE, Black RE, et al. Children who avoid drinking cow's milk are at increased risk for prepubertal bone fractures. J Am Diet Assoc 2004;104(2):250-253.
527. Abrams SA, Griffin IJ, Hicks PD, et al. Pubertal girls only partially adapt to low dietary calcium intakes. J Bone Miner Res 2004;19(5):759-763.
528. Anderson JJ, Pollitzer WS. Ethnic and genetic differences in susceptibility to osteoporotic fractures. Adv Nutr Res 1994;9: 129-149.
529. Gilsanz V, Roe TF, Mora S, et al. Changes in vertebral bone density in black girls and white girls during childhood and puberty. Am J Med Genet 1991;41:313-318.
530. Chan GM, Hoffman K, McMurry M. Effects of dairy products on bone and body composition in pubertal girls. J Pediatr 1995;126: 551-556.
531. Anderson JJ, Metz JA. Contributions of dietary calcium and physical activity to primary prevention of osteoporosis in females. J Am Coll Nutr 1993;12:378-383.
532. Johnston CCJ, Miller JZ, Slemenda CW, et al. Calcium supplementation and increases in bone mineral density in children. N Engl J Med 1992;327:82-87.
533. Matkovic V. Calcium and peak bone mass. J Intern Med 1992; 231:151-160.
534. Teegarden D, Lyle RM, Proulx WR, et al. Previous milk consumption is associated with greater bone density in young women. Am J Clin Nutr 1999;69(5):1014-1017.
535. Lee WT, Leung SS, Leung DM, et al. A follow-up study on the effects of calcium-supplement withdrawal and puberty on bone acquisition of children. Am J Clin Nutr 1996;64:71-77.

536. Bonjour JP, Chevalley T, Ammann P, et al. Gain in bone mineral mass in prepubertal girls 3.5 years after discontinuation of calcium supplementation: a follow-up study. Lancet 2001; 358(9289):1208-1212.
537. Abrams SA, Copeland KC, Gunn SK, et al. Calcium absorption, bone mass accumulation, and kinetics increase during early pubertal development in girls. J Clin Endocrinol Metab 2000; 85(5):1805-1809.
538. Rozen GS, Rennert G, Dodiuk-Gad RP, et al. Calcium supplementation provides an extended window of opportunity for bone mass accretion after menarche. Am J Clin Nutr 2003;78(5): 993-998.
539. Courteix D, Jaffre C, Lespessailles E, et al. Cumulative effects of calcium supplementation and physical activity on bone accretion in premenarchal children: a double-blind randomised placebo-controlled trial. Int J Sports Med 2005;26(5):332-338.
540. Bonofiglio D, Garofalo C, Catalano S, et al. Low calcium intake is associated with decreased adrenal androgens and reduced bone age in premenarcheal girls in the last pubertal stages. J Bone Miner Metab 2004;22(1):64-70.
541. Chevalley T, Rizzoli R, Hans D, et al. Interaction between calcium intake and menarcheal age on bone mass gain: an eight-year follow-up study from prepuberty to postmenarche. J Clin Endocrinol Metab 2005;90(1):44-51.
542. Bounds W, Skinner J, Carruth BR, Ziegler P. The relationship of dietary and lifestyle factors to bone mineral indexes in children. J Am Diet Assoc 2005;105(5):735-741.
543. Bougle DL, Sabatier JP, Guaydier-Souquieres G, et al. Zinc status and bone mineralisation in adolescent girls. J Trace Elem Med Biol 2004;18(1):17-21.
544. Winzenberg TM, Shaw K, Fryer J, et al. Calcium supplementation for improving bone mineral density in children. Cochrane Database Syst Rev 2006;(2):CD005119.
545. Hopper JL, Green RM, Nowson CA, et al. Genetic, common environment, and individual specific components of variance for bone mineral density in 10- to 26-year-old females: a twin study. Am J Epidemiol 1998;147(1):17-29.
546. Nowson CA, Green RM, Hopper JL, et al. A co-twin study of the effect of calcium supplementation on bone density during adolescence. Osteoporos Int 1997;7(3):219-225.
547. Cameron MA, Paton LM, Nowson CA, et al. The effect of calcium supplementation on bone density in premenarcheal females: a co-twin approach. J Clin Endocrinol Metab 2004;89(10): 4916-4922.
548. Van Langendonck L, Claessens AL, Vlietinck R, et al. Influence of weight-bearing exercises on bone acquisition in prepubertal monozygotic female twins: a randomized controlled prospective study. Calcif Tissue Int 2003;72(6):666-674.
549. Lonzer MD, Imrie R, Rogers D, et al. Effects of heredity, age, weight, puberty, activity, and calcium intake on bone mineral density in children. Clin Pediatr (Phila) 1996;35:185-189.
550. McKay HA, Bailey DA, Wilkinson AA, et al. Familial comparison of bone mineral density at the proximal femur and lumbar spine. Bone Miner 1994;24:95-107.
551. Cheng S, Tylavsky F, Kroger H, et al. Association of low 25-hydroxyvitamin D concentrations with elevated parathyroid hormone concentrations and low cortical bone density in early pubertal and prepubertal Finnish girls. Am J Clin Nutr 2003; 78(3):485-492.
552. Abrams SA, Griffin IJ, Hawthorne KM, et al. Vitamin D receptor Fok1 polymorphisms affect calcium absorption, kinetics, and bone mineralization rates during puberty. J Bone Miner Res 2005;20(6):945-953.
553. Strandberg S, Nordstrom P, Lorentzon R, et al. Vitamin D receptor start codon polymorphism (FokI) is related to bone mineral density in healthy adolescent boys. J Bone Miner Metab 2003;21(2):109-113.
554. Suuriniemi M, Mahonen A, Kovanen V, et al. Association between exercise and pubertal BMD is modulated by estrogen receptor alpha genotype. J Bone Miner Res 2004;19(11):1758-1765.
555. Gustavsson A, Thorsen K, Nordstrom P. A 3-year longitudinal study of the effect of physical activity on the accrual of bone mineral density in healthy adolescent males. Calcif Tissue Int 2003;73(2):108-114.
556. Vicente-Rodriguez G, Jimenez-Ramirez J, Ara I, et al. Enhanced bone mass and physical fitness in prepubescent footballers. Bone 2003;33(5):853-859.
557. Remer T, Boye KR, Hartmann M, et al. Adrenarche and bone modeling and remodeling at the proximal radius: weak androgens make stronger cortical bone in healthy children. J Bone Miner Res 2003;18(8):1539-1546.
558. Moreira-Andres MN, Canizo FJ, de la Cruz FJ, et al. Bone mineral status in prepubertal children with constitutional delay of growth and puberty. Eur J Endocrinol 1998;139(3):271-275.
559. Finkelstein JS, Neer RM, Biller BM, et al. Osteopenia in men with a history of delayed puberty. N Engl J Med 1992;326:600-604.
560. Finkelstein JS, Klibanski A, Neer RM. A longitudinal evaluation of bone mineral density in adult men with histories of delayed puberty. J Clin Endocrinol Metab 1996;81:1152-1155.
561. Finkelstein JS, Klibanski A, Neer RM. Evaluation of lumber spine bone mineral density (BMD) using dual energy x-ray absorptiometry (DXA) in 21 young men with histories of constitutionally-delayed puberty. J Clin Endocrinol Metab 1999;84(9):3400-3401.
562. Behre HM, Simoni M, Nieschlag E. Strong association between serum levels of leptin and testosterone in men. Clin Endocrinol (Oxf) 1997;47(2):237-240.
563. Bertelloni S, Baroncelli GI, Battini R, et al. Short-term effect of testosterone treatment on reduced bone density in boys with constitutional delay of puberty. J Bone Miner Res 1995;10: 1488-1495.
564. Bertelloni S, Baroncelli GI, Ferdeghini M, et al. Normal volumetric bone mineral density and bone turnover in young men with histories of constitutional delay of puberty. J Clin Endocrinol Metab 1998;83(12):4280-4283.
565. Bertelloni S, Baroncelli GI, Saggese G. Normal volumetric bone mineral density in young men with histories of constitutional delay of puberty—author's response. J Clin Endocrinol Metab 1999;84:3403.
566. Yap F, Hogler W, Briody J, et al. The skeletal phenotype of men with previous constitutional delay of puberty. J Clin Endocrinol Metab 2004;89(9):4306-4311.
567. Krupa B, Miazgowski T. Bone mineral density and markers of bone turnover in boys with constitutional delay of growth and puberty. J Clin Endocrinol Metab 2005;90(5):2828-2830.
568. Mauras N, Haymond MW, Darmaun D, et al. Calcium and protein kinetics in prepubertal boys. Positive effects of testosterone. J Clin Invest 1994;93:1014-1019.
569. Arisaka O, Arisaka M, Nakayama Y, et al. Effect of testosterone on bone density and bone metabolism in adolescent male hypogonadism. Metabolism 1995;44:419-423.
570. Simberg N, Titinen A, Silfvast A, et al. High bone density in hyperandrogenic women: effect of gonadotropin-releasing hormone agonist alone or in conjunction with estrogen-progestin replacement. J Clin Endocrinol Metab 1995;80:646-651.
571. Buchanan JR, Hospodar C, Myers Pea. Effect of excess androgens on bone density in young women. J Clin Endocrinol Metab 1988;67:937-943.
572. Orwel ES. Androgens as anabolic agents for bone. Trends Endocrinol Metab 1996;7:77-84.
573. Kubler A, Schulz G, Cordes U, et al. The influence of testosterone substitution on bone mineral density in patients with Klinefelter's syndrome. Exp Clin Endocrinol 1992;100:129-132.
574. Hergenroeder AC. Bone mineralization, hypothalamic amenorrhea, and sex steroid therapy in female adolescents and young adults. J Pediatr 1995;126:683-689.
575. Fabbri G, Petraglia F, Segre A, et al. Reduced spinal bone density in young women with amenorrhoea. Eur J Obstet Gynecol Reprod Biol 1991;41:117-122.
576. Grinspoon S, Thomas E, Pitts S, et al. Prevalence and predictive factors for regional osteopenia in women with anorexia nervosa. Ann Intern Med 2000;133(10):790-794.
577. Saggese G, Bertelloni S, Baroncelli GI, et al. Reduction of bone density: an effect of gonadotropin releasing hormone analogue treatment in central precocious puberty. Eur J Pediatr 1993; 152:717-720.
578. Saggese G, Bertelloni S, Baroncelli GI, et al. Bone loss during gonadotropin-releasing hormone agonist treatment in girls with true precocious puberty is not due to an impairment of calcitonin secretion. J Endocrinol Invest 1991;14:231-236.

579. Verrotti A, Chiarelli F, Montanaro AF, et al. Bone mineral content in girls with precocious puberty treated with gonadotropin-releasing hormone analog. Gynecol Endocrinol 1995;9:277-281.
580. Neely EK, Bachrach LK, Hintz RL, et al. Bone mineral density during treatment of central precocious puberty. J Pediatr 1995;127:819-822.
581. Antoniazzi F, Bertoldo F, Zamboni G, et al. Bone mineral metabolism in girls with precocious puberty during gonadotrophin-releasing hormone agonist treatment. Eur J Endocrinol 1995; 133:412-417.
582. Blumsohn A, Hannon RA, Wrate R, et al. Biochemical markers of bone turnover in girls during puberty. Clin Endocrinol (Oxf) 1994;40:663-670.
583. Jarvinen TL, Kannus P, Sievanen H. Estrogen and bone—a reproductive and locomotive perspective. J Bone Miner Res 2003; 18(11):1921-1931.
584. Braillon PM. Annual changes in bone mineral content and body composition during growth. Horm Res 2003;60(6): 284-290.
585. Rolland-Cachera MF. Body composition during adolescence: methods, limitations and determinants. Horm Res 1993;39 Suppl 3:25-40.
586. Rosenthal M, Bain SH, Bush A, et al. Weight/height$^{2.88}$ as a screening test for obesity or thinness in schoolage children. Eur J Pediatr 1994;153:876-883.
587. Dietz WH, Bellizzi MC. Introduction: the use of body mass index to assess obesity in children. Am J Clin Nutr 1999;70(1): 123S-125S.
588. Brambilla P, Manzoni P, Sironi S, et al. Peripheral and abdominal adiposity in childhood obesity. Int J Obes Relat Metab Disord 1994;18:795-800.
589. Gidding SS. Preventive pediatric cardiology. Tobacco, cholesterol, obesity, and physical activity. Pediatr Clin North Am 1999;46(2):253-262.
590. Roemmich JN, Rogol AD. Hormonal changes during puberty and their relationship to fat distribution. Am J Human Biol 1999;11(2):209-224.
591. Goran MI. Energy expenditure, body composition, and disease risk in children and adolescents. Proc Nutr Soc 1997;56(1B): 195-209.
592. Goran MI, Kaskoun M, Shuman WP. Intra-abdominal adipose tissue in young children. Int J Obes Relat Metab Disord 1995;19(4):279-283.
593. Fernandez JR, Redden DT, Pietrobelli A, et al. Waist circumference percentiles in nationally representative samples of African-American, European-American, and Mexican-American children and adolescents. J Pediatr 2004;145(4):439-444.
594. Neovius M, Linne Y, Rossner S. BMI, waist-circumference and waist-hip-ratio as diagnostic tests for fatness in adolescents. Int J Obes Relat Metab Disord 2005;29(2):163-169.
595. Kissebah AH, Krakower GR. Regional adiposity and morbidity. Physiol Rev 1994;74:761-811.
596. Caserta F, Tchkonia T, Civelek VN, et al. Fat depot origin affects fatty acid handling in cultured rat and human preadipocytes. Am J Physiol Endocrinol Metab 2001;280(2):E238-E247.
597. He Q, Horlick M, Thornton J, et al. Sex-specific fat distribution is not linear across pubertal groups in a multiethnic study. Obes Res 2004;12(4):725-733.
598. Ellis KJ, Shypailo RJ, Pratt JA, et.al. Accuracy of dual-energy x-ray absorptiometry for body-composition measurements in children. Am J Clin Nutr 1994;60:660-665.
599. Fox KR, Peters DM, Sharpe P, et al. Assessment of abdominal fat development in young adolescents using magnetic resonance imaging. Int J Obes Relat Metab Disord 2000;24:1653-1659.
600. Goran MI. Measurement issues related to studies of childhood obesity: assessment of body composition, body fat distribution, physical activity and food intake. Pediatrics 1998;101:505-518.
601. Goran MI, Gower BA, Treuth M, et al. Prediction of intra-abdominal and subcutaneous abdominal adipose tissue in healthy pre-pubertal children and subcutaneous abdominal adipose tissue SAwith body composition and anthropometry in children. Int J Obes Relat Metab Disord 1998;22(6):549-558.
602. Molina RM, Bouchard C. Growth, Maturation and Physical Activity. Champaign, IL: Human Kinetics, 1991.
603. Dore E, Martin R, Ratel S, et al. Gender differences in peak muscle performance during growth. Int J Sports Med 2005;26(4): 274-280.
604. Ogden CL, Carroll MD, Curtin LR, et al. Prevalence of overweight and obesity in the United States, 1999-2004. JAMA 2006;295(13): 1549-1555.
605. Styne DM. Childhood and adolescent obesity. Prevalence and significance. Pediatr Clin North Am 2001;48(4):823-54, vii.
606. Must A, Jacques PF, Dallal GE, et al. Long-term morbidity and mortality of overweight adolescents. A follow-up of the Harvard Growth Study of 1922 to 1935. N Engl J Med 1992;327(19): 1350-1355.
607. DiPietro L, Mossberg HO, Stunkard AJ. A 40-year history of overweight children in Stockholm: life-time overweight, morbidity, and mortality. Int J Obes Relat Metab Disord 1994;18:585-590.
608. Nieto FJ, Szklo M, Comstock GW. Childhood weight and growth rate as predictors of adult mortality [see comments]. Am J Epidemiol 1992;136(2):201-213.
609. Mossberg HO. 40-year follow-up of overweight children. Lancet 1989;2(8661):491-493.
610. Hoffmans MD, Kromhout D, Coulander CD. Body mass index at the age of 18 and its effects on 32-year-mortality from coronary heart disease and cancer. A nested case-control study among the entire 1932 Dutch male birth cohort. J Clin Epidemiol 1989; 42(6):513-520.
611. Hoffmans MD, Kromhout D, de Lezenne CC. The impact of body mass index of 78,612 18-year old Dutch men on 32-year mortality from all causes. J Clin Epidemiol 1988;41(8):749-756.
612. Gunnell DJ, Frankel SJ, Nanchahal K, et al. Childhood obesity and adult cardiovascular mortality: a 57-y follow-up study based on the Boyd Orr cohort. Am J Clin Nutr 1998;67(6):1111-1118.
613. Lawlor DA, Martin RM, Gunnell D, et al. Association of body mass index measured in childhood, adolescence, and young adulthood with risk of ischemic heart disease and stroke: findings from 3 historical cohort studies. Am J Clin Nutr 2006;83(4): 767-773.
614. Kirkland RT, Keenan BS, Probstfield JL, et al. Decrease in plasma high-density lipoprotein cholesterol levels at puberty in boys with delayed adolescence. Correlation with plasma testosterone levels. JAMA 1987;257:502-507.
615. LaRosa JC. Lipids and cardiovascular disease: do the findings and therapy apply equally to men and women? Womens Health Issues 1992;2:102-11; discussion 111-113.
616. Sorva R, Kuusi T, Dunkel L, et al. Effects of endogenous sex steroids on serum lipoproteins and postheparin plasma lipolytic enzymes. J Clin Endocrinol Metab 1988;66:408-413.
617. Srinivasan SR, Myers L, Berenson GS. Changes in metabolic syndrome variables since childhood in prehypertensive and hypertensive subjects: the Bogalusa Heart Study. Hypertension 2006;48(1):33-39.
618. Sinaiko AR, Steinberger J, Moran A, et al. Influence of insulin resistance and body mass index at age 13 on systolic blood pressure, triglycerides, and high-density lipoprotein cholesterol at age 19. Hypertension 2006;48(4):730-736.
619. Frontini MG, Srinivasan SR, Berenson GS. Longitudinal changes in risk variables underlying metabolic syndrome X from childhood to young adulthood in female subjects with a history of early menarche: the Bogalusa Heart Study. Int J Obes Relat Metab Disord 2003;27(11):1398-1404.
620. Freedman DS, Dietz WH, Srinivasan SR, et al. The relation of overweight to cardiovascular risk factors among children and adolescents: the Bogalusa Heart Study. Pediatrics 1999;103(6 Pt 1):1175-1182.
621. Csabi G, Torok K, Jeges S, et al. Presence of metabolic cardiovascular syndrome in obese children. Eur J Pediatr 2000;159(1-2): 91-94.
622. Wilcken DE, Lynch JF, Marshall MD, et al. Relevance of body weight to apolipoprotein levels in Australian children. Med J Aust 1996;164:22-25.
623. Cameron JL. Metabolic cues for the onset of puberty. Horm Res 1991;36:97-103.
624. Berenson GS, Srinivasan SR, Bao W, et al. Association between multiple cardiovascular risk factors and atherosclerosis in children and young adults. The Bogalusa Heart Study. N Engl J Med 1998;338(23):1650-1656.

625. McGill HJ, McMahan CA, Zieske AW, et al. Association of Coronary Heart Disease Risk Factors with microscopic qualities of coronary atherosclerosis in youth. Circulation 2000;102(4):374-379.
626. Lauer RM, Lee J, Clarke WR. Factors affecting the relationship between childhood and adult cholesterol levels: the Muscatine Study. Pediatrics 1988;82(3):309-318.
627. Nicklas TA, von Duvillard SP, Berenson GS. Tracking of serum lipids and lipoproteins from childhood to dyslipidemia in adults: the Bogalusa Heart Study. Int J Sports Med 2002;23(Suppl 1):S39-S43.
628. Srinivasan SR, Wattigney W, Webber LS, et al. Race and gender differences in serum lipoproteins of children, adolescents, and young adults—emergence of an adverse lipoprotein pattern in white males: the Bogalusa Heart Study. Prev Med 1991;20:671-684.
629. Hulman S, Kushner H, Katz S, et al. Can cardiovascular risk be predicted by newborn, childhood, and adolescent body size? An examination of longitudinal data in urban African Americans. J Pediatr 1998;132(1):90-97.
630. Chen W, Bao W, Begum S, et al. Age-related patterns of the clustering of cardiovascular risk variables of syndrome X from childhood to young adulthood in a population made up of black and white subjects: the Bogalusa Heart Study. Diabetes 2000;49(6):1042-1048.
631. Schur EA, Sanders M, Steiner H. Body dissatisfaction and dieting in young children. Int J Eat Disord 2000;27(1):74-82.
632. Neumark-Sztainer D, Hannan PJ. Weight-related behaviors among adolescent girls and boys: results from a national survey. Arch Pediatr Adolesc Med 2000;154(6):569-577.
633. Schreiber GB, Robins M, Striegel-Moore R, et al. Weight modification efforts reported by black and white preadolescent girls: National Heart, Lung, and Blood Institute Growth and Health Study. Pediatrics 1996;98:63-70.
634. Neumark-Sztainer D, Rock CL, Thornquist MD, et al. Weight-control behaviors among adults and adolescents: associations with dietary intake. Prev Med 2000;30(5):381-391.
635. Reaven GM. The metabolic syndrome: is this diagnosis necessary? Am J Clin Nutr 2006;83(6):1237-1247.
636. McFarlane SI, Banerji M, Sowers JR. Insulin resistance and cardiovascular disease. J Clin Endocrinol Metab 2001;86(2):713-718.
637. Goran MI, Gower BA. Longitudinal study on pubertal insulin resistance. Diabetes 2001;50(11):2444-2450.
638. Arslanian SA. Type 2 diabetes mellitus in children: pathophysiology and risk factors. J Pediatr Endocrinol Metab 2000;13(Suppl 6):1385-1394.
639. Travers SH, Jeffers BW, Bloch CA, et al. Gender and Tanner stage differences in body composition and insulin sensitivity in early pubertal children. J Clin Endocrinol Metab 1995;80:172-178.
640. Svec F, Nastasi K, Hilton C, et al. Black-white contrasts in insulin levels during pubertal development. The Bogalusa Heart Study. Diabetes 1992;41:313-317.
641. Cruz ML, Weigensberg MJ, Huang TT, et al. The metabolic syndrome in overweight Hispanic youth and the role of insulin sensitivity. J Clin Endocrinol Metab 2004;89(1):108-113.
642. Goran MI, Bergman RN, Gower BA. Influence of total vs. visceral fat on insulin action and secretion in African American and white children. Obes Res 2001;9(8):423-431.
643. Caprio S, Amiel SA, Merkel P, et al. Insulin-resistant syndromes in children. Horm Res 39 Suppl 1993;3:112-114.
644. Radetti G, Pasquino B, Gottardi E, et al. Insulin sensitivity in Turner's syndrome: influence of GH treatment. Eur J Endocrinol 2004;151(3):351-354.
645. Type 2 diabetes in children and adolescents. American Diabetes Association. Diabetes Care 2000;23(3):381-389.
646. Kibirige M, Metcalf B, Renuka R, et al. Testing the accelerator hypothesis: the relationship between body mass and age at diagnosis of type 1 diabetes. Diabetes Care 2003;26(10):2865-2870.
647. Gillespie KM, Nolsoe R, Betin VM, et al. Is puberty an accelerator of type 1 diabetes in IL6-174CC females? Diabetes 2005;54(4):1245-1248.
648. Amiel SA, Caprio S, Sherwin RS, et al. Insulin resistance of puberty: a defect restricted to peripheral glucose metabolism. J Clin Endocrinol Metab 1991;72:277-282.
649. Rosenbloom AL, Wheeler L, Bianchi R, et al. Age-adjusted analysis of insulin responses during normal and abnormal glucose tolerance tests in children and adolescents. Diabetes 1975;4:820-828.
650. Hindmarsh P, Di Silvio L, Pringle PJ, et al. Changes in serum insulin concentration during puberty and their relationship to growth hormone. Clin Endocrinol (Oxf) 1988;28:381-388.
651. Arslanian SA, Kalhan SC. Correlations between fatty acid and glucose metabolism. Potential explanation of insulin resistance of puberty. Diabetes 1994;43:908-914.
652. Radetti G, Pasquino B, Gottardi E, et al. Insulin sensitivity in growth hormone-deficient children: influence of replacement treatment. Clin Endocrinol (Oxf) 2004;61(4):473-477.
653. Holl RW, Heinze E, Seifert M, et al. Longitudinal analysis of somatic development in paediatric patients with IDDM: genetic influences on height and weight. Diabetologia 1994;37:925-929.
654. Kokkonen J, Laatikainen L, van Dickhoff K, et al. Ocular complications in young adults with insulin-dependent diabetes mellitus since childhood. Acta Paediatr 1994;83:273-278.
655. Algvere P. Prepubertal diabetes duration increases the risk of retinopathy. Acta Paediatr 1994;83:341.
656. Flack A, Kaar ML, Laatikainen L. A prospective, longitudinal study examining the development of retinopathy in children with diabetes. Acta Paediatr 1996;85:313-319.
657. Fairchild JM, Hing SJ, Donaghue KC, et al. Prevalence and risk factors for retinopathy in adolescents with type 1 diabetes. Med J Aust 1994;160:757-762.
658. Flack AA, Kaar ML, Laatikainen LT. Prevalence and risk factors of retinopathy in children with diabetes. A population-based study on Finnish children. Acta Ophthalmol (Copenh) 1993;71:801-809.
659. McNally PG, Raymond NT, Swift PG, et al. Does the prepubertal duration of diabetes influence the onset of microvascular complications? Diabet Med 1993;10:906-908.
660. Goldstein DE, Blinder KJ, Ide CH, et al. Glycemic control and development of retinopathy in youth-onset insulin-dependent diabetes mellitus. Results of a 12-year longitudinal study. Ophthalmology 1993;100:1125-31; discussion 1131.
661. de Abreu JR, Silva R, Cunha-Vaz JG. The blood-retinal barrier in diabetes during puberty. Arch Ophthalmol 1994;112:1334-1338.
662. Janner M, Knill SE, Diem P, et al. Persistent microalbuminuria in adolescents with type I (insulin-dependent) diabetes mellitus is associated to early rather than late puberty. Results of a prospective longitudinal study. Eur J Pediatr 1994;153:403-408.
663. Gungor N, Bacha F, Saad R, et al. Youth type 2 diabetes: insulin resistance, beta-cell failure, or both? Diabetes Care 2005;28(3):638-644.
664. Todd JA. Transcribing diabetes. Nature 1996;384:407-408.
665. Glaser NS. Non-insulin-dependent diabetes mellitus in childhood and adolescence. Pediatr Clin North Am 1997;44:307-337.
666. Glaser N, Jones KL. Non-insulin-dependent diabetes mellitus in children and adolescents. Adv Pediatr 1996;43:359-396.
667. Musso C, Shawker T, Cochran E, et al. Clinical evidence that hyperinsulinaemia independent of gonadotropins stimulates ovarian growth. Clin Endocrinol (Oxf) 2005;63(1):73-78.
668. Musso C, Cochran E, Javor E, et al. The long-term effect of recombinant methionyl human leptin therapy on hyperandrogenism and menstrual function in female and pituitary function in male and female hypoleptinemic lipodystrophic patients. Metabolism 2005;54(2):255-263.
669. Ibanez L, Potau N, Zampolli M, et al. Hyperinsulinemia in postpubertal girls with a history of premature pubarche and functional ovarian hyperandrogenism. J Clin Endocrinol Metab 1996;81(3):1237-1243.
670. Ibanez L, Potau N, Marcos MV, et al. Adrenal hyperandrogenism in adolescent girls with a history of low birthweight and precocious pubarche. Clin Endocrinol (Oxf) 2000;53(4):523-527.
671. Ibanez L, Potau N, de Zegher F. Endocrinology and metabolism after premature pubarche in girls. Acta Paediatrica Supplement 1999;88(433):73-77.
672. Ibanez L, de Zegher F, Potau N. Premature pubarche, ovarian hyperandrogenism, hyperinsulinism and the polycystic ovary syndrome: from a complex constellation to a simple sequence of prenatal onset. J Endocrinol Invest 1998;21(9):558-566.

673. Stoll BA. Obesity and breast cancer. Int J Obes Relat Metab Disord 1996;20:389-392.
674. Stoll BA. Timing of weight gain in relation to breast cancer risk. Ann Oncol 1995;6:245-248.
675. Stoll BA, Secreto G. New hormone-related markers of high risk to breast cancer. Ann Oncol 1992;3:435-438.
676. Stoll BA. Breast cancer risk in Japanese women with special reference to the growth hormone-insulin-like growth factor axis. Jpn J Clin Oncol 1992;22:1-5.
677. Shankar RR, Eckert GJ, Saha C, et al. The change in blood pressure during pubertal growth. J Clin Endocrinol Metab 2005;90(1): 163-167.
678. Voors AW, Webber LS, Frerichs RR, et al. Body height and body mass as determinants of basal blood pressure in children—the Bogalusa Heart Study. Am J Epidemiol 1977;106:101-108.
679. Lurbe E, Alvarez V, Liao Y, et al. The impact of obesity and body fat distribution on ambulatory blood pressure in children and adolescents. Am J Hypertens 1998;11(4 Pt 1):418-424.
680. Martins JM, Carreiras F, Falcaao J, et al. Dyslipidaemia in female overweight and obese patients. Relation to anthropometric and endocrine factors. Int J Obes Relat Metab Disord 1998;22(2): 164-170.
681. Berkey CS, Gardner J, Colditz GA. Blood pressure in adolescence and early adulthood related to obesity and birth size. Obes Res 1998;6(3):187-195.
682. Deckelbaum RJ, Williams CL. Childhood obesity: the health issue. Obes Res 2001;9(Suppl 4):239S-243S.
683. Feld LG, Springate JE, Waz WR. Special topics in pediatric hypertension. Semin Nephrol 1998;18(3):295-303.
684. Flynn JT. What's new in pediatric hypertension? Curr Hypertens Rep 2001;3(6):503-510.
685. He Q, Ding ZY, Fong DY, et al. Blood pressure is associated with body mass index in both normal and obese children. Hypertension 2000;36(2):165-170.
686. Modesti PA, Pela I, Cecioni I, et al. Changes in blood pressure reactivity and 24-hour blood pressure profile occurring at puberty. Angiology 1994;45:443-450.
687. Nelson MJ, Ragland DR, Syme SL. Longitudinal prediction of adult blood pressure from juvenile blood pressure levels. Am J Epidemiol 1992;136:633-645.
688. Resnicow K, Futterman R, Vaughan RD. Body mass index as a predictor of systolic blood pressure in a multiracial sample of US schoolchildren. Ethn Dis 1993;3(4):351-361.
689. Rocchini AP, Katch V, Anderson J, et al. Blood pressure in obese adolescents: effect of weight loss. Pediatrics 1988;82(1):16-23.
690. Rosner B, Prineas R, Daniels SR, et al. Blood pressure differences between blacks and whites in relation to body size among US children and adolescents. Am J Epidemiol 2000;151(10): 1007-1019.
691. Dietz WH. Health consequences of obesity in youth: childhood predictors of adult disease. Pediatrics 1998;101:518-525.
692. Bao W, Threefoot SA, Srinivasan SR, et al. Essential hypertension predicted by tracking of elevated blood pressure from childhood to adulthood: the Bogalusa Heart Study. Am J Hypertens 1995;8(7):657-665.
693. Pankow JS, Jacobs DR Jr, Steinberger J, et al. Insulin resistance and cardiovascular disease risk factors in children of parents with the insulin resistance (metabolic) syndrome. Diabetes Care 2004;27(3):775-780.
694. Liker HR, Barnes KM, Comite F, et al. Blood pressure and body size in precocious puberty. Acta Paediatr Scand 1988;77: 294-298.
695. Charmandari E, Kino T, Souvatzoglou E, et al. Pediatric stress: hormonal mediators and human development. Horm Res 2003;59(4):161-179.
696. Sowell ER, Trauner DA, Gamst A, et al. Development of cortical and subcortical brain structures in childhood and adolescence: a structural MRI study. Dev Med Child Neurol 2002;44(1):4-16.
697. Sowell ER, Thompson PM, Leonard CM, et al. Longitudinal mapping of cortical thickness and brain growth in normal children. J Neurosci 2004;24(38):8223-8231.
698. Sowell ER, Thompson PM, Toga AW. Mapping changes in the human cortex throughout the span of life. Neuroscientist 2004;10(4):372-392.
699. Sowell ER, Thompson PM, Tessner KD, et al. Mapping continued brain growth and gray matter density reduction in dorsal frontal cortex: Inverse relationships during postadolescent brain maturation. J Neurosci 2001;21(22):8819-8829.
700. Huttenlocher PR. Synaptic density in human frontal cortex-developmental changes and effects of aging. Brain Res 1979;163(2): 195-205.
701. Sowell ER, Delis D, Stiles J, et al. Improved memory functioning and frontal lobe maturation between childhood and adolescence: a structural MRI study. J Int Neuropsychol Soc 2001;7(3): 312-322.
702. Gogtay N, Giedd JN, Lusk L, et al. Dynamic mapping of human cortical development during childhood through early adulthood. Proc Natl Acad Sci U S A 2004;101(21):8174-8179.
703. Thompson PM, Sowell ER, Gogtay N, et al. Structural MRI and brain development. Int Rev Neurobiol 2005;67:285-323.
704. Giedd JN, Clasen LS, Lenroot R, et al. Puberty-related influences on brain development. Mol Cell Endocrinol 2006;254-255: 154-162.
705. Feinberg I, Carlson VR. Sleep variables as a function of age in man. Arch Gen Psychiatry 1968;18:18239-18250.
706. Yun AJ, Bazar KA, Lee PY. Pineal attrition, loss of cognitive plasticity, and onset of puberty during the teen years: is it a modern maladaptation exposed by evolutionary displacement? Med Hypotheses 2004;63(6):939-950.
707. Feinberg I, Thode HC J., Chugani HT, et al. Gamma distribution model describes maturational curves for delta wave amplitude, cortical metabolic rate and synaptic density. J Theor Biol 1990; 142(2):149-161.
708. Heyman I, Fombonne E, Simmons H, et al. Prevalence of obsessive-compulsive disorder in the British nationwide survey of child mental health. Int Rev Psychiatry 2003;15(1-2):178-184.
709. Dahl RE, Lewin DS. Pathways to adolescent health sleep regulation and behavior. J Adolesc Health 2002;31(Suppl 6):175-184.
710. Anokhin AP, Birbaumer N, Lutzenberger W, et al. Age increases brain complexity. Electroencephalogr Clin Neurophysiol 1996; 99:63-68.
711. Feinberg I. Changes in sleep cycle patterns with age. J Psychiatr Res 1974;10(3-4):283-306.
712. Jenni OG, Carskadon MA. Spectral analysis of the sleep electroencephalogram during adolescence. Sleep 2004;27(4):774-783.
713. Roenneberg T, Daan S, Merrow M. The art of entrainment. J Biol Rhythms 2003;18(3):183-194.
714. Crowley SJ, Acebo C, Carskadon MA. Sleep, circadian rhythms, and delayed phase in adolescence. Sleep Med 2007.
715. Carskadon MA, Acebo C, Richardson GS, et al. An approach to studying circadian rhythms of adolescent humans. J Biol Rhythms 1997;12(3):278-289.
716. Andrade MM, Benedito-Silva AA, Domenice S, et al. Sleep characteristics of adolescents: a longitudinal study. J Adolesc Health 1993;14:401-406.
717. Carskadon MA, Wolfson AR, Acebo C, et al. Adolescent sleep patterns, circadian timing, and sleepiness at a transition to early school days. Sleep 1998;21(8):871-881.
718. Knutson KL. The association between pubertal status and sleep duration and quality among a nationally representative sample of U. S. adolescents. Am J Hum Biol 2005;17(4):418-424.
719. Carskadon MA, Vieira C, Acebo C. Association between puberty and delayed phase preference. Sleep 1993;16(3):258-262.
720. Abbott A. Physiology: an end to adolescence. Nature 2005; 433(7021):27.
721. Roenneberg T, Kuehnle T, Pramstaller PP, et al. A marker for the end of adolescence. Curr Biol 2004;14(24):R1038-R1039.
722. Hamburg BA. Development of Sexual Behavior. In Freidman SB, Fisher M, Schonberg SK, eds. St Louis: Quality Medical Publishing, 1992.
723. Michael RP, Zumpke D. Behavioral changes associated with puberty in higher primates and the human. In Grumbach MM, Sizonenko PC, Aubert ML, eds. Control of the Onset of Puberty. Baltimore: Williams & Wilkins, 1990:574-587.
724. Remschmidt H. Psychosocial milestones in normal puberty and adolescence. Horm Res 1994;41(Suppl 2):19-29.
725. Slap GB, Khalid N, Paikoff RL, et al. Evolving self-image, pubertal manifestations, and pubertal hormones: preliminary findings in young adolescent girls. J Adolesc Health 1994;15:327-335.

726. Brooks-Gunn J, Graber JA. Puberty as a biological and social event: implications for research on pharmacology. J Adolesc Health 1994;15:663-671.
727. Steinberg L, Morris AS. Adolescent development. Annu Rev Psychol 2001;52:83-110.
728. Hall GS. Adolescence; Its Psychology and Its Relations to Physiology, Anthropology, Sociology, Sex, Crime, Religion and Education. New York: Appleton, 1904.
729. Udry RR, Billy JOG, Morris NM, et al. Serum androgenic hormones motivate sexual behavior in boys. Fertil Steril 1985;43: 90-94.
730. Offer D. The Psychological World of the Teenager: A Study of Normal Adolescent Boys. New York: Basic Books, 1969.
731. Masterson JFJ. The psychiatric significance of adolescent turmoil. Am J Psychiatry 1968;124:1549-1554.
732. Offer D, Schonert-Reichl KA. Debunking the myths of adolescence: findings from recent research. J Am Acad Child Adolesc Psychiatry 1992;31:1003-1014.
733. Slap GB, Khalid N, Paikoff RL, et al. Evolving self-image, pubertal manifestations, and pubertal hormones: preliminary findings in young adolescent girls. J Adolesc Health 1994;15(4): 327-335.
734. Warren MP, Brooks-Gunn J. Mood and behavior at adolescence: evidence for hormonal factors. J Clin Endocrinol Metab 1989;69(1):77-83.
735. Graber JA, Seeley JR, Brooks-Gunn J, et al. Is pubertal timing associated with psychopathology in young adulthood. J Am Acad Child Adolesc Psychiatry 2004;43(6):718-726.
736. Patton GC, McMorris BJ, Toumbourou JW, et al. Puberty and the onset of substance use and abuse. Pediatrics 2004;114(3): e300-e306.
737. Blyth DA, Simmons RG, Blucroft R, et al. The effects of physical development on self-image and satisfaction with body-image for early adolescent males. In Simmon RG, ed. Research in Community and Mental Health. Norwalk, CT: JAI Press, 1981:43-73.
738. Mobbs EJ. The psychological outcome of constitutional delay of growth and puberty. Horm Res 2005;63(Suppl 1):1-66.
739. Lewis VG, Money J, Bobrow NA. Idiopathic pubertal delay beyond age fifteen: psychologic study of twelve boys. Adolescence 1977;12(45):1-11.
740. Koivusilta L, Rimpela A. Pubertal timing and educational careers: a longitudinal study. Ann Hum Biol 2004;31(4):446-465.
741. Hayward C, Killen JD, Wilson DM, et al. Psychiatric risk associated with early puberty in adolescent girls. J Am Acad Child Adolesc Psychiatry 1997;36(2):255-262.
742. Obeidallah D, Brennan RT, Brooks-Gunn J, et al. Links between pubertal timing and neighborhood contexts: implications for girls' violent behavior. J Am Acad Child Adolesc Psychiatry 2004;43(12):1460-1468.
743. Newcombe N, Dubas JS. Individual differences in cognitive ability: Are they related to timing of puberty? In Lerner RM, Foch TT, eds. Biological-Pschosocial Interactions in Early Adolescence. Hillsdale, NJ: Lawrence Erlbaum Associates, 1987: 249-302.
744. McCabe MP, Ricciardelli LA. A longitudinal study of pubertal timing and extreme body change behaviors among adolescent boys and girls. Adolescence 2004;39(153):145-166.
745. Brooks-Gunn J, Warren MP. Mother-daughter differences in menarcheal age in adolescent girls attending national dance company schools and non-dancers. Ann Hum Biol 1988;15(1):35-43.
746. Brooks-Gunn J. Pubertal processes and girls' psychological adaptation. In Lerner RM, Foch TT, eds. Biological-Psychosocial Interactions in Early Adolescence. Hillsdale, NJ: Lawrence Erlbaum Associates, 1987:123-153.
747. Walker EF, Sabuwalla Z, Huot R. Pubertal neuromaturation, stress sensitivity, and psychopathology. Dev Psychopathol 2004;16(4): 807-824.
748. Weiner IB, del Gaudio AC. Psychopathology in adolescence. An epidemiological study. In Chess S, Thomas A, eds. Annual Progress in Child Psychiatry and Child Development. New York: Brunner/Mazel, 1977:471-488.
749. Rao U, Weissman MM, Martin JA, Hammond RW. Childhood depression and risk of suicide: a preliminary report of a longitudinal study. J Am Acad Child Adolesc Psychiatry 1993; 32:21-27.
750. Angold A, Costello EJ, Worthman CM. Puberty and depression: the roles of age, pubertal status and pubertal timing. Psychological Medicine 1998;28(1):51-61.
751. Angold A, Worthman CW. Puberty onset of gender differences in rates of depression: a developmental, epidemiologic and neuroendocrine perspective. J Affect Disord 1993;29:145-158.
752. Angold A, Costello EJ, Erkanli A, et al. Pubertal changes in hormone levels and depression in girls. Psychological Medicine 1999;29(5):1043-1053.
753. Herva A, Jokelainen J, Pouta A, et al. Age at menarche and depression at the age of 31 years: findings from the Northern Finland 1966 Birth Cohort Study. J Psychosom Res 2004;57(4): 359-362.
754. Ryan ND. Psychoneuroendocrinology of children and adolescents. Psychiatr Clin North Am 1998;21(2):435-441.
755. Stroud LR, Papandonatos GD, Williamson DE, et al. Sex differences in the effects of pubertal development on responses to a corticotropin-releasing hormone challenge: the Pittsburgh psychobiologic studies. Ann N Y Acad Sci 2004;1021:348-351.
756. Dorn LD, Chrousos GP. The neurobiology of stress: understanding regulation of affect during female biological transitions. Semin Reprod Endocrinol 1997;15(1):19-35.
757. Swedo SE, Pleeter JD, Richter DM, et al. Rates of seasonal affective disorder in children and adolescents. Am J Psychiatry 1995;152: 1016-1019.
758. Birmaher B, Dahl RE, Williamson DE, et al. Growth hormone secretion in children and adolescents at high risk for major depressive disorder. Arch Gen Psychiatry 2000;57(9):867-872.
759. Hayward C, Killen JD, Hammer LD, et al. Pubertal stage and panic attack history in sixth- and seventh-grade girls. Am J Psychiatry 1992;149:1239-1243.
760. Hafner H, an der HW, Behrens S, et al. Causes and consequences of the gender difference in age at onset of schizophrenia. Schizophr Bull 1998;24(1):99-113.
761. Lewis DA. Schizophrenia and peripubertal refinements in prefronatal cortical circuitry. In Bourguignon JP, Plant TM, eds. The onset of puberty in perspective. Amsterdam: Elsevier, 2000: 165-183.
762. Orr DP, Ingersoll GM. The contribution of level of cognitive complexity and pubertal timing to behavioral risk in young adolescents. Pediatrics 1995;95:528-533.
763. Steinberg L. Risk taking in adolescence: what changes, and why? Ann N Y Acad Sci 2004;1021:51-58.
764. Wilson DM, Killen JD, Hayward C, et al. Timing and rate of sexual maturation and the onset of cigarette and alcohol use among teenage girls. Arch Pediatr Adolesc Med 1994;148:789-795.
765. Tschann JM, Adler NE, Irwin CEJ, et al. Initiation of substance use in early adolescence: the roles of pubertal timing and emotional distress. Health Psychol 1994;13:326-333.
766. Rodgers JL. Development of sexual behavior. In Freidman SB, Fisher M, Schonberg SK, es. Comprehensive Adolescent Health. St Louis: Quality Medical Publishing, 1997.
767. Brindis CD, Irwin Jr CE, Millstein SG. United States profile. In McAnarney ER, Kreipe RE, Irr DP, et al, eds. Textbook of Adolescent Medicine. Philadelphia: WB Saunders, 1992:12.
768. Hayes CD. Risking the Future: Adolescent Sexuality, Pregnancy and Childbearing. Washington, DC: National Academy Press, 1987.
769. Garriguet D. Early sexual intercourse. Health Rep 2005;16(3): 9-18.
770. Halpern CT, Udry JR, Campbell B, et al. Testosterone and pubertal development as predictors of sexual activity: a panel analysis of adolescent males. Psychosom Med 1993;55:436-447.
771. Udry JR, Billy JO, Morris NM, et al. Serum androgenic hormones motivate sexual behavior in adolescent boys. Fertil Steril 1985;43:90-94.
772. Halpern CT, Udry JR, Campbell B, et al. Testosterone and pubertal development as predictors of sexual activity: a panel analysis of adolescent males. Psychosom Med 1993;55(5): 436-447.
773. Halpern CT, Udry JR, Suchindran C. Monthly measures of salivary testosterone predict sexual activity in adolescent males. Arch Sex Behav 1998;27(5):445-465.
774. Udry JR, Talbert LM, Morris NM. Biosocial foundations for adolescent female sexuality. Demography 1986;23(2):217-230.

775. Halpern CT, Udry JR, Suchindran C. Testosterone predicts initiation of coitus in adolescent females. Psychosom Med 1997;59(2):161-171.
776. Hutchinson KA. Androgens and sexuality. Am J Med 1995;98: 111S-115S.
777. Money J. Sexual revolution and counter-revolution. Horm Res 1994;41(Suppl 2):44-48.
778. Friedman HL. Changing patterns of adolescent sexual behavior: consequences for health and development. J Adolesc Health 1992;13:345-350.
779. Finkelstein JW, Susman EJ, Chinchilli VM, et al. Effects of estrogen or testosterone on self-reported sexual responses and behaviors in hypogonadal adolescents. J Clin Endocrinol Metab 1998;83(7):2281-2285.
780. Halpern CT, Joyner K, Udry JR, et al. Smart teens don't have sex (or kiss much either). J Adolesc Health 2000;26(3):213-225.
781. Wolf P. Epilepsy and puberty. In Bourguignon JP, Plant TM, eds. The Onset of Puberty in Perspective. Amsterdam: Elsevier, 2000:157-164.
782. Klein P, Passel-Clark LM, Pezzullo JC. Onset of epilepsy at the time of menarche. Neurology 2003;60(3):495-497.
783. Wu FC. Neurosignaling and the onset of puberty-integration. In Bourguignon JP, Plant TM, eds. The onset of puberty in perspective. Amsterdam: Elsevier, 2001:179-183.
784. Lipton RB, Bigal ME. Migraine: epidemiology, impact, and risk factors for progression. Headache 2005;45(Suppl 1):S3-S13.
785. Rhee H. Relationships between physical symptoms and pubertal development. J Pediatr Health Care 2005;19(2):95-103.
786. Grumbach MM, Roth JC, Kaplan SL, et al. Hypothalamic-pituitary regulation of puberty in man: evidence and concepts derived from clinical research. In Grumbach MM, Grave GD, Mayer FE, eds. Control of the Onset of Puberty. New York: John Wiley & Sons, 1974:115-166.
787. Grumbach MM, Kaplan SL. The neuroendocrinology of human puberty: an ontogenetic perspective. In Grumbach MM, Sizonenko PC, Aubert ML, eds. Control of the Onset of Puberty. Baltimore: Williams & Wilkins, 1990:1-68.
788. Dunkel L, Alfthan H, Stenman U, et al. Pulsatile secretion of LH and FSH in prepubertal and early pubertal boys revealed by ultrasensitive time-resolved immunofluorometric assays. Pediatr Res 1990;27:215-219.
789. Dunkel L, Alfthan H, Stenman U, et al. Gonadal control of pulsatile secretion of luteinizing hormone and follicle-stimulating hormone in prepubertal boys evaluated by ultrasensitive time-resolved immunofluorometric assays. J Clin Endocrinol Metab 1990;70:107-114.
790. Albertsson-Wikland K, Rosberg S, Lannering B, et al. Twenty-four-hour profiles of luteinizing hormone, follicle-stimulating hormone, testosterone, and estradiol levels: a semilongitudinal study throughout puberty in healthy boys. J Clin Endocrinol Metab 1997;82:541-549.
791. Wu FC, Butler GE, Kelnar CJ, et al. Ontogeny of pulsatile gonadotropin releasing hormone secretion from midchildhood, through puberty, to adulthood in the human male: a study using deconvolution analysis and an ultrasensitive immunofluorometric assay. J Clin Endocrinol Metab 1996;81:1798-1805.
792. Apter D, Butzow TL, Laughlin GA, et al. Gonadotropin-releasing hormone pulse generator activity during pubertal transition in girls: pulsatile and diurnal patterns of circulating gonadotropins. J Clin Endocrinol Metab 1993;76:940-949.
793. Mitamura R, Yano K, Suzuki N, et al. Diurnal rhythms of luteinizing hormone, follicle-stimulating hormone, and testosterone secretion before the onset of male puberty. J Clin Endocrinol Metab 1999;84(1):29-37.
794. Mitamura R, Yano K, Suzuki N, et al. Diurnal rhythms of luteinizing hormone, follicle-stimulating hormone, testosterone, and estradiol secretion before the onset of female puberty in short children. J Clin Endocrinol Metab 2000;85(3):1074-1080.
795. Corley KP, Valk TW, Kelch RP, et al. Estimation of GnRH pulse amplitude during pubertal development. Pediatr Res 1981;15: 157-162.
796. Jakacki RI, Kelch RP, Sauder SE, et al. Pulsatile secretion of luteinizing hormone in children. J Clin Endocrinol Metab 1982;55: 453-458.
797. Kelch RP, Clemens LE, Markovs M, et al. Metabolism and effects of synthetic gonadotropin-releasing hormone (GnRH) in children and adults. J Clin Endocrinol Metab 1975;40:53-61.
798. Hassing JM, Padmanabhan V, Kelch RP, et al. Differential regulation of serum immunoreactive luteinizing hormone and bioactive follicle-stimulating hormone by testosterone in early pubertal boys. J Clin Endocrinol Metab 1990;70:1082-1089.
799. Kaplan SL, Grumbach MM, Aubert ML. The ontogenesis of pituitary hormones and hypothalamic factors in the human fetus: maturation of central nervous system regulation of anterior pituitary function. Recent Prog Horm Res 1976;32: 161-243.
800. Spratt DI, Crowley WFJ. Pituitary and gonadal responsiveness is enhanced during GnRH-induced puberty. Am J Physiol 1988;254: E652-E657.
801. Beitins IZ, Padmanabhan V. Bioactivity of gonadotropins. Endocrinol Metab Clin North Am 1991;20:85-120.
802. Clark PA, Iranmanesh A, Veldhuis JD, Rogol AD. Comparison of pulsatile luteinizing hormone secretion between prepubertal children and young adults: evidence for a mass/amplitude-dependent difference without gender or day/night contrasts. J Clin Endocrinol Metab 1997;82(9):2950-2955.
803. Rifkind AB. Sleep and puberty: who wakes the bugler? N Engl J Med 1972;287:613-614.
804. Boyar RM, Rosenfeld RS, Kapen S, et al. Simultaneous augmented secretion of luteinizing hormone and testosterone during sleep. J Clin Invest 1974;54:609-618.
805. Boyar RM, Finkelstein J, Roffwarg H, et al. Synchronization of augmented luteinizing hormone secretion with sleep during puberty. N Engl J Med 1972;287:582-586.
806. Hale PM, Khoury S, Foster CM, et al. Increased luteinizing hormone pulse frequency during sleep in early to midpubertal boys: effects of testosterone infusion. J Clin Endocrinol Metab 1988;66:785-791.
807. Wennink JM, Delemarre-Van deWaal HA, van Kessel H, et al. Luteinizing hormone secretion patterns in boys at the onset of puberty measured using a highly sensitive immunoradiometric assay. J Clin Endocrinol Metab 1988;67:924-928.
808. Kapen S, Boyar RM, Hellman L, Weitzman ED. Twenty-four-hour patterns of luteinizing hormone secretion in humans: ontogenetic and sexual considerations. Prog Brain Res 1975;42: 103-113.
809. Reiter EO, Biggs DE, Veldhuis JD, et al. Pulsatile release of bioactive luteinizing hormone in prepubertal girls: discordance with immunoreactive luteinizing hormone pulses. Pediatr Res 1987;21: 409-413.
810. Apter D, Cacciatore B, Alfthan H, et al. Serum luteinizing hormone concentrations increase 100-fold in females from 7 years to adulthood, as measured by time-resolved immunofluorometric assay. J Clin Endocrinol Metab 1989;68:53-57.
811. Burr IM, Sizonenko PC, Kaplan SL, et al. Hormonal changes in puberty. I. Correlation of serum luteinizing hormone and follicle stimulating hormone with stages of puberty, testicular size, and bone age in normal boys. Pediatr Res 1970;4:25-35.
812. Sizonenko PC, Burr IM, Kaplan SL, et al. Hormonal changes in puberty. II. Correlation of serum luyteinizing hormone and follicle stimulating hormone with stages of puberty and bone age in normal girls. Pediatr Res 1970;4:36-45.
813. August GP, Grumbach MM, Kaplan SL. Hormonal changes in puberty. 3. Correlation of plasma testosterone, LH, FSH, testicular size, and bone age with male pubertal development. J Clin Endocrinol Metab 1972;34:319-326.
814. Jenner MR, Kelch RP, Kaplan SL, et al. Hormonal changes in puberty. IV. Plasma estradiol, LH, and FSH in prepubertal children, pubertal females, and in precocious puberty, premature thelarche, hypogonadism, and in a child with a feminizing ovarian tumor. J Clin Endocrinol Metab 1972;34:521-530.
815. Belgorosky A, Chahin S, Chaler E, Maceiras M, et al. Serum concentrations of follicle stimulating hormone and luteinizing hormone in normal girls and boys during prepuberty and at early puberty. J Endocrinol Invest 1996;19:88-91.
816. Faiman C, Winter JSD. Gonadotropins and sex hormone patterns in puberty: clinical data. In Grumbach MM, Grave GD, Mayer FE, eds. Control of the Onset of Puberty. New York: John Wiley & Sons, 1974:32-61.

817. Veldhuis JD, Pincus SM, Mitamura R, et al. developmentally delimited emergence of more orderly luteinizing hormone and testosterone secretion during late prepuberty in boys. J Clin Endocrinol Metab 2001;86(1):80-89.
818. Yen SS, Apter D, Butzow T, Laughlin GA. Gonadotrophin releasing hormone pulse generator activity before and during sexual maturation in girls: new insights. Hum Reprod 1993;8(Suppl 2):66-71.
819. Roth JC, Kelch RP, Kaplan SL, et al. FSH and LH response to luteinizing hormone-releasing factor in prepubertal and pubertal children, adult males and patients with hypogonadotropic and hypertropic hypogonadism. J Clin Endocrinol Metab 1972;35: 926-930.
820. Cavallo A, Zhou XH. LHRH test in the assessment of puberty in normal children. Horm Res 1994;41:10-15.
821. Ghai K, Rosenfield RL. Maturation of the normal pituitary-testicular axis, as assessed by gonadotropin-releasing hormone agonist challenge. J Clin Endocrinol Metab 1994;78:1336-1340.
821a. Potau N, Ibanez L, Sentis M, Carrascosa A. Sexual dimorphism in the maturation of the pituitary-gonadal axis, assessed by GnRH agonist challenge. Eur J Endocrinol 1999;141:27-34.
821b. Street ME, Bandello MA, Terzi C, et al. Leuteinizing hormone responses to leuprolide acetate discriminate between hypogonadotropic hypogonadism and constitutional delay of puberty. Fertil Steril 2002;77:555-560.
822. Ghai K, Cara JF, Rosenfield RL. Gonadotropin releasing hormone agonist (nafarelin) test to differentiate gonadotropin deficiency from constitutionally delayed puberty in teen-age boys—a clinical research center study. J Clin Endocrinol Metab 1995;80: 2980-2986.
822a. Elsholz DD, Padmanabhan V, Rosenfield RL, et al. GnRH agonist stimulation of the pituitary-gonadal axis in children: age and sex differences in circulating inhibin-B and activin-A. Hum Reprod 2004;19:2748-2758.
823. Garibaldi LR, Picco P, Magier S, et al. Serum luteinizing hormone concentrations, as measured by a sensitive immunoradiometric assay, in children with normal, precocious or delayed pubertal development. J Clin Endocrinol Metab 1991;72:888-898.
824. Demir A, Voutilainen R, Juul A, et al. Increase in first morning voided urinary luteinizing hormone levels precedes the physical onset of puberty. J Clin Endocrinol Metab 1996;81:2963-2967.
825. Huhtaniemi IT, Haavisto AM, Anttila R, et al. Sensitive immunoassay and in vitro bioassay demonstrate constant bioactive/immunoreactive ratio of luteinizing hormone in healthy boys during the pubertal maturation. Pediatr Res 1996;39:180-184.
826. Baenziger JU. Editorial: Glycosylation: to what end for the glycoprotein hormones? Endocrinology 1996;137:1520-1522.
827. Ulloa-Aguirre A, Midgley Jr AR, Beitins IZ, et al. Follicle-stimulating isohormones: characterization and physiological relevance. Endocr Rev 1995;16:765-787.
828. Wide L, Albertsson-Wikland K, Phillips DJ. More basic isoforms of serum gonadotropins during gonadotropin-releasing hormone agonist therapy in pubertal children. J Clin Endocrinol Metab 1996;81:216-221.
829. Kasa-Vubu JZ, Padmanabhan V, Kletter GB, et al. Serum bioactive luteinizing and follicle-stimulating hormone concentrations in girls increase during puberty. Pediatr Res 1993;34:829-833.
830. Kletter GB, Padmanabhan V, Brown MB, et al. Serum bioactive gonadotropins during male puberty: a longitudinal study. J Clin Endocrinol Metab 1993;76:432-438.
831. Dunger DB, Villa AK, Matthews DR, et al. Pattern of secretion of bioactive and immunoreactive gonadotrophins in normal pubertal children. Clin Endocrinol (Oxf) 1991;35:267-275.
832. Phillips DJ, Wide L. Serum gonadotropin isoforms become more basic after an exogenous challenge of gonadotropin-releasing hormone in children undergoing pubertal development. J Clin Endocrinol Metab 1994;79:814-819.
833. Wang C, Zhong CQ, Leung A, et al. Serum bioactive follicle-stimulating hormone levels in girls with precocious sexual development. J Clin Endocrinol Metab 1990;70:615-619.
834. Reiter EO, Beitins IZ, Ostrea T, et al. Bioassayable luteinizing hormone during childhood and adolescence and in patients with delayed pubertal development. J Clin Endocrinol Metab 1982;54: 155-161.
835. Zoppi G. [Physiology of pubertal maturation] Fisiologia della maturazione puberale. Pediatr Med Chir 1992;14:375-379.
836. Schroor EJ, van Weissenbruch MM, Engelbregt M, et al. Bioactivity of luteinizing hormone during normal puberty in girls and boys. Hormone Research 1999;51(5):230-237.
837. Olivares A, Soderlund D, Castro-Fernandez C, et al. Basal and gonadotropin-releasing hormone-releasable serum follicle-stimulating hormone charge isoform distribution and in vitro biological-to-immunological ratio in male puberty. Endocrine 2004; 23(2-3):189-198.
838. Weinstein RL, Kelch RP, Jenner MR, et al. Secretion of unconjugated androgens and estrogens by the normal and abnormal human testis before and after hCG. J Clin Invest 1974;53:1.
839. Wang C, Catlin DH, Demers LM, et al. Measurement of total serum testosterone in adult men: comparison of current laboratory methods versus liquid chromatography-tandem mass spectrometry. J Clin Endocrinol Metab 2004;89(2):534-543.
840. Taieb J, Mathian B, Millot F, et al. Testosterone measured by 10 immunoassays and by isotope-dilution gas chromatography-mass spectrometry in sera from 116 men, women, and children. Clin Chem 2003;49(8):1381-1395.
841. Herold DA, Fitzgerald RL. Immunoassays for testosterone in women: better than a guess? Clin Chem 2003;49(8):1250-1251.
842. Albrecht L, Styne DM. Pitfalls of Gonadal steroid assays. Pediatr Endocr Rev. In press.
843. Knoor D, Bidlingmaier F, Butenandt O, et al. Plasma testosterone in male puberty. I. Physiology of plasma testosterone. Acta Endocrinol 1974;75:181-194.
844. Corbier P, Edwards DA, Roffi J. The neonatal testosterone surge: a comparative study. Arch Int Physiol Biochim Biophys 1992;100(2):127-131.
845. Forest MG, Sizonenko PC, Cathiard AM, et al. Hypophyso-gonadal function in humans during the first year of life. 1. Evidence for testicular activity in early infancy. J Clin Invest 1974;53(3): 819-828.
846. Gendrel D, Chaussain JL, Roger M, et al. Simultaneous postnatal rise of plasma LH and testosterone in male infants. J Pediatr 1980;97(4):600-602.
847. Judd HL, Parker DC, Yen SS. Sleep-wake patterns of LH and testosterone release in prepubertal boys. J Clin Endocrinol Metab 1977;44:865-869.
848. Goji K, Tanikaze S. Spontaneous gonadotropin and testosterone concentration profiles in prepubertal and pubertal boys: temporal relationship between luteinizing hormone and testosterone. Pediatr Res 1993;34:229-236.
849. Kratzsch J, Keller E, Hoepffner W, et al. The DSL analog free testosterone assay: serum levels are not related to sex hormone-binding globulin in normative data throughout childhood and adolescence. Clin Lab 2001;47(1-2):73-77.
850. Raivio T, Palvimo JJ, Dunkel L, Wickman S, et al. Novel assay for determination of androgen bioactivity in human serum. J Clin Endocrinol Metab 2001;86(4):1539-1544.
851. Raivio T, Dunkel L, Wickman S, et al. Serum androgen bioactivity in adolescence: a longitudinal study of boys with constitutional delay of puberty. J Clin Endocrinol Metab 2004;89(3):1188-1192.
852. Roy P, Franks S, Read M, et al. Determination of androgen bioactivity in human serum samples using a recombinant cell based in vitro bioassay. J Steroid Biochem Mol Biol 2006;101(1): 68-77.
853. Chen J, Sowers MR, Moran FM, et al. Circulating bioactive androgens in mid-life women. J Clin Endocrinol Metab 2006; 91(11):4387-4394.
854. Boas SR, Cleary DA, Lee PA, et al. Salivary testosterone levels in male adolescents with cystic fibrosis. Pediatrics 1996;97: 361-363.
855. Ohzeki T, Manella B, Gubelin-De Campo C, et al. Salivary testosterone concentrations in prepubertal and pubertal males: comparison with total and free plasma testosterone. Horm Res 1991;36:235-237.
856. Bruno-Ambrosius K, Yucel-Lindberg T, Twetman S. Salivary buffer capacity in relation to menarche and progesterone levels in saliva from adolescent girls: a longitudinal study. Acta Odontol Scand 2004;62(5):269-272.
857. Netherton C, Goodyer I, Tamplin A, et al. Salivary cortisol and dehydroepiandrosterone in relation to puberty and gender. Psychoneuroendocrinology 2004;29(2):125-140.

858. Granger DA, Shirtcliff EA, Zahn-Waxler C, et al. Salivary testosterone diurnal variation and psychopathology in adolescent males and females: individual differences and developmental effects. Dev Psychopathol 2003;15(2):431-449.
859. Inkster S, Yue W, Brodie A. Human testicular aromatase: immunocytochemical and biochemical studies. J Clin Endocrinol Metab 1995;80:1941-1947.
860. Brodie A., Inkster S. Aromatase in the human testis. J Steroid Biochem Mol Biol 1993;44:549-555.
861. Norjavaara E, Ankarberg C, Albertsson-Wikland K. Diurnal rhythm of 17 beta-estradiol secretion throughout pubertal development in healthy girls: evaluation by a sensitive radioimmunoassay. J Clin Endocrinol Metab 1996;81:4095-4102.
862. Paris F, Servant N, Terouanne B, et al. A new recombinant cell bioassay for ultrasensitive determination of serum estrogenic bioactivity in children. J Clin Endocrinol Metab 2002;87(2): 791-797.
863. Goji K. Twenty-four-hour concentration profiles of gonadotropin and estradiol (E2) in prepubertal and early pubertal girls: the diurnal rise of E2 is opposite the nocturnal rise of gonadotropin. J Clin Endocrinol Metab 1993;77:1629-1635.
864. Angsusingha K, Kenny FM, Nankin HR, et al. Unconjugated estrone, estradiol and FSH and LH in prepubertal and pubertal males and females. J Clin Endocrinol Metab 1974;39: 63-68.
865. Apter D, Bolton NJ, Hammond GL, et al. Serum sex hormone-binding globulin during puberty in girls and in different types of adolescent menstrual cycles. Acta Endocrinol (Copenh) 1984;107:413-419.
866. Lee IR, Lawder LE, Townend DC, et al. Plasma sex hormone binding globulin concentration and binding capacity in children before and during puberty. Acta Endocrinol (Copenh) 1985; 109(2):276-280.
867. Pugeat M, Cousin P, Baret C, et al. Sex hormone-binding globulin during puberty in normal and hyperandrogenic girls. J Pediatr Endocrinol Metab 2000;13(Suppl 5):1277-1279.
868. Derman O, Kanbur NO, Tokur TE. The effect of tamoxifen on sex hormone binding globulin in adolescents with pubertal gynecomastia. J Pediatr Endocrinol Metab 2004;17(8):1115-1119.
869. Maruyama Y, Aoki N, Suzuki Y, et al. Sex-steroid-binding plasma protein (SBP), testosterone, oestradiol and dehydroepiandrosterone (DHEA) in prepuberty and puberty. Acta Endocrinol (Copenh) 1987;114:60-67.
870. August GP, Tkachuk M, Grumbach MM. Plasma testosterone-binding affinity and testosterone in umbilical cord plasma, late pregnancy, prepubertal children and adults. J Clin Endocrinol Metab 1969;29:891-899.
871. Anderson DC. Sex hormone-binding globulin. Clin Endocrinol 1974;3:69-95.
872. Horst HJ, Bartsch W, Dirksen-Thiedens I. Plasma testosterone, sex hormone binding globulin binding capacity and per cent binding of testosterone and 5alpha-dihydrotestosterone in prepubertal, pubertal and adult males. J Clin Endocrinol Metab 1977;45: 522-527.
873. Cunningham SK, Loughlin T, Culliton M, McKenna TJ. The relationship between sex steroids and sex-hormone-binding globulin in plasma in physiological and pathological conditions. Ann Clin Biochem 1985;22(Pt 5):489-497.
874. Cunningham SK, McKenna TJ. Evaluation of an immunoassay for plasma sex hormone-binding globulin: comparison with steroid-binding assay under physiological and pathological conditions. Ann Clin Biochem 1988;25:360-366.
875. Cunningham SK, Loughlin T, Culliton M, et al. Plasma sex hormone-binding globulin levels decrease during the second decade of life irrespective of pubertal status. J Clin Endocrinol Metab 1984;58:915-918.
876. Rudd BT, Rayner PH, Thomas PH. Observations on the role of GH/IGF-1 and sex hormone binding globulin (SHBG) in the pubertal development of growth hormone deficient (GHD) children. Acta Endocrinol Suppl 1986;279:164-169.
877. Holly JM, Dunger DB, al-Othman SA, et al. Sex hormone binding globulin levels in adolescent subjects with diabetes mellitus. Diabet Med 1992;9:371-374.
878. Aubert ML, Sizonenko PC, Kaplan SL, et al. The ontogenesis of human prolactin from fetal life to puberty. In Crosignani PG, Robyn C, eds. Prolactin and Human Reproduction. New York: Academic Press, 1977:9-20.
879. Vale W, Bilezikjian LM, Rivier C. Reproductive and other roles of inhibins and activins. In Knobil E, Neil JD, eds. Physiology of Reproduction. New York: Raven Press, 1994:1861-1878.
880. Mather JP. Follistatins and alpha 2-macroglobulin are soluble binding proteins for inhibin and activin. Horm Res 1996;45: 207-210.
881. Groome NP, Evans LW. Does measurement of inhibin have a clinical role? Ann Clin Biochem 2000;37(Pt 4):419-431.
882. Hayes FJ, Pitteloud N, DeCruz S, et al. Importance of inhibin B in the regulation of FSH secretion in the human male. J Clin Endocrinol Metab 2001;86(11):5541-5546.
883. Welt CK, Smith ZA, Pauler DK, et al. Differential regulation of inhibin A and inhibin B by luteinizing hormone, follicle-stimulating hormone, and stage of follicle development. J Clin Endocrinol Metab 2001;86(6):2531-2537.
884. McLachlan RI, Robertson DM, Burger HG, et al. The radioimmunoassay of bovine and human follicular fluid and serum inhibin. Mol Cell Endocrinol 1986;46:175-185.
885. Groome NP, Illingworth PJ, O'Brien M, et al. Measurement of dimeric inhibin B throughout the human menstrual cycle. J Clin Endocrinol Metab 1996;81:1401-1405.
886. Robertson DM, Cahir N, Findlay JK, et al. The biological and immunological characterization of inhibin A and B forms in human follicular fluid and plasma. J Clin Endocrinol 1997;82: 889-896.
887. Meachem SJ, Nieschlag E, Simoni M. Inhibin B in male reproduction: pathophysiology and clinical relevance. Eur J Endocrinol 2001;145(5):561-571.
888. Wallace E, Riley SM, Crossley JA, et al. Dimeric inhibins in amniotic fluid, maternal serum, and fetal serum in human pregnancy. J Clin Endocrinol Metab 1997;82:218-222.
889. Fowler PA, Evans LW, Groome NP, et al. A longitudinal study of maternal serum inhibin-A, inhibin-B, activin-A, activin-AB, pro-alphaC and follistatin during pregnancy. Hum Reprod 1998;13(12): 3530-3536.
890. Majdic G, McNeilly AS, Sharpe RM, et al. Testicular expression of inhibin and activin subunits and follistatin in the rat and human fetus and neonate and during postnatal development in the rat. Endocrinology 1997;138:2136-2147.
891. Debieve F, Beerlandt S, Hubinont C, et al. Gonadotropins, prolactin, inhibin A, inhibin B, and activin A in human fetal serum from midpregnancy and term pregnancy. J Clin Endocrinol Metab 2000;85(1):270-274.
892. Burger HG, McLachlan RI, Bangah M, et al. Serum inhibin concentrations rise throughout normal male and female puberty. J Clin Endocrinol Metab 1988;67:689-694.
893. Manasco PK, Umbach DM, Muly SM, et al. Ontogeny of gonadotropin, testosterone, and inhibin secretion in normal boys through puberty based on overnight serial sampling. J Clin Endocrinol Metab 1995;80:2046-2052.
894. Bergada I, Rojas G, Ropelato G, et al. Sexual dimorphism in circulating monomeric and dimeric inhibins in normal boys and girls from birth to puberty. Clin Endocrinol 1999;51(4):455-460.
895. Andersson A-M, Juul A, Petersen JH, et al. Serum inhibin B in healthy pubertal and adolescent boys: relation to age, stage of puberty and FSH, LH, testosterone, and estradiol levels. J Clin Endocrinol Metab 1997;82(12):3976-3981.
896. Byrd W, Bennett MJ, Carr BR, et al. Regulation of biologically active dimeric inhibin A and B from infancy to adulthood in the male. J Clin Endocrinol Metab 1998;83(8):2849-2854.
897. Groome NP, Tsigou A, Cranfield M, et al. Enzyme immunoassays for inhibins, activins and follistatins. Mol Cell Endocrinol 2001;180(1-2):73-77.
898. Anawalt BD, Bebb RA, Matsumoto AM, et al. Serum inhibin B levels reflect Sertoli cell function in normal men and in men with testicular dysfunction. J Clin Endocrinol Metab 1996;81:3341-3345.
899. Andersson A, Skakkebaek NE. Serum inhibin B levels during male childhood and puberty. Mol Cell Endocrinol 2001;180(1-2): 103-107.
900. Raivio T, Perheentupa A, McNeilly AS, et al. Biphasic increase in serum inhibin B during puberty: a longitudinal study of healthy Finnish boys. Pediatric Research 1998;44(4):552-556.

901. Radicioni AF, Anzuini A, De Marco E, et al. Changes in serum inhibin B during normal male puberty. Eur J Endocrinol 2005; 152(3):403-409.
902. Crofton PM, Evans AE, Groome NP, et al. Inhibin B in boys from birth to adulthood: relationship with age, pubertal stage, FSH and testosterone. Clin Endocrinol (Oxf) 2002;56(2):215-221.
903. Chada M, Prusa R, Bronsky J, et al. Inhibin B, follicle stimulating hormone, luteinizing hormone and testosterone during childhood and puberty in males: changes in serum concentrations in relation to age and stage of puberty. Physiol Res 2003;52(1): 45-51.
904. Crofton PM, Evans AE, Groome NP, et al. Dimeric inhibins in girls from birth to adulthood: relationship with age, pubertal stage, FSH and oestradiol. Clin Endocrinol (Oxf) 2002;56(2): 223-230.
905. Foster CM, Phillips DJ, Wyman T, et al. Changes in serum inhibin, activin and follistatin concentrations during puberty in girls. Hum Reprod 2000;15(5):1052-1057.
906. Chada M, Prusa R, Bronsky J, et al. Inhibin B, follicle stimulating hormone, luteinizing hormone, and estradiol and their relationship to the regulation of follicle development in girls during childhood and puberty. Physiol Res 2003;52(3):341-346.
907. Foster CM, Olton PR, Padmanabhan V. Diurnal changes in FSH-regulatory peptides and their relationship to gonadotrophins in pubertal girls. Hum Reprod 2005;20(2):543-548.
908. Crofton PM, Evans AE, Wallace AM, et al. Nocturnal secretory dynamics of inhibin B and testosterone in pre- and peripubertal boys. J Clin Endocrinol Metab 2004;89(2):867-874.
909. Young J, Chanson P, Salenave S, et al. Testicular anti-mullerian hormone secretion is stimulated by recombinant human FSH in patients with congenital hypogonadotropic hypogonadism. J Clin Endocrinol Metab 2005;90(2):724-728.
910. Elsholz DD, Padmanabhan V, Rosenfield RL, et al. GnRH agonist stimulation of the pituitary-gonadal axis in children: age and sex differences in circulating inhibin-B and activin-A. Hum Reprod 2004;19(12):2748-2758.
911. Foster CM, Olton PR, Racine MS, et al. Sex differences in FSH-regulatory peptides in pubertal age boys and girls and effects of sex steroid treatment. Hum Reprod 2004;19(7):1668-1676.
912. Mitchell R, Schaefer F, Morris ID, et al. Elevated serum immunoreactive inhibin levels in peripubertal boys with chronic renal failure. Cooperative Study Group on Pubertal Development in Chronic Renal Failure (CSPCRF). Clin Endocrinol (Oxf) 1993; 39:27-33.
913. Lee PA, Coughlin MT, Bellinger MF. No relationship of testicular size at orchiopexy with fertility in men who previously had unilateral cryptorchidism. J Urol 2001;166(1):236-239.
914. Dunkel L, Siimes MA, Bremner WJ. Reduced inhibin and elevated gonadotropin levels in early pubertal boys with testicular defects. Pediatr Res 1993;33:514-518.
915. Andersson AM, Muller J, Skakkebaek NE. Different roles of prepubertal and postpubertal germ cells and Sertoli cells in the regulation of serum inhibin B levels. J Clin Endocrinol Metab 1998;83(12):4451-4458.
916. Kubini K, Zachmann M, Albers N, et al. Basal inhibin B and the testosterone response to human chorionic gonadotropin correlate in prepubertal boys. J Clin Endocrinol Metab 2000;85(1): 134-138.
917. Josso N, Legeai L, Forest MG, Chaussain JL, Brauner R. An enzyme linked immunoassay for anti-mullerian hormone: a new tool for the evaluation of testicular function in infants and children. J Clin Endocrinol Metab 1990;70:23-27.
918. Donahoe PK. Mullerian inhibiting substance in reproduction and cancer. Mol Reprod Dev 1992;32:168-172.
919. Lee MM, Donahoe PK, Hasegawa T, et al. Mullerian inhibiting substance in humans: normal levels from infancy to adulthood. J Clin Endocrinol Metab 1996;81:571-576.
920. Hudson PL, Dougas I, Donahoe PK, et al. An immunoassay to detect human mullerian inhibiting substance in males and females during normal development. J Clin Endocrinol Metab 1990;70:16-22.
921. Rey R, Mebarki F, Forest MG, et al. Anti-mullerian hormone in children with androgen insensitivity. J Clin Endocrinol Metab 1994;79:960-964.
922. Baker ML, Hutson JM. Serum levels of mullerian inhibiting substance in boys throughout puberty and in the first two years of life. J Clin Endocrinol Metab 1993;76:245-247.
923. Josso N. Paediatric applications of anti-mullerian hormone research. Horm Res 1995;43:243-248.
924. Josso N, Picard JY, Rey R, di Clemente N. Testicular anti-Mullerian hormone: history, genetics, regulation and clinical applications. Pediatr Endocrinol Rev 2006;3(4):347-358.
925. Lee MM, Donahoe PK, Silverman BL, et al. Measurements of serum Mullerian inhibiting substance in the evaluation of children with nonpalpable gonads. N Engl J Med 1997;336: 1480-1486.
926. Schreiber L, Lifschitz-Mercer B, Paz G, et al. Lack of RBM expression as a marker for carcinoma in situ of prepubertal dysgenetic testis. J Androl 2003;24(1):78-84.
927. Wikstrom AM, Bay K, Hero M, et al. Serum INSL3 levels during puberty in healthy boys and boys with Klinefelter syndrome. J Clin Endocrinol Metab. In press.
928. Randell EW, Diamandis EP, Ellis G. Serum prostate-specific antigen measured in children from birth to age 18 years. Clin Chem 1996;42:420-423.
929. Vieira JG, Nishida SK, Pereira AB, et al. Serum levels of prostate-specific antigen in normal boys throughout puberty. J Clin Endocrinol Metab 1994;78:1185-1187.
930. Kim MR, Gupta MK, Travers SH, et al. Serum prostate specific antigen, sex hormone binding globulin and free androgen index as markers of pubertal development in boys. Clin Endocrinol 1999;50(2):203-210.
931. Dhanasekaran SM, Dash A, Yu J, et al. Molecular profiling of human prostate tissues: insights into gene expression patterns of prostate development during puberty. FASEB J 2005;19(2): 243-245.
932. Kiess W, Meidert A, Dressendorfer RA, et al. Salivary cortisol levels throughout childhood and adolescence: relation with age, pubertal stage, and weight. Pediatr Res 1995;37:502-506.
933. Grumbach MM. The neuroendocrinology of puberty. In Krieger DT, Hughes JC, et al, eds. Neuroendocrinology. Sunderland, MA: Sinauer Associates, 1980:249-258.
934. Grumbach MM, Kaplan SL. Fetal pituitary hormones and the maturation of central nervous system regulation of anterior pituitary function. In Gluck L, ed. Modern Perinatal Medicine. Chicago: Year Book Medical, 1974:247-271.
935. Reiter EO, Grumbach MM. Neuroendocrine control mechanisms and the onset of puberty. Annu Rev Physiol 1982;44:595-613.
936. Ibanez L, DiMartino-Nardi J, Potau N, et al. Premature adrenarche—normal variant or forerunner of adult disease? Endocr Rev 2000;21(6):671-696.
937. Grumbach MM. A window of opportunity: the diagnosis of gonadotropin deficiency in the male infant. J Clin Endocrinol Metab 2005;90(5):3122-3127.
938. Terasawa E, Fernandez DL. Neurobiological mechanisms of the onset of puberty in primates. Endocr Rev 2001;22(1):111-151.
939. Critchlow V, Bar-Sela ME. Control of the onset of puberty. In Martini L, Ganong WF, eds. Neuroendocrinology. New York: Academic, 1967:101-162.
940. Donovan BT, van der Werff JJ. Physiology of Puberty. Baltimore: Williams & Wilkins, 1965.
941. Germak JA, Knobil E. Control of puberty in the rhesus monkey. In Grumbach MM, Sizonenko PC, Aubert ML, eds. Control of the Onset of Puberty. Baltimore: Williams & Wilkins, 1990:69-81.
942. Plant TM. Control of puberty in non-human primates. In Pescovitz OH, Walvoord EC, eds. When Puberty is Precocious: Scientific and Clinical Aspects. Totowa, NJ: Humana Press, 2007:35-50.
943. Plant TM. Neurobiological bases underlying the control of the onset of puberty in the rhesus monkey: a representative higher primate. Front Neuroendocrinol 2001;22(2):107-139.
944. Kaplan SL, Grumbach MM. Pituitary and placental gonadotropins and sex steroids in the human and sub-human primate fetus. Clin Endocrinol Metab 1978;7:487-511.
945. Wilkins L. The Diagnosis and Treatment of Endocrine Disorders in Childhood and Adolescence. Springfield, IL: Charles C Thomas, 1965.
946. King JC, Anthony ELP, Fitzgerald DM, et al. Luteinizing hormone-releasing hormone neurons in human preoptic/hypothalamus:

differential intraneuronal localization of immunoreactive forms. J Clin Endocrinol Metab 1985;60:88-97.
947. Knobil E. The neuroendocrine control of the menstrual cycle. Recent Prog Horm Res 1980;36:53-88.
948. Knobil E. On the control of gonadotropin secretion in the rhesus monkey. Recent Prog Horm Res 1974;30:1-46.
949. Martinez de la Escalera G, Clapp C. Regulation of gonadotropin-releasing hormone secretion: insights from GT1 immortal GnRH neurons. Arch Med Res 2001;32(6):486-498.
950. Mellon PL, Windle JJ, Goldsmith PC, et.al. Immortalization of hypothalamic GnRH neurons by genetically targeted tumorigenesis. Neuron 1990;5:1-10.
951. Knobil E. The GnRH pulse generator. Am J Obstet Gynecol 1990;163:1721-1727.
952. Martinez de la Escalera G, Choi ALH, Weiner RI. Generation and synchronization of gonadotropin-releasing hormone (GnRH) pulses: intrinsic properties of the GT1-1 gonadotropin-releasing hormone (GnRH) neuronal cell line. Proc Natl Acad Sci USA 1992;89:1852-1855.
953. Adelman JP, Mason AJ, Hayflick JS, et al. Isolation of the gene and hypothalamic cDNA for the common precursor of gonadotropin-releasing hormone and prolactin release-inhibiting factor in human and rat. Proc Natl Acad Sci U S A 1986;83: 179-183.
954. Shacham S, Harris D, Ben-Shlomo H, et al. Mechanism of GnRH receptor signaling on gonadotropin release and gene expression in pituitary gonadotrophs. Vitam Horm 2001;63:63-90.
955. Themmen APN, Huhtaniemi IT. Mutations of gonadotropins and gonadotropin receptors: elucidating the physiology and pathophysiology of pituitary-gonadal function. Endocr Rev 2000;21(5): 551-583.
956. Huckle W, Conn PM. Molecular mechanisms of gonadotropin releasing hormone action. II. The effector system. Endocr Rev 1988;9:387-395.
957. Hazum E, Conn PM. Molecular mechanism of gonadotropin releasing hormone (GnRH) action. I. The GnRH receptor. Endocr Rev 1988;9:379-386.
958. Sealfon SC, Weinstein H, Millar RP. Molecular mechanisms of ligand interaction with the gonadotropin-releasing hormone receptor. Endocr Rev 1997;18:180-205.
959. Short RV. The evolution of human reproduction. Proc R Soc Med 1976;195:3-24.
960. Bronson FH, Rissman EF. The biology of puberty. Biol Rev 1986;61:157-195.
961. Blackman BE, Yoshida H, Paruthiyil S, Weiner RI. Frequency of intrinsic pulsatile GnRH secretion is regulated by the expression of cyclic nucleotide gate (CNS) channels in GT1 cells. Endocrinology 2007;148(7):3299-3306.
962. Wetsel W, ValenHa MM, Merchenthaler I. Intrinsic pulsatile secretory activity of immortalized luteinizing hormone-releasing hormone-secreting neurons. Proc Natl Acad Sci U S A 1992;89: 4149-4153.
963. Abe H, Terasawa E. Firing pattern and rapid modulation of activity by estrogen in primate luteinizing hormone releasing hormone-1 neurons. Endocrinology 2005;146(10):4312-4320.
964. Wildt L, Hausler A, Marshall G, et al. Frequency and amplitude of gonadotropin-releasing hormone stimulation and gonadotropin secretion in the rhesus monkey. Endocrinology 1981;109: 376-385.
965. Gross KM, Matsumoto AM, Brenner WJ. Differential control of luteinizing hormone and follicle-stimulating hormone secretion by luteinizing hormone-releasing hormone pulse frequency in man. J Clin Endocrinol Metab 1987;64:675-680.
966. Finkelstein JS, Budger TM, O'Dea SStL, et al. Effects of decreasing the frequency of gonadotropin-releasing hormone stimulation on gonadotropin secretion in gonadotropin-releasing hormone-deficient men and perifused rat pituitary cells. J Clin Invest 1988;81:1725-1733.
967. Belchetz PE, Plant TM, Nakai Y, et al. Hypophyseal responses to continuous and intermittent delivery of hypothalamic gonadotropin-releasing hormone. Science 1978;202:631-633.
968. Nett TM, Crowder ME, Moss GE, et al. GnRH-receptor interaction. v. Down-regulation of pituitary receptors for GnRH in ovariectomized ewes by infusion of homologous hormone. Biol Reprod 1981;24:1145-1155.
969. Wetsel WC. Immortalized hypothalamic luteinizing hormone-releasing hormone (LHRH) neurons: a new tool for dissecting the molecular and cellular basis of LHRH physiology. Cell Molec Neurobiol 1995;15:43-78.
970. Martinez de la Escalera G, Choi ALH, Weiner RI. Signaling pathways involved in GnRH Secretion in GT1 Cells. Neuroendocrinology 1995;61:310-317.
971. Krsmanovic LZ, Stojilkovic SS, Catt KJ. Pulsatile gonadotropin-releasing hormone release and its regulation. Trends Endocrinol Metab 1996;7:56-59.
972. Kusano K, Fueshke S, Gainer H, Wray S. Electrical and synaptic properties of embryonic luteinizing hormone-releasing hromone neurons in explant cultures. Proc Natl Acad Sci U S A 1995;92: 3918-3922.
973. Grumbach MM. The neuroendocrinology of human puberty revisited. Horm Res 2002;57(suppl 2):2-14.
974. Marshall PE, Goldsmith PC. Neuroregulatory and neuroendocrine GnRH pathways in the hypothalamus and forebrain of the baboon. Brain Res 1980;193:353-372.
975. Witkin JW, Silverman AJ. Synaptology of LHRH neurons in rat preoptic area. Peptides 1985;6:263-271.
976. Costantin JL, Charles AC. Modulation of Ca(2+) signaling by K(+) channels in a hypothalamic neuronal cell line (GT1-1). J Neurophysiol 2001;85(1):295-304.
977. Vitalis EA, Costantin JL, Tsai PS, et al. Role of the cAMP signaling pathway in the regulation of gonadotropin-releasing hormone secretion in GT1 cells. Proc Natl Acad Sci U S A 2000;97(4): 1861-1866.
978. Vazquez-Martinez R, Shorte SL, Faught WJ, et al. Pulsatile exocytosis is functionally associated with GnRH gene expression in immortalized GnRH-expressing cells. Endocrinology 2001; 142(12):5364-5370.
979. Vazquez-Martinez R, Shorte SL, Boockfor FR, et al. Synchronized exocytotic bursts from gonadotropin-releasing hormone-expressing cells: dual control by intrinsic cellular pulsatility and gap junctional communication. Endocrinology 2001;142(5):2095-2101.
980. Charles A, Weiner R, Costantin J. cAMP modulates the excitability of immortalized H=hypothalamic (GT1) neurons via a cyclic nucleotide gated channel. Mol Endocrinol 2001;15(6):997-1009.
981. Hu L, Olson AJ, Weiner RI, et al. Connexin 26 expression and extensive gap junctional coupling in cultures of GT1-7 cells secreting gonadotropin-releasing hormone. Neuroendocrinology 1999;70(4):221-227.
982. Pitts GR, Nunemaker CS, Moenter SM. Cycles of transcription and translation do not comprise the gonadotropin-releasing hormone pulse generator in GT1 cells. Endocrinology 2001;142: 1858-1864.
983. Mahachoklertwattana P, Black SM, Kaplan SL, et al. Nitric oxide synthesized by gonadotropin-releasing hormone neurons is a mediator of N-methyl-D-aspartate (NMDA)-induced GnRH secretion. Endocrinology 1994;135:1709-1712.
984. Morreto M, Lopez FJ, Negro-Villar A. Nitric oxide regulates luteinizing hormone-releasing hormone secretion. Endocrinology 1993;133:2399-2402.
985. Schwanzel-Fukuda M, Pfaff DW. Origin of luteinizing hormone-releasing hormone neurons. Nature 1989;338:161-164.
986. Wray S, Grant P, Gainer H. Evidence that cells expressing luteinizing hormone-releasing hormone mRNA in the mouse are derived from progenitor cells in the olfactory placode. Proc Natl Acad Sci U S A 1989;86:8132-8136.
987. Wray S, Nieburgs A, Elkabes S. Spatiotemporal cell expression for luteinizing hormone-releasing hormone in the prenatal mouse: evidence for an embryonic origin in the olfactory placode. Dev Brain Res 1989;46:309-318.
988. Moore JP Jr, Wray S. Luteinizing hormone-releasing hormone (LHRH) biosynthesis and secretion in embryonic LHRH. Endocrinology 2000;141(12):4486-4495.
988a. Charlton H. Neural transplantation in hypogonadal (hpg) mice – physiology and neurobiology. Reproduction 2004;127:3-12.
989. Ronnekleiv OK, Resko JA. Ontogeny of gonadotropin-releasing hormone-containing neurons in early fetal development of rhesus macaques. Endocrinology 1990;126:498-511.
990. Terasawa E, Schanhofer WK, Keen KL, Luchansky L. Intracellular Ca(2+) oscillations in luteinizing hormone-releasing hormone

neurons derived from the embryonic olfactory placode of the rhesus monkey. J Neurosci 1999;19(14):5898-5909.
991. Schwanzel-Fukuda M, Bick D, Pfaff DW. Luteinizing hormone-releasing hormone (LHRH)-expressing cells do not migrate normally in an inherited hypogonadal (Kallmann) syndrome. Mol Brain Res 1989;6:311-326.
992. Schwanzel-Fukuda M, Crossin KL, Pfaff DW, et al. Migration of luteinizing hormone-releasing hormone (LHRH) neurons in early human embryos. J Comp Neurol 1996;366:547-557.
993. Parhar I, Pfaff D, Schwanzel-Fukuda M. Genes and behavior as studied through gonadotropin-releasing hormone (GnRH) neurons: comparative and functional aspects. Cell Mol Neurobiol 1995;15:107-116.
994. Tobet SA, Schwarting GA. Minireview: recent progress in gonadotropin-releasing hormone neuronal migration. Endocrinology 2006;147(3):1159-1165.
995. Spitzer NC. Electrical activity in early neuronal development. Nature 2006;444(7120):707-712.
996. Cottrell EC, Campbell RE, Han SK, et al. Postnatal remodeling of dendritic structure and spine density in gonadotropin-releasing hormone neurons. Endocrinology 2006;147(8):3652-3661.
997. Clarkson J, Herbison AE. Development of GABA and glutamate signaling at the GnRH neuron in relation to puberty. Mol Cell Endocrinol 2006;254-255:32-38.
998. Castellano JM, Navarro VM, Fernandez-Fernandez R, et al. Changes in hypothalamic KiSS-1 system and restoration of pubertal activation of the reproductive axis by kisspeptin in undernutrition. Endocrinology 2005;146(9):3917-3925.
999. Terasawa E. Postnatal remodeling of gonadotropin-releasing hormone I neurons: toward understanding the mechanism of the onset of puberty. Endocrinology 2006;147(8):3650-3651.
1000. Gluckman PD, Grumbach MM, Kaplan SL. The neuroendocrine regulation and function of growth hormone and prolactin in the mammalian fetus. Endocr Rev 1981;2:363-395.
1001. Thliveris JA, Currie RW. Observations on the hypothalamo-hypophyseal portal vasculature in the developing human fetus. Am J Anat 1980;157:441-444.
1002. Clark SJ, Ellis N, Styne DM, et al. Hormone ontogeny in the ovine fetus. XVII. Demonstration of pulsatile luteinizing hormone secretion by the fetal pituitary gland. Endocrinology 1984;115:1774-1779.
1003. Clark SJ, Hauffa BP, Rodens KP, et al. Hormone ontogeny in the ovine fetus. XIX. The effect of a potent luteinizing hormone-releasing factor agonist on gonadotropin and testosterone release in the fetus and neonate. Pediatr Res 1989;25:347-352.
1004. Huhtaniemi I, Lautala P. Stimulation of steroidogenesis in human fetal testes by the placenta during perifusion. J Steroid Biochem 1979;10:109-113.
1005. Molsberry RL, Carr BR, Mendelson CR, et al. Human chorionic gonadotropin binding to human fetal testes as a function of gestational age. J Clin Endocrinol Metab 1982;55:791-794.
1006. Huhtaniemi IT, Yamamoto M, Ranta T, et al. Follicle-stimulating hormone receptors appear earlier in the primate fetal testis than in the ovary. J Clin Endocrinol Metab 1987;65:1210-1214.
1007. Huhtaniemi I, Pelliniemi J. Fetal Leydig cells: cellular origin, morphology, life span and special functional feature. Proc Soc Exp Biol Med 1992;201:125-140.
1008. Huhtaniemi I. Ontogeny of luteinizing homrone action in the male. In Payne AH, Jardy MP, Russel LD, eds. The Leydig Cell. Vienna, IL: Cache River Press, 1996:366-382.
1009. Saez JM. Leydig cells: endocrine, paracrine and autocrine regulation. Endocr Rev 1994;15:574-626.
1010. Habert R, Lejeune H, Saez JM. Origin, differentiation and regulation of fetal and adult Leydig cells. Mol Cell Endocrinol 2001;179(1-2):47-74.
1011. Baker RG, Scrimgeour JB. Development of the gonad in normal and anencephalic human fetuses. J Reprod Fertil 1980;68:193-199.
1012. Beck-Peccoz P, Padmanabhan V, Baggiani AM, et al. Maturation of hypothalamic-pituitary-gonadal function in normal human fetuses: circulating levels of gonadotropins, their common alpha subunit and free testosterone, and discrepancy between immunological and biological activities of circulating follicle-stimulating hormone. J Clin Endocrinol Metab 1991;73:525-532.
1013. Massa G, de Zegher F, Vanderschueren-Lodeweyckx M. Serum levels of immunoreactive inhibin, FSH and LH in human infants at preterm and term birth. Biol Neonate 1992;61:150-155.
1014. Gluckman PD, Marti Henneberg C, Kaplan SL, et al. Hormone ontogeny in the ovine fetus. XIV. The effect of 17β-estradiol infusion on fetal plasma gonadotropins and prolactin and the maturation of sex steroid-dependent negative feedback. Endocrinology 1983;112:1618-1623.
1015. Groom GV, Boyns AR. Effect of hypothalamic releasing factor and steroids on release of gonadotrophins by organ culture of human fetal pituitary glands. J Endocrinol 1973;59:511-522.
1016. Jaffe AB, Mulcahey JJ, DiBabio AM, et al. Peptide regulation of pituitary and target tissue function and growth in the primate fetus. Recent Prog Horm Res 1988;44:431-544.
1017. Takagi ST, Yoshida T, Tsubata K, et al. Sex differences in fetal gonadotropins and androgens. J Steroid Biochem 1977;8:609-620.
1018. Davies JL, Naftolin F, Ryan KJ, et al. A specific high affinity limited capacity estrogen binding component in the cytosol of human fetal pituitary and brain tissues. J Clin Endocrinol Metab 1975;40:909.
1019. Mesiano S, Hart CS, Heyer BW, et al. Hormone ontogeny in the ovine fetus XXVI. A sex difference in the effect of castration on the hypothalamic-pituitary gonadotropin unit in the ovine fetus. Endocrinology 1991;129:3073-3079.
1020. Cuttler L, Egli CA, Styne DM, et al. Hormone ontogeny in the ovine fetus. XVIII. The effect of an opioid antagonist on luteinizing hormone secretion. Endocrinology 1985;116:1997-2002.
1021. Bettendorf M, de Zegher F, Albers N, et al. Acute N-methyl-D,L-aspartate administration stimulates the luteinizing hormone releasing hormone pulse generator in the ovine fetus. Horm Res 1999;51(1):25-30.
1022. Van den Pol AN, Wuarin JP, Dudek FE. Glutamate, the dominant excitatory transmitter in neuroendocrine regulation. Science 1990;250(4985):1276-1278.
1023. Dhandapani KM, Brann DW. The role of glutamate and nitric oxide in the reproductive neuroendocrine system. Biochem Cell Biol 2000;78(3):165-179.
1024. Albers N, Bettendorf M, Hart CS, et al. Hormone ontogeny in the ovine fetus. XXIII. Pulsatile administration of follicle-stimulating hormone stimulates inhibin production and decreases testosterone synthesis in the ovine fetal gonad. Endocrinology 1989;124:3089-3094.
1025. Albers N, Hart CS, Kaplan SL, et al. Hormone ontogeny in the ovine fetus. XXIV. Porcine follicular fluid "inhibins" selectively suppress plasma follicle-stimulating hormone in the ovine fetus. Endocrinology 1989;125:675-678.
1026. Corbier P, Dehenin L, Castanier M, et al. Sex differences in serum luteinizing hormone and testosterone in the human neonate during the first few hours after birth. J Clin Endocrinol Metab 1990;71:1347-1348.
1027. Lustig RH, Conte FA, Kogan BA, et.al. Ontogeny of gonadotropin secretion in congenital anorchism: sexual dimorphism versus syndrome of gonadal dysgenesis and diagnostic considerations. J Urol 1987;138:587-591.
1028. Plant TM. The effects of neonatal orchidectomy on the developmental pattern of gonadotropin secretion in the male rhesus monkey (*Macaca mulatta*). Endocrinology 1980;106:1451-1454.
1029. Terasawa E, Fernandez DL. Neurobiological mechanisms of the onset of puberty in primates. Endocr Rev 2001;22(1):111-151.
1030. Muller J, Skakkebaek NE. Fluctuations in the number of germ cells during the late foetal and early postnatal periods in boys. Acta Endocrinol (Copenh) 1984;105(2):271-274.
1031. Winter JSD, Faiman C, Hobson WC, et al. Pituitary-gonadal regulations in infancy. I. Patterns of serum gonadotropin concentrations from birth to four years of age in man and chimpanzee. J Clin Endocrinol Metab 1975;40:545-551.
1032. Forest MG. Pituitary gonadotropin and sex steroid secretion during the first two years of life. In Grumbach MM, Sizonenko PC, Aubert AU, eds. Control of the Onset of Puberty. Baltimore: Williams & Wilkins, 1990:451-478.
1033. Grumbach MM. The central nervous system and the onset of puberty. In Falkner F, Tanner JM, eds. Human Growth. New York: Plenum, 1978:215-238.

1034. Sharpe RM, Fraser HM, Brougham MF, et al. Role of the neonatal period of pituitary-testicular activity in germ cell proliferation and differentiation in the primate testis. Hum Reprod 2003; 18(10):2110-2117.
1035. Sharpe RM, McKinnell C, Kivlin C, et al. Proliferation and functional maturation of Sertoli cells, and their relevance to disorders of testis function in adulthood. Reproduction 2003;125(6): 769-784.
1036. Pitteloud N, Hayes FJ, Dwyer A, et al. Predictors of outcome of long-term GnRH therapy in men with idiopathic hypogonadotropic hypogonadism. J Clin Endocrinol Metab 2002;87(9): 4128-4136.
1037. Odell WD, Swerdloff RS. Etiologies of sexual maturation: a model system based on the sexually maturing rat. Recent Prog Horm Res 1976;32:245-288.
1038. Davidson JM. Hypothalamic-pituitary regulation of puberty: evidence from animal experimentation. In Grumbach MM, Grave GD, Mayer FE, eds. Control of the Onset of Puberty. New York: John Wiley & Sons, 1974:79-103.
1039. Ramirez VD. Endocrinology of puberty. Female reproductive system. Part 1. In Greep RO, Astwood EB, eds. Handbook of Physiology. Sect 7: Endocrinology. Washington, DC: American Physiological Society, 1973:1-28.
1040. Lenko HL, Lang U, Aubert ML, et al. Hormonal changes in puberty. VII. Lack of variation of daytime plasma melatonin. J Clin Endocrinol Metab 1982;54:1056-1058.
1041. Cohen HN, Hay ID, Annesley TM, et al. Serum immunoreactive melatonin in boys with delayed puberty. Clin Endocrinol 1982;17:517-521.
1042. Reppert SM, Weaver DR. Melatonin madness. Cell 1995;83: 1059-1062.
1043. Luboshitzky R, Lavi S, Thuma I, et al. Increased nocturnal melatonin secretion in male patients with hypogonadotropic hypogonadism and delayed puberty. J Clin Endocrinol Metab 1995; 80:2144-2148.
1044. Cavallo A. Melatonin and human puberty: current perspectives. J Pineal Res 1993;15:115-121.
1045. Cavallo A. Melatonin secretion during adrenarche in normal human puberty and in pubertal disorders. J Pineal Res 1992; 12:71-78.
1046. Cavallo A. Plasma melatonin rhythm in normal puberty: interactions of age and pubertal stages. Neuroendocrinology 1992;55: 372-379.
1047. Cavallo A, Ritschel WA. Pharmacokinetics of melatonin in human sexual maturation. J Clin Endocrinol Metab 1996;81: 1882-1886.
1048. Luboshitzky R, Lavi S, Thuma I, et al. Testosterone treatment alters melatonin concentrations in male patients with gonadotropin-releasing hormone deficiency. J Clin Endocrinol Metab 1996;81:770.
1049. Okatani Y, Sagara Y. Amplification of nocturnal melatonin secretion in women with functional secondary amenorrhoea: relation to endogenous oestrogen concentration. Clin Endocrinol 1994;41: 763-770.
1050. Salti R, Galluzzi F, Bindi G, et al. Nocturnal melatonin patterns in children. J Clin Endocrinol Metab 2000;85(6):2137-2144.
1051. Ojeda SR, Lomniczi A, Mastronardi C, et al. Minireview: the neuroendocrine regulation of puberty: is the time ripe for a systems biology approach? Endocrinology 2006;147(3):1166-1174.
1052. Hirschhorn JN, Lindgren CM, Daly MJ, et al. Genomewide linkage analysis of stature in multiple populations reveals several regions with evidence of linkage to adult height. Am J Hum Genet 2001;69(1):106-116.
1053. Perola M, Ohman M, Hiekkalinna T, et al. Quantitative-trait-locus analysis of body-mass index and of stature, by combined analysis of genome scans of five Finnish study groups. Am J Hum Genet 2001;69(1):117-123.
1054. Lander ES, Schork NJ. Genetic dissection of complex traits. Science 1994;265:2037-2048.
1055. Frankel WN, Schork N. Who's afraid of epistasis? Nature Genet 1996;14:371-373.
1056. Paterson AH. Molecular dissection of quantitative traits: progress and prospects. Genome Res 1995;5:321-333.
1057. Risch N, Merikangas K. The future of genetic studies of complex human diseases. Science 1996;273:1516-1517.
1058. Mackay TF. The genetic architecture of quantitative traits. Annu Rev Genet 2001;35:303-339.
1059. Brookes AJ. Rethinking genetic strategies to study complex diseases. Trends Mol Med 2001;7(11):512-516.
1060. Guo Y, Shen H, Xiao P, et al. Genomewide linkage scan for quantitative trait loci underlying variation in age at menarche. J Clin Endocrinol Metab 2006;91(3):1009-1014.
1061. Sedlmeyer IL, Pearce CL, Trueman JA, et al. Determination of sequence variation and haplotype structure for the gonadotropin-releasing hormone (GnRH) and GnRH receptor genes: investigation of role in pubertal timing. J Clin Endocrinol Metab 2005;90(2):1091-1099.
1062. Sedlmeyer IL, Hirschhorn JN, Palmert MR. Pedigree analysis of constitutional delay of growth and maturation: determination of familial aggregation and inheritance patterns. J Clin Endocrinol Metab 2002;87(12):5581-5586.
1063. Kennedy GC, Mitra J. Body weight and food intake as initiating factors for puberty in the rat. J Physiol 1963;166:408-418.
1064. Frisch RE. Body fat, puberty and fertility. Biol Rev Camb Philos Soc 1984;59:161-188.
1065. Frisch RE, McArthur JW. Menstrual cycles: fatness as a determinant of minimum weight for height necessary for their maintenance or onset. Science 1974;185:949-951.
1066. Frisch RE. Pubertal adipose tissue: is it necessary for normal sexual maturation? Evidence from the rat and human female. Fed Proc 1980;39:2395-2400.
1067. Boyar RM, Katz J, Finkelstein JW, et al. Anorexia nervosa. Immaturity of the 24-hour luteinizing hormone secretory pattern. N Engl J Med 1974;291:861-865.
1068. Frisch RE, Wyshak G, Vincent L. Delayed menarche and amenorrhea in ballet dancers. N Engl J Med 1980;303:17-19.
1069. de Souza MJ, Metzger DA. Reproductive dysfunction in amenorrheic athletes and anorexic patients: a review. Med Sci Sports Exerc 1991;23:995-1007.
1070. Frisch RE, Gotz-Welbergen AV, McArthur JW, et al. Delayed menarche and amenorrhea of college athletes in relation to age of onset of training. JAMA 1981;246:1559-1564.
1071. McArthur JW, Bullen BA, Beitins IZ, et al. Hypothalamic amenorrhea in runners of normal body composition. Endocr Res Commun 1980;7:13-25.
1072. Frisch RE. Fatness of girls from menarche to age 18 with a nomogram. Hum Biol 1976;48:353-359.
1073. Fellier H, Frisch H, Gleispach H. [LH-, estrogen- and testosterone excretion in correlation with the testicle size (author's transl)] Untersuchung der LH-, Ostrogen- und Testosteronausscheidung im Vergleich zur Testesgrosse. Z Kinderheilkd 1974;116:319-324.
1074. Frisch RE, Revelle R. Height and weight at menarche and a hypothesis of critical body weights and adolescent events. Science 1970;169:397-399.
1075. Garn SM, LaVelle M. Reproductive histories of low weight girls and women. Am J Clin Nutr 1983;37(5):862-866.
1076. Garn SM, LaVelle M, Pilkington JJ. Comparison of fatness in premenarchial and postmenarchial girls of the same age. J Pediatr 1983;103:328-331.
1077. Forbes GB. Body size and composition of perimenarchal girls. Am J Dis Child 1992;146(1):63-66.
1078. Bronson FH, Manning JM. Minireview: the energetic regulation of ovulation; a realistic role of body fat. Biol Reprod 1991;44: 945-950.
1079. Malina RM. Menarche in athletes: a synthesis and hypothesis. Ann Hum Biol 1983;10:1-24.
1080. Wellens R, Malina RM., Roche AF, et al. Body size and fatness in young adults in relation to age of menarche. Am J Hum Biol 1992;4:783-787.
1081. Johnston FE, Roche AF, Schell LM, et al. Critical weight at menarche. Am J Dis Child 1975;129:19-23.
1082. Cameron N. Weight and skinfold variation at menarche and the critical body weight hypothesis. Ann Hum Biol 1976;3:279-282.
1083. Billewicz WS, Fellowes HM, Hytten CA. Comments on the critical metabolic mass and the enage of menarche. Ann Hum Biol 1976;3:51-59.
1084. Vizmanos B, Marti-Henneberg C. Puberty begins with a characteristic subcutaneous body fat mass in each sex. Eur J Clin Nutr 2000;54(3):203-208.

1085. Legro RS, Lin HM, Demers LM, et al. Rapid maturation of the reproductive axis during perimenarche independent of body composition. J Clin Endocrinol Metab 2000;85(3):1021-1025.
1086. Zhang Y, Proenca R, Maffel M, et al. Positional cloning of the mouse obese gene and its human analogue. Nature 1994; 372:425-432.
1087. Campfield LA, Smith FJ, Guisez Y, et al. Recombinant mouse OB protein: evidence for a peripheral signal linking adiposity and central neural networks. Science 1995;269:546-549.
1088. Halaas JL, Gajiwala KS, Maffei M, et al. Weight-reducing effects of the plasma protein encoded by the obese gene. Science 1995;269:543-549.
1089. Spiegelman BM, Flier JS. Adipogenesis and obesity: rounding out the big picture. Cell 1996;87:377-389.
1090. Pelleymounter MA, Cullen MJ, Baker MB, et al. Effects of the obese gene product on body weight regulation in ob/ob mice. Science 1995;269:540-543.
1091. Caro JF, Sinha MK, Kolacznski JW, et al. Leptin: the tale of an obesity gene. Diabetes 1996;45:1455-1462.
1092. Tartaglia LA, Dembski M, Weng X, et al. Identification and expression cloning of a leptin receptor, OB-R. Cell 1995;83: 1263-1271.
1093. Lee GH, Proenca R, Montez JM, et al. Abnormal splicing of the leptin receptor in diabetic mice. Nature 1996;379(6566): 632-635.
1094. Coleman DL. Obese and diabetes: two mutant genes causing diabetes-obesity syndromes in mice. Diabetologia 1978;14(3):141-148.
1095. Chehab FF, Lim ME, Lu R. Correction of the sterility defect in homozygous obese female mice by treatment with the human recombinant leptin. Nature Genet 1996;12:318-320.
1096. Chehab FF, Qiu J, Mounzih K, et al. Leptin and reproduction. Nutr Rev 2002;60(10 Pt 2):S39-S46.
1097. Chehab FF. Leptin as a regulator of adipose mass and reproduction. Trends Pharmacol Sci 2000;21(8):309-314.
1098. Mounzih K, Lu R, Chehab FF. Leptin treatment rescues the sterility of genetically obese ob/ob males. Endocrinology 1997;138: 1190-1193.
1099. Cheung CC, Thornton JE, Kuijper JL, et al. Leptin is a metabolic gate for the onset of puberty in the female rat. Endocrinology 1997;138:855-858.
1100. Gruaz NM, Lalaoui M, Pierroz DD, et al. Chronic administration of leptin into the lateral ventricle induces sexual maturation in severely food-restricted female rats. J Neuroendocrinol 1998; 10(8):627-633.
1101. Cheung CC, Clifton DK, Steiner RA. Perspectives on leptin's role as a metabolic signal for the onset of puberty. Front Horm Res 2000;26:87-105.
1102. Cheung CC, Thornton JE, Nurani SD, et al. A reassessment of leptin's role in triggering the onset of puberty in the rat and mouse. Neuroendocrinology 2001;74(1):12-21.
1103. Magni P, Vettor R, Pagano C, et al. Expression of a leptin receptor in immortalized gonadotropin-releasing hormone-secreting neurons. Endocrinology 1999;140(4):1581-1585.
1104. Zamorano PL, Mahesh VB, De Sevilla L, et al. Excitatory amino acid receptors and puberty. Steroids 1998;63(5-6):268-270.
1105. Woller M, Tessmer S, Neff D, et al. Leptin stimulates gonadotropin releasing hormone release from cultured intact hemihypothalami and enzymatically dispersed neurons. Exp Biol Med (Maywood) 2001;226(6):591-596.
1106. Yu WH, Kimura M, Walczewska A, et al. Role of leptin in hypothalamic-pituitary function. Proc Natl Acad Sci U S A 1997;94: 1023-1028.
1107. Parent AS, Lebrethon MC, Gerard A, et al. Leptin effects on pulsatile gonadotropin releasing hormone secretion from the adult rat hypothalamus and interaction with cocaine and amphetamine regulated transcript peptide and neuropeptide Y. Regul Pept 2000;92(1-3):17-24.
1108. Plant TM, Durrant AR. Circulating leptin does not appear to provide a signal for triggering the initiation of puberty in the male rhesus monkey (*Macaca mulatta*). Endocrinology 1997; 138(10):4505-4508.
1109. Urbanski HF, Pau KY. A biphasic developmental pattern of circulating leptin in the male rhesus macaque *Macaca mulatta*. Endocrinology 1998;139(5):2284-2286.
1110. Finn PD, Cunningham MJ, Pau KY, et al. The stimulatory effect of leptin on the neuroendocrine reproductive axis of the monkey. Endocrinology 1998;139(11):4652-4662.
1111. Ahima RS, Saper CB, Flier JS, et al. Leptin regulation of neuroendocrine systems. Front Neuroendocrinol 2000;21(3): 263-307.
1112. Wauters M, Considine RV, Van Gaal LF. Human leptin: from an adipocyte hormone to an endocrine mediator. Eur J Endocrinol 2000;143(3):293-311.
1113. Caprio M, Fabbrini E, Isidori AM, et al. Leptin in reproduction. Trends Endocrinol Metab 2001;12(2):65-72.
1114. Licinio J, Mantzoros C, Negrno AB, et al. Human leptin levels are pulsatile and inversely related to pituitary-adrenal function. Nature Med 1997;3:575-579.
1115. Klein KO, Larmore KA, de Lancey E, et al. Effect of obesity on estradiol level, and its relationship to leptin, bone maturation, and bone mineral density in children. J Clin Endocrinol Metab 1998;83(10):3469-3475.
1116. Clayton PE, Gill MS, Hall CM, Tillmann V, et al. Serum leptin through childhood and adolescence. Clin Endocrinol 1997;46(6): 727-733.
1117. Blum WF, Englaro P, Hanitsch S, et al. Plasma leptin levels in healthy children and adolescents: dependence on body mass index, body fat mass, gender, pubertal stage, and testosterone. J Clin Endocrinol Metab 1997;82(9):2904-2910.
1118. Ahmed ML, Ong KK, Morrell DJ, et al. Longitudinal study of leptin concentrations during puberty: sex differences and relationship to changes in body composition. J Clin Endocrinol Metab 1999;84(3):899-905.
1119. Palmert MR, Radovick S, Boepple PA. The impact of reversible gonadal sex steroid suppression on serum leptin concentrations in children with central precocious puberty. J Clin Endocrinol Metab 1998;83(4):1091-1096.
1120. Andreelli F, Hanaire-Broutin H, Laville M, et al. Normal reproductive function in leptin-deficient patients with lipoatropic diabetes. J Clin Endocrinol Metab 2000;85(2):715-719.
1121. Clayton PE, Trueman JA. Leptin and puberty. Arch Dis Child 2000;83(1):1-4.
1122. Grasemann C, Wessels HT, Knauer-Fischer S, et al. Increase of serum leptin after short-term pulsatile GnRH administration in children with delayed puberty. Eur J Endocrinol 2004;150(5): 691-698.
1123. Sinha MK, Opentanova I, Ohannesian JP, et al. Evidence of free and bound leptin in human circulation. Studies in lean and obese subjects and during short-term fasting. J Clin Invest 1996;98(6): 1277-1282.
1124. Quinton ND, Smith RF, Clayton PE, et al. Leptin binding activity changes with age: the link between leptin and puberty. J Clin Endocrinol Metab 1999;84(7):2336-2341.
1125. Mann DR, Johnson AO, Gimpel T, et al. Changes in circulating leptin, leptin receptor, and gonadal hormones from infancy until advanced age in humans. J Clin Endocrinol Metab 2003;88(7): 3339-3345.
1126. Li HJ, Ji CY, Wang W, et al. A twin study for serum leptin, soluble leptin receptor, and free insulin-like growth factor-I in pubertal females. J Clin Endocrinol Metab 2005;90(6):3659-3664.
1127. Banerjee I, Trueman JA, Hall CM, et al. Phenotypic variation in constitutional delay of growth and puberty: relationship to specific leptin and leptin receptor gene polymorphisms. Eur J Endocrinol 2006;155(1):121-126.
1128. Ozata M, Ozdemir IC, Licinio J. Human leptin deficiency caused by a missense mutation: multiple endocrine defects, decreased sympathetic tone, and immune system dysfunction indicate new targets for leptin action, greater central than peripheral resistance to the effects of leptin, and spontaneous correction of leptin-mediated defects. J Clin Endocrinol Metab 1999;84(10): 3686-3695.
1129. Clement K, Vaisse C, Lahlou N, et al. A mutation in the human leptin receptor gene causes obesity and pituitary dysfunction. Nature 1998;392(6674):398-401.
1130. Farooqi IS, Jebb SA, Langmack G, et al. Effects of recombinant leptin therapy in a child with congenital leptin deficiency. N Engl J Med 1999;341(12):879-884.
1131. Apter D. The role of leptin in female adolescence. Ann N Y Acad Sci 2003;997:64-76.

1132. Brown DC, Kelnar CJ, Wu FC. Energy metabolism during male human puberty. I. Changes in energy expenditure during the onset of puberty in boys. Ann Hum Biol 1996;23:273-279.
1133. Brown DC, Kelnar CJ, Wu FC. Energy metabolism during male human puberty. II. Use of testicular size in predictive equations for basal metabolic rate. Ann Hum Biol 1996;23:281-284.
1134. Korbonits M, Grossman AB. Ghrelin: update on a novel hormonal system. Eur J Endocrinol 2004;151(Suppl 1):S67-S70.
1135. Fernandez-Fernandez R, Martini AC, Navarro VM, et al. Novel signals for the integration of energy balance and reproduction. Mol Cell Endocrinol 2006;254-255:127-132.
1136. Bottner A, Kratzsch J, Muller G, et al. Gender differences of adiponectin levels develop during the progression of puberty and are related to serum androgen levels. J Clin Endocrinol Metab 2004;89(8):4053-4061.
1137. Tsou PL, Jiang YD, Chang CC, et al. Sex-related differences between adiponectin and insulin resistance in schoolchildren. Diabetes Care 2004;27(2):308-313.
1138. Gerber M, Boettner A, Seidel B, et al. Serum resistin levels of obese and lean children and adolescents: biochemical analysis and clinical relevance. J Clin Endocrinol Metab 2005;90(8): 4503-4509.
1139. Foster DL, Ryan KD. Puberty in the lamb: sexual maturation of a seasonal breeder in a changing environment. In Grumbach MM, Sizonenko PC, Aubert ML, eds. Control of the Onset of Puberty Control of the Onset of Puberty. Baltimore: Williams & Wilkins, 1990:143-155.
1140. Ojeda SR, Smith-White S, Advis JP, et al. First preovulatory gonadotropin surge in the rodent. In Grumbach MM, Sizonenko PC, Aubert ML, eds. Control of the Onset of Puberty. Baltimore: Williams & Wilkins, 1990:156-182.
1141. Donovan BT. Puberty in the guinea pig and rabbit. In Grumbach MM, Sizonenko PC, Aubert ML, eds. Control of the Onset of Puberty. Baltimore: Williams & Wilkins, 1990:143-144.
1142. Vandenbergh JG. Pheromones and mammalian reproduction. In Knobil E, Neill JD, eds. The Physiology of Reproduction. New York: Raven, 1994:1679-1696.
1143. Grumbach MM, Conte FA. Disorders of sexual differentiation. In Wilson JD, Foster DW, Kroneberg HM, et al, eds. Willliams Textbook of Endocrinology. Philadelphia: WB Saunders, 1998: 1509-1626.
1144. Conte FA, Grumbach MM, Kaplan SL, et al. Correlation of luteinizing hormone-releasing factor-induced luteinizing hormone and follicle-stimulating hormone release from infancy to 19 years with the changing pattern of gonadotropin secretion in agonadal patients: relation to the restraint of puberty. J Clin Endocrinol Metab 1980;50:163-168.
1145. Conte FA, Grumbach MM, Kaplan SL. A diphasic pattern of gonadotropin secretion in patients with the syndrome of gonadal dysgenesis. J Clin Endocrinol Metab 1975;40:670-674.
1146. Kelch RP, Kaplan SL, Grumbach MM. Suppression of urinary and plasma follicle-stimulating hormone by exogenous estrogens in prepubertal and pubertal children. J Clin Invest 1973;52: 1122-1128.
1147. Grumbach MM, Kaplan SL. Recent advances in the diagnosis and management of sexual precocity. Acta Paediatr Jpn (Overseas Ed) 1988;30:155-175.
1148. Voigt P, Ma YJ, Gonazalez D, et al. Neural and glial mediated effects of growth factors acting via tyrosine kinase receptors on luteinizing hormone-releasing hormone neurons. Endocrinology 1997;137:2593-2605.
1149. Wetsel WC, Hill DF, Ojeda SR. Basic fibroblast growth factor regulates the conversion of pro-luteinizing hormone releasing hormone (pro-LHRH) to LHRH in immortalized hypothalamic neurons. Endocrinology 1997;137:2606-2616.
1150. Junier MP, Ma YJ, Costa ME, et al. Transforming growth factor alpha contributes to the mechanism by which hypothalamic injury induces precocious puberty. Proc Natl Acad Sci U S A 1991;88:9743-9747.
1151. Olson BR, Scott DC, Wetsel WC, et al. Effects of insulin-like growth factors I and II and insulin on the immortalized hypthalamic GTI-7 cell line. Neuroendocrinology 1995;62:155-165.
1152. Ojeda SR, Dissen GA, Junier M-P. Neutrophilic factors and female sexual development. In Frontiers in Neuroendocrinology. New York: Raven Press, 1992:120-162.
1153. Hiney JK, Srivastava V, Nyberg CL, et al. Insulin-like growth factor I of peripheral origin acts centrally to accelerate the initiation of female puberty. Endocrinology 1996;137:3717-3728.
1154. Gallo F, Morale MC, Avola R, et al. Cross-talk between luteinizing hormone-releasing hormone (LHRH) neurons and astroglia cells: developing glia release factors that accelerate neuronal differentiation and stimulate LHRH release from GT neuronal cell line and LHRH neurons induce astroglia proliferation. Endocrine 1995;3:863-874.
1155. Watanabe G, Terasawa E. In vivo luteinizing hormone releasing hormone increases with puberty in the female rhesus monkey. Endocrinology 1989;125:92-99.
1156. Mitsushima D, Hei DL, Terasawa E. Gamma-Aminobutyric acid is an inhibitory neurotransmitter restricting the release of luteinizing hormone-releasing hormone before the onset of puberty. Proc Natl Acad Sci U S A 1994;91:395-399.
1157. Mitsushima D, Marzban F, Luchansky LL, et al. Role of glutamic acid decarboxylase in the prepubertal inhibition of the luteinizing hormone releasing hormone release in female rhesus monkeys. J Neurosci 1996;16:2563-2573.
1158. Terasawa E, Noonan JJ, Nass TE, et al. Posterior hypothalamic lesions advance the onset of puberty in the female rhesus monkey. Endocrinology 1984;115:2241-2250.
1159. Schultz NJ, Terasawa E. Posterior hypothalamic lesions advance the time of the pubertal changes in luteinizing hormone release in ovariectomized female rhesus monkeys. Endocrinology 1988; 123:445.
1160. Hochman HI, Judge DM, Reichlin S. Precocious puberty and hypothalamic hamartoma. Pediatrics 1981;67:236-244.
1161. Judge DM, Kulin HE, Santen R, et al. Hypothalamic hamartoma: a source of luteinizing-hormone-releasing factor in precocious puberty. N Engl J Med 1977;296:7-10.
1162. Mahachoklertwattana P, Kaplan SL, Grumbach MM. The luteinizing hormone-releasing hormone-secreting hypothalamic hamartoma is a congenital malformation: natural history. J Clin Endocrinol Metab 1993;77:118-124.
1163. Krieger DT, Perlow MJ, Gibson MJ, et al. Brain grafts reverse hypogonadism of gonadotropin-releasing hormone deficiency. Nature 1982;298:468-472.
1164. Silverman AJ, Gibson M. Hypothalamic transplantation. Repair of defects in hypogonadal mice. Trends Endocrinol Metab 1990; 1:403-408.
1165. Arslan M, Pohl CR, Plant TM. DL-2-Amino-5-phosphonopentanoic acid, a specific N-methyl-D-aspartic acid receptor antagonist, suppresses pulsatile LH release in the rat. Neuroendocrinology 1988;47:465-468.
1166. Bettendorf M, Albers N, de Zegher F, et al. A neuroexcitatory amino acid analogue, N-methyl-D,L-aspartate (NMDA), elicits LH and FSH release in the ovine fetus by a central mechanism. Endocr Soc Abstr 288, 1988 (abstract).
1166a. Bettendorf M, de Zegher F, Albers N, et al. Acute N-Methyl-D,L-Aspartate administration stimulates the luteinizing hormone releasing hormone pulse generator in the ovine fetus. Horm Res 1999;51:25-30.
1167. Gambacciani M, Yen SS, Rasmussen D. GnRH release from the mediobasal hypothalamus: in vitro inhibition by corticotropin releasing factor. Neuroendocrinology 1986;43:533-536.
1168. Kuljis RO, Advis JP. Immunocytochemical and physiological evidence of a synapse between dopamine- and luteinizing hormone releasing hormone-containing neurons in the ewe median eminence. Endocrinology 1989;124:1579-1581.
1169. MacLusky NJ, Naftolin F, Leranth C. Immunocytochemical evidence for direct synaptic connections between corticotrophin-releasing factor (CRF) and gonadotrophin-releasing hormone (GnRH)-containing neurons in the preoptic area of the rat. Brain Res 1988;439:391-395.
1170. Plant TM, Gay VL, Marshall GR, et al. Puberty in monkeys is triggered by chemical stimulation of the hypothalamus. Proc Natl Acad Sci U S A 1989;86:2506-2510.
1171. Thind KK, Goldsmith PC. Infundibular gonadotropin-releasing hormone neurons are inhibited by direct opioid and autoregulatory synapses in juvenile monkeys. Neuroendocrinology 1988; 47:203-216.

1172. Wilson RC, Kesner JS, Kaufman JM, et al. Central electrophysiologic correlates of pulsatile luteinizing hormone secretion in the rhesus monkey. Neuroendocrinology 1984;39:256-260.
1173. Ozata M, Bulur M, Bingol N, et al. Daytime plasma melatonin levels in male hypogonadism. J Clin Endocrinol Metab 1996; 81:1877-1881.
1174. Kelch RP , Foster CM, Kletter GB. Neuroendocrine regulation of puberty in boys. In Sizonenko PC, Aubert ML, eds. Developmental Endocrinology. New York: PB-Raven, 1990:103-115.
1175. Fraioli F, Cappa M, Fabbri A, et al. Lack of endogenous opioid inhibitory tone on LH secretion in early puberty. Clin Endocrinol (Oxf) 1984;20:299-305.
1176. Petraglia F, Bernasconi S, Iughetti L, et al. Naloxone-induced luteinizing hormone secretion in normal, precocious, and delayed puberty. J Clin Endocrinol Metab 1986;63:1112-1116.
1177. Mauras N, Veldhuis JD, Rogol AD. Role of endogenous opiates in pubertal maturation: opposing actions of naltrexone in prepubertal and late pubertal boys. J Clin Endocrinol Metab 1986;62: 1256-1263.
1178. Saunder SE, Case GD, Hopwood NJ, et al. the effects of opiate antagonism on gonadotropin secretion in children and in women with hypothalamic amenorrhea. Pediatr Res 1984;18:322-328.
1179. Mitsushima D, Marzban F, Luchansky LL, et al. Role of glutamic acid decarboxylase in the prepubertal inhibition of the luteinizing hormone releasing hormone release in female rhesus monkeys. J Neuroscience 1996;16:2563-2573.
1180. Terasawa E. Control of luteinizing hormone-releasing hormone pulse generation in nonhuman primates. Cell Molec Neurobiol 1995;15:141-164.
1181. Kasuya E, Nyberg CL, Mogi K, et al. A role of gamma-amino butyric acid (GABA) and glutamate in control of puberty in female rhesus monkeys: effect of an antisense oligodeoxynucleotide for GAD67 messenger ribonucleic acid and MK801 on luteinizing hormone-releasing hormone release. Endocrinology 1999; 140(2):705-712.
1182. Keen KL, Burich AJ, Mitsushima D, et al. Effects of pulsatile infusion of the GABA(A) receptor blocker bicuculline on the onset of puberty in female rhesus monkeys. Endocrinology 1999;140(11): 5257-5266.
1183. Martinez de la Escalera, Choi ALH, Weinter RI. Biphasic gabaergic regulation of GnRH secretion in GT1 cell lines. Neuroendocrinology 1994;59:420-425.
1184. Hales TG, Sanderson MJ, Charles AC. GABA has excitatory actions on GnRH-secreting immortalized hypothalamic (GT1-7) neurons. Neuroendocrinology 1994;59(3):297-308.
1185. El Etr M, Akwa Y, Fiddes RJ, et al. A progesterone metabolite stimulates the release of gonadotropin-releasing hormone from GT1-1 hypothalamic neurons via the gamma-aminobutyric acid type A receptor. Proc Natl Acad Sci U S A 1995;92(9): 3769-3773.
1186. Cherubini E, Gaiarsa JL, Ben Ari Y. GABA: an excitatory transmitter in early postnatal life. Trends Neurosci 1991;14(12):515-519.
1187. Ganguly K, Schinder AF, Wong ST, et al. GABA itself promotes the developmental switch of neuronal GABAergic responses from excitation to inhibition. Cell 2001;105(4):521-532.
1188. Terasawa E, Luchansky LL, Kasuya E, et al. An increase in glutamate release follows a decrease in gamma aminobutyric acid and the pubertal increase in luteinizing hormone releasing hormone release in the female rhesus monkeys. J Neuroendocrinol 1999;11(4):275-282.
1189. Van den Pol AN, Trombley PQ. Glutamate neurons in hypothalamus regulate excitatory transmission. J Neurosci 1993;13(7): 2829-2836.
1190. Gay VL, Plant TM. N-methyl-D,L-aspartate elicits hypothalamic gonadotropin-releasing hormone release in prepubertal male rhesus monkeys (*Macaca mulatta*). Endocrinology 1987;120: 2289-2296.
1191. Claypool LE, Kasuya E, Saitoh Y, et al. N-methyl D,L-aspartate induces the release of luteinizing hormone-releasing hormone in the prepubertal and pubertal female rhesus monkey as measured by in vivo push-pull perfusion in the stalk-median eminence. Endocrinology 2000;141(1):219-228.
1192. Ottem EN, Godwin JG, Krishnan S, et al. Dual-phenotype GABA/ glutamate neurons in adult preoptic area: sexual dimorphism and function. J Neurosci 2004;24(37):8097-8105.
1193. Urbanski HF, Ojeda SR. Activation of luteinizing hormone-releasing hormone release advances the onset of female puberty. Neuroendocrinology 1987;46:273-276.
1194. Price MT, Olney JW, Cicero TJ. Acute elevations of serum luteinizing hormone induced by kainic acid, N-methyl aspartic acid or homocystic acid. Neuroendocrinology 1978;26:352-358.
1195. Wilson RC, Knobil E. Acute effects of N-methyl-DL-aspartate on the release of pituitary gonadotropins and prolactin in the adult female rhesus monkey. Brain Res 1982;248:177-179.
1196. Bourguignon JP, Gerard A, Mathieu J, et al. Pulsatile release of gonadotropin-releasing hormone from hypothalamic explants is restrained by blockade of N-methyl-D,L-aspartate receptors. Endocrinology 1989;125:1090-1096.
1197. Hardelin JP, Levilliers J, Young J, et al. Xp22.3 deletions in isolated familial Kallmann's syndrome. J Clin Endocrinol Metab 1993; 76:827-831.
1198. Mahachoklertwattana P, Sanchez J, Kaplan SL, et al. N-methyl-D-aspartate (NMDA) receptors mediate the release of hormone (GnRH) by NMDA in a hypothalamic neuronal cell line (GT1-1). Endocrinology 1994;134:1023-1030.
1199. Terasawa E. Hypothalamic control of the onset of puberty. Curr Opin Endocrinol Diabet 1999;6:44-49.
1200. Smith JT, Clifton DK, Steiner RA. Regulation of the neuroendocrine reproductive axis by kisspeptin-GPR54 signaling. Reproduction 2006;131(4):623-630.
1201. Tena-Sempere M. Hypothalamic KiSS-1: the missing link in gonadotropin feedback control? Endocrinology 2005;146(9):3683-3685.
1202. Aparicio SA. Kisspeptins and GPR54—the new biology of the mammalian GnRH axis. Cell Metab 2005;1(5):293-296.
1203. de Roux N. GnRH receptor and GPR54 inactivation in isolated gonadotropic deficiency. Best Pract Res Clin Endocrinol Metab 2006;20(4):515-528.
1204. Muir AI, Chamberlain L, Elshourbagy NA, et al. AXOR12, a novel human G protein-coupled receptor, activated by the peptide KiSS-1. J Biol Chem 2001;276(31):28969-28975.
1205. Ohtaki T, Shintani Y, Honda S, et al. Metastasis suppressor gene KiSS-1 encodes peptide ligand of a G-protein-coupled receptor. Nature 2001;411(6837):613-617.
1206. Shahab M, Mastronardi C, Seminara SB, et al. Increased hypothalamic GPR54 signaling: a potential mechanism for initiation of puberty in primates. Proc Natl Acad Sci U S A 2005;102(6): 2129-2134.
1207. Gottsch ML, Cunningham MJ, Smith JT, et al. A role for kisspeptins in the regulation of gonadotropin secretion in the mouse. Endocrinology 2004;145(9):4073-4077.
1208. Messager S, Chatzidaki EE, Ma D, et al. Kisspeptin directly stimulates gonadotropin-releasing hormone release via G protein-coupled receptor 54. Proc Natl Acad Sci U S A 2005;102(5): 1761-1766.
1209. Han SK, Gottsch ML, Lee KJ, et al. Activation of gonadotropin-releasing hormone neurons by kisspeptin as a neuroendocrine switch for the onset of puberty. J Neurosci 2005;25(49): 11349-11356.
1210. Smith JT, Popa SM, Clifton DK, et al. Kiss1 neurons in the forebrain as central processors for generating the preovulatory luteinizing hormone surge. J Neurosci 2006;26(25):6687-6694.
1210a. Dungan HM, Clifton DK, Steiner RA. Minireview: kisspeptin neurons as central processors in the regulation of gonadotropin-releasing hormone secretion. Endocrinology 2006;147:1154-1158.
1211. Seminara SB, Messager S, Chatzidaki EE, et al. The GPR54 gene as a regulator of puberty. N Engl J Med 2003;349(17): 1614-1627.
1212. Patterson M, Murphy KG, Thompson EL, et al. Administration of kisspeptin-54 into discrete regions of the hypothalamus potently increases plasma luteinising hormone and testosterone in male adult rats. J Neuroendocrinol 2006;18(5):349-354.
1213. Navarro VM, Castellano JM, Fernandez-Fernandez R, et al. Characterization of the potent luteinizing hormone-releasing activity of KiSS-1 peptide, the natural ligand of GPR54. Endocrinology 2005;146(1):156-163.
1214. Navarro VM, Castellano JM, Garcia-Galiano D, Tena-Sempere M. Neuroendocrine factors in the initiation of puberty: The emergent role of kisspeptin. Rev Endocr Metab Disord 2007;8:11-20.

1215. Navarro VM, Castellano JM, Fernandez-Fernandez R, et al. Developmental and hormonally regulated messenger ribonucleic acid expression of KiSS-1 and its putative receptor, GPR54, in rat hypothalamus and potent luteinizing hormone-releasing activity of KiSS-1 peptide. Endocrinology 2004;145(10):4565-4574.
1216. Navarro VM, Fernandez-Fernandez R, Castellano JM, et al. Advanced vaginal opening and precocious activation of the reproductive axis by KiSS-1 peptide, the endogenous ligand of GPR54. J Physiol 2004;561(Pt 2):379-386.
1217. Matsui H, Takatsu Y, Kumano S, et al. Peripheral administration of metastin induces marked gonadotropin release and ovulation in the rat. Biochem Biophys Res Commun 2004;320(2):383-388.
1217a. Smith JT, Acohido BV, Clifton DK, et al: Kiss-1 neurones are direct targets for leptin in the ob/ob mouse. J Neuroendocrinol 2006;18(4):298-303.
1218. Seminara SB, Dipietro MJ, Ramaswamy S, et al. Continuous human metastin 45-54 infusion desensitizes G protein-coupled receptor 54-induced gonadotropin-releasing hormone release monitored indirectly in the juvenile male Rhesus monkey (*Macaca mulatta*): a finding with therapeutic implications. Endocrinology 2006;147(5):2122-2126.
1219. Colledge WH. GPR54 and puberty. Trends Endocrinol Metab 2004;15(9):448-453.
1219a. Dhillo WS, Chaudhri OB, Patterson M, et al. Kisspeptin-54 stimulates the hypothalamic-pituitary gonadal axis in human males. J Clin Endocrinol Metab 2005;90:6609-6615.
1220. Smith JT, Clarke IJ. Kisspeptin expression in the brain: Catalyst for the initiation of puberty. Rev Endocr Metab Disord 2007;8:1-9.
1220a. d'Anglemont de Tassigny X, Fagg LA, Dixon JP, et al. Hypogonadotropic hypogonadism in mice lacking a functional Kiss1 gene. Proc Natl Acad Sci USA 2007;104(25):10714-10719.
1221. Smith JT, Clifton DK, Steiner RA: Regulation of the neuroendocrine reproductive axis by kisspeptin-GPR54 signaling. Reproduction 2006;131:623-630.
1221a. Han SK, Gottsch ML, Lee KJ, et al. Activation of gonadotropin-releasing hormone neurons by kisspeptin as a neuroendocrine switch for the onset of puberty. J Neurosci 2005;25:11349-11356.
1221b. Smith JT, Popa SM, Clifton DK, et al. Kiss1 neurons in the forebrain as central processors for generating the preovulatory luteinizing hormone surge. J Neurosci 2006;26:6687-6694.
1221c. Clarkson J, Herbison AE: Development of GABA and glutamate signaling at the GnRH neuron in relation to puberty. Mol Cell Endocrinol 2006;254-255:32-38.
1222. Ma YJ, Costa ME, Ojeda SR. Developmental expression of the genes encoding transforming growth factor alpha and its receptor in the hypothalamus of female rhesus macaques. Neuroendocrinology 1994;60:346-359.
1222a. Heger S, Mastronardi C, Dissen GA, et al. Enhanced at puberty 1 (EAP1) is a new transcriptional regulator of the female neuroendocrine reproductive axis. J Clin Invest 2007;Jul 12:[Epub ahead of print].
1223. Plant TM. Neurobiological bases underlying the control of the onset of puberty in the rhesus monkey: a representative higher primate. Front Neuroendocrinol 2001;22(2):107-139.
1224. Clarkson J, Herbison AE. Postnatal development of kisspeptin neurons in mouse hypothalamus; sexual dimorphism and projections to gonadotropin-releasing hormone neurons. Endocrinology 2006;147:5817-5825.
1225. Kelch RP, Marshall JC. Pulsatile gonadotropin-releasing hormone and the induction of puberty in human beings. In Grumbach MM, Sizonenko PC, Aubert ML, eds. Control of the Onset of Puberty. Baltimore: Williams & Wilkins, 1990:82-107.
1226. Penny R, Olambiwonnu NO, Frasier SD. Episodic fluctuations of serum gonadotropins in pre- and post-pubertal girls and boys. J Clin Endocrinol Metab 1977;45:307-311.
1227. Boyar RM, Finkelstein JW, Roffwarg H, et al. Twenty-four patterns of luteinizing hormone and follicle-stimulating hormone secretory patterns in gonadal dysgenesis. J Clin Endocrinol Metab 1973;37:521-525.
1228. Boyar R, Finkelstein JW, David R, et al. Twenty-four hour patterns of plasma luteinizing hormone and follicle-stimulating hormone in sexual precocity. N Engl J Med 1973;289:282-286.
1229. Kulin HE, Moore RGJ, Santner SJ. Circadian rhythms in gonadotropin excretion in prepubertal and pubertal children. J Clin Endocrinol Metab 1976;42:770-773.
1230. Kletter GB, Foster CM, Brown MB, et al. Nocturnal naloxone fails to reverse the suppressive effects of testosterone infusion on luteinizing hormone secretion in pubertal boys. J Clin Endocrinol Metab 1994;79:1147-1151.
1231. Grumbach MM, Sizonenko PC, Aubert ML, eds. Control of the Onset of Puberty. Baltimore: Williams & Wilkins, 1990:1-710.
1232. Watanabe G, Terasawa E. In vivo release of luteinizing hormone releasing hormone increases with puberty in the female rhesus monkey. Endocrinology 1989;125:92-99.
1233. Roth JC, Grumbach MM, Kaplan SL. Effect of synthetic luteinizing hormone-releasing factor on serum testosterone and gonadotropins in prepubertal, pubertal, and adult males. J Clin Endocrinol Metab 1973;37:680-686.
1234. Job JC, Garnier PE, Chaussain JL, et al. Elevation of serum gonadotropins (LH and FSH) after releasing hormone (LH-RH) injection in normal children and in patients with disorders of puberty. J Clin Endocrinol Metab 1972;35:473-476.
1235. Yen SSC, Lasley BL, Wang FC, et al. The operating characteristics of the hypothalamic-pituitary system during the menstrual cycle and observations of biological action of somatostatin. Recent Prog Horm Res 1975;31:321-363.
1236. Keye WR, Jaffe RB. Strength-duration characteristics of estrogen effects on gonadotropin response to gonadotropin-releasing hormone in women. I. Effects of varying duration of estradiol administration. J Clin Endocrinol Metab 1975;41:1003-1008.
1237. Reiter EO, Kaplan SL, Conte FA, et al. Responsivity of pituitary gonadotropes to luteinizing hormone-releasing factor in idiopathic precocious puberty, precocious thelarche, precocious adrenarche, and in patients treated with medroxyprogesterone acetate. Pediatr Res 1975;9:111-116.
1238. Crowley WF, Filicori M, Spratt DI. The physiology of gonadotropin releasing hormone (GnRH) secretion in men and women. Recent Prog Horm Res 1985;41:473-526.
1239. Crowley WF Jr, McArthur JW. Stimulation of the normal menstrual cycle in Kallmann's syndrome by pulsatile administration of luteinizing hormone-releasing hormone (LHRH). J Clin Endocrinol Metab 1980;51:173-175.
1240. Yoshimoto Y, Moridera K, Imura H. Restoration of normal pituitary gonadotropin reserve by administration of luteinizing hormone releasing hormone in patients with hypogonadotropic hypogonadism. N Engl J Med 1975;292:242-245.
1241. Jacobson RI, Seyler LE, Tamborlane WV, et al. Pulsatile subcutaneous nocturnal administration of Gn-RH by portable infusion pump in hypogonadotropic hypogonadism: initiation of gonadotropin responsiveness. J Clin Endocrinol Metab 1979;49:652-654.
1242. Marshall JC, Kelch RP. Low dose pulsatile gonadotropin-releasing hormone in anorexia nervosa: a model of human pubertal development. J Clin Endocrinol Metab 1979;49:712-718.
1243. Valk TW, Corley KP, Kelch RP, et al. Hypogonadotropic hypogonadism: hormonal responses to low dose pulsatile administration of gonadotropin-releasing hormone. J Clin Endocrinol Metab 1980;51:730-737.
1244. Pohl GR, Knobil E. The role of the central nervous system in the control of ovarian function in higher primates. Annu Rev Physiol 1982;44:583-593.
1245. Knobil E, Plant TM. The neuroendocrine control of gonadotropin secretion in the female rhesus monkey. Front Neuroendocrinol 1978;4:249-264.
1246. Wildt L, Marshall G, Knobil E. Experimental induction of puberty in the infantile female rhesus monkey. Science 1980;207:1373-1375.
1247. Boyar RM, Finkelstein JW, Witkin M, et al. Studies of endocrine function in "isolated" gonadotropin deficiency. J Clin Endocrinol Metab 1973;36:64-72.
1248. Winter JS, Taraska S, Faiman C. The hormonal response to HCG stimulation in male children and adolescents. J Clin Endocrinol Metab 1972;34:348-353.
1249. Sizonenko PC, Cuendet A, Paunier L. FSH. 1. Evidence for its mediating role on testosterone secretion in cryptorchidism. J Clin Endocrinol Metab 1973;37:68-73.

1250. Reiter EO, Kulin HE, Hamwood SM. The absence of positive feedback between estrogen and luteinizing hormone in sexually immature girls. Pediatr Res 1974;8:740-745.
1251. Presl J, Horejsi J, Strouflova A, et al. Sexual maturation in girls and the development of estrogen-induced gonadotropic hormone release. Ann Biol Anim Biochim Biophys 1976;16:377-383.
1252. Ross GT, Cargille CM, Lipsett MB, et al. Pituitary and gonadal hormones in women during spontaneous and induced ovulatory cycles. Recent Prog Horm Res 1970;26:1-62.
1253. Hayes FJ, Seminara SB, DeCruz S, et al. Aromatase inhibition in the human male reveals a hypothalamic site of estrogen feedback. J Clin Endocrinol Metab 2000;85(9):3027-3035.
1253a. Wintermantel TM, Campbell RE, Porteous R, et al. Definition of estrogen receptor pathway critical for estrogen positive feedback to gonadotropin-releasing hormone neurons and fertility. Neuron 2006;52(2):271-280.
1254. Knobil E, Plant TM, Wildt L, et al. Control of the rhesus monkey menstrual cycle: permissive role of the hypothalamic gonadotropin-releasing hormone. Science 1980;207:1371-1373.
1255. Doring GK. Uber die relativ Sterilitat in den Jahren nach der Menarche. Geburtsh Frauenheilkd 1963;23:30-36.
1256. Hansen JW, Hoffman HJ, Ross GT. Monthly gonadotropin cycles in premenarcheal girls. Science 1975;190:161-163.
1257. Winter JSD, Faiman C. Pituitary-gonadal relations in female children and adolescents. Pediatr Res 1973;7:948-953.
1258. Cutler GBJ, Loriaux DL. Andrenarche and its relationship to the onset of puberty. Fed Proc 1980;39:2384-2390.
1259. Sklar CA, Kaplan SL, Grumbach MM. Evidence for dissociation between adrenarche and gonadarche: studies in patients with idiopathic precocious puberty, gonadal dysgenesis, isolated gonadotropin deficiency, and constitutionally delayed growth and adolescence. J Clin Endocrinol Metab 1980;51:548-556.
1260. Hopper BR, Yen SSC. Circulating concentrations of dehydroepiandrosterone and dehydroepiandrosterone sulfate during puberty. J Clin Endocrinol Metab 1975;40:458-461.
1261. Sizonenko PC, Paunier LC. Correlation of plasma dehydroepiandrosterone, testosterone, FSH, and LH with stages of puberty and bone age in normal boys and girls and in patients with Addison's disease or hypogonadism or with premature or late adrenarche. J Clin Endocrinol Metab 1975;41:894-904.
1262. Reiter EO, Fuldauer VG, Root AW. Secretion of the adrenal androgen, dehydroepiandrosterone sulfate, during normal infancy, childhood, and adolescence, in sick infants, and in children with endocrinologic abnormalities. J Pediatr 1977;90:766-770.
1263. Apter D, Pakarinen A, Hammond GL, et al. Adrenocortical function in puberty. serum ACTH, cortisol and dehydroepiandrosterone in girls and boys. Acta Paediatr Scand 1979;68:599-604.
1264. Dhom G. The prepuberal and puberal growth of the adrenal (adrenarche). Beitr Pathol 1973;150:357-377.
1265. Endoh A, Kristiansen SB, Casson PR, et al. The zona reticularis is the site of biosynthesis of dehydroepiandrosterone and dehydroepiandrosterone sulfate in the adult human adrenal cortex resulting from its low expression of 3-8 hydroxysteroid dehydrogenase. J Clin Endocrinol Metab 1996;81:3558-3565.
1266. Kennerson AR, McDonald DA, Adams JB. Dehydroepiandrosterone sulfotransferase localization in human adrenal glands: a light and electron microscope study. J Clin Endocrinol Metab 1983;56:786-790.
1267. Gell JS, Carr BR, Sasano H, et al. Adrenarche results from development of a 3beta-hydroxysteroid dehydrogenase-deficient adrenal reticularis. J Clin Endocrinol Metab 1998;83(10):3695-3701.
1268. Dupont E, Luu-The V, Labrie F, et al. Ontogeny of 3 beta-hydroxysteroid dehydrogenase/delta 5-delta 4 isomerase (3 beta-HSD) in human adrenal gland performed by immunocytochemistry.
1269. Parker Jr CR, Stankovic AK, Falany CN, et al. Immunocytochemical analyses of dehydroepiandrosterone sulfotransferase in cultured human fetal adrenal cells. J Clin Endocrinol Metab 1995;80: 1027-1031.
1270. Khoury EL, Greenspan JS, Greenspan FS. Adrenocortical cells of the zona reticularis normally express HLA-DR antigenic determinants. Am J Pathol 1987;127:580-591.
1271. Marx C, Bornstein SR, Wolkersdorfer GW. Relevance of MHC class II expression as a hallmark for the cellular differentiation in the human adrenal cortex. J Clin Endocrinol Metab 1997;82(9): 3136-3140.
1272. Miller WL, Auchus RJ, Geller DH. The regulation of 17,20 lyase activity. Steroids 1997;62:133-142.
1273. Geller DH, Auchus RJ, Mendonca BB, et al. The genetic and functional basis of isolated 17,20-lyase deficiency. Nat Genet 1997;17(2):201-205.
1274. Zhang L, Rodriguez H, Ohno S, et al. Serine phosphorylation of human P450c17 increases 17,20 lyase activity: implications for adrenarche and for the polycystic ovary syndrome. Proc Natl Acad Sci U S A 1995;92:10619-10623.
1275. Auchus RJ, Miller WL. Molecular modeling of human P450c17 (17alpha-hydroxylase/17,20-lyase): insights into reaction mechanisms and effects of mutations. Mol Endocrinol 1999;13(7): 1169-1182.
1276. Miller WL. The molecular basis of premature adrenarche: an hypothesis. Acta Paediatrica Supplement 1999;88(433): 60-66.
1277. Weber A, Clark AJ, Perry LA, et al. Diminished adrenal androgen secretion in familial glucocorticoid deficiency implicates a significant role for ACTH in the induction of adrenarche. Clin Endocrinol 1997;46(4):431-437.
1278. Ibanez L, Potau N, Marcos MV, et al. Corticotropin-releasing hormone as adrenal androgen secretagogue. Pediatr Res 1999; 46(3):351-353.
1279. Ibanez L, Potau N, Marcos MV, et al. Corticotropin-releasing hormone: a potent androgen secretagogue in girls with hyperandrogenism after precocious pubarche. J Clin Endocrinol Metab 1999;84(12):4602-4606.
1280. Smith R, Mesiano S, Chan EC, et al. Corticotropin-releasing hormone directly and preferentially stimulates dehydroepiandrosterone sulfate secretion by human fetal adrenal cortical cells. J Clin Endocrinol Metab 1998;83(8):2916-2920.
1281. Karteris E, Randeva HS, Grammatopoulos DK, et al. Expression and coupling characteristics of the CRH and orexin type 2 receptors in human fetal adrenals. J Clin Endocrinol Metab 2001;86(9):4512-4519.
1282. Biason-Lauber A, Zachmann M, Schoenle EJ. Effect of leptin on CYP17 enzymatic activities in human adrenal cells: new insight in the onset of adrenarche. Endocrinology 2000;141(4): 1446-1454.
1283. Auchus RJ, Rainey WE. Adrenarche-physiology, biochemistry and human disease. Clin Endocrinol (Oxf) 2004;60(3):288-296.
1284. Remer T, Manz F. Role of nutritional status in the regulation of adrenarche. J Clin Endocrinol Metab 1999;84(11):3936-3944.
1285. Reiter EO, Grumbach MM, Kaplan SL, et al. The response of pituitary gonadotropes to synthetic LRF in children with glucocorticoid-treated congenital adrenal hyperplasia: lack of effect of intrauterine and neonatal androgen excess. J Clin Endocrinol Metab 1975;40:318-325.
1286. Butler GE, McKie M, Ratcliffe SG. The cyclical nature of prepubertal growth [see comments]. Ann Hum Biol 1990;17: 177-198.
1287. Remer T, Manz F. The midgrowth spurt in healthy children is not caused by adrenarche. J Clin Endocrinol Metab 2001;86(9): 4183-4186.
1288. Prader A. Delayed adolescence. Clin Endocrinol Metab 1975;4: 143-155.
1289. Sedlmeyer IL, Palmert MR. Delayed puberty: analysis of a large case series from an academic center. J Clin Endocrinol Metab 2002;87(4):1613-1620.
1290. Counts DR, Pescovitz OH, Barnes KM, et al. Dissociation of adrenarche and gonadarche in precocious puberty and in isolated hypogonadotropic hypogonadism. J Clin Endocrinol Metab 1987;64:1174-1178.
1291. Nathan BM, Sedlmeyer IL, Palmert MR. Impact of body mass index on growth in boys with delayed puberty. J Pediatr Endocrinol Metab 2006;19(8):971-977.
1292. Wu FC, Brown DC, Butler GE, et al. Early morning plasma testosterone is an accurate predictor of imminent pubertal development in prepubertal boys. J Clin Endocrinol Metab 1993;76: 26-31.
1293. Du Caju MV, op de Beeck L, Sys SU, Hagendorens MM, et al. Progressive deceleration in growth as an early sign of delayed puberty in boys. Horm Res 2000;54(3):126-130.
1294. Apter D. Self-image in adolescents with delayed puberty and growth retardation. J Youth Adolesc 1981;10:501-505.

1295. Mussen PH, Jones MC. Self conceptions, motivations and interpersonal attitudes of late and early maturing boys. Child Dev 1957;28:243-256.
1296. Gordon M, Crouthamel C, Post EM. Psychosocial aspects of constitutional short stature: social competence, behavior problems, self esteem and family functioning. J Pediatr 1982;101: 477-480.
1297. Crowne EC, Shalet SM, Wallace WH, et al. Final height in boys with untreated constitutional delay in growth and puberty. Arch Dis Child 1990;65:1109-1112.
1298. Rikken B, Wit JM. Prepubertal height velocity references over a wide age range. Arch Dis Child 1992;67:1277-1280.
1299. Bierich JR. Serum growth hormone levels in provocation tests and during nocturnal spontaneous secretion: a comparative study. Acta Paediatr Scand Suppl 1987;337:48-59.
1300. Saggese G, Cesaretti G, Giannessi N, et al. Stimulated growth hormone (GH) secretion in children with delays in pubertal development before and after the onset of puberty: relationship with peripheral plasma GH-releasing hormone and somatostatin levels. J Clin Endocrinol Metab 1992;74:272-278.
1301. Clayton PE, Shalet SM, Price DA, et al. Growth and growth hormone responses to oxandrolone in boys with constitutional delay of growth and puberty (CDGP). Clin Endocrinol (Oxf) 1988;29:123-130.
1302. Stanhope R, Hindmarsh P, Pringle PJ, et al. Oxandrolone induces a sustained rise in physiological growth hormone secretion in boys with constitutional delay of growth and puberty. Pediatrician 1987;14:183-188.
1303. Loche S, Corda R, Lampis A, et al. The effect of oxandrolone on the growth hormone response to growth hormone releasing hormone in children with constitutional growth delay. Clin Endocrinol 1986;25:195-200.
1304. Stolecke H, Gilessen G. Oxandrolone and spontaneous hGH secretion. Pediatr Res 1984;18:1216 (abstract).
1305. Cara JF, Rosenfield RL. Insulin-like growth factor I and insulin potentiate luteinizing hormone-induced androgen synthesis by rat ovarian theca-interstitial cells. Endocrinology 1988;123: 733-739.
1306. Blethen SL, Gaines S, Weldon V. Comparison of predicted and adult heights in short boys: effect of androgen therapy. Pediatr Res 1984;18(5):467-469.
1307. Crowne EC, Shalet SM, Wallace WH, et al. Final height in girls with untreated constitutional delay in growth and puberty. Eur J Pediatr 1991;150:708-712.
1308. LaFranchi S, Hanna CE, Mandel SH. Constitutional delay of growth: expected versus final adult height. Pediatrics 1991;87: 82-87.
1309. Butenandt O, Bechtold S, Meidert A. Final height in patients with constitutional delay of growth and development from tall statured families. J Pediatr Endocrinol Metab 2005;18(2): 165-169.
1310. Albanese A, Stanhope R. Predictive factors in the determination of final height in boys with constitutional delay of growth and puberty. J Pediatr 1995;126:545-550.
1311. Albanese A, Stanhope R. Does constitutional delayed puberty cause segmental disproportion and short stature? Eur J Pediatr 1993;152:293-296.
1312. Rensonnet C, Kanen F, Coremans C, et al. Pubertal growth as a determinant of adult height in boys with constitutional delay of growth and puberty. Horm Res 1999;51(5):223-229.
1313. Moreira-Andres MN, Canizo FJ, de la Cruz FJ, et al. Bone mineral status in prepubertal children with constitutional delay of growth and puberty. Eur J Endocrinol 1998;139(3):271-275.
1314. Finkelstein JS, Klibanski A, Neer RM. A longitudinal evaluation of bone mineral density in adult men with histories of delayed puberty [see comments]. J Clin Endocrinol Metab 1996;81(3): 1152-1155.
1315. Finkelstein JS, Klibanski A, Neer RM. Evaluation of lumber spine bone mineral density (BMD) using dual energy x-ray absorptiometry (DXA) in 21 young men with histories of constitutionally-delayed puberty [letter]. J Clin Endocrinol Metab 1999;84(9): 3400-3401.
1316. Yap F, Hogler W, Briody J, et al. The skeletal phenotype of men with previous constitutional delay of puberty. J Clin Endocrinol Metab 2004;89(9):4306-4311.
1317. Krupa B, Miazgowski T. Bone mineral density and markers of bone turnover in boys with constitutional delay of growth and puberty. J Clin Endocrinol Metab 2005;90(5):2828-2830.
1318. Carel JC. Can we increase adolescent growth? Eur J Endocrinol 2004;151(Suppl 3):U101-U108.
1319. Yanovski JA, Rose SR, Municchi G, et al. Treatment with a luteinizing hormone-releasing hormone agonist in adolescents with short stature. N Engl J Med 2003;348(10):908-917.
1320. Lee MM. Is treatment with a luteinizing hormone-releasing hormone agonist justified in short adolescents? N Engl J Med 2003;348(10):942-945.
1321. Bierich JR, Nolte K, Drews K, et al. Constitutional delay of growth and adolescence. Results of short-term and long-term treatment with GH. Acta Endocrinol (Copenh) 1992;127:392-396.
1322. Carel JC, Ecosse E, Nicolino M, et al. Adult height after long term treatment with recombinant growth hormone for idiopathic isolated growth hormone deficiency: observational follow up study of the French population based registry. BMJ 2002;325(7355): 70.
1323. Ranke MB, Lindberg A, Martin DD, et al. The mathematical model for total pubertal growth in idiopathic growth hormone (GH) deficiency suggests a moderate role of GH dose. J Clin Endocrinol Metab 2003;88(10):4748-4753.
1324. Volta C, Bernasconi S, Tondi P, et al. Combined treatment with growth hormone and luteinizing hormone releasing hormone-analogue (LHRHa) of pubertal children with familial short stature. J Endocrinol Invest 1993;16:763-767.
1325. Mericq MV, Eggers M, Avila A, et al. Near final height in pubertal growth hormone (GH)-deficient patients treated with GH alone or in combination with luteinizing hormone-releasing hormone analog: results of a prospective, randomized trial. J Clin Endocrinol Metab 2000;85(2):569-573.
1326. Tuvemo T, Jonsson B, Gustafsson J, et al. Final height after combined growth hormone and GnRH analogue treatment in adopted girls with early puberty. Acta Paediatr 2004;93(11): 1456-1462.
1327. Kamp GA, Mul D, Waelkens JJ, et al. A randomized controlled trial of three years growth hormone and gonadotropin-releasing hormone agonist treatment in children with idiopathic short stature and intrauterine growth retardation. J Clin Endocrinol Metab 2001;86(7):2969-2975.
1328. Municchi G, Rose SR, Pescovitz OH, et al. Effect of deslorelin-induced pubertal delay on the growth of adolescents with short stature and normally timed puberty: preliminary results. J Clin Endocrinol Metab 1993;77:1334-1339.
1329. Saggese G, Cesaretti G, Andreani G, et al. Combined treatment with growth hormone and gonadotropin-releasing hormone analogues in children with isolated growth hormone deficiency. Acta Endocrinol (Copenh) 1992;127:307-312.
1330. Carel JC, Hay F, Coutant R, et al. Gonadotropin-releasing hormone agonist treatment of girls with constitutional short stature and normal pubertal development. J Clin Endocrinol Metab 1996; 81:3318-3322.
1331. Yanovski JA, Rose SR, Filmer KM. Deslorelin-induced delay of puberty increases adult height of adolescents with short stature: results of randomized, placebo-controlled trial. Pediatr Res 1996;39:101A (abstract).
1332. Saggese G, Federico G, Barsanti S, et al. Is there a place for combined therapy with GnRH agonist plus growth hormone in improving final height in short statured children? J Pediatr Endocrinol Metab 2000;13(Suppl 1):821-826.
1333. Carel JC. Management of short stature with GnRH agonist and co-treatment with growth hormone: a controversial issue. Mol Cell Endocrinol 2006;254-255:226-233.
1334. Reiter EO. A brief review of the addition of gonadotropin-releasing hormone agonists (GnRH-Ag) to growth hormone (GH) treatment of children with idiopathic growth hormone deficiency: Previously published studies from America. Mol Cell Endocrinol 2006;254-255:221-225.
1335. Finkelstein BS, Imperiale TF, Speroff T, et al. Effect of growth hormone therapy on height in children with idiopathic short stature: a meta-analysis. Arch Pediatr Adolesc Med 2002;156(3): 230-240.
1336. Kaplowitz PB. If gonadotropin-releasing hormone plus growth hormone (GH) really improves growth outcomes in short non-

GH-deficient children, then what? J Clin Endocrinol Metab 2001;86(7):2965-2968.

1337. Finkelstein BS, Silvers JB, Marrero U, et al. Insurance coverage, physician recommendations, and access to emerging treatments: growth hormone therapy for childhood short stature [see comments]. JAMA 1998;279(9):663-668.
1338. Bryant J, Cave C, Milne R. Recombinant growth hormone for idiopathic short stature in children and adolescents. Cochrane Database Syst Rev 2003;(4):CD004440.
1339. Wickman S, Sipila I, Ankarberg-Lindgren C, et al. A specific aromatase inhibitor and potential increase in adult height in boys with delayed puberty: a randomised controlled trial. Lancet 2001;357(9270):1743-1748.
1340. Wickman S, Kajantie E, Dunkel L. Effects of suppression of estrogen action by the p450 aromatase inhibitor letrozole on bone mineral density and bone turnover in pubertal boys. J Clin Endocrinol Metab 2003;88(8):3785-3793.
1341. Dunkel L, Wickman S. Novel treatment of short stature with aromatase inhibitors. J Steroid Biochem Mol Biol 2003;86(3-5): 345-356.
1342. Dunkel L. Use of aromatase inhibitors to increase final height. Mol Cell Endocrinol 2006;254-255:207-216.
1343. Mauras N, Welch S, Rini A, et al. An open label 12-month pilot trial on the effects of the aromatase inhibitor anastrozole in growth hormone (GH)-treated GH deficient adolescent boys. J Pediatr Endocrinol Metab 2004;17(12):1597-1606.
1344. Lin L, Conway GS, Hill NR, et al. A homozygous R262Q mutation in the gonadotropin-releasing hormone receptor (GNRHR) presenting as constitutional delay of growth and puberty with subsequent borderline oligospermia. J Clin Endocrinol Metab 2006;91(12):5117-5121.
1345. Spratt DI, O'Dea LS, Schoenfeld D. Neuroendocrine-gonadal axis in men: frequent sampling of LH, FSH, and testosterone. Am J Physiol 1988;254:E658-E666.
1346. Spratt DI, Carr DH, Merriam GR, et al. The spectrum of abnormal patterns of gonadotropin-releasing hormone secretion in men with idiopathic hypogonadotropic hypogonadism: clinical and laboratory correlations. J Clin Endocrinol 1987;64: 283-291.
1347. Byrne MN, Sessions DG. Nasopharyngeal craniopharyngioma. Case report and literature review. Ann Otol Rhinol Laryngol 1990;99:633-639.
1348. Fukushima T, Hirakawa K, Kimura M. Intraventricular craniopharyngioma: its characteristics in magnetic resonance imaging and successful total removal. Surg Neurol 1990;33:22-27.
1349. DeVile CJ, Grant DB, Hayward RD, et al. Growth and endocrine sequelae of craniopharyngioma. Arch Dis Child 1996;75(2): 108-114.
1350. Banna M. Craniopharyngioma: based on 160 cases. Br J Radiol 1976;49:206-223.
1351. Banna M, Hoare RD, Stanley P. Craniopharyngioma in children. J Pediatr 1973;83:781-785.
1352. Thomsett MJ, Conte FA, Kaplan SL, et al. Endocrine and neurologic outcome in childhood craniopharyngioma: review of effect of treatment in 42 patients. J Pediatr 1980;97:728-735.
1353. De Vries L, Lazar L, Phillip M. Craniopharyngioma: presentation and endocrine sequelae in 36 children. J Pediatr Endocrinol Metab 2003;16(5):703-710.
1354. Baumgartner JE, Wilson CB, Edwards MSB, et al. Management of craniopharyngioma in children. Part 1. The effect of surgery and radiation therapy on outcome magnetic resonance imaging of pituitary and parasellar abnormalities. J Neurosurg 1989;27: 265-281.
1355. Chakeres DW, Curtin A, Ford G. Magnetic resonance imaging of pituitary and parasellar abnormalities. Radiol Clin North Am 1989;27:265-281.
1356. Fahlbusch R, Honegger J, Paulus W, et al. Surgical treatment of craniopharyngiomas: experience with 168 patients. J Neurosurg 1999;90(2):237-250.
1357. Curtis J, Daneman D, Hoffman HJ, et al. The endocrine outcome after surgical removal of craniopharyngiomas. Pediatr Neurosurg 1994;21(Suppl 1):24-27.
1358. Weiss M, Sutton L, Marcial V. The role of radiation therapy in the management of childhood craniopharyngioma. Int J Radiat Oncol Biol Phys 1989;17:1313-1321.
1359. Fischer EG, Welch K, Shillito J Jr. Craniopharyngiomas in children: long term effects of conservative surgical procedures combined with radiation therapy. J Neurosurg 1990;73:534-540.
1360. Warnick RE, Edwards MSB. Pediatric brain tumors. Curr Probl Pediatr 1991;21:129-173.
1361. Paja M, Lucas T, GarcRa-UrRa J. Hypothalamic-pituitary dysfunction in patients with craniopharyngioma. Clin Endocrinol 1995;42:467-473.
1362. De Vile CJ, Grant DB, Hayward RD. Obesity in childhood craniopharyngioma: relation to post-operative hypothalamic damage shown by magnetic resonance imaging. J Clin Endocrinol Metab 1996;81:2734-2737.
1363. Bray GA. Genetic, hypothalamic, and endocrine features of clinical and experimental obesity. Prog Brain Res 1992;93: 333-341.
1364. Preeyasombat C, Bacchetti P, Lazar AA, et al. Racial and etiopathologic dichotomies in insulin hypersecretion and resistance in obese children. J Pediatr 2005;146(4):474-481.
1365. Lustig RH, Greenway F, Velasquez-Mieyer P, et al. A multicenter, randomized, double-blind, placebo-controlled, dose-finding trial of a long-acting formulation of octreotide in promoting weight loss in obese adults with insulin hypersecretion. Int J Obes (Lond) 2006;30(2):331-341.
1366. Ismail D, O'Connell MA, Zacharin MR. Dexamphetamine use for management of obesity and hypersomnolence following hypothalamic injury. J Pediatr Endocrinol Metab 2006;19(2):129-134.
1367. Kalapurakal JA, Goldman S, Hsieh YC, et al. Clinical outcome in children with craniopharyngioma treated with primary surgery and radiotherapy deferred until relapse. Med Pediatr Oncol 2003;40(4):214-218.
1368. Marcus CL, Trescher WH, Halbower AC, et al. Secondary narcolepsy in children with brain tumors. Sleep 2002;25(4): 435-439.
1369. Muller HL, Handwerker G, Wollny B, et al. Melatonin secretion and increased daytime sleepiness in childhood craniopharyngioma patients. J Clin Endocrinol Metab 2002;87(8):3993-3996.
1370. Poretti A, Grotzer MA, Ribi K, et al. Outcome of craniopharyngioma in children: long-term complications and quality of life. Dev Med Child Neurol 2004;46(4):220-229.
1371. Rehman HU, Atkin SL. Sleep disturbances and cardiac arrhythmia after treatment of a craniopharyngioma. J R Soc Med 1999;92(11):585-586.
1372. Tachibana N, Taniike M, Okinaga T, et al. Hypersomnolence and increased REM sleep with low cerebrospinal fluid hypocretin level in a patient after removal of craniopharyngioma. Sleep Med 2005;6(6):567-569.
1373. Muller HL, Handwerker G, Gebhardt U, et al. Melatonin treatment in obese patients with childhood craniopharyngioma and increased daytime sleepiness. Cancer Causes Control 2006;17(4): 583-589.
1374. Cohan P, Foulad A, Esposito F, et al. Symptomatic Rathke's cleft cysts: a report of 24 cases. J Endocrinol Invest 2004;27(10): 943-948.
1375. Monzavi R, Kelly DF, Geffner ME. Rathke's cleft cyst in two girls with precocious puberty. J Pediatr Endocrinol Metab 2004;17(5): 781-785.
1376. Mukherjee S, Louie SG, Campbell M, et al. Ductal growth is impeded in mammary glands of C-neu transgenic mice. Oncogene 2000;19(52):5982-5987.
1377. Dayan AD, Marshall AHE, Miller AA. Atypical teratomas of the pineal and hypothalamus. J Pathol Bacteriol 1966;92:1-28.
1378. Schneider DT, Calaminus G, Koch S, et al. Epidemiologic analysis of 1,442 children and adolescents registered in the German germ cell tumor protocols. Pediatr Blood Cancer 2004;42(2):169-175.
1379. Mootha SL, Barkovich AJ, Grumbach MM, et al. Idiopathic hypothalamic diabetes insipidus, pituitary stalk thickening and the occult intracranial germinoma in children and adolescents. J Clin Endocrinol Metab 1997;82:1362-1367.
1380. Sklar CA, Grumbach MM, Kaplan SL. Hormonal and metabolic abnormalities associated with central nervous system germinoma in children and adolescents and the effect of therapy: report of 10 patients. J Clin Endocrinol Metab 1981;52:9-16.
1381. Kitanaka C, Matsutani M, Sora S, et al. Precocious puberty in a girl with an hCG-secreting suprasellar immature teratoma. Case report. J Neurosurg 1994;81:601-604.

1382. Schmidt F, Penka B, Trauner M, et al. Lack of pineal growth during childhood. J Clin Endocrinol Metab 1995;80:1221-1225.
1383. Dickerman RD, Stevens QE, Steide JA, et al. Precocious puberty associated with a pineal cyst: is it disinhibition of the hypothalamic-pituitary axis? Neuro Endocrinol Lett 2004;25(3):173-175.
1384. Wara WM, Fellows FC, Sheline GE. Radiation therapy for pineal tumors and suprasellar germinomas. Radiology 1977;124:221-223.
1385. Saxena KM. Endocrine manifestations of neurofibromatosis in children. Am J Dis Child 1970;120:265-272.
1386. Fienman NL, Yakovac WC. Neurofibromatosis in childhood. J Pediatr 1970;76:339-346.
1387. Kibirige MS, Birch JM, Campbell RH. A review of astrocytoma in childhood. Pediatr Hematol Oncol 1989;6:319-329.
1388. De Menis E, Visentin A, Billeci D, et al. Pituitary adenomas in childhood and adolescence. Clinical analysis of 10 cases. J Endocrinol Invest 2001;24(2):92-97.
1389. Mindermann T, Wilson CB. Pediatric pituitary adenomas. Neurosurgery 1995;36:259-268.
1390. Cannavo S, Venturino M, Curto L, et al. Clinical presentation and outcome of pituitary adenomas in teenagers. Clin Endocrinol (Oxf) 2003;58(4):519-527.
1391. Job JC, Chaussain JL, Toublanc JE. Delayed puberty. In Grumbach MM, Sizonenko PC, Aubert ML, eds. Control of the Onset of Puberty. Baltimore: Williams & Wilkins, 1990:588-619.
1392. Cheyne KL, Lightner ES, Comerci GD. Bromocriptine-unresponsive prolactin macroadenoma in a prepubertal female. J Adolesc Health Care 1988;9:331-334.
1393. Patton ML, Woolf PD. Hyperprolactinemia and delayed puberty: a report of three cases and their response to therapy. Pediatrics 1983;71:572-575.
1394. Mahachoklertwattana P, Conte FA, Grumbach MM, et al. Prolactinomas in children and adolescents: affect on pubertal onset and long term outcome following selective transsphenoidal adenomectomy. unpublished data, 1997.
1395. Koenig MP, Zuppinger K, Liechti B. Hyperprolactinemia as a cause of delayed puberty: successful treatment with bromocriptine. J Clin Endocrinol Metab 1977;45:825-828.
1396. Knoepfelmacher M, Gomes MC, Melo ME, et al. Pituitary apoplexy during therapy with cabergoline in an adolescent male with prolactin-secreting macroadenoma. Pituitary 2004;7(2): 83-87.
1397. Yuen YP, Lai JP, Au KM, et al. Macroprolactin-a cause of pseudo-hyperprolactinaemia. Hong Kong Med J 2003;9(2):119-121.
1398. Willman CL, Busque L, Griffith BB. Langerhans'-cell histiocytosis (histiocytosis X)—a clonal proliferative disease. N Engl J Med 1994;331:154-160.
1399. Herzog KM, Tubbs RR. Langerhans cell histiocytosis. Adv Anat Pathol 1998;5(6):347-358.
1400. Vogel JM, Vogel P. Idiopathic histiocytosis: a discussion of eosinophilic granuloma, the Hand-Sch[umlaut-u]ller-Christian syndrome, and the Letterer-Siwe syndrome. Semin Hematol 1972;9:349-364.
1401. Sims DG. Histocytosis X: follow-up of 43 cases. Arch Dis Child 1977;52:433-440.
1402. Egeler RM, Nesbit ME. Langerhans cell histiocytosis and other disorders of monocyte-histiocyte lineage. Crit Rev Oncol Hematol 1995;18:9-35.
1403. Maghnie M, Cosi G, Genovese E, et al. Central diabetes insipidus in children and young adults. N Engl J Med 2000;343(14): 998-1007.
1404. Nanduri VR, Bareille P, Pritchard J, et al. Growth and endocrine disorders in multisystem Langerhans' cell histiocytosis. Clin Endocrinol (Oxf) 2000;53(4):509-515.
1405. Kaltsas GA, Powles TB, Evanson J, et al. Hypothalamo-pituitary abnormalities in adult patients with Langerhans cell histiocytosis: clinical, endocrinological, and radiological features and response to treatment. J Clin Endocrinol Metab 2000;85(4): 1370-1376.
1406. Willis B, Ablin A, Weinberg V, et al. Disease course and late sequelae of Langerhans' cell histiocytosis: 25-year experience at the University of California, San Francisco. J Clin Oncol 1996;14(7):2073-2082.
1407. Gadner H, Grois N, Arico M, et al. A randomized trial of treatment for multisystem Langerhans' cell histiocytosis. J Pediatr 2001; 138(5):728-734.
1408. Lavin PT, Osband ME. Evaluating the role of therapy in histiocytosis X: clinical studies, staging, and scoring. Hematol Oncol Clin North Am 1987;1:35-47.
1409. Egeler RM, D'Angio GJ. Langerhans cell histiocytosis. J Pediatr 1995;127:1-11.
1410. Asherson RA, Jackson WPU, Lewis B. Abnormalities of development associated with hypothalamic calcification after tuberculous meningitis. Br Med J 1965;2:839-843.
1411. Fiedler R, Krieger DT. Endocrine disturbances in patients with congenital aqueductal stenosis. Acta Endocrinol 1975;80: 1-13.
1412. Cholley F, Trivin C, Sainte-Rose C, et al. Disorders of growth and puberty in children with non-tumoral hydrocephalus. J Pediatr Endocrinol Metab 2001;14(3):319-327.
1413. Richards GE, Wara WM, Grumbach MM, et al. Delayed onset of hypopituitarism: sequelae of therapeutic irradiation of central nervous system, eye, and middle ear tumors. J Pediatr 1976;89: 553-559.
1414. Schmiegelow M, Lassen S, Poulsen HS, et al. Gonadal status in male survivors following childhood brain tumors. J Clin Endocrinol Metab 2001;86(6):2446-2452.
1415. Gurney JG, Kadan-Lottick NS, Packer RJ, et al. Endocrine and cardiovascular late effects among adult survivors of childhood brain tumors: Childhood Cancer Survivor Study. Cancer 2003;97(3):663-673.
1416. Shalet SM, Crowne EC, Didi MA, et al. Irradiation-induced growth failure. Baillieres Clin Endocrinol Metab 1992;6:513-526.
1417. Oberfield SE, Soranno D, Nirenberg A, et al. Age at onset of puberty following high-dose central nervous system radiation therapy. Arch Pediatr Adolesc Med 1996;150:589-592.
1418. Hokken-Koelega AC, van Doorn JW, Hahlen KST, et al. Long-term effects of treatment for acute lymphoblastic leukemia with and without cranial irradiation on growth and puberty: a comparative study. Pediatr Res 1993;33:577-582.
1419. Stubberfield TG, Byrne GC, Jones TW. Growth and growth hormone secretion after treatment for acute lymphoblastic leukemia in childhood. 18-Gy versus 24-Gy cranial irradiation. J Pediatr Hematol Oncol 1995;17:167-171.
1420. Bath LE, Anderson RA, Critchley HO, Kelnar CJ, Wallace WH. Hypothalamic-pituitary-ovarian dysfunction after prepubertal chemotherapy and cranial irradiation for acute leukaemia. Hum Reprod 2001;16(9):1838-1844.
1421. Xu W, Janss A, Packer RJ, et al. Endocrine outcome in children with medulloblastoma treated with 18 Gy of craniospinal radiation therapy. Neuro-oncol 2004;6(2):113-118.
1422. Byrne J, Fears TR, Mills JL, et al. Fertility in women treated with cranial radiotherapy for childhood acute lymphoblastic leukemia. Pediatr Blood Cancer 2004;42(7):589-597.
1423. Frisk P, Arvidson J, Gustafsson J, et al. Pubertal development and final height after autologous bone marrow transplantation for acute lymphoblastic leukemia. Bone Marrow Transplant 2004; 33(2):205-210.
1424. Duffner PK. Long-term effects of radiation therapy on cognitive and endocrine function in children with leukemia and brain tumors. Neurologist 2004;10(6):293-310.
1425. Rose SR, Schreiber RE, Kearney NS, et al. Hypothalamic dysfunction after chemotherapy. J Pediatr Endocrinol Metab 2004; 17(1):55-66.
1426. Seminara SB, Hayes FJ, Crowley WJ. Gonadotropin-releasing hormone deficiency in the human (idiopathic hypogonadotropic hypogonadism and Kallmann's syndrome): pathophysiological and genetic considerations. Endocr Rev 1998;19(5):521-539.
1427. Seminara SB, Hayes FJ, Crowley WFJ. Gonadotropin-releasing hormone deficiency in the human (idiopathic hypogonadotropic hypogonadism and Kallmann's syndrome): pathophysiological and genetic considerations. Endocr Rev 1999; 19(5):521-539.
1428. Layman LC. Mutations in human gonadotropin genes and their physiologic significance in puberty and reproduction. Fertility and Sterility 1999;71(2):201-218.
1429. Seminara SB, Oliveira LM, Beranova M, et al. Genetics of hypogonadotropic hypogonadism. J Endocrinol Invest 2000;23(9): 560-565.
1430. Weinstein RL, Reitz RE. Pituitary-testicular responsiveness in male hypogonadotropic hypogonadism. J Clin Invest 1974;53: 408-415.

1431. Van Dop C, Burstein S, Conte FA, et al. Isolated gonadotropin deficiency in boys: clinical characteristics and growth. J Pediatr 1987;111:684-692.
1432. Pitteloud N, Hayes FJ, Boepple PA, et al. The role of prior pubertal development, biochemical markers of testicular maturation, and genetics in elucidating the phenotypic heterogeneity of idiopathic hypogonadotropic hypogonadism. J Clin Endocrinol Metab 2002;87(1):152-160.
1433. Van Dop C, Burstein S, Conte FA, et al. Isolated gonadotropin deficiency in boys: clinical characteristics and growth. J Pediatr 1987;111(5):684-692.
1434. Uriarte MM, Baron J, Garcia HB, et al. The effect of pubertal delay on adult height in men with isolated hypogonadotropic hypogonadism [published erratum appears in J Clin Endocrinol Metab 1992 Oct;75(4):1009]. J Clin Endocrinol Metab 1992;74: 436-440.
1435. Kallmann F, Schonfeld WA, Barrera SW. Genetic aspects of primary eunuchoidism. Am J Ment Defic 1944;48:203-236.
1436. Munoz A, Dieguez E. A plea for proper recognition: the syndrome of Maestre de San Juan-Kallman. AJNR Am J Neuroradiol 1997;18(7):1395-1396.
1437. Wortsman J, Hughes LF. Case report: olfactory function in a fertile eunuch with Kallmann syndrome. Am J Med Sci 1996;311: 135-138.
1438. Doty RL, Shaman P, Dann M. The development of the University of Pennsylvania smell I dentification test: a standardized micro-encapsulated test of olfactory function. Physiol Behav 1984; 32:501-507.
1439. Bauman A. Markedly delayed puberty or Kallmann's syndrome variant. J Androl 1986;7(4):224-227.
1440. Quinton R, Cheow HK, Tymms DJ, et al. Kallmann's syndrome: is it always for life? Clin Endocrinol 1999;50(4):481-485.
1441. Wu FC, Butler GE, Kelnar CJ, et al. Patterns of pulsatile luteinizing hormone and follicle-stimulating hormone secretion in prepubertal (midchildhood) boys and girls and patients with idiopathic hypogonadotropic hypogonadism (Kallmann's syndrome): a study using an ultrasensitive time-resolved immunofluorometric assay. J Clin Endocrinol Metab 1991;72:1229-1237.
1442. Santen RJ, Paulsen CA. Hypogonadotropic eunuchoidism. I. Clinical study of the mode of inheritance. J Clin Endocrinol Metab 1973;36:47-54.
1443. Massin N, Pecheux C, Eloit C, et al. X chromosome-linked Kallmann syndrome: clinical heterogeneity in three siblings carrying an intragenic deletion of the KAL-1 gene. J Clin Endocrinol Metab 2003;88(5):2003-2008.
1444. Prager D, Braunstein GD. Editorial: X-chromosome-linked Kallmann's syndrome: pathology at the molecular level. J Clin Endocrinol Metab 1993;76:824-826.
1445. Kirk JMW, Grant DB, Besser GM, et al. Unilateral renal aplasia in X-linked Kallmann's syndrome. Clin Genet 1994;46:260-262.
1446. Dunek A, Heye B, Schroedter R. Cortically evoked motor responses in patients with Xp22.3-linked Kallmann's syndrome and in female gene carriers. Am J Neuroradiol 1992;31:299-304.
1447. Ballabio A, Bardoni B, Carrozzo R, et al. Contiguous gene syndromes due to deletions in the distal short arm of the human X chromosome. Proc Natl Acad Sci U S A 1989;86:10001-10005.
1447a. Pitteloud N, Quinton R, Pearce S, et al. Digenic mutations account for variable phenotypes in idiopathic hypogonadotropic hypogonadism. J Clin Invest 2007;117:457-463.
1447b. Pitteloud N, Cole LW, Sidis Y, Plummer L, et al. Mutations in the gene for prokinectin 2 receptor (PROKR2) cause both Kallmann's syndrome (KS) and normosmic idiopathic hypogonadotropic hypogonadism (nIHH). Endo 07 (OR8-3).
1448. Hardelin JP, Julliard AK, Moniot B, et al. Anosmin-1 is a regionally restricted component of basement membranes and interstitial matrices during organogenesis: implications for the developmental anomalies of X chromosome-linked Kallmann syndrome. Dev Dyn 1999;215(1):26-44.
1448a. Gonzalez-Martinez D, Kim SH, Hu Y, et al. Anosmin-1 modulates fibroblast growth factor receptor 1 signaling in human gonadotropin-releasing hormone olfactory neuroblasts through a heparan sulfate-dependent mechanism. J Neurosci 2004; 24:10384-10392.
1449. Duke VM, Winyard PJ, Thorogood P, et al. KAL, a gene mutated in Kallmann's syndrome, is expressed in the first trimester of human development. Mol Cell Endocrinol 1995;110(1-2):73-79.
1450. Legouis R, Hardelin J-P, Levilliers J, et al. The candidate gene for the X-linked Kallmann syndrome encodes a protein related to adhesion molecules. Cell 1991;67:423-435.
1451. Quinton R, Duke VM, de Zoysa PA, et al. The neuroradiology of Kallmann's syndrome: a genotypic and phenotypic analysis. J Clin Endocrinol Metab 1996;81:3010-3017.
1452. Hardelin JP. Kallmann syndrome: towards molecular pathogenesis. Mol Cell Endocrinol 2001;179(1-2):75-81.
1453. Sato N, Katsumata N, Kagami M, et al. Clinical assessment and mutation analysis of Kallmann syndrome 1 (KAL1) and fibroblast growth factor receptor 1 (FGFR1, or KAL2) in five families and 18 sporadic patients. J Clin Endocrinol Metab 2004;89(3):1079-1088.
1454. Cohen-Salmon M, Tronche F, del Castillo, et al. Characterization of the promotor of the human KAL gene responsible for the X-chromosome-linked Kallmann syndrome. Gene 1995;164:235-242.
1455. Maya-Nuanez G, Torres L, Ulloa-Aguirre A, et al. An atypical contiguous gene syndrome: molecular studies in a family with X-linked Kallmann's syndrome and X-linked ichthyosis. Clin Endocrinol 1999;50(2):157-162.
1456. Oliveira LM, Seminara SB, Beranova M, et al. The importance of autosomal genes in Kallmann syndrome: genotype-phenotype correlations and neuroendocrine characteristics. J Clin Endocrinol Metab 2001;86(4):1532-1538.
1457. Lee SH, Han JH, Cho SW, et al. Mutation analysis of the KAL gene in female patients with gonadotropin-releasing hormone deficiency. Yonsei Med J 2004;45(1):107-112.
1458. Santen RJ, Paulsen CA. Hypogonadotropic eunuchoidism. II. Gonadal responsiveness to exogenous gonadotropins. J Clin Endocrinol Metab 1973;36:55-63.
1459. Merriam GR, Beitins IZ, Bode HH. Father to son transmission of hypogonadism with anosmia. Am J Dis Child 1977;131:1216-1219.
1460. Dode C, Levilliers J, Dupont JM, et al. Loss-of-function mutations in FGFR1 cause autosomal dominant Kallmann syndrome. Nat Genet 2003;33(4):463-465.
1461. Pitteloud N, Acierno JS Jr, Meysing AU, et al. Reversible Kallmann syndrome, delayed puberty, and isolated anosmia occurring in a single family with a mutation in the fibroblast growth factor receptor 1 gene. J Clin Endocrinol Metab 2005;90(3):1317-1322.
1462. Zenaty D, Bretones P, Lambe C, et al. Paediatric phenotype of Kallmann syndrome due to mutations of fibroblast growth factor receptor 1 (FGFR1). Mol Cell Endocrinol 2006;254-255:78-83.
1463. White BJ, Rogol AD, Brown KS, et al. The syndrome of anosmia with hypogonadotropic hypogonadism: a genetic study of 18 new families and a review. Am J Med Genet 1983;15:417-435.
1464. Hipkin LJ, Casson IF, Davis JC. Identical twins discordant for Kallmann's syndrome. J Med Genet 1990;27:198-199.
1465. Truwit CL, Barkovich AJ, Grumbach MM, et al. Magnetic resonance imaging of Kallmann syndrome, a genetic disorder of neuronal migration affecting the olfactory and genital systems. Am J Neuroradiol 1993;14:827-838.
1466. Quinton R, Duke VM, de Zoysa PA, et al. The neuroradiology of Kallmann's syndrome: a genotypic and phenotypic analysis [published erratum appears in J Clin Endocrinol Metab 1996 Oct;81(10):3614]. J Clin Endocrinol Metab 1996;81(8):3010-3017.
1467. Klingmhller D, Dewes W, Krahe T, et al. Magnetic resonance imaging of the brain in patients with anosmia and hypothalamic hypogonadism (Kallmann's syndrome). J Clin Endocrinol Metab 1987;65:581-584.
1468. Pinto G, Abadie V, Mesnage R, et al. CHARGE syndrome includes hypogonadotropic hypogonadism and abnormal olfactory bulb development. J Clin Endocrinol Metab 2005;90(10):5621-5626.
1468a. Azoulay R, Fallet-Bianco C, Garel C, et al. MRI of the olfactory bulbs and sulci in human fetuses. Pediatr Radiol 2006; 36:97-107.
1469. Layman LC. Genetics of human hypogonadotropic hypogonadism. Am J Med Genet 1999;89(4):240-248.
1470. Achermann JC, Weiss J, Lee EJ, et al. Inherited disorders of the gonadotropin hormones. Mol Cell Endocrinol 2001;179(1-2): 89-96.
1471. de Roux N, Milgrom E. Inherited disorders of GnRH and gonadotropin receptors. Mol Cell Endocrinol 2001;179(1-2):83-87.
1472. Seeburg PH, Mason AJ, Steward TA, et al. The mammalian GnRH gene and its pivotal role in reproduction. Recent Prog Horm Res 1987;43:69-107.

1473. de Roux N, Genin E, Carel JC, et al. Hypogonadotropic hypogonadism due to loss of function of the KiSS1-derived peptide receptor GPR54. Proc Natl Acad Sci U S A 2003;100(19):10972-10976.
1474. Cerrato F, Seminara SB. Human genetics of GPR54. Rev Endocr Metab Disord 2007;8:47-55.
1474a. Semple RK, Achermann JC, Ellery J, et al. Two novel missense mutations in g protein-coupled receptor 54 in a patient with hypogonadotropic hypogonadism. J Clin Endocrinol Metab 2005;90(3):1849-1855.
1475. Miura K, Acierno JS Jr, Seminara SB. Characterization of the human nasal embryonic LHRH factor gene, NELF, and a mutation screening among 65 patients with idiopathic hypogonadotropic hypogonadism (IHH). J Hum Genet 2004;49(5):265-268.
1476. Bo-Abbas Y, Acierno JS Jr, Shagoury JK, et al. Autosomal recessive idiopathic hypogonadotropic hypogonadism: genetic analysis excludes mutations in the gonadotropin-releasing hormone (GnRH) and GnRH receptor genes. J Clin Endocrinol Metab 2003;88(6):2730-2737.
1477. de Roux N, Young J, Misrahi M, et al. A family with hypogonadotropic hypogonadism and mutations in the gonadotropin-releasing hormone receptor. N Engl J Med 1997;337(22):1597-1602.
1478. de Roux N, Young J, Misrahi M, et al. Loss of function mutations of the GnRH receptor: a new cause of hypogonadotropic hypogonadism. J Pediatr Endocrinol Metab 1999;12(Suppl 1): 267-275.
1479. de Roux N, Young J, Brailly-Tabard S, et al. The same molecular defects of the gonadotropin-releasing hormone receptor determine a variable degree of hypogonadism in affected kindred. J Clin Endocrinol Metab 1999;84(2):567-572.
1480. Beranova M, Oliveira LM, Bedecarrats GY, et al. Prevalence, phenotypic spectrum, and modes of inheritance of gonadotropin-releasing hormone receptor mutations in idiopathic hypogonadotropic hypogonadism. J Clin Endocrinol Metab 2001; 86(4):1580-1588.
1481. Kottler ML, Chauvin S, Lahlou N, et al. A new compound heterozygous mutation of the gonadotropin-releasing hormone receptor (L314X, Q106R) in a woman with complete hypogonadotropic hypogonadism: chronic estrogen administration amplifies the gonadotropin defect. J Clin Endocrinol Metab 2000;85(9): 3002-3008.
1482. Pralong FP, Gomez F, Castillo E, et al. Complete hypogonadotropic hypogonadism associated with a novel inactivating mutation of the gonadotropin-releasing hormone receptor. J Clin Endocrinol Metab 1999;84(10):3811-3816.
1483. Bedecarrats GY, Linher KD, Janovick JA, et al. Four naturally occurring mutations in the human GnRH receptor affect ligand binding and receptor function. Mol Cell Endocrinol 2003; 205(1-2):51-64.
1484. Janovick JA, Maya-Nunez G, Conn PM. Rescue of hypogonadotropic hypogonadism-causing and manufactured GnRH receptor mutants by a specific protein-folding template: misrouted proteins as a novel disease etiology and therapeutic target. J Clin Endocrinol Metab 2002;87(7):3255-3262.
1485. Maya-Nunez G, Janovick JA, Ulloa-Aguirre A, et al. Molecular basis of hypogonadotropic hypogonadism: restoration of mutant (E(90)K) GnRH receptor function by a deletion at a distant site. J Clin Endocrinol Metab 2002;87(5):2144-2149.
1486. Leanos-Miranda A, Janovick JA, Conn PM. Receptor-misrouting: an unexpectedly prevalent and rescuable etiology in gonadotropin-releasing hormone receptor-mediated hypogonadotropic hypogonadism. J Clin Endocrinol Metab 2002;87(10):4825-4828.
1487. Pitteloud N, Boepple PA, DeCruz S, et al. The fertile eunuch variant of idiopathic hypogonadotropic hypogonadism: spontaneous reversal associated with a homozygous mutation in the gonadotropin-releasing hormone receptor. J Clin Endocrinol Metab 2001;86(6):2470-2475.
1488. Seminara SB, Beranova M, Oliveira LM, et al. Successful use of pulsatile gonadotropin-releasing hormone (GnRH) for ovulation induction and pregnancy in a patient with GnRH receptor mutations. J Clin Endocrinol Metab 2000;85(2):556-562.
1489. Bin-Abbas B, Conte FA, Grumbach MM, et al. Congenital hypogonadotropic hypogonadism and micropenis: effect of testosterone treatment on adult penile size why sex reversal is not indicated. Journal of Pediatrics 1999;134(5):579-583.
1490. Zanarla E, Muscatelli F, Bardoni B, et al. An unusual member of the nuclear hormone receptor superfamily responsible for X-linked adrenal hypoplasia congenita. Nature 1994;372:635-641.
1491. Muscatelli F, Strom TM, Walker AP, et al. Mutations in the dax1 gene give rise to both X-linked adrenal hypoplasia congenita and hypogonadotropic hypogonadism. Nature 1994;372:672-676.
1492. Guo W, Burris TP, Zhang Y-H, et al. Genomic sequence of the DAX1 gene: an orphan nuclear receptor responsible for X-linked adrenal hypoplasia congenita and hypogonadotropic hypogonadism. J Clin Endocrinol Metab 1996;81:2481-2486.
1493. Burris TP, Guo W, McCabe ERB. The gene responsible for adrenal hypoplasia congenita, dax1, encodes a nuclear hormone receptor that defines a new class within the superfamily. Rec Prog Horm Res 1996;51:241-260.
1494. McCabe ERB. Adrenal hypoplasias and aplasias. In Scriver CR, Beaudet AL, Sly WS, et al., eds. The Metabolic and Molecular Basis of Inherited Diseases. New York: McGraw Hill, 2001: 4263-4274.
1495. Ito M, Yu R, Jameson JL. dax1 inhibits sf1-mediated transactivation via a carboxy-terminal domain that is deleted in adrenal hypoplasia congenita. Mol Cell Biol 1997;17(3):1476-1483.
1496. Lalli E, Bardoni B, Zazopoulos E, et al. A transcriptional silencing domain in dax1 whose mutation causes adrenal hypoplasia congenita. Mol Endocrinol 1997;11(13):1950-1960.
1497. Burris TP, Guo W, Le T, McCabe ERB. Identification of a putative steroidogenic fa tor-1 response element in the dax1 promoter. Biochem Biophys Res Communications 1995;214:576-581.
1498. Vilain E, Guo W, Zhang YH, et al. DAX1 gene expression upregulated by steroidogenic factor 1 in an adrenocortical carcinoma cell line. Biochem Mol Med 1997;61(1):1-8.
1499. Ingraham HA, Lala DS, Ikeda Y, et al. The nuclear receptor steroidogenic factor 1 acts at multiple levels of the reproductive axis. Genes Dev 1994;8:2302-2312.
1500. Prader A, Zachmann M, Illig KR. Luteinizing hormone deficiency in hereditary congenital adrenal hypoplasia. J Pediatr 1975; 86:421-422.
1501. Kruse K, Sippell WG, Schnakenburg KV. Hypogonadism in congenital adrenal hypoplasia: evidence for a hypothalamic origin. J Clin Endocrinol Metab 1984;58:12-17.
1502. Hay ID, Smail PJ, Forsyth CC. Familial cytomegalic adrenocortical hypoplasia: an X-linked syndrome of pubertal failure. Arch Dis Child 1981;56:715-721.
1503. Kikuchi K, Kaji M, Momoi T, et al. Failure to induce puberty in a man with X-linked congenital adrenal hypoplasia and hypogonadotropic hypogonadism by pulsatile administration of low-dose gonadotropin-releasing hormone. Acta Endocrinol (Copenh) 1987;114:153-160.
1504. Kletter GB, Gorski JL, Kelch RP. Congenital adrenal hypoplasia and isolated gonadotropin deficiency. Trends Endocrinol Metab 1991;2:123-128.
1505. Achermann JC, Wen-xia G, Kotlar J, et.al. Mutational Analysis of DAX1 in patients with hypogonadotropic hypogonadism or pubertal delay. J Clin Endocrinol Metab 1999;84:4497-4500.
1506. Uttley WS. Familial congenital adrenal hypoplasia. Arch Dis Child 1968;43:724-730.
1507. Seltzer WK, Firminger H, Klein L, et al. Adrenal dysfunction in glycerol kinase deficiency. Biochem Med 1985;33:189-199.
1508. Reutens AT, Achermann JC, Ito M, et al. Clinical and functional effects of mutations in the dax1 gene in patients with adrenal hypoplasia congenita. J Clin Endocrinol Metab 1999;84(2): 504-511.
1509. Peter M, Viemann M, Partsch CJ, et al. Congenital adrenal hypoplasia: clinical spectrum, experience with hormonal diagnosis, and report on new point mutations of the dax1 gene. J Clin Endocrinol Metab 1998;83(8):2666-2674.
1510. Mantovani G, Ozisik G, Achermann JC, et al. Hypogonadotropic hypogonadism as a presenting feature of late-onset X-linked adrenal hypoplasia congenita. J Clin Endocrinol Metab 2002; 87(1):44-48.
1511. Tabarin A, Achermann JC, Recan D, et al. A novel mutation in DAX1 causes delayed-onset adrenal insufficiency and incomplete hypogonadotropic hypogonadism. J Clin Invest 2000;105(3): 321-328.

1512. Merke DP, Tajima T, Baron J, et al. Hypogonadotropic hypogonadism in a female caused by an X-linked recessive mutation in the DAX1 gene. N Engl J Med 1999;340(16):1248-1252.
1513. McCabe ER. Editorial: Vulnerability within a robust complex system-dax1 mutations and steroidogenic axis development. J Clin Endocrinol Metab 2002;87(1):41-43.
1514. Seminara SB, Achermann JC, Genel M, et al. X-linked adrenal hypoplasia congenita: a mutation in DAX1 expands the phenotypic spectrum in males and females. J Clin Endocrinol Metab 1999;84(4501):4509.
1515. Guo W, Mason JS, Stone Jr CG, et al. Diagnosis of X-linked adrenal hypoplasia congenita by mutation analysis of the DAX1 gene. JAMA 1995;274:324-330.
1516. Yanase T, Takayanagi R, Oba K, et al. New mutations of dax1 genes in two Japanese patients with X-linked congenital adrenal hypoplasia and hypogonadotropic hypogonadism. J Clin Endocrinol Metab 1996;81:530-535.
1517. Phelan JK, McCabe ER. Mutations in NR0B1 (DAX1) and NR5A1 (SF1) responsible for adrenal hypoplasia congenita. Hum Mutat 2001;18(6):472-487.
1518. Habiby RL, Boepple P, Nachtigall L, et al. Adrenal hypoplasia congenita with hypogonadotropic hypogonadism. Evidence that dax1 mutations lead to combined hypothalamic and pituitary defects in gonadotropin production. J Clin Invest 1996;98: 1055-1062.
1519. Guo W, Burris TP, McCabe ERB. Expression of dax1, the gene responsible for X-linked adrenal hypoplasia congenita and hypogonadotropic hypogonadism, in the hypothalamic-pituitary-adrenal/gonadal axis. Biochem Mol Med 1995;56:8-13.
1520. Takahashi T, Shoji Y, et al. Active hypothalamic-pituitary-gonadal axis in an infant with X-linked adrenal hypoplasia congenita. J Pediatr 1997;130:485-488.
1521. Kaiserman KB, Nakamoto JM, Geffner ME, et al. Minipuberty of infancy and adolescent pubertal function in adrenal hypoplasia congenita. Journal of Pediatrics 1998;133(2):300-302.
1522. Takahashi I, Takahashi T, Shoji Y, et al. Prolonged activation of the hypothalamus-pituitary-gonadal axis in a child with X-linked adrenal hypoplasia congenita. Clin Endocrinol (Oxf) 2000;53(1): 127-129.
1523. Domenice S, Latronico AC, Brito VN, et al. Adrenocorticotropin-dependent precocious puberty of testicular origin in a boy with X-linked adrenal hypoplasia congenita due to a novel mutation in the DAX1 gene. J Clin Endocrinol Metab 2001;86(9): 4068-4071.
1524. Argente J, Ozisik G, Pozo J, et al. A novel single base deletion at codon 434 (1301delT) of the DAX1 gene associated with prepubertal testis enlargement. Mol Genet Metab 2003;78(1): 79-81.
1525. Worley KC, Ellison KA, Zhang Y-H, et al. Yeast artificial chromosome cloning in the glycerol kinase and adrenal hypoplasia congenita region of Xp21. Genomics 1993;16:407-416.
1526. Talaban R, Sellick GS, Spendlove HE, et al. Inherited pericentric inversion (X)(p11.4q11.2) associated with delayed puberty and obesity in two brothers. Cytogenet Genome Res 2005;109(4): 480-484.
1527. Jackson RS, Creemers JW, Ohagi S, et al. Obesity and impaired prohormone processing associated with mutations in the human prohormone convertase 1 gene. Nat Genet 1997;16(3): 303-306.
1528. O'Rahilly S, Gray H, Humphreys PJ, et al. Brief report: impaired processing of prohormones associated with abnormalities of glucose homeostasis and adrenal function. N Engl J Med 1995;333(21):1386-1390.
1529. Jackson RS, Creemers JW, Farooqi IS, et al. Small-intestinal dysfunction accompanies the complex endocrinopathy of human proprotein convertase 1 deficiency. J Clin Invest 2003;112(10): 1550-1560.
1530. Smals AGH, Kloppenborg PWC, Van Haelst UJG, et al. Fertile eunuch syndrome versus classic hypogonadotrophic hypogonadism. Acta Endocrinol 1978;87:389-399.
1531. Weiss J, Axelrod L, Whitcomb RW, et al. Hypogonadism caused by a single amino acid substitution in the beta subunit of luteinizing hormone. N Engl J Med 1992;326:179-183.
1532. Lovinger RD, Kaplan SL, Grumbach MM. Congenital hypopituitarism associated with neonatal hypoglycemia and microphallus: four cases secondary to hypothalamic hormone deficiencies. J Pediatr 1975;87(6 PT 2):1171-1181.
1533. Layman LC, Lee EJ, Peak DB, et al. Delayed puberty and hypogonadism caused by mutations in the follicle-stimulating hormone beta-subunit gene. N Engl J Med 1997;337(9):607-611.
1534. Matthews C, Chatterjee VK. Isolated deficiency of follicle-stimulating hormone re-revisited. N Engl J Med 1997;337(9):642.
1535. Matthews CH, Borgato S, Beck-Peccoz P, et al. Primary amenorrhoea and infertility due to a mutation in the beta-subunit of follicle-stimulating hormone. Nat Genet 1993;5(1):83-86.
1536. Rabin D, Spitz I, Bercovici B, et al. Isolated deficiency of follicle-stimulating hormone: clinical and laboratory features. N Engl J Med 1972;287:1313-1317.
1537. Lindstedt G, Nystrom E, Matthews C, et al. Follitropin (FSH) deficiency in an infertile male due to FSHbeta gene mutation. A syndrome of normal puberty and virilization but underdeveloped testicles with azoospermia, low FSH but high lutropin and normal serum testosterone concentrations. Clin Chem Lab Med 1998; 36(8):663-665.
1538. Phillip M, Arbelle JE, Segev Y, et al. Male hypogonadism due to a mutation in the gene for the beta-subunit of follicle-stimulating hormone. N Engl J Med 1998;338(24):1729-1732.
1539. Hanna CE, Mandel SH, LaFranchi SH. Puberty in the syndrome of septo-optic dysplasia. Am J Dis Child 1989;143:186-189.
1540. Kaplan SL, Grumbach MM, Hoyt WF. A syndrome of hypopituitary dwarfism, hypoplasia of optic nerves, and malformation of prosencephalon: report of 6 patients. Pediatr Res 1970;4:480-481 (abstract).
1541. Badawy SZ, Pisarska MD, Wasenko JJ, et al. Congenital hypopituitarism as part of suprasellar dysplasia. A case report. J Reprod Med 1994;39:643-648.
1542. Wales JK, Quarrell OW. Evidence for possible Mendelian inheritance of septo-optic dysplasia. Acta Paediatr 1996;85(3): 391-392.
1543. Dattani MT, Martinez-Barbera JP, Thomas PQ, et al. Mutations in the homeobox gene HESX1/Hesx1 associated with septo-optic dysplasia in human and mouse. Nat Genet 1998;19(2):125-133.
1544. Parks JS, Brown MR, Hurley DL, et al. Heritable disorders of pituitary development. J Clin Endocrinol Metab 1999;84(12): 4362-4370.
1545. Birkebaek NH, Patel L, Wright NB, et al. Endocrine status in patients with optic nerve hypoplasia: relationship to midline central nervous system abnormalities and appearance of the hypothalamic-pituitary axis on magnetic resonance imaging. J Clin Endocrinol Metab 2003;88(11):5281-5286.
1546. Brodsky MC, Conte FA, Taylor D, et al. Sudden death in septo-optic dysplasia. Report of 5 cases. Arch Ophthalmol 1997; 115(1):66-70.
1547. Rappaport EB, Ulstrom RA, Gorlin RJ, et al. Solitary maxillary central incisor and short stature. J Pediatr 1977;91(6):924-928.
1548. Nanni L, Ming JE, Du Y, et al. SHH mutation is associated with solitary median maxillary central incisor: a study of 13 patients and review of the literature. Am J Med Genet 2001; 102(1):1-10.
1549. Nanni L, Ming JE, Bocian M, et al. The mutational spectrum of the sonic hedgehog gene in holoprosencephaly: SHH mutations cause a significant proportion of autosomal dominant holoprosencephaly. Hum Mol Genet 1999;8(13):2479-2488.
1550. Kollias SS, Ball WS, Prenger EC. Review of the embryologic development of the pituitary gland and report of a case of hypophyseal duplication detected by MRI. Neuroradiology 1995;37:3-12.
1551. Perrone L, Del Gaizo D, D'Angelo E, et al. Endocrine studies in children with myelomeningocele. J Pediatr Endocrinol 1994;7: 219-223.
1552. Elias ER, Sadeghi-Nejad A. Precocious puberty in girls with myelodysplasia. Pediatrics 1994;93:521-522.
1553. Reynaud R, Saveanu A, Barlier A, et al. Pituitary hormone deficiencies due to transcription factor gene alterations. Growth Horm IGF Res 2004;14(6):442-448.
1554. Wu W, Cogan JD, Pfeaffle RW, et al. Mutations in PROP1 cause familial combined pituitary hormone deficiency. Nat Genet 1998;18(2):147-149.
1555. Fluck C, Deladoey J, Rutishauser K, et al. Phenotypic variability in familial combined pituitary hormone deficiency caused by a

PROP1 gene mutation resulting in the substitution of Arg->Cys at codon 120 (R120C). J Clin Endocrinol Metab 1998;83(10): 3727-3734.

1556. Deladoey J, Fluck C, Buyukgebiz A, et al. "Hot spot" in the PROP1 gene responsible for combined pituitary hormone deficiency. J Clin Endocrinol Metab 1999;84(5):1645-1650.
1557. Reynaud R, Chadli-Chaieb M, Vallette-Kasic S, et al. A familial form of congenital hypopituitarism due to a PROP1 mutation in a large kindred: phenotypic and in vitro functional studies. J Clin Endocrinol Metab 2004;89(11):5779-5786.
1558. Asteria C, Oliveira JH, Abucham J, et al. Central hypocortisolism as part of combined pituitary hormone deficiency due to mutations of Prop1 gene. Eur J Endocrinol 2000;143(3):347-352.
1559. Netchine I, Sobrier ML, Krude H, et al. Mutations in LHX3 result in a new syndrome revealed by combined pituitary hormone deficiency. Nat Genet 2000;25(2):182-186.
1560. Phillips JA III. Inherited defects in growth hormone synthesis and action. In Scriver CR, Beaudet AI, Sly WS, et al, eds. The Metabolic Basis of Inherited Disease, 6th ed. New York: McGraw-Hill, 1989:1965-1983.
1561. Rosenbloom AL, Almonte AS, Brown MR, et al. Clinical and biochemical phenotype of familial anterior hypopituitarism from mutation of the PROP1 gene. J Clin Endocrinol Metab 1999;84(1): 50-57.
1562. Pernasetti F, Toledo SP, Vasilyev VV, et al. Impaired adrenocorticotropin-adrenal axis in combined pituitary hormone deficiency caused by a two-base pair deletion (301-302delAG) in the prophet of Pit-1 gene. J Clin Endocrinol Metab 2000;85(1):390-397.
1563. Solomon NM, Ross SA, Morgan T, et al. Array comparative genomic hybridisation analysis of boys with X linked hypopituitarism identifies a 3.9 Mb duplicated critical region at Xq27 containing SOX3. J Med Genet 2004;41(9):669-678.
1564. Goodman HG, Grumbach MM, Kaplan SL. Growth and growth hormone. II A comparison of isolated growth-hormone deficiency and multiple pituitary-hormone deficiencies in 35 patients with idiopathic hypopituitary dwarfism N Engl J Med 1968;278: 57-68.
1565. Tanner JM, Whitehouse RH. A note on the bone age at which patients with true isolated growth hormone deficiency enter puberty. J Clin Endocrinol Metab 1975;41:788-790.
1566. Arrigo T, Crisafulli G, Salamone A, et al. Adult height exceeding target height in a patient with congenital panhypopituitarism diagnosed after the age of 25 years. J Pediatr Endocrinol 1994;7:269-272.
1567. Saggese G, Federico G, Barsanti S, et al. The effect of administering gonadotropin-releasing hormone agonist with recombinant-human growth hormone (GH) on the final height of girls with isolated GH deficiency: results from a controlled study. J Clin Endocrinol Metab 2001;86(5):1900-1904.
1568. Albanese A, Stanhope R. Treatment of growth delay in boys with isolated growth hormone deficiency. Eur J Endocrinol 1994;130: 65-69.
1569. Bray GA, Dahms WT, Swerdloff RS, et.al. The Prader-Willi syndrome: a study of 40 patients and a review of the literature. Medicine (Baltimore) 1983;62:59-80.
1570. Prader A, Labhart A, Willi H. Ein syndrom von Adipositas, Kleinwuchs, Kryptorchidismus und Oligophrenie nach Myatonieartigem Zustad im Neugeborenalter. Schweiz Med Wochenschr 1956;86:1260-1261.
1571. Tolis G, Lewis W, Verdy M, et al. Anterior pituitary function in the Prader-Labhart-Willi (PLW) syndrome. J Clin Endocrinol Metab 1974;39:1061-1066.
1572. Linde R, McNeil L, Rabin D. Induction of menarche by clomiphene citrate in a fifteen-year-old girl with the Prader-Labhart-Willi syndrome. Fertil Steril 1982;37:118-120.
1573. Holm VA, Cassidy SB, Butler MG, et al. Prader-Willi syndrome: consensus diagnostic criteria. Pediatrics 1993;91:398-402.
1574. Cassidy SB, Schwartz S. Prader-Willi and Angelman syndromes. Disorders of genomic imprinting. Medicine (Baltimore) 1998;77(2):140-151.
1575. Crino A, Schiaffini R, Ciampalini P, et al. Hypogonadism and pubertal development in Prader-Willi syndrome. Eur J Pediatr 2003;162(5):327-333.
1576. Eiholzer U, Bachmann S, l'Allemand D. Is there growth hormone deficiency in Prader-Willi Syndrome? Six arguments to support the presence of hypothalamic growth hormone deficiency in Prader-Willi syndrome. Horm Res 2000;53(Suppl 3):44-52.
1577. Lindgren AC, Ritzen EM. Five years of growth hormone treatment in children with Prader-Willi syndrome. Swedish National Growth Hormone Advisory Group. Acta Paediatr Suppl 1999;88(433): 109-111.
1578. Lindgren AC, Hagenas L, Muller J, et al. Growth hormone treatment of children with Prader-Willi syndrome affects linear growth and body composition favourably. Acta Paediatr 1998;87(1): 28-31.
1579. Carrel AL, Myers SE, Whitman BY, et al. Sustained benefits of growth hormone on body composition, fat utilization, physical strength and agility, and growth in Prader-Willi syndrome are dose-dependent. J Pediatr Endocrinol Metab 2001;14(8): 1097-1105.
1580. Zaglia F, Zaffanello M, Biban P. Unexpected death due to refractory metabolic acidosis and massive hemolysis in a young infant with Prader-Willi syndrome. Am J Med Genet A 2005;132(2): 219-221.
1581. Schrander-Stumpel CT, Curfs LM, Sastrowijoto P, et al. Prader-Willi syndrome: causes of death in an international series of 27 cases. Am J Med Genet A 2004;124(4):333-338.
1582. Stevenson DA, Anaya TM, Clayton-Smith J, et al. Unexpected death and critical illness in Prader-Willi syndrome: report of ten individuals. Am J Med Genet A 2004;124(2):158-164.
1583. Vogels A, Van Den EJ, Keymolen K, et al. Minimum prevalence, birth incidence and cause of death for Prader-Willi syndrome in Flanders. Eur J Hum Genet 2004;12(3):238-240.
1584. Oiglane E, Ounap K, Bartsch O, et al. Sudden death of a girl with Prader-Willi syndrome. Genet Couns 2002;13(4):459-464.
1585. Nordmann Y, Eiholzer U, l'Allemand D, et al. Sudden death of an infant with Prader-Willi syndrome—not a unique case? Biol Neonate 2002;82(2):139-141.
1586. Sacco M, Di Giorgio G. Sudden death in Prader-Willi syndrome during growth hormone therapy. Horm Res 2005;63(1):29-32.
1587. Van Vliet G, Deal CL, Crock PA, et al. Sudden death in growth hormone-treated children with Prader-Willi syndrome. J Pediatr 2004;144(1):129-131.
1588. Eiholzer U, Nordmann Y, l'Allemand D. Fatal outcome of sleep apnoea in PWS during the initial phase of growth hormone treatment. A case report. Horm Res 2002;58(Suppl 3):24-26.
1589. Cassidy SB, Ledbetter DH. Prader-Willi syndrome. Neurol Clin 1989;7:37-54.
1590. Knoll JHM, Nicholls RD, Magenis RE, et al. Angleman and Prader-Willi share a common chromosome 15 deletion but differ in parental origin of the deletion. Am J Med Genet 1989;32: 285-290.
1591. Nicholls RD. Imprinting mechanisms and genes involved in Prader-Willi and Angelman syndromes. Dev Biol 1994;5:311-322.
1592. Saitoh S, Buiting K, Rogan PK, et al. Minimal definition of the imprinting region center and fixation of a chromosome 15q11-q13 epigenotype by imprinting mutations. Proc Natl Acad Sci U S A 1996;93:7811-7815.
1593. Nicholls RD, Knoll JHM, Butler MG, et al. Genetic imprinting suggested by maternal hetero-disomy in non-deletion Prader-Willi syndrome. Nature 1989;342:281-285.
1594. OzHelik R, Leff S, Robinson W, et al. Small nuclear ribonucleoprotein polypeptide N (SNRPN), an expressed gene in the Prader-Willi syndrome critical region. Nature Genet 1992;2: 259-269.
1595. Lalande M. In and around SNRPN. Nature Genet 1994;8:5-6.
1596. Swaab DF, Purba JS, Hoffman MA. Alterations in the paraventricular nucleus and its oxytocin neurons (putative satiety cells) in Prader-Willi syndrome: a study of five cases. J Clin Endocrinol Metab 1995;80:573-579.
1597. DelParigi A, Tschop M, Heiman ML, et al. High circulating ghrelin: a potential cause for hyperphagia and obesity in prader-willi syndrome. J Clin Endocrinol Metab 2002;87(12):5461-5464.
1598. Haqq AM, Farooqi IS, O'Rahilly S, et al. Serum ghrelin levels are inversely correlated with body mass index, age, and insulin concentrations in normal children and are markedly increased in Prader-Willi syndrome. J Clin Endocrinol Metab 2003;88(1): 174-178.
1599. Haqq AM, Stadler DD, Rosenfeld RG, et al. Circulating ghrelin levels are suppressed by meals and octreotide therapy in chil-

dren with Prader-Willi syndrome. J Clin Endocrinol Metab 2003;88(8):3573-3576.
1600. Laurence JZ, Moon RC. Four cases of "retinitis pigmentosa," occurring in the same family, and accompanied by general imperfections of development. Ophthalamic Rev 1866;2:32-41.
1601. Bell J. The Laurence-Moon syndrome. The Treasury of Human Inheritance. Cambridge: Cambridge University Press, 1958:51.
1602. Blacque OE, Leroux MR. Bardet-Biedl syndrome: an emerging pathomechanism of intracellular transport. Cell Mol Life Sci 2006;63(18):2145-2161.
1603. Katsanis N, Ansley SJ, Badano JL, et al. Triallelic inheritance in Bardet-Biedl syndrome, a Mendelian recessive disorder. Science 2001;293(5538):2256-2259.
1604. Nishimura DY, Searby CC, Carmi R, et al. Positional cloning of a novel gene on chromosome 16q causing Bardet-Biedl syndrome (BBS2). Hum Mol Genet 2001;10(8):865-874.
1605. Burghes AH, Vaessin HE, de La CA. Genetics. The land between Mendelian and multifactorial inheritance. Science 2001; 293(5538):2213-2214.
1606. Moore SJ, Green JS, Fan Y, et al. Clinical and genetic epidemiology of Bardet-Biedl syndrome in Newfoundland: a 22-year prospective, population-based, cohort study. Am J Med Genet A 2005;132(4):352-360.
1607. Verloes A, Temple IK, Bonnet S, et al. Coloboma, mental retardation, hypogonadism, and obesity: critical review of the so-called Biemond syndrome type 2, updated nosology, and delineation of three "new" syndromes. Am J Med Genet 1997;69(4):370-379.
1608. Maki M, Kallonen K, Lahdeaho ML, et al. Changing pattern of childhood coeliac disease in Finland. Acta Paediatr Scand 1988;77:408-412.
1609. Vigersky R, Anderson AE, Thompson RH. Hypothalamic dysfunction in secondary amenorrhea associated with simple weight loss. N Engl J Med 1977;297:1141-1145.
1610. Swenne I. Weight requirements for return of menstruations in teenage girls with eating disorders, weight loss and secondary amenorrhoea. Acta Paediatr 2004;93(11):1449-1455.
1611. Landon C, Rosenfeld RG. Short stature and pubertal delay in male adolescents with cystic fibrosis. Androgen treatment. Am J Dis Child 1984;138:388-391.
1612. Reiter EO, Stern RC, Root AW. The reproductive endocrine system in cystic fibrosis. I Basal gonadotropin and sex steroid levels Am J Dis Child 1981;135:422-426.
1613. Stern RC, Boat TF, Doershuk CF, et al. Course of cystic fibrosis in 95 patients. J Pediatr 1976;89:406-411.
1614. Aswani N, Taylor CJ, McGaw J, et al. Pubertal growth and development in cystic fibrosis: a retrospective review. Acta Paediatr 2003;92(9):1029-1032.
1615. Arrigo T, De Luca F, Lucanto C, et al. Nutritional, glycometabolic and genetic factors affecting menarcheal age in cystic fibrosis. Diabetes Nutr Metab 2004;17(2):114-119.
1616. Taussig LM, Lobeck CC, di Sant'Agnese PA, et al. Fertility in males with cystic fibrosis. N Engl J Med 1972;287:586-589.
1617. Tizzano EF, Silver MM, Chitayat D, et al. Differential cellular expression of cystic fibrosis transmembrane regulator in human reproductive tissues. Clues for the infertility in patients with cystic fibrosis. Am J Pathol 1994;144:906-914.
1618. Johannesson M, Gottlieb C, Hjelte L. Delayed puberty in girls with cystic fibrosis despite good clinical status. Pediatrics 1997;99: 29-34.
1619. Serjeant GR, Hambleton I, Thame M. Fecundity and pregnancy outcome in a cohort with sickle cell-haemoglobin C disease followed from birth. BJOG 2005;112(9):1308-1314.
1620. Olatunji Olambiwonnu N, Penny R, Frasier SD. Sexual maturation in subjects with sickle cell anemia: studies of serum gonadotropin concentration, height, weight, and skeletal age. J Pediatr 1975;87:459-464.
1621. Chatterjee R, Katz M. Evaluation of gonadotrophin insufficiency in thalassemic boys with pubertal failure: spontaneous versus provocative test. J Pediatr Endocrinol Metab 2001;14(3):301-312.
1622. Chatterjee R, Katz M. Reversible hypogonadotrophic hypogonadism in sexually infantile male thalassaemic patients with transfusional iron overload. Clin Endocrinol 2000;53(1):33-42.
1623. Wang C, Tso SC, Todd D. Hypogonadotropic hypogonadism in severe beta-thalassemia: effect of chelation and pulsatile gonadotropin-releasing hormone therapy. J Clin Endocrinol Metab 1989;68(3):511-516.
1624. Grundy RG, Woods KA, Savage MO, et al. Relationship of endocrinopathy to iron chelation status in young patients with thalassaemia major. Arch Dis Child 1994;71:128-132.
1625. Shalitin S, Carmi D, Weintrob N, et al. Serum ferritin level as a predictor of impaired growth and puberty in thalassemia major patients. Eur J Haematol 2005;74(2):93-100.
1626. Yesilipek MA, Bircan I, Oygur N, et al. Growth and sexual maturation in children with thalassemia major. Haematologica 1993;78: 30-33.
1627. Kwan EY, Lee AC, Li AM, et al. A cross-sectional study of growth, puberty and endocrine function in patients with thalassaemia major in Hong Kong. J Paediatr Child Health 1995;31:83-87.
1628. Chern JP, Lin KH, Tsai WY, et al. Hypogonadotropic hypogonadism and hematologic phenotype in patients with transfusion-dependent beta-thalassemia. J Pediatr Hematol Oncol 2003; 25(11):880-884.
1629. Borgna Pignatti C, De Stefano P, Zonta L, et al. Growth and sexual maturation in thalassemia major. J Pediatr 1985;106:150-155.
1630. Italian Working Group on Endocrine Complications in Non-endocrine Diseases. Multicentre study on prevalence of endocrine complications in thalassemia major. Clin Endocrinol 1995;42:581-586.
1631. Balducci R, Toscano V, Finocchi G, et al. Effect of hCG or hCG+ treatments in young thalassemic patients with hypogonadotropic hypogonadism. J Endocrinol Invest 1990;13:1-7.
1632. De Sanctis V, Vullo C, Katz M, et al. Gonadal function in patients with beta thalassaemia major. J Clin Pathol 1988;41:133-137.
1633. Sklar CA, Lew LQ, Yoon DJ, et al. Adrenal function in thalassemia major following long-term treatment with multiple transfusions and chelation therapy. Evidence for dissociation of cortisol and adrenal androgen secretion Am J Dis Child 1987;141: 327-330.
1634. Soliman AT, elZalabany MM, Ragab M, et al. Spontaneous and GnRH-provoked gonadotropin secretion and testosterone response to human chorionic gonadotropin in adolescent boys with thalassaemia major and delayed puberty. J Trop Pediatr 2000;46(2):79-85.
1635. Caruso-Nicoletti M, De S, V, Raiola G, et al. No difference in pubertal growth and final height between treated hypogonadal and non-hypogonadal thalassemic patients. Horm Res 2004; 62(1):17-22.
1636. Benigno V, Bertelloni S, Baroncelli GI, et al. Effects of thalassemia major on bone mineral density in late adolescence. J Pediatr Endocrinol Metab 2003;16(Suppl 2):337-342.
1637. Bielinski BK, Darbyshire PJ, Mathers L, et al. Impact of disordered puberty on bone density in beta-thalassaemia major. Br J Haematol 2003;120(2):353-358.
1638. De Sanctis V, Galimberti M, Lucarelli G, et al. Pubertal development in thalassaemic patients after allogenic bone marrow transplantation [published erratum appears in Eur J Pediatr 1994;153(6):470]. Eur J Pediatr 1993;152:993-997.
1639. Vlachopapadopoulou E, Kitra V, Peristeri J, et al. Gonadal function of young patients with beta-thalassemia following bone marrow transplantation. J Pediatr Endocrinol Metab 2005;18(5): 477-483.
1640. Hovi L, Saarinen-Pihkala UM, Taskinen M, et al. Subnormal androgen levels in young female bone marrow transplant recipients with ovarian dysfunction, chronic GVHD and receiving glucocorticoid therapy. Bone Marrow Transplant 2004;33(5): 503-508.
1641. Li CK, Chik KW, Wong GW, et al. Growth and endocrine function following bone marrow transplantation for thalassemia major. Pediatr Hematol Oncol 2004;21(5):411-419.
1642. Gertner JM, Kaufman FR, Donfield SM, et al. Delayed somatic growth and pubertal development in human immunodeficiency virus-infected hemophiliac boys: Hemophilia Growth and Development Study. J Pediatr 1994;124:896-902.
1643. Chiarelli F, Galli L, Pomilio M, et al. Early detection and treatment of altered growth and puberty in children and adolescents with vertically-acquired HIV-1 infection: It's time to think about it. Int J Immunopathol Pharmacol 2001;14(1):45-47.
1644. Buchacz K, Rogol AD, Lindsey JC, et al. Delayed onset of pubertal development in children and adolescents with perinatally

acquired HIV infection. J Acquir Immune Defic Syndr 2003; 33(1):56-65.
1645. Chantry CJ, Frederick MM, Meyer WA III, et al. Endocrine abnormalities and impaired growth in human immunodeficiency virus-infected children. Pediatr Infect Dis J 2007;26(1):53-60.
1646. Brain CE, Savage MO. Growth and puberty in chronic inflammatory bowel disease. Baillieres Clin Gastroenterol 1994;8:83-100.
1647. Cacciari E, Corazza GR, Salardi S, et al. What will be the adult height of coeliac patients? Eur J Pediatr 1991;150:407-409.
1648. Ferraris J, Saenger P, Levine L, et al. Delayed puberty in males with chronic renal failure. Kidney Int 1980;18:344-350.
1649. Schaefer F, Stanhope R, Scheil H, et al. Pulsatile gonadotropin secretion in pubertal children with chronic renal failure. Acta Endocrinol 1989;120:14-19.
1650. Kulin H, Demers L, Chinchilli V, et al. Usefulness of sequential urinary follicle-stimulating hormone and luteinizing hormone measurements in the diagnosis of adolescent hypogonadotropism in males. J Clin Endocrinol Metab 1994;78:1208-1211.
1651. van Diemen-Steenvoorde R, Donckerwolcke RA, Brackel H, et al. Growth and sexual maturation in children after kidney transplantation. J Pediatr 1987;110:351-356.
1652. Martin LW, McEnery PT, Rosenkrantz JG, et al. Renal homotransplantation in children. J Pediatr Surg 1979;14:571-576.
1653. Ferraris JR, Domene HM, Escobar ME, et al. Hormonal problems in pubertal females with chronic renal failure: before and under hemodialysis and after renal transplantation. Acta Endocrinol 1987;115:289-296.
1654. van Diemen-Steevoorde MD, Donckerwolcke RA, Brakel H, et al. Growth and sexual maturation in children after kidney transplantation. J Pediatr 1987;110:351-356.
1655. Belgorosky A, Ferraris JR, Ramirez JA, et al. Serum sex hormone-binding globulin and serum nonsex hormone-binding globulin-bound testosterone fractions in prepubertal boys with chronic renal failure. J Clin Endocrinol Metab 1991;73:107-110.
1656. Rees L, Greene SA, Adlard P, et al. Growth and endocrine function in steroid sensitive nephrotic syndrome. Arch Dis Child 1988;63:484-490.
1657. Hokken-Koelega AC, Stijnen T, De Muinck Keizer-Schrama SM, et al. Levels of growth hormone, insulin-like growth factor-I (IGF-I) and -II, IGF-binding protein-1 and -3, and cortisol in prednisone-treated children with growth retardation after renal transplantation. J Clin Endocrinol Metab 1993;77:932-938.
1658. Polito C, Di Toro R. Delayed pubertal growth spurt in glomerulopathic boys receiving alternate-day prednisone. Child Nephrol Urol 1992;12:202-207.
1659. Siris ES, Leventhal BG, Vaitukaitis JL. Effects of childhood leukemia and chemotherapy on puberty and reproductive function in girls. N Engl J Med 1976;294:1143-1146.
1660. Vilska S, Lahteenmaki P, Kaihola HL, et al. Endocrine status and growth after malignancy treated in childhood or adolescence. Int J Fertil 1988;33:283-290.
1661. Wikstrom AM, Hovi L, Dunkel L, et al. Restoration of ovarian function after chemotherapy for osteosarcoma. Arch Dis Child 2003;88(5):428-431.
1662. Lannering B, Rosberg S, Marky I, et al. Reduced growth hormone secretion with maintained periodicity following cranial irradiation in children with acute lymphoblastic leukaemia. Clin Endocrinol (Oxf) 1995;42:153-159.
1663. Cicognani A, Cacciari E, Rosito P, et al. Longitudinal growth and final height in long-term survivors of childhood leukaemia. Eur J Pediatr 1994;153:726-730.
1664. Ochs J, Mulhern R. Long-term sequelae of therapy for childhood acute lymphoblastic leukaemia. Baillieres Clin Haematol 1994;7: 365-376.
1665. Follin C, Thilen U, Ahren B, et al. Improvement in cardiac systolic function and reduced prevalence of metabolic syndrome after two years of growth hormone (GH) treatment in GH-deficient adult survivors of childhood-onset acute lymphoblastic leukemia. J Clin Endocrinol Metab 2006;91(5):1872-1875.
1666. Jarfelt M, Lannering B, Bosaeus I, et al. Body composition in young adult survivors of childhood acute lymphoblastic leukaemia. Eur J Endocrinol 2005;153(1):81-89.
1667. Didi M, Didcock E, Davies HA, et al. High incidence of obesity in young adults after treatment of acute lymphoblastic leukemia in childhood. Multiple hormone deficiencies in children with hemochromatosis. J Clin Endocrinol Metab. J Pediatr 1993; 76:357-361.
1668. Mauriac P. Hepatomalie de l'enfance avec troubles de la croissance et du mJtabolisme des glucides. Paris Mjd 1987;2: 206-208.
1669. Arreola F, Junco E, Partida-Hernandez G, et al. HbA1, height velocity and weight gain as indicators of metabolic control in type I diabetic children. A 5 year survey. Arch Invest Med (Mex) 1991;22:303-307.
1670. Wise JE, Kolb EL, Sauder SE. Effect of glycemic control on growth velocity in children with IDDM. Diabetes Care 1992;15:826-830.
1671. Travis LB. Diabetes Mellitus in Children and Adolescents. Philadelphia: WBSaunders, 1987.
1672. Styne DM, Grumbach MM, Kaplan SL, et al. Treatment of Cushing's disease in childhood and adolescence by transsphenoidal microadenomectomy. N Engl J Med 1984;310:889-893.
1673. Devoe DJ, Miller WL, Conte FA, et al. Long-term outcome in children and adolescents after transsphenoidal surgery for Cushing's disease. J Clin Endocrinol Metab 1997;82(10):3196-3202.
1674. Diagnostic and statistical manual of mental disorders: DSM-IV. Washington: American Psychiatric Association, 1994.
1675. Crisp AH. The dyslipophobias: a view of the psychopathologies involved and the hazards of construing anorexia nervosa and bulimia nervosa as 'eating disorders'. Proc Nutr Soc 1996;54: 701-709.
1676. Graber JA, Brooks-Gunn J, Warren MP. The vulnerable transition: puberty and the development of eating pathology and negative mood. Womens Health Issues 1999;9(2):107-114.
1677. Schwabe AD, Lippe BM, Chang RJ, et al. Anorexia nervosa. Ann Intern Med 1981;94(3):371-381.
1678. Silverman JA. Anorexia nervosa: clinical and metabolic observations in a successful treatment plan. In Vigersky RA, ed. Anorexia Nervosa. New York: Raven, 1977:331-339.
1679. Warren MP, Vande Wile RL. Clinical and metabolic features of anorexia nervosa. Am J Obstet Gynecol 1973;117:435-449.
1680. Polivy J, Herman CP. Causes of eating disorders. Annu Rev Psychol 2002;53:187-213.
1681. Kaye WH, Klump KL, Frank GK, et al. Anorexia and bulimia nervosa. Annu Rev Med 2000;51:299-313.
1682. Danziger Y, Mukamel M, Zeharia A, et al. Stunting of growth in anorexia nervosa during the prepubertal and pubertal period. Isr J Med Sci 1994;30:581-584.
1683. De Lange WE, Sluiter WJ, Van Zanten AK, et al. The effect of injection and infusion of LH-RH on serum LH and FSH in normal males and in boys with delayed puberty. Neth J Med 1974;17: 196-201.
1684. van Binsbergen CJM, Coelingh Bennink HJT, Odink J, et al. A comparative and longitudinal study on endocrine changes related to ovarian function in patients with anorexia nervosa. J Clin Endocrinol Metab 1990;71:705-711.
1685. Beaumont PJV, George GCW, Pimstone BL, et al. Body weight and the pituitary response to hypothalamic releasing hormones in patients with anorexia nervosa. J Clin Endocrinol Metab 1976;43:487-496.
1686. Grinspoon S, Gulick T, Askari H, et al. Serum leptin levels in women with anorexia nervosa. J Clin Endocrinol Metab 1996;81: 3861-3863.
1687. Ferron F, Considine RV, Peino R, et al. Serum leptin concentrations in patients with anorexia nervosa, bulimia nervosa and non-specific eating disorders correlate with the body mass index but are independent of the respective disease. Clin Endocrinol 1997;46:289-293.
1688. Casanueva FF, Dieguez C, Popovic V, et al. Serum immunoreactive leptin concentrations in patients with anorexia nervosa before and after partial weight recovery. Biochem Mol Med 1997;60:116-120.
1689. Waldhauser F, Toifl K, Spona J, et al. Diminished prolactin response to thyrotropin and insulin in anorexia nervosa. J Clin Endocrinol Metab 1984;59:538-544.
1690. Stoving RK, Hangaard J, Hagen C. Update on endocrine disturbances in anorexia nervosa. J Pediatr Endocrinol Metab 2001;14(5):459-480.
1691. Misra M, Aggarwal A, Miller KK, et al. Effects of anorexia nervosa on clinical, hematologic, biochemical, and bone density param-

eters in community-dwelling adolescent girls. Pediatrics 2004;114(6):1574-1583.
1692. Misra M, Miller KK, Almazan C, et al. Hormonal and body composition predictors of soluble leptin receptor, leptin, and free leptin index in adolescent girls with anorexia nervosa and controls and relation to insulin sensitivity. J Clin Endocrinol Metab 2004;89(7):3486-3495.
1693. Warren MP. Metabolic factors and the onset of puberty. In: Grumbach MM, Sizonenko PC, Aubert ML, editors. Control of the Onset of Puberty. Baltimore: Williams & Wilkins, 1990:553-573.
1694. Yen SSC, Rebar R, VandenBerg G, et al. Hypothalamic amenorrhea and hypogonadotropinism: responses to synthetic LRF. J Clin Endocrinol Metab 1973;36:816.
1695. Couzinet B, Young J, Brailly S, et al. Functional hypothalamic amenorrhoea: a partial and reversible gonadotrophin deficiency of nutritional origin. Clin Endocrinol (Oxf) 1999;50(2):229-235.
1696. Warren MP, Voussoughian F, Geer EB, et al. Functional hypothalamic amenorrhea: hypoleptinemia and disordered eating. J Clin Endocrinol Metab 1999;84(3):873-877.
1697. Shapiro JR, Berkman ND, Brownley KA, et al. Bulimia nervosa treatment: a systematic review of randomized controlled trials. Int J Eat Disord 2007;40(4):321-336.
1698. Russell GFM. Bulimia nervosa: an ominous variant of anorexia nervosa. Psychol Med 1979;9:429-448.
1699. Eisenstein TD, Gerson MJ. Psychosocial growth retardation in adolescence. A reversible condition secondary to severe stress. J Adolesc Health Care 1988;9:436-440.
1700. Warren MP, Shantha S. The female athlete. Baillieres Best Pract Res Clin Endocrinol Metab 2000;14(1):37-53.
1701. Warren MP, Perlroth NE. The effects of intense exercise on the female reproductive system. J Endocrinol 2001;170(1):3-11.
1702. Kaga M, Takahashi K, Ishihara T, et al. Bone assessment of female long-distance runners. J Bone Miner Metab 2004;22(5): 509-513.
1703. Claessens AL, Bourgois J, Beunen G, et al. Age at menarche in relation to anthropometric characteristics, competition level and boat category in elite junior rowers Ann Hum Biol 2003;30(2): 148-159.
1704. Warren MP, Brooks-Gunn J, Fox RP, et al. Persistent osteopenia in ballet dancers with amenorrhea and delayed menarche despite hormone therapy: a longitudinal study. Fertil Steril 2003;80(2): 398-404.
1705. Baxter-Jones A, Maffulli N, Helms P. Low injury rates in elite athletes. Arch Dis Child 1993;68:130-132.
1706. Lucas JA, Lucas PR, Vogel S, et al. Effect of sub-elite competitive running on bone density, body composition and sexual maturity of adolescent females. Osteoporos Int 2003;14(10):848-856.
1707. Sundgot-Borgen J. Risk and trigger factors for the development of eating disorders in female elite athletes. Med Sci Sports Exerc 1994;26:414-419.
1708. Torstveit MK, Sundgot-Borgen J. Participation in leanness sports but not training volume is associated with menstrual dysfunction: a national survey of 1276 elite athletes and controls. Br J Sports Med 2005;39(3):141-147.
1709. Constantini NW, Warren MP. Special problems of the female athlete. Baillieres Clin Rheumatol 1994;8:199-219.
1710. Loucks AV, Horvath SB. Athletic amenorrhea: a review. Med Sci Sports Exerc 1985;17:56-72.
1711. Baxter-Jones AD, Helms P, Baines-Preece J, et al. Menarche in intensively trained gymnasts, swimmers and tennis players. Ann Hum Biol 1994;21:407-415.
1712. Damsgaard R, Bencke J, Matthiesen G, et al. Is prepubertal growth adversely affected by sport? Med Sci Sports Exerc 2000;32(10): 1698-1703.
1713. Damsgaard R, Bencke J, Matthiesen G, et al. Body proportions, body composition and pubertal development of children in competitive sports. Scand J Med Sci Sports 2001;11(1):54-60.
1714. Claessens AL, Malina RM, Lefevre J, et al. Growth and menarcheal status of elite female gymnasts. Med Sci Sports Exerc 1992;24(7): 755-763.
1715. Georgopoulos N, Markou K, Theodoropoulou A, et al. Growth and pubertal development in elite female rythmic gymansts. J Clin Endocrinol Metab 1999;84:4525-4530.
1716. Theodoropoulou A, Markou KB, Vagenakis GA, et al. Delayed but normally progressed puberty is more pronounced in artistic compared with rhythmic elite gymnasts due to the intensity of training. J Clin Endocrinol Metab 2005;90(11):6022-6027.
1717. Klentrou P, Plyley M. Onset of puberty, menstrual frequency, and body fat in elite rhythmic gymnasts compared with normal controls. Br J Sports Med 2003;37(6):490-494.
1718. Munoz MT, de la PC, Barrios V, et al. Changes in bone density and bone markers in rhythmic gymnasts and ballet dancers: implications for puberty and leptin levels. Eur J Endocrinol 2004; 151(4):491-496.
1719. Warren MP. The effects of exercise on pubertal progression and reproductive function in girls. J Clin Endocrinol Metab 1980;51: 1150-1157.
1720. Constantini NW, Warren MP. Menstrual dysfunction in swimmers: a distinct entity. J Clin Endocrinol Metab 1995;80:2740-2744.
1721. Theintz GE, Howald H, Weiss U, et al. Evidence for a reduction of growth potential in adolescent female gymnasts [see comments]. J Pediatr 1993;122:306-313.
1722. Georgopoulos NA, Theodoropoulou A, Leglise M, et al. Growth and skeletal maturation in male and female artistic gymnasts. J Clin Endocrinol Metab 2004;89(9):4377-4382.
1723. Lindholm C, Hagenfeldt K, Ringertz BM. Pubertal development in elite juvenile gymnasts. Effects of physical training. Acta Obstet Gynecol Scand 1994;73:269-273.
1724. Adiyaman P, Ocal G, Berberoglu M, et al. Alterations in serum growth hormone (GH)/GH dependent ternary complex components (IGF-I, IGFBP-3, ALS, IGF-I/IGFBP-3 molar ratio) and the influence of these alterations on growth pattern in female rhythmic gymnasts. J Pediatr Endocrinol Metab 2004;17(6): 895-903.
1725. Brisson GR, Volle MA, Desharnais M, et al. Exercise induced dissociation of the blood prolactin response in young women according to their sports habits. Horm Metab Res 1980;21: 201-205.
1726. Eliakim A, Beyth Y. Exercise training, menstrual irregularities and bone development in children and adolescents. J Pediatr Adolesc Gynecol 2003;16(4):201-206.
1727. Hagglund G, Karlberg J, Willner S. Growth in girls with adolescent idiopathic scoliosis. Spine 1992;17:108-111.
1728. Goldberg CJ, Dowling FE, Fogarty EE. Adolescent idiopathic scoliosis—early menarche, normal growth. Spine 1993;18: 529-535.
1729. Carr AJ, Jefferson RJ, Turner-Smith AR. Family stature in idiopathic scoliosis. Spine 1993;18:20-23.
1730. Gurd B, Klentrou P. Physical and pubertal development in young male gymnasts. J Appl Physiol 2003;95(3):1011-1015.
1731. Harmon J, Aliapoulios MA. Gynecomastia in marihuana user. N Engl J Med 1972;287:936.-1080.
1732. Copeland KC, Underwood LE, Van Wyk JJ. Marihuana smoking and pubertal arrest. J Pediatr 1980;96:1079-1080.
1733. Granovsky-Grisaru S, Aboulafia Y, Diamant YZ, et al. Gynecologic and obstetric aspects of Gaucher's disease: a survey of 53 patients. Am J Obstet Gynecol 1995;172:1284-1290.
1734. Maayan C, Sela O, Axelrod F, et al. Gynecological aspects of female familial dysautonomia. Isr Med Assoc J 2000;2(9): 679-683.
1735. Rosenfeld RG, Northcraft GB, Hintz RL. A prospective, randomized study of testosterone treatment of constitutional delay of growth and development in male adolescents. Pediatrics 1982;69(6):681-687.
1736. Susman EJ, Finkelstein JW, Chinchilli VM, et al. The effect of sex hormone replacement therapy on behavior problems and moods in adolescents with delayed puberty. J Pediatr 1998;133(4): 521-525.
1737. Hsueh AJ, Eisenhauer K, Chun SY, et al. Gonadal cell apoptosis. Recent Prog Horm Res 1996;51:433-455; discussion 455-456.
1738. Klinefelter HF Jr, Reifenstein EC Jr, Albright F. Syndrome characterized by gynecomastia, aspermatogenesis without A-leydigism, and increased excretion of follicle-stimulating hormone. J Clin Endocrinol 1942;2:615-627.
1739. Bojesen A, Juul S, Gravholt CH. Prenatal and postnatal prevalence of Klinefelter syndrome: a national registry study. J Clin Endocrinol Metab 2003;88(2):622-626.
1740. Caldwell PD, Smith DW. The XXY (Klinefelter's) syndrome in childhood: detection and treatment. J Pediatr 1972;80: 250-258.

1741. Wittenberg DF, Padayachi T, Norman RJ. Hypogonadotrophic variant of Klinefelter's syndrome. A case report. S Afr Med J 1988;74:181-183.
1742. Mikamo K, Aguercif M, Hazeghi P, et al. Chromatin-positive Klinefelter's syndrome. A quantitative analysis of spermatogonial deficiency at 3, 4, and 12 months of age. Fertil Steril 1968;19(5): 731-739.
1743. Meuller J, Skakkebaek NE, Ratcliffe SG. Quantified testicular histology in boys with sex chromosome abnormalities. Int J Androl 1995;18(2):57-62.
1744. Wikstrom AM, Raivio T, Hadziselimovic F, et al. Klinefelter syndrome in adolescence: onset of puberty is associated with accelerated germ cell depletion. J Clin Endocrinol Metab 2004;89(5): 2263-2270.
1745. Wikstrom AM, Painter JN, Raivio T, et al. Genetic features of the X chromosome affect pubertal development and testicular degeneration in adolescent boys with Klinefelter syndrome. Clin Endocrinol (Oxf) 2006;65(1):92-97.
1746. Christiansen P, Andersson AM, Skakkebaek NE. Longitudinal studies of inhibin B levels in boys and young adults with Klinefelter syndrome. J Clin Endocrinol Metab 2003;88(2): 888-891.
1747. Aksglaede L, Wikstrom M, Meyts ER, et al. Natural history of seminiferous tubule degeneration in Klinefelter syndrome. Hum Reprod Update 2005.
1748. Sagawa I, Kazama T, Terada T, et al. Hormonal profiles in Klinefelters syndrome with and without testicular epidermoid cyst. Arch Androl 1988;21:205-209.
1749. Salbenblatt JA, Bender BG, Puck MH, et al. Pituitary-gonadal function in Klinefelter syndrome before and during puberty. Pediatr Res 1985;19:82-86.
1750. Wikstrom AM, Dunkel L, Wickman S, et al. Are adolescent boys with Klinefelter syndrome androgen deficient? A longitudinal study of Finnish 47,XXY boys. Pediatr Res 2006;59(6): 854-859.
1751. Plymate SR, Leonard JM, Paulsen CA. Sex hormone-binding globulin changes with androgen replacement. J Clin Endocrinol Metab 1983;57:645-648.
1752. Wieland RG, Zorn EM, Johnson MW. Elevated testosterone-binding globulin in Klinefelter's syndrome. J Clin Endocrinol Metab 1980;51:1199-1200.
1753. Eberle AJ, Sparrow JT, Keenan BS. Treatment of persistent pubertal gynecomastia with dihydrotestosterone heptanoate. J Pediatr 1986;109:144-149.
1754. Zinn AR, Ramos P, Elder FF, et al. Androgen receptor CAGn repeat length influences phenotype of 47,XXY (Klinefelter) syndrome. J Clin Endocrinol Metab 2005;90(9):5041-5046.
1755. Zitzmann M, Depenbusch M, Gromoll J, et al. X-chromosome inactivation patterns and androgen receptor functionality influence phenotype and social characteristics as well as pharmacogenetics of testosterone therapy in Klinefelter patients. J Clin Endocrinol Metab 2004;89(12):6208-6217.
1756. Kleczkowska A, Fryns JP, Van den Berghe H. X-chromosome polysomy in the male: the Leuven experience 1966-1987. Hum Genet 1988;80:16-22.
1757. Nielsen J, Pelsen B. Follow-up 20 years later of 34 Klinefelter males with karyotype 47,XXY and 16 hypogonadal males with karyotype 46,XY. Hum Genet 1987;77:188-192.
1758. Sorenson K, Porter ME, Gardner HA, et al. Verbal deficits in Klinefelter (XXY) adults living in the community. Clin Genet 1988; 33:246-253.
1759. Rovet J, Netley C, Keenan M, et al. The psychoeducational profile of boys with Klinefelter syndrome. J Learn Disabil 1996;29(2): 180-196.
1760. Boone KB, Swerdloff RS, Miller BL, et al. Neuropsychological profiles of adults with klinefelter syndrome. J Int Neuropsychol Soc 2001;7(4):446-456.
1761. Rovet J, Netley C, Bailey J, et al. Intelligence and achievement in children with extra X aneuploidy: a longitudinal perspective. Am J Med Genet 1995;60(5):356-363.
1762. Collaer ML, Hines M. Human behavioral sex differences: a role for gonadal hormones during early development? Psychol Bull 1995;118(1):55-107.
1763. Netley C, Rovet J. Hemispheric lateralization in 47,XXY Klinefelter's syndrome boys. Brain Cogn 1984;3(1):10-18.
1764. Netley C, Rovet J. Relations between a dermatoglyphic measure, hemispheric specialization, and intellectual abilities in 47,XXY males. Brain Cogn 1987;6(2):153-160.
1765. Stewart DA, Bailey JD, Netley CT, et al. Growth and development of children with X and Y chromosome aneuploidy from infancy to pubertal age: the Toronto study. Birth Defects Orig Artic Ser 1982;18(4):99-154.
1766. Geschwind N, Galaburda AM. Cerebral lateralization. Biological mechanisms, associations, and pathology: I. A hypothesis and a program for research. Arch Neurol 1985;42(5):428-459.
1767. Geschwind DH, Boone KB, Miller BL, et al. Neurobehavioral phenotype of Klinefelter syndrome. Ment Retard Dev Disabil Res Rev 2000;6(2):107-116.
1768. Nielsen J, Pelsen B, Sorensen K. Follow-up of 30 Klinefelter males treated with testosterone. Clin Genet 1988;33(4):262-269.
1769. Price WH, Clayton JF, Wilson J. Causes of death in X chromatin positive males (Klinefelter's syndrome). J Epidemiol Community Health 1985;39:330-336.
1770. Scheike O, Visfeldt J, Peterson B. Male breast cancer: III Breast carcinoma in association with the Kllinefelter sydrome. Acta Pathol Microbiol Scand Suppl 1973;81:352-358.
1771. Bizzarro A, Valentini G, DiMartino G. Influence of testosterone therapy on clinical and immunological features of autoimmune diseases associated with Klinefelter's syndrome. J Clin Endocrinol Metab 1987;64:32-36.
1772. Fialkow PJ. Genetic aspects of autoimmunity. Prog Med Genet 1969;6:117-167.
1773. Foresta C, Busnardo B, Zanatta G. Lower calcitonin levels in young hypogonadic men with osteoporosis. Horm Metab Res 1983;15:206-207.
1774. Dexeus FH, Logothetis CJ, Chong C, et al. Genetic abnormalities in men with germ cell tumors. J Urol 1988;140(1):80-84.
1775. Billmire D, Vinocur C, Rescorla F, et al. Malignant mediastinal germ cell tumors: an intergroup study. J Pediatr Surg 2001;36(1): 18-24.
1776. Derenoncourt AN, Castro-Magana M, Jones KL. Mediastinal teratoma and precocious puberty in a boy with mosaic Klinefelter syndrome. Am J Med Genet 1995;55:38-42.
1777. Von Muhlendahl KE, Heinrich U. Sexual precocity in Klinefelter syndrome: report on two new cases with idiopathic central precocious puberty. Eur J Pediatr 1994;153:322-324.
1778. Hasle H, Jacobsen BB, Asschenfeldt P, et al. Mediastinal germ cell tumour associated with Klinefelter syndrome. A report of case and review of the literature. Eur J Pediatr 1992;151:735-739.
1779. Bramswig JH, Heimes U, Heiermann E, et al. The effects of different cumulative doses of chemotherapy on testicular function. Results in 75 patients treated for Hodgkin's disease during childhood or adolescence. Cancer 1990;65:1298-1302.
1780. Afify Z, Shaw PJ, Clavano-Harding A, et al. Growth and endocrine function in children with acute myeloid leukaemia after bone marrow transplantation using busulfan/cyclophosphamide. Bone Marrow Transplant 2000;25(10):1087-1092.
1781. Zaletel LZ, Bratanic N, Jereb B. Gonadal function in patients treated for leukemia in childhood. Leuk Lymphoma 2004;45(9): 1797-1802.
1782. Kenney LB, Laufer MR, Grant FD, et al. High risk of infertility and long term gonadal damage in males treated with high dose cyclophosphamide for sarcoma during childhood. Cancer 2001;91(3): 613-621.
1783. Garolla A, Pizzato C, Ferlin A, et al. Progress in the development of childhood cancer therapy. Reprod Toxicol 2006;22(2): 126-132.
1784. Mustieles C, Munoz A, Alonso M, et al. Male gonadal function after chemotherapy in survivors of childhood malignancy. Med Pediatr Oncol 1995;24:347-351.
1785. Penso J, Lippe B, Ehrlich R, et al. Testicular function in prepubertal and pubertal male patients treated with cyclophosphamide for nephrotic syndrome. J Pediatr 1974;84:831-836.
1786. Callis L, Nieto J, Vila A, et al. Chlorambucil treatment in minimal lesion nephrotic syndrome: a reappraisal of its gonadal toxicity. J Pediatr 1980;97:653-656.
1787. Hoorweg-Nijman JJ, Delemarre-van de Waal HA, de Waal FC, et al. Cyclophosphamide-induced disturbance of gonadotropin secretion manifesting testicular damage. Acta Endocrinol (Copenh) 1992;126:143-148.

1788. Dhabhar BN, Malhotra H, Joseph R, et al. Gonadal function in prepubertal boys following treatment for Hodgkin's disease. Am J Pediatr Hematol Oncol 1993;15:306-310.
1789. van den BH, Furstner F, van den BC, Behrendt H. Decreasing the number of MOPP courses reduces gonadal damage in survivors of childhood Hodgkin disease. Pediatr Blood Cancer 2004; 42(3):210-215.
1790. Bramswig JH, Heimes U, Heiermann E, et al. The effects of different cumulative doses of chemotherapy on testicular function. Cancer 1990;65:1298-1302.
1791. Ben Arush MW, Solt I, Lightman A, et al. Male gonadal function in survivors of childhood Hodgkin and non-Hodgkin lymphoma. Pediatr Hematol Oncol 2000;17(3):239-245.
1792. Barrett A, Nicholls J, Gibson B. Late effects of total body irradiation. Radiother Oncol 1987;9:131-135.
1793. Ogilvy-Stuart AL, Shalet SM. Effect of radiation on the human reproductive system. Environ Health Perspect 1993;101(Suppl 2):109-116.
1794. Aslam I, Fishel S, Moore H, et al, Thornton S. Fertility preservation of boys undergoing anti-cancer therapy: a review of the existing situation and prospects for the future. Hum Reprod 2000;15(10): 2154-2159.
1795. Muller J, Sonksen J, Sommer P, et al. Cryopreservation of semen from pubertal boys with cancer. Medical and Pediatric Oncology 2000;34(3):191-194.
1796. Schover LR, Agarwal A, Thomas AJ Jr. Cryopreservation of gametes in young patients with cancer. J Pediatr Hematol Oncol 1998;20(5):426-428.
1797. Tesarik J, Bahceci M, Ozcan C, et al. Restoration of fertility by in-vitro spermatogenesis. Lancet 1999;353(9152):555-556.
1798. Antinori S, Versaci C, Dani G, et al. Successful fertilization and pregnancy after injection of frozen-thawed round spermatids into human oocytes. Hum Reprod 1997;12(3):554-556.
1799. Brougham MF, Kelnar CJ, Sharpe RM, et al. Male fertility following childhood cancer: current concepts and future therapies. Asian J Androl 2003;5(4):325-337.
1800. Martin RM, Lin CJ, Costa EM, et al. P450c17 deficiency in Brazilian patients: biochemical diagnosis through progesterone levels confirmed by CYP17 genotyping. J Clin Endocrinol Metab 2003;88(12):5739-5746.
1801. Bosson D, Wolter R, Toppet M, et al. Partial 17, 20-desmolase and 17 alpha-hydroxylase deficiencies in a 16-year-old boy. J Endocrinol Invest 1988;11:527-533.
1802. Bose HS, Sugawara T, Strauss JF 3rd, et al. The pathophysiology and genetics of congenital lipoid adrenal hyperplasia. International Congenital Lipoid Adrenal Hyperplasia Consortium. N Engl J Med 1996;335:1870-1878.
1803. Bose HS, Pescovitz OH, Miller WL. Spontaneous feminization in a 46,XX female patient with congenital lipoid adrenal hyperplasia due to a homozygous frameshift mutation in the steroidogenic acute regulatory protein. J Clin Endocrinol Metab 1997;82: 1511-1515.
1804. Fujieda K, Tajima T, Nakae J, et al. Spontaneous puberty in 46,XX subjects with congenital lipoid adrenal hyperplasia. Ovarian steroidogenesis is spared to some extent despite inactivating mutations in the steroidogenic acute regulatory protein (StAR) gene. J Clin Invest 1997;99:1265-1271.
1805. Dufau ML. The luteinizing hormone receptor. Annu Rev Physiol 1998;60:461-496.
1806. Huhtaniemi I, Alevizaki M. Gonadotrophin resistance. Best Pract Res Clin Endocrinol Metab 2006;20(4):561-576.
1807. David R, Yoon DJ, Landin L, et al. A syndrome of gonadotropin resistance possibly due to a luteinizing hormone receptor defect. J Clin Endocrinol Metab 1984;59:156-160.
1808. Gromoll J, Eiholzer U, Nieschlag E, et al. Male hypogonadism caused by homozygous deletion of exon 10 of the luteinizing hormone (LH) receptor: differential action of human chorionic gonadotropin and LH. J Clin Endocrinol Metab 2000;85(6): 2281-2286.
1809. Latronico AC, Anasti J, Arnhold IJ, et al. Brief report: testicular and ovarian resistance to luteinizing hormone caused by inactivating mutations of the luteinizing hormone-receptor gene. N Engl J Med 1996;334(8):507-512.
1810. Martens JW, Verhoef-Post M, Abelin N, et al. A homozygous mutation in the luteinizing hormone receptor causes partial Leydig cell hypoplasia: correlation between receptor activity and phenotype. Molecular Endocrinology 1998;12(6):775-784.
1811. Winkler L, Offner G, Krull F, et al. Growth and pubertal development in nephropathic cystinosis. Eur J Pediatr 1993;152:244-249.
1812. Chik CL, Friedman A, Merriam GR, et al. Pituitary-testicular function in nephropathic cystinosis. Ann Intern Med 1993;119: 568-575.
1813. Lee P. Fertility in cryptorchidism: does treatment make a difference? Enodocrinol Metab Clin North Am 1993;22,479-490.
1814. Hutson JM, Hasthorpe S, Heyns CF. Anatomical and functional aspects of testicular descent and cryptorchidism. Endocr Rev 1997;18:259-280.
1814a. Pettersson A, Richiardi L, Nordenskjold A, et al. Age at surgery for undescended testis and risk of testicular cancer. N Engl J Med 2007;356:1835-1841.
1815. Lee PA, Coughlin MT. Fertility after bilateral cryptorchidism. Evaluation by paternity, hormone, and semen data. Horm Res 2001;55(1):28-32.
1815a. Virtanen HE, Bjerknes R, Cortes D, et al. Cryptorchidism: classification, prevalence and long-term consequences. Acta Paediatr 2007;96:611-616.
1816. Saez J, Forest MG. Kinetics of human chorionic gonadotropin-induced steroidogenic reponse of the human testis. I. Plasma testosterone: implications for human chorionic gonadotropin stimulation test. J Clin Endocrinol Metab 1979;49:278-283.
1817. Hurwitz RS, Kaptein JS. How well does contralateral testis hypertrophy predict the absence of the nonpalpable testis? J Urol 2001;165(2):588-592.
1818. Laron Z, Dickerman Z, Ritterman I, et al. Follow-up of boys with unilateral compensatory testicular hypertrophy. Fertil Steril 1980;33:297-301.
1819. Pyorala S, Huttunen N-P, Uhari M. A review and meta analysis of hormonal treatment of cryptorchidism. J Clin Endocrinol Metab 1995;80:2795-2799.
1820. Lala R, Matarazzo P, Chiabotto P, et al. Early hormonal and surgical treatment of cryptorchidism. J Urol 1997;157(5):1898-1901.
1821. Bertelloni S, Baroncelli GI, Ghirri P, et al. Hormonal treatment for unilateral inguinal testis: comparison of four different treatments. Horm Res 2001;55(5):236-239.
1822. Esposito C, De Lucia A, Palmieri A, et al. Comparison of five different hormonal treatment protocols for children with cryptorchidism. Scand J Urol Nephrol 2003;37(3):246-249.
1823. Fedder J, Boesen M. Effect of a combined GnRH/hCG therapy in boys with undescended testicles: evaluated in relation to testicular localization within the first week after birth. Arch Androl 1998;40(3):181-186.
1824. Cortes D, Thorup J, Visfeldt J. Hormonal treatment may harm the germ cells in 1 to 3-year-old boys with cryptorchidism. J Urol 2000;163(4):1290-1292.
1824a. Thorsson AV, Christiansen P, Ritzen M. Efficacy and safety of hormonal treatment of cryptorchidism: current state of the art. Acta Paediatr 2007;96:628-630.
1825. Hamza AF, et al. Testicular descent: when to interfere? Eur J Pediatr Surg 2001;11(3):173-176.
1826. Huff DS, Fenig DM, Canning DA, et al. Abnormal germ cell development in cryptorchidism. Horm Res 2001;55(1):11-17.
1827. Grasso M, Buonaguidi A, Lania C, et al. Postpubertal cryptorchidism: review and evaluation of the fertility. Eur Urol 1991;20: 126-128.
1828. Docimo SG. The resultts of surgical therapy for cryptorchidism: a literature review and analysis. J Urol 1995;154:1148-1152.
1829. Lee PA. Fertility in cryptorchidism. Does treatment make a difference? Endocrinol Metab Clin North Am 1993;22:479-490.
1830. Mininberg DT, Rodger JC, Bedford JM. Ultrastructural evidence of the onset of testicular pathological conditions in the cryptorchid human testis within the first year of life. J Urol 1982; 128(4):782-784.
1831. Cendron M, Keating MA, Huff DS, et al. Cryptorchidism, orchiopexy and infertility: a critical long-term retrospective analysis. J Urol 1989;142(2 Pt 2):559-562.
1832. Huff DS, Hadziselimovic F, Snyder HM III, et al. Postnatal testicular maldevelopment in unilateral cryptorchidism. J Urol 1989;142(2 Pt 2):546-548.

1833. Lin YM, Hsu CC, Lin JS. Successful testicular sperm extraction and fertilization in an azoospermic man with postpubertal mumps orchitis. BJU Int 1999;83(4):526-527.
1834. Heaton ND, Davenport M, Pryor JP. Fertility after correction of bilateral undescended testes at the age of 23 years. Br J Urol 1993;71(4):490-491.
1835. Shin D, Lemack GE, Goldstein M. Induction of spermatogenesis and pregnancy after adult orchiopexy. J Urol 1997;158(6): 2242.
1836. Giwercman A, Hansen LL, Skakkebaek NE. Initiation of sperm production after bilateral orchiopexy: clinical and biological implications. J Urol 2000;163(4):1255-1256.
1837. Moller H, Jorgensen N, Forman D. Trends in incidence of testicular cancer in boys and adolescent men. Int J Cancer 1995;61: 761-764.
1838. Moller H, Evans H. Epidemiology of gonadal germ cell cancer in males and females. APMIS 2003;111(1):43-46.
1839. Skakkebaek NE, Rajpert-De Meyts E, Main KM. Testicular dysgenesis syndrome: an increasingly common developmental disorder with environmental aspects. Hum Reprod 2001;16(5): 972-978.
1840. Cortes D, Thorup JM, Visfeldt J. Cryptorchidism: aspects of fertility and neoplasms. A study including data of 1,335 consecutive boys who underwent testicular biopsy simultaneously with surgery for cryptorchidism. Horm Res 2001;55(1):21-27.
1841. United Kingdom Testicular Cancer Study Group. Aetiology of testicular cancer: association with congenital abnormalities, age at puberty, infertility, and exercise. BMJ 1994;308:1393-1399.
1842. Parkinson MC, Swerdlow AJ, Pike MC. Carcinoma in situ in boys with cryptorchidism: when can it be detected? Br J Urol 1994; 73:431-435.
1843. Giwercman A, von der Maase H, Skakkebaek NE. Epidemiological and clinical aspects of carcinoma in situ of the testis. Eur Urol 1993;23:104-10; discussion 111-114.
1844. Sinisi AA, Pasquali D, Papparella A, et al. Antisperm antibodies in cryptorchidism before and after surgery. J Urol 1998;160(5): 1834-1837.
1845. Mirilas P, Mamoulakis C, De Almeida M. Puberty does not induce serum antisperm surface antibodies in patients with previously operated cryptorchidism. J Urol 2003;170(6 Pt 1):2432-2435.
1846. Hack WW, Meijer RW, Van Der Voort-Doedens LM, et al. Natural course of acquired undescended testis in boys. Br J Surg 2003;90(6):728-731.
1847. La Scala GC, Ein SH. Retractile testes: an outcome analysis on 150 patients. J Pediatr Surg 2004;39(7):1014-1017.
1848. Thomas DB, Jimenez LM, McTiernan A, et al. Breast cancer in men: risk factors with hormonal implications. Am J Epidemiol 1992;135:734-748.
1849. Rosenfeld RG, Grumbach MM. Turner Syndrome. New York: Marcel Decker, 1990.
1850. Turner Syndrome: Growth Promoting Therapies. Amsterdam: Excerpta Medica, 1991.
1851. Basic and Clinical Approach to Turner Syndrome. Amsterdam: Excerpta Medica, 1993.
1852. Turner Syndrome in a Life Span Perspective: Research and Clinical Aspects. Amsterdam, Elsevier, 1995.
1853. Elsheikh M, Dunger DB, Conway GS, et al. Turner's syndrome in adulthood. Endocr Rev 2002;23(1):120-140.
1854. Ranke MB, Saenger P. Turner's syndrome. Lancet 2001; 358(9278):309-314.
1855. Hook EB, Warburton D. The distribution of chromosomal genotypes associated with Turner's syndrome: livebirth prevalence rates and evidence for diminished fetal mortality and severity in genotypes associated with structural X abnormalities or mosaicism. Hum Genet 1983;64:24-27.
1856. Turner HH. A syndrome of infantilism, congenital webbed neck and cubitus valgus. Endocrinology 1938;23:566-574.
1857. Carr DH, Gedeon M. Population cytogenetics in human abortuses. In Hook EB, Porter IH, editors. Population Cytogenetics. New York: Academic Press, 1977:1-9.
1858. Warburton D, Kline J, Stein I. Monosomy X: a chromosomal anomaly associated with young maternal age. Lancet 1980;1: 167-169.
1859. Saenger P, Wikland KA, Conway GS, et al. Recommendations for the diagnosis and management of Turner syndrome. J Clin Endocrinol Metab 2001;86(7):3061-3069.
1860. Roa E, Weiss B, Fukami M, et al. Pseudoautosomal deletions encompassing a novel homeobox gene cause growth failure in idiopathic short stature and Turner syndrome. Nature Genet 1997;16:54-62.
1861. Ellison JW, Wardak Z, Young M, et al. PHOG, a candidate gene for involvement in the short stature of Turner syndrome. Hum Mol Genet 1997, in press 449 Palmer CG, Reichman A Chromosomal and clinical findings in 110 females with Turner syndrome Hum Genet 1976;35:35-49.
1862. Belin V, Cusin V, Viot G, et al. SHOX mutations in dyschondrosteosis (Leri-Weill syndrome). Nat Genet 1998;19(1):67-69.
1863. Kosho T, Muroya K, Nagai T, et al. Skeletal features and growth patterns in 14 patients with haploinsufficiency of SHOX: implications for the development of Turner syndrome. J Clin Endocrinol Metab 1999;84(12):4613-4621.
1864. Blaschke RJ, Rappold GA. SHOX: Growth, Leri-Weill and Turner syndromes. Trends Endocinol Metab 2000;11:227-230.
1865. Ogata T, Muroya K, Matsuo N, et al. Turner syndrome and Xp deletions: clinical and molecular studies in 47 patients. J Clin Endocrinol Metab 2001;86(11):5498-5508.
1866. Ogata T, Matsuo N, Nishimura G. SHOX haploinsufficiency and overdosage: impact of gonadal function status. J Med Genet 2001;38(1):1-6.
1867. Clement-Jones M, Schiller S, Rao E, et al. The short stature homeobox gene SHOX is involved in skeletal abnormalities in Turner syndrome. Hum Mol Genet 2000;9(5):695-702.
1868. Ogata T, Kosho T, Wakui K, et al. Short stature homeobox-containing gene duplication on the der(X) chromosome in a female with 45,X/46,X, der(X), gonadal dysgenesis, and tall stature. J Clin Endocrinol Metab 2000;85(8):2927-2930.
1869. Rappold G, Blum WF, Shavrikova EP, et al. Genotypes and phenotypes in children with short stature: clinical indicators of SHOX haploinsufficiency. J Med Genet 2006;44(5):306-313.
1870. Barrenas ML, Landin-Wilhelmsen K, Hanson C. Ear and hearing in relation to genotype and growth in Turner syndrome. Hear Res 2000;144:21-28.
1871. Palmer CG, Reichman A. Chromosomal and clinical findings in 110 females with Turner syndrome. Human Genetics 1976;35: 35-49.
1872. Lin AE, Lippe BM, Geffner ME, et al. Aortic dilation, dissection, and rupture in patients with Turner syndrome. J Pediatr 1986; 109:820-826.
1873. Lippe BM, Geffner ME, Dietrich RB, et al. Renal malformations in patients with Turner syndrome: imaging in 141 patients. Pediatrics 1988;82:852-856.
1874. Gravholt CH, Juul S, Naeraa RW, et al. Morbidity in Turner syndrome. J Clin Epidemiol 1998;51(2):147-158.
1875. Elsheikh M, Wass JA, Conway GS. Autoimmune thyroid syndrome in women with Turner's syndrome—the association with karyotype. Clin Endocrinol (Oxf) 2001;55(2):223-226.
1876. Savendahl L, Davenport ML. Delayed diagnoses of Turner's syndrome: proposed guidelines for change. J Pediatr 2000;137(4): 455-459.
1877. Wilson CA, Heinrichs C, Larmore KA, et al. Estradiol levels in girls with Turner's syndrome compared to normal prepubertal girls as determined by an ultrasensitive assay. J Pediatr Endocrinol Metab 2003;16(1):91-96.
1878. Doerr HG, Bettendorf M, Hauffa BP, et al. Uterine size in women with Turner syndrome after induction of puberty with estrogens and long-term growth hormone therapy: results of the German IGLU Follow-up Study 2001. Hum Reprod 2005;20(5):1418-1421.
1879. Livadas S, Xekouki P, Kafiri G, et al. Spontaneous pregnancy and birth of a normal female from a woman with Turner syndrome and elevated gonadotropins. Fertil Steril 2005;83(3):769-772.
1880. Cools M, Rooman RP, Wauters J, et al. A nonmosaic 45,X karyotype in a mother with Turner's syndrome and in her daughter. Fertil Steril 2004;82(4):923-925.
1881. Timmreck LS, Reindollar RH. Contemporary issues in primary amenorrhea. Obstet Gynecol Clin North Am 2003;30(2):287-302.
1882. Karnis MF, Zimon AE, Lalwani SI, et al. Risk of death in pregnancy achieved through oocyte donation in patients with Turner syndrome: a national survey. Fertil Steril 2003;80(3):498-501.
1883. Even L, Cohen A, Marbach N, et al. Longitudinal analysis of growth over the first 3 years of life in Turner's syndrome. J Pediatr 2000;137(4):460-464.

1884. Lyon AJ, Preece MA, Grant DB. Growth curve for girls with Turner syndrome. Arch Dis Child 1985;60:932-935.
1885. Ranke MB, Stubbe P, Majewski F, et al. Spontaneous growth in Turner's syndrome. Acta Paediatr Scand Suppl 1988;343:22-30.
1886. Hochberg Z, Khaesh-Goldberg I, Partsch CJ, et al. Differences in infantile growth patterns in Turner syndrome girls with and without spontaneous puberty. Horm Metab Res 2005;37(4): 236-241.
1887. Ranke MB, Grauer ML. Adult height in Turner syndrome: results of a multinational survey 1993. Horm Res 1994;42(3):90-94.
1888. Massa G, Vanderschueren-Lodeweyckx M, Malvaux P. Linear growth in patients with Turner syndrome: influence of spontaneous puberty and parental height. Eur J Pediatr 1990;149:246-250.
1889. Sas TC, de Muinck Keizer-Schrama S, Stijnen T, et al. Normalization of height in girls with Turner syndrome after long-term growth hormone treatment: results of a randomized dose-response trial. J Clin Endocrinol Metab 1999;84(12):4607-4612.
1890. Carel JC, Mathivon L, Gendrel C, et al. Near normalization of final height with adapted doses of growth hormone in Turner's syndrome. J Clin Endocrinol Metab 1998;83(5):1462-1466.
1891. Cacciari E, Mazzanti L. Final height of patients with Turner's syndrome treated with growth hormone (GH): indications for GH therapy alone at high doses and late estrogen therapy. Italian Study Group for Turner Syndrome. J Clin Endocrinol Metab 1999;84(12):4510-4515.
1892. Cave CB, Bryant J, Milne R. Recombinant growth hormone in children and adolescents with Turner syndrome. Cochrane Database Syst Rev 2003;(3).
1893. Rosenfeld RG, Attie KM, Frane J, et al. Growth hormone therapy of Turner's syndrome: beneficial effect on adult height. J Pediatr 1998;132(2):319-324.
1894. Ranke MB, Lindberg A, Chatelain P, et al. Prediction of long-term response to recombinant human growth hormone in Turner syndrome: development and validation of mathematical models. KIGS International Board. Kabi International Growth Study. J Clin Endocrinol Metab 2000;85(11):4212-4218.
1895. Betts PR, Butler GE, Donaldson MD, et al. A decade of growth hormone treatment in girls with Turner syndrome in the UK. UK KIGS Executive Group. Arch Dis Child 1999;80(3):221-225.
1896. Takano K, Ogawa M, Tanaka T, et al. Clinical trials of GH treatment in patients with Turner's syndrome in Japan—a consideration of final height. The Committee for the Treatment of Turner's Syndrome. Eur J Endocrinol 1997;137(2):138-145.
1897. Sas TC, Gerver WJ, De Bruin R, et al. Body proportions during long-term growth hormone treatment in girls with Turner syndrome participating in a randomized dose-response trial. J Clin Endocrinol Metab 1999;84(12):4622-4628.
1898. Parvin M, Roche E, Costigan C, et al. Treatment outcome in Turner syndrome. Ir Med J 2004;97(1):12, 14-12, 15.
1899. Massa G, Heinrichs C, Verlinde S, et al. Late or delayed induced or spontaneous puberty in girls with Turner syndrome treated with growth hormone does not affect final height. J Clin Endocrinol Metab 2003;88(9):4168-4174.
1900. Chernausek SD, Attie KM, Cara JF, et al. Growth hormone therapy of Turner syndrome: the impact of age of estrogen replacement on final height. Genentech, Inc., Collaborative Study Group. J Clin Endocrinol Metab 2000;85(7):2439-2445.
1901. Jospe N, Orlowski CC, Furlanetto RW. Comparison of transdermal and oral estrogen therapy in girls with Turner's syndrome. J Pediatr Endocrinol Metab 1995;8(2):111-116.
1902. Stephure DK. Impact of growth hormone supplementation on adult height in turner syndrome: results of the Canadian randomized controlled trial. J Clin Endocrinol Metab 2005;90(6): 3360-3366.
1903. van Pareren YK, de Muinck Keizer-Schrama SM, Stijnen T, et al. Final height in girls with turner syndrome after long-term growth hormone treatment in three dosages and low dose estrogens. J Clin Endocrinol Metab 2003;88(3):1119-1125.
1904. Sas TC, de Muinck Keizer-Schrama SM, Stijnen T, et al. Bone mineral density assessed by phalangeal radiographic absorptiometry before and during long-term growth hormone treatment in girls with turner's syndrome participating in a randomized dose-response study. Pediatr Res 2001;50(3):417-422.
1905. Bechtold S, Rauch F, Noelle V, et al. Musculoskeletal analyses of the forearm in young women with Turner syndrome: a study using peripheral quantitative computed tomography. J Clin Endocrinol Metab 2001;86(12):5819-5823.
1906. Bertelloni S, Cinquanta L, Baroncelli GI, et al. Volumetric bone mineral density in young women with Turner's syndrome treated with estrogens or estrogens plus growth hormone. Horm Res 2000;53(2):72-76.
1907. Ari M, Bakalov VK, Hill S, et al. The effects of GH treatment on bone mineral density and body composition in girls with Turner syndrome. J Clin Endocrinol Metab 2006;91(11):4302-4305.
1908. Bakalov VK, Van PL, Baron J, et al. Growth hormone therapy and bone mineral density in Turner syndrome J Clin Endocrinol Metab 2004;89(10):4886-4889.
1909. Nilsson KO, Albertsson-Wikland K, Alm J, et al. Improved final height in girls with Turner's syndrome treated with growth hormone and oxandrolone. J Clin Endocrinol Metab 1996;81: 635-640.
1910. Schweizer R, Ranke MB, Binder G, et al. Experience with growth hormone therapy in Turner syndrome in a single centre: low total height gain, no further gains after puberty onset and unchanged body proportions. Horm Res 2000;53(5):228-238.
1911. Takano K, Shizume K, Hibi IO, et al. Growth hormone treatment in Turner syndrome: results of a multicentre study in Japan. The Committee for the Treatment of Turner Syndrome. Horm Res 1993;39(Suppl 2):37-41.
1912. Rovet J, Holland J. Psychological aspects of the Canadian randomized controlled trial of human growth hormone and low-dose ethinyl oestradiol in children with Turner syndrome. The Canadian Growth Hormone Advisory Group. Horm Res 1993;39(Suppl 2):60-64.
1913. Knudtzon J, Aarskog D. Results of two years of growth hormone treatment followed by combined growth hormone and oestradiol in Turner syndrome. The Norwegian Turner Study Group. Horm Res 1993;39(Suppl 2):7-17.
1914. Attanasio A, James D, Reinhardt R, et al. Final height and long-term outcome after growth hormone therapy in Turner syndrome: results of a German multicentre trial. Horm Res 1995;43: 147-149.
1915. Massa G, Maes M, Heinrichs C, et al. Influence of spontaneous or induced puberty on the growth promoting effect of treatment with growth hormone in girls with Turner's syndrome. Clin Endocrinol (Oxf) 1993;38:253-260.
1916. Rosenfeld RG, Hintz RL, Johanson AJ, et al. Growth hormone therapy in Turner's syndrome. In Rosenfeld RG, Grumbach MM, eds. Turner Syndrome. New York: Marcel Dekker, 1990:393-405.
1917. Johnston DI, Betts P, Dunger D, et al. A multicentre trial of recombinant growth hormone and low dose oestrogen in Turner syndrome: near final height analysis. Arch Dis Child 2001;84(1): 76-81.
1918. Reiter EO, Blethen SL, Baptista J, et al. Early initiation of growth hormone treatment allows age-appropriate estrogen use in Turner's syndrome. J Clin Endocrinol Metab 2001;86(5):1936-1941.
1919. Nielsen J. Mental aspects of Turner syndrome and the importance of information and Turner contact groups. In Rosenfeld RG, Grumbach MM, eds. Turner Syndrome. New York: Marcel Dekker, 1946:451-467.
1920. Gravholt CH, Vestergaard P, Hermann AP, et al. Increased fracture rates in Turner's syndrome: a nationwide questionnaire survey. Clin Endocrinol (Oxf) 2003;59(1):89-96.
1921. Lagrou K, Xhrouet-Heinrichs D, Heinrichs C, et al. Age-related perception of stature, acceptance of therapy, and psychosocial functioning in human growth hormone-treated girls with Turner's syndrome. J Clin Endocrinol Metab 1998;83(5):1494-1501.
1922. van Pareren YK, Duivenvoorden HJ, Slijper FM, et al. Psychosocial functioning after discontinuation of long-term growth hormone treatment in girls with turner syndrome. Horm Res 2005;63(5):238-244.
1923. Ross JL, Feuillan P, Kushner H, et al. Absence of growth hormone effects on cognitive function in girls with Turner syndrome [see comments]. J Clin Endocrinol Metab 1997;82(6):1814-1817.
1924. Siegel PT, Clopper R, Stabler B. The psychological consequences of Turner syndrome and review of the National Cooperative Growth Study psychological substudy. Pediatrics 1998;102: 488-491.
1925. Carel JC, Ecosse E, Bastie-Sigeac I, et al. Quality of life determinants in young women with turner's syndrome after growth

hormone treatment: results of the StaTur population-based cohort study. J Clin Endocrinol Metab 2005;90(4):1992-1997.

1926. van Pareren YK, Duivenvoorden HJ, Slijper FM, et al. Psychosocial functioning after discontinuation of long-term growth hormone treatment in girls with turner syndrome. Horm Res 2005;63(5):238-244.
1927. Cicognani A, Mazzanti L, Tassinari D, et al. Differences in carbohydrate tolerance in Turner syndrome depending on age and karyotype. Eur J Pediatr 1988;148:64-68.
1928. Nielsen J, Johansen K, Yde H. The frequency of diabetes mellitus in patients with Turner's syndrome and pure gonadal dysgenesis. Acta Endocrinol 1969;62:251-269.
1929. Sas TC, de Muinck Keizer-Schrama S, Stijnen T, et al. Carbohydrate metabolism during long-term growth hormone (GH) treatment and after discontinuation of GH treatment in girls with Turner syndrome participating in a randomized dose-response study. Dutch Advisory Group on Growth Hormone. J Clin Endocrinol Metab 2000;85(2):769-775.
1930. Ross JL, Feuillan P, Long LM, et al. Lipid abnormalities in Turner syndrome. J Pediatr 1995;126:242-245.
1931. Martin DD, Schweizer R, Schwarze CP, et al. The early dehydroepiandrosterone sulfate rise of adrenarche and the delay of pubarche indicate primary ovarian failure in Turner syndrome. J Clin Endocrinol Metab 2004;89(3):1164-1168.
1932. Sklar CA, Kaplan SL, Grumbach MM. Lack of effect of oestrogens on adrenal androgen secretion in children and adolescents with a comment on oestrogens and pubic hair growth. Clin Endocrinol 1981;14:311-320.
1933. Mazzocco MM. A process approach to describing mathematics difficulties in girls with Turner syndrome. Pediatrics 1998;102: 492-496.
1934. Van Dyke DL, Wiktor A, Palmer CG, et al. Ullrich-Turner syndrome with a small ring X chromosome and presence of mental retardation. Am J Med Genet 1992;43(6):996-1005.
1935. Silbert A, Wolffe PH, Lilienthal J. Spatial and temporal processing in patients with Turner's syndrome. Behav Genet 1977;7:11-21.
1936. Swillen A, Fryns JP, Kleczkowska A, et al. Intelligence, behaviour and psychosocial development in Turner syndrome. A cross-sectional study of 50 pre-adolescent and adolescent girls (4-20 years). Genet Couns 1993;4:7-18.
1937. Garron DC. Intelligence among persons with Turner's syndrome. Behav Genet 1977;7:105-127.
1938. Temple CM, Carney R. Reading skills in children with Turner's syndrome: an analysis of hyperplexia. Cortex 1996;32(2): 335-345.
1939. Ross JL, Kushner H, Roeltgen DP. Developmental changes in motor function in girls with Turner syndrome. Pediatr Neurol 1996;15(4):317-322.
1940. Ross JL, Stefanatos G, Roeltgen D, et al. Ullrich-Turner syndrome: neurodevelopmental changes from childhood through adolescence. Am J Med Genet 1995;58(1):74-82.
1941. Reiss AL, Mazzocco MM, Greenlaw R, et al. Neurodevelopmental effects of X monosomy: a volumetric imaging study. Ann Neurol 1995;38(5):731-738.
1942. Murphy DG, Mentis MJ, Pietrini P, et al. A PET study of Turner's syndrome: effects of sex steroids and the X chromosome on brain. Biol Psychiatry 1997;41(3):285-298.
1943. Murphy DG, DeCarli C, Daly E, et al. X-chromosome effects on female brain: a magnetic resonance imaging study of Turner's syndrome. Lancet 1993;342(8881):1197-1200.
1944. Voeller KK. Right-hemisphere deficit syndrome in children. Am J Psychiatry 1986;143(8):1004-1009.
1945. McCauley E, Kay T, Ito J, et al. The Turner syndrome: cognitive deficits, affective discrimination, and behavior problems. Child Dev 1987;58(2):464-473.
1946. Albertsson-Wiklund K., Ranke MB. Turner Syndrome in a Life Span Perspective: Research and Clinical Aspects. Amsterdam: Elsevier Science BV, 1995.
1947. Skuse DH, James RS, Bishop DVM, et al. Evidence from Turner's syndrome of an imprinted X-linked locus affecting cognitive function. Nature 1997;387:705-708.
1948. Mazzocco MM, Baumgardner T, Freund LS, et al. Social functioning among girls with fragile X or Turner syndrome and their sisters. J Autism Dev Disord 1998;28(6):509-517.
1949. Rovet J, Ireland L. Behavioral phenotype in children with Turner syndrome. J Pediatr Psychol 1994;19:779-790.
1950. Jani MM, Torchia BS, Pai GS, et al. Molecular characterization of tiny ring X chromosomes from females with functional X chromosome disomy and lack of cis X inactivation. Genomics 1995; 27(1):182-188.
1951. Ross JL, Roeltgen D, Kushner H, et al. The Turner syndrome-associated neurocognitive phenotype maps to distal Xp. Am J Hum Genet 2000;67(3):672-681.
1952. McGuffin P, Scourfield J. A father's imprint on his daughter's thinking. Nature 1997;387:652-653.
1953. Ross J, Roeltgen D, Zinn A. Cognition and the sex chromosomes: studies in Turner syndrome. Horm Res 2006;65(1):47-56.
1954. Skuse DH. Genomic imprinting of the X chromosome: a novel mechanism for the evolution of sexual dimorphism. J Lab Clin Med 1999;133(1):23-32.
1955. Bishop DV, Canning E, Elgar K, et al. Distinctive patterns of memory function in subgroups of females with Turner syndrome: evidence for imprinted loci on the X-chromosome affecting neurodevelopment. Neuropsychologia 2000;38(5):712-721.
1956. Rickert VI, Hassed SJ, Hendon AE, et al. The effects of peer ridicule on depression and self-image among adolescent females with Turner syndrome. J Adolesc Health 1996;19(1): 34-38.
1957. Ross JL, Roeltgen D, Feuillan P, et al. Use of estrogen in young girls with Turner syndrome: effects on memory. Neurology 2000;54(1):164-170.
1958. Phillips SM, Sherwin BB. Effects of estrogen on memory function in surgically menopausal women. Psychoneuroendocrinology 1992;17(5):485-495.
1959. Phillips SM, Sherwin BB. Variations in memory function and sex steroid hormones across the menstrual cycle. Psychoneuroendocrinology 1992;17(5):497-506.
1960. Karnis MF, Reindollar RH. Turner syndrome in adolescence. Obstet Gynecol Clin North Am 2003;30(2):303-320.
1961. Mazzanti L, Nizzoli G, Tassinari D, et al. Spontaneous growth and pubertal development in Turner's syndrome with different karyotypes. Acta Paediatr 1994;83:299-304.
1962. Cuseen LJ, MacMahan RA. Germ cells and ova in dysgenetic gonads of a 46-XY female dizygotic twin. Am J Dis Child 1979;133:373-375.
1963. Scully RE. Gonadoblastoma: a review of 74 cases. Cancer 1970; 25:1340-1356.
1964. Hoepffner W, Horn LC, Simon E, et al. Gonadoblastomas in 5 patients with 46,XY gonadal dysgenesis. Exp Clin Endocrinol Diabetes 2005;113(4):231-235.
1965. Khodr GS, Cadena GD, Ong TC. Y-autosome translocation, gonadal dysgenesis, and gonadoblastoma. Am J Dis Child 1979;133:277-282.
1966. Jamieson CR, van der Burgt I, Brady AF, et al. Mapping a gene for Noonan syndrome to the long arm of chromosome 12. Nature Genet 1994;8:357-360.
1967. Umehara F, Tate G, Itoh K, et al. A novel mutation of desert hedgehog in a patient with 46,XY partial gonadal dysgenesis accompanied by minifascicular neuropathy. Am J Hum Genet 2000;67(5):1302-1305.
1968. Thibaud E, Ramirez M, Brauner R, et al. Preservation of ovarian function by ovarian transposition performed before pelvic irradiation during childhood. J Pediatr 1992;121:880-884.
1969. Quigley C, Cowell C, Jimenez M, et al. Normal or early development of puberty despite gonadal damage in children treated for acute lymphoblastic leukemia. N Engl J Med 1989;321:143-151.
1970. Lahteenmaki PM, Toppari J, Ruokonen A, et al. Low serum inhibin B concentrations in male survivors of childhood malignancy. Eur J Cancer 1999;35(4):612-619.
1971. Paulino AC, Wen BC, Brown CK, et al. Late effects in children treated with radiation therapy for Wilms' tumor. Int J Rad Oncol Biol Phys 2000;46(5):1239-1246.
1972. Byrne J, Fears TR, Gail MH, et al. Early menopause in long-term survivors of cancer during adolescence. Am J Obstet Gynecol 1992;166(3):788-793.
1973. Longhi A, Porcu E, Petracchi S, et al. Reproductive functions in female patients treated with adjuvant and neoadjuvant chemotherapy for localized osteosarcoma of the extremity. Cancer 2000;89(9):1961-1965.

1974. Hoek A, Schoemaker J, Drexhage HA. Premature ovarian failure and ovarian autoimmunity. Endocr Rev 1997;18:107-134.
1975. Irvine WJ. Autoimmunity in endocrine disease. Recent Prog Horm Res 1980;36:509-556.
1976. Ahonen P, Myllarniemi S, Sipila I, et al. Clinical variation of autoimmune polyendocrinopathy-candidiasis-ectodermal dystrophy (APECED) in a series of 68 patients. N Engl J Med 1990;322: 1829-1836.
1976a. Perheentupa J. Autoimmune polyendocrinopathy-candidiasis-ectodermal dystrophy. J Clin Endocrinol Metab 2006;91: 2843-2850.
1977. Lucky AW, Rebar RW, Blizzard RM, et al. Pubertal progression in the presence of elevated serum gonadotropins in girls with multiple endocrine deficiencies. J Clin Endocrinol Metab 1977;45:673-678.
1978. Betterle C, Rossi A, Dalla Pria S, et al. Premature ovarian failure: autoimmunity and natural history. Clin Endocrinol 1993;39: 35-43.
1979. Chen S, Sawicka J, Betterle C, et al. Autoantibodies to steroidogenic enzymes in autoimmune polyglandular syndrome, Addison's disease, and premature ovarian failure. J Clin Endocrinol Metab 1996;81:1871-1876.
1980. Scott HS, Heino M, Peterson P, et al. Common mutations in autoimmune polyendocrinopathy-candidiasis-ectodermal dystrophy patients of different origins. Mol Endocrinol 1998;12(8): 1112-1119.
1981. Halonen M, Eskelin P, Myhre AG, et al. AIRE mutations and human leukocyte antigen genotypes as determinants of the autoimmune polyendocrinopathy-candidiasis-ectodermal dystrophy phenotype. J Clin Endocrinol Metab 2002;87(6):2568-2574.
1982. Flora S, Bottazzo GF, Doniach D. Immunofluorescence studies on antibodies to steroid producing cells, and to germ line cells in endocrine disease and infertility. Clin Exp Immunol 1980;39: 97-111.
1983. Arif S, Underhil JA, Donaldson P, et al. J Clin Endocrinol Metab 1999;84:1056-1060.
1984. Dewhurst CJ, Dekoos EB, Ferreira HP. The resistant ovary syndrome. Br J Obstet Gynaecol 1975;82:341-345.
1985. Evers JLH, Rolland RT. The gonadotropin resistant ovary syndrome: a curable disease? Clin Endocrinol 1981;14:99-103.
1986. Davis CJ, Davison RM, Payne NN, et al. Female sex preponderance for idiopathic familial premature ovarian failure suggests an X chromosome defect: opinion. Hum Reprod 2000;15(11): 2418-2422.
1987. Gibson JB. Gonadal function in galactosemics and in galactose-intoxicated animals. Eur J Pediatr 1995;154(Suppl 2):S14-S20.
1988. Schweitzer S, Shin Y, Jakobs C, et al. Long-term outcome in 134 patients with galactosaemia. Eur J Pediatr 1993;152:36-43.
1989. Forges T, Monnier-Barbarino P, Leheup B, et al. Pathophysiology of impaired ovarian function in galactosaemia. Hum Reprod Update 2006;12(5):573-584.
1990. Kaufman FR, Kogut MD, Donnell GN, et al. Hypergonadotropic hypogonadism in female patients with galactosemia. N Engl J Med 1981;304:994-998.
1991. Crisponi L, Deiana M, Loi A, et al. The putative forkhead transcription factor FOXL2 is mutated in blepharophimosis/ptosis/epicanthus inversus syndrome. Nat Genet 2001;27(2):159-166.
1992. Nicolino M, Bost M, David M, et al. Familial blepharophimosis: an uncommon marker of ovarian dysgenesis. J Pediatr Endocrinol Metab 1995;8(2):127-133.
1993. Jaeken J, Matthijs G. Congenital disorders of glycosylation. Annu Rev Genomics Hum Genet 2001;2:129-151.
1994. Kristiansson B, Stibler H, Wide L. Gonadal function and glycoprotein hormones in the carbohydrate-deficient glycoprotein (CDG) syndrome. Acta Paediatr 1995;84:655-660.
1995. de Zegher F, Jaeken J. Endocrinology of the carbohydrate-deficient glycoprotein syndrome type 1 from birth through adolescence. Pediatr Res 1995;37:395-401.
1996. Sprengel R, Braun T, Nikolics K, et al. The testicular receptor for follicle-stimulating hormone: structure and functional expression of cloned DNA. Mol Endocrinol 1990;4:525-530.
1997. Simoni M, Gromoll J, Nieschlag E. The follicle-stimulating hormone receptor: biochemistry, molecular biology, physiology, and pathophysiology. Endocr Rev 1997;18(6):739-773.
1998. Aittomaki K. The genetics of XX gonadal dysgenesis. Am J Hum Genet 1994;54:844-851.
1999. Aittomaki K, Herva R, Stenman U-Hea. Clinical features of primary ovarian failure caused by a point mutation in the follicle-stimulating hormone receptor gene. J Clin Endocrinol Metab 1996;81:3722-3726.
2000. Kumar TR, Wang Y, Lu N. Follicle stimulating hormone is required for ovarian follicle maturation but not male fertility. Nature Genet 1997;15:201-204.
2001. Aittomaki K, Dieguez Lucena JL, Pakarinen P, et al. Mutation in the follicle-stimulating hormone receptor gene causes hereditary hypergonadotropic ovarian failure. Cell 1995;82: 959-968.
2002. Tapanainen JS, Aittomaki K, Min J, et al. Men homozygous for an inactivating mutation of the follicle-stimulating hormone (FSH) receptor gene present variable suppression of spermatogenesis and fertility. Nature Genet 1997;15:205-206.
2003. Latronico AC, Anasti J, Arnhold IJP, et al. Testicular and ovarian resistance to luteinizing hormone caused by inactivating mutations of the luteinizing hormone receptor gene. N Engl J Med 1996;344:507-512.
2004. Stanhope R, Adams J, Brook CG. Evolution of polycystic ovaries in a girl with delayed menarche. A case report. J Reprod Med 1988;33:482-484.
2005. Porcu E, Venturoli S, Magrini O, et al. Circadian variation of luteinizing hormone can have two different profiles in adolescent anovulation. J Clin Endocrinol Metab 1987;65:488-493.
2006. Dunaif A, Thomas A. Current concepts in the polycystic ovary syndrome. Annu Rev Med 2001;52:401-419.
2007. Azziz R, Carmina E, Dewailly D, et al. Position statement: criteria for defining polycystic ovary syndrome as a predominantly hyperandrogenic syndrome: an androgen excess society guideline. J Clin Endocrinol Metab 2006;91(11):4237-4245.
2008. Codner E, Mook-Kanamori D, Bazaes RA, et al. Ovarian function during puberty in girls with type 1 diabetes mellitus: response to leuprolide. J Clin Endocrinol Metab 2005;90(7): 3939-3945.
2009. Dunaif A. Insulin resistance in women with polycystic ovary syndrome. Fertil Steril 2006;86(Suppl 1):S13-S14.
2010. Elsawi MM, Pryor JP, Klufio G, et al. Genital tract function in men with Noonan syndrome. J Med Genet 1994;31:468-470.
2011. Witt DR, Keena BA, Hall JG, et al. Growth curves for height in Noonan syndrome. Clin Genet 1986;30(3):150-153.
2012. Kelnar CJ. Growth hormone therapy in noonan syndrome. Horm Res 2000;53(Suppl 1):77-81.
2013. Brown DC, Macfarlane CE, McKenna WJ, et al. Growth hormone therapy in Noonan's syndrome: non-cardiomyopathic congenital heart disease does not adversely affect growth improvement. J Pediatr Endocrinol Metab 2002;15(6):851-852.
2014. Macfarlane CE, Brown DC, Johnston LB, et al. Growth hormone therapy and growth in children with Noonan's syndrome: results of 3 years' follow-up. J Clin Endocrinol Metab 2001;86(5): 1953-1956.
2015. Takagi M, Miyashita Y, Koga M, et al. Estrogen deficiency is a potential cause for osteopenia in adult male patients with Noonan's syndrome. Calcif Tissue Int 2000;66(3):200-203.
2016. Carrascosa A, Gussinye M, Terradas P, et al. Spontaneous, but not induced, puberty permits adequate bone mass acquisition in adolescent Turner syndrome patients. J Bone Miner Res 2000; 15(10):2005-2010.
2017. Gwin K, Cajaiba M, Caminoa-Lizarralde A, et al. Expanding the clinical spectrum of frasier syndrome. Pediatr Dev Pathol 2007;1.
2018. Bailey WA, Zwingman TA, Reznik VM, et al. End-stage renal disease and primary hypogonadism associated with a 46,XX karyotype. Am J Dis Child 1992;146:1218-1223.
2019. Gilger JW, Geary DC, Eisele LM. Reliability and validity of retrospective self-reports of the age of pubertal onset using twin, sibling, and college student data. Adolescence 1991;26:41-53.
2020. Carskadon MA, Acebo C. A self-administered rating scale for pubertal development. J Adolesc Health 1993;14:190-195.
2021. John H, Schmid C. Kallmann's syndrome: clues to clinical diagnosis. Int J Impot Res 2000;12(5):269-271.
2022. Fleischer AC, Shawker TH. The role of sonography in pediatric gynecology. Clin Obstet Gynecol 1987;30:735-746.

2023. Zevenhuijzen H, Kelnar CJ, Crofton PM. Diagnostic utility of a low-dose gonadotropin-releasing hormone test in the context of puberty disorders. Horm Res 2004;62(4):168-176.
2024. Eckert KL, Wilson DM, Bachrach LK, et al. A single-sample, subcutaneous gonadotropin-releasing hormone test for central precocious puberty. Pediatrics 1996;97:517-519.
2025. Rosenfield RL, Burstein S, Cuttler L. Use of nafarelin for testing pituitary-ovarian function. J Reprod Med 1989;34:1044-1050.
2026. Zamboni G, Antoniazzi F, Tato L. Use of the gonadotropin-releasing hormone agonist triptorelin in the diagnosis of delayed puberty in boys. J Pediatr 1995;126:756-758.
2027. Degros V, Cortet-Rudelli C, Soudan B, et al. The human chorionic gonadotropin test is more powerful than the gonadotropin-releasing hormone agonist test to discriminate male isolated hypogonadotropic hypogonadism from constitutional delayed puberty. Eur J Endocrinol 2003;149(1):23-29.
2028. Mainieri AS, Elnecave RH. Usefulness of the free alpha-subunit to diagnose hypogonadotropic hypogonadism. Clin Endocrinol (Oxf) 2003;59(3):307-313.
2029. Cohen HN, Wallace AM, Beastall GH, et al. Clinical value of adrenal androgen measurement in the diagnosis of delayed puberty. Lancet 1981;1:689-692.
2030. Copeland KC, Paunier L, Sizonenko PC. The secretion of adrenal androgens and growth patterns of patients with hypogonadotropic hypogonadism and idiopathic delayed puberty. J Pediatr 1977;91:985-990.
2031. Bonneville JF, Cattin F. The role of magnetic resonance imaging in the diagnosis of endocrine tumours of the sellar region in children. Horm Res 1995;43:151-153.
2032. Hedlund GL, Royal SA, Parker KL. Disorders of puberty: a practical imaging approach. Semin Ultrasound CT MR 1994;15: 49-77.
2033. Lee PDK, Rosenfeld RG. Psychosocial correlates of short stature and delayed puberty. Pediatr Adolesc Endocrinol 1987;4: 851-863.
2034. Ehrhardt AA, Meyer-Bahlburg HFL. Psychologic correlates of abnormal pubertal development. Clin Endocrinol Metab 1975;4: 207-222.
2035. Apter A, Galatzer A, Weizman A, et al. Psychological aspects of developmental endocrinopathies in adolescence. Isr J Psychiatry Relat Sci 1994;31:246-253.
2036. Kaplowitz PB. Diagnostic value of testosterone therapy in boys with delayed puberty. Am J Dis Child 1989;143:116-120.
2037. Wilson DM, Kei J, Hintz RL, et al. Effects of testosterone therapy for pubertal delay [published erratum appears in Am J Dis Child 1988 Mar;142(3):286]. Am J Dis Child 1988;142:96-99.
2038. Richman RA, Kirsch LR. Testosterone treatment in adolescent boys with constitutional delay in growth and development. N Engl J Med 1988;319:1563-1567.
2039. Kelly BP, Paterson WF, Donaldson MD. Final height outcome and value of height prediction in boys with constitutional delay in growth and adolescence treated with intramuscular testosterone 125 mg per month for 3 months. Clin Endocrinol (Oxf) 2003;58(3): 267-272.
2040. Lampit M, Hochberg Z. Androgen therapy in constitutional delay of growth. Horm Res 2003;59(6):270-275.
2041. Morrison JA, Barton BA, Biro FM, et al. Sex hormones and the changes in adolescent male lipids: longitudinal studies in a biracial cohort. J Pediatr 2003;142(6):637-642.
2042. Ishak KG, Zimmerman HJ. Hepatotoxic effects of the anabolic/androgenic steroids. Semin Liver Dis 1987;7(3):230-236.
2043. Soe KL, Soe M, Gluud C. Liver pathology associated with the use of anabolic-androgenic steroids. Liver 1992;12(2):73-79.
2044. Stanhope R, Buchanan CR, Fenn GC, et al. Double blind placebo controlled trial of low dose oxandrolone in the treatment of boys with constitutional delay of growth and puberty. Arch Dis Child 1988;63:501-505.
2045. Malhotra A, Poon E, Tse WY, et al. The effects of oxandrolone on the growth hormone and gonadal axes in boys with constitutional delay of growth and puberty. Clin Endocrinol (Oxf) 1993;38:393-398.
2046. Papadimitriou A, Wacharasindhu S, Pearl K, et al. Treatment of constitutional growth delay in prepubertal boys with a prolonged course of low dose oxandrolone. Arch Dis Child 1991;66: 841-843.
2047. Bassi F, Neri AS, Gheri RG, et al. Oxandrolone in constitutional delay of growth: analysis of the growth patterns up to final stature. J Endocrinol Invest 1993;16:133-137.
2048. Uruena M, Pantsiotou S, Preece MA, et al. Is testosterone therapy for boys with constitutional delay of growth and puberty associated with impaired final height and suppression of the hypothalamo-pituitary-gonadal axis? Eur J Pediatr 1992;151:15-18.
2049. Albanese A, Kewley GD, Long A, et al. Oral treatment for constitutional delay of growth and puberty in boys: a randomised trial of an anabolic steroid or testosterone undecenoate. Arch Dis Child 1994;71:315-317.
2050. Brown DC, Butler GE, Kelnar CJ, et al. A double blind, placebo controlled study of the effects of low dose testosterone undecanoate on the growth of small for age, prepubertal boys. Arch Dis Child 1995;73(2):131-135.
2051. Butler GE, Sellar RE, Walker RF, et al. Oral testosterone undecenoate in the management of delayed puberty in boys: pharmacokinetics and effects on sexual maturation and growth. J Clin Endocrinol Metab 1992;75:37-44.
2052. De Sanctis V, Vullo C, Urso L, et al. Clinical experience using the Androderm testosterone transdermal system in hypogonadal adolescents and young men with beta-thalassemia major. J Pediatr Endocrinol Metab 1998;11(Suppl 3):891-900.
2053. Mayo A, Macintyre H, Wallace AM, et al. Transdermal testosterone application: pharmacokinetics and effects on pubertal status, short-term growth, and bone turnover. J Clin Endocrinol Metab 2004;89(2):681-687.
2054. Adan L, Souberbielle JC, Brauner R. Management of the short stature due to pubertal delay in boys. J Clin Endocrinol Metab 1994;78:478-482.
2055. Zadik Z, Sinai T, Zung A, et al. Vitamin A and iron supplementation is as efficient as hormonal therapy in constitutionally delayed children. Clin Endocrinol (Oxf) 2004;60(6):682-687.
2056. Zachmann M, Studer S, Prader A. Short-term testosterone treatment at bone age of 12 to 13 years does not reduce adult height in boys with constitutional delay of growth and adolescence. Helv Paediatr Acta 1987;42:21-28.
2057. Rosenfield RL. Clinical review 6: diagnosis and management of delayed puberty. J Clin Endocrinol Metab 1990;70:559-562.
2058. Ankarberg-Lindgren C, Elfving M, Wikland KA, et al. Nocturnal application of transdermal estradiol patches produces levels of estradiol that mimic those seen at the onset of spontaneous puberty in girls. J Clin Endocrinol Metab 2001;86(7):3039-3044.
2059. Cisternino M, Nahoul K, Bozzola M, et al. Transdermal estradiol substitution therapy for the induction of puberty in female hypogonadism. J Endocrinol Invest 1991;14:481-488.
2060. Gussinye M, Terrades P, Yeste D, et al. Low areal bone mineral density values in adolescents and young adult Turner syndrome patients increase after long-term transdermal estradiol therapy. Horm Res 2000;54(3):131-135.
2061. Illig R, DeCampo C, Lang-Muritano MR, et al. A physiological mode of puberty induction in hypogonadal girls by low dose transdermal 17 beta-oestradiol. Eur J Pediatr 1990;150:86-91.
2062. Turgeon JL, McDonnell DP, Martin KA, et al. Hormone therapy: physiological complexity belies therapeutic simplicity. Science 2004;304(5675):1269-1273.
2063. Stanhope R, Albanese A, Hindmarsh P, et al. The effects of growth hormone therapy on spontaneous sexual development. Horm Res 1992;38(Suppl 1):9-13.
2064. Rikken B, Massa GG, Wit JM. Final height in a large cohort of Dutch patients with growth hormone deficiency treated with growth hormone. Dutch Growth Hormone Working Group. Horm Res 1995;43:135-137.
2065. Frisch H, Birnbacher R. Final height and pubertal development in children with growth hormone deficiency after long-term treatment. Horm Res 1995;43:132-134.
2066. Toublanc JE, Couprie C, Garnier P, et al. The effects of treatment combining an agonist of gonadotropin-releasing hormone with growth hormone in pubertal patients with isolated growth hormone deficiency. Acta Endocrinol (Copenh) 1989;120: 795-799.
2067. Burstein S, Grumbach MM, Kaplan SL. Early determination of androgen-responsiveness is important in the management of microphallus. Lancet 1979;2:983-986.

2068. Reilly JM, Woodhouse CR. Small penis and the male sexual role. J Urol 1989;142:569-71; discussion 572.
2069. Lee PA, Houk CP. Outcome studies among men with micropenis. J Pediatr Endocrinol Metab 2004;17(8):1043-1053.
2070. Levy JB, Husmann DA. Micropenis secondary to growth hormone deficiency: does treatment with growth hormone alone result in adequate penile growth? J Urol 1996;156:214-216.
2071. Aulitzky W, Frick J, Galvan G. Pulsatile luteinizing hormone-releasing hormone treatment of male hypogonadotropic hypogonadism. Fertil Steril 1988;50:480-486.
2072. Stanhope R, Brook CG, Pringle PJ, et al. Induction of puberty by pulsatile gonadotropin releasing hormone. Lancet 1987;2: 552-555.
2073. Delemarre-van de Waal HA, Odink RJ. Pulsatile GnRH treatment in boys and girls with idiopathic hypogonadotrophic hypogonadism. Hum Reprod 1993;8(Suppl 2):180-183.
2074. Iwatani N, Kodama M, Miike T. Pulsatile LH-RH administration induces puberty in hypogonadotropic GH-deficient patients. Endocr J 1993;40:191-196.
2075. Santoro N, Filicori M, Crowley WFJ. Hypogonadotropic disorders in men and women: diagnosis and therapy with pulsatile gonadotropin-releasing hormone. Endocr Rev 1986;7:11-23.
2076. Delemarre-van de Waal HA. Application of gonadotropin releasing hormone in hypogonadotropic hypogonadism—diagnostic and therapeutic aspects. Eur J Endocrinol 2004;151(Suppl 3): U89-U94.
2077. Stanhope R, Adams J, Jacobs HS, et al. Ovarian ultrasound assessment in normal children, idiopathic precocious puberty, and during low dose pulsatile gonadotrophin releasing hormone treatment of hypogonadotrophic hypogonadism. Arch Dis Child 1985;60:116-119.
2078. Schoemaker J, van Kessel H, Simons AH, et al. Induction of first cycles in primary hypothalamic amenorrhea with pulsatile luteinizing hormone-releasing hormone: a mirror of female pubertal development. Fertil Steril 1987;48:204-212.
2079. Marshall JC, Griffin ML. The role of changing pulse frequency in the regulation of ovulation. Hum Reprod 1993;8(Suppl 2): 57-61.
2080. Bridges NA, Hindmarsh PC, Matthews DR, et al. The effect of changing gonadotropin-releasing hormone pulse frequency on puberty. J Clin Endocrinol Metab 1994;79:841-847.
2081. Tato L, Zamboni G, Antoniazzi F, et al. Gonadal function and response to growth hormone (GH) in boys with isolated GH deficiency and to GH and gonadotropins in boys with multiple pituitary hormone deficiencies. Fertil Steril 1996;65:830-834.
2082. Buchter D, Behre HM, Kliesch S, et al. Pulsatile GnRH or human chorionic gonadotropin/human menopausal gonadotropin as effective treatment for men with hypogonadotropic hypogonadism: a review of 42 cases. Eur J Endocrinol 1998;139(3):298-303.
2083. Gambineri A, Pasquali R. Testosterone therapy in men: clinical and pharmacological perspectives. J Endocrinol Invest 2000; 23(3):196-214.
2084. Mazer NA. New clinical applications of transdermal testosterone delivery in men and women. J Controlled Release 2000;65(1-2): 303-315.
2085. Arisaka O, Hoshi M, Kanazawa S, et al. Systemic effects of transdermal testosterone for the treatment of microphallus in children. Pediatr Int 2001;43(2):134-136.
2086. Kunz GJ, Klein KO, Clemons RD, et al. Virilization of young children after topical androgen use by their parents. Pediatrics 2004;114(1):282-284.
2087. Franklin SL, Geffner ME. Precocious puberty secondary to topical testosterone exposure. J Pediatr Endocrinol Metab 2003;16(1): 107-110.
2088. Creatsas G, Arefetz N, Adamopoulos PN, et al. Transdermal estradiol plus oral medroxyprogesterone acetate replacement therapy in primary amenorrheic adolescents. Clinical, hormonal and metabolic aspects. Maturitas 1994;18(2):105-114.
2089. Jospe N, Orlowski CC, Furlanetto RW. Comparison of transdermal and oral estrogen therapy in girls with Turner's syndrome. J Pediatr Endocrinol Metab 1995;8(2):111-116.
2090. Piippo S, Lenko H, Kainulainen P, et al. Use of percutaneous estrogen gel for induction of puberty in girls with Turner syndrome. J Clin Endocrinol Metab 2004;89(7):3241-3247.
2091. Rubin K. Turner syndrome and osteoporosis: mechanisms and prognosis. Pediatrics 1998;102:481-485.
2092. Naeraa RW, Brixen K, Hansen RM, et al. Skeletal size and bone mineral content in Turner's syndrome: relation to karyotype, estrogen treatment, physical fitness, and bone turnover. Calcif Tissue Int 1991;49(2):77-83.
2093. Balducci R, Toscano V, Mangiantini A, et al. The effect of growth hormone administration on testicular response during gonadotropin therapy in subjects with combined gonadotropin and growth hormone deficiencies. Acta Endocrinol (Copenh) 1993;128:19-23.
2094. Padova G, Finocchiaro C, Briguglia G, et al. Pubarche induction with testosterone treatment in women with panhypopituitarism. Fertil Steril 1996;65:437-439.
2095. Wit JM, Langenhorst VJ, Jansen M, et al. Dehydroepiandrosterone sulfate treatment for atrichia pubis. Horm Res 2001;56(3-4): 134-139.
2096. Didi M, Morris-Jones PH, Gattamaneni HR, et al. Pubertal growth in response to testosterone replacement therapy for radiation-induced Leydig cell failure. Med Pediatr Oncol 1994;22:250-254.
2097. Kaplan SL, Grumbach MM. Pathogenesis of sexual precocity. In Grumbach MM, Sizonenko PC, Aubert ML, eds. Control of the Onset of Puberty. Baltimore: Williams & Wilkins, 1990: 620-660.
2098. Paul D, Conte FA, Grumbach MM, et al. Long-term effect of gonadotropin-releasing hormone agonist therapy on final and near-final height in 26 children with true precocious puberty treated at a median age of less than 5 years. J Clin Endocrinol Metab 1995;80:546-551.
2099. Thamdrup E. Precocious Sexual Development: A Clinical Study of 100 Patients. Springfield, IL: Charles C Thomas, 1961.
2100. Thamdrup E. [Somatic development in puberty. A survey] Den somatiske udvikling i pubertetsarene. En oversigt. Nord Med 1965;74:1013-1018.
2101. Kaplan SL, Grumbach MM. Clinical review 14: pathophysiology and treatment of sexual precocity. J Clin Endocrinol Metab 1990;71:785-789.
2102. Sigurjonsdottir TJ, Hayles AB. Precocious puberty. A report of 96 cases. Am J Dis Child 1968;115:309-321.
2103. Lee PA. Medroxyprogesterone therapy for sexual precocity in girls. Am J Dis Child 1981;135:443-445.
2104. Sorgo W, Kiraly E, Homoki J, et al. The effects of cyproterone acetate on statural growth in children with precocious puberty. Acta Endocrinol (Copenh) 1987;115:44-56.
2105. Werder EA, Murset G, Zachmann M, et al. Treatment of precocious puberty with cyproterone acetate. Pediatr Res 1974;8: 248-256.
2106. Schiele F, Henny J, Hitz J, et al. Total bone and liver alkaline phosphatases in plasma: biological variations and reference limits. Clin Chem 1983;29:634-641.
2107. Hertel NT, Stoltenberg M, Juul A, et al. Serum concentrations of type I and III procollagen propeptides in healthy children and girls with central precocious puberty during treatment with gonadotropin-releasing hormone analog and cyproterone acetate. J Clin Endocrinol Metab 1993;76:924-927.
2108. Saggese G, Bertelloni S, Baroncelli GI, et al. Growth velocity and serum aminoterminal propeptide of type III procollagen in precocious puberty during gonadotropin-releasing hormone analogue treatment. Acta Paediatr 1993;82:261-266.
2109. Trivedi P, Risteli J, Risteli L, et al. Serum concentrations of the type I and III procollagen propeptides as biochemical markers of growth velocity in healthy infants and children and in children with growth disorders. Pediatr Res 1991;30:276-280.
2110. National High Blood Pressure Education Program Working Group on High Blood Pressure in Children and Adolescents. The fourth report on the diagnosis, evaluation, and treatment of high blood pressure in children and adolescents. Pediatrics 2004;114(2 Suppl 4th Report):555-576.
2111. Palmert MR, Boepple PA. Variation in the timing of puberty: clinical spectrum and genetic investigation. J Clin Endocrinol Metab 2001;86(6):2364-2368.
2112. Cisternino M, Arrigo T, Pasquino AM, et al. Etiology and age incidence of precocious puberty in girls: a multicentric study. J Pediatr Endocrinol Metab 2000;13(Suppl 1):695-701.

2113. Chemaitilly W, Trivin C, Adan L, et al. Central precocious puberty: clinical and laboratory features. Clin Endocrinol (Oxf) 2001;54(3):289-294.
2114. Lenz J. Vorzeitige Mestruation, Geschlechtsreife und Entwicklung. Arch Gynaekol 1913;99:67.
2115. Muram D, Dewhurst J, Grant DB. Precocious puberty: a follow-up study. Arch Dis Child 1984;59:77-78.
2116. Benedict PH. Endocrine features in Albright's syndrome (fibrous dysplasia of bone). Metabolism 1962;11:30-45.
2117. Danon M, Crawford JD. The McCune-Albright syndrome. Ergeb Inn Med Kinderheilkd 1987;55:81-115.
2118. Heger S, Muller M, Ranke M, et al. Long-term GnRH agonist treatment for female central precocious puberty does not impair reproductive function. Mol Cell Endocrinol 2006;254-255: 217-220.
2119. Palmert MR, Boepple PA. Variation in the timing of puberty: clinical spectrum and genetic investigation. J Clin Endocrinol Metab 2001;86(6):2364-2368.
2120. Bierich JR. Sexual precocity. Clin Endocrinol Metab 1975;4: 107-142.
2121. Liu N, Grumbach MM, De Napoli RA, et al. Prevalence of electroencephalographic abnormalities in idiopathic precocious puberty and premature pubarche: bearing on pathogenesis and neuroendocrine regulation of puberty. J Clin Endocrinol Metab 1965;25:1296-1308.
2122. Palmert MR, Malin HV, Boepple PA. Unsustained or slowly progressive puberty in young girls: initial presentation and long-term follow-up of 20 untreated patients. J Clin Endocrinol Metab 1999;84(2):415-423.
2123. Fontoura M, Brauner R, Prevot C, et al. Precocious puberty in girls: early diagnosis of a slowly progressing variant. Arch Dis Child 1989;64:1170-1176.
2124. Celani MF, Rota C, Messori A, et al. Effect of increased haemoglobin levels on growth hormone (GH) secretion in beta-thalassaemia major: differences between prepubertal subjects and patients with delayed puberty. Exp Clin Endocrinol 1988;92:225-230.
2125. Kreiter M, Burstein S, Rosenfield RL, et al. Preserving adult height potential in girls with idiopathic true precocious puberty. J Pediatr 1990;117:364-370.
2126. Rosenfield RL. Selection of children with precocious puberty for treatment with gonadotropin releasing hormone analogs. J Pediatr 1994;124:989-991.
2127. Bridges NA, Cooke A, Healy MJ, et al. Ovaries in sexual precocity. Clin Endocrinol (Oxf) 1995;42:135-140.
2128. Ehrhardt AA, Meyer-Bahlburg HF. Psychosocial aspects of precocious puberty. Horm Res 1994;41(Suppl 2):30-35.
2129. Money J, Alexander D. Psychosexual development and absence of homosexuality in males with precocious puberty. Review of 18 cases. J Nerv Ment Dis 1969;148:111-123.
2130. Kastrup KW. Growth and development in girls with Turner's syndrome during early therapy with low doses of estradiol. Acta Endocrinol Suppl (Copenh) 1986;279:157-163.
2131. Kao SC, Cook JS, Hansen JR, et al. MR imaging of the pituitary gland in central precocious puberty. Pediatr Radiol 1992;22: 481-484.
2132. Sharafuddin MJ, Luisiri A, Garibaldi LR, et al. MR imaging diagnosis of central precocious puberty: importance of changes in the shape and size of the pituitary gland. AJR Am J Roentgenol 1994;162:1167-1173.
2133. Gupta R, Ammini AC. Precocious puberty with pituitary gland hyperplasia: two cases in one family. Pediatr Radiol 1996;26: 418-420.
2134. Cacciari E, Zucchini S, Ambrosetto P, et al. Empty sella in children and adolescents with possible hypothalamic-pituitary disorders. J Clin Endocrinol Metab 1994;78:767-771.
2135. Rapaport R, Logrono R. Primary empty sella syndrome in childhood: association with precocious puberty. Clin Pediatr (Phila) 1991;30:466-471.
2136. Zucchini S, Ambrosetto P, Carla G, et al. Primary empty sella: differences and similarities between children and adults. Acta Paediatr 1995;84:1382-1385.
2137. Neely EK, Wilson DM, Lee PA, et al. Spontaneous serum gonadotropin concentrations in the evaluation of precocious puberty. J Pediatr 1995;127:63-67.
2138. Lawson ML, Cohen N. A single sample subcutaneous luteinizing hormone (LH)-releasing hormone (LHRH) stimulation test for monitoring LH suppression in children with central precocious puberty receiving LHRH agonists. J Clin Endocrinol Metab 1999;84:4536-4540.
2139. Brito VN, Batista MC, Borges MF, et al. Diagnostic value of fluorometric assays in the evaluation of precocious puberty. J Clin Endocrinol Metab 1999;84(10):3539-3544.
2140. Schwarz HP, Tschaeppeler H, Zuppinger K. Case report: unsustained central sexual precocity in four girls. Med Sci 1990;299: 260-264.
2141. Zipf WB, Kelch RP, Hopwood NJ, et al. Suppressed responsiveness to gonadotropin-releasing hormone in girls with unsustained isosexual precocity. J Pediatr 1979;95:38-43.
2142. Pescovitz OH, Hench KD, Barnes KM, et al. Premature thelarche and central precocious puberty: the relationship between clinical presentation and the gonadotropin response to luteinizing hormone-releasing hormone. J Clin Endocrinol Metab 1988;67: 474-479.
2143. Bridges NA, Christopher JA, Hindmarsh PC, et al. Sexual precocity: sex incidence and aetiology. Arch Dis Child 1994;70:116-118.
2143a. Latronico AC. Role of GPR54 mutations in pubertal disorders. Endo 2007 (Abstract S18-3).
2144. Janss AJ, Grundy R, Cnaan A, et al. Optic pathway and hypothalamic/chiasmatic gliomas in children younger than age 5 years with a 6-year follow-up. Cancer 1995;75:1051-1059.
2145. Leiper AD, Stanhope R, Kitching P, et al. Precocious and premature puberty associated with treatment of acute lymphoblastic leukaemia. Arch Dis Child 1987;1107-1112.
2146. Rappaport R, Brauner R. Growth and endocrine disorders secondary to cranial irradiation. Pediatr Res 1989;25:561-567.
2147. Nicholl RM, Kirk JM, Grossman AB, et al. Acceleration of pubertal development following pituitary radiotherapy for Cushing's disease. Clin Oncol (R Coll Radiol) 1993;5:393-394.
2148. Sklar CA, Constine LS. Chronic neuroendocrinological sequelae of radiation therapy. Int J Radiat Oncol Biol Phys 1995;31: 1113-1121.
2149. Cara JF, Kreiter ML, Rosenfield RL. Height prognosis of children with true precocious puberty and growth hormone deficiency: effect of combination therapy with gonadotropin releasing hormone agonist and growth hormone. J Pediatr 1992;120: 709-715.
2150. Kamp GA, Manasco PK, Barnes KM, et al. Low growth hormone levels are related to increased body mass index and do not reflect impaired growth in luteinizing hormone-releasing hormone agonist-treated children with precocious puberty. J Clin Endocrinol Metab 1991;72:301-307.
2151. Zuniga OF, Tanner SM, Wild WO, et al. Hamartoma of CNS associated with precocious puberty. Am J Dis Child 1983;137: 127-133.
2152. Price RA, Lee PA, Albright AL, et al. Treatment of sexual precocity by removal of a luteinizing hormone-releasing hormone secreting hamartoma. JAMA 1984;251:2247-2249.
2153. Nishio S, Fujiwara S, Aiko Y, et al. Hypothalamic hamartoma. Report of two cases J Neurosurg 1989;70:640-645.
2154. Sato M, Ushio Y, Arita N, et al. Hypothalamic hamartoma: report of two cases. Neurosurgery 1985;16:198-206.
2155. Turjman F, Xavier JL, Froment JC, et al. Late MR follow-up of hypothalamic hamartomas. Childs Nerv Syst 1996;12:63-68.
2156. Feuillan PP, Jones JV, Barnes K, et al. Reproductive axis after discontinuation of gonadotropin-releasing hormone analog treatment of girls with precocious puberty: long term follow-up comparing girls with hypothalamic hamartoma to those with idiopathic precocious puberty. J Clin Endocrinol Metab 1999; 84(1):44-49.
2157. Freeman JL, Coleman LT, Wellard RM, et al. MR imaging and spectroscopic study of epileptogenic hypothalamic hamartomas: analysis of 72 cases. AJNR Am J Neuroradiol 2004;25(3): 450-462.
2158. Diebler C, Ponsot G. Hamartomas of the tuber cinereum. Neuroradiology 1983;25:93-101.
2159. Lin SR, Bryson MM, Gobien R, et al. Neuroradiologic study of hamartomas of the tuber cinereum and hypothalamus. Neuroradiology 1978;16:17-19.

2160. Kizilkilic O, Yalcin O, Yildirim T, et al. Hypothalamic hamartoma associated with a craniopharyngeal canal. AJNR Am J Neuroradiol 2005;26(1):65-67.
2161. Jung H, Neumaier PE, Hauffa BP, et al. Association of morphological characteristics with precocious puberty and/or gelastic seizures in hypothalamic hamartoma. J Clin Endocrinol Metab 2003;88(10):4590-4595.
2162. Nakagawa N, Takahashi M, Kohrogi Y. Neuroradiologic findings of hypothalamic hamartoma with emphasis on computed tomography. J Comput Tomogr 1986;10:77-83.
2163. Peterman SB, Steiner RE, Bydder GM. Magnetic resonance imaging of intracranial tumors in children and adolescents. AJNR Am J Neuroradiol 1984;5:703-709.
2164. Hahn FJ, Leibrock LG, Huseman CA, et al. The MR appearance of hypothalamic hamartoma. Neuroradiology 1988;30:65-68.
2165. Booth TN, Timmons C, Shapiro K, et al. Pre- and postnatal MR imaging of hypothalamic hamartomas associated with arachnoid cysts. AJNR Am J Neuroradiol 2004;25(7):1283-1285.
2166. Jung H, Carmel P, Schwartz MS, et.al. Some hypothalamic hamartomas contain transforming growth factor α, a puberty-inducing growth factor, not luteinizing hormone releasing hormone neurons. J Clin Endocrinol Metab 1999;84:4695-4701.
2167. Jung H, Parent AS, Ojeda SR. Hypothalamic hamartoma: a paradigm/model for studying the onset of puberty. Endocr Dev 2005;8:81-93.
2168. Styne DM, Harris DA, Egli CA, et al. Treatment of true precocious puberty with a potent luteinizing hormone-releasing factor agonist: effect on growth, sexual maturation, pelvic sonography, and the hypothalamic-pituitary-gonadal axis. J Clin Endocrinol Metab 1985;61:142-151.
2169. Feuillan PP, Jones JV, Barnes KM, et al. Boys with precocious puberty due to hypothalamic hamartoma: reproductive axis after discontinuation of gonadotropin-releasing hormone analog therapy. J Clin Endocrinol Metab 2000;85(11):4036-4038.
2170. Albright AL, Lee PA. Neurosurgical treatment of hypothalamic hamartomas causing precocious puberty. J Neurosurg 1993;78:77-82.
2171. Rosenfeld JV, Harvey AS, Wrennall J, et al. Transcallosal resection of hypothalamic hamartomas, with control of seizures, in children with gelastic epilepsy. Neurosurgery 2001;48(1):108-118.
2172. Grumbach MM. True or central precocious puberty. In Kreiger DT, Bardin CW, eds. Current Therapy in Endocrinology and Metabolism. Toronto: BC Decker, 1985:4-8.
2173. Valdueza JM, Cristante L, Dammann O, et al. Hypothalamic hamartomas: with special reference to gelastic epilepsy and surgery. Neurosurgery 1994;34:949-58; discussion 958.
2174. Starceski PJ, Lee PA, Albright AL, et al. Hypothalamic hamartomas and sexual precocity. Evaluation of treatment options. Am J Dis Child 1990;144:225-228.
2175. Cacciari E, Frejaville E, Cicognani A, et al. How many cases of true precocious puberty in girls are idiopathic? J Pediatr 1983; 102:357-360.
2176. Pescovitz OH, Comite F, Hench K, et al. The NIH experience with precocious puberty: diagnostic subgroups and response to short-term luteinizing hormone releasing hormone analogue therapy. J Pediatr 1986;108:47-54.
2177. Daly D, Mulder D. Gelastic epilepsy. Neurology 1957;7:189-192.
2178. Minns RA, Stirling HF, Wu FC. Hypothalamic hamartoma with skeletal malformations, gelastic epilepsy and precocious puberty. Dev Med Child Neurol 1994;36:173-176.
2179. Deonna T, Ziegler AL. Hypothalamic hamartoma, precocious puberty and gelastic seizures: a special model of "epileptic" developmental disorder. Epileptic Disord 2000;2(1):33-37.
2180. Kuzniecky R, Guthrie B, Mountz J, et al. Intrinsic epileptogenesis of hypothalamic hamartomas in gelastic epilepsy. Ann Neurol 1997;42(1):60-67.
2181. Striano S, Striano P, Sarappa C, et al. The clinical spectrum and natural history of gelastic epilepsy-hypothalamic hamartoma syndrome. Seizure 2005;14(4):232-239.
2182. Brandberg G, Raininko R, Eeg-Olofsson O. Hypothalamic hamartoma with gelastic seizures in Swedish children and adolescents. Eur J Paediatr Neurol 2004;8(1):35-44.
2183. Arzimanoglou AA, Hirsch E, Aicardi J. Hypothalamic hamartoma and epilepsy in children: illustrative cases of possible evolutions. Epileptic Disord 2003;5(4):187-199.
2184. Delalande O, Fohlen M. Disconnecting surgical treatment of hypothalamic hamartoma in children and adults with refractory epilepsy and proposal of a new classification. Neurol Med Chir (Tokyo) 2003;43(2):61-68.
2185. Fohlen M, Lellouch A, Delalande O. Hypothalamic hamartoma with refractory epilepsy: surgical procedures and results in 18 patients. Epileptic Disord 2003;5(4):267-273.
2186. Barajas MA, Ramirez-Guzman MG, Rodriguez-Vazquez C, et al. Gamma knife surgery for hypothalamic hamartomas accompanied by medically intractable epilepsy and precocious puberty: experience in Mexico. J Neurosurg 2005;102(Suppl):53-55.
2187. Regis J, Hayashi M, Eupierre LP, et al. Gamma knife surgery for epilepsy related to hypothalamic hamartomas. Acta Neurochir Suppl 2004;91:33-50.
2188. Freeman JL, Zacharin M, Rosenfeld JV, et al. The endocrinology of hypothalamic hamartoma surgery for intractable epilepsy. Epileptic Disord 2003;5(4):239-247.
2189. Boudreau EA, Liow K, Frattali CM, et al. Hypothalamic hamartomas and seizures: distinct natural history of isolated and Pallister-Hall syndrome cases. Epilepsia 2005;46(1):42-47.
2190. Wacharasindhu S, Shotelersuk V, Srivuthana S, et al. Pallister-Hall syndrome with hypoparathyroidism. J Pediatr Endocrinol Metab 2004;17(5):801-803.
2191. Lopponen T, Saukkonen AL, Serlo W, et al. Accelerated pubertal development in patients with shunted hydrocephalus. Arch Dis Child 1996;74:490-496.
2192. Robertson CM, Morrish DW, Wheler GH, et al. Neonatal encephalopathy: an indicator of early sexual maturation in girls. Pediatr Neurol 1990;6:102-108.
2193. Blendonohy PM, Philip PA. Precocious puberty in children after traumatic brain injury. Brain Inj 1991;5:63-68.
2194. Tubiana-Rufi N, Thizon-de Gaulle I, et al. Hypothalamopituitary deficiency and precocious puberty following hyperhydration in diabetic ketoacidosis. Horm Res 1992;37:60-63.
2195. Brauner R, Rappaport R, Nicod C, et al. [True precocious puberty in non-tumor hydrocephalus. An analysis of 16 cases] Pubertes precoces vraies au cours de l'hydrocephalie non tumorale. Analyse de 16 observations. Arch Fr Pediatr 1987;44:433-436.
2196. Lopponen T, Saukkonen AL, Serlo W, et al. Slow prepubertal linear growth but early pubertal growth spurt in patients with shunted hydrocephalus. Pediatrics 1995;95:917-923.
2197. Brauner R, Pierre-Kahn A, Nemedy-Sandor E. Precocious puberty caused by a suprasellar arachnoid cyst.Analysis of 6 cases. Arch Fr Pediatr 1987;44:489-493.
2198. Huang HP, Tung YC, Tsai WY, et al. Arachnoid cyst with GnRH-dependent sexual precocity and growth hormone deficiency. Pediatr Neurol 2004;30(2):143-145.
2199. Okamoto K, Nakasu Y, Sato M, et al. Isosexual precocious puberty associated with multilocular arachnoid cysts at the cranial base. Report of a case. Acta Neurochir (Wien) 1981;57:87-93.
2200. Clark SJ, Van Dop C, Conte FA, et al. Reversible true precocious puberty secondary to a congenital arachnoid cyst. Am J Dis Child 1988;142:255-256.
2201. Habiby R, Silverman B, Listernick R, et al. Precocious puberty in children with neurofibromatosis type 1. J Pediatr 1995;126:364-367.
2202. Zacharin M. Precocious puberty in two children with neurofibromatosis type I in the absence of optic chiasmal glioma. J Pediatr 1997;130:155-157.
2203. Listernick R, Charrow J, Greenwald M, et al. Natural history of optic pathway tumors in children with neurofibromatosis type 1: a longitudinal study [see comments]. J Pediatr 1994;125:63-66.
2204. Riccardi VM., Heim RA, Kam-Morgan LNW, et al. Distribution of 13 truncating mutations in the neurofibromatosis 1 gene. Hum Mol Genet 1995;4:975-981.
2205. Xu GF, Lin B, Tanaka K, et al. The catalytic domain of the neurofibromatosis type 1 gene product stimulates ras GTPase and complements ira mutants of Scerevisiae. Cell 1990;63:835-841.
2206. Ballester R, Marchuk D, Boguski M, et al. The NF1 locus encodes a protein functionally related to mammalian GAP and yeast IRA proteins. Cell 1990;63:851-859.
2207. Martin GA, Viskochil D, Bollag G, et al. The GAP-related domain of the neurofibromatosis type 1 gene product interacts with ras p21. Cell 1990;63:843-849.

2208. Stephens K, Keyes L, Riccardi VM, et al. Preferential mutation of the neurofibromatosis type 1 gene in paternally-derived chromosomes. Hum Genet 1992;88(3):279-282.
2209. Mashour GA, Driever PH, Hartmann M, et al. Circulating growth factor levels are associated with tumorigenesis in neurofibromatosis type 1. Clin Cancer Res 2004;10(17):5677-5683.
2210. Riccardi VM. Neurofibromatosis: Phenotype, Natural History and Pathogenesis. Baltimore: Johns Hopkins Press, 1992.
2211. Listernick R, Charrow J. Neurofibromatosis type 1 in childhood. J Pediatr 1990;116:845-853.
2212. Nichols JC, Amato JE, Chung SM. Characteristics of Lisch nodules in patients with neurofibromatosis type 1. J Pediatr Ophthalmol Strabismus 2003;40(5):293-296.
2213. Mulvihill JJ, Parry DM, Sherman JL, et al. NIH conference. Neurofibromatosis 1 (Recklinghausen disease) and neurofibromatosis 2 (bilateral acoustic neurofibromatosis). An Update. Ann Intern Med 1990;113:39-52.
2214. Cohen BH, Rothner AD. Incidence, types, and management of cancer in patients with neurofibromatosis. Oncology 1989;3: 23-30.
2215. Boulanger JM, Larbrisseau A. Neurofibromatosis type 1 in a pediatric population: Ste-Justine's experience. Can J Neurol Sci 2005;32(2):225-231.
2216. Huguenin M, Trivin C, Zerah M, et al. Adult height after cranial irradiation for optic pathway tumors: relationship with neurofibromatosis. J Pediatr 2003;142(6):699-703.
2217. Samuelsson B, Riccardi VM. Neurofibromatosis in Gothenburg, Sweden. II. Intellectual compromise. Neurofibromatosis 1989;2: 78-83.
2218. Samuelsson B, Riccardi VM. Neurofibromatosis in Gothenburg, Sweden. III. Psychiatric and social aspects. Neurofibromatosis 1989;2:84-106.
2219. Money J, Hosta G. Laughing seizures with sexual precocity. Johns Hopkins Med J 1967;120:326-336.
2220. Sockalosky JJ, Kriel RL, Krach LE, et al. Precocious puberty after traumatic brain injury. J Pediatr 1987;110:373-377.
2221. Freude S, Frisch H, Wimberger D, et al. Septo-optic dysplasia and growth hormone deficiency: accelerated pubertal maturation during GH therapy. Acta Paediatr 1992;81:641-645.
2222. LaFranchi SH. Sexual precocity with hypothalamic hypopituitarism. Am J Dis Child 1979;133:739-742.
2223. Virdis R, Street ME, Zampolli M, et al. Precocious puberty in girls adopted from developing countries. Arch Dis Child 1998;78(2): 152-154.
2224. Tuvemo T, Proos LA. Girls adopted from developing countries: a group at risk of early pubertal development and short final height. Implications for health surveillance and treatment [editorial]. Ann Med 1993;25:217-219.
2225. Proos LA, Hofvander Y, Tuvemo T. Menarcheal age and growth pattern of Indian girls adopted in Sweden. II. Catch-up growth and final height. Indian J Pediatr 1991;58:105-114.
2226. Krstevska-Konstantinova M, Charlier C, Craen M, et al. Sexual precocity after immigration from developing countries to Belgium: evidence of previous exposure to organochlorine pesticides. Hum Reprod 2001;16(5):1020-1026.
2227. Fredriks AM, van Buuren S, Jeurissen SE, et al. Height, weight, body mass index and pubertal development reference values for children of Turkish origin in the Netherlands. Eur J Pediatr 2003;162(11):788-793.
2228. Mul D, Oostdijk W, Waelkens JJ, et al. Final height after treatment of early puberty in short adopted girls with gonadotrophin releasing hormone agonist with or without growth hormone. Clin Endocrinol (Oxf) 2005;63(2):185-190.
2229. Dacou-Voutetakis C, Karidis N. Congenital adrenal hyperplasia complicated by central precocious puberty: treatment with LHRH-agonist analogue. Ann N Y Acad Sci 1993;250-254.
2230. Erkula G, Jones KB, Sponseller PD, et al. Growth and maturation in Marfan syndrome. Am J Med Genet 2002;109(2): 100-115.
2231. Ehrhardt AA, Meyer-Bahlburg HF. Idiopathic precocious puberty in girls: long-term effects on adolescent behavior. Acta Endocrinol Suppl (Copenh) 1986;279:247-253.
2232. Boulgourdjian E, Escobar ME, Martinez A, et al. Bone age at discontinuation of medroxyprogesterone acetate therapy in girls with precocious puberty: effect on final height. Horm Res 1995;44:12-16.
2233. Lee TC, Miller WL, Auchus RJ. Medroxyprogesterone acetate and dexamethasone are competitive inhibitors of different human steroidogenic enzymes. J Clin Endocrinol Metab 1999;84(6): 2104-2110.
2234. Sadeghi-Nejad A, Kaplan SL, Grumbach MM. The effect of medroxyprogesterone acetate on adrenocortical function in children with precocious puberty. J Pediatr 1971;78:616-624.
2235. Stanhope R, Huen KF, Buzi F, et al. The effect of cyproterone acetate on the growth of children with central precocious puberty. Eur J Pediatr 1987;146:500-503.
2236. Conn PM, Crowley WFJ. Gonadotropin-releasing hormone and its analogs. Annu Rev Med 1994;45:391-405.
2237. Partsch CJ, Heger S, Sippell WG. Management and outcome of central precocious puberty. Clin Endocrinol (Oxf) 2002;56(2): 129-148.
2238. Conn PM, Janovick JA, Stanisloaus K, et al. Molecular and cellular bases of gonadotropin -releasing hormone action in the pituitary and central nervous system. In Vitamins and Hormones. New York: Academic Press, 1995.
2239. Karten MJ, Rivier JE. Gonadotropin-releasing hormone analog design. Structure-function studies toward the development of agonists and antagonists: rationale and perspective. Endocr Rev 1986;7:44-66.
2240. Lemay A. Clinical appreciation of LHRH analogue formulation. Horm Res 1989;32:93-101.
2241. Handelsman DJ, Swerdloff RS. Pharmacokinetics of gonadotropin-releasing hormone and its analogs. Endocr Rev 1986;7: 95-105.
2242. Boepple PA, Mansfield MJ, Wierman ME, et al. Use of a potent, long acting agonist of gonadotropin-releasing hormone in the treatment of precocious puberty. Endocr Rev 1986;7: 24-33.
2243. Comite F, Cutler GBJ, Rivier J, et al. Short-term treatment of idiopathic precocious puberty with a long-acting analogue of luteinizing hormone-releasing hormone. A preliminary report. N Engl J Med 1981;305:1546-1550.
2244. Drop SL, Odink RJ, Rouwe C, et al. The effect of treatment with an LH-RH agonist (Buserelin) on gonadal activity growth and bone maturation in children with central precocious puberty. Eur J Pediatr 1987;146:272-278.
2245. Crowley WF Jr, et al. Therapeutic use of pituitary desensitization with a long-acting LHRH agonist: a potential new treatment for idiopathic precocious puberty. J Clin Endocrinol Metab 1981;52:370-372.
2246. Comite F, Cassorla F, Barnes KM, et al. Luteinizing hormone releasing hormone analogue therapy for central precocious puberty. Long term effect on somatic growth, bone maturation, and predicted height. JAMA 1986;255:2613-2616.
2247. Bourguignon JP, Van Vliet G, Vandeweghe M, et al. Treatment of central precocious puberty with an intranasal analogue of GnRH (buserelin). Eur J Pediatr 1987;146:555-560.
2248. Kaplan SL, Grumbach MM. True precocious puberty: treatment with GnRH-agonists. In Delemarre-Van de Waal H, Plant TM, van Rees GP, et al, eds. Control of the Onset of Puberty. Amsterdam: Elsevier, 1989:357-373.
2249. Neely EK, Hintz RL, Parker B, et al. Two-year results of treatment with depot leuprolide acetate for central precocious puberty. J Pediatr 1992;121:634-640.
2250. Carel JC, Lahlou N, Guazzarotti L, et al. Treatment of central precocious puberty with depot leuprorelin. French Leuprorelin Trial Group. Eur J Endocrinol 1995;132:699-704.
2251. Tanaka T, Hibi I, Kato K, et al. A dose finding study of a super long-acting luteinizing hormone-releasing hormone analog (leuprolide acetate depot, TAP-144-SR) in the treatment of central precocious puberty. The TAP-144-SR CPP Study Group. Endocrinol Jpn 1991;38:369-376.
2252. Holland FJ, Fishman L, Costigan DC, et al. Pharmacokinetic characteristics of the gonadotropin-releasing hormone analog D-Ser (tBU)6Pro9NEt luteinizing hormone-releasing hormone (buserelin) after subcutaneous and intranasal administration in children with central precocious puberty. J Clin Endocrinol Metab 1986;63:1065-1070.
2253. Antoniazzi F, Cisternino M, Nizzoli G, et al. Final height in girls with central precocious puberty: comparison of two different luteinizing hormone-releasing hormone agonist treatments. Acta Paediatr 1994;83:1052-1056.

2254. Stasiowska B, Vannelli S, Benso L. Final height in sexually precocious girls after therapy with an intranasal analogue of gonadotrophin-releasing hormone (buserelin). Horm Res 1994;42:81-85.
2255. Cacciari E, Cassio A, Balsamo A, et al. Long-term follow-up and final height in girls with central precocious puberty treated with luteinizing hormone-releasing hormone analogue nasal spray. Arch Pediatr Adolesc Med 1994;148:1194-1199.
2256. Heinrichs C, Craen M, Vanderschueren-Lodeweyckx M, et al. Variations in pituitary-gonadal suppression during intranasal buserelin and intramuscular depot-triptorelin therapy for central precocious puberty. Belgian Study Group for Pediatric Endocrinology. Acta Paediatr 1994;83:627-633.
2257. Partsch CJ, Hummelink R, Peter M, et al. Comparison of complete and incomplete suppression of pituitary-gonadal activity in girls with central precocious puberty: influence on growth and predicted final height. The German-Dutch Precocious Puberty Study Group. Horm Res 1993;39:111-117.
2258. Hummelink R, Oostdijk W, Partsch CJ, et al. Growth, bone maturation and height prediction after three years of therapy with the slow release GnRH-agonist Decapeptyl-Depot in children with central precocious puberty. Horm Metab Res 1992;24:122-126.
2259. Sklar CA, Rothenberg S, Blumberg D, et al. Suppression of the pituitary-gonadal axis in children with central precocious puberty: effects on growth, growth hormone, insulin-like growth factor-I, and prolactin secretion. J Clin Endocrinol Metab 1991;73:734-738.
2260. Kletter GB, Kelch RP. Clinical review 60: Effects of gonadotropin-releasing hormone analog therapy on adult stature in precocious puberty. J Clin Endocrinol Metab 1994;79:331-334.
2261. Arrigo T, Cisternino M, Galluzzi F, et al. Analysis of the factors affecting auxological response to GnRH agonist treatment and final height outcome in girls with idiopathic central precocious puberty. Eur J Endocrinol 1999;141(2):140-144.
2262. Heger S, Partsch CJ, Sippell WG. Long-term outcome after depot gonadotropin-releasing hormone agonist treatment of central precocious puberty: final height, body proportions, body composition, bone mineral density, and reproductive function. J Clin Endocrinol Metab 1999;84(12):4583-4590.
2263. Kauli R, Galatzer A, Kornreich L, et al. Final height of girls with central precocious puberty, untreated versus treated with cyproterone acetate or GnRH analogue. A comparative study with re-evaluation of predictions by the Bayley-Pinneau method. Horm Res 1997;47:54-61.
2264. Tanaka T, Niimi H, Matsuo N, Fujieda K, Tachibana K, Ohyama K, et al. Results of long-term follow-up after treatment of central precocious puberty with leuprorelin acetate: evaluation of effectiveness of treatment and recovery of gonadal function. The TAP-144-SR Japanese Study Group on Central Precocious Puberty. J Clin Endocrinol Metab 2005;90(3):1371-1376.
2265. Oerter KE, Manasco PK, Barnes KM, et al. Effects of luteinizing hormone-releasing hormone agonists on final height in luteinizing hormone-releasing hormone-dependent precocious puberty. Acta Paediatr Suppl 1993;388:62-68; discussion 69.
2266. Crawford JD, et.al. Analysis of growth data in children with central precocious puberty: the impact of long term GnRH agonist therapy. In Grave GD, Cutler GBJ, eds. Sexual Precocity: Etiology, Diagnosis, and Management. New York: Raven Press, 1993:69-83.
2267. Carel JC, Lahlou N, Roger M, et al. Precocious puberty and statural growth. Hum Reprod Update 2004;10(2):135-147.
2268. Cassio A, Cacciari E, Balsamo A, et al. Randomised trial of LHRH analogue treatment on final height in girls with onset of puberty aged 7.5-8.5 years. Arch Dis Child 1999;81(4):329-332.
2269. Bouvattier C, Coste J, Rodrigue D, et al. Lack of effect of GnRH agonists on final height in girls with advanced puberty: a randomized long-term pilot study. J Clin Endocrinol Metab 1999;84(10):3575-3578.
2270. Tanaka T, Niimi H, Matsuo N, et al. Results of long-term follow-up after treatment of central precocious puberty with leuprorelin acetate: evaluation of effectiveness of treatment and recovery of gonadal function. The TAP-144-SR Japanese Study Group on Central Precocious Puberty. J Clin Endocrinol Metab 2005;90(3):1371-1376.
2271. Carel JC, Roger M, Ispas S, et al. Final height after long-term treatment with triptorelin slow release for central precocious puberty: importance of statural growth after interruption of treatment. French Study Group of Decapeptyl in Precocious Puberty. J Clin Endocrinol Metab 1999;84(6):1973-1978.
2272. Mul D, Oostdijk W, Otten BJ, et al. Final height after gonadotrophin releasing hormone agonist treatment for central precocious puberty: the Dutch experience. J Pediatr Endocrinol Metab 2000;13(Suppl 1):765-772.
2273. Pasquino AM, Pucarelli I, Segni M, et al. Adult height in girls with central precocious puberty treated with gonadotropin-releasing hormone analogues and growth hormone. J Clin Endocrinol Metab 1999;84(2):449-452.
2274. Roth CL, Brendel L, Ruckert C, et al. Antagonistic and agonistic GnRH analogue treatment of precocious puberty: tracking gonadotropin concentrations in urine. Horm Res 2005;63(5):257-262.
2275. Wu MH, Lin SJ, Wu LH, et al. Clinical suppression of precocious puberty with cetrorelix after failed treatment with GnRH agonist in a girl with gonadotrophin-independent precocious puberty. Reprod Biomed Online 2005;11(1):18-21.
2276. Boot AM, De Muinck K, Pols HA et al. Bone mineral density and body composition before and during treatment with gonadotropin-releasing hormone agonist in children with central precocious and early puberty. J Clin Endocrinol Metab 1998;83(2):370-373.
2277. Palmert MR, Mansfield MJ, Crowley WFJ, et al. Is obesity an outcome of gonadotropin-releasing hormone agonist administration? Analysis of growth and body composition in 110 patients with central precocious puberty. J Clin Endocrinol Metab 1999;84:4480-4488.
2278. Paterson WF, McNeill E, Young D, et al. Auxological outcome and time to menarche following long-acting goserelin therapy in girls with central precocious or early puberty. Clin Endocrinol (Oxf) 2004;61(5):626-634.
2279. Unal O, Berberoglu M, Evliyaoglu O, et al. Effects on bone mineral density of gonadotropin releasing hormone analogs used in the treatment of central precocious puberty. J Pediatr Endocrinol Metab 2003;16(3):407-411.
2280. Arrigo T, De Luca F, Antoniazzi F, et al. Reduction of baseline body mass index under gonadotropin-suppressive therapy in girls with idiopathic precocious puberty. Eur J Endocrinol 2004;150(4):533-537.
2281. Verrotti A, Basciani F, Trotta D, et al. Serum leptin levels in girls with precocious puberty. Diabetes Nutr Metab 2003;16(2):125-129.
2282. Costin G, Kaufman FR. Growth hormone secretory patterns in children with short stature. J Pediatr 1987;110:362-368.
2283. Eshet R, Silbergeld A, Kauli R, et al. GH and GHBP activity and not IGF-1 and its receptor activity express growth velocity reduction during treatment of central precocious puberty by a superactive GNRH analogue. Isr J Med Sci 1994;30:592-595.
2284. Eshet R, Silbergeld A, et al. Erythrocytes from patients with low concentrations of IGF1 have an increase in receptor sites of IGF1. Acta Endocrinol 1991;125:354-358.
2285. Chaussain JL, Roger M, Couprie C, et al. Treatment of precocious puberty with a long-acting preparation of D-Trp6-LHRH. Horm Res 1987;28:155-163.
2286. Kappy M, Stuart T, Perelman A, et al. Suppression of gonadotropin secretion by a long-acting gonadotropin-releasing hormone analog (leuprolide acetate, Lupron Depot) in children with precocious puberty. J Clin Endocrinol Metab 1989;69:1087-1089.
2287. Roger M, Chaussain JL, Berlier P, et al. Long term treatment of male and female precocious puberty by periodic administration of a long-acting preparation of D-Trp6-luteinizing hormone-releasing hormone microcapsules. J Clin Endocrinol Metab 1986;62:670-677.
2288. Ambrosino MM, Hernanz-Schulman M, Genieser NB, et al. Monitoring of girls undergoing medical therapy for isosexual precocious puberty. J Ultrasound Med 1994;13:501-508.
2289. Bhatia S, Neely EK, Wilson DM. Serum luteinizing hormone rises within minutes after depot leuprolide injection: implications for monitoring therapy. Pediatrics 2002;109(2):E30.
2290. Brito VN, Latronico AC, Arnhold IJ, et al. A single luteinizing hormone determination 2 hours after depot leuprolide is useful for therapy monitoring of gonadotropin-dependent precocious puberty in girls. J Clin Endocrinol Metab 2004;89(9):4338-4342.

2291. Manasco PK, Pescovitz OH, Feuillan PP, et al. Resumption of puberty after long term luteinizing hormone-releasing hormone agonist treatment of central precocious puberty. J Clin Endocrinol Metab 1988;67:368-372.
2292. Jay N, Mansfield MJ, Blizzard RM, et al. Ovulation and menstrual function of adolescent girls with central precocious puberty after therapy with gonadotropin-releasing hormone agonists. J Clin Endocrinol Metab 1992;75:890-894.
2293. Schroor EJ, van Weissenbruch MM, Delemarre-van de Waal HA. Long-term GnRH-agonist treatment does not postpone central development of the GnRH pule generator in girls with idiopathic precocious puberty. J Clin Endocrinol Metab 1995;80:1696-1701.
2294. Bassi F, Bartolini O, Neri AS, et al. Precocious puberty: auxological criteria discriminating different forms. J Endocrinol Invest 1994;17:793-797.
2295. Brauner R, Adan L, Malandry F, et al. Adult height in girls with idiopathic true precocious puberty. J Clin Endocrinol Metab 1994;79:415-420.
2296. Garibaldi LR, Aceto T Jr, Weber C. The pattern of gonadotropin and estradiol secretion in exaggerated thelarche. Acta Endocrinol 1993;128:345-350.
2297. Pasquino AM, Pucarelli I, Passeri F, et al. Progression of premature thelarche to central precocious puberty. J Pediatr 1995; 126:11-14.
2298. Brauner R, Malandry F, Rappaport R. Predictive factors for the effect of gonadotrophin releasing hormone analogue therapy on the height of girls with idiopathic central precocious puberty. Eur J Pediatr 1992;151:728-730.
2299. Neely EK, Wilson DM. Letter to the Editor (reply) 1995;126: 159-160.
2300. Kauschansky A, Nussinovitch M, Frydman M, et al. Hyperprolactinemia after treatment of long-acting gonadotropin-releasing hormone analogue Decapeptyl in girls with central precocious puberty. Fertil Steril 1995;64:285-287.
2301. van der Sluis I, Boot AM, Krenning EP, et al. Longitudinal follow-up of bone density and body composition in children with precocious or early puberty before, during and after cessation of GnRH agonist therapy. J Clin Endocrinol Metab 2002;87(2): 506-512.
2302. Antoniazzi F, Zamboni G, Bertoldo F, et al. Bone mass at final height in precocious puberty after gonadotropin-releasing hormone agonist with and without calcium supplementation. J Clin Endocrinol Metab 2003;88(3):1096-1101.
2303. Antoniazzi F, Zamboni G, Bertoldo F, et al. Bone development during GH and GnRH analog treatment. Eur J Endocrinol 2004;151(Suppl 1):S47-S54.
2304. Tylavsky FA, Holliday K, Danish R, et al. Fruit and vegetable intakes are an independent predictor of bone size in early pubertal children. Am J Clin Nutr 2004;79(2):311-317.
2305. Kempers MJ, Noordam C, Rouwe CW, et al. Can GnRH-agonist treatment cause slipped capital femoral epiphysis? J Pediatr Endocrinol Metab 2001;14(6):729-734.
2306. van Puijenbroek E, Verhoef E, de Graaf L. Slipped capital femoral epiphyses associated with the withdrawal of a gonadotrophin releasing hormone. BMJ 2004;328(7452):1353.
2307. Puylaert D, DiMeglio A, Bentahar T. Staging puberty in slipped capital femoral epiphysis: importance of the triradiate cartilage. J Pediatr Orthop 2004;24(2):144-147.
2308. Mouridsen SE, Larsen FW. Psychological aspects of precocious puberty. An overview. Acta Paedopsychiatr 1992;55:45-49.
2309. Gleeson HK, Stoeter R, Ogilvy-Stuart AL, et al. Improvements in final height over 25 years in growth hormone (GH)-deficient childhood survivors of brain tumors receiving GH replacement. J Clin Endocrinol Metab 2003;88(8):3682-3689.
2310. Pucarelli I, Segni M, Ortore M, et al. Effects of combined gonadotropin-releasing hormone agonist and growth hormone therapy on adult height in precocious puberty: a further contribution. J Pediatr Endocrinol Metab 2003;16(7):1005-1010.
2311. Saggese G, Cesaretti G, Barsanti S, et al. Combination treatment with growth hormone and gonadotropin-releasing hormone analogs in short normal girls. J Pediatr 1995;126:468-473.
2312. Pasquino AM, Pucarelli I, Roggini M, et al. Adult height in short normal girls treated with gonadotropin-releasing hormone analogs and growth hormone. J Clin Endocrinol Metab 2000;85(2):619-622.
2313. Balducci R, Toscano V, Mangiantini A, et al. Adult height in short normal adolescent girls treated with gonadotropin-releasing hormone analog and growth hormone. J Clin Endocrinol Metab 1995;80:3596-3600.
2314. Lanes R, Palacios A, Avendano E, et al. The metoclopramide test: a useful tool with the luteinizing hormone-releasing hormone test in distinguishing between constitutional delay of puberty and hypogonadotropic hypogonadism. Fertil Steril 1989;52: 55-59.
2315. Pescovitz OH, Comite F, Cassorla F, et al. True precocious puberty complicating congenital adrenal hyperplasia: treatment with a luteinizing hormone-releasing hormone analog. J Clin Endocrinol Metab 1984;58:857-861.
2316. Markin RS, Leibrock LG, Huseman CA, et al. Hypothalamic hamartoma: a report of 2 cases. Pediatr Neurosci 1987;13:19-26.
2317. Roosen N, Cras P, Van Vyve M. Hamartoma of the tuber cinereum in a six-month-old boy, causing isosexual precocious puberty. Neurochirurgia (Stuttg) 1987;30:56-60.
2318. Nishio S, Shigeto H, Fukui M. Hypothalamic hamartoma: the role of surgery. Neurosurg Rev 1993;16:157-160.
2319. Romner B, Trumpy JH, Marhaug G, et al. Hypothalamic hamartoma causing precocious puberty treated by surgery: case report. Surg Neurol 1994;41:306-309.
2320. Faglia G, Arosio M, Porretti S. Delayed closure of epiphyseal cartilages induced by the aromatase inhibitor anastrozole. Would it help short children grow up? J Endocrinol Invest 2000;23(11): 721-723.
2321. Rochira V. Aromatase inhibitors in pubertal boys: clinical implications. J Clin Endocrinol Metab 2001;86(4):1836-1838.
2322. Stanhope R. Use of a specific aromatase inhibitor in delayed puberty. Lancet 2001;357(9270):1723-1724.
2323. Sklar CA, Conte FA, Kaplan SL, et al. Human chorionic gonadotropin-secreting pineal tumor;relation to pathogenesis and sex limitation of sexual precocity. J Clin Endocrinol Metab 1981;53: 656-660.
2324. van der HM, Niggli FK, Willi UV, et al. Solitary infantile choriocarcinoma of the liver: MRI findings. Pediatr Radiol 2004;34(10): 820-823.
2325. Morinaga S, Yamaguchi M, Watanabe I, et al. An immunohistochemical study of hepatoblastoma producing human chorionic gonadotropin. Cancer 1983;51:1647-1652.
2326. McArthur JW, Toll GD, Russfield AB, et al. Sexual precocity attributable to ectopic gonadotropin secretion by hepatoblastoma. Am J Med 1973;54:390-403.
2327. Braunstein GD, Bridson WE, Glass A, et al. In vivo and in vitro production of human chorionic gonadotropin and alpha-fetoprotein by a virilizing hepatoblastoma. J Clin Endocrinol Metab 1972;35:857-862.
2328. Heimann A, White PF, Riely CA, et al. Hepatoblastoma presenting as isosexual precocity. The clinical importance of histologic and serologic parameters. J Clin Gastroenterol 1987;9:105-110.
2329. Blohm ME, Gobel U. Unexplained anaemia and failure to thrive as initial symptoms of infantile choriocarcinoma: a review. Eur J Pediatr 2004;163(1):1-6.
2330. Chaussain J-L, Lemerle J, Roager M, et al. Klinefelter's syndrome, tumor and sexual precocity. J Pediatr 1980;97(4):607-609.
2331. Hasle H, Jacobsen BB, Asschenfeldt P, et al. Mediastinal germ cell tumor associated with Klinefelter's syndrome. Eur J Pediatr 1992;151:735-739.
2332. Englund AT, Geffner ME, Nagel RA, et al. Pediatric germ cell and human chorionic gonadotropin-producing tumors. Clinical and laboratory features. Am J Dis Child 1991;145:1294-1297.
2333. Starzyk J, Starzyk B, Bartnik-Mikuta A, et al. Gonadotropin releasing hormone-independent precocious puberty in a 5 year-old girl with suprasellar germ cell tumor secreting beta-hCG and alpha-fetoprotein. J Pediatr Endocrinol Metab 2001;14(6):789-796.
2334. O'Marcaigh AS, Ledger GA, Roche PC, et al. Aromatase expression in human germinomas with possible biological effects. J Clin Endocrinol Metab 1995;80:3763-3766.
2335. Reuben MS, Manning GR. Precocious puberty. Arch Pediatr 1923;40:27-44.
2336. Cohen AR, Wilson JA, Sadeghi-Nejad A. Gonadotropin-secreting pineal teratoma causing precocious puberty. Neurosurgery 1991;28:597-602; discussion 602.

2337. Marx M, Beck JD, Grabenbauer GG, et al. Gonadotrophin-independent puberty in a boy with a beta-HCG-secreting brain tumour. Horm Res 2000;54(1):44-48.
2338. Kretschmar CS. Germ cell tumors of the brain in children: a review of current literature and new advances in therapy. Cancer Invest 1997;15(2):187-198.
2339. Bjornsson J, Scheithauer BW, Okazaki H, et al. Intracranial germ cell tumors: pathobiological and immunohistochemical aspects of 70 cases. J Neuropathol Exp Neurol 1985;44(1):32-46.
2340. Shinoda J, Sakai N, Yano H, et al. Prognostic factors and therapeutic problems of primary intracranial choriocarcinoma/germ-cell tumors with high levels of HCG. J Neurooncol 2004;66(1-2): 225-240.
2341. Haupt C, Ancker U, Muller M, et al. Intracranial germ-cell tumours—treatment results and residuals. Eur J Pediatr 1996;155(3):230-236.
2342. Faggiano M, Criscuolo T, Perrone L, et al. Sexual precocity in a boy due to hypersecretion of LH and prolactin by a pituitary adenoma. Acta Endocrinol (Copenh) 1983;102:167-172.
2343. Ambrosi B, Bassetti M, Ferrario R, et al. Precocious puberty in a boy with a PRL-, LH- and FSH-secreting pituitary tumour: hormonal and immunocytochemical studies. Acta Endocrinol (Copenh) 1990;122:569-576.
2344. White PC, Speiser PW. Congenital adrenal hyperplasia due to 21-hydroxylase deficiency. Endocr Rev 2000;21(3):245-291.
2345. Charmandari E, Brook CG, Hindmarsh PC. Classic congenital adrenal hyperplasia and puberty. Eur J Endocrinol 2004;151(Suppl 3):U77-U82.
2346. Schmitt K, Frisch H, Neuhold N, et al. Aldosterone and testosterone producing adrenal adenoma in childhood. J Endocrinol Invest 1995;18:69-73.
2347. Makino S, Oda S, Saka T, et al. A case of aldosterone-producing adrenocortical adenoma associated with preclinical Cushing's syndrome and hypersecretion of parathyroid hormone. Endocr J 2001;48(1):103-111.
2348. Walker BR, Skoog SJ, Winslow BH, et al. Testis sparing surgery for steroid unresponsive testicular tumors of the adrenogenital syndrome. J Urol 1997;157(4):1460-1463.
2348a. Claahsen-van der Grinten HL, Otten BJ, Takahashi S, et al. Testicular adrenal rest tumors in adult males with congenital adrenal hyperplasia: evaluation of pituitary-gonadal function before and after successful testis-sparing surgery in eight patients. J Clin Endocrinol Metab 2007;92:612-615.
2349. Pabon JE, Li X, Lei ZM, et al. Novel presence of luteinizing hormone/chorionic gonadotropin receptors in human adrenal glands. J Clin Endocrinol Metab 1996;81(6):2397-2400.
2350. Lacroix A, Ndiaye N, Tremblay J, et al. Ectopic and abnormal hormone receptors in adrenal Cushing's syndrome. Endocr Rev 2001;22(1):75-110.
2351. Bourdeau I, D'Amour P, Hamet P, et al. Aberrant membrane hormone receptors in incidentally discovered bilateral macronodular adrenal hyperplasia with subclinical Cushing's syndrome. J Clin Endocrinol Metab 2001;86(11):5534-5540.
2352. Benvenga S, Smedile G, Lo Giudice F, et al. Testicular adrenal rests: evidence for luteinizing hormone receptors and for distinct types of testicular nodules differing for their autonomization. Eur J Endocrinol 1999;141(3):231-237.
2353. Leung AC, Kogan SJ. Focal lobular spermatogenesis and pubertal acceleration associated with ipsilateral Leydig cell hyperplasia. Urology 2000;56(3):508-509.
2354. Liu G, Duranteau L, Carel JC, et al. Leydig-cell tumors caused by an activating mutation of the gene encoding the luteinizing hormone receptor. N Engl J Med 1999;341(23):1731-1736.
2355. Barnes RB, Rosenfield RL, Ehrmann DA, et al. Ovarian hyperandrogenism as a result of congenital adrenal virilizing disorders: evidence for perinatal masculinization of neuroendocrine function in women. J Clin Endocrinol Metab 1994;79:1328-1333.
2356. Schedewie HK, Reiter EO, Beitins IZ. Testicular Leydig cell hyperplasia as a cause of familial sexual precocity. J Clin Endocrinol Metab 1981;52:271-278.
2357. Rosenthal SM, Grumbach MM, Kaplan SL. Gonadotropin-independent familial sexual precocity with premature Leydig and germinal cell maturation (familial testotoxicosis): effects of a potent luteinizing hormone-releasing factor agonist and medroxyprogesterone acetate therapy in four cases. J Clin Endocrinol Metab 1983;57:571-579.
2358. Egli CA, Rosenthal SM, Grumbach MM, et al. Pituitary gonadotropin-independent male-limited autosomal dominant sexual precocity in nine generations: familial testotoxicosis. J Pediatr 1985;106:33-40.
2359. Gondos B, Egli CA, Rosenthal SM, et al. Testicular changes in gonadotropin-independent familial male sexual precocity. Familial testotoxicosis. Arch Pathol Lab Med 1985;109:990-995.
2360. Holland FJ. Gonadotropin-independent precocious puberty. Endocrinol Metab Clin North Am 1991;20:191-210.
2361. Wierman ME, Beardsworth DE, Mansfield MJ, et al. Puberty without gonadotropins. A unique mechanism of sexual development. N Engl J Med 1985;312:65-72.
2362. Huhtaniemi I. The Parkes lecture. Mutations of gonadotrophin and gonadotrophin receptor genes: what do they teach us about reproductive physiology? J Reprod Fertil 2000;119(2):173-186.
2363. Stone RK. Extraordinary precocity in the development of male sexual organs and muscular system in a child four years old. Am J Med Sciences 1852;24:561-564.
2364. Soriano-Guillen L, Mitchell V, Carel JC, et al. Activating mutations in the luteinizing hormone receptor gene: a human model of non-follicle-stimulating hormone-dependent inhibin production and germ cell maturation. J Clin Endocrinol Metab 2006;91(8): 3041-3047.
2365. Rosenthal IM, Refetoff S, Rich B, et al. Response to challenge with gonadotropin-releasing hormone agonist in a mother and her two sons with a constitutively activating mutation of the luteinizing hormone receptor—a clinical research center study. J Clin Endocrinol Metab 1996;81:3802-3806.
2366. Shenker A, Laue L, Kosugi S, et al. A constitutively activating mutation of the luteinizing hormone receptor in familial male precocious puberty. Nature 1993;365:652-654.
2367. Kremer H, Mariman E, Otten BJ, et al. Cosegregation of missense mutations of the luteinizing hormone receptor gene with familial male-limited precocious puberty. Hum Mol Genet 1993;2: 1779-1783.
2368. Minegishi T, Nakamura K, Takakura Y, et al. Cloning and sequencing of porcine LH-hCG receptor cDNA. Biochem Biophys Res Comm 1990;172:1049-1054.
2369. Atger M, Misrahi M, Sar S, et al. Structure of the human luteininzing hormone/choriogonadotropin receptor gene:unusual promoter and 5' non-coding regions. Mol Cell Biol 1995;111:113-123.
2370. Dufau ML. The leutinizing hormone receptor. The Leydig Cell. Vienna, IL: Cache River Press, 1994:334-350.
2371. Baldwin JM. Stucture and function of receptors coupled to G protein. Curr Opinion Cell Biol 1994;6:180-190.
2372. Dufau ML. The luteinizing hormone receptor. Curr Op Endo Diabetes 1995;2:365-374.
2373. Evans BA, Bowen DJ, Smith PJ, et al. A new point mutation in the luteinising hormone receptor gene in familial and sporadic male limited precocious puberty: genotype does not always correlate with phenotype. J Med Genet 1996;33:143-147.
2374. Yano K, Kohn LD, Saji M, et al. A case of male-limited precocious puberty caused by a point mutation in the second transmembrane domain of the luteinizing hormone choriogonadotropin receptor gene. Biochem Biophys Res Commun 1996;220: 1036-1042.
2375. Latronico AC, Segaloff DL. Naturally occurring mutations of the luteinizing-hormone receptor: lessons learned about reproductive physiology and G protein-coupled receptors. Am J Hum Genet 1999;65(4):949-958.
2376. Latronico AC, Shinozaki H, Guerra G Jr, et al. Gonadotropin-independent precocious puberty due to luteinizing hormone receptor mutations in Brazilian boys: a novel constitutively activating mutation in the first transmembrane helix. J Clin Endocrinol Metab 2000;85(12):4799-4805.
2377. Gromoll J, Partsch CJ, Simoni M, et al. A mutation in the first transmembrane domain of the lutropin receptor causes male precocious puberty. J Clin Endocrinol Metab 1998;83(2): 476-480.
2378. Laue L, Chan WY, Hsueh AJ, et al. Genetic heterogeneity of constitutively activating mutations of the human luteinizing hormone receptor in familial male-limited precocious puberty. Proc Natl Acad Sci U S A 1995;92(6):1906-1910.

2379. Kremer H, Martens JW, van Reen M, et al. A limited repertoire of mutations of the luteinizing hormone (LH) receptor gene in familial and sporadic patients with male LH-independent precocious puberty. J Clin Endocrinol Metab 1999;84(3):1136-1140.
2380. Lin Z, Shenker A, Pearlstein R. A model of the lutropin/choriogonadotropin receptor: insights into the structural and functional effects of constitutively activating mutations. Protein Eng 1997;10(5):501-510.
2381. Wu SM, Leschek EW, Rennert OM, et al. Luteinizing hormone receptor mutations in disorders of sexual development and cancer. Front Biosci 2000;5:D343-D352.
2382. Ignacak M, Hilczer M, Zarzycki J, et al. Substitution of M398T in the second transmembrane helix of the LH receptor in a patient with familial male-limited precocious puberty. Endocr J 2000; 47(5):595-599.
2383. Feldman D. Ketoconazole and other imidazole derivatives as inhibitors of steroidogenesis. Endocr Rev 1986;7:409-420.
2384. Holland FJ, Fishman L, Bailey JD, et al. Ketoconazole in the management of precocious puberty not responsive to LHRH-analogue therapy. N Engl J Med 1985;312:1023-1028.
2385. Babovic-Vuksanovic D, Donaldson MD, Gibson NA, et al. Hazards of ketoconazole therapy in testotoxicosis. Acta Paediatr 1994;83: 994-997.
2386. Soriano-Guillen L, Lahlou N, Chauvet G, et al. Adult height after ketoconazole treatment in patients with familial male-limited precocious puberty. J Clin Endocrinol Metab 2005;90(1): 147-151.
2387. Laue L, Kenigsberg D, Pescovitz OH, et al. The treatment of familial male precocious puberty with spironolactone and testolactone. N Engl J Med 1989;320:496-502.
2387a. Kreher NC, Pescovitz OH, Delameter P, et al. Treatment of familial male-limited precocious puberty with bicalutamide and anastrozole. J Pediatr 2006;149:416-420.
2388. Laue L, Chan WY, Hsueh AJ, et al. Genetic heterogeneity of constitutively activating mutations of the human luteinizing hormone receptor in familial male-limited precocious puberty. Proc Natl Acad Sci U S A 1995;92:1906-1910.
2389. Kuhn JM, Billebaud T, Navratil H. Prevention of the transient adverse effects of a gonadotropin-releasing hormone analogue (buserelin) in metastatic prostatic carcinoma by administration of an antiandrogen (nilutamide). N Engl J Med 1989;321: 413-418.
2390. Lipton A, Demers LM, Harvey HA, et al. Letrozole (CGS 20267). A phase I study of a new potent oral aromatase inhibitor of breast cancer. Cancer 1995;75(8):2132-2138.
2391. Bhatnagar AS, Hausler A, Schieweck M, et al. Highly selective inhibition of estrogen biosynthesis by CGS 20267, a new non-steroidal aromatase inhibitor. J Ster Biochem 1990;Mol Biol 3.
2392. Partsch CJ, Krone N, Riepe FG, et al. Long-term follow-up of spontaneous development in a boy with familial male precocious puberty. Horm Res 2004;62(4):177-181.
2393. Spiegel AM, Shenker A, Weinstein LS. Receptor-effector coupling by G proteins: implications for normal and abnormal signal transduction. Endocr Rev 1992;13:536-565.
2394. Nakamoto JM, Zimmerman D, Jones EA, et al. Concurrent hormone resistance (pseudohypoparathyroidism type Ia) and hormone independence (testotoxicosis) caused by a unique mutation in the G alpha s gene. Biochem Mol Med 1996;58: 18-24.
2395. Ringel MD, Schwindinger WF, Levine MA. Clinical implications of genetic defects in G proteins. Medicine (Baltimore) 1996;75:171-184.
2396. Iiri T, Herzmark P, Nakamoto JM, et al. Rapid GDP release from Gs" in patients with gain and loss of endocrine function. Nature 1994;371:164-167.
2397. de Silva KS, Kanumakala S, Grover SR, et al. Ovarian lesions in children and adolescents—an 11-year review. J Pediatr Endocrinol Metab 2004;17(7):951-957.
2398. Polhemus DW. Ovarian maturation and cyst formation in children. Pediatrics 1953;11:588-594.
2399. Peters H. The human ovary in childhood and early maturity. Eur J Obstet Gynecol Reprod Biol 1979;3:137-144.
2400. de Sa DJ. Follicular ovarian cysts in stillbirths and neonates. Arch Dis Child 1975;50:45-50.
2401. Zachariou Z, Roth H, Boos R, et al. Three years' experience with large ovarian cysts diagnosed in utero. J Pediatr Surg 1989;24: 478-482.
2402. Sedin G, Bergquist C, Lindgren PG. Ovarian hyperstimulation syndrome in preterm infants. Pediatr Res 1985;19:548-551.
2403. Lee PA, Migeon CJ, Bias WB, et al. Familial hypersecretion of adrenal androgens transmitted as a dominant, non-HLA linked trait. Obstet Gynecol 1987;69:259-264.
2404. Arisaka O, Hosaka A, Shimura N, et al. Effect of neonatal ovarian cysts on infant growth. Clin Pediatr Endocrinol 1995;4:155-162.
2405. Lyon AJ, De Bruyn R, Grant DB. Transient sexual precocity and ovarian cysts. Arch Dis Child 1985;60:819-822.
2406. Liapi C, Evain-Brion D. Diagnosis of ovarian follicular cysts from birth to puberty: a report of twenty cases. Acta Paediatr Scand 1987;76:91-96.
2407. Richards GE, Kaplan SL, Grumbach MM. Sexual precocity associated with functional follicular cysts, prepubertal gonadotropins and LRF response and fluctuating estrogen levels. Pediatr Res 1977;11:431 (abstract).
2408. Fakhry J, Khoury A, Kotval PS, et al. Sonography of autonomous follicular ovarian cysts in precocious pseudopuberty. J Ultrasound Med 1988;7:597-603.
2409. Salardi S, Orsini LF, Cacciari E, et al. Pelvic ultrasonography in girls with precocious puberty, congenital adrenal hyperplasia, obesity, or hirsutism. J Pediatr 1988;112:880-887.
2410. Tonetta SA, di Zerega GS. Intragonadal regulation of follicular maturation. Endocr Rev 1989;10:205-229.
2411. Butler MG, Najjar JL. Do some patients with fragile X syndrome have precocious puberty. Am J Med Genet 1988;31:779-781.
2412. Natarajan A, Wales JK, Marven SS, et al. Precocious puberty secondary to massive ovarian oedema in a 6-month-old girl. Eur J Endocrinol 2004;150(2):119-123.
2413. Feuillan PP, Jones J, Oerter KE, et al. Luteinizing hormone-releasing hormone (LHRH)-independent precocious puberty unresponsive to LHRH agonist therapy in two girls lacking the features of the McCune-Albright syndrome. J Clin Endocrinol Metab 1991;73:1370-1373.
2414. Hassan E, Creatsas G, Michalas S. Genital tumors during childhood and adolescence. A clinical and pathological study of 71 cases. Clin Exp Obstet Gynecol 1999;26(1):20-21.
2415. Cass DL, Hawkins E, Brandt ML, et al. Surgery for ovarian masses in infants, children, and adolescents: 102 consecutive patients treated in a 15-year period. J Pediatr Surg 2001;36(5):693-699.
2416. Skinner MA, Schlatter MG, Heifetz SA, et al. Ovarian neoplasms in children. Arch Surg 1993;128:849-853.
2417. Abell MR, Holtz F. Ovarian neoplasms in childhood and adolescence. II. Tumors of non-germ cell origin. Am J Obstet Gynecol 1965;93(6):850-866.
2418. Schultz KA, Sencer SF, Messinger Y, et al. Pediatric ovarian tumors: a review of 67 cases. Pediatr Blood Cancer 2005;44(2): 167-173.
2419. Shankar KR, Wakhlu A, Kokai GK, et al. Ovarian adenocarcinoma in premenarchal girls. J Pediatr Surg 2001;36(3):511-515.
2420. Lack EE, Young RH, Scully RE. Pathology of ovarian neoplasms in childhood and adolescence. Pathol Annu 1992;27(Pt 2): 281-356.
2421. Imai A, Furui T, Tamaya T. Gynecologic tumors and symptoms in childhood and adolescence; 10-years' experience. Int J Gynaecol Obstet 1994;45:227-234.
2422. Young RH, Dickersin GR, Scully RE. Juvenile granulosa cell tumor of the ovary. A clinicopathologic analysis of 125 cases. Am J Surg Pathol 1984;8:575-596.
2423. Eberlein WR, Bongiovanni AM, Jones IT, et al. Ovarian tumors and cysts associated with sexual precocity. J Pediatr 1960;57: 484-497.
2424. Biscotti CV, Hart WR. Juvenile granulosa cell tumors of the ovary. Arch Pathol Lab Med 1989;113:40-46.
2425. Kalfa N, Patte C, Orbach D, et al. A nationwide study of granulosa cell tumors in pre- and postpubertal girls: missed diagnosis of endocrine manifestations worsens prognosis. J Pediatr Endocrinol Metab 2005;18(1):25-31.
2426. Abell MR. Undifferentiated malignant germ cell neoplasm (embryonal carcinoma) of ovary with stromal luteinization and masculinization. Am J Obstet Gynecol 1968;101(4):570-572.

2427. Lee MM, Donahoe PK, Hasegawa T, et al. Mhllerian inhibiting substance in humans: normal levels from infancy to adulthood. J Clin Endocrinol Metab 1996;81:571-576.
2428. Silverman LA, Gitelman SE. Immunoreactive inhibin, mullerian inhibitory substance, and activin as biochemical markers for juvenile granulosa cell tumors. J Pediatr 1996;129:918-921.
2429. Gustafson ML, Lee MM, Scully RE, et al. Mullerian inhibiting substance as a marker for sex-cord tumor. N Engl J Med 1992;326:466-471.
2430. Lapp'hn RE, Burger HC, Bouma J, et al. Inhibin as a marker for granulosa-cell tumors. N Engl J Med 1989;321:790-793.
2431. Burger HG, Fuller PJ. The inhibin/activin family and ovarian cancer. Trends Endocrinol Metab 1996;7:197-202.
2432. Masson P. Pflugerome. Bull Soc Anat (Paris) 1912;14:403-404.
2433. Talerman A. The pathology of gonadal neoplasm composed of germ cells and sex cord stroma derivatives. Pathol Res Pract 1980;170:24-38.
2434. Bhathena D, Haning RV, Shapiro S. Coexistence of a gonadoblastoma and mixed germ-cell cord stroma tumor. Pathol Res Pract 1985;180:203-206.
2435. Lacson AG, Gillis DA, Shawwa A. Malignant mixed germ-cell-sex cord-stromal tumors of the ovary associated with isosexual precocious puberty. Cancer 1988;61:2122-2133.
2436. Solh HM, Azoury RS, Najjar SS. Peutz-Jeghers syndrome associated with precocious puberty. J Pediatr 1983;103:593-595.
2437. Coen P, Kulin H, Ballantine T, et al. An aromatase-producing sex-cord tumor resulting in prepubertal gynecomastia. N Engl J Med 1991;324:317-322.
2438. Young RH, Dickersin GR, Scully RE. A distinctive ovarian sex cord-stromal tumor causing sexual precocity in the Peutz-Jeghers syndrome. Am J Surg Pathol 1983;7:233-243.
2439. Young S, Gooneratne S, Straus FH, et al. Feminizing Sertoli cell tumors in boys with Peutz-Jeghers syndrome. Am J Surg Pathol 1995;19:50-58.
2440. Berensztein E, Belgorosky A, de Davila MT, et al. Testicular steroid biosynthesis in a boy with a large cell calcifying Sertoli cell tumor producing prepubertal gynecomastia. Steroids 1995; 60:220-225.
2441. Jenne DE, Reimann H, Nezu J, et al. Peutz-Jeghers syndrome is caused by mutations in a novel serine threonine kinase. Nat Genet 1998;18(1):38-43.
2442. Karuman P, Gozani O, Odze RD, et al. The Peutz-Jegher gene product LKB1 is a mediator of p53-dependent cell death. Mol Cell 2001;7(6):1307-1319.
2443. Abed AA, Gunther K, Kraus C, et al. Mutation screening at the RNA level of the STK11/LKB1 gene in Peutz-Jeghers syndrome reveals complex splicing abnormalities and a novel mRNA isoform (STK11 c.597(insertion mark)598insIVS4). Hum Mutat 2001;18(5):397-410.
2444. Ylikorkala A, Avizienyte E, Tomlinson IP, et al. Mutations and impaired function of LKB1 in familial and non-familial Peutz-Jeghers syndrome and a sporadic testicular cancer. Hum Mol Genet 1999;8(1):45-51.
2445. Outwater EK, Wagner BJ, Mannion C, et al. Sex cord-stromal and steroid cell tumors of the ovary. Radiographics 1998;18(6): 1523-1546.
2446. Rishi M, Howard LN, Bratthauer GL, et al. Use of monoclonal antibody against human inhibin as a marker for sex cord-stromal tumors of the ovary. Am J Surg Pathol 1997;21(5): 583-589.
2447. Zumkeller W, Krause U, Holzhausen HJ, et al. Ovarian sex cord tumor with annular tubules associated with precocious puberty. Medical and Pediatric Oncology 2000;35(2):144-146.
2448. Phornphutkul C, Okubo T, Wu K, et al. Aromatase p450 expression in a feminizing adrenal adenoma presenting as isosexual precocious puberty. J Clin Endocrinol Metab 2001;86(2): 649-652.
2449. McCune DJ, Bruch H. Osteodystrophia fibrosa: report of a case in which the condition was combined with true precocious puberty, pathologic pigmentation of the skin and hyperthyroidism, with a review of the literature. Am J Dis Child 1937;54: 806-848.
2450. Albright F, Butler AM, Hampton AO, et al. Syndrome characterized by osteitis fibrosa disseminata, areas of pigmentation and endocrine dysfunction, with precocious puberty in females. N Engl J Med 1937;216:727-746.
2451. Danon MS, Robboy SH, Kin S, et al. Cushing syndrome, sexual precocity and polyostotic fibrous dysplasia. J Pediatr 1975;87: 917-921.
2452. Feuillan PP, Jones J, Ross JL. Growth hormone hypersecretion in a girl with McCune-Albright syndrome: comparison with controls and response to a dose of long-acting somatostatin analog. J Clin Endocrinol Metab 1995;80:1357-1360.
2453. Eons MJ, Drezner MK. Tumor-induced osteomalacia-unveiling a new hormone. N Engl J Med 1994;330:1679-1681.
2454. Zung A, Chalew SA, Schwindinger WF, et al. Response to PTH (1-34) is altered in patients with McCune-Albright syndrome. J Bone Miner Res 1993;8:S228.
2455. Shenker A, Weinstein LS, Moran A, etal. Severe endocrine and nonendocrine manifestations of the McCune-Albright syndrome associated with activating mutations of stimulatory G protein Gs. J Pediatr 1993;123:509-518.
2456. Endo M, Yamada Y, Matsuura N, et al. Monozygotic twins discordant for the major signs of McCune-Albright syndrome. Am J Med Genet 1991;41:216-220.
2457. Lumbroso S, Paris F, Sultan C. Activating Gsalpha mutations: analysis of 113 patients with signs of McCune-Albright syndrome—a European Collaborative Study. J Clin Endocrinol Metab 2004;89(5):2107-2113.
2458. Mantovani G, Bondioni S, Lania AG, et al. Parental origin of Gsalpha mutations in the McCune-Albright syndrome and in isolated endocrine tumors. J Clin Endocrinol Metab 2004;89(6): 3007-3009.
2459. Roman R, Johnson MC, Codner E, et al. Activating GNAS1 gene mutations in patients with premature thelarche. J Pediatr 2004;145(2):218-222.
2460. De Sanctis C, Lala R, Matarazzo P, et al. McCune-Albright syndrome: a longitudinal clinical study of 32 patients. J Pediatr Endocrinol Metab 1999;12(6):817-826.
2461. Nager GT, Kennedy DW, Kopstein E. Fibrous dysplasia: a review of the disease and its manifestations in the temporal bone. Ann Otol Rhinol Laryngol Suppl 1982;92:1-52.
2462. Leet AI, Chebli C, Kushner H, et al. Fracture incidence in polyostotic fibrous dysplasia and the McCune-Albright syndrome. J Bone Miner Res 2004;19(4):571-577.
2463. Hannon TS, Noonan K, Steinmetz R, et al. Is McCune-Albright syndrome overlooked in subjects with fibrous dysplasia of bone? J Pediatr 2003;142(5):532-538.
2464. Akintoye SO, Otis LL, Atkinson JC, et al. Analyses of variable panoramic radiographic characteristics of maxillo-mandibular fibrous dysplasia in McCune-Albright syndrome. Oral Dis 2004; 10(1):36-43.
2465. Galland F, Kamenicky P, Affres H, et al. McCune-Albright syndrome and acromegaly: effects of hypothalamo-pituitary radiotherapy and/or pegvisomant in somatostatin analogue-resistant patients. J Clin Endocrinol Metab. In press.
2466. Carani C, Pacchioni C, Baldini A, et al. Effects of cyproterone acetate, LHRH agonist and ovarian surgery in McCune-Albright syndrome with precocious puberty and galactorrhea. J Endocrinol Invest 1988;11:419-423.
2467. Reith KG, Comite F, Shawker T, et al. Pituitary and ovarian abnormalities demonstrated by CT and ultrasound in children with features of the McCune-Albright syndrome. Radiology 1984;153: 389-393.
2468. Foster CM, Comite F, Pescovitz OH, et al. Variable response to a long-acting agonist of luteinizing hormone-releasing hormone in girls with McCune-Albright syndrome. J Clin Endocrinol Metab 1984;59:801-805.
2469. Foster CM, Ross JL, Shawker T, et al. Absence of pubertal gonadotropin secretion in girls with McCune-Albright syndrome. J Clin Endocrinol Metab 1984;58:1161-1165.
2470. Pasquino AM, Tebaldi L, Cives C, et al. Precocious puberty in the McCune-Albright syndrome. Progression from gonadotrophin-independent to gonadotrophin-dependent puberty in a girl. Acta Paediatr Scand 1987;76:841-843.
2471. Feuillan PP, Foster CM, Pescovitz OH, et al. Treatment of precocious puberty in the McCune-Albright syndrome with the aromatase inhibitor testolactone. N Engl J Med 1986;315: 1115-1119.

2472. Hauffa BP, Havers W, Stolecke H. Short term effects of testolactone compared to other treatment modalities on longitudinal growth and ovarian activity in a girl with McCune Albright syndrome. Helv Paediatr Acta 1987;42:471-480.
2473. Feuillan PP, Jones J, Cutler GBJ. Long-term testolactone therapy for precocious puberty in girls with the McCune-Albright syndrome. J Clin Endocrinol Metab 1993;77:647-651.
2474. Nunez SB, Calis K, Cutler GB Jr, et al. Lack of efficacy of fadrozole in treating precocious puberty in girls with the McCune-Albright syndrome. J Clin Endocrinol Metab 2003;88(12):5730-5733.
2475. Eugster EA, Shankar R, Feezle LK, et al. Tamoxifen treatment of progressive precocious puberty in a patient with McCune-Albright syndrome. J Pediatr Endocrinol Metab 1999;12(5 Suppl 2): 681-686.
2476. Eugster EA, Rubin SD, Reiter EO, et al. Tamoxifen treatment for precocious puberty in McCune-Albright syndrome: a multicenter trial. J Pediatr 2003;143(1):60-66.
2477. Giovanelli G, Bernasconi S, Banchini G. McCune-Albright syndrome in a male child: a clinical and endocrinologic enigma. J Pediatr 1978;92:220-226.
2478. Coutant R, Lumbroso S, Rey R, et al. Macroorchidism due to autonomous hyperfunction of Sertoli cells and G(s)alpha gene mutation: an unusual expression of McCune-Albright syndrome in a prepubertal boy. J Clin Endocrinol Metab 2001;86(4): 1778-1781.
2479. Wasniewska M, De Luca F, Bertelloni S, et al. Testicular microlithiasis: an unreported feature of McCune-Albright syndrome in males. J Pediatr 2004;145(5):670-672.
2480. Happle R. The McCune Albright syndrome: a lethal gene surviving by mosaicism. Clin Genet 1986;29:321-324.
2481. Lyons J, Landis CA, Harsh G, et al. Two G protein oncogenes in human endocrine tumors. Science 1990;249:655-659.
2482. Neer EJ. Heterotrimeric G proteins: organizers of transmembrane signals. Cell 1995;80:249-257.
2483. Spiegel AM. The molecular basis of disorders caused by defects in G proteins. Horm Res 1997;47:89-96.
2484. Bourne HR. Trimeric G proteins: surprise witness tells a tale. Science 1995;270:933-934.
2485. Clapham DE. The G-protein nanomachine. Nature 1996;379: 297-299.
2486. Neer EJ, Smith TF. G protein heterodimers: new structures propel new questions. Cell 1996;84:175-178.
2487. Coleman DE, Sprang SR. How G proteins work: a continuing story. TIBS 1996;21:41-44.
2488. Dhanasekaran N, Heasley LE, Johnson GL. G protein-coupled receptor systems involved in cell growth and oncogenesis. Endocr Rev 1995;16:259-270.
2489. Weinstein LS, Shenker A, Gejman PV, et al. Activating mutations of the stimulatory G protein in the McCune-Albright syndrome. N Engl J Med 1991;325:1688-1695.
2490. Schwindinger WF, Francomano CA, Levine MA. Identification of a mutation in the gene encoding the "subunit of the stimulatory G protein of adenylyl cyclase in McCune-Albright syndrome. Proc Natl Acad Sci U S A 1992;89:5152-5156.
2491. Spiegel AM. Mutations in G proteins and G protein-coupled receptors in endocrine disease. J Clin Endocrinol Metab 1996;81: 2434-2442.
2492. Lania A, Mantovani G, Spada A. G protein mutations in endocrine diseases. Eur J Endocrinol 2001;145(5):543-559.
2493. Shenker A, et al. An activating Gs" mutation is present in fibrous dysplasia of bone in the McCune-Albright syndrome. J Clin Endocrinol Metab 1994;79:750-755.
2494. Candeliere GA, Gloueux FH, Prud' homme J, et al. Increased expression of the C-fos proto-oncogene in bone from patients with fibrous dysplasia. N Engl J Med 1995;332:1546-1551.
2495. Kendle FW. Case of precocious puberty in a female cretin. Br Med J 1905;1:246.
2496. Suter SN, Kaplan SL, Aubert ML, et al. Plasma prolactin and thyrotropin and the response to throtropin-releasing factor in children with primary and tertiary hypothyroidism. J Clin Endocrinol Metab 1978;47:1015-1020.
2497. Hemady ZS, Siler-Khodr TM, Najjar S. Precocious puberty in juvenile hypothyroidism. J Pediatr 1978;92:55-59.
2498. Piziak VK, Hahn HBJ. Isolated menarche in juvenile hypothyroidism. Clin Pediatr (Phila) 1984;23:177-179.
2499. Wood LC, Olichney M, Locke H, et al. Syndrome of juvenile hypothyroidism associated with advanced sexual development: report of two new cases and comment on the management of an associated ovarian mass. J Clin Endocrinol Metab 1965;25:1289-1295.
2500. Rakover Y, Weiner E, Shalev E, et al. Vaginal bleeding: presenting symptom of acquired primary hypothyroidism in a seven year-old girl. J Pediatr Endocrinol 1993;6:197-200.
2501. Phupong V, Aribarg A. Vaginal bleeding in a young girl due to primary hypothyroidism. Arch Gynecol Obstet 2003;268(3): 217-218.
2502. Chemaitilly W, Thalassinos C, Emond S, et al. Metrorrhagia and precocious puberty revealing primary hypothyroidism in a child with Down's syndrome. Arch Dis Child 2003;88(4): 330-331.
2503. Radaideh AM, Nusier M, El Akawi Z, Jaradat D. Precocious puberty with congenital hypothyroidism. Neuro Endocrinol Lett 2005;26(3):253-256.
2504. Takeuchi K, Deguchi M, Takeshima Y, et al. A case of multiple ovarian cysts in a prepubertal girl with severe hypothyroidism due to autoimmune thyroiditis. Int J Gynecol Cancer 2004;14(3): 543-545.
2505. Chattopadhyay A, Kumar V, Marulaiah M. Polycystic ovaries, precocious puberty and acquired hypothyroidism: The Van Wyk and Grumbach syndrome. J Pediatr Surg 2003;38(9):1390-1392.
2506. Laron Z, Karp M, Dolberg L. Juvenile hypothyroidism with testicular enlargement. Acta Paediatr Scand 1970;59:317-322.
2507. Jannini EA, Ulisse S, D'Aromiento M. Thyroid hormone and male gonadal function. Endocrine Rev 1995;16:443-459.
2508. Pringle PJ, Stanhope R, Hindmarsh P, et al. Abnormal pubertal development in primary hypothyroidism. Clin Endocrinol (Oxf) 1988;28:479-486.
2509. Buchanan CR, Stanhope R, Adlard P, et al. Gonadotropin, growth hormone and prolactin secretion in children with primary hypothyroidism. Clin Endocrinol 1988;29:427-436.
2510. Bruder JM, Samuels MH, Bremner WJ, et al. Hypothyroidism-induced macroorchidism: use of a gonadotropin-releasing hormone agonist to understand its mechanism and augment adult stature. J Clin Endocrinol Metab 1995;80:11-16.
2511. Hess RA, Cooke PS, Bunick D, et al. Adult testicular enlargement induced by neonatal hypothyroidism is accompanied by increased Sertoli and germ cell numbers. Endocrinology 1993;132:2607-2613.
2512. Marshall GR, Plant TM. Puberty occurring either spontaneously or induced precociously in rhesus monkey (Macaca mulatta) is associated with a marked proliferation of Sertoli cells. Biol Reprod 1996;54:1192-1199.
2513. Anasti JN, Flack MR, Froehlich J, et al. A potential novel mechanism for precocious puberty in juvenile hypothyroidism [see comments]. J Clin Endocrinol Metab 1995;80:276-279.
2514. Money J, Lamacz M. Genital examination and exposure experienced as nosocomial sexual abuse in childhood. J Nerv Ment Dis 1987;175:713-721.
2515. Ivarsson SA, Nilsson KO, Persson PH. Ultrasonography of the pelvic organs in prepubertal and postpubertal girls. Arch Dis Child 1983;58:352-354.
2516. Griffin IJ, Cole TJ, Duncan KA, et al. Pelvic ultrasound measurements in normal girls. Acta Paediatr 1995;84:536-543.
2517. Haber HP, Mayer EI. Ultrasound evaluation of uterine and ovarian size from birth to puberty. Pediatr Radiol 1994;24:11-13.
2518. Gadelha DC, Filho FM, Ferreira AC, et al. Uterine volume in adolescents. Ultrasound Med Biol 2004;30(1):7-10.
2519. Garibaldi LR, Aceto TJ, Weber C, et al. The relationship between luteinizing hormone and estradiol secretion in female precocious puberty: evaluation by sensitive gonadotropin assays and the leuprolide stimulation test. J Clin Endocrinol Metab 1993;76:851-856.
2520. Oberman AS, Flatau E, Luboshitzky R. Bilateral testicular adrenal rests in a patient with 11-hydroxylase deficient congenital adrenal hyperplasia. J Urol 1993;149:350-352.
2521. Rieth KG, Comite F, Dwyer AJ, et al. CT of cerebral abnormalities in precocious puberty. AJR 1987;148:1231-1238.
2522. Burton EM, Ball WSJ, Crone K, et al. Hamartoma of the tuber cinereum: a comparison of MR and CT findings in four cases. AJNR Am J Neuroradiol 1989;10:497-501.

2523. Robben SG, Oostdijk W, Drop SL, et al. Idiopathic isosexual central precocious puberty: magnetic resonance findings in 30 patients. Br J Radiol 1995;68:34-38.
2524. Ng SM, Kumar Y, Cody D, et al. Cranial MRI scans are indicated in all girls with central precocious puberty. Arch Dis Child 2003;88(5):414-418.
2525. Argyropoulou M, Perignon F, Brunelle F, et al. Height of normal pituitary gland as a function of age evaluated by magnetic resonance imaging in children. Pediatr Radiol 1991;21:247-249.
2526. Perignon F, Brauner R, Argyropoulou M, et al. Precocious puberty in girls: pituitary height as an index of hypothalamo-pituitary activation. J Clin Endocrinol Metab 1992;75:1170-1172.
2527. Van Beek JT, Sharafuddin MJ, Kao SC, et al. Prospective assessment of pituitary size and shape on MR imaging after suppressive hormonal therapy in central precocious puberty. Pediatr Radiol 2000;30(7):444-446.
2528. Ghazi AA, Mofid D, Rahimi F, et al. Cortisol and estradiol secretion by a benign virilizing adrenocortical tumor in a prepubertal girl. J Pediatr Endocrinol Metab 2004;17(2):235-238.
2529. Segal DG, DiMeglio LA, Ryder KW, et al. Assay interference leading to misdiagnosis of central precocious puberty. Endocrine 2003;20(3):195-199.
2530. Cook CD, McArthur JW, Berenberg W. Pseudoprecocious puberty in girls as a result of estrogen ingestion. N Engl J Med 1953; 248:671-674.
2531. Landolt R, Murset G. [Premature puberty sigsns as result of unintensional estrogen administration] Vorzeitige Pubertatsmerkmale als Folge unbeabsichtigyer Ostrogenverabreichung. Schweiz Med Wochenschr 1968;98:638-641.
2532. Partsch CJ, Sippell WG. Pathogenesis and epidemiology of precocious puberty. Effects of exogenous oestrogens. Hum Reprod Update 2001;7(3):292-302.
2533. Zimmerman PA, Francis GL, Poth M. Hormone-containing cosmetics may cause signs of early sexual development. Mil Med 1995;160:628-630.
2534. Peter M, Krolikowski I, Sippell WG. Transient pseudoprecocious puberty caused by a dermal ointment containing oestrogens. Monatssch Kinderheilkd 1995;143:485-488.
2534a. Henley DV, Lipson N, Korach KS, et al. Prepubertal gynecomastia linked to lavender and tea tree oils. N Engl J Med 2007;356:479-485.
2535. Svoren BM, Wolfsdorf JI. Sexual development in a 21 month-old boy caused by testosterone contamination of a topical hydrocortisone cream. J Pediatr Endocrinol Metab 2005;18(5):507-510.
2536. Andersson AM, Skakkebaek NE. Exposure to exogenous estrogens in food: possible impact on human development and health. Eur J Endocrinol 1999;140(6):477-485.
2537. Scaglioni S, Di Pietro C, Bigatello A, et al. Breast enlargement at an Italian school. Lancet 1978;1(8063):551-552.
2538. Fara GM, Del Corvo G, Bernuzzi S, et al. Epidemic of breast enlargement in an Italian school. Lancet 1979;2:295-297.
2539. Pasquino AM, Balducci R, Manca Bitti ML, et al. Transient pseudoprecocious puberty by probable oestrogen intake in 3 girls. Arch Dis Child 1982;57:954-956.
2540. Nizzoli G, Del Corno G, Fara GM, et al. Gynaecomastia and premature thelarche in a schoolchildren population of northern Italy. Acta Endocrinol Suppl (Copenh) 1986;279:227-231.
2541. Bongiovanni AM. An epidemic of premature thelarche in Puerto Rico. J Pediatr 1983;103:245-246.
2542. Precocious development in Puerto Rican children. Lancet 1986;1:721-722 (editorial).
2543. Larriuz-Serrano MC, Perez-Cardona CM, Ramos-Valencia G, et al. Natural history and incidence of premature thelarche in Puerto Rican girls aged 6 months to 8 years diagnosed between 1990 and 1995. P R Health Sci J 2001;20(1):13-18.
2544. Mills JL. Endocrinology of premature thelarche. In McLachlan JA, ed. Estrogens in the Environment. II. Influences on Development. New York: Elsevier, 1985:412-427.
2545. US Food and Drug Administration. Guideline 3, part 2: Guideline for toxicological testing. *www. fda. gov* 1999.
2546. Giampietro PG, Bruno G, Furcolo G, et al. Soy protein formulas in children: no hormonal effects in long-term feeding. J Pediatr Endocrinol Metab 2004;17(2):191-196.
2547. Colon I, Caro D, Bourdony CJ, et al. Identification of phthalate esters in the serum of young Puerto Rican girls with premature breast development. Environ Health Perspect 2000;108(9): 895-900.
2548. McKee RH. Phthalate exposure and early thelarche. Environ Health Perspect 2004;112(10):A541-A543.
2549. Blanck HM, Marcus M, Tolbert PE, et al. Age at menarche and tanner stage in girls exposed in utero and postnatally to polybrominated biphenyl. Epidemiology 2000;11(6):641-647.
2550. Hormones and Endocrine Disrupters in Food and Water. Copenhagen: Munkogaard, 2001.
2551. Berkowitz GS, Wolff MS, Matte T, et al. The rationale for a national prospective cohort study of environmental exposure and childhood development. Environ Res 2001;85(2):59-68.
2552. Massart F, Seppia P, Pardi D, et al. High incidence of central precocious puberty in a bounded geographic area of northwest Tuscany: an estrogen disrupter epidemic? Gynecol Endocrinol 2005;20(2):92-98.
2553. Denham M, Schell LM, Deane G, et al. Relationship of lead, mercury, mirex, dichlorodiphenyldichloroethylene, hexachlorobenzene, and polychlorinated biphenyls to timing of menarche among Akwesasne Mohawk girls. Pediatrics 2005;115(2): e127-e134.
2554. Scheele J, Teufel M, Niessen KH. A comparison of the concentrations of certain chlorinated hydrocarbons and polychlorinated biphenyls in bone marrow and fat tissue of children and their concentrations in breast milk. J Environ Pathol Toxicol Oncol 1995;14(1):11-14.
2555. Selevan SG, Rice DC, Hogan KA, et al. Blood lead concentration and delayed puberty in girls. N Engl J Med 2003;348(16): 1527-1536.
2556. Wu T, Buck GM, Mendola P. Blood lead levels and sexual maturation in U.S. girls: the Third National Health and Nutrition Examination Survey, 1988-1994. Environ Health Perspect 2003;111(5): 737-741.
2557. Rais-Bahrami K, Nunez S, Revenis ME, et al. Follow-up study of adolescents exposed to di(2-ethylhexyl) phthalate (DEHP) as neonates on extracorporeal membrane oxygenation (ECMO) support. Environ Health Perspect 2004;112(13):1339-1340.
2558. Saiyed H, Dewan A, Bhatnagar V, et al. Effect of endosulfan on male reproductive development. Environ Health Perspect 2003;111(16):1958-1962.
2559. Warner M, Samuels S, Mocarelli P, et al. Serum dioxin concentrations and age at menarche. Environ Health Perspect 2004;112(13): 1289-1292.
2560. Wolff MS, Britton JA, Russo JC. TCDD and puberty in girls. Environ Health Perspect 2005;113(1):A17.
2561. Visfeldt J, Jorgensen N, Muller J, et al. Testicular germ cell tumours of childhood in Denmark, 1943-1989: incidence and evaluation of histology using immunohistochemical techniques. J Pathol 1994;174:39-47.
2562. Boisen KA, Chellakooty M, Schmidt IM, et al. Hypospadias in a cohort of 1072 Danish newborn boys: prevalence and relationship to placental weight, anthropometrical measurements at birth, and reproductive hormone levels at three months of age. J Clin Endocrinol Metab 2005;90(7):4041-4046.
2563. Boisen KA, Kaleva M, Main KM, et al. Difference in prevalence of congenital cryptorchidism in infants between two Nordic countries. Lancet 2004;363(9417):1264-1269.
2564. Main KM, Toppari J, Suomi AM, et al. Larger testes and higher inhibin B levels in Finnish than in Danish newborn boys. J Clin Endocrinol Metab 2006;91(7):2732-2737.
2565. Main KM, Mortensen GK, Kaleva MM, et al. Human breast milk contamination with phthalates and alterations of endogenous reproductive hormones in infants three months of age. Environ Health Perspect 2006;114(2):270-276.
2566. Hsu PC, Lai TJ, Guo NW, et al. Serum hormones in boys prenatally exposed to polychlorinated biphenyls and dibenzofurans. J Toxicol Environ Health A 2005;68(17-18):1447-1456.
2567. Gladen BC, Klebanoff MA, Hediger ML, et al. Prenatal DDT exposure in relation to anthropometric and pubertal measures in adolescent males. Environ Health Perspect 2004;112(17):1761-1767.
2568. Guo YL, Lambert GH, Hsu CC, et al. Yucheng: health effects of prenatal exposure to polychlorinated biphenyls and dibenzofurans. Int Arch Occup Environ Health 2004;77(3):153-158.
2569. Howard CP, Takahashi H, Hayles AB. Feminizing adrenal adenoma in a boy. Mayo Clin Proc 1977;52:354-357.

2570. MacLaren NL, Migeon CH, Raiti S. Gynecomastia with congenital virilizing adrenal hyperplasia (11-β-hydroxylase deficiency). J Pediatr 1975;86:579-581.
2571. Hemsell DL, Edman CD, Marks JF, et al. Massive extranglandular aromatization of plasma androstenedione resulting in feminization of a prepubertal boy. J Clin Invest 1977;60:455-464.
2572. Berkovitz GD, Guerami A, Brown TR, et al. Familial gynecomastia with increased extraglandular aromatization of plasma carbon19-steroids. J Clin Invest 1985;75:1763-1769.
2573. Stratakis CA, Vottero A, Brodie A, et al. The aromatase excess syndrome is associated with feminization of both sexes and autosomal dominant transmission of aberrant P450 aromatase gene transcription. J Clin Endocrinol Metab 1998;83(4):1348-1357.
2574. Sebastian S, Shozu M, Hsu W, et.al. Estrogen excess by gain-of-function mutations of the CYP19 (aromatase) gene involving the chromosome 15q21.2-q21.3 region. The Endocrine Society 83rd Annual Meeting 2001;127(abstract).
2575. Binder G, Iliev DI, Dufke A, et al. Dominant transmission of prepubertal gynecomastia due to serum estrone excess: hormonal, biochemical, and genetic analysis in a large kindred. J Clin Endocrinol Metab 2005;90(1):484-492.
2576. Tiulpakov A, Kalintchenko N, Semitcheva T, et al. A potential rearrangement between CYP19 and TRPM7 genes on chromosome 15q21.2 as a cause of aromatase excess syndrome. J Clin Endocrinol Metab 2005;90(7):4184-4190.
2577. Wilson DM, Pitts WC, Hintz RL, et al. Testicular tumors with Peutz-Jeghers syndrome. Cancer 1986;57:2238-2240.
2578. Harigopal M, Murray MP, Rosen PP, et al. Prepubertal gynecomastia with lobular differentiation. Breast J 2005;11(1):48-51.
2579. Einav-Bachar R, Phillip M, Aurbach-Klipper Y, et al. Prepubertal gynaecomastia: aetiology, course and outcome. Clin Endocrinol (Oxf) 2004;61(1):55-60.
2580. Arai K, Chrousos GP. Syndromes of glucocorticoid and mineralocorticoid resistance. Steroids 1995;60:173-179.
2581. Malchoff CD, Reardon G, Javier EC, et al. Dexamethasone therapy for isosexual precocious pseudopuberty caused by generalized glucocorticoid resistance. J Clin Endocrinol Metab 1994;79:1632-1636.
2582. Young RH, Scully RE. Ovarian Sertoli cell tumors: a report of 10 cases. Int J Gynecol Pathol 1984;2:349-363.
2583. Tavassoli FA, Norris HJ. Sertoli tumors of the ovary. A clinicopathologic study of 28 cases with ultrastructural observations. Cancer 1980;46:2282-2297.
2584. Ilicki A, Lewin P, Kauli LR, et al. Premature thelarche—natural history and sex hormone secretion in 68 girls. Acta Paediatr Scand 1984;73:756-762.
2585. Volta C, Bernasconi S, Cisternino M, et al. Isolated premature thelarche and thelarche variant: clinical and auxological follow-up of 119 girls. J Endocrinol Invest 1998;21(3):180-183.
2586. Van Winter JT, Noller KL, Zimmerman D, et al. Natural history of premature thelarche in Olmsted County, Minnesota, 1940 to 1984. J Pediatr 1990;116:278-280.
2587. McKiernan J, Coyne J, Cahalane S. Histology of breast development in early life. Arch Dis Child 1988;63:136-139.
2588. Dresch PC, Arnal M, Prader A. A premature thelarche. Helv Paediatr Acta 1960;15:585-593.
2589. Caparo VJ, Bayonet-Rivera NP, Thomas A, et al. Premature thelarche. Obstet Gynecol Surg 1971;26:2-7.
2590. Ferrier P, Shepard TH, Smith FK. Growth disturbances and values for hormone excretion in various forms of precocious sexual development. Pediatrics 1961;28:258-275.
2591. Rosenfield RL. Normal and almost normal precocious variations in pubertal development premature pubarche and premature thelarche revisited. Horm Res 1994;41(Suppl 2):7-13.
2592. Simmons PS. Diagnostic considerations in breast disorders of children and adolescents. Obstet Gynecol Clin North Am 1992;19:91-102.
2593. Klein KO, Mericq V, Brown-Dawson JM, et al. Estrogen levels in girls with premature thelarche compared with normal prepubertal girls as determined by an ultrasensitive recombinant cell bioassay. J Pediatr 1999;134(2):190-192.
2594. Wenick GB, Chasalow FI, Blethen SL. Sex hormone-binding globulin and thyroxine-binding globulin levels in premature thelarche. Steroids 1988;52:543-550.
2595. Collett-Solberg PR, Grumbach MM. A simplified procedure for evaluating estrogenic effects and the sex chromatin pattern in exfoliated cells in urine: studies in premature thelarche and gynecomastia of adolescence. J Pediatr 1965;66:883-890.
2596. Stanhope R, Abdulwahid NA, Adams J, et al. Studies of gonadotrophin pulsatility and pelvic ultrasound examinations distinguish between isolated premature thelarche and central precocious puberty. Eur J Pediatr 1986;145:190-194.
2597. Caufriez H, Wolter R, Gouaerts M, et al. Gonadotropins and prolactin pituitary reserve in premature thelarche. J Pediatr 1977;91:751-753.
2598. Crofton PM, Evans NE, Wardhaugh B, et al. Evidence for increased ovarian follicular activity in girls with premature thelarche. Clin Endocrinol (Oxf) 2005;62(2):205-209.
2599. Verrotti A, Ferrari M, Morgese G, et al. Premature thelarche: a long-term follow-up. Gynecol Endocrinol 1996;10:241-247.
2600. Garibaldi LR, Aceto TJ, Weber C. The pattern of gonadotropin and estradiol secretion in exaggerated thelarche. Acta Endocrinol (Copenh) 1993;128:345-350.
2601. Murram D, Dewhurst J, Grant DB. Premature menarche: a follow-up study. Arch Dis Child 1983;58:142-143.
2602. Blanco-Garcia M, Eva-Brion D, Roger M, et al. Isolated menses in prepubertal girls. Pediatrics 1985;76:43-47.
2603. Heller ME, Dewhurst J, Grant DB. Premature menarche without other evidence of precocious puberty. Arch Dis Child 1979;54:472-475.
2604. Saggese G, Ghirri P, Del Vecchio A, et al. Gonadotropin pulsatile secretion in girls with premature menarche. Horm Res 1990;33:5-10.
2605. Fishman A, Paldi E. Vaginal bleeding in premenarchal girls: a review. Obstet Gynecol Surv 1991;46:457-460.
2606. Hill NCW, Oppenheimer LW, Morton KE. The aetiology of vaginal bleeding in children. A 20-year review Br J Obstetr Gynaecol 1989;96:467-470.
2607. David L, Betand B, Berlier P, et al. Les hJmorragie gJnitales de la fille avant la pubert. J Ann Pediatr (Paris) 1984;31:55-61.
2608. Silverman SH, Migeon CJ, Rosenberg E, et al. Precocious growth of sexual hair without other secondary sexual development; "premature pubarche," a constitutional variation of adolescence. Pediatrics 1952;10:426-431.
2609. Thamdrup E. Premature pubarche, a hypothalamic disorder? Acta Endocrinol 1955;18:564-567.
2610. Rappaport R. Plasma androgens and LH in scoliotic patients with premature pubarche. J Clin Endocrinol Metab 1974;38:401-406.
2611. Reichlin S. Neuroendocrinology. In Wilson JD, Foster DW, eds. Williams Textbook of Endocrinology. Philadelphia: WB Saunders, 1992:135-219.
2612. Lee PA, Migeon CJ, Bias WB, et al. Familial hypersecretion of adrenal androgens transmitted as a dominant, non-HLA linked trait. Obstet Gynecol 1987;69(2):259-264.
2613. Ibanez L, Potau N, de Zegher F. Recognition of a new association: reduced fetal growth, precocious pubarche, hyperinsulinism and ovarian dysfunction. Ann Endocrinol (Paris) 2000;61(2):141-142.
2614. Ferrier P, Shepard TH, Smith FK. Growth disturbances and values for hormone excretion in various forms of precocious sexual development. Pediatrics 1961;28:258-275.
2615. Korth-Schutz S, Levine LS, New MI. Serum androgens in normal prepubertal and pubertal children and in children with precocious adrenarche. J Clin Endocrinol Metab 1976;42:117-124.
2616. Rosenfield RL. Plasma 17-ketosteroids and 17-beta-hydroxysteroid in girls with premature development of sexual hair. J Pediatr 1971;79:260-266.
2617. Miller WL, Auchus RJ, Geller DH. The regulation of 17,20 lyase activity. Steroids 1997;62:133-142.
2618. Apter D, Bhtzow T, Laughlin GA, et al. Metabolic features of polycystic ovary syndrome are found in adolescent girls with hyperandrogenism. J Clin Endocrinol Metab 1995;80:2966-2973.
2619. Ibanez L, Ong KK, Mongan N, et al. Androgen receptor gene CAG repeat polymorphism in the development of ovarian hyperandrogenism. J Clin Endocrinol Metab 2003;88(7):3333-3338.
2620. Lee PA, Gareis FJ. Gonadotropin and sex steroid response to luteinizing hormone-releasing hormone in patients with premature adrenarche. J Clin Endocrinol Metab 1976;43:195-197.

2621. Ibanez L, Virdio R, Potau N, et al. Natural history of premature pubarche: an auxological study. J Clin Endocrinol Metab 1992;74:254-257.
2622. Pere A, Perheentupa J, Peter M, et al. Follow up of growth and steroids in premature adrenarche. Eur J Pediatr 1995;154: 346-352.
2623. Accetta SG, Di Domenico K, Ritter CG, et al. Anthropometric and endocrine features in girls with isolated premature pubarche or non-classical congenital adrenal hyperplasia. J Pediatr Endocrinol Metab 2004;17(5):767-773.
2624. Diamanti-Kandarakis E, Dunaif A. New perspectives in polycystic ovary syndrome. Trends Endocrinol Metab 1996;7:267-271.
2625. Oberfield SE, Mayes DM, Levine LS. Adrenal steroidogenic function in a black and Hispanic population with precocious pubarche. J Clin Endocrinol Metab 1990;70:76-82.
2626. Wilson R, Mercado A, Cheng K, et al. Steroid 21-hydroxylase deficiency: genotype may not predict phenotype. J Clin Endocrinol Metab 1995;80:2322-2329.
2627. Likitmaskul S, Cowell CT, Donaghue K, et al. "Exaggerated adrenarche" in children presenting with premature adrenarche. Clinical Endocrinol 1995;42:265-272.
2628. Morris AH, Reiter EO, Geffner ME, et al. Absence of nonclassical congenital adrenal hyperplasia in patients with precocious adrenarche. J Clin Endocrinol Metab 1989;69:709-715.
2629. Speiser PW, Dupont B, Rubenstein P, et al. High frequency of nonclassical steroid 21-hydroxylase deficiency. Am J Hum Genet 1985;35:650-667.
2630. Temeck JW, Pang S, Nelson C, et al. Genetic defects of steroidogenesis in premature pubarche. J Clin Endocrinol Metab 1987;64: 609-617.
2631. Balducci R, Boscherini B, Mangiantini A, et al. Isolated precocious pubarche: an approach. J Clin Endocrinol Metab 1994;79: 582-589.
2632. Zerah M, RhJaume E, Mani P, et al. No evidence of mutations in the genes for type I and type II β-hydroxysteroid dehydrogenase (38-HSD) in nonclassical β-HSD deficiency. J Clin Endocrinol Metab 1994;79:1811-1817.
2633. Chang YT, Zhang L, Alkaddour HS, et al. Absence of molecular defect in type II β-hydroxysteroid dehydrogenase (38-HSD) gene in premature pubarche children and hirsute female patients with moderately decreased adrenal β-HSD activity. Pediatr Res 1995;37:820-824.
2634. Morel Y, MJbarki F, RhJaume E, et al. Structure-function relationships of β-hydroxysteroid dehydrogenase: contribution made by the molecular genetics of β-hydroxysteroid dehydrogenase deficiency. Steroids 1997;62:176-184.
2635. Mendonca BB, Russell AJ, Vasconcelos-Leite M, et al. Mutation in 3 beta-hydroxysteroid dehydrogenase type II associated with pseudohermaphroditism in males and premature pubarche or cryptic expression in females. J Mol Endocrinol 1994;12:119-122.
2636. Carbunaru G, Prasad P, Scoccia B, et al. The hormonal phenotype of nonclassic 3 beta-hydroxysteroid dehydrogenase (HSD3B) deficiency in hyperandrogenic females is associated with insulin-resistant polycystic ovary syndrome and is not a variant of inherited HSD3β deficiency. J Clin Endocrinol Metab 2004; 89(2):783-794.
2637. Mermejo LM, Elias LL, Marui S, et al. Refining hormonal diagnosis of type II 3beta-hydroxysteroid dehydrogenase deficiency in patients with premature pubarche and hirsutism based on HSD3B2 genotyping. J Clin Endocrinol Metab 2005;90(3): 1287-1293.
2638. Deplewski D, Rosenfield RL. Role of hormones in pilosebaceous unit development. Endocr Rev 2000;21(4):363-392.
2639. Lucky AW, Biro FM, Huster GA, et al. Acne vulgaris in premenarchal girls. An early sign of puberty associated with rising levels of dehydroepiandrosterone. Arch Dermatol 1994;130:308-314.
2640. Yamamoto A, Ito M. Sebaceous gland activity and urinary androgen levels in children. J Dermatol Sci 1992;4:98-104.
2641. Stewart ME, Downing DT, Cook JS, et al. Sebaceous gland activity and serum dehydroepiandrosterone sulfate levels in boys and girls. Arch Dermatol 1992;128:1345-1348.
2642. Yen SCC. The polycystic ovary syndrome. Clin Endocrinol 1980;12:177-207.
2643. Franks S. Polycystic ovary syndrome. N Engl J Med 1995;333: 853-861.
2644. Ehrman DA, Barnes RB, Rosenfield RL. Polycystic ovary syndrome as a form of functional ovarian hyperandrogenism due to dysregulation of androgen secretion. Endocr Rev 1995;16: 322-353.
2645. Morales AJ, Laughlin GA, Bhtzow T, et al. Insulin somatotropic and luteinizing hormone axes in lean and obese women with polycystic ovary syndrome: common and distinct features. J Clin Endocrinol Metab 1996;81:2854-2864.
2646. Dunaif A, Segal KR, Shelley DR, et al. Evidence for distinctive and intrinsic defects in insulin action in polycystic ovary syndrome. Diabetes 1992;41:1257-1266.
2647. Dunaif A, Xia J, Book CB, et al. Excessive insulin receptor serine phosphorylation in cultured fibroblasts and in skeletal muscle: a potential mechanism for insulin resistance in the polycystic ovary syndrome. J Clin Invest 1995;96:801-810.
2648. Banerjee S, Raghavan S, Wasserman EJ, et al. Hormonal findings in African-American and Caribbean Hispanic girls with premature adrenarche: implications for polycystic ovarian syndrome. Pediatrics 1998;102(3):E36.
2649. Ibanez L, Ong K, de Zegher F, et al. Fat distribution in non-obese girls with and without precocious pubarche: central adiposity related to insulinaemia and androgenaemia from prepuberty to postmenarche. Clin Endocrinol (Oxf) 2003;58(3):372-379.
2650. Biro FM. Body morphology and its impact on adolescent and pediatric gynecology, with a special emphasis on polycystic ovary syndrome. Curr Opin Obstet Gynecol 2003;15(5):347-351.
2651. Driscoll DA. Polycystic ovary syndrome in adolescence. Semin Reprod Med 2003;21(3):301-307.
2652. Ibanez L, Potau N, Francois I, et al. Precocious pubarche, hyperinsulinism, and ovarian hyperandrogenism in girls: relation to reduced fetal growth. J Clin Endocrinol Metab 1998;83(10): 3558-3562.
2653. Ibanez L, de Zegher F, Potau N. Anovulation after precocious pubarche: early markers and time course in adolescence. J Clin Endocrinol Metab 1999;84(8):2691-2695.
2654. Veening MA, van Weissenbruch MM, Roord JJ, et al. Pubertal development in children born small for gestational age. J Pediatr Endocrinol Metab 2004;17(11):1497-1505.
2655. Boonstra VH, Mulder PG, De Jong FH, et al. Serum dehydroepiandrosterone sulfate levels and pubarche in short children born small for gestational age before and during growth hormone treatment. J Clin Endocrinol Metab 2004;89(2):712-717.
2656. Lazar L, Pollak U, Kalter-Leibovici O, et al. Pubertal course of persistently short children born small for gestational age (SGA) compared with idiopathic short children born appropriate for gestational age (AGA). Eur J Endocrinol 2003;149(5):425-432.
2657. Boonstra V, van Pareren Y, Mulder P, et al. Puberty in growth hormone-treated children born small for gestational age (SGA). J Clin Endocrinol Metab 2003;88(12):5753-5758.
2658. Neville KA, Walker JL. Precocious pubarche is associated with SGA, prematurity, weight gain, and obesity. Arch Dis Child 2005;90(3):258-261.
2659. Ibanez L, Aulesa C, Potau N, et al. Plasminogen activator inhibitor-1 in girls with precocious pubarche: a premenarcheal marker for polycystic ovary syndrome? Pediatr Res 2002;51(2):244-248.
2660. Ibaenez L, Potau N, Zampolli M, et al. Source localization of androgen excess in adolescent girls. J Clin Endocrinol Metab 1994;79:1778-1784.
2661. Oppenheimer E, Linder B, DiMartino-Nardi J. Decreased insulin sensitivity in prepubertal girls with premature adrenarche and acanthosis nigricans. J Clin Endocrinol Metab 1995;80:614-618.
2662. Ibaenez L, Potau N, Zampolli M, et al. Hyperinsulinemia in postpubertal girls with a history of premature pubarche and functional ovarian hyperandrogenism. J Clin Endocrinol Metab 1996;81:1237-1243.
2663. Ibanez L, Potau N, de Zegher F. Ovarian hyporesponsiveness to follicle stimulating hormone in adolescent girls born small for gestational age. J Clin Endocrinol Metab 2000;85(7): 2624-2626.
2664. Ibanez L, Valls C, Potau N, et al. Sensitization to insulin in adolescent girls to normalize hirsutism, hyperandrogenism, oligomenorrhea, dyslipidemia, and hyperinsulinism after precocious pubarche. J Clin Endocrinol Metab 2000;85(10):3526-3530.
2665. Arslanian SA, Lewy V, Danadian K, Saad R. Metformin therapy in obese adolescents with polycystic ovary syndrome and impaired

glucose tolerance: amelioration of exaggerated adrenal response to adrenocorticotropin with reduction of insulinemia/insulin resistance. J Clin Endocrinol Metab 2002;87(4):1555-1559.

2666. Jones KL, Arslanian S, Peterokova VA, et al. Effect of metformin in pediatric patients with type 2 diabetes: a randomized controlled trial. Diabetes Care 2002;25(1):89-94.
2667. Ibanez L, Valls C, Marcos MV, et al. Insulin sensitization for girls with precocious pubarche and with risk for polycystic ovary syndrome: effects of prepubertal initiation and postpubertal discontinuation of metformin treatment. J Clin Endocrinol Metab 2004;89(9):4331-4337.
2668. Ibanez L, Ferrer A, Ong K, et al. Insulin sensitization early after menarche prevents progression from precocious pubarche to polycystic ovary syndrome. J Pediatr 2004;144(1):23-29.
2669. Azziz R, Ehrmann D, Legro RS, et al. Troglitazone improves ovulation and hirsutism in the polycystic ovary syndrome: a multicenter, double blind, placebo-controlled trial. J Clin Endocrinol Metab 2001;86(4):1626-1632.
2670. Arlt W, Auchus RJ, Miller WL. Thiazolidinediones but not metformin directly inhibit the steroidogenic enzymes P450c17 and 3beta-hydroxysteroid dehydrogenase. J Biol Chem 2001;276(20): 16767-16771.
2671. Biro FM, Lucky AW, Huster GA, et al. Hormonal studies and physical maturation in adolescent gynecomastia. J Pediatr 1990;116: 450-455.
2672. Nydick M, Bustos J, Dale JH, et al. Gynecomastia in adolescent boys. JAMA 1961;178:449-454.
2673. Large DM, Anderson DC. Twenty-four hour profiles of circulating androgens and oestrogens in male puberty with and without gynaecomastia. Clin Endocrinol (Oxf) 1979;11:505-521.
2674. Carlson SE. Gynecomastia. N Engl J Med 1980;404:795-799.
2675. LaFranchi SH, Parlow AF, Lippe BM, et al. Pubertal gynecomastia and transient elevation of serum estradiol level. Am J Dis Child 1975;129:927-931.
2676. Siiteri PK, MacDonald PC. The role of extraglandular estrogen in human endocrinology. In Greep RO, Astwood EB, eds. Handbook of Physiology. Sect 7: Endocrinology. Vol II. Part 1. Female Reproductive System. Washington, DC: American Physiological Society, 1973:615-629.
2677. Moore DC, Schlaepfer LV, Punier L, et al. Hormonal changes during puberty. V. Transient pubertal gynecomastia: abnormal androgen-estrogen ratios. J Clin Endocrinol Metab 1997;58: 492-499.
2678. Villalpando S, Mondragon L, Barron C, et al. Role of testosterone and dihydrotestosterone in spontaneous gynecomastia of adolescents. Arch Androl 1992;28:171-176.
2679. Sasano H, Kimura M, Shizawa S, et al. Aromatase and steroid receptors in gynecomastia and male breast carcinoma: an immunohistochemical study. J Clin Endocrinol Metab 1996;81: 3063-3067.
2680. Riepe FG, Baus I, Wiest S, et al. Treatment of pubertal gynecomastia with the specific aromatase inhibitor anastrozole. Horm Res 2004;62(3):113-118.
2681. Lawrence SE, Faught KA, Vethamuthu J, et al. Beneficial effects of raloxifene and tamoxifen in the treatment of pubertal gynecomastia. J Pediatr 2004;145(1):71-76.
2682. Derman O, Kanbur NO, Kutluk T. Tamoxifen treatment for pubertal gynecomastia. Int J Adolesc Med Health 2003;15(4):359-363.
2683. McGrath MH, Mukerji S. Plastic surgery and the teenage patient. J Pediatr Adolesc Gynecol 2000;13(3):105-118.
2684. Mohoney J, Hynes B. Concurrent Poland's syndrome and gynecomastia: a case report. Can J Surg 1990;33:58-60.
2685. Glass AR. Gynecomastia. Endocrinol Metab Clin North Am 1994;23:825-837.
2686. Meschede D, Behre HM, Nieschlag E. Endocrine and spermatologic characteristics of 135 patients with bilateral megalotestis. Andrologia 1995;27(4):207-212.
2687. Chudley AE, Hagerman RJ. Fragile X syndrome. J Pediatr 1987;110: 821-830.
2688. Lachiewicz AM, Dawson DV. Do young boys with fragile X syndrome have macroorchidism? Pediatrics 1994;93:992-995.
2689. Marshall WA, Tanner JM. Variations in pattern of pubertal changes in girls. Arch Dis Child 1969;44:291-303.
2690. Dupertuis CW, Atkinson WB, Elftman H. Sex differences in pubic hair distribution. Hum Biol 1945;17:137-142.
2691. Marshall WA, Tanner JM. Variations in the pattern of pubertal changes in boys. Arch Dis Child 1970;45:13-23.
2692. Billewicz WZ, Fellowes HM, Thomson AM. Menarche in Newcastle upon Tyne girls. Ann Hum Biol 1981;8:313-320.
2693. Roy MP, Sempe M, Orssaud E, et al. [Clinical course of puberty in girls (somatic longitudinal study of 80 adolescents)] Evolution clinique de la puberte de la fille (etude longitudinale somatique de 80 adolescentes. Arch Fr Pediatr 1972;29:155-168.
2694. Taranger J, Engstrom I, Lichtenstein H, et al. VI. Somatic pubertal development. Acta Paediatr Scand Suppl 1976;121-135.
2695. Van Wieringen JD, Wafelbakker F, Verbrugge HP. Growth Diagrams 1965 Netherlands: Second National Survey on 0-24 Year Olds. Netherlands Institute for Preventative Medicine TNO. Groningen: Wolters-Noordhoof Publishing, 1971.
2696. Neyzi O, Alp H, Orhon A. Sexual maturation in Turkish girls. Ann Hum Biol 1975;2(1):49-59.
2697. Villarreal SF, Martorell R, Mendoza F. Sexual maturation of Mexican-American adolescents. American Journal of Human Biology 1989;1:87-95.
2698. Largo RH, Prader A. Pubertal development in Swiss boys. Helv Paediatr Acta 1983;38:211-228.
2699. Neyzi O, Alp H, Yalcindag A, et al. Sexual Maturation in Turkish boys. Annals of Human Biology 1975;2(3):251-259.
2700. Oerter KE, Manasco P, Barnes KM, et al. Adult height in precocious puberty after long-term treatment with deslorelin. J Clin Endocrinol Metab 1991;73:1235-1240.
2701. Boepple PA, Crowley WFJ. Gonadotrophin-releasing hormone analogues as therapeutic probes in human growth and development: evidence from children with central precocious puberty. Acta Paediatr Scand Suppl 1991;372:33-38.
2702. Rappaport R, Fontoura M, Brauner R. Treatment of central precocious puberty with an LHRH agonist (Buserelin): effect on growth and bone maturation after three years of treatment. Horm Res 1987;28:149-154.
2703. Suwa S, Hibi I, Kato K, Nakazima H. LH-RH agonistic analog (buserelin) treatment of precocious puberty: collaborative study in Japan. Acta Paediatr Jpn 1988;30 Suppl:176-184.
2704. Luder AS, Holland FJ, Costigan DC, et al. Intranasal and subcutaneous treatment of central precocious puberty in both sexes with a long-acting analog of luteinizing hormone-releasing hormone. J Clin Endocrinol Metab 1984;58:966-972.
2705. Donaldson MD, Stanhope R, Lee TJ, et al. Gonadotrophin responses to GnRH in precocious puberty treated with GnRH analogue. Clin Endocrinol (Oxf) 1984;21:499-503.
2706. Rime JL, Zumsteg U, Blumberg A, et al. Long-term treatment of central precocious puberty with an intranasal LHRH analogue: control of pituitary function by urinary gonadotropins. Eur J Pediatr 1988;147:263-269.
2707. Stanhope R, Pringle PJ, Brook CG. Growth, growth hormone and sex steroid secretion in girls with central precocious puberty treated with a gonadotrophin releasing hormone (GnRH) analogue. Acta Paediatr Scand 1988;77:525-530.
2708. Kauli R, Pertzelan A, Ben-Zeev Z, et al. Treatment of precocious puberty with LHRH analogue in combination with cyproterone acetate-further experience. Clin Endocrinol (Oxf) 1984;20:377-387.
2709. Mantzoros CS, Flier JS, Rogol AD: A longitudinal assessment of hormonal and physical alterations during normal puberty in boys. J Clin Endocrinol Metab 1997;82:1066-1070.
2710. Horlick MB, Rosenbaum M, Nicolson M, et al: Effects of puberty on the relationship between circulating leptin and body composition. J of Clin Endocrinol Metab 2000;85(7):2509-2518.

CHAPTER 25

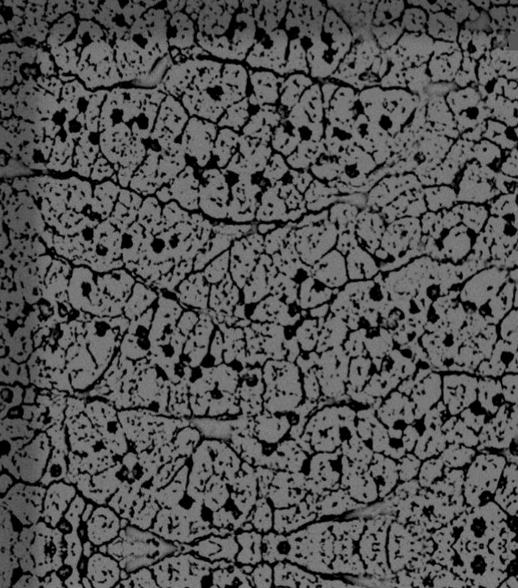

HORMONES AND ATHLETIC PERFORMANCE

Fabio Lanfranco, Ezio Ghigo, and Christian J. Strasburger

EFFECT OF ATHLETIC PERFORMANCE ON HORMONAL SYSTEMS

Catecholamines

The two catecholamines norepinephrine and epinephrine are closely coupled in their actions. Catecholamines respond rapidly to exercise. Norepinephrine increases from a resting level of 1.2 to 3.0 nmol/L to levels as high as 12.0 nmol/L at maximal exercise.[1] Resting concentrations of epinephrine are 380 to 655 pmol/L. With maximal exercise, epinephrine concentrations can increase up to 3300 pmol/L. Both these hormones progressively increase as workload increases. Following exercise, resting concentrations are achieved within 30 minutes after exercise.[1]

Mild exercise produces little or no response in catecholamines, whereas at moderate exercise levels norepinephrine significantly increases with minimal change in circulating epinephrine. At intense or prolonged exercise levels, both hormones increase significantly.[2] Acute, short duration maximal exercise can significantly increase norepinephrine and epinephrine levels. This rapid response suggests that the levels are primarily regulated via neural release mediated by activation of the sympathetic nervous system. Spillover from active muscle during exercise appears to be the primary contributor, but the kidneys are a possible other source.[1] Moreover, alteration in the ratio of norepinephrine to epinephrine, with a greater increase in the release of epinephrine from the adrenal medulla during exercise, suggests a possible hypothalamic mediation in the response to exercise.

Graded exercise produces a lower response than continuous prolonged exercise. The responses are directly related to workload and oxygen uptake and are greater with small muscle groups than with large muscle groups. Training results in a diminished catecholamine response to the same absolute level of physical activity, but may increase the ability to secrete epinephrine in response to other stimuli.[2]

The effects of catecholamine release include increased glycogenolysis and increased free fatty acid (FFA) concentrations. Cardiovascular adaptations to exercise are mediated at least in part by catecholamines. Redistribution of circulation to working muscles and to the skin for heat loss and sweating is mediated through changes in catecholamines directly or indirectly via other intermediate hormones. Moreover, catecholamines may mediate mental performance improvement, which occurs through exercise.[3]

Summary

Catecholamines respond rapidly to exercise. Acute, short duration maximal exercise as well as intense or prolonged exercise can significantly increase norepinephrine and epinephrine levels. The effects of catecholamine release include increased glycogenolysis and increased FFA concentrations, cardiovascular adaptations to exercise, redistribution of circulation to working muscles and to the skin, and mental performance improvement that occurs through exercise.

Fluid Homeostasis—Vasopressin—Renin-Angiotensin-Aldosterone System

During physical exercise, there is a considerable loss of water and electrolytes in sweat, which is necessary to maintain body temperature by dissipating heat generated from muscle use. The rate of fluid loss owing to sweating may be as high as 1500 mL/hr.[4] The loss of fluids is replaced by the subsequent ingestion of liquids, which is modulated by thirst. The replacement of electrolyte is the result of the normal intake of food. Renal function is the major mechanism by which electrolytes are conserved following exercise.

The maintenance of fluid and electrolyte homeostasis depends on the action of vasopressin (AVP), natriuretic peptides, the renin-angiotensin-aldosterone (RAA) axis, and catecholamines. These hormonal systems are modified in response to exercise, with different patterns depending on the amount of relative work performed, the duration of exercise, and the training status. Other factors influencing the response of hormones to exercise include the mode of exercise, environmental factors, age and gender of the subjects, and several medical/physiologic conditions.[1]

Hormones involved in the regulation of fluid and electrolyte homeostasis show a relatively consistent response among individuals. AVP concentrations increase during exercise and persist elevated for more than 60 minutes following maximal exercise. The stimulus for the increase in AVP during exercise is the increase in plasma osmolality and reduction in blood volume.[5]

Atrial natriuretic peptide (ANP) and brain natriuretic peptide (BNP), which may be altered by exercise,[1] also elicit a natriuretic effect. ANP increase is transitory in exercise of extended duration, with hormone values returning to resting levels over time.[6] Sodium intake may affect the ANP response to exercise: the ANP increase has been shown to be higher on a high-sodium diet (300 mmol/day) than in the same subjects during a low-sodium regimen (40 mmol/day).[7]

BNP response to exercise is modulated by sodium intake and by the hydration status.[1] Interestingly, BNP levels have been found to increase in hypertensive subjects during exercise, whereas no changes have been described in normal subjects in several study protocols.[8,9]

The RAA system is closely coupled and responds to exercise. Increased values of plasma renin activity (PRA) are reported following maximal exercise.[1] The increase in PRA occurs at submaximal workloads of greater than 60% to 70%. With the increase in PRA during exercise, there is a concomitant increase in angiotensin II (A-II), which partially mediates the increase in circulating aldosterone concentrations.[1] Elevated levels of aldosterone may persist for days after the end of exercise depending on water and sodium intake.[1]

The primary activator of the RAA system during exercise is the sympathetic nervous system. Stimulation of the release of renin is modulated by changes in renal sympathetic nerve activity, resulting in an increase in local norepinephrine.[10] During exercise, the increase in renin activity is correlated with the increase in norepinephrine concentration in the renal vein.[10] The increase in aldosterone with exercise is assumed to be mediated by the increase in A-II in response to activation of the RAA system. However, inhibition of angiotensin-converting enzyme does not attenuate the increase in aldosterone with maximal exercise in healthy subjects.[11] Other factors involved in the activation of aldosterone production include sodium intake, potassium balance, and levels of adrenocorticotropin hormone (ACTH). The persistent increase of aldosterone long after the end of exercise may be associated with reductions in plasma osmolality and sodium concentrations due to ingestion of water to replace total body water losses.[1] Thus, the interaction of a number of regulating factors is involved in mediating the response of aldosterone.

Summary

The maintenance of fluid and electrolyte homeostasis depends on the action of AVP, natriuretic peptides, the RAA axis, and catecholamines. AVP concentrations increase following the increase in plasma osmolality and reduction in blood volume. ANP and BNP transiently increase during exercise. PRA, A-II, and aldosterone increment is modulated by the sympathetic nervous system, sodium intake, potassium balance, and levels of ACTH.

Hypothalamus-Pituitary-Adrenal Axis

Glucocorticoids

Since the pioneering studies of Davies and Few,[12] it has been known that exercise of an appropriate intensity is a potent stimulus for cortisol secretion. Physical exercise induces an effect on ACTH and cortisol secretion greater than that which can be accounted for by corticotropin releasing hormone (CRH) alone. In humans, exercise is accompanied by increases in AVP release into the systemic circulation, which occur in proportion to the intensity of the exercise. Pulses of ACTH and AVP secretion are concordant during exercise in humans.[13]

Increases in plasma lactate have been implicated as one of the mechanisms responsible for activation of the hypothalamus-pituitary-adrenal (HPA) axis during exercise. Other humoral mediators like A-II and interleukins, which increase during exercise, are also capable of activating the HPA axis. However, their role in humans during exercise has not been defined. Afferent nerve signals from working muscles have been shown to be essential for the activation of the HPA axis during exercise.[14] Furthermore, signals generated from peripheral nerves originating in muscle tissue contribute to the increase in plasma AVP, which occurs during exercise. Changes in plasma volume and osmolality also occur during exercise accompanied by proportional changes in plasma AVP.

Cortisol response is dependent on the relative exercise workload for both aerobic and strength exercise, and the rise of plasma cortisol is associated with an increase in ACTH concentration.[15] Activation of the HPA axis was initially described to occur during aerobic physical activity that exceeded 60% of the maximum aerobic power.[16] However, when evaluated relative to the circadian baseline rather than to the preexercise baseline, responses of plasma cortisol to 90 minutes of exercise at 55% and even 25% maximal oxygen uptake (VO_{2max}) may be substantial.[17]

Activation of the HPA axis during aerobic exercise is proportional to the relative intensity of the exercise and is independent of the fitness level of the subject.[18] Prolonged submaximal physical activity and very brief high-intensity exercise result in activation of the HPA axis.[19,20] Interestingly, brief high-intensity exercise produces an increase in plasma ACTH levels that is greater than that found during prolonged submaximal exercise but less than that seen following graded exercise to exhaustion.[19,20]

Duration of the physical activity may be important in determining the response of plasma cortisol to exercise. Plasma cortisol has been shown to increase more after a 42-km than a 19-km kayak race.[21] During a 6-day Nordic ski race, plasma ACTH levels increased and then remained similar throughout the race, whereas plasma cortisol was highest on the initial 2 days.[22]

The cortisol response is influenced by the type of exercise. In contrast to sustained aerobic activity, intermittent exercise of varying intensities, such as matchplay tennis, does not appear to induce activation of the HPA axis.[23] Isometric exercise induces activation of the HPA axis, which is intensity-dependent.[24] Anaerobic exercise induces a greater increase in plasma cortisol than aerobic exercise of the same total work output.[25]

The response of the HPA axis to physical activity is independent of age. In elderly males, the cortisol response to heavy-resistance exercise is diminished,[26] although a reduced effort may be involved. An earlier activation of the HPA axis accompanied by a more pronounced increase in the activity of the sympathetic nervous system has been demonstrated in elderly subjects during submaximal aerobic exercise.[27] However, no significant difference in cortisol response to aerobic exercise at the same relative intensity has been observed in young and elderly subjects.[28]

Gender does not affect cortisol response to physical activity. Although males show predominantly increased autonomic, cardiovascular, and carbohydrate oxidation counterregulatory responses to exercise, and on the contrary females have predominantly increased lipolytic and ketogenic responses, plasma cortisol levels respond similarly in men and women.[29]

Compared with sedentary women, both amenorrheic athletic women and athletic women with regular menstrual cycles were demonstrated to have blunted cortisol response to CRH.[30] Female sex steroids could play a crucial role in mediating the adrenocortical response to external stimulation: estradiol may impair the glucocorticoid receptor–mediated slow negative feedback. A reduction in free cortisol levels after physical exercise has been demonstrated in women using estrogen-containing contraceptives compared with women who do not.[31] Kirschbaum and colleagues[32] demonstrated that short-term estradiol administration resulted in hyperresponses of the HPA axis to a standardized psychosocial stress task in healthy men. Altogether, estrogens are potent regulators of the HPA axis.[33]

Repeated stress, either acute or chronic, reduces the sensitivity of the rat HPA axis to glucocorticoid negative feedback.[34] Endurance training has been compared to chronic stress in humans.[35] ACTH and cortisol responses to exercise are attenuated in trained subjects for a given absolute workload, and moreover, highly trained athletes have diminished responses of ACTH and cortisol to CRH, which are consistent with a sustained hypercortisolism state.

Using this model of repeated physical stress, Duclos and colleagues[33] have shown that in long-distance runners the recovery after a muscle exercise regardless of its duration and intensity modifies ACTH production. During this period, plasma ACTH is increased without noticeable change on plasma cortisol when compared with a control resting day, supporting the hypothesis of a decreased pituitary sensitivity to the cortisol negative feedback and counterarguing the hypothesis of a decreased adrenal sensitivity to ACTH. A reduction of cortisol levels during a training program without significant changes in ACTH concentrations have been described by some authors, indicating that the ACTH receptors in the adrenal gland may be down-regulated.[36] The reductions in cortisol are thought to provide one possible mechanism by which protein accretion is enhanced by reduced degradation in type I muscle fibers.[37]

As a condition of overtraining develops, the pituitary ACTH release starts to decrease.[38] The overtraining syndrome (OTS) is a neuroendocrine disorder characterized by poor performance in competition, inability to maintain training loads, persistent fatigue, reduced catecholamine excretion, frequent illness such as upper respiratory tract infections, disturbed sleep, and alterations in mood state.[39] A hallmark feature of OTS is the inability to sustain intense exercise and recover for the next training or competition session. This complex condition affects a large percentage of elite athletes. Common, however, is a short-term overtraining or "overreaching," which is reversible within days to weeks.[39]

A number of factors modify the response of the HPA axis to physical activity. Cortisol responses to exercise are blunted when exercise is initiated at the peak of the cortisol response to a meal.[17] During exercise at low altitude, the response of plasma ACTH, but not cortisol, is increased compared with when exercise is undertaken at a moderate level of altitude. At high altitude, both ski-training[40] and marathon running[41] produce greater increases in plasma cortisol than training at moderate or low altitude. Mild dehydration does not affect the response of plasma cortisol to prolonged low-intensity exercise.[42] The response of plasma cortisol to short-duration, high-intensity exercise is not modified by an increase in environmental temperature.[43]

During prolonged, low-intensity exercise in humans, decreased blood glucose concentrations result in activation of the HPA axis, which can be prevented by maintaining the blood glucose constant.[44] The ingestion of carbohydrate during acute exercise attenuates the cortisol response, whereas during prolonged running exercise, it has been shown to result in either no change[45] or an increased serum cortisol compared with ingestion of placebo in control subjects.[46]

Mineralocorticoids

The RAA system is closely coupled and responds to exercise. PRA values increase following maximal exercise.[1] Progressively higher increases in aldosterone levels have been observed with increasing degrees of exertion. Elevated levels of aldosterone may persist for days after the end of exercise depending on water and sodium intake.[1]

The interaction of a number of regulating factors is involved in mediating the response of aldosterone. These include the sympathetic nervous system, renin activity, A-II, sodium intake, potassium balance, blood volume reductions, and levels of ACTH.[1]

Endorphins

Exercise is able to influence the release of β-endorphin depending on intensity and duration of the physical activity. If a threshold intensity is exceeded, endogenous opiate levels start to increase. Incremental graded exercise tests elevate β-endorphin levels 1.5- to 7-fold. Short bouts of anaerobic exercise induce a twofold to fourfold increase of β-endorphin depending on the duration of exercise stress.[47] Lactate and catecholamine concentrations are the main factors being correlated with these responses. Duration of aerobic exercise seems to be an independent factor that stimulates β-endorphin release after about 1 hour if a threshold intensity—around 55% to 60% VO_{2max}—is reached. Very little is known about the influence of training status on the release of β-endorphin and study results are often inconsistent.

A physiologic purpose of endogenous opiate increase in athletes can be the modulation of pain and the improvement of mood.[48] Sudden cessation of regular training is supposed to induce a depressed mood, which is considered to be part of the "detraining syndrome."[47] Altogether, the action of endogenous opiates can be described as a rewarding system that makes the athlete continue physical activity.

Summary

Exercise is accompanied by increases in ACTH and cortisol release. Activation of the HPA axis during aerobic exercise is proportional to the relative intensity of the exercise and is independent of the fitness level of the subject. Intermittent exercise of varying intensities does not appear to induce activation of the HPA axis. Anaerobic exercise induces a greater increase in plasma cortisol than aerobic exercise of the same total work output. The response of the HPA axis to physical activity is independent of age and gender, and is affected by altitude and carbohydrate ingestion.

The RAA system is closely coupled and responds to exercise. PRA, A-II, and aldosterone increase during exercise following the interaction of a number of regulating factors, such as the activity of the sympathetic nervous system, sodium intake, potassium balance, and levels of ACTH.

Exercise is able to influence the release of β-endorphin depending on intensity and duration of the physical activity. β-endorphin increases are also induced by anaerobic exercise and by incremental exercise that reaches anaerobic stages. The purpose of endogenous opiate increase in athletes can be the modulation of pain and the improvement of mood.

Hypothalamus-Pituitary-Gonadal Axis

Male Gonadal Axis

The effects of physical activity on the male reproductive axis vary with the intensity and duration of the activity, the fitness of the individual, and his nutritional-metabolic status. Relatively short, intense exercise usually increases while more prolonged exercise usually decreases serum testosterone levels. Endurance and other forms of training can induce subclinical inhibition of normal reproductive function, although clinical expression of reproductive dysfunction with exercise is uncommon in men.[49]

Increased serum testosterone levels have been reported during relatively strenuous free and treadmill running, weight training, and ergometer cycling.[49] The testosterone response has been reported to increase with increased exercise load.[50] Similar workloads produce similar responses, regardless of whether the load is aerobic or anaerobic.[25] Dietary intake may influence basal testosterone levels, but not the exercise response to high-intensity, resistance exercise.[51] Increased and decreased ambient temperature, altitude, and dehydration have no effect on testosterone response to intense exercise.[42,43] Acute exercise-induced testosterone increments are also seen in older men, despite their different hormonal milieu.[26]

There is conflicting evidence about gonadotropin response to exercise, because luteinizing hormone (LH) and follicle-stimulating hormone (FSH) levels have been reported to be unchanged, increased, or decreased by short-term strenuous exercise.[49] Because the LH response to exercise is inconsistent and because testosterone levels increase in response to exercise more quickly than their response to LH, it is accepted that the exercise-associated increment in circulating testosterone is not mediated by LH. Possible mechanisms such as hemoconcentration, reduced clearance, and/or increased testosterone synthesis may be involved. For nonspecific mechanisms to be responsible for the acute serum testosterone increase, a similar increase would be expected for all circulating steroids.[49] However, the timing of testosterone increase differs from that of androstenedione and dehydroepiandrosterone,[52] thus suggesting that specific testicular mechanisms are involved.

In contrast to the short-term testosterone increment, a suppression of serum testosterone levels occurs during and subsequent to more prolonged exercise, and to some extent in the hours following intense short-term exercise. A variety of systems could influence the decrease of testosterone synthesis, including decreased gonadotropins, increased cortisol or catecholamine levels, or even an accumulation of metabolic waste materials.[53] The fall in serum testosterone must result from decreased production rates, decreased binding, or increased clearance.

Acute submaximal, repeated exercise alters the secretion of gonadotropins. It has been observed in healthy males that prolonged walking provokes a reduction in the plasma concentration of FSH, LH, and testosterone in the first 3 days, but the acute response of LH and testosterone to exercise disappears within 4 days.[54] Prolonged exposure to exercise also disturbs the balance of the pituitary-gonadal axis. A reduction in LH activity that could be responsible for the reductions in total and free testosterone associated with prolonged exercise can be expected. However, evidence for altered LH pulsatile release is conflicting. Gonadotropin response to gonadotropin-releasing hormone (GnRH) has been reported both reduced and increased following prolonged, exhaustive exercise.[55]

Endurance training induces changes in the function of the reproductive axis in men in a similar manner to the changes in women. There is a subclinical inhibition of normal reproductive function but it is unclear whether clinical expression of reproductive suppression is common in men. Although measures of sperm function are generally normal in runners with very strenuous training regimens even with very low physiologic androgen levels,[56] there is evidence that males with a high level of physical activity have some abnormalities of semen analysis.[57,58] Libido may also be reduced in some athletes during intense endurance training periods; reduced testosterone levels but also chronic fatigue may play a role.[49,56]

Alterations in circulating β-endorphin levels have been considered responsible for short-term and chronic exercise-associated suppression of the gonadal axis.[59]

Prolactin is a hormone also associated with causing perturbations in the gonadal axis. At either excessively low or high circulating levels, prolactin can result in suppression of testosterone levels in men.[60] It has been speculated that the absence of prolactin at the testicle alters the effectiveness of LH to stimulate testosterone production. This theory is based upon the proposed synergistic effects of prolactin upon testicular LH receptors.[61] However, not all investigators reporting low resting testosterone in endurance-trained men have reported the concomitant existence of low resting prolactin levels.[60]

Some investigations have looked at a potential relationship between high prolactin levels and low testosterone. Hackney and colleagues[62] indicated that elevations in resting prolactin levels occur with endurance training in men and that this change corresponds with low resting testosterone. In this study, however, the testosterone levels did not remain chronically suppressed in response to the exercise training. Serum prolactin levels are chronically depressed rather than elevated and not likely involved in the change in testosterone in highly trained male runners.[61]

Another potential disruptive hormone to the gonadal axis is cortisol. Cumming and colleagues[63] have demonstrated that the direct infusion of cortisol in men results in concurrent declines in testosterone levels. However, in the hormonal profile studies reporting the existence of low testosterone in trained men, none have reported elevated resting cortisol levels.[61,64,65] Thus, at this time, the role of cortisol to the changes found in the gonadal axis of trained men is in need of further study.

Summary

Short, intense exercise usually increases while prolonged exercise usually decreases serum testosterone levels. The exercise-associated increment in circulating testosterone does not seem to be mediated by LH. Possible mechanisms such as hemoconcentration, reduced clearance, and/or increased testosterone synthesis may be involved. A variety of systems could influence the testosterone decrease during and subsequent to more prolonged exercise, including decreased gonadotropins, increased cortisol or catecholamine levels, or even an accumulation of metabolic waste materials. The fall in serum testosterone results from decreased production rates, decreased binding, or increased clearance.

Endurance and other forms of training can induce subclinical inhibition of normal reproductive function. Libido may also be reduced in some athletes during intense endurance training periods, due to reduced testosterone levels and to chronic fatigue.

Female Gonadal Axis

The endocrine equilibrium that regulates reproductive function in women can be affected by physical and psychological factors. Blood levels of hormones depend on a balance between production, metabolism, and clearance rates. Intensive physical exercise may affect this balance via different mechanisms, such as stress associated with competition, dieting, reduction of body fat and body weight, production of heat, or hypoxia. Women who engage in regular high-intensity exercise may be at risk, as a consequence of these hormonal changes, of developing menstrual disturbances such as delayed menarche, oligomenorrhea, and amenorrhea. Impaired production of gonadotropins, which leads to luteal phase deficiency and anovulation, is a common hormonal finding with exercise-induced menstrual disturbances, but several other hormones may show significant alterations.[66]

Many female athletes develop oligomenorrhea, amenorrhea, and luteal phase defects.[67] Although factors such as physical and/or psychological stress of competition have been postulated to underlie the exercise-induced reproductive disorder, evidence accumulated to date indicates that negative energy balance is the primary cause of the impairment of normal reproductive function commonly observed in female athletes.[68-70] In 1980, Warren was the first to suggest that menstrual disorders in dancers are disrupted by an "energy drain."[68] In 1984, Winterer and colleagues[71] hypothesized that lack of sufficient metabolic fuels to meet the energy requirements of the brain causes and alteration in brain function that disrupts the GnRH pulse generator, although the mechanism of this alteration was unknown. The energy availability hypothesis is supported by endocrine observations of athletes. Amenorrheic athletes display low 24-hour blood glucose, low 24-hour insulin, and high 24-hour insulin-like growth factor binding protein 1 (IGFBP-1),[72] loss of the leptin diurnal rhythm,[73] and low T_3 levels in the morning.[74] Loucks and colleagues[69] found that low-energy availability reduced LH pulse frequency and increased LH pulse amplitude, and that exercise stress had no suppressive effect on LH pulsatility beyond the impact of the energy cost of exercise on energy availability. LH pulsatility was disrupted regardless of whether energy availability was reduced by extreme energy restriction alone, by extreme exercise energy expenditure alone, or by a combination of moderate dietary energy restriction and moderate exercise energy expenditure. Dietary supplementation prevented the suppression of LH pulsatility by exercise energy expenditure.

The discovery of leptin in 1994[75] was fundamental in clarifying the relationship between negative energy balance and reproductive dysfunction. Leptin acts as a peripheral signal that gives adequate information to the central nervous system (CNS) about body energy reserves, leading the individual to increase energy intake when fat stores diminish, and vice versa.[76] In reproduction, leptin is implicated in fertility regulation and appears as a permissive factor for puberty. In particular, various sets of data suggest that leptin may serve as a signal to the CNS with information on the critical amount of adipose tissue stores that is necessary for GnRH secretion and pubertal activation of the hypothalamic-pituitary-gonadal axis. Several unfavorable metabolic situations are associated with low plasma leptin, increased secretion of hypothalamic neuropeptide Y (NPY), and hypogonadism, and a causal relationship has been evoked. Severe dietary restriction in juvenile female rats is associated with low plasma leptin and sexual immaturity. Cessation of food restriction leads to immediate increase in plasma leptin followed by sexual maturation.[77] Leptin administration for the relative leptin deficiency in women with hypothalamic amenorrhea improves reproductive, thyroid, and growth hormone axes and markers of bone formation, confirming that leptin is required for normal reproductive and neuroendocrine function.[78,79]

The stress hypothesis holds that exercise activates the hypothalamic-pituitary-adrenal axis, which disrupts the GnRH pulse generator by another unknown mechanism. Both central and peripheral mechanisms may be involved in this dysregulation. Amenorrheic athletes may display mildly elevated cortisol levels[72,80] and this observation is the basis for attributing their amenorrhea to stress. Mild hypercortisolism is also associated with amenorrhea in patients with functional hypothalamic amenorrhea and anorexia nervosa.[81] However, because cortisol is a glucoregulatory hormone activated by low blood glucose levels, the mild hypercortisolism observed in amenorrheic athletes may reflect a chronic energy deficiency rather than exercise stress.[82]

The involvement of endogenous opioid peptides and catecholestrogens in provoking menstrual irregularities in women athletes has also been suggested.[83] In basal circumstances, β-endorphin may decrease LH levels by suppressing hypothalamic GnRH; some catecholestrogens may suppress LH levels, while others seem to potentiate and induce LH surge. Both the activities of β-endorphin and catecholestrogens depend on the essential presence of a sufficiently estrogenic environment. In addition, both endogenous opioid peptides and some of the catecholestrogens appear to be able to suppress prolactin release, probably by interfering with its inhibiting factor dopamine. The increased plasma concentrations of β-endorphin, which are found after physical exercise, give rise to speculations as to their involvement in the frequently appearing menstrual irregularities in women athletes.[83]

Circulating levels of testosterone, dehydroepiandrosterone, dehydroepiandrosterone sulphate, estradiol, growth hormone (GH), and cortisol have been shown to increase in response to an acute bout of endurance exercise in women. However, only GH, estradiol, and cortisol have been reported to increase following resistance exercise.[84]

Hyperandrogenism has been suggested as a possible alternative mechanism underlying oligomenorrhea or amenorrhea in some female athletes with menstrual disturbances.[85] Interestingly, hyperandrogenic female athletes have a more anabolic body composition and higher VO_{2max} and performance values in comparison with female athletes with menstrual disturbances but normal androgen concentrations.[85]

Summary

The endocrine equilibrium that regulates reproductive function in women can be affected by physical and psychological factors. Many female athletes develop oligomenorrhea, amenorrhea, and luteal phase defects. Negative energy balance is the primary cause of the impairment of normal reproductive function commonly observed in female athletes. The link between negative energy balance and reproductive dysfunction is represented by leptin, which serves as a signal to the CNS with information on the critical amount of adipose tissue stores that is necessary for GnRH secretion and pubertal activation of the hypothalamic-pituitary-gonadal axis. Possible alternative mechanisms underlying oligomenorrhea or amenorrhea in some female athletes include the stress-induced activation of the hypothalamic-pituitary-adrenal axis, endogenous opioid peptides, catecholestrogens, and hyperandrogenism.

Prolactin

Elevated prolactin levels are associated with causing perturbations in the gonadal axis function both in males and in females.[60] PRL levels increase with exercise in sedentary control subjects and in recreational and competitive runners, and this response appears proportional to the exercise intensity.[2,60] However, exercise-induced PRL increases are rather transitory in nature and last only a few hours into the recovery from activity. The effect of training appears negligible, in that equivalent exercise loads produce generally similar serum PRL increases in trained and untrained individuals.[2,86] However, Hackney and colleagues[87] have demonstrated that an endurance exercise training session results in a greatly enhanced nocturnal rise in the PRL levels of trained men during sleep. Yet, no direct relationship was found to exist between the changes in nighttime PRL and testosterone responses as brought about by the daytime endurance-exercise session.

The mechanisms of PRL increase with exercise are unclear. PRL levels may increase when the anaerobic threshold is reached, perhaps concomitantly with a GH increase.[88] Even prolonged (90 minutes) exercise below this threshold fails to elicit any response.[89] PRL increments with exercise appear to be correlated with levels of pro-opiomelanocortin derivatives, ACTH, and β-endorphins.[18] Moreover, the PRL increase may be related to changes in body temperature and dehydration, is exaggerated by stress, is reduced with habituation and hypoxia, and is unresponsive to metabolic events.[2]

Some studies[61,65] indicate that trained men who exhibit lower testosterone levels also seem to have low resting PRL levels, in that the absence of PRL at the testicle may alter the effectiveness of LH to stimulate testosterone production. On the other hand, some investigations have focused on the potential relationship between high PRL levels and low testosterone. Only one study has indicated that elevations in resting PRL levels occur with endurance training in men and the change corresponded with low resting testosterone.[62] In this study, however, the testosterone levels did not remain chronically suppressed in response to the exercise training. Interestingly, a study by Hackney and colleagues[64] showed that the metoclopramide-stimulated release of PRL from the pituitary of endurance-trained men (i.e., with low resting testosterone) is greater than that in sedentary men.

Summary

Prolactin levels transiently increase with exercise, and this response is proportional to the exercise intensity. PRL increments occur when the anaerobic threshold is reached and appear to be correlated with levels of pro-opiomelanocortin derivatives, ACTH, and β-endorphins. Moreover, the PRL increase may be related to changes in body temperature and dehydration, is exaggerated by stress, is reduced with habituation and hypoxia, and is unresponsive to metabolic events.

GH/IGF-I Axis

Physical exercise is an important environmental regulator of the GH/IGF-I axis activity. It was first shown by Roth and colleagues[90] that exercise increases circulating GH levels. This observation was among the earliest identified endocrine responses to exercise, and this effect has been used clinically to examine GH release, particularly in children.[2] GH response to strenuous exercise is low in GH-deficient children, although even well-controlled strenuous exercise fails to release GH in one third of children who have a response to other stimuli. The GH response to exercise is dependent on the duration and intensity of the exercise bout, the fitness level of the exercising subject, the refractoriness of pituitary somatotroph cells to the exercise stimuli, and other environmental factors.[91,92] Lactate and nitric oxide are suggested to be afferent stimulation for the exercise-induced GH response.[93]

Several investigators have demonstrated that circulating GH levels increase only when the lactic/anaerobic threshold (LAT) is reached lactic/anaerobic threshold (LAT).[91] Other reports demonstrate that loads of 75% to 90% of maximal aerobic power yielded a greater GH rise than milder loads.[94] Thus, considering the GH response to exercise at a fixed work rate would lead to the conclusion that fitter subjects have smaller rather than larger GH responses.

Given the influence of intensity of exercise, few studies investigate the effect of duration of exercise on the GH response, with longer duration exercise increasing the GH response.[95] The exercise duration should be at least 10 minutes,[96] because exercise of shorter duration both below and above the lactate threshold was not accompanied by increases in circulating GH levels.[91] Exercise-induced GH peak occurs 25 to 30 minutes after the start of exercise, regardless of the exercise duration.[91,97] Thus, when the task is brief, a peak may be reached after its cessation, but when the task is long (e.g., 45 minutes), the GH peak occurs while the individual is still exercising.[92,98]

The interaction of duration and intensity of exercise also influences GH responses to endurance type exercise. Short-duration, high-intensity exertion (7 minutes of rowing races for Olympic athletes) has been shown to provoke remarkable GH responses.[99]

The nature of the exercise may also influence the GH response. While the continuous exercise protocols may be comparable to competition events, the endurance-type training undertaken by many athletes involves intermittent or interval exertion. Comparing exercise at equivalent total workloads, GH levels are lower with continuous (40% to 45% VO_{2max}) as opposed to interval protocols with twice the work rate for half the time reflecting the greater metabolic stress and lactate levels in the latter.[100] With resistance exercise, incremental GH responses have also been described.[101] The important determinants appear to be the relationship between load and frequency of individual repetitions. Greater GH increments have been reported following "hypertrophy" protocols (moderate loads, high number of repetitions) than "strength" protocols (heavy loads, low repetitions) in both men and women.[95]

There is conflicting evidence regarding the neuroendocrine pathways that regulate GH secretion during exercise. Mechanisms involving cholinergic, serotoninergic, α-adrenergic, dopaminergic, and opioidergic pathways have been proposed.[2,102,103] There may be interactions among the pathways and they may operate at different exercise intensities. In young males, regular but not acute exercise is associated with higher growth hormone production and also augments GH stimulation of GH release by growth hormone–releasing hormone.[104] It has been hypothesized that this is due to decreased hypothalamic somatostatinergic activity and higher growth hormone pulsatility.

Fluid intake influences exercise-induced GH release. The increased rate of sweating during physical activity performed without water ingestion results in dehydration and lower GH response to exercise.[105]

Environmental and nutritional factors as well as some pathologic states may interfere with GH response to exercise. Cappon and colleagues[106] showed that a high-fat meal could inhibit the magnitude of GH response to exercise, the inhibition of the exercise-induced GH response being correlated with circulating levels of somatostatin. High ambient temperature may in itself increase circulating GH levels,[107] whereas low temperature attenuates GH release.[108] Obesity and/or polycystic ovarian syndrome are characterized by attenuated GH response to exercise.[109]

Gender governs the relationship between exercise intensity and GH release, because for each incremental increase in exercise intensity, the fractional stimulation of GH secretion is greater in women than in men. Moreover, women have greater basal (nonpulsatile) GH secretion across all conditions, more frequent GH secretory pulses, a greater GH secretory pulse amplitude, a greater production rate, and a trend for a greater mass of GH secreted per pulse than men.[110] The more intense GH secretion in women is related to estrogens. Both oral and transdermal estrogen administration increase GH release in postmenopausal women,[111] and young females under oral contraceptive therapy exhibit greater GH responses to exercise than nontreated women.[112]

The acute GH response to aerobic or resistance exercise is reduced with age.[103] Basal and exercise-stimulated plasma IGF-I levels are higher in physically conditioned versus sedentary young men. Because of the general decline in physical activity with advancing age, a decrease in aerobic capacity may contribute to diminished serum IGF-I levels in elderly persons.

Kelley and colleagues[113] found a significant positive correlation between VO_{2max} and both circulating GH and IGF-I levels in healthy premenopausal and postmenopausal females. They found that both VO_{2max} and IGF-I concentrations decline with age. However, when the influence of both age and fitness was analyzed using multiple regression, VO_{2max} remained the only independent predictor of IGF-I concentrations. Therefore, they concluded that the decrease in serum IGF-I with age is not related to aging per se, but probably to age-related decline in physical activity and fitness.

The effect of exercise on circulating IGF-I has been examined by several investigators with differing results. Wilson and Horowitz[114] reported no increase in serum IGF-I in children after 15 minutes of cycle ergometer exercise protocol. Hagberg and colleagues[115] did not find an increase in IGF-I after 60 minutes of treadmill exercise at 70% of the subjects's VO_{2max} in young and old adults. Moreover, the effect of exercise on IGF-I appears to depend on the type of the exercise performed.[92] Schwarz and coworkers[116] demonstrated IGF-I increases following 10 minutes of exercise at both less than and greater than LAT. This study suggests that the increase in IGF-I accompanying exercise is not related to GH.

The transient nature of IGF increases suggests that hemodynamic or metabolic effects of exercise per se might play a role. Exercise in humans is accompanied by the rapid "hemotransfusion" of hemoconcentrated blood from the spleen into the circulation by increased blood flow to the exercising muscle and by loss of plasma water. These phenomena might explain, at least in part, an increased IGF concentration by changes in IGF flux and/or volume of distribution.

Longer periods of exercise training, however, are able to stimulate IGF-I gene expression both in the central neuroendocrine and local tissue components of the GH/IGF-I system. Zanconato and colleagues[117] found that by 4 weeks of endurance training in young rats, hepatic and muscle IGF-I gene expression as well as muscle IGF-I protein were increased. Eliakim and colleagues[118] showed that muscle IGF-I protein concentrations in rats can increase with endurance training, despite the lack of change in muscle IGF-I mRNA or serum IGF-I.

Few studies have investigated the response of IGF binding proteins (IGFBPs) to exercise. IGFBP-1 levels have been shown not to change during 30 minutes of moderate exercise,[95] but to increase transiently after acute exercise.[119] The physiologic role of the postexercise increase in IGFBP-1, given IGFBP-1 inhibition of IGF-I metabolic actions, may be to prevent late hypoglycemia.[119]

Schwarz and colleagues[116] have demonstrated that IGFBP-3 levels increased with both low- and high-intensity exercise and that high-intensity exercise increased IGFBP-3 proteolysis. A transient increase in IGFBP-3 levels in response to an acute exercise has been confirmed also by Wallace and colleagues[119] who described an acute increase of all components of the ternary complex, IGF-I, IGFBP-3, and acid labile subunit (ALS).

Eliakim and colleagues[120] have described that functional and structural indices of fitness were correlated with mean overnight GH levels, growth hormone binding protein (GHBP), and serum IGF-I levels in late pubertal adolescent girls. Moreover, thigh muscle volume was inversely correlated with IGFBP-2 and IGFBP-4.

The acute increase in serum GHBP in response to acute exercise has been described also by Wallace and colleagues[119]; because GHBP at rest acts as a damper on GH oscillation, these authors speculate that the postexercise GHBP increase may prolong the GH signal, increasing the GH-mediated signal for postexercise protein synthesis, tissue repair, and muscle glycogen replenishment. The increment in the serum GHBP concentration may represent either increased synthesis from the liver or reduced clearance.[119]

Summary

Physical exercise is an important environmental regulator of the GH/IGF-I axis activity. The GH response to exercise is dependent on the duration and intensity of the exercise bout, the fitness level of the exercising subject, the refractoriness of pituitary somatotroph cells to the exercise stimuli, and other environmental factors. The neuroendocrine pathways that regulate GH secretion during exercise include the cholinergic, serotoninergic, α-adrenergic, dopaminergic, and opioidergic systems. The exercise-induced GH release is influenced by fluid intake, environmental and nutritional factors, as well as some pathologic states. Gender governs the relationship between exercise intensity and GH release, in that GH secretion is greater in women than in men. The acute GH response to aerobic or resistance exercise is reduced with age.

Exercise leads to increases in IGF-I levels, which are likely to occur via GH-independent mechanisms. Hemodynamic or metabolic effects of exercise per se might play a role, although long periods of exercise training are able to stimulate IGF-I gene expression.

Hypothalamus-Pituitary-Thyroid Axis

Exercise has effects on thyroid function, either secondary to acute alterations in the integrity of the pituitary-thyroid axis or to more long-lasting changes noted in well-trained athletes. Alterations in thyroid function in athletes can be viewed as an adaptive mechanism associated with enhanced performance, possibly serving to provide a better balance between energy consumption and expenditure.

In at least one study, TSH was noted to rise just in anticipation of strenuous exercise, although the response disappeared with repetitive testing, suggesting the implication of a psychological influence on the TSH rise.[121] Sawhney and colleagues[122] showed a drop in T_4 and T_3 levels at 20 and 40 minutes postexercise in healthy men undergoing bicycle ergometry for 20 minutes. A free T_4 increase of 25% was seen postexercise.[123] A progressive rise in TSH levels was observed both during short-duration graded exercise with increasing workload and with prolonged exercise.[124] Comparing the effects of submaximal and maximal exercise on thyroid hormone levels, Schmid and colleagues[125] showed a decrease in TSH, FT_4, stable rT_3 and a rise in T_3 during maximal exercise, and an increase in TSH but unchanged levels of T_3, rT_3, and fT_4 in submaximal exercise.

Semple and colleagues[126] found no change in TSH, T_4, T_3, or rT_3 levels in marathon runners before and after the marathon. However, a prolonged increase in TSH and free T4 postmarathon, with a decrease in fT_3 and a rise in T_4 to free r T_3 conversion was shown by Sander and Rocker.[127] A significant increase in T_4, fT_4 and fT_3 with no change in TSH and T_3 concentrations has been described in professional cyclists during a 3-week stage competition.[128]

The training level has been shown to influence the thyroid hormone response to acute exercise in athletes. An increase in rT_3 in well-trained athletes has been observed and explained as an adaptive mechanism expressing a more efficient cellular oxidation process.[129]

Variations in ambient temperature appear to alter the thyroid hormone response to exercise. TSH and fT_4 levels rose in swimmers exercising in cold water (22° C), were unchanged at 26° C, and fell at warm (32° C) water temperature.[130]

The chronic effects on thyroid hormone parameters have also been studied in endurance athletes, with conflicting results with regard to whether or not baseline hormonal levels are shifted in well-trained athletes. Regular bicycle ergometry training in recreational athletes over 6 weeks did not change TSH or TSH response to TRH stimulation.[131]

Energy balance plays a role in the body thyroid hormone response to exercise. Loucks and colleagues[132] found a decrease in T_3 and fT_3 along with an increase in rT_3 in healthy women undergoing aerobic exercise testing with low caloric intake. This "low T_3 syndrome" was not seen in individuals receiving a higher caloric diet. Even mild energy deficiencies may influence thyroid hormone levels. Female gymnasts with borderline energy deficit had a decrease in T_3 and increase in T_4 during 3 days of heavy workouts.[133] Energy balance in women runners has also been investigated. Subjects with negative energy balance had a decrease in T_3 and fT_3, but an increase in rT_3.[132]

Summary

The thyroid function changes secondary to physical exercise represent a complex physiologic response, which is influenced by several individual and environmental factors. One of the more consistent findings is rT_3 increase, particularly when a caloric energy deficiency is associated with exercise. TSH, T_4, fT_4, T_3, and fT_3 levels have been reported to be unaffected, increased, or decreased, varying with the type and duration of exercise, ambient temperature, and energy intake.

Insulin and Glucose Metabolism

Physical activity affects the metabolism of glucose and other intermediate substrates in normal subjects and in subjects with diabetes mellitus.[134] The effects of exercise on carbohydrate metabolism are complex and involve type, intensity, and duration of exercise, changes in body composition, alterations in other behaviors, such as food intake, degree of insulin deficiency, and a complex time-course of the glucose-insulin response.[135]

During moderate exercise, insulin levels remain unchanged over the first 40 to 60 minutes of exercise. More prolonged or strenuous exercise induces a decline in insulin levels.[136] Counterregulatory hormones, catecholamines, glucagon, GH, and cortisol tend to increase, inducing hepatic glycogenolysis, gluconeogenesis, and lipolysis to provide increased FFA for use as a metabolic fuel. During short-term strenuous exercise, when the counterregulatory hormones rise, glucose levels may transiently increase. After exercise, insulin levels may rapidly return to baseline.

Glucose uptake by exercising muscles is remarkably increased, due to an increase in blood flow to the muscle during activity, an increase in the number of insulin receptors, and an increase in the number and intrinsic activity of glucose transporter proteins present in plasma membrane of skeletal muscle.[137] The muscle glucose uptake, which is not directly mediated by insulin, requires the presence of at least basal insulin levels.[138] Increased insulin availability above basal levels has little effect on glucose transport, and the supply of glucose to the muscle is maintained during exercise despite decreased insulin levels.

Insulin also plays a role in controlling the sensitivity of hepatic glucose production.[139] Both insulin and glucose changes are needed for optimal activity to occur.[2] Glucagon levels increase during strenuous exercise, while the response is variable at lesser intensities.[2] During prolonged mild-intensity exercise in healthy subjects, the rise in glucagon is essential for the increase in hepatic glucose production and the increase in gluconeogenesis.[140] Decreasing blood glucose levels stimulate glucagon, and the glucagon response is generally blunted by preloading with glucose. Levels of glucagon usually correspond significantly with epinephrine and norepinephrine levels, although the sympathoadrenal system seems more important in maintaining euglycemia and enhanced hepatic production of glucose.[141]

In normal individuals, no major alterations in blood glucose levels are usually seen during exercise, despite the increase in glucose utilization by skeletal muscle. With the onset of activity, activation of the α-adrenergic system results in inhibition of insulin release from the pancreas. This results in an increased rate of lipolysis in the periphery as well as a stimulation of hepatic glucose output. As glucose levels begin to fall, glucagon levels rise, further stimulating hepatic glucose output. Finally, as plasma glucose drops toward hypoglycemic levels, epinephrine is released, further stimulating hepatic glucose production and increasing lipolysis in the periphery. The increased availability of FFA for muscle metabolism helps restrain the rate of glucose utilization. It has been shown that when one of these mechanisms fails, the others can largely compensate, preventing hypoglycemia from developing.[135]

Training induces a reduction in basal insulin levels and in the exercise-associated changes in glucagon and insulin, increases insulin sensitivity at rest and in response to a glucose load, and reduces insulin decline during acute exercise.[2,142]

Regular exercise has become an integral part of the treatment recommendations for type 2 diabetes patients, because it improves insulin sensitivity and reduces average blood glucose concentrations.[143] Physical training results in an increase in insulin-stimulated glucose disposal and improves glucose control in type 2 diabetes. However, the increase in insulin sensitivity is rapidly lost if exercise is not performed on a regular basis. Exercise may also be effective in delaying or preventing the development of type 2 diabetes.[143]

Summary

Physical activity affects the metabolism of glucose and other intermediate substrates in normal subjects and in subjects with diabetes mellitus. The effects of exercise on carbohydrate metabolism are complex and involve type, intensity, and duration of exercise, changes in body composition, alterations in other behaviors, such as food intake, degree of insulin deficiency, and a complex time-course of the glucose-insulin response.

PERFORMANCE-ENHANCING (AB)USE OF HORMONES

Anabolic Steroids

Anabolic-androgenic steroids (AASs) are chemically modified analogues of testosterone. First isolated in 1935, AASs have been modified many times to maximize the anabolic effects of the drug and to minimize the androgenic effects by alkylation of the 17α position or carboxylation of the 17β hydroxyl group on the sterol D ring. These analogues are degraded much more slowly than endogenous testosterone is, resulting in a higher prolonged concentration of the analogue.[144,145] The AASs used for nontherapeutic purposes are (1) endogenous androgens (e.g., androstenedione, DHEA); (2) 17β-esters of testosterone (e.g., cypionate, enanthate, heptylate, propionate, undecanoate, bucyclate); (3) 17α-alkyl derivatives of testosterone (e.g., methyltestosterone, fluoxymesterone, oxandrolone, stanozol); (4) 19-nortestosterone (nandrolone); (5) 17β-esters of 19-nortestosterone (e.g., decanoate, phenpropionate); (6) 19-norandrostenedione and 19-norandrostenediol; tetrahydrogestrinone. More than 100 different AASs have been developed, with most of them being used illegally, synthesized in clandestine laboratories, commercialized without medical prescription or safety controls, and sometimes unknown to the scientific world (Table 25–1).[145]

AASs have been used in sport for more than 50 years. Although their use is most common among weight lifters and heavy throwers, almost all types of athletes whose event requires explosive strength, including football players, swimmers, and track and field athletes, have been known to use steroids. Steroid hormones or synthetic analogues of steroid hormones promote both tissue growth and masculinization; the androgenic compounds are widely used to enhance lean body mass and to improve sport performance. The anabolic-androgenic activity of each steroid compound is a function of its chemical structure and/or metabolites, and its activity can vary considerably. These drugs may act by binding with androgen and glucocorticoid receptors, by exerting central and peripheral effects on neurotransmitters, and by interacting with IGF-I or its binding proteins in the circulation and/or in the muscles.[145]

TABLE 25–1 PERFORMANCE-ENHANCING HORMONES

Anabolic Androgenic Steroids
17β-ESTERS OF TESTOSTERONE
Cypionate, enanthate, heptylate, propionate, undecanoate, bucylate
17α-ALKYL DERIVATIVES OF TESTOSTERONE
Methyltestosterone Fluoxymesterone Oxandrolone Stanozolol 19-Nortestosterone (nandrolone) 17β-esters of 19-nortestosterone Decanoate, phenpropionate 19-Norandrostenedione 19-Norandrostenediol Tetrahydrogestrinone
PEPTIDE HORMONES
GH IGF-I Insulin Erythropoietin

In 1991, data from the National Household Survey on Drug Abuse indicated that there were more than 1 million AAS users in the United States and that the lifetime use was 0.9% for males and 0.1% for females.[146] Current estimates indicate that there are as many as 3 million AAS users in the United States and that 2.7% to 2.9% of young American adults have taken an AAS at least once in their lives.[147] Surveys in the field indicate that AAS use among community weight trainers attending gyms and health clubs is 15% to 30%.[148] Two thirds of AAS users are noncompetitive recreational body builders or nonathletes who use these drugs for cosmetic purposes rather than to enhance sports performance.[145,148]

During the past decade, careful scientific study of suprapharmacologic doses supports the anabolic efficacy of these AAS regimens. Furthermore, recent years have seen an increasing interest in the medical use of AAS for the treatment of hypogonadal men, age-related sarcopenia, and HIV-related muscle wasting.[148]

The positive effects of steroids on body composition include increased fat-free mass, decreased total body fat, and a decrease in the percentage of body fat located in the gluteal, femoral, and triceps regions in women.[149] The effects of anabolic steroids on lipolysis and skeletal muscle mass are potentiated by caloric restriction[149] and mechanical loading.[150]

Skeletal muscle is a primary target tissue for the anabolic effects of AAS. The action of AAS in stimulating growth of skeletal muscles in subjects with low circulating testosterone, such as women and children, is undisputed. However, an early and comprehensive review of previous results concluded that there was little evidence for supraphysiologic doses of testosterone or synthetic AAS having any appreciable effect on muscle size or strength in healthy men.[151]

More recent reviews suggest that the administration of AAS can consistently result in significant increases in strength if male athletes satisfy certain criteria, including the timing of doses and dietary factors.[152,153] Bhasin and colleagues[150] demonstrated that the administration of supraphysiologic doses of testosterone in combination with exercise in male weight lifters induces a greater increase in muscle size and strength compared with exercise alone or testosterone treatment alone, that is, the effects of combining supraphysiologic doses of testosterone with exercise are additive. Subsequent work showed that increases in fat-free mass, muscle size, strength, and power are highly dose-dependent and correlated with serum testosterone concentrations.[154]

The anabolic effect of testosterone is dose dependent, and significant increases in muscle size and strength occur only with doses of 300 mg per week and higher.[154,155] The increase in muscle size is due to a hypertrophy that results from an increase in cross-sectional areas of both type I and type II muscle fibers and from an increase in myonuclear number.[155]

In postmenopausal women undergoing caloric restriction, administration of 30 mg of nandrolone decanoate every 2 weeks for 9 months increased fat-free mass, decreased body fat, redistributed abdominal body fat from subcutaneous to visceral stores, and increased thigh muscle cross-sectional area in comparison with a control group.[149] Evidence of the effects of anabolic steroids on body fat distribution in young adult females has been accumulated in studies of women undergoing gender reassignment and women athletes. Women ingesting high doses of androgens experience a shift of body fat from a gynoid to an android distribution and a decrease of subcutaneous body fat in the abdomen, hip and thigh regions.[156] In contrast, postmenopausal women treated with estrogens maintain a gynoid fat pattern, suggesting that fat distribution patterns are controlled by the ratio of circulating estrogens to androgens.

Investigations into the performance-enhancing effects of anabolic steroids began in the late 1960s and continued into the early 1980s. Some studies demonstrated a positive effect of steroids on strength when drug abuse was combined with resistance training, whereas others did not. Since 1994, a few studies have documented the performance-enhancing effects of anabolic steroids in athletes and healthy men.[150,157] However, several issues remain unresolved regarding the use of AAS for athletic enhancement. In fact, it is unknown what minimal doses of a steroid or combination of steroids are necessary to produce significant increases in strength and muscle mass in healthy, resistance-trained men and women. Moreover, the belief that several different anabolic steroids used concurrently will elicit a significantly greater anabolic effect than any single drug has not been evaluated in controlled studies. Finally, it has been speculated that gains in lean mass and strength acquired while using steroids are maintained indefinitely following cessation of drug treatment.[145]

AASs have also been shown to improve exercise tolerance and the adaptability of muscle to overload by protecting against muscle fiber damage and increasing the rate of protein synthesis during recovery.[158]

The types and doses of AAS used by athletes are not easy to define because it is difficult to obtain accurate drug-use information from athletes. In a survey conducted in Great Britain, the majority of male anabolic steroid users reported that testosterone or nandrolone esters were the drugs of choice, whereas women preferred oxandrolone, stanozolol, and methandienone.[159] Testing by International Olympic Committee laboratories in 1993 revealed that the most commonly detected steroids were testosterone (32.5%), nandrolone (23.9%), stanozolol (11.4%), metandienone (10.7%), and methenolone preparations (7.7%).[160] A recent study suggested that the drugs methyltestosterone and norethandrolone were those most commonly used by athletes.[161]

The dose of AAS used by athletes varies considerably and is often thought to exceed 10 to 40 times the recommended therapeutic dose.[161] In a survey of 100 male AAS users, the drug dosages ranged from 250 mg to 3200 mg per week of testosterone or its equivalent.[162] Fifty percent of the AAS users in this sample reported using a weekly dose of at least 500 mg. To achieve these supraphysiologic doses, 88% of AAS users in this sample combined two or more different types of AAS—a process known as *stacking*.

In most surveys, the duration of steroid administration or steroid cycle lasts between 4 and 12 weeks.[148] The time interval between steroid cycles is more variable. Regular users allow a 4- to 6-week drug holiday, whereas less frequent users may remain drug free for months.[148] In one survey, approximately half of the sample reported that their total annual AAS use was less than 6 months, whereas the other half used AAS for more than 6 months each year.[162] Three of the 100 AAS users surveyed admitted to continuously use steroids for 52 weeks of the year.

The side effects associated with AAS use are numerous and involve multiple organ systems.[145,163] With the exception of the association between hepatic dysfunction and the use of some oral AASs,[164] many of the reports of serious side effects in otherwise healthy individuals have come from anecdotal case studies.[165] Confounding factors, such as undiagnosed preexisting conditions, family history, and concurrent use of other drugs, further dampen the credibility of case reports. Moreover, because most anabolic steroids are obtained on the black market and are of dubious quality, there is potential for adverse medical events to occur independent of steroid use. However, data from larger observational studies[162,166] suggest that the majority (88% to 96%) of AAS users experience at least one minor subjective side effect, including acne (40% to 54%), testicular atrophy (40% to 51%), gynecomastia (10% to 34%), cutaneous striae (34%), and injection site pain (36%) (Table 25–2).

Dyslipidemia and cardiovascular disease have been reported to be linked with the use of AAS. In general, the ingestion of

TABLE 25–2 SIDE EFFECTS OF ANABOLIC ANDROGENIC STEROIDS

CARDIOVASCULAR
Cardiomyopathy Lipid disorders (decreased high-density lipoprotein, increased low-density lipoprotein) Increased platelet aggregation Increased hematocrit Elevated blood pressure
COSMETIC
Gynecomastia Acne Hair loss Cutaneous striae
REPRODUCTIVE-ENDOCRINE
Libido changes Subfertility *In males* Testicular atrophy Impaired spermatogenesis Erectile dysfunction Prostate diseases *In females* Hirsutism Breast atrophy Voice deepening Virilization (clitoromegaly) Menstrual disturbances
HEPATIC
Cholestasis Steatosis Tumors Hepatocellular adenoma and carcinoma Hepatic angiosarcoma and cholangiocarcinoma
PSYCHOLOGICAL
Aggression Mood swings Anxiety Psychosis Irritability Dependence Withdrawal Depression
INJECTION RELATED
Infection Bruising Fibrosis Injection site pain

oral C-17 α-alkylated anabolic steroids causes an average 30% decrease in high-density lipoprotein (HDL) and an average 30% increase in low-density lipoprotein (LDL).[167] The mechanisms for this effect are unknown, but apparently include an increase in the activity of hepatic triglyceride lipase that catabolizes HDL particles. Most studies indicate that injectable non–C-17 α-alkylated anabolic steroids, such as testosterone and nandrolone esters, exert minimal adverse effects on blood lipids.[150,167] Anabolic-androgenic steroids may also influence platelet aggregation and the myocardium, although the relationship between these effects and cardiovascular disease is unclear.[168] Occasional reports of cardiomyopathies and arrhythmias associated with steroid use have been published, and several mechanisms have been proposed.[168] It is unclear if the adverse changes in blood lipids as a function of testosterone use actually lead to an increase in the incidence of coronary artery disease.

Liver disease is a well-documented side effect of most, but not all, C-17 α-alkylated anabolic-androgenic steroids, the exception being oxandrolone. In contrast, most non–C-17 α-alkylated steroids exert minimal hepatotoxicity. Liver pathologies associated with anabolic steroids include cholestasis, peliosis hepatis, hepatocellular adenoma and carcinoma, and hepatic angiosarcoma and cholangiocarcinoma.[148,164]

Potential effects on the reproductive system include infertility and testicular atrophy in men and menstrual and genital tract alterations in women.[148] Although all AASs suppress the hypothalamic-pituitary axis to some extent, the resulting infertility in males is generally reversible. Benign prostatic hyperplasia and prostate cancer are also possible side effects of anabolic steroid use, but this has been reported only once in otherwise healthy steroid users.[169] The effects on the prostate likely depend on the chemical structure and androgenicity of the drugs.

The effects of AAS use on fertility in women is unknown. High doses of androgens decrease circulating FSH and sex hormone binding globulin (SHBG) concentrations in eugonadal women,[170] whereas no changes are observed in mean nadir and LH pulse amplitude and in circulating concentrations of estradiol, estrone, and adrenal steroids.[171] Menstruation is either diminished or absent in steroid users, but ovulation may occur.[172]

All anabolic-androgenic steroids may cause some degree of acne if taken in a high enough dose.[169] This is particularly true with strong androgen preparations, which may cause severe scarring acne.

With the exception of oxandrolone and perhaps of methenolone, if used intermittently in modest doses, most women will experience some form of permanent virilization by use of anabolic steroids. The degree of virilization depends on the drug, the dose, the duration of use, and the individual response. Body composition changes during steroid use are similar to those experienced in young boys during puberty. In addition to irreversible side effects, such as deepened voice, increased terminal facial hair, and a hypertrophied clitoris, some of the hypertrophic effects of anabolic steroids on skeletal muscle in women may be permanent.

Balding is common in those who use AAS that undergo 5α reduction to potent androgens.

In some male steroid users, gynecomastia may be caused by increased circulating estrogen associated with the use of aromatizable androgens and/or hCG, with decreased clearance of circulating estrogens as a result of impaired hepatic function, and/or with a temporary state of hypotestosteronemia following anabolic-androgenic steroid withdrawal.[148]

Ruptured tendons have been associated with AAS use on the basis of a small number of published case reports, and it has been suggested that these drugs predispose to tendon rupture by altering collagen structure.[173] It is possible that the rapid strength adaptations produced by AAS in skeletal muscle are not simultaneously matched by slower adapting, less vascular tendon structures, making tendons the weakest link in the chain.[174]

Several studies have suggested that anabolic steroid use may lead to significant psychological morbidity. Psychological pathologies associated with anabolic steroids include anxiety, psychosis, irritability, increased aggression, and antisocial and violent behavior.[175] In addition to behavioral problems, dependence, withdrawal symptoms, and depression have been reported with and following the nonmedical use of anabolic steroids.[162,176]

All known AASs can be detected via urinalysis (gas chromatography–mass spectrometry) for a period of time following the last dose.[177,178] The detection of these drugs depends on several factors, including their chemical structures, metabolism, the form in which they were administered, pattern of dosing, and concomitant use of other drugs. The assessment of illegal testosterone use is based on the urinary ratio of testosterone to epitestosterone, with a ratio of six being the upper legal cutoff limit. Because testosterone is not readily converted to epitestosterone, exogenous use of testosterone will increase this ratio. Some athletes inject epitestosterone before drug testing in an effort to mask exogenous testosterone use. To counteract this strategy, urine epitestosterone concentrations above 200 ng/mL are considered proof of epitestosterone manipulation. Furthermore, short-lasting forms of testosterone can raise serum testosterone for only a few hours, after which the testosterone-to-epitestosterone ratio may return rapidly to baseline. Detection of testosterone use represents a significant challenge for doping control laboratories.

Summary

AASs are chemically modified analogues of testosterone that act by binding with androgen and glucocorticoid receptors, by exerting central and peripheral effects on neurotransmitters, and by interacting with IGF-I or its binding proteins in the circulation and/or in the muscles. Skeletal muscle is a primary target tissue for the anabolic effects of AAS. The anabolic effect of testosterone is dose dependent, and significant increases in muscle size and strength occur only with supraphysiologic doses. The dose of AAS used by athletes varies considerably and is often thought to exceed 10 to 40 times the recommended therapeutic dose. The side effects associated with AAS use are numerous and involve multiple organ systems. They include acne, testicular atrophy, infertility, gynecomastia, cutaneous striae, dyslipidemia, cardiovascular disease, liver disease, menstrual alterations, and various degrees of virilization in women, and psychological pathologies.

Growth Hormone

GH has been used as a drug of abuse in sport since the early 1980s, although the first scientific studies demonstrating a clear cut physiologic role for GH in adults was only published in the peer-reviewed medical literature in 1989.[179,180] There are currently no proper scientific studies providing GH to be performance enhancing in normal subjects, but GH has been shown to have a very important role in regulating body composition in adult humans and in other species. In cattle, GH is known as a "partitioning agent": it specifically diverts calories in food toward protein synthesis and away from fat synthesis. Animals made transgenic for GH have greatly increased lean tissues and reduced fat. Similar changes in body composition are seen in humans with acromegaly. On the other hand, GH-deficient (GHD) adults have reduced lean body mass and increased fat mass, especially at the abdominal level. Physiologic replacement therapy with recombinant GH (rhGH) in GHD adults results in significant changes in body composition with, on average, a 5-kg increase in lean body mass within the first month and a comparable loss of 5 kg of fat.[180]

Adults with GHD show significantly reduced muscle mass, strength, and exercise performance.[181] Furthermore, the discontinuation of GH supplementation in patients with GHD leads to a reduction in isometric muscle strength and muscle size by 5% after 1 year.[182]

There is a lack of general agreement whether GH replacement improves physical performance in GHD patients. In fact, exercise capacity is reported to increase in some[179,183] but not all placebo-controlled trials conducted in hypopituitary adult patients.[184] Moreover, GH replacement therapy in GHD patients has been shown to increase lean body mass but not aerobic capacity.[185] The mechanisms through which GH acts on exercise performance are more complex than the simple increase in lean body mass. For instance, GH stimulates erythropoiesis under various conditions[186] and exerts significant cardiovascular effects, increasing plasma volume and peripheral blood flow and enhancing left ventricular stroke volume and cardiac output.[187,188] All these factors may well contribute to improve aerobic capacity. Evidence suggests that GH therapy alone, in the absence of some form of exercise program, may increase the lean body mass but not its functional capacity, thus indicating that training may have to be combined with GH replacement in these patients to increase physical performance.[185]

The only controlled studies on the effects of GH on muscle function in experienced weight lifters or power athletes have not been able to show a significant positive effect of GH on muscular protein biosynthesis or strength.[189-191] Only one study has demonstrated an increase in fat-free mass and a decrease in fat mass in healthy men and women undergoing intensive exercise.[192] Two recent studies in obese men[193] and women[194] found that GH treatment augmented fat loss in conjunction with dietary restriction and/or exercise.

Moreover, Lange and colleagues[195] have demonstrated that rhGH combined with endurance training in healthy elderly women increases muscle oxidative enzymes activity in comparison to exercise alone. GH administration for 3 to 6 months in healthy elderly individuals increased IGF-I levels to those observed in younger control individuals, while muscle mass, skin thickness, and bone mineral content significantly increased and fat mass decreased.[196] Physiologic doses of GH given for 6 months to healthy older men with well-preserved functional abilities have been shown able to improve body composition, increasing lean tissue mass and decreasing fat mass. However, functional ability was not improved, while frequent side effects were reported.[197]

Two different strategies have been proposed to detect GH doping in sports. For the marker method "pharmacodynamical endpoints of GH-use," the consortium GH 2000 identified biochemical parameters of the IGF-system such as IGF-I, IGFBP-3, and the acid labile subunit (ALS) as suitable markers of GH use in combination with procollagen cleavage products that also show a clear-cut increase following GH use. The combination of IGFBP-3 and the procollagen III N-terminal extension peptide (PIIIP)[198] is proposed to provide a set of markers that allow the detection of GH abuse in athletes for up to 2 weeks after the last injection. During the initial phase of GH application, however, these pharmacodynamic markers are not expected to indicate the GH abuse by athletes. The "GH-isoform method"[199] exploits the difference in isoform composition between recombinant growth hormone consisting mostly of monomeric 22 kd hGH while the pituitary secrets a variety of GH isoforms including a 20-kd form lacking 14 amino acids as well as amidated and acylated isoforms. After peripheral injection of recombinant 22 kDa hGH, the pituitary's production of GH isoforms is reduced by negative feedback via IGF-I (Fig. 25–1). Subjecting serum samples to two immunoassay analyses, one of which is specific for 22-kd monomeric hGH while the other recognizes the majority of isoforms released from the pituitary, allows the calculation of an isoform ratio. This approach for the detection of GH doping has been applied since the 2004 Olympic Games but at this point in time still has not led to a positive case of GH doping. It is foreseeable that both strategies will be used side by side in the future and will primarily have their place in unannounced sampling out of competition. The isoform test has a window of opportunity to detect GH abuse during the first 36 hours after the last injection and the pharmacodynamic end-point method provides a longer window of opportunity.

Summary

GH has been used as a drug of abuse in sport since the early 1980s, although there are no proper scientific studies providing GH to be performance enhancing in normal subjects. GH has a very important role in regulating body composition in adult humans. Physiologic replacement therapy with rhGH in GHD adults results in significant changes in body composition with an increase in lean body mass and a loss of fat. However, GH therapy alone, in the absence of some form of exercise program, may increase the lean body mass but not its functional capacity, thus indicating that training may have to be combined with GH replacement in these patients to increase physical performance. The only controlled studies on the effects of GH on muscle function in experienced weight lifters or power athletes have not been able to show a significant positive effect of GH on muscular protein biosynthesis or strength. Two different strategies have been proposed to detect GH doping in sports: parameters of the IGF system such as IGF-I, IGFBP-3, and ALS are suitable markers of GH use in combination with procollagen cleavage products; the "GH isoform method" exploits the difference in isoform composition between recombinant and endogenous growth hormone.

Erythropoietin and EPO System

Erythropoietin (EPO), a glycoprotein hormone naturally produced in the kidney and the liver, is an essential growth factor for the erythrocytic progenitors in the bone marrow. Once released, it serves to stimulate an increase in hemoglobin. In this way, it increases the oxygen-carrying capacity of the blood.[200]

The effects of physical exercise on circulating EPO levels have been studied in various disciplines including cross-country skiing, cycling, long-distance running, and biathlon.[200] The results indicate that the level of EPO is not significantly affected by single bouts of strenuous exercise, although slight increases were occasionally observed a few hours after long-distance running.[201] Despite the lack of EPO response to acute physical exercise, the number of reticulocytes may increase within 1 or 2 days after exercise.[202] It is likely that stress hormones such as catecholamines and cortisol stimulate the release of young red blood cells from bone marrow. Sustained training is associated with increased reticulocyte counts.[202] Hemoglobin levels and hematocrit may nevertheless be below normal. This so-called sports anemia is a pseudoanemia, in that the plasma volume is increased.[200]

Lavoie and colleagues[203] investigated the effects of recombinant EPO on metabolism in rats. The authors found that 15 days of rEPO administration resulted in a significant increase in hematocrit. In addition, they found that exercised rats in the

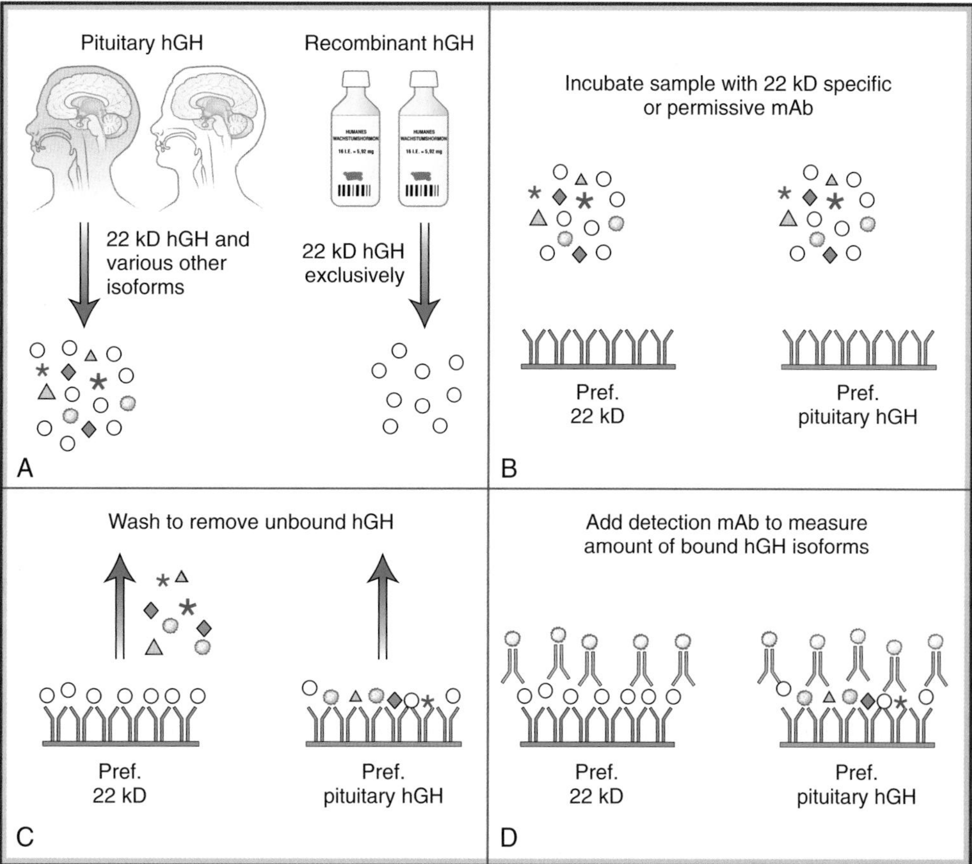

Figure 25–1 ▪ Differential immunoassays for growth hormone isoform composition.

rEPO group had higher muscle glycogen and free fatty acids and lower lactate levels compared with those of controls. The results suggest that energy substrate use during exercise is affected by enhanced oxygen availability. They concluded that supplementation with rEPO resulted in a lower contribution of anaerobic metabolism to energy production.

Because endurance athletes are particularly sensitive to the oxygen-carrying capacity in their blood, any substance that increases this capacity provides a tremendous aerobic advantage. This advantage is evidenced by the long-recognized practices of living at altitude and sleeping in altitude tents.[144] Another method of accomplishing this increase is through blood doping, which involves an autologous transfusion of previously donated blood after a period of hematocrit recovery or through a homologous transfusion from a cross-matched donor. These transfusions artificially increase the hematocrit mass and thus the oxygen-carrying capacity of blood.

An alternative to doping, the drug EPO increases hematocrit when administered in a recombinant form.[203] RhEPO has been imputed to be abused by athletes in aerobic sports early after its marketing as an erythropoiesis-stimulating drug.[204] This drug is effective and does not require the initial donation of blood or potential risks of transfusion to achieve the increase in hematocrit. It is perceived to be effective enough that many cyclists and other aerobic athletes consider EPO to be an occupational necessity at their sport's highest levels.

Although few studies on the ergogenic potential of rhEPO have been done, some investigations have come to similar conclusions to those achieved in studies of blood doping. Birkeland and colleagues[205] performed a double-blind, placebo-controlled study of 4 weeks of rhEPO supplementation using a cycle ergometer to measure effects. The authors reported that in rhEPO subjects, hematocrit increased from 42.7% to 50.8%. In addition, VO_{2max} significantly increased from 63.6 to 68.1 mL/kg/min, a 7% increase. Neither outcome measure showed a significant increase in the placebo group. Similar findings were noted by Ekblom and Berglund.[206] They reported a 6% to 11% increase in hematocrit and increases in VO_{2max} in time to exhaustion after 7 weeks of rhEPO administration.

Williams and Branch[207] reported that an increase of 1 g/dL of hemoglobin in an athlete with an exercise cardiac output of 25 L/min would increase oxygen transport by 335 mL, which extrapolates to an 8% increase given a normal VO_{2max} of 4000 mL O_2/min. Artificially raising hemoglobin levels can have dangerous consequences. In 1987, the first year of EPO release in Europe, five Dutch cyclists died of unexplained reasons. Between 1997 and 2000, 18 cyclists died of stroke, myocardial infarction, or pulmonary embolism.[144]

In contrast to the effect of endurance training, which results in an increased plasma volume, the administration of rhEPO produces a selective increase in red cell mass. If hematocrit exceeds 0.50, blood viscosity and cardiac afterload increase significantly. The main risk of erythrocytosis with hematocrit greater than 0.55 include heart failure, myocardial infarction, seizures, peripheral thromboembolic events, and pulmonary embolism.[200]

Since the 1996 Atlanta Olympics, gas chromatography–mass spectrometry evaluations have been used for screening of exogenous EPO in the urine.[144] Recently, high-performance liquid chromatography has also been used to detect subtle peptides in the urine.[178] Despite these recent advances, exogenous EPO remains a particularly difficult substance to detect through tests.

Two teams of scientists developed tests for EPO that were used at the 2000 Sydney Olympic Games. An indirect test based on the measurement of five blood parameters including reticulocyte hematocrit, serum EPO, hematocrit, soluble transferrin receptor, and the percentage macrocytes was developed by Parisotto and coworkers.[208] Two models were developed. The "on" model used all parameters to detect recent use of EPO. The "off" model used three parameters to detect EPO use with more retrospectivity. The "on" model was used as a screening test at the Sydney Olympic Games. Confirmation of rhEPO use was accomplished through the use of an isoelectric focusing/immunoblotting/chemiluminescence technique that was able to detect the different glycoforms of recombinant versus native EPO.[209] This method can also be applied to detect the use of the novel erythropoiesis-stimulating drug darbepoetin alpha.[210] The limitation of this technique is that it allows detection of EPO for only a few days after use. At the Sydney Olympic Games both tests were required to be positive to confirm EPO use, and no positive cases were detected.

Despite the development of a test for rhEPO, numerous questions remain to be resolved. The development of additional rhEPO products may have different, and indistinguishable, glycoforms and isoforms. In addition, other approaches to improving oxygen transport can be envisioned including polymerized and cross-linked hemoglobins (hemoglobin-based oxygen carriers; HBOCs), blood substitutes such as perfluorohydrocarbons, and 2,3-diphosphoglycerate (2,3-DPG) mimetics. The latter group, including RSR 13, work by shifting the oxygen saturation curve to the left and delivering more oxygen to the tissue per molecule of hemoglobin.[211]

Advances in science related to doping require further research.

Summary

EPO is an essential growth factor for the erythrocytic progenitors in the bone marrow. Once released, it serves to stimulate an increase in hemoglobin thus increasing the oxygen-carrying capacity of the blood. EPO increases hematocrit when administered in a recombinant form. RhEPO has been imputed to be abused by athletes in aerobic sports early after its marketing as an erythropoiesis-stimulating drug.

Artificially raising hemoglobin levels can have dangerous consequences. The administration of rhEPO produces a selective increase in red cell mass. The main risk of erythrocytosis include heart failure, myocardial infarction, seizures, peripheral thromboembolic events, and pulmonary embolism.

REFERENCES

1. Wade CE. Hormonal regulation of fluid homeostasis during and following exercise. In Warren MP, Constantini NW, eds. Contemporary Endocrinology: Sports Endocrinology. Totowa, NJ: Humana Press, 2000:207-225.
2. Cumming DC. Hormones and athletic performance. In Felig P, Baxter JD, Frohman LA, eds. Endocrinology and Metabolism, 3rd ed. New York: McGraw-Hill, 1995:1837-1885.
3. Peyrin L, Pequignot JM, Lacour JR, et al. Relationships between catecholamine or 3-methoxy 4-hydroxy phenylglycol changes and the mental performance under submaximal exercise in man. Psychopharmacology 1987;93:188-192.
4. Rogers G, Goodman C, Rosen C. Water budget during ultra-endurance exercise. Med Sci Sports Exerc 1997;29:1477-1481.
5. Wade CE, Claybaugh J. Renin activity, vasopressin concentration, and urinary excretory responses to exercise in men. J Appl Physiol 1980;49:930-936.
6. Nose H, Takamata A, Mack GW, et al. Right atrial pressure and ANP release during prolonged exercise in a hot environment. J Appl Physiol 1994;76:1882-1887.
7. Cuneo RC, Espiner EA, Nicholls MG, et al. Renal, hemodynamic, and hormonal responses to atrial natriuretic peptide infusions in normal man, and effect of sodium intake. J Clin Endocrinol Metab 1986;63:946-953.
8. Mudambo KS, Coutie W, Rennie MJ. Plasma arginine vasopressin, atrial natriuretic peptide and brain natriuretic peptide responses to long-term field training in the heat: effects of fluid ingestion and acclimatization. Eur J Appl Physiol Occup Physiol 1997;75: 219-225.
9. Nishikimi T, Morimoto A, Ishikawa K, et al. Different secretion patterns of adrenomedullin, brain natriuretic peptide, and atrial natriuretic peptide during exercise in hypertensive and normotensive subjects. Clin Exp Hypertens 1997;19:503-518.
10. Tidgren B, Hjemdahl P, Theodorsson E, et al. Renal neurohormonal and vascular responses to dynamic exercise in humans. J Appl Physiol 1991;70:2279-2286.
11. Wade CE, Ramee SR, Hunt MM, et al. Hormonal and renal responses to converting enzyme inhibition during maximal exercise. J Appl Physiol 1987;63:1796-1800.
12. Davies CT, Few JD. Effects of exercise on adrenocortical function. J Appl Physiol 1973;35:887-891.
13. Wittert GA, Stewart DE, Graves MP, et al. Plasma corticotrophin releasing factor and vasopressin responses to exercise in normal man. Clin Endocrinol 1991;35:311-317.
14. Kjaer M, Secher NH, Bangsbo J, et al. Hormonal and metabolic responses to electrically induced cycling during epidural anesthesia in humans. J Appl Physiol 1996;80:2156-2162.
15. Raastad T, Bjoro T, Hallen J. Hormonal responses to high- and moderate-intensity strength exercise. Eur J Appl Physiol 2000; 82:121-128.
16. Few JD. Effect of exercise on the secretion and metabolism of cortisol in man. J Endocrinol 1974;62:341-353.
17. Brandenberger G, Follenius M. Influence of timing and intensity of muscular exercise on temporal patterns of plasma cortisol levels. J Clin Endocrinol Metab 1975;40:845-849.
18. Oleshansky MA, Zoltick JM, Herman RH, et al. The influence of fitness on neuroendocrine responses to exhaustive treadmill exercise. Eur J Appl Physiol Occup Physiol 1990;59:405-410.
19. Farrell PA, Garthwaite TL, Gustafson AB. Plasma adrenocorticotropin and cortisol responses to submaximal and exhaustive exercise. J Appl Physiol 1983;55:1441-1444.
20. Buono MJ, Yeager JE, Hodgdon JA. Plasma adrenocorticotropin and cortisol responses to brief high-intensity exercise in humans. J Appl Physiol 1986;61:1337-1339.
21. Lutoslawska G, Obminski Z, Krogulski A, et al. Plasma cortisol and testosterone following 19-km and 42-km kayak races. J Sports Med Phys Fitness 1991;31:538-542.
22. Fellmann N, Bedu M, Boudet G, et al. Inter-relationships between pituitary-adrenal hormones and catecholamines during a 6-day Nordic ski race. Eur J Appl Physiol Occup Physiol 1992;64: 258-265.
23. Bergeron MF, Maresh CM, Kraemer WJ, et al. Tennis: a physiological profile during match play. Int J Sports Med 1991;12:474-479.
24. Häkkinen K, Pakarinen A. Acute hormonal responses to two different fatiguing heavy-resistance protocols in male athletes. J Appl Physiol 1993;74:882-887.
25. Hackney AC, Premo MC, McMurray RG. Influence of aerobic versus anaerobic exercise on the relationship between reproductive hormones in men. J Sports Sci 1995;13:305-311.
26. Häkkinen K, Pakarinen A. Acute hormonal responses to heavy resistance exercise in men and women at different ages. Int J Sports Med 1995;16:507-513.
27. Korkushko OV, Frolkis MV, Shatilo VB, et al. Hormonal and autonomic reactions to exercise in elderly healthy subjects and patients with ischemic heart disease. Acta Clin Belg 1990;45: 164-175.
28. Silverman HG, Mazzeo RS. Hormonal responses to maximal and submaximal exercise in trained and untrained men of various ages. J Gerontol A Biol Sci Med Sci 1996;51:B30-37.
29. Davis SN, Galassetti P, Wasserman DH, et al. Effects of gender on neuroendocrine and metabolic counterregulatory responses to exercise in normal man. J Clin Endocrinol Metab 2000;85: 224-230.
30. Loucks AB, Mortola JF, Girton L, et al. Alterations in the hypothalamic-pituitary-ovarian and the hypothalamic-pituitary-adrenal axes in athletic women. J Clin Endocrinol Metab 1989;68: 402-411.

31. Bonen A, Haynes FW, Graham TE. Substrate and hormonal responses to exercise in women using oral contraceptives. J Appl Physiol 1991;70:1917-1927.
32. Kirschbaum C, Schommer N, Federenko I, et al. Short-term estradiol treatment enhances pituitary-adrenal axis and sympathetic responses to psychosocial stress in healthy young men. J Clin Endocrinol Metab 1996;81:3639-3643.
33. Duclos M, Corcuff J-B, Rashedi M, et al. Trained versus untrained men: different immediate post-exercise responses of pituitary-adrenal axis. A preliminary study. Eur J Appl Physiol 1997;75:343-350.
34. Akana SF, Dallman MF. Feedback and facilitation in the adrenocortical system: unmasking facilitation by partial inhibition of the glucocorticoid response to prior stress. Endocrinology 1992;131:57-68.
35. Heuser IJE, Wark HJ, Keul J, et al. Hypothalamic-pituitary-adrenal axis function in elderly endurance athletes. J Clin Endocrinol Metab 1991;73:485-488.
36. Kreaemer WJ, Fleck SJ, Callister R, et al. Training responses of plasma β-endorphin, adrenocorticotropin, and cortisol. Med Sci Sports Exerc 1989;21:146-153.
37. Kraemer WJ, Fleck SJ, Evans WJ. Strength and power training: physiological mechanisms of adaptation. In Holloszy JO, ed. Exercise and Sport Sciences Reviews. Baltimore, MD: Williams & Wilkins, 1996:363-397.
38. Lehmann M, Foster C, Dickhuth HH, et al. Autonomic imbalance hypothesis and overtraining. Med Sci Sports Exerc 1998;30:1140-1145.
39. Kuipers H, Keizer HA. Over-training in elite athletes. Review and directions for the future. Sports Med 1988;6:82-97.
40. Vasankari TJ, Rusko H, Kujala UM, et al. The effect of ski training at altitude and racing on pituitary, adrenal and testicular function in men. Eur J Appl Physiol Occup Physiol 1993;66:221-225.
41. Marinelli M, Roi GS, Giacometti M, et al. Cortisol, testosterone, and free testosterone in athletes performing a marathon at 4,000 m altitude. Horm Res 1994;41:225-229.
42. Hoffman JR, Maresh CM, Armstrong LE, et al. Effects of hydration state on plasma testosterone, cortisol and catecholamine concentrations before and during mild exercise at elevated temperature. Eur J Appl Physiol Occup Physiol 1994;69:294-300.
43. Hoffman JR, Falk B, Radom-Isaac S, et al. The effect of environmental temperature on testosterone and cortisol responses to high intensity, intermittent exercise in humans. Eur J Appl Physiol Occup Physiol 1997;75:83-87.
44. Tabata I, Ogita F, Miyachi M, et al. Effect of low blood glucose on plasma CRF, ACTH, and cortisol during prolonged physical exercise. J Appl Physiol 1991;71:1807-1812.
45. Tsintzas OK, Williams C, Wilson W, et al. Influence of carbohydrate supplementation early in exercise on endurance running capacity. Med Sci Sports Exerc 1996;28:1373-1379.
46. Vasankari TJ, Kujala UM, Viljanen TT, et al. Carbohydrate ingestion during prolonged running exercise results in an increase of serum cortisol and decrease of gonadotrophins. Acta Physiol Scand 1991;141:373-377.
47. Meyer T, Schwarz L, Kindermann W. Exercise and endogenous opiates. In Warren MP, Constantini NW, eds. Contemporary Endocrinology: Sports Endocrinology. Totowa, NJ: Humana Press, 2000:31-42.
48. Allen M. Activity-generated endorphins: a review of their role in sports science. Can J Appl Sport Sci 1983;8:115-133.
49. Cumming DC. The male reproductive system, exercise, and training. In Warren MP, Constantini NW, eds. Contemporary Endocrinology: Sports Endocrinology. Totowa, NJ: Humana Press, 2000:119-131.
50. Gotshalk LA, Loebel CC, Nindl BC, et al. Hormonal responses of multiset versus single-set heavy-resistance exercise protocols. Can J Appl Physiol 1997;22:244-255.
51. Volek JS, Kraemer WJ, Bush JA, et al. Testosterone and cortisol in relationship to dietary nutrients and resistance exercise. J Appl Physiol 1997;82:49-54.
52. Cumming DC, Brunsting LA 3rd, Strich G, et al. Reproductive hormone increases in response to acute exercise in men. Med Sci Sports Exerc 1986;18:369-373.
53. Cumming DC, Wheeler GD, McColl EM. The effects of exercise on reproductive function in men. Sports Med 1989;7:1-17.
54. Vaananen I, Vasankari T, Mantysaari M, et al. Hormonal responses to daily strenuous walking during 4 successive days. Eur J Appl Physiol 2002;88:122-127.
55. Kujala UM, Alen M, Huhtaniemi IT. Gonadotrophin-releasing hormone and human chorionic gonadotrophin tests reveal that both hypothalamic and testicular endocrine functions are suppressed during acute prolonged physical exercise. Clin Endocrinol 1990;33:219-225.
56. Ayers WT, Komesu Y, Romani T, et al. Anthropomorphic, hormonal, and psychologic correlates of semen quality in endurance-trained male athletes. Fertil Steril 1985;43:917-921.
57. De Souza MJ, Arce JC, Pescatello LS. Gonadal hormones and semen quality in male runners. A volume threshold effect of endurance training. Int J Sports Med 1994;15:383-391.
58. Gebreegziabher Y, Marcos E, McKinon W, et al. Sperm characteristics of endurance trained cyclists. Int J Sports Med 2004;25:247-251.
59. Elias AN, Fairshter R, Pandian MR, et al. Beta-endorphin/beta-lipotropin release and gonadotropin secretion after acute exercise in physically conditioned males. Eur J Appl Physiol Occup Physiol 1989;58:522-527.
60. Hackney AC. The male reproductive system and endurance exercise. Med Sci Sports Exerc 1996;28:180-189.
61. Wheeler GD, Wall SR, Belcastro AN, et al. Reduced serum testosterone and prolactin levels in male distance runners. JAMA 1984;252:514-516.
62. Hackney AC, Sharp RL, Runyan WS, et al. Relationship of resting prolactin and testosterone in males during intensive training. Br J Sports Med 1989;23:194.
63. Cumming DC, Quigley ME, Yen SS. Acute suppression of circulating testosterone levels by cortisol in men. J Clin Endocrinol Metab 1983;57:671-673.
64. Hackney AC, Sinning WE, Bruot BC. Hypothalamic-pituitary-testicular function of endurance-trained and untrained males. Int J Sports Med 1990;11:298-303.
65. Wheeler GD, Singh M, Pierce WD, et al. Endurance training decreases serum testosterone levels in men without change in luteinizing hormone pulsation release. J Clin Endocrinol Metab 1991;72:422-425.
66. Arena B, Maffulli N, Maffulli F, et al. Reproductive hormones and menstrual changes with exercise in female athletes. Sports Med 1995;19:278-287.
67. Loucks AB, Vaitukaitis J, Cameron JL, et al. The reproductive system and exercise in women. Med Sci Sports Exerc 1992;24:288-293.
68. Warren MP. The effects of exercise on pubertal progression and reproductive function in girls. J Clin Endocrinol Metab 1980;51:1150-1157.
69. Loucks AB, Verdun M, Heath EM. Low energy availability, not stress of exercise, alters LH pulsatility in exercising women. J Appl Physiol 1998;84:37-46.
70. Stafford DE. Altered hypothalamic-pituitary-ovarian axis function in young female athletes: implications and recommendations for management. Treat Endocrinol 2005;4:147-154.
71. Winterer J, Cutler GB Jr, Loriaux DL. Caloric balance, brain to body ratio, and the timing of menarche. Med Hypotheses 1984;15:87-91.
72. Laughlin GA, Yen SS. Nutritional and endocrine-metabolic aberrations in amenorrheic athletes. J Clin Endocrinol Metab 1996;81:4301-4309.
73. Laughlin GA, Yen SS. Hypoleptinemia in women athletes: absence of a diurnal rhythm with amenorrhea. J Clin Endocrinol Metab 1997;82:318-321.
74. Loucks AB, Laughlin GA, Mortola JF, et al. Hypothalamic-pituitary-thyroidal function in eumenorrheic and amenorrheic athletes. J Clin Endocrinol Metab 1992;75:514-518.
75. Zhang Y, Proenca R, Maffei M, et al. Positional cloning of the mouse obese gene and its human homologue. Nature 1994;372:425-432.
76. Considine RV, Sinha MK, Heiman ML, et al. Serum immunoreactive-leptin concentrations in normal-weight and obese humans. N Engl J Med 1996;334:292-295.
77. Aubert ML, Pierroz DD, Gruaz NM, et al. Metabolic control of sexual function and growth: role of neuropeptide Y and leptin. Mol Cell Endocrinol 1998;140:107-113.

78. Welt CK, Chan JL, Bullen J, et al. Recombinant human leptin in women with hypothalamic amenorrhea. N Engl J Med 2004;351:987-997.
79. Chan JL, Mantzoros CS. Role of leptin in energy-deprivation states: normal human physiology and clinical implications for hypothalamic amenorrhoea and anorexia nervosa. Lancet 2005;366: 74-85.
80. De Souza MJ, Maguire MS, Maresh CM, et al. Adrenal activation and the prolactin response to exercise in eumenorrheic and amenorrheic runners. J Appl Physiol 1991;70:2378-2387.
81. Stoving RK, Hangaard J, Hagen C. Update on endocrine disturbances in anorexia nervosa. J Pediatr Endocrinol Metab 2001; 14:459-480.
82. Loucks AB. Exercise training in the normal female. Effects of exercise stress and energy availability on metabolic hormones and LH pulsatility. In Warren MP, Constantini NW, eds. Contemporary Endocrinology: Sports Endocrinology. Totowa, NJ: Humana Press, 2000:165-180.
83. De Cree C. The possible involvement of endogenous opioid peptides and catecholestrogens in provoking menstrual irregularities in women athletes. Int J sports Med 1990;11:329-348.
84. Consitt LA, Copeland JL, Tremblay MS. Endogenous anabolic hormone responses to endurance versus resistance exercise and training in women. Sports Med 2002;32:1-22.
85. Rickenlund A, Carlstrom K, Ekblom B, et al. Hyperandrogenicity is an alternative mechanism underlying oligomenorrhea or amenorrhea in female athletes and may improve physical performance. Fertil Steril 2003;79:947-955.
86. Odink J, Van der Beek EJ, Van den Berg H, et al. Effect of work load on free and sulfate-conjugated plasma catecholamines, prolactin, and cortisol. Int J Sports Med 1986;7:352-357.
87. Hackney AC, Ness RJ, Schrieber A. Effects of endurance exercise on nocturnal hormone concentration in males. Chronobiol Int 1989;6:341-346.
88. De Meirleir KL, Baeyens L, L'Hermite-Baleriaux M, et al. Exercise-induced prolactin release is related to anaerobiosis. J Clin Endocrinol Metab 1985;60:1250-1252.
89. Mastrogiacomo I, Toderini D, Bonanni G, et al. Gonadotropin decrease induced by prolonged exercise at about 55% of the VO2max in different phases of the menstrual cycle. Int J Sports Med 1990;11:198-203.
90. Roth J, Glick SM, Yalow RS. Hypoglycemia: a potent stimulus to the secretion of growth hormone. Science 1963;140:987-988.
91. Felsing NE, Brasel JA, Cooper DM. Effect of low and high intensity exercise on circulating growth hormone in men. J Clin Endocrinol Metab 1992;75:157-162.
92. Eliakim A, Brasel JA, Cooper DM. Exercise and the growth hormone-insulin-like growth factor-1 axis. In Warren MP, Constantini NW, eds. Contemporary Endocrinology: Sports Endocrinology. Totowa, NJ: Humana Press, 2000:77-95.
93. Godfrey R, Madgwick Z, Whyte G. The exercise-induced growth hormone response in athletes. Sports Med 2003;33:599-613.
94. Sutton JR, Lazarus L. Growth hormone and exercise comparison of physiological and pharmacological stimuli. J Appl Physiol 1976;41:523-527.
95. Cuneo RC, Wallace JD. Growth hormone, insulin-like growth factors and sport. Endocrinol Metab 1994;1:3-13.
96. Bar-Or O. Growth hormone deficiency-using exercise in the diagnosis. In Bar-Or O, ed. Pediatric Sports Medicine for the Practitioner. New York: Springer-Verlag, 1983:182-191.
97. Eliakim A, Brasel JA, Cooper DM. GH response to exercise: assessment of the pituitary refractory period, and relationship with circulating components of the GH-IGF-I axis in adolescent females. J Pediatr Endocrinol Metab 1999;12:47-55.
98. Ehrnborg C, Lange KHW, Dall R, et al. The growth hormone/insulin-like growth factor-I axis hormones and bone markers in elite athletes in response to a maximum exercise test. J Clin Endocrinol Metab 2003;88:394-401.
99. Snegovskeya V, Viru A. Elevation of cortisol and growth hormone levels in the courses of further improvement of performance capacity in trained rowers. Int J Sports Med 1993;14:202-206.
100. Karagiorgos A, Garcia JF, Brooks GA. Growth hormone response to continuous and intermittent exercise. Med Sci Sports 1979;11:302-307.
101. Häkkinen K, Pakarinen A, Alen M, et al. Neuromuscular and hormonal responses in elite athletes to two successive strength training sessions in one day. Eur J Appl Physiol 1988;57:133-139.
102. Weltman A, Weltman JY, Womack CJ, et al. Exercise training decreases the growth hormone (GH) response to acute constant-load exercise. Med Sci Sports Exerc 1997;29:669-676.
103. Wideman L, Weltman JY, Hartman ML, et al. Growth hormone release during acute and chronic aerobic and resistance exercise: recent findings. Sports Med 2002;32:987-1004.
104. Kanaley JA, Weltman JY, Veldhuis JD, et al. Human growth hormone response to repeated bouts of aerobic exercise. J Appl Physiol 1997;83:1756-1761.
105. Peyreigne C, Bouix D, Fedou C, et al. Effect of hydration on exercise-induced growth hormone response. Eur J Endocrinol 2001;145:445-450.
106. Cappon JP, Ipp E, Brasel JA, et al. Acute effect of high-fat and high-glucose meals on the growth hormone response to exercise. J Clin Endocrinol Metab 1993;76:1418-1422.
107. Okada Y, Hikita T, Ishitobi K, et al. Human growth hormone secretion during exposure to hot air in normal adult male subjects. J Clin Endocrinol Metab 1972;34:759-763.
108. Buckler JM. The relationship between changes in plasma growth hormone levels and body temperature occurring with exercise in man. Biomedicine 1973;19:193-197.
109. Wilkinson PW, Parkin JM. Growth hormone response to exercise in obese children. Lancet 1974;2:55.
110. Pritzlaff-Roy CJ, Widemen L, Weltman JY, et al. Gender governs the relationship between exercise intensity and growth hormone release in young adults. J Appl Physiol 2002;92:2053-2060.
111. Friend KE, Hartman ML, Pezzoli SS, et al. Both oral and transdermal estrogen increase growth hormone release in postmenopausal women: a clinical research center study. J Clin Endocrinol Metab 1996;81:2250-2256.
112. Bernardes RP, Radomski MW. Growth hormone responses to continuous and intermittent exercise in females under oral contraceptive therapy. Eur J Appl Physiol Occup Physiol 1998;79:24-29.
113. Kelley PJ, Eisman JA, Stuart MC, et al. Somatomedin-C, physical fitness, and bone density. J Clin Endocrinol Metab 1990;70: 718-723.
114. Wilson DP, Horowitz JL. Exercise-induced changes in growth hormone and somatomedine-C. Am J Med Sci 1987;293:216-217.
115. Hagberg JM, Seals DR, Yerg JE, et al. Metabolic responses to exercise in young and older athletes and sedentary men. J Appl Physiol 1988;65:900-908.
116. Schwarz AJ, Brasel JA, Hintz RL, et al. Acute effect of brief low- and high-intensity exercise on circulating IGF-I, II, and IGF binding protein-3 and its proteolysis in young healthy men. J Clin Endocrinol Metab 1996;81:3492-3497.
117. Zanconato S, Moromisato DY, Moromisato MY, et al. Effect of training and growth hormone suppression on insulin-like growth factor-I mRNA in young rats. J Appl Physiol 1994;76:2204-2209.
118. Eliakim A, Moromisato M, Moromisato D, et al. Increase in muscle IGF-I protein but not IGF-I mRNA after 5 days of endurance training in young rats. J Appl Physiol 1997;42:1557-1561.
119. Wallace JD, Cuneo RD, Baxter R, et al. Responses of the growth hormone (GH) and insulin-like growth factor axis to exercise, GH administration, and GH withdrawal in trained adult males: a potential test for GH abuse in sport. J Clin Endocrinol Metab 1999;84:3591-3601.
120. Eliakim A, Brasel JA, Mohan S, et al. Physical fitness, endurance training, and the GH-IGF-1 system in adolescent females. J Clin Endocrinol Metab 1996;81:3986-3992.
121. Mason JW, Hartley LH, Kotchen TA, et al. Plasma thyroid-stimulating hormone response in anticipation of muscular exercise in the human. J Clin Endocrinol Metab 1973;37:403-406.
122. Sawhney RC, Malhotra AS, Gupta RB, et al. A study of pituitary-thyroid function during exercise in man. Indian J Physiol Pharmacol 1984;28:153-158.
123. Liewendahl K, Helenius T, Naveri H, et al. Fatty acid–induced increase in serum dialyzable free thyroxine after physical exercise: implication for nonthyroidal illness. J Clin Endocrinol Metab 1992;74:1361-1365.
124. Galbo H, Hummer L, Peterson IB, et al. Thyroid and testicular hormone responses to graded and prolonged exercise in man. Eur J Appl Physiol Occup Physiol 1977;36:101-106.

125. Schmid P, Wolf W, Pilger E, et al. TSH, T3, rT3 and fT4 in maximal and submaximal physical exercise. Eur J Appl Physiol Occup Physiol 1982;48:31-39.
126. Semple CG, Thomson JA, Beastall GH. Endocrine responses to marathon running. Br J Sports Med 1985;19:148-151.
127. Sander M, Rocker L. Influence of marathon running on thyroid hormones. Int J Sports Med 1988;9:123-126.
128. Chicharro JL, Hoyos J, Bandres F, et al. Thyroid hormone levels during a 3-week professional road cycling competition. Horm Res 2001;56:159-164.
129. Limanova Z, Sonka J, Kratochvil O, et al. Effects of exercise on serum cortisol and thyroid hormones. Exp Clin Endocrinol 1983;81:308-314.
130. Deligiannis A, Karamouzis M, Kouidi E, et al. Plasma TSH, T3, T4 and cortisol responses to swimming at varying water temperatures. Br J Sports Med 1993;27:247-250.
131. Lehmann M, Knizia K, Gastmann U, et al. Influence of 6-week, 6 days per week, training on pituitary function in recreational athletes. Br J Sports Med 1993;27:186-192.
132. Loucks AB, Heath EM. Induction of low-T3 syndrome in exercising women occurs at a threshold of energy availability. Am J Physiol 1994;266:R817-R823.
133. Jahreis G, Kauf E, Frohner G, et al. Influence of intensive exercise on insulin-like growth factor I, thyroid and steroid hormones in female gymnasts. Growth Regul 1991;1:95-99.
134. Task Force on Community Preventive Services. Increasing Physical Activity. A Report on Recommendations of the Task Force on Community Preventive Services: Morbidity and Mortality Weekly Reports Recommendations and Reports 2001. Centers for Disease Control 2001, Vol 50, RR-18.
135. Schneider SH, Guleria PS. Diabetes and exercise. In Warren MP, Constantini NW, eds. Contemporary Endocrinology: Sports Endocrinology. Totowa, NJ: Humana Press, 2000:227-238.
136. Felig P, Wahren J. Fuel homeostasis in exercise. N Engl J Med 1975;293:1078-1084.
137. Rodnick KJ, Henriksen EJ, James DE, et al. Exercise training, glucose transporters, and glucose transport in rat skeletal muscles. Am J Physiol 1992;262:C9-C14.
138. DeFronzo RA, Ferrannini E, Sato Y, et al. Synergistic interaction between exercise and insulin on peripheral glucose uptake. J Clin Invest 1981;68:1468-1474.
139. Jenkins AB, Furler SM, Chisholm DJ, et al. Regulation of hepatic glucose output during exercise by circulating glucose and insulin in humans. Am J Physiol 1986;250:R411-R417.
140. Lavoie C, Ducros F, Bourque J, et al. Glucose metabolism during exercise in man: the role of insulin and glucagon in the regulation of hepatic glucose production and gluconeogenesis. Can J Physiol Pharmacol 1997;75:26-35.
141. Naveri H, Kuoppasalmi K, Harkonen M: Plasma glucagon and catecholamines during exhaustive short-term exercise. Eur J Appl Physiol Occup Physiol 1985;53:308-311.
142. O'Rahilly SO, Hosker JP, Rudenski AS, et al. The glucose stimulus-response curve of the beta-cell in physically trained humans, assessed by hyperglycemic clamps. Metabolism 1988;37:919-923.
143. Roberts CK, Barnard RJ. Effects of exercise and diet on chronic disease. J Appl Physiol 2005;98:3-30.
144. Tokish JM, Kocher MS, Hawkins RJ. Ergogenic aids: a review of basic science, performance, side effects, and status in sports. Am J Sports Med 2004;32:1543-1553.
145. Di Luigi L, Romanelli F, Lenzi A. Androgenic-anabolic steroids abuse in males. J Endocrinol Invest 2005;28:81-84.
146. Yesalis CE III, Kennedy NJ, Kopstein AN, et al. Anabolic-androgenic steroid use in the United States. JAMA 1993;270:1217-1221.
147. National Institute on Drug Abuse. About anabolic steroid abuse. NIDA Notes 2000;15:15.
148. Evans NA. Current concepts in anabolic-androgenic steroids. Am J Sports Med 2004;32:534-542.
149. Lovejoy JC, Bray GA, Bourgeois MO, et al. Exogenous androgens influence body composition and regional body fat distribution in obese postmenopausal women—a clinical research center study. J Clin Endocrinol Metab 1996;81:2198-2203.
150. Bhasin S, Storer TW, Berman N, et al. The effects of supraphysiological doses of testosterone on muscle size and strength in normal men. N Engl J Med 1996;335:1-7.
151. Ryan AJ. Athletics. In Kochakian CD, ed. Anabolic-Androgenic Steroids, Vol 43. Berlin: Springer-Verlag, 1976:515-534.
152. Haupt HA, Rovere GD: Anabolic steroids: a review of the literature. Am J Sports Med 1984;12:469-484.
153. Strauss RH, Yesalis CE. Anabolic steroids in the athlete. Annu Rev Med 1991;42:449-457.
154. Bhasin S, Woodhouse L, Casaburi R, et al. Testosterone dose-response relationships in healthy young men. Am J Physiol Endocrinol Metab 2001;281:E1172-E1181.
155. Sinha-Hikim I, Artaza J, Woodhouse L, et al. Testosterone-induced increase in muscle size in healthy young men is associated with muscle fiber hypertrophy. Am J Physiol Endocrinol Metab 2002;283:E154-E164.
156. Elbers JMH, Asscheman H, Seidell JC, et al. Effects of sex steroid hormones on regional fat depots as assessed by magnetic resonance imaging in transexuals. Am J Physiol 1999;276:E317-E325.
157. Alway SE. Characteristics of the elbow flexors in women bodybuilders using androgenic-anabolic steroids. J Strength Cond Res 1994;8:161-169.
158. Tamaki T, Uchiyama S, Uchiyama Y, et al. Anabolic steroids increase exercise tolerance. Am J Physiol Endocrinol Metab 2001;280:E973-E981.
159. Korkia P, Stimson GV. Indications of prevalence, practice and effects of anabolic steroid use in Great Britain. Int J Sports Med 1997;18:557-562.
160. Catlin DH. Androgen abuse by athletes. In Bhasin S, Gabelnick HL, Spieler JM, et al, eds. Pharmacology, Biology, and Clinical Applications of Androgens. New York: Wiley-Liss, 1996:289-295.
161. Bronson FH, Matherne CM. Exposure to anabolic-androgenic steroids shortens life span of male mice. Med Sci Sports Exerc 1997;29:615-619.
162. Evans NA. Gym & tonic: a profile of 100 male steroid users. Br J Sports Med 1997;31:54-58.
163. Hall RC, Hall RC. Abuse of supraphysiologic doses of anabolic steroids. South Med J 2005;98:550-555.
164. Ishak KG, Zimmerman HJ. Hepatotoxic effects of the anabolic/androgenic steroids. Semin Liver Dis 1987;7:230-236.
165. Street C, Antonio J, Cudlipp D. Androgen use by athletes: a reevaluation of the health risks. Can J Appl Physiol 1996;21:421-440.
166. Bolding G, Sherr L, Elford J. Use of anabolic steroids and associated health risks among gay men attending London gyms. Addiction 2002;97:195-201.
167. Thompson PD, Cullinane EM, Sady SP, et al. Contrasting effects of testosterone and stanozolol on serum lipoprotein levels. JAMA 1989;261:1165-1168.
168. Parssinen M, Seppala T. Steroid use and long term health risks in former athletes. Sports Med 2002;32:83-94.
169. Freidl KE. Effects of anabolic steroids on physical health. In Yesalis CE III, ed. Anabolic Steroids in Sports and Exercise. Champaign, IL: Human Kinetics, 1993:107-150.
170. Malarkey WB, Strauss RH, Leizman DJ, et al. Endocrine effects in female weight lifters who self-administer testosterone and anabolic steroids. Am J Obstet Gynecol 1991;165:1385-1390.
171. Spinder T, Spijkstra JJ, Van Den Tweel JG, et al. The effects of long term testosterone administration on pulsatile luteinizing hormone secretion and on ovarian histology in eugonadal female to male transsexual subjects. J Clin Endocrinol Metab 1989; 69:151-157.
172. Strauss RH, Liggett M, Lanese RR. Anabolic steroid use and perceived effects in ten weight-trained women athletes. JAMA 1985;253:2871-2873.
173. Lasseter JT, Russell JA. Anabolic steroid induced tendon pathology: a review of the literature. Med Sci Sports Exerc 1991;23:1-3.
174. Evans NA, Bowrey DJ, Newman DR. Ultrastuctural analysis of ruptured tendon from anabolic steroid users. Injury 1998;29:769-773.
175. Pope HG, Katz DL. Psychiatric and medical effects of anabolic-androgenic steroid use. Arch Gen Psychiatry 1998;51:375-382.
176. Brower KJ, Eliopulos GA, Blow FC, et al. Evidence for physical and psychological dependence on anabolic androgenic steroids in eight weight lifters. Am J Psychiatry 1990;147:510-512.
177. Catlin DH, Hatton CK, Starcevic SH. Issues in detecting abuse of xenobiotic anabolic steroids and testosterone by analysis of athletes' urine. Clin Chem 1997;43:1280-1288.
178. Bowers LD. Analytical advances in detection of performance-enhancing compounds. Clin Chem 1997;43:1299-1304.

179. Jorgensen JOL, Pedersen SA, Thuesen L, et al. Beneficial effects of growth hormone treatment in GH deficient adults. Lancet 1989;1:1221-1225.
180. Salomon F, Cuneo RC, Hesp R, et al. The effects of treatment with recombinant human growth hormone on body composition and metabolism in adults with growth hormone deficiency. N Engl J Med 1989;321:1797-1803.
181. De Boer H, Blok GJ, van der Veen EA. Clinical aspects of growth hormone deficiency in adults. Endocr Rev 1995;16:63-86.
182. Rutherford OM, Jones DA, Round JM, et al. Changes in skeletal muscle after discontinuation of growth hormone treatment in young adults with hypopituitarism. Acta Paediatr Scand Suppl 1989;356:61-63.
183. Svensson J, Stibrant Sunnerhagen K, Johannsson G. Five years of growth hormone replacement therapy in adults: age- and gender-related changes in isometric and isokinetic muscle strength. J Clin Endocrinol Metab 2003;88:2061-2069.
184. Degerblad M, Almkvist O, Grunditz Hall K, et al. Physical and psychological capabilities during substitution therapy with recombinant growth hormone deficiency. Acta Endocrinol 1990;123: 185-193.
185. Rodriguez-Arnao J, Jabbar A, Fulcher K, et al. Effects of growth hormone replacement on physical performance and body composition in GH deficient adults. Clin Endocrinol 1999;51:53-60.
186. Christ ER, Cummings MH, Westwood NB, et al. The importance of growth hormone in the regulation of erythropoiesis, red cell mass, and plasma volume in adults with growth hormone deficiency. J Clin Endocrinol Metab 1997;82:2985-2990.
187. Thuesen L, Jorgensen JOL, Muller JR, et al. Short and long term cardiovascular effects of growth hormone therapy in growth hormone deficient adults. Clin Endocrinol 1994;41:615-620.
188. Boger RH, Skamira C, Bode-Boger SM, et al. Nitric oxide may mediate the hemodynamic effects of recombinant growth hormone in patients with acquired growth hormone deficiency. A double-blind, placebo-controlled study. J Clin Invest 1996; 98:2706-2713.
189. Yarasheski KE, Zachwieja JJ, Angelopoulos TJ, et al. Short-term growth hormone treatment does not increase muscle protein synthesis in experienced weightlifters. J Appl Physiol 1993;74:3073-3076.
190. Deyssig R, Frisch H, Blum WF, et al. Effect of growth hormone treatment on hormonal parameters, body composition and strength in athletes. Acta Endocrinol 1993;128:313-318.
191. Ehrnborg C, Bengtsson BA, Rosen T. Growth hormone abuse. Best Pract Res Clin Endocrinol Metab 2000;14:71-77.
192. Crist DM, Peake GT, Egan PA, et al. Body composition response to exogenous GH during training in highly conditioned adults. J Appl Physiol 1988;65:579-584.
193. Johannsson G, Mårin P, Lönn L, et al. Growth hormone treatment of abdominally obese man reduces abdominal fat mass, improves glucose and lipoprotein metabolism, and reduces diastolic blood pressure. J Clin Endocrinol Metab 1997;82:727-734.
194. Thompson JL, Butterfield GE, Gylfadottir UK, et al. Effects of human growth hormone, insulin-like growth factor I, and diet and exercise on body composition of obese postmenopausal women. J Clin Endocrinol Metab 1998;83:1477-1484.
195. Lange KH, Isaksson F, Juul A, et al. Growth hormone enhances effects of endurance training on oxidative muscle metabolism in elderly women. Am J Physiol Endocrinol Metab 2000;279: E989-E996.
196. Rudman D, Feller AG, Nagraj HS, et al. Effects of human growth hormone in men over 60 years old. N Engl J Med 1990;323: 1-6.
197. Papadakis MA, Grady D, Black D, et al. Growth hormone replacement in healthy older men improves body composition but not functional ability. Ann Intern Med 1996;124:708-716.
198. Wallace JD, Cuneo RD, Lundberg PA, et al. Responses of markers of bone and collagen turnover to exercise, growth hormone (GH) administration and GH withdrawal in trained adult males. J Clin Endocrinol Metab 1999;85:124-133.
199. Wu Z, Bidlingmaier M, Dall R, et al. Detection of doping with human growth hormone. Lancet 1999;353:895.
200. Jelkmann W. Erythropoietin. J Endocrinol Invest 2003;26: 832-837.
201. Schobersberger W, Hobisch-Hagen P, Fries P, et al. Increase in immune activation, vascular endothelial growth factor and erythropoietin after an ultramarathon run at moderate altitude. Immunobiology 2000;201:611-620.
202. Schmidt W, Maassen N, Trost F, et al. Training induced effects on blood volume, erythrocyte turnover and haemoglobin oxygen binding properties. Eur J Appl Physiol Occup Physiol 1988; 57:490-498.
203. Lavoie C, Diguet A, Milot M, et al. Erythropoietin (rHuEPO) doping: effects of exercise on anaerobic metabolism in rats. Int J Sports Med 1998;19:281-286.
204. Spalding BJ. Black-market biotechnology: athletes abuse EPO and HGH. Biotechnology NY 1991;9:1050-1053.
205. Birkeland KI, Stray-Gundersen J, Hemmersbach P, et al. Effect of rhEPO administration on serum levels of sTfR and cycling performance. Med Sci Sports Exerc 2000;32:1238-1243.
206. Ekblom B, Berglund B. Effect of erythropoietin administration on maximal aerobic power. Scand J Med Sci Sports 1991;1:88-93.
207. Williams MH, Branch JD. Ergogenic aids for improved performance. In Garrett WE, Kirkendall DT, eds. Exercise and Sport Science. Philadelphia: Lippincott Williams & Wilkins, 2000: 373-384.
208. Parisotto R, Gore CJ, Emslie KR, et al. A novel method utilising markers of altered erythropoiesis for the detection of recombinant human erythropoietin abuse in athletes. Hematologica 2000; 85:564-572.
209. Lasne J, de Ceaurriz J. Recombinant erythropoietin in urine. Nature 2000;405:635.
210. Egrie JK, Browne JK. Development and characterization of novel erythropoiesis stimulating protein (NESP). Br J Cancer 2001; 84:3-10.
211. Bowers LD. Abuse of performance-enhancing drugs in sport. Ther Drug Monit 2002;24:178-181.

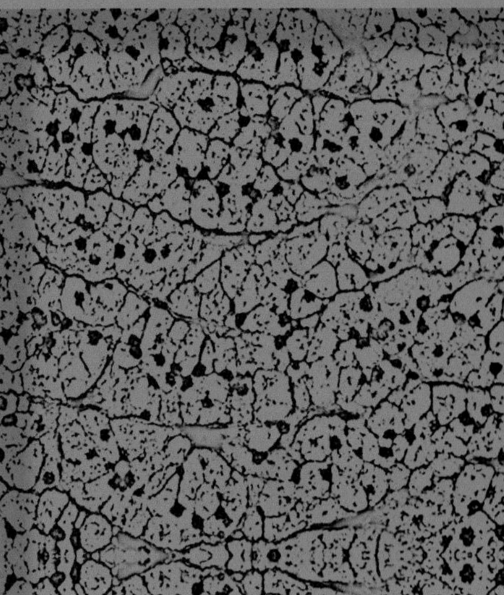

CHAPTER 26

ENDOCRINOLOGY AND AGING

Steven W. J. Lamberts

The average length of human life is currently 75 to 78 years and may increase to 85 years during the coming 10 years,[1] but it is not clear whether these additional years will be satisfactory. Most data indicate a modest gain in the number of healthy years lived but a far greater increase in years of compromised physical, mental, and social function.[2] The number of days with restricted activity and admissions to hospitals and nursing homes increases sharply after 70 years of age.[3] The U.S. National Health Interview Survey indicated that more than 25 million aging people suffer from physical impairment and the number of persons requiring assistance with activities of daily living increases from 14% at ages 65 to 75 years to 45% in people older than age 85 years.[4,5]

Aging and Physical Frailty

Throughout adult life, all physiologic functions start to decline gradually.[6] There is a diminished capacity for cellular protein synthesis, a decline in immune function, an increase in fat mass, a loss of muscle mass and strength, and a decrease in bone mineral density.[6] Most older adults die of atherosclerosis, cancer, or dementia, but in an increasing number of the "healthy" oldest old, loss of muscle strength is the limiting factor that determines their chances of an independent life until death.

Age-related disability is characterized by generalized weakness, impaired mobility and balance, and poor endurance. In the oldest old, this state is termed *physical frailty,* defined as "a state of reduced physiological reserves associated with increased susceptibility to disability."[7] Clinical correlates of physical frailty include falls, fractures, impairment in activities of daily living, and loss of independence. Falls contribute to 40% of admissions to nursing homes.[8]

Loss of muscle strength is an important factor in the development of frailty. Muscle weakness can be caused by aging of muscle fibers and their innervation, osteoarthritis, and chronic debilitating diseases.[9] A sedentary lifestyle, decreased physical activity, and disuse, however, are also important determinants of the decline in muscle strength.

In a study of 100 frail nursing home residents (average age 87 years), lower extremity muscle mass and strength were closely related.[10] Supervised resistance exercise training (45 minutes three times a week for 10 weeks) doubled muscle strength and significantly increased gait velocity and stair-climbing power. This finding demonstrates that frailty in the elderly population is not an irreversible effect of aging and disease but can be influenced and perhaps even prevented.[10] Furthermore, in nondisabled elderly persons living in the community, objective measures of lower extremity function are highly predictive of subsequent disability.[11] Prevention of frailty can be achieved only by working (training). However, exercise is difficult to implement in the daily routine of the aging population, and the number of dropouts from exercise programs is very high.

Part of the aging process involving body composition (i.e., loss of muscle [strength] and bone, increase in fat mass) might also be related to changes in the endocrine system.[6] Current knowledge has shed light on the effects of long-term hormonal replacement therapy on body composition as well as on atherosclerosis, cancer formation, and cognitive function.

THE ENDOCRINOLOGY OF AGING

The two most important clinical changes in endocrine activity during aging involve the pancreas and the thyroid gland.

Approximately 40% of individuals age 65 to 74 years and 50% of those older than 80 years have impaired glucose tolerance or diabetes mellitus, and in nearly 50% of elderly adults with diabetes, the disease is undiagnosed.[12] These adults are at risk for development of secondary, mainly macrovascular, complications at an accelerated rate. Pancreatic, insulin receptor, and postreceptor changes associated with aging are critical components of the endocrinology of aging. Apart from decreased (relative) insulin secretion by the β cells, peripheral insulin resistance related to poor diet, physical inactivity, increased abdominal fat mass, and decreased lean body mass contributes to the deterioration of glucose metabolism.[12] Dietary management, exercise, oral hypoglycemic agents, and insulin are the four components of treatment for these patients, whose medical care is costly and intensive (see Chapter 26).

Age-related thyroid dysfunction is also common.[13] Lowered plasma thyroxine (T_4) and increased thyrotropin concentrations occur in 5% to 10% of elderly women.[13] These abnormalities are mainly caused by autoimmunity and are thus an expression of age-associated disease rather than a consequence of the aging process. Normal aging is accompanied by a slight decrease in pituitary thyrotropin release but especially by decreased peripheral degradation of T_4, which results in a gradual age-dependent decline in serum triiodothyronine (T_3) concentrations without changes in T_4 levels.[13] This slight decrease in plasma T_3 concentration occurs largely within the broad normal range of the healthy elderly population and has not been convincingly related to functional changes during the aging process. At present, the question of whether healthy aging subjects might benefit from T_3 replacement therapy remains unresolved.

Changes in insulin sensitivity and thyroid function that occur in the aging population are frequently of clinical importance and recognized and treated as diseases. Three other hormonal systems exhibit lowered circulating hormone concentrations during normal aging, and these changes have thus far been considered mainly physiologic (Figs. 26–1 and 26–2). Hormone replacement strategies have been developed, but many aspects remain controversial, and replenishing hormone blood levels to those found in 30- to 50-year-old patients has not yet uniformly proved beneficial and safe.

The most dramatic and rapidly occurring change in women around age 50 years is *menopause.*[14] Cycling estradiol production during the reproductive years is replaced by very low, constant estradiol levels. For many years, the prevailing view was that menopause resulted from exhaustion of ovarian follicles. An alternative perspective is that age-related changes in the central nervous system and the h ypothalamic-pituitary unit initiate the menopausal transition. The evidence that both the ovary and the brain are key pacemakers in menopause is compelling.[14]

Changes in the activity of the hypothalamic-pituitary-gonadal axis in men are slower and more subtle. During aging, a gradual decline in serum total and free testosterone levels occurs.[15] *Andropause* is characterized by a decrease in testicular Leydig cell numbers and their secretory capacity as well as by an age-related decrease in episodic and stimulated gonadotropin secretion.[16,17] The primary site of the aging effect appears to be the Leydig cell's ability to respond to LH with increased testosterone production.

The second hormonal system demonstrating age-related changes is *adrenopause,* a term that describes the gradual decline in circulating levels of dehydroepiandrosterone (DHEA) and its sulfate (DHEAS).[18,19] Adrenal secretion of DHEA gradually decreases over time, while corticotropin secretion, which is physiologically linked to plasma cortisol levels, remains largely unchanged. The decline in DHEA and DHEAS levels in both sexes, therefore, contrasts with the maintenance of plasma cortisol levels and seems to be caused by a selective decrease in the number of functional zona reticularis cells in the adrenal cortex instead of being regulated by a central (hypothalamic) pacemaker of aging.[20]

The third endocrine system that gradually declines in activity during aging is the growth hormone (GH)–insulin-like growth factor I (IGF-I) axis (see Fig. 26–2).[6,21] Mean pulse amplitude and duration and fraction of GH secreted, but not pulse frequency, gradually decrease during aging. In parallel, a progressive drop in circulating IGF-I levels occurs in both sexes.[21,22] There is no evidence for a peripheral factor in this process of *somatopause,* and its triggering pacemaker seems mainly localized in the hypothalamus because pituitary somatotropes, even of the oldest old, can be restored to their youthful secretory capacity by treatment with GH-releasing peptides (see later discussion).

It is unclear whether changes in gonadal function (menopause, andropause) are interrelated with the processes of adrenopause and somatopause, which occur in both men and women. Also, functional correlates (muscle size and function, fat and bone mass, progression of atherosclerosis, and changes in cognitive function) have not been related to these changes in endocrine activity. However, a number of effects of normal aging closely resemble features of (isolated) hormonal deficiency (hypogonadism, GH deficiency), which in subjects in middle adulthood are successfully reversed by replacement of the appropriate hormone.[23,24] Although aging does not simply result from a variety of hormone deficiency states, medical intervention in the processes of menopause, andropause,

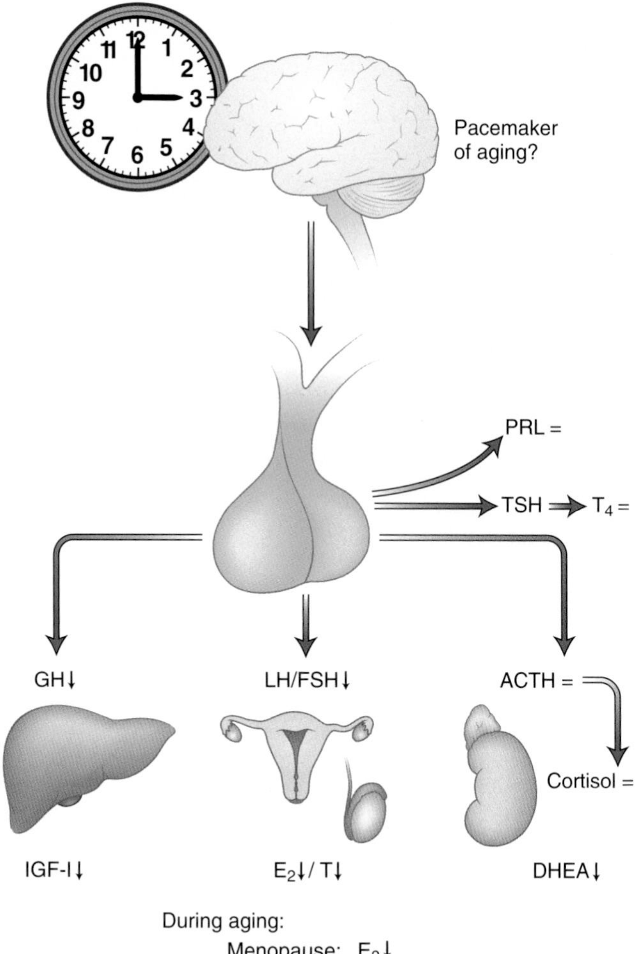

Figure 26–1 ▪ During aging, declines in the activities of a number of hormonal systems occur. **Left,** A decrease in growth hormone (GH) release by the pituitary gland causes a decrease in the production of insulin-like growth factor I (IGF-I) by the liver and other organs (somatopause). **Middle,** A decrease in release of gonadotropin luteinizing hormone (LH) and follicle-stimulating hormone (FSH) and decreased secretion at the gonadal level (from the ovaries, decreased estradiol [E_2]; from the testicle, decreased testosterone [T]) cause menopause and andropause, respectively. (Immediately after the initiation of menopause, serum LH and FSH levels increase sharply.) **Right,** The adrenocortical cells responsible for the production of dehydroepiandrosterone (DHEA) decrease in activity (adrenopause) without clinically evident changes in corticotropin (adrenocorticotropic hormone; ACTH) and cortisol secretion. A central pacemaker in the hypothalamus or higher brain areas (or both) is hypothesized, which together with changes in the peripheral organs (the ovaries, testicles, and adrenal cortex) regulates the aging process of these endocrine axes. *PRL,* Prolactin; *T_4,* thyroxine; *TSH,* thyrotropin.

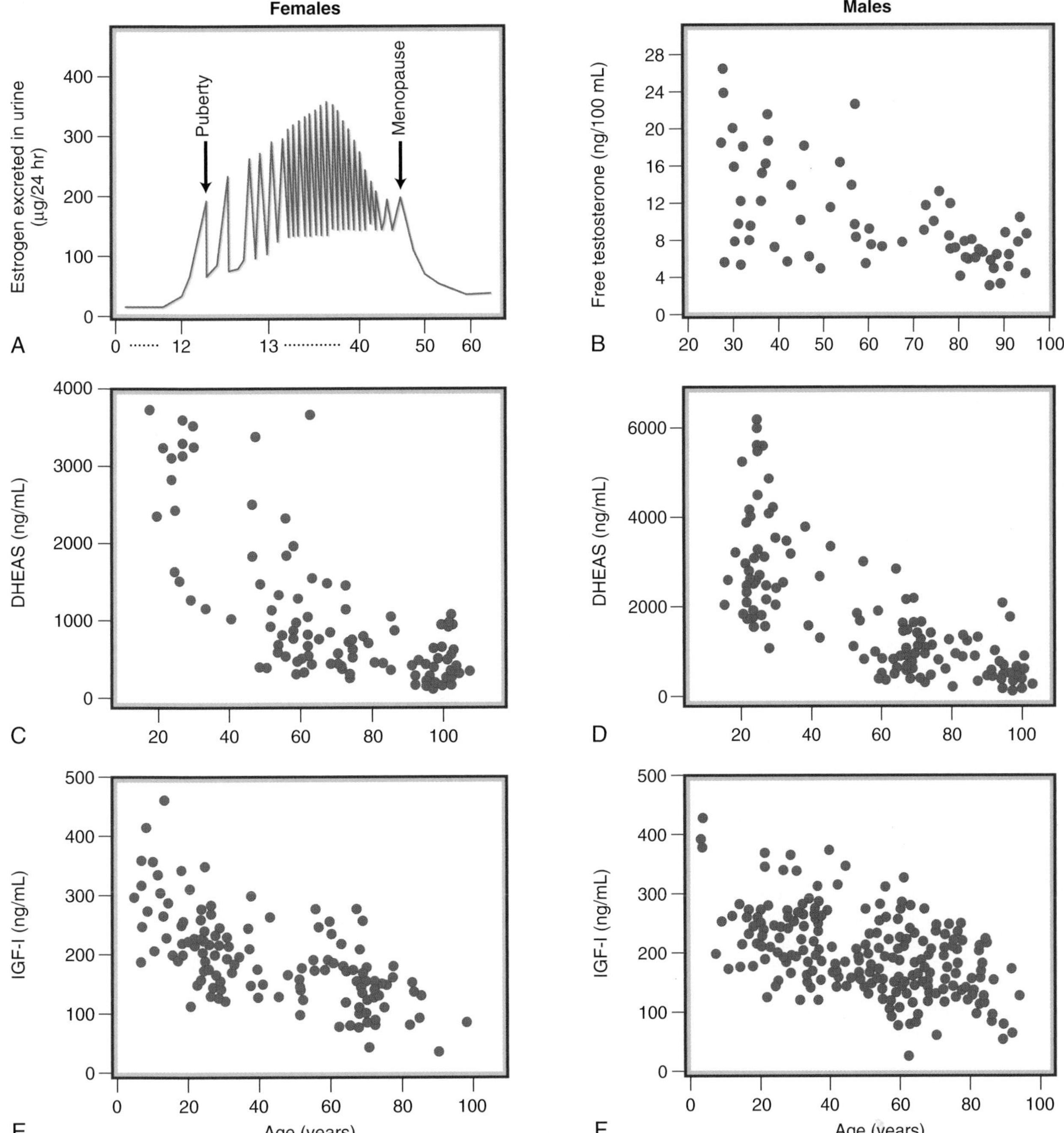

Figure 26–2 ▪ Changes in the hormone levels of normal women *(left)* and men *(right)* during the aging process. Estrogen secretion throughout an individual normal woman's life (expressed as urinary estrogen excretion) **(A)** and mean free testosterone (T) index (the ratio of serum total T to sex hormone–binding globulin levels) during the life span of healthy men **(B).** (From Guyton A. Textbook of Medical Physiology, 8th ed. Philadelphia: WB Saunders, 1991:899.)

Serum dehydroepiandrosterone sulfate (DHEAS) concentrations in 114 healthy women **(C)** and 163 healthy men **(D).** (Adapted from Ravaglia G, Forti P, Maioli F, et al. The relationship of dehydroepiandrosterone sulfate [DHEAS] to endocrine-metabolic parameters and functional status in the oldest-old. Results from an Italian study on healthy free-living over-ninety-year-olds. J Clin Endocrinol Metab 1996;81[3]:1173.)

The course of serum insulin-like growth factor I (IGF-I) concentrations in 131 healthy women **(E)** and 223 healthy men **(F)** during aging. Note the difference in the distribution of ages in the different panels. (Adapted from Corpas E, Harman SM, Blackman MR. Human growth hormone and human aging. Endocr Rev 1993;14[1]:20.)

adrenopause, or somatopause might prevent or delay some aspects of the aging process.

Menopause

Menopause is the permanent cessation of menstruation resulting from the loss of ovarian follicular function and is diagnosed retrospectively after 12 months of amenorrhea.

In most women, vasomotor reactions, depressed mood, and urogenital complaints accompany this period of estrogen decline. In the subsequent years, the loss of estrogens is followed by a high incidence of cardiovascular disease, loss of bone mass, and cognitive impairment. The average age of menopause (51.4 years) has not changed over time and seems to be largely determined by genetic factors.

Perimenopausal Use of Hormone Therapy

Typical symptoms that result from the sudden decrease in estrogen production around menopause are menstrual cycle disorders, vasomotor changes (hot flushes, night sweats), and urogenital complications (atrophic vaginal irritation and dryness, dyspareunia, atrophic urethral epithelium leading to micturition disorders). Additional symptoms are irritability, mood swings, joint pain, and sleep disturbances. Frequency, severity, onset, and duration of symptoms vary widely between individuals and between ethnic groups. About 75% of women in Western societies experience so few troublesome symptoms during the menopausal transition that hormone therapy (HT) is not needed or requested.[25]

HT rapidly alleviates the symptoms of menopause. Hot flushes and vasomotor instability as well as symptoms of urogenital atrophy rapidly disappear upon the start of HT.

Long-Term Hormone Replacement Therapy

Because life expectancy is increasing, the time a woman spends after menopause constitutes more than one third of her life. Until recently long-term use of HT (5 to 10 years) was considered to offer advantages with regard to the prevention of the three chronic disorders most common in the elderly: cardiovascular diseases, osteoporosis, and dementia. In the early 1990s, a number of cross-sectional and prospective studies demonstrated a statistically significant reduction in coronary heart disease in menopausal women taking HT. Grady and colleagues[26] presented a meta-analysis of published observational studies and reported that HT was associated with one-third less fatal coronary heart disease. A meta-analysis of 25 observational studies conducted between 1976 and 1996 showed that the relative risk for coronary heart disease in women who ever used HT compared with never-users was 0.70.[27]

The Nurse's Health Study was a comprehensive investigation conducted in 121,700 female nurses age 30 to 55 years. In the latest report, compiled with data from 70,533 postmenopausal nurses followed up for 20 years, the overall risk of coronary heart disease in current users of HT was reduced, with a relative risk of 0.61.[28]

Over the past 5 years, however, findings from a number of prospective, randomized, controlled trials have fully changed the attitudes concerning benefits and harms of HT. The Women's Health Initiative (WHI) trial comprised two large randomized placebo-controlled clinical trials, including estrogen-only and combined estrogen-progestin studies in more than 161,000 "healthy" postmenopausal women age 50 to 79 years.[29] It was expected that the WHI, which was scheduled to be completed in 2005, would definitely answer whether or not estrogen is cardioprotective. However, the estrogen-progestin versus placebo trial, which involved more than 16,000 women, was discontinued in 2002, because of an increase in cardiovascular complications (coronary heart disease, stroke, and venous thromboembolism) as well as an increased incidence of breast cancer in the treatment group.[29] Although important benefits were also seen (risk reduction for fractures and colon cancer), there was concern that the risks of combined estrogen-progestin outweighed the benefits. The estrogen-only versus placebo trial included nearly 11,000 women who had undergone hysterectomy and therefore did not require a progestin. This trial was also stopped early because a small increase in breast cancer and coronary heart disease risk was seen, while hip fracture risk was reduced.[30]

Three other randomized controlled trials supported the absence of benefit of HT for prevention of coronary heart disease and ischemic stroke.[31-33] These studies were carried out in postmenopausal women with documented ischemic stroke or transient ischemic attack,[31] in women after documented myocardial infarction,[32] or in women with documented coronary heart disease.[33]

Taken together, the WHI, which studied women presumed healthy at recruitment, and the three other trials carried out in women with documented cardiovascular disorders argue strongly against the earlier assumptions made on the basis of observational studies that estrogen users had a 30% to 40% reduced risk of coronary heart disease mortality and morbidity relative to nonusers.

A series of commentaries has addressed the differences in findings between the observational studies and the randomized trials[34,35]: healthy user bias, the age at which study participants started HT, the different estrogen and progestin preparations, and dose all have been mentioned as possible confounders.

Subsequently, a number of studies have confirmed the risk of breast cancer, which increases with longer duration of HT.[36-38] In the Million Women Study, current users of estrogen had an increased risk of incident invasive breast cancer of 30%, whereas in women using estrogen plus progestin this risk had doubled. Past users of HT had no increased risk, however.[39]

Also the earlier expectations from observational studies that estrogen use might prevent cognitive decline were not confirmed by randomized placebo-controlled trials. Estrogen therapy alone did not reduce dementia or mild cognitive impairment in women 65 years of age or older, whereas the estrogen-progestin combination resulted in slightly increased risks for both end-points.[40]

The efficacy of HT in the prevention of osteoporotic fractures remains undisputed, although only few prospective controlled trials have been carried out.[29]

The findings of the WHI trial are so important and have been so broadly publicized that they have created the perception that HT, in general, carries risks that exceed its benefits. Pending further evidence, it is now generally recommended not to use estrogen plus progestin in the prevention of chronic conditions in postmenopausal women. Also the use of estrogen alone in women who have had a hysterectomy is not recommended.

Several authors have summarized the extensive experimental evidence concerning the endothelial, cardiac, and neurologic protective actions of estrogens, and they suggest that more clinical trials should be carried out, mainly involving women participating at the start of menopause. Some evidence supports the concept that the start of menopause is a critical time for initiation of HT.[41]

Given the noted uncertainties, HT is currently only recommended in the perimenopausal period in women suffering from menopausal symptoms. HT is highly effective in alleviating hot flushes and night sweats. An association between endometrial cancer and estrogen use was observed many years ago. Ten years of unopposed estrogen use increases the risk for endometrial cancer 10-fold.[26] For this reason, the HT regimens were supplemented with progestagens, which almost completely prevented this excess risk for endometrial cancer.

Presently advised doses of estrogen were originally designed to prevent bone loss, and progestagen regimens were opposed to prevent endometrial cancer. Several estrogen and progestagen preparations are available for HT.[25] Components of available preparations vary in their effects on different target tissues. Commercial preparations differ in their clinical effect by design, and individual women differ in their responses. HT can be administered orally, transdermally, topically, intranasally, or as subcutaneous implants.

Although HT in the perimenopausal state can cause some symptoms (e.g., vaginal discharge, uterine bleeding, and breast tenderness), it relieves many others including hot flashes and the severity of night sweats.[42] Grady has estimated that about one serious adverse event will occur among every one thousand 50-year-old women using HT for 1 year.[43] The HT regimen used in the WHI trial combined 0.625 mg/day of conjugated equine estrogen and 2.5 mg/day of medroxyprogesterone acetate. The dose of estrogen necessary to diminish perimenopausal symptoms might be lower in many women. Therefore down-titration of the estrogen dose during the 1 or 2 years of HT in the perimenopausal transition is recommended.[44]

Selective Estrogen Receptor Modulators

In the search for optimal hormone replacement therapy during menopause came observations that tamoxifen has variable antiestrogenic and estrogenic actions in different tissues.[45,46] Tamoxifen suppresses the growth of estrogen receptor–positive breast cancer cells. Long-term treatment of menopausal patients with breast cancer with tamoxifen also lowered the incidence of new (contralateral) breast cancer by 40%. In addition, the number of cardiovascular incidents decreased by 70%, and the age-related decrease in bone mineral density was partially prevented.[47-49]

These initially puzzling observations were explained by the fact that tamoxifen and other compounds such as raloxifene have selective estrogen receptor–modulating effects, exerting antiestrogenic actions on normal and cancerous breast tissue but agonistic actions on bone, lipids, and blood vessel walls.[50-52] These effects of tamoxifen and raloxifene may be explained by differential stabilization of the conformation of the estrogen receptor but might also be related to the activation of different estrogen receptor forms, in which the α form is the classical estrogen receptor and the β form mediates the vascular and bone effects of estrogens.[53,54]

Raloxifene is the second selective estrogen receptor modulator (SERM) available for clinical use in menopausal women. It demonstrates estrogen agonist activity on bone and lipid metabolism and has estrogen antagonist activity in uterine and breast tissue. The 60-mg dose is currently approved for the prevention and treatment of postmenopausal osteoporosis.

The efficacy and safety of raloxifene for the prevention of osteoporosis in postmenopausal women were proved in a study that demonstrated a 2.5% increase in bone mineral density in the lumbar spine and hip in a group of postmenopausal nonosteoporotic women treated with raloxifene for 2 years.[55] A significant reduction of vertebral fracture risk by raloxifene was subsequently demonstrated.[56] A total of 7705 postmenopausal women with existing osteoporosis were studied. After 36 months, bone mineral density at the hip and spine increased in the women treated with 60 mg of raloxifene by 2.1% and 2.6%, respectively, compared with those receiving placebo. At 36 months, 7.4% of women had at least one new vertebral fracture, including 10.1% of women receiving placebo and 6.6% of those receiving raloxifene at 60 mg/day. Compared with the placebo group, those receiving 60 mg of raloxifene had a relative risk for fracture of 0.7 ($P < .001$). Forty-six subjects needed raloxifene at 60 mg for 3 years to prevent one vertebral fracture in menopausal women without an existing fracture; for those with an existing fracture, 16 subjects required treatment.

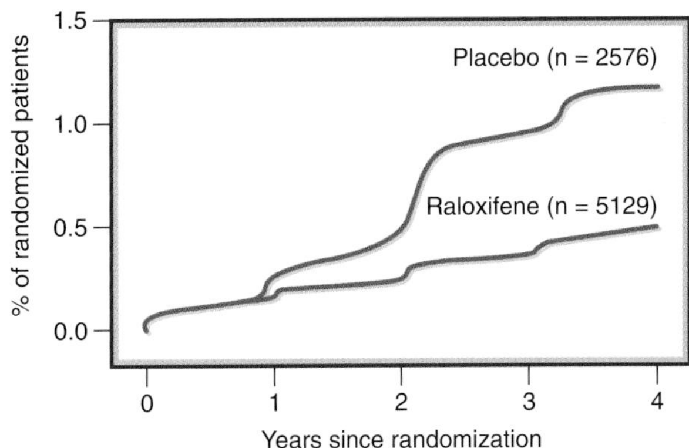

Figure 26–3 ▪ Effect of raloxifene administration (60 to 120 mg/day) on the cumulative incidence of breast cancer in 7705 postmenopausal women (mean age, 66.5 years) with osteoporosis. Statistical significance of the difference between the groups was $P < .001$. (From Cummings SR, Eckert S, Krueger KA, et al. The effect of raloxifene on risk of breast cancer in postmenopausal women: results from the MORE randomized trial. Multiple Outcomes of Raloxifene Evaluation. JAMA 1999;281[23]:2189.)

Raloxifene has effects on lipids similar to those of estrogen, except for a relatively small effect on high-density lipoprotein cholesterol and no significant effect on triglycerides.[55,57] Data on cardiovascular event rates and on cognitive function are not yet available.

Raloxifene, in contrast to tamoxifen and estrogen, does not stimulate endometrial thickness or vaginal bleeding.[55,57] With regard to side effects, raloxifene causes an increased incidence of leg cramps and hot flashes.[58]

A most promising effect of raloxifene is its chemoprotective action against breast cancer. Cummings and colleagues[59] reported the effects in 7705 postmenopausal women (mean age, 66.5 years) with osteoporosis who were treated for a median of 40 months with placebo or raloxifene at 60 or 120 mg/day. Thirteen cases of breast cancer were confirmed among the women assigned to raloxifene compared with 27 among the women assigned to placebo (relative risk 0.24; $P < .001$). To prevent one case of breast cancer, 126 women would need to be treated. Raloxifene decreased the risk of estrogen receptor–positive breast cancer by 90% but did not affect the risk of estrogen receptor–negative invasive breast cancer. This important study demonstrated that among postmenopausal women with osteoporosis, the risk of invasive breast cancer was decreased by 76% during 3 years of treatment with raloxifene (Fig. 26–3).

Androgen Replacement

In premenopausal women, androgen production originates equally from the adrenal glands and the ovaries. Androgen production in women declines with aging. After menopause, circulating androgen levels decrease by more than 50%.

At present there is increasing awareness of the impact of low androgen levels on emotional and sexual well-being in perimenopausal women. No single androgen level is predictive of low female sexual function and, in a study of 1423 women age 18 to 75 years with low DHEAS levels, the majority had normal sexual function.[60]

No large, randomized, placebo-controlled studies with androgens to determine the efficacy and safety in healthy menopausal women with low sexual desire have been reported. Smaller studies in oophorectomized women indeed point to improved sexual function and decreased distress, for example, after 24 weeks of therapy with concomitant estrogen and testosterone (300 μg/day in a patch).[61]

Hormone Therapy, Selective Estrogen Receptor Modulators, or No Treatment?

The issue of hormonal therapy in postmenopausal women is controversial, and many aspects remain unresolved. The idea that HT is a global risk reduction strategy has been abandoned. Although the general benefits of HT in the short term during and after the menopausal transition are present in women suffering from estrogen-withdrawal symptoms, the balance of the effects of long-term HT after menopause points to a negative outcome with more harm than benefits.

Currently, a vast armamentarium of pharmacologic treatments to reduce cardiovascular and bone risks is available; these include cholesterol-lowering statins, β-blockers, SERMs, and bisphosphonates. An optimal choice of these different lifestyle drugs for menopausal women requires individualization of the treatment decision. Coronary artery disease, for example, is a complex disorder, resulting from an interaction of genetic predisposition and environmental factors. Risk factor modification (diet, smoking, physical activity) should be advised. Secondary prevention of coronary artery disease and atherosclerosis includes lipid-lowering drugs, aspirin, nitrates, and β-blockers.[62]

For women with existing osteoporosis, HT is effective. However, SERMs and bisphosphonates come close in their fracture-reducing effects. Recognition of an increased risk for breast cancer in menopausal women is an important consideration in the choice for SERMs. If the impressive preventive effect of raloxifene on breast cancer is confirmed to last longer than 3 years, chemoprevention of breast cancer will probably become a major consideration in the pharmacologic choice for risk reduction in the long-term preventive treatment of postmenopausal women.

Andropause

Role of Testosterone During Aging

Age-associated hypogonadism does not develop as clearly in men at andropause as in women at menopause. The key difference is the gradual, often subtle change in androgen levels in men versus the precipitate fall of estrogen production in women. It is generally agreed that as men age, there is a decline in serum total testosterone concentration that begins after the age of 40 years. In cross-sectional studies, the annual decline in total and free testosterone is 1.0% and 1.2%, respectively. The higher decline in free testosterone levels is related to the increase in sex hormone–binding globulin (SHBG) levels with age.[15,63]

It remains unclear whether the well-known biologic changes occurring during aging in men (e.g., reduced sexual activity, reduced muscle mass and strength, and skeletal mineralization) are causally related to these changes in testosterone bioactivity. The decline in testosterone levels, when associated with signs and symptoms of androgen deficiency, has been called *andropause,* but this term might be better replaced by *(partial) androgen deficiency of the aging male* ([P]ADAM), because androgen production in the elderly male does not cease, but gradually decreases.

In recent years there has been major disagreement on how to define androgen deficiency in the elderly male. Investigators have generally taken two approaches: one is purely biochemical, whereas the other is clinical.

The biochemical approach consists of defining androgen deficiency with the use of testosterone measurements, choosing percentile cutoff values (e.g., 2.5th percentile) from young normal males to determine prevalence.[64,65] Harman and colleagues[65] measured total testosterone and SHBG levels in a study in 890 men in the Baltimore Longitudinal Study on Aging. They observed significant health factor–independent age-related decrease in both total and free testosterone levels, with an average of −0.124 nmol testosterone per year. Using total testosterone criteria of less than 11.3 nmol/L (<325 ng/dL) about 20% of men older than 60 years, 30% older than 70 years, and 50% older than 80 years of age were hypogonadal. Using the free testosterone index, even greater percentages of hypogonadal elderly men were diagnosed. The most important problem with this biochemical statistical approach is that men with low testosterone levels may not exhibit clinically significant symptoms, raising the possibility that large numbers of men, simply by virtue of falling below an arbitrary threshold, are diagnosed as candidates for testosterone replacement therapy.

Also the clinical approach to the diagnosis of androgen deficiency of the aging male has important drawbacks.[66] All symptoms and signs of androgen deficiency are nonspecific and readily accounted for by comorbidities. Lethargy, reduced concentration, sleep disturbance, irritability, and depressed mood may relate to physical illness (and side effects of treatment), obesity, and/or lack of physical exercise, and other lifestyle issues (e.g., alcohol or drug use), relationship difficulties, and occupational or financial stresses. Indeed, existing screening tools for androgen deficiency lack adequate specificity and sensitivity to be reliably employed directing clinical diagnosis and treatment.

Araujo and colleagues[67] recently for the first time attempted to estimate the prevalence and incidence of androgen deficiency in healthy elderly males in a prospective longitudinal study using diagnostic criteria based on clinical as well as biochemical parameters. Their study included eight clinical features (loss of libido, erectile dysfunction, depression, lethargy, inability to concentrate, sleep disturbance, irritability, and depressed mood), along with serum total and (calculated) free testosterone concentrations. Data on androgen deficiency (defined using both signs and symptoms plus total and free testosterone) were at baseline for 1691 men and at follow-up after a mean of 8.8 years for 1087 men. Crude and age-specific prevalence and incidence rates were calculated. Based on these estimates, projections for the number of cases of androgen deficiency in the 40- to 69-year-old U.S. male population were computed. Estimates of the crude prevalence of androgen deficiency at baseline and follow-up were 6.0% and 12.3%, respectively. Prevalence increased significantly with age. From baseline age-specific prevalence data, it is estimated that there are approximately 2.4 million 40- to 69-year-old U.S. males with androgen deficiency, whereas 481,000 new cases of androgen deficiency per year can be expected in U.S. men age 40 to 69 years old.

Testosterone Replacement Therapy

Many persuasive reports in the literature demonstrate that testosterone replacement in men of all ages (young, adult, and old) with clear clinical and biochemical hypogonadism instantly reverses vasomotor activity (flushes and sweats); improves libido, sexual activity, and mood; increases muscle mass, strength, and bone mineralization; prevents fractures; decreases fat mass; and decreases fatigue and poor concentration.[23,63,68]

Also, the treatment of normal adult men with supraphysiologic doses of testosterone, especially when combined with resistance exercise training, increased fat-free mass and muscle size and strength.[69]

Most studies reporting the results of androgen therapy in older men were small, short-term, noncontrolled, and without uniform end-points. The results of a large randomized study in healthy elderly men have now been published and seem representative for effects expected of androgen therapy.[70,71] Ninety-six men (mean age, 73 years) wore a testosterone patch on their scrotum (6 mg of testosterone per 24 hours) or a placebo patch for 36 months. Mean serum testosterone concentrations in the men treated with testosterone increased from 12.7 ± 2.9 nmol/L (367 ± 7.9 ng/dL) before treatment to 21.7 ± 8.6 nmol/L (625 ± 249 ng/dL; $P < .001$) at 6 months of treatment and remained at that level for the duration of the study. The decrease in fat mass (−3.0 ± 0.5 kg) in the testosterone-treated men during the 36 months of treatment was significantly different from the decrease (−0.7 ± 0.5 kg) in the placebo-treated men ($P < .001$) (Fig. 26–4). The increase in lean mass (1.9 ± 0.3 kg) in the testosterone-treated men was significantly different from that in the placebo-treated men (0.2 ± 0.2 kg; $P < .001$).

Changes in knee extension and flexion strength, handgrip, walking speed, and other parameters of muscle strength and function were not significantly different in the two groups. Bone mineral density in the lumbar spine increased in both the testosterone-treated (4.2% ± 0.8%) and placebo-treated (2.5% ± 0.6%) groups, but mean changes did not differ between groups (see Fig. 26–4). However, the lower the pretreatment serum testosterone concentration, the greater the effects of testosterone treatment on lumbar spine bone density after 36 months ($P = .02$). A minimal effect (0.9 ± 1.0%) of testosterone treatment on bone mineral density was observed in men with a pretreatment serum testosterone concentration of 13.9 nmol/L (400 ng/dL), but an increase of 5.9% ± 2.2% was found in men with a pretreatment testosterone concentration of 6.9 nmol/L (200 ng/dL).

The subjective perception of physical functioning decreased significantly during the 36 months of treatment in the placebo-treated ($P < .001$) but not in the testosterone-treated group. Interestingly, the effect of testosterone treatment on the perception of physical functioning varied inversely with the pretreatment serum testosterone concentration ($P < .01$). There was no significant difference between the two treatment groups with regard to the subjective perception of energy or sexual functions.

With regard to the potential adverse effects of testosterone treatment in healthy elderly men, again the study by Snyder and colleagues[70] seems representative. The mean serum prostate-specific antigen (PSA) concentration did not change during the 36 months of treatment in the placebo-treated group but increased by a relatively small but statistically significant ($P < .001$) amount by 6 months of treatment in the testosterone-treated group and remained relatively stable for the remainder of the study. The urine flow rate, volume of urine in the bladder after voiding, and number of clinically significant prostate events during the 3 years of the study were similar in the two groups. Hemoglobin and hematocrit did not change in the placebo-treated group during treatment, but both increased significantly ($P < .001$) in the testosterone-treated group within 6 months and remained relatively stable for the remainder of the study. Three men treated with testosterone developed persistent erythrocytosis (hemoglobin >17.5 g/dL; hematocrit >52%) during treatment.

Numerous studies of large populations of healthy men have shown a marked rise in the incidence of impotence to more than 50% in men 60 to 70 years old.[72] Although this increased rate occurs in the same age group who show a clear decline in serum (free) testosterone levels, no causal relationships have been demonstrated. In most instances, testosterone replacement therapy in elderly men is not effective for the treatment of loss of libido or impotence in individuals with serum testosterone concentrations within the normal range in age-matched subjects. Other factors, such as atherosclerosis, alcohol consumption, smoking, and the quality of personal relationships, seem to be more important.[73,74] Only in the case of clear

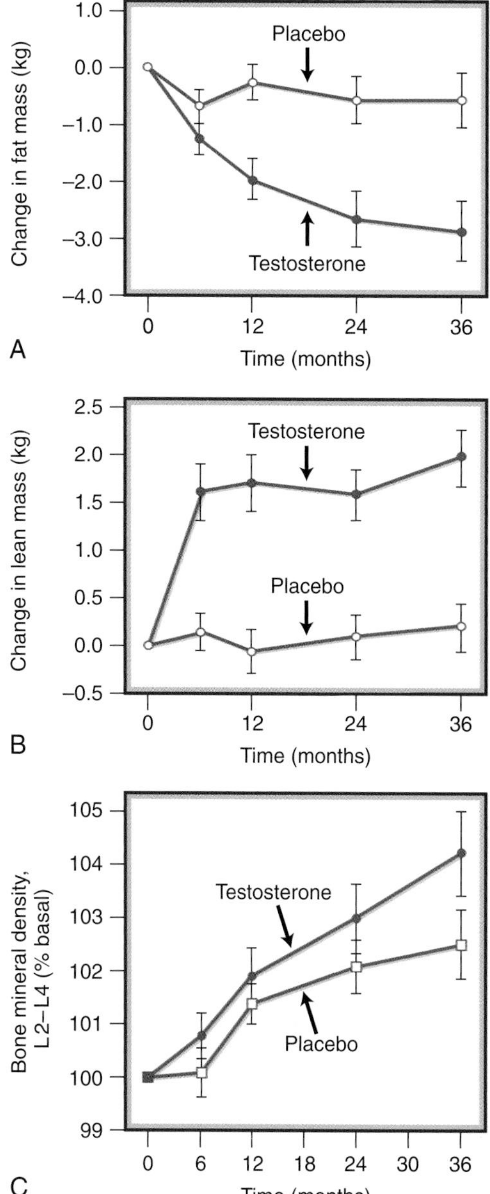

Figure 26–4 ▪ Mean (± standard error) change from baseline in fat mass, lean mass, and bone mineral density of the lumbar spine (L2 to L4) as determined by dual-energy x-ray absorptiometry in 108 men older than 65 years of age who were treated with either testosterone or placebo (54 men each). The decrease in fat mass ($P < .005$) and the increase in lean mass ($P < .01$) in the testosterone-treated subjects were significantly different from those in placebo-treated subjects at 36 months. Bone mineral density increased significantly in both groups. (**A** and **B** from Snyder PJ, Peachey H, Hannoush P, et al. Effect of testosterone treatment on bone mineral density in men over 65 years of age. J Clin Endocrinol Metab 1999;84[6]:1966; **C** from Snyder PJ, Peachey H, Hannoush P, et al. Effect of testosterone treatment on body composition and muscle strength in men over 65 years of age. J Clin Endocrinol Metab 1999;84[8]:2647.)

hypogonadism is the decrease in libido and testosterone restored by potency therapy.[23,68] This result suggests that there is a threshold level of testosterone in the low-normal range below which libido and sexual function are impaired and above which there is no further enhancement of response.[75]

In a review, Liu and colleagues[76] reported the results of a Medline search (years 1966 through January 2004, using search terms *random* and *androgen*) to identify randomized placebo-controlled studies of androgen therapy. These studies show that androgen replacement in unselected older healthy men increases muscle and reduces fat mass to a small degree, but in general has not improved muscle strength, physical function, or insulin sensitivity, nor does it convincingly improve bone density, although the latter effect is particularly dose-responsive.[76] However, idiosyncratic adverse effects, such as disordered sleep and breathing as well as polycythemia, are also dose responsive, suggesting that dose escalation to increase efficacy may create or aggravate undesirable side effects. The authors conclude that, with the current knowledge, androgen supplementation in otherwise healthy elderly males is not recommended.

However, detailed analysis of a number of studies in elderly men selected on the basis of low pretreatment serum testosterone concentrations indicated a beneficial effect of testosterone replacement therapy on muscle strength, bone density, mood, and (subjective) aspects of quality of life.[77-79]

One randomized placebo-controlled trial in 70 men age 65 years or older, who were selected on the basis of a serum testosterone concentration of less than 12.1 nmol/L (less than 350 ng/dL), is particularly relevant. Amory and colleagues[80] and Page and colleagues[81] compared testosterone therapy with or without the administration of finasteride, a 5a-reductase inhibitor that blocks the conversion of testosterone to dihydrotestosterone, particularly in the prostate. Testosterone enanthate, 200 mg intramuscularly every 2 weeks for 36 months with or without 5 mg finasteride daily were compared with placebo administration. After 3 years, testosterone (with or without finasteride) significantly improved functional performance and handgrip strength, while lean body mass (+3.8 kg) as well as bone mineral density at lumbar spine (+10.2 ± 1.4%), and at the hip (+2.7 ± 0.7%) had also significantly increased. Total low-density lipoprotein (LDL) cholesterol levels significantly decreased, without affecting high-density lipoprotein cholesterol.

Although the administration of finasteride in combination with testosterone did not influence these positive effects of testosterone, the 5a-reductase inhibitor prevented the deleterious effects of testosterone on the prostate gland: the small but statistically significant increase in PSA levels after 36 months of testosterone administration was completely prevented by finasteride. Prostate volume increased in all groups over the 3-year study period. The increase in prostate volume in the testosterone-only group was similar to the increase seen in the placebo treatment group, whereas the increase in prostate volume in the testosterone-finasteride group was significantly less than in the testosterone-only group ($P = 0.02$).

These studies[80,81] underline the concept of a beneficial effect of testosterone replacement therapy on muscle strength, physical functioning, and bone mineral density in elderly men with (partial) androgen deficiency. The simultaneous administration of finasteride seemed to protect the effects of testosterone on PSA levels. This proof of principle study, however, needs to be commented upon in further detail. First, the injectable testosterone enanthate used in this study achieves higher average and peak testosterone levels than those achieved in most previous studies, including that by Snyder and colleagues.[70,71] The testosterone regimen used in this trial was associated with a high frequency of erythrocytosis (hematocrit >52%), necessitating to lower the dose of testosterone enanthate from 200 tot 150 mg/2 weeks in 30% of the men assigned to the testosterone group.

Also, despite the improvement in grip strength, no consistent beneficial effect of testosterone administration was measured on lower extremity strength, making the improvement in physical performance difficult to interpret.

In the past there has been concern that testosterone replacement may negatively impact cardiovascular risk in elderly men. In contrast, despite substantial increases in serum testosterone levels, Page and colleagues[81] demonstrate a lowering of total and LDL cholesterol in the testosterone treatment groups. In line with this, Muller and colleagues[82] reported in a group of nearly 200 elderly independently living men (mean age, 78 years) that higher serum free testosterone concentrations were inversely related to the mean progression of the intima-media-thickness of the common carotid artery during a 4-year follow-up. This association was independent of body mass index, waist-to-hip ratio, presence of hypertension and diabetes, smoking, and serum cholesterol levels.

Which Elderly Man Should Be Treated?

A key lesson from the Heart and Estrogen/Progestin Replacement and Women's Health Initiative studies is that conventional medical practice should not precede substantiation with reliable clinical evidence of safety and efficacy.[76] Androgen replacement in older men is the male counterpart of hormonal therapy in postmenopausal women, but differs crucially in that a clear syndrome of androgen deficiency is lacking. The Endocrine Society of Australia and the U.S. Endocrine Society have independently formulated similar recommendations for the biochemical diagnosis of androgen deficiency of older men as well as guidelines for diagnosis and therapy.[76] On the basis of a number of suggestive clinical features collected from the history, symptoms, or signs in an elderly man, the biochemical confirmation of androgen deficiency is sought.

In previous discussions of testosterone replacement in older men,[73,78] it was suggested that the biochemical diagnosis of hypogonadism seems certain if the serum total testosterone concentration is less than 7.0 nmol/L (200 ng/dL). This cutoff remains arbitrary and does not answer the question of whether healthy elderly men with testosterone levels between 7.0 and 10.4 nmol/L are hypogonadal or whether such men would benefit from replacement therapy with testosterone. Also, it has been demonstrated that intercurrent diseases frequently result in a transient, sharp drop in serum testosterone concentrations,[83] whereas frail, elderly men in general tend to have testosterone levels 10% to 15% lower than those of healthy, age-matched control subjects.[84]

When a serum testosterone concentration is found to be below 7.0 nmol/L (200 ng/dL), an additional evaluation with measurements of serum gonadotropins and prolactin is mandatory in order to exclude pituitary pathology.

If one decides to start testosterone replacement, the major goal of therapy is to return testosterone levels to values as close to "physiologic" levels in age-matched controls as possible. The dose should thus be titrated according to serum levels. Considerations concerning the choice of testosterone preparation as well as the route of administration (oral, injectable, implantable, or transdermal) are discussed in Chapter 8.

At present, the duration of testosterone administration is uncertain. Control of prostate size, PSA levels, and hematocrit is mandatory. The identification of elderly men who might benefit most from testosterone treatment remains uncertain, and the risks to the prostate and possible effects on the process of atherosclerosis require further study. The development of androgenic compounds with variable biologic action in different organs (selective androgen receptor modulation) is currently being pursued.[85]

Testosterone effects are mediated via the androgen receptor, and the considerable variation in testosterone responsiveness that is observed between aging males receiving therapy might be related to variations in the androgen receptor gene. A candidate for this variability is the CAG repeat polymorphism in exon 1 of the androgen receptor gene, which is localized on the X chromosome.[86] The CAG repeat encodes for a polyglutamine tract in the androgen receptor protein and ranges normally from about 6 to 37 repeats with an average of between 20 and 22. The number of CAG repeats is inversely associated with the transcriptional activity in testosterone target genes.[86] Krithivas and colleagues[87] demonstrated that the CAG repeat in the androgen receptor gene is associated with the age-related decline in serum testosterone levels in men: the lower the number of repeats, the sharper the decline in serum testosterone concentrations. Also, the lower the number of CAG repeats in normal healthy men, the earlier and higher the degree of prostate hyperplasia during the aging process.[88] Testosterone substitution of hypogonadal adult men for 36 months with a fixed dose showed that prostate size increased significantly more as the number of CAG repeats in the androgen receptor gene was lower.[86] This first pharmacogenetic study demonstrating that the effect of androgen replacement therapy on prostate growth in hypogonadal men is greatly influenced by the genetic background has important implications to its use in otherwise healthy elderly males. Supposedly, androgen sensitivity as determined by variations in the androgen receptor gene of muscle, fat, brain, vessel walls, and the prostate will within one individual be similar. In future selection of aging males for testosterone therapy, the genetic background should probably be taken into account. The same applies to the androgen dose prescribed.

Adrenopause

Role of Dehydroepiandrosterone during Aging

Humans are unique among primates and rodents because the human adrenal cortex secretes large amounts of the steroid precursor DHEA and its sulfate derivative DHEAS.[89] Serum DHEAS concentrations in adult men and women are 100 to 500 times higher than those of testosterone and 1000 to 10,000 times higher than those of estradiol. In normal subjects, serum concentrations of DHEA and its sulfate are highest in the third decade of life, after which the concentrations of both gradually decrease, so that by the age of 70 to 80 years, the values are about 20% of peak values in men and 30% of peak values in women (see Fig. 26–2).[19]

DHEA and DHEAS seem to be inactive precursors that are transformed within human tissues by a complicated network of enzymes into androgens or estrogens, or both (Fig. 26–5). The key enzymes are aromatase, steroid sulfatase, 3β-hydroxysteroid dehydrogenases (3β-HSD-1, -2), and at least seven organ-specific 17β-hydroxysteroid dehydrogenases (17β-HSD-1 to -7). Labrie and colleagues[89] introduced the term *intracrinology* to describe this synthesis of active steroids in peripheral target tissues in which the action is exerted in the same cells in which synthesis takes place, without release into the extracellular space and general circulation.

In postmenopausal women, nearly 100% of sex steroids are synthesized in peripheral tissues from precursors of adrenal origin except for a small contribution from ovarian or adrenal testosterone and androstenedione. Thus, in postmenopausal women, virtually all active sex steroids are made in target tissues by an intracrine mechanism. In elderly men, the intracrine production of androgens is also important; less than 50% of the androgen supply is derived from testicular production.

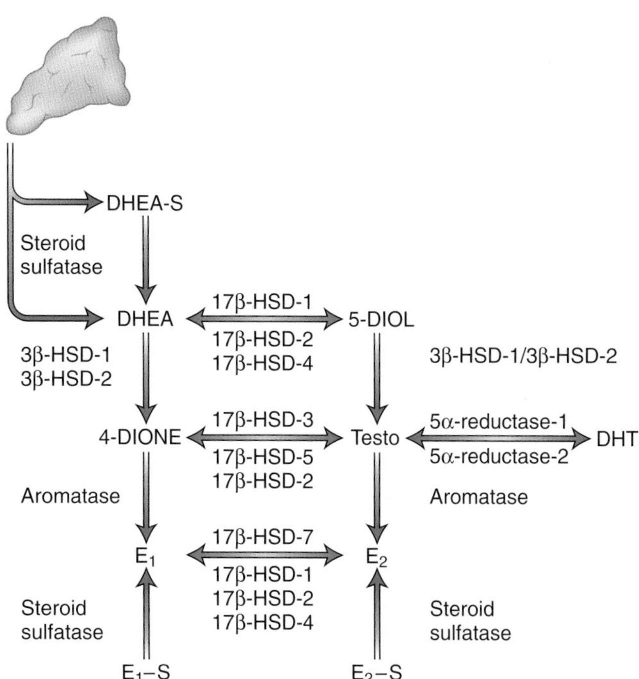

Figure 26–5 ▪ Human steroidogenic enzymes in peripheral intracrine tissues. *DHEA,* Dehydroepiandrosterone; *DHEAS,* DHEA sulfate; *DHT,* dihydrotestosterone; *5-DIOL,* androsterone-5-ene-3β,17β-diol; *4-Dione,* androstenedione; E_1, estrone; E_2, estradiol; *3β-HSD,* 3β-hydroxysteroid dehydrogenase; *17β-HSD,* 17β-hydroxysteroid dehydrogenase; *Testo,* testosterone. (Modified and adapted from Labrie F, Luu-The V, Lin SX, et al. Intracrinology: role of the family of 17 beta-hydroxysteroid dehydrogenases in human physiology and disease. J Mol Endocrinol 2000;25[1]:1.)

The high secretion rate of adrenal precursor sex steroids in men and women differs from that in laboratory animal models, in which the secretion of sex steroids occurs exclusively in the gonads. In rats and mice, long-term administration of DHEA prevented obesity, diabetes mellitus, cancer, and heart disease and enhanced immune function.[18,20,90]

These experimental animal data have been used to argue that DHEA administration in adult or elderly individuals prolongs life span and might be an "elixir of youth." Supportive data in humans are few, however, and highly controversial. Epidemiologic studies indeed point to a mild cardioprotective effect of higher DHEAS levels in both men and women.[91] Functional parameters of activities of daily living in men older than 90 years were lowest in those with the lowest serum DHEAS concentrations,[19] and in healthy elderly individuals there was an association between the ratio of cortisol to DHEAS levels and cognitive impairment.[92]

Dehydroepiandrosterone Replacement Therapy

Several randomized placebo-controlled studies demonstrated that oral administration of DHEA was beneficial.[93-95] Three months of daily treatment with 50 mg of DHEA in 20 healthy adults, most of whom were not elderly, increased serum DHEA and DHEAS concentrations to young adult levels, increased androgen and IGF-I concentrations, and induced a remarkable increase in perceived physical and psychological well-being in both sexes without an effect on libido (Fig. 26–6).[94] In a subsequent study, treatment with 100 mg of DHEA for 6 months in eight adult men and eight adult women increased lean body

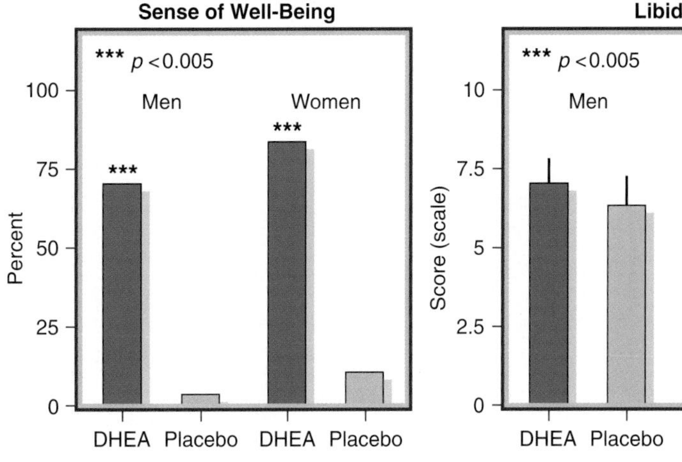

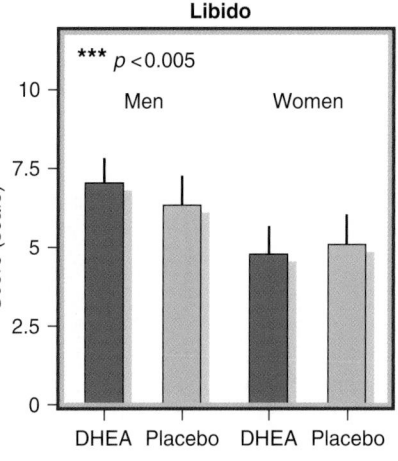

Figure 26–6 ▪ Percentage of healthy adult men and women who reported an improved sense of well-being after 12 weeks of oral administration of 50 mg of DHEA nightly in comparison with placebo: ***$P < .005$ compared with placebo values. Scored values of libido on a Visual Analogue Scale in men and women did not change during DHEA administration. (From Morales AJ, Nolan JJ, Nelson JC, et al. Effects of replacement dose of dehydroepiandrosterone in men and women of advancing age. J Clin Endocrinol Metab 1994;78[6]:1360.)

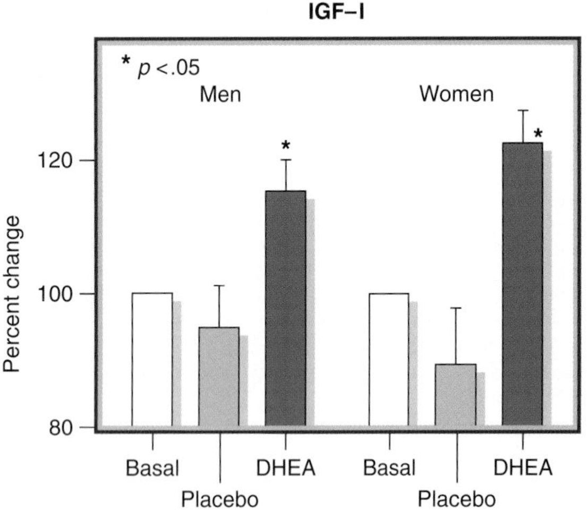

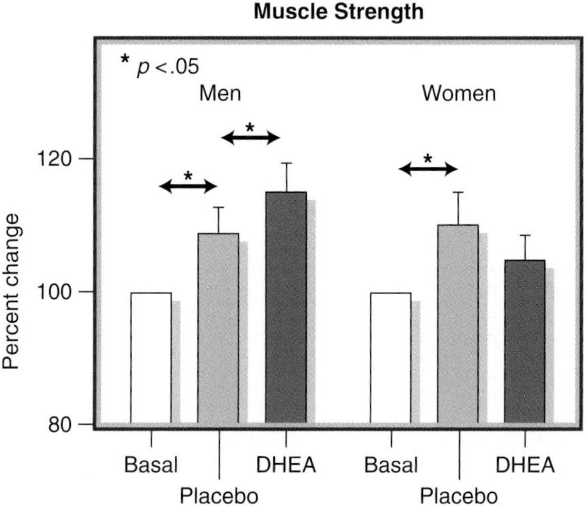

Figure 26–7 ▪ Knee extension-flexion muscle strength at baseline (100%) and percentage change in response to placebo and DHEA (100 mg/day) in aging men (n = 8) and women (n = 8), expressed as number of feet. *$P < .05$, placebo versus baseline; *$P < .05$, DHEA versus placebo. (From Yen SS, Morales AJ, Khorram O. Replacement of DHEA in aging men and women. Potential remedial effects. Ann N Y Acad Sci 1995;774:128.)

mass in both sexes but increased muscle strength only in the men (Fig. 26–7).[95] A number of shorter, well-controlled trials with DHEA subsequently did not demonstrate a clinically significant effect on the parameters just mentioned.[96]

After 280 healthy elderly women and men, age 60 to 79 years, were given DHEA at 50 mg or placebo orally daily for 1 year in a randomized trial, no adverse effects were noted. A significant increase in most parameters related to libido was observed in older women. Improved skin status, including hydration, epidermal thickness, serum production, and pigmentation, was also noted, particularly in women. In women older than 70 years, bone turnover slightly improved as a result of a decrease in osteoclast activity.[97] In another randomized placebo-controlled trial in 56 healthy persons, 6 months of administration of 50 mg/day of DHEA moderately but significantly decreased the visceral fat area (–13 cm^2 vs +3 cm^2, respectively, after placebo; $P = .001$) and subcutaneous fat (–13 cm^2 vs +2 cm^2; $P = .003$).[98]

A physiologic functional role of DHEA in women has been ascertained in a careful double-blind study. In women with adrenal insufficiency,[99] DHEA administration (50 mg/day) normalized serum concentrations of DHEA, DHEAS, androstenedione, and testosterone. DHEA significantly improved overall well-being as well as scores for depression and anxiety, the frequency of sexual thoughts, sexual interest, and satisfaction with both mental and physical aspects of sexuality.

Conclusions

No prospective, long-term, randomized studies of DHEA administration have been carried out in frail elderly people or in the elderly individuals with the lowest serum DHEA and DHEAS concentrations. DHEAS is a universal precursor for the peripheral local production and action of estrogens and androgens in elderly people. The data suggest that serum estradiol concentrations (which might be a surrogate marker for tissue concentrations) and serum luteinizing hormone concentrations (which reflect serum androgen and estrogen activity) demonstrate important positive relations with bone mineral density, quality of life, cognitive decline, and degree of atherosclerosis.[100-102]

The addition of DHEA (50 mg) to the existing large pool of DHEA and DHEAS in unselected elderly individuals has limited clinical effects, especially in elderly women. It is not known whether the increase in sex steroid levels induced by long-term DHEA administration is safe with regard to development of ovarian, prostate, or other types of steroid-dependent cancers. DHEA is currently widely used in the United States as an unapproved treatment against aging. With the scientific verdict still out, without further confirmation of the reported beneficial actions of DHEA in humans, and without a better understanding of its potential risks, it is premature to recommend the routine use of DHEA for delaying or preventing the physiologic consequences of aging.[103,104]

Somatopause

Role of Growth Hormone and Insulin-like Growth Factor I during Aging

Elderly men and women secrete GH less frequently and at lower amplitude than do young people.[21] In fact, GH secretion declines approximately 14% per decade in normal individuals.[105,106] In parallel, serum levels of IGF-I (see Fig. 26–2) are 20% to 80% lower in healthy elderly individuals than in healthy young adults.[107] The concept that this decline in GH and IGF-I secretion contributes to the decline of functional capacity in elderly people (somatopause) is mainly derived from studies in which GH replacement therapy in GH-deficient adults was shown to increase muscle mass, muscle strength, bone mass, and the quality of life. A beneficial effect on the lipid profile and an important decrease in fat mass were also observed in these patients.[24,108,109] As in hypogonadal individuals, adult GH deficiency can thus be considered a model of normal aging because a number of catabolic processes that are central in the biology of aging can be reversed by GH replacement.

Several studies of the relationship between body composition and functional capacity and serum IGF-I concentrations demonstrated contradictory results. In a study of healthy individuals of a broad age range, an association was observed between the maximum aerobic capacity and circulating IGF-I levels.[110] However, no relationship with IGF-I was demonstrated in a group of highly active older people when grip strength, physical performance, and cognitive state were measured.[111,112]

Growth Hormone Replacement Therapy

Rudman and colleagues,[113] after a ground-breaking randomized controlled trial in healthy men 61 to 81 years old with serum IGF-I concentrations in the lower third for their age, reported in 1990 that GH treatment (30 μg/kg three times weekly for 6 months) restored the men's IGF-I levels to "normal." In the treatment group, lean body mass rose by 8.8% and lumbar vertebral density increased by 1.6%. The magnitudes of these initial changes were equivalent to a reversal of the age-related changes by 10 to 20 years. However, during continuation of this study to 12 months, the significant positive effect on bone mineral density at any site was lost.[114]

In the subsequent years, it became clear that GH administration in healthy elderly individuals frequently caused acute adverse effects such as carpal tunnel syndrome, gynecomastia, fluid retention, and hyperglycemia, which were severe enough for an appreciable number of individuals to drop out of these studies. The most disappointing aspect, however, was that no positive effects of GH administration were observed on muscle strength, maximal oxygen consumption, or functional capacity. (In contrast, when GH was administered in combination with resistance exercise training, a significant positive effect on muscle mass and muscle strength was recorded that did not differ from that seen with placebo treatment, which suggests that GH does not add to the beneficial effects of exercise.[115,116] A representative example of a well-controlled study[117] of GH administration in unselected elderly men is given in Table 26–1.

Recently Blackman and colleagues[118] studied in a randomized controlled trial the effect of a combination of GH and sex steroids in healthy elderly women and men. A slight increase in lean body mass and muscle strength was observed in elderly men, but side effects were numerous.

Earlier studies demonstrated that pharmacologic doses of GH prevent the *autocannibalistic* effects of acute diseases on muscle mass.[119] Confirmation is needed, however, before GH can gain a place in the treatment of acute catabolic states in frail elderly people.

Other components in the regulation of the GH-IGF-I axis are effective in activating GH and IGF-I secretion. Long-acting derivatives of the hypothalamic peptide growth hormone-releasing hormone (GHRH), given twice daily subcutaneously for 14 days to healthy 70-year-old men, increased GH and IGF-I levels to those encountered in 35-year-olds.[21] These studies suggest that

TABLE 26–1 EFFECTS OF GROWTH HORMONE ADMINISTRATION (30 μg/kg THREE TIMES A WEEK) FOR 6 MONTHS IN 52 HEALTHY MEN (69 YEARS) WITH WELL-PRESERVED FUNCTIONAL ABILITY BUT LOW LEVELS OF INSULIN-LIKE GROWTH FACTOR I

	Mean Change In Variable		
	GH (n = 26)	**Placebo (n = 26)**	***P* Value**
IGF-I (ng/mL)	119.2	7.6	<.0001
Body weight and composition			
Weight, kg	0.5	1.0	>.2
Lean mass, %	4.3	−0.1	<.001
Fat mass, %	−13.1	−0.3	<.001
Bone mineral content, %	0.9	−0.1	.05
Skin thickness, %	13.4	1.1	.09
Muscle strength, %			
Knee extension	3.8	1.3	>.2
Knee flexion	10.0	8.2	>.2
Hand grip	−1.5	3.8	.11
Maximum oxygen consumption, %	2.5	−2.0	>.2

GH, growth hormone; IGF-I, insulin-like growth factor I.
From Papadakis MA, Grady D, Black D, et al. Growth hormone replacement in healthy older men improves body composition but not functional ability. Ann Intern Med 1996;124:708-716.

somatopause is driven primarily by the hypothalamus and that pituitary somatotropes retain their capacity to synthesize and secrete high levels of GH.

GH-releasing peptides (GHRPs) are oligopeptides with even more powerful GH-releasing effects.[120] They were originally developed by design. Their effects on GH secretion are mediated through endogenous specific receptors.[121,122] Nonpeptide analogues (e.g., MK-677 and L-692,429) have powerful GH-releasing effects, restoring IGF-I secretion in older adults to levels typical of young adults.[123,124] Long-term oral administration of MK-677 to healthy elderly individuals increased lean body mass but not muscle strength. If proven to be GH-specific, these orally active GHRP derivatives might be important alternatives to subcutaneously administered GH for studies of the reversal of somatopause, prevention of frailty, and reversal of acute catabolism.[125]

The long-term safety of activating GH and IGF-I levels in older people has become a concern because of reports of an association between serum IGF-I concentrations and cancer risk. Individuals with high IGF-I levels (or low IGF-binding protein 3 levels) within the broad normal range have an increased risk of prostate, colon, and breast cancer.[126-128] These epidemiologic studies, together with experimental data, suggest that the IGF-I system is involved in tumor development and progression. However, no causal relationship between IGF-I levels and cancer risk has yet been established, and possible medical intervention directed at increasing IGF-I bioactivity in elderly people will in most instances be given toward the end of life, presumably not allowing enough time to affect tumor development or progression.

Conclusions

During the aging process, GH–IGF-I axis activity declines. It is unclear whether changes in body composition and functional capacity are directly related. GH administration in older adults causes an increase in lean body mass and an appreciable loss of fat mass. However, the very limited ability of GH treatment to improve muscle strength and functional capacity in elderly people, despite restoration of circulating IGF-I concentrations to young adult levels, limits its application. Furthermore, most dose regimens of GH cause appreciable adverse effects, and long-term safety with regard to tumor development and progression remains uncertain. GHRP and its orally active analogues are capable of restoring GH and IGF-I levels in the elderly population.

In the near future, clinical trials with such orally active molecules in frail elderly people or in elderly individuals with clearly lowered IGF-I levels, or both, should be able to delineate the precise role of the GH-IGF-I axis in the aging process. In such trials, much emphasis must be given to safety aspects. At present, there is insufficient evidence to recommend medical intervention in the GH-IGF-I axis to rejuvenate healthy elderly people.[125,129,130] Only elderly patients with GH deficiency caused by organic diseases, such as pituitary adenomas, clearly benefit from GH replacement therapy.[131]

The Concept of Successful Aging

There is considerable variation in the effects of aging on healthy individuals, with some people exhibiting greater and others evidencing few or no age-related alterations in physiologic functions. It has been suggested that it might be useful to distinguish between usual and successful patterns of aging.[132] Genetic factors, lifestyle, and societal investments in a safe and healthful environment are important aspects of successful aging.[133] Traditionally, the aging process, including the development of physical frailty toward the end of life, has been considered physiologic and unavoidable.

It has recently become evident, however, that it might not be necessary to accept the grim stereotype of aging as an unalterable process of decline and loss.[132] As life expectancy rises further in the coming decades, the overarching goal should be "an increase in years of healthy life with a full range of functional capacity at each stage of life."[134] Such a compression of morbidity can be achieved by adapting lifestyle measures, but a number of aspects of the aging process of the endocrine system invite the development of routine medical intervention programs offering long-term replacement therapy with one or more hormones in order to delay the aging process and to allow humans to live for a longer period in a relatively intact state.[135]

REFERENCES

1. Fries JF. Aging, natural death, and the compression of morbidity. N Engl J Med 1980;303(3):130.
2. Campion EW. The oldest old. N Engl J Med 1994;330(25):1819.
3. Kosorok MR, Omenn GS, Diehr P, et al. Restricted activity days among older adults. Am J Public Health 1992;82(9):1263.
4. Moss AJ, Parsons VL. Current estimates from the National Health Interview Survey. United States, 1985. Vital Health Stat 1986; 10(160):i.
5. Brody JA. Prospects for an ageing population. Nature 1985; 315(6019):463.
6. Rudman D, Rao MP. Serum insulin-like growth factor I in healthy older men in relation to physical activity. In Morley JE, Korenman SG, eds. Endocrinology and Metabolism in the Elderly. Oxford: Blackwell Scientific, 1992:50.
7. Buchner DM, Wagner EH. Preventing frail health. Clin Geriatr Med 1992;8(1):1.
8. Tinetti ME, Speechley M, Ginter SF. Risk factors for falls among elderly persons living in the community. N Engl J Med 1988;319(26):1701.
9. Kallman DA, Plato CC, Tobin JD. The role of muscle loss in the age-related decline of grip strength: cross-sectional and longitudinal perspectives. J Gerontol 1990;45(3):M82.
10. Fiatarone MA, O'Neill EF, Ryan ND, et al. Exercise training and nutritional supplementation for physical frailty in very elderly people. N Engl J Med 1994;330(25):1769.
11. Guralnik JM, Ferrucci L, Simonsick EM, et al. Lower-extremity function in persons over the age of 70 years as a predictor of subsequent disability. N Engl J Med 1995;332(9):556.
12. Peters AL. Aging and diabetes. In Alberti KGMM ZP, Defrozo RA, eds. International Textbook of Diabetes Mellitus. Chichester, UK: John Wiley & Sons, 1997:1151.
13. Mariotti S, Franceschi C, Cossarizza A, et al. The aging thyroid. Endocr Rev 1995;16(6):686.
14. Wise PM, Krajnak KM, Kashon ML. Menopause: the aging of multiple pacemakers. Science 1996;273(5271):67.
15. Vermeulen A. Clinical review 24: androgens in the aging male. J Clin Endocrinol Metab 1991;73(2):221.
16. Harman SM, Tsitouras PD. Reproductive hormones in aging men. I. Measurement of sex steroids, basal luteinizing hormone, and Leydig cell response to human chorionic gonadotropin. J Clin Endocrinol Metab 1980;51(1):35.
17. Harman SM, Tsitouras PD, Costa PT, et al. Reproductive hormones in aging men. II. Basal pituitary gonadotropins and gonadotropin responses to luteinizing hormone-releasing hormone. J Clin Endocrinol Metab 1982;54(3):547.
18. Herbert J. The age of dehydroepiandrosterone. Lancet 1995; 345(8959):1193.
19. Ravaglia G, Forti P, Maioli F, et al. The relationship of dehydroepiandrosterone sulfate (DHEAS) to endocrine-metabolic parameters and functional status in the oldest-old. Results from an Italian study on healthy free-living over-ninety-year-olds. J Clin Endocrinol Metab 1996;81(3):1173.
20. Hornsby PJ. Biosynthesis of DHEAS by the human adrenal cortex and its age-related decline. Ann N Y Acad Sci 1995;774:29.
21. Corpas E, Harman SM, Pineyro MA, et al. Growth hormone (GH)-releasing hormone-(1-29) twice daily reverses the decreased GH

and insulin-like growth factor-I levels in old men. J Clin Endocrinol Metab 1992;75(2):530.
22. Blackman MR. Pituitary hormones and aging. Endocrinol Metab Clin North Am 1987;16(4):981.
23. Wang C, Swedloff RS, Iranmanesh A, et al. Transdermal testosterone gel improves sexual function, mood, muscle strength, and body composition parameters in hypogonadal men. Testosterone Gel Study Group. J Clin Endocrinol Metab 2000;85(8):2839.
24. Attanasio AF, Lamberts SW, Matranga AM, et al. Adult growth hormone (GH)-deficient patients demonstrate heterogeneity between childhood onset and adult onset before and during human GH treatment. Adult Growth Hormone Deficiency Study Group. J Clin Endocrinol Metab 1997;82(1):82.
25. Barrett-Connor E. Hormone replacement therapy. BMJ 1998; 317(7156):457.
26. Grady D, Rubin SM, Petitti DB, et al. Hormone therapy to prevent disease and prolong life in postmenopausal women. Ann Intern Med 1992;117(12):1016.
27. Barrett-Connor E, Grady D. Hormone replacement therapy, heart disease, and other considerations. Annu Rev Public Health 1998;19:55.
28. Grodstein F, Manson JE, Colditz GA, et al. A prospective, observational study of postmenopausal hormone therapy and primary prevention of cardiovascular disease. Ann Intern Med 2000; 133(12):933.
29. Rossouw JE, Anderson GL, Prentice RL, et al. Risks and benefits of estrogen plus progestin in healthy postmenopausal women: principal results from the Women's Health Initiative randomized controlled trial. JAMA 2002;288(3):321.
30. Anderson GL, Limacher M, Assaf AR, et al. Effects of conjugated equine estrogen in postmenopausal women with hysterectomy: the Women's Health Initiative randomized controlled trial. JAMA 2004;291(14):1701.
31. Viscoli CM, Brass LM, Kernan WN, et al. A clinical trial of estrogen-replacement therapy after ischemic stroke. N Engl J Med 2001; 345(17):1243.
32. Cherry N, Gilmour K, Hannaford P, et al. Oestrogen therapy for prevention of reinfarction in postmenopausal women: a randomised placebo controlled trial. Lancet 2002;360(9350): 2001.
33. Hulley S, Grady D, Bush T, et al. Randomized trial of estrogen plus progestin for secondary prevention of coronary heart disease in postmenopausal women. Heart and Estrogen/progestin Replacement Study (HERS) Research Group. JAMA 1998; 280(7):605.
34. Dubey RK, Imthurn B, Zacharia LC, et al. Hormone replacement therapy and cardiovascular disease: what went wrong and where do we go from here? Hypertension 2004;44(6):789.
35. Peterson HB, Thacker SB, Corso PS, et al. Hormone therapy: making decisions in the face of uncertainty. Arch Intern Med 2004;164(21):2308.
36. Weiss LK, Burkman RT, Cushing-Haugen KL, et al. Hormone replacement therapy regimens and breast cancer risk. Obstet Gynecol 2002;100(6):1148.
37. Li CI, Malone KE, Porter PL, et al. Relationship between long durations and different regimens of hormone therapy and risk of breast cancer. JAMA 2003;289(24):3254.
38. Chlebowski RT, Hendrix SL, Langer RD, et al. Influence of estrogen plus progestin on breast cancer and mammography in healthy postmenopausal women: the Women's Health Initiative Randomized Trial. JAMA 2003;289(24):3243.
39. Beral V. Breast cancer and hormone-replacement therapy in the Million Women Study. Lancet 2003;362(9382):419.
40. Shumaker SA, Legault C, Kuller L, et al. Conjugated equine estrogens and incidence of probable dementia and mild cognitive impairment in postmenopausal women: Women's Health Initiative Memory Study. JAMA 2004;291(24):2947.
41. Hodis HN, Mack WJ, Lobo RA, et al. Estrogen in the prevention of atherosclerosis. A randomized, double-blind, placebo-controlled trial. Ann Intern Med 2001;135(11):939.
42. Hays J, Ockene JK, Brunner RL, et al. Effects of estrogen plus progestin on health-related quality of life. N Engl J Med 2003; 348(19):1839.
43. Grady D. Postmenopausal hormones—therapy for symptoms only. N Engl J Med 2003;348(19):1835.
44. Hickey M, Davis SR, Sturdee DW. Treatment of menopausal symptoms: what shall we do now? Lancet 2005;366(9483):409.
45. Santen RJ. Long-term tamoxifen therapy: can an antagonist become an agonist? J Clin Endocrinol Metab 1996;81(6):2027.
46. Grainger DJ, Metcalfe JC. Tamoxifen: teaching an old drug new tricks? Nat Med 1996;2(4):381.
47. Love RR, Mazess RB, Barden HS, et al. Effects of tamoxifen on bone mineral density in postmenopausal women with breast cancer. N Engl J Med 1992;326(13):852.
48. Grey AB, Stapleton JP, Evans MC, et al. The effect of the antiestrogen tamoxifen on bone mineral density in normal late postmenopausal women. Am J Med 1995;99(6):636.
49. Rutqvist LE, Mattsson A. Cardiac and thromboembolic morbidity among postmenopausal women with early-stage breast cancer in a randomized trial of adjuvant tamoxifen. The Stockholm Breast Cancer Study Group. J Natl Cancer Inst 1993;85(17):1398.
50. Black LJ, Sato M, Rowley ER, et al. Raloxifene (LY139481 HCI) prevents bone loss and reduces serum cholesterol without causing uterine hypertrophy in ovariectomized rats. J Clin Invest 1994; 93(1):63.
51. Draper MW, Flowers DE, Huster WJ, et al. A controlled trial of raloxifene (LY139481) HCl: impact on bone turnover and serum lipid profile in healthy postmenopausal women. J Bone Miner Res 1996;11(6):835.
52. Yang NN, Bryant HU, Hardikar S, et al. Estrogen and raloxifene stimulate transforming growth factor-beta 3 gene expression in rat bone: a potential mechanism for estrogen- or raloxifene-mediated bone maintenance. Endocrinology 1996;137(5):2075.
53. McDonnell DP, Clemm DL, Hermann T, et al. Analysis of estrogen receptor function in vitro reveals three distinct classes of antiestrogens. Mol Endocrinol 1995;9(6):659.
54. Korach KS, Couse JF, Curtis SW, et al. Estrogen receptor gene disruption: molecular characterization and experimental and clinical phenotypes. Recent Prog Horm Res 1996;51:159.
55. Delmas PD, Bjarnason NH, Mitlak BH, et al. Effects of raloxifene on bone mineral density, serum cholesterol concentrations, and uterine endometrium in postmenopausal women. N Engl J Med 1997;337(23):1641.
56. Ettinger B, Black DM, Mitlak BH, et al. Reduction of vertebral fracture risk in postmenopausal women with osteoporosis treated with raloxifene: results from a 3-year randomized clinical trial. Multiple Outcomes of Raloxifene Evaluation (MORE) Investigators. JAMA 1999;282(7):637.
57. Walsh BW, Kuller LH, Wild RA, et al. Effects of raloxifene on serum lipids and coagulation factors in healthy postmenopausal women. JAMA 1998;279(18):1445.
58. Davies GC, Huster WJ, Lu Y, et al. Adverse events reported by postmenopausal women in controlled trials with raloxifene. Obstet Gynecol 1999;93(4):558.
59. Cummings SR, Eckert S, Krueger KA, et al. The effect of raloxifene on risk of breast cancer in postmenopausal women: results from the MORE randomized trial. Multiple Outcomes of Raloxifene Evaluation. JAMA 1999;281(23):2189.
60. Davis SR, Davison SL, Donath S, et al. Circulating androgen levels and self-reported sexual function in women. JAMA 2005; 294(1):91.
61. Simon J, Braunstein G, Nachtigall L, et al. Testosterone patch increases sexual activity and desire in surgically menopausal women with hypoactive sexual desire disorder. J Clin Endocrinol Metab 2005;90(9):5226.
62. Nabel EG. Coronary heart disease in women—an ounce of prevention. N Engl J Med 2000;343(8):572.
63. Tenover JS. Androgen administration to aging men. Endocrinol Metab Clin North Am 1994;23:877.
64. Vermeulen A, Kaufman JM. Diagnosis of hypogonadism in the aging male. Aging Male 2002;5(3):170.
65. Harman SM, Metter EJ, Tobin JD, et al. Longitudinal effects of aging on serum total and free testosterone levels in healthy men. Baltimore Longitudinal Study of Aging. J Clin Endocrinol Metab 2001;86(2):724.
66. McLachlan RI, Allan CA. Defining the prevalence and incidence of androgen deficiency in aging men: where are the goal posts? J Clin Endocrinol Metab 2004;89(12):5916.
67. Araujo AB, O'Donnell AB, Brambilla DJ, et al. Prevalence and incidence of androgen deficiency in middle-aged and older men:

estimates from the Massachusetts Male Aging Study. J Clin Endocrinol Metab 2004;89(12):5920.
68. Wang C, Eyre DR, Clark R, et al. Sublingual testosterone replacement improves muscle mass and strength, decreases bone resorption, and increases bone formation markers in hypogonadal men—a clinical research center study. J Clin Endocrinol Metab 1996;81(10):3654.
69. Bhasin S, Storer TW, Berman N, et al. The effects of supraphysiologic doses of testosterone on muscle size and strength in normal men. N Engl J Med 1996;335(1):1.
70. Snyder PJ, Peachey H, Hannoush P, et al. Effect of testosterone treatment on bone mineral density in men over 65 years of age. J Clin Endocrinol Metab 1999;84(6):1966.
71. Snyder PJ, Peachey H, Hannoush P, et al. Effect of testosterone treatment on body composition and muscle strength in men over 65 years of age. J Clin Endocrinol Metab 1999;84(8):2647.
72. Pearlman CK, Kobashi LI. Frequency of intercourse in men. J Urol 1972;107(2):298.
73. Bhasin S, Bremner WJ. Clinical review 85: emerging issues in androgen replacement therapy. J Clin Endocrinol Metab 1997;82(1):3.
74. Bagatell CJ, Bremner WJ. Androgens in men—uses and abuses. N Engl J Med 1996;334(11):707.
75. Hayes FJ: Testosterone—fountain of youth or drug of abuse? J Clin Endocrinol Metab 2000;85(9):3020.
76. Liu PY, Swerdloff RS, Veldhuis JD. Clinical review 171: the rationale, efficacy and safety of androgen therapy in older men: future research and current practice recommendations. J Clin Endocrinol Metab 2004;89(10):4789.
77. Tenover JL. Testosterone and the aging male. J Androl 1997;18(2):103.
78. Bhasin S, Bagatell CJ, Bremner WJ, et al. Issues in testosterone replacement in older men. J Clin Endocrinol Metab 1998; 83(10):3435.
79. Sih R, Morley JE, Kaiser FE, et al. Testosterone replacement in older hypogonadal men: a 12-month randomized controlled trial. J Clin Endocrinol Metab 1997;82(6):1661.
80. Amory JK, Watts NB, Easley KA, et al. Exogenous testosterone or testosterone with finasteride increases bone mineral density in older men with low serum testosterone. J Clin Endocrinol Metab 2004;89(2):503.
81. Page ST, Amory JK, Bowman FD, et al. Exogenous testosterone (T) alone or with finasteride increases physical performance, grip strength, and lean body mass in older men with low serum T. J Clin Endocrinol Metab 2005;90(3):1502.
82. Muller M, van den Beld AW, Bots ML, et al. Endogenous sex hormones and progression of carotid atherosclerosis in elderly men. Circulation 2004;109(17):2074.
83. Morley JE, Melmed S. Gonadal dysfunction in systemic disorders. Metabolism 1979;28(10):1051.
84. Gray A, Feldman HA, McKinlay JB, et al. Age, disease, and changing sex hormone levels in middle-aged men: results of the Massachusetts Male Aging Study. J Clin Endocrinol Metab 1991; 73(5):1016.
85. Negro-Vilar A. Selective androgen receptor modulators (SARMs): a novel approach to androgen therapy for the new millennium. J Clin Endocrinol Metab 1999;84(10):3459.
86. Zitzmann M, Nieschlag E. The CAG repeat polymorphism within the androgen receptor gene and maleness. Int J Androl 2003;26(2):76.
87. Krithivas K, Yurgalevitch SM, Mohr BA, et al. Evidence that the CAG repeat in the androgen receptor gene is associated with the age-related decline in serum androgen levels in men. J Endocrinol 1999;162(1):137.
88. Giovannucci E, Platz EA, Stampfer MJ, et al. The CAG repeat within the androgen receptor gene and benign prostatic hyperplasia. Urology 1999;53(1):121.
89. Labrie F, Luu-The V, Lin SX, et al. Intracrinology: role of the family of 17 beta-hydroxysteroid dehydrogenases in human physiology and disease. J Mol Endocrinol 2000;25(1):1.
90. Labrie F, Belanger A, Simard J, et al. DHEA and peripheral androgen and estrogen formation: intracrinology. Ann N Y Acad Sci 1995;774:16.
91. Barrett-Connor E, Goodman-Gruen D. The epidemiology of DHEAS and cardiovascular disease. Ann N Y Acad Sci 1995;774:259.
92. Kalmijn S, Launer LJ, Stolk RP, et al. A prospective study on cortisol, dehydroepiandrosterone sulfate, and cognitive function in the elderly. J Clin Endocrinol Metab 1998;83(10):3487.
93. Baulieu EE. Studies on dehydroepiandrosterone (DHEA) and its sulphate during aging. C R Acad Sci III 1995;318(1):7.
94. Morales AJ, Nolan JJ, Nelson JC, et al. Effects of replacement dose of dehydroepiandrosterone in men and women of advancing age. J Clin Endocrinol Metab 1994;78(6):1360.
95. Yen SS, Morales AJ, Khorram O. Replacement of DHEA in aging men and women. Potential remedial effects. Ann N Y Acad Sci 1995;774:128.
96. Flynn MA, Weaver-Osterholtz D, Sharpe-Timms KL, et al. Dehydroepiandrosterone replacement in aging humans. J Clin Endocrinol Metab 1999;84(5):1527.
97. Baulieu EE, Thomas G, Legrain S, et al. Dehydroepiandrosterone (DHEA), DHEA sulfate, and aging: contribution of the DHE Age Study to a sociobiomedical issue. Proc Natl Acad Sci U S A 2000;97(8):4279.
98. Villareal DT, Holloszy JO. Effect of DHEA on abdominal fat and insulin action in elderly women and men: a randomized controlled trial. JAMA 2004;292(18):2243.
99. Arlt W, Callies F, van Vlijmen JC, et al. Dehydroepiandrosterone replacement in women with adrenal insufficiency. N Engl J Med 1999;341(14):1013.
100. Barrett-Connor E, Mueller JE, von Muhlen DG, et al. Low levels of estradiol are associated with vertebral fractures in older men, but not women: the Rancho Bernardo Study. J Clin Endocrinol Metab 2000;85(1):219.
101. van den Beld A, Huhtaniemi IT, Pettersson KS, et al. Luteinizing hormone and different genetic variants, as indicators of frailty in healthy elderly men. J Clin Endocrinol Metab 1999;84(4):1334.
102. Yaffe K, Lui LY, Grady D, et al. Cognitive decline in women in relation to non–protein-bound oestradiol concentrations. Lancet 2000;356(9231):708.
103. Nestler JE. Regulation of human dehydroepiandrosterone metabolism by insulin. Ann N Y Acad Sci 1995;774:73.
104. Skolnick AA. Scientific verdict still out on DHEA. JAMA 1996; 276(17):1365.
105. Toogood AA, O'Neill PA, Shalet SM. Beyond the somatopause: growth hormone deficiency in adults over the age of 60 years. J Clin Endocrinol Metab 1996;81(2):460.
106. Toogood AA, Jones J, O'Neill PA, et al. The diagnosis of severe growth hormone deficiency in elderly patients with hypothalamic-pituitary disease. Clin Endocrinol (Oxf) 1998;48(5):569.
107. Borst SE, Millard WJ, Lowenthal DT. Growth hormone, exercise, and aging: the future of therapy for the frail elderly. J Am Geriatr Soc 1994;42(5):528.
108. Nass R, Huber RM, Klauss V, et al. Effect of growth hormone (hGH) replacement therapy on physical work capacity and cardiac and pulmonary function in patients with hGH deficiency acquired in adulthood. J Clin Endocrinol Metab 1995;80(2):552.
109. Salomon F, Cuneo RC, Hesp R, et al. The effects of treatment with recombinant human growth hormone on body composition and metabolism in adults with growth hormone deficiency. N Engl J Med 1989;321(26):1797.
110. Poehlman ET, Copeland KC. Influence of physical activity on insulin-like growth factor-I in healthy younger and older men. J Clin Endocrinol Metab 1990;71(6):1468.
111. Papadakis MA, Grady D, Tierney MJ, et al. Insulin-like growth factor 1 and functional status in healthy older men. J Am Geriatr Soc 1995;43(12):1350.
112. Rudman D. Growth hormone, body composition, and aging. J Am Geriatr Soc 1985;33(11):800.
113. Rudman D, Feller AG, Nagraj HS, et al. Effects of human growth hormone in men over 60 years old. N Engl J Med 1990;323(1):1.
114. Rudman D, Feller AG, Cohn L, et al. Effects of human growth hormone on body composition in elderly men. Horm Res 1991;36(suppl 1):73.
115. Taaffe DR, Pruitt L, Reim J, et al. Effect of recombinant human growth hormone on the muscle strength response to resistance exercise in elderly men. J Clin Endocrinol Metab 1994; 79(5):1361.
116. Yarasheski KE, Zachwieja JJ, Campbell JA, et al. Effect of growth hormone and resistance exercise on muscle growth and strength in older men. Am J Physiol 1995;268(2 Pt 1):E268.

117. Papadakis MA, Grady D, Black D, et al. Growth hormone replacement in healthy older men improves body composition but not functional ability. Ann Intern Med 1996;124(8):708.
118. Blackman MR, Sorkin JD, Munzer T, et al. Growth hormone and sex steroid administration in healthy aged women and men: a randomized controlled trial. JAMA 2002;288(18):2282.
119. Herndon DN, Barrow RE, Kunkel KR, et al. Effects of recombinant human growth hormone on donor-site healing in severely burned children. Ann Surg 1990;212(4):424.
120. Bowers CY, Momany FA, Reynolds GA, et al. On the in vitro and in vivo activity of a new synthetic hexapeptide that acts on the pituitary to specifically release growth hormone. Endocrinology 1984;114(5):1537.
121. Howard AD, Feighner SD, Cully DF, et al. A receptor in pituitary and hypothalamus that functions in growth hormone release. Science 1996;273(5277):974.
122. Pong SS, Chaung LY, Dean DC, et al. Identification of a new G-protein–linked receptor for growth hormone secretagogues. Mol Endocrinol 1996;10(1):57.
123. Chapman IM, Hartman ML, Pezzoli SS, et al. Enhancement of pulsatile growth hormone secretion by continuous infusion of a growth hormone-releasing peptide mimetic, L-692,429, in older adults—a clinical research center study. J Clin Endocrinol Metab 1996;81(8):2874.
124. Chapman IM, Bach MA, Van Cauter E, et al. Stimulation of the growth hormone (GH)-insulin-like growth factor I axis by daily oral administration of a GH secretogogue (MK-677) in healthy elderly subjects. J Clin Endocrinol Metab 1996;81(12):4249.
125. Chapman IM. Hypothalamic growth hormone-IGF-I axis. In Morley JE, van den Berg L, eds. Endocrinology of Aging. Totowa, NJ: Humana Press, 2000:23.
126. Chan JM, Stampfer MJ, Giovannucci E, et al. Plasma insulin-like growth factor-I and prostate cancer risk: a prospective study. Science 1998;279(5350):563.
127. Hankinson SE, Willett WC, Colditz GA, et al. Circulating concentrations of insulin-like growth factor-I and risk of breast cancer. Lancet 1998;351(9113):1393.
128. Ma J, Pollak MN, Giovannucci E, et al. Prospective study of colorectal cancer risk in men and plasma levels of insulin-like growth factor (IGF)-I and IGF-binding protein-3. J Natl Cancer Inst 1999;91(7):620.
129. Martin F. Frailty and the somatopause. Growth Horm IGF Res 1999;9(1):3.
130. Rosen CJ. Growth hormone and aging. Endocrine 2000;12(2): 197.
131. Shalet SM. GH deficiency in the elderly: the case for GH replacement. Clin Endocrinol (Oxf) 2000;53(3):279.
132. Rowe JW, Kahn RL. Human aging: usual and successful. Science 1987;237(4811):143.
133. Hazzard WR. Weight control and exercise. Cardinal features of successful preventive gerontology. JAMA 1995;274(24):1964.
134. Healthy People 2000. National and Health Promotion and Disease Prevention Objectives. Washington, DC: Government Printing Office, 1991.
135. Lamberts SW, van den Beld AW, van der Lely AJ. The endocrinology of aging. Science 1997;278(5337):419.

SECTION VII

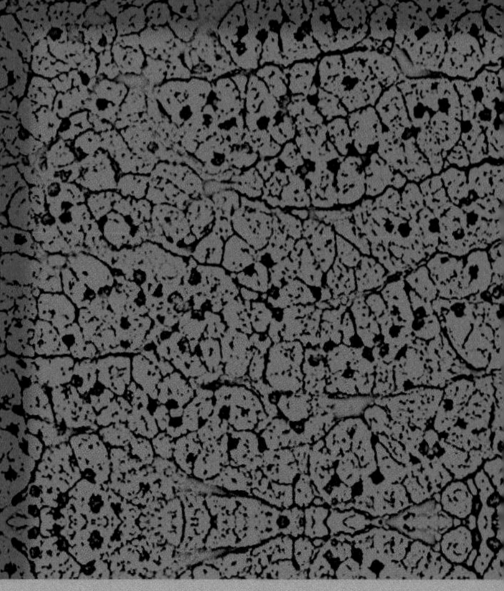

Mineral Metabolism

CHAPTER 27

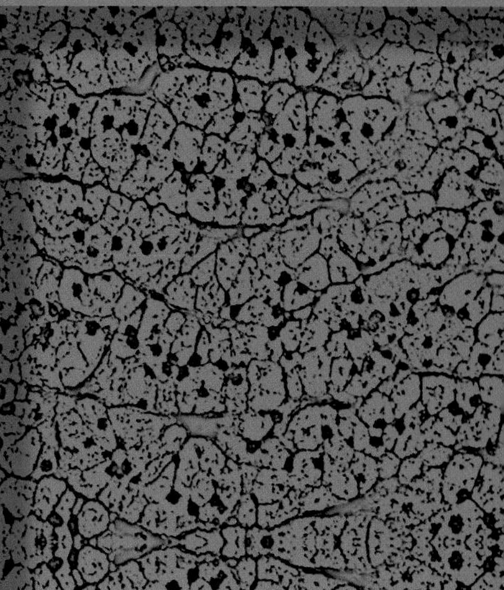

HORMONES AND DISORDERS OF MINERAL METABOLISM

F. Richard Bringhurst, Marie B. Demay, and Henry M. Kronenberg

BASIC BIOLOGY OF MINERAL METABOLISM

Roles of the Mineral Ions

Calcium (Ca) and phosphorus (P) are the principal constituents of bone, and together they comprise 65% of its weight. Bone, in turn, contains nearly all of the calcium and phosphorus and more than half of the magnesium in the human body. The quantitatively minor amounts of each of these ions in the extracellular fluid and within cells play crucial roles in normal physiology (Fig. 27–1).

Ninety-nine percent of total body calcium resides in bone, of which 99% is located within the crystal structure of the mineral phase. The remaining 1% of bone calcium is rapidly exchangeable with extracellular calcium; this calcium is equally distributed between the intracellular and extracellular fluids. Extracellular calcium is the principal substrate for the mineralization of cartilage and bone, but it also serves as a cofactor for many extracellular enzymes, most notably the enzymes of the coagulation cascade, and as a source of calcium ions for a great diversity of cellular processes. These processes include automaticity of nerve and muscle; contraction of cardiac, skeletal, and smooth muscle; release of neurotransmitters; and secretion of endocrine and exocrine hormones.

In blood, approximately 50% of total calcium is bound to proteins, mainly albumin and globulins. The ionized calcium concentration in serum is approximately 1.2 mM (5 mg/dL), and it is this ionized fraction that is biologically active and that is tightly controlled by hormonal mechanisms. Because intracellular cytosolic free calcium concentrations typically are in the range of only 100 nM, a very large chemical gradient (10,000 : 1), augmented by the large negative electrical potential, favors calcium entry into cells through calcium channels. This gradient is maintained by the limited conductance of resting calcium channels and by the energy-dependent extrusion of calcium into the extracellular fluid via high-affinity Ca^{2+}/H^+/ATPases and low-affinity sodium-calcium (Na^+/Ca^{2+}) exchangers.

More than 99% of intracellular calcium exists in the form of complexes within the mitochondrial compartment, bound to the inner plasma membrane, or associated with the inner membranes of the endoplasmic reticulum and other compartments. Release of calcium from membrane-bound compartments transduces cellular signals and is tightly regulated. The mechanisms responsible for translocations of intracellular calcium between the cytosol and these sequestered regions are becoming better understood with the identification of specific receptors for calciotropic signaling molecules such as the inositol triphosphate (IP_3) receptor and ryanodine receptors.

Phosphate is more widely distributed to nonosseous tissues than is calcium. Eighty-five percent of body phosphate is in the mineral phase of bone, and the remainder is located in inorganic or organic form throughout the extracellular and intracellular compartments. In human serum, inorganic phosphate (P_i) is present at a concentration of approximately 1 mM and exists almost entirely in ionized form as either $H_2PO_4^-$ or HPO_4^{2-}. Only 12% of serum phosphate is protein-bound, and an additional small fraction is loosely complexed with calcium, magnesium, and other cations. Intracellular free phosphate concentrations are generally comparable to those in the extracellular fluid (1-2 mM), although the inside-negative electrical potential of the cell creates a significant energy requirement for translocation of phosphate into cells. This process generally is accomplished through sodium-phosphate cotransport driven by the transmembrane sodium gradient. A number of sodium-phosphate cotransporters have been cloned; various cells and tissues employ different species of such transporters with distinctive regulatory characteristics.

Organic phosphate is a key component of virtually all classes of structural, informational, and effector molecules that are

	Calcium ions	Phosphate ions
Extracellular		
Concentration		
total, in serum	2.5×10^{-3} M	1.00×10^{-3} M
free	1.2×10^{-3} M	0.85×10^{-3} M
Functions	Bone mineral Blood coagulation Membrane excitability	Bone mineral
Intracellular		
Concentration	10^{-7} M	$1–2 \times 10^{-3}$ M
Functions	**Signal for:** • Neuron activation • Hormone secretion • Muscle contraction	• Structural role • High energy bonds • Regulation of proteins by phosphorylation

Figure 27–1 ▪ Distribution and function of calcium and phosphate. Note the dramatic differences between intracellular and extracellular concentrations of calcium ion and the dramatically different functions of calcium and phosphate inside cells.

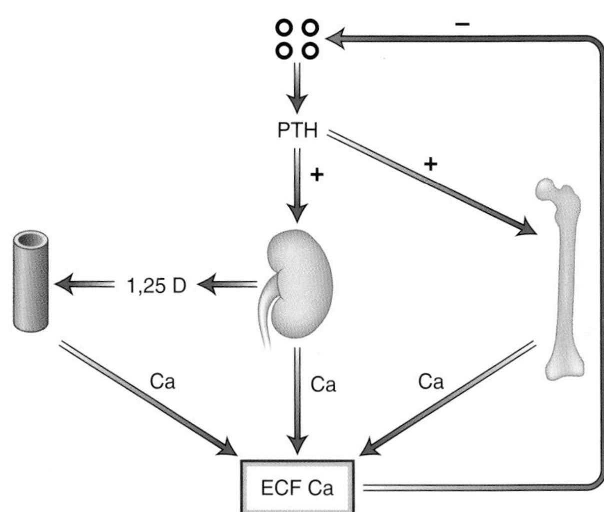

Figure 27–2 ▪ Parathyroid hormone–calcium feedback loop that controls calcium homeostasis. Four organs—the parathyroid glands, intestine, kidney, and bone—together determine the parameters of calcium homeostasis. +, positive effect; –, negative effect; 1,25 D, 1,25-dihydroxy vitamin D; ECF, extracellular fluid; PTH, parathyroid hormone.

essential for normal genetic, developmental, and physiologic processes. Phosphate is an integral constituent of nucleic acids; phospholipids; complex carbohydrates; glycolytic intermediates; structural, signaling, and enzymatic phosphoproteins; and nucleotide cofactors for enzymes and G proteins. Of particular importance are the high-energy phosphate ester bonds present in molecules such as adenosine triphosphate (ATP), diphosphoglycerate, and creatine phosphate that store chemical energy. Phosphate plays a particularly prominent role as the key substrate or recognition site in numerous kinase and phosphatase regulatory cascades. Cytosolic phosphate per se also directly regulates a number of crucial intracellular reactions, including those involved in glucose transport, lactate production, and synthesis of ATP. In light of these diverse roles, it is not surprising that disorders of phosphate homeostasis associated with severe depletion of intracellular phosphate lead to profound and global impairment of organ function.

Magnesium is the fourth most abundant cation in the body. Roughly half is found in bone and half in muscle and other soft tissues. As much as half of the magnesium in bone is not sequestered in the mineral phase but is freely exchangeable with the extracellular fluid and, therefore, may serve as a buffer against changes in extracellular magnesium concentration. Less than 1% of all magnesium in the body is present in the extracellular fluid, where the magnesium concentration is approximately 0.5 mM. The concentration of magnesium in serum normally is 0.7 to 1.0 mM, of which roughly one third is protein bound, 15% is loosely complexed with phosphate or other anions, and 55% is present as the free ion. More than 95% of intracellular magnesium is bound to other molecules, most notably ATP, whose concentration is approximately 5 mM. The intracellular cytosolic free magnesium concentration is approximately 0.5 mM—i.e., 1000-fold higher than that of calcium—and is maintained by an active sodium-magnesium antiporter. The mechanism whereby magnesium enters cells, presumably down a favorable electrochemical gradient, is unknown, although some evidence for regulated channels has been obtained.[1]

Intracellular magnesium, like phosphate, is necessary for a wide range of cellular functions. It is an essential cofactor in enzymatic reactions, including most of the same glycolytic, kinase, and phosphatase pathways that also involve phosphate. Magnesium serves to directly stabilize the structures of a variety of macromolecules and complexes, including DNA, RNA, and ribosomes; is a key activator of the many ATPase-coupled ion transporters; and it plays a direct role in mitochondrial oxidative metabolism. As a result, magnesium is critical for energy metabolism and the maintenance of a normal intracellular environment. Extracellular magnesium is crucial for normal neuromuscular excitability and nerve conduction, and many of the clinical consequences of magnesium deficiency or excess reflect abnormalities in this sphere.

The levels of extracellular calcium and phosphate are regulated in a coordinated way that reflects the roles of calcium and phosphate in mineralization of bone. The concentrations of these ions in body fluids are together close to the concentrations that could lead to spontaneous precipitation in soft tissues. In fact, elaborate mechanisms, most of them poorly understood, have evolved to prevent calcium and phosphate precipitation in tissues and yet to allow the controlled deposition of calcium and phosphate in bone.[2] The importance of the mineral ions for normal cellular physiology as well as skeletal integrity is reflected in the powerful endocrine control mechanisms that have evolved to maintain their extracellular concentrations within relatively narrow limits. The following topics describe the structures, secretory controls, actions, and interactions of parathyroid hormone, calcitonin, 1,25-dihydroxyvitamin D [$1,25(OH)_2D_3$ or calcitriol], and fibroblast growth factor 23 (FGF23)—the major hormones involved in mineral ion homeostasis. Subsequent topics cover the wide variety of clinical disorders that accompany abnormalities in this hormonal network.

Parathyroid Hormone

Parathyroid hormone (PTH) is the peptide hormone that controls the minute-to-minute level of ionized calcium in the blood and extracellular fluids. PTH binds to cell surface receptors in bone and kidney, thereby triggering responses that increase blood calcium (Fig. 27–2). PTH also increases renal synthesis of $1,25(OH)_2D_3$, the hormonally active form of vitamin D, which then acts on the intestine to augment absorption of dietary calcium in addition to promoting calcium fluxes into blood from bone and kidney. The resulting increase in blood calcium and in $1,25(OH)_2D_3$ feeds back on the parathyroid glands to decrease the secretion of PTH. The parathyroid glands, bones, kidney,

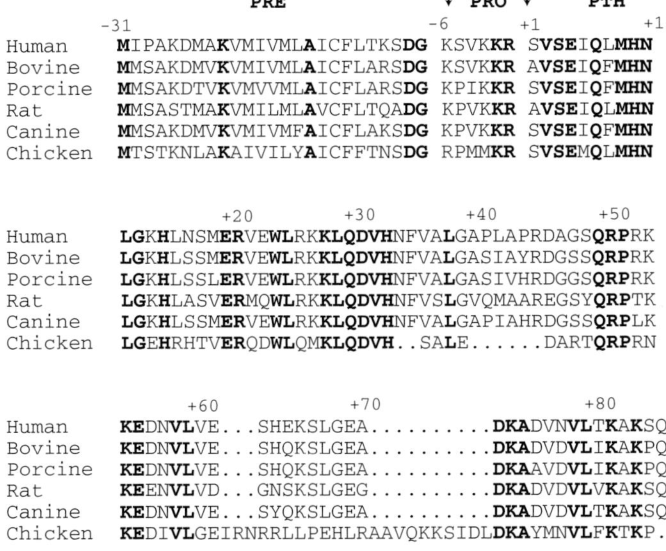

Figure 27–3 ▪ Sequences of pre-proparathyroid hormone from six species. Completely conserved residues are in *boldface*. *Arrows* indicate the sites of signal sequence ("pre") and "pro" sequence cleavage. Numbers start at residue +1 of mature parathyroid hormone (PTH); because of gaps, the numbers correspond only to the mammalian and not to the chicken sequence. Amino acids are indicated by the single-letter code: A, Ala; R, Arg; N, Asn; D, Asp; C, Cys; Q, Gln; E, Glu; G, Gly; H, His; I, Ile, L, Leu; K, Lys; M, Met; F, Phe; P, Pro; S, Ser; T, Thr; W, Trp; Y, Tyr; V, Val.

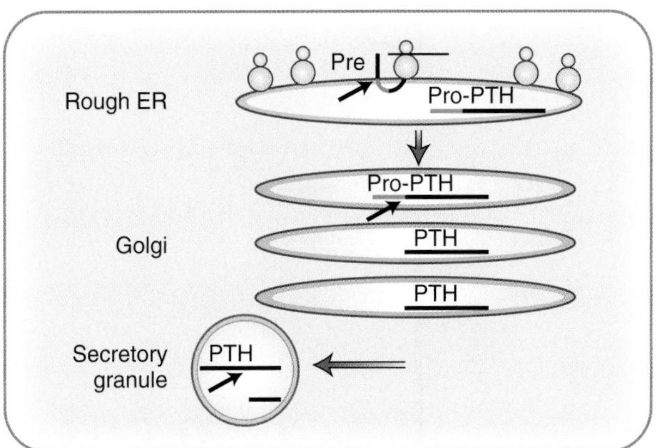

Figure 27–4 ▪ Intracellular processing of pre-proparathyroid hormone (pre-pro-PTH). *Diagonal arrows* indicate sites of cleavage by enzymes that generate pro-PTH in the rough endoplasmic reticulum (ER), PTH in the Golgi, and carboxy-terminal fragments of PTH in the secretory granule.

and gut are thus the crucial organs that participate in PTH-mediated calcium homeostasis.

Parathyroid Gland Biology

Parathyroid glands first appeared in evolutionary history with the exit of amphibians from the sea and a switch from dependence on gills to sole dependence on bone, intestine, and kidney to maintain extracellular calcium homeostasis. Reptiles, birds, and mammals all have parathyroid glands that develop as epithelial specializations from the endoderm of the pharyngeal pouches. Although fish have no discrete parathyroid glands, they do synthesize PTH.[3,4] The physiologic role of this PTH in fish is not yet defined.

Parathyroid chief cells have three properties vital to their homeostatic function: They rapidly secrete hormone in response to changes in blood calcium; they can synthesize, process, and store large amounts of PTH in a regulated manner; and parathyroid cells replicate when chronically stimulated. These functional attributes allow for short-term, intermediate-term, and long-term adaptation, respectively, to changes in calcium availability.

Parathyroid Hormone Biosynthesis

PTH, a protein of 84 amino acids, is synthesized as a larger precursor, pre-proparathyroid hormone (pre-pro-PTH). Figure 27–3 illustrates the reported pre-pro-PTH sequences. These pre-pro-PTH sequences share a 25-residue *pre* or signal sequence and a 6-residue *pro* sequence. The signal sequence, along with the short pro sequence, functions to direct the protein into the secretory pathway (Fig. 27–4). During transit across the membrane of the endoplasmic reticulum, the signal sequence is cleaved off and rapidly degraded. The importance of the signal sequence for normal secretion of PTH is illustrated by the hypoparathyroidism inherited in families carrying mutations in the signal sequence of pre-pro-PTH.[5,6]

The role of the short pro sequence is not completely understood; it might help the signal sequence to work efficiently and ensure accurate cleavage of the precursor.[7] After cleavage of the pro sequence, the mature PTH(1-84) is concentrated in secretory vesicles and granules. One morphologically distinct subtype of granule contains both PTH and the proteases cathepsin B and cathepsin H. This colocalization of proteases and PTH in secretory granules probably explains the observation that a portion of the PTH secreted from parathyroid glands consists of carboxy-terminal PTH fragments. No amino-terminal fragments of PTH are secreted. Although the possible functions of carboxy-terminal fragments of PTH are still poorly characterized, these fragments do not activate the PTH/PTHrP (parathyroid hormone–related protein) receptor and might even block bone resorption[8] (see later). The intracellular degradation of newly synthesized PTH thus provides an important regulatory mechanism. Under conditions of hypercalcemia, the secretion of PTH is substantially decreased, and most of what is secreted consists of carboxy-terminal fragments.[9,10]

Parathyroid Hormone Secretion

Although catecholamines, magnesium, and other stimuli can affect PTH secretion, the major regulator of PTH secretion is the concentration of ionized calcium in blood. Increased serum ionized calcium leads to a decrease in PTH secretion (Fig. 27–5A). The shape of the dose-response curve is sigmoid. Properties of the parathyroid cell determine the conformation of the sigmoid curve but do not alone determine the point on the curve that represents a physiologic steady state for an individual person. This point, usually between the midpoint and the bottom of the curve, is determined by how vigorously target organs respond to PTH.[11] Figure 27–5C *(solid line)* shows how a person's calcium level rises in response to increases in PTH; the parathyroid gland's sigmoid curve is the *dotted line.* In the steady state, a person's blood levels of PTH and calcium represent the intersection of the two lines.

The sigmoid curve reveals several important physiologic properties of the parathyroid gland. The minimal secretory rate is low but not zero. The maximal secretory rate represents the reserve of the parathyroid's capacity to respond to hypocalcemia. Because values from normal persons in the steady state are located in the lower portion of the sigmoid curve, the system

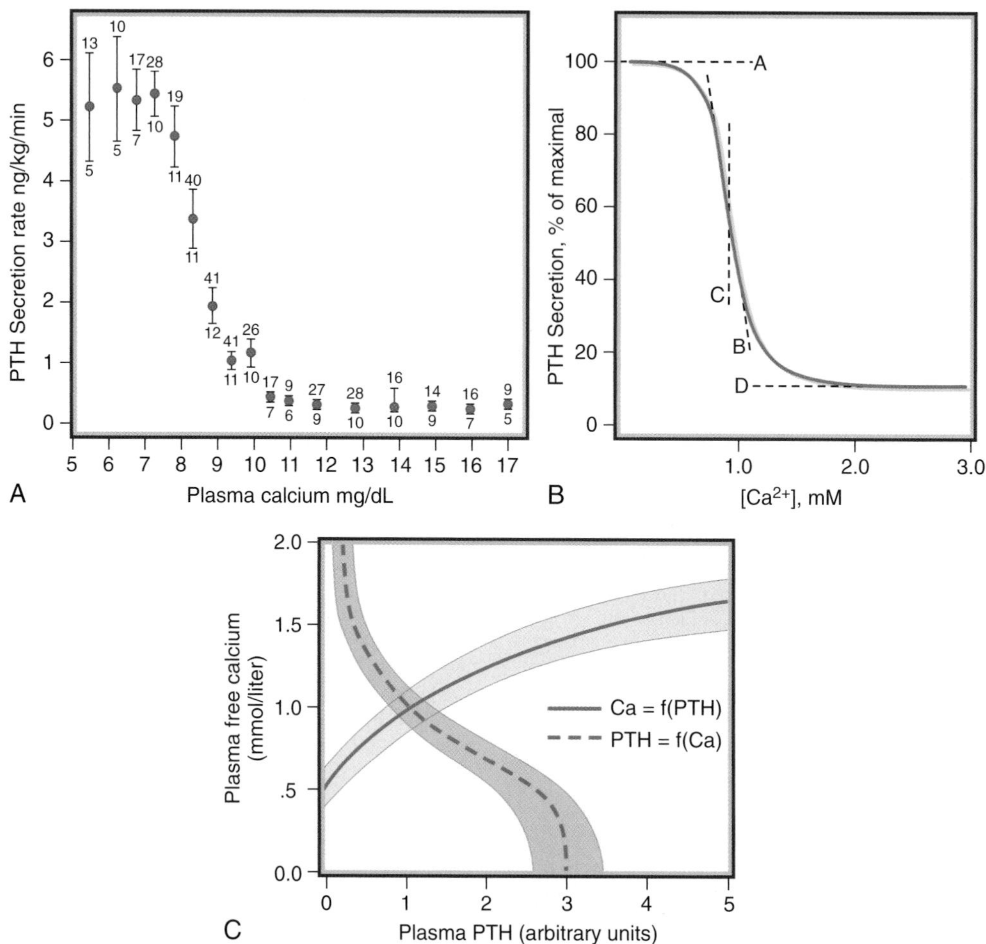

Figure 27–5 ▪ Parathyroid hormone (PTH) secretion. **A,** Secretory response of bovine parathyroid glands to induced alterations of plasma calcium concentration. Calves were infused with calcium chloride or ethylenediaminetetraacetic acid (EDTA), and PTH secretion was assessed by measuring PTH levels in the parathyroid venous effluent. The symbols and *vertical bars* indicate the secretory rate (mean ±SE) in calcium concentration ranges of 1.0 or 0.5 mg/100 mL. The number of calves and samples are indicated, respectively, by numbers below and above the bars. **B,** Sigmoidal curve generated by the equation $Y=\{[A-D]/[1+(X/C)^B]\}+D$. Such a curve can be defined by four parameters: the maximal secretory rate *(A)*, the slope of the curve at its midpoint *(B)*, the level of calcium at the midpoint (often called the set-point) *(C)*, and the minimal secretory rate *(D)*; the significance of *A, B, C,* and *D* is described in the text. **C,** Relationships between calcium and PTH levels when each in turn is treated as an independent variable. The *dashed line* represents the sigmoidal relationship between calcium and PTH, when calcium is the independent variable. This curve is the same as that in **A** and **B,** but it is turned on its side, because the axes are reversed. The *solid line* represents the relationship between calcium and PTH when PTH is considered the independent variable; values for this curve result from measurements made during PTH infusion into parathyroidectomized animals. Actual data are limited; thus, the curves should be viewed as illustrative. (**A** from Mayer GP, Hurst JG. Sigmoidal relationship between parathyroid hormone secretion rate and plasma calcium concentration in calves. Endocrinology 1978;10:1037-1042. **B** modified from Brown EM. Four-parameter model of the sigmoidal relationship between parathyroid hormone release and extracellular calcium concentration in normal and abnormal parathyroid tissue. J Clin Endocrinol Metab 1983;56:572-581. **C** from Parfitt AM. Calcium homeostasis. In Mundy GR, Martin TJ [eds]. Physiology and Pharmacology of Bone. Berlin, Springer-Verlag, 1993.)

seems designed to respond more dramatically to hypocalcemia than to hypercalcemia.

Physiologic studies in humans confirmed this sigmoid relationship and have also revealed that the parathyroid cell responds both to the absolute level of blood calcium and to the rate of fall of calcium level. Thus, PTH levels briefly rise higher during a sudden drop in blood calcium than they do during a more gradual fall in calcium. This property of the parathyroid cell offers an additional protection against sudden hypocalcemia.

The biochemical and cellular determinants of the parathyroid gland's sigmoid response curve are beginning to be defined. A parathyroid calcium-sensing receptor[12] on the parathyroid cell surface is a member of the G protein–coupled family of receptors. The sequence of the receptor suggests that it spans the plasma membrane seven times, like other receptors in the G protein–linked receptor family (Fig. 27–6). A large extracellular domain resembles similar domains in brain metabotropic glutamate receptors as well as bacterial periplasmic proteins designed to bind small ligands, including cations. The receptor has been expressed in a number of cell types and has been shown to activate phospholipase C and to block stimulation of cyclic adenosine monophosphate (cAMP) production, just as it does in normal parathyroid cells.

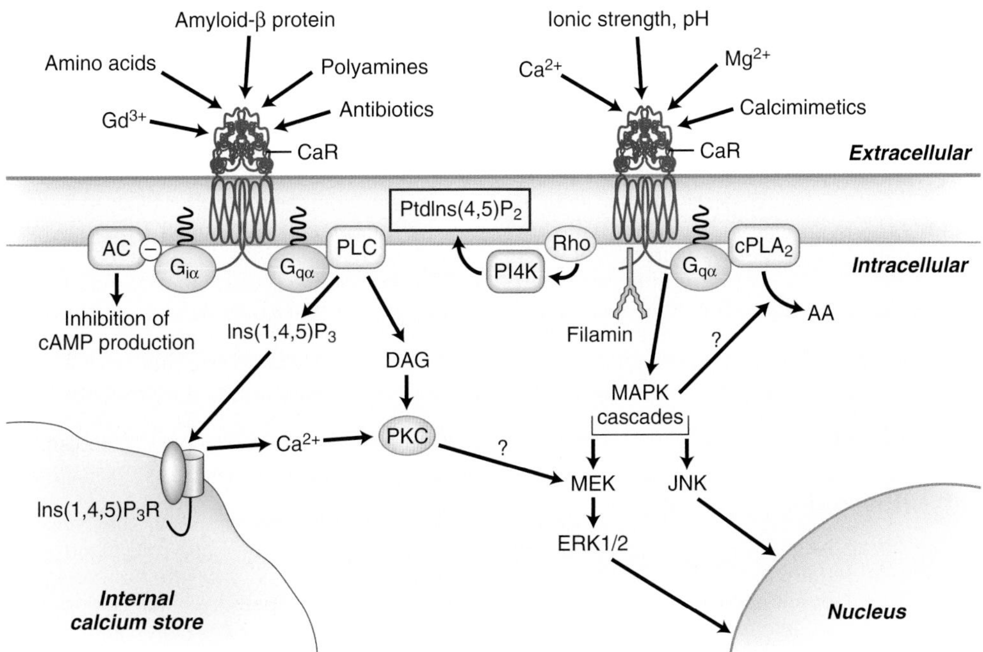

Figure 27–6 ▪ Signaling by the calcium-sensing receptor. Numerous agonists activate the calcium-sensing receptor (CaR) and trigger intracellular pathways. AA, arachidonic acid; AC, adenylate cyclase; cAMP, cyclic adenosine monophosphate; $cPLA_2$, cytosolic phospholipase A_2; DAG, diacylglycerol; ERK, extracellular signal-regulated kinase; Gia and Gqa, a subunits of the i- and q-type heterotrimeric G proteins, respectively; Ins(1,4,5)P3, inositol-1,4,5-trisphosphate; Ins(1,4,5)P3R, inositol-1,4,5-trisphosphate receptor; JNK, Jun amino-terminal kinase; MAPK, mitogen-activated protein kinase; MEK, MAPK kinase; PI4K, phosphatidylinositol 4-kinase; PKC, protein kinase C; PLC, phospholipase C; $PtdIns(4,5)P_2$, phosphatidylinositol-4,5-bisphosphate. (From Hofer AM, Brown EM. Extracellular calcium sensing and signaling. Nat Rev Molec Cell Biol 2003;4:530-538.)

The most convincing proof of the identity of the parathyroid calcium–sensing receptor has been the observation that mutations in the receptor gene cause characteristic human diseases. Inactivating mutations cause familial hypocalciuric hypercalcemia (FHH), a disease of defective calcium sensing (see later),[13] whereas activating mutations cause familial hypoparathyroidism with hypercalciuria.[14] Furthermore, mice genetically engineered to have only one functioning copy of the calcium-sensing receptor gene also have the expected defects in parathyroid calcium sensing.[15] Calcimimetic compounds that activate the cloned calcium-sensing receptor have been shown to inhibit PTH secretion in humans and are useful in the treatment of secondary hyperparathyroidism.[16] Despite the enormous increase in understanding how extracellular calcium activates the parathyroid calcium-sensing receptor, the mechanism whereby this activation leads to a decrease in PTH secretion is poorly understood.

The calcium-sensing receptor is expressed widely. Expression in the renal tubules and calcitonin-producing cells of the thyroid contributes to calcium homeostasis, whereas expression in organs such as the brain points to multiple roles for calcium signaling. The observation that the calcium-sensing receptor also responds to physiologic levels of certain amino acids[17] suggests that the expression of the calcium-sensing receptor in the gut, parathyroid, and other sites might facilitate the assimilation of multiple nutrients.

Regulation of the Parathyroid Hormone Gene

The minute-to-minute regulation of PTH blood levels can be explained by the two mechanisms already discussed: regulation of PTH secretion by the calcium-sensing receptor and amplification of this regulation by intracellular degradation of stored hormone. Over a longer time frame, the parathyroid cell regulates the expression of the PTH gene as well.

Although $1,25(OH)_2D_3$—the active form of vitamin D—has no direct effect on PTH secretion, it dramatically suppresses PTH gene transcription.[18] This suppression of transcription does not occur when $1,25(OH)_2D_3$ is administered to chronically hypocalcemic animals, however, perhaps because hypocalcemia leads to a fall in parathyroid cell vitamin D receptors or because hypocalcemia increases the expression of calreticulin in the parathyroid.[19] The ability of hypocalcemia to override the effects of high levels of $1,25(OH)_2D_3$ represents an important defense, because it provides a way for the parathyroid cell to synthesize large amounts of PTH and $1,25(OH)_2D_3$ at the same time, when both are needed.

Calcium also regulates the biosynthesis of PTH. In vivo studies show that acute hypocalcemia in rats leads, within an hour, to an increase in PTH messenger RNA (mRNA).[20] In contrast, hypercalcemia leads to little or no change in PTH mRNA. Thus, under normal conditions, the inhibition by calcium of PTH biosynthesis already is nearly maximal, just as it is for PTH secretion. The parathyroid gland is poised to respond to a fall in calcium much more readily than to a rise. The mechanism for the increase in PTH mRNA in response to hypocalcemia is uncertain; differing experimental paradigms suggest regulation at the levels of gene transcription, mRNA translation, and mRNA stability. The latter mechanism is the one best understood at the molecular level.[21]

For decades it has been known that phosphate elevation stimulates PTH secretion largely by lowering blood calcium and $1,25(OH)_2D_3$ levels. More recently, a series of studies in vitro[22,23] and in vivo[24] have demonstrated that phosphate can increase

PTH secretion directly, independent of effects on blood calcium and $1,25(OH)_2D_3$. Phosphate increases PTH secretion acutely only after a delay and probably works largely through regulation of PTH mRNA levels.

The regulation of the PTH gene has particular clinical relevance in patients with renal failure. Hypocalcemia, low levels of $1,25(OH)_2D_3$, hyperphosphatemia, and, possibly, uremic toxins disrupt normal calcium homeostasis in this setting. Therapy with $1,25(OH)_2D_3$ and calcium increases calcium absorption and also inhibits PTH synthesis by direct effects on the parathyroid gland. Cinecalcet, an activator of the calcium-sensing receptor, lowers PTH secretion and thereby lowers both calcium and phosphorus levels. (In renal failure, the role of PTH to increase release of phosphorus from bone dominates any action of PTH to increase phosphaturia.) Prevention of hyperphosphatemia avoids the direct and indirect actions of phosphate to stimulate PTH secretion.

Regulation of Parathyroid Cell Number

Parathyroid cells divide during the growth of young animals but replicate little in adulthood.[25] Parathyroid cell number can dramatically increase, however, in the setting of hypocalcemia, low levels of $1,25(OH)_2D_3$, hyperphosphatemia, and uremia as well as during neoplastic growth.

Calcium, acting through the parathyroid calcium-sensing receptor, restrains parathyroid proliferation. This effect has been demonstrated clinically in patients who lack both copies of the calcium-sensing receptor gene. These neonates exhibit severe primary hyperparathyroidism with large, diffusely hyperplastic glands that presumably have developed because of insufficient activation of the parathyroid calcium-sensing receptor by extracellular calcium. Furthermore, administration of the calcimimetic compound NPS R-568, which activates the calcium-sensing receptor directly, prevents parathyroid cell proliferation in experimental uremia.

The role of $1,25(OH)_2D_3$, independent of blood calcium, in regulating parathyroid cell proliferation is less well established than that of calcium. That $1,25(OH)_2D_3$ can dramatically affect parathyroid cell number has been shown in vivo in many settings, but such studies cannot rigorously eliminate effects of transient changes in blood calcium. The suppression of proliferation of cultured parathyroid cells by $1,25(OH)_2D_3$ certainly suggests that $1,25(OH)_2D_3$ can directly inhibit parathyroid cell replication.[26] In experimental renal failure, the action of $1,25(OH)_2D_3$ to decrease parathyroid cell TGF-α expression might partly explain the dampening of parathyroid cell proliferation.[27] Nevertheless, vitamin D action is not essential for control of parathyroid cell number, because calcium alone can prevent parathyroid cell hyperplasia in mice engineered to lack vitamin D receptors.[28]

Although the ability to increase parathyroid cell number in response to physiologic challenge represents an important defense against hypocalcemia, it is a slow response that is not easily reversible. When the need for an increased number of parathyroid cells disappears (e.g., after renal transplantation for uremia), persistent hyperparathyroidism can cause vexing clinical problems for months and years thereafter. The mechanisms for decreasing parathyroid cell number, if they exist, are poorly understood. Apoptosis of normal parathyroid cells in response to experimental manipulation has not been demonstrated.[29]

Parathyroid Gland Development

Genes involved in making parathyroid cells during development might also regulate PTH synthesis and parathyroid cell number throughout life; thus, an understanding of parathyroid cell development could have broad clinical implications.

Although the genetic mechanisms used to generate parathyroid chief cells during development are largely unknown, the importance of several specific genes has become clear. Studies of knockout mice have shown that the hoxa3,[30] pax1,[31] pax9,[32] and Eya1[33] transcription factors are needed to form parathyroid glands as well as many other pharyngeal pouch derivatives, such as the thymus. In humans and mice, haploinsufficiency for the transcription factor Tbx1 is likely to be responsible for many of the abnormalities found in DiGeorge syndrome, including hypoparathyroidism.[34]

Sox3 is another transcription factor expressed in the pharyngeal pouches that give rise to parathyroid cells. Humans with X-linked hypoparathyroidism manifest a deletion-insertion near the end of the *SOX3* gene, a finding that suggests an important role for Sox3 in parathyroid development.[35] People with mutations in the gene encoding the transcription factor GATA3 exhibit a syndrome of hypoparathyroidism, sensorineural deafness, and renal anomalies when only one copy of the gene is mutated.[36]

Mice[37] or humans[38] missing the *gcm2* and *GCMB* genes, respectively, have no parathyroid glands. In both species, the deletion of *gcm2* or *GCMB* (the human equivalent) is very specific for controlling parathyroid development because no abnormalities in other tissues have been noted. Mice, which have only two parathyroid glands normally, still make PTH in a small number of cells in the thymus after *gcm2* gene ablation and secrete this PTH into the circulation. Humans without *GCMB* have little detectable circulating PTH at birth and low levels of PTH several years later.

Peripheral Metabolism of Parathyroid Hormone

The earliest radioimmunoassays for PTH demonstrated that the molecular forms of PTH in the circulation differ from those in the parathyroid gland.[39] Characterization of the metabolism of PTH and its fragments has clarified the origins and significance of immunoreactive PTH molecules in the bloodstream.[40] As noted previously, both PTH(1-84) and carboxy-terminal fragments of PTH are secreted from the parathyroid gland; the ratio of inactive PTH to active PTH secretion increases with increasing blood calcium. Secreted intact PTH(1-84) is extensively metabolized by liver (70%) and kidney (20%) and disappears from the circulation with a half-life of 2 minutes. This rapid peripheral metabolism of PTH is unaffected by widely varying levels of blood calcium or $1,25(OH)_2D_3$. Less than 1% of the secreted hormone finds its way to PTH receptors on physiologic target organs. These features of PTH metabolism ensure that the blood level of PTH is determined principally by the activity of the parathyroid glands and that the PTH level can respond rapidly to small changes in the rate of secretion of the hormone.

In the liver, a small amount of PTH binds to physiologically relevant PTH receptors, but most of the intact PTH is cleaved, initially after residues 33 and 36, probably by cathepsins. In the kidney, a small amount of intact PTH binds to physiologic PTH receptors, but most of the intact PTH is filtered at the glomerulus and subsequently bound by a large, membrane-bound luminal protein, megalin20; this binding leads to internalization and degradation of PTH by the tubules.[42] Carboxy-terminal fragments are also cleared efficiently by glomerular filtration. In fact, the kidney is the only known site of clearance of carboxy-terminal PTH fragments; these fragments thus accumulate dramatically when the glomerular filtration rate (GFR) falls. Even in the presence of normal renal function, the half-life of carboxy-terminal fragments of PTH exceeds that of PTH(1-84) by several-fold. Consequently, the concentration of carboxy-terminal fragments in the circulation exceeds that of intact PTH, even though intact PTH usually is the major form of PTH secreted from the parathyroid gland.

Careful analysis of PTH fragments using high-performance liquid chromatography (HPLC) and immunologic methods have revealed almost full-length PTH fragments that are missing the first several amino acids of the hormone but that contain most or all of the remaining hormone sequence.[43] These still incompletely characterized fragments are secreted from the parathyroid gland and are generated by peripheral metabolism of the hormone. Because they are missing the amino-terminal portion of PTH, they cannot stimulate cyclic adenosine monophosphate (cAMP) production by the PTH–parathyroid hormone–related protein (PTHrP) receptor, and except in renal failure, they circulate in small amounts. Nevertheless, the possible biologic activity of these and other PTH fragments, possibly through novel receptors, remains an area of active investigation. Experiments with PTH(7-84) suggest that such extended carboxyl fragments might exert potent effects in vivo, antagonistic to those of intact PTH (see later).[44-46]

Actions of Parathyroid Hormone

Actions of Parathyroid Hormone on the Kidney

Stimulation of Calcium Reabsorption

Almost all of the calcium in the initial glomerular filtrate is reabsorbed by the renal tubules. Sixty five percent is reabsorbed by the proximal convoluted and straight tubules via a passive, paracellular route.[47,48] Changes in the transepithelial voltage gradient, determined largely by the rate of sodium reabsorption, control the rate of calcium transport in the proximal tubule, and PTH does little to affect calcium flux in this region. The remaining calcium is largely reabsorbed more distally—20% of the initial filtrate in the cortical thick ascending limb (cTAL) of Henle's loop and 10% in the distal convoluted and connecting tubules.

In the cTAL, calcium reabsorption also is mainly passive and paracellular, although some transcellular, active calcium transport may occur as well.[49] Efficient paracellular calcium and magnesium movement requires expression of a unique tight-junction protein, paracellin-1; mutant paracellin-1 genes underlie a rare renal calcium- and magnesium-wasting disorder.[50] Because paracellular cation transport in the cTAL is driven by the lumen-positive transepithelial voltage gradient that is established by active $Na/K/Cl_2$ reabsorption, calcium reabsorption there is strongly inhibited by loop diuretics like furosemide.

The calcium-sensing receptor, initially characterized in the parathyroid, also is expressed in the cTAL.[51] When activated by high blood calcium or magnesium, this receptor inhibits $Na/K/Cl_2$ reabsorption in the cTAL and thereby inhibits paracellular calcium reabsorption as well. This provides a parathyroid-independent mechanism for controlling renal calcium handling in direct response to changes in blood calcium concentration.

Although PTH modestly stimulates paracellular calcium reabsorption in the cTAL, the primary site for hormonal regulation of renal calcium reabsorption is the distal nephron, which normally reabsorbs nearly all of the remaining 10% of filtered calcium by a unique transcellular active transport mechanism. As depicted in Figure 27–1, the intracellular level of calcium is extremely low, about 150 nM, compared with the millimolar levels in the glomerular filtrate and the blood. Calcium enters distal tubular cells from the tubular lumen down a highly favorable electrochemical gradient via selective channels (TRPV5 and TRPV6) present on the apical membrane of cells in the distal convoluted tubule (DCT) and connecting tubule (CNT). Intracellular calcium inhibits the activity of these channels, but this inhibition is minimized by the avid binding of calcium to calbindin-D28K, which effectively buffers cytosolic calcium and transports it to the basolateral membrane. There, calcium is ejected via active processes involving mainly the sodium-calcium exchanger NCX1 and an ATP-driven calcium pump (PMCA).[52] PTH stimulates DCT and CNT active calcium transport by up-regulating several of these components, including TRPV5, calbindin-D28K and NCX1, both directly and indirectly, via increased synthesis of $1,25(OH)_2D$.[52,53]

The amount of calcium in the final urine reflects all of the tubular reabsorption processes just enumerated but also depends crucially on the initial filtered load of calcium. All of PTH's actions serve to raise the blood calcium level, so that the filtered load of calcium is high in states of PTH excess. In that setting, even though the rate of distal tubular calcium reabsorption is increased by PTH, the total amount of calcium in the final urine is likely to be high because of the high initial filtered load.

Inhibition of Phosphate Transport

Phosphate reabsorption occurs mainly in the proximal renal tubules, which reclaim roughly 80% of the filtered load. Some additional phosphate (8% to 10%) is reabsorbed in the distal tubule (but not in Henle's loop), leaving about 10% to 12% for excretion in the urine. The normal overall fractional tubular reabsorption of phosphate (TRP), therefore, is about 90%, although a more reliable measure of renal phosphate handling is the *phosphate threshold* (TmP/GFR), which can be derived from the TRP through the use of a nomogram (Fig. 27–7) based on studies of experimental phosphate infusions in healthy persons and in patients with a variety of diseases that affect phosphate excretion.

Phosphate reabsorption in both proximal and distal tubules is strongly inhibited by PTH, although the proximal effect is

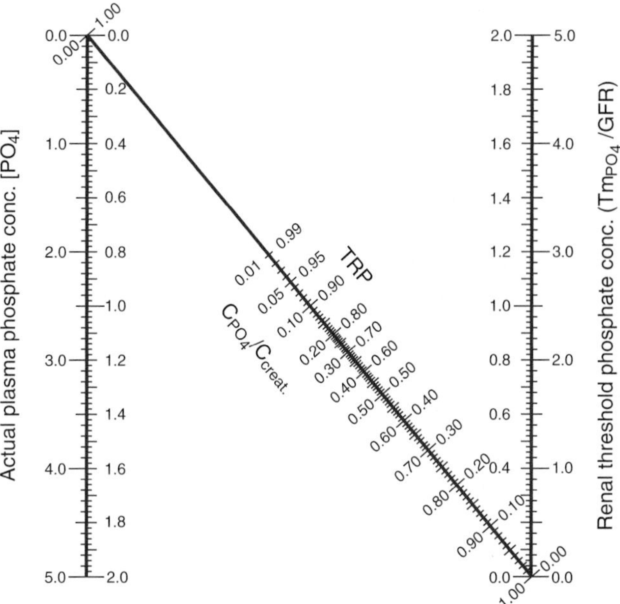

Figure 27–7 ■ Nomogram for determining renal threshold phosphate concentration (Tm_{PO_4}/GFR) from the plasma phosphate concentration and the fractional reabsorption of filtered phosphate (TRP) or fractional excretion of filtered phosphate (1-TRP, or C_{PO_4}/C_{creat}). Because the blood level of phosphate influences the renal handling of phosphate, the renal threshold phosphate concentration best separates normal from abnormal renal phosphate handling. C, clearance; creat, creatinine; GFR, glomerular filtration rate; TRP, tubular resorption of phosphate. (From Walton RJ, Bijvoet OLM. Nomogram of derivation of renal threshold phosphate concentration. Lancet 1975;2:309-310.)

quantitatively most important. Phosphate is reabsorbed by a transepithelial route. Transport from the glomerular filtrate into the cell is mediated by specific sodium-phosphate (NaPi) cotransporters, several types of which have been cloned and extensively characterized.[54] The low level of sodium within the cell drives the cotransport of sodium and phosphate, even though the phosphate travels up an electrochemical gradient. In response to PTH, the V_{max} for sodium-phosphate cotransport decreases because NaPi cotransporters are rapidly (15 min) sequestered within subapical endocytic vesicles, after which they are delivered to lysosomes and undergo proteolysis.[55] Conversely, in hypoparathyroidism, expression of NaPi protein and mRNA is strongly up-regulated.[56]

Dietary intake of phosphate also reciprocally regulates the expression and activity of NaPi cotransporters and, thus, the proximal tubular absorption of phosphate by a mechanism that is independent of PTH. Deprivation of dietary phosphate, for example, leads to a stimulation of phosphate reabsorption that can override the effects of PTH on the proximal tubule. It is likely that this dietary regulation of NaPi expression is mediated by FGF23[57] (see later).

Other Renal Effects of Parathyroid Hormone

PTH stimulates the synthesis of $1,25(OH)_2D$ in the proximal tubule by rapidly inducing transcription of the 25(OH)D 1α-hydroxylase gene, an effect that can be overridden by hypercalcemia or by $1,25(OH)_2D$.[58] PTH inhibits proximal tubular transcription of the 25(OH)D 24-hydroxylase gene and antagonizes the up-regulation of 24-hydroxylase activity by $1,25(OH)_2D$[59] (see "Metabolism of Vitamin D"). PTH inhibits proximal tubular sodium, water, and bicarbonate reabsorption, mainly via inhibition of the apical Na^+/H^+ exchanger (NHE3) and the basolateral Na^+/K^+/ATPase.[60] PTH also stimulates proximal tubular gluconeogenesis and acts directly on glomerular podocytes to decrease the single nephron and the whole kidney glomerular filtration rate.

Actions of Parathyroid Hormone on Bone

The actions of PTH on bone are complicated because PTH acts on a number of cell types both directly and indirectly. For years, the release of calcium from bone through stimulation of bone resorption has been considered the major action of PTH on bone. This is only part of the story, however. In fact, PTH administration by any route increases both bone resorption and bone formation. Which action dominates depends on the dose of PTH and the route of administration. When PTH is administered continuously, the effect of PTH on bone resorption dominates, and the net result is release of calcium from bone and a decrease in bone mass. This action of PTH thus contributes to the increase in blood calcium seen upon administration of PTH. In contrast, administration of low doses of PTH or active amino-terminal fragments of PTH by once-daily subcutaneous injection leads to a net increase in bone mass, with only transient effects on blood calcium.

Explanations for these divergent effects of PTH are incompletely understood, but they certainly reflect the variety of cell types in bone that respond directly to PTH, the varying time courses of these responses, and the indirect effects of PTH caused by autocrine and paracrine responses to PTH.

Figure 27–8 illustrates the cells of the osteoblast lineage (see also Chapter 28). Osteoblasts are probably derived from pluripotent mesenchymal stem cells that can differentiate into chondrocytes, adipocytes, osteoblasts, and other cell types.[61] Within the osteoblast lineage, committed osteoprogenitor cells divide, become preosteoblastic stromal cells (which can divide further), and then become osteoblasts. Osteoblasts no longer divide and are cuboidal cells found on the bone surface actively laying down new bone. When these cells become surrounded by bone, they become stellate osteocytes. If, instead, osteoblasts stop synthesizing matrix and remain on the bone surface, they flatten out as bone lining cells. Not all preosteoblasts and osteoblasts mature; a variable number die by apoptosis.[62]

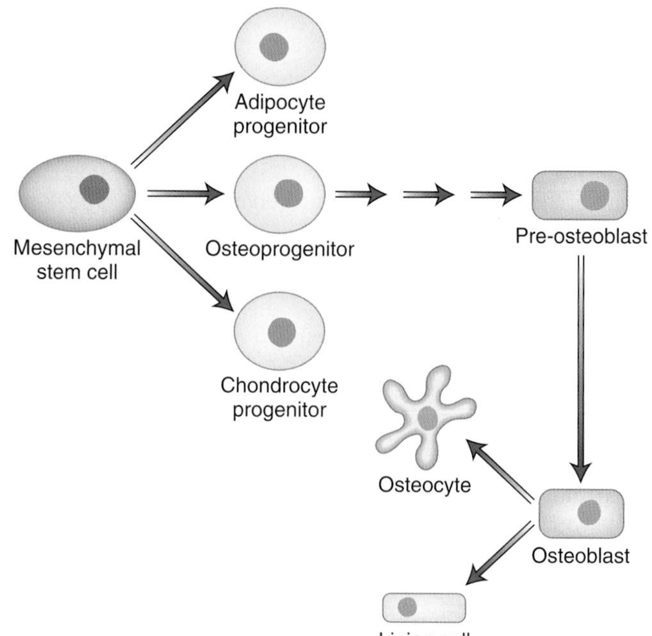

Figure 27–8 ▪ Osteoblast lineage. All precursors of osteoblasts can proliferate; osteoblasts are transformed to osteocytes and lining cells without further proliferation. Some data suggest that lining cells might revert to osteoblast function after parathyroid hormone stimulation. At each stage in the lineage, apoptotic cell death is probably an alternative fate.

Receptors for PTH are found on preosteoblasts, osteoblasts, lining cells, and osteocytes. A variety of actions of PTH on these cells change the numbers and activities of these cells. PTH changes the osteoblast lineage cell population by stimulating[63] or inhibiting[64] cell proliferation (depending on the conditions); by decreasing apoptosis of preosteoblasts and osteoblasts,[65] thereby increasing the number of osteocytes; and perhaps by converting inactive lining cells to osteoblasts.[66] When added to cells in culture, PTH stops preosteoblastic cells from becoming mature osteoblasts.[67] Furthermore, PTH changes the activity of mature osteoblasts by a variety of mechanisms. When PTH is added to calvariae in vitro, the osteoblasts decrease their synthesis of collagen I[68] and other matrix proteins. This action might reflect, in part, the action of PTH to steer the essential transcription factor core-binding factor-α1 (CBFA1) toward proteosomal destruction.[69]

In vivo, however, the most obvious effects of PTH are to increase bone formation, probably by indirect actions on autocrine and paracrine pathways. PTH stimulation of osteoblastic cells leads to release of growth factors such as IGF-1, FGF-2, and amphiregulin from these cells.[70] PTH also decreases the synthesis of dickkopf-1[71] and SOST,[72] inhibitors of Wnt signaling[73]; these actions are expected to increase the anabolic actions of Wnts on osteoblasts. These paracrine actions of PTH might not only stimulate osteoblastic cells with PTH receptors but might also activate osteoblast precursors too immature to express PTH receptors. Further, because bone matrix is a rich source of osteoblast growth factors, the release of these growth factors from this matrix following PTH-induced bone resorption might increase bone formation. Thus, a variety of both direct and indirect actions of PTH can lead to increased production of bone.

Surprisingly, osteoclasts, the bone-resorbing cells derived from hematopoietic precursors, have no PTH receptors on their surfaces. Instead, preosteoblasts and osteoblasts signal to osteoclast precursors to cause them to fuse and form mature osteoclasts. This signaling also serves to stimulate mature osteoclasts to resorb bone and to avoid apoptosis (Fig. 27–9). Two osteoblast surface proteins, macrophage colony–stimulating factor (M-CSF) and RANK (receptor activator of nuclear factor κB) ligand (RANKL), are essential for stimulation of osteoclastogenesis,[74] and RANKL is essential for activation of mature osteoclasts. The growth factor M-CSF (or CSF1), is expressed both as a secreted protein and as a cell surface protein; the production of both forms is stimulated by PTH.[75] RANKL—also named *osteoprotegerin ligand* (OPGL), *osteoclast-differentiating factor* (ODF), and TRANCE—is a membrane-bound member of the tumor necrosis factor (TNF) family; its synthesis is also increased by PTH.[76] RANKL binds to its receptor, RANK, a member of the TNF receptor family. RANK is found both on osteoclast precursors and on mature osteoclasts. The binding of RANKL to RANK can be blocked by osteoprotegerin (OPG), another member of the TNF receptor family. OPG (also called OCIF and TR1) circulates and is also secreted by cells of the osteoblastic lineage. PTH decreases the synthesis and secretion of OPG from these cells. Thus, PTH, by increasing RANK and decreasing OPG locally in bone, serves to increase bone resorption.

Because PTH can increase both formation and resorption of bone, the net effect of PTH on bone mass varies from one part of bone to another and also varies dramatically according to whether PTH is administered continuously or intermittently. Intermittent administration of low doses of PTH causes a dramatic net increase in trabecular bone mass with little effect on cortical bone mass in humans. Continuous administration of PTH, in contrast, leads to a decrease in cortical bone mass; the net effect of PTH on trabecular bone depends on the dose. In mild primary hyperparathyroidism, there is little net effect of PTH on trabecular bone and a decrease in cortical bone. In all of these settings, the rate of bone formation is increased. The varying rate of osteoclastic resorption determines the net effect of PTH on bone mass.

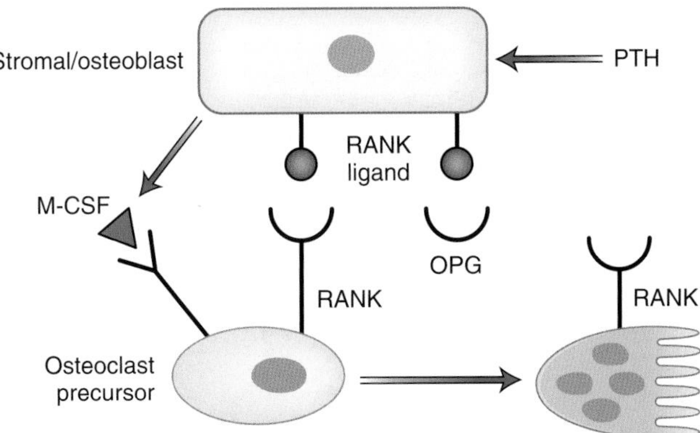

Figure 27–9 ▪ Stromal cell control of osteoclastogenesis and osteoclast activity. Parathyroid hormone (PTH) acts on PTH/PTH-related protein (PTHrP) receptors on precursors of osteoblasts to increase the production of macrophage colony–stimulating factor (M-CSF) and RANK (receptor activator of nuclear factor κB) ligand and to decrease the production of osteoprotegerin (OPG). M-CSF and RANK ligand stimulate the production of osteoclasts and increase the activity of mature osteoclasts by binding to the receptor RANK. OPG blocks the interaction of RANK ligand and RANK.

Molecular Basis of Parathyroid Hormone Action

Ever since the discovery that PTH stimulates the secretion of cAMP into the urine,[77] PTH has been thought to act by triggering a cascade of intracellular second messengers. This guiding hypothesis, in its current form, postulates that all of the actions of PTH result from the binding of the hormone to a receptor on the plasma membrane of target tissues. This receptor is a member of a large family of G protein–linked receptors that span the plasma membrane seven times (Fig. 27–10). The binding of hormone on the outside of the membrane causes conformational changes in the receptor molecule that activate the receptor's ability to release guanosine diphosphate (GDP) from the α subunit of a G protein bound to the receptor. The G protein then binds guanosine triphosphate (GTP) in place of GDP. The GTP-binding α subunit of the G protein then separates from the βγ subunits, and the separate subunits of the G protein then modulate the activity of enzymes and channels. The activity of these enzymes and channels then affects proteins farther downstream, eventually leading to the physiologic responses of bone and kidney cells.

Parathyroid Hormone and Parathyroid Hormone-Related Receptors

DNA encoding a PTH/PTHrP receptor has been isolated from rat, opossum, human, pig, *Xenopus* (toad), and zebrafish cells and tissues.[78] The receptor mediates actions of both PTH and PTHrP (see discussion of PTHrP later). The predicted amino acid sequence of the receptor and direct mapping of inserted epitopes suggest that the receptor spans the plasma membrane seven times, but the sequence does not closely resemble the sequences of most known G protein–linked receptors. Instead, it is a member of a distinct subfamily of closely related receptors. Most of these receptors bind peptides of 30 to 40 amino acids in length. Known members include receptors for the secretin family of peptides (secretin, vasoactive intestinal peptide [VIP], glucagon, glucagon-like peptide, growth hormone–releasing hormone, pituitary adenylate cyclase–activating peptide, gastric inhibitory peptide), corticotropin-releasing hormone,

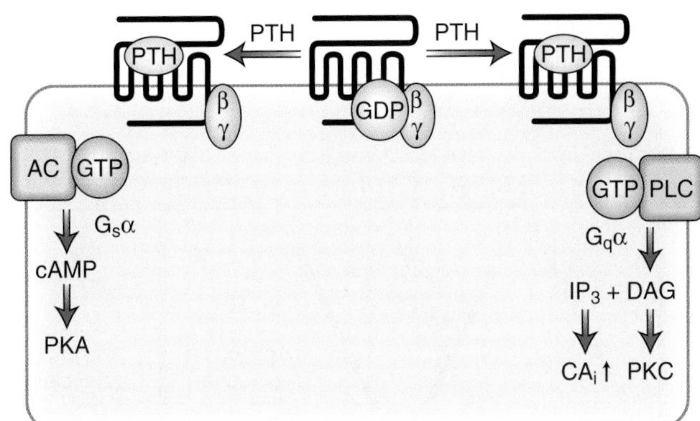

Figure 27–10 ▪ Parathyroid hormone (PTH)/PTH-related protein (PTHrP) receptors act as nucleotide exchangers. PTH binding to the receptor leads to exchange of guanosine triphosphate (GTP) for guanosine diphosphate (GDP) bound to Gα subunits. Gα subunits bound to GTP are released from the receptor and from the βγ subunits and then activate effectors. $G_s\alpha$ activates adenylate cyclase (AC), leading to the formation of cyclic adenosine monophosphate (cAMP), which then activates protein kinase A (PKA). $G_q\alpha$ and related α subunits activate phospholipase C (PLC). PLC hydrolyzes phosphotidyl inositol (1,4,5)trisphosphate to generate diacyl glycerol (DAG) and inositol (1,4,5)trisphosphate (IP_3). The DAG then activates protein kinase C (PKC), and the IP_3 activates a receptor on microsomal vesicles that directs the movement of calcium from microsomal vesicles into the cytosol. CA_i, intracellular calcium.

calcitonin, and insect diuretic hormones related to corticotropin-releasing hormone. The PTH/PTHrP receptor most closely resembles receptors of the secretin group. The gene encoding the PTH/PTHrP receptor has a complicated structure, with 13 introns interrupting the coding sequence.

The cloned PTH/PTHrP receptor binds amino-terminal fragments of PTH and PTHrP with equal affinity. The receptor is expressed at high levels in kidney and in osteoblasts of bone but is also expressed in a wide variety of tissues, such as smooth muscle, brain, and a variety of fetal tissues, which are thought to be target tissues more for PTHrP than for PTH. In response to binding of PTH or PTHrP, the receptor activates several G proteins, including G_s, G_q, G_{11}, G_i, G_{12}, and G_{13}.[79]

The PTH/PTHrP receptor mediates many of the actions of both PTH and PTHrP. The ligand-binding and signaling properties of the receptor, the pattern of expression of the receptor, and the consequences of mutation of the receptor sequence (see later) are persuasive evidence in this regard. Nevertheless, the scheme of PTH action illustrated in Figure 27–10 should be considered a simplified outline. It is unlikely that all of the actions of PTH can be explained by interactions with the cloned PTH/PTHrP receptor: Fragments of PTH that seem not to bind the receptor may be biologically active[21]; some cells respond to PTH in ways not mimicked by the cloned receptor.[22] Furthermore, the carboxyl-terminal portion of PTH(1-84) binds a cell surface protein distinct from the PTH/PTHrP receptor.

A second PTH receptor, which can be activated by PTH but not by PTHrP, called the PTH2 receptor (PTH2R), has been cloned.[82] This receptor is expressed in multiple tissues, including brain, vascular endothelium and smooth muscle, endocrine cells of the gastrointestinal tract, and sperm. Expression is not seen in osteoblasts or renal tubules, however. Although PTH activates the human PTH2R well, PTH only poorly activates the rat and other species of PTH2R. Furthermore, a novel ligand called TIP39 has been characterized and shown to be a potent activator of PTH2R. TIP39 bears only a weak resemblance to PTH or PTHrP and is likely to be a physiologically relevant activator of the PTH2. The functional role of the PTH2R is unknown, but it appears to mediate many actions of TIP39 in the brain; this receptor may well not normally mediate actions of PTH in vivo. The two cloned PTHRs, as well as distinct receptors for fragments of PTHrP (see later), probably are part of a complex network of ligands and receptors (Fig. 27–11).

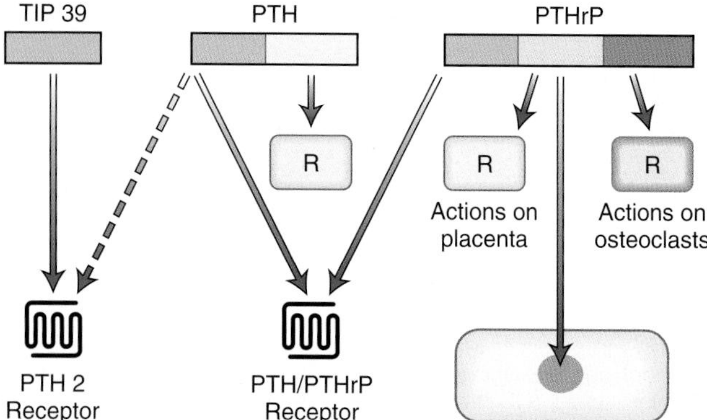

Figure 27–11 ▪ Network of parathyroid hormone (PTH) ligands and receptors (R). PTH and PTH-related protein (PTHrP) closely resemble each other at the amino-terminal region; TIP39 (39-residue tuberoinfundibular peptide) is more distantly related. Although only the PTH/PTHrP receptor and the PTH2 receptors have been cloned, biologic actions suggest receptors specific for the carboxy-terminal portion of PTH, as well as distinct receptors for the mid-region of PTHrP and for a more distal region of PTHrP. PTHrP is also found in nuclei and may act directly there.

Functional Implications of Parathyroid Hormone Structure

Amino-terminal fragments of PTH as short as PTH(1-34) have potency at least as great as that of the full-length PTH(1-84).[78] Several discrete portions of the PTH(1-34) peptide interact with the receptor. The first several residues of PTH are particularly important for triggering the conformational change in the receptor that results in activation of G_s and adenylate cyclase. Sequences responsible for transmembrane activation of G_s make up most of the first 13 residues of PTH; it is these residues that are highly conserved between PTH and PTHrP. At high concentrations, PTH(1-14) by itself can activate the PTH/PTHrP receptor. This activation domain interacts with the receptor's transmembrane domains and extracellular loops. When the first nine residues of PTH are covalently linked to the receptor's transmembrane domains and extracellular loops, they can activate the receptor. An analogue of PTH(1-14) can trigger G_q activation, thus activating phospholipase C.[83] These data, plus the observation that a PTH analogue modified at position 1 selectively loses its ability to activate phospholipase C,[84] demonstrate that the amino-terminal portion of PTH is essential for activation of both G_s and G_q. More distal regions of PTH(1-34) can activate protein kinase C and can raise intracellular calcium levels by mechanisms that have not been fully clarified.

The more carboxy-terminal portions of PTH(1-34) contribute importantly to the specificity and tight binding of PTH to the PTH/PTHrP receptor, at least partly through interactions with the receptor's amino-terminal extracellular domain (Fig. 27–12). A variety of studies of genetically altered receptors and biochemical studies using photoactivated crosslinks between PTH and the receptor have reinforced each other and show that the carboxy-terminal portion of PTH makes multiple contacts with the amino-terminal extension of the receptor and with its extracellular loops. This interaction of PTH with the amino-terminal portion of the receptor occurs extremely rapidly, with a time constant of 140 msec.[85] In contrast, the subsequent interaction of the amino-terminal portion of PTH with the so-called J

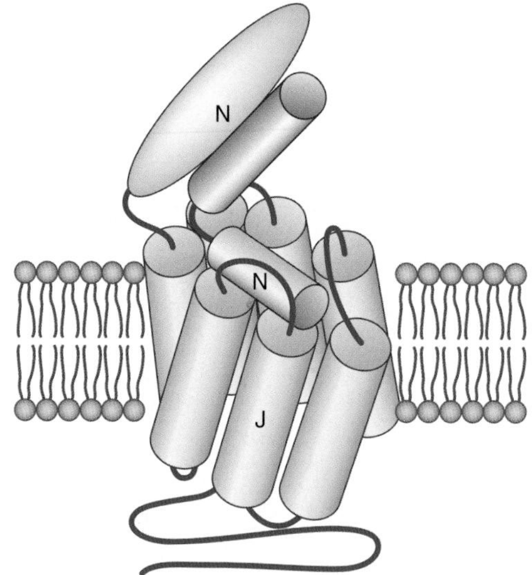

Figure 27–12 ▪ Binding of parathyroid hormone (PTH)1-34 to the PTH/PTH-related protein (PTHrP) receptor. The amino-terminal extracellular domain of the receptor binds rapidly to the carboxy-terminal portion of the ligand. The "J" domain of the receptor, containing the transmembrane domains and associated loops, binds to the amino-terminal domain of the ligand. This binding is slower and might require conformational changes in both the ligand and receptor. These conformational changes then trigger G protein activation, receptor internalization, and other actions. (Figure courtesy of Tom Gardella.)

domain of the receptor (the transmembrane domains and associated extracellular loops) occurs more slowly, with a time constant of 1 sec. Presumably, this extra time is needed for the amino-terminus of PTH to form an α helix and for the receptor to attain an optimal conformation for binding. When this slow interaction occurs, then the receptor changes the relationships of its transmembrane domains and activates G proteins.[86]

Studies of the structure of PTH by nuclear magnetic resonance (NMR) spectroscopy[87,88] suggest that the activation domain and the carboxy-terminal domain are discrete entities dominated by α-helices separated by a flexible loop of variable size, depending on the hydrophobicity of the solvent. In the crystal structure of human PTH(1-34), the flexible loop is entirely replaced with helical structure.[89] Taken together, these studies suggest that the carboxy-terminal portion of PTH makes multiple contacts with the receptor that allow high-affinity binding and position the amino-terminal portion of PTH to activate the receptor through contacts with transmembrane domains and associated loops.

Activation of Second Messengers

Precisely how binding of PTH to the extracellular domains of the PTH/PTHrP receptor leads to activation of G proteins is not understood. The crystal structure of rhodopsin, another member of the seven-transmembrane receptor family, as well as the behavior of certain mutant PTH/PTHrP receptors,[90,91] suggests that the seven transmembrane domains of the PTH/PTHrP receptors form a ring, with the seventh transmembrane domain adjacent to the first and second domains. Presumably, binding of PTH to several different regions of the receptor changes the relationships of the transmembrane domains[86] such that the receptor's three intracellular loops and carboxy-terminal tail interact with G proteins in an altered way.

Receptors with certain point mutations in the second, sixth, and seventh transmembrane domains can activate G_s even without stimulation by hormone. These mutant receptors were discovered by analyzing the PTH/PTHrP receptors in patients with Jansen's metaphyseal chondrodystrophy.[92] Patients with this disorder have signs of parathyroid overactivity (hypercalcemia, hypophosphatemia, high levels of $1,25(OH)_2D_3$, and urinary cAMP) but low PTH and PTHrP levels. The mutations must change the conformation of the intracellular face of the receptor in a way that resembles the effect of binding of PTH to the normal receptor. The observation that inappropriate activation of the PTH/PTHrP receptor in Jansen's chondrodystrophy leads to all of the metabolic abnormalities found in primary hyperparathyroidism is one of the most persuasive pieces of evidence that the cloned PTH/PTHrP receptor does, in fact, mediate the actions of PTH in bone and kidney in vivo.

Second Messengers and Distal Effects of Parathyroid Hormone

The activation of multiple G proteins by PTH raises questions about the individual roles of each second messenger and their possible interactions. The importance of cAMP as a mediator of the physiologic actions of PTH has been demonstrated by studies in vivo[23] and in vitro.[93,94] Furthermore, patients with pseudohypoparathyroidism type 1, who cannot increase urinary cAMP levels in response to PTH, show clear renal resistance to PTH (see later).

Activation of phospholipase C, with concomitant activation of protein kinase C and synthesis of IP_3, might contribute to physiologic actions of PTH as well, such as inhibition of sodium-phosphate cotransport[95] and stimulation of the renal 25(OH)D 1α-hydroxylase.[96] Some actions of PTH might require activation of both adenylate cyclase and phospholipase C for optimal activity.

The stimulation of one G protein or another by the PTH/PTHrP receptor can vary in different types of cells and even in differing regions of the same cell.[24] In some settings, this choice may be influenced by the interactions of the PTH/PTHrP receptor with intracellular scaffolding proteins, such as NHERF1 and NHERF2 (Na^+/H^+ exchanger regulatory factor). Binding of the PTH/PTHrP receptor to NHERFs is directed by the last four amino acids in the receptor sequence. This binding—which is particularly prominent at the apical surface of the proximal tubular cells of the kidney, for example—changes the G protein activated by the PTH/PTHrP receptor from predominantly G_s to predominantly G_i.[97,98]

Target Cell Responsiveness to Parathyroid Hormone

Physiologic responses to PTH depend not only on the concentration of PTH in blood but also on the responsiveness of target cells to PTH. This responsiveness can be modified by previous exposure to PTH or by exposure to a variety of other hormones and paracrine factors. Responsiveness can be changed by alterations at virtually every step in the cellular response to PTH.

Major regulators of PTH/PTHrP receptor gene expression include, not surprisingly, PTH and $1,25(OH)_2D_3$, both of which can decrease PTH/PTHrP receptor mRNA in certain target cells.[99] In some settings, PTH decreases the amount of immunoreactive and functional receptor on the cell surface without changing the levels of PTH/PTHrP mRNA. This decrease reflects ligand-induced internalization and degradation of receptors. Internalization of receptor is stimulated by PTH binding, which leads to phosphorylation of specific serines found in the receptor's cytoplasmic tail and subsequent internalization directed by binding of arrestin to the receptor.[100,101] Even without change in receptor number, the binding of arrestin to the PTH/PTHrP receptor decreases the efficiency of activation of G proteins (desensitization).

Parathyroid Hormone–Related Protein

PTHrP was discovered because the secretion of PTHrP by a wide variety of tumors contributes to the humoral hypercalcemia of malignancy. For this reason, the initial studies of PTHrP in humans and animals stressed the PTH-like structure and properties of the molecule. Subsequent studies soon showed, however, that PTHrP, unlike PTH, is made by a wide variety of tissues, in which it acts locally in ways that might have little relevance to the control of blood calcium.

Gene and Protein Structure

PTHrP sequences from human, rat, mouse, dog, cow, chicken, fugu fish, zebra fish, and sea bream have been cloned (Fig. 27–13).[3,102,103] In humans, alternative RNA splicing yields transcripts that encode three distinct proteins of 139, 141, and 173 residues that differ only after residue 139.

Inspection of these sequences suggests that PTHrP has several functionally distinct domains. Eight or nine of the first 13 residues of PTHrP are identical to those in known mammalian PTH sequences. These sequences encompass the known activation domain of PTH (see earlier) and are instrumental in the ability of PTHrP to activate PTH/PTHrP receptors. The conserved histidine at position 5 of all PTHrP molecules, which differs from the hydrophobic residue found at the corresponding position of all PTHs, allows PTHrP to activate the PTH/PTHrP receptor but not the PTH2 receptor.

The sequences in PTHrP(14-34) are also highly conserved. Although these sequences little resemble the corresponding

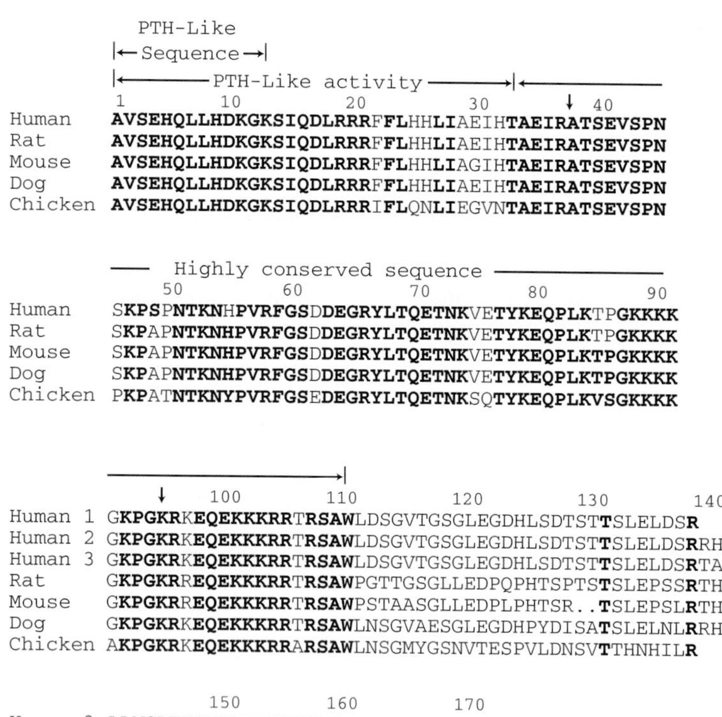

Figure 27–13 ▪ Sequences of parathyroid hormone–related protein (PTHrP) from five species. Completely conserved residues are in *boldface;* note the high level of conservation through residue 111. *Arrows* indicate sites of internal cleavage after residues 37 and 95, which lead to generation of PTHrP(38-94) amide and PTHrP(38-95). Another site of cleavage, generating PTHrP(38-101) and, perhaps, PTHrP(107-139) is not shown.[103] The three human sequences represent proteins synthesized from alternatively spliced mRNAs and differ only after residue 139. Amino acids are indicated by the single letter code; see the legend to Figure 26-3 for code.

region of PTH, they can displace PTH from the PTH/PTHrP receptor. Studies of the secondary and tertiary structures of PTHrP(1-34) and PTH(1-37) suggest that they have similar structures dominated by α-helices connected by a flexible hinge.

The remaining portion of the PTHrP molecule bears no resemblance to corresponding sequences in PTH. Nevertheless, residues 35 to 111 of PTHrP are strikingly well conserved, and only nine residues differ between mammalian and chicken PTHrP sequences. This sequence conservation is considerably greater than that found in the carboxyl-terminal portion of PTH, suggesting that this region of PTHrP has unique and important functions. After residue 111, the PTHrP sequences vary considerably from species to species.

Interspersed within the PTHrP sequences are multiple sites containing one or several basic residues that might serve as post-translational cleavage sites (see Fig. 27–13). Extensive analysis of PTHrP fragments in tumors, cell lines, and transfected cells has shown that several of these sites are, in fact, functional cleavage signals. PTHrP is cleaved after the arginine at residue 37; this cleavage, followed by carboxypeptidase cleavage, generates a PTH-like PTHrP(1-36) fragment as well as the fragments PTHrP(38-94)amide, PTHrP(38-95), and PTHrP(38-101).[104] More carboxy-terminal fragments of PTHrP have been detected in cells as well.

In the blood of patients with humoral hypercalcemia of malignancy, multiple immunoreactive species of PTHrP have been found that may well correspond to the fragments of PTHrP in cells and tissue culture media, although precise characterization of these various immunoreactive species is incomplete (see later). Full-length PTHrP may well not circulate, because an amino-terminal–specific immunoaffinity column was unable to extract carboxy-terminal immunoreactivity from the serum of patients with malignant hypercalcemia.[105]

Functions of Parathyroid Hormone–Related Protein

The first actions of PTHrP to be defined were the PTH-like actions associated with the humoral hypercalcemia of malignancy. In this pathologic entity, PTHrP acts as a hormone; it is secreted from the tumor into the bloodstream and then acts on bone and kidney to raise the calcium level (see "Hypercalcemia of Malignancy" later).[106] Whether or not PTHrP circulates at high enough levels in normal adults to contribute to normal calcium homeostasis is an unanswered question. With metastases of breast cancer to bone, locally produced PTHrP can raise serum calcium without necessarily raising blood levels of PTHrP.[107]

PTHrP acts as a calciotropic hormone during fetal life and in lactation. PTHrP secreted from the fetal parathyroid gland stimulates transport of calcium across the placenta in sheep.[108] PTH, in contrast, has no effect on placental calcium transport. Furthermore, fetal mice missing the PTHrP gene transport ^{45}Ca across the placenta inefficiently.[109] This action of PTHrP requires only the mid-region of PTHrP and probably involves a receptor distinct from the PTH/PTHrP receptor.

The second possible setting for humoral actions of PTHrP is lactation. In mice, secretion of PTHrP from the breast into the bloodstream leads to an increase in bone resorption.[110] Calcium then activates the calcium-sensing receptor in breast tissue, increases the movement of calcium into milk, and down-regulates expression of PTHrP in the breast.[111] PTHrP, therefore, probably contributes to the dramatic but largely reversible bone loss during lactation in humans, which is only minimally affected by calcium supplementation.[112,113] An exaggeration of this lactational role of PTHrP might explain the rare presentation of hypercalcemia and high PTHrP levels in pregnant and lactating women.[114] Large amounts of PTHrP are also secreted into breast milk, although the role of PTHrP in milk is unknown.

Most of the actions of PTHrP are likely to be paracrine or autocrine.[115] PTHrP is synthesized at one time or another during fetal life in virtually every tissue. Its role in the development of fetal bone has been demonstrated through the striking abnormalities found in PTHrP knockout mice. These abnormalities suggest that PTHrP normally keeps chondrocytes proliferating in orderly columns, thereby delaying chondrocyte differentiation.[116] The role of PTHrP in many other fetal tissues might analogously involve regulation of proliferation and differentiation. The widespread expression of the PTHrP in fetal life probably underlies the expression of PTHrP in a wide variety of malignancies. As is often the case in malignancy, the expression of PTHrP represents the reinitiation of a fetal pattern of gene expression.

PTHrP is synthesized by many adult tissues. In tissues such as skin, hair, and breast, it is likely that PTHrP regulates cell proliferation and differentiation. PTHrP is also synthesized in response to stretch in the smooth muscle of blood vessels and of the gastrointestinal tract, uterus, and bladder and acts in an autocrine fashion to relax the smooth muscle.[117] PTHrP is also widely expressed in neurons of the central nervous system; its function in the brain is unknown, but it might protect neurons from excitotoxicity by decreasing flux through voltage-gated calcium channels[118]; an analogous mechanism might explain the role of PTHrP in smooth muscle relaxation.

Many of the actions of PTHrP are mediated by the PTH/PTHrP receptor. Others, such as the activation of placental calcium transport, are probably mediated by a distinct receptor, and other actions on bone cells probably involve yet another receptor responsive to more distal portions of PTHrP. Increasing evidence suggests, furthermore, that some actions of PTHrP involve direct nuclear actions of PTHrP.[119] Thus, both PTH and PTHrP are likely to use multiple mechanisms to stimulate cells (see Fig. 27–11).

Calcitonin

Calcitonin has an important role in regulating blood calcium in fish and a demonstrable role in rodents; however, the importance of calcitonin in human calcium homeostasis remains uncertain.

The existence of a second calcium-regulating hormone, in addition to PTH, was first demonstrated during perfusion studies of the thyroid and parathyroid glands of dogs.[120] High calcium perfusion resulted in a rapid decrease in plasma calcium, even more rapid than after parathyroidectomy. This suggested that calcium had stimulated the secretion of a hormone that lowered blood calcium. It was subsequently demonstrated that this missing hormone, named *calcitonin* for its role in regulating the "tone" or level of calcium, was elaborated by the thyroid gland, not the parathyroids.

Calcitonin is found in the nonfollicular cells of the thyroid, called *C cells,* which originate from the neural crest. In fish, the location of the C cells in discrete organs led to the rapid isolation of calcitonin from these ultimobranchial bodies in dogfish, salmon, and several other species. The identification of the glandular origin of calcitonin enabled the isolation of sufficient quantities of calcitonin for sequence analysis and studies of its structure and biologic function.

Synthesis and Secretion

Calcitonin consists of a 32-amino-acid polypeptide with an intrachain disulfide bond provided by the cysteines at positions 1 and 7 (Fig. 27–14). These two cysteine residues, along with the carboxy-terminal proline-amide and six additional residues are the only amino acids conserved among the calcitonins isolated from various species. The disulfide linkage and proline-amide residues are important for the function of the molecule, although biologically active analogues lacking disulfide bonds have been developed.

Interestingly, fish calcitonin is more potent in mammals than is the mammalian hormone. The mature peptide is derived from the middle of a 136-amino-acid precursor. The human calcitonin gene, located on the short arm of chromosome 11, contains 6 exons that are alternately spliced in a tissue-specific manner to yield the mRNAs encoding calcitonin or calcitonin gene–related peptide (CGRP) (Fig. 27–15). The mRNA encoding calcitonin is derived by splicing together the first four exons [121] and represents more than 95% of mature transcripts in the thyroid C cells. The splicing of the first three exons to exons 5 and 6 results in an mRNA that encodes the 37 amino acid α-CGRP peptide. The mRNA encoding α-CGRP is expressed in multiple tissues and is the only mature transcript of the calcitonin gene detected in neural tissue. A second CGRP gene encodes the closely related β-CGRP. In humans, the predicted sequence of the mature peptide differs from that of α-CGRP by only three amino acids (see Fig. 27–14). The β-CGRP gene is also found on chromosome 11; its tissue distribution is the same as that of α-CGRP.

Synthesis and secretion of calcitonin are tightly regulated. Studies in a porcine model reveal a linear relationship between the secretion of calcitonin and ambient calcium levels.[122] Cell culture studies with calcium ionophores and calcium channel blockers demonstrate that the calcium ion concentration within the C cell determines this secretion rate.[123] The calcium-sensing receptor cloned from parathyroid cells is also expressed in C cells, and it contributes to the regulation of calcitonin secretion.[124] Other calcitonin secretagogues include glucocorticoids, CGRP, glucagon, enteroglucagon, gastrin, pentagastrin, pancreozymin, and β-adrenergic agents.[125] The physiologic role of the gastrointestinal hormones in regulating calcitonin remains unclear; however, they have been postulated to play a role in the regulation of postprandial hypercalcemia. The secretion of calcitonin is inhibited by somatostatin, which is also secreted by the thyroid C cells. In vivo[126] and in vitro[127] studies have dem-

Peptide	Species	Sequence	
CT	Human	**C**GNLST**C**MLGTYTQDFNKFHTFPQTAIGVGAP	-NH2
	Salmon-1	**C**S----**C**V--KLS-ELH-LQTY-R-NT-SGT-	-NH2
	Salmon-2	**C**S----**C**V--KLS-DLH-LQTF-R-NT-AGV-	-NH2
	Salmon-3	**C**S----**C**M--KLS-DLH-LQTF-R-NT-AGV-	-NH2
CGRP	Human α	A**C**DTAT**C**VTHRLAGLLSRSGGVVKNNFVPTNVGSKAF	-NH2
	Human β	-**C**N---**C**-----------------S------------	-NH2
	Salmon	-**C**N---**C**------DF-N-----GNS------------	-NH2
Amylin	Human	A**C**DTAT**C**VTHRLAGLLSRSGGVVKNNFVPTNVGSKAF	-NH2
ADM	Human	YRQSMNNFQGLRSFG**C**RFGT**C**TVQKLAHQIYQFTDKDKDNVAPRSKISPQGY	-NH2
IMD	Human	TQAQLLRVG**C**VLGT**C**QVQNLSHRLWQLMGPAGRQDSAPVDPSSPHSYG	-NH2
CRSP-1	Porcine	S**C**NTAT**C**MTHRLVGLLSRSGSMVRSNLLPTKMGFKVFG	-NH2
CRSP-2	Porcine	-**C**---S**C**V--KMT-W------VAKN-FM--NVDS-IL	-NH2
CRSP-3	Porcine	-**C**---I**C**V--KMA-W------V-KN-FM-IN--S-VL	-NH2

Figure 27–14 ▪ The amino acid sequences of calcitonin (CT), calcitonin gene–related peptide (CGRP), amylin, adrenomedullin (ADM), intermedin (IDM), and calcitonin receptor–stimulating proteins (CSRP) from selected species. The *bold Cs* represent the cysteine residues that form the disulfide linkages critical for the secondary structure of these peptides. The other conserved residues are indicated by a *dashed line.* See the legend to Figure 27–3 for the single-letter amino acid codes.

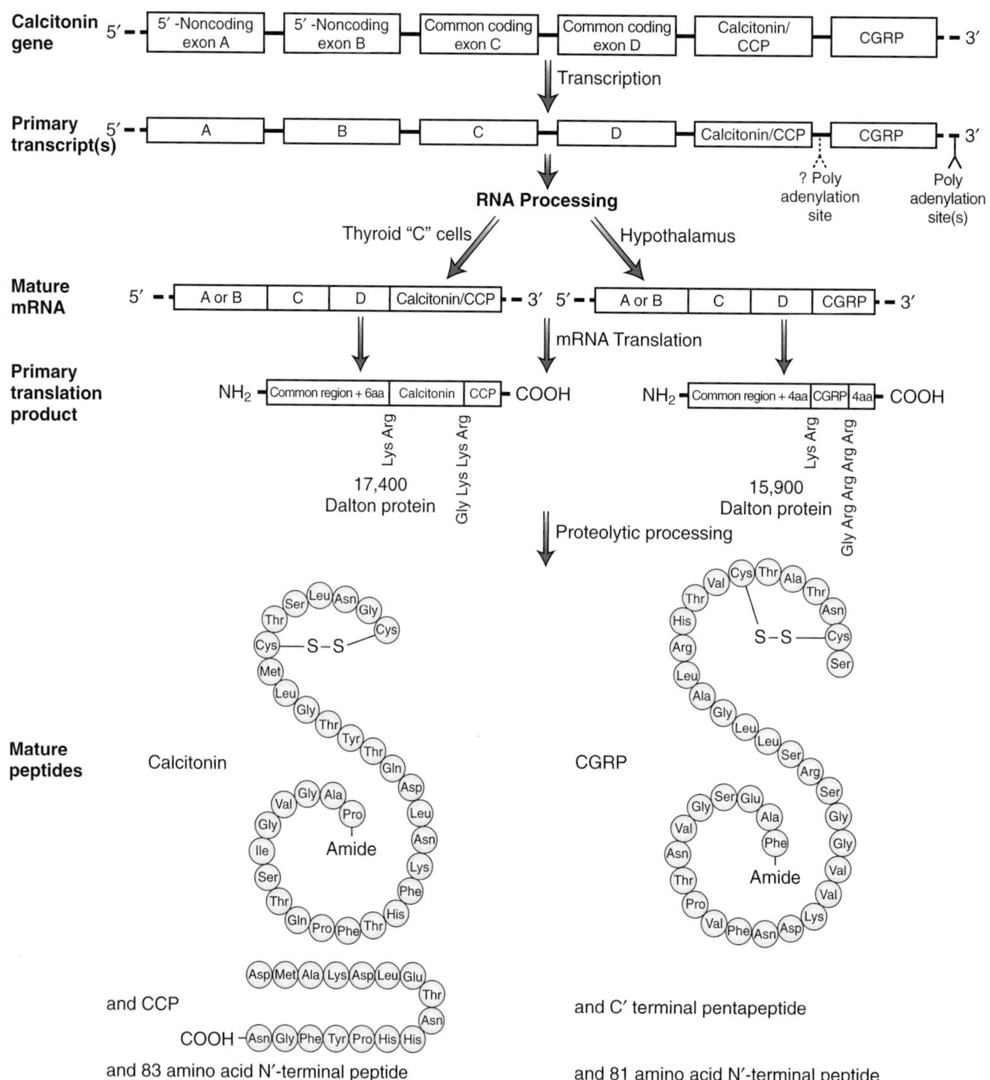

Figure 27–15 ▪ Tissue-specific expression of the calcitonin gene. Splicing of alternative exons leads to two different messenger RNAs (mRNAs). The mRNA encoding calcitonin is found predominantly in the thyroid C cell; the mRNA encoding calcitonin gene related–peptide (CGRP) is found predominantly in the hypothalamus and other nervous tissue. CCP, calcitonin carboxyl-terminal peptide. (From Amara SG, Jones V, Rosenfeld MG, et al. Alternative RNA processing in calcitonin gene expression generates mRNAs encoding different polypeptide products. Nature 1982;298:240-244.)

onstrated that $1,25(OH)_2D_3$ decreases calcitonin mRNA levels by a transcriptional mechanism.

Calcitonin, when administered acutely, decreases tubular resorption of calcium[49] and impairs osteoclast-mediated bone resorption by a direct action on osteoclasts.[128] In rodents, calcitonin has been shown to play a role in the regulation of postprandial hypercalcemia.[129] Studies in calcitonin knockout mice reveal a doubling of bone formation rate in the absence of hormone, accompanied by resistance to ovariectomy-induced bone loss[130]; a similar increase in bone formation is found in mice heterozygous for ablation of the calcitonin receptor.[131] The mechanism of this apparent effect of calcitonin on bone formation is not understood.

The physiologic role of calcitonin in humans, however, remains elusive. The effect of calcitonin on bone density was examined in patients with long-term hypercalcitoninemia secondary to medullary carcinoma of the thyroid (MCT) and in patients with subtotal thyroidectomy resulting in lack of calcitonin secretory reserve.[132] Bone density at the lumbar spine and distal radius were not influenced by the abnormal calcitonin levels. Furthermore, no physiologic abnormalities have been reported with long-term high-dose administration of exogenous calcitonin.

Many of the effects of calcitonin are mediated by a G protein–coupled cell surface receptor in the PTH/secretin receptor family.[133,134] The mRNA encoding this receptor has been found in several tissues including kidney, brain, and osteoclasts. The coupling of this receptor to different G proteins results in the activation of either adenylate cyclase or phospholipase C; in some settings, this is cell cycle–dependent.[135]

Calcitonin Family: Calcitonin Gene-Related Peptide, Amylin, Adrenomedullin, and Intermedin

CGRP, amylin, adrenomedullin, CSRP-1, and intermedin have all been shown to have high-affinity binding sites on cell membranes, and displacement studies suggest that several receptor subtypes for these related ligands are present. However, cloning of specific receptors for these ligands proved difficult, because the functional receptors consist of heterodimers between G protein–coupled receptors and single *trans*-membrane proteins of the RAMP (receptor activity modifying proteins) family.[136,137] Interaction of the calcitonin receptor–like receptor, a relative of the calcitonin receptor, with RAMP1 results in a CGRP receptor, whereas RAMP2 and RAMP3 interactions with the same calcitonin receptor–like receptor generate adrenomedullin receptors. Interaction of RAMP1 with the calcitonin receptor creates an amylin receptor.[138]

CGRP is thought to act as a neurotransmitter and vasodilator rather than as a hormone. In support of this hypothesis, mice lacking α-CGRP have been shown to have an increase in mean arterial pressure.[139] Immunohistochemical studies of CGRP in the brain and peripheral nervous system suggest that this neuropeptide also plays an important role in sensory and integrative motor functions.

Three structurally related peptides have been isolated from porcine brain (see Fig. 27–14). These calcitonin receptor–stimulating peptides (CRSP) are also expressed in the thyroid gland. CRSP-1, which is 60% homologous to α-CGRP at the amino acid level, binds to the calcitonin receptor and dose-dependently stimulates cAMP production. Consistent with this observation, administration of CRSP-1, like administration of calcitonin, results in a decrease in serum calcium. The receptors for CRSP-2 and CRSP-3 have not been identified.[140]

Amylin is highly homologous to CGRP and calcitonin (see Fig. 27–14). Although amylin has been shown to have skeletal actions, the presence of amylin in the pancreas of patients with type 2 diabetes mellitus suggests an etiologic role for this peptide in this disorder.[141,142] Amylin administration inhibits bone loss associated with ovariectomy[143] and streptozotocin-induced diabetes mellitus in rats.[144] Targeted ablation of amylin in mice results in low bone mass due to an increase in bone resorption.[131] Amylin has also been shown to decrease food intake and inhibit gastric acid secretion, protecting against ulcer development in numerous models.[145]

Adrenomedullin (see Fig. 27–14) has vasodilative effects similar to those of CGRP. In addition to activating CGRP receptors, adrenomedullin binds to specific receptors in the vascular system.[146] Mice missing DNA coding adrenomedullin die in midgestation[147]; the physiologic roles of adrenomedullin in adults remain to be clarified.

Intermedin, the newest member of this family (see Fig. 27–14), was identified by homology screening of expressed sequence tags. It is expressed primarily in the pituitary and the gastrointestinal tract. Intermedin can signal through CGRP receptors and competes with CGRP for receptor binding.[148] However, unlike CGRP and adrenomedullin, intermedin is a nonselective agonist for the RAMP coreceptors.

Calcitonin in Human Disease

Calcitonin is secreted by several endocrine malignancies and therefore can serve as a tumor marker. Basal and pentagastrin-stimulated calcitonin levels have been used to identify and follow those at risk for, or affected by, medullary carcinoma of the thyroid (see Chapter 40), although abnormal basal and stimulated levels may be observed in patients on chronic hemodialysis.[149] Calcitonin may also be ectopically secreted by other tumors, including insulinomas, VIPomas, and lung cancers. Severely ill patients, including those with burn inhalation injury,[150] toxic shock syndrome, and pancreatitis, might also have elevated calcitonin levels.

Therapeutic Uses

The observation that calcitonin inhibits osteoclastic bone resorption has led to its therapeutic use for the treatment of several disorders associated with excess bone resorption, including osteoporosis and Paget's disease (see Chapter 28). However, paradoxically, mice lacking the gene that encodes calcitonin/α-CGRP have an increase in bone formation rate and demonstrate protection against ovariectomy-induced bone loss.[130] This effect is thought to be specifically due to lack of calcitonin, because mice lacking α-CGRP have a reduction in bone formation,[151] and mice heterozygous for knockout of the calcitonin receptor also have increased bone formation.[131] Calcitonin has also been used for its analgesic effect in the treatment of patients with vertebral crush fractures, osteolytic metastases, or phantom limb.[152,153]

Vitamin D

Metabolism of Vitamin D

Vitamin D is not a true vitamin, because nutritional supplementation is not required in humans who have adequate sun exposure. When exposed to ultraviolet irradiation, the cutaneous precursor of vitamin D, 7-dehydrocholesterol, undergoes photochemical cleavage of the carbon bond between carbons 9 and 10 of the steroid ring (Fig. 27–16). The resultant product, previtamin D, is thermally labile, and over a period of 48 hours it undergoes a temperature-dependent molecular rearrangement that results in the production of vitamin D.[154] Alternatively, this thermally labile product can isomerize to two biologically inert products, luminosterol and tachysterol. This alternative photoisomerization prevents production of excessive amounts of vitamin D with prolonged sun exposure. The degree of skin pigmentation, which increases in response to solar exposure, also regulates the conversion of 7-dehydrocholesterol to vitamin D by blocking the penetration of ultraviolet rays.

The alternative source of vitamin D is the diet. The elderly, the institutionalized, and those living in northern climates likely obtain most of their vitamin D from dietary sources. However, with increasing avoidance of sun exposure by the general population, ensuring adequate dietary intake of vitamin D has become important for the population at large. Vitamin D deficiency is prevalent[155] and has been shown to contribute significantly to osteopenia and fracture risk. The major dietary sources of vitamin D are fortified dairy products, although the lack of monitoring of this supplementation results in marked variation in the amount of vitamin D provided.[156] Other dietary sources include egg yolks, fish oils, and fortified cereal products. Vitamin D provided by plant sources is in the form of vitamin D_2, whereas that provided by animal sources is in the form of vitamin D_3 (see Fig. 27–16). These two forms have equivalent biologic potencies and are activated equally efficiently by the hydroxylases in humans.

Vitamin D is absorbed into the lymphatics and enters the circulation bound primarily to vitamin D binding protein, although a fraction of vitamin D circulates bound to albumin. The human vitamin D binding protein is a 52-kd globulin synthesized in the liver. The protein has a high affinity for 25(OH)D but also binds vitamin D and $1,25(OH)_2D$. Approximately 88% of 25(OH)D circulates bound to the vitamin D binding protein, 0.03% is free, and the rest circulates bound to albumin.[157] In contrast, 85% of the circulating $1,25(OH)_2D_3$ binds to the vitamin D binding protein, 0.4% is free, and the rest binds to albumin.[158] Mice lacking vitamin D binding protein have increased susceptibility to $1,25(OH)_2D_3$ toxicity as well as to dietary vitamin D deficiency.[159] Thus, the role of vitamin D binding protein is to

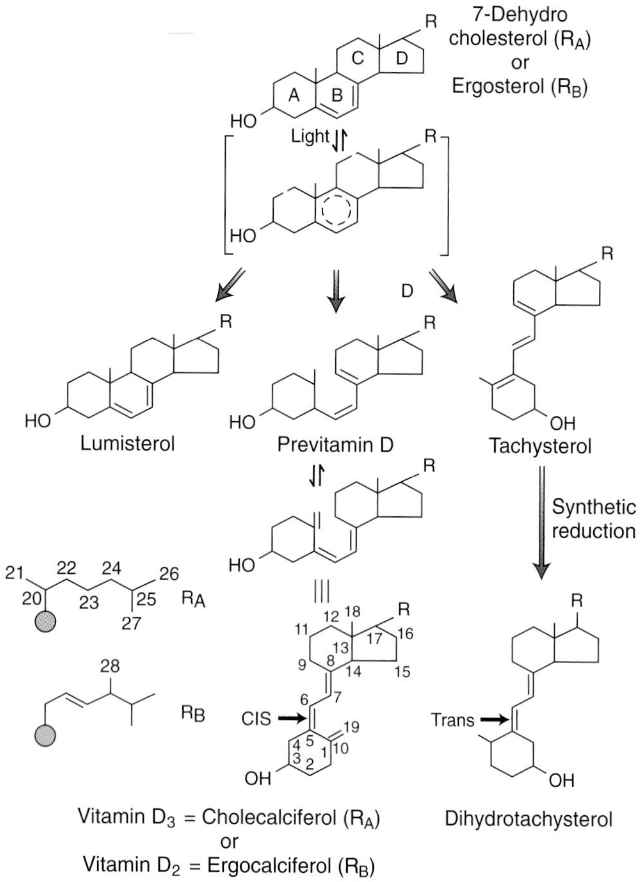

Figure 27–16 ▪ Vitamin D precursors and alternative reaction products. The numbering system for vitamin D carbons and the distinct structures of vitamin D_2 (ergocalciferol) and D_3 (cholecalciferol) are noted, as is the structure of dihydrotachysterol, a synthetic product not produced in vivo. Note that the 3-hydroxyl group of dihydrotachysterol is in a pseudo-1-hydroxyl configuration. This may explain the relatively high potency of dihydrotachysterol in conditions associated with low 1α-hydroxylase activity.

maintain a serum reservoir and to modulate the activity of vitamin D metabolites. Studies in megalin null mice suggest that vitamin D binding protein is filtered by the glomerulus and reabsorbed by a megalin-dependent pathway in the proximal renal tubule.[160] Further investigations will be required to determine the importance of this pathway in vitamin D metabolism and the tissues in which megalin-dependent endocytosis plays an important role.

In the liver, vitamin D undergoes 25-hydroxylation by a cytochrome P450-like enzyme present in the mitochondria and microsomes. The half-life of 25(OH)D is approximately 2 to 3 weeks. The 25-hydroxylation of vitamin D is not tightly regulated; therefore, the blood levels of 25(OH)D reflect the amount of vitamin D entering the circulation. When levels of vitamin D binding protein are low, such as in the nephrotic syndrome, circulating levels of 25(OH)D are also reduced. The half-life of 25(OH)D is shortened by increases in levels of its active metabolite, $1,25(OH)_2D_3$.

The final step in the production of the active hormone is the renal 1α-hydroxylation of 25(OH)D to $1,25(OH)_2D_3$. The half-life of this hormone is approximately 6 to 8 hours. Like the 25-hydroxylase, the 1α-hydroxylase in the proximal convoluted tubule is a cytochrome P450-like mixed function oxidase,[161-163] but unlike the 25-hydroxylase, the 1α-hydroxylase is tightly regulated. PTH and hypophosphatemia are the major inducers of this microsomal enzyme, whereas calcium and the enzyme's product, 1,25(OH)2D, repress it.[58] FGF23 has also been shown to repress 1α-hydroxylase mRNA production.[164] Analogous to mice lacking FGF23, mice with inactivating mutations of klotho, a type 1 membrane protein with homology to β-glycosidases, develop hypercalcemia due to increased levels of $1,25(OH)_2D_3$. Like the FGF23 null mice, klotho null mice have increased levels of the 1α-hydroxylase[165] and their phenotype is alleviated with impairment of $1,25(OH)_2D_3$ action.[166] Klotho binds to FGF receptor 1 and substantially increases the activation of FGF receptors by FGF23.[167] These findings suggest that FGF23 and klotho cooperate in suppressing the synthesis of 1α-hydroxylase. In animal models and in vitro studies, other hormones such as estrogen, calcitonin, growth hormone, and prolactin have been shown to increase 1α-hydroxylase activity; however, the clinical importance of these observations has not been established. Ketoconazole has been shown to decrease levels of $1,25(OH)_2D_3$ in a dose-dependent manner, presumably by interfering with 1α-hydroxylase activity.

The 1α-hydroxylase enzyme is also expressed in keratinocytes,[161] the trophoblastic layer of the placenta,[168] and granulomata, including sarcoid granulomata.[169] In granulomatous tissue, the 1α-hydroxylase gene that is expressed is identical to that expressed in the kidney but is not regulated by PTH, phosphate, calcium, or vitamin D metabolites in these cells. Activation of macrophages with interferon γ (IFN-γ)[170] or with ligands that activate the heterodimer of toll-like receptors 1 and 2,[171] however, increases the expression of the 1α-hydroxylase in macrophages, whereas treatment of sarcoidosis-associated hypercalcemia with glucocorticoids, ketoconazole,[172] or chloroquine[173] has been shown to lower serum $1,25(OH)_2D_3$ levels. Activation of the vitamin D receptor in human macrophages induces the antimicrobial peptide cathelicidin and increases killing of intracellular *Mycobacterium tuberculosis*.[171] Thus, the pathologic excess of $1,25(OH)_2D_3$ in sarcoidosis might represent an exaggeration of a healthy paracrine response of tissue macrophages.

25(OH)D and $1,25(OH)_2D_3$ can also be hydroxylated by the vitamin D 24-hydroxylase, which is present in most tissues including kidney, cartilage, and intestine. $1,25(OH)_2D_3$ increases the activity of the 24-hydroxylase, thereby inducing its own metabolism. The 24-hydroxylated vitamin D metabolites, $24,25(OH)_2D_3$ and $1,24,25(OH)_3D_3$, are not thought to play major biologic roles other than inactivation of $1,25(OH)_2D_3$. Mice null for the 24-hydroxylase gene demonstrate hypercalcemia, hypercalciuria, and nephrocalcinosis due to vitamin D toxicity.[174] Although $24,25(OH)_2D_3$ has been shown to have unique actions in a number of biologic systems,[175,176] no unique receptor for this metabolite has been identified and the physiologic role of $24,25(OH)_2D_3$ is unclear.

$1,25(OH)_2D_3$ is also metabolized to several inactive products by 23- or 26-hydroxylation and side chain oxidation and cleavage. This latter side chain cleavage, resulting in the formation of calcitroic acid occurs in the liver and intestine, whereas inactivation of $1,25(OH)_2D_3$ in a wide variety of target tissues occurs by 24-hydroxylation. In addition, polar metabolites of $1,25(OH)_2D_3$ are excreted in the bile. Some of these metabolites are deconjugated in the intestine and reabsorbed into the enterohepatic circulation.

Actions of Vitamin D

Vitamin D Receptors

$1,25(OH)_2D_3$ exerts its biologic functions by binding to a nuclear receptor, which then regulates transcription of DNA into RNA. Among the other nuclear receptors, the vitamin D receptor most closely resembles the retinoic acid, triiodothyronine, and

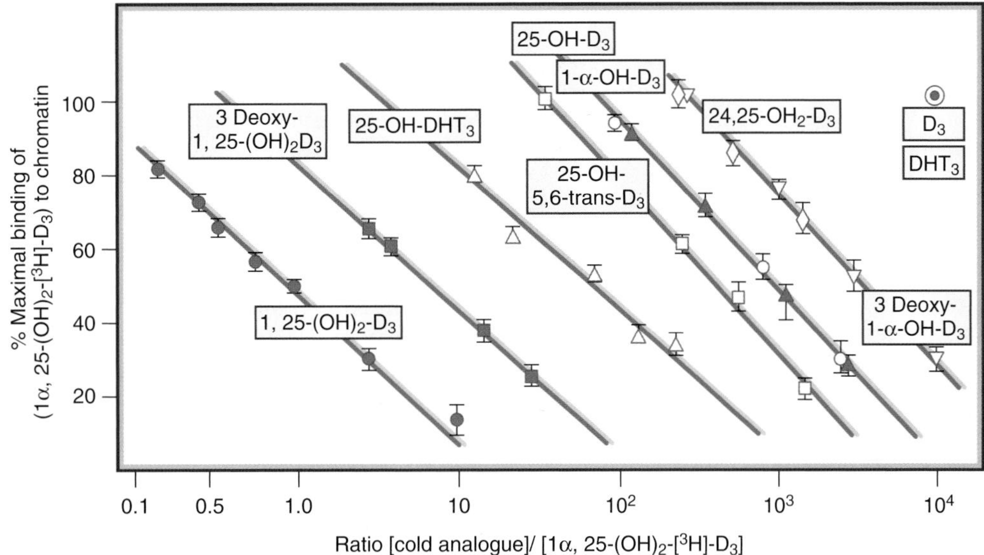

Figure 27–17 ▪ Relative potency of analogues of $1,25(OH)_2D_3$ (1,25-dihydroxyvitamin D_3) in competitive binding to vitamin D receptors of chick intestinal mucosa. Slopes are plotted for *(left to right)*: $1,25(OH)_2D_3$, 1,25-dihydroxyvitamin D_3; 3 deoxy-$1,25(OH)_2D_3$, 3 deoxy-1,25-dihydroxyvitamin D_3; 25-OH-DHT_3, 25-hydroxydihydrotachysterol; 25-OH-5,6-*trans* D_3, 25-hydroxy-5,6 transvitamin D_3; 25-OH-D_3, 25-hydroxyvitamin D_3; 1-α-OH-D_3, 1-α-hydroxyvitamin D_3; 24,25-OH_2D_3, 24,25-dihydroxyvitamin D_3; 3-deoxy-1α-OH-D_3, 3-deoxy-1α-hydroxyvitamin D_3; D_3, vitamin D_3; DHT_3, dihydrotachysterol. (From Proscal DA, Okamura WH, Norman AW. Structural requirements for the interaction of 1α,25-$(OH)_2$-vitamin D_3 with its chick intestinal system. J Biol Chem 1975; 250:8382-8388.)

retinoid-X receptors. The affinity of the receptor for $1,25(OH)_2D_3$ is approximately three orders of magnitude higher than that for other vitamin D metabolites (Fig. 27–17). Although $25(OH)D_3$ is less potent on a molar basis, its concentration in the serum is approximately three orders of magnitude higher than that of $1,25(OH)_2D_3$. However, its free concentration is only two orders of magnitude greater than that of $1,25(OH)_2D_3$. Therefore, under normal circumstances it is unlikely that $25(OH)D_3$ contributes importantly to calcium homeostasis.

Because the affinity of the vitamin D binding protein for $25(OH)_2D_3$ is greater than for $1,25(OH)_2D_3$, in states of vitamin D intoxication (with its associated high levels of $25(OH)D_3$), the free levels of $1,25(OH)_2D_3$ increase[177] because 25(OH)D displaces it from the vitamin D binding protein. $25(OH)D_3$ might, therefore, play a role in the clinical syndrome of vitamin D intoxication both by its direct biologic effects, when present at toxic levels, as well as by increasing free levels of $1,25(OH)_2D_3$.

The vitamin D receptor acts by forming a heterodimer with the retinoid-X receptor, binding to DNA elements, and recruiting coactivators in a ligand-dependent fashion.[178] These coactivators link the receptor complex to the basal transcription apparatus, thereby regulating transcription of target genes. In most cases, the up-regulatory response elements for vitamin D contain hexameric repeats separated by three bases (Fig. 27–18). However, vitamin D also promotes the DNA-protein interactions of other transcription factors, such as SP1 and NF-Y, in genes lacking classical response elements, by uncertain mechanisms.[179]

The mechanism of transcriptional repression by vitamin D is varied. For example, VDR-RXR heterodimers repress the 1α-hydroxylase gene by binding to and blocking the function of another transcription factor.[180] Interaction of the vitamin D receptor with the Ku antigen, acting as a transcription factor, is required for transcriptional repression of the hPTHrP gene.[181]

Glucocorticoids have been shown to decrease the expression of the vitamin D receptor gene in osteosarcoma cell lines,[182]

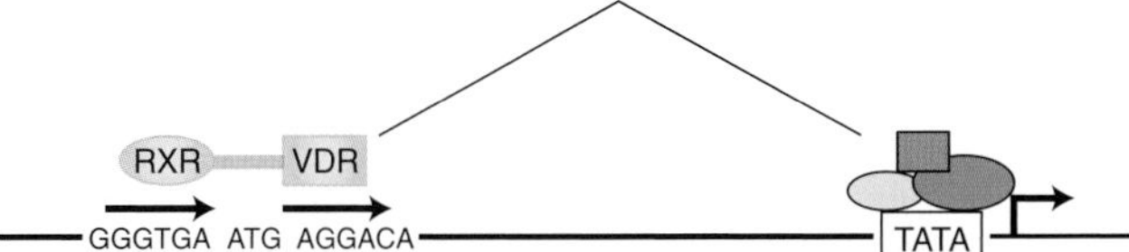

Figure 27–18 ▪ Transcriptional activation by 1,25-dihydroxyvitamin D_3 [$1,25(OH)_2D_3$]. A heterodimer of retinoid X receptor (RXR) and vitamin D receptor (VDR) binds to a pair of hexameric sequences separated by three intervening bases (ATG). *Arrows* indicate that the hexamers found in the up-regulated rat osteocalcin gene are variants of a consensus sequence, repeated here with identical orientations (direct repeats). Upon binding to DNA, the RXR-VDR heterodimer facilitates formation of a transcription initiation complex, which binds to DNA at and near the TATA sequence.

whereas $1,25(OH)_2D_3$ increases its expression in many cells. In the renal proximal convoluted tubule, however,$1,25(OH)_2D_3$ decreases the levels of vitamin D receptors. This decrease has been postulated to lead to decreased activation of the renal 24-hydroxylase by $1,25(OH)_2D_3$, thereby protecting the newly synthesized 1,25-dihydroxyvitamin D from local inactivation.[183]

$1,25(OH)_2D_3$ also has some biologic effects that occur too rapidly for transcriptional mechanisms to be implicated. These nongenomic actions—including a rapid increase in intracellular calcium, activation of phospholipase C, and opening of calcium channels—are observed in several cell types within minutes of exposure to $1,25(OH)_2D_3$.[184] Additional data supporting the hypothesis that nongenomic actions do not depend on the classical receptor include identification of specific binding sites for $1,25(OH)_2D_3$ on the antiluminal surface of intestinal cells[185] and a disparity between the affinity of the various vitamin D analogues for the nuclear receptor and their potency in these nongenomic actions. However, both the rapid intracellular accumulation of cGMP in association with the vitamin D receptor and the rapid increase in intracellular calcium in response to 1,25-dihydroxyvitamin D depend on the presence of an intact nuclear receptor, because these effects are not observed in cells derived from patients and mice with vitamin D receptor mutations.[186,187] The physiologic importance of the nongenomic actions of vitamin D metabolites has not yet been established.

The vitamin D receptor is expressed in most tissues and has been shown to regulate cellular differentiation and function in many cell types. Nevertheless, the most dramatic physiologic effects of vitamin D, acting through the vitamin D receptor, involve regulation of intestinal calcium transport. This is most clearly demonstrated by the phenotype of patients and mice with mutant vitamin D receptors (hereditary vitamin D–resistant rickets)[28,188]; dramatic abnormalities in bone mineralization can be reversed by bypassing the defect in intestinal calcium absorption.[189-191]

Intestinal Calcium Absorption

Under normal diet conditions, calcium intake is in the range of 700 to 900 mg daily. Approximately 30% to 35% of this calcium is absorbed; however, losses from intestinal secretion of calcium lead to a net daily uptake of approximately 200 mg.[192] Though vitamin D is the major hormonal determinant of intestinal calcium absorption, the bioavailability of mineral ions in the intestinal lumen may be affected by a number of local factors and dietary constituents. Absorption of calcium and magnesium is impaired by bile salt deficiency, unabsorbed free fatty acids in steatorrheic states, and high dietary content of fiber or phytate. Gastric acid is needed to promote dissociation of calcium from anionic components of food or therapeutic preparations of calcium salts. Administration of calcium salts with meals, especially in patients with achlorhydria, and use of divided doses or more soluble salts such as calcium citrate are commonly employed strategies to increase calcium bioavailability.

Calcium is thought to be absorbed by three pathways: the transcellular route, vesicular calcium transport, and paracellular transport. The first two pathways have been shown to depend on $1,25(OH)_2D_3$. Although the necessity of vitamin D for paracellular calcium absorption remains controversial, substantial evidence exists that the hormone enhances this pathway, as well.[193]

The most extensively studied mechanism of intestinal calcium absorption involves the transcellular route. This pathway is thought to involve three steps: entry of calcium into the enterocyte (which is the rate-limiting step), transport across the cell, and extrusion across the basolateral membrane.

Entry into the Enterocyte

A number of brush border proteins, including the intestinal membrane calcium binding protein, brush border alkaline phosphatase, and low affinity Ca/Mg ATPase, have been shown to be induced by $1,25(OH)_2D_3$. The activity of these proteins correlates with active calcium transport; however, a causal relationship remains to be established. Two calcium channels, TRPV5 and TRPV6,[194,195] members of the transient receptor potential vanilloid receptor subfamily containing six membrane-spanning domains, are expressed in the duodenum, the jejunum, and the kidney as well as in other tissues. TRPV6 is thought to play a critical role in intestinal calcium absorption, and its expression is increased by 1,25-dihydroxyvitamin D, as is that of TRP5.[196] Studies in mice lacking TRPV5 demonstrate that this channel is primarily responsible for renal calcium reabsorption, because mice lacking TRPV5 have enhanced, rather than impaired, intestinal calcium absorption, due to their high circulating levels of 1,25-dihydroxyvitamin D.[197] Upon entering the enterocyte, calcium binds to components of the brush border complex subjacent to the plasma membrane. Calmodulin is redistributed to the brush border in response to $1,25(OH)_2D_3$ and might play a role in this process, as might the $1,25(OH)_2D_3$-inducible calcium binding protein, calbindin 9K.[198]

Transcellular Transport

The best-studied effect of Vitamin D on the enterocyte is the induction of synthesis of the intestinal calcium-binding protein, calbindin 9K. This protein has an EF hand structure that permits the binding of two calcium ions per molecule. The affinity of calbindin for calcium is approximately four times that of the brush border calcium-binding components, so calcium is preferentially transferred to calbindin. Calbindin serves to buffer the intracellular free calcium concentration during calcium absorption. It associates with microtubules and might play a role in the transport of calcium across the enterocyte. Organelles such as the mitochondria, Golgi complex, and endoplasmic reticulum also serve as repositories for intracellular calcium.

Exit from the Enterocyte

The transport of calcium across the antiluminal surface of the enterocyte, the final process involved in intestinal calcium absorption, depends on $1,25(OH)_2D_3$. The main mechanism of calcium extrusion is the $1,25(OH)_2D_3$-inducible[199] ATP-dependent Ca^{2+} pump (PMCA1b). The affinity of the pump for calcium is approximately 2.5 times that of calbindin.[200] With high calcium intake, a $1,25(OH)_2D_3$-independent Na^+/Ca^{2+} ion exchanger might play a role in the transfer of calcium across the basolateral membrane, as well.

Actions on the Parathyroid Gland

$1,25(OH)_2D_3$ has been shown to regulate gene transcription and cell proliferation in the parathyroids. The hormone also inhibits the proliferation of dispersed parathyroid cells in culture, although the relative contribution of calcium and $1,25(OH)_2D_3$ in the regulation of parathyroid cell proliferation in vivo has not been established. Normocalcemic mice lacking functional vitamin D receptors have normal serum PTH levels and normal sized parathyroid glands, demonstrating that the genomic actions of $1,25(OH)_2D_3$ are not essential for parathyroid cellular homeostasis.[191] $1,25(OH)_2D_3$ has, however, been shown to decrease the transcription of the PTH gene both in vivo and in vitro. This action has been exploited in the use of $1,25(OH)_2D_3$ in treating the secondary hyperparathyroidism associated with chronic renal failure (see "Parathyroid Hormone Biosynthesis" and "Vitamin D Deficiency" sections).

Actions on Bone

The effects of $1,25(OH)_2D_3$ on bone are numerous. $1,25(OH)_2D_3$ is a major transcriptional regulator of the two most abundant bone matrix proteins: it represses synthesis of type 1 collagen[201] and induces synthesis of osteocalcin.[202] $1,25(OH)_2D_3$ promotes differentiation of osteoclasts from monocyte-macrophage stem cell precursors in vitro and also increases osteoclastic bone resorption in high doses in vivo by stimulating production of RANK ligand (also called osteoclast differentiating factor) by osteoblasts.[203] Despite the multiple effects of $1,25(OH)_2D_3$ on the biology of bone in vitro, in vivo studies in $1,25(OH)_2D_3$-deficient rats and in mice lacking functional vitamin D receptors[189] suggest that the major osseous consequences of hormone and receptor deficiency can be reversed when mineral ion homeostasis is normalized. In addition, parenteral calcium infusions have been shown to heal the osteomalacic lesions in children with mutant vitamin D receptors.[190] These observations suggest that the major role of $1,25(OH)_2D_3$in bone is to provide the proper microenvironment for bone mineralization through stimulation of the intestinal absorption of calcium and phosphate.

Vitamin D Analogues

The recognition that 1,25$(OH)_2D_3$ promotes cellular differentiation and inhibits cellular proliferation has led to efforts directed at producing new analogues that retain these effects but do not cause hypercalcemia. Several analogues have been shown to have antiproliferative effects on normal cells as well as on malignant cells in vitro and in xenografts in immunosuppressed mice.[204,205] In addition, analogues of vitamin D have been shown to synergize with cyclosporine in preventing rejection of transplanted islet cells in a murine model[206] One nonhypercalcemic analogue, 22-oxacalcitriol, has been shown to suppress PTH synthesis and secretion in rats[207] at doses that stimulate intestinal calcium absorption less than 1,25$(OH)_2D_3$. This suggests that such analogues may be useful in preventing and treating hyperparathyroidism. The antiproliferative effects of vitamin D have been exploited clinically in treating psoriasis.[208] Although analogues with reduced calcemic activity are predominantly used, hypercalcemic crisis after excessive topical use of such compounds can occur.[209]

The physiology underlying the differential biological effects of these analogues is not completely understood. Altered affinity for the vitamin D binding protein, metabolism by target tissues,[210] and effects on recruitment of coactivators by the vitamin D receptor might contribute to the unique properties of vitamin D analogues.[211]

Fibroblast Growth Factor-23

Fibroblast Growth Factor 23 in Human Disease

The search for the hormonal factor responsible for the hypophosphatemia in patients with tumor-induced osteomalacia (TIO; see Chapter 28) was brought to a close with the identification of the molecular basis for the human disorder autosomal dominant hypophosphatemic rickets (ADHR).[212] Linkage analyses of affected kindreds identified mutation of the gene encoding FGF23 as the basis for ADHR. The mutation in affected persons abolishes an RXXR protease recognition motif that is thought to be responsible for the cleavage and inactivation of FGF23.[213,214] The cDNA encoding FGF23 predicts a peptide of 251 amino acids, the first 24 of which compose a signal peptide. Studies using recombinant FGF23 demonstrate that the full-length mature peptide is required for its biologic activity and that the cleavage site mutated in the ADHR patients is responsible for its inactivation. Cleavage of FGF23 is inhibited by furin inhibition, suggesting that the enzyme responsible is a subtilisin-like proprotein convertase.

Analyses of tumors isolated from patients with TIO reveal a dramatic increase in mRNA expression of FGF23.[215] Serum levels of FGF23 have been found to be elevated in several patients with TIO and have been shown to normalize after removal of the tumor, correlating with resolution of the hypophosphatemia that characterizes this disorder.[216,217] Conversely, patients with the rare syndrome tumoral calcinosis present with hyperphosphatemia and soft tissue calcium-phosphate deposits. Some of these patients have point mutations in the FGF23 gene that cause abnormal processing of the protein, with low levels of the active hormone in the blood and high levels of inactive fragments.[218-220] Thus, human diseases of both increased and decreased FGF23 activity suggest that this "new" factor represents an important regulator of phosphate metabolism.

Actions of Fibroblast Growth Factor-23

Evidence that FGF23 is a novel hormone that plays a key role in normal phosphate homeostasis has been obtained in murine models of overexpression and ablation. Overexpression of FGF23 or administration of FGF23 to animals results in development of hypophosphatemia[214] and impaired 1-α hydroxylation of 25(OH)D,[164,221] thus recapitulating the findings observed in patients affected by TIO. Investigations in mice with targeted ablation of FGF23 have proved that endogenous production of this hormone is critical for normal phosphate homeostasis and regulation of vitamin D metabolism.[222,223] Absence of FGF23 results in impaired renal phosphate excretion, leading to the development of hyperphosphatemia within the first 2 weeks of life. Affected mice also develop hypercalcemia due to high levels of 1,25-dihydroxyvitamin D, a result of the lack of the normal suppressive effect of FGF23 on the renal 25-hydroxyvitamin D 1α-hydroxylase.[164] Ablation of FGF23 results in premature death associated with ectopic mineralization of soft tissues, including the kidney. Impairing 1,25-dihydroxyvitamin D action in these animals prevents the development of hypercalcemia and improves survival, suggesting that the premature death is a direct consequence of impaired mineral ion homeostasis rather than a specific developmental or maturational effect of FGF23.[224]

FGF23 impairs sodium-dependent phosphate transport in both intestinal and renal brush border membrane vesicles.[225] It has been shown to decrease the levels of the types IIa, IIb, and IIc sodium-dependent phosphate transporters, thereby regulating both intestinal and renal phosphate transport.[226-228] FGF23 decreases circulating levels of 1,25-dihydroxyvitamin D, both by decreasing mRNA levels for the renal 25 hydroxyvitamin D 1α-hydroxylase and by increasing expression of the 24-hydroxylase, the key enzyme involved in inactivation of 1,25-dihydroxyvitamin D.[164] The receptors mediating these actions of FGF23 are currently unknown. FGF23 can activate FGF receptor 1in the presence of klotho, a single-pass transmembrane protein.[167] Because the klotho knockout mouse exhibits the same hyperphosphatemia and high 1,25$(OH)_2D_3$ levels seen in the FGF23 knockout mouse,[165] klotho may be part of the cellular apparatus mediating the actions of FGF23.

Regulation of Fibroblast Growth Factor-23

Circulating FGF23 levels are increased by dietary phosphorus, serum phosphorus, serum calcium, and 1,25-dihydroxyvitamin D.[57,229,230] In patients with chronic renal failure, an increase in FGF23 levels has been shown to antedate the development of secondary hyperparathyroidism and thus may be beneficial in predicting which patients will develop this disorder.[231]

Treatment of dialysis patients with sevalamar hydrochloride and calcium carbonate decreases phosphate and FGF23 levels in parallel, implicating increases in serum phosphate or intestinal absorption as the pathophysiologic basis for the increased FGF23 levels in this population.[232] Thus, FGF23 has emerged as an essential regulator of normal phosphate and 1,25$(OH)_2D_3$ homeostasis. Phosphate and 1,25$(OH)_2D_3$ increase FGF23 levels; FGF23 then acts on the renal proximal tubule to suppress synthesis of 1,25$(OH)_2D_3$ and to decrease the reabsorption of phosphate.

Calcium and Phosphate Homeostasis

The cytosolic concentrations of intracellular calcium, phosphorus, and magnesium differ markedly, as reviewed previously, and their physiologic roles within cells are diverse and largely unrelated (see Fig. 27–1). In contrast, the concentrations of these mineral ions in extracellular fluid are quite comparable (i.e., 1-2 mM), and it is here that they exert important interactions, both with cells and with one another, that are critical for bone mineralization, neuromuscular function, and normal mineral ion homeostasis. Extracellular calcium and phosphate, in particular, exist so close to the limits of their mutual solubility that stringent regulation of their concentrations is required to prevent diffuse precipitation of calcium phosphate crystals in tissues.

Serum concentrations and total body balances of the mineral ions are maintained within narrow limits by powerful interactive homeostatic mechanisms. PTH, $1,25(OH)_2D$, and FGF-23 regulate mineral ion levels; mineral ion levels, in turn, regulate PTH, $1,25(OH)_2D$, and FGF-23 secretion; and these hormones can regulate the production of one another. Calcium sensors in the parathyroid glands control PTH secretion by monitoring the blood concentration of ionized calcium, and those in the kidney act to adjust tubular calcium reabsorption independently of PTH or $1,25(OH)_2D$. In contrast, the mechanisms of the phosphate sensing needed for normal homeostasis are not understood. The operation of these homeostatic mechanisms can be appreciated by considering the following examples of how the organism adapts to changes in calcium loads (Fig. 27–19).

Dietary calcium restriction, for example, is followed by an increase in the efficiency of intestinal calcium absorption. This increased efficiency results from a sequence of homeostatic responses in which lowered blood ionized calcium activates secretion of PTH, PTH augments synthesis of $1,25(OH)_2D_3$ by the proximal tubules of the kidney, and $1,25(OH)_2D_3$ then acts directly upon enterocytes to increase active transcellular transport of calcium. Enhanced intestinal calcium absorption is quantitatively the most important response to calcium deprivation, but a series of other homeostatic events also occur that limit the impact of this stress. Renal tubular calcium reabsorption is increased by PTH, an effect that is enhanced by increased $1,25(OH)_2D_3$-stimulated expression of calbindin-D28K in the distal tubules. Calcium reabsorption is also enhanced directly by any tendency to hypocalcemia, which is detected by calcium-sensing receptors in Henle's loop (and possibly also in the distal nephron) that control transepithelial calcium movements independent of PTH or $1,25(OH)_2D_3$.

The impact of dietary calcium deprivation is reduced by approximately 15% through release of calcium from bone in response to PTH and $1,25(OH)_2D_3$. The concomitant increase in net bone resorption causes release of phosphate as well as calcium into the extracellular fluid. Intestinal phosphate absorption also is increased by $1,25(OH)_2D_3$. These phosphate loads are problematic, in that phosphate directly lowers ionized calcium in extracellular fluid, suppresses renal synthesis of $1,25(OH)_2D_3$, and directly inhibits bone resorption. These potentially negative effects of phosphate are obviated by the powerful phosphaturic action of PTH and of FGF-23, the secretion of which is promoted by phosphate, calcium, and $1,25(OH)_2D$.

Finally, the possibility of unrestrained secretion of PTH, leading to excessive bone resorption and severe hypophosphatemia, is prevented by the effects of calcium on PTH secretion and by the direct suppressive effect of $1,25(OH)_2D_3$ on the synthesis of PTH and of PTH receptors. As a result of these homeostatic responses, calcium-deprived people maintain near-normal serum calcium and phosphate concentrations but display increased intestinal calcium absorption, increased bone resorption and progressive osteopenia, increased renal tubular calcium reabsorption, decreased renal tubular phosphate reabsorption, low urinary calcium excretion, elevated urinary phosphate excretion, and high serum concentrations of PTH and $1,25(OH)_2D_3$.

Calcium loads induce an opposite series of adaptations: parathyroid suppression, inhibition of renal $1,25(OH)_2D_3$ synthesis, decreased intestinal active transport of calcium, increased renal excretion of calcium and decreased renal excretion of phosphate (secondary to functional hypoparathyroidism), and a decrease in bone resorption sufficient to allow positive skeletal calcium balance. The decline in intestinal calcium absorption is the major safeguard against calcium overload, although this mechanism may be overridden with extraordinarily high intakes of calcium because of the persistence of the passive, non–vitamin D-dependent mode of calcium absorption. Moreover, nonenteral sources of calcium, such as intravenous calcium infusion or excessive net bone resorption (as from immobilization or malignancy), can readily overwhelm the limited homeostatic adaptations that remain once suppressed intestinal calcium absorption is bypassed. In such situations, the kidney

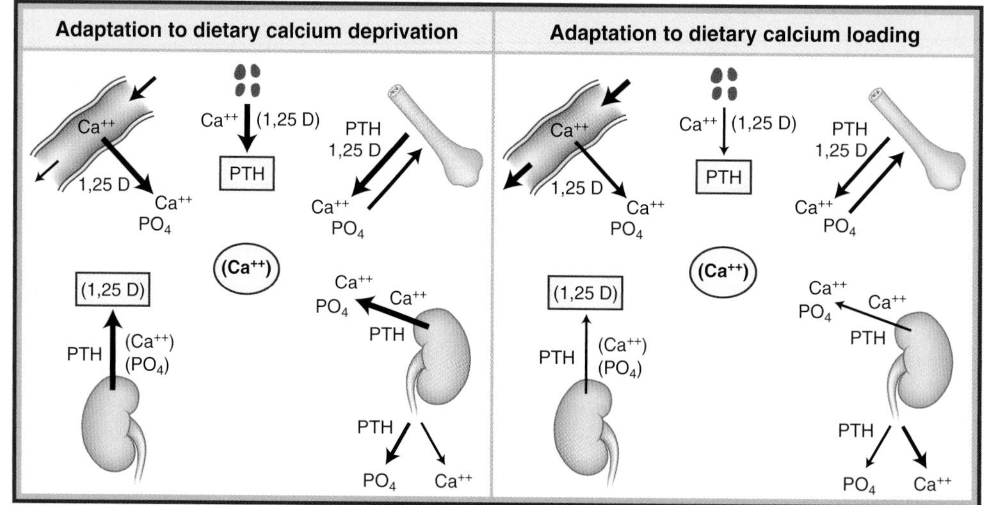

Figure 27–19 ▪ Homeostatic responses to variations in dietary calcium content. Major homeostatic responses to dietary calcium deprivation or loading are depicted. Arrow thickness indicates relative activity of transport or secretory mechanisms, whereas amounts of hormones or transported ions are related to the size of their notations. Parentheses indicate an inhibitory regulation. Note that the extracellular calcium concentration is well maintained, although different underlying mechanisms are involved in the two circumstances (see text for details). PTH, parathyroid hormone.

rather than the intestine becomes the principal defense against hypercalcemia, and calcium homeostasis becomes critically dependent on adequate renal function. If renal function is impaired in these settings, as often occurs clinically, severe hypercalcemia and pathologic calcium deposition in extraskeletal sites can ensue.

Laboratory Assessment of Mineral Metabolism

Parathyroid Hormone

The major challenges in the measurement of blood PTH have been the low levels of circulating PTH and the presence of inactive PTH fragments in far greater abundance than for the intact, biologically active PTH molecule. The measurement of inactive fragments would not be a concern if the ratio of inactive to active PTH molecules remained constant. However, this ratio does change in response to changes in GFR and in parathyroid gland secretory activity (see "Parathyroid Hormone Secretion" and "Peripheral Metabolism of Parathyroid Hormone" earlier). Consequently, radioimmunoassays of PTH have suffered from lack of sensitivity and from the inability to measure the biologically active hormone directly.

For these reasons, two-site assays that require the presence of amino-terminal and carboxy-terminal sequences of full-length PTH(1-84) on the same molecule have replaced older radioimmunoassay.[233] The assays are sensitive enough to detect PTH in all normal persons. The assays have demonstrated modest circadian variation in PTH levels and some pulsatility in PTH secretion, but these variations have not interfered with the diagnostic usefulness of randomly drawn PTH measurements. Some studies have reported modest increases of PTH levels with age, although others have not. Unlike older radioimmunoassays, the two-site assays demonstrate virtually no overlap in PTH levels between patients with primary hyperparathyroidism and those with nonparathyroid hypercalcemia (Fig. 27–20). Because this distinction represents the most important challenge in the clinical setting, the use of the two-site assay has dramatically facilitated the clinician's task.

This straightforward picture has been complicated by the realization that most two-site assays detect small amounts of PTH fragments that are large but do not extend to the hormone's amino-terminus.[234] These fragments accumulate in significant amounts in patients with renal failure. These observations have prompted the development of two-site PTH assays that use antibodies specific for the first four amino acids of PTH and thus do not detect large fragments of PTH. Although it seems plausible that such assays might prove particularly useful in some clinical situations, their role is at present unclear. They offer no advantage over older two-site assays, for example, in diagnosing primary hyperparathyroidism.[235]

Parathyroid Hormone–Related Protein

The measurement of PTHrP in serum presents a series of challenges. The concentration of PTHrP in the bloodstream, even in some patients with PTHrP-mediated malignant hypercalcemia, is not high, and the molecular definition of circulating, biologically active fragments is incomplete. Despite these problems, several groups of investigators have developed assays for PTHrP that can be helpful in evaluating a subset of hypercalcemic patients. Radioimmunoassays for amino-terminal portions of PTHrP and two-site assays for amino-terminal and mid-region PTHrP[105] separate healthy persons and patients with nonmalignant hypercalcemia from most patients with the humoral hypercalcemia of malignancy (Fig. 27–21). When measured with the most recently developed assays, PTHrP levels are elevated in almost all patients with malignant hypercalcemia without bone metastases and in most patients with hypercalcemia and bone metastases.

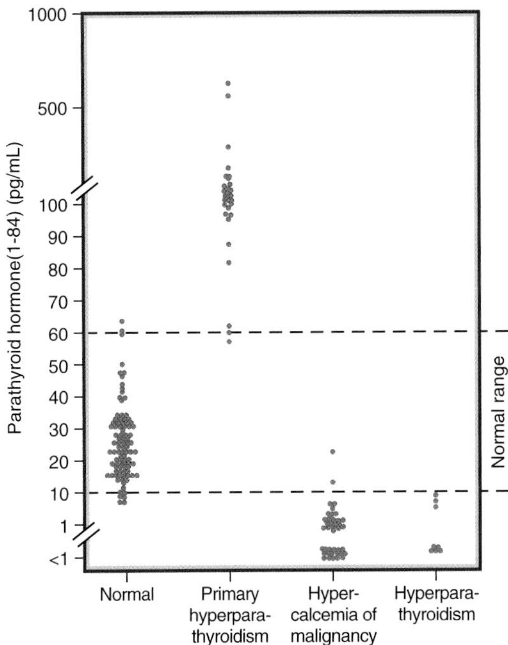

Figure 27–20 ▪ Intact immunoreactive parathyroid hormone (PTH) determined using a two-site immunoradiometric assay in normal and three different patient groups. Note there is some overlap between normal subjects and patients with primary hyperparathyroidism, but there is no overlap between hypercalcemic patients with primary hyperparathyroidism and those with hypercalcemia of malignancy. (From Segre GV. Advances in techniques for measurement of parathyroid hormone: current applications in clinical medicine and directions for future research. Trends Endocrinol Metab 1990;1:243-247.)

In occasional patients, the PTHrP assay has helped distinguish an occult malignancy from other causes of non–PTH-dependent hypercalcemia.[236] Nevertheless, because the diagnosis of malignancy as the cause of hypercalcemia is usually clinically obvious, and the PTH assay can be used to diagnose primary hyperparathyroidism, the role of PTHrP assays in clinical practice is limited.

Calcitonin

Several assays for measuring serum calcitonin are commercially available. The measurements are based on single or double antibody radioimmunoassays or enzyme immunoassays, several of which are sufficiently sensitive to detect calcitonin deficiency.[237,238] The calcitonin monomer is thought to be the biologically active molecule; therefore, some investigators think that extraction of the multimeric forms prior to radioimmunoassay provides a more sensitive and specific measurement of serum calcitonin levels. However, the double antibody radioimmunoassay is thought by others to provide the same information with less sample manipulation. The only clinical use of the calcitonin assay is as a tumor marker, primarily in medullary carcinoma of the thyroid.

Vitamin D Metabolites

The radioligand assays for determining the levels of vitamin D metabolites require fractionation and extraction of the hormone from serum proteins by HPLC or silica cartridges.[239] These

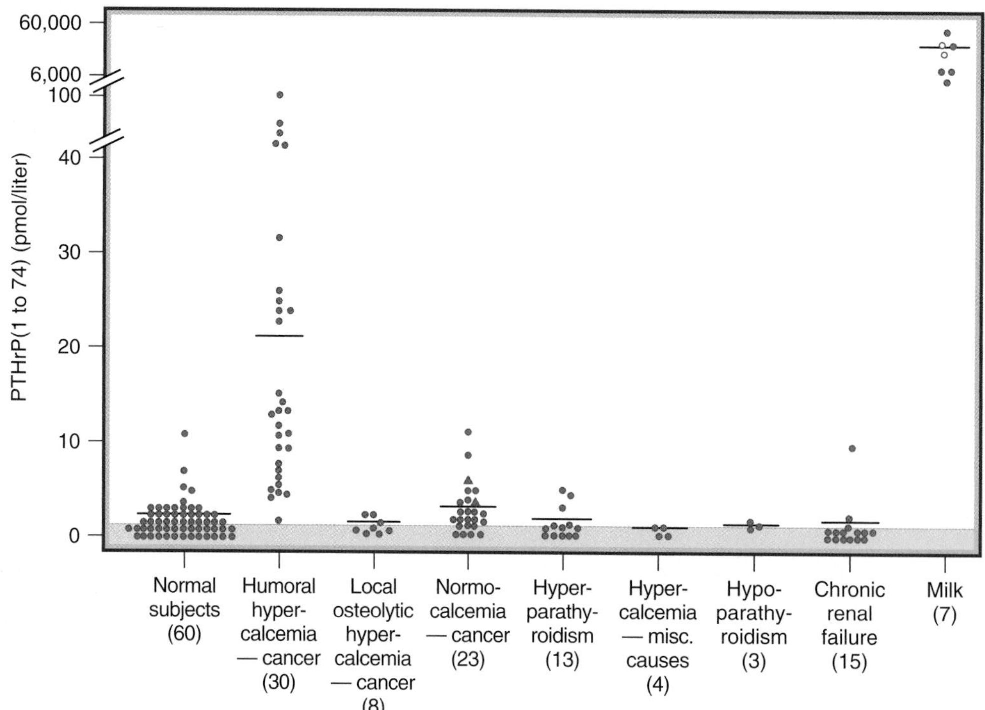

Figure 27–21 ▪ Plasma PTHrP(1-74) determined by two-site immunoradiometric assay in selected patient groups and normal subjects. Also shown are concentrations of PTHrP in human milk *(filled circles)* and in bovine milk *(open circles)*. Two normocalcemic patients with cancer *(filled triangles)* subsequently became hypercalcemic. *Hatched area* denotes levels too low to detect with this assay. PTHrP, parathyroid hormone–related protein. (Adapted from Burtis WJ, Brady TG, Orloff JJ, et al. Immunochemical characterization of circulating parathyroid hormone related protein in patients with humoral hypercalcemia of cancer. N Engl J Med 1990;322:1106-1112.)

assays are sufficiently sensitive to detect subnormal values. Because the assays measure both protein-bound and unbound vitamin D metabolites, results might not always reflect the levels of biologically relevant (free) metabolites. This limitation can lead to misleading results in patients with the nephrotic syndrome and vitamin D intoxication. With the move away from using radioligand-based assays, other methods for measuring vitamin D metabolites, including chemiluminescent assays have been pioneered.[240] Although these assays have not withstood the test of time, they have proved as accurate as the currently available radioimmunoassay.

The levels of 25(OH)D correlate better with the clinical signs and symptoms of vitamin D deficiency than do the levels of $1,25(OH)_2D_3$. Because the 25-hydroxylation of vitamin D is not tightly regulated, measurements of 25(OH)D more accurately reflect body stores of vitamin D. This metabolite should be measured, therefore, when vitamin D deficiency is suspected.

Measurements of $1,25(OH)_2D_3$ should be reserved for cases when excessive or impaired 1α-hydroxylation is suspected. High $1,25(OH)_2D_3$ levels can be seen in sarcoidosis, lymphomas, William's syndrome, and intoxication with 1α-hydroxylated metabolites (see "Parathyroid-Independent Hypercalcemia" later). Impaired 1α-hydroxylation can contribute to the hypocalcemia of patients with renal dysfunction, oncogenic osteomalacia, and hereditary defects of vitamin D metabolism (see "Hypocalcemic Disorders" later).

Fibroblast Growth Factor-23

Currently two types of immunoassays are available for the measurement of serum FGF23 in humans. An assay using two polyclonal antibodies directed against C-terminal epitopes[241] detects most, if not all, circulating forms of FGF23 but does not discriminate between the intact active hormone and the cleaved fragment, which is not thought to have biologic activity. An assay for the intact hormone is a classic sandwich assay with antibodies directed against both the N and C termini of the hormone.[242] This sandwich assay has been shown to be more useful for studying the effects of dietary phosphate on FGF23 levels in humans and thus is thought to provide a more precise determination of the biologically active levels of the hormone in the circulation.[243]

CLINICAL DISORDERS

Hypercalcemic Disorders

Parathyroid-Dependent Hypercalcemia

It is useful to delineate two categories of hypercalcemia: hypercalcemia associated with dysfunction of the parathyroid cells and hypercalcemia that occurs despite appropriate parathyroid suppression. This distinction is particularly useful clinically, because it emphasizes the centrality of the PTH assay in the diagnostic approach to the hypercalcemic patient. Abnormal parathyroid glands are associated with hypercalcemia in three settings: primary hyperparathyroidism, familial hypocalciuric hypercalcemia (FHH), and lithium-induced hypercalcemia.

Primary Hyperparathyroidism

In primary hyperparathyroidism, a primary abnormality of parathyroid tissue leads to inappropriate secretion of PTH. In contrast, increased secretion of PTH that is an appropriate response to hypocalcemia is called *secondary hyperparathyroidism.* The inappropriately high serum concentration of PTH in primary hyperparathyroidism, in turn, sustains excessive renal calcium reabsorption, phosphaturia, and $1,25(OH)_2D$ synthesis, as well as increased bone resorption. These actions of PTH produce the characteristic biochemical phenotype of hypercalcemia and hypophosphatemia, loss of cortical bone, hypercalciuria, and the various clinical sequelae of chronic hypercalcemia. Primary hyperparathyroidism results most often (75%-80%) from the occurrence of one or more adenomas in previously normal parathyroid glands, although in 20% of cases diffuse hyperplasia of all parathyroid glands may be present or, rarely, parathyroid carcinoma may be found (less than 1%-2%).[244,245]

Classic Primary Hyperparathyroidism

The bone disease osteitis fibrosa cystica first was described by von Recklinghausen in 1891, but the etiologic link between this disease and parathyroid neoplasms was not established until 1925, when Mandl observed clinical improvement following removal of a parathyroid adenoma from a young male patient with severe bone disease. In early clinical descriptions of primary hyperparathyroidism, the disease emerged as a distinctly uncommon disorder with significant morbidity and mortality, in which nearly all affected patients manifested radiographically significant or symptomatic skeletal or renal involvement, or both.

The skeletal involvement in classic primary hyperparathyroidism reflects a striking and generalized increase in osteoclastic bone resorption, which is accompanied by fibrovascular marrow replacement and increased osteoblastic activity. The radiographic appearance (Fig. 27–22) features

- *generalized demineralization* of bone, with coarsening of the trabecular pattern (due to osteoclastic resorption of the smaller trabeculae)
- characteristic *subperiosteal resorption,* often most evident in the phalanges of the hands, which gives an irregular, serrated appearance to the outer, subperiosteal cortex and can progress to extensive cortical resorption
- *bone cysts,* usually multiple, which contain a brownish serous or mucoid fluid, tend to occur in the central medullary portions of the shafts of the metacarpals, ribs, or pelvis, and can expand into and disrupt the overlying cortex
- *osteoclastomas,* or *brown tumors,* composed of numerous multinucleated osteoclasts (giant cells) admixed with stromal cells and matrix, which are found most often in trabecular portions of the jaw, long bones, and ribs
- pathologic *fractures*

The skull can exhibit a finely mottled salt-and-pepper radiographic appearance, with loss of definition of the inner and outer cortices. Dental radiographs typically show erosion or disappearance of the lamina dura due to subperiosteal resorption, often with extension into the adjacent mandibular bone. The erosion and demineralization of cortical bone can lead to radiographic disappearance of some bones, most notably the tufts of the distal phalanges of the hands, the inferolateral cortex of the distal third of the clavicles, the distal ulna, the inferior margin of the femoral neck and pubis, and the medial aspect of the proximal tibia. The clinical correlates of these changes can include aching bone pain and tenderness, bowing of the shoulders, kyphosis and loss of height, and collapse of lateral ribs and pelvis with pigeon breast and triradiate deformities, respectively.

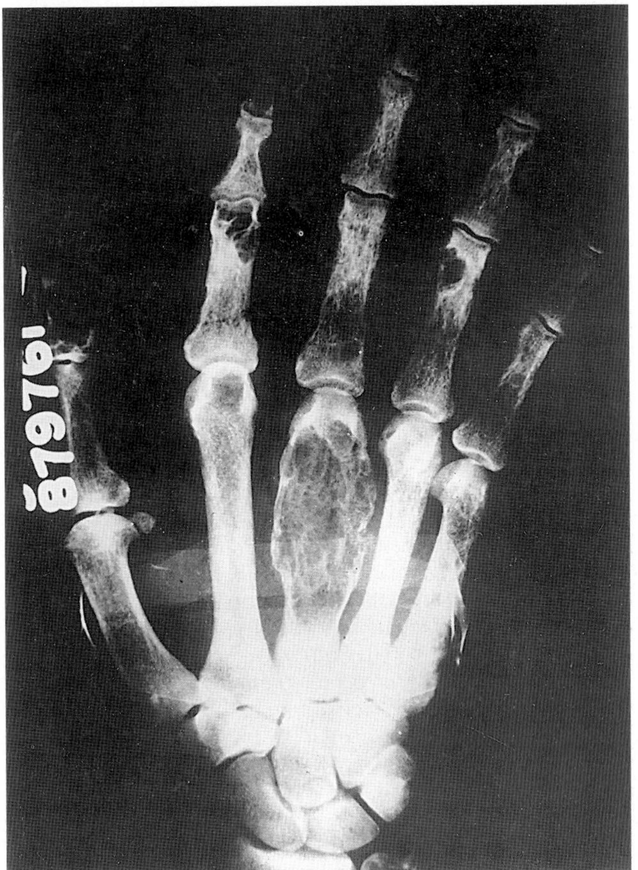

Figure 27–22 ▪ Radiograph of hand from a patient with severe primary hyperparathyroidism. Note the dramatic remodeling associated with the intense region of high bone turnover in the third metacarpal in addition to widespread evidence of subperiosteal, endosteal, and trabecular resorption. (Courtesy of Fuller Albright Collection, Massachusetts General Hospital.)

The renal manifestations of classic severe primary hyperparathyroidism include recurrent calcium nephrolithiasis, nephrocalcinosis, and renal functional abnormalities that range from impaired concentrating ability to end-stage renal failure. Associated signs and symptoms include recurrent flank pain, polyuria, and polydipsia. No unique features of the stone disease in primary hyperparathyroidism serve to distinguish it from disease associated with other, more common causes of calcium kidney stones. The stone disease more often may be recurrent and severe, and in some patients, the stones may be composed entirely of calcium phosphate, instead of the pure oxalate or mixtures of oxalate and phosphate more commonly encountered in other disorders. In cases diagnosed before 1965, the frequency with which nephrolithiasis complicated primary hyperparathyroidism was as high as 60% to 80% (the frequency is currently less than 25%), yet in studies of unselected patients conducted since 1965, primary hyperparathyroidism has accounted for fewer than 5% of all calcium kidney stones.

Other clinical features that have been reported in association with classic severe primary hyperparathyroidism are conjunctival calcifications, band keratopathy, hypertension (50%), gastrointestinal signs and symptoms (anorexia, nausea, vomiting, constipation, or abdominal pain), peptic ulcer disease, and acute or chronic pancreatitis. The issue of whether primary hyperparathyroidism increases the risk of peptic ulcer disease and pancreatitis remains controversial. Although hyperparathyroidism is associated with a higher risk of hypertension, successful parathyroidectomy has not been shown to correct the hypertension.

Signs and symptoms in primary hyperparathyroidism can result from the involvement of bone (fracture, bone pain) or kidneys (renal colic, renal failure), peptic ulcer disease, pancreatitis, or hypercalcemia per se (weakness, apathy, depression, polyuria, constipation, coma). The presence and severity of neuropsychiatric symptoms, in particular, correlate poorly with the serum calcium concentration, although few patients with severe hypercalcemia are entirely asymptomatic. Elderly persons are most likely to exhibit such symptoms. A peculiar neuromuscular syndrome, first described in 1949 and rarely encountered now, includes symmetrical proximal weakness and gait disturbance, with muscle atrophy, characteristic electromyographic abnormalities, generalized hyperreflexia, and tongue fasciculations.[246]

Modern Primary Hyperparathyroidism

The clinical spectrum of primary hyperparathyroidism was changed dramatically in the early 1970s by the introduction of routine multichannel serum chemistry screening, which unearthed a large population of patients with previously unsuspected, asymptomatic disease. In Rochester, Minnesota, for example, the annual incidence of the disease increased abruptly from 0.15 to 1.12 per 1000 persons between the prescreening era (1965-1974) and 1975, the year after routine screening was introduced.[247] The peak incidence occurs in the sixth decade of life, and the disease rarely is encountered in patients younger than 15 years. It is two to three times more common in women, who are slightly older at diagnosis than are men.

Annual incidence rates, widely reported to be 0.1 to 0.3 per 1000 persons in the wake of this surge of ascertainment in Europe and the United States, appear to have declined substantially since the 1990s to levels as low as 0.04 per 1000.[247] This might represent a true decline in disease incidence or simply the residual effect of sweeping the population of prevalent subclinical disease since the 1970s.

Ascertainment of mild or asymptomatic disease might decline even further in the future because of prevalent economic disincentives to routine serum chemistry screening in the primary care setting. On the other hand, insistence upon overt hypercalcemia as a diagnostic criterion might underestimate the true incidence of the disease. For example, when serum calcium and iPTH were measured in a large population of Swedish women undergoing routine mammographic screening, the prevalence of unsuspected primary hyperparathyroidism, defined by criteria that included the combination of high-normal serum calcium plus elevated or high-normal iPTH, was 2.1%.[248] Two-thirds of these women (72/109) were normocalcemic (10.0-10.4 mg/dL), yet bone density was reduced in the group as a whole and the disease was confirmed histologically in 98% of the 61 who had surgery.

Not surprisingly, given that primary hyperparathyroidism now usually is diagnosed incidentally, few patients are found to have overt signs or symptoms of the classic disease and thus are considered to be asymptomatic. For example, only 2% of patients with primary hyperparathyroidism residing in Olmsted County, Minnesota, and only 17% of 121 patients studied at an academic referral center in New York City had classic disease symptoms.[247,249] In most of these, the relevant symptom was urolithiasis. Many clinicians argue, however, that most patients regarded as having asymptomatic primary hyperparathyroidism and only minimally elevated serum calcium actually suffer from various neuropsychiatric or other symptoms that might improve following curative surgery.[250-252] These symptoms, however, which include fatigability, weakness, forgetfulness, depression, somatization, polydipsia, polyuria, and bone and joint pain, are common in otherwise normal persons.

The difficulties in designing appropriately controlled studies to determine if these symptoms can be confidently ascribed to the parathyroid disorder are well described.[253] While as yet unresolved, this is a critical issue, because the advent of less-invasive operative approaches and concerns regarding fracture, cancer, and mortality risk have lowered the threshold for considering surgery in many patients with the disease (see later). Throughout this chapter, "asymptomatic primary hyperparathyroidism" refers to patients who lack signs or symptoms of the classic disease, whether or not they experience any of the subtle symptoms mentioned.

The natural history of untreated asymptomatic primary hyperparathyroidism, as currently detected, remains incompletely understood. Few patients seem to experience progression of disease, as measured by extreme elevations of serum or urinary calcium, appearance of renal dysfunction or nephrocalcinosis, or worsening osteopenia, over many years of observation.[249] On the other hand, an excess risk of mortality, mainly from cardiovascular disease, has been noted during extended follow-up of large cohorts of patients with chronic hypercalcemia (and presumed primary hyperparathyroidism) identified by population health screening in Sweden,[254] and similar observations have been made during extended follow-up of postsurgical patients with hyperparathyroidism.[252,255] Associations of hypertension, hyperuricemia, and glucose intolerance with primary hyperparathyroidism have been implicated, together with hypercalcemia per se, as contributors to this elevated risk.[256] Abnormal cardiac calcification and left ventricular hypertrophy (reversible by successful parathyroidectomy) have been reported in primary hyperparathyroidism as well.[257]

Increased cardiovascular mortality may be a feature only of severe hyperparathyroidism, because it was restricted to those in the highest quartile of serum calcium in the Olmsted County study, which otherwise showed an overall decreased risk of death.[258] A 40% excess risk of malignancy also was reported among 4163 Swedish patients who had undergone surgery more than a year earlier for (presumably symptomatic) primary hyperparathyroidism.[259] It has been argued that these increased risks of mortality and malignancy, even if confirmed, might apply only to those with primary hyperparathyroidism that is more severe than the asymptomatic version typically encountered today.[256]

Abnormalities of bone in modern mild primary hyperparathyroidism are far subtler than those associated with the classic disease. Histologically, the rate at which new bone remodeling cycles are activated is increased. Because the phase of restorative bone formation at each remodeling site takes much more time than does the initial resorptive phase, such an increase in remodeling rate inevitably increases the ambient volume of the remodeling space and, thus, the porosity of bone. Depending upon the rate and extent of the accompanying increase in osteoblastic activity and the resulting local balance between net bone formation and resorption, mineralized bone volume can decrease further, remain stable, or even increase (despite an increased remodeling space). For reasons not yet understood, the balance achieved between increased resorption and formation of bone in primary hyperparathyroidism depends not only upon the severity of the hyperparathyroidism but also upon skeletal location. Thus, net resorption of endosteal bone can predominate in cortical sites, whereas net apposition of mineral can occur in trabecular bone (Fig. 27–23).[260]

In mild primary hyperparathyroidism, osteopenia generally is not evident radiographically, although bone mineral density may be reduced, particularly at sites of predominantly cortical bone such as the mid-radius, by as much as 10% to 20%.[261,262] The mass of trabecular or cancellous bone, as represented in the vertebral bodies, is preferentially preserved and often is normal.[263] Curiously, the reduced cortical bone density at the

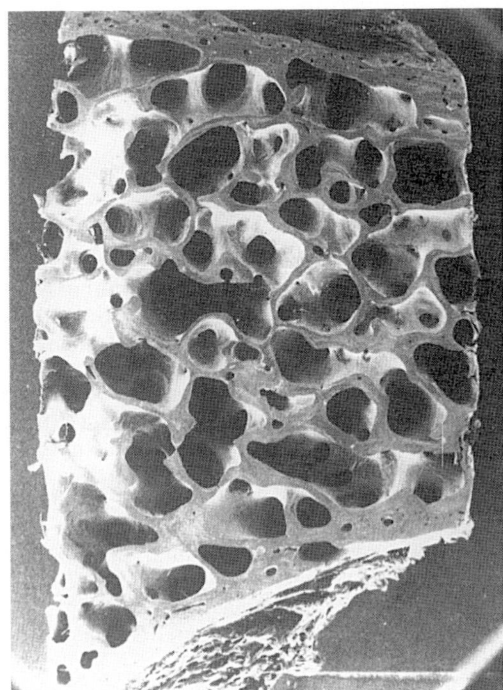
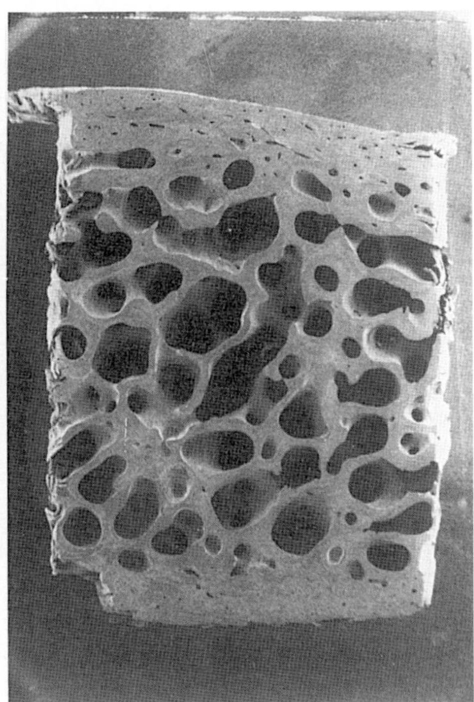

Figure 27–23 ▪ Iliac crest biopsy specimens from a patient with primary hyperparathyroidism *(left)* and a normal control *(right)*, viewed by scanning electron microscopy. Note the thin cortices and contrasting maintenance of trabecular bone in the patient. (From Parisien M, Silverberg SJ, Shane E, et al. The histomorphometry of bone in primary hyperparathyroidism: preservation of cancellous bone structure. J Clin Endocrinol Metab 1990;70:930-938.)

forearm is not improved by successful parathyroidectomy, whereas density at trabecular-rich sites such as the hip and spine can increase by 10% to 15% over several years postoperatively.[249]

The critical issue of whether fracture risk is increased in patients with primary hyperparathyroidism was addressed by a retrospective analysis of fracture incidence within a cohort of 407 residents of Rochester, Minnesota, whose disease was diagnosed between 1965 and 1992.[264] Compared to the expected age- and sex-adjusted rates of incident fractures in that community, the relative risk among those with hyperparathyroidism was significantly elevated at the vertebrae (3.2-fold), distal forearm (2.2-fold) and ribs (2.7-fold), although not at the hip (1.4-fold). Overall risk of fracture at any site was significantly increased as well (1.3-fold) and was as high in patients with disease diagnosed incidentally (following the institution of automated chemistry screening in 1974) as in those with disease diagnosed before then. Similar findings were reported in 674 Danish patients prior to undergoing parathyroidectomy.[265]

These results are consistent with several previous studies involving smaller cohorts of patients and, in the absence of data from an appropriately controlled prospective study, strongly support the conclusion that patients with primary hyperparathyroidism should be considered to be at increased risk for fracture. This presumably is true of those with both symptomatic and asymptomatic disease, because less than 10% of the post-screening Rochester cohort had symptoms or complications of primary hyperparathyroidism.[247] What is not yet known is whether fracture risk is reduced by successful parathyroidectomy, although in the Danish series, risk of vertebral and lower-extremity fractures was no longer increased postoperatively.[265]

Kidney stones now are reported in only 10% to 25% of patients with primary hyperparathyroidism, although some degree of renal dysfunction, either a significant reduction in creatinine clearance or impaired concentrating or acidifying ability, may be found in up to one third of those with asymptomatic disease.[266] As with the reduction in cortical bone mineral density, these renal abnormalities are not progressive in the majority of affected patients.[249,267] The association of kidney stones with primary hyperparathyroidism generally is viewed as an indication for parathyroidectomy, however, because successful surgery usually prevents further symptomatic stone disease.[249,252] On the other hand, it is not possible at present to confidently predict, from biochemical measurements in blood or urine, which asymptomatic patients with hyperparathyroidism will go on to develop new stone disease. Stone formers are more likely to be hypercalciuric than not, but less than one third of hypercalciuric patients with hyperparathyroidism actually develop stones. As noted later, however, marked hypercalciuria (>400 mg/day) generally is viewed as an indication for surgery in otherwise asymptomatic patients.[268]

Etiology and Pathogenesis

Parathyroid adenomas are caused by mutations in the DNA of parathyroid cells; these mutations confer a proliferative or survival advantage for affected cells over their normal neighbors.[269,270] As a consequence of this advantage, the descendants of one particular parathyroid cell, a clone of cells, undergo clonal expansion to produce an adenoma.

Multiple chromosomal regions are missing in the parathyroid cells of individual parathyroid adenomas. These genetic deletions probably reflect the deletion of tumor suppressor genes. These chromosomal loci include portions of chromosome 1p-pter (in 40% of adenomas), 6q (in 32% of adenomas), 15q (in 30% of adenomas), and 11q (in 25% to 30% of adenomas). Many of the 11q deletions are associated, in the undeleted chromosome 11, with mutations in the gene encoding the transcription factor menin, the gene mutated in multiple endocrine neoplasia type 1 (MEN-1). Thus, this gene is also commonly involved in somatic mutations in patients with sporadic parathyroid adenomas. The widespread presence of somatic mutations in sporadic parathyroid adenomas, which are detectable only because large numbers of cells in any one tumor contain the same deletion, constitutes the strongest evidence that parathyroid adenomas are clonal expansions of mutant cells.

One parathyroid proto-oncogene, the *PRAD 1* or cyclin D1 gene, has been identified.[271] This gene was discovered at the breakpoint of an inversion on chromosome 11 in a parathyroid adenoma. This inversion led to the juxtaposition of the PTH gene's regulatory region and the DNA encoding cyclin D1. As a consequence, the cyclin D1 gene was overexpressed. Cyclin D1 is an important regulator of the transition from the G_1 phase of the cell cycle (which follows mitosis) to the S phase (associated with DNA synthesis) and is mutated or amplified in a wide variety of malignancies. Cyclin D1 is overexpressed in about 20% of parathyroid adenomas, though cyclin D1 gene rearrangements have been documented in only 5% of adenomas. Overexpression of cyclin D1 in the parathyroids of transgenic mice leads to formation of parathyroid adenomas and hypercalcemia over many months.[272] The phenotype of these mice demonstrates that cyclin D1 overexpression can cause primary hyperparathyroidism.

As expected for a disease caused by mutations in DNA, parathyroid adenomas occur more often in patients who underwent neck irradiation decades earlier, and greater radiation exposure leads to higher risk.[273] Most patients have no definite history of exposure to specific mutagens, however. An intriguing clue that abnormalities of vitamin D physiology might predispose to primary hyperparathyroidism has come from the observation that patients with parathyroid adenomas are more likely than others to inherit a particular allele of the vitamin D receptor gene.[274] These patients have tumors with particularly low levels of mRNA encoding the vitamin D receptor.

The cause of sporadic primary parathyroid hyperplasia is unknown. The known stimulus for parathyroid cell proliferation—low levels of blood calcium or $1,25(OH)_2D_3$—is not present in this disease. Presumably, some other stimulus outside the parathyroid glands or a genetic abnormality present in all four parathyroid glands leads to inappropriate cell proliferation. Such abnormalities have been found in several inherited forms of parathyroid hyperplasia (see later), but most cases of parathyroid hyperplasia are not found in familial clusters.

The theoretical distinction between adenoma as a clonal proliferation and hyperplasia as a polyclonal growth is clear. In some settings, however, clonal expansion can occur in the context of preexisting nonclonal proliferation. The clearest example of this complication has been found in the large glands associated with severe renal failure. In many such glands removed surgically because of hypercalcemia or severe parathyroid-dependent bone disease, evidence for clonal proliferation complicating secondary hyperplasia has been found. Interestingly, the pattern of chromosomal abnormalities in these clonal tumors differs from that found in parathyroid adenomas in the absence of renal failure.[275] Analogous mechanisms may be operative in a number of settings associated with stimuli to parathyroid cell proliferation, such as X-linked hypophosphatemia[276] and long-term lithium therapy.[277] Furthermore, just as clonal tumors can arise in the setting of *secondary* parathyroid hyperplasia, they can also arise in the setting of sporadic *primary* parathyroid hyperplasia[278] and in MEN.[269,279]

The distinction between adenoma and hyperplasia is clinically important, because removal of the one abnormal gland can be expected to cure a parathyroid adenoma, whereas removal of multiple glands is required to cure parathyroid hyperplasia. Unfortunately, differentiating adenoma from hyperplasia from normal parathyroid tissue at pathologic examination is not straightforward. Pathologists distinguish normal from abnormal parathyroid glands by the increase in size and the paucity of fat in abnormal glands. Attempts have been made to distinguish an adenoma from an individual hyperplastic gland on the basis of morphologic features, but no criteria have proved completely reliable.[280] The formation of clonal neoplasms in originally hyperplastic tumors might explain some of the difficulty in pathologic diagnosis.

An increase in cell number is not the only abnormality in primary hyperparathyroidism. The ability of the normal parathyroid cell to suppress PTH secretion in response to hypercalcemia might be expected to protect the patient from sustained hypercalcemia, even if the number of parathyroid cells increased moderately. Unfortunately, parathyroid cells in parathyroid adenomas usually demonstrate abnormalities in their responsiveness to calcium, with a shift in set-point to the right (Fig. 27–24). This set-point shift, combined with the nonsuppressible component of PTH secretion, leads to a new steady state in which both the PTH level and the blood calcium level are higher than normal.

The molecular underpinning of the abnormal parathyroid cell responsiveness is beginning to be understood. Parathyroid cells from adenomas respond to changes in extracellular calcium with smaller-than-normal increases in intracellular

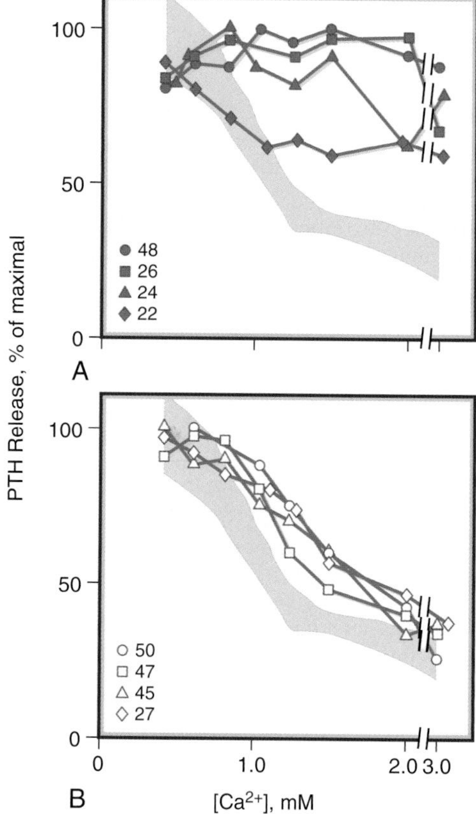

Figure 27–24 ▪ Abnormal patterns of parathyroid hormone (PTH) secretion from cells prepared from adenomatous glands and stimulated with varying levels of calcium in tissue culture. The *shaded area* shows the pattern of PTH release (±1 standard deviation) from normal human parathyroid cells. **A,** The pattern from four patients with little suppression of PTH secretion by calcium. **B,** The pattern from four patients with relatively intact mechanism of suppression of PTH secretion by calcium. Even in this group, the set-point for calcium suppression is shifted to the right. (From Brown, EM. Calcium-regulated parathyroid hormone release in primary hyperparathyroidism, studies in vitro with dispersed parathyroid cells. Am J Med 1979;66:923-931.)

calcium, and the amount of calcium-sensing receptor protein on the cell surface is reduced.[281] Perhaps surprisingly, no mutations in genes encoding the calcium-sensing receptor have been found in parathyroid adenomas. In the experimental model in which overexpression of cyclin D1 results in primary hyperparathyroidism, reduced expression of the calcium-sensing receptor occurs only after cell proliferation has been increased for some time. Thus, the decreased expression of the calcium-sensing receptor in parathyroid adenomas is likely to be a secondary response that occurs during tumor formation.

Inherited Primary Hyperparathyroidism

Although uncommon, inherited forms of primary hyperparathyroidism are clinically important for several reasons. The management of the parathyroid tumors found in familial parathyroid syndromes often differs from that of sporadic primary hyperparathyroidism. Furthermore, extra-parathyroidal manifestations of inherited syndromes may need treatment, and awareness of familial clustering should prompt systematic family screening.

Multiple Endocrine Neoplasia Type 1

MEN-1 (see also Chapter 40) is caused by inactivating mutations in the tumor-suppressor gene encoding menin.[282] Menin is a ubiquitously expressed transcription factor that is part of a complex that targets histone H3 for methylation[283] and thereby leads to expression of cell cycle inhibitors in pancreatic islets and other tissues.[284] Although MEN-1 includes tumors of the parathyroid, anterior pituitary, and pancreatic islets, the parathyroid tumors are far more prevalent than the others; 95% of affected patients eventually develop hyperparathyroidism. Most of the parathyroid tumors harbor mutations in both copies of the menin gene; one mutation is inherited and the second occurs in the parathyroid cell whose progeny form the tumor.

The onset of hypercalcemia occurs in the second and third decades of life, though occasional patients present in the first decade. Hypercalcemia never appears at birth or in infancy. The disease involves all four parathyroid glands, although the involvement can be asymmetrical and apparently asynchronous. Apart from the earlier age at diagnosis, the presenting clinical picture generally resembles that of sporadic primary hyperparathyroidism. One common complicating feature is that hypercalcemia can dramatically increase the gastrin levels and symptoms of patients who also have gastrinomas.

Treatment of the parathyroid disease in this setting can greatly simplify the management of the gastric hyperacidity. After parathyroid surgery, hypoparathyroidism and recurrent hyperparathyroidism are more common than in other forms of hyperparathyroidism. The timing and type of surgery are therefore more complicated issues than in sporadic primary hyperparathyroidism. Most authorities agree that parathyroid disease recurs eventually, particularly if fewer than three glands are removed. Some surgeons prefer subtotal parathyroidectomy, whereas others prefer total parathyroidectomy with forearm implantation of a small amount of parathyroid tissue.

Multiple Endocrine Neoplasia Type 2a

Parathyroid disease is a usually late and infrequent (5% to 20%) occurrence in MEN-2a (see also Chapter 40), a disease defined by the clustering of medullary carcinoma of the thyroid, pheochromocytoma, and hyperparathyroidism. In some families, hyperparathyroidism is more common; however, these families have the same mutations in the *RET* gene that are found in families without frequent hyperparathyroidism.[199] Both parathyroid hyperplasia and adenoma have been noted at surgery. Because asymptomatic parathyroid hyperplasia has been noted at the time of thyroid surgery, a progression from hyperplasia to adenoma in MEN-2a has been suggested.

The approach to diagnosis and treatment of hyperparathyroidism is similar to that in sporadic primary hyperparathyroidism, but hyperplasia is more commonly the underlying disorder. The pathogenesis of the hyperparathyroidism is uncertain, but the *RET* gene, mutated in virtually all cases of MEN-2a, is expressed in parathyroid cells,[200] so abnormal ret expression in parathyroid cells might directly cause parathyroid tumorigenesis. Hyperparathyroidism does not occur in MEN-2b, the variant associated with mucosal neuromas.

Hyperparathyroidism–Jaw Tumor Syndrome

Patients with hereditary hyperparathyroidism–jaw tumor syndrome[191] present with parathyroid adenomas that can be multiple and that are usually cystic. These tumors are often but not invariably associated with fibrous jaw tumors that are unrelated to the hyperparathyroidism. Importantly, the parathyroid tumors are often malignant, in contrast to the findings in MEN-1 and MEN-2. Wilms' tumor and polycystic renal disease also have occurred in affected families. The gene mutated in this syndrome, *HRPT2,* encodes the nuclear protein, parafibromin.[201] Parafibromin is part of an evolutionarily highly conserved complex that binds RNA polymerase II and regulates gene expression.[202,203] Parafibromin binds beta-catenin and can mediate Wnt pathway signaling, though whether this property of parafibromin is related to its tumor-suppressor function is unknown.[189] Inactivating mutations in parafibromin are found in a high number of patients with apparently sporadic parathyroid cancer.[206] Because some of these patients have subsequently proved to be members of families with inherited *HPRT2* mutations, perhaps all patients with parathyroid cancer should be screened for germline mutations in *HPRT2.*

Management of Primary Hyperparathyroidism

The strategy for managing primary hyperparathyroidism has evolved in parallel with the changing presentation of the disease. The only opportunity for permanent cure is surgical removal of the abnormal gland(s), an approach that clearly was appropriate for virtually all patients in whom the classic, severe form of the disease was diagnosed four to five decades ago. It still is the treatment of choice for patients who present with recurrent kidney stones, nephrocalcinosis, clinically overt bone disease, or severe hypercalcemia.

In contrast, the choice of surgical versus medical management for patients with asymptomatic primary hyperparathyroidism remains an open and hotly debated question. Those who favor surgery point to the expected improvement in bone mineral density (at the hip and spine) and left ventricular hypertrophy following successful surgical intervention; evidence of increased risk of fracture, cardiovascular mortality, malignancy, and neuropsychiatric symptoms associated with primary hyperparathyroidism; and the recent successful development of effective minimally invasive surgical procedures (see later). Those who favor an observational approach emphasize the evidence for lack of disease progression in most asymptomatic patients; the small but definite risk of surgical failure and postoperative complications; the probability that excess mortality and cancer risks documented in patients with relatively severe disease might not apply to those with mild, asymptomatic primary hyperparathyroidism; the difficulty in assigning vague neuropsychiatric symptoms to the parathyroid disorder; the lack of evidence (or negative evidence) that hypertension and increased risk of cancer, fracture, or cardiovascular mortality, even if present, are improved by successful parathyroidectomy; and the availability of sensitive techniques for monitoring disease status in nonsurgical patients.[256]

Unfortunately, no large prospective studies have compared outcomes in patients with asymptomatic primary hyperparathyroidism randomly assigned to surgery or to medical management. One small study involving 53 patients demonstrated a significant improvement in hip (but not vertebral or forearm) bone density and modest effects upon quality of life measures attributable to parathyroidectomy but not medical management,[285] but more data are needed. Further, no large trials of differing strategies in medical management of the disease have been conducted. Surgical series generally reflect outcomes in patients preselected to receive interventional treatment, and results thus might not be readily extrapolated to those with mild, asymptomatic disease. The puzzling disparities between the severity of preoperative deficits in bone density of cortical versus trabecular bone and the subsequent responses of these sites to successful parathyroidectomy, in particular, as well as the apparently uniform increase in fracture risk at both cortical- and trabecular-rich sites, confound attempts to interpret the benefits of surgery on the skeletal manifestations of the disease. For all of these reasons, and given the evolution of surgical approaches to this disease, opinion in this area is divided, and all recommendations thus should be considered provisional.

One set of such provisional recommendations was issued by a National Institutes of Health (NIH)-sponsored consensus development conference held in 1990 and updated in 2002.[268] The major conclusion of that group was that surgery should always be considered an appropriate option, but many patients with asymptomatic primary hyperparathyroidism can be safely monitored without surgery. These patients were defined as those who lacked "significant bone, renal, gastrointestinal, or neuromuscular symptoms typical of primary hyperparathyroidism" and who also did not meet the other criteria listed in Table 27–1. Such patients compose at least 50% of those who currently present with primary hyperparathyroidism.

On the other hand, surgery could be preferable if the patient desired surgery even when asymptomatic, if the probability of consistent monitoring seemed low, if concomitant illness seemed likely to complicate management or obscure significant disease progression, or if the patient was relatively young (younger than 50 years). The latter recommendation reflects the absence of reliable information about the natural history of the disease over many decades of follow-up, the cumulative cost of medical monitoring, which begins to exceed that of surgery by 5 to 10 years, and some data suggesting that young people are more likely than others to have progressive disease.[286] On the other hand, age alone was not viewed as a contraindication to parathyroidectomy. The procedure has been accomplished with excellent results, with a perioperative mortality of 15% to 3%, in large numbers of appropriately selected patients older than 75 years. Because hypertension is not thought to be a feature of mild primary hyperparathyroidism, and because hypertension generally is not improved by parathyroidectomy, hypertension was not viewed as an indication for surgery.

TABLE 27–1 INDICATIONS FOR SURGERY IN PRIMARY HYPERPARATHYROIDISM

Overt clinical manifestations of disease
- Kidney stones or nephrocalcinosis
- Fractures or classic radiographic findings of osteitis fibrosa
- Classic neuromuscular disease
- Symptomatic or life-threatening hypercalcemia

Serum calcium >1 mg/dL above the upper limit of normal
Urinary calcium excretion >400 mg/day
Creatinine clearance <70% of predicted
Bone mineral density low (T score <2.5) at any site
Young age (<50 years)
Uncertain prospects for adequate medical monitoring

Indications based upon recommendations of the 2002 NIH-sponsored "Workshop on Asymptomatic Primary Hyperparathyroidism." Modified from Bilezikian JP, Potts JT Jr, Fuleihan Gel H, et al. Summary statement from a workshop on asymptomatic primary hyperparathyroidism: a perspective for the 21st century. J Clin Endocrinol Metab 2002;87(12):5353-5361.

Although the consensus conference recommendations and subsequent modifications provide a useful framework for decision making, supporting data from large clinical trials are lacking. In a series of 52 asymptomatic patients selected for nonoperative management mainly on the basis of the consensus conference criteria and whose course was followed for 10 years, approximately 25% developed one or more new indications for surgery (see Table 27–1).[249] Patients who do not meet the consensus conference criteria for surgery might nevertheless experience the same postsurgical increase in bone density as those who do.[287] Some have emphasized that evidence of baseline vertebral osteopenia, an unusual finding in primary hyperparathyroidism, should be considered among the consensus criteria for surgery (see Table 27–1)[263] and that surgery also should be considered for menopausal women who exhibit vertebral bone loss in the setting of primary hyperparathyroidism.[249,256]

A common dilemma is the inability to ascertain whether vague but troublesome symptoms such as fatigue, lethargy, weakness (without objective muscle weakness) or depression are due to hyperparathyroidism and thus qualify as "significant" in the context of considering the decision for surgery. Most clinicians do not routinely recommend parathyroidectomy on the basis of such symptoms alone, although dramatic responses to surgery are occasionally seen. With the availability of improved, minimally invasive surgical approaches, the threshold for considering surgery in patients who are significantly disabled by such symptoms clearly is lower now than in the past. Some have advocated, in selected cases, a limited trial of medical therapy to reduce serum calcium (calcimimetics—see later) and thereby attempt to predict the symptomatic response to surgical cure.

Medical Monitoring of Primary Hyperparathyroidism

The NIH consensus conference recommended that patients be followed carefully, at least semiannually initially and at longer intervals if the disease remains stable. Patients should be monitored at 1- to 2-year intervals for appearance of symptoms; appearance of adverse effects on blood pressure and on serum or urinary calcium or creatinine; and serial determination of bone mineral density. The most appropriate bone densitometric site is one that reflects mainly changes in cortical bone (distal forearm or total body), although the importance of following vertebral bone density as well has been emphasized,[249,263] and the revised criteria acknowledge the importance of significant bone loss at any site.[268]

Patients undergoing nonoperative medical management must be cautioned to maintain adequate hydration, to avoid diuretics and prolonged immobilization, and to seek prompt medical attention in the event of illnesses accompanied by significant vomiting or diarrhea. Dietary calcium probably should not exceed the RDA of 800 mg/day even though short-term studies in highly selected patients with elevated serum $1,25(OH)_2D$ levels have demonstrated that a high-calcium diet can reduce serum $1,25(OH)_2D$ and PTH, albeit at the expense of a mild increase in serum and urinary calcium.[288]

The goal of an effective medical therapy for primary hyperparathyroidism remains elusive, though study of sex hormones and selective estrogen-receptor modulators (SERMs), bisphosphonates, and calcimimetics continue. Estrogens and progestins might reduce serum calcium and phosphorus, urinary calcium and hydroxyproline, and histologic evidence of active bone resorption in women with primary hyperparathyroidism, although safety concerns have limited these therapeutic options in postmenopausal women. Limited data with raloxifene suggest that it may be useful in controlling serum calcium and lowering bone turnover in women with primary hyperparathyroidism.[289]

Intravenous bisphosphonates have been employed successfully in the urgent therapy of hypercalcemia due to primary hyperparathyroidism, and several trials have shown that treatment with oral alendronate for 1 year or more improves bone density at the spine and hip, with only transient effects on serum calcium and PTH.[290,291] The calcimimetics represent a new class of agents that, by sensitizing the calcium-sensing receptor to extracellular calcium, can reduce PTH secretion. Cinacalcet, the first calcimimetic approved for control of secondary hyperparathyroidism in renal disease, was shown to lower serum calcium and PTH in primary hyperparathyroidism (and in some patients with parathyroid carcinoma), although improvement in bone density has not been documented in this population.[292]

Thus, in patients for whom surgery for asymptomatic primary hyperparathyroidism is not an option, therapy with oral bisphosphonates can improve bone density without worsening other features of the disease, at least over 2 years of follow-up. Whether this or any other medical therapy offers a beneficial long-term alternative to surgery is unknown.

Surgical Treatment of Primary Hyperparathyroidism

Parathyroidectomy is a safe and highly effective approach to definitive treatment of primary hyperparathyroidism. The most serious potential complications of parathyroid surgery—vocal cord paralysis and permanent hypoparathyroidism—occur after fewer than 1% and 4%, respectively, of procedures performed by highly skilled surgeons, although these rates can be much higher in less-experienced hands. Such complications occur most often in patients who require subtotal parathyroid resections for hyperplasia or resection of carcinoma. The surgical cure rate for primary hyperparathyroidism in the best hands is at least 95%.[293,294]

Apart from operator inexperience, the usual cause of initial surgical failure ("persistent disease") is the presence of either unrecognized (often very asymmetrical) parathyroid hyperplasia or ectopic parathyroid tissue (intrathyroidal, undescended, retroesophageal, or mediastinal glands) (Fig. 27–25).[295,296] Up to one in five parathyroid glands is located ectopically, and this is especially true of supernumerary glands.[244,297] Recurrent disease, defined as that occurring after an interval of at least 6 to 12 months of normocalcemia, varies in incidence from 2% to 16%. Recurrent hyperparathyroidism usually arises in unresected hyperplastic glands, but rarely it is due to parathyroid carcinoma, to a second adenoma, or to a multicentric or miliary parathyromatosis engendered by inadvertent local seeding of parathyroid tissue (usually hyperplastic) into the neck during previous parathyroid surgery.[244]

Until very recently, there was broad agreement that the best approach is a bilateral neck exploration in which all four parathyroids are identified and all enlarged glands removed.[297] With this procedure, preoperative parathyroid localization studies prior to initial cervical exploration are superfluous, because the positive predictive value of even the best technique (^{99m}Tc-sestamibi scanning) falls well short of the success rate of experienced surgeons unaided by prior imaging.[244,298,299]

With the advent of preoperative ^{99m}Tc-sestamibi scanning, which can accurately localize 80% to 90% of the single adenomas that account for 75% to 85% of cases, there has been renewed interest in performance of directed unilateral explorations, which reduce operative and recovery-room time, minimize the number of frozen sections required, are associated with significantly fewer postoperative complications, and can more readily be performed using minimally invasive techniques (including local anesthesia and intravenous sedation) that enable same-day discharge.[300,301] Sestamibi scanning also can

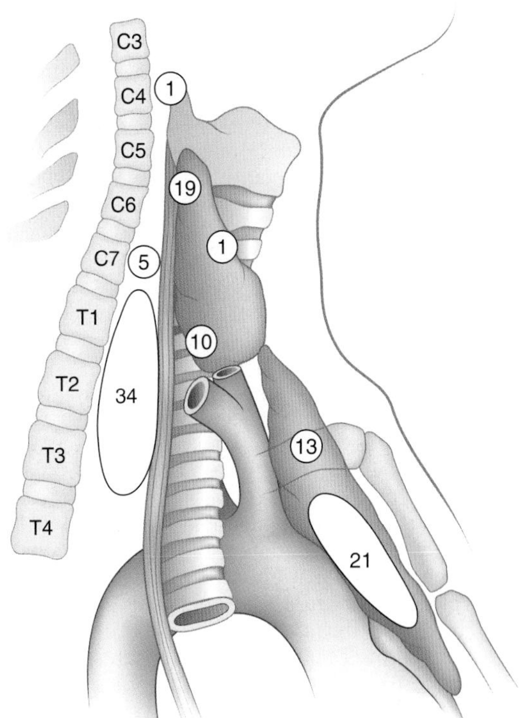

Figure 27–25 ▪ Sites of ectopic location of 104 parathyroid glands found at reoperation for primary hyperparathyroidism. (From Wang C-A. A clinical and pathological study of 112 cases. Ann Surg 1977;186:140-145.)

identify the occasional mediastinal adenoma and thereby allow the surgeon to forgo an unnecessary neck exploration.

On the other hand, the sensitivity and positive predictive value of sestamibi scanning is poor (<50%) in the presence of multiglandular disease (hyperplasia or double adenomas), and thus the test can miss bilateral disease.[294,302] To reduce this failure rate, which is unacceptably high in comparison to bilateral exploration, supplemental preoperative ultrasonic imaging (with or without needle biopsy) is often employed, and rapid intraoperative PTH assays have been developed to verify successful excision.[303] Because the half-life of intact PTH in blood is very short (<2 min), a decline of 50% or more from baseline within 10 minutes or so can signal successful removal of all hyperfunctioning parathyroid tissue. This approach has functioned well in patients with single adenomas, but it can be misleading in those with multiglandular disease unless more stringent criteria for cure are applied (>90% decline, or even normalization, of iPTH).[304]

At present, preoperative imaging enables consideration of a minimally invasive unilateral parathyroidectomy in approximately 70% of patients thought preoperatively to have sporadic primary hyperparathyroidism due to a solitary adenoma. Surgical cure rates in appropriately selected patients are comparable to those after bilateral neck exploration (95%-97%).[293,294] Patients known or suspected to have muliglandular disease, such as those with MEN-1 and those younger than 30 years, should undergo bilateral neck exploration.[305-307] Options for patients with hyperplasia include resection limited to visibly abnormal glands, subtotal parathyroidectomy with cryopreservation of tissue, and total parathyroidectomy with immediate transplantation in the forearm of some of the excised tissue. In patients with MEN-1, considerations of recurrence rates (30%-50% or higher with long-term follow-up) and the timing thereof versus the potential morbidity of surgical hypoparathyroidism tend to favor subtotal parathyroidectomy as the preferred approach at present.[305]

The incidence of parathyroid carcinoma in primary hyperparathyroidism is less than 1%,[245] but this possibility should be strongly considered in patients with unusually severe hyperparathyroidism, a palpable neck mass, hoarseness, evidence of local invasion at surgery, or recurrent hypercalcemia (see later). Even so, parathyroid carcinoma rarely is suspected preoperatively and often eludes diagnosis at the time of initial surgery. When the disease is recognized, vigorous attempts should be made to remove the tumor en bloc. The incidence of local recurrence approaches 50%, however, and distant metastases, particularly to lung, may be heralded by recurrent, severe hyperparathyroidism.[297]

Immediate postoperative management of parathyroidectomy focuses upon establishing the success of the surgery and monitoring the patient closely for symptomatic hypocalcemia and for uncommon but potentially serious acute complications such as bleeding, vocal cord paralysis, or laryngospasm. After successful resection of a parathyroid adenoma, serum intact PTH levels decline rapidly, often to undetectable concentrations, with a disappearance half-time of about 2 minutes, whereas serum calcium typically reaches a nadir between 24 and 36 hours. Serum PTH returns to the normal range within 30 hours, although measurements of the parathyroid secretory response to hypocalcemia suggest that it does not fully normalize for at least several weeks.[308]

In the past, patients generally were maintained on a low-calcium diet until normalization of serum calcium was clearly documented, ampoules of injectable calcium and other seizure precautions were maintained at the bedside, serum calcium was measured at least every 12 hours until levels were stable, and symptomatic hypocalcemia was promptly treated with calcium, either intravenously (90-mg bolus, 50-100 mg/hr) or orally (1.5-3.0 g/day). This approach is no longer appropriate for most patients, who are discharged within a few hours after limited surgery. Instead, oral calcium supplements routinely are provided as soon as oral intake is reestablished, and moderate doses of $1,25(OH)_2D_3$ (0.5-1.0 μg daily) are added for those with large adenomas and severe hyperparathyroidism or for those in whom alkaline phosphatase had been elevated preoperatively, namely, patients in whom an impressive calcium requirement can be anticipated, often for many weeks postoperatively, as they remineralize their skeletons. This hungry bone syndrome is associated with hypocalcemia, hypophosphatemia, and low urinary calcium excretion.

Serum calcium should be checked at intervals of several days initially to guide adjustment of calcium and vitamin D therapy as needed to achieve a stable result. In those in whom hypocalcemia persists for more than several days, serum PTH should be measured to exclude the possibility of postoperative hypoparathyroidism. Given evidence that bone mineral density continues to increase for at least 1 year after successful parathyroidectomy,[249] it is prudent to continue calcium supplementation for at least that long.

The approach to patients with persistent or recurrent hyperparathyroidism is informed by the recognition that parathyroid hyperplasia or carcinoma, ectopic or supernumerary parathyroid tissue, and postoperative hypoparathyroidism and other complications of further surgery all are more common in this population.[296,299] The first issue to address is whether surgery is indicated. When a presumed adenoma had not been identified initially, the original indications for surgery generally still exist, although some patients might not be suitable candidates for more extensive surgery, such as a median sternotomy, because of concurrent medical illness. Patients with parathyroid hyperplasia may have experienced significant clinical improvement, even after incomplete parathyroidectomy, although those with MEN-1 are very likely to experience further progression of their disease.[305]

Preoperative localization studies are recommended for patients with persistent or recurrent disease after a first operation. Scanning with ^{99m}Tc-sestamibi offers the highest sensitivity and accuracy, although other studies (ultrasonography, CT, MRI) can provide additional or confirmatory information.[309] Sestamibi does localize to thyroid nodules, which can accompany parathyroid disease in 20% to 40% of patients, although it tends to wash out of thyroid tissue much more rapidly than from parathyroids. ^{99m}Tc-sestamibi can be combined with ^{123}I scanning to improve distinction of parathyroids from thyroid nodules or with single photon emission CT (SPECT) imaging to achieve accuracy in localization not possible with planar imaging. (Fig. 27–26). On the other hand, sestamibi scanning can fail to reveal small glands (uptake is related to gland size and PTH levels[310]) or to demonstrate multiple abnormal glands in cases of parathyroid hyperplasia, the most common cause of persistent postoperative hyperparathyroidism.[294,302]

More-invasive techniques have been employed as well, including angiography and selective venous sampling for measuring PTH.[311,312] Ultrasound- or CT-guided fine-needle aspiration of suspected parathyroid tissue may be used to obtain cytologic or immunochemical confirmation before surgery,[313] and intraoperative ultrasonography has been useful in some cases to locate cervical or intrathyroidal glands.[299] Success with video-assisted thoracoscopic resection of documented mediastinal lesions[314] offers a less-invasive alternative to median sternotomy for this relatively common cause of persistent hyperparathyroidism.

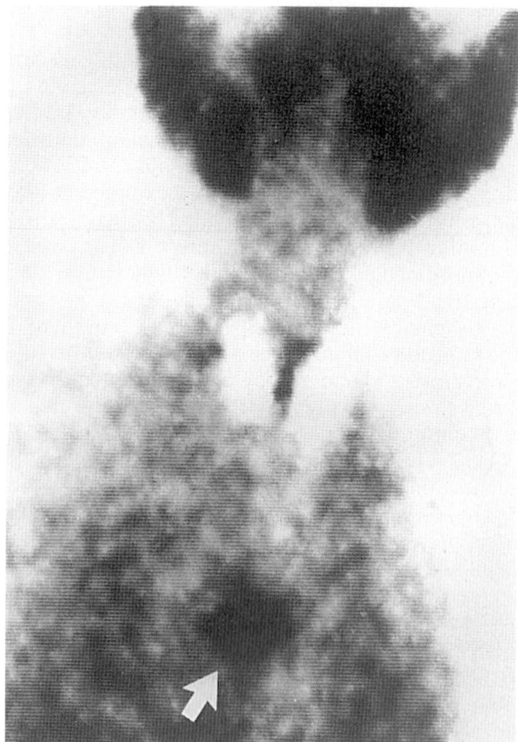

Figure 27–26 ▪ Technetium Tc 99m sestamibi ^{123}I subtraction scanning of a patient with persistent hyperparathyroidism after two previous unsuccessful operations. *Arrow* points to parathyroid adenoma, shown as increased tracer uptake in the aortopulmonary window. (From Thule P, Thakore K, Vansant J, et al. Preoperative localization of parathyroid tissue with technetium-99m sestamibi ^{123}I subtraction scanning. J Clin Endocrinol Metab 1994;78:77-82.)

The need for these procedures depends upon the experience of the original surgeon and the confidence that the neck was adequately explored initially. For example, among reoperations at one center, more than half of the "missed" hyperplastic parathyroid glands in those cases previously explored by a highly experienced parathyroid surgeon were found by the surgeon in the mediastinum or another ectopic location, whereas more than 90% of those referred by less-experienced surgeons were discovered in a normal anatomic location in the neck.[244]

Following successful surgery for primary hyperparathyroidism, bone mass generally improves by as much as 5% to 10% in the first year at sites rich in trabecular bone (spine, femoral neck), whereas improvement at cortical sites (distal radius) is less predictable.[15,315] Increases at trabecular sites can continue for several years, to as much as 12% to 15% after 10 years, although normal bone mineral density might not be achieved.[262,316] This improvement, which is most apparent in those with the greatest preoperative reductions in bone mass, may be related in part to rapid remineralization of the previously enlarged bone remodeling volume,[287] but the continued improvement over years suggests a more sustained increase in net bone formation and total bone volume, as well.[249]

Familial Hypocalciuric Hypercalcemia

Familial hypocalciuric hypercalcemia (FHH), also appropriately called *familial benign hypercalcemia,* is, in most families, a disorder of autosomal dominant inheritance caused by mutations of the calcium-sensing receptor gene found in parathyroid glands, kidney, and other organs[317] (see the earlier discussion of calcium sensing). The mutations, which cause complete or partial loss of function of the calcium-sensing receptor, lead to a shift in the parathyroid cell's set-point for calcium. As a consequence, higher than normal levels of blood calcium are needed to suppress PTH secretion. Furthermore, abnormal function of the calcium-sensing receptor in the renal thick ascending limb leads to increased, PTH-independent calcium reabsorption and consequent hypocalciuria.

The presence of one normal sensing receptor gene with the abnormal one usually leads to a very mild clinical disorder, although the receptor functions as a dimer, and certain mutations can worsen the function of the normal allele. Rare patients who inherit mutant calcium-sensing receptor genes from both parents present at birth with severe, life-threatening primary hyperparathyroidism and almost always require immediate parathyroid surgery. In another genetic variation, a familial form of calcium-sensing receptor-dependent hypercalcemia has been described in association with other autoimmune disorders such as Hashimoto's hypothyroidism and celiac sprue, in which autoantibodies directed against the sensor apparently antagonize calcium recognition by the parathyroids and renal tubules.[318,319]

FHH is manifested at birth by hypercalcemia. Although some controversy exists, most observers note that the condition is asymptomatic and that apparent symptoms represent ascertainment bias. Possible exceptions include the occurrence of chondrocalcinosis and perhaps pancreatitis. The blood calcium level is usually less than 12 mg/dL but can be higher. Phosphate measurements are low, as in primary hyperparathyroidism. Blood magnesium levels are high normal or slightly elevated. PTH levels are inappropriately normal for the degree of hypercalcemia and are occasionally modestly elevated. Urine calcium is usually low, though one novel mutation in the receptor's intracellular tail has been associated with hypercalciuria, possibly because of only mild dysfunction in the kidney.[320]

When patients present as adults, the distinction from mild primary hyperparathyroidism can be difficult. The distinction between FHH and primary hyperparathyroidism is a crucial one, however. Young patients with primary hyperparathyroidism are usually treated surgically and cured. In contrast, hypercalcemia always recurs after surgery for FHH, unless the patient is rendered hypoparathyroid by the removal of all parathyroid tissue. Therefore, surgery is contraindicated as therapy for FHH, except in the very rare patient with severe symptomatic hypercalcemia. No blood or urine measurements are completely reliable for distinguishing between the two conditions, though the ratio of calcium clearance to creatinine clearance distinguishes most patients with FHH from those with primary hyperparathyroidism.[321] Figure 27–27 shows, however, that this ratio separates the two groups, with modest overlap between the groups. However, because primary hyperparathyroidism is much more common than FHH, most patients with values near the cut-off value of 0.01 for the ratio of calcium clearance to creatinine clearance have primary hyperparathyroidism and not FHH. The most helpful diagnostic information is the presence of hypercalcemia in an infant relative; such early hypercalcemia does not occur in MEN-1. Furthermore, a past history of clearly normal blood calcium, considerably lower than current measurements, makes FHH unlikely in the absence of another reason for a change in blood calcium.

Lithium Toxicity

Treatment of bipolar affective disorders with lithium commonly leads to mild, persistent increases in blood calcium[277,322] occasionally out of the normal range, in affected persons. After several years of therapy, clear elevations of PTH levels and modest increases in parathyroid gland size, detected by ultrasonography, often occur. Usually, when lithium therapy is stopped, the blood calcium and PTH normalize within several

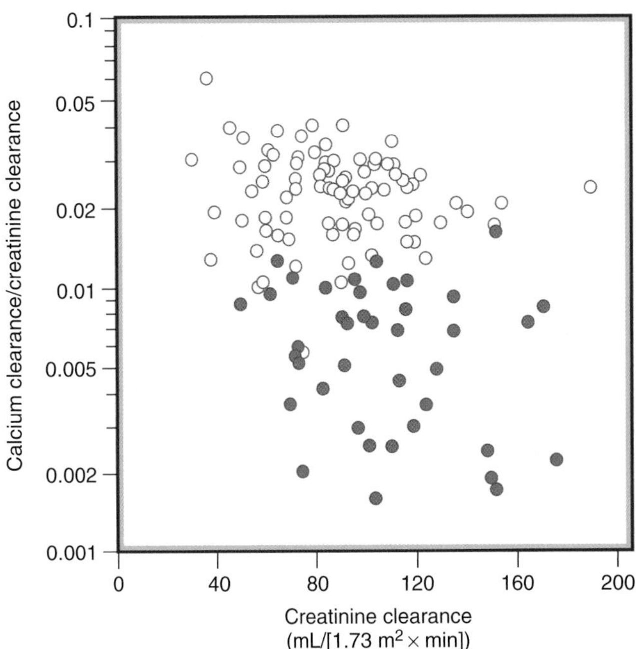

Figure 27–27 ▪ Index of urinary excretion rate for calcium as a function of creatinine clearance. Each point represents the mean of multiple determinations for a hypercalcemic patient with familial hypocalciuric hypercalcemia *(filled circles)* or with typical primary hyperparathyroidism *(open circles)*. The data are based on average 24-hour urinary excretion values and average fasting serum samples. (From Marx SJ, Attie MF, Levine MA, et al. The hypocalciuric or benign variant of familial hypercalcemia: clinical and biochemical features in fifteen kindreds. Medicine (Baltimore) 1981;60(6):397-412.)

months. Uncommonly, substantial hypercalcemia and clear hyperparathyroidism ensue. At surgery, parathyroid hyperplasia and, sometimes, parathyroid adenomas have been found.[323]

Management of patients with mild lithium-induced hypercalcemia is somewhat complex. Like patients with mild primary hyperparathyroidism, patients taking lithium usually tolerate mild hypercalcemia without obvious symptoms. These patients can be monitored with protocols similar to those for patients with asymptomatic primary hyperparathyroidism. Close attention must be paid to urine-concentrating ability in these patients, however, because the nephrogenic diabetes insipidus associated with lithium therapy can lead to dehydration and sudden worsening of hypercalcemia. Substantial hypercalcemia should lead to withdrawal of lithium therapy, if possible, with substitution of newer psychopharmacologic agents. If hypercalcemia persists after withdrawal of lithium, decisions about surgery follow the same guidelines as those for patients with primary hyperparathyroidism.

Lithium increases the set-point for PTH secretion when it is added to isolated parathyroid cells in vitro. The set-point for PTH secretion in vivo is shifted to the right in patients who have received lithium for several years as well. A corresponding shift in the concentration of extracellular calcium needed to raise intracellular calcium levels suggests that lithium interferes with the action of the parathyroid calcium-sensing receptor, perhaps by interfering with inositol phosphate metabolism.

Parathyroid-Independent Hypercalcemia

In parathyroid-independent hypercalcemia, PTH secretion is appropriately suppressed. PTH levels, measured using two-site assays, are invariably lower than 25 pg/mL and are usually lower than normal or undetectable. Most affected patients have malignant hypercalcemia, although parathyroid-independent hypercalcemia occurs in a number of other settings as well.[324]

Hypercalcemia of Malignancy

The diagnosis of malignant hypercalcemia is seldom a subtle one.[106] Most malignancies produce hypercalcemia only when they are far advanced; the diagnosis becomes evident after routine studies, guided by the history and physical examination. Patients with malignant hypercalcemia usually die a month or two after hypercalcemia is discovered. Patients present with the classic signs and symptoms of hypercalcemia: confusion, polydipsia, polyuria, constipation, nausea, and vomiting. Perhaps because of the acuteness of the hypercalcemia and the elderly patient population involved, dramatic changes in mental status, culminating in coma, are relatively common. The diagnosis can be missed because the manifestations often overlap those of the underlying malignancy and because low blood albumin can lead to an apparently normal total blood calcium, despite an elevated blood ionized calcium. Even though the overall prognosis is grim, the diagnosis of malignant hypercalcemia is important to make.

Treatment is usually simple and effective in the short term; such treatment can importantly reverse the patient's symptoms for several weeks and even provide time for a fundamental attack on the underlying tumor, if it is treatable. Only effective treatment of the underlying neoplasm can significantly influence the long-term prognosis for patients with malignant hypercalcemia.

Although mechanisms in a given patient may be multiple, it is still useful to distinguish hypercalcemia associated with local involvement of bone from that caused by humoral mechanisms. In all cases, resorption of bone plays a pivotal role in the pathogenesis.

Local Osteolytic Hypercalcemia

Hypercalcemia resulting from tumors invading bone occurs most clearly in patients with multiple myeloma and in some patients with breast cancer. There is little evidence that the tumor cells themselves resorb bone. Instead, active osteoclasts found near the tumor cells are thought to be the proximate mediators of bone resorption.[325] Myeloma cells and marrow cells associated with myeloma cells secrete numerous cytokines and chemokines capable of stimulating bone resorption, including MIP-1α, lymphotoxin (tumor necrosis factor β [TNF-β]), and interleukin (IL)-1β,IL-3, and IL-6. These factors lead to increased expression of RANK ligand on the surface of marrow stromal cells and stimulation of osteoclast formation and activity. RANK ligand is also found on the surface of myeloma cells and therefore might stimulate the production and activity of osteoclasts. In patients with myeloma, treatment with intermittent intravenous bisphosphonates inhibits this resorption and reduces the incidence of bone pain, fracture, and hypercalcemia.

The pathogenesis of hypercalcemia in breast cancer is not completely understood. Extensive metastases to bone are detected in most patients with hypercalcemia and breast cancer; this finding suggests that factors produced in bone by the metastatic tumor cells may be important. Breast cancer cells make a host of cytokines capable of resorbing bone. The role of tumor-produced PTHrP may be particularly important.[326] A majority of breast cancer patients with hypercalcemia have elevated blood levels of PTHrP. This circulating PTHrP, as well as PTHrP produced in bone by metastatic tumor cells, might generate the hypercalcemia. Primary breast tumors that stain for PTHrP are more likely to result in bone metastases than are those that do not stain for PTHrP; this PTHrP may be instrumental in the establishment of lytic metastases. Animal models indicate that transforming growth factor β (TGF-β), released from bone matrix by PTHrP-stimulated osteoclastic resorption, may further augment PTHrP secretion by the tumor cells. PTHrP secretion may be further promoted by estrogen, which might explain the occasional occurrence of hypercalcemia following institution of estrogen or tamoxifen therapy in breast cancer.[326]

Humoral Hypercalcemia of Malignancy

Albright, in 1941, was the first to propose that a PTH-like humoral factor caused the hypercalcemia in patients with malignancy but few or no bone metastases.[327] Four decades later biochemical analysis demonstrated that such patients have high blood calcium levels, low blood phosphate levels, and high urinary cAMP levels like those found in primary hyperparathyroidism, but no elevation in iPTH levels.[328] The stimulation of cAMP production was used as an assay to eventually purify PTHrP from human tumors associated with the humoral hypercalcemia of malignancy.[102]

The evidence that PTHrP mediates the humoral hypercalcemia of malignancy in most patients is substantial. PTHrP binds to the PTH/PTHrP receptor and mimics all of the actions of amino-terminal fragments of PTH. Blood levels of PTHrP are elevated in most patients with solid tumors and hypercalcemia. In animal models of the humoral hypercalcemia of malignancy, antibodies against PTHrP can reverse the hypercalcemia.[329]

The acute actions of PTHrP cannot explain all of the findings in patients with the hypercalcemia of malignancy, however. Acutely administered PTHrP increases blood levels of $1,25(OH)_2D_3$ by stimulating the renal 1α-hydroxylase, though the stimulation is less than that induced by PTH.[330] Nevertheless, patients with the humoral hypercalcemia of malignancy usually have low levels of $1,25(OH)_2D_3$.[328] This finding is particularly puzzling, because human tumors associated with low $1,25(OH)_2D_3$ levels stimulate $1,25(OH)_2D_3$ synthesis after they are transplanted into nude mice.[331] Possible explanations for the low $1,25(OH)_2D_3$ levels in patients include the weak activation of the renal 1α-hydroxylase in humans by PTHrP, combined with the inhibition of the 1α-hydroxylase by hypercalcemia[332] or by tumor products.[333]

A second disparity between the acute actions of PTHrP and the findings in patients with malignant hypercalcemia involves the rate of bone formation. Acutely, PTHrP, like PTH, leads to increased bone formation. Nevertheless, in patients with malignant hypercalcemia, bone formation is markedly lower than normal. The explanation for this effect may well lie in the action of other cytokines, immobilization, or particular fragments of PTHrP with novel properties.

The tumors most commonly associated with humoral hypercalcemia include squamous cell cancers of the lung, head and neck, esophagus, cervix, vulva, and skin; breast cancer; renal cell cancer; and bladder cancer. Benign or malignant pheochromocytomas, islet cell tumors, and carcinoids can also overproduce PTHrP, causing hypercalcemia. The aggressive T-cell lymphoma associated with human T-cell lymphotropic virus-1 (HTLV-1) infection is the only hematologic malignancy commonly associated with PTHrP overproduction and hypercalcemia.

It is unlikely that PTHrP is the sole cause of the humoral hypercalcemia of malignancy. As noted previously, many cytokines produced by tumors can stimulate bone resorption. The actions of these cytokines have been shown to synergize with those of PTHrP in a number of experimental models. Furthermore, in hypercalcemic patients with non-Hodgkin's lymphoma, blood levels of $1,25(OH)_2D_3$ were found to be higher than otherwise expected,[334] and such patients show abnormal sensitivity to 25(OH)D administration.[335] In these hypercalcemic patients, the relative importance of $1,25(OH)_2D_3$ cytokines, PTHrP, and immobilization needs to be clarified.

In a few reported cases, malignant tumors secrete PTH and not PTHrP.[106] Although this phenomenon has now been well documented, in almost all patients with cancer and high PTH levels, concurrent primary hyperparathyroidism, not ectopic PTH production, is the cause of the hyperparathyroidism.

Vitamin D Intoxication

Because the synthesis of $1,25(OH)_2D_3$ is so tightly regulated, extremely large doses of vitamin D, on the order of 100,000 units per day, are required to cause hypercalcemia. Such doses are available in the United States only by prescription; therefore, most cases of vitamin D intoxication are iatrogenic. Occasionally, inadvertent ingestion occurs. Patients present with nausea, vomiting, weakness, and altered level of consciousness. Hypercalcemia can be severe and prolonged, because of the storage of vitamin D in fat. As expected, PTH levels are suppressed, and levels of 25(OH)D, which are poorly regulated and reflect levels of ingested vitamin D, are dramatically elevated. In contrast, the levels of $1,25(OH)_2D_3$ are only modestly elevated or can be normal or even low. The modest changes in $1,25(OH)_2D_3$ levels result from the down-regulation of the renal 1α-hydroxylase by low levels of PTH and high levels of phosphate, calcium, and $1,25(OH)_2D_3$ itself. The cause of the hypercalcemia, when it occurs in the face of normal levels of $1,25(OH)_2D_3$, is uncertain but might reflect the direct action of 25(OH)D and possibly other vitamin D metabolites, which are capable of binding the $1,25(OH)_2D_3$ receptor weakly. Also, the weaker vitamin D metabolites can displace $1,25(OH)_2D_3$ from the circulating D-binding protein and increase the concentration of active, free $1,25(OH)_2D_3$.[177]

The hypercalcemia of vitamin D intoxication results from increased intestinal absorption of calcium and from the direct effect of $1,25(OH)_2D_3$ to increase resorption of bone. In severe cases, therefore, bisphosphonate therapy can be usefully added to the therapeutic regimen of hydration and omission of dietary calcium.[336]

Sarcoidosis and Other Granulomatous Diseases

Sarcoidosis may be associated with hypercalcemia and, even more commonly, hypercalciuria.[337] Hypercalcemic patients have high levels of $1,25(OH)_2D_3$; the high level of $1,25(OH)_2D_3$ probably causes the hypercalcemia, although overproduction of bone-resorbing cytokines and PTHrP might contribute in some patients. As expected in $1,25(OH)_2D_3$-dependent hypercalcemia, intestinal absorption of calcium is increased and PTH levels are suppressed. Furthermore, the hypercalcemia and high levels of $1,25(OH)_2D_3$ decrease when treated with glucocorticoids. The unregulated synthesis of $1,25(OH)_2D_3$, found even in an anephric patient, occurs not in the kidney but rather in the sarcoid granulomas. Removal of a large amount of granulomatous tissue can reverse hypercalcemia.[338] Furthermore, isolated sarcoid macrophages can synthesize $1,25(OH)_2D_3$ from 25(OH)D, as can normal macrophages stimulated with IFN-γ. IFN-γ also suppresses the macrophage's metabolism of $1,25(OH)_2D_3$ to inactive $1,24,25(OH)_2D_3$.[339] Such macrophages express the gene encoding the identical 25(OH)D 1α-hydroxylase found in the kidney.

The unregulated synthesis of $1,25(OH)_2D_3$ by activated macrophages explains many of the findings in sarcoid patients. These patients have unusual sensitivity to vitamin D and can become hypercalcemic in response to ultraviolet radiation or oral vitamin D intake. Abnormalities in calcium metabolism are usually found only in patients with active disease and large, clinically obvious total-body burdens of granulomas. Nevertheless, hypercalcemia can occur in patients without obvious pulmonary disease. Furthermore, subtle abnormalities of vitamin D metabolism can be demonstrated even in patients with mildly active sarcoidosis.

Hypercalcemia is also associated with other granulomatous diseases, such as tuberculosis, fungal infections, and berylliosis. It has been reported in Wegener's granulomatosis, in acquired immunodeficiency syndrome (AIDS)-related *Pneumocystis jiroveci (formerly called carinii)* infection, and even in association with extensive granulomatous foreign body reactions.[324] Patients with Crohn's disease occasionally have hypercalcemia with elevations of $1,25(OH)_2D_3$ levels, but they often have elevated $1,25(OH)_2D_3$ levels with normal calcium levels and low bone mass, associated with increased production of $1,25(OH)_2D_3$ in intestinal macrophages.[340]

Hyperthyroidism

Mild hypercalcemia can result from thyrotoxicosis. Blood calcium levels seldom exceed 11 mg/dL, but mild elevations are found in a quarter of patients. Patients have low PTH levels, low $1,25(OH)_2D_3$ levels, and hypercalciuria. The hypercalcemia is caused by a direct action of thyroid hormone to stimulate bone resorption.[341] β-Adrenergic blocking agents can reverse the hypercalcemia.[342]

Vitamin A Intoxication

Excess ingestion of vitamin A (retinol) results in a syndrome of dry skin, pruritus, headache from pseudotumor cerebri, bone pain, and, occasionally, hypercalcemia. Hypercalcemia occurs only with the ingestion of 10 times the RDA (5000 IU/day). The identical syndrome can result from ingestion of the vitamin A derivatives isotretinoin (13-*cis*-retinoic acid [Accutane]) and tretinoin (all-*trans*-retinoic acid [Retin-A]), used to treat acne.[343] Bones can show characteristic periosteal calcification on radiographs. The hypercalcemia is probably caused by the action of retinoids to directly stimulate bone resorption. The diagnosis is made by the association of a history of excess ingestion of retinoids with the characteristic syndrome and abnormal results of liver function tests; elevated vitamin A levels confirm the diagnosis. Treatment involves hydration and, if necessary, glucocorticoids or bisphosphonates.

Adrenal Insufficiency

Hypercalcemia occurs in the setting of adrenal insufficiency. Blood calcium is elevated partly as a result of hemoconcentration and increased albumin levels, but the level of ionized calcium can be increased as well.[344] The hypercalcemia in this study resulted from a combination of influx of calcium into the vascular space, probably from bone, combined with low renal clearance.

Thiazide Diuretics

Thiazide diuretics do not cause hypercalcemia by themselves, but they can exacerbate the hypercalcemia of primary hyperparathyroidism or any other cause of increased input of calcium into the bloodstream. The mechanism of the hypercalcemia might involve the action of thiazide diuretics to increase proximal tubular calcium reabsorption as a secondary consequence of direct action of thiazides on the distal tubule.[345] Decreased renal clearance of calcium alone would be expected to raise blood calcium in the normal human only transiently because the transient hypercalcemia would be expected to suppress PTH secretion and lead to return of the blood calcium to normal. However, in the presence of primary hyperparathyroidism, sarcoidosis, excess calcium intake, or any other cause of high, fixed calcium load, thiazide administration increases the level of calcium in blood.

As predicted by this model, thiazide administration leads to chronic hypercalcemia in patients with abnormal parathyroid physiology but not in normal patients. In primary hyperparathyroidism, thiazide administration exacerbates the hypercalcemia, and in hypoparathyroidism, thiazide administration facilitates the maintenance of normocalcemia when given in conjunction with $1,25(OH)_2D_3$ and calcium.

Milk-Alkali Syndrome

The triad of hypercalcemia, metabolic alkalosis, and renal failure can be the consequence of massive ingestion of calcium and absorbable alkali. This syndrome was first described when milk and sodium bicarbonate were used in large amounts to treat peptic ulcer disease. With the change in ulcer treatment to nonabsorbable antacids and suppression of acid secretion, milk-alkali syndrome became rare. In the last several years, however, the increased use of calcium carbonate to treat dyspepsia and osteoporosis has led to the reappearance of milk-alkali syndrome.[346]

In most cases, a history of ingestion of several grams per day of calcium in the form of calcium carbonate can be elicited. The pathogenesis of the syndrome is not understood in detail but might involve a vicious cycle in which alkalosis decreases renal calcium clearance and hypercalcemia helps maintain alkalosis. Nephrocalcinosis, nephrogenic diabetes insipidus, decrease in GFR associated with hypercalcemia, and hypovolemia from vomiting all lead to renal failure, which can be severe. PTH levels, measured with currently available two-site assays, are invariably low in hypercalcemic patients, as are levels of $1,25(OH)_2D_3$. After clearance of the calcium by hydration or dialysis, if necessary, renal function generally returns to normal, unless the disorder has been severe and long-standing.

Immobilization

Immobilization can lead to bone resorption sufficient to cause hypercalcemia. The immobilization is usually caused by spinal cord injury or extensive casting after fractures, though it can occur in patients with Parkinson's disease.[347] Hypercalcemia of immobilization occurs predominantly in the young or in patients with other reasons for a high rate of bone turnover, such as Paget's disease or extensive fractures. Hypercalciuria and substantial bone loss are more common than hypercalcemia is. After spinal cord injury, the hypercalciuria is maximal at 4 months and can persist for more than a year. PTH and $1,25(OH)_2D_3$ levels are suppressed; bone biopsies show increased resorption and decreased formation of bone. Bisphosphonates have been used to reverse the hypercalcemia and hypercalciuria of spinal cord injury.

Renal Failure

Following rhabdomyolysis, during the oliguric phase of acute renal failure, severe hypocalcemia can result from acute hyperphosphatemia and calcium deposition in muscle.[348] PTH levels are high. In the diuretic phase that follows, hypercalcemia can occur. The hypercalcemia results from the high $1,25(OH)_2D_3$ levels observed in some patients and from mobilization of the calcium deposits.[349]

In chronic renal failure, hypercalcemia can result from tertiary hyperparathyroidism or may appear during therapy of aplastic bone disease associated with low PTH levels and sometimes with aluminum toxicity.

Williams' Syndrome

Williams' syndrome is a developmental disorder in which supravalvular aortic stenosis is associated with elfin facies and mental retardation.[350] Hypercalcemia can occur transiently in the first four years of life. Affected hypercalcemic infants have been found to have increased intestinal absorption of calcium and associated elevations of $1,25(OH)_2D_3$ that fall to normal as the blood calcium normalizes.[351] Levels of 25(OH)D are normal. The hypercalcemia can generally be controlled by manipulating the diet.

Molecular analysis has clarified the origin of the connective tissue component of Williams' syndrome. Isolated supravalvular aortic stenosis is associated with deletion or translocation of the distal portion of the elastin gene. Williams' syndrome, with more protean connective tissue abnormalities and mental retardation, is associated with large deletions that include the elastin gene and a gene encoding the protein kinase LIM-kinase 1.[352] A gene within the Williams' syndrome deletion region encodes a nuclear protein, Williams' syndrome transcription factor, that is part of a large chromatin remodeling complex that can bind the vitamin D receptor and influence the transcription of VDR-responsive genes.[353] For this reason, this gene is a strong candidate for the gene associated with transient hypercalcemia in this disorder. Genetic proof that this gene is responsible for the hypercalcemia, however, is still lacking.

Jansen's Metaphyseal Chondrodysplasia

Jansen's metaphyseal chondrodysplasia is a rare disease in which affected persons present in childhood with short stature and hypercalcemia (Fig. 27–28). Blood chemistry studies suggest hyperparathyroidism, with high calcium, low normal phosphate, high $1,25(OH)_2D_3$, high alkaline phosphatase, and high urinary hydroxyproline, but PTH levels are suppressed.[354] A generalized defect in endochondral bone formation results from abnormally organized chondrocytes in growth plates. Metaphyses appear disordered and rachitic on radiographs. The bones can show signs of osteitis fibrosa cystica.

Constitutive activation of the PTH/PTHrP receptor, caused by point mutations in the transmembrane domains of the receptor, explains the findings in this disorder.[92,355] The abnormalities

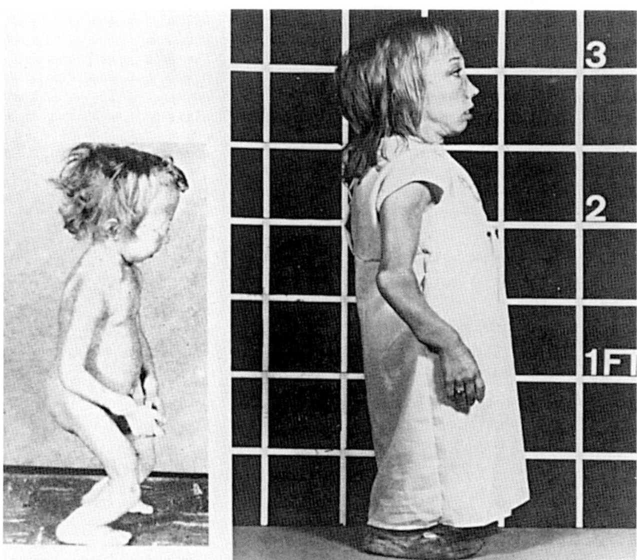

Figure 27–28 ▪ A patient with Jansen's metaphyseal chondrodysplasia at ages 5 years and 22 years. Note the short stature, characteristic facies, and misshapen metaphyseal region of long bones. (From Frame B, Poznanski AK. Conditions that may be confused with rickets. In DeLuca HF, Anastas CS [eds]. Pediatric Diseases Related to Calcium. New York, Elsevier, 1980:269-289.)

on serum chemistry studies result from PTH-like actions of the receptor in bone and kidney. The growth plate disorder results from PTHrP-like actions of the receptor on the growth plate.[356]

Approach to the Hypercalcemic Patient

The diagnostic approach to the hypercalcemic patient is strongly influenced by the clinical setting and the knowledge that primary hyperparathyroidism is at least twice as common as all other causes combined (Table 27–2). These considerations are particularly significant in the patient who seems otherwise well and in whom the hypercalcemia is detected incidentally or is mild, stable, or known to be of long duration (i.e., years). Among outpatients referred to endocrinologists for evaluation of hypercalcemia, for example, more than 90% are found to have primary hyperparathyroidism. In ill or hospitalized patients, malignant disease is the cause in more than 50% of cases. The differential diagnosis is seldom complicated, however, because malignant hypercalcemia usually manifests in the context of advanced, clinically obvious disease.

Because hypercalcemia usually is first detected as an elevation of total serum calcium, it is important to distinguish hemoconcentration or rare instances of calcium-binding paraproteinemia or thrombocythemia-associated hypercalcemia (due to release of intracellular calcium in vitro) from a true increase in serum ionized calcium (Fig. 27–29). The presence of hypercalcemia should be confirmed by direct measurement of ionized calcium, and total calcium should be repeated, together with albumin, globulin electrolytes, BUN, creatinine, and phosphate. Especially when hypercalcemia is mild, it is prudent to repeat the serum total or ionized calcium measurement at least twice, preferably fasting and without venous occlusion, before proceeding with more costly studies directed at its etiology.

A careful history and physical examination, combined with efforts to assess chronicity by seeking prior results of routine multichannel serum chemistry determinations, most often will point to the likely diagnosis. Serum phosphate often is low in hyperparathyroidism, but as this often is true also of PTHrP-

TABLE 27–2 CAUSES OF HYPERCALCEMIA

PARATHYROID-DEPENDENT HYPERCALCEMIA
Primary hyperparathyroidism
Tertiary hyperparathyroidism
Familial hypocalciuric hypercalcemia
Lithium-associated hypercalcemia
Antagonistic autoantibodies to the calcium-sensing receptor
PARATHYROID-INDEPENDENT HYPERCALCEMIA
Neoplasms
• PTHrP dependent
• Other humoral syndromes
• Local osteolytic disease (including metastases)
PTHrP excess (non-neoplastic)
Excess vitamin D action
• Ingestion of excess vitamin D or vitamin D analogues
• Topical vitamin D analogues
• Granulomatous disease
• Williams' syndrome
Thyrotoxicosis
Adrenal insufficiency
Renal failure
• Acute renal failure
• Chronic renal failure with aplastic bone disease
Immobilization
Jansen's disease
Drugs
• Vitamin A intoxication
• Milk-alkali syndrome
• Thiazide diuretics
• Theophylline

PTHrP, parathyroid hormone–releasing hormone.

secreting malignancies, the presence of hypophosphatemia is not helpful in distinguishing these possibilities. When serum phosphate is normal or high despite correction of dehydration, the possibility of PTH- or PTHrP-independent hypercalcemia should be considered more strongly, however. Elevations in serum chloride and alkaline phosphatase often observed in primary hyperparathyroidism cannot be reliably employed in the differential diagnosis of hypercalcemia. Important elements of the medical history of hypercalcemic patients include inquiries about kidney stones, fractures, weight loss, back or bone pain, fatigue or weakness, cough or dyspnea, ulcer disease, and pancreatitis; ingestion of vitamins, calcium preparations, lithium or thiazides; dates of most recent mammograms and chest x-rays; and a family history of hypercalcemia, kidney stones, ulcer disease, endocrinopathy, or tumors of the head or neck. Because malignancy is a common cause of hypercalcemia and can occur concomitantly with primary hyperparathyroidism, clinical findings strongly suggesting malignancy should be acted upon by proceeding directly to a search for an underlying tumor, regardless of serum PTH.

The single most important test in the differential diagnosis of hypercalcemia is the measurement of serum PTH, preferably in a two-site assay specific for the intact, biologically active molecule (see Fig. 27–20). New PTH assays have been introduced that ignore the long, circulating fragments of the hormone that lack the amino-terminal residues required for activity at the PTH/PTHrP receptor. Whether these assays will be more useful than standard "intact PTH" assays remains to be established.[357,358] A consistently elevated serum PTH in the presence of true hypercalcemia always is abnormal and almost always indicates primary hyperparathyroidism. The exceptions that also can be

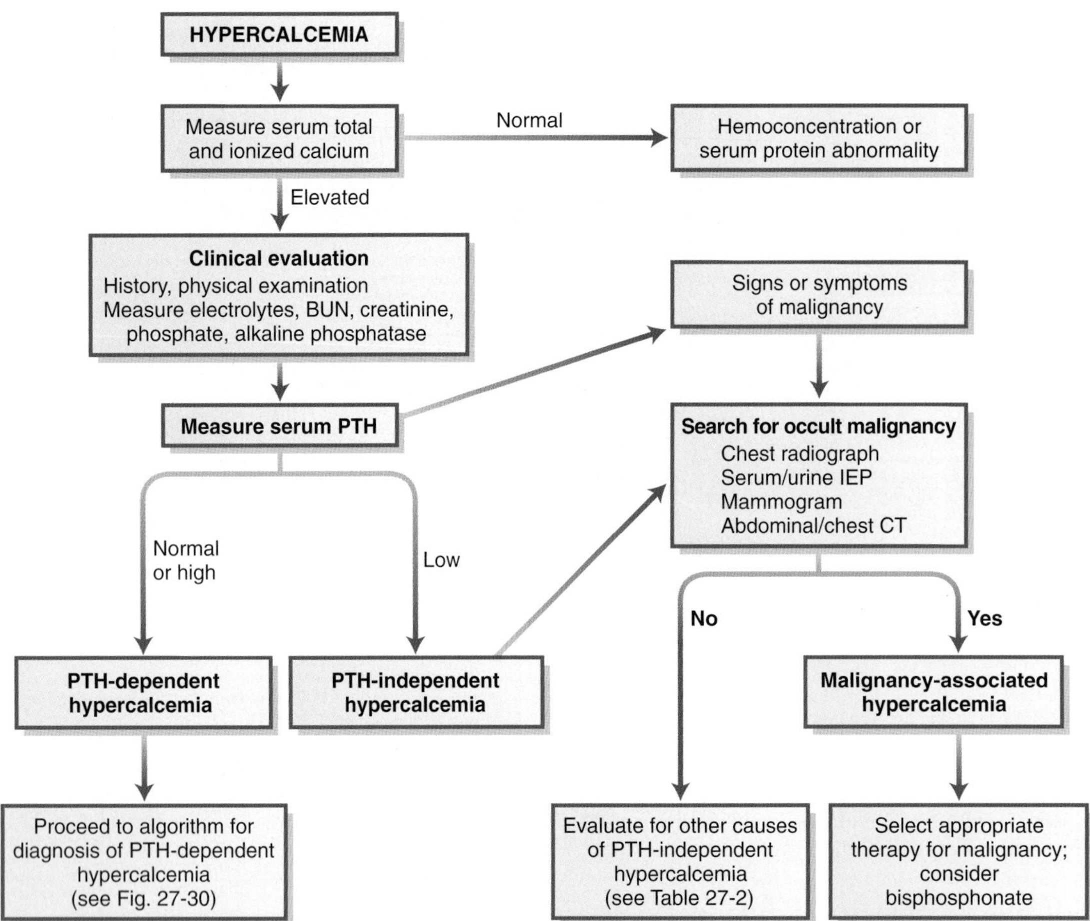

Figure 27–29 ▪ Approach to the management of the hypercalcemic patient. BUN, blood urea nitrogen; CT, computed tomography; IEP, immunoelectrophoresis; PTH, parathyroid hormone.

associated with elevated PTH levels are FHH, autonomous parathyroid secretion complicating secondary hyperparathyroidism (tertiary hyperparathyroidism), lithium-associated hyperparathyroidism, and, very rarely, ectopic PTH secretion by a malignant neoplasm or antagonizing autoantibodies directed against the calcium-sensing receptor in patients with other autoimmune disease(s)—an acquired condition that mimics FHH.[318,319]

Diagnosis of primary hyperparathyroidism is complicated, however, by the fact that some patients fail to exhibit both hypercalcemia and elevated iPTH. In up to 10% of patients with hypercalcemia and primary hyperparathyroidism, PTH levels can fall within the (high) normal range with current PTH assays. Such PTH levels are inappropriate in the face of hypercalcemia, however, and support the diagnosis of PTH-dependent hypercalcemia. In fact, many such patients manifest frankly elevated serum PTH if retested, especially if dietary calcium is restricted beforehand. Some patients present with serum calcium in the high-normal range (>10.0 mg/dL) and an elevated or high-normal PTH.[248] This may be discovered incidentally in an otherwise asymptomatic subject or in the course of evaluating recurrent urolithiasis or osteopenia. Those with persistently high-normal serum calcium and high-normal iPTH should be retested at intervals and, meanwhile, given a provisional diagnosis of hyperparathyroidism and evaluated accordingly.

In patients with PTH-dependent hypercalcemia (Fig. 27–30), calcium and creatinine should be measured in a 24-hour urine collection and simultaneous serum sample to measure total urinary calcium output (mg/day) and the clearance ratio of calcium-to-creatinine. A daily calcium excretion of less than 100 mg/day, or a clearance ratio less than 0.01, should prompt consideration of FHH, especially in patients who are younger than 40 years, who have a family history of FHH, or whose serum iPTH levels are within the normal range. A urinary calcium excretion greater than 4 mg/kg/day or clearance ratio greater than 0.02 effectively excludes FHH. In FHH, serum phosphate is normal or slightly low, serum magnesium may be slightly high, and serum $1,25(OH)_2D_3$ is normal or low (unlike in primary hyperparathyroidism).

A definite diagnosis of FHH, as in the MEN syndromes, may be provided by confirming the presence of mutations in the relevant genes, although such studies are not invariably informative (presumably because of mutations in introns and other unchecked regions) and usually are unnecessary. The identification of *RET* gene mutations is now an essential part of the management of families with MEN-2, because this information most effectively guides the decision for preventive thyroidectomy to prevent medullary cancer of the thyroid. In contrast, the identification of *MENIN* gene mutations has not yet led to any effective preventive strategies; thus, genetic analysis may be useful only for genetic counseling in families with MEN-1. Even for this purpose, the incomplete ascertainment of mutations limits the effectiveness of such analysis.

In patients with suspected lithium-induced hyperparathyroidism, a trial off lithium, if feasible clinically, can confirm the diagnosis or indicate the presence of persistent primary hyperparathyroidism. Patients with primary hyperparathyroidism

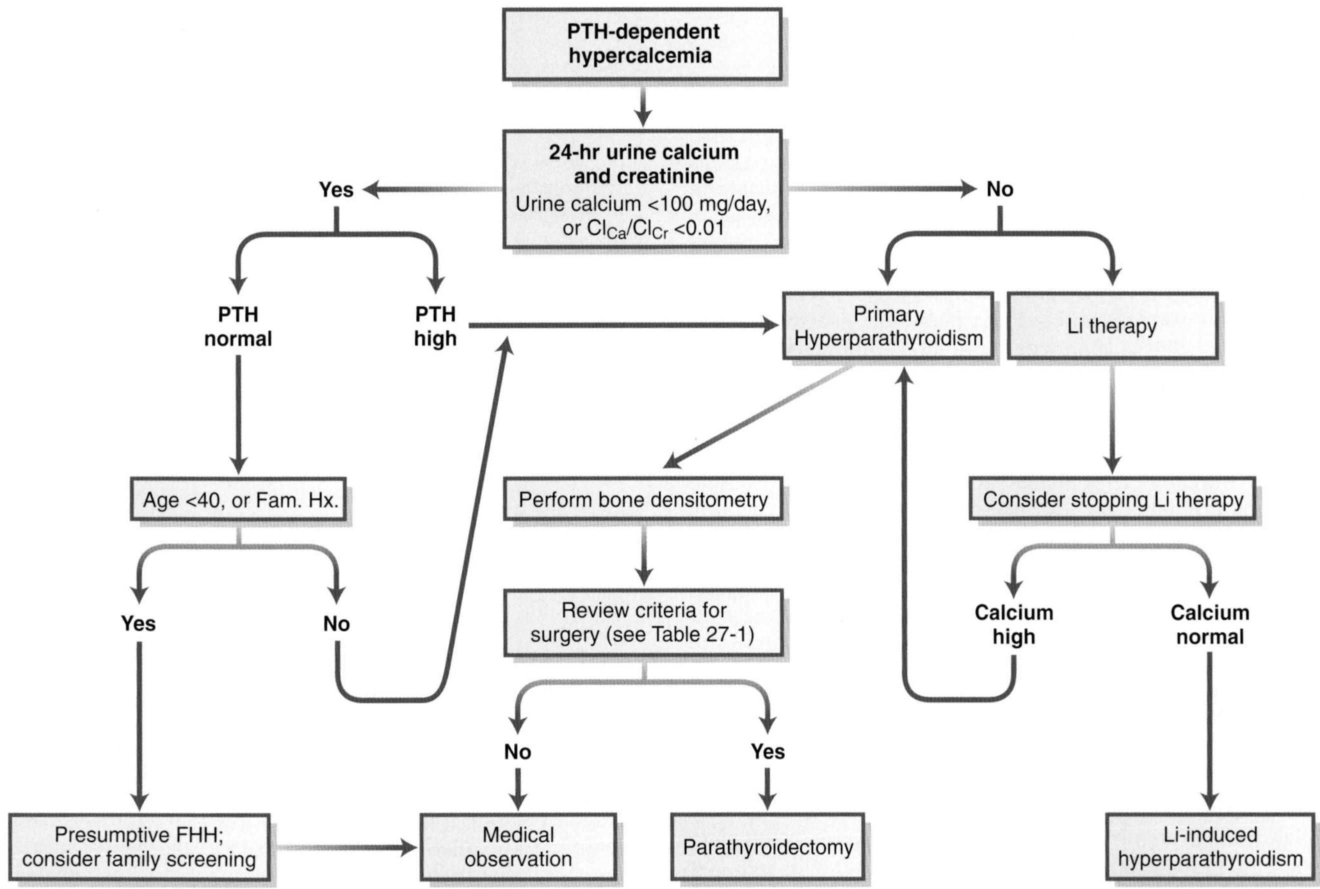

Figure 26-30 ■ Approach to the management of the hypercalcemic patient with parathyroid hormone–dependent hypercalcemia. Cl, clearance; FHH, familial hypocalciuric hypercalcemia; Li, lithium; PTH, parathyroid hormone; Fam. Hx., family history.

should undergo bone densitometry, preferably at both cortical- and trabecular-rich sites (forearm or hip and lumbar spine, respectively) to assist in the decision about surgery. Those younger than 40 years or having a family history of hypercalcemia (or other MEN manifestations) should be evaluated for these syndromes as well. Patients not meeting criteria for parathyroidectomy should be followed medically, as should those with FHH. In rare patients with calcium-sensing receptor–blocking autoantibodies, hypercalcemia might respond to glucocorticoids.[319]

A low or undetectable serum PTH level signifies the presence of nonparathyroid hypercalcemia and should prompt a detailed evaluation for malignancy or other causes of PTH-independent hypercalcemia (see Table 27–2). Breast and lung cancers alone account for more than 50% of all malignancy-associated hypercalcemias. Mammography, chest radiography with or without CT, abdominal CT, and serum and urinary immunoelectrophoresis are among the more useful tests for detecting the cause of nonparathyroid hypercalcemia. Although humoral mechanisms, especially secretion of PTHrP, are implicated in the pathogenesis of most cancer-associated hypercalcemias, bone metastases are common, particularly in breast cancer. Technetium-99m bone scanning, therefore, generally is useful for detecting this syndrome and identifying bones vulnerable to fracture. The utility of serum PTHrP measurements probably is limited to the unusual situation in which serum PTH is suppressed but an underlying malignancy cannot readily be demonstrated. PTHrP-associated hypercalcemia can occur rarely during pregnancy and lactation, via secretion from benign neoplasms, or in association with lymphoid hyperplasia in lupus erythematosus or HIV.[324]

In the absence of evident malignancy, unusual causes of hypercalcemia should be sought.[324] Vitamin D and vitamin A intoxication can be excluded by measurement of serum 25(OH)D and retinoids, respectively. Elevated $1,25(OH)_2D_3$ and hypercalcemia can occur in several settings, including sarcoidosis and other granulomatous diseases, B-cell and T-cell lymphomas (including AIDS-associated lymphomas), and, uncommonly, in epithelial neoplasms such as lung cancer. Very rarely, patients with severe idiopathic hypercalciuria and excessive absorption of dietary calcium manifest mild, dietary-dependent hypercalcemia. Overtreatment of hypoparathyroidism or other conditions with oral $1,25(OH)_2D_3$ or topical use of analogues of the active metabolite in psoriasis should be obvious from the history. Because hypercalcemia and hypercalciuria are observed in up to 10% and 30%, respectively, of patients with thyrotoxicosis, measurement of serum thyroid-stimulating hormone (TSH) may be helpful, especially in older patients who may be less overtly symptomatic. Adrenal insufficiency and pheochromocytoma usually are accompanied by characteristic clinical features, but a definite diagnosis may be sought with appropriate studies. Granulomatous diseases are among the more common disorders that underlie initially unexplained hypercalcemia.

Therapy of Severe Hypercalcemia

Causes of Severe Hypercalcemia

The need for urgent therapy of acute, severe hypercalcemia, usually defined as a serum calcium concentration greater than 14 mg/dL (3.5 mM), is unusual. This is because most patients with hypercalcemia have primary hyperparathyroidism, in which hypercalcemia is typically chronic and mild. Episodes of acute, severe hypercalcemia can occur occasionally in primary hyperparathyroidism (parathyroid crisis), usually in patients with large parathyroid adenomas and very high PTH levels. The severe hypercalcemia appears in patients with dehydration due to diarrheal illness, protracted vomiting, protracted diuretic therapy, recovery from major surgery, immobilization, ingestion of large amounts of oral calcium salts, or parathyroid carcinoma.

Most often, acute, severe hypercalcemia is encountered in patients with underlying malignancy, in whom accelerated bone resorption dramatically increases the filtered load of calcium. The ensuing profound hypercalciuria impairs renal tubular sodium reabsorption, which induces progressive extracellular volume depletion, reduces GFR, impairs renal calcium clearance, and further aggravates the hypercalcemia. In many such patients, elevated circulating levels of PTHrP compound the problem by mimicking the action of PTH to enhance distal tubular calcium reabsorption.

Clinical Features of Severe Hypercalcemia

The indications for urgent therapy of hypercalcemia usually relate more to the presence of clinical symptoms of hypercalcemia than to the absolute level of serum calcium, although few clinicians would hesitate to treat patients in whom total serum calcium exceeded 14 mg/dL (3.5 mM). Many patients with previously mild hypercalcemia become symptomatic when serum calcium concentrations exceed 12 mg/dL (3.0 mM). It is important to remember that hypoalbuminemia can mask significant elevations of ionized calcium. The most common symptoms of severe hypercalcemia are referable to disturbances of nervous system and gastrointestinal function: fatigue, weakness, lethargy, confusion, coma (rarely), anorexia, nausea, abdominal pain (rarely due to pancreatitis), and constipation. Polyuria, nocturia, and polydipsia commonly are present also.

Bone pain is often present but is usually due to underlying metastatic disease. Cardiac arrhythmias can occur, particularly bradyarrhythmias or heart block, and digitalis toxicity may be potentiated. Patients who suffer a fatal outcome from acute severe hypercalcemia can manifest coma, hypotension, acute pancreatitis, acute renal failure, widespread soft tissue calcification, heart failure, or venous thrombosis, particularly of the renal veins.

Management of Severe Hypercalcemia

The first decision to be made in the management of acute, severe hypercalcemia is whether or not to treat the problem at all. This may become an issue for the patient with an untreatable, widely disseminated malignancy, when all other approaches to controlling the neoplasm have been exhausted, and the patient has chosen not to have complications treated. Otherwise, as noted earlier, patients who are symptomatic or have serum calcium greater than 14 mg/dL ordinarily should be treated aggressively. Treatment most often entails rehydration and administration of a bisphosphonate intravenously (Table 27–3). Calcitonin can be useful as a temporary measure early in therapy, and glucocorticoids or dialysis may be indicated in some patients.[106]

TABLE 27–3 Therapy of Severe Hypercalcemia

Therapy	Usual Dose	Frequency
Rehydration	2-4 L/day of 0.9% NaCl IV	qd×1-5 days
Furosemide	20-40 mg IV (after rehydration)	q12-24 hr
Pamidronate	60-90 mg IV over 2-4 hr	Once
Zoledronate	4 mg IV over 15-30 min	Once
Calcitonin	4-8 IU/kg SC	q12-24 hr
Gallium nitrate	200 mg/m^2 IV over 24 hr	qd×5 days
Plicamycin	15-25 μg/kg IV over 4-6 hr	qd or qod×1-5 doses
Glucocorticoids	200-300 mg hydrocortisone IV	qd×3-5 days
	40-60 mg prednisone PO	qd×3-5 days
Dialysis		

Volume Repletion

When treatment is indicated, the first priority is to correct the extracellular volume depletion that almost invariably is present, usually by infusing isotonic saline at a rate of 2 to 4 L/day. The aggressiveness with which the individual patient is rehydrated must be considered in relation to both the patient's volume status and the risk of precipitating or aggravating congestive heart failure or ascites. Diuretics, particularly thiazides, should be discontinued. The use of furosemide or other potent loop diuretics to promote calciuresis can exacerbate extracellular volume depletion if used too early in the course of treatment. In light of the availability of highly effective alternatives for the therapy of hypercalcemia, such drugs probably are best avoided, except in circumstances in which vigorous rehydration fails to improve severe hypercalcemia or might precipitate congestive heart failure. In any case, prolonged use of saline-induced calciuresis without the early introduction of an effective antiresorptive agent is ill advised and ultimately futile.

Bisphosphonates

Intravenous bisphosphonates rapidly inhibit bone resorption and currently are the agents of first choice in managing severe hypercalcemia that is known or suspected to be driven mainly by osteoclastic bone resorption.[106] Bisphosphonates should not be used in patients with milk-alkali syndrome, for example, in whom they are likely to induce post-treatment hypocalcemia.[346]

Pamidronate and zoledronate are most widely used in the United States, although ibandronate and clodronate have been successfully deployed elsewhere. These drugs generally are well tolerated, although local pain or swelling at the infusion site, low grade fever 1 to 2 days after the infusion, transient lymphopenia, and mild hypophosphatemia or hypomagnesemia can occur. Serum calcium usually declines within 24 hours and reaches a nadir within a week following a single infusion, at which point calcium may be normal in 70% to 90% of treated patients.

Intravenous bisphosphonates may be nephrotoxic, but clinical data to guide their use in patients with renal insufficiency are not yet available. Most clinicians employ the standard dose (see Table 27–3)—perhaps at half or less of the usual rate of administration—in patients with moderate renal insufficiency (GFR>30 mL/min), which is common in the setting of severe hypercalcemia. In patients with more severe renal insufficiency, bisphosphonates probably are best avoided and dialysis may be a more appropriate alternative (see below).

The duration of the response to intravenous bisphosphonate treatment is quite variable, between a week or two and several months. Depending upon clinical circumstances, repeated courses of therapy may be indicated and effective.

Calcitonin

Calcitonin, which directly inhibits osteoclast function, may be used with other antiresorptive agents to achieve more rapid control of severe hypercalcemia. Calcitonin rarely produces a decline in serum calcium of more than 1 to 2 mg/dL, however, and its efficacy typically is limited to a few days at most, possibly because of receptor down-regulation in target cells of bone and kidney. Its major advantages are a more rapid onset of action than bisphosphonates (several hours) and its potential to augment renal calcium excretion directly. Calcitonin generally is well tolerated, although transient nausea, vomiting, abdominal cramps, flushing, and local skin reactions can occur.

Other Approaches to Treatment of Severe Hypercalcemia

Because of their potential toxicity, other antiresorptives such as gallium nitrate, plicamycin (mithramycin), and intravenous phosphate (in patients with severe hypophosphatemia) have largely been abandoned in the treatment of severe hypercalcemia. Oral or enteral phosphate repletion is appropriate for patients with significant hypophosphatemia (<2.5 mg/dL), provided that serum phosphate and renal function are closely monitored. Intravenous or oral glucocorticoids should be considered early in patients with suspected vitamin D–dependent hypercalcemia, including those with lymphoma or granulomatous disease. The response to glucocorticoids may be more delayed than that to bisphosphonates.

In patients with severe renal insufficiency, with or without complicating heart disease, in whom saline rehydration and associated calciuresis might not be feasible and bisphosphonates probably are best avoided, dialytic therapy against a low-calcium or zero-calcium dialysate may be the most appropriate tactic. In patients with known primary hyperparathyroidism and intercurrent severe hypercalcemia (parathyroid storm), urgent parathyroidectomy (following initial medical stabilization) should be considered.

Novel approaches to the treatment of severe hypercalcemia currently are in development. One available therapy for parathyroid carcinoma is the calcimimetic cinacalcet, which may be effective in some patients.[359] Monoclonal antibodies directed against PTHrP could prove useful in controlling PTHrP-dependent hypercalcemia,[360] and other novel antiresorptives (monoclonals against the osteoclastogenic factor RANKL or recombinant osteoprotegerin, which neutralizes RANKL) are on the horizon.

Hypocalcemic Disorders

Clinical Presentation

The predominant clinical symptoms and signs of hypocalcemia are those of neuromuscular irritability, including perioral paresthesias, tingling of the fingers and toes, and spontaneous or latent tetany. Tetany can be elicited by percussion of the facial nerve below the zygoma, resulting in ipsilateral contractions of the facial muscle (Chvostek's sign) or by 3 minutes of occlusive pressure with a blood pressure cuff resulting in carpal spasm, which, on occasion, can be very painful (Trousseau's sign) (Fig. 27–31). The usefulness of these signs in diagnosing hypocalcemia and in following therapeutic responses cannot be overemphasized.

Electrocardiographic abnormalities also result from hypocalcemia, including prolonged QT intervals and marked QRS and ST changes that may mimic acute myocardial infarction or

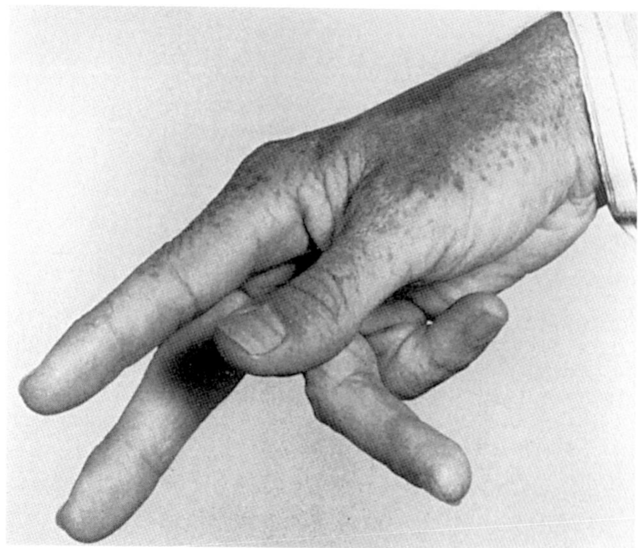

Figure 27–31 ▪ Trousseau's sign. (From Burnside JW, McGlynn TJ. Physical Diagnosis, 17th ed. Baltimore, Williams & Wilkins, 1987:63.)

conduction abnormalities. Ventricular arrhythmias are a rare complication of hypocalcemia, although congestive heart failure, corrected by normalization of serum calcium, has been reported.[361]

In profound hypocalcemia or during acute falls in serum calcium, grand mal seizures or laryngospasm also may be observed. Chronic hypocalcemia is associated with milder symptoms and signs of neuromuscular irritability and can even be asymptomatic. Long-standing hypocalcemia associated with hyperphosphatemia (observed with PTH deficiency or resistance) can lead to calcification of the basal ganglia and occasional extrapyramidal disorders. In addition, mineral ion deposits in the lens can lead to cataract formation.

Chronic hypocalcemia, particularly when associated with hypophosphatemia, as in vitamin D deficiency, is associated with growth plate abnormalities in children (rickets) and defects in the mineralization of new bone (osteomalacia) (see Chapter 28). Severe symptomatic hypocalcemia constitutes an emergency that requires immediate attention to prevent seizures and death from laryngospasm or cardiac causes.

Total calcium in serum includes both the free (biologically active) and protein-bound components; the major binding protein is albumin (see "Roles of the Mineral Ions"). Therefore, measurements of total calcium cannot be interpreted without concurrent measurement of albumin. Studies of hypoalbuminemic patients with cirrhosis have led to a formula for correction of total calcium based on concurrent albumin levels (a decrease in calcium of 0.8 mg/dL for every 1 g/dL decrease in albumin). No formula has proved accurate, however, for assessment of calcium in acutely ill patients. This probably relates to the variety of factors that can increase protein binding and decrease the fraction of total calcium present as the free ion, including alkalosis, elevated circulating free fatty acids, and lipid infusions.[362] Consequently, ionized calcium should be measured when the diagnosis of hypocalcemia is considered in the setting of acute illness or severe hypoalbuminemia.

Chronic hypocalcemia is most often due to deficiency of PTH or $1,25(OH)_2D_3$ or to resistance to the biologic effects of these calcium-regulating hormones (Table 27–4).

TABLE 27–4 CAUSES OF HYPOCALCEMIA

PARATHYROID-RELATED DISORDERS
Absence of the parathyroid glands or of PTH
Congenital
DiGeorge's syndrome
X-linked or autosomally inherited hypoparathyroidism
Autoimmune polyglandular syndrome type I
PTH gene mutations
Postsurgical hypoparathyroidism
Infiltrative disorders
Hemochromatosis
Wilson's disease
Metastases
Hypoparathyroidism following radioactive iodine thyroid ablation
Impaired secretion of PTH
Hypomagnesemia
Respiratory alkalosis
Activating mutations of the calcium sensor
Target organ resistance
Hypomagnesemia
Pseudohypoparathyroidism
Type I
Type II
VITAMIN D–RELATED DISORDERS
Vitamin D deficiency
Dietary absence
Malabsorption
Accelerated loss
Impaired enterohepatic recirculation
Anticonvulsant medications
Impaired 25-hydroxylation
Liver disease
Isoniazid
Impaired 1α-hydroxylation
Renal failure
Vitamin D–dependent rickets type I
Oncogenic osteomalacia
Target organ resistance
Vitamin D–dependent rickets type II
Phenytoin
OTHER CAUSES
Excessive deposition into the skeleton
Osteoblastic malignancies
Hungry bone syndrome
Chelation
Foscarnet
Phosphate infusion
Infusion of citrated blood products
Infusion of EDTA-containing contrast reagents
Fluoride
Neonatal hypocalcemia
Prematurity
Asphyxia
Diabetic mother
Hyperparathyroid mother
HIV infection
Drug therapy
Vitamin D deficiency
Hypomagnesemia
Impaired PTH responsiveness
Critical illness
Pancreatitis
Toxic shock syndrome
Intensive care unit patients

EDTA, ethylenediaminetetraacetic acid; HIV, human immunodeficiency virus; PTH, parathyroid hormone.

Parathyroid-Related Disorders

Hypocalcemia associated with parathyroid dysfunction can be differentiated from other causes of hypocalcemia by routine laboratory tests. Serum calcium is low owing to lack of PTH-mediated bone resorption and urinary calcium reabsorption. Serum phosphate is increased owing to impaired renal clearance. Serum $1,25(OH)_2D_3$ is low because PTH and hypophosphatemia stimulate the renal 25(OH)D 1α-hydroxylase. Consequently, $1,25(OH)_2D_3$-mediated intestinal calcium absorption is markedly decreased, further exacerbating the hypocalcemia. PTH levels measured using sensitive two-site PTH assays (see Fig. 27–20) are usually low or undetectable but may be inappropriately normal if some degree of PTH production is preserved. Elevated levels of PTH are found in syndromes associated with resistance to the biologic effects of PTH.

Congenital or Inherited Parathyroid Disorders

Several rare syndromes associated with congenital or inherited hypoparathyroidism appear sporadically or in a variety of inheritance patterns, suggesting multiple etiologies. Mutation of a transcription factor, glial cell missing *(GCMB)* (6p23), which is expressed in the PTH-secreting cells of the developing parathyroids, has been shown to be a cause of familial hypoparathyroidism in humans and mice.[38] The genetic abnormality responsible for X-linked recessive hypoparathyroidism has been identified as a deletion/insertion of DNA near the *SOX3* gene at Xq26-Xq27.[35]

In a number of diseases, hypoparathyroidism is associated with multiple abnormalities in embryonic development in the neck and chest region. DiGeorge's syndrome occurs sporadically and is associated with an embryologic defect in the formation of the third, fourth, and fifth branchial pouches, resulting in the absence of parathyroid glands. DiGeorge's syndrome may, in fact, be a neurocrestopathy, because ablation of the premigratory cephalic neural crest in chick embryos produces the same phenotype.[363] The contribution of homeobox genes to parathyroid development and their potential relationship to DiGeorge's syndrome also has been demonstrated by the absence of thymic and parathyroid tissue, accompanied by cardiac and craniofacial abnormalities, in mice lacking the homeobox gene *hoxa3*.[364]

DiGeorge's syndrome is often associated with other congenital abnormalities in a syndrome referred to by the acronym CATCH 22 (*c*ardiac defect, *a*bnormal facies, *t*hymic hypoplasia, *c*left palate, *h*ypocalcemia, and 22q11 deletions).[365] Microdeletion of 22q11.21-q11.23[366] and a t(2;22)(q14;q11) balanced translocation suggest that a gene at chromosome 22q11 may be pathogenetic in this syndrome.[367] Hypoparathyroidism also has been reported in two patients with a 22q11 deletion.[368] Although deletion of the *TBX1* gene has been shown to be responsible for the cardiovascular defects in this syndrome,[369] the molecular basis for impaired parathyroid gland development has not yet been elucidated.

A number of cases of DiGeorge and velocardiofacial syndromes have been shown to have no detectable abnormality at 22q11 but instead have terminal 10p deletions or interstitial 10p13/10p14 deletions, suggesting that two loci may be critical for development of branchial pouch structures.[370] Terminal deletions of 10p accompanied by hypoparathyroidism can be further subdivided into DiGeorge critical region II (10p13-14) and a more telomeric region (10p14-10pter), wherein mutation of the transcription factor GATA3 causes the syndrome of hypoparathyroidism, sensorineural deafness, and renal anomaly (HDR).[371] The genetic basis for some cases of HDR and the related disorder, Kenny-Caffey syndrome (which, in addition, is associated with recurrent bacterial infections), has been shown to be linked to 1q43-44. These disorders involve mutations in the chaperone protein, TBCE, which is required for the proper folding of α tubulin and the formation of α-β tubulin heterodimers.[372]

Familial hypoparathyroidism is seen in conjunction with mucocutaneous candidiasis, Addison's disease, and other immune disorders in autosomal recessive autoimmune polyglandular syndrome, Type 1, caused by mutations in the autoimmune regulatory gene *(AIRE)* (see Chapter 41).[373] Hypoparathyroidism may also be observed in association with mitochondrial myopathies such as mitochondrial trifunctional protein and the Kearns-Sayre syndrome.[374] Other inherited forms of hypoparathyroidism may be observed as an isolated defect[375] or can manifest with other features such as lymphedema, dysmorphism, and renal and cardiac abnormalities.[376]

Abnormalities in the Parathyroid Hormone Gene

Specific defects have been found in the PTH gene in a small number of kindreds affected by congenital hypoparathyroidism. These include point mutations in the signal peptide[5,6] and in an intron border, leading to aberrant splicing.[377] No abnormalities in the sequences encoding PTH (1-84) have been discovered in familial hypoparathyroidism.

Destruction of the Parathyroid Glands

The most common cause of chronic hypocalcemia is postsurgical hypoparathyroidism. This can occur after removal of all parathyroid tissue during thyroidectomy and radical neck dissection for malignancies, or it can occur after inadvertent interruption of the blood supply to the parathyroid glands during head and neck surgery. Transient hypoparathyroidism, attributed to reversible damage to the remaining normal glands, is common after parathyroidectomy; permanent hypoparathyroidism can occur after vascular or surgical injury or inadvertent removal of all parathyroid tissue. Rarely, transient hypoparathyroidism follows spontaneous infarction of autonomous tissue in primary hyperparathyroidism.[378] Hypoparathyroidism is a rare complication of radioactive iodine ablation of the thyroid gland for Graves' disease.[379]

Hypoparathyroidism also can occur as a result of infiltrative diseases of the parathyroids. This is seen in diseases of iron overload such as hemochromatosis and in patients with thalassemia major who have received heavy transfusions.[380] Copper deposition in Wilson's disease[381] can also cause parathyroid dysfunction. Metastatic disease to the parathyroids can cause hypoparathyroidism, but rarely, presumably because of the need for four gland involvement before significant hypoparathyroidism is observed.

Impaired Parathyroid Hormone Secretion

Impaired secretion of PTH from the parathyroid glands can lead to functional hypoparathyroidism. This is commonly seen in profound hypomagnesemia,[382] in which target organ resistance to PTH can also occur. Both of these abnormalities are reversible upon magnesium repletion (See "Disorders of Magnesium Metabolism").[383]

Chronic respiratory alkalosis leads to hyperphosphatemia and decreased ionized calcium levels accompanied by impaired renal calcium resorption and inappropriately normal PTH levels.[384] This biochemical phenotype suggests both an abnormality of PTH secretion and renal resistance to PTH. Acute alkalosis in dogs also suppresses PTH secretion.[385]

Activating mutations in the calcium sensing receptor cause autosomal dominant hypocalcemia (ADH) associated with inappropriately normal PTH levels. The clinical syndrome is variable; patients present with hypocalcemia and seizures, whereas their affected relatives may be only subsequently found to have asymptomatic hypocalcemia.[14] Unlike patients with inactivating mutations of the calcium sensor, homozygously affected persons do not appear to have a more severe phenotype. The presence of hypercalciuria in these patients makes medical management uniquely challenging. Treatment with vitamin D metabolites often results in a marked increase in renal calcium excretion, associated with renal calcification and resultant renal impairment. Based on these observations, it has been suggested that asymptomatic persons be left untreated and that the goal of therapy in patients with symptomatic hypocalcemia be solely to relieve symptoms, not to achieve normocalcemia. Treatment with calcium and vitamin D metabolites should be accompanied by the use of thiazide diuretics to decrease urinary calcium excretion as well as to ensure adequate urinary volume to decrease urinary calcium concentration.

Pseudohypoparathyroidism

The idiopathic and inherited forms of PTH resistance are referred to as pseudohypoparathyroidism (PHP). The first cases of documented PTH resistance were described by Albright in 1942.[386] The patients were hypocalcemic and hyperphosphatemic, and they also exhibited a number of features that are now called *Albright's hereditary osteodystrophy* (AHO). These features include short stature, rounded face, foreshortened fourth and other metacarpals, obesity, and subcutaneous calcifications (Figs. 27–32 and 27–33).

PTH administration to these patients failed to provoke a phosphate diuresis or an increase in serum calcium. It was subsequently demonstrated that hypocalcemic patients with features of AHO had elevated PTH levels and that PTH infusions failed to stimulate renal production of cAMP. Failure of stimulation of cyclic AMP production suggested a defect in the PTH receptor or in its cAMP-mediated signal transduction.[387] The measurement of cAMP in the urine following an infusion of synthetic PTH(1-34) is now used to establish the diagnosis of PTH resistance.[388]

The variable presence of AHO and renal resistance to PTH in PHP has led to the subclassification of pseudohypoparathyroidism (Table 26–5). PHP type 1a is characterized by AHO and diminished $G_s\alpha$ activity (approximately 50% of normal). Diminished $G_s\alpha$ activity has been demonstrated in several tissues, including kidney, fibroblasts, transformed lymphocytes, platelets, and erythrocytes. Decreased amounts of $G_s\alpha$ mRNA (50%) are present in fibroblasts of many patients with PHP1a,[389,390] and inactivating mutations in the $G_s\alpha$ gene have been identified in several kindreds.[391]

Impaired mentation is seen in approximately half of the patients with PHP1a and appears to be related to the $G_s\alpha$ deficiency rather than to chronic hypocalcemia, because patients with other forms of PHP and hypocalcemia have normal mentation.[392] The $G_s\alpha$ deficiency in PHP1a may be associated not only with PTH resistance but also with resistance to other hormones such as TSH, glucagon, and gonadotropins, resulting in thyroid and gonad dysfunction. Paradoxically, two unrelated male patients with both PHP1a and gonadotropin-independent precocious puberty have been described. The $G_s\alpha$ point mutation found in these patients is thought to lead to a protein that is unstable at 37° C and, therefore, to confer renal resistance to PTH. At the lower temperature of the testes, however, the protein is not degraded. In this setting, the stable but mutated protein is constitutively active and stimulates the Leydig cell in a manner similar to the skeletal effects of the G_s mutations in McCune-Albright syndrome (see Chapter 24).[393]

Pseudo-pseudohypoparathyroidism (pseudo-PHP) refers to phenotypical AHO with normal biochemical parameters. Patients with pseudo-PHP often are found in the same kindreds

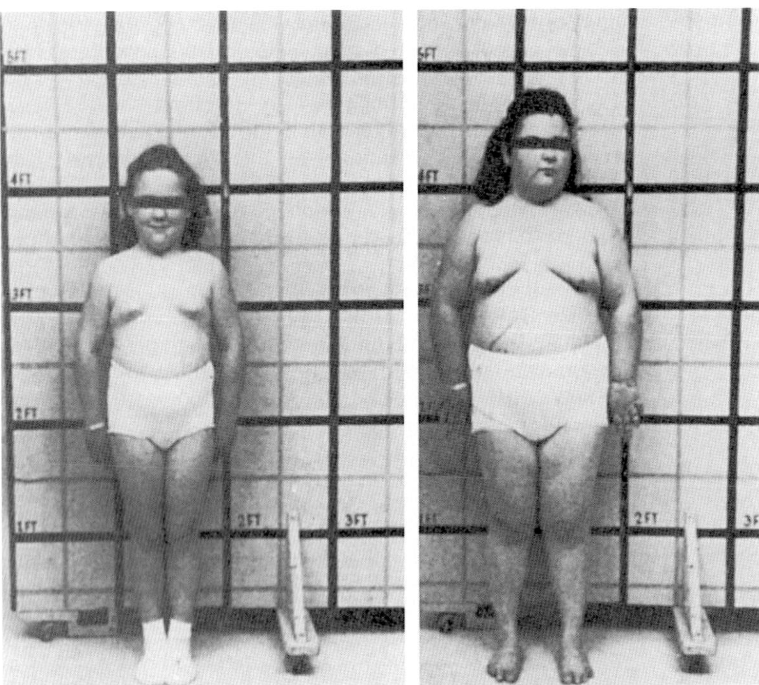

Figure 27–32 ▪ Daughter *(left)* and mother *(right)* with pseudohypoparathyroidism and Albright's hereditary osteodystrophy.

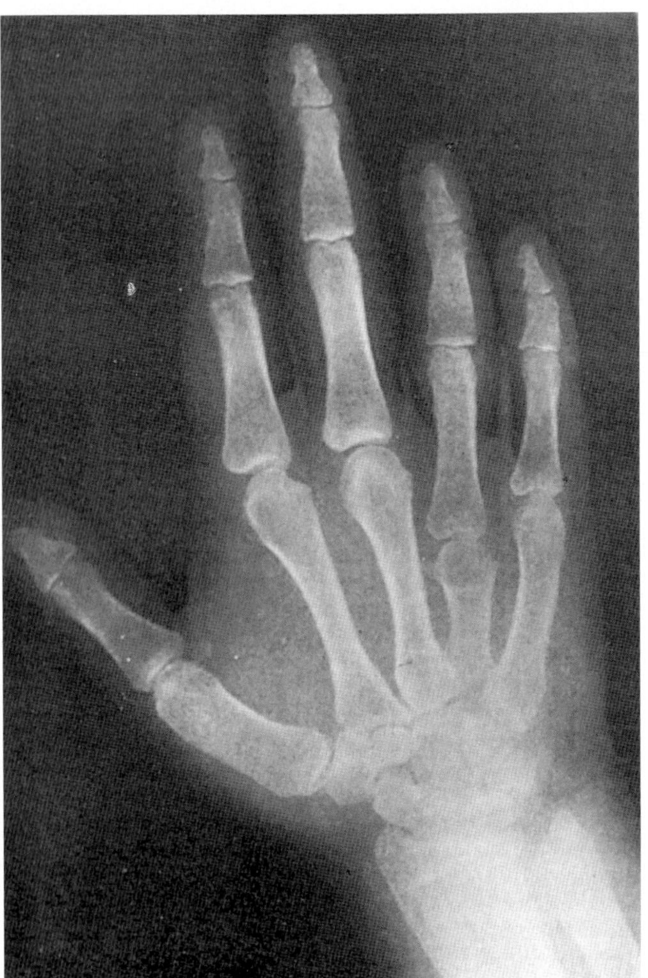

Figure 27–33 ▪ Radiograph of hand from a patient with pseudohypoparathyroidism and Albright's hereditary osteodystrophy. Note the shortened fourth metacarpal.

as those with PHP1a, and they invariably inherit the same abnormal $G_s\alpha$ gene found in their PTH-resistant relatives.[390] When patients inherit the mutant $G_s\alpha$ gene from their fathers, they exhibit pseudo-pseudohypoparathyroidism; when they inherit the mutant $G_s\alpha$ gene from their mothers, they exhibit pseudohypoparathyroidism.[394] This pattern, in which the phenotype depends on the parent of origin, is termed *genetic imprinting;* mice with targeted ablation of the Gsα gene *(GNAS1)* also display such imprinting.[395]

The observation of a phenotype in a heterozygous "loss of function" mutation in $G_s\alpha$ is in contrast to the findings in mice with targeted deletions of the other Gα genes ($G_i2\alpha$, $G_o\alpha$, Gqα, $G_{13}\alpha$), in which a phenotype is observed only in the homozygous state.[396] The fact that the *GNAS1* gene is imprinted has partly resolved the dilemma of this dominant phenotype. Notably, mice with targeted ablation of one *GNAS1* gene fail to express Gsα mRNA in the renal cortex when the mutant gene is inherited from the mother, but they have normal expression in the cortex when the mutant gene is inherited from the father. No such imprinting pattern is seen in the inner medulla; this correlates with the mice (and patients) exhibiting PTH, but not vasopressin, resistance.[395]

Pseudohypoparathyroidism type 1b (PHP1b) manifests with hypocalcemia, high PTH levels, and failure of PTH infusions to increase urinary cAMP production. However, it is not accompanied by any of the clinical features of AHO, nor is it associated with abnormal $G_s\alpha$ levels in fibroblasts. Although mild TSH resistance has been reported,[397-399] renal resistance to PTH is the only consistent feature of PHP1b. Therefore, several investigators had postulated that this syndrome was due to an isolated abnormality of the PTH receptor. However, a search for mutations in the coding exons of the receptor gene failed to reveal a functional receptor abnormality. The target organ manifestations of PHP1b are variable, with some affected persons having manifestations of PTH overactivity in bone and PTH resistance in kidney. Cultured osteoblast-like cells from a patient with this disorder demonstrated normal cAMP responsiveness to PTH, despite the lack of renal responsiveness.[400]

The locus responsible for PHP1b has been found to reside on chromosome 20q13.3,[401] the same region that contains the

TABLE 27–5 TYPES OF PSEUDOHYPOPARATHYROIDISM

Disorder	Urinary cAMP Response to PTH	Urinary PO_4 Response to PTH	Other Hormonal Resistance	AHO	Pathophysiology
Pseudohypoparathyroidism IA	Decreased	Decreased	Yes	Yes	Gsα mutation
Pseudo-pseudohypoparathyroidism	Normal	Normal	No	Yes	Gsα mutation
Pseudohypoparathyroidism IB	Decreased	Decreased	No	No	20q13.3 defect (GNAS1 locus)
Pseudohypoparathyroidism IC	Decreased	Decreased	Yes	Yes	Gsα function normal
Pseudohypoparathyroidism II	Normal	Decreased	No	No	Vitamin D deficiency Myotonic dystrophy in some cases

AHO, Albright's hereditary osteodystrophy; cAMP, cyclic adenosine monophosphate; PO_4, phosphate; PTH, parathyroid hormone.

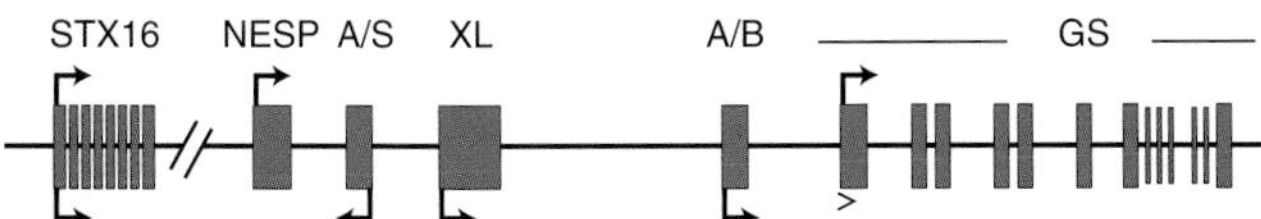

Figure 27–34 ▪ The GNAS locus and adjacent STx16 locus. A schematic representation of the GNAS locus is shown, with the black boxes indicating exons for STX-16, NESP55 (NESP), the antisense (A/S) NESP55 transcript, XLas (XL), A/B and $G_s\alpha$(Gs). The start site of and direction (sense versus antisense) of transcription is indicated by the arrows. Genes that are maternally transcribed are indicated by arrows above the relevant genes, and those that are paternally transcribed are indicated below. The expression of XLas, A/B, and A/S is from the paternal allele, whereas the maternal NESP 55 transcript is expressed. Expression of STX-16 is biallelic. The arrowhead below the $G_s\alpha$ locus indicates that only the maternal allele is expressed in the renal tubules.

GNAS1 gene, encoding $G_s\alpha$. The disease is inherited with the imprinting characteristic of PHP1a, but mapping studies suggest that the disease-causing mutations are close to but distinct from the Gsα coding region. The mutations in these patients do not involve the $G_s\alpha$ coding region, and the molecular basis for the PTH resistance remains to be defined. However, most affected persons have imprinting abnormalities of the GNAS locus.[398-402]

The GNAS locus gives rise to multiple transcripts (Fig. 27–34), including $G_s\alpha$, which is biallelically expressed in most tissues, but only the maternal transcript is expressed in the renal proximal tubules, thyroid, gonads, and pituitary. In contrast, expression of the XLαs, A/B, and antisense (A/S) transcripts are paternally expressed, whereas the NESP55 transcript is maternally expressed. The methylation defect found in all patients with PHP1b is a loss of methylation at exon A/B, which results in biallelic expression of the transcript. This abnormality might play a role in the hormone resistance observed.[402]

Linkage analyses in multiple kindreds point to deletion of a 3-kb region, approximately 220 kb centromeric of GNAS, in most such families, along with an overlapping deletion in another family.[403,404] These deletions remove several exons of the STX16 locus, which encodes syntaxin-16, a protein that plays a role in intracellular trafficking. Although the development of PHP1b correlates with maternal inheritance of this gene defect, STX16 itself is not imprinted.[404] However, deletions in this locus result in a loss of methylation at the distant A/B locus.

Deletions in the region of DNA encoding NESP55, a chromogranin-like neurosecretory peptide, have also been found in PHP1b.[404,405] These deletions also cause abnormal imprinting of exon A/B and presumably define a distinct imprint control region within GNAS.

Although most sporadic cases of PHP1b are not associated with STX16 or NESP55 deletions, they are uniformly associated with impaired methylation of exon A/B. In addition to the methylation defects in the A/B region, gain of methylation of NESP55 and loss of methylation of XL and of the promoter of the A/S transcript have been reported. Whether multiple genetic loci underlie the methylation abnormalities in these sporadic patients or whether a common locus will be identified as the genetic basis for the majority of cases of PHP1b remains to be determined.

Several patients with AHO and PTH resistance have been found to have normal $G_s\alpha$ activity; this subgroup has been designated PHP1c. Biochemical characterization in one case[406] revealed a significant decrease in the manganese-stimulated adenylate cyclase activity in fibroblast membranes of the affected patient, raising the possibility that a second defect in the cAMP pathway might lead to the phenotype of PHP1c. Another PCP1c patient was found to have a short deletion at the carboxy terminus of $G_s\alpha$, leading to normal levels of $G_s\alpha$ activity when assayed in erythrocytes, but defective activation by receptors.[407]

In PHP2, PTH infusions increase urinary cAMP normally; however, PTH does not elicit a phosphaturic response.[408] This syndrome, like PHP1b, lacks signs of AHO or resistance to other hormones, but unlike PHP1b, it is not familial in origin. The age of onset in patients with this disorder is variable, ranging from infancy to senescence, suggesting that it is an acquired defect or that the biochemical phenotype may be unmasked by intercurrent abnormalities. A subset of patients with myotonic dystrophy display the biochemical features of PHP2, the degree of PTH resistance correlating with the degree of expansion of the pathogenetic CTG repeats in the myotonin protein kinase gene.[409] A similar biochemical phenotype can also be observed in vitamin D deficiency, and some authors have suggested that PHP2 is a manifestation of vitamin D deficiency rather than a distinct clinical entity.[410] Minagawa and colleagues reported cases of three neonates with no signs of rickets and with normal levels of vitamin D who presented with transient PHP2 that resolved at about 6 months of age.[411] They postulated that PTH responsiveness is subject to maturation during fetal and neonatal development. PHP2, therefore, seems to reflect a heterogeneous clinical disorder associated with defects in PTH responsiveness distal to cAMP or involving a separate signal transduction pathway.[412]

The resistance to PTH in PHP has not been documented in bone cells; rather, several patients with PHP IB have been reported to have skeletal changes consistent with hyperparathyroidism.[413] Patients with PHP have lower bone density than normal persons and hypoparathyroid controls. Basal urinary hydroxyproline excretion in patients with PHP is twice that of hypoparathyroid controls, and they have similar increases in response to parathyroid extract.[414] Because the markers of bone turnover in patients with PHP are not as high as those of hyperparathyroid patients with similar or lower PTH levels, some authors have postulated that the PTH resistance in bone is relative.[1] However, normal cAMP response has been documented in osteoblasts isolated from patients with PHP1a[415] and PHP1b.[400] This suggests that the hypocalcemia in PHP is not secondary to skeletal resistance but is a consequence of the renal resistance to PTH and the associated low levels of $1,25(OH)_2D_3$. The hypocalcemia occurs in the face of relatively normal bone and renal distal (hypocalciuric) tubular responses to PTH.[416] The lack of activation of vitamin D results in diminished intestinal calcium absorption and osteomalacia, both of which further exacerbate the hypocalcemia. Deficiency of $1,25(OH)_2D_3$ and the resultant hypocalcemia can, in turn, impair the phosphaturic but not the urinary cAMP responses to PTH[417]; therefore, it is imperative that studies to confirm the diagnosis of PHP2 be performed in normocalcemic patients who have normal vitamin D status.

Vitamin D–Related Disorders

Hypocalcemia secondary to vitamin D deficiency or resistance to the biologic effects of $1,25(OH)_2D_3$ is easily differentiated from the hypocalcemia of hypoparathyroidism by routine clinical and laboratory evaluation. The primary cause of hypocalcemia in vitamin D deficiency is decreased intestinal absorption of calcium. In the setting of normal renal function, the hypocalcemia of vitamin D deficiency, unlike that of hypoparathyroidism, is accompanied by hypophosphatemia and increased renal phosphate clearance. This increase in phosphate clearance is a direct result of compensatory (secondary) hyperparathyroidism. The hyperparathyroidism is a consequence of the hypocalcemic stimulus to PTH secretion and the stimulation of PTH gene expression and parathyroid cell proliferation caused by hypocalcemia (see "Parathyroid Hormone Biosynthesis" earlier). Therefore, measurement of serum phosphate and PTH are very useful in distinguishing these disorders from hypoparathyroidism. The secondary hyperparathyroidism results in increased calcium mobilization from the skeleton, increased renal reabsorption of calcium, and increased renal 1α-hydroxylation of 25(OH)D. In severe vitamin D deficiency, the increased levels of PTH no longer lead to increased bone resorption, perhaps because osteoclasts appear not to resorb unmineralized osteoid.

In profound vitamin D deficiency, the level of $1,25(OH)_2D_3$ is usually low; in moderate vitamin D deficiency, the stimulation of the renal 1α-hydroxylase by PTH can result in a normal or even elevated $1,25(OH)_2D_3$ level. These high levels of $1,25(OH)_2D_3$ reflect the action of PTH on the renal 1α-hydroxylase. The ineffectiveness of the high levels of total $1,25(OH)_2D_3$ to normalize serum calcium may be explained by increased binding of this metabolite to vitamin D–binding protein when the levels of 25(OH)D are very low.

Vitamin D Deficiency

Because the two sources of vitamin D are the diet and cutaneous synthesis after UV irradiation, lack of solar irradiation and decreased intake or impaired absorption of vitamin D can lead to vitamin D deficiency. As the population has become increasingly educated about the risks of skin cancer from solar irradiation, the avoidance of long periods of intense sun exposure and the use of high SPF (solar protective factor) sun blocks have resulted in increased reliance on dietary sources of vitamin D. The recommended daily allowance for vitamin D is 200 IU; however, in the absence of solar exposure, this recommendation is two to three times lower than that required to prevent vitamin D deficiency.[418]

Vitamin D is present in many food sources, both vegetable and animal. In addition, many prepared foods, especially cereal products, are fortified with vitamin D. Although dairy products have been fortified with vitamin D as well, the actual amount of vitamin D provided does not correlate well with the purported content.[156] The vitamin D derived from vegetable sources is vitamin D_2 and that from animal sources is vitamin D_3. These two forms of vitamin D are metabolized identically and have equivalent biologic potency in humans. Both forms have been used to fortify foods.

Early vitamin D deficiency can be detected when the serum level of 25(OH)D falls below 15 ng/dL, because this level has been shown to be associated with the development of secondary hyperparathyroidism. Although elderly, homebound persons are at high risk, several studies have demonstrated that vitamin D deficiency is prevalent in the general population (reviewed in reference 471). The clinical relevance of this vitamin D deficiency has been confirmed by a study demonstrating that vitamin D administration (800 IU/day) to an ambulatory elderly population decreases serum PTH levels as well as the incidence of hip fracture.[419] Malabsorption also remains an important cause of vitamin D deficiency in all age groups.

Because vitamin D is a fat-soluble vitamin, its absorption is dependent upon emulsification by bile acids. Any cause of fat malabsorption or short bowel syndrome can result in vitamin D deficiency; therefore, malabsorption should be ruled out in patients with low 25(OH)D levels (<8 ng/dL).

Accelerated Loss of Vitamin D

25(OH)D and $1,25(OH)_2D_3$ are secreted with bile salts and undergo enterohepatic circulation; therefore, intestinal disease can also result in vitamin D deficiency due to excessive losses. Increased metabolism of vitamin D, leading to low blood levels of 25(OH)D, is seen in patients taking anticonvulsant medications and antituberculous therapy. Phenobarbital, primidone, phenytoin, rifampin, and glutethimide have all been reported to accelerate the hepatic inactivation of vitamin D.

Impaired 25-Hydroxylation of Vitamin D

The vitamin D that is absorbed undergoes 25-hydroxylation in the liver; therefore, severe hepatic parenchymal damage can result in 25(OH)D deficiency. Clinically, severe vitamin D deficiency as a consequence of liver disease is rare, because the degree of hepatic destruction necessary to impair 25-hydroxylation is incompatible with long-term survival. However, isoniazid has been shown to decrease the 25-hydroxylation of vitamin D.[420] Two kindreds have been described in whom the clinical and biochemical presentations and therapeutic responses suggest an inherited 25-hydroxylation defect.[421]

Impaired 1α-Hydroxylation of 25-Hydroxyvitamin D

The final step in the activation of vitamin D is the hydroxylation of 25(OH)D by the renal 1α-hydroxylase to yield $1,25(OH)_2D_3$. Renal parenchymal damage, therefore, can result in deficiency of the active metabolite of vitamin D. Impaired 1α-hydroxylation is observed once creatinine clearance decreases to approximately 30 to 40 mL/min. Unlike with liver failure, with renal failure, dialysis permits long-term survival; therefore, deficiency of $1,25(OH)_2D_3$ as a result of impaired renal 1α-hydroxylation is a common and important clinical entity.

The metabolic consequences of chronic renal failure on the parathyroid glands and the skeleton are complex (see Chapter 28). Impaired renal 1α-hydroxylation leads to decreased intestinal absorption of calcium, resulting in hypocalcemia. The diminished phosphate clearance associated with renal failure leads to elevated levels of blood phosphate and consequently increases in circulating FGF23; this, in turn, further lowers levels of $1,25(OH)_2D_3$ and calcium. The resultant secondary hyperparathyroidism increases release of calcium and phosphate from bone; however, because of the renal insufficiency, PTH does not have a phosphaturic effect. As a result, the increased serum phosphate rises further.

Oral phosphate binders are used to lower blood phosphate. Calcium-containing antacids, which replaced the more toxic aluminum-containing antacids (see Chapter 28), are being supplemented or replaced with the phosphate-binding exchange resin sevelamer.

Calcium administration also attenuates the hypocalcemic stimulus to parathyroid secretion. $1,25(OH)_2D_3$ therapy is critical for the absorption of this calcium and should be administered early in the course of renal failure (when the creatinine clearance falls below 30-40 mL/min) to prevent development of secondary hyperparathyroidism, with careful monitoring to avoid hypercalcemia. Once secondary hyperparathyroidism has developed, pharmacologic doses of $1,25(OH)_2D_3$, delivered intravenously or orally, or calcimimetics[422] may be required to suppress PTH gene transcription and parathyroid cellular proliferation.

Efforts are under way to develop nonhypercalcemic analogues of $1,25(OH)_2D_3$ that maintain their PTH suppressing and antiproliferative effects. Such analogues would be invaluable for preventing and treating secondary hyperparathyroidism in the setting of chronic renal failure and perhaps in the treatment of malignancies whose proliferation is inhibited by pharmacologic doses of $1,25(OH)_2D_3$.

Decreased levels of $1,25(OH)_2D_3$ can also be observed in patients taking ketoconazole[172] and in X-linked hypophosphatemia and TIO, diseases associated with high FGF23 levels (see Chapter 28).[164]

A rare heritable defect of vitamin D activation has been described in several kindreds. Biochemically, pseudo–vitamin D deficiency rickets (PDDR) is characterized by hypocalcemia and secondary hyperparathyroidism. The only metabolic abnormalities that differentiate it from dietary vitamin D deficiency are the presence of normal or elevated levels of vitamin D and 25(OH)D accompanied by low levels of $1,25(OH)_2D_3$.[423] The disease is inherited in an autosomal recessive fashion and manifests in infancy with rickets, osteomalacia, and seizures. Cloning of the 1α-hydroxylase gene has confirmed that mutation of this gene is the molecular basis for the disorder[424,425] and, as expected, physiologic replacement doses of 1α-hydroxylated metabolites of vitamin D result in clinical remission.

Target Organ Resistance to 1,25-Dihydroxyvitamin D_3

A second rare inherited disorder, characterized by resistance to the biologic actions of $1,25(OH)_2D_3$, has been described in several kindreds. This disorder, referred to as *hereditary vitamin D resistant rickets* (HVDRR), is also characterized by autosomal recessive inheritance. Its biochemical presentation, with hypocalcemia, hypophosphatemia, and secondary hyperparathyroidism, resembles that of vitamin D deficiency, but it is accompanied by elevated levels of $1,25(OH)_2D_3$. The molecular basis for this disease is mutation of the vitamin D receptor gene, resulting in impaired target organ responsiveness. Most of the mutations that have been described involve the DNA binding domain of the receptor. These mutations result in a decreased affinity of the receptor for its response elements on target genes, leading to impaired regulation of these genes. Mutations in the hormone binding and nuclear receptor coactivator binding domains of the receptor have also been described in kindreds with HVDRR.[426]

The clinical presentation of HVDRR is variable; however, most patients present in infancy with rickets, hypophosphatemia, and seizures, although presentation in late adolescence has also been described. Alopecia totalis, developing in the first two years of life, is present in some kindreds.[427] The finding of alopecia in mice with VDR mutations[28,187] confirms the association of alopecia with disruption of the VDR gene.

Because of the target organ resistance to the active metabolite of vitamin D, there is no ideal treatment for HVDRR. Pharmacologic doses of vitamin D, 25(OH)D, $24,25(OH)_2D$ and $1,25(OH)_2D_3$ have been administered in an attempt to overcome this target organ resistance, with variable effects. In patients in whom the hypocalcemia and osteomalacia are resistant to such therapeutic interventions, parenteral calcium infusions have been used to heal osteomalacic lesions.[190] Studies in VDR-ablated mice have demonstrated that maintenance of normal mineral ion homeostasis prevents all the complications of VDR ablation except alopecia.[189,191] Based on these observations, patients with VDR mutations should be treated early and aggressively to prevent skeletal abnormalities and parathyroid hyperplasia. Lifelong therapy is usually required, although spontaneous remissions off therapy have been described.[428] The pathophysiology of the spontaneous remissions is not well understood, because the underlying genetic defect still exists. It is likely that these "remissions" reflect compensated calcium homeostasis once the needs of the growing skeleton are met. In support of this hypothesis is a report of a relapse in a pregnant woman, followed by a remission post partum.[429]

Phenytoin causes target organ resistance to the biologic effects of $1,25(OH)_2D_3$, in addition to its acceleration of the hepatic catabolism of vitamin D metabolites. Phenytoin has been shown to impair intestinal calcium absorption in vivo in rats and impair PTH and $1,25(OH)_2D_3$-mediated bone resorption in vitro. Combination chemotherapy with 5-fluorouracil and low-dose leucovorin has been reported to cause hypocalcemia in 65% of patients, which is associated with an acute decrease in plasma $1,25(OH)_2D_3$ levels.[430]

Other Causes

Excessive Deposition into the Skeleton

Excessive deposition of calcium into the skeleton can occur in association with osteoblastic metastases, with chondrosarcomas, or in the hungry bone syndrome. This syndrome manifests as prolonged hypocalcemia, hypocalciuria, and hypophosphatemia following parathyroidectomy for primary hyperparathyroidism (see "Primary Hyperparathyroidism"). The hypocalcemia is a consequence of remineralization of a skeleton that has been subjected to the bone-resorbing effects of PTH over a prolonged period. Hungry bone syndrome can also be observed after treatment of other diseases that are associated with excessive bone resorption. It has been described following radioactive iodine treatment of a patient with Graves' disease.[431]

Chelation

Decreases in ionized calcium have been reported with foscarnet, a pyrophosphate analogue that is used as an antiviral agent,[432] perhaps because of complex formation between ionized calcium and the drug.

Hyperphosphatemia due to phosphate administration or rapid destruction of soft tissue (i.e., rhabdomyolysis, chemotherapy of hematologic malignancies) can produce profound hypocalcemia by directly complexing and precipitating calcium in bone or soft tissues, by inhibiting bone resorption, and by blocking renal synthesis of $1,25(OH)_2D_3$ (see "Hyperphosphatemia").

Massive infusions of citrated blood products can cause hypocalcemia, presumably because citrate complexes calcium in the recipient's plasma.[433] Large doses of radiographic contrast dyes containing ethylenediaminetetraacetic acid (EDTA) have also been reported to cause hypocalcemia. Hypocalcemia, due to complexes of calcium and fluoride, has been reported with hydrofluoric acid burns or ingestion.[434]

Neonatal Hypocalcemia

Neonatal hypocalcemia is seen in infants of hyperparathyroid mothers, infants of diabetic mothers, premature infants, and infants with birth asphyxia. The cause of hypocalcemia in infants of diabetic mothers is likely multifactorial. Prematurity per se does not account for the higher incidence.[435] The response of premature infants and infants of diabetic mothers to exogenous PTH suggests that functional hypoparathyroidism might, in part, account for the increased hypocalcemia in these two populations.[435] The hypocalcemia in infants of hyperparathyroid mothers is presumably secondary to the maternal hypercalcemia that, in turn, suppresses fetal parathyroid function.[436]

Human Immunodeficiency Virus Infection

Hypocalcemia is sixfold more prevalent in HIV-infected patients than in the general population.[437] Although hypocalcemia is often a consequence of antiretroviral and antibiotic or antimycotic therapy, vitamin D deficiency and hypomagnesemia are also common in patients with AIDS. Impaired parathyroid responsiveness to hypocalcemia has also been documented (see Chapter 37).

Critical Illness

Hypocalcemia is commonly seen in critically ill patients and is thought to be a reflection of parathyroid gland suppression, failure to activate vitamin D, calcium chelation or sequestration, or hypomagnesemia. However, an increased basal level and secretory response of PTH to lowering of serum calcium has been observed in some septic and nonseptic ICU patients, emphasizing the multifactorial origin of the hypocalcemia.[438] There was a correlation between cytokine levels and hypocalcemia in this and other studies, suggesting that these inflammatory agents might play a role in redistribution of calcium to the intracellular or other pools. IL- has been shown to increase the expression of the calcium sensing receptor on parathyroid cells and lower PTH secretion and blood calcium in rats injected with the cytokine.[439]

Severe acute pancreatitis is often associated with hypocalcemia, and this association is a negative prognostic indicator. The hypocalcemia occurs shortly after the onset of the pancreatitis and is associated with an increase in PTH levels, suggesting that parathyroid function is normal. It has long been thought that this hypocalcemia is secondary to deposition of calcium soaps consisting of calcium and fatty acids. Supporting this hypothesis, studies in a patient with a pancreatic fistula have demonstrated hypocalcemia (4.3 mg/dL) in the setting of high levels of calcium (26 mg/dL) and fatty acids in ascitic fluid.[440] Subsequent studies in a rat model have supported this finding and demonstrated that oleate has a high binding capacity for calcium.[441] However, other investigations in a porcine model of experimental pancreatitis have demonstrated that hypocalcemia does not occur if the animals are subjected to thyroidectomy prior to the induction of pancreatitis.[442] This finding suggests a role for calcitonin in the development of hypocalcemia with acute pancreatitis, although several clinical studies have documented normal calcitonin levels in hypocalcemic individuals with pancreatitis.[443]

Severe hypocalcemia with hypercalcitoninemia and hypophosphatemia has been reported in the toxic shock syndrome sepsis and in critically ill patients.[444] As in acute pancreatitis, this hypocalcemia is usually accompanied by increases in serum levels of PTH, and the degree of hypocalcemia is a negative prognostic indicator. The mechanism of hypocalcemia in these patients is likely to be heterogeneous and has not been clearly defined.

Treatment

Acute hypocalcemia is an emergency that requires prompt attention. If symptoms of neuromuscular irritability are present and carpopedal spasm is elicited on physical examination, treatment with intravenous calcium is indicated until the signs and symptoms of hypocalcemia subside. Approximately 100 mg of elemental calcium should be infused over a period of 10 to 20 minutes (Table 27–6). If this is not sufficient to alleviate the clinical findings of hypocalcemia, an infusion of 100 mg/hr can be given to adults for several hours, with close monitoring of calcium levels.

In hypocalcemia associated with hypomagnesemia, magnesium replacement also is required. Magnesium should be given intravenously, 100 mEq over 24 hours in the acute setting. Because most of the parenteral magnesium is excreted in the urine, oral magnesium oxide should be instituted as soon as possible to replete body stores. Special caution and reduced doses are necessary when administering magnesium to patients in renal failure (see "Magnesium Disorders").

Treatment of hypocalcemia should be directed at the underlying disorder. In all cases, replacement with exogenous calcium (1-3 g elemental calcium daily, given orally) should be instituted. Calcium carbonate is the least expensive formulation, but it requires acidification for efficient absorption. This becomes important in patients with achlorhydria and those in whom gastric acid production is being suppressed with pharmacologic agents. Notable in this respect is the acid buffering capacity of calcium carbonate. Because of this, it is recommended that patients take their calcium carbonate supplements in divided doses of 1 g or less. In these cases, the calcium should be taken with food or citrus drinks to promote maximal absorption.

In cases of vitamin D deficiency or resistance, the metabolite of vitamin D chosen depends on the underlying disorder. If impaired renal 1α-hydroxylation is present, such as in renal failure, hypoparathyroidism (or PTH resistance), or the vitamin D–dependent rickets syndromes, metabolites that do not require this modification should be administered (calcitriol 0.25 to 1 μg/day or dihydrotachysterol 0.2 to 1 mg/day). If decreased intake or increased losses are the problem, vitamin D should be administered and the treatment directed at the underlying disorder. Initial repletion of stores can be undertaken with 50,000 IU of vitamin D daily for 2 to 3 weeks, followed by weekly or bimonthly administration until the underlying disorder has been treated. In patients with resistance to vitamin D, such as those taking phenytoin, high doses (50,000 IU one to three times weekly) should be used as maintenance therapy. In other patients, once treatment of the underlying disorder and repletion of body stores have been addressed, two multivitamins (800 IU) should provide sufficient maintenance therapy. In cases of severe malabsorption, vitamin D can be administered parenterally.

Patients should be monitored closely to assess response to therapy and to prevent therapeutic complications. Serum calcium should be monitored frequently (daily in profound hypocalcemia, weekly in moderate hypocalcemia) for the first month of therapy. Concomitant with resolution of hypocalcemia, one should observe a decline in the serum PTH level as the secondary hyperparathyroidism resolves. Measurement of serum PTH and assessment of 24-hour urinary calcium excretion should be performed within 2 to 4 weeks of institution of therapy.

TABLE 27–6 THERAPEUTIC MINERAL ION PREPARATIONS

				Available Formulations					
				Oral Preparations			Parenteral Preparations		
Compound	**MW***	**Mineral Ion Content**		**Compound**	**Mineral Ion Content**		**Compound**	**Mineral Ion Content**	
		mg/g	**mM/g**		**mg/g**	**mM/g**		**mg/g**	**mM/g**
				CALCIUM					
Ca carbonate	100	400	10.0	1250 mg[‡]	500 mg	12.5 mM			
Ca phosphate	310	383	9.6	1565 mg	600 mg	15.0 mM			
Ca acetate	158	253	6.3	668 mg[‡]	167 mg	4.2 mM			
Ca citrate	498	210	6.0	950 mg[‡]	200 mg	5.0 mM			
Ca lactate	218	130	4.6	650 mg[‡]	84 mg	2.1 mM			
Ca glubionate		64	1.7	5 mL	115 mg	2.0 mM			
Ca gluconate	430	93	2.3	1000 mg[‡]	93 mg	2.3 mM	10% soln	93 mg/10 mL	2.3 mM/10 mL
Ca gluceptate	488	82	2.0				22% soln	90 mg/5 mL	2.3 mM/10 mL
Ca chloride	147	273	6.8				10% soln	273 mg/10 mL	11.2 mM/10 mL
				MAGNESIUM					
Mg oxide	40	603	24.8	400 mg[‡]	241 mg	9.9 mM			
Mg gluconate	450	54	2.2	500 mg	27 mg	1.1 mM			
Mg chloride	203	120	4.9	535 mg	64 mg	2.6 mM	20% soln	24 mg/mL	1.0 mM/mL
Mg sulfate	246	99	4.1				50% soln	49 mg/mL	2.0 mM/mL
				PHOSPHORUS[†]					
Na/K phosphate (neutral)				capsule	250 mg	8.1 mM			
K phosphate (neutral)				capsule	250 mg	8.1 mM	soln	94 mg/mL	3.0 mM/mL
Na phosphate (neutral)							soln	94 mg/mL	3.0 mM/mL

Note: Other formulations exist. Those shown are among those approved in the United States.
*Molecular weights of compounds shown are for the usual chemical forms, including water molecules (e.g., MgSO4 • 7 H_2O).
[†]Phosphate preparations contain buffered mixtures of monobasic (H_2PO4) and dibasic (HPO_4) ions; the P content therefore is specified in millimoles. Oral phosphates contain 7 mEq Na and K per capsule (Na/K form) or 14 mEq K per capsule (K form). Parenteral solutions typically contain 4 mEq of Na or K per milliliter.
[‡]Other formulations exist. Those shown are those approved in the United States.
mM, millimole; MW, molecular weight; soln, solution.
Data from Olin B. Drug Facts and Comparisons. St. Louis: Facts and Comparisons, 2007.

The urinary calcium measurement reflects the effect of therapy on the patient's ability to absorb calcium and the net uptake of calcium by bone. A low urine calcium indicates poor adherence to a regimen, poor absorption of calcium, or increased uptake by bone. In addition, the urine calcium provides important information on which to base therapeutic modifications to avoid nephrolithiasis.

Once normalization of serum and urinary calcium and a decrease in PTH levels are observed, aggressive replacement therapy should be shifted to maintenance therapy to prevent hypercalcemia and nephrolithiasis. These same parameters should be monitored 1 and 3 months after a dose change to assess the effect of the therapeutic intervention. Monitoring of the alkaline phosphatase can also be performed at this time. Alkaline phosphatase levels can actually increase soon after starting treatment because of healing of the osteomalacic lesions; however, by 3 to 4 months after institution of therapy, a clear downward trend should be observed. Alkaline phosphatase and PTH values can remain elevated for 6 to 12 months after therapy is instituted and should not be a cause for alarm, provided that they are declining and that the other parameters suggest that therapy is effective.

All patients receiving vitamin D metabolites and calcium need to be aware of potential therapeutic complications. Importantly, the mild symptoms of hypercalcemia should be emphasized to the patient. It is essential that these patients be aware that their calcium should be monitored more frequently during intercurrent illnesses that can affect the absorption of calcium or their hydration status in order to prevent the development of hypocalcemia or severe hypercalcemia.

Disorders of Phosphate Metabolism

Hyperphosphatemia

Serum phosphate levels are controlled primarily by the rate of proximal renal tubular phosphate reabsorption, which is due, in turn, to the integrated activity of the major sodium-dependent cotransporters (NaPi-2a and NaPi-2c). The latter are strongly down-regulated by parathyroid hormone and FGF-23, both of which are stimulated by phosphate. Thus, in the absence of extraordinary filtered loads of phosphate, the capacity of normal kidneys to excrete phosphate is not easily exceeded. Consequently, the occurrence of hyperphosphatemia usually signifies impaired renal function, hypoparathyroidism, defective FGF-23 action, a huge flux of phosphate into the extracellular fluid, or some combination of these factors (Table 27–7).

The most common cause of hyperphosphatemia is acute or chronic renal failure in which GFR is so reduced that the usual daily load of phosphate cannot be excreted at a normal level of serum phosphate, despite maximal inhibition of phosphate reabsorption in the remaining functional nephrons. In hypoparathyroidism (or pseudohypoparathyroidism), serum phosphate can rise to levels as high as 6 to 8 mg/dL due to loss of the tonic inhibitory effect of PTH on phosphate reabsorption, although elevated FGF-23 levels can prevent even further increases in serum phosphate.[446] The hyperphosphatemia of hypoparathyroidism is only partly due to the absence of PTH per se. Hypocalcemia can further impair phosphate clearance in this setting, and correction of hypocalcemia by treatment with vitamin D metabolites and oral calcium can reduce serum phosphate, for example, even though PTH levels remain low.[447]

Other circumstances in which renal tubular phosphate excretion is decreased, in the absence of renal failure, include acromegaly,[448,449] chronic therapy with heparin, and familial tumoral calcinosis.[450] Familial tumoral calcinosis can result from inactivating mutations in either FGF-23 or the *O*-linked glycosyltransferase GALNT3, which can glycosylate and activate FGF-23.[451,452] The choice of FGF-23 assay is important, because the responsible FGF-23 mutations can render the molecule more susceptible to proetolyic degradation, such that the blood levels of (inactive) carboxyl fragments may be quite high in contrast to low levels of (bioactive) intact FGF-23.[451]

TABLE 27–7 CAUSES OF HYPERPHOSPHATEMIA

IMPAIRED RENAL PHOSPHATE EXCRETION
Renal insufficiency
Familial tumoral calcinosis
Endocrinopathies
• Acromegaly
• Hypoparathyroidism
• Pseudohypoparathyroidism
Heparin
INCREASED EXTRACELLULAR PHOSPHATE
Rapid administration of phosphate (IV, oral, rectal)
Phosphate salts
Fosphenytoin
Liposomal amphotericin B
Rapid cellular catabolism or lysis
Catabolic states
Tissue injury
• Hyperthermia
• Crush injuries
• Fulminant hepatitis
Cellular lysis
• Hemolytic anemia
• Rhabdomyolysis
• Tumor lysis syndrome
Transcellular shifts of phosphate
Metabolic acidosis
Respiratory acidosis

Affected patients can display focal hyperostosis; large, lobulated periarticular ectopic calcifications, especially around shoulders or hips; hyperphosphatemia due to increased renal tubular reabsorption of phosphate; increased serum $1,25(OH)_2D$ despite normal or low serum PTH; and increased intestinal calcium absorption, consistent with the elevated serum $1,25(OH)_2D$ concentration. The disorder can appear in childhood or adulthood, is more common in blacks, and is lifelong, with a tendency for the tumoral calcifications to progress at affected sites. In contrast to the elevated serum $1,25(OH)_2D$, hyperphosphatemia is not a constant feature of tumoral calcinosis, although it tends to be most severe in those with prominent calcifications. Despite their chronic hyperphosphatemia, secondary hyperparathyroidism does not develop in these patients, presumably because of the high $1,25(OH)_2D$ levels and intestinal hyperabsorption of calcium. Treatment is problematic, although some success has been reported with phosphate-binding antacids, calcium deprivation, and calcitonin therapy.

Hyperphosphatemia can result from overly rapid administration of therapeutic phosphate preparations or phosphate-rich drugs (fosphenytoin, liposomal amphotericin B), especially if renal function is compromised,[453,454] or from rapid shifts of phosphate out of cells, most often provoked by mechanical injury or metabolic insult. Most cases of hyperphosphatemia associated with intestinal phosphate loads have involved children who received phosphate-containing laxatives or enemas or older adults with impaired renal function receiving phosphate-based cathartics in preparation for colonoscopy.[455] Hyperphosphatemia due to cytolytic release of intracellular phosphate can be quite dramatic, with serum phosphate concentrations up to or exceeding 20 mg/dL. This was described initially as a complication of rapid induction chemotherapy for certain hematologic malignancies (tumor lysis syndrome), although it also can occur from cellular injury associated with trauma, hyperthermia, overwhelming infection, hemolysis, rhabdomyolysis, or metabolic acidosis.[456,457]

Rarely, apparent hyperphosphatemia reflects measurement artifact caused by paraproteins in myeloma.[458]

Most often, hyperphosphatemia is mild and asymptomatic, although chronic hyperphosphatemia is an important factor in the development of secondary hyperparathyroidism in progressive renal failure. The clinical manifestations of acute severe hyperphosphatemia are related mainly to those of the accompanying hypocalcemia, caused by formation of insoluble calcium phosphate precipitates. Thus, tetany, muscle cramps, paresthesias, and seizures can occur, and these may be compounded by other metabolic disturbances (hyperkalemia, acidosis, hyperuricemia) that often coexist. Generalized precipitation of calcium phosphate into soft tissues can produce organ dysfunction, notably renal failure.[455]

Therapeutic options for hyperphosphatemia are limited. Volume expansion may be helpful to improve GFR in acute syndromes. Identification and removal of any exogenous sources of phosphate is important, and phosphate-binding aluminum hydroxide antacids may be useful in limiting intestinal phosphate absorption and chelating phosphate secreted into the intestine. Hemodialysis is the most effective approach and should be considered early in severe hyperphosphatemia, especially in the tumor-lysis syndrome and particularly if symptomatic hypocalcemia cannot be adequately treated for fear of inducing widespread soft-tissue calcification.

Hypophosphatemia

Etiology

Hypophosphatemia can result from one or more of three general mechanisms (Table 27–8): increased urinary losses due to

TABLE 27–8 CAUSES OF HYPOPHOSPHATEMIA

Reduced Renal Tubular Phosphate Reabsorption	
Excess PTH or PTHrP	
Primary hyperparathyroidism	
PTHrP-dependent hypercalcemia of malignancy	
Secondary hyperparathyroidism	
Vitamin D deficiency/resistance	
Calcium starvation or malabsorption	
Imatinib	
Rapid, selective correction of severe hypomagnesemia	
Excess FGF-23 or other "phosphatonins"	
Familial hypophosphatemic rickets (XLH)	
Autosomal dominant hypophosphatemic rickets (ADHR)	
Tumor-induced osteomalacia syndrome (TIO)	
McCune–Albright syndrome (fibrous dysplasia)	
Epidermal nevus syndrome	
Idiopathic hypercalciuria	
Intrinsic renal disease	
Fanconi syndrome(s), other renal tubular disorders	
Cystinosis	Wilson's disease
Amyloidosis	Multiple myeloma
Hemolytic uremic syndrome	Heavy metal toxicity
Magnesium deficiency	Rewarming or hyperthermia
Npt 2a mutations	
Npt 2c mutations (HHRH)	
Other	
Poorly controlled diabetes, alcoholism	
Hyperaldosteronism	
Post partial hepatectomy	
Post renal transplantation	
Drugs or toxins	
Ethanol	High-dose estrogens
Acetazolamide, other diuretics	Ifosfamide
High-dose glucocorticoids	Cisplatin
Bicarbonate	Suramin
Toluene	Foscarnet
Heavy metals (Pb, Cd)	N-methyl formamide
Calcitonin	Bisphosphonates
Tenofovir	Paraquat
Shifts of Extracellular Phosphate into Cells or Bone	
Acute Intracellular Shifts	
Intravenous glucose, fructose, glycerol	
Insulin therapy for hyperglycemia, diabetic ketoacidosis	
Catecholamines (epinephrine, albuterol, terbutaline, dopamine)	
Thyrotoxic periodic paralysis	
Acute respiratory alkalosis, salicylate intoxication, acute gout	
Gram-negative sepsis, toxic shock syndrome	
Recovery from acidosis, starvation, anorexia nervosa, hepatic failure	
Rapid cellular proliferation	
Leukemic blast crisis	
Intensive erythropoetin, G-CSF therapy	
Accelerated Net Bone Formation	
Post-parathyroidectomy	
Osteoblastic metastases	
Treatment of vitamin D deficiency	
Antiresorptive therapy of severe Paget's disease	
Impaired Intestinal Phosphate Absorption	
Aluminum-containing antacids	

FGF, fibrablast growth factor; G-CSF, granulocyte-wlony stimulating factor; PTH, parathyriod hormone, PTHrP, parathyroid hormone-related protein.

decreased net renal tubular phosphate reabsorption; rapid shifts of phosphate from extracellular fluid into the intracellular space or the mineral phase of bone; or, rarely, severe and selective deprivation of dietary phosphate, as can occur with chronic ingestion of large amounts of nonabsorbable aluminum-containing antacids. Fasting or starvation does not lead directly to hypophosphatemia, apparently because phosphate is mobilized from catabolized bone and soft tissue in amounts sufficient to maintain serum phosphate, even during prolonged caloric deprivation.[459] Starvation does induce phosphate deficiency and, therefore, predisposes to subsequent hypophosphatemia.[460]

Chronic hypophosphatemia usually can be traced to ongoing renal phosphate wasting. Elevation of serum PTH for any reason (other than renal failure), as in primary hyperparathyroidism or secondary hyperparathyroidism due to vitamin D or calcium deficiency, results in inhibition of tubular phosphate reabsorption and fasting hypophosphatemia. Phosphate clearance also is increased in PTHrP-associated hypercalcemia of malignancy, although when such patients develop severe hypercalcemia, hypophosphatemia may be masked initially by underlying volume depletion and compromised GFR. Therapy with the tyrosine kinase inhibitor imatinib appears to cause hypophosphatemia, at least in part, by inhibiting bone turnover, lowering serum calcium, and stimulating secondary hyperparathyroidism.[461] When PTH secretion is compromised by severe hypomagnesemia, rapid intravenous administration of magnesium alone, without concurrent attention to coexisting hypocalcemia, can provoke massive phosphaturia and hypophosphatemia in patients with underlying phosphate depletion.

The discovery that gain-of-function mutations in FGF-23 cause autosomal dominant hypophosphatemic rickets (ADHR) inaugurated a new era in understanding of phosphate homeostasis.[462-464] Immunoassays for FGF-23[465] have pointed to elevated circulating FGF-23 as at least one "phosphatonin" responsible for reduction of phosphate reabsorption and serum $1,25(OH)_2D$ levels in the more common disorder, X-linked hypophosphatemic rickets (XLH), in the rare but distinctive tumor-induced osteomalacia (TIO) and epidermal nevus syndromes, and in the approximately 50% of patients with McCune-Albright syndrome (fibrous dysplasia of bone) who manifest hypophosphatemia.[462-464,466-468] These disorders share a common biochemical phenotype, which can include a more generalized proximal tubular dysfunction, with modest proteinuria and aminoaciduria. Serum calcium usually is normal or low-normal, urinary calcium often is low, PTH is normal or only slightly elevated, and $1,25(OH)_2D$ is inappropriately normal. The clinical picture is dominated by weakness, bone pain, and other features attributable to the associated rickets or osteomalacia (see Chapter 28). Increased FGF-23 also can play a role in impaired phosphate reabsorption seen in the 20% or so of patients with calcium kidney stones and idiopathic hypercalciuria who exhibit fasting hypophosphatemia,[469] although a few such patients might harbor mutations in the Npt-2a sodium phosphate cotransporter.[470]

Renal phosphate clearance may be impaired in the context of a more generalized renal tubular disorder such as Fanconi's syndrome(s) or others associated with systemic diseases such as amyloidosis, Wilson's disease, or cystinosis (see Table 27–8). In addition to Npt-2a mutations, inactivating mutations in the

Npt-2c cotransporter, also expressed in the proximal tubule and known to be regulated by both PTH and FGF-23, have been shown to account for hereditary hypophosphatemic rickets with hypercalciuria, a rare disorder in which primary renal tubular phosphate wasting causes appropriate elevation of serum $1,25(OH)_2D$ and resulting hypercalciuria.[471,472] Other causes of impaired renal tubular phosphate reabsorption include the osmotic diuresis associated with poorly controlled diabetes, alcoholism, hyperaldosteronism, and exposure to any of a wide variety of drugs or toxins (see Table 27–8). The pathogenesis of phosphate wasting that often follows partial hepatectomy or renal transplantation remains unclear, but humoral mechanisms seem to be involved.[473,474]

Rapid egress of extracellular phosphate into cells is the cause of hypophosphatemia that develops acutely during administration of intravenous glucose, insulin therapy for hyperglycemia, administration of catecholamines (pressors or bronchodilators), thyrotoxic periodic paralysis, profound respiratory alkalosis, refeeding syndrome in the wake of severe acidosis or starvation, recovery from acute hepatic failure (where hypophosphatemia is a recognized favorable prognostic factor[475]), or other circumstances involving rapid cellular proliferation such as leukemic blast crisis or responsiveness to hematopoietic growth factors. Hypophosphatemia in these situations is most pronounced when there is underlying phosphate depletion, as in hyperparathyroidism or vitamin D deficiency, or following prolonged malnutrition, alcoholism, or glycosuria. Accelerated uptake of phosphate into cells is particularly common in postsurgical, burn, or trauma patients, where it may be promoted by high levels of circulating catecholamines and exacerbated by concurrent respiratory alkalosis, fever, volume expansion, sepsis, and hypokalemia. Situations of greatly accelerated net bone formation, such as hungry bone syndrome immediately following parathyroidectomy for primary or tertiary hyperparathyroidism, during initial treatment of severe vitamin D deficiency or Paget's disease, or in occasional patients with extensive osteoblastic bone metastases, can manifest hypophosphatemia as well as hypocalcemia.

Clinical Features

The clinical significance of hypophosphatemia depends upon the presence and severity of underlying phosphate depletion. Unfortunately, the status of the total-body phosphorus pool, and more particularly the critical intracellular pool, is reflected only indirectly by the concentration of phosphate in the extracellular fluid, which contains less than 0.5% of body phosphorus. Thus, although serum phosphate concentrations generally are used to characterize hypophosphatemia as severe (<1-1.5 mg % or <0.3-0.5 mM), moderate (1.5-2.2 mg %, 0.5-0.7 mM) or mild (2.2-3.0 mg %, 0.75-1.0 mM), serum phosphate may be normal or even high (depending upon renal function) in the presence of profound intracellular phosphate deficiency. Conversely, it may be low when intracellular phosphate is relatively normal, such as following a sudden movement of extracellular phosphate into cells.

The prevalence of severe hypophosphatemia among hospitalized patients overall is less than 1%, whereas mild or moderate hypophosphatemia may be detected in 2% to 5%.[476] Hypophosphatemia is recognized most often in critically ill patients, alcoholics or other malnourished persons, decompensated diabetics, and those with acute infectious or pulmonary disorders.[477]

The clinical manifestations of severe hypophosphatemia are protean. Among the most common are various neuromuscular symptoms, ranging from progressive lethargy, muscle weakness, and paresthesias to paralysis, coma, and even death, depending upon the severity of the phosphate depletion. Confusion, profound weakness, paralysis, seizures, and other major sequelae generally are limited to patients with serum phosphate concentrations less than 0.8-1.0 mg/dL.[478] Biochemical evidence of muscle injury is observed within 1 to 2 days in more than one third of patients whose serum phosphate concentrations fall to less than 2 mg %.[479] Overt rhabdomyolysis also can occur, especially in the setting of chronic alcoholism with underlying malnutrition and phosphate depletion.[480] However, by the time this is recognized, the serum phosphate often has been increased by the large amounts of cellular phosphate released from damaged muscle. Reversible respiratory failure due to respiratory muscle weakness can preclude successful weaning from ventilatory support.[481] Left ventricular dysfunction, heart failure, and ventricular arrhythmias can result from profound hypophosphatemia but might not be significant if serum phosphate is greater than 1.5 mg %.[482,483] Correction of moderate hypophosphatemia (<2 mg %) in patients with septic shock led to a significant increase in blood pressure as well as left ventricular function and arterial pH.[482]

Hematologic sequelae of severe hypophosphatemia include hemolysis, platelet dysfunction with bleeding, and impaired leukocyte function (phagocytosis and killing).[484] Erythrocytes demonstrate increased fragility; altered membrane composition, rigidity, and microspherocytosis; and reduced levels of ATP and 2,3-diphosphoglycerate (2,3-DPG).[485] The reduction in erythrocyte 2,3-DPG impairs oxyhemoglobin dissociation and thereby can reduce oxygen delivery to tissues. This problem, together with accelerated hemolysis, can provoke a substantial increase in cardiac output. The blockade in cellular glycolysis becomes demonstrable at levels of serum phosphate between 1 and 2 mg %.[486] Glucose intolerance and insulin resistance also have been demonstrable in these patients.[487]

Treatment

Hypophosphatemia appears most often in acutely or critically ill patients. Accordingly, it often is difficult to discern whether hypophosphatemia is responsible for features of the multiple organ dysfunction commonly encountered in this population. For example, although depression of intracellular high-energy organophosphates has been demonstrated during treatment of diabetic ketoacidosis and phosphate repletion leads to more rapid recovery of erythrocyte 2,3-DPG concentrations, opinion is divided as to whether phosphate therapy in this setting hastens recovery, prevents complications, or improves mortality.[488,489] Nevertheless, because severe hypophosphatemia has been associated, in a variety of clinical settings, with serious neuromuscular, cardiovascular, and hematologic dysfunction that is at least partially reversible with phosphate repletion, most now agree that one should adopt a relatively low threshold for treatment.[482]

The decision to correct hypophosphatemia urgently should be guided by the estimated severity of the cellular phosphate deficit, the presence of signs or symptoms suggesting phosphate depletion, and the overall clinical status of the patient. The presence of renal insufficiency (a risk for iatrogenic hyperphosphatemia), concomitant administration of intravenous glucose (alone or as a component of hyperalimentation solutions), and the potential for aggravating coexistent hypocalcemia also should be considered.

Limited data are available from clinical trials to predict the appropriate dose and rate of phosphate administration. In patients without severe renal insufficiency or hypocalcemia, administration of intravenous phosphate at rates of 2 to 8 mM/hr of elemental phosphorus over 4 to 8 hours often corrects hypophosphatemia without provoking hyperphosphatemia or hypocalcemia.[490-493] Suggested guidelines based upon serum phosphate are shown in Table 27–9. It is essential that serum

TABLE 27–9 URGENT THERAPY OF HYPOPHOSPHATEMIA

CONSIDER

Severity of hypophosphatemia
Likelihood of underlying phosphate depletion
Clinical condition of the patient
Renal function
Serum calcium
Concurrent parenteral therapy (glucose, hyperalimentation)

GUIDELINES

Serum PO4 (mg/dL)	Rate of Infusion (mM/hr)	Duration (hr)	Total PO4 (mM)
<2.5	2.0	6	12
<1.5	4.0	6	24
<1.0	8.0	6	48

Rates shown are normalized for a 70-kg person. Most formulations available in the United States provide 3 mM/mL of sodium or potassium phosphate.

calcium and phosphate be monitored every 6 to 12 hours during and after phosphate therapy, both to detect untoward consequences and because many patients require additional infusions for recurrent hypophosphatemia within 24 to 48 hours of apparently successful repletion.[492] Less acute or severe hypophosphatemia should be managed with oral (or enteral) phosphate supplements if possible, generally given as a total of 1.0 to 2.0 gm/day (as elemental phosphate) of neutral sodium or potassium phosphate in divided doses three to four times a day (see Table 27–6). In many patients, however, oral phosphate therapy is limited by gastrointestinal symptoms such as nausea or diarrhea.

Disorders of Magnesium Metabolism

The fourth most abundant extracellular cation, magnesium, like calcium, plays a critical physiologic role, particularly in neuromuscular function but also as a component of the mineral phase of bone. Intracellular magnesium is crucial for normal energy metabolism as a cofactor for ATP and numerous enzymes and transporters, which is reflected in the global clinical effects that accompany disorders of magnesium homeostasis. Hypomagnesemia and hypermagnesemia are among the most common electrolyte disturbances; one or the other of these abnormalities is observed in as many as 20% of hospitalized patients and even more often (30%-40%) among those admitted to intensive care units.[494]

Hypermagnesemia

Magnesium homeostasis is achieved mainly through highly efficient regulation of tubular magnesium reabsorption in the loop of Henle.[1] Because normal kidneys can readily excrete even large amounts of magnesium (500 mEq/day), high filtered loads of magnesium rarely cause hypermagnesemia except in patients with significant renal insufficiency.[495] Increased magnesium loads in such cases can arise from ingestion of large amounts of oral magnesium salts, typically given as cathartics or antacids, or from extensive soft-tissue ischemia or necrosis in patients with trauma, sepsis, cardiopulmonary arrest, burns, or shock (Table 27–10). Hypermagnesemia can result from parenteral administration of magnesium salts, as when magnesium is used to treat preeclampsia or as a tocolytic.[496] The infants of such hypermagnesemic mothers can manifest transient hypermagnesemia as well, along with parathyroid suppression and neurobehavioral symptoms.[497] The use of oral magnesium preparations as laxatives can lead to hypermagnesemia if absorption is increased by intestinal ileus, obstruction, or perforation.[498]

TABLE 27–10 CAUSES OF HYPERMAGNESEMIA

EXCESSIVE MAGNESIUM INTAKE

Cathartics, antacids, enemas
Dead Sea drowning
Intestinal obstruction or perforation following magnesium ingestion
Magnesium-rich urologic irrigants
Parenteral magnesium

RAPID MOBILIZATION FROM SOFT TISSUES

Burns
Cardiac arrest
Shock, sepsis
Trauma

IMPAIRED MAGNESIUM EXCRETION

Familial hypocalciuric hypercalcemia
Renal failure

OTHER

Adrenal insufficiency
Hypothermia
Hypothyroidism

The most prominent clinical manifestations of hypermagnesemia are vasodilation and neuromuscular blockade, which can involve both pre- and postsynaptic inhibition of neuromuscular transmission.[499] Signs and symptoms generally do not appear unless the serum magnesium exceeds 4 mEq/L.[495] Hypotension, often refractory to pressors and volume expansion, may be one of the earliest signs of progressive hypermagnesemia.[500] Lethargy, nausea, and weakness, accompanied by reduction or loss of deep tendon reflexes, can progress to stupor or coma with respiratory insufficiency or quadriparesis at serum concentrations in excess of 8 to 10 mEq/L. Gastrointestinal hypomotility or ileus is common. Facial flushing and pupillary dilation may be observed. Hypotension may be complicated by a paradoxical relative bradycardia, and other cardiac effects may be evident, including prolongation of the PR, QRS, and QTc intervals, appearance of heart block, and, ultimately, asystole as serum concentrations approach 20 mEq/L.

Hypermagnesemia activates calcium-sensing receptors (CaSRs) in the parathyroids, thereby suppressing PTH secretion,[501] and in the renal distal tubules, thereby reducing tubular calcium and magnesium reabsorption. Severe hypocalcemia opposes the effect of hypermagnesemia on PTH secretion, so that serum PTH can remain within the normal range but still be inappropriate for the level of serum calcium.[502]

Successful treatment of hypermagnesemia requires identification and interruption of the source of magnesium, together with measures to increase clearance of magnesium from the extracellular fluid. Use of magnesium-free cathartics or enemas to accelerate clearance of ingested magnesium from the gastrointestinal tract, together with vigorous intravenous hydration, generally have been successful in reversing hypermagnesemia. Refractory cases, especially those with advanced renal insufficiency, can require hemodialysis. Intravenous calcium (100-200 mg) infusions have been advocated as an effective antidote to hypermagnesemia, and there are examples in which this has apparently been successful, at least temporarily.[495,499,503]

Hypomagnesemia

Hypomagnesemia can occur because of impaired intestinal magnesium absorption or, more commonly, excessive gastrointestinal losses due to diarrhea, preprocedural bowel preparation, or prolonged drainage. Most often, hypomagnesemia reflects defective renal tubular reabsorption of magnesium, although rapid shifts into cells, other extrarenal losses, or incorporation into new bone can occur (Table 27–11). Because only 1% of the body's magnesium content is present in extracellular fluid, measurements of serum total or ionized magnesium concentration might not adequately reflect total-body magnesium or the magnesium status of the intracellular compartment in critical tissues such as muscle. Thus, patients with deficiency of tissue magnesium can fail to manifest overt hypomagnesemia while exhibiting abnormal retention (>50% in 24 hr) of infused magnesium, a maneuver that may be employed to assess magnesium status.[504]

Etiology

Intestinal Causes of Hypomagnesemia

Selective dietary magnesium deficiency does not occur, and it is remarkably difficult, in fact, to induce magnesium depletion experimentally by feeding magnesium-deficient diets, probably

TABLE 27–11 CAUSES OF HYPOMAGNESEMIA

IMPAIRED INTESTINAL MAGNESIUM ABSORPTION	
Hypomagnesemia with secondary hypocalcemia Malabsorption syndromes	
INCREASED INTESTINAL MAGNESIUM LOSSES	
Bowel preparation (procedures, surgery) Intestinal drainage or fistula Protracted vomiting or diarrhea	
IMPAIRED RENAL TUBULAR MAGNESIUM REABSORPTION	
Genetic Magnesium-Wasting Syndromes Autosomal dominant hypocalcemia Bartter's syndrome(s) Familial hypomagnesemia with hypercalciuria and nephrocalcinosis Gitelman's syndrome Hypomagnesemia with hypertension and hypercholesterolemia Hypomagnesemia with secondary hypocalcemia Isolated renal magnesium wasting **Acquired Renal Disease** Postobstruction acute tubular necrosis (diuretic phase) Renal transplantation Tubulointerstitial disease **Drugs and Toxins** Aminoglycosides Amphotericin B Cetuximab Cyclosporine Digoxin Diuretics (loop, thiazide, osmotic) Ethanol	Foscarnet Interleukin-2 Pentamidine *cis*-Platinum Tacrolimus **Endocrine and Metabolic Abnormalities** Diabetes mellitus Extracellular fluid volume expansion Hypercalcemia Hyperaldosteronism (primary, secondary) Hyperthyroidism Inappropriate ADH secretion Metabolic acidosis Phosphate depletion **Other** Acute brain injury Hydrogen fluoride burns Hypothermia Sézary syndrome
RAPID SHIFTS OF MAGNESIUM OUT OF EXTRACELLULAR FLUID	
Intracellular Redistribution Catecholamines Correction of respiratory acidosis Recovery from diabetic ketoacidosis Refeeding syndrome Thyrotoxic periodic paralysis **Accelerated Net Bone Formation** After parathyroidectomy Calcitonin therapy	Osteoblastic metastases Treatment of vitamin D deficiency **Other Losses** Blood transfusions Excessive sweating Extensive burns Pancreatitis Pregnancy (third trimester) and lactation

ADH, antidiuretic hormone.

because renal magnesium conservation is so efficient. Large amounts of magnesium may be lost in chronic diarrheal states (this fluid can contain more than 10 mEq/L of magnesium) or via intestinal fistulae or prolonged gastrointestinal drainage. More commonly, magnesium becomes trapped within fatty acid soaps in disorders associated with chronic malabsorption. Investigation of a rare autosomal recessive disorder, hypomagnesemia with secondary hypocalcemia (HSH), has led to the identification of the transient receptor potential channel protein TRPM6, in the form of a hetero-oligomer with the closely related channel protein TRPM7, as a key molecular mediator of intestinal (and renal tubular) transepithelial magnesium transport [505]

Renal Causes of Hypomagnesemia

Roughly 60% of renal magnesium reabsorption occurs in the thick ascending limb of Henle's loop, and another 5% to 10% is reabsorbed in the distal tubules.[1] Investigation of the pathogenesis of several genetic disorders associated with renal magnesium wasting have identified key pathways of magnesium reabsorption at these sites (see Table 27–11).

In familial hypomagnesemia with hypercalciuria and nephrocalcinosis, loss-of-function mutations in the claudin 16 gene encoding the paracellin-1 protein, a component of the tight junctions between adjacent epithelial cells, selectively impair paracellular magnesium (and calcium) reabsorption in response to the (lumen-positive) transepithelial voltage gradient.[50] In Bartter's syndrome(s), inactivating mutations in any of several transporters involved in sodium chloride reabsorption in the ascending limb cause salt wasting, compromise the voltage gradient, and similarly impair paracellular magnesium and calcium reabsorption.[506-508] In autosomal dominant hypocalcemia, mutations causing increased sensitivity of CaSRs to cationic agonists can cause hypomagnesemia, as well as hypocalcemia, through inappropriate CaSR-dependent suppression of PTH secretion and of renal tubular cation reabsorption.[509]

In Gitelman's syndrome, inactivating mutations in the luminal thiazide-sensitive NaCl cotransporter (NCC) expressed in the distal convoluted tubules lead to sodium chloride and magnesium wasting, in this case with hypocalciuria.[506-508,510] The manner whereby impaired NCC activity compromises (transcellular) magnesium reabsorption in this segment is unclear, although NCC-knockout mice (or normal mice treated with thiazides) display reduced distal tubular expression of the TRPM6 channel protein required for normal magnesium transport across the apical membrane.[345] Mutations in the FXYD2 γ-subunit of the distal tubular basolateral Na^+/K^+/ATPase[511] similarly impair salt and magnesium reabsorption at that site and account for some, but not all, cases of isolated renal magnesium wasting.[512] Another genetic syndrome featuring renal magnesium wasting and hypocalciuria (as in Gitelman's syndrome), and thus presumably involving a defect in distal tubular function as well, in association with hypertension and hypercholesterolemia, is linked to a mutation in mitochondrial tRNA DNA.[513]

Most often, renal magnesium wasting is attributable to an acquired abnormality in tubular magnesium reabsorption. In normal subjects, magnesium reabsorption is virtually complete within several days of instituting experimental dietary magnesium deficiency, even before serum magnesium has declined substantially.[514] Thus, the finding of more than 1 mEq/day of urinary magnesium in a frankly hypomagnesemic patient indicates a defect in renal tubular magnesium reabsorption. The causes of acquired primary tubular magnesium wasting include various tubulointerstitial disorders, recovery from acute tubular necrosis or obstruction, renal transplantation, various endocrinopathies, alcoholism, and exposure to certain drugs (see Table 27–11).

Hypomagnesemia or magnesium depletion due to subnormal renal reabsorption can complicate a variety of endocrinopathies, including hyperaldosteronism, hyperthyroidism, and disorders associated with hypercalcemia, hypercalciuria, or phosphate depletion.[504] In primary hyperparathyroidism, PTH stimulates increased tubular magnesium reabsorption, but this is opposed by a direct tubular effect of hypercalcemia. As a result, serum magnesium in primary hyperparathyroidism generally is normal or only slightly reduced. In hypoparathyroidism, serum and urinary magnesium are low. The magnesium depletion in hypoparathyroidism is consistent with loss of both the magnesium-retaining renal action of PTH and the stimulatory effect of $1,25(OH)_2D$ on intestinal magnesium absorption.

Diabetes is among the most common disorders associated with hypomagnesemia.[515] The severity of the hypomagnesemia in diabetics correlates with indices of glycosuria and poor glycemic control,[516] which suggests that urinary losses of magnesium on the basis of glycosuria partly explain the magnesium depletion. Rapid correction of hyperglycemia with insulin therapy causes magnesium to enter cells and might further lower the extracellular magnesium concentration during treatment.

Alcoholism is another very common clinical setting in which hypomagnesemia occurs. Magnesium depletion in alcoholism can result in part from nutritional deficiency of magnesium, overall caloric starvation and ketosis, and gastrointestinal losses due to vomiting or diarrhea, but an acute magnesuric effect of alcohol ingestion likely plays the major role.[517] This effect of alcohol is most evident during the rising limb of the blood ethanol curve and may be related to transient suppression of PTH secretion.[517] Other factors that can contribute to hypomagnesemia in alcoholism include pancreatitis, malabsorption, secondary hyperaldosteronism, respiratory alkalosis, and elevated plasma catecholamines, which increase intracellular sequestration of magnesium.[504]

A number of drugs have been identified as causes of defective renal tubular magnesium reabsorption and hypomagnesemia.[504] These include diuretics (especially loop diuretics), digoxin, cisplatin, cetuximab, pentamidine, cyclosporine, tacrolimus, interleukin-2, aminoglycosides, foscarnet, and amphotericin B. Most often, drug-induced hypomagnesemia is mild and reversible, particularly that associated with diuretic therapy. In more than half of patients treated with cisplatin, hypomagnesemia occurs within days or weeks, and roughly half of those who develop it exhibit persistent hypomagnesemia many months or even years later. The median duration of hypomagnesemia in cisplatin-treated patients is about 2 months, but recovery has been observed for up to 2 years after treatment.[518] Cisplatin can induce a more global nephropathy and azotemic renal failure, but the magnesium wasting appears to be an isolated functional abnormality. There is some evidence that the renal magnesium-wasting syndrome can be prevented by intravenous magnesium administration (24-40 mEq) before or during cisplatin infusion.[519] Such findings suggest that cisplatin selectively impairs magnesium reabsorption by binding competitively to sites or cells involved in binding and transport of magnesium.

Magnesium, like phosphate, is a major intracellular ion, and significant shifts of magnesium from the extracellular compartment therefore can occur during recovery from chronic respiratory acidosis or acute ketoacidosis, during refeeding, during administration of hyperalimentation solutions, and in response to elevations of circulating catecholamines.[504] Other rapid losses of extracellular magnesium can occur during periods of greatly accelerated net bone formation (following parathyroidectomy, during recovery from vitamin D deficiency, or with osteoblastic metastases) or with large losses due to pancreatitis, cardiopulmonary bypass surgery, massive transfusion, extensive burns, excessive sweating, pregnancy, or lactation.

Consequences

Most of the signs and symptoms of hypomagnesemia reflect alterations in neuromuscular function: tetany, hyperreflexia, positive Chvostek and Trousseau signs, tremors, fasciculations, seizures, ataxia, nystagmus, vertigo, choreoathetosis, muscle weakness, apathy, depression, irritability, delirium, and psychosis.[504] Patients usually are not symptomatic unless serum magnesium falls below 1 mEq/L, although occurrence of symptoms, like intracellular magnesium, might not correlate well with serum magnesium. Atrial or ventricular arrhythmias may occur, as may various electrocardiographic abnormalities—prolonged PR or QT intervals, T wave flattening or inversion, or ST straightening. Hypomagnesemia also increases myocardial sensitivity to digitalis intoxication.[520]

Hypomagnesemia evokes important alterations in mineral ion and potassium homeostasis that often aggravate the clinical syndrome. Magnesium-deprived humans or animals develop hypocalcemia, hypocalciuria, hypokalemia (due to impaired tubular reabsorption of potassium), and positive calcium and sodium balance.[514] Sustained correction of hypocalcemia or hypokalemia cannot be achieved by administration of calcium or potassium alone, respectively, whereas both abnormalities respond to administration of magnesium.[521]

The mechanism of hypocalcemia in this setting may be multifactorial. Inappropriately normal or low serum PTH, despite hypocalcemia, is common and indicates a defect in PTH secretion,[522] which is due to augmented signaling by CaSR-associated G proteins, normally inhibited by magnesium, within the parathyroid cell.[523] Other evidence indicates that hypomagnesemia also may impair PTH action on target cells in bone and kidney, although some have observed normal responsiveness, and the issue remains controversial.[383,522,524]

Vitamin D resistance also is a feature of hypomagnesemic states.[525] This appears to be due mainly to impaired renal 1α-hydroxylation of 25(OH)D, although tissue resistance to $1,25(OH)_2D$ also may play a role.[526] The serum $1,25(OH)_2D$ concentration usually is low during hypomagnesemia, which can result from magnesium depletion per se, parathyroid insufficiency, or coexistent vitamin D deficiency.[527,528] Deficiency of $1,25(OH)_2D$ probably is not the main cause of hypocalcemia in these patients, however, because hypocalcemia can be rapidly corrected (within hours to days) by magnesium therapy alone, well in advance of any increase in the serum $1,25(OH)_2D$ concentration.[527]

Therapy

Patients with mild, asymptomatic hypomagnesemia may be treated with oral magnesium salts ($MgCl_2$, MgO, $Mg(OH)_2$), usually given in divided doses totaling 40 to 60 mEq (480-720 mg) per day (see Table 27–6). Diarrhea sometimes occurs with larger doses but generally is not a problem. The gluconate form (54 mg Mg/g) is said to cause less diarrhea.[504] Patients with malabsorption or ongoing urinary magnesium losses might require chronic oral therapy to prevent recurrent magnesium depletion. Although intestinal magnesium absorption is severely impaired in renal failure,[529] oral magnesium must be administered with great caution in this setting, especially in patients receiving concomitant therapy with $1,25(OH)_2D_3$.

Symptomatic or severe (<1 mEq/L) hypomagnesemia, especially if complicated by hypocalcemia, usually signifies magnesium deficits of at least 1 to 2 mEq/kg and is best treated promptly with parenteral magnesium salts. The use of intramuscular $MgSO_4$ is to be discouraged, because the injections are painful and provide relatively little magnesium (2 mL of 50% $MgSO_4$ supplies only 8 mEq of magnesium, compared with typical magnesium deficits in excess of 100 mEq). Moreover, because unretained sulfate ions also can increase urinary calcium excretion, intravenous magnesium chloride or gluconate probably is the most logical approach to initial parenteral therapy for patients who also may be hypocalcemic.

In adult hypomagnesemic patients with normal renal function, rates of infusion of 2 to 4 mEq/h (50-100 mEq/d) generally are needed to maintain serum magnesium in the range of 2 to 3 mEq/L.[521,527] Up to 100 mEq/d for 2 days can be safely administered without elevating serum magnesium above 4 mEq/L, whereas doses of 200 mEq/day can increase serum magnesium to 4.5 to 5.5 mEq/L and thus are excessive. In patients with active seizures or other urgent indications, the infusion may be preceded by a slowly administered bolus of 10 to 20 mEq, followed by a higher rate of infusion (10-15 mEq/hr) for the first 1 to 2 hours only. Patients with normal renal function can readily excrete more than 400 mEq/day of magnesium in the urine without becoming hypermagnesemic, but even mild renal failure can greatly limit magnesium excretion. Therefore, doses of magnesium supplements should be reduced two- to threefold and careful serial monitoring of serum magnesium should be performed in patients with compromised renal function.

It is important to appreciate that a large fraction of parenterally administered magnesium may be excreted in the urine, even in patients with profound magnesium deficiency. Many such patients excrete as much as 50% to 75% of infused magnesium, whereas in normal subjects this approaches 100%.[521] Moreover, because equilibration of the intracellular and extracellular magnesium pools is relatively slow, it is generally necessary to continue magnesium therapy for 3 to 5 days to achieve adequate repletion of the typical 1 to 2 mEq/kg deficit. Because serum magnesium can become normal well before tissue stores are repleted, monitoring of urinary magnesium excretion is a more reliable measure of the approach to full repletion, especially after patients are switched to oral therapy.

The need for calcium, potassium, and phosphate supplementation should be considered in the usual clinical setting of hypomagnesemia. Vitamin D deficiency also commonly coexists and should be treated with oral or parenteral vitamin D or 25(OH)D. Use of $1,25(OH)_2D_3$ is not necessary, does not hasten recovery, and can actually worsen hypomagnesemia by suppressing PTH secretion and thereby promoting renal magnesium excretion.[530] Initial parenteral magnesium therapy in hypocalcemic patients can produce dramatic hypophosphatemia via the rapid stimulation of PTH secretion. This is most likely to be problematic in those with underlying phosphate depletion (malabsorption, alcoholism, diabetes), in whom it can provoke acute neuromuscular dysfunction. Hypophosphatemia may be avoided by concomitant intravenous calcium therapy.

REFERENCES

1. de Rouffignac C, Quamme G. Renal magnesium handling and its hormonal control. Physiol Rev 1994;74(2):305-322.
2. Murshed M, Harmey D, Millan JL, et al. Unique coexpression in osteoblasts of broadly expressed genes accounts for the spatial restriction of ECM mineralization to bone. Genes Dev 2005;19(9):1093-1104.
3. Gensure RC, Ponugoti B, Gunes Y, et al. Identification and characterization of two parathyroid hormone–like molecules in zebrafish. Endocrinology 2004;145(4):1634-1639.
4. Hogan BM, Danks JA, Layton JE, et al. Duplicate zebrafish *pth* genes are expressed along the lateral line and in the central nervous system during embryogenesis. Endocrinology 2005; 146(2):547-551.
5. Arnold A, Horst SA, Gardella TJ, et al. Mutation of the signal peptide-encoding region of the preproparathyroid hormone gene in familial isolated hypoparathyroidism. J Clin Invest 1990; 86(4):1084-1087.
6. Sunthornthepvarakul T, Churesigaew S, Ngowngarmratana S. A novel mutation of the signal peptide of the preproparathyroid

hormone gene associated with autosomal recessive familial isolated hypoparathyroidism. J Clin Endocrinol Metab 1999;84(10): 3792-3796.

7. Wiren KM, Potts JT Jr, Kronenberg HM. Importance of the propeptide sequence of human preproparathyroid hormone for signal sequence function. J Biol Chem 1988;263(36):19771-19777.
8. Divieti P, John MR, Juppner H, Bringhurst FR. Human PTH-(7-84) inhibits bone resorption in vitro via actions independent of the type 1 PTH/PTHrP receptor. Endocrinology 2002;143(1):171-176.
9. Mayer GP, Keaton JA, Hurst JG, Habener JF. Effects of plasma calcium concentration on the relative proportion of hormone and carboxyl fragments in parathyroid venous blood. Endocrinology 1979;104(6):1778-1784.
10. D'Amour P, Rakel A, Brossard JH, et al. Acute regulation of circulating parathyroid hormone (PTH) molecular forms by calcium: utility of PTH fragments/PTH(1-84) ratios derived from three generations of PTH assays. J Clin Endocrinol Metab 2006;91(1): 283-389.
11. Parfitt AM. Calcium homeostasis. In Mundy GR, Martin TJ, eds. Physiology and Pharmacology of Bone. Berlin: Springer-Verlag, 1993:1-65.
12. Hofer AM, Brown EM. Extracellular calcium sensing and signalling. Nat Rev Mol Cell Biol 2003;4(7):530-538.
13. Pollak MR, Brown EM, Chou YH, et al. Mutations in the human Ca^{2+}-sensing receptor gene cause familial hypocalciuric hypercalcemia and neonatal severe hyperparathyroidism. Cell 1993;75: 1297-1303.
14. Pearce SH, Williamson C, Kifor O, et al. A familial syndrome of hypocalcemia with hypercalciuria due to mutations in the calcium-sensing receptor. N Eng J Med 1996;335(15):1115-1122.
15. Ho C, Conner DA, Pollack MR, et al. A mouse model of human familial hypocalciuric hypercalcemia and neonatal severe hyperparathyroidism. Nat Genet 1995;11:389-394.
16. Moe SM, Cunningham J, Bommer J, et al. Long-term treatment of secondary hyperparathyroidism with the calcimimetic cinacalcet HCl. Nephrol Dial Transplant 2005;20(10):2186-2193.
17. Conigrave AD, Mun HC, Delbridge L, et al. L-Amino acids regulate parathyroid hormone secretion. J Biol Chem 2004;279(37): 38151-38159.
18. Silver J, Naveh-Many T, Mayer H, et al. Regulation by vitamin D metabolites of parathyroid hormone gene transcription in vivo in the rat. J Clin Invest 1986;78(5):1296-1301.
19. Sela-Brown A, Russell J, Koszewski NJ, et al. Calreticulin inhibits vitamin D's action on the PTH gene in vitro and may prevent vitamin D's effect in vivo in hypocalcemic rats. Mol Endocrinol 1998;12:1193-1200.
20. Naveh-Many T, Friedlaender MM, Mayer H, Silver J. Calcium regulates parathyroid hormone messenger ribonucleic acid (mRNA), but not calcitonin mRNA in vivo in the rat. Dominant role of 1,25-dihydroxyvitamin D. Endocrinology 1989;125(1):275-280.
21. Bell O, Gaberman E, Kilav R, et al. The protein phosphatase calcineurin determines basal parathyroid hormone gene expression. Mol Endocrinol 2005;19(2):516-526.
22. Almaden Y, Canalejo A, Hernandez A, et al. Direct effect of phosphorus on PTH secretion from whole rat parathyroid glands in vitro. J Bone Miner Res 1996;11(7):970-976.
23. Slatopolsky E, Finch J, Denda M, et al. Phosphorus restriction prevents parathyroid gland growth. J Clin Invest 1996;97(11): 2534-2540.
24. Kilav R, Silver J, Naveh-Many T. Parathyroid hormone gene expression in hypophosphatemic rats. J Clin Invest 1995;96:327–333.
25. Parfitt AM. Parathyroid growth: normal and abnormal. In Bilezikian JP, ed. The Parathyroids, 2nd ed. San Diego: Academic Press, 2001:293-329.
26. Kremer R, Bolivar I, Goltzman D, Hendy GN. Influence of calcium and 1,25-dihydroxycholecalciferol on proliferation and proto-oncogene expression in primary cultures of bovine parathyroid cells. Endocrinology 1989;125:935-941.
27. Dusso A, Cozzolino M, Lu Y, et al. 1,25-Dihydroxyvitamin D down-regulation of TGFα/EGFR expression and growth signaling: a mechanism for the antiproliferative actions of the sterol in parathyroid hyperplasia of renal failure. J Steroid Biochem Mol Biol 2004;89-90(1-5):507-511.
28. Li YC, Pirro AE, Amling M, et al. Targeted ablation of the vitamin D receptor: an animal model of vitamin D–dependent rickets type II with alopecia. Proc Nat Acad Sci U S A 1997;94(18):9831-9835.
29. Naveh-Many T, Rahamimov R, Livni N, Silver J. Parathyroid cell proliferation in normal and chronic renal failure rats: the effects of calcium, phosphate and vitamin D. J Clin Invest 1995;96: 1786-1793.
30. Manley NR, Capecchi MR. Hox group 3 paralogs regulate the development and migration of the thymus, thyroid, and parathyroid glands. Dev Biol 1998;195(1):1-15.
31. Su D, Ellis S, Napier A, et al. *Hoxa3* and *pax1* regulate epithelial cell death and proliferation during thymus and parathyroid organogenesis. Dev Biol 2001;236(2):316-329.
32. Peters H, Neubuser A, Kratochwil K, Balling R. *Pax9*-deficient mice lack pharyngeal pouch derivatives and teeth and exhibit craniofacial and limb abnormalities. Genes Dev 1998;12(17):2735-2747.
33. Xu PX, Zheng W, Laclef C, et al. *Eya1* is required for the morphogenesis of mammalian thymus, parathyroid and thyroid. Development 2002;129(13):3033-3044.
34. Baldini A. Dissecting contiguous gene defects: *TBX1*. Curr Opin Genet Dev 2005;15(3):279-284.
35. Bowl MR, Nesbit MA, Harding B, et al. An interstitial deletion-insertion involving chromosomes 2p25.3 and Xq27.1, near *SOX3*, causes X-linked recessive hypoparathyroidism. J Clin Invest 2005; 115(10):2822-2831.
36. Zahirieh A, Nesbit MA, Ali A, et al. Functional analysis of a novel *GATA3* mutation in a family with the hypoparathyroidism, deafness, and renal dysplasia syndrome. J Clin Endocrinol Metab 2005;90(4):2445-2450.
37. Gunther T, Chen ZF, Kim J, Pet al. Genetic ablation of parathyroid glands reveals another source of parathyroid hormone. Nature 2000;406(6792):199-203.
38. Ding C, Buckingham B, Levine MA. Familial isolated hypoparathyroidism caused by a mutation in the gene for the transcription factor GCMB. J Clin Invest 2001;108(8):1215-1220.
39. Berson SA, Yallow RS. Immunochemical heterogeneity of parathyroid hormone in plasma. J Clin Endocrinol Metab 1968;28: 1037-1047.
40. Bringhurst FR. Circulating forms of parathyroid hormone: peeling back the onion. Clin Chem 2003;49(12):1973-1975.
41. Hilpert J, Nykjaer A, Jacobsen C, et al. Megalin antagonizes activation of the parathyroid hormone receptor. J Biol Chem 1999; 274(9):5620-5625.
42. Martin KJ, Hruska KA, Freitag JJ, et al. The peripheral metabolism of parathyroid hormone. N Engl J Med 1979;301(20):1092-1098.
43. D'Amour P, Brossard JH, Rousseau L, et al. Structure of non-(1-84) PTH fragments secreted by parathyroid glands in primary and secondary hyperparathyroidism. Kidney Int 2005;68(3):998-1007.
44. Slatopolsky E, Finch J, Clay P, et al. A novel mechanism for skeletal resistance in uremia. Kidney Int 2000;58(2):753-761.
45. D'Amour P, Brossard JH. Carboxyl-terminal parathyroid hormone fragments: role in parathyroid hormone physiopathology. Curr Opin Nephrol Hypertens 2005;14(4):330-336.
46. Divieti P, John MR, Juppner H, Bringhurst FR. Human PTH-(7-84) inhibits bone resorption in vitro via actions independent of the type 1 PTH/PTHrP receptor. Endocrinology 2002;143(1):171-176.
47. Friedman PA, Gesek FA. Calcium transport in renal epithelial cells. Am J Physiol 1993;264:F181-F198.
48. Bourdeau JE. Mechanisms and regulation of calcium transport in the nephron. Semin Nephrol 1993;13:191-201.
49. Friedman PA, Gesek FA. Cellular calcium transport in renal epithelia: measurement, mechanisms and regulation. Physiol Rev 1995;75:429-471.
50. Simon DB, Lu Y, Choate KA, et al. Paracellin-1, a renal tight junction protein required for paracellar Mg^{2+} resorption. Science 1999;285:103-106.
51. Brown EM, Pollak M, Hebert SC. The extracellular calcium-sensing receptor: its role in health and disease. Ann Rev Med 1998; 49:15-29.
52. Hoenderop JG, Nilius B, Bindels RJ. Calcium absorption across epithelia. Physiol Rev 2005;85(1):373-422.
53. van Abel M, Hoenderop JG, van der Kemp AW, et al. Coordinated control of renal Ca^{2+} transport proteins by parathyroid hormone. Kidney Int 2005;68(4):1708-1721.
54. Murer H, Forster I, Biber J. The sodium phosphate cotransporter family SLC34. Pflugers Arch 2004;447(5):763-767.

55. Lotscher M, Scarpetta Y, Levi M, et al. Rapid downregulation of rat renal Na/P_i cotransporter in response to parathyroid hormone involves microtubule rearrangement. J Clin Invest 1999;104(4):483-494.
56. Kilav R, Silver J, Biber J, et al. Coordinate regulation of rat renal parathyroid hormone receptor mRNA and Na-Pi cotransporter mRNA and protein. Am J Physiol 1995;268(6 Pt 2):F1017-F1022.
57. Saito H, Maeda A, Ohtomo S, et al. Circulating FGF-23 is regulated by 1α,25-dihydroxyvitamin D_3 and phosphorus in vivo. J Biol Chem 2005;280(4):2543-2549.
58. Murayama A, Takeyama K, Kitanaka S, et al. Positive and negative regulations of the renal 25-hydroxyvitamin D_3 1α-hydroxylase gene by parathyroid hormone, calcitonin, and 1α,25$(OH)_2D_3$ in intact animals. Endocrinology 1999;140(5):2224-2231.
59. Yang W, Friedman PA, Kumar R, et al. Expression of 25$(OH)D_3$ 24-hydroxylase in distal nephron: coordinate regulation by 1,25$(OH)_2D_3$ and cAMP or PTH. Am J Physiol 1999;276(4 Pt 1):E793-E805.
60. Derrickson BH, Mandel LJ. Parathyroid hormone inhibits Na^+-K^+-ATPase through Gq/G11 and the calcium-independent phospholipase A_2. Am J Physiol 1997;272(6 Pt 2):F781-F788.
61. Aubin JE, Triffitt JT. Mesenchymal stem cells and osteoblast differentiation. In Bilezikian JP, Raisz LG, Rodan GA, eds. Principles of Bone Biology, 2nd ed. San Diego: Academic Press, 2002:59-81.
62. Manolagas SC. Birth and death of bone cells: basic regulatory mechanisms and implications for the pathogenesis and treatment of osteoporosis. Endocr Rev 2000;21(2):115-137.
63. Canalis E, Centrella M, Burch W, McCarthy TL. Insulin-like growth factor I mediates selective anabolic effects of parathyroid hormone in bone cultures. J Clin Invest 1989;83(1):60-65.
64. Qin L, Li X, Ko JK, Partridge NC. Parathyroid hormone uses multiple mechanisms to arrest the cell cycle progression of osteoblastic cells from G_1 to S phase. J Biol Chem 2005;280(4):3104-3111.
65. Jilka RL, Weinstein RS, Bellido T, et al. Increased bone formation by prevention of osteoblast apoptosis with parathyroid hormone. [see comments]. J Clin Invest 1999;104(4):439-446.
66. Dobnig H, Turner RT. Evidence that intermittent treatment with parathyroid hormone increases bone formation in adult rats by activation of bone lining cells. Endocrinology 1995;136(8):3632-3638.
67. Bellows CG, Ishida H, Aubin JE, Heersche JN. Parathyroid hormone reversibly suppresses the differentiation of osteoprogenitor cells into functional osteoblasts. Endocrinology 1990;127(6):3111-3116.
68. Bogdanovic Z, Huang YF, Dodig M, et al. Parathyroid hormone inhibits collagen synthesis and the activity of rat *col1a1* transgenes mainly by a cAMP-mediated pathway in mouse calvariae. J Cell Biochem 2000;77(1):149-158.
69. Bellido T, Ali AA, Plotkin LI, et al. Proteasomal degradation of *Runx2* shortens parathyroid hormone–induced anti-apoptotic signaling in osteoblasts. A putative explanation for why intermittent administration is needed for bone anabolism. J Biol Chem 2003;278(50):50259-50272.
70. Qin L, Tamasi J, Raggatt L, et al. Amphiregulin is a novel growth factor involved in normal bone development and in the cellular response to parathyroid hormone stimulation. J Biol Chem 2005;280(5):3974-3981.
71. Kulkarni NH, Halladay DH, Miles RR, et al. Wnt signaling pathway: A target for PTH action in bone and bone cells. J. Bone Mineral Res. 2003;18(suppl 2):S100 (abstract).
72. Bellido T, Ali AA, Gubrij I, et al. Chronic elevation of parathyroid hormone in mice reduces expression of sclerostin by osteocytes: a novel mechanism for hormonal control of osteoblastogenesis. Endocrinology 2005;146(11):4577-4583.
73. Semenov M, Tamai K, He X. SOST is a ligand for LRP5/LRP6 and a Wnt signaling inhibitor. J Biol Chem 2005;280(29):26770-26775.
74. Teitelbaum SL, Ross FP. Genetic regulation of osteoclast development and function. Nat Rev Genet 2003;4(8):638-649.
75. Yao GQ, Sun B, Hammond EE, et al. The cell-surface form of colony-stimulating factor-1 is regulated by osteotropic agents and supports formation of multinucleated osteoclast-like cells. J Biol Chem 1998;273(7):4119-4128.
76. Huang JC, Sakata T, Pfleger LL, et al. PTH differentially regulates expression of RANKL and OPG. J Bone Miner Res 2004;19(2):235-244.
77. Chase LR, Aurbach GD. Parathyroid function and the renal excretion of 3'5'-adenylic acid. Proc Natl Acad Sci U S A 1967;58(2):518-525.
78. Gensure RC, Gardella TJ, Juppner H. Parathyroid hormone and parathyroid hormone–related peptide, and their receptors. Biochem Biophys Res Commun 2005;328(3):666-678.
79. Singh AT, Gilchrist A, Voyno-Yasenetskaya T, et al. Gα12/Gα13 subunits of heterotrimeric G proteins mediate parathyroid hormone activation of phospholipase D in UMR-106 osteoblastic cells. Endocrinology 2005;146(5):2171-2175.
80. Murray TM, Rao LG, Divieti P, Bringhurst FR. Parathyroid hormone secretion and action: evidence for discrete receptors for the carboxyl-terminal region and related biological actions of carboxyl-terminal ligands. Endocr Rev 2005;26(1):78-113.
81. Gaich G, Orloff JJ, Atillasoy EJ, et al. Amino-terminal parathyroid hormone–related protein: specific binding and cytosolic calcium responses in rat insulinoma cells. Endocrinology 1993;132(3):1402-1409.
82. Usdin TB, Bonner TI, Hoare SR. The parathyroid hormone 2 (PTH2) receptor. Receptors Channels 2002;8(3-4):211-218.
83. Shimizu M, Potts JT Jr, Gardella TJ. Minimization of parathyroid hormone. J Biol Chem 2000;275(29):21836-21843.
84. Takasu H, Gardella TJ, Luck MD, et al. Amino-terminal modifications of human parathyroid hormone (PTH) selectively alter phospholipase C signaling via the type 1 PTH receptor: implications for design of signal-specific PTH ligands. Biochemistry 1999;38(41):13453-13460.
85. Castro M, Nikolaev VO, Palm D, et al. Turn-on switch in parathyroid hormone receptor by a two-step parathyroid hormone binding mechanism. Proc Natl Acad Sci U S A 2005;102(44):16084-16089.
86. Vilardaga JP, Bunemann M, Krasel C, et al. Measurement of the millisecond activation switch of G protein–coupled receptors in living cells. Nat Biotechnol 2003;21(7):807-812.
87. Pellegrini M, Royo M, Rosenblatt M, et al. Addressing the tertiary structure of human parathyroid hormone-(1-34). J Biol Chem 1998;273(17):10420-10427.
88. Marx UC, Adermann K, Bayer P, et al. Solution structures of human parathyroid hormone fragments hPTH(1-34) and hPTH(1-39) and bovine parathyroid hormone fragment bPTH(1-37). Biochem Biophys Res Commun 2000;267(1):213-220.
89. Jin L, Briggs SL, Chandrasekhar S, et al. Crystal structure of human parathyroid hormone 1-34 at 0.9-A resolution. J Biol Chem 2000;275(35):27238-27244.
90. Gardella TJ, Luck MD, Fan MH, Lee C. Transmembrane residues of the parathyroid hormone (PTH)/PTH-related peptide receptor that specifically affect binding and signaling by agonist ligands. J Biol Chem 1996;271(22):12820-12825.
91. Sheikh SP, Vilardarga JP, Baranski TJ, et al. Similar structures and shared switch mechanisms of the β_2-adrenoceptor and the parathyroid hormone receptor. Zn(II) bridges between helices III and VI block activation. J Biol Chem 1999;274(24):17033-17041.
92. Bastepe M, Raas-Rothschild A, Silver J, et al. A form of Jansen's metaphyseal chondrodysplasia with limited metabolic and skeletal abnormalities is caused by a novel activating parathyroid hormone (PTH)/PTH-related peptide receptor mutation. J Clin Endocrinol Metab 2004;89(7):3595-3600.
93. Bringhurst FR, Zajac JD, Daggett AS, et al. Inhibition of parathyroid hormone responsiveness in clonal osteoblastic cells expressing a mutant form of 3',5'-cyclic adenosine monophosphate–dependent protein kinase. Mol Endocrinol 1989;3:60-67.
94. Segal JH, Pollock AS. Transfection-mediated expression of a dominant cAMP-resistant phenotype in the opossum-kidney (OK) cell line prevents parathyroid hormone–induced inhibition of Na-phosphate cotransport. J Clin Invest 1990;86:1442-1450.
95. Traebert M, Volkl H, Biber J, et al. Luminal and contraluminal action of 1-34 and 3-34 PTH peptides on renal type IIa Na-P_i cotransporter. Am J Physiol Renal Physiol 2000;278(5):F792-F798.
96. Janulis M, Tembe V, Favus MJ. Role of protein kinase C in parathyroid hormone stimulation of renal 1,25-dihydroxyvitamin D_3 secretion. J Clin Invest 1992;90(6):2278-2283.
97. Mahon MJ, Donowitz M, Yun CC, Segre GV. Na^+/H^+ exchanger regulatory factor 2 directs parathyroid hormone 1 receptor signalling. Nature 2002;417(6891):858-861.

98. Mahon MJ, Segre GV. Stimulation by parathyroid hormone of a NHERF-1-assembled complex consisting of the parathyroid hormone I receptor, phospholipase Cβ, and actin increases intracellular calcium in opossum kidney cells. J Biol Chem 2004; 279(22):23550-23558.
99. Xie LY, Leung A, Segre GV, et al. Downregulation of the PTH/PTHrP receptor by vitamin D_3 in the osteoblast-like ROS 17/2.8 cells. Am J Physiol 1996;270(4 Pt 1):E654-E660.
100. Vilardaga JP, Krasel C, Chauvin S, et al. Internalization determinants of the parathyroid hormone receptor differentially regulate β-arrestin/receptor association. J Biol Chem 2002;277(10): 8121-8129.
101. Tawfeek HA, Qian F, Abou-Samra AB. Phosphorylation of the receptor for PTH and PTHrP is required for internalization and regulates receptor signaling. Mol Endocrinol 2002;16(1):1-13.
102. Suva LJ, Winslow GA, Wettenhall RE, et al. A parathyroid hormone–related protein implicated in malignant hypercalcemia: cloning and expression. Science 1987;237(4817):893-896.
103. Orloff JJ, Reddy D, de Papp AE, et al. Parathyroid hormone–related protein as a prohormone: posttranslational processing and receptor interactions. Endocr Rev 1994;15(1):40-60.
104. Wu TL, Vasavada RC, Yang KH, et al. Structural and physiologic characterization of the mid-region secretory species of parathyroid hormone–related protein. J Biol Chem 1996;271(40): 24371-24381.
105. Burtis WJ, Brady TG, Orloff JJ, et al. Immunochemical characterization of circulating parathyroid hormone–related protein in patients with humoral hypercalcemia of cancer. N Engl J Med 1990;322:1106-1112.
106. Stewart AF. Clinical practice. Hypercalcemia associated with cancer. N Engl J Med 2005;352(4):373-379.
107. Guise TA, Yin JJ, Taylor SD, et al. Evidence for a causal role of parathyroid hormone–related protein in the pathogenesis of human breast cancer–mediated osteolysis. J Clin Invest 1996; 98(7):1544-1549.
108. Abbas SK, Pickard DW, Rodda CP, et al. Stimulation of ovine placental calcium transport by purified natural and recombinant parathyroid hormone–related protein (PTHrP) preparations. Q J Exp Physiol 1989;74:549-552.
109. Kovacs CS, Lanske B, Hunzelman JL, et al. Parathyroid hormone–related peptide (PTHrP) regulates fetal-placental calcium transport through a receptor distinct from the PTH/PTHrP receptor. Proc Nat Acad Sci U S A 1996;93(26):15233-15238.
110. VanHouten JN, Dann P, Stewart AF, et al. Mammary-specific deletion of parathyroid hormone–related protein preserves bone mass during lactation. J Clin Invest 2003;112(9):1429-436.
111. VanHouten J, Dann P, McGeoch G, et al. The calcium-sensing receptor regulates mammary gland parathyroid hormone–related protein production and calcium transport. J Clin Invest 2004; 113(4):598-608.
112. Kalkwarf HJ, Specker BL, Bianchi DC, et al. The effect of calcium supplementation on bone density during lactation and after weaning. [see comments]. N Engl J Med 1997;337(8):523-528.
113. Kalkwarf HJ, Specker BL, Ho M. Effects of calcium supplementation on calcium homeostasis and bone turnover in lactating women. J Clin Endocrinol Metab 1999;84(2):464-470.
114. Khosla S, Johansen KL, Ory SJ, et al. Parathyroid hormone–related peptide in lactation and in umbilical cord blood. Mayo Clin Proc 1990;65:1408-1414.
115. Strewler GJ. The physiology of parathyroid hormone–related protein. N Engl J Med 2000;342(3):177-185.
116. Kronenberg HM. Developmental regulation of the growth plate. Nature 2003;423(6937):332-336.
117. Maeda S, Sutliff RL, Qian J, et al. Targeted overexpression of parathyroid hormone–related protein (PTHrP) to vascular smooth muscle in transgenic mice lowers blood pressure and alters vascular contractility. Endocrinology 1999;140(4):1815-1825.
118. Chatterjee O, Nakchbandi IA, Philbrick WM, et al. Endogenous parathyroid hormone–related protein functions as a neuroprotective agent. Brain Res 2002;930(1-2):58-66.
119. Clemens TL, Cormier S, Eichinger A, et al. Parathyroid hormone–related protein and its receptors: nuclear functions and roles in the renal and cardiovascular systems, the placental trophoblasts and the pancreatic islets. Br J Pharmacol 2001;134(6):1113-1136.
120. Copp DH, Cameron EC, Cheney B, et al. Evidence for calcitonin—a new hormone from the parathyroid that lowers blood calcium. Endocrinology 1962;70:638-649.
121. Amara SG, Jones V, Rosenfeld MG, et al. Alternative RNA processing in calcitonin gene expression generates mRNAs encoding different polypeptide products. Nature 1982;298:240-244.
122. Care AD, Cooper CW, Duncan T, Orimo H. A study of thyrocalcitonin secretion by direct measurement of in vivo secretion rates in pigs. Endocrinology 1968;83:161-169.
123. Cooper CW, Borosky SA, Farrell PE, Steinsland OS. Effects of the calcium channel activator BAY-K-8644 on in vitro secretion of calcitonin and parathyroid hormone. Endocrinology 1986;118: 545-549.
124. Garrett JE, Tamir H, Kifor O, et al. Calcitonin-secreting cells of the thyroid express and extracellular calcium receptor gene. Endocrinology 1995;136(11):5202-5211.
125. Care AD. The regulation of the secretion of calcitonin. Bone Miner 1992;16:182-185.
126. Naveh-Many T, Raue F, Grauer A, Silver J. Regulation of calcitonin gene expression by hypocalcemia, hypercalcemia, and vitamin D in the rat. J Bone Miner Res 1992;7:1233-1237.
127. Peleg S, Abruzzese RV, Cooper CW, Gagel RF. Down-regulation of calcitonin gene transcription by vitamin D requires two widely separated enhancer sequences. Mol Endocrinol 1993;7:999-1008.
128. Chambers TJ, McSheehy PM, Thomson BM, Fuller K. The effect of calcium-regulating hormones and prostaglandins on bone resorption by osteoclasts disaggregated from neonatal rabbit bones. Endocrinology 1985;116(1):234-239.
129. Talmage RV, Vanderwiel CJ, Decker SA, Grubb SA. Changes produced in postprandial urinary calcium excretion by thyroidectomy and calcitonin administration in rats on different calcium regimes. Endocrinology 1979;105:459-464.
130. Hoff AO, Catala-Lehnen P, Thomas PM, et al. Increased bone mass is an unexpected phenotype associated with deletion of the calcitonin gene. J Clin Invest 2002;110(12):1849-1857.
131. Dacquin R, Davey RA, Laplace C, et al. Amylin inhibits bone resorption while the calcitonin receptor controls bone formation in vivo. J Cell Biol 2004;164(4):509-514.
132. Hurley DL, Tiegs RD, Wahner HW, Heath H. Axial and appendicular bone mineral density in patients with long-term deficiency or excess of calcitonin. N Engl J Med 1987;317:537-541.
133. Lin HY, Harris TL, Flannery MS, et al. Expression cloning of an adenylate cyclase–coupled calcitonin receptor. Science 1991;254: 1022-1024.
134. Purdue BW, Tilakaratne N, Sexton PM. Molecular pharmacology of the calcitonin receptor. Receptors Channels 2002;8(3-4):243-255.
135. Chakraborty M, Chatterjee D, Kellokumpu S, et al. Cell cycle–dependent coupling of the calcitonin receptor to different G proteins. Science 1991;251:1078-1082.
136. McLatchie L, Fraser N, Main M, et al. RAMPs regulate the transport and ligand specificity of the calcitonin-receptor–like receptor. Nature 1998;393(May 28):333-339.
137. Udawela M, Hay DL, Sexton PM. The receptor activity modifying protein family of G protein coupled receptor accessory proteins. Semin Cell Dev Biol 2004;15(3):299-308.
138. Zumpe E, Tilakaratne N, Fraser N, et al. Multiple ramp domains are required for generation of amylin receptor phenotype from the calcitonin receptor gene product. Biochem Biophys Res Commun 2000;267:368-372.
139. Gangula P, Zhao H, Supowit S, et al. Increased blood presure in α-calcitonin gene-related peptide/calcitonin gene knockout mice. Hypertension 2000;35(1 Pt 2):470-475.
140. Katafuchi T, Minamino N. Structure and biological properties of three calcitonin receptor–stimulating peptides, novel members of the calcitonin gene–related peptide family. Peptides 2004;25(11): 2039-2045.
141. Lorenzo A, Razzaboni B, Weir GC, Yankner BA. Pancreatic islet cell toxicity of amylin associated with type-2 diabetes mellitus. Nature 1994;368:756-757.
142. Wilding JPH, Khandan-Nia N, Bennet WM, et al. Lack of acute effect of amylin (islet associated polypeptide) on insulin sensitivity during hyperinsulinaemic euglycaemic clamp in humans. Diabetologia 1994;37:166-169.

143. Horcajada-Molteni MN, Davicco MJ, Lebecque P, et al. Amylin inhibits ovariectomy-induced bone loss in rats. J Endocrinol 2000;165(3):663-668.
144. Horcajada-Molteni MN, Chanteranne B, Lebecque P, et al. Amylin and bone metabolism in streptozotocin-induced diabetic rats. J Bone Miner Res 2001;16(5):958-965.
145. Samonina GE, Kopylova GN, Lukjanzeva GV, et al. Antiulcer effects of amylin: a review. Pathophysiology 2004;11(1):1-6.
146. Hinson JP, Kapas S, Smith DM. Adrenomedullin, a multifunctional regulatory peptide. Endocr Rev 2000;21(2):138-167.
147. Shimosawa T, Shibagaki Y, Ishibashi K, et al. Adrenomedullin, an endogenous peptide, counteracts cardiovascular damage. Circulation 2002;105(1):106-111.
148. Roh J, Chang CL, Bhalla A, Klein C, Hsu SY. Intermedin is a calcitonin/calcitonin gene–related peptide family peptide acting through the calcitonin receptor–like receptor/receptor activity–modifying protein receptor complexes. J Biol Chem 2004;279(8): 7264-7274.
149. Niccoli P, Brunet P, Roubicek C, et al. Abnormal calcitonin basal levels and pentagastrin response in patients with chronic renal failure on maintenance hemodialysis. Eur J Endocrinol 1995;132: 75-81.
150. O'Neill WJ, Jordan MH, Lewis MS, et al. Serum calcitonin may be a marker for inhalation injury in burns. J Burn Care Rehabil 1992;13:605-616.
151. Schinke T, Liese S, Priemel M, et al. Decreased bone formation and osteopenia in mice lacking α-calcitonin gene–related peptide. J Bone Miner Res 2004;19(12):2049-2056.
152. Szanto J, Ady N, Jozsef S. Pain killing with calcitonin nasal spray in patients with malignant tumors. Oncology 1992;49:180-182.
153. Jaeger H, Maier C. Calcitonin in phantom limb pain: a double-blind study. Pain 1992;48:21-27.
154. Holick MF, MacLaughlin JA, Clark MB, et al. Photosynthesis of previtamin D_3 in human skin and the physiologic consequences. Science 1980;210:203-205.
155. Thomas M, Demay M. Vitamin D deficiency and disorders of vitamin D metabolism. Endocrinol Metab Clin North AM 2000; 29(3):611-627.
156. Holick MF, Shao Q, Liu WW, Chen TC. The vitamin D content of fortified milk and infant formula. N Engl J Med 1992;326: 1178-1181.
157. Bikle DD, Gee E, Halloran B, et al. Assessment of the free fraction of 25-hydroxyvitamin D in serum and its regulation by albumin and the vitamin D–binding protein. J Clin Endocrinol Metab 1986;63:954-959.
158. Bikle DD, Siiteri PK, Ryzen E, Haddad JG. Serum protein binding of 1,25-dihydroxyvitamin D: A reevaluation by direct measurement of free metabolite levels. J Clin Endocrinol Metab 1985;61:969-975.
159. Safadi F, Thornton P, Magiera H, et al. Osteopathy and resistance to vitamin D toxicity in mice null for vitamin D binding protien. J Clin Invest 1999;103(2):239-251.
160. Nykjaer A, Dragun D, Walther D, et al. An endocytic pathway essential for renal uptake and activation of the steroid 25-(OH) vitamin D_3. Cell 1999;96(4):507-515.
161. Fu G, Lin D, Zang M, et al. Cloning of human 25-hydroxyvitamin D-1α-hydroxylase and mutations causing vitamin D–dependent rickets type 1. Mol Endocrinol 1997(11):1961-1970.
162. St-Arnaud R, Messerlian S, Moir J, et al. The 25-hydroxyvitamin D 1α-hydroxylase gene maps to the pseudovitamin D–deficiency rickets (PDDR) disease locus. J Bone Miner Res 1997;12(10): 1552-1559.
163. Takeyama K, Kitanaka S, Sato T, et al. 25-Hydroxyvitamin D_3 1α-hydroxylase and vitamin D synthesis. Science 1997;277(5333): 1827-1830.
164. Shimada T, Hasegawa H, Yamazaki Y, et al. FGF-23 is a potent regulator of vitamin D metabolism and phosphate homeostasis. J Bone Miner Res 2004;19(3):429-435.
165. Yoshida T, Fujimori T, Nabeshima Y. Mediation of unusually high concentrations of 1,25-dihydroxyvitamin D in homozygous klotho mutant mice by increased expression of renal 1α-hydroxylase gene. Endocrinology 2002;143(2):683-689.
166. Tsujikawa H, Kurotaki Y, Fujimori T, et al. Klotho, a gene related to a syndrome resembling human premature aging, functions in a negative regulatory circuit of vitamin D endocrine system. Mol Endocrinol 2003;17(12):2393-403.
167. Kurosu H, Ogawa Y, Miyoshi M, et al. Regulation of fibroblast growth factor–23 signaling by klotho. J Biol Chem 2006;281(10): 6120-6123.
168. Tanaka Y, Halloran B, Schnoes HK, DeLuca HF. In vitro production of 1,25-dihydroxyvitamin D_3 by rat placental tissue. Proc Nat Acad Sci U S A 1979;76:5033-5035.
169. Barbour GL, Coburn JW, Slatopolsky E, et al. Hypercalcemia in an anephric patient with sarcoidosis: evidence for extrarenal generation of 1,25-dihydroxyvitamin D. N Engl J Med 1981;305:440-443.
170. Overbergh L, Decallonne B, Valckx D, et al. Identification and immune regulation of 25-hydroxyvitamin D-1α-hydroxylase in murine macrophages. Clin Exp Immunol 2000;120(1):139-146.
171. Liu PT, Stenger S, Li H, et al. Toll-like receptor triggering of a vitamin D–mediated human antimicrobial response. Science 2006;311(5768):1770-1773.
172. Adams JS, Sharma OP, Diz MM, Endres DB. Ketoconazole decreases the serum 1,25-dihydroxyvitamin D and calcium concentration in sarcoidosis-associated hypercalcemia. J Clin Endocrinol Metab 1990;70:1090-1095.
173. Adams JS, Diz MM, Sharma OP. Effective reduction in the serum 1,25-dihydroxyvitamin D and calcium concentration in sarcoidosis-associated hypercalcemia with short-course chloroquine therapy. Ann Intern Med 1989;111:437-438.
174. St-Arnaud R, Arabian A, Travers R, et al. Deficient mineralization of intramembranous bone in vitamin D–24-hydroxylase–ablated mice is due to elevated 1,25-dihydroxyvitamin D and not to the absence of 24,25-dihydroxyvitamin D. Endocrinology 2000;141(7): 2658-2666.
175. Canterbury JM, Gavellas G, Bourgoignie JJ, Reiss E. Metabolic consequences of oral administration of 24,25-dihydroxycholecalciferol to uremic dogs. J Clin Invest 1980;65:571-576.
176. Schwartz Z, Brooks B, Swain L, Del Toro F, et al. Production of 1,25-dihydroxyvitamin D_3 and 24, 25-dihydroxyvitamin D_3 by growth zone and resting zone chondrocytes is dependent on cell maturation and is regulated by hormones and growth factors. Endocrinology 1992;130:2495-2504.
177. Pettifor JM, Bikle DD, Cavaleros M, et al. Serum levels of free 1,25-dihydroxyvitamin D in vitamin D toxicity. Ann Intern Med 1995;122:511-513.
178. Rachez C, Freedman LP. Mechanisms of gene regulation by vitamin D_3 receptor a network of coactivator interactions. Gene 2000; 246(9/21):9-21.
179. Inoue T, Kamiyama J, Sakai T. Sp1 and NF-Y synergistically mediate the effect of vitamin D_3 in the $p27^{Kip1}$ gene promotor that lacks vitamin D response elements. J Biol Chem 1999;274(45): 32309-32317.
180. Murayama A, Takeyama K, Asahina T, et al. Cloning of a novel transcription factor mediating the negative vitamin D responsiveness through the human 25-hydroxyvitamin D 1α-hydroxylase nVDRE. J Bone Miner Res 2000;15 S1:A1244.
181. Nishishita T, Okazaki T, Ishikawa T, et al. A Negative vitamin D response DNA element in the human parathyroid hormone–related peptide gene binds to vitamin D receptor along with Ku antigen to mediate negative gene regulation by vitamin D. J Biol Chem 1998;273(18):10901-10907.
182. Godschalk M, Levy JR, Downs RW Jr. Glucocorticoids decrease vitamin D receptor number and gene expression in human osteosarcoma cells. J Bone Miner Res 1992;7:21-27.
183. Iida K, Shinki T, Yamaguchi A, et al. A possible role of vitamin D receptors in regulating vitamin D activation in the kidney. Proc Natl Acad Sci U S A 1995;92:6112-6116.
184. Caffrey JM, Farach-Carson MC. Vitamin D_3 metabolites modulate dihydropyridine-sensitive calcium currents in clonal rat osteosarcoma cells. J Biol Chem 1989;264:20265-20274.
185. Nemere I, Dormanen MC, Hammond MW, et al. Identification of a specific binding protein for 1a,25-dihydroxyvitamin D_3 in basal-lateral membranes of chick intestinal epithelium and relationship to transcaltachia. J Biol Chem 1994;269:23750-23756.
186. Barsony J, Marx SJ. Rapid accumulation of cyclic GMP near activated vitamin D receptors. Proc Natl Acad Sci U S A 1991; 88:1436-1440.
187. Erben RG, Soegiarto DW, Weber K, et al. Deletion of deoxyribonucleic acid binding domain of the vitamin D receptor abrogates

genomic and nongenomic functions of vitamin D. Mol Endocrinol 2002;16(7):1524-1537.

188. Hughes MR, Malloy PJ, Kieback DG, Ket al. Point mutations in the human vitamin D receptor gene associated with hypocalcemic rickets. Science 1988;242:1702-1705.
189. Amling M, Priemel M, Holzmann T, et al. Rescue of the skeletal phenotype of vitamin D receptor–ablated mice in the setting of normal mineral ion homeostasis: formal histomorphometric and biomechanical analyses. Endocrinology 1999;140(11):4982-4987.
190. Balsan S, Garabedian M, Larchet M, et al. Long-term nocturnal calcium infusions can cure rickets and promote normal mineralization in hereditary resistance to 1,25-dihydroxyvitamin D. J Clin Invest 1986;77:1661-1667.
191. Li YC, Amling M, Pirro AE, et al. Normalization of mineral ion homeostasis by dietary means prevents hyperparathyroidism, rickets, and osteomalacia, but not alopecia in vitamin D receptor–ablated mice. Endocrinology 1998;139(10):4391-4396.
192. van Os CH. Transcellular calcium transport in intestinal and renal epithelial cells. Biochim Biophys Acta 1987;906:195-222.
193. Karbach U. Paracellular calcium transport across the small intestine. J Nutr 1992;122:672-677.
194. Hoenderop JG, van der Kemp AWCM, Hartog A, et al. Molecular identification of the Apical Ca^{2+} channel in 1,25-dihydroxyvitamin D_3-responsive epithelia. J Biol Chem 1999;274(13):8375-8378.
195. Peng J, Chen X, Berger UV, et al. Molecular cloning and characterization of a channel-like transporter mediating intestinal calcium absorption. J Biol Chem 1999;274(32):22739-22746.
196. van de Graaf SF, Boullart I, Hoenderop JG, Bindels RJ. Regulation of the epithelial Ca^{2+} channels TRPV5 and TRPV6 by 1α,25-dihydroxy vitamin D_3 and dietary Ca^{2+}. J Steroid Biochem Mol Biol 2004;89-90(1-5):303-308.
197. Hoenderop JG, van Leeuwen JP, van der Eerden BC, et al. Renal Ca^{2+} wasting, hyperabsorption, and reduced bone thickness in mice lacking TRPV5. J Clin Invest 2003;112(12):1906-1914.
198. Kaune R, Munson S, Bikle DD. Regulation of calmodulin binding to the ATP extractable 110 kDa protein (myosin I) from chicken duodenal brush border by $1,25(OH)_2D_3$. Biochim Biophys Acta 1994;1190:329-336.
199. Cai Q, Chandler JS, Wasserman RH, et al. Vitamin D and adaptation to dietary calcium and phosphate deficiencies increase intestinal plasma membrane calcium pump gene expression. Proc Natl Acad Sci U S A 1993;90:1345-1349.
200. Wasserman RH, Chandler JS, Meyer SA, et al. Intestinal calcium transport and calcium extrusion processes at the basolateral membrane. J Nutr 1992;122:662-671.
201. Harrison JR, Petersen DN, Lichtler AC, et al. 1,25-dihydroxyvitamin D_3 inhibits transcription of type I collagen genes in the rat osteosarcoma line ROS 17/2.8. Endocrinology 1989;125:327–333.
202. Price PA. Vitamin K–dependent formation of bone Gla protein (osteocalcin) and its function. Vitam Horm 1985;42:65-108.
203. Yasuda H, Shima N, Nakagawa N, et al. Osteoclast differentiation factor is a ligand for osteoprotegerin/osteoclastogenesis-inhibitory factor and is identical to TRANCE/RANKL. Proc Natl Acad Sci U S A 1998;95(7):3597-3602.
204. Halline AG, Davidson NO, Skarosi SF, et al. Effects of 1,25-dihydroxyvitamin D_3 on proliferation and differentiation of Caco-2 cells. Endocrinology 1994;134:1710-1717.
205. Shabahang M, Buras RR, Davoodi F, et al. Growth inhibition of HT-29 human colon cancer cells by analogues of 1,25-dihydroxyvitamin D_3. Cancer Res 1994;54:4057-4064.
206. Mathieu C, Laureys J, Waer M, Bouillon R. Prevention of autoimmune destruction of transplanted islets in spontaneously diabetic NOD mice by KH1060, a 20-epi analog of vitamin D: synergy with cyclosporine. Transplant Proc 1994;26:3128-3129.
207. Brown AJ, Ritter CR, Finch JL, et al. The noncalcemic analogue of vitamin D, 22-oxacalcitriol, suppresses parathyroid hormone synthesis and secretion. J Clin Invest 1989;84:728-732.
208. Holick MF, Smith E, Pincus S. Skin as the site of vitamin D synthesis and target tissue for 1,25-dihydroxyvitamin D_3. Use of calcitriol (1,25-dihydroxyvitamin D_3) for treatment of psoriasis. Arch Dermatol 1987;123:1677-1683.
209. Hoeck HC, Laurberg G, Laurberg P. Hypercalcemia crisis after excessive topical use of a vitamin D derivative. J Intern Med 1994;235:281-282.
210. Kamimura S, Gallieni M, Kubodera N, et al. Differential catabolism of 22-oxacalcitriol and 1,25-dihydroxyvitamin D_3 by normal human peripheral monocytes. Endocrinology 1993;133:2719-2722.
211. Peleg S, Sastry M, Collins ED, et al. Distinct conformational changes induced by 20-epi analogues of 1α,25-dihydroxyvitamin D_3 are associated with enhanced activation of the vitamin D receptor. J Biol Chem 1995;270:10551-10558.
212. Autosomal dominant hypophosphataemic rickets is associated with mutations in FGF23. Nat Genet 2000;26(3):345-348.
213. White KE, Carn G, Lorenz-Depiereux B, et al. Autosomal-dominant hypophosphatemic rickets (ADHR) mutations stabilize FGF-23. Kidney Int 2001;60(6):2079-2086.
214. Shimada T, Muto T, Urakawa I, et al. Mutant FGF-23 responsible for autosomal dominant hypophosphatemic rickets is resistant to proteolytic cleavage and causes hypophosphatemia in vivo. Endocrinology 2002;143(8):3179-3182.
215. Shimada T, Mizutani S, Muto T, et al. Cloning and characterization of FGF23 as a causative factor of tumor-induced osteomalacia. Proc Natl Acad Sci U S A 2001;98(11):6500-6505.
216. White KE, Jonsson KB, Carn G, et al. The autosomal dominant hypophosphatemic rickets (ADHR) gene is a secreted polypeptide overexpressed by tumors that cause phosphate wasting. J Clin Endocrinol Metab 2001;86(2):497-500.
217. Ward LM, Rauch F, White KE, et al. Resolution of severe, adolescent-onset hypophosphatemic rickets following resection of an FGF-23-producing tumour of the distal ulna. Bone 2004;34(5): 905-911.
218. Araya K, Fukumoto S, Backenroth R, et al. A novel mutation in fibroblast growth factor 23 gene as a cause of tumoral calcinosis. J Clin Endocrinol Metab 2005;90(10):5523-5527.
219. Chefetz I, Heller R, Galli-Tsinopoulou A, et al. A novel homozygous missense mutation in FGF23 causes familial tumoral calcinosis associated with disseminated visceral calcification. Hum Genet 2005;118(2):261-266.
220. Larsson T, Yu X, Davis SI, et al. A novel recessive mutation in fibroblast growth factor-23 causes familial tumoral calcinosis. J Clin Endocrinol Metab 2005;90(4):2424-2427.
221. Larsson T, Marsell R, Schipani E, et al. Transgenic mice expressing fibroblast growth factor 23 under the control of the $\alpha1$(I) collagen promoter exhibit growth retardation, osteomalacia, and disturbed phosphate homeostasis. Endocrinology 2004;145(7):3087-3094.
222. Shimada T, Kakitani M, Yamazaki Y, et al. Targeted ablation of Fgf23 demonstrates an essential physiological role of FGF23 in phosphate and vitamin D metabolism. J Clin Invest 2004;113(4): 561-568.
223. Sitara D, Razzaque MS, Hesse M, et al. Homozygous ablation of fibroblast growth factor-23 results in hyperphosphatemia and impaired skeletogenesis, and reverses hypophosphatemia in Phex-deficient mice. Matrix Biol 2004;23(7):421-432.
224. Razzaque M, Sitara D, Taguchi T, et al. Premature aging–like phenotype in fibroblast growth factor 23 null mice is a vitamin D–mediated process. FASEB J 2006;20:720-722.
225. Saito H, Kusano K, Kinosaki M, et al. Human fibroblast growth factor-23 mutants suppress Na^+-dependent phosphate co-transport activity and 1α,25-dihydroxyvitamin D_3 production. J Biol Chem 2003;278(4):2206-2211.
226. Segawa H, Kawakami E, Kaneko I, et al. Effect of hydrolysis-resistant FGF23-R179Q on dietary phosphate regulation of the renal type-II Na/Pi transporter. Pflugers Arch 2003;446(5): 585-592.
227. Yan X, Yokote H, Jing X, et al. Fibroblast growth factor 23 reduces expression of type IIa Na^+/Pi co-transporter by signaling through a receptor functionally distinct from the known FGFRs in opossum kidney cells. Genes Cells 2005;10(5):489-502.
228. Miyamoto K, Ito M, Kuwahata M, et al. Inhibition of intestinal sodium-dependent inorganic phosphate transport by fibroblast growth factor 23. Ther Apher Dial 2005;9(4):331-335.
229. Yu X, Sabbagh Y, Davis SI, et al. Genetic dissection of phosphate- and vitamin D–mediated regulation of circulating Fgf23 concentrations. Bone 2005;36(6):971-977.
230. Perwad F, Azam N, Zhang MY, et al. Dietary and serum phosphorus regulate fibroblast growth factor 23 expression and 1,25-dihydroxyvitamin D metabolism in mice. Endocrinology 2005;146(12): 5358-5364.

231. Nakanishi S, Kazama JJ, Nii-Kono T, et al. Serum fibroblast growth factor-23 levels predict the future refractory hyperparathyroidism in dialysis patients. Kidney Int 2005;67(3):1171-1178.
232. Koiwa F, Kazama JJ, Tokumoto A, et al. Sevelamer hydrochloride and calcium bicarbonate reduce serum fibroblast growth factor 23 levels in dialysis patients. Ther Apher Dial 2005;9(4):336-339.
233. Nussbaum SR, Zahradnik RJ, Lavigne JR, et al. Highly sensitive two-site immunoradiometric assay of parathyrin and its clinical utility in evaluating patients with hypercalcemia. Clin Chem 1987;33:1364-1367.
234. Gao P, D'Amour P. Evolution of the parathyroid hormone (PTH) assay—importance of circulating PTH immunoheterogeneity and of its regulation. Clin Lab 2005;51(1-2):21-29.
235. Boudou P, Ibrahim F, Cormier C, et al. Third- or second-generation parathyroid hormone assays: a remaining debate in the diagnosis of primary hyperparathyroidism. J Clin Endocrinol Metab 2005; 90(12):6370-6372.
236. Ratcliffe WA, Hutchesson ACJ, Bundred NJ, Ratcliffe JG. Role of assays for parathyroid-hormone–related protein in investigation of hypercalcaemia. Lancet 1992;339:164-167.
237. Isomura M, Honda N, Kawada A, et al. Development of a highly sensitive enzyme immunoasay for human calcitonin using solid phase coupled with multiple antibodies. Ann Clin Biochem 1999;36(5):629-635.
238. Lavigne JR, Zahradnik RJ, Conklin RL, et al. Stimulation of calcitonin secretion by calcium receptor activators: evaluation using a new, highly sensitive, homologous immunoradiometric assay for rat calcitonin. Endocrine 1998;9(3):293-301.
239. Hollis B. Quantitation of 25-hydroxyvitamin D and 1,25-dihydroxyvitamin D by radioimmunoassay using radioiodinated tracers. Methods Enzymol 1997;282:174-186.
240. Ersfeld DL, Rao DS, Body JJ, et al. Analytical and clinical validation of the 25 OH vitamin D assay for the LIAISON automated analyzer. Clin Biochem 2004;37(10):867-874.
241. Jonsson KB, Zahradnik R, Larsson T, et al. Fibroblast growth factor 23 in oncogenic osteomalacia and X-linked hypophosphatemia. N Engl J Med 2003;348(17):1656-1663.
242. Yamazaki Y, Okazaki R, Shibata M, et al. Increased circulatory level of biologically active full-length FGF-23 in patients with hypophosphatemic rickets/osteomalacia. J Clin Endocrinol Metab 2002;87(11):4957-4960.
243. Burnett SA, Gunawardene SC, Bringhurst FR, et al. Regulation of C-terminal and intact FGF-23 by dietary phosphate in men and women. J Bone Miner Res 2006;21(8):1187-1196.
244. Weber CJ, Sewell CW, McGarity WC. Persistent and recurrent sporadic primary hyperparathyroidism: histopathology, complications, and results of reoperation. Surgery 1994;116(6):991-998.
245. Shane E, Bilezikian JP. Parathyroid carcinoma: a review of 62 patients. Endocr Rev 1982;3:218-226.
246. Patten BM, Bilezikian JP, Mallette LE, et al. Neuromuscular disease in hyperparathyroidism. Ann Intern Med 1974;80:182-193.
247. Wermers RA, Khosla S, Atkinson EJ, et al. The rise and fall of primary hyperparathyroidism: a population-based study in Rochester, Minnesota, 1965-1992. Ann Intern Med 1997;126(6):433-440.
248. Lundgren E, Rastad J, Thrufjell E, et al. Population-based screening for primary hyperparathyroidism with serum calcium and parathyroid hormone values in menopausal women. Surgery 1997;121(3):287-294.
249. Silverberg SJ, Shane E, Jacobs TP, et al. A 10-year prospective study of primary hyperparathyroidism with or without parathyroid surgery [see comments]. N Engl J Med 1999;341(17):1249-1255.
250. Clark OH. Presidential address: "Asymptomatic" primary hyperparathyroidism: is parathyroidectomy indicated? Surgery 1994; 116:947-953.
251. Pasieka JL, Parsons LL. Prospective surgical outcome study of relief of symptoms following surgery in patients with primary hyperparathyroidism. World J Surg 1998;22(6):513-518; discussion 518-519.
252. Walgenbach S, Hommel G, Junginger T. Outcome after surgery for primary hyperparathyroidism: ten-year prospective follow-up study. World J Surg 2000;24(5):564-569.
253. Kleerekoper M, Bilezkian JP. A cure in search of a disease: parathyroidectomy for nontraditional features of primary hyperparathyroidism [editorial; comment]. Am J Med 1994;96(2):99-100.
254. Palmer M, Adami HO, Bergstrom R, et al. Mortality after surgery for primary hyperparathyroidism: a followup of 441 patients operated on from 1956-1979. Surgery 1987;102:1-7.
255. Hedback G, Tisell LE, Bengtsson BA, et al. Premature death in patients operated on for primary hyperparathyroidism. World J Surgery 1990;14:829-836.
256. Silverberg SJ, Bilezikian JP, Bone HG, et al. Therapeutic controversies in primary hyperparathyroidism. J Clin Endocrinol Metab 1999;84(7):2275-2285.
257. Stefenelli T, Abela C, Frank H, et al. Cardiac abnormalities in patients with primary hyperparathyroidism: implications for follow-up. J Clin Endocrinol Metab 1997;82(1):106-112.
258. Wermers RA, Khosla S, Atkinson EJ, et al. Survival after the diagnosis of hyperparathyroidism: a population-based study. Am J Med 1998;104(2):115-122.
259. Palmer M, Adami HO, Krusemo UB, Ljunghall S. Increased risk of malignant diseases after surgery for primary hyperparathyroidism. A nationwide cohort study. Am J Epidemiol 1988;127:1031-1040.
260. Parisien M, Silverberg SJ, Shane E, et al. The histomorphometry of bone in primary hyperparathyroidism: preservation of cancellous bone structure. J Clin Endocrinol Metab 1990;70:930-938.
261. Alhava EM. Bone mineral density and surgical treatment of primary hyperparathyroidism. Acta Chir Scand 1988;154:345-347.
262. Silverberg SJ, Gartenberg F, Jacobs TP, et al. Longitudinal measurements of bone density and biochemical indices in untreated primary hyperparathyroidism. J Clin Endocrinol Metab 1995; 80(3):723-728.
263. Silverberg SJ, Locker FG, Bilezikian JP. Verterbral osteopenia: a new indication for surgery in primary hyperparathyroidism. J Clin Endocrinol Metab 1996;81:4007-4012.
264. Khosla S, Melton LJI, Wermers RA, et al. Primary hyperparathyroidism and the risk of fracture: a population-based study. J Bone Miner Res 1999;14:1700-1707.
265. Vestergaard P, Mollerup CL, Frokjaer VG, et al. Cohort study of risk of fracture before and after surgery for primary hyperparathyroidism. BMJ 2000;321(7261):598-602.
266. Mitlak B, Daly M, Potts JJ, et al. Asymptomatic primary hyperparathyroidism. J Bone Miner Res 1991;6:S103-S110.
267. Rao DS, Wilson RJ, Kleerekoper M, Parfitt AM. Lack of biochemical progression or continuation of accelerated bone loss in mild asymptomatic primary hyperparathyroidism: evidence for biphasic disease course. J Clin Endocrinol Metab 1988;67:1294-1298.
268. Bilezikian JP, Potts JT Jr, Fuleihan Gel H, et al. Summary statement from a workshop on asymptomatic primary hyperparathyroidism: a perspective for the 21st century. J Clin Endocrinol Metab 2002;87(12):5353-5361.
269. Arnold A, Staunton CE, Kim HG, et al. Monoclonality and abnormal parathyroid hormone genes in parathyroid adenomas. N Engl J Med 1988;318:658-662.
270. Arnold A, Shattuck TM, Mallya SM, et al. Molecular pathogenesis of primary hyperparathyroidism. J Bone Miner Res 2002;17(suppl 2):N30-N36.
271. Motokura T, Bloom T, Kim HG, et al. A BCL1-linked candidate oncogene which is rearranged in parathyroid tumors encodes a novel cyclin. Nature 1991;350:512-515.
272. Mallya SM, Gallagher JJ, Wild YK, et al. Abnormal parathyroid cell proliferation precedes biochemical abnormalities in a mouse model of primary hyperparathyroidism. Mol Endocrinol 2005; 19(10):2603-2609.
273. Schneider AB, Gierlowski TC, Shore-Freedman E, et al. Dose-response relationships for radiation-induced hyperparathyroidism. J Clin Endocrinol Metab 1995;80(1):254-257.
274. Carling T. Molecular pathology of parathyroid tumors. Trends Endocrinol Metab 2001;12(2):53-58.
275. Imanishi Y, Tahara H, Palanisamy N, et al. Clonal chromosomal defects in the molecular pathogenesis of refractory hyperparathyroidism of uremia. J Am Soc Nephrol 2002;13(6):1490-1498.
276. Davies M. Hyperparathyroidism in X-linked hypophosphataemic osteomalacia. Clin Endocrinol 1995;42:205-206.
277. Mallette LE, Khouri K, Zengotita H, et al. Lithium treatment increases intact and midregion parathyroid hormone and parathyroid volume. J Clin Endocrinol Metab 1989;68(3):654-660.
278. Arnold A, Brown MF, Urena P, et al. Monoclonality of parathyroid tumors in chronic renal failure and in primary parathyroid hyperplasia. J Clin Invest 1995;95:2047-2053.

279. Friedman E, Sakaguchi K, Bale AE, et al. Clonality of parathyroid tumors in familial multiple endocrine neoplasia type I. N Engl J Med 1989;321:213-218.
280. Livolsi V. Parathyroids: morphology and pathology. In Bilezikian J (ed). The Parathyroids: Basic and Clinical Concepts, 2nd ed. San Diego: Academic Press, 2001:1-16.
281. Kifor O, Moore FD, Wang P, et al. Reduced immunostaining for the extracellular Ca^{2+}-sensing receptor in primary and uremic secondary hyperparathyroidism. J Clin Endocrinol Metab 1996;81(4): 1598-1606.
282. Marx SJ. Molecular genetics of multiple endocrine neoplasia types 1 and 2. Nat Rev Cancer 2005;5(5):367-375.
283. Hughes CM, Rozenblatt-Rosen O, Milne TA, et al. Menin associates with a trithorax family histone methyltransferase complex and with the hoxc8 locus. Mol Cell 2004;13(4):587-597.
284. Karnik SK, Hughes CM, Gu X, et al. Menin regulates pancreatic islet growth by promoting histone methylation and expression of genes encoding p27Kipl and pl8INK4c. Proc Natl Acad Sci U S A 2005;102(41):14659-14664.
285. Rao DS, Phillips ER, Divine GW, Talpos GB. Randomized controlled clinical trial of surgery versus no surgery in patients with mild asymptomatic primary hyperparathyroidism. J Clin Endocrinol Metab 2004;89(11):5415-5422.
286. Silverberg SJ, Brown I, Bilezikian JP. Age as a criterion for surgery in primary hyperparathyroidism. Am J Med 2002;113(8):681-684.
287. Nakaoka D, Sugimoto T, Kobayashi T, et al. Prediction of bone mass change after parathyroidectomy in patients with primary hyperparathyroidism. J Clin Endocrinol Metab 2000;85(5): 1901-1907.
288. Insogna KL, Mitnick ME, Stewart AF, et al. Sensitivity of the parathyroid hormone–1,25-dihydroxyvitamin D axis to variations in calcium intake in patients with primary hyperparathyroidism. N Engl J Med 1985;313:1126-1130.
289. Rubin MR, Lee KH, McMahon DJ, Silverberg SJ. Raloxifene lowers serum calcium and markers of bone turnover in postmenopausal women with primary hyperparathyroidism. J Clin Endocrinol Metab 2003;88(3):1174-1178.
290. Khan AA, Bilezikian JP, Kung AW, et al. Alendronate in primary hyperparathyroidism: a double-blind, randomized, placebo-controlled trial. J Clin Endocrinol Metab 2004;89(7):3319-3325.
291. Chow CC, Chan WB, Li JK, et al. Oral alendronate increases bone mineral density in postmenopausal women with primary hyperparathyroidism. J Clin Endocrinol Metab 2003;88(2):581-587.
292. Peacock M, Bilezikian JP, Klassen PS, et al. Cinacalcet hydrochloride maintains long-term normocalcemia in patients with primary hyperparathyroidism. J Clin Endocrinol Metab 2005;90(1): 135-141.
293. Grant CS, Thompson G, Farley D, van Heerden J. Primary hyperparathyroidism surgical management since the introduction of minimally invasive parathyroidectomy: Mayo Clinic experience. Arch Surg 2005;140(5):472-478; discussion 478-479.
294. Ruda JM, Hollenbeak CS, Stack BC Jr. A systematic review of the diagnosis and treatment of primary hyperparathyroidism from 1995 to 2003. [Review] [225 refs]. Otolaryngol Head Neck Surg 2005;132(3):359-372.
295. Gaz R, Doubler PB, Wang C. The management of 50 unusual hyperfunctioning parathyroid glands. Surgery 1987;102:949-957.
296. Akerstrom G, Rundberg C, Grimelius L, et al. Causes of failed primary exploration and technical aspects of reoperation in primary hyperparathyroidism. World J Surg 1992;16:562-569.
297. Oertli D, Richter M, Kraenzlin M, et al. Parathyroidectomy in primary hyperparathyroidism: preoperative localization and routine biopsy of unaltered glands are not necessary. Surgery 1995;117(4):392-396.
298. Doppman JL, Miller DL. Localization of parathyroid tumors in patients with asymptomatic hyperparathyroidism and no previous surgery. J Bone Miner Res 1991;6 (suppl):S153-S158.
299. Mitchell BK, Merrell RC, Kinder BK. Localization studies in patients with hyperparathyroidism. Surg Clin N Am 1995;75(3):483-498.
300. Udelsman R, Donovan PI. Open minimally invasive parathyroid surgery. World J Surg 2004;28(12):1224-1226.
301. Irvin GL 3rd, Carneiro DM, Solorzano CC. Progress in the operative management of sporadic primary hyperparathyroidism over 34 years. Ann Surg 2004;239(5):704-708; discussion 708-711.
302. Milas M, Wagner K, Easley KA, Siperstein A, Weber CJ. Double adenomas revisited: nonuniform distribution favors enlarged superior parathyroids (fourth pouch disease). Surgery 2003;134(6): 995-1003; discussion 1003-1004.
303. Inabnet WB. Intraoperative parathyroid hormone monitoring. World J Surg 2004;28(12):1212-1215.
304. Weber KJ, Misra S, Lee JK, et al. Intraoperative PTH monitoring in parathyroid hyperplasia requires stricter criteria for success. Surgery 2004;136(6):1154-1159.
305. Elaraj DM, Skarulis MC, Libutti SK, et al. Results of initial operation for hyperparathyroidism in patients with multiple endocrine neoplasia type 1. Surgery 2003;134(6):858-864; discussion 864-865.
306. Cupisti K, Raffel A, Dotzenrath C, et al. Primary hyperparathyroidism in the young age group: particularities of diagnostic and therapeutic schemes. World J Surg 2004;28(11):1153-1156.
307. Lambert LA, Shapiro SE, Lee JE, et al. Surgical treatment of hyperparathyroidism in patients with multiple endocrine neoplasia type 1. Arch Surg 2005;140(4):374-382.
308. Bergenfelz A, Valdermarsson S, Ahren B. Functional recovery of the parathyroid glands after surgery for primary hyperparathyroidism. Surgery 1994;116(5):827–836.
309. Gross ND, Weissman JL, Veenker E, Cohen JI. The diagnostic utility of computed tomography for preoperative localization in surgery for hyperparathyroidism. Laryngoscope 2004;114(2):227–231.
310. Biertho LD, Kim C, Wu HS, et al. Relationship between sestamibi uptake, parathyroid hormone assay, and nuclear morphology in primary hyperparathyroidism. J Am Coll Surg 2004;199(2): 229-233.
311. Estella E, Leong MS, Bennett I, et al. Parathyroid hormone venous sampling prior to reoperation for primary hyperparathyroidism. A N Z J Surg 2003;73(10):800-805.
312. Chaffanjon PC, Voirin D, Vasdev A, et al. Selective venous sampling in recurrent and persistent hyperparathyroidism: indication, technique, and results. World J Surg 2004;28(10):958-961.
313. MacFarlane MP, Fraker DL, Shawker TH, et al. Use of preoperative fine-needle aspiration in patients undergoing reoperation for primary hyperparathyroidism. Surgery 1994;116(6):959-964.
314. Smythe WR, Bavaria JE, Hall RA, et al. Thoracoscopic removal of mediastinal parathyroid adenoma. Ann Thorac Surg 1995;59(1): 236-238.
315. Nomura R, Sugimoto T, Tsukamoto T, et al. Marked and sustained increase in bone mineral density after parathyroidectomy in patients with primary hyperparathyroidism; a six-year longitudinal study with or without parathyroidectomy in a Japanese population. Clin Endocrinol 2004;60(3):335-342.
316. Martin P. Long-term irreversibility of bone loss after surgery. Arch Intern Med 1990;150:1495-1497.
317. Pollak MR, Brown EM, Chou YH, et al. Mutations in the human Ca^{2+}-sensing receptor gene cause familial hypocalciuric hypercalcemia and neonatal severe hyperparathyroidism. Cell 1993;75(7): 1297-1303.
318. Kifor O, Moore FD Jr, Delaney M, et al. A syndrome of hypocalciuric hypercalcemia caused by autoantibodies directed at the calcium-sensing receptor. J Clin Endocrinol Metab 2003;88(1): 60-72.
319. Pallais JC, Kifor O, Chen YB, et al. Acquired hypocalciuric hypercalcemia due to autoantibodies against the calcium-sensing receptor. N Engl J Med 2004;351(4):362-369.
320. Carling T, Szao E, Bai M, et al. Familial hypercalcemia and hypercalciuria caused by a novel mutation in the cytoplasmic tail of the calcium receptor. J Clin Endocrinol Metab 2000;85(5):2042-2047.
321. Marx SJ, Attie MF, Levine MA, et al. The hypocalciuric or benign variant of familial hypercalcemia: clinical and biochemical features in fifteen kindreds. Medicine (Baltimore) 1981;60(6): 397-412.
322. Bendz H, Sjodin I, Toss G, Berglund K. Hyperparathyroidism and long-term lithium therapy—a cross-sectional study and the effect of lithium withdrawal. J Intern Med 1996;240(6):357-365.
323. Hundley JC, Woodrum DT, Saunders BD, et al. Revisiting lithium-associated hyperparathyroidism in the era of intraoperative parathyroid hormone monitoring. Surgery 2005;138(6):1027–1031; discussion 1031-1032.
324. Jacobs TP, Bilezikian JP. Clinical review: rare causes of hypercalcemia. J Clin Endocrinol Metab 2005;90(11):6316-622.

325. Ehrlich LA, Roodman GD. The role of immune cells and inflammatory cytokines in Paget's disease and multiple myeloma. Immunol Rev 2005;208:252-266.
326. Guise TA. Molecular mechanisms of osteolytic bone metastases. Cancer 2000;88(12 Suppl):2892-2898.
327. Case records of the Massachusetts General Hospital (case 27461). New Eng J Med 1941;225:789-791.
328. Stewart AF, Horst R, Deftos LJ, et al. Biochemical evaluation of patients with cancer-associated hypercalcemia: evidence for humoral and nonhumoral groups. N Engl J Med 1980;303(24): 1377-1383.
329. Kukreja SC, Shevrin DH, Wimbiscus SA, et al. Antibodies to parathyroid hormone–related protein lower serum calcium in athymic mouse models of malignancy-associated hypercalcemia due to human tumors. J Clin Invest 1988;82:1798-1802.
330. Horwitz MJ, Tedesco MB, Sereika SM, et al. Continuous PTH and PTHrP infusion causes suppression of bone formation and discordant effects on 1,25$(OH)_2$ vitamin D. J Bone Miner Res 2005;20(10): 1792-1803.
331. Strewler GJ, Wronski TJ, Halloran BP. Pathogenesis of hypercalcemia in nude mice bearing a human renal carcinoma. Endocrinology 1986;119:303-309.
332. Bushinsky DA, Riera GS, Favus MJ, Coe FL. Evidence that blood ionized calcium can regulate serum 1,25$(OH)_2D_3$ independently of parathyroid hormone and phosphorus in the rat. J Clin Invest 1985;76:1599-1604.
333. Ikeda K, Ogata E. Humoral hypercalcemia of malignancy: some enigmas on the clinical features. J Cell Biochem 1995;57:384-391.
334. Seymour JF, Gagel RF, Hagemeister FB, et al. Calcitriol production in hypercalcemic and normocalcemic patients with non-Hodgkin lymphoma. Ann Intern Med 1994;121:633-640.
335. Davies M, Hayes ME, Yin JA, et al. Abnormal synthesis of 1,25-dihydroxyvitamin D in patients with malignant lymphoma. J Clin Endocrinol Metab 1994;78(5):1202-1207.
336. Selby PL, Davies M, Marks JS, Mawer EB. Vitamin D intoxication causes hypercalcaemia by increased bone resorption which responds to pamidronate. Clin Endocrinol (Oxf) 1995;43(5): 531-536.
337. Conron M, Young C, Beynon HL. Calcium metabolism in sarcoidosis and its clinical implications. Rheumatology (Oxf) 2000;39(7): 707-713.
338. Kruithoff KL, Gyetko MR, Scheiman JM. Giant splenomegaly and refractory hypercalcemia due to extrapulmonary sarcoidosis. Arch Intern Med 1993;153:2793-2796.
339. Vidal M, Ramana CV, Dusso AS. Stat1–vitamin D receptor interactions antagonize 1,25-dihydroxyvitamin D transcriptional activity and enhance stat1-mediated transcription. Mol Cell Biol 2002; 22(8):2777-2787.
340. Abreu MT, Kantorovich V, Vasiliauskas EA, et al. Measurement of vitamin D levels in inflammatory bowel disease patients reveals a subset of Crohn's disease patients with elevated 1,25-dihydroxyvitamin D and low bone mineral density. Gut 2004;53(8):1129-136.
341. Bassett JH, Williams GR. The molecular actions of thyroid hormone in bone. Trends Endocrinol Metab 2003;14(8):356-364.
342. Mallette LE, Rubenfeld S, Silverman V. A controlled study of the effects of thyrotoxicosis and propranolol treatment on mineral metabolism and parathyroid hormone immunoreactivity. Metabolism 1985;34:999-1006.
343. Valentic JP, Elias AN, Weinstein GD. Hypercalcemia associated with oral isotretinoin in the treatment of severe acne. J Am Med Assoc 1986;250:1899-1900.
344. Muls E, Bouillon R, Boelaert J, et al. Etiology of hypercalcemia in a patient with Addison's disease. Calcif Tissue Int 1982;34: 523-526.
345. Nijenhuis T, Vallon V, van der Kemp AW, et al. Enhanced passive Ca^{2+} reabsorption and reduced Mg^{2+} channel abundance explains thiazide-induced hypocalciuria and hypomagnesemia. J Clin Invest 2005;115(6):1651-1658.
346. Picolos MK, Lavis VR, Orlander PR. Milk-alkali syndrome is a major cause of hypercalcaemia among non–end-stage renal disease (non-ESRD) inpatients. Clin Endocrinol (Oxf) 2005;63(5): 566-576.
347. Sato Y, Honda Y, Iwamoto J, et al. Abnormal bone and calcium metabolism in immobilized Parkinson's disease patients. Mov Disord 2005;20(12):1598-603.
348. Llach F, Felsenfeld AJ, Haussler MR. The pathophysiology of altered calcium metabolism in rhabdomyolysis-induced acute renal failure. N Engl J Med 1981;305:117-123.
349. Shrestha SM, Berry JL, Davies M, Ballardie FW. Biphasic hypercalcemia in severe rhabdomyolysis: serial analysis of PTH and vitamin D metabolites. A case report and literature review. Am J Kidney Dis 2004;43(3):e31-e35.
350. Williams JCP, Barratt-Boyes BG, Lowe JB. Supravalvular aortic stenosis. Circulation 1961;24:1311-1318.
351. Garabedian M, Jacqz E, Guillozo H, et al. Elevated plasma 1,25-dihydroxyvitamin D concentrations in infants with hypercalcemia and an elfin facies. N Engl J Med 1985;312:948-952.
352. Frangiskakis JM, Ewart AK, Morris CA, et al. LIM-kinase 1 hemizygosity implicated in impaired visuospacial constructive cognition. Cell 1996;86:59-69.
353. Kitagawa H, Fujiki R, Yoshimura K, et al. The chromatin-remodeling complex WINAC targets a nuclear receptor to promoters and is impaired in Williams syndrome. Cell 2003;113(7):905-917.
354. Kruse K, Schutz C. Calcium metabolism in the Jansen type of metaphyseal dysplasia. Eur J Pediatr 1993;152(11):912-915.
355. Schipani E, Kruse K, Juppner H. A constitutively active mutant PTH-PTHrP receptor in Jansen-type metaphyseal chondrodysplasia. Science 1995;268(5207):98-100.
356. Schipani E, Lanske B, Hunzelman J, et al. Targeted expression of constitutively active receptors for parathyroid hormone and parathyroid hormone–related peptide delays endochondral bone formation and rescues mice that lack parathyroid hormone–related peptide. Proc Nat Acad Sci U S A 1997;94(25):13689-13694.
357. Silverberg SJ, Gao P, Brown I, et al. Clinical utility of an immunoradiometric assay for parathyroid hormone (1-84) in primary hyperparathyroidism. J Clin Endocrinol Metab 2003;88(10): 4725-4730.
358. Carnevale V, Dionisi S, Nofroni I, et al. Potential clinical utility of a new IRMA for parathyroid hormone in postmenopausal patients with primary hyperparathyroidism. Clinical Chemistry 2004; 50(3):626-631.
359. Barman Balfour JA, Scott LJ. Cinacalcet hydrochloride. Drugs 2005;65(2):271-281.
360. Onuma E, Sato K, Saito H, et al. Generation of a humanized monoclonal antibody against human parathyroid hormone–related protein and its efficacy against humoral hypercalcemia of malignancy. Anticancer Res 2004;24(5A):2665-2673.
361. Connor TB, Rosen BL, Blaustein MP, et al. Hypocalcemia precipitating congestive heart failure. N Engl J Med 1982;307:869-872.
362. Zaloga GP, Willey S, Tomasic P, Chernow B. Free fatty acids alter calcium binding: A cause for misinterpretation of serum calcium values and hypocalcemia in critical illness. J Clin Endocrinol Metab 1987;64:1010-1014.
363. Bockman DE, Kirby ML. Dependence of thymus development on derivatives of the neural crest. Science 1984;223:498-500.
364. Chisaka O, Capecchi MR. Regionally restricted developmental defects resulting from targeted disruption of the mouse homeobox gene *hox-1.5*. Nature 1991;350:473-479.
365. Garabedian M. Hypocalcemia and chromosome 22q11 microdeletion. Genet Couns 1999;10(4):389-394.
366. Karayiorgou M, Morris MA, Morrow B, et al. Schizophrenia susceptibility associated with interstitial deletions of chromosome 22q11. Proc Natl Acad Sci U S A 1995;92:7612-7616.
367. Budarf ML, Collins J, Gong W, et al. Cloning a balanced translocation associated with DiGeorge syndrome and identification of a disrupted candidate gene. Nat Genet 1995;10:269-278.
368. Scire G, Dallapiccola B, Iannetti P, et al. Hypoparathyroidism as the major manifestation in two patients with 22q11 deletions. Am J Med Genet 1994;52:478-482.
369. Merscher S, Funke B, Epstein JA, et al. *TBX1* is responsible for cardiovascular defects in velo-cardio-facial/DiGeorge syndrome. Cell 2001;104(4):619-629.
370. Daw S, Taylor C, Kraman M, et al. A common region of 10p deleted and velocardiofacial syndromes. Nat Gen 1996;13(4):458-460.
371. Van Esch H, Groenen P, Nesbit MA, et al. *GATA3* haplo-insufficiency causes human HDR syndrome. Nature 2000;406:419-422.
372. Parvari R, Hershkovitz E, Grossman N, et al. Mutation of TBCE causes hypoparathyroidism-retardation-dysmorphism and autosomal recessive Kenny-Caffey syndrome. Nat Genet 2002;32(3): 448-452.

373. Su MA, Anderson MS. Aire: an update. Curr Opin Immunol 2004;16(6):746-752.
374. Papadimitriou A, Hadjigeorgiou G, Divari R, et al. The influence of coenzyme Q10 on total serum calcium concentration in two patients with Kearns-Sayre syndrome ana hypoparathyroidism. Neuromuscul Disord 1996;6(1):49-53.
375. Ahn TG, Antonarakis SE, Kronenberg HM, et al. Familial isolated hypoparathyroidism: a molecular genetic analysis of 8 families with 23 affected persons. Medicine 1986;65:73-81.
376. Baldellou A, Bone J, Tamparillas M, et al. Congenital hypoparathyroidism, ocular colobomata, unilateral renal agenesis and dysmorphic features. Genet Couns 1991;2:245-247.
377. Parkinson DB, Thakker RV. A donor splice site mutation in the parathyroid hormone gene is associated with autosomal recessive hypoparathyroidism. Nat Genet 1992;2:149-152.
378. Hammes M, DeMory A, Sprague SM. Hypocalcemia in end-stage renal disease: a consequence of spontaneous parathyroid gland infarction. Am J Kidney Dis 1994;24:519-522.
379. Burch WM, Posillico JT. Hypoparathyroidism after I-131 therapy with subsequent return of parathyroid function. J Clin Endocrinol Metab 1983;57:398-401.
380. Gertner JM, Broadus AE, Anast CS, et al. Impaired parathyroid response to induced hypocalcemia in thalassemia major. J Pediatr 1979;95:210-213.
381. Carpenter TO, Carnes DL, Anast CS. Hypoparathyroidism in Wilson's disease. N Engl J Med 1983;309:873-877.
382. Suh SM, Tashjian AH, Matsuo N, et al. Pathogenesis of hypocalcemia in primary hypomagnesemia: normal end-organ responsiveness to parathyroid hormone, impaired parathyroid gland function. J Clin Invest 1973;52:153-160.
383. Rude RK, Oldham SB, Singer FR. Functional hypoparathyroidism and parathyroid hormone end-organ resistance in human magnesium deficiency. Clin Endocrinol 1976;5:209-224.
384. Krapf R, Jaeger P, Hulter HN, et al. Chronic respiratory alkalosis induces renal PTH-resistance, hyperphosphatemia and hypocalcemia in humans. Kidney Int 1992;42:727-734.
385. Lopez I, Rodriguez M, Felsenfeld AJ, et al. Direct suppressive effect of acute metabolic and respiratory alkalosis on parathyroid hormone secretion in the dog. J Bone Miner Res 2003;18(8): 1478-1485.
386. Albright F, Aub J, Bauer W. Hyperparathyroidism. A common and polymorphic condition as illustrated by seventeen proved cases from one clinic. J Am Med Assoc 1934;102:1276-1287.
387. Farfel Z, Brickman AS, Kaslow HR, et al. Defect of receptor-cyclase coupling protein in pseudohypoparathyroidism. N Engl J Med 1980;303:237-242.
388. Mallette LE, Kirkland JL, Gagel RF, et al. Synthetic human parathyroid hormone-(1-34) for the study of pseudohypoparathyroidism. J Clin Endocrinol Metab 1988;67:964-972.
389. Carter A, Bardin C, Collins R, et al. Reduced expression of multiple forms of the α subunit of the stimulatory GTP-binding protein in pseudohypoparathyroidism type 1a. Proc Natl Acad Sci USA 1987;84:7266-7269.
390. Levine MA, Ahn TG, Klupt SF, et al. Genetic deficiency of the α subunit of the guanine nucleotide-binding protein Gs as the molecular basis for Albright hereditary osteodystrophy. Proc Natl Acad Sci U S A 1988;85:617-621.
391. Weinstein LS, Gejman PV, de Mazancourt P, et al. A heterozygous 4-bp deletion mutation in the Gsα gene *(GNAS1)* in a patient with Albright hereditary osteodystrophy. Genomics 1992;13:1319-1321.
392. Farfel Z, Friedman E. Mental deficiency in pseudohypoparathyroidism type I is associated with Ns-protein deficiency. Ann Intern Med 1986;105:197-199.
393. Iiri T, Herzmark P, Nakamoto JM, et al. Rapid GDP release from Gsα in patients with gain and loss of endocrine function. Nature 1994;371:164-168.
394. Wilson LC, Oude Luttikhuis ME, et al. Parental origin of Gsα gene mutations in Albright's hereditary osteodystrophy. J Med Genet 1994;31:835-839.
395. Yu S, Yu D, Lee E, et al. Variable and tissue-specific hormone resistance in heterotrimeric G_s protein α-subunit ($G_s\alpha$) knockout mice is due to tissue-specific imprinting of the $G_s\alpha$ gene. Proc Natl Acad Sci U S A 1998;95:8715-8720.
396. Farfel Z, Bourne H, Iiri T. The expanding spectrum of G protein diseases. N Engl J Med 1999;340(13):1012-1020.
397. Bastepe M, Lane AH, Juppner H. Paternal uniparental isodisomy of chromosome 20q—and the resulting changes in *GNAS1* methylation—as a plausible cause of pseudohypoparathyroidism. Am J Hum Genet 2001;68(5):1283-1239.
398. Bastepe M, Pincus JE, Sugimoto T, et al. Positional dissociation between the genetic mutation responsible for pseudohypoparathyroidism type Ib and the associated methylation defect at exon A/B: evidence for a long-range regulatory element within the imprinted *GNAS1* locus. Hum Mol Genet 2001;10(12):1231-1241.
399. Liu J, Erlichman B, Weinstein LS. The stimulatory G protein alpha-subunit Gs alpha is imprinted in human thyroid glands: implications for thyroid function in pseudohypoparathyroidism types 1A and 1B. J Clin Endocrinol Metab 2003;88(9):4336-4341.
400. Murray TM, Rao LG, Wong MM, et al. Pseudohypoparathyroidism with osteitis fibrosa cystica: direct demonstration of skeletal responsiveness to parathyroid hormone in cells cultured from bone. J Bone Miner Res 1993;8:83-91.
401. Jüppner H, Schipani E, Bastepe M, et al. The gene responsible for pseudohypoparathyroidism type Ib is paternally imprinted and maps in four unrelated kindreds to chromosome 20q13.3. Proc Natl Acad Sci U S A 1998;95:11798-11803.
402. Liu J, Litman D, Rosenberg MJ, et al. A *GNAS1* imprinting defect in pseudohypoparathyroidism type Ib. J Clin Invest 2000;106(9): 1167-1174.
403. Bastepe M, Frohlich LF, Hendy GN, et al. Autosomal dominant pseudohypoparathyroidism type Ib is associated with a heterozygous microdeletion that likely disrupts a putative imprinting control element of *GNAS*. J Clin Invest 2003;112(8):1255-1263.
404. Linglart A, Gensure RC, Olney RC, et al. A novel *STX16* deletion in autosomal dominant pseudohypoparathyroidism type Ib redefines the boundaries of a *cis*-acting imprinting control element of *GNAS*. Am J Hum Genet 2005;76(5):804-814.
405. Bastepe M, Frohlich LF, Linglart A, et al. Deletion of the *NESP55* differentially methylated region causes loss of maternal GNAS imprints and pseudohypoparathyroidism type Ib. Nat Genet 2005;37(1):25-27.
406. Barrett D, Breslau NA, Wax MB, et al. New form of pseudohypoparathyroidism with abnormal catalytic adenylate cyclase. Am J Physiol 1989;257:E277-E283.
407. Linglart A, Carel JC, Garabedian M, et al. GNAS1 lesions in pseudohypoparathyroidism Ia and Ic: genotype phenotype relationship and evidence of the maternal transmission of the hormonal resistance. J Clin Endocrinol Metab 2002;87(1):189-197.
408. Drezner M, Neelon FA, Lebovitz HE. Pseudohypoparathyroidism type II: a possible defect in the reception of the cyclic AMP signal. N Engl J Med 1973;289:1056-1060.
409. Konoshita M, Komori T, Ohtake T, et al. Abnormal calcium metabolism in myotonic dystrophy as shown by the Ellsworth-Howard test and its relation to CTG triplet repeat length. J Neurol 1997;244: 613-622.
410. Koo BB, Schwindinger WF, Levine MA. Characterization of Albright hereditary osteodystrophy and related disorders. Acta Pediatr Sin 1995;36:3-13.
411. Minagawa M, Yasuda T, Kobayashi Y, Niimi H. Transient pseudohypoparathyroidism of the neonate. Eur J Endocrinol 1995; 133:151-155.
412. Silve C. Pseudohypoparathyroidism syndromes: the many faces of parathyroid hormone resistance. Eur J Endocrinol 1995; 133:145-146.
413. Kruse K, Kracht U, Wohlfart K, Kruse U. Biochemical markers of bone turnover, intact serum parathyroid hormone and renal calcium excretion in patients with pseudohypoparathyroidism and hypoparathyroidism before and during vitamin D treatment. Eur J Pediatr 1989;148:535-539.
414. Breslau NA, Moses AM, Pak CYC. Evidence for bone remodeling but lack of calcium mobilization response to parathyroid hormone in pseudohypoparathyroidism. J Clin Endocrinol Metab 1983;57: 638-644.
415. Ish-Shalom S, Rao LG, Levine MA, et al. Normal parathyroid hormone responsiveness of bone-derived cells from a patient with pseudohypoparathyroidism. J Bone Miner Res 1996;11:8-14.
416. Yamamoto M, Takuwa Y, Masuko S, Ogata E. Effects of endogenous and exogenous parathyroid hormone on tubular reabsorption of calcium in pseudohypoparathyroidism. J Clin Endocrinol Metab 1988;66(3):618-625.

417. Rao DS, Parfitt AM, Kleerekoper M, et al. Dissociation between the effects of endogenous parathyroid hormone on adenosine 3',5'-monophosphate generation and phosphate reabsorption in hypocalcemia due to vitamin D depletion: an acquired disorder resembling pseudohypoparathyroidism type II. J Clin Endocrinol Metab 1985;61:285-290.
418. Thomas MK, Lloyd-Jones DM, Thadhani RI, et al. Hypovitaminosis D in medical patients. N Engl J Med 1998;338(12):777-783.
419. Chapuy MC, Arlot ME, Duboeuf F, et al. Vitamin D_3 and calcium to prevent hip fractures in elderly women. N Engl J Med 1992; 327:1637-1642.
420. Brodie MJ, Boobis AR, Hillyard CJ, et al. Effect of rifampicin and isoniazid on vitamin D metabolism. Clin Pharmacol Ther 1982; 32:525-530.
421. Casella SJ, Reiner BJ, Chen TC, et al. A possible genetic defect in 25-hydroxylation as a cause of rickets. J Pediatr 1994;124: 929-932.
422. Goodman WG. Calcimimetic agents for the treatment of secondary hyperparathyroidism. Semin Nephrol 2004;24(5):460-463.
423. Delvin EE, Glorieux FH, Marie PJ, Pettifor JM. Vitamin D dependency: replacement therapy with calcitriol. Pediatrics 1981;99: 26-34.
424. Kitanaka S, Takeyama K, Murayama A, et al. Inactivating mutations in the 25-hydroxyvitamin D, 1α-hydroxylase gene in patients with pseudovitamin D–deficiency rickets. N Engl J Med 1998;338(10): 653-661.
425. Wang J, Lin C-J, Burridge S, et al. Genetics of vitamin D 1α-hyroxylase deficiency in 17 families. Am J Hum Gen 1998(63): 1694-1702.
426. Malloy PJ, Pike JW, Feldman D. The vitamin D receptor and the syndrome of hereditary 1,25-dihydroxyvitamin D–resistant rickets. Endocr Rev 1999;20(2):156-188.
427. Fraher LJ, Karmali R, Hinde FRJ, et al. Vitamin D–dependent rickets type II: extreme end organ resistance to 1,25-dihydroxy vitamin D_3 in a patient without alopecia. Eur J Pediatr 1986;145: 389-395.
428. Takeda E, Yokota I, Kawakami I, et al. Two siblings with vitamin-D–dependent rickets type II: no recurrence of rickets for 14 years after cessation of therapy. Eur J Pediatr 1989;149:54-57.
429. Marx SJ, Liberman UA, Eil C, et al. Hereditary resistance to 1,25-dihydroxyvitamin D. Recent Prog Horm Res 1984;40:589-615.
430. Kido Y, Okamura T, Tomikawa M, et al. Hypocalcemia associated with 5-fluorouracil and low dose leucovorin in patients with advanced colorectal or gastric carcinomas. Cancer 1996;78(8): 1794-1797.
431. Dembinski TC, Yatscoff RW, Blandford DE. Thyrotoxicosis and hungry bone syndrome—a cause of posttreatment hypocalcemia. Clin Biochem 1994;27:69-74.
432. Jacobson MA, Gambertoglio JG, Aweeka FT, et al. Foscarnet-induced hypocalcemia and effects of foscarnet on calcium metabolism. J Clin Endocrinol Metab 1991;72:1130-1135.
433. Aggeler PM, Perkins HA, Watkins HB. Hypocalcemia and defective hemostasis after massive blood transfusion. Report of a case. Transfusion 1967;7:35-39.
434. Kao W, Dart R, Kuffner E, Bogdan G. Ingestion of low-concentration hydrofluoric acid: an insidious and potentially fatal poisoning. Ann Emerg Med 1999;34(1):35-41.
435. Tsang RC, Kleinman LI, Sutherland JM, Light IJ. Hypocalcemia in infants of diabetic mothers. J Pediatr 1972;80:384-395.
436. Kaplan EL, Burrington JD, Klementschitsch P, et al. Primary hyperparathyroidism, pregnancy and neonatal hypocalcemia. Surgery 1984;96:717-722.
437. Kuehn E, Anders H, Bogner J, et al. Hypocalcemia in HIV infection and AIDS. J Intern Med 1999(245):69-73.
438. Lind L, Carlstedt F, Rastad J, et al. Hypocalcemia and parathyroid hormone secretion in critically ill patients. Crit Care Med 2000;28(1):93-99.
439. Canaff L, Hendy GN. Calcium-sensing receptor gene transcription is up-regulated by the proinflammatory cytokine, interleukin-1β. Role of the NF-κB pathway and κB elements. J Biol Chem 2005;280(14):14177-14188.
440. Stewart AF, Longo W, Kreutter D, et al. Hypocalcemia associated with calcium-soap formation in a patient with a pancreatic fistula. N Engl J Med 1986;315:496-498.
441. Dettelbach MA, Deftos LJ, Stewart AF. Intraperitoneal free fatty acids induce severe hypocalcemia in rats: a model for the hypocalcemia of pancreatitis. J Bone Miner Res 1990;5:1249-1255.
442. Norberg HP, DeRoos J, Kaplan EL. Increased parathyroid hormone secretion and hypocalcemia in experimental pancreatitis: Necessity for an intact thyroid gland. Surgery 1975;77:773-779.
443. Weir GC, Lesser PB, Drop LJ, et al. The hypocalcemia of acute pancreatitis. Ann Intern Med 1975;83:185-189.
444. Desai TK, Carlson RW, Geheb MA. Prevalence and clinical implications of hypocalcemia in acutely ill patients in a medical intensive care setting. Am J Med 1988;84:209-214.
445. Winer KK, Ko CW, Reynolds JC, et al. Long-term treatment of hypoparathyroidism: a randomized controlled study comparing parathyroid hormone-(1-34) versus calcitriol and calcium. J Clin Endocrinol Metab 2003;88(9):4214-4220.
446. Gupta A, Winer K, Econs MJ, et al. FGF-23 is elevated by chronic hyperphosphatemia. J Clin Endocrinol Metab 2004;89(9): 4489-4492.
447. Okano K, Furukawa Y, Hirotoshi M, Fujita T. Comparative efficacy of various vitamin D metabolites in the treatment of various types of hypoparathyroidism. J Clin Endocrinol Metab 1982;55:238-242.
448. Corvilain J, Abramow M. Growth and renal control of plasma phosphate. J Clin Endocrinol Metab 1972;34:452-459.
449. Schwartz E, Wiedman E, Simon S, Schiffer M. Estrogenic antagonism of metabolic effects of administered growth hormone. J Clin Endocrinol Metab 1969;29:1176.
450. Lyles KW, Halsey DL, Friedman NE, Lobaugh B. Correlations of serum concentrations of 1,25-dihydroxyvitamin D, phosphorous, and parathyroid hormone in tumoral calcinosis. J Clin Endocrinol Metab 1988;67:88-92.
451. Larsson T, Davis SI, Garringer HJ, et al. Fibroblast growth factor-23 mutants causing familial tumoral calcinosis are differentially processed. Endocrinology 2005;146(9):3883-3891.
452. Topaz O, Shurman DL, Bergman R, et al. Mutations in *GALNT3*, encoding a protein involved in *O*-linked glycosylation, cause familial tumoral calcinosis. Nat Genet 2004;36(6):579-581.
453. Chernow B, Rainey TG, Georges LP, O'Brian JT. Iatrogenic hyperphosphatemia: a metabolic consideration in critical care medicine. Crit Care Med 1981;9:772-774.
454. McBryde KD, Wilcox J, Kher KK. Hyperphosphatemia due to fosphenytoin in a pediatric ESRD patient. Pediatric Nephrology 2005;20(8):1182-1185.
455. Markowitz GS, Stokes MB, Radhakrishnan J, D'Agati VD. Acute phosphate nephropathy following oral sodium phosphate bowel purgative: an underrecognized cause of chronic renal failure. J Am Soc Nephrol 2005;16(11):3389-3396.
456. O'Connor LR, Klein KL, Bethune JE. Hyperphosphatemia in lactic acidosis. N Engl J Med 1977;297:707-709.
457. Miller PD, Heinig RE, Waterhouse C. Treatment of alcoholic ketoacidosis. Arch Intern Med 1978;138:57-72.
458. Marcu CB, Hotchkiss M. Pseudohyperphosphatemia in a patient with multiple myeloma. Conn Med 2004;68(2):71-72.
459. Spencer H, Lewin I, Samachson J, Lazlo J. Changes in metabolism in obese persons during starvation. Am J Med 1966;40:27–37.
460. Silvis SE, Paragas PU Jr. Paresthesias, weakness, seizures and hypophosphatemia in patients receiving hyperalimentation. Gastroenterology 1972;62:513-520.
461. Berman E, Nicolaides M, Maki RG, et al. Altered bone and mineral metabolism in patients receiving imatinib mesylate. N Engl J Med 2006;354(19):2006-2013.
462. Quarles LD. FGF23, PHEX, and MEPE regulation of phosphate homeostasis and skeletal mineralization. Am J Physiol Endocrinol Metab 2003;285(1):E1-E9.
463. Schiavi SC, Kumar R. The phosphatonin pathway: new insights in phosphate homeostasis. Kidney Int 2004;65(1):1-14.
464. Berndt TJ, Schiavi S, Kumar R. "Phosphatonins" and the regulation of phosphorus homeostasis. Am J Physiol Renal Physiol 2005;289(6):F1170-F1182.
465. Ito N, Fukumoto S, Takeuchi Y, et al. Comparison of two assays for fibroblast growth factor (FGF)-23. J Bone Miner Metab 2005;23(6): 435-440.
466. Yamamoto T, Imanishi Y, Kinoshita E, et al. The role of fibroblast growth factor 23 for hypophosphatemia and abnormal regulation of vitamin D metabolism in patients with McCune-Albright syndrome. J Bone Miner Metab 2005;23(3):231-237.

467. Riminucci M, Collins MT, Fedarko NS, et al. FGF-23 in fibrous dysplasia of bone and its relationship to renal phosphate wasting. J Clin Invest 2003;112(5):683-692.
468. Hoffman WH, Jueppner HW, Deyoung BR, et al. Elevated fibroblast growth factor-23 in hypophosphatemic linear nevus sebaceous syndrome. Am J Med Genet 2005;134(3):233-236.
469. Rendina D, Mossetti G, De Filippo G, et al. Fibroblast growth factor 23 is increased in calcium nephrolithiasis with hypophosphatemia and renal phosphate leak. J Clin Endocrinol Metab 2006;91(3): 959-963.
470. Prie D, Huart V, Bakouh N, et al. Nephrolithiasis and osteoporosis associated with hypophosphatemia caused by mutations in the type 2a sodium-phosphate cotransporter. N Engl J Med 2002; 347(13):983-991.
471. Bergwitz C, Roslin NM, Tieder M, et al. *SLC34A3* mutations in patients with hereditary hypophosphatemic rickets with hypercalciuria predict a key role for the sodium phosphate cotransporter NaPi IIc in maintaining phosphate homeostasis. Am J Hum Genet 2006;78(2):179-192.
472. Lorenz-Depiereux B, Benet-Pages A, Eckstein G, et al. Hereditary hypophosphatemic rickets with hypercalciuria is caused by mutations in the sodium phosphate cotransporter gene *SLC34A3*. Am J Hum Genet 2006;78(2):193-201.
473. Green J, Debby H, Lederer E, et al. Evidence for a PTH-independent humoral mechanism in post-transplant hypophosphatemia and phosphaturia. Kidney Int 2001;60(3):1182-1196.
474. Salem RR, Tray K. Hepatic resection-related hypophosphatemia is of renal origin as manifested by isolated hyperphosphaturia. Ann Surg 2005;241(2):343-348.
475. Chung PY, Sitrin MD, Te HS. Serum phosphorus levels predict clinical outcome in fulminant hepatic failure. Liver Transpl 2003;9(3):248-253.
476. Daily WH, Tonnesen AS, Allen SJ. Hypophosphatemia. Incidence, etiology and prevention in the trauma patient. Crit Care Med 1990;18:1210-1214.
477. Fiaccadori E, Coffrini E, Ronda N, et al. Hypophosphatemia in course of chronic obstructive pulmonary disease. Prevalence, mechanisms, and relationships with skeletal muscle phosphorus content. Chest 1990;97:857-868.
478. Vanneste J, Hage J. Acute severe hypophosphatemia mimicking Wernicke's encephalopathy. Lancet 1986;1:44.
479. Singhal PC, Kumar A, Desroches L, et al. Prevalence and predictors of rhabdomyolysis in patients with hypophosphatemia. Am J Med 1992;92:458-464.
480. Gabow PA, Kaehny WD, Kelleher SP. The spectrum of rhabdomyolysis. Medicine (Baltimore)1982;61:141-152.
481. Aubier M, Murciano D, Lecocguic Y, et al. Effect of hypophosphatemia on diaphragmatic contractility in patients with acute respiratory failure. N Engl J Med 1985;3131:420-424.
482. Bollaert PE, Levy B, Nace L, et al. Hemodynamic and metabolic effects of rapid correction of hypophosphatemia in patients with septic shock. Chest 1995;107(6):1698-1701.
483. Rasmussen A, Buus S, Hessov I. Postoperative myocardial performance during glucose-induced hypophosphatemia. Acta Chir Scand 1985;151:13-15.
484. Yawata Y, Hebbel RP, Silvis S, et al. Blood cell abnormalities complicating the hypophosphatemia of hyperalimentation: erythrocyte and platelet ATP deficiency associated with hemolytic anemia and bleeding in hyperalimented dogs. J Lab Clin Med 1974;84: 643-653.
485. Lichtman MA, Miller DR, Cohen J, Waterhouse C. Reduced red cell glycolysis, 2,3-diphosphoglycerate and adenosine triphosphate concentration and increased hemoglobin oxygen affinity caused by hypophosphatemia. Ann Intern Med 1971;74:562-568.
486. Travis SF, Sugerman HJ. Alterations in red-cell glycolytic intermediates and oxygen transport as a consequence of hypophosphatemia in patients receiving intravenous hyperalimentation. N Engl J Med 1971;285:763-768.
487. DeFronzo RA, Lang R. Hypophosphatemia and glucose interolerance: evidence for tissue insensitivity to insulin. N Engl J Med 1980;202:1259-1263.
488. Wilson HK, Keuer SP, Lea AS, et al. Phosphate therapy in diabetic ketoacidosis. Arch Intern Med 1982;142:517-520.
489. Keller U, Berger W. Prevention of hypophosphatemia by phosphate infusion during treatment of diabetic ketoacidosis and hypersmolar coma. Diabetes 1980;29:87-95.
490. Rosen GH, Boullata JI, O'Rangers EA, et al. Intravenous phosphate repletion regimen for critically ill patients with moderate hypophosphatemia. Crit Care Med 1995;23(7):1204-1210.
491. Clark CL, Sacks GS, Dickerson RN, et al. Treatment of hypophosphatemia in patients receiving specialized nutrition support using a graduated dosing scheme: results from a prospective clinical trial. Crit Care Med 1995;23:1504-1511.
492. Charron T, Bernard F, Skrobik Y, et al. Intravenous phosphate in the intensive care unit: more aggressive repletion regimens for moderate and severe hypophosphatemia. Intensive Care Med 2003;29(8):1273-1278.
493. Taylor BE, Huey WY, Buchman TG, et al. Treatment of hypophosphatemia using a protocol based on patient weight and serum phosphorus level in a surgical intensive care unit. J Am Coll Surg 2004;198(2):198-204.
494. Broner CW, Stidham GL, Westenkirchner DF, Tolley EA. Hypermagnesemia and hypocalcemia as predictors of high mortality in critically ill pediatric patients. Crit Care Med 1990;18(9):921-928.
495. Mordes JP, Wacker WE. Excess magnesium. Pharmacol Rev 1978;29:273-300.
496. Cao Z, Bideau R, Valdes R Jr, Elin RJ. Acute hypermagnesemia and respiratory arrest following infusion of $MgSO_4$ for tocolysis. Clin Chim Acta 1999;285(1-2):191-193.
497. Rasch DK, Huber PA, Richardson CJ, et al. Neurobehavioral effects of neonatal hypermagnesemia. J Pediatr 1982;100(2):272-276.
498. Brand JM, Greer FR. Hypermagnesemia and intestinal perforation following antacid administration in a premature infant. Pediatrics 1990;85(1):121-124.
499. Mordes JP, Swartz R, Arky RA. Extreme hypermagnesemia as a cause of refractory hypotension. Ann Intern Med 1975;83(5): 657-658.
500. Ferdinandus J, Pederson JA, Whang R. Hypermagnesemia as a cause of refractory hypotension, respiratory depression, and coma. Arch Intern Med 1981;141(5):669-670.
501. Cholst IN, Steinberg SF, Tropper PJ, et al. The influence of hypermagnesemia on serum calcium and parathyroid hormone levels in human subjects. N Engl J Med 1984;310:1221-1225.
502. Cruikshank DP, Pitkin RM, Donnelly E, Reynolds WA. Urinary magnesium, calcium, and phosphate excretion during the magnesium sulfate infusion. Obstet Gynecol 1981;58:430-434.
503. Fassler CA, Rodriguez RM, Badesch DB, et al. Magnesium toxicity as a cause of hypotension and hypoventilation. Occurrence in patients with normal renal function. Arch Intern Med 1985;145(9): 1604-1606.
504. Al-Ghamdi SMG, Cameron EC, Sutton RAL. Magnesium deficiency: pathophysiologic and clinical overview. [Review]. Am J Kid Dis 1994;24(5):737-752.
505. Schmitz C, Perraud AL, Fleig A, Scharenberg AM. Dual-function ion channel/protein kinases: novel components of vertebrate magnesium regulatory mechanisms. Pediatr Res 2004;55(5):734-737.
506. Ellison DH. Divalent cation transport by the distal nephron: insights from Bartter's and Gitelman's syndromes. Am J Physiol Renal Physiol 2000;279(4):F616-F625.
507. Konrad M, Schlingmann KP, Gudermann T. Insights into the molecular nature of magnesium homeostasis. Am J Physiol Renal Physiol 2004;286(4):F599-F605.
508. Schlingmann KP, Konrad M, Seyberth HW. Genetics of hereditary disorders of magnesium homeostasis. Pediatr Nephrol 2004;19(1): 13-25.
509. Nagase T, Murakami T, Tsukada T, et al. A family of autosomal dominant hypocalcemia with a positive correlation between serum calcium and magnesium: identification of a novel gain of function mutation (Ser(820)Phe) in the calcium-sensing receptor. J Clin Endocrinol Metab 2002;87(6):2681-2687.
510. Simon DB, Nelson-Williams C, Bia MJ, et al. Gitelman's variant of Bartter's syndrome, inherited hypokalaemic alkalosis, is caused by mutations in the thiazide-sensitive Na-Cl cotransporter. Nature Genetics 1996;12(1):24-30.
511. Meij IC, Koenderink JB, De Jong JC, et al. Dominant isolated renal magnesium loss is caused by misrouting of the N^{a+},K^+-ATPase gamma-subunit. Ann N Y Acad Sci 2003;986:437-443.

512. Kantorovich V, Adams JS, Gaines JE, et al. Genetic heterogeneity in familial renal magnesium wasting. J Clin Endocrinol Metab 2002;87(2):612-617.
513. Wilson FH, Hariri A, Farhi A, et al. A cluster of metabolic defects caused by mutation in a mitochondrial tRNA. Science 2004; 306(5699):1190-1194.
514. Shils ME. Experimental human magnesium depletion. Medicine (Baltimore) 1969;48:61-85.
515. Mather HM, Nisbet JA, Burton GH, et al. Hypomagnesemia in diabetes. Clin Chim Acta 1979;95:235-242.
516. Martin HE. Clinical magnesium deficiency. Ann N Y Acad Sci 1969;162:891-900.
517. Laitinen K, Lamberg-Allardt C, Tunninen R, et al. Transient hypoparathyroidism during acute alcohol intoxication. N Engl J Med 1991;324:721-727.
518. Schilsky RI, Anderson T. Hypomagnesemia and renal magnesium wasting in patients receiving cisplatin. Ann Intern Med 1979;90:929-931.
519. Martin M, Diaz RE, Casado A, et al. Intravenous and oral magnesium supplementations in the prophylaxis of cisplatin-induced hypomagnesemia. Results of a controlled trial. Am J Clin Oncol 1992;15(4):348-351.
520. Beller GA, Hood DB, Smith TW, et al. Correlation of serum magnesium levels and cardiac digitalis intoxication. Am J Cardiol 1974;33:225-229.
521. Rude RK, Singer FR. Magnesium deficiency and excess. Ann Rev Med 1981;32:245-259.
522. Allgrove J, Adami S, Fraher L, et al. Hypomagnesemia: studies of parathyroid hormone secretion and function. Clin Endocrinol 1984;21:435-449.
523. Quitterer U, Hoffmann M, Freichel M, Lohse MJ. Paradoxical block of parathormone secretion is mediated by increased activity of G alpha subunits. J Biol Chem 2001;276(9):6763-6769.
524. Johannesson AJ, Raisz LG. Effects of low media magnesium concentration on bone resorption in response to parathyroid hormone and 1,25-dihydroxyvitamin D in organ culture. Endocrinology 1983;113:2294-2298.
525. Medalle R, Waterhouse C, Hahn TJ. Vitamin D resistance in magnesium deficiency. Am J Clin Nutr 1976;29:854-858.
526. Rosler A, Rabinowitz D. Magnesium induced reversal of vitamin D resistance in hypoparathyroidism. Lancet 1973;1:803-805.
527. Rude RK, Adams JS, Ryzen E, et al. Low serum concentrations of 1,25-dihydroxyvitamin D in human magnesium deficiency. J Clin Endocrinol Metab 1985;61:933-940.
528. Fuss M, Bergmann P, Bergans A, et al. Correction of low circulating levels of 1,25-dihydroxyvitamin D by 25-hydroxyvitamin D during reversal of hypomagnesaemia. Clin Endocrinol 1989;31:31-38.
529. Brannan PG, Vergne-Marini P, Pak CYC, et al. Magnesium absorption in the human small intestine. J Clin Invest 1976;57:1412-1418.
530. Sutton RAL, Walker VR, Halabe A, et al. Chronic hypomagnesemia caused by cisplatin: effect of calcitriol. J Lab Clin Med 1991;117:40-43.

CHAPTER 28

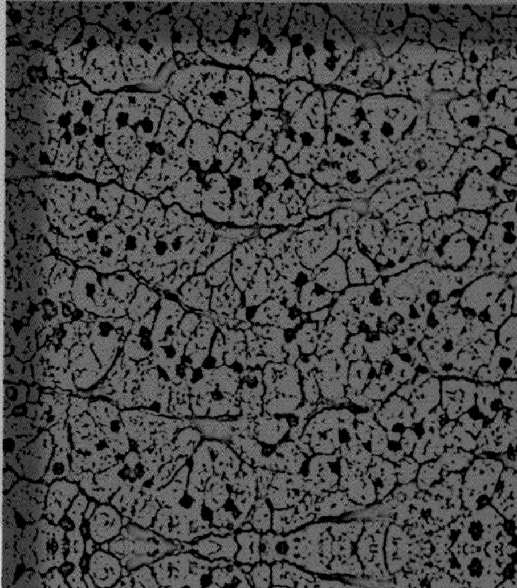

METABOLIC BONE DISEASE

Joseph A. Lorenzo, Ernesto Canalis and Lawrence G. Raisz

STRUCTURE AND FUNCTION OF THE SKELETON

The skeleton is one of the largest organ systems in the body. It consists of a mineralized matrix with a small, but highly active cellular fraction. The skeleton serves a structural function and also serves as a storehouse of minerals, and as such it plays an essential role in the maintenance of serum calcium levels. Imbalance between the structural and the metabolic functions of the skeleton can be important in the pathogenesis of bone diseases.[1]

Embryology and Anatomy

In the embryo, skeletal development begins with the condensation of mesenchyme into an anlagen of future bones. Bone formation then occurs through either endochondral or intramembranous bone formation.[2] The growth of long bones and of the vertebrae involves endochondral bone formation (Fig. 28–1). This process begins when mesenchymal condensations differentiate into cartilage, which then generates a characteristic matrix and directs the invasion of blood vessels and osteoblasts. The osteoblasts replace the dying chondrocytes and lay down a bone matrix to replace that generated by the chondrocytes. Throughout bone lengthening, cartilage remains in an area called the growth plate, where this process of endochondral bone formation repeats itself. The cartilage cells in the growth plate proliferate and undergo hypertrophy; this is followed by partial degradation of the matrix, which then mineralizes. The cartilage is invaded by vessels, and the spicules of mineralized cartilage are covered by osteoblasts to form a cancellous or trabecular bone termed the primary spongiosa. These structures are then resorbed and replaced by trabecular plates made up entirely of bone, termed the *secondary spongiosa*. In the adult, it is most abundant at the ends of the long bones and in the bodies of the vertebrae.

Intramembranous bone formation occurs in two settings. In the skull and a few other areas, mesenchymal condensations transform directly into cells of the osteoblast lineage and form flat bones. In the bone collar adjacent to the cartilage template of endochondral bones, such as the long bones of the extremities, bone also forms by periosteal apposition. This bone, too, because it does not replace a cartilage mold, is intramembranous. Initially, relatively disorganized woven bone is formed, but this rapidly converts into more organized lamellar bone produced by oriented layers of osteoblasts. The main difference between endochondral and intramembranous bone formation is that the latter does not use a calcified cartilage matrix as a direct template upon which osteoblasts lay down a true bone matrix.

Cortical bone is the dense bone that is found in the shafts of long bones. It makes up 80% of the mass of the skeleton, determines its shape, and provides much of its strength. Modeling of cortical bone alters skeletal shape (see Fig. 28–1). During longitudinal skeletal growth, endochondral and periosteal apposi-

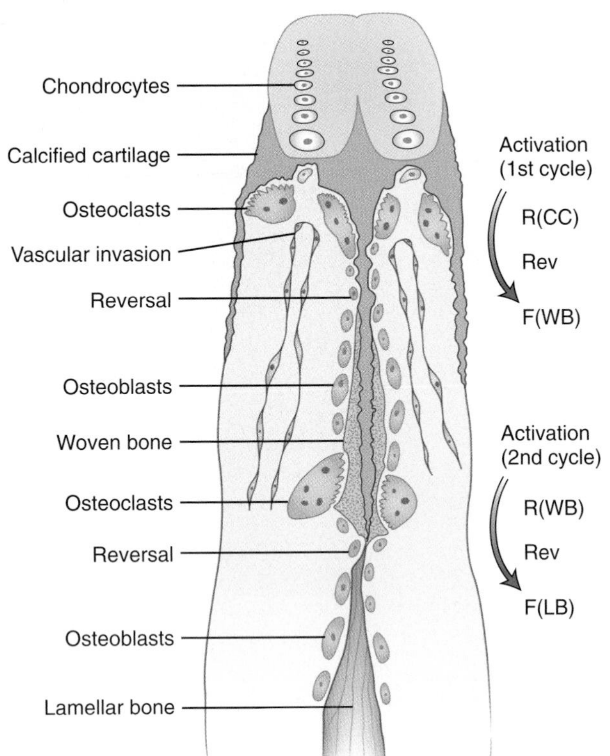

Figure 28–1 ▪ Steps in endochondral bone formation. *CC,* Calcified cartilage; *F,* formation; *LB,* lamellar bone; *R,* resorption; *Rev,* reversal; *WB,* woven bone. (Redrawn from Baron R. Anatomy and ultrastructure of bone. In Favus MJ, ed. Primer on the Metabolic Bone Diseases and Disorders of Mineral Metabolism, 2nd ed. New York: Lippincott-Raven, 1993:3-9. Copyright 1993, American Society for Bone and Mineral Research.)

tional bone formation determine the length and width of the bones.[3] As new bone is formed, it is shaped by a process called *modeling*, which is carried out by osteoblasts and osteoclasts in a way that leads to a net increase in bone mass, with a shape that is partly carved out by bone-resorbing osteoclasts. Modeling is influenced by mechanical forces, and is increased during the adolescent growth spurt.[4] The wide cortex at the epiphyseal plate of long bones must be resorbed by the modeling process because these bones elongate to maintain the narrow tubular structure of the diaphysis.

In contrast to bone modeling, bone remodeling is a closely regulated process, which results in the coordinated resorption and formation of bone. It is carried out in basic multicellular units throughout life. Remodeling is more active and occurs earlier in cancellous or trabecular bone, than in cortical bone.[5] In smaller animals, such as rodents, cortical bone can remain in a simple lamellar system. In large animals and humans, simple lamellar cortical bone is gradually replaced through haversian remodeling to form cylindrical osteons of lamellar bone surrounding blood vessels.

Chemistry of Bone Matrix and Mineral

The bone matrix consists of fibers of type I collagen laid down as orderly arrays (lamellae) in layers that have various orientations, which may add to the strength of the matrix. The matrix contains many additional proteins, including small amounts of other collagen types that may be important in determining the size and orientation of collagen fibers and the interaction of type I collagen with noncollagen proteins. The noncollagen proteins represent about 10% of the total protein in bone and may serve to direct the formation of fibers, mineralize bone, regulate the attachment of bone cells to its matrix, and play a role in the function of bone forming and resorbing cells (Table 28–1).

The protein composition of the matrix may vary, particularly between woven and lamellar bone.[6] These proteins range from the large cell-attachment proteins (e.g., thrombospondin and fibronectin) with molecular masses higher than 400 kd, to the small, vitamin K–dependent gamma-carboxylated proteins, matrix Gla protein, and osteocalcin, which is a 6-kd calcium-binding protein. A number of the noncollagen proteins (e.g., biglycan, decorin, bone sialoprotein, osteopontin, and osteoadherin) are highly acidic. In addition to cell-attachment sequences, these proteins contain varying amounts of carbohydrate and

TABLE 28–1 NONCOLLAGEN PROTEINS OF BONE

Name	Possible Function
γ-CARBOXYGLUTAMIC ACID–CONTAINING PROTEINS	
Osteocalcin	May regulate bone mineral maturation; negative regulator of bone formation and osteoblast function
Matrix Gla protein	Inhibits mineralization
RGD-CONTAINING GLYCOPROTEINS	
Fibronectin	Binds to cells; binds to gelatin and collagen
Thrombospondins	Cell attachment; binds to heparin, type I collagen, thrombin, laminin
Vitronectin	Cell attachment; binds to collagen and heparin
Fibrillin	May regulate elastic fiber formation
Osteopontin	Binds to cells; mediates effect of mechanical stress on osteoclasts and osteoblasts
Bone sialoprotein	Binds cells, binds calcium; may initiate mineralization
GLYCOPROTEINS	
Alkaline phosphatase	Hydrolyzes mineralization inhibitors
Osteonectin	Binds to growth factors; may regulate mineralization
Tetranectin	May regulate mineralization
GAG-CONTAINING	
Biglycan	May bind to collagen and TGF-β
Decorin	Binds to collagen and may regulate fibril diameter; binds to TGF-β
Fibromodulin	Binds to collagen and may regulate fibril diameter; binds to TGF-β
Osteoadherin	Promotes integrin-mediated cell attachment
Hyaluronan	Synthesized during early bone formation; may capture space destined to become bone

TGF-β, Transforming growth factor β.
Adapted from Liam JB, Stein GS, Canalis E, et al. Bone formation osteoblast lineage cells, growth factors, matrix proteins, and the mineralization process. In Favus MJ, ed. Primer on the Metabolic Bone Disorders of Mineral Metabolism, 4th ed. Philadelphia: Lippincott Williams and Wilkins, 1999:14-29.

may be termed *glycoproteins* or *proteoglycans*. Noncollagen proteins of bone are often highly phosphorylated; this enables them to bind calcium and may regulate mineralization. The use of targeted gene deletion in experimental murine models has provided important information about the function of noncollagenous proteins. For example, null mutations of the osteonectin gene lead to osteopenia, indicating that this matrix protein is important for the maintenance of a normal bone structure.[7]

Collagen Synthesis

Type I collagen is the most abundant protein of the bone matrix, and it is a rigid, rodlike, insoluble molecule composed of two α1 chains and one α2 chain.[8,9] Collagen chains consist of repeating triplets of amino acids with glycine in every third position and a high content of proline and lysine (Fig. 28–2). The two a1 and the a2 collagen chains form a triple helix that is stabilized by the hydroxylation of certain proline and lysine residues; this process requires ascorbic acid. Collagen is synthesized as a soluble propeptide with large nonhelical extensions at both the carboxy- and amino-terminal ends. Procollagen also contains carboxy-terminal interchain disulfide bonds that help initiate the formation of the triple helical structure. Procollagen is released into the cisternae of the rough endoplasmic reticulum, packaged in the Golgi vesicles, and secreted extracellularly. The procollagen peptide ends are then removed by specific peptidases to produce mature insoluble collagen molecules, which are further stabilized by intramolecular and intermolecular cross-links. The major cross-links are formed by lysine and hydroxylysine residues that ultimately form pyridinium ring structures.

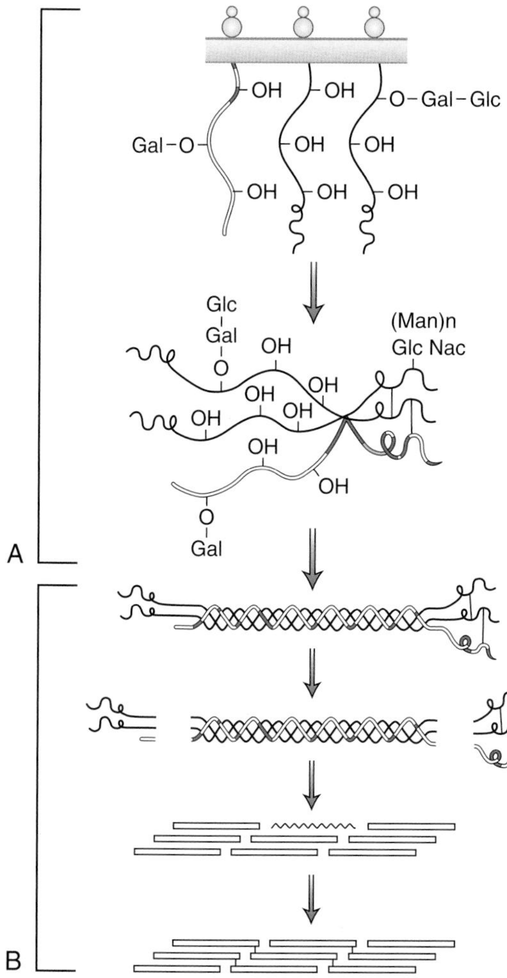

Figure 28–2 ▪ Synthesis and assembly of collagen fibrils. **A,** Intracellular posttranslational modifications of pro alpha chains, association of pro-peptide domains, and folding into triple-helical conformation. *Gal,* Galactose; *Glc,* glucose; *Glc Nac, N*-acetylglucosamine; *(Man)n,* mannose. **B,** Enzymatic cleavage of procollagen to collagen, self-assembly of collagen monomers into fibrils, and cross-linking of fibrils. (Modified from Prockop DJ, Kivirikko K. Heritable diseases of collagen. N Engl J Med 1984;311:376-386.)

Mineralization

Bone mineral is formed by small imperfect hydroxyapatite crystals, which contain carbonate, magnesium, sodium, and potassium. Mineralization occurs by two distinct mechanisms. The initial mineralization of calcified cartilage and woven bone probably occurs by means of matrix vesicles.[10] These membrane-bound bodies are released from chondrocytes and osteoblasts, contain alkaline phosphatase, and can form a nidus for crystallization. In contrast, in lamellar bone, the collagen fibers are tightly packed and matrix vesicles are rarely seen. Mineralization does not occur immediately after collagen deposition, and there is a layer of 10 to 100 μm of unmineralized osteoid between the mineralization front and the osteoblast. Perhaps changes in the packing of the fibrils and in the composition of the noncollagen proteins are required for mineralization. Mineralization of collagen fibrils begins in the hole zones, where there is more room for inorganic ions to accumulate (Fig. 28–3). Mineralization requires calcium, phosphate, and alkaline phosphatase. The alkaline phosphatase probably functions to hydrolyze local inhibitors of mineralization, such as pyrophosphate. The mineralization process is impaired in vitamin D deficiency, with its low calcium-phosphate product and hypophosphatasia, a disorder of mutated alkaline phosphatase genes.

Collagen Degradation

As part of the bone remodeling process, collagen is cleaved and degraded by a group of proteases, termed *collagenases*. These are matrix metalloproteases (MMP) that can initiate cleavage of collagen fibrils at neutral pH and are central to the process of collagen degradation, matrix breakdown, and bone remodeling. Three collagenases have been described: collagenase 1 (MMP-1), 2 (MMP-8), and 3 (MMP-13).[11,12] Human osteoblasts express the collagenase 1 and 3 genes. Unstimulated osteoblasts secrete limited amounts of collagenase and changes in the synthesis of collagenase correlate with changes in bone resorption. Collagenase plays a critical function in bone remodeling. Mice with deletions of the collagenase 3 gene or with mutations of the α1[1] type I collagen gene, which cause resistance to collagenase 3 cleavage, fail to resorb bone following exposure to parathyroid hormone (PTH).[13] The synthesis of collagenase by osteoblasts is regulated by hormones and by cytokines present in the bone microenvironment acting by transcriptional and posttranscriptional mechanisms.[14] Collagenases cause the initial cleavage of the collagen molecule, but complete collagen degradation requires the action of additional proteases, such as cathepsins.

Osteoblast Differentiation and Function

Bone is formed by osteoblasts, which are highly differentiated cells that have many unique features (Fig. 28–4).[15] Osteoblasts are derived from mesenchymal cells, present in the skeletal microenvironment.[16] Osteogenic precursors may appear in the

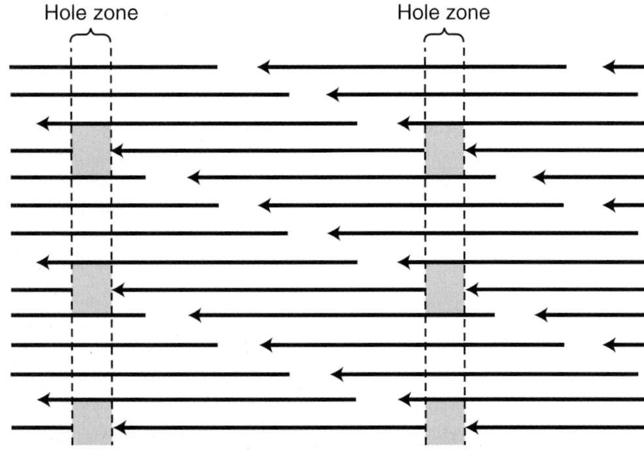

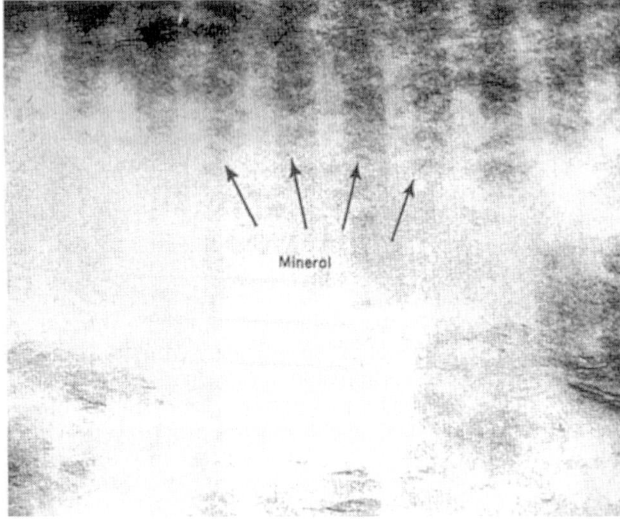

Figure 28–3 ▪ The staggered arrangement of individual molecules in collagen fibers results in hole zones between the head of one molecule and the tail of the next. Mineral deposition (*bottom*) begins within the hole zones. (From Glimcher MJ, Krane SM. Treatise on Collagen 2, part B. New York: Academic Press, 1968:67-251.)

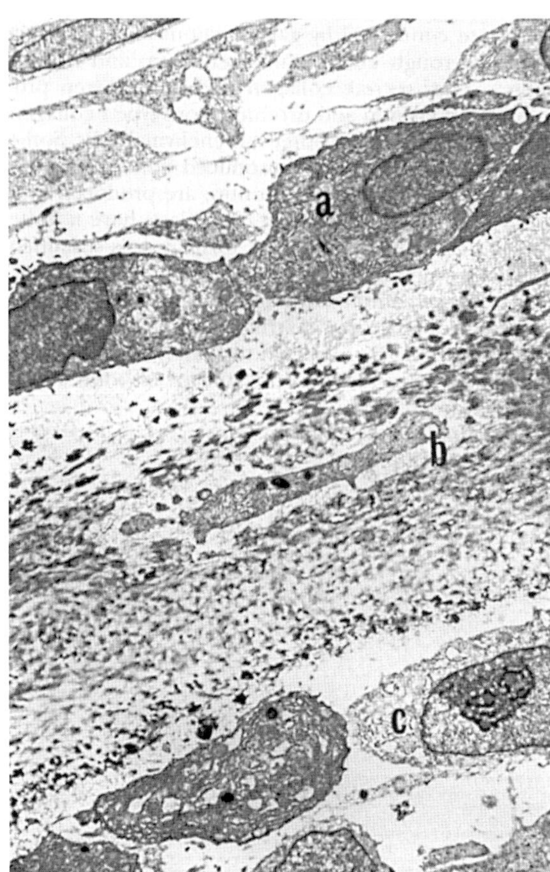

Figure 28–4 ▪ Electron micrograph of rat calvarial bone showing mature osteoblasts with their dense, rough endoplasmic reticulum and large Golgi apparatus **(A)**, an osteocyte embedded in the bone **(B)**, and a less differentiated cell that may represent a preosteoblast **(C)**. (Courtesy of Dr. Marijke E. Holtrop.)

circulation, but these originate from skeletal tissue and their contribution to bone formation is not well documented.[17] Osteoprogenitor cells or preosteoblasts replicate and differentiate into active osteoblasts that may exhibit varying phenotypic characteristics.[15] For example, osteoblasts in early development and during repair produce woven bone, whereas more mature osteoblasts produce lamellar bone. The activity of osteoblasts can vary during bone formation. Some cells are tall and closely packed and produce a large amount of matrix in a small area; others are flatter and produce matrix at a slower rate over a larger area. Nevertheless, all differentiated osteoblasts share certain features. They are connected by gap junctions and contain a dense network of rough endoplasmic reticulum and a large Golgi complex. They secrete collagen and noncollagen proteins in an oriented fashion and produce more type I collagen and alkaline phosphatase than other mesenchymal cells. Some products, such as osteocalcin, are produced almost uniquely by osteoblasts; consequently changes in serum levels of osteocalcin reflect changes in osteoblast activity.

Mature osteoblasts have a finite capacity to produce matrix, and bone formation is sustained by the arrival of new populations of cells at the bone surface. The number and the function of osteoblasts is determined by hormones and local signals. Some act as classic cell mitogens and increase the population of preosteoblastic cells, some determine their differentiation into mature osteoblasts, and others modify the function of mature cells.[18] The ultimate fate of a mature osteoblast is death by apoptosis. However, an osteoblast may become embedded in the matrix as an osteocyte, or may be converted to flattened lining cells, which cover a large percentage of the surface of bone with a thin cytoplasmic layer.

Bone marrow stroma contain pluripotential cells with the potential to differentiate into diverse cells of mesenchymal lineage, including osteoblasts, chondrocytes, myoblasts, and adipocytes.[16] The ultimate cellular phenotype depends on signals present in the cellular microenvironment and their effects on intracellular signals and gene expression. Transcription factors are nuclear proteins, and some play a role in determining the fate of undifferentiated cells. CCAAT-enhancer binding protein (C/EBP) β and δ play an essential role in the differentiation of cells toward the adipocyte lineage, whereas runt-related transcription factor (Runx-2) plays a central role in the differentiation of cells toward the osteoblast lineage.[19,20] Gene-targeted disruption of Runx-2 results in disorganized chondrocyte maturation and a complete lack of bone formation due to an arrest of osteoblast development.[21] Osterix is an additional transcription factor required for endochondral and intramembranous bone formation, and osterix null mice fail to develop a mineralized skeleton because of an arrest of late stages of osteoblast differentiation. Interactions between nuclear factors are common steps in the regulation of transcription and differentiation.[22] Osterix associates and acts cooperatively with nuclear factor of activated T cells (NFAT), a factor that regulates osteoblastogenesis and osteoclastogenesis.[23] C/EBPs can interact with Runx-2 and with the activator of transcription (ATF)/cyclic adenosine monophosphate (AMP) response element binding protein (CREB) family of proteins. ATF 4 plays a central role in later osteoblastic function and its activity is regulated by a nuclear matrix attachment region binding protein, SATB2, which interacts both with ATF 4 and Runx-2 to regulate osteoblast differentiation.[24]

The conversion of osteoblasts to osteocytes involves a reduction, but not a complete loss of, metabolic activity.[25] A critical feature of osteocyte differentiation is the development of an extensive network of cytoplasmic connections. The osteoblasts have multiple cell processes that are connected to underlying osteocytes through small canaliculi. After mineralization is complete, the processes persist as connections between osteocytes (Fig. 28–5). This extended syncytium is probably important in maintaining the viability of the osteocytes, which otherwise would be separated from the extracellular fluid, and for signaling by osteocytes.

Initially, osteocytes may continue to synthesize collagen and play a role in mineralization. Later, the major role of the osteocyte-osteoblast syncytium may be to sense mechanical forces.[26] Osteocytes probably sense bone deformation and provide signals for adaptive remodeling of bone size and shape.[27] One hypothesis is that small strains produce fluid shear stress in the canaliculi between osteocytes. This effect may result in intracellular signaling through changes in ion channels or in the production of biologically active molecules. Regions of bone microdamage contain apoptotic osteocytes, which may provide signals for the initiation of bone remodeling by osteoclasts and the consequent removal of damaged bone.[8] Osteocytes also express regulators of osteoblast function, such as sclerostin, an inhibitor of Wnt signaling.

Cells of the osteoblastic lineage are important not only in forming bone but also in initiating resorption. Both mature osteoblasts and osteocytes may play a role in activating resorption. Most of the hormonal factors that stimulate bone resorption act on cells of the osteoblastic lineage, which release receptor activator of nuclear factor κB ligand (RANKL) and colony stimulating factor-1 (CSF-1) that are essential for osteoclastogenesis. Osteoblasts also produce factors that regulate bone resorption, including cytokines, prostaglandins, and growth factors. In cell culture, contact between osteoblastic cells and hematopoietic cells appears to be necessary for osteoclast formation (Fig. 28–6). Osteoblasts may also play a role in initiating bone resorption by releasing collagenases, other metalloproteinases, and plasminogen activator. These enzymes may remove the surface proteins of bone, which prevent the access of osteoclasts to the mineralized matrix. Osteoblasts may also influence the development and maintenance of the marrow because cells of the osteoblast lineage are sources of growth factors, cytokines, and chemokines that may act on hematopoietic cells.

Osteoclast Differentiation and Function

Osteoclasts are derived from hematopoietic progenitors and appear to be myeloid in origin. Hematopoietic stem cells under the direction of cytokines and possibly cell-cell interactions express transcription factors that define their commitment to the osteoclast lineage. Granulocyte-macrophage colony-stimulating factor (GM-CSF) and colony-stimulating factor 1 (macrophage colony-stimulating factor [M-CSF]) appear to be important cytokines that regulate the replication and development of bone marrow progenitor cells that are capable of differentiating into osteoclasts. In addition, expression of the transcription factor PU.1 is also necessary for the osteoclast precursor cell to develop.[28] In bone marrow, the osteoclast precursor cell is multipotential and can differentiate into monocyte-macrophages, dendritic cells, or preosteoclasts.[29] The latter fuse to form highly differentiated multinucleated osteoclasts that resorb bone (see Fig. 28–6). Progression through the osteoclast pathway probably involves multiple local and systemic hormones that may include 1,25-dihydroxyvitamin D (1,25[OH]2D), prostaglandins, and the cytokines interleukin-1 (IL-1), IL-6, and tumor necrosis factor (TNF).

The nature of the osteoblast-lineage cell products, which directly regulate osteoclast formation and function, has been

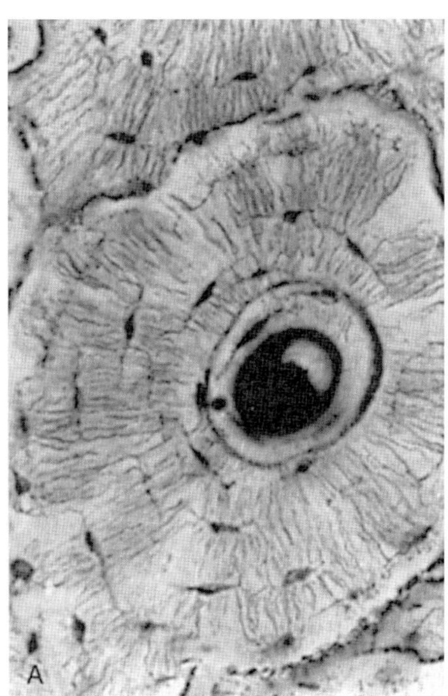

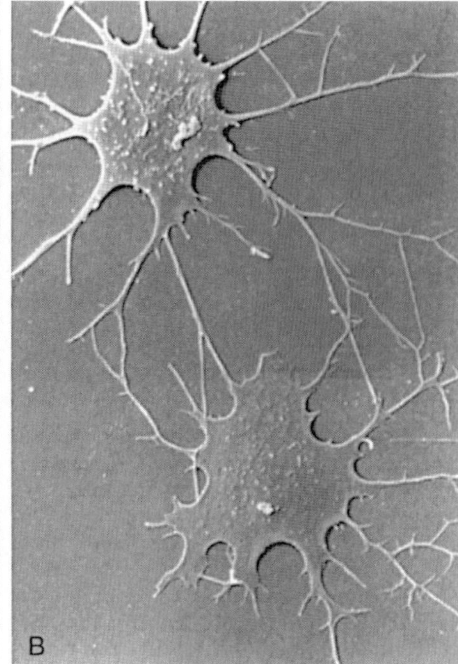

Figure 28–5 ■ **A,** Cross-section of an osteon. **B,** Cultured cells from avian bone, showing osteocytes and their cytoplasmic connections. (From Aarden EM, Burger EH, Nijweide PJ. Function of osteocytes and bone. J Cell Biochem 1994; 55:287-299. Reprinted by permission of Wiley-Liss, Inc., a subsidiary of John Wiley & Sons, Inc.)

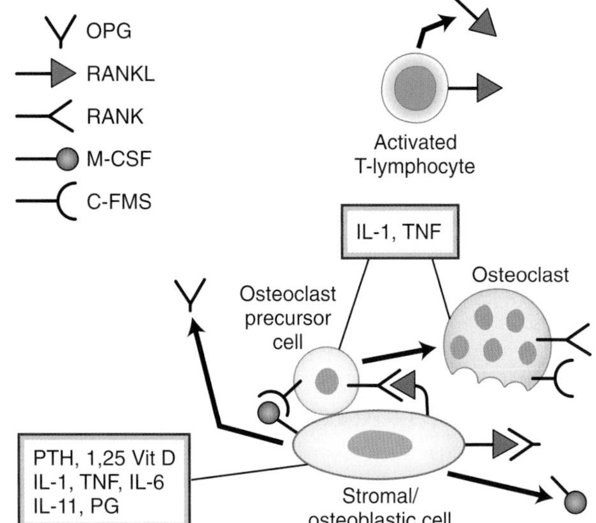

Figure 28–6 ▪ Osteoclast formation. Osteoclasts form from osteoclast precursor cells, which are derived from hematopoietic lineage cells. These express C-FMS (the receptor for M-CSF) and RANK and attach to stromal/osteoblastic cells, which express M-CSF (both membrane-bound and soluble), membrane-bound RANKL, and OPG under the influence of stimulators of resorption (PTH, 1,25-Vit D, IL-1, TNF, IL-6, IL-11, or PGs). If stromal or osteoblastic cells produce more RANKL than OPG, osteoclasts are formed and activated, which increases bone resorption. If stromal or osteoblastic cells produce more OPG than RANKL, OPG binds the available RANKL and new osteoclast formation is prevented. During states of inflammation, T lymphocytes are activated and produce both membrane-bound and soluble RANKL, which can, in turn, stimulate osteoclast-mediated bone resorption. It has also been shown that IL-1 and TNF can augment the effects of RANKL and M-CSF on osteoclast formation and bone resorption by directly stimulating osteoclast precursor cells and mature osteoclasts. *IL,* Interleukin; *M-CSF,* macrophage colony-stimulating factor; *OPG,* osteoprotegerin; *PG,* prostaglandin; *PTH,* parathyroid hormone; RANK, receptor activator of nuclear factor κB; RANKL; RANK ligand; *TNF,* tumor necrosis factor; *1,25 Vit D,* 1,25-dihydroxyvitamin D.

clarified.[30] The principal stimulator of osteoclast formation is a member of the TNF protein superfamily, termed receptor activator of nuclear factor κB ligand (RANKL). This protein was originally identified as a product of activated T lymphocytes but is also recognized as a critical stimulator of osteoclastogenesis.

Production of RANKL in osteoblast-lineage cells is stimulated by essentially all agents that enhance osteoclast formation, including parathyroid hormone (PTH), 1,25(OH)2D, prostaglandins, and many cytokines. Mice deficient in RANKL do not form osteoclasts and have osteopetrosis. In contrast, injection of RANKL into mice stimulates osteoclast formation and bone resorption. RANKL is produced as a membrane protein. In activated T lymphocytes. however, RANKL is cleaved from the cell membrane and is released as a soluble factor.[31] It is unclear whether similar events occur in osteoblast-lineage cells, although there is some evidence that cleavage and release of soluble RANKL occur in malignant cells that metastasize to bone.

In addition to RANKL, osteoblast-lineage cells produce an inhibitor of osteoclastogenesis, called osteoprotegerin (OPG). OPG is a soluble receptor for RANKL that binds this ligand and prevents interaction of RANKL with its cognate receptor, RANK. OPG is produced widely. In bone marrow cultures, a number of stimulators of resorption, including PTH, 1,25(OH)2D, and prostaglandin E2 (PGE2), inhibit OPG production. Hence, for these factors there is a reciprocal relationship between RANKL stimulation and OPG inhibition that causes activation of osteoclastogenesis and enhanced resorption. Mice deficient in OPG have osteoporosis, whereas mice that overexpress OPG have increased bone mass. These results, together with those for RANKL-deficient mice or mice injected with RANKL, demonstrate that osteoclast-mediated bone resorption is tightly regulated by the combined actions of RANKL and OPG.

The active receptor for RANKL is RANK, a member of the TNF receptor superfamily. Osteoclasts and their immediate precursor cells express RANK, which is induced by M-CSF.[32] Binding of RANKL to RANK activates a series of intracellular pathways that activate nuclear factor κB (NF-κB) and mitogen-activated protein (MAP) kinases as well as nuclear factor of activated T cells (NFAT) and the activator protein-1 (AP-1) family of transcription factors. The TNF receptor-associated factors (TRAFs) and particularly TRAF-6 bind RANK intracellularly and are involved in RANK responses. Mice deficient in TRAF-6, like those deficient in RANK, develop osteopetrosis. In addition to its effects on bone, the RANKL-RANK system is involved in lymphocyte function, as well as breast and lymph node development. Mature osteoclasts express RANK, and treatment of these cells with RANKL inhibits programmed cell death (apoptosis) and stimulates resorptive activity.[33]

In addition to RANKL, M-CSF is essential for osteoclast formation. Mice deficient in M-CSF have osteopetrosis and few osteoclasts.[34] In cultures of isolated osteoclast precursor cells, both M-CSF and RANKL must be present for mature osteoclasts to form. M-CSF enhances RANK production in osteoclast precursors and inhibits apoptosis of both osteoclast precursors and mature osteoclasts. The receptor for M-CSF, c-fms, is present on both osteoclast precursors and mature osteoclasts.[32,35] Binding of c-fms by M-CSF activates tyrosine kinase activity in the receptor, which initiates a series of intracellular events.

It has also become clear that there are a series of coactivator molecules that are critical for osteoclast development. These include members of the immunoreceptor tyrosine-based activation motif (ITAM) family, named FC-receptor common γ subunit (FCRγ) and DNAX activator protein 12 (DAP-12). These intracellular proteins interact with the membrane receptor proteins: osteoclast associated receptor (OSCAR) and triggering receptor expressed on myeloid cells-2 (TREM-2), respectively, in osteoclast precursor cells. Mice deficient in both FCRγ and DAP-12 have osteopetrosis and deficient osteoclast formation despite their ability to express RANKL, RANK, M-CSF, and c-fms.[23,36]

The formation of multinucleated osteoclast-like cells in vitro requires both hematopoietic precursors and cells of the osteoblastic lineage. In vivo or in cultures with devitalized bone, mononuclear preosteoclasts attach to the bone surface and form multinucleated osteoclasts by fusion. The accumulation of additional nuclei into osteoclasts by fusion probably continues while the cell is actively resorbing. The life span of the osteoclast is limited. As osteoclasts become inactive, they die by apoptosis. Hormones that enhance bone resorption may delay apoptosis, and inhibitors of resorption can accelerate it. The mechanisms that limit the extent of osteoclastic resorption are incompletely understood and may involve inhibition by calcium ions, which accumulate under the osteoclast resorbing surface, or by local inhibitory factors, such as transforming growth factor β (TGF-β), which are released and activated during resorption.

The mature osteoclast is a unique and highly specialized cell (Fig. 28–7). It usually contains 10 to 20 nuclei, but giant osteoclasts with up to 100 nuclei can be seen in Paget's disease or giant cell tumors of bone. The large size of osteoclasts is probably essential for their resorptive function. The best evidence for this comes from studies of dendritic cell specific transmembrane protein (DC-STAMP), since inhibition of this protein or its complete deficiency in mouse models results in the generation of only mononuclear osteoclasts that have impaired resorptive activity.[37,38] The capacity of osteoclasts to resorb bone depends on their ability to isolate a region of the bone surface from the

extracellular fluid and produce a local environment that can dissolve bone mineral and degrade matrix. It is also critical that the osteoclast polarize and produce a basolateral membrane opposite the resorption space, which facilitates the excretion of resorption products. The resorbing apparatus consists of a central ruffled border area, which secretes hydrogen ions and proteolytic enzymes, surrounded by a clear or sealing zone in a structure called the *podosome*. The podosome contains filamentous actin linked to $\alpha v\beta 3$ integrin, and anchors the cell to the bone surface. The osteoclast attaches to bone through the interaction of integrins in the podosome with noncollagenous proteins like vitronectin and osteopontin in the matrix.

Acidification of the resorption space adjacent to the ruffled border membrane requires that osteoclasts have a vacuolar proton pump (H^+-ATPase) and a chloride channel that is charge-coupled to H^+ secretion across the ruffled membrane to preserve electron neutrality. These osteoclast H^+-ATPase pumps are similar to the vacuolar proton pumps that acidify intracellular organelles, but in the osteoclast they are exteriorized to increase the extracellular hydrogen ion concentration in the resorption space.[39] The hydrogen ions dissociate from carbonic acid, which is synthesized by carbonic anhydrase II; the bicarbonate generated by this dissociation is removed from the cell by chloride-bicarbonate exchange at the basolateral membrane of the osteoclast. Ion pumps can transport the dissolved calcium from the bone surface through the cell to the extracellular fluid.

However, calcium can also reach the extracellular fluid directly if the sealing zone is disrupted. The proteolytic enzymes produced by the osteoclast include lysosomal enzymes and metalloproteinases. Lysosomal proteases can degrade collagen at the low pH present in the ruffled border area. Cathepsin K is probably the most important of these.[40] Metalloproteinases, which are active at neutral pH, have also been detected at the resorption site.[41] The products of resorption are transported across the ruffled boarder membrane and excreted through the basolateral membrane of the osteoclast by a process termed transcytosis.[42] In trabecular bone, osteoclasts characteristically resorb to a limited depth and then move laterally to produce irregular, platelike resorption areas that are termed Howship's lacunae. In cortical remodeling, the path of directed resorption is longer, possibly because of renewal of osteoclasts from hematopoietic cells brought to the site through the haversian canal.

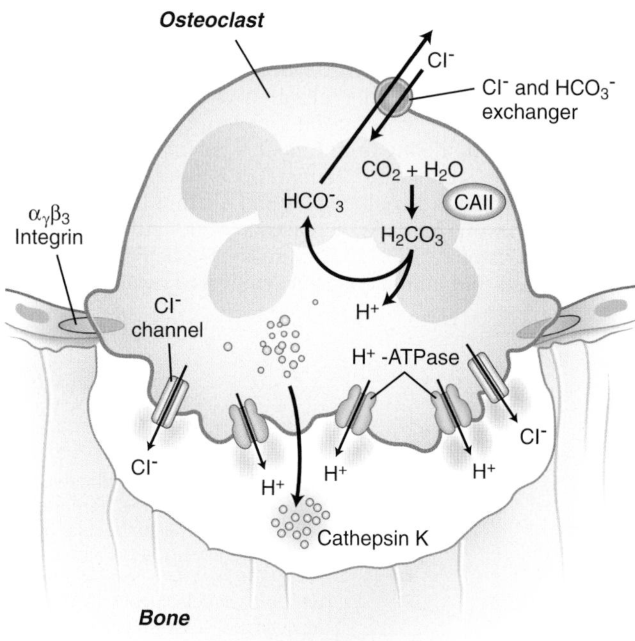

Figure 28–7 ▪ Functional elements of the fully differentiated osteoclast. Osteoclasts attach to bone via podosomes containing $\alpha v\beta 3$ integrin. Protons are generated through the actions of carbonic anhydrase II (CA II), which is transported into the resorption space by the vacuolar-type H^+-ATPase "proton pump." A chloride channel coupled to the proton pump facilitates charge neutrality across the membrane while passive exchange of chloride for bicarbonate in the basolateral membrane removes excess bicarbonate. Cathepsin K is an important enzyme for the removal of the organic components of bone in the acid environment of the resorption space. (Redrawn from Tolar J, Teitelbaum SL, Orchard PJ. Osteopetrosis. N Engl J Med 2004;351:2839-2849.)

BONE REMODELING AND ITS REGULATION

Bone remodeling is a temporally regulated process resulting in the coordinated resorption and formation of skeletal tissue carried out in basic multicellular units.[5] Bone remodeling occurs throughout life. Signals determining the fate, function, and death of cells of the osteoclast and osteoblast lineages define the populations of cells that resorb and form bone in basic multicellular units. There, osteoblasts appear at sites vacated by osteoclasts, a process called coupling. As resorption by osteoclasts is terminated, the resorptive surface is covered by a thin layer of cement, where osteoblasts assemble to form bone and fill the cavity.[3,5] The remodeling cycle can be divided into four steps: (1) activation, (2) resorption, (3) reversal, and (4) formation (Figs. 28–8 and 28–9).

Similar sequences are seen in trabecular and cortical remodeling, although remodeling is more active in trabecular bone.[9] In young adults, this cycle is tightly coupled and the amount of new bone formed by osteoblasts is equal to the amount resorbed by osteoclasts. However, when resorption increases and formation no longer keeps up, bone loss and eventually osteoporosis occurs. During the menopausal years, women remodel bone at a higher rate than in the premenopause. However, because these remodeling cycles are unbalanced, with resorption exceeding formation, they result in progressive bone loss.[43]

Although 80% of skeletal mass is cortical bone, the surface area of cortical bone is only about one fifth that of cancellous bone. Moreover, more osteoclast precursor cells are available in cancellous bone and on the endosteal surfaces of cortical bone than within cortical bone or the periosteal surface. Consequently, turnover is greater on these surfaces than on those of periosteal bone, which normally undergoes little remodeling. However, subperiosteal resorption can be activated in hyperparathyroidism, and the periosteal surface contains preosteoblasts that may become active late in life and cause an age-related increase in the periosteal diameter of long bones. This periosteal expansion may maintain bone strength and compensate for losses at the endosteal surfaces and in cancellous bone.

Remodeling can be activated by both systemic and local factors. It is necessary to maintain skeletal strength and contributes to the maintenance of the serum levels of calcium. Changes in mechanical force can activate remodeling to improve skeletal strength, and remodeling serves to remove and repair bone that has undergone microdamage. This occurs particularly in cortical bone and may account for the fact that remodeling is sustained in the aging skeleton.[44] However, loss of osteocytes with age may impair this response.[45] Systemic hormones influence bone remodeling to regulate the movement of mineral from

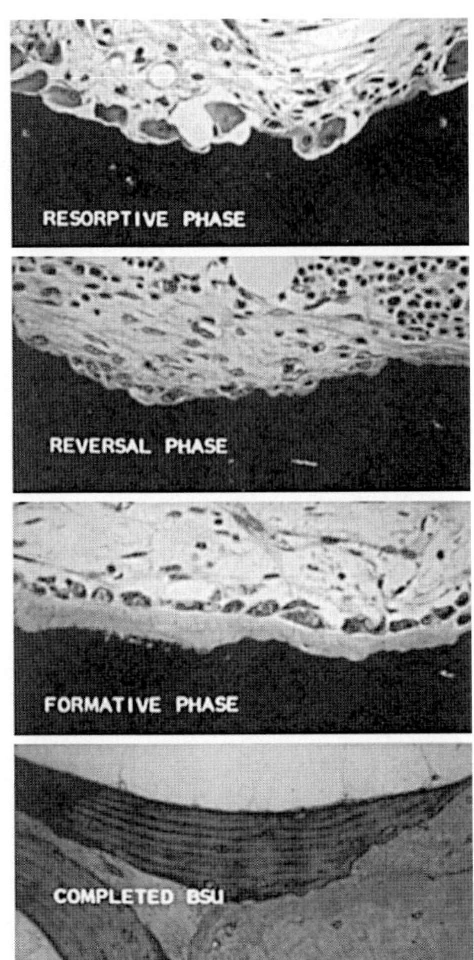

Figure 28–8 ▪ Stages of bone remodeling. The resorptive, reversal, and formative phases of bone remodeling and a completed bone structural unit (BSU) on a trabecular surface are illustrated. The morphologic features of the activation step have not been defined. (Courtesy of Dr. Robert E. Schenk, University of Berne, Switzerland.)

bone to extracellular fluid to maintain serum calcium levels and as part of their overall effects on growth. During pubertal growth, bone modeling and remodeling intensifies, correlating with serum levels of insulin-like growth factor (IGF) I.[4] Studies performed in mice lacking molecular clock genes suggest that bone remodeling is subject to circadian regulation.[46]

Calcium-Regulating Hormones

(see also Chapter 27)

Parathyroid Hormone

Parathyroid hormone (PTH) acts on bone to stimulate resorption but does not act on osteoclasts in the absence of cells of the osteoblastic lineage; moreover, PTH receptors are abundant on osteoblasts, but not on osteoclasts.[47] PTH acts on osteoblasts to cause cell contraction; to induce immediate-early response genes, including c-fos and the inducible form of prostaglandin G/H synthase (cyclooxygenase); and to increase the synthesis of local mediators, IGF-I and IL-6.[47,48] High concentrations of PTH in vitro inhibit the expression of type I collagen, but intermittent administration of PTH in vivo or in vitro can stimulate bone formation.[48] PTH induces the production of RANKL and inhibits the production of osteoprotegerin by cells of the osteoblast lineage, thereby increasing osteoclastogenesis and the activity of osteoclasts. In some settings, PTH increases proliferation of cells of the osteoblast lineage and decreases their death by apoptosis.[49]

Vitamin D

The hormonal form of vitamin D-1,25(OH)2D3 is necessary for normal amounts of intestinal calcium and phosphorus absorption and, therefore, for mineralization of bone. This form of vitamin D also has effects on the skeleton, but its physiologic role in bone remodeling is not clear.[50] By increasing RANKL production by osteoblasts, vitamin D is a potent stimulator of osteoclast formation in cell culture and vitamin D intoxication is associated with dramatic increases in bone resorption. High concentrations of 1,25(OH)2D3 increase osteocalcin synthesis by osteoblasts and inhibit collagen synthesis. Lower concentra-

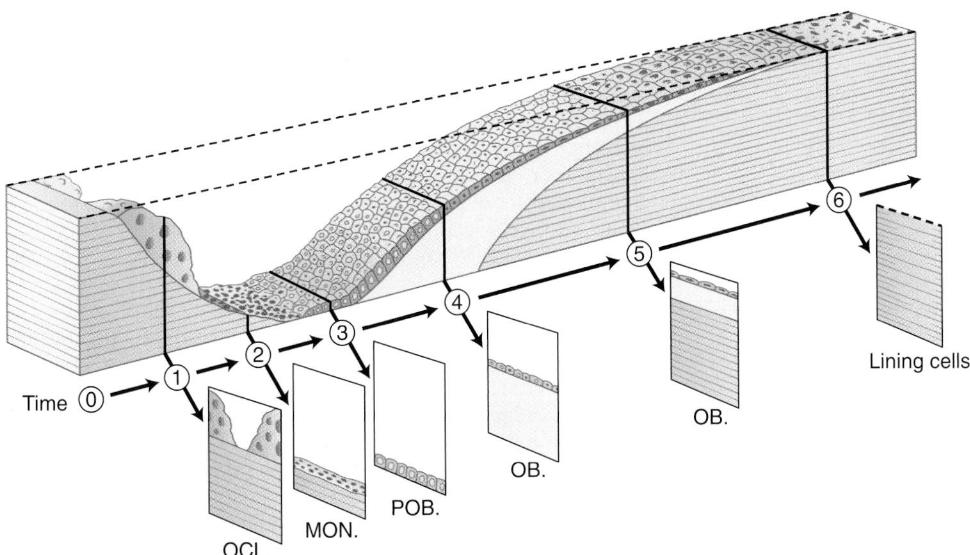

Figure 28–9 ▪ Three-dimensional reconstruction of the remodeling sequence in human trabecular bone. *1,* Early bone resorption with osteoclasts (OCL); *2,* late bone resorption with mononuclear cells (MON); *3,* reversal phase with preosteoblasts (POB); *4,* early matrix formation by osteoblasts (OB); *5,* late bone formation with mineralization; *6,* completed remodeling cycle with reversion to lining cells. (From Eriksen EF. Normal and pathological remodeling of human trabecular bone: three dimensional reconstruction of the remodeling sequence in normals and in metabolic bone disease. Endocr Rev 1986;7:379-408. Copyright 1986 by The Endocrine Society.)

tions may increase bone formation, but not to the extent seen with intermittent administration of PTH.

Calcitonin

Calcitonin inhibits bone resorption by acting directly on the osteoclast, but it appears to play a small role in the regulation of bone turnover in adults. Bone mass is not greatly altered in patients with medullary thyroid carcinoma, who have an excess of calcitonin production, or in athyreotic patients receiving adequate thyroid hormone replacement, who have low calcitonin levels.[51] In fact, bone turnover is increased in patients with medullary thyroid carcinoma.[52] In addition, mice with a deletion of the gene responsible for the production of both calcitonin and its alternate transcript, calcitonin gene-related peptide, have increased bone mass and enhanced rates of bone formation.[53] In contrast, mice with a deletion of only the calcitonin gene-related peptide have decreased bone mass.[54] These results imply that calcitonin influences bone formation as well as bone resorption. However, the mechanisms by which calcitonin affects bone growth are unknown.

Other Systemic Hormones

Growth Hormone

Deficiency and excess of growth hormone have marked effects on skeletal growth.[55] Growth hormone increases both circulating and local levels of IGF-I, which mediates the skeletal effects of growth hormone. Both exogenous growth hormone and IGF-I increase bone remodeling. Growth hormone also stimulates cartilage growth, probably through an increase in local and systemic IGF-I production and possibly by direct stimulation of cartilage cell proliferation, in that low levels of growth hormone receptors are present in skeletal cells and ablation of these receptors synergizes with loss of IGF-I signaling to regulate postnatal bone growth.[56]

Glucocorticoids

Glucocorticoids exert profound effects on bone remodeling.[57] Glucocorticoids decrease the intestinal absorption of calcium and have the potential to induce osteoclastogenesis and bone resorption because they increase the expression of RANKL in osteoblasts.[58] However, the most significant effect of glucocorticoids is the suppression of bone remodeling secondary to a depletion of the osteoblastic cell population.[57] Glucocorticoids inhibit the replication of osteoblast precursors and their differentiation into mature osteoblasts by suppressing Wnt signaling.[59] Glucocorticoids induce the apoptosis of osteoblasts and osteocytes, contributing to the decrease in bone-forming cells.[60] In addition, glucocorticoids inhibit the differentiated function of the osteoblast and bone formation. This is secondary to direct effects of glucocorticoids on the osteoblast and to a suppression of igf 1 gene transcription.[61]

Thyroid Hormones

In children, hyperthyroidism is associated with increased skeletal growth, and hypothyroidism results in decreased growth.[62] Thyroid hormones are crucial for cartilage growth and differentiation and enhance the response to growth hormone. Thyroid hormones increase bone resorption and turnover, although their effects on bone formation are less clear.[63] Coupled with their effects on bone resorption, thyroid hormones increase the transcription of collagenase and other metalloproteinases by osteoblasts.[64] As thyroid hormones increase bone remodeling, there may be a secondary increase in bone formation in vivo.

Insulin

Normal skeletal growth depends on an adequate amount of insulin.[65] Excess insulin production by the fetuses of mothers with uncontrolled diabetes results in excessive growth of the skeleton and other tissues, and undertreated diabetes mellitus impairs skeletal growth and mineralization. In vitro, insulin at physiologic concentrations selectively stimulates osteoblastic collagen synthesis by a pretranslational mechanism. Insulin can mimic the effects of IGF-I, but only at supraphysiological levels.[66] Mice deficient in insulin receptor substrate 1, a major substrate of both insulin and IGF-I receptor tyrosine kinases, exhibit impaired osteoblastic function and low bone turnover osteopenia, documenting the central role of insulin/IGF-I signaling in the maintenance of bone remodeling.[67]

Gonadal Hormones

Both estrogens and androgens are critical for skeletal development and maintenance. Bone cells contain estrogen and androgen receptors. Gonadal hormones are crucial for the pubertal growth spurt, and estrogen is necessary for epiphyseal closure.[68] Deficiency of estrogen or androgen increases bone resorption in vivo, possibly by increasing the local synthesis or sensitivity to cytokines, such as IL-1 and IL-6 or TNF-α, and to prostaglandins. Estrogens may also act by decreasing RANK signaling in osteoclasts and their precursor cells.[69,70] Androgens can increase bone formation in vivo.[71] The effect of estrogens on bone formation is less clear. The absolute rate of bone formation is increased in estrogen deficiency states, because of an increase in bone remodeling. However, estrogen deficiency causes bone loss, implying a relative deficiency in bone formation that is not sufficient to compensate for the increased resorption.[43]

Local Regulators

Characterization of local regulators produced within the bone itself represents a major advance in bone biology.[72,73] These local factors can be synthesized by bone cells or by adjacent hematopoietic cells and can interact both with each other and with systemic hormones. They are critical in the repair of skeletal damage and in the response to mechanical forces.

Cytokines

IL-1α, IL-1-β, TNF-α, and TNF-β are potent stimulators of bone resorption and inhibitors of bone formation and may mediate bone loss after estrogen withdrawal.[74,75] IL-6 increases osteoclastogenesis in cell cultures and may mediate some of the resorbing activity of PTH. IL-6 is produced by osteoblasts, and its production is stimulated by PTH,[76] PGE2, and other factors that increase resorption. IL-11, another member of the IL-6 cytokine family, also stimulates resorption. Another IL-6 family member, leukemia inhibitory factor (LIF), has biphasic effects on bone formation.[77] As noted previously, colony-stimulating factors are probably important in the early stages of osteoclast formation.

IL-4 and IL-13 inhibit resorption and prostaglandin synthesis in bone cells,[78] IL-7 stimulates B lymphopoiesis, which may be involved in osteoclastogenesis.[79] IL-10[80] is an inhibitor of osteoclastogenesis and bone resorption. IL-15 and IL-17 stimulate it, whereas IL-18 is inhibitory through its ability to increase production of granulocyte-macrophage colony-stimulating factor.[81]

Interferon β and γ inhibit resorption by blocking RANK signaling pathways.[82] In addition to direct effects, responses to cytokines can be blocked by inhibitors, such as the IL-1 receptor antagonist and the soluble TNF receptor, or they can be enhanced by activators such as the soluble IL-6 receptor.

Transforming Growth Factor α and Epidermal Growth Factor

These peptides stimulate bone resorption through the same receptor and act by both prostaglandin-dependent and prostaglandin-independent pathways. TGF-α and epidermal growth factor (EGF) are potent mitogens in bone that probably act on both mesenchymal and hematopoietic precursors.[83,84] TGF-α is produced by neoplasms and may play a role in the increased bone resorption that occurs in certain malignancies.

Prostaglandins

Prostaglandins are potent regulators of bone cell metabolism and are synthesized by many cell types in the skeleton.[85] Prostaglandin production in bone is regulated by the effects of local and systemic hormones and mechanical forces on the inducible cyclooxygenase (COX-2). Increased prostaglandin production may contribute to the increase in bone resorption with immobilization, the increase in bone formation with impact loading, and the changes after estrogen withdrawal. Many of the hormones, cytokines, and growth factors that stimulate bone resorption also increase prostaglandin production.

Prostaglandins have biphasic effects on bone formation. Stimulation of bone formation is seen in vivo, and inhibition of collagen synthesis occurs in osteoblast cultures. Bone cells produce PGE2, PGF2α, prostacyclin, and lipoxygenase products (e.g., leukotriene B4), which may also stimulate bone resorption.

Growth Factors

Skeletal cells synthesize a variety of growth factors that regulate the replication, differentiation, and function of bone cells. These growth factors are not synthesized specifically by skeletal cells and some are present in the systemic circulation, and can act both as local and systemic regulators of bone remodeling. Skeletal cells also synthesize growth factor binding proteins. These regulate the activity and storage of specific factors and their interactions with other proteins present in the extracellular matrix.[86]

Fibroblast Growth Factors

Fibroblast growth factors (FGF) form a large family of polypeptides characterized by their affinity for glycosaminoglycan heparin binding sites.[87] FGF-1 and -2 have been studied extensively and have mitogenic properties for cells of the osteoblastic lineage, which eventually differentiate into mature osteoblasts, but FGFs do not stimulate the differentiation or the function of the osteoblast.[66] FGF-2 inhibits Wnt signaling, and the synthesis of IGF-I, explaining a decrease in osteoblastogenesis and in osteoblastic function.[88] In vivo experiments have confirmed this action of FGF, and mice overexpressing FGF-2 are osteopenic.[89] However, studies in fgf-2 null mice indicate that FGF-2 is necessary for optimal osteoblast formation, possibly because of its effects on cell replication.[90] FGF can stimulate bone resorption by prostaglandin-dependent and independent pathways.[91]

Platelet-Derived Growth Factor/Vascular Endothelial Growth Factor

Platelet derived growth factor (PDGF) was originally isolated from human platelets, and four members of the pdgf gene family have been identified: pdgf a, pdgf b, pdgf c, and pdgf d.[92] Vascular endothelial growth factor (VEGF) shares a high degree of sequence homology with PDGF, and these factors are often referred as members of the PDGF/VEGF family.[93]

PDGFs must form homodimers or heterodimers to exhibit activity. PDGF AA, AB, and BB are the isoforms studied more extensively in skeletal cells, and they exert similar biologic actions. The primary function of PDGF in bone is the stimulation of cell replication, and PDGF impairs the differentiation and the function of osteoblasts.[94] PDGF also stimulates bone resorption. Null mutations of pdfg a or b and pdfg α and β receptors cause embryonic lethality or perinatal death, not allowing the study of the function of PDGF in the postnatal skeleton.[95] Although skeletal cells express the pdfg a, pdfg b, and pdfg c genes, the major source of PDGF is the systemic circulation, and skeletal cells become exposed to PDGF following platelet aggregation.

VEGF A is essential for angiogenesis and vegf a and vegf receptor genes are expressed by chondrocytes and osteoblasts.[96] VEGF A is required for blood vessel formation and vessel invasion into cartilage during the process of endochondral bone formation, and for chondrocyte survival during skeletal development.[97] VEGF A is required for intramembranous bone formation and osteoblastic maturation.[98] The expression of PDGF and VEGF by osteoblasts is regulated by other growth factors.

Insulin-Like Growth Factors

IGFs increase bone matrix synthesis and bone formation.[99] Both the systemic circulating as well as the locally synthesized IGF-I contribute to bone formation.[100] Transgenic mice overexpressing IGF-I have increased bone mass, whereas igf-1 null mice exhibit decreased bone formation and decreased cortical bone.[101,102] IGF-I increases osteoclastogenesis and bone remodeling.[103] Both IGF-I and IGF-II are synthesized by bone cells and are stored in the bone matrix, but IGF-I is a more potent stimulator of osteoblastic function.[99] There are six known IGF-binding proteins that have been identified in bone. IGF-binding proteins can inhibit or enhance IGF responses. PTH and PGE2 are major inducers of skeletal IGF-I synthesis and glucocorticoids suppress IGF-I transcription.[99] IGFs mediate selected effects of these hormones on bone formation.

Transforming Growth Factor β

Transforming growth factor β (TGF-β) belongs to a family of closely related polypeptides with various degrees of structural homology and important effects on cell function.[104] Skeletal cells express TGF-β1, 2, and 3. TGF-β has complex and somewhat contradictory actions in bone cells. TGF-β can stimulate osteoblastic cell replication and bone formation, but it does not favor osteoblastic cell differentiation.[105,106] The effects of TGF-β are dependent on the target cell and experimental conditions. The actions of TGF-β on bone resorption have been a source of controversy. TGF-β has a biphasic effect on osteoclastogenesis, but it decreases bone resorption.[107] Targeted gene disruption of the mouse tgf β 1 gene is lethal, but does not result in abnormal skeletal development.[108] TGF-β is secreted as a latent high-molecular-weight complex consisting of the carboxy-terminal remnant of the TGF-β precursor and a TGF-β–binding protein.[79] The biologically active levels of TGF-β depend on changes in its synthesis and in the activation of its latent form.

Bone Morphogenetic Proteins and Wnts

Bone morphogenetic proteins (BMPs) are members of the TGF-β superfamily of polypeptides and were originally identified because of their ability to induce endochondral bone formation when implanted subcutaneously. BMPs are expressed by osteoblasts and play an autocrine role in osteoblastic differentiation and function.[109] The fundamental function of BMPs is the

induction of osteoblastic cell differentiation, endochondral ossification, and chondrogenesis.[109,110] The genesis and differentiation of osteoblasts and of osteoclasts are coordinated events, and BMPs also induce osteoclastogenesis and osteoclast survival.[111]

BMP activity is regulated by a large group of secreted polypeptides that bind and limit BMP action. These extracellular BMP antagonists prevent BMP signaling. Extracellular BMP antagonists include, but are not limited to, noggin, follistatin, twisted gastrulation, the chordin family, and the Dan/Cerberus family of proteins.[109]

The Wnt family of secreted glycoproteins, like BMPs, play a critical role in cell fate and osteoblastogenesis. In skeletal cells, certain Wnts use the canonical Wnt/β-catenin signaling pathway.[112] In the absence of Wnt, axin, adenomatous polyposis coli (APC), and β-catenin form a complex in which β-catenin is phosphorylated and degraded. The binding of Wnts to specific Frizzled membrane receptors and to co-receptors, leads to the stabilization of β-catenin, its nuclear translocation, and subsequent transcriptional regulation of target genes. The Wnt/β-catenin signaling pathway is central to osteoblastogenesis and bone formation, and Wnts and BMPs act in concert to regulate cell differentiation. Gene deletions of Wnts or β-catenin result in the inhibition of osteogenesis and of skeletal tissue, and inactivating mutations of Wnt co-receptors result in osteopenia.[113] Wnt/β-catenin signaling induces osteoprotegerin and through this mechanism Wnts are negative regulators of osteoclastogenesis.[114,115]

CLINICAL EVALUATION OF METABOLIC BONE DISEASE

Bone Densitometry

The most widely used procedure for measuring bone mass is dual-energy x-ray absorptiometry (DXA).[116,117] Other methods include quantitative computed tomography (QCT), quantitative radiography, single-energy x-ray absorptiometry, and ultrasonography.[118-121] The correlations among these methods are quite variable.

Both densitometry and ultrasound data are reported in terms of T-scores (standard deviations from the young adult norm for that instrument) or Z-scores (standard deviations from the expected value for individuals of the same sex, age, and body size). These values depend on the normative data that have been obtained for each specific instrument. Moreover, the normative data are likely to be different for different populations, not only for men and women but also for members of different racial and ethnic groups. Methods of assessing microarchitecture using magnetic resonance imaging (MRI) and QCT are being developed but are not yet available for routine clinical use.[122,123]

Dual-Energy X-Ray Absorptiometry

DXA can provide accurate and reproducible values for bone mineral content (BMC) and bone mineral density (BMD) in the lumbar spine, the proximal femur, the distal radius, and the whole body. BMD is calculated from the BMC and the area of bone scanned (g/cm^2); hence, it represents a real bone density rather than true volumetric density.

DXA has many advantages. Radiation exposure is minimal (<10 mrem), and scanning time is short (5 to 20 minutes). If quality control is maintained, variability of repeated readings is less than 1% for phantom standards; less than 2% for lumbar spine, total body, and radius; and less than 3% for proximal femur.

The major disadvantages of DXA are as follows: Changes with disease progression or therapy are small in relation to the variability of the measurement.[124] The test is moderately expensive. Anteroposterior measurements of the lumbar spine in older patients are subject to errors caused by aortic calcification and osteoarthritic changes.

The last disadvantage can be overcome by performing lateral densitometry of the lumbar spine, but this measurement is less precise. Newer DXA systems may also have sufficient resolution to measure changes in vertebral body height in thoracic as well as the lumbar vertebrae. Detection of new vertebral compressions by this method may be particularly useful in patients with prior vertebral fractures, height loss, or thoracic back pain (Fig. 28–10).[125,126]

Quantitative Computed Tomography

QCT, which employs instruments available in most radiology departments, can be used to assess true bone density (g/cm^3) and to separate cancellous and cortical bone in the vertebral body. Thus, it can measure trabecular BMD in the presence of osteoarthritis.[127] QCT has also been used to measure cortical and trabecular bone density in the appendicular skeleton. The radiation exposure (100 to 300 mrem) is larger than for DXA, and the precision and accuracy are lower but within the acceptable range. A major disadvantage may be cost, but this varies widely.

Peripheral Densitometry

A number of methods to measure bone mass and density in the appendicular skeleton have been developed that are less expensive, faster, and more portable than DXA or QCT.[128] Measurement of cortical bone in the shaft of the radius and ulna and trabecular bone in the distal radius or calcaneus by radiography, x-ray absorptiometry, or CT scanning is precise and can be used to predict fracture risk in populations, but it cannot predict BMD of the spine and hip in individual patients. The advantages of ultrasonography, particularly of the calcaneus, are that (1) it does not use x-rays, (2) it is rapid and portable, and (3) it has the capability of predicting fracture risk.[129] These measurements may be particularly useful for large-scale screening programs.

Biochemical Measurements

One of the most important advances in metabolic bone disease has been the development of more accurate biochemical measurements that can assess rates of bone formation and resorption. In population studies, these methods have been used to show that increased turnover (i.e., high rates of both resorption and formation) correlates inversely with bone mass and may predict a high rate of bone loss and an increased risk of fracture.[130] However, markers currently available are characterized by a wide normal range and considerable variability, which limit their use in individual patients.[131] The most common current clinical use of these assays in care of patients is to obtain a more rapid assessment of the response to antiresorptive agents, which can be detected at 3 to 6 months, before changes in BMD.[132,133]

Markers of Bone Formation

Alkaline Phosphatase

Total serum alkaline phosphatase is measured to assess osteoblastic activity in Paget's disease, primary hyperparathyroidism,

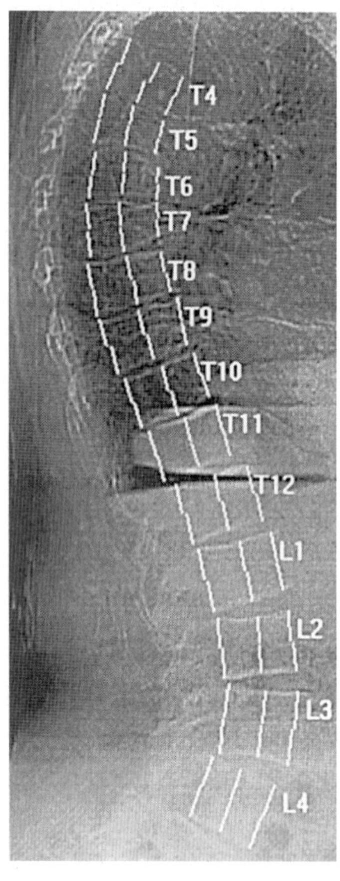

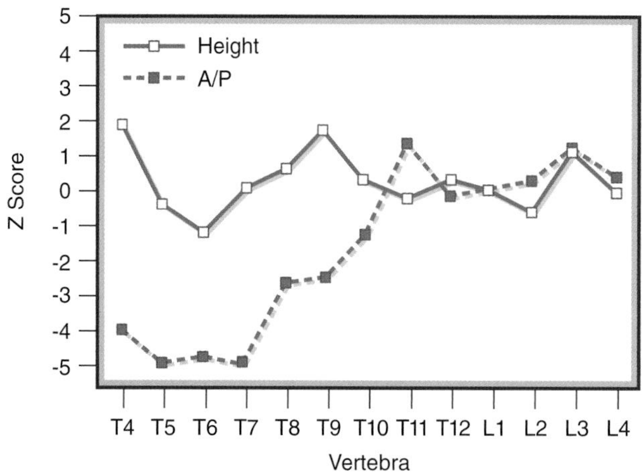

Region		Height (mm)	Height Z	A/P Ratio	A/P Z
T4	>	18.6	+1.9	0.74	-4.0
T5	>	16.2	-0.5	0.69	-4.9
T6	>	15.6	-1.4	0.66	-4.8
T7	>	17.6	+0.2	0.64	-5.0
T8		18.7	+0.7	0.77	-2.6
T9		20.7	+1.8	0.81	-2.5
T10		20.0	+0.2	0.88	-1.2
T11		20.5	-0.3	1.00	+1.4
T12		23.5	+0.4	0.93	-0.2
L1		24.4	+0.1	0.96	+0.2
L2		23.9	0.7	1.01	+0.4
L3		28.8	+1.5	1.07	+1.1
L4		25.7	+0.1	1.07	+0.5

Figure 28–10 ■ Use of dual-energy x-ray absorptiometry for vertebral body morphometry. Posterior vertebral body heights and the ratio of anterior to posterior (A/P) height are presented in terms of standard deviation scores. Note that minor anterior wedging alone may not indicate an osteoporotic fracture. (Courtesy of Dr. Richard B. Mazess.)

osteomalacia, and rickets.[134,135] An immunoassay that selectively measures the bone isoenzyme may increase the usefulness of this test in osteoporosis, in which changes in osteoblastic activity are smaller. High bone-specific alkaline phosphatase values have been shown to predict bone loss and fractures.[136]

Osteocalcin

Osteocalcin, a bone carboxyglutamic acid–containing protein, is one of the few proteins that are relatively specific for skeletal tissue. A fraction of the osteocalcin synthesized by osteoblasts is released into the circulation. Carboxyl-terminal cleavage of the molecule may occur after release, but both the intact and amino-terminal portions can be measured by specific immunoassays. Serum osteocalcin correlates with skeletal growth rates in childhood and puberty and is increased when bone turnover is accelerated (e.g., in hyperparathyroidism and hyperthyroidism).[134,135] In Paget's disease, osteocalcin is elevated to a lesser degree than alkaline phosphatase.

Because osteocalcin production is increased by 1,25(OH)2D, the levels may be low in osteomalacia and rickets even when alkaline phosphatase is elevated. Conversely, osteocalcin levels may be selectively reduced in patients given glucocorticoids to a greater degree than other formation markers. Under-carboxylated osteocalcin is present in vitamin K and vitamin D deficiency, increases with age, and is associated with increased fracture risk.[137]

Procollagen Peptides

The amino-terminal and carboxyl-terminal extension peptides of procollagen (see Fig. 28–2), which are removed during processing of collagen, are released into the circulation. Their measurement is an index of total body synthesis of collagen, the bulk of which is derived from bone. Procollagen peptide levels correlate with histologic measures of bone formation. They may be useful in predicting the response to anabolic agents such as teriparatide.[138] Levels of procollagen peptides are high in infants and may provide a clinically useful index of growth.

Markers of Bone Resorption

Calcium

Measurement of fasting urinary calcium excretion is convenient but shows wide variation, reflecting the net result of intestinal absorption, bone resorption, and mineralization as well as renal tubular handling of calcium. Markedly increased urinary calcium occurs with a marked increase in osteoclastic activity with little change in formation, for example, in some patients with osteolytic bone metastases.

Hydroxyproline

Collagen degradation releases hydroxyproline into the circulation in both free and peptide-bound forms. Because bone resorption is by far the largest contributor to collagen breakdown, urinary hydroxyproline excretion has been used as a measure of bone resorption. However, 80% to 90% of the released hydroxyproline is metabolized, and hydroxyproline from collagen or gelatin in the diet is excreted in urine. Because cross-link excretion can also be used in these conditions, hydroxyproline assays are used less frequently in clinical assessment.

Collagen Cross-Links

Unlike hydroxyproline, the pyridinoline and deoxypyridinoline cross-links that stabilize collagen in the extracellular matrix (Fig. 28–11) are not metabolized but are excreted in the urine in either a free or peptide-bound form. The deoxypyridinoline cross-link is almost entirely derived from skeletal tissue and therefore is a more sensitive indicator of bone resorption than pyridinoline, which is also found in skin and other connective tissues.

Measurement of total urinary pyridinoline and particularly deoxypyridinoline by high-performance liquid chromatography (HPLC) probably provides the best measure of bone resorption but is expensive and time-consuming. Immunoassays have been developed for free pyridinoline and deoxypyridinoline as well as for peptides that include these cross-links and are released during resorption. These assays can now be carried out in serum as well as urine, and this may increase precision.[139,140] Measurements correlate with bone turnover and change in response to agents that affect resorption. Hence, they are useful in assessing changes in resorption in the course of disease or in response to therapy. They may also be valuable in identifying patients with high bone turnover, who not only have low bone mass but also lose bone rapidly and are more likely to develop osteoporosis.

All of these assays have shown diurnal variation and may also be affected by meals.[141] For urine assays, a fasting, second-voided morning urine sample is probably the most reliable.

Other Assays

Tartrate-resistant acid phosphatase is secreted by osteoclasts into serum and may be useful as a measure of bone resorption.[142] Measurements of other enzymes such as cathepsin K and other products of bone matrix are being developed.

Bone Biopsy

Transiliac bone biopsy can provide direct information about cancellous bone volume, the density of connections between trabecular plates (connectivity), and the function of bone cells.[143] The rate of bone formation and mineralization can be measured by this technique with the use of dynamic histomorphometry after tetracycline labeling (Fig. 28–12), but bone resorption is more difficult to assess by bone biopsy. Bone biopsy necessitates the use of a large needle with a 7- to 9-mm internal bore and the technical skill to obtain a sample that is not crushed or distorted. The sample must be processed without decalcification and stained appropriately. Unstained sections are needed in order for one to see fluorescent tetracycline labels. Special stains may be used to identify mast cells in mastocytosis or aluminum in renal osteodystrophy.

Bone biopsies are rarely indicated in the clinical care of patients with osteoporosis but may be indicated for patients with unusual skeletal lesions or for young men or women who have fragility fractures with no evident secondary cause. However, therapeutic decisions can generally be made without biopsies. Biopsies may be indicated more frequently in renal osteodystrophy because the different forms of this disorder are managed differently.[144]

Skeletal Imaging

The use of radiographs, CT, bone scans, and MRI in diagnosis is covered under the discussions of specific disorders. All of these methods are useful in detecting fractures.[145] CT and MRI may also be used to assess bone structure.[122,123] High-resolution radiographs and CT images have also been used to assess cortical porosity.

Bone scans using technetium-99m linked to a bisphosphonate are useful in localization of bone lesions. Uptake is a

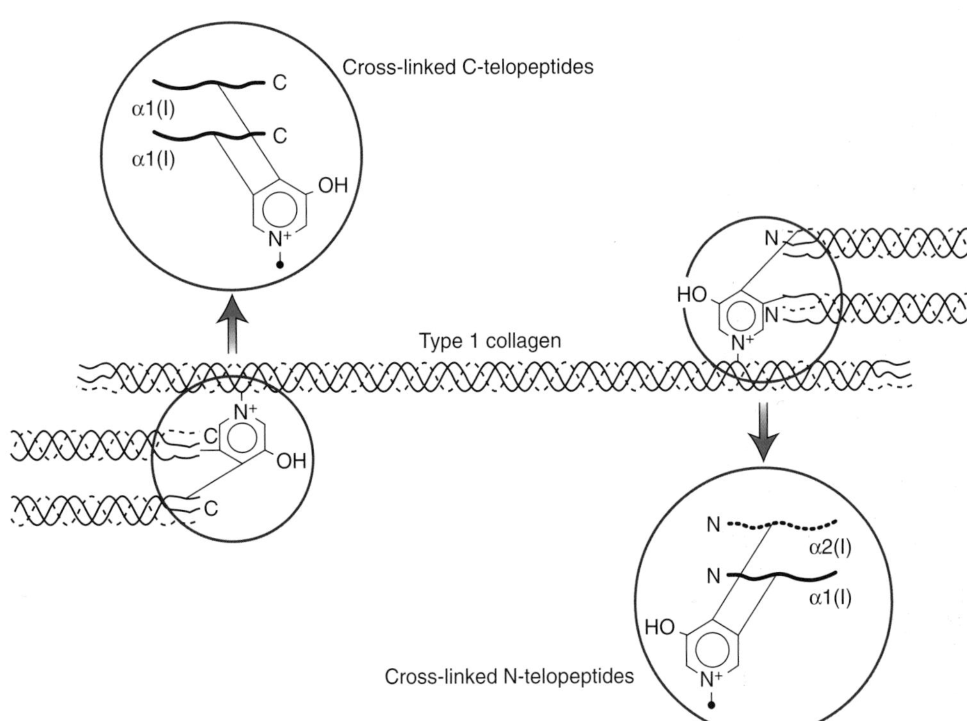

Figure 28–11 ▪ Collagen cross-links. Cross-links are formed between the COOH-terminal and NH2-terminal nonhelical portions of collagen and adjacent helical molecules. Immunoassays are available for the pyridinoline and deoxypyridinoline molecules themselves and for the adjacent nonhelical peptides. (Redrawn from Eyre DR. The specificity of collagen crosslinks as markers of bone and connective tissue degradation. Acta Orthop Scand 1995;266:166-170.)

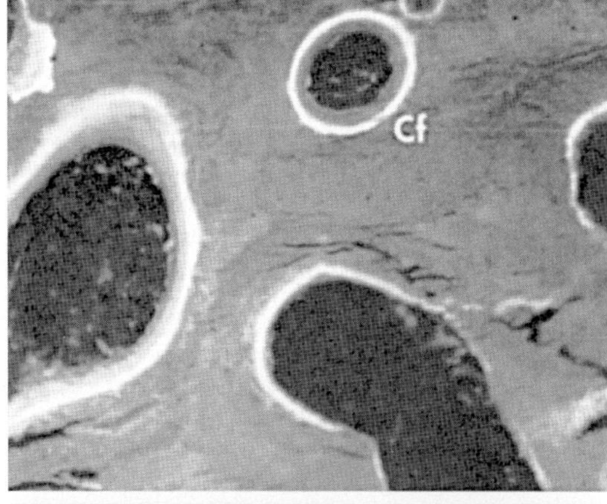

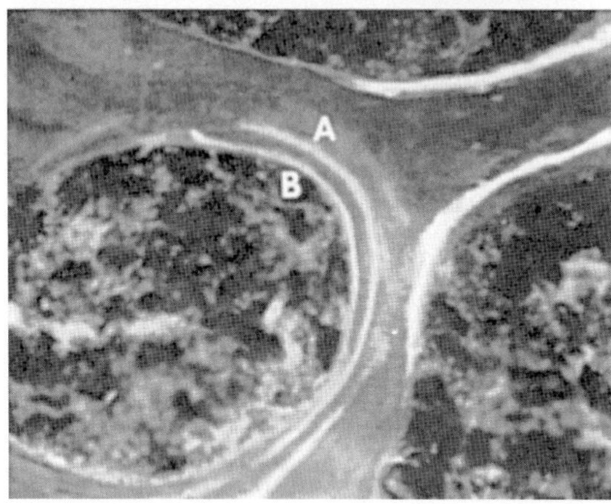

Figure 28–12 ▪ Tetracycline labels sites of active mineralization and is deposited at the calcification front (Cf) (*top*). A double-label technique can be used to measure the rate of mineralization; label A was administered about 10 days before label B (*bottom*). Undecalcified iliac crest, ultraviolet light, ×113. (From Aaron J. Histology and microanatomy of bone. In Nordin BEC, ed. Calcium, Phosphate and Magnesium Metabolism. Edinburgh: Churchill Livingstone, 1976:298-356.)

function of blood flow to the region and the amount of mineralizing bone. The test does not give information about the nature of the lesion but may serve as a guide for further studies. Radiographs or CT scans cannot distinguish old from new fractures, but increased uptake on bone scan or edema on MRI can indicate that the fracture is relatively recent.

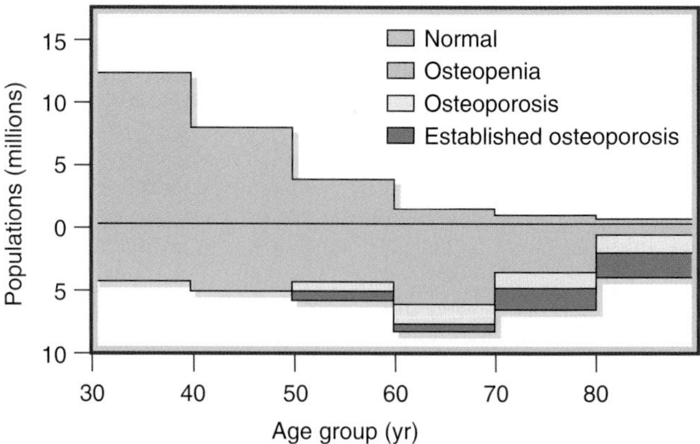

Figure 28–13 ▪ Estimation of the current prevalence of osteoporosis in the United States. On the basis of World Health Organization criteria, more than 9 million women in the United States have osteoporosis; more than half of these women have established osteoporosis with fractures. In addition, 17 million postmenopausal women have osteopenia (low bone mass) and are at risk for development of osteoporosis. (From Melton LJ. How many women have osteoporosis now? J Bone Miner Res 1995;10:175-177.)

TABLE 28–2 DIAGNOSTIC CATEGORIES FOR OSTEOPOROSIS BASED ON MEASUREMENTS OF BONE MINERAL DENSITY AND BONE MINERAL CONTENT

Category	Definition
Normal	A value for BMD or BMC ± 1 SD of the young adult reference mean
Low bone mass (osteopenia)	A value for BMD or BMC > 1 SD and < 2.5 SD lower than the young adult mean
Osteoporosis	A value for BMD or BMC > 2.5 SD lower than the young adult mean
Severe osteoporosis (established osteoporosis)	A value for BMD or BMC > 2.5 SD lower than the young adult mean in the presence of one or more fragility fractures

BMC, Bone mineral content; *BMD,* bone mineral density; *SD,* standard deviation.

OSTEOPOROSIS

Primary Osteoporosis

Definition

Osteoporosis is by far the most common metabolic bone disease. One in two white and Asian postmenopausal women and at least one in eight older men and women of other racial backgrounds are likely to have an osteoporotic fracture at some time during their lifetime (Fig. 28–13). Osteoporosis has been better defined by the Consensus Development Conference[146] as "a disease characterized by low bone mass and microarchitectural deterioration of bone tissue, leading to enhanced bone fragility and a consequent increase in fracture risk."

Currently, diagnostic categories for postmenopausal women are based on measurements of BMD (Table 28–2). These categories are clearly arbitrary but do give some indication of fracture risk. However, the risk of fracture at any given BMD increases markedly with age and can be affected by a number of other factors.[147,148]

A more rational approach to diagnosis and management might be to obtain an estimate of fracture risk based on all factors in individual patients. The use of T-scores to categorize BMD measurements as indicating the presence or absence of osteoporosis is complicated by the fact that the estimation of fracture risk is both site- and method-specific.[149]

Epidemiology

Osteoporosis has been considered a disorder of postmenopausal women of Northern European descent because they have high rates of fractures.[150,151] However, the frequency of osteoporotic fractures is also high in other populations and is likely to increase further as life expectancy increases. Moreover, the age-adjusted incidence of hip fractures around the world is rising, possibly related to increasing industrialization and decreasing physical activity. Most of the epidemiologic data are for hip fractures, but vertebral fractures are equally common. In one study, the lifetime risk of osteoporotic fractures of the hip, spine, or wrist after age 50 years was about 40% in women and 13% in men (Table 28–3). The temporal pattern of the increase in fracture incidence differs for the hip, spine, and wrist (Fig. 28–14).

Pathogenesis

Understanding of the pathogenesis of primary osteoporosis remains largely descriptive.[152] Decreased bone mass and increased fragility can occur because of (1) failure to achieve optimal peak bone mass, (2) bone loss caused by increased bone resorption, or (3) inadequate replacement of lost bone as a result of decreased bone formation. Moreover, an analysis of the pathogenesis of osteoporosis must take into account the heterogeneity of clinical expression.

Inadequate Peak Bone Mass and Strength

Studies of twins suggest that genetic determinants are responsible for up to 85% of the variation in peak bone mass and may also determine bone turnover and fracture risk.[153] Polymorphisms of candidate genes, including vitamin D and estrogen receptors, collagen, cytokines, neurotransmitters, and growth regulators, have been analyzed to assess their possible roles in determining peak bone mass, remodeling, and fracture risk.[153-160] The results generally show small effects or are inconsistent. This problem may reflect the fact that the sample sizes are too small, that it is difficult to determine the appropriate control population, or that these polymorphisms may reflect effects of linked genes.[161] Moreover, gene effects may be influenced by environmental factors.

A broader search for quantitative trait loci associated with differences in bone mass has identified a number of chromosomes that may be involved, not only in determining peak bone mass but also architecture and turnover. These may differ in men and women.[162-164]

While the major determinants of peak bone mass and strength are genetic, there are major factors during childhood and adolescence that can affect the ability to achieve optimal peak bone mass.[165] These include nutrition, particularly of calcium, physical activity, and a wide variety of intercurrent illnesses. Estrogen plays a critical role in both men and women, not only in regulating bone remodeling, but also in determining the time of epiphyseal closure.

TABLE 28–3 ESTIMATED LIFETIME FRACTURE RISK IN WOMEN AND MEN FROM ROCHESTER, MINNESOTA, AT AGE 50 YEARS

Fracture Site	Women (% [95% Confidence Interval])	Men (% [95% Confidence Interval])
Proximal femur	17.5 (16.8-18.2)	6.0 (5.6-6.5)
Vertebra*	15.6 (14.8-16.3)	5.0 (4.6-5.4)
Distal forearm	16.0 (15.7-16.7)	2.5 (2.2-3.1)
Any of the above	39.7 (38.7-40.6)	13.1 (12.4-13.7)

*Clinically diagnosed fractures.
From Melton LJ III, Chrischilles EA, Cooper C, et al. How many women have osteoporosis? J Bone Miner Res 1992;7:1005-1010.

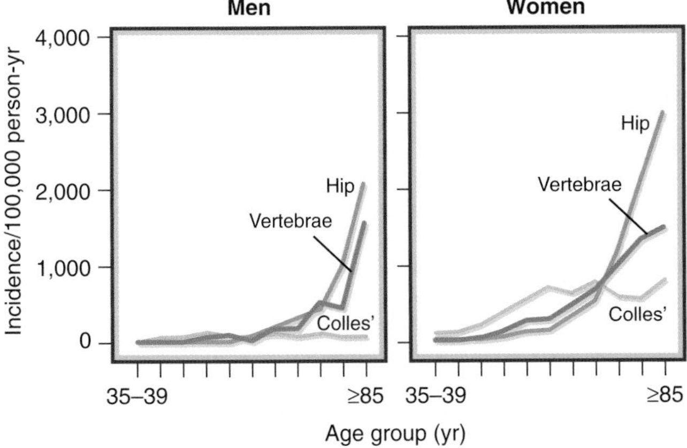

Figure 28–14 ▪ Age-specific incidence rates for hip, vertebral, and Colles' fractures in Rochester, Minnesota. (From Cooper C, Melton LJ. Epidemiology of osteoporosis. Trends Endocrinol Metab 1992;3:224. Copyright 1992 by Elsevier Science Inc.)

Increased Resorption

Peak bone mass is probably achieved in the third decade. Over the next three decades there is some bone loss, particularly of trabecular bone, but fragility fractures are rare, even in those who have low peak bone mass.[166] An increase in the rate of Colles' fractures occurs before the menopause in women, while the increase in vertebral and hip fractures begins in women in their 60s and in men in their 80s (see Fig. 28–14). Increased bone resorption is the major mechanism for increased skeletal fragility. The time required for resorption is much shorter than that for formation in the bone remodeling cycle; hence, any increase in the number of resorption sites will result not only in decreased bone mass, but also in changes in microarchitecture that result in a more fragile skeleton.[167] High rates of bone remodeling, as reflected in the high values for the biochemical markers of bone turnover, persist into old age, and are associated with an increased risk of fracture independent of BMD.[168]

Decreased Bone Formation

Skeletal bone mass increases during puberty and young adult life, even though the rate of resorption is high. Thus, menopausal and age-related bone loss must involve relative impairment of bone formation. With age, the amount of bone formed decreases with each bone structural unit, as evidenced by a decrease in mean wall thickness. This decrease may be due to an age-related decline in skeletal growth factors. Thus, biopsies of patients with established osteoporosis often show decreased bone formation.[169]

Biochemical Abnormalities

Classically, osteoporosis is differentiated from disorders such as osteomalacia and osteogenesis imperfecta by the fact that there is no obvious defect in mineralization or the structure of collagen. However, polymorphisms in the collagen gene COL1A1 or differences in circulating homocysteine levels can result in an increased risk of fracture independent of BMD.[170,171] This could be due to subtle alterations in the collagenous matrix. Differences in crystal structure and alignment have also been described, but these may simply be the consequence of differences in turnover.[172] The further possibility that one or more of the many noncollagen proteins in bone is abnormal in osteoporosis has not been adequately explored.

Pathogenetic Factors

Systemic Hormones

In the past, the search for pathogenetic factors in osteoporosis focused primarily on systemic hormones. A critical role for estrogen deficiency is supported by the fact that postmenopausal women have the highest incidence of osteoporosis and the lowest levels of estradiol. Estrogen levels correlate most strongly with BMD in elderly men, and low estrogen levels are associated with osteoporosis in men.[173,174]

Osteoporosis can occur, albeit rarely, in the absence of any evidence of gonadal hormone deficiency, but defects in receptors for these hormones and other downstream events may be involved. Low BMD and osteoporosis are also associated with high levels of sex hormone–binding globulin (SHBG).[175,176] This association may reflect decreased availability of sex hormones to the tissues when SHBG levels are high.

Other systemic hormones may play a role in age-related bone loss. PTH levels increase with age. The increase is probably due to decreased dietary intake and impaired intestinal absorption of calcium, often associated with vitamin D deficiency. Secondary hyperparathyroidism and vitamin D deficiency can not only accelerate bone loss, but also impair neuromuscular functions. This increases the risk of falls and consequently of fractures.[177,178] However, PTH levels in patients with vertebral fractures are not different from those in age-matched control subjects. 25(OH)D levels are often decreased in the elderly and particularly in osteoporotic patients.[179] Calcitonin deficiency does not appear to play a role in osteoporosis,[180] although pharmacologic doses of calcitonin can prevent bone loss or increase bone mass in patients with high bone turnover.

Glucocorticoid excess can produce secondary osteoporosis but does not appear to play a major role in primary osteoporosis. Growth hormone secretion and circulating IGF-I decrease with age, and differences in IGF-I levels have been associated with fracture risk.[181] Thyroid hormone excess may exacerbate bone loss, and both hyperthyroidism and hypothyroidism are associated with increased fracture risk.[182,183]

Local Factors

Two features of osteoporosis suggest a role for local factors in pathogenesis. (1) Systemic hormones that influence the skeleton, including estrogen and PTH, alter the production of local factors (e.g., cytokines, prostaglandins, and growth factors). (2) Differential bone loss occurs in different parts of the skeleton.

There are limited genetic and biochemical data supporting a role for cytokines in human osteoporosis.[184-186] The most striking evidence for the role of cytokines in the bone loss of estrogen deficiency comes from rodent models. The loss of bone after ovariectomy in rats can be blocked by inhibiting the activity of IL-1 and TNF-α .[187] Ovariectomy does not cause bone loss in mice lacking the biologically active IL-1-receptor.[188] PGE2 production is increased in bones from oophorectomized animals and decreased by estrogen administration.[189] Studies in rodent models suggest the existence of an important interaction between cytokines produced by cells in the marrow, possibly both hematopoietic and mesenchymal, and osteoblasts.[184] These local factors act through the RANKL-RANK system, including OPG, but defects in this system have not yet been identified in osteoporotic patients.[190] In fact, OPG levels may be negatively rather than positively associated with BMD and fracture risk.[191,192]

It is likely that skeletal as well as systemic production of IGF or IGF-binding proteins play a role in osteoporosis.[181] Other growth factors, including BMP-2, have been implicated in genetic studies.

Nutrition and Lifestyle

Calcium deficiency and decreased physical activity in early life can lead to failure to achieve optimal peak bone mass and can accelerate bone loss later in life.[165] Calcium and vitamin D supplementation can slow bone loss and reduce fractures in older adults.[193-195]

Low protein intake is associated with increased fractures in a U.S. study, although in worldwide epidemiologic studies high animal protein intakes are associated with increased risk.[196,197] Vitamin K deficiency is associated with increased hip fracture risk.[198] There are positive correlations between body fat, lean body mass, and bone density. One mechanism of protection of bone density in overweight people may be conversion of adrenal androgens to estrogens in fat. Another pathway may be the decrease in sex hormone globulin associated with increased body mass index.[199] In addition, increased fat and muscle mass would lead to increased impact loading and mechanical stress on bone. Finally, it has become clear that smoking, through a variety of mechanisms, significantly increases the risk for the development of osteoporosis.[200,201]

Nonskeletal Factors

Low body weight and weight loss are important risk factors for osteoporotic fractures. This association may be due in part to nonskeletal effects, such as decreased padding of the hip and decreased muscle strength. Neuromuscular factors, such as loss of muscle strength, impaired balance, and impaired vision, are important, particularly in increasing the risk of falls that result in hip fracture.[202] Drugs that affect the central nervous system or that decrease vascular volume and cause postural hypotension are likely to increase this risk, particularly in older adults.

Clinical Features

Vertebral Crush Fractures

Compression fractures of the vertebrae, which occur spontaneously or with minimal trauma, are the most common manifestation of osteoporosis. The terms postmenopausal osteoporosis and type I osteoporosis have been applied to vertebral crush fracture at a younger age and mainly in women, whereas senile osteoporosis and type II osteoporosis have been used for hip fractures in older women and men.[203] These distinctions may not be helpful clinically. The disorders certainly are not separate, because patients with any type of osteoporotic fracture are more likely to have subsequent fractures of either the spine or the hip.

The clinical course of the vertebral crush fracture syndrome varies. Some patients exhibit compression of only one vertebra and others show collapse of multiple vertebrae. Nevertheless, the risk of additional fractures is high.[204] Vertebrae may show extensive loss of trabecular structure before they collapse (Fig. 28–15). Radiologically, fractures can vary from mild end-plate deformities or anterior wedging to complete vertebral collapse (Fig. 28–16). The most frequent fractures are in the thoracic vertebrae below T6 and in the lumbar vertebrae.

Patients with vertebral crush fractures often have back pain that leads to radiologic assessment. Pain in the lumbar or sacral area, compared with pain in the thoracic area, is less likely to be associated with vertebral compression. Height loss is a sensitive indicator of compression, but height loss can occur without fractures as a result of narrowing of vertebral discs and postural changes.[205] Many patients are asymptomatic. Silent vertebral fractures are still an indication of increased risk and can be assessed by DXA or radiographs.[125,126,206] However, anterior wedging in the upper thoracic vertebrae (T5 to T8) is common

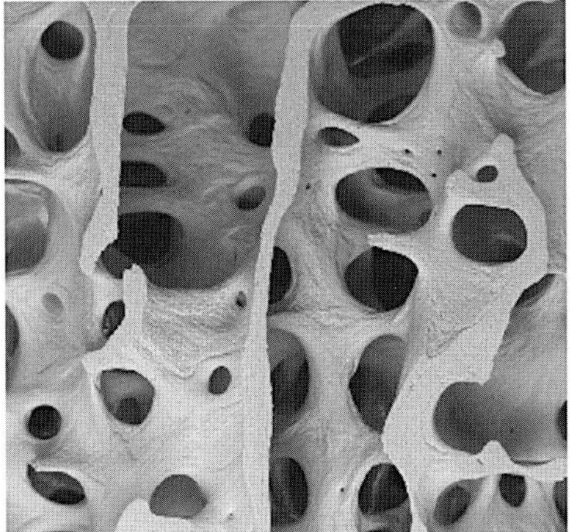

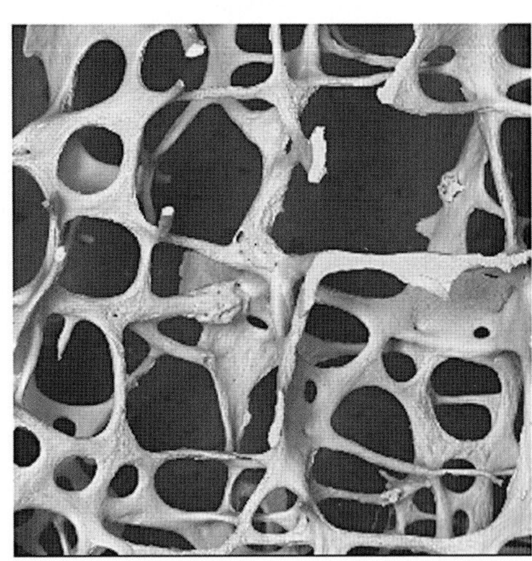

Figure 28–15 ▪ Scanning electron micrographs of a normal vertebrae from a 31-year-old man and an osteoporotic vertebrae from an 89-year-old woman showing extensive loss of trabecular bone architecture with conversion of plates to rods and a microfracture. (From Boyd A. Morphologic detail of aging bone in human vertebrae. Endocrine 2002;17:5-14.)

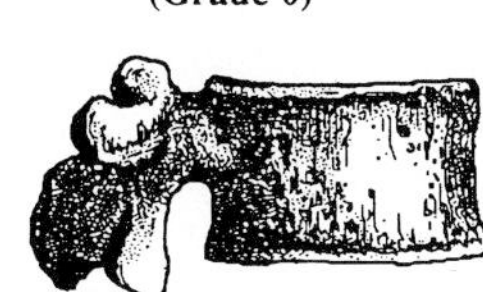

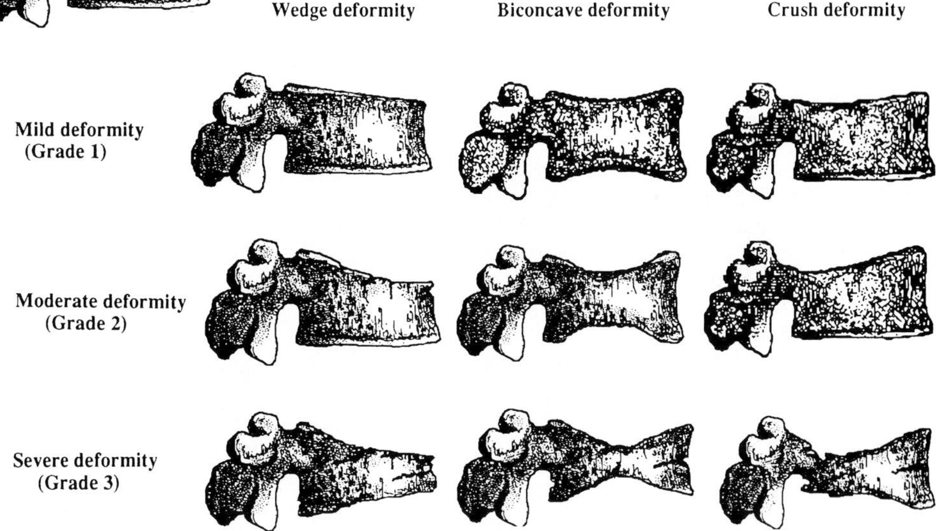

Figure 28–16 ▪ Types of vertebral compression fractures. Changes in vertebral height can be quantitated by measuring percent change or standard deviations from expected normal heights. (From Genant HK, Wu CY, van Kuijk C, et al. Vertebral fracture assessment using a semiquantitative technique. J Bone Miner Res 1993;8:1137-1148.)

in older men and women and is not necessarily due to compression fractures. Bone density measurements can help predict fracture risk in these patients. Anterior wedging may also develop early in life, probably during pubertal growth, as a genetic disorder called Scheuermann's disease.[207]

Multiple vertebral crush fractures cause severe impairment. Kyphosis and loss of the lumbar lordosis are deforming and can exacerbate back pain. Impairment of chest wall function may reduce vital capacity.[208] Compression of abdominal contents may be disfiguring and uncomfortable. Ultimately, impingement of the ribs on the iliac crest is another source of pain. Many patients have additional spinal abnormalities, including spondylolisthesis, intervertebral disc disease, and osteoarthritis, particularly in the spinal facets. Osteoporosis itself rarely compresses nerve roots or the spinal cord. Although patients with severe osteoarthritis are somewhat less likely to have osteoporosis, these two disorders commonly occur in the same patient.

Hip Fracture

Fractures of the proximal femur are a major cause of morbidity and mortality in older people. Most fractures are in the femoral neck or at the base of the greater trochanter and are associated with trauma, although the trauma may be minimal. The risk is influenced by factors that increase the risk of falling and by the type of fall as well as the structure of the skeleton and surrounding soft tissue. The increased incidence of hip fractures with age is caused both by increased falls and by continued bone loss.[209]

Hip fracture is usually treated surgically, and the costs are substantial. In addition, perioperative and postoperative complications are associated with a 5% to 20% mortality rate. Many older patients cannot return to their previous level of activity after hip fracture and require long-term nursing home care. It is important to perform a diagnostic evaluation and to develop a prevention plan for these patients because a second hip fracture or a fragility fracture at another site is likely to occur. Unfortunately, most patients with hip fractures do not undergo evaluation or treatment to prevent progression of osteoporosis and additional fractures.[210]

Colles' Fracture

Colles' fractures of the distal radius, which is composed largely of trabecular bone, are caused by falling on the outstretched hand. The incidence in women begins to increase after age 40 years and may be associated with premenopausal and perimenopausal bone loss and with genetic factors.[211] Unlike that of vertebral and hip fractures, the incidence of Colles' fractures in men does not increase with age. Colles' fractures usually heal well and only occasionally result in long-term morbidity. Women with a Colles' fracture should be assessed for osteoporosis so that an appropriate treatment plan can be provided.

Other Fractures

Fractures at any site, with the possible exception of the face and skull, can be associated with osteoporosis. Measurements of bone mass and further diagnostic workup are indicated for all fractures that occur with minimal trauma.

Osteoporosis in Men

The incidence of hip and spine fractures in men increases with age and is about one third that in women. Men often have vertebral deformities associated with trauma earlier in life. In men, the increase in hip fractures tends to occur later in life, and a higher proportion of men have definable secondary causes.[212] Bone histomorphometry shows both increased resorption and decreased formation.[213]

Osteoporosis in men is associated with low androgen and estrogen and high SHBG levels.[214,215] Abnormalities of the IGF system and particular polymorphisms of the LRP-5 gene are also implicated.[215,216] A diagnostic workup and therapeutic plan should be provided for men with fragility fractures, but this is rarely carried out in practice. Screening for osteoporosis in older men who do not have fractures has not yet been evaluated but may be justified now that preventive therapy is available.

Juvenile Osteoporosis

Juvenile osteoporosis is a rare, self-limiting disease that can begin between the ages of 8 and 14 years with back pain and vertebral compression.[217] Antiresorptive agents may be beneficial.[218] However, deficient bone formation may be the critical defect leading to fractures in these children.[219] Spontaneous remission usually occurs, and the disorder usually does not lead to permanent deformity. Mutation in type I collagen and LRP-5 have been reported in this disorder.[220,221]

Idiopathic Osteoporosis

Osteoporosis with no obvious secondary cause in premenopausal women or younger men is called idiopathic osteoporosis. The term is not used consistently, and patients so defined include individuals with both high and low bone turnover.[222] Some patients have a transient, self-limited condition, whereas others have a progressive and disabling disease. Idiopathic osteoporosis can be associated with nonspecific inflammatory changes, and these cases may be caused by abnormal cytokine activity. A careful evaluation, including consideration of bone biopsy, should be made to search for secondary causes.

Osteoporosis in Pregnancy

Osteoporosis in pregnancy is rare and may represent a genetically determined bone disease that has been present before pregnancy.[223] Bone loss can occur during pregnancy and lactation, but this is transient and not a risk factor for osteoporosis.[224]

Localized Osteoporosis

Immobilization is the most common cause of localized osteoporosis (see later). Transient osteoporosis of the hip has been reported in middle-aged men and in pregnancy.[225] Regional migratory osteoporosis can occur without immobilization, particularly in the lower extremities.[226] This phenomenon may be associated with local inflammation or autonomic dysfunction with vasomotor changes and hyperesthesia, a syndrome called reflex sympathetic dystrophy or complex regional pain syndrome.[227]

Secondary Osteoporosis

The division of osteoporosis into primary and secondary forms is somewhat arbitrary. For example, patients with diseases that lead to hypogonadism early in life are considered to have *secondary* osteoporosis, whereas osteoporosis in women with natural menopause and older men with low sex hormone levels is termed *primary.* Moreover, many patients have a combination of primary and secondary causes. Although most postmenopausal women and older men do not have a definable secondary cause, the few who do can be treated more effectively. Therefore, this possibility should be considered in every patient. There are many causes of secondary osteoporosis (Table 28–4), only a few of which are discussed here.[228]

Glucocorticoid-Induced Osteoporosis

The most common form of secondary osteoporosis is that induced by exogenous glucocorticoids.[229] Cushing's syndrome, caused by an excess of endogenous glucocorticoids, is less common but may also involve osteoporosis at presentation. Patients with rheumatoid arthritis, chronic pulmonary disease, or gastrointestinal disease who receive exogenous glucocorticoids are at additional risk because disease-associated inflammation, poor nutrition, and immobilization can worsen bone loss. Glucocorticoid-induced osteoporosis is particularly common in postmenopausal women, presumably because they also have primary osteoporosis. However, fragility fractures can occur in any patient receiving moderate to high doses of glucocorticoids. The increased fracture risk appears within a few months of initiating therapy and rapidly declines after cessation of treatment.[230]

Glucocorticoid-induced osteoporosis is a result of both increased bone resorption and decreased bone formation. Increased resorption may be in part indirectly caused by decreased calcium absorption and the resulting secondary hyperparathyroidism. Decreased bone formation is probably caused by direct inhibition of osteoblasts, which are highly sensitive to glucocorticoids. For example, as little as 2.5 mg of prednisone given at bedtime can block the normal nocturnal rise in osteocalcin.[231] Glucocorticoids can decrease osteoblast and osteocyte function by increasing apoptosis,[232] but may increase osteoclast formation by preventing apoptosis.[233] Glucocorticoids also increase urinary calcium and phosphate and can inhibit gonadal hormone production by blocking gonadotropin release. Levels of testosterone are low in men receiving prednisone, 20 mg/day or more.[234] Exogenous glucocorticoids

TABLE 28–4 CAUSES OF SECONDARY OSTEOPOROSIS
ENDOCRINE DISORDERS
Hyperparathyroidism Cushing's syndrome Hypogonadism Hyperthyroidism Prolactinoma Diabetes mellitus Acromegaly Pregnancy and lactation
HEMATOPOIETIC DISORDERS
Plasma cell dyscrasias: multiple myeloma and macroglobulinemia Systemic mastocytosis Leukemias and lymphomas Sickle cell disease and thalassemia minor Lipidoses: Gaucher's disease Myeloproliferative disorders: polycythemia
CONNECTIVE TISSUE DISORDERS
Osteogenesis imperfecta Ehlers-Danlos syndrome Marfan's syndrome Homocystinuria and lysinuria Menkes' syndrome Scurvy
DRUG-INDUCED DISORDERS
Glucocorticoids Heparin Anticonvulsants Methotrexate, cyclosporine Luteinizing hormone–releasing hormone (LHRH) agonist or antagonist therapy Aluminum-containing antacids
IMMOBILIZATION
RENAL DISEASE
Chronic renal failure Renal tubular acidosis
NUTRITIONAL AND GASTROINTESTINAL DISORDERS
Malabsorption Total parenteral nutrition Gastrectomy Hepatobiliary disease Chronic hypophosphatemia
MISCELLANEOUS
Familial dysautonomia (Riley-Day syndrome) Reflex sympathetic dystrophy

decrease secretion of corticotropin, thereby decreasing the production of adrenal androgens, which are the major precursors for estrogen formation in postmenopausal women.

Clinically, glucocorticoid-induced osteoporosis is similar to primary osteoporosis. Initial bone loss is predominantly trabecular and is best assessed in the spine or distal radius. However, rib fractures and aseptic necrosis of the femoral or humeral heads or the vertebrae are common in glucocorticoid-induced osteoporosis, although they are rare in primary osteoporosis. Glucocorticoid-induced osteoporosis can be reversible, particularly in young patients who are cured of Cushing's syndrome.[235] In patients who cannot discontinue glucocorticoid therapy, early preventive therapy may be effective. Bisphosphonates and PTH prevent bone loss in patients with glucocorticoid-induced osteoporosis.[236-238] Bisphosphonates also decrease fracture risk[239]. They may act in part by suppressing osteoblast and osteocyte apoptosis.[240]

Hypogonadism

Hypogonadism can occur in either men or women and has multiple causes. Patients with primary hypogonadism related to ovarian or testicular failure or secondary hypogonadism related to hypothalamic or pituitary disease lose bone rapidly and often have fragility fractures. The hypogonadotropic group includes patients with anorexia nervosa, athletic amenorrhea, prolactinoma, or lesions of the pituitary gland or hypothalamus, including tumors. Undernutrition and hypercortisolism may also contribute to bone loss in anorexia nervosa and athletic amenorrhea.[241,242] Loss of growth hormone may play a role in the osteoporosis of pituitary tumors.

Drug-induced hypogonadism is increasing in frequency. Long-acting progestins used for contraception in young women cause bone loss that is usually reversible.[243] Gonadotropin-releasing hormone (GnRH) analogues and aromatase inhibitors used to block sex hormone production in women with breast cancer or endometriosis and men with prostate cancer can cause rapid bone loss.[244,245]

Other Endocrine Causes

Hyperthyroidism can produce bone loss[182]; however, the increase in formation in young persons is usually adequate, and, if the disease is treated early, changes in bone mass are small.[246] Both hormone excess and deficiency may increase the risk of fractures.[183] In individuals at risk for osteoporosis, primary hyperthyroidism may be missed or excessive amounts of exogenous thyroid hormone may be administered for many years. Osteoporosis has been seen in patients with growth hormone deficiency and can respond to growth hormone replacement.[247] A large pituitary tumor may cause gonadotropin deficiency and bone loss.[248] Decreased estradiol levels may be the main determinant of low BMD in both sexes.

Patients with insulin-dependent diabetes mellitus often have low bone mass and diminished bone formation, perhaps because they lack an anabolic effect of insulin.[249] The role of non–insulin-dependent diabetes mellitus in the pathogenesis of osteoporosis is unclear. BMD is usually normal or high, but fracture incidence is increased, suggesting that there is an independent effect of diabetes on bone fragility or on the frequency of falls.[250,251]

Malignancy

Multiple myeloma and other lymphoproliferative malignancies can produce a clinical picture that resembles primary osteoporosis. It is particularly important to exclude myeloma in patients with rapidly progressive vertebral crush fracture syndrome. Myeloma may cause rapid bone loss because the malignant cells produce both stimulators of resorption and inhibitors of formation.[252,253] Metastases to the spine may also cause vertebral compression and should be considered in the differential diagnosis, particularly for patients with normal bone density. These lesions can usually be differentiated from osteoporotic fractures by MRI.[254]

Other Diseases

The incidence and severity of osteoporosis are increased in patients with chronic hepatic and intestinal disorders, not only for nutritional reasons or because these patients often receive glucocorticoids or other drugs that affect the skeleton, but also because of increased cytokine production.[255,256] Impaired absorption of calcium and vitamin D also occurs in celiac disease.[257] Although it was initially thought that impairment of vitamin D function in hepatic and intestinal disease would cause osteomalacia, the most common lesion in such patients is osteoporosis. Unfortunately, these patients often do not respond to vitamin D supplementation. People with severe alcoholism can also have osteoporosis; however, lower intakes of ethanol may be associated with increased bone mass and a decreased fracture risk.[258]

Mastocytosis causes both osteoporosis and osteosclerosis, and the number of mast cells may be increased in the marrow of patients with primary osteoporosis.[259-261] The functional significance of the mast cells is not known, although they do produce heparin, which can cause bone loss. Hyperplastic anemias, such as thalassemia, can also cause bone loss,[262] partly because of bone erosion by the marrow and partly because of hypogonadism associated with transfusion-induced hemochromatosis.[263] Osteoporosis after organ transplantation is common and results both from the underlying disease and from the drugs used to prevent graft rejection.[264]

Drugs

A number of drugs can produce osteoporosis.[228,265] Heparin stimulates bone resorption and inhibits bone formation and can cause osteoporosis. Patients receiving anticonvulsants, including phenytoin, barbiturates, and carbamazepine, often have low bone mass. Impairment of vitamin D metabolism has been described, but most patients have osteoporosis with normal mineralization. Immunosuppressive agents, such as cyclosporine and FK506, are associated with bone loss. GnRH analogues, which decrease production of gonadal hormones and aromatase inhibitors, which block formation of estrogen from androgen, can lead to osteoporosis.[266,267] Some agents used in cancer chemotherapy probably act both by inhibiting osteoblasts and by suppressing gonadal hormones.

Diagnosis

As indicated by the World Health Organization, osteoporosis can be diagnosed before fracture occurs by measuring bone density. The frequency of diagnosis, therefore, depends on the frequency, site, and timing of bone density measurements.[268,269] While there is not yet complete agreement about who should be screened or when screening should be done, a suggested approach is illustrated in Figure 28-17.

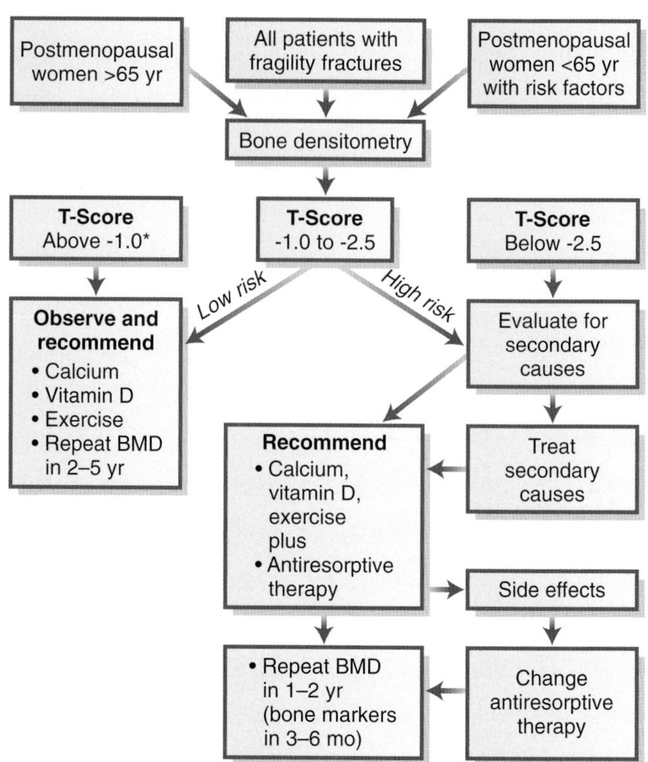

*Patients with fragility fractures and a T-score above -1.0 should be evaluated for other causes of pathologic fracture.

Figure 28–17 ■ Diagnosis and management of osteoporosis. The diagram outlines an approach based largely on evidence from studies of postmenopausal white women, with dual-energy x-ray absorptiometry used to measure bone mineral density (BMD). Its application to other populations, including patients with secondary osteoporosis and other methods of assessing BMD, is not established.

Universal screening of postmenopausal women after age 65 years has been recommended as cost-effective.[116] Earlier screening is recommended for women who have multiple risk factors, such as low body weight or a personal or family history of fragility fractures (appendicular or axial fractures after a fall from standing height or less). Bone density should also be measured in men and premenopausal women with fragility fractures. BMD measurements may also be useful in early postmenopausal women under consideration for hormone replacement therapy. Bone density measurements not only establish the severity of bone loss but also provide a baseline for monitoring the patient's therapeutic response. The test may also enhance health-related behavior.[270] The subsequent workup should be the same whether osteoporosis is diagnosed on the basis of screening or after the finding of a fragility fracture.

The history should include a detailed analysis of calcium intake and nutrition, changes in height or weight, physical activity and lifestyle, smoking history, menstrual and reproductive history, and personal or family history of fragility fractures or other metabolic or endocrine disorders that may affect the skeleton. Physical examination should include a careful height measurement, assessment of the spine, and evaluation for thyroid or adrenal disease.

Radiologic assessment of fractures may be possible using DXA as well as ordinary radiographs. In addition, MRI or CT may be indicated if there are neurologic changes or if fractures are associated with normal bone density, raising the possibility of malignancy.

A minimal laboratory screen should include measurement of serum calcium, preferably as ionized calcium or with albumin to permit correction for protein-bound calcium and fasting calcium excretion (most easily measured as the calcium/creatinine ratio in the second-voided morning specimen). Appropriate tests to exclude secondary causes of osteoporosis should be based on the history and physical findings. Serum phosphorus and alkaline phosphatase are useful in ruling out hyperparathyroidism and osteomalacia. Measurements of 25-hydroxyvitamin D and PTH are indicated if the screening test results are abnormal. Routine measurement of 25-hydroxyvitamin D may be indicated in areas where deficiency is common. Serum electrophoresis, blood count, and erythrocyte sedimentation rate can help to rule out myeloma, and thyroid function should be assessed. Laboratory studies for Cushing's syndrome are indicated in patients with suggestive clinical features. Measurements of gonadal and pituitary hormones are indicated for younger patients with osteoporosis. Gluten-sensitive enteropathy should be ruled out in patients with weight loss or frequent bowel movements.

Despite the inverse correlation between markers of bone resorption and formation and bone mass, these measurements have wide variations and cannot substitute for measurements of BMD in the diagnosis of osteoporosis. Because elevated values of both resorption and formation markers do indicate increased risk for bone loss and fractures, these measurements may become useful in determining the need for therapy, particularly if they can be made more accurate and less expensive.[271]

Prevention and Therapy

Although it is important to relieve pain and to limit the impact of deformities in established osteoporosis, the primary goal of treatment is to prevent fractures. Therefore, prevention and therapy are considered together.

Nutrition and Calcium Supplementation

The calcium intakes recommended for prevention and treatment of osteoporosis range from 1 to 2 g/day.[272,273] In children and adolescents, intakes of 1000 to 1200 mg/day are recommended. Most studies indicate that calcium supplementation slows bone loss,[274] but there is limited evidence that calcium supplementation alone can decrease fracture risk. Moreover, low calcium intakes in the presence of low calcium absorption increase the risk of hip fractures.[275] High calcium intakes are generally safe, although it may be worthwhile to check urinary calcium levels.

There is no clear advantage for any particular calcium formulation. Calcium carbonate is inexpensive and, when taken with meals, is usually well absorbed, even in patients with achlorhydria.[276] Calcium citrate and other salts may be absorbed better than calcium carbonate in the fasting state.

It is also worthwhile to include foods high in calcium in the diet. Patients should be informed about the calcium content of the major food sources, such as dairy products.

Vitamin D intake should be at least 400 U/day, and up to 2000 U/day has been suggested; higher levels may produce hypercalciuria or hypercalcemia. Calcium and vitamin D increase bone mass, decrease seasonal bone loss,[274] and can decrease the incidence of fractures, particularly in populations likely to have deficient intakes or limited sun exposure.[277] Other forms of vitamin D have been used, including calcidiol (25[OH]D), calcitriol (1,25[OH]2D), and 1α (OH)D, but, except in renal disease, there is little direct evidence that these are superior to ordinary vitamin D, which is less expensive.[278,279] Dietary intakes of other minerals and of vitamins C and K, which are important for bone matrix synthesis, as well as protein should be adequate.

Exercise, Lifestyle, and Prevention of Falls

The role of exercise in treatment of osteoporosis has not been defined. On the basis of limited data, ½-hour of weight-bearing exercise per day is recommended for patients who can tolerate it.[280] Epidemiologic data suggest that lifetime leisure exercise is associated with higher BMD at the hip but may have no effect on fracture incidence.[281] Patients are often better able to develop and maintain a suitable exercise program under the supervision of a physical therapist. Patients should also be instructed in body mechanics and posture in order to minimize musculoskeletal damage and the likelihood of falls. They should stop smoking and limit their intake of alcohol.

Medicines that cause prolonged sedation[282] or postural hypertension should be avoided in older adults. Help should be provided for coping with osteoporosis and for designing a lifestyle that maintains function and minimizes fracture risk.[283,284] Excessive sodium and protein intake should be avoided because they can increase urinary calcium excretion.[197]

Management of Fractures

Fractures of the hip as well as other appendicular fractures are generally treated surgically. Vertebral fractures may require transient bed rest. A careful but intensive program of rehabilitation is critical in patients with fractures of the hip and spine.[280] Pain relief for patients with vertebral crush fractures can usually be achieved with mild analgesics and local physical therapy. Calcitonin has analgesic effects and may be useful in patients with severe pain.

Surgical treatment of individual vertebral fractures by injection of methacrylate resin has been used to relieve pain and expand the compressed vertebral body. Kyphoplasty employs a balloon to create a space for the resin, whereas in vertebroplasty the resin is injected directly.[285]

Hormone Replacement Therapy

The role of hormone replacement therapy for the prevention and treatment of osteoporosis has been altered substantially by the findings of the large Women's Health Initiative (WHI) clinical trial as well as a number of other controlled trials. The finding that the risk of cardiovascular disease as well as breast cancer was increased, although fracture risk was decreased, has shifted the risk/benefit ratio and substantially decreased the use of HRT.[286-289] Thus, while HRT is still considered appropriate for the treatment of menopausal symptoms, prevention of osteoporosis is no longer considered an appropriate indication. An approach that deserves further exploration is the use of much lower doses of estrogen which have been shown to prevent bone loss with minimal side effects.[290,291] Both oral and transdermal ultra low dose estrogen produce minimal stimulation of the uterus and breast, but their effect on cardiovascular disease and on fracture risk have not yet been assessed. In contrast to bisphosphonate therapy (see later), there is often accelerated bone loss after withdrawal of estrogen therapy[292]; therefore, many patients who have discontinued estrogen because of the findings of the WHI need to be carefully monitored and alternative therapy considered.

Bisphosphonates

Bisphosphonates are pyrophosphate analogues that bind to bone mineral are then taken up by osteoclasts and rapidly inhibit resorption.[293,294] The first compound available for clinical use, etidronate, inhibits bone mineralization at high doses but increases bone mass without impairing mineralization when given intermittently.[295] Another first generation compound, clodronate, does not inhibit mineralization.[296] Second-generation bisphosphonates, such as alendronate, risedronate, and ibandronate, do not impair mineralization and are more potent. The inhibitory effects on osteoclast function differ for the first-generation compounds, which lower adenosine triphosphate levels at high concentrations, and the second-generation compounds, which impair isoprenylation of proteins at low concentrations.[297]

Alendronate, risedronate, and ibandronate are approved for prevention and treatment of osteoporosis in the United States on the basis of evidence that they decrease bone resorption, increase bone mass in the spine and hip, and decrease the incidence of fractures.[298-300] Bisphosphonates can prevent bone loss in patients receiving glucocorticoids[301] and in men.[302] There is no consensus on the duration of therapy, but continued benefit has been observed in patients treated for up to 10 years.[303]

Bisphosphonates are poorly absorbed orally and must be taken on an empty stomach with no food or other medication. The major side effects are gastrointestinal, particularly esophageal irritation. Gastrointestinal side effects may also be reduced by giving bisphosphonates weekly instead of daily.[304] This problem may be circumvented by using parenteral bisphosphonates. Pamidronate and zoledronic acid are available for intravenous use in malignancy, although not yet approved for osteoporosis therapy.[305] Most recently there has been significant concern about the development of osteonecrosis of the jaw in bisphosphonate-treated patients. The incidence of this syndrome is currently unknown but it appears to be most prevalent in individuals who have received high-dose intravenous bisphosphonate therapy for treatment of complications from malignant disease.[306]

Calcitonin

Calcitonin, an inhibitor of bone resorption, can increase bone mass, particularly in association with high turnover rates. Calcitonin also has some analgesic properties and may be particularly useful in patients with recent painful vertebral fractures. It is available either for subcutaneous injection or as a nasal spray. The former preparation is probably more effective but is less well tolerated, often producing gastrointestinal side effects. In a 3-year randomized trial, nasal calcitonin at 200 U/day was found to decrease fracture incidence significantly, although the effects on bone turnover and bone mass were diminished by the end of the study.[307] However, the fact that doses of 100 or 400 U/day did not significantly decrease fractures and other concerns have raised questions about the efficacy of calcitonin.[308] Nasal calcitonin is less effective in increasing BMD than alendronate.[309] Calcitonin has been used acutely to reduce pain in patients with vertebral fractures.[310]

Selective Estrogen Receptor Modulators

A number of compounds have had effects similar to those of estrogen on bone, but they act as antagonists in the breast and hence have been called selective estrogen receptor modulators (SERMs).

Tamoxifen has been shown to diminish bone loss in women with breast cancer.[311] Another SERM, raloxifene, has not only prevented bone loss but has also reduced the risk of vertebral fracture in osteoporotic patients.[312] Its effects on bone turnover and mass are somewhat less than those of estrogen.[313] Raloxifene does not stimulate the breast or uterus and appears to decrease the risk of breast cancer.[314] It reduces low-density lipoprotein (LDL) levels but does not increase high-density lipoprotein (HDL).[315] However, it is associated with an increased risk of thromboembolism and may produce hot flashes.

New SERMS with potentially greater effects in bone are currently being studied.[316,317]

Anabolic Therapy

Parathyroid Hormone

Many years ago, PTH given intermittently in low doses was shown to increase bone mass in animals. The use of intermittent low-dose synthetic PTH (teriparatide) in both men and women with osteoporosis has produced a substantial increase in trabecular bone mass with little loss or even a gain in cortical bone in the femur and has reduced the incidence of fractures.[318,319] Treatment with PTH is likely to be the most effective approach in patients who lose bone or continue to have fractures on antiresorptive therapy. PTH may be particularly useful in glucocorticoid-induced osteoporosis.[238] PTH must be given by injection, and patients must be monitored carefully for hypercalcemia and hypercalciuria.

Prior or concomitant therapy with bisphosphonates may blunt or delay the anabolic response to PTH, but certainly does not abrogate it.[320-322] In addition, treatment with bisphosphonates after a course of PTH may help maintain the gains of PTH therapy.[323]

Strontium Ranelate

Strontium ranelate has been proposed as an anabolic agent that also may be antiresorptive. It has been shown to reduce the incidence of both vertebral and nonvertebral fractures in large clinical trials.[324] It has not been approved for the treatment of osteoporosis in the United States.

Anabolic Steroids

Anabolic androgenic steroids (e.g., testosterone) may increase bone as well as muscle mass. However, high doses produce unacceptable androgenic side effects in many women. Testosterone therapy can increase bone mass and improves trabecular architecture in hypogonadal men.[325-327]

Testosterone can also increase bone and muscle mass in older men, particularly those with low levels of bioavailable testosterone.

Thiazides

Thiazides can decrease urinary calcium excretion and increase bone mass in patients with hypercalciuria and may reduce cortical bone loss in normal postmenopausal women and decrease the incidence of hip fractures.[328,329] Thiazide therapy is particularly appropriate in patients with osteoporosis who have high fasting urinary calcium excretion due to a renal load.

Other Osteoclast Inhibitors

There are several critical aspects of osteoclast function, including RANKL-RANK interactions, the secretion of acid and proteolytic enzymes, and the expression of integrins that could be potential sites for effective intervention in osteoporosis. Selective antagonists for these processes have been developed and are currently being explored in the laboratory and the clinic.[330,331]

RICKETS AND OSTEOMALACIA

Rickets and osteomalacia are disorders of the mineralization of newly synthesized organic matrix. In adults, the disorder involves only bone; in children, however, abnormalities also occur in the growth plate and in the mineralization of cartilage, leading to characteristic deformities.

Pathogenesis

To understand the pathogenesis of rickets and osteomalacia, we should recognize that vitamin D is a prohormone that can be synthesized in the skin or supplied in the diet. Vitamin D deficiency is usually the combined result of deficient sun exposure and decreased dietary intake or intestinal malabsorption. Rickets and osteomalacia can also be caused by metabolic defects in the vitamin D hormone system, including inadequate activation in the liver and kidney and abnormalities of the vitamin D receptor (see Chapter 27). Mineralization can also be impaired when the supply or transport of mineral, particularly phosphate, is impaired in renal, intestinal, or bone cell disorders.[332]

Nutritional and Gastrointestinal Disorders

Inadequate vitamin D intake is less common in the United States than in other countries because many foods are supplemented with this vitamin. However, the combination of inadequate sunlight or lack of the appropriate ultraviolet wavelengths, which occurs during the winter in the northern half of the United States, and failure to provide vitamin D supplements in the diet can lead to rickets in infants and osteomalacia in older persons. Individuals with darker pigmentation of the skin are more susceptible to vitamin D deficiency because they are less efficient in converting 7-dehydrocholesterol to vitamin D.[333,334] For example, nutritional rickets occurs in black infants who are breastfed without vitamin D supplementation. Adult Asiatic Indians in the United States and Europe have low 25(OH)D levels and are more likely to have osteomalacia. Intestinal malabsorption of fat can also cause deficiency of vitamin D and of other fat-soluble vitamins.[335] Inability to produce adequate amounts of 25(OH)D can occur in advanced liver disease and with the use of antiepileptic drugs.

Calcium deficiency rickets may differ from other forms of rickets and osteomalacia, particularly in adolescents, who may have genu valgum without end-plate deformities.[336,337] In contrast, phosphate deficiency causes typical rickets. Because most foods contain phosphate, this form of rickets requires markedly unbalanced nutrition, such as can occur with prolonged intravenous feeding, removal of phosphate by dialysis with a low-phosphate solution, or use of aluminum-containing antacids, which bind phosphate in the intestine.

Renal Defects

Impairment of 1α-hydroxylase can occur because of loss of renal mass or in renal tubular disorders such as the Fanconi syndrome. A hereditary deficiency of 1α-hydroxylase, termed vitamin D–dependent rickets type I or pseudo-vitamin D deficiency, is a rare autosomal recessive disorder in which rickets develops during the first year of life. It occurs in rodents with homozygous inactivating mutations of the 1α-hydroxylase gene and responds to physiologic doses of calcitriol.[338,339]

Hereditary Resistance to Vitamin D (Vitamin D–Dependent Rickets Type II)

This severe form of rickets occurs in members of families who are homozygous for defects in the vitamin D receptor gene. These patients also often have alopecia. They show improvement in mineralization in response to high doses of calcium and phosphorus, but this does not reverse the alopecia.[340]

Familial X-Linked Hypophosphatemia

Originally termed *vitamin D–resistant rickets*, this syndrome is caused by a defect in phosphate transport. Although the most apparent abnormality is decreased renal tubular reabsorption of phosphate, phosphate transport may be impaired in other cells, particularly osteoblasts. Inactivating mutations in a gene (PHEX), which encodes a protein that is a member of the M13 family of membrane-bound metalloproteases, have been found in this disorder.[341-343] While the exact mechanism by which PHEX mutations mediate this condition is unknown, one explanation for how this syndrome develops revolves around the hypothesis that PHEX normally either directly or indirectly modifies one or more phosphate transport regulating hormones (phosphatonins). In individuals with mutations in PHEX, modification of phosphatonins may be abnormal, leading to the clinical syndrome. These patients may also have some impairment in 1α-hydroxylase activity, and treatment involves a combination of calcitriol and phosphate.[344] However, it is difficult to achieve normal growth rates in this disorder.

The condition exhibits genetic and phenotypic heterogeneity. Autosomal dominant and recessive as well as X-linked transmission has been described.[345] At present there are four proteins that may act as phosphatonins: fibroblast growth factor 23 (FGF-23), FGF-7, secreted frizzle related protein-4 (SFRP-4), and matrix extracellular phosphoglycoprotein (MEPE). All have been shown to decrease renal sodium phosphate transport, and FGF-23 and sSFRP-4 can also inhibit syntheses of 1,25 dihydroxy vitamin D.[286]

Oncogenic Osteomalacia

This severe form of osteomalacia is presumably caused by production of one or more phosphatonins by fibrous and mesenchymal tumors that are often small and difficult to identify. Removal of the tumor causes rapid reversal of the osteomalacia. The phosphatonin that has been most frequently identified is FGF-23, but FGF-7 and MEPE may also be involved.[346,347]

Hypophosphatasia

A rare autosomal recessive disorder, hypophosphatsia is characterized by mutations in the gene for the tissue-nonspecific (liver-bone-kidney) isoenzyme of alkaline phosphatase.[348] Clinical manifestations vary from death in utero related to severe deformities through infantile and childhood rickets to adult-onset osteomalacia.[349] Premature loss of deciduous teeth and impaired dentition in adults are common. Levels of organic phosphate compounds, such as pyridoxal 5-phosphate, in plasma are increased.[350] Infusion of normal alkaline phosphatase has provided only temporary improvement, but prolonged response has been observed after transplantation of marrow cells which express the normal enzymes.[351]

Drug-Induced Osteomalacia

High doses of sodium fluoride or of first-generation bisphosphonates (e.g., etidronate) can produce osteomalacia. Anticonvulsant therapy in patients with a marginal vitamin D supply can cause osteomalacia by decreasing 25(OH)D levels.[352]

Clinical Features

Rickets differs from osteomalacia in that it occurs before closure of the epiphyses. Enlargement of cartilage at the growth plate causes the so-called rachitic rosary at the costochondral junctions of the ribs and widening of the cartilaginous ends of the long bones. Impaired mineralization results in bowing of long bones. Radiologically, widening, cupping, and fraying of the metaphyses are seen (Fig. 28–18). Severe vitamin D deficiency causes muscle weakness, and this weakness, combined with the deformity of the chest wall, causes an increased incidence of pneumonia. The clinical expression of osteomalacia in adults varies widely. The most common deformity is bowing of the

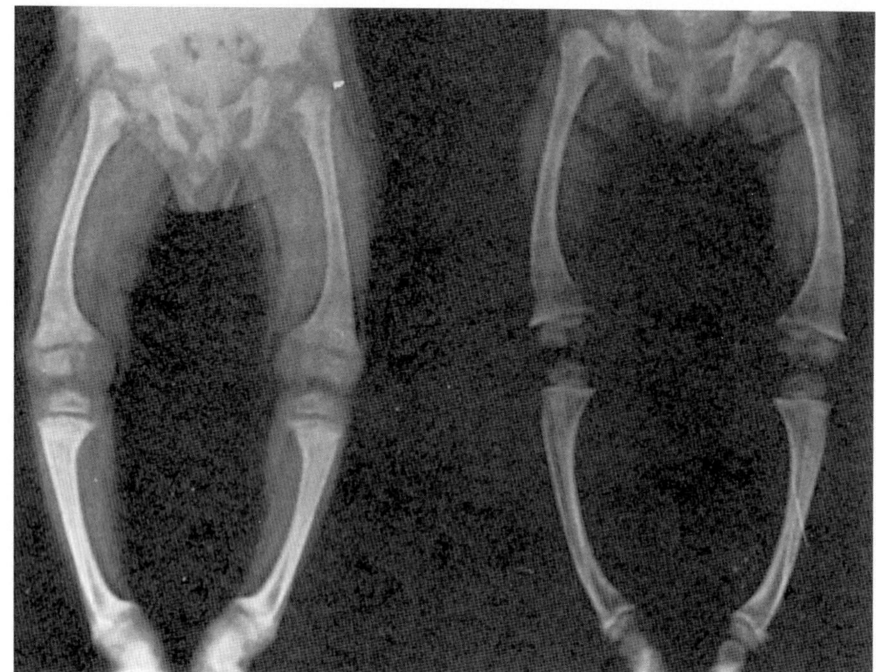

Figure 28–18 ▪ Rickets. *Left,* Active rickets in a patient with tissue resistance to 1,25-dihydroxyvitamin D at age 21 months with genu varum, irregular metaphyses, and widened growth plates. *Right,* Inactive rickets in the same patient at age 27 months after treatment with massive doses of ergocalciferol. (From Marx SJ, Spiegel AM, Brown EM, et al. Familial syndrome of decrease in sensitivity to 1,25-hydroxyvitamin D. J Clin Endocrinol Metab 1978;47:1303-1310. Copyright © 1978 by The Endocrine Society.)

legs, and in severe cases bone pain and weakness may cause the patient to be bedridden.[353]

Radiographic changes include subperiosteal erosions caused by marked secondary hyperparathyroidism and a virtually pathognomonic but relatively uncommon lesion, the so-called pseudofracture (Looser's zones or Milkman's syndrome) of the long bones, ribs, scapulae, or pubic rami (Fig. 28–19). Coarsening of the trabecular pattern in the spine may be present, but it is also seen in osteoporosis.

Diagnosis

Although clinical features may point to rickets or osteomalacia, the diagnosis depends on laboratory studies. The biochemical picture can vary with different pathogenetic mechanisms and with different stages of disease. In infants with vitamin D deficiency, serum calcium may be low and the serum phosphorus concentration may be normal initially; as secondary hyperparathyroidism develops, however, calcium concentrations usually return to the low-normal range and serum phosphorus levels fall further. In advanced stages, the serum calcium concentration may fall again. This fall has been attributed to the inability of secondary hyperparathyroidism to maintain the serum calcium level when the bone surface is covered by osteoid and is resistant to attack by osteoclasts.

In adults, the characteristic picture is a low-normal or slightly decreased serum calcium level, a decreased urinary calcium level, and a low serum phosphate level. Increased alkaline phosphatase levels reflect the activity of the osteoblasts, which form unmineralized matrix. PTH levels may be markedly increased. The key diagnostic test in vitamin D deficiency is demonstration of a decreased serum 25(OH)D value. The 25(OH)D levels may also be decreased in hepatic disease or with drugs that impair 25-hydroxylase. The 1,25(OH)2D levels may be normal in vitamin D deficiency, presumably because of a maximal stimulation of 1α-hydroxylase by the low serum phosphorus and high PTH levels. Nevertheless, the amount of this hormone is inadequate to activate the receptors in intestine and bone. Because of the high activity of 1α-hydroxylase, administration of vitamin

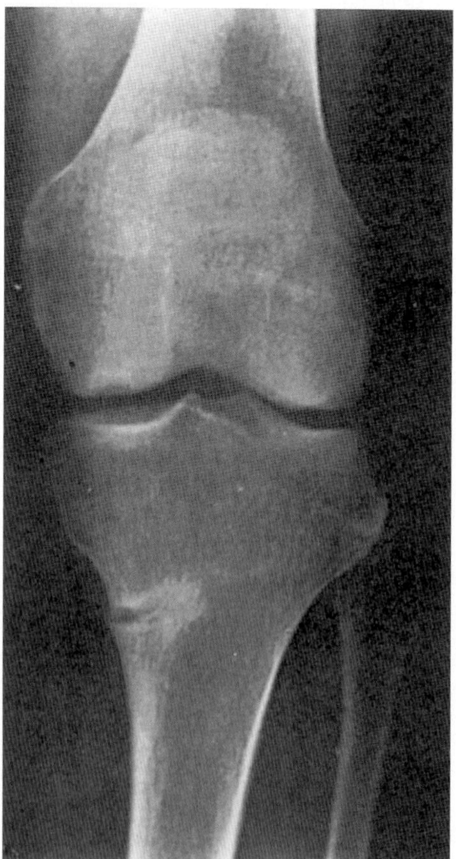

Figure 28–19 ▪ Active osteomalacia in a patient (a sibling of the patient in Fig. 28–18) with hereditary tissue resistance to 1,25-dihydroxyvitamin D at age 18 with pseudofracture of the left tibia. (From Marx SJ, Spiegel AM, Brown EM, et al. Familial syndrome of decrease in sensitivity to 1,25-hydroxyvitamin D. J Clin Endocrinol Metab 1978;47:1303-1310. Copyright © 1978 by The Endocrine Society.)

D to these patients causes a further increase in 1,25(OH)2D to supranormal levels.

The diagnosis of other forms of rickets and osteomalacia can be made by measuring vitamin D metabolite levels. For example, low values of 1,25(OH)2D and normal levels of 25(OH)D suggest a defect in 1α-hydroxylase that may be genetic or acquired as a result of loss of renal function or tumor-induced osteomalacia. High levels of 1,25(OH)2D and normal levels of 25(OH)D are seen in patients with vitamin D receptor defects. In X-linked hypophosphatemia, serum phosphorus levels are low and levels of serum calcium and vitamin D metabolites are normal. If alkaline phosphatase levels are low, a definitive diagnosis of hypophosphatasia should be sought by measuring pyridoxal 5-phosphate; elevated levels are relatively specific for hypophosphatasia and correlate with clinical severity.

Although the diagnosis of osteomalacia can usually be made on the basis of clinical findings and laboratory studies, a bone biopsy is sometimes needed for a definitive diagnosis. The characteristic finding is markedly widened osteoid seams and impaired mineralization with diffuse or absent tetracycline labeling. The bone also shows great variation in trabecular width and resorption lacunae resulting from secondary hyperparathyroidism. A modest increase in osteoid width can occur in a high-turnover state, such as hyperparathyroidism, thyrotoxicosis, or Paget's disease; however, tetracycline labeling shows a normal mineralization front in these conditions.

Therapy

Vitamin D is effective in the treatment of nutritional and malabsorptive rickets and osteomalacia. High doses (50,000 to 100,000 U/day) may be given initially, but it is important not to overtreat patients because vitamin D is stored in the fat and excessive amounts can cause prolonged hypercalcemia and hypercalciuria. Monitoring of urinary calcium excretion is useful to determine when the vitamin D dose should be decreased. Patients with malabsorption may require large doses or parenteral vitamin D. Patients with defects in 1α-hydroxylase can be treated with calcitriol. If the cause is tumor-induced osteomalacia, the treatment is to find and remove the lesion. Oral or intravenous phosphate and calcitriol can be used to heal the skeletal lesions, but this may lead to tertiary hyperparathyroidism.[354]

Severe defects in the vitamin D receptor are most difficult to treat. Massive doses of calcium and phosphorus have been given to these patients, but normal growth is rarely achieved and alopecia persists.[340,355] Intravenous calcium therapy may be necessary and is effective in restoring bone mineralization. Similarly, normal growth may not occur despite repletion of phosphorus and administration of calcitriol in patients with X-linked hypophosphatemia, although bone mineralization can be restored. Growth hormone has been used to help achieve normal height.[356] Careful monitoring of levels of calcium, phosphorus, and vitamin D metabolites is important to prevent impairment of renal function. At present, there is no effective therapy for hypophosphatasia.

HYPERPARATHYROID BONE DISEASE

In the past, severe cases of primary hyperparathyroidism showed osteitis fibrosa cystica generalisata, manifested by generalized bone loss with increased bone resorption, including both subperiosteal and endosteal surfaces.[357] The formation of fibrotic cystic lesions (brown tumors) in the long bones and jaw caused swelling, pathologic fractures, and bone pain. This bone disease is now rarely seen in primary hyperparathyroidism but may occur in poorly managed secondary hyperparathyroidism.

With the common forms of relatively mild, asymptomatic hyperparathyroidism, the major finding is an increased rate of remodeling in bone. Bone density is low in the cortical bone of the radius, but bone density in the metaphyses and vertebrae, which represent largely trabecular bone, may be normal or only moderately decreased.[358] Vitamin D insufficiency is common and associated with lower BMD.[359] Patients with mild to moderate disease do not have progressive bone loss; however, when these patients are cured surgically, bone density in the spine can increase by as much as 15%,[360] even in postmenopausal women who are at the highest risk for fracture. Bone density also increases in the radius and hip. Moreover, bone loss is attenuated in postmenopausal women with hypoparathyroidism.[361] On the basis of these results, patients with primary hyperparathyroidism and low bone density who are at risk for fractures, are candidates for parathyroid surgery.

Renal Osteodystrophy

In view of the central role of the kidney in regulating mineral metabolism, it is not surprising that patients with chronic renal failure frequently have skeletal abnormalities. The most frequent form of osteodystrophy in renal failure is due to the decreased capacity to synthesize 1,25(OH)2D and to excrete phosphate. The lowering of serum calcium by phosphate, the impairment of calcium absorption in the intestine, and the loss of the feedback inhibitory effect of 1,25(OH)2D on PTH production produces severe secondary hyperparathyroidism and ultimately leads to osteitis fibrosis cystica.

Development of bone disease can be slowed or prevented by phosphate restriction or by treatment with phosphate binders and calcitriol or analogues of calcitriol that are less likely to cause hypercalcemia.[362] When this fails, it is possible to reduce PTH levels with a calcimimetic.[363] In the past, aluminum hydroxide was used to bind phosphate, a therapy that sometimes caused aluminum-induced adynamic bone disease. This condition is less common with the use of calcium salts sevelamer or lanthanum to decrease phosphate absorption. Adynamic bone disease can occur without aluminum excess, particularly in patients in whom secondary hyperparathyroidism has been reversed; however, the relation of PTH levels and bone turnover is variable and biopsies are needed for a definitive diagnosis.[364] Osteomalacia can occur in patients receiving dialysis if they have an inadequate supply of vitamin D and calcium, but this is unusual. Osteoporosis is common in chronic renal failure and is often aggravated after transplantation.[365]

Renal osteodystrophy causes growth retardation and skeletal deformities in children, and both children and adults have bone pain and muscle weakness. Soft issue calcifications are particularly dangerous when they occur in blood vessels and lead to ischemia and gangrene. Calcification may be the result of a high calcium-phosphorus product and of vessel wall changes secondary to renal failure or direct effects of PTH. To prevent calcification, it is important to avoid a high serum calcium-phosphorus ion product and to minimize secondary hyperparathyroidism.[364]

Diagnosis

The diagnosis of a specific form of renal osteodystrophy can often be made on biochemical grounds. Levels of PTH are high in patients with severe secondary hyperparathyroidism. Plasma aluminum levels may be elevated in patients with aluminum-induced osteodystrophy but do not necessarily reflect the stores in bone. Deferoxamine chelates aluminum, and this agent can be used to measure the body burden and to treat aluminum overload. The interpretation of biochemical markers of bone turnover is difficult in renal disease because their clearance may be altered.

A bone biopsy is often needed to clarify the pathogenesis of renal osteodystrophy.[366] Using double tetracycline labeling, it is possible to determine whether mineralization is impaired. Sections that have not been decalcified show the extent of osteoid seams and resorption surfaces. Aluminum can be identified by special stains. Amyloid deposits, which consist largely of β2-microglobulin, may be seen in the bone. Amyloidosis of the bone is associated with cystic lesions but not necessarily with bone pain.

Therapy

The treatment of renal osteodystrophy can be highly successful if it is correctly focused on specific pathogenetic mechanisms. The goal should be to maintain normal serum calcium and phosphorus levels and minimize exposure to aluminum. Phosphate restriction should be instituted relatively early in renal failure, but diets low in phosphorus are difficult to achieve. Therefore, after the filtration rate is reduced below 25% of normal, it is usually necessary to administer phosphate binders such as calcium salts, sevelamer, or lanthanum. The ability of citrate to increase aluminum absorption is a concern. Correction of acidosis is also important in preventing bone disease.

Early in renal failure, modest supplementation with vitamin D may be sufficient to maintain 1,25(OH)2D levels, but eventually calcitriol itself should be administered. Low doses (0.25 to 0.5 μg/day) are well tolerated, but higher doses can lead to hypercalcemia and hypercalciuria. Vitamin D analogues that produce less hypercalcemia are now available.[144]

In some cases, parathyroidectomy may be required. Persistent hypercalcemia in patients with renal failure, intractable pruritus, extracellular calcifications, and severe skeletal lesions are all indications for surgery. However, parathyroidectomy should be avoided in patients with adynamic bone disease because symptoms may be worsened.

Renal transplantation corrects many of the biochemical disturbances that lead to renal osteodystrophy, but bone disease may progress. Usually, secondary hyperparathyroidism slowly resolves, but patients with persistent hypercalcemia or autonomy of the parathyroid glands (tertiary hyperparathyroidism) may require surgery. A major concern, particularly in older patients, is progressive osteoporosis; glucocorticoids and immunosuppressants worsen bone loss in these patients. Optimal therapy has not been defined but bisphosphonates and vitamin D analogues may slow bone loss.[362,365] Finally, osteonecrosis or avascular necrosis, particularly of the proximal femur, is common after renal transplantation.

PAGET'S DISEASE

Paget's disease may affect as many as 3% of adults older than 40 years of age; it is often asymptomatic and usually progresses slowly.[367]

Pathogenesis

The primary abnormality in Paget's disease is the localized, uncontrolled formation of large, highly active osteoclasts. The initial lesion is an increase in bone resorption. The response to this resorption, particularly in bones that are subject to mechanical force, is an intense but chaotic increase in osteoblastic activity. The characteristic histologic appearance is of focal lesions with many giant osteoclasts and active osteoblasts. The bone that forms in the lesions is disorganized and has a mosaic pattern with loss of the usual lamellar structure. The marrow shows a pattern of fibrosis and increased vascularity.[368]

The concept of a viral origin of Paget's disease is based on the finding of nuclear inclusion bodies in osteoclasts (Fig. 28–20) and the detection of viral transcripts in hematopoietic cells from patients with the disease. Several paramyxoviruses have been suggested, including measles and canine distemper virus.[369] Expression of the measles virus nucleocapsid protein gene in osteoclast precursor cells was found to enhance the ability of these cells to form osteoclasts.[370] However, further work is needed to establish pathogenetic links between viral sequences and production of abnormal osteoclasts in this condition. Pagetic osteoclasts differ from normal osteoclasts not only in their greater size and the presence of viral inclusions but also because they express IL-6, which may play a role in pathogenesis.[371] Expression of resorption stimulators by osteoblast-lineage cells is probably also involved in the development of Paget's disease.

Pagetic bone often distributes in a heterogeneous pattern throughout the skeleton. In addition, when lesions appear, they remain stationary within a particular bone over many years; although they may advance within an involved bone over time. A description of the pathogenetic mechanisms in Paget's disease must elucidate how the spotty distribution of this condition develops. Some insight into this puzzle was provided by studies of bone marrow stromal cells from pagetic lesions. These cells, believed to be stationary in bone, have been shown to produce enhanced RANKL mRNA compared with marrow stromal cells from uninvolved areas in the same patient.[372]

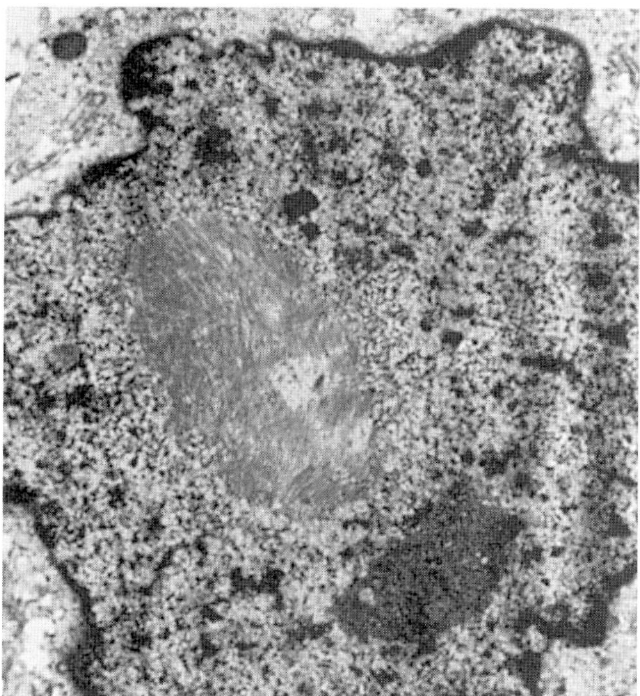

Figure 28–20 ▪ Electron micrograph of an osteoclast nucleus from a patient with Paget's disease showing characteristic intranuclear inclusion (consisting of microfilaments 125 nm in diameter). Decalcified bone, × 32,400. (Courtesy of Dr. Barbara G. Mills and Dr. Frederick R. Singer.)

There may also be a genetic component in Paget's disease.[373] As many as 15% to 30% of patients have a positive family history, and first-degree relatives of patients with Paget's disease have a sevenfold greater relative risk of having the disorder than individuals with no affected relatives. There is also ethnic and geographic clustering. The incidence is high in some areas of northern Europe, particularly in northern England, but low in Norway and Sweden. A rare related illness, familial expansile osteolysis, which is seen in young adults as a generalized increase in osteoclastic activity and bone turnover, has been found to result from an activating mutation of RANK, the receptor for RANKL.[366]

Mutations in the ubiquitin-associated (UBA) domain of the gene sequestosome 1 (SQSTM1/p62) have now been linked to the development of both familial and sporadic Paget's disease.[374,375] At least 11 separate UBA mutations have been identified as predisposing individuals to Paget's disease. SQSTM1/p62 appears involved in RANK signaling through its role in the activation of NF-κB, but the exact mechanism by which it leads to the development of Paget's disease has yet to be defined.

Clinical Features

Paget's disease affects men and women almost equally, but men tend to be more symptomatic. The disease is usually not clinically apparent until age 50 to 60 years. It usually progresses slowly and does not develop in new sites. Many different bones can be affected, and the lesions can vary from single, monostotic lesions to involvement of almost the entire skeleton. The pelvis, femur, spine, skull, and tibia are most commonly involved, whereas hands and feet are rarely affected.

Paget's disease is often discovered in asymptomatic patients because of an elevated serum alkaline phosphatase measurement obtained on routine screening or because of a radiograph taken for an unrelated problem. The most common symptom is bone pain at the site of pagetic involvement. Pain also commonly occurs in adjacent joints as a result of secondary degenerative arthritis. Bowing of the legs is common (Fig. 28–21), and pathologic fractures can occur. Vertebral involvement can cause kyphosis and compression of the spinal cord. Neural changes can also result from vascular steal because of the high blood flow to the lesion. The most common consequence of Paget's disease of the skull is hearing loss, which can be both conductive and neurosensory. Extensive involvement of the base of the skull can produce basilar impression and, rarely, brain stem compression (Fig. 28–22). Facial and skull deformities and dental problems are common.

The incidence of osteosarcoma is increased but is less than 1%. When osteosarcoma does occur, it is highly malignant. Most patients do not live longer than 1 to 3 years. Fibrosarcomas, chondrosarcomas, and benign giant cell tumors are also occasionally seen. The giant cell tumors, termed *reparative granulomas*, may represent an extension of pagetic tissue outside the skeleton. These tumors are sensitive to antipagetic therapy and may also respond to glucocorticoids.

Patients with Paget's disease may have an increased incidence of primary hyperparathyroidism. Angioid streaks are often seen in the fundus. Pseudogout, gout, and osteoarthritis occur. Patients with heart disease may show worsening of heart failure, which has been attributed to the increase in blood flow in pagetic lesions.

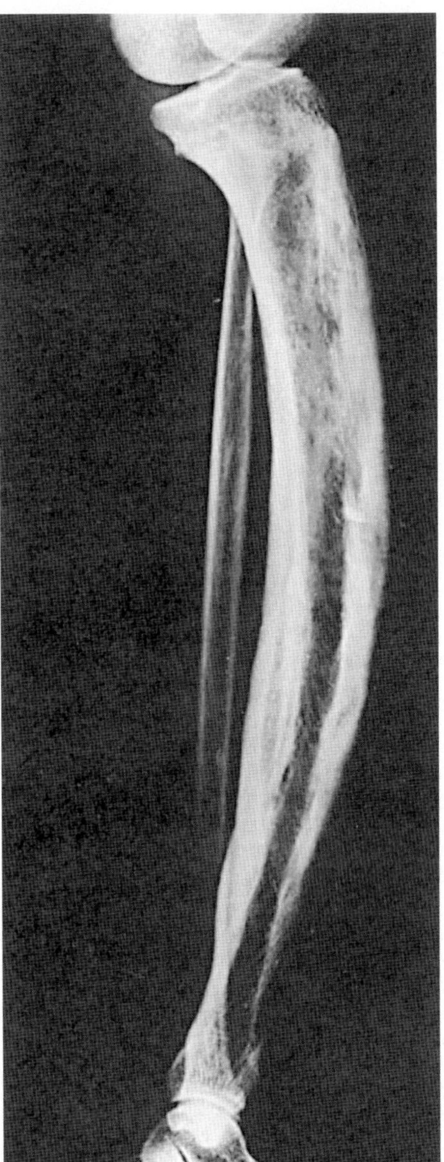

Figure 28–21 ▪ Paget's disease of the tibia. Note the bowing, marked irregularity of the anterior cortex and the flame-shaped lytic lesion of the posterior cortex. (Courtesy of Dr. Ethel S. Siris.)

Diagnosis

As noted previously, the diagnosis of Paget's disease may be made by the finding of an elevated alkaline phosphatase concentration or after a routine radiograph. In older persons with deformities or bone pain, the diagnosis should be considered, and a careful family history and review of the musculoskeletal system by both history and physical examination should be obtained. A bone scan should be carried out to localize possible pagetic sites. Positive scans do not necessarily indicate Paget's disease, and radiographs should be obtained to confirm that Paget's disease is the cause of the increased uptake. Rarely, pagetic sites in bone are not evident on bone scan because there is a minimal formation response in the lesion. Such pagetic lesions in the skull are termed *osteoporosis circumscripta*.

An audiogram should be obtained in patients with involvement of the petrous bone or in those with complaints of hearing loss. Because of the possible increased incidence of hyperparathyroidism, ionized calcium levels should be measured in the initial workup. Monostotic Paget's disease, particularly in the vertebrae, may be difficult to distinguish from metastatic disease. In males it is prudent to rule out the diagnosis of metastatic

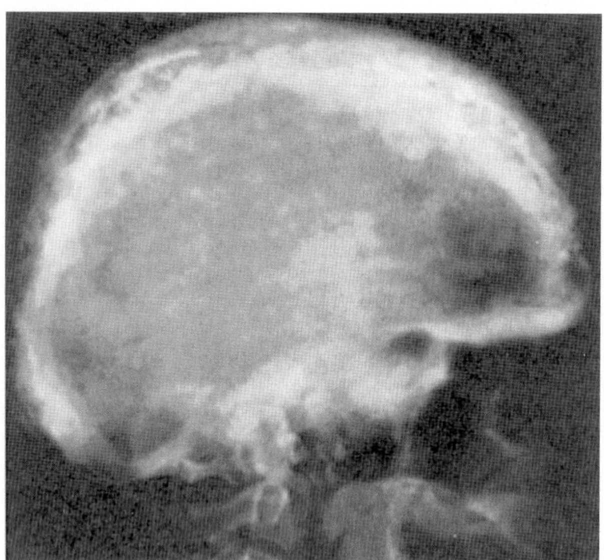

Figure 28–22 ▪ Radiograph of the skull of a patient with advanced Paget's disease showing thickening, disordered new bone formation (cotton-wool patches), and basilar impression. (From Singer FR. Paget's Disease of Bone. New York: Plenum, 1977.)

prostate cancer, which can mimic many of the laboratory, radiographic, and bone scan findings of Paget's disease. Some patients with vertebral disease may have impingement on the spinal canal. In these individuals, the area should be examined by CT or MRI. Bone biopsies can be useful in atypical cases. An ordinary aspiration biopsy sometimes yields the giant osteoclasts that are pathognomonic of Paget's disease. Samples of bone that show the irregular marble bone pattern can also be diagnostic.

After the initial evaluation has been completed, the patient can usually be monitored biochemically by serial measurements of total or bone-specific alkaline phosphatase and a marker of bone resorption.[376] Urinary hydroxyproline measurements may be used, as may serum or urinary levels of type I collagen breakdown products, such as C-telopeptide or N-telopeptide, or measurements of pyridinoline or deoxypyridinoline in the urine.

Therapy

In the past, patients with Paget's disease were often simply observed until symptoms were clear-cut or until there was evidence of progression in critical areas of the skeleton. With the newer bisphosphonates, treatment is instituted earlier. Pamidronate is available for intravenous use. Patients with more extensive disease may require retreatment and should be evaluated by measuring levels of bone turnover markers at regular intervals. Intravenous pamidronate is generally safe, although transient fever and a transient increase in bone pain may occur. Rare idiosyncratic reactions include uveitis.

Other bisphosphonates are given orally. Alendronate, risedronate, and tiludronate are approved in the United States. As with pamidronate, patients may require repeated therapy with oral bisphosphonates after a drug-free period that varies with each agent. Oral bisphosphonates need to be taken in a manner that minimizes the development of esophagitis or interactions with food and other therapeutics in the stomach. Osteonecrosis of the jaw has been detected occasionally in this condition in patients treated with bisphosphonates. Treatments with the newer bisphosphonates have largely replaced therapy with calcitonin, etidronate, or plicamycin. All of these agents act by inhibiting osteoclastic activity, and the earliest indication of therapeutic response is a drop in resorption markers followed by a decrease in formation markers.

The indications for treatment are pain that can be attributed to Paget's disease and deformities that might produce neurologic changes or are likely to lead to fracture, such as the osteolytic flame lesion or blade of grass lesion in weight-bearing bones (see Fig. 28–20). Hearing loss may be an indication for therapy, although most patients do not show major improvement after treatment.

Patients with heart disease and extensive Paget's disease should be treated in the hope that decreased pagetic activity will improve management. With the advent of safe and effective therapy, patients with mild to moderate disease, particularly those with the potential for complications (i.e., those with lesions in weight-bearing bone, the vertebral bodies, or the base of the skull), can be considered for treatment before symptoms develop. Early treatment is logical in young patients with Paget's disease because it is hoped that therapy may prevent progression. However, proof of this hypothesis is not conclusive.

Many patients with Paget's disease have pain associated with joint damage that does not respond to antipagetic therapy. These patients may respond to anti-inflammatory drugs. If osteoarthritis is advanced, knee and hip replacement may be appropriate but biochemical remission of the Paget's disease should be obtained before surgery.

A high calcium intake may be useful in Paget's disease. Bisphosphonate therapy can lower the serum calcium level and cause secondary hyperparathyroidism, which is probably not advantageous; increased calcium intake may prevent this development. Moreover, calcium loading can produce an increase in endogenous calcitonin secretion that may have beneficial effects. It is also important to monitor serum 25(OH)D levels periodically in patients with Paget's disease who are treated with bisphosphonates, as osteomalacia is not uncommon in the older population at risk for this condition and low serum vitamin D levels may exacerbate the potential of bisphosphonates to cause hypocalcemia. Urinary calcium should be checked before calcium or vitamin D supplementation is given because an increase in the incidence of renal stones has been reported in pagetic patients.

Hereditary Hyperphosphatasia

Although hereditary hyperphosphatasia has been termed juvenile Paget's disease, it involves all of the skeleton and develops in infants.[377] The serum alkaline phosphatase levels are very high. There are severe bone deformities, and the histologic appearance resembles that of Paget's disease with high bone turnover, although the osteoclasts are not enlarged. Treatment with bisphosphonates or calcitonin may be effective in reducing bone turnover and improving bone lesions. A new familial form with expansile long bone lesions has been described.[378,379]

OSTEOGENESIS IMPERFECTA

Osteogenesis imperfecta, or brittle bone disease, is a heterogeneous, congenital disorder in which increased bone fragility leads to fractures and deformity.[380] It ranges in severity from a lethal perinatal form to a mild disorder that results only in increased fractures.

Pathogenesis

Most patients with osteogenesis imperfecta have defects in the genes for type I collagen. Bones, ligaments, skin, sclerae, and teeth are affected. The incidence of osteogenesis imperfecta is estimated to be 1 in 200,000 to 500,000. The heterogeneity of the features is caused by the variety of genetic defects, although phenotypic variation occurs even with the same genetic abnormality (Table 28–5). The more severe forms, type II and type III, involve mutations in the helical portion of the collagen molecule that prevent normal assembly and produce unstable triple helices. Point mutations in this portion of the collagen gene can be associated with mild disease (type IV). An autosomal recessive form of osteogenesis imperfecta is caused by mutations in two different genes required for the unique 3-hydroxylation of proline 986 in the α1 chain of type I collagen.[380a,380b]

Type I osteogenesis imperfecta differs from the other forms in that there is usually a deletion of one allele of the α1(I) procollagen gene, resulting in decreased collagen production but a normal molecular structure.[381] This disorder is of particular interest because familial osteoporosis may also exhibit such defects.[382,383] Bone biopsies show decreased cortical width and trabecular bone volume, increased turnover, and decreased bone formation in patients with type I disease.[384] The disorder in a subgroup of patients with low turnover and ligamentous calcifications has been designated type V osteoporosis imperfecta.[385]

Classification and Clinical Features

The classification devised by Sillence and modified by Byers[380] is summarized in Table 28–5. In addition to the bone involvement, there may be ligament laxity, joint hypermobility, and easy bruising. Dentin formation is often abnormal, and the teeth are fragile and discolored. The finding of blue sclerae is a variable manifestation and does not correlate with severity. Because of the thoracic deformities, patients with severe manifestations are predisposed to pulmonary infections and usually have a shortened life span. Intelligence is not affected, and individuals with marked deformities can be highly productive if appropriate conditions are provided.

Diagnosis

In patients with moderate to severe disease, the clinical features make the diagnosis relatively straightforward; in patients with the milder forms, however, the diagnosis may be missed. In children without deformities, multiple fractures are usually attributed to trauma; in infants, the presence of such fractures may lead to an accusation of parental abuse. In the absence of typical clinical features, the diagnosis can be made only biochemically. Culture of fibroblasts from skin biopsies and analysis of the collagen by gel electrophoresis can point to a defect, and the techniques of molecular biology can identify the mutation more specifically. This analysis is useful for families because specific deoxyribonucleic acid (DNA) polymorphisms may allow prenatal diagnosis if the mutation has already been identified in other affected family members.

In children and adolescents with multiple fractures but no deformity, measurements of bone density and turnover may point toward the diagnosis. In the type I disorder, both bone density and serum type I procollagen peptide levels are likely to be decreased. However, because excretion of collagen crosslinks is increased in most types of osteogenesis imperfecta, increased bone resorption may play a role in pathogenesis.[386]

Therapy

Antiresorptive therapy with intravenous pamidronate has been shown to decrease fractures in children with severe osteogenesis imperfecta, even before 3 years of age.[387,388] Oral bisphosphonates may be effective in older children and adults.[389] Supportive treatment is important. The Osteogenesis Imperfecta Foundation works with patients and families to improve the quality of life. Orthopedic and rehabilitation services can be helpful in

TABLE 28–5 CLASSIFICATION OF OSTEOGENESIS IMPERFECTA

Type	Clinical Features	Inheritance	Common Biochemical Abnormality
I	Normal stature, little or no deformity, blue sclerae, hearing loss in 50% of families Dentinogenesis imperfecta may distinguish a subset.	AD	Nonfunctional allele of the α1(I) procollagen gene (*COL1A1*)
II	Lethal in the perinatal period; minimal calvarial mineralization, beaded ribs, compressed femurs, marked long bone deformity, platyspondyly	AD (new mutations) AR (rare)	Substitution of glycine in triple helix of *COL1A1* or *COL1A2*
III	Progressively deforming bones, usually with moderate deformity at birth Scleral hue varies, often lightening with age Dentinogenesis imperfecta common, hearing loss common Stature very short	AD AR (uncommon)	Substitution of glycine in triple helix of *COL1A1* or *COL1A2*
IV	Normal sclerae, mild to moderate bone deformity, and variable short stature; dentinogenesis imperfecta is common and hearing loss occurs in some families	AD	Substitution of glycine in triple helix of *COL1A1* or *COL1A2;* exon skipping in *COL1A2*

AD, Autosomal dominant; *AR,* autosomal recessive.
Classification from Sillence et al, as modified from Byers PH. Osteogenesis imperfecta. In Royce PM, Steinman B, eds. Connective Tissue and Its Heritable Disorders: Molecular, Genetic and Medical Aspects. New York: Wiley-Liss, 1993:317-350.

dealing with deformities. Genetic counseling and prenatal diagnosis, including ultrasound examination and testing for informative DNA polymorphisms, are important for the family. Gene therapy is being explored.[390]

Other Connective Tissue Disorders Affecting the Skeleton

Other inherited disorders of connective tissue with impairment of skeletal development or increased bone fragility include Ehlers-Danlos syndrome, Menkes' disease, lysinuric protein intolerance, and homocystinuria.[228] In these disorders, abnormalities of collagen cross-linking can affect bone and other connective tissues. In Ehlers-Danlos syndrome, the cross-linking enzyme lysyl oxidase is deficient, and in Menkes' disease, copper deficiency impairs the function of the enzyme. Lysinuric protein intolerance and homocystinuria probably also impair cross-linking of collagen.

OSTEOPETROSIS

Osteopetrosis, or marble bone disease, is a heterogeneous group of disorders characterized by a generalized increase in bone density caused by defective osteoclastic bone resorption.[391] These syndromes must be distinguished from a variety of disorders in which osteosclerosis occurs due to increased bone formation. There may even be disorders in which both decreased resorption and increased formation play a role such as the skeletal abnormalities associated with mutations in the LDL receptor-related protein-5 (LRP-5). In contrast to the murine models, in which formation as well as function of osteoclasts can be impaired, the genes identified in human osteopetrosis have been largely associated with the function of mature osteoclasts. It is likely that severe defects in osteoclast formation are embryonically lethal.

Osteopetrotic rats and mice with specific defects in osteoclasts have been found as a result of spontaneous mutations and developed using gene knockout techniques. The op/op mouse has a genetic defect in the production of M-CSF that results in failure of osteoclast formation. This can be corrected by treatment with M-CSF.[392] Knockouts of the proto-oncogenes c-src and c-fos, of TRAF-6, a mediator of RANK action, of osteoclast integrins, and of osteoclast cathepsin K and tartrate-resistant acid phosphatase also cause osteopetrosis.[393-397]

Infantile Osteopetrosis

Infantile osteopetrosis is a rare, autosomal recessive disorder in which failure to resorb bone and calcified metaphyseal cartilage causes near obliteration of the marrow spaces.[342,398-402] Extramedullary hematopoiesis occurs in the liver and spleen. The cranial nerve foramina do not form normally, causing optic atrophy and other cranial nerve defects. The bones, although dense, are brittle, and pathologic fractures can occur.

The impaired function of the hematopoietic system causes death in the first decade from hemorrhage or infection. On the basis of studies in animal models in which transfer of hematopoietic tissue resulted in cure, patients have been treated with total body radiation and grafting of marrow from human leukocyte antigen-identical donors (Fig. 28–23).[399] When suitable donors could not be found, therapy with high doses of interferon have improved bone resorption.[403] The majority of these patients (about 60%) have been shown to have genetic defects

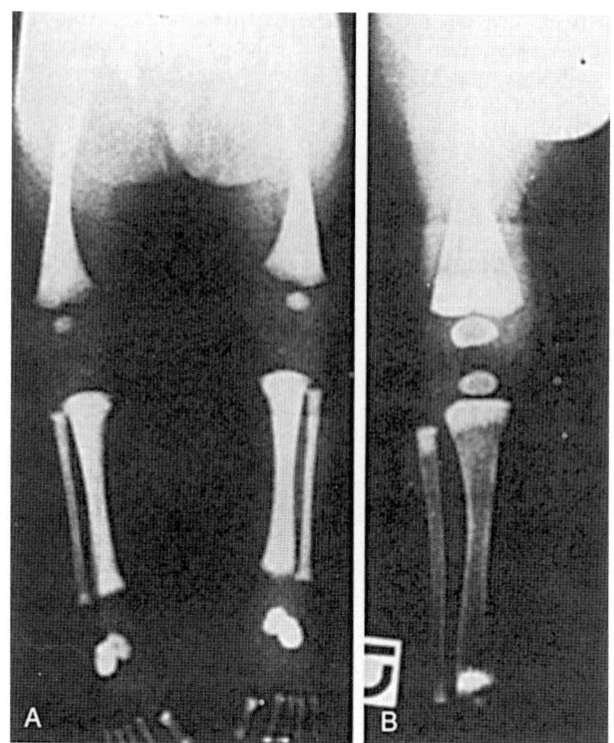

Figure 28–23 ▪ Radiographs of the lower limb of a patient with osteopetrosis at age 2 months **(A)** before bone marrow transplantation and at age 9 months after transplantation **(B)** showing formation of normal medullary bone. (From Ballet JJ, Griscelli C. Lymphoid cell transplantation in human osteopetrosis. In Horton JE, Tarpley TM, Davis WF, eds. Mechanisms of Localized Bone Loss. London: IRI, 1978:399-414, by permission of Oxford University Press.)

of subunits of the vascular-type H^+-adenosine triphosphatase that acts as a proton pump in osteoclasts (TCIRG1, also termed *ATP6i* and *OC116*) or in the osteoclast chloride channel (CLCN7) (about 15%),[391] but others may have different mutations.[404]

Carbonic Anhydrase II Deficiency

Carbonic anhydrase II deficiency, a nonlethal autosomal recessive disorder, is associated with a complete deficiency of the type II carbonic anhydrase that provides carbonic acid for hydrogen ion secretion by osteoclasts and by the distal tubules.[405] Hence, osteopetrosis is accompanied by renal tubular acidosis that may involve both distal and proximal lesions. Affected individuals are shorter than their siblings and may have calcification of the basal ganglia. Bone marrow transplantation can correct the skeletal abnormalities.[406]

Albers-Schönberg Disease (Autosomal Dominant Osteopetrosis Type II)

Classic Albers-Schönberg disease is now called *autosomal dominant osteopetrosis type II.* It is characterized by generalized osteosclerosis with thickening of the vertebral end-plates (sandwich vertebrae) and bone within bone in the pelvis. Although ADO II has been termed "benign osteoporosis," the majority of patients have clinical problems, presumably related to impaired bone remodeling. These include fractures, osteoarthritis, skeletal deformities, and cranial nerve involvement.[407] Most patients with ADO II have a milder form of mutation in the chloride transport gene ClCN-7 than that seen in the more severe forms of infantile osteopetrosis,[391] although other genes may be involved. Decreased bone resorption is presumably due to impaired acidification and tartrate resistant acid phosphatase activity in the serum is actually increased.[408-410]

OTHER SCLEROSING BONE DISORDERS

There are a number of rare, skeletal disorders that cause irregular bone structure and varying degrees of sclerosis. Some of these are associated with increased bone formation rather than decreased resorption although both processes may be affected. Acquired osteosclerosis related to increased bone formation occurs in fluorosis[411] and in rare cases of hepatitis C infection,[412] and a localized form is seen in certain metastatic malignancies, particularly cancers of the prostate and breast.

Pyknodysostosis

Pyknodysostosis is an autosomal recessive disorder characterized by short stature, a large cranium, and small facies and skeletal fragility.[413] Unlike patients with osteopetrosis, these patients do not demonstrate loss of the marrow cavity and are not anemic. Histologically, trabecular bone volume is increased despite an increase in the number of osteoclasts. There is a defect in osteoclast function due to a mutation of the cathepsin K gene.[414-416]

Progressive Diaphyseal Dysplasia

Known as *Camurati-Engelmann disease*, progressive diaphyseal dysplasia consists of patchy thickening of the bone on both periosteal and endosteal surfaces and is associated with pain in the extremities, gait abnormalities, and muscle wasting. The histologic picture is one of increased bone formation rather than decreased resorption.[417] The disease can be inherited as an autosomal dominant disorder, and is associated with mutations in the TGF-β1 gene mainly in the latency-associated peptide region.[418,419] Glucocorticoid therapy relieves bone pain and reverses the histologic abnormalities in some cases.

Autosomal Dominant Osteopetrosis Type I and Skeletal Abnormalities Associated with LRP-5

Following the initial identification of an activating mutation of LRP-5 in two families with autosomal dominant high bone mass,[420,421] a number of other families have been found to have missense mutations in the LRP-5 gene with somewhat variable phenotypic expression.[422] In the original families there was little evidence of deformity, but in other families the picture described as autosomal dominant osteopetrosis type I, which can result in cranial nerve involvement has been found. While the increase in bone mass appears to be attributable to increased bone formation in these patients as well as in a mouse model of this disorder,[423] that may also be an abnormality of osteoclast function in vivo, although isolated osteoclasts from these patients are still active in vitro.[424]

Endosteal Hyperostosis

The term *van Buchem's disease* is applied to both severe and mild forms of hyperostosis. The disorder begins in infancy, and progressive enlargement of the jaw commences at puberty. Some subjects have cranial nerve deficits caused by impingement of the foramina. This disorder may be related to sclerosteosis and autosomal recessive disorder, in which there also may be syndactyly. Subjects with both disorders are usually tall and heavy. Mutations in the SOST gene, which codes for sclerostin, an inhibitor of Wnt signaling, has recently been identified in these disorders.[425] Heterozygotes in families with sclerosteosis have increased BMD.[426]

Other Disorders

Three disorders characterized by irregular increases in bone density, osteopoikilosis, the Buschke-Ollendorff syndrome, and melorheostosis, may all represent different phenotypes of a common genetic abnormality. A loss of function mutation of LEMD-3, a gene that encodes an inner nuclear membrane protein, has been found in families with these disorders.[427] Osteopathia striata with cranial sclerosis is a rare syndrome characterized by longitudinal striations in metaphyses of long bones. It is more common in females and may have an X-linked dominant inheritance.[428] Axial osteomalacia is a disorder characterized by back pain and osteosclerosis of the spine and pelvis which may respond to antiinflammatory agents.[429,430] Fibrogenesis imperfecta ossium is another rare condition characterized by both increased bone density and patchy areas of bone loss which may represent a defect in bone matrix synthesis.[431]

More localized periosteal new bone formation can occur in a number of different syndromes. Caffey's disease or cortical hyperostosis can vary from a severe and lethal disorder to mild increases in periosteal bone formation.[432] Recently a mutation in Col1A1 has been identified in a family with an autosomal dominant form of this disorder.[433] However, this disorder can be mimicked by prolonged infusion of PGE1 in neonates and such infusions can also cause hypertrophic osteoarthropthy in adults.[434,435] Pachydermoperiostosis is a rare congenital disorder with skin changes and digital clubbing.[436] Secondary hypertrophic osteoarthropathy and clubbing can occur with pulmonary disease or as a paraneoplastic syndrome, possibly related to overproduction of vascular endothelial growth factor.[437-439] If the underlying disorder cannot be treated effectively, bisphosphonates may provide relief from pain.[437]

FIBROUS DYSPLASIA

Clinical Features

Fibrous dysplasia is characterized by expanding lesions within the bone that contain both fibroblastic and osteoblastic elements. The disorder can occur as a monostotic lesion without any associated abnormalities or in a polyostotic form, which may occur as part of the McCune-Albright syndrome, associated with functional abnormalities of one or more endocrine glands and irregular hyperpigmented macules called café-au-lait spots.

The most common endocrine manifestation is precocious puberty, particularly in girls.[440] The molecular defect in the McCune-Albright syndrome is somatic mosaicism for an activating mutation of the Gs α subunit of the nucleotide-binding regulatory protein that couples receptors to adenylyl cyclase. Similar defects have been found in bone lesions in the absence of McCune-Albright syndrome.[441] Local production of PTHrP may also be involved in pathogenesis.[442] Hypophosphatemia may occur associated with increased FGF-23 production.[443,444]

Diagnosis

Monostotic fibrous dysplasia is usually diagnosed in the second or third decade of life as an expanding bone lesion that can cause fracture, deformity, or nerve entrapment. Sarcomatous degeneration can occur. In fibrous dysplasia, any skeletal site can be affected but the femur, tibia, ribs, and face are most often involved. Histologically, the lesions contain many spindle-shaped fibroblasts and islands of woven bone. Bone lesions can worsen during pregnancy, and estrogen receptors have been identified in the bone lesions of patients with McCune-Albright syndrome.[445]

Therapy

The course of both monostotic and polyostotic fibrous dysplasia is variable. Patients who show progression, nerve compression, or pathologic fractures may require surgery. Careful assessment of the endocrine system is critical in the McCune-Albright syndrome because early intervention can prevent irreversible changes resulting from precocious puberty. The bone lesions may respond to bisphosphonate.[446] Treatment with 1,25(OH)2D may reduce PTHrP production and decrease activity of the bone lesions.[442]

EXTRASKELETAL CALCIFICATION AND OSSIFICATION

Mineral deposition in soft tissues is a common consequence of tissue damage and of a local elevation of the extracellular calcium-phosphate product. Ectopic or heterotopic bone formation can occur at sites of injury or surgical trauma and may be related to the presence of an inductive protein matrix.[447] This form of bone induction stimulated the search for BMPs. The frequency of heterotopic ossification after hip replacement or spinal cord injury can be decreased by treatment with local irradiation or nonsteroidal antiinflammatory drugs that inhibit prostaglandin synthesis.[448] Extensive subcutaneous calcium deposition may be crippling in inflammatory disorders such as dermatomyositis.

The term *myositis ossificans* is used when bone formation occurs in traumatized muscle, but similar masses can be formed in tendon, ligaments, joint capsules, and fascia without trauma.[447]

Tumoral Calcinosis

Primary tumoral calcinosis is an inherited disorder characterized by periarticular calcification and hyperphosphatemia. It is associated with defective phosphate transport and sometimes with excessive activity of renal 1α-hydroxylase. An inactivating mutation in the FGF-23 gene may cause this disorder.[449] The primary disorder must be differentiated from secondary tumoral calcinosis, which occurs in association with renal failure and with hypercalcemic disorders.

Treatment by phosphate depletion using phosphate-binding antacids or diuretics, parathyroidectomy, and dialysis has been attempted.[450]

Fibrodysplasia Ossificans Progressiva

This rare congenital disorder is most often sporadic but can be transmitted as an autosomal dominant disorder.[451] Characteristic short phalanges and soft tissue swelling can be detected at birth. Abnormal regulation of the BMP has been implicated.[452] Painful, tender lesions caused by true ectopic bone can develop in connective tissues. Severe progressive deformities may include scoliosis and ankylosis of the spine and rib cage. There is no known therapy. However, its genetic mutation was recently identified in the gene for BMP type I receptor ACVR1.[453]

Progressive osseous heteroplasia is another genetic disorder in which ossification occurs largely in the skin. It may be caused by an inactivating mutation of GSα.[451]

REFERENCES

1. Raisz L, Shoukri KC. Pathogeneis of Osteoporosis in Physiology and Pharmacology of Bone. New York: Springer-Verlag, 1993.
2. Baron R. Anatomy and Ultrastructure of Bone. New York: Lippincott Williams & Wilkins, 1999.
3. Parfitt AM. The mechanism of coupling: a role for the vasculature. Bone 2000;26:319-323.
4. Canalis E. The fate of circulating osteoblasts. N Engl J Med 2005;352:2014-2016.
5. Parfitt AM. The bone remodeling compartment: a circulatory function for bone lining cells. J Bone Miner Res 2001;16:1583-1585.
6. Gorski JP. Is all bone the same? Distinctive distributions and properties of non-collagenous matrix proteins in lamellar vs. woven bone imply the existence of different underlying osteogenic mechanisms. Crit Rev Oral Biol Med 1998;9:201-223.
7. Delany AM, Amling M, Priemel M, et al. Osteopenia and decreased bone formation in osteonectin-deficient mice. J Clin Invest 2000;105:1325.
8. Seeman E, Delmas PD. Bone quality—the material and structural basis of bone strength and fragility. N Engl J Med 2006;354: 2250-2261.
9. Viguet-Carrin S, Garnero P, Delmas PD. The role of collagen in bone strength. Osteoporos Int 2006;17:319-336.
10. Anderson HC. Molecular biology of matrix vesicles. Clin Orthop Relat Res 1995;314:266-280.
11. Mauviel A. Cytokine regulation of metalloproteinase gene expression. J Cell Biochem 1993;53:288-295.
12. Rajakumar RA, Quinn CO. Parathyroid hormone induction of rat interstitial collagenase mRNA in osteosarcoma cells is mediated through an AP-1-binding site. Mol Endocrinol 1996;10:867-878.
13. Zhao W, Byrne MH, Boyce BF, et al. Bone resorption induced by parathyroid hormone is strikingly diminished in collagenase-resistant mutant mice. J Clin Invest 1999;103:517-524.
14. Rydziel S, Delany AM, Canalis E. AU-rich elements in the collagenase 3 mRNA mediate stabilization of the transcript by cortisol in osteoblasts. J Biol Chem 2004;279:5397-5404.
15. Liu F, Malaval L, Aubin JE. The mature osteoblast phenotype is characterized by extensive plasticity. Exp Cell Res 1997;232: 97-105.
16. Bianco P, Gehron Robey P. Marrow stromal stem cells. J Clin Invest 2000;105:1663-1668.
17. Eghbali-Fatourechi GZ, Lamsam J, Fraser D, et al. Circulating osteoblast-lineage cells in humans. N Engl J Med 2005;352:1959-1966.
18. Canalis E, Deregowski V, Pereira RC, et al. Signals that determine the fate of osteoblastic cells. J Endocrinol Invest 2005;28:3-7.
19. Karsenty G. Minireview: transcriptional control of osteoblast differentiation. Endocrinology 2001;142:2731-2733.
20. Tanaka T, Yoshida N, Kishimoto T, et al. Defective adipocyte differentiation in mice lacking the C/EBPbeta and/or C/EBPdelta gene. Embo J 1997;16:7432-7443.
21. Ducy P, Zhang R, Geoffroy V, et al. Osf2/Cbfal: a transcriptional activator of osteoblast differentiation. Cell 1997;89:747-754.

22. Nakashima K, Zhou X, Kunkel G, et al. The novel zinc finger–containing transcription factor osterix is required for osteoblast differentiation and bone formation. Cell 2002;108:17-29.
23. Koga T, Inui M, Inoue K, et al. Costimulatory signals mediated by the ITAM motif cooperate with RANKL for bone homeostasis. Nature 2004;428:758-763.
24. Dobreva G, Chahrour M, Dautzenberg M, et al. SATB2 is a multifunctional determinant of craniofacial patterning and osteoblast differentiation. Cell 2006;125:971-986.
25. Aarden EM, Burger EH, Nijweide PJ. Function of osteocytes in bone. J Cell Biochem 1994;55:287-299.
26. Burger EH, Klein-Nulend J. Mechanotransduction in bone—role of the lacuno-canalicular network. FASEB J 1999;13(suppl): S101-S112.
27. Han Y, Cowin SC, Schaffler MB, et al. Mechanotransduction and strain amplification in osteocyte cell processes. Proc Natl Acad Sci U S A 2004;101:16689-16694.
28. Tondravi MM, McKercher SR, Anderson K, et al. Osteopetrosis in mice lacking haematopoietic transcription factor PU.1. Nature 1997;386:81-84.
29. Miyamoto T, Ohneda O, Arai F, et al. Bifurcation of osteoclasts and dendritic cells from common progenitors. Blood 2001;98: 2544-2554.
30. Suda T, Takahashi N, Udagawa N, et al. Modulation of osteoclast differentiation and function by the new members of the tumor necrosis factor receptor and ligand families. Endocr Rev 1999; 20:345-357.
31. Lorenzo J. Interactions between immune and bone cells: new insights with many remaining questions. J Clin Invest 2000;106: 749-752.
32. Arai F, Miyamoto T, Ohneda O, et al. Commitment and differentiation of osteoclast precursor cells by the sequential expression of c-Fms and receptor activator of nuclear factor kappaB (RANK) receptors. J Exp Med 1999;190:1741-1754.
33. Lacey DL, Tan HL, Lu J, et al. Osteoprotegerin ligand modulates murine osteoclast survival in vitro and in vivo. Am J Pathol 2000;157:435-448.
34. Yoshida H, Hayashi S, Kunisada T, et al. The murine mutation osteopetrosis is in the coding region of the macrophage colony stimulating factor gene. Nature 1990;345:442-444.
35. Hofstetter W, Wetterwald A, Cecchini MG, et al. Detection of transcripts and binding sites for colony-stimulating factor-1 during bone development. Bone 1995;17:145-151.
36. Mocsai A, Humphrey MB, Van Ziffle JA, et al. The immunomodulatory adapter proteins DAP12 and Fc receptor gamma-chain (FcRgamma) regulate development of functional osteoclasts through the Syk tyrosine kinase. Proc Natl Acad Sci U S A 2004;101: 6158-6163.
37. Kukita T, Wada N, Kukita A, et al. RANKL-induced DC-STAMP is essential for osteoclastogenesis. J Exp Med 2004;200:941-946.
38. Yagi M, Miyamoto T, Sawatani Y, et al. DC-STAMP is essential for cell-cell fusion in osteoclasts and foreign body giant cells. J Exp Med 2005;202:345-351.
39. Ravesloot JH, Eisen T, Baron R, et al. Role of Na-H exchangers and vacuolar H^+ pumps in intracellular pH regulation in neonatal rat osteoclasts. J Gen Physiol 1995;105:177-208.
40. Blair HC, Sidonio RF, Friedberg RC, et al. Proteinase expression during differentiation of human osteoclasts in vitro. J Cell Biochem 2000;78:627-637.
41. Delaisse JM, Eeckhout Y, Neff L, et al. (Pro)collagenase (matrix metalloproteinase-1) is present in rodent osteoclasts and in the underlying bone-resorbing compartment. J Cell Sci 1993;106 (Pt 4):1071-1082.
42. Salo J, Lehenkari P, Mulari M, et al. Removal of osteoclast bone resorption products by transcytosis. Science 1997;276:270-273.
43. Recker R, Lappe J, Davies KM, et al. Bone remodeling increases substantially in the years after menopause and remains increased in older osteoporosis patients. J Bone Miner Res 2004;19: 1628-1633.
44. Hirano T, Turner CH, Forwood MR, et al. Does suppression of bone turnover impair mechanical properties by allowing microdamage accumulation? Bone 2000;27:13-20.
45. Verborgt O, Gibson GJ, Schaffler MB. Loss of osteocyte integrity in association with microdamage and bone remodeling after fatigue in vivo. J Bone Miner Res 2000;15:60-67.
46. Fu L, Patel MS, Bradley A, et al. The molecular clock mediates leptin-regulated bone formation. Cell 2005;122:803-815.
47. Dempster DW, Cosman F, Parisien M, et al. Anabolic actions of parathyroid hormone on bone. Endocr Rev 1993;14:690-709.
48. Canalis E, Centrella M, Burch W, et al. Insulin-like growth factor I mediates selective anabolic effects of parathyroid hormone in bone cultures. J Clin Invest 1989;83:60-65.
49. Manolagas SC. Birth and death of bone cells: basic regulatory mechanisms and implications for the pathogenesis and treatment of osteoporosis. Endocr Rev 2000;21:115-137.
50. Shiraishi A, Takeda S, Masaki T, et al. Alfacalcidol inhibits bone resorption and stimulates formation in an ovariectomized rat model of osteoporosis: distinct actions from estrogen. J Bone Miner Res 2000;15:770-779.
51. Hurley DL, Tiegs RD, Wahner HW, et al. Axial and appendicular bone mineral density in patients with long-term deficiency or excess of calcitonin. N Engl J Med 1987;317:537-541.
52. Eriksen EF, Kudsk H, Emmertsen K, et al. Bone remodeling during calcitonin excess: reconstruction of the remodeling sequence in medullary thyroid carcinoma. Bone 1993;14:399-401.
53. Hoff AO, Catala-Lehnen P, Thomas PM, et al. Increased bone mass is an unexpected phenotype associated with deletion of the calcitonin gene. J Clin Invest 2002;110:1849-1857.
54. Schinke T, Liese S, Priemel M, et al. Decreased bone formation and osteopenia in mice lacking alpha-calcitonin gene-related peptide. J Bone Miner Res 2004;19:2049-2056.
55. Ohlsson C, Bengtsson BA, Isaksson OG, et al. Growth hormone and bone. Endocr Rev 1998;19:55-79.
56. Lupu F, Terwilliger JD, Lee K, et al. Roles of growth hormone and insulin-like growth factor 1 in mouse postnatal growth. Dev Biol 2001;229:141-162.
57. Canalis E, Bilezikian JP, Angeli A, et al. Perspectives on glucocorticoid-induced osteoporosis. Bone 2004;34:593-598.
58. Hofbauer LC, Gori F, Riggs BL, et al. Stimulation of osteoprotegerin ligand and inhibition of osteoprotegerin production by glucocorticoids in human osteoblastic lineage cells: potential paracrine mechanisms of glucocorticoid-induced osteoporosis. Endocrinology 1999;140:4382-4389.
59. Smith E, Frenkel B. Glucocorticoids inhibit the transcriptional activity of LEF/TCF in differentiating osteoblasts in a glycogen synthase kinase-3beta-dependent and -independent manner. J Biol Chem 2005;280:2388-2394.
60. Weinstein RS, Jilka RL, Parfitt AM, et al. Inhibition of osteoblastogenesis and promotion of apoptosis of osteoblasts and osteocytes by glucocorticoids. Potential mechanisms of their deleterious effects on bone. J Clin Invest 1998;102:274-282.
61. Delany AM, Durant D, Canalis E. Glucocorticoid suppression of IGF I transcription in osteoblasts. Mol Endocrinol 2001;15: 1781-1789.
62. Greenspan SL, Greenspan FS. The effect of thyroid hormone on skeletal integrity. Ann Intern Med 1999;130:750-758.
63. Engler H, Oettli RE, Riesen WF. Biochemical markers of bone turnover in patients with thyroid dysfunctions and in euthyroid controls: a cross-sectional study. Clin Chim Acta 1999;289: 159-172.
64. Pereira RC, Jorgetti V, Canalis E. Triiodothyronine induces collagenase-3 and gelatinase B expression in murine osteoblasts. Am J Physiol 1999;277:E496-E504.
65. Bouillon R, Bex M, Van Herck E, et al. Influence of age, sex, and insulin on osteoblast function: osteoblast dysfunction in diabetes mellitus. J Clin Endocrinol Metab 1995;80:1194-1202.
66. Canalis E. Effect of insulinlike growth factor I on DNA and protein synthesis in cultured rat calvaria. J Clin Invest 1980;66:709-719.
67. Ogata N, Chikazu D, Kubota N, et al. Insulin receptor substrate-1 in osteoblast is indispensable for maintaining bone turnover. J Clin Invest 2000;105:935-943.
68. Bilezikian JP, Morishima A, Bell J, et al. Increased bone mass as a result of estrogen therapy in a man with aromatase deficiency. N Engl J Med 1998;339:599-603.
69. Srivastava S, Toraldo G, Weitzmann MN, et al. Estrogen decreases osteoclast formation by down-regulating receptor activator of NF-kappa B ligand (RANKL)-induced JNK activation. J Biol Chem 2001;276:8836-8840.
70. Shevde NK, Bendixen AC, Dienger KM, et al. Estrogens suppress RANK ligand-induced osteoclast differentiation via a stromal cell

independent mechanism involving c-Jun repression. Proc Natl Acad Sci U S A 2000;97:7829-7834.

71. Falahati-Nini A, Riggs BL, Atkinson EJ, et al. Relative contributions of testosterone and estrogen in regulating bone resorption and formation in normal elderly men. J Clin Invest 2000;106: 1553-1560.
72. Raisz LG. Local and systemic factors in the pathogenesis of osteoporosis. N Engl J Med 1988;318:818-828.
73. Raisz LG. Osteoporosis: current approaches and future prospects in diagnosis, pathogenesis, and management. J Bone Miner Metab 1999;17:79-89.
74. Lorenzo JA. The role of cytokines in the regulation of local bone resorption. Crit Rev Immunol 1991;11:195-213.
75. Pacifici R. Cytokines, estrogen, and postmenopausal osteoporosis—the second decade. Endocrinology 1998;139:2659-2661.
76. Grey A, Mitnick MA, Masiukiewicz U, et al. A role for interleukin-6 in parathyroid hormone-induced bone resorption in vivo. Endocrinology 1999;140:4683-4690.
77. Malaval L, Gupta AK, Aubin JE. Leukemia inhibitory factor inhibits osteogenic differentiation in rat calvaria cell cultures. Endocrinology 1995;136:1411-1418.
78. Onoe Y, Miyaura C, Kaminakayashiki T, et al. IL-13 and IL-4 inhibit bone resorption by suppressing cyclooxygenase-2-dependent prostaglandin synthesis in osteoblasts. J Immunol 1996;156: 758-764.
79. Miyaura C, Onoe Y, Inada M, et al. Increased B-lymphopoiesis by interleukin 7 induces bone loss in mice with intact ovarian function: similarity to estrogen deficiency. Proc Natl Acad Sci U S A 1997;94:9360-9365.
80. Owens J, Chambers TJ. Differential regulation of osteoclast formation: interleukin 10 (cytokine synthesis inhibitory factor) suppresses formation of osteoclasts but not macrophages in murine bone marrow cultures. J Bone Miner Res 1995;10:S220.
81. Horwood NJ, Udagawa N, Elliott J, et al. Interleukin 18 inhibits osteoclast formation via T cell production of granulocyte macrophage colony-stimulating factor. J Clin Invest 1998;101: 595-603.
82. Takayanagi H, Ogasawara K, Hida S, et al. T-cell-mediated regulation of osteoclastogenesis by signalling cross-talk between RANKL and IFN-gamma. Nature 2000;408:600-605.
83. Guise TA, Yoneda T, Yates AJ, et al. The combined effect of tumor-produced parathyroid hormone-related protein and transforming growth factor-alpha enhance hypercalcemia in vivo and bone resorption in vitro. J Clin Endocrinol Metab 1995;77:40-45.
84. Lorenzo JA, Quinton J, Sousa S, et al. Effects of DNA and prostaglandin synthesis inhibitors on the stimulation of bone resorption by epidermal growth factor in fetal rat long-bone cultures. J Clin Invest 1986;77:1897-1902.
85. Pilbeam CC, Harrision J, Raisz LG. Prostaglandins and Bone Metabolism. In Billezikian JP, Raisz LG, Rodan GA, eds. Principles of Bone Biology. San Diego: Academic Press, 1997:715-728.
86. Canalis E. Skeletal Growth Factors, 3rd ed. San Diego: Elsevier, 2006.
87. Itoh N, Ornitz DM. Evolution of the Fgf and Fgfr gene families. Trends Genet 2004;20:563-569.
88. Mansukhani A, Ambrosetti D, Holmes G, et al. Sox2 induction by FGF and FGFR2 activating mutations inhibits Wnt signaling and osteoblast differentiation. J Cell Biol 2005;168:1065-1076.
89. Sobue T, Naganawa T, Xiao L, et al. Over-expression of fibroblast growth factor-2 causes defective bone mineralization and osteopenia in transgenic mice. J Cell Biochem 2005;95:83-94.
90. Montero A, Okada Y, Tomita M, et al. Disruption of the fibroblast growth factor-2 gene results in decreased bone mass and bone formation. J Clin Invest 2000;105:1085-1093.
91. Okada Y, Montero A, Zhang X, et al. Impaired osteoclast formation in bone marrow cultures of Fgf2 null mice in response to parathyroid hormone. J Biol Chem 2003;278:21258-21266.
92. Fredriksson L, Li H, Eriksson U. The PDGF family: four gene products form five dimeric isoforms. Cytokine Growth Factor Rev 2004;15:197-204.
93. Ferrara N, Davis-Smyth T. The biology of vascular endothelial growth factor. Endocr Rev 2004;18:4-25.
94. Hock JM, Canalis E. Platelet-derived growth factor enhances bone cell replication, but not differentiated function of osteoblasts. Endocrinology 1994;134:1423-1428.
95. Betsholtz C. Insight into the physiological functions of PDGF through genetic studies in mice. Cytokine Growth Factor Rev 2004;15:215-228.
96. Zelzer E, Olsen BR. Multiple roles of vascular endothelial growth factor (VEGF) in skeletal development, growth, and repair. Curr Top Dev Biol 2005;65:169-187.
97. Gerber HP, Vu TH, Ryan AM, et al. VEGF couples hypertrophic cartilage remodeling, ossification and angiogenesis during endochondral bone formation. Nat Med 1999;5:623-628.
98. Street J, Bao M, deGuzman L, et al. Vascular endothelial growth factor stimulates bone repair by promoting angiogenesis and bone turnover. Proc Natl Acad Sci U S A 2002;99:9656-9661.
99. Gazzerro E, Canalis E. Skeletal actions of insulin-like growth factors. Exp Rev Endocrinol Metab 2006;1:47.
100. Yakar S, Bouxsein ML, Canalis E, et al. The ternary IGF complex influences postnatal bone acquisition and the skeletal response to intermittent parathyroid hormone. J Endocrinol 2006;189:289-299.
101. Bikle D, Majumdar S, Laib A, et al. The skeletal structure of insulin-like growth factor I-deficient mice. J Bone Miner Res 2001;16: 2320-2329.
102. Zhao G, Monier-Faugere MC, Langub MC, et al. Targeted overexpression of insulin-like growth factor I to osteoblasts of transgenic mice: increased trabecular bone volume without increased osteoblast proliferation. Endocrinology 2000;141:2674-2682.
103. Hill PA, Reynolds JJ, Meikle MC. Osteoblasts mediate insulin-like growth factor-I and -II stimulation of osteoclast formation and function. Endocrinology 1995;136:124-131.
104. Barnard JA, Lyons RM, Moses HL. The cell biology of transforming growth factor beta. Biochim Biophys Acta 1990;1032:79-87.
105. Hock JM, Canalis E, Centrella M. Transforming growth factor-beta stimulates bone matrix apposition and bone cell replication in cultured fetal rat calvariae. Endocrinology 1990;126:421-426.
106. Spinella-Jaegle S, Roman-Roman S, Faucheu C, et al. Opposite effects of bone morphogenetic protein-2 and transforming growth factor-beta1 on osteoblast differentiation. Bone 2001;29:323-330.
107. Pfeilschifter J, Seyedin SM, Mundy GR. Transforming growth factor beta inhibits bone resorption in fetal rat long bone cultures. J Clin Invest 1988;82:680-685.
108. Shull MM, Ormsby I, Kier AB, et al. Targeted disruption of the mouse transforming growth factor-beta 1 gene results in multifocal inflammatory disease. Nature 1992;359:693-699.
109. Canalis E, Economides AN, Gazzerro E. Bone morphogenetic proteins, their antagonists, and the skeleton. Endocr Rev 2003;24: 218-235.
110. Leboy P, Grasso-Knight G, D'Angelo M. Smad-Runx interactions during chondrocyte maturation. J Bone Joint Surg Am 2001;83-A(suppl):S15-S22.
111. Kaneko H, Arakawa T, Mano H, et al. Direct stimulation of osteoclastic bone resorption by bone morphogenetic protein (BMP)-2 and expression of BMP receptors in mature osteoclasts. Bone 2000;27:479-486.
112. Johnson ML, Harnish K, Nusse R, et al. LRP5 and Wnt signaling: a union made for bone. J Bone Miner Res 2004;19:1749-1757.
113. Glass DA 2nd, Karsenty G. Molecular bases of the regulation of bone remodeling by the canonical Wnt signaling pathway. Curr Top Dev Biol 2006;73:43-84.
114. Glass DA 2nd, Bialek P, Ahn JD, et al. Canonical Wnt signaling in differentiated osteoblasts controls osteoclast differentiation. Dev Cell 2005;8:751-764.
115. Holmen SL, Zylstra CR, Mukherjee A, et al. Essential role of beta-catenin in postnatal bone acquisition. J Biol Chem 2005;280:21162-21168.
116. Lewiecki EM, Watts NB, McClung MR, et al. Official positions of the international society for clinical densitometry. J Clin Endocrinol Metab 2004;89:3651-3655.
117. Cummings SR, Bates D, Black DM. Clinical use of bone densitometry: scientific review. JAMA 2002;288:1889-1897.
118. Bauer DC, Gluer CC, Genant HK, et al. Quantitative ultrasound and vertebral fracture in postmenopausal women. Fracture Intervention Trial Research Group. J Bone Miner Res 1995;10: 353-358.
119. Williams ED, Daymond TJ. Evaluation of calcaneus bone densitometry against hip and spine for diagnosis of osteoporosis. Br J Radiol 2003;76:123-128.

120. Kroger H, Lunt M, Reeve J, et al. Bone density reduction in various measurement sites in men and women with osteoporotic fractures of spine and hip: the European quantitation of osteoporosis study. Calcif Tissue Int 1999;64:191-199.
121. Faulkner KG, von Stetten E, Miller P. Discordance in patient classification using T-scores. J Clin Densitom 1999;2:343-350.
122. Benito M, Gomberg B, Wehrli FW, et al. Deterioration of trabecular architecture in hypogonadal men. J Clin Endocrinol Metab 2003;88:1497-1502.
123. Boutroy S, Bouxsein ML, Munoz F, et al. In vivo assessment of trabecular bone microarchitecture by high-resolution peripheral quantitative computed tomography. J Clin Endocrinol Metab 2005;90:6508-6515.
124. Cummings SR, Palermo L, Browner W, et al. Monitoring osteoporosis therapy with bone densitometry: misleading changes and regression to the mean. Fracture Intervention Trial Research Group. JAMA 2000;283:1318-1321.
125. Rea JA, Li J, Blake GM, et al. Visual assessment of vertebral deformity by X-ray absorptiometry: a highly predictive method to exclude vertebral deformity. Osteoporos Int 2000;11:660-668.
126. Binkley N, Krueger D, Gangnon R, et al. Lateral vertebral assessment: a valuable technique to detect clinically significant vertebral fractures. Osteoporos Int 2005;16:1513-1518.
127. Guglielmi G, Floriani I, Torri V, et al. Effect of spinal degenerative changes on volumetric bone mineral density of the central skeleton as measured by quantitative computed tomography. Acta Radiol 2005;46:269-275.
128. Masud T, Francis RM. The increasing use of peripheral bone densitometry. BMJ 2000;321:396-398.
129. Siris ES, Miller PD, Barrett-Connor E, et al. Identification and fracture outcomes of undiagnosed low bone mineral density in postmenopausal women: results from the National Osteoporosis Risk Assessment. JAMA 2001;286:2815-2822.
130. Chapurlat RD, Garnero P, Breart G, et al. Serum type I collagen breakdown product (serum CTX) predicts hip fracture risk in elderly women: the EPIDOS study. Bone 2000;27:283-286.
131. Rogers A, Hannon RA, Eastell R. Biochemical markers as predictors of rates of bone loss after menopause. J Bone Miner Res 2000;15:1398-1404.
132. Eastell R, Barton I, Hannon RA, et al. Relationship of early changes in bone resorption to the reduction in fracture risk with risedronate. J Bone Miner Res 200318:1051-1056.
133. Greenspan SL, Rosen HN, Parker RA. Early changes in serum N-telopeptide and C-telopeptide cross-linked collagen type 1 predict long-term response to alendronate therapy in elderly women. J Clin Endocrinol Metab 2000;85:3537-3540.
134. Gundberg CM. Biochemical markers of bone formation. Clin Lab Med 2000;20:489-501.
135. Gundberg CM, Looker AC, Nieman SD, et al. Patterns of osteocalcin and bone specific alkaline phosphatase by age, gender, and race or ethnicity. Bone 2002;31:703-708.
136. Ross PD, Kress BC, Parson RE, et al. Serum bone alkaline phosphatase and calcaneus bone density predict fractures: a prospective study. Osteoporos Int 2000;11:76-82.
137. Booth SL, Broe KE, Peterson JW, et al. Associations between vitamin K biochemical measures and bone mineral density in men and women. J Clin Endocrinol Metab 2004;89:4904-4909.
138. Chen P, Satterwhite JH, Licata AA, et al. Early changes in biochemical markers of bone formation predict BMD response to teriparatide in postmenopausal women with osteoporosis. J Bone Miner Res 2005;20:962-970.
139. Fall PM, Kennedy D, Smith JA, et al. Comparison of serum and urine assays for biochemical markers of bone resorption in postmenopausal women with and without hormone replacement therapy and in men. Osteoporos Int 2000;11:481-485.
140. Huber F, Traber L, Roth HJ, et al. Markers of bone resorption—measurement in serum, plasma or urine? Clin Lab 2003;49:203-207.
141. Henriksen DB, Alexandersen P, Bjarnason NH, et al. Role of gastrointestinal hormones in postprandial reduction of bone resorption. J Bone Miner Res 2003;18:2180-2189.
142. Obrant KJ, Ivaska KK, Gerdhem P, et al. Biochemical markers of bone turnover are influenced by recently sustained fracture. Bone 2005;36:786-792.
143. Trueba D, Sawaya BP, Mawad H, et al. Bone biopsy: indications, techniques, and complications. Semin Dial 2003;16:341-345.
144. Martin KJ, Olgaard K, Coburn JW, et al. Diagnosis, assessment, and treatment of bone turnover abnormalities in renal osteodystrophy. Am J Kidney Dis 2004;43:558-565.
145. Lenchik L, Rogers LF, Delmas PD, et al. Diagnosis of osteoporotic vertebral fractures: importance of recognition and description by radiologists. AJR Am J Roentgenol 2004;183:949-958.
146. Consensus development conference: diagnosis, prophylaxis, and treatment of osteoporosis. Am J Med 1993;94:646-650.
147. Kanis JA, Melton LJ 3rd, Christiansen C, et al. The diagnosis of osteoporosis. J Bone Miner Res 1994;9:1137-1141.
148. Kanis JA, Borgstrom F, De Laet C, et al. Assessment of fracture risk. Osteoporos Int 2005;16:581-589.
149. Melton LJ 3rd, Khosla S, Achenbach SJ, et al. Effects of body size and skeletal site on the estimated prevalence of osteoporosis in women and men. Osteoporos Int 2000;11:977-983.
150. Johnell O, Kanis JA. An estimate of the worldwide prevalence, mortality and disability associated with hip fracture. Osteoporos Int 2004;15:897-902.
151. Kannus P, Palvanen M, Niemi S, et al. Osteoporotic fractures of the proximal humerus in elderly Finnish persons: sharp increase in 1970-1998 and alarming projections for the new millennium. Acta Orthop Scand 2000;71:465-470.
152. Raisz L. Pathogenesis of osteoporosis. J Clin Invest 2005;115:3318-3325.
153. Ralston SH. Genetic determinants of osteoporosis. Curr Opin Rheumatol 2005;17:475-479.
154. Brown MA, Haughton MA, Grant SF, et al. Genetic control of bone density and turnover: role of the collagen 1 alpha 1, estrogen receptor, and vitamin D receptor genes. J Bone Miner Res 2001;16:758-764.
155. Nguyen TV, Esteban LM, White CP, et al. Contribution of the collagen I alpha 1 and vitamin D receptor genes to the risk of hip fracture in elderly women. J Clin Endocrinol Metab 2005;90:6575-6579.
156. Styrkarsdottir U, Cazier JB, Kong A, et al. Linkage of osteoporosis to chromosome 20p12 and association to BMP2. PLoS Biol 2003;1:E69.
157. Gennari L, Merlotti D, De Paola V, et al. Estrogen receptor gene polymorphisms and the genetics of osteoporosis: a HuGE review. Am J Epidemiol 2005;161:307-320.
158. Ichikawa S, Koller DL, Peacock M, et al. Polymorphisms in the estrogen receptor beta (ESR2) gene are associated with bone mineral density in Caucasian men and women. J Clin Endocrinol Metab 2005;90:5921-5927.
159. Karsak M, Cohen-Solal M, Freudenberg J, et al. The cannabinoid receptor type 2 (CNR2) gene is associated with human osteoporosis. Hum Mol Genet 2005;14:3389-3396.
160. Bollerslev J, Wilson SG, Dick IM, et al. LRP5 gene polymorphisms predict bone mass and incident fractures in elderly Australian women. Bone 2005;36:599-606.
161. Shen H, Liu Y, Liu P, et al. Nonreplication in genetic studies of complex diseases—lessons learned from studies of osteoporosis and tentative remedies. J Bone Miner Res 2005;20:365-376.
162. Ralston SH, Galwey N, MacKay I, et al. Loci for regulation of bone mineral density in men and women identified by genome wide linkage scan: the FAMOS study. Hum Mol Genet 2005;14:943-951.
163. Peacock M, Koller DL, Lai D, et al. Sex-specific quantitative trait loci contribute to normal variation in bone structure at the proximal femur in men. Bone 2005;37:467-473.
164. Peacock M, Koller DL, Fishburn T, et al. Sex-specific and non-sex-specific quantitative trait loci contribute to normal variation in bone mineral density in men. J Clin Endocrinol Metab 2005;90:3060-3066.
165. Heaney RP, Abrams S, Dawson-Hughes B, et al. Peak bone mass. Osteoporos Int 2000;11:985-1009.
166. Riggs BL, Melton LJ III, Robb RA, et al. Population-based study of age and sex differences in bone volumetric density, size, geometry, and structure at different skeletal sites. J Bone Miner Res 2004;19:1945-1954.
167. Aaron JE, Shore PA, Shore RC, et al. Trabecular architecture in women and men of similar bone mass with and without vertebral fracture: II. Three-dimensional histology. Bone 2000;27:277-282.

168. Sornay-Rendu E, Munoz F, Garnero P, et al. Identification of osteopenic women at high risk of fracture: The OFELY Study. J Bone Miner Res 2005;20:1813-1819.
169. Parfitt AM, Villanueva AR, Foldes J, et al. Relations between histologic indices of bone formation: implications for the pathogenesis of spinal osteoporosis. J Bone Miner Res 1995;10:466-473.
170. Mann V, Ralston SH. Meta-analysis of COL1A1 Sp1 polymorphism in relation to bone mineral density and osteoporotic fracture. Bone 2003;32:711-717.
171. van Meurs JB, Dhonukshe-Rutten RA, Pluijm SM, et al. Homocysteine levels and the risk of osteoporotic fracture. N Engl J Med 2004;350:2033-2041.
172. Boskey AL, Dicarlo E, Paschalis E, et al. Comparison of mineral quality and quantity in iliac crest biopsies from high- and low-turnover osteoporosis: an FT-IR microspectroscopic investigation. Osteoporos Int 2005;16:2031-2038.
173. Khosla S, Melton LJ 3rd, Robb RA, et al. Relationship of volumetric BMD and structural parameters at different skeletal sites to sex steroid levels in men. J Bone Miner Res 2005;20:730-740.
174. Van Pottelbergh I, Goemaere S, Zmierczak H, et al. Perturbed sex steroid status in men with idiopathic osteoporosis and their sons. J Clin Endocrinol Metab 2004;89:4949-4953.
175. Lormeau C, Soudan B, d'Herbomez M, et al. Sex hormone-binding globulin, estradiol, and bone turnover markers in male osteoporosis. Bone 2004;34:933-939.
176. Rapuri PB, Gallagher JC, Haynatzki G. Endogenous levels of serum estradiol and sex hormone binding globulin determine bone mineral density, bone remodeling, the rate of bone loss, and response to treatment with estrogen in elderly women. J Clin Endocrinol Metab 2004;89:4954-4962.
177. Bischoff-Ferrari HA, Dawson-Hughes B, Willett WC, et al. Effect of Vitamin D on falls: a meta-analysis. JAMA 2004;291:1999-2006.
178. Sambrook PN, Chen JS, March LM, et al. Serum parathyroid hormone is associated with increased mortality independent of 25-hydroxy vitamin d status, bone mass, and renal function in the frail and very old: a cohort study. J Clin Endocrinol Metab 2004;89:5477-5481.
179. Gaugris S, Heaney RP, Boonen S, et al. Vitamin D inadequacy among post-menopausal women: a systematic review. QJM 2005;98:667-676.
180. Tiegs RD, Body JJ, Wahner HW, et al. Calcitonin secretion in postmenopausal osteoporosis. N Engl J Med 1985;312:1097-1100.
181. Niu T, Rosen CJ. The insulin-like growth factor-I gene and osteoporosis: A critical appraisal. Gene 2005;361:38-56.
182. Murphy E, Williams GR. The thyroid and the skeleton. Clin Endocrinol (Oxf) 2004;61:285-298.
183. Vestergaard P, Rejnmark L, Mosekilde L. Influence of hyper- and hypothyroidism, and the effects of treatment with antithyroid drugs and levothyroxine on fracture risk. Calcif Tissue Int 2005; 77:139-144.
184. Teitelbaum SL. Postmenopausal osteoporosis, T cells, and immune dysfunction. Proc Natl Acad Sci U S A 2004;101:16711-16712.
185. Ferrari SL, Karasik D, Liu J, et al. Interactions of interleukin-6 promoter polymorphisms with dietary and lifestyle factors and their association with bone mass in men and women from the Framingham Osteoporosis Study. J Bone Miner Res 2004;19:552-559.
186. Moffett SP, Zmuda JM, Oakley JI, et al. Tumor necrosis factor-alpha polymorphism, bone strength phenotypes, and the risk of fracture in older women. J Clin Endocrinol Metab 2005;90:3491-3497.
187. Kimble RB, Matayoshi AB, Vannice JL, et al. Simultaneous block of interleukin-1 and tumor necrosis factor is required to completely prevent bone loss in the early postovariectomy period. Endocrinology 1995;136:3054-3061.
188. Lorenzo JA, Naprta A, Rao Y, et al. Mice lacking the type I interleukin-1 receptor do not lose bone mass after ovariectomy. Endocrinology 1998;139:3022-3025.
189. Kawaguchi H, Pilbeam CC, Vargas SJ, et al. Ovariectomy enhances and estrogen replacement inhibits the activity of bone marrow factors that stimulate prostaglandin production in cultured mouse calvariae. J Clin Invest 1995;96:539-548.
190. Hofbauer LC, Heufelder AE. Role of receptor activator of nuclear factor-kappaB ligand and osteoprotegerin in bone cell biology. J Mol Med 2001;79:243-253.
191. Rogers A, Eastell R. Circulating osteoprotegerin and receptor activator for nuclear factor kappaB ligand: clinical utility in metabolic bone disease assessment. J Clin Endocrinol Metab 2005;90: 6323-6331.
192. Mezquita-Raya P, de la Higuera M, Garcia DF, et al. The contribution of serum osteoprotegerin to bone mass and vertebral fractures in postmenopausal women. Osteoporos Int 2005;16: 1368-1374.
193. Chapuy MC, Pamphile R, Paris E, et al. Combined calcium and vitamin D3 supplementation in elderly women: confirmation of reversal of secondary hyperparathyroidism and hip fracture risk: the Decalyos II study. Osteoporos Int 2002;13:257-264.
194. Lilliu H, Pamphile R, Chapuy MC, et al. Calcium-vitamin D3 supplementation is cost-effective in hip fractures prevention. Maturitas 2003;44:299-305.
195. Bischoff-Ferrari HA, Willett WC, Wong JB, et al. Fracture prevention with vitamin D supplementation: a meta-analysis of randomized controlled trials. JAMA 2005;293:2257-2264.
196. Wengreen HJ, Munger RG, West NA, et al. Dietary protein intake and risk of osteoporotic hip fracture in elderly residents of Utah. J Bone Miner Res 2004;19:537-545.
197. Frassetto LA, Todd KM, Morris RC Jr, et al. Worldwide incidence of hip fracture in elderly women: relation to consumption of animal and vegetable foods. J Gerontol A Biol Sci Med Sci 2000;55: M585-M592.
198. Bugel S. Vitamin K and bone health. Proc Nutr Soc 2003;62: 839-843.
199. Heiss CJ, Sanborn CF, Nichols DL, et al. Associations of body fat distribution, circulating sex hormones, and bone density in postmenopausal women. J Clin Endocrinol Metab 1995;80:1591-1596.
200. Kapoor D, Jones TH. Smoking and hormones in health and endocrine disorders. Eur J Endocrinol 2005;152:491-499.
201. Tziomalos K, Charsoulis F. Endocrine effects of tobacco smoking. Clin Endocrinol (Oxf) 2004;61:664-674.
202. Tinetti ME, Williams CS. Falls, injuries due to falls, and the risk of admission to a nursing home. N Engl J Med 1997;337:1279-1284.
203. Riggs BL, Melton LJ 3rd. Involutional osteoporosis. N Engl J Med 1986;314:1676-1686.
204. Lindsay R, Silverman SL, Cooper C, et al. Risk of new vertebral fracture in the year following a fracture. JAMA 2001;285:320-323.
205. Siminoski K, Warshawski RS, Jen H, et al. The accuracy of historical height loss for the detection of vertebral fractures in postmenopausal women. Osteoporos Int 2005;17:290-296.
206. Schousboe JT, Ensrud KE, Nyman JA, et al. Potential cost-effective use of spine radiographs to detect vertebral deformity and select osteopenic post-menopausal women for amino-bisphosphonate therapy. Osteoporos Int 2005;16:1883-1893.
207. Axenovich TI, Zaidman AM, Zorkoltseva IV, et al. Segregation analysis of Scheuermann disease in ninety families from Siberia. Am J Med Genet 2001;100:275-279.
208. Lombardi I Jr, Oliveira LM, Mayer AF, et al. Evaluation of pulmonary function and quality of life in women with osteoporosis. Osteoporos Int 2005;16:1247-1253.
209. Nguyen ND, Pongchaiyakul C, Center JR, et al. Identification of high-risk individuals for hip fracture: a 14-year prospective study. J Bone Miner Res 2005;20:1921-1928.
210. Solomon DH, Finkelstein JS, Katz JN, et al. Underuse of osteoporosis medications in elderly patients with fractures. Am J Med 2003;115:398-400.
211. Deng HW, Chen WM, Recker S, et al. Genetic determination of Colles' fracture and differential bone mass in women with and without Colles' fracture. J Bone Miner Res 2000;15:1243-1252.
212. Orwoll ES, Klein RF. Osteoporosis in men. Endocr Rev 1995;16: 87-116.
213. Chavassieux P, Meunier PJ. Histomorphometric approach of bone loss in men. Calcif Tissue Int 2001;69:209-213.
214. Center JR, Nguyen TV, Sambrook PN, et al. Hormonal and biochemical parameters in the determination of osteoporosis in elderly men. J Clin Endocrinol Metab 1999;84:3626-3635.
215. Rucker D, Ezzat S, Diamandi A, et al. IGF-I and testosterone levels as predictors of bone mineral density in healthy, community-dwelling men. Clin Endocrinol (Oxf) 2004;60:491-499.
216. Ferrari SL, Deutsch S, Baudoin C, et al. LRP5 gene polymorphisms and idiopathic osteoporosis in men. Bone 2005;37:770-775.
217. Bachrach LK. Osteoporosis and measurement of bone mass in children and adolescents. Endocrinol Metab Clin North Am 2005;34:521-535, vii.

218. Gandrud LM, Cheung JC, Daniels MW, et al. Low-dose intravenous pamidronate reduces fractures in childhood osteoporosis. J Pediatr Endocrinol Metab 2003;16:887-892.
219. Rauch F, Travers R, Norman ME, et al. Deficient bone formation in idiopathic juvenile osteoporosis: a histomorphometric study of cancellous iliac bone. J Bone Miner Res 2000;15:957-963.
220. Dawson PA, Kelly TE, Marini JC. Extension of phenotype associated with structural mutations in type I collagen: siblings with juvenile osteoporosis have an alpha2(I)Gly436 →Arg substitution. J Bone Miner Res 1999;14:449-455.
221. Hartikka H, Makitie O, Mannikko M, et al. Heterozygous mutations in the LDL receptor-related protein 5 (LRP5) gene are associated with primary osteoporosis in children. J Bone Miner Res 2005;20:783-789.
222. Khosla S, Lufkin EG, Hodgson SF, et al. Epidemiology and clinical features of osteoporosis in young individuals. Bone 1994;15: 551-555.
223. Peris P, Guanabens N, Monegal A, et al. Pregnancy associated osteoporosis: the familial effect. Clin Exp Rheumatol 2002;20: 697-700.
224. Javaid MK, Crozier SR, Harvey NC, et al. Maternal and seasonal predictors of change in calcaneal quantitative ultrasound during pregnancy. J Clin Endocrinol Metab 2005;90:5182-5187.
225. Schapira D, Braun Moscovici Y, Gutierrez G, et al. Severe transient osteoporosis of the hip during pregnancy. Successful treatment with intravenous biphosphonates. Clin Exp Rheumatol 2003;21: 107-110.
226. Toms AP, Marshall TJ, Becker E, et al. Regional migratory osteoporosis: a review illustrated by five cases. Clin Radiol 2005;60: 425-438.
227. Manicourt DH, Brasseur JP, Boutsen Y, et al. Role of alendronate in therapy for posttraumatic complex regional pain syndrome type I of the lower extremity. Arthritis Rheum 2004;50:3690-3697.
228. Stein E, Shane E. Secondary osteoporosis. Endocrinol Metab Clin North Am 2003;32:115-134, vii.
229. Shaker JL, Lukert BP. Osteoporosis associated with excess glucocorticoids. Endocrinol Metab Clin North Am 2005;34:341-356, viii-ix.
230. Van Staa TP, Leufkens HG, Abenhaim L, et al. Use of oral corticosteroids and risk of fractures. J Bone Miner Res 2000;15:993-1000.
231. Nielsen HK, Charles P, Mosekilde L. The effect of single oral doses of prednisone on the circadian rhythm of serum osteocalcin in normal subjects. J Clin Endocrinol Metab 1988;67:1025-1030.
232. O'Brien CA, Jia D, Plotkin LI, et al. Glucocorticoids act directly on osteoblasts and osteocytes to induce their apoptosis and reduce bone formation and strength. Endocrinology 2004;145: 1835-1841.
233. Weinstein RS, Chen JR, Powers CC, et al. Promotion of osteoclast survival and antagonism of bisphosphonate-induced osteoclast apoptosis by glucocorticoids. J Clin Invest 2002;109:1041-1048.
234. Reid IR, Heap SW. Determinants of vertebral mineral density in patients receiving long-term glucocorticoid therapy. Arch Intern Med 1990;150:2545-2548.
235. Hermus AR, Smals AG, Swinkels LM, et al. Bone mineral density and bone turnover before and after surgical cure of Cushing's syndrome. J Clin Endocrinol Metab 1995;80:2859-2865.
236. Saag KG, Emkey R, Schnitzer TJ, et al. Alendronate for the prevention and treatment of glucocorticoid-induced osteoporosis. Glucocorticoid-Induced Osteoporosis Intervention Study Group. N Engl J Med 1998;339:292-299.
237. Lane NE, Sanchez S, Modin GW, et al. Parathyroid hormone treatment can reverse corticosteroid-induced osteoporosis. Results of a randomized controlled clinical trial. J Clin Invest 1998;102: 1627-1633.
238. Lane NE, Sanchez S, Modin GW, et al. Bone mass continues to increase at the hip after parathyroid hormone treatment is discontinued in glucocorticoid-induced osteoporosis: results of a randomized controlled clinical trial. J Bone Miner Res 2000;15: 944-951.
239. Wallach S, Cohen S, Reid DM, et al. Effects of risedronate treatment on bone density and vertebral fracture in patients on corticosteroid therapy. Calcif Tissue Int 2000;67:277-285.
240. Plotkin LI, Weinstein RS, Parfitt AM, et al. Prevention of osteocyte and osteoblast apoptosis by bisphosphonates and calcitonin. J Clin Invest 1999;104:1363-1374.
241. Grinspoon S, Thomas E, Pitts S, et al. Prevalence and predictive factors for regional osteopenia in women with anorexia nervosa. Ann Intern Med 2000;133:790-794.
242. Birch K. Female athlete triad. BMJ 2005;330:244-246.
243. Scholes D, LaCroix AZ, Ichikawa LE, et al. Change in bone mineral density among adolescent women using and discontinuing depot medroxyprogesterone acetate contraception. Arch Pediatr Adolesc Med 2005;159:139-144.
244. Hoff AO, Gagel RF. Osteoporosis in breast and prostate cancer survivors. Oncology (Williston Park) 2005;19:651-658.
245. Eastell R, Hannon R. Long-term effects of aromatase inhibitors on bone. J Steroid Biochem Mol Biol 2005;95:151-154.
246. Karga H, Papapetrou PD, Korakovouni A, et al. Bone mineral density in hyperthyroidism. Clin Endocrinol (Oxf) 2004;61: 466-472.
247. Biermasz NR, Hamdy NA, Pereira AM, et al. Long-term skeletal effects of recombinant human growth hormone (rhGH) alone and rhGH combined with alendronate in GH-deficient adults: a seven-year follow-up study. Clin Endocrinol (Oxf) 2004;60:568-575.
248. Colao A, Loche S, Cappa M, et al. Prolactinomas in children and adolescents. Clinical presentation and long-term follow-up. J Clin Endocrinol Metab 1998;83:2777-2780.
249. Thrailkill KM, Lumpkin CK, Bunn RC, et al. Is insulin an anabolic agent in bone? Dissecting the diabetic bone for clues. Am J Physiol Endocrinol Metab 2005;289:E735-E745.
250. Strotmeyer ES, Cauley JA, Schwartz AV, et al. Nontraumatic fracture risk with diabetes mellitus and impaired fasting glucose in older white and black adults: the health, aging, and body composition study. Arch Intern Med 2005;165:1612-1617.
251. de Liefde II, van der Klift M, de Laet CE, et al. Bone mineral density and fracture risk in type-2 diabetes mellitus: the Rotterdam Study. Osteoporos Int 2005;16:1713-1720.
252. Oyajobi BO, Mundy GR. Receptor activator of NF-kappaB ligand, macrophage inflammatory protein-1alpha, and the proteasome: novel therapeutic targets in myeloma. Cancer 2003;97:813-817.
253. Tian E, Zhan F, Walker R, et al. The role of the Wnt-signaling antagonist DKK1 in the development of osteolytic lesions in multiple myeloma. N Engl J Med 2003;349:2483-2494.
254. Tehranzadeh J, Tao C. Advances in MR imaging of vertebral collapse. Semin Ultrasound CT MR 2004;25:440-460.
255. Hay JE, Guichelaar MM. Evaluation and management of osteoporosis in liver disease. Clin Liver Dis 2005;9:747-766.
256. Sylvester FA. IBD and skeletal health: children are not small adults! Inflamm Bowel Dis 2005;11:1020-1023.
257. Collin P. Should adults be screened for celiac disease? What are the benefits and harms of screening? Gastroenterology 2005;128: S104-S108.
258. Cauley JA, Fullman RL, Stone KL, et al. Factors associated with the lumbar spine and proximal femur bone mineral density in older men. Osteoporos Int 2005;16:1525-1537.
259. Brumsen C, Papapoulos SE, Lentjes EG, et al. A potential role for the mast cell in the pathogenesis of idiopathic osteoporosis in men. Bone 2002;31:556-561.
260. Chines A, Pacifici R, Avioli LV, et al. Systemic mastocytosis presenting as osteoporosis: a clinical and histomorphometric study. J Clin Endocrinol Metab 1991;72:140-144.
261. Pardanani A. Systemic mastocytosis: bone marrow pathology, classification, and current therapies. Acta Haematol 2005;114: 41-51.
262. Wonke B, Jensen C, Hanslip JJ, et al. Genetic and acquired predisposing factors and treatment of osteoporosis in thalassaemia major. J Pediatr Endocrinol Metab 1998;11(suppl 3):795-801.
263. Diamond T, Stiel D, Posen S. Effects of testosterone and venesection on spinal and peripheral bone mineral in six hypogonadal men with hemochromatosis. J Bone Miner Res 1991;6:39-43.
264. Maalouf NM, Shane E. Osteoporosis after solid organ transplantation. J Clin Endocrinol Metab 2005;90:2456-2465.
265. Tannirandorn P, Epstein S. Drug-induced bone loss. Osteoporos Int 2000;11:637-659.
266. Shahinian VB, Kuo YF, Freeman JL, et al. Risk of fracture after androgen deprivation for prostate cancer. N Engl J Med 2005;352: 154-164.
267. Lester J, Coleman R. Bone loss and the aromatase inhibitors. Br J Cancer 2005;93(suppl 1):S16-S22.

268. Hannan MT, Felson DT, Dawson-Hughes B, et al. Risk factors for longitudinal bone loss in elderly men and women: the Framingham Osteoporosis Study. J Bone Miner Res 2000;15:710-720.
269. Raisz LG. Clinical practice. Screening for osteoporosis. N Engl J Med 2005;353:164-171.
270. Marci CD, Anderson WB, Viechnicki MB, et al. Bone mineral densitometry substantially influences health-related behaviors of postmenopausal women. Calcif Tissue Int 2000;66:113-118.
271. Weisman SM, Matkovic V. Potential use of biochemical markers of bone turnover for assessing the effect of calcium supplementation and predicting fracture risk. Clin Ther 2005;27:299-308.
272. Heaney RP, Weaver CM. Calcium and vitamin D. Endocrinol Metab Clin North Am 2003;32:181-194, vii-viii.
273. Heaney RP. The vitamin D requirement in health and disease. J Steroid Biochem Mol Biol 2005;97:13-19.
274. Storm D, Eslin R, Porter ES, et al. Calcium supplementation prevents seasonal bone loss and changes in biochemical markers of bone turnover in elderly New England women: a randomized placebo-controlled trial. J Clin Endocrinol Metab 1998;83: 3817-3825.
275. Ensrud KE, Duong T, Cauley JA, et al. Low fractional calcium absorption increases the risk for hip fracture in women with low calcium intake. Study of Osteoporotic Fractures Research Group. Ann Intern Med 2000;132:345-353.
276. Recker RR. Calcium absorption and achlorhydria. N Engl J Med 1985;313:70-73.
277. Chapuy MC, Arlot ME, Delmas PD, et al. Effect of calcium and cholecalciferol treatment for three years on hip fractures in elderly women. BMJ 1994;308:1081-1082.
278. Andress DL. Vitamin D treatment in chronic kidney disease. Semin Dial 2005;18:315-321.
279. Avenell A, Gillespie W, Gillespie L, et al. Vitamin D and vitamin D analogues for preventing fractures associated with involutional and post-menopausal osteoporosis. Cochrane Database Syst Rev 2005:CD000227.
280. Bonner FJ Jr, Sinaki M, Grabois M, et al. Health professional's guide to rehabilitation of the patient with osteoporosis. Osteoporos Int 2003;14(suppl 2):S1-S22.
281. Bonaiuti D, Shea B, Iovine R, et al. Exercise for preventing and treating osteoporosis in postmenopausal women. Cochrane Database Syst Rev 2002:CD000333.
282. Pierfitte C, Macouillard G, Thicoipe M, et al. Benzodiazepines and hip fractures in elderly people: case-control study. BMJ 2001;322: 704-708.
283. Gold DT. Osteoporosis and quality of life psychosocial outcomes and interventions for individual patients. Clin Geriatr Med 2003;19:271-280, vi.
284. Gold DT, Shipp KM, Pieper CF, et al. Group treatment improves trunk strength and psychological status in older women with vertebral fractures: results of a randomized, clinical trial. J Am Geriatr Soc 2004;52:1471-1478.
285. Mathis JM, Ortiz AO, Zoarski GH. Vertebroplasty versus kyphoplasty: a comparison and contrast. AJNR Am J Neuroradiol 2004;25:840-845.
286. Nelson HD, Humphrey LL, Nygren P, et al. Postmenopausal hormone replacement therapy: scientific review. JAMA 2002;288: 872-881.
287. Anderson GL, Limacher M, Assaf AR, et al. Effects of conjugated equine estrogen in postmenopausal women with hysterectomy: the Women's Health Initiative randomized controlled trial. JAMA 2004;291:1701-1712.
288. Majumdar SR, Almasi EA, Stafford RS. Promotion and prescribing of hormone therapy after report of harm by the Women's Health Initiative. JAMA 2004;292:1983-1988.
289. Lindsay R. Hormones and bone health in postmenopausal women. Endocrine 2004;24:223-230.
290. Prestwood KM, Kenny AM, Kleppinger A, et al. Ultralow-dose micronized 17beta-estradiol and bone density and bone metabolism in older women: a randomized controlled trial. JAMA 2003;290:1042-1048.
291. Ettinger B, Ensrud KE, Wallace R, et al. Effects of ultralow-dose transdermal estradiol on bone mineral density: a randomized clinical trial. Obstet Gynecol 2004;104:443-451.
292. Greenspan SL, Emkey RD, Bone HG, et al. Significant differential effects of alendronate, estrogen, or combination therapy on the rate of bone loss after discontinuation of treatment of postmenopausal osteoporosis. A randomized, double-blind, placebo-controlled trial. Ann Intern Med 2002;137:875-883.
293. Leu CT, Luegmayr E, Freedman LP, et al. Relative binding affinities of bisphosphonates for human bone and relationship to antiresorptive efficacy. Bone 2005;38:628-636.
294. Raisz L, Smith JA, Trahiotis M, et al. Short-term risedronate treatment in postmenopausal women: effects on biochemical markers of bone turnover. Osteoporos Int 2000;11:615-620.
295. Kherani RB, Papaioannou A, Adachi JD. Long-term tolerability of the bisphosphonates in postmenopausal osteoporosis: a comparative review. Drug Saf 2002;25:781-790.
296. Saarto T, Taube T, Blomqvist C, et al. Three-year oral clodronate treatment does not impair mineralization of newly formed bone—a histomorphometric study. Calcif Tissue Int 2005;77: 84-90.
297. Rogers MJ, Gordon S, Benford HL, et al. Cellular and molecular mechanisms of action of bisphosphonates. Cancer 2000;88: 2961-2978.
298. Harris ST, Watts NB, Genant HK, et al. Effects of risedronate treatment on vertebral and nonvertebral fractures in women with postmenopausal osteoporosis: a randomized controlled trial. Vertebral Efficacy with Risedronate Therapy (VERT) Study Group. JAMA 1999;282:1344-1352.
299. McClung MR, Geusens P, Miller PD, et al. Effect of risedronate on the risk of hip fracture in elderly women. Hip Intervention Program Study Group. N Engl J Med 2001;344:333-340.
300. Felsenberg D, Miller P, Armbrecht G, et al. Oral ibandronate significantly reduces the risk of vertebral fractures of greater severity after 1, 2, and 3 years in postmenopausal women with osteoporosis. Bone 2005;37:651-654.
301. Reid DM, Hughes RA, Laan RF, et al. Efficacy and safety of daily risedronate in the treatment of corticosteroid-induced osteoporosis in men and women: a randomized trial. European Corticosteroid-Induced Osteoporosis Treatment Study. J Bone Miner Res 2000;15:1006-1013.
302. Orwoll E, Ettinger M, Weiss S, et al. Alendronate for the treatment of osteoporosis in men. N Engl J Med 2000;343:604-610.
303. Bone HG, Hosking D, Devogelaer JP, et al. Ten years' experience with alendronate for osteoporosis in postmenopausal women. N Engl J Med 2004;350:1189-1199.
304. Schnitzer T, Bone HG, Crepaldi G, et al. Therapeutic equivalence of alendronate 70 mg once-weekly and alendronate 10 mg daily in the treatment of osteoporosis. Alendronate Once-Weekly Study Group. Aging (Milano) 2000;12:1-12.
305. Reid IR, Brown JP, Burckhardt P, et al. Intravenous zoledronic acid in postmenopausal women with low bone mineral density. N Engl J Med 2002;346:653-661.
306. Woo SB, Hellstein JW, Kalmar JR. Narrative [corrected] review: bisphosphonates and osteonecrosis of the jaws. Ann Intern Med 2006;144:753-761.
307. Chesnut CH 3rd, Silverman S, Andriano K, et al. A randomized trial of nasal spray salmon calcitonin in postmenopausal women with established osteoporosis: the prevent recurrence of osteoporotic fractures study. PROOF Study Group. Am J Med 2000;109: 267-276.
308. Cummings SR, Chapurlat RD. What PROOF proves about calcitonin and clinical trials. Am J Med 2000;109:330-331.
309. Downs RW Jr, Bell NH, Ettinger MP, et al. Comparison of alendronate and intranasal calcitonin for treatment of osteoporosis in postmenopausal women. J Clin Endocrinol Metab 2000;85: 1783-1788.
310. Knopp JA, Diner BM, Blitz M, et al. Calcitonin for treating acute pain of osteoporotic vertebral compression fractures: a systematic review of randomized, controlled trials. Osteoporos Int 2005;16: 1281-1290.
311. Baum M, Buzdar A, Cuzick J, et al. Anastrozole alone or in combination with tamoxifen versus tamoxifen alone for adjuvant treatment of postmenopausal women with early-stage breast cancer: results of the ATAC (Arimidex, Tamoxifen Alone or in Combination) trial efficacy and safety update analyses. Cancer 2003;98: 1802-1810.
312. Ettinger B, Black DM, Mitlak BH, et al. Reduction of vertebral fracture risk in postmenopausal women with osteoporosis treated with raloxifene: results from a 3-year randomized clinical trial.

Multiple Outcomes of Raloxifene Evaluation (MORE) Investigators. JAMA 1999;282:637-645.
313. Prestwood KM, Gunness M, Muchmore DB, et al. A comparison of the effects of raloxifene and estrogen on bone in postmenopausal women. J Clin Endocrinol Metab 2000;85:2197-2202.
314. Martino S, Cauley JA, Barrett-Connor E, et al. Continuing outcomes relevant to Evista: breast cancer incidence in postmenopausal osteoporotic women in a randomized trial of raloxifene. J Natl Cancer Inst 2004;96:1751-1761.
315. Johnston CC Jr, Bjarnason NH, Cohen FJ, et al. Long-term effects of raloxifene on bone mineral density, bone turnover, and serum lipid levels in early postmenopausal women: three-year data from 2 double-blind, randomized, placebo-controlled trials. Arch Intern Med 2000;160:3444-3450.
316. Ke HZ, Foley GL, Simmons HA, et al. Long-term treatment of lasofoxifene preserves bone mass and bone strength and does not adversely affect the uterus in ovariectomized rats. Endocrinology 2004;145:1996-2005.
317. Komm BS, Kharode YP, Bodine PV, et al. Bazedoxifene acetate: a selective estrogen receptor modulator with improved selectivity. Endocrinology 2005;146:3999-4008.
318. Neer RM, Arnaud CD, Zanchetta JR, et al. Effect of parathyroid hormone (1-34) on fractures and bone mineral density in postmenopausal women with osteoporosis. N Engl J Med 2001;344:1434-1441.
319. Kurland ES, Cosman F, McMahon DJ, et al. Parathyroid hormone as a therapy for idiopathic osteoporosis in men: effects on bone mineral density and bone markers. J Clin Endocrinol Metab 2000;85:3069-3076.
320. Ettinger B, San Martin J, Crans G, et al. Differential effects of teriparatide on BMD after treatment with raloxifene or alendronate. J Bone Miner Res 2004;19:745-751.
321. Black DM, Greenspan SL, Ensrud KE, et al. The effects of parathyroid hormone and alendronate alone or in combination in postmenopausal osteoporosis. N Engl J Med 2003;349:1207-1215.
322. Cosman F, Nieves J, Zion M, et al. Daily and cyclic parathyroid hormone in women receiving alendronate. N Engl J Med 2005;353:566-575.
323. Black DM, Bilezikian JP, Ensrud KE, et al. One year of alendronate after one year of parathyroid hormone (1-84) for osteoporosis. N Engl J Med 2005;353:555-565.
324. Meunier PJ, Roux C, Seeman E, et al. The effects of strontium ranelate on the risk of vertebral fracture in women with postmenopausal osteoporosis. N Engl J Med 2004;350:459-468.
325. Snyder PJ, Peachey H, Berlin JA, et al. Effects of testosterone replacement in hypogonadal men. J Clin Endocrinol Metab 2000;85:2670-2677.
326. Kenny AM, Prestwood KM, Gruman CA, et al. Effects of transdermal testosterone on bone and muscle in older men with low bioavailable testosterone levels. J Gerontol A Biol Sci Med Sci 2001;56:M266-M272.
327. Snyder PJ, Peachey H, Hannoush P, et al. Effect of testosterone treatment on bone mineral density in men over 65 years of age. J Clin Endocrinol Metab 1999;84:1966-1972.
328. Schoofs MW, van der Klift M, Hofman A, et al. Thiazide diuretics and the risk for hip fracture. Ann Intern Med 2003;139:476-482.
329. Reid IR, Ames RW, Orr-Walker BJ, et al. Hydrochlorothiazide reduces loss of cortical bone in normal postmenopausal women: a randomized controlled trial. Am J Med 2000;109:362-370.
330. Murphy MG, Cerchio K, Stoch SA, et al. Effect of L-000845704, an alphaVbeta3 integrin antagonist, on markers of bone turnover and bone mineral density in postmenopausal osteoporotic women. J Clin Endocrinol Metab 2005;90:2022-2028.
331. Rodan GA, Martin TJ. Therapeutic approaches to bone diseases. Science 2000;289:1508-1514.
332. Godsall JW, Baron R, Insogna KL. Vitamin D metabolism and bone histomorphometry in a patient with antacid-induced osteomalacia. Am J Med 1984;77:747-750.
333. Awumey EM, Mitra DA, Hollis BW, et al. Vitamin D metabolism is altered in Asian Indians in the southern United States: a clinical research center study. J Clin Endocrinol Metab 1998;83:169-173.
334. Kreiter SR, Schwartz RP, Kirkman HN Jr, et al. Nutritional rickets in African American breast-fed infants. J Pediatr 2000;137:153-157.
335. Basha B, Rao DS, Han ZH, et al. Osteomalacia due to vitamin D depletion: a neglected consequence of intestinal malabsorption. Am J Med 2000;108:296-300.
336. Schnitzler CM, Pettifor JM, Patel D, et al. Metabolic bone disease in black teenagers with genu valgum or varum without radiologic rickets: a bone histomorphometric study. J Bone Miner Res 1994;9:479-486.
337. Pettifor JM. Rickets and vitamin D deficiency in children and adolescents. Endocrinol Metab Clin North Am 2005;34:537-553, vii.
338. Kitanaka S, Takeyama K, Murayama A, et al. Inactivating mutations in the 25-hydroxyvitamin D3 1alpha-hydroxylase gene in patients with pseudovitamin D-deficiency rickets. N Engl J Med 1998;338:653-661.
339. Kato S, Yoshizazawa T, Kitanaka S, et al. Molecular genetics of vitamin D-dependent hereditary rickets. Horm Res 2002;57:73-78.
340. Kruse K, Feldmann E. Healing of rickets during vitamin D therapy despite defective vitamin D receptors in two siblings with vitamin D-dependent rickets type II. J Pediatr 1995;126:145-148.
341. Berndt TJ, Schiavi S, Kumar R. "Phosphatonins" and the regulation of phosphorus homeostasis. Am J Physiol Renal Physiol 2005;289:F1170-F1182.
342. Quarles LD. FGF23, PHEX, and MEPE regulation of phosphate homeostasis and skeletal mineralization. Am J Physiol Endocrinol Metab 2003;285:E1-9.
343. Dixon PH, Christie PT, Wooding C, et al. Mutational analysis of PHEX gene in X-linked hypophosphatemia. J Clin Endocrinol Metab 1998;83:3615-3623.
344. Petersen DJ, Boniface AM, Schranck FW, et al. X-linked hypophosphatemic rickets: a study (with literature review) of linear growth response to calcitriol and phosphate therapy. J Bone Miner Res 1992;7:583-597.
345. Consortium A. Autosomal dominant hypophosphataemic rickets is associated with mutations in FGF23. Nat Genet 2000;26:345-348.
346. Carpenter TO, Ellis BK, Insogna KL, et al. Fibroblast growth factor 7: an inhibitor of phosphate transport derived from oncogenic osteomalacia-causing tumors. J Clin Endocrinol Metab 2005;90:1012-1020.
347. Jonsson KB, Zahradnik R, Larsson T, et al. Fibroblast growth factor 23 in oncogenic osteomalacia and X-linked hypophosphatemia. N Engl J Med 2003;348:1656-1663.
348. Whyte MP. Hypophosphatasia and the role of alkaline phosphatase in skeletal mineralization. Endocr Rev 1994;15:439-461.
349. Pauli RM, Modaff P, Sipes SL, et al. Mild hypophosphatasia mimicking severe osteogenesis imperfecta in utero: bent but not broken. Am J Med Genet 1999;86:434-438.
350. Iqbal SJ, Brain A, Reynolds TM, et al. Relationship between serum alkaline phosphatase and pyridoxal-5'-phosphate levels in hypophosphatasia. Clin Sci (Lond) 1998;94:203-206.
351. Whyte MP, Kurtzberg J, McAlister WH, et al. Marrow cell transplantation for infantile hypophosphatasia. J Bone Miner Res 2003;18:624-636.
352. Xu Y, Hashizume T, Shuhart M, et al. Intestinal and hepatic CYP3A4 catalyze hydroxylation of 1 alpha,25-dihydroxyvitamin D3: implications for drug-induced osteomalacia. Mol Pharmacol 2005;69:56-65.
353. Reginato AJ, Falasca GF, Pappu R, et al. Musculoskeletal manifestations of osteomalacia: report of 26 cases and literature review. Semin Arthritis Rheum 1999;28:287-304.
354. Huang QL, Feig DS, Blackstein ME. Development of tertiary hyperparathyroidism after phosphate supplementation in oncogenic osteomalacia. J Endocrinol Invest 2000;23:263-267.
355. Li YC, Amling M, Pirro AE, et al. Normalization of mineral ion homeostasis by dietary means prevents hyperparathyroidism, rickets, and osteomalacia, but not alopecia in vitamin D receptor-ablated mice. Endocrinology 1998;139:4391-4396.
356. Wilson DM. Growth hormone and hypophosphatemic rickets. J Pediatr Endocrinol Metab 2000;13(suppl 2):993-998.
357. Albright F, Reifenstein EC Jr. The Parathyroid Glands and Metabolic Bone Disease: Selected Studies. Baltimore: Williams & Wilkins, 1948.
358. Bilezikian JP, Silverberg SJ. Clinical practice. Asymptomatic primary hyperparathyroidism. N Engl J Med 2004;350:1746-1751.
359. Moosgaard B, Vestergaard P, Heickendorff L, et al. Vitamin D status, seasonal variations, parathyroid adenoma weight and bone

mineral density in primary hyperparathyroidism. Clin Endocrinol (Oxf) 2005;63:506-513.
360. Silverberg SJ, Gartenberg F, Jacobs TP, et al. Increased bone mineral density after parathyroidectomy in primary hyperparathyroidism. J Clin Endocrinol Metab 1995;80:729-734.
361. Chan FK, Tiu SC, Choi KL, et al. Increased bone mineral density in patients with chronic hypoparathyroidism. J Clin Endocrinol Metab 2003;88:3155-3159.
362. Palmer S, McGregor DO, Strippoli GF. Interventions for preventing bone disease in kidney transplant recipients. Cochrane Database Syst Rev 2005:CD005015.
363. Lindberg JS. Calcimimetics: a new tool for management of hyperparathyroidism and renal osteodystrophy in patients with chronic kidney disease. Kidney Int Suppl 2005:S33-S36.
364. Gal-Moscovici A, Popovtzer MM. New worldwide trends in presentation of renal osteodystrophy and its relationship to parathyroid hormone levels. Clin Nephrol 2005;63:284-289.
365. Cunningham J, Sprague SM, Cannata-Andia J, et al. Osteoporosis in chronic kidney disease. Am J Kidney Dis 2004;43:566-571.
366. Hughes AE, Ralston SH, Marken J, et al. Mutations in TNFRSF11A, affecting the signal peptide of RANK, cause familial expansile osteolysis. Nat Genet 2000;24:45-48.
367. Siris ES. Extensive personal experience: Paget's disease of bone. J Clin Endocrinol Metab 1995;80:335-338.
368. Singer FR. Paget's disease of bone: classical pathology and electron microscopy. Semin Arthritis Rheum 1994;23:217-218.
369. Reddy SV, Singer FR, Roodman GD. Bone marrow mononuclear cells from patients with Paget's disease contain measles virus nucleocapsid messenger ribonucleic acid that has mutations in a specific region of the sequence. J Clin Endocrinol Metab 1995;80:2108-2111.
370. Kurihara N, Reddy SV, Menaa C, et al. Osteoclasts expressing the measles virus nucleocapsid gene display a pagetic phenotype. J Clin Invest 2000;105:607-614.
371. Roodman GD, Kurihara N, Ohsaki Y, et al. Interleukin 6. A potential autocrine/paracrine factor in Paget's disease of bone. J Clin Invest 1992;89:46-52.
372. Menaa C, Reddy SV, Kurihara N, et al. Enhanced RANK ligand expression and responsivity of bone marrow cells in Paget's disease of bone. J Clin Invest 2000;105:1833-1838.
373. Siris ES. Epidemiological aspects of Paget's disease: family history and relationship to other medical conditions. Semin Arthritis Rheum 1994;23:222-225.
374. Laurin N, Brown JP, Morissette J, et al. Recurrent mutation of the gene encoding sequestosome 1 (SQSTM1/p62) in Paget disease of bone. Am J Hum Genet 2002;70:1582-1588.
375. Layfield R, Ciani B, Ralston SH, et al. Structural and functional studies of mutations affecting the UBA domain of SQSTM1 (p62) which cause Paget's disease of bone. Biochem Soc Trans 2004;32:728-730.
376. Alvarez L, Guanabens N, Peris P, et al. Discriminative value of biochemical markers of bone turnover in assessing the activity of Paget's disease. J Bone Miner Res 1995;10:458-465.
377. Chosich N, Long F, Wong R, et al. Post-partum hypercalcemia in hereditary hyperphosphatasia (juvenile Paget's disease). J Endocrinol Invest 1991;14:591-597.
378. Demir E, Bereket A, Ozkan B, et al. Effect of alendronate treatment on the clinical picture and bone turnover markers in chronic idiopathic hyperphosphatasia. J Pediatr Endocrinol Metab 2000;13:217-221.
379. Whyte MP, Mills BG, Reinus WR, et al. Expansile skeletal hyperphosphatasia: a new familial metabolic bone disease. J Bone Miner Res 2000;15:2330-2344.
380. Byers PH. Osteogenesis imperfecta. In Royce PaSB, ed. Connective tissue and its heritable disorders: molecular, genetic, and medical aspects. Wiley-Liss, New York, 1993:317-350.
380a. Barnes AM, Chang W, Morello R, Cabral WA, Weis M, Eyre DR, et al. Deficiency of cartilage-associated protein in recessive lethal osteogenesis imperfecta. N Engl J Med 2006;355(26): 2757-2764.
380b. Cabral WA, Chang W, Barnes AM, Weis M, Scott MA, Leikin S, et al. Prolyl 3-hydroxylase 1 deficiency causes a recessive metabolic bone disorder resembling lethal/severe osteogenesis imperfecta. Nat Genet 2007;39(3):359-365.
381. Redford-Badwal DA, Stover ML, Valli M, et al. Nuclear retention of COL1A1 messenger RNA identifies null alleles causing mild osteogenesis imperfecta. J Clin Invest 1996;97:1035-1040.
382. Spotila LD, Colige A, Sereda L, et al. Mutation analysis of coding sequences for type I procollagen in individuals with low bone density. J Bone Miner Res 1994;9:923-932.
383. Spotila LD, Constantinou CD, Sereda L, et al. Mutation in a gene for type I procollagen (COL1A2) in a woman with postmenopausal osteoporosis: evidence for phenotypic and genotypic overlap with mild osteogenesis imperfecta. Proc Natl Acad Sci U S A 1991;88: 5423-5427.
384. Rauch F, Travers R, Parfitt AM, et al. Static and dynamic bone histomorphometry in children with osteogenesis imperfecta. Bone 2000;26:581-589.
385. Glorieux FH, Rauch F, Plotkin H, et al. Type V osteogenesis imperfecta: a new form of brittle bone disease. J Bone Miner Res 2000;15:1650-1658.
386. Braga V, Gatti D, Rossini M, et al. Bone turnover markers in patients with osteogenesis imperfecta. Bone 2004;34:1013-1016.
387. Glorieux FH, Bishop NJ, Plotkin H, et al. Cyclic administration of pamidronate in children with severe osteogenesis imperfecta. N Engl J Med 1998;339:947-952.
388. Munns CF, Rauch F, Travers R, et al. Effects of intravenous pamidronate treatment in infants with osteogenesis imperfecta: clinical and histomorphometric outcome. J Bone Miner Res 2005;20: 1235-1243.
389. Vyskocil V, Pikner R, Kutilek S. Effect of alendronate therapy in children with osteogenesis imperfecta. Joint Bone Spine 2005;72:416-423.
390. Chamberlain JR, Schwarze U, Wang PR, et al. Gene targeting in stem cells from individuals with osteogenesis imperfecta. Science 2004;303:1198-201.
391. Tolar J, Teitelbaum SL, Orchard PJ. Osteopetrosis. N Engl J Med 2004;351:2839-2849.
392. Abboud SL, Woodruff K, Liu C, et al. Rescue of the osteopetrotic defect in op/op mice by osteoblast-specific targeting of soluble colony-stimulating factor-1. Endocrinology 2002;143:1942-1949.
393. Gowen M, Lazner F, Dodds R, et al. Cathepsin K knockout mice develop osteopetrosis due to a deficit in matrix degradation but not demineralization. J Bone Miner Res 1999;14:1654-1663.
394. Grigoriadis AE, Wang ZQ, Cecchini MG, et al. c-Fos: a key regulator of osteoclast-macrophage lineage determination and bone remodeling. Science 1994;266:443-448.
395. Hollberg K, Hultenby K, Hayman A, et al. Osteoclasts from mice deficient in tartrate-resistant acid phosphatase have altered ruffled borders and disturbed intracellular vesicular transport. Exp Cell Res 2002;279:227-238.
396. McHugh KP, Hodivala-Dilke K, Zheng MH, et al. Mice lacking beta3 integrins are osteosclerotic because of dysfunctional osteoclasts. J Clin Invest 2000;105:433-440.
397. Naito A, Azuma S, Tanaka S, et al. Severe osteopetrosis, defective interleukin-1 signalling and lymph node organogenesis in TRAF6-deficient mice. Genes Cells 1999;4:353-362.
398. Chalhoub N, Benachenhou N, Rajapurohitam V, et al. Grey-lethal mutation induces severe malignant autosomal recessive osteopetrosis in mouse and human. Nat Med 2003;9:399-406.
399. Fasth A, Porras O. Human malignant osteopetrosis: pathophysiology, management and the role of bone marrow transplantation. Pediatr Transplant 1999;3(suppl 1):102-107.
400. Frattini A, Orchard PJ, Sobacchi C, et al. Defects in TCIRG1 subunit of the vacuolar proton pump are responsible for a subset of human autosomal recessive osteopetrosis. Nat Genet 2000;25: 343-346.
401. Frattini A, Pangrazio A, Susani L, et al. Chloride channel ClCN7 mutations are responsible for severe recessive, dominant, and intermediate osteopetrosis. J Bone Miner Res 2003;18:1740-1747.
402. Ramirez A, Faupel J, Goebel I, et al. Identification of a novel mutation in the coding region of the grey-lethal gene OSTM1 in human malignant infantile osteopetrosis. Hum Mutat 2004;23:471-476.
403. Key LL Jr, Rodriguiz RM, Willi SM, et al. Long-term treatment of osteopetrosis with recombinant human interferon gamma. N Engl J Med 1995;332:1594-1599.
404. Quarello P, Forni M, Barberis L, et al. Severe malignant osteopetrosis caused by a GL gene mutation. J Bone Miner Res 2004;19: 1194-1199.

405. Cotter M, Connell T, Colhoun E, et al. Carbonic anhydrase II deficiency: a rare autosomal recessive disorder of osteopetrosis, renal tubular acidosis, and cerebral calcification. J Pediatr Hematol Oncol 2005;27:115-117.
406. McMahon C, Will A, Hu P, et al. Bone marrow transplantation corrects osteopetrosis in the carbonic anhydrase II deficiency syndrome. Blood 2001;97:1947-1950.
407. Benichou OD, Laredo JD, de Vernejoul MC. Type II autosomal dominant osteopetrosis (Albers-Schonberg disease): clinical and radiological manifestations in 42 patients. Bone 2000;26: 87-93.
408. Alatalo SL, Ivaska KK, Waguespack SG, et al. Osteoclast-derived serum tartrate-resistant acid phosphatase 5b in Albers-Schonberg disease (type II autosomal dominant osteopetrosis). Clin Chem 2004;50:883-890.
409. Del Fattore A, Peruzzi B, Rucci N, et al. Clinical, genetic and cellular analysis of forty-nine osteopetrotic patients: implications for diagnosis and treatment. J Med Genet 2005;43:315-325.
410. Henriksen K, Gram J, Schaller S, et al. Characterization of osteoclasts from patients harboring a G215R mutation in ClC-7 causing autosomal dominant osteopetrosis type II. Am J Pathol 2004;164:1537-1545.
411. Wang YZ, Gilula LA. Endemic florosis of the skeleton: radiographic features in 127 patients. AJR Am J Roentgenol 1994;162:93-98.
412. Khosla S, Hassoun AA, Baker BK, et al. Insulin-like growth factor system abnormalities in hepatitis C-associated osteosclerosis. Potential insights into increasing bone mass in adults. J Clin Invest 1998;101:2165-2173.
413. Fratzl-Zelman N, Valenta A, Roschger P, et al. Decreased bone turnover and deterioration of bone structure in two cases of pycnodysostosis. J Clin Endocrinol Metab 2004;89:1538-1547.
414. Hou WS, Bromme D, Zhao Y, et al. Characterization of novel cathepsin K mutations in the pro and mature polypeptide regions causing pycnodysostosis. J Clin Invest 1999;103:731-738.
415. Fujita Y, Nakata K, Yasui N, et al. Novel mutations of the cathepsin K gene in patients with pycnodysostosis and their characterization. J Clin Endocrinol Metab 2000;85:425-431.
416. Haagerup A, Hertz JM, Christensen MF, et al. Cathepsin K gene mutations and 1q21 haplotypes in patients with pycnodysostosis in an outbred population. Eur J Hum Genet 2000;8:431-436.
417. Hernandez MV, Peris P, Guanabens N, et al. Biochemical markers of bone turnover in Camurati-Engelmann disease: a report on four cases in one family. Calcif Tissue Int 1997;61:48-51.
418. Janssens K, Vanhoenacker F, Bonduelle M, et al. Camurati-Engelmann disease: review of the clinical, radiological and molecular data of 24 families and implications towards diagnostics and treatment. J Med Genet 2005;43:1-11.
419. Wallace SE, Lachman RS, Mekikian PB, et al. Marked phenotypic variability in progressive diaphyseal dysplasia (Camurati-Engelmann disease): report of a four-generation pedigree, identification of a mutation in TGFB1, and review. Am J Med Genet A 2004;129:235-247.
420. Boyden LM, Mao J, Belsky J, et al. High bone density due to a mutation in LDL-receptor-related protein 5. N Engl J Med 2002;346:1513-1521.
421. Little RD, Carulli JP, Del Mastro RG, et al. A mutation in the LDL receptor-related protein 5 gene results in the autosomal dominant high-bone-mass trait. Am J Hum Genet 2002;70:11-19.
422. Van Wesenbeeck L, Cleiren E, Gram J, et al. Six novel missense mutations in the LDL receptor-related protein 5 (LRP5) gene in different conditions with an increased bone density. Am J Hum Genet 2003;72:763-771.
423. Babij P, Zhao W, Small C, et al. High bone mass in mice expressing a mutant LRP5 gene. J Bone Miner Res 2003;18:960-974.
424. Henriksen K, Gram J, Hoegh-Andersen P, et al. Osteoclasts from patients with autosomal dominant osteopetrosis type 1 caused by a T253I mutation in low-density lipoprotein receptor-related protein 5 are normal in vitro, but have decreased resorption capacity in vivo. Am J Pathol 2005;167:1341-1348.
425. Balemans W, Patel N, Ebeling M, et al. Identification of a 52 kb deletion downstream of the SOST gene in patients with van Buchem disease. J Med Genet 2002;39:91-97.
426. Gardner JC, van Bezooijen RL, Mervis B, et al. Bone mineral density in sclerosteosis; affected individuals and gene carriers. J Clin Endocrinol Metab 2005;90:6392-6395.
427. Hellemans J, Preobrazhenska O, Willaert A, et al. Loss-of-function mutations in LEMD3 result in osteopoikilosis, Buschke-Ollendorff syndrome and melorheostosis. Nat Genet 2004; 36:1213-1218.
428. Viot G, Lacombe D, David A, et al. Osteopathia striata cranial sclerosis: non-random X-inactivation suggestive of X-linked dominant inheritance. Am J Med Genet 2002;107:1-4.
429. Bagur A, Dobrovsky V, Mautalen C. Bone densitometry of a patient with osteosclerosis. J Clin Densitom 2003;6:67-71.
430. Demiaux-Domenech B, Bonjour JP, Rizzoli R. Axial osteomalacia: report of a new case with selective increase in axial bone mineral density. Bone 1996;18:633-637.
431. Sissons HA. Fibrogenesis imperfecta ossium (Baker's disease): a case studied at autopsy. Bone 2000;27:865-873.
432. Schweiger S, Chaoui R, Tennstedt C, et al. Antenatal onset of cortical hyperostosis (Caffey disease): case report and review. Am J Med Genet A 2003;120:547-552.
433. Gensure RC, Makitie O, Barclay C, et al. A novel COL1A1 mutation in infantile cortical hyperostosis (Caffey disease) expands the spectrum of collagen-related disorders. J Clin Invest 2005;115: 1250-1257.
434. Crevenna R, Quittan M, Hulsmann M, et al. Hypertrophic osteoarthropathy caused by PGE1 in a patient with congestive heart failure during cardiac rehabilitation. Wien Klin Wochenschr 2002;114:115-118.
435. Gardiner JS, Zauk AM, Donchey SS, et al.1995; Prostaglandin-induced cortical hyperostosis. Case report and review of the literature. J Bone Joint Surg Am 1995;77:932-936.
436. Castori M, Sinibaldi L, Mingarelli R, et al. Pachydermoperiostosis: an update. Clin Genet 2005;68:477-486.
437. Amital H, Applbaum YH, Vasiliev L, et al. Hypertrophic pulmonary osteoarthropathy: control of pain and symptoms with pamidronate. Clin Rheumatol 2004;23:330-332.
438. Atkinson S, Fox SB. Vascular endothelial growth factor (VEGF)-A and platelet-derived growth factor (PDGF) play a central role in the pathogenesis of digital clubbing. J Pathol 2004;203: 721-728.
439. Olan F, Portela M, Navarro C, et al. Circulating vascular endothelial growth factor concentrations in a case of pulmonary hypertrophic osteoarthropathy. Correlation with disease activity. J Rheumatol 2004;31:614-616.
440. DiCaprio MR, Enneking WF. Fibrous dysplasia. Pathophysiology, evaluation, and treatment. J Bone Joint Surg Am 2005;87: 1848-1864.
441. Bianco P, Riminucci M, Majolagbe A, et al. Mutations of the GNAS1 gene, stromal cell dysfunction, and osteomalacic changes in non-McCune-Albright fibrous dysplasia of bone. J Bone Miner Res 2000;15:120-128.
442. Fraser WD, Walsh CA, Birch MA, et al. Parathyroid hormone-related protein in the aetiology of fibrous dysplasia of bone in the McCune Albright syndrome. Clin Endocrinol (Oxf) 2000;53: 621-628.
443. Kobayashi K, Imanishi Y, Koshiyama H, et al. Expression of FGF23 is correlated with serum phosphate level in isolated fibrous dysplasia. Life Sci 2005;78:2295-2301.
444. Yamamoto T, Imanishi Y, Kinoshita E, et al. The role of fibroblast growth factor 23 for hypophosphatemia and abnormal regulation of vitamin D metabolism in patients with McCune-Albright syndrome. J Bone Miner Metab 2005;23:231-237.
445. Kaplan FS, Fallon MD, Boden SD, et al. Estrogen receptors in bone in a patient with polyostotic fibrous dysplasia (McCune-Albright syndrome). N Engl J Med 1988;319:421-425.
446. Chapurlat RD, Hugueny P, Delmas PD, et al. Treatment of fibrous dysplasia of bone with intravenous pamidronate: long-term effectiveness and evaluation of predictors of response to treatment. Bone 2004;35:235-242.
447. McCarthy EF, Sundaram M. Heterotopic ossification: a review. Skeletal Radiol 2005;34:609-619.
448. Pakos EE, Ioannidis JP. Radiotherapy vs. nonsteroidal anti-inflammatory drugs for the prevention of heterotopic ossification after major hip procedures: a meta-analysis of randomized trials. Int J Radiat Oncol Biol Phys 2004;60:888-895.
449. Araya K, Fukumoto S, Backenroth R, et al. A novel mutation in fibroblast growth factor 23 gene as a cause of tumoral calcinosis. J Clin Endocrinol Metab 2005;90:5523-5527.

450. Mockel G, Buttgereit F, Labs K, et al. Tumoral calcinosis revisited: pathophysiology and treatment. Rheumatol Int 2005;25:55-59.
451. Kaplan FS, Glaser DL, Hebela N, et al. Heterotopic ossification. J Am Acad Orthop Surg 2004;12:116-125.
452. de la Pena LS, Billings PC, Fiori JL, et al. Fibrodysplasia ossificans progressiva (FOP), a disorder of ectopic osteogenesis, misregulates cell surface expression and trafficking of BMPRIA. J Bone Miner Res 2005;20:1168-1176.
453. Shore EM, Xu M, Feldman GJ, et al. A recurrent mutation in the BMP type I receptor ACVR1 causes inherited and sporadic fibrodysplasia ossificans progressiva. Nat Genet 2006;38:525-527.

CHAPTER 29

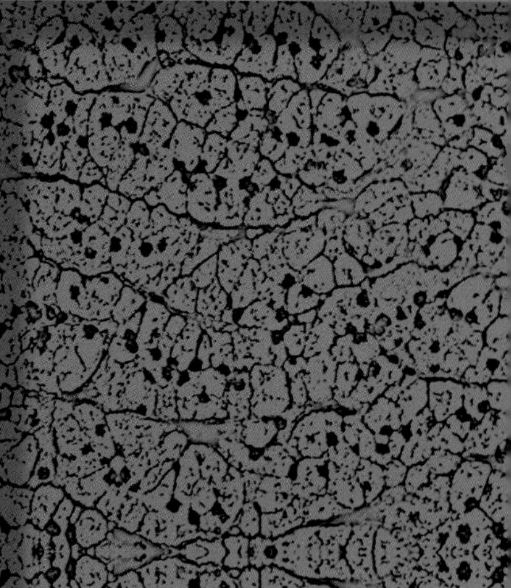

KIDNEY STONES

Rebeca D. Monk and David A. Bushinsky

Nephrolithiasis is a common disorder with an incidence greater than one case per 1000 patients per year. The prevalence in industrialized nations is approximately 6% to 12% and appears to be rising over time.[1] The incidence peaks in the third and fourth decades, and prevalence increases with age until approximately age 70 years.[1-4] In general, stones may be composed of calcium oxalate, calcium phosphate, uric acid, magnesium ammonium phosphate (struvite), or cystine, alone or in combination. A variety of pathogenic mechanisms determine the type of stone formed.

Stones tend to localize in the renal tubules and collecting system but are also commonly found within the ureters and bladder.[5] Nephrolithiasis rarely results in renal insufficiency or life-threatening illness but is responsible for substantial morbidity. Overweight stone formers (those with a body mass index [BMI] >27) are more likely to have reduced renal function than those with a BMI less than 27.[6] The severe pain of renal colic can lead to frequent hospitalization, shock wave lithotripsy, or invasive surgical procedures. Insight into the mechanisms involved in stone formation can help direct appropriate therapy, which is known to decrease the incidence of stone formation and its associated morbidity.

Stone Formation

Epidemiology

Numerous factors determine the prevalence of stones, including sex, age, race, and geographic distribution. Nephrolithiasis is more common in men than women at a ratio of 2:1 to 4:1.[1-4] In the United States, blacks, Latin Americans, and Asian Americans are much less likely to have stones than whites. Geography also appears to influence stone formation in the United States, with a decreasing prevalence from south to north and, to some degree, from east to west.

The greater exposure to sunlight in the southeastern United States may be responsible for the increased rates of nephrolithiasis in that area. Sun exposure can lead to more concentrated urine by increasing insensible fluid losses due to sweating. In addition, it can stimulate vitamin D production, resulting in intestinal calcium absorption and urinary calcium excretion.[7]

Geographic location and genetic predisposition can also influence the type of stone formed.[7,8] Uric acid stones, for example, predominate in Mediterranean and Middle Eastern countries, where they constitute up to 75% of all the stones formed. In the United States, however, less than 10% are pure uric acid stones, and more than 70% of stones formed are composed of calcium and an associated anion. Less common are magnesium ammonium phosphate (struvite or infection) stones, which account for about 10% to 15% of stones formed, and cystine stones, which are due to an autosomal recessive disorder and constitute only about 1% of all stones formed (Table 29–1).[2,8,9]

Pathogenesis of Stone Formation

Physiology

Kidney stones form when urine becomes oversaturated with respect to the specific components of the stone. Saturation is dependent on chemical free ion activities of the stone constituents. Factors that affect chemical free ion activity include urinary ion concentration, pH, and combination with other substances. For example, an increase in the urinary calcium concentration or a decrease in urine volume increases the free ion activity of calcium ions in the urine. Urinary pH can also modify chemical free ion activity. A low urinary pH increases the free ion activity of uric acid ions but decreases the activity of calcium and phosphate ions. Citrate combines with calcium ions to form soluble complexes and can thereby decrease their free ion activity. When the chemical free ion activities are increased, the urine becomes oversaturated. In this setting new stones may form and established stones may grow. In the setting of decreased free ion activity, urine becomes undersaturated and stones do not grow and can even dissolve. The *equilibrium solubility product* is the degree of chemical free ion activity of stone components in a solution in which the stone neither grows nor dissolves.

TABLE 29–1 PERCENTAGE OF PATIENTS WITH VARIOUS STONE TYPES IN THE UNITED STATES

Type	Percentage
Mixed calcium oxalate and calcium phosphate	37
Calcium oxalate	26
Calcium phosphate	7
Uric acid	5
Struvite	22
Cystine	2

Adapted from Bushinsky DA. Renal lithiasis. In Humes HD, ed: Kelly's Textbook of Medicine. Philadelphia: Lippincott Williams & Wilkins, 2000:1243-1248.

Formation of stones occurs through either *homogeneous* or *heterogeneous* nucleation. In homogeneous nucleation, progressive oversaturation can eventually result in the complexing of identical ions into small clusters; these clusters grow to form a permanent solid phase, or crystals. Heterogeneous nucleation refers to crystal formation on the surface of a different crystal type or on other dissimilar substances, such as cells. In vivo, this type of nucleation is more common than homogeneous nucleation because crystals form at a lower level of oversaturation in the presence of a solid phase.

The crystals must then aggregate into clinically significant stones, a process that takes longer than the passage of urine through the renal tubules. For stone formation to occur before the crystals are eliminated, the crystals must somehow anchor themselves to renal tubular epithelium in order to allow more time for growth. This *anchoring* of crystals occurs at the renal papillae, over areas of interstitial calcium phosphate in the form of apatite, termed *Randall's plaques.*[11-13] The apatite crystals appear to originate at the basement membrane of tubular cells in the thin loop of Henle and extend into the interstitium without damaging the cells themselves or filling the tubular lumens. A combination of apatite crystal and organic material extends from the loop of Henle tubular basement membrane to the papillary uroepithelial surface, where calcium oxalate crystals or other crystals can adhere and form stones.

An important factor in the development of kidney stones may be the absence of adequate levels or activity of crystallization inhibitors in patients with stones. Uropontin, pyrophosphate, and nephrocalcin are endogenously produced substances that have been shown to inhibit calcium crystallization. Differences in the amount or activity of inhibitors might account for the variability in stone formation among people with similar degrees of urinary oversaturation.[9,10]

Clinically, most physicians evaluate the lithogenic potential of the urine from stone formers by measuring the rate of excretion of the principal stone-forming elements in mass per unit time (e.g., milligrams or millimoles per 24 hours). It is clear, however, that the lithogenic potential of urine is better determined by the degree of oversaturation. Computer programs that calculate saturation from concentrations of various elements in the urine and the urinary pH are now available and more accurately determine the risk of stone formation. Any calculation of mean saturation underestimates the maximum oversaturation because of hourly variations in water and solute excretion throughout the day.

Diet

Dietary factors have a great influence on the concentration of excreted ions. Simply informing patients to increase fluid intake can have a great impact on reducing stone growth and formation.[14-16] Renal calcium excretion is augmented by increased sodium excretion,[17] and hypercalciuric patients tend to have a greater calciuric response to a sodium load than control subjects.[5] Dietary sodium restriction with the consequent decrease in urinary sodium thus reduces calcium excretion. Patients are therefore counseled to limit their daily sodium intake to 3000 mg (~130 mEq) in an attempt to reduce hypercalciuria.[2,17,18]

A moderate reduction in animal protein (~1.0 mg/kg per day) is beneficial in patients with nephrolithiasis because of the multiple mechanisms by which animal protein can contribute to stone formation.[18] A mild metabolic acidosis develops when animal proteins are metabolized. In order to buffer the excess hydrogen ions, calcium is resorbed from bone, which increases the filtered load of calcium.[19,20] Metabolic acidosis also diminishes renal tubular calcium reabsorption, which further enhances hypercalciuria.[19] In addition, metabolism of amino acids contained in animal protein generates sulfate ions, which couple with calcium ions to form insoluble complexes.[19,21]

Citrate, a base, forms soluble complexes with calcium and is beneficial in lowering calcium oxalate and calcium phosphate oversaturation and in reducing stone formation. During metabolic acidosis, citrate is reabsorbed proximally, reducing the amount of citrate excreted in the urine.[22] Hypokalemia can also lead to reduced citrate excretion. A protein-induced reduction in citrate can promote formation of both calcium oxalate and uric acid stones.[5,20]

Studies have demonstrated the apparently paradoxical benefits of a diet containing an age- and gender-appropriate amount of calcium in patients with kidney stones.[15,18,23] Ingested calcium binds intestinal oxalate, reducing its absorption and consequent renal excretion.[15] In a long-term prospective trial, Borghi and colleagues randomized hypercalciuric male stone patients to either a low-calcium diet or to a diet with a normal amount of calcium but low in sodium and animal protein.[18] Both groups of men were instructed to restrict oxalate intake and drink 2 to 3 liters of water daily. The group of men on a normal-calcium, low-sodium, low–animal-protein diet had a significantly lower recurrence of nephrolithasis and a greater reduction in oxalate excretion and calcium oxalate supersaturation compared with the men on the low-calcium diet.[18] In a retrospective review, Pak and colleagues demonstrated that stone-forming patients with elevated urinary calcium excretion (>275 mg/day) could be prescribed a low-calcium diet without a resultant elevation in urinary oxalate when provided adequate instruction on a low-oxalate diet.[24] They contend that patients with no evidence of bone loss, excessive absorption of calcium, and severe hypercalciuria might benefit from dietary calcium restriction.

Our contention remains that patients should be maintained on an age- and gender-appropriate intake of calcium and that dietary calcium restriction should not be prescribed unless nephrolithiasis is poorly controlled with other therapeutic interventions and the patient is not at risk for osteopenia. The recommended dietary intake for men and women is 1000 mg of elemental calcium from ages 19 through 50 years and then 1200 mg of calcium thereafter.[25] Teenagers should consume 1300 mg of calcium per day. Excess calcium should be avoided, because the combination of calcium and vitamin D supplementation has recently been shown to significantly increase the risk of kidney stones in postmenopausal women.[26]

Pathogenesis of Idiopathic Hypercalciuria

Idiopathic hypercalciuria (IH) is the most common cause of calcium-containing kidney stones. Hypercalciuria is defined as excessive urinary calcium excretion. IH is excessive urinary calcium excretion in the setting of normocalcemia and in the absence of secondary causes of hypercalciuria. The disorder is familial; it was initially thought to exhibit an autosomal dominant pattern of inheritance but is almost certainly polygenetic.[27]

The mechanism by which IH leads to hypercalciuria is not known. It has been postulated that IH comprises three distinct disorders: excessive intestinal calcium absorption, decreased renal tubular calcium reabsorption, and enhanced bone demineralization. Recent observations have led many to believe that IH is a systemic disorder of calcium homeostasis with dysregulation of calcium transport at all of these sites.[28] An understanding of calcium homeostasis helps elucidate the potential mechanisms involved in IH.

Calcium Homeostasis

Urinary calcium homeostasis is regulated by the gastrointestinal (GI) tract, the kidneys and bone, and the hormones parathyroid hormone (PTH) and 1,25-dihydroxyvitamin D_3 (1,25[OH]$_2D_3$). Approximately 99% of the calcium in the body is contained within the bone mineral. Daily bone resorption and bone formation, which in healthy, nonpregnant adults should be equal, allow less than 1% of bone calcium to be exchanged with that in the extracellular fluid.

Both PTH and 1,25(OH)$_2D_3$, at high concentrations, stimulate release of calcium from the bone mineral through osteoclast-mediated bone resorption. Net calcium influx into the extracellular fluid is achieved principally by absorption from the GI tract, which occurs through 1,25(OH)$_2D_3$-dependent and -independent mechanisms. Although PTH appears to have no direct effect on GI calcium absorption, increased levels of the hormone can stimulate production of 1,25(OH)$_2D_3$, which in turn leads to enhanced absorption. Increased serum levels of calcium and 1,25(OH)$_2D_3$ provide negative feedback to the parathyroid glands, resulting in reduced PTH secretion.

The roughly 60% of calcium in the extracellular fluid that is not protein bound is freely filtered by the renal glomeruli. Approximately 80% to 85% of this amount is passively reabsorbed in the proximal tubule. Most of the remaining calcium is reabsorbed in the distal cortical tubules under PTH stimulation. Ultimately, these reabsorptive mechanisms result in a urinary calcium concentration that is less than 2% of the daily filtered load of calcium.[29] Except during pregnancy and lactation, in healthy, nonosteoporotic adults, urinary calcium excretion precisely equals net intestinal calcium absorption.

Potential Mechanisms for Development of Idiopathic Hypercalciuria

Dysregulation of calcium flux at any of these sites can lead to hypercalciuria. For example, excessive calcium absorption by the GI tract leads to a transient increase in the serum calcium. This increase in serum calcium suppresses secretion of PTH which, along with the increased filtered load of calcium to the kidneys, results in hypercalciuria. Excessive 1,25(OH)$_2D_3$ has a similar effect of increasing intestinal calcium absorption, but it also results in an influx of calcium into the extracellular fluid because of enhanced bone resorption. The result is hypercalciuria even in the setting of a low-calcium diet or an overnight fast. The excess 1,25(OH)$_2D_3$ also suppresses PTH secretion, thereby further reducing renal tubular reabsorption of calcium.

If a primary defect in renal calcium reabsorption has led directly to hypercalciuria, there is a fall in the serum calcium concentration that stimulates synthesis of PTH and 1,25(OH)$_2D_3$. Increased 1,25(OH)$_2D_3$ results in enhanced intestinal calcium absorption and bone resorption. The renal loss of calcium persists even with a low-calcium diet or overnight fast.

Hypercalciuria can also develop as a result of a defect in renal phosphorus reabsorption. The resultant hypophosphatemia leads to enhanced 1,25(OH)$_2D_3$ production, which stimulates intestinal absorption of phosphorus and calcium. The increased serum calcium and 1,25(OH)$_2D_3$ suppresses PTH synthesis and release. The increased filtered load of calcium in the setting of suppressed PTH leads to hypercalciuria. Enhanced bone resorption increases the serum calcium concentration, which in turn suppresses PTH production further. The increase in the filtered load of calcium in this setting results in hypercalciuria.

Thus, there are several potential mechanisms for hypercalciuria.[28] Do human or animal data support one mechanism above all others? From a clinical therapeutic standpoint, is it worth differentiating among the various potential mechanisms in each patient with suspected IH?

Human Data

Lemann[30] compiled the results of numerous calcium balance studies on patients with IH and normocalciuric control subjects and normalized the results for calcium intake. He found that intestinal calcium absorption was significantly higher in the subjects with IH.

Asplin and colleagues,[5] also collecting data from published metabolic balance studies, compared net intestinal calcium absorption and urinary calcium excretion in hypercalciuric and normocalciuric adults. They also noted an increase in intestinal calcium absorption in subjects with IH but found that urinary excretion of calcium was increased to an even greater degree, placing many of these patients in net negative calcium balance.

Although these data confirm that enhanced intestinal absorption of calcium probably plays a role in the pathogenesis of IH, the investigators could not clarify whether this is the *primary* defect or is secondary to another lesion, such as a primary defect in renal handling of calcium. Others suggested that the increase in intestinal calcium absorption, in combination with excessive renal calcium excretion, indicated a more generalized defect in calcium homeostasis. Nonetheless, the finding of enhanced calcium absorption makes enhanced bone resorption an unlikely primary mechanism of IH, because the increase in serum calcium concentration resulting from bone resorption would suppress 1,25(OH)$_2D_3$-mediated intestinal calcium absorption.

In most published studies, patients with IH have higher serum levels of 1,25(OH)$_2D_3$ than normocalciuric control subjects.[5,28,31] Kaplan and colleagues[31] determined that 1,25(OH)$_2D_3$ levels were higher than control values in approximately one third of patients with IH and that intestinal calcium absorption was inappropriately high for the level of 1,25(OH)$_2D_3$. These studies support either 1,25(OH)$_2D_3$-mediated intestinal calcium absorption or a primary defect in renal tubular calcium reabsorption as a primary mechanism for hypercalciuria in IH.

PTH levels in patients with IH have been reported as normal or slightly lower than those in controls.[20,32] This finding argues against a reduction in renal tubular calcium reabsorption as the primary defect in IH, because with this mechanism the hypercalciuria would lead to low serum calcium levels and stimulation of PTH secretion. This finding also does not support the hypothesis that elevated levels of PTH are the stimulus for the increased levels of serum 1,25(OH)$_2D_3$ observed in many studies. It is, however, consistent with the other potential mechanisms for IH.

Bone mass in patients with IH has been assessed by a number of methods, including radiologic densitometry, quantitative computed tomography (CT), dual-energy x-ray absorptiometry (DEXA), single-photon absorptiometry, and others. Studies of patients with IH have generally shown only a mild reduction of bone mineral density compared with values in controls.[20,32] The studies were unable to reveal a unifying mechanism for the mild reduction in bone mineral density, but primary net bone resorption is unlikely because a much greater decrease in bone density would be expected in this setting. Altered $1,25(OH)_2D_3$ regulation would be consistent with this finding because the effects of $1,25(OH)_2D_3$ on bone resorption would be mitigated by the increased intestinal calcium absorption stimulated by the hormone.

Until recently, it was considered essential to determine whether a patient with IH tended to have excessive GI calcium absorption *(absorptive hypercalciuria)* or excessive renal excretion *(renal leak)*.[24,33] Patients with excessive renal calcium excretion were prescribed thiazide diuretics, and those thought to have a predominantly absorptive defect were prescribed a low-calcium diet. Coe and colleagues[32] undermined the validity of this approach in a study in which 24 patients with IH and nine control subjects were given a low-calcium diet (2 mg/kg per day) for more than 1 week. Urine and blood tests revealed normal serum calcium levels, a mild decrease in PTH levels in the patients with IH, and no difference in $1,25(OH)_2D_3$ levels.

The striking finding was that whereas all the normocalciuric subjects excreted less calcium than they ingested on the low-calcium diet, 16 of the 24 subjects with IH had urinary calcium excretion that exceeded their intake. Thus, most of the patients with IH receiving a low-calcium diet were in net negative calcium balance. No clear demarcation was noted between the patients who tended to excrete excessive amounts of calcium and those who did not. Instead, there was a smooth continuum of urinary calcium excretion among patients with IH that appeared not to be influenced by calcemic hormones. From a therapeutic standpoint, these findings have rendered insignificant not only the need to clinically distinguish IH mechanisms in humans but also the prescription of a low-calcium diet in any of these patients. This approach to diet is important because a low-calcium diet can result in a dangerous reduction in bone mineral density, especially in women.[28,32,34,35] As mentioned earlier (see Pathogenesis of Stone Formation), there also appears to be no benefit of such a diet in the prevention of stones.[15,18]

Genetic Hypercalciuric Stone-Forming Rats

To explain more fully the mechanism of IH in humans, we have developed an animal model of this disorder.[36-40] Through more than 65 generations of successive inbreeding of the most hypercalciuric progeny of hypercalciuric Sprague-Dawley rats, we have established a strain of rats that excrete 8 to 10 times as much urinary calcium as control Sprague-Dawley rats (Fig. 29–1).

Compared with control Sprague-Dawley rats, these genetic hypercalciuric rats absorb far more calcium at lower dietary levels of $1,25(OH)_2D_3$.[38,41] When these hypercalciuric rats were fed a diet very low in calcium, their urinary calcium excretion remained elevated compared with that of similarly treated control rats, indicating a defect in renal calcium reabsorption or an increase in bone resorption, or both,[42] again similar to observations in humans.[32,43] Bone from these hypercalciuric rats released more calcium than the bone of control rats when exposed to increasing amounts of $1,25(OH)_2D_3$,[44] and the administration of a bisphosphonate to rats fed a low-calcium diet significantly reduced urinary calcium excretion.[45] In addition, a primary defect in renal calcium reabsorption was observed during clearance studies.[46] We have shown that besides the intestine, both the bone and kidney of the hypercalciuric rats have an increased number of vitamin D receptors.[36,44,47,48]

Thus, hypercalciuric rats appear to have a systemic abnormality in calcium homeostasis; they absorb more intestinal calcium, they resorb more bone, and they do not adequately reabsorb filtered calcium. Because every one of the hypercalciuric rats forms renal stones, we have described them as *genetic hypercalciuric stone-forming* (GHS) rats.[38,39] These studies suggest that an increased number of vitamin D receptors may be the underlying mechanism for hypercalciuria in these rats[48] and perhaps in humans, as well.[38,40,47] In a recent clinical study, circulating monocytes from humans with idiopathic hypercalciuria were shown to have an increased number of vitamin D receptors.[49]

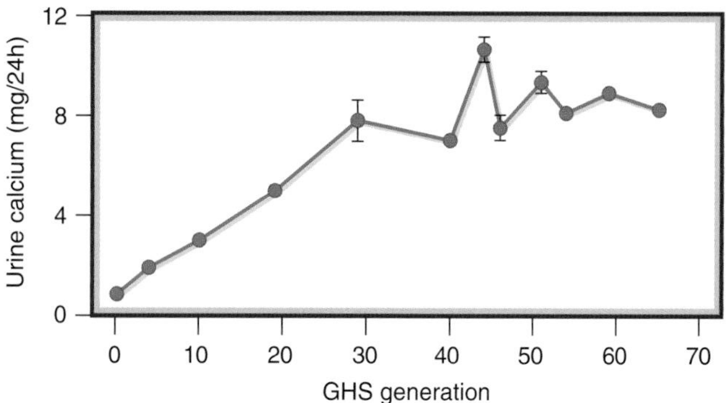

Figure 29–1 ▪ Genetic hypercalciuric stone-forming (GHS) rats.

Genetics of Idiopathic Hypercalciuria in Humans

The difficulty in ascertaining the genetics of IH arises, in part, from the numerous other factors that influence stone formation such as diet, environment, sun exposure, and gender. Because half of patients with IH report a family history of stones and male patients often have fathers or sons with the disorder, inheritance is not believed to be recessive or X-linked. A multitude of monogenic hereditary disorders (see later) can lead to hypercalciuria by causing a variety of mutations resulting in changes in calcium handling at the level of kidney, bone, gut, and the calcium-sensing receptor in the kidneys and parathyroid glands. Given the evidence discussed earlier that IH is a complex trait that as a phenotype can develop in multiple ways, it is most likely a polygenic disorder, with hereterogeneity of loci, and most likely with polygenic modifiers. Although attempts at diagnosing the exact cause of IH in a particular patient might not be critical from a therapeutic standpoint, determining the etiology of IH in a particular family is essential to researchers attempting to clarify the genetics of IH.[12,27,50,51]

Other Genetic Causes of Stones and Nephrocalcinosis

Numerous monogenic disorders cause hypercalciuria and subsequent nephrolithiasis or nephrocalcinosis.[12,27,50-54] Disorders that lead to hypercalciuria by augmenting bone resorption include osteogenesis imperfecta type 1, multiple endocrine neoplasia type 1 (MEN-1) syndrome with hyperparathyroidism, McCune-Albright syndrome, and infantile hypophosphatemia. Disorders that result in hypercalciuria via intestinal hyperabsorption of calcium include hypophosphatemia and absorptive hypercalciuria type 3, Down's syndrome, and congenital lactate deficiency. Next we describe in more detail several disorders that result in hypercalciuria via their effect on the kidney. Others include autosomal dominant hypocalcemia (which is caused by an activating mutation of the calcium-sensing receptor), Lowe oculocerebrorenal syndrome, and Wilson's disease.

X-Linked Hypercalciuric Nephrolithiasis (Dent's Disease and Others)

Several families around the world were discovered to have a variable combination of disorders including hypercalciuria, low-molecular-weight proteinuria, nephrocalcinosis or stones, hypophosphatemic rickets, and renal failure.[52,53] Some affected persons demonstrate evidence of defects in proximal tubular reabsorption of amino acids, glucose, or phosphate. PTH tends to be quite low and $1,25(OH)_2D_3$ high in the majority of patients. The abnormalities completely resolve in the patients who receive renal transplants, a finding that suggests a renal tubular disorder rather than a systemic process. In all families, the pattern of inheritance is consistent with an x-linked recessive disorder, with male patients affected to a greater extent than female patients. The latter are often minimally affected but transmit the disorder to half of their male offspring.

Over time, the various disorders—X-linked recessive nephrolithiasis in the United States, Dent's disease in the United Kingdom, X-linked recessive hypophosphatemic rickets in Italy, and low-molecular-weight proteinuria with hypercalciuria and nephrocalcinosis in Japan—have all been linked to mutations affecting the *CLCN5* gene on the Xp11.22 locus of the X chromosome. This gene encodes the CLC-5 protein, which is one of the nine members of the CLC family of voltage-gated chloride channels. How defects in this channel lead to the array of disorders listed here, including hypercalciuria, stones, and renal failure, is not yet understood.

Bartter's Syndrome

Bartter's syndrome comprises approximately five genetic mutations, predominantly autosomal recessive, that lead to sodium chloride wasting at the thick ascending limb (TAL) of the loop of Henle.[12,13,27,54,55]

Defects can arise in the NKCC2 (sodium potassium chloride cotransporter), the ROMK (renal outer medullary potassium channel), the CLC-Kb (basolateral chloride channel), or in a chloride channel subunit known as Barttin. The resultant defect in sodium transport leads to a reduction in the transtubular potential difference, resulting in a decrease in paracellular calcium reabsorption in the TAL. The ensuing reduction in intravascular volume also induces an aldosterone-mediated metabolic alkalosis. Bartter's syndrome, therefore, resembles high-dose furosemide administration and differs from Gitleman's syndrome in that hypercalciuria, nephrocalcinosis, and nephrolithiasis are seen with Bartter's but not with Gitleman's. An autosomal dominant form of Bartter's results from a gain-of-function mutation in the calcium sensing receptor in renal tubular cells. This mutation leads to reduced calcium reabsorption, hypocalcemia, and low PTH levels. Therapy with vitamin D and calcium supplementation can exacerbate stone disease in this disorder. For unknown reasons, the Barttin defects leads to deafness but not to nephrocalcinosis or stones.

Familial Hypomagnesemia with Hypercalciuria and Nephrocalcinosis

Familial hypomagnesemia with hypercalciuria and nephrocalcinosis is an autosomal recessive disorder that results in defective production of paracellin-1, a tight-junction claudin family protein that facilitates calcium and magnesium reabsorption in the TAL. Hypomagnesemia, hypercalciuria, nephrolithiasis, distal renal tubular acidosis (RTA), polyuria, and severe nephrocalcinosis ensue, with progressive renal failure evident by late childhood.[12,13]

Distal Renal Tubular Acidosis

Distal RTA (dRTA) is caused by dysfunctional α-intercalated cells, resulting in defective acid excretion.[12,13,27,50,56] This inability to adequately acidify the urine results in metabolic acidosis, hypocitraturia, hypokalemia, hypercalciuria, and nephrocalcinosis and stones. The metabolic acidosis leads to resorption of both calcium and phosphate from bone. The increased filtered load of calcium and phosphate, along with the elevated urine pH and hypocitraturia, results in favorable conditions for calcium phosphate stone formation. Although there are secondary causes of dRTA such as Sjögren's syndrome and carbonic anhydrase inhibitors (e.g., acetazolamide), there are also a number of hereditary causes of dRTA. Some are autosomal recessive and can also result in hearing loss; others are autosomal dominant. One form of dRTA that targets carbonic anhydrase II results in osteopetrosis and brain calcifications. Patients with dRTA fail to lower their urine pH below 5.5 following ingestion of an acid load. Their urine citrate is extremely low, despite often mildly reduced or even normal serum bicarbonate levels.

Hereditary Hypophosphatemic Rickets with Hypercalciuria

Hereditary hypophosphatemic rickets with hypercalciuria is an autosomal form of hypophosphatemic rickets that is clinically manifested by hypophosphatemia secondary to renal phosphate wasting.[57,58] These patients have hypophosphatemia-induced increase in levels of $1,25(OH)_2D_3$, which leads to increased intestinal calcium absorption and results in hypercalciuria. The bone pain, muscle weakness, limb deformities, and rickets remit completely with administration of oral phosphate. This disorder has been mapped to a region of chromosome 9 that contains the gene for the renal sodium phosphate cotransporter NaPi-IIc. Mutations of this gene likely result in a complete loss of function of this protein in patients who have a homozygous single-nucleotide deletion.

Primary Hyperoxaluria

Primary hyperoxaluria is discussed under Specific Therapy —Hyperoxaluria.

Presentation and Evaluation

Clinical Presentation

Kidney stones vary in clinical presentation from asymptomatic ones to large, obstructing staghorn calculi that can significantly impair renal function and lead to end-stage renal disease.[4,59] The severity of stone disease depends on the pathogenetic factors contributing to the rate of stone formation in addition to the stone type, size, and location.

In its most classic form, nephrolithiasis is manifested as renal colic. This discomfort of abrupt onset intensifies over time into an excruciating, severe flank pain that resolves only with stone passage or removal. The pain might migrate anteriorly along the abdomen and inferiorly to the groin, testicles, or labia majora as the stone moves toward the ureterovesical junction. Gross hematuria, urinary urgency and frequency, nausea, and vomiting may be present. Stones smaller than 5 mm are likely to pass spontaneously with hydration, whereas larger stones often necessitate urologic intervention.

Certain disorders can lead to small, diffuse renal parenchymal calcifications termed *nephrocalcinosis*.[4,13,56,60] The calcifications, usually calcium phosphate or calcium oxalate, may be present in the cortex or medulla. Among the most common causes of stone-related nephrocalcinosis are primary hyperoxaluria and medullary sponge kidney.

Metabolic Evaluation of Stone Formers

Although it is uniformly accepted that patients with multiple stones merit a thorough investigation into the cause of nephrolithiasis, evaluation of the patient with a single stone is controversial. This is probably due to the difficulty in determining the cost-to-benefit ratio of stone evaluations and wide differences in reported rates of stone recurrence.

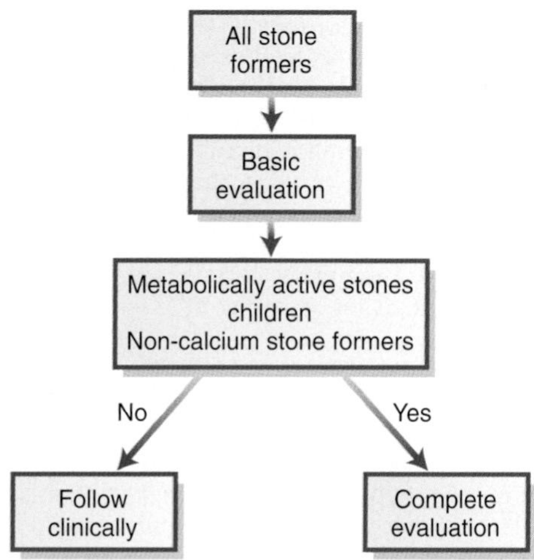

Figure 29–2 ▪ Evaluation of stone formers.

The National Institutes of Health has convened several consensus conferences to resolve such issues related to the prevention and treatment of kidney stones.[3] These panels determined that all patients, even those with a single stone, should undergo at least a basic evaluation in order to rule out a systemic etiologic mechanism. Patients with an increase in number or size of stones (metabolically active stones), all children, all non-calcium oxalate stone formers, and those in demographic groups not typically susceptible to stone formation (nonwhites) warrant a more complete metabolic evaluation (Fig. 29–2).[3]

The Basic Evaluation

Elements of the basic evaluation are listed in Table 29–2.

History

In addition to the medical history typically obtained from new patients, the evaluation of the stone former includes a stone history and a thorough review of diet, fluid intake, and lifestyle. Specific laboratory studies and radiographic tests are also required.

Stone History

The stone history begins with a chronology of stone events: age of incidence of first stone, size and number of stones formed, frequency of passage, stone type if known, and whether the stones occur equally in both kidneys or unilaterally. Also helpful is a report of the patient's symptoms with each episode as well as the need for and response to surgical intervention.

This information imparts not only the severity of the stone disease but also clues to the origin of the patient's nephrolithiasis. For example, nephrolithiasis that begins at a young age may be attributable to an inherited metabolic disorder such as primary hyperoxaluria or cystinuria. Large staghorn calculi that are difficult to eradicate and that recur despite frequent surgical intervention are more likely to be composed of struvite instead of calcium oxalate. Cystine stones are not crushed thoroughly with the use of lithotripsy, and alternative surgical modalities are generally required for stone removal. In patients who tend to form stones in only one kidney, the possibility of congenital abnormalities of that kidney, such as megacalyx or medullary sponge kidney, should be explored.

Medical History

Systemic disorders that can contribute to nephrolithiasis are sought in the medical history. For example, any disorder that can result in hypercalcemia, such as sarcoidosis or certain malignancies, may also lead to hypercalciuria. A variety of GI disorders associated with malabsorption (e.g., sprue, Crohn's disease) can cause calcium oxalate nephrolithiasis on the basis of enteric hyperoxaluria. Patients with gout or insulin resistance are more likely to have uric acid stones[8,51] (Tables 29–3 and 29–4).

TABLE 29–2 THE BASIC EVALUATION

HISTORY
Stone history Medical history Family history
MEDICATIONS
OCCUPATION AND LIFESTYLE
DIET AND FLUID INTAKE
PHYSICAL EXAMINATION
LABORATORY TESTS
Urinalysis Urine culture and sensitivity Cystine screening
BLOOD TESTS
Sodium, potassium, chloride, bicarbonate Calcium, phosphorus, uric acid, creatinine Intact parathyroid hormone if calcium is elevated or at upper limit of normal Tetrahydrodeoxycortisol, urinary free cortisol, and 25(OH)D levels as appropriate
STONE ANALYSIS
RADIOLOGY (CHOOSE APPROPRIATE STUDY AS INDICATED; SEE TEXT)
Unenhanced helical (spiral) computed tomography Kidneys, ureter, and bladder examination Intravenous pyelography Ultrasonography

Adapted from Monk RD. Clinical approach to adults. Semin Nephrol 1996;16:375-388; Monk RD, Bushinsky DA. Nephrolithiasis and nephrocalcinosis. In Johnson R, Feehally J, eds: Comprehensive Clinical Nephrology. London: Mosby, 2000:973-989.

Family History

A number of stone disorders are inherited, making the family history an important component of the basic evaluation. IH appears to be a familial disorder. Although the exact chromosomes and genes have not yet been identified, the pattern of inheritance is almost certainly polygenic.

Stones arising in childhood or young adulthood can be related to autosomal recessive disorders such as cystinuria and primary oxaluria, although the latter tends to affect younger children. Cystinuria is caused by a variety of mutations in either of two genes: *SLC3A1* on chromosome 2 and *SLC7A9* on chromosome 19. Rare families inherit mutations in both genes. Primary hyperoxaluria (PH) is another familiar disorder. Type I PH is due to mutations the *AGXT* gene on chromosome 2 whereas the milder type II PH results from mutations in the *GRHPR* gene on chromosome 9. The high prevalence of uric

TABLE 29–3 CAUSES OF CALCIUM STONE FORMATION

HYPERCALCIURIA
Cushing's syndrome Granulomatous diseases Hypercalcemic disorders Idiopathic hypercalciuria Immobilization Malignancy Milk-alkali syndrome Primary hyperparathyroidism Sarcoid Thyrotoxicosis
MEDICATIONS
See Table 29–5
HYPEROXALURIA
Biliary obstruction Chronic pancreatitis Crohn's disease Dietary hyperoxaluria (urine oxalate 40-60 mg/day) Enteric oxaluria (urine oxalate 60-100 mg/day) Jejunoileal bypass Malabsorptive disorders Primary hyperoxaluria types 1 and 2 (oxalate 80-300 mg/day) Sprue (celiac disease)
HYPERURICOSURIA
See Table 29–4
HYPOCITRATURIA
Androgens Exercise Hypokalemia Hypomagnesemia Infection Metabolic acidosis Starvation
RENAL TUBULAR ACIDOSIS (DISTAL, TYPE 1)
ANATOMIC GENITOURINARY TRACT ABNORMALITIES
Congenital megacalyx Medullary sponge kidney Tubular ectasia

Adapted from Monk RD. Clinical approach to adults. Semin Nephrol 1996;16:375-388; Monk RD, Bushinsky DA. Nephrolithiasis and nephrocalcinosis. In Johnson R, Feehally J, eds: Comprehensive Clinical Nephrology. London: Mosby, 2000:973-989; Bushinsky DA, Monk RD. Calcium. Lancet 1998;352:306-311.

TABLE 29–4 FACTORS ASSOCIATED WITH NONCALCIUM STONE FORMATION

URIC ACID STONES
Cushing's syndrome Diarrhea Diet high in animal protein Excessive dietary purine Excessive insensible losses Genetic predisposition Glucose-6-phosphatase deficiency Gout Hemolytic anemia Hyperuricemia Hyperuricosuria Inadequate fluid intake Inborn errors of metabolism Insulin resistance Intracellular to extracellular uric acid shift Lesch-Nyhan syndrome Low urine pH (<5.5) Low urine volume Malabsorptive disorders Medications (see Table 29–5) Metabolic syndrome Myeloproliferative disorders Obesity Tumor lysis
STRUVITE STONES
Urease-producing bacteria *Proteus, Pseudomonas, Haemophilus, Yersinia, Ureaplasma, Klebsiella, Corynebacterium, Serratia, Citrobacter, Staphylococcus,* and others Never *Escherichia coli*—not a urease producer High urine pH (>6.5) Indwelling urinary catheter Neurogenic bladder
CYSTINE STONES
Autosomal recessive trait Excessive excretion of cystine, ornithine, lysine, and arginine Low solubility of cystine (<250 mg/L)

Adapted from Monk RD. Clinical approach to adults. Semin Nephrol 1996;16:375-388; Monk RD, Bushinsky DA. Nephrolithiasis and nephrocalcinosis. In Johnson R, Feehally J, eds: Comprehensive Clinical Nephrology. London: Mosby, 2000:973-989.

acid stones in certain areas of the world is suggestive of genetic as well as environmental risk factors. Genes that cause either excessively acidic urine or hyperuricosuria have been implicated.[2,4,8,12,60-63]

Medications

Medications can contribute to stone formation in several ways. Calcium-containing supplements, for example, can increase the amount of calcium absorbed and subsequently excreted.[26] Loop diuretics, on the other hand, can directly promote renal tubular excretion of calcium. Acetazolamide, a weak diuretic, induces a mild metabolic acidosis and alkaline urine, favorable conditions for the development of calcium phosphate stones. Other medications, such as salicylates and probenecid, are implicated in uric acid lithiasis.

Certain crystals or stones can consist completely of precipitated medication. Such medications include intravenously administered acyclovir, triamterene, indinavir, and various sulfonamides, such as sulfadiazine. Although oxalate is a metabolic end product of vitamin C, there has been no obvious correlation between vitamin C ingestion and calcium oxalate nephrolithiasis. Nonetheless, patients are counseled to avoid large doses of the vitamin (Table 29–5).[64]

Lifestyle and Diet

Occupation and lifestyle are aspects of the social history that can contribute to stone formation. Surgeons and traveling sales-

TABLE 29–5 MEDICATIONS ASSOCIATED WITH RENAL LITHIASIS AND NEPHROCALCINOSIS

MEDICATIONS THAT PROMOTE CALCIUM STONE FORMATION
Acetazolamide
Amphotericin B
Antacids (calcium and noncalcium antacids)
Calcium supplements
Glucocorticoids
Loop diuretics
Theophylline
Vitamin C?
Vitamin D
MEDICATIONS THAT PROMOTE URIC ACID LITHIASIS
Allopurinol (associated with xanthene stones)
Probenecid
Salicylates
MEDICATIONS THAT CAN PRECIPITATE INTO STONES OR CRYSTALS
Acyclovir (when infused rapidly intravenously)
Indinavir
Nelfinavir
Sulfonamides
Triamterene

Adapted from Monk RD. Clinical approach to adults. Semin Nephrol 1996;16:375-388; Monk RD, Bushinsky DA. Nephrolithiasis and nephrocalcinosis. In Johnson R, Feehally J, eds: Comprehensive Clinical Nephrology. London: Mosby, 2000:973-989.

people, for example, tend to minimize fluid intake in order to avoid frequent micturition throughout the day. Loss of insensible fluid can also exacerbate nephrolithiasis and may be related to employment (e.g., construction work) or hobbies (running, gardening).

The evaluation proceeds with a thorough review of the patient's diet and fluid intake. Patients are asked to review what they eat at all meals and snacks. Particular attention is paid to ingestion of foods high in sodium (fast foods, canned foods, added salt or soy sauce) and the quantity of animal protein consumed (see later). Patients are also asked to list four or five favorite foods or snacks to assess whether they may be consuming foods high in oxalate or purine as well. Many patients are erroneously counseled by physicians to avoid calcium-containing foods. Doing so not only results in bone demineralization, a grave concern in women with stones, but also appears to be associated with increased stone formation.[15,18,23]

Physical Examination

For most patients with nephrolithiasis, physical findings are normal; in some patients, however, the findings may reveal a systemic disorder related to the stone disease. An enterocutaneous fistula, for example, may be associated with Crohn's disease, a common cause of enteric oxaluria. A paraplegic patient with an indwelling catheter may be susceptible to frequent urinary tract infections with urease-producing organisms and consequent struvite stone formation. Hyperuricosuria and uric acid stone formation may be seen in patients with tophi related to gout.[2,4]

Laboratory Tests

Although valuable information is gleaned from the history and physical examination, it is often difficult to determine the metabolic cause of a patient's nephrolithiasis without laboratory data. The urinalysis is an easy and inexpensive test that provides a great deal of information. Uric acid and calcium oxalate stones, for example, grow more favorably at an acidic pH, and a consistently high urinary pH may suggest calcium phosphate or struvite nephrolithiasis. The specific gravity, if high, can confirm suspicions of inadequate fluid intake.

Hematuria is often present in active stone disease. Microscopic examination of the urine in this case might reveal characteristic crystals. Bacteria and pyuria noted in conjunction with a high urinary pH (>6.5) are characteristic of struvite stone disease. Urine specimens for culture should be obtained in this setting. Because enough urease may be produced to form struvite stones even when colony counts are low (<50,000 colony-forming units), the microbiology laboratory should be instructed specifically to identify the organism and to check for urease despite low colony counts.[65]

Qualitative cystine screening should be performed on a urine specimen. Urine turns purple-red when sodium nitroprusside is added to a specimen containing cystine at a concentration greater than 75 mg/L.[61]

Recommended blood tests in the basic evaluation include electrolytes (sodium, potassium, chloride, bicarbonate), serum creatinine to determine the overall renal function, uric acid, calcium, and phosphorus.[2,3] If the calcium level is elevated or at the upper limit of normal or if the serum phosphorus level is reduced or at the lower limit of normal, a serum intact PTH level is also determined to rule out primary hyperparathyroidism. Low serum bicarbonate levels suggest a hypocitraturic disorder such as renal tubular acidosis (RTA) or acetazolamide ingestion.

Stone Analysis

Stone analysis should be performed, whenever possible, in patients with a new history of nephrolithiasis or in patients with long-standing stone disease who note a difference in clinical presentation or in the color, shape, or texture of any stone passed. Knowing the constituents of a stone can help the physician target certain elements of the medical history and specific urine studies. In most cases, the stone must be sent to an outside laboratory for examination. X-ray diffraction crystallography and infrared spectroscopy are currently the most accurate methods available for stone analysis.[66]

Radiologic Evaluation

Various radiologic tests can help determine the location and extent of the stone burden and might elucidate genitourinary abnormalities contributing to stone formation. For acute renal colic, spiral (or helical) computed tomography (CT) without contrast (unenhanced) has replaced intravenous pyelogram (IVP) as the gold standard study for detection and localization of kidney stones. Helical CT has proved to be at least as sensitive and specific as IVP in detecting stones of all types in both the kidneys and ureters. In addition, it can more accurately reveal causes of flank pain and hematuria not related to stones and requires no exposure to intravenous contrast material. Radiation exposure is a disadvantage of both CT and IVP, and the exposure to patients undergoing helical CT may be triple that of IVP. Helical CT takes less time to perform, a potential advantage in an emergency department setting, but it tends to be more costly.[59,67-69]

CT should be followed by a plain film (radiograph) of the abdomen that includes the kidneys, ureter, and bladder (KUB). Plain films can assist in determining stone composition. Stones composed of calcium, cystine, and struvite are radiopaque and visible on KUB, whereas radiolucent stones, such as those composed of uric acid and xanthine, are not.

IVPs are useful in detecting certain genitourinary abnormalities that can predispose to nephrolithiasis, such as medullary sponge kidney and caliceal abnormalities. Another advantage of IVP is that the osmotic diuresis generated by the contrast agent administered might flush out the offending stone during an episode of acute renal colic. A major disadvantage of IVP is exposure to radiographic contrast material. Administration of contrast should be avoided in patients who are at high risk for developing nephrotoxicity from the contrast, such as the elderly; those with diabetes mellitus, proteinuria, or preexisting kidney disease; and patients with significant intravascular volume depletion. Renal ultrasound is a useful test for patients who must avoid exposure to radiation or contrast, such as pregnant women and children. It is fairly specific, but not as sensitive as spiral CT for detecting stones within the kidney. Visualization of ureteral stones is poor with ultrasound.

Once a patient is known to have a certain type of stone, specific tests may be used in follow-up. For example, a patient known to have asymptomatic calcium stones can have a KUB test 6 to 12 months later to assess for any increase in stone size or number.[2,4]

The Complete Evaluation

The complete evaluation (see Table 29–3) comprises the entire basic examination as well as a 24-hour urine collection to determine volume and levels of calcium, oxalate, citrate, sodium, urate, phosphorus, and creatinine (Table 29–6). Creatinine is used to assess the adequacy of the collection; men should excrete at least 15 to 20 mg/kg of creatinine per day, and women should excrete 10 to 15 mg/kg of creatinine per day. In patients known to have cystine stones or in whom prior urine studies have been unrevealing, cystine should also be measured.

Patients should be instructed to collect the urine on a day when they perform usual activities and have their typical fluid and dietary intake. The first morning's urine specimen is discarded, and all urine for the next 24 hours (including the next morning's specimen) is collected in the jug. The ideal 24-hour urine collection provides 24-hour urine analysis for supersaturation of calcium oxalate, calcium phosphate, and uric acid, in addition to the various constituents listed in Table 29–3. Patients should be instructed to discontinue multivitamins approximately 5 days before the collection to prevent any antioxidant effect of the vitamins on the urine sample. In most cases, an acid or antibiotic is included in the collection jug or added with the first urine sample as a preservative. Certain laboratories require various preservatives for the different factors measured. Physicians should ask their laboratory how many 24-hour urine collections and which preservatives are required for the complete evaluation. Clearly, simplifying this process to a single urine collection that provides all the information required improves patient compliance.[2,70]

Patients who require the complete evaluation are as follows: all children, nonwhite patients (demographic groups not typically prone to nephrolithiasis), non–calcium stone formers, and patients with metabolically active stone disease (metabolically active stones are those that grow in size or number within 1 year).[2-4]

TABLE 29–6 OPTIMAL 24-HOUR URINE VALUES IN PATIENTS WITH NEPHROLITHIASIS

Parameter	Value
Volume	>2-2.5 L
pH	>5.5, <7.0 (24-h specimen not required)
Calcium	<~300 mg or <3.5-4.0 mg/kg in men <~250 mg or <3.5-4.0 mg/kg in women
Oxalate	<40 mg
Sodium	<3000 mg or <130 mEq
Uric acid	<800 mg in men <750 mg in women
Phosphorus	<1100 mg
Citrate	>320 mg
Creatinine	>15 mg/kg in men >10 mg/kg in women in order to ensure adequacy of collection
Supersaturation of calcium oxalate	<5
Supersaturation of calcium phosphate	0.5-2* (ideally less than 1)
Supersaturation of uric acid	0-1*

*Ideal values can vary between laboratories that perform supersaturation analysis.

Therapy

Nonspecific Therapy

Most patients, irrespective of stone type, are given general advice about fluid and dietary modification to prevent further stone formation. These nonpharmacologic interventions, which include an increase in fluid intake as well as restriction of dietary sodium and animal protein, can reduce the incidence of stone formation, a result termed the *stone clinic effect.*[16] In one study, such interventions resulted in a 60% decrease in stone recurrence over 5 years.[71]

The mainstay of nonspecific therapy involved dietary measures (see "Diet" under "Pathogenesis of Stone Formation"): increased fluid intake to raise urine volume to approximately 2 to 2.5 L, a reduction in sodium intake to less than 3000 mg/day (130 mEq), moderate reduction in animal protein ingestion to approximately 1.0 mg/kg per day, and, perhaps, eating certain fruits or juices high in citrate.[2,15-18,71-73] Dietary calcium restriction is no longer recommended because it not only reduces bone mineral but also tends to exacerbate stone formation by causing excess urinary oxalate excretion. On retrospective studies of dietary intake, both women and men have been found to have reduced stone formation with increased dietary calcium ingestion. Calcium *supplements,* however, were associated with an increased risk of stones in women. Thus, patients should be advised to maintain an age- and gender-appropriate intake of dietary calcium without supplements.[15,18,23,26,74]

Specific Therapy and Etiology

The optimal therapy for patients with metabolically active stone disease is directed at the particular metabolic abnormality. Before medications for nephrolithiasis are prescribed, all patients should be treated with the nonspecific measures just noted.

Prior to any therapeutic intervention, it is also worth assessing the patient's existing stone burden with a radiologic examination (KUB, spiral CT, IVP, or ultrasonography). If stones are seen, the subsequent passage of stones would not necessarily indicate therapeutic failure. The basic and complete evaluations help direct the clinician to the specific treatments discussed here.

Calcium Stones

Most kidney stones (~70%) contain calcium (see Table 29–1). More than one third of these are composed of calcium oxalate alone, and another 7% are composed of calcium phosphate alone. The remainder are composed of a combination of calcium oxalate and either urate or calcium phosphate. The stones tend to be gray, brown, or tan and rarely grow larger than 1 to 2 cm.[2,10,66]

The main causes of calcium stone formation are hypercalciuria (excessive urinary calcium excretion), hyperoxaluria (excessive oxalate excretion), hyperuricosuria (excessive uric acid excretion), hypocitraturia (insufficient citrate excretion), renal tubular acidosis, congenital abnormalities of the genitourinary tract, and certain medications.

Hypercalciuria

Patients with persistent hypercalciuria despite a low-sodium diet often benefit from a thiazide diuretic. This class of drugs is inexpensive and extremely effective at reducing urinary calcium excretion and stone formation.[2,75]

To maximize the efficacy of thiazides, patients must consume a sodium-restricted diet. Whereas hydrochlorothiazide is more commonly used for hypertension, chlorthalidone is favored for treating hypercalciuria because it has a longer half-life and requires only once-daily dosing. The starting dose is 25 mg and can be increased to 50 mg. In petite patients or those with low blood pressure, therapy can be initiated with 12.5 mg.

Side effects of thiazides include an increase in serum lipid levels and hyperglycemia. For patients in whom this is a concern, such as those with hypercholesterolemia, other cardiac risk factors, or elevated blood glucose levels, indapamide (1.25 to 2.5 mg) is a good alternative. This agent has less of an effect on serum lipids and blood sugar than thiazides.

Hypokalemia is another common side effect of thiazide therapy. Patients should be advised to increase their dietary intake of potassium-rich foods, and the potassium level should be checked 7 to 10 days after starting the medication. Hypokalemia can result not only in cardiac and neuromuscular problems but also in hypocitraturia, another risk factor for stone formation. The supplement of choice, therefore, is potassium with a base, such as citrate or bicarbonate, as the accompanying anion.

Potassium citrate is available as a liquid or as a wax-matrix tablet. The wax-matrix form is preferable because patients find the liquid unpalatable. Patients with malabsorption disorders, however, absorb potassium citrate better in the liquid form. Potassium citrate in the wax matrix formulation is available as 5- and 10-mEq tablets; 20 to 40 mEq/day in single or divided doses is usually adequate supplementation. Determination of follow-up potassium and bicarbonate levels may be required for further dose adjustment. Because citrate is a base, metabolic alkalosis can result with this medication, and an alternative potassium supplement (e.g., potassium chloride) may be required. If hypokalemia persists or if large doses of supplemental medication are required, the patient might benefit from the addition of a potassium-sparing diuretic. Triamterene is generally avoided because it can precipitate into stones. Amiloride, however, may be initiated at a starting dose of 5 mg or in a combination tablet with thiazide.

After at least 4 weeks of the new medication, the 24-hour urine test should be repeated to assess the efficacy of therapy in reducing calcium levels; 24-hour urinary sodium and citrate levels should also be measured. The thiazide dose may need to be increased to decrease calcium excretion to less than 3 to 4 mg/kg per day. If sodium excretion remains high in conjunction with elevated urinary calcium excretion, further dietary counseling aimed at reducing dietary sodium may be required. Additional potassium citrate may be required if urinary citrate or serum potassium levels remain low.[2,76]

Hyperoxaluria

Oxalate is produced predominantly by endogenous metabolism of glyoxylate and, to a lesser extent, by ascorbic acid.[5,60] Some urinary oxalate is derived from dietary sources, such as rhubarb, cocoa, nuts, tea, and certain leafy green vegetables. Absorbed oxalate is excreted unchanged in the urine and raises urinary supersaturation with respect to calcium oxalate. Hyperoxaluria accounts for the formation of approximately 5% of all calcium stones.[12,77,78]

The three main causes of hyperoxaluria are excessive oxalate ingestion *(dietary oxaluria)*, malabsorptive GI disorders *(enteric oxaluria)*, and excessive endogenous metabolism of oxalate related to a hepatic enzyme deficiency *(primary hyperoxaluria)*.

Because ethylene glycol (used as antifreeze in automobiles) is metabolized to oxalate, nephrolithiasis, in conjunction with severe metabolic acidosis and renal failure, is often observed in patients after ingestion of ethylene glycol.

Dietary Oxaluria

Dietary oxaluria results in urinary oxalate levels that are mildly elevated (40 to 60 mg/day). Patients with hyperoxaluria should be given detailed lists of high-oxalate foods to avoid (Table 29–7). In addition, calcium carbonate (500 to 650 mg per tablet, two or three tablets with each meal and snack) might further help reduce the amount of oxalate absorbed. Alternatively, patients can be advised to drink a glass of milk with meals, especially meals that might be high in oxalate. The calcium in milk binds the dietary oxalate and helps prevent its absorption.[12,15]

Enteric Oxaluria

Enteric oxaluria results in higher urinary oxalate levels (60 to 100 mg/day). Gastrointestinal malabsorptive conditions associ-

TABLE 29–7 FOODS HIGH IN OXALATE

Beans (green and dried)
Beer: Draft, stout, lager, pilsner
Beets
Berries (blackberries, blueberries, raspberries, strawberries, juice containing berries)
Black tea
Black pepper
Celery
Chocolate, cocoa
Eggplant
Figs, dried
Greens (collard greens, dandelion greens, endive, escarole, kale, leeks, mustard greens, parsley, sorrel, spinach, Swiss chard, watercress)
Green peppers
Lemon, lime, and orange peel
Nuts
Pecans, peanuts, peanut butter
Okra
Rhubarb
Sweet potato
Tofu

Adapted from Monk RD, Bushinsky DA. Nephrolithiasis and nephrocalcinosis. In Johnson R, Feehally J, eds: Comprehensive Clinical Nephrology. London: Mosby, 2000:973-989; Wainer L, Resnik BA, Resnik MI. Nutritional Aspects of Stone Disease. Boston: Martinus Nijhoff, 1987.

ated with normal colonic function, such as Crohn's disease, celiac sprue, jejunoileal bypass, chronic pancreatitis, and biliary obstruction, can lead to enteric oxaluria. In these disorders, malabsorbed fatty acids bind calcium in the intestinal lumen, making more free oxalate available for absorption in the colon. In addition, the colonic mucosa becomes more permeable to oxalate as a result of exposure to malabsorbed bile salts.

The mainstay of treatment, whenever possible, is therapy for the underlying disorder. A gluten-free diet, for example, can significantly reduce hyperoxaluria associated with sprue; for other conditions (e.g., surgical short-bowel syndrome), no specific therapy is feasible. In such cases, reduction of malabsorption and oxalate absorption may be achieved by instituting general therapy for steatorrhea, such as a low-fat diet, cholestyramine, and medium-chain triglycerides. As in patients with dietary oxaluria, an oxalate-restricted diet and calcium carbonate with meals should be prescribed (Fig. 29-3).[15,80] Because of chronic diarrhea, these patients are also at risk for low urine volumes, hypocitruria, hypokalemia, and hypomagnesuria. The acidic, concentrated urine also predisposes to development of uric acid stones.[81,82] Additional fluid intake must be stressed, and potassium citrate (the liquid form is generally better absorbed in these patients) and magnesium supplementation are often prescribed. Magnesium appears to be an inhibitor of stone formation and is supplied as magnesium oxide at 400 mg by mouth twice a day or magnesium gluconate at 0.5 to 1 g by mouth three times a day.[83]

Primary Hyperoxaluria

Primary hyperoxaluria (PH) leads to nephrolithiasis, because hepatic enzyme deficiencies in these patients lead to massive endogenous oxalate production.[60,62,84] PH results not only in severe hyperoxaluria (80 to 300 mg/day) but also in widespread deposition of oxalate in numerous organs and tissues such as the heart, bone marrow, muscle, and renal parenchyma at a young age. Cardiomyopathy, bone marrow suppression, and renal failure can ensue. In type 1 PH, the deficient hepatic enzyme is alanine : glyoxylate aminotransferase (AGT), and deficiency is caused by one of several mutations found in the AGT gene *AGXT.* In type 2 PH, which is an even more uncommon disorder, patients lack D-glycerate reductase and glyoxylate reductase due to mutations in the gene *GRHPR.* In some patients with type 1 PH pyridoxine (vitamin B_6) can increase enzyme activity, thereby reducing oxalate production.

All patients with PH should be treated with measures that reduce calcium oxalate precipitation, such as large fluid supplementation, potassium citrate, magnesium, and orthophosphate. Orthophosphate is an effective inhibitor of calcium oxalate crystallization but should be avoided in patients with a glomerular filtration rate less than 50 mL/minute. Patients with renal failure might benefit from renal transplantation because dialysis is not as effective as a functioning kidney in oxalate removal.

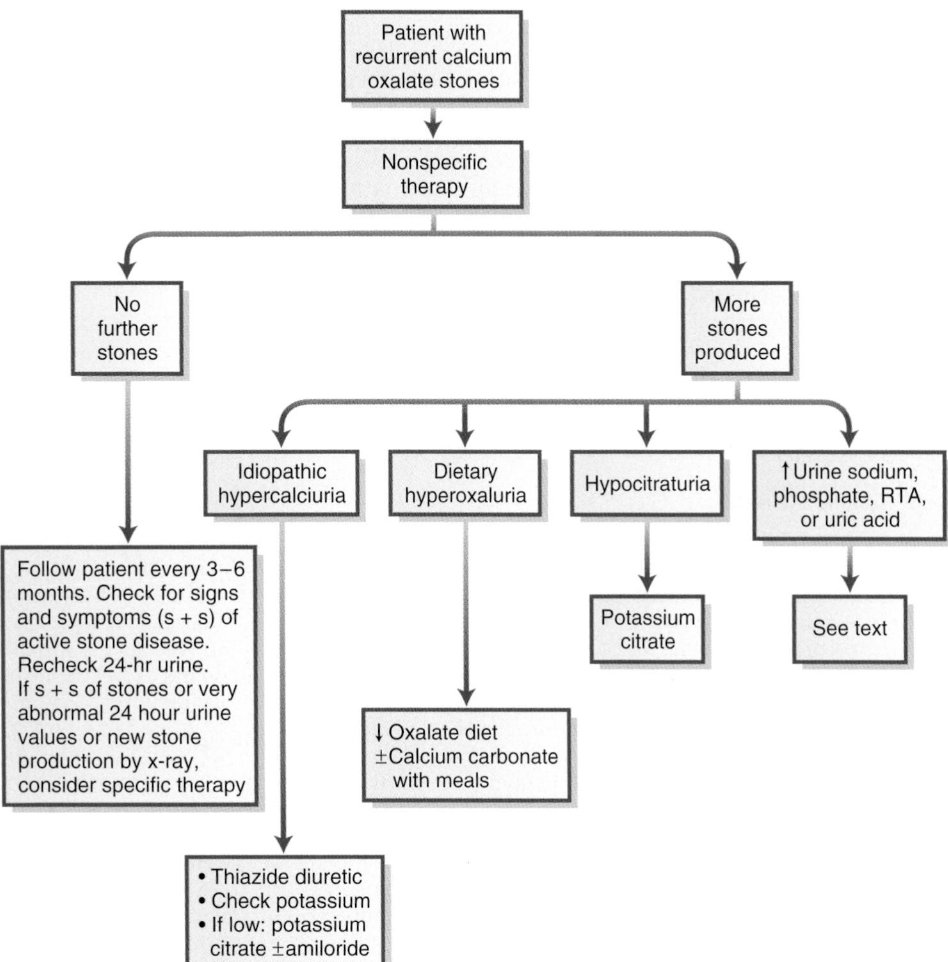

Figure 29–3 ▪ Treatment of the patient with recurrent calcium oxalate stones. *RTA,* Renal tubular acidosis.

These measures should be continued after renal transplantation to prevent rapid loss of the allograft caused by calcium oxalate deposition. Ultimately, for patients with type 1 PH, liver transplantation can supply the missing AGT and may be curative, especially if it is performed before the development of end-stage renal failure. Some patients require combined liver and kidney transplantation.[60,62,85]

Hyperuricosuria

Calcium oxalate crystals in the urine preferentially nucleate around other types of crystals or sloughed cells (heterogeneous nucleation). Uric acid crystals often form the nidus or internal core of calcium oxalate stones. In fact, up to 15% of calcium stones are found in patients with hyperuricosuria. In contrast to patients with pure calcium oxalate stones, these patients typically have elevated urinary uric acid levels but normal urinary calcium and oxalate levels.[86,87] They also differ from patients with pure uric acid stones in that they tend to have a higher urinary pH (>5.5).

Therapy consists of dietary purine restriction and increased fluid intake. If urinary uric acid levels remain uncontrolled with these measures, allopurinol, 100 to 300 mg/day, may be added.[86,87]

Hypocitraturia

Citrate combines with calcium to form a soluble complex that reduces calcium oxalate and calcium phosphate precipitation. In some patients, hypocitraturia is the principal metabolic abnormality found in the 24-hour urine collection. Risk factors for hypocitraturia include high protein intake, hypokalemia, metabolic acidosis, exercise, infection, starvation, androgens, and acetazolamide. Men tend to have lower urinary citrate concentrations than women, which may be responsible for the higher incidence of stone formation in men. Furthermore, women with nephrolithiasis have lower urinary citrate concentrations than non–stone-forming women.[88]

Along with therapy for the underlying condition, such as moderating dietary protein intake, potassium citrate is prescribed. This salt is preferable to sodium citrate because sodium excretion promotes calcium excretion. Again, potassium citrate in the wax-matrix formulation is preferred to the liquid preparation because of increased palatability. Large amounts may be required (30 to 75 mEq/day) in divided doses in order to raise the urinary citrate concentration to more than 320 mg/day. Potassium and bicarbonate levels should be closely monitored, especially in patients with renal insufficiency. If metabolic alkalosis ensues, partial supplementation with potassium chloride may be necessary.[76,89]

Renal Tubular Acidosis

Distal (type 1) RTA is a disorder in which distal tubular hydrogen ion excretion is impaired, resulting in a non–anion gap metabolic acidosis and a persistently alkaline urine. The acidosis leads to calcium and phosphate release from bone as well as enhanced proximal tubular reabsorption of citrate and diminished tubular reabsorption of calcium. The net result is an increased filtered load and excretion of calcium and phosphate, severe hypocitraturia, and an elevated urinary pH, all of which promote calcium phosphate precipitation. Nephrocalcinosis, or renal parenchymal calcification, is frequently seen in this setting.

Twenty-four–hour urinary citrate levels are commonly less than 100 mg in patients with distal RTA. Therapy consists of potassium citrate or potassium bicarbonate supplementation in order to treat both the metabolic acidosis and hypocitraturia. Large doses of these medications are often required: 1 to 3 mEq/kg per day in two or three divided doses.[10,62,86]

Nephrocalcinosis

Nephrocalcinosis is a process in which calcium is deposited in the renal parenchyma. There are two forms: dystrophic calcification and metastatic calcification.

In *dystrophic calcification,* calcium deposition arises from tissue necrosis secondary to neoplasm, infarction, or infection. It may be seen in the setting of renal transplant rejection, renal cortical necrosis, chronic glomerulonephritis, ethylene glycol toxicity, acquired immunodeficiency syndrome (AIDS)-related infections, and Alport's syndrome. In general, serum calcium and phosphorus levels are normal and calcium phosphate deposition occurs predominantly in the renal cortex.

In *metastatic calcification,* patients can have elevated serum calcium and phosphate levels or an elevated urinary pH. Calcification in this setting occurs more commonly in the renal medulla. Common causes include RTA, primary hyperparathyroidism (or any disorder resulting in elevated serum calcium levels), medullary sponge kidney, papillary necrosis, primary hyperoxaluria and administration of acetazolamide, amphotericin B, or triamterene. Primary hyperoxaluria can result in both medullary and cortical calcifications.

Both medullary and cortical parenchymal calcifications are easily noted with ultrasonography and CT scanning, even before they can be detected on plain radiographs. Therapy consists of treating the underlying disorder whenever possible. Otherwise, measures aimed at reducing hypercalcemia, oxalosis, and hyperphosphatemia should be attempted.[13,27,90]

Uric Acid Stones

Although uric acid stones make up only about 5% to 10% of all calculi formed in the United States, the prevalence of uric acid lithiasis is much greater in Mediterranean countries. These stones tend to be round, smooth, and yellow-orange. Because they are radiolucent, they are not visible on plain films but can be detected by ultrasonography or CT or as filling defects on IVP. Uric acid is a purine metabolite and is also found in large quantities within cells. The three main causes of uric acid stone formation are low urine volume, low urinary pH, and elevated urinary uric acid levels. Factors associated with uric acid stones are listed in Table 29–4.

Urine Volume and pH

Any disorder that results in low urine volume (e.g., diarrheal disorders, diaphoresis, reduced fluid intake) can contribute to uric acid lithiasis. Diarrhea and diets high in animal protein can also contribute to an acidic urinary pH. Uric acid is increasingly soluble at an alkaline urinary pH such that urine with a pH of 6.5 can contain more than five times more uric acid than urine at pH 5.3 without inducing precipitation and can actually dissolve existing stones.[8,87] There is evidence that uric acid stone formers have greater body weight and a higher incidence of insulin resistance and type 2 diabetes mellitus. The vast majority of these patients have significantly lower urinary pH compared with non–uric acid stone formers. Researchers theorize that insulin resistance can lead to impaired ammoniagenesis and ammonium excretion, resulting in excretion of more unbuffered hydrogen ion.[8,51,91,92]

Hyperuricosuria

Hyperuricosuria may be evident in patients who ingest large quantities of dietary purine or animal protein. Foods high in purine include organ meats, shellfish, certain fish, meat extracts, yeast, gravy, and stock (Table 29–8). Hyperuricemic disorders such as gout, myeloproliferative disorders, tumor lysis syndrome, and certain inborn errors of metabolism (e.g., glucose-6-phosphatase deficiency, Lesch-Nyhan syndrome) can also contribute to an increased urinary filtered load of uric acid.

TABLE 29–8 FOODS HIGH IN PURINE

Organ meats: Brain, heart, kidney, liver, sweetbreads
Meat extracts: Bouillon, consomme, stock, gravy
Meat: Beef, chicken, goose, lamb, pork
Shellfish: Clams, mussels, scallops, shrimp, oysters
Fish: Anchovies, fish roe, herring, mackerel, sardines, others
Certain vegetables: Asparagus, cauliflower, kidney beans, lentils, lima beans, mushrooms, peas, spinach

Adapted from Monk RD, Bushinsky DA. Nephrolithiasis and nephrocalcinosis. In Johnson R, Feehally J, eds: Comprehensive Clinical Nephrology. London: Mosby, 2000:973-989; Wainer L, Resnik BA, Resnik MI. Nutritional Aspects of Stone Disease. Boston: Martinus Nijhoff, 1987.

Certain medications such as salicylates and probenecid can be hyperuricosuric as well.[4,8,64]

Therapy for patients with uric acid stones begins with nonspecific measures such as increasing fluid intake to maintain urine volume at about 3 L/day. Patients are prescribed a low-purine diet to decrease uric acid production. Despite dietary intervention, hyperuricemia often persists, especially in patients with disorders of cellular catabolism. In this setting, allopurinol should be prescribed at a starting dose of 100 mg/day, increasing to 300 mg/day as needed.[5,93]

A diet low in animal protein is also beneficial because the decreased endogenous acid production raises urinary pH.[19] Ideally, the urinary pH should be elevated to approximately 6.5 to 7.0, a level that can dissolve existing crystals and stones. A urinary pH higher than 7.0 should be avoided, however, because calcium phosphate deposition can result. Potassium citrate at doses of 30 mEq by mouth twice a day or greater may be required to raise the urinary pH sufficiently. (See "Hypercalciuria" and "Hypocitraturia" on available potassium citrate preparations.) Prescription of nitrazine paper allows patients to monitor the urinary pH at various times of day and adjust their potassium citrate intake accordingly.

Although sodium bicarbonate can effectively alkalinize the urine, it should be avoided because the additional sodium excretion encourages sodium urate formation. Sodium urate in the setting of alkaline urine can serve as a nidus for calcium oxalate precipitation. If the urinary pH cannot be raised adequately despite high doses of potassium citrate or if the dose prescribed results in hyperkalemia, the carbonic anhydrase inhibitor acetazolamide may be initiated. Use of this medication results in an alkaline urine and mild systemic metabolic acidosis, a pattern similar to that in type 1 RTA. Again, the urinary pH should be maintained at less than 7.0 in order to avoid calcium phosphate precipitation.[86]

Struvite Stones

Struvite stones have also been termed *triple phosphate stones, magnesium ammonium phosphate stones,* and *infection stones.* Although they make up only about 10% to 15% of all stones formed, most staghorn calculi (large stones that extend beyond a single renal calix) are composed of struvite. The propensity of these stones to grow rapidly to a large size, to recur despite therapy, and to result in significant morbidity (and potential mortality) has also led to the appellation *stone cancer.* Infection with urease-producing bacteria must be present for these stones to form, and therefore severe renal infections as well as sepsis and loss of renal function can develop. Factors associated with struvite stones are listed in Table 29–4.

In contrast to other stone types, struvite stones occur with a higher incidence in women than in men, largely because of women's increased susceptibility to urinary tract infections. Other groups at risk for development of struvite stones because of urinary stasis or infection include elderly people and patients with neurogenic bladders, indwelling urinary catheters, spinal cord lesions, or genitourinary abnormalities. Even in the absence of stone analysis, struvite stones should be suspected in patients with large stones, an alkaline urinary pH (>7), and the presence of urease-producing bacteria in the urine. Early detection and therapy are essential to prevent great potential morbidity.[65]

Urease-Producing Bacteria

The formation of struvite stones depends on the presence of both ammonium ions and an alkaline urinary pH, conditions met clinically only through the actions of urease-producing bacteria. Ammonium, magnesium, and carbonate apatite $[Ca_{10}(PO_4)_6CO_3]$ in the urine combine with phosphate, which is present in this setting in its trivalent form.

Numerous bacteria, both gram-negative and gram-positive, as well as *Mycoplasma* and yeast species have been implicated in urease production. Bacteria species in which urease is frequently isolated include *Proteus, Haemophilus, Corynebacterium,* and *Ureaplasma. Escherichia coli,* despite its frequent role as a urinary tract pathogen, has not been shown to produce urease. Urease production adequate to stimulate stone formation may be present despite low bacterial colony counts. For this reason, the microbiology laboratory should be asked specifically to perform bacteria identification and to determine sensitivities even with colony counts lower than 100,000 colony-forming units. If no bacteria are isolated but a urease producer is suspected, special cultures for *Ureaplasma urealyticum,* a mycobacterium, should be ordered.[94]

Therapy

To eradicate struvite stones, early and aggressive medical and urologic management is required. Appropriate antibiotic therapy is essential but must be combined with long-term bacterial suppression and complete surgical or medical stone removal. Extracorporeal shock wave lithotripsy is often adequate for fragmentation of stones smaller than 2 cm, but percutaneous nephrostolithotomy or a combination of the two procedures is usually required for larger stones. Antibiotics should be continued on the basis of cultures of any stone fragments retrieved. After approximately 2 weeks of antibiotic therapy, when the urine culture is sterile, the dose of antibiotic should be halved. Suppressive antibiotics should continue at this dose as long as monthly surveillance cultures remain sterile for three consecutive months. At this point, antibiotics may be discontinued as long as surveillance urine cultures are obtained monthly for 1 year.[94,95]

In addition to antimicrobial therapy, medical treatment may involve urease inhibition and chemolysis. In chemolysis, the kidney is irrigated with an acidic solution through a nephrostomy tube or ureteral catheter. Although rarely used today with the advent of less-invasive surgical techniques, it can still play a role in dissolution of residual stone fragments. Ten percent hemiacidrin, the solution most commonly used, is composed of carbonic acid, citric acid, D-gluconic acid, and magnesium at a pH of 3.9. The use of chemolysis was controversial in the past because high mortality rates were reported, but with close monitoring of serum magnesium levels, intrapelvic pressures, infection, and obstruction to flow, it is now thought to be relatively safe.[94,96]

Urease inhibition has been shown to retard stone growth and to prevent new stone formation. It does not decrease bacterial counts and cannot eradicate existing stones. Combined with antimicrobial therapy, it serves primarily as palliative care for patients who cannot undergo definitive surgical management. The agent most commonly used is acetohydroxamic acid (AHA).

These medications require adequate renal clearance for therapeutic efficacy and are contraindicated in patients with a serum creatinine level higher than 2 mg/dL (176 μM/L). Chronic kidney disease can increase the incidence of side effects of the medications, which are numerous and limit their use. Side effects that result in discontinuation of the drug include neurologic symptoms, GI upset, hair loss, hemolytic anemia, and rash. Fortunately, the side effects all resolve with discontinuation of the drug. AHA is also teratogenic. The starting dose of AHA is 250 mg by mouth twice a day. If it is well tolerated for about 1 month, the dose is increased to 250 mg by mouth three times a day.[94]

Cystine Stones

Cystinuria is an autosomal disorder that may be recessive or dominant with incomplete penetrance.[63] The disorder is due to mutations of the *SL3A1* gene on chromosome 2 or to mutations of the *SCLC7A9* gene on chromosome 19, both resulting in decreased renal tubular reabsorption and excessive urinary excretion of the dibasic amino acids cystine, ornithine, lysine, and arginine. The genetic defect would probably go unnoticed were it not for the low solubility of cystine, approximately 300 mg/L. Factors associated with cystine stones are listed in Table 29–4.

Cystinuria should not be confused with *cystinosis*, a more serious and debilitating disorder that results in extensive intracellular cystine accumulation. Whereas people with no tubular defect in cystine transport excrete approximately 30 to 50 mg of cystine per day, heterozygotes excrete about 400 mg/day and homozygotes often excrete larger amounts (>600 mg/day).[61]

Stones usually develop in patients within the second or third decade. The stones can grow to large size and can appear as staghorn calculi or multiple stones. They are radiopaque because of the sulfur content of cystine molecules. The disease should be suspected in any patient with stone onset in childhood, frequent recurrence of nephrolithiasis, and a strong family history of the disease. The presence of the classic hexagonal cystine crystals in the urine can verify the diagnosis. Because these crystals might not be evident in dilute or alkaline urine, qualitative screening with the sodium nitroprusside test better confirms the presence of cystinuria at a concentration greater than 75 mg/L. Quantitative cystine measures with a 24-hour urine sample should follow to determine the risk of stone formation and to guide therapy.

Therapy

The aim of treatment is to lower the urinary cystine concentration below the limits of solubility (<300 mg/L). Patients are advised to drink large quantities of fluids. A patient with a cystine excretion of 750 mg/day, for example, should ideally drink enough fluid to increase urine output to more than 3 L/day. Large quantities of milk should be avoided because dairy products and foods high in protein contain large amounts of methionine, an essential amino acid that is a precursor of cystine.[97] Because cystine is more soluble at a higher pH, juices are encouraged because they tend to alkalinize the urine. Potassium citrate (see "Hypercalciuria" and "Hypocitraturia" for details) is also prescribed to maintain the urinary pH between 6.5 and 7.0.

Approximately 50% of cystine stones are mixed stones. Patients with cystinuria often have other metabolic defects such as hypercalciuria, hypocitraturia, and hyperuricosuria. Therefore, a complete 24-hour urine collection for all stone-forming elements is necessary to treat nephrolithiasis fully in this setting.

If these measures are inadequate in controlling stone formation or if the urinary cystine concentration is too high to make adequate fluid intake practical, chelating agents may be added. D-Penicillamine is a chelating agent that reduces the cystine concentration by forming a more soluble compound with cystine. The medication is associated with numerous serious side effects that limit its use. Second-generation and third-generation chelating agents such as α-mercaptoproprionylglycine and bucillamine are now available that reduce the cystine concentration with fewer side effects.[61,98,99]

ACKNOWLEDGMENTS

This work was supported in part by grants DK 56788 and AR 46289 from National Institutes of Health and grants from the Renal Research Institute (all to David A. Bushinsky).

REFERENCES

1. Stamatelou KK, Francis ME, Jones CA, et al. Time trends in reported prevalence of kidney stones in the United States: 1976-1994. Kidney Int 2003;63:1817-1823.
2. Monk RD. Clinical approach to adults. Semin Nephrol 1996;16: 375-388.
3. Consensus Conference: Prevention and treatment of kidney stones. JAMA 1988;260:977-981.
4. Monk RD, Bushinsky DA. Nephrolithiasis and nephrocalcinosis. In Johnson R, Frehally J, eds: Comprehensive Clinical Nephrology. London: Mosby, 2003:731-744.
5. Coe FL, Favus MJ, Asplin JR. Nephrolithiasis. In Brenner BM, ed. Brenner and Rector's The Kidney. Philadelphia: WB Saunders, 2004:1819-1866.
6. Gillen DL, Worcester EM, Coe FL. Decreased renal function among adults with a history of nephrolithiasis: a study of NHANES III. Kidney Int 2005;67:685-690.
7. Soucie JM, Thun MJ, Coates RJ, et al. Demographic and geographic variability of kidney stones in the United States. Kidney Int 1994;46:893-899.
8. Maalouf NM, Cameron MA, Moe OW, Sakhaee K. Novel insights into the pathogenesis of uric acid nephrolithiasis. Curr Opin Nephrol Hypertens 2004;13:181-189.
9. Mandel N. Mechanism of stone formation. Semin Nephrol 1996;16:364-374.
10. Bushinsky DA. Renal lithiasis. In Humes HD, ed. Kelly's Textbook of Internal Medicine. Philadelphia: Lippincott Williams & Wilkins, 2000:1243-1248.
11. Evan AP, Lingeman JE, Coe FL, et al. Randall plaque of patients with nephrolithiasis begins in basement membranes of thin loops of Henle. J Clin Invest 2003;111:607-616.
12. Coe FL, Evan A, Worcester E. Kidney stone disease. J Clin Invest 2005;115:2598-2608.
13. Sayer JA, Carr G, Simmons NL. Nephrocalcinosis: molecular insights into calcium precipitation within the kidney. Clin Sci 2004;106: 549-561.
14. Borghi L, Meschi T, Amato F, et al. Urinary volume, water, and recurrences in idiopathic calcium nephrolithiasis: A 5-year randomized prospective study. J Urol 1996;155:839-843.
15. Lemann J Jr, Pleuss JA, Worcester EM, et al. Urinary oxalate excretion increases with body size and decreases with increasing dietary calcium intake among healthy adults. Kidney Int 1996;49:200-208. Erratum in Kidney Int 1996;50:341.
16. Hosking DH, Erickson SB, Van Den Berg CJ, et al. The stone clinic effect in patients with idiopathic calcium urolithiasis. J Urol 1983;130:1115-1118.
17. Muldowney FP, Freaney R, Moloney MF. Importance of dietary sodium in the hypercalciuria syndrome. Kidney Int 1972;22: 292-296.
18. Borghi L, Schianchi T, Meschi T, et al. Comparison of two diets for the prevention of recurrenct stones in idiopathic hypercalciuria. N Engl J Med 2002;346:77-84.
19. Lemann J Jr, Bushinsky DA, Hamm LL. Bone buffering of acid and base in humans. Am J Physiol Renal Physiol 2003;285:F811-F832.
20. Bataille P, Achard JM, Fournier A, et al. Diet, vitamin D and vertebral mineral density in hypercalciuric calcium stone formers. Kidney Int 1991;39:1193-1205.

21. Bushinsky DA. Acid-base balance and bone health. In Holick MF, Dawson-Hughes B, eds. Nutrition and Bone Health. Totowa, NJ: Humana Press, 2004:279-304.
22. Hamm LL. Renal handling of citrate. Kidney Int 1990;38:728-735.
23. Curhan GC, Willett WC, Rimm EB, Stampfer MJ. A prospective study of dietary calcium and other nutrients and the risk of symptomatic kidney stones. N Engl J Med 1993;328:833-838.
24. Pak CYC, Odvina CV, Pearle MS, et al. Effect of dietary modification on urinary stone risk factors. Kidney Int 2005;68:2264-2273.
25. Committee on Dietary Reference Intakes. Dietary Reference Intakes for Calcium, Phosphorus, Magnesium, Vitamin D and Fluoride. Washington, DC: National Academy Press, 1997.
26. Jackson RD, LaCroix AZ, Gass M, et al. Calcium plus vitamin D supplementation and the risk of fractures. N Engl J Med 2006;354: 669-683.
27. Moe OW, Bonny O. Genetic hypercalciuria. J Am Soc Nephrol 2005;16:729-745.
28. Monk RD, Bushinsky DA: Pathogenesis of idiopathic hypercalciuria. In Coe F, Favus M, Pak C, et al, eds. Kidney Stones: Medical and Surgical Management. Philadelphia: Lippincott-Raven, 1996: 759-772.
29. Bushinsky DA, Monk RD. Calcium. Lancet 1998;352:306-311.
30. Lemann J Jr. Pathogenesis of idiopathic hypercalciuria and nephrolithiasis. In Coe FL, Favus MJ, eds. Disorders of Bone and Mineral Metabolism. Philadelphia: Lippincott Williams & Wilkins, 1992: 685-706.
31. Kaplan RA, Haussler MR, Deftos LJ, et al. The role of 1,25 dihydroxyvitamin D in the mediation of intestinal hyperabsorption of calcium in primary hyperparathyroidism and absorptive hypercalciuria. J Clin Invest 1977;59:756-760.
32. Coe FL, Favus MJ, Crockett T, et al. Effects of low-calcium diet on urine calcium excretion, parathyroid function and serum $1,25(OH)_2D_3$ levels in patients with idiopathic hypercalciuria and in normal subjects. Am J Med 1982;72:25-32.
33. Pak CYC, Ohata M, Lawrence EC, Snyder W. The hypercalciurias: causes, parathyroid functions, and diagnostic criteria. J Clin Invest 1974;54:387-400.
34. Asplin JR, Bauer KA, Kinder J, et al. Bone mineral density and urine calcium excretion among subjects with and without nephrolithiasis. Kidney Int 2003;63:662-669.
35. Freundlich M, Alonzo E, Bellorin-Font E, Weisinger JR. Reduced bone mass in children with idiopathic hypercalciuria and in their asymptomatic mothers. Nephrol Dial Transplant 2002;17:1396-1401.
36. Yao J, Karnauskas AJ, Bushinsky DA, Favus MJ. Regulation of renal calcium-sensing receptor gene expression in response to $1,25(OH)_2D_3$ in genetic hypercalciuric stone forming rats. J Am Soc Nephrol 2005;16:1300-1308.
37. Bushinsky DA, Asplin JR. Thiazides reduce brushite, but not calcium oxalate, supersaturation and stone formation in genetic hypercalciuric stone-forming rats. J Am Soc Nephrol 2005;16:417-424.
38. Bushinsky DA, Frick KK, Nehrke K. Genetic hypercalciuric stone-forming rats. Curr Opinion Nephrol Hypertens 2006;15:403-418.
39. Bushinsky DA, Parker WR, Asplin JR. Calcium phosphate supersaturation regulates stone formation in genetic hypercalciuric stone-forming rats. Kidney Int 2000;57:550-560.
40. Bushinsky DA, Asplin JR, Grynpas MD, et al. Calcium oxalate stone formation in genetic hypercalciuric stone-forming rats. Kidney Int 2002;61:975-987.
41. Bushinsky DA, Favus MJ. Mechanism of hypercalciuria in genetic hypercalciuric rats: inherited defect in intestinal calcium transport. J Clin Invest 1988;82:1585-1591.
42. Kim M, Sessler NE, Tembe V, et al. Response of genetic hypercalciuric rats to a low calcium diet. Kidney Int 1993;43:189-196.
43. Pak CY. Nephrolithiasis. Current Ther Endocrinol Metab 1997;6: 572-576.
44. Krieger NS, Stathopoulos VM, Bushinsky DA. Increased sensitivity to $1,25(OH)_2D_3$ in bone from genetic hypercalciuric rats. Am J Physiol (Cell Physiol) 1996;271:C130-C135.
45. Bushinsky DA, Neumann KJ, Asplin J, Krieger NS. Alendronate decreases urine calcium and supersaturation in genetic hypercalciuric rats. Kidney Int 1999;55:234-243.
46. Tsuruoka S, Bushinsky DA, Schwartz GJ. Defective renal calcium reabsorption in genetic hypercalciuric rats. Kidney Int 1997;51: 1540-1547.
47. Karnauskas AJ, van Leeuwen JP, van den Bemd GJ, et al. Mechanism and function of high vitamin D receptor levels in genetic hypercalciuric stone–forming rats. J Bone Min Res 2005;20: 447-454.
48. Li X-Q, Tembe V, Horwitz GM, et al. Increased intestinal vitamin D receptor in genetic hypercalciuric rats: a cause of intestinal calcium hyperabsorption. J Clin Invest 1993;91:661-667.
49. Favus MJ, Karnauskas AJ, Parks JH, Coe FL. Peripheral blood monocyte vitamin D receptor levels are elevated in patients with idiopathic hypercalciuria. J Clin Endocrinol Metab 2004;89:4937-4943.
50. Gambaro G, Vezzoli G, Casari G, et al. Genetics of hypercalciuria and calcium nephrolithiasis: from the rare monogenic to the common polygenic forms. Am J Kid Dis 2004;44:963-986.
51. Moe OW. Kidney stones: pathophysiology and medical management. Lancet 2006;367:333-344.
52. Scheinman SJ, Guay-Woodford LM, Thakker RV, Warnock DG. Genetic disorders of renal electrolyte transport. N Engl J Med 1999; 340:1177-1187.
53. Lloyd SE, Pearce SH, Fisher SE, et al. A common molecular basis for three inherited kidney stone diseases. Nature 1996;379: 445-449.
54. Frick KK, Bushinsky DA. Molecular mechanisms of primary hypercalciuria. J Am Soc Neph 2003;14:1082-1095.
55. Naesens M, Steels P, Verberckmoes R, et al. Bartter's and Gitelmans' syndromes: from gene to clinic. Nephron Phys 2004;96:65-78.
56. Nicoletta JA, Schwartz GJ. Distal renal tubular acidosis. Current Opin Pediatr 2004;16:194-198.
57. Bergwitz C, Roslin NM, Tieder M, et al. SLC34A3 mutations in patients with hereditary hypophosphatemic rickets with hypercalciuria predict a key role for the sodium-phosphate cotransporter NaP i -IIc in maintaining phosphate homeostasis. Am J Hum Genet 2006;78:179-192.
58. Levi M, Blaine J, Breusegem S, et al. Renal phosphate-wasting disorders. Adv Chronic Kidney Dis 2006;13:155-165.
59. Teichman JMH. Acute renal colic from ureteral calculus. N Engl J Med 2004;350:684-693.
60. Milliner DS. The primary hyperoxalurias: an algorithm for diagnosis. Am J Nephrol 2005;25:154-160.
61. Sakhaee K. Pathogenesis and medical management of cystinuria. Semin Nephrol 1996;16:435-447.
62. Danpure CJ. Molecular etiology of primary hyperoxaluria type 1: New direction for treatment. Am J Nephrol 2005;25:303-310.
63. Font-Llitjos M, Jimenez-Vidal M, Bisceglia L, et al. New insights into cystinuria: 40 new mutations, genotype-phenotype correlation, and digenic inheritance causing partial phenotype. J Med Genet 2005;42:58-68.
64. Daudon M, Jungers P. Drug-induced renal calculi: epidemiology, prevention and management. Drugs 2004;64:245-275.
65. Rodman JS. Struvite stones. Nephron 1999;81:50-59.
66. Mandel GS, Mandel N. Analysis of stones. In Coe F, Favus M, Pak C, et al, eds. Kidney Stones: Medical and Surgical Management. Philadelphia: Lippincott-Raven, 1996:323-335.
67. Denton ER, Mackenzie A, Greenwell T, et al. Unenhanced helical CT for renal colic—is the radiation dose justifiable? Clin Radiol 1999;54:444-447.
68. Smith RC, Coll DM. Helical computed tomography in the diagonosis of ureteric colic. BJU Int 2000;86:33-41.
69. Nakada SY, Hoff DG, Attai S, et al. Determination of stone composition by noncontrast spiral computed tomography in the clinical setting. Urology 2000;55:816-819.
70. Parks JH, Coward M, Coe FL. Correspondence between stone composition and urine supersaturation in nephrolithiasis. Kidney Int 1997;51:894-900.
71. Uribarri J, Oh MS, Carroll HJ. The first kidney stone. Kidney Int 1989;111:1006-1009.
72. Meschi T, Schianchi T, Ridolo E, et al. Body weight, diet and water intake in preventing stone disease. Urol Int 2004;72:29-33.
73. Meschi T, Maggiore U, Fiaccadori E, et al. The effect of fruits and vegetables on urinary stone risk factors. 2004;66:2402-2410.
74. Curhan GC, Willett WC, Speizer FE, et al. Comparison of dietary calcium with supplemental calcium and other nutrients as factors affecting the risk for kidney stones in women. Ann Intern Med 1997;126:497-504.

75. Coe FL, Parks JH, Bushinsky DA, et al. Chlorthalidone promotes mineral retention in patients with idiopathic hypercalciuria. Kidney Int 1988;33:1140-1146.
76. Pak CYC, Fuller C, Sakhaee K, et al. Long-term treatment of calcium oxalate nephrolithiasis with potassium citrate. J Urol 1985;134: 11-19.
77. Holmes RP, Goodman HO, Assimos DG. Contribution of dietary oxalate to urinary oxalate excretion. Kidney Int 2006;59:270-276.
78. Parks JH, Worcester EM, O'Connor RC, Coe FL. Urine stone risk factors in nephrolithiasis patients with and without bowel disease. Kidney Int 2003;63:255-265.
79. Wainer L, Resnik BA, Resnick MI. Nutritional Aspects of Stone Disease. Boston: Martinus Nijhoff, 1987:143-164.
80. Nordenvall B, Backman L, Larsson L, Tiselius HG. Effects of calcium, aluminum, magnesium and cholestyramine on hyperoxaluria in patients with jejunoileal bypass. Acta Chir Scand 1983;149:93-98.
81. Clarke AM, McKenzie RG. Ileostomy and the risk of urinary uric acid stones. Lancet 1969;2:395-397.
82. Rudman D, Dedonis JL, Fountain MT, et al. Hypocitraturia in patients with gastrointestinal malabsorption. N Engl J Med 1980; 303:657-661.
83. Worcester EM. Stones due to bowel disease. In Coe F, Favus M, Pak C, et al, eds. Kidney Stones: Medical and Surgical Management. Philadelphia: Lippincott-Raven, 1996:883-903
84. Petrarulo M, Vitale C, Facchini P, Marangella M. Biochemical approach to diagnosis and differentiation of primary hyperoxalurias: an update. J Nephrol 1998;11:23-28.
85. Watts RWE, Danpure CJ, de Pauw L, et al. Combined liver-kidney and isolated liver transplantations for primary hyperoxaluria type 1. The European experience. Nephrolol Dial Transplant 1991: 502-511.
86. Coe FL, Parks JH, Asplin JR. The pathogenesis and treatment of kidney stones. N Engl J Med 1992;327:1141-1152.
87. Millman S, Strauss AL, Parks JH, Coe FL. Pathogenesis and clinical course of mixed calcium oxalate and uric acid nephrolithiasis. Kidney Int 1982;22:366-370.
88. Pak CY. Citrate and renal calculi: an update. Min Electrolyte Metab 1994;20:371-377.
89. Pak CYC, Fuller C. Idiopathic hypocitraturic calcium oxalate nephrolithiasis successfully treated with potassium citrate. Ann Intern Med 1986;104:33-37.
90. Ramchandani P, Pollack HM. Radiologic evaluation of patients with urolithiasis. In Coe F, Favus M, Pak C, et al, eds. Kidney Stones: Medical and Surgical Management. Philadelphia: Lippincott-Raven, 1996:369-435.
91. Sakhaee K, Adams-Huet B, Moe OW, Pak CY. Pathyophysiologic for normouricosuric uric acid nephrolithiasis. Kidney Int 2002;62: 971-979.
92. Maalouf NM, Sakhaee K, Parks JH, et al. Association of urinary pH with body weight in nephrolithiasis. Kidney Int 2004;65:1422-1425.
93. Ettinger B, Tang A, Citron JT, et al. Randomized trial of allopurinol in the prevention of calcium oxalate calculi. N Engl J Med 1986;315:1386-1389.
94. Wong HY, Riedl CR, Griffith DP. Medical management and prevention of struvite stones. In Coe F, Favus M, Pak C, et al, eds. Kidney Stones: Medical and Surgical Management. Philadelphia: Lippincott-Raven, 1996:941-950.
95. Michaels EK. Surgical management of struvite stones. In Coe F, Favus M, Pak C, et al, eds. Kidney Stones: Medical and Surgical Management. Philadelphia: Lippincott-Raven, 1996:951-970.
96. Sant GR, Blaivas JG. Hemiacidrin irrigation in the management of struvite calculi: long-term results. J Urol 1983;130:1048-1050.
97. Kolb FO, Earll JM, Harper HA. "Disappearance" of cystinuria in a patient treated with prolonged low methionine diet. Metabolism 1967;16:378-381.
98. Pak CYC. Prevention of recurrent nephrolithiasis. In Pak CYC, ed. Renal Stone Disease: Pathogenesis, Prevention, and Treatment. Boston: Kluwer Academic, 1987:165-199.
99. Pak CYC. Cystine lithiasis. In Resnick MI, Pak CYC, eds. Urolithiasis: A Medical and Surgical Reference. Philadelphia: Saunders, 1990:133-143.

SECTION VIII

Disorders of Carbohydrate and Metabolism

CHAPTER 30

TYPE 2 DIABETES MELLITUS

John B. Buse, Kenneth S. Polonsky, and Charles F. Burant

EPIDEMIOLOGY AND DIAGNOSIS

Epidemiology

Type 2 diabetes mellitus (T2DM) is the predominant form of diabetes worldwide, accounting for 90% of cases globally.[1,2] An epidemic of T2DM is under way in both developed and developing countries, although the brunt of the disorder is felt disproportionately in non-European populations as evidenced by studies in Latin American populations, Native American and Canadian communities, Pacific and Indian Ocean island populations, and in India and Australian Aboriginal communities.[3-5] In the Pacific island of Nauru, diabetes was virtually unknown 50 years ago and is now present in approximately 40% of adults. Globally, the number of people with diabetes is expected to rise from the current estimate of 150 million to 220 million in 2010 and 300 million in 2025. Alarming increases in the prevalence of diabetes have occurred in various Chinese populations. Type 2 diabetes has become one of the world's most important public health problems.

Considerable information is available on the factors that are responsible for the development of T2DM, and these are summarized in Table 30–1.

Type 2 diabetes is currently thought to occur in genetically predisposed persons who are exposed to a series of environmental influences that precipitate the onset of clinical disease. The genetic basis of T2DM is discussed in detail later in this chapter, but the syndrome consists of monogenic and polygenic forms that can be differentiated both on clinical grounds and in terms of the genes that are involved in the pathogenesis of these disorders.

Sex, age, and ethnic background are important factors in determining risk of developing T2DM.[6-8] The disorder is more common in women, and the increased prevalence in certain racial and ethnic groups has already been alluded to. Age is also a critical factor. Type 2 diabetes has been viewed in the past as a disorder of aging, with an increasing prevalence with age. This remains true today. However, a disturbing trend has become apparent in which the prevalence of obesity and T2DM in children is rising dramatically. In the past, it was believed that the overwhelming majority of children with diabetes had type 1 diabetes (T1DM), and only 1% to 2% of diabetic children were considered to have type 2 or other rare forms of diabetes.[9] Later reports suggest that as many as 8% to 45% of children with newly diagnosed diabetes have non–immune-mediated diabetes. The majority of these children have T2DM, but other types are being increasingly identified.

Data relating to the alarming increase in the prevalence of T2DM in children and adolescents has recently been reviewed.[10] The National Health and Nutrition Examination Study (NHANES) data for 1999 to 2000 suggest that 15.5% of 12- to 19-year-olds, 15.3% of 6- to 11-year-olds, and 10.4% of 2- to 5-year-olds have a body mass index (BMI) above the 95th percentile adjusted for age and sex. This represents an approximately 30% increase over the prevalence previously determined for 1988 to 1994. The increases are particularly striking in Hispanic and African-American children. Of even greater concern, impaired glucose tolerance and T2DM have now emerged as critical health issues in overweight children, particularly overweight African-American, Latin American, and Native American adolescents.

In a clinic-based study, 25% of 55 obese children and 21% of 112 obese adolescents had impaired glucose tolerance and 45 had undiagnosed T2DM.[11] An idiopathic non–immune-mediated form of diabetes has been reported particularly in the black population.

Diagnostic Criteria for Diabetes Mellitus

The diagnosis of diabetes rests on the measurement of plasma glucose levels. The diagnostic criteria for diabetes were changed in 1997.[12] The most significant changes were the level of fasting plasma glucose (FPG) that is recognized as diagnostic for diabetes, which was decreased from 140 to 126 mg/dL, and the introduction of a category of impaired fasting glucose (IFG). Current criteria for the diagnosis of diabetes, impaired fasting glucose, and impaired glucose tolerance (IGT) are shown in Table 30–2.

Because plasma glucose concentrations range as a continuum, the criteria are based on estimates of the threshold for the complications of diabetes. The primary end-point used to evaluate the relationship between glucose levels and complications is retinopathy. The prevalence of retinopathy in comparison with FPG and 2-hour plasma glucose has been evaluated in two relatively large studies.[13,14] Both diagnostic criteria were able to predict the presence of retinopathy and, by inference, glucose levels that are diagnostic of diabetes (Fig. 30–1). There is also an association between FPG and 2-hour plasma glucose and risk of macrovascular and cardiovascular disease.[15-17] For instance, the Paris Prospective Study showed that the incidence of fatal coronary heart disease was related to both FPG and 2-hour plasma glucose that were determined at a baseline examination.[18] Rates of disease were markedly increased at FPG greater than 125 mg/dL (6.9 mM/L) or 2-hour plasma glucose greater than 140 mg/dL (7.8 mM/L).

Reproducibility of the plasma glucose concentration is an important issue for interpreting the results of diagnostic tests for diabetes. There is significant variation in the results of repeated tests in adults after a 2- to 6-week interval. The intraindividual coefficient of variation in one study was 6.4% for the FPG and 16.7% for the 2-hour plasma glucose value. Thus, it is essential that abnormal results be confirmed by a repeated test. Although the oral glucose tolerance test (OGTT) is an invaluable tool in research, it is not recommended for routine use in diagnosing diabetes. It is inconvenient for patients, and in the vast majority of cases the diagnosis can be made on the basis of either an elevated fasting glucose concentration or an elevated random glucose determination in the presence of hyperglycemic symptoms.

Levels of hemoglobin A_{1c} (HbA_{1c}) are not currently recommended for diagnosing diabetes. The major reasons are the lack of standardization of the assays for HbA_{1c}, false positive and false negative results related to hemoglobinopathy and altered red cell survival and the imperfect correlation between HbA_{1c} and FPG and 2-hour plasma glucose. However, HbA_{1c} remains the preferred method for monitoring the effectiveness of diabetes treatment.

TABLE 30–1 EPIDEMIOLOGIC DETERMINANTS AND RISK FACTORS OF TYPE 2 DIABETES

GENETIC FACTORS
Genetic markers Family history "Thrifty gene(s)"
DEMOGRAPHIC CHARACTERISTICS
Sex Age Ethnicity
BEHAVIORAL AND LIFESTYLE-RELATED RISK FACTORS
Obesity (including distribution of obesity and duration) Physical inactivity Diet Stress Westernization, urbanization, modernization
METABOLIC DETERMINANTS AND INTERMEDIATE-RISK CATEGORIES OF TYPE 2 DIABETES
Impaired glucose tolerance Insulin resistance Pregnancy-related determinants • Parity • Gestational diabetes • Diabetes in offspring of women with diabetes during pregnancy • Intrauterine malnutrition or overnutrition

From Zimmer P, Alberti KG, Shaw J. Global and societal implications of the diabetes epidemic. Nature 2001;414:782-787.

Screening for Type 2 Diabetes

Undiagnosed T2DM is common, with an estimated lag of 5 to 7 years between the onset of diabetes and diagnosis.[19-21] It is estimated that in up to 30% of affected people the disease are

TABLE 30–2 CRITERIA FOR THE DIAGNOSIS OF DIABETES

Test	Normoglycemia (mg/dL)	IFG (mg/dL)	IGT (mg/dL)	Diabetes*
FPG	<100	100-125		≥126 mg/dL
2-hr PG	<140		140-199 mg/dL	≥200 mg/dL
Casual plasma glucose concentration				≥200 mg/dL plus symptoms of diabetes

*A diagnosis of diabetes must be confirmed on a subsequent day by measuring FPG, 2-hr PG, or random plasma glucose (if symptoms are present). The FPG test is greatly preferred because of ease of administration, convenience, acceptability to patients, and lower cost. Fasting is defined as no caloric intake for at least 8 hours.
FPG, fasting plasma glucose; IFG, impaired fasting glucose; IGT, impaired glucose tolerance; PG, plasma glucose.

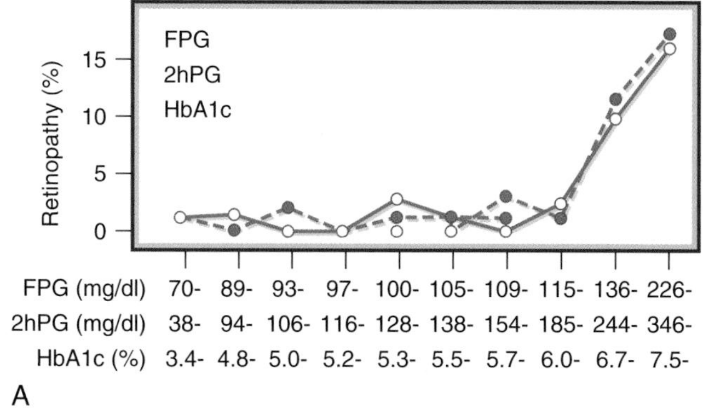

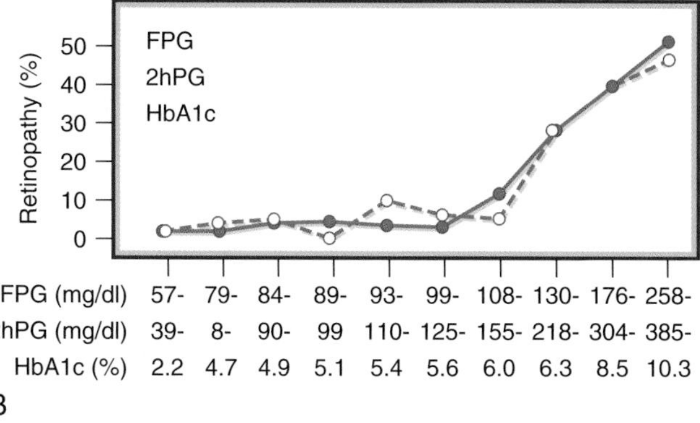

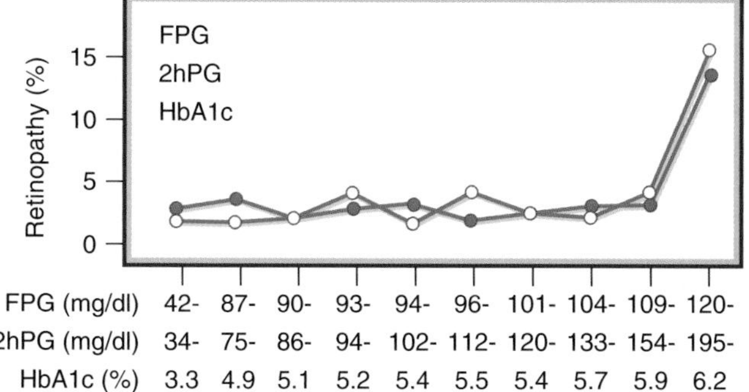

Figure 30–1 ▪ American Diabetes Association consensus. FPG, fasting plasma glucose; 2hPG, 2-hour plasma glucose; HbA1c, hemoglobin A_{1c}.

undiagnosed.[22] Subjects with IGT and undiagnosed T2DM are at significantly increased risk for coronary heart disease, stroke, and peripheral vascular disease. Thus, this delay in the diagnosis of T2DM causes an increase in microvascular and macrovascular disease. In addition, affected individuals have a greater likelihood of having dyslipidemia, hypertension, and obesity. Therefore, it is important for the clinician to screen for diabetes in a cost-effective manner in subjects who demonstrate major risk factors for diabetes as summarized in Table 30–3. Recommendations for screening are summarized in Table 30–4.

PATHOGENESIS

The pathogenesis of T2DM is complex and involves the interaction of genetic and environmental factors. A number of environmental factors have been shown to play a critical role in the development of the disease, particularly excessive caloric intake leading to obesity and a sedentary lifestyle. The clinical presentation is also heterogeneous, with a wide range in age of onset, severity of associated hyperglycemia, and degree of obesity. From a pathophysiologic standpoint, persons with T2DM consistently demonstrate three cardinal abnormalities: resistance to the action of insulin in peripheral tissues, particularly muscle and fat but also liver; defective insulin secretion, particularly in response to a glucose stimulus; and increased glucose production by the liver.

Although the precise way these genetic, environmental, and pathophysiologic factors interact to lead to the clinical onset of T2DM is not known, our understanding of these processes has increased substantially. With the exception of specific monogenic forms of the disease that might result from defects largely confined to the pathways that regulate insulin action in muscle, liver, and fat or defects in insulin secretory function in the pancreatic beta cell, there is an emerging consensus that the common forms of T2DM are polygenic in nature and are due to a combination of insulin resistance and abnormal insulin secretion. From a pathophysiologic standpoint, it is the inability of the pancreatic beta cell to adapt to the reductions in insulin sensitivity that occur over the lifetime of human subjects that precipitates the onset of T2DM. The most common factors that place an increased secretory burden on the beta cell are puberty,

TABLE 30–3 MAJOR RISK FACTORS FOR TYPE 2 DIABETES

Overweight (BMI ≥25 kg/m^2)
Habitual physical inactivity
Race/ethnicity (e.g., African American, Latin American, Native American, Asian American, Pacific Islander)
Previously identified IFG or IGT
Hypertension (≥140/90 mm Hg in adults)
HDL cholesterol ≤35 mg/dL (0.90 mmol/L) and/or a triglyceride level ≥250 mg/dL (2.82 mmol/L)
History of GDM or delivery of a baby weighing >9 lb (4.1 kg)
Polycystic ovary syndrome

BMI, body mass index; GDM, gestational diabetes mellitus; HDL, high-density lipoprotein; IFG, impaired fasting glucose; IGT, impaired glucose tolerance.

From American Diabetes Association. Standards of medical care in diabetes—2006. Diabetes Care 2006;29:s4-s42.

TABLE 30–4 SUMMARY OF MAJOR RECOMMENDATIONS FOR SCREENING

Evaluation for type 2 diabetes should be performed within the health care setting. Patients should be screened at 3-year intervals beginning at age 45 years; testing should be considered at an earlier age or be carried out more frequently if diabetes risk factors are present (see Table 30–3).
The FPG is the recommended screening test. The OGTT may be necessary for diagnosing diabetes when the FPG is normal. The FPG is preferred for screenings because it is faster and easier to perform, more convenient, acceptable to patients, and less expensive.
Diagnostic testing should be performed in any clinical situation in which such testing is warranted
Screening outside of health care settings (community screening) has not been shown to be beneficial and can result in some harm; this type of screening is not recommended.

pregnancy, a sedentary lifestyle, and overeating leading to weight gain. An underlying genetic predisposition appears to be a critical factor in determining the frequency with which beta cell failure occurs.

Genetic Factors in the Development of Type 2 Diabetes

Genetically, T2DM consists of monogenic and polygenic forms.[23,24] The monogenic forms, although relatively uncommon, are nevertheless important, and a number of the genes involved have been identified and characterized. The genes involved in the common polygenic form or forms of the disorder have been far more difficult to identify and characterize.

Monogenic Forms of Diabetes

In the monogenic forms of diabetes, the gene involved is both necessary and sufficient to cause disease. In other words, environmental factors play little or no role in determining whether or not a genetically predisposed person develops clinical diabetes. The monogenic forms of diabetes generally occur in young patients, often in the first two to three decades of life, although if only mild asymptomatic elevations in blood glucose occur the diagnosis may be missed until later in life.

The monogenic forms of diabetes are summarized in Table 30–5 and can be divided into those in which the mechanism is a defect in insulin secretion and those that involve defective responses to insulin or insulin resistance.

Monogenic Forms of Diabetes Associated with Insulin Resistance

Mutations in the Insulin Receptor

More than 70 mutations have been identified in the insulin receptor gene in various insulin-resistant patients.[25] There are at least three clinical syndromes caused by mutations in the insulin receptor gene. Type A insulin resistance is defined by the presence of insulin resistance, acanthosis nigricans, and hyperandrogenism.[26] Patients with leprechaunism have multiple abnormalities, including intrauterine growth retardation, fasting hypoglycemia, and death within the first 1 to 2 years of life.[27-29] The Rabson-Mendenhall syndrome is associated with short stature, protuberant abdomen, and abnormalities of teeth and nails; pineal hyperplasia was a characteristic in the original description of this syndrome.[30]

These mutations might impair receptor function by a number of different mechanisms, including decreasing the number of receptors expressed on the cell surface, for example, by decreasing the rate of receptor biosynthesis (class 1), accelerating the rate of receptor degradation (class 5), or inhibiting the transport of receptors to the plasma membrane (class 2). The intrinsic function of the receptor may be abnormal if the affinity of insulin binding is reduced (class 3) or if receptor tyrosine kinase is inactivated (class 4). The insulin resistance that is associated with insulin receptor mutations may be severe and present in the neonatal period, as with leprechaunism and the Rabson-Mendenhall syndrome, or it can occur in a milder form in adulthood, leading to insulin-resistant diabetes with marked hyperinsulinemia, acanthosis nigricans, and hyperandrogenism.

TABLE 30–5 MONOGENIC FORMS OF DIABETES

ASSOCIATED WITH INSULIN RESISTANCE
Mutations in the insulin receptor gene
• Type A insulin resistance
• Leprechaunism
• Rabson-Mendenhall syndrome
Lipoatrophic diabetes
Mutations in the PPARγ gene
ASSOCIATED WITH DEFECTIVE INSULIN SECRETION
Mutations in the insulin or proinsulin genes
Mitochondrial gene mutations
Maturity-onset Diabetes of the Young (MODY)
HNF-4α (MODY 1)
Glucokinase (MODY 2)
HNF-1α (MODY 3)
IPF-1 (MODY 4)
HNF-1β (MODY 5)
NeuroD1/Beta2 (MODY 6)

HNF, hepatocyte nuclear factor; IPF, insulin promoter factor; NeuroD1/Beta2, neurogenic differentiation 1/beta cell E-box *trans*-activator 2; PPAR, peroxisome proliferator-activated receptor.

Lipoatrophic Diabetes

In another monogenic form of diabetes, lipoatrophic diabetes, severe insulin resistance is associated with lipoatrophy and lipodystrophy. This form of diabetes is characterized by a paucity of fat, insulin resistance, and hypertriglyceridemia.[31] The disease has several genetic forms, including face-sparing partial lipoatrophy (the Dunnigan syndrome or the Koberling-Dunnigan syndrome), an autosomal dominant form caused by mutations in the lamin A/C gene,[32] and congenital generalized lipoatrophy (the Seip-Berardinelli syndrome), an autosomal recessive form that appears to be due to mutations in either 1-acyl-*sn*-glycerol-3-phosphate acyltransferase-2 (AGPAT2) or in the Seipin gene product.[33,34]

Mutations in Peroxisome Proliferator-Activated Receptorn–γ

It has been demonstrated that mutations in the transcription factor peroxisome proliferator-activated receptor–γ (PPARγ) can cause T2DM of early onset (familial lipodystrophy type 3).[35] Two different heterozygous mutations were identified in the ligand-binding domain of PPARγ in three subjects with severe insulin resistance. In the PPARγ crystal structure, the mutations destabilize helix 12, which mediates *trans*-activation. Both receptor mutants showed markedly decreased transcriptional activation and inhibited the action of coexpressed wild-type PPARγ in a dominant negative manner. A Dutch kindred with a –14A → G mutation within the promoter of the PPARγ4 isoform, which results in decreased expression but no qualitative protein abnormalities, has been described.[36]

A common amino acid polymorphism (Pro12Ala) in PPARγ has been associated with T2DM. People homozygous for the Pro12 allele are more insulin resistant than those having one Ala12 allele and have a 1.25-fold increased risk of diabetes. There is also evidence for interaction between this polymorphism and fatty acids, linking this locus with diet. A second polymorphism, C161 → T, has been linked to insulin resistance in Hispanic and non-Hispanic white women.[37]

Monogenic Forms of Diabetes Associated with Defects in Insulin Secretion

Mutant Insulin Syndromes

The first syndrome associated with diabetes to be characterized in terms of the clinical picture, genetic mechanisms, and clinical pathophysiology was that associated with mutant insulin or proinsulin.[38] Persons with this disorder present clinically with a mild non–insulin-dependent form of diabetes. Affected persons characteristically have marked hyperinsulinemia on routine insulin assays. Increases in the concentration of insulin in association with diabetes usually indicate insulin resistance, but in this syndrome, insulin resistance can be easily excluded because the patients respond normally to administration of exogenous insulin. Characterization of the insulin by high-performance liquid chromatography (HPLC) reveals that the hyperinsulinemia is due to the presence of the abnormal insulin or proinsulin and related breakdown products. The increased concentrations of insulin appear to be related to the presence of mutations in regions of the insulin molecule that are important for receptor binding, particularly the COOH terminus of the insulin B chain.

Because the liver is the major site of insulin clearance and the first-pass hepatic insulin uptake and degradation are mediated by the insulin receptor, mutant forms of insulin with diminished insulin receptor binding ability are cleared more slowly from the circulation, and this reduction in insulin clearance leads to hyperinsulinemia. Alternatively, mutations in proinsulin can reduce the conversion of proinsulin to insulin, leading to accumulation of proinsulin.[39,40] Because proinsulin is cleared more slowly from the circulation than insulin, proinsulin levels increase. Proinsulin cross-reacts in most commercially available assays, and this insulin-like immunoreactivity can be characterized as related to the presence of proinsulin rather than insulin only by HPLC or by the use of assays that are specific for insulin and proinsulin.

A patient with a mutation in prohormone convertase 1, one of the enzymes responsible for the conversion of proinsulin to insulin, has been described.[41]

Mitochondrial Diabetes

An A-to-G transition in the mitochondrial tRNALeu(UUR) gene at base pair 3243 has been shown to be associated with maternally transmitted diabetes and sensorineural hearing loss.[42] In other subjects, this mutation is associated with diabetes and the syndrome of mitochondrial myopathy, encephalopathy, lactic acidosis, and strokelike episodes (MELAS syndrome). The mitochondrion plays a key role in the regulation of insulin secretion, particularly in response to glucose. We have documented abnormal insulin secretion on at least one of a battery of tests in subjects with this mitochondrial mutation, even in subjects with normal or impaired glucose tolerance who have not developed overt diabetes.[43]

Maturity-Onset Diabetes of the Young

Maturity-onset diabetes of the young (MODY) is a genetically and clinically heterogeneous group of disorders characterized by nonketotic diabetes mellitus, an autosomal dominant mode of inheritance, onset usually before 25 years of age and often in childhood or adolescence, and a primary defect in pancreatic beta cell function. A detailed review of MODY has been published,[44] and the information contained in that review is summarized.

MODY can result from mutations in any one of at least six different genes. One of these genes encodes the glycolytic enzyme glucokinase (*MODY2*),[45] and the other five encode transcription factors, hepatocyte nuclear factor (HNF)-4α (*MODY1*),[46] HNF-1α (*MODY3*),[47] insulin promoter factor-1 (IPF-1) (*MODY4*),[48] HNF-1β (*MODY5*),[49] and neurogenic differentiation 1/beta cell E-box *trans*-activator 2 (NeuroD1/BETA2) (*MODY6*).[50] All of these genes are expressed in the insulin-producing pancreatic beta cell, and heterozygous mutations cause diabetes related to beta cell dysfunction. Abnormalities in liver and kidney function occur in some forms of MODY, reflecting expression of the transcription factors in these tissues. Nongenetic factors that affect insulin sensitivity (infection, puberty, pregnancy, and rarely obesity) can trigger diabetes onset and affect the severity of hyperglycemia in MODY but do not play a significant role in the development of MODY.

The most common clinical presentation of MODY is a mild asymptomatic increase in blood glucose in a child, adolescent, or young adult with a prominent family history of diabetes often in successive generations, suggesting an autosomal dominant mode of inheritance. Some patients have mild hyperglycemia for many years, whereas others have varying degrees of glucose intolerance for several years before the onset of persistent hyperglycemia.[44] The diagnosis may be made only in adulthood even though the elevation in plasma glucose has been present for many years. Prospective testing indicates that in most patients the disease onset occurs in childhood or adolescence. In some patients, there may be a rapid progression to overt asymptomatic or symptomatic hyperglycemia, necessitating therapy with an oral hypoglycemic drug or insulin. The presence of persistently normal plasma glucose levels in subjects with mutations in any of the known MODY genes is unusual, and the majority eventually experience diabetes (with the exception of many patients with glucokinase mutations; see later).

Although the exact prevalence of MODY is not known, current estimates suggest that MODY might account for 1% to 5% of all cases of diabetes in the United States and other industrialized countries.[44] Several clinical characteristics distinguish patients with MODY from those with T2DM, including a prominent family history of diabetes in three or more generations, young age at presentation, and absence of obesity.

Functional Effects of MODY Genes

The identification of several genes associated with diabetes has provided a unique opportunity to characterize the pathophysiologic mechanisms by which genetic mutations can lead to an increase in the plasma glucose concentration. All the susceptibility genes identified to date cause impaired insulin secretory responses to glucose, although the mechanisms differ.

Glucokinase. Glucokinase is expressed at its highest levels in the pancreatic beta cell and the liver. It catalyzes the transfer of phosphate from adenosine triphosphate (ATP) to glucose to generate glucose-6-phosphate (Fig. 30–2).

This reaction is the first rate-limiting step in glucose metabolism. Glucokinase functions as the glucose sensor in the beta cell by controlling the rate of entry of glucose into the glycolytic pathway (glucose phosphorylation) and its subsequent metabolism. In the liver glucokinase plays a key role in the ability to store glucose as glycogen, particularly in the postprandial state. Heterozygous mutations leading to partial deficiency of glucokinase are associated with MODY, and homozygous mutations resulting in complete deficiency of this enzyme lead to permanent neonatal diabetes mellitus.[51] As predicted by the physiologic functions of glucokinase, the increase in plasma glucose concentrations seen in patients with this form of diabetes is due to a combination of reduced glucose-induced insulin secretion from the pancreatic beta cell and reduced glycogen storage in the liver after glucose ingestion.

Liver-Enriched Transcription Factors. The transcription factors HNF-1α, HNF-1β, and HNF-4α play a key role in the tissue-specific regulation of gene expression in the liver[52] and are also expressed in other tissues including pancreatic islets, kidney, and genital tissues. HNF-1α and HNF-1β are members of the homeodomain-containing family of transcription factors, and HNF-4α is an orphan nuclear receptor.[52,53]

HNF-1α, HNF-1β, and HNF-4α make up part of an interacting network of transcription factors that function together to control gene expression during embryonic development and in adult

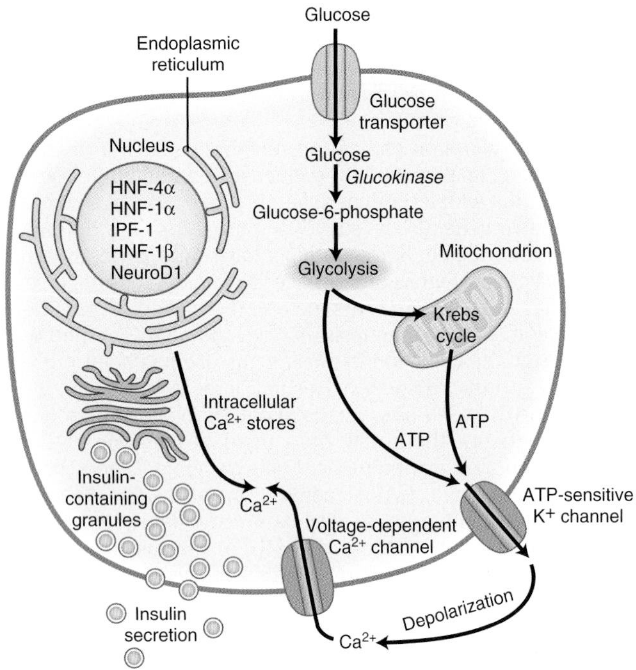

Figure 30–2 ▪ Model of a pancreatic beta cell and the proteins implicated in maturity-onset diabetes of the young. ATP, adenosine triphosphate; HNF, hepatocyte nuclear factor, IPF, insulin promoter factor. (From Fajans SS, Bell GI, Polonsky KS. Molecular mechanisms and clinical pathophysiology of maturity-onset diabetes of the young. N Engl J Med 2001;345:973.)

tissues in which they are coexpressed. In the pancreatic beta cell, these transcription factors regulate the expression of the insulin gene as well as proteins involved in glucose transport and metabolism and mitochondrial metabolism (all linked to insulin secretion) and lipoprotein metabolism.[54] The expression of HNF-1α is regulated at least in part by HNF-4α.

Persons with diabetes related to mutations in these genes have defects in insulin secretory responses to a variety of secretagogues, particularly glucose, that are present before the onset of hyperglycemia, suggesting that they represent the primary functional defect in the syndrome. Reduced glucagon responses to arginine have also been observed, suggesting that the pancreatic alpha cell is also involved in a broader pancreatic developmental abnormality.

Insulin Promoter Factor-1. IPF-1 is a homeodomain-containing transcription factor that was originally isolated as a transcriptional regulator of the insulin and somatostatin genes. It also plays a central role in the development of the pancreas as well as in regulating expression of a variety of pancreatic islet genes including, besides insulin, glucokinase, islet amyloid polypeptide, and glucose transporter 2 genes. IPF-1 also appears to mediate glucose-induced stimulation of insulin gene transcription.[55]

A child born with pancreatic agenesis was shown to have a mutation in IPF-1 that lacked the homeodomain required for DNA binding and nuclear localization. Heterozygous carriers of an IPF-1 mutation from the same kindred developed an early-onset autosomal dominant form of diabetes (i.e., MODY) caused by dominant negative inhibition of transcription of the insulin gene and other beta cell–specific genes regulated by the mutant IPF-1.[56] Additional IPF-1 mutations have been discovered in pedigrees with late-onset T2DM.[57] Thus, mutations in IPF-1 can cause a range of phenotype manifestations, depending on whether the subjects have homozygous or heterozygous mutations and the severity of the functional effects.

Neurogenic Differentiation-1 Transcription Factor. The basic helix-loop-helix transcription factor neurogenic differentiation–1 (NeuroD1/BETA2) was isolated on the basis of its ability to activate transcription of the insulin gene and is required for normal pancreatic islet development. Two patients with heterozygous mutations in NeuroD1 and diabetes have been described,[50] and a third has been identified in an Icelandic population.[58] Studies in other populations have failed to detect mutations in NeuroD1 even in subjects with a MODY phenotype. It therefore appears that mutations in NeuroD1 are a rare cause of MODY.

Genetics of the Polygenic Forms of Type 2 Diabetes

As alluded to earlier, the common polygenic form of T2DM has complex pathophysiology, and genetic and environmental factors both play a major role. The phenotypic manifestations of the disease are also complex and include resistance to the action of insulin in muscle, fat, and liver; defects in insulin secretory responses from the pancreatic beta cell; and increases in hepatic glucose production. However, the primary defect or defects responsible for the development of the syndrome remain elusive and are likely not to be defined until more is known about the genes responsible for diabetes and the nature of the gene-environment interactions that are ultimately responsible for the development of the disorder in predisposed persons.

Insulin resistance is present in persons predisposed to T2DM before the onset of hyperglycemia, and this finding has been interpreted by some to indicate that insulin resistance is the primary abnormality that is responsible for the development of T2DM. However, defective beta cell function is also present before the onset of T2DM when IGT is present and in first-degree relatives of persons with T2DM who have completely normal plasma glucose concentrations. Thus, although there is still controversy about whether insulin resistance or abnormal insulin secretion represents the primary defect in T2DM, there is general consensus that both defects are present in essentially all subjects with the disorder, often from an early preclinical stage.

The identification and characterization of the genes responsible for T2DM will add an essential level to our understanding of the pathophysiology of the disorder. Because the candidate gene approach has not been productive in identifying the genes for the common forms of T2DM, linkage analysis has been applied.[59] This approach involves defining regions of chromosomal DNA shared to excess by affected family members. Parents are genotyped at a particular marker, and the offspring are scored for sharing of zero, one, or two alleles inherited from their parents. Markers are genotyped in family members in the regions of polymorphic repeats called microsatellites or simple tandem repeats. Because in the case of T2DM (as well as other common polygenic human diseases) there is no prior knowledge of the gene defect, microsatellites at defined chromosomal locations are typed either in family members or in affected sibling pairs. To screen the whole genome, 300 to 400 microsatellites are genotyped in the study subjects at roughly 10-centimorgan (cM) intervals. This is generally adequate to define chromosomal regions sharing single gene defects. The evidence for linkage usually extends over a broad region, which may be 10 to 20 cM, and positional cloning strategies are then used to find the gene within this broad region.

As a result of recent progress, a number of genes have been shown to determine risk for T2DM. The most extensively studied are *calpain-10, PPARγ2,* and *Kir6.2.* Their roles as diabetes genes have been confirmed in many but not all studies, and their presence in predisposed persons increases risk of diabetes by approximately 20%. With all three genes, meta-analyses and large case-control studies have confirmed that they are diabetes genes. However, individual contributions of genetic variation in these genes alone does not appear to be sufficient to account for the development of diabetes.

Calpain-10 *Gene*

The linkage between *calpain-10* and T2DM first observed by a group headed by Graeme Bell[60] was completely unexpected and was based purely on the application of sophisticated methods of analysis in a genetic study rather than on any novel physiologic insights. A number of studies have corroborated the initial observation that genetic variation in the *calpain-10* gene increases the risk of T2DM, but others have not. However, two recent meta-analyses of all the published data support a role for this gene in diabetes susceptibility. Song's group,[61] after analyzing 11 studies, have shown an odds ratio for T2DM of 1.19 comparing persons with the G/G genotype of UCSNP43 in *calpain-10* versus all carriers of the A allele. Weedon's group[62] calculated an odds ratio of 1.17 for UCSNP-44.

Calpains are Ca^{2+}-dependent cysteine proteases. The first calpain was purified in 1976, and although the understanding of calpain biology has increased substantially, the regulation of calpain activity and the roles these enzymes play in normal physiology and disease states are still poorly understood.[63] It has been suggested that calpains contribute to a number of disease states. The best characterized of these is limb girdle muscular dystrophy type 2A, which is due to disruption of the gene for calpain-3. It has also been proposed that calpains contribute to ischemic tissue damage following stroke, myocardial infarction, and traumatic brain and spinal cord injuries as well as a number of other diverse conditions including cataracts and Alzheimer's disease.

The precise physiologic mechanisms by which genetic variation in the *calpain-10* gene leads to altered susceptibility to diabetes is still being characterized. Pharmacologic inhibition of calpain activity results in insulin resistance and impaired insulin secretion.[64,65] The insulin secretory response to glucose in mouse pancreatic islets was increased by a 4-hour exposure to the cell-permeable calpain inhibitors ALLM and E-64-d. In muscle strips and adipocytes, calpain inhibitor II and E-64-d both reduced insulin-mediated glucose transport. Incorporation of glucose into glycogen in muscle also was reduced.[64] Exposure of mouse islets to calpain inhibitors of different structure and mechanism of action for 48 hours reversibly suppresses glucose-induced insulin secretion by 40% to 80%.[65]

Transgenic mice overexpressing calpastatin (an endogenous inhibitor of calpain activity) in muscle (CsTg) demonstrate a more than threefold increase in the levels of the glucose transporter GLUT4 in soleus, triceps, and tibialis anterior muscles.[66] The magnitude of insulin- or contraction-stimulated muscle glucose transport is normally directly proportional to muscle GLUT4 content. Surprisingly, the marked increase in GLUT4 was not associated with an increase in insulin-mediated glucose transport into muscle or glucose transport stimulated by electrically induced muscle contraction. Increased GLUT4 in muscle due to reduced metabolism by calpains is associated with a state of relative insulin resistance due to GLUT4 dysfunction. There is also evidence that calpain-10 plays a role in regulating apoptosis in the pancreatic beta cell.[67] Thus, calpains play a role in regulating insulin secretion and insulin action.

Kir6.2 *Gene*

The beta cell ATP-sensitive K+ channel (K_{ATP}) is composed of two subunits: a high-affinity sulfonylurea receptor (SUR1) and an inward rectifier (Kir6.2).[68] The missense mutation Glu23Lys (E23K) in the *Kir6.2* gene has been associated with increased risk of T2DM in some but not all studies,[62,69-71] similar to what was observed with *calpain-10*. Meta-analyses have shown that the E23K variant affects diabetes risk.[62,72] The study by Love-Gregory's group[72] suggested that the K allele of the E23K polymorphism increases the risk of T2DM by an average of 13% and that the KK homozygote is at greatest risk (relative risk 1.28). 't Hart and colleagues have examined the influence of the E23K variant of *Kir6.2* on the insulin secretory responses to glucose and found no effect. However, they did not consider the confounding effect of insulin resistance.[73]

Peroxisome Proliferator-Activated Receptor–γ

PPARγ is a member of the PPAR subfamily of nuclear receptors. It is an important regulator of lipid and glucose homeostasis and cellular differentiation. Although PPARγ is most abundantly expressed in adipose tissue, it is also expressed in the pancreatic beta cell, and targeted elimination of the receptor in the beta cell leads to a blunting of the normal increase in beta cell mass that occurs on a high-fat diet.[74] Meta-analyses of all published studies performed by Altshuler and colleagues[75] have shown that the missense mutation Pro12Ala (P12A) in *PPARγ2* is associated with decreased risk for T2DM (estimated risk ratio of 0.79 for the alanine allele).

Hepatocyte Nuclear Factor–4α Gene

The role of *HNF-4α* in the development of MODY has already been clearly documented. Mutations in this gene lead to abnormalities in insulin secretion. Recently studies involving different populations[76-78] have demonstrated that genetic variation in the region of an alternative promoter for the *HNF-4α* gene is associated with increased risk of T2DM. It is likely that these at-risk polymorphisms alter expression of the *HNF-4α* gene, thereby causing increased susceptibility to T2DM.

Transcription Factor 7–like 2 Gene

Grant and colleagues[79] have genotyped 228 microsatellite markers in Icelandic patients with T2DM and in controls. A microsatellite, DG10S478, within intron 3 of the transcription factor 7–like 2 gene (*TCF7L2;* formerly *TCF4*) was associated with T2DM. This was replicated in a Danish cohort and in a U.S. cohort. Compared with noncarriers, heterozygous and homozygous carriers of the at-risk alleles (38% and 7% of the population, respectively) have relative risks of 1.45 and 2.41. This corresponds to a population attributable risk of 21%. The TCF7L2 gene product is a high mobility group box containing transcription factors previously implicated in blood glucose homeostasis. It is thought to act through regulation of proglucagon gene expression in enteroendocrine cells via the Wnt signaling pathway.

In a follow-up study to this observation, Florez and colleagues[80] observed that specific polymorphisms in the *TCF7L2* gene increase the risk of progression from impaired glucose tolerance to T2DM, and this effect is mediated through a reduction of glucose-induced insulin secretion.

Insulin Resistance and the Risk of Type 2 Diabetes

Insulin Resistance

A substantial amount of data indicates that insulin resistance plays a major role in the development of glucose intolerance and diabetes. Insulin resistance is a consistent finding in patients with T2DM, and resistance is present years before the onset of diabetes.[81-86] Prospective studies show that insulin resistance predicts the onset of diabetes.[82,83]

The term *insulin resistance* indicates the presence of an impaired biologic response to either exogenously administered or endogenously secreted insulin. Insulin resistance is manifested by decreased insulin-stimulated glucose transport and metabolism in adipocytes and skeletal muscle and by impaired suppression of hepatic glucose output.

Insulin sensitivity is influenced by a number of factors including age,[87] weight, ethnicity, body fat (especially abdominal), physical activity, and medications. Insulin resistance is associated with the progression to IGT and T2DM,[88] although diabetes is rarely seen in insulin-resistant persons without some degree of beta cell dysfunction.[86] First-degree relatives of type 2 diabetics have insulin resistance even at a time when they are not obese, implying a strong genetic component in the development of insulin resistance.[82,88,89] There is also a strong influence of environmental factors on the genetic predisposition to insulin resistance and therefore to diabetes.[90,91]

Obesity and Type 2 Diabetes

The association of obesity with T2DM has been recognized for decades. A close association between obesity and insulin resistance is seen in all ethnic groups and is found across the full range of body weights, across all ages, and in both sexes (Fig. 30–3).[92-94] A number of large epidemiologic studies showed that the risk of diabetes, and presumably insulin resistance, rises as body fat content increases from the very lean to the very obese, implying that the absolute amount of body fat has an effect on insulin sensitivity across a broad range (Fig. 30–4A).[95-97] However, central (intra-abdominal) adiposity is more strongly linked to insulin resistance (Fig. 30–4B) and a number of important metabolic variables, including plasma glucose, insulin, total plasma cholesterol and triglyceride concentrations, and decreased plasma high-density lipoprotein (HDL) cholesterol concentration, than is total adiposity.[98-104] In addition, the effect of accumulation of abdominal fat on glucose tolerance is independent of total adiposity.[105,106]

The reason for the relationship to intra-abdominal fat with abnormal metabolism is not clearly defined, but a number of hypotheses, which are not mutually exclusive, have been proposed. First, abdominal fat is more lipolytically active than subcutaneous fat, perhaps because of its greater complement of adrenergic receptors.[107,108] In addition, the abdominal adipose store is resistant to the antilipolytic effects of insulin,[109] including alterations in lipoprotein lipase activity, which leads to increased lipase activity and a greater flux of fatty acids into the circulation, with the portal circulation receiving the greatest fatty acid load. Finally, the high levels of 11β-hydroxysteroid dehydrogenase type 1 (11βHSD1) in mesenteric fat could result in enhanced conversion of inactive cortisone to active cortisol, resulting in increased local cortisol production. This might change adipocytes to increase lipolysis and alter the production of adipokines, which might directly modulate glucose metabolism. The role of the liver in insulin resistance and hyperglycemia is discussed later.

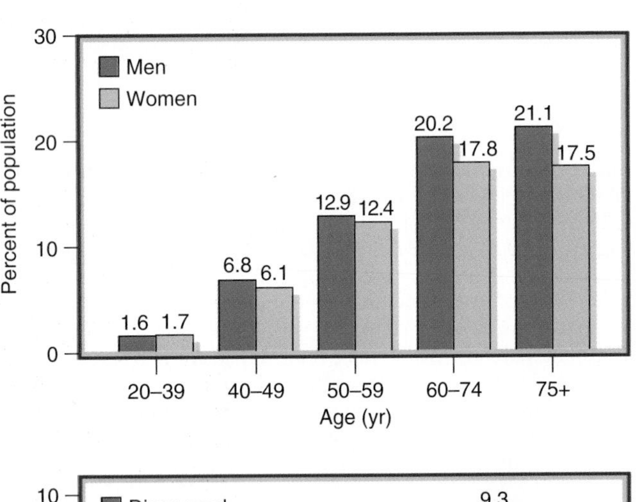

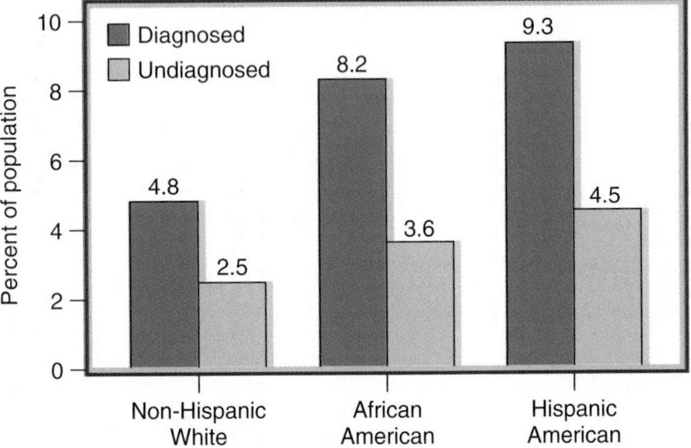

Figure 30–3 ■ Prevalence of diabetes by age *(top panel)* and by ethnicity *(bottom panel)*. (From Harris MI, Flegal KM, Cowie CC, et al. Prevalence of diabetes, impaired fasting glucose, and impaired glucose tolerance in U.S. adults. The Third National Health and Nutrition Examination Survey, 1988-1994. Diabetes Care 1998;21:518-524.)

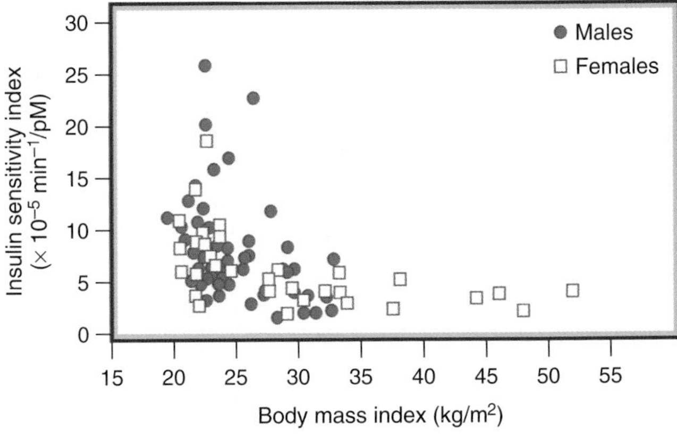

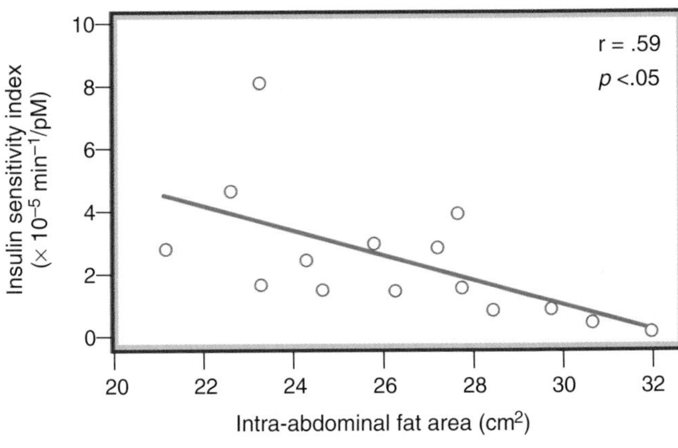

Figure 30–4 ■ Relationship between body mass index *(top panel)* or intra-abdominal fat *(bottom panel)* and insulin sensitivity. (*Top*, From Fujimoto WY, Bergstrom RW, Boyko EJ, et al. Susceptibility to development of central adiposity among populations. Obesity Res 1995;3(suppl 2):179S–186S; *bottom*, from Kahn SE, Prigeon RL, McCulloch DK, et al. Quantification of the relationship between insulin sensitivity and beta-cell function in human subjects: evidence for a hyperbolic function. Diabetes 1993;42:1663-1672.)

Skeletal Muscle Insulin Resistance

The primary site of glucose disposal after a meal is skeletal muscle, and the primary mechanism of glucose storage is through its conversion to glycogen. Studies using the hyperinsulinemic-euglycemic clamp technique have demonstrated that in insulin-resistant people with and without T2DM, there is a deficiency in the nonoxidative disposal of glucose related primarily to a defect in glycogen synthesis (Fig. 30–5).[110,111]

Fatty Acids and Insulin Resistance

Free Fatty Acids

Elevated free fatty acids (FFAs) predict the progression from IGT to diabetes.[112,113] In the periphery, FFAs might not be markedly elevated because of efficient extraction by the liver and skeletal muscle. Thus, normal or minimally elevated FFA levels might not reflect the true exposure of fatty acids to peripheral tissues. Increases in fatty acid flux to skeletal muscle related to the increased visceral lipolysis have been implicated in the inhibition of muscle glucose uptake.

The Randle hypothesis, or the glucose–fatty acid cycle, was originally proposed to account for the ability of FFAs to inhibit muscle glucose utilization. Randle and colleagues[114] demonstrated that fatty acids compete with glucose for substrate oxidation in isolated muscle. The increase in fatty acid metabolism leads to an increase in the intramitochondrial acetyl coenzyme A (CoA)/CoA and reduced nicotinamide adenine dinucleotide (NADH)/NAD+ ratios, with subsequent inhibition of pyruvate dehydrogenase. The resulting increased intracellular mitochondrial (and cytosolic) citrate concentrations result in allosteric inhibition of phosphofructokinase, the key rate-controlling enzyme in glycolysis. Subsequent accumulation of glucose-6-phosphate would inhibit hexokinase II activity, resulting in an increase in intracellular glucose concentrations and decreased glucose uptake.

More recent studies have suggested that the primary effect of fatty acids, at least in the presence of elevated insulin levels, is a decrease in glucose transport as measured by a reduction in the rate of accumulation of intracellular glucose and glycogen using ^{13}C and ^{31}P nuclear magnetic resonance (NMR) spectroscopy. In normal subjects, elevated fatty acids, achieved by infusion of triglyceride emulsions and heparin (to activate lipoprotein lipase), resulted in a fall in intracellular glucose and glucose-6-phosphate concentrations that preceded the fall in glycogen accumulation.[115,116] These results challenge the Randle hypothesis (which predicts a rise in intracellular glucose-6-phosphate concentrations) as the basis of the reduction in insulin sensitivity seen with elevated fatty acids. Similar decreases in glucose transport have been seen in patients with T2DM[117] and in lean, normoglycemic, insulin-resistant offspring of type 2 diabetics.[118,119] These studies also found a decrease in the activity of phosphatidylinositol 3-phosphate kinase (PI 3-kinase) and increased protein kinase C–θ (PKCθ) activity that might, in part, mediate the effect of elevated FFAs.[120,121]

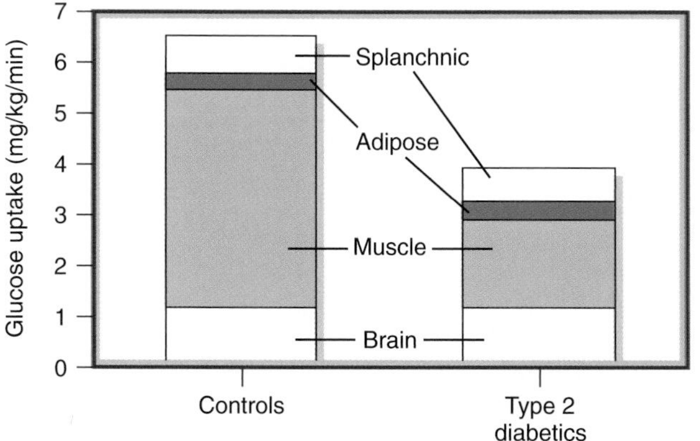

Figure 30–5 ▪ Tissue uptake of glucose in nondiabetic and insulin-resistant diabetic subjects during a hyperinsulinemic-euglycemic clamp. (From DeFronzo RA. Lilly lecture 1987. The triumvirate: beta-cell, muscle, liver. A collusion responsible for NIDDM. Diabetes 1988;37:667-687.)

More recent evidence has suggested that the mammalian target of rapamycin (mTOR) may be part of the integration of excess nutrient accumulation and insulin resistance. Mice with ablation of S6 kinase 1, an effector within the mTOR nutrient signaling pathway, are protected from developing obesity and insulin resistance when given a high-fat diet.[122] Like PKC, S6 kinase can phosphorylate insulin receptor substrate–1 (IRS-1) and result in down-regulation of insulin signaling. Studies also suggest that PKC-mediated serine phosphorylation of inhibitor of κB kinase (IKK) β subunit (IKKβ), leading to its degradation and the unregulated translocation of nuclear factor–κB (NF-κB) into the nucleus, might also be important to fatty acid–induced insulin resistance.[123] This is the mechanism by which high-dose aspirin therapy improves glucose metabolism in T2DM.[123] Disruption of the IKKβ inflammatory pathway by high-dose aspirin therapy in a small human trial resulted in an improvement in insulin sensitivity.

Intramuscular Triglycerides

Insulin-stimulated glucose uptake is inversely related to the amount of intramuscular triglycerides. A strong correlation between intramuscular triglyceride concentration and insulin resistance has been demonstrated by evaluating intramuscular triglyceride with biopsy,[124] computed tomography (CT) scanning,[125] and magnetic resonance imaging (MRI) measurements.[126] MRI has been a valuable addition because the magnetic resonance signal can distinguish intramyocellular from extramyocellular fat and demonstrates the increased triglyceride accumulation within the myofiber itself.[127] First-degree relatives of type 2 diabetics have an increase in intramyocellular fat, and in this group there is also a correlation with insulin resistance.[126]

The mechanism for accumulation of triglyceride in the skeletal muscle of obese and insulin-resistant persons is probably related to the mismatching of FFA uptake and oxidation. During resting postabsorptive conditions, about 30% of fatty acid flux in the plasma pool is accounted for by oxidation, and the remaining 70% of flux is recycled into triglyceride, indicating a physiologic reserve that exceeds immediate tissue needs for oxidative substrates. The equilibrium between oxidation and reesterification within muscle is paramount in determining fatty acid storage within tissue. The uptake, transport, and metabolism of fatty acids are highly regulated processes (Fig. 30–6), and alteration of the balance between uptake and oxidation in skeletal muscle leads to increased intramyocellular triglycerides. The increased lipolysis associated with obesity provides an increased amount of FFA presented to muscle.

Increased muscle triglyceride content is not invariably linked to insulin resistance because exercise training is associated with increased muscle triglyceride content,[128] and chronic exercise increases insulin sensitivity as well as the capacity for fatty acid oxidation.[129-133]

Fatty Acid Metabolism in Skeletal Muscle

The uptake of fatty acid from the serum, where it is mostly bound to albumin, is mediated by at least three families of proteins: fatty acid translocase, plasma membrane fatty acid binding protein (FABP-pm), and fatty acid transport protein.[134-136] The levels of the putative transport proteins are regulated by exercise,[137] are correlated with body weight (at least in women), and can be modulated by insulin infusion.[138]

FABPs are capable of binding multiple hydrophobic ligands, including fatty acids, eicosanoids, and retinoids with high affinity.[139] FABPs are thought to facilitate uptake of fatty acids and promote subsequent intracellular transport to subcellular organelles.[140] There is a direct correlation between heart-type FABP content and oxidative capacity observed during development and among different muscle types.[141,142] In mice with a disruption of the heart[143] or adipocyte[144] isoform of FABP, plasma fatty acid concentrations were significantly elevated and plasma glucose was decreased, suggesting a key role in normal regulation in fatty acid oxidation. Some[145] but not all[146] studies have shown a decrease in heart-type FABP in insulin-resistant humans.

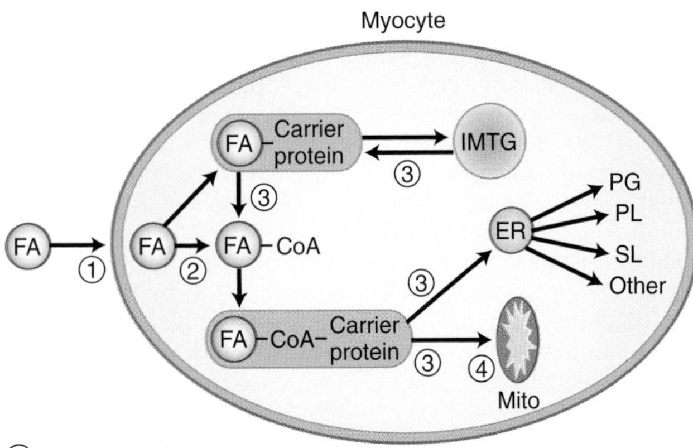

Figure 30–6 ▪ Simplified schematic diagram demonstrating fatty acid (FA) uptake, activation (formation of FA-coenzyme A [CoA]), and intracellular transport to different organelles within a muscle cell. ER, endoplasmic reticulum; IMTG, intramuscular triglyceride; Mito, mitichondrion; PG, prostaglandin; PL, phospholipid; SL, sphingolipid.

Carnitine palmitoyltransferase I (CPT-I) has been the subject of intense scrutiny for many years because of its central role in the balance between mitochondrial glucose and fatty acid metabolism, primarily because of inhibition of mitochondrial fatty acid uptake by malonyl CoA.[147,148] A specific isoform contributes 97% of the CPT-I in muscle and has 100-fold lower sensitivity to inhibition by malonyl CoA.[149] This lower sensitivity to malonyl CoA inhibition suggests that the levels of CPT-I itself may be important in the balance of uptake and oxidation of fatty acids. Evidence for this in skeletal muscle stems from the finding that as with other fatty acid-oxidizing enzymes, muscle CPT-I mRNA is regulated by PPARα activators, fat feeding, and exercise in rodents and is inversely correlated with obesity in humans.[150-153]

Long-chain fatty acids, after passing through the inner mitochondrial membrane as acylcarnitines, are metabolized at the surface of the inner mitochondrial membrane by CPT-II and the long chain–specific oxidation system consisting of very-long-chain acyl CoA dehydrogenase (VLCAD) and the trifunctional protein (TFP) oxidation complex (Fig. 30–7). Transfer of the acyl chain from carnitine to CoA catalyzed by CPT-II is followed by one cycle of oxidation catalyzed by VLCAD and TFP to yield a chain-shortened acyl CoA that can recycle through the same oxidation system.[154] In actuality, four different acyl CoA dehydrogenase enzymes catalyze the initial dehydrogenation of straight-chain fatty acids in mitochondria. Three of them—short-chain acyl CoA dehydrogenase (SCAD), medium-chain acyl CoA dehydrogenase (MCAD), and long-chain acyl CoA dehydrogenase (LCAD)—are soluble enzymes located in the mitochondrial matrix as homotetramers. A fourth, VLCAD, is attached to the inner membrane as a homodimer. Their names derive from the length of the fatty acids that they process. VLCAD and LCAD shorten the long-chain fatty acids into medium-chain fatty

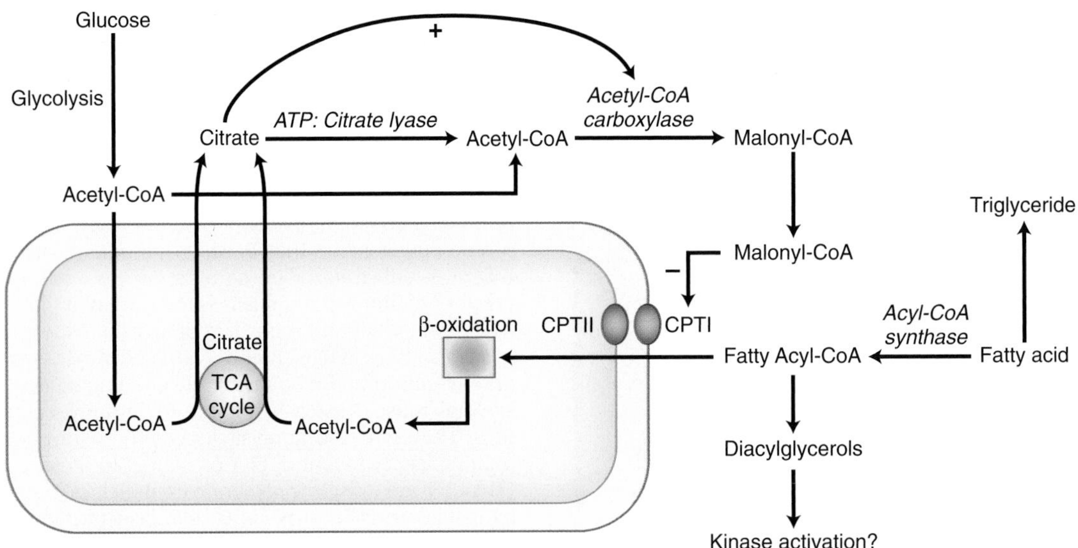

Figure 30–7 ▪ Glucose effect on triglyceride metabolism. Increased uptake of glucose results in an increase in the production of acetyl coenzyme A (CoA) as a product of glycolysis. The increased tricarboxylic acid (TCA) cycle activity associated with oxidation of triglycerides and glucose increases the production of citrate, which is shuttled to the cytoplasm, activates the enzyme acetyl-CoA carboxylase (ACC) by allosteric mechanisms, and increases the susceptibility of ACC to phosphatases. This leads to increased ACC activity, converting acetyl CoA to malonyl CoA. Malonyl CoA is a potent inhibitor of carnitine palmitoyltransferase (CPT) I on the outer mitochondrial membrane, which leads to accumulation of fatty acyl CoAs in the cytoplasm. This can result in the production of signaling molecules that can increase the activity of kinases and other enzymes and lead to insulin resistance.

acids that can then be processed by MCAD and SCAD.[155] The SCAD, MCAD, and LCAD monomers share a high degree of homology but do not share homology with VLCAD. At least some of these enzymes can be regulated in humans during exercise training.[156]

Uncoupling protein-1 (UCP1) is clearly related to the uncoupling of oxidative phosphorylation in brown adipose tissue.[117] UCP2 and UCP3 have structural similarities to UCP1, but it is not clear that they are actually uncouplers of oxidative phosphorylation.[157] Newer members of the family, brain mitochondrial carrier protein 1 (BMCP1) and UCP4, have an even more distant sequence relationship.[158] BMCP1 and UCP4 are predominantly expressed in neural tissues, namely the brain. UCP3 mRNA is found primarily in skeletal muscle and in brown adipose tissue. UCP2 has a ubiquitous tissue distribution. UCP2 and UCP3 mRNA levels have been correlated with different physiologic states, and numerous studies indicate that expression of UCP2 and UCP3 is stimulated by thyroid hormones and in the presence of high levels of fatty acids.[159] In humans, the levels of UCP2 and UCP3 mRNAs were up-regulated by a high-fat diet, and the up-regulation was more pronounced in humans with high percentages of type IIA fibers.[160] In a small study, exercise training in humans increased mitochondrial oxidative capacity but did not change UCP2 or UCP3 levels.[161] Obesity itself was shown to be positively correlated with a splice isoform of UCP3.[162] A unique polymorphism in the promoter region of UCP3 correlated with the expression of UCP3 in skeletal muscle.[163]

Mitochondrial Abnormalities and Insulin Resistance

A decrease in oxidative capacity is seen in both humans and animals with insulin resistance, obesity, and T2DM.[164,165] Recent studies have suggested that increases in intramyocellular fat content in skeletal muscle associated with insulin resistance (see earlier) may be due to alterations in mitochondrial mass. In one study, young insulin-resistant offspring of parents with T2DM demonstrated a 60% reduction in insulin-stimulated skeletal muscle glucose uptake compared to control subjects that correlated with an increase of approximately 80% in the intramyocellular lipid content.[166] The elevated intramyocellular lipid content was attributable to the 30% reduction in mitochondrial oxidative capacity. Interestingly, the insulin-resistant subjects showed a lower ratio of type 1 to type 2 muscle fibers. Type 1 fibers are mostly oxidative and contain more mitochondria than type 2 muscle fibers, which are more glycolytic.

Decreased expression of nuclear-encoded genes that regulate mitochondrial biogenesis, such as peroxisome proliferator–activated receptor γ (PPARγ)-coactivator-1α and -1β (PGC-1α and PGC-1β), have been shown to be important for mitochondrial biogenesis and for fiber type selection during development.[167] PGC-1α transcriptionally activates the nuclear respiratory factors (NRF)-1 and -2, which are known to be important for mitochondrial biogenesis.[168] PGC-1α–responsive genes are down-regulated in obese white patients with impaired glucose tolerance and T2DM.[169,170] In obese diabetic and nondiabetic Mexican-Americans, PGC-1α and PGC-1β expression levels are reduced compared to levels in nonobese persons.[171] The activity of the electron transport chain is reduced and intramyofibrillar mitochondria are smaller in T2DM and both size of intramyofibrillar mitochondria and electron transport chain activity in muscle homogenates correlated with severity of insulin resistance.[172]

The remaining question is whether the correlations between altered mitochondrial mass and fiber type with alterations in oxidative metabolism are inherited or acquired. One study has shown that young insulin-resistant persons without diabetes also have a reduction in mitochondrial area, but they do not have a reduction in PGC-1α or -1β levels in skeletal muscle.[173] An emerging concept, nonexercise activity thermogenesis (NEAT), which is the energy expended for everything that is not sleeping, eating, or sportslike exercise, suggests that subtle differences in activity throughout the day can result in up to a 350-calorie-per-day difference in caloric expenditure.[174] It is known that exercise can alter muscle fiber types and mitochondrial density, though this is usually of high intensity and this may be in part due to an up-regulation of PGC-1α.[175] Thus, long-term differences in NEAT could potentially result in alteration in skeletal muscle.

In addition, because insulin itself can up-regulate mitochondrial biogenesis, muscle insulin resistance could provide a mechanism for the reduction in mitochondria. Thus, the cause-and-effect relationship among mitochondrial biogenesis, oxidative capacity, and insulin resistance in humans remain unclear. In one study, rats bred for differences in oxidative capacity as determined by their intrinsic ability to run were described. The skeletal muscle of the animals with a low capacity for aerobic exercise showed a reduction in mitochondrial gene expression and PGC-1α, similar to that seen in humans. When multiple metabolic parameters were assessed, it was determined that the group with poor aerobic capacity had several significant abnormalities including obesity, insulin resistance, hypertension, and dyslipidemia, suggesting that the defects found in humans could have a genetic basis.

Glucose Influence on Fatty Acid Metabolism

An emerging concept that could couple the increased fatty acid flux into skeletal muscle with impaired insulin action is the central role of malonyl CoA in regulating fatty acid and glucose oxidation (see Fig. 30–7).[176] Malonyl CoA is an allosteric inhibitor of CPT-I, the enzyme that controls the transfer of long-chain fatty acyl CoAs into the mitochondria.[147,177,178] Even in insulin-resistant skeletal muscle, glucose uptake into the skeletal muscle is higher, especially at the elevated levels of glucose found in T2DM.[179,180] The glucose is shunted toward the glycolytic pathway, generating acetyl CoA that can be converted to malonyl CoA in the cytoplasm by the action of the highly regulated enzyme acetyl CoA carboxylase (ACC).

In humans, an infusion of insulin and glucose at a high rate leads to increases in the concentration of malonyl CoA in skeletal muscle and to decreases in whole-body and, presumably, muscle fatty acid oxidation.[181] In the presence of elevated glucose and insulin levels, the tricarboxylic acid (TCA) cycle is activated, resulting in an increase in citrate in the cytoplasm through increased malate cycling in the mitochondria. The increased citrate is converted to acetyl CoA through citrate lyase and thus provides an indirect substrate for ACC. Citrate also allosterically activates ACC and makes ACC a better substrate for phosphatases that activate the enzyme.[182,183] ACC is also regulated by a phosphorylation-dephosphorylation cycle, with adenosine monophosphate (AMP)-dependent protein kinase an important kinase, which inhibits ACC basal activity and activation by citrate.[184] ACC then generates malonyl CoA, which in turn allosterically inhibits CPT-I residing on the outer mitochondrial membrane, inhibiting uptake of acyl CoA. The resulting buildup of long-chain acyl CoAs and diacylglycerols is proposed to activate one or more PKC isoforms or other lipid-activated proteins, resulting in insulin resistance.[176] Support for this hypothesis is the finding that exercise, which activates AMP-dependent kinase, inactivates ACC, lowers intracellular long-chain acyl CoA levels, and has an acute insulin-sensitizing effect.[185]

Hyperinsulinemia and Insulin Resistance

Hyperinsulinemia per se has been proposed to cause insulin resistance. Elevated concentrations of insulin can cause insulin resistance by down-regulating insulin receptors and desensitizing postreceptor pathways.[186] Del Prato and associates showed that 24 and 72 hours of sustained physiologic hyperinsulinemia in normal persons specifically inhibited the ability of insulin to increase nonoxidative glucose disposal in association with an impaired ability of insulin to stimulate glycogen synthase activity.[187] Suppression of insulin secretion in obese, insulin-resistant persons results in increased insulin sensitivity.[188,189]

Insulin-Signaling Abnormalities in Insulin Resistance

The pathways that are critical for insulin regulation of glucose and lipid metabolism are being clarified. However, the complete cascade of events remains to be determined. Besides intermediary metabolism of glucose and lipid, signaling by insulin affects other cellular processes such as amino acid transport and metabolism, protein synthesis, cell growth, differentiation, and apoptosis.

Insulin Signaling

Insulin signaling is initiated through the binding to and activation of its cell-surface receptor and initiates a cascade of phosphorylation and dephosphorylation events, second messenger generation, and protein-protein interactions that result in the diverse metabolic events in nearly every tissue (Fig. 30–8). The insulin receptor consists of two insulin-binding α subunits and two catalytically active β subunits that are disulfide linked into an $\alpha_2\beta_2$ heterotetrameric complex. Insulin binds to the extracellular α subunits, activating the intracellular tyrosine kinase domain of the β subunit.[190] One receptor β subunit phosphorylates its partner on specific tyrosine residues that may have distinct functions such as stimulation of intermolecular association of signaling molecules such as Shc and Grb, members of the insulin receptor substrate family (IRS1, 2, 3, 4), Shc adapter protein isoforms, and SIRP (signal regulatory protein) family members, Gab-1, Cbl, CAP, and APS[191,192]; stimulation of mitogenesis[193]; and receptor internalization.[194]

The insulin receptor β subunit has also been shown to undergo serine-threonine phosphorylation, which might decrease the ability of the receptor to autophosphorylate. The activities of a number of PKC isoforms that catalyze the serine or threonine phosphorylation of the insulin receptor are elevated in animal models of insulin resistance and in insulin-resistant humans.[195,196] Interventions that decrease serine phosphorylation of the insulin receptor result in increased insulin signaling.[197] Termination of the insulin signaling event occurs by internalization and dephosphorylation of the receptor by protein tyrosine phosphatases. Increased activity of protein tyrosine phosphatase can attenuate insulin signaling. Two protein tyrosine phosphatases that have been shown to negatively regulate insulin signaling, PTP1B and LAR (leukocyte antigen related), have been reported to be elevated in insulin-resistant patients.[198,199] Conversely, disruption of PTB1B in mice resulted in a marked increase in insulin sensitivity and resistance to diet-induced obesity.[200]

Mutations in the insulin receptor are associated with rare forms of insulin resistance. These mutations affect insulin receptor number, splicing, trafficking, binding, and phosphorylation. The affected patients demonstrate severe insulin resistance, manifest as clinically diverse syndromes including the type A syndrome, leprechaunism, Rabson-Mendenhall syndrome, and lipoatrophic diabetes.[201,202]

Downstream Events Following Insulin Receptor Phosphorylation

The insulin receptor substrates (IRSs) act as multifunctional docking proteins activated by tyrosine phosphorylation.[203] The IRS proteins have multiple functional domains, including Pleckstrin homology (PH) and phosphotyrosine binding (PTB), and SH domains that interact with other proteins to mediate the

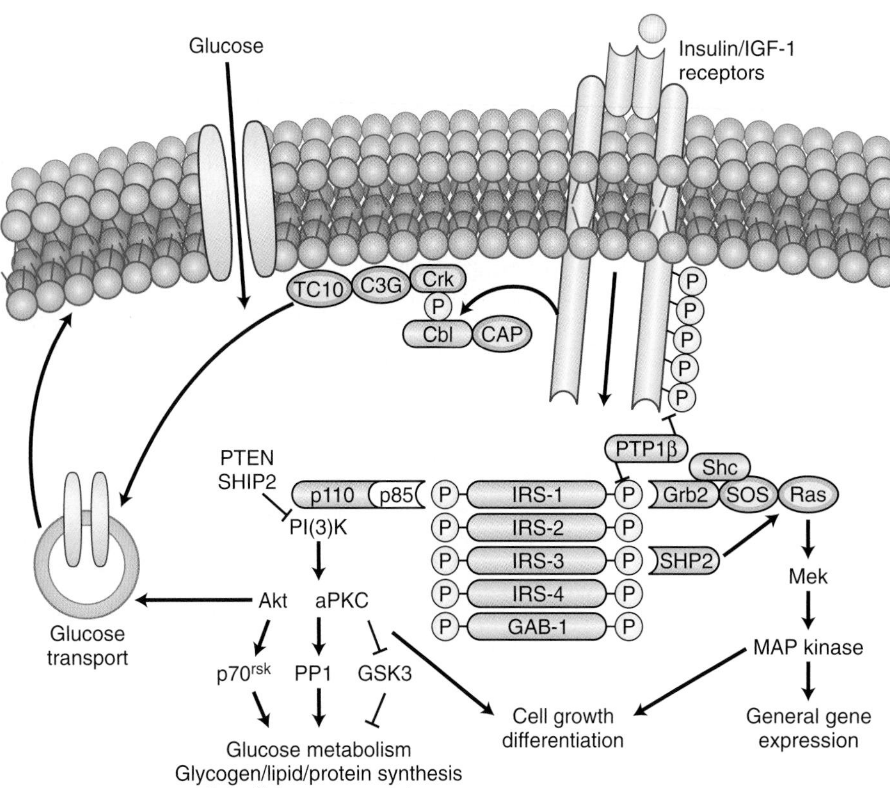

Figure 30–8 ■ Insulin signaling. The insulin receptor is autophosphorylated on multiple tyrosine residues, allowing the docking and activation of multiple signaling molecules, which mediates the increases in glucose uptake and metabolism as well as changes in protein and lipid metabolism. aPKC, atypical protein kinase C; GSK3, glycogen synthase kinase-3; IGF, insulin-like growth factor; MAP, mitogen-activated protein; PI(3)K, PtdIns-3-kinase; PP1, protein phosphatase 1; PTEN, Phosphatase and tensin homologue deleted on chromosome 10; SHIP2, SH2-domain-containing inositol 5-phosphatase. (From Saltiel AR, Kahn CR. Insulin signalling and the regulation of glucose and lipid metabolism. Nature 2001;414:799-806.)

insulin signaling events. Disruption of IRS1 in mice resulted in mild insulin resistance and growth retardation, whereas disruption of IRS2 resulted in beta cell failure and secondary insulin resistance.[204] Alterations in the phosphorylation and levels of IRS-1 and IRS-2 are found in many insulin-resistant tissues. Serine phosphorylation on IRS proteins is mediated by a variety of kinases, including PKC isoforms and mTOR/S6 kinase. Serine phosphorylation on appropriate residues might increase ubiquination and down-regulation of the protein, which would result in decreased downstream signaling.[205]

PI 3-kinase, which is regulated by interaction with IRS proteins, is necessary but not sufficient for the stimulation of the glucose transporter GLUT4-mediated increase in glucose transport in insulin-sensitive tissues.[206] In addition, inhibition of PI 3-kinase activity with the fungal inhibitor wortmannin inhibited insulin-stimulated glucose uptake, glycogen synthesis, triglyceride accumulation, protein synthesis, and modulation of gene expression.[207] PI 3-kinase generates 3,4,5-phosphoinositol, which activates several PIP3 (phosphatidylinositol-3,4,5 triphosphate)-dependent serine-threonine kinases, such as PI-dependent protein kinases 1 and 2, which in turn activates Akt, salt- and glucocorticoid-induced kinases,[137] PKC, wortmannin-sensitive and insulin-stimulated serine kinase, and others.

Akt kinase (also known as protein kinase B) exists as three distinct isoforms that are activated by phosphorylation on specific threonine and serine residues.[208,209] Activated Akt has the ability to phosphorylate proteins that regulate lipid synthesis, glycogen synthesis, protein synthesis, and apoptosis. Disruption of Akt2 resulted in insulin resistance and diabetes in mice.[210] Several investigators have examined the role of PI 3-kinase and Akt in persons with insulin resistance. Studies have shown a decrease in IRS-associated PI 3-kinase[211] and Akt[212] activity in insulin-resistant skeletal muscle; however, in some patients with reduced PI 3-kinase activity there was normal activation of Akt.[213]

A primary effect of insulin is to stimulate translocation of the glucose transporter GLUT4 from an intracellular pool to the surface of cells, primarily in skeletal muscle and adipose tissue and heart.[214] The mechanism by which the signaling pathways converge on the intracellular GLUT4-containing vesicles to cause GLUT4 translocation is not well understood. It appears that the number of glucose transporters in skeletal muscle of insulin-resistant persons is not changed, but the ability of insulin to effect this translocation is disrupted.[215-217]

Glucocorticoid-Induced Insulin Resistance

Cushing's syndrome and exogenous glucocorticoid treatment have long been known to induce significant insulin resistance in humans. The exact mechanism is unknown, but it is associated with redistribution of fat from the periphery to the central compartment. Elevations in triglyceride and FFA levels also occur. At a molecular level, dexamethasone has differential effects on the proteins involved in the early steps in insulin action in liver and muscle. In both tissues, dexamethasone treatment results in a reduction in insulin-stimulated IRS1-associated PI 3-kinase, which may play a role in the pathogenesis of insulin resistance at the cellular level in these animals. On the basis of studies performed in mice it has been suggested that the effects of glucocorticoids to raise glucose concentrations and cause hypertension are mediated through activation of PPARα receptors in the liver.[218] This is an interesting suggestion, although the relevance of the observation to humans is not currently known.

Tumor Necrosis Factor-α

Studies in humans and in animal models of obesity have identified changes in the expression and activity of key molecules involved in the insulin-signaling pathway. Decreases in the number and the kinase activity of insulin receptors[219] and impairment in the activation of IRS1,[220] PI 3-kinase,[221,222] and protein kinase B[223] have been observed. Although the basis for the changes is, in general, unknown, a tumor necrosis factor α (TNF-α)–mediated mechanism for the decreased activity in the initial steps of the insulin signaling cascade has been proposed. TNF-α, made and secreted by adipocytes, is elevated in a variety of experimental models of obesity.[224] The kinase activity of the insulin receptor in rats[225] or in 3T3-L1 adipocytes[224] treated with TNF-α was reduced, possibly by increased serine phosphorylation.[226] Fat-fed mice with genetic ablation of TNF-α production had increased kinase activity of the insulin receptor compared with control mice and demonstrated increased insulin sensitivity.[227] In addition, rats treated with neutralizing antisera or soluble TNF receptors demonstrated an amelioration of their insulin resistance. As described later, other interventions to decrease TNF-α action result in increased insulin sensitivity.

Glucotoxicity, Glucosamine

Hyperglycemia is a primary factor in the development of the complications of diabetes, and decreases in average blood glucose have a profound effect to prevent complications in both T1DM[228] and T2DM.[229] Hyperglycemia itself can cause insulin resistance. In Pima Indians, the level of fasting glycemia is the primary determinant of insulin sensitivity.[230] The defect is primarily in skeletal muscle[231] and is related to the degree of hyperglycemia.

Entry of glucose into the cell results in its phosphorylation to glucose-6-phosphate, which has multiple metabolic fates. The hexosamine pathway is a relatively minor branch of the glycolytic pathway, encompassing ~3% of total glucose used. The first and rate-limiting enzyme glutamine:fructose 6-phosphate (F-6-*P*) amidotransferase (GFAT), converts F-6-*P* and glutamine to glucosamine 6-phosphate (GlcN-6-*P*) and glutamate. Subsequent steps metabolize GlcN-6-*P* to UDP-*N*-acetylglucosamine (UDP-GlcNAc), UDP-*N*-acetylgalactosamine (UDP-GalNAc), and CMP-syalic acid, essential building blocks of the glycosyl side chains of glycoproteins, glycolipids, proteoglycans, and gangliosides.[232] Evidence suggests that the hexosamine pathway underlies the defect in glucose utilization associated with hyperglycemia. Increased flux through the hexosamine pathway appears to be required for some of the metabolic effects of sustained, increased glucose flux, which promotes the complications of diabetes including diminished expression of sarcoplasmic reticulum Ca^{2+}-ATPase in cardiomyocytes and induction of TGF-β and plasminogen activator inhibitor-1 in vascular smooth muscle cells, mesangial cells, and aortic endothelial cells.[233]

Hexosamines, such as glucosamine, when incubated with adipose tissue, induce insulin resistance in fat cells[234] and in skeletal muscle.[235] Infusion of glucosamine into rats resulted in a dose-dependent increase in insulin resistance of skeletal muscle.[235] Finally, transgenic mice that overexpress GFAT specifically in skeletal muscle acquired severe insulin resistance.[236] By a pathway that is unclear, glucosamine overproduction resulted in a disruption of the ability of insulin to cause translocation of GLUT4 to the cell surface.[237] Through its anti-insulin action, the hexosamine pathway has been hypothesized to be a glucose sensor that allows the cell to sense and adapt to the prevailing level of glucose.[231]

Insulin Resistance and Lipodystrophy Associated with Human Immunodeficiency Virus Infection

A syndrome with many of the clinical and metabolic features of insulin resistance is increasingly being recognized in patients with human immunodeficiency virus (HIV) infection.[238] An unusual form of lipodystrophy is observed in certain of these patients in whom there is significant fat redistribution from the extremities and face to the torso with accumulation of intra-abdominal and intrascapular fat. This form of lipodystrophy is associated with significant insulin resistance and T2DM, dyslipidemia with elevated total and low-density lipoprotein (LDL) cholesterol and suppressed HDL cholesterol concentrations, and a susceptibility to lactic acidemia.[239]

Epidemiologic studies have associated this syndrome with previous or current treatment with antiretroviral protease inhibitors or nucleoside reverse transcriptase inhibitors. There is also an association with increased age.[238] Other possible contributing factors are male sex, diagnosis of the acquired immunodeficiency syndrome (AIDS), responsiveness to antiretroviral treatment, and increases in CD4 T-cell counts. An increased emphasis has been placed on the role of protease inhibitors in the pathogenesis of the syndrome. Administration of these drugs or ritonavir to normal subjects caused increases in plasma triglyceride and very-low-density lipoprotein (VLDL) cholesterol and decreased plasma HDL cholesterol levels.[240] Indinavir administration for 4 weeks resulted in small increases in serum glucose and insulin levels and decreased insulin-mediated glucose disposal as assessed with a hyperinsulinemic euglycemic clamp. In this study there were no changes in lipoprotein, triglycerides, or FFA levels.[241]

The molecular basis of the metabolic syndrome is not clear. A number of protease inhibitors can inhibit glucose transport in vitro and in vivo, and there is evidence for a direct interaction with the GLUT4 glucose transporter[242] that could inhibit glucose uptake specifically in insulin-responsive tissue. Mitochondrial abnormalities have been described in subcutaneous adipose tissue biopsy specimens of HIV-infected patients with lipodystrophy compared with those without the syndrome.[243] A direct effect of protease inhibitors on differentiation of adipocytes has also been described.[244-246] At present, the precise mechanism for the lipodystrophy associated with HIV infection is not known.

Treatment of HIV-associated lipodystrophy is at present inadequate. Using alternative protease inhibitors might improve metabolic abnormalities, particularly those induced or increased by protease inhibitor therapy. However, changing protease inhibitors has little impact on body fat. Switching thymidine analogues has been the only intervention to improve lipoatrophy in different independent studies.[247] Insulin-sensitizing thiazolidinediones have shown mixed results, with improvement in insulin sensitivity but little alteration in fat distribution.[248] More than 75% of patients with HIV who have acute myocardial infarction are older than 55 years. Because of the increased risk of cardiovascular disease, treatment of hyperlipidemia is essential in these patients with HMG-CoA reductase inhibitors and fibrates alone or in combination as first-line drugs.[249,250]

MEASURES TO IMPROVE INSULIN SENSITIVITY

Mechanisms of Reducing Insulin Resistance

The most effective measures to improve insulin sensitivity are weight loss and exercise. Both modalities are effective and can be additive in their ability to improve insulin action. Later in this chapter, the role of these interventions in the treatment of patients with T2DM is discussed. The scientific basis and molecular mechanisms responsible for the improvements in insulin sensitivity seen with these interventions are now summarized.

Mechanisms for Improved Insulin Sensitivity with Weight Loss

Weight loss can be a highly effective treatment for overweight patients with T2DM and other cardiovascular risk factors, and indeed it is advocated as the first line of therapy. Weight loss might also play a role in preventing T2DM.[95,251] In overweight patients with T2DM, weight loss can reduce hepatic glucose production, insulin resistance, and fasting hyperinsulinemia and can improve glycemic control. Weight loss in T2DM is also associated with a reduction in blood pressure and an improvement in the lipid profile. These benefits can occur with as little as 5% to 10% weight loss.[252-254] Moreover, preventing obesity in primates with long-term caloric restriction attenuates the development of insulin resistance.

One possible mechanism for improvements in insulin sensitivity through weight loss may be effects on the pattern of muscle fatty acid metabolism and the accumulation of lipid within muscle. In this context, it would be important to know whether alterations in the pathways of fatty acid utilization in skeletal muscle represent primary defects in obese persons or arise secondarily, after a person has become obese. This question cannot be answered by cross-sectional comparisons of lean and obese subjects. One prospective clinical study indicated that lower rates of lipid oxidation were a predisposing factor for greater weight gain,[163] and collateral studies implicated altered skeletal muscle enzyme activities in impaired lipid oxidation.[176,177] A reduced reliance on lipid oxidation has also been identified as a risk factor for weight regain after weight loss.[178] These data raise the possibility that a potential impairment in the capacity for lipid oxidation may be a primary defect in obesity.

Weight loss can markedly improve insulin-resistant glucose metabolism in skeletal muscle. When the patient's response indicates a substantial acquired or secondary component of obesity-related insulin-resistant glucose metabolism, it is important to determine whether weight loss can modulate patterns of skeletal muscle metabolism of fatty acids, including the content of fat within muscle.

Mechanisms for Improved Insulin Sensitivity with Exercise

Exercise is clearly effective in increasing insulin sensitivity in animals and in humans. There appear to be two separable but related effects of exercise on insulin action. A single bout of exercise can result in an acute increase in insulin-independent glucose transport measurable during and for a relatively short period after exercise.[255-259] Like insulin, exercise and muscle contractions increase glucose transport by translocation of intracellular GLUT4 glucose transporters to the cell surface.[260-262]

Acute Exercise

The signaling pathway leading to the exercise-induced increase in glucose transporter translocation and glucose transport is unknown, although there is ample evidence that the pathway is independent of the insulin-stimulated, receptor-mediated pathway. The effect of exercise and contractions on translocation and transport is additive to the maximal effect of insulin.[255,262-265] Insulin-stimulated glucose transport in muscle is inhibited by specific inhibitors of PI 3-kinase, such as wortmannin, whereas transport or translocation stimulated by muscle contractions is insensitive to these inhibitors.[262-266,267] Stimulation of muscle contractions in situ and exercise do not increase insulin receptor phosphorylation or tyrosine kinase activity, IRS phosphorylation, or PI 3-kinase activity.[261,268] In addition, in many insulin-resistant states the acute exercise-stimulated (but not insulin-stimulated) glucose transport and GLUT4 translocation is normal. This has been demonstrated in the obese, insulin-resistant Zucker rat[269] and in type 2 diabetic patients.[217] Finally, hypoxia, a stimulus for glucose transport that is also independent of the insulin receptor–mediated pathway, is effective in increasing glucose transport in muscle strips from obese, insulin-resistant patients and in patients with T2DM.[270]

The acute effect of exercise and hypoxia may be mediated by AMP-dependent protein kinase (AMPK). AMPK is thought to be a sensor of intracellular energy stores and is activated by increases in intracellular AMP. A stable AMP analogue, 5-amino-4-imidazole carboxamide ribotide (ZMP), can be generated intracellularly from 5-aminoimidazole-4-carboxamide ribonucleoside (AICAR) and can activate AMPK in cells, leading to increased phosphorylation of known substrates for AMPK including 3-hydroxy-3-methylglutaryl CoA reductase, acyl-CoA carboxylase, and creatine kinase.[271] Treatment of incubated skeletal muscle with AICAR resulted in increased glucose uptake and glucose transporter translocation.[272] Similarly, the inclusion of 2 mM AICAR in the perfusate of the rat hind limb resulted in inactivation of ACC, decreases in malonyl CoA levels, and a twofold increase in glucose uptake.[273,274]

The euglycemic clamp technique has been used in conscious rats to demonstrate that infusion of AICAR resulted in a more than twofold increase in glucose utilization. Uptake of the glucose analogue 2-deoxyglucose was also increased twofold in vivo in soleus and gastrocnemius muscles. As with previous studies, this uptake was not associated with PI 3-kinase activation, again indicating a separate pathway from that of insulin.

A second effect of exercise, which becomes evident as the acute effect on glucose transport reverses, is a large increase in the sensitivity of glucose transport to stimulation by insulin.[275-278] This effect is due to translocation of more GLUT4 glucose transporters to the cell surface for any given dose of insulin.[279,280] As with the acute stimulation of transport by exercise, the cellular mechanisms leading to enhanced translocation in response to submaximally effective stimuli are unknown. However, several studies have shown that steps in the insulin-signaling cascade leading to activation of PI 3-kinase are not enhanced after a bout of exercise. There is no change in insulin binding to its receptor,[268,281] insulin stimulation of receptor tyrosine kinase activity,[268,282] increase in insulin-stimulated tyrosine phosphorylation of IRS1,[279] or PI 3-kinase activity associated with IRS1.[261,282]

Exercise Training

Exercise training also results in increases in insulin sensitivity[283,284] and can delay or prevent the onset of T2DM in those at high risk.[285] Using the hyperinsulinemic-euglycemic clamp, Perseghin and coworkers[286] compared exercise training for 45 minutes on a stair-climbing machine 4 days per week for 6 weeks in normal insulin-sensitive subjects and a group of high-risk, insulin-resistant relatives of type 2 diabetics. A 100% increase in insulin sensitivity was seen in both groups without a significant change in body weight. Interestingly, the higher basal and glucose-stimulated insulin release seen in the insulin-resistant subjects was not altered after exercise training. The effect of exercise training on insulin sensitivity has been proposed to be due to up-regulation.

A primary effect of exercise training is to increase glucose transporter number, changes in capillary density, and increases in the number of red, glycolytic (type IIa) fibers as well as the density of mitochondria.[287,288] A reduction in mitochondrial oxidative capacity could underlie the dysregulation of lipid metabolism that results in reduced skeletal muscle glucose metabolism. Expression of nuclear-encoded genes that regulate mitochondrial biogenesis, such as nuclear respiratory factors (NRFs) and PPARγ-coactivator 1α (PGC-1α and PGC-1β), have been shown to be important for both mitochondrial biogenesis and for fiber type selection during development.[167,289] In muscle-specific transgenic mice, PGC-1α promotes muscle fiber-type switching from fast-twitch fibers (glycolytic; type IIa and IIb) to slow-twitch (oxidative; type I), increases mitochondrial density, and improves oxidative capacity.[290] These changes are also observed following exercise training.

Indeed, many of the changes observed following exercise are likely mediated in part through PGC-1α levels and activity. Exercise-induced expression of PGC-1α in skeletal muscle is thought to be mediated through myocyte enhancer factor 2 (MEF2),[291] possibly through its interaction with MEF2[292] and cyclic AMP (cAMP)-response element–binding protein (CREB).[291] PGC-1α itself regulates its own promoter activity in a positive autoregulation loop. Activation of estrogen-related receptor α (Errα) and GA repeat-binding protein α (Gabpa) by PGC-1α appears to mediate much of the effect to increase oxidative phosphorylation gene expression in muscle.[169] Nitric oxide produced by endothelial nitric oxide synthase controls mitochondrial biogenesis,[293] possibly through increased expression of PGC-1α as well as other transcription factors. This process is mediated by cyclic guanosine 3′,5′-phosphate, resulting from activation of "soluble" guanylate cyclase.

The pathway from exercise to activation of PGC-1α has been partially elucidated. Increases in calcium levels activate calcium/calmodulin dependent kinase IV (CaMKIV) and calcineurin. Activated CaMKIV phosphorylates CREB, which increases transcription at CREB-responsive elements in the PGC-1α promoter.[294] Exercise also increases PGC-1α activity via phosphorylation through p38 mitogen-activated protein kinase (MAPK).[295,296] AMP-activated protein kinase (AMPK), which is activated by exercise-induced changes in AMP levels, also increases mitochondrial biogenesis and PGC-1α activity in skeletal muscle,[297-299] but at present there is no evidence that PGC-1α is an AMPK substrate. Other conditions that induce mitochondrial biogenesis also increase PGC-1α promoter activity.

MECHANISMS THAT LINK CARDIOVASCULAR DISEASE AND INSULIN RESISTANCE

The Metabolic Syndrome or Syndrome X

Myocardial infarction, stroke, and nonischemic cardiovascular disease are the cause of death in up to 80% of patients with T2DM. Independent of other risk factors, T2DM increases the risk of cardiovascular morbidity and mortality but also provides a synergistic interaction with other risk factors such as smoking, hypertension, and dyslipidemia.[300] In a Finnish population, diabetes increased the risk of myocardial infarction fivefold,[301] and insulin resistance as measured by elevated fasting insulin levels increased the risk of death from heart disease.[302] Women are particularly vulnerable to the cardiovascular effects of T2DM because they appear to lose the protective effects of estrogen in the premenopausal period.[303,304]

A constellation of metabolic derangements that are often seen in patients with insulin resistance and T2DM are individually associated with an increased risk of cardiovascular disease. These metabolic derangements have been variously designated syndrome X; the dysmetabolic syndrome; hypertension, obesity, non–insulin-dependent diabetes mellitus (NIDDM), dyslipidemia, and atherosclerotic cardiovascular disease (HONDA); or the "deadly quartet."[305,306] The syndrome has also been associated with easily oxidized, small LDL particles; heightened blood-clotting activity (e.g., increased plasminogen activator inhibitor 1); and elevated serum uric acid concentration. The proposed central abnormality associated with syndrome X is insulin resistance. Some of the abnormalities have also been proposed to contribute *to* insulin resistance.

Controversy surrounding the metabolic syndrome has not called into question the clustering of cardiovascular risk factors such as central obesity, dyslipidemia, and hypertension and the association of this clustering with the risk of developing diabetes and cardiovascular disease. The controversy largely focuses on the etiology of the syndrome, how best to define its presence, how clinical decision making should be modified based on those definitions, and whether there are not more effective ways to screen for diabetes and cardiovascular risk.[307]

Perhaps the overriding risk factor for coronary artery disease in insulin resistance and T2DM is the associated dyslipidemia. The profile includes hypertriglyceridemia, low plasma HDL, and small, dense LDL particle concentrations. The percentage of men with T2DM who have abnormal cholesterol levels is not different from that of nondiabetic men with abnormal cholesterol. However, diabetic women have nearly double the rate of hypercholesterolemia[308] and greater changes in other lipid parameters that increase the risk of cardiovascular disease (Fig. 30–9). The physiologic basis for this abnormal lipid profile appears to be overproduction of apolipoprotein B–containing VLDL particles. The apolipoprotein B production by the liver is primarily post-translational[309] and augmented by insulin and by the increased availability of FFAs in the portal circulation,[310-314] probably as a result of increased lipolysis in the visceral adipose tissue.[315-317] Part of the post-translational regulation may be due to insulin and fatty acid–mediated increases in microsomal triglyceride transfer protein levels that catalyze the transfer of lipids to apolipoprotein B and decrease the ubiquination-dependent degradation of apolipoprotein B.[318-320]

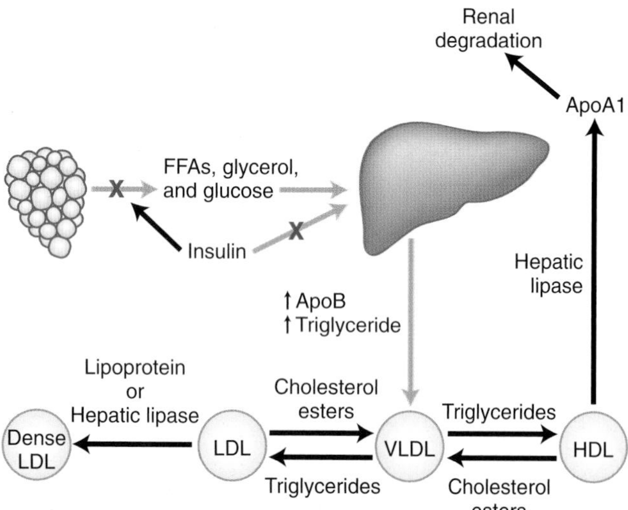

Figure 30–9 ▪ Insulin resistance and dyslipidemia. The suppression of lipoprotein lipase and very-low-density lipoprotein (VLDL) production by insulin is defective in insulin resistance, leading to increased free fatty acid (FFA) flux to the liver and increased VLDL production, which results in increased circulating triglyceride concentrations. The triglycerides are transferred to low-density lipoprotein (LDL) and high-density lipoprotein (HDL), and the VLDL particle gains cholesterol esters by the action of the cholesterol ester transfer protein (CETP). This leads to increased catabolism of HDL particles by the liver and loss of apolipoprotein (Apo) A, resulting in low HDL concentrations. The triglyceride-rich LDL particle is stripped of the triglycerides, resulting in the accumulation of atherogenic small, dense LDL particles.

The overproduction of VLDL triglyceride results in increased transfer of VLDL triglyceride to HDL particles in exchange for HDL cholesterol esters mediated by the cholesterol ester transfer protein.[321] The triglyceride-rich HDL is hydrolyzed by hepatic lipase, which results in the generation of small HDL, which is degraded more readily by the kidney, resulting in low HDL levels in serum. Cholesterol ester transfer protein–mediated exchange of VLDL triglyceride for LDL cholesterol esters and subsequent triglyceride hydrolysis by hepatic lipase probably result in generation of the small, dense LDL particles found in insulin-resistant subjects.[322-325]

The increased risk of heart disease in patients with diabetes has prompted the recommendation that persons with diabetes be treated for their dyslipidemia as aggressively as persons who have had a previous myocardial infarction. In addition, patients with the metabolic syndrome of insulin resistance and obesity are considered to be in a higher risk category and should also be aggressively treated to lower lipids.[326]

Hypertension and overt diabetes double the risk of cardiovascular disease. Defects in vasodilation and alterations in blood flow might provide a link to hypertension in insulin-resistant subjects. The normal vasodilative response of insulin is disrupted in obese, insulin-resistant, and diabetic persons,[327] perhaps through insulin's inability to increase the production of the potent vasodilator nitric oxide by endothelial cells.[328,329] The defect may be magnified by increases in plasma FFAs.[330] Other proposed mechanisms for insulin resistance leading to hypertension are the activation of the sympathetic nervous system by insulin[331-333] and the intrinsic ability of insulin to cause salt and water readsorption in the kidney, resulting in expanded plasma volume.[334-336]

Hypertension itself, independent of other risk factors, has been associated with the propensity to become diabetic.[337] A prospective cohort study found that T2DM was nearly 2.5 times more likely to develop in subjects with hypertension than in subjects with normal blood pressure.[338] A possible mechanism is that an intrinsic defect in vasodilation might contribute to insulin resistance by decreasing the surface area of the vasculature perfusing skeletal muscle, decreasing the efficiency of glucose uptake.[330] Conversely, vasodilative agents might improve glucose uptake and might even prevent the onset of diabetes, as has been observed with angiotensin-converting enzyme (ACE) inhibitor therapy.[339]

Several factors involved in clotting and fibrinolysis, including fibrinogen, factor VII, and plasminogen activator inhibitor 1 (PAI-1), have been shown to be increased in persons with insulin resistance.[340-345] PAI-1 has been extensively studied, and there is a clear relationship between elevated PAI-1 levels and risk of coronary artery disease.[346] Insulin increased PAI-1 expression in hepatocytes, endothelial cells, and abdominal adipose tissue,[347-349] and insulin-sensitizing thiazolidinediones decreased PAI-1 activity.[350]

Upper-body rather than lower-body obesity (the apple rather than the pear shape) is highly correlated with insulin resistance and risk for T2DM. Thus, the anatomic distribution of fat, rather than the overall degree of obesity, appears to determine risk for the metabolic syndrome. The reported association between increased abdominal (upper-body) fat and an increased risk of coronary heart disease is related to visceral fat, for which the waist-to-hip ratio is a convenient index. A waist-to-hip ratio greater than 1.0 in men and greater than 0.8 in women indicates abdominal obesity.[351] The National Cholesterol Education Program (NCEP) has suggested that a waist circumference greater than 40 inches (101.5 cm) in men and greater than 35 inches (89 cm) in women is a marker for the metabolic syndrome.[352]

The Role of Increased Hepatic Glucose Production

The disposal of glucose after meals depends on the ability of insulin to increase peripheral glucose uptake and simultaneously decrease endogenous glucose production. Although studies have suggested that the kidney can contribute up to 25% of endogenous glucose production,[353,354] the defect in T2DM is primarily in defective regulation of glucose production from the liver (hepatic glucose output [HGO]). Two routes of glucose production by the liver are glycogenolysis of stored glycogen and gluconeogenesis from two- and three-carbon substrates derived primarily from skeletal muscle.[355,356] Under different conditions and at different times postprandially, the contribution of each of these to maintenance of glucose levels may vary. Using ^{13}C NMR spectroscopy combined with measurement of whole-body glucose production in normal human subjects at different intervals after fasting, it was found that gluconeogenesis accounted for 50% to 96% of glucose production, and the percentage increased with increasing duration of fasting.[357,358]

The production of glucose by the liver is regulated primarily by the relative actions of glucagon and insulin to activate or suppress glucose production, respectively, although the nervous system[359] and glucose autoregulation of hepatic glucose production probably play less important roles.[360] The ability of insulin to reduce HGO is an important mechanism for maintaining normal glucose tolerance.[361,362] Under normal circumstances, insulin suppresses up to 85% of glucose production in normal persons by directly inhibiting glycogenolysis, especially at lower insulin concentrations.[363] Under circumstances in which glycogenolysis is enhanced by glucagon, the effects of insulin to suppress hepatic glucose production may be even greater.[364] Glucagon increases glycogenolysis by activation of the classic protein kinase cascade involving cAMP-dependent protein kinase and phosphorylase and also increases gluconeogenesis in part by increasing the transcription of phosphoenolpyruvate carboxykinase through the cAMP response element binding protein (CREB).[362,365,366]

Data suggest that the regulatory mechanisms triggered by cAMP are much more complex, with the CREB transcriptional coactivator Torc2 playing an important role. Torc2 is specifically dephosphorylated in response to cAMP, resulting in the translocation of the Torc2 protein to the nucleus, allowing activation of CREB-dependent transcription of gluconeogenic enzymes.[367] In addition, CREB might increase transcription of PGC-1α, which serves as a critical coactivator of the transcription factor Foxol, which also plays a role in the transcriptional activation of various genes associated with gluconeogenesis.[365]

Insulin decreases endogenous glucose production by direct and indirect mechanisms (Fig. 30–10).[368] In its direct action, portal insulin suppresses glucose production by inhibiting glycogenolysis through an increase in phosphodiesterase activity[369,370] or changes in the assembly of protein phosphatase complexes.[371,372] Insulin can also directly suppress gluconeogenesis by inhibiting the activation of phosphoenolpyruvate carboxykinase transcription through the insulin-dependent phosphorylation of the forkhead transcription factor (Foxol and perhaps FoxoA2), sequestering it in the cytoplasm.[373-376]

The indirect or peripheral effect of insulin in controlling glucose production by the liver is twofold. First, insulin has a profound effect on decreasing glucagon secretion by the alpha cell of the pancreas through systemic and paracrine effects.[377,378] The decrease in glucagon secretion decreases the activation of glycogenolysis and gluconeogenesis. The second important peripheral action of insulin is decreasing FFA levels by suppressing lipolysis. FFAs increase hepatic glucose production by stimulating gluconeogenesis.[379] When the reduction in plasma FFAs during a hyperinsulinemic clamp was prevented by infusion of triglyceride emulsions with heparin (which results in increased FFA levels by activation of lipoprotein lipase), insulin-mediated suppression of HGO was reduced.[355,380] The suppression of glucagon secretion and decrease in FFA delivery to the liver are additive in reducing liver glucose production.[381]

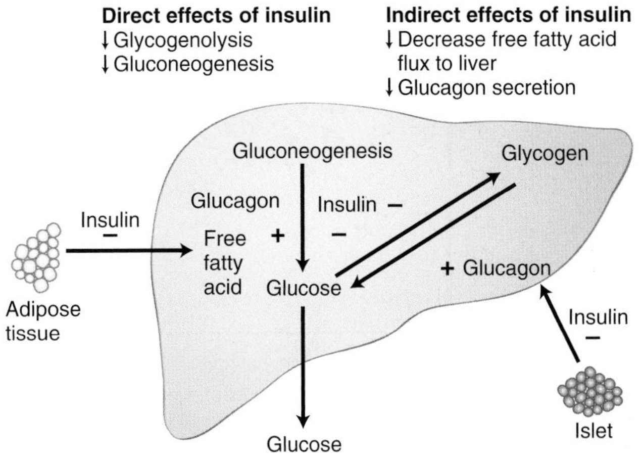

Direct effects of insulin
↓ Glycogenolysis
↓ Gluconeogenesis

Indirect effects of insulin
↓ Decrease free fatty acid flux to liver
↓ Glucagon secretion

Gluconeogenesis
Glycogen
Glucagon
Insulin –
Insulin
–
Free fatty acid +
–
+ Glucagon
Glucose
Adipose tissue
Insulin
–
Islet
Glucose

Figure 30–10 ▪ Insulin suppresses hepatic glucose production by direct and indirect mechanisms. In insulin resistance, insulin's ability to suppress lipolysis in adipose tissue and glucagon secretion by alpha cells in the islet results in increased gluconeogenesis. In addition, insulin inhibition of glycogenolysis is impaired. Thus, both hepatic and peripheral insulin resistance results in abnormal glucose production by the liver.

Hepatic insulin resistance plays an important role in the hyperglycemia of T2DM,[382-385] and the impairment in suppression of HGO appears to be quantitatively similar to or even larger than the defect in the stimulation of peripheral glucose disposal.[383,386] There is a direct relationship between increases in HGO and fasting hyperglycemia (Fig. 30–11).[86] Insulin-mediated suppression of HGO is impaired at both low and high plasma insulin levels in type 2 diabetic patients,[386,387-389] and hepatic glucose production is elevated early in the course of the disease[390] but it may be normal in lean, relatively insulin-sensitive type 2 diabetics.[390] Treatment of patients with metformin, which suppresses hepatic glucose production, results in improvements in glucose tolerance.[391]

Alterations in both the direct and indirect effects of insulin in type 2 diabetics appear to play a role in the elevation in hepatic glucose production. Defects in the direct effect of insulin to suppress hepatic glucose production that have been demonstrated in humans[392] appear to be due to a large rightward shift in the steep dose-response curve for insulin's inhibition of glycogenolysis.[393] However, peripheral insulin resistance might play the bigger role in elevated hepatic glucose production in T2DM. The resistance of adipose tissue, especially visceral fat, to suppression of lipolysis by insulin is responsible for part of insulin's inability to suppress hepatic glucose production by the indirect route, resulting in enhanced gluconeogenesis.[394,395] In addition, the suppression of glucagon levels in humans with insulin resistance may be impaired, again leading to an increase in endogenous glucose production.[396]

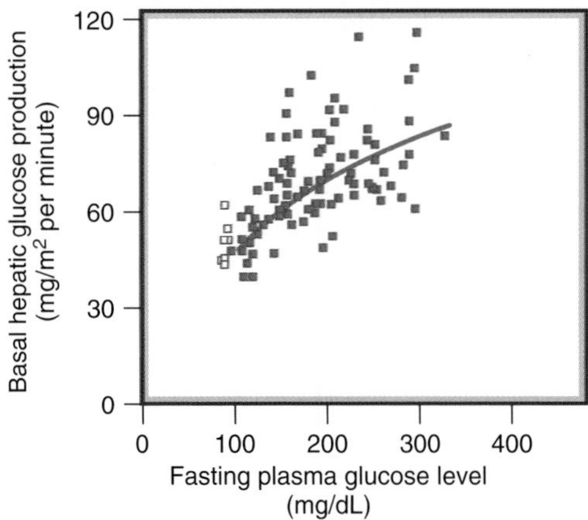

Figure 30–11 ▪ Relationship between fasting hepatic glucose output and fasting plasma glucose levels. *Open squares* represent nondiabetic control subjects; *closed squares* represent diabetic subjects. (From Maggs DG, Buchanan TA, Burant CF, et al. Metabolic effects of troglitazone monotherapy in type 2 diabetes mellitus: a randomized, double-blind, placebo-controlled trial. Ann Intern Med 1998;128:176-185.)

Central Control of Glucose Metabolism

The hypothalamus and perhaps other brain regions can sense metabolic requirements and change peripheral metabolism. Studies by Rossetti and colleagues suggest that uptake of fatty acids by the mediobasal hypothalamus decreases feeding behavior and decreases hepatic glucose production via central nervous system (CNS) efferents.[397] Inhibition of fatty acid oxidation results in decreased food intake and reduction in glucose production, suggesting that buildup of long-chain fatty acids or their derivatives change feeding and hepatic glucose production.

AMPK might also play a role in integrating CNS nutrient supply. AMPK is activated by cellular AMP levels and is thus a sensor of energy supply.[398] Higher cellular energy, due to glucose or fatty acid surfeit, would lead to decreased activation of AMPK and its downstream target acetyl-CoA carboxylase (ACC). ACC generates malonyl CoA (an allosteric inhibitor of CPT-1), which would decrease the entry of long-chain fatty acids into the mitochondria, resulting in their buildup in the cytoplasm.

Cytokines and Insulin Sensitivity

Adipose tissue is classically viewed as simply the site for storage of excess energy in the form of triglycerides. However, it is now clear that adipose tissue secretes a variety of endocrine and paracrine factors that have significant effects on metabolism.[399] These adipokines regulate a diverse array of actions, including alterations in feeding behavior; changes in liver, muscle, and adipose tissue insulin sensitivity; vascular reactivity; and atherosclerosis progression.

Leptin

Leptin is a 16-kd protein synthesized mainly in adipose tissue and is mutated in ob/ob mice. Leptin suppresses feeding behavior, and humans with mutations in leptin are morbidly obese and insulin resistant. However, studies from a number of laboratories, using in vitro and in vivo models, indicate a direct role for leptin in lipid metabolism, including increased metabolic rate, lipolysis, stimulation of fatty acid oxidation, inhibition of lipogenesis, and increases in AMPK activity.

Adiponectin

Adiponectin (ACRP30, adipoQ, apM1, or GBP28) is a 30-kd protein that is synthesized and secreted from adipocytes and circulates as a trimer and as multimeric complexes (called the *HMW form*). The HMW form may be further cleaved to forms that may be the active transducer of signaling. The purported receptor for adiponectin is controversial, so its exact signaling mechanism remains uncertain. In the mouse, adiponectin can increase fatty acid oxidation, perhaps through the activation of AMPK.[400,401] Disruption of adiponectin in mice predisposes them to high-fat diet–induced insulin resistance, though there little alteration in mice consuming a normal diet.[402] Adiponectin levels are low in humans with obesity and insulin resistance and are increased by insulin-sensitizing PPARγ agonists.

Resistin

Resistin is a 12-kd protein that is synthesized and secreted from adipose tissue and is a member of the FIZZ family of proteins, which are C-terminal cysteine-rich proteins.[403,404] As with adiponectin, resistin circulates in both trimeric and hexameric forms, with the smaller form having greater activity.[142] Resistin levels are elevated in both diet-induced obesity and genetic mouse models of obesity and diabetes. Leptin causes hepatic insulin resistance, and disruption of resitin results in lowered ambient glucose levels. The role of resistin in human physiology remains uncertain.[405]

Tumor Necrosis Factor-α

TNF-α is a 26-kd transmembrane protein, which is cleaved and circulates in a 17-kd soluble form. Elaborated by multiple tissues, including adipocytes, its role in insulin resistance is unclear. It might work primarily as a paracrine effector to induce tissue insulin resistance.[406] Data suggest that much of TNF-α, along with other inflammatory cytokines associated with adipose tissue, is elaborated by resident macrophages as well as adipocytes.[407,408] TNF-α has two main receptors, type 1 and type 2, which signal through the p44/42 and JNK pathway. Systemic effects on TNF-α include the induction of lipogenesis in the liver and insulin resistance in skeletal muscle.

Monocyte Chemotactic Protein-1

Monocyte chemotatic protein-1 (MCP-1) C-C motif chemokine ligand-2 (CCL2) is increased in proportion to adipose tissue mass and correlates with insulin resistance.[409] CCL2 inhibits insulin action and adipocyte differentiation.[410] The receptor for MCP-1 C-C motif chemokine receptor-2 (CCR2) regulates monocyte and macrophage recruitment and is necessary for macrophage-dependent inflammatory responses. Disruption of CCR2 in mice reduced their food intake, attenuated the development of obesity following a high-fat diet, and attenuated the infiltration of macrophages into adipose tissue, further supporting the concept that adipose-resident macrophages are important for their systemic effect of adipocity.[411]

Interleukin-6

IL-6 is a glycoprotein of 22 to 27 kd that circulates at relatively high concentrations. Circulating levels correlate with the degree of adiposity.[412] Humans receiving IL-6 infusions show increases in insulin resistance, hepatic glucose production, lipolysis, and fatty acid oxidation.[413] About a third of circulating IL-6 is secreted by adipocytes; however, a significant amount is elaborated by skeletal muscle and is increased by exercise. The lipolytic effect of IL-6 might link exercise to the mobilization of fatty acids.[166]

INSULIN SECRETION AND TYPE 2 DIABETES

Normal insulin secretory function is essential for maintaining normal glucose tolerance, and abnormal insulin secretion is invariably present in patients with T2DM. In this section, the physiology of normal insulin and the alterations that are present in persons with T2DM are reviewed.

Quantitation of Beta Cell Function

The measurement of peripheral insulin concentrations by radioimmunoassay is still the most widely used method for quantifying beta cell functions in vivo.[414] Although this approach provides valuable information, it is limited because 50% to 60% of the insulin produced by the pancreas is extracted by the liver without ever reaching the systemic circulation.[415,416] The standard radioimmunoassay for measuring insulin concentrations is also unable to distinguish between endogenous and exogenous insulin, making it ineffective as a measure of endogenous beta cell reserve in the insulin-treated diabetic patient. Anti-insulin antibodies that may be present in patients treated with insulin interfere with the insulin radioimmunoassay, making insulin measurements in insulin-treated patients inaccurate. Conventional insulin radioimmunoassays are also unable to distinguish between levels of circulating proinsulin and true levels of circulating insulin.

Insulin is derived from a single-chain precursor, proinsulin.[417] Within the Golgi apparatus of the pancreatic beta cell, proinsulin is cleaved by convertases to form insulin, C peptide, and two pairs of basic amino acids. Insulin is subsequently released into the circulation at concentrations equimolar with those of C peptide.[418,419] In addition, small amounts of intact proinsulin and proinsulin conversion intermediates are released. Proinsulin and its related conversion intermediates can be detected in the circulation, where they constitute 20% of the total circulating insulin-like immunoreactivity.[420] In vivo, proinsulin has a biologic potency that is only about 10% of that of insulin[421,422] and the potency of split proinsulin intermediates is between those of proinsulin and insulin.[423,424] C peptide has no known conclusive effects on carbohydrate metabolism,[425,426] although certain physiologic effects of C peptide have been proposed.[427] Unlike insulin, C peptide is not extracted by the liver[418,428,429] and is excreted almost exclusively by the kidneys. Its plasma half-life of approximately 30 minutes[430] contrasts sharply with that of insulin, which is approximately 4 minutes.

Because C peptide is secreted in equimolar concentrations with insulin and is not extracted by the liver, many investigators have used levels of C peptide as a marker of beta cell function. The use of plasma C peptide levels as an index of beta cell function depends on the critical assumption that the mean clearance rates of C peptide are constant over the range of C peptide levels observed under normal physiologic conditions. This assumption has been shown to be valid for both dogs and humans,[416,431] and this approach can be used to derive rates of insulin secretion from plasma concentrations of C peptide under steady-state conditions.[431] However, because of the long plasma half-life of C peptide, under non–steady-state conditions (e.g., after a glucose infusion) peripheral plasma levels of C peptide do not change in proportion to the changing insulin secretion rate.[431,432] Thus, under these conditions, insulin secretion rates are best calculated with use of the two-compartment model initially proposed by Eaton and coworkers.[433]

Modifications to the C peptide model of insulin secretion have been introduced. This approach combines the minimal model of insulin action with the two-compartment model of C peptide kinetics and allows insulin secretion and insulin sensitivity to be derived after either intravenous or oral administration of glucose.[434-437]

Signaling Pathways in the Beta Cell and Insulin Secretion

The signaling pathways in the pancreatic beta cell that are involved in the stimulus-secretion coupling of insulin release. These pathways provide the mechanism whereby insulin secretion rates respond to changes in blood glucose concentrations (Figure 30–12). Glucose enters the pancreatic beta cell by a process of facilitated diffusion mediated by the glucose transporter GLUT2. Although levels of GLUT2 on the beta cell membrane are reduced in diabetic states for various reasons, it is not currently believed that this is a rate-limiting step in the regulation of insulin secretion.

The first rate-limiting step in this process is the phosphorylation of glucose to glucose-6-phosphate. This reaction is mediated by the enzyme glucokinase.[438,439] There is considerable evidence that glucokinase, by determining the rate of glycolysis, functions as the glucose sensor of the beta cell and that this is the primary mechanism whereby the rate of insulin secretion adapts to changes in blood glucose. According to this view, as blood glucose levels increase, more glucose enters the beta cell, the rate of glycolysis increases, and the rate of insulin secretion increases. A fall in blood glucose levels results in a fall in the rate of glycolysis and a reduction in the rate of insulin secretion.

Glucose metabolism produces an increase in cytosolic ATP, the key signal that initiates insulin secretion by causing blockade of the ATP-dependent K+ channel (K_{ATP}) on the beta cell membrane. Blockade of this channel induces membrane depolarization, which leads to an increase in cytosolic Ca^{2+} and insulin secretion. The biochemical events that link the increase in glycolysis to an increase in ATP are complex. Dukes and coworkers[440] proposed the glycolytic production of NADH during the oxidation of glyceraldehyde-3-phosphate as the key process because NADH is subsequently processed into ATP by mitochondria through the operation of specific shuttle systems.

The rate of pyruvate generation has also been proposed as an explanation for the link between glucose metabolism and the increase in insulin secretion.[441] According to this view, pyruvate generated by the glycolytic pathway enters the mitochondria and is metabolized further in the TCA cycle. Electron transfer from the TCA cycle to the respiratory chain by NADH and reduced flavin adenine dinucleotide ($FADH_2$) promotes the generation of ATP, which is exported into the cytosol. The increase in ATP closes ATP-sensitive K^+ channels, which depolarizes the beta cell membrane and opens the voltage-dependent Ca^{2+} channels, leading to an increase in intracellular Ca^{2+}. The increase in cytosolic Ca^{2+} is the main trigger for exocytosis, the process by which insulin-containing secretory granules fuse with the plasma membrane, leading to the release of insulin into the circulation. The increase in ATP not only closes K_{ATP} channels but also serves as a major permissive factor for movement of insulin granules and for priming of exocytosis.

Cyclic AMP also plays an important role in beta cell signal transduction pathways. This second messenger is generated at the plasma membrane from ATP and potentiates glucose-stimulated insulin secretion, particularly in response to glucagon, glucagon-like peptide 1 (GLP-1), and gastric inhibitory polypeptide. The cAMP-dependent pathways appear to be particularly important in the exocytotic machinery.

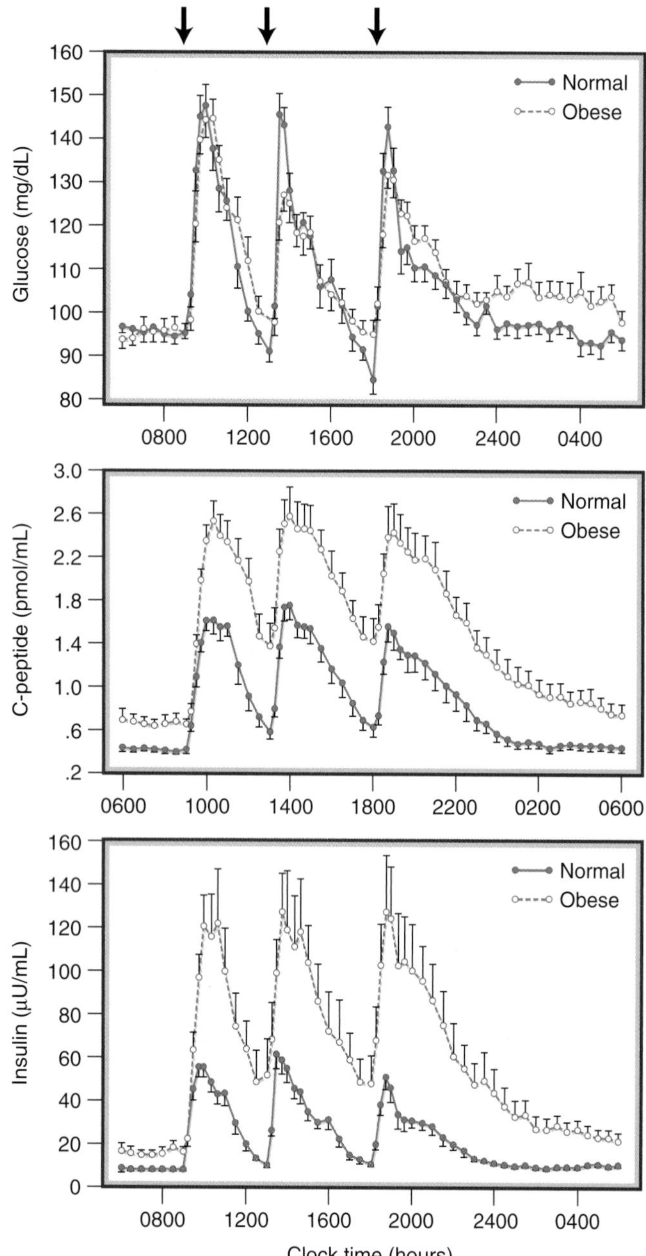

Figure 30–12 ▪ Mean 24-hour profiles of plasma concentrations of glucose *(top panel)*, C peptide *(middle panel)*, and insulin *(bottom panel)* in normal and obese subjects. (From Polonsky KS, Given BD, van Cauter E. Twenty-four-hour profiles and pulsatile patterns of insulin secretion in normal and obese subjects. J Clin Invest 1988;81: 442-448.)

K_{ATP} channels play an essential role in beta cell stimulus-secretion coupling. The reader is directed to an excellent review for more complete information.[442] K_{ATP} channels include sulfonylurea receptors (SURs) and potassium inward rectifiers, KIR6.1 and KIR6.2, which assemble to form a large octameric channel with a (SUR/KIR6.x) stoichiometry. In the pancreatic beta cell, the SUR1/KIR6.2 pairs constitute the K_{ATP} channel. K_{ATP} channels control the flux of potassium ions driven by an electrochemical potential. Opening these channels can set the resting membrane potential of beta cells below the threshold for activation of voltage-gated Ca^{2+} channels when plasma glucose levels are low, thus reducing insulin secretion. Changes in the cytosolic concentrations of ATP and adenosine diphosphate (ADP) as summarized earlier lead to closure of the channels and depolarization of the beta cell membrane. Mutations in both components of the beta cell K_{ATP}, SUR1, and KIR6.2 have been shown to lead to hypersecretion of insulin, resulting clinically in either a recessive form of familial hyperinsulinemia or persistent hyperinsulinemic hypoglycemia of infancy.

Physiologic Factors Regulating Insulin Secretion

Carbohydrate Nutrients

The most important physiologic substance involved in the regulation of insulin release is glucose.[443-445] The effect of glucose on the beta cell is dose related. Dose-dependent increases in concentrations of insulin and C peptide and in rates of insulin secretion have been observed after oral and intravenous glucose loads, with 1.4 units of insulin, on average, being secreted in response to an oral glucose load as small as 12 g.[446-449] The insulin secretory response is greater after oral than after intravenous glucose administration.[450-452] Known as the incretin effect,[448,453] this enhanced response to oral glucose has been interpreted as an indication that absorption of glucose by way of the gastrointestinal tract stimulates the release of hormones and other mechanisms that ultimately enhance the sensitivity of the beta cell to glucose (see following discussion of hormonal factors). In a study involving nine normal volunteers in whom glucose was infused at a rate designed to achieve levels previously attained after an oral glucose load, the amount of insulin secreted in response to the intravenous load was 26% less than that secreted in response to the oral load.[452]

Insulin secretion does not respond as a linear function of glucose concentration. The relationship of glucose concentration to the rate of insulin release follows a sigmoidal curve, with a threshold corresponding to the glucose levels normally seen under fasting conditions and with the steep portion of the dose-response curve corresponding to the range of glucose levels normally achieved postprandially.[454-456] The sigmoidal nature of the dose-response curve has been attributed to a gaussian distribution of thresholds for stimulation among the individual beta cells.[456-458]

When glucose is infused intravenously at a constant rate, an initial biphasic secretory response is observed that consists of a rapid, early insulin peak followed by a second, more slowly rising peak.[443,459,460] The significance of the first-phase insulin release is unclear, but it might reflect the existence of a compartment of readily releasable insulin within the beta cell or a transient rise and fall of a metabolic signal for insulin secretion.[461] Despite early suggestions to the contrary,[462,463] a subsequent study demonstrated that the first-phase response to intravenous glucose is highly reproducible within subjects.[464] After the acute response, a second phase of insulin release occurs that is directly related to the level of glucose elevation. In vitro studies of isolated islet cells and the perfused pancreas have identified a third phase of insulin secretion commencing 1.5 to 3.0 hours after exposure to glucose and characterized by a spontaneous decline in secretion to 15% to 25% of the amount released during peak secretion, a level subsequently maintained for more than 48 hours.[465-468]

In addition to its acute secretagogue effects on insulin secretion, glucose has intermediate- and longer-term effects that are physiologically and clinically relevant. In the intermediate term, exposure of the pancreatic beta cell to a high concentration of glucose primes its response to a subsequent glucose stimulus, leading to a shift to the left in the dose-response curve relating glucose and insulin secretion.[469,470] However, when pancreatic islets are exposed to high concentrations for prolonged periods, a reduction of insulin secretion is seen. Although all the precise mechanisms responsible for these adverse effects that have been termed *glucotoxicity* are not known, there is evidence that long-term exposure to high glucose reduces expression of a number of genes that are critical to normal beta cell function, including the insulin gene.[471,472]

Noncarbohydrate Nutrients

Amino acids have been shown to stimulate insulin release in the absence of glucose, the most potent secretagogues being the essential amino acids leucine, arginine, and lysine.[473,474] The effects of arginine and lysine on the beta cell appear to be more potent than that of leucine. The effects of amino acids on insulin secretion are potentiated by glucose.[475,476]

In contrast to amino acids, various lipids and their metabolites appear to have only minor effects on insulin release in vivo. Although carbohydrate-rich fat meals stimulate insulin secretion, carbohydrate-free fat meals have minimal effects on beta cell function.[477] Ketone bodies and short- and long-chain fatty acids have been shown to stimulate insulin secretion acutely both in islet cells and in humans.[478-482] The effects of elevated FFAs in the insulin secretory responses to glucose are related to the duration of the exposure. Zhou and Grill[483] first suggested that long-term exposure of pancreatic islets to FFAs inhibited glucose-induced insulin secretion and biosynthesis. This observation has been confirmed in rats.[484] In humans, it was demonstrated that the insulin resistance induced by an acute (90-minute) elevation in FFAs was compensated for by an appropriate increase in insulin secretion.[485] After chronic elevation of FFAs (48 hours), the beta cell compensatory response for insulin resistance was not adequate. Additional studies have demonstrated that the adverse effects of prolonged FFAs on glucose-induced insulin secretion are not seen in subjects with T2DM. From these results, it appears that elevated FFAs might contribute to the failure of beta cell compensation for insulin resistance.

Hormonal Factors

The release of insulin from the beta cell after a meal is facilitated by a number of gastrointestinal peptide hormones, including glucose-dependent insulinotropic peptide (GIP), cholecystokinin, and GLP-1.[453,486-493] These hormones are released from small intestinal endocrine cells postprandially and travel in the bloodstream to reach the beta cells, where they act through second messengers to increase the sensitivity of these islet cells to glucose. In general, these hormones are not themselves secretagogues, and their effects are evident only in the presence of hyperglycemia.[486-488] The release of these peptides might explain why the modest postprandial glucose levels achieved in normal subjects in vivo have such a dramatic effect on insulin production, whereas similar glucose concentrations in vitro elicit a much smaller response.[493] Similarly, this incretin effect could account for the greater beta cell response observed after oral as opposed to intravenous glucose administration.

Whether impaired postprandial secretion of incretin hormones plays a role in the inadequate insulin secretory response to oral glucose and to meals in IGT or diabetes is controversial,[494-501] but pharmacologic doses of these peptides might have future therapeutic benefit. Subcutaneous administration of GLP-1, the most potent of the incretin peptides, lowers glucose in type 2 diabetic patients by stimulating endogenous insulin secretion and perhaps by inhibiting glucagon secretion and gastric empyting.[502,503] Because of its short half-life, however, its longer-acting analogue, exendin-4, has greater therapeutic promise.[504] Treatment with supraphysiologic doses of GIP during hyperglycemia has been shown to augment insulin secretion in normal humans[505,506] but not in diabetic humans.[497,506] Although cholecystokinin has the ability to augment insulin secretion in humans, whether it is an incretin at physiologic levels is not firmly established.[507-510] Its effects are also seen largely at pharmacologic doses.[511]

The postprandial insulin secretory response may also be influenced by other intestinal peptide hormones, including vasoactive intestinal polypeptide,[512] secretin,[513-516] and gastrin,[513,517] but the precise role of these hormones remains to be elucidated.

The hormones produced by pancreatic alpha and beta cells also modulate insulin release. Whereas glucagon has a stimulatory effect on the beta cell,[518] somatostatin suppresses insulin release.[519] It is currently unclear whether these hormones reach the beta cell by traveling through the islet cell interstitium (thus exerting a paracrine effect) or through islet cell capillaries. Indeed, the importance of these two hormones in regulating basal and postprandial insulin levels under normal physiologic circumstances is in doubt. Paradoxically, the low insulin levels observed during prolonged periods of starvation have been attributed to the elevated glucagon concentrations seen in this setting.[477,520-523] Other hormones that exert a stimulatory effect on insulin secretion include growth hormone,[524] glucocorticoids,[525] prolactin,[526-528] placental lactogen,[529] and the sex steroids.[530]

Whereas all of the preceding hormones might stimulate insulin secretion indirectly by inducing a state of insulin resistance, some might also act directly on the beta cell, possibly to augment its sensitivity to glucose. Thus, hyperinsulinemia is associated with conditions in which these hormones are present in excess, such as acromegaly, Cushing's syndrome, and the second half of pregnancy. Furthermore, treatments with placental lactogen,[531] hydrocortisone,[532] and growth hormone[532,533] are all effective in reversing the reduction in insulin response to glucose that is observed in vitro after hypophysectomy. Although hyperinsulinemia after an oral glucose load has been observed in patients with hyperthyroidism,[534,535] the increased concentration of immunoreactive insulin in this setting might reflect elevations in serum proinsulin rather than a true increase in serum insulin.[536]

Neural Factors

The islets are innervated by both the cholinergic and adrenergic limbs of the autonomic nervous system. Although both sympathetic stimulation and parasympathetic stimulation enhance secretion of glucagon,[537,538] the secretion of insulin is stimulated by vagal nerve fibers and inhibited by sympathetic nerve fibers.[537-542] Adrenergic inhibition of the beta cell appears to be mediated by the α-adrenoceptor because its effect is attenuated by the α-antagonist phentolamine[538] and reproduced by the α_2-agonist clonidine.[543] There is also considerable evidence that many indirect effects of sympathetic nerve stimulation play a role in regulating beta cell function through stimulation or inhibition of somatostatin, β_2-adrenoceptors, and neuropeptides galanin and neuropeptide Y.[544]

Parasympathetic stimulation of islets results in stimulation of insulin, glucagon, and pancreatic polypeptide directly and through the neuropeptides vasoactive intestinal polypeptide (VIP), gastrin-releasing polypeptide, and pituitary adenylate cyclase–activating polypeptide.[544] In addition, sensory innervation of islets might play a role in tonic inhibition of insulin secretion through the neuropeptides calcitonin gene–related peptide[545-547] and, less clearly, substance P.[548,549]

The importance of the autonomic nervous system in regulating insulin secretion in vivo is unclear. The neural effects on beta cell function cannot be entirely dissociated from the hormonal effects because some of the neurotransmitters of the autonomic nervous system are, in fact, hormones. Furthermore, the secretion of insulinotropic hormones such as GIP and GLP-1 postprandially has been shown to be under vagal[550,551] and adrenergic[552,553] control.

Temporal Pattern of Insulin Secretion

It has been estimated that in any 24-hour period, 50% of the total insulin secreted by the pancreas is secreted under basal conditions and the remainder is secreted in response to meals.[554,555] The estimated basal insulin secretion rates range from 18 to 32 units per 24 hours (0.7 to 1.3 mg).[431,433,446,554] After meal ingestion, the insulin secretory response is rapid, and insulin secretion increases approximately fivefold over baseline to reach a peak within 60 minutes (Fig. 30–13; see Fig. 30–12). In these studies, subjects consumed 20% of calories with breakfast and 40% with lunch and dinner, respectively. However, the amount of insulin secreted after each meal did not differ significantly. The rapidity of the insulin secretory response to breakfast is underscored by the fact that 71.6% ± 1.6% of the insulin secreted in the 4 hours after the meal was produced in the first 2 hours and the remainder in the next 2 hours. Insulin secretion did not decrease as rapidly after lunch and dinner, and 62.8% ± 1.6% and 59.6% ± 1.4% of the total meal response was secreted in the first 2 hours after these meals.

The normal insulin secretory profile is characterized by a series of insulin secretory pulses. After breakfast, 1.8 ± 0.2 secretory pulses were identified in normal volunteers, and the peaks of these pulses occurred 42.8 ± 3.4 minutes after the meal. Multiple insulin secretory pulses were also identified after lunch and dinner. After these meals, up to four pulses of insulin secretion were identified in both groups of subjects. Thus, in the 5-hour time interval between lunch and dinner, an average of 2.5 ± 0.3 secretory pulses were identified, and 2.6 ± 0.2 were identified in the same period after dinner.

Pulses of insulin secretion that did not appear to be meal-related were also identified. Between 11:00 PM and 6:00 AM and in the 3 hours before breakfast, on average 3.9 ± 0.3 secretory pulses were present in normal subjects. Thus, over the 24-hour period of observation, a total of 11.1 ± 0.5 pulses were identified in normal subjects. Close to 90% (87% ± 3%) of postmeal pulses in insulin secretion, but only 47% ± 8% of non–meal-related pulses, were concomitant with a pulse in glucose.

In vivo studies of beta cell secretory function have demonstrated that insulin is released in a pulsatile manner. This behavior is characterized by rapid oscillations occurring every 8 to 15 minutes that are superimposed on slower (ultradian) oscillations occurring at a periodicity of 80 to 150 minutes.[556] The rapid oscillations persist in vitro and are therefore likely to be the result of metabolic pathways in the pancreatic beta cell that involve negative feedback loops with time lags.

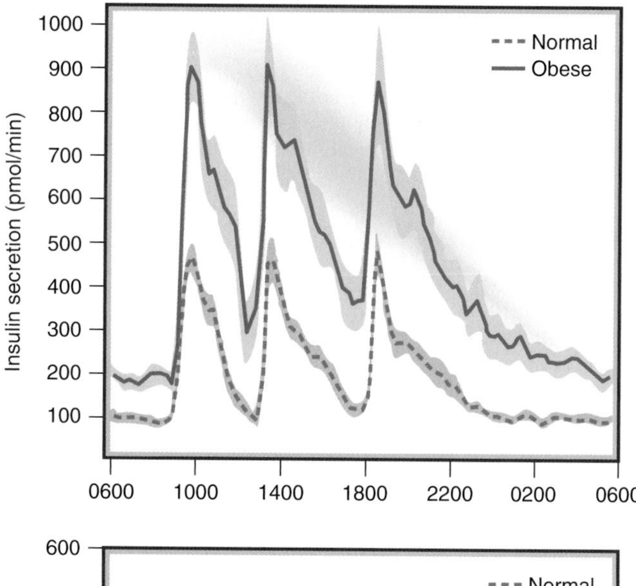

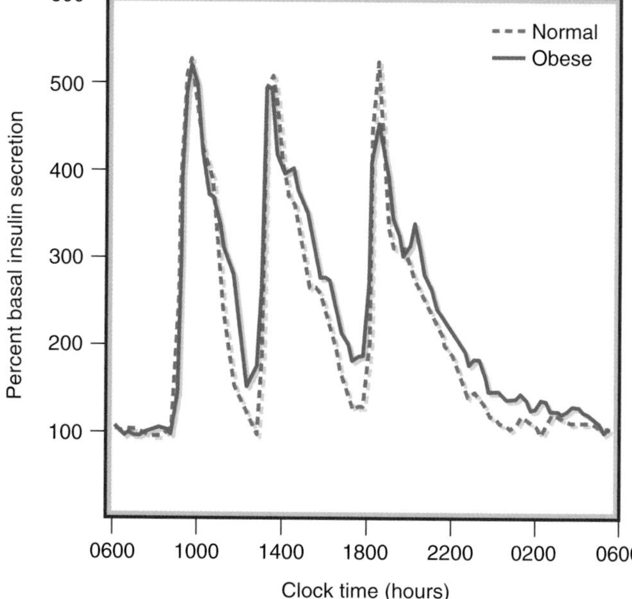

Figure 30–13 ▪ Mean 24-hour profiles of insulin secretion rates in normal and obese subjects *(top)*. The *hatched areas* represent ±1 standard error of the mean. The curves in the *lower panel* were derived by dividing the insulin secretion rate measured in each subject by the basal secretion rate derived in the same subject. Mean data for the normal *(dashed line)* and obese *(solid line)* subjects are shown. (From Polonsky KS, Given BD, van Cauter E. Twenty-four-hour profiles and pulsatile patterns of insulin secretion in normal and obese subjects. J Clin Invest 1988;81:442-448.)

Rapid Oscillations

The rapid oscillations of insulin are of small amplitude in the systemic circulation, averaging between 0.4 and 3.2 μU/mL in several published human studies.[557-559] Because these values are close to the limits of sensitivity of most standard insulin radioimmunoassays, the characterization of these oscillations is subject to considerable pitfalls,[560] not the least of which is the need to differentiate between true oscillations of small amplitude and random assay noise. The latter problem has been overcome by the development of extremely sensitive enzyme-linked immunosorbent assays that allow the detection of extremely small changes in peripheral insulin concentrations. The application of these assays in studies involving frequent sampling from the peripheral circulation has led to a series of studies of the role of these oscillations in the overall regulation of insulin secretion.[561-565]

These studies have suggested that increases in overall insulin secretion seen in response to a variety of secretagogues in various physiologic and pathophysiologic states are due to an increase in the amplitude of the bursts of insulin secretion. The studies have proposed that 75% of insulin secretion is accounted for by secretory bursts and that the responses to GLP-1, sulfonylureas, and oral glucose are all mediated by an increase in the amplitude of insulin secretory pulses. Furthermore, consistent with observations made by O'Rahilly and colleagues,[566] relatives of patients with T2DM demonstrate a disorderly profile of the insulin secretory oscillations. A number of mathematical programs have been developed that allow these insulin secretory oscillations to be evaluated and studied.[567] The latest addition to the list is ApEn and cross ApEn, which are statistics that measure temporal regularity of the oscillations in the insulin secretory profile.[568]

The low amplitude of the rapid oscillations in the systemic circulation contrasts sharply with observations in the portal vein, where pulse amplitudes of 20 to 40 μU/mL have been recorded in dogs.[569] Although the physiologic importance of these low-amplitude rapid pulses in the periphery is unclear, they are likely to be of physiologic importance in the portal vein. It is possible that the liver responds more readily to insulin delivered in a pulsatile fashion than to insulin delivered at a constant rate.[570-572]

Ultradian Oscillations

In contrast to the rapid oscillations, the slower (ultradian) oscillations are of much larger amplitude in the peripheral circulation. They are present under basal conditions but are amplified postprandially (Fig. 30–14) and have been observed in subjects receiving intravenous glucose, suggesting that they are not generated by intermittent absorption of nutrients from the gut. Furthermore, they do not appear to be related to fluctuations in glucagon or cortisol levels[465] and are not regulated by neural factors because these oscillations are also present in recipients of successful pancreas transplants.[573,574] Many of these ultradian insulin and C peptide pulses are synchronous with pulses of similar oscillatory period in glucose, raising the possibility that these oscillations are a product of the insulin-glucose feedback mechanism. Ultradian oscillations are self-sustained during constant glucose infusion at various rates, they are increased in amplitude after stimulation of insulin secretion without change in frequency, and there is a slight temporal advance of the glucose versus the insulin oscillation.

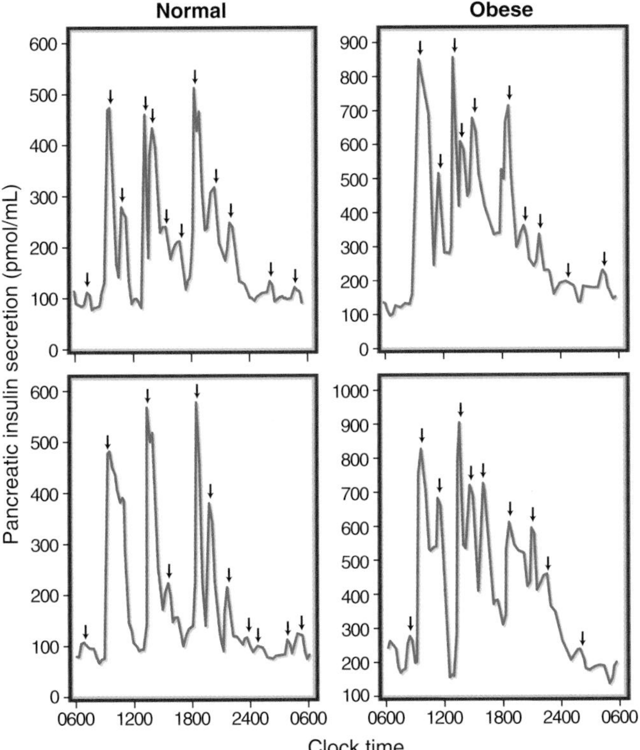

Figure 30–14 ▪ Patterns of insulin secretion in normal and obese subjects. Four representative 24-hour profiles are shown from two normal-weight subjects *(left)* and two obese subjects *(right)*. Meals were consumed at 0900, 1300, and 1800 hours. Statistically significant pulses of secretion are shown by the *arrows*. (From Polonsky KS, Given BD, van Cauter E. Twenty-four-hour profiles and pulsatile patterns of insulin secretion in normal and obese subjects. J Clin Invest 1988;81: 442-448.)

These findings suggest that the ultradian oscillations may be entirely accounted for by the major dynamic characteristics of the insulin-glucose feedback system, with no need to postulate the existence of an intrapancreatic pacemaker.[575] In support of this hypothesis, Sturis and colleagues[576] demonstrated that when glucose is administered in an oscillatory pattern, ultradian oscillations in plasma glucose and insulin secretion are generated that are 100% concordant with the oscillatory period of the exogenous glucose infusion. This close relationship between the ultradian oscillations in insulin secretion and similar oscillations in plasma glucose was further exemplified in a series of dose-response studies in which the largest amplitude oscillations in insulin secretion were observed in the subjects exhibiting the largest amplitude glucose oscillations, which in turn were directly related to the infusion dose of glucose. It has been shown that in normal humans, insulin is more effective in reducing plasma glucose levels when administered intravenously as a 120-minute oscillation than when delivered at a constant rate. These results indicate that the ultradian oscillations have functional significance.

Circadian Oscillations

Circadian variations in the secretion of insulin have also been reported. When insulin secretory responses were measured during a 24-hour period during which subjects received three standard meals, the maximal postprandial responses were observed after breakfast.[555,557] These findings are mirrored by the results of studies in which subjects were tested for oral glucose tolerance at different times of the day and were found to exhibit maximal insulin secretory responses in the morning and lower responses in the afternoon and evening.[578-580] These diurnal differences are also noted in tests for intravenous glucose tolerance. Furthermore, although ultradian glucose and insulin oscillations are closely correlated during a constant 24-hour glucose infusion, the nocturnal rise in mean glucose levels is not accompanied by a similar increase in the insulin secretory rate.[581] It has been postulated that these diurnal differences might reflect diminished responsiveness of the beta cell to glucose in the afternoon and evening.[580]

Insulin Secretion in Obesity and Insulin Resistance

Obesity and other insulin-resistant states are associated with a substantially greater risk of developing T2DM. The ability of the pancreatic beta cell to compensate for insulin resistance determines whether blood glucose levels remain normal in insulin-resistant subjects or whether the subjects develop glucose intolerance or diabetes.

The nature of the beta cell's compensation for insulin resistance involves hypersecretion of insulin even in the presence of normal glucose concentrations. This can occur only if beta cell sensitivity to glucose is increased. The increase in beta cell sensitivity to glucose seen in obesity appears to be mediated by two factors. First, increased beta cell mass is observed in obesity and other insulin-resistant states.[582] Second, insulin resistance appears to be associated with increased expression of hexokinase in the beta cell relative to the expression of glucokinase.[583] Because hexokinase has a significantly lower Michaelis constant (K_m) for glucose than glucokinase, the functional effect of increased hexokinase expression is to shift the glucose-insulin secretion dose-response curve to the left, leading to increased insulin secretion across a wide range of glucose concentrations.

Assessment of the adequacy of the beta cell compensation for insulin resistance is important because this is the major determinant of the development of diabetes. In insulin-resistant states it is important to evaluate beta cell function in relation to the degree of insulin resistance. Kahn and coworkers[584] studied the relationship between insulin sensitivity and beta cell function in 93 relatively young, apparently healthy human subjects of varying degrees of obesity. The sensitivity index (SI) was calculated using the minimal model of Bergman as a measure of insulin sensitivity and was then compared with various measures of insulin secretion.[436,585] The relationship between the SI and the beta cell measures was curvilinear and reciprocal for fasting insulin ($P < .0001$), first-phase insulin response (AIR [acute insulin response] glucose; $P < .0001$), glucose potentiation slope ($n = 56$; $P < .005$), and beta cell secretory capacity (AIR_{max}; $n = 43$; $P < .0001$). The curvilinear relationship between SI and the beta cell measures could not be distinguished from a hyperbola, that is:

$$SI \times \text{beta cell function} = \text{constant}$$

The nature of this relationship is consistent with a regulated feedback loop control system such that for any difference in SI, a proportionate reciprocal difference occurs in insulin levels and responses in subjects with similar carbohydrate tolerance. Thus, in human subjects with normal glucose tolerance and varying degrees of obesity, beta cell function varies quantitatively with differences in insulin sensitivity. The increase in insulin secretion that is observed with a fall in SI should be viewed as the beta cell compensation that allows normal glucose tolerance to be maintained in the presence of insulin resistance.

The insulin resistance of obesity is characterized by hyperinsulinemia. Hyperinsulinemia in this setting reflects a combination of increased insulin production and decreased insulin clearance, but most evidence suggests that increased insulin secretion is the predominant factor.[586,587] Both basal and 24-hour insulin secretory rates are three to four times higher in obese subjects and are strongly correlated with BMI. Insulin secretory responses to intravenous glucose have been studied in otherwise healthy insulin-resistant subjects in comparison with insulin-sensitive subjects by means of a graded glucose infusion.

Figure 30–15 depicts insulin concentrations and insulin secretion rates at each level of plasma glucose achieved, thereby constructing a glucose-insulin concentration or glucose-insulin secretion rate dose-response relationship. Both insulin concentrations and insulin secretion rates are increased in insulin-resistant subjects, resulting from a combination of increased insulin secretion and decreased insulin clearance. For each level of glucose, insulin secretion rates are higher in the insulin-resistant subjects, reflecting an adaptive response of the beta cell to peripheral insulin resistance. Similar compensatory hyperinsulinemia has been demonstrated using other clinical techniques, such as the frequently sampled intravenous glucose tolerance test, in obesity and in other insulin-resistant states such as late pregnancy.[584,588]

The temporal pattern of insulin secretion is unaltered in obese subjects compared with normal subjects. Basal insulin secretion in obese subjects accounts for 50% of the total daily production of insulin, and secretory pulses of insulin occur every 1.5 to 2 hours.[557,586] However, the amplitude of these pulses postprandially is greater in obese subjects. Nevertheless, when these postprandial secretory responses are expressed as a percentage of the basal secretory rate, the postprandial responses in obese and normal subjects are identical.

Insulin Secretion in Subjects with Impaired Glucose Tolerance

It has been suggested that insulin secretion may be normal in subjects with IGT. However, substantial defects in insulin secretion have been demonstrated in people who have normal fasting glucose and normal glycosylated hemoglobin concentrations with glucose values greater than 140 mg/dL or 7.8 mM/L 2 hours after ingestion of 75 g of glucose orally. Thus, defects in insulin secretion can be detected before the onset of overt hyperglycemia.

Detailed study of insulin secretion in patients with IGT has demonstrated that consistent quantitative and qualitative defects are seen in this group. During oral glucose tolerance testing, there is a delay in the peak insulin response.[85,589,590] The glucose-

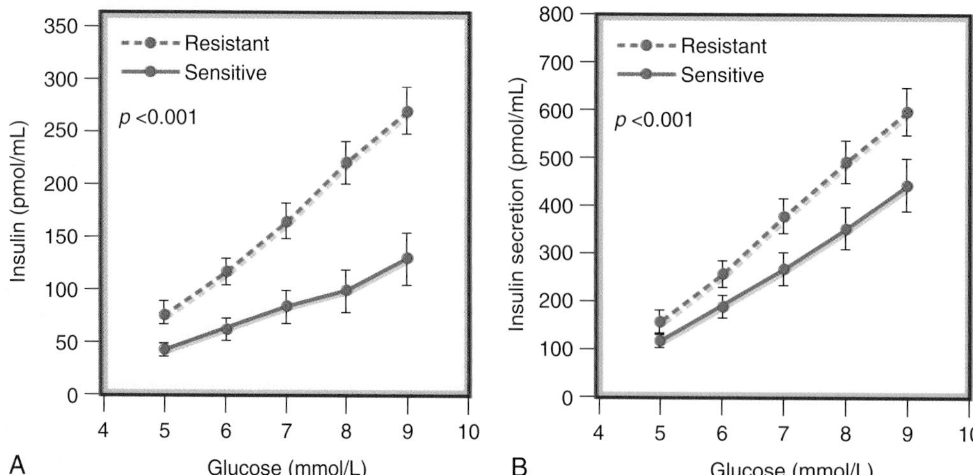

Figure 30–15 ▪ Plasma insulin concentrations **(A)** and insulin secretion rates **(B)** in response to molar increments in the plasma glucose concentration during the graded glucose infusion in the insulin-resistant *(dotted line)* and insulin-sensitive *(solid line)* groups. (From Jones CNO, Pei D, Staris P, et al. Alterations in the glucose-stimulated insulin secretory dose-response curve and in insulin clearance in nondiabetic insulin-resistant individuals. J Clin Endocrinol Metab 1997;82:1834-1838.)

insulin secretion dose-response relationship is flattened and shifted to the right (Fig. 30–16), and first-phase insulin responses to an intravenous glucose bolus are consistently decreased in relation to ambient insulin sensitivity.[591,592] Further, abnormalities in first-phase insulin secretion were observed in first-degree relatives of patients with T2DM who exhibited only mild intolerance to glucose,[593] and an attenuated insulin response to oral glucose was observed in normoglycemic twins of patients with T2DM.[594] This pattern of insulin secretion during the prediabetic phase was also seen in subjects with IGT who later developed T2DM[478,595,596] and in normoglycemic obese subjects with a recent history of gestational diabetes,[597] another group at high risk for T2DM.[598] Beta cell abnormalities can therefore precede the development of overt T2DM by many years.

The temporal pattern of insulin secretory responses is altered in IGT and is similar to but not as pronounced as that seen in diabetic subjects (see later). There is a loss of coordinated insulin secretory responses during oscillatory glucose infusion, indicating that the ability of the beta cell to sense and respond appropriately to parallel changes in the plasma glucose level is impaired (Fig. 30–17). Abnormalities in rapid oscillations of insulin secretion have also been observed in first-degree relatives of patients with T2DM who have only mild glucose intolerance,[566] further suggesting that abnormalities in the temporal pattern of beta cell function may be an early manifestation of beta cell dysfunction preceding the development of T2DM. Because an elevation in serum proinsulin is seen in subjects with diabetes, the contribution of proinsulin to the hyperinsulinemia of IGT has been questioned. The hyperinsulinemia of IGT has not been accounted for by an increase in proinsulin, although elevations in fasting and stimulated proinsulin or proinsulin-to-insulin ratios have been found by many, although not all, investigators.[599-604] Correlation of elevated proinsulin levels in IGT as a predictor of future conversion to diabetes has also been observed.[605-607]

Insulin Secretion in Type 2 Diabetes Mellitus

Because of the presence of concomitant insulin resistance, patients with T2DM are often hyperinsulinemic, but the degree of hyperinsulinemia is inappropriately low for the prevailing glucose concentrations. Nevertheless, many of these patients have sufficient beta cell reserve to maintain a euglycemic state by diet restriction with or without an oral agent. The beta cell defect in patients with T2DM mellitus is characterized by an absent first-phase insulin and C peptide response to an intravenous glucose load and a reduced second-phase response.[608] Although hyperglycemia can play a role in mediating these changes, the abnormal first-phase response to intravenous glucose persists in patients whose diabetic control has been

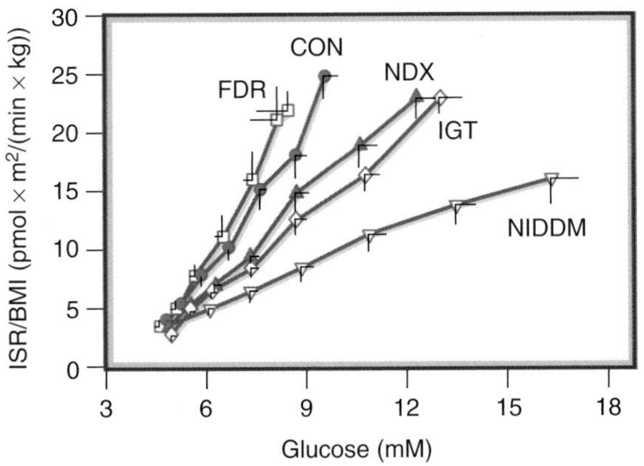

Figure 30–16 ▪ Dose-response relationship between glucose and insulin secretory rate (ISR) after an overnight fast in control subjects (CON), normoglycemic subjects with a family history of non–insulin-dependent diabetes mellitus (FDR), subjects with a nondiagnostic oral glucose tolerance test (NDX), subjects with impaired glucose tolerance (IGT), and subjects with non–insulin-dependent diabetes mellitus (NIDDM). BMI, body mass index. (From Byrne MM, Sturis J, Sobel RJ, Polonsky KS. Elevated plasma glucose 2 h postchallenge predicts defects in beta-cell function. Am J Physiol 1996;270:E572-E579. Copyright 1996, the American Physiological Society.)

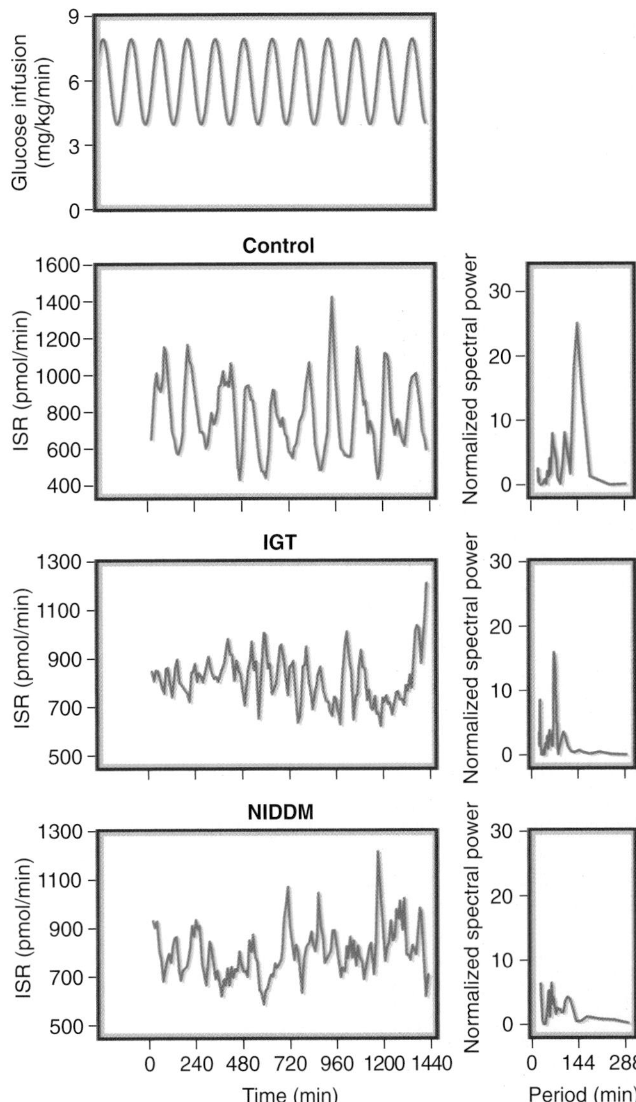

Figure 30–17 ▪ Oscillatory glucose infusions *(first panel)* were administered with a periodicity of 144 minutes in representative subjects with normal glucose tolerance (Control; *second panels*), impaired glucose tolerance (IGT; *third panels*), and type 2 diabetes (NIDDM; *fourth panels*). In the control subject, the insulin secretion rate (ISR) adjusts and responds to the 144-minute oscillations in glucose, resulting in sharp spectral peak at 144 minutes. In the subjects with IGT and type 2 diabetes, the ISR does not respond to the oscillatory glucose stimulus, and although oscillations in insulin secretion are evident, they are irregular, resulting in markedly reduced spectral peaks at 144 minutes and small-amplitude high-frequency spectral peaks. (Adapted from O'Meara NM, Sturis J, Van Cauter E, Polonsky KS. Lack of control by glucose of ultradian insulin secretory oscillations in impaired glucose tolerance and in non–insulin-dependent diabetes mellitus. J Clin Invest 1993;92:262-271.)

greatly improved,[609,610] consistent with the idea that patients with T2DM have an intrinsic defect in the beta cell. Furthermore, abnormalities in first-phase insulin secretion have also been observed in first-degree relatives of patients with T2DM who have only mild glucose intolerance, and an attenuated insulin response to oral glucose has been observed in normoglycemic twins of patients with T2DM, a group at high risk for T2DM and who can legitimately be classified as prediabetic.[611] This pattern of insulin secretion during the prediabetic phase is also seen in subjects with IGT who later develop T2DM and in normoglycemic obese subjects with a recent history of gestational diabetes, who are also at high risk for T2DM. Beta cell abnormalities can therefore precede the development of overt T2DM by many years.

Type 2 diabetes also affects proinsulin levels in serum. Increased levels of proinsulin are consistently seen in association with increases in the proinsulin-to-insulin molar ratio.[608] The amount of proinsulin produced in this setting appears to be related to the degree of glycemic control rather than to the duration of the diabetic state, and in one series proinsulin levels contributed almost 50% of the total insulin immunoreactivity in T2DM patients who had marked hyperglycemia. In addition to intact proinsulin, the beta cell secretes one or more of the four major proinsulin conversion products (split 32,33-, split 65,66-, des-31,32-, and des-64,65-proinsulin) into the circulation. These conversion products are produced within the secretory granules of the islet as a result of the activity of specific conversion enzymes at the two cleavage sites in proinsulin linking the C peptide to the A and B chains.

The composition of the elevated proinsulin-like immunodeficiency (PLI) in patients with T2DM compared with control subjects has not been fully characterized. Hales and colleagues[612] have developed immunoradiometric assays for this purpose. Using these assays, split 32,33-proinsulin was reported to be the predominant proinsulin conversion product in the circulation, although des-31,32-proinsulin levels can also be elevated. Insulin, proinsulin, and conversion product concentrations were also measured with these assays 30 minutes after oral glucose in patients with T2DM. Insulin was reduced in all patients, with no overlap between patients and controls, and concentrations of proinsulin and conversion products were elevated in the diabetic patients. These data highlight the importance of the potentially confounding effects of proinsulin and proinsulin conversion products in the interpretation of circulating immunoreactive insulin in patients with T2DM and emphasize the need to measure the concentrations of the individual peptides.

Abnormalities in the temporal pattern of insulin secretion have also been demonstrated in patients with T2DM. In contrast to normal subjects, in whom equal amounts of insulin are secreted basally and postprandially in a given 24-hour period, patients with T2DM secrete a greater proportion of their daily insulin under basal conditions (Fig. 30–18).[613] This reduction in the proportion of insulin secreted postprandially appears to be related in part to a reduction in the amplitude of the secretory pulses of insulin occurring after meals rather than to a reduction in the number of pulses. In contrast to normal subjects, patients with T2DM have ultradian oscillations in insulin secretion that are less tightly coupled with oscillations in plasma glucose (Fig. 30–19). Similar findings were observed in patients with IGT studied under the same experimental conditions and in a further group of type 2 diabetic patients studied under fasting conditions. The rapid insulin pulses are also abnormal in T2DM because the persistent regular rapid oscillations present in normal subjects are not observed. Instead, the cycles are shorter and irregular. Similar findings were observed in a group of first-degree relatives of patients with T2DM who had only mild glucose intolerance, suggesting that abnormalities in oscillatory activity may be an early manifestation of beta cell dysfunction.[591]

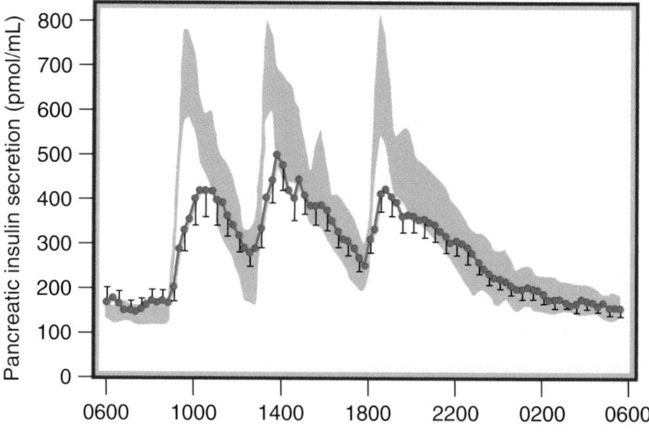

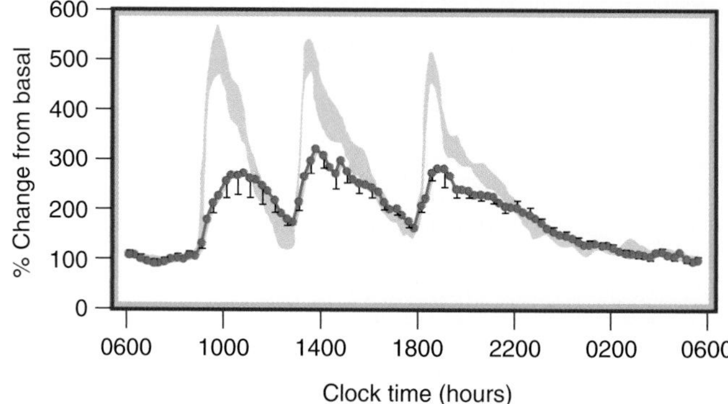

Figure 30–18 ■ Mean (±•• [standard error of the mean]) rates of insulin secretion in type 2 diabetic patients compared with control subjects. The *shaded area* corresponds to 1 SEM above and below the mean in control subjects. The curves in the lower panel were derived by dividing, for each subject, the insulin secretion rate at each sampling time by the average fasting secretion rate measured between 6 AM and 9 AM in the same subject.

The effects of therapy on beta cell function in patients with T2DM have also been investigated. Although interpretation of the results in many instances is limited because beta cell function was not always studied at comparable levels of glucose before and during therapy, the majority of the studies indicated that improvements in diabetic control are associated with an enhancement of beta cell secretory activity. This increased endogenous production of insulin appears to be independent of the mode of treatment and is in particular associated with increases in the amount of insulin secreted postprandially.[610,614] The enhanced beta cell secretory activity after meals reflects an increase in the amplitude of existing secretory pulses rather than an increased number of pulses. Despite improvements in glycemic control, beta cell function is not normalized after therapy, suggesting that the intrinsic defect in the beta cell persists.

Treatment with the sulfonylurea glyburide increases the amount of insulin secreted in response to meals but does not correct the underlying abnormalities in the pattern of insulin secretion. In particular, the abnormalities in the pulsatile pattern of ultradian insulin secretory oscillations persist on treatment with glyburide despite the increase in the amount of insulin secreted.

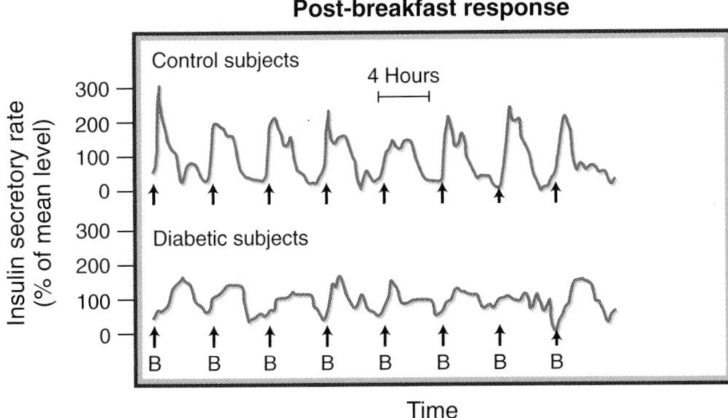

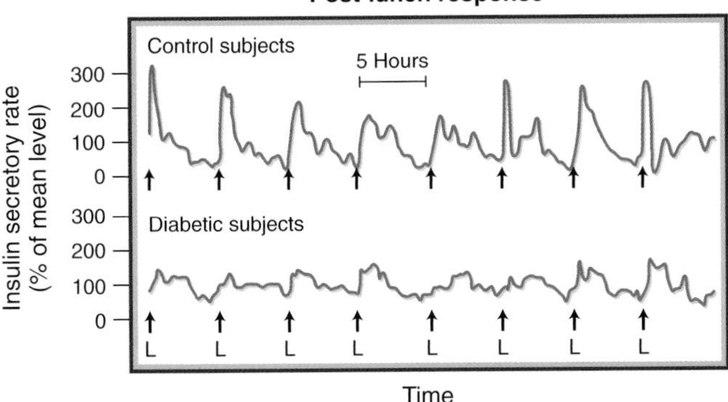

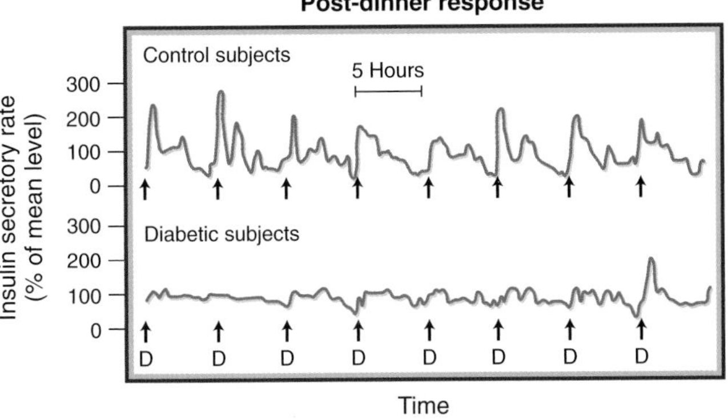

Figure 30–19 ▪ Temporal variations in postbreakfast *(top panel)*, postlunch *(middle panel)*, and postdinner *(bottom panel)* rates of insulin secretion in control and diabetic subjects. In each subject, the secretion rates during the 30 minutes before the meal and the 4 hours after breakfast or the 5 hours after lunch or dinner were expressed as a percentage of the mean rate of insulin secretion during that interval. The curves were obtained by concatenating the resulting postmeal profiles in eight representative subjects. The times when the meals were served to successive subjects in the series are indicated by *arrows*. (From Polonsky KS, Given BD, Hirsch LJ, et al. Abnormal patterns of insulin secretion in non–insulin-dependent diabetes mellitus. N Engl J Med 1988;318:1231-1239.)

We have also investigated the effects on insulin secretion of improving insulin resistance in subjects with IGT by using the insulin-sensitizing agent troglitazone, a thiazolidinedione. Troglitazone therapy improved insulin sensitivity, and this was associated with enhanced ability of the pancreatic beta cell to respond to a glucose stimulus as judged by improvements in the dose-response relationships between glucose and insulin secretion as well as enhanced ability of the pancreatic beta cell to detect and respond to small oscillations in the plasma glucose concentration.[615]

RODENT MODELS OF TYPE 2 DIABETES

A number of spontaneous and genetically selected animal models of T2DM have been identified. Most of the models combine the two main features of T2DM, obesity-associated insulin resistance and beta cell dysfunction with or without diminished beta cell mass. As with diabetes in humans, the different rodent models of T2DM have similarities, but a number of overt and subtle differences make them useful surrogates for intensive study of the syndromes associated with T2DM.

An interesting observation is the striking sexual dimorphism in most rodent models of T2DM, with the male most often being affected exclusively, earlier, or more severely in most instances. In this regard, it is not like the human situation. The advent of transgenic and knockout technology in mice has produced a wide range of models of insulin resistance and beta cell dysfunction that results in hyperglycemia. It is beyond the scope of this chapter to review each of these, and the reader is referred to the primary literature for review of these animals. We limit our discussion to the well-documented spontaneous or derived models of the disease in rodents.

Mouse Models of Type 2 Diabetes

Leptin (*Lep*^{ob}) and the Leptin Receptor (*db*)

The *ob* mutation, now designated *Lep*^{ob}, was first described in 1950,[616] but the gene mutation responsible for the syndrome was not described until the *ob* mutation was found to be in the gene for leptin.[617] Mice homozygous for the *ob* mutation do not produce the satiety factor leptin and become markedly hyperphagic, obese, insulin resistant, and hyperinsulinemic. They have a multitude of other hypothalamic dysfunctions that render them hypometabolic, contribute to the obesity, and also result in infertility.[618,619] Leptin treatment of these mice results in decreased food intake and reverses many of their other metabolic defects.[620-624] The *ob* mice develop obesity at weaning that becomes progressive because of hyperphagia. Insulin resistance is seen in muscle, adipose tissue, and liver, with a variety of signaling defects that are also reversible with insulin administration.[625] The *ob* mouse becomes hyperglycemic and has a profound hyperinsulinemia associated with beta cell hyperplasia with up to a 10-fold increase in islet mass.[626,627]

Parabiotic experiments between the *ob* and *db* mice suggested that the *db* mutation would be in the receptor for ob. This was confirmed with the identification of multiple mutations in the leptin receptor in *db*.[628,629] Like *ob* mice, *db* mice are hyperphagic and begin to surpass their littermates in weight at weaning. They are progressively hyperinsulinemic, become hyperglycemic at 6 to 8 weeks, and, because of a decline in beta cell function,[630-633] become markedly hyperglycemic at 4 to 6 months. The reason for the more severe diabetes in the *db* mouse is not clear, but it may be due to background strain differences, because similar defects in insulin signaling are seen in this animal model as well.[634-636] Treatment of both *ob* and *db* mice with insulin-sensitizing agents such as thiazolidinediones reversed the insulin resistance and ameliorated or prevented the onset of diabetes.[637,638]

Agouti Mouse

Dominant "yellow" mutations in the *agouti* gene produce obesity and hyperglycemia. Depending on the background strain, the *agouti* mutation has a variable phenotype. In susceptible strains, the onset of hyperinsulinemia begins at 6 weeks of age and insulin levels continue to increase with age with beta cell hyperplasia and hypertrophy.[639,640] The *agouti* mutation results in systemic production of a protein normally expressed in the skin, most frequently because of a retrotransposon insertion into the promoter region of the gene.[641] Interestingly, a number of genes, including the fatty acid synthase gene, have both insulin and agouti response elements, which result in a marked increase in expression leading to increased hepatic fatty acid synthesis and enhanced fat deposition in adipocytes.[629,642,643] The hyperglycemia is postprandial, and the fasting glucose levels are usually normal. The exact function of the *agouti* gene is unknown, but the animals are hyperphagic and show enhanced growth.

KK Mouse

These mice were originally bred for enhanced size but are not as obese as most other obese mice (usually less than 60 g). Breeding the KK into various background strains has produced variable insulin resistance, hyperinsulinemia, and hyperglycemia. The most studied strain is the KKA^y produced in Japan.[644] This mouse has markedly increased insulin levels (>1000 μU/mL) when fed a high-fat diet.[645,646] As the male mouse ages, glucose levels fall toward the normal range. The mutation responsible for the KK phenotype is unknown.

NZO Mouse

New Zealand obese (NZO) mice were derived by inbreeding of abdominally obese outbred mice.[627,647-649] NZO neonates have high birth weights, and mice of both sexes are large and at weaning exhibit an elevated carcass fat content.[647] Approximately 40% to 50% of group-caged NZO males, but not females, develop type 2 diabetes between 12 and 20 weeks of age when maintained with a chow diet containing 4.5% fat.[650] Obesity in NZO mice is characterized by widespread accumulation of subcutaneous as well as visceral fat. The obesity in these mice is accompanied by glucose intolerance in males associated with increased hepatic and peripheral insulin resistance. In contrast to those in *ob* and *db* mice, genes encoding certain gluconeogenic and glycolytic enzymes in the liver retain normal responsiveness to insulin, although there is evidence for an inappropriately active fructose-1,6-biphosphatase.[651-653] Defective beta cell insulin secretion from NZO islets in vitro and in vivo has been described.[647] There appears be a defect in the glycolytic pathway in beta cells leading to defective glucose-stimulated insulin release.[654]

The genetics of NZO mice show a polygenic disorder, and none of the allelic variants have been discovered. Complicating the analysis of the model is the susceptibility of the mice to autoimmune disorders including a lupus-like syndrome[655,656] and insulin receptor autoantibodies.[657] There is also a maternal influence in the peripartum period in the development of the disorder, which might reflect substances in the maternal milk.[658]

Gold Thioglucose–Induced Diabetes

Gold thioglucose induces specific lesions in the ventromedial hypothalamus and induces an initial chronic hyperinsulinemia that leads to hypoglycemia, hyperphagia, obesity, and the development of insulin resistance and hyperglycemia.[659] This model has been used as an example of pancreatic dysfunction preceding the induction of insulin resistance as opposed to pancreatic compensation for insulin resistance.

Diabetes Induced by Fat Ablation

Three models of insulin-resistant diabetes have been created in which adipose tissue has been genetically eliminated by overproduction of foreign genes using the fat-specific promoter aP2. Expression of an attenuated diphtheria toxin in adipose tissue resulted in an age-dependent loss of fat, progressive insulin resistance, hyperinsulinemia, and significant diabetes.[660,661] Adipose-specific expression of a constitutively active form of the sterol regulatory element-binding protein SREBP-1c also resulted in fat ablation.[662] Lipoatrophy has also been induced by fat-specific overexpression of a dominant-negative form of the transcription factor A-ZIP/F.[663,664] The A-ZIP/F protein heterodimerizes with and inactivates basic zipper (B-ZIP) transcription factors, including activating protein-1 (AP-1) and CCAAT/enhancer binding protein (C/EBP) isoforms, probably disrupting normal fat development.

The lack of fat in the various models leads to hepatomegaly, insulin resistance with hyperinsulinemia, hypoleptinemia and significant glucose intolerance, and diabetes. These mice represent a model of the human condition lipodystrophic diabetes and demonstrate the importance of fat in normal glucose homeostasis. It has been suggested that the lack of fat depots results in elevated fatty acid delivery to liver and muscle and the development of insulin resistance. The diabetes in these animals can be variously treated by thiazolidinediones,[660] leptin administration,[665] and fat transplantation.[664] Interestingly, human lipodystrophy also responds to thiazolidinedione treatment,[666] suggesting that some of the effects of these compounds are not wholly dependent upon adipose tissue.

C57BL/6J Mice Fed a High-Fat Diet

Male C57BL/6J (also know as B6) mice fed a high-fat, high-carbohydrate diet (a "Western" diet, 58% fat by kilocalories) developed hyperglycemia, hyperinsulinemia, hyperlipidemia, and increased adiposity.[667,668] Glucose-stimulated insulin secretion was blunted, and there was significant insulin resistance.[669,670] Despite obesity, plasma leptin levels in the Western diet–fed B6 mice were significantly lower than in control mice in the absence of hyperphagia.[667,671] The weight gain is due primarily to an increase in mesenteric adiposity, which makes this a good model for adult-onset T2DM.

Nagoya-Shibata-Yasuda Mice

The Nagoya-Shibata-Yasuda (NSY) mouse shows male-specific mild IGT, and only a minority of the females become diabetic.[672] An impairment in beta cell function and obesity are present. These mice do not show the typical islet hyperplasia associated with insulin resistance.

TallyHo Mice

The TallyHo mouse also has a male-only development of diabetes associated with beta cell hyperplasia. Both male and female TallyHo mice are obese, hyperinsulinemic, and hyperlipidemic, and the males have glucose levels greater than 500 mg/dL.[673]

Rat Models of Type 2 Diabetes

Zucker Diabetic Fatty (ZDF) Rat

The orthologue of the *db* mouse, the obese Zucker rat (*fa/fa*), has a mutation in the leptin receptor that results in significant hyperphagia.[674] The *fa* mutation is distinct from the mutations in *db* in that it does not disrupt leptin receptor gene expression and does not affect ligand binding.[674,675] This mutation results in a constitutive intracellular signaling domain, which might induce a desensitization of the leptin signaling pathways.[676]

The selection of the inbred ZDF strain used Zucker (*fa/fa*) rats that had progressed to a diabetic phenotype. Brother-sister mating resulted in nearly 100% diabetes in the male rats receiving a 5% fat diet.[677] Hyperglycemia begins to develop in males at 7 weeks of age, with serum glucose levels rising to 500 mg/dL by 12 weeks of age. The hyperinsulinemia precedes hyperglycemia with marked islet hyperplasia with dysmorphogenesis,[678] but by 19 weeks of age insulin levels drop concomitantly with islet atrophy, in part because of an imbalance of hyperplasia and apoptosis.[582] The islets of prediabetic ZDF rats secrete significantly more insulin in response to glucose, with elevated basal levels of insulin secretion and a leftward shift, but a blunted glucose dose-response curve.[583,679] Islets of prediabetic male ZDF rats also have defects in the normal oscillatory pattern of insulin secretion.[684]

In contrast to the male ZDF rat, the female rat has significant insulin resistance but does not become diabetic unless given a proprietary high-fat diet (GMI 13004).[680] The high-fat diet appears to have a direct effect on the beta cell because there is no change in peripheral insulin sensitivity (P. Hansen and C. F. Burant, unpublished observations). Interestingly, there is a decrease in peripheral triglyceride and FFA levels in the female rat after the institution of the high-fat diet.

The underlying genetic defect that results in beta cell failure in the ZDF rat is unknown. The beta cell number and insulin content are not different from those in homozygous normal animals, but insulin promoter activity is doubled in the ZDF rat.[681] Insulin promoter mapping studies suggest that a critical region in the promoter of the insulin gene is affected. A number of other gene expression differences have been described in ZDF islets, including decreases in the expression of GLUT2[682,683]; increases in glucokinase and hexokinase activity[679]; decreases in mitochondrial metabolism[679]; accumulation of intraislet lipid and long-chain fatty acyl CoA, which is associated with abnormal beta cell secretion[684-686]; and increases in nitric oxide and ceramide accumulation,[687,688] which is associated with apoptosis. Other gene expression changes are also found in the prediabetic rat islet.[689] Which of these defects are important for the development of the diabetes is not clear. Despite the fixed genetic defect in the male animal that leads to diabetes, this defect interacts with the insulin resistance because treatment with insulin-sensitizing agents can prevent the onset of diabetes in the male and female.[686,690] These agents are not effective in the male after establishment of diabetes; however, the female rat can respond to thiazolidinediones, even after significant hyperglycemia.

Goto-Kakizaki (GK) Rats

The GK inbred rat strain was derived from outbred Wistar rats by selection for IGT.[691] Early in the development of diabetes, there are mild elevations of both glucose and insulin levels in the GK rat, but as the animals age, reduced beta cell mass is evident, with markedly diminished insulin stores and abnormal secretory responses to glucose.[692,693] A number of biochemical defects have been described in the islets of these animals, including decreased energy production,[694-696] expression of proteins involved in insulin granule movement,[697] and decreased adenylate cyclase activity.[698] Defects in peripheral signaling include decreased maximal and submaximal insulin-stimulated IRS1 tyrosine phosphorylation, IRS1-associated PI3-kinase activity, and Akt activation in muscle[699] and defective regulation of protein phosphatase-1 (PP-1), PP-2A, and mitogen-activated protein kinase activation by upstream insulin signaling components in adipocytes.[700] Some of these defects may be due to hyperglycemia, because they can be reversed by phlorizin-induced normalization of serum glucose.[699]

Bureau of Home Economics (BHE/Cdb) Rats

The Bureau of Home Economics (BHE/Cdb) rat is a subline of the parent BHE obtained by selection for hyperglycemia and dyslipidemia without obesity.[701] Glucose-stimulated insulin secretion is markedly diminished in these rats, a trait that is maternally inherited.[702] A significant defect appears to be in the liver, where increased gluconeogenesis and lipogenesis precede the hyperglycemia, which may be due to defects in mitochondrial respiration associated with mitochondrial DNA mutations.[703,704]

Psammomys obesus (Sand Rat)

This is a nutritionally induced obesity model of T2DM. Genetically, the sand rat is in reality a gerbil, and the animal usually lives on a low-calorie vegetable diet.[705] When given a high-carbohydrate diet, the sand rat rapidly becomes hyperglycemic secondary to weight gain associated with significant insulin resistance[706] and enhanced hepatic glucose production.[707] When a relatively hypocaloric diet is restored, the metabolic syndrome reverts to normoglycemia. A subpopulation of the sand rat develops frank beta cell failure and becomes ketotic.

Otsuka Long-Evans Tokushima Fatty (OLETF) Rats

The Otsuka Long-Evans Tokushima Fatty (OLETF) rat strain was derived from the Long-Evans rat with polyuria, polydipsia, and mild obesity.[708] About 90% of the male animals become diabetic by 1 year of age. Statistical tests have determined that the locus containing the cholecystokinin A receptor is responsible for about 50% of the T2DM in the OLETF rats.[709] The receptor is disrupted in the OLETF rat because of a 165-bp deletion in exon 1.[710,711] Genetic segregation analysis has also shown interaction with a second locus, *Obd2*, which acts in a synergistic fashion to result in NIDDM, and both of these loci are required in homozygous OLETF rats to cause elevated plasma glucose.[712]

The role of sex hormones is pronounced in this strain. Orchiectomy markedly reduces the incidence of diabetes and oophorectomy increases hyperglycemia to 30% in the female. Further, treatment of castrated males with testosterone restores the incidence to 89%. The islets undergo a progressive inflammatory reaction with progressive fibrosis. This reaction is associated with the impairment of beta cell function.[713] Obesity and insulin resistance appear to precede the development of beta cell failure.[714] Studies have also shown that obesity is necessary for the development of T2DM in OLETF males and that insulin resistance may be closely related to fat deposition in the abdominal cavity.[715] Troglitazone and metformin have been used successfully to treat the diabetes in the OLETF rat, and troglitazone completely prevents the morphologic and functional deterioration of the beta cells.[716]

Neonatal Streptozotocin

Two models have been described in which a single dose of the beta cell toxin streptozotocin is given to 2-day-old female Wistar[717,718] or male Sprague-Dawley rats.[719,720] These animals have a transient hyperglycemia but develop IGT at 4 to 6 weeks of age. There is an initial reduction of beta cell mass, but subsequent regeneration results restoration of the beta cell mass to a level approximately 50% below normal adult level.

MANAGEMENT OF TYPE 2 DIABETES

Over the last decade, a conceptual transformation in the principles of management of T2DM has occurred. Fundamentally, there has been a change in the level of concern about diabetes as a public health issue as well as in attitudes toward its treatment. Dramatic advances in the spectrum of pharmacologic agents and monitoring technology available for the treatment of diabetes have made it possible to lower glucose safely to the near-normal range in the majority of patients. Great strides have been made in establishing an evidence base for guidelines regarding glycemic control and efforts to reduce the risk of complications. Both corporate and government health insurance providers have greatly improved the extent to which diabetes equipment and supplies are covered.

A comprehensive review of all the subtleties of diabetes management in the 21st century is beyond the scope of this chapter. In the following pages, we deal with the salient features of the epidemiology of the complications of T2DM, diagnostic strategies, treatment guidelines, lifestyle interventions, and pharmacotherapy before turning briefly to a discussion of preventive measures for T2DM and its complications. An excellent source of information on these issues that is updated annually is the American Diabetes Association's Clinical Practice Recommendations, which is published as the first supplement to the journal *Diabetes Care* each January and is available at www.diabetes.org.

Scope of the Problem

In 2005, the prevalence of T2DM in the United States was estimated to be 20.8 million or 7.0% of the population, including 14.6 million diagnosed cases and 6.2 million undiagnosed cases. There is an epidemic of diabetes nationwide, with more than 1.5 million cases diagnosed in people older than 20 years in 2005 alone. Worldwide, the prevalence of diabetes is increasing even faster. This increase is driven by population aging; population growth, particularly among ethnic groups with greater susceptibility to the disease; and dramatic increases in rates of obesity as a consequence of increasingly sedentary lifestyles and greater consumption of simple sugars and calorie-dense foods. At least in the United States, opportunistic screening for diabetes in high-risk populations is recommended by professional societies and many insurers, resulting in an increase in the fraction of affected persons with diagnosed diabetes from approximately one half in the 1990s to about two thirds in the first decade of the 21st century.[7,8,721-723]

The morbidity, mortality, and expense associated with diabetes are staggering. In Western society, people with diabetes are three times more likely to be hospitalized than nondiabetic persons. In the United States, diabetes is the leading cause of blindness and accounts for more than 40% of the new cases of end-stage renal disease. The risk of heart disease and stroke is 2 to 4 times higher and the risk of lower extremity amputation is approximately 20 times higher for people with diabetes than for those without. Life expectancy is reduced by approximately 10 years in people with diabetes, and although diabetes is the sixth leading cause of death in the United States, this is clearly an underestimate. Only about 35% to 40% of those who die with diabetes have the disease listed anywhere on the death certificate, and only 10% to 15% have it listed as the underlying cause of death.[723]

Tragically, this enormous burden of death and disability has not been reduced by huge health care expenditures. In fact, the epidemic of diabetes is one of the drivers of increasing health care costs, with annual disbursements for people with diabetes approximately three to five times higher per capita than those for persons without diabetes. In the United States, at least 15% of health care expenditures are related to the treatment of people with diabetes. Nevertheless, whereas rates of coronary artery disease are declining in the United States in general, this is not the case for people with diabetes. However, there is evidence that increased effort to control diabetes and its comorbidities can even reduce costs associated with diabetes and that a public health approach to diabetes can reduce the burden of complications of diabetes.[1,724-729]

Screening and Diagnosis

The role of screening to make the diagnosis of diabetes in asymptomatic persons is an area of substantial controversy. No prospective randomized trials have examined the benefit of such a screening program. On the other hand, it seems self-evident that early diagnosis and intervention have at least the potential to reduce complications in a disease in which 20% to 50% of patients have a complication at the time of diagnosis. The cost-effectiveness of universal approaches to diabetes screening has been called into question. The American Diabetes Association (ADA) recommendations[730] for screening are based on a review that concludes, "Periodic, targeted, and opportunistic screening within the existing health care system seems to offer the greatest yield and likelihood of appropriate follow-up and treatment."[731] The ADA suggests that patients (i.e., screening should be performed only in the context of a routine health care setting) should be screened at 3-year intervals beginning at age 45 and that testing should be considered at an earlier age or be carried out more frequently if diabetes risk factors are present. Those risk factors are listed in Table 30–3.

Most groups recommend FPG as the most practical screening test, although its sensitivity is substantially lower than that of the OGTT. More recent data suggest that alternative screening strategies might have advantages. In a study employing glucose meters to measure random capillary blood glucose, values of 120 mg/dL or higher obtained at random without regard to meals were 75% to 84% sensitive and 86% to 90% specific for detecting diabetes as defined by either FPG or OGTT.[732] In the future, it is possible that well-validated models will allow us to predict diabetes risk from standard biologic measures such as BMI, blood pressure, and lipids with greater precision than today.[733]

Classically, diabetes has been diagnosed on the basis of prospective epidemiologic data associating circulating glucose levels with the future development of diabetic retinopathy. In 1997, recommendations were made by an expert committee to change the diagnostic criteria for diabetes to improve the sensitivity of FPG for the diagnosis of diabetes.[734] They determined, from a review of several large data sets, that FPG 126 mg/dL (7.0 mM/L) or higher identified a population with a risk of retinopathy similar to that of those with a 2-hour value in an OGTT of 200 mg/dL or higher. In an effort to simplify the OGTT, only the 2-hour plasma glucose after a 75-g oral glucose load needs to be measured for diagnostic purposes. Furthermore, patients with classic symptoms of diabetes in association with a random glucose level of 200 mg/dL or higher also meet diagnostic criteria for diabetes. To avoid misclassification, it is further suggested that patients should meet one of the three diagnostic criteria on at least two separate days before diabetes is diagnosed.

Because macrovascular disease accounts for the majority of the morbidity and almost all the mortality associated with diabetes and the diagnosis of diabetes is associated with more stringent guidelines for the treatment of comorbidities such as dyslipidemia and hypertension, it seems likely that the diagnostic criteria for diabetes will be lowered again to make the fasting glucose cut points more sensitive. This seems appropriate, because it is clear that glucose levels above normal but below the current thresholds for diabetes are associated with increased cardiovascular risk. A debate unlikely to be resolved soon is whether it is acceptable to measure only fasting glucose as an index of glucose intolerance or whether it is cost-effective to use an oral challenge to fully ascertain glucose-related risks.[735-738]

Glucose Treatment Guidelines

Study Results and Recommendations

Prospective randomized clinical trials have documented improved rates of microvascular complications in patients with T2DM treated to lower glycemic targets. In the UK Prospective Diabetes Study (UKPDS),[739] patients with new-onset diabetes were treated with diet and exercise for 3 months with an average reduction in glycosylated hemoglobin (HbA_{1c}) from approximately 9% to 7% (upper limit of normal is 6%). Those with FPG greater than 108 mg/dL (6 mM/L) were randomly assigned to two treatment policies. In the standard intervention, subjects continued the lifestyle intervention. Pharmacologic therapy was initiated only if the FPG reached 15 mM/L (270 mg/dL) or the patient became symptomatic.

In the more intensive treatment program, all patients were randomly assigned and treated with either sulfonylurea, metformin, or insulin as initial therapy, with the dose increased to try to achieve an FPG less than 108 mg/dL. Combinations of agents were used only if the patients became symptomatic or FPG rose to greater than 270 mg/dL (15 mM/L). As a consequence of the design, although the HbA_{1c} fell initially to about 6%, over the average 10 years of follow-up it rose to approximately 8%. The average HbA_{1c} in the standard treatment group was approximately 1 percentage point higher. The risk of severe hypoglycemia was small—on the order of 1% to 5% per year in the insulin-treated group—and weight gain was modest; both were higher in patients randomly assigned to insulin and lower in those receiving metformin.[740] Associated with this improvement in glycemic control, there was a reduction in the risk of microvascular complications (retinopathy, nephropathy, and neuropathy) in the intensive group. Although there was a trend toward reduced rates of macrovascular events in the more intensively treated group, it did not reach statistical significance.[739]

Similar reductions in microvascular events were observed in another trial of entirely different design and much smaller size. In the Kumamoto study, Japanese patients of normal weight with T2DM treated with insulin were randomly assigned to standard treatment or an intensive program of insulin therapy designed to achieve normal glycemia. The control group maintained HbA_{1c} values at approximately 9%, whereas the HbA_{1c} in the intensive group was reduced to approximately 7% and the separation was maintained for 6 years. Again, there was a modest increased risk of hypoglycemia and weight gain, a reduction in microvascular complications, and a non–statistically significant trend toward reduced rates of vascular end-points.[741]

Although no interventional studies in T2DM have documented a reduced risk of vascular end-points associated with an improvement in glycemic control, multiple epidemiologic studies have suggested that there is an association between cardiovascular risk and HbA_{1c}, FPG, and the 2-hour level in the OGTT.[738,742,743] In the UKPDS epidemiologic analysis, there was a 16% reduction in cardiovascular disease rates for each percentage point reduction in HbA_{1c} without evidence of a threshold or lower limit of benefit all the way into the normal range.[743]

Blood Glucose Treatment Targets

In Table 30–6, guidelines from the ADA and the American College of Endocrinology (ACE) are presented. The ADA suggests that the goal of treatment in the management of diabetes should be an HbA_{1c} value less than 7% in general, but for the individual patient the A_{1c} should be as close to normal (<6%) as possible without significant hypoglycemia.[744,745] The ACE has recommended an HbA_{1c} goal of less than 6.5%.[746] Because the average HbA_{1c} in the United States is estimated to be in the 7.5% to 9.5% range, the argument about whether the HbA_{1c} target should be 6.0%, 6.5% or 7% is of limited practical significance.

However, it should be recognized that there are potential adverse events related to pursuit of more aggressive targets: hypoglycemia, long-term exposure to poorly studied combinations of medications, expense, life disruption caused by greater attention and effort to achieve lower glycemic targets, and the potential that great efforts expended in achieving extremely stringent glycemic goals will result in less attention to other health risks by patient or provider. No patient cohort of substantial size has ever been reported in which an average HbA_{1c} level less than 7% has been achieved over a time frame that exceeds more than a few months. Several adequately powered, randomized, controlled clinical trials are under way or being planned to explore the effects of seeking more intensive glycemic targets (HbA_{1c} <6%).[747] Although it is clear that many patients can achieve lower glucose levels with currently available drugs and lifestyle interventions, it remains theoretically possible that the risks would exceed the benefits of seeking glucose targets less than 7%.

With respect to fasting, premeal, or postprandial targets, there is little support for any particular level of glycemic control in the management of T2DM because no large-scale outcome study has targeted particular levels of glucose with home glucose monitoring. The ADA target of fasting and premeal plasma glucose levels of 70 to 130 mg/dL was initially developed based on an estimate of the range of average glucose values that would be associated with a low risk of hypoglycemia and HbA_{1c} less than 7%. It was modified based on recognition that to routinely achieve an HbA_{1c} less than 7%, many patients will have moderate hypoglycemic events with glucose levels in the 70 to 90 mg/dL range.[744,745] The ACE target of less than 110 mg/dL is an effort to achieve normal levels of glycemia.[746] However, consistent fasting and premeal glucose levels less than 110 mg/dL would be expected to be associated with an HbA_{1c} of approximately 5.5%.[748]

TABLE 30–6 GLYCEMIC TARGETS

Parameter	Normal	ADA	ACE
Premeal plasma glucose (mg/dL)	<100 (mean ~90)	70-130	<110
Postprandial plasma glucose (mg/dL)	<140	<180	<140
HbA_{1c}	4%-6%	<7%	<6.5%

ACE, American College of Endocrinology; ADA, American Diabetes Association.

From American Diabetes Association. Standards of medical care in diabetees—2006. Diabetes Care 2006;29:s4-s42; American College of Endocrinology. American College of Endocrinology consensus statement onf guidelines for glycemic control. Endocr Pract 2002;8(suppl1):5-11; Nathan DM, Buse JB, Davidson MG, et al. Management of hyperglycemia in type 2 diabetes mellitus: a consensus algorithy for the initiation and adjustment of therapy. Diabetes Care 2006;29:1963-1972 and Diabetologia 2006;49:1711-21 (published simultaneously).

The ADA treatment target for peak postprandial glucose levels is set at <180 mg/dL in part because those levels would be generally associated with an A_{1c} of <7% and because nondiabetic persons who have a large evening meal have been demonstrated to exhibit transient elevations of glucose to that level.[749] There are no published studies in which even safety, much less outcome, is documented for targeting a particular level of postprandial glucose. However, it is clear that there are effective HbA_{1c}-lowering agents that primarily target postprandial glucose levels and that monitoring postprandial glucose levels may be necessary to optimize dose adjustment of these agents. Furthermore, there are patients with diabetes who have average fasting glucose levels within targets but whose HbA_{1c} is elevated. In these patients, monitoring and specifically treating postprandial elevations can provide improvements in HbA_{1c}, perhaps with a lower risk of hypoglycemia and weight gain than further lowering fasting and premeal glucose levels.[744,750] The ACE recommends targeting a 2-hour postprandial glucose less than 140 mg/dL (7.8 mM/L) in an effort to achieve near-normal glycemia.[746] Consistent postprandial glucose values less than 140 mg/dL would be associated with average HbA_{1c} levels of approximately 5%.[748]

Lifestyle Intervention

The components of lifestyle intervention include medical nutrition counseling, exercise recommendations, and comprehensive diabetes education with the purpose of changing the paradigm of care in diabetes from provider-focused to patient-focused. Arguably, since the turn of the 21st century, nothing has changed more fundamentally than the emphasis on lifestyle intervention. For decades, physicians and patients have paid lip service to the notion that lifestyle intervention is important. Now we have significant clinical trial evidence that each component of lifestyle intervention, when appropriately administered, can contribute to improved outcomes. Furthermore, since the Balanced Budget Act of 1997 and the passage of complementary legislation in most state governments, lifestyle intervention has been a covered benefit for most people. Although full implementation of these regulations is still in progress, they have dramatically expanded the fraction of the population with diabetes with insurance coverage for these essential services.

Education of Patients

Diabetes is a lifelong disease, and health care providers have almost no control over the extent to which patients adhere to the day-to-day treatment regimen. The appropriate role of the health care provider is to serve as a coach to the patient, who has primary responsibility for the delivery of daily care.

As a result, health care providers must carefully engage patients as partners in the therapeutic process. It is critical for the health care professional to understand the context in which patients are taking care of their disease. Using a prescriptive approach in which patients are told what to do can work in some situations but fails more often than not because of unrecognized barriers to the execution of a particular plan. For long-term success, diabetes self-management education is critical.

As defined by the ADA,[751] diabetes self-management education is the process of providing the person with diabetes with the knowledge and skills needed to perform self-care, manage crises, and make lifestyle changes. As a result of this process, the patient must become a knowledgeable and active participant in the management of his or her disease. To achieve this task, patients and providers work together in a long-term, ongoing process. Minimal diabetes education should be universally provided and individualized with emphasis on the issues highlighted in Table 30–7. There are many more specialized topics relevant to almost all patients, such as how to adjust therapy when eating out or during travel as well as review of available local health care resources such as support groups and insurance issues. Although there are only limited studies, they do provide support for the concept that diabetes education can be cost-effective and can improve outcomes.[752-754]

A team of providers is generally required to fully implement the process of diabetes self-management education because the amount of information that needs to be exchanged is large and the needed range of expertise is broad. It is generally not possible to cover the recommended content fully in the context of several or even many brief encounters with a physician in an office setting. Potential providers in a team care approach could include nurses, dietitians, exercise specialists, behavioral therapists, pharmacists, and other medical specialists including diabetologists or endocrinologists, podiatrists, medical subspecialists, obstetrician-gynecologists, psychiatrists, and surgeons. The potential role of the community in which the patient lives and works in the diabetes self-care process is enormous, including family, friends, employers, and health insurance providers. Each potential member of the team has a role to play in the process, which must be reviewed and assessed frequently (Table 30–8). The primary role of the providers in this process is to provide guidance in goal setting to manage the risk of complications, suggest strategies to achieve goals and techniques to overcome barriers, provide training in skills, and help screen for complications. For this process to be a success, the patient must commit to the principles of self-care, participate fully in the development of a treatment plan, make ongoing decisions regarding self-care from day to day, and communicate honestly and with sufficient frequency with the team.

Fortunately, barriers to providing team care are becoming less daunting. Diabetes education programs are being rapidly established. The American Association of Diabetes Educators (800-TEAM-UP4) and the ADA (800-DIABETES) can provide information regarding diabetes educators and education programs in your area.

For team care to be most effective, communication, trust, and mutual respect are critical. Unfortunately, in many communities, the full benefit of the consultation and ongoing care with diabetes educators, nurses, dietitians, pharmacists, or

TABLE 30–7 CURRICULAR AREAS THAT SHOULD BE ADDRESSED IN DIABETES SELF-MANAGEMENT EDUCATION

- Pathophysiology of the patient's diabetes and its relationship to treatment options
- Incorporating appropriate nutritional management
- Incorporating physical activity into lifestyle
- Using medications (if applicable) for therapeutic effectiveness
- Monitoring blood glucose and (when appropriate) urine ketones and using the results to improve control
- Preventing, detecting, and treating acute complications including sick day rules and hypoglycemia
- Preventing (through risk detection), detecting, and treating chronic complications
- Goal-setting to promote health and problem solving for daily living
- Integrating psychosocial adjustment to daily life
- Promoting preconception care, management during pregnancy, and gestational diabetes management (if applicable)

Adapted from Mensing C, Boucher J, Cypress M, et al. National standards for diabetes self-management education. Diabetes Care 2006;29:S78-S85.

TABLE 30–8 TEAM CARE ROLES OF THE PLAYERS

PRIMARY CARE PROVIDER
To be a source of accurate information and to refer to and coordinate with other sources of information as necessary To provide guidance in developing goals of treatment To screen for complications and evaluate progress in meeting treatment goals To help develop strategies to achieve treatment goals and avoid complications
OTHER PROVIDERS
To be a source of accurate information, to communicate with the primary care provider, and to coordinate with other sources of information as necessary To provide guidance in developing goals of treatment and to help the primary care provider develop strategies to achieve treatment goals and avoid complications
PATIENT
To commit to diabetes self-management as defined above To be an active participant in the process To communicate with other team members when goals are not achieved or barriers or problems are encountered
COMMUNITY
To provide support to encourage ongoing diabetes self-care

others is not achieved because of overly hierarchic approaches to care. Nonphysicians, including patients, ought to provide suggestions regarding medication and lifestyle adjustments and help in the process of identifying barriers to effective management such as lack of knowledge, lack of time, and lack of resources and strategies to overcome those barriers.

Perhaps some of the most overlooked contributors to ineffective care in the setting of T2DM are the relatively common barriers created by psychiatric, neurocognitive function, and adjustment disorders, which are largely responsive to psychosocial therapies.[755]

Nutrition

With respect to self-management education, a technical review documents the effect of medical nutrition therapy and specific advice on diabetes-related outcomes such as HbA_{1c}, weight, and proteinuria.[756] These are summarized in Table 30–9. A comprehensive, individually negotiated nutrition program in which each patient's circumstances, preferences, and cultural background as well as the overall treatment program are considered is most likely to result in optimal outcomes. Because of the complexity of both the medical and nutritional issues for most patients, it is recommended that a registered dietitian, with specific skill and experience in implementing nutrition therapy in diabetes management, work collaboratively with the patient and other health care team members in providing medical nutrition therapy.

Structured programs that emphasize lifestyle changes including education, reduced fat and energy intake, regular physical activity, and regular participant contact can produce long-term weight loss of 5% to 7% of starting weight and reduce the risk of developing diabetes. Everyone, especially family members of persons with T2DM, should be encouraged to engage in regular physical activity to decrease the risk of developing T2DM.

TABLE 30–9 MAJOR NUTRITION RECOMMENDATIONS FOR DIABETES

People with diabetes should receive individualized medical nutrition therapy (MNT) as needed to achieve treatment goals, preferably provided by a registered dietitian familiar with the components of diabetes MNT.
Both the amount (grams) of carbohydrate as well as the type of carbohydrate in a food influence blood glucose level. Monitoring total grams of carbohydrate, whether by use of exchanges or carbohydrate counting, remains a key strategy in achieving glycemic control.
The use of the glycemic index or glycemic load may provide an additional benefit over that observed when total carbohydrate is considered alone.
Low-carbohydrate diets (restricting total carbohydrate to <130 g/day) are not recommended in the management of diabetes.
To reduce the risk of nephropathy, protein intake should be limited to the recommended dietary allowance (RDA) (0.8 g/kg) in those with any degree of chronic kidney disease.
Saturated fat intake should be <7% of total calories.
Intake of *trans* fat should be minimized.
Weight loss is recommended for all overweight (BMI 25.0-29.9 kg/m^2) or obese (BMI ≥30.0 kg/m^2) adults who have, or are at risk for developing, type 2 diabetes.
The primary approach for achieving weight loss is therapeutic lifestyle change, which includes a reduction in energy intake and an increase in physical activity. A moderate decrease in caloric balance (500-1000 kcal/day) will result in a slow but progressive weight loss (1-2 lb/week). For most patients, weight loss diets should supply at least 1000 to 1200 kcal/day for women and 1200 to 1600 kcal/day for men.
Initial physical activity recommendations should be modest and based on the patient's willingness and ability, gradually increasing the duration and frequency to 30 to 45 min of moderate aerobic activity, 3 to 5 days/week (goal at least 150 min/wk). Greater activity levels of at least 1 hr/day of moderate (walking) or 30 min/day of vigorous (jogging) activity may be needed to achieve successful long-term weight loss.
Drug therapy for obesity and surgery to induce weight loss may be appropriate in selected patients.
Nonnutritive sweeteners are safe when consumed within the acceptable daily intake levels established by the Food and Drug Administration (FDA).
If adults with diabetes choose to use alcohol, daily intake should be limited to a moderate amount (one drink per day or less for women and two drinks per day or less for men); one drink is defined as 12 oz beer, 5 oz wine, or 1.5 oz distilled spirits.
Routine supplementation with antioxidants, such as vitamins E and C and β-carotene, is not advised because of lack of evidence of efficacy and concern related to long-term safety.
Benefit from chromium supplementation in people with diabetes or obesity has not been conclusively demonstrated and therefore cannot be recommended.

Adapted from American Diabetes Association. Standards of Medical Care in Diabetes 2006. Diabetes Care 2006;29:s4-s42.

Analogously, physicians and other members of the health care team need to understand the major issues in diabetes and nutrition and to support the nutritional plan developed collaboratively. Individualized dietary advice can be developed by a physician from a brief diet history obtained by asking: "What do you eat for breakfast? Lunch? Dinner? Do you have snacks between breakfast and lunch? Lunch and dinner? Dinner and bedtime? What do you drink during the day?" Ideally, this information should be obtained at each visit, with specific suggestions for change that both patient and provider agree are important and achievable.

Easy issues to address include caloric beverages, which tend to elevate glucose levels dramatically and can generally be replaced quite painlessly by artificially sweetened alternatives. Juices are generally perceived as healthful but can significantly affect glycemic control and total calorie intake. Substituting low-fat products for higher fat alternatives is often suggested but needs to be done with the recognition that they are generally higher in carbohydrates. Fat-free and sugar-free foods need to be recognized as food that is not "free." Portion control and recipe modification are excellent techniques, particularly for meats and fried foods.

Adequate spacing between meals is usually good advice for patients with T2DM because postprandial glucose levels generally peak 2 hours after a meal, when a snack would normally be taken. Eating approximately every 4 hours while awake is the most practical dietary plan for most overweight people. Frequent small meals have been shown to be of benefit when used in a controlled inpatient setting, but in general when overweight patients are encouraged to eat more frequently they often overeat more frequently. At a minimum, avoiding high-calorie snacks is reasonable advice for most people with diabetes. A repeated diet history and additional modest changes negotiated every few weeks to months by all health care providers (doctor, nurse, or dietitian) allow assessment of whether previously agreed to changes were enacted, reinforcement of the importance of diet efforts, and slow enticement of patients into more healthful dietary choices.

In general, the critical nutrient for glycemic consistency is carbohydrate. Essentially every molecule of carbohydrate consumed is converted to glucose in the gut and requires the action of insulin to be cleared from the circulation. The carbohydrate-counting technique can be used in patients with T2DM to facilitate consistent carbohydrate intake or to allow insulin dose adjustment in response to changes in carbohydrates consumed.[757] Whereas the beta cell in T2DM has generally lost its responsiveness to glucose, the second phase of insulin secretion is largely spared in T2DM and is in part driven by amino acids and fatty acids. Therefore, including some protein and fat in each meal and snack is useful.

Dietary fat is the nutrient most closely associated in epidemiologic studies with the risk of developing T2DM. Although dietary fats clearly have an impact on total caloric intake related to their caloric density and on circulating lipids, they have a minimal impact on glycemia acutely. Fat intake is a contributor to obesity and the critical nutrient for cardiovascular risk management. It is generally recommended that people with diabetes (and everyone in general) consume a diet that is modestly restricted in calories (if they are overweight) containing less than 10% of total calories as saturated fat and less than 10% as polyunsaturated fat. Some advocate substituting foods high in monounsaturated fatty acids—seeds, nuts, avocado, olives, olive oil, and canola oil—for carbohydrate, but most patients do not find adequate variety in the monounsaturated fatty acid category and often overeat these high-calorie foods. Higher-carbohydrate diets can raise postprandial glucose and triglycerides but are much less calorically dense and have a higher thermic effect, both of which tend to promote weight loss.

Dietary protein similarly has a minimal impact on glucose levels, although amino acids do promote insulin secretion, which may be advantageous in patients with T2DM. Metabolism of protein results in the formation of acids and nitrogenous waste, which can lead to bone demineralization and glomerular hyperfiltration. At least 0.8 g of high-quality dietary protein per kilogram of body weight is generally recommended; otherwise, restriction of protein intake to 10% to 20% of total calories minimizes potential adverse long-term effects of high protein intake.

The role of vitamins, trace minerals, and nutritional supplements in the treatment of diabetes is poorly understood. Some are absolutely convinced of the utility of soluble fiber, magnesium, chromium, zinc, folic acid, pyridoxine, cyanocobalamin, vitamin A, vitamin C, vitamin E, vanadium, selenium, garlic, and others. Clinical trial data to support their safety and efficacy are inconclusive at best. Many patients are convinced that nutritional supplementation is healthful, and it is often counterproductive to engage in scholarly discussion of the nature of the evidence base for their decision. At a minimum, discussion should include the documented efficacy of more classic lifestyle and pharmacologic intervention and the idea that these efforts should not be left by the wayside when budget constraints affect potentially more effective interventions.[758,759] A small randomized, controlled trial has demonstrated that a multivitamin and mineral supplement reduced the incidence of participant-reported infection and related absenteeism among patients with T2DM mellitus, perhaps related to a high prevalence of subclinical micronutrient deficiency.[760]

Although there are proponents of a wide range of dietary composition, there are few data to support these recommendations from long-term outcome studies of prescribed diets. Mixed meals containing 10% to 20% of calories from protein, no more than 10% of calories from saturated fat, and the remainder largely from monounsaturated fats (seeds, nuts, avocados, olives, olive oil, canola oil) and carbohydrates, particularly whole grains, fruit, vegetables, and low-fat milk, are probably most reasonable. There is evidence to suggest that a diet rich in complex carbohydrates and low in fat and animal protein is a beneficial component of comprehensive lifestyle management in the setting of cardiovascular disease.[761] On the other hand, a number of studies suggest that diets lower in carbohydrate and higher in protein and fat reduce caloric intake and provide improvements in insulin sensitivity, glycemia, and cardiovascular risk markers.

Weight loss is a goal of many patients with and without diabetes and certainly is associated with improvements in glycemic control, insulin resistance, circulating lipids, and blood pressure. Numerous clinical studies document that certain changes can produce modest weight loss that can be largely maintained with sustained effort. These changes include intensive lifestyle programs involving frequent contact with patients, individualized counseling, and education aimed at reducing calorie intake. Additional, complementary changes by the patient include regular physical activity and efforts to understand and control behaviors that result in overeating.[96,762-765]

Exercise

There is a substantial body of literature supporting exercise as a modality of treatment in T2DM.[96,762-767] Exercise is perhaps the single most important lifestyle intervention in diabetes because it is associated with improved glycemic control, insulin sensitivity, cardiovascular fitness, and remodeling. Aerobic exercise and resistance (strength) training both have a positive impact on glucose control. Improvements in glycemic control are generally apparent immediately and become maximal after a few weeks of consistent exercise. However, they might persist for only 3 to 6 days after the cessation of training; hence the rationale for negotiating a minimum of three exercise sessions a week to maintain the benefit of the intervention.

The key concept is to promote an increase in activity using an approach similar to the one discussed for diet. Goals, methods, intensity, and frequency have to be negotiated with patients with great sensitivity to recognizing barriers and helping patients discover solutions. The role of educators, exercise specialists, physical therapists, and social supports in this process is critical. The major role for the physician is to screen for complications (neuropathy, nephropathy, retinopathy, vascular disease) and discover ways for patients to be able to exercise safely. Exercise in the presence of uncontrolled diabetes, hypertension, retinopathy, nephropathy, neuropathy, and cardiovascular disease can create devastating problems. These can all be addressed creatively and should never present an insurmountable barrier to increasing physical activity.

Some authorities recommend that all patients older than 35 years have stress tests before exercise. The utility of stress tests is potentially limited by their poor sensitivity and specificity.[724,768] If the exercise program contemplated does not involve more strenuous (intensity and duration) activity than the patient has engaged in recently but merely involves more frequent activity, screening cardiovascular stress testing is unlikely to be useful. However, when sedentary patients plan to embark on a program of strenuous exercise, stress testing is prudent to evaluate for subclinical coronary disease. Stress testing should be seriously considered in patients with an estimated 10-year risk of cardiovascular disease greater than 10%. Even when stress testing is employed and negative results are obtained, it is reasonable to encourage patients not to overexert and to recognize exertional chest, jaw, or arm discomfort as well as palpitations and dyspnea as symptoms of cardiac dysfunction.

Over time, improved exercise tolerance should be viewed as a measure of improving cardiorespiratory function. For aerobic exercise to improve insulin sensitivity, glycemic control, and cardiovascular risk, the patient must engage in at least 150 minutes per week of moderate-intensity aerobic physical activity (50%-70% of maximum heart rate) or 90 minutes per week of vigorous aerobic exercise (>70% of maximum heart rate).[649] Exercise should be regular, at least every 48 hours. Patients with T2DM should be encouraged to perform resistance exercise targeting all major muscle groups three times a week.[649]

For the average patient with T2DM starting an exercise program, this equates to quite low level activity initially, such as walking at a pace of 2 miles an hour. Initially, it may even be advantageous to negotiate once-weekly walks or shorter-duration exercise sessions, or both, and proceed from there. Over time, patients are encouraged to pick up the pace as tolerated and increase the duration and frequency of exercise sessions slowly to avoid overuse injuries. It is not unreasonable to suggest to patients that if they are going to incorporate exercise in their diabetes management program, they must think of exercise as a treatment that takes the place of a pill and thus requires adherence to produce benefit.

Self-Monitoring of Blood Glucose

Self-monitoring of blood glucose (SMBG) has not been demonstrated in clinical trials to change outcomes in T2DM when evaluated in isolation.[769] However, many diabetes self-management programs have been demonstrated to help reduce complications. In all of these, SMBG is an integral part of the process, suggesting that SMBG is at least a component of effective therapy. The frequency and type of monitoring in diabetes therapy should be determined in consultation with the patient, taking into account the nature of the diabetes, the overall treatment plan and goals, and the patient's abilities. SMBG is particularly recommended for all patients with T2DM taking insulin or sulfonylureas because it allows patients to identify minimal or asymptomatic episodes of hypoglycemia.

Although severe hypoglycemia is relatively rare in T2DM, it can have devastating consequences such as trauma or self-injury or change in the perceived ability of a patient to continue to live independently as a result of confusion or loss of consciousness. Also, it is essential to have patients critically assess the nature of any hypoglycemic symptoms that may occur. Many patients are fearful or overconcerned about hypoglycemia and routinely consume extra calories in response to a variety of life's circumstances, such as when they are hungry, sweaty, nervous, or upset. Monitoring studies generally document that most symptoms in patients with T2DM are not related to hypoglycemia and should not be treated with excessive calorie consumption.

Timing of SMBG varies depending on the diabetes therapy. It is important to advise patients to vary the time of the day at which blood glucose levels are checked. For some patients, the highest blood glucose of the day is the morning glucose, whereas for others the highest is before bed. Particularly in early diabetes, gestational diabetes, and well-controlled diabetes, monitoring 1 to 2 hours after meals allows patients to assess the effect of their lifestyle and pharmacologic efforts in controlling postprandial glucose levels, which are usually the only glycemic abnormality present. Monitoring and thus targeting therapy at just one time of day can leave the patient with a less than ideal overall response to therapy.

When glucose control is poor, having patients concentrate on premeal glucose levels is adequate. Once the premeal glucose levels reach the low 100s, many advocate that patients switch to checking 1- to 2-hour postprandial glucose levels because it amplifies the observed effect of diet on glycemic control and enables patients to see that moderate changes in meal plan, activity, and medications have a significant impact on glycemic control. Even after substantial inappropriate changes in food intake, activity, or timing or dose of medication, blood sugar values often return to near-normal levels overnight or by the time of the next meal.

The frequency of glucose monitoring needs to be matched to individual patients' needs and treatment. Many clinicians ask patients to monitor at least once a day, varying among before breakfast, lunch, dinner, bedtime, and midsleep as well as with hypoglycemic symptoms. Others ask intensively insulin-treated patients to monitor with intensity similar to that described for patients with T1DM (four times per day before meals, with weekly checks at least once after breakfast, lunch, dinner, and at midsleep, as well as with symptoms). Some ask for sets of glycemic readings more infrequently (e.g., fasting and 1 hour after the biggest meal). In the subset of patients who achieve stable blood glucose levels without significant hypoglycemia, it is generally appropriate to decrease the frequency of SMBG to a few times a week. It is critical that SMBG be frequent enough that both patient and provider have a good understanding of both the adequacy of the treatment regimen and the stability of glycemic control.

It has been widely assumed that the benefits of SMBG stem from the effect of putting patients in a situation in which they can be in control of their own therapy. If patients are aware of the glycemic targets associated with the outcomes they seek to achieve, SMBG enables them to critically evaluate their response to therapy and assure themselves that they are reaching their goals. It is generally useful for patients to keep a daily diary of their SMBG results, not only so that they can assess their results periodically but also so that they can share them with the health care team. Unfortunately, many patients faithfully perform daily or more frequent SMBG, record the results as instructed, and discuss them with their health care team only at quarterly or semiannual visits even though their control is inadequate. Unless SMBG results are entirely within agreed-to targets, they should be communicated and reviewed at least monthly with a member of the health care team by telephone, fax, mail, or e-mail or at an interim visit to trigger changes in therapy as the need arises. Unfortunately, such services are generally not reimbursed and can become an unsustainable burden on health care teams.

One of the most difficult areas in which to keep current is the area of available equipment and supplies, particularly for glucose monitoring. A useful resource in this regard is the annual *Resource Guide*, which comes out as the January issue of *Diabetes Forecast*, a magazine for lay people with diabetes and their families. It is available on line at the ADA Web site (www.diabetes.org) by clicking on "Community and Resources" and then on "Diabetes Forecast" and finally on "Back Issues" to find the most recent January issue.

Pharmacotherapy of Type 2 Diabetes

The revolution in the treatment of T2DM since 1995 in the United States has been driven by the release of several new classes of drugs that independently address different pathophysiologic mechanisms that contribute to the development of diabetes. The available oral antidiabetic agents can be divided by mechanism of action into insulin sensitizers with primary action in the liver, insulin sensitizers with primary action in peripheral tissues, insulin secretagogues, and agents that slow the absorption of carbohydrates. Insulin therapy in patients with T2DM effectively is a supplement to endogenous insulin secretion. The relative benefits of lifestyle intervention and the nine classes of drugs available for the management of T2DM are shown in Table 30–10. This area has been the subject of extensive reviews.[770-773] In the following discussion the principles outlined in these reviews are summarized, and limited additional references are provided.

Insulin Sensitizers with Predominant Action in the Liver

Metformin is the only biguanide available in the United States. Phenformin was removed from the United States market in the 1970s because of deaths associated with lactic acidosis. Phenformin and buformin remain available in some countries. Although metformin has been available in Europe for almost 40 years, it has been approved in the United States only since 1995. The precise mechanism of action of metformin is unknown; recent studies suggest that it activates AMP-activated protein kinase, an intracellular signal of depleted cellular energy stores implicated in the stimulation of skeletal muscle glucose uptake and in the inhibition of hepatic gluconeogenesis.[774] The major clinical activity of metformin is to reduce hepatic insulin resistance and thereby gluconeogenesis and glucose production. It has more inconsistently demonstrated effects to improve insulin sensitivity in peripheral tissues. Because of its limited duration of action, it is generally taken at least twice daily, although a sustained-release formulation is now available.

Because biguanides do not increase insulin levels, they are not associated with a significant risk of hypoglycemia. The most common adverse events are gastrointestinal: nausea, diarrhea, crampy abdominal pain, and dysgeusia. About one third of patients have some gastrointestinal distress, particularly early in their course of treatment. This distress can be minimized by starting with a low dose once daily with meals and titrating upward slowly (over weeks) to effective doses. Sustained-release metformin is associated with less-frequent and less-severe upper GI symptoms, the more common of the adverse effects of metformin, but it can increase the frequency of diarrhea, a much less common adverse effect overall. The vast majority of patients note no adverse effects with metformin therapy, and at least 90% tolerate it adequately with long-term use. Perhaps as a result of clinical or subclinical GI effects, metformin is associated with less weight gain than other antidiabetic agents, and in some studies it is associated with a modest mean weight loss.

The other side effect of metformin is lactic acidosis, which is quite rare and occurs almost exclusively in patients who are at high risk for developing lactic acidosis apart from metformin therapy. As a result, it is recommended that high-risk patients not use metformin.[775] The package insert states that metformin is absolutely contraindicated in patients with renal insufficiency because the drug is cleared renally. Metformin should not be used in male patients with a serum creatinine 1.5 mg/dL or higher and in female patients with a serum creatinine 1.4 mg/dL or higher.

Obviously, there is a complex relationship between serum creatinine and renal function. Thus, reasonable practice generally involves not using metformin in patients with an estimated glomerular filtration rate (GFR) based on the MDRD equation[776] of less than 40 mL/min (estimated GFR for a 79-year-old white woman with a creatinine of 1.3 mg/dL) and avoiding greater than half-maximal doses of metformin in patients with an estimated GFR between 40 and 60 mL/min. An MDRD GFR calculator is available at nephron.com. Metformin is also contraindicated in patients with congestive heart failure requiring drug treatment, in those with hepatic insufficiency, and in the setting of alcohol abuse. Caution is required in elderly people, patients with acute illness or poorly controlled chronic illness, and in the setting of simultaneous treatment with nephrotoxic drugs (e.g., contrast dye).

The glucose-lowering efficacy and the prevalence of adverse gastrointestinal effects increase proportionately in the dose range 500 to 2000 mg/day. The maximal dose of 2550 mg does not generally provide additional benefit beyond that seen at 2000 mg daily. Newer formulations of metformin combined with glipizide, glyburide, pioglitazone, and rosiglitazone have been developed to maximize glucose-lowering effectiveness with a single prescription through the synergy of using two classes of agents with different actions.

Arguably, metformin has the best record among oral antidiabetic agents in outcome studies. In the UKPDS, among overweight subjects, those randomly assigned to metformin not only had improvements in microvascular complications similar to those of subjects randomly assigned to insulin and sulfonylurea but also demonstrated a reduction in diabetes-related deaths and myocardial infarction.[740] The validity of this observation has been challenged because of unusual responses in a subsequent subrandomization. The beneficial effect of metformin on macrovascular complications through mechanisms independent of glycemic control is certainly plausible and supported by such observations as metformin-associated modest reductions in LDL, triglycerides, blood pressure, and procoagulant factors. The ADA has recently published a consensus statement on medical management that suggests metformin be initiated in all patients with T2DM, absent contraindications, at or near the time of diagnosis of diabetes.[745]

Insulin Sensitizers with Predominant Action in Peripheral Insulin-Sensitive Tissues

The thiazolidinedione class of drugs (TZDs or glitazones), has engendered great enthusiasm and controversy since the first agent, troglitazone, was approved in 1997.[777] Rare fatal hepatotoxicity was associated with troglitazone and it was withdrawn from the United States market in 2000, largely because the other TZDs (pioglitazone and rosiglitazone) were thought to be safer. These agents are believed to work through binding and modulation of the activity of a family of nuclear transcription factors termed *peroxisome proliferator-activated receptors* (PPARs). They are associated with slow improvement in glycemic control over weeks to months in parallel with an improvement in insulin sensitivity and reduction of FFA levels.

Each of these agents varies in important ways with regard to potency, pharmacokinetics, metabolism, binding characteris-

TABLE 30–10 COMPARISONS OF THERAPIES FOR TYPE 2 DIABETES

Property	Lifestyle	Insulins	Sulfonylureas	Metformin	α-Glucosidase Inhibitors	Glitazones	Glinides	Exenatide	Pramlintide
Target tissue	Muscle or fat	Beta cell supplement	Beta cell	Liver	Gut	Muscle	Beta cell	Various	Brain
Δ HbA_{1c} (monotherapy)	Variable	1%->2%	1%-2%	1%-2%	0.5%-1%	0.5%-2%	Re: 1%-2% N: 0.5%-1%	~1%	~0.5%
Fasting effect	Good	Excellent	Good	Good	Poor	Good	Re: Mod N: Poor	Poor	Poor
Postprandial effect	Good	Excellent	Good	Good	Excellent	Good	Re: Good N: Exc	Excellent	Excellent
Severe hypoglycemia	No	Yes	Yes	No	No	No	Re: Yes N: No	No	No
Dosing interval	Continuous	qd to continuous	qd to tid	bid or tid	bid to qid	P: qd Ro: qd or bid	tid to qid with meals	bid	tid
Δ Weight (lb/yr)	+1	+3	+1-3	0 to −6	0 to −10	+1-13	+1-3	−6 to −12	−3 to −6
Δ Insulin	Variable	Increase	Increase	Modest decrease	Modest decrease	Decrease	Increase	Increase	None
Δ LDL	Minimal decrease	Minimal decrease	None	Decrease	Mnimal decrease	Increase	None	None	None
Δ HDL	Minimal increase	None	None	Increase	None	Increase	None	Decrease	None
Δ TG	Minimal decrease	Decrease	None	Decrease	Minimal decrase	P: Decrease Ro: None	None	Decrease	None
Common problem	Recidivism, injury	Hypoglycemia, weight gain	Hypoglycemia, weight gain	Transient GI	Flatulence	Weight gain, edema, anemia	Hypoglycemia	GI	GI
Rare problem				Lactic acidosis		Hepatotoxicity?			
Contraindications	None	None	Allergy	Renal failure Liver failure CHF >80 yr old	Intestinal disease	Hepatocellular disease		None	None
Cost ($/mo)	0-200	30-450	10-15	30-60	40-80	75-180	70-110	170-200	200-400
Maximum effective dose		1-2 U/kg/day	½ max or double starting	1000 mg bid	50 mg tid	P: 45 mg qd Ro: 4 mg bid	Re: 2 mg tid N: 120 mg tid	10 μg bid	120 μg ac

Exc, excellent; HDL, high-density lipoprotein; LDL, low-density lipoprotein; max, maximum; Mod, moderate; N, nateglinide; P, pioglitazone; Re, repaglinide; Ro, rosiglitazone; TG, triglycerides.

tics, and demonstrated lipid effects. At the same time, all are effective glucose-lowering agents that are remarkably well tolerated. The only significant adverse effects are weight gain and fluid retention (and associated edema formation and hemodilution). There is no substantial evidence that these newer agents are associated with hepatotoxicity, but this record of safety has been established in appropriate patients. Patients should have liver function tests before beginning TZD therapy. TZDs are contraindicated in patients with active hepatocellular disease and in patients with unexplained serum alanine aminotransferase (ALT) levels greater than 2.5 times the upper limit of normal.

Pioglitazone and rosiglitazone are equally effective glucose-lowering agents, and they have similar extent of weight gain and incidence of edema formation. They also provide equivalent improvements in markers of insulin resistance and inflammation. In a head-to-head study among dyslipidemic patients, pioglitazone reduced triglycerides approximately 20%, whereas rosiglitazone increased triglycerides on average by 5%. Pioglitazone is associated with a modestly greater improvement in HDL particle number and size and with an improvement in both LDL particle size and number. Rosiglitazone was associated with an increase in LDL particle number and an improvement in LDL particle size.[778]

The promise of the glitazone class to reverse or prevent the negative cardiovascular associations of insulin resistance in parallel with its demonstrated effect of improving insulin sensitivity was suggested by a series of associations: reduced carotid intimal medial thickness, normalization of vascular endothelial function, improvements in dyslipidemia, lower blood pressure, and improved fibrinolytic and coagulation parameters. The PROactive Study was a randomized, double-blind, placebo-controlled trial in 5238 patients who had T2DM and documented macrovascular disease. Subjects were randomized to placebo or to 45 mg/day of pioglitazone and otherwise treated according to guidelines for hyperglycemia and major cardiovascular risk factors. The primary end-point was the time from randomization to a broad set of macrovascular end-points. Pioglitazone was associated with a 10% reduction in the primary end-point, but the reduction was not statistically significant. However, for the principal secondary end-point, time from randomization to one of all-cause mortality, nonfatal MI (excluding silent MI), and stroke, pioglitazone therapy was associated with a 16% reduction, which was marginally statistically significant. Subsequent analysis and discussion of this technically negative and somewhat flawed trial has been extensive and supports the notion that pioglitazone therapy is associated with reductions in cardiovascular events that are largely accounted for by improvements in glycemia, lipids. and blood pressure. The benefits were in part mitigated by an increased incidence of heart failure, weight gain, and edema.[779] This issue will be further addressed by a number of trials under way.[747]

A second attribute of the glitazones that has generated great enthusiasm is an improvement in insulin secretory dynamics in subjects with diabetes and IGT. These observations provide hope that glitazone therapy may be useful in preventing diabetes or in halting the progression of established diabetes, thereby reducing the need for additional drug therapy. It is critical to recognize that the proven effects of pioglitazone and rosiglitazone to date are limited to improvements in glycemic control and changes in lipid parameters. A number of studies reported in 2006 and subsequently will address this issue robustly.[780,781]

The adverse effects that have engendered the greatest concern regarding this class of drugs is weight gain and fluid retention, which can manifest as heart failure. Careful study indicates that the weight gain is a result of subcutaneous and not visceral fat accumulation and that there is, in fact, a reduction in visceral fat, hepatic fat, and intramyocellular fat. Thus, the weight gain observed with glitazones, while having obvious negative consequences from the cosmetic standpoint, is perhaps less likely to cause significant adverse cardiovascular effects. Both weight gain and fluid retention are more common and severe in patients with the greatest glycemic responses, making expectant management of these adverse effects mandatory. All patients prescribed glitazones should be counseled to redouble lifestyle efforts to minimize weight gain.

With regard to edema, with appropriate caution almost no one should need to withdraw from therapy as a result of fluid retention. The patients most likely to experience edema are those treated with insulin and those with preexisting edema. Thus, women, overweight patients, and those with diastolic dysfunction or renal insufficiency are at greatest risk. It is prudent to teach patients with preexisting edema how to assess pitting pretibial edema at home and suggest that they make a habit of checking nightly. If they note a pattern of increasing edema at home, patients can be instructed to restrict sodium intake, to start a diuretic, or to increase their diuretic by some specified quantity on their own as needed.

In the previously edematous patient and in patients treated with insulin, it is prudent to initiate therapy with the lowest available dose of glitazone. In 1 to 3 months, if the glycemic response has been inadequate and significant edema has not developed, consider increasing the dose of glitazone further with continued expectant home evaluation for edema. Most patients with mild edema respond to a low-dose thiazide diuretic (e.g., 25 mg hydrochlorothiazide). In patients with more extensive edema, a combination of low-dose thiazide diuretic with moderate-dose loop diuretic is sometimes required. Anecdotal reports suggest that avoidance of nonsteroidal antiinflammatory agents and dihydropyridine calcium channel blockers can reduce the frequency of edema as an adverse event. Fluid retention to the point of congestive heart failure and anasarca has been reported; in the PROactive study, an excess of approximately 2% of patients treated with high-dose pioglitazone required hospitalization for heart failure as compared with placebo. In some patients, edema is refractory to diuretic therapy. In some of these patients, edema resolves with a reduction of glitazone dose, and some patients require drug withdrawal. Preclinical studies suggest that amiloride may be effective in minimizing edema, although human trials have not been reported.[782]

A series of nonthiazolidinedione drugs with activity in the PPAR system were under development worldwide. Their development has largely stopped due to concerns regarding mitogenicity, increased cardiovascular events, and edema. We still have a great deal to learn regarding the activity and regulation of the PPAR system and the risks and benefits of its modulation.

Insulin Secretagogues

Currently available insulin secretagogues all bind to the sulfonylurea receptor (SUR1), a subunit of the ATP-sensitive potassium channel (K_{ATP}) on plasma membrane of pancreatic beta cells. The SUR1 subunit regulates the activity of the channel and also binds ATP and ADP, effectively functioning as a glucose sensor and trigger for insulin secretion. Sulfonylurea binding leads to closing of the channel; increases in intracellular ATP and decreases in ADP as a result of fuel metabolism also lead to closing of the channel. The membrane depolarization that ensues causes the opening of voltage-dependent L-type calcium channels. Subsequent calcium influx results in an increase in intracellular calcium, which leads to insulin secretion. Differences in pharmacokinetic and binding properties of the various insulin secretagogues result in the specific responses that each agent produces. The major difference between them seems to be related to duration of action and to fairly subtle variations in their hypoglycemic potential.

Sulfonylureas

The sulfonylureas have been available since the 1950s. They have a relatively slow onset of action and variable duration of action. There are numerous choices available (Table 30–11), which can be divided into first- and second-generation agents. In general, the second-generation agents are more potent and as a result have fewer adverse effects and drug-drug interactions. Extended-release glipizide and glimepiride are preferred agents because they can be given once daily in the vast majority of patients and involve a relatively low risk of hypoglycemia and weight gain. Almost all oral secretagogues have been shown to have a significantly lower hypoglycemic potential than glyburide. Nonetheless, glyburide is one of the most commonly prescribed insulin secretagogues, even in the face of concerns about its potential cardiovascular toxicity.[783]

An unusual characteristic of sulfonylureas is that the maximum marketed dose is generally two to four times higher than the maximum effective dose. There has been concern that sulfonylureas might cause increased arrhythmic cardiovascular events in patients with diabetes as a result of their activity on vascular and cardiac SUR2 receptors, with an effect of blunting ischemic preconditioning, a protective autoregulatory mechanism in the heart. There is some evidence that this may be less likely with glimepiride than with glyburide, but it is also a good reason to avoid high-dose sulfonylurea therapy.[784]

Sulfonylureas are arguably the most cost-effective glucose-lowering agents and therefore are clearly worthy of their widespread use. In general, limiting the dose to one-fourth the maximum marketed dose, unless higher doses are clearly demonstrated to provide significant benefits in glycemic control, minimizes costs and adverse events. Small doses of sulfonylurea (e.g., 0.5 to 1 mg of glimepiride or 2.5 mg of extended-release glipizide) are remarkably effective, particularly in patients on concomitant insulin-sensitizing therapy, and are almost uniformly well tolerated.

Repaglinide

Repaglinide is a member of the meglitinide family of insulin secretagogues, distinct from the sulfonylureas. It has a short half-life and a distinct SUR1 binding site. As a result of more rapid absorption, it produces a generally faster and briefer stimulus to insulin secretion. As a result, it is generally taken with each meal and provides better postprandial control and generally less hypoglycemia and weight gain than glyburide. Repaglinide does seem to have a long residence time on the sulfonylurea receptor and a prolonged effect on fasting glucose, even though its pharmacologic half-life is quite short. Repaglinide is available in 0.5, 1, and 2 mg tablets. The maximum dose is 4 mg with each meal. As is the case with the sulfonylureas, there is only a modest glucose-lowering advantage of high doses versus moderate doses of repaglinide.

Nateglinide

Nateglinide is a derivative of phenylalanine, structurally distinct from both sulfonylureas and the meglitinides. It has a quicker onset and shorter duration of action than repaglinide. Its interaction with SUR1 is fleeting. As a result, its effect in lowering postprandial glucose is quite specific, and it has little effect in lowering fasting glucose. This provides advantages (less hypoglycemia) and disadvantages (less overall glucose-lowering effectiveness). Therefore, nateglinide is most appropriately used when fasting glucose levels are modestly elevated in early diabetes or in combination with insulin sensitizers or long-acting evening insulin. Nateglinide is available as 120-mg tablets and is taken with each meal. A 60-mg tablet is available but is not generally used except in patients with minimal hyperglycemia.

The rationale for stimulating insulin secretion in a way that minimizes fasting hyperinsulinemia and maximizes postprandial control is compelling. Furthermore, these newer agents demonstrate little binding to the vascular smooth muscle and cardiac SUR2 receptors. However, the use in the United States of these newer glinide agents has been modest, in part because of the need for multiple daily doses, greater expense than with

TABLE 30–11 CHARACTERISTICS OF SULFONYLUREAS

Drug	Initial Daily Dose	Maximum Daily Dose	Equivalent Doses (mg)	Duration of Action	Comments
Acetohexamide	250 mg	1500 mg, div bid	500	Int: 12-18 hr	Metabolized by liver to active metabolite twice as potent as parent compound. Has diuretic activity. Has uricosuric activity.
Chlorpropamide	100 mg	750 mg (500 mg in older patients)	250	Very long: 60 hr	70% metabolized by liver to less active metabolites; 30% excreted intact by kidneys. Can potentiate ADH. Disulfiram-like reaction with alcohol occurs in nearly 1/3 of patients.
Tolazamide	100 mg	1000 mg, div bid	250	Int: 12-24 hr	Metabolized by liver to less active and inactive products. Has diuretic activity.
Tolbutamide	250-500 mg	3000 mg, div bid or tid	1000	Short: 6-12 hr	Metabolized by liver to inactive product.
Glipizide	5 mg	40 mg, div bid	5	Int: 12-24 hr	Metabolized by liver to inactive products that are excreted in the urine and, to a lesser extent, in the bile. Mild diuretic activity.
Glipizide ER	5 mg	20 mg qd	5	Long: >24 hr	
Glyburide	2.5 mg	20 mg, div bid	5	Int: 16-24 hr	Metabolized by liver to weakly active and inactive products, excreted in urine and bile. Mild diuretic activity. Highest risk of hypoglycemia.
Micronized glyburide	3 mg	6 mg bid	3	Shorter	
Glimepiride	1 mg	8 mg qd	2	Long: >24 hr	Metabolized to inactive metabolites by liver, excreted in urine and bile.

div, divided; int, intermediate.

sulfonylureas, and lack of head-to-head comparative studies that demonstrate superiority over newer sulfonylureas, which are already perceived as having low potential for producing hypoglycemia and weight gain.

Carbohydrate Absorption Inhibitors: α-Glucosidase Inhibitors

α-Glucosidase inhibitors (AGIs) work to inhibit the terminal step of carbohydrate digestion at the brush border of the intestinal epithelium. As a result, carbohydrate absorption is shifted more distally in the intestine and is therefore delayed, allowing the sluggish insulin secretory dynamics characteristic of T2DM to catch up with carbohydrate absorption.

There are two currently available agents, acarbose and miglitol. Their use in the United States has been limited by a number of factors, including the need to administer the medication at the beginning of each meal, flatulence as a common side effect, and only modest reductions in blood glucose. These factors should be balanced against the AGI's ability to lower postprandial glucose, thereby improving glycemia without increasing weight or hypoglycemic risk. Even though they potentially lower glucose in everyone, the extent of the lowering is generally modest, calling into question their utility in the presence of substantial expense and side effects.

To maximize the potential for these agents to be well tolerated, start with a low dose such as one fourth of the maximum dose just once daily and increase over a period of weeks to months to one-fourth to one-half the maximum dose with each meal.

Insulins

Insulin has been commercially available since the early 1920s and is arguably still the mainstay of therapy for most people with T2DM worldwide. Subcutaneous injection of insulin in T2DM is designed to supplement endogenous production of insulin both in the basal state to modulate hepatic glucose production and in the postprandial state, in which a surge in insulin release normally facilitates glucose clearance into muscle and fat for storage to allow intraprandial metabolism. Currently, almost all insulin used worldwide is of recombinant human origin or analog. The available formulations largely differ in their pharmacokinetics as shown in Table 30–12.

Insulin lispro, insulin aspart, and insulin glulisine are rapid-acting insulin analogues that have an onset of action in 5 to 15 minutes, peak activity in approximately 1 hour, and a duration of activity of approximately 4 hours. Regular insulin is approximately half as fast as the rapid-acting analogue, with onset in 30 minutes, a peak at 2 to 4 hours, and a duration of action of 6 to 8 hours or longer. Regular human insulin when administered IV is instantly effective, with a half-life on the order of 10 minutes. Administered IM, regular human insulin has a half-life of approximately 20 minutes. Rapid-acting insulin analogues do not exhibit discernible advantages on IV or IM administration.

Neutral protamine Hagedorn (NPH) is the only intermediate-acting insulin available since Lente insulin was withdrawn from the market. It is approximately twice as slow as regular insulin, with an onset of action in 1 to 2 hours, a peak at 4 to 8 hours, and a duration of action of 12 to 16 hours.

Ultralente insulin is no longer available as a human long-acting insulin. Insulin glargine is a long-acting insulin analogue that is solubilized in acid but precipitates when neutralized in tissues upon injection, producing no distinctive peak in activity and a duration of action of more than 24 hours in most patients. Insulin detemir is a long-acting analogue in which a fatty-acid side chain has been covalently bound to the insulin molecule; it remains soluble both in the vial and in tissues and has a duration of action of approximately 24 hours except at low doses (<20-30 units).

Premixed insulin formulations provide greater convenience and accuracy of mixing than those mixed by patients but at the expense of reduced flexibility. Premixed formulations available in the United States are 70/30 and 50/50 mixtures of NPH and regular insulin, a 75/25 and 50/50 mixture of lispro insulin in its NPH-like formulation with insulin lispro, and a 70/30 mixture of insulin aspart with its NPH-like congener. Premixed insulin provides a profile of activity as expected from the addition of the activities of its components.

The tactics in insulin administration in the setting of T2DM are the focus of great debate and strong opinion. Remaining great debates revolve around whether the relative benefits of analogue insulins are justified in light of the approximately threefold greater expense and whether the greater convenience of low-complexity regimens is justifiable in light of the greater risk associated with lesser flexibility in dosing.[785-787]

Adverse events associated with insulin are well known and include weight gain and hypoglycemia. Both fast-acting and long-acting insulin analogues have been shown to provide a modest reduction in hypoglycemia. Insulin allergies are rare, as are chronic skin reactions, which include lipodystrophy and lipohypertrophy. The absolute risk of severe hypoglycemia in patients with T2DM is relatively small, approximately one third to one tenth as high as in similarly treated patients with T1DM. This risk can be further minimized with appropriate education of patients and expectant home glucose monitoring at times when unrecognized hypoglycemia is most likely to occur, such as midsleep or during unplanned or strenuous activity.

Newer insulin needles cause less discomfort than those previously available because of a finer gauge, shorter length, sharper points, and smoother surfaces. Insulin pen technology makes teaching a patient to take insulin much easier and provides greater convenience and accuracy of dosing. Insulin pump

TABLE 30–12 PHARMACOLOGY OF INSULIN

Duration	Insulin	Peak (hr)	Duration (hr)	Forms and Modifiers	Variability in Absorption
Rapid	Lispro, aspart, glulisine	~1	3-4	Analogue, monomeric	Minimal
Short	Regular	2-4	6-8	None	Moderate
Intermediate	NPH	4-8	12-16	Protamine	High
Long	Glargine	No distinct peak	~24	Analogue, precipitates at neutral pH	Moderate
	Detemir	No distinct peak	~24 (less at doses <20-30 units)	Analogue with fatty-acid side chain	Minimal

therapy has been used in patients with T2DM but is not widely accepted as cost-effective in routine use.

Inhaled insulin has recently been approved for use in patients with T1DM and T2DM. Clearly, this advance removes the barrier of injection but is associated with a bulkier and somewhat cumbersome device. The activity of human insulin on inhalation varies by formulation. The currently available formulation has an onset and peak of action similar to rapid-acting analogues but with a bit longer duration or tail in activity. It can be administered in combination with oral agents and with or without long-acting insulin in patients with T2DM. It is equally effective as injected insulin, although there are substantial barriers to high-dose inhaled insulin therapy. The question remains whether inhaled insulin will increase the use of what is arguably the most effective antihyperglycemic agent.[788]

Incretin-Related Therapies

The incretin effect is the process by which oral glucose has a greater stimulatory effect on insulin secretion than intravenous glucose does. In humans, this effect seems to be primarily mediated by GLP-1 and GIP. GLP-1 is produced from the proglucagon gene in intestinal L cells and is secreted in response to nutrients. GLP-1 stimulates insulin secretion in a glucose-dependent fashion, inhibits inappropriate hyperglucagonemia, slows gastric emptying, reduces appetite and improves satiety, and has beta cell–proliferative, antiapoptotic, and differentiation effects. GLP-1 has a very short half-life in plasma of 1 to 2 minutes due to N-terminal degradation by the enzyme dipeptidyl peptidase IV (DPP-IV). A variety of pharmacologic techniques have been developed to harness the potential of GLP-1 signaling to treat diabetes. This include incretin mimetics, GLP-1 analogues, and DPP-IV inhibition.[789,790]

Exendin-4 is a naturally occurring component of the saliva of the Gila monster *(Heloderma suspectum)* and shares 53% sequence identity with GLP-1; it is resistant to DPP-IV degradation. Exenatide is synthetic exendin-4 and is the first GLP-1–based therapy to be approved for human use in the United States. When injected subcutaneously, it produces the effects listed earlier and has a peak of action and half-life of approximately 2 hours. It is indicated for therapy of patients with T2DM inadequately controlled on metformin, sulfonylurea, TZD or combinations of the two.

In the registration trials, exenatide was studied at doses of 5 µg and 10 µg injected subcutaneously twice daily and was associated with approximately a 1% reduction in HbA_{1c}, predominant lowering of postprandial glucose levels, and about 0.5 to 1 pound per month of weight loss as compared to placebo. Open-label extension studies have demonstrated sustained lowering of HbA_{1c} and continuous weight loss averaging about 12 pounds at 2 years. With prolonged use, the greater weight loss has been associated with expected improvements in blood pressure and lipids.

The most common adverse effect is nausea, which occurs in 40% to 50% of patients, generally early in the course of therapy. The intensity is mild to moderate, and the nausea wanes over time. Nausea leads to withdrawal of therapy in about 5% of patients. Nausea is reduced in frequency and intensity by dose titration, beginning with a 5-µg twice-daily dose for the first month in clinical practice. Though hypoglycemia does not occur at higher rates than seen with placebo when exenatide is combined with metformin, mild to moderate hypoglycemia is observed with exenatide in combination with sulfonylureas. Reducing the dose of sulfonylurea down to the smallest available tablet size reduces hypoglycemia without substantially sacrificing efficacy.

Two DPP-IV inhibitors, vildagliptin and sitagliptin, are under review by the FDA. They produce sustained inhibition of DPP-IV when administered orally and produce moderate increases in GLP-1 and GIP with subsequent HbA_{1c} reduction of approximately 0.7%. They are not associated with weight loss or nausea. A DPP-IV–resistant analogue of GLP-1, liraglutide, is now in phase III trials. With once-daily subcutaneous injection, it is associated with similar efficacy on HbA_{1c} and weight as exenatide, though it causes greater lowering of fasting glucose and less nausea. A once-weekly formulation of exenatide is also in phase III trials. Many other DPP-IV inhibitors and GLP-1 analogues are under development.

Amylinomimetics

Amylin is a neuroendocrine hormone cosecreted with insulin by pancreatic beta cells. As would be expected, in parallel with the insulin deficiencies of T1DM and T2DM, amylin deficiencies are evident. Amylin and insulin have complementary actions in regulating plasma glucose. Amylin binds to brain nuclei. It promotes satiety and reduces appetite, and through vagal efferents it mediates a decrease in the rate of gastric emptying. It also regulates suppression of glucagon secretion in a glucose-dependent fashion, thus regulating the rate of glucose appearance from the GI tract and the liver. Insulin, on the other hand, regulates the rate of glucose disappearance from the circulation by stimulating glucose uptake in muscle and fat.[790,791]

However, amylin is relatively insoluble in aqueous solution and aggregates on plastic and glass. Pramlintide was developed as a soluble, nonaggregating, equipotent amylin analogue. It is indicated for use in patients with T1DM and insulin-treated patients with T2DM for mealtime subcutaneous injection. In patients with T2DM, when pramlintide was added to insulin therapy with or without a sulfonylurea or metformin, HbA_{1c} was reduced by about 0.5 to 0.7 percentage points and patients lost about 0.5 pounds per month.

Mild nausea, which wanes with continued therapy, is the most common adverse effect. It is minimized by titrating from 60 µg with meals to the usual 120 µg dose over 3 to 7 days as tolerated. Hypoglycemia is less frequent in patients with T2DM than in patients with T1DM, who do occasionally exhibit severe hypoglycemia. Prandial insulin should be reduced by 50% when initiating therapy in both clinical situations.

Oral medications that require rapid absorption for effectiveness should be administered either 1 hour before or 2 hours after injection of pramlintide.

Practical Aspects of Initiating and Progressively Managing Type 2 Diabetes

A significant challenge in clinical decision making in diabetes is that the increased availability of therapeutic options for antidiabetic therapy is ahead of adequate prospective outcome studies. Currently available clinical trial data have not identified the preferred agents in T2DM, either as initial therapy or in subsequent care. Each class of drugs and even agents within each class have advantages and limitations, and individual issues can significantly affect the appropriate choice of therapy in particular patients. Table 30–10 highlights some of the relative advantages and disadvantages of various agents and classes.

A general approach in the absence of any patient-specific factors is suggested in the algorithm presented in Figure 30–20. A growing body of experience indicates that the use of metformin as initial therapy in combination with diet and exercise can provide impressive lowering of glucose with essentially no risk of hypoglycemia.[745] Because this agent is available as a generic preparation, relative cost is low, and if the response is judged to

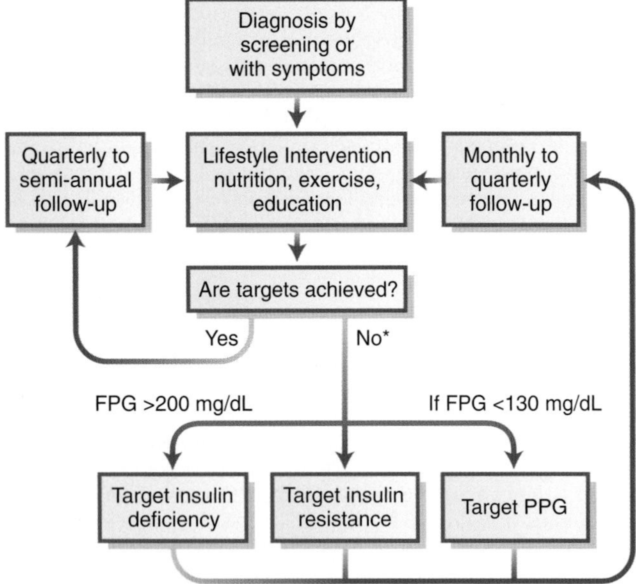

Figure 30–20 ▪ Treatment algorithm for type 2 diabetes. FPG, fasting plasma glucose; PPG, postprandial plasma glucose.

be inadequate, essentially any other agent can be added. It has been proposed that the use of metformin alone or in combination with a thiazolidinedione can lead to a greater reduction in cardiovascular risk than similarly effective (with respect to glycemia) approaches that increase insulin levels. At present, the data are not definitive on this point.

Patients with higher levels of glucose (generally FPG >200 mg/dL) almost always require agents to increase insulin levels. Because insulin, sulfonylureas, and glinides provide much faster improvements in overall control than metformin, glitazones, or AGIs, they are preferred in patients with higher blood glucose levels either as monotherapy or as part of initial combined therapy. Starting a patient with a low dose of a glimepiride, glipizide-GITS, or insulin combined with either metformin or glitazone is a reasonable initial approach to the poorly controlled condition.

In patients who have reasonable control of fasting and preprandial plasma glucose levels (more than 50% of values <130 mg/dL) whose overall control as assessed by HbA_{1c} is still higher than desired, monitoring may be either inaccurate or ineffective or postprandial plasma glucose (PPG) levels may be elevated. As it can be more difficult to have patients monitor in the postprandial state, it is important to remember that without specific therapy, almost all patients with T2DM have elevated PPG. Thus, in such patients, targeting presumed PPG elevations with the use of AGIs, glinides, exenatide, or rapid-acting insulin analogues can theoretically lower average glucose with a lower risk of weight gain and hypoglycemia than with sulfonylureas or long-acting insulin.

The most critical issue in long-term glycemic management is that of continuously reassessing with patients the adequacy of their control, examining glucose monitoring logs and HbA_{1c} values, and refining treatment regimens to achieve optimal control with the lowest doses of the fewest medications. Most patients in specialty care require two or more drugs to achieve recommended targets. Many patients require three or more (particularly if you consider long-acting and short-acting insulin as two agents). Fortunately, almost all the possible two-drug combinations and many of the three-drug combinations have been examined in modest-sized studies and have been shown to be safe and effective. Generally, it is preferred to add agents if there was an improvement in control with the first agent selected and to continue to add agents as needed to achieve goals. Subsequent back-titration to optimize treatment is often possible when glycemic goals are achieved. The selection of initial therapy should be based on mutually (patient and provider) recognized priorities. Increasingly, practitioners are using submaximal doses of agents in combination to increase the ratio of efficacy to adverse effects and in recognition of the potential synergy of sensitizers and secretagogues as well as the value of treatment of postprandial glucose and fasting glucose in combination therapy.

When adding insulin in the management of inadequately controlled T2DM, some practitioners prefer to stop the oral antidiabetic agents and switch to insulin. Most generally continue the oral agents and add an evening dose of insulin. Classically, bedtime NPH insulin and more lately bedtime long-acting insulin analogues have been preferred for initiating insulin therapy. In more overweight patients (>120% of ideal body weight), the use of mixed insulin (or premixed insulin) at dinner (evening meal) can help clear glucose elevations after the evening meal, generally the largest meal of the day. This works quite well in most patients, although some experience nocturnal hypoglycemia, which is less common with mixtures employing rapid-acting insulin analogues. There are data suggesting that glargine given at bedtime can similarly provide lower morning glucose values with less nocturnal hypoglycemia than NPH insulin, particularly in more overweight patients. Many patients eventually require more complex regimens, such as twice-daily injections or multiple injection regimens, and only rarely require insulin pump therapy. A minority of patients with T2DM have a better response to insulin administered in the morning than in the evening. Studies suggest that to achieve HbA_{1c} levels under 7%, many if not most patients require insulin doses on the order of 1 to 2 units per kilogram per day in addition to insulin sensitizers.

It is important that both patient and health care provider agree on how to reach the goals of therapy. Therefore, biases and concerns of the patient should be addressed when trying to determine which agent should be prescribed. These biases can be elucidated in interviews with patients through discussions of various strategies.

Strategies

Minimal Cost Strategy

For a large fraction of patients, particularly those who are elderly, drug costs are an overwhelming issue. Diet and exercise can be extremely effective and almost free.

The least expensive drugs for the treatment of diabetes are the sulfonylureas. Metformin and human insulin are relatively inexpensive. Thus, a minimum-cost strategy could start with a sulfonylurea and progress to the addition of generic metformin or bedtime or predinner insulin and finally two or more insulin injections per day, if necessary. In the Veterans Administration Cooperative Study, excellent control was achieved in the context of a comprehensive program of diabetes education using a combination of daytime sulfonylurea and evening insulin.

Although insulin is relatively inexpensive, at high doses (1 U/kg or more) the costs begin to rise, creating a rationale for adding metformin or a thiazolidinedione. Most pharmaceutical companies have programs to provide no-cost or low-cost medication to the poor. Many of these are listed with links at www.needymeds.com. Furthermore, for increasing numbers of patients, the major driving force in their drug expenses is the number of prescriptions, because each is associated with a copayment, providing a rationale for using combination agents.

Minimum Weight Gain Strategy

Weight gain associated with the treatment of diabetes is of concern to most clinicians and is often an overriding issue with patients. A strategy to minimize weight gain would emphasize diet and exercise and would almost certainly employ metformin as initial therapy. Exenatide is associated with substantial weight loss in most patients with long-term use and would almost always be used as second-line therapy if weight was truly the driving and only consideration. Because sulfonylureas and repaglinide seem to have a modest weight-sparing effect in combination therapy with insulin, one or the other could be added before insulin administration in such a strategy. As discussed earlier, the weight gain associated with thiazolidinediones, although certainly a cosmetic issue, might not be associated with increased cardiovascular risk.

Minimal Injection Strategy

Too many patients are determined to avoid insulin injections at any cost. The minimal injection strategy involves sulfonylureas, metformin, AGIs, thiazolidinediones, and inhaled insulin, which can be added in any order. Injected insulin, probably as a bedtime or predinner dose to minimize the inconvenience, would be added only if absolutely necessary. The strategy of using thiazolidinediones early in the course of diabetes in the hope that this might reduce the rate of progressive beta cell dysfunction remains unproved.

It is important to try to dispel notions that insulin therapy is difficult, ominous, or fraught with peril by highlighting its efficacy and the great strides that have been made in insulin formulations and delivery devices. Most diabetic patients require insulin at some point in their lifetime.

Quite a few patients who have resisted the use of insulin have not balked at exenatide therapy. This suggests that although patients have identified the needle as the predominant barrier to insulin therapy, they really had other biases driving their fears.

Minimal Insulin Resistance Strategy

The possible atherogenic effects of insulin have been widely touted in the lay press and by marketing programs within the pharmaceutical industry. The relationship between circulating insulin levels and cardiovascular risk in nondiabetic populations is incontrovertible but probably related to the presence of insulin resistance rather than the insulin concentrations per se. Furthermore, in essentially all studies of intensive management with insulin, improved outcomes were observed with insulin treatment. There are no clinical data to suggest that exogenous insulin is associated with adverse side effects or long-term complications beyond its hypoglycemic effects and the associated weight gain.

In any case, this strategy is analogous to the minimal injection strategy except that the order of introduction of agents is perhaps important. The thiazolidinediones have the greatest efficacy in reducing insulin resistance, metformin is second, and AGIs are third. Exenatide has been demonstrated in animal models to produce modest improvement in insulin sensitivity and would be assumed to reduce insulin resistance in parallel with weight; however, exenatide does increase postprandial insulin levels. Nateglinide is associated with more specific stimulation of insulin levels after meals than the other insulin secretagogues, which all increase peripheral insulin levels less than injected insulin.

Minimal Effort Strategy

Many patients are capable of making only a minimal effort with regard to their diabetes. Questioning patients about their pill-taking history and their realistic ability to comply with a prescribed frequency of therapy is important. Taking a once-a-day sulfonylurea or thiazolidinedione requires the least effort by the patient. At least one combination tablet taking advantage of this concept is available: rosiglitazone 4 mg in combination with either 1 or 2 mg of glimepiride. Taking bedtime insulin is actually relatively well accepted by patients to whom this consideration is important. Developing strategies to improve adherence and increase motivation is certainly a long-term goal in this population.

Hypoglycemia Avoidance Strategy

This is another important consideration for many patients. The AGIs and glitazones have been reported in small studies to reduce reactive hypoglycemia. Theoretically, exenatide and metformin should not be associated with hypoglycemia. Other oral agents could be added in any order, with the exception that insulin secretagogues would be added last, their dose minimized, and glyburide avoided. Nateglinide in particular among the secretagogues is associated with an exceptionally low risk of significant hypoglycemia. The rapid-acting insulin analogues are associated with a lower risk of hypoglycemia than human insulin. The long-acting insulin analogue detemir seems to be associated with a substantially lower risk of hypoglycemia than NPH and perhaps modestly hypoglycemic risk than glargine.

Postprandial Targeting Strategy

Achieving postprandial glucose targets is generally associated with better control than just meeting premeal targets.[792] On the basis of epidemiologic studies, it has been suggested that PPG is more highly correlated with cardiovascular disease risk than fasting glucose levels. Correction for confounding variables such as components of the multiple metabolic syndrome has not been performed, however. Furthermore, there are no outcome studies that have demonstrated the superiority of these approaches in patients with T2DM.

Control of postprandial glycemia can be achieved only with specific lifestyle efforts and pharmacologic agents that target postprandial glucose. Postprandial glucose monitoring is helpful in this regard because it reinforces the goals and is the most effective measure to assess the effectiveness of treatment. Nonpharmacologic techniques that can improve postprandial control include lowering the carbohydrate content of meals, adding fiber, substituting monounsaturated fats for carbohydrates, and encouraging physical activity after meals. The pharmacologic approach includes AGIs, exenatide, and rapid-acting insulin analogues. Nateglinide and repaglinide provide a theoretical advantage in this situation compared with other secretagogues, although formal head-to-head studies have not been completed comparing the glinides with glimepiride and glipizide-GITS.

Preventing Type 2 Diabetes

The possibility that T2DM can be prevented in high-risk persons has been formally tested in a series of large-scale clinical trials. The Da Qing study randomly assigned clinics in an industrial city in China to dietary intervention, exercise intervention, combined diet and exercise, or no intervention at all. Among the clinics, 577 subjects with IGT were studied. In this study, the interventions were quite modest and conducted largely in group settings. All three interventions led to reductions in the risk of conversion to diabetes of 31% to 46% compared with the control groups.[765] In a Finnish study, a similar number of middle-aged obese subjects with IGT were randomly assigned to a control group that received minimal lifestyle advice or to intensive, individualized instruction on food intake, increased physical activity, and weight reduction. The intensive lifestyle therapy group demonstrated a 58% relative risk reduction compared with the control group in the incidence of diabetes.[96]

In the United States, the Diabetes Prevention Program enrolled more than 3000 middle-aged, overweight subjects with IGT including substantial representation from high-risk minority groups. The intensive lifestyle group in this study also demonstrated a 58% relative risk reduction in the progression to diabetes.[251] In the Diabetes Prevention Program, there was another arm of the study that evaluated the ability of metformin at 500 mg twice a day to prevent the development of diabetes. It was moderately successful, with a 31% relative reduction in the progression of diabetes, although the benefit seemed to be greater in younger, more overweight, and more hyperglycemic subjects. In other studies, other oral antidiabetic agents—troglitazone in the Troglitazone in the Prevention of Diabetes (TRIPOD) study[763] and acarbose in the STOP-NIDDM study[764]—have been reported to reduce the risk of developing diabetes. Additional studies with currently available glitazones and nateglinide are underway. Patients and families as well as health care professionals are excited about the possibilities of preventing the disease.

The success of the lifestyle interventions is impressive, demonstrating conclusively that with a variety of techniques it is possible for patients to achieve physiologically relevant changes in body weight. Medications overall had less positive impact than lifestyle intervention, although troglitazone did perform remarkably well in diabetes prevention. The questions that arise from these results are how to screen for people at risk and what intervention should be initiated in those with an interest in prevention.

It seems reasonable to screen on the basis of current recommendations, as outlined earlier primarily for case finding, but also recognizing that patients with abnormal glucose values (fasting >100 mg/dL or IGT with an OGTT) would be ideal candidates for preventive strategies. Certainly, high-risk persons should be counseled on nutritional approaches to achieve weight loss, instructed to increase physical activity, and observed prospectively to determine whether progression of hyperglycemia has occurred. Treatment for other cardiovascular risk factors should also be considered if they are present. In the absence of outcome studies, it is difficult to recommend drug therapy to prevent diabetes because significant diabetes complications are unlikely to develop in the short window of time during which glucose levels increase from a fasting glucose of 100 to 126 mg/dL. An extension phase of the Diabetes Prevention Program that is under way should provide evidence concerning whether prevention or delay in the development of diabetes will prevent death or disability.

Future Directions

The present-day management of T2DM is significantly more effective and easier for patients than the situation that prevailed even in the 1990s. A better understanding of the barriers to effective diabetes management and how to overcome them would be of great benefit. The epidemic in diabetes and obesity that is under way, coupled with the predicted early death and disability that follow, threatens to overwhelm our health care system. Practical, cost-effective public health approaches to stem this tide are desperately needed.[793]

The pipeline of novel pharmaceutical agents for the treatment of diabetes and its complications is full. Earlier we touched on the PPAR system and incretin-related therapies under development. Near at hand, rimonabant has received an approvable letter from the FDA as a weight-loss agent with glucose and lipid-lowering effects; numerous other weight loss agents are under development.[794]

There is continued interest in glucagon-receptor antagonists, glucokinase activators, inhibitors of gluconeogenic and glycogenolytic pathways, activators of the insulin-signaling pathways, inhibitors of active glucose transport molecules, modifiers of lipid metabolism, and many other areas in early pharmaceutical development.[795,796] Substantial development in insulin delivery and glucose-monitoring technologies should be expected before 2010.[797] Finally, there are a huge number of large outcomes studies under way in diabetes that should mold treatment paradigms and algorithms of care in the near term.[747]

REFERENCES

1. Zimmet P, Alberti KG, Shaw J. Global and societal implications of the diabetes epidemic. Nature 2001;414:782-787.
2. King H, Aubert RE, Herman WH. Global burden of diabetes, 1995-2025: prevalence, numerical estimates, and projections. Diabetes Care 1998;21:1414-1431.
3. Boyko EJ, de Cowten M, Zimmer PZ, et al. Features of the metabolic syndrome predict higher risk of diabetes and impaired glucose tolerance: a prospective study in Mauritius. Diabetes Care 2000;23:1242-1248.
4. Ramachandran A, Snehalatha C, Latha E, et al. Rising prevalence of NIDDM in an urban population in India. Diabetologia 1997; 40:232-237.
5. O'Dea K. Westernisation, insulin resistance and diabetes in Australian aborigines. Med J Aust 1991;155:258-264.
6. Harris MI, Flegal KM, Cowie CC, et al. Prevalence of diabetes, impaired fasting glucose, and impaired glucose tolerance in U.S. adults. The Third National Health and Nutrition Examination Survey, 1988-1994. Diabetes Care 1998;21:518-524.
7. Harris MI, Eastman RC, Cowie CC, et al. Comparison of diabetes diagnostic categories in the U.S. population according to the 1997 American Diabetes Association and 1980-1985 World Health Organization diagnostic criteria. Diabetes Care 1997;20:1859-1862.
8. Mokdad AH, Bowman BA, Ford ES, et al. The continuing epidemics of obesity and diabetes in the United States. JAMA 2001;286: 1195-1200.
9. American Diabetes Association. Type 2 diabetes in children and adolescents. Diabetes Care 2000;23:381-389.
10. Goran MI, Ball GD, Cruz ML. Obesity and risk of type 2 diabetes and cardiovascular disease in children and adolescents. J Clin Endocrinol Metab 2003;88(4):1417-1427.
11. Sinha, R, Fisch G, Teague B, et al. Prevalence of impaired glucose tolerance among children and adolescents with marked obesity. N Engl J Med 2002;346(11):802-810.
12. Report of the Expert Committee on the Diagnosis and Classification of Diabetes Mellitus. Diabetes Care 1997;20:1183-1197.
13. McCance DR, Hanson RL, Charles MA, et al. Comparison of tests for glycated haemoglobin and fasting and two hour plasma glucose concentrations as diagnostic methods for diabetes. BMJ 1994; 308:1323-1328.
14. Engelgau MM, Thompson TJ, Herman WH, et al. Comparison of fasting and 2-hour glucose and HbA_{1c} levels for diagnosing diabetes: diagnostic criteria and performance revisited. Diabetes Care 1997;20:785-791.
15. Jackson CA, Yudkin JS, Forrest RD. A comparison of the relationships of the glucose tolerance test and the glycated haemoglobin assay with diabetic vascular disease in the community. The Islington Diabetes Survey. Diabetes Res Clin Pract 1992;17:111-123.
16. Beks PH, Mackaay AJ, de Vries H, et al. Carotid artery stenosis is related to blood glucose level in an elderly Caucasian population: the Hoorn Study. Diabetologia 1997;40:290-298.
17. Fuller JH, Shipley MJ, Rose G, et al. Coronary-heart-disease risk and impaired glucose tolerance: the Whitehall study. Lancet 1980; 1:1373-1376.
18. Charles MA, Shipley MJ, Rose G, et al. Risk factors for NIDDM in white population: Paris prospective study. Diabetes 1991;40: 796-799.

19. Harris MI, Klein R, Welbom JA, Knuiman MW. Onset of NIDDM occurs at least 4-7 yr before clinical diagnosis. Diabetes Care 1992;15:815-819.
20. Harris MI. Undiagnosed NIDDM: clinical and public health issues. Diabetes Care 1993;16:642-652.
21. Harris MI, Eastman RC. Early detection of undiagnosed diabetes mellitus: a US perspective. Diabetes Metab Res Rev 2000;16: 230-236.
22. Harris MI, Hadden WC, Knowler WC, Bennett PH. Prevalence of diabetes and impaired glucose tolerance and plasma glucose levels in U.S. population aged 20-74 yr. Diabetes 1987;36:523-534.
23. Almind K, Doria A, Kahn CR. Putting the genes for type II diabetes on the map. Nat Med 2001;7:277-279.
24. Bell GI, Polonsky KS. Diabetes mellitus and genetically programmed defects in beta-cell function. Nature 2001;414:788-791.
25. Taylor SI, Arioglu E. Genetically defined forms of diabetes in children. J Clin Endocrinol Metab 1999;84:4390-4396.
26. Kahn CR, Flier JS, Bar RS, et al. The syndromes of insulin resistance and acanthosis nigricans: insulin-receptor disorders in man. N Engl J Med 1976;294:739-745.
27. Donohue W. Leprechaunism: a euphemism for a rare familial disorder. J Pediatr 1954;45:505-519.
28. Elders MJ, Schedewie HK, Olefsky J, et al. Endocrine-metabolic relationships in patients with leprechaunism. J Natl Med Assoc 1982;74:1195-1210.
29. Rosenberg AM, Haworth JC, Degroot GW, et al. A case of leprechaunism with severe hyperinsulinemia. Am J Dis Child 1980; 134:170-175.
30. Rabson S, Mendenhall E. Familial hypertrophy of pineal body, hyperplasia of adrenal cortex and diabetes mellitus. Am J Clin Pathol 1956;26:283-290.
31. Garg A. Lipodystrophies. Am J Med 2000;108:143-152.
32. Vigouroux C, Magre J, Vantyghem MC, et al. Lamin A/C gene: sex-determined expression of mutations in Dunnigan-type familial partial lipodystrophy and absence of coding mutations in congenital and acquired generalized lipoatrophy. Diabetes 2000;49: 1958-1962.
33. Garg A. Acquired and inherited lipodystrophies. N Engl J Med 2004;350(12):1220-1234.
34. Magre J, Delepine M, Khallouf E, et al. Identification of the gene altered in Berardinelli-Seip congenital lipodystrophy on chromosome 11q13. Nat Genet 2001;28:365-370.
35. Barroso I, Gurnell M, Crowley VE, et al. Dominant negative mutations in human PPARγ associated with severe insulin resistance, diabetes mellitus and hypertension. Nature 1999;402: 880-883.
36. Hegele RA, Pollex RL. Genetic and physiological insights into the metabolic syndrome. Am J Physiol Regul Integr Comp Physiol 2005;289(3):R663-R669.
37. Moffett SP, Feingold E, Barmada MM, et al. The C161 → T polymorphism in peroxisome proliferator-activated receptor gamma, but not P12A, is associated with insulin resistance in Hispanic and non-Hispanic white women: evidence for another functional variant in peroxisome proliferator-activated receptor gamma. Metabolism 2005;54(11):1552-1556.
38. Haneda M, Polonsky KS, Bergenstal RM, et al. Familial hyperinsulinemia due to a structurally abnormal insulin: definition of an emerging new clinical syndrome. N Engl J Med 1984;310: 1288-1294.
39. Gruppuso PA, Gorden P, Kahn CR, et al. Familial hyperproinsulinemia due to a proposed defect in conversion of proinsulin to insulin. N Engl J Med 1984;311:629-634.
40. Shibasaki Y, Kawakami T, Kanazawa Y, et al. Posttranslational cleavage of proinsulin is blocked by a point mutation in familial hyperproinsulinemia. J Clin Invest 1985;76:378-380.
41. O'Rahilly S, Gray H, Humphreys PJ, et al. Brief report: impaired processing of prohormones associated with abnormalities of glucose homeostasis and adrenal function. N Engl J Med 1995; 333:1386-1390.
42. Ballinger SW, Shoffner JM, Hedaya EV, et al. Maternally transmitted diabetes and deafness associated with a 10.4 kb mitochondrial DNA deletion. Nat Genet 1992;1:11-15.
43. Velho G, Byrne MM, Clement K, et al. Clinical phenotypes, insulin secretion, and insulin sensitivity in kindreds with maternally inherited diabetes and deafness due to mitochondrial tRNALeu(UUR) gene mutation. Diabetes 1996;45:478-487.
44. Fajans SS, Bell GI, Polonsky KS. Molecular mechanisms and clinical pathophysiology of maturity-onset diabetes of the young. N Engl J Med 2001;345:971-980.
45. Froguel P, Zouali H, Vionnet N, et al. Familial hyperglycemia due to mutations in glucokinase: definition of a subtype of diabetes mellitus. N Engl J Med 1993;328:697-702.
46. Yamagata K, Furuta H, Oda N, et al. Mutations in the hepatocyte nuclear factor–4α gene in maturity-onset diabetes of the young (MODY1). Nature 1996;384:458-460.
47. Yamagata K, Oda N, Kaisaki PJ, et al. Mutations in the hepatocyte nuclear factor–1α gene in maturity-onset diabetes of the young (MODY3). Nature 1996;384:455-458.
48. Stoffers DA, Ferrer J, Clarke WL, Habener N. Early-onset type-II diabetes mellitus (MODY4) linked to IPF1. Nat Genet 1997;17: 138-139.
49. Horikawa Y, Iwasaki N, Hara N, et al. Mutation in hepatocyte nuclear factor–1β gene (TCF2) associated with MODY. Nat Genet 1997;17:384-385.
50. Malecki MT, Jhala US, Antonellis A, et al. Mutations in NEUROD1 are associated with the development of type 2 diabetes mellitus. Nat Genet 1999;23:323-328.
51. Njolstad PR, Sovik O, Cuesta-Munoz A, et al. Neonatal diabetes mellitus due to complete glucokinase deficiency. N Engl J Med 2001;344:1588-1592.
52. Cereghini S. Liver-enriched transcription factors and hepatocyte differentiation. FASEB J 1996;10:267-282.
53. Duncan SA, Navas MA, Dufort D, et al. Regulation of a transcription factor network required for differentiation and metabolism. Science 1998;281:692-695.
54. Stoffel M, Duncan SA. The maturity-onset diabetes of the young (MODY1) transcription factor HNF4α regulates expression of genes required for glucose transport and metabolism. Proc Natl Acad Sci U S A 1997;94:13209-13214.
55. Edlund H. Factors controlling pancreatic cell differentiation and function. Diabetologia 2001;44:1071-1079.
56. Stoffers DA, Stanojevic V, Habener JF. Insulin promoter factor–1 gene mutation linked to early-onset type 2 diabetes mellitus directs expression of a dominant negative isoprotein. J Clin Invest 1998;102:232-241.
57. Hani EH, Stoffers DA, Chevre JC, et al. Defective mutations in the insulin promoter factor–1 (IPF-1) gene in late-onset type 2 diabetes mellitus. J Clin Invest 1999;104:R41-R48.
58. Kristinsson SY, Thorolfsdottir ET, Talseth B, et al. MODY in Iceland is associated with mutations in HNF-1α and a novel mutation in NeuroD1. Diabetologia 2001;44:2098-2103.
59. Permutt MA, Hattersley AT. Searching for type 2 diabetes genes in the post-genome era. Trends Endocrinol Metab 2000;11:383-393.
60. Horikawa Y, Oda N, Cox NJ, et al. Genetic variation in the gene encoding calpain-10 is associated with type 2 diabetes mellitus. Nat Genet 2000;26(2):163-175.
61. Song Y, Niu T, Manson JE, et al. Are variants in the CAPN10 gene related to risk of type 2 diabetes? A quantitative assessment of population and family-based association studies. Am J Hum Genet 2004;74(2):208-222.
62. Gloyn AL, Weedon MN, Owen KR, et al. Large-scale association studies of variants in genes encoding the pancreatic beta-cell KATP channel subunits Kir6.2 (KCNJ11) and SUR1 (ABCC8) confirm that the KCNJ11 E23K variant is associated with type 2 diabetes. Diabetes 2003;52(2):568-572.
63. Goll DE, Thompson VF, Li H, et al. The calpain system. Physiol Rev 2003;83(3):731-801.
64. Sreenan SK, Zhou YP, Otani K, et al. Calpains play a role in insulin secretion and action. Diabetes 2001;50(9):2013-2020.
65. Zhou YP, Sreenan S, Pan CY, et al. A 48-hour exposure of pancreatic islets to calpain inhibitors impairs mitochondrial fuel metabolism and the exocytosis of insulin. Metabolism 2003;52(5): 528-534.
66. Otani K, Han DH, Ford EL, et al. Calpain system regulates muscle mass and glucose transporter GLUT4 turnover. J Biol Chem 2004;279(20):20915-20920.
67. Johnson JD, Han Z, Otani K, et al. RyR2 and calpain-10 delineate a novel apoptosis pathway in pancreatic islets. J Biol Chem 2004;279(23):24794-24802.

68. Aguilar-Bryan L, Bryan J. Molecular biology of adenosine triphosphate–sensitive potassium channels. Endocr Rev 1999;20(2): 101-135.
69. Nielsen EM, Hansen L, Carstensen B, et al. The E23K variant of Kir6.2 associates with impaired post-OGTT serum insulin response and increased risk of type 2 diabetes. Diabetes 2003;52(2): 573-577.
70. Gloyn AL, Hashim Y, Ashcroft SJ, et al. Association studies of variants in promoter and coding regions of beta-cell ATP-sensitive K-channel genes SUR1 and Kir6.2 with type 2 diabetes mellitus (UKPDS 53). Diabet Med 2001;18(3):206-212.
71. Hani EH, Boutin P, Durand E, et al. Missense mutations in the pancreatic islet beta cell inwardly rectifying K+ channel gene (KIR6.2/BIR): a meta-analysis suggests a role in the polygenic basis of Type II diabetes mellitus in Caucasians. Diabetologia 1998;41(12):1511-1515.
72. Love-Gregory L, Wasson J, Lin J, et al. E23K single nucleotide polymorphism in the islet ATP-sensitive potassium channel gene (Kir6.2) contributes as much to the risk of Type II diabetes in Caucasians as the PPARγ Pro12Ala variant. Diabetologia 2003; 46(1):136-137.
73. 't Hart, LM, van Haeften TW Dekker JM, et al. Variations in insulin secretion in carriers of the E23K variant in the KIR6.2 subunit of the ATP-sensitive K(+) channel in the beta-cell. Diabetes 2002;51(10):3135-3138.
74. Rosen ED, Kulkarni RN, Sarraf P, et al. Targeted elimination of peroxisome proliferator-activated receptor gamma in beta cells leads to abnormalities in islet mass without compromising glucose homeostasis. Mol Cell Biol 2003;23(20):7222-7229.
75. Altshuler D, Hirschhorn JN, Klannemark M, et al. The common PPARγ Pro12Ala polymorphism is associated with decreased risk of type 2 diabetes. Nat Genet 2000;26(1):76-80.
76. Love-Gregory, LD, Wasson J, Ma J, et al. A common polymorphism in the upstream promoter region of the hepatocyte nuclear factor-4α gene on chromosome 20q is associated with type 2 diabetes and appears to contribute to the evidence for linkage in an Ashkenazi Jewish population. Diabetes 2004;53(4):1134-1140.
77. Silander K, Mohlke KL, Scott LJ, et al. Genetic variation near the hepatocyte nuclear factor-4α gene predicts susceptibility to type 2 diabetes. Diabetes 2004;53(4):1141-1149.
78. Weedon MN, Owen KR, Shields B, et al. Common variants of the hepatocyte nuclear factor-4α P2 promoter are associated with type 2 diabetes in the U.K. population. Diabetes 2004;53(11): 3002-3006.
79. Grant SF, Thorleifsson G, Reynisdottir I, et al. Variant of transcription factor 7–like 2 (TCF7L2) gene confers risk of type 2 diabetes. Nat Genet 2006;38(3):320-323.
80. Florez JC, Jablonski KA, Bayley N, et al. TCF7L2 polymorphisms and progression to diabetes in the Diabetes Prevention Program. N Engl J Med 2006;355(3):241-250.
81. Himsworth H, Kerr RB. Insulin-sensitive and insulin-insensitive types of diabetes mellitus. Clin Sci 1939;4:119-152.
82. Warram JH, Martin BC, Krowelski AS, et al. Slow glucose removal rate and hyperinsulinemia precede the development of type II diabetes in the offspring of diabetic parents. Ann Intern Med 1990;113:909-915.
83. Lillioija S, Mott DM, Howard BV, et al. Impaired glucose tolerance as a disorder of insulin action: longitudinal and cross-sectional studies in Pima Indians. N Engl J Med 1988; 318:1217-1225.
84. Haffner SM, Stern MP, Dunn J, et al. Diminished insulin sensitivity and increased insulin response in nonobese, nondiabetic Mexican Americans. Metabolism 1990;39:842-847.
85. Reaven GM, Bernstein R, Davis B, Olefsky JM. Nonketotic diabetes mellitus: insulin deficiency or insulin resistance? Am J Med 1976;60:80-88.
86. DeFronzo RA. Lilly lecture 1987. The triumvirate: beta-cell, muscle, liver. A collusion responsible for NIDDM. Diabetes 1988;37: 667-687.
87. Paolisso G, Tagliamonte MR, Rizzo MR, Giugliano D. Advancing age and insulin resistance: new facts about an ancient history. Eur J Clin Invest 1999;29:758-769.
88. Groop L. Genetics of the metabolic syndrome. Br J Nutr 2000; 83(suppl 1):S39-S48.
89. Lehtovirta M, Kaprio J, Forsblom C, et al. Insulin sensitivity and insulin secretion in monozygotic and dizygotic twins. Diabetologia 2000;43:285-293.
90. Mayer EJ, Newman B, Austin MA, et al. Genetic and environmental influences on insulin levels and the insulin resistance syndrome: an analysis of women twins. Am J Epidemiol 1996;143:323-332.
91. Hong Y, Pedersen NL, Brismar K, de Faire U. Genetic and environmental architecture of the features of the insulin-resistance syndrome. Am J Hum Genet 1997;60:143-152.
92. Fujioka S, Matsuzawa Y, Tokunaga K, Tarui S. Contribution of intra-abdominal fat accumulation to the impairment of glucose and lipid metabolism in human obesity. Metabolism 1987;36:54-59.
93. Brambilla P, Manzoni P, Sironi S, et al. Peripheral and abdominal adiposity in childhood obesity. Int J Obes Relat Metab Disord 1994;18:795-800.
94. Berman DM, Rodriguez LM, Nicklas BJ, et al. Racial disparities in metabolism, central obesity, and sex hormone–binding globulin in postmenopausal women. J Clin Endocrinol Metab 2001;86: 97-103.
95. Hu FB, Manson JE, Stampfer MJ, et al. Diet, lifestyle, and the risk of type 2 diabetes mellitus in women. N Engl J Med 2001;345: 790-797.
96. Tuomilehto J, Lindstrom J, Eriksson G, et al. Prevention of type 2 diabetes mellitus by changes in lifestyle among subjects with impaired glucose tolerance. N Engl J Med 2001;344:1343-1350.
97. Must A, Spadano J, Coakley EH, et al. The disease burden associated with overweight and obesity. JAMA 1999;282:1523-1529.
98. Cefalu WT, Werbel S, Bell-Farrow AD, et al. Insulin resistance and fat patterning with aging: relationship to metabolic risk factors for cardiovascular disease. Metabolism 1998;47:401-408.
99. Larsson B, Svardsudd K, Welin L, et al. Abdominal adipose tissue distribution, obesity, and risk of cardiovascular disease and death: 13 year follow up of participants in the study of men born in 1913. Br Med J (Clin Res Ed) 1984;288:1401-1404.
100. Despres JP, Tremblay A, Perusse L, et al. Abdominal adipose tissue and serum HDL-cholesterol: association independent from obesity and serum triglyceride concentration. Int J Obes 1988;12:1-13.
101. Landin K, Krotkiewski M, Smith U. Importance of obesity for the metabolic abnormalities associated with an abdominal fat distribution. Metabolism 1989;38:572-576.
102. Heitmann BL. The variation in blood lipid levels described by various measures of overall and abdominal obesity in Danish men and women aged 35-65 years. Eur J Clin Nutr 1992;46:597-605.
103. Reeder BA, Senthilselvan A, Despres JP, et al. The association of cardiovascular disease risk factors with abdominal obesity in Canada. Canadian Heart Health Surveys Research Group. Can Med Assoc J 1997;157(suppl 1):S39-S45.
104. Lamarche B. Abdominal obesity and its metabolic complications: implications for the risk of ischaemic heart disease. Coron Artery Dis 1998;9:473-481.
105. Evans DJ, Hoffmann RG, Kalkhoff RK, Kissebah AH. Relationship of body fat topography to insulin sensitivity and metabolic profiles in premenopausal women. Metabolism 1984;33:68-75.
106. Peiris AN, Mueller RA, Smith GA, et al. Splanchnic insulin metabolism in obesity. Influence of body fat distribution. J Clin Invest 1986;78:1648-1657.
107. Arner P, Hellstrom L, Wahrenberg H, Bronnegard M. Beta-adrenoceptor expression in human fat cells from different regions. J Clin Invest 1990;86:1595-1600.
108. Nicklas BJ, Rogus EM, Colman EG, Goldberg AP. Visceral adiposity, increased adipocyte lipolysis, and metabolic dysfunction in obese postmenopausal women. Am J Physiol 1996;270:E72-E78.
109. Mittelman SD, Van Citters GW, Kim SP, et al. Longitudinal compensation for fat-induced insulin resistance includes reduced insulin clearance and enhanced beta-cell response. Diabetes 2000;49: 2116-2125.
110. Del Prato S, Bonadonna RC, Bonora E, et al. Characterization of cellular defects of insulin action in type 2 (non–insulin-dependent) diabetes mellitus. J Clin Invest 1993;91:484-494.
111. Freymond D, Bogardus C, Okubo M, et al. Impaired insulin-stimulated muscle glycogen synthase activation in vivo in man is related to low fasting glycogen synthase phosphatase activity. J Clin Invest 1988;82:1503-1509.
112. Charles MA, Eschwege E, Thibult N, et al. The role of non-esterified fatty acids in the deterioration of glucose tolerance in Caucasian

subjects: results of the Paris Prospective Study. Diabetologia 1997;40:1101-1106.
113. Paolisso G, Tataranni PA, Foley JE, et al. A high concentration of fasting plasma non-esterified fatty acids is a risk factor for the development of NIDDM. Diabetologia 1995;38:1213-1217.
114. Garland PB, Newsholme EA, Randle PJ. Regulation of glucose uptake by muscle. 9. Effects of fatty acids and ketone bodies, and of alloxan-diabetes and starvation, on pyruvate metabolism and on lactate-pyruvate and L-glycerol 3-phosphate-dihydroxyacetone phosphate concentration ratios in rat heart and rat diaphragm muscles. Biochem J 1964;93:665-678.
115. Roden M, Price TB, Perseghin G, et al. Mechanism of free fatty acid–induced insulin resistance in humans. J Clin Invest 1996; 97:2859-2865.
116. Jucker BM, Rennings AJ, Cline GW, Shulman GI. ^{13}C and ^{31}P NMR studies on the effects of increased plasma free fatty acids on intramuscular glucose metabolism in the awake rat. J Biol Chem 1997;272:10464-10473.
117. Adams SH. Uncoupling protein homologs: emerging views of physiological function. J Nutr 2000;130:711-714.
118. Rothman DL, Magnusson I, Cline G, et al. Decreased muscle glucose transport/phosphorylation is an early defect in the pathogenesis of non–insulin-dependent diabetes mellitus. Proc Natl Acad Sci U S A 1995;92:983-987.
119. Price TB, Parseghin G, Duleba A, et al. NMR studies of muscle glycogen synthesis in insulin-resistant offspring of parents with non–insulin-dependent diabetes mellitus immediately after glycogen-depleting exercise. Proc Natl Acad Sci U S A 1996;93: 5329-5334.
120. Itani SI, Pories WJ, Macdonald KG, Dohm GL. Increased protein kinase C theta in skeletal muscle of diabetic patients. Metabolism 2001;50:553-557.
121. Griffin ME, Marcucci MJ, Cline GW, et al. Free fatty acid–induced insulin resistance is associated with activation of protein kinase C theta and alterations in the insulin signaling cascade. Diabetes 1999;48:1270-1274.
122. Um SH, Frigerio F, Watanabe M, et al. Absence of S6K1 protects against age- and diet-induced obesity while enhancing insulin sensitivity. Nature 2004;431(7005):200-205.
123. Hundal RS, Petersen KF, Mayerson AB, et al. Mechanism by which high-dose aspirin improves glucose metabolism in type 2 diabetes. J Clin Invest 2002;109(10):1321-1326.
124. Pan DA, Lillioja S, Kriketos AD, et al. Skeletal muscle triglyceride levels are inversely related to insulin action. Diabetes 1997;46: 983-988.
125. Goodpaster BH, Thaete FL, Simoneau JA, Kelley DE. Subcutaneous abdominal fat and thigh muscle composition predict insulin sensitivity independently of visceral fat. Diabetes 1997;46: 1579-1585.
126. Perseghin G, Scifo P, De Cobelli F, et al. Intramyocellular triglyceride content is a determinant of in vivo insulin resistance in humans: a ^{1}H-^{13}C nuclear magnetic resonance spectroscopy assessment in offspring of type 2 diabetic parents. Diabetes 1999;48:1600-1606.
127. Boesch C, Slotboom J, Hoppeler H, Kreis R. In vivo determination of intra-myocellular lipids in human muscle by means of localized ^{1}H-MR-spectroscopy. Magn Reson Med 1997;37:484-493.
128. Carlson LA, Ekelund LG, Froberg SO. Concentration of triglycerides, phospholipids and glycogen in skeletal muscle and of free fatty acids and beta-hydroxybutyric acid in blood in man in response to exercise. Eur J Clin Invest 1971;1:248-254.
129. Laws A, Reaven GM. Effect of physical activity on age-related glucose intolerance. Clin Geriatr Med 1990;6:849-863.
130. Gollnick PD, Saltin B. Significance of skeletal muscle oxidative enzyme enhancement with endurance training. Clin Physiol 1982;2:1-12.
131. Turcotte LP, Richter EA, Kiens B. Increased plasma FFA uptake and oxidation during prolonged exercise in trained vs. untrained humans. Am J Physiol 1992;262:E791-E799.
132. Romijn JA, Klein S, Coyle EF, et al. Strenuous endurance training increases lipolysis and triglyceride-fatty acid cycling at rest. J Appl Physiol 1993;75:108-113.
133. Phillips SM, Green HJ, Tamopolsky MA, et al. Effects of training duration on substrate turnover and oxidation during exercise. J Appl Physiol 1996;81:2182-2191.
134. Stremmel W, Strohmeyer G, Borchard F, et al. Isolation and partial characterization of a fatty acid binding protein in rat liver plasma membranes. Proc Natl Acad Sci U S A 1985;82:4-8.
135. Abumrad NA, el-Maghrabi MR, Amri EZ, et al. Cloning of a rat adipocyte membrane protein implicated in binding or transport of long-chain fatty acids that is induced during preadipocyte differentiation: homology with human CD36. J Biol Chem 1993; 268:17665-17668.
136. Stahl A, Gimeno RE, Tartaglia LA, Lodish HF. Fatty acid transport proteins: a current view of a growing family. Trends Endocrinol Metab 2001;12:266-273.
137. Luiken JJ, Glatz JF, Bonen A. Fatty acid transport proteins facilitate fatty acid uptake in skeletal muscle. Can J Appl Physiol 2000;25: 333-352.
138. Binnert C, Koistinen HA, Martin G, et al. Fatty acid transport protein-1 mRNA expression in skeletal muscle and in adipose tissue in humans. Am J Physiol 2000;279:E1072-E1079.
139. Veerkamp JH. Fatty acid transport and fatty acid–binding proteins. Proc Nutr Soc 1995;54:23-37.
140. Schaap FG, van der Vusse GJ, Glatz JF. Fatty acid–binding proteins in the heart. Mol Cell Biochem 1998;180:43-51.
141. Van Nieuwenhoven FA, Verstijnen CP, Abumrad NA, et al. Putative membrane fatty acid translocase and cytoplasmic fatty acid–binding protein are co-expressed in rat heart and skeletal muscles. Biochem Biophys Res Commun 1995;207:747-752.
142. Linssen MC, Vork MM, de Jong YF, et al. Fatty acid oxidation capacity and fatty acid–binding protein content of different cell types isolated from rat heart. Mol Cell Biochem 1990;98:19-25.
143. Binas B, Danneberg H, McWhir J, et al. Requirement for the heart-type fatty acid binding protein in cardiac fatty acid utilization. FASEB J 1999;13:805-812.
144. Hotamisligil GS, Johnson RS, Distel RJ, et al. Uncoupling of obesity from insulin resistance through a targeted mutation in aP2, the adipocyte fatty acid binding protein. Science 1996;274:1377-1379.
145. Blaak EE, Wagenmakers AJ, Glatz JF, et al. Plasma FFA utilization and fatty acid–binding protein content are diminished in type 2 diabetic muscle. Am J Physiol 2000;279:E146-E154.
146. Simoneau JA, Veerkamp JH, Turcotte LP, Kelley DE. Markers of capacity to utilize fatty acids in human skeletal muscle: relation to insulin resistance and obesity and effects of weight loss. FASEB J 1999;13:2051-2060.
147. McGarry JD. Glucose–fatty acid interactions in health and disease. Am J Clin Nutr 1998;67(3 suppl):500S-504S.
148. McGarry JD. Malonyl-CoA and satiety? Food for thought. Trends Endocrinol Metab 2000;11:399-400.
149. Zammit VA, Price NT, Fraser F, Jackson VN. Structure-function relationships of the liver and muscle isoforms of carnitine palmitoyltransferase I. Biochem Soc Trans 2001;29:287-292.
150. Minnich A, Tian N, Byan L, Bilder G. A potent PPARα agonist stimulates mitochondrial fatty acid beta-oxidation in liver and skeletal muscle. Am J Physiol 2001;280:E270-E279.
151. Power GW, Newsholme EA. Dietary fatty acids influence the activity and metabolic control of mitochondrial carnitine palmitoyltransferase I in rat heart and skeletal muscle. J Nutr 1997;127: 2142-2150.
152. Hildebrandt AL, Neufer PD. Exercise attenuates the fasting-induced transcriptional activation of metabolic genes in skeletal muscle. Am J Physiol 2000;278:E1078-E1086.
153. Kim JY, Hickner RC, Cartright RL, et al. Lipid oxidation is reduced in obese human skeletal muscle. Am J Physiol 2000;279: E1039-E1044.
154. Eaton S, Bartlett K, Pourfarzam M. Mammalian mitochondrial beta-oxidation. Biochem J 1996;320:345-357.
155. Nada MA, Rhead WJ, Sprecher H, et al. Evidence for intermediate channeling in mitochondrial beta-oxidation. J Biol Chem 1995; 270:530-535.
156. Horowitz JF, Leone TC, Feng W, et al. Effect of endurance training on lipid metabolism in women: a potential role for PPARα in the metabolic response to training. Am J Physiol 2000;279: E348-E355.
157. Porter RK. Mitochondrial proton leak: a role for uncoupling proteins 2 and 3? Biochim Biophys Acta 2001;1504:120-127.
158. Bouillaud F, Couplan E, Pecqueur C, Rigquier D. Homologues of the uncoupling protein from brown adipose tissue (UCP1): UCP2,

UCP3, BMCP1 and UCP4. Biochim Biophys Acta 2001;1504: 107-119.
159. Boss O, Muzzin P, Giacobino JP. The uncoupling proteins, a review. Eur J Endocrinol 1998;139:1-9.
160. Schrauwen P, Hoppeler H, Billeter R, et al. Fiber type dependent upregulation of human skeletal muscle UCP2 and UCP3 mRNA expression by high-fat diet. Int J Obes Relat Metab Disord 2001;25:449-456.
161. Tonkonogi M, Krook A, Walsh B, Sahlin K. Endurance training increases stimulation of uncoupling of skeletal muscle mitochondria in humans by non-esterified fatty acids: an uncoupling-protein-mediated effect? Biochem J 2000;351:805-810.
162. Bao S, Kennedy A, Wojciechowski B, et al. Expression of mRNAs encoding uncoupling proteins in human skeletal muscle: effects of obesity and diabetes. Diabetes 1998;47:1935-1940.
163. Schrauwen P, Xia J, Wakler K, et al. A novel polymorphism in the proximal UCP3 promoter region: effect on skeletal muscle UCP3 mRNA expression and obesity in male non-diabetic Pima Indians. Int J Obes Relat Metab Disord 1999;23:1242-1245.
164. Schrauwen P, Hesselink MK. Oxidative capacity, lipotoxicity, and mitochondrial damage in type 2 diabetes. Diabetes 2004;53(6): 1412-1417.
165. Boirie Y. Insulin regulation of mitochondrial proteins and oxidative phosphorylation in human muscle. Trends Endocrinol Metab 2003;14(9):393-394.
166. Pedersen BK, Steensberg A, Fischer C, et al. The metabolic role of IL-6 produced during exercise: is IL-6 an exercise factor? Proc Nutr Soc 2004;63(2):263-267.
167. Puigserver P, Spiegelman BM. Peroxisome proliferator-activated receptor-γ coactivator 1α (PGC-1α): transcriptional coactivator and metabolic regulator. Endocr Rev 2003;24(1):78-90.
168. Puigserver P, Wu Z, Park CW, et al. A cold-inducible coactivator of nuclear receptors linked to adaptive thermogenesis. Cell 1998; 92(6):829-839.
169. Mootha VK, Handschin C, Arow D, et al. Erralpha and Gabpa/b specify PGC-1α–dependent oxidative phosphorylation gene expression that is altered in diabetic muscle. Proc Natl Acad Sci U S A, 2004;101(17):6570-6575.
170. Mootha VK, Lindgren CM, Eriksson KF, et al. PGC-1α–responsive genes involved in oxidative phosphorylation are coordinately downregulated in human diabetes. Nat Genet 2003;34(3): 267-273.
171. Patti ME, Butte AJ, Crunkhorn S, et al. Coordinated reduction of genes of oxidative metabolism in humans with insulin resistance and diabetes: potential role of PGC1 and NRF1. Proc Natl Acad Sci U S A 2003;100(14):8466-8471.
172. Kelley DE, He J, Menshikova EV, Ritov VB. Dysfunction of mitochondria in human skeletal muscle in type 2 diabetes. Diabetes 2002;51(10):2944-2950.
173. Morino K, Petersen KF, Dufour S, et al. Reduced mitochondrial density and increased IRS-1 serine phosphorylation in muscle of insulin-resistant offspring of type 2 diabetic parents. J Clin Invest 2005;115(12):3587-3593.
174. Levine JA, Lanningham-Foster LM, McCrady SK, et al. Interindividual variation in posture allocation: possible role in human obesity. Science 2005;307(5709):584-586.
175. Baar K. Involvement of PPARγ co-activator-1, nuclear respiratory factors 1 and 2, and PPARα in the adaptive response to endurance exercise. Proc Nutr Soc 2004;63(2):269-273.
176. Ruderman NB, Saha AK, Vavvas D, Witters LA. Malonyl-CoA, fuel sensing, and insulin resistance. Am J Physiol 1999;276:E1-E18.
177. McGarry JD. Malonyl-CoA and carnitine palmitoyltransferase I: an expanding partnership. Biochem Soc Trans 1995;23:481-485.
178. Swanson ST, Foster DW, McGarry JD, Brown NF. Roles of the N- and C-terminal domains of carnitine palmitoyltransferase I isoforms in malonyl-CoA sensitivity of the enzymes: insights from expression of chimaeric proteins and mutation of conserved histidine residues. Biochem J 1998;335:513-519.
179. Kelley DE, Simoneau JA. Impaired free fatty acid utilization by skeletal muscle in non–insulin-dependent diabetes mellitus. J Clin Invest 1994;94:2349-2356.
180. Kelley DE, Mandarino LJ. Hyperglycemia normalizes insulin-stimulated skeletal muscle glucose oxidation and storage in noninsulin-dependent diabetes mellitus. J Clin Invest 1990;86: 1999-2007.
181. Bavenholm PN, Pigon J, Saha AK, et al. Fatty acid oxidation and the regulation of malonyl-CoA in human muscle. Diabetes 2000;49:1078-1083.
182. Jamil H, Madsen NB. Phosphorylation state of acetyl-coenzyme A carboxylase. I. Linear inverse relationship to activity ratios at different citrate concentrations. J Biol Chem 1987;262:630-637.
183. Jamil H, Madsen NB. Phosphorylation state of acetyl-coenzyme A carboxylase. II. Variation with nutritional condition. J Biol Chem 1987;262:638-642.
184. Winder WW, Wilson HA, Hardie DG, et al. Phosphorylation of rat muscle acetyl-CoA carboxylase by AMP-activated protein kinase and protein kinase A. J Appl Physiol 1997;82:219-225.
185. Dean D, Daugaard JR, Young ME, et al. Exercise diminishes the activity of acetyl-CoA carboxylase in human muscle. Diabetes 2000;49:1295-1300.
186. Olefsky JM, Revers RR, Prince M, et al. Insulin resistance in non–insulin dependent (type II) and insulin dependent (type I) diabetes mellitus. Adv Exp Med Biol 1985;189:176-205.
187. Del Prato S, Leonetti F, Simonson DC, et al. Effect of sustained physiologic hyperinsulinaemia and hyperglycaemia on insulin secretion and insulin sensitivity in man. Diabetologia 1994; 37:1025-1035.
188. Ratzmann KP, Ruhnke R, Kohnert KD. Effect of pharmacological suppression of insulin secretion on tissue sensitivity to insulin in subjects with moderate obesity. Int J Obes 1983;7:453-458.
189. Alemzadeh R, Langley G, Upchurch L, et al. Beneficial effect of diazoxide in obese hyperinsulinemic adults. J Clin Endocrinol Metab 1998;83:1911-1915.
190. White MF, Kahn CR. The insulin signaling system. J Biol Chem 1994;269:1-4.
191. Ward CW, Gough KH, Rashke M, et al. Systematic mapping of potential binding sites for Shc and Grb2 SH2 domains on insulin receptor substrate–1 and the receptors for insulin, epidermal growth factor, platelet-derived growth factor, and fibroblast growth factor. J Biol Chem 1996;271:5603-5609.
192. Pessin JE, Saltiel AR. Signaling pathways in insulin action: molecular targets of insulin resistance. J Clin Invest 2000;106:165-169.
193. McClain DA, Maegawa H, Thies RS, Olefsky JM. Dissection of the growth versus metabolic effects of insulin and insulin-like growth factor–I in transfected cells expressing kinase-defective human insulin receptors. J Biol Chem 1990;265:1678-1682.
194. McClain DA. Mechanism and role of insulin receptor endocytosis. Am J Med Sci 1992;304:192-201.
195. Formisano P, Beguinot F. The role of protein kinase C isoforms in insulin action. J Endocrinol Invest 2001;24:460-467.
196. Itani SI, Zhou Q, Pories WJ, et al. Involvement of protein kinase C in human skeletal muscle insulin resistance and obesity. Diabetes 2000;49:1353-1358.
197. Peraldi P, Xu M, Spiegelman BM. Thiazolidinediones block tumor necrosis factor–α–induced inhibition of insulin signaling. J Clin Invest 1997;100:1863-1869.
198. Goldstein BJ, Ahmad F, Ding W, et al. Regulation of the insulin signalling pathway by cellular protein-tyrosine phosphatases. Mol Cell Biochem 1998;182:91-99.
199. Drake PG, Bevan AP, Burgess JW, et al. A role for tyrosine phosphorylation in both activation and inhibition of the insulin receptor tyrosine kinase in vivo. Endocrinology 1996;137:4960-4968.
200. Elchebly M, Payette P, Michaliszyn E, et al. Increased insulin sensitivity and obesity resistance in mice lacking the protein tyrosine phosphatase–1B gene. Science 1999;283:1544-1548.
201. Krook A, O'Rahilly S. Mutant insulin receptors in syndromes of insulin resistance. Baillieres Clin Endocrinol Metab 1996;10: 97-122.
202. Taylor SI, Arioglu E. Syndromes associated with insulin resistance and acanthosis nigricans. J Basic Clin Physiol Pharmacol 1998; 9:419-439.
203. White MF. The IRS-signaling system: a network of docking proteins that mediate insulin and cytokine action. Recent Prog Horm Res 1998;53:119-138.
204. Previs SF, Withers DJ, Ren JM, et al. Contrasting effects of IRS-1 versus IRS-2 gene disruption on carbohydrate and lipid metabolism in vivo. J Biol Chem 2000;275:38990-38994.
205. White MF. IRS proteins and the common path to diabetes. Am J Physiol Endocrinol Metab, 2002;283(3):E413-E422.

206. Czech MP, Corvera S. Signaling mechanisms that regulate glucose transport. J Biol Chem 1999;274:1865-1868.
207. Kido Y, Nakae J, Accili D. Clinical review 125: the insulin receptor and its cellular targets. J Clin Endocrinol Metab 2001;86:972-979.
208. Kohn AD, Barthel A, Kovacina KS, et al. Construction and characterization of a conditionally active version of the serine/threonine kinase Akt. J Biol Chem 1998;273:11937-11943.
209. Sarbassov DD, Guertin DA, Ali SM, Sabatini DM. Phosphorylation and regulation of Akt/PKB by the rictor-mTOR complex. Science 2005;307(5712):1098-1101.
210. Cho H, Mu J, Kim JK, et al. Insulin resistance and a diabetes mellitus–like syndrome in mice lacking the protein kinase Akt2 (PKB beta). Science 2001;292:1728-1731.
211. Zierath JR, Krook A, Wallberg-Henriksson H. Insulin action in skeletal muscle from patients with NIDDM. Mol Cell Biochem 1998;182:153-160.
212. Krook A, Roth RA, Jiang XJ, et al. Insulin-stimulated Akt kinase activity is reduced in skeletal muscle from NIDDM subjects. Diabetes 1998;47:1281-1286.
213. Kim YB, Nikoulina SE, Ciaraldi TP, et al. Normal insulin-dependent activation of Akt/protein kinase B, with diminished activation of phosphoinositide 3-kinase, in muscle in type 2 diabetes. J Clin Invest 1999;104:733-741.
214. Zorzano A, Sevilla L, Tomas E, et al. Trafficking pathway of GLUT4 glucose transporters in muscle. Int J Mol Med 1998;2:263-271.
215. Davidson MB. Role of glucose transport and GLUT4 transporter protein in type 2 diabetes mellitus. J Clin Endocrinol Metab 1993;77:25-26.
216. Garvey WT, Maianu L, Zhu JH, et al. Multiple defects in the adipocyte glucose transport system cause cellular insulin resistance in gestational diabetes: heterogeneity in the number and a novel abnormality in subcellular localization of GLUT4 glucose transporters. Diabetes 1993;42:1773-1785.
217. Kennedy JW, Hirshman MF, Gervino EV, et al. Acute exercise induces GLUT4 translocation in skeletal muscle of normal human subjects and subjects with type 2 diabetes. Diabetes 1999;48:1192-1197.
218. Bernal-Mizrachi C, Weng S, Feng C, et al. Dexamethasone induction of hypertension and diabetes is PPARα-dependent in LDL receptor-null mice. Nat Med 2003;9(8):1069-1075.
219. Gumbiner B, Mucha JF, Lindstrom JE, et al. Differential effects of acute hypertriglyceridemia on insulin action and insulin receptor autophosphorylation. Am J Physiol 1996;270:E424-E429.
220. Saad MJ, Araki E, Miralpeix M, et al. Regulation of insulin receptor substrate–1 in liver and muscle of animal models of insulin resistance. J Clin Invest 1992;90:1839-1849.
221. Zierath JR, Houseknecht KL, Gnudi L, Kahn BB. High-fat feeding impairs insulin-stimulated GLUT4 recruitment via an early insulin-signaling defect. Diabetes 1997;46:215-223.
222. Anai M, Funaki M, Ogihara T, et al. Altered expression levels and impaired steps in the pathway to phosphatidylinositol 3-kinase activation via insulin receptor substrates 1 and 2 in Zucker fatty rats. Diabetes 1998;47:13-23.
223. Krook A, Kawano Y, Song XM, et al. Improved glucose tolerance restores insulin-stimulated Akt kinase activity and glucose transport in skeletal muscle from diabetic Goto-Kakizaki rats. Diabetes 1997;46:2110-2114.
224. Hotamisligil GS, Spiegelman BM. Tumor necrosis factor alpha: a key component of the obesity-diabetes link. Diabetes 1994;43:1271-1278.
225. Miles PD, Romeo OM, Higo K, et al. TNF-α–induced insulin resistance in vivo and its prevention by troglitazone. Diabetes 1997;46:1678-1683.
226. Hotamisligil GS, Peraldi P, Budavari A, et al. IRS-1-mediated inhibition of insulin receptor tyrosine kinase activity in TNF-α– and obesity-induced insulin resistance. Science 1996;271:665-668.
227. Uysal KT, Wiesbrock SM, Marino MW, Hotamisligil GS. Protection from obesity-induced insulin resistance in mice lacking TNF-α function. Nature 1997;389:610-614.
228. The effect of intensive treatment of diabetes on the development and progression of long-term complications in insulin-dependent diabetes mellitus. The Diabetes Control and Complications Trial Research Group. N Engl J Med 1993;329:977-986.
229. Turner RC. The U.K. Prospective Diabetes Study. A review. Diabetes Care 1998;21(suppl 3):C35-C38.
230. Sakul H, Pratley R, Cardon L, et al. Familiality of physical and metabolic characteristics that predict the development of non–insulin-dependent diabetes mellitus in Pima Indians. Am J Hum Genet 1997;60:651-656.
231. Yki-Jarvinen H, Sahlin K, Ren JM, Koivisto VA. Localization of rate-limiting defect for glucose disposal in skeletal muscle of insulin-resistant type I diabetic patients. Diabetes 1990;39:157-167.
232. Kornfeld R. Studies on L-glutamine D-fructose 6-phosphate amidotransferase. I. Feedback inhibition by uridine diphosphate-*N*-acetylglucosamine. J Biol Chem 1967;242:3135-3141.
233. Buse MG. Hexosamines, insulin resistance, and the complications of diabetes: current status. Am J Physiol Endocrinol Metab 2006;290(1):E1-E8.
234. Marshall S, Bacote V, Traxinger RR. Discovery of a metabolic pathway mediating glucose-induced desensitization of the glucose transport system: role of hexosamine biosynthesis in the induction of insulin resistance. J Biol Chem 1991;266:4706-4712.
235. Robinson KA, Weinstein ML, Lindenmayer GE, Buse MG. Effects of diabetes and hyperglycemia on the hexosamine synthesis pathway in rat muscle and liver. Diabetes 1995;44:1438-1446.
236. Hebert LF Jr, Daniels MC, Zhou J, et al. Overexpression of glutamine: fructose-6-phosphate amidotransferase in transgenic mice leads to insulin resistance. J Clin Invest 1996;98:930-936.
237. Baron AD, Zhu JS, Zhu JH, et al. Glucosamine induces insulin resistance in vivo by affecting GLUT 4 translocation in skeletal muscle: implications for glucose toxicity. J Clin Invest 1995;96:2792-2801.
238. Mallon PW, Cooper DA, Carr A. HIV-associated lipodystrophy. HIV Med 2001;2:166-173.
239. Shevitz A, Wanke CA, Falutz J, Kotler DP. Clinical perspectives on HIV-associated lipodystrophy syndrome: an update. AIDS 2001;15:1917-1930.
240. Purnell JQ, Zambon A, Knopp RH, et al. Effect of ritonavir on lipids and post-heparin lipase activities in normal subjects. AIDS 2000;14:51-57.
241. Noor MA, Lo JC, Mulligan K, et al. Metabolic effects of indinavir in healthy HIV-seronegative men. AIDS 2001;15:F11-F18.
242. Murata H, Hruz PW, Mueckler M. The mechanism of insulin resistance caused by HIV protease inhibitor therapy. J Biol Chem 2000;275:20251-20254.
243. Shikuma CM, Hu N, Milne C, et al. Mitochondrial DNA decrease in subcutaneous adipose tissue of HIV-infected individuals with peripheral lipoatrophy. AIDS 2001;15:1801-1809.
244. Caron M, Auclair M, Vigouroux C, et al. The HIV protease inhibitor indinavir impairs sterol regulatory element-binding protein-1 intranuclear localization, inhibits preadipocyte differentiation, and induces insulin resistance. Diabetes 2001;50:1378-1388.
245. Dowell P, Flexner C, Kwiterovich PO, Lane MD. Suppression of preadipocyte differentiation and promotion of adipocyte death by HIV protease inhibitors. J Biol Chem 2000;275:41325-41332.
246. Carr A, Samaras K, Chisholm DJ, Cooper DA. Pathogenesis of HIV-1-protease inhibitor–associated peripheral lipodystrophy, hyperlipidaemia, and insulin resistance. Lancet 1998;351:1881-1883.
247. Milinkovic A, Martinez E. Current perspectives on HIV-associated lipodystrophy syndrome. J Antimicrob Chemother 2005;56(1):6-9.
248. Grinspoon SK. Metabolic syndrome and cardiovascular disease in patients with human immunodeficiency virus. Am J Med 2005;118(suppl 2):23S-28S.
249. Mauss S. HIV-associated and antiretroviral-induced hyperlipidaemia: an update. J HIV Ther 2003;8(2):29-31.
250. Chuck SK, Penzak SR. Risk-benefit of HMG-CoA reductase inhibitors in the treatment of HIV protease inhibitor–related hyperlipidaemia. Expert Opin Drug Saf 2002;1(1):5-17.
251. Knowler WC, Barrett-Connor E, Fowler SE, et al. Reduction in the incidence of type 2 diabetes with lifestyle intervention or metformin. N Engl J Med 2002;346:393-403.
252. Kelley DE, Mandarino LJ. Fuel selection in human skeletal muscle in insulin resistance: a reexamination. Diabetes 2000;49:677-683.
253. Long SD, O'Brien K, MacDonald KG Jr, et al. Weight loss in severely obese subjects prevents the progression of impaired glucose tolerance to type II diabetes: a longitudinal interventional study. Diabetes Care 1994; 17:372-375.

254. Wing RR, Venditti E, Jakicic JM, et al. Lifestyle intervention in overweight individuals with a family history of diabetes. Diabetes Care 1998;21:350-359.
255. Nesher R, Karl IE, Kipnis DM. Dissociation of effects of insulin and contraction on glucose transport in rat epitrochlearis muscle. Am J Physiol 1985;249:C226-C232.
256. Wallberg-Henriksson H, Holloszy JO. Activation of glucose transport in diabetic muscle: responses to contraction and insulin. Am J Physiol 1985;249:C233-C237.
257. Wallberg-Henriksson H, Constable SH, Young DA, Holloszy JO. Glucose transport into rat skeletal muscle: interaction between exercise and insulin. J Appl Physiol 1988;65:909-913.
258. Young DA, Wallberg-Henriksson H, Sleeper MD, Holloszy JO. Reversal of the exercise-induced increase in muscle permeability to glucose. Am J Physiol 1987;253:E331-E335.
259. Douen AG, Ramlal T, Rastogi S, et al. Exercise induces recruitment of the "insulin-responsive glucose transporter." Evidence for distinct intracellular insulin- and exercise-recruitable transporter pools in skeletal muscle. J Biol Chem 1990;265:13427-13430.
260. Goodyear LJ, Hirshman MF, King PA, et al. Skeletal muscle plasma membrane glucose transport and glucose transporters after exercise. J Appl Physiol 1990;68:193-198.
261. Goodyear LJ, Giorgino F, Balon TW, et al. Effects of contractile activity on tyrosine phosphoproteins and PI3-kinase activity in rat skeletal muscle. Am J Physiol 1995;268:E987-E995.
262. Lund S, Holman GD, Schmitz O, Pedersen O. Contraction stimulates translocation of glucose transporter GLUT4 in skeletal muscle through a mechanism distinct from that of insulin. Proc Natl Acad Sci U S A 1995;92:5817-5821.
263. Zorzano A, Balon TW, Goodman MN, Ruderman NB. Additive effects of prior exercise and insulin on glucose and AIB uptake by rat muscle. Am J Physiol 1986;251:E21-E26.
264. Henriksen EJ, Bourey RE, Rodnick KJ, et al. Glucose transporter protein content and glucose transport capacity in rat skeletal muscles. Am J Physiol 1990;259:E593-E598.
265. Gao J, Ren J, Gulve EA, Holloszy JO. Additive effect of contractions and insulin on GLUT-4 translocation into the sarcolemma. J Appl Physiol 1994;77:1597-1601.
266. Lee AD, Hansen PA, Holloszy JO. Wortmannin inhibits insulin-stimulated but not contraction-stimulated glucose transport activity in skeletal muscle. FEBS Lett 1995;361:51-54.
267. Yeh JI, Gulve EA, Rameh L, Birnbaum MJ. The effects of wortmannin on rat skeletal muscle: dissociation of signaling pathways for insulin- and contraction-activated hexose transport. J Biol Chem 1995;270:2107-2111.
268. Treadway JL, James DE, Burcel E, Ruderman B. Effect of exercise on insulin receptor binding and kinase activity in skeletal muscle. Am J Physiol 1989;256:E138-E144.
269. Brozinick JT Jr, Etgen GJ Jr, Yaspelkis BB 3rd, Ivy JL. Contraction-activated glucose uptake is normal in insulin-resistant muscle of the obese Zucker rat. J Appl Physiol 1992;73:382-387.
270. Azevedo JL Jr, Carey JO, Pories WJ, et al. Hypoxia stimulates glucose transport in insulin-resistant human skeletal muscle. Diabetes 1995;44:695-698.
271. Winder WW, Hardie DG. AMP-activated protein kinase, a metabolic master switch: possible roles in type 2 diabetes. Am J Physiol 1999;277:E1-E10.
272. Hayashi T, Hirshman MF, Kurth EJ, et al. Evidence for 5′ AMP-activated protein kinase mediation of the effect of muscle contraction on glucose transport. Diabetes 1998;47:1369-1373.
273. Merrill GF, Kurth EJ, Hardie DG, Winder WW. AICA riboside increases AMP-activated protein kinase, fatty acid oxidation, and glucose uptake in rat muscle. Am J Physiol 1997;273:E1107-E1112.
274. Bergeron R, Russell RR 3rd, Young LH, et al. Effect of AMPK activation on muscle glucose metabolism in conscious rats. Am J Physiol 1999;276:E938-E944.
275. Richter EA, Garetto LP, Goodman MN, Ruderman NB. Muscle glucose metabolism following exercise in the rat: increased sensitivity to insulin. J Clin Invest 1982;69:785-793.
276. Garetto LP, Richter EA, Goodman MN, Ruderman NB. Enhanced muscle glucose metabolism after exercise in the rat: the two phases. Am J Physiol 1984;246:E471-E475.
277. Cartee GD, Young DA, Sleeper MD, et al. Prolonged increase in insulin-stimulated glucose transport in muscle after exercise. Am J Physiol 1989;256:E494-E499.
278. Richter EA, Young DA, Sleeper MD, et al. Effect of exercise on insulin action in human skeletal muscle. J Appl Physiol 1989; 66:876-885.
279. Hansen PA, Nolte LA, Chen MM, Holloszy JO. Increased GLUT-4 translocation mediates enhanced insulin sensitivity of muscle glucose transport after exercise. J Appl Physiol 1998;85: 1218-1222.
280. Thorell A, Hirshman MF, Nygren J, et al. Exercise and insulin cause GLUT-4 translocation in human skeletal muscle. Am J Physiol 1999;277:E733-E741.
281. Zorzano A, Balon TW, Garetto LP, et al. Muscle α-aminoisobutyric acid transport after exercise: enhanced stimulation by insulin. Am J Physiol 1985;248:E546-E552.
282. Wojtaszewski JF, Hansen BF, Kiens B, Richter EA. Insulin signaling in human skeletal muscle: time course and effect of exercise. Diabetes 1997;46:1775-1781.
283. Oshida Y, Yamanouchi K, Hayamizu S, Sato Y. Long-term mild jogging increases insulin action despite no influence on body mass index or VO_2 max. J Appl Physiol 1989;66:2206-2210.
284. DeFronzo RA, Sherwin RS, Kraemer N. Effect of physical training on insulin action in obesity. Diabetes 1987;36:1379-1385.
285. Helmrich SP, Rayland DR, Leung RW, Paffenbarger RS Jr. Physical activity and reduced occurrence of non–insulin-dependent diabetes mellitus. N Engl J Med 1991;325:147-152.
286. Perseghin G, Price TB, Petersen KF, et al. Increased glucose transport–phosphorylation and muscle glycogen synthesis after exercise training in insulin-resistant subjects. N Engl J Med 1996; 335:1357-1362.
287. Ebeling P, Bourey R, Koranyi L, et al. Mechanism of enhanced insulin sensitivity in athletes. Increased blood flow, muscle glucose transport protein (GLUT-4) concentration, and glycogen synthase activity. J Clin Invest 1993;92:1623-1631.
288. Houmard JA, Egan PC, Neufer PD, et al. Elevated skeletal muscle glucose transporter levels in exercise-trained middle-aged men. Am J Physiol 1991;261:E437-E443.
289. Hood DA. Invited review: contractile activity-induced mitochondrial biogenesis in skeletal muscle. J Appl Physiol, 2001;90(3): 1137-1157.
290. Lin J, Wu H, Tarr PT, et al. Transcriptional co-activator PGC-1 alpha drives the formation of slow-twitch muscle fibres. Nature 2002;418(6899):797-801.
291. Handschin C, Rhee J, Lin J, et al. An autoregulatory loop controls peroxisome proliferator–activated receptor γ coactivator 1α expression in muscle. Proc Natl Acad Sci U S A 2003; 100(12):7111-7116.
292. Michael LF, Wu Z, Cheatham RB, et al. Restoration of insulin-sensitive glucose transporter (GLUT4) gene expression in muscle cells by the transcriptional coactivator PGC-1. Proc Natl Acad Sci U S A 2001;98(7):3820-3825.
293. Nisoli E, Tonello C, Cardile A, et al. Calorie restriction promotes mitochondrial biogenesis by inducing the expression of eNOS. Science 2005;310(5746):314-317.
294. Wu H, Kanatous SB, Thurmond, et al. Regulation of mitochondrial biogenesis in skeletal muscle by CaMK. Science 2002;296(5566): 349-352.
295. Puigserver P, Rhee J, Lin J, et al. Cytokine stimulation of energy expenditure through p38 MAP kinase activation of PPARγ coactivator-1. Mol Cell 2001;8(5):971-982.
296. Cao W, Medvedev AV, Daniel KW, Collins S. β-Adrenergic activation of p38 MAP kinase in adipocytes: cAMP induction of the uncoupling protein 1 (UCP1) gene requires p38 MAP kinase. J Biol Chem 2001;276(29):27077-27082.
297. Terada S, Tabata I. Effects of acute bouts of running and swimming exercise on PGC-1α protein expression in rat epitrochlearis and soleus muscle. Am J Physiol Endocrinol Metab 2004;286(2): E208-E216.
298. Terada S, Goto M, Kato M, et al. Effects of low-intensity prolonged exercise on PGC-1 mRNA expression in rat epitrochlearis muscle. Biochem Biophys Res Commun 2002;296(2):350-354.
299. Zong H, Ren JM, Young LH, et al. AMP kinase is required for mitochondrial biogenesis in skeletal muscle in response to chronic energy deprivation. Proc Natl Acad Sci U S A 2002;99(25): 15983-15987.
300. Stamler J, Vaccaro O, Neaton JD, Wentworth D. Diabetes, other risk factors, and 12-yr cardiovascular mortality for men screened

in the Multiple Risk Factor Intervention Trial. Diabetes Care 1993;16:434-444.

301. Haffner SM, Lehto S, Ronnemaa T, et al. Mortality from coronary heart disease in subjects with type 2 diabetes and in nondiabetic subjects with and without prior myocardial infarction. N Engl J Med 1998;339:229-234.

302. Fontbonne AM, Eschwege EM. Insulin and cardiovascular disease. Paris Prospective Study. Diabetes Care 1991;14:461-469.

303. Willeit J, Kiechl S, Egger G, et al. The role of insulin in age-related sex differences of cardiovascular risk profile and morbidity. Atherosclerosis 1997;130:183-189.

304. Hu FB, Stampfer MJ, Soloman CG, et al. The impact of diabetes mellitus on mortality from all causes and coronary heart disease in women: 20 years of follow-up. Arch Intern Med 2001;161:1717-1723.

305. Reaven GM. Banting Lecture 1988. Role of insulin resistance in human disease. Nutrition 1997;13:65; discussion 64, 66.

306. Reaven GM. Role of insulin resistance in human disease (syndrome X): an expanded definition. Annu Rev Med 1993;44:121-131.

307. Kahn R, Buse J, Ferrannini E, et al. The metabolic syndrome: time for a critical appraisal: joint statement from the American Diabetes Association and the European Association for the Study of Diabetes. Diabetes Care 2005;28(9):2289-2304.

308. Siegel RD, Cupples A, Schaefer EJ, Wilson PW. Lipoproteins, apolipoproteins, and low-density lipoprotein size among diabetics in the Framingham offspring study. Metabolism 1996;45:1267-1272.

309. Davidson NO, Shelness GS. Apolipoprotein B: mRNA editing, lipoprotein assembly, and presecretory degradation. Annu Rev Nutr 2000;20:169-193.

310. Lewis GF, Steiner G. Acute effects of insulin in the control of VLDL production in humans: implications for the insulin-resistant state. Diabetes Care 1996;19:390-393.

311. Riches FM, Watts GF, Naoumova RP, et al. Hepatic secretion of very-low-density lipoprotein apolipoprotein B-100 studied with a stable isotope technique in men with visceral obesity. Int J Obes Relat Metab Disord 1998;22:414-423.

312. Wang SL, Du EZ, Martin TD, Davis RA. Coordinate regulation of lipogenesis, the assembly and secretion of apolipoprotein B–containing lipoproteins by sterol response element binding protein 1. J Biol Chem 1997;272:19351-19358.

313. Moberly JB, Cole TG, Alpers DH, Schonfeld G. Oleic acid stimulation of apolipoprotein B secretion from HepG2 and Caco-2 cells occurs post-transcriptionally. Biochim Biophys Acta 1990;1042:70-80.

314. Ellsworth JL, Erickson SK, Cooper AD. Very low and low density lipoprotein synthesis and secretion by the human hepatoma cell line Hep-G2: effects of free fatty acid. J Lipid Res 1986;27:858-874.

315. Kobatake T, Matsuzawa Y, Tokunaga K, et al. Metabolic improvements associated with a reduction of abdominal visceral fat caused by a new α-glucosidase inhibitor, AO-128, in Zucker fatty rats. Int J Obes 1989;13:147-154.

316. Matsuzawa Y, Shimomura I, Nakamura T, et al. Pathophysiology and pathogenesis of visceral fat obesity. Diabetes Res Clin Pract 1994;24(suppl):S111-S116.

317. Nguyen TT, Mijares AH, Johnson CM, Jensen MD. Postprandial leg and splanchnic fatty acid metabolism in nonobese men and women. Am J Physiol 1996;271:E965-E972.

318. Gordon DA, Jamil H, Sharp D, et al. Secretion of apolipoprotein B–containing lipoproteins from HeLa cells is dependent on expression of the microsomal triglyceride transfer protein and is regulated by lipid availability. Proc Natl Acad Sci U S A 1994;91:7628-7632.

319. Gordon DA, Jamil H. Progress towards understanding the role of microsomal triglyceride transfer protein in apolipoprotein-B lipoprotein assembly. Biochim Biophys Acta 2000;1486:72-83.

320. Liao W, Kobayashi K, Chan L. Adenovirus-mediated overexpression of microsomal triglyceride transfer protein (MTP): mechanistic studies on the role of MTP in apolipoprotein B-100 biogenesis. Biochemistry 1999;38:7532-7544.

321. Horowitz BS, Goldberg IJ, Merab J, et al. Increased plasma and renal clearance of an exchangeable pool of apolipoprotein A-I in subjects with low levels of high density lipoprotein cholesterol. J Clin Invest 1993;91:1743-1752.

322. Lemieux I, Couillard C, Pascot A, et al. The small, dense LDL phenotype as a correlate of postprandial lipemia in men. Atherosclerosis 2000;153:423-432.

323. Tan KC, Cooper MB, Ling KL, et al. Fasting and postprandial determinants for the occurrence of small dense LDL species in non–insulin-dependent diabetic patients with and without hypertriglyceridaemia: the involvement of insulin, insulin precursor species and insulin resistance. Atherosclerosis 1995;113:273-287.

324. Austin MA, Selby JV. LDL subclass phenotypes and the risk factors of the insulin resistance syndrome. Int J Obes Relat Metab Disord 1995;19(suppl 1):S22-S26.

325. Stewart MW, Laker MF, Dyer RG, et al. Lipoprotein compositional abnormalities and insulin resistance in type II diabetic patients with mild hyperlipidemia. Arterioscler Thromb 1993;13:1046-1052.

326. Alexander JK. Obesity and coronary heart disease. Am J Med Sci 2001;321:215-224.

327. Laakso M, Edelman SV, Brechtel G, Baron AD. Impaired insulin-mediated skeletal muscle blood flow in patients with NIDDM. Diabetes 1992;41:1076-1083.

328. Steinberg HO, Brechtel G, Johnson A, et al. Insulin-mediated skeletal muscle vasodilation is nitric oxide dependent. A novel action of insulin to increase nitric oxide release. J Clin Invest 1994;94:1172-1179.

329. Baron AD, Zhu JS, Marshall S, et al. Insulin resistance after hypertension induced by the nitric oxide synthesis inhibitor L-NMMA in rats. Am J Physiol 1995;269:E709-E715.

330. Steinberg HO, Paradisi G, Hook G, et al. Free fatty acid elevation impairs insulin-mediated vasodilation and nitric oxide production. Diabetes 2000;49:1231-1238.

331. Landsberg L. Insulin resistance, energy balance and sympathetic nervous system activity. Clin Exp Hypertens A 1990;12:817-830.

332. Weidmann P, de Courten M, Bohlen L. Insulin resistance, hyperinsulinemia and hypertension. J Hypertens Suppl 1993;11(suppl 5):S27-S38.

333. Masuo K, Mikami H, Itoh M, et al. Sympathetic activity and body mass index contribute to blood pressure levels. Hypertens Res 2000;23:303-310.

334. DeFronzo RA. Insulin and renal sodium handling: clinical implications. Int J Obes 1981;5(suppl 1):93-104.

335. DeFronzo RA, Goldberg M, Agus ZS. The effects of glucose and insulin on renal electrolyte transport. J Clin Invest 1976;58:83-90.

336. DeFronzo RA, Cooke CR, Andres R, et al. The effect of insulin on renal handling of sodium, potassium, calcium, and phosphate in man. J Clin Invest 1975;55:845-855.

337. Welborn TA, Breckenridge A, Rubinstein AH, et al. Serum-insulin in essential hypertension and in peripheral vascular disease. Lancet 1966;1:1336-1337.

338. Gress TW, Nieto FJ, Shahar E, et al. Hypertension and antihypertensive therapy as risk factors for type 2 diabetes mellitus. Atherosclerosis Risk in Communities Study. N Engl J Med 2000;342:905-912.

339. Yusuf S, Sleight P, Pogue J, et al. Effects of an angiotensin-converting-enzyme inhibitor, ramipril, on cardiovascular events in high-risk patients. The Heart Outcomes Prevention Evaluation Study Investigators. N Engl J Med 2000;342:145-153.

340. Sebestjen M, Zegura B, Guzic-Salobir B, Keber I. Fibrinolytic parameters and insulin resistance in young survivors of myocardial infarction with heterozygous familial hypercholesterolemia. Wien Klin Wochenschr 2001;113:113-118.

341. Juhan-Vague I, Alessi MC, Morange PE. Hypofibrinolysis and increased PAI-1 are linked to atherothrombosis via insulin resistance and obesity. Ann Med 2000;32(suppl 1):78-84.

342. Fujii S, Goto D, Zaman T, et al. Diminished fibrinolysis and thrombosis: clinical implications for accelerated atherosclerosis. J Atheroscler Thromb 1998;5:76-81.

343. Sobel BE. The potential influence of insulin and plasminogen activator inhibitor type 1 on the formation of vulnerable atherosclerotic plaques associated with type 2 diabetes. Proc Assoc Am Physicians 1999;111:313-318.

344. Festa A, D'Agostino R Jr, Mykkanan L, et al. Relative contribution of insulin and its precursors to fibrinogen and PAI-1 in a large population with different states of glucose tolerance. The Insulin

Resistance Atherosclerosis Study (IRAS). Arterioscler Thromb Vasc Biol 1999;19:562-568.

345. Lormeau B, Aurousseau MH, Valensi P, et al. Hyperinsulinemia and hypofibrinolysis: effects of short-term optimized glycemic control with continuous insulin infusion in type II diabetic patients. Metabolism 1997;46:1074-1079.
346. Hamsten A, Eriksson P, Karpe F, Silveira A. Relationships of thrombosis and fibrinolysis to atherosclerosis. Curr Opin Lipidol 1994; 5:382-389.
347. Grenett HE, Benza RL, Li XN, et al. Expression of plasminogen activator inhibitor type I in genotyped human endothelial cell cultures: genotype-specific regulation by insulin. Thromb Haemost 1999;82:1504-1509.
348. Chomiki N, Henry M, Alessi MC, et al. Plasminogen activator inhibitor-1 expression in human liver and healthy or atherosclerotic vessel walls. Thromb Haemost 1994;72:44-53.
349. Koistinen HA, Dusserre E, Ebeling P, et al. Subcutaneous adipose tissue expression of plasminogen activator inhibitor-1 (PAI-1) in nondiabetic and type 2 diabetic subjects. Diabetes Metab Res Rev 2000;16:364-369.
350. Kruszynska YT, Yu JG, Olefsky JM, Sobel BE. Effects of troglitazone on blood concentrations of plasminogen activator inhibitor 1 in patients with type 2 diabetes and in lean and obese normal subjects. Diabetes 2000;49:633-639.
351. Stunkard AJ. Current views on obesity. Am J Med 1996;100: 230-236.
352. Expert Panel on Detection, Evaluation and Treatment of High Blood Cholesterol in Adults. Executive Summary of the Third Report of the National Cholesterol Education Program (NCEP) Expert Panel on Detection, Evaluation and Treatment of High Blood Cholesterol in Adults (Adult Treatment Panel III). JAMA 2001;285:2486-2497.
353. Gerich JE, Meyer C, Woerle HJ, Stumvoll M. Renal gluconeogenesis: its importance in human glucose homeostasis. Diabetes Care 2001;24:382-391.
354. Meyer C, Stumvoll M, Nadkami V, et al. Abnormal renal and hepatic glucose metabolism in type 2 diabetes mellitus. J Clin Invest 1998;102:619-624.
355. Rebrin K, Steil GM, Mittelman SD, Bergman RN. Causal linkage between insulin suppression of lipolysis and suppression of liver glucose output in dogs. J Clin Invest 1996;98:741-749.
356. Mittelman SD, Fu YY, Rebrin K, et al. Indirect effect of insulin to suppress endogenous glucose production is dominant, even with hyperglucagonemia. J Clin Invest 1997;100:3121-3130.
357. Rothman DL, Magnusson I, Katz LD, et al. Quantitation of hepatic glycogenolysis and gluconeogenesis in fasting humans with ^{13}C NMR. Science 1991;254:573-576.
358. Petersen KF, Price T, Cline GW, et al. Contribution of net hepatic glycogenolysis to glucose production during the early postprandial period. Am J Physiol 1996;270:E186-E191.
359. Nonogaki K. New insights into sympathetic regulation of glucose and fat metabolism. Diabetologia 2000;43:533-549.
360. Moore MC, Connolly CC, Cherrington AD. Autoregulation of hepatic glucose production. Eur J Endocrinol 1998;138:240-248.
361. Bavenholm PN, Pigon J, Ostenson CG, Efendic S. Insulin sensitivity of suppression of endogenous glucose production is the single most important determinant of glucose tolerance. Diabetes 2001;50:1449-1454.
362. Mitrakou A, Kelley D, Mokan M, et al. Role of reduced suppression of glucose production and diminished early insulin release in impaired glucose tolerance. N Engl J Med 1992;326:22-29.
363. McCall RH, Wiesenthal SR, Shi ZQ, et al. Insulin acutely suppresses glucose production by both peripheral and hepatic effects in normal dogs. Am J Physiol 1998;274:E346-E356.
364. Lewis GF, Vranic M, Giacca A. Glucagon enhances the direct suppressive effect of insulin on hepatic glucose production in humans. Am J Physiol 1997;272:E371-E378.
365. Herzig S, Long F, Jhala US, et al. CREB regulates hepatic gluconeogenesis through the coactivator PGC-1. Nature 2001;413:179-183.
366. Yoon JC, Puigserver P, Chen G, et al. Control of hepatic gluconeogenesis through the transcriptional coactivator PGC-1. Nature 2001;413:131-138.
367. Koo SH, Flechner L, Qi L, et al. The CREB coactivator TORC2 is a key regulator of fasting glucose metabolism. Nature 2005; 437(7062):1109-1111.
368. Cherrington AD, Edgerton D, Sindelar DK. The direct and indirect effects of insulin on hepatic glucose production in vivo. Diabetologia 1998;41:987-996.
369. Chiasson JL, Liljenquist JE, Finger FE, Lacy WW. Differential sensitivity of glycogenolysis and gluconeogenesis to insulin infusions in dogs. Diabetes 1976;25:283-291.
370. Rossetti L, Giaccari A, Barzilai N, et al. Mechanism by which hyperglycemia inhibits hepatic glucose production in conscious rats: implications for the pathophysiology of fasting hyperglycemia in diabetes. J Clin Invest 1993;92:1126-1134.
371. Gasa R, Jansen PB, Berman HK, et al. Distinctive regulatory and metabolic properties of glycogen-targeting subunits of protein phosphatase-1 (PTG, GL, GM/RGl) expressed in hepatocytes. J Biol Chem 2000;275:26396-26403.
372. Newgard CB, Brady MJ, O'Doherty RM, Saltiel AR. Organizing glucose disposal: emerging roles of the glycogen targeting subunits of protein phosphatase-1. Diabetes 2000;49:1967-1977.
373. Yeagley D, Guo S, Unterman T, Quinn PG. Gene- and activation-specific mechanisms for insulin inhibition of basal and glucocorticoid-induced insulin-like growth factor binding protein-1 and phosphoenolpyruvate carboxykinase transcription: roles of forkhead and insulin response sequences. J Biol Chem 2001;276: 33705-33710.
374. Jackson JG, Kreisberg JI, Koterba AP, et al. Phosphorylation and nuclear exclusion of the forkhead transcription factor FKHR after epidermal growth factor treatment in human breast cancer cells. Oncogene 2000;19:4574-4581.
375. Hall RK, Yamasaki T, Kucera T, et al. Regulation of phosphoenolpyruvate carboxykinase and insulin-like growth factor-binding protein-1 gene expression by insulin: the role of winged helix/forkhead proteins. J Biol Chem 2000;275:30169-30175.
376. Wolfrum C, Asilmaz E, Luca E, et al. Foxa2 regulates lipid metabolism and ketogenesis in the liver during fasting and in diabetes. Nature 2004;432(7020):1027-1032.
377. Asplin CM, Paquette TL, Palmer JP. In vivo inhibition of glucagon secretion by paracrine beta cell activity in man. J Clin Invest 1981;68:314-318.
378. Shi ZQ, Wasserman D, Vranic M. Metabolic implications of exercise and physical fitness in physiology and diabetes. In Porte D, Sherwin R, eds. Ellenberg and Rifkin Diabetes Mellitus. Norwalk, Conn: Appleton & Lange, 1997:653-687.
379. Chen X, Iqbal N, Boden G. The effects of free fatty acids on gluconeogenesis and glycogenolysis in normal subjects. J Clin Invest 1999;103:365-372.
380. Boden G. Fatty acids and insulin resistance. Diabetes Care 1996;19: 394-395.
381. Lewis GF, Vranic M, Giacca A. Role of free fatty acids and glucagon in the peripheral effect of insulin on glucose production in humans. Am J Physiol 1998;275:E177-E186.
382. Perriello G, Pampanelli S, Del Sindaco P, et al. Evidence of increased systemic glucose production and gluconeogenesis in an early stage of NIDDM. Diabetes 1997;46:1010-1016.
383. DeFronzo RA, Bonadonna RC, Ferrannini E. Pathogenesis of NIDDM: a balanced overview. Diabetes Care 1992;15:318-368.
384. DeFronzo RA, Simonson D, Ferrannini E. Hepatic and peripheral insulin resistance: a common feature of type 2 (non–insulin-dependent) and type 1 (insulin-dependent) diabetes mellitus. Diabetologia 1982;23:313-319.
385. Bogardus C, Lillioja S, Howard BV, et al. Relationships between insulin secretion, insulin action, and fasting plasma glucose concentration in nondiabetic and noninsulin-dependent diabetic subjects. J Clin Invest 1984;74:1238-1246.
386. Hother-Nielsen O, Beck-Nielsen H. Insulin resistance, but normal basal rates of glucose production in patients with newly diagnosed mild diabetes mellitus. Acta Endocrinol (Copenh) 1991; 124:637-645.
387. Hother-Nielsen O, Beck-Nielsen H. On the determination of basal glucose production rate in patients with type 2 (non–insulin-dependent) diabetes mellitus using primed-continuous 3-^{3}H-glucose infusion. Diabetologia 1990;33:603-610.
388. Firth R, Bell P, Rizza R. Insulin action in non–insulin-dependent diabetes mellitus: the relationship between hepatic and extrahepatic insulin resistance and obesity. Metabolism 1987;36: 1091-1095.

389. Groop LC, Bonadonna RC, Shank M, et al. Role of free fatty acids and insulin in determining free fatty acid and lipid oxidation in man. J Clin Invest 1991;87:83-89.
390. Pigon J, Giacca A, Ostenson CG, et al. Normal hepatic insulin sensitivity in lean, mild noninsulin-dependent diabetic patients. J Clin Endocrinol Metab 1996;81:3702-3708.
391. Stumvoll M, Nurjhan N, Perriello G, et al. Metabolic effects of metformin in non–insulin-dependent diabetes mellitus. N Engl J Med 1995;333:550-554.
392. Lewis GF, Carpentier A, Vranic N, Giacca A. Resistance to insulin's acute direct hepatic effect in suppressing steady-state glucose production in individuals with type 2 diabetes. Diabetes 1999; 48:570-576.
393. Staehr P, Hother-Nielsen O, Levin K, et al. Assessment of hepatic insulin action in obese type 2 diabetic patients. Diabetes 2001; 50:1363-1370.
394. Magnusson I, Rothman DL, Gerard DP, et al. Contribution of hepatic glycogenolysis to glucose production in humans in response to a physiological increase in plasma glucagon concentration. Diabetes 1995;44:185-189.
395. Magnusson I, Rothman DL, Katz LD, et al. Increased rate of gluconeogenesis in type II diabetes mellitus: a ^{13}C nuclear magnetic resonance study. J Clin Invest 1992;90:1323-1327.
396. Baron AD, Schaeffer L, Shragg P, Kolterman OG. Role of hyperglucagonemia in maintenance of increased rates of hepatic glucose output in type II diabetics. Diabetes 1987;36:274-283.
397. Lam TK, Pocai A, Gutierrez-Juarez R, et al. Hypothalamic sensing of circulating fatty acids is required for glucose homeostasis. Nat Med 2005;11(3):320-327.
398. Minokoshi Y, Alquier T, Furukawa N, et al. AMP-kinase regulates food intake by responding to hormonal and nutrient signals in the hypothalamus. Nature 2004;428(6982):569-574.
399. Yu YH, Ginsberg HN. Adipocyte signaling and lipid homeostasis: sequelae of insulin-resistant adipose tissue. Circ Res 2005;96(10): 1042-1052.
400. Yamauchi T, Kamon J, Minokoshi Y, et al. Adiponectin stimulates glucose utilization and fatty-acid oxidation by activating AMP-activated protein kinase. Nat Med 2002;8(11):1288-1295.
401. Tomas E, Tsao TS, Saha AK, et al. Enhanced muscle fat oxidation and glucose transport by ACRP30 globular domain: acetyl-CoA carboxylase inhibition and AMP-activated protein kinase activation. Proc Natl Acad Sci U S A 2002;99(25):16309-16313.
402. Maeda N, Shimomura I, Kishida K, et al. Diet-induced insulin resistance in mice lacking adiponectin/ACRP30. Nat Med 2002;8(7): 731-737.
403. Steppan CM, Brown EJ, Wright CM, et al. A family of tissue-specific resistin-like molecules. Proc Natl Acad Sci U S A 2001;98(2): 502-506.
404. Steppan CM, Bailey ST, Bhat S, et al. The hormone resistin links obesity to diabetes. Nature 2001;409(6818):307-312.
405. Kusminski CM, McTernan PG, Kumar S. Role of resistin in obesity, insulin resistance and type II diabetes. Clin Sci (Lond) 2005; 109(3):243-256.
406. Ruan H, Lodish HF. Insulin resistance in adipose tissue: direct and indirect effects of tumor necrosis factor-α. Cytokine Growth Factor Rev 2003;14(5):447-455.
407. Weisberg SP, McCann D, Desai M, et al. Obesity is associated with macrophage accumulation in adipose tissue. J Clin Invest 2003;112(12):1796-1808.
408. Fain JN, Madan AK, Hiler ML, et al. Comparison of the release of adipokines by adipose tissue, adipose tissue matrix, and adipocytes from visceral and subcutaneous abdominal adipose tissues of obese humans. Endocrinology 2004;145(5):2273-2282.
409. Takahashi K, Mizuarai S, Araki H, et al. Adiposity elevates plasma MCP-1 levels leading to the increased CD11b-positive monocytes in mice. J Biol Chem 2003;278(47):46654-46660.
410. Sartipy P, Loskutoff DJ. Monocyte chemoattractant protein 1 in obesity and insulin resistance. Proc Natl Acad Sci U S A 2003; 100(12):7265-7270.
411. Weisberg SP, Hunter D, Huber R, et al. CCR2 modulates inflammatory and metabolic effects of high-fat feeding. J Clin Invest 2006;116(1):115-124.
412. Kern PA, Ranganathan S, Li C, et al. Adipose tissue tumor necrosis factor and interleukin-6 expression in human obesity and insulin resistance. Am J Physiol Endocrinol Metab 2001;280(5): E745-E751.
413. van Hall G, Steensberg A, Sacchetti M, et al. Interleukin-6 stimulates lipolysis and fat oxidation in humans. J Clin Endocrinol Metab 200388(7):3005-3010.
414. Yalow R, Berson S. Immunoassay of endogenous plasma insulin in man. J Clin Invest 1960;39:1157-1175.
415. Polonsky K, Jaspan J, Emmanouel D, et al. Differences in the hepatic and renal extraction of insulin and glucagon in the dog: evidence for saturability of insulin metabolism. Acta Endocrinol (Copenh) 1983;102:420-427.
416. Polonsky K, Jaspan J, Pugh W, et al. Metabolism of C-peptide in the dog: in vivo demonstration of the absence of hepatic extraction. J Clin Invest 1983;72:1114-1123.
417. Steiner DF, James DE. Cellular and molecular biology of the beta cell. Diabetologia 1992;35(suppl 2):S41-S48.
418. Melani F, Ryan WG, Rubenstein AH, Steirer DF. Proinsulin secretion by a pancreatic beta-cell adenoma. Proinsulin and C-peptide secretion. N Engl J Med 1970;283:713-719.
419. Horwitz D, Starr JI, Mako ME, et al. Proinsulin, insulin, and C-peptide concentrations in human portal and peripheral blood. J Clin Invest 1975;55:1278-1283.
420. Melani F, Rubenstein A, Steiner D. Human serum proinsulin. J Clin Invest 1970;49:497-507.
421. Bergenstal R, Cohen RM, Lever E, et al. The metabolic effects of biosynthetic human proinsulin in individuals with type I diabetes. J Clin Endocrinol Metab 1984;58:973-979.
422. Revers R, Henry R, Schmeiser L, et al. The effects of biosynthetic human proinsulin on carbohydrate metabolism. Diabetes 1984;33:762-770.
423. Peavy D, Brunner MR, Duckworth W, et al. Receptor binding and biological potency of several split forms (conversion intermediates) of human proinsulin: studies in cultured IM-9 lymphocytes and in vivo and in vitro in rats. J Biol Chem 1985;260: 13989-13994.
424. Gruppuso P, Frank B, Schwartz R. Binding of proinsulin and proinsulin conversion intermediates to human placental insulin-like growth factor 1 receptors. J Clin Endocrinol Metab 1988;67: 197.
425. Polonsky K, Rubenstein A. C-peptide as a measure of the secretion and hepatic extraction of insulin: pitfalls and limitations. Diabetes 1984;33:486-494.
426. Wojcikowski C, Blackman J, Ostrega D, et al. Lack of effect of high-dose biosynthetic human C-peptide on pancreatic hormone release in normal subjects. Metabolism 1990;39:827-832.
427. Wahren J, Ekberg K, Johansson J, et al. Role of C-peptide in human physiology. Am J Physiol 2000;278:E759-E768.
428. Polonsky K, Pugh W, Jaspan JB, et al. C-peptide and insulin secretion: relationship between peripheral concentrations of C-peptide and insulin and their secretion rates in the dog. J Clin Invest 1984;74:1821-1829.
429. Bratusch-Marrain P, Waldhausl WK, Gasic S, Hofer A. Hepatic disposal of biosynthetic human insulin and porcine C-peptide in humans. Metabolism 1984;33:151-157.
430. Faber O, Hagen C, Binder C, et al. Kinetics of human connecting peptide in normal and diabetic subjects. J Clin Invest 1978;62: 197-203.
431. Polonsky K, Licinio-Paixas J, Given BD, et al. Use of biosynthetic human C-peptide in the measurement of insulin secretion rates in normal volunteers and type I diabetic patients. J Clin Invest 1986;77:98-105.
432. Shapiro E, Tillil H, Rubenstein H, Polonsky KS. Peripheral insulin parallels changes in insulin secretion more closely than C-peptide after bolus intravenous glucose administration. J Clin Endocrinol Metab 1988;67:1094-1099.
433. Eaton R, Allen RC, Schade DS, et al. Prehepatic insulin production in man: kinetic analysis using peripheral connecting peptide behavior. J Clin Endocrinol Metab 1980;51:520-528.
434. Welch S, Gebhart SS, Bergman RN, Phillips LS. Minimal model analysis of intravenous glucose tolerance test-derived insulin sensitivity in diabetic subjects. J Clin Endocrinol Metab 1990;71: 1508-1518.
435. Breda E, Cavaghan MK, Toffolo G, et al. Oral glucose tolerance test minimal model indexes of beta-cell function and insulin sensitivity. Diabetes 2001;50:150-158.

436. Bergman R, Phillips L, Cobelli C. Physiologic evaluation of factors controlling glucose tolerance in man: measurement of insulin sensitivity and beta-cell glucose sensitivity from the response to intravenous glucose. J Clin Invest 1981;68:1456-1467.
437. Caumo A, Bergman R, Cobelli C. Insulin sensitivity from meal tolerance tests in normal subjects: a minimal model index. J Clin Endocrinol Metab 2000;85:4396-4402.
438. Davis EA, Cuesta-Munoz A, Raoul M, et al. Mutants of glucokinase cause hypoglycaemia and hyperglycaemia syndromes and their analysis illuminates fundamental quantitative concepts of glucose homeostasis. Diabetologia 1999;42:1175-1186.
439. Matschinsky FM, Glaser B, Magnuson MA. Pancreatic beta-cell glucokinase: closing the gap between theoretical concepts and experimental realities. Diabetes 1998;47:307-315.
440. Dukes ID, McIntyre MS, Mertz RJ, et al. Dependence on NADH produced during glycolysis for beta-cell glucose signaling. J Biol Chem 1994;269:10979-10982.
441. Maechler P, Wollheim CB. Mitochondrial function in normal and diabetic beta-cells. Nature 2001;414:807-812.
442. Aguilar-Bryan L, Bryan J, Nakazaki M. Of mice and men: K_{ATP} channels and insulin secretion. Recent Prog Horm Res 2001;56: 47-68.
443. Porte DJ, Pupo A. Insulin responses to glucose: evidence for a two-pooled system in man. J Clin Invest 1969;48:2309-2319.
444. Chen M, Porte DJ. The effect of rate and dose of glucose infusion on the acute insulin response in man. J Clin Endocrinol Metab 1976;42:1168-1175.
445. Ward W, Beard JC, Halter JB, et al. Pathophysiology of insulin secretion in non–insulin-dependent diabetes mellitus. Diabetes Care 1984;7:491-502.
446. Waldhäus W, Bratusch-Marrain P, Gasic S, et al. Insulin production rate following glucose ingestion estimated by splanchnic C-peptide output in normal man. Diabetologia 1979;17:221-227.
447. Eaton R, Allen R, Schade D. Hepatic removal of insulin in normal man: dose response to endogenous insulin secretion. J Clin Endocrinol Metab 1983;56:1294-1300.
448. Nauck M, Homberger E, Siegel EG, et al. Incretin effects of increasing glucose loads in man calculated from venous insulin and C-peptide responses. J Clin Endocrinol Metab 1986;63:492-498.
449. Tillil H, Shapiro ET, Miller MA, et al. Dose-dependent effects of oral and intravenous glucose on insulin secretion and clearance in normal humans. Am J Physiol 1988;254:E349-E357.
450. Faber O, Madsbad S, Kehlet H, Binder C. Pancreatic beta cell secretion during oral and intravenous glucose administration. Acta Med Scand Suppl 1979;624:61-64.
451. Madsbad S, Kehlet H, Hilsted J, Tronier B. Discrepancy between plasma C-peptide and insulin response to oral and intravenous glucose. Diabetes 1983;32:436-438.
452. Shapiro E, Tillil H, Miller MA, et al. Insulin secretion and clearance: comparison after oral and intravenous glucose. Diabetes 1987;93:1120-1130.
453. Creutzfeldt W, Ebert R. New developments in the incretin concept. Diabetologia 1985;28:565-576.
454. Pagliara A, Stillings SN, Hover B, et al. Glucose modulation of amino acid–induced glucagon and insulin release in the isolated perfused rat pancreas. J Clin Invest 1974;54:819-832.
455. Gerich J, Charles M, Grodsky G. Characterization of the effects of arginine and glucose on glucagon and insulin release from the perfused rat pancreas. J Clin Invest 1974;54:833-847.
456. Grodsky G. The kinetics of insulin release. In Hasselblatt A, Bruchhausen F. eds. Handbook of Experimental Pharmacology, vol 32. Berlin, Springer-Verlag, 1975:1-19.
457. Salomon D, Meda P. Heterogeneity and contact-dependent regulation of hormone secretion by individual β cells. Exp Cell Res 1986;162:507-520.
458. Schmitz O, Porksen N, Nyholm B, et al. Disorderly and nonstationary insulin secretion in relatives of patients with NIDDM. Am J Physiol 1997;272:E218-E226.
459. Cerasi E, Luft R. The plasma insulin response to glucose infusion in healthy subjects and in diabetes mellitus. Acta Endocrinol (Copenh) 1967;55:278-304.
460. Bennett L, Grodsky G. Multiphasic aspects of insulin release after glucose and glucagon. Diabetes. Proceedings of the Sixth Congress of the International Diabetes Federation. Amsterdam, Excerpta Medica, 1967:000-000.
461. Grodsky G. A threshold distribution hypothesis for packet storage of insulin and its mathematical modeling. J Clin Invest 1972;51: 2047-2059.
462. Smith C, Tam AC, Thomas JM, et al. Between and within subject variation of the first phase insulin response to intravenous glucose. Diabetologia 1988;31:123-125.
463. Bardet S, Pasqual C, Maugendre D, et al. Inter and intra individual variability of acute insulin response during intravenous glucose tolerance tests. Diabetes Metab 1989;15:224-232.
464. Rayman G, Clark P, Schneider AE, Hales CN. The first phase insulin response to intravenous glucose is highly reproducible. Diabetologia 1990;33:631-634.
465. Bolaffi J, Haldt A, Lewis LD, Grodsky GM. The third phase of in vitro insulin secretion: evidence for glucose insensitivity. Diabetes 1986;35:370-373.
466. Curry D. Insulin content and insulinogenesis by the perfused rat pancreas: effects of long term glucose stimulation. Endocrinology 1986;118:170-175.
467. Hoenig M, MacGregor L, Matschinsky F. In vitro exhaustion of pancreatic β-cells. Am J Physiol 1986;250:E502-E511.
468. Grodsky G. A new phase of insulin secretion: how will it contribute to our understanding of β-cell function? Diabetes 1989;38: 673-678.
469. Cerasi E. Potentiation of insulin release by glucose in man. Acta Endocrinol (Copenh) 1975;79:511-534.
470. Grill V. Time and dose dependencies for priming effect of glucose on insulin secretion. Am J Physiol 1981;240:E24-E31.
471. Poitout V, Robertson RP. Minireview: secondary beta-cell failure in type 2 diabetes—a convergence of glucotoxicity and lipotoxicity. Endocrinology 2002;143:339-342.
472. Leahy JL. Natural history of beta-cell dysfunction in NIDDM. Diabetes Care 1990;13:992-1010.
473. Levin S, Karam JH, Hane S, et al. Enhancement of arginine-induced insulin secretion in man by prior administration of glucose. Diabetes 1971;20:171-176.
474. Fajans S, Floyd J. Stimulation of islet cell secretion by nutrients and by gastrointestinal hormones released during digestion. In Steiner D, Freinkel N, eds. Handbook of Physiology. Section 7. Endocrinology. Washington, DC: American Physiological Society, 1972:473-493.
475. Ward W, Bolgiano DC, McKnight B, et al. Diminished β-cell secretory capacity in patients with non–insulin dependent diabetes mellitus. J Clin Invest 1984;74:1318-1328.
476. Kadowaki T, Miyake Y, Hagura R, et al. Risk factors for worsening to diabetes in subjects with impaired glucose tolerance. Diabetologia 1984;26:44-49.
477. Muller W, Faloona G, Unger R. The influence of the antecedent diet upon glucagon and insulin secretion. N Engl J Med 1971;285: 1450-1454.
478. Goberna R, Tamarit J Jr, Osorio J, et al. Action of β-hydroxybutyrate, acetoacetate and palmitate on the insulin release from the perfused isolated rat pancreas. Horm Metab Res 1974;6:256-260.
479. Crespin S, Greenough D, Steinberg D. Stimulation of insulin secretion by long-chain free fatty acids. J Clin Invest 1973;52: 1979-1984.
480. Crespin S, Greenough W, Steinberg D. Stimulation of insulin secretion by infusion of fatty acids. J Clin Invest 1969;48:1934-1943.
481. Paolisso G, Gambardella M, Amato L, et al. Opposite effects of short- and long-term fatty acid infusion on insulin secretion in healthy subjects. Diabetologia 1995;38:1295-1299.
482. Boden G, Chen X. Effects of fatty acids and ketone bodies on basal insulin secretion in type 2 diabetes. Diabetes 1999;48:577-583.
483. Zhou Y-P, Grill V. Long term exposure of rat pancreatic islets to fatty acids inhibits glucose-induced insulin secretion and biosynthesis through a glucose fatty acid cycle. J Clin Invest 1994;93: 870-876.
484. Mason T, Goh T, Tchipashvili V, et al. Prolonged elevation of plasma free fatty acids desensitizes the insulin secretory response to glucose in vivo in rats. Diabetes 1999;48:524-530.
485. Carpentier A, Mittelman SD, Lamarche B, et al. Acute enhancement of insulin secretion by FFA in humans is lost with prolonged FFA elevation. Am J Physiol 1999;276:E1055-E1066.
486. Dupre J, Ross SA Watson D, Brown JC. Stimulation of insulin secretion by gastric inhibitory polypeptide in man. J Clin Endocrinol Metab 1973;37:826-828.

487. Andersen D, Elahi D, Brown JC, et al. Oral glucose augmentation of insulin secretion: interactions of gastric inhibitory polypeptide with ambient glucose and insulin levels. J Clin Invest 1978;62: 152-161.
488. Schmidt W, Siegel E, Creutzfeldt W. Glucagon-like peptide-2 stimulates insulin release from isolated rate pancreatic islets. Diabetologia 1985;28:704-707.
489. Kreymann B, Williams G, Ghatei MA, Bloom SR. Glucagon-like peptide-1 7-36: a physiological incretin in man. Lancet 1987;2: 1300-1304.
490. Zawalich W, Diaz V. Prior cholecystokinin exposure sensitizes islets of Langerhans to glucose stimulation. Diabetes 1987;36: 118-227.
491. Zawalich W. Synergistic impact of cholecystokinin and gastric inhibitory polypeptide on the regulation of insulin secretion. Metabolism 1988;37:778-781.
492. Weir G, Mojsovs S, Hendrick GK, Habener JF. Glucagon-like peptide 1(7-37) actions on endocrine pancreas. Diabetes 1989;38: 338-342.
493. Rasmussen H, Zawalich KC, Ganesan S, et al. Physiology and pathophysiology of insulin secretion. Diabetes Care 1990;13: 655-666.
494. Fukase N, Manaka H, Sugiyama K, et al. Response of truncated glucagon-like peptide-1 and gastric inhibitory polypeptide to glucose ingestion in non–insulin dependent diabetes mellitus. Effect of sulfonylurea therapy. Acta Diabetol 1995;32:165-169.
495. Groop P. The influence of body weight, age and glucose tolerance on the relationship between GIP secretion and beta-cell function in man. Scand J Clin Lab Invest 1989;49:367-379.
496. Creutzfeldt W, Ebert R, Nauck M, Stockmann F. Disturbances of the entero-insulin axis. Scand J Gastroenterol 1983;83(suppl):111-119.
497. Nauck M, Heimesaat MM, Orskov C, et al. Preserved incretin activity of glucagon-like peptide 1(7-36 amide) but not of synthetic human gastric inhibitory polypeptide in patients with type 2 diabetes mellitus. J Clin Invest 1993;91:301-307.
498. Ahrén B, Larsson H, Holst J. Reduced gastric inhibitory polypeptide but normal glucagon-like peptide 1 response to oral glucose in postmenopausal women with impaired glucose tolerance. Eur J Endocrinol 1997; 137:127-131.
499. Rushakoff R, Goldfine ID, Beccaria LJ, et al. Reduced postprandial cholecystokinin (CCK) secretion in patients with noninsulin-dependent diabetes mellitus: evidence for a role for CCK in regulating postprandial hyperglycemia. J Clin Endocrinol Metab 1993;76:489-493.
500. Meguro T, Shimosegawa T, Satoh A, et al. Gallbladder emptying and cholecystokinin and pancreatic polypeptide responses to a liquid meal in patients with diabetes mellitus. J Gastroenterol 1997;32:628-634.
501. Hasegawa H, Shirohara H, Okabayashi Y, et al. Oral glucose ingestion stimulates cholecystokinin release in normal subjects and patients with non–insulin-dependent diabetes mellitus. Metabolism 1996;45:196-202.
502. Nauck M, Wollschlager D, Werner J, et al. Effects of subcutaneous glucagon-like peptide 1 (GLP-1 (7-36 amide)) in patients with NIDDM. Diabetologia 1996;39:1546-1553.
503. Creutzfeldt W, Kleine N, Willms B, et al. Glucagonostatic actions and reduction of fasting hyperglycemia by exogenous glucagon-like peptide I(7-36) amide in type I diabetic patients. Diabetes Care 1996;19:580-586.
504. Young A, Gedulin BR, Bhavsar S, et al. Glucose-lowering and insulin-sensitizing actions of exendin-4: studies in obese diabetic *(ob/ob, db/db)* mice, diabetic fatty Zucker rats, and diabetic rhesus monkeys *(Macaca mulatta)*. Diabetes 1999;48:1026-1034.
505. Nauck M, Bartels E, Orskov C, et al. Additive insulinotropic effects of exogenous synthetic human gastric inhibitory polypeptide and glucagon-like peptide-1-(7-36) amide infused at near-physiological insulinotropic hormone and glucose concentrations. J Clin Endocrinol Metab, 1993;76:912-917.
506. Elahi D, McAloon-Dyke M, Fukagawa NK, et al. The insulinotropic actions of glucose-dependent insulinotropic polypeptide (GIP) and glucagon-like peptide-1 (7-37) in normal and diabetic subjects. Regul Pept 1994;51:63-74.
507. Niederau C, Schwarzendrube J, Luthen R, et al. Effects of cholecystokinin receptor blockade in circulating concentrations of glucose, insulin, C-peptide, and pancreatic polypeptide after various meals in healthy human volunteers. Pancreas 1992;7: 1-10.
508. Fieseler P, Bridenbaugh S, Nustede R, et al. Physiological augmentation of amino acid–induced insulin secretion by GIP and GLP-I but not by CCK-8. Am J Physiol 1995;268:E949-E955.
509. Reimers J, Nauck M, Creutzfeldt W, et al. Lack of insulinotropic effect of endogenous and exogenous cholecystokinin in man. Diabetologia 1988;31:271-280.
510. Rushakoff R, Goldfine ID, Carter JD, Liddle RA. Physiological concentrations of cholecystokinin stimulate amino acid–induced insulin release in humans. J Clin Endocrinol Metab 1987;65: 395-401.
511. Ahrén B, Holst J, Efendic S. Antidiabetogenic action of cholecystokinin-8 in type 2 diabetes. J Clin Endocrinol Metab 2000;85: 1043-1048.
512. Schebalin M, Said S, Makhlouf G. Stimulation of insulin and glucagon secretion by vasoactive intestinal peptide. Am J Physiol 1977;232:E197-E200.
513. Dupre J, Curtis JD, Unger RH, et al. Effects of secretin, pancreozymin, or gastrin on the response of the endocrine pancreas to administration of glucose or arginine in man. J Clin Invest 1969;48:745-757.
514. Halter J, Porte DJ. Mechanisms of impaired acute insulin release in adult onset diabetes: studies with isoproterenol and secretin. J Clin Endocrinol Metab 1978;46:952-960.
515. Glaser B, Shapiro B, Glowniak J, et al. Effects of secretin on the normal and pathological beta-cell. J Clin Endocrinol Metab 1988;66:1138-1143.
516. Bertrand G, Puech R, Maisonnasse Y, et al. Comparative effects of PACAP and VIP on pancreatic endocrine secretions and vascular resistance in rat. Br J Pharmacol 1996;117:764-770.
517. Rehfeld J, Stadil F. The effect of gastrin on basal- and glucose-stimulated insulin secretion in man. J Clin Invest 1973;52: 1415-1426.
518. Samols E, Marri G, Marks V. Promotion of insulin secretion by glucagon. Lancet 1965;2:15-16.
519. Alberti K, Christensen NJ, Christensen SE, et al. Inhibition of insulin secretion by somatostatin. Lancet 1973;2:1299-1301.
520. Aguilar-Parada E, Eisentraut A, Unger R. Effects of starvation on plasma pancreatic glucagon in normal man. Diabetes 1969;18: 717-723.
521. Marliss E, Aoki TT, Unger RH, et al. Glucagon levels and metabolic effects in fasting man. J Clin Invest 1970;49:2256-2270.
522. Malaisse W, Malaisse L, Wright P. Effect of fasting upon insulin secretion in the rat. Am J Physiol 1967;213:843-848.
523. Zawalich W, Dye ES, Pagliara AS, et al. Starvation diabetes in the rat: onset, recovery and specificity of reduced responsiveness of pancreatic β-cells. Endocrinology 1979;104:1344-1351.
524. Felig P, Marliss E, Cahill JG. Metabolic response to human growth hormone during prolonged starvation. J Clin Invest 1971;50: 411-421.
525. Kalhan S, Adam P. Inhibitory effect of prednisone on insulin secretion in man: model for duplication of blood glucose concentration. J Clin Endocrinol Metab 1975;41:600-610.
526. Landgraf R, Landgraf-Luers MM, Weissmann A, et al. Prolactin: a diabetogenic hormone. Diabetologia 1977;13:99-104.
527. Gustafson A, Banasiak MF, Kalkhoff RK, et al. Correlation of hyperprolactinemia with altered plasma insulin and glucagon: similarity to effects of late human pregnancy. J Clin Endocrinol Metab 1980;51:242-246.
528. Brelje T, Sorenson R. Nutrient and hormonal regulation of the threshold of glucose-stimulated insulin secretion in isolated rat pancreases. Endocrinology 1988;123:1582-1590.
529. Beck P, Daughaday W. Human placental lactogen: studies of its acute metabolic effects and disposition in normal man. J Clin Invest 1967;46:103-110.
530. Ensinck J, Williams R. Hormonal and nonhormonal factors modifying man's response to insulin. In Steiner D, Freinkel N, eds. Handbook of Physiology. Section 7. Endocrinology. Washington, DC: American Physiological Society, 1972:665-669.
531. Martin J, Friesen H. Effect of human placental lactogen on the isolated islets of Langerhans in vitro. Endocrinology 1969;84: 619-621.
532. Curry D, Bennett L. Dynamics of insulin release by perfused rat pancreases: effects of hypophysectomy, growth hormone, adreno-

corticotropic hormone and hydrocortisone. Endocrinology 1973;93:602-609.
533. Malaisse W, Malaisse-Lagae F, King S, Wright PH. Effect of growth hormone on insulin secretion. Am J Physiol 1968;215:423-428.
534. Randin J, Scazziga B, Jequier E, Felber JP. Study of glucose and lipid metabolism by continuous indirect calorimetry in Graves' disease: effect of an oral glucose load. J Clin Endocrinol Metab 1985;61:1165-1171.
535. Foss M, Paccola GM, Saad MJ, et al. Peripheral glucose metabolism in human hyperthyroidism. J Clin Endocrinol Metab 1990;70: 1167-1172.
536. Sestoft L, Heding L. Hypersecretion of proinsulin in thyrotoxicosis. Diabetologia 1981;21:103-107.
537. Nishi S, Seino Y, Ishida H, et al. Vagal regulation of insulin, glucagon, and somatostatin secretion in vitro in the rat. J Clin Invest 1987;79:1191-1196.
538. Kurose T, Seino Y, Nishi S, et al. Mechanism of sympathetic neural regulation of insulin, somatostatin, and glucagon secretion. Am J Physiol 1990;251:E220-E227.
539. Woods S, Porte DJ. Neural control of the endocrine pancreas. Physiol Rev 1974;54:596-619.
540. Bloom SR, Edwards A. Certain pharmacological characteristics of the release of pancreatic glucagon in response to stimulation of the splanchnic nerves. J Physiol (Lond) 1978;280:25-35.
541. Porte D Jr, Girardier L, Seydoux J, et al. Neural regulation of insulin secretion in the dog. J Clin Invest 1973;52:210-214.
542. Roy M, Lee KC, Jones MS, Miller RE. Neural control of pancreatic insulin and somatostatin secretion. Endocrinology 1984;115: 770-775.
543. Skoglund G, Lundquist I, Ahren B. Selective α_2-adrenoceptor activation by clonidine: effects on $^{45}Ca^{2}$+ efflux and insulin secretion from isolated rat islets. Acta Physiol Scand 1988;132:289-296.
544. Ahrén B. Autonomic regulation of islet hormone secretion: implications for health and disease. Diabetologia 2000;43:393-410.
545. Pettersson M, Ahrén B. Calcitonin gene–related peptide inhibits insulin secretion: studies on ion fluxes and cyclic AMP in isolated rat islets. Diabetes Res Clin Pract 1990;15:9-14.
546. Pettersson M, Ahrén B, Bottcher G, Sundler F. Calcitonin gene–related peptide: occurrence in pancreatic islets in the mouse and the rat and inhibition of insulin secretion in the mouse. Diabetologia 1986;119:865-869.
547. Ahrén B, Mårtensson H, Nobin A. Effects of calcitonin gene–related peptide (CGRP) on islet hormone secretion in the pig. Diabetologia 1987;30:354-359.
548. Lundquist I, Sundler F, Ahrén B, et al. Somatostatin, pancreatic polypeptide, substance P, and neurotensin: cellular distribution and effects on stimulated insulin secretion in the mouse. Endocrinology 1979;104:832-838.
549. Hermansen K. Effects of substance P and other peptides on the release of somatostatin, insulin and glucagon in vitro. Endocrinology 1980;107:256-261.
550. Larrimer J, Mazzaferri EL, Cataland S, Mekhjian HS. Effect of atropine on glucose-stimulated gastric inhibitory polypeptide. Diabetes 1978;27:638-642.
551. Rocca A, Brubaker P. Role of the vagus nerve in mediating proximal nutrient-induced glucagon-like peptide-1 secretion. Endocrinology 1999;140:1687-1694.
552. Flaten O, Sand T, Myren J. β-Adrenergic stimulation and blockade of the release of gastric inhibitory polypeptide and insulin in man. Scand J Gastroenterol 1982;17:283-288.
553. Claustre J, Brechet S, Plaisancie P, et al. Stimulatory effect of β-adrenergic agonists on ileal L cell secretion and modulation by α-adrenergic activation. J Endocrinol 1999;162:271-278.
554. Kruszynska Y, Home PD, Hanning I, Alberti KG. Basal and 24-h C-peptide and insulin secretion rate in normal man. Diabetologia 1987;30:16-21.
555. Polonsky KS, Given BD, Van Cauter E. Twenty-four-hour profiles and pulsatile patterns of insulin secretion in normal and obese subjects. J Clin Invest 1988;81:442-448.
556. Polonsky KS. Lilly Lecture 1994. The beta-cell in diabetes: from molecular genetics to clinical research. Diabetes 1995;44: 705-717.
557. Lang DA, Matthews DR, Peto J, Turner RC. Cyclic oscillations of basal plasma glucose and insulin concentrations in human beings. N Engl J Med 1979;301:1023-1027.
558. Hansen BC, Jen KC, Belbez Pek S, Wolfe RA. Rapid oscillations in plasma insulin, glucagon, and glucose in obese and normal weight humans. J Clin Endocrinol Metab 1982;54:785-792.
559. Matthews DR, Lang DA, Burnett MA, Turner RC. Control of pulsatile insulin secretion in man. Diabetologia 1983;24:231-237.
560. O'Meara NM, Sturis J, Van Cauter E, Polonsky KS. Lack of control by glucose of ultradian insulin secretory oscillations in impaired glucose tolerance and in non–insulin-dependent diabetes mellitus. J Clin Invest 1993;92:262-271.
561. Porksen N, Grafte B, Nyholm B, et al. Glucagon-like peptide 1 increases mass but not frequency or orderliness of pulsatile insulin secretion. Diabetes 1998;47:45-49.
562. Porksen N, Nyholm B, Veldhuis JD, et al. In humans at least 75% of insulin secretion arises from punctuated insulin secretory bursts. Am J Physiol 1997;273:E908-E914.
563. Porksen N, Hussain MA, Bianda TL, et al. IGF-I inhibits burst mass of pulsatile insulin secretion at supraphysiological and low IGF-I infusion rates. Am J Physiol 1997;272:E352-E358.
564. Porksen NK, Munn SR, Steers JL, et al. Mechanisms of sulfonylurea's stimulation of insulin secretion in vivo: selective amplification of insulin secretory burst mass. Diabetes 1996;45:1792-1797.
565. Porksen N, Munn S, Steers J, et al. Effects of glucose ingestion versus infusion on pulsatile insulin secretion. The incretin effect is achieved by amplification of insulin secretory burst mass. Diabetes 1996;45:1317-1323.
566. O'Rahilly S, Turner RC, Matthews DR. Impaired pulsatile secretion of insulin in relatives of patients with non–insulin-dependent diabetes. N Engl J Med 1988;318:1225-1230.
567. Van Cauter E. Estimating false-positive and false-negative errors in analyses of hormonal pulsatility. Am J Physiol 1988;254: E786-E794.
568. Pincus SM. Quantification of evolution from order to randomness in practical time series analysis. Methods Enzymol 1994;240: 68-89.
569. Jaspan JB, Lever E, Polonsky KS, Van Cauter E. In vivo pulsatility of pancreatic islet peptides. Am J Physiol 1986;251:E215-E226.
570. Matthews DR, Naylor BA, Jones RG, et al. Pulsatile insulin has greater hypoglycemic effect than continuous delivery. Diabetes 1983;32:617-621.
571. Bratusch-Marrain PR, Komjati M, Waldhausl WK. Efficacy of pulsatile versus continuous insulin administration on hepatic glucose production and glucose utilization in type I diabetic humans. Diabetes 1986;35:922-926.
572. Ward GM, Walters JM, Aitken PM, et al. Effects of prolonged pulsatile hyperinsulinemia in humans. Enhancement of insulin sensitivity. Diabetes 1990;39:501-507.
573. Sonnenberg GE, Hoffmann RG, Johnson CP, Kissebah AH. Low- and high-frequency insulin secretion pulses in normal subjects and pancreas transplant recipients: role of extrinsic innervation. J Clin Invest 1992;90:545-553.
574. Blackman JD, Polonsky KS, Jaspan JB, et al. Insulin secretory profiles and C-peptide clearance kinetics at 6 months and 2 years after kidney-pancreas transplantation. Diabetes 1992;41:1346-1354.
575. Sturis J, Polonsky KS, Mosekilde E, Van Cauter E. Computer model for mechanisms underlying ultradian oscillations of insulin and glucose. Am J Physiol 1991;260:E801-E809.
576. Sturis J, Van Cauter E, Blackman JD, Polonsky KS. Entrainment of pulsatile insulin secretion by oscillatory glucose infusion. J Clin Invest 1991;87:439-445.
577. Malherbe C, De Gasparo M, De Hertogh R, Hoet JJ. Circadian variations of blood sugar and plasma insulin levels in man. Diabetologia 1969;5:397-404.
578. Jarrett RJ, Baker IA, Keen H, Oakley NW. Diurnal variation in oral glucose tolerance: blood sugar and plasma insulin levels morning, afternoon, and evening. Br Med J 1972;1:199-201.
579. Carroll KF, Nestel PJ. Diurnal variation in glucose tolerance and in insulin secretion in man. Diabetes 1973;22:333-348.
580. Aparicio NJ, Puchulu FE, Gagliardino JJ, et al. Circadian variation of the blood glucose, plasma insulin and human growth hormone levels in response to an oral glucose load in normal subjects. Diabetes 1974;23:132-137.
581. Van Cauter E, Desir D, Decoster C, et al. Nocturnal decrease in glucose tolerance during constant glucose infusion. J Clin Endocrinol Metab 1989;69:604-611.

582. Pick A, Clark J, Kubstrup P, et al. Role of apoptosis in failure of beta-cell mass compensation for insulin resistance and beta-cell defects in the male Zucker diabetic fatty rat. Diabetes 1998; 47:358-364.
583. Cockburn BN, Ostrega DM, Sturis J, et al. Changes in pancreatic islet glucokinase and hexokinase activities with increasing age, obesity, and the onset of diabetes. Diabetes 1997;46:1434-1439.
584. Kahn SE, Prigeon RL, McCulloch DK, et al. Quantification of the relationship between insulin sensitivity and beta-cell function in human subjects: evidence for a hyperbolic function. Diabetes 1993;42:1663-1672.
585. Toffolo G, Bergman RN, Finegood DT, et al. Quantitative estimation of beta cell sensitivity to glucose in the intact organism: a minimal model of insulin kinetics in the dog. Diabetes 1980; 29:979-990.
586. Polonsky KS, Given BD, Hirsch L, et al. Quantitative study of insulin secretion and clearance in normal and obese subjects. J Clin Invest 1988;81:435-441.
587. Jones CN, Pei D, Staris P, et al. Alterations in the glucose-stimulated insulin secretory dose-response curve and in insulin clearance in nondiabetic insulin-resistant individuals. J Clin Endocrinol Metab 1997;82:1834-1838.
588. Buchanan TA, Metzger BE, Freinkel N, Bergman RN. Insulin sensitivity and B-cell responsiveness to glucose during late pregnancy in lean and moderately obese women with normal glucose tolerance or mild gestational diabetes. Am J Obstet Gynecol 1990;162:1008-1014.
589. Bergstrom RW, Wahl PW, Leonetti DL, Fujimoto WY. Association of fasting glucose levels with a delayed secretion of insulin after oral glucose in subjects with glucose intolerance. J Clin Endocrinol Metab 1990;71:1447-1453.
590. Phillips DI, Clark PM, Hales CN, Osmond C. Understanding oral glucose tolerance: comparison of glucose or insulin measurements during the oral glucose tolerance test with specific measurements of insulin resistance and insulin secretion. Diabet Med 1994;11:286-292.
591. Byrne MM, Sturis J, Sobel RJ, Polonsky KS. Elevated plasma glucose 2 h postchallenge predicts defects in beta-cell function. Am J Physiol 1996;270:E572-E579.
592. Ahrén B, Pacini G. Impaired adaptation of first-phase insulin secretion in postmenopausal women with glucose intolerance. Am J Physiol 1997;273:E701-E707.
593. O'Rahilly SP, Nugent Z, Rudenski AS, et al. Beta-cell dysfunction, rather than insulin insensitivity, is the primary defect in familial type 2 diabetes. Lancet 1986;2:360-364.
594. Barnett AH, Spiliopoulos AJ, Pyke DA, et al. Metabolic studies in unaffected co-twins of non–insulin-dependent diabetics. Br Med J (Clin Res Ed) 1981;282:1656-1658.
595. Kosaka K, Hagura R, Kuzuya T. Insulin responses in equivocal and definite diabetes, with special reference to subjects who had mild glucose intolerance but later developed definite diabetes. Diabetes 1977;26:944-952.
596. Efendic S, Luft R, Wajngot A. Aspects of the pathogenesis of type 2 diabetes. Endocr Rev 1984;5:395-410.
597. Ward WK, Johnston CL, Beard JC, et al. Insulin resistance and impaired insulin secretion in subjects with histories of gestational diabetes mellitus. Diabetes 1985;34:861-869.
598. O'Sullivan JB. Body weight and subsequent diabetes mellitus. JAMA 1982;248:949-952.
599. Yoshioka N, Kuzuya T, Matsuda A, et al. Serum proinsulin levels at fasting and after oral glucose load in patients with type 2 (non–insulin-dependent) diabetes mellitus. Diabetologia 1988;31: 355-360.
600. Saad MF, Kahn SE, Nelson RG, et al. Disproportionately elevated proinsulin in Pima Indians with noninsulin-dependent diabetes mellitus. J Clin Endocrinol Metab 1990;70: 1247-1253.
601. Reaven GM, Chen YD, Hollenbeck CB, et al. Plasma insulin, C-peptide, and proinsulin concentrations in obese and nonobese individuals with varying degrees of glucose tolerance. J Clin Endocrinol Metab 1993;76:44-48.
602. Larsson H, Ahren B. Relative hyperproinsulinemia as a sign of islet dysfunction in women with impaired glucose tolerance. J Clin Endocrinol Metab 1999;84:2068-2074.
603. Snehalatha C, Ramachandran A, Satyavani K, et al. Specific insulin and proinsulin concentrations in nondiabetic South Indians. Metabolism 1998;47:230-233.
604. Birkeland KI, Torjesen PA, Eriksson J, et al. Hyperproinsulinemia of type II diabetes is not present before the development of hyperglycemia. Diabetes Care 1994;17:1307-1310.
605. Inoue I, Takahashi K, Katayama S, et al. A higher proinsulin response to glucose loading predicts deteriorating fasting plasma glucose and worsening to diabetes in subjects with impaired glucose tolerance. Diabet Med 1996;13:330-336.
606. Kahn SE, Leonetti DL, Prigeon RL, et al. Proinsulin levels predict the development of non-insulin-dependent diabetes mellitus (NIDDM) in Japanese-American men. Diabet Med 1996;13(9 suppl 6):S63-S66.
607. Heine RJ, Nijpels G, Mooy JM. New data on the rate of progression of impaired glucose tolerance to NIDDM and predicting factors. Diabet Med 1996;13(3 suppl 2):S12-S14.
608. Porte D Jr. Clinical importance of insulin secretion and its interaction with insulin resistance in the treatment of type 2 diabetes mellitus and its complications. Diabetes Metab Res Rev 2001; 17:181-188.
609. Ferner RE, Ashworth L, Tronier B, Alberti KG. Effects of short-term hyperglycemia on insulin secretion in normal humans. Am J Physiol 1986;250:E655-E661.
610. O'Meara NM, Shapiro ET, Van Cauter E, Polonsky KS. Effect of glyburide on beta cell responsiveness to glucose in non–insulin-dependent diabetes mellitus. Am J Med 1990;89:11S–16S; discussion 51S–53S.
611. Gerich JE. The genetic basis of type 2 diabetes mellitus: impaired insulin secretion versus impaired insulin sensitivity. Endocr Rev 1998;19:491-503.
612. Clark PM, Levy JL, Cox L, et al. Immunoradiometric assay of insulin, intact proinsulin and 32-33 split proinsulin and radioimmunoassay of insulin in diet-treated type 2 (non–insulin-dependent) diabetic subjects. Diabetologia 1992;35:469-474.
613. Polonsky KS, Given BD, Hirsch LJ, et al. Abnormal patterns of insulin secretion in non–insulin-dependent diabetes mellitus. N Engl J Med 1988;318:1231-1239.
614. Block MB, Rosenfield RL, Mako ME, et al. Sequential changes in beta-cell function in insulin-treated diabetic patients assessed by C-peptide immunoreactivity. N Engl J Med 1973;288:1144-1148.
615. Cavaghan MK, Ehrmann DA, Byrne MM, Polonsky KS. Treatment with the oral antidiabetic agent troglitazone improves beta cell responses to glucose in subjects with impaired glucose tolerance. J Clin Invest 1997;100:530-537.
616. Ingalls AM, Dickie MM, Snell GD. Obese, a new mutation in the house mouse. Obes Res 1996;4:101.
617. Zhang Y, Proenca R, Maffei M, et al. Positional cloning of the mouse obese gene and its human homologue. Nature 1994;372: 425-432.
618. Pelleymounter MA, Cullen MJ, Baker MB, et al. Effects of the obese gene product on body weight regulation in ob/ob mice. Science 1995;269:540-543.
619. Halaas JL, Gajiwala KS, Maffei M, et al. Weight-reducing effects of the plasma protein encoded by the obese gene. Science 1995; 269:543-546.
620. Friedman JM, Halaas JL. Leptin and the regulation of body weight in mammals. Nature 1998;395:763-770.
621. Friedman JM. Leptin and the regulation of body weight. Harvey Lect 1999;95:107-136.
622. Halaas JL, Boozer C, Blair-West J, et al. Physiological response to long-term peripheral and central leptin infusion in lean and obese mice. Proc Natl Acad Sci U S A 1997;94:8878-8883.
623. Friedman JM. The alphabet of weight control. Nature 1997;385: 119-120.
624. Friedman JM. Leptin, leptin receptors and the control of body weight. Eur J Med Res 1997;2:7-13.
625. Kerouz NJ, Horsch D, Pons S, Kahn CR. Differential regulation of insulin receptor substrates-1 and -2 (IRS-1 and IRS-2) and phosphatidylinositol 3-kinase isoforms in liver and muscle of the obese diabetic (ob/ob) mouse. J Clin Invest 1997;100:3164-3172.
626. Genuth SM, Przybylski RJ, Rosenberg DM. Insulin resistance in genetically obese, hyperglycemic mice. Endocrinology 1971;88: 1230-1238.

627. Herberg L, Coleman DL. Laboratory animals exhibiting obesity and diabetes syndromes. Metabolism 1977;26:59-99.
628. Lee GH, Proenca R, Montez JM, et al. Abnormal splicing of the leptin receptor in diabetic mice. Nature 1996;379:632-635.
629. Chen H, Charlat O, Tartaglia LA, et al. Evidence that the diabetes gene encodes the leptin receptor: identification of a mutation in the leptin receptor gene in db/db mice. Cell 1996;84:491-495.
630. Coleman DL, Hummel KP. Hyperinsulinemia in pre-weaning diabetes (db) mice. Diabetologia 1974;10(suppl):607-610.
631. Like AA, Chick WL. Studies in the diabetic mutant mouse. I. Light microscopy and radioautography of pancreatic islets. Diabetologia 1970;6:207-215.
632. Lavine RL, Chick WL, Like AA, Makdisi TW. Glucose tolerance and insulin secretion in neonatal and adult mice. Diabetes 1971;20: 134-139.
633. Like AA, Chick WL. Studies in the diabetic mutant mouse. II. Electron microscopy of pancreatic islets. Diabetologia 1970;6: 216-242.
634. Shargill NS, Tatoyan A, el-Rafai MF, et al. Impaired insulin receptor phosphorylation in skeletal muscle membranes of db/db mice: the use of a novel skeletal muscle plasma membrane preparation to compare insulin binding and stimulation of receptor phosphorylation. Biochem Biophys Res Commun 1986;137:286-294.
635. Hummel KP, Coleman DL, Lane PW. The influence of genetic background on expression of mutations at the diabetes locus in the mouse. I. C57BL-KsJ and C57BL-6J strains. Biochem Genet 1972;7:1-13.
636. Coleman DL, Hummel KP. The influence of genetic background on the expression of the obese (Ob) gene in the mouse. Diabetologia 1973;9:287-293.
637. Cantello BC, Cawthorne MA, Cottam GP, et al. ((ω-(Heterocyclylamino)alkoxy)benzyl)-2,4-thiazolidinediones as potent antihyperglycemic agents. J Med Chem 1994;37:3977-3985.
638. Lohray BB, Bhushan V, Rao BP, et al. Novel euglycemic and hypolipidemic agents. 1. J Med Chem 1998;41:1619-1630.
639. Frigeri LG, Wolff GL, Robel G. Impairment of glucose tolerance in yellow (Avy/A) (BALB/c X VY) F-1 hybrid mice by hyperglycemic peptide(s) from human pituitary glands. Endocrinology 1983; 113:2097-2105.
640. Warbritton A, Gill AM, Yen TT, et al. Pancreatic islet cells in preobese yellow Avy/-mice: relation to adult hyperinsulinemia and obesity. Proc Soc Exp Biol Med 1994;206:145-151.
641. Michaud EJ, Bultman SJ, Klebig ML, et al. A molecular model for the genetic and phenotypic characteristics of the mouse lethal yellow (Ay) mutation. Proc Natl Acad Sci U S A 1994;91: 2562-2566.
642. Claycombe KJ, Wang Y, Jones BH, et al. Transcriptional regulation of the adipocyte fatty acid synthase gene by agouti: interaction with insulin. Physiol Genomics 2000;3:157-162.
643. Claycombe KJ, Wang Y, Jones BH, et al. Regulation of leptin by agouti. Physiol Genomics 2000;2:101-105.
644. Kondo ZK, Nozawa K, Tomito T, Ezaki K. Inbred strains resulting from Japanese mice. Bull Exp Anim 1957;5:107-116.
645. Iwatsuka H, Shino A, Suzuoki Z. General survey of diabetic features of yellow KK mice. Endocrinol Jpn 1970;17:23-35.
646. Matsuo T, Shino A, Iwatsuka H, Suzuoki Z. Induction of overt diabetes in KK mice by dietary means. Endocrinol Jpn 1970;17: 477-488.
647. Veroni MC, Proietto J, Larkins RG. Evolution of insulin resistance in New Zealand obese mice. Diabetes 1991;40:1480-1487.
648. Cameron DP, Opat F, Insch S. Studies of immunoreactive insulin secretion in NZO mice in vivo. Diabetologia 1974;10(suppl): 649-654.
649. Bielschowsky M, Bielschowsky F. A new strain of mice with hereditary obesity. Proc Univ Otago Med Sch 1953;31:29-31.
650. Leiter EH, Reifsnyder PC, Flurkey K, et al. NIDDM genes in mice: deleterious synergism by both parental genomes contributes to diabetogenic thresholds. Diabetes 1998;47:1287-1295.
651. Thorburn A, Andrikopoulos S, Proietto J. Defects in liver and muscle glycogen metabolism in neonatal and adult New Zealand obese mice. Metabolism 1995;44:1298-1302.
652. Andrikopoulos S, Proietto J. The biochemical basis of increased hepatic glucose production in a mouse model of type 2 (non–insulin-dependent) diabetes mellitus. Diabetologia 1995;38: 1389-1396.
653. Andrikopoulos S, Rosella G, Kacmarczyk SJ, et al. Impaired regulation of hepatic fructose-1,6-biphosphatase in the New Zealand obese mouse: an acquired defect. Metabolism 1996;45:622-626.
654. Larkins RG, Simeonova L, Veroni MC. Glucose utilization in relation to insulin secretion in NZO and C57Bl mouse islets. Endocrinology 1980;107:1634-1638.
655. Melez KA, Harrison LC, Gilliam JN, Steinberg AD. Diabetes is associated with autoimmunity in the New Zealand obese (NZO) mouse. Diabetes 1980;29:835-840.
656. Melez KA, Reeves JP, Steinberg AD. Regulation of the expression of autoimmunity in NZB × NZW F1 mice by sex hormones. J Immunopharmacol 1978;1:27-42.
657. Harrison LC, Itin A. A possible mechanism for insulin resistance and hyperglycaemia in NZO mice. Nature 1979;279:334-336.
658. Reifsnyder PC, Churchill G, Leiter EH. Maternal environment and genotype interact to establish diabesity in mice. Genome Res 2000;10:1568-1578.
659. Blair SC, Caterson ID, Cooney GJ. Glucose and lipid metabolism in the gold-thioglucose injected mouse model of diabesity. In Shafir E (ed). Lessons from Animal Diabetes VI. Boston, Birkhauser, 1996:239-267.
660. Burant CF, Sreenan S, Hirano K, et al. Troglitazone action is independent of adipose tissue. J Clin Invest 1997;100:2900-2908.
661. Ross SR, Graves RA, Choy L, et al. Transgenic mouse models of disease: altering adipose tissue function in vivo. Ann NY Acad Sci 1995;758:297-313.
662. Shimomura I, Hammer RE, Richardson JA, et al. Insulin resistance and diabetes mellitus in transgenic mice expressing nuclear SREBP-1c in adipose tissue: model for congenital generalized lipodystrophy. Genes Dev 1998;12:3182-3194.
663. Reitman ML, Gavrilova O. A-ZIP/F-1 mice lacking white fat: a model for understanding lipoatrophic diabetes. Int J Obes Relat Metab Disord 2000;24(suppl 4):S11-S14.
664. Gavrilova O, Marcus-Samuels B, Graham D, et al. Surgical implantation of adipose tissue reverses diabetes in lipoatrophic mice. J Clin Invest 2000;105:271-278.
665. Shimomura I, Hammer RE, Ikemoto S, et al. Leptin reverses insulin resistance and diabetes mellitus in mice with congenital lipodystrophy. Nature 1999;401:73-76.
666. Arioglu E, Duncan-Marin J, Sebring N, et al. Efficacy and safety of troglitazone in the treatment of lipodystrophy syndromes. Ann Intern Med 2000;133:263-274.
667. Surwit RS, Feinglos MN, Rodin J, et al. Differential effects of fat and sucrose on the development of obesity and diabetes in C57BL/6J and A/J mice. Metabolism 1995;44:645-651.
668. Rebuffe-Scrive M, Surwit R, Feinglos M, et al. Regional fat distribution and metabolism in a new mouse model (C57BL/6J) of non–insulin-dependent diabetes mellitus. Metabolism 1993;42: 1405-1409.
669. Wencel HE, Smothers C, Opara ED, et al. Impaired second phase insulin response of diabetes-prone C57BL/6J mouse islets. Physiol Behav 1995;57:1215-1220.
670. Lee SK, Opara EC, Surwit RS, et al. Defective glucose-stimulated insulin release from perifused islets of C57BL/6J mice. Pancreas 1995;11:206-211.
671. Parekh PI, Petro AE, Tiller JM, et al. Reversal of diet-induced obesity and diabetes in C57BL/6J mice. Metabolism 1998;47: 1089-1096.
672. Shibata M, Yasuda B. (Spontaneously occurring diabetes in NSY mice). Jikken Dobutsu 1979;28:584-590.
673. Kim JH, Sen S, Avery CS, et al. Genetic analysis of a new mouse model for non–insulin-dependent diabetes. Genomics 2001;74: 273-286.
674. Phillips MS, Liu Q, Hammond HA, et al. Leptin receptor missense mutation in the fatty Zucker rat. Nat Genet 1996;13:18-19.
675. Chua SC Jr, White DW, Wu-Peng XS, et al. Phenotype of fatty due to Gln269Pro mutation in the leptin receptor (Lepr). Diabetes 1996;45:1141-1143.
676. White DW, Wang DW, Chua SC Jr, et al. Constitutive and impaired signaling of leptin receptors containing the Gln → Pro extracellular domain fatty mutation. Proc Natl Acad Sci U S A 1997;94: 10657-10662.
677. Peterson RG, et al. Zucker diabetic fatty rat as a model for non–insulin-dependent diabetes mellitus. ILAR News 1990;32: 16-19.

678. Janssen SW, Hermus AR, Lange WP, et al. Progressive histopathological changes in pancreatic islets of Zucker diabetic fatty rats. Exp Clin Endocrinol Diabetes 2001;109:273-282.
679. Zhou YP, Cockburn BN, Pugh W, Polonsky KS. Basal insulin hypersecretion in insulin-resistant Zucker diabetic and Zucker fatty rats: role of enhanced fuel metabolism. Metabolism 1999;48:857-864.
680. Corsetti JP, Sparks JD, Peterson RG, et al. Effect of dietary fat on the development of non–insulin dependent diabetes mellitus in obese Zucker diabetic fatty male and female rats. Atherosclerosis 2000;148:231-241.
681. Griffen SC, Wang J, German MS. A genetic defect in beta-cell gene expression segregates independently from the fa locus in the ZDF rat. Diabetes 2001;50:63-68.
682. Johnson JH, Ogawa A, Chen L, et al. Underexpression of beta cell high K_m glucose transporters in noninsulin-dependent diabetes. Science 1990;250:546-549.
683. Orci L, Ravazzola M, Baetens D, et al. Evidence that down-regulation of beta-cell glucose transporters in non–insulin-dependent diabetes may be the cause of diabetic hyperglycemia. Proc Natl Acad Sci U S A 1990;87:9953-9957.
684. Unger RH. Lipotoxicity in the pathogenesis of obesity-dependent NIDDM: genetic and clinical implications. Diabetes 1995;44:863-870.
685. Lee Y, Hirose H, Zhou YT, et al. Increased lipogenic capacity of the islets of obese rats: a role in the pathogenesis of NIDDM. Diabetes 1997;46:408-413.
686. Sreenan S, Keck S, Fuller T, et al. Effects of troglitazone on substrate storage and utilization in insulin-resistant rats. Am J Physiol 1999;276:E1119-E1129.
687. Shimabukuro M, Ohneda M, Lee Y, Unger RH. Role of nitric oxide in obesity-induced beta cell disease. J Clin Invest 1997;100:290-295.
688. Shimabukuro M, Higa M, Zhou YT, et al. Lipoapoptosis in beta-cells of obese prediabetic fa/fa rats: role of serine palmitoyltransferase overexpression. J Biol Chem 1998;273:32487-32490.
689. Tokuyama Y, Sturis J, DePaoli AM, et al. Evolution of beta-cell dysfunction in the male Zucker diabetic fatty rat. Diabetes 1995;44:1447-1457.
690. Sreenan S, Sturis J, Pugh W, et al. Prevention of hyperglycemia in the Zucker diabetic fatty rat by treatment with metformin or troglitazone. Am J Physiol 1996;271:E742-E747.
691. Goto Y, Kakizaki M, Masaki N. Spontaneous diabetes produced by selective breeding of normal Wistar rats. Proc Jpn Acad 1975;51:80-85.
692. Movassat J, Saulnier C, Serradas P, Portha B. Impaired development of pancreatic beta-cell mass is a primary event during the progression to diabetes in the GK rat. Diabetologia 1997;40:916-925.
693. Movassat J, Saulnier C, Portha B. Beta-cell mass depletion precedes the onset of hyperglycaemia in the GK rat, a genetic model of non-insulin-dependent diabetes mellitus. Diabet Metab 1995;21:365-370.
694. Ostenson CG, Khan A, Abdel-Halim SM, et al. Abnormal insulin secretion and glucose metabolism in pancreatic islets from the spontaneously diabetic GK rat. Diabetologia 1993;36:3-8.
695. Ostenson CG, Abdel-Halim SM, Rasschaert J, et al. Deficient activity of FAD-linked glycerophosphate dehydrogenase in islets of GK rats. Diabetologia 1993;36:722-726.
696. Abdel-Halim SM, Guenifi A, Efendic S, Ostenson CG. Both somatostatin and insulin responses to glucose are impaired in the perfused pancreas of the spontaneously noninsulin-dependent diabetic GK (Goto-Kakizaki) rats. Acta Physiol Scand 1993;148:219-226.
697. Nagamatsu S, Nakamichi Y, Yamamura C, et al. Decreased expression of t-SNARE, syntaxin 1, and SNAP-25 in pancreatic beta-cells is involved in impaired insulin secretion from diabetic GK rat islets: restoration of decreased t-SNARE proteins improves impaired insulin secretion. Diabetes 1999;48:2367-2373.
698. Guenifi A, Portela-Gomes GM, Grimelius L, et al. Adenylyl cyclase isoform expression in non-diabetic and diabetic Goto-Kakizaki (GK) rat pancreas: evidence for distinct overexpression of type-8 adenylyl cyclase in diabetic GK rat islets. Histochem Cell Biol 2000;113:81-89.
699. Song XM, Kawano Y, Krook A, et al. Muscle fiber type-specific defects in insulin signal transduction to glucose transport in diabetic GK rats. Diabetes 1999;48:664-670.
700. Begum N, Ragolia L. Altered regulation of insulin signaling components in adipocytes of insulin-resistant type II diabetic Goto-Kakizaki rats. Metabolism 1998;47:54-62.
701. Berdanier CD. The BHE strain to rat: an example of the role of inheritance in determining metabolic controls. Fed Proc 1976;35:2295-2299.
702. Berdanier CD, Tobin RB, DeVore V. Effects of age, strain, and dietary carbohydrate on the hepatic metabolism of male rats. J Nutr 1979;109:261-271.
703. Mathews CE, McGraw RA, Dean R, Berdanier CD. Inheritance of a mitochondrial DNA defect and impaired glucose tolerance in BHE/Cdb rats. Diabetologia 1999;42:35-40.
704. McCusker RH, Deaver OE Jr, Berdanier CD. Effect of sucrose or starch feeding on the hepatic mitochondrial activity of BHE and Wistar rats. J Nutr 1983;113:1327-1334.
705. Borenshtein D, Ofri R, Werman M, et al. Cataract development in diabetic sand rats treated with alpha-lipoic acid and its gamma-linolenic acid conjugate. Diabetes Metab Res Rev 2001;17:44-50.
706. Ikeda Y, Olsen GS, Ziv E, et al. Cellular mechanism of nutritionally induced insulin resistance in *Psammomys obesus:* overexpression of protein kinase Cepsilon in skeletal muscle precedes the onset of hyperinsulinemia and hyperglycemia. Diabetes 2001;50:584-592.
707. Kanety H, Moshe S, Shafrir E, et al. Hyperinsulinemia induces a reversible impairment in insulin receptor function leading to diabetes in the sand rat model of non–insulin-dependent diabetes mellitus. Proc Natl Acad Sci U S A 1994;91:1853-1857.
708. Kawano K, Hirashima T, Mori S, et al. Spontaneous long-term hyperglycemic rat with diabetic complications: Otsuka Long-Evans Tokushima Fatty (OLETF) strain. Diabetes 1992;41:1422-1428.
709. Moralejo DH, Ogino T, Zhu M, et al. A major quantitative trait locus co-localizing with cholecystokinin type A receptor gene influences poor pancreatic proliferation in a spontaneously diabetogenic rat. Mamm Genome 1998;9:794-798.
710. Takiguchi S, Takata Y, Takahashi N, et al. A disrupted cholecystokinin A receptor gene induces diabetes in obese rats synergistically with *ODB1* gene. Am J Physiol 1998;274:E265-E270.
711. Takiguchi S, Takata Y, Funakoshi A, et al. Disrupted cholecystokinin type-A receptor (CCKAR) gene in OLETF rats. Gene 1997;197:169-175.
712. Hirashima T, Kawano K, Mori S, Natori T. A diabetogenic gene, ODB2, identified on chromosome 14 of the OLETF rat and its synergistic action with ODB1. Biochem Biophys Res Commun 1996;224:420-425.
713. Shi K, Mizuno A, Sano T, et al. Sexual difference in the incidence of diabetes mellitus in Otsuka-Long-Evans-Tokushima-Fatty rats: effects of castration and sex hormone replacement on its incidence. Metabolism 1994;43:1214-1220.
714. Ishida K, Mizuno A, Murakami T, Shima K. Obesity is necessary but not sufficient for the development of diabetes mellitus. Metabolism 1996;45:1288-1295.
715. Okauchi N, Mizuno A, Zhu M, et al. Effects of obesity and inheritance on the development of non–insulin-dependent diabetes mellitus in Otsuka-Long-Evans-Tokushima fatty rats. Diabetes Res Clin Pract 1995;29:1-10.
716. Kosegawa I, Chen S, Awata T, et al. Troglitazone and metformin, but not glibenclamide, decrease blood pressure in Otsuka Long Evans Tokushima fatty rats. Clin Exp Hypertens 1999;21:199-211.
717. Triadou N, Portha B, Picon L, Rosselin G. Experimental chemical diabetes and pregnancy in the rat: evolution of glucose tolerance and insulin response. Diabetes 1982;31:75-79.
718. Portha B, Picon L, Rosselin G. Chemical diabetes in the adult rat as the spontaneous evolution of neonatal diabetes. Diabetologia 1979;17:371-377.
719. Kodama T, Iwase M, Nunoi K, et al. A new diabetes model induced by neonatal alloxan treatment in rats. Diabetes Res Clin Pract 1993;20:183-189.
720. Iwase M, Nunoi K, Wakisaka M, et al. Spontaneous recovery from non–insulin-dependent diabetes mellitus induced by neonatal streptozotocin treatment in spontaneously hypertensive rats. Metabolism 1991;40:10-14.

721. Bjork S. The cost of diabetes and diabetes care. Diabetes Res Clin Pract 2001;54(suppl 1):S13-S18.
722. Boyle JP, Honeycutt AA, Narayan KM, et al. Projection of diabetes burden through 2050: impact of changing demography and disease prevalence in the U.S. Diabetes Care 2001;24:1936-1940.
723. Centers for Disease Control and Prevention. National diabetes fact sheet: general information and national estimates on diabetes in the United States, 2005. Atlanta, U.S. Department of Health and Human Services, Centers for Disease Control and Prevention, 2005.
724. American Diabetes Association. Consensus development conference on the diagnosis of coronary heart disease in people with diabetes: 10-11 February 1998, Miami, Florida. Diabetes Care 1998;21:1551-1559.
725. Bojestig M, Arnqvist HJ, Hermansson G, et al. Declining incidence of nephropathy in insulin-dependent diabetes mellitus. N Engl J Med 1994;330:15-18.
726. Gu K, Cowie CC, Harris MI. Mortality in adults with and without diabetes in a national cohort of the U.S. population, 1971-1993. Diabetes Care 1998;21:1138-1145.
727. Gu K, Cowie CC, Harris MI. Diabetes and decline in heart disease mortality in US adults. JAMA 1999;281:1291-1297.
728. Rubin RJ, Altman WM, Mendelson DN. Health care expenditures for people with diabetes mellitus, 1992. J Clin Endocrinol Metab 1994;78:809A–809F.
729. Wagner EH, Sandhu N, Newton KM, et al. Effect of improved glycemic control on health care costs and utilization. JAMA 2001;285:182-189.
730. American Diabetes Association. Screening for diabetes. Diabetes Care 2002;25(suppl 1):S21-S24.
731. Engelgau MM, Narayan KM, Herman WH. Screening for type 2 diabetes. Diabetes Care 2000;23:1563-1580.
732. Rolka DB, Narayan KM, Thompson TJ, et al. Performance of recommended screening tests for undiagnosed diabetes and dysglycemia. Diabetes Care 2001;24:1899-1903.
733. Stern M, Williams K, Haffner S. Identification of individuals at high risk of type 2 diabetes: do we need the oral glucose tolerance test? Ann Intern Med 2002;136:575-581.
734. Expert Committee on the Diagnosis and Classification of Diabetes Mellitus. Report on the diagnosis and classification of diabetes mellitus. American Diabetes Association. Diabetes Care 2002; 25(suppl 1):S5-S20.
735. Bjornholt JV, Erikssen G, Aaser E, et al. Fasting blood glucose: an underestimated risk factor for cardiovascular death. Results from a 22-year follow-up of healthy nondiabetic men. Diabetes Care 1999;22:45-49.
736. Khaw KT, Wareham N, Luben R, et al. Glycated haemoglobin, diabetes, and mortality in men in Norfolk cohort of European prospective investigation of cancer and nutrition (EPIC-Norfolk). BMJ 2001;322:15-18.
737. Saydah SH, Miret M, Sung J, et al. Postchallenge hyperglycemia and mortality in a national sample of U.S. adults. Diabetes Care 2001;24:1397-1402.
738. Glucose tolerance and cardiovascular mortality: comparison of fasting and 2-hour diagnostic criteria. Arch Intern Med 2001; 161:397-405.
739. UK Prospective Diabetes Study (UKPDS) Group. Intensive blood-glucose control with sulphonylureas or insulin compared with conventional treatment and risk of complications in patients with type 2 diabetes (UKPDS 33). Lancet 1998;352:837-853.
740. UK Prospective Diabetes Study (UKPDS) Group. Effect of intensive blood-glucose control with metformin on complications in overweight patients with type 2 diabetes (UKPDS 34). Lancet 1998; 352:854-865.
741. Ohkubo Y, Kishikawa H, Araki E, et al. Intensive insulin therapy prevents the progression of diabetic microvascular complications in Japanese patients with non–insulin-dependent diabetes mellitus: a randomized prospective 6-year study. Diabetes Res Clin Pract 1995;28:103-117.
742. Smith NL, Barzilay JI, Shaffer D, et al. Fasting and 2-hour postchallenge serum glucose measures and risk of incident cardiovascular events in the elderly: the Cardiovascular Health Study. Arch Intern Med 2002;162:209-216.
743. Stratton IM, Adler AI, Neil HA, et al. Association of glycaemia with macrovascular and microvascular complications of type 2 diabetes (UKPDS 35): prospective observational study. BMJ 2000; 321:405-412.
744. American Diabetes Association. Standards of medical care in diabetes—2006. Diabetes Care 2006;29(suppl 1):S4-S42.
745. Nathan DM, Buse JB, Davidson MB, et al. Management of hyperglycemia in type 2 diabetes mellitus: a consensus algorithm for the initiation and adjustment of therapy. Diabetes Care 2006;29: 1963-1972.
746. American College of Endocrinologists. American College of Endocrinologists consensus statement on guidelines for glycemic control. Endocr Pract 2002;8(suppl 1):5-11.
747. Buse JB, Rosenstock J. Prevention of cardiovascular outcomes in type 2 diabetes mellitus: trials on the horizon. Endocrinol Metab Clin North Am 2005;34(1):221-235.
748. Rohlfing CL, Wiedmeyer HM, Little RR, et al. Defining the relationship between plasma glucose and HbA_{1c}: analysis of glucose profiles and HbA_{1c} in the Diabetes Control and Complications Trial. Diabetes Care 2002;25:275-278.
749. Service FJ, Hall LD, Westland RE, et al. Effects of size, time of day and sequence of meal ingestion on carbohydrate tolerance in normal subjects. Diabetologia 1983;25(4):316-321.
750. American Diabetes Association. Postprandial blood glucose. Diabetes Care 2001;24:775-778.
751. Mensing C, Boucher J, Cypress M, et al. National Standards for Diabetes Self-Management Education. Diabetes Care 2006;29: S78-S85.
752. Klonoff DC, Schwartz DM. An economic analysis of interventions for diabetes. Diabetes Care 2000;23:390-404.
753. Norris SL, Engelgau MM, Narayan KM. Effectiveness of self-management training in type 2 diabetes: a systematic review of randomized controlled trials. Diabetes Care 2001;24:561-587.
754. Norris SL, Nichols PJ, Caspersen CJ, et al. Increasing diabetes self-management education in community settings. A systematic review. Am J Prev Med 2002;22(4 Suppl):39-66.
755. Delamater AM, Jacobson AM, Anderson B, et al. Psychosocial therapies in diabetes: report of the Psychosocial Therapies Working Group. Diabetes Care 2001;24:1286-1292.
756. Evidence-based nutrition principles and recommendations for the treatment and prevention of diabetes and related complications. Diabetes Care 2002;25:202-212.
757. Gillespie SJ, Kulkarni KD, Daly AE. Using carbohydrate counting in diabetes clinical practice. J Am Diet Assoc 1998;98:897-905.
758. Egede LE, Ye K, Zhang D, Silverstein MD. The prevalence and pattern of complementary and alternative medicine use in individuals with diabetes. Diabetes Care 2002;25:324-329.
759. Ernst E. Complementary medicine: its hidden risks. Diabetes Care 2001;24:1486-1488.
760. Barringer TA, Kirk JK, Santaniello AC, et al. Effect of a multivitamin and mineral supplement on infection and quality of life. A randomized, double-blind, placebo-controlled trial. Ann Intern Med. 2003;138(5):365-371.
761. Connor WE, Connor SL. Should a low-fat, high-carbohydrate diet be recommended for everyone? The case for a low-fat, high-carbohydrate diet. N Engl J Med 1997;337:562-563; discussion, 566-567.
762. Kanaley J, Weinstock R. Nonpharmacologic therapy in the treatment of insulin resistance. Curr Opin Endocrinol Diabetes 2001;8:219-225.
763. Buchanan TA, Xiang AH, Peters RK, et al. Preservation of pancreatic β-cell function and prevention of type 2 diabetes by pharmacological treatment of insulin resistance in high-risk Hispanic women. Diabetes 2002;51:2796-2803.
764. Chiasson JL, Josse RG, Gomis R, et al; STOP-NIDDM Trial Research Group. Acarbose for the prevention of type 2 diabetes, hypertension and cardiovascular disease in subjects with impaired glucose tolerance: facts and interpretations concerning the critical analysis of the STOP-NIDDM Trial data. Diabetologia 2004;47:969-977.
765. Pan XR, Li GW, Hu YH, et al. Effects of diet and exercise in preventing NIDDM in people with impaired glucose tolerance. The Da Qing IGT and Diabetes Study. Diabetes Care 1997;20:537-544.
766. American Diabetes Association. Diabetes mellitus and exercise. Diabetes Care 2002;25(suppl 1):S64-S68.
767. Boule NG, Haddad E, Kenny GP, et al. Effects of exercise on glycemic control and body mass in type 2 diabetes mellitus: a meta-analysis of controlled clinical trials. JAMA 2001;286:1218-1227.

768. Inzucchi SE. Noninvasive assessment of the diabetic patient for coronary artery disease. Diabetes Care 2001;24:1519-1521.
769. Faas A, Schellevis FG, Van Eijk JT. The efficacy of self-monitoring of blood glucose in NIDDM subjects: a criteria-based literature review. Diabetes Care 1997;20:1482-1486.
770. Buse JB. Overview of current therapeutic options in type 2 diabetes: rationale for combining oral agents with insulin therapy. Diabetes Care 1999;22(suppl 3):C65-C70.
771. DeFronzo RA. Pharmacologic therapy for type 2 diabetes mellitus. Ann Intern Med 2000;133:73-74.
772. Inzucchi SE. Oral antihyperglycemic therapy for type 2 diabetes: scientific review. JAMA 2002;287:360-372.
773. Lebovitz HE. Oral therapies for diabetic hyperglycemia. Endocrinol Metab Clin North Am 2001;30:909-933.
774. Long YC, Zierath JR. AMP-activated protein kinase signaling in metabolic regulation. J Clin Invest 2006;116(7):1776-1783.
775. Chan NN, Brain HP, Feher MD. Metformin-associated lactic acidosis: a rare or very rare clinical entity? Diabet Med 1999;16: 273-281.
776. Levey AS, Bosch JP, Lewis JB, et al. A more accurate method to estimate glomerular filtration rate from serum creatinine: a new prediction equation. Modification of Diet in Renal Disease Study Group. Ann Intern Med 1999;130(6):461-70.
777. Parulkar AA, Pendergrass ML, Granda-Ayala R, et al. Nonhypoglycemic effects of thiazolidinediones. Ann Intern Med 2001;134: 61-71.
778. Goldberg RB, Kendall DM, Deeg MA, et al; GLAI Study Investigators. A comparison of lipid and glycemic effects of pioglitazone and rosiglitazone in patients with type 2 diabetes and dyslipidemia. Diabetes Care 2005;28:1547-54.
779. Dormandy JA, Charbonnel B, Eckland DJ, et al. Secondary prevention of macrovascular events in patients with type 2 diabetes in the PROACTIVE Study (PROspective pioglitAzone Clinical Trial In macroVascular Events): a randomised controlled trial. Lancet 2005;366(9493):1279-1289.
780. Viberti G, Kahn SE, Greene DA, et al. A diabetes outcome progression trial (ADOPT): an international multicenter study of the comparative efficacy of rosiglitazone, glyburide, and metformin in recently diagnosed type 2 diabetes. Diabetes Care 2002;25(10): 1737-1743.
781. Gerstein HC, Yusuf S, Holman R, et al. Rationale, design and recruitment characteristics of a large, simple international trial of diabetes prevention: the DREAM trial. Diabetologia 2004;47(9): 1519-1527.
782. Guan Y, Hao C, Cha DR, et al. Thiazolidinediones expand body fluid volume through PPARγ stimulation of ENaC-mediated renal salt absorption. Nat Med 2005;11(8):861-866.
783. Riddle MC. Editorial: sulfonylureas differ in effects on ischemic preconditioning—is it time to retire glyburide? J Clin Endocrinol Metab 2003;88(2):528-530.
784. Klepzig H, Kober G, Matter C, et al. Sulfonylureas and ischaemic preconditioning; a double-blind, placebo-controlled evaluation of glimepiride and glibenclamide. Eur Heart J 1999;20:439-446.
785. Hirsch IB, Bergenstal RM, Parkin CG, et al. A real-world approach to insulin therapy in primary care practice. Clinical Diabetes 2005;23:78-86.
786. Bergenstal RM. Treatment models from the International Diabetes Center: advancing from oral agents to insulin therapy in type 2 diabetes. Endocr Pract 2006;12(suppl 1):98-104.
787. Heise T, Nosek L, Ronn BB, et al. Lower within-subject variability of insulin detemir in comparison to NPH insulin and insulin glargine in people with type 1 diabetes. Diabetes, 2004;53(6): 1614-1620.
788. Freemantle N, Strack T. Will availability of inhaled human insulin (Exubera) improve management of type 2 diabetes? The design of the Real World trial. Trials 2006;7(1):25.
789. Dungan K, Buse JB. Glucagon-like peptide 1–based therapies for type 2 diabetes: a focus on exenatide. Clinical Diabetes 2005; 23:56-62.
790. Dungan K, Buse J. Amylin and GLP-1-based therapies for the treatment of diabetes. 2006. UpToDate. Subscription required. Available at http://www.uptodateonline.com (accessed May 23, 2007).
791. Young A. Clinical studies. Adv Pharmacol 2005;52:289-320.
792. Buse JB, Hroscikoski M. The case for a role for postprandial glucose monitoring in diabetes management. J Fam Pract 1998;47(5 suppl):S29-S36.
793. Narayan KM, Gregg EW, Engelgau MM, et al. Translation research for chronic disease: the case of diabetes. Diabetes Care 2000;23:1794-1798.
794. Halford JC. Obesity drugs in clinical development. Curr Opin Investig Drugs 2006;7(4):312-318.
795. Moller DE. New drug targets for type 2 diabetes and the metabolic syndrome. Nature 2001;414:821-827.
796. Lebovitz H. Diabetes: assessing the pipeline. Atheroscler Suppl 2006;7(1):43-49.
797. Garg S, Zisser H, Schwartz S, et al. Improvement in glycemic excursions with a transcutaneous, real-time continuous glucose sensor: a randomized controlled trial. Diabetes Care 2006;29(1):44-50.

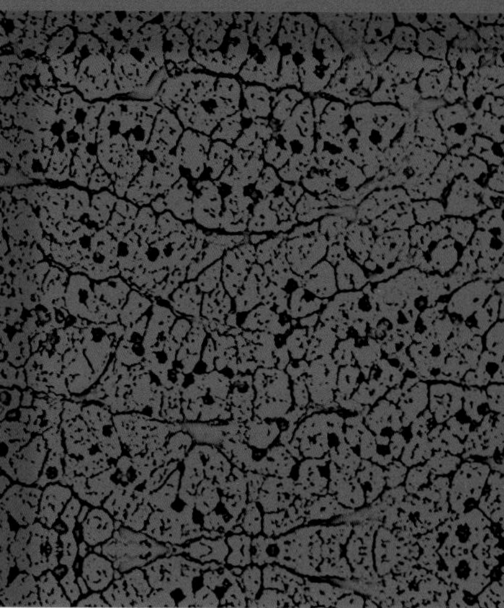

CHAPTER 31

TYPE 1 DIABETES MELLITUS

George S. Eisenbarth, Kenneth S. Polonsky, and John B. Buse

In 1984, Sutherland and coworkers[1] transplanted the tail of the pancreas from nondiabetic identical twins to their twin mates who had type 1 diabetes mellitus (T1DM). In contrast to the transplantation of organs such as kidneys, in which the transplants are accepted between identical twins, pancreatic islets but not acinar pancreas were rapidly destroyed.[1] The diabetes of the twin transplant recipients was cured for only a matter of weeks. In retrospect, the results of these transplants were predictable, given the autoimmune nature of type 1A diabetes and similar results in animal models of the disorder.[2] Following this clinical study, T1DM became one of the most intensively studied autoimmune disorders, and the National Institutes of Health has designated type 1A diabetes a Priority One target for the development of a preventive immunologic vaccine. Knowledge of the immunogenetics and immunopathogenesis of type 1A diabetes is beginning to influence clinical care,[3] greatly influences current clinical research, and will, we hope, lead to disease prevention.[4]

Differential Diagnosis of Type 1 Diabetes

An expert committee of the American Diabetes Association, with its etiologic diagnostic criteria (Table 31–1), has recommended dividing T1DM into type 1A (immune-mediated) and type 1B (other forms of diabetes with severe insulin deficiency).[5] At the onset of diabetes, distinguishing type 1A diabetes from type 2 diabetes, let alone type 1B diabetes, is not always a simple task. The best current criterion for diagnosis of type 1A diabetes is the presence of anti-islet autoantibodies measured with highly specific (and reasonably sensitive) autoantibody radioassays.[6]

The presence of autoantibodies with assays defined as positive in less than 1 of 100 control subjects (specificity ≥99%) is reasonably diagnostic of type 1A diabetes. Non-Hispanic white children presenting with diabetes usually have type 1A diabetes, whereas adults older than 40 years usually have type 2 diabetes.[7]

TABLE 31–1 DIFFERENTIAL DIAGNOSIS OF TYPE 1A DIABETES

Diabetes Type	Islet Autoantibodies	Genetics	Comments
Type 1A	Positive >90%	30%-50% DR3 *and* DR4 90% DR3 *or* DR4 <3% DQB1*0602	90% non-Hispanic white children 50% black children 50% Latin American children
Type 1B	Negative	Unknown	Rare in whites
Type 2	Negative	Unknown	If Ab^+, likely LADA, and HLA is similar to type 1A
Other	Negative	MODY mutations, other syndromes	

Ab, antibody; HbA_{1c}, hemoglobin A_{1c}; HLA, human leukocyte antigen; LADA, latent autoimmune diabetes adult; MODY, maturity-onset diabetes of the young.

More than 90% of such children presenting with diabetes express one of three commonly measured autoantibodies (see later). In contrast, among black or Latin American children, almost one half lack any autoantibody.[8-10] Most of these children appear to have an early age of onset of type 2 diabetes mellitus, and many have attendant risk factors such as obesity and lack human leukocyte antigen (HLA) alleles associated with type 1A diabetes (see later).

Imagawa and coworkers[11] described an unusual form of diabetes. The patients had normal hemoglobin A_{1c} (HbA_{1c}) despite severe hyperglycemia, suggesting that the diabetes had been present for only a short time. Histologic examination of pancreatic sections demonstrated pancreatitis but no insulitis, and anti-islet autoantibodies were not detected. It is not clear whether this represents one of the first examples of type 1B diabetes, although a fulminant type 1A is possible and studies indicate a large fraction of these patients have HLA alleles associated with type 1A diabetes.

Obesity does not protect a person from developing type 1A diabetes, although it is usually associated with insulin-resistant forms of diabetes. It is also important to realize that patients can have both insulin resistance and type 1A diabetes, and such autoantibody-positive patients with both can present with diabetes with high levels of fasting insulin or C peptide but loss of stimulated insulin secretion. With current assays for anti-islet autoantibodies, a subset of children with type 1A diabetes is negative for the autoantibodies. Some children (relatively uncommon), as they progress to diabetes, lose expression of all autoantibodies by the time of diagnosis.[12] Such type 1A autoantibody-negative children typically have HLA alleles associated with type 1A diabetes, are not insulin resistant, might present with ketoacidosis, and, with time, lose C peptide secretion. The diagnosis is not, however, clear at diabetes onset, and perhaps designations such as anti-islet autoantibody positive and negative are more accurate with current laboratory tests.

Animal Models of Type 1A Diabetes

In relation to other autoimmune disorders, type 1A diabetes is unusual in having a series of spontaneous animal models of the disease.[13-16] These animal models provide clues to potential mechanisms of pathogenesis and allow testing of therapies for disease prevention. As for most animal models, only some therapeutic results translate into efficacy in humans.[14] It should also be recognized that many of the spontaneous animal models are inbred and thus not diallelic at any locus, whereas all humans have different alleles at tens of thousands of loci. Thus, each animal model might or might not provide insights into one of the forms of human diabetes.

Despite the preceding caveats, the animal models are remarkably similar to humans in a number of key immunologic parameters. The most notable include the importance of the major histocompatibility complex (MHC) for disease and the presence of lymphocytic islet invasion followed by specific destruction of islet beta cells. For reasons that are currently unclear, given specific HLA molecules, humans, rats, and mice have a marked propensity for autoimmunity directed at islet beta cells. This propensity may be related to a specific lack of tolerance to a single islet molecule such as insulin, to specific sensitivity of islet beta cells to immune-mediated destruction, or to factors not currently appreciated. It is likely that understanding this propensity will lead to effective therapies.

Polygenic Spontaneous Animal Models: Nonobese Diabetic Mouse

The nonobese diabetic (NOD) mouse is the most intensively studied animal model.[17] As with type 1A diabetes of humans, specific HLA class II and class I (see later) molecules are central for disease pathogenesis.[18,19] The NOD mouse has mutations that cause absence of the I-E (histocompatibility) molecule (similar to human DR) and an unusual I-A (similar to human DQ).[20] The I-A molecule in the NOD mouse is termed $I\text{-}A^{g7}$, which designates a specific amino acid sequence. HLA class II molecules (in humans there are three, DP, DQ, and DR) function to bind peptides and present these peptides to the T-cell receptor of CD4 (helper) T lymphocytes. The genes were termed *immune response genes* because common variations in their sequences (allelic variation) determine the peptides to which an individual mouse or person can mount a T-cell response. Thus, a central role for these molecules in immune function and autoimmunity is expected. If the lack of I-E expression is corrected in the NOD mouse with introduction of an I-E transgene, diabetes is prevented.[21] If a different I-A sequence is introduced as a transgene into the NOD mouse, diabetes is also prevented.[22] In addition to these class II molecules determining diabetes susceptibility, more than 15 other genetic loci contribute to disease, each with a relatively small contribution, each neither necessary nor sufficient.[23-26] Thus, inheritance of diabetes in the NOD mouse is polygenic. One way the NOD mouse differs from humans is that more female than male NOD mice develop diabetes.

NOD mice, like humans, produce anti-insulin autoantibodies before developing diabetes.[27] Autoantibodies usually appear at between 6 and 8 weeks of age, and diabetes usually develops after 16 weeks of age. Studies of islet beta cell mass indicate islet beta cell destruction and beta cell regeneration months before the onset of diabetes,[28] although there is convincing evidence of an acceleration of beta cell destruction at disease onset.[29-31] T cells and not autoantibodies mediate islet beta cell destruction, and clones of T cells reacting with several antigens are able to transfer disease.[32-35] A large number of T cell clones reacting with insulin[36] and reacting with unknown antigens have been characterized. There is debate about whether any given autoantigen is primary, although recent studies have provided evidence for a central role of T-cell autoimmunity directed at insulin. In addition, lymphocytes and autoantibodies contribute to pathogenesis.

Diabetes can be prevented in the NOD mouse with more than 100 different therapies.[14] Most, but not all, of these therapies target the immune system, and a number of these therapies are now in clinical trials in humans. Consistent with diabetes being mediated by T lymphocytes, immunosuppression or genes that block T-cell function prevent disease. Administration of high doses of nicotinamide delays the development of diabetes in NOD mice.

Some of the most interesting therapies use autoantigens as vaccines; in particular both glutamic acid decarboxylase (GAD) and insulin, when administered to the mice, prevented diabetes.[37-40] The insulin molecule does not have to be metabolically active, and a dominant insulin peptide, insulin peptide B:9-23, given as a single subcutaneous injection, prevented diabetes in 90% of susceptible NOD mice.[32] It is thought that vaccination prevents diabetes by generating T lymphocytes (e.g., TH2 type, transforming growth factor β [TGFβ] producing) that target an islet molecule (e.g., insulin) but that produce protective cytokines (e.g., interleukin [IL]-4, IL-10, TGFβ) when they home to the islets.

Oligogenic Animal Models

BioBreeding Rat

The BB (BioBreeding) rat was the first intensively studied animal model of type 1A diabetes. The diabetes in this model differs from human diabetes in that diabetes-prone BB rats have an autosomal recessive mutation that produces a severe T-cell lymphopenia.[41] One can induce diabetes in a related strain of rat, termed *BB diabetes resistant* (BB-DR), by administering a monoclonal antibody that depletes T lymphocytes. As in humans and the NOD mouse, the disease depends upon specific class II alleles (similar to human HLA-DR and HLA-DQ) of the histocompatibility complex, in particular RT1-U. Diabetes can be induced to develop in a series of rat strains with RT1-U (see later). Additional genes segregate to create diabetes susceptibility, but the number of genes is much less than for NOD mice.[41-43]

Prevention of diabetes in BB rats is more difficult than in NOD mice, which may be related to the severe T-cell lymphopenia, which results from a mutation of an *Ian* gene inherited in an autosomal recessive manner.[44] For example, insulin administration to BB rats prevented both diabetes and insulitis, but, in contrast to NOD mice, metabolically active insulin and insulin doses that induce hypoglycemia were usually required for prevention.[45,46]

Long-Evans Tokushima Lean Rat

Like BB rats, the Long-Evans Tokushima Lean (LETL) rat strain has the RT-1U alleles and has an oligogenic inheritance of diabetes with mutation of a gene (*Cbl-b*) that alters T-cell signaling.[47-49]

Induced Models of Type 1A Diabetes

Diabetes or insulitis can be induced in several strains of animals with drugs that induce islet destruction and broadly activate immune responses or with specific islet antigens. The drug streptozotocin is directly toxic to islet beta cells. In high doses, it rapidly induces diabetes. In low doses, a more chronic diabetes develops that is likely to have some immunologic derivation.[50,51] Surprisingly, administration of copolymer of polyinosinic and polycytidylic acids (poly-IC), a simple polynucleotide that activates interferon (IFN)-α production when administered to a number of rat strains with the diabetes-susceptible RT1-U alleles, induced insulitis and diabetes.[52] This suggests that many animals are susceptible to diabetes or insulitis given a strong immunologic stimulus. A ubiquitous heat shock protein has been administered to produce a transient form of diabetes in mice.[53] Peptides of this heat shock protein are in clinical trials as a diabetes vaccine.[54]

Histopathology of Type 1A Diabetes

As in animal models, type 1A diabetes of humans is characterized by selective destruction of the beta cells within islets.[55-58] The non–insulin-producing cells of the islets remain in patients with long-standing T1DM, and these remaining islets lacking insulitis and beta cells are termed *pseudoatrophic*. A remarkable feature of the pancreas of patients with new-onset diabetes is heterogeneity of islet lesions. Within the same section of pancreas, a normal islet with no infiltrate can coexist with an islet containing beta cells with intense infiltration and a pseudoatrophic islet that has no infiltrate. This spottiness of the pathologic process is reminiscent of the destruction of areas of the skin in patients with vitiligo, in which melanocytes are destroyed in patches. Such heterogeneity of lesions might underlie the chronic development of type 1A diabetes in humans.

Islets of patients with type 1A diabetes overexpress class I HLA antigens, relatively rarely express class II HLA molecules on beta cells, express IFN-α, and up-regulate Fas molecules on all islet cells.[56,59-61] The hypothesis that class II HLA expression contributes directly to beta cell autoimmunity is controversial. There is evidence that such expression in animal models does not activate autoimmunity, and some researchers think insulin-positive and class II–positive islet cells might be macrophages that have ingested dead beta cells. Antigen presentation requires costimulatory molecules in addition to class II molecules, and beta cells do not express these costimulatory molecules.[62] The specific way the immune system destroys beta cells is not known, and molecules such as Fas may be important because T cells expressing Fas ligand might induce apoptosis of beta cells.[63-65] Cytokines and CD8 cytotoxic lymphocytes are also likely to contribute to beta cell destruction.[66-71]

Searches for viral particles and viral RNA within islets of patients with new-onset diabetes have been unrewarding, but newer technologies and concepts should facilitate additional studies, and it is likely that there is heterogeneity among patients.[72,73] In contrast to the islets of patients with new-onset diabetes, the pancreata of identical twin donors have been described as normal and the pancreata from patients (the few studied) with long-standing diabetes are composed of pseudoatrophic islets without markers of immune activation. A subset of patients with diabetes of several years' duration still has beta cells and insulitis, however.[55]

Genetics of Type 1A Diabetes

It has long been recognized that diabetes is a heterogeneous group of disorders. It is also becoming apparent that type 1A diabetes is heterogeneous. There are probably many genetic forms of type 1A diabetes, and most forms are influenced by HLA class II molecules.[74] This group of disorders is likely to be linked by the presence of immunologic abnormalities that foster loss of tolerance to self antigens. Patients with specific HLA class I and class II molecules with immune dysfunction are susceptible to target islet autoantigens.

Many of the genes underlying diabetes susceptibility are similar in diverse countries, although specific alleles of those genes differ in their frequency.[75] Several monogenic forms of type 1A diabetes can now be identified. It is not clear whether these genetically characterized forms of diabetes should now be included in the group of other defined causes of diabetes.[5] For the great majority of patients with type 1A diabetes, most of the genes causing diabetes susceptibility remain to be identified.

Monogenic Forms of Type 1A Diabetes

Autoimmune Polyendocrine Syndrome Type I (AIRE Gene)

The autoimmune polyendocrine syndrome type I (APS-I) is rare, with an increased incidence in Finland and Sardinia and among Iranian Jews, but it has a worldwide occurrence. The disorders of the syndrome such as T1DM, mucocutaneous candidiasis, hypoparathyroidism, Addison's disease, and hepatitis (see Chapter 37 for a more detailed discussion) identify a unique syndrome, and patients with this group of disorders almost always have mutations of the *AIRE* (autoimmune regulator) gene on chromosome 21. This gene apparently encodes a DNA binding protein. Studies of this gene with its expression in the thymus indicate that it might play an important role in maintaining self tolerance and influences the expression of what are termed *peripheral antigens,* such as insulin, in the thymus. It is hypothesized that greater expression of insulin and other tissue-specific antigens leads to tolerance and disease suppression.[76]

There is considerable variability in the diseases expressed even for siblings with the same mutation. Some of this variability is likely to be influenced by genetic loci other than the *AIRE* gene. One example is the observation that although 18% of patients with APS-I develop T1DM, those with the common diabetes-protective HLA allele DQB*10602 appear to have some protection from diabetes but not from Addison's disease.

X-Linked Polyendocrinopathy, Immune Dysfunction, and Diarrhea (Scurfy Gene)

The syndrome of X-linked polyendocrinopathy, immune dysfunction, and diarrhea (XPID) is associated with overwhelming neonatal autoimmunity, and most children die in the first few days of life or in infancy.[77-80] In this syndrome, lymphocytes invade multiple organs. It is associated with insulitis and beta cell destruction as well as lymphocytic intestinal inflammation with flattened villi and severe malabsorption. It is inherited as an X-linked recessive disease affecting only boys, with a frequent clinical history of lack of male births.

The disease apparently results from mutations of the *FOXp3* gene, whose function as transcription factor has been elucidated.[77,81,82] This gene appears to function as a master switch for regulatory (suppressor) $CD4^{+}/CD25^{+}$ T lymphocytes. Lack of such regulatory T cells leads to overwhelming autoimmunity in humans and mice. This is an important syndrome to recognize because bone marrow transplantation with restoration of T regulatory cells (even with partial chimerism) is therapeutic.

Idiopathic Type 1A Diabetes

Descriptive Genetics

In the United States, the risk of childhood diabetes is approximately 1 in 300.[83] This is 15-fold less than the diabetes risk for a first-degree relative of a patient with T1DM (Table 31–2). It is 150-fold less than the risk for a monozygotic twin of a patient with T1DM.[84,85] Although the population risk of T1DM in Japan is 15-fold less than in the United States, the risk for an identical twin in Japan is similar to that for an identical twin in the United States.[86,87] This suggests that when genetic susceptibility is present, either in Japan or in the United States, the diabetes risk is extremely high.

Although the risk of diabetes is much greater for relatives of patients with type 1A diabetes, it is important to realize that most (>85%) persons in whom type 1A diabetes develops do not have a first-degree relative with the disease. The incidence of sporadic cases results in part because almost 40% of persons in the general population carry high-risk HLA alleles for type 1A diabetes (see "The Major Histocompatibility Complex").

The highest known incidence of type 1A diabetes is found in Finland and Sardinia. Finland now has an annual incidence approaching 50 per 100,000 children. Since the 1960s the incidence has increased almost threefold, suggesting a dramatic environmental change (either an increase of causative factors or a decrease of protective factors).

Twin Studies

Twin studies of diabetes have an impressive pedigree. The study of monozygotic twins of patients with diabetes by Pyke and coworkers[88] contributed to the recognition of distinct forms of diabetes, initially termed adult-onset and juvenile-onset, subsequently termed insulin-dependent and non–insulin-dependent, and now termed type 1 and type 2 diabetes.[5] The concordance rate for monozygotic and dizygotic twins provides important information regarding genetic factors contributing to a disease because monozygotic twins share all germ line–inherited poly-

TABLE 31–2 RISK OF TYPE 1A DIABETES

Proband with DM	% Childhood DM (incidence/yr)	Islet Autoantibody	Comment
General population, United States	0.3% (15-25/100,000)	3% single Ab 0.3% multiple Abs	Japanese incidence 1/100,000 Incidence increasing in United States and many European countries Colorado now 25/100,000
Offspring	1%	4.1%	
Sibling	3.2%, 6% lifetime	7.4%	
Dizygotic twin	6%	10%	
Mother	2%	5%	Lower risk than offspring of father with DM
Father	4.6%	6.5%	
Both parents	10%?	?	
Monozygotic twin	50%, but incidence varies w/age of index twin	50%	MZT in Japan, 40% risk of DM

Ab, antibody; DM, diabetes mellitus; MZT, monozygotic twin.

morphisms or mutations, whereas dizygotic twins are similar to siblings of patients with a disease and have only one half of genes in common. For a locus that contributes to disease in a recessive manner, only one fourth of dizygotic twins would be homozygous to a sibling with diabetes at that locus, but all monozygotic twins would be homozygous for all recessive loci of their diabetic twin mate. Although overall concordance rates of monozygotic twins for T1DM are calculated, it is likely that type 1 diabetes is heterogeneous and that groups of monozygotic twins have different genetic etiologies for their diabetes. With such genetic heterogeneity, one would expect different concordance rates for different genetic diseases.

Redondo and coworkers[89] have analyzed prospective follow-up data from a large series of initially discordant monozygotic twins from Great Britain combined with a series from the United States. Progression to diabetes was identical for both series of twins. There was no length of time of discordance beyond which a monozygotic twin mate did not have a risk of T1DM. Nevertheless, the hazard rate for development of diabetes decreased as the period of discordance increased. There was also a marked variation in the risk of diabetes relative to the age at which diabetes developed in the index twin. The overall rate of concordance for monozygotic twins was 50%. However, if T1DM developed in the index twin after age 25 years, the concordance rate by life table analysis was less than 10% (Fig. 31–1). If diabetes developed in the index twin before age 5 years, the concordance rate was 70% by 40 years of follow-up. This analysis of monozygotic twins suggests genetic heterogeneity but also confirms that a significant subset of monozygotic twins do not progress to diabetes. This suggests that environmental factors, random factors, or non–germ line-inherited variations (e.g., imprinting, T-cell receptor polymorphisms, somatic mutations) contribute to diabetes risk.

An important unanswered question (given the limited number and size of studies) is whether dizygotic twins of patients with type 1A diabetes have a diabetes risk greater than that of siblings. If the risk is identical, it suggests that environmental factors whose presence is time-dependent (e.g., uncommon infections) have little influence on the development of diabetes. Dizygotic twins differ from siblings in terms of a greater commonality of environment over time (e.g., common pregnancy). Studies of dizygotic twins suggest that their risk of diabetes might not differ from that of siblings or at most is increased by a factor of two compared with the 10-fold increase for monozygotic twins.

Genetic factors influence not only the development of diabetes but also the expression of anti-islet autoantibodies. For identical twins, the expression of anti-islet autoantibodies is tightly linked to the eventual progression to overt diabetes, and monozygotic twins have a high prevalence of expression of autoantibodies. Dizygotic twins much less often express anti-islet autoantibodies, and the prevalence is similar to that of siblings.[90]

Associated Autoimmune Disorders

Because type 1A diabetes is an immune-mediated illness that develops in a genetically susceptible person, it is not surprising that most patients with type 1A diabetes have one or more additional autoimmune diseases. The most common associated disorders are thyroid autoimmunity (Graves' disease or Hashimoto's thyroiditis) and celiac disease (Table 31–3).

The Major Histocompatibility Complex

The most important loci determining the risk of T1DM are within the MHC on chromosome 6p21 (Fig. 31–2), in particular HLA class II molecules (DR, DQ, and DP).[19,94-96] In addition, standard class I loci (HLA A, B, and C) influence disease, and it is likely

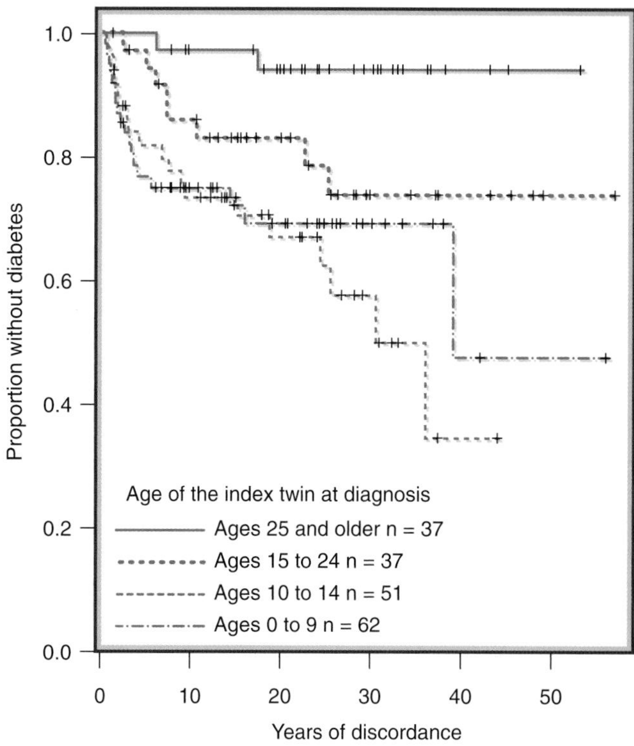

Figure 31–1 ■ Progression to diabetes of initially discordant monozygotic twins of patients with type 1 diabetes subdivided by the age of diabetes onset of the first twin to develop diabetes (proband). Late progression to diabetes is evident, with some twins becoming diabetic more than 20 years after their twin mate. For discordant twins whose twin mate developed diabetes after age 25 years, the risk of diabetes is less than 10%. (From Redondo MJ, Yu L, Hawa M, et al. Heterogeneity of type 1 diabetes: analysis of monozygotic twins in Great Britain and the United States. Diabetologia 2001;44:354-362.)

TABLE 31–3 ASSOCIATED AUTOIMMUNE DISEASES

Disease	Autoantibody		Disease Prevalence (%)
	Type	Percentage	
Addison's disease[92]	21-hydroxylase	1.5%	0.5
Celiac disease[91]	Transglutaminase	12%	6
Pernicious anemia[93]	Parietal cell	21%	2.6
Thyroiditis or Graves' disease	Peroxidase or thyroglobulin	25%	4

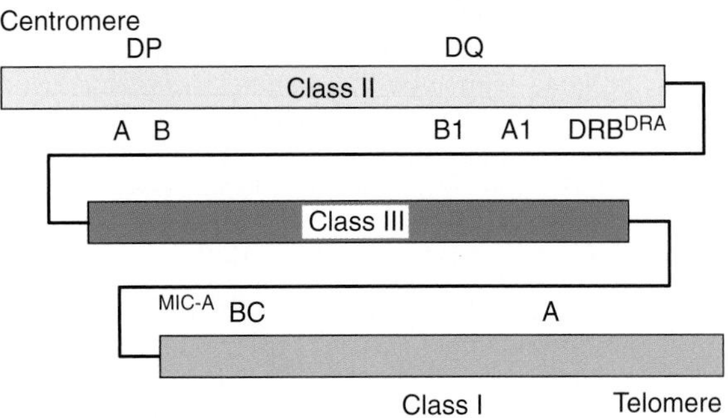

Figure 31–2 ▪ Genes within the human leukocyte antigen (HLA) region (major histocompatibility complex) with HLA class I, class II, and class III regions illustrated. Each class II molecule is made up of two chains. DRB alleles are polymorphic; DRA does not vary. DQA and DQB molecules are both polymorphic. DPA and DPB are both also polymorphic. The class III region contains important genes such as complement components as well as the tumor necrosis factor-α gene. The class I region includes MIC-A and MIC-B genes as well as the classic histocompatibility HLA genes, A, B, and C.

TABLE 31–4 DIABETES RISK OF REPRESENTATIVE DR AND DQ HAPLOTYPES

DRB1	DQA1	DQB1
	HIGH RISK	
0401 or 0403 or 0405	0301	0302 (DQ8)
0301	0501	0201 (DQ2)
	MODERATE RISK	
0801	0401	0402
0404	0301	0302
0101	0101	0501
0901	0301	0303
	MODERATE PROTECTION	
0403	0301	0302
0701	0201	0201
1101	0501	0301
	STRONG PROTECTION	
1501	0102	0602 (DQ6)
1401	0101	0503
0701	0201	0303

that additional loci within or linked to the MHC that influence immune function contribute to diabetes risk.[97] Figure 31–2 illustrates the MHC. The nomenclature for alleles of this region is somewhat daunting, but with definitions of several terms and a description of the basis for classification it is comprehensible.

The function of HLA molecules is to present peptides to T lymphocytes. Each molecule is made up of two chains, and each chain is encoded by a separate gene. These molecules are extremely polymorphic in amino acid sequence. Each polymorphic variant of each chain is designated with a gene locus name (e.g., DRB1) followed by an asterisk (*), followed by two digits referring to the serologic specificity (from the time when typing was performed with antibodies), followed by two digits for the specific allele (now determined with DNA-based typing), followed by a single digit to distinguish silent nucleotide polymorphisms (nucleotide differences that do not change amino acid sequence). For example, the designated allele DRB1*0405 has DR4 serologic specificity and is associated with high diabetes risk. For DR alleles, one usually specifies only the DRB chain because the DRA chain is not polymorphic. For the class I molecules (A, B, and C) one also specifies only a single chain because the other chain, β_2-microglobulin, is minimally polymorphic. There are more than 240 different known alleles of DRB1. Each person inherits two DRB1 alleles, one from each parent.

Because HLA gene loci are in close proximity to each other on the sixth chromosome, one usually inherits a group of alleles as a unit, and this is termed a *haplotype*. For example, the alleles A*0101, B*0801, DRB1*0301, and DQA1*0501, DQB1*0201 constitute a common haplotype associated with diabetes risk. When specific alleles of different genes are nonrandomly associated with each other on a haplotype (such as the alleles A1, B8, and DR3), the alleles are said to be in linkage dysequilibrium. Linkage dysequilibrium is not the same as linkage, although to have linkage dysequilibrium, genes must be linked. Genes are linked when they are close together on the same chromosome and thus are transmitted from parents to children as a haplotype group. Alleles of genes that are linked if the alleles are nonrandomly associated with each other in a population are in linkage dysequilibrium.

Two MHC haplotypes, one inherited from each parent, constitute the MHC genotype. This genotype ultimately determines the MHC-encoded risk of type 1A diabetes. For DQ molecules, both of the chains (DQA and DQB) are polymorphic. This adds an important level of diversity in that the protein chains encoded by the alleles of one haplotype can combine with the chains encoded by the other haplotype. For example, persons with the highest risk genotype DRB1*0301,DQA1*0501,DQB1*0201 and DRB1*0405,DQA1*0301,DQB1*0302 can produce four different DQ molecules: DQA1*0501,DQB1*0201 and DQA1*0301, DQB1*0302 as expected but also DQA1*0501,DQB1*0302 and DQA1*0301,DQB1*0201. The DQ molecule DQA1*0501, DQB1*0201 is also called DQ2 and DQA1*0301,DQB1*0302 is called DQ8. A common DQ molecule, DQA1*0102,DQB1*0602, provides dominant protection from T1DM and is termed DQ6.

The major determinants of diabetes susceptibility are DR and DQ molecules, and specific alleles of both DR and DQ can either increase or decrease the risk of diabetes. Table 31–4 summarizes the diabetes risk associated with a number of DR and DQ haplotypes.

In a number of studies, children at birth, either from the general population or relatives of patients with T1DM, have been HLA typed.[27,98,99] The typing is relatively straightforward and either is based on direct DNA sequencing of polymerase chain reaction (PCR)-amplified DNA fragments or uses DNA probes that hybridize specifically to different allelic sequences. In Denver, Colorado, 2.4% of newborns have the highest risk DR-DQ genotype for type 1A diabetes, namely DR3-DQ2 with DR4-DQ8 (DR3/4 DQ8/2 heterozygotes). Fifty percent of children younger than 10 years and approximately 30% of older children who develop diabetes have this highest risk genotype. One can estimate that approximately 1 of 16 children with the highest risk HLA genotype from the general population progress to diabetes (versus a population risk of 1 per 300). Alternatively, 15 of 16 children from the general population who are DQ8/DQ2 heterozygotes do not develop diabetes. Recent studies indicate that newborn siblings of patients with T1DM, with DQ2, and DQ8 have a risk of expressing islet autoantibodies exceeding 40% by age 6 years, and of those, 50% develop diabetes by age 10 years.

This suggests that a genetic risk, especially MHC encoded, is extremely high.

Ninety-five percent of persons who develop diabetes have either DR3-DQ2 or DR4-DQ8, as do approximately 40% of the general population. The protective haplotype DRB1*1501,DQA1 *0102,DQB1*0602 is present in 20% of the general population and in less than 3% of patients with type 1A diabetes. A DR allele, DRB1*1401, also appears to provide dominant protection.[100] There are additional high-risk haplotypes that are not common, such as DQA1*0401,DQB1*0402.[101] It was proposed as a simple rule that the presence of aspartic acid at position 57 of the DQβ chain and arginine at DQα 52 is associated with diabetes risk.[102] As illustrated before, there are many exceptions to this rule, and knowledge of the complete sequences (allele) rather than dependence on this rule is essential.

Insulin Locus

In 1984, Bell and colleagues[103] published their discovery that variations in the number of nucleotide repeat elements 5′ of the insulin gene were associated with the development of type 1A diabetes. The longest group of repeats was associated with decreased diabetes risk. These studies have been replicated, and the locus of importance is clearly limited to the insulin gene.[104] The protective insulin gene polymorphism is associated with greater insulin messenger RNA (mRNA) expression within the thymus.[105,106] Hannahan[107] advanced the hypothesis that within lymphoid organs there are "peripheral antigen expressing cells," which, for example, produce insulin, and that such expression leads to tolerance and thereby decreases the risk of diabetes.

PTPN22 *Gene*

PTPN22, a gene encoding a lymphoid-specific phosphatase that influences T-cell receptor signaling, is the third confirmed gene influencing T1DM risk.[108] This gene influences T-cell receptor signaling, and the polymorphism associated with diabetes (TRP for ARG) blocks binding to a signaling molecule CSK. Nevertheless, the relative risk associated with this polymorphism for T1DM and other autoimmune disorders, such as rheumatoid arthritis, is only 1.7.

Other Loci

There is an international effort to define additional genes that contribute to the development of type 1A diabetes. The genes associated with the two monogenic forms of polyendocrinopathy (*AIRE* gene and *FOXp3* gene), HLA genes, and the insulin gene are to date the only clearly identified genes. Much of the effort PTPN22 and CTLA-4 in searching for relevant genes has analyzed the common inheritance of genetic regions for pairs of diabetic siblings. With such an analysis, a long list of genes for T1DM, termed *iddm loci,* have been proposed, each with a specific number (e.g., iddm1 is the MHC, iddm2 the insulin gene, and iddm15 a locus on chromosome 6q).[109,110] Such studies are likely to generate at least as many false-positive loci as true loci, and the difficulty in replicating findings attests to the problems.[111]

Polymorphisms of the *CTLA4* gene (iddm12) contribute to Graves' disease and apparently to diabetes in some but not all populations with relative risks less than 1.3.[112] A locus associated with the IL-2 receptor has a statistical association with analysis of thousands of persons.[113] Conflicting reports are available for the gene *SUM04.*[114] One locus, iddm17, was identified not through analysis of sibling pairs but by intensive study of a single family with 21 members with type 1A diabetes.[115] It appears that this locus, in combination with high-risk HLA alleles within the initial family studied, creates a risk of diabetes approaching 40%.

In summary, many putative diabetes loci have been identified outside the HLA region, but at present only the insulin gene can materially influence the prediction of genetic risk in populations; the PTPN22 polymorphism is the next strongest association. To date, other genes and loci have negligible or nonpublished effects. In contrast, HLA typing is being used to define the risk of diabetes at birth. The defined risk can be extremely high, depending on the relationship to a proband with diabetes and the specific HLA genotype. For example, siblings of patients with type 1A diabetes with the DR3-DQ2/DR4-DQ8 genotype appear to have a diabetes risk that exceeds 50%.[116] In contrast, children from the general population with the same HLA DR and DQ genotype have a risk of less than 6%. There is evidence that this extreme additional risk is due to genes linked to DR and DQ alleles, and thus siblings who can share both HLA haplotypes with a proband in addition to having DQ8-DQ2 alleles have a much higher risk than offspring of patients with T1DM and the general population. In addition to influencing diabetes risk, specific HLA genotypes contribute to risk of associated autoimmune disorders. It is remarkable that one third of DR3-DQ2 homozygous patients with type 1A diabetes express transglutaminase autoantibodies and half of them have celiac disease on biopsy.[117]

Environmental Factors

Despite more than three decades of research, there is only one environmental factor clearly associated with type 1A diabetes, namely congenital rubella infection (see later).[118] The association of only one factor is probably related to the long prodromal phase that precedes type 1A diabetes, which makes the discovery of relevant environmental factors particularly difficult.

A number of factors can induce type 1A diabetes in animal models, one of the most interesting being the Kilham rat virus infection of BB-DR rats.[119] In this model, which lacks the lymphopenia of the related BB strain, diabetes does not develop unless the animals are infected with Kilham virus (a parvovirus) or injected with poly-IC.[52] Poly-IC mimics double-stranded RNA and induces high levels of IFN-α. The Kilham virus apparently does not directly infect islets and is thought to be an immune activator similar to poly-IC. Diabetes induction depends on specific class II alleles termed RT1-U, and a number of animal strains with RT1-U are susceptible to diabetes.[52] If these animal models are relevant to humans, it may be that many environmental stimuli in a genetically susceptible host activate autoimmunity.

In countries throughout the world the incidence of type 1A diabetes is increasing, particularly for children in whom the disease develops before age 5 years.[120-122] This is strong evidence that environmental factors related to diabetes risk have changed since the 1960s. Factors that increase diabetes risk may be increasing, or, just as likely, factors that suppress the development of diabetes may be decreasing. For example, in animal models of type 1A diabetes (NOD mouse and BB rat), infections with common viruses usually decrease the development of diabetes.

Infections

Congenital rubella, but not noncongenital infection, greatly increases the development of type 1A diabetes.[123] Children with diabetes usually have high-risk HLA alleles,[124] and these children commonly have thyroid autoimmunity.[125] The way this congenital infection increases diabetes development is currently unknown. Hypotheses have ranged from potential molecular mimicry[126] to long-term alteration in T-cell function secondary to the congenital insult.[127]

Enteroviruses are small RNA viruses that often infect young children. Initial anecdotal reports that coxsackievirus infections might cause diabetes evaluated children who had severe infections and who died at diabetes onset.[128,129] These studies preceded the realization that type 1A diabetes is not an acute disease, and it is likely that viral infection at the onset of T1DM is most often incidental. At the time of presentation with diabetes, almost all children have elevated HbA_{1c}, reflecting probably months of hyperglycemia preceding diagnosis. A description from Japan of persons with acute-onset diabetes and normal HbA_{1c}, elevated amylase, and infiltrates within the exocrine but not endocrine pancreas appears to represent a form of type 1B diabetes.[11]

The potential importance of enteroviral infection has been emphasized by studies from Scandinavia in which enteroviral infection was evaluated during pregnancy and in infancy. Infection is usually detected by changes in antiviral antibodies or detection of enteroviral RNA by molecular techniques.[118] Although some studies have reported increased enteroviral infection during pregnancy in mothers whose children have developed diabetes, others have not.[130,131] As infants with a genetic risk for the development of diabetes are followed from birth, it becomes possible to analyze prospectively the expression of enterovirus RNA. Enteroviral infection is associated with the appearance of anti-islet autoantibodies.[130] Similar studies from Denver, Colorado, did not find an association.[131] The major difference between the two studies appears to be the lower rate of enteroviral infection in Finnish control subjects compared with Colorado control subjects.

Other viruses are being evaluated for association with the triggering of autoimmunity. One study from Australia found an association with rotavirus infection.[132] Rotavirus infection is common in young children. The Australian study did not find an increase in rotavirus infection compared with that in control subjects, but it reported an association of rotavirus infection with increases of anti-islet autoantibodies. Studies from Denver did not indicate an increase in rotavirus infection in infants developing autoantibodies.

Vaccination

It has been claimed that the timing of routine childhood vaccinations influences the development of type 1A diabetes.[133] This is an important health concern if parents alter their family's childhood vaccination because of concern about development of diabetes. A series of studies have been carried out[134-136] and do not provide evidence that childhood vaccinations influence the development of diabetes.

Diet

A disease such as celiac disease is critically dependent on the ingestion of a specific food, namely the wheat protein gliadin.[137] In addition, a number of dietary modifications altered the development of diabetes in NOD mice and BB rats.[138] Investigators have championed the hypothesis that early introduction of bovine milk increases the development of diabetes. This hypothesis is primarily based on retrospective studies associating early or increased bovine milk ingestion (or less breastfeeding) with an increased risk of type 1A diabetes.[139] Several prospective studies in which infants are observed until the development of anti-islet autoantibodies have failed to find an association or have found a weak association with either breastfeeding or bovine milk ingestion.[140-143] Pilot studies of an infant formula lacking bovine milk proteins have been initiated in Finland. Preliminary data suggest that such a restricted diet might produce a small decrease of cytoplasmic islet cell autoantibodies but not of GAD65 autoantibodies.[144] Recently studies from Germany and Denver have provided evidence that early (<3 months) introduction of cereals might increase the development of islet autoimmunity.[145,146]

Natural History of Type 1A Diabetes

We typically divide the development of type 1A diabetes into a series of stages beginning with genetic susceptibility and ending with essentially complete beta cell destruction (Fig. 31–3). It is, however, likely that both genes and environmental factors influ-

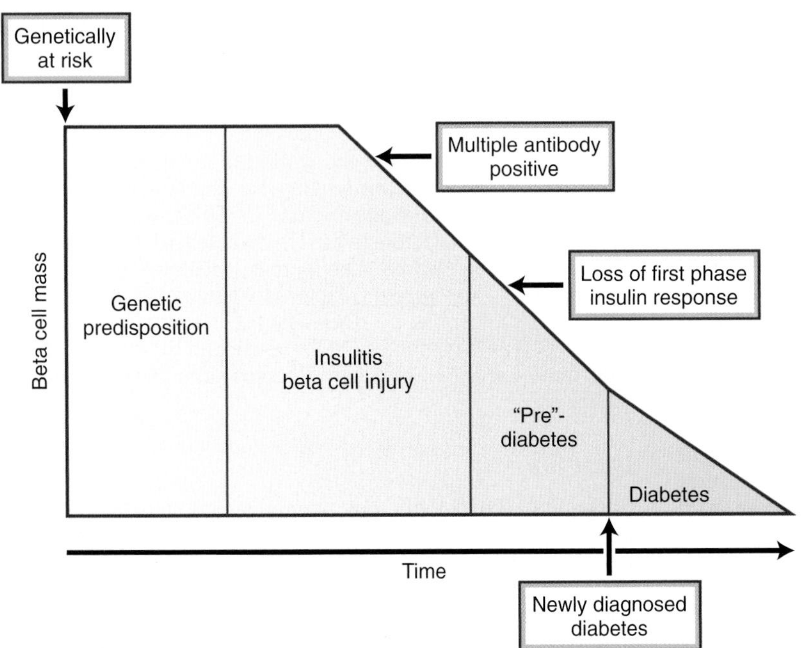

Figure 31–3 ▪ Hypothetical stages in the development of type 1A diabetes beginning with genetic susceptibility and ending with complete beta cell destruction. (Modified from Eisenbarth GS. Type 1 diabetes mellitus: a chronic autoimmune disease. N Engl J Med 1986;314:360-368; modifications by Jay Skyler, University of Miami.)

ence the course of development of type 1A diabetes during the complete prediabetic period. For instance, injection of immunostimulants such as Freund's adjuvant can prevent progression to diabetes in animals with insulitis. Mathis and coworkers[147] have proposed the existence of checkpoints in the development of diabetes, and such checkpoints might have a strong genetic component. As discussed later, type 1A diabetes is quite predictable given specific immunologic, genetic, and metabolic characteristics, and it is such characteristics that set the stage for preventive trials.

Genetic and Immunologic Heterogeneity by Age of Onset

Type 1A diabetes can develop at any age, from the neonatal period to the sixth decade of life. In that identical twins can become concordant 30 years after their twin mate, not all age heterogeneity can be ascribed to different genetic syndromes.[90] Nevertheless, there is an overall correlation between the age at which diabetes develops in one twin or sibling and the age of development of diabetes in his or her relative. Children in whom type 1A diabetes develops at an early age more often are DR3/4,DQ8/2 heterozygotes. In addition, there is evidence that class I HLA alleles (or other non–class II genes with the HLA region) can influence the age of diabetes onset (e.g., the A24 allele).[148] At the other end of the age spectrum, there is evidence that the protective HLA allele DQA*10102,DQB1*0602 is not as protective for young adults as it is for children.[149]

The most characteristic difference related to the age of diabetes onset is the presence of higher levels of insulin autoantibodies in children who develop the disease at an early age (e.g., younger than 5 years).[150,151] The high levels and frequent positivity of insulin autoantibodies make measurement of IAA (insulin autoantibodies) the best single marker for diabetes development in young children. For children in whom autoantibodies arise in the first 3 years of life, insulin autoantibodies often appear first. In contrast, GAD65 autoantibodies are more often positive in adults developing type 1A diabetes. The correlation of levels of insulin autoantibodies and age of diabetes onset may be related to children with higher levels progressing more rapidly to diabetes.[152] Such rapid progression, however, occurs only if insulin autoantibodies are present with another islet autoantibody (see "Combinatorial Autoantibody Prediction" next) (Fig. 31–4).

Combinatorial Autoantibody Prediction

The most specific anti-islet autoantibody assays are usually set with cutoffs above the 99th percentile of control populations. Thus, with three major autoantibody assays (GAD65, ICA512 [islet cell antibody], and insulin) one would predict that approximately three of 100 normal persons would express one or more of the three autoantibodies. Because approximately 3 of 1000 children develop type 1A diabetes, this suggests that in the great majority of antibody-positive persons, diabetes never develops or can develop late in life.

A relatively low positive predictive value for single antibodies may be due to methodologic limitations or the presence of autoantibodies identical to those in patients with prediabetes but found in some persons who do not progress to diabetes. It is likely that both occur. For example, a low positive (but >99th percentile) autoantibody result of a control subject is often not confirmed on repeated testing. Autoantibodies of prediabetic persons usually react with multiple epitopes of the ICA512 molecule, whereas false-positive autoantibodies often react with only one or no clearly defined epitope of the molecule, suggesting that false-positive and diabetes-associated anti-ICA512 auto-

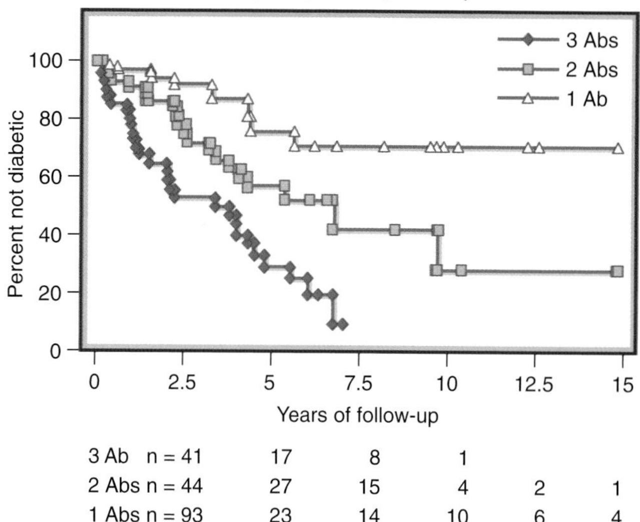

Figure 31–4 ▪ Progression to type 1 diabetes of first-degree relatives of patients with diabetes. Patients are subdivided by the number of anti-islet autoantibodies of insulin, GAD65 (glutamic acid decarboxylase), and ICA512 (IA-2) expressed. (From Verge CF, Gianani R, Kawasaki E, et al. Prediction of type 1 diabetes in first-degree relatives using a combination of insulin, GAD, and ICA512 bdc/IA-2 autoantibodies. Diabetes 1996;45:926-933.)

antibodies differ. There are, however, some persons, usually adult relatives of patients with type 1A diabetes (often with DQB1*0602), who have extremely high levels of GAD65 autoantibodies that react with multiple GAD epitopes with no evidence of progression to diabetes.[153]

Bonifacio and coworkers analyzed the affinity of insulin autoantibodies in children of the BabyDiab study from Germany. Insulin autoantibodies of high affinity measured in offspring of patients with type 1 diabetes were associated with progression to diabetes.[154]

Assessment of the significance of an autoantibody result (as for any diagnostic test) is improved by taking into account the prior probability of disease. A patient with overt diabetes and expression of a single anti-islet autoantibody has a high probability of type 1A diabetes. A person from the general population or even a relative expressing a single autoantibody (and not developing more than that one autoantibody) has a much lower risk of progressing to type 1A diabetes.[155]

Usually, in attempting to improve the specificity of a test, one sacrifices sensitivity. For prediction of type 1A diabetes, because three biochemical autoantibodies are measurable, one can combine the tests with the observation that the presence of two or more autoantibodies is associated with a very high risk of diabetes.[156,157] Approximately 1 of 350 persons from the general population express two or more of the GAD65, ICA512, or insulin autoantibodies, which approaches population estimates of type 1A diabetes. Among first-degree relatives of patients with type 1A diabetes, two or more autoantibodies indicate a risk of more than 90% over 10 years, whereas a single autoantibody is associated with a risk of less than 20% over 10 years.[156]

Metabolic Progression before Hyperglycemia

The intravenous glucose tolerance test (GTT) aids in evaluating the time to onset of diabetes among persons expressing anti-islet autoantibodies.[158] Most commonly, glucose is given at 0.5 g/kg over 5 minutes (maximum 35 g, 25 g/dL) and insulin levels are measured before and 1 and 3 minutes after the glucose infusion.[159,160] Most persons within a year of overt diabetes have no first-phase insulin secretion after intravenous glucose.

The diagnosis of type 1A diabetes usually relies upon the presence of fasting hyperglycemia, but with prospective evaluation, many persons have diabetes by the 120-minute criteria on oral glucose tolerance with nondiagnostic fasting glucose. Impaired fasting glucose or impaired glucose tolerance (glucose at 120 minutes or oral GTT) is usually abnormal within 6 months of the onset of overt diabetes.

C-Peptide Loss after Hyperglycemia

Following the diagnosis of diabetes, levels of C peptide can be used to assess remaining beta cell function. C-peptide levels are usually measured in the fasting state or after intravenous glucagon or with a standard liquid meal. Such measurements are primarily of importance for trials of therapies to alleviate loss of insulin secretion after diagnosis. Determination of C peptide provides the best current measure for assessing the impact of new therapies. As shown in the Diabetes Control and Complications Trial (DCCT), a small amount of remaining C peptide is associated with impressive metabolic benefit.[161,162]

Type 1A Diabetes with Pregnancy

Approximately 5% of women with gestational diabetes (diabetes diagnosed during pregnancy) have an early form of type 1A diabetes that is discovered during pregnancy.[163] These women express anti-islet autoantibodies and progress to overt diabetes more rapidly after pregnancy.

Latent Autoimmune Diabetes of Adults

Type 1A diabetes can occur at any age. Depending on the population, between 5% and 15% of persons with what appears to be type 2 diabetes express anti-islet autoantibodies.[164,165] Multiple studies have demonstrated that such persons progress relatively rapidly (within 3 years) to insulin-requiring diabetes. The HLA alleles of such persons reflect that of type 1A diabetes.[166]

Transient Hyperglycemia

A significant number of children are evaluated by endocrinologists for transient hyperglycemia. The usual history is of severe stress associated with hyperglycemia that resolves within days to a month. Such children may be in the honeymoon phase of type 1A diabetes or might truly have a transient episode of hyperglycemia. Rarely, diabetes in children is misdiagnosed (e.g., we have seen a child with normal HbA_{1c} values for several years who stopped insulin and was subsequently found to have renal glucosuria and not diabetes). Children without severe stress with transient hyperglycemia or with a relative with type 1A diabetes are more likely to have early type 1A diabetes. Absence of anti-islet autoantibodies and a normal intravenous glucose tolerance test strongly indicate transient hyperglycemia and not type 1A diabetes.[167] It is not known whether children with transient hyperglycemia are at increased risk for type 2 diabetes later in life.

Immunotherapy of Type 1A Diabetes

At the onset of type 1A diabetes, a major clinical research goal is the prevention of further beta cell destruction. At present there is no proven safe and effective therapy to prevent such further destruction or to prevent the development of type 1A diabetes in those at risk (e.g., genetically at-risk persons with anti-islet autoantibodies). A number of clinical trials have been completed and a large number of trials are under way or about to be initiated.

Immunosuppression

The earliest studies of therapies to prevent beta cell destruction used immunosuppressive agents. Large trials of cyclosporine indicated that while it was administered it prevented further loss of C-peptide secretion and improved metabolic function.[168-171] It did not, however, maintain a nondiabetic state when therapy was instituted after the onset of diabetes, and with discontinuation of the drug, persons rapidly lost C-peptide reserve. The combination of inability to cure diabetes and toxicities associated with cyclosporine (in particular nephrotoxicity and concern about increased risk of malignancy) has ruled out its use. Other immunosuppressive agents such as prednisone or azathioprine had relatively little effect.[172-174] A small study suggested that methotrexate, another common immunotherapeutic agent, is ineffective.[175] Thus, at present, although type 1A diabetes is an immune-mediated disorder, it is not treated with common immunotherapeutic agents.

Two studies of modified antibodies to CD3 have been reported and additional trials are likely.[176] A single course of anti-CD3 therapy decreases loss of C-peptide secretion of new-onset patients, but it appears that after 1 year progressive loss of secretion resumes.[177] Concerns related to the activation of EBV infection and the lack of information relative to the duration of C-peptide preservation cautions against nonresearch application of such therapy at present.

The TrialNet group has begun a randomized multicenter trial of anti-IL2 receptor antibody with continuous mycophenolate mofetil therapy, two medications with extensive use in humans. Subjects for similar trials in the setting of new onset T1DM may be referred by contacting TrialNet at 1-800-HALT-DM1 or www.diabetestrialnet.org.

Immunologic Vaccination

In animal models (especially the NOD mouse), it is relatively easy to prevent T1DM.[14] Potentially the most exciting modalities use forms of immunologic vaccination. Much of the excitement derives from the specificity of the therapy and the relatively low risk compared with immunosuppression and not from demonstrated efficacy in humans. The basic concept behind the bulk of such therapies is the induction of lymphocytes that target a given islet antigen and, upon encountering their target antigen (e.g., insulin), produce cytokines that suppress autoimmunity and tissue destruction.[38,178]

A general class of T lymphocytes termed TH2 T cells produce the cytokine IL-4 rather than IFN-γ and IL-2 (TH1 T cells) and decrease cell-mediated immune destruction. Induction of a protective immune response might depend upon the route of administration of the given antigen (e.g., oral tolerance) or the use of an altered antigen (e.g., altered peptide ligands). For example, insulin given either orally or by subcutaneous injection prevented diabetes in NOD mice.[179,180] Intact insulin is not necessary because insulin B chain and an immunodominant B:9-23 peptide of insulin were also effective.[40] The latter molecules have no insulin-like metabolic effect but are able to activate T lymphocytes that target insulin.

The Diabetes Prevention Trial Type 1 studied both oral insulin and parenteral injections of low doses of insulin. The results of the parenteral trial did not demonstrate a reduction in the risk of developing diabetes.[181] The oral trial did not document an overall benefit of insulin, but in the subgroup with higher levels of insulin autoantibodies at entry, a statistically significant delay in progression to diabetes was observed.[182] Because this was a subgroup analysis, replication of this potentially exciting finding is imperative. Relatives of patients with T1DM can be tested for anti-islet autoantibodies by TrialNet (1-800-HALT-DM1 or www.diabetestrialnet.org).

Other Therapies

A review by Atkinson and Leiter[14] pointed out that more than 100 different interventions prevent diabetes in NOD mice. The relative ease of diabetes prevention in this animal model provides the basis for a number of trials initiated in humans. The largest such European trial (ENDIT, European Nicotinamide Trial) uses nicotinamide in gram doses. Nicotinamide can prevent diabetes induced by the drug streptozotocin and probably acts by preserving nicotinamide adenine dinucleotide levels in islet cells or blocking cytokine-induced destruction. Nicotinamide did not delay progression to diabetes.

Immunology of Pancreatic Islet Transplantation

Pancreatic transplantation for patients requiring a kidney transplant is an accepted clinical procedure.[183] Patients with a kidney transplant receive immunosuppressive drugs, and results for pancreatic transplantation in this setting have progressively improved. With a successful pancreas transplant, hyperglycemia is immediately reversed and there is some evidence of improved long-term outcomes,[183,184] although there is considerable debate concerning pancreas transplant without the transplantation of a kidney.[185] Nevertheless, the surgery is extensive and there are multiple potential complications associated with the transplant. Diabetes can recur because of either recurrent autoimmunity or, more often, allograft rejection.[186] It is difficult to monitor specific islet destruction, and with the development of hyperglycemia it is usually not possible to restore euglycemia.

Up until studies from Edmonton, the results of islet transplantation have been poor: less than 10% of patients with type 1A diabetes achieved insulin independence at 1 year.[187] In contrast, with autotransplants of patients with pancreatitis, most patients become insulin independent and remain so. The Edmonton group has used meticulous islet isolation techniques, transplantation of islets from two pancreata, and an immunosuppressive regimen using the drug rapamycin.[187]

The Edmonton protocol has been tested in a series of specialized centers throughout North America and Europe. It is clear that multiple centers with varying success rates can successfully transplant islets, and for patients with severe hypoglycemia there is long-term prevention of severe hypoglycemic episodes. For the majority of patients who achieve insulin independence, resumption of use of low doses of insulin is necessary within 2 years.[188] Even if the Edmonton results are reproduced at multiple centers, the number of islets available from cadaveric donors for transplantation is limited. Further research to allow xenogeneic transplantation or production of islets from stem cells is essential.

Insulin Autoimmune Syndrome

The insulin autoimmune syndrome, also termed *Hirata syndrome,* is rare and typically associated with hypoglycemia.[189] These patients have extremely high concentrations of autoantibodies reacting with human insulin. It is thought that inappropriate (nonregulated) release of autoantibody-bound insulin produces the hypoglycemia. The disease occurs most commonly in Asian persons. Among 50 Japanese patients with the syndrome and the typical polyclonal anti-insulin autoantibodies, 96% had a DRB1,DR4 allele and 84% (42 of 50) had the DRB1*0406 allele.[190] In contrast, patients with monoclonal anti-insulin autoantibodies do not have such a remarkable HLA association. Most patients develop the disease in association with treatment with sulfhydryl-containing medications, in particular methimazole. Treatment usually consists of stopping these medications, and for more than 75% the disease remits.[190]

Insulin Allergy

Mild forms of immune reactivity to insulin are not uncommon. Essentially all patients treated with human insulin produce anti-insulin autoantibodies that are measurable with sensitive fluid phase radioassays. The levels of these autoantibodies are relatively low, and they do not appear to interfere with insulin therapy, although there are reports correlating insulin antibodies with macrosomia.[191] With the introduction of recombinant human insulin replacing animal insulins, symptomatic immune responses to insulin such as immediate hypersensitivity, delayed hypersensitivity, lipoatrophy, and lipohypertrophy have decreased.[192] Allergic reactions can occur with insulin analogues, although this is uncommon. More common perhaps are allergies to protamine used to complex insulin in neutral protamine Hagedorn (NPH) formulations as well as to the lubricants, preservatives, and plastics in bottles, stoppers, syringes, and needles.

The usual therapy consists of switching the type or formulation of insulin followed by oral antihistamines for immunoglobulin E–mediated local reactions, followed by insulin desensitization or addition of small amounts of glucocorticoids to the insulin injected for local delayed hypersensitivity reactions. Whether inhaled insulin will provide a safe alternative in patients with insulin allergy is completely unknown.

Anti-Insulin Receptor Autoantibodies

Anti-insulin receptor autoantibodies (type B insulin resistance) are associated with both hypoglycemia and insulin resistance.[193] It appears that anti-insulin receptor autoantibodies can act as either antagonists or agonists. This syndrome is rare and is often associated with non–organ-specific autoimmunity.[194]

Clinical Presentation

The peak age of presentation of T1DM in children is around the age of puberty. The symptoms and signs are related to the presence of hyperglycemia and the resulting effects on fluid and electrolyte balance. They generally include polyuria, polydipsia, polyphagia, weight loss, and blurred vision. Because infection might have precipitated the initial presentation, symptoms of infection might also be present, such as fever, sore throat, cough, or dysuria. In children in particular, the onset of symptoms can occur over a brief period and families may be able to date their onset with considerable accuracy. Onset of symptoms can also be insidious, particularly in older persons with T1DM, and can occur over a time frame of weeks or even months.

If onset of T1DM is associated with ketoacidosis, which is not uncommon, additional symptoms related to this acute metabolic complication of diabetes are also present. These symptoms can include abdominal pain, nausea, and vomiting. Variable effects on mental status may be seen, ranging from slight drowsiness to profound lethargy and even coma if the condition has been untreated for a significant period.

Laboratory Findings

Plasma glucose concentrations at presentation are elevated, usually in the range 300 to 500 mg/dL. If the presentation is uncomplicated, the remainder of the fluid and electrolyte measurements may be completely normal. On the other hand, if diabetic ketoacidosis is present, the measurements reflect the presence of an acidosis as well as more severe dehydration. Thus, in diabetic ketoacidosis, the serum sodium value is often at the lower limit of normal or even mildly reduced, reflecting the osmotic effect of hyperglycemia and on occasion the presence of vomiting with continued water intake. A sodium value less than 120 mM/L is usually associated with severe hypertriglyceridemia that can lead to spurious hyponatremia.

Despite significant losses of potassium in the urine and total-body potassium deficits, acidosis usually leads to an elevated serum potassium concentration at the time of the initial presentation. Serum bicarbonate concentrations are usually less than 10 mg/dL, and elevations in serum concentrations of triglyceride and free fatty acids are found. Levels of ketone bodies are also elevated. Because dehydration is invariably present, this leads to increases in the concentrations of blood urea nitrogen (BUN) and creatinine. In conjunction with the increase in serum glucose, the increases in BUN invariably increase the serum osmolality, often to greater than 300 mM/kg.

Treatment of Type 1 Diabetes

Importance of Tight Glucose Control

The overriding principle in the treatment of most patients with T1DM is that a health care team that includes a physician, diabetes nurse educator, nutritionist, and other health care professionals as appropriate should work closely with the patient to achieve blood glucose concentrations as close to normal as possible because these are associated with a reduced risk of diabetic complications. Although studies in animal models[195-197] and epidemiologic studies[198-200] suggested that tighter glucose control was associated with better long-term outcomes for the diabetic patient in terms of a reduced risk of complications, the most definitive study in this regard has been the Diabetes Control and Complications Trial (DCCT) that was completed in 1993.[201] This landmark study was performed in a total of 1441 patients with T1DM—726 with no retinopathy at baseline (the primary prevention cohort) and 715 with mild retinopathy (the secondary intervention cohort) who were randomly assigned to intensive therapy or conventional therapy.

Intensive therapy consisted of insulin administration by an external pump or by three or more daily insulin injections. The dosage was adjusted according to the results of self-monitoring of the blood glucose performed at least four times per day as well as in response to dietary intake and anticipated exercise. The goals of intensive therapy were to achieve blood glucose concentrations between 70 and 120 mg/dL before meals, values less than 180 mg/dL after meals, a weekly 3 AM measurement greater than 65 mg/dL, and an HbA_{1c} value within the normal range (6.05% or less). Patients in the intensive treatment group visited their centers each month and had more frequent contacts with a member of the health care team, generally weekly, to review and adjust their regimens.

Conventional therapy consisted of one or two daily injections of insulin, including mixed intermediate and rapid-acting insulins, daily self-monitoring of urine or blood glucose, and education about diet and exercise. The goals of conventional therapy included absence of symptoms of hyperglycemia; absence of ketonuria; maintenance of normal growth, development, and ideal body weight; and freedom from frequent severe hypoglycemia.

The entire cohort of patients was observed for a mean of 6.5 years, and 99% of the patients completed the study. Although only 5% of the subjects in the intensive treatment group were able to sustain the goal of a normal HbA_{1c} over time, they nevertheless did have significantly lower average values (approximately 7%) over time than the subjects in the conventional treatment group (approximately 9%). Average capillary blood glucose profiles in the intensive treatment group were 155±30 mg/dL compared with 231±55 mg/dL in the conventional therapy group ($P < .0001$). These differences in glucose control formed the basis of analyses to determine the effects of lower levels of glycemia on diabetic complications.

When both the primary prevention and secondary intervention cohorts were considered, intensive therapy reduced the risk of proliferative or severe nonproliferative retinopathy by 47% and the need for treatment by photocoagulation by 56%. Intensive therapy reduced the mean adjusted risk of microalbuminuria (defined as urinary albumin excretion >40 mg/24 hr) by 34% in the primary prevention cohort and by 43% in the secondary intervention cohort. The risk of albuminuria was reduced by 56% in the secondary intervention cohort. Intensive therapy reduced the appearance of neuropathy by 69% in the primary prevention cohort and by 57% in the secondary intervention cohort.

Some have suggested potential adverse effects of aggressive insulin therapy in exacerbating the predisposition to macrovascular disease in diabetes. In the DCCT study, intensive insulin therapy reduced the development of macrovascular disease by 41%, although the difference was not statistically significant.[202] Ninety-three percent of DCCT participants were followed after the randomized portion of the trial in the Epidemiology of Diabetes Interventions and Complications (EDIC) study. Glycemic control in both groups drifted toward just under an A_{1c} of 8% within the first year or so after conclusion of the randomized trial. With 17 years of follow-up after randomization, despite similar glycemic control in both groups for 10 years, cardiovascular disease (defined as nonfatal myocardial infarction [MI], stroke, death from cardiovascular disease [CVD], confirmed angina, or the need for coronary-artery revascularization) was reduced 42% and nonfatal MI, stroke, and CVD death were reduced by 57%. The authors concluded that "the decrease in glycosylated hemoglobin values during the DCCT was significantly associated with most of the positive effects of intensive treatment on the risk of cardiovascular disease. . . . Intensive diabetes therapy has long-term beneficial effects on the risk of cardiovascular disease in patients with type 1 diabetes."[203]

Were there any adverse events associated with the intensive treatment regimen in the DCCT? Overall mortality did not differ in the two treatment groups and was actually less than expected on the basis of population-based mortality studies. However, the incidence of severe hypoglycemia was approximately three times higher in the intensive therapy group than in the conventional therapy group ($P < .001$). Some of the episodes of hypoglycemia were quite severe, resulting in motor vehicle accidents or the need for hospitalization. Severe hypoglycemia occurred more often during sleep,[204] and of episodes that occurred while the patients were awake, a significant fraction (approximately one third) were not associated with warning symptoms. In intensively treated subjects, predictors of hypoglycemia included a history of severe hypoglycemia, longer duration of diabetes, higher baseline HbA_{1c}, and a lower recent HbA_{1c}.

Weight gain also occurred in more of the intensively treated patients. Intensive therapy was associated with a 33% increase in risk of becoming overweight, defined as a body weight more than 120% above the ideal. Five years into the trial, patients being treated intensively had gained a mean of 4.6 kg more than patients receiving conventional therapy. Among subjects in the top quartile of weight gain, changes in plasma lipids, blood pressure, and body fat distribution were observed that were similar to those seen with insulin resistance.[205]

Goals of Treatment

On the basis of these results, the authors of the DCCT study recommended that most patients with T1DM be treated with an intensive treatment regimen under the close supervision of a health care team consisting of a physician, nurses, nutritionist, and behavioral and exercise specialists as needed. However, for certain groups of patients this recommendation may need to be modified because the risk-to-benefit ratio might not be as favorable as it was in the cohorts with mild or no diabetic complications that were studied in the DCCT.

Patients for whom it may be appropriate to be more cautious about instituting intensive treatment regimens include children younger than 13 years, elderly people, and patients with advanced complications such as end-stage renal disease or significant cardiovascular or cerebrovascular disease. It has also been reported[206-208] that instituting aggressive insulin therapy in subjects with proliferative or severe nonproliferative retinopathy can lead to accelerated progression of retinopathy after the start of intensive therapy. Treatment of the eye disease should be considered before instituting an aggressive insulin regimen. Patients who do not experience warning adrenergic symptoms of hypoglycemia (hypoglycemia unawareness) are at significantly greater risk for severe recurrent hypoglycemia, and this may prevent the safe institution of tight glucose control.[209]

In Table 31–5, guidelines from the American Diabetes Association (ADA) and the American College of Endocrinology (ACE) are presented. The ADA suggests that the goal of treatment in the management of diabetes should be an HbA_{1c} value less than 7% in general, but for the individual patient the A_{1c} should be as close to normal (<6%) as possible without significant hypoglycemia.[210,211] The ACE has recommended an HbA_{1c} goal of less than 6.5%.[212] Because the average HbA_{1c} in the United States is estimated to be in the 7.5% to 9.5% range, the argument about whether the HbA_{1c} target should be 6.0%, 6.5%, or 7% has limited practical significance.

It is recognized that to achieve glucose control at this level, patients need to monitor glucose frequently and receive nutritional counseling and training in self-management of the insulin doses and problem solving to allow them to deal with the problems that they encounter in their daily lives.

TABLE 31–5 GLYCEMIC TARGETS

Parameter	Normal	ADA	ACE
Premeal plasma glucose (mg/dL)	<100 (mean ~90)	90-130	<110
Postprandial plasma glucose (mg/dL)	<140	<180	<140
Hb A_{1c}	4%-6%	<7%	<6.5%

ACE, American College of Endocrinologists; ADA, American Diabetes Association; Hb A_{1c}, hemoglobin A_{1c}.
From American Diabetes Association. Standards of Medical Care in Diabetes—2006. Diabetes Care 2006; 29:s4-42; American College of Endocrinologists. American College of Endocrinology consensus statement on guidelines for glycemic control. Endocr Pract 2002;8(suppl 1):5-11.

Team Approach to Treatment

The DCCT trial validated the use of: continuous subcutaneous insulin infusion (CSII; insulin pump) and multiple daily injections (MDI), which are titrated based on frequent glucose monitoring. Several companies are developing continuous glucose sensors, and pramlintide, an amylin analogue, is the first fundamentally new treatment for patients with T1DM to become available since 1922. Because of the complex nature of modern intensive diabetes treatment regimens and the need for regular feedback and modification of the parameters of treatment, it has now become generally accepted that intensive insulin regimens can be instituted more effectively by a health care team than by a physician alone. Members of the team can include diabetes nurse educators, nutritionists, psychologists, medical social workers, and others, such as exercise physiologists, depending on the needs of a particular patient. A critical aspect of intensive diabetes treatment is the need for continuous monitoring of the effectiveness of specific components of the regimen and to make adjustments in response to changing life circumstances of the patient.

Pharmacokinetics of Available Insulin Preparations

In the past, insulin for human use was obtained from animal sources: cows and pigs. With advances in recombinant DNA technology, it is now possible to produce large quantities of insulin with an amino acid structure identical to that of human insulin or to modify the human amino acid sequence to produce desirable pharmacodynamic properties. The various formulations of insulin differ in the rapidity of the onset of action, the time from injection to peak action, and the duration of action, depending on the chemical nature of the particular insulin preparation. These data are summarized in Table 31–6. The available insulins can be divided into three broad categories on a pharmacokinetic basis: rapid acting, intermediate, and long acting.

Rapid-Acting Insulins

These insulins have an onset of action within an hour or less and are used to reduce the peak of glycemia that occurs after meal ingestion.

TABLE 31–6 PHARMACOKINETIC PROPERTIES OF INSULIN PREPARATION

Preparation	Onset (hr)	Peak (hr)	Duration (hr)
RAPID ACTING			
Regular	0.5-1	2-4	6-8
Lispro	0.25	1	3-4
Aspart	0.25	1	3-4
Glulisine	0.25	1	3-4
INTERMEDIATE ACTING			
NPH	1-3	6-8	12-16
LONG ACTING			
Glargine	1	NA	11-24
Detemir	1	3-9	6-23

NPH, neutral protamine Hagedorn.

Regular Insulin

Regular insulin consists of zinc-insulin crystals dissolved in a clear fluid. After subcutaneous injection regular insulin tends to dissociate from its normal hexameric form, first into dimers and then into monomers; only the monomeric and dimeric forms can pass through the endothelium into the circulation to any appreciable degree.[213] This feature determines the pharmacokinetic profile of regular insulin. The resulting relative delay in the onset and duration of action of regular insulin limits its effectiveness in controlling postprandial glucose and results in dose-dependent pharmacokinetics, with prolonged onset, peak, and duration of action with higher doses.

Insulin Analogues

Insulin Lispro

Insulin lispro, of recombinant DNA origin, is a human insulin analogue created when amino acids at positions 28 and 29 on the human insulin B chain are reversed. Insulin lispro was the first insulin analogue to receive approval by the United States Food and Drug Administration. It is chemically Lys(B28), Pro(B29) insulin and is created in a special nonpathogenic laboratory strain of *Escherichia coli* that has been genetically altered by the addition of the gene for insulin lispro.

The effect of this amino acid rearrangement is to reduce the capacity of the insulin to self-aggregate in subcutaneous tissues, resulting in behavior similar to that of monomeric insulin. This leads to lispro's more rapid absorption and shorter duration of action compared with regular insulin when given by subcutaneous injection. However, lispro is not intrinsically more active and on a molar basis is equipotent to human insulin. When they are given by intravenous injection, the pharmacokinetic profiles of lispro and human regular insulin are similar. Because of its rapid onset of action within 5 to 15 minutes of administration and peak action within 1 to 2 hours, lispro was the first insulin that mimics the time course of the increase in plasma glucose seen after ingestion of a carbohydrate-rich meal.

Insulin Aspart

Insulin aspart differs from human insulin by substitution of aspartic acid for proline in position B28.

Insulin Glulisine

Insulin glulisine involves substitution of the asparagine at position B3 with lysine and the lysine in position B29 with glutamic acid.

Advantages of Analogues

Lispro, aspart, and glulisine seem to have similar pharmacokinetics and clinical effects in the setting of T1DM. Although little difference is observed in most cases by either patients or providers, there certainly may be differences, at least in subsets of patients, that could be exploited to improve glycemic control.

In general, treatment with monomeric insulin analogues (lispro, aspart, and glulisine) is associated with a lower risk of hypoglycemia, particularly in sleep, than treatment with regular insulin. It is quite easy to document improved glycemic control in the postprandial state. Finally, patients may inject these insulin analogues immediately before or after meals instead of 30 to 60 minutes before meals, as is classically recommended with regular insulin, providing greater convenience. These features have been exploited in clinical trials to produce modest improvements in overall control with monomeric insulin analogues versus regular insulin.

Intermediate and Long-Acting Insulins

Intermediate and long-acting insulins have a significantly longer delay in their onset and duration of action. In the setting of T1DM they should be always used in combination with a rapid-acting form of insulin. They are generally administered before bedtime and titrated to produce normal glucose levels through the night and in the fasting state.

NPH Insulin

NPH insulin is a crystalline suspension of insulin with protamine and zinc, providing an intermediate-acting insulin with onset of action in 1 to 3 hours, duration of action up to 24 hours, and peak action from 6 to 8 hours. NPH insulin usually cannot be administered once daily in the setting of T1DM, at least in combination with rapid acting monomeric analogue insulin. In the pre-analogue era, NPH insulin was used successfully in combination with regular insulin, though this human insulin–based regimen has been largely supplanted by analogue insulin because of perceived lower risk of hypoglycemia.[214]

Insulin Glargine

Insulin glargine is a recombinant human insulin analogue that does provide a 24-hour duration of action in most, but not all, patients with T1DM. It differs from human insulin in that the amino acid asparagine at position A21 is replaced by glycine, and two arginines are added to the C-terminus of the B chain. In the injection solution at pH 4, insulin glargine is completely soluble. However, it has low solubility at neutral pH.

After injection into the subcutaneous tissue, the acidic solution is neutralized, leading to the formation of microprecipitates from which small amounts of insulin glargine are slowly released, resulting in absorption over an approximately 24-hour period with no pronounced peak. It thus simulates the basal production of insulin. In other respects the mechanism of action of glargine insulin is similar to that of human insulin, and on a molar basis its glucose-lowering effects are similar to those of human insulin when given intravenously.

Because this insulin is provided in an acid vehicle, it cannot be mixed with other forms of insulin or intravenous fluids, and some patients have greater discomfort with injection at least some of the time. In general, glargine is less variably absorbed than NPH insulin, and in clinical trials in patients with T1DM it has been associated with a reduced risk of hypoglycemia, particularly nocturnal hypoglycemia.

In about 10% of patients, insulin glargine must be taken twice daily to provide 24-hour coverage of basal insulin needs. In a smaller percentage of patients, there may be a modest peak in effect approximately 2 to 6 hours after injection, which can produce nocturnal hypoglycemia.

Insulin Detemir

Insulin detemir differs from human insulin in that the threonine in position B30 has been eliminated and a C14 fatty acid chain has been attached to amino acid B29. It is unique among insulins of prolonged duration in that it is soluble both in the vial and under the skin. This may be the cause of its more consistent absorption after subcutaneous injection.[215] In comparison to NPH insulin in the setting of T1DM, detemir is associated with less weight gain (in some trials patients have experienced weight loss) and reduced risk of hypoglycemia.[214]

Alternative Routes of Insulin Administration

Numerous alternative routes of insulin administration are being examined.[216,217] There is tremendous interest on the part of patients in inhaled insulin. Some studies suggest that there is substantial preference, at least among most research volunteers, for the pulmonary versus the subcutaneous route of insulin administration.

However, the currently available formulation and delivery system (Exubera) has several limitations to wholesale substitution in the setting of T1DM. Most importantly, insulin for inhalation will only be available in 1-mg and 3-mg packets, which respectively provide approximately 3 units and approximately 8 units of insulin activity. The packet size sets clinically important limitations on the precise titration of insulin possible with syringes, pens, and, particularly, pumps. Secondly, there are concerns that greater variability in absorption from the intrapulmonary than subcutaneous site will amplify the glycemic instability inherent in T1DM, particularly in the setting of intercurrent respiratory illness or exposures such as tobacco smoke.

That said, there are a small number of clinical trials in T1DM that suggest that the pulmonary route of insulin administration is adequate to provide at least moderate control of T1DM. After inhalation, the onset of glucose-lowering activity in healthy volunteers occurs within 10 to 20 minutes, with a peak effects at approximately 2 hours and duration of approximately 6 hours. Thus its onset is akin to rapid-acting analogues and the duration more like the regular insulin from which it is formulated.

The long-term safety of the pulmonary route of insulin administration is unknown, particularly in the setting of T1DM, in which insulin is likely to be administered three or more times a day potentially for 50 or more years.

Approach to the Treatment of Type 1 Diabetes

Levels of glucose control equivalent to those achieved in the intensive treatment group in the DCCT are not possible in the vast majority of patients unless the insulin regimen uses a multiple daily injection (MDI) regimen combining rapid and long-acting insulin or a continuous subcutaneous infusion of insulin (CSII) via an insulin pump with the patient adjusting the insulin dose depending on the results of self-monitoring of glucose as well as on the basis of dietary intake and physical activity. The reason for this is relatively simple. In patients with little or no endogenous insulin production, the exogenous insulin regimen needs to simulate the multiphasic profile of insulin secretory responses to meals and snacks present in normal subjects if levels of glycemia approaching normal are to be achieved.

A number of regimens have been used to achieve these ends. Three basic approaches are reviewed, although it is clear that other possible approaches may be effective in individual patients. Achieving the glycemic goals of therapy is far more important than the details of the insulin regimen. Nevertheless, one of the following three general approaches to therapy is most likely to lead to the desired outcome.

Combination of Rapid-Acting and Intermediate-Acting Insulin with Breakfast and Dinner and Intermediate-Acting Insulin at Bedtime

The rationale for these regimens is that the rapid-acting insulin limits the postprandial glucose rise after breakfast and dinner, the intermediate-acting insulin administered before breakfast limits glycemia in the afternoon, and the intermediate-acting insulin before dinner limits glycemia in the early hours of the morning. Although such a regimen may be sufficient to achieve glucose targets in some patients, in many persons the intermediate-acting insulin given before dinner is insufficient to control elevations in blood glucose commonly seen in the early morning (dawn phenomenon). Attempts to increase the dose of intermediate-acting insulin at dinner expose the patient to a greater risk of hypoglycemia in the middle of the night, hence the need for a smaller dose at bedtime to provide sufficient insulin to restrain the dawn phenomenon the following morning while moderating the risk of nocturnal hypoglycemia. This three-injection regimen was the mainstay of therapy in the DCCT but is rapidly being supplanted by regimens that take greater advantage of the availability of insulin analogues.

Combination of Rapid-Acting Insulin Given with Meals and Long-Acting Insulin at Bedtime

This combination of insulins can also simulate the pattern of insulin production that occurs normally. Use of monomeric insulin analogues provides excellent meal coverage. Use of long-acting insulin at bedtime provides excellent control of the fasting plasma glucose. This combination of rapid-acting monomeric insulin analogues with long-acting analogues has largely supplanted human insulin–based treatment regimens because it seems to be associated with less variability in glycemic control associated with lower risks of hypoglycemia. When long-acting insulin is administered once a day in the evening, an unexplained and consistent rise in glucose can occur just before the evening injection of long-acting insulin because the analogue's duration is less than 24 hours. This is more common in patients who require low doses (<20 units) of long-acting analogue and arguably is more common with detemir than glargine.

Insulin Administration by an External Insulin Pump

An alternative method of delivering insulin is by an external mechanical pump. This approach involves administering a rapidly acting insulin preparation delivered by continuous subcutaneous infusion through a catheter usually inserted into the subcutaneous tissues of the anterior abdominal wall. The pump delivers insulin as a preprogrammed basal infusion as well as patient-directed boluses given before meals or snacks or in response to elevations in the blood glucose concentration outside the desired range. With currently available pumps, the basal insulin infusion rate (usually approximately 1 U/hr) can be programmed either to continue at a constant rate over the 24-hour period or more commonly to increase and decrease at predetermined times of the day to prevent anticipated excursions in the blood glucose concentration, for example, morning rises in glucose. Newer pumps allow multiple basal profiles to deal with recurrent patterns (e.g., menstruation, weekends, activity). Protocols for insulin administration by the pump usually require approximately half the insulin to be administered as a basal infusion and the remainder as premeal boluses.

Insulin administration by an external pump has some advantages over regimens that use multiple insulin injections. Only rapidly acting insulin is used in the insulin pump. Consequently, adjustments to the basal insulin infusion rate or changes in the size and timing of the insulin boluses result in more rapid changes in the blood glucose concentration than are possible when adjustments are made to the dose of intermediate-acting or long-acting insulin. This leads to greater flexibility for the patient. It has been suggested that use of analogue insulin can lead to a lower risk of hypoglycemia.[218,219]

However, there are also disadvantages of insulin pump therapy. There is a significant initial cost of the pump itself. Furthermore, the tubing, which needs to be changed every 24 to 72 hours, and other supplies are expensive. The risk of infection at the site of insulin administration is significant. Infections occur on average once per year per patient even in the best of practices, and although these can usually be treated by changing the site of infusion and giving a short course of oral antibiotics, if an abscess develops, surgical drainage may be necessary. In addition, because only rapidly acting insulin is used, pump failure as a result of mechanical malfunction or catheter-related problems can quickly result in severe hyperglycemia and even ketoacidosis. Patients treated with insulin pump therapy must monitor glucose frequently and always be alert to the possibility of failure of the infusion system.

Controlled clinical trials have indicated that on average, intensive insulin regimens that use multiple insulin injections lead to levels of glucose control similar to those achieved with the insulin pump. On the other hand, some patients never achieve adequate control with multiple daily injections but experience dramatic improvements with pump therapy. According to the Clinical Practice Recommendations of the American Diabetes Association,[220] the insulin pump should be used only by candidates strongly motivated to improve glucose control and willing to work with their health care provider in assuming substantial responsibility for their day-to-day care. They must also understand and demonstrate use of the insulin pump and self-monitoring of blood glucose and be able to use the data obtained in an appropriate fashion.

Algorithms of Insulin Administration

An essential component of intensive regimens of insulin replacement is the need to make regular adjustments to the insulin dose depending on the prevailing blood glucose concentration, planned activity, and food intake. Algorithms have been developed to guide these adjustments that aim to simulate the normal feedback control of insulin secretion whereby hyperglycemia stimulates and hypoglycemia inhibits insulin secretion. They all involve frequent monitoring of the blood glucose concentration, generally four times per day or more; increases in the insulin dose if glucose levels are above the target upper level that is judged to be acceptable; reductions in the insulin dose if glucose levels are below the acceptable lower level; and techniques for adjusting insulin doses for changes in diet. Several are referenced for convenience.[221-223]

Pramlintide

Amylin is a neuroendocrine hormone cosecreted with insulin by pancreatic beta cells. It was originally identified as a major constituent of pancreatic amyloid deposits. Its biologically active form is a 37–amino acid peptide that is extensively post-translationally processed, including carboxy-terminal amidation and glycosylation. As would be expected, in parallel with insulin deficiency, amylin deficiency develops in T1DM. Amylin and insulin have complementary actions in regulating plasma glucose. Insulin can be thought of as regulating the rate of glucose disappearance from the circulation. Amylin is thought to exert its major antihyperglycemic actions through central mechanisms after binding to brain nuclei such as the nucleus accumbens, dorsal raphe, and area postrema, promoting satiety and reducing appetite. It also is thought to act via vagal efferents, mediating a decrease in the rate of gastric emptying and a suppressesion of glucagon secretion in a glucose-dependent fashion. Effectively, amylin plays a role in regulating the rate of glucose appearance from the GI tract and the liver.[224,225]

However, amylin is relatively insoluble in aqueous solution and aggregates on plastic and glass. Pramlintide was developed as a soluble, nonaggregating, equipotent amylin analogue. In 2005, pramlintide was approved for human use in the United States. As expected, when injected before meals, pramlintide slows gastric emptying, suppresses glucagon, and promotes satiety, with a subsequent reduction in postprandial glucose. In T1DM, pramlintide therapy is usually initiated at a dose of 15 μg before meals (0.025 mL or "2.5 units" in a U-100 insulin syringe of the marketed pramlintide acetate 0.6 mg/dL). Slow titration from there to the usual dose in patients with T1DM of 60 μg before meals as tolerated is recommended to minimize nausea and insulin-induced hypoglycemia. The maximally labeled dose in the setting of T2DM is 120 μg before meals.

In T1DM, the addition of pramlintide can be expected to produce modest reductions in A_{1c} and weight, 0.3 percentage points and 1.5 kg, respectively, as compared to placebo in controlled trials. Weight loss is more prevalent in overweight patients compared to those with normal body weight, and it is generally independent of nausea. Severe insulin hypoglycemia can develop as a complication, particularly upon initiation, because the effect of pramlintide on satiety can be robust, effectively stopping some patients from eating midmeal. To minimize this risk, it is suggested that patients reduce rapid-acting insulin at meals by approximately 50% on initiating pramlintide; this is optimally accomplished by reducing the insulin-to-carbohydrate ratio and in many cases by administering pramlintide before the meal and insulin after the meal so that insulin dose reduction can be accomplished if the meal is not finished. Despite its role in glucagon regulation, pramlintide does not interfere with recovery from insulin-induced hypoglycemia.

Pramlintide is an agent whose role in the routine management of T1DM is evolving. The additional injections and expense certainly constitute a burden to patients and the health care system. Most patients note a dramatic improvement in postprandial glucose, Many find the appetite-suppressing effects quite helpful even in the absence of substantial weight gain. Some report an improvement in sense of well-being and energy. What is absolutely certain is that initiating and titrating pramlintide is complex and fraught with potential pitfalls. Perhaps more so than any other treatment for diabetes, it absolutely requires careful collaboration of patients and diabetes educators.

Complications of Intensive Management of Type 1 Diabetes

Hypoglycemia

The most serious complication of intensive regimens of insulin replacement is hypoglycemia, and this is generally the factor that limits patients' ability to achieve tight glucose control. In the DCCT, patients in the intensive treatment group had an approximately threefold greater risk of hypoglycemia than those in the conventional treatment group. Hypoglycemia may be life-threatening, leading to motor vehicle accidents, serious falls with fractures, and seizures. Patients with T1DM have serious defects in mechanisms responsible for glucose counterregulation, and this is a major underlying reason for the predisposition to hypoglycemia. Glucose counterregulation is reviewed in detail in Chapter 32.

The risk of hypoglycemia can be reduced if all patients treated with intensive regimens of insulin replacement are carefully educated about recognizing hypoglycemia symptoms and about the measures that should be taken to prevent more serious hypoglycemia after symptoms are initially experienced. Certain patients, particularly those with long-standing diabetes and autonomic neuropathy, might not subjectively sense symptoms of hypoglycemia even in the presence of low glucose concentrations. Glycemic targets of therapy should be adjusted upward in these patients because they are at particularly high risk for hypoglycemia. Similarly, patients with advanced end-stage microvascular or macrovascular diabetic complications in whom the benefit of intensive glucose control is likely to be less should not be exposed to the increased risk of hypoglycemia that is inherent in extremely intensive insulin-treatment regimens.

In addition to the availability of glucose tablets, hard candy, or other sources of a readily absorbable form of carbohydrate, virtually all patients with T1DM should have emergency glucagon kits at home and at work, assuming that there are people in those settings who can be trained to use them. The administration of 0.5 to 1 mg of glucagon intramuscularly to a severely symptomatic person with hypoglycemia rapidly increases the plasma glucose concentration to an acceptable range and prevents the difficulties and dangers associated with attempting to get a stuporous or disoriented person to ingest glucose by mouth. Nevertheless, because of occasional failures of glucagon to reverse hypoglycemia fully, friends and family members should always be instructed to call for medical assistance as soon as the injection is provided.

The recent availability of continuous glucose sensors with alarms can reduce the time that patients spend with glucose in the hypoglycemic range. Early experience suggests that this can be particularly valuable in the setting of hypoglycemia unawareness.[226]

Weight Gain

Improvement in glucose control with a reduction in glycosuria is invariably associated with weight gain as the leakage of calories into the urine is reduced or eliminated. In addition, increased food intake to treat or prevent hypoglycemia can contribute to weight gain. Insulin itself can stimulate appetite. As a result of the combination of all these effects, weight gain is common, particularly with intensive regimens of insulin replacement. As discussed earlier, this can be minimized or partially reversed with the addition of pramlintide.

Worsening of Retinopathy

Institution of regimens of tight glucose control has been reported to exacerbate the underlying retinopathy. Thus, if a patient with serious background of proliferative retinopathy presents in poor glucose control, ophthalmologic treatment of the retinopathy should be considered before instituting tight glucose control.

Insulin Allergy

Insulin allergy has become much less common with the use of human insulin. Most manifestations of allergic reactions to insulin consist of local wheal-and-flare reactions at the site of injection. The allergic reaction can be to the insulin itself or to other components of the insulin preparation, such as the protamine in NPH insulin. Occasionally, more generalized allergic reactions occur, and even more rarely anaphylactic reactions take place. In general, mild local allergic reactions to insulin can be treated with antihistamines. More severe reactions require desensitization or coadministration of glucocorticoids. Admission to the hospital is necessary, and under close supervision of a physician with access to equipment for emergency resuscitation, a protocol is followed in which the patient is exposed to gradually increasing amounts of insulin administered according to a set schedule.[227]

Acute Diabetic Emergencies: Diabetic Ketoacidosis

Diabetic ketoacidosis (DKA) is a life-threatening condition in which severe insulin deficiency leads to hyperglycemia, excessive lipolysis, and unrestrained fatty acid oxidation, producing the ketone bodies acetone, β-hydroxybutyrate, and acetoacetate. This results in metabolic acidosis, dehydration, and deficits in fluid and electrolytes. Excess secretion of primarily glucagon as well as catecholamines, glucocorticoids, and growth hormone in combination with insulin deficiency produces hyperglycemia by stimulating glycogenolysis and gluconeogenesis and impairing glucose disposal. DKA is a far more characteristic feature of T1DM than of T2DM but may be seen in persons with T2DM under conditions of stress such as occurs with serious infections, trauma, and cardiovascular or other emergencies.

Clinical Presentation

Patients with uncontrolled diabetes present with nonspecific complaints. If the disease follows an indolent course over months to years, patients can manifest profound wasting, cachexia, and prostration similar in degree to those of patients with long-standing malignancy or chronic infection. With significant physical or emotional stress, sudden metabolic decompensation can occur. The cases of DKA that are misdiagnosed usually occur in patients with new-onset diabetes. Polyuria (or at least nocturia) and weight loss are almost always present, although they are often not reported by the patient. Any patient with severe illness (acute or chronic) or neurologic changes should have glucose and electrolytes measured.

In DKA, metabolic decompensation usually develops over a period of hours to a few days. Patients with DKA classically present with lethargy and a characteristic hyperventilation pattern with deep slow breaths (Kussmaul respirations) associated with the fruity odor of acetone. They often complain of nausea and vomiting, and abdominal pain is somewhat less frequent. The abdominal pain can be quite severe and may be associated with distention, ileus, and tenderness without rebound but usually resolves relatively quickly with therapy unless there is underlying abdominal pathology. Most patients are normotensive, tachycardic, and tachypneic and have signs of mild to moderate volume depletion. Hypothermia has been described in DKA, and patients with underlying infection might not manifest fever. Cerebral edema does occur, generally during therapy. Patients with DKA can have stupor and obvious profound dehydration, and they often demonstrate focal neurologic deficits such as Babinski reflexes, asymmetrical reflexes, cranial nerve findings, paresis, fasciculations, and aphasia.

Laboratory Test Results and Differential Diagnosis

Laboratory Tests

Laboratory tests that are routinely monitored in the setting of DKA include hemoglobin, white blood cell and differential count, glucose, electrolytes, blood urea nitrogen (BUN), and creatinine. Changes in Na, K, Cl, P, BUN, and creatinine are also monitored.

The sine qua non of DKA is acidosis, and the serum HCO_3 concentration is usually less than 10 mEq/L. The acidosis is due to production and accumulation of ketones in the serum. Three ketones are produced in DKA: two ketoacids (β-hydroxybutyrate and acetoacetate) and the neutral ketone acetone. Ketones can be detected in serum and urine using the nitroprusside reaction on diagnostic strips for use at the patient's bedside or in the clinical laboratory. This test detects acetoacetate more effectively than acetone and does not detect an increased concentration of β-hydroxybutyrate. Particularly in severe DKA, β-hydroxybutyrate is the predominant ketone, and it is possible although unusual to have a negative serum nitroprusside reaction in the presence of severe ketosis. However, under these circumstances the serum HCO_3 is still markedly reduced and the anion gap is increased, indicating metabolic acidosis. The urinary β-hydroxybutyrate can be measured at many centers and commercially but is not usually readily available.

The anion gap is a readily available index for unmeasured anions in the blood (normal <14 mEq/L):

$$\text{Anion gap} = \text{sodium} - (\text{chloride} + \text{bicarbonate})$$

Most patients with DKA present with an anion gap greater than 20 mEq/L, and some present with a gap greater than 40 mEq/L. However, occasional patients have a hyperchloremic metabolic acidosis without a significant anion gap.[228]

Patients with DKA almost invariably have large amounts of ketones in their urine. The serum glucose in DKA is usually in the 500 mg/dL range. However, an entity known as euglycemic DKA has been described, particularly in the presence of decreased oral intake or in pregnancy, in which the serum glucose is normal or near normal but the patient requires insulin therapy for the clearance of ketoacidosis.[229] The arterial pH is commonly less than 7.3 and can be as low as 6.5. There is partial respiratory compensation with hypocarbia. Patients are often mildly hyperosmolar, although osmolalities greater than 330 mOsm/kg are unusual without mental status changes.

Differential Diagnosis

Not all patients with hyperglycemia and an anion gap metabolic acidosis have DKA, and other causes of metabolic acidosis must be considered in these patients, particularly if the serum or urine ketone measurements are not elevated. The following causes of metabolic acidosis need to be considered in the differential diagnosis of DKA.

Lactic acidosis is the most common cause of metabolic acidosis in hospitalized patients and can be seen in patients with uncomplicated diabetes as well as those with DKA. Lactic acidosis usually occurs in the setting of decreased tissue oxygen delivery, resulting in the nonoxidative metabolism of glucose to lactic acid. Lactic acidosis complicates other primary metabolic acidoses as a consequence of dehydration or shock, and assessing its relative contribution can be difficult. The presentation is identical to that of DKA. In pure lactic acidosis, the serum glucose and ketones should be normal and the serum lactate concentration should be greater than 5 mM. The therapy of lactic acidosis is directed at the underlying cause and optimizing tissue perfusion.[230]

Starvation ketosis is caused by inadequate carbohydrate availability, resulting in physiologically appropriate lipolysis and ketone production to provide fuel substrates for muscle. The blood glucose is usually normal. Although the urine can have large amounts of ketones, the blood rarely does. Arterial pH is normal, and the anion gap is at most mildly elevated.

Alcoholic ketoacidosis is a more severe form of starvation ketosis wherein the appropriate ketogenic response to poor carbohydrate intake is increased through as yet poorly defined effects of alcohol on the liver. Classically, these patients are long-standing alcoholics for whom ethanol has been the main caloric source for days to weeks. The ketoacidosis occurs when for some reason alcohol and caloric intake decreases. In isolated alcoholic ketoacidosis, the metabolic acidosis is usually mild to moderate. The anion gap is elevated. Serum and urine ketones are always present. However, alcoholic ketoacidosis produces an even higher ratio of β-hydroxybutyrate to acetoacetate than DKA does, and negative or weakly positive nitroprusside reactions are common. Respiratory alkalosis associated with delirium tremens, agitation, or pulmonary processes often normalizes the pH but should be evident with careful analysis of acid-base status. Usually, the patient is normoglycemic or hypoglycemic, although mild hyperglycemia is occasionally present. Patients who are significantly hyperglycemic should be treated as if they have DKA. The therapy of alcoholic ketoacidosis consists of thiamine, carbohydrates, fluids, and electrolytes, with special attention to the more severe consequences of alcohol toxicity, alcohol withdrawal, and chronic malnutrition. In more severely ill patients in whom alcoholic ketoacidosis is considered a possibility, there is usually another underlying illness such as pancreatitis, gastrointestinal bleeding, hepatic encephalopathy, delirium tremens, or infection complicated by concomitant lactic acidosis.[231,232]

Uremic acidosis is characterized by extremely large elevations in the BUN (often >200 mg/dL) and creatinine (>10 mg/dL) with normoglycemia. The pH and anion gap are usually only mildly abnormal. The treatment is supportive, with careful attention to fluid and electrolytes until dialysis can be performed. Rhabdomyolysis is a cause of renal failure in which the anion gap can be significantly elevated and acidosis can be severe. There should be marked elevation of creatine phosphokinase and myoglobin. Mild rhabdomyolysis is not uncommon in DKA, but the presence of hyperglycemia and ketonemia leaves no doubt about the primary etiology of the acidosis.[233]

Toxic ingestions can be differentiated from DKA by history and laboratory investigation. Salicylate intoxication produces an anion gap metabolic acidosis usually with a respiratory alkalosis. The plasma glucose is normal or low, the osmolality is normal, ketones are negative, and salicylates can be detected in the urine or blood. Salicylates can cause a false-positive glucose determination when using the cupric sulfate method and a false-negative result when using the glucose oxidase reaction. Methanol and ethylene glycol also produce an anion gap metabolic acidosis without hyperglycemia or ketones but need to be kept in mind primarily because they produce an increase in the measured serum osmolality but not in the calculated serum osmolality—an osmolar gap. Their serum levels can also be measured. Isopropyl alcohol does not cause a metabolic acidosis but should be remembered because it is metabolized to acetone, which can produce a positive result in the nitroprusside reaction commonly used for the detection of ketoacids. These intoxications must be appropriately treated.[234-236] Rare cases of anion gap acidoses have been reported with other ingestions including toluene, iron, hydrogen sulfide, nalidixic acid, papaverine, paraldehyde, strychnine, isoniazid, and outdated tetracycline.

When DKA is considered, the diagnosis can be made quickly with routine laboratory tests. Blood and urine glucose and ketones can be obtained in minutes with glucose oxidase–impregnated strips and the nitroprusside reaction, respectively.

Osmolarity

The increase in osmolarity (mOsm/L) that occurs in DKA must be differentiated from the increase in osmolarity seen in hyperosmolar-hyperglycemic nonketotic (diabetic) coma (HHNC). The osmolarity can be measured by freezing point depression or estimated using the following formula:

$$\text{Osmolarity} = (2 \times \text{sodium}) + (\text{glucose}/18) + (\text{BUN}/2.8) + (\text{ethanol}/4.6)$$

Patients with DKA not uncommonly present with hyperosmolarity and coma. In HHNC, the osmolarity is generally greater than 350 mOsm/L and can exceed 400 mOsm/L. The serum sodium and potassium can be high, normal, or low and do not reflect total-body levels, which are uniformly depleted. The glucose is usually greater than 600 mg/dL, and levels higher than 1000 mg/dL are quite common. In pure HHNC, there is not a significant metabolic acidosis or anion gap.

Patients often present with combinations of the preceding findings. HHNC can involve mild to moderate ketonemia and acidosis. Alcoholic ketoacidosis can contribute to either DKA or HHNC. Lactic acidosis is common in severe DKA and HHNC. Any patient with hyperglycemia greater than 250 mg/dL and an anion gap metabolic acidosis should be treated by the general principles outlined in the next section, with special consideration of other possible contributing metabolic acidoses.

Therapy

The optimal management of DKA has been the source of considerable controversy since the 1950s. Only recently have prospective studies of various therapeutic approaches been performed. The guidelines we propose rely heavily on prospective studies of DKA by Kitabchi and coworkers.[237,238] The general approach is to provide necessary fluids to restore the circulation, treat insulin deficiency with continuous insulin, treat electrolyte disturbances, observe the patient closely and carefully, and search for underlying causes of metabolic decompensation.

Fluids

Volume contraction is one of the hallmarks of DKA. It can contribute to acidosis through lactic acid production as well as decreased renal clearance of organic and inorganic acids. It contributes to hyperglycemia by decreasing renal clearance of glucose. If decreased tissue perfusion is significant, it causes insulin resistance by decreasing insulin delivery to the sites of insulin-mediated glucose disposal, namely muscle and adipose tissue, as well as through stimulation of catecholamine and glucocorticoid secretion. Fluid deficits on the order of 5 to 10 L are common in DKA. The urine produced during the osmotic diuresis of hyperglycemia is approximately half-normal with respect to sodium. Therefore, water deficits are in excess of sodium deficits. Historically, large quantities of isotonic intravenous fluids have been administered rapidly to patients in DKA. For patients with a history of congestive heart failure, chronic or acute renal failure, severe hypotension, or significant pulmonary disease, early invasive hemodynamic monitoring should be considered.

When there is physical evidence of dehydration—that is, hypotension, decreased skin turgor, or dry mucous membranes—generally administer 1 L of normal saline over the first hour and 200 to 500 mL/hour in subsequent hours until hypotension resolves and adequate circulation is maintained. If hypotension is severe, there is clinical evidence of hypoperfusion, and hypotension does not respond to crystalloid, therapy with colloid is considered, often in combination with invasive hemodynamic monitoring. If there is no hypotension and no concern about renal failure, administer 1 L of half-normal saline over the first hour.

During that first hour, the laboratory data usually return and can be quite helpful in planning further therapy. Despite the excess of water losses over sodium, the measured sodium is usually low because of osmotic effects of glucose. These osmotic effects can be corrected using a simple formula:

$$\text{Corrected sodium concentration} = \text{measured sodium} + 0.016 \times (\text{glucose} - 100)$$

Severe hypertriglyceridemia, which is common in severe diabetes, can cause a false decrease in the serum sodium concentration by approximately 1.0 mEq/L at a serum lipid concentration of 460 mg/dL.[227] An estimated water deficit can be calculated using the corrected sodium:

$$\text{Water deficit in liters} = 0.6 \times \text{weight in kg} \times [(\text{sodium}/140) - 1]$$

Using these formulas, a 70-kg patient with a measured sodium level of 140 mEq/L and a glucose concentration of 1000 mg/dL has a calculated water deficit of 4.3 L. If the patient is normotensive after the first liter of fluids, it is reasonable to aim to replace urinary losses with one-half normal saline and also provide approximately one half the water deficit as 5% dextrose over the first 12 to 24 hours (using the preceding example, 2 L) and the remainder over the subsequent 24 hours. The plan for fluid therapy should be continuously reevaluated in light of the clinical and laboratory response of the patient. When the serum glucose reaches 250 to 300 mg/dL, all fluids should contain 5% dextrose and therapy should be aimed at maintaining the serum glucose in that range for 24 hours to allow slow equilibration of osmotically active substances across cell membranes.

The primary goal of fluid therapy is to maintain an adequate circulation, and the secondary goal is to maintain a brisk diuresis. Beyond that, pulmonary edema, hyperchloremic metabolic acidosis, and a rapid fall in the serum osmolality should be prevented by frequent monitoring of the patient, glucose, and electrolytes. It has been demonstrated that fluid administration and subsequent continued osmotic diuresis are responsible for a large portion of the initial decline in glucose during therapy.

Insulin

Insulin is the mainstay of therapy of DKA because DKA is essentially an insulin-deficient state. In the past, high doses of insulin (upward of 50 U/hr) were favored. In later studies, low-dose insulin therapy (0.1 U/kg per hour) has been shown to be as effective as higher doses in producing a decrease in serum glucose and clearance of ketones. Furthermore, low-dose therapy results in a reduction in the major morbidity of intensive insulin therapy, namely hypoglycemia and hypokalemia.

Studies have also shown that intravenous insulin is significantly more effective than intramuscular or subcutaneous insulin in lowering the ketone body concentration over the first 2 hours of therapy. The subcutaneous route is probably inappropriate for the critically ill patient because of the possibility of tissue hypoperfusion and slower kinetics of absorption; however, a study has documented that subcutaneous rapid-acting insulin analogue administered every 1 to 2 hours was as safe and effective as intravenous regular insulin in the treatment of patients with uncomplicated DKA.[239] Numerous studies attest to the efficacy of intramuscular therapy in severe DKA. When there is insufficient nursing monitoring or intravenous access to allow safe intravenous administration, intramuscular therapy would be the route of choice.

Lastly, it has been shown that a 10-U intravenous insulin priming dose when insulin therapy is started significantly improves the glycemic response to the first hour of therapy. The rationale is to saturate insulin receptors fully before beginning continuous therapy and to avoid the lag time necessary to achieve steady-state insulin levels. When mixing insulin in normal saline, it does not seem to be necessary to add albumin to prevent insulin adsorption to the infusion set. However, the intravenous tubing should be flushed with the insulin infusate before use.

In the rare instances in which the glucose does not decrease at least 10% or 50 mg/dL in an hour, the insulin infusion rate should be increased by 50% to 100% and a second bolus of intravenous insulin should be administered. As the glucose level decreases, it is usually necessary to decrease the rate of infusion. After the glucose reaches approximately 250 mg/dL, it is prudent to decrease the insulin infusion rate and administer dextrose. It usually takes an additional 12 to 24 hours to clear ketones from the circulation after hyperglycemia is controlled. With resolution of ketosis, the rate of infusion approaches the physiologic range of 0.3 to 0.5 U/kg per day.

When the decision is made to feed the patient, the patient should be switched from intravenous or intramuscular therapy to subcutaneous therapy. Subcutaneous insulin should be administered before a meal and the insulin drip discontinued approximately 30 minutes later. The glucose should be checked in 2 hours and at least every 4 hours subsequently until a relatively stable insulin regimen is determined. Early conversion to oral feeding and subcutaneous insulin therapy is associated with a shorter hospital stay.

Potassium

Potassium losses during the development of DKA are usually quite high (3-10 mEq/kg) and are mediated by shifts to the extracellular space secondary to acidosis and protein catabolism compounded by hyperaldosteronism and osmotic diuresis. Although most patients with DKA or HHNC have normal or even high serum potassium at presentation, the initial therapy with fluids and insulin causes it to fall.

Our approach has been to monitor the electrocardiogram (ECG) for signs of hyperkalemia (peaked T wave, QRS widening) initially and to administer potassium if these are absent and the serum potassium is less than 5.5 mEq/L. If the patient is oliguric, we do not administer potassium unless the serum concentration is less than 4 mEq/L or there are ECG signs of hypokalemia (U wave), and even then potassium is administered with extreme caution. With therapy of DKA, the potassium level always falls, usually reaching a nadir after several hours. We usually replace potassium at 10 to 20 mEq/hr (half as potassium chloride and half as potassium phosphate), monitor serum levels at least every 2 hours initially, and follow ECG morphology. Occasionally, patients with DKA who have had protracted courses that include vomiting, hypokalemia, and acidosis require 40 to 60 mEq/hr by central line to prevent further decreases in the serum potassium.

Phosphate

Like potassium, phosphate is depleted in patients with DKA. Although patients usually present with elevated serum phosphate, the serum level declines with therapy. No well-documented clinical significance of these findings has been determined and no benefit of phosphate administration has been demonstrated, but most authorities recommend phosphate therapy as before and monitoring for its possible complications, which include hypocalcemia and hypomagnesemia.

Bicarbonate

Serum bicarbonate is always low in DKA, but a true deficit is not present because the ketoacid and lactate anions are metabolized to bicarbonate during therapy. The use of bicarbonate in the therapy of DKA is highly controversial. No benefit of bicarbonate therapy has been demonstrated in clinical trials. In fact, in two trials, hypokalemia was more common in bicarbonate-treated patients. There are theoretical considerations against the use of bicarbonate. Cellular levels of 2,3-diphosphoglycerate are depleted in DKA, causing a shift in the oxyhemoglobin dissociation curve to the left and thus impairing tissue oxygen delivery. Acidemia has the opposite effect, and therefore reversing acidosis acutely could decrease tissue oxygen delivery. In addition, in vitro data suggest that pH is a regulator of cellular lactate metabolism and correction of acidosis could increase lactate production. These observations are of questionable clinical relevance, however.

We reserve bicarbonate therapy for patients with severe acidosis (pH < 6.9), for patients with hemodynamic instability if the pH is less than 7.1, or in cases of hyperkalemia with ECG findings. When bicarbonate is used, it should be used sparingly and considered a temporizing measure while definitive therapy with insulin and fluids is under way. Approximately 1 mEq/kg of bicarbonate is administered as a rapid infusion over 10 to 15 minutes, and further therapy is based on repeated arterial blood gases every 30 to 120 minutes. Potassium therapy should be considered before treatment with bicarbonate because transient hypokalemia is not an uncommon complication of the administration of alkali.

Monitoring

It is possible to manage many cases of mild DKA without admitting the patient to the intensive care unit, depending on staff availability. We routinely admit patients with DKA to the intensive care unit if they have a pH less than 7.3. If mental status is compromised, prophylactic intubation is considered and nasogastric suctioning is always performed because of frequent ileus and danger of aspiration. If the patient cannot void at will, bladder catheterization is necessary to follow urine output adequately. ECG monitoring is continuous, with hourly documentation of QRS intervals and T-wave morphology. Initially, serum glucose, electrolytes, BUN, creatinine, calcium, magnesium, phosphate, ketones, lactate, creatine phosphokinase, and liver function tests as well as urinalysis, ECG, upright chest radiograph, complete blood count, and arterial blood gases are obtained. If there is any concern about possible toxic ingestions, toxicology screening is also performed. Subsequently, glucose and electrolytes are measured at least hourly; calcium, magnesium, and phosphate every 2 hours; and BUN, creatinine, and ketones every 6 to 24 hours.

It is often not necessary to monitor arterial blood gases routinely because bicarbonate and anion gap are relatively good indices of the response to therapy. Monitoring venous pH has also been shown to reflect acidemia and response to therapy adequately. Usually, frequent blood work is necessary only for the first 12 hours or so. In the severely ill patient with obvious underlying disease, the course is often more protracted and, particularly when venous access is a problem, early consideration should be given to placement of an arterial line. A flow sheet tabulating these findings as well as mental status, vital signs, insulin dose, fluid and electrolytes administered, and urine output allows easy analysis of response to therapy. When the acidosis begins to resolve and the response to therapy becomes predictable, it is reasonable to curtail laboratory testing. If cardiovascular status is unclear or troublesome, invasive hemodynamic monitoring is an appropriate guide for fluid therapy. The goals should be to achieve hemodynamic stability rapidly and to correct DKA fully in 12 to 36 hours.

Search for Underlying Causes

After stabilizing the patient, a careful history and physical examination and a diagnostic strategy should be aimed at determining the precipitating event. In most inner-city practices, the most common cause of DKA is noncompliance with insulin therapy and is usually easily treated. The second most common cause is infection, with viral syndromes, urinary tract infection, pelvic inflammatory disease, and pneumonia predominating. It is often difficult to determine initially whether the patient is infected. Fever is absent in a significant fraction of patients with diabetic emergencies. The white blood cell count is not uncommonly elevated in the range of 20,000 or higher even in the absence of infection.[240] As a result, cultures should be performed for most patients, and if there is significant concern about infection, empirical broad antibiotic coverage should be considered pending microbiologic findings.

Special consideration should be given to ruling out meningitis in the patient with altered mental status. In this regard, most would perform lumbar punctures in all patients with meningismus and in patients with disproportionate mental status changes. If the index of suspicion is lower, gear the antibiotic therapy to cover bacterial meningitis and perform a lumbar puncture if the mental status does not improve quickly with therapy. The cerebrospinal fluid glucose is not particularly useful in determining whether the fluid is infected, and a cerebrospinal fluid glucose level less than 100 mg/dL is unusual when the serum glucose is greater than 250 mg/dL.[241] The relative frequency of sinus infection (particularly with *Mucor*), foot infection, bacterial arthritis, cholecystitis, cellulitis, and necrotizing fasciitis should also be considered.

Pneumonia can be difficult to diagnose in patients with dehydration because the alveolar edema fluid that shows up as an infiltrate on chest radiographs is often not present but develops along with progressive hypoxia during hydration. To prevent this occurrence, we administer intravenous fluid judiciously to patients we suspect have pneumonia. Pancreatitis and pregnancy are common precipitants and should be especially considered when assessing the abdominal pain that is almost ubiquitous at presentation. Abdominal guarding and tenderness associated with vomiting are common, and rebound is occasionally present. These symptoms and findings usually resolve quickly with therapy in the absence of intra-abdominal pathology. The serum amylase is often elevated without pathologic significance, although lipase is usually more specific.[242] Acute myocardial infarction and stroke as well as thromboembolic phenomena are frequent precipitants and complications of DKA.

The more insulin resistant the patient seems to be, the more likely one is to find a precipitating cause. If a precipitating cause is found, treatment is essential if adequate metabolic control is to be achieved.

Complications and Prognosis

It should now be possible to treat almost all cases of DKA successfully. The most troublesome complication is cerebral edema. It is common particularly in children and can be fatal. In most series, specific causes could not be assigned, although aggressive hydration, particularly with hypotonic fluids, can contribute.[243] In 50% of patients who subsequently had a respiratory arrest, there were premonitory symptoms, and despite early intervention only half of them avoided severe or fatal brain damage.

Other complications of life-threatening severity that have been reported include the acute respiratory distress syndrome and bronchial mucous plugging.[244-246] Arterial and venous thromboembolic events are quite common. Standard prophylactic low-dose heparin is certainly reasonable in patients with DKA, but currently no indication exists for full anticoagulation.

Two studies show that specialists (endocrinologists) provide more cost-effective care compared with nonspecialists. Patients under the care of specialists have a shorter hospital stay, fewer medical procedures, and lower medical costs.[247,248]

REFERENCES

1. Sutherland DE, Sibley R, Xu XA, et al. Twin-to-twin pancreas transplantation: reversal and reenactment of the pathogenesis of type I diabetes. Trans Assoc Am Physicians 1984;97:80-87.
2. Wang YO, Ponteselli RG, Gill RG, et al. The role of CD4 and CD8 T cells in the destruction of islet grafts by diabetic NOD mice. Proc Natl Acad Sci U S A 1991;88:527-531.
3. Devendra D, Liu E, Eisenbarth GS. Type 1 diabetes: recent developments. Brit Med J 2004;328(7442):750-754.
4. Glandt M, Herold KC. Treatment of type 1 diabetes with anti-T-cell agents: from T-cell depletion to T-cell regulation. Curr Diab Rep 2004;4(4):291-297.
5. American Diabetes Association. Clinical practice recommendations 2002. Diabetes Care 2002;25(suppl 1):S1-147.
6. Leslie RD, Atkinson MA, Notkins AL. Autoantigens IA-2 and GAD in type I (insulin-dependent) diabetes. Diabetologia 1999;42: 3-14.
7. Rewers M, Norris JM, Dabela D. Epidemiology of type I diabetes. In Eisenbarth GS, Lafferty KJ, eds. Type 1 Diabetes: Molecular, Cellular, and Clinical Immunology, 2nd ed. New York: Kluwer Academic, 2005:219-246.
8. Pinhas-Hamiel O, Dolan LM, Daniels SR, et al. Increased incidence of non–insulin dependent diabetes mellitus among adolescents. J Pediatr 1996;128:608-615.
9. Pinhas-Haniel O, Dolan LM, Zeitlers PS. Diabetic ketoacidosis among obese African-American adolescents with NIDDM. Diabetes Care 1997;20:484-486.
10. Rosenbloom AL, House DV, Winter WE. Non–insulin dependent diabetes mellitus (NIDDM) in minority youth: research priorities and needs. Clin Pediatr (Phila) 1998;37:143-152.
11. Imagawa A, Hanafusa T, Miyagawa J. A novel subtype of type 1 diabetes mellitus characterized by a rapid onset and an absence of diabetes-related antibodies. N Engl J Med 2000;342:301-307.
12. Ziegler A-G, Hummel M, Schenker M, Bonifacio E. Autoantibody appearance and risk for development of childhood diabetes in offspring of parents with type 1 diabetes: the 2-year analysis of the German BABYDIAB study. Diabetes 1999;48:460-468.
13. Mordes JP, Bortell R, Doukas J, et al. The BB/Wor rat and the balance hypothesis of autoimmunity. Diabetes Metab Rev 1996; 12:103-109.
14. Roep BO, Atkinson M, von Herrath M. Satisfaction (not) guaranteed: re-evaluating the use of animal models of type 1 diabetes. Nat Rev Immunol 2004;4(12):989-997.
15. Thomas HE, Kay TW. Beta cell destruction in the development of autoimmune diabetes in the non-obese diabetic (NOD) mouse. Diabetes Metab Res Rev 2000;16:251-261.
16. Wong FS, Janeway CAJ. Insulin-dependent diabetes mellitus and its animal models. Curr Opin Immunol 1999;11:643-647.
17. Eisenbarth GS. Animal models of type 1 diabetes: genetics and immunological function. In Eisenbarth GS, Lafferty KJ, eds. Type 1 Diabetes: Molecular, Cellular, and Clinical Immunology, 2nd ed. New York: Kluwer Academic, 2005:91-116.
18. Hattori M, Buse JB, Jackson RA, et al. The NOD mouse: recessive diabetogenic gene within the major histocompatibility complex. Science 1986;231:733-735.
19. Noble JA, Valdes AM, Cook M, et al. The role of HLA class II genes in insulin-dependent diabetes mellitus: molecular analysis of 180 caucasian, multiplex families. Am J Hum Genet 1996;59: 1134-1148.
20. Todd JA, Bell JI, McDevitt HO. HLA-DQB gene contributes to susceptibility and resistance to insulin-dependent diabetes mellitus. Nature 1987;329:599-604.
21. Nishimoto H, Kikutani H, Yamamura K, Kishimoto T. Prevention of autoimmune insulitis by expression of I-E molecules in NOD mice. Nature 1987;328:432-434.
22. Singer SM, Tisch R, Yang XD, et al. Prevention of diabetes in NOD mice by a mutated I-Ab transgene. Diabetes 1998;47:1570-1577.
23. Lyons PA, Hancock WW, Denny P, et al. The NOD Idd9 genetic interval influences the pathogenicity of insulitis and contains molecular variants of Cd30, Tnfr2, and Cd137. Immunity 2000; 13:107-115.
24. Mathews CE, Graser RT, Serreze DV, Leiter EH. Reevaluation of the major histocompatibility complex genes of the NOD-progenitor CTS/Shi strain. Diabetes 2000;49:131-134.
25. Yui MA, Muralidharan K, Moreno-Altamirano B, et al. Production of congenic mouse strains carrying NOD-derived diabetogenic genetic intervals: an approach for the genetic dissection of complex traits. Mamm Genome 1996;7:331-334.
26. Wicker LS, Miller BJ, Coker LZ, et al. Genetic control of diabetes and insulitis in the nonobese diabetic (NOD) mouse. J Exp Med 1987;165:1639-1654.
27. Yu L, Robles DT, Abiru N, et al. Early expression of anti-insulin autoantibodies of man and the NOD mouse: evidence for early determination of subsequent diabetes. Proc Natl Acad Sci U S A 2000;97:1701-1706.
28. Sreenan S, Pick AJ, Levisetti M, et al. Increased β-cell proliferation and reduced mass before diabetes onset in the nonobese diabetic mouse. Diabetes 1999;48:989-996.
29. Dilts SM, Lafferty KJ. Autoimmune diabetes: the involvement of benign and malignant autoimmunity. J Autoimmun 1999;12: 229-232.
30. Shimada A, Charlton B, Taylor-Edwards C, Fathman CG. β-Cell destruction may be a late consequence of the autoimmune process in nonobese diabetic mice. Diabetes 1996;45:1063-1067.
31. Chatenoud L, Primo J, Bach JF. CD3 antibody-induced dominant self tolerance in overtly diabetic NOD mice. J Immunol 1997;158:2947-2954.
32. Wegmann DR, Eisenbarth GS. It's Insulin. J Autoimmun 2000;15: 286-291.
33. Nagata M, Santamaria P, Kawamura T, et al. Evidence for the role of $CD8^+$ cytotoxic T cells in the destruction of pancreatic β-cells in nonobese diabetic mice. J Immunol 1994;152:2042-2050.

34. Schmidt D, Amrani A, Verdaguer J, et al. Autoantigen-independent deletion of diabetogenic CD4+ thymocytes by protective MHC class II molecules. J Immunol 1999;162:4627-4636.
35. Haskins K. T cell receptor gene usage in autoimmune diabetes. Int Rev Immunol 1999;18:61-81.
36. Nakayama M, Abiru N, Moriyama H, et al. Prime role for an insulin epitope in the development of type 1 diabetes in NOD mice. Nature 2005;435(7039):220-223.
37. Tian J, Atkinson M, Clare-Salzer M, et al. Nasal administration of glutamate decarboxylase (GAD65) peptides induces Th2 responses and prevents murine insulin dependent diabetes. J Exp Med 1996;183:1561-1567.
38. Muir A, Peck A, Clare-Salzler M, et al. Insulin immunization of nonobese diabetic mice induces a protective insulitis characterized by diminished intraislet interferon-gamma transcription. J Clin Invest 1995;95:628-634.
39. Cetkovic-Cvrlje M, Gerling IC, Muir A, et al. Retardation or acceleration of diabetes in NOD/Lt mice mediated by intrathymic administration of candidate β-cell antigens. Diabetes 1997;46:1975-1982.
40. Daniel D, Wegmann DR. Protection of nonobese diabetic mice from diabetes by intranasal or subcutaneous administration of insulin peptide B-(9-23). Proc Natl Acad Sci U S A 1996;93:956-960.
41. Awata T, Guberski DL, Like AA. Genetics of the BB rat: association of autoimmune disorders (diabetes, insulitis, and thyroiditis) with lymphopenia and major histocompatibility complex class II. Endocrinology 1995;136:5731-5735.
42. Achenbach P, Koczwara K, Knopff A, et al. Mature high-affinity immune responses to (pro)insulin anticipate the autoimmune cascade that leads to type 1 diabetes. J Clin Invest 2004;114(4):589-597.
43. Jacob HJ, Pettersson A, Wilson D, et al. Genetic dissection of autoimmune type I diabetes in the BB rat. Nat Genet 1992;2:56-60.
44. Hornum L., Romer J, Markholst H. The diabetes-prone BB rat carries a frameshift mutation in *Ian4*, a positional candidate of *Iddm1*. Diabetes 2002;51(6):1972-1979.
45. Gottlieb PA, Handler ES, Appel MC, et al. Insulin treatment prevents diabetes mellitus but not thyroiditis in RT 6–depleted diabetes resistant BB/Wor rats. Diabetologia 1991;34:296-300.
46. Song HY, Abad MM, Mahoney CP, McEvoy RC. Human insulin B chain but not A chain decreases the rate of diabetes in BB rats. Diabetes Res Clin Pract 1999;46:109-114.
47. Yokoi N, Komeda K, Wang HY, et al. Cblb is a major susceptibility gene for rat type 1 diabetes mellitus. Nat Genet 2002;31(4):391-394.
48. Kawano K, Hirashima T, Mori S, et al. New inbred strain of Long-Evans Tokushima lean rats with IDDM without lymphopenia. Diabetes 1991;40:1375-1381.
49. Yokoi N, Kanazawa M, Kitada K, et al. A non-MHC locus essential for autoimmune type I diabetes in the Komeda diabetes-prone rat. J Clin Invest 1997;100:2015-2021.
50. Uchigata Y, Yamamoto H, Nagai H, Okamoto H. Effect of poly(ADP-ribose) synthetase inhibitor administration to rats before and after injection of alloxan and streptozotocin on islet proinsulin synthesis. Diabetes 1983;32:316-318.
51. Tanaka SI, Nakajima AS, Inoue S, et al. Genetic control by I-A subregion in H-2 complex of incidence of streptozotocin-induced autoimmune diabetes in mice. Diabetes 1990;39:1298-1304.
52. Ellerman KE, Like AA. Susceptibility to diabetes is widely distributed in normal class IIu haplotype rats. Diabetologia 2000;43:890-898.
53. Birk OS, Elias D, Weiss AS, et al. NOD mouse diabetes: the ubiquitous mouse hsp60 is a beta-cell target antigen of autoimmune T cells. J Autoimmun 1996;9:159-166.
54. Ablamunits V, Elias D, Reshef T, Cohen IR. Islet T cells secreting IFN-γ in NOD mouse diabetes: arrest by p277 peptide treatment. J Autoimmun 1998;11:73-81.
55. Pipeleers D, Ling Z. Pancreatic beta cells in insulin-dependent diabetes. Diabetes Metab Rev 1992;8:209-227.
56. Foulis AK, Clark A. Pathology of the pancreas in diabetes mellitus. In Kahn CR, Weir GC, eds. Joslin's Diabetes Mellitus, 13th ed. Philadelphia: Lea & Febiger, 1994:265-281.
57. Doniach D, Morgan AG. Islets of Langerhans in juvenile diabetes mellitus. Clin Endocrinol (Oxf) 1973;2:233-248.
58. Gepts W, LeCompte PM. The pancreatic islets in diabetes. Am J Med 1981;70:105-115.
59. Foulis AK, Liddle CN, Farquharson MA, et al. The histopathology of the pancreas in type I diabetes (insulin dependent) mellitus: a 25-year review of deaths in patients under 20 years of age in the United Kingdom. Diabetologia 1986;29:267-274.
60. Foulis AK, Farquharson MA, Hardman R. Aberrant expression of class II major histocompatibility complex molecules by β cells and hyperexpression of class I major histocompatibility complex molecules by insulin containing islets in type 1 (insulin dependent) diabetes mellitus. Diabetologia 1987;30:333-343.
61. Huang X, Yuan J, Goddard A, et al. Interferon expression in the pancreases of patients with type I diabetes. Diabetes 1995;44:658-664.
62. Milton MJ, Poulin M, Mathews C, Piganelli JD. Generation, maintenance, and adoptive transfer of diabetogenic T-cell lines/clones from the nonobese diabetic mouse. Methods Mol Med 2004;102:213-225.
63. Amrani A, Verdaguer J, Thiessen S, et al. IL-1α, IL-1β, and IFN-γ mark beta cells for fas-dependent destruction by diabetogenic CD4+ T lymphocytes. J Clin Invest 2000;105:459-468.
64. Itoh N, Imagawa A, Hanafusa T, et al. Requirement of Fas for the development of autoimmune diabetes in nonobese diabetic mice. J Exp Med 1997;186:613-618.
65. Chervonsky AV, Wang Y, Wong FS, et al. The role of Fas in autoimmune diabetes. Cell 1997;89:17-24.
66. Thomas HE, Kay TW. How beta cells die in type 1 diabetes. Curr Dir Autoimmun 2001;4:144-70.
67. Marleau AM, Sarvetnick N. T cell homeostasis in tolerance and immunity. J Leukoc Biol 2005;78(3):575-584.
68. Lo D. Immune regulation: susceptibility and resistance to autoimmunity. Immunol Res 2000;21:239-246.
69. Wong FS, Janeway CAJ. The role of CD4 vs. CD8 T cells in IDDM. J Autoimmun 1999;13:290-295.
70. Lieberman SM, Takaki T, Han B, et al. Individual nonobese diabetic mice exhibit unique patterns of CD8+ T cell reactivity to three islet antigens, including the newly identified widely expressed dystrophia myotonica kinase. J Immunol 2004;173(11):6727-6734.
71. Wong FS, Dittel BN, Janeway CAJ. Transgenes and knockout mutations in animal models of type 1 diabetes and multiple sclerosis. Immunol Rev 1999;169:93-104.
72. Ylipaasto P, Klingel K, Lindberg AM, et al. Enterovirus infection in human pancreatic islet cells, islet tropism in vivo and receptor involvement in cultured islet beta cells. Diabetologia 2004;47(2):225-239.
73. Foulis AK, McGill M, Farquharson MA, Hilton DA. A search for evidence of viral infection in pancreases of newly diagnosed patients with IDDM. Diabetologia 1997;40:53-61.
74. Thorsby E. Invited anniversary review: HLA associated diseases. Hum Immunol 1997;53:1-11.
75. Yu J, Shin CH, Yang SW, et al. Analysis of children with type 1 diabetes in Korea: high prevalence of specific anti-islet autoantibodies, immunogenetic similarities to Western populations with "unique" haplotypes, and lack of discrimination by aspartic acid at position 57 of DQB. Clin Immunol 2004;113(3):318-325.
76. Anderson MS, Venanzi ES, Klein L, et al. Projection of an immunological self shadow within the thymus by the aire protein. Science 2002;298(5597):1395-1401.
77. Clark LB, Appleby MW, Brunkow ME, et al. Cellular and molecular characterization of the scurfy mouse mutant. J Immunol 1999;162:2546-2554.
78. Powell BR, Buist NR, Stenzel P. An X-linked syndrome of diarrhea, polyendocrinopathy, and fatal infection in infancy. J Pediatr 1982;100:731-737.
79. Roberts J, Searle J. Neonatal diabetes mellitus associated with severe diarrhea, hyperimmunoglobulin E syndrome, and absence of islets of Langerhans. Pediatr Pathol Lab Med 1995;15:477-483.
80. Cilio CM, Bosco A, Moretti C, et al. Congenital autoimmune diabetes mellitus (letter). N Engl J Med 2000;342:1529-1531.
81. Kanangat S, Blair P, Reddy R, et al. Disease in the scurfy (sf) mouse is associated with overexpression of cytokine genes. Eur J Immunol 1996;26:161-165.

82. Fontenot JD, Gavin MA, Rudensky AY. Foxp3 programs the development and function of CD4+CD25+ regulatory T cells. Nat Immunol 2003;4(4):330-336.
83. Rewers M, Norris J, Dabelea D. Epidemiology of Type 1 Diabetes Mellitus. Adv Exp Med Biol 2004;552:219-246.
84. Redondo MJ, Yu L, Hawa M, et al. Late progression to type 1 diabetes of discordant twins of patients with type 1 diabetes: combined analysis of two twin series (United States and United Kingdom) (abstract). Diabetes 1999;48:780.
85. Kyvik KO, Green A, Beck-Nielsen H. Concordance rates of insulin dependent diabetes mellitus: a population based study of young Danish twins. BMJ 1995;311:913-917.
86. Committee on Diabetic Twins, Japan Diabetes Society. Diabetes mellitus in twins: a cooperative study in Japan. Diabetes Res Clin Pract 1988;5:271-280.
87. Ikegami H, Ogihara T. Genetics of insulin-dependent diabetes mellitus. Endocr J 1996;43:605-613.
88. Barnett AH, Eff C, Leslie RD, Pyke DA. Diabetes in identical twins: a study of 200 pairs. Diabetologia 1981;20:87-93.
89. Redondo MJ, Yu L, Hawa M, et al. Heterogeneity of type 1 diabetes: analysis of monozygotic twins in Great Britain and the United States. Diabetologia 2001;44:354-362.
90. Bowden DW, Akots G, Rothschild CB, et al. Linkage analysis of maturity-onset diabetes of the young (MODY): genetic heterogeneity and nonpenetrance. Am J Hum Genet 1992;50:607-618.
91. Bao F, Yu L, Babu S, et al. One third of HLA DQ2 homozygous patients with type 1 diabetes express celiac disease associated transglutaminase autoantibodies. J Autoimmun 1999;13:143-148.
92. Yu L, Brewer KW, Gates S, et al. DRB104 and DQ alleles: expression of 21-hydroxylase autoantibodies and risk of progression to Addison's disease. J Clin Endocrinol Metab 1999;84:328-335.
93. De Block CE, De Leeuw IH, Van Gaal LF. High prevalence of manifestations of gastric autoimmunity in parietal cell antibody-positive type 1 (insulin-dependent) diabetic patients. The Belgian Diabetes Registry. J Clin Endocrinol Metab 1999;84:4062-4067.
94. Nepom GT, Kwok WW. Perspectives in diabetes: molecular basis for HLA-DQ associations with IDDM. Diabetes 1998;47:1177-1184.
95. McDevitt HO. The role of MHC class II molecules in susceptibility and resistance to autoimmunity. Curr Opin Immunol 1998;10:677-681.
96. Eisenbarth GS. Genetic counseling for type 1 diabetes. In Lebovitz H ed. Therapy for Diabetes Mellitus and Related Disorders. Alexandria, VA: American Diabetes Association, 2004:000-000.
97. Nakanishi K, Kobayashi T, Murase T, et al. Human leukocyte antigen-A24 and -DQA10301 in Japanese insulin-dependent diabetes mellitus: independent contributions to susceptibility to the disease and additive contributions to acceleration of beta-cell destruction. J Clin Endocrinol Metab 1999;84:3721-3725.
98. Rewers M, Bugawan TL, Norris JM, et al. Newborn screening for HLA markers associated with IDDM: diabetes autoimmunity study in the young (DAISY). Diabetologia 1996;39:807-812.
99. Kulmala P, Savola K, Reijonen H, et al. Genetic markers, humoral autoimmunity, and prediction of type 1 diabetes in siblings of affected children. Childhood Diabetes in Finland Study Group. Diabetes 2000;49:48-58.
100. Redondo MJ, Kawasaki E, Mulgrew CL, et al. DR and DQ associated protection from type 1 diabetes: comparison of DRB11401 and DQA*10102-DQB*10602. J Clin Endocrinol Metab 2000;85:3793-3797.
101. Kawasaki E, Noble J, Erlich H, et al. Transmission of DQ haplotypes to patients with type 1 diabetes. Diabetes 1998;47:1971-1973.
102. Morel PA, Dorman JS, Todd JA, et al. Aspartic acid at position 57 of the HLA-DQ beta chain protects against type I diabetes: a family study. Proc Natl Acad Sci U S A 1988;85:8111-8115.
103. Bell GI, Horita S, Karam JH. A polymorphic locus near the human insulin gene is associated with insulin-dependent diabetes mellitus. Diabetes 1984;33:176-183.
104. Bennett ST, Lucassen AM, Gough SCL, et al. Susceptibility to human type I diabetes at *IDDM2* is determined by tandem repeat variation at the insulin gene minisatellite locus. Nat Genet 1995;9:284-292.
105. Pugliese A, Zeller M, Fernandez A, et al. The insulin gene is transcribed in the human thymus and transcription levels correlate with allelic variation at the INS VNTR-IDDM2 susceptibility locus for type I diabetes. Nat Genet 1997;15:293-297.
106. Vafiadis P, Bennett ST, Todd JA, et al. Insulin expression in human thymus is modulated by INS VNTR alleles at the IDDM2 locus. Nat Genet 1997;15:289-292.
107. Hanahan D. Peripheral-antigen-expressing cells in thymic medulla: factors in self-tolerance and autoimmunity. Curr Opin Immunol 1998;10:656-662.
108. Bottini N, Musumeci L, Alonso A, et al. A functional variant of lymphoid tyrosine phosphatase is associated with type I diabetes. Nat Genet 2004;36(4):337-338.
109. Todd JA, Farrall M. Panning for gold: genome-wide scanning for linkage in type I diabetes. Hum Mol Genet 1996;5:1443-1448.
110. Concannon P, Gogolin-Ewens KJ, Hinds DA, et al. A second-generation screen of the human genome for susceptibility to insulin-dependent diabetes mellitus. Nat Genet 1998;19:292-296.
111. Pugliese A, Eisenbarth GS. Type 1 diabetes mellitus of man: genetic susceptibility and resistance. In Eisenbarth GS, Lafferty KJ, eds. Type 1 Diabetes: Molecular, Cellular, and Clinical Immunology, 2nd ed. New York: Kluwer Academic, 2005:170-203.
112. Larsen ZM, Kristiansen OP, Mato E, et al. *IDDM12* (CTLA4) on 2q33 and *IDDM13* on 2q34 in genetic susceptibility to type 1 diabetes (insulin-dependent). Autoimmunity 1999;31:35-42.
113. Vella A, Cooper JD, Lowe CE, et al. Localization of a type 1 diabetes locus in the IL2RA/CD25 region by use of tag single-nucleotide polymorphisms. Am J Hum Genet 2005;76(5):773-779.
114. Smyth DJ, Howson JM, Lowe CE, et al. Assessing the validity of the association between the SUMO4 M55V variant and risk of type 1 diabetes. Nat Genet 2005;37(2):110-111; author reply 112-113.
115. Verge CF, Vardi P, Babu S, et al. Evidence for oligogenic inheritance of type 1A diabetes in a large Bedouin Arab family. J Clin Invest 1998;102:1569-1575.
116. Eisenbarth GS, Elsey C, Yu L, Rewers M. Infantile anti-islet autoimmunity: DAISY study (abstract). Diabetes 1998;47:A210.
117. Schenker M, Hummel M, Ferber K, et al. Early expression and high prevalence of islet autoantibodies for DR3/4 heterozygous and DR4/4 homozygous offspring of parents with type I diabetes: the German BABYDIAB study. Diabetologia 1999;42:671-677.
118. Robles DT, Eisenbarth GS. Type 1A diabetes induced by infection and immunization. J Autoimmun 2001;16:355-362.
119. Ellerman KE, Richards CA, Guberski DL, et al. Kilham rat virus triggers T cell-dependent autoimmune diabetes in multiple strains of rat. Diabetes 1996;45:557-562.
120. Gardner SG, Bingley PJ, Sawtell PA, et al. Rising incidence of insulin dependent diabetes in children aged under 5 years in the Oxford region: time trend analysis. BMJ 1997;315:713-717.
121. Tuomilehto J, Karvonen M, Pitkaniemi J, et al. Record-high incidence of type I (insulin-dependent) diabetes mellitus in Finnish children. The Finnish Childhood Type I Diabetes Registry Group. Diabetologia 1999;42:655-660.
122. Feltbower RG, McKinney PA, Bodansky HJ. Rising incidence of childhood diabetes is seen at all ages and in urban and rural settings in Yorkshire, United Kingdom (letter). Diabetologia 2000;43:682-684.
123. Shaver KA, Boughman JA, Nance WE. Congenital rubella syndrome and diabetes: a review of epidemiologic, genetic, and immunologic factors. Am Ann Deaf 1985;130:526-532.
124. Rubenstein P. The HLA system in congenital rubella patients with and without diabetes. Diabetes 1982;31:1088-1091.
125. Clarke WL, Shaver KA, Bright GM, et al. Autoimmunity in congenital rubella syndrome. J Pediatr 1984;104:370-373.
126. Ou D, Jonsen LA, Metzger DL, Tingle AJ. CD4+ and CD8+ T cell clones from congenital rubella syndrome patients with IDDM recognize overlapping GAD65 protein epitopes: implications for HLA class I and II allelic linkage to disease susceptibility. Hum Immunol 1999;60:652-664.
127. Rabinowe SL, George KL, Loughlin R, et al. Congenital rubella: monoclonal antibody-defined T cell abnormalities in young adults. Am J Med 1986;81:779-782.
128. Yoon JW, Austin M, Onodera T, Notkins A. Isolation of a virus from the pancreas of a child with diabetic ketoacidosis. N Engl J Med 1979;300:1173-1179.
129. Nigro G, Pacella ME, Patane E, Midulla M. Multi-system Coxsackie virus B-6 infection with findings suggestive of diabetes mellitus. Eur J Pediatr 1986;145:557-559.

130. Lonnrot M, Korpela K, Knip M, et al. Enterovirus infection as a risk factor for beta-cell autoimmunity in a prospectively observed birth cohort: the Finnish Diabetes Prediction and Prevention Study. Diabetes 2000;49:1314-1318.
131. Graves PM, Rewers M. The role of enteroviral infections in the development of IDDM: limitations of current approaches. Diabetes 1997;46:161-168.
132. Honeyman MC, Coulson BS, Stone NL, et al. Association between rotavirus infection and pancreatic islet autoimmunity in children at risk of developing type 1 diabetes. Diabetes 2000;49:1319-1324.
133. Classen DC, Classen JB. The timing of pediatric immunization and the risk of insulin-dependent diabetes mellitus. Infect Dis Clin Pract 1997;6:449-454.
134. Karvonen M, Cepaitis Z, Tuomilehto J. Association between type 1 diabetes and *Haemophilus influenzae* type b vaccination: birth cohort study. BMJ 1999;318:1169-1172.
135. Lindberg B, Ahlfors K, Carlsson A, et al. Previous exposure to measles, mumps, and rubella—but not vaccination during adolescence—correlates to the prevalence of pancreatic and thyroid autoantibodies. Pediatrics 1999;104:e12.
136. Graves PM, Barriga KJ, Norris JM, et al. Lack of association between early childhood immunizations and beta-cell autoimmunity. Diabetes Care 1999;22:1694-1697.
137. Bao F, Rewers M, Scott F, Eisenbarth GS. Celiac disease. In Eisenbarth GS ed. Endocrine and Organ Specific Autoimmunity. Austin, TX: RG Landes, 1999:85-96.
138. Scott FW, Cloutier HE, Kleemann R, et al. Potential mechanisms by which certain foods promote or inhibit the development of spontaneous diabetes in BB rats. Diabetes 1997;46:589-598.
139. Akerblom HK, Savilahti E, Saukkonen TT, et al. The case for elimination of cow's milk in early infancy in the prevention of type 1 diabetes: the Finnish experience. Diabetes Metab Rev 1993;9: 269-278.
140. Virtanen SM, Laara E, Hypponen E, et al. Cow's milk consumption, HLA-DQB1 genotype, and type 1 diabetes: a nested case-control study of siblings of children with diabetes. Childhood Diabetes in Finland Study Group. Diabetes 2000;49:912-917.
141. Virtanen SM, Rasanen L, Aro A, et al. Infant feeding in Finnish children less than 7 yr of age with newly diagnosed IDDM. Childhood Diabetes in Finland Study Group. Diabetes Care 1991;14: 415-417.
142. Couper JJ, Steele C, Beresford S, et al. Lack of association between duration of breast-feeding or introduction of cow's milk and development of islet autoimmunity. Diabetes 1999;48:2145-2149.
143. Norris JM, Beaty B, Klingensmith G, et al. Lack of association between early exposure to cow's milk protein and β-cell autoimmunity: Diabetes Autoimmunity Study in the Young (DAISY). JAMA 1996;276:609-614.
144. Akerblom HK, Virtanen SM, Ilonen J, et al. Dietary manipulation of beta cell autoimmunity in infants at increased risk of type 1 diabetes: a pilot study. Diabetologia 2005;48(5):829-837.
145. Norris JM, Barriga K, Klingensmith G, et al. Timing of initial cereal exposure in infancy and risk of islet autoimmunity. JAMA 2003;290(13):1713-1720.
146. Ziegler AG, Schmid S, Huber D, et al. Early infant feeding and risk of developing type 1 diabetes-associated autoantibodies. JAMA 2003;290(13):1721-1728.
147. Andre I, Gonzalez A, Wong B, et al. Checkpoints in the progression of autoimmune disease: lessons from diabetes models. Proc Natl Acad Sci U S A 1996;93:2260-2263.
148. Fennessy M, Metcalfe K, Hitman GA, et al. A gene in the HLA class I region contributes to susceptibility to IDDM in the Finnish population. Childhood Diabetes in Finland (DiMe) Study Group. Diabetologia 1994;37:937-944.
149. Kockum I, Sanjeevi CB, Eastman S, et al. Population analysis of protection by HLA-DR and DQ genes from insulin-dependent diabetes mellitus in Swedish children with insulin-dependent diabetes and controls. Eur J Immunogenet 1995;22:443-465.
150. Vardi P, Ziegler AG, Matthews JH, et al. Concentration of insulin autoantibodies at onset of type I diabetes: inverse log-linear correlation with age. Diabetes Care 1988;11:736-739.
151. Arslanian SL, Becker DJ, Rabin B, et al. Correlates of insulin antibodies in newly diagnosed children with insulin-dependent diabetes before insulin therapy. Diabetes 1985;34:926-930.
152. Eisenbarth GS, Gianani R, Yu L, et al. Dual-parameter model for prediction of type 1 diabetes mellitus. Proc Assoc Am Physicians 1998;110:126-135.
153. Pugliese A, Kawasaki E, Zeller M, et al. Sequence analysis of the diabetes-protective human leukocyte antigen-DQB*10602 allele in unaffected, islet cell antibody-positive first degree relatives and in rare patients with type 1 diabetes. J Clin Endocrinol Metab 1999;84: 1722-1728.
154. Achenbach P, Koczwara K, Knopff A, et al. Mature high-affinity immune responses to (pro)insulin anticipate the autoimmune cascade that leads to type 1 diabetes. J Clin Invest 2004;114(4): 589-597.
155. Barker JM, Barriga KL, Yu L, et al. Prediction of autoantibody positivity and progression to type 1 diabetes: Diabetes Autoimmunity Study in the Young (DAISY). J Clin Endocrinol Metab 2004;89(8):3896-3902.
156. Verge CF, Gianani R, Kawasaki E, et al. Prediction of type I diabetes in first-degree relatives using a combination of insulin, GAD, and ICA512bdc/IA-2 autoantibodies. Diabetes 1996;45:926-933.
157. Bingley PJ, Bonifacio E, Williams AJK, et al. Prediction of IDDM in the general population: strategies based on combinations of autoantibody markers. Diabetes 1997;46:1701-1710.
158. Chase HP, Cuthbertson DD, Dolan LM, et al. First phase insulin release during the intravenous glucose tolerance test as a risk factor for type 1 diabetes. J Pediatr 2001;138:244-249.
159. Bingley PJ, Colman P, Eisenbarth GS, et al. Standardization of IVGTT to predict IDDM. Diabetes Care 1992;15:1313-1316.
160. Bingley PJ. Interactions of age, islet cell antibodies, insulin autoantibodies, and first-phase insulin response in predicting risk of progression to IDDM in ICA$^+$ relatives: the ICARUS data set. Diabetes 1996;45:1720-1728.
161. The DCCT Research Group. Epidemiology of severe hypoglycemia in the diabetes control and complications trial. Am J Med 1991;90:450-459.
162. Palmer JP, Fleming GA, Greenbaum CJ, et al. C-peptide is the appropriate outcome measure for type 1 diabetes clinical trials to preserve beta-cell function: report of an ADA workshop, 21-22 October 2001. Diabetes 2004;53(1):250-264.
163. Füchtenbusch M, Ferber K, Standl E, et al. Prediction of type I diabetes postpartum in patients with gestational diabetes mellitus by combined islet cell autoantibody screening: a prospective multicenter study. Diabetes 1997;46:1459-1467.
164. Zimmet PZ, Tuomi T, Mackay IR, et al. Latent autoimmune diabetes mellitus in adults (LADA): the role of antibodies to glutamic acid decarboxylase in diagnosis and prediction of insulin dependency. Diabet Med 1994;11:299-303.
165. Turner R, Stratton I, Horton V, et al. UKPDS 25: autoantibodies to islet-cell cytoplasm and glutamic acid decarboxylase for prediction of insulin requirement in type 2 diabetes. UK Prospective Diabetes Study Group. Lancet 1997;350:1288-1293.
166. Horton V, Stratton I, Bottazzo GF, et al. Genetic heterogeneity of autoimmune diabetes: age of presentation in adults is influenced by HLA DRB1 and DQB1 genotypes (UKPDS 43). UK Prospective Diabetes Study (UKPDS) Group. Diabetologia 1999;42: 608-616.
167. Ricker AT, Herskowitz R, Wolfsdorf JI, et al. Prognostic factors in children and young adults presenting with transient hyperglycemia or impaired glucose tolerance (abstract). Diabetes 1986; 35(suppl 1):93A.
168. Assan R, Feutren G, Debray-Sachs M, et al. Metabolic and immunological effects of cyclosporine in recently diagnosed type I diabetes mellitus. Lancet 1985;1:67-71.
169. Chase HP, Butler-Simon N, Garg SK, et al. Cyclosporine A for the treatment of new-onset insulin-dependent diabetes mellitus. Pediatrics 1990;85:241-245.
170. Stiller CR, Dupre J, Gent M, et al. Effects of cyclosporine immunosuppression in insulin-dependent diabetes mellitus of recent onset. Science 1984;223:1362-1367.
171. Carel J-C, Boitard C, Eisenbarth G, et al. Cyclosporine delays but does not prevent clinical onset in glucose intolerant pre-type 1 diabetic children. J Autoimmun 1996;9:739-745.
172. Cook JJ, Hudson I, Harrison LC, et al. Double-blind controlled trial of azathioprine in children with newly diagnosed type I diabetes. Diabetes 1989;38:779-783.

173. Silverstein J, Maclaren N, Riley W, et al. Immunosuppression with azathioprine and prednisone in recent-onset insulin-dependent diabetes mellitus. N Engl J Med 1988;319:599-604.
174. Eisenbarth GS, Srikanta S, Jackson R, et al. Anti-thymocyte globulin and prednisone immunotherapy of recent onset type I diabetes mellitus. Diabetes Res 1985;2:271-276.
175. Buckingham BA, Sandborg CI. A randomized trial of methotrexate in newly diagnosed patients with type 1 diabetes mellitus. Clin Immunol 2000;96:86-90.
176. Herold KC, Hagopian W, Auger JA, et al. Anti-CD3 monoclonal antibody in new-onset type 1 diabetes mellitus. N Engl J Med 2002;346:1692-1698.
177. Herold KC, Gitelman SE, Masharani U, et al. A single course of anti-CD3 monoclonal antibody hOKT3γ1(Ala-Ala) results in improvement in C-peptide responses and clinical parameters for at least 2 years after onset of type 1 diabetes. Diabetes 2005; 54(6):1763-1769.
178. Weiner HL, Miller A, Khoury SJ, et al. Suppression of organ-specific autoimmune diseases by oral administration of autoantigens. In Proceedings of the 8th International Congress on Immunology. Heidelberg: Springer-Verlag, 1992:627-634.
179. Zhang ZJ, Davidson L, Eisenbarth G, Weiner HL. Suppression of diabetes in nonobese diabetic mice by oral administration of porcine insulin. Proc Natl Acad Sci U S A 1991;88:10252-10256.
180. Atkinson MA, Maclaren NK, Luchetta R. Insulitis and diabetes in NOD mice reduced by prophylactic insulin therapy. Diabetes 1990;39:933-937.
181. Diabetes Prevention Trial—Type 1 Diabetes Study Group. Effects of insulin in relatives of patients with type 1 diabetes mellitus. N Engl J Med 2002;346(22):1685-1691.
182. Skyler JS, Krischer JP, Wolfsdorf J, et al. Effects of oral insulin in relatives of patients with type 1 diabetes: The Diabetes Prevention Trial—Type 1. Diabetes Care 2005;28(5):1068-1076.
183. Robertson RP, Sutherland DER, Kendall DM, et al. Metabolic characterization of long-term successful pancreas transplants in type I diabetes. J Investig Med 1996;44:549-555.
184. Robertson RP, Kendall D, Teuscher A, Sutherland DER. Long-term metabolic control with pancreatic transplantation. Transplant Proc 1994;26:386-387.
185. Naftanel MA, Harlan DM. Pancreatic islet transplantation. PLoS Med 2004;1(3):e58; quiz e75.
186. Nakhleh RE, Gruessner RWG, Swanson PE, et al. Pancreas transplant pathology: a morphologic, immunohistochemical, and electron microscopic comparison of allogeneic grafts with rejection, syngeneic grafts, and chronic pancreatitis. Am J Surg Pathol 1991;15:246-256.
187. Shapiro AM, Lakey JR, Ryan EA, et al. Islet transplantation in seven patients with type 1 diabetes mellitus using a glucocorticoid-free immunosuppressive regimen. N Engl J Med 2000;343:230-238.
188. Nanji SA, Shapiro AM. Advances in pancreatic islet transplantation in humans. Diabetes Obes Metab 2006;8(1):15-25.
189. Uchigata Y, Kuwata S, Tsushima T, et al. Patients with Graves' disease who developed insulin autoimmune syndrome (Hirata disease) possess HLA-Bw62/Cw4/DR4 carrying DRB*10406. J Clin Endocrinol Metab 1993;77:249-254.
190. Uchigata Y, Hirata Y. Insulin autoimmune syndrome (IAS, Hirata disease). In Eisenbarth G ed. Molecular Mechanisms of Endocrine and Organ Specific Autoimmunity. Austin, Tex: RG Landes, 1999:133-148.
191. Menon RK, Cohen RM, Sperling MA, et al. Transplacental passage of insulin in pregnant women with insulin-dependent diabetes mellitus: its role in fetal macrosomia. N Engl J Med 1990;323: 309-315.
192. Schernthaner G. Immunogenicity and allergenic potential of animal and human insulins. Diabetes Care 1993;16:155-165.
193. Taylor SI, Grunberger G, Marcus-Samuels B, et al. Hypoglycemia associated with antibodies to the insulin receptor. N Engl J Med 1982;307:1422-1426.
194. Dons RF, Havlik R, Taylor SI, et al. Clinical disorders associated with autoantibodies to the insulin receptor: simulation by passive transfer of immunoglobulins to rats. J Clin Invest 1983;72: 1072-1080.
195. Engerman R, Bloodworth JM Jr, Nelson S. Relationship of microvascular disease in diabetes to metabolic control. Diabetes 1977;26:760-769.
196. Engerman RL, Kern TS. Progression of incipient diabetic retinopathy during good glycemic control. Diabetes 1987;36:808-812.
197. Cohen AJ, McGill PD, Rossetti RG, et al. Glomerulopathy in spontaneously diabetic rat: impact of glycemic control. Diabetes 1987;36:944-951.
198. Klein R, Klein BE, Moss SE, et al. The Wisconsin epidemiologic study of diabetic retinopathy. II. Prevalence and risk of diabetic retinopathy when age at diagnosis is less than 30 years. Arch Ophthalmol 1984;102:520-526.
199. Klein R, Klein BE, Moss SE, et al. Glycosylated hemoglobin predicts the incidence and progression of diabetic retinopathy. JAMA 1988;260:2864-2871.
200. Chase HP, Jackson WE, Hoops SL, et al. Glucose control and the renal and retinal complications of insulin-dependent diabetes. JAMA 1989;261:1155-1160.
201. The effect of intensive treatment of diabetes on the development and progression of long-term complications in insulin-dependent diabetes mellitus. The Diabetes Control and Complications Trial Research Group. N Engl J Med 1993;329:977-986.
202. Effect of intensive diabetes management on macrovascular events and risk factors in the Diabetes Control and Complications Trial. Am J Cardiol 1995;75:894-903.
203. Nathan DM, Cleary PA, Backlund JY, et al. Intensive diabetes treatment and cardiovascular disease in patients with type 1 diabetes. N Engl J Med 2005;353(25):2643-2653.
204. Sherwin R, Felig P. Hypoglycemia. In Felig P ed. Endocrinology and Metabolism, 2nd ed. New York: McGraw-Hill, 1987:1043-1178.
205. Purnell JQ, Hokanson JE, Marcovina SM, et al. Effect of excessive weight gain with intensive therapy of type 1 diabetes on lipid levels and blood pressure: results from the DCCT. Diabetes Control and Complications Trial. JAMA 1998;280:140-146.
206. Blood glucose control and the evolution of diabetic retinopathy and albuminuria: a preliminary multicenter trial. The Kroc Collaborative Study Group. N Engl J Med 1984;311:365-372.
207. Lauritzen T, Frost-Larsen K, Larsen HW, Deckert T. Effect of 1 year of near-normal blood glucose levels on retinopathy in insulin-dependent diabetics. Lancet 1983;1:200-204.
208. Dahl-Jorgensen K, Brinchmann-Hansen O, Hansen KF, et al. Rapid tightening of blood glucose control leads to transient deterioration of retinopathy in insulin dependent diabetes mellitus: the Oslo study. Br Med J (Clin Res Ed) 1985;290:811-815.
209. Cryer PE. Hypoglycemia-associated autonomic failure in diabetes. Am J Physiol 2001;281:E1115-E1121.
210. American Diabetes Association. Standards of medical care for patients with diabetes mellitus. Diabetes Care 2002;25(suppl 1):33-49.
211. American Diabetes Association. Standards of Medical Care in Diabetes—2006. Diabetes Care 2006;29:s4-s42.
212. American College of Endocrinologists. American College of Endocrinology consensus statement on guidelines for glycemic control. Endocr Pract 2002;8(suppl 1):5-11.
213. Hirsch IB. Intensive treatment of type 1 diabetes. Med Clin North Am 1998;82:689-719.
214. Home P, Kurtzhals P. Insulin detemir: from concept to clinical experience. Expert Opin Pharmacother 2006;7(3):325-343.
215. Heise T, Nosek L, Ronn BB, et al. Lower within-subject variability of insulin detemir in comparison to NPH insulin and insulin glargine in people with type 1 diabetes. Diabetes 2004;53(6): 1614-1620.
216. Cefalu WT. Evolving strategies for insulin delivery and therapy. Drugs 2004;64(11):1149-1161.
217. Pfizer Labs: Exubera prescribing information. New York: Pfizer, 2007. Available at http://www.pfizer.com/pfizer/download/uspi_exubera.pdf (accessed January 29, 2007).
218. Lougheed WD, Zinman B, Strack TR, et al. Stability of insulin lispro in insulin infusion systems. Diabetes Care 1997;20:1061-1065.
219. Bode BW, Steed RD, Davidson PC. Reduction in severe hypoglycemia with long-term continuous subcutaneous insulin infusion in type I diabetes. Diabetes Care 1996;19:324-327.
220. American Diabetes Association. Continuous subcutaneous insulin infusion. Diabetes Care 2002;25(suppl 1):116.
221. Hirsch IB, Edelman SV. Practical Management of Type 1 Diabetes. Caddo, OK: Professional Communications, 2005.

222. American Diabetes Association. Medical Management of Type 1 Diabetes, 4th ed. Alexandria, VA: American Diabetes Association, 2003.
223. American Diabetes Association. Intensive Diabetes Management, 3rd ed. Alexandria, VA: American Diabetes Association, 2003.
224. Dungan K, Buse J. Amylin and GLP-1-based therapies for the treatment of diabetes. UpToDate, 2006 (subscription required).
225. Young, A. Clinical studies. Adv Pharmacol 2005;52:289-320.
226. Garg S, Zisser H, Schwarz S, et al. Improvement in glycemic excursions with a transcutaneous, real-time continuous glucose sensor: a randomized controlled trial. Diabetes Care 2006;29(1):44-50.
227. Weisberg LS. Pseudohyponatremia: A reappraisal. Am J Med 1989;86:315-318.
228. Adrogue HJ, Wilson H, Boyd AE 3rd, et al. Plasma acid-base patterns in diabetic ketoacidosis. N Engl J Med 1982;307:1603-1610.
229. Munro JF, Campbell IW, McCuish AC, Duncan LJ. Euglycaemic diabetic ketoacidosis. BMJ 1973;2:578-580.
230. Madias NE. Lactic acidosis. Kidney Int 1986;29:752-774.
231. Fulop M. Alcoholism, ketoacidosis, and lactic acidosis. Diabetes Metab Rev 1989;5:365-378.
232. Duffens K, Marx JA. Alcoholic ketoacidosis: a review. J Emerg Med 1987;5:399-406.
233. Moller-Petersen J, Andersen PT, Hjorne N, Ditzel J. Nontraumatic rhabdomyolysis during diabetic ketoacidosis. Diabetologia 1986;29:229-234.
234. Brenner BE, Simon RR. Management of salicylate intoxication. Drugs 1982;24:335-340.
235. Turk J, Morrell L. Ethylene glycol intoxication. Arch Intern Med 1986;146:1601-1603.
236. Rich J, Scheife RT, Katz N, Caplan LR. Isopropyl alcohol intoxication. Arch Neurol 1990;47:322-324.
237. Kitabchi AE. Low-dose insulin therapy in diabetic ketoacidosis: fact or fiction? Diabetes Metab Rev 1989;5:337-363.
238. Kitabchi AE, Umpierrez GE, Murphy MB, et al. Hyperglycemic crises in diabetes. Diabetes Care 2004;27(Suppl 1):S94-S102.
239. Umpierrez GE, Guervo R, Karabell A, et al. Treatment of diabetic ketoacidosis with subcutaneous insulin aspart. Diabetes Care 2004;27(8):1873-1878.
240. Burris AS. Leukemoid reaction associated with severe diabetic ketoacidosis. South Med J 1986;79:647-648.
241. Powers WJ. Cerebrospinal fluid to serum glucose ratios in diabetes mellitus and bacterial meningitis. Am J Med 1981;71:217-220.
242. Campbell IW, Duncan LJ, Innes JA, et al. Abdominal pain in diabetic metabolic decompensation: clinical significance. JAMA 1975;233:166-168.
243. Rosenbloom AL. Intracerebral crises during treatment of diabetic ketoacidosis. Diabetes Care 1990;13:22-33.
244. Brun-Buisson CJ, Bonnet F, Bergeret S, et al. Recurrent high-permeability pulmonary edema associated with diabetic ketoacidosis. Crit Care Med 1985;13:55-56.
245. Brandstetter RD, Tamarin FM, Washington D, et al. Occult mucous airway obstruction in diabetic ketoacidosis. Chest 1987;91: 575-578.
246. Hansen LA, Prakash UB, Colby TV. Pulmonary complications in diabetes mellitus. Mayo Clin Proc 1989;64:791-799.
247. Levetan CS, Salas JR, Wilets JF, Zumoff B. Impact of endocrine and diabetes team consultation on hospital length of stay for patients with diabetes. Am J Med 1995;99(1):22-28.
248. Levetan CS, Passaro MD, Jablonski KA, Ratner RE. Effect of physician specialty on outcomes in diabetic ketoacidosis. Diabetes Care 1999;22(11):1790-1795.

CHAPTER 32

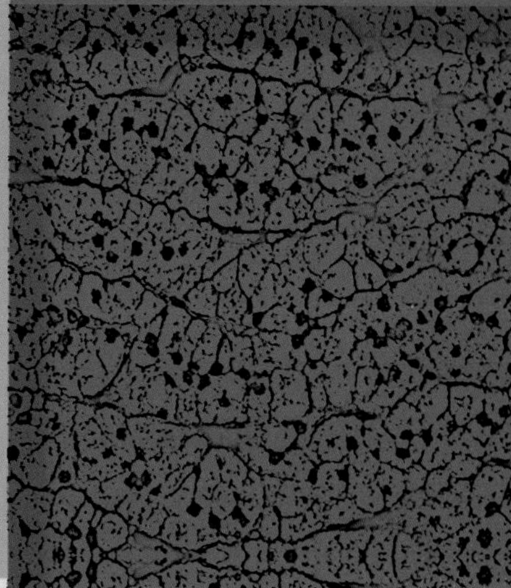

COMPLICATIONS OF DIABETES MELLITUS

Michael Brownlee, Lloyd P. Aiello,
Mark E. Cooper, Aaron I. Vinik,
Richard W. Nesto, and Andrew J. M. Boulton

BIOCHEMISTRY AND MOLECULAR CELL BIOLOGY

All forms of diabetes, both inherited and acquired, are characterized by hyperglycemia, a relative or absolute lack of insulin, and the development of diabetes-specific microvascular pathology in the retina, renal glomerulus, and peripheral nerve. Diabetes is also associated with accelerated atherosclerotic macrovascular disease affecting arteries that supply the heart, brain, and lower extremities. Pathologically, this condition resembles macrovascular disease in nondiabetic patients, but it is more extensive and progresses more rapidly. As a consequence of its microvascular pathology, diabetes mellitus is now the leading cause of new blindness in people 20 to 74 years of age and the leading cause of end-stage renal disease (ESRD).

People with diabetes mellitus are the fastest growing group of renal dialysis and transplant recipients. The life expectancy of patients with diabetic end-stage renal failure is only 3 or 4 years. More than 60% of diabetic patients are affected by neuropathy, which includes distal symmetrical polyneuropathy (DSPN), mononeuropathies, and a variety of autonomic neuropathies causing erectile dysfunction, urinary incontinence, gastroparesis, and nocturnal diarrhea. Accelerated lower extremity arterial disease in conjunction with neuropathy makes diabetes mellitus account for 50% of all nontrauma amputations in the United States. The risk of cardiovascular complications is increased by twofold to sixfold in subjects with diabetes. Overall, life expectancy is about 7 to 10 years shorter than for people without diabetes mellitus because of increased mortality from diabetic complications.[1]

Large prospective clinical studies show a strong relationship between glycemia and diabetic microvascular complications in both type 1 diabetes mellitus (T1DM) and type 2 diabetes (T2DM).[2,3] There is a continuous, though not linear, relationship between level of glycemia and the risk of development and progression of these complications (Fig. 32–1).[4,5] Hyperglycemia and the consequences of insulin resistance both appear to play important roles in the pathogenesis of macrovascular complications.[6-10]

Shared Pathophysiologic Features of Microvascular Complications

In the retina, glomerulus, and vasa nervorum, diabetes-specific microvascular disease is characterized by similar pathophysiologic features.

Requirement for Intracellular Hyperglycemia

Clinical and animal model data indicate that chronic hyperglycemia is the central initiating factor for all types of diabetic microvascular disease. Duration and magnitude of hyperglycemia are both strongly correlated with the extent and rate of progression of diabetic microvascular disease. In the Diabetes Control and Complications Trial (DCCT), for example, T1DM patients whose intensive insulin therapy resulted in hemoglobin A_{1c} (Hb A_{1c}) levels 2% lower than those receiving conventional insulin therapy had a 76% lower incidence of retinopathy, a 54% lower incidence of nephropathy, and a 60% reduction in neuropathy.[2,3]

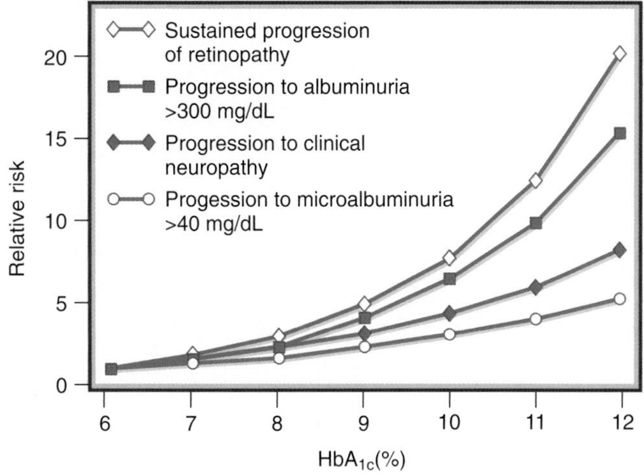

Figure 32–1 ▪ Relative risks for the development of diabetic complications at different levels of mean hemoglobin A_{1c} (HbA_{1c}, glycated hemoglobin) obtained from the Diabetes Control and Complications Trial. (Adapted from Skyler J: Diabetic complications: the importance of glucose control. Endocrinol Metab Clin North Am 1996;25:243-254.)

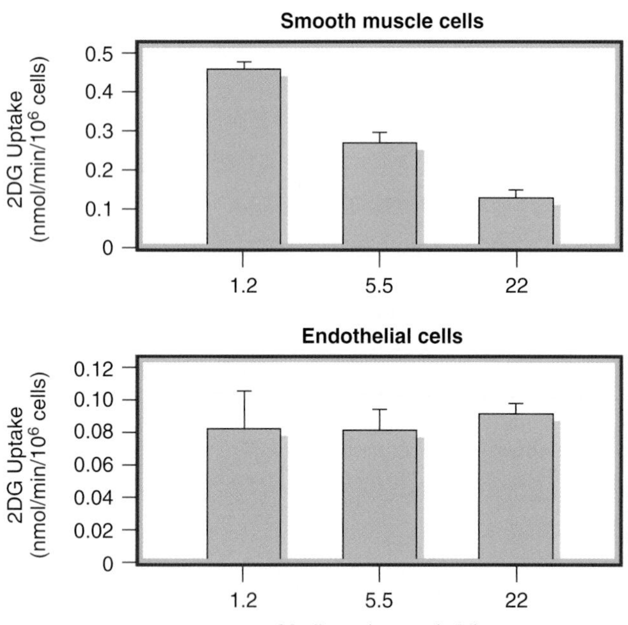

Figure 32–2 ▪ Lack of down-regulation of glucose transport in cells affected by diabetic complications. *Upper panel,* 2-deoxyglucose (2DG) uptake in vascular smooth muscle cells pre-exposed to 1.2, 5.5, or 22 mM glucose. *Lower panel,* 2DG uptake in bovine endothelial cells pre-exposed to 1.2, 5.5, or 22 mM glucose. (From Kaiser N, Feener EP, Boukobza-Vardi N, et al. Differential regulation of glucose transport and transporters by glucose in vascular endothelial and smooth muscle cells. Diabetes 1993;42:80-89.)

Although all diabetic cells are exposed to elevated levels of plasma glucose, hyperglycemic damage is limited to those cell types (e.g., endothelial cells) that develop intracellular hyperglycemia. Endothelial cells develop intracellular hyperglycemia because, unlike many other cells, they cannot down-regulate glucose transport when exposed to extracellular hyperglycemia. As illustrated in Figure 32–2, vascular smooth muscle cells, which are not damaged by hyperglycemia, show an inverse relationship between extracellular glucose concentration and

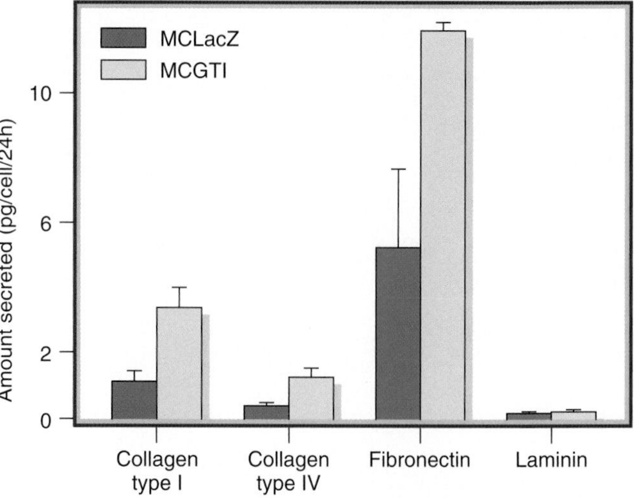

Figure 32–3 ▪ Overexpression of *GLUT1* in mesangial cells cultured in normal glucose mimics the diabetic phenotype. Mesangial cells transfected with either *LacZ* (MCLacZ)- or *GLUT1* (MCGT1)-expressing constructs were cultured in 5-mM glucose, and the amount of the indicated matrix components secreted was determined. (From Heilig CW, Concepcion LA, Riser BL, et al. Overexpression of glucose transporters in rat mesangial cells cultured in a normal glucose milieu mimics the diabetic phenotype. J Clin Invest 1995;96:1802-1814.)

subsequent rate of glucose transport measured as 2-deoxyglucose uptake (Fig. 32–2, *upper part*). In contrast, vascular endothelial cells show no significant change in subsequent rate of glucose transport after exposure to elevated glucose concentrations (see Fig. 32–2, *lower part*).[11] That intracellular hyperglycemia is necessary and sufficient for the development of diabetic pathology is further demonstrated by the fact that overexpression of the GLUT1 glucose transporter in mesangial cells cultured in a normal glucose milieu mimics the diabetic phenotype, inducing the same increases in collagen type IV, collagen type I, and fibronectin gene expression as diabetic hyperglycemia (Fig. 32–3).[12]

Abnormal Endothelial Cell Function

Early in the course of diabetes mellitus, before structural changes are evident, hyperglycemia causes abnormalities in blood flow and vascular permeability in the retina, glomerulus, and peripheral nerve vasa nervorum.[13,14] The increase in blood flow and intracapillary pressure is thought to reflect hyperglycemia-induced decreased nitric oxide (NO) production on the efferent side of capillary beds and possibly an increased sensitivity to angiotensin II. As a consequence of increased intracapillary pressure and endothelial cell dysfunction, retinal capillaries exhibit increased leakage of fluorescein and glomerular capillaries have an elevated albumin excretion rate (AER). Comparable changes occur in the vasa vasorum of peripheral nerve. Early in the course of diabetes, increased permeability is reversible; as time progresses, however, it becomes irreversible.

Increased Vessel Wall Protein Accumulation

The common pathophysiologic feature of diabetic microvascular disease is progressive narrowing and eventual occlusion of vascular lumina, which results in inadequate perfusion and function of the affected tissues. Early hyperglycemia-induced microvascular hypertension and increased vascular permeability contribute to irreversible microvessel occlusion by three processes.

The first process is an abnormal leakage of periodic acid–Schiff (PAS)-positive, carbohydrate-containing plasma proteins, which are deposited in the capillary wall and can stimulate perivascular cells such as pericytes and mesangial cells to elaborate growth factors and extracellular matrix.

The second is extravasation of growth factors, such as transforming growth factor β_1 (TGF-β_1), which directly stimulates overproduction of extracellular matrix components[15] and can induce apoptosis in certain complication-relevant cell types.

The third is hypertension-induced stimulation of pathologic gene expression by endothelial cells and supporting cells, which include GLUT1 glucose transporters, growth factors, growth factor receptors, extracellular matrix components, and adhesion molecules that can activate circulating leukocytes.[16] The observation that unilateral reduction in the severity of diabetic microvascular disease occurs on the side with ophthalmic or renal artery stenosis is consistent with this concept.[17,18]

Microvascular Cell Loss and Vessel Occlusion

The progressive narrowing and occlusion of diabetic microvascular lumina are also accompanied by microvascular cell loss. In the retina, diabetes mellitus induces programmed cell death of Müller cells and ganglion cells,[19] pericytes, and endothelial cells.[20] In the glomerulus, declining renal function is associated with widespread capillary occlusion and podocyte loss, but the mechanisms underlying glomerular cell loss are not yet known. In the vasa nervorum, endothelial cell and pericyte degeneration occur,[21] and these microvascular changes appear to precede the development of diabetic peripheral neuropathy.[22] The multifocal distribution of axonal degeneration in diabetes supports a causal role for microvascular occlusion, but hyperglycemia-induced decreases in neurotrophins might contribute by preventing normal axonal repair and regeneration.[23]

Development of Microvascular Complications during Posthyperglycemic Euglycemia

Another common feature of diabetic microvascular disease has been termed *hyperglycemic memory,* or the persistence or progression of hyperglycemia-induced microvascular alterations during subsequent periods of normal glucose homeostasis. The most striking example of this phenomenon is the development of severe retinopathy in histologically normal eyes of diabetic dogs that occurred entirely during a 2.5-year period of normalized blood glucose that followed 2.5 years of hyperglycemia (Fig. 32–4).[24] Normal dogs were compared to diabetic dogs with either poor control for 5 years, good control for 5 years, or poor control for 2.5 years ($P \rightarrow G_a$) followed by good control for the next 2.5 years ($P \rightarrow G_b$). Hb A_1 values for both the good control group and the $P \rightarrow G_b$ group were identical to the normal group. Hyperglycemia-induced increases in selected matrix gene transcription also persist for weeks after restoration of normoglycemia in vivo, and a less pronounced, but qualitatively similar, prolongation of hyperglycemia-induced increase in selected matrix gene transcription occurs in cultured endothelial cells.[25]

Data from the DCCT study suggested that hyperglycemic memory occurs in patients. In the secondary-intervention cohort, there was no difference in the incidence of sustained progression of retinopathy for the first 3 years, no difference in development of clinical albuminuria for 4 years, and no difference in the rate of change in creatinine clearance during the

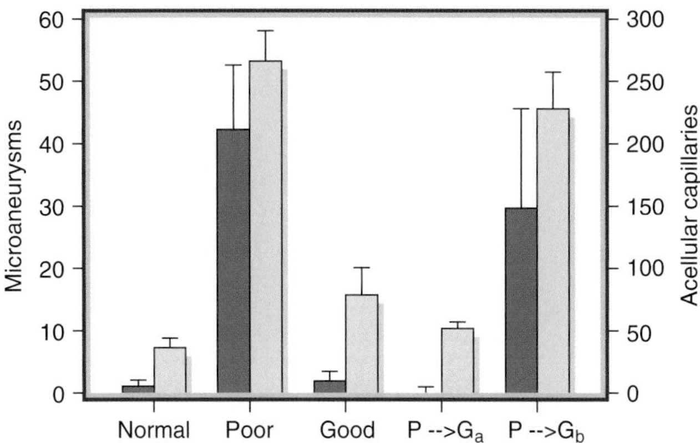

Figure 32–4 ▪ Development of retinopathy during posthyperglycemic normoglycemia (hyperglycemic memory). Quantitation of retinal microaneurysms and acellular capillaries in normal dogs, dogs with poor glycemic control for 5 years, dogs with good glycemic control for 5 years, dogs with poor glycemic control for 2.5 years ($P \rightarrow G_a$), and the same dogs after a subsequent 2.5 years of good glycemic control ($P \rightarrow G_b$). (Adapted from Engerman RL, Kern TS. Progression of incipient diabetic retinopathy during good glycemic control. Diabetes 1987;36:808-812.)

entire study. For neuropathy, the sural nerve sensory conduction velocity did not differ between the groups for 4 years, and intensive therapy did not slow the rate of decline of autonomic function at all.[2,26-28]

Data from the post-DCCT long-term follow-up study, the Epidemiology of Diabetes Interventions and Complications (EDIC) study, proved that the effects of former intensive and conventional therapy persist for 12 years. In the conventional therapy group, the effects of previous high Hb A_{1c} on post-study retinopathy, nephropathy, and cardiovascular disease persisted as if there had been no improvement in Hb A_{1c} at all. Atherosclerotic changes not even present at the end of the DCCT have appeared subsequently in the previously higher Hb A_{1c} group, followed by a twofold increase in heart attacks, strokes, and cardiovascular death, even though their Hb A_{1c} since the end of the DCCT was identical to that of the formerly intensive control group during the entire time that these arterial changes developed (Fig. 32–5).[29,30] On the other hand, the beneficial effects of previous lower Hb A_{1c} also persisted in the intensive treatment group after their Hb A_{1c} went up, as if there had been no deterioration in their Hb A_{1c}.

Thus, the phenomenon of hyperglycemic memory presents a paradox: Patients in the DCCT with long-term exposure to a higher level of hyperglycemia became more susceptible to damage from subsequent lower levels of hyperglycemia than they were when they first started the trial. In contrast, lower levels of hyperglycemia made patients more resistant to damage from subsequent higher levels.

Genetic Determinants of Susceptibility to Microvascular Complications

Clinicians have long observed that different patients with similar duration and degree of hyperglycemia differ markedly in their susceptibility to microvascular complications. Such observations suggested that genetic differences exist that affected the pathways by which hyperglycemia damaged microvascular cells. The leveling of risk of overt proteinuria after 30 years' duration of T1DM at 27% is evidence that only a subset of patients are susceptible to development of diabetic nephropathy.[31]

A role for genetic determinant of susceptibility to diabetic nephropathy is most strongly supported by familial clustering,

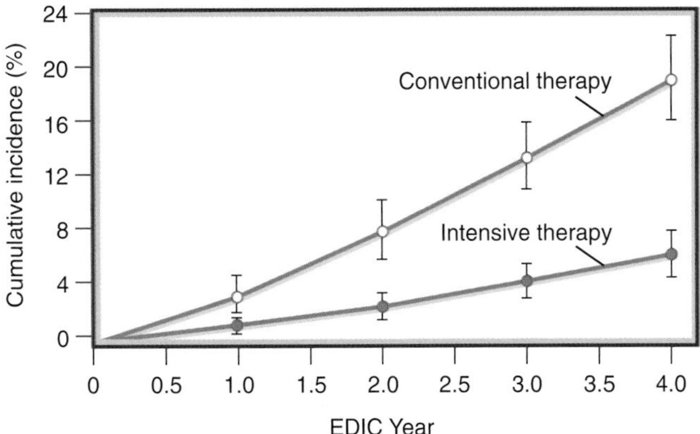

Figure 32–5 ▪ Cumulative incidence of further progression of retinopathy 4 years after the end of the Diabetes Control and Complications Trial. Median glycosylated hemoglobin was 8.2% for the conventional therapy group and 7.9% for the intensive therapy group. EDIC, Epidemiology of Diabetes Interventions and Complications [Research Group]. (From Retinopathy and nephropathy in patients with type 1 diabetes four years after a trial of intensive therapy. The Diabetes Control and Complications Trial/Epidemiology of Diabetes Interventions and Complications Research Group. N Engl J Med 2000;342:381-389.)

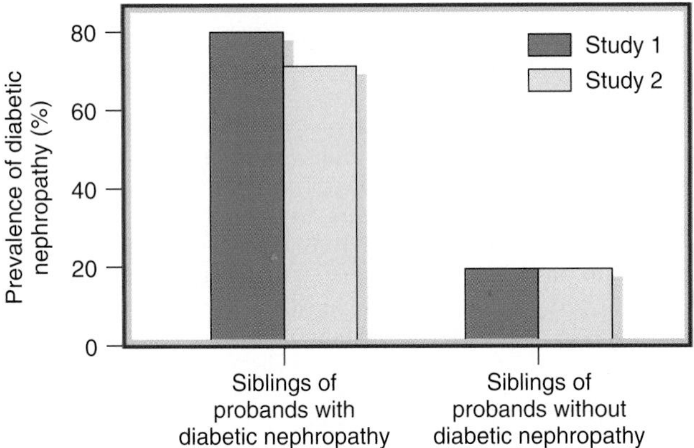

Figure 32–6 ▪ Familial clustering of diabetic nephropathy. Prevalence of diabetic nephropathy in two studies of diabetic siblings of probands with or without diabetic nephropathy. (Adapted from Seaquist ER, Goetz FC, Rich S, Barbosa J. Familial clustering of diabetic kidney disease: evidence for genetic susceptibility to diabetic nephropathy. N Engl J Med 1989;320:1161-1165; and Quinn M, Angelico MC, Warram JH, Krolewski AS. Familial factors determine the development of diabetic nephropathy in patients with IDDM. Diabetologia 1996;39: 940-945.)

with an estimated heritability of at least 40%.[32] In two studies of families that have two or more siblings with T1DM, if one diabetic sibling had advanced diabetic nephropathy, the other diabetic sibling had a nephropathy risk of 83% or 72%. In contrast, the risk was only 17% or 22% if the index patient did not have diabetic nephropathy (Fig. 32–6),[33,34] or retinopathy. The DCCT reported familial clustering as well, with an odds ratio of 5.4 for the risk of severe retinopathy in diabetic relatives of positive versus negative subjects from the conventional treatment group.[35] Coronary artery calcification, an indicator of subclinical atherosclerosis, also shows familiar clustering.

Numerous associations have been made between various genetic polymorphisms and the risk of various diabetic complications. Examples include the 5′ insulin gene polymorphism,[36] the G2m23+ immunoglobulin allotype,[37] angiotensin-converting enzyme (ACE) insertion/deletion polymorphisms,[38,39] HLA-DQB10201/0302 alleles,[40] polymorphisms of the aldose reductase gene,[41] and a polymorphic CCTTT (n) repeat of nitric oxide synthetase (NOS) 2A.[42] In all of these studies, there is no indication that the polymorphic gene actually plays a functional role rather than simply being in linkage disequilibrium with the locus encoding the unidentified relevant genes.

A whole genome linkage analysis using families of Pima Indians showed susceptibility loci for diabetic nephropathy on chromosome 3, 7, and 20. Another linkage analysis using discordant sib-pairs of white families with T1DM identified a critical area on chromosome3q. Evidence for linkage to kidney disease has been detected and replicated at several loci on chromosomes 3q (types 1 and 2 diabetic nephropathy), 10q (diabetic and nondiabetic kidney disease), and 18q (type 2 diabetic nephropathy).[43]

Family-based studies with simple tandem repeat polymorphisms (STRPs) and single nucleotide polymorphisms (SNPs) in 115 candidate genes for linkage and association with diabetic nephropathy in type 1 diabetic families of European descent have shown a positive association with polymorphisms in 20 genes, including 12 that have not been studied previously. Three genes code for components of the extracellular matrix *(COL4A1, LAMA4,* and *LAMC1),* and two are involved in its metabolism *(MMP9* and *TIMP3).* Five genes code for transcription factors or signaling molecules *(HNF1B1/TCF2, NRP1, PRKCB1, SMAD3,* and *USF1).* Three genes code for growth factors or growth factor receptors *(IGF1, TGFBR2,* and *TGFBR3).* The other genes *(AGTR1, AQP1, BCL2, CAT, GPX1, LPL,* and *p22phox)* code for a variety of products likely to be relevant in kidney function.[44]

As genes are identified that affect susceptibility to diabetic complications, a new area of research has emerged that will make it possible to identify genetic modifiers of the clinical manifestation of complications. With the completion of the genetic map known as the International HapMap Project, and new high-throughput genotyping technologies, this promising area of research holds great potential for understanding genetic determinants of the varying clinical severity of diabetic complications. These modifying genes are genetic variants that are distinct from disease-susceptibility genes and that modify the phenotypic and clinical expression of the disease genes.[45] Because complications are likely to result not only from hyperglycemia but also from a susceptibility to later pathophysiologic steps, such as inflammation or aberrant angiogenesis, a number of modifier genes may be relevant to diabetic complications.

Pathophysiologic Features of Macrovascular Complications

Unlike microvascular disease, which occurs only in patients with diabetes mellitus, macrovascular disease resembles that in subjects without diabetes. However, subjects with diabetes have more rapidly progressive and extensive cardiovascular disease (CVD), with a greater incidence of multivessel disease and a greater number of diseased vessel segments than nondiabetic persons.[46] Although dyslipidemia and hypertension occur with great frequency in type 2 diabetic populations, there is still excess risk in diabetic subjects after adjusting for these other risk factors.[47,48] Diabetes itself can confer 75% to 90% of the excess risk of coronary disease in these diabetic subjects, and it enhances the deleterious effects of the other major cardiovascular risk factors (Fig. 32–7).[49,50] The importance of hyperglycemia in the pathogenesis of diabetic macrovascular disease is suggested by the observation that glycohemoglobin A_1 is an independent risk factor for CVD[51] in T1DM, and numerous correlational studies show that hyperglycemia is a continuous risk factor for macrovascular disease.[52-56]

However, data from the United Kingdom Prospective Diabetes Study (UKPDS) show that hyperglycemia is not nearly as central a determinant of diabetic macrovascular disease as it is in microvascular disease. For microvascular disease end-points, there is a nearly 10-fold increase in risk as Hb A_{1c} increases from 5.5% to 9.5%, whereas over the same Hb A_{1c} range, macrovascular risk increases only about twofold.[3]

Insulin resistance occurs in the majority of patients with T2DM and in two thirds of subjects with impaired glucose tolerance.[57] Both these groups have a significantly higher risk of developing CVD.[58-61] To isolate the effects of insulin resistance from those of hyperglycemia and diabetes, several studies have evaluated subjects with normal glucose tolerance. In T1DM, hyperglycemia itself causes secondary insulin resistance in nearly all patients. In nonobese subjects without diabetes, insulin resistance predicted the development of CVD independently of other known risk factors.[62] In another group of subjects without diabetes or impaired glucose tolerance, those in the highest quintile of insulin resistance had a 2.5-fold increase in CVD risk compared with those in the lowest quintile.[63] These data indicate that insulin resistance itself promotes atherogenesis.

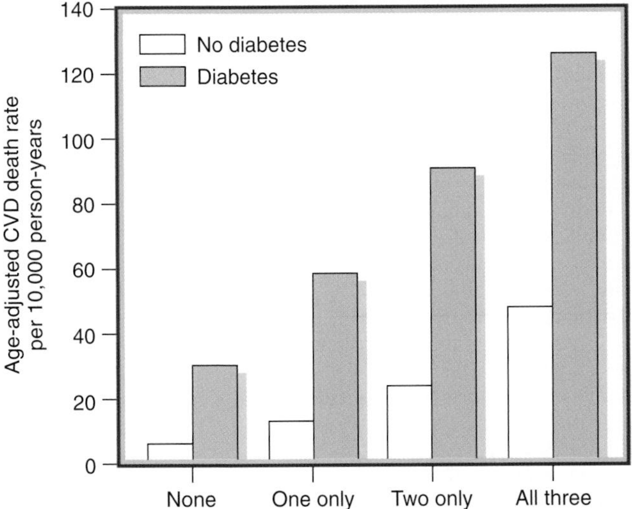

Figure 32–7 ▪ Adjusted death rates by number of cardiovascular disease (CVD) risk factors for diabetic and nondiabetic men. Subjects are participants from the Multiple Risk Factor Intervention Trial (MRFIT) study; risk factors are hypercholesterolemia, hypertension, and cigarette smoking. (From Stamler J, Vaccaro O, Neaton JD, Wentworth D. Diabetes, other risk factors, and 12-year cardiovascular mortality for men screened in the Multiple Risk Factor Intervention Trial. Diabetes Care 1993;2:434-444.)

Insulin resistance is commonly associated with a proatherogenic dyslipidemia, which data from Brown, Goldstein, and colleagues suggest results from hyperinsulinemia-induced activation of SREBP-1c transcription in the liver by a mechanism that is not affected by the defects in hepatic phosphatidylinositol 3-kinase (PI3K)-mediated insulin signaling.[64,65] Insulin resistance is associated with a characteristic lipoprotein profile that includes a high very-low-density lipoprotein (VLDL), a low high-density lipoprotein (HDL), and small, dense LDL. Both low HDL and small, dense LDL are each independent risk factors for macrovascular disease. This profile arises as a direct result of increased net free fatty acid (FFA) release by insulin-resistant adipocytes (Fig. 32–8).[10] Increased FFA flux into hepatocytes stimulates VLDL secretion. In the presence of cholesteryl ester transfer protein, excess VLDL transfers significant amounts of triglyceride to both HDL and LDL while depleting HDL and LDL of cholesteryl ester. The resultant triglyceride-enriched HDL carries less cholesteryl ester for reverse cholesterol transport to the liver, and loss of ApoIA-1 from these particles reduces the total concentration of HDL available for reverse cholesterol transport. The triglyceride-enriched, cholesteryl ester-depleted LDL is smaller and denser than normal LDL, allowing it to penetrate the vessel wall and be oxidized more easily.

In vitro studies suggest that at the level of the vessel wall, insulin has both antiatherogenic and proatherogenic effects (Fig. 32–9)[66,67] One major antiatherogenic effect is the stimulation of endothelial NO production. NO released from endothelial cells is a potent inhibitor of platelet aggregation and adhesion to the vascular wall. Endothelial NO also controls the expression of genes involved in atherogenesis. It decreases expression of monocyte chemoattractant protein (MCP)-1 and of surface adhesion molecules such as CD11/CD18, P-selectin, vascular cell adhesion molecule-1 (VCAM-1), and intercellular adhesion molecule-1 (ICAM-1). Endothelial cell NO also reduces vascular permeability and decreases the rate of oxidation of low-density lipoprotein (LDL) to its proatherogenic form. Finally, endothelial cell NO inhibits proliferation of vascular smooth muscle cells.[68]

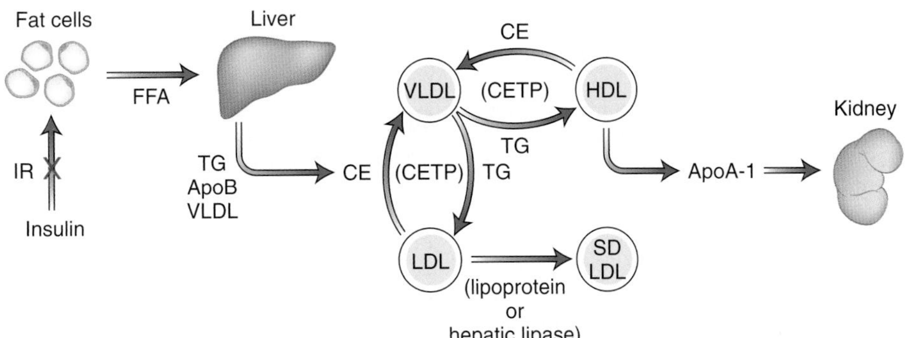

Figure 32–8 ▪ Schematic summary relating insulin resistance (IR) to the characteristic dyslipidemia of type 2 diabetes mellitus. IR at the adipocyte results in increased free fatty acid (FFA) release. Increased FFA flux stimulates very-low-density lipoprotein (VLDL) secretion, causing hypertriglyceridemia (TG). VLDL stimulates a reciprocal exchange of TG to cholesteryl ester (CE) from both high-density lipoprotein (HDL) and low-density lipoprotein (LDL), catalyzed by CE transfer protein (CETP). TG-enriched HDL dissociates from ApoA-1, leaving less HDL for reverse cholesterol transport. TG-enriched LDL serves as a substrate for lipases that convert it to atherogenic small, dense LDL particles (SD LDL). (From Ginsberg HN. Insulin resistance and cardiovascular disease. J Clin Invest 2000;106:453-458.)

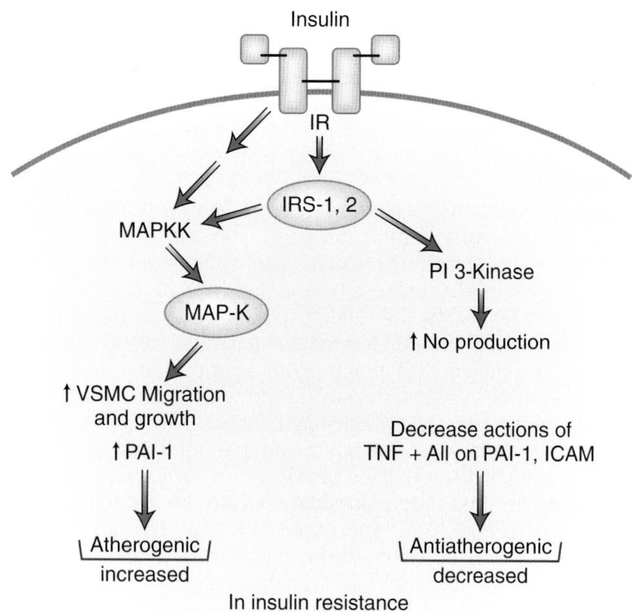

Figure 32–9 ▪ Schematic summary of proatherosclerotic and antiatherosclerotic actions of insulin on vascular cells. ICAM, intercellular adhesion molecule; IRS, insulin resistance syndrome; MAP-K, mitogen-activated protein kinase; MAPKK, MAPK kinase; PAI, plasminogen activator inhibitor; PI, phosphatidylinositol; TNF, tumor necrosis factor. (Adapted from King G, Brownlee M. The cellular and molecular mechanisms of diabetic complications. Endocrinol Metab Clin North Am 1996;2:255-270; and Hsueh WA, Law RE. Cardiovascular risk continuum: implications of insulin resistance and diabetes. Am J Med 1998;105:4S-14S.)

Two major proatherogenic effects of insulin are the potentiation of platelet-derived growth factor (PDGF)-induced vascular smooth muscle cell (VSMC) proliferation and the stimulation of VSMC plasminogen activator inhibitor 1 (PAI-1) production.[69,70] Because insulin-induced NO production is mediated by the insulin receptor substrate–PI3K signal transduction pathway, and the effects on smooth muscle cells are mediated by the Ras/Raf/MEKK/MAPK (mitogen-activated protein kinase [MAPK]; MAPK/extracellular-signal-regulated kinase [ERK] kinase [MEK] kinase) signal transduction pathway,[66,67] it has been proposed that pathway-selective insulin resistance in arterial cells might contribute to diabetic atherosclerosis. Evidence of such selective vascular resistance to insulin has been demonstrated in the obese Zucker rat.[71]

Hyperglycemia also inhibits arterial endothelial NO production, both in vivo and in vitro.[72-75] Similarly, hyperglycemia potentiates PDGF-induced VSMC proliferation and stimulates endothelial cell PAI-1 production.[74,76] In addition, hyperglycemia has a variety of other proatherogenic effects on endothelial cells, platelets, and monocyte/macrophages. These include increased expression of MCP-1,[77] up-regulation of adhesion molecules such as ICAM-1 and VCAM-1,[78-80] potentiation of collagen-induced platelet activation, and increased secretion of collagen type IV and fibronectin.[81,82]

Surprisingly, however, in subjects without diabetes or impaired glucose tolerance, after adjustment for 11 known cardiovascular risk factors, including LDL, triglycerides, HDL, systolic blood pressure (BP), and smoking, the most insulin-resistant subjects still have a twofold increase in the risk of CVD.[63] This observation suggests that a significant part of the increased CVD risk due to insulin resistance reflects a consequence of insulin resistance not previously identified as being proatherogenic. Recent data suggest that increased oxidation of FFAs by insulin-resistant aortic endothelial cells inactivates two important antiatherosclerotic enzymes: prostacyclin synthase, and endothelial NOS (eNOS). This inactivation is reversed by inhibition of the rate-limiting enzyme of fatty acid oxidation, carnitine palmitoyltransferase I, and by inhibition of FFA release from insulin-resistant adipose tissue.[83]

Impaired Collateral Blood Vessel Formation from Bone Marrow Progenitor Cells

It has become apparent that diabetic complications result not only from damage to vascular cells but also from a defective repair process. Normally, in response to acute ischemia, new blood vessel growth rescues stunned areas of the heart or central nervous system, reducing morbidity and mortality. In response to chronic ischemia, collateral vessel development reduces the size and severity of subsequent infarction. In response to ischemia, circulating endothelial progenitor cells from the bone marrow promote the regeneration of blood vessels, acting in concert with cells and extracellular matrix at the site of injury. In experimental diabetes, however, these circulating endothelial progenitor cells are depleted and dysfunctional. As a result, diabetic animals have decreased vascular density following hind limb ischemia. Similarly, in human diabetes, endothelial progenitor cells are also depleted and dysfunctional.[84]

Many of the diabetic patients who have impaired blood vessel growth after ischemic events also have increased retinal neovascularization (diabetic retinopathy). This diabetic paradox is at present poorly understood.[85,86] The question of how endothelial progenitor cell dysfunction can participate in diabetic retinopathy is especially intriguing, given the recent findings by Grant and colleagues[87] that bone marrow–derived endothelial progenitor cells play a role in a model of adult retinal revascularization. A plausible explanation may be that the retina responds differently to ischemic events when compared with tissue outside of the central nervous system. Vascular endothelial growth factor (VEGF) is known to be significantly elevated in the ocular fluid of diabetic patients but has also been shown to be decreased in ischemic nonretinal tissues.[88] Because VEGF has a stimulatory effect on endothelial progenitor cell proliferation and is a potent stimulator of vasculogenesis,[89] unique retinal pathways for VEGF regulation may be sufficient to overcome endothelial progenitor cell dysfunction that results in diabetic retinopathy.

Mechanisms of Hyperglycemia-Induced Damage

Four major hypotheses about how hyperglycemia causes diabetic complications have generated a large amount of data as well as several clinical trials based on specific inhibitors of these mechanisms. Until recently, there was no unifying hypothesis linking these four mechanisms together, nor was there an obvious connection between any of these mechanisms, each of which responds quickly to normalization of hyperglycemia, and the phenomenon of hyperglycemic memory (see earlier).

Increased Polyol Pathway Flux

Aldose reductase [alditol:NAD(P)$^+$ 1-oxidoreductase, EC 1.1.1.21] is a cytosolic, monomeric oxidoreductase that catalyzes the nicotinamide adenine dinucleotide phosphate (NADPH)-dependent reduction of a wide variety of carbonyl compounds, including glucose. Triphosphopyridine nucleotide, the reduced form of NADP (NADPH), is the cofactor in both this reaction and in the regeneration of glutathione by glutathione reductase. Aldose reductase has a low affinity (high Michaelis constant [K_m]) for glucose, and at the normal glucose concentrations found in nondiabetic patients, metabolism of glucose by this pathway constitutes a small percentage of total glucose utilization. In a hyperglycemic environment, however, increased intracellular glucose results in increased enzymatic conversion to the polyalcohol sorbitol, with concomitant decreases in NADPH. In the polyol pathway, sorbitol is oxidized to fructose by the enzyme sorbitol dehydrogenase, with nicotinamide adenine dinucleotide (NAD^+) reduced to NADH (Fig. 32–10). Flux through this pathway during hyperglycemia varies from 33% of total glucose utilization in the rabbit lens to 11% in human erythrocytes. Thus, the contribution of this pathway to diabetic complications may be very much species, site, and tissue dependent.

A number of mechanisms have been proposed to explain the potential detrimental effects of hyperglycemia-induced increases in polyol pathway flux. These include sorbitol-induced osmotic stress, decreased Na^+/K^+-ATPase activity, increased cytosolic $NADH/NAD^+$, and decreased cytosolic NADPH. Sorbitol does not diffuse easily across cell membranes, and it was originally suggested that this resulted in osmotic damage to microvascular cells. However, sorbitol concentrations measured in diabetic vessels and nerves are far too low to cause osmotic damage.

Another early suggestion was that increased flux through the polyol pathway decreased Na^+/K^+-ATPase activity. Although this was originally thought to be mediated by polyol-pathway-linked decreases in phosphatidylinositol synthesis, it has been shown to result from activation of protein kinase C (PKC) (see later). Hyperglycemia-induced activation of PKC increases cytosolic phospholipase A_2 activity, which increases the production of two inhibitors of Na^+/K^+-ATPase, arachidonate and prostaglandin E_2 (PGE_2).[90]

More recently, it has been proposed that oxidation of sorbitol by NAD^+ increases the cytosolic ratio of $NADH/NAD^+$, thereby inhibiting activity of the enzyme glyceraldehyde-3-phosphate dehydrogenase (GADPH) and increasing concentrations of triose phosphate.[91] Elevated triose phosphate concentrations could increase formation of both methylglyoxal, a precursor of advanced glycation end products (AGEs), and diacylglycerol (DAG) (via α-glycerol-3-phosphate), thus activating PKC (discussed in later sections). Although increased NADH production is supported by the observation that hyperglycemia increases both lactate concentration and the lactate-to-pyruvate ratio, there is no direct evidence that the concentrations of NADH and NAD^+, as opposed to NADH and NAD^+ flux, are altered. In endothelial cells, where aldose reductase activity is low, increased NADH production might also reflect hyperglycemia-induced increased flux through glycolysis[92] and through the glucuronic acid pathway.[93]

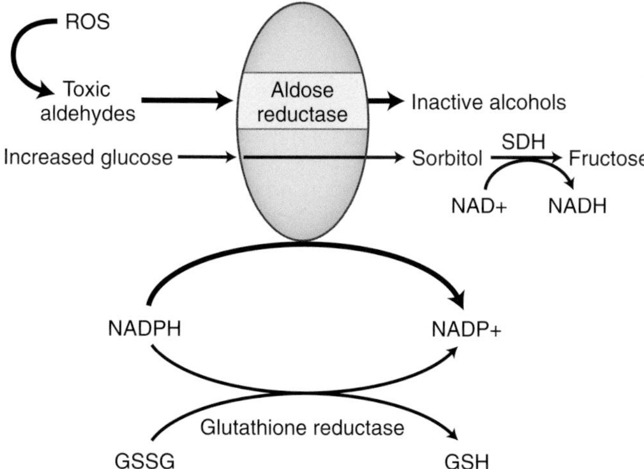

Figure 32–10 ■ Aldose reductase and the polyol pathway. Aldose reductase reduces reactive oxygen species (ROS)-generated toxic aldehydes to inactive alcohols, and glucose to sorbitol, using triphosphopyridine nucleotide (NADPH), the reduced form of nicotinamide adenine dinucleotide phosphate (NADP) as a cofactor. In cells where aldose reductase activity is sufficient to deplete reduced glutathione (GSH), oxidative stress would be augmented. Sorbitol dehydrogenase (SDH) oxidizes sorbitol to fructose using nicotinamide-adenine dinucleotide (NAD^+) as a cofactor. GSSG, oxidized glutathione.

Other evidence presented in support of this hypothesis includes the observation that administration of pyruvate can prevent diabetes-related endothelial dysfunction in some systems. However, the observed effects of pyruvate on microvascular function might reflect its potent antioxidant properties rather than effects on the $NADH/NAD^+$ ratio, because reactive oxygen species (ROS) also partially inhibit GADPH and increase glyceraldehyde-3-phosphate levels.[94,95] The source of hyperglycemia-induced ROS is discussed later in this section.

It has also been proposed that reduction of glucose to sorbitol by NADPH consumes the cofactor NADPH. Because NADPH is required for regenerating reduced glutathione (GSH), this could induce or exacerbate intracellular oxidative stress. Less reduced glutathione has in fact been found in the lens of transgenic mice that overexpress aldose reductase, and this is the most likely mechanism by which increased flux through the polyol pathway has deleterious consequences.[96] This conclusion is further supported by recent experiments with aldose reductase–deficient homozygous knockout mice, showing that in contrast to wild-type mice, diabetes neither decreases sciatic nerve GSH content nor reduces motor nerve conduction velocity (S.K. Chung, personal communication).

Recent observations suggest that NO maintains aldose reductase in an inactive state and that this repression is relieved in diabetic tissues[97] Aldose reductase appears to be inhibited by NO-derived adduct formation on active-site Cys-298.[98,99] These observations suggest that diabetes-induced decreases in NO might further activate the polyol pathway.

In vivo studies of polyol pathway inhibition have yielded inconsistent results. In a 5-year study in dogs, aldose reductase inhibition prevented diabetic neuropathy but failed to prevent retinopathy or capillary basement membrane thickening in the retina, kidney, or muscle.[100] Several negative clinical trials have questioned the relevance of this mechanism in humans.[101] However, the positive effect of aldose reductase inhibition on diabetic neuropathy has been confirmed in humans in a rigorous multidose, placebo-controlled trial with the potent aldose reductase inhibitor zenarestat.[102]

Increased Intracellular Advanced Glycation End Product Formation

Advanced Glycation End Products are Formed from Intracellular Dicarbonyl Precursors

AGEs are found in increased amounts in extracellular structures of diabetic retinal vessels[103-105] and renal glomeruli,[106-108] where they can cause damage by mechanisms described later in this section. These AGEs were originally thought to arise from nonenzymatic reactions between extracellular proteins and glucose. However, the rate of AGE formation from glucose is orders of magnitude slower than the rate of AGE formation from glucose-derived dicarbonyl precursors generated intracellularly, and it now seems likely that intracellular hyperglycemia is the primary initiating event in the formation of both intracellular and extracellular AGEs.[109] AGEs can arise from intracellular autooxidation of glucose to glyoxal,[110] decomposition of the Amadori product to 3-deoxyglucosone (perhaps accelerated by an amadoriase), and fragmentation of glyceraldehyde-3-phosphate to methylglyoxal[111] (Fig. 32–11). These reactive intracellular dicarbonyls react with amino groups of intracellular and extracellular proteins to form AGEs. Methylglyoxal and glyoxal are detoxified by the glyoxalase system.[111] All three AGE precursors are also

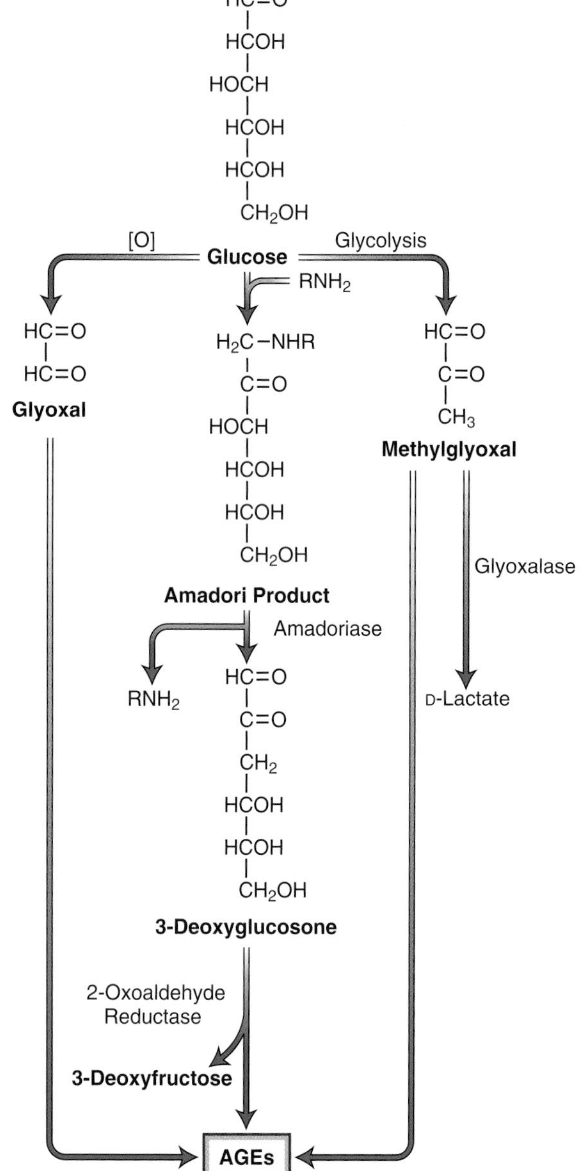

Figure 32–11 ▪ Potential pathways leading to the formation of advanced glycation end product (AGE) from intracellular dicarbonyl precursors. Glyoxal arises from the auto-oxidation of glucose, 3-deoxyglucosone arises from decomposition of the Amadori product, and methylglyoxal arises from fragmentation of glyceraldehyde 3-phosphate. These reactive dicarbonyls react with amino groups of proteins to form AGEs. Methylglyoxal and glyoxal are detoxified by the glyoxalase system. (Adapted from Shinohara M, Thornalley PJ, Giardino I, et al. Overexpression of glyoxalase-I in bovine endothelial cells inhibits intracellular advanced glycation end-product formation and prevents hyperglycemia-induced increases in macromolecular endocytosis. J Clin Invest 1998;101:1142-1147.)

substrates for other reductases.[112,113] In vascular endothelial cells, methylglyoxal accounts for nearly all the hyperglycemia-induced increase in reactive AGE precursors.

The potential importance of AGEs in the pathogenesis of diabetic complications is suggested by the observation in animal models that two structurally unrelated AGE inhibitors partially prevented various functional and structural manifestations of diabetic microvascular disease in retina, kidney, and nerve.[114,115] In the human diabetic retina, AGEs might contribute to both macular edema and retinal neovascularization by increasing expression of VEGF through activation of the MAP kinase ERK1/2 and concomitant activation of the transcription factor hypoxia inducible factor-1 (HIF-1).[116] In the early phase of diabetic nephropathy, AGEs induce hyperfiltration and microalbuminuria by stimulating the secretion of VEGF and MCP-1.[117] AGEs contribute to more advanced lesions of diabetic nephropathy by inducing apoptosis in glomerular mesangial cells and by inducing epithelial-myofibroblast transdifferentiation via ligation of the AGE receptor RAGE (receptor for advanced glycation end products; see later), ultimately leading to tubulointerstitial fibrosis.[118]

Intracellular production of AGE precursors damages target cells by three general mechanisms (Fig. 32–12): Intracellular proteins modified by AGEs have altered function. Extracellular matrix components modified by AGE precursors interact abnormally with other matrix components and with matrix receptors (integrins) on cells. Plasma proteins modified by AGE precursors bind to AGE receptors on cells such as macrophages, inducing receptor-mediated ROS production. This AGE-receptor ligation activates the pleiotropic transcription factor nuclear factor κB (NFκB), causing pathologic changes in gene expression.[119]

Advanced Glycation End Products Alter Intracellular Protein Function

It has recently been shown that AGE modification of intracellular proteins can regulate expression of genes involved in the pathogenesis of diabetic retinopathy. In diabetic retinal capillaries, the earliest morphologic changes are pericyte loss and acellular capillary formation. The primary pathologic processes of retinal pericyte loss and acellular capillary formation are regulated by complex context-dependent interactions among a number of pro- and antiangiogenic factors,[120-122] including angiopoietin-2 (Ang-2). When insufficient levels of VEGF and other angiogenic signals are present, Ang-2 causes endothelial cell death and vessel regression.[123-125]

Diabetes induces a significant increase in retinal expression of Ang-2 in rats,[126] and diabetic Ang-$2^{+/-}$ mice have both decreased pericyte loss and reduced acellular capillary formation.[127] In retinal Müller cells, increased glycolytic flux causes increased methylglyoxal modification of the corepressor mSin3A. Methylglyoxal modification of mSin3A results in increased Ang-2 expression. A similar mechanism involving methylglyoxal modification of other coregulator proteins might play a role in a variety of other diabetes-induced changes in gene expression.[128]

Advanced Glycation End Products Interfere with Normal Matrix-Matrix and Matrix-Cell Interactions

Methylglyoxal also leaks out of cells and is increased threefold to fivefold in the blood of diabetic patients, circulating at a concentration as high as 8 μM.[129] Methylglyoxal at this level greatly enhances apoptosis caused by agents that induce oxidative stress and DNA damage.[130] Methylglyoxal also can act as an antiapoptotic modulator by direct modification of heat-shock protein 27 (HSP27) at amino acid Arg-188, which allows HSP 27 to repress cytochrome c-mediated caspase activation.[131]

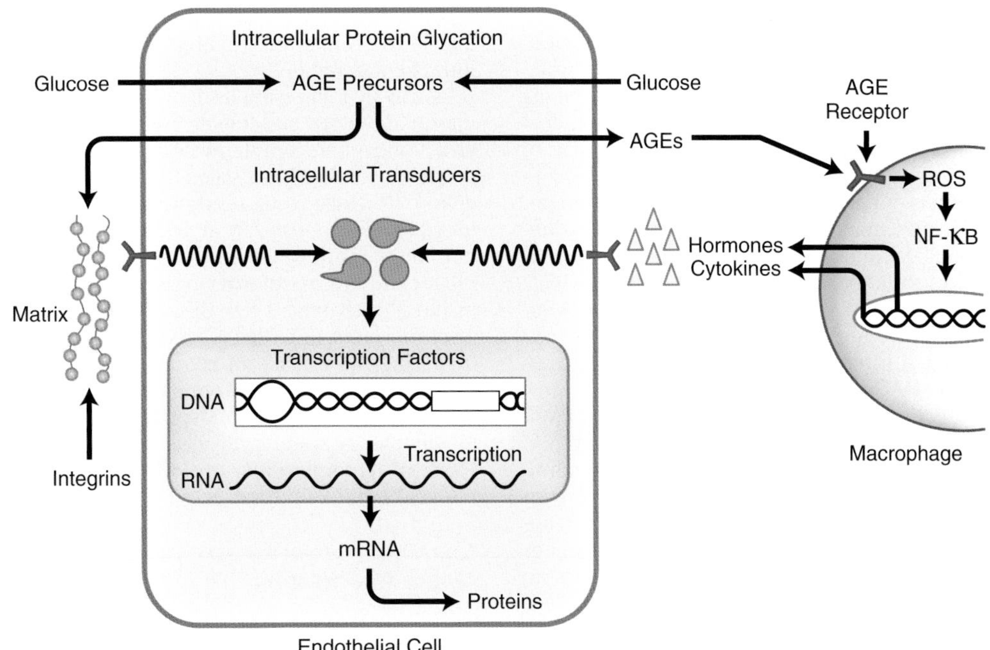

Figure 32–12 ▪ Potential mechanisms by which intracellular production of advanced glycation end-product (AGE) precursors damages vascular cells. First, intracellular protein modification alters protein function. Second, extracellular matrix modified by AGE precursors has abnormal functional properties. Third, plasma proteins modified by AGE precursors bind to AGE receptors on adjacent cells such as macrophages, thereby inducing receptor-mediated production of deleterious gene products such as cytokines. mRNA, messenger RNA; NFκB, neurotropic factor-κB; ROS, reactive oxygen species. (Adapted from Brownlee M. Lilly Lecture 1993: Glycation and diabetic complications. Diabetes 1994;43:836-841.)

AGE formation from circulating methylglyoxal and other AGE precursors alters the functional properties of several important matrix molecules. On type I collagen, this cross-linking induces an expansion of the molecular packing.[132] These AGE-induced cross-links alter the function of intact vessels. For example, AGEs decrease elasticity in large vessels from diabetic rats, even after vascular tone is abolished, and increase fluid filtration across the carotid artery.[133] AGE formation on type IV collagen from basement membrane inhibits lateral association of these molecules into a normal network-like structure by interfering with binding of the noncollagenous NC1 domain to the helix-rich domain.[134] AGE formation on laminin causes decreased polymer self-assembly, decreased binding to type IV collagen, and decreased binding of heparan sulfate proteoglycan.[135] In vitro AGE formation on intact glomerular basement membrane increases its permeability to albumin in a manner that resembles the abnormal permeability of diabetic nephropathy.[136,137]

AGE formation on extracellular matrix interferes not only with matrix-matrix interactions but also with matrix-cell interactions. For example, AGE modification of type IV collagen's cell-binding domains decreases endothelial cell adhesion,[138] and AGE modification of a six-amino-acid growth-promoting sequence in the A chain of the laminin molecule markedly reduces neurite outgrowth[139] AGE modification of vitronectin reduces cell attachment-promoting activity.[140] Research has shown that increased modification of vascular basement membrane type IV collagen by methylglyoxal, at hotspot modification sites in RGD and GFOGER integrin-binding sites of collagen, causes endothelial cell detachment and inhibition of angiogenesis.[141] In addition, matrix glycation impairs agonist-induced Ca^{2+} increases, which might adversely affect regulatory functions of the endothelium.[142]

Advanced Glycation End Product Receptors Mediate Pathologic Changes in Gene Expression

Several cell-associated binding proteins for AGEs have been identified, including OST-48, 80K-H, galectin-3, macrophage scavenger receptor type II, and RAGE.[143-147] Some of these are more likely to contribute to clearance of AGEs, whereas others can cause sustained cellular perturbations mediated by AGE ligand binding. In cell culture systems, the receptors identified to date appear to mediate long-term effects of AGEs on key cellular targets of diabetic complications such as macrophages, glomerular mesangial cells, and vascular endothelial cells, although not all these receptors bind proteins with physiologic AGE-modified levels. These effects include expression of cytokines and growth factors by macrophages and mesangial cells (interleukin [IL]-1, insulin-like growth factor [IGF]-I, tumor necrosis factor α [TNF-α], TGF-β, macrophage colony-stimulating factor [M-CSF], granulocyte-macrophage colony-stimulating factor [GM-CSF], and PDGF)[148-162] and expression of procoagulatory or proinflammatory molecules by endothelial cells (thrombomodulin, tissue factor, and VCAM-1).[163-166] In addition, endothelial AGE receptor binding appears to mediate in part the hyperpermeability induced by diabetes, probably through the induction of VEGF.[167-169]

Blockade of RAGE, a member of the pattern-recognition receptor class of the innate immune system, suppresses macrovascular disease in an atherosclerosis-prone type 1 diabetic mouse model in a glucose- and lipid-independent fashion.[170] Blockade of RAGE has also been shown to inhibit the development of diabetic vasculopathy,[171] nephropathy,[118] and periodontal disease[172] and to enhance wound repair in murine models via suppression of cytokines, TNF-α, IL-6, and metalloproteinases 2, 3, and 9.[173] In models of diabetic atherosclerosis (diabetic apolipoprotein E [apoE]-null mice), RAGE plays an important role in accelerated lesion formation and in lesion regression. Blockade of RAGE significantly reduced lesion size and structure and decreased parameters of inflammation as well as mononuclear phagocyte and smooth muscle cell activation.[170,174] In human saphenous vein endothelial cells, engagement of RAGE by heterogeneous AGEs or *N*-(carboxymethyl)lysine (CML)-modified adducts enhanced levels of mRNA and antigen for VCAM-1, ICAM-1, and E-selectin, leading to increased adhesion of polymorphonuclear leukocytes to stimulated endothelial cells. These effects were markedly reduced by blocking RAGE.[175] RAGE has been shown to mediate signal transduction via generation of ROS, which activates both NFκB, and p21 ras.[176-178] AGE signaling is blocked in cells by expression of RAGE antisense cDNA[176,179] or antiRAGE ribozyme.[177,180]

Vascular endothelial cells and pericytes have been demonstrated to express two splice variants of full-length RAGE mRNA. One codes for an isoform that lacks the N-terminal V-type immunoglobulin-like domain (N-truncated), and one codes for an isoform lacking the C-terminal transmembrane domain (C-truncated). The C-truncated type lacks the transmembrane domain and is secreted extracellularly and detected in human sera as endogenous secretory (es) RAGE. Circulating esRAGE levels are significantly lower in type 1 diabetic patients than in nondiabetic subjects, and plasma esRAGE levels are inversely correlated with carotid intima-media thickness (CIMT) and with increased risk of CVD.[181,182] Thus, it is possible that individual differences in esRAGE expression influence the development of diabetic vascular complications.

Activation of Protein Kinase C

Mechanism of Hyperglycemia-Induced Protein Kinase C Activation

PKCs are a family of at least 11 isoforms, nine of which are activated by the lipid second messenger DAG. Intracellular hyperglycemia increases DAG content in cultured microvascular cells and in the retina and renal glomeruli of diabetic animals.[183-185] Intracellular hyperglycemia appears to increase DAG content primarily by increasing its de novo synthesis from the glycolytic intermediate glyceraldehyde-3-phosphate via reduction to glycerol-3-phosphate and stepwise acylation.[184,186] Increased de novo synthesis of DAG activates PKC both in cultured vascular cells[185,187-189] and in retina and glomeruli of diabetic animals.[184,185,187] Increased DAG primarily activates the β and δ isoforms of PKC, but increases in other isoforms have also been found, such as PKC-α and PKC-ε isoforms in the retina[190] and PKC-α and PKC-δ in the glomerulus[191,192] of diabetic rats. DAG, its mimetics, the phorbol esters, and reactive oxygen all activate PKC isoforms by triggering the release of zinc ions from the cysteine-rich zinc finger of the regulatory domain. PKC isoforms can also be activated through tyrosine phosphorylation in a manner unrelated to receptor-coupled hydrolysis of inositol phospholipids. The effect of hyperglycemia on PKC tyrosine phosphorylation has not yet been examined.[193,194]

Consequences of Hyperglycemia-Induced Protein Kinase C Activation

In early experimental diabetes, activation of PKC-β isoforms has been shown to mediate retinal and renal blood flow abnormalities,[195] perhaps by depressing NO production and increasing endothelin-1 activity (Fig. 32–13). Abnormal activation of PKC has been implicated in the decreased glomerular production of NO induced by experimental diabetes[196] and in the decreased smooth muscle cell NO production induced by hyperglycemia.[197] PKC activation also inhibits insulin-stimulated expression of eNOS messenger RNA (mRNA) in cultured endothelial cells.[203] Hyperglycemia increases endothelin 1–stimulated MAPK activity in glomerular mesangial cells by activating PKC isoforms.[199] The increased endothelial cell permeability induced by high glucose concentrations in cultured cells is mediated by activation of PKC-β, however.[200] Activation of PKC by elevated glucose

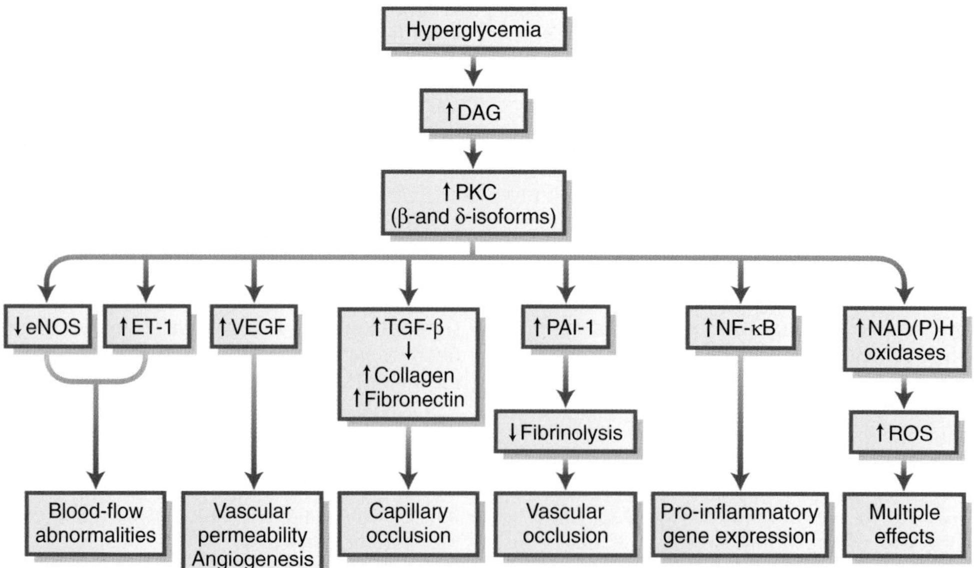

Figure 32–13 ■ Potential consequences of hyperglycemia-induced protein kinase C (PKC) activation. Hyperglycemia increases diacylglycerol (DAG) content, which activates PKC, primarily the β and δ isoforms. Activated PKC has a number of pathogenic consequences. eNOS, endothelial nitric oxide synthetase; ET-1, endothelin 1; NAD(P)H, nicotinamide adenine dinucleotide phosphate; PAI, plasminogen activator inhibitor; ROS, reactive oxygen species; TGF, transforming growth factor; VEGF, vascular endothelial growth factor. (Adapted from Koya D, Jirousek MR, Lin YW, et al. Characterization of protein kinase C beta isoform activation on the gene expression of transforming growth factor-beta, extracellular matrix components, and prostanoids in the glomeruli of diabetic rats. J Clin Invest 1997;100:115-126.)

levels also induces expression of the permeability-enhancing factor VEGF in smooth muscle cells.[201]

In addition to affecting hyperglycemia-induced abnormalities of blood flow and permeability, activation of PKC contributes to increased microvascular matrix protein accumulation by inducing the expression of TGF-β_1, fibronectin, and α1(IV) collagen in cultured mesangial cells[202,203] and in the glomeruli of diabetic rats.[196] This effect appears to be mediated through PKC's inhibition of NO production.[204] Hyperglycemia-induced expression of laminin C1 in cultured mesangial cells is independent of PKC activation, however.[205] Hyperglycemia-induced activation of PKC has also been implicated in the overexpression of the fibrinolytic inhibitor PAI-1[206] and in the activation of the pleiotrophic transcription factor NF-κB in cultured endothelial cells and vascular smooth muscle cells.[207,208]

In early experimental diabetes, activation of PKC-β isoforms has been shown to mediate retinal and renal blood flow abnormalities,[196] perhaps by depressing NO production or by increasing endothelin-1 activity. Abnormal activation of PKC has been implicated in the decreased glomerular production of NO induced by experimental diabetes[197] and in the decreased smooth muscle cell NO production induced by hyperglycemia.[198] PKC activation also inhibits insulin-stimulated expression of eNOS mRNA in cultured endothelial cells.[198] Hyperglycemia increases endothelin-1-stimulated MAPK activity in glomerular mesangial cells by activating PKC isoforms.[200] The increased endothelial cell permeability induced by high glucose in cultured cells is mediated by activation of PKC-α and is independent of the intracellular calcium concentration–NO pathway. [209]

In vascular smooth muscle cells, activation of PKC by elevated glucose increases p38 MAPK activity and induces expression of the permeability-enhancing factor VEGF.[202,210] PKC activation also activates various membrane-associated NAD(P)H-dependent oxidases.[211] Treatment of human blood vessels ex vivo from diabetic patients with coronary artery disease with a PKC inhibitor reduced diabetes-induced vascular superoxide production by NAD(P)H oxidases and superoxide-induced uncoupling of eNOS.[212] In normal subjects, the reduction in endothelium-dependent vasodilation induced by acute hyperglycemia is normalized by inhibition of PKC-β consistent with prevention of hyperglycemia-induced eNOS uncoupling.[213]

In addition to affecting hyperglycemia-induced abnormalities of blood flow and permeability, activation of PKC contributes to increased microvascular matrix protein accumulation by inducing expression of TGF-β_1, fibronectin, and α1(IV) collagen in both cultured mesangial cells[203] and in glomeruli of diabetic rats.[204] This effect appears to be mediated through PKC's inhibition of NO production.[205] Hyperglycemia-induced expression of laminin C1 in cultured mesangial cells is independent of PKC activation.[206] Hyperglycemia-induced activation of PKC has also been implicated in the overexpression of the fibrinolytic inhibitor PAI-1[207] and in the activation of the pleiotrophic transcription factor NFκB in cultured endothelial cells and vascular smooth muscle cells.[198,208] When PKC-β_2 is selectively overexpressed in the myocardium of diabetic mice, connective tissue growth factor (CTGF) and TGF-β_1 expression increases, and the mice develop cardiomyopathy and cardiac fibrosis.[214]

Increased Hexosamine Pathway Flux

A fourth hypothesis about how hyperglycemia causes diabetic complications has recently been formulated,[215-218] in which glucose is shunted into the hexosamine pathway (Fig. 32–14). In this pathway, fructose-6-phosphate is diverted from glycolysis to provide substrates for reactions that require uridine diphosphate-*N*-acetylglucosamine (UDP-GlcNAc), such as proteoglycan synthesis and the formation of *O*-linked glycoproteins. Inhibition of the rate-limiting enzyme in the conversion of glucose to glucosamine, glutamine: fructose-6-phosphate amidotransferase (GFAT), blocks hyperglycemia-induced increases in the transcription of both TGF-α_1[215] and TGF-β_1.[216] This pathway has previously been shown to play an important role in hyperglycemia-induced and fat-induced insulin resistance[219-221] by impairing activation of the insulin resistance/IRS/PI3K/Akt pathway.[222]

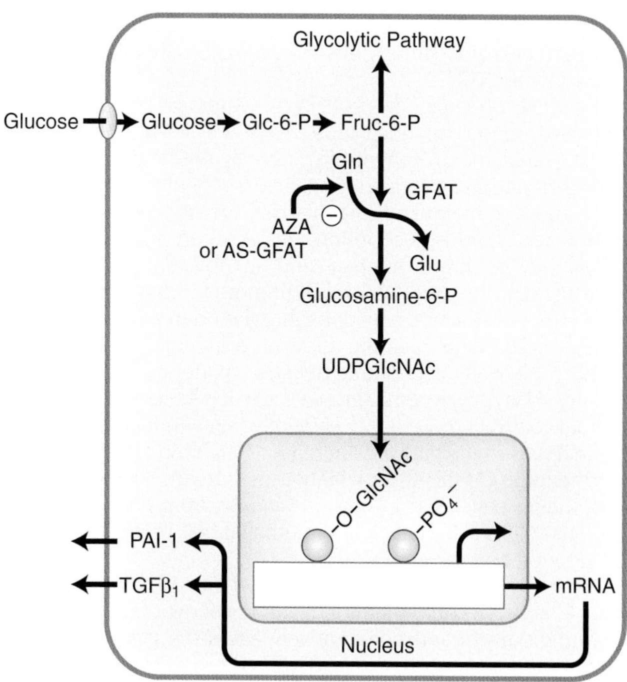

Figure 32–14 ▪ Schematic representation of the hexosamine pathway. The glycolytic intermediate fructose-6-phosphate (Fruc-6-P) is converted to glucosamine-6-phosphate (Glc-6-P) by the enzyme glutamine: fructose 6-phosphate amidotransferase (GFAT). Increased donation of *N*-acetylglucosamine moieties to serine and threonine residues of transcription factors such as Sp1 increases production of such complication-promoting factors as plasminogen activator inhibitor 1 (PAI-1) and transforming growth factor β_1 (TGF-β_1). AZA, azaserine; GlcNAc, -*N*-acetylglucosamine; UDP, uridine diphosphate. (Adapted from Du XL, Edelstein D, Rossetti L, et al. Hyperglycemia-induced mitochondrial superoxide overproduction activates the hexosamine pathway and induces plasminogen activator inhibitor-1 expression by increasing Sp1 glycosylation. Proc Natl Acad Sci U S A 2000;97: 12222-12226.)

The mechanism by which increased flux through the hexosamine pathway mediates hyperglycemia-induced increases in gene transcription has not been clear, but the observation that Sp1 sites regulate hyperglycemia-induced activation of the PAI-1 promoter in vascular smooth muscle cells[223] suggested that covalent modification of Sp1 by GlcNAc might explain the link between hexosamine pathway activation and hyperglycemia-induced changes in gene transcription. Glucosamine itself subsequently was shown to activate the PAI-1 promoter through Sp1 sites in glomerular mesangial cells.[224] Hyperglycemia has been shown to induce a 2.4-fold increase in hexosamine pathway activity in aortic endothelial cells, resulting in a 1.7-fold increase in Sp1 *O*-linked GlcNAc and a 70% to 80% decrease in Sp1 *O*-linked phosphothreonine and phosphoserine.[75] Concomitantly, hyperglycemia increased expression from an 85-bp truncated PAI-1 promoter luciferase reporter containing two Sp1 sites by 3.8-fold, but failed to increase expression when the two Sp1 sites were mutated.[75] In endothelial cells, signal transduction by the hexosamine pathway requires PKC-β_1 and PKC-δ activation for regulation of the PAI-1 promoter.[225] GlcNAc modification of Sp1 also regulates glucose-responsive expression of the prosclerotic growth factor TGF-β_1.

Because virtually every RNA polymerase II transcription factor examined has been found to be *O*-GlcNAcylated,[226] it is possible that reciprocal modification by *O*-GlcNAcylation and phosphorylation of transcription factors other than Sp1 function as a more generalized mechanism for regulating glucose-responsive gene transcription. In addition to transcription factors, many other nuclear and cytoplasmic proteins are dynamically modified by *O*-GlcNAc moieties and might exhibit reciprocal modification by phosphorylation in a manner analogous to Sp1.[174] One example relevant to diabetic complications is the inhibition of endothelial nitric oxide synthase (eNOS) activity by hyperglycemia-induced *O*-GlcNAcylation at the Akt site of the eNOS protein.[76,226] Hyperglycemia-induced activation of the hexosamine pathway increases activation of matrix metalloproteinase (MMP)-2 and MMP-9 in human coronary artery endothelial cells, and in carotid plaques from type 2 diabetic patients, *O*-GlcNAcylation of endothelial cell proteins is significantly increased.[222]

Hyperglycemia increases GFAT activity in aortic smooth muscle cells, and biochemical analyses show that hyperglycemia qualitatively and quantitatively alters the glycosylation or expression of many *O*-GlcNAc-modified proteins in the nucleus of these cells.[227] Thus, activation of the hexosamine pathway by hyperglycemia can result in many changes in gene expression and in protein function that together contribute to the pathogenesis of diabetic complications.

Different Hyperglycemia-Induced Pathogenic Mechanisms Reflect a Single Process

Although specific inhibitors of aldose reductase activity, AGE formation, and PKC activation each ameliorate various diabetes-induced abnormalities in animal models, there has been no apparent common element linking the four mechanisms of hyperglycemia-induced damage discussed in the preceding section.[100,196,229-231] It has also been conceptually difficult to explain the phenomenon of hyperglycemic memory (discussed earlier) as a consequence of four processes that quickly normalize when euglycemia is restored. These issues have now been resolved by the discovery that each of the four different pathogenic mechanisms reflects a single hyperglycemia-induced process: overproduction of superoxide by the mitochondrial electron transport chain.[75,232,233]

Hyperglycemia increases ROS production inside cultured bovine aortic endothelial cells. To understand how this occurs, a brief overview of glucose metabolism is helpful. Intracellular glucose oxidation begins with glycolysis in the cytoplasm, which generates NADH and pyruvate. Cytoplasmic NADH can donate reducing equivalents to the mitochondrial electron transport chain via two shuttle systems, or it can reduce pyruvate to lactate, which exits the cell to provide substrate for hepatic gluconeogenesis. Pyruvate can also be transported into the mitochondria, where it is oxidized by the tricarboxylic acid (TCA) cycle to produce CO_2, H_2O, four molecules of NADH, and one molecule of $FADH_2$. Mitochondrial NADH and $FADH_2$ (flavin adenine dinucleotide) provide energy for adenosine triphosphate (ATP) production via oxidative phosphorylation by the electron transport chain.

Electron flow through the mitochondrial electron transport chain is carried out by four inner membrane–associated enzyme complexes, plus cytochrome-*c* and the mobile carrier ubiquinone.[234] NADH derived from both cytosolic glucose oxidation and mitochondrial TCA cycle activity donates electrons to NADH: ubiquinone oxidoreductase *(Complex I)*. Complex I ultimately transfers its electrons to ubiquinone. Ubiquinone can also be reduced by electrons donated from several $FADH_2$-containing dehydrogenases, including succinate: ubiquinone oxidoreductase *(Complex II)* and glycerol-3-phosphate dehydrogenase. Electrons from reduced ubiquinone are then transferred to ubiquinol: cytochrome-*c* oxidoreductase *(Complex III)* by the ubisemiquinone radical–generating Q cycle.[235] Electron transport then proceeds through cytochrome-*c*, cytochrome-*c* oxidase *(Complex IV)*, and, finally, molecular oxygen.

Electron transfer through Complexes I, III, and IV generates a proton gradient that drives ATP synthase *(Complex V)*. When the electrochemical potential difference generated by this proton gradient is high, the life of superoxide-generating electron transport intermediates such as ubisemiquinone is prolonged. There appears to be a threshold value above which superoxide production is markedly increased (Fig. 32–15).[236]

Using inhibitors of both the shuttle that transfers cytosolic NADH into mitochondria and the transporter that transfers cytosolic pyruvate into the mitochondria, the TCA cycle was shown to be the source of hyperglycemia-induced ROS in endothelial cells. Overexpression of uncoupling protein 1 (UCP-1), a specific protein uncoupler of oxidative phosphorylation capable of collapsing the proton electrochemical gradient,[237] also prevented the effect of hyperglycemia. These results demonstrate that hyperglycemia-induced intracellular ROS are produced by the proton electrochemical gradient generated by the mitochondrial electron transport chain. Overexpression of manganese superoxide dismutase (MnSOD), the mitochondrial form of this antioxidant enzyme,[238] also prevents the effect of hyperglycemia. Prevention of mitochondrial superoxide production also completely prevents activation of the polyol pathway, AGE formation, PKC, and the hexosamine pathway (Fig. 32–16). In endothelial cells, PKC also activates NFκB, a transcription factor that itself activates many proinflammatory genes in the vasculature. As expected, hyperglycemia-induced NFκB activation is also prevented by either UCP-1 or MnSOD, both in cells and in animals.

In addition, diabetes-induced loss of vascular cyclic adenosine monophosphate (cAMP)-responsive element-binding protein (CREB) and enhanced expression of platelet-derived growth factor receptor (PDGFR)-α in nonobese diabetic (NOD) mice are both reversed by treatment with an SOD mimetic,[239] and hyperglycemia-mediated interference with neuronal CREB and bcl-2 expression can be restored by treatment of the neurons in vitro with an SOD mimetic.[228]

Thus, hyperglycemia-induced mitochondrial production of ROS is both necessary and sufficient for activation of each of these pathways.

After hyperglycemia induces mitochondrial ROS production, these ROS can activate a number of other superoxide production pathways that might amplify the original damaging effect of hyperglycemia (M. Brownlee, unpublished observations).

How does hyperglycemia-induced ROS activate AGE formation, PKC, the hexosamine pathway, and the polyol pathway? It does this by inhibiting activity of the key glycolytic enzyme GAPDH (Fig. 32–17). When GAPDH activity is inhibited, the level of all the glycolytic intermediates that are upstream of GAPDH increase. An increased level of the upstream glycolytic metabolite glyceraldehyde-3 phosphate activates two of the four pathways. It activates the AGE pathway because the major intracellular AGE precursor methylglyoxal is formed from glyceraldehyde-3 phosphate. It also activates the classic PKC pathway, because the activator of PKC, diacylglycerol, is also formed from glyceraldehyde-3 phosphate. Farther upstream, levels of the glycolytic metabolite fructose-6 phosphate increase, which increases flux

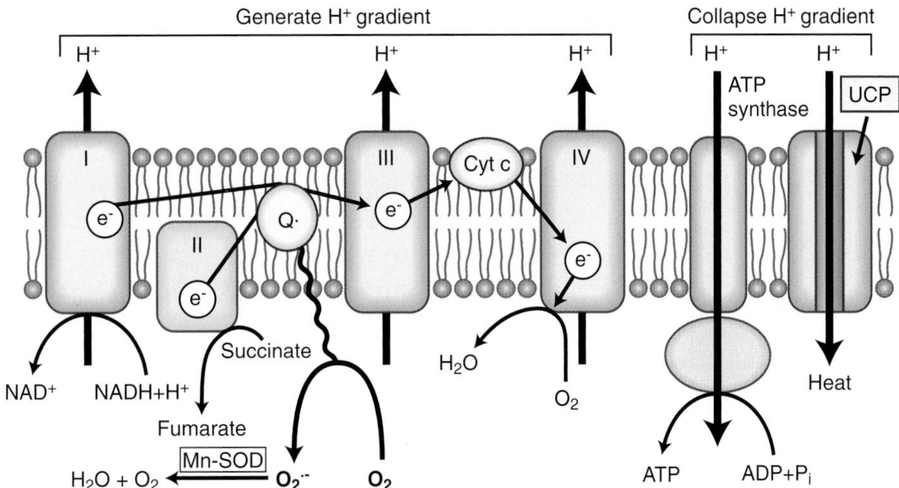

Figure 32–15 ▪ Production of superoxide by the mitochondrial electron transport chain. Increased hyperglycemia-derived electron donors from the tricarboxylic acid cycle (NADH and $FADH_2$) generate a high mitochondrial membrane potential ($\Delta\mu$ H^+) by pumping protons across the mitochondrial inner membrane. This inhibits electron transport at complex III and increases the half-life of free radical intermediates of coenzyme Q, which reduce O_2 to superoxide. ADP, adenosine diphosphate; ATP, adenosine triphosphate; Mn-SOD, manganese superoxide dismutase; NAD^+, nicotinamide adenine dinucleotide; NADH, reduced nicotinamide adenine dinucleotide; UCP, uncoupling protein. (From Boss O, Hagen T, Lowell BB. Uncoupling proteins 2 and 3: potential regulators of mitochondrial energy metabolism. Diabetes 2000;49:143-156.)

through the hexosamine pathway, where fructose-6 phosphate is converted by the enzyme GFAT to UDP-GlcNAc. Finally, inhibition of GAPDH increases intracellular levels of the first glycolytic metabolite, glucose. This increases flux through the polyol pathway, where the enzyme aldose reductase reduces it, consuming NADPH in the process. Inhibition of GAPDH using DNA antisense activates each of these pathways to the same extent as diabetes, when glucose concentrations are physiologic.[240]

Hyperglycemia-induced mitochondrial superoxide itself can directly inactivate GAPDH, but only at concentrations that far exceed levels found in hyperglycemic cells. In vivo, hyperglycemia-induced superoxide inhibits GAPDH activity by modifying the enzyme with polymers of adenosine diphosphate (ADP)-ribose.[241] Inhibition of mitochondrial superoxide production with either UCP-1 or MnSOD prevents both modification of GAPDH by ADP-ribose and reduction of its activity by hyperglycemia. Most importantly, both modifications of GAPDH by ADP-ribose and reduction of its activity by hyperglycemia are also prevented by a specific inhibitor of the enzyme poly(ADP-ribose) polymerase (PARP). PARP is a nuclear DNA-repair enzyme that is activated by DNA strand breaks. Increased intracellular glucose generates increased ROS in the mitochondria, and these free radicals cause DNA strand breaks, thereby activating PARP (Fig. 32–18). Once activated, PARP splits the NAD molecule into its two component parts: nicotinic acid and ADP-ribose. PARP then generates polymers of ADP-ribose, which accumulate on GAPDH and other nuclear proteins. Although GAPDH is commonly thought to reside exclusively in the cytosol, in fact, it normally shuttles in and out of the nucleus, where it plays a critical role in DNA repair.[242,243]

A schematic summary showing the elements of the unified mechanism of hyperglycemia-induced cellular damage is shown in (Fig. 32–19). When intracellular hyperglycemia develops in target cells of diabetic complications, it causes increased mitochondrial production of ROS. The ROS causes strand breaks in nuclear DNA, which activates PARP. PARP then modifies GAPDH, thereby reducing its activity. Finally, decreased GAPDH activity activates the polyol pathway, increases intracellular AGE formation, activates PKC and subsequently NFκB, and activates hexosamine pathway flux.

In cultured glomerular mesangial cells, overexpression of MnSOD suppresses the increase in collagen synthesis induced by high glucose.[243] In dorsal root ganglion (DRG) neurons from both wild-type and $MnSOD^{+/-}$ mice, overexpression of MnSOD decreases hyperglycemia-induced programmed cell death, and in embryonic rat DRG neurons, overexpression of UCP-1 inhibits cleavage of programmed cell death effector caspases.[244] In aortic endothelial cells, overexpression of either UCP-1 or MnSOD completely blocks hyperglycemia-induced monocyte adhesion to endothelial cells (J.L. Nadler and C.C. Hedrick, personal communication). Overexpression of UCP-1 or MnSOD also prevents hyperglycemia-induced inhibition of the antiatherogenic enzyme prostacyclin synthetase (M. Brownlee, et al, unpublished observation). In diabetes, inhibition of prostacyclin synthetase causes accumulation of the precursor prostaglandin PGI_2, which activates thromboxane receptors that trigger vasoconstriction, platelet aggregation, increased expression of leukocyte adhesion molecules, and apoptosis.[245]

Overexpression of either MnSOD or UCP-1 also prevents inhibition of eNOS activity by hyperglycemia.[76] In platelets, chemical uncouplers or SOD mimetics both prevent potentiation by hyperglycemia of collagen-induced platelet activation and aggregation.[77] Antioxidant treatment prevents hyperglycemia-induced activity of matrix metalloproteinase-9 (MMP-9) in VSMC.[246]

In streptozotocin diabetic transgenic mice overexpressing human cytoplasmic Cu^{2+}/Zn^{2+} SOD, albuminuria, glomerular hypertrophy, and glomerular content of TGF-β and collagen α1(IV) were all attenuated compared to wild-type littermates after 4 months of diabetes.[247] Overexpression of the human *SOD1* transgene in db/db diabetic mice similarly normalized the extensive expansion of the glomerular mesangial matrix that was otherwise evident by age 5 months in the nontransgenic db/db littermates.[248] Similarly, transgenic overexpression of the antioxidant enzymes MnSOD and catalase reduced ROS and prevented diabetes-induced abnormalities in cardiac contractility in an animal model of diabetic cardiomyopathy[249,250] In humans, skin fibroblast gene expression profiles from two groups of type 1 diabetic patients—20 with very fast (fast-track) versus 20 with very slow (slow-track) rates of development of

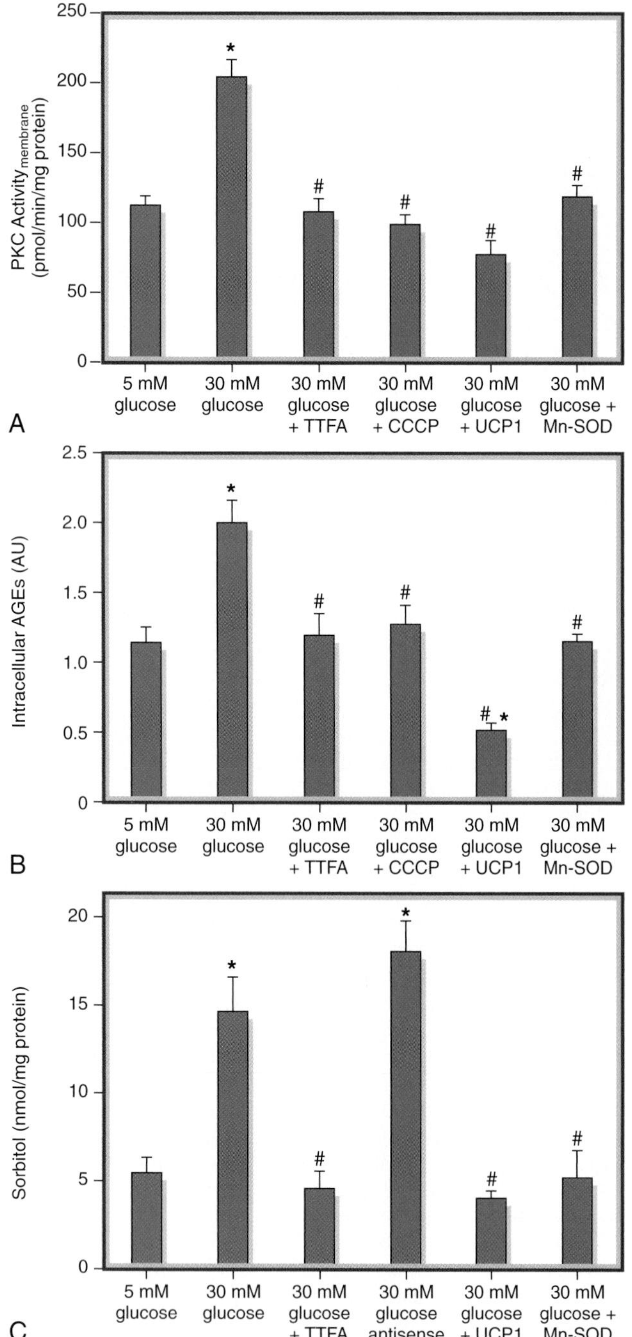

Figure 32–16 ▪ Effect of agents that alter mitochondrial electron transport chain function on the three main pathways of hyperglycemic damage. **A,** Hyperglycemia-induced protein kinase C (PKC) activation. **B,** Intracellular advanced glycation end-product (AGE) formation. **C,** Sorbitol accumulation. Cells were incubated in 5-mM glucose, 30-mM glucose alone, and 30-mM glucose plus either agents that uncouple oxidative phosphorylation and reduce the high mitochondrial membrane potential (TTFA, CCCP, UCP-1), or dismutate superoxide (Mn-SOD). CCCP, carbonyl cyanide *m*-chlorophenylhydrazone; TTFA, thenoyltrifluoroacetone; UCP-1, uncoupling protein-1. (From Nishikawa T, Edelstein D, Du XL, et al. Normalizing mitochondrial superoxide production blocks three pathways of hyperglycaemic damage. Nature 2000;404:787-790.)

diabetic nephropathy lesions—showed that the fast-track group has increased expression of oxidative phosphorylation genes, mitochondrial electron transport system complex III, and TCA cycle genes. These associations are consistent with a central role for mitochondrial reactive oxygen production in the pathogenesis of diabetic nephropathy.[251]

Free Fatty Acid–Induced Proatherogenic Changes Are Also Caused by Mitochondrial ROS Production

Insulin resistance causes increased FFA release from adipocytes. In macrovascular, but not in microvascular, endothelial cells, the resultant increased flux of FFA results in increased FFA oxidation by the mitochondria. Because both oxidation of fatty acids and oxidation of FFA-derived acetyl CoA by the TCA cycle generate the same electron donors (NADH and $FADH_2$) generated by glucose oxidation, increased FFA oxidation causes mitochondrial overproduction of ROS by exactly the same mechanism described for hyperglycemia. As with hyperglycemia, this FFA-induced increase in ROS activates the same damaging pathways: AGEs, PKC, the hexosamine pathway (GlcNAc), and NFκB, which together activate a variety of proinflammatory signals previously implicated in hyperglycemia-induced vascular damage (Fig. 32–20). In addition, these ROS directly inactivate two important antiatherogenic enzymes, prostacyclin synthase and eNOS, independent of the pathways just discussed. In two insulin-resistant nondiabetic animal models, inhibition of either FFA release from adipocytes or FFA oxidation in arterial endothelium prevents the increased production of ROS and its damaging effects.[84]

Possible Molecular Basis For Hyperglycemic Memory

Continued mitochondrial superoxide production might explain the occurrence of complications during posthyperglycemic normoglycemia. In the retina of diabetic rats with poor glycemic control for 2 months, subsequent normalization of Hb A_1 for 7 months only lowered elevated retinal lipid peroxides by approximately 50% and failed to have any beneficial effects on levels of the oxidative marker 3-nitrotyrosine. In the retinas of diabetic animals with poor glycemic control for 6 months, subsequent normalization of Hb A_1 for 6 months had no effect on elevated retinal oxidative stress levels and only a small effect on elevated levels of 3-nitrotyrosine.[252]

Although the molecular changes that result in continuous overproduction of ROS in normoglycemic animals and humans have not yet been identified, several hypotheses are being tested. One hypothesis involves induction of stable epigenetic changes such as DNA methylation and histone acetylation. Such changes can alter levels of gene expression for many years. Another hypothesis concerns changes in mitochondrial biology. It is now recognized that mitochondria are not all the same, but rather have important functional differences. Furthermore, mitochondria are not static structures in the cell. Rather, they continuously fuse to form larger organelles or pull apart to form smaller organelles. The processes underlying these changes are beginning to be understood, but aberrations induced by diabetes and different degrees of hyperglycemia are important new areas that will likely yield new insights into hyperglycemic memory.[253]

The third hypothesis currently being evaluated is altered regulation of the antioxidant response element. Perhaps not

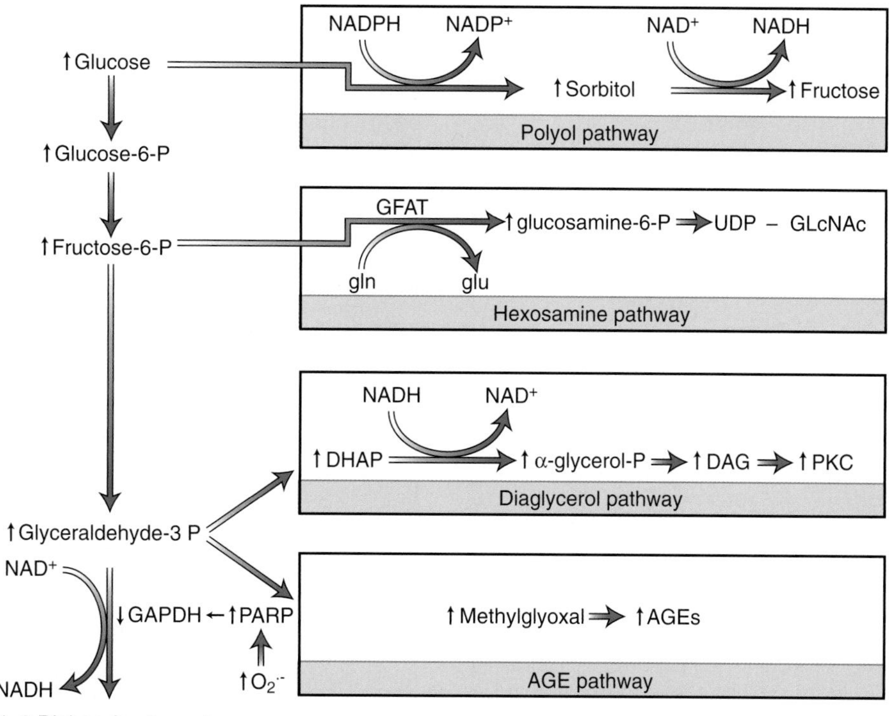

Figure 32–17 ▪ Potential mechanism by which hyperglycemia-induced mitochondrial superoxide overproduction activates four pathways of hyperglycemic damage. Excess superoxide partially inhibits the glycolytic enzyme glyceraldehyde-3-phosphate dehydrogenase by activating PARP and causing ADP-ribosylation of GADPH. Decreased GADPH activity increases concentration of upstream metabolites and diverts them from glycolysis into pathways of glucose overutilization. This results in increased flux of triose phosphate to diacylglycerol (DAG), an activator of protein kinase C (PKC), and to methylglyoxal, the major intracellular advanced glycation end product (AGE) precursor. Increased flux of fructose-6-phosphate to UDP-*N*-acetylglucosamine increases modification of proteins by hexosamine, and increased glucose flux through the polyol pathway consumes NADPH and depletes GSH. ADP, adenosine diphosphate; DHAP, dihydroxyacetone phosphate; GAPDH, glyceraldehyde-3-phosphate dehydrogenase; GSH, reduced glutathione; NAD^+, nicotinamide adenine dinucleotide; NADH, reduced nicotinamide adenine dinucleotide; PARP, poly(ADP-ribose) polymerase; NADPH, nicotinamide adenine dinucleotide phosphate; UDP, uridine diphosphate.

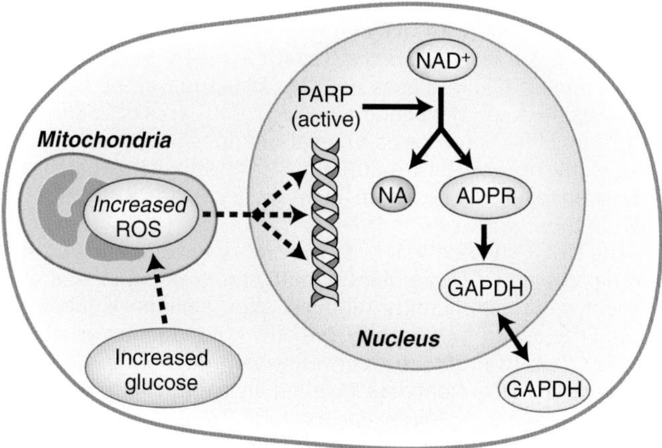

Figure 32–18 ▪ Schematic representation of the mechanism by which hyperglycemia-induced mitochondrial superoxide overproduction activates PARP and modifies GAPDH. Hyperglycemia-induced mitochondrial superoxide overproduction causes DNA strand breaks, thereby activating the nuclear DNA-repair enzyme PARP. Activated PARP splits the NAD molecule into its two component parts: nicotinic acid and ADP-ribose. PARP then generates polymers of ADP-ribose, which accumulate on GAPDH, inactivating the enzyme. ADP, adenosine diphosphate; GAPDH, glyceraldehyde-3-phosphate dehydrogenase; PARP, poly(ADP-ribose) polymerase. (Adapted from Brownlee M. Banting Lecture 2004. The pathobiology of diabetic complications: a unifying mechanism. Diabetes 2005;54:1615-1625.)

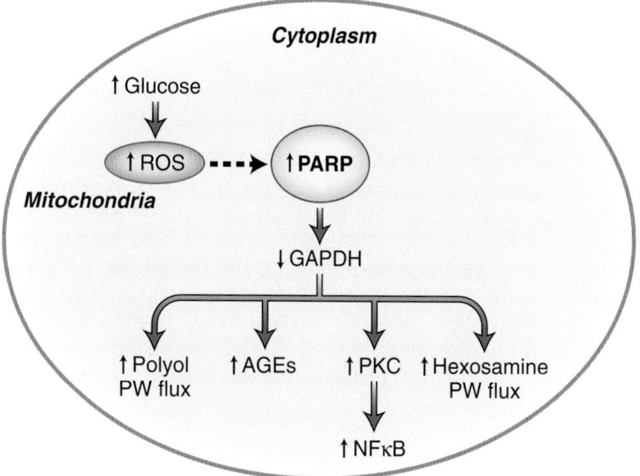

Figure 32–19 ▪ Unifying mechanism of hyperglycemia-induced cellular damage. Intracellular hyperglycemia causes increased mitochondrial production of reactive oxygen species (ROS). The ROS cause strand breaks in nuclear DNA, which activates PARP. PARP then modifies GAPDH, thereby reducing its activity. Decreased GAPDH activity activates the polyol pathway, increases intracellular AGE formation, activates PKC and subsequently NFκB, and activates hexosamine pathway (PW) flux. AGE, advanced glycation end product; GAPDH, glyceraldehyde-3-phosphate dehydrogenase; NFκB, nuclear factor κB; PARP, poly(ADP-ribose) polymerase; PKC, protein kinase C. (Adapted from Brownlee M. Banting Lecture 2004. The pathobiology of diabetic complications: a unifying mechanism. Diabetes 2005;54:1615-1625.)

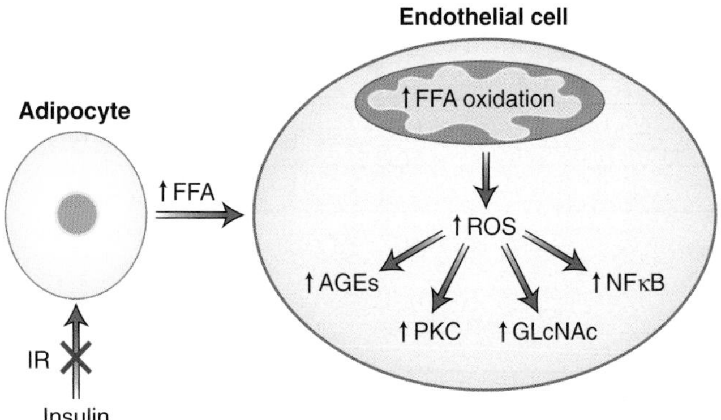

Figure 32–20 ▪ Schematic mechanism by which insulin resistance (IR) causes increased oxidation of free fatty acids (FFA) in arterial endothelial cells, which activates proatherogenic signals and inhibits key antiatherogenic enzymes. IR causes increased FFA release from adipocytes. In macrovascular endothelial cells, the increased flux of FFA results in increased FFA oxidation by the mitochondria, thereby causing mitochondrial overproduction of reactive oxygen species (ROS). FFA-induced increase in ROS activates advanced glycation end products (AGEs), protein kinase C (PKC), the hexosamine pathway (GlcNAc), and nuclear factor κB (NFκB), which together activate a variety of proinflammatory signals. In addition, ROS directly inactivate two important antiatherogenic enzymes, prostacyclin synthase and endothelial nitric oxide synthase (eNOS). GlcNAc, -*N*-acetylglucosamine. (Adapted from Du, X., et al. Insulin resistance reduces arterial prostacylcin synthase and eNOS activities by increasing endothelial fatty acid oxidation. J Clin Invest 2006;116:1071-1080.)

surprisingly, cells have their own protective antioxidant machinery. Cells responded to oxidative stress by activating a previously sequestered transcription factor (Nrf2), which controls the expression of a diverse set of genes involved in decreasing ROS in the cell. An important research focus is the identification and regulation of proteins in this pathway, including proteins that bind to a special promoter element called the antioxidant response element (ARE) after activation by ROS.

RETINOPATHY, MACULAR EDEMA, AND OTHER OCULAR COMPLICATIONS*

Diabetic retinopathy is a well-characterized sight-threatening chronic microvascular complication that eventually afflicts virtually all patients with diabetes mellitus.[60] Diabetic retinopathy is characterized by gradually progressive alterations in the retinal microvasculature, leading to areas of retinal nonperfusion, increased vascular permeability, and pathologic intraocular proliferation of retinal vessels. The complications associated with the increased vascular permeability, termed *macular edema,* and uncontrolled neovascularization, termed *proliferative diabetic retinopathy* (PDR), can result in severe and permanent vision loss.

*Portions of this section draw on, among others, Aiello LM, Cavallerano JD, Aiello LP. Diagnosis, management, and treatment of nonproliferative diabetic retinopathy and diabetic macular edema. In Albert DM, Jokobiec FA, eds. Principles and Practice of Ophthalmology, 2nd ed. Philadelphia: WB Saunders, 2000:1900-1914; Aiello LP, Cavallerano J, Klein R. Diabetic eye disease. In DeGroot LJ, James JL, eds. Endocrinology, 5th ed. Philadelphia, WB Saunders, 2005:1305-1317. Aiello LP, Gardner TW, King GL, et al. Diabetic retinopathy: Technical review. American Diabetes Association. Diabetes Care 1998;21:143-156; and Aiello LP, Cavallerano J. Diabetic retinopathy. In Johnstone MT, Veves A, eds. Contemporary Cardiology: Diabetes and Cardiovascular Disease. Totowa, NJ: Humana Press, 2001:385-398.

Despite decades of research, there is currently no known means of preventing diabetic retinopathy and, despite effective therapies, diabetic retinopathy remains the leading cause of new-onset blindness in working-aged persons in most developed countries of the world.[60] With appropriate medical and ophthalmologic care, however, more than 90% of vision loss resulting from proliferative diabetic retinopathy can be prevented.[254] Thus, until a cure for diabetes is discovered, the primary clinical care emphasis for the prevention of vision loss is appropriately directed at early identification, accurate classification, and timely treatment of retinopathy.

However, the increased understanding of the mechanistic pathways underlying hyperglycemia-induced retinal changes has provided new targets against which novel therapies have been devised. These novel therapies, such as VEGF inhibitors, corticosteroids, and PKC-β inhibitors,[255-263] have entered clinical trials with promising initial results and are likely to increase therapeutic options for patients with diabetic eye disease. Emphasis must also be placed on adhering to lifelong routine ophthalmologic follow-up of the diabetic patient and optimization of associated systemic disorders.

Epidemiology and Impact

By 2030, it is estimated that 366 million persons worldwide will have diabetes.[264] More than 20 million Americans currently have diabetes mellitus, but only half are aware that they have the disease.[60,265] Diabetic retinopathy is the leading cause of new cases of legal blindness among Americans between the ages of 20 and 74 years.[266] There is a higher risk of more frequent and severe ocular complications in T1DM.[265] Approximately 25% of patients with T1DM have retinopathy after 5 years, and this figure increases to 60% and 80% after 10 and 15 years, respectively. Because T2DM accounts for 90% to 95% of the diabetic population in the United States, type 2 disease accounts for a higher fraction of patients with vision loss. The most threatening form of retinopathy (PDR) is present in approximately 25% of T1DM patients who have had diabetes for 15 years.[268]

An estimated 700,000 persons have PDR, 130,000 with high-risk PDR, 500,000 with macular edema, and 325,000 with *clinically significant macular edema* (CSME) in the United States.[269-273] An estimated 63,000 cases of PDR, 29,000 cases of high-risk PDR, 80,000 cases of macular edema, 56,000 cases of CSME, and 12,000 to 24,000 new cases of legal blindness occur each year as a result of diabetic retinopathy.[269,270,274] Blindness has been estimated to be 25 times more common in persons with diabetes than in those without the disease.[275,276]

The DCCT showed that both the rate of development of any retinopathy and the rate of retinopathy progression once it was present were significantly reduced after 3 years of intensive insulin therapy.[277] Interestingly, the effect of reducing the Hb A_{1c} in this group from 9.1% for conventional treatment to the 7.3% for intensive treatment has resulted in a benefit maintained through 7 years of follow-up, even though the difference in mean Hb A_{1c} levels of the two former randomized treatment groups was only 0.4% at 1 year ($P<.001$), continued to narrow, and became statistically nonsignificant by 5 years (8.1% vs. 8.2%, $P=.09$). The further rate of progression of complications from their levels at the end of the DCCT remains less in the former intensive treatment group. Thus, the benefits of 6.5 years of intensive treatment extend well beyond the period of its most intensive implementation..[26,29,278,279] Applying DCCT intensive insulin therapy to all persons in the United States with T1DM would result in a gain of 920,000 person-years of sight,[280] although the costs of intensive therapy are three times that of conventional therapy.[281]

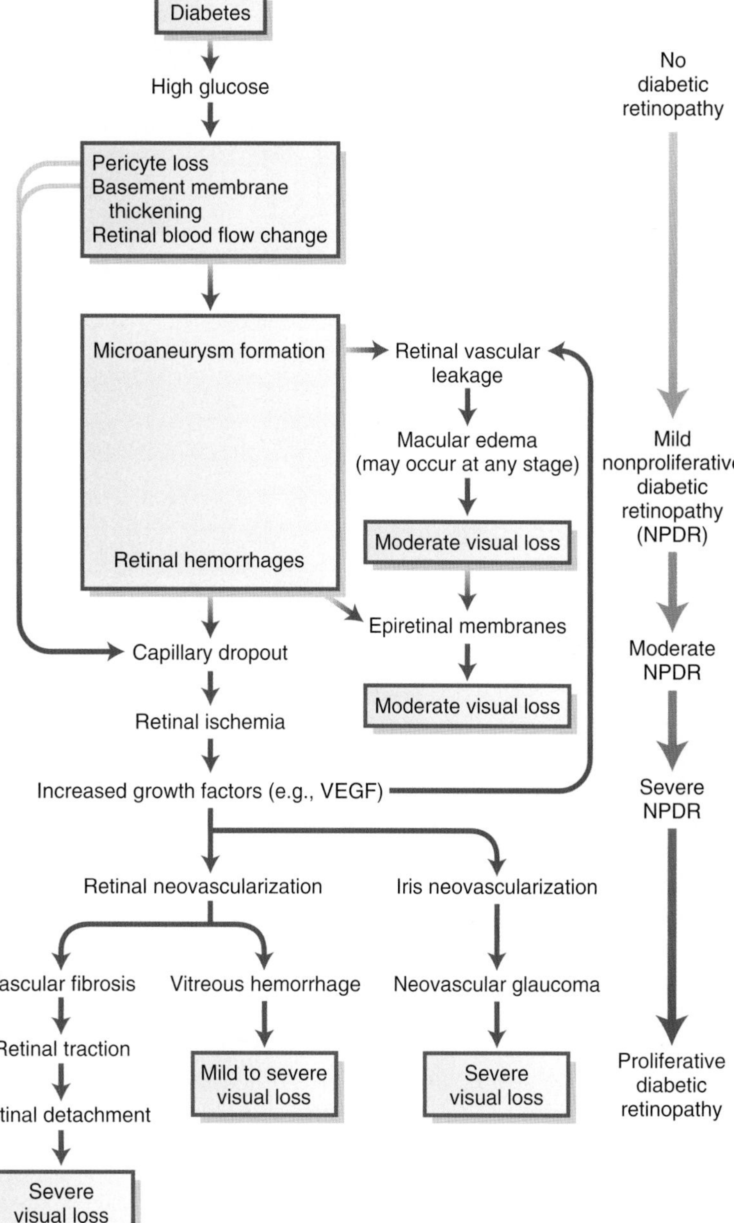

Figure 32–21 ▪ Diabetic retinopathy pathogenesis flow chart. The schematic flow chart represents the major preclinical and clinical findings associated with the full spectrum of diabetic retinopathy and macular edema. NPDR, nonproliferative diabetic retinopathy; VEGF, vascular endothelial growth factor.

Pathophysiology

A detailed discussion of the pathophysiologic mechanisms underlying diabetic retinopathy and other diabetes-related complications has been presented earlier in this chapter. The earliest histologic effects of diabetes mellitus in the eye include loss of retinal vascular pericytes (supporting cells for retinal endothelial cells), thickening of vascular endothelium basement membrane, and alterations in retinal blood flow (Fig. 32–21).[24,282-287] With increasing loss of retinal pericytes, the retinal vessel wall develops outpouchings (microaneurysms) and becomes fragile.

Clinically, microaneurysms and small retinal hemorrhages might not always be readily distinguishable and are usually evaluated together as "hemorrhages and microaneurysms" (Fig. 32–22A). Rheologic changes occur in diabetic retinopathy and result from increased platelet aggregation, integrin-mediated leukocyte adhesion, and endothelial damage.[288-290] Disruption of the blood-retina barrier can ensue, characterized by increased vascular permeability.[291-292] The subsequent leakage of blood and serum from the retinal vessels results in retinal hemorrhages, retinal edema, and hard exudates (see Fig. 32–22A and C). Moderate vision loss follows if the fovea is affected by the leakage.[293]

With time, increasing sclerosis and endothelial cell loss lead to narrowing of the retinal vessels, which decreases vascular perfusion and can ultimately lead to obliteration of the capillaries and small vessels (see Fig. 32–22B). The resulting retinal ischemia is a potent inducer of angiogenic growth factors. Several angiogenic growth factors have been isolated from eyes with diabetic retinopathy, including insulin-like growth factors, basic fibroblast growth factor (bFGF), hepatocyte growth factor (HGF), and VEGF.[294-297] These factors promote the development of new vessel growth and retinal vascular permeability.[298-302] Indeed, inhibition of molecules such as VEGF and their signaling pathways can suppress the development of retinal neovascularization and retinal vascular permeability.[299,303-307] Endogenous inhibitors of angiogenesis such as pigment

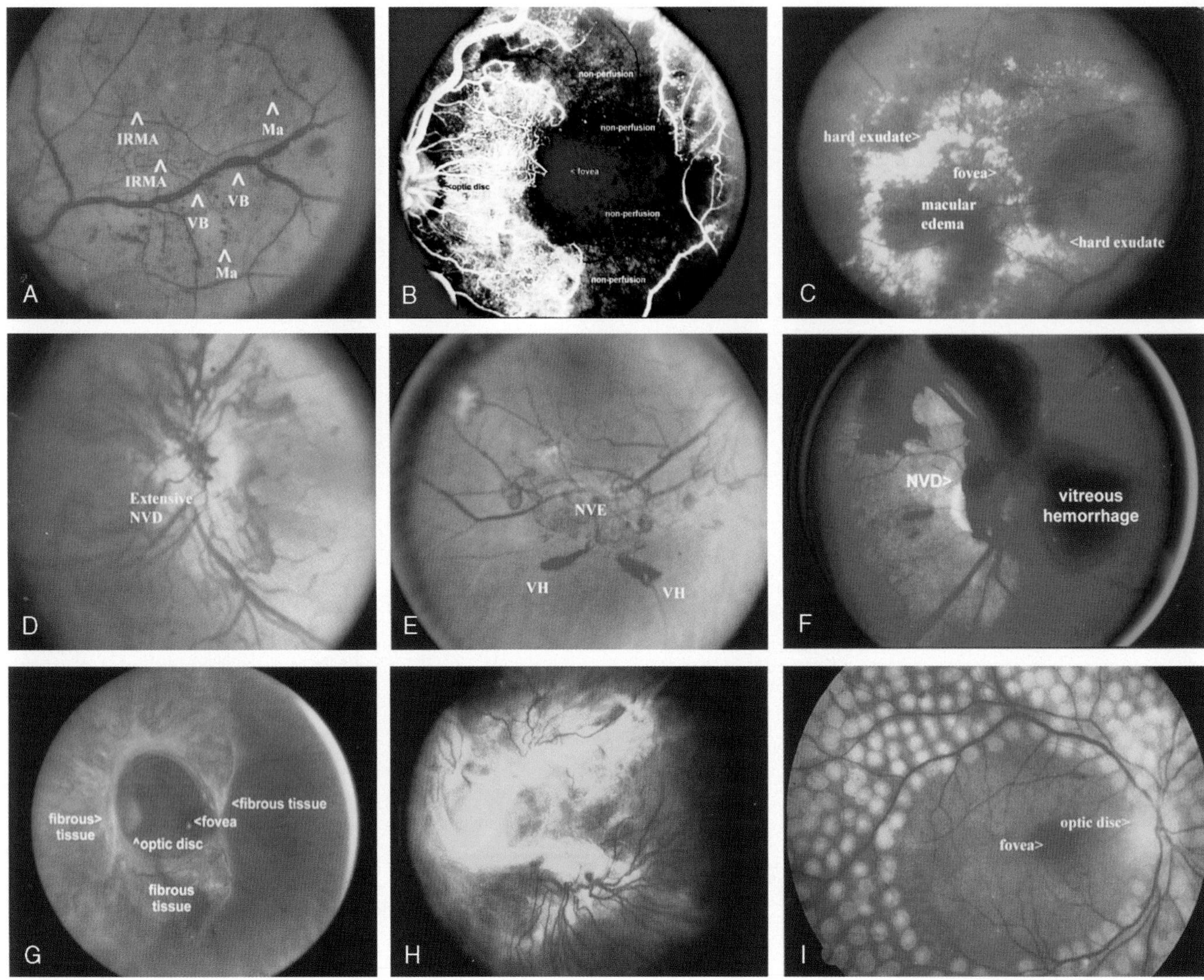

Figure 32–22 ▪ Clinical features of diabetic retinopathy: Some typical findings in human diabetic retinopathy. **A,** Findings in severe nonproliferative diabetic retinopathy, including microaneurysms (Ma), venous beading (VB), and intraretinal microvascular abnormalities (IRMA). **B,** Fluorescein angiogram showing marked capillary nonperfusion. **C,** Clinically significant macular edema with retinal thickening and hard exudates involving the fovea. **D,** Extensive neovascularization of the optic disc (NVD), illustrating high-risk proliferative diabetic retinopathy. **E,** Neovascularization elsewhere (NVE) and two small vitreous hemorrhages (VH), also illustrating high-risk proliferative diabetic retinopathy. **F,** Extensive vitreous hemorrhage arising from severe neovascularization of the disc (NVD). **G,** Severe fibrovascular proliferation surrounding the fovea. **H,** Traction retinal detachment from extensive fibrovascular proliferation. **I,** Scars from scatter (panretinal) laser photocoagulation. The macula and fovea and optic disc are not treated to preserve central vision. Laser burns are evident as white retinal lesions. (Adapted from Aiello LP. Eye complications of diabetes. In Korenman SG, Kahn CR [eds]. Atlas of Clinical Endocrinology. Vol 2: Diabetes. Philadelphia, Blackwell Scientific, 1999.)

epithelial-derived factor (PEDF) have also been found in the eye, and these have physiologic and therapeutic potential.[308]

New vessels tend to grow in regions of strong vitreous adhesion to the retina, such as at the optic disc and major vascular arcades (see Fig. 32–22D and E). The posterior vitreous face also serves as a scaffold for pathologic neovascularization, and the new vessels commonly arise at the junctions between perfused and nonperfused retina. When the retina is severely ischemic, the concentration of angiogenic growth factors can reach sufficient concentration in the anterior chamber to cause abnormal new vessel proliferation on the iris and the anterior chamber angle.[296,309] Uncontrolled anterior segment neovascularization can result in neovascular glaucoma because the fibrovascular proliferation in the angle of the eye causes blockage of aqueous outflow through the trabecular meshwork.[310]

Proliferating new vessels in diabetic retinopathy are fragile and have a tendency to bleed, which results in preretinal and vitreous hemorrhages (see Fig. 32–22E and F). Although the presence of a large amount of blood in the preretinal space or vitreous cavity per se is not damaging to the retina, these intraocular hemorrhages often cause prolonged vision loss by blocking the visual axis. Membranes on the retinal surface can be induced by blood and result in wrinkling and traction on the retina. Although all retinal neovascularization eventually becomes quiescent, as with most scarring processes there is progressive fibrosis of the new vessel complexes that is associated with contraction. In the eye, such forces can exert traction on the retina, leading to tractional retinal detachment and retinal tears that can result in severe and permanent vision loss if left untreated (see Fig. 32–22G and H).

In short, causes of vision loss from complications of diabetes mellitus include retinal ischemia involving the fovea, macular edema at or near the fovea, preretinal or vitreous hemorrhages, retinal detachment, and neovascular glaucoma. Vision loss can also result from more indirect effects of disease progression in diabetic patients, such as retinal vessel occlusion, accelerated atherosclerotic disease, and embolic phenomena.

Clinical Features

Risk Factors

Duration of diabetes is closely associated with the onset and severity of diabetic retinopathy. Diabetic retinopathy is rare in prepubescent patients with T1DM, but nearly all patients with T1DM and more than 60% of patients with T2DM develop some degree of retinopathy after 20 years.[60,268,311] In U.S. reports of patients with T2DM, approximately 20% had retinopathy at the time of diabetes diagnosis[311] and most had some degree of retinopathy over subsequent decades. In the UKPDS study of T2DM, 35% of female subjects and 39% of male subjects had some level of diabetic retinopathy at the time of diabetes diagnosis.[312]

Diabetic retinopathy is the most common cause of new-onset blindness among American adults aged 20 to 74 years. In the Wisconsin Epidemiologic Study of Diabetic Retinopathy, approximately 4% of patients younger than 30 years of age at diagnosis and nearly 2% of patients older than 30 years of age at diagnosis were legally blind. In the younger-onset group, 86% of blindness was attributable to diabetic retinopathy. In the older-onset group, where other eye diseases were also common, 33% of the cases of legal blindness were due to diabetic retinopathy.[268,311] Currently, diabetes is thought to account for 12,000 to 24,000 new cases of blindness in the United States each year.[274]

Lack of appropriate glycemic control is another significant risk factor for the onset and progression of diabetic retinopathy. The DCCT demonstrated a clear relationship between hyperglycemia and diabetic microvascular complications, including retinopathy in 1441 patients with T1DM.[26,27,279,280,313]

In patients monitored for 4 to 9 years, the DCCT showed that intensive insulin therapy reduced or prevented the development of retinopathy by 27% as compared with conventional therapy. Additionally, intensive insulin therapy reduced the progression of diabetic retinopathy by 34% to 76% and had a substantial beneficial effect over the entire range of retinopathy severity. This improvement was achieved with an average 10% reduction in Hb A_{1c} from 8% to 7.2%. These results underscore that although intensive therapy might not prevent retinopathy completely, it reduces the risk of retinopathy onset and progression.

Renal disease, as manifested by microalbuminuria and proteinuria, is yet another significant risk factor for onset and progression of diabetic retinopathy.[314,315] Hypertension is associated with proliferative diabetic retinopathy (PDR) and is an established risk factor for the development of macular edema.[316] Additionally, elevated serum lipid levels are associated with extravasated lipid in the retina (hard exudates) and vision loss.[317]

Clinical Findings

Clinical findings associated with early and progressing diabetic retinopathy include hemorrhages or microaneurysms, cotton-wool spots, hard exudates, intraretinal microvascular abnormalities, and venous caliber abnormalities such as venous loops, venous tortuosity, and venous beading (see Fig. 32–22A and C). Microaneurysms are saccular outpouchings of the capillary walls that can leak fluid and result in intraretinal edema and hemorrhages. The intraretinal hemorrhages can be flame-shaped or dot-blot–like in appearance, reflecting the architecture of the layer of the retina in which they occur. Flame-shaped hemorrhages occur in inner retina closer to the vitreous, and dot-blot hemorrhages occur deeper in the retina. Intraretinal microvascular abnormalities are either new vessel growth within the retinal tissue itself or shunt vessels through areas of poor vascular perfusion. It is common for intraretinal microvascular abnormalities to be located adjacent to cotton-wool spots. Cotton-wool spots are caused by microinfarcts in the nerve fiber layer of the retina. Venous caliber abnormalities are generally a sign of severe retinal hypoxia. In some cases of extensive vascular loss, however, the retina might actually appear free of nonproliferative lesions. Such areas are termed *featureless retina* and are a sign of severe retinal hypoxia.

Vision loss from diabetic retinopathy generally results from persistent nonclearing vitreous hemorrhage, traction retinal detachment, or diabetic macular edema (see Figs. 32–21 and 32–22). Neovascularization with fibrous tissue contraction can distort the retina and lead to traction retinal detachment. The new vessels can bleed, causing preretinal or vitreous hemorrhage. The most common cause of vision loss from diabetes, however, is macular disease and macular edema. Macular edema is more likely to occur in patients with T2DM, which represents 90% to 95% of the diabetic population. In diabetic macular disease, macular edema involving the fovea or nonperfusion of the capillaries in the central macula is responsible for the loss of vision.

Classification Systems

Classification of Diabetic Retinopathy

Diabetic retinopathy is broadly classified into *nonproliferative diabetic retinopathy* (NPDR) and *proliferative diabetic retinopathy* (PDR) categories.[318,319] Macular edema can coexist with either group and is not used in the classification of level of retinopathy. The historical terms *background retinopathy* and *preproliferative diabetic retinopathy* have been replaced to reflect the specific characteristics and risk stratification of the prognostically important subgroups in NPDR (Table 32–1).

Generally, diabetic retinopathy progresses from no retinopathy through mild, moderate, severe, and very severe nonproliferative diabetic retinopathy and eventually on to PDR. The level of NPDR is determined by the extent and location of clinical manifestations of retinopathy. Mild NPDR is characterized by limited microvascular abnormalities such as hemorrhages or microaneurysms, cotton-wool spots, and increased vascular permeability. Moderate and severe NPDR are characterized by increasing severity of hemorrhages or microaneurysms, venous caliber abnormalities, intraretinal microvascular abnormalities, and vascular closure. The level of NPDR establishes the risk of progression to sight-threatening retinopathy and dictates appropriate clinical management and follow-up.

PDR is characterized by vasoproliferation of the retina and its complications, including new vessels on the optic disc (NVD), new vessels elsewhere on the retina (NVE), preretinal hemorrhage (PRH), vitreous hemorrhage, and fibrous tissue proliferation (FP). On the basis of the extent and location of these lesions, PDR is classified as *early PDR* or *high-risk PDR*. Larger areas of these complications as well as new vessels that are near the optic disc are associated with greater risks of vision loss.

Classification of Diabetic Macular Edema

Diabetic macular edema can be present with any level of diabetic retinopathy. When edema involves or threatens the center of the macula, it is called *CSME*. CSME exists if there is retinal thickening at or within 500 μm of the fovea, hard exudates with adjacent retinal thickening at or within 500 μm of the fovea, or an area of retinal thickening 1500 μm or more in diameter, any

TABLE 32–1 GLOSSARY AND ABBREVIATIONS PERTINENT TO DIABETIC EYE DISEASE

Background diabetic retinopathy (BDR): An outdated term referring to some stages of nonproliferative diabetic retinopathy. Because this terminology is not closely associated with disease progression, it has been replaced by the various levels of nonproliferative diabetic retinopathy.
Clinically significant macular edema (CSME): Thickening of the retina in the macular region of sufficient extent and location to threaten central visual function.
Cotton wool spot: A gray or white area lesion in the nerve fiber layer of the retina resulting from stasis of axoplasmic flow as a result of microinfarcts of the retinal nerve fiber layer.
Diabetes Control and Complications Trial (DCCT): A multicenter randomized clinical trial designed to address whether intensive insulin therapy could prevent or slow the progression of systemic complications of diabetes mellitus.
Diabetic retinopathy (DR): Retinal pathology related to the underlying systemic disease of diabetes mellitus.
Diabetic Retinopathy Study (DRS): The first multicenter randomized clinical trial to demonstrate the value of scatter (panretinal) photocoagulation in reducing the risk of vision loss among patients with all levels of diabetic retinopathy.
Diabetic Retinopathy Vitrectomy Study (DRVS): A multicenter clinical trial evaluating early vitrectomy for patients with very advanced diabetic retinopathy or nonresolving vitreous hemorrhage.
Early Treatment Diabetic Retinopathy Study (ETDRS): A multicenter randomized clinical trial that addressed at what stage of retinopathy scatter (panretinal) photocoagulation was indicated, whether focal photocoagulation was effective for preventing moderate vision loss from clinically significant macular edema, and whether aspirin therapy altered the progression of diabetic retinopathy.
Focal or grid laser photocoagulation: A type of laser treatment whose main goal is to reduce vascular leakage either by focal treatment of leaking retinal microaneurysms or by application of therapy in a grid-like pattern for patients with clinically significant macular edema.
Hard exudate: Lipid accumulation within the retina as a result of increased vasopermeability.
High-risk-characteristic proliferative diabetic retinopathy (HRC-PDR): Proliferative diabetic retinopathy of defined extent, location, and/or clinical findings that is particularly associated with severe vision loss.
Microaneurysm: An early vascular abnormality consisting of an outpouching of the retinal microvasculature.
Neovascular glaucoma (NVG): Elevation of intraocular pressure caused by the development of neovascularization in the anterior segment of the eye.
Neovascularization at the disc (NVD): Retinal neovascularization occurring at or within 1500 µm of the optic disc.
Neovascularization elsewhere (NVE): Retinal neovascularization that is located more than 1500 µm away from the optic disc.
Neovascularization of the iris (NVI): Neovascularization occurring on the iris (rubeosis iridis), usually as a result of extensive retinal ischemia.
No light perception (NLP): The inability to perceive light.
Nonproliferative diabetic retinopathy (NPDR): Severities of clinically evident diabetic retinopathy that precede the development of proliferative diabetic retinopathy.
Preproliferative diabetic retinopathy (PPDR): An outdated term referring to more advanced levels of nonproliferative diabetic retinopathy. Because this term is not closely associated with disease progression, it has been replaced by the various levels of nonproliferative diabetic retinopathy.
Proliferative diabetic retinopathy (PDR): An advanced level of diabetic retinopathy, where proliferation of new vessels or fibrous tissue occurs on or within the retina.
Rubeosis iridis: see Neovascularization of the iris (NVI).

TABLE 32–2 LEVELS OF DIABETIC RETINOPATHY

International Classification Level	ETDRS Level
No apparent retinopathy	Level 10: DR absent
Mild NPDR	Level 20; very mild NPDR
Moderate NPDR	Levels 35, 43, 47; moderate NPDR
Severe NPDR	Levels 53A-E; severe to very severe NPDR
PDR	Levels 61,65,71,75,81,85; PDR, high-risk PDR, very severe or advanced PDR

DR, diabetic retinopathy; ETDRS, Early Treatment Diabetic Retinopathy Study; NPDR, nonproliferative diabetic retinopathy; PDR, proliferative diabetic retinopathy.

part of which is within 1500 µm of the fovea.[318,320,321] CSME is a clinical diagnosis that is not dependent on visual acuity or results of ancillary testing such as fluorescein angiography and can be present even when vision is 20/20 or better.

International Classification of Diabetic Retinopathy

The American Academy of Ophthalmology initiated a project to establish a consensus International Classification of Diabetic Retinopathy and Diabetic Macular Edema in an effort to simplify classification and standardize communication among diabetes health care providers.[322,323] This international classification describes five clinical levels of diabetic retinopathy: no apparent retinopathy (no abnormalities), mild NPDR (microaneurysms only), moderate NPDR (more than microaneurysms only but less than severe NPDR), severe NPDR (any of the following: more than 20 intraretinal hemorrhages in each of four quadrants, definite venous beading in two or more quadrants, prominent intraretinal microvascular abnormalities in one or more quadrants, and no PDR), and PDR (one or more of retinal neovascularization, vitreous hemorrhage, or preretinal hemorrhage). Table 32–2 compares levels of retinopathy in the international classification to those defined by the landmark ETDRS.

In regard to diabetic macular edema, the international classification identifies two broad categories: macular edema apparently absent (no apparent retinal thickening or hard exudates in the posterior pole) and macular edema apparently present (some apparent retinal thickening or hard exudates in the posterior pole). Macular edema is subclassified as mild (some retinal thickening or hard exudates in the posterior pole but distant from the center of the macula), moderate (retinal thickening or hard exudates approaching the center of the macula but not involving the center), or severe (retinal thickening or hard exudates involving the center of the macula). Table 32–3 compares levels of diabetic macular edema in the international classification to ETDRS levels of diabetic macular edema.

As compared with ETDRS retinopathy grading, the International Classification of Diabetic Retinopathy and Diabetic Macular Edema reduces the number of levels of diabetic retinopathy, simplifies descriptions of the categories, and describes the levels without relying on reference to the standard photographs of the Airlie House Classification of diabetic retinopathy. This makes clinical use easier and more uniform among practitioners not versed in the complexities of the ETDRS grading system. However, because of this simplification, the International Classification of Diabetic Retinopathy and Diabetic Macular Edema is not a replacement for ETDRS levels of diabetic retinopathy in large-scale clinical trials or studies where precise retinopathy classification is required.

TABLE 32–3 CLASSIFICATION OF DIABETIC MACULAR EDEMA

Disease Severity Level	Findings
DME apparently absent	No apparent retinal thickening or HE in posterior pole
DME apparently present	Some apparent retinal thickening or HE in posterior pole
International Classification Scale	**ETDRS Scale**
Mild DME: some retinal thickening or HE in posterior pole but distant from center of the macula	DME but not CSME
Moderate DME: retinal thickening or HE approaching the center but not involving the center	CSME
Severe DME: retinal thickening or HE involving the center of the macula	CSME

CSME, clinically significant macular edema; DME, diabetic macular edema; ETDRS, Early Treatment Diabetic Retinopathy Study; HE, hard exudates.

Other Ocular Manifestations of Diabetes

All structures of the eye are susceptible to complications of diabetes. The consequence of these changes can range from being unnoticed by both patient and physician, to symptomatic but not sight-threatening, to requiring evaluation to rule out potentially life-threatening underlying causes other than diabetes.

Mononeuropathies of the third, fourth, or sixth cranial nerves can arise in association with diabetes; mononeuropathy of the fourth cranial nerve is least likely associated with diabetes.[326-328] Nerve palsies present a significant diagnostic challenge because misdiagnosis can result in a life-threatening lesion remaining untreated. In one review of cranial nerve palsies treated in a diabetic patient population in 1967, 42% of mononeuropathies were not diabetic in origin.[327] This finding underscores the danger of routinely attributing mononeuropathies to the diabetic condition itself without carefully ruling out other potential causes. The percentage of all extraocular muscle palsies attributable to diabetes mellitus is estimated at 4.5% to 6%.[328] Mononeuropathies may be the initial presenting sign of new-onset diabetes, and diabetes should therefore be considered in the differential diagnosis of any mononeuropathy affecting the extraocular muscles, even in patients who do not claim a history of diabetes. Diabetes-induced third-, fourth-, and sixth-nerve palsies are usually self-limited and should resolve spontaneously in 2 to 6 months. Palsies can recur or subsequently develop in the contralateral eye.

The optic disc can be affected by diabetes in a variety of ways other than vasoproliferation. Diabetic papillopathy must be distinguished from other causes of disc swelling such as true papilledema from increased intracranial pressure, pseudopapilledema such as optic nerve head drusen, toxic optic neuropathies, neoplasms of the optic nerve, and hypertension.[339] Optic disc pallor can occur following spontaneous remission of proliferative retinopathy or remission following scatter (panretinal) laser photocoagulation (see Fig. 32–22I). Because diabetes poses an increased risk for developing open-angle glaucoma, the disc pallor following remission of retinopathy or laser photocoagulation must be considered when evaluating the optic nerve head for glaucoma.

A potentially serious diabetic ocular complication is neovascularization of the iris. Usually the new iris vessels are first observed at the pupillary border, followed by a fine network of vessels over the iris tissue progressing into the filtration angle of the eye. Closure of the angle by the fibrovascular network results in neovascular glaucoma.[330] Neovascular glaucoma is difficult to manage and requires aggressive treatment. Diabetes is the second leading cause of neovascular glaucoma, accounting for 32% of cases.[331] Neovascularization of the iris occurs in 4% to 7% of diabetic eyes and may be present in up to 40% to 60% of eyes with proliferative retinopathy.[332,333] When possible, scatter (panretinal) laser photocoagulation is the principal therapy for neovascularization of the iris, although other approaches such as goniophotocoagulation, topical or systemic antiglaucoma medications, and antiglaucomatous filtration surgery are available when needed.[334-336] VEGF inhibitors have been tried in small-scale uncontrolled studies with resultant transient regression of the neovascularization.[337]

The cornea of the diabetic person is more susceptible to injury and slower to heal after injury than is the nondiabetic cornea.[338,339] The diabetic cornea is also more prone to infectious corneal ulcers, which can lead to rapid loss of vision, need for corneal transplant, or loss of the eye if it is not treated aggressively. Consequently, diabetic patients using contact lenses should exercise caution and maintain careful monitoring.

Open-angle glaucoma is 1.4 times more common in the diabetic population than in the nondiabetic population.[340] The prevalence of glaucoma increases with age and duration of diabetes, but medical therapy for open-angle glaucoma is generally effective. In a study of 76,318 women enrolled in the Nurses' Health Study, Pasquale and coworkers found that T2DM is associated with an increased risk of primary open-angle glaucoma in women.[341]

Diabetes effects on the crystalline lens can result in transitory refractive changes, alterations in accommodative ability,[342] and cataracts. Refractive change can be significant and is related to fluctuation of blood glucose levels with osmotic lens swelling.[331] Cataracts can occur earlier in life and progress more rapidly in the presence of diabetes.[343,344] Cataracts are 1.6 times more common in people with diabetes than in those without diabetes.[343,344] In patients with earlier-onset diabetes, duration of diabetes, retinopathy status, diuretic use, and Hb A_{1c} levels are risk factors.[345] In patients with later-onset diabetes, age of the patient, lower intraocular pressure, smoking, and lower diastolic BP may be additional risk factors.[346,347] Diabetic patients undergoing simultaneous kidney or pancreas transplantation are at an increased risk of developing all types of cataract, independent of the use of corticosteroids after transplantation.[348] Both phacoemulsification and extracapsular cataract extraction with intraocular lens implantation are appropriate surgical therapies. The principal determinant of postoperative vision and progression of retinopathy is related to the preoperative presence of diabetic macular edema and level of NPDR.[349,350]

Other findings with higher incidence among patients with diabetes include xanthelasma,[326] microaneurysms of the bulbar conjunctiva,[351] posterior vitreous detachment,[352] and the rare but often fatal orbital fungal infection Mucorales phycomycosis.[332,333] Prompt diagnosis and treatment of phycomycosis caused by *Mucor* species is crucial, although the survival rate still remains at only 57%.[333,353]

Monitoring and Treatment of Diabetic Retinopathy

Appropriate clinical management of diabetic retinopathy has been defined by results of major randomized, multicenter

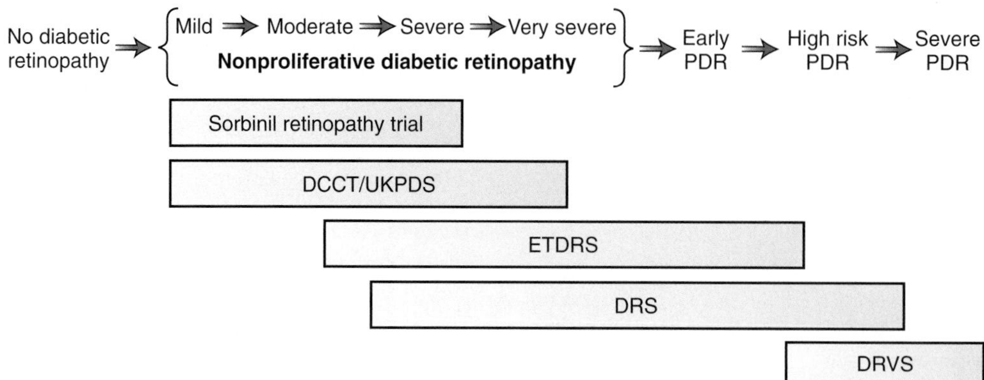

Figure 32–23 ▪ Major multicenter clinical trials of diabetic retinopathy. Schematic representation of the major multicenter clinical trials of diabetic retinopathy and the levels of diabetic retinopathy that they primarily addressed. DCCT, Diabetes Control and Complications Trial; DRS, Diabetic Retinopathy Study; DRVS, Diabetic Retinopathy Vitrectomy Study; ETDRS, Early Treatment Diabetic Retinopathy Study; PDR, proliferative diabetic retinopathy; UKPDS, United Kingdom Prospective Diabetes Study.

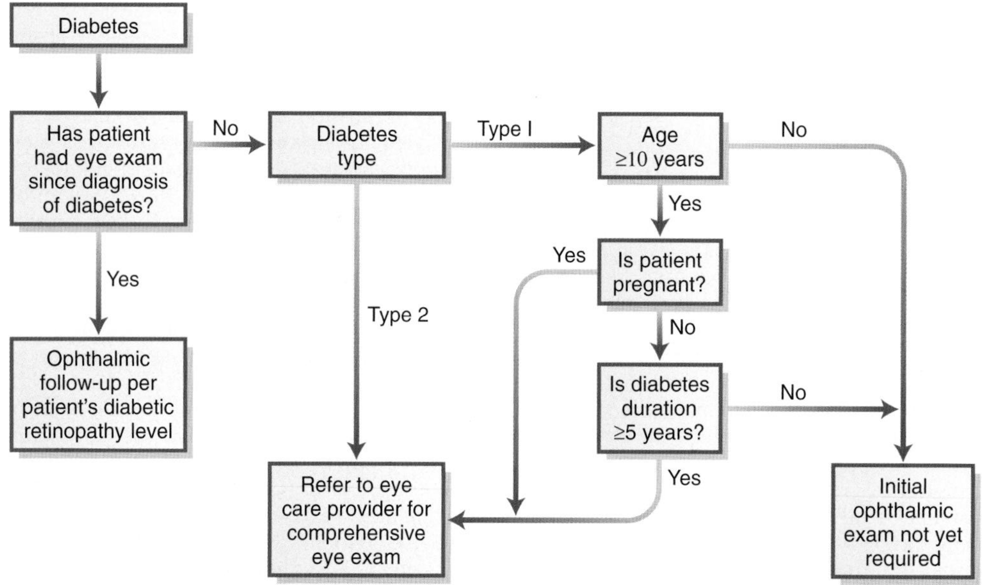

Figure 32–24 ▪ Initial ophthalmic examination flow chart. Schematic flow chart of major principles involved in determining the timing of initial ophthalmic examination following diagnosis of diabetes mellitus. These are minimal recommended frequencies. Ocular symptoms, complaints, or other associated medical issues can necessitate earlier evaluation. Guidelines are regularly reevaluated based on new study results.

clinical trials (Fig. 32–23): the Diabetic Retinopathy Study (DRS),[354] the ETDRS,[293] the Diabetic Retinopathy Vitrectomy Study (DRVS),[355] the DCCT,[356] and the UKPDS.[3] These studies have elucidated the progression rates of each level of diabetic retinopathy, guided follow-up intervals, and elucidated the proper delivery, timing, and resulting effectiveness of glycemic control and laser photocoagulation surgery (Figs. 32–24 to 32–27). They have also established recommendations for vitrectomy surgery.

Comprehensive Eye Examination

An accurate ocular examination detailing the extent and location of retinopathy-associated findings is critical for making monitoring and treatment decisions in patients with diabetic retinopathy. As detailed later, most of the blindness associated with advanced stages of retinopathy can be averted with appropriate and timely diagnosis and therapy. Unfortunately, many diabetic patients do not receive adequate eye care at an appropriate stage in their disease.[357,358] In one study, 55% of patients with high-risk PDR or CSME had never had laser photocoagulation.[357] In fact, 11% of T1DM and 7% of T2DM patients with high-risk PDR necessitating prompt treatment had not been examined by an ophthalmologist within the past 2 years.[358]

The comprehensive eye examination is the mainstay of such evaluation and is necessary on a repetitive, life-long basis for patients with diabetes.[318,359] Such an evaluation has four major components: history, examination, diagnosis, and treatment. Annual retinal evaluation to asses the presence and level of diabetic retinopathy and diabetic macular edema is essential to guide patient care. The fundamentals of a comprehensive eye examination for the nondiabetic patient have been detailed by the American Academy of Ophthalmology [359] and the American Optometric Association.[360] The examination of the patient with

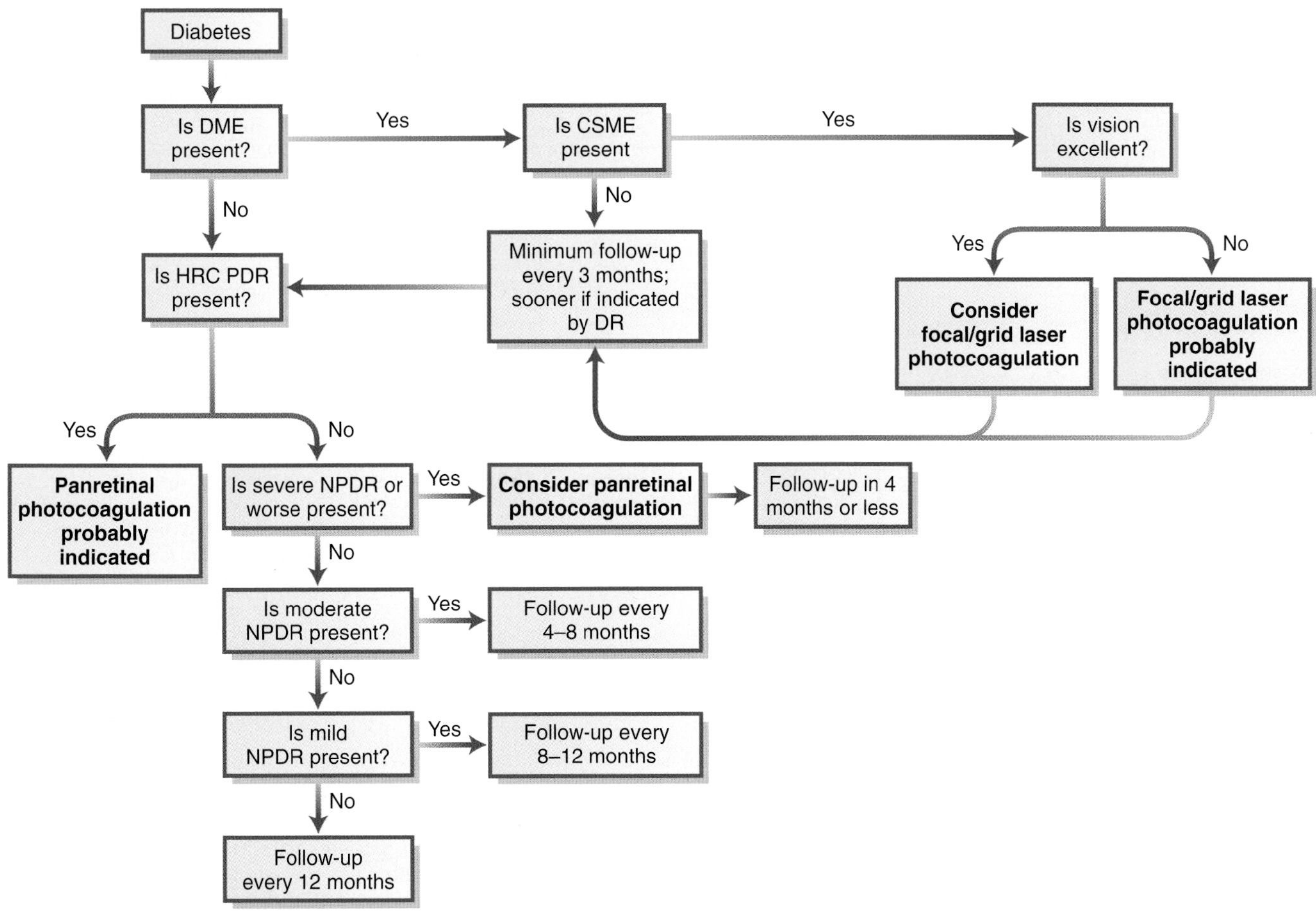

Figure 32–25 ▪ Diabetic retinopathy and macular edema examination and treatment flow chart: nonpregnant patients. The schematic flow chart presents major principles involved in determining routine ophthalmic follow-up and indications for treatment in nonpregnant patients with diabetes. These are only general, minimal recommended frequencies. Ocular symptoms, complaints, or other associated ophthalmic or medical issues can necessitate earlier evaluation and/or an altered approach. Guidelines are regularly reevaluated based on new study results. CSME, clinically significant macular edema; DME, diabetic macular edema; DR, diabetic retinopathy; HRC PDR, high-risk characteristic proliferative diabetic retinopathy; NPDR, nonproliferative diabetic retinopathy; PDR, proliferative diabetic retinopathy.

diabetes should be similar, with additional emphasis on portions of the examination that relate to problems particularly relevant to diabetes.

Dilated ophthalmic examination is superior to undilated evaluation because only 50% of eyes are correctly classified as to presence and severity of retinopathy through undilated pupils.[361,362] Appropriate ophthalmic evaluation entails pupillary dilation, slit-lamp biomicroscopy, examination of the retinal periphery with indirect ophthalmoscopy or mirrored contact lens, and sometimes gonioscopy.[359,360] Because of the complexities of the diagnosis and treatment of PDR and CSME, ophthalmologists with specialized knowledge and experience in the management of diabetic retinopathy are required to determine and provide appropriate surgical intervention.[363] Thus, it is recommended that all patients with diabetes should have dilated ocular examinations by an experienced eye care provider (ophthalmologist or optometrist), and diabetic patients should be under the direct or consulting care of an ophthalmologist experienced in the management of diabetic retinopathy at least by the time severe diabetic retinopathy or diabetic macular edema is present.[318] Retinal imaging that has demonstrated equivalency to dilated retinal fundus examination or the accepted standard of seven-standard-field stereoscopic retinal imaging can also be appropriate.[364]

Initial Ophthalmic Evaluation

The recommendation for initial ocular examination in persons with diabetes is based on prevalence rates of retinopathy (see Fig. 32–24). Approximately 80% of T1DM patients have retinopathy after 15 years of disease, but only about 25% have any retinopathy after 5 years.[362] The prevalence of PDR is less than 2% at 5 years and 25% by 15 years. For T2DM, the onset date of diabetes is usually unknown, and more severe disease can be observed at diagnosis. Up to 3% of patients whose diabetes is first diagnosed after age 30 years (T2DM) have CSME or high-risk PDR at the time of initial diagnosis of diabetes.[365] Thus, in patients older than 10 years, initial ophthalmic examination is recommended beginning 5 years after the diagnosis of T1DM and on diagnosis of T2DM (see Fig. 32–24).[318,367]

Puberty and pregnancy can accelerate retinopathy progression. The onset of vision-threatening retinopathy is rare in children prior to puberty, regardless of the duration of diabetes;[268,367-369] however, significant retinopathy can arise within 6 years of disease if diabetes is diagnosed between the ages of 10 and 30 years.[269] Diabetic retinopathy can become particularly aggressive during pregnancy in patients with diabetes.[370,371] In the past, the prognosis for pregnancy in the diabetic patient with microvascular complications was so poor that pregnant diabetic

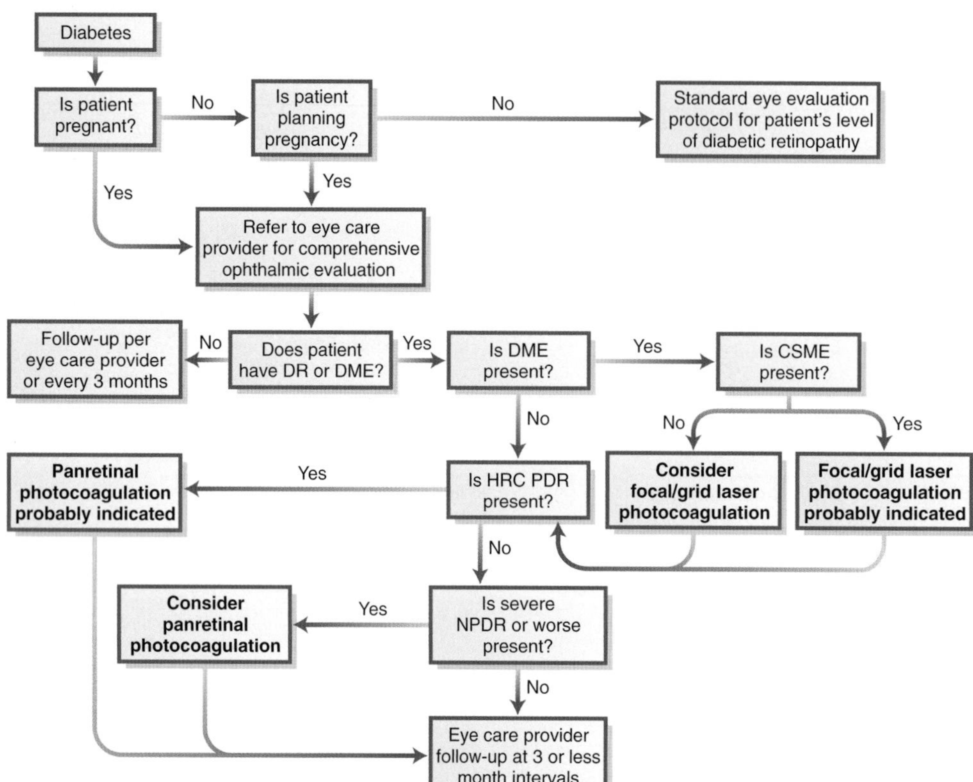

Figure 32–26 ▪ Diabetic retinopathy and macular edema examination and treatment flow chart: pregnant patients. The schematic flow chart shows major principles involved in determining routine ophthalmic follow-up and indications for treatment in pregnant patients with diabetes. These are only general, minimal recommended frequencies. Ocular symptoms, complaints, or other associated ophthalmic or medical issues can necessitate earlier evaluation and/or an altered approach. Because retinopathy can progress rapidly in pregnant patients with diabetes, careful and more frequent evaluation is often indicated. Guidelines are regularly reevaluated based on new study results. CSME, clinically significant macular edema; DME, diabetic macular edema; DR, diabetic retinopathy; HRC PDR, high-risk characteristic proliferative diabetic retinopathy; NPDR, nonproliferative diabetic retinopathy.

patients were commonly advised to avoid or terminate pregnancies.[372] With recognition of the importance of glycemic control, many diabetic patients in the child-bearing age now experience safe pregnancy and childbirth with minimal risk to both the mother and the baby. There are excellent reviews on this subject.[373]

Ideally, patients with diabetes who are planning pregnancy should have a comprehensive eye examination within 1 year before conception (see Fig. 32–26). Patients who become pregnant should have a comprehensive eye examination in the first trimester of pregnancy. Close follow-up throughout pregnancy is indicated, with subsequent examinations determined by the

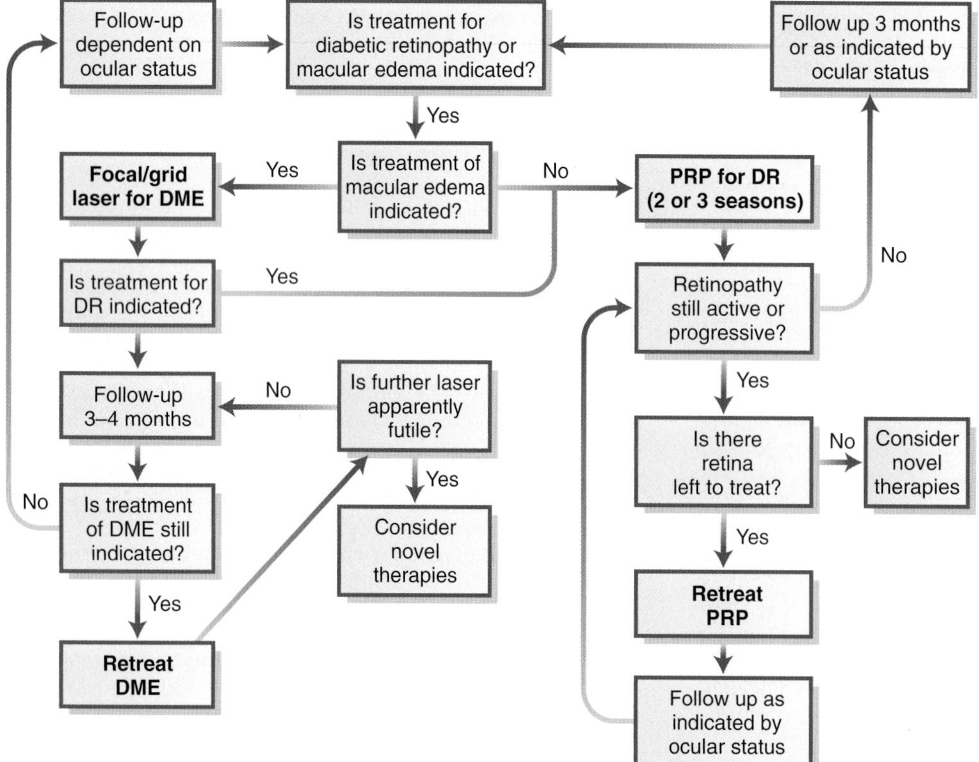

Figure 32–27 ▪ Photocoagulation flow chart. The schematic flow chart details general photocoagulation treatment approaches in patients with diabetic retinopathy and/or diabetic macular edema. These are only general guidelines, and actual treatment choices can be affected by numerous other factors, including findings in the same eye, contralateral eye, systemic issues, etc. DR, diabetic retinopathy; DME, diabetic macular edema; PRP, scatter (panretinal) photocoagulation.

findings present at the first-trimester examination.[318] This recommendation does not apply to women who develop gestational diabetes, because such women are not at increased risk of developing diabetic retinopathy.

Follow-Up Ophthalmic Examination

Follow-up ocular examination is determined from the risk of disease progression at any particular retinopathy level (see Fig. 32–25). NPDR is categorized into four levels of severity based on clinical findings compared to stereo fundus photographic standards: mild, moderate, severe, and very severe.[325] Progression of nonproliferative retinopathy to the visually threatening level of high-risk PDR is closely correlated with NPDR level (Table 32–4). Progression rates from each individual NPDR level to any other retinopathy level are also known. These are used to define standard minimal follow-up intervals as detailed in Figure 32–25 and Table 32–5. Because significant sight-threatening retinopathy can initially occur with no or minimal symptoms, patients with no clinically evident diabetic retinopathy and no known ocular problems require annual comprehensive ophthalmic examinations even if they are totally asymptomatic.

Proliferative Diabetic Retinopathy

The extent and location of neovascularization determine the level of PDR.[374,375] PDR is best evaluated by dilated examination using slit-lamp biomicroscopy combined with indirect ophthalmoscopy or stereo fundus photography. Without photocoagulation, eyes with high-risk PDR have a 28% risk of severe vision loss within 2 years. This risk compares with a 7% risk of severe vision loss after 2 years for eyes with PDR but without high-risk characteristics.[374]

Severe vision loss is defined as best-corrected acuity of 5/200 or worse on two consecutive visits 4 months apart. This represents vision loss substantially worse than the 20/200 or worse limit for legal blindness. The DRS demonstrated that scatter (panretinal) laser photocoagulation was effective in reducing the risk of severe vision loss from PDR by 50% or more. The ETDRS demonstrated that scatter (panretinal) laser photocoagulation applied when an eye approaches or just reaches high-risk PDR reduces the risk of severe vision loss to less than 4%. Prompt scatter photocoagulation is thus indicated for all patients with high-risk PDR, usually indicated for patients with PDR less than high risk, and may be advisable for patients with severe or very severe NPDR, especially in the setting of T2DM (see Fig. 32–25).[293,374-377] Recent progression of eye disease, status of the fellow eye, compliance with follow-up, concurrent health concerns such as hypertension or kidney disease, and other factors must be considered in determining if laser surgery should be performed in these patients. In particular, patients with T2DM should be considered for scatter photocoagulation before high-risk PDR develops because the risk of severe vision loss and the need for pars plana vitrectomy (PPV) can be reduced by 50% in these patients, especially when macular edema is present.[377]

In scatter coagulation, 1200 to 1800 laser burns are applied to the peripheral retinal tissue, actually focally destroying the outer photoreceptor and retinal pigment epithelium of the retina (see Fig. 32–22I). Large vessels are avoided, as are areas of preretinal hemorrhage. The treatment is thought to exert its effect by increasing oxygen delivery to the inner retina, decreasing viable hypoxic growth factor–producing cells, and increasing the relative perfusion per area of viable retina. The total treatment is usually applied over two or three sessions, spaced 1 to 2 weeks apart. Follow-up evaluation usually occurs at 3 months.

The response to scatter photocoagulation varies. The most desirable effect is to see a regression of the new vessels, although stabilization of the neovascularization with no further growth can result. This latter situation requires careful clinical monitoring. In some cases, new vessels continue to proliferate, requiring additional scatter photocoagulation (see Fig. 32–27). As discussed later, novel therapeutic approaches are now being used in some clinical settings, especially in cases where response to scatter photocoagulation is inadequate. Definitive multicenter randomized, controlled clinical trials have not yet been performed using these new therapeutic approaches.

The DRVS, completed in 1989, demonstrated that early PPV in persons with severe fibrovascular proliferation was more likely to result in better vision and less likely to result in poor vision, particularly in patients with T1DM.[355] PPV is surgery within the eye aimed primarily at removing abnormal fibrovascular tissue, alleviating retinal traction, allowing the retina to obtain a more anatomically normal position, and removing vitreous opacities such as vitreous hemorrhage. The actual outcome data from this study might not be totally applicable today due to the dramatic advances in surgical techniques and the advent of laser endophotocoagulation that have occurred in the intervening years. It is clear that PPV can save and restore vision in many cases of severe retinal disease not amenable or not responsive to laser photocoagulation.

TABLE 32–4 PROGRESSION TO PDR BY NPDR LEVEL

Retinopathy Level	CHANCE (%) OF HIGH-RISK PDR	
	1 Year	5 Years
Mild NPDR	1	16
Moderate NPDR	3-8	27-39
Severe NPDR	15	56
Very severe NPDR	45	71
PDR with fewer high-risk characteristics	22-46	64-75

NPDR, nonproliferative diabetic retinopathy; PDR, proliferative diabetic retinopathy.

From Aiello LP, Gardner TW, King GL, et al. Diabetic retinopathy: technical review. Diabetes Care 1998;21:143-156.

Macular Edema

Untreated CSME is associated with an approximately 25% chance of moderate vision loss after 3 years (defined as at least doubling the visual angle; e.g., 20/40 reduced to 20/80).[293] Macular edema is best evaluated by dilated examination using slit-lamp biomicroscopy or stereo fundus photography. Focal laser photocoagulation is generally indicated for patients with CSME (see Figs. 32–22C and 32–25). The ETDRS demonstrated that focal laser photocoagulation for CSME reduced the 5-year risk of moderate vision loss from nearly 30% to less than 15%.[321] In focal laser photocoagulation, lesions from 500 to 3000 μm from the center of the macula that are contributing to thickening of the macular area are generally directly photocoagulated. These lesions are identified clinically or by fluorescein angiography and consist primarily of leaking microaneurysms. When leakage is diffuse or microaneurysms are extensive, photocoagulation may be applied to the macula in a grid configuration, avoiding the fovea region.

Although fluorescein angiography is useful for guiding therapy once CSME has been diagnosed, it is not required for the diagnosis of CSME or PDR because these findings should be

TABLE 32–5 RECOMMENDED GENERAL MANAGEMENT OF DIABETIC RETINOPATHY

Level of DR	RISK (%) OF PROGRESSION TO		EVALUATION		TREATMENT		Follow-up (mo)
	PDR (1 yr)	High-Risk PDR (5 yr)	Color Photo	FA	Scatter Laser (PRP)	Focal Laser	
MILD NPDR							
All	5	15					
No ME			No	No	No	No	12
ME			Yes	Occ	No	No	4-6
CSME			Yes	Yes	No	Yes	2-4
MODERATE NPDR							
All	12-27	33					
No ME			Yes	No	No	No	6-8
ME			Yes	Occ	No	Occ	4-6
CSME			Yes	Yes	No	Yes	2-4
SEVERE NPDR							
All	52	60					
No ME			Yes	No	Rarely	No	3-4
Me			Yes	Occ	Occ AF	Occ	2-3
CSME			Yes	Yes	Occ AF	Yes	2-3
VERY SEVERE NPDR							
All	75	75					
No ME			Yes	No	Occ	No	2-3
Me			Yes	Occ	Occ AF	Occ	2-3
CSME			Yes	Yes	Occ AF	Yes	2-3
PDR<HIGH RISK							
All	—	75					
No ME			Yes	No	Occ	No	2-3
Me			Yes	Occ	Occ AF	Occ	2-3
CSME			Yes	Yes	Occ AF	Yes	2-3
All	—	—					
No ME			Yes	No	Yes	No	2-3
Me			Yes	Yes	Yes	Usually	1-2
CSME			Yes	Yes	Yes	Yes	1-2

AF, after focal; CSME, clinically significant macular edema; FA, fluorescein angiography; ME macular edema; NPDR, nonproliferative diabetic retinopathy; Occ, occasionally; PDR, proliferative diabetic retinopathy.

Courtesy of Lloyd M. Aiello, MD.

clinically evident in most cases (Fig. 32–28). Fluorescein angiography is a valuable test for guiding treatment of CSME, identifying macular capillary nonperfusion, and evaluating unexplained vision loss. Because there are risks associated with fluorescein angiography, including nausea, urticaria, hives, and rarely death (1 in 222,000 patients) or severe medical sequelae (1 in 2000 patients),[378-380] fluorescein angiography is not part of the examination of an otherwise normal patient with diabetes, and the procedure is usually contraindicated in patients with known allergy to fluorescein dye or during pregnancy.

Follow-up evaluation of focal laser surgery generally occurs after 3 months (see Fig. 32–25). In the cases where macular edema persists, further treatment may be necessary. In the presence of macular edema, patients with severe or very severe NPDR should be considered for focal treatment of macular edema whether or not the macular edema is clinically significant because they are likely to require scatter laser photocoagulation in the near future and because scatter photocoagulation, while beneficial for proliferative diabetic retinopathy, can exacerbate existing macular edema. As discussed below, novel therapeutic approaches are now being used in some clinical settings to treat diabetic macular edema. These therapies are becoming more commonly employed in cases where response to focal/grid laser has been inadequate or cannot be performed. Definitive multicenter randomized, controlled clinical trials are under way for most of these new approaches.

Control of Systemic Disorders

In addition to the importance of intensive glycemic control in reducing the onset and progression of diabetic retinopathy as discussed earlier, it is critical for optimal ocular health of diabetic patients that several other systemic considerations be optimized.

Patients with diabetes mellitus commonly suffer from concomitant hypertension. Patients with T1DM have a 17% prevalence of hypertension at baseline and a 25% incidence after 10 years.[381] There is a 38% to 68% prevalence in T2DM.[382-384] In most

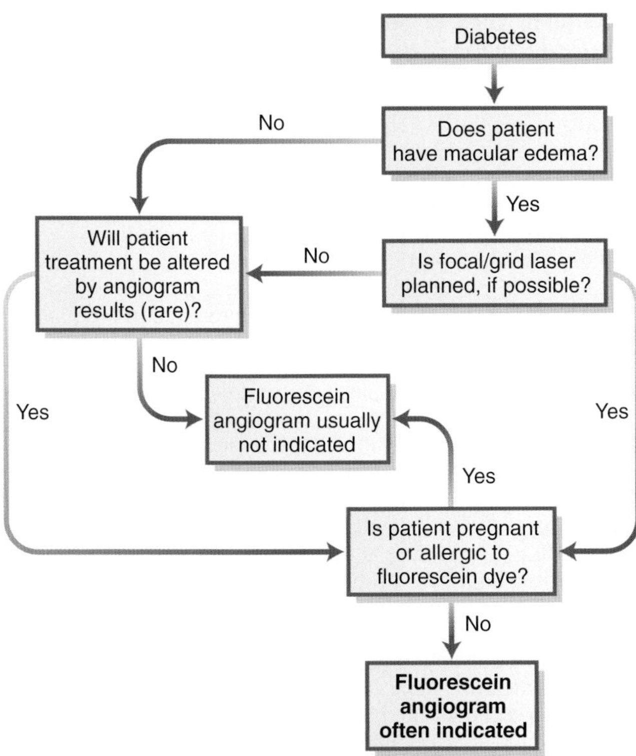

Figure 32–28 ▪ Fluorescein angiogram flow chart. The schematic flow chart details a general algorithm for appropriate use of fluorescein angiography in the ocular evaluation of patients with diabetes mellitus. In unusual cases, confounding factors can alter the appropriate approach.

studies, hypertension is correlated to the duration of diabetes, higher Hb A_{1c} level, presence of gross proteinuria, and male gender. Elevated BP exacerbates the development and progression of diabetic retinopathy. The risk of PDR is associated with the presence of hypertension at the baseline visit, higher glycosylated hemoglobin levels, and presence of more severe levels of retinopathy at the initial visit.[385] Patients with hypertension are more likely to develop retinopathy, diffuse macular edema, and more severe levels of retinopathy[385-387] and have more rapid progression of retinopathy when compared with diabetic patients who do not have hypertension.[388-390]

The large randomized, prospective UKPDS in 1148 patients with T2DM demonstrated a 34% (P = .0004) and 47% (P = .004) reduction in risk of diabetic retinopathy progression and moderate visual acuity loss, respectively, in patients assigned to intensive BP control.[391] These effects were independent of glycemic control, and the risk reductions were similar, regardless of whether the hypertension was controlled with an ACE inhibitor (captopril) or a β-blocker (atenolol). Overall, hypertension appears to be a significant risk factor in the development and progression of diabetic retinopathy and should be rigorously controlled. Until the results of specific trials investigating the BP levels required to minimize end organ damage in patients with diabetes are known,[392] target BP should most likely be maintained as low as safely possible.

Associations between renal and retinal angiopathy are numerous. Proteinuria or microalbuminuria is associated with retinopathy.[393-405] The presence and severity of diabetic retinopathy are indicators of the risk of gross proteinuria,[397,406] and, conversely, proteinuria predicts PDR.[395,407,451] Half of all patients with T1DM with PDR and 10 or more years of diabetes have concomitant proteinuria.[393] In T1DM, the prevalence of PDR increases from 7% at onset of microalbuminuria to 29% 4 years after onset of albuminuria as compared with 3% and 8%, respectively, in patients without persistent microalbuminuria.[396] The Appropriate Blood Pressure Control in Diabetes (ABCD) Trial found both the severity and progression of retinopathy were associated with overt albuminuria.[408-410] The presence of gross proteinuria at baseline is associated with 95% increased risk of developing macular edema among patients with T1DM,[385] and dialysis can improve macular edema in diabetic patients with renal failure.[335]

Despite these associations, the frequent coexistence of retinal and renal microangiopathies and factors such as associated hypertension and disease duration can confound these results.[411] Overall, it is important to carefully consider the renal status of any patient with diabetes mellitus and to ensure that the patient is receiving optimal care in this regard. In addition, rapidly progressive retinopathy, especially in a patient with long history of diabetes mellitus and where retinopathy has been previously stable, should suggest the need for renal evaluation.

Low hematocrit was an independent risk factor in the ETDRS analysis of baseline risk factors for development of high-risk PDR and of severe vision loss.[412] A cross-sectional study involving 1691 patients revealed a twofold increased risk of any retinopathy in patients with a hemoglobin level less than 12 g/dL as compared to those with a higher hemoglobin concentration using multivariate analyses controlling for serum creatinine, proteinuria, and other factors.[413] In patients with retinopathy, those with low hemoglobin levels have a fivefold increased risk of severe retinopathy compared with those with higher hemoglobin levels. There have been limited reports of resolution of macular edema and hard exudate with improvement or stabilization of visual acuity in erythropoietin-treated patients after an increase in mean hematocrit.[414] In view of the potential association of low hematocrit and diabetic retinopathy, it is important to ensure that patients with diabetic retinopathy and anemia are receiving appropriate management.

In summary, diabetes is clearly a multisystem disease requiring a comprehensive medical team approach. Even with regard to ocular health, this necessitates the involvement of multiple health care specialists for optimal patient care.

DIABETIC NEPHROPATHY

Diabetic nephropathy remains a major cause of morbidity and mortality for persons with either T1DM or T2DM. In Western countries, diabetes is the leading single cause of end-stage renal disease (ESRD).[415] Indeed, in many countries such as the United States, more than 50% of patients in renal replacement therapy programs have diabetes as the major cause of their renal failure.[416] However, the full impact of diabetic nephropathy is far greater.[417] Globally most patients with diabetes are in developing countries[418] that do not have the resources or health infrastructure to provide universal renal replacement therapy. Even in developed countries, for every 20 patients with diabetes and chronic kidney disease, less than one will survive to ESRD, succumbing instead to cardiovascular disease, heart failure, or infection, to which the presence and severity of diabetic renal disease significantly contributes. For example, almost all of the excess in cardiovascular deaths in persons with diabetes younger than 50 years can be attributed to nephropathy.[419] In patients with T2DM, microalbuminuria is associated with a twofold to fourfold increase in the risk of death. In patients with overt proteinuria and hypertension, the risk is even higher.[420] Consequently, the goal to reduce ESRD in patients with diabetes is only one component as part of the overall benefit in preventing diabetic kidney disease.

It is estimated that 25% to 40% of patients with T1DM and 5% to 40% of patients with T2DM ultimately develop diabetic kidney disease.[421,422] Up to 20% of patients with T2DM already have diabetic kidney disease when they are diagnosed with diabetes,[423] and a further 30% to 40% develop diabetic nephropathy, mostly within 10 years of diagnosis.[424] Although nephropathy appears be more common in T1DM, because of the large and increasing number of persons with T2DM,[425] more than 80% of diabetic patientts in renal replacement programs have T2DM.

Natural History of Nephropathy in Type 1 Diabetes

Nephropathy and specifically proteinuria in the setting of diabetes have been known for more than 100 years, and the classic structural features of glomerulosclerosis were described more than 70 years ago.[426] However, it is only since the 1980s that the natural history of this condition has been extensively delineated. This is partly because significantly more patients are surviving to see the full presentation of this condition. For example, in 1971, the median survival of patients with T1DM and overt nephropathy was 5 years, with less than 10% surviving more than 10 years.[427] Consequently, few patients were able to survive the course of their renal disease. By comparison, in 1996, the median survival in an equivalent population was more than 17 years. Not surprisingly, nearly 10 times more patients with T1DM are now entering ESRD programs.

Diabetic nephropathy is characterized clinically as a triad of hypertension, proteinuria, and, ultimately, renal impairment.[428] The classic five stages of nephropathy as described by Mogensen,[429] although not totally accurate, remain the best way of describing this condition (Fig. 32–29). This description relies on functional evaluation of the renal disease and is based on serial measurements of glomerular filtration rate and albuminuria.

Stage 1: Hyperfiltration

The initial phase has been termed the *hyperfiltration* phase. It is associated with an elevation of glomerular filtration rate (GFR)[430] and an increase in capillary glomerular pressure. Although invariably present in animal models of T1DM,[431] an elevation in GFR occurs in only a significant minority of type 1 diabetic patients. Hyperfiltration is considered to occur as a result of concomitant renal hypertrophy[432] as well as being partly due to a range of intrarenal hemodynamic abnormalities that occur in the diabetic milieu that contribute to glomerular hypertension.[433] The pathophysiology of renal hypertrophy associated with diabetes remains unexplained, although specific growth factors such as the GH-IGF-1 system and TGF-β have been implicated.[434,435] Notably, there is not only glomerular but also tubular hypertrophy. Indeed, the tubular hypertrophy explains the increased kidney weight in diabetes because tubules make up more than 90% of the kidney weight.[436] In addition, increased salt reabsorption associated with proximal tubular hypertrophy can also contribute to glomerular hyperfiltration via tubuloglomerular feedback.[432]

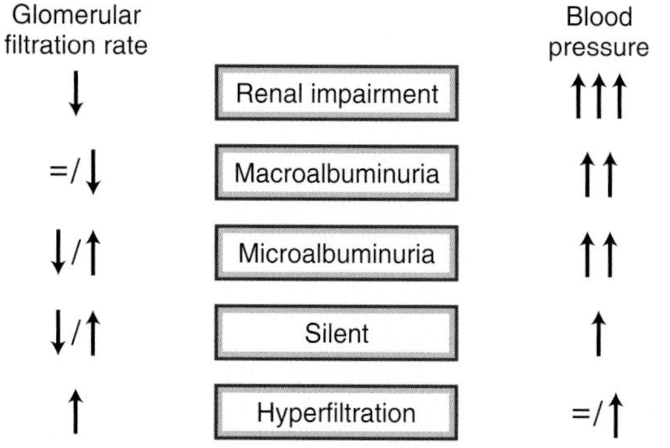

Figure 32–29 ■ The phases (natural history) of diabetic nephropathy.

The second explanation for the increase in GFR associated with diabetes relates to hemodynamic changes within the kidney. Although not directly tested in humans, micropuncture studies in rodents, particularly by Brenner's group in the 1980s, revealed that experimental diabetes was associated with a range of intrarenal hemodynamic changes.[433] Alongside hyperfiltration, there is an increase in effective renal plasma flow, and thus some investigators call this the *hyperperfusion-hyperfiltration* phase of diabetic nephropathy. At the same time, increased intraglomerular capillary pressure is increased, reflecting relative efferent versus afferent arteriolar vasoconstriction[433] with activation of the intrarenal renin-angiotensin system and reduced synthesis of the vasodilator NO.

The importance of this hyperfiltration phase as predicting and leading to diabetic nephropathy remains controversial. Several groups have confirmed the initial relationship between elevated GFR and later development of proteinuria described by Mogensen.[437] However, this has not been a universal finding. Nevertheless, subsequent studies with antihypertensive agents, and in particular agents that interrupt the renin-angiotensin system, have shown attenuation of some of these glomerular hemodynamic abnormalities. This provides justification to consider that at least some of these intrarenal hemodynamic changes in diabetes play a role in the development and progression of nephropathy.

Stage 2: The Silent Stage

The next stage is known as the *silent stage*, where, from a clinical point of view, there is no overt evidence of any form of renal dysfunction. Patients usually have normal GFR with no evidence of albuminuria. However, this phase is associated with significant structural changes including basement membrane thickening and mesangial expansion. It is only by performing detailed quantitative studies of renal morphology that one can postulate that there will be subsequent renal damage.[438] This is a very important phase clinically because it is hoped that investigators will be able to develop new tests, such as biomarkers in plasma or urine or sophisticated assessments from renal biopsy material to identify which patients will progress to more advanced renal disease. Because overall less than 40% of type 1 diabetic subjects will progress, it is critical that we detect those who are the potential progressors and could be candidates for early prevention and treatment strategies to avoid ESRD. As yet, no such surrogate markers or predictors have been identified at this silent phase of the disease.

Extensive studies using various plasma markers such as prorenin[439] or DNA studies to identify certain gene polymorphisms such as the ACE genotype[38] have been promising. The measurement of albumin fragments (ghost albumin) in the urine of patients with diabetes may be another approach.[440] Serial prospective ambulatory blood pressure monitoring studies have also demonstrated modest rises in blood pressure in patients in this silent phase up to 5 years before urinary albumin excretion begins to increase.[441] However, none of these markers have been proved to be sensitive or specific enough on further clinical evaluation for widespread clinical application.

Stage 3: Microalbuminuria

The third phase is known as *microalbuminuria* or the stage of *incipient nephropathy*. At this stage, often 5 to 15 years after the initial diagnosis of T1DM, the urinary albumin excretion rate has increased into the microalbuminuric range of 20 to 200 µg/min or 30 to 300 mg/24 hours.[442] In the past, microalbuminuria was considered to be a predictor rather than a manifestation of diabetic kidney disease. Increasingly it has been appreciated, particularly when based on interpretation of renal morphologic studies, that in the microalbuminuric phase there is already widespread evidence of advanced glomerular structural changes.[443] Concomitant with these changes, systolic and diastolic blood pressure are increased. Furthermore, the nocturnal dip in blood pressure seen in normal persons is often lost with the development of microalbuminuria.[444] Renal function during this phase may be increased, normal, or reduced.

The best approach to screen for microalbuminuria remains controversial. The original studies used 24-hour or overnight urine sampling methods. However, a spot urine albumin-to-creatinine ratio in an early morning urine specimen has been validated and appears to be a practical option for routine clinical practice.[442] Because the onset of persistent microalbuminuria, if left untreated, is often a reliable harbinger of overt nephropathy,[437] it is incumbent on clinicians to perform serial measurements of this parameter and to repeat the measurement if there is an isolated elevation in urinary albumin excretion.

Studies suggest that in many patients with T1DM, microalbuminuria can be transient and can reverse to normoalbuminuria.[445] Thus, the onset of microalbuminuria does not irrevocably seal the fate of the patient. A study of 386 patients with persistent microalbuminuria showed that regression of microalbuminuria occurred in 58% of patients,[445] although other groups have reported much lower rates of this phenomenon.[446] Notably, in that study, microalbuminuria of short duration, optimal levels of Ab A_{1c} (<8%), low systolic blood pressure (<115 mm Hg), and low levels of both cholesterol and triglycerides were independently associated with the regression of microalbuminuria. Therefore, screening of diabetic patients for nephropathy is now recommended to include at least twice-annual measurements of urinary albumin concentrations in type 1 diabetic patients.

Stage 4: Macroalbuminuria

The next stage is the macroalbuminuria phase or overt nephropathy. This stage represents the phase that has been previously described as diabetic nephropathy and is highly predictive of subsequent renal failure if left untreated. It is characterized by a urinary albumin excretion rate greater than 300 mg/24 hours (200 µg/min). This phase usually occurs after 10 to 15 years of diabetes, but the risk of overt renal disease never truly disappears and can appear after 40 or 50 years of T1DM.

There are at least two peaks of incidence of overt nephropathy, and this has been termed by some investigators as representing slow and fast trackers.[447] The key contributors of this marked variation in the timing of onset of proteinuria, independent of glycemia or blood pressure control, remains elusive, although a range of genetic, molecular, and environmental factors have been proposed. In association with this increase in proteinuria, more than two thirds of patients have overt systemic hypertension.[448] During this phase, if left untreated, BP continues to rise, accelerating the decline in GFR, which promotes a further rise in BP, creating a vicious cycle of progressive renal impairment that ultimately leads to ESRD.

Stage 5: Uremia

The final uremic phase, which can occur in up to 40% of type 1 diabetic subjects, requires the institution of renal replacement therapy. As recently as the 1970s, patients with diabetes were not considered candidates for renal replacement therapy because of their abysmal prognosis. However, improvements in the management of cardiovascular disease and renal replacement options have seen the survival on dialysis approach that of patients with renal disease from other causes. Many patients with diabetes and ESRD are also now considered candidates for renal transplantation, which is associated with better outcomes than remaining on dialysis. However, there is evidence that the renal lesions of diabetes often recur in the transplanted kidney, though the lead time to develop ESRD means that few kidneys are lost through recurrent disease.

Increasingly, single pancreas-kidney (SPK) and pancreas-after-kidney (PAK) transplantation have become therapeutic options for patients with T1DM and ESRD, and they appear to offer advantages over kidney-alone transplantation. In particular there is some evidence that maintaining euglycemia following pancreas transplantation can lead to resolution of many diabetes-related renal lesions such as mesangial expansion.[449] This reversal is often not apparent till after 10 years of euglycemia, emphasizing the slow turnover of matrix and the potential long-term effects of hyperglycemic memory in the kidney.

Natural History of Nephropathy in Type 2 Diabetes

The natural history of diabetic nephropathy in patients with T2DM is less well understood than in patients with T1DM. This partly reflects the fact that T2DM is largely a disease of an older population, with associated obesity, hypertension, and dyslipidemia and high rates of cardiovascular disease that restrict the manifestation of diabetic renal disease. In addition, approximately 7% of patients with T2DM already have microalbuminuria at the time of diagnosis. This may be partly related to the fact that most of these patients have had untreated diabetes for 10 years (on average) before diagnosis. Within 5 years of a diagnosis of T2DM, up to 18% of patients have microalbuminuria, especially those with poor metabolic control and high BP levels. This has led some investigators to suggest that nephropathy in T2DM is different from that seen in patients with T1DM.

However, the natural history of nephropathy in T2DM has more similarities than differences from that seen in T1DM. Hyperfiltration does occur in T2DM,[450] although it has been reported to be less common than in T1DM. This observation must be interpreted with caution, because GFR normally declines with age, and hyperfiltration can still exist although the GFR remains in the normal adult range. Microalbuminuria also occurs in T2DM. However, the finding of microalbuminuria in T2DM might not be as specific for diabetic renal disease as described in the seminal studies in T1DM. In the context of a very high prevalence of cardiovascular disease, microalbuminuria may be more closely associated with nonrenal events such as stroke and myocardial infarction.[451] Furthermore, incipient or overt cardiac failure, urinary tract infection, and urinary obstruction (e.g., enlarged prostate) can also lead to microalbuminuria.[433]

Many patients with T2DM and microalbuminuria also progress to overt proteinuria. However, it is increasingly appreciated that the situation has become much more complex, and several groups have described subjects with T1DM[452] as well as T2DM[453] who develop renal impairment in the absence of significant proteinuria. The exact explanation for this phenomenon is unknown, and ongoing studies are exploring if these patients have different renal morphologic changes from those with the more classic syndrome of diabetic nephropathy: overt proteinuria and declining GFR. Preliminary studies suggest a prominent vascular component for this form of nonproteinuric renal dysfunction. Nonetheless, it appears that the risk of ESRD in patients with T2DM and renal impairment is similar in the presence or absence of microalbuminuria, underlining the importance of an estimated GFR in the management of patients with T2DM.

Pathogenesis

It is likely that many of the mechanisms implicated in diabetic microvascular complications, in general, play a central role in the development and progression of diabetic nephropathy (Fig. 32–30).[232] It is clearly evident that hyperglycemia is necessary for the initiation of renal injury, because patients without diabetes do not develop this type of nephropathy. Moreover, intensive therapy designed to achieve improved glycemic control is able to attenuate the development of nephropathy, as assessed by urinary albumin excretion, although it is not fully prevented.[278] However, it is now clear that other factors must also be involved because continuous florid hyperglycemia is not necessarily required for diabetic hyperfiltration and kidney growth to occur. Indeed, glomerular hyperfiltration and tubular hypertrophy can persist in patients with T1DM even after euglycemia is achieved through aggressive insulin therapy.[454]

Other pathways that may be involved in diabetic nephropathy include generation of mitochondrial ROS, accumulation of AGEs, and activation of intracellular signaling molecules such as PKC.[232] Many of the seminal studies performed in endothelial cells demonstrating a central role of mitochondrial ROS in activating pathways implicated in diabetic vascular complications have been reproduced in mesangial cells.[455] Advanced glycation, which occurs at an accelerated rate in diabetic patients, is a prominent phenomenon in the kidney. Not only is the kidney the major site for excretion of AGEs, but also many of the proteins with a long life, such as collagen, are extensively glycated in patients with diabetes.[456] Furthermore, various AGE receptors such as RAGE have been described in the kidney, which appear to play a role in mediating some of the deleterious effects of AGEs, such as stimulation of growth factor expression and induction of important phenotypic changes within certain renal cell populations to promote scarring.[118]

Preliminary studies using various approaches to inhibit renal AGE accumulation and action including a soluble RAGE (sRAGE). A range of pharmacologic agents have shown promising results, but clinical translation of these findings remains to be fully defined.[456] Selective PKC isoform inhibitors are in clinical trial but their role in renal disease remains to be clarified. Some exciting pilot studies evaluating a number of cytosolic sources of oxidative stress, such as NADPH oxidase, suggest that certain NADPH oxidase isoforms such as Nox4 may be excellent targets for new renoprotective therapies.[457]

In addition to the mechanisms described above, the diabetic kidney appears to be readily modulated by a range of vasoactive hormones. Indeed, it is increasingly appreciated that there may be important interactions between metabolic pathways and various hemodynamic factors including vasoactive hormones such as angiotensin II in mediating renal injury in diabetes (see Fig. 32–30).[458,459] Although many drugs that modulate hormone levels or action might not be specific for diabetic kidney disease, interruption of the renin-angiotensin system appears to be an excellent approach not only for reducing BP but also for correcting many of the cellular, biochemical, hemodynamic, and structural abnormalities seen in the diabetic kidney. These agents appear to be very powerful antiproteinuric agents, although the exact mechanism of action remains to be fully defined. Based on the discovery in the late 1990s that proteinuria in a range of nephropathies could occur as a result of molecular and structural abnormalities in a highly specialized structure known as the slit diaphragm within the glomerular epithelial cell (podocyte), a number of experimental studies, subsequently confirmed in humans, showed that depletion of one of these slit pore proteins, nephrin, could be attenuated or prevented by agents that interrupt the renin-angiotensin system.[460]

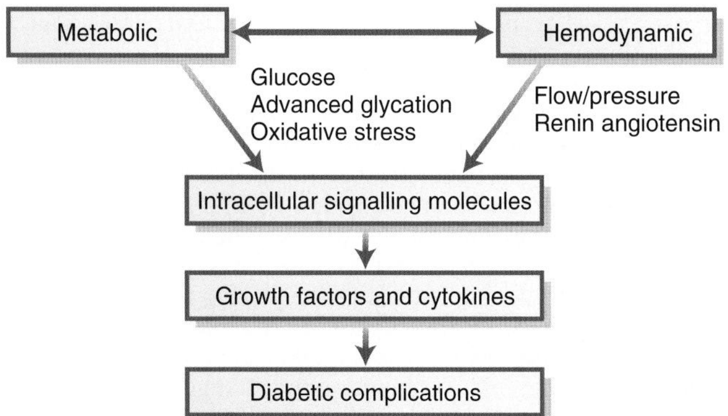

Figure 32–30 ▪ Interactions between metabolic and hemodynamic factors in promoting diabetic complications including nephropathy.

In addition to promoting glomerular nephrin depletion, angiotensin II also appears to have other actions that promote the development of proteinuria, including trophic effects on the kidney and increasing glomerular membrane pore size.[461] Although many investigators have focused on the renin-angiotensin system and, in particular, the vasoconstrictor angiotensin II, it is increasingly appreciated that other vasoconstrictors may be important. These include endothelin and a number of vasodilators such as nitric oxide, bradykinin, atrial natriuretic peptide, and vasodilative angiotensins, such as angiotensin 1-7.[462] This exploration of the role of vasoactive hormones and their respective receptors in the diabetic kidney is critical for designing new treatments for this condition, because these pathways are ideal targets for drug development. This point has already been demonstrated for agents that interrupt the renin-angiotensin system, including ACE inhibitors and angiotensin II receptor blockers (ARBs).

Pathology

Diabetic renal disease was originally described as a glomerulopathy associated with diffuse or nodular glomerulosclerosis.[426] Subsequent studies using electron microscopy have revealed that glomerular basement membrane thickening and mesangial expansion are prominent glomerular abnormalities in diabetes[438] (Fig. 32–31). Indeed, prospective studies have shown that these changes predict to a certain degree the development of overt renal disease in patients with T1DM. However, fewer than one third of diabetic patients with microalbuminuria have the typical glomerulopathy described by Kimmelsteil and Wilson in 1936.[426,463] Although initial studies emphasized the mesangial cell changes in the glomerulus, glomerular epithelial cell abnormalities represent new areas of active research.[54] Podocyte dysfunction and subsequent apoptosis ultimately leading to depletion of podocytes within the glomerulus appears to play a pivotal role in the development of proteinuria in diabetes.

Although most of the focus has been on glomerular changes in the diabetic kidney, more recent studies have identified important changes in the other sites within the kidney, including the tubules, interstitium, medulla, and papilla.[436] *Diabetic tubulopathy* is characterized by a variety of structural and functional changes including tubuloepithelial cell hypertrophy, tubular basement membrane thickening. epithelial-mesenchymal transition,[118] and the accumulation of glycogen (see Fig. 32–31). There is also an expansion of the interstitial space with infiltration of various cell types, including myofibroblasts and macrophages.

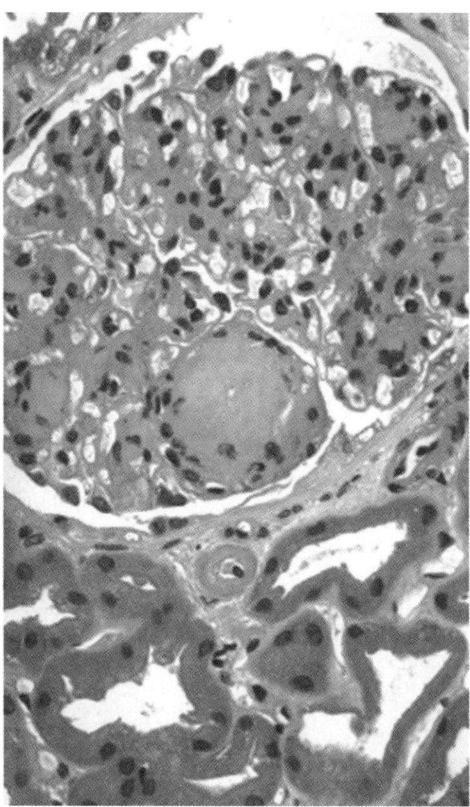

Glomerulopathy
Mesangial expansion
Glomerular hypertension
Diffuse thickening of the GBM
Broadening of foot processes
Podocyte loss
Reduced slit pore proteins
Glomerulomegaly
Kimmelstiel-Wilson lesion
Adhesions to Bowman's capsule
Neovascularization
Nodular and diffuse glomerulosclerosis
Tubulopathy
Tubular hyperplasia and hypertrophy
Progressive and cumulative atrophy
Thickening of the TBM
Epithelial mesenchymal transition
Accumulation of lysosomal bodies
Armani-Ebstein lesion
Reduced tubular brush border
Increased tubular salt reabsorption
Increased Na+/H+ antiporter activity
Impaired tubular acidification
Abnormal tubuloglomerular feedback
Decreased endocytosis of protein
Abnormal lysosomal processing
Impaired uptake of organic ions

Figure 32–31 ▪ Glomerular and tubular manifestations of diabetic nephropathy. GBM, glomerular basement membrane; TBM, tubular basement membrane.

These tubular changes represent more than just the aftermath of diabetic nephropathy. The dysregulation of tubular functions in diabetes can precede or at least accompany the changes in the renal glomerulus and the onset of albuminuria.[463] Indeed, the functional and structural changes in the proximal tubule may be a key to the contributor to the development and progression of diabetic nephropathy.[436] For example, it has been suggested that tubuloglomerular feedback mechanisms can drive hyperfiltration associated with diabetes[432] and that tubular dysfunction can contribute to albuminuria due to defective uptake and lysosomal processing.[440] Indeed, renal function and prognosis correlate better with structural lesions in the tubules and cortical interstitium than with classic glomerular changes of diabetic nephropathy.

Renal Artery Stenosis

Because diabetic patients have, in general, an increased burden of atherosclerosis, they appear to have a higher risk of renal artery stenosis. However, although angiographic studies have demonstrated a high prevalence of renal artery stenosis in diabetic patients, these lesions are often of no hemodynamic significance. Nevertheless, a small subgroup will have a hemodynamically significant stenosis enhancing hypertension, increasing the risk of acute pulmonary edema, and inducing progressive renal impairment.[464] In such subjects, specific interventions such as surgery or angioplasty need to be considered.[465] Furthermore, some patients have bilateral renal artery stenosis that, on commencement of an agent such as an ACE inhibitor, can lead to acute renal failure.[466] Fortunately, in most patients, if the renal failure is diagnosed early, cessation of the ACE inhibitor leads to rapid restoration of renal function in this situation.

Renal Papillary Necrosis

Renal papillary necrosis involves a severe destructive process, presumably as a result of ischemia to the medulla and papilla.[467] Beethoven's final illness might have been papillary necrosis in the context of diabetes.[468] The papilla is very sensitive to these ischemic changes because even in the normal setting it is exposed to a relatively hypoxic environment. Concomitant exacerbating factors include urinary tract infection and analgesic abuse. The importance of ischemia and possibly angiotensin II in this disorder has been suggested in experimental studies in transgenic rats that overexpress renin and angiotensin II in their kidney after induction of diabetes.[469] In these rats, diabetes was associated with development of papillary necrosis; development of papillary necrosis was prevented by blockade of the renin-angiotensin system. Clinically, papillary necrosis often manifests as flank pain, hematuria, and fever. Urinalysis reveals red and white blood cells, bacteria, and papillary fragments. Ureteric obstruction can occur as a result of these fragments and must be addressed as an emergency.

Renal Tubular Acidosis

A well-known functional abnormality associated with diabetic tubulopathy is *renal tubular acidosis,* manifesting as hyperkalemia and hyperchloremic metabolic acidosis.[470] This is thought to be a manifestation of hyporeninemic hypoaldosteronism associated with diabetes, resulting in proximal tubule ammonia production reduced to levels inadequate to buffer acid in the distal nephron. The precise causes of this abnormality remain to be established. In some patients there appears to be a defect in the conversion of prorenin to active renin.[471] It has also been suggested that damage to the tubular cells of the juxtaglomerular apparatus associated with diabetes can contribute to impaired renin release, possibly due to reduced renal prostaglandin production and elevated vasopressin levels.[472]

A major risk associated with hyporeninemic hypoaldosteronism is the development of life-threatening hyperkalemia. This is an increasingly important issue with the widespread use of ACE inhibitors and ARBs, often in combination, in this population. This is further exacerbated by the use of potassium-sparing diuretics (such as spironolactone) and β-blockers.

Other Renal Manifestations

Because many diabetic subjects have impaired renal function, they are at high risk for increased renal impairment from certain nephrotoxic agents. One of the most important risks relates to radiocontrast dyes.[473] Where possible, patients with diabetes and renal impairment should avoid imaging studies that involve contrast and, in particular, multiple studies performed in rapid succession. Where intravenous contrast forms an indispensable tool to management, low-osmolality, nonionic or gadolinium-based contrast media may be less nephrotoxic in patients with renal failure.[474] It is also critical to ensure that patients who require such procedures are well hydrated before, during, and after the procedure. The role of *N*-acetylcysteine, a thiol-containing antioxidant, shows promise to protect against contrast-induced nephropathy.[475] The oral hypoglycemic drug metformin should also be discontinued before contrast procedures to prevent life-threatening lactic acidosis.

Management

Blood pressure and glycemic control represent the major cornerstones for preventing and treating diabetic nephropathy (Figs. 32–32 and 32–33). In the early 1980s a number of Scandinavian researchers found that aggressive BP reduction reduces the rate of progression of diabetic nephropathy,[476,477] and in the 1990s other researchers found that intensified glycemic control has a similar benefit in both T1DM (DCCT)[278] and T2DM (UKPDS) diabetic subjects.[479] These findings have led to the view that optimization of BP and plasma glucose levels should be the mainstay of therapy for diabetic nephropathy.

Glycemic Control

The importance of glucose as a factor in the progression of diabetic kidney disease, as initially suggested from epidemiologic and preclinical studies, was clearly demonstrated in the DCCT study in patients with T1DM.[278] In both the primary and secondary prevention aim of the study, any decrease in Hb A_{1c} was strongly associated with a reduction in the risk of development of microalbuminuria as well as a decrease in the risk of progression to overt nephropathy. The follow-up EDIC study has confirmed long-lasting benefits of this therapeutic approach.

It remains to be determined how useful intensification of glycemic control is in the setting of overt nephropathy as a last-ditch strategy to delay the onset of ESRD. Aggressive management of hypertension is clearly more important than glycemic control in reducing cardiovascular events and slowing renal disease progression at this stage of relatively advanced disease, although some studies suggest that poor glycemic control can accelerate the loss of renal function in diabetic nephropathy.[479] However, a number of large studies have failed to show any evidence that strict glycemic control per se retards renal progression once overt nephropathy is present.[480] In addition, as renal function fails, tight glycemic control becomes more hazardous, with an increased risk of hypoglycemia. Nonetheless, because there is sufficient evidence that glycemic control can

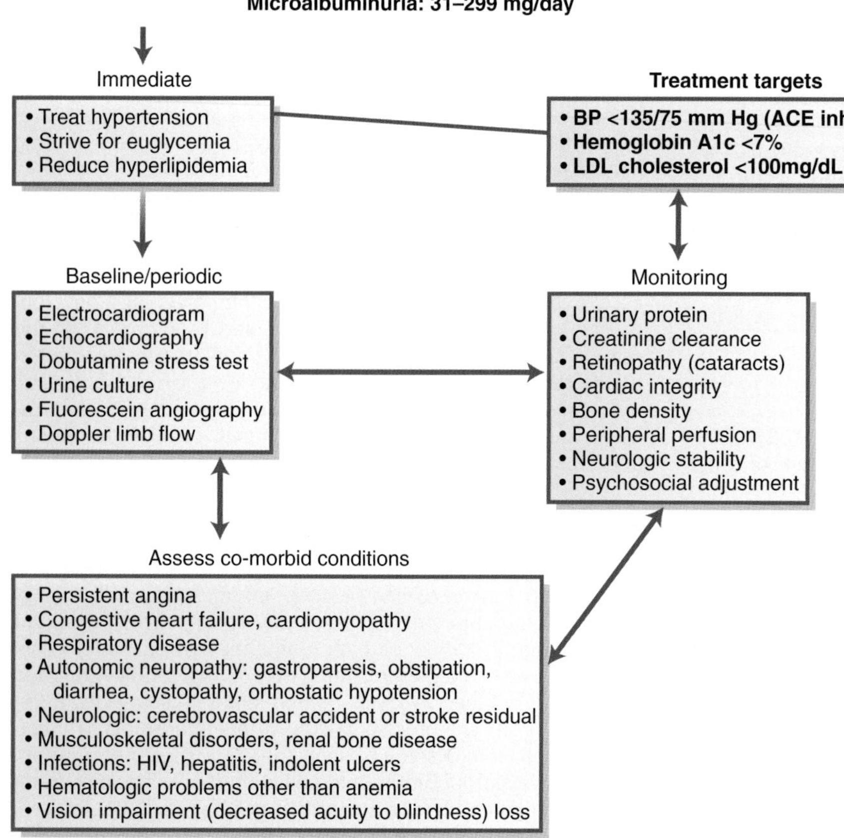
Microalbuminuria: 31–299 mg/day
Immediate
• Treat hypertension
• Strive for euglycemia
• Reduce hyperlipidemia
Treatment targets
• BP <135/75 mm Hg (ACE inhibitor)
• Hemoglobin A1c <7%
• LDL cholesterol <100mg/dL (statin)
Baseline/periodic
• Electrocardiogram
• Echocardiography
• Dobutamine stress test
• Urine culture
• Fluorescein angiography
• Doppler limb flow
Monitoring
• Urinary protein
• Creatinine clearance
• Retinopathy (cataracts)
• Cardiac integrity
• Bone density
• Peripheral perfusion
• Neurologic stability
• Psychosocial adjustment
Assess co-morbid conditions
• Persistent angina
• Congestive heart failure, cardiomyopathy
• Respiratory disease
• Autonomic neuropathy: gastroparesis, obstipation, diarrhea, cystopathy, orthostatic hypotension
• Neurologic: cerebrovascular accident or stroke residual
• Musculoskeletal disorders, renal bone disease
• Infections: HIV, hepatitis, indolent ulcers
• Hematologic problems other than anemia
• Vision impairment (decreased acuity to blindness) loss

Figure 32–32 ▪ Flow chart illustrating the management of patients with diabetic nephropathy before the onset of renal failure. ACE, angiotensin-converting enzyme; HIV, human immunodeficiency virus; LDL, low-density lipoprotein.

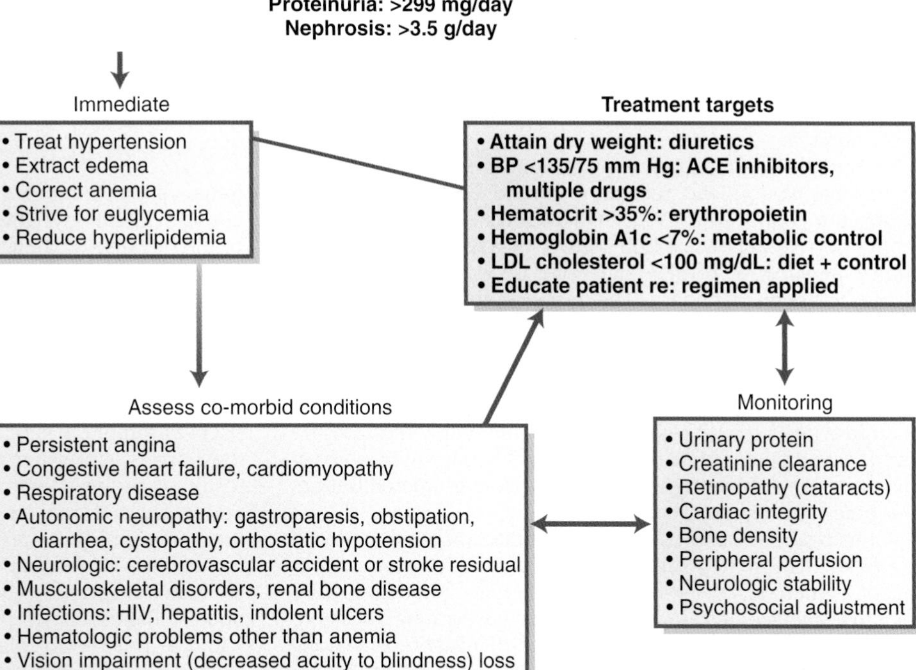
Proteinuria: >299 mg/day
Nephrosis: >3.5 g/day
Immediate
• Treat hypertension
• Extract edema
• Correct anemia
• Strive for euglycemia
• Reduce hyperlipidemia
Treatment targets
• Attain dry weight: diuretics
• BP <135/75 mm Hg: ACE inhibitors, multiple drugs
• Hematocrit >35%: erythropoietin
• Hemoglobin A1c <7%: metabolic control
• LDL cholesterol <100 mg/dL: diet + control
• Educate patient re: regimen applied
Assess co-morbid conditions
• Persistent angina
• Congestive heart failure, cardiomyopathy
• Respiratory disease
• Autonomic neuropathy: gastroparesis, obstipation, diarrhea, cystopathy, orthostatic hypotension
• Neurologic: cerebrovascular accident or stroke residual
• Musculoskeletal disorders, renal bone disease
• Infections: HIV, hepatitis, indolent ulcers
• Hematologic problems other than anemia
• Vision impairment (decreased acuity to blindness) loss
Monitoring
• Urinary protein
• Creatinine clearance
• Retinopathy (cataracts)
• Cardiac integrity
• Bone density
• Peripheral perfusion
• Neurologic stability
• Psychosocial adjustment

Figure 32–33 ▪ Flow chart illustrating the management of patients with diabetic nephropathy after the onset of clinical proteinuria. ACE, angiotensin-converting enzyme; HIV, human immunodeficiency virus; LDL, low-density lipoprotein.

reduce both macrovascular events and microvascular complications of diabetes at other sites, it is reasonable to suggest that optimization of metabolic control in patients with overt nephropathy remains worthwhile.

Similar benefits on renal disease in the context of T2DM are seen following optimization of glycemic control.[3] However, the choice of agent remains controversial. Certainly, several types of drugs are able improve glycemic control in the patients with T2DM; however, the particular advantages of once class over another for preventing and treatng diabetic nephropathy remains to be established.

A number of differences in the side effect profiles should influence prescribing habits. In patients with renal impairment, particular care must be exercised in selecting and dosing oral diabetic therapy because an accumulation of either the drug or active metabolites can lead to hypoglycemia (e.g., with glyburide) and other serious adverse effects such as lactic acidosis (with metformin). Thiazolodinediones, such as pioglitazone and rosiglitazone, should be used with caution in patients at risk for heart failure.

Other agents that directly inhibit glucose-induced changes in various biochemical pathways will likely become available. These include benfotiamine, a thiamine alternative that appears to inhibit the downstream effects of mitochondrial ROS generation[481] and various antiglycation strategies,[482] as outlined previously.

Blood Pressure Control

A sustained reduction in BP appears to be the most important single intervention to prevent progressive nephropathy in T1DM and T2DM. For example, in the UKPDS, a reduction in BP from 154 to 144 mm Hg was associated with a 30% reduction in microalbuminuria.[478] All national and international guidelines now emphasize the importance of BP reduction in the diabetic patient. Although many guidelines suggest specific targets should be achieved, no such threshold appears to exist for any renal end-point in patients with diabetes. In particular, the risk of progressive diabetic nephropathy continues to decrease with BP reductions into the normal range and below, meaning that the lowest achievable BP is associated with the best clinical outcomes. This is particularly important in those with the greatest risk of renal damage, patients with overt nephropathy. In these patients, it has been suggested that optimal BP control is less than 125/75 mm Hg.[483]

There is good evidence that tight BP control, no matter how it was achieved, is associated with a significant reduction in the risk of microalbuminuria (primary prevention). Although BP reduction appears paramount, there is also evidence that ACE inhibitors[484] have renoprotective actions beyond their antihypertensive effects for primary prevention.[485-487] However, if treatment should commence in the normoalbuminuric stage, such a strategy would involve treating the majority of patients who are not at risk of nephropathy. Ideally, it would be useful to be able to identify patients, still normoalbuminuric, whose likelihood of progression is increased. As yet no such markers of predisposition to renal disease are available, although serum prorenin[439] and modest elevations in urinary albumin excretion albeit still within the normal range (borderline microalbuminuria)[445] might ultimately be such markers.

In secondary prevention studies, the additional benefits achieved from blocking the renin-angiotensin system are clearer.[488] A meta-analysis incorporating the findings of more than 10 studies in patients with microalbuminuria has demonstrated the ability of ACE inhibitors not only ot retard the development of overt proteinuria but also to decrease urinary albumin excretion by more than 30%. In some patients with microalbuminuria, ACE inhibition can reduce urinary albumin excretion into the normoalbuminuric range.[485] In patients with T1DM and overt proteinuria, aggressive BP reduction reduced proteinuria by up to 50% and retarded the rate of decline in renal function.[476,477]

Similar studies have been performed in type 2 diabetic patients. Two landmark trials, RENAAL (Reduction in Endpoints in patients with Non–insulin-dependent diabetes mellitus with the Angiotensin II Antagonist Losartan) and IDNT (Irbesartan in Diabetic Nephropathy Trial), examined the renoprotective effects of the ARBs losartan and irbesartan, respectively.[489,490] In both studies, when compared to various alternative antihypertensive agents such as calcium antagonists (but not ACE inhibitors), ARB treatment was associated with a reduction in end-stage renal failure, a greater than 30% decrease in proteinuria, and a major reduction in hospitalization for heart failure. As a result of these studies, ARBs are recommended as first-line treatment for BP reduction in type 2 diabetic patients with overt proteinuria.[491]

Although ACE inhibitors have not been as extensively studied in this population, the recently reported DETAIL (Diabetics Exposed to Telmisartan And EnalaprIL) trial suggested similar renoprotective actions of both drug classes.[492] Indeed, from a clinical perspective, no clear difference between these two drug classes has been identified. (The one exception is cough, which occurs in 5% to 30% of patients taking ACE inhibitors, depending on ethnicity [higher in Asian subjects]). In microalbuminuric type 2 diabetic subjects, ARBs have also been demonstrated to have a role. For example, in the IRMA2 (IRbesartan MicroAlbuminuria type 2) trial, irbesartan dose-dependently reduced the risk of development of macroproteinuria,[493] confirming the findings seen predominantly with ACE inhibitors in microalbuminuric type 1 diabetic subjects.[485]

Other approaches focusing on BP reduction continue to be examined in these populations. This includes mineralocorticoid receptor antagonists such as spironolactone[494] and the more selective agent epleronone, which has fewer antiandrogenic side effects.[495] Furthermore, a number of agents, at various stages of preclinical and early clinical development, are under investigation, including endothelin antagonists and vasopeptidase (dual ACE/NEP) inhibitors.[496]

Other Approaches

Low-protein diets (0.75 g/kg per day) have been shown to retard the progression of renal disease, although the data are not totally convincing for diabetic nephropathy per se. A meta-analysis of five studies in type 1 diabetic subjects supported a minor renoprotective role for these diets,[497] but this has not been a universal finding.[498] There are even fewer data in type 2 diabetic subjects with overt nephropathy.[499] However, the expected benefits that can be achieved through protein restriction in patients with diabetic nephropathy are at best modest in comparison with adequate BP control and blockade of the renin-angiotensin system. Moreover, the nutritional impact of such interventions must be carefully considered, particularly in patients with brittle glycemic control.

The role of lipid-lowering agents as renoprotective drugs remains controversial. Although in rodents a large body of evidence suggests that lipids promote renal injury and that various lipid-lowering drugs reduce nephropathy, even in the setting of no or minimal effect on lipids,[500] the data in humans are variable.[501] However, in a study of fenofibrate in T2DM, there was an impressive reduction in albuminuria.[502] Furthermore, in the Heart Protection Study, simvastatin appeared to retard the decline in renal function, although this analysis was not confined to the diabetic subgroup.[503] Another group has also reported a potential renoprotective effect of a statin,[504] although this effect has not been observed in all studies. Nevertheless, because cardiovascular disease is so prominent in diabetic patients, particularly those with incipient or overt renal disease, lipid-lowering treatment should be considered in most patients independent of its putative renoprotective actions.[505]

Other approaches to consider include correction of anemia with agents such as erythropoietin.[506] The role of these agents as renoprotective drugs remains to be clarified,[507] but the potential benefits on general patient well-being and in reducing left ventricular hypertrophy[508] provide a rationale for using such agents judiciously in diabetic patients.

With respect to likely new agents for diabetic nephropathy in the near future, a number of clinical trials are in progress. These include protein kinase C inhibitors[509] and sulodexide, an agent postulated to restore the glomerular charge by repleting the loss of glycosaminoglycans,[510] thus acting as an antiproteinuric and ultimately renoprotective drug.

Treatment of the Diabetic Uremic Patient

Renal impairment in a patient with diabetes necessitates changes in therapy. Often blood glucose control becomes more brittle because the half-life of insulin is prolonged and the renal response to hypoglycemia is impaired. High swinging blood glucose levels in a patient with nephropathy can often mistakenly lead to an increase in oral therapy. However, in patients with renal impairment, particular care must be exercised in the selection and dosing of oral hypoglycemic therapy. Nonsteroidal antiinflammatory drugs (NSAIDs) and cyclooxgenase-2 (COX-2) inhibitors should be avoided where possible because their use is associated with inadequate BP control, often as a result of reduced efficacy of antihypertensive drug therapy. Patients at high risk for progressive deterioration in their renal function should be considered for an early referral to a nephrology service for management of renal failure (Fig. 32–34). This facilitates access to erythropoietin and control of calcium phosphate balance and to planning for renal replacement therapy with the preemptive placement of access catheters and lines. Delay in referral can result in a more precipitous start to renal replacement and usually a bad prognostic outcome.[511]

Many options are now available for the diabetic patient requiring renal replacement therapy.[512] These include home or facility hemodialysis, peritoneal dialysis, renal transplantation (cadaveric or living related), or combined pancreas-kidney transplantation. Most patients choose hemodialysis rather than peritoneal dialysis, although data conflict regarding which approach leads to better survival (Table 32–6). Some patients opt for withdrawal of treatment because their quality of life, with advanced cardiovascular disease, visual impairment, and amputations, is poor.

The Burden of Nephropathy

One must never consider renal disease in a diabetic patient in isolation. Proteinuria per se is strongly associated with other complications such as macrovascular disease, heart failure, and retinopathy, and treatments directed toward one complication may be useful for the other complications. Indeed, intensified glycemic control has been shown to be particularly useful for other microvascular complications,[2] and the various antihypertensive regimens, particularly those using agents that interrupt the renin-angiotensin system, also confer important cardiovascular benefits such as reducing heart failure.[489] Thus, as clearly expounded in the Steno-2 study, the multifactorial approach in microalbuminuric subjects will not only lead to renal benefits but will also confer other advantages to the diabetic patient.[513] Because those with renal disease have the greatest risk for nonrenal complications, it stands to reason that they also are likely to have the greatest absolute benefit from risk-reduction strategies.

DIABETIC NEUROPATHIES

Diabetic neuropathies are a heterogeneous group of disorders and present a wide range of abnormalities. They are among the most common long-term complications of diabetes and are a significant source of morbidity and mortality.[514,515] Estimates of the prevalence of neuropathy vary substantially, depending on

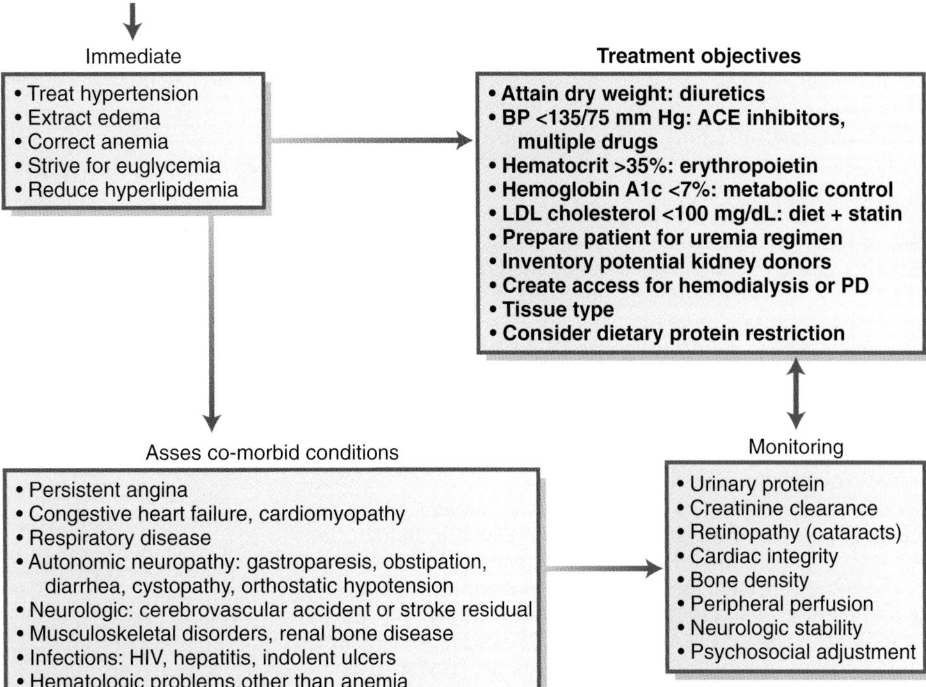

Azotemia: Serum creatinine >2.0 mg/dL
Immediate
• Treat hypertension
• Extract edema
• Correct anemia
• Strive for euglycemia
• Reduce hyperlipidemia
Treatment objectives
• Attain dry weight: diuretics
• BP <135/75 mm Hg: ACE inhibitors, multiple drugs
• Hematocrit >35%: erythropoietin
• Hemoglobin A1c <7%: metabolic control
• LDL cholesterol <100 mg/dL: diet + statin
• Prepare patient for uremia regimen
• Inventory potential kidney donors
• Create access for hemodialysis or PD
• Tissue type
• Consider dietary protein restriction
Asses co-morbid conditions
• Persistent angina
• Congestive heart failure, cardiomyopathy
• Respiratory disease
• Autonomic neuropathy: gastroparesis, obstipation, diarrhea, cystopathy, orthostatic hypotension
• Neurologic: cerebrovascular accident or stroke residual
• Musculoskeletal disorders, renal bone disease
• Infections: HIV, hepatitis, indolent ulcers
• Hematologic problems other than anemia
• Vision impairment (decreased acuity to blindness) loss
Monitoring
• Urinary protein
• Creatinine clearance
• Retinopathy (cataracts)
• Cardiac integrity
• Bone density
• Peripheral perfusion
• Neurologic stability
• Psychosocial adjustment

Figure 32–34 ▪ Flow chart illustrating the management of patients after onset of renal failure. ACE, angiotensin-converting enzyme; HIV, human immunodeficiency virus; LDL, low-density lipoprotein; PD, peritoneal dialysis.

TABLE 32–6 OPTIONS IN THERAPY FOR END-STAGE RENAL DISEASE IN DIABETIC PATIENTS

Variable	Peritoneal Dialysis	Hemodialysis	Kidney Transplant
Extensive extrarenal disease	No limitation	No limitation except for hypotension	Excluded in cardiovascular insufficiency
Geriatric patients		No limitation	Arbitrary exclusion as determined by program
Complete rehabilitation	Rare, if ever	Very few patients	Common so long as graft functions
Death rate	Much higher than for nondiabetic patients	Much higher than for nondiabetic patients	About the same as for nondiabetic patients
First-year survival	~75%	~75%	>90%
Morbidity during first year	~15 days in hospital	~12 days in hospital	Weeks to months hospitalized
Survival to second decade	Almost never	<5%	~1 in 5
Progression of complications	Usual and unremitting; hyperglycemia and hyperlipidemia	Usual and unremitting; might benefit from metabolic control	Interdicted by functioning pancreas plus kidney; partially ameliorated by correction of azotemia
Special advantage	Can be self-performed; Avoids swings in solute and intravascular volume level	Can be self-performed; efficient extraction of solute and water in hours	Cures uremia; freedom to travel
Disadvantages	Peritonitis; hyperinsulinemia; hyperglycemia, hyperlipidemia; long hours of treatment; more days hospitalized than with either hemodialysis or transplant	Blood access a hazard for clotting, hemorrhage, and infection; cyclical hypotension, weakness, aluminum toxicity, amyloidosis	Cosmetic disfigurement, hypertension, personal expense for cototoxic drugs; induced malignancy; HIV transmission
Patient acceptance	Variable, usual compliance with passive tolerance for regimen	Variable, often noncompliant with dietary, metabolic or antihypertensive components of regimen	Enthusiastic during periods of good renal allograft function; exalted when pancreas proffers euglycemia
Relative cost	Most expensive over long run	Less expensive than kidney transplant in the first year; subsequent years more expensive	Pancreas plus kidney engraftment most expensive uremia therapy for diabetic; after first year, kidney transplant alone is lowest-cost option

specific diagnostic criteria.[516,517] In the United States, prevalence estimates have ranged from 5% to 100%.[514,516,517-519] In Pirart's classic study of a cohort of 4400 patients, prevalence was found to reach approximately 45% after 25 years.[520] Using this estimate, about 7 million persons in the United States alone are likely to be afflicted with diabetic neuropathy and about 2.7 million have painful neuropathy.[521] Furthermore, it is now evident that neuropathy can occur with impaired glucose tolerance[522] and with the metabolic syndrome in the absence of hyperglycemia.[523] It is the most common form of neuropathy in the developed countries of the world, accounts for more hospitalizations than all the other diabetic complications combined, and is responsible for 50% to 75% of nontrauma amputations.[518,519] Diabetic peripheral neuropathy is also responsible for weakness and ataxia, with an estimated increase in likelihood of falling that is 15 times that of unaffected population.[524,525]

Diabetic neuropathy is a set of clinical syndromes that affect distinct regions of the nervous system, singly or combined. Clinical signs and symptoms can be nonspecific and insidious, and progression can be slow. Neuropathy may be silent and go undetected while exercising its ravages, or it can manifest with clinical symptoms and signs that mimic those seen in many other diseases. It is, therefore, diagnosed by exclusion.

The true prevalence is not known and depends on the criteria and methods used to define neuropathy. Of patients attending a diabetes clinic, 25% volunteered symptoms, but 50% were found to have neuropathy after a simple clinical test such as the ankle jerk or vibration perception test. Almost 90% tested positive to sophisticated tests of autonomic function or peripheral sensation.[526] Neuropathy is grossly underdiagnosed by endocrinologists and nonendocrinologists.[527] Neurologic complications occur equally in T1DM and T2DM and additionally in various forms of acquired diabetes.[517]

The major morbidity associated with somatic neuropathy is foot ulceration, the precursor of gangrene and limb loss. Neuropathy increases the risk of amputation 1.7-fold, 12-fold if there is deformity (itself a consequence of neuropathy), and 36-fold if there is a history of previous ulceration.[528] There are 86,000 amputations in the United States each year, one every 10 minutes, and neuropathy is the major contributor in 87% of cases.[515] It is also the most life-spoiling of the diabetic complications and has tremendous ramifications for the quality of life of the person with diabetes.[529] Once autonomic neuropathy sets in, life can become quite dismal, and the mortality rate approximates 25% to 50% within 5 to 10 years.[530-533]

Classification

Diabetic neuropathy is not a single entity but a number of different syndromes with subclinical or clinical manifestations depending on the classes of nerve fibers involved. According to the San Antonio Convention,[534] the main groups of neurologic disturbance in diabetes mellitus include:

- Subclinical neuropathy, which is determined by abnormalities in electrodiagnostic and quantitative sensory testing
- Diffuse clinical neuropathy with distal symmetric sensorimotor and autonomic syndromes
- Focal syndromes

Subclinical neuropathy is diagnosed on the basis of abnormal electrodiagnostic tests with decreased nerve conduction velocity (NCV) or decreased amplitudes; abnormal quantitative sensory tests (QST) for vibration, tactile, thermal warming, and cooling thresholds; and quantitative autonomic function tests (QAFT) revealing diminished heart rate variation with deep breathing, Valsalva maneuver, and postural testing. The different clinical presentations of diabetic neuropathy are schematically illustrated in Figure 32–35.

Natural History

The natural history of neuropathies separates them into two very distinct entities, namely those that progress gradually with increasing duration of diabetes and those that remit, usually completely. Sensory and autonomic neuropathies generally progress, and mononeuropathies, radiculopathies, and acute painful neuropathies, although symptoms are severe, are short-lived, and patients tend to recover.[535]

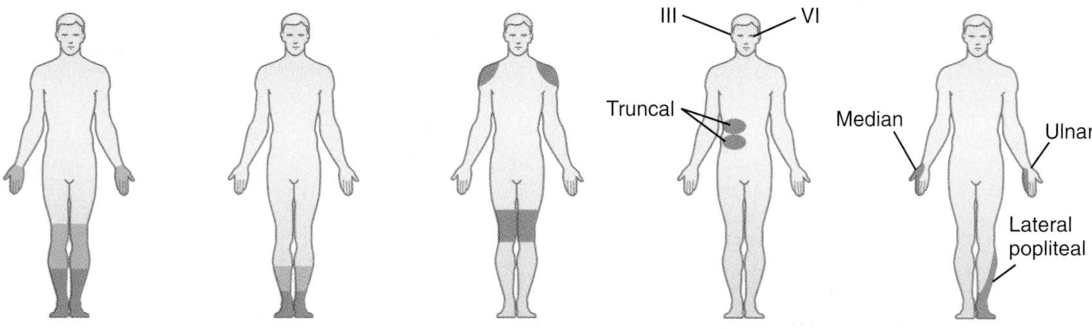

Large-fiber Neuropathy	Small-fiber Neuropathy	Proximal motor neuropathy	Acute mononeuropathies	Entrapments
Sensory loss: 0→+++ (Touch, vibration) Pain: +→ +++ Tendon reflex: N→↓↓↓ Motor deficit 0→ +++	Sensory loss: 0→ + (thermal, allodynia) Pain: +→ +++ Tendon reflex: N→↓ Motor deficit: 0	Sensory loss: 0→ + Pain: +→ +++ Tendon reflex: ↓↓ Proximal motor deficit: +→ +++	Sensory loss: 0→ + Pain: +→ +++ Tendon reflex: N Motor deficit: +→ +++	Sensory loss in Nerve distribution: +→ +++ Pain: +→ + Tendon reflex: N Motor deficit: +→ +++

Figure 32–35 ▪ Different clinical presentations of diabetic neuropathies. (Modified from Pickup J, Williams G [eds]. Textbook of Diabetes, Vol 1. Oxford, UK, Blackwell Scientific, 1997.)

Progression of neuropathy is related to glycemic control in both T1DM and T2DM.[536,537] It appears that the most rapid deterioration of nerve function occurs soon after the onset of T1DM, and within 2 to 3 years there is a slowing of the progression, with a shallower slope in the curve of dysfunction. In contrast, in T2DM, slowing of NCVs may be one of the earliest neuropathic abnormalities and often is present even at diagnosis.[538] After diagnosis, slowing of NCV generally progresses at a steady rate of approximately 1 m/sec per year, and the level of impairment is positively correlated with duration of diabetes. Although most studies have documented that symptomatic patients are more likely to have slower NCVs than patients without symptoms, these do not relate to the severity of symptoms. In a long-term follow-up study of T2DM patients,[539] electrophysiologic abnormalities in the lower limb increased from 8% at baseline to 42% after 10 years.

A decrease in sensory and motor amplitudes, indicating axonal destruction, was more pronounced than the slowing of the NCVs. An increase of about 2 points in an 80-point clinical scale can be expected per year. These scales contain information on motor, sensory, and autonomic signs and symptoms. Using objective measures of sensory function, such as the vibration perception threshold test, the rate of decline in function has been reported as 1 to 2 vibration units per year. However, there now appears to be a decline in this rate of evolution. For example, in the recent nerve growth factor (NGF) study, the vibration perception threshold at the beginning of the study in the placebo group was identical to that at the end of 1 year.[540,541]

It appears that host factors pertaining to general health and nerve nutrition are changing. This is particularly important in doing studies on treatment of diabetic neuropathy, which have always relied on differences between drug treatment and placebo and have apparently been successful because of the decline in placebo-treated patients.[542] Based upon the earlier estimates of change, clinically meaningful loss of vibration perception and conduction velocity was estimated to take at least 3 years, dictating a future need to carry out studies over a longer period of time.

It is also important to recognize that diabetic neuropathy is a disorder wherein the prevailing abnormality is loss of axons that electrophysiologically translates to a reduction in amplitudes and not conduction velocities, and changes in NCV might not be an appropriate means of monitoring progress or deterioration of nerve function. It has always been assumed that diabetes affects the longest fibers first—hence, the increased predisposition in taller persons.[543] Now it seems that small-fiber involvement can herald the onset of neuropathy and even diabetes. Small-fiber function is not detectable using standard electrophysiology and requires measurement of sensory, neurovascular, and autonomic thresholds and cutaneous nerve fiber density.[523,544-546] There are few data on the longitudinal trends in small-fiber dysfunction, although it appears that the nerve fiber loss in prediabetic neuropathy might respond to lifestyle changes.[547]

Much remains to be learned of the natural history of diabetic autonomic neuropathy. Karamitsos and colleagues[548] have reported that the progression of diabetic autonomic neuropathy is significant during the 2 years subsequent to its discovery. The mortality rate for diabetic autonomic neuropathy has been estimated to be 44% within 2.5 years of diagnosing symptomatic autonomic neuropathy.[530] A meta-analysis[549] revealed that the mortality rate after 5.8 years of diabetes with symptomatic autonomic neuropathy was 29%. In a meta-analysis of 12 published studies, reduced cardiovascular function as measured by heart rate variability was shown to be associated with an increased risk of silent myocardial infarction.[533]

Similarly, a meta-analysis of prospective studies has demonstrated increased mortality in patients with cardiac autonomic neuropathy, with the risk ratio increasing in direct proportion to the number of autonomic abnormalities.[532,533] The relative risk of mortality from 15 studies (N=2900; 95% CI) was increased in patients with cardiac autonomic neuropathy by 2.14 (CI 1.83-2.51).[533] However, if cardiac autonomic neuropathy is defined by the presence of at least two abnormal autonomic function tests, this risk increases to 3.45 (CI 2.66-4.47).[532]

Clinical Presentation

An international consensus meeting on the outpatient diagnosis and management of diabetic neuropathy agreed that a simple definition of diabetic neuropathy was "the presence of symptoms and/or signs of peripheral nerve dysfunction in people with diabetes after the exclusion of other causes."[534] It was also agreed that neuropathy cannot be diagnosed without a careful clinical examination; absence of symptoms cannot be equated with absence of neuropathy because asymptomatic neuropathy is common. The American Diabetes Association has recently endorsed these recommendations.[550] The importance of excluding nondiabetic causes was emphasized in the Rochester Diabetic Neuropathy Study, in which up to 10% of peripheral neuropathy in diabetic patients was deemed to be of nondiabetic etiology.[517] Many conditions need to be excluded before the diagnosis of diabetic neuropathy can be made.[515] A more detailed definition of neuropathy had previously been agreed on at the San Antonio Consensus Conference: "Diabetic neuropathy is a descriptive term meaning a demonstrable disorder, either clinically evident or sub-clinical, that occurs in the setting of diabetes mellitus without other causes for peripheral neuropathy. The neuropathic disorder includes manifestations in the somatic and/or autonomic parts of the peripheral nervous system."[534]

It is generally agreed that diabetic neuropathy should not be diagnosed on one symptom, sign, or test alone. A minimum of two abnormalities (from symptoms, signs, nerve conduction abnormalities, quantitative sensory tests, or quantitative autonomic tests) is recommended.[551] Diabetic neuropathy is, however, woefully underdiagnosed by endocrinologists as well as nonendocrinologists. In the goal A_{1c} study,[527] identification of the absence of neuropathy in 7000 patients was fairly adequate but was only accurate in the presence of mild neuropathy one third of the time, and it reached 75% only if neuropathy was severe. Clearly there is a need for education of the means whereby neuropathy may be diagnosed.

The spectrum of clinical neuropathic syndromes described in patients with diabetes mellitus includes dysfunction of almost every segment of the somatic peripheral and autonomic nervous system.[552] Thus, as the saying goes, knowing neuropathy means to know the whole of medicine. Each syndrome can be distinguished by its pathophysiologic, therapeutic, and prognostic features.

Focal Neuropathies

Mononeuropathies occur primarily in the older population. Their onset is generally acute and associated with pain, and their course is self-limiting, resolving within 6 to 8 weeks. Mononeuropathies result from vascular obstruction after which adjacent neuronal fascicles take over the function of those infarcted by the clot.[553] Mononeuropathies must be distinguished from entrapment syndromes that start slowly, progress, and persist without intervention, as shown in Table 32–7. Common entrapment sites in diabetic patients involve median, ulnar, and radial nerves; femoral nerves, lateral cutaneous nerves of the thigh, and peroneal nerves; and the medial and lateral plantar nerves.

TABLE 32–7 MONONEURITIS AND ENTRAPMENT SYNDROMES

Feature	Nononeuritis	Entrapment
Onset	Sudden	Gradual
Nerves	Usually single but may be multiple	Single nerves exposed to trauma
Common nerves	C3, C6, C7, ulnar, median, peroneal	Median, ulnar, peroneal, medial and lateral plantar
Progression	Not progressive; resolves spontaneously	Progressive
Treatment	Symptomatic	Rest, splints, diuretics, steroid injections, surgery for paralysis

Adapted from Vinik A, Mehrabyan A. Diabetic neuropathies. Med Clin North Am 2004;88(4):947-999.

Carpal tunnel syndrome occurs three times as often in persons with diabetes compared with a normal, healthy population,[554,555] and its increased prevalence in diabetes may be related to diabetic cheiroarthropathy,[556] repeated undetected trauma, metabolic changes, or accumulation of fluid or edema within the confined space of the carpal tunnel.[552] It is found in up to one third of patients with diabetes.[557] If carpal tunnel syndrome is recognized, the diagnosis can be confirmed by electrophysiologic study, and therapy is simple, with surgical release. The mainstays of nonsurgical treatment are resting the wrist, aided by the placement of a wrist splint in a neutral position for day and night use, and the addition of antiinflammatory medications. Surgical treatment consists of sectioning the volar carpal ligament.[558] The decision to proceed with surgery should be based on several considerations, including severity of symptoms, appearance of motor weakness, and failure of nonsurgical treatment.[559]

Diffuse Neuropathies

Proximal Motor Neuropathies

For many years, proximal neuropathy has been considered a component of diabetic neuropathy, although its pathogenesis was ill understood.[560] The condition has a number of synonyms; proximal neuropathy, femoral neuropathy, diabetic amyotrophy, and diabetic neuropathic cachexia.

Proximal motor neuropathy has certain common features. It primarily affects the elderly. Its onset, which can be gradual or abrupt, begins with pain in the thighs and hips or buttocks, followed by significant weakness of the proximal muscles of the lower limbs with inability to rise from the sitting position (positive Gower's maneuver). The neuropathy begins unilaterally and spreads bilaterally and coexists with distal symmetric polyneuropathy and spontaneous muscle fasciculation. It can be provoked by percussion.

The condition is now recognized as secondary to a variety of causes that are unrelated to diabetes but that have a greater incidence in patients with diabetes than in the general population. This includes patients with chronic inflammatory demyelinating polyneuropathy (CIDP), monoclonal gammopathy, circulating GM1 antibodies and antibodies to neuronal cells, and inflammatory vasculitis.[561,562] Proximal motor neuropathy was formerly thought to resolve spontaneously in 1.5 to 2 years. However, immune-mediated neuropathy can resolve within days on immunotherapy.

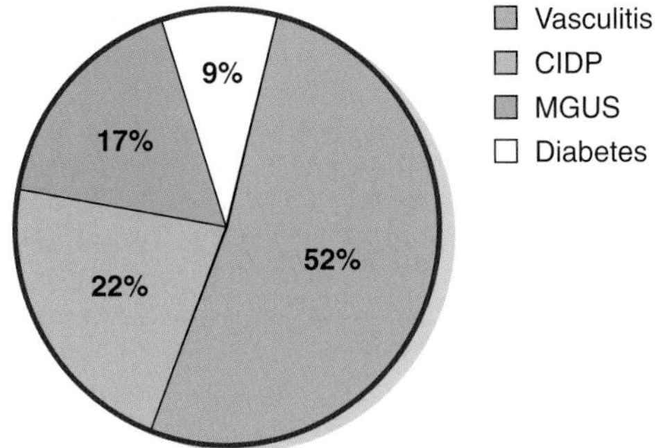

Figure 32–36 ▪ Obturator nerve biopsy. CIDP, chronic inflammatory demyelinating polyradiculoneuropathy; MGUS, monoclonal gammopathy of undetermined significance. (Adapted from Vinik A: Diagnosis and management of diabetic neuropathy. Clin Geriatr Med 1999;15: 293-319.)

The condition is readily recognizable clinically with prevailing weakness of the iliopsoas, obturator, and adductor muscles, together with relative preservation of function of the gluteus maximus and minimus and hamstrings.[563] Patients have great difficulty rising out of chairs unaided and often use their arms to assist themselves. Heel or toe standing is surprisingly good. In the classic form of diabetic amyotrophy, axonal loss is the predominant process, and the condition coexists with DSPN.[564] Electrophysiologic evaluation reveals lumbosacral plexopathy.[563]

If demyelination predominates and the motor deficit affects proximal and distal muscle groups, the diagnosis of CIDP, monoclonal gammopathy of unknown significance (MGUS), and vasculitis should be considered.[565,566] It seems probable that these conditions occur more commonly in people with diabetes.[567,568] Vinik and colleagues[525,569-571] have pointed out that almost half the patients with proximal neuropathies have a vasculitis and all but 9% have CIDP or MGUS or a ganglioside antibody syndrome.[572] Sharma examined more than 1000 patients with neurologic disorders and found that CIDP was 11 times more common among their diabetic than the nondiabetic population.[568]

Biopsy of the obturator nerve reveals demyelination, deposition of immunoglobulin, and inflammatory cell infiltrate of the vasa nervorum[573] (Fig. 32–36). Cerebrospinal fluid (CSF) protein content is high and there is an increase in the lymphocyte count. Treatment options include intravenous immunoglobulin for CIDP, plasma exchange for MGUS, steroids and azathioprine for vasculitis, and withdrawal from drugs or other agents that might have caused a vasculitis. It is important to divide proximal syndromes into these subcategories, because the CIDP variant responds dramatically to intervention,[565,574] whereas amyotrophy runs its own course over months to years. Until more evidence is available, they should be considered separate syndromes.

These conditions need to be distinguished from spinal stenosis syndromes (Fig. 32–37). In spinal stenosis there is encroachment on nerve roots as they emerge from the spinal cord, and osteophytes can cause compression. With aging there is hypertrophy of the ligamentum flavum and disk dehydration, and there might even be some form of arachnoiditis.

When the compression involves the vascular system, claudication typically occurs upon walking downhill, is relieved by bending forward, and originates at the watershed level between T12 and L1-2. Nerve root compression is more typical at L5-S1, and thus in difficult cases it may be necessary to obtain an MRI of the lumbosacral spine. Diagnosis is critical because therapy may be simple physical therapy or surgical decompression if symptoms are severe or there is motor paralysis.

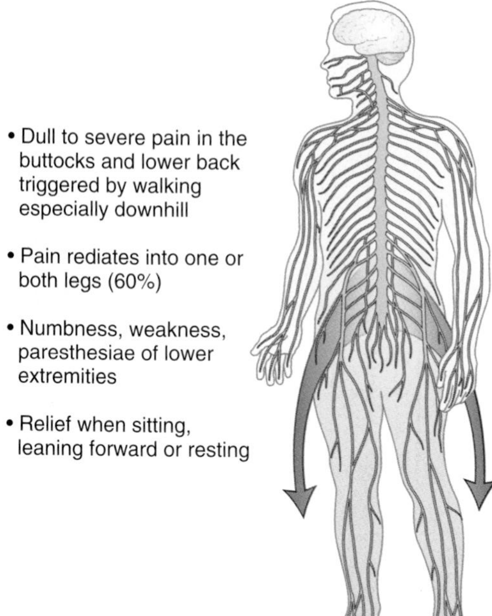

Spinal stenosis/claudication
• Dull to severe pain in the buttocks and lower back triggered by walking especially downhill
• Pain rediates into one or both legs (60%)
• Numbness, weakness, paresthesiae of lower extremities
• Relief when sitting, leaning forward or resting

Figure 32–37 ▪ Spinal stenosis syndromes.

Distal Symmetric Polyneuropathy

Distal symmetric polyneuropathy (DSPN) is the most common and widely recognized form of diabetic neuropathy. The onset is usually insidious but occasionally is acute, following stress or initiation of therapy for diabetes. DSPN may be either sensory or motor and can involve small fibers, large fibers, or both.[575] Figure 32–38 is a simplified version of the peripheral nervous system. Also shown in Figure 32–38 is the usual clinical presentation of the large and small fiber neuropathies.

Small nerve fiber dysfunction usually occurs early and often is present without objective signs or electrophysiologic evidence of nerve damage.[576] It is manifested early with symptoms of pain and hyperalgesia in the lower limbs, followed by a loss of thermal sensitivity and reduced light touch and pinprick sensation.[552]

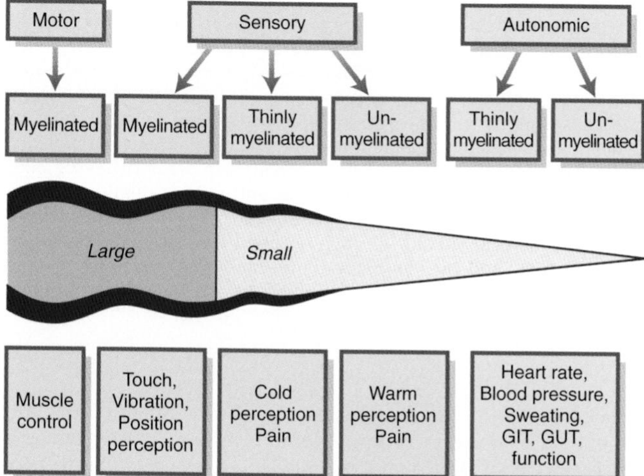

Figure 32–38 ▪ Simplified view of the peripheral nervous system. GIT, gastrointestinal tract; GUT, genitourinary tract. (Vinik A, Ullal J, Parson H, Casellini C. Diabetic neuropathies: clinical manifestations and current treatment options. Nat Clin Pract Endocrinol Metab 2006;2:269-281.)

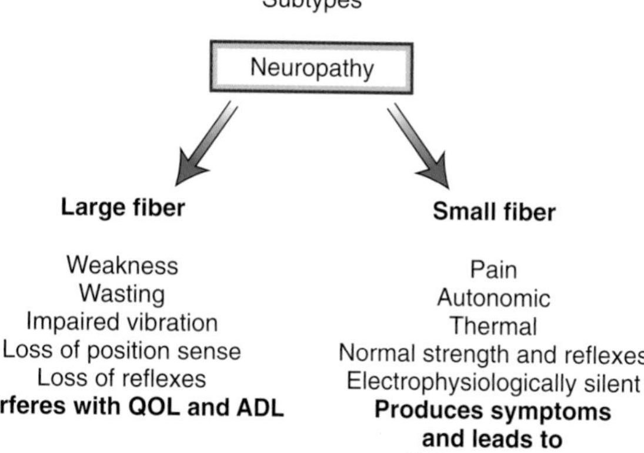

Figure 32–39 ▪ Differences in clinical presentations of large- and small-fiber neuropathies. ADL, activities of daily living; QOL, quality of life. (Adapted from Vinik AI, Mehrabyan A. Diabetic neuropathies. Med Clin North Am 2004;88:947-999.)

There is now evidence that DSPN may be accompanied by loss of cutaneous nerve fibers that stain positive for the neuronal antigen panaxonal marker protein gene product 9.5 (PGP 9.5)[577] (Fig. 32–39) and by impaired neurovascular blood flow.[578] The importance of the skin biopsy as a diagnostic tool for diabetic peripheral neuropathy is increasingly being recognized.[523,544,579,580] This technique quantitates small epidermal nerve fibers through antibody staining of PGP 9.5.[573,581,582] Though minimally invasive (3-mm–diameter punch biopsies), it enables a direct study of small fibers that cannot be evaluated by NCV studies (see Fig. 32–35).

Pain in Diabetic Neuropathies

Overall, approximately 10% of patients with diabetes experience persistent pain from neuropathy.[583] Pain syndromes that last less than 6 months to a year are classified as acute. These include the insulin neuritis syndrome, which occurs often at the beginning of therapy for diabetes and is self-limiting. Pain syndromes lasting longer than 6 months to a year are classified as chronic.[584] The pain may be ongoing, spontaneous, or hyperalgesic (increased response to a painful stimulus). It can be severe and sometimes intractable.

Management of painful diabetic neuropathy, as well as other pain syndromes, is changing as research elucidates underlying pathophysiologic mechanisms. The complexities of pain syndromes and advances in basic pain research have contributed to an evolving concept of pain and strategies for its management. Backonja defined neuropathic pain as "a group of disorders characterized by pain due to dysfunction or disease of the nervous system at a peripheral level, a central level, or both."[585]

Acute Painful Neuropathy

Some patients develop a predominantly *small-fiber neuropathy,* which is manifested by pain and paresthesias early in the course of diabetes (Fig. 32–40). It may be associated with the onset of insulin therapy and has been termed *insulin neuritis.*[586] By definition it has been there for less than 6 months.

Symptoms often are exacerbated at night and are manifested in the feet more than the hands. Spontaneous episodes of pain

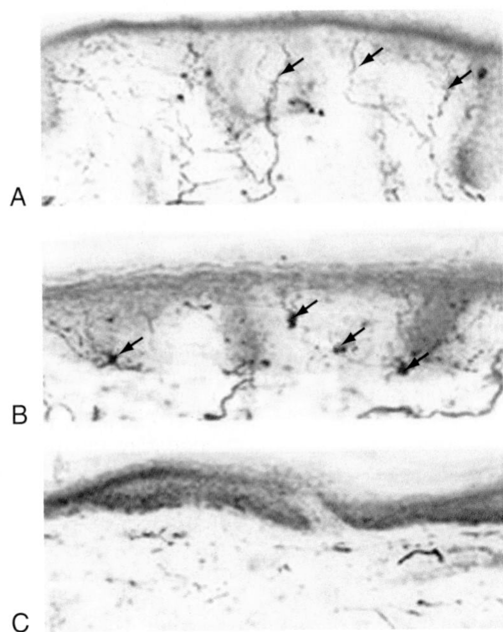

Figure 32–40 ▪ Loss of cutaneous nerve fibers that stain positive for the neuronal antigen protein gene product 9.5 in sensory neuropathy. **A,** Normal epidermal fibers in the back. **B,** Slightly reduced density and swelling in the proximal thigh. **C,** Complete clearance in calf. (From McArthur JC, Stocks EA, Hauer P. Epidermal nerve fiber density: normative reference range and diagnostic efficiency. Arch Neurol 1998;55: 1513-1520.)

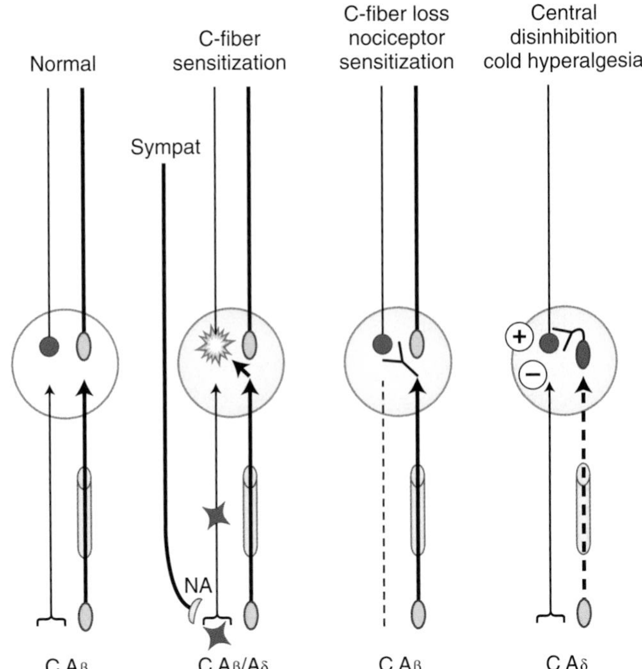

Figure 32–41 ▪ Schematic representation of the generation of pain. *Left panel,* Normal situation, no pain. Central terminals of unmyelinated primary C-afferents project into the dorsal horn and make contact with secondary pain-signaling neurons. Low-threshold mechanoreceptive primary Aβ-afferents project without synaptic transmission into the dorsal columns (not shown) and also contact secondary afferent dorsal horn neurons. *Left-center panel,* Peripheral sensitization and central sensitization processes in peripheral nociceptors (peripheral sensitization, star in the periphery) leading to spontaneous burning pain, static mechanical hyperalgesia, and heat hyperalgesia. This spontaneous activity in nociceptors induces secondary changes in the central sensory processing, leading to spinal cord hyperexcitability (central sensitization, star in spinal cord) that causes input from mechanoreceptive Aβ-fibers (light touching) and Aδ-fibers (punctuate stimuli) to be perceived as pain (dynamic and punctuate mechanical allodynia). Moreover, afferent terminals in the periphery or afferent somata in the dorsal root ganglion acquire sensitivity to norepinephrine (NE) by expressing A-receptors at their membrane. Activity in postganglionic sympathetic neurons is now capable of activating afferent neurons by the release of NA. *Center right panel,* Synaptic reorganization after C-nociceptor degeneration. Nociceptor function may be selectively impaired and the fibers degenerate after nerve lesion. Accordingly, the synaptic contacts between central nociceptor terminals and secondary nociceptive neurons are reduced. Central terminals from intact mechanoreceptive Aβ-fibers start to sprout to form novel synaptic contacts with the free central nociceptive neurons. This anatomic reorganization in the dorsal horn causes input from mechanoreceptive Aβ-fibers (light touching) to be perceived as pain (dynamic mechanical allodynia). In such patients, temperature sensation is profoundly impaired in areas of severe allodynia. *Right panel,* Central disinhibition and cold hyperalgesia. Normally, cold stimuli are conveyed by Aδ-fibers and cold pain by C-fibers. A selective damage of cold-sensitive Aδ-fibers leads to a loss of central inhibition mediated by interneurons (disinhibition), resulting in cold hyperalgesia. NA, noradrenaline (norepinephrine). (Adapted from Vinik A, Mehrabyan A. Diabetic neuropathies. Med Clin North Am 2004; 88(4):947-999.)

can be severely disabling. The pain varies in intensity and character. In some patients, the pain has been variably described as burning, lancinating, stabbing, or sharp. Paresthesias or episodes of distorted sensation, such as pins and needles, tingling, coldness, numbness, or burning often accompany the pain.[575] The lower legs may be exquisitely tender to touch, with any disturbance of the hair follicles resulting in excruciating pain. Because pain can be aggravated by repeated contact of the lower limbs with foreign objects, even basic daily activities such as sitting at a desk may be disrupted. Pain often occurs at the onset of the disease and is often worsened by initiation of therapy with insulin or sulfonylureas.[586]

Neuropathy may be associated with profound weight loss and severe depression that has been termed *diabetic neuropathic cachexia.*[587] This syndrome occurs predominantly in male patients and can occur at any time in the course of T1DM or T2DM. It is self-limiting and invariably responds to simple symptomatic treatment. Conditions such as Fabry's disease, amyloid, HIV infection, heavy metal poisoning (such as arsenic), and excess alcohol consumption should be excluded. Acute painful neuropathy does overlap with the idiopathic variety of acute painful small fiber neuropathy that is also a diagnosis by exclusion.[588]

Chronic Painful Neuropathy

Chronic painful neuropathy is another variety of painful polyneuropathy. Onset is later, often years into the course of the diabetes, and which the pain persists for longer than 6 months and becomes debilitating (see Fig. 32–38). This condition can result in tolerance to narcotics and analgesics, finally resulting in addiction. It is extremely resistant to all forms of intervention and is most frustrating to both patient and physician.

Pathophysiologic changes in the nervous system can produce symptoms defined as either negative, such as loss of sensory quality, or positive, such as spontaneous pain. Patients with neuropathic pain usually present with both. Absence of pain sometimes is not due to improvement in neuropathy but is a consequence of neuronal loss. Physicians must exclude progression of neuropathy when patients report loss of pain. Neuropathic pain can manifest as stimulus-independent pain or as stimulus-evoked or stimulus-dependent pain, whose underlying mechanisms are likely to differ. A simplified scheme of pain generation is shown in Figure 32–41.

Similarly, the mechanisms responsible for hyperalgesia and allodynia differ. Hyperalgesia is defined as increased pain response to a normally painful stimulus. Allodynia occurs when pain is provoked by a stimulus not normally painful. This is related to the different nerve pathways implicated in these various categories. For example, aberrations of the C and Aδ fibers can result in the burning and prickling sensations of stimulus-independent pain or of hyperalgesia. Under pathologic conditions, touch-sensitive Aβ fibers can cause stimulus-independent dysesthesias or paresthesias or stimulus-evoked allodynia.

Small-Fiber Neuropathies

Symptoms are prominent in small-fiber neuropathies. Pain is of the C-fiber type. It is burning and superficial and is associated with allodynia (interpretation of all stimuli as painful). Patients have defective autonomic function with decreased sweating, dry skin, impaired vasomotion and blood flow, and cold feet. There are abnormalities in thresholds for warm thermal perception, neurovascular function, pain, quantitative sudorimetry, and quantitative autonomic function tests. Late in the condition there is hypoalgesia. However, there is remarkable intactness of reflexes and motor strength.

Clinical diagnosis is by reduced sensitivity to 1.0-g Semmes-Weinstein monofilament and pricking sensation using the Waardenberg wheel or similar instrument. These neuropathies are electrophysiologically silent, but there is loss of cutaneous nerve fibers that stain for PGP 9.5.

The prominent risk is foot ulceration and subsequent gangrene. There are 86,000 foot amputations in diabetic patients in the United States each year, one every 10 minutes. Half of these are preventable.

Large-Fiber Neuropathies

Large fiber neuropathies can involve sensory or motor nerves, or both. These tend to be the neuropathies of signs rather than symptoms. Large fibers subserve motor function, vibration perception, position sense, and cold thermal perception. Unlike the small nerve fibers, these are the myelinated, rapidly conducting fibers that begin in the toes and have their first synapse in the medulla oblongata. They tend to be affected first because of their length and the tendency in diabetes for nerves to die back. Because they are myelinated, they are the fibers represented in the EMG, and subclinical abnormalities in nerve function are readily detected. The symptoms may be minimal and include a sensation of walking on cotton, floors feeling strange, inability to turn the pages of a book, or inability to discriminate among coins.

Clinical Presentation

Signs and symptoms of larg-fiber neuropathy include impaired vibration perception (often the first objective evidence) and position sense, depressed tendon reflexes, and sensory ataxia (waddling like a duck). Aδ-fiber pain is deep-seated gnawing, dull, like a toothache in the bones of the feet, or even crushing or cramp-like pain. Signs in the distal lower extremities include wasting of the small muscles of the feet, with hammertoes (intrinsic minus feet and hands) and weakness of the feet; shortening of the Achilles tendon with pes equinus, and increased blood flow (hot foot). Patients also have weakness in the hands.

Most patients with DSPN, however, have a mixed variety of neuropathy, with both large and small nerve fiber damage. In the case of DSPN, a glove-and-stocking distribution of sensory loss is almost universal.[552] Early in the course of the neuropathic process, multifocal sensory loss also might be found. In some patients, severe distal muscle weakness can accompany the sensory loss, resulting in an inability to stand on the toes or heels. Some grading systems use this as a definition of severity.

Diagnosis and Differential Diagnosis of Peripheral Neuropathy

The diagnosis of diabetic neuropathy rests heavily on a careful history, for which a number of questionnaires have been developed by Young and colleagues,[516] Dyck,[589] Vinik,[590] and others.[591,592] The initial neurologic evaluation should be directed toward detecting the specific part of the nervous system affected by diabetes (Fig. 32–42). Bedside neurologic examination is quick and easy but provides nominal or ordinal measures and contains substantial inter-and intraindividual variation. For example, it is useless to measure vibration perception with a tuning fork other than one that has a frequency of 128 Hz. Similarly, using a 10-g monofilament is good for predicting foot ulceration, as is the Achilles reflex, but both are insensitive to the early detection of neuropathy, and a 1.0-g monofilament increases the sensitivity from 60% to 90%.[593]

Sensory function must be evaluated on both sides of the feet and hands if one wants to be sure not to miss entrapment syndromes.[594] Tinel's sign is not only useful for carpal tunnel problems but can also be applied to the ulnar notch, the head of the fibula, and below the medial tibial epicondyle for ulnar, peroneal, and medial plantar entrapments, respectively.

The 1988 San Antonio conference on diabetic neuropathy and the 1992 conference of the American Academy of Neurology[534] recommended that at least one parameter from each of the following five categories are measured to classify diabetic neuropathy: symptom profiles, neurologic examination, QST, nerve conduction study, and autonomic function testing. A number of simple symptom screening questionnaires are available to record symptom quality and severity. A simplified neuropathy symptom score that was used in the European prevalence studies could also be useful in clinical practice.[516,595] The Michigan Neuropathy Screening Instrument (MNSI) is a 15-item questionnaire that can be administered to patients as a screening tool for neuropathy.[592] Other similar symptom-scoring systems have also been described, such as the nerve impairment score of the lower limbs (NIS-LL).[596]

Simple visual analogue or verbal descriptive scales may be used to follow patients' responses to treatment of their neuropathic symptoms.[195,597,598] However, it must always be remembered that identification of neuropathic symptoms is not useful as a diagnostic or screening tool in assessing diabetic neuropathy, as shown by Franse and colleagues.[599] The QST and QAFT are objective indices of neurologic functional status. Combined, these tests cover vibratory, proprioceptive, tactile, pain, thermal, and autonomic function.

An international group of experts in diabetic neuropathy held a consensus meeting to develop guidelines for managing diabetic peripheral neuropathy by the practicing clinician.[534] This clinical staging is in general agreement with that proposed by Dyck[551] for use in both clinical practice and epidemiologic studies or controlled clinical trials. The clinical *no neuropathy* is equivalent to Dyck's N0 (no objective evidence of diabetic neuropathy) or N1a (no symptoms or signs but neuropathic test abnormalities). *Clinical neuropathy* is equivalent to N1b (test abnormalities plus neuropathic impairment on neurologic exam), N2a (symptoms, signs, and test abnormalities), and N2b (N2a plus significant ankle dorsiflexor weakness). *Late complications* is equivalent to Dyck N3 (disabling polyneuropathy).

There have been a number of other relevant reports, including two on measures for use in clinical trials to assess symptoms[600] and QST.[601] The strengths of QST are well documented,[601]

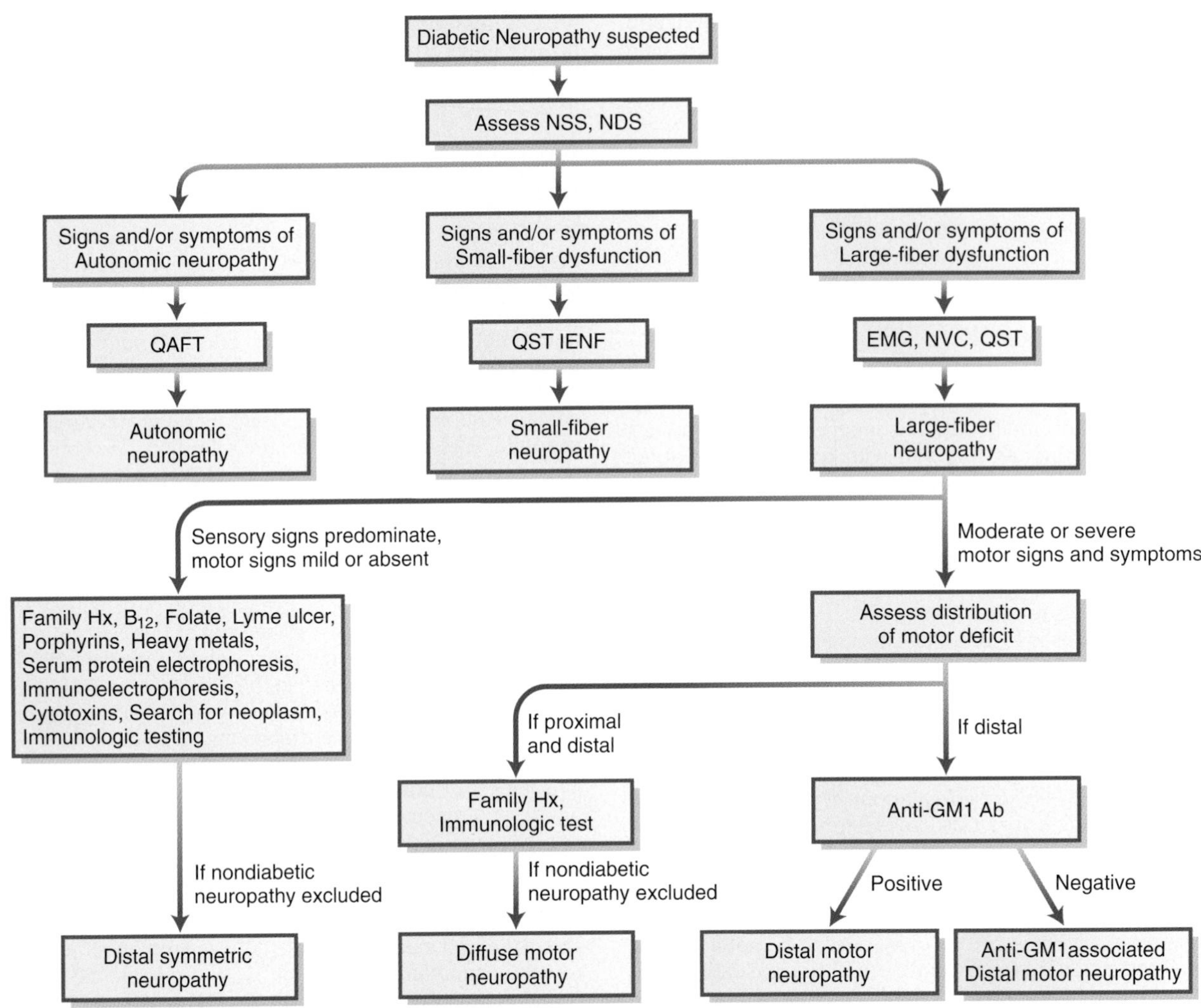

Figure 32–42 ▪ A diagnostic algorithm for assessing neurologic deficit and classification of neuropathic syndrome. EMG, electromyogram; GM1, monosialoganglioside; Hx, history; IENF, MGUS, monoclonal gammopathy of unknown significance; NCV, nerve conduction velocity; NDS, nerve disability (sensory and motor evaluation); NSS, neurologic symptom score; QAFT, quantitative autonomic function tests; QST, quantitative sensory tests. (Adapted with permission from Vinik A, Mehrabyan A. Diabetic neuropathies. Med Clin North Am 2004;88(4):947-999.).

but the limitations of QST are also clear. No matter what the instrument or procedure used, QST is only a semiobjective measure, because it is affected by the subject's attention, motivation, and cooperation, as well as by anthropometric variables such as age, gender, body mass, and history of smoking and alcohol consumption.[602,603] Expectancy and subject bias are additional factors that can exert a powerful influence on QST findings.[604] Further, QST is sensitive to changes in structure or function along the entire neuroaxis from nerve to cortex; it is not a specific measure of peripheral nerve function.[605] The American Academy of Neurology reported on the use of QST for clinical and research purposes,[601] suggesting that it could be used as an ancillary test but was not sufficiently robust for routine clinical use.

A number of simple symptom screening questionnaires are available to record symptom quality and severity. A simplified neuropathy symptom score that was used in the European prevalence studies could also be useful in clinical practice.[516] The Michigan Neuropathy Screening Instrument (MNSI) is a brief 15-item questionnaire that can be administered to patients as a screening tool for neuropathy.[606] Other similar symptom scoring systems have also been described.[607] Simple visual analogue or verbal descriptive scales may be used to follow patients' responses to treatment of their neuropathic symptoms[607,608]; however, it must always be remembered that identification of neuropathic symptoms is not useful as a diagnostic or screening tool in the assessment of diabetic neuropathy, as shown by Franse and Coworkers.[599]

Peripheral Testing Devices

A number of relatively inexpensive devices allow suitable assessment of somatosensory function, including vibration, thermal, light touch, and pain perception.[609] These types of instruments allow cutaneous sensory functions to be assessed noninvasively, and their measurements are correlated with specific neural fiber function.

The most widely used device in clinical practice is the Semmes-Weinstein monofilament.[610-612] The filament assesses pressure perception when gentle pressure is applied to the handle sufficient to buckle the nylon filament. Although filaments of many different sizes are available, the one that exerts 10 g of pressure is most commonly used to assess pressure sensation in the diabetic foot. It is also referred to as the 5.07 monofilament because, during calibration, the filaments are calibrated to exert a force measured in grams that is 10 times the log of the force exerted at the tip: hence 5.07 exerts 10 g force.

A number of cross-sectional studies have assessed the sensitivity of the 10-g monofilament to identify feet at risk for ulceration. Sensitivities vary from 86% to 100%,[613,614] although there is no consensus as to how many sites should be tested. The commonest algorithm recommends four sites per foot, generally the hallux and the first, third, and fifth metatarsal heads.[611] However, there is little advantage to multiple site assessments.[609] There is also no universal agreement about what constitutes an abnormal result (one, two, three, or four abnormal results from the sites tested). Despite these problems, the 10-g monofilament is widely used to clinically asses risk of foot ulceration, but as we pointed out, one needs to use a 1-g or less monofilament to detect neuropathy with a high sensitivity.[609] A final caution on the use of the filaments[615]: Filaments manufactured by certain companies do not actually buckle at 10 g of force. Indeed, several tested filaments buckled at less than 8 g. In our practice we use 25-lb strain fishing line and cut it into 1000 pieces at a total cost of $5. We provide patients with these to test themselves at home, thus using them to assist in behavior modification. This has reduced the incidence of foot ulcers in our practice by more than 50%.[612]

The graduated Rydel-Seifer tuning fork is used in some centers to assess neuropathy.[616,617] This fork uses a visual optical illusion to allow the assessor to determine the intensity of residual vibration on a 0 to 8 scale at the point of threshold (disappearance of sensation). Liniger and colleagues reported that results with this instrument correlated well with other QST measures.[616] The tactile circumferential discriminator assesses the perception of calibrated change in the circumference of a probe (a variation of two-point discrimination).[618] Vileikyte and coworkers[619] reported a 100% sensitivity in identifying patients at risk for foot ulceration.[619] Similarly, this device also demonstrated good agreement with other measures of QST. Neuropen is a clinical device that assesses pain using a pin (Neurotip) at one end of the pen and a 10-g monofilament at the other end. This was shown to be a sensitive device for assessing nerve function when compared to the simplified neuropathy disability score.[620]

Cardiovascular Testing Devices

QAFT consists of a series of simple noninvasive tests for detecting cardiovascular autonomic neuropathy.[576,621] These tests are based on detection of heart rate and BP response to a series of maneuvers. Specific tests are used in evaluating disordered regulation of gastrointestinal, genitourinary, and sudomotor function and peripheral skin blood flow induced by autonomic diabetic neuropathy.[593]

Biopsy

Biopsy of nerve tissue may be helpful for excluding other causes of neuropathy and in determining predominant pathologic changes in patients with complex clinical findings as a means of dictating choice of treatment.[564,622] Skin biopsy has some clinical advantages in diagnosing small-fiber neuropathies by quantification of PGP9.5 when all other measures are negative.[544,623]

Differential Diagnosis

Diabetes as the cause of neuropathy is diagnosed by excluding various other causes of neuropathy.[552,624] Patients presenting with painful feet might have impaired glucose tolerance[625,626] or the metabolic syndrome.[627] Quantitation of intraepidermal nerve fiber density has also been used to demonstrate the ability to induce nerve regeneration and correlates with indices of neuropathy relevant to function of small unmyelinated C fibers.[628] More recently, confocal corneal microscopy has been used in assessing peripheral neuropathy. This is a completely noninvasive technique that offers the future potential of assessing nerve structure in vivo without the need for biopsy.[629]

Nerve Conduction Studies

Whole nerve electrophysiologic procedures (e.g., NCV, F-waves, sensory amplitudes, motor amplitudes) have emerged as important methods of tracing the onset and progression of peripheral neuropathy.[630] An appropriate battery of electrophysiologic tests supports the measurement of the speed of sensory and motor conduction, the amplitude of the propagating neural signal, the density and synchrony of muscle fibers activated by maximal nerve stimulation, and the integrity of neuromuscular transmission (see references 657, 658). These are objective, parametric, noninvasive and highly reliable measures. However, standard procedures, such as maximal NCV, reflect only a limited aspect of neural activity, and then only in a small subset of large-diameter and heavily myelinated axons. Even in large-diameter fibers, NCV is insensitive to many pathologic changes known to be associated with peripheral neuropathy.

However, a key role for electrophysiologic assessment is to rule out other causes of neuropathy or to identify neuropathies superimposed on peripheral neuropathy. Unilateral conditions, such as entrapments, are far more common in the patients with diabetes.[555] The principal factors that influence the speed of NCV are the integrity and degree of myelination of the largest diameter fibers, the mean cross-sectional diameter of the responding axons, the representative internodal distance in the segment under study, and the microenvironment at the nodes, including the distribution of ion channels.[631] Thus, demyelinating conditions affect conduction velocities whereas diabetes primarily reduces amplitudes. Therefore, the finding of a profound reduction in conduction velocity strongly supports the occurrence in a diabetic patient of an alternative condition. Indeed, the odds of occurrence of chronic inflammatory demyelinating polyradiculoneuropathy) were 11 times higher among diabetic than nondiabetic patients.[632] NCV is only gradually diminished by peripheral neuropathy, with estimates of a loss of approximately 0.5 m/sec per year.[630]

In a 10-year natural history study of 133 patients with newly diagnosed T2DM, NCV deteriorated in all six nerve segments evaluated, but the largest deficit was 3.9 m/sec for the sural nerve (48.3 m/sec slowed to 44.4 m/sec); peroneal motor NCV was decreased by 3.0 m/sec over the same period.[539] A similar slow rate of decline was demonstrated in the DCCT. A simple rule is that a decrease in HB A_{1c} of one percentage point improves conduction velocity about 1.3 m/sec.[633] There is, however, a strong correlation ($r = 0.74$; $P < 0.001$) between myelinated fiber density and whole nerve sural amplitude.[634]

Management

Once neuropathy is diagnosed, therapy can then be instituted with the goal of both ameliorating symptoms and preventing the progression of neuropathy. Successful management of these syndromes must be geared to individual pathogenic processes (Fig. 32–43).

Control of Hyperglycemia

Retrospective and prospective studies have suggested a relationship between hyperglycemia and the development and severity of diabetic neuropathy. Pirart[520] followed 4400 diabetic patients over 25 years and showed an increase in prevalence of clinically detectable diabetic neuropathy from 12% of patients at the time of diagnosis of diabetes to almost 50% after 25 years. The highest prevalence occurred in the people with poorest diabetes control.

The DCCT Research Group[536] reported significant effects of intensive insulin therapy on prevention of neuropathy. The prevalence rates for clinical or electrophysiologic evidence of neuropathy were reduced by 50% in those treated by intensive insulin therapy during 5 years. At that stage of the study, only

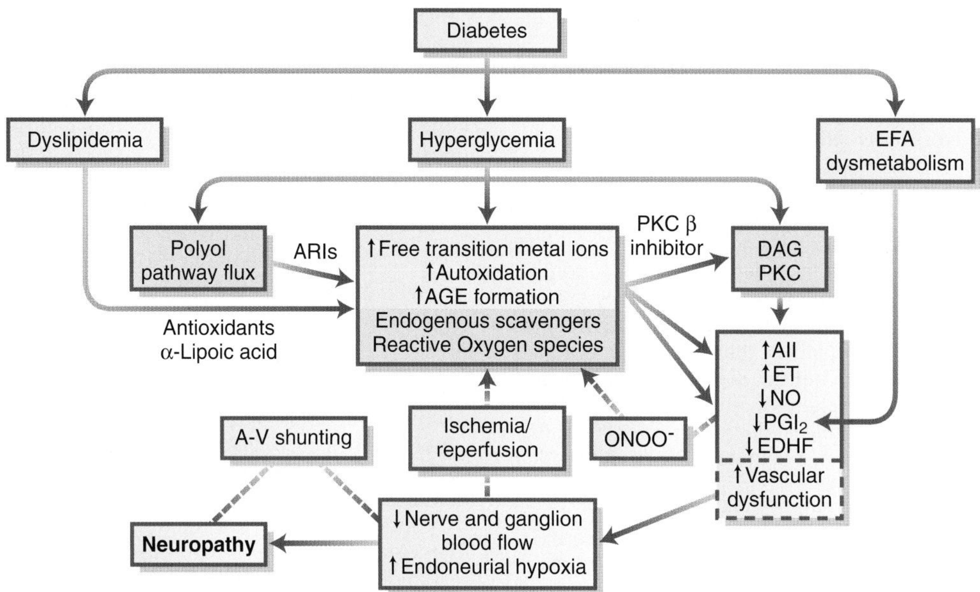

Figure 32–43 ▪ Management aimed at pathogenic mechanisms. AII, angiotensin II; A-V, arteriovenous; EDHF, endothelium-derived hyperpolarizing factor; EFA, essential fatty acid; ET, endothelin; NO, nitric oxide; PGI_2, prostaglandin I_2. (Adapted from Vinik A, Mehrabyan A. Diabetic neuropathies. Med Clin North Am 2004;88(4):947-999.)

3% of the patients in the primary prevention cohort treated by intensive insulin therapy showed minimal signs of diabetic neuropathy, compared to 10% of those treated by the conventional regimen. In the secondary prevention cohort, intensive insulin therapy significantly reduced the prevalence of clinical neuropathy by 56% (7% in intensive insulin therapy group vs. 16% in conventional therapy group). The results of the DCCT study support the necessity for strict glycemic control, but the effect of insulin as a growth factor and immunomodulator, aside from its metabolic effects, must also be investigated.

In the UKPDS, control of blood glucose was associated with improvement in vibration perception.[3,478,635] In the Steno trial,[636] a reduction of the odds ratio for the development of autonomic neuropathy to 0.32 was reported. This was a stepwise, progressive study that involved treating T2DM patients with hypotensive drugs, including ACE inhibitors, calcium-channel antagonists, hypoglycemic agents, aspirin, hypolipidemic agents, and antioxidants. These findings argue strongly for the multifactorial nature of neuropathy and for the need to address the multiple metabolic abnormalities.

Pharmacologic Therapy

Aldose Reductase Inhibitors

Aldose reductase inhibitors (ARIs) reduce the flux of glucose through the polyol pathway, inhibiting tissue accumulation of sorbitol and fructose and preventing reduction of redox potentials.

In a placebo-controlled, double-blind study of tolrestat, 219 diabetic patients with symmetrical polyneuropathy, as defined by at least one pathologic cardiovascular reflex, were treated for 1 year.[636] Patients who received tolrestat showed significant improvement in autonomic function tests and in vibration perception, whereas placebo-treated patients showed deterioration in most of the parameters measured.[638]

There is a dose-dependent improvement in nerve fiber density, particularly small unmyelinated nerve fibers, in a 12 month study of zenarestat.[102] This was accompanied by an increase in NCV, although the changes in NCV occurred at a dose of the drug that did not change the nerve fiber density.[102] Impaired cardiac ejection fractions can be improved with zopolrestat.[639] Clinical improvement has been reported for fidarestat and epalrestat in Japan.[640,641]

The promise shown with the newer ARIs is being exploited by other companies, and promising results have now been reported in a phase II study in the United States.[642] It is also becoming clear that aldose reductase inhibition may be insufficient in its own right to achieve the desirable degree of metabolic enhancement in patients with a multitude of biochemical abnormalities. Combinations of therapy with ARIs and antioxidants may become critical if we are to curb the relentless progress of diabetic neuropathy.

α-Lipoic Acid

Lipoic acid (1,2-dithiolane-3-pentanoic acid), a derivative of octanoic acid, is present in food and is also synthesized by the liver. It is a natural cofactor in the pyruvate dehydrogenase complex, where it binds acyl groups and transfers them from one part of the complex to another. α-Lipoic acid, which also known as thioctic acid, has generated considerable interest as a thiol-replenishing and redox-modulating agent. It has been shown to be effective in ameliorating the somatic and autonomic neuropathies in diabetes.[643-645] It is undergoing extensive trials in the United States for treating diabetes and diabetic neuropathy.

γ-Linolenic Acid

Linoleic acid, an essential fatty acid, is metabolized to dihomo-γ-linolenic acid, which serves as an important constituent of neuronal membrane phospholipids and as a substrate for prostaglandin E formation, which appears to be important for preserving nerve blood flow. In diabetes, conversion of linoleic acid to γγlinolenic acid and subsequent metabolites is impaired, possibly contributing to the pathogenesis of diabetic neuropathy.[646] A recent multicenter double-blind, placebo-controlled trial, patients using GLA for 1 year showed significant improvements in clinical measures and in electrophysiologic testing.[647]

Protein Kinase C-β Inhibition

Neural vascular insufficiency has been proposed as a contributing factor to development of diabetic neuropathy.[648] PKC activation is a critical step in the pathway to diabetic microvascular complications[649] It is hyperactivated by hyperglycemia and disordered fatty acid metabolism, resulting in increased production of vasoconstrictive, angiogenic, and chemotactic cytokines including TGF-β, VEGF, endothelin, and ICAMs. Nonselective PKC inhibitors normalize hyperglycemia-induced decreases in endoneurial blood flow and abrogate the neuronal abnormalities seen in diabetic rodents.[62,597,650] Preclinical studies in animal diabetes models using ruboxistaurin mesylate (LY333531), a PKC-β inhibitor, have shown improvement in many diabetes-related changes in vascular function such as retinal blood flow,[195] endoneurial blood flow, and NCV.[651,652]

Preliminary results of a multinational randomized, double-blind, placebo-controlled phase II trial showed a statistically significant improvement in symptoms, measured by the Neuropathy Total Symptom Score 6 (NTSS-6), in ruboxistaurin-treated neuropathy groups as compared with placebo.[653] In patients with symptomatic neuropathy (NTSS-6 >6) and a sural nerve action potential (SNAP) greater than 0 μV at baseline, a measure that has been show to define a responsive subpopulation of peripheral neuropathy,[550] the frequency and intensity of symptoms and the change from baseline for vibratory detection threshold were statistically significantly improved in the treated groups. Vibratory detection threshold changes correlated well with the improvement in symptoms; the drug was well tolerated and there were few adverse events.

Aminoguanidine

Animal studies using aminoguanidine, an inhibitor of the formation of AGEs, show improvement in nerve conduction velocity in streptozotocin-induced diabetic neuropathy in rats. Controlled clinical trials to determine its efficacy in humans[654,655] have been discontinued because of toxicity. There are, however, successors to aminoguanidine that hold promise for this approach.[656]

Human Intravenous Immunoglobulin

Immune intervention with IVIG has become appropriate in some patients with forms of peripheral diabetic neuropathy that are associated with signs of antineuronal autoimmunity.[565,574] Treatment with immunoglobulin is well tolerated and is considered safe, especially with respect to viral transmission.[657] The major toxicity of IVIG has been an anaphylactic reaction, but the frequency of these reactions is now low and confined mainly to patients with immunoglobulin (usually IgA) deficiency. Patients might experience severe headache due to aseptic meningitis, which resolves spontaneously. In some instances, it may be necessary to combine treatment with prednisone or azathioprine. Relapses can occur, requiring repeated courses of therapy. However, new data support a predictive role of the presence of antineuronal antibodies on the later development of neuropathy,[658] which might not be innocent bystanders but neurotoxins.[659] Some patients, particularly those with autonomic neuropathy and antineuronal autoimmunity, and CIDP, might benefit from IVIG.[563,574]

Neurotrophic Therapy

There is now considerable evidence in animal models of diabetes that decreased expression of NGF and its receptors, TrkA and p75, reduces retrograde axonal transport of NGF and diminishes support of small unmyelinated neurons and their neuropeptides, such as substance P and calcitonin gene–related peptide (CGRP)—both potent vasodilators.[521,659-661] Furthermore, administration of recombinant human NGF (rhNGF) restores these neuropeptide levels toward normal and prevents the manifestations of sensory neuropathy in animals.[662]

In a 15-center double-blind, placebo-controlled study of the safety and efficacy of rhNGF in 250 subjects with symptomatic small-fiber neuropathy,[540] rhNGF improved the neurologic impairment score of the lower limbs and improved small nerve fiber function cooling threshold (Aδ-fibers) and the ability to perceive heat pain (C-fiber) compared with placebo. These results were consistent with the postulated actions of NGF on TrkA receptors present on small-fiber neurons. This led to two large multicenter studies conducted in the United States and the rest of the world. Subsequently, a phase III trial in 1019 diabetic patients with sensory polyneuropathy failed to demonstrate a significant benefit.[663]

Results of these NGF studies were presented at the ADA meetings in June 1999.[541] Regrettably, rhNGF was not found to have beneficial effects over placebo. The reason for this dichotomy has not been resolved, but this has somewhat dampened the enthusiasm for growth factor therapy of diabetic neuropathy.

More recently, a randomized, double blind, placebo-controlled study of brain-derived neurotrophic factor (rhBDNF) in 30 diabetic patients demonstrated no significant improvement in nerve conduction and quantitative sensory and autonomic function tests, including the cutaneous axon reflex.[664] A small trial of neurotrophin 3 (NT3) for safety was interpreted as negative for efficacy, and IGF1 and IGF11 have not been considered to be safe for administration to humans. Possible a more promising therapy is to be found with the proinsulin C-peptide.[665]

Pain Control

Control of pain constitutes one of the most difficult management issues in diabetic neuropathy. In essence, simple measures are tried first. If no distinction is made for pain syndromes, then the number needed to treat (NNT) to reduce pain by 50% is 1.4 for optimal-dose tricyclic antidepressants, 1.9 for dextromethorphan, 3.3 for carbamazepine, 3.4 for tramadol, 3.7 for gabapentin, 5.9 for capsaicin, 6.7 for selective serotonin reuptake inhibitors, and 10.0 for mexiletine.[666] If, however, pain is divided according to its derivation from different nerve fiber type (Aδ vs C-fiber), spinal cord, or cortical, then different types of pain respond to different therapies (Fig. 32–44).

C-Fiber Pain

Initially, when there is ongoing damage to the nerves, the patient experiences pain of the burning, lancinating, dysesthetic type often accompanied by hyperalgesia and allodynia. Because the peripheral sympathetic nerve fibers are also small unmyelinated C-fibers, sympathetic blocking agents (clonidine) can improve the pain. Loss of sympathetic regulation of sweat glands and arteriovenous shunt vessels in the foot creates a favorable environment for bacteria to penetrate, multiply, and wreak havoc with the foot. These fibers use the neuropeptide substance P as their neurotransmitter, and depletion of axonal substance P (capsaicin) often leads to amelioration of the pain. However, when the destructive forces persist, the patient becomes pain free and develops impaired warm temperature and pain thresholds. Disappearance of pain in these circumstances should be hailed as a warning that the neuropathy is progressing. Targeting higher levels of pain transmission also helps with C-fiber pain..[667,668]

Capsaicin

Capsaicin is extracted from chili peppers, and a simple, cheap mixture is to add one to three teaspoons 15-45 mL) of cayenne pepper to a jar of cold cream and apply to the area of pain. It has high selectivity for a subset of sensory neurons, which have

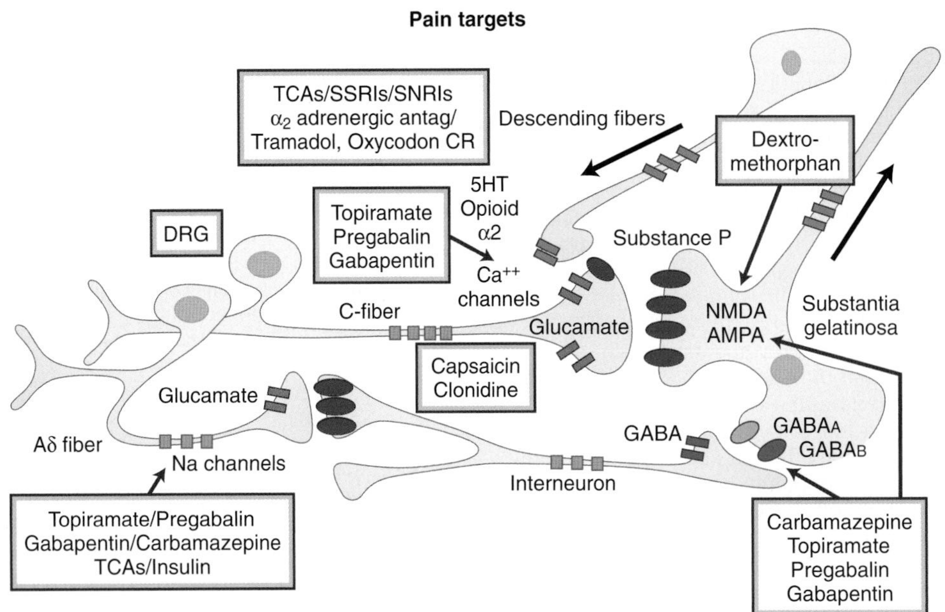

Figure 32–44 ▪ Pain response to various therapies. C fibers are modulated by sympathetic input with spontaneous firing of different neurotransmitters to the dorsal root ganglia, spinal cord, and cerebral cortex. Sympathetic blockers (e.g., clonidine) and depletion of axonal substance P used by C fibers as their neurotransmitter (e.g., by capsaicin) can relieve pain. In contrast, Aδ fibers use Na^+ channels for their conduction. Agents that inhibit Na^+ exchange, such as antiepileptic drugs, tricyclic antidepressants, and insulin, can ameliorate this form of pain. Anticonvulsants (carbamazepine, gabapentin, pregabalin, topiramate) potentiate activity of γ-aminobutyric acid, inhibit Na^+ and Ca^{2+} channels, and inhibit *N*-methyl-D-aspartate receptors and α-amino-3-hydroxy-5-methyl-4-isoxazole propionic acid receptors Dextromethorphan blocks *N*-methyl-D-aspartate receptors in the spinal cord. Tricyclic antidepressants, selective serotonin reuptake inhibitors (e.g., fluoxetine), and serotonin and norepinephrine reuptake inhibitors inhibit serotonin and norepinephrine reuptake, enhancing their effect in endogenous pain-inhibitory systems in the brain. Tramadol is a central opioid analgesic. α_2 antag, α_2 antagonists; 5HT, 5-hydroxytryptamine; AMPA, α-amino-3-hydroxy-5-methyl-4-isoxazole propionic acid; DRG, dorsal root ganglia; GABA, γ-aminobutyric acid; NMDA, *N*-methyl-D-aspartate; SNRIs, serotonin and norepinephrine reuptake inhibitors; SP, substance P; SSRIs, selective serotonin reuptake inhibitors; TCA, tricyclic antidepressants. (Adapted from Vinik AI, Ullal J, Parson H, Cassellini C. Diabetic neuropathies: clinical manifestations and current treatment options. Nature Clin Pract Endocrinol Metab 2006;2:269-281.)

been identified as unmyelinated C-fiber afferent or thin-myelinated (Aδ) fibers. Prolonged application of capsaicin depletes stores of substance P, and possibly other neurotransmitters, from sensory nerve endings. This reduces or abolishes the transmission of painful stimuli from the peripheral nerve fibers to the higher centers.[669] Care must be taken to avoid eyes and genitals, and gloves must be worn. Because of capsaicin's volatility, it is safer to cover affected areas with plastic wrap. There is initial exacerbation of symptoms followed by relief in 2 to 3 weeks.

Clonidine

There is an element of sympathetic-mediated C-fiber type pain that can be overcome with clonidine (α_2-adrenergic agonist) or phentolamine. Clonidine can be applied topically,[670] but the dose titration may be more difficult. If clonidine fails, the local anesthetic agent mexiletine warrants a trial. Unresponsive patients are treated as outlined in Figure 32–45.

Aδ fiber pain

Aδ fiber pain is a more deep-seated, dull, and gnawing ache that often does not respond to the previously described measures. A number of different agents have been used for the pain associated with these fibers with varying success.

Insulin

Continuous intravenous insulin infusion without resort to blood glucose lowering may be useful in these patients. A response with reduction of pain usually occurs within 48 hours,[671] and the insulin infusion can be discontinued. If this measure fails several medications are available that might abolish the pain.

Nerve Blocking

Lidocaine given by slow infusion has been shown to provide relief of intractable pain for 3 to 21 days. This form of therapy may be of most use in self-limited forms of neuropathy. If successful, therapy can be continued with oral mexiletine. These compounds target the pain caused by hyperexcitability of superficial free nerve endings.[672]

Tramadol and Dextromethorphan

There are two possible targeted therapies. Tramadol is a centrally acting weak opioid analgesic for use in treating moderate to severe pain. Tramadol was shown to be better than placebo in a randomized, controlled trial[673] of only 6 weeks' duration, but a subsequent follow-up study suggested that symptomatic relief could be maintained for at least 6 months.[674] Side effects are, however, relatively common and are similar to those of other opioid-like drugs.

Another spinal cord target for pain relief is the excitatory glutaminergic *N*-methyl-D-aspartate (NMDA) receptor. Blockade of NMDA receptors is believed to be one mechanism by which dextromethorphan exerts analgesic efficacy.[675] An accomplished pharmacist can procure a sugar-free solution of dextromethorphan.

Antidepressants

Antidepressants inhibit reuptake of norepinephrine or serotonin, or both. Their use is limited by anticholinergic effects, orthostatic hypotension, and sexual side effects. Clinical trials

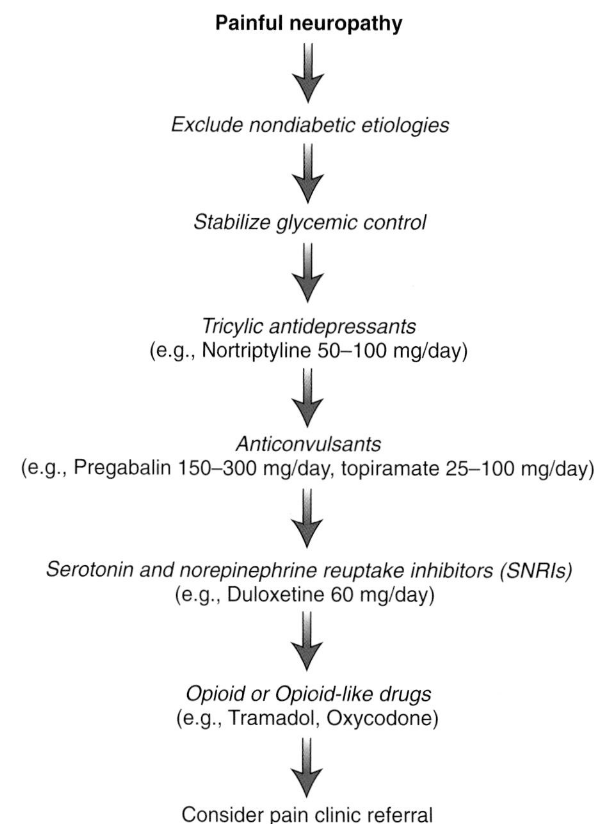
Painful neuropathy
Exclude nondiabetic etiologies
Stabilize glycemic control
Tricylic antidepressants
(e.g., Nortriptyline 50–100 mg/day)
Anticonvulsants
(e.g., Pregabalin 150–300 mg/day, topiramate 25–100 mg/day)
Serotonin and norepinephrine reuptake inhibitors (SNRIs)
(e.g., Duloxetine 60 mg/day)
Opioid or Opioid-like drugs
(e.g., Tramadol, Oxycodone)
Consider pain clinic referral
*Nonpharmacological, topical, or physical therapies can be useful at any time (capsaicin, acupuncture, etc.).

Figure 32–45 ▪ Algorithm for managing painful diabetic neuropathy. Nonpharmacologic, topical, or physical therapies can be useful at any time (capsaicin, acupuncture, etc.). SNRIs, serotonin and norepinephrine reuptake inhibitors. (Modified from Boulton AJ, Vinik AI, Arezzo JC, et al. Diabetic neuropathies: a statement by the American Diabetes Association. Diabetes Care 2005;28:956-962.)

have focused on interrupting pain transmission with antidepressant drugs that inhibit the reuptake of norepinephrine or serotonin. This central action accentuates the effects of these neurotransmitters in activation of endogenous pain–inhibitory systems in the brain that modulate pain-transmission cells in the spinal cord.[676] Side effects, including dysautonomia and dry mouth, can be troublesome. Switching to nortriptyline can lessen some of the anticholinergic effects of amitriptyline.

They remain first-line agents in many centers, but consideration of their safety and tolerability is important in avoiding adverse effects, a common result of treatment of neuropathic pain. Dosages must be titrated based on positive responses, treatment adherence, and adverse events.[677] Among the norepinephrine reuptake inhibitors, desipramine, amitriptyline, and imipramine have been shown to be of benefit.[678,679]

Selective serotonin reuptake inhibitors (SSRIs) that have been used for neuropathic pain are paroxetine, fluoxetine, sertraline, and citalopram. Paroxetine appears to be associated with more pain relief.[680] Fluoxetine failed a placebo-controlled trial.[676] Duloxetine has been approved for neuropathic pain in the United States. It is a selective, balanced and potent inhibitor of serotonin noradrenalin reuptake in the brain and spinal, cord leading to increased neuronal activity in efferent inhibitory pathways. Physicians must be alert to suicidal ideation, exacerbation of autonomic symptoms, and aggravation of depression and should stop drug immediately if patients experience any of these.

Other antidepressants, such as venlafaxine, have proved to be of greater efficacy than placebo.[181] Nortriptyline-fluphenazine has also been shown to reduce pain. However, adverse events are fairly common with nortriptyline-fluphenazine.[681]

Antiepileptic Drugs

For a detailed discussion of the subject, refer to the review by Vinik.[682]

Anticonvulsants have stood the test of time in treatment of diabetic neuropathy.[683,684] Principal mechanisms of action include sodium channel blockade (felbamate, lamotrigine, oxcarbazepine, topiramate, zonisamide), potentiation of γ-aminobutyric acid (GABA) activity (tiagabine, topiramate), calcium-channel blockade (felbamate, lamotrigine, topiramate, zonisamide), antagonism of glutamate at NMDA receptors (felbamate) or α-amino-3-hydroxy-5-methyl-4-isoxazole propionic acid (AMPA) (felbamate, topiramate).[685]

Carbamazepine is useful for patients with shooting or electric-shock–like pain. Several double-blind, placebo-controlled studies have demonstrated carbamazepine to be effective in the management of pain in diabetic neuropathy.[686] Toxic side effects can limit its use in some patients.

Phenytoin has long been used in the treatment of painful neuropathies. Double-blind crossover studies do not demonstrate a therapeutic benefit of phenytoin compared with placebo in diabetic neuropathy.[683] Phenytoin is associated with significant side effects, and it must be administered as much as three or four times daily. Some studies have reported positive findings, with 24% of patients reporting improvement,[687] but in others it failed to show any benefit.[688] Also, side effects mitigate its use in people with diabetes. Its ability to suppress insulin secretion has resulted in precipitation of hyperosmolar diabetic coma. Valproic acid failed to prove superior to placebo on any outcome measures.[689]

Gabapentin is an effective anticonvulsant whose mechanism is not well understood, but it holds additional promise as an analgesic agent in painful neuropathy.[690] In a multicenter study in the United States,[691] gabapentin monotherapy appeared to be efficacious for treating pain and sleep interference associated with diabetic peripheral neuropathy. It also exhibits positive effects on mood and quality of life.[692] Effective dosing can require 1800 to 3600 mg/day, and this is associated with untoward side effects. In a placebo-controlled trial, gabapentin-treated patients had significantly lower mean daily pain scores and improvement of all secondary efficacy parameters.[691] In another study on diabetic neuropathy, gabapentin was found to be equivalent to amitriptyline.[693] Gabapentin has the additional benefit of improving sleep,[691] which is often compromised in patients with chronic pain.[677] In the long term, it is known to produce weight gain, which can complicate diabetes management. Gabapentin has not been successful in all trials.[694]

Lamotrigine is an antiepileptic agent with at least two antinociceptive properties. In a randomized, placebo-controlled study, Eisenberg and colleagues[695] confirmed the efficacy of this agent in patients with neuropathic pain. However, titration needs to be inordinately slow to prevent Stevens-Johnson syndrome. Bradycardia has been reported. Lamotrigine caused a significant decrease in pain intensity in two controlled studies.[695,696]

Topiramate is a fructose analogue that was initially examined because of its ant-diabetic possibilities. Unfortunately it was first examined only in normal animals and had no hypoglycemic properties. It has now undergone extensive testing for epilepsy, migraine, involuntary movements, CNS injury, and neuropathic pain. Unfortunately, the first two studies used a titration to 400 mg/day, which was associated with fairly severe CNS side effects, which were prohibitive. The studies failed to establish an effect in diabetic neuropathic pain. A third study using different end-points, with specificity for the nature and site of the pain and recognizing that paresthesias were a side effect of the drug and were not mistaken for pain, was successful.[697] What has emerged from all the studies is that the drug lowers BP, improves lipid profiles, decreases insulin resistance, and increases nerve fiber regeneration in the skin.[550] It thus has the potential to relieve pain by altering the biology of the disease and has now been shown to increase intraepidermal nerve fiber density. Further trials are under way. One must start with no more than 15 mg/day, preferably at night and then increase the dose only after the patient can tolerate the drug. A maximum of 200 mg was sufficient to induce nerve fiber recovery.

Pregabalin produced significant improvements on pain scores within 1 week of treatment ($P < 0.01$), and these improvements persisted for 8 weeks ($P < 0.01$). For the patient global impression of change (PGIC), there was a 67% improvement versus 39% in patients given placebo ($P = 0.001$). Furthermore, 40% of patients receiving pregabalin reported a 50% reduction in pain, compared with 14.5% of the placebo group ($P = 0.001$). There is, however, concern with the labeling as a narcotic drug.[667]

In trials with topiramate, a fructose analogue, 50% of patients on topiramate versus 34% on placebo responded to treatment, defined as a greater than 30% reduction in pain score ($P < 0.004$). Topiramate also reduced pain intensity compared with placebo ($P < 0.003$) as well as sleep-disruption scores ($P < 0.02$).[697] This drug also lowers BP, has a favorable impact on lipids, decreases insulin resistance, and causes growth of intraepidermal nerve fibers.[682,697]

Pain symptoms in neuropathy significantly affect quality of life. Neuropathic pain therapy is challenging, and selection of pain medication and dosages must be individualized, with attention to potential side effects and drug interactions.

Adjunct Management and Treatment of Complications

Although small-fiber neuropathy manifests as different forms of pain, large-fiber neuropathy is manifested by reduced vibration perception and position sense, weakness, muscle wasting, and depressed deep tendon reflexes. Diabetic patients with large-fiber neuropathies are uncoordinated and ataxic and are 17 times more likely to fall than their non-neuropathic counterparts.[698] Therefore, it is important to improve strength and balance in patients with large-fiber neuropathy. Patients can benefit from high-intensity strength training by increasing muscle strength and improving coordination and balance, thus reducing fall and fracture risks.[699,700] Low-impact activities, which emphasize muscle strength and coordination and challenge the vestibular system, such as Pilates, yoga, and tai chi, can also be particularly helpful. In addition, options to prevent and correct foot deformities are available, including orthotics, surgery, and reconstruction.

Prevention

Basic management of small-fiber neuropathies by the patient should be encouraged. These include foot protection and ulcer prevention by wearing padded socks; daily foot inspection using a mirror to examine the soles of the feet; selection of proper footwear; scrutiny of shoes for the presence of foreign objects that lodge themselves in closed shoes; and avoidance of sun-heated surfaces, hot bathwater, and sleeping with feet in front of fireplaces or heaters. Patient education should reinforce these strategies and should also discourage soaking feet in water. Education also promotes foot care by encouraging emollient creams to help skin retain moisture and prevent cracking and infection.

Stimulation

Transcutaneous nerve stimulation (electrotherapy) occasionally is helpful and certainly represents one of the more benign therapies for painful neuropathy.[701] Care should be taken to move the electrodes around to identify sensitive areas and obtain maximum relief. Static magnetic field therapy[702] has been reported to be of benefit, but it is difficult to blind such studies. Similarly, the use of infrared light has reportedly had benefit but, this remains to be proved. A case series of patients with severe painful neuropathy unresponsive to conventional therapy suggested efficacy of using an implanted spinal cord stimulator.[586] However, this cannot be generally recommended except in very resistant cases because it is invasive, expensive, and unproven in controlled studies. Even stochastic resonance therapy can improve sensation.[634] There is no support for the notion that surgical decompression can be used to treat common diabetic neuropathy.[703]

Pharmacologic Therapy

Analgesics

Analgesics are rarely of much benefit in the treatment of painful neuropathy, although they may be of some use on a short-term basis for some of the self-limited syndromes, such as painful diabetic third nerve palsy. Narcotics are generally avoided in the setting of chronic pain because of the risk of addiction.

Calcitonin

In a placebo-controlled study, 10 patients with painful diabetic neuropathy were treated with 100 IU of calcitonin per day. About 39% of patients had near-complete relief of symptom. The improvement was seen after only 2 weeks of treatment.[704]

Management of Small-Fiber Neuropathies

Patients must be instructed on foot care with daily foot inspection. They must have a mirror in the bathroom for inspecting the soles of the feet. Providing patients with a monofilament for self-testing reduces ulcers.

All diabetic patients should wear padded socks. Shoes must fit well and have adequate support, and they must be inspected for the presence of foreign bodies (e.g., nails, pins, teeth) before donning.

Patients must exercise care with exposure to heat (no falling asleep in front of fires). Emollient creams should be used for the drying and cracking. After bathing feet should be thoroughly dried and powdered between the toes. Nails should be cut transversely, preferably by a podiatrist.

Management of Large-Fiber Neuropathies

Patients with large-fiber neuropathies are uncoordinated and ataxic. As a result, they are more likely to fall than non-neuropathic age-matched persons.[705] High-intensity strength training in older people increases muscle strength in a variety of muscles. More importantly, the strength training results in improved coordination and balance quantifiable with backward tandem walking.[699] Thus it is vital to embark on a program of strength training and improvement of balance to include gait and strength training, tendon lengthening for Achilles tendon shortening, orthotics and proper shoes for the deformities, pain management as detailed earlier, bisphophonates for osteopenia, and surgical reconstruction and full-length casting as necessary.

Autonomic Neuropathies

The autonomic nervous system (ANS) supplies all organs in the body and consists of an afferent and an efferent system, with long efferents in the vagus (cholinergic) and short postganglionic unmyelinated fibers in the sympathetic system (adrenergic). A third component is the neuropeptidergic system, with its neurotransmitters substance P, vasoactive intestinal polypeptide (VIP), and CGRP, among others.

Diabetic autonomic neuropathy can cause dysfunction of every part of the body. Diabetic autonomic neuropathy often goes completely unrecognized by patient and physician alike because of its insidious onset and protean multiple organ involvement. Alternatively, the appearance of complex and confusing symptoms in a single organ system due to diabetic autonomic neuropathy can cause profound symptoms and receive intense diagnostic and therapeutic attention. Subclinical involvement may be widespread, whereas clinical symptoms and signs may be focused within a single organ. The organ systems that most often exhibit prominent clinical autonomic signs and symptoms in diabetes include the ocular pupil, sweat glands, genitourinary system, gastrointestinal system, adrenal medullary system, and cardiovascular system (Table 32–8).

Diabetic autonomic neuropathy can involve any system in the body. It has been said that to know autonomic neuropathy is to know the whole of medicine. Involvement of the autonomic nervous system can occur as early as the first year after diagnosis. Major manifestations are cardiovascular, gastrointestinal, and genitourinary system dysfunction.[552,706] Reduced exercise tolerance, edema, paradoxical supine or nocturnal hypertension, and intolerance to heat due to defective thermoregulation are consequences of autonomic neuropathy.

TABLE 32–8 CLINICAL MANIFESTATIONS OF AUTONOMIC NEUROPATHY

CARDIOVASCULAR
Alterations in skin blood flow Cardiac denervation, painless myocardial infarction Heat intolerance Orthostatic hypotension Tachycardia, exercise intolerance
GASTROINTESTINAL
Constipation Diarrhea Esophageal dysfunction Fecal incontinence Gastroparesis diabeticorum
GENITOURINARY
Cystopathy Erectile dysfunction Neurogenic bladder Retrograde ejaculation
METABOLIC
Hypoglycemia unawareness Hypoglycemia unresponsiveness
PUPILLARY
Argyll-Robertson–type pupil Decreased diameter of dark adapted pupil
SWEATING DISTURBANCES
Areas of symmetrical anhydrosis Gustatory sweating

Defective blood flow in the small capillary circulation is found with decreased responsiveness to mental arithmetic, cold pressor, hand grip, and heating.[578] The defect is associated with a reduction in the amplitude of vasomotion[698] that resembles premature aging.[578] There are differences in the glabrous and hairy skin circulations. In hairy skin, a functional defect is found before neuropathy develops,[707] and it is correctable with antioxidants.[708] The clinical counterpart is skin that is dry and cold, loses ability to sweat, and develops fissures and cracks that are portals of entry for organisms leading to infectious ulcers and gangrene. Silent myocardial infarction, respiratory failure, amputations, and sudden death are hazards for diabetic patients with cardiac autonomic neuropathy.[549,709] Therefore, it is vitally important to make this diagnosis early so that appropriate intervention can be instituted.[710]

Disturbances in autonomic nervous system may be functional and include gastroparesis with hyperglycemia and ketoacidosis. In organic disturbances, nerve fibers are actually lost. This creates inordinate difficulties in diagnosing, treating, and prognosticating as well as establishing true prevalence rates.

Tests of autonomic function generally stimulate entire reflex pathways. Furthermore, autonomic control for each organ system is usually divided between opposing sympathetic and parasympathetic innervation, so that heart rate acceleration, for example, might reflect either decreased parasympathetic or increased sympathetic nervous system stimulation.

Because many conditions affect the autonomic nervous system and autonomic neuropathy is not unique to diabetes, the diagnosis of diabetic autonomic neuropathy rests with establishing the diagnosis and excluding other causes. The best studied tests, and those for which there are large databases and evidence to support their use in clinical practice, relate to the evaluation of cardiovascular reflexes. Evaluation of orthostasis is fairly straightforward and is readily done in clinical practice, as are establishing the causes of gastrointestinal symptoms and erectile dysfunction. The evaluation of pupillary abnormalities, hypoglycemia unawareness and unresponsiveness, neurovascular dysfunction, and sweating disturbances are for the most part done only in research laboratories, require specialized equipment and familiarity with the diagnostic procedures, and are best left in the hands of those who have a special interest in the area.

Tables 32–9 and 32–10 present the diagnostic tests that apply to the diagnosis of cardiovascular autonomic neuropathy. These tests can be used as a surrogate for the diagnosis of autonomic neuropathy of any system because it is generally rare to find involvement (although it does occur) of any other division of the ANS in the absence of cardiovascular autonomic dysfunction. For example, if one entertains the possibility that the patient's erectile dysfunction is due to autonomic neuropathy, then before embarking upon a sophisticated and expensive evaluation of erectile status one should measure the heart rate and its variability in response to deep breathing. If this measurement is normal, it excludes autonomic neuropathy as a cause of erectile dysfunction, and the cause should be sought elsewhere. Similarly, it is extremely unusual to find gastroparesis secondary to autonomic neuropathy in a patient with normal cardiovascular autonomic reflexes.

Prevention and Reversibility

It has now become clear that strict glycemic control[537] and stepwise progressive management of hyperglycemia, lipids, and BP and use of antioxidants[644] and ACE inhibitors[711] reduce the odds

TABLE 32–9 DIFFERENTIAL DIAGNOSIS OF DIABETIC AUTONOMIC NEUROPATHY

Clinical Manifestations	Differential Diagnosis
CARDIOVASCULAR	
Cardiac denervation Exercise intolerance Orthostatic hypotension Painless myocardial infarction Tachycardia	Carcinoid syndrome Congestive heart disease Hyperadrenergic hypotension Hypovolemia Idiopathic orthostatic hypotension Multiple system atrophy with parkinsonism Panhypopituitarism Pheochromocytoma Orthostatic tachycardia Shy-Drager syndrome
GASTROINTESTINAL	
Constipation Diarrhea Esophageal dysfunction Fecal incontinence Gastroparesis diabeticorum	Bezoars Biliary disease Medications Obstruction Psychogenic vomiting Secretory diarrhea (endocrine tumors)
GENITOURINARY	
Cystopathy Erectile dysfunction Neurogenic bladder Retrograde ejaculation	Alcohol abuse Atherosclerotic vascular disease Genital and pelvic surgery Medications
NEUROVASCULAR	
Dry skin Gustatory sweating Heat intolerance Impaired skin blood flow	Amyloidosis Arsenic Chagas' disease
METABOLIC	
Hypoglycemia-associated autonomic failure Hypoglycemia unawareness Hypoglycemia unresponsiveness	Drugs that mask hypoglycemia Other cause of hypoglycemia Intensive glycemic control
PUPILLARY	
Argyll-Robertson–type pupil Decreased diameter of dark adapted pupil	Syphilis

ratio for autonomic neuropathy to 0.32.[627] It has also been shown that mortality is a function of loss of beat-to-beat variability with MI. This can be reduced by 33% with acute administration of insulin.[712] Kendall and coworkers[713] reported that successful pancreas transplantation improves epinephrine response and normalizes hypoglycemia symptom recognition in patients with longstanding diabetes and established autonomic neuropathy. Burger's group[714] showed a reversible metabolic component in patients with early cardiac autonomic neuropathy (Table 32–11).

TABLE 32–10 DIAGNOSTIC TESTS OF CARDIOVASCULAR AUTONOMIC NEUROPATHY

RESTING HEART RATE
Rate >100 beats/min is abnormal.
BEAT-TO-BEAT HEART RATE VARIATION*
With the patient at rest and supine (no overnight coffee or hypoglycemic episodes), breathing 6 breaths/min, heart rate monitored by ECG or Anscore device, a difference in heart rate of >15 beats/min is normal and <10 beats/min is abnormal, R-R inspiration to R-R expiration >1.17. All indices of HRV are age-dependent.†
HEART RATE RESPONSE TO STANDING*
During continuous ECG monitoring, the R-R interval is measured at beats 15 and 30 after standing. Normally, a tachycardia is followed by reflex bradycardia. The 30:15 ratio is normally >1.03.
HEART RATE RESPONSE TO VALSALVA MANEUVER*
The subject forcibly exhales into the mouthpiece of a manometer to 40 mm Hg for 15 seconds during ECG monitoring. Healthy subjects develop tachycardia and peripheral vasoconstriction during strain and an overshoot bradycardia and rise in blood pressure with release. The ratio of longest R-R shortest R-R should be >1.2.
SYSTOLIC BLOOD PRESSURE RESPONSE TO STANDING
Systolic blood pressure is measured in the supine subject. The patient stands and the systolic blood pressure is measured after 2 min. Normal response is a fall of <10 mm Hg, borderline is a fall of 10-29 mm Hg, and abnormal is a fall of >30 mm Hg with symptoms.
DIASTOLIC BLOOD PRESSURE RESPONSE TO ISOMETRIC EXERCISE
The subject squeezes a handgrip dynamometer to establish a maximum. Grip is then squeezed at 30% maximum for 5 min. The normal response for diastolic blood pressure is a rise of >16 mm Hg in the other arm.
ECG QT/QTC INTERVALS
The QTc (corrected QT intevval on EKG) should be <440 ms.
SPECTRAL ANALYSIS
HF peak ↓ (parasympathetic dysfunction) LF peak ↓ (sympathetic dysfunction) LH/HF ratio ↓ (sympathetic imbalance) VLF peak ↓ (sympathetic dysfunction)
NEUROVASCULAR FLOW
Noninvasive laser Doppler measures peripheral sympathetic responses to nociception.

*These can now be performed quickly (<15 min) in the practitioner's office, with a central reference laboratory providing quality control and normative values. These are now readily available in most cardiologist's practice.

†Lowest normal value of E/I ratio: Age 20-24 yr: 1.17; 25-29 yr: 1.15; 30-34 yr: 1.13; 35-30 yr: 1.12; 40-44 yr: 1.10; 45-49 yr: 1.08; 50-54 yr: 1.07; 55-59 yr: 1.06; 60-64 yr: 1.04; 65-69 yr: 1.03; 70-75 yr: 1.02.

ECG, electrocardiogram; HF, high frequency; HRV, heart rate variation; LF, low frequency; VLF, very low frequency.

TABLE 32–11 CLINICAL FEATURES, DIAGNOSIS, AND TREATMENT OF DIABETIC AUTONOMIC NEUROPATHY

Symptoms	Tests	Treatments
	CARDIAC	
Resting tachycardia, exercise intolerance	HRV, MUGA thallium scan, MIBG scan	Graded supervised exercise, ACE inhibitors, β-blockers
Postural hypotension, dizziness, weakness, fatigue, syncope	HRV, supine and standing BP, catecholamines	Mechanical measures, clonidine, midodrine, octreotide, erythropoietin
	GASTROINTESTINAL	
Gastroparesis, erratic glucose control	Gastric emptying study, barium study	Frequent small meals, prokinetic agents (metoclopramide, domperidone, erythromycin)
Abdominal pain, early satiety, nausea, vomiting, bloating, belching	Endoscopy, manometry, electrogastrogram	Antibiotics, antiemetics, bulking agents, tricyclic antidepressants, pyloric botulinum toxin, gastric pacing
Constipation	Endoscopy	High-fiber diet, bulking agents, osmotic laxatives, lubricating agents
Diarrhea (often nocturnal alternating with constipation)		Soluble fiber, gluten and lactose restriction, anticholinergic agents, cholestyramine, antibiotics, somatostatin, pancreatic enzyme supplements
	SEXUAL DYSFUNCTION	
Erectile dysfunction	H&P, HRV, penile-brachial pressure index, nocturnal penile tumescence	Sex therapy, psychological counseling, phosphodiesterase inhibitors, PGE_1 injections, devices or prostheses
Vaginal dryness		Vaginal lubricants
	BLADDER DYSFUNCTION	
Frequency, urgency, nocturia, urinary retention, incontinence	Cystometrogram, postvoid sonography	Bethanechol, intermittent catheterization
	SUDOMOTOR DYSFUNCTION	
Anhidrosis, heat intolerance, dry skin, hyperhidrosis	Quantitative sudomotor axon reflex, sweat test, skin blood flow	Emollients and skin lubricants, scopolamine, glycopyrrolate, botulinum toxin, vasodilators
	PUPILLOMOTOR AND VISCERAL DYSFUNCTION	
Blurred vision, impaired adaptation to ambient light, Argyll- Robertson pupil	Pupillometry, HRV	Care with driving at night
Impaired visceral sensation: silent MI, hypoglycemia unawareness		Recognition of unusual presentation of MI, control of risk factors, control of plasma glucose levels

ACE, acetylcholinesterase; BP, blood pressure; H&P, history and physical examination; HRV, heart rate variability; MI, myocardial infarction; MIBG: metaiodobenzlyguanidine; MUGA, multigated angiography.

Management

Postural Hypotension

The syndrome of postural hypotension is posture-related dizziness and syncope (Fig. 42-46). Patients who have T2DM and orthostatic hypotension are hypovolemic and have sympathoadrenal insufficiency; both factors contribute to the pathogenesis of orthostatic hypotension.[715] Postural hypotension in the patient with diabetic autonomic neuropathy can present a difficult management problem. Elevating the BP in the standing position must be balanced against preventing hypertension in the supine position.

Supportive Garments

Whenever possible, attempts should be made to increase venous return from the periphery using total body stockings. Leg compression alone is less effective, presumably reflecting the large capacity of the abdomen relative to the legs.[716] Patients should be instructed to put these garments on while lying down and to not remove them until returning to the supine position.

Drug Therapy

Some patients with postural hypotension benefit from treatment with 9-fluorohydrocortisone. Unfortunately, symptoms do not improve until edema occurs, and there is a significant risk of developing congestive heart failure and hypertension. If 9-fluorohydrocortisone does not work satisfactorily, various adrenergic agonists and antagonists may be used. If the adrenergic receptor status is known, then therapy can be guided to the appropriate agent. Metoclopromide may be helpful in patients with dopamine excess or increased sensitivity to dopaminergic stimulation. Patients with α_2-adrenergic receptor excess might respond to the α_2-antagonist yohimbine. Those few patients in whom β-receptors are increased may be helped with propranolol. α_2-Adrenergic receptor deficiency can be

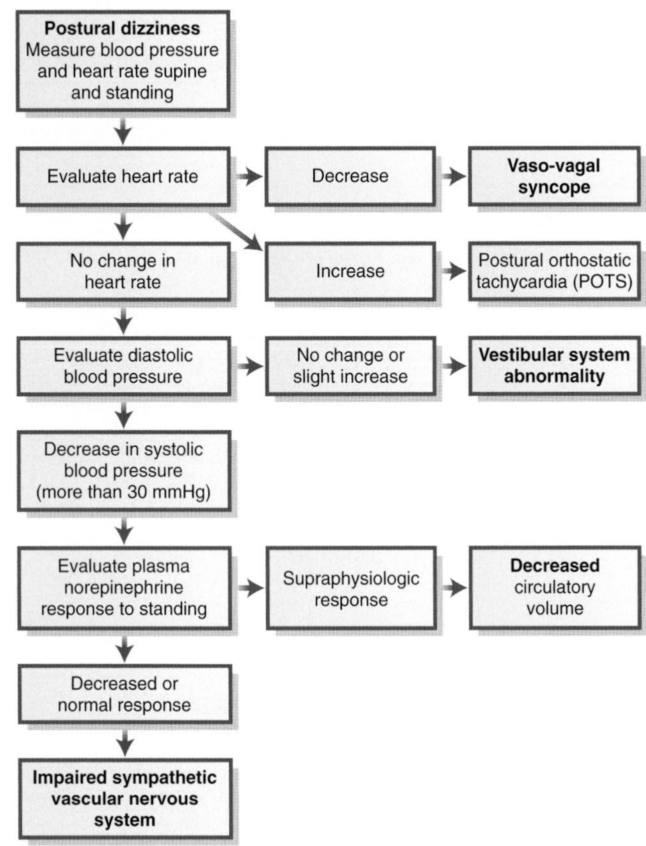

Figure 32–46 ▪ Evaluation of postural dizziness in diabetic patients. (Modified from Vinik A, Mehrabyan A. Diabetic neuropathies. Med Clin North Am 2004;88:947-999.)

treated with the α_2-agonist clonidine, which in this setting can paradoxically increase BP. One should start with small doses and gradually increase the dose. If these measures fail, midodrine (an α_1-adrenergic agonist) or dihydroergotamine in combination with caffeine can help. A particularly refractory form of postural hypotension occurs in some patients postprandially and might respond to therapy with octreotide given subcutaneously in the mornings.

Gastropathy

Gastrointestinal motor disorders (Fig. 42-47) are frequent and widespread in type 2 diabetic patients, regardless of symptoms,[717] and there is a poor correlation between symptoms and objective evidence of functional or organic defects. The first step in management of diabetic gastroparesis consists of multiple small feedings. The amount of fat should be decreased, because it tends to delay gastric emptying. Maintenance of glycemic control is important.[718,719] Metoclopromide may be used. Cisapride and domperidone[720,721] have been shown to be effective in some patients, although probably no more so than metoclopromide (cisapride has been withdrawn from the market). Erythromycin given as either a liquid or suppository also may be helpful. Erythromycin acts on the motilin receptor (the sweeper of the gut) and shortens gastric emptying time.[722] If medications fail and severe gastroparesis persists, jejunostomy placement into normally functioning bowel may be needed.

Enteropathy

Enteropathy involving the small bowel and colon can produce both chronic constipation and explosive diabetic diarrhea, making treatment of this particular complication difficult.

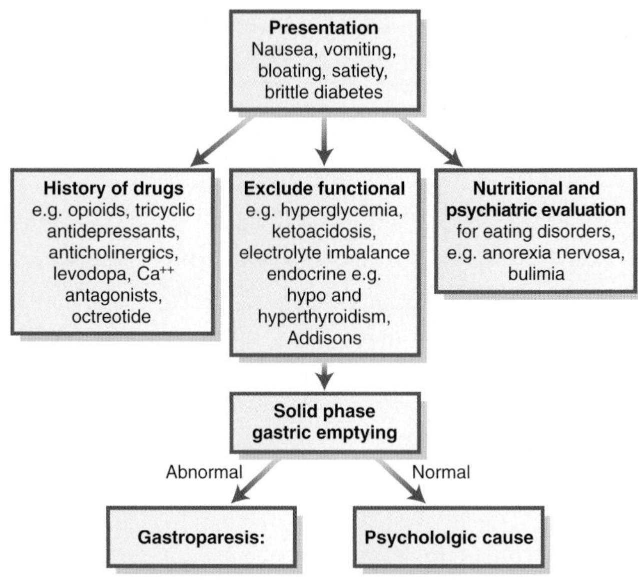

Figure 32–47 ▪ Evaluation of the patient with suspected gastroparesis. (Adapted with permission from Vinik A, Mehrabyan A. Diabetic neuropathies. Med Clin North Am 2004;88:947-999.)

Antibiotics

Stasis of bowel contents with bacterial overgrowth can contribute to the diarrhea. Treatment with broad-spectrum antibiotics is the mainstay of therapy, including tetracycline or trimethoprim-sulfamethoxazole. Metronidazole appears to be the most effective and should be continued for at least 3 weeks.

Cholestyramine

Retention of bile can occur and can be highly irritating to the gut. Chelation of bile salts with cholestyramine 4 g mixed with fluid three times a day can relieve symptoms.

Diphenoxylate plus Atropine

Diphenoxylate plus atrophine can help to control the diarrhea. However, toxic megacolon can occur, and extreme care should be used.

Diet

Patients with poor digestion can benefit from a gluten-free diet. Beware of certain fibers in the neuropathic patient that can lead to bezoar formation because of bowel stasis in gastroparetic or constipated patients.

Cystopathy

Patients with neurogenic bladder should be instructed to palpate the bladder and, if they are unable to initiate micturition when their bladder is full, use Crede's maneuver to start the flow of urine. Parasympathomimetics such as bethanechol are sometimes helpful, although often they do not help to fully empty the bladder. Extended sphincter relaxation can be achieved with an α_1-blocker, such as doxazosin.[552] Self-catheterization can be particularly useful in this setting, with the risk of infection generally being low.

Sexual Dysfunction

Male Sexual Dysfunction

Erectile dysfunction (ED) occurs in 50% to 75% of diabetic men, and it tends to occur at an earlier age than in the general population. The incidence of ED in diabetic men aged 20 to 29 years is 9% and increases to 95% by age 70 years. It may be the presenting symptom of diabetes. More than 50% notice the onset of ED within 10 years of the diagnosis, but it can precede the other complications of diabetes.

The etiology of ED in diabetes is multifactorial. Neuropathy, vascular disease, diabetes control, nutrition, endocrine disorders, psychogenic factors, and drugs used to treat diabetes and its complications play a role.[723,724] The diagnosis of the cause of ED is made by a logical stepwise progression in all instances.[723,724] An approach to therapy has been presented and is discussed later.[723]

Diagnosis

A thorough workup for impotence includes medical and sexual history; physical and psychological evaluations; blood test for diabetes and a check of levels of testosterone, prolactin, and thyroid hormones; test for nocturnal erections; tests to assess penile, pelvic, and spinal nerve function; and test to assess penile blood supply and BP. The flow chart provided is intended as a guide to assist in defining the problem.

The health care provider should initiate questions that will help distinguish the various forms of organic ED from those that are psychogenic. Physical examination must include an evaluation of the ANS, vascular supply, and hypothalamic-pituitary-gonadal axis.

Autonomic neuropathy causing ED is almost always accompanied by loss of ankle jerks and absence or reduction of vibration sense over the large toes. More direct evidence of impairment of penile autonomic function can be obtained by demonstrating normal perianal sensation, assessing the tone of the anal sphincter during a rectal exam, and ascertaining the presence of an anal wink when the area of the skin adjacent to the anus is stroked or contraction of the anus when the glans penis is squeezed (the bulbo-cavernosus reflex). These measurements are easily and quickly done at the bedside and reflect the integrity of sacral parasympathetic divisions.

Vascular disease is usually manifested by buttock claudication but may be due to stenosis of the internal pudendal artery. A penile-brachial index of less than 0.7 indicates diminished blood supply. A venous leak manifests as unresponsiveness to vasodilators and needs to be evaluated by penile Doppler sonography.

In order to distinguish psychogenic from organic erectile dysfunction, nocturnal penile tumescence (NPT) can be tested. Normal NPT defines psychogenic ED, and a negative response to vasodilators implies vascular insufficiency. Application of NPT is not so simple. It is much like having a sphygmomanometer cuff inflate over the penis many times during the night while one is trying to have a normal night's sleep. The patient might have to take home the device and become familiar with it over several nights before one has a reliable estimate of the failure of NPT.

Treatment

A number of treatment modalities are available, and each treatment has positive and negative effects. Patients must be made aware of positive and negative aspects before a therapeutic decision is made. Before considering any form of treatment, every effort should be made to have the patient withdraw from alcohol and eliminate smoking. The patient should be removed, if possible, from drugs that are known to cause erectile dysfunction. Metabolic control should be optimized.

According to more recent research, relaxation of the corpus cavernosus smooth-muscle cells is caused by NO and cyclic guanosine monophosphate (cGMP), and the ability to have and maintain an erection depends on NO and cGMP. Sildenafil (Viagra) exerts its effect by transiently increasing NO and cGMP levels. Sildenafil is a GMP type-5 phosphodiesterase inhibitor that enhances blood flow to the corpora cavernosa with sexual stimulation. A 50 mg tablet (Table 42-12) is the usual starting dose and is taken 60 minutes before sexual activity. Lower doses should be considered in patients with renal failure and hepatic dysfunction. The duration of the drug effect is 4 hours. Before it is prescribed, it is important to exclude ischemic heart disease. Sildenafil is absolutely contraindicated in patients being treated with nitroglycerine or other nitrate-containing drugs because severe hypotension and fatal cardiac events can occur.[725]

Direct injection of prostacyclin into the corpus cavernosum induces satisfactory erections in a significant number of men. Also, surgical implantation of a penile prosthesis may be appropriate. The less expensive type of prosthesis is a semirigid, permanently erect type that is embarrassing and uncomfortable for some patients. The inflatable type is three times more expensive and subject to mechanical failure, but it avoids the embarrassment caused by other devices.

Female Sexual Dysfunction

Women with diabetes mellitus can experience decreased sexual desire and more pain on sexual intercourse, but they are also at risk for decreased sexual arousal, with inadequate lubrication.[726] Diagnosis of female sexual dysfunction using vaginal plethysmography to measure lubrication and vaginal flushing has not been well established.

Cystopathy

In diabetic autonomic neuropathy, the motor function of the bladder is unimpaired, but afferent fiber damage results in diminished bladder sensation. The urinary bladder can be enlarged to more than three times its normal size. Patients are seen with bladders filled to their umbilicus, yet they feel no discomfort. Loss of bladder sensation occurs with diminished voiding frequency, and the patient is no longer able to void completely. Consequently, dribbling and overflow incontinence are common complaints. A postvoid residual of greater than 150 mL diagnoses cystopathy. Cystopathy can put the patients at risk for urinary infections.

Patients with cystopathy should be instructed to palpate the bladder and, if they are unable to initiate micturition when their bladder is full, use Crede's maneuver (massage or pressure on the lower portion of abdomen just above the pubic bone) to start the flow of urine. The principal aim of the treatment should be to improve bladder emptying and to reduce the risk of urinary tract infection. Parasympathomimetics such as bethanechol are sometimes helpful, although often they do not help to fully empty the bladder. Extended sphincter relaxation can be achieved with an α_1-blocker, such as doxazosin. Self-catheterization can be particularly useful in this setting, and the risk of infection generally is low.

Sweating Disturbances

Hyperhidrosis of the upper body, often related to eating (gustatory sweating) is a characteristic feature of autonomic neuropathy. Gustatory sweating accompanies the ingestion of certain foods, particularly spicy foods and cheeses. Gustatory sweating is more common than previously believed, and topically applied glycopyrrolate (an antimuscarinic compound) is a very effective treatment in reducing both the severity and frequency.[727,728] Symptoms are avoided by avoiding the inciting food.

Anhidrosis of the lower body is also common in autonomic neuropathy. Loss of lower body sweating can cause dry, brittle skin that cracks easily, predisposing one to ulcer formation that can lead to loss of the limb. Special attention must be paid to foot care.

TABLE 32–12 PHARMACOLOGIC TREATMENT OF AUTONOMIC NEUROPATHY

Drug	Class	Dosage	Side Effects
		ORTHOSTATIC HYPOTENSION	
9α Fluorohydrocortisone	Mineralocorticoid	0.5-2 mg/day	Congestive heart failure, hypertension
Clonidine	α_2-Adrenergic agonist	0.1-0.5 mg at bedtime	Hypotension, sedation, dry mouth
Octreotide	Somatostatin analogue	0.1-0.5 μg/kg/day	Injection site pain, diarrhea
		GASTROPARESIS	
Metoclopromide	D_2-Receptor antagonist	10 mg 30-60 min before meals and at bedtime	Galactorrhea, extrapyramidal symptoms
Domperidon	D_2-Receptor antagonist	10-20 mg 30-60 min before meals and at bedtime	Galactorrhea
Erythromycin	Motilin receptor agonist	250 mg 30 minutes before meals	Abdominal cramp, nausea, diarrhea, rash
Levosulfide	D_2-Receptor antagonist	25 mg tid	Galactorrhea
		DIABETIC DIARRHEA	
Metranidazole	Broad-spectrum antibiotic	250 mg tid, minimum 3 weeks	Orthostatic hypotension
Clonidine	α_2-Adrenergic agonist	0.1 mg bid or tid	Toxic megacolon
Cholestyramine	Bile acid sequestrant	4 g 1-6 times/day	Aggravate nutrient malabsorption (at higher doses)
Loperamide	Opiate-receptor agonists	2 mg qid	
Octreotide	Somatostatin analogue	50 μg tid	
		CYSTOPATHY	
Bethanechol	Acetylcholine receptor agonist	10 mg, 4 times/day	
Doxazosin	α_1-Adrenergic antagonist	1-2 mg, 2-3 times/day	Hypotension, headache, palpitations
		ERECTILE DYSFUNCTION	
Sildenafil	GMP type-5 phosphodiesterase inhibitor	50 mg before sexual activity, only once per day	Hypotension and fatal cardiac event (with nitrate-containing drugs), headache, flushing, nasal congestion, dyspepsia, musculoskeletal pain, blurred vision

Metabolic Dysfunction

Blood glucose concentration is normally maintained during starvation or increased insulin action by an asymptomatic parasympathetic response with bradycardia and mild hypotension, followed by a sympathetic response with glucagon and epinephrine secretion for short-term glucose counterregulation and growth hormone and cortisol in long-term regulation. Blood glucose concentration is normally maintained during starvation or increased insulin action by an asymptomatic parasympathetic response with bradycardia and mild hypotension, followed by a sympathetic response with glucagon and epinephrine secretion for short-term glucose counterregulation and growth hormone and cortisol in long-term regulation. The release of catecholamine alerts the patient to take the required measures to prevent coma due to low blood glucose. The absence of warning signs of impending neuroglycopenia is known as *hypoglycemic unawareness*. The failure of glucose counterregulation can be confirmed by the absence of glucagon and epinephrine responses to hypoglycemia induced by a standard controlled dose of insulin.[729]

In patients with T1DM, the glucagon response is impaired with diabetes duration of 1 to 5 years, and after 14 to 31 years of diabetes, the glucagon response is almost undetectable. It is not present in those with autonomic neuropathy. However, a syndrome of hypoglycemic autonomic failure occurs with intensification of diabetes control and repeated episodes of hypoglycemia. The exact mechanism is not understood, but it does represent a real barrier to physiologic glycemic control. In the absence of severe autonomic dysfunction, hypoglycemic awareness associated with hypoglycemia at least in part reversible.

Patients with hypoglycemia unawareness and unresponsiveness pose a significant management problem for the physician. Although autonomic neuropathy can improve with intensive therapy and normalization of blood glucose, there is a risk to the patient, who may become hypoglycemic without being aware of it and who cannot mount a counterregulatory response. It is our recommendation that if a pump is used, boluses of smaller than calculated amounts should be used. If intensive conventional therapy is used, long-acting insulin with very small boluses should be given. In general, too prevent hypoglycemia in these patients, normal glucose and Hb A_{1c} levels should not be goals.[730]

Further complicating management of some diabetic patients is the development of a functional autonomic insufficiency associated with intensive insulin treatment, which resembles autonomic neuropathy in all relevant aspects. In these instances, it is prudent to relax therapy, as for the patient with bona fide autonomic neuropathy. If hypoglycemia occurs in these patients at a certain glucose level, it will take a lower glucose level to trigger the same symptoms in the next 24 to 48 hours. Avoidance of hypoglycemia for a few days will result in recovery of the adrenergic response.

CORONARY HEART DISEASE

The last decades have been witness to substantial declines in coronary heart disease (CHD) mortality in the general population in the United States. The improvement in CHD mortality has been significantly lower in diabetic men and women.[731] More than 90% of all patients with diabetes have T2DM, and it is this population (mostly middle-aged and elderly) that has been evaluated in the most studies of CHD risk. In these studies, the excess morbidity and mortality associated with diabetes and elevated glucose remained even after adjustment for traditional CHD risk factors.

Effect of Diabetes on Risk of Coronary Heart Disease

The Framingham Study showed a twofold to threefold elevation in the risk of clinically evident atherosclerotic disease in patients with T2DM compared to those without diabetes.[608] Diabetic men in the Multiple Risk Factor Intervention Trial (MRFIT) had an absolute risk of CHD death more than three times higher than that in the nondiabetic cohort, even after adjustment for established risk factors.[47] Seminal work from Finland showed that patients with T2DM without a previous myocardial infarction have a risk of myocardial infarction (MI) over 7 years as high as nondiabetic patients with an MI (Fig. 32–48).[58] In this study, the case fatality rate following an MI was also substantially higher in patients with diabetes. In women, diabetes mitigates the cardioprotective effects of the premenopausal period, and women with diabetes had a CHD mortality rate as high as that in diabetic men.

The risk of cardiovascular mortality and events conferred by T2DM has been examined in several prospective and observational trials with varying populations of patients.[732-735] Prospective data from the Organization to Assess Strategies for Ischemic Syndromes (OASIS) registry was analyzed to determine the effect of diabetes on outcomes of patients with unstable angina and non–Q-wave MI.[732] Patients with diabetes had a significantly increased adjusted relative risk (RR) for total mortality (RR 1.57, 95% CI 1.38-1.81, $P < 0.001$), death due to cardiovascular disease (CVD) (RR 1.49, 95% CI 1.27-1.74, $P < 0.001$), new MI (RR 1.34, 95% CI 1.14-1.57, $P < 0.001$), stroke (RR 1.45, 95% CI 1.09-1.92, $P = 0.009$), and new congestive heart failure (CHF) (RR 1.41, 95% CI 1.24-1.60, $P < 0.001$). Diabetic patients without prior CVD had the same event rates for all outcomes as nondiabetic patients with previous vascular disease.

In another prospective cohort trial,[733] the adjusted hazard ratio (HR) for overall mortality in diabetic patients (n = 393) following a first MI was 1.5 (95% CI 1.1-2.0) compared with equivalent nondiabetic patients (n = 1132). The HR for cardiovascular mortality in diabetic patients was similar to that seen in nondiabetic patients who had experienced a previous MI. The risk of mortality from all causes was significantly higher in women than in men (adjusted HR 2.7 vs. 1.3, $P = 0.01$).

In contrast to these findings, two large observational trials have failed to find that diabetes confers equivalent or greater risk of mortality than previous MI.[735,736]

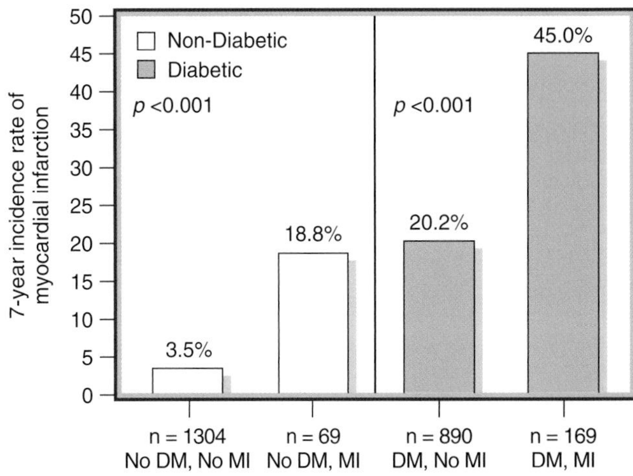

Figure 32–48 ■ Marked increase in the risk of coronary artery disease in patients with type 2 diabetes mellitus compared to nondiabetic subjects, in a population-based study in Finland, over a 7-year follow-up period. Patients with diabetes without a history of previous myocardial infarction had a risk of first myocardial infarction approximately equal to that of nondiabetic subjects who had already sustained a myocardial infarction. These data support recommendations from the American Diabetes Association to treat diabetic subjects as if they already have established coronary artery disease. DM, diabetes mellitus; MI, myocardial infarction. (From Haffner SM, Lehto S, Ronnemaa T, et al. Mortality from coronary heart disease in subjects with type 2 diabetes and in nondiabetic subjects with and without prior myocardial infarction. N Engl J Med 1998;339:229-234.)

In the cross-sectional study, RR for all-cause mortality was 1.33 (95% CI 1.14-1.55) for patients with MI compared to patients with type 2 diabetes. In the cohort study, patients with MI also had significantly higher risk of all-cause death (adjusted RR 1.35, 95% CI 1.25-1.44), cardiovascular death (RR 2.93, 95% CI 2.54-3.41), and hospital admission for MI (RR 3.1, 95% CI 2.57-3.73). Based on these findings, the authors concluded that established CVD confers greater risk than diabetes[734]

The risk of mortality conferred by diabetes has also been assessed in the Atherosclerosis Risk in Communities (ARIC) study, a population-based cohort study that has investigated the etiology of atherosclerosis in a biracial population in the United States.[735] Patients with prior MI had an adjusted RR of 1.9 (95% CI 1.35-2.56, $P<0.001$) for fatal CHD or nonfatal MI and adjusted RR of 1.8 (95% CI 1.22-2.72, $P=0.003$) for fatal CHD or nonfatal MI when compared to the patients with diabetes and no previous MI. There was no significant difference in the risk of stroke in the two groups.

Thus all these studies have demonstrated that diabetes alone results in a significantly increased risk of CVD. The strategy of considering diabetes as a CHD risk equivalent for purposes of assessing risk and defining a treatment regimen is appropriate.

The risk of CHD has also been evaluated in small subsets of patients with T1DM. In the Framingham study, the cumulative coronary artery disease mortality in patients with T1DM was approximately four times that of nondiabetic patients by age 55 years[736] Similar to patients with T2DM, the first deaths related to coronary artery disease in patients with T1DM generally occur by the fourth decade of life, and the cumulative mortality increases at a similar rate in both groups in the subsequent 20 years. The rise in coronary artery disease mortality with age in patients with T1DM is substantially higher in patients with nephropathy. In these patients, the risk of coronary artery disease can be as much as 15 times higher than in patients without persistent proteinuria. Thus, persistent proteinuria is a strong predictor of the development of coronary artery disease in this population. These findings suggest that proteinuria is a marker of generalized vascular damage that predisposes to CVD.

Two prospective epidemiologic studies, the Pittsburgh Epidemiology of Diabetes Complications study (EDC)[737] and Eurodiab,[738] a multicenter, clinic-based study in Europe, confirmed the Framingham findings and reported an incidence of total coronary events of 16% over 10 years and 9% over 7 years of follow-up in patients with T1DM. These incidence rates presumably reflect patients in their late 30s, 10 years beyond baseline age in the studies. In EDC, total coronary artery disease (CAD) incidence (including angina and ischemic ECG changes) was more than 2% per year for those older than 35 years. A more recent report, using 12-year follow-up data,[739] proposed that the annual rate of major CAD events (MI, fatal CAD, or revascularization) is 0.98% for those with diabetes duration of 20 to 30 years (aged, on average, 28-38 years). The event rates are identical for both genders, consistent with a loss of the protection from CHD mortality in premenopausal women with diabetes.

The recent follow-up of the Diabetes UK cohort, a group of 23,751 subjects with insulin-treated diabetes diagnosed at younger than 30 years, also shows similar mortality rates for men and women, and the size of this cohort permits robust gender-specific estimates of standardized mortality ratios (SMRs).[740] In those aged 20 to 29 years, the SMR for ischemic heart disease mortality was 11.8 in men and 44.8 in women; for those aged 30 to 39 years, the SMR was 8.0 and 41.6 in men and women, respectively. Other forms of CVD such as hypertension, valvular disease, cardiomyopathy, heart failure, and stroke were also increased.

It is unclear whether there has been any recent decline in mortality or morbidity from CHD associated with T1DM. The Pittsburgh EDC reported no difference in the cumulative incidence of CAD by 20, 25, or 30 years' duration according to year of diagnosis (1950-1980).[739] The benefits of improved diabetes care therefore do not appear to have reduced CAD mortality associated with T1DM.

Aggregation of Traditional Coronary Heart Disease Risk Factors in Diabetes

It is now well established that a number of traditional CHD risk factors (e.g., hypertension, dyslipidemia, obesity, insulin resistance) tend to occur together in patients with diabetes.[741] Approximately 50% of patients with diabetes have hypertension, and more than 30% have hypercholesterolemia at the time of diagnosis. As in nondiabetic patients, these risk factors independently predict the risk of CVD mortality[47] However, even in the presence of one or more concomitant risk factors, diabetes increases the CVD death rate (Fig. 32–49). It also appears that diabetes interacts synergistically with other risk factors to more sharply increase risk as the number of total risk factors increases.

There are data suggesting that the cardiovascular risk associated with T2DM is a consequence of insulin-resistance during the prediabetic state.[742] A population-based study of diabetes and cardiovascular disease followed Mexican American and non–Latin American white subjects for 7 years. These subjects who converted to diabetes from a prediabetic state and who were insulin resistant had higher BP, triglyceride levels, and lower HDL cholesterol levels. These CVD risk factors suggest that the atherogenic changes seen during the prediabetic state are primarily associated with increased insulin resistance and

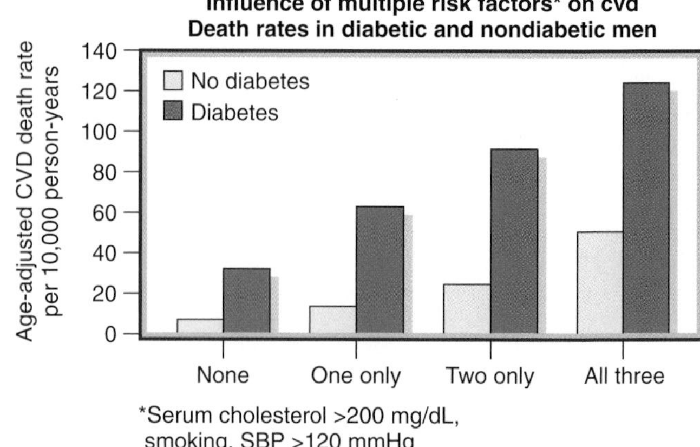

Figure 32–49 ■ Age-adjusted cardiovascular disease (CVD) death rates by presence of number of risk factors for men with and without diabetes at baseline screened for the Multiple Risk Factor Intervention Trial. In the presence of diabetes, the cardiovascular death rate steeply rises at any level of concomitant risk factors. SBP, systolic blood pressure. (From Stamler J, Vaccaro O, Neaton JD, et al. Diabetes, other risk factors, and 12-year cardiovascular mortality for men screened in the Multiple Risk Factor Intervention Trial. Diabetes Care 1993;16:434-444.)

that treatment strategies that increase insulin secretion in these patients can reduce cardiovascular risk.

Other studies have also concluded that impaired insulin sensitivity during the prediabetic state contributes to atherogenic risk.[743] Prediabetic subjects who were insulin resistant had higher levels of inflammatory markers (C-reactive protein [CRP], plasminogen activator inhibitor [PAI-1], and fibrinogen) than convertors with predominant low insulin secretion or nonconvertors. Thus a proinflammatory state can contribute to the atherogenic risk profile in prediabetic patients with increased insulin resistance. Evidence of inflammation is not seen in prediabetic patients with a primary defect in insulin secretion.

The UKPDS further confirms the importance of risk factor aggregation in diabetic patients. In this large population of patients with newly diagnosed T2DM, the development of coronary artery disease during follow-up was significantly associated with increased concentrations of LDL cholesterol, decreased concentrations of HDL cholesterol, increased levels of Hb A_{1c} and SBP, and a history of smoking as measured at baseline.[744]

Given the multifactorial nature of atherogenic risk in patients with T2DM, it is reasonable to conclude that an aggressive multifactorial intervention could significantly reduce cardiovascular risk. The value of such a treatment regimen has been tested in a recent study[513] In the Steno-2 study, 80 patients with T2DM and microalbuminuria were randomized to receive conventional treatment in accordance with national guidelines, and the outcomes compared with those of 80 similar patients who received intensive therapy that included behavior modification and targeted pharmacologic therapy for hyperglycemia, hypertension, dyslipidemia, and microalbuminuria along with secondary prevention of CVD with aspirin.

Over a mean follow-up period of 7.8 years, patients who received intensive treatment had greater improvements in glycosylated hemoglobin values, BP, fasting serum cholesterol and triglyceride values, and urinary albumin excretion than patients receiving conventional therapy. The greater degree of improvement in risk factors with intensive therapy was also reflected in outcomes. Patients receiving intensive therapy had a significantly lower risk of CVD (HR 0.47, 95% CI 0.24-0.73), nephropathy (HR 0.39, 95% CI 0.17-0.87), retinopathy (HR 0.42, 95% CI 0.21-0.86), and autonomic neuropathy (HR 0.37, 95% CI 0.18-

0.79). Overall, long-term intensive treatment of risk factors reduces the risk of CVD and microvascular events by about 50%.[513]

Plasma Glucose and Insulin Resistance as Independent Risk Factors for Atherosclerosis

Hyperglycemia may be responsible for the high excess risk of CHD that cannot be accounted for by the interaction of multiple risk factors alone. This association appears to be graded and continuous, without a clear threshold below which the relationship ends. One study showed that mortality from all causes, CVD, and ischemic heart disease increases progressively across quintiles of fasting blood glucose levels in patients with T2DM (Fig. 32–50).[745] Other data suggest a dose-response relationship between hyperglycemia and CVD mortality in diabetes, with patients with the highest levels of fasting blood glucose having a CVD mortality rate almost five times higher than patients with the two lowest levels combined.[746]

In the most recent study of the relationship of blood glucose and cardiovascular mortality, 17,869 male civil servants enrolled in the Whitehall Study in 1967 to 1969 were followed and outcomes were correlated with measurements of 2-hour postload blood glucose (2hBG) following a 50-g oral glucose load that were taken at baseline.[747] In these subjects, the HR for CHD mortality increased as a linear function of 2hBG for all values of 2hBG above 83 mg/dL. Between 2hBG values of 83 mg/dL and 200 mg/dL. the age-adjusted HR for CHD was 3.62 (95% CI 2.3-5.6).

Tominaga and colleagues examined survival rates in a cohort of participants in a diabetes prevalence trial in Japan[748] and concluded that the risk of cardiovascular mortality is based on impaired glucose tolerance rather than impaired fasting glucose.

Further substantiation of the role of impaired glucose tolerance in cardiovascular mortality risk was provided by an analysis of data from the Diabetes Epidemiology: Collaborative analysis of Diagnostic criteria in Europe (DECODE) study.[749] In this study, more than 25,000 men and women were followed for a mean of 7.3 years, and outcomes were correlated with measurements of fasting glucose and 2hBG following a 75-mg glucose load at baseline. The results indicated that the oral glucose tolerance test provides the best index of risk of mortality associated with impaired glucose tolerance.

The Nurses' Health Study also implicated the prediabetic state as a risk factor for cardiovascular disease.[750] In this large cohort of women, 5894 developed diabetes over a 20-year follow-up. In this group, the age-adjusted RR for MI was 3.75 (95% CI 3.10-4.53) in the period prior to diagnosis of diabetes and 4.57 (95% CI 3.87-5.39) after diagnosis compared to women who did not develop diabetes even after adjustment for other cardiovascular risk factors. The risk of stroke was also increased before onset of diabetes.

The continuum of CVD risk with rising glucose levels has also been identified in patients with T1DM[751] and in subjects without clinically overt diabetes but with varying levels of glucose intolerance.[752] Hyperglycemia also has adverse effects on the vessel wall as judged by objective assessment of carotid artery intima-media thickness (CIMT).[6,753-755]

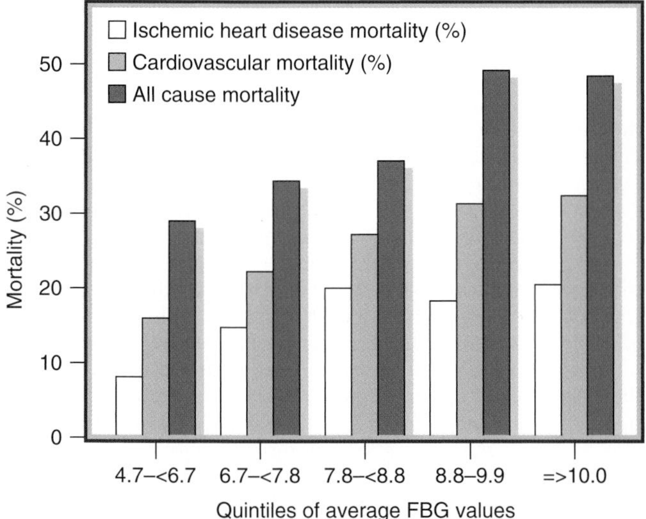

Figure 32–50 ▪ All-cause mortality, cardiovascular mortality, and ischemic heart disease mortality in patients with type 2 diabetes mellitus by quintiles of average fasting blood glucose (FBG). Cardiovascular mortality and all-cause mortality increase throughout the range of fasting plasma glucose in a graded fashion. (From Andersson DK, Svardsudd K. Long-term glycemic control relates to mortality in type II diabetes. Diabetes Care 1995;18:1534-1543.)

The Metabolic Syndrome

Definitions and Diagnosis

Almost all patients with diabetes and the concomitant CVD risk factors of hypertension, obesity, and dyslipidemia also have insulin resistance.[57] This clustering of these risk factors in a single patient has been termed *the metabolic syndrome.* Although there is general agreement on the components of the metabolic syndrome (obesity, hypertension, dyslipidemia, and dysfunctional glucose metabolism), the criteria for clinical diagnosis are still under discussion. Separate sets of diagnostic criteria for the metabolic syndrome have been published by the National Cholesterol Education Program (NCEP) Adult Treatment Panel III (ATP III),[756] by the World Health Organization (WHO),[757] and by the International Diabetes Federation (IDF).[758]

According to the NCEP guidelines, the metabolic syndrome is based on the presence of three of the following five risk factors[756]:

- Abdominal obesity (waist circumference >40 inches in men, >35 inches in women)
- Plasma triglycerides 150 mg/dL
- Plasma HDL cholesterol less than 40 mg/dL in men and less than 50 mg/dL in women
- Blood pressure 130/85 mm Hg
- Fasting plasma glucose 110 mg/dL

The NCEP criteria give precedence to obesity as a contributor to the metabolic syndrome and apply cutpoints for triglycerides and HDL that are probably less stringent than would be used to identify a categorical risk factor, reflecting the fact that many marginal risk factors can result in a significant risk for CVD. The NCEP criteria do not require explicit demonstration of insulin resistance for diagnosis of the metabolic syndrome, and patients with diabetes are not excluded from the diagnosis.[757] There are modest differences between the NCEP criteria and those developed by the WHO[757] and the IDF.[758]

Epidemiology

The prevalence of the metabolic syndrome in the Unites States, as defined by the NCEP criteria, has been estimated using the National Health and Nutrition Examination Survey (NHANES) database.[759] Based on data from the third NHANES (1988-1994) survey, the overall age-adjusted prevalence of the metabolic syndrome was 23.7%. The prevalence increased with age, ranging from 6.7% in subjects aged 20 to 29 years to 43.5% in subjects aged 60 to 69 years. There were also differences in prevalence based on ethnicity, with the highest prevalence in Mexican Americans (31.9%).

The Metabolic Syndrome and Cardiovascular Disease

The impact of metabolic syndrome on incidence and mortality of cardiovascular disease has been examined in several studies.[760-762] A Finnish prospective cohort study showed the age-adjusted RR for CHD mortality was 2.96 (95% CI1.30-6.76) compared to those without this condition. Similar increases in risk were also noted for CVD mortality (RR 2.76, 95% CI 1.45-5.24) and all-cause mortality (RR 2.05, 95% CI 1.31-3.21). Similar degrees of increase in risk with the metabolic syndrome were also seen when other diagnostic criteria were used.

In the United States, NHANES II studied the impact of the metabolic syndrome on CVD mortality.[763] The HRs for CHD mortality and CVD mortality were 1.65 (95% CI1.10-2.47, P = 0.02) and 1.56 (95% CI 1.15-2.12, P = 0.005), respectively, compared to subjects without the metabolic syndrome.

The West of Scotland Coronary Prevention Study[846] also demonstrated increased risk of CHD in the metabolic syndrome. In this study, elevated CRP was more common in subjects with the metabolic syndrome and added to prognostic value for both CHD and diabetes.

A summary of all of the studies that assessed the increased risk of mortality, cardiovascular disease, and diabetes associated with the metabolic syndrome has also been published.[763] Studies that used NCEP and WHO diagnostic criteria for defining the metabolic syndrome were analyzed separately. For three studies that used the exact NCEP definition of the metabolic syndrome, the increased risk of all-cause mortality was not significant. For seven studies that used the NCEP definition, the RR for CVD was 1.65 (95% CI 1.38-1.99). Inclusion of four other studies that used a modified NCEP definition did not appreciably change the RR. In four studies that used the NCEP definition, the RR for diabetes was 2.99 (95% CI 1.96-4.57). For studies that used the most exact WHO definition of the metabolic syndrome, the fixed-effects estimates of RR were 1.37 (95% CI 1.09-1.74) for all-cause mortality, 1.93 (95% CI 1.39-2.67) for cardiovascular disease, and 6.08 (95% CI 4.76-7.76) for diabetes.

Clinical guidelines for diagnosis and management of the metabolic syndrome have been addressed in a recent joint statement by the American Heart Association and the National Heart, Lung, and Blood Institute summarizing currently available steps for managing the risk factors associated with the metabolic syndrome.[764]

It has been hypothesized that hyperinsulinemia is the underlying link between hyperglycemia and CVD in these patients.[765] A number of studies have shown hyperinsulinemia to be an independent predictor of CVD risk. Furthermore, in patients spanning the spectrum of glucose tolerance, from normal to hyperglycemic to diabetic, insulin resistance positively correlates with atherosclerosis as assessed by CIMT.[766]

The San Antonio Heart Study, a population-based study of diabetes and CVD in Mexican Americans and non–Latin American whites, confirmed the relationship between insulin resistance and plasma insulin to CVD.[63]

The Role of Glycemic Control

The UKPDS confirmed the positive association between plasma glucose levels and CHD risk for Hb A_{1c} levels greater than 6.2% in patients with diabetes.[765] CHD risk increased by 11% with each one percentage point elevation in Hb A_{1c} (Table 32–13). The question remains, however, whether intensive glycemic control can modify the cardiovascular risk profile of patients with diabetes.

TABLE 32–13 TREATMENT GOALS FOR PREVENTION OF CORONARY HEART DISEASE IN PATIENTS WITH DIABETES

Hemoglobin A_{1c} ≤6.2%
Low-density lipoprotein cholesterol ≤100 mg/dL
Blood pressure ≤130/85 mm Hg
Aspirin 81-325 mg/day

Earlier studies, such as the DCCT and the smaller Veterans Affairs (VA) study, did not show a reduction in cardiovascular end-points with intensive metabolic control. These studies had limitations, however. Although relatively large (N = 1441), the DCCT followed a relatively young (mean age, 27 years) population of patients with T1DM for more than 6 years. At the end of follow-up, few events had occurred.[2] Intensive therapy reduced the risk of cardiovascular and peripheral vascular by 41% compared to conventional therapy, although the difference was not statistically significant. Similarly, in the VA study, intensive blood glucose control in patients with T2DM did not significantly reduce cardiovascular end-points.[767] Both studies lacked adequate power to detect a difference in macrovascular events between treatment groups because of the small number of events in each group, small patient populations, and relatively short follow-up.

A recent follow-up for 17 years of 1441 patients from the DCCT trial more unambiguously demonstrated the benefit of intensive glycemic control in T1DM.[768] This is part of the observational Epidemiology of Diabetes Interventions and Complications (EDIC) study. During follow-up, intensive treatment reduced the risk of cardiovascular disease by 42% (P = 0.02) and the risk of nonfatal MI, stroke, or death from CVD by 57% (P = 0.02). After 11 years of follow-up, both treatment groups were virtually identical in terms of Hb A_{1c}, BP, and lipid risk factors. Patients in the conventional treatment group had more albuminuria and microalbuminuria than intensively treated patients, but the differences in risk remained significant after adjusting for these factors. These findings indicate that intensive glycemic control reduced the long-term risk of CVD in patients with T1DM.

The UKPDS was larger and adequately powered to detect a difference between groups in macrovascular events.[3] Intensive glycemic control trended toward demonstrating a lower rate of myocardial infarction than conventional treatment (P = .052).[3] As in the DCCT, intensive therapy in the UKPDS significantly improved the rate of microvascular disease.

Despite the lack of overall efficacy of intensive treatment for managing macrovascular complications of diabetes in the UKPDS, there are indications that specific therapies may be effective.[3] In a retrospective analysis of an overweight subset (n = 342) of the UKPDS cohort who were treated with metformin, there were significant reductions in the occurrence of any diabetes-related end-point (32%), diabetes-related death (42%), and all-cause mortality (36%) compared with conventionally treated patients.

Two studies have suggested that thiazolidinediones can also prevent macrovascular events associated with T2DM. Sidhu and colleagues demonstrated that 8 weeks of treatment with rosiglitazone 4 mg daily significantly reduced progression of thickening of the common carotid intima-media, a surrogate index of atherosclerotic disease progression, compared to placebo treatment in nondiabetic patients with established coronary artery disease.[766]

In the PROactive study (PROspective pioglitAzone Clinical Trial In macroVascular Events), 5238 patients with T2DM and evidence of macrovascular disease were randomized to receive pioglitazone in addition to glucose-lowering drugs and other medications.[769] After a mean of 34.5 months there was no significant difference in the two treatment groups in terms of the primary end-point of the study, a composite of all-cause mortality, nonfatal MI, stroke, acute coronary syndrome, surgical intervention in the leg or coronary arteries, or amputation above the ankle. Patients treated with pioglitazone had significantly lower risk for the secondary end-point of composite all-cause mortality, nonfatal MI, and stroke, however (HR 0.84, 95% CI 0.80-1.02, $P = 0.027$). Pioglitazone also significantly reduced the need to add insulin to glucose-lowering regimens compared to placebo-treated patients.

Dyslipidemia and Its Treatment in Patients with Diabetes Mellitus

Dyslipidemia is the best-characterized risk factor for increasing atherosclerosis in patients with T2DM. A number of features of dyslipidemia are uniquely associated with diabetes and appear to increase the predisposition to atherogenesis. Although patients with diabetes tend not to have marked elevations in plasma LDL cholesterol levels, LDL cholesterol particles in patients with diabetes are generally smaller and more dense than typical LDL cholesterol particles. These small, dense LDL cholesterol particles are more susceptible to oxidation, particularly in the setting of poor glucose control. Other evidence suggests that glycation of LDL may be enhanced in diabetes, impairing recognition of the lipoprotein by its hepatoreceptor and extending its half-life. Conversely, levels of the cardioprotective lipid fraction, HDL cholesterol, are decreased in patients with diabetes. The HDL cholesterol of these patients might also be less effective at protecting LDL cholesterol from oxidative stress, one of the proposed mechanisms for the cardioprotective effect of HDL cholesterol.[770]

Undoubtedly, the key feature of diabetic dyslipidemia is an increase in the production of very low density lipoprotein (VLDL) by the liver in response to elevations in FFAs. Although insulin mediates the uptake of FFAs by striated muscle, reducing the levels presented to the liver, insulin resistance results in the opposite effect, increasing the levels of FFAs available to the liver. The metabolic syndrome, with its characteristic abdominal obesity, also increases the delivery of FFAs to the liver. In addition, reduced lipoprotein lipase activity in T2DM leads to an accumulation of triglyceride-rich lipoproteins in the plasma of these patients. Triglyceride-rich lipoproteins also play a role in the reduced levels of HDL cholesterol by increasing the transfer of cholesterol from these particles.

A number of landmark trials have proved that lowering lipid levels produces major clinical benefits in terms of reducing cardiovascular events in patients with and without a history of CHD at baseline. These findings have now been extended to the population of subjects with T2DM and dyslipidemia. For example, even though LDL levels are often within the average range in these patients, treatment with hydroxymethylglutaryl coenzyme A reductase inhibitors (statins) has been shown to improve outcomes. In the Cholesterol and Recurrent Events (CARE) trial, diabetic patients treated with pravastatin had a significant 25% reduction in the incidence of CHD death, nonfatal myocardial infarction, coronary artery bypass graft surgery, and revascularization procedures.[7] In the Long-term Intervention with Pravastatin in Ischemic Disease (LIPID) study, patients with diabetes had a 19% reduction in major CHD (fatal CHD and nonfatal myocardial infarction).[771]

In a post hoc subgroup analysis of secondary prevention in a large cohort of patients with diabetes, impaired glucose tolerance, or normal glucose tolerance, simvastatin normalized associated elevations in total cholesterol and triglycerides across the range of glucose values.[772] Treatment also significantly reduced major coronary events and revascularizations in patients with diabetes and reduced major coronary events, revascularizations, and total and coronary mortality in patients with impaired glucose tolerance.

Several more-recent studies have further verified the use of statins in patients with diabetes and related conditions.[773-777] In the Heart Protection Study, a large (N = 20,536) randomized, placebo-controlled trial of the use of simvastatin 40 mg in high-risk patients, roughly 29% of the study participants had T2DM.[778] Over the 5-year course of the study, treatment with simvastatin resulted in a significant reduction in the occurrence of major vascular events in type 2 diabetics who had previous MI or other coronary heart disease (33.4% versus 37.8% in simvastatin- and placebo-treated patients, respectively), in diabetics with no prior CHD (13.8% vs. 18.6%), and in both categories combined (20.2% versus 25.1%). Overall, the study also demonstrated a highly significant 12% relative risk reduction in all-cause mortality and 18% relative risk reduction in coronary mortality in all subjects treated with simvastatin.

The Collaborative Atorvastatin Diabetes Study (CARDS) was a large (N = 2838) randomized, placebo-controlled trial that assessed the benefit of atorvastatin 10 mg/day for preventing acute coronary heart disease events, coronary revascularization, or stroke in patients with T2DM who had no documented history of CVD and plasma LDL levels of <160 mg/dL.[779] The trial was terminated 2 years early because prespecified efficacy criteria were met. After a median of 3.9 years follow-up, patients treated with atorvastatin had a relative risk reduction of first cardiovascular events of 37% (95% CI -52, -17; $P = 0.001$) compared with placebo-treated patients. Assessed separately, acute coronary heart disease, coronary revascularizations, and stroke were significantly reduced by 36%, 31%, and 48%, respectively. Based on these results, the CARDS investigators concluded that in patents with T2DM, a threshold LDL cholesterol level should not be the sole determinant of whether a statin is prescribed.

A post hoc study compared major coronary events, total mortality, and revascularization rates in two subsets of patients who received simvastatin 20 to 40 mg/day for a median of 5.4 years in the Scandinavian Simvastatin Survival Study (4S).[773] Treatment with simvastatin resulted in a 52% RR reduction of major coronary events, a greater treatment effect than was seen in the patients with isolated high LDL cholesterol. Reanalysis of the data after exclusion of the patients with diabetes did not substantially alter the findings.

The Treating to New Targets (TNT) study compared the effects of atorvastatin 10 mg or 80 mg daily for a median follow-up period of 4.9 years in patients with clinically evident CHD who also met the NCEP criteria for diagnosis of the metabolic syndrome.[774] The study included 778 patients with T2DM, who constituted 22% of the study population. Treatment with atorvastatin 80 mg was significantly more effective for reducing major cardiovascular events than atorvastatin 10 mg (HR = 0.71, 95% CI 0.61-0.84, $P < 0.0001$), presumably due to the significantly greater reduction in LDL cholesterol seen with the higher dosing of atorvastatin.

The Arterial Biology for the Investigation of the Treatment Effects of Reducing Cholesterol (ARBITER)[775] was a randomized, double-blind study in which patients were assigned to receive extended-release niacin 500 mg titrated to 1000 mg qd (n = 87) or placebo (n = 80) on a background statin therapy. The primary end-point of the study was change in CIMT after 1 year of niacin treatment. Despite a significant 21% increase in HDL cholesterol levels in the patients receiving niacin, the overall difference in CIMT progression between the niacin- and placebo-treated groups only tended toward significance (P = 0.08).

Fibric acid derivatives might also be beneficial in patients with diabetes, because these agents address the low HDL cholesterol and high triglyceride levels typically associated with diabetes. In the VA High-Density Lipoprotein Cholesterol Intervention Trial (VA-HIT), men given gemfibrozil had lower rates of coronary events and strokes.[776] A fibric acid derivative in combination with a statin may be the optimal approach in patients with diabetes and CHD who have hypercholesterolemia in association with elevated triglycerides and reduced HDL cholesterol levels.

The Fenofibrate Intervention and Event Lowering in Diabetes (FIELD) study assessed the effect of long-term fenofibrate therapy on cardiovascular events in patients with T2DM.[777] Patients were randomized to receive either micronized fenofibrate 200 mg qd (n = 4895) or placebo (n = 4900). During 5-year follow-up, 5.9% of the placebo patients and 5.2 % of the fenofibrate patients had a coronary event, a difference that was not significantly different. Fenofibrate therapy significantly reduced total CVD events (HR 0.89, 95% CI 0.75-1.05, P = 0.035), progression of albuminuria, and the need for laser treatment of retinopathy. Statistical significance for the primary end-point of the study might have been missed because a greater percentage of patients in the placebo group initiated lipid-lowering therapy during the study period, and this masked the treatment effect.

The importance of dyslipidemia as a contributor to cardiovascular risk in patients with diabetes is reflected in the new guidelines of the NCEP ATP III.[756] For the first time, diabetes is considered a CHD risk equivalent, meaning that patients with diabetes have a risk of CHD that is similar to that in patients with clinically manifest CHD (>20% risk of an event in the following 10 years). In addition, the presence of multiple CHD risk factors, theh metabolic syndrome, and mixed hyperlipidemia (high triglyceride and low HDL cholesterol levels) all should be taken into account when estimating a patient's global risk.

According to the NCEP ATP III guidelines, diabetic patients are candidates for cholesterol-lowering therapy if the LDL cholesterol level is higher than 3.36 mM/L (130 mg/dL) (with the goal of reducing LDL cholesterol to <2.57 mM/L [100 mg/dL]),[758] although many clinicians consider it prudent to approach therapy more aggressively by instituting drug treatment if the LDL cholesterol level is higher than 2.57 mM/L (100 mg/dL). Based on new trial information, these guidelines have been modified to state that when risk is very high, an LDL cholesterol goal of lower than 70 mg/dL is a reasonable clinical strategy, even when the high-risk patient has a baseline LDL cholesterol of less than 100 mg/dL.[780] Additionally, when a high-risk patient has low HDL cholesterol or high triglycerides, combining niacin or a fibrate with an LDL-lowering drug should be considered. However, regardless of the drug regimen employed, patients with diabetes should maintain tight glycemic control, which in itself can help reverse the dyslipidemic profile prevalent in diabetes. As with all patients, lifestyle modification, including weight reduction and regular exercise, remains an important cornerstone of treating dyslipidemia in patients with diabetes.

Signature Features and Treatment of Hypertension in Diabetic Patients

It has been estimated that up to 50% of patients with newly diagnosed diabetes also have high BP. As with dyslipidemia, hypertension interacts with diabetes to amplify the risk of cardiac mortality (see Fig. 32–49). Although the etiology of hypertension is multifactorial, the insulin-resistant state is one factor postulated to predispose patients to develop hypertension. In addition to its negative effects on the cardiovascular system, high BP is a key contributor to the development of microvascular disease in diabetes. Based on the guidelines of the Joint National Committee on Prevention, Detection, Evaluation, and Treatment of High Blood Pressure (JNC VII), BP should be reduced to be less than 130/85 mm Hg in patients with diabetes.[781]

Results of the most recent clinical trials underscore the benefits of aggressive treatment of hypertension in patients with diabetes, although none of these studies achieved mean BP reductions to currently recommended targets. A long-acting dihydropyridine calcium channel blocker in the Systolic Hypertension in Europe (Syst-Eur) study resulted in substantial reductions in total mortality (55%), cardiovascular mortality (76%), and cardiovascular events (69%) in the diabetic subgroup, greater benefits than were seen in the subgroup without diabetes.[782]

In the Heart Outcomes Prevention Evaluation (HOPE) study, in which almost 40% of patients had diabetes and one other cardiovascular risk factor, ramipril reduced the primary outcome by 24% and total mortality by 25%.[783] Even in normotensive patients with diabetes, some benefit was seen, with a 2- to 4-mm Hg drop in BP with ACE inhibitor therapy.

Other rigorously designed studies, such as the UKPDS[784] and the Hypertension Optimal Treatment (HOT) study,[785] suggest even greater benefits from tight BP control in patients with diabetes.

In the Losartan Intervention for Endpoint Reduction in Hypertension (LIFE) study, patients with diabetes, hypertension, and signs of left ventricular hypertrophy (LVH) were randomly assigned to treatment with losartan-based (n=586) or atenolol-based (n=609) treatment for hypertension.[786] Despite similar BP reductions, losartan was more effective than atenolol for reducing cardiovascular morbidity and mortality, mortality from cardiovascular disease, and mortality from all causes. The ability of losartan to reduce events more effectively than atenolol may be related to the ability of ARBs to reverse LVH more effectively than β-blockers.

Although β-blockers are thought to worsen glycemic control in patients with diabetes, it is not clear if this is a property of all members of this drug class and if this property persists if β-blockers are given in combination with renin-angiotensin system inhibitors that are known to increase insulin sensitivity. In the Glycemic Effects in Diabetes Mellitus: Carvdeilol-Metoprolol Comparison in Hypertensives (GEMINI) trial, patients with documented T2DM and hypertension who were taking a stable dose of either an ARB or an ACE inhibitor were randomized to receive either carvedilol or metoprolol. Although the degree of BP control was similar with both β-blockers, Hb A_{1c} and insulin sensitivity increased significantly with metoprolol but not with carvedilol. Thus, carvedilol can prevent the adverse effects of metoprolol on glucose levels when used in combination with renin-angiotensin system inhibitors, although this conclusion needs to be tested in a longer-term outcome trial.

The investigators of the Antihypertensive and Lipid-Lowering Treatment to Prevent Heart Attack Trial (ALLHAT) have recently compared outcomes during first-step treatment of hypertension in 31,512 patients with T2DM, IFG, or normoglycemia with a calcium channel blocker (CCB; amlodipine 2.5-10 mg/day) or ACE inhibitor (lisinopril 10-40 mg/day) compared with a thiazide-type diuretic (chlorthalidone 12.5-25 mg/day).[786] There was no significant difference in the occurrence of the primary outcome (fatal coronary heart disease or nonfatal MI) in patients with T2DM treated with CCB or ACE inhibitor compared with chlorthalidone. Patients with IFG treated with CCB had a significantly higher RR for the primary outcome than patients receiving chlorthalidone.

Acute Coronary Syndromes in Diabetes Mellitus

The case fatality rate from MI is nearly twice as high in patients with diabetes as in nondiabetic patients. This excess risk is seen both during the acute phase of MI and in the early and late postinfarction period. A number of mechanisms have been responsible for worse outcomes in patients with diabetes, including:

- Increased risk of congestive failure (CHF) due to maladaptive remodeling of the left ventricle[787-789]
- Increased risk of sudden death due to sympathovagal imbalance as a consequence of autonomic neuropathy[790-792]
- Increased likelihood of early reinfarction due to impaired fibrinolysis[793-795]
- Extensive underlying coronary artery disease[796,797]
- Changes in myocardial cell metabolism, including a shift from glucose oxidation to FFA oxidation, with less generation of ATP at any level of oxygen consumption[798,799]
- Associated cardiomyopathy.[706]

Collective data provide strong evidence that a variety of treatment modalities can improve outcomes from myocardial infarction in patients with diabetes. In terms of interventions, patients with diabetes experiencing an acute myocardial infarction respond as favorably to fibrinolytic therapy as do nondiabetic patients.[41,796,797] Excellent glycemic control is an essential component of overall management. Glucose levels at hospital admission have been independently correlated with early and late mortality after MI in patients both with and without diabetes mellitus.[800-803]

Studies such as the Diabetes and Insulin-Glucose Infusion in Acute Myocardial Infarction (DIGAMI) study have assessed the impact of intensive glycemic control in patients with diabetes during the acute phase of MI. Patients in this study were randomized to either intensive insulin therapy (insulin-glucose infusion for 24 hours, followed by subcutaneous insulin injection for 3 months) or standard glycemic control.[804] The intensive insulin regimen lowered blood glucose level during the first hour after admission and at discharge compared with conventional therapy. One-year mortality was significantly reduced with the insulin infusion compared with control, a difference that was maintained after 3.4 years of follow-up.

A recent follow-up to DIGAMI, DIGAMI 2, a prospective randomized open-label trial, compared outcomes in patients with either T1DM or T2DM and failed to corroborate the improvement in outcomes with intensive insulin treatment.[805] The lack of effect of long-term insulin treatment on outcomes may be at least partially explained by the fact that 14% of the patients in the conventional treatment group received insulin-glucose infusions in violation of the protocol, and as many as 41% had extra glucose injections. As a result, the blood glucose levels in all three groups were not significantly different following treatment.

Although the mechanism(s) responsible for the potential benefit shown in the original DEGAMI study are not entirely clear, experimental data suggest that strict glycemic control can improve myocardial cell metabolism by increasing the availability of glucose as a substrate for ATP generation and reducing the formation of FFAs, thereby shifting cardiac metabolism from FFA oxidation to glycolysis and glucose oxidation. Intensive glycemic control can also reverse the impaired fibrinolysis that is typically seen in patients with diabetes.

The CREATE-ECLA (Clinical Trial of Reviparin and Metabolic Modulation in Acute Myocardial Infarction Treatment Evaluation—Estudios Cardiologicos Latin America) randomized, controlled trial randomized 20,201 patients who presented with ST-segment elevation MI within 12 hours of onset of symptoms to treatment with high-dose GIK (25% glucose, 50 U/L regular insulin, and 80 m/Eq KCl) infused over 24 hours or to usual care.[806] Roughly 18% of the patients in both treatment arms had T2DM. After 30 days, there were no differences in the rate of occurrence of mortality, cardiac arrest, cardiogenic shock, or reinfarction in the two treatment groups.

Sulfonylureas have been implicated in an increase in cardiovascular mortality, particularly in patients undergoing revascularization for acute MI.[807] The UKPDS did not show a deleterious effect of these agents on the incidence of sudden death or MI over 10 years of follow-up.[3] The sulfonylureas act through the sulfonylurea receptor component of ATP-sensitive potassium channels in the pancreatic beta cell. In the heart, ATP-sensitive potassium channels are involved in ischemic preconditioning and coronary vasodilation.[808-810] It is not clear if the sulfonylureas modulate these channels in the heart or vascular system or if they significantly increase risk in diabetic patients with an acute MI.

ACE inhibitors dramatically reduce mortality following an MI in patients with diabetes, ostensibly through their effects to reduce infarct size and limit ventricular remodeling. In addition to these hemodynamic benefits, ACE inhibitors can also improve outcomes in diabetes by improving endothelial function,[811] improving fibrinolysis,[812] and decreasing insulin resistance.[813]

In a retrospective analysis of the Gruppo Italiano per lo Studio della Sopravvivenza nell'Infarto Miocardico (GISSI-3) study,[814] lisinopril administration within 24 hours of hospital admission substantially reduced both 6-week and 6-month mortality in patients with diabetes compared with the nondiabetic group. Similarly, a subgroup analysis from the Trandolapril Cardiac Evaluation Study (TRACE) showed that patients with diabetes suffering an anterior myocardial infarction treated with trandolapril had greatly improved outcomes over 5 years compared with patients without diabetes, including a nearly 50% reduction in the risk of sudden death, reinfarction, and progression of CHF.[815]

β-Blockers are now widely accepted for the treatment of acute coronary syndrome in patients with diabetes. Older, noncardioselective β-blockers might have adversely affected the lipid profile and inhibited the metabolic response to hypoglycemia, but more recent data with cardioselective β-blockers suggest these agents have less negative effect on metabolic indices, perhaps because they increase peripheral blood flow and improve glucose delivery.[816,817] Clinical trial data confirm that β-blockers reduce the rates of mortality and reinfarction in patients with myocardial infarction in the presence of diabetes. In fact, their effects in patients with diabetes appear to exceed those seen in nondiabetic patients. A large review of data from more than 45,000 patients, 26% of whom had diabetes, showed that β-blocker therapy was associated with a lower 1-year mortality rate in patients with diabetes than in those without diabetes, with no evidence of an increase in diabetes-related complications.[818]

Postulated mechanisms for the benefit of β-blockers in patients with diabetes include dampening of the sympathetic nervous system overactivity that arises as a consequence of autonomic neuropathy. β-Blockers can also reduce FFA levels and thereby reduce myocardial oxygen requirements. Carvedilol, although not cardioselective, is a β-blocker that decreases insulin resistance and also has antioxidant effects, both of which may be of particular benefit in patients with T2DM.[819]

Aspirin is a cornerstone of therapy for the primary or secondary prevention of acute coronary syndrome in patients with T1DM and T2DM who do not have contraindications to its use. Aspirin significantly lowers the risk of myocardial infarction without increasing the risk of vitreous or retinal bleeding, even in patients with retinopathy.[820] Enteric-coated aspirin, 81 to

325 mg/day, is currently recommended by the American Diabetes Association.[821] The benefits of this therapy are likely due to effects on the enhanced platelet aggregation evident in patients with either T1DM or T2DM.[822]

Antiplatelet therapy with clopidogrel also benefits patients with diabetes. The CAPRIE trial compared outcomes in patients with non-ST-segment elevation MI treated with aspirin or clopidogrel and included 3866 patients with diabetes.[823] Although the event rate was higher in the diabetic patients than in the overall study population, the response to treatment was also better. The event rate for the primary end-point (vascular death, ischemic stroke, MI, or rehospitalization for ischemia or bleeding) was 17.7% for diabetic patients treated with aspirin and 15.6% for those randomized to clopidogrel, a significant relative risk reduction of 12.5%.

Newer adjunct therapies, such as the platelet glycoprotein IIb/IIIa receptor antagonists that antagonize platelet action, have also been assessed in diabetic patients who present with unstable angina or non–Q-wave infarction. Overall, these agents appear to work equally well, or perhaps slightly better, in patients with diabetes as in nondiabetic patients.

In the Platelet Receptor Inhibition in Ischemic Syndrome Management in Patients Limited by Unstable Signs and Symptoms (PRISM-PLUS) study, the addition of tirofiban to heparin therapy reduced the 7-day composite end-point compared with heparin alone. This effect was greater in patients with diabetes than in patients without diabetes.[824]

In one study of patients undergoing percutaneous transluminal coronary angioplasty (PTCA), glycoprotein IIb/IIIa antagonist therapy was associated with fewer acute events but a higher rate of target-vessel revascularization in the long term in the diabetic cohort compared with the nondiabetic cohort.[825] In another trial, however, in which stents were used, the rate of target vessel revascularization at 6 months was significantly decreased with the addition of a glycoprotein IIb/IIIa antagonist compared with placebo.[826]

Results of the Bypass Angioplasty Revascularization Investigation (BARI) showed that coronary bypass graft surgery provides better outcomes than PTCA in patients with diabetes, possibly as a result of addressing the extensive coronary vascular disease in these patients[827] This study did not employ stents or glycoprotein IIb/IIIa inhibitors, two modalities that, when used together, appear to improve outcomes after PTCA in patients with diabetes.

Cardiomyopathy in Patients with Diabetes Mellitus

Diabetes is associated with a fourfold increase in the risk of CHF, even after adjustment for other cardiovascular risk factors such as age, BP, cholesterol level, obesity, and history of coronary artery disease.[828] Patients with diabetes experience higher rates of CHF than nondiabetic patients following an acute MI, regardless of the size of the infarct zone.[788,829] These findings suggest that diabetes itself causes deleterious effects on the myocardium, leading to poorer outcomes.

A number of key structural, functional, and metabolic factors in diabetes have been implicated in the increased risk of maladaptive remodeling that leads to CHF. For example, evidence of silent myocardial infarction is found in up to 40% of patients with diabetes presenting with a clinically apparent MI and can lead to unrecognized regional and global ventricular dysfunction.[814,830] As many as 50% of patients with diabetes and coronary artery disease have cardiac autonomic neuropathy, which is known to contribute to both systolic and diastolic dysfunction.[706] Like hypertension, diabetes can cause fibrosis of the myocardium and increased collagen deposition.[831,832] These effects are even more pronounced in patients with coexisting hypertension and diabetes. Enhanced endothelial dysfunction in diabetes has also been described as a pathophysiologic pathway to impaired microvascular perfusion and ischemia.[833,834]

On a cellular level, both hyperglycemia and insulin resistance have direct negative effects on myocardial metabolism. Depression of myocardial GLUT4 transporter protein levels in the setting of diabetes and ischemia inhibits glucose entry and glycolysis in the heart. As a result, intracellular metabolism shifts from glycolysis to FFA oxidation, thereby suppressing glycolytic ATP generation, a major source of energy under anaerobic (i.e., ischemic) conditions.[798] The production of oxygen free radicals can also be enhanced in this situation, further depressing myocardial contractile function.[834]

Collectively, these various abnormalities potentiate the characteristic left ventricular remodeling of diabetes, clinically manifested as serial wall motion changes, reduced regional ejection fraction, and increased end-diastolic and end-systolic volumes.[835,836]

THE DIABETIC FOOT

Of all the late complications of diabetes, foot problems are probably the most preventable. Thus, Joslin, who wrote in 1934 that "diabetic gangrene is not heaven-sent, but earth-born," was correct: The development of foot ulceration mostly results from the way we care for our patients or the way patients care for themselves.

Increasing interest in the diabetic foot has resulted in a better understanding of the factors that interact to cause ulceration and amputation. The neuropathic foot does not spontaneously ulcerate; insensitivity in combination with other factors, such as deformity and unperceived trauma (e.g., inappropriate footwear), leads to skin breakdown. This increase in the knowledge of pathogenesis should permit the design of appropriate screening programs for risk and preventive education. Much progress has been made, but it has not yet resulted in a universal decrease in amputation rates. In the VA system, for example, amputation rates in diabetic patients[837] have not declined; certain European countries have, however, reported a significant reduction in amputation rates following implementation of foot screening programs.[838,839] Thus, much research is still needed to implement strategies to reduce ulceration and amputation, and this is particularly required in the fields of behavioral and psychosocial aspects of the diabetic foot.[840]

Two major texts on the diabetic foot were published in 2006.[840,841] The reader is referred to these sources together with other major recent review articles[842,843] for more detailed discussion of this topic.

Epidemiology and Pathogenesis of Diabetic Foot Ulceration

Foot ulceration is common and occurs in both T1DM and T2DM. Approximately 5% to 10% of diabetic patients have had past or present foot ulceration, and 1% have undergone amputation.[840] Diabetes is the most common cause of nontrauma lower limb amputation in the United States, and rates are15 times those in the nondiabetic population. More than 80% of amputations are preceded by foot ulcers. A large community-based study in the United Kingdom showed an annual incidence of ulceration of approximately 2%; this rises to 7% in those with known diabetic neuropathy and is as high as 50% in those with a past history of ulceration.[842] The lifetime risk of a diabetic patient developing a foot ulcer is estimated to be as high as 25%.[843]

Pathway to Ulceration

Foot ulceration results from an interaction of a number of component causes, none of which alone is sufficient to cause ulceration but, when combined, complete the causal pathway to skin breakdown. Knowledge of these component causes and their potential to interact facilitates the design of preventive foot care programs.

Diabetic Neuropathy

All three components of neuropathy—sensory, motor, and autonomic—can contribute to ulceration in the foot. Chronic sensorimotor neuropathy is common, affecting at least one third of older patients in Western countries. Its onset is gradual and insidious, and symptoms may be so minimal that they go unnoticed by some patients. Although in some patients uncomfortable, painful, and paresthetic symptoms predominate, some patients never experience symptoms. Clinical examination usually reveals a sensory deficit in a glove-and-stocking distribution, with signs of motor dysfunction, such as small muscle wasting in the feet and absent ankle reflexes. Thus, although a history of typical symptoms strongly suggests a diagnosis of neuropathy, *absence of symptoms does not exclude the diagnosis* and must *never* be equated with a lack of foot ulcer risk. Therefore, assessment of the foot ulcer risk must always include a careful foot examination, whatever the history.

Sympathetic autonomic neuropathy affecting the lower limbs results in reduced sweating, dry skin, and development of cracks and fissures. In the absence of large-vessel arterial disease, there may be increased blood flow to the foot, with arteriovenous shunting leading to the warm but at-risk foot.

The importance of neuropathy as a contributory cause to foot ulceration has been confirmed. The risk in patients with neuropathy is sevenfold higher than in those without.[844]

Peripheral Vascular Disease

Peripheral vascular disease itself in isolation rarely causes ulceration. However, the common combination of vascular disease with minor trauma can lead to ulceration. Thus, minor injury and subsequent infection increase the demand for blood supply beyond the circulatory capacity, and ischemic ulceration and risk of amputation develop. Early identification of those at risk for peripheral vascular disease is essential, and appropriate investigation involving noninvasive studies, together with arteriography, often leads to bypass surgery to improve blood flow to the extremities. Distal bypass surgery is often performed, with good short-term and long-term results in limb salvage.[845] Doppler-derived ankle pressure can be misleadingly high in longstanding diabetes, but the presence or absence of a dorsalis pedis or posterior tibial pulse is the simplest and most reliable indicator of significant ischemia that can be elicited at the bedside.[838]

Past Foot Ulceration or Foot Surgery

Foot ulceration is most common in patients with a history of similar problems, and even in experienced diabetic foot clinics, more than 50% of patients with new foot ulcers give a past ulcer history.

Other Diabetic Complications

Patients with retinopathy and renal dysfunction are at increased risk for foot ulceration.

Callus, Deformity, and High Foot Pressures

Motor neuropathy, with imbalance of the flexor and extensor muscles in the foot, commonly results in foot deformity, with prominent metatarsal heads and clawing of the toes (Fig. 32–51). In turn, the combination of the proprioceptive loss due to neuropathy and the prominence of metatarsal heads leads to increases in the pressures and loads under the diabetic foot.

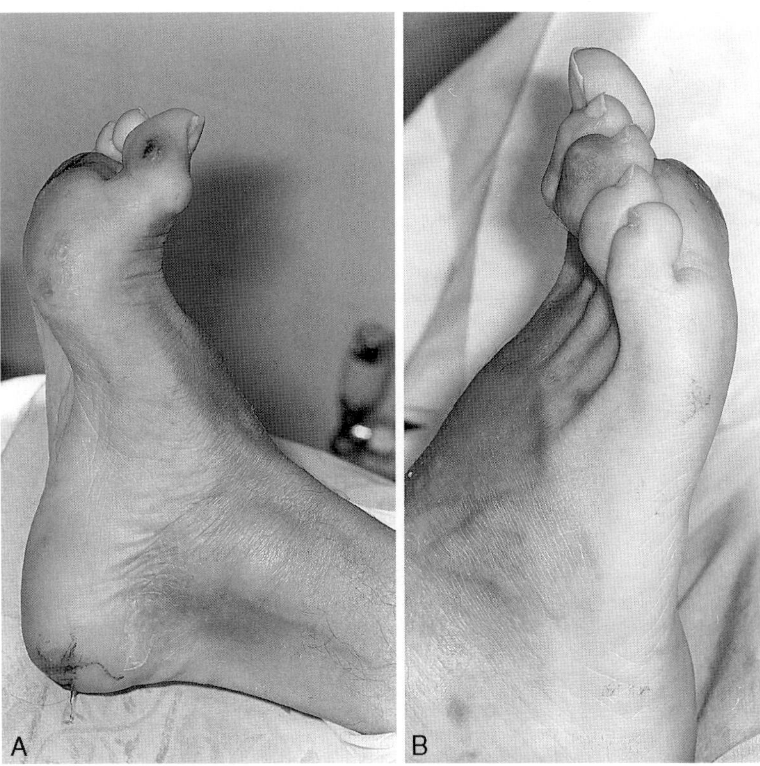

Figure 32–51 ▪ **A** and **B**, The high-risk neuropathic foot. Two lateral views of a patient with typical signs of a high-risk neuropathic foot. Note the small muscle wasting, clawing of the toes, and marked prominence of the metatarsal heads. At presentation of type 2 diabetes mellitus, this patient had severe neuropathy with foot ulceration on both right (as noted in these figures) and left feet. (From Andersson DK, Svardsudd K. Long-term glycemic control relates to mortality in type II diabetes. Diabetes Care 1995;18:1534-1543.)

High pressures, together with dry skin, often result in the formation of callus under weight-bearing areas of the metatarsal heads. The presence of such plantar callus has been shown in cross-sectional and prospective studies to be a highly significant marker of foot ulcer risk. Conversely, removal of plantar callus is associated with a reduction in foot pressures and thus a reduction in foot ulcer risk.[846]

It is the combination of two or more of the earlier described risk factors that ultimately results in diabetic foot ulceration. In 1999, a North American/United Kingdom collaborative study[847] assessed the risk factors that resulted in ulceration in more than 150 consecutive foot ulcer cases. From this study, a number of causal pathways were identified, but the most common triad of component causes was present in 63% of incident ulcers and comprised neuropathy, deformity, and trauma. Edema and ischemia were also common component causes.

Prevention of Foot Ulceration and Amputation

That diabetic foot ulceration is largely preventable is not disputed; small, mostly single-center studies have shown that relatively simple interventions can reduce amputations by up to 80%. Thus, strategies for the earlier identification of patients at potential risk for ulceration are required, and education programs that can be adapted for widespread application need to be developed. Because foot ulcers precede most amputations, are among the most common causes of hospital admission for patients with diabetes, and account for much morbidity and even mortality, the widespread application of preventive foot care strategies is urgently required.

All patients with all types of diabetes require regular review and screening of the feet for evidence of risk factors for foot ulceration irrespective of disease duration. At a minimum, such screening should be carried out annually. Of all the long-term complications of diabetes, foot problems and their risk factors are probably the easiest to detect. No expensive equipment is required, and the feet can be examined for evidence of neuropathic and vascular deficits in the office setting using simple equipment. It must be remembered that neuropathy, vascular disease, and even foot ulceration may be the presenting feature of T2DM, and thus there can be no exception to the rule of screening.

A simple algorithm for the diabetic foot screen is provided in Figure 32–52. The most important message to practitioners is to have the patient remove the shoes and socks and to look at the feet for risk factors (e.g., presence of callus, deformity, muscle wasting, and dry skin), all of which are clearly visible on clinical inspection. A simple neurologic examination that might include a modified neuropathy disability score is recommended; in the large UK community study,[844] this simple clinical exam was the best predictor of foot ulcer risks Absence of the ability to perceive pressure from a 10-g monofilament, inability to perceive a vibrating 128-Hz tuning fork over the hallux, and absent ankle reflexes all have been shown to be predictors of foot ulceration.[841,842,846]

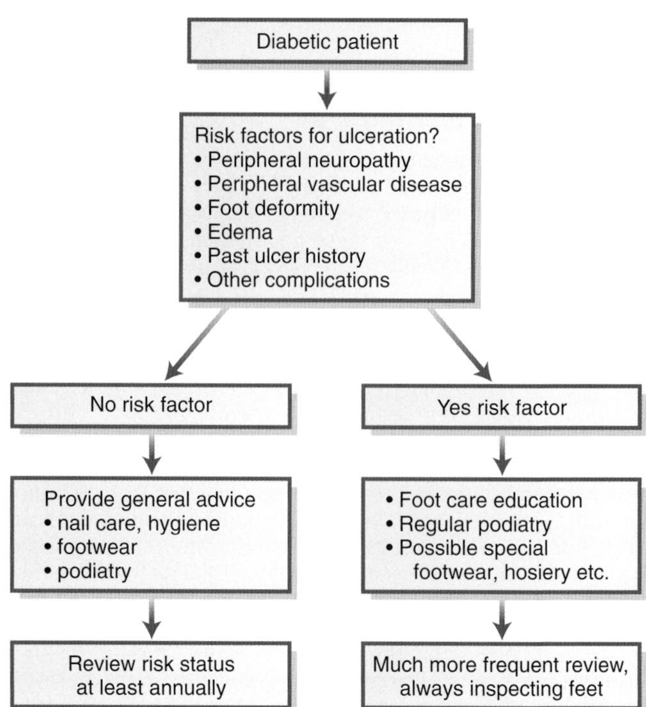

Figure 32–52 ▪ Simple algorithm for risk screening in the diabetic foot.

TABLE 32–14 WAGNER DIABETIC FOOT ULCER CLASSIFICATION SYSTEM

Grade	Description
0	No ulcer, but high-risk foot (e.g., deformity, callus, insensitivity)
1	Superficial full-thickness ulcer
2	Deeper ulcer, penetrating tendons, no bone involvement
3	Deeper ulcer with bone involvement, osteitis
4	Partial gangrene (e.g., toes, forefoot)
5	Gangrene of whole foot

Modified from Oyibo S, Jude EB, Tarawneh I, et al: A comparison of two diabetic foot ulcer classification systems: the Wagner and the 32001;24:84-88.

The Diabetic Foot Care Team

Patients identified as being at high risk for foot ulceration should be managed by a team of specialists with interest and expertise in the diabetic foot. The podiatrist generally takes responsibility for follow-up and care of the skin and nails and, together with the specialist nurse or diabetes educator, provides foot care education. The orthotist, or shoe fitter, is invaluable for advising about and sometimes designing footwear to protect high-risk feet, and these members of the team should work closely with the diabetologist and the vascular and orthopedic surgeons. Patients with risk factors for ulceration require preventive foot care education and frequent review.[848]

Classification of Foot Ulcers

Many different classification systems have been reported in the literature,[842,843] but the one developed by Wagner (Table 32–14) for grading diabetic foot ulcers has been widely used and accepted. More recently, the University of Texas (UT) group has developed an alternative classification system that, in addition to depth (as in the Wagner system), takes into account the presence or absence of infection and ischemia (Table 32–15).[849] A prospective study from 2001 has assessed and compared these two wound classification systems and concludes that the

TABLE 32-15 UNIVERSITY OF TEXAS WOUND CLASSIFICATION SYSTEM

Stage	Grade 0	Grade 1	Grade 2	Grade 3
A	Preulcer or postulcer lesion No skin break	Superficial ulcer	Deep ulcer to tendon or capsule	Wound penetrating bone or joint
B	+ Infection	+ Infection	+ Infection	+ Infection
C	+ Ischemia	+ Ischemia	+ Ischemia	+ Ischemia
D	+ Infection and ischemia	+ Infection and ischemia	+ Infection and ischemia	+ Infection and ischemia

Modified from Armstrong DG, Lavery LA, Harkless LB. Validation of a diabetic wound classification system. Diabet Med 1998;14:855-859.

University of Texas scheme is a better predictor of outcome than the older Wagner system.[850]

Management of Diabetic Foot Ulcers

Basic principles of wound healing apply equally to diabetic foot ulcers as to wounds in any other site or condition. Basically, a diabetic foot ulcer will heal if the following three conditions are satisfied:

- Arterial inflow is adequate.
- Infection is treated appropriately.
- Pressure is removed from the wound and the immediate surrounding area.

Although this approach might seem simplistic, failure of diabetic foot ulcers to heal is usually a result of failure to pay sufficient attention to one or more contributing conditions, including pressure on the wound, infection, ischemia, and inadequate debridement.

The most common cause of nonhealing of neuropathic foot ulcers is the failure to remove pressure from the wound and immediate surrounding area. Medical practitioners forget that patients advised not to put pressure over an ulcer find it difficult to adhere to such advice if peripheral sensation is lost or reduced. Pain results in protection of an injured area; the lack of pain permits pressure to be put directly onto the ulcer and results in nonhealing. A patient with normal sensation and a foot wound will limp to avoid putting pressure on the wound because this is painful; hence the observation made initially in leprosy, and more recently in diabetic neuropathy, that a patient who walks on a plantar wound without limping must have neuropathy.

The effects of pressure relief on the histopathologic features of neuropathic ulcers was assessed in a randomized study.[851] Patients with chronic neuropathic diabetic foot ulcers were randomized to have a biopsy either at presentation or after 20 days of offloading in a total contact cast (TCC). Although histologic features of chronic inflammation, with mononuclear infiltration, cellular debris, and scarce evidence of angiogenesis or granulation were seen in patients who underwent biopsy at presentation, granulation, neoangiogenesis, and a predominance of fibroblasts were seen in patients treated with TCC before biopsy. These important observations strongly suggest that repetitive pressure on a neuropathic wound contributes to the chronicity of the wound, whereas pressure relief results in the wound appearing, in several respects, more like an acute wound in the reparative phase.

The next most common error is inappropriate management of infection. Topical applications are generally unhelpful, and if clinical infection is present, it must be treated appropriately (see later).

Another common error is the failure to appreciate ischemic symptoms that are atypical due to altered pain sensation as a result of neuropathy. The most difficult ulcer to heal is the neuroischemic ulcer, and symptoms and even signs of ischemia may be altered in the diabetic state. Thus, appropriate noninvasive investigation and arteriography are indicated in the nonhealing diabetic foot ulcer where there is any question about the vascular status.

Finally, inappropriate wound debridement is another reason for slow healing or nonhealing of a diabetic foot ulcer. When patients with neuropathy put pressure on active ulcer areas, the pressure leads to an often extensive buildup of callus tissue. Appropriate debridement and removal of all dead and macerated tissue is essential in the local treatment of a diabetic foot ulcer. Steed and colleagues have demonstrated that aggressive debridement of neuropathic foot ulcers leads to a more rapid healing of ulcers compared with wounds that are inadequately debrided.[852]

The principles of management of neuropathic and neuroischemic foot ulcers are considered next. Because it is not possible to provide complete details on the individual stages and grades of ulcers, we refer to both the University of Texas and the Wagner grading systems.

Neuropathic Foot Ulcer without Osteomyelitis (Wagner Grades 1, 2; University of Texas Grades 1a, 2a)

The most important feature in the management of neuropathic foot ulcers that typically occur under weight-bearing areas such as the metatarsal heads and great toe is to provide adequate pressure relief. This is usually achieved by a cast such as a TCC or a removable Scotch cast boot.[842,843]

The TCC was recognized as the gold standard for off-loading a foot wound in the 1999 consensus statement on diabetic foot wounds by the American Diabetes Association.[853] This endorsement was subsequently confirmed as correct in a randomized, controlled trial in which Armstrong and colleagues compared three off-loading techniques and found that the TCC was associated with the shortest healing time.[843,854] When any cast device is used, regular removal of the cast is essential because regular debridement of the wound by a podiatrist is essential, and any casting device might injure insensitive skin, especially over bony prominences. For this reason, and because the TCC requires a specially trained casting technician to apply it, recent research has been directed to alternative irremovable devices that might be equally efficacious.

In the aforementioned trial by Armstrong's group,[854] the removable cast walker (RCW) resulted in slower healing than the TCC even though prior gait laboratory studies suggested that both are equally efficacious at offloading. The reason for this disparity was identified in an observational study of patients using RCWs in the treatment of their plantar neuropathic ulcers. Although patients were instructed to wear the RCW at all times, careful monitoring showed that RCWs were only used for 28% of all footsteps during a 24-hour period.[854] It was therefore suggested that the RCW, which can be applied by any clinic personnel and does not require specialist training, might be rendered irremovable by wrapping it in casting material. A controlled trial has shown that the irremovable RCW was as effective at healing neuropathic foot wounds as the TCC.[855]

Theoretically, complete healing of all superficial and neuropathic ulcers should be possible without the need for amputation. In neuropathic ulcers with a good peripheral circulation, antibiotics are not indicated unless there are clear clinical signs of infection, including prominent discharge, local erythema, and cellulitis. The presence of any of these features in Wagner's grade 1 or 2 ulcers would warrant reclassification in the University of Texas system to 1b or 2b. In such cases, deep wound swabs should be taken and broad-spectrum oral antibiotic treatment started with either an amoxicillin–clavulanic acid combination (Augmentin) or clindamycin. The antibiotic might need to be altered when sensitivity results become available.[856]

Neuroischemic Ulcers (Wagner Grades 1, 2; University of Texas Grades 1c, 1d)

The principles of management of neuroischemic Wagner grades 1 and 2 ulcers are similar to those for neuropathic ulcers with the following important exceptions: Total contact casts are not usually recommended for management of neuroischemic ulcers, although removable casts and pneumatic cast boots (Aircast) may be used. Antibiotic therapy is usually recommended for all neuroischemic ulcers. Investigation of the circulation (including noninvasive assessment and, when required, arteriography with appropriate subsequent surgical management or angioplasty) is indicated.

Osteomyelitis (Wagner Grade 3; University of Texas Grades 3b, 3d)

Wagner or University of Texas grade 3 ulcers are deeper and involve underlying bone, often with abscess formation. Osteomyelitis is a serious complication of foot ulceration and may be present in as many as 50% of diabetic patients with moderate to severe foot infections.[843] If the physician can probe down to bone in a deep ulcer, the presence of osteomyelitis is strongly suggested. Plain radiographs are indicated in any nonhealing foot ulcer and are useful in the diagnosis of osteomyelitis in more than two thirds of patients, although it should be kept in mind that the radiologic changes may be delayed. In difficult cases, further investigation, such as magnetic resonance imaging, bone scans, or an ^{111}In-labeled white blood cell scan can be useful in diagnosing bone infection.

Although the treatment of osteomyelitis is commonly surgical and involves resecting the infected bone, there have been reports of successful long-term treatment with antibiotics that treat the underlying bacterium, most commonly *Staphylococcus aureus*. Thus, agents such as clindamycin (which penetrates bone well) or flucloxacillin are often used.

Gangrene (Wagner Grades 4, 5)

Gangrene or areas of tissue death is always a serious sign in the diabetic foot. However, localized areas of gangrene, especially in the toes, without cellulitis, spreading infection, or discharge, can occasionally be left to spontaneously autoamputate. The presence of more extensive gangrene requires urgent hospital admission; treatment of infection, often with multiple antibiotics; control of the diabetes, usually with intravenous insulin; and detailed vascular assessment. It is in this area that the team approach is most important, with close collaboration among the diabetes specialist, the vascular surgeon, and the radiologist.

Adjunct Treatments for Foot Ulcers

Platelet-Derived Growth Factors

Several controlled trials of becaplermin, a recombinant human PDGF β-chain homodimer, have confirmed the efficacy of this topically applied agent in promoting healing of neuropathic foot ulcers. In a combined analysis of randomized, controlled studies, Smiell and coworkers[857] showed that active treatment was associated with a significant increase in the probability of complete healing compared to placebo gel.

The use of such an agent should probably be reserved for managing difficult-to-heal neuropathic ulcers that do not respond to standard treatment, such as off-loading or regular debridement. Widespread use of becaplermin is somewhat limited by its cost. When used selectively, however, this agent can accelerate the wound healing of neuropathic foot ulcers.

Tissue-Engineered Skin

The development of living human skin equivalents produced by tissue-engineering techniques has produced new possibilities for wound-healing therapies and chronic ulcers, such as those caused by venous disease or diabetic neuropathy. However, both living skin equivalents and topically applied growth factors are expensive treatments that must be seen not as a replacement but as an addition to good wound care,[842] which must always include adequate off-loading and regular debridement.

Intermittent Negative Pressure

Negative-pressure wound therapy, also known as vacuum-assisted closure (VAC), is being used increasingly to treat large, complex diabetic foot wounds. This treatment stimulates the development of granulation tissue in previously nonhealing wounds, and it is particularly helpful in postoperative management of diabetic foot wounds. Evidence suggests that this treatment can speed wound closure in certainly carefully chosen cases.[858]

Charcot's Neuroarthropathy

Charcot's neuroarthropathy is a rare and disabling condition affecting the joints and bones of the feet. Permissive features for the development of this condition include the presence of severe peripheral neuropathy, together with autonomic dysfunction, with increased blood flow to the foot; the peripheral circulation is usually intact. In the Western world, diabetes is the most common cause of a Charcot's foot, and increased awareness of this condition can enable earlier diagnosis and treatment to prevent severe deformity and disability.

The actual pathogenesis of the Charcot process is poorly understood; however, the patient with peripheral insensitivity and autonomic dysfunction with increased blood flow to the foot is vulnerable to unrecognized trauma that may be so trivial that the patient cannot recall the event. Repetitive trauma results in increased blood flow through the bone, increased osteoclastic activity, and remodeling of bone. In certain cases, patients walk on a fracture that leads to continuing destruction of bones and joints in that area.

Charcot's neuropathy is sometimes difficult to distinguish from osteomyelitis or an inflammatory arthropathy. However, a unilateral swollen, hot foot is a patient with neuropathy must be considered to be Charcot's foot until proved otherwise.

Charcot's arthropathy can be diagnosed in most patients by plain radiograph and a high index of suspicion. Radiographs might reveal bone and joint destruction, fragmentation, and remodeling, although in the early stages, the radiographic finding may be normal. In such cases, the three-phase bisphosphonate bone scan shows increased bone uptake, although the ^{111}In-labeled bone scan will be negative in the absence of infection.

After diagnosis, management of the acute phase involves immobilization, usually in a TCC. Evidence suggests that treatment with bisphosphonates, which reduce osteoclastic activity, can reduce swelling, discomfort, and bone turnover markers.[842]

Although rare, Charcot's neuroarthropathy should be suspected in any patient with unexplained swelling and heat in a neuropathic foot, and early intervention with immobilization and possibly bisphosphonate treatment might halt progression that in the untreated state can lead to marked foot deformity and require local or major amputations.

REFERENCES

1. Skyler J. Diabetic complications: the importance of glucose control. Endocrinol Metab Clin North Am 1996;25:243-254.
2. Diabetes Control and Complications Trial Research Group. The effect of intensive treatment of diabetes on the development and progression of long-term complications in insulin-dependent diabetes mellitus. N Engl J Med 1993;329:977-986.
3. UK Prospective Diabetes Study (UKPDS) Group. Intensive blood-glucose control with sulphonylureas or insulin compared with conventional treatment and risk of complications in patients with type 2 diabetes (UKPDS 33). Lancet 1998;352:837-853.
4. Krolewski AS, Laffel LM, Krolewski M, et al. Glycosylated hemoglobin and the risk of microalbuminuria in patients with insulin-dependent diabetes mellitus. N Engl J Med 1995;332: 1251-1255.
5. The absence of a glycemic threshold for the development of long-term complications: the perspective of the Diabetes Control and Complications Trial. Diabetes 1996;45:1289-1298.
6. Wagenknecht LE, D'Agostino RB Jr, Haffner SM, et al. Impaired glucose tolerance, type 2 diabetes, and carotid wall thickness: the Insulin Resistance Atherosclerosis Study. Diabetes Care 1998; 21:1812-1818.
7. Goldberg RB, Mellies MJ, Sacks FM, et al. Cardiovascular events and their reduction with pravastatin in diabetic and glucose-intolerant myocardial infarction survivors with average cholesterol levels: subgroup analyses in the cholesterol and recurrent vents (CARE) trial. The Care Investigators. Circulation 1998;98: 2513-2519.
8. Haffner SM. The Scandinavian Simvastatin Survival Study (4S) subgroup analysis of diabetic subjects: implications for the prevention of coronary heart disease. Diabetes Care 1997;20:469-471.
9. Ebara T, Conde K, Kako Y, et al. Delayed catabolism of apoB-48 lipoproteins due to decreased heparan sulfate proteoglycan production in diabetic mice. J Clin Invest 2000;105:1807-1818.
10. Ginsberg HN. Insulin resistance and cardiovascular disease. J Clin Invest 2000;106:453-458.
11. Kaiser N, Feener EP, Boukobza-Vardi N, et al. Differential regulation of glucose transport and transporters by glucose in vascular endothelial and smooth muscle cells. Diabetes 1993;42:80-89.
12. Heilig CW, Concepcion LA, Riser BL, et al. Overexpression of glucose transporters in rat mesangial cells cultured in a normal glucose milieu mimics the diabetic phenotype. J Clin Invest 1995;96:1802-1814.
13. Shore AC, Tooke JE. Microvascular function and haemodynamic disturbances in diabetes mellitus and its complications. In Pickup J, Williams G, eds. Textbook of Diabetes, vol 1. Oxford, UK: Blackwell Scientific, 1997:43.1-43.13.
14. Kihara M, Schmelzer JD, Poduslo JF, et al. Aminoguanidine effects on nerve blood flow, vascular permeability, electrophysiology, and oxygen free radicals. Proc Natl Acad Sci U S A 1991;88: 6107-6111.
15. Kopp JB, Factor VM, Mozes M, et al. Transgenic mice with increased plasma levels of TGF-β_1 develop progressive renal disease. Lab Invest 1996;74:991-1003.
16. Chien S, Li S, Shyy YJ. Effects of mechanical forces on signal transduction and gene expression in endothelial cells. Hypertension 1998;(1 Pt 2):162-169.
17. Walker JD, Viberti GC. Pathophysiology of microvascular disease: an overview. In Pickup J, Williams G, eds. Textbook of Diabetes, vol 1. Oxford, UK: Blackwell Scientific, 1991:526-533.
18. Brownlee M. Advanced products of nonenzymatic glycosylation and the pathogenesis of diabetic complications. In Rifkin H, Porte D Jr, eds. Diabetes Mellitus: Theory and Practice. New York: Elsevier, 1990:279-291.
19. Hammes HP, Federoff HJ, Brownlee M. Nerve growth factor prevents both neuroretinal programmed cell death and capillary pathology in experimental diabetes. Mol Med 1995;(5):527-534.
20. Mizutani M, Kern TS, Lorenzi M. Accelerated death of retinal microvascular cells in human and experimental diabetic retinopathy. J Clin Invest 1996;97:2883-2890.
21. Giannini C, Dyck PJ. Ultrastructural morphometric features of human sural nerve endoneurial microvessels. J Neuropathol Exp Neurol 1993;52:361-369.
22. Giannini C, Dyck PJ. Basement membrane reduplication and pericyte degeneration precede development of diabetic polyneuropathy and are associated with its severity. Ann Neurol 1995;37: 498-504.
23. Tomlinson DR, Fernyhough P, Diemel LT. Role of neurotrophins in diabetic neuropathy and treatment with nerve growth factors. Diabetes 1997;46(supp 12):S43-S49.
24. Engerman RL, Kern TS. Progression of incipient diabetic retinopathy during good glycemic control. Diabetes 1987;36:808-812.
25. Roy S, Sala R, Cagliero E, Lorenzi M. Overexpression of fibronectin induced by diabetes or high glucose phenomenon with a memory. Proc Natl Acad Sci U S A 1990;87:404-408.
26. Diabetes Control and Complications Trial Research Group. The effect of intensive treatment of diabetes on the development and progression of long-term complications in insulin-dependent diabetes mellitus. N Engl J Med 1993;329(14):977-986.
27. Diabetes Control and Complications Trial (DCCT) Research Group. Effect of intensive therapy on the development and progression of diabetic nephropathy in the Diabetes Control and Complications Trial. Kidney Int 1995;47:1703-1702.
28. Diabetes Control and Complications Trial Research Group. The effect of intensive diabetes therapy on the development and progression of neuropathy. Ann Intern Med 1995;122(8):561-568.
29. Writing Team for the Diabetes Control and Complications Trial/ Epidemiology of Diabetes Interventions and Complications Research Group. Effect of intensive therapy on the microvascular complications of type 1 diabetes mellitus. JAMA 2002;287:2563-2569.
30. Writing Team for the Diabetes Control and Complications. Trial/ Epidemiology of Diabetes Interventions and Complications Research Group. Sustained effect of intensive treatment of type 1 diabetes mellitus on development and progression of diabetic nephropathy: the Epidemiology of Diabetes Interventions and Complications (EDIC) study. JAMA 2003;290:2159-2167.
31. Krolewski AS, Warram JH, Freire MB. Epidemiology of late diabetic complications: a basis for the development and evaluation of preventive programs. Endocrinol Metab Clin North Am 1996;25: 217-242.
32. Wagenknecht LE, Bowden DW, Carr JJ, et al. Familial aggregation of coronary artery calcium in families with type 2 diabetes. Diabetes 2001;50:861-866.
33. Seaquist ER, Goetz FC, Rich S, Barbosa J. Familial clustering of diabetic kidney disease. Evidence for genetic susceptibility to diabetic nephropathy. N Engl J Med 1989;32018:1161-1165.
34. Quinn M, Angelico MC, Warram JH, Krolewski AS. Familial factors determine the development of diabetic nephropathy in patients with IDDM. Diabetologia 1996;39:940-945.
35. Diabetes Control and Complications Trial Research Group. Clustering of long-term complications in families with diabetes in the Diabetes Control and Complications Trial. Diabetes 1997;46: 1829-1839.
36. Raffel LJ, Vadheim CM, Roth MP, et al. The 5′ insulin gene polymorphism and the genetics of vascular complications in type 1 (insulin-dependent) diabetes mellitus. Diabetologia 1991;34: 680-683.

37. Stewart LL, Field LL, Ross S, McArthur RG. Genetic risk factors in diabetic retinopathy. Diabetologia 1993;36:1293-1298.
38. Marre M, Bernadet P, Gallois Y, et al. Relationships between angiotensin I converting enzyme gene polymorphism, plasma levels, and diabetic retinal and renal complications. Diabetes 1994;43: 384-388.
39. Marre M, Jeunemaitre X, Gallois Y, et al. Contribution of genetic polymorphism in the renin-angiotensin system to the development of renal complications in insulin-dependent diabetes: Genetique de la Nephropathie Diabetique (GENEDIAB) study group. J Clin Invest 1997;99:1585-1595.
40. Agardh D, Gaur LK, Agardh E, et al. LADQB1*0201/0302 is associated with severe retinopathy in patients with IDDM. Diabetologia 1996;39:1313-1317.
41. Oates PJ, Mylari BL. Aldose reductase inhibitors: therapeutic implications for diabetic complications. Exp Opin Invest Drugs 1999;8: 1-25.
42. Warpeha KM, Xu W, Liu L, et al. Genotyping and functional analysis of a polymorphic (CCTTT)(n) repeat of NOS2A in diabetic retinopathy. FASEB J.1999;13:1825-1832.
43. Satko SG, Freedman BI, Moossavi S. Genetic factors in end-stage renal disease. Kidney Int Suppl 2005;94:S46-S49.
44. Ewens KG, George RA, Sharma K, et al. Assessment of 115 candidate genes for diabetic nephropathy by transmission/disequilibrium test. Diabetes 2005;54:3305-3318.
45. Haston CK, Hudson TJ. Finding genetic modifiers of cystic fibrosis. N Engl J Med 2005;353:1509-1511.
46. Granger CB, Califf RM, Young S. Outcome of patients with diabetes mellitus and acute myocardial infarction treated with thrombolytic agents. The Thrombolysis and Angioplasty in Myocardial Infarction (TAMI) Study Group. J. Am Coll Cardiol 1993;21: 920-925.
47. Stamler J, Vaccaro O, Neaton JD, Wentworth D. Diabetes, other risk factors, and 12-yr cardiovascular mortality for men screened in the Multiple Risk Factor Intervention Trial. Diabetes Care 1993;16:434-444.
48. Fitzgerald AP, Jarrett RJ. Are conventional risk factors for mortality relevant in type 2 diabetes? Diabet Med 1991;8:475-480.
49. Fuller JH, Shipley MJ, Rose G, et al. Coronary-heart-disease risk and impaired glucose tolerance. The Whitehall study. Lancet 1980;1:1373-1376.
50. Rosengren A, Welin L, Tsipogianni A, Wilhelmsen. Impact of cardiovascular risk factors on coronary heart disease and mortality among middle aged diabetic men: a general population study. BMJ 1989;299:1127-1131.
51. Lehto S, Ronnemma T, Pyorala K, Laakso M. Poor glycemic control predicts coronary heart disease events in patients with type I diabetes without nephropathy. Arterioscler Thromb Vasc Biol 1999;19:1014-1019.
52. Gerstein HC. Is glucose a continuous risk factor for cardiovascular mortality? Diabetes Care 1999;22:659-660.
53. Gall MA, Borch-Johnsen K, Hougaard P, et al. Albuminuria and poor glycemic control predict mortality in NIDDM. Diabetes 1995;44:1303-1309.
54. Kuusisto J, Mykkanen L, Pyorala K, Laakso M. NIDDM and its metabolic control predict coronary heart disease in elderly subjects. Diabetes 1994;43:960-967.
55. Salomaa V, Riley W, Kark JD, et al. Non–insulin-dependent diabetes mellitus and fasting glucose and insulin concentrations are associated with arterial stiffness indexes. The ARIC Study. Atherosclerosis Risk in Communities Study. Circulation 1995;91: 1432-1443.
56. Laakso M, Kuusisto J. Epidemiological evidence for the association of hyperglycaemia and atherosclerotic vascular disease in non–insulin-dependent diabetes mellitus. Ann Med 1996;28: 415-418.
57. Bonora, E, Kiechl S, Willeit J, et al. Prevalence of insulin resistance in metabolic disorders: the Bruneck Study. Diabetes. 1998;47: 1643-1649.
58. Haffner SM, Lehto S, Ronnemaa T, et al. Mortality from coronary heart disease in subjects with type 2 diabetes and in nondiabetic subjects with and without prior myocardial infarction. N Engl J Med 1998;339:229-234.
59. Saydah SH, Miret M, Sung J, et al. Postchallenge hyperglycemia and mortality in a national sample of U.S. adults. Diabetes Care 2001;24:1397-1402.
60. National Diabetes Data Group. Diabetes in America, 2nd ed. Bethesda, Maryland: National Institute of Diabetes and Digestive and Kidney Diseases, 1995.
61. DECODE Study Group, the European Diabetes Epidemiology Group. Glucose tolerance and cardiovascular mortality: comparison of fasting and 2-hour diagnostic criteria. Arch Intern Med 2001;161:397-405.
62. Yip J, Facchini FS, Reaven GM. Resistance to insulin-mediated glucose disposal as a predictor of cardiovascular disease. J Clin Endocrinol Metab 1998;83:2773-2776.
63. Hanley AJ, Williams K, Stern MP, Haffner S.M. Homeostasis model assessment of IR in relation to the incidence of cardiovascular disease: the San Antonio Heart Study. Diabetes Care 2002;25: 1177-1184.
64. Shimomura I, Bashmakov Y, Ikemoto S, et al. Insulin selectively increases SREBP-1c mRNA in the livers of rats with streptozotocin-induced diabetes. Proc Natl Acad Sci U S A 1999;96:13656-13661.
65. Chen G, Liang G, Ou J, et al. Central role for liver X receptor in insulin-mediated activation of Srebp-1c transcription and stimulation of fatty acid synthesis in liver. Proc Natl Acad Sci U S A 2004;101:11245-11250.
66. King G, Brownlee M. The cellular and molecular mechanisms of diabetic complications. Endocrinol Metab Clin North Am 1996;2:255-270.
67. Hsueh WA, Law RE. Cardiovascular risk continuum: implications of insulin resistance and diabetes. Am J Med 1998;105:4S-14S.
68. Li H, Forstermann U. Nitric oxide in the pathogenesis of vascular disease. J Pathol 2000;190:244-254.
69. Banskota NK, Taub R, Zellner K, King GL. Insulin, insulin-like growth factor I and platelet-derived growth factor interact additively in the induction of the protooncogene c-myc and cellular proliferation in cultured bovine aortic smooth muscle cells. Mol Endocrinol 1989;8:1183-1190.
70. Stolar MW. Atherosclerosis in diabetes: the role of hyperinsulinemia. Metabolism 1988;7(suppl 1):1-9.
71. Jiang ZY, Lin YW, Clemont A, et al. Characterization of selective resistance to insulin signaling in the vasculature of obese Zucker (fa/fa) rats. J Clin Invest 1999;104:447-457.
72. Akbari CM, Saouaf R, Barnhill DF, et al. Endothelium-dependent vasodilatation is impaired in both microcirculation and macrocirculation during acute hyperglycemia J Vasc Surg 1998;28: 687-694.
73. Williams SB, Goldfine AB, Timimi FK, et al. Acute hyperglycemia attenuates endothelium-dependent vasodilation in humans in vivo. Circulation 1998;97:1695-1701.
74. Du XL, Edelstein D, Rossetti L, et al. Hyperglycemia-induced mitochondrial superoxide overproduction activates the hexosamine pathway and induces plasminogen activator inhibitor-1expression by increasing Sp1 glycosylation. Proc Natl Acad Sci U S A 2000;97:12222-12226.
75. Du XL, Edelstein D, Dimmler S, et al. Hyperglycemia inhibits endothelial nitric oxide synthase activity by altering its post-translational modification at the akt site of the eNOS protein. J Clin Invest 2001;108:1341-1348.
76. Yamagishi S, Edelstein D, Du XD, Brownlee M. Hyperglycemia potentiates platelet-derived growth factor induced proliferation of smooth muscle cells through mitochondrial superoxide overproduction. Diabetes 2001;50:1491-1494.
77. Sassy-Prigent C, Heudes D, Mandet C, et al. Early glomerular macrophage recruitment in streptozotocin-induced diabetic rats Diabetes 2000;49:466-475.
78. Gilcrease MZ, Hoover RL. Examination of monocyte adherence to endothelium under hyperglycemic conditions. Am J Pathol 1991;139:1089-1097.
79. Ceriello A, Falleti E, Motz E. Hyperglycemia-induced circulating ICAM-1 increased in diabetes mellitus: the possible role of oxidative stress. Horm Metab Res 1998;30:146-149.
80. Kim JA, Berliner JA, Natarajan RD, Nadler JL. Evidence that glucose increases monocyte binding to human aortic endothelial cells. Diabetes 1994;43:1103-1107.
81. Cagliero E, Maiello M, Boeri D, et al. Increased expression of basement membrane components in human endothelial cells cultured in high glucose. J Clin Invest 1988;82:735-738.
82. Cagliero E, Roth T, Roy S, et al. Expression of genes related to the extracellular matrix in human endothelial cells. Differential modu-

lation by elevated glucose concentrations, phorbol esters, and cAMP. J Biol Chem 1991;266:14244-14250.
83. Du XD, Edelstein D, Obici S, et al. Insulin resistance reduces arterial prostacyclin synthase and eNOS activities by increasing endothelial fatty acid oxidation J Clin Invest 2006;116:1071-1080.
84. Tepper OM, Galiano RD, Capla JM, et al. Human endothelial progenitor cells from type II diabetics exhibit impaired proliferation, adhesion, and incorporation into vascular structures. Circulation 2002;106:2781-2786.
85. Duh E, Aiello LP. Vascular endothelial growth factor and diabetes: the agonist versus antagonist paradox. Diabetes 1999;48:1899-1906.
86. Waltenberger J. Impaired collateral vessel development in diabetes: potential cellular mechanisms and therapeutic implications. Cardiovasc Res 2001;49:554-560.
87. Grant MB, May WS, Caballero S, et al. Adult hematopoietic stem cells provide functional hemangioblast activity during retinal neovascularization. Nat Med 2002;8:607-612.
88. Rivard A, Silver M, Chen D, et al. Rescue of diabetes-related impairment of angiogenesis by intramuscular gene therapy with adeno-VEGF. Am J Pathol 1999;154:355-363.
89. Iwaguro H, Yamaguchi J, Kalka C, et al. Endothelial progenitor cell vascular endothelial growth factor gene transfer for vascular regeneration. Circulation 2002;105:732-738.
90. Xia P, Kramer RM, King GL. Identification of the mechanism for the inhibition of Na^+,K^+-adenosine triphosphatase by hyperglycemia involving activation of protein kinase C and cytosolic phospholipase A2. J. Clin Invest 1995;96:733-740.
91. Williamson JR, Chang K, Frangos M, et al. Hyperglycemic pseudohypoxia and diabetic complications. Diabetes 1993;42:801-813.
92. Nishikawa T, Edelstein D, Du XL, et al. Normalizing mitochondrial superoxide production blocks three pathways of hyperglycaemic damage. Nature 2000;404:787-790.
93. Marano CW, Szwergold BS, Kapper F, et al. Human retinal pigment epithelial cells cultured in hyperglycemic media accumulate increased amounts of glycosaminoglycan precursors. Invest Ophthalmol Vis Sci 1992;33:2619-2625.
94. Beyer-Mears A, Diecke FP, Mistry K, et al. Effect of pyruvate lens myo-inositol transport and polyol formation in diabetic cataract. Pharmacology 1997;55:78-86.
95. Knight RJ, Koefoed KF, Schelbert HR, Buxton DB. Inhibition of glyceraldehyde-3-phosphate dehydrogenase in post-ischaemic myocardium. Cardiovasc Res 1996;32:1016-1023.
96. Lee AY, Chung SS. Contributions of polyol pathway to oxidative stress in diabetic cataract. FASEB J 1999;13:23-30.
97. Chandra D, Jackson EB, Ramana KV, et al. Nitric oxide prevents aldose reductase activation and sorbitol accumulation during diabetes. Diabetes 2002;51:3095-3101.
98. Petrash JM, Harter TM, Devine CS, et al. Involvement of cysteine residues in catalysis and inhibition of human aldose reductase. Site-directed mutagenesis of Cys-80, -298, and -303. J Biol Chem 1992;267:24833-24840.
99. Chandra A, Srivastava S, Petrash JM, et al. Active site modification of aldose reductase by nitric oxide donors. Biochim Biophys Acta 1997;1341:217-222.
100. Engerman RL, Kern TS, Larson ME. Nerve conduction and aldose reductase inhibition during 5 years of diabetes or galactosaemia in dogs. Diabetologia 1994;37:141-144.
101. Sorbinil Retinopathy Trial Research Group. A randomized trial of sorbinil, an aldose reductase inhibitor, in diabetic retinopathy. Arch Ophthalmol 1990;108:1234-1244.
102. Greene DA, Arezzo JC, Brown MB. Effect of aldose reductase inhibition on nerve conduction and morphometry in diabetic neuropathy. Zenarestat Study Group. Neurology 1999;53:580-591.
103. Hammes H-P, Martin S, Federlin K, et al. Aminoguanidine treatment inhibits the development of experimental diabetic retinopathy. Proc Natl Acad Sci U S A 1991;88:11555-1559.
104. Stitt AW, Moore JE, Sharkey JA, Murphy G, et al. Advanced glycation end products in vitreous: Structural and functional implications for diabetic vitreopathy. Invest Ophthalmol Vis Sci 1998;39:2517-2521.
105. Stitt AW, Li YM, Gardiner TA, et al. Advanced glycation end products (AGEs) co-localize with AGE receptors in the retinal vasculature of diabetic and of AGE- infused rats. Am J Pathol 1997;150: 523-528.
106. Nishino T, Horri Y, Shikki H, et al. Immunohistochemical detection of advanced glycosylation end products within the vascular lesions and glomeruli in diabetic nephropathy. Hum Pathol 1995;26:308-312.
107. Horie K, Miyata T, Maeda K, et al. Immunohistochemical colocalization of glycoxidation products and lipid peroxidation products in diabetic renal glomerular lesions. Implication for glycoxidative stress in the pathogenesis of diabetic nephropathy. J Clin Invest 1997;100:2995-2999.
108. Niwa T, Katsuzaki T, Miyazaki S, et al. Immunohistochemical detection of imidazolone, a novel advanced glycation end product, in kidneys and aortas of diabetic patients. J Clin Invest 1997;99: 1272-1276.
109. Degenhardt TP, Thorpe SR, Baynes JW. Chemical modification of proteins by methylglyoxal. Cell Mol Biol 1998;44:1139-1145.
110. Wells-Knecht KJ, Zyzak DV, Litchfield JE, et al. Mechanism of autoxidative glycosylation: identification of glyoxal and arabinose as intermediates in the autoxidative modification of proteins by glucose. Biochemistry 1995;34:3702-3709.
111. Thornalley PJ. The glyoxalase system: new developments towards functional characterization of a metabolic pathway fundamental to biological life. Biochem J 1990;269:1-11.
112. Takahashi M, Fujii J, Teshima T, et al. Identity of a major 3-deoxyglucosone reducing enzyme with aldehyde reductase in rat liver established by amino acid sequencing and cDNA expression. Gene 1993;127:249-253.
113. Suzuki K, Koh YH, Mizuno H, et al. Overexpression of aldehyde reductase protects PC12 cells from the cytotoxicity of methylglyoxal or 3-deoxyglucosone. J Biochem 1998;123:353-357.
114. Nakamura S, Makita Z, Ishikawa S, et al. Progression of nephropathy in spontaneous diabetic rats is prevented by OPB-9195, a novel inhibitor of advanced glycation. Diabetes 1997;46:895-899.
115. Soulis-Liparota T, Cooper M, Papazoglou D, et al. Retardation by aminoguanidine of development of albuminuria, mesangial expansion, and tissue fluorescence in streptozocin-induced diabetic rat. Diabetes 1991;40:1328-1334.
116. Treins C, Giorgetti-Peraldi S, Murdaca J, Van Obberghen E. Regulation of vascular endothelial growth factor expression by advanced glycation end products. J Biol Chem 2001;276:43836-4341.
117. Yamagishi S, Inagaki Y, Okamoto T, et al. Advanced glycation end product–induced apoptosis and overexpression of vascular endothelial growth factor and monocyte chemoattractant protein-1 in human-cultured mesangial cells. J Biol Chem 2002;277: 20309-20315.
118. Oldfield MD, Bach LA, Forbes JM, et al. Advanced glycation end products cause epithelial-myofibroblast transdifferentiation via the receptor for advanced glycation end products (RAGE). J Clin Invest 2001;108:1853-1863.
119. Chang EY, Szallasi Z, Acs P, et al. Functional effects of overexpression of protein kinase C-alpha, -beta, -delta, -epsilon, and -eta in the mast cell line RBL-2H3. J Immunol 1997;1159:2624-2632.
120. Carmeliet P. Angiogenesis in health and disease. Nat Med. 2003;9:653-660.
121. Hanahan D. Signaling vascular morphogenesis and maintenance. Science 1997;277:48-50.
122. Jain RK. Molecular regulation of vessel maturation. Nat Med 2003;9:685-693.
123. Gale NW, Thurston G, Hackett SF, et al. Angiopoietin-2 is required for postnatal angiogenesis and lymphatic patterning, and only the latter role is rescued by angiopoietin-1. Dev Cell 2003;3: 411-423.
124. Hackett SF, Wiegand S, Yancopoulos G, Campochiaro PA. Angiopoietin-2 plays an important role in retinal angiogenesis. J Cell Physiol 2002;192:182-187.
125. Maisonpierre PC, Suri C, Jones PF, et al. Angiopoietin-2, a natural antagonist for Tie2 that disrupts in vivo angiogenesis. Science 1997;277:55-60.
126. Hammes HP, Lin J, Wagner P, et al. Angiopoietin-2 causes pericyte dropout in the normal retina: evidence for involvement in diabetic retinopathy. Diabetes 2004;53:1104-1110.
127. Hammes HP, Lin J, Renner O, et al. Pericytes and the pathogenesis of diabetic retinopathy. Diabetes 2002;51:3107-3112.
128. Yao D, Taguchi T, Matsumura T, et al. Methylglyoxal modification of mSin3A links glycolysis to angiopoietin-2 transcription. Cell 2006;124: 275-286.

129. McLellan AC, Thornalley PJ, Benn J, Sonksen PH. Glyoxalase system in clinical diabetes mellitus and correlation with diabetic complications. Clin Sci (Lond) 1994;87:21-29.
130. Godbout JP, Pesavento J, Hartman ME, et al. Methylglyoxal enhances cisplatin-induced cytotoxicity by activating protein kinase Cδ. J Biol Chem 2002;277:2554-2561.
131. Sakamoto H, Mashima T, Yamamoto K, Tsuruo T. Modulation of heat-shock protein 27 (Hsp27) anti-apoptotic activity by methylglyoxal modification. J Biol Chem 2002;277:45770-45775.
132. Tanaka S, Avigad G, Brodsky B, Eikenberry EF. Glycation induces expansion of the molecular packing of collagen. J Mol Biol 1988;203:495-505.
133. Huijberts MS, Wolffenbuttel BH, Boudier HA, et al. Aminoguanidine treatment increases elasticity and decreases fluid filtration of large arteries from diabetic rats. J Clin Invest 1993;92:1407-1411.
134. Tsilibary EC, Charonis AS, Reger LA, et al. The effect of nonenzymatic glucosylation the binding of the main noncollagenous NC1 domain to type IV collagen. J Biol Chem 1990;263:4302-4308.
135. Charonis AS, Reger LA, Dege JE, et al. Laminin alterations after in vitro nonenzymatic glycosylation. Diabetes 1988;39:807-814.
136. Cochrane SM, Robinson GB. In vitro glycation of a glomerular basement membrane alters its permeability: a possible mechanism in diabetic complications. FEBS Lett 1995;375:41-44.
137. Boyd-White J, Williams JC Jr. Effect of cross-linking on matrix permeability. A model for AGE-modified basement membranes. Diabetes 1996;45:348-353.
138. Haitoglou CS, Tsilibary EC, Brownlee M, Charonis AS. Altered cellular interactions between endothelial cells and nonenzymatically glucosylated laminin/type IV collagen. J Biol Chem 1992;267: 12404-12407.
139. Federoff HJ, Lawrence D, Brownlee M. Nonenzymatic glycosylation of laminin and the laminin peptide CIKVAVS inhibits neurite outgrowth. Diabetes 1993;42:509-513.
140. Hammes HP, Weiss A, Hess S, et al. Modification of vitronectin by advanced glycation alters functional properties in vitro and in the diabetic retina. Lab Invest 1996;75:325-338.
141. Dobler D, Ahmed N, Song L, et al. Increased dicarbonyl metabolism in endothelial cells in hyperglycemia induces anoikis and impairs angiogenesis by RGD and GFOGER motif modification. Diabetes 2006;55:1961-1969.
142. Bishara NB, Dunlop ME, Murphy TV, et al. Matrix protein glycation impairs agonist-induced intracellular Ca^{2+} signaling in endothelial cells. J Cell Physiol 2002;193:80-92.
143. Li YM, Mitsuhashi T, Wojciechowicz D, et al. Molecular identity and cellular distribution of advanced glycation end product receptors: relationship of p60 to OST-48 and p90 to 80K-H membrane proteins. Proc Natl Acad Sci U S A 1996;93:11047-11052.
144. Yang Z, Makita Z, Horii Y, et al. Two novel rat liver membrane proteins that bind advanced glycosylation end products: Relationship to macrophage receptor for glucose-modified proteins. J Exp Med 1991;174:515-524.
145. Schmidt AM, Vianna M, Gerlach M, et al. Isolation and characterization of two binding proteins for advanced glycosylation end products from bovine lung which are present on the endothelial cell surface. J Biol Chem 1992;267:14987-14997.
146. Neeper M, Schmidt AM, Brett J, et al. Cloning and expression of a cell surface receptor for advanced glycosylation end products of proteins. J Biol Chem 1992;267:14998-15004.
147. Schmidt AM, Mora R, Cao R, et al. The endothelial cell binding site for advanced glycation endproducts consists of a complex: an integral membrane protein and a lactoferrin-like polypeptide. J Biol Chem 1994;269:9882-9888.
148. Vlassara H, Brownlee M, Manogue K, et al. Cachectin/TNF and IL-1 induced by glucose-modified proteins: role in normal tissue remodeling. Science 1988;240:1546-1548.
149. Kirstein M, Aston C, Hintz R, Vlassara H. Receptor-specific induction of insulin-like growth factor I in human monocytes by advanced glycosylation end product–modified proteins. J Clin Invest 1992;90:439-446.
150. Yui S, Sasaki T, Araki N, et al. Induction of macrophage growth by advanced glycation end products of the Maillard reaction. J Immunol 1994;152:1943-1949.
151. Higashi T, Sano H, Saishoji T, et al. The receptor for advanced glycation end products mediates the chemotaxis of rabbit smooth muscle cells. Diabetes 1997;46:463-472.
152. Westwood ME, Thornalley PJ. Induction of synthesis and secretion of interleukin 1 beta in the human monocytic THP-1 cells by human serum albumins modified with methylglyoxal and advanced glycation endproducts. Immunol Lett 1996;50:17-21.
153. Abordo EA, Westwood ME, Thornalley PJ. Synthesis and secretion of macrophage colony stimulating factor by mature human monocytes and human monocytic THP-1 ells induced by human serum albumin derivatives modified with methylglyoxal and glucose-derived advanced glycation endproducts. Immunol Lett 1996;53: 7-13.
154. Abordo EA, Thornalley PJ. Synthesis and secretion of tumour necrosis factor-alpha by human monocytic THP-1 cells and chemotaxis induced by human serum albumin derivatives modified with methylglyoxal and glucose-derived advanced glycation endproducts. Immunol Lett 1997;58:139-147.
155. Webster L, Abordo EA, Thornalley PJ, Limb GA. Induction of TNF alpha and IL-beta mRNA in monocytes by methylglyoxal- and advanced glycated endproduct-modified human serum albumin. Biochem Soc Trans 1997;25:250S.
156. Pugliese G, Pricci F, Romeo G, et al. Upregulation of mesangial growth factor and extracellular matrix synthesis by advanced glycation end products via a receptor-mediated mechanism. Diabetes 1997;46:1881-1887.
157. Smedsrod B, Melkko J, Araki N, et al. Advanced glycation end products are eliminated by scavenger-receptor-mediated endocytosis in hepatic sinusoidal kupffer and endothelial cells. Biochem J 1997;322:567-573.
158. Horiuchi S, Higashi T, Ikeda K, et al. Advanced glycation end products and their recognition by macrophage and macrophage-derived cells. Diabetes 1996;45:S73-S76.
159. Sano H, Higashi T, Matsumoto K, et al. Insulin enhances macrophage scavenger receptor-mediated endocytic uptake of advanced glycation end products. Biol Chem 1998;273:8630-8637.
160. Vlassara H, Li YM, Imani F, et al. Identification of galectin-3 as a high-affinity binding protein for advanced glycation end products (AGE): a new member of the AGE-receptor complex. Mol Med 1995;1:634-646.
161. Skolnik EY, Yang Z, Makita Z, et al. Human and rat mesangial cell receptors for glucose-modified proteins: potential role in kidney tissue remodelling and diabetic nephropathy. J Exp Med 1991;174:931-939.
162. Doi T, Vlassara H, Kirstein M, et al. Receptor-specific increase in extracellular matrix productions in mouse mesangial cells by advanced glycosylation end products is mediated via platelet derived growth factor. Proc Natl Acad Sci U S A 1992;89: 2873-2877.
163. Vlassara H, Fuh H, Donnelly T, Cybulsky M. Advanced glycation endproducts promote adhesion molecule (VCAM-1, ICAM-1) expression and atheroma formation in normal rabbits. Mol Med 1995;1:447-456.
164. Schmidt AM, Hori O, Chen JX, et al. Advanced glycation endproducts interacting with their endothelial receptor induce expression of vascular cell adhesion molecule-1 (VCAM-1) in cultured human endothelial cells and in mice: a potential mechanism for the accelerated vasculopathy of diabetes. J Clin Invest 1995;96: 1395-1403.
165. Sengoelge G, Fodinger M, Skoupy S, et al. Endothelial cell adhesion molecule and PMNL response to inflammatory stimuli and AGE-modified fibronectin. Kidney Int 1998;54:1637-1651.
166. Schmidt AM, Crandall J, Hori O, et al. Elevated plasma levels of vascular cell adhesion molecule-1 (VCAM-1) in diabetic patients with microalbuminuria: a marker of vascular dysfunction and progressive vascular disease. Br J Haematol 1996;92:747-750.
167. Wautier JL, Zoukourian C, Chappey O, et al. Receptor-mediated endothelial cell dysfunction in diabetic vasculopathy: soluble receptor for advanced glycation end products blocks hyperpermeability in diabetic rats. J Clin Invest 1996;97:238-243.
168. Lu M, Kuroki M, Amano S, et al. Advanced glycation end products increase retinal vascular endothelial growth factor expression. J Clin Invest 1998;101:1219-1224.
169. Hirata C, Nakano K, Nakamura N, et al. Advanced glycation end products induce expression of vascular endothelial growth factor by retinal Muller cells. Biochem Biophys Res Commun 1997;236: 712-715.

170. Park L, Raman KG, Lee KJ, et al. Suppression of accelerated diabetic atherosclerosis by the soluble receptor for advanced glycation end products. Nat Med 1998;4:1025-1031.
171. Kislinger T, Tanji N, Wendt T, et al. Receptor for advanced glycation end products mediates inflammation and enhanced expression of tissue factor in vasculature of diabetic apolipoprotein E-null mice. Arterioscler Thromb Vasc Biol 2001;21:905-910.
172. Lalla E, Lamster IB, Feit M, et al. Blockade of RAGE suppresses periodontitis-associated bone loss in diabetic mice. J Clin Invest 2000;105:1117-1124.
173. Goova MT, Li J, Kislinger T, Qu W, et al. Blockade of receptor for advanced glycation end-products restores effective wound healing in diabetic mice. Am J Pathol 2001;159:513-525.
174. Bucciarelli LG, Wendt T, Qu W, et al. RAGE blockade stabilizes established atherosclerosis in diabetic apolipoprotein E-null mice. Circulation 2002;106:2827-2835.
175. Basta G, Lazzerini G, Massaro M, et al. Advanced glycation end products activate endothelium through signal-transduction receptor RAGE: a mechanism for amplification of inflammatory responses. Circulation 2002;105:816-822.
176. Yan SD, Schmidt AM, Anderson GM, et al. Enhanced cellular oxidant stress by the interaction of advanced glycation end products with their receptors/binding proteins. J Biol Chem 1994;269:9889-9897.
177. Lander HM, Tauras JM, Ogiste JS, et al. Activation of the receptor for advanced glycation end products triggers a p21(ras)-dependent mitogen-activated protein kinase pathway regulated by oxidant stress. J Biol Chem 1997;272:17810-17814.
178. Li J, Schmidt AM. Characterization and functional analysis of the promoter of RAGE, the receptor for advanced glycation end products. J Biol Chem 1997;272:16498-16506.
179. Yamagishi S, Fujimori H, Yonekura H, et al. Advanced glycation end products inhibit prostacyclin production and induce plasminogen activator inhibitor-1 in human microvascular endothelial cells. Diabetologia 1998;41:1435-1441.
180. Tsuji H, Iehara N, Masegi T, et al. Ribozyme targeting of receptor for advanced glycation end products in mouse mesangial cells. Biochem Biophys Res Commun 1998;245:583-588.
181. Basta G, Sironi AM, Lazzerini G, et al. Circulating soluble receptor for advanced glycation end products is inversely associated with glycemic control and S100A12 protein. J Clin Endocrinol Metab 2006;91:4628-4634.
182. Naoto K, Munehide M, Hideaki K, et al. Decreased endogenous secretory advanced glycation end product receptor in type 1 diabetic patients: its possible association with diabetic vascular complications Diabetes Care 2005;28:2716-2721.
183. Inoguchi T, Battan R, Handler E, et al. Preferential elevation of protein kinase C isoform beta II and diacylglycerol levels in the aorta and heart of diabetic rats: differential reversibility to glycemic control by islet cell transplantation. Proc Natl Acad Sci U S A 1992;89:11059-1063.
184. Craven PA, Davidson CM, DeRubertis FR. Increase in diacylglycerol mass in isolated glomeruli by glucose from de novo synthesis of glycerolipids. Diabetes 1990;39:667-674.
185. Shiba T, Inoguchi T, Sportsman JR, et al. Correlation of diacylglycerol level and protein kinase C activity in rat retina to retinal circulation. Am J Physiol 1993;265(5 Pt 1):E783-E793.
186. Inoguchi T, Xia P, Kunisaki M, et al. Insulin's effect on protein kinase C and diacylglycerol induced by diabetes and glucose in vascular tissues. Am J Physiol 1994;267(3 Pt 1):E369-E379.
187. Derubertis FR, Craven PA. Activation of protein kinase C in glomerular cells in diabetes. Mechanisms and potential links to the pathogenesis of diabetic glomerulopathy. Diabetes 1994;43:1-8.
188. Xia P, Inoguchi T, Kern TS, et al. Characterization of the mechanism for the chronic activation of diacylglycerol–protein kinase C pathway in diabetes and hypergalactosemia. Diabetes 1994;43:1122-1129.
189. Ayo SH, Radnik R, Garoni JA, et al. High glucose increases diacylglycerol mass and activates protein kinase C in mesangial cell cultures. Am J Physiol 1991;261(4 Pt 2):F571-F577.
190. Koya D, King GL. Protein kinase C activation and the development of diabetic complications. Diabetes 1998;47:859-866.
191. Koya D, Jirousek MR, Lin YW, et al. Characterization of protein kinase C beta isoform activation on the gene expression of transforming growth factor-beta, extracellular matrix components, and prostanoids in the glomeruli of diabetic rats. J Clin Invest 1997;100:115-126.
192. Kikkawa R, Haneda M, Uzu T, et al. Translocation of protein kinase C alpha and zeta in rat glomerular mesangial cells cultured under high glucose conditions. Diabetologia 1994;37:838-841.
193. Knapp LT, Klann E. Superoxide-induced stimulation of protein kinase C via thiol modification and modulation of zinc content. J Biol Chem 2000;275:24136-24145.
194. Konishi H, Tanaka M, Takemura Y, et al. Activation of protein kinase C by tyrosine phosphorylation in response to H_2O_2. Proc Natl Acad Sci U S A 1997;94:11233-11237.
195. Ishii H, Jirousek MR, Koya D, et al. Amelioration of vascular dysfunctions in diabetic rats by an oral PKC-β inhibitor. Science 1996;272:728-731.
196. Craven PA, Studer RK, DeRubertis FR. Impaired nitric oxide–dependent cyclic guanosine monophosphate generation in glomeruli from diabetic rats. Evidence for protein kinase C–mediated suppression of the cholinergic response. J Clin Invest 1994;93:311-320.
197. Ganz MB, Seftel A. Glucose-induced changes in protein kinase C and nitric oxide are prevented by vitamin E. Am J Physiol 2000;278:E146-152.
198. Kuboki K, Jiang ZY, Takahara N, et al. Regulation of endothelial constitutive nitric oxide synthase gene expression in endothelial cells and in vivo: a specific vascular action of insulin. Circulation 2000;101:676-681.
199. Glogowski EA, Tsiani E, Zhou X, et al. High glucose alters the response of mesangial cell protein kinase C isoforms to endothelin-1. Kidney Int 1999;55:486-499.
200. Hempel A, Maasch C, Heintze U, et al. High glucose concentrations increase endothelial cell permeability via activation of protein kinase C alpha. Circ Res 1997;81:363-371.
201. Williams B, Gallacher B, Patel H, Orme C. Glucose-induced protein kinase C activation regulates vascular permeability factor mRNA expression and peptide production by human vascular smooth muscle cells in vitro. Diabetes 1997;46:1497-1503.
202. Studer RK, Craven PA, DeRubertis FR. Role for protein kinase C in the mediation of increased fibronectin accumulation by mesangial cells grown in high-glucose medium. Diabetes 1993;42:118-126.
203. Pugliese G, Pricci F, Pugliese F, et al. Mechanisms of glucose-enhanced extracellular matrix accumulation in rat glomerular mesangial cells. Diabetes 1994;43:478-490.
204. Craven PA, Studer RK, Felder J, et al. Nitric oxide inhibition of transforming growth factor-beta and collagen synthesis in mesangial cells Diabetes 1997;46:671-681.
205. Phillips SL, DeRubertis FR, Craven PA. Regulation of the laminin C1 promoter in cultured mesangial cells. Diabetes 1999;48:2083-2089.
206. Feener EP, Xia P, Inoguchi T, Shiba T, et al. Role of protein kinase C in glucose- and angiotensin II-induced plasminogen activator inhibitor expression. Contrib Nephrol 1996;118:180-187.
207. Pieper GM, Riaz-ul-Haq J. Activation of nuclear factor-κB in cultured endothelial cells by increased glucose concentration: prevention by calphostin C. Cardiovasc Pharmacol 1997;30:528-532.
208. Yerneni KK, Bai W, Khan BV, et al. Hyperglycemia-induced activation of nuclear transcription factor κB in vascular smooth muscle cells. Diabetes 1999;48:855-864.
209. Dang L, Seale JP, Qu X. High glucose-induced human umbilical vein endothelial cell hyperpermeability is dependent on protein kinase C activation and independent of the Ca^{2+}-nitric oxide signalling pathway. Clin Exp Pharmacol Physiol 2005;32:771-776.
210. Igarashi M, Wakasaki H, Takahara N, et al. Glucose or diabetes activates p38 mitogen-activated protein kinase via different pathways. J Clin Invest 1999;103:185-195.
211. Fontayne A, Dang PM, Gougerot-Pocidalo MA, El Benna J. Phosphorylation of p47phox sites by PKC-alpha, beta II, delta, and zeta: effect on binding to p22phox and on NADPH oxidase activation. Biochemistry 2002;41:7743-7750.
212. Guzik TJ, Mussa S, Gastaldi D, et al. Mechanisms of increased vascular superoxide production in human diabetes mellitus: role of NAD(P)H oxidase and endothelial nitric oxide synthase. Circulation 2002;105:1656-1662.
213. Beckman JA, Goldfine AB, Gordon MB, et al. Inhibition of protein kinase Cβ prevents impaired endothelium- dependent vasodila-

tion caused by hyperglycemia in humans. Circ Res 2002;90(1): 107-111.
214. Way KJ, Isshiki K, Suzuma K, et al. Expression of connective tissue growth factor is increased in injured myocardium associated with protein kinase C β2 activation and diabetes. Diabetes 2002;51: 2709-2718.
215. Sayeski PP, Kudlow JE. Glucose metabolism to glucosamine is necessary for glucose stimulation of transforming growth factor-alpha gene transcription. J Biol Chem 1996;271:15237-15243.
216. Kolm-Litty V, Sauer U, Nerlich A, Lehmann R, Schleicher ED. High glucose-induced transforming growth factor beta1 production is mediated by the hexosamine pathway in porcine glomerular mesangial cells. J Clin Invest 1998;101:160-169.
217. Daniels MC, Kansal P, Smith TM, et al. Glucose regulation of transforming growth factor-alpha expression is mediated by products of the hexosamine biosynthesis pathway. Mol Endocrinol 1993;7: 1041-1048.
218. McClain DA, Paterson AJ, Roos MD, et al. Glucose and glucosamine regulate growth factor gene expression in vascular smooth muscle cells. Proc Natl Acad Sci U S A 1992;89:8150-8154.
219. Marshall S, Bacote V, Traxinger RR. Discovery of a metabolic pathway mediating glucose-induced desensitization of the glucose transport system. Role of hexosamine biosynthesis in the induction of insulin resistance. J Biol Chem 1991;266: 4706-4712.
220. Rossetti L, Hawkins M, Chen W, et al. In vivo glucosamine infusion induces insulin resistance in normoglycemic but not in hyperglycemic conscious rats. J Clin Invest 1995;96:132-140.
221. Hawkins M, Barzilai N, Liu R, et al. Role of the glucosamine pathway in fat-induced insulin resistance. J Clin Invest 1997;99: 2173-2182.
222. Federici M, Menghini R, Mauriello A, et al. Insulin-dependent activation of endothelial nitric oxide synthase is impaired by *O*-linked glycosylation modification of signaling proteins in human coronary endothelial cells. Circulation 2002;106:466-472.
223. Chen YQ, Su M, Walia RR, et al. Sp1 sites mediate activation of the plasminogen activator inhibitor-1 promoter by glucose in vascular smooth muscle cells. J Biol Chem 1998;273:8225-8231.
224. Goldberg HJ, Scholey J, Fantus IG. Glucosamine activates the plasminogen activator inhibitor 1 gene promoter through Sp1 DNA binding sites in glomerular mesangial cells. Diabetes 2000;49: 863-871.
225. Goldberg HJ, Whiteside CI, Fantus IG. The hexosamine pathway regulates the plasminogen activator inhibitor-1 gene promoter and Sp1 transcriptional activation through protein kinase C-beta I and -delta. J Biol Chem 2002;277:33833-33841.
226. Hart GW. Dynamic *O*-linked glycosylation of nuclear and cytoskeletal proteins. Annu Rev Biochem 1997;66:315-335.
227. Akimoto Y, Kreppel LK, Hirano H, Hart GW. Hyperglycemia and the *O*-GlcNAc transferase in rat aortic smooth muscle cells: elevated expression and altered patterns of *O*-GlcNAcylation. Arch Biochem Biophys 2001;389:166-175.
228. Pugazhenthi S, Nesterova A, Jambal P, et al. Oxidative stress-mediated down-regulation of bcl-2 promoter in hippocampal neurons. J Neurochem 2003;84:982-996.
229. Sima AA, Prashar A, Zhang WX, et al. Preventive effect of long-term aldose reductase inhibition (ponalrestat) on nerve conduction and sural nerve structure in the spontaneously diabetic Bio-Breeding rat. J. Clin Invest 1990;85:1410-1420.
230. Lee, AY, Chung, SK, and Chung, SS. Demonstration that polyol accumulation is responsible for diabetic cataract by the use of transgenic mice expressing the aldose reductase gene in the lens. Proc Natl Acad Sci U S A 1995;92:2780-2784.
231. Brownlee M. Advanced protein glycosylation in diabetes and aging. Annu Rev Med 1995;46:223-234.
232. Brownlee M Biochemistry and molecular cell biology of diabetic complications Nature 2001;414:813-820.
233. Giardino, I, Edelstein, D, Brownlee, M. BCL-2 expression or antioxidants prevent hyperglycemia-induced formation of intracellular advanced glycation end products in bovine endothelial cells. J Clin Invest 1996;97:1422-1428.
234. Wallace DC. Diseases of the mitochondrial DNA. Annu Rev Biochem 1992;61:1175-1212.
235. Trumpower BL. The proton motive Q cycle. J Biol Chem 1990;265: 11409-11412.
236. Korshunov SS, Skulachev VP, Starkov AA. High protonic potential actuates a mechanism of production of reactive oxygen species in mitochondria. FEBS Lett 1997;416:15-18.
237. Casteilla L, Blondel,O, Klaus S, et al. Stable expression of functional mitochondrial uncoupling protein in Chinese hamster ovary cells. Proc Natl Acad Sci U S A 1990;87:5124-5128.
238. Manna SK, Zhang HJ, Yan T, et al. Overexpression manganese superoxide dismutase suppresses tumor necrosis factor–induced apoptosis and activation of nuclear transcription factor-κB and activated protein-1. J Biol Chem 1998;273:13245-13254.
239. Haskins K, Bradley B, Powers K, et al. Oxidative stress in type 1 diabetes. Ann N Y Acad Sci 2003;1005:43-54.
240. Du X, Matsumura T, Edelstein D, et al. Inhibition of GAPDH activity by poly(ADP-ribose) polymerase activates three major pathways of hyperglycemic damage in endothelial cells. J Clin Invest 2003;112:1049-1057.
241. Sawa A, Khan AA, Hester LD, Snyder SH. Glyceraldehyde-3-phosphate dehydrogenase: nuclear translocation participates in neuronal and nonneuronal cell death. Proc Natl Acad Sci U S A 1997;94:11669-11674.
242. Schmidtz HD. Reversible nuclear translocation of glyceraldehyde-3-phosphate dehydrogenase upon serum depletion. Eur J Cell Biol 2001;80:419-427.
243. Craven PA, Phillips SL, Melhem MF, et al. Overexpression of manganese superoxide dismutase suppresses increases in collagen accumulation induced by culture of mesangial cells in high-media glucose. Metabolism 2001;50:1043-1048.
244. Vincent AM, Brownlee M, Russell JW. Oxidative stress and programmed cell death in diabetic neuropathy. Ann N Y Acad Sci 2002;959:368-383.
245. Zou MH, Shi C, Cohen RA. High glucose via peroxynitrite causes tyrosine nitration and inactivation of prostacyclin synthase that is associated with thromboxane/prostaglandin H_2 receptor–mediated apoptosis and adhesion molecule expression in cultured human aortic endothelial cells. Diabetes 2002;51:198-203.
246. Uemura S, Matsushita H, Li W, et al. Diabetes mellitus enhances vascular matrix metalloproteinase activity: role of oxidative stress. Circ Res 2001;88:1291-1298.
247. Craven PA, Melhem MF, Phillips SL, Derubertis FR. Overexpression of Cu^{2+}/Zn^{2+} superoxide dismutase protects against early diabetic glomerular injury in transgenic mice. Diabetes 2001;50: 2114-2125.
248. DeRubertis FR, Craven PA, Melhem MF, Salah EM. Attenuation of renal injury in db/db mice overexpressing superoxide dismutase: evidence for reduced superoxide–nitric oxide interaction. Diabetes 2004;53:762-768.
249. Ye G, Metreveli NS, Donthi RV, et al. Catalase protect cardiomyocyte function in models of type 1 and type 2 diabetes. Diabetes 2004;53:1336-1343.
250. Shen X, Zheng S, Metreveli NS, Epstein PN. Protection of cardiac mitochondria by overexpression of MnSOD reduces diabetic cardiomyopathy. Diabetes 2006;55:798-805.
251. Huang C, Kim Y, Caramori ML, et al. Diabetic nephropathy is associated with gene expression levels of oxidative phosphorylation and related pathways. Diabetes 2006;55:1826-1831.
252. Kowluru RA. Effect of reinstitution of good glycemic control on retinal oxidative stress and nitrative stress in diabetic rats. Diabetes 2003;52(3):818-823.
253. Yu T, Robotham JL, Yoon Y. Increased production of reactive oxygen species in hyperglycemic conditions requires dynamic change of mitochondrial morphology Proc Natl Acad Sci U S A 2006;103:2653-2658.
254. Ferris FL. How effective are treatments for diabetic retinopathy? JAMA 1993;269:1290-1291.
255. The PKC-DRS Study Group. The effect of ruboxistaurin on visual loss in patients with moderately severe to very severe nonproliferative diabetic retinopathy: initial results of the PKC-DRS Multicenter Randomized Clinical Trial. Diabetes 2005;54:2188-2197.
256. Strøm C, Sander B, Klemp K, et al. Effect of ruboxistaurin on blood-retinal barrier permeability in relation to severity of leakage in diabetic macular edema. Invest Ophthalmol Vis Sci 2005;46: 3855-3858.
257. Aiello LP, Clermont A, Arora V, et al. Inhibition of PKC-β by oral administration of ruboxistaurin (LY333531) mesylate is well-tolerated and ameliorates diabetes-induced retinal hemodynamic

abnormalities in patients. Invest Ophthalmol Vis Sci 2005;47:86-92.

258. The PKC-DMES Study Group. Effect of ruboxistaurin, a PKCβ isoform-selective inhibitor, in patients with diabetic macular edema: 30-month results of the randomized PKC-DMES clinical trial. Arch Opthalmal 2007;125:318-324.
259. The PKC-DRS2 Study Group. Effect of ruboxistaurin on visual loss in patients with diabetic retinopathy. Ophthalmology 2006;113:2221-2230.
260. Tuttle KR, Bakris GL, Toto RD, et al. The effect of ruboxistaurin on nephropathy in type 2 diabetes. Diabetes Care 2005;28:2686-2690.
261. Cunningham ET, Adamis AP, Altaweel M, et al, and the Macugen Diabetic Retinopathy Study Group. A phase ii randomized double-masked trial of pegaptanib, an anti-vascular endothelial growth factor aptamer, for diabetic macular edema. Ophthalmology 2005;46:3855-3858.
262. Chun DW, Heier JS, Topping TM, et al. A pilot study of multiple intravitreal injections of ranibizumab in patients with center-involving clinically significant diabetic macular edema. Ophthalmology 2006;113:1706-1712.
263. Jager RD, Aiello LP, Patel SC, Cunningham ET. Risks of intravitreal injection: a comprehensive review. Retina 2004;24:676-698.
264. Wild S, Roglic G, Green A, et al. Global prevalence of diabetes: estimates for the year 2000 and projections for 2030. Diabetes Care 2004;27:1047-1053.
265. Harris MI, Hadden WC, Knowler WC, Bennett PH. Prevalence of diabetes and impaired glucose tolerance and plasma glucose levels in US population aged 20-74 years. Diabetes 1998;36:523-534.
266. Operational Research Department of the National Society to Prevent Blindness. Vision problems in the United States. A statistical analysis. New York: National Society to Prevent Blindness, 1980.
267. Klein R, Klein BE, Moss SE. Visual impairment in diabetes. Ophthalmology 1984;91:1-9.
268. Klein R, Klein BE, Moss SE, et al. The Wisconsin Epidemiologic Study of Diabetic Retinopathy: II. Prevalence and risk of diabetic retinopathy when age at diagnosis is less than 30 years. Arch Ophthalmol 1984;102:520-536.
269. Klein R, Klein BE, Moss SE, Cruickshanks KJ. The Wisconsin Epidemiologic Study of Diabetic Retinopathy: XV. The long-term incidence of macular edema. Ophthalmology 1995;102:7-16.
270. Javitt JC, Canner JK, Sommer A. Cost effectiveness of current approaches to the control of retinopathy in type 1 diabetics. Ophthalmology 1989;96:255-264.
271. Javitt JC, Aiello LP, Bassi LJ, et al. Detecting and treating retinopathy in patients with type I diabetes mellitus: savings associated with improved implementation of current guidelines. American Academy of Ophthalmology. Ophthalmology 1991;98:1565-1573.
272. Javitt JC, Aiello LP, Chiang Y, et al. Preventive eye care in people with diabetes is cost-saving to the federal government: implications for health-care reform. Diabetes Care 1994;17:909-917.
273. Javitt JC, Aiello LP. Cost-effectiveness of detecting and treating diabetic retinopathy (see comments). Ann Intern Med 1996;124(1 Pt 2):164-169.
274. Centers for Disease Control and Prevention. National Diabetes Fact Sheet. National Estimate on Diabetes. Available at http://www.cdc.gov/diabetes/pubs/estimates.htm (accessed March 21, 2007).
275. Kahn HA, Hiller R. Blindness caused by diabetic retinopathy. Am J Ophthalmol 1974;78:58-67.
276. Palmberg PF. Diabetic retinopathy. Diabetes 1977;26:703-709.
277. DCCT Research Group. The Diabetes Control and Complications Trial (DCCT). Design and methodologic considerations for the feasibility phase. Diabetes 1986;35:530-545.
278. Diabetes Control and Complications Trial/Epidemiology of Diabetes Interventions and Complications Research Group. Retinopathy and nephropathy in patients with type 1 diabetes four years after a trial of intensive therapy. N Engl J Med 2000;342:381-389.
279. The relationship of glycemic exposure (Hb A_{1c}) to the risk of development and progression of retinopathy in the Diabetes Control and Complications trial. Diabetes 1995;44:968-983.
280. Diabetes Control and Complications Trial Research Group. Lifetime benefits and costs of intensive therapy as practiced in the Diabetes Control and Complications Trial (see comments) (published erratum appears in JAMA 1997;278:25). JAMA 1996;276: 1409-1415.
281. Resource utilization and costs of care in the diabetes control and complications trial. Diabetes Care 1995;18:1468-1478.
282. Cogan DG, Toussaint D, Kuwabara T. Retinal vascular patterns: IV. Diabetic retinopathy. Arch Ophthalmol 1961;66:366-378.
283. Konno S, Feke GT, Yoshida A, et al. Retinal blood flow changes in type I diabetes: a long-term follow-up study. Invest Ophthalmol Vis Sci 1996;37:1140-1148.
284. Grunwald JE, Riva CE, Sinclair SH, et al. Laser Doppler velocimetry study of retinal circulation in diabetes mellitus. Arch Ophthalmol 1986;104:991-996.
285. Bursell SE, Clermont AC, Kinsley BT, et al. Retinal blood flow changes in patients with insulin-dependent diabetes mellitus and no diabetic retinopathy. Am J Physiol 1996;270(1 Pt 2):R61-R70.
286. Sosula L, Beaumont P, Hollows FC, Jonson KM. Dilatation and endothelial proliferation of retinal capillaries in streptozotocin-diabetic rats: quantitative electron microscopy. Invest Ophthalmol 1972;11:926-935.
287. Speiser P, Gittelsohn AM, Patz A. Studies on diabetic retinopathy: III. Influence of diabetes on intramural pericytes. Arch Ophthalmol 1968;80:332-337.
288. Barouch FC, Miyamoto K, Allport JR, et al. Integrin-mediated neutrophil adhesion and retinal leukostasis in diabetes. Invest Ophthalmol Vis Sci 2000;41:1153-1158.
289. Miyamoto K, Khosrof S, Bursell SE, et al. Vascular endothelial growth factor (VEGF)-induced retinal vascular permeability is mediated by intercellular adhesion molecule-1 (ICAM-1). Am J Pathol 2000;156:1733-1739.
290. Miyamoto K, Khosrof S, Bursell SE, et al. Prevention of leukostasis and vascular leakage in streptozotocin-induced diabetic retinopathy via intercellular adhesion molecule-1 inhibition. Proc Natl Acad Sci U S A 1999;96:10836-10841.
291. Stitt AW, Gardiner TA, Archer DB. Histological and ultrastructural investigation of retinal microaneurysm development in diabetic patients. Br J Ophthalmol 1995;79:362-367.
292. Cunha-Vaz J, Faria DA Jr, Campos AJ. Early breakdown of the blood-retinal barrier in diabetes. Br J Ophthalmol 1975;59: 649-656.
293. The Early Treatment Diabetic Retinopathy Study Research Group. Early photocoagulation for diabetic retinopathy. ETDRS Report No. 9. Ophthalmology 1991;98(5 Suppl):766-785.
294. Meyer-Schwickerath R, Pfeiffer A, Blum WF, et al. Vitreous levels of the insulin-like growth factors I and II, and the insulin-like growth factor-binding proteins 2 and 3, increase in neovascular eye disease: studies in nondiabetic and diabetic subjects. J Clin Invest 1993;92:2620-2625.
295. Nishimura M, Ikeda T, Ushiyama M, et al. Increased vitreous concentrations of human hepatocyte growth factor in proliferative diabetic retinopathy. J Clin Endocrinol Metab 1999;84:659-662.
296. Aiello LP, Avery RL, Arrigg PG, et al. Vascular endothelial growth factor in ocular fluid of patients with diabetic retinopathy and other retinal disorders (see comments). N Engl J Med 1994;331: 1480-1487.
297. Adamis AP, Miller JW, Bernal MT, et al. Increased vascular endothelial growth factor levels in the vitreous of eyes with proliferative diabetic retinopathy. Am J Ophthalmol 1994;118:445-450.
298. Aiello LP, Hata Y. Molecular mechanisms of growth factor action in diabetic retinopathy. Curr Opin Endocrinol Diabetes 1999;6: 146-156.
299. Aiello LP, Bursell SE, Clermont A, et al. Vascular endothelial growth factor–induced retinal permeability is mediated by protein kinase C in vivo and suppressed by an orally effective beta isoform–selective inhibitor. Diabetes 1997;46:1473-1480.
300. Miller JW, Adamis AP, Aiello LP. Vascular endothelial growth factor in ocular neovascularization and proliferative diabetic retinopathy. Diabetes Metab Rev 1997;13:37-50.
301. Okamoto N, Tobe T, Hackett SF, et al. Transgenic mice with increased expression of vascular endothelial growth factor in the retina: a new model of intraretinal and subretinal neovascularization (see comments). Am J Pathol 1997;151:281-291.
302. Ozaki H, Hayashi H, Vinores SA, et al. Intravitreal sustained release of VEGF causes retinal neovascularization in rabbits and breakdown of the blood-retinal barrier in rabbits and primates. Exp Eye Res 1997;64:505-517.

303. Aiello LP, Pierce EA, Foley ED, et al. Suppression of retinal neovascularization in vivo by inhibition of vascular endothelial growth factor (VEGF) using soluble VEGF-receptor chimeric proteins. Proc Natl Acad Sci U S A 1995;92:10457-10461.
304. Robinson GS, Pierce EA, Rook SL, et al. Oligodeoxynucleotides inhibit retinal neovascularization in a murine model of proliferative retinopathy. Proc Natl Acad Sci USA 1996;93:4851-4856.
305. Adamis AP, Shima DT, Tolentino MJ, et al. Inhibition of vascular endothelial growth factor prevents retinal ischemia–associated iris neovascularization in a nonhuman primate. Arch Ophthalmol 1996;114:66-71.
306. Danis RP, Bingaman DP, Jirousek M, Yang Y. Inhibition of intraocular neovascularization caused by retinal ischemia in pigs by PKC-β inhibition with LY333531. Invest Ophthalmol Vis Sci 1998;39: 171-179.
307. Ozaki H, Seo MS, Ozaki K, et al. Blockade of vascular endothelial cell growth factor receptor signaling is sufficient to completely prevent retinal neovascularization. Am J Pathol 2000;156:697-707.
308. Duh EJ, Yang HS, Suzuma I, et al. Pigment epithelium–derived factor (PEDF) suppresses ischemia-induced retinal neovascularization and VEGF-induced migration and growth. Invest Ophthalmol Vis Sci 2002;43(3):821-829.
309. Tripathi RC, Li J, Tripathi BJ, et al. Increased level of vascular endothelial growth factor in aqueous humor of patients with neovascular glaucoma. Ophthalmology 1998;105:232-237.
310. Tolentino MJ, Miller JW, Gragoudas ES, et al. Vascular endothelial growth factor is sufficient to produce iris neovascularization and neovascular glaucoma in a nonhuman primate. Arch Ophthalmol 1996;114:964-970.
311. Klein R, Klein BE, Moss SE, et al. The Wisconsin Epidemiologic Study of Diabetic Retinopathy: III. Prevalence and risk of diabetic retinopathy when age at diagnosis is 30 or more years. Arch Ophthalmol 1984;102:527-532.
312. Kohner EM, Aldington SJ, Stratton IM, et al; for the United Kingdom Prospective Diabetes Study. United Kingdom Prospective Diabetes Study, 30: Diabetic retinopathy at diagnosis of non–insulin-dependent diabetes mellitus and associated risk factors. Arch Ophthalmol 1998;116:297-303.
313. Diabetes Control and Complications Trial Research Group. Progression of retinopathy with intensive versus conventional treatment in the Diabetes Control and Complications Trial. Ophthalmology 1995;102:647-661.
314. Kroc Collaborative Study Group. Blood glucose control and the evolution of diabetic retinopathy and albuminuria: a preliminary multicenter trial. N Engl J Med 1984;311:365-372.
315. Chase HP, Jackson WE, Hoops SL, et al. Glucose control and the renal and retinal complications of insulin-dependent diabetes. JAMA 1989;261:1155-1160.
316. Krolewski AS, Canessa M, Warram JH, et al. Predisposition to hypertension and susceptibility to renal disease in insulin-dependent diabetes mellitus. N Engl J Med 1988;318:140-145.
317. Stern MP, Patterson JK, Haffner SM, et al. Lack of awareness and treatment of hyperlipidemia in type II diabetes in a community survey. JAMA 1989;262:360-364.
318. Aiello LP, Gardner TW, King GL, et al. Diabetic retinopathy: technical review. Diabetes Care 1998;21:143-156.
319. Diabetic Retinopathy Study Research Group. Four risk factors for severe visual loss in diabetic retinopathy. The Third Report from the Diabetic Retinopathy Study. Arch Ophthalmol 1979;97: 654-655.
320. The Early Treatment Diabetic Retinopathy Study Research Group. Treatment techniques and clinical guidelines for photocoagulation of diabetic macular edema. Early Treatment Diabetic Retinopathy Study Report No. 2. Ophthalmology 1987;94:761-774.
321. The Early Treatment Diabetic Retinopathy Study Research Group. Photocoagulation for diabetic macular edema: Early Treatment Diabetic Retinopathy Study Report No. 4. Int Ophthalmol Clin 1987;27:265-272.
322. Wilkinson CP, Ferris FL III, Klein RE, et al. Proposed International Clinical Diabetic Retinopathy and Diabetic Macular Edema Disease Severity Scales. Ophthalmology 2003;110(9):1677-1682.
323. Chew E.Y. A simplified diabetic retinopathy scale. Ophthalmology 2003;110(9):1675-1676.
324. Early Treatment Diabetic Retinopathy Study Research Group. Fundus photographic risk factors for progression of diabetic retinopathy. ETDRS Report Number 12. Ophthalmology 1991;98(5 suppl):823-833.
325. Early Treatment Diabetic Retinopathy Study Research Group. Grading diabetic retinopathy from stereoscopic color fundus photographs—an extension of the modified Airlie House classification. ETDRS Report Number 10. Ophthalmology 1991;98(5 suppl):786-806.
326. Waite JH, Beetham WP. Visual mechanisms in diabetes mellitus: comparative study of 2002 diabetics and 437 nondiabetics for control. N Engl J Med 1935;212:367-379.
327. Zorrilla E, Kozak GP. Ophthalmoplegia in diabetes mellitus. Ann Intern Med 1967;67:968-976.
328. Rush JA, Younge BR. Paralysis of cranial nerves III, IV, and VI: cause and prognosis in 1000 cases. Arch Ophthalmol 1981;99: 76-79.
329. Barr CC, Glaser JS, Blankenship G. Acute disc swelling in juvenile diabetes: clinical profile and natural history of 12 cases. Arch Ophthalmol 1980;98:2185-2192.
330. Gartner S, Henkind P. Neovascularization of the iris (rubeosis iridis). Surv Ophthalmol 1978;22:291-312.
331. Brown GC, Magargal LE, Schachat A, Shah H. Neovascular glaucoma: etiologic considerations. Ophthalmology 1984;91: 315-320.
332. Schwartz JN, Donnelly EH, Klintworth GK. Ocular and orbital phycomycosis. Surv Ophthalmol 1977;22:3-28.
333. Blitzer A, Lawson W, Meyers BR, Biller HF. Patient survival factors in paranasal sinus mucormycosis. Laryngoscope 1980;90: 635-648.
334. Wand M, Dueker DK, Aiello LM, Grant WM. Effects of panretinal photocoagulation on rubeosis iridis, angle neovascularization, and neovascular glaucoma. Am J Ophthalmol 1978;86:332-339.
335. Aiello LM, Wand M, Liang G. Neovascular glaucoma and vitreous hemorrhage following cataract surgery in patients with diabetes mellitus. Ophthalmology 1983;90:814-820.
336. Simmons RJ, Dueker DK, Kimbrough RL, Aiello LM. Goniophotocoagulation for neovascular glaucoma. Trans Am Acad Ophthalmol Otolaryngol 1977;83:80-89.
337. Mason JO 3rd, Albert MA Jr, Mays A, Vail R. Regression of neovascularization iris vessels by intravitreal injection of bevacizumab. Retina 2006;26(7):839-841.
338. Hyndiuk RA, Kazarian EL, Schultz RO, Seideman S. Neurotrophic corneal ulcers in diabetes mellitus. Arch Ophthalmol 1977;95: 2193-2196.
339. Khodadoust AA, Silverstein AM, Kenyon DR, Dowling JE. Adhesion of regenerating corneal epithelium: the role of basement membrane. Am J Ophthalmol 1968;65:339-348.
340. Klein BE, Klein R, Moss SE. Intraocular pressure in diabetic persons. Ophthalmology 1984;91:1356-1360.
341. Pasquale LR, Kang JH, Manson JE, et al. Prospective study of type 2 diabetes mellitus and risk of primary open-angle glaucoma in women. Ophthalmology 2006;113:1081-1086.
342. Marmor MF. Transient accommodative paralysis and hyperopia in diabetes. Arch Ophthalmol 1973;89:419-421.
343. Klein BE, Klein R, Moss SE. Prevalence of cataracts in a population-based study of persons with diabetes mellitus. Ophthalmology 1985;92:1191-1196.
344. Ederer F, Hiller R, Taylor HR. Senile lens changes and diabetes in two population studies. Am J Ophthalmol 1981;91:381-395.
345. Bursell SE, Baker RS, Weiss JN, et al. Clinical photon correlation spectroscopy evaluation of human diabetic lenses. Exp Eye Res 1989;49:241-258.
346. Klein BE, Klein R, Moss SE. Incidence of cataract surgery in the Wisconsin Epidemiologic Study of Diabetic Retinopathy. Am J Ophthalmol 1995;119:295-300.
347. Klein BE, Klein R, Wang Q, Moss SE. Older-onset diabetes and lens opacities: the Beaver Dam Eye Study. Ophthalmic Epidemiol 1995;2:49-55.
348. Pai RP, Mitchell P, Chow VC, et al. Posttransplant cataract: lessons from kidney-pancreas transplantation (see comments). Transplantation 2000;69:1108-1114.
349. Dowler JG, Hykin PG, Hamilton AM. Phacoemulsification versus extracapsular cataract extraction in patients with diabetes. Ophthalmology 2000;107:457-462.
350. Borrillo JL, Mittra RA, Dev S, et al. Retinopathy progression and visual outcomes after phacoemulsification in patients with diabe-

tes mellitus. Trans Am Ophthalmol Soc 1999;97:435-445. Am J Ophthalmol 2000;129:832.
351. Funahashi T, Fink AI. The pathology of the bulbar conjunctiva in diabetes mellitus: I. Microaneurysms. Am J Ophthalmol 1963;55: 504-511.
352. Tagawa H, McMeel JW, Trempe CL. Role of the vitreous in diabetic retinopathy: II. Active and inactive vitreous changes. Ophthalmology 1986;93:1188-1192.
353. Fleckner RA, Goldstein JH. Mucormycosis. Br J Ophthalmol 1969; 53:542-548.
354. Diabetic Retinopathy Study Research Group. Photocoagulation treatment of proliferative diabetic retinopathy: clinical application of Diabetic Retinopathy Study (DRS) findings, DRS Report No. 8. Ophthalmology 1981;88:583-600.
355. Diabetic Retinopathy Vitrectomy Study Group. Two-year course of visual acuity in severe proliferative diabetic retinopathy with conventional management. Diabetic Retinopathy Vitrectomy Study (DRVS) Report No. 1. Ophthalmology 1985;92:492-502.
356. Diabetes Control and Complications Trial Research Group. The effect of intensive diabetes treatment on the progression of diabetic retinopathy in insulin-dependent diabetes mellitus: the Diabetes Control and Complications Trial. Arch Ophthalmol 1995;113:36-51.
357. Klein R, Klein BE, Moss SE, et al. The Wisconsin Epidemiologic Study of Diabetic Retinopathy: VI. Retinal photocoagulation. Ophthalmology 1987;94:747-753.
358. Witkin SR, Klein R. Ophthalmologic care for persons with diabetes. JAMA 1984;251:2534-2537.
359. American Academy of Ophthalmology. Comprehensive Adult Medical Eye Evaluation: Preferred Practice Pattern, 2005. PDF available for download at http://www.aao.org/education/library/ppp/camee.cfm (accessed March 21, 2007).
360. American Optometric Association. Comprehensive Adult Eye and Vision Examination: Optometric Clinical Practice Guideline, 2005. PDF available at http://www.aoa.org/documents/CPG-1.pdf (accessed March 21, 2007).
361. Klein R, Klein BE, Neider MW, et al. Diabetic retinopathy as detected using ophthalmoscopy, a nonmydriatic camera, and a standard fundus camera. Ophthalmology 1985;92:485-491.
362. Moss SE, Klein R, Kessler SD, Richie KA. Comparison between ophthalmoscopy and fundus photography in determining severity of diabetic retinopathy. Ophthalmology 1985;92:62-67.
363. Sussman EJ, Tsiaras WG, Soper KA. Diagnosis of diabetic eye disease. JAMA 1982;247:3231-3234.
364. Cavallerano JD, Aiello LP, Cavallerano AA, et al, and the Joslin Vision Network Team. Nonmydriatic digital imaging alternative for annual retinal exam in persons with previously documented no or mild diabetic retinopathy. Am J Ophthalmol 2005;140(4):667.
365. Klein R, Moss SE, Klein BE. New management concepts for timely diagnosis of diabetic retinopathy treatable by photocoagulation. Diabetes Care 1987;10:633-638.
366. Klein R, Klein BE, Moss SE, et al. Retinopathy in young-onset diabetic patients. Diabetes Care 1985;8:311-315.
367. Krolewski AS, Warram JH, Rand LI, et al. Risk of proliferative diabetic retinopathy in juvenile-onset type I diabetes: a 40-year follow-up study. Diabetes Care 1986;9:443-452.
368. Klein BE, Moss SE, Klein R. Is menarche associated with diabetic retinopathy? Diabetes Care 1990;13:1034-1038.
369. Kostraba JN, Klein R, Dorman JS, et al. The epidemiology of diabetes complications study: IV. Correlates of diabetic background and proliferative retinopathy. Am J Epidemiol 1991;133:381-391.
370. Sunness JS. The pregnant woman's eye. Surv Ophthalmol 1988;32:219-238.
371. Klein BE, Moss SE, Klein R. Effect of pregnancy on progression of diabetic retinopathy. Diabetes Care 1990;13:34-40.
372. White P. Diabetes mellitus in pregnancy. Clin Perinatol 1974;1: 331-347.
373. Best RM, Chakravarthy U. Diabetic retinopathy in pregnancy. Br J Ophthalmol 1997;81:249-251.
374. Diabetic Retinopathy Study Research Group. Indications for photocoagulation treatment of diabetic retinopathy: Diabetic Retinopathy Study Report No. 14. Int Ophthalmol Clin 1987;27: 239-253.
375. Diabetic Retinopathy Study Research Group. Photocoagulation treatment of proliferative diabetic retinopathy: the second report of diabetic retinopathy study findings. Ophthalmology 1978;85: 82-106.
376. The Early Treatment Diabetic Retinopathy Study Research Group. Photocoagulation for diabetic macular edema. Early Treatment Diabetic Retinopathy Study Report No. 1. Arch Ophthalmol 1985; 103:1796-1806.
377. Ferris F. Early photocoagulation in patients with either type 1 or type 2 diabetes. Trans Am Ophthalmol Soc 1996;94:505-537.
378. LaPiana FG, Penner R. Anaphylactoid reaction to intravenously administered fluorescein. Arch Ophthalmol 1968;79:161-162.
379. Butner RW, McPherson AR. Adverse reactions in intravenous fluorescein angiography. Ann Ophthalmol 1983;15:1084-1086.
380. Wittpenn JR, Rapoza P, Sternberg P, et al. Respiratory arrest following retrobulbar anesthesia. Ophthalmology 1986;93:867-870.
381. Klein R, Klein BE, Lee KE, et al. The incidence of hypertension in insulin-dependent diabetes. Arch Intern Med 1996;156:622-627.
382. Thai Multicenter Research Group on Diabetes Mellitus. Vascular complications in non–insulin-dependent diabetics in Thailand. Diabetes Res Clin Pract 1994;25:61-69.
383. Klein R, Klein BE, Moss SE, DeMets DL. Blood pressure and hypertension in diabetes. Am J Epidemiol 1985;122:75-89.
384. Fujimoto WY, Leonetti DL, Kinyoun JL, et al. Prevalence of complications among second-generation Japanese-American men with diabetes, impaired glucose tolerance, or normal glucose tolerance. Diabetes 1987;36:730-739.
385. Klein R, Klein BE, Moss SE, Cruickshanks KJ. The Wisconsin Epidemiologic Study of Diabetic Retinopathy: XVII. The 14-year incidence and progression of diabetic retinopathy and associated risk factors in type 1 diabetes (see comments). Ophthalmology 1998;105:1801-1815.
386. Zander E, Heinke P, Herfurth S, et al. Relations between diabetic retinopathy and cardiovascular neuropathy: a cross-sectional study in IDDM and NIDDM patients. Exp Clin Endocrinol Diabetes 1997;105:319-326.
387. Diabetes Drafting Group. Prevalence of small vessel and large vessel disease in diabetic patients from 14 centres: the World Health Organization Multinational Study of Vascular Disease in Diabetes. Diabetologia 1985;28:615-640.
388. Agardh CD, Agardh E, Torffvit O. The association between retinopathy, nephropathy, cardiovascular disease, and long-term metabolic control in type 1 diabetes mellitus: a 5-year follow-up study of 442 adult patients in routine care. Diabetes Res Clin Pract 1997;35:113-121.
389. Lopes de Faria JM, Jalkh AE, Trempe CL, McMeel JW. Diabetic macular edema: risk factors and concomitants. Acta Ophthalmol Scand 1999;77:170-175.
390. Marshall G, Garg SK, Jackson WE, et al. Factors influencing the onset and progression of diabetic retinopathy in subjects with insulin-dependent diabetes mellitus. Ophthalmology 1993;100: 1133-1139.
391. UK Prospective Diabetes Study Group. Tight blood pressure control and risk of macrovascular and microvascular complications in type 2 diabetes: UKPDS 38 (see comments) (published erratum appears in BMJ 1999;318:29). BMJ 1998;317:703-713.
392. Schrier RW, Estacio RO, Jeffers B. Appropriate Blood Pressure Control in NIDDM (ABCD) Trial. Diabetologia 1996;39:1646-1654.
393. Klein R, Klein BE, Moss SE, et al. The Wisconsin Epidemiology Study of Diabetic Retinopathy: V. Proteinuria and retinopathy in a population of diabetic persons diagnosed prior to 30 years of age. In Friedman EA, L'Esperance FA Jr, eds. Diabetic Renal-Retinal Syndrome, 3rd ed. Orlando: Grune & Stratton, 1986:245-264.
394. Kullberg CE, Arnqvist HJ. Elevated long-term glycated haemoglobin precedes proliferative retinopathy and nephropathy in type 1 (insulin-dependent) diabetic patients. Diabetologia 1993;36:961-965.
395. Klein R, Moss SE, Klein BE. Is gross proteinuria a risk factor for the incidence of proliferative diabetic retinopathy? Ophthalmology 1993;100:1140-1146.
396. Mathiesen ER, Ronn B, Storm B, et al. The natural course of microalbuminuria in insulin-dependent diabetes: a 10-year prospective study. Diabet Med 1995;12:482-487.
397. Park JY, Kim HK, Chung YE, et al. Incidence and determinants of microalbuminuria in Koreans with type 2 diabetes. Diabetes Care 1998;21:530-534.

398. Hasslacher C, Bostedt-Kiesel A, Kempe HP, Wahl P. Effect of metabolic factors and blood pressure on kidney function in proteinuric type 2 (non–insulin-dependent) diabetic patients. Diabetologia 1993;36:1051-1056.
399. Collins VR, Dowse GK, Plehwe WE, et al. High prevalence of diabetic retinopathy and nephropathy in Polynesians of Western Samoa. Diabetes Care 1995;18:1140-1149.
400. Lee ET, Lee VS, Kingsley RM, et al. Diabetic retinopathy in Oklahoma Indians with NIDDM: incidence and risk factors. Diabetes Care 1992;15:1620-1627.
401. Esmatjes E, Castell C, Gonzalez T, et al. Epidemiology of renal involvement in type II diabetics (NIDDM) in Catalonia. The Catalan Diabetic Nephropathy Study Group. Diabetes Res Clin Pract 1996;32:157-163.
402. Savage S, Estacio RO, Jeffers B, Schrier RW. Urinary albumin excretion as a predictor of diabetic retinopathy, neuropathy, and cardiovascular disease in NIDDM. Diabetes Care 1996;19:1243-1248.
403. Fujisawa T, Ikegami H, Yamato E, et al. Association of plasma fibrinogen level and blood pressure with diabetic retinopathy, and renal complications associated with proliferative diabetic retinopathy, in type 2 diabetes mellitus. Diabet Med 1999;16:522-526.
404. Cruickshanks KJ, Ritter LL, Klein R, Moss SE. The association of microalbuminuria with diabetic retinopathy. The Wisconsin Epidemiologic Study of Diabetic Retinopathy. Ophthalmology 1993;100:862-867.
405. Roy MS. Diabetic retinopathy in African Americans with type 1 diabetes—the New Jersey 725: II. Risk factors. Arch Ophthalmol 2000;118:105-115.
406. Klein R, Klein BE, Moss SE, Cruickshanks KJ. Ten-year incidence of gross proteinuria in people with diabetes. Diabetes 1995;44: 916-923.
407. Mogensen CE, Chachati A, Christensen CK, et al. Microalbuminuria: an early marker of renal involvement in diabetes. Uremia Invest 1985;9:85-95.
408. Villarosa IP, Bakris GL. The Appropriate Blood Pressure Control in Diabetes (ABCD) Trial. J Hum Hypertens 1998;12:653-655.
409. Nelson RG, Knowler WC, Pettitt DJ, et al. Incidence and determinants of elevated urinary albumin excretion in Pima Indians with NIDDM. Diabetes Care 1995;18:182-187.
410. Gomes MB, Lucchetti MR, Gazzola H, et al. Microalbuminuria and associated clinical features among Brazilians with insulin-dependent diabetes mellitus. Diabetes Res Clin Pract 1997;35: 143-147.
411. The Microalbuminuria Collaborative Study Group. Predictors of the development of microalbuminuria in patients with type 1 diabetes mellitus: a seven-year prospective study (see comments). Diabet Med 1999;16:918-925.
412. Davis MD, Fisher MR, Gangnon RE, et al. Risk factors for high-risk proliferative diabetic retinopathy and severe visual loss: Early Treatment Diabetic Retinopathy Study Report No. 18. Invest Ophthalmol Vis Sci 1998;39:233-252.
413. Qiao Q, Keinanen-Kiukaanniemi S, Laara E. The relationship between hemoglobin levels and diabetic retinopathy. J Clin Epidemiol 1997;50:153-158.
414. Friedman EA, Brown CD, Berman DH. Erythropoietin in diabetic macular edema and renal insufficiency. Am J Kidney Dis 1995; 26:202-208.
415. Gilbertson DT, Liu J, Xue JL, et al. Projecting the number of patients with end-stage renal disease in the United States to the year 2015. J Am Soc Nephrol 2005;16:3736-3741.
416. U.S. Renal Data System. USRDS 2006 Annual Data Report: Atlas of End-Stage Renal Disease in the United States. Bethesda, MD: National Institutes of Health, National Institute of Diabetes and Digestive and Kidney Diseases, 2006.
417. Cooper ME, Jandeleit-Dahm K, Thomas MC. Targets to retard the progression of diabetic nephropathy. Kidney Int 2005;68: 1439-1445.
418. Atkins RC. The epidemiology of chronic kidney disease. Kidney Int Suppl 2005;(94) S14-S18.
419. Muhlhauser I, Sawicki PT, Blank M, et al. Reliability of causes of death in persons with type I diabetes. Diabetologia 2002;45: 1490-1497.
420. Stephenson JM, Kenny S, Stevens LK, et al. Proteinuria and mortality in diabetes: the WHO Multinational Study of Vascular Disease in Diabetes. Diabet Med 1995;12:149-155.
421. Ismail N, Becker B, Strzelczyk P, et al. Renal disease and hypertension in non–insulin-dependent diabetes mellitus. Kidney Int 1999;55:1-28.
422. Parving HH, Hommel E, Mathiesen E, et al. Prevalence of microalbuminuria, arterial hypertension, retinopathy and neuropathy in patients with insulin dependent diabetes. Br Med J (Clin Res Ed) 1988;296:156-160.
423. Standl E, Stiegler H. Microalbuminuria in a random cohort of recently diagnosed type 2 (non–insulin-dependent) diabetic patients living in the greater Munich area. Diabetologia 1993;36: 1017-1020.
424. Schmitz A, Vaeth M, Mogensen CE. Systolic blood pressure relates to the rate of progression of albuminuria in NIDDM. Diabetologia 1994;37:1251-1258.
425. Zimmet P, Alberti KG, Shaw J. Global and societal implications of the diabetes epidemic. Nature 2001;414:782-787.
426. Kimmelsteil P, Wilson C. Intercapillary lesions in the glomeruli in the kidney. Am J Path 1936;12:83-97.
427. Ghavamian M, Gutch CF, Kopp KF, et al. The sad truth about hemodialysis in diabetic nephropathy. JAMA 1972;222:1386-1389.
428. Cooper ME. Pathogenesis, prevention and treatment of diabetic nephropathy. Lancet 1998;352:213-219.
429. Mogensen CE, Christensen, C K, Vittinghus E. The stages in diabetic renal disease. With emphasis in the stage of incipient diabetic nephropathy. Diabetes 1983;32:64-78.
430. Cambien F. Application de la théorie de Rehberg a l'étude clinique des affections rénales and du diabète. Annu Med 1934;35: 273-299.
431. Allen TJ, Cooper ME, Lan HY. Use of genetic mouse models in the study of diabetic nephropathy. Curr Diab Rep 2004;4: 435-440.
432. Thomson SC, Vallon V, Blantz RC. Kidney function in early diabetes: the tubular hypothesis of glomerular filtration. Am J Physiol Renal Physiol 2004;286:F8-F15.
433. Hostetter TH, Troy JL, Brenner BM. Glomerular hemodynamics in experimental diabetes mellitus. Kidney Int 1981;19:410-415.
434. Sharma K, Jin Y, Guo J, et al. Neutralization of TGF-β by anti-TGF-β antibody attenuates kidney hypertrophy and the enhanced extracellular matrix gene expression in STZ-induced diabetic mice. Diabetes 1996;45:522-530.
435. Segev Y, Landau D, Rasch R, et al. Growth hormone receptor antagonism prevents early renal changes in nonobese diabetic mice. J Am Soc Nephrol 1999;10:2374-2381.
436. Thomas MC, Burns WC, Cooper ME. Tubular changes in early diabetic nephropathy. Adv Chronic Kidney Dis 2005;12:177-186.
437. Mogensen CE, Christensen CK. Predicting diabetic nephropathy in insulin-dependent diabetic patients. N Engl J Med 1984;311: 89-93.
438. Mauer S, Steffes M, Ellis E, et al. Structural-functional relationships in diabetic nephropathy. J Clin Invest 1984;74:1143-1155.
439. Allen TJ, Cooper ME, Gilbert RG, et al. Serum total renin is increased before microalbuminuria in diabetes (IDDM). Kidney Int 1996;50:902-907.
440. Comper WD, Osicka TM, Clark M, et al. Earlier detection of microalbuminuria in diabetic patients using a new urinary albumin assay. Kidney Int 2004;65:1850-1855.
441. Poulsen PL, Hansen KW, Mogensen CE. Ambulatory blood pressure in the transition from normo- to microalbuminuria. A longitudinal study in IDDM patients. Diabetes 1994;43:1248-1253.
442. Mogensen CE, Keane WF, Bennett PH, et al. Prevention of diabetic renal disease with special reference to microalbuminuria. Lancet 1995;346:1080-1084.
443. Steinke JM, Sinaiko AR, Kramer MS, et al. The early natural history of nephropathy in type 1 diabetes: III. Predictors of 5-year urinary albumin excretion rate patterns in initially normoalbuminuric patients. Diabetes 2005;54:2164-2171.
444. Lurbe E, Redon J, Kesani A, et al. Increase in nocturnal blood pressure and progression to microalbuminuria in type 1 diabetes. N Engl J Med 2002;347:797-805.
445. Perkins BA, Ficociello LH, Silva KH, et al. Regression of microalbuminuria in type 1 diabetes. N Engl J Med 2003;348:2285-2293.
446. Hovind P, Tarnow L, Rossing P, et al. Predictors for the development of microalbuminuria and macroalbuminuria in patients with type 1 diabetes: inception cohort study. BMJ 2004;328:1105.

447. Bilous RW, Mauer SM, Sutherland DE, et al. Mean glomerular volume and rate of development of diabetic nephropathy. Diabetes 1989;38:1142-1147.
448. Parving H-H, Andersen AR, Smidt VM, et al. Diabetic nephropathy and arterial hypertension. Diabetologia 1983;24:10-12.
449. Fioretto P, Steffes MW, Sutherland DE, et al. Reversal of lesions of diabetic nephropathy after pancreas transplantation. N Engl J Med 1998;339:69-75.
450. Vora JP, Leese GP, Peters JR, et al. Longitudinal evaluation of renal function in non-insulin dependent diabetic patients with early nephropathy. J Diabetes Complications 1996;10:88-93.
451. Damsgaard EM, Froland A, Jorgensen OD, et al. Prognostic value of urinary albumin excretion rate and other risk factors in elderly diabetic patients and non-diabetic control subjects surviving the first 5 years after assessment. Diabetologia 1993;36:1030-1036.
452. Lane PH, Steffes MW, Mauer SM. Glomerular structure in IDDM women with low glomerular filtration rate and normal urinary albumin excretion. Diabetes 1992;41:581-586.
453. Tsalamandris C, Allen TJ, Gilbert RE, et al. Progressive decline in renal function in diabetic patients with and without albuminuria. Diabetes 1994;43:649-655.
454. Wiseman MJ, Mangili R, Alberetto M, et al. Glomerular response mechanisms to glycemic changes in insulin-dependent diabetics. Kidney Int 1987;31:1012-1018.
455. Kiritoshi S, Nishikawa T, Sonoda K, et al. Reactive oxygen species from mitochondria induce cyclooxygenase-2 gene expression in human mesangial cells: potential role in diabetic nephropathy. Diabetes 2003;52:2570-2577.
456. Forbes JM, Cooper ME, Oldfield MD, et al. Role of advanced glycation end products in diabetic nephropathy. J Am Soc Nephrol 2003;14:S254-S258.
457. Gorin Y, Block K, Hernandez J, et al. Nox4 NAD(P)H oxidase mediates hypertrophy and fibronectin expression in the diabetic kidney. J Biol Chem 2005;280:39616-39626.
458. Cooper ME. Interaction of metabolic and haemodynamic factors in mediating experimental diabetic nephropathy. Diabetologia 2001;44:1957-1972.
459. Thomas MC, Tikellis C, Burns WM, et al. Interactions between renin angiotensin system and advanced glycation in the kidney. J Am Soc Nephrol 2005;16:2976-2984.
460. Cooper ME, Mundel P, Boner G. Role of nephrin in renal disease including diabetic nephropathy. Semin Nephrol 2002;22:393-398.
461. Andersen S, Blouch K, Bialek J, et al. Glomerular permselectivity in early stages of overt diabetic nephropathy. Kidney Int 2000; 58:2129-2137.
462. Wassef L, Langham RG, Kelly DJ. Vasoactive renal factors and the progression of diabetic nephropathy. Curr Pharm Des 2004;10: 3373-3384.
463. Gilbert RE, Cooper ME. The tubulointerstitium in progressive diabetic kidney disease: More than an aftermath of glomerular injury? Kidney Int 1999;56:1627-1637.
464. Gilbert RE, Cooper ME, Krum H. Drug administration in patients with diabetes mellitus. Safety considerations. Drug Safety 1998;18:441-455.
465. Salifu MO, Haria DM, Badero O, et al. Challenges in the diagnosis and management of renal artery stenosis. Curr Hypertens Rep 2005;7:219-227.
466. Hricik DE, Browning PJ, Kopelman R, et al. Captopril-induced functional renal insufficiency in patients with bilateral renal-artery stenoses or renal-artery stenosis in a solitary kidney. N Engl J Med 1983;308:373-376.
467. Griffin MD, Bergstralhn EJ, Larson TS. Renal papillary necrosis—a sixteen-year clinical experience. J Am Soc Nephrol 1995;6: 248-256.
468. Davies PJ. Beethoven's nephropathy and death: discussion paper. J R Soc Med 1993;86:159-161.
469. Kelly DJ, Wilkinson-Berka JL, Allen TJ, et al. A new model of diabetic nephropathy with progressive renal impairment in the transgenic (mRen-2)27 rat (tgr). Kidney Int 1998;54:343-352.
470. DeFronzo RA. Hyperkalemia and hyporeninemic hypoaldosteronism. Kidney Int 1980;17:118-134.
471. Lush DJ, King JA, Fray JC. Pathophysiology of low renin syndromes: sites of renal renin secretory impairment and prorenin overexpression. Kidney Int 1993;43:983-999.
472. Nadler JL, Lee FO, Hsueh W, et al. Evidence of prostacyclin deficiency in the syndrome of hyporeninemic hypoaldosteronism. N Engl J Med 1986;314:1015-1020.
473. Parfrey PS, Griffiths SM, Barrett BJ, et al. Contrast material–induced renal failure in patients with diabetes mellitus, renal insufficiency, or both. A prospective controlled study. N Engl J Med 1989;320:143-149.
474. Weisberg LS, Kurnik PB, Kurnik BR. Risk of radiocontrast nephropathy in patients with and without diabetes mellitus. Kidney Int 1994;45:259-265.
475. Tepel M, van der Giet M, Schwarzfeld C, et al. Prevention of radiographic-contrast-agent–induced reductions in renal function by acetylcysteine. N Engl J Med 2000;343:180-184.
476. Mogensen CE. Long-term antihypertensive treatment inhibiting progression of diabetic nephropathy. BMJ 1982;285:685-688.
477. Parving H-H, Andersen, AR, Smidt, VM, et al. Effect of antihypertensive treatment on kidney function in diabetic nephropathy. Br Med J 1987;294:1443-1447.
478. UK Prospective Diabetes Study (UKPDS) Group. Tight blood pressure control and risk of macrovascular and microvascular complications in type 2 diabetes: UKPDS 38. BMJ 1998;317:703-713.
479. Björck S. Clinical trials in overt diabetic nephropathy. In Mogensen CE, ed. The Kidney and Hypertension in Diabetes Mellitus, 3rd ed. London: Kluwer Academic, 1996:375-384.
480. Parving HH. Renoprotection in diabetes: genetic and non-genetic risk factors and treatment. Diabetologia 1998;41:745-759.
481. Babaei-Jadidi R, Karachalias N, Ahmed N, et al. Prevention of incipient diabetic nephropathy by high-dose thiamine and benfotiamine. Diabetes 2003;52:2110-2120.
482. Thallas-Bonke V, Lindschau C, Rizkalla B, et al. Attenuation of extracellular matrix accumulation in diabetic nephropathy by the advanced glycation end product cross-link breaker ALT-711 via a protein kinase C-alpha-dependent pathway. Diabetes 2004;53: 2921-2930.
483. Chobanian AV, Bakris GL, Black HR, et al. Seventh report of the Joint National Committee on Prevention, Detection, Evaluation, and Treatment of High Blood Pressure. Hypertension 2003;42: 1206-1252.
484. Strippoli G, Craig M, Craig J. Antihypertensive agents for preventing diabetic kidney disease. Cochrane Database Syst Rev 2005;4: CD004136.
485. The ACE Inhibitors in Diabetic Nephropathy Trialist Group. Should all patients with type 1 diabetes mellitus and microalbuminuria receive angiotensin-converting enzyme inhibitors? A meta-analysis of individual patient data. Ann Intern Med 2001;134:370-379.
486. The EUCLID study group. Randomised placebo-controlled trial of lisinopril in normotensive patients with insulin-dependent diabetes and normoalbuminuria or microalbuminuria. Lancet 1997; 349:1787-1792.
487. Kvetny J, Gregersen G, Pedersen RS. Randomized placebo-controlled trial of perindopril in normotensive, normoalbuminuric patients with type 1 diabetes mellitus. QJM 2001;94:89-94.
488. Hommel E, Parving HH, Mathiesen E, et al. Effect of captopril on kidney function in insulin-dependent diabetic patients with nephropathy. Br Med J 1986;293:467-470.
489. Brenner BM, Cooper ME, de Zeeuw D, et al. Effects of losartan on renal and cardiovascular outcomes in patients with type 2 diabetes and nephropathy. N Engl J Med 2001;345:861-869.
490. Lewis EJ, Hunsicker LG, Clarke WR, et al. Renoprotective effect of the angiotensin-receptor antagonist irbesartan in patients with nephropathy due to type 2 diabetes. N Engl J Med 2001;345: 851-860.
491. Arauz-Pacheco C, Parrott MA, Raskin P. Treatment of hypertension in adults with diabetes. Diabetes Care 2003;26(suppl 1):S80-S82.
492. Barnett AH, Bain SC, Bouter P, et al. Angiotensin-receptor blockade versus converting-enzyme inhibition in type 2 diabetes and nephropathy. N Engl J Med 2004;351:1952-1961.
493. Parving HH, Lehnert H, Brochner-Mortensen J, et al. The effect of irbesartan on the development of diabetic nephropathy in patients with type 2 diabetes. N Engl J Med 2001;345:870-878.
494. Schjoedt KJ, Rossing K, Juhl TR, et al. Beneficial impact of spironolactone in diabetic nephropathy. Kidney Int 2005;68:2829-2836.
495. Epstein M. Aldosterone as a mediator of progressive renal disease: pathogenetic and clinical implications. Am J Kidney Dis 2001;37: 677-688.

496. Tikkanen I, Tikkanen T, Cao Z, et al. Combined inhibition of neutral endopeptidase with angiotensin converting enzyme or endothelin converting enzyme in experimental diabetes. J Hypertens 2002;20:707-714.
497. Pedrini MT, Levey AS, Lau J, et al. The effect of dietary protein restriction on the progression of diabetic and nondiabetic renal diseases—a meta-analysis. Ann Int Med 1996;124:627-632.
498. Hansen HP, Tauber-Lassen E, Jensen BR, et al. Effect of protein restriction on prognosis in type 1 diabetic patients with diabetic nephropathy. Kidney Int 2002;62:220-228.
499. Waugh NR, Robertson AM. Protein restriction for diabetic renal disease. Cochrane Database Syst Rev 2000;2:CD002181.
500. Jandeleit-Dahm K, Cao ZM, Cox AJ, et al. Role of hyperlipidemia in progressive renal disease: Focus on diabetic nephropathy. Kidney Int 1999;56:S31-S36.
501. Fried LF, Forrest KY, Ellis D, et al. Lipid modulation in insulin-dependent diabetes mellitus: effect on microvascular outcomes. J Diabetes Complications 2001;15:113-119.
502. Keech A, Simes RJ, Barter P, et al. Effects of long-term fenofibrate therapy on cardiovascular events in 9795 people with type 2 diabetes mellitus (the FIELD study): randomised controlled trial. Lancet 2005;366:1849-1861.
503. Collins R, Armitage J, Parish S, et al. MRC/BHF Heart Protection Study of cholesterol-lowering with simvastatin in 5963 people with diabetes: a randomised placebo-controlled trial. Lancet 2003;361: 2005-2016.
504. Athyros VG, Papageorgiou AA, Elisaf M, et al. Statins and renal function in patients with diabetes mellitus. Curr Med Res Opin 2003;19:615-617.
505. Colhoun HM, Betteridge DJ, Durrington PN, et al. Primary prevention of cardiovascular disease with atorvastatin in type 2 diabetes in the Collaborative Atorvastatin Diabetes Study (CARDS): multicentre randomised placebo-controlled trial. Lancet 2004;364: 685-696.
506. Thomas MC, Cooper ME, Tsalamandris C, et al. Anemia with impaired erythropoietin response in diabetic patients. Arch Intern Med 2005;165:466-469.
507. Jungers P, Choukroun G, Oualim Z, et al. Beneficial influence of recombinant human erythropoietin therapy on the rate of progression of chronic renal failure in predialysis patients. Nephrol Dial Transplant 2001;16:307-312.
508. Mix TC, Brenner RM, Cooper ME, et al. Rationale—Trial to Reduce Cardiovascular Events with Aranesp Therapy (TREAT): evolving the management of cardiovascular risk in patients with chronic kidney disease. Am Heart J 2005;149:408-413.
509. Williams ME, Tuttle KR. The next generation of diabetic nephropathy therapies: an update. Adv Chronic Kidney Dis 2005;12: 212-222.
510. Achour A, Kacem M, Dibej K, et al. One year course of oral sulodexide in the management of diabetic nephropathy. J Nephrol 2005;18:568-574.
511. Jungers P, Zingraff J, Page B, et al. Detrimental effects of late referral in patients with chronic renal failure: a case-control study. Kidney Int Suppl 1993;41:S170-S173.
512. Pirson Y. The diabetic patient with ESRD: how to select the modality of renal replacement. Nephrol Dial Transplant 1996;11: 1511-1513.
513. Gaede P, Vedel P, Larsen N, et al. Multifactorial intervention and cardiovascular disease in patients with type 2 diabetes. N Engl J Med 2003;348:383-393.
514. Vinik AI, Mitchell BD, Leichter SB, et al: Epidemiology of the complications of diabetes. In Leslie RDG, Robbins DC, eds. Diabetes: Clinical Science in Practice. Cambridge, UK: Cambridge University Press, 1995:221-287.
515. Vinik A, Mehrabyan A. Diabetic neuropathies. Med Clin North Am 2004;88(4):947-999.
516. Young MJ, Boulton AJM, MacLeod AF, et al. A multicentre study of the prevalence of diabetic peripheral neuropathy in the United Kingdom hospital clinic population. Diabetologia 1993; 36:1-5.
517. Dyck PJ, Kratz KM, Karnes JL, et al. The prevalence by staged severity of various types of diabetic neuropathy, retinopathy, and nephropathy in a population-based cohort: The Rochester Diabetic Neuropathy Study. Neurology 1993;43:817-824.
518. Holzer SE, Camerota A, Martens L, et al. Costs and duration of care for lower extremity ulcers in patients with diabetes. Clin Ther 1998;20:169-181.
519. Caputo GM, Cavanagh PR, Ulbrecht JS, et al. Assessment and management of foot disease in patients with diabetes. N Engl J Med 1994;331:854-860.
520. Pirart J. [Diabetes mellitus and its degenerative complications: a prospective study of 4,400 patients observed between 1947 and 1973 (3rd and last part) (author's transl)]. Diabete Metab 1977;3:245-256.
521. Vinik A, Ullal J, Parson H, Casellini C. Diabetic neuropathies: clinical manifestations and current treatment options. Nat Clin Pract Endocrinol Metab 2006;2:269-281.
522. Smith A, Ramachandran P, Tripp S, Singleton J. Epidermal nerve innervation in impaired glucose tolderance and diabetes-associated neuropathy. Neurology 2001;57:1701-1704.
523. Pittenger GL, Ray M, Burcus NI, et al: Intraepidermal nerve fibers are indicators of small-fiber neuropathy in both diabetic and nondiabetic patients. Diabetes Care 2004;27:1974-1979.
524. Vinik AI. Diabetic neuropathy, mobility and balance. Geriatric Times 2003;4(1):13-15.
525. Resnick HE, Stansberry KB, Harris TB, et al: Diabetes, peripheral neuropathy, and old age disability. Muscle Nerve 2002;25:43-50.
526. Vinik A. Diabetic neuropathy: pathogenesis and therapy. Am J Med 1999;107:17S-26S.
527. Herman WH, Kennedy L. Underdiagnosis of peripheral neuropathy in type 2 diabetes. Diabetes Care 2005;28:1480-1481.
528. Armstrong DG, Lavery LA, Harkless LB: Validation of a diabetic wound classification system. The contribution of depth, infection, and ischemia to risk of amputation. Diabetes Care 1998;21: 855-859.
529. Vinik EJ, Hayes RP, Oglesby A, et al. The development and validation of the Norfolk QOL-DN, a new measure of patients' perception of the effects of diabetes and diabetic neuropathy. Diabetes Technol Ther 2005;7:497-508.
530. Levitt NS, Stansberry KB, Wychanck S, Vinik AI. Natural progression of autonomic neuropathy and autonomic function tests in a cohort of IDDM. Diabetes Care 1996;19:751-754.
531. Rathmann W, Ziegler D, Jahnke M, et al. Mortality in diabetic patients with cardiovascular autonomic neuropathy. Diabet Med 1993;10:820-824.
532. Maser RE, Mitchell BD, Vinik AI, Freeman R. The association between cardiovascular autonomic neuropathy and mortality in individuals with diabetes: a meta-analysis. Diabetes Care 2003; 26(6):1895-1901.
533. Vinik AI, Maser RE, Mitchell BD, Freeman R. Diabetic autonomic neuropathy. Diabetes Care 2003;26(5):1553-1579.
534. American Diabetes Association and American Academy of Neurology. Consensus statement: report and recommendations of the San Antonio conference on diabetic neuropathy. Diabetes Care 1988;11:592-597.
535. Watkins PJ. Progression of diabetic autonomic neuropathy. Diabet Med 1993;10(Suppl 2):77S-78S.
536. DCCT Research Group. The effect of intensive treatment of diabetes on the development and progression of long-term complications in insulin-dependent diabetes mellitus. N Engl J Med 1993;329:977-986.
537. DCCT Research Group. The effect of intensive diabetes therapy on the development and progression of neuropathy. Ann Intern Med 1995;122:561-568.
538. Ziegler D, Cicmir I, Mayer P, Wiefels K, Gries FA. Somatic and autonomic nerve function during the first year after diagnosis of type 1 (insulin-dependent) diabetes. Diabetes Res 1988;7:123-127.
539. Partanen J, Niskanen L, Lehtinen J, et al. Natural history of peripheral neuropathy in patients with non–insulin-dependent diabetes mellitus. N Engl J Med 1995;333:89-94.
540. Apfel SC, Kessler JA, Adornato BT, et al; NGF Study Group. Recombinant human nerve growth factor in the treatment of diabetic polyneuropathy. Neurology 1998;51:695-702.
541. Vinik AI. Treatment of diabetic polyneuropathy (DPN) with recombinant human nerve growth factor (rhNGF). (Abstract). Diabetes 1999;48(Suppl 1):A54-A55.
542. Dyck PJ, Kratz KM, Lehman KA, et al. The Rochester Diabetic Neuropathy Study: design, criteria for types of neuropathy, selec-

tion bias, and reproducibility of neuropathic tests. Neurology. 1991;41:799-807.

543. Oh SJ: Clinical electromyelography: nerve conduction studies. In Oh SJ, ed. Nerve Conduction in Polyneuropathies, 2nd ed. Baltimore: Williams & Wilkins, 1993:579-591.
544. Kennedy WR, Wendelschafer-Crabb G, Johnson T. Quantitation of epidermal nerves in diabetic neuropathy. Neurology 1996;47: 1042-1048.
545. Herrmann DN, Griffin JW, Hauer P, et al. Epidermal nerve fiber density and sural nerve morphometry in peripheral neuropathies. Neurology 1999;53:1634-1640.
546. Vinik A, Erbas T, Park T, et al. Dermal neurovascular dysfunction in type 2 diabetes. Diabetes Care 2001;24:1468-1475.
547. Smith AG, Russell J, Feldman EL, et al. Lifestyle intervention for pre-diabetic neuropathy. Diabetes Care 2006;29:1294-1299.
548. Karamitsos DT, Didangelos TP, Athyros VG, Kontopoulos AG:.The natural history of recently diagnosed autonomic neuropathy over a period of 2 years. Diabetes Res Clin Pract 1998;42:55-63.
549. Ziegler D. Diabetic cardiovascular autonomic neuropathy: prognosis, diagnosis and treatment. Diabetes Metab Rev 1994;10: 339-383.
550. Boulton AJ, Vinik AI, Arezzo JC, et al. Diabetic neuropathies: a statement by the American Diabetes Association. Diabetes Care 2005;28:956-962.
551. Dyck PJ. Severity and staging of diabetic polyneuropathy. In Gries FA, Cameron NE, Low PA, Ziegler D, eds. Textbook of Diabetic Neuropathy. Stuttgart: Thieme, 2003:170-175.
552. Vinik AI, Holland MT, LeBeau JM, et al. Diabetic neuropathies. Diabetes Care 1992;15:1926-1975.
553. Vinik AI, Suwanwalaikorn S. Autonomic neuropathy. In DeFronzo RA, ed. Current Therapy of Diabetes Mellitus. St. Louis: Mosby, 1997:165-176.
554. Karpitskaya Y, Novak CB, Mackinnon SE. Prevalence of smoking, obesity, diabetes mellitus and thyroid disease in patients with carpal tunnel syndrome. Am Plast Surg 2002;48:269-273.
555. Perkins B, Olaleye D, Bril V. Carpal tunnel syndrome in patients with diabetic polyneuropathy. Diabetes Care 2002;25: 565-569.
556. Chaudhuri KR, Davidson AR, Morris IM. Limited joint mobility and carpal tunnel syndrome in insulin dependent diabetes. Br J Rheumatol 1989;28:191-194.
557. Wilbourn AJ. Diabetic entrapment and compression neuropathies. In Dyck PJ, Thomas PK, eds. Diabetic Neuropathy. Philadelphia, Saunders, 1999;481-508.
558. Dawson DM. Entrapment neuropathies of the upper extremities. N Engl J Med 1993;329:2013-2018.
559. Vinik A, Mehrabyan A, Colen L, Boulton A. Focal entrapment neuropathies in diabetes. Diabetes Care 2004;27(7):1783-1788.
560. Sima AAF, Sugimoto K. Experimental diabetic neuropathy: an update. Diabetologia 1999;42:773-788.
561. Vinik AI, Pittenger GL, Milicevic Z, Knezevic-Cuca J. Autoimmune mechanisms in the pathogenesis of diabetic neuropathy. In Eisenbarth RG, ed. Molecular Mechanisms of Endocrine and Organ Specific Autoimmunity. Georgetown, Landes, 1998:217-251.
562. Steck AJ, Kappos L. Gangliosides and autoimmune neuropathies: classification and clinical aspects of autoimmune neuropathies. J Neurol Neurosurg Psychiatry 1994;57(suppl):26-28.
563. Sander HW, Chokroverty S. Diabetic amyotrophy: current concepts. Semin Neurol 1996;16:173-178.
564. Said G, Goulon-Goreau C, Lacroix C, Moulonguet A. Nerve biopsy findings in different patterns of proximal diabetic neuropathy. Ann Neurol 1994;35:559-569.
565. Krendel DA, Costigan DA, Hopkins LC. Successful treatment of neuropathies in patients with diabetes mellitus. Arch Neurol 1995;52:1053-1061.
566. Britland ST, Young RJ, Sharma AK, Clarke BF. Acute and remitting painful diabetic polyneuropathy: a comparison of peripheral nerve fibre pathology. Pain 1992;48:361-370.
567. Stewart JD, McKelvey R, Durcan L, et al. Chronic inflammatory demyelinating polyneuropathy (CIDP). J Neurol Sci 1996;142: 59-64.
568. Sharma K, Cross J, Ayyar D, et al. Diabetic demyelinating polyneuropathy responsive to intravenous immunoglobulin therapy. Arch Neurol 2002;59:751-757.
569. Witzke K, Vinik A: Diabetic neuropathy in older adults (abstract). Rev Endocr & Metab Disord 2005;6:117-127.
570. Resnick HE, Vinik AI, Schwartz AV, et al. Independent effects of peripheral nerve dysfunction on lower-extremity physical function in old age: the Women's Health and Aging Study. Diabetes Care 2000;23:1642-1647.
571. Witzke KA, Vinik AI. Diabetic neuropathy in older adults. Rev Endocrin Metab Disord 2005;6:117-127.
572. Milicevic Z, Newlon PG, Pittenger GL, et al. Anti-ganglioside GM1 antibody and distal symmetric "diabetic polyneuropathy" with dominant motor features. Diabetologia 1997;40:1364-1365.
573. Griffin JW, McArthur JC, Polydefkis M. Assessment of cutaneous innervation by skin biopsies. Curr Opin Neurol 2001;14:655-659.
574. Barada A, Reljanovic M, Milicevic Z, et al. Proximal diabetic neuropathy-response to immunotherapy (abstract). Diabetes 1999;48(Suppl 1):A148.
575. Bird SJ, Brown MJ. The clinical spectrum of diabetic neuropathy. Semin Neurol 1996;16:115-122.
576. Hanson PH, Schumaker P, Debugne TH, Clerin M. Evaluation of somatic and autonomic small fibers neuropathy in diabetes. Am J Phys Med Rehabil 1992;71:44-47.
577. McArthur JC, Stocks EA, Hauer P, et al. Epidermal nerve fiber density: normative reference range and diagnostic efficiency. Arch Neurol 1998;55:1513-1520.
578. Stansberry KB, Hill MA, Shapiro SA, et al. Impairment of peripheral blood flow responses in diabetes resembles an enhanced aging effect. Diabetes Care 1997;20:1711-1716.
579. Hirai A, Yasuda H, Joko M, et al. Evaluation of diabetic neuropathy through the quantitation of cutaneous nerves. J Neurol Sci 2000;172:55-62.
580. Polydefkis M, Hauer P, Griffin JW, McArthur JC. Skin biopsy as a tool to assess distal small fiber innervation in diabetic neuropathy. Diabetes Technol Ther 2001;3:23-28.
581. Dalsgaard CJ, Rydh M, Haegerstrand A. Cutaneous innervation in man visualized with protein gene product 9.5 (PGP 9.5) antibodies. Histochemistry 1989;92:385-390.
582. McCarthy BG, Hsieh ST, Stocks A, et al. Cutaneous innervation in sensory neuropathies: evaluation by skin biopsy. Neurology 1995; 45:1848-1855.
583. Low P, Dotson R. Symptom treatment of painful neuropathy. JAMA 1998;280:1863-1864.
584. Vinik AI, Park TS, Stansberry KB, Pittenger GL. Diabetic neuropathies. Diabetologia 2000;43:957-973.
585. Backonja M. Anticonvulsants (antineuropathics) for neuropathic pain syndromes. Clin J Pain 2000;16(2 Suppl):S67-S72.
586. Tesfaye S, Malik R, Harris N, et al. Arterio-venous shunting and proliferating new vessels in acute painful neuropathy of rapid glycaemic control (insulin neuritis). Diabetologia 1996;39:329-335.
587. Van Heel DA, Levitt NS, Winter TA. Diabetic neuropathic cachexia: the importance of positive recognition and early nutritional support. Int J Clin Pract 1998;52:591-592.
588. Holland NR, Crawford TO, Hauer P, et al. Small-fiber sensory neuropathies: clinical course and neuropathology of idiopathic cases. Ann Neurol 1998;44:47-59.
589. Dyck PJ. Detection, characterization and staging of polyneuropathy: assessed in diabetes. Muscle Nerve 1988;11:21-32.
590. Vinik AI, Mitchell B. Clinical aspects of diabetic neuropathies. Diabetes Metab Rev 1988;4:223-253.
591. Ziegler D, Hanefeld M, Ruhnau KJ, et al. Treatment of symptomatic diabetic peripheral neuropathy with the anti-oxidant alpha-lipoic acid. A 3-week multicentre randomized controlled trial (ALADIN Study). Diabetologia 1995;38:1425-1433.
592. Feldman EL, Stevens MJ, Thomas PK, et al. A practical two-step quantitative clinical and electrophysiological assessment for the diagnosis and staging of diabetic neuropathy. Diabetes Care 1994;17:1281-1289.
593. Vinik AI, Newlon P, Milicevic Z, et al. Diabetic neuropathies: an overview of clinical aspects. In LeRoith D, Taylor SI, Olefsky JM, eds. Diabetes Mellitus: A Fundamental and Clinical text. Philadelphia; Lippincot-Raven, 1996:737-751.
594. Vinik A, Mehrabyan A, Colen L, Boulton A. Focal entrapment neuropathies in diabetes. Diabetes Care 2004;27(7):1783-1788.
595. Cabezas-Cerrato, J. The prevalence of diabetic neuropathy in Spain: a study in primary care and hospital clinic groups. Diabeteologia 1998;41:1263-1269.
596. Bril V. NIS-LL: the primary measurement scale for clinical trial endpoints in diabetic peripheral neuropathy. Eur Neurol 1999; 41(suppl 1):8-13:8-13.

597. Hermenegildo C, Felipo V, Minana MD, et al. Sustained recovery of Na^+-K^+-ATPase activity in sciatic nerve of diabetic mice by administration of H7 or calphostin C, inhibitors of PKC. Diabetes 1993;42:257-262.
598. Cameron NE, Cotter MA, Basso M, Hohman TC. Comparison of the effects of inhibitors of aldose reductase and sorbitol dehydrogenase on neurovascular function, nerve conduction and tissue polyol pathway metabolites in streptozotocin-diabetic rats. Diabetologia 1997;40(3):271-281.
599. Franse LV, Valk GD, Dekker JH, et al. Numbness of the feet is a poor indicator for polyneuropathy in type 2 diabetic patients. Diabetes Care 2000;17:105-110.
600. Apfel SC, Asbury A, Bril V, et al. Positive neuropathic sensory symptoms as endpoints in diabetic neuropathy trials (abstract). J Neurol Sci 2001;189:3-5.
601. Shy ME, Frohman EM, So YT, et al; Subcommittee of the American Academy of Neurology. Quantitative sensory testing. Neurology 2003;602:898-906.
602. Gerr F, Letz R. Covariates of human peripheral function: vibrotactile and thermal thresholds. Neurotoxicol Teratol 1994;16:102-112.
603. Gelber DA, Pfeifer MA, Broadstone VL, et al. Components of variance for vibratory and thermal threshold testing in normal and diabetic subjects. J Diabetes Complications 1995;9:170-176.
604. Dyck PJ, Dyck PJ, Larson TS, et al. Patterns of quantitative sensation testing of hypoesthesia and hyperalgesia are predictive of diabetic polyneuropathy: a study of three cohorts. Nerve growth factor study group. Diabetes Care 2000;23:510-517.
605. Maser RE, Nielsen VK, Bass EB, et al. Measuring diabetic neuropathy. Assessment and comparison of clinical examination and quantitative sensory testing. Diabetes Care 1989;12:270-275.
606. Feldman EL. Oxidative stress and diabetic neuropathy: a new understanding of an old problem. J Clin Invest 2003;111:431-433.
607. Meijer JW, Smit AJ, Sondersen EV, et al. Symptom scoring systems to diagnose distal polyneuropathy in diabetes; the Diabetic Neuropathy Symptom Score. Diabetic Med 2002;19:962-965.
608. Scott J, Huskisson EC. Graphic representation of pain. Pain 1976;2:175-186.
609. Vinik AI, Suwanwalaikorn S, Stansberry KB, et al. Quantitative measurement of cutaneous perception in diabetic neuropathy. Muscle Nerve 1995;18:574-584.
610. Valk GD, de Sonnaville JJ, van Houtum WH, et al. The assessment of diabetic polyneuropathy in daily clinical practice: reproducibility and validity of Semmes Weinstein monofilaments examination and clinical neurological examination. Muscle Nerve 1997;20:116-118.
611. Mayfield JA, Sugarman JR. The use of Semmes-Weinstein monofilament and other threshold tests for preventing foot ulceration and amputation in people with diabetes. J Fam Pract 2000;49(suppl): 517-529.
612. Bourcier ME, Ullal J, Parson HK, et al. Diabetic peripheral neuropathy: how reliable is a homemade 1-g monofilament for screening? J Fam Pract 2006;55:505-508.
613. Kumar S, Fernando DJ, Veves A, et al. Semmes-Weinstein monofilaments: a simple, effective and inexpensive screening device for identifying diabetic patients at risk of foot ulceration. Diabetes Res Clin Pract 1991;13:63-67.
614. Armstrong D, Lavery L, Vela S, et al. Choosing a practical screening instrument to identify patients at risk for diabetic foot ulceration. Arch Intern Med 1998;158:289-292.
615. Booth J, Young MJ. Differences in the performance of commercially available 10-g monofilaments. Diabetes Care 2000;23: 984-988.
616. Liniger C, Albeanu A, Bloise D, Assal JP. The tuning fork revisited. Diabetic Med 1990;7:859-864.
617. Shin JB, Seong YJ, Lee HJ, et al. Foot screening technique in diabetic populations. J Korean Med Sci 2000;15:78-82.
618. Katoulis EC, Ebdon-Parry M, Lanshammar H, et al. Gait abnormalities in diabetic neuropathy. Diabetes Care 1997;20:1904-1907.
619. Vileikyte L, Hutchings G, Hollis S, Boulton AJM. The tactile circumferential discriminator: a new simple screening device to identify diabetic patients at risk of foot ulceration. Diabetes Care 1997;20:623-626.
620. Paisley AN, Abbott CA, van Schie CHM, Boulton AJM. A comparison of the Neuropen against standard quantitative sensory threshold measures for assessing peripheral nerve function. Diabetic Med 2002;19:400-405.
621. Ducher M, Thivolet C, Cerutti C, et al. Noninvasive exploration of cardiac autonomic neuropathy. Diabetes Care 1999;22:388-393.
622. Jaradeh SS, Prieto TE, Lobeck LJ. Progressive polyradiculoneuropathy in diabetes: correlation of variables and clinical outcome after immunotherapy. J Neurol Neurosurg Psychiatry 1999;67: 607-612.
623. Periquet MI, Novak V, Collins MP, et al. Painful sensory neuropathy: prospective evaluation using skin biopsy. Neurology 1999;53: 1641-1647.
624. Krendel DA, Zacharias A, Younger DS. Autoimmune diabetic neuropathy. Neurol Clin 1997;15:959-971.
625. Singleton J, Smith AG, Bromberg MB. Painful sensory polyneuropathy associated with impaired glucose tolerance. Muscle Nerve 2001;24:1225-1228.
626. Sumner C, Sheth S, Griffin J, et al. The spectrum of neuropathy in diabetes and impaired glucose tolerance. Neurology 2003;60: 108-111.
627. Mehrabyan A, Pittenger G, Burcus N, et al. Polyneuropathy in patients with dysmetabolic syndrome and newly diagnosed. Diabetes 2004;53(suppl 2):A510.
628. Vinik A, Pittenger G, Anderson A, et al. Topiramate improves c-fiber neuropathy and features of the dysmetabolic syndrome in type 2 diabetes. Diabetes 2003;52(suppl 1):A130.
629. Quattrini C, Jeziorska M, Malik RA. Small fiber neuropathy in diabetes: clinical consequence and assessment. Int J Low Extrem-Wounds 2004;3:16-21.
630. Arezzo JC. The use of electrophysiology for the assessment of diabetic neuropathy. Neurosci Res Comm 1997;21:13-22.
631. Arezzo JC, Zotova E. Electrophysiologic measures of diabetic neuropathy: mechanism and meaning. Intern Rev Neurobiol 2002;50: 229-255.
632. Sharma K, Cross J, Farronay O, et al. Demyelinating neuropathy in diabetes mellitus. Arch Neurol 2002;59:758-765.
633. Amthor KF, Dahl-Jorgensen K, Berg TJ, et al. The effect of 8 years of strict glycaemic control on peripheral nerve function in IDDM patients: the Oslo Study. Diabetologia 1994;37:579-584.
634. Veves A, Malik RA, Lye RH, et al. The relationship between sural nerve morphometric findings and measures of peripheral nerve function in mild diabetic neuropathy. Diabet Med 1991;8: 917-921.
635. UK Prospective Diabetes Study (UKPDS) Group. Effect of intensive blood-glucose control with metformin on complications in overweight patients with type 2 diabetes (UKPDS 34). Lancet 1998;352:854-865.
636. Gaede P, Vedel P, Parving HH, Pedersen O. Intensified multifactorial intervention in patients with type 2 diabetes mellitus and microalbuminuria: the Steno type 2 randomised study. Lancet 1999;353:617-622.
637. Boulton AJM, Levin S, Comstock J. A multicentre trial of the aldose reductase inhibitor, tolrestat, in patients with symptomatic diabetic neuropathy. Diabetologia 1990;33:431-437.
638. Didangelos TP, Karamitsos DT, Athyros VG, Kourtoglou GI: Effect of aldose reductase inhibition on cardiovascular reflex tests in patients with definite diabetic autonomic neuropathy. J Diabetes Complications 1998;12:201-207.
639. Johnson BF, Law G, Nesto R, et al. Aldose reductase inhibitor zopolrestat improves systolic function in diabetics (abstract). Diabetes 1999;48(suppl 1):A133.
640. Hotta, N, Toyota, T, Matsuoka, K, et al, and the SNK-860 Diabetic Neuropathy Study Group. Clinical efficacy of fidarestat, a novel aldose reductase inhibitor, for diabetic peripheral neuropathy. Diabetes Care 2001;24:1776-1782.
641. Hotta N, Akanuma Y, Kawamori R, et al. Long-term clinical effects of epalrestat, an aldose reductase inhibitor, on diabetic peripheral neuropathy: the 3-year, multicenter, comparative Aldose Reductase Inhibitor-Diabetes Complications Trial. Diabetes Care 2006;29:1538-1544.
642. Bril V, Buchanan RA. Aldose reductase inhibition by AS-3201 in sural nerve from patients with diabetic sensorimotor polyneuropathy. Diabetes Care 2004;27:2369-2375.
643. Ziegler D, Schatz H, Conrad F, et al. Effects of treatment with the antioxidant alpha-lipoic acid on cardiac autonomic neuropathy in NIDDM patients. A 4-month randomized controlled multicenter

trial (DEKAN Study). Deutsche Kardiale Autonome Neuropathie. Diabetes Care 1997;20:369-373.
644. Ziegler D, Gries FA. Alpha-lipoic acid in the treatment of diabetic peripheral and cardiac autonomic neuropathy. Diabetes 1997; 46(suppl 2):S62-S66.
645. Ziegler D, Hanefeld M, Ruhnau KJ, et al. Treatment of symptomatic diabetic polyneuropathy with the antioxidant alpha-lipoic acid: a 7-month multicenter randomized controlled trial (ALADIN III Study). ALADIN III Study Group. Alpha-Lipoic Acid in Diabetic Neuropathy. Diabetes Care 1999;22:1296-1301.
646. Jamal GA. The use of gamma linolenic acid in the prevention and treatment of diabetic neuropathy. Diabet Med 1994;11:145-149.
647. Keen H, Payan J, Allawi J, et al. Treatment of diabetic neuropathy with γ- linolenic acid. Diabetes Care 1993;16:8-15.
648. Dyck PJ. Hypoxic neuropathy: does hypoxia play a role in diabetic neuropathy? The 1988 Robert Wartenberg lecture. Neurology 1989;39:111-118.
649. Kles KA, Vinik AI. Pathophysiology and treatment of diabetic peripheral neuropathy: the case for diabetic neurovascular function as an essential component. Curr Diabetes Rev 2006;2: 131-145.
650. Hermenegildo C, Felipo V, Minana MD, Grisolia S: Inhibition of protein kinase C restores Na^+,K^+-ATPase activity in sciatic nerve of diabetic mice. J Neurochem 1992;58:1246-1249.
651. Nakamura J, Koh N, Hamada Y, et al. Effect of a protein kinase C-β specific inhibitor on diabetic neuropathy in rats. Diabetes 1998;47(suppl 1):A70.
652. Granberg V, Ejskjaer N, Peakman M, Sundkvist G. Autoantibodies to autonomic nerves associated with cardiac and peripheral autonomic neuropathy. Diabetes Care 2005;28:1959-1964.
653. Vinik A, Bril V, Kempler P, et al, for the MBBQ Study: Treatment of symptomatic diabetic peripheral neuropathy with protein kinase Cβ inhibitor ruboxistaurin mesylate during a 1-year randomized, placebo-controlled, double-blind clinical trial. Clin Ther 2005;27:1164s-1180s.
654. Miyauchi Y, Shikama H, Takasu T, et al. Slowing of peripheral motor nerve conduction was ameliorated by aminoguanidine in streptozocin-induced diabetic rats. Eur J Endocrinol 1996;134: 467-473.
655. Schmidt RE, Dorsey DA, Beaudet LN, et al. Effect of aminoguanidine on the frequency of neuroaxonal dystrophy in the superior mesenteric sympathetic autonomic ganglia of rats with streptozotocin-induced diabetes. Diabetes 1996;45:284-290.
656. Nargi SE, Colen LB, Liuzzi F, et al. PTB Treatment restores joint mobility in a new model of diabetic cheirothropathy (abstract). Diabetes 1999;48(suppl 1):A17.
657. Suez D. Intravenous immunoglobulin therapy: indication, potential side effects and treatment guidelines. J Intraven Nurs 1995;18: 178-190.
658. Vinik AI, Anandacoomaraswamy D, Ullal J. Antibodies to neuronal structures: innocent bystanders or neurotoxins? Diabetes Care 2005;28:2067-2072.
659. Diemel LT, Stevens JC, Willars GB, Tomlinson DR. Depletion of substance P and calcitonin gene-related peptide in sciatic nerve of rats with experimental diabetes: effects of insulin and aldose reductase inhibition. Neurosci Lett 1992;137:253-256.
660. Hellweg R, Wohrle M, Hartung HD. Diabetes mellitus associated decrease in nerve growth factor levels is reversed by allogenetic pancreatic islet transplantation. Neurosci Lett 1991;125:1-4.
661. Tomlinson DR, Fernyhough P, Diemel LT. Neurotrophins and peripheral neuropathy. Philos Trans R Soc Lond B Biol Sci 1996;351:455-462.
662. Apfel SC, Kessler JA. Neurotropic factors in the therapy of peripheral neuropathy. Bailliere Clin Neuropathy 1995;4:593-606.
663. Apfel SC, Schwartz S, Adornato B, et al. Efficacy and safety of recombinant human nerve growth factor in patients with diabetic polyneuropathy. JAMA 2000;284:2215-2221.
664. Wellmer, A, Misra, V, Sharief, M, et al. A double-blind placebo-controlled clinical trial of recombinant human brain-derived neurotrophic factor (rhBDNF) in diabetic polyneuropathy. J Peripheral Nerv Syst 2001;6(4):204-210.
665. Wahren J, Ekberg K, Samnegard B, Johansson BL. C-peptide: a new potential in the treatment of diabetic nephropathy. Curr Diab Rep 2001;1:261-266.
666. Sindrup SH, Jensen TS. Efficacy of pharmacological treatments of neuropathic pain: an update and effect related to mechanism of drug action. Pain 1999;83:389-400.
667. Rosenstock J, Tuchman M, LaMoreaux L, Sharma U: Pregabalin for the treatment of painful diabetic peripheral neuropathy: a double-blind, placebo-controlled trial. Pain 2004;110:628-638.
668. Goldstein DJ, Lu Y, Detke MJ, et al: Duloxetine vs. placebo in patients with painful diabetic neuropathy. Pain 2005;116:109-118.
669. Rains C, Bryson HM. Topical capsaicin. A review of its pharmacological properties and therapeutic potential in post-herpetic neuralgia, diabetic neuropathy and osteoarthritis. Drugs Aging 1995;7:317-328.
670. Bays-Smith MG, Max MB, Muir J, Kingman A. Transdermal clonidine compared to placebo in painful diabetic neuropathy using a two-stage "enriched enrollment" design. Pain 1995;60:267-274.
671. Said G, Bigo A, Ameri A, et al. Uncommon early-onset neuropathy in diabetic patients. J Neurol 1998;245:61-68.
672. Jarvis B, Coukell AJ. Mexiletine. A review of its therapeutic use in painful diabetic neuropathy. Drugs 1998;56:691-707.
673. Harati Y, Gooch C, Swenson M, et al. Double-blind randomized trial of tramadol for the treatment of the pain of diabetic neuropathy. Neurology 1998;50:1842-1846.
674. Harati Y, Gooch C, Swenson M, et al. Maintenance of the long-term effectiveness of tramadol in treatment of the pain of diabetic neuropathy. J Diabetes Complications 2000;14:65-70.
675. Nelson KA, Park KM, Robinovitz E, et al. High-dose oral dextromethorphan versus placebo in painful diabetic neuropathy and postherpetic neuralgia. Neurology 1997;48:1212-1218.
676. Max M, Lynch S, Muir J: Effects of desipramine, amitryptiline and fluoxetine on pain in diabetic neuropathy. N Engl J Med 1992;326:1250-1256.
677. Dworkin RH, Backonja M, Rowbotham MC, et al. Advances in neuropathic pain: diagnosis, mechanisms, and treatment recommendations. Arch Neurol 2003;60:1524-1534.
678. McQuay H, Tramer M, Nye B, et al. A systematic review of antidepressants in neuropathic pain. Pain 1996;68:217-227.
679. Joss JD. Tricyclic antidepressant use in diabetic neuropathy. Ann Pharmacother 1999;33:996-1000.
680. Sindrup S, Gram L, Brosen K, et al. The selective serotonin reuptake inhibitor paroxetine is effective in treatment of diabetic neuropathy symptoms. Pain 1990;42:135-144.
681. Gomez-Perez FJ, Choza R, Rios JM, et al. Nortriptyline-fluphenazine vs. carbamazepine in the symptomatic treatment of diabetic neuropathy. Arch Med Res 1996;27:525-529.
682. Vinik A. Use of antiepileptic drugs in the treatment of chronic painful diabetic neuropathy. J Clin Endocrinol Metab 2005;90(8):4936-4945.
683. McQuay H, Carroll D, Jadad AR, et al. Anticonvulsant drugs for management of pain: a systematic review. BMJ 1995;311: 1047-1052.
684. Vinik AI. Advances in diabetes for the millennium: new treatments for diabetic neuropathies. MedGenMed 2004;6(3 suppl):13.
685. LaRoche SM, Helmers SL. The new antiepileptic drugs: scientific review. JAMA 2004;291:605-614.
686. Jensen TS. Anticonvulsants in neuropathic pain: rationale and clinical evidence. Eur J Pain 2002;6(suppl A):61-68.
687. Chadda VS, Mathur MS. Double blind study of the effects of diphenylhydantoin sodium on diabetic neuropathy. J Assoc Physicians India 1978;26:403-406.
688. Saudek CD, Werns S, Reidenberg MM. Phenytoin in the treatment of diabetic symmetrical polyneuropathy. Clin Pharmacol Ther 1977;22:196-199.
689. Otto M, Bach FW, Jensen TS, Sindrup SH. Valproic acid has no effect on pain in polyneuropathy: a randomized, controlled trial. Neurology 2004;62:285-288.
690. Gorson KC, Schott C, Herman R, et al. Gabapentin in the treatment of painful diabetic neuropathy: a placebo controlled, double blind, crossover trial. J Neurol Neurosurg Psychiatry 1999;66: 251-252.
691. Backonja M, Beydoun A, Edwards KR, et al. Gabapentin for the symptomatic treatment of painful neuropathy in patients with diabetes mellitus. JAMA 1998;280:1831-1836.
692. Vinik A, Fonseca V, LaMoreaux L, et al. Neurontin (gabapentin, GBP) improves quality of life (QOL) in patients with painful diabetic peripheral neuropathy (abstract). Diabetes 1998;(suppl 1):47:A374.

693. Morello CM, Leckband SG, Stoner CP, et al. Randomized double-blind study comparing the efficacy of gabapentin with amitriptyline on diabetic peripheral neuropathy pain. Arch Intern Med 1999;159:1931-1937.
695. DeToledo JC, Toledo C, DeCerce J, Ramsay RE. Changes in body weight with chronic, high-dose gabapentin therapy. Ther Drug Monit 1997;19:394-396.
695. Eisenberg E, Lurie Y, Braker C, et al. Lamotrigine reduces painful diabetic neuropathy: a randomized, controlled study. Neurology 2001;57:505-509.
696. Eisenberg E, Alon N, Ishay A, et al. Lamotrigine in the treatment of painful diabetic neuropathy. Eur J Neurol 1998;5:167-173.
697. Raskin, P, Donofrio, P, Rosenthal, N, et al. Topiramate vs placebo in painful diabetic neuropathy: analgesic and metabolic effects. Neurology 2004;63:865-873.
698. Stansberry KB, Shapiro SA, Hill MA, et al. Impaired peripheral vasomotion in diabetes. Diabetes Care 1996;19:715-721.
699. Nelson ME, Fiatarone MA, Morganti CM, et al. Effects of high-intensit strength training on multiple risk factors for osteoporotic fractures. A randomized controlled trial. JAMA 1994;272: 1909-1914.
700. Liu-Ambrose T, Khan KM, Eng JJ, et al. Resistance and agility training reduce fall risk in women aged 75 to 85 with low bone mass: a 6-month randomized, controlled trial. J Am Geriatr Soc 2004;52:657-665.
701. Somers DL, Somers MF. Treatment of neuropathic pain in a patient with diabetic neuropathy using transcutaneous electrical nerve stimulation applied to the skin of the lumbar region. Phys Ther 1999;79:767-775.
702. Weintraub M. Preliminary findings: alternative medicine. Am J Pain Manage 1998;8:12-16.
703. Chaudry V, Corse AM, Cornblath DR, et al. Multifocal motor neuropathy: response to human immune globulin. Ann Neurol 1993;33:237-242.
704. Zieleniewski W: Calcitonin nasal spray for painful diabetic neuropathy. Lancet 1990;336:449.
705. Cavanagh PR, Derr JA, Ulbrecht JS, et al. Problems with gait and posture in neuropathic patients with insulin-dependent diabetes mellitus. Diabet Med 1992;9:469-474.
706. Zola BE, Vinik AI. Effects of autonomic neuropathy associated with diabetes mellitus on cardiovascular function. Coron Artery Dis 1992;3:33-41.
707. Stansberry KB, Peppard HR, Babyak LM, et al. Primary nociceptive afferents mediate the blood flow dysfunction in non-glabrous (hairy) skin of type 2 diabetes. Diabetes Care 1999;22:1549-1554.
708. Haak ES, Usadel KH, Kohleisen M, et al. The effect of alpha-lipoic acid on the neurovascular reflex arc in patients with diabetic neuropathy assessed by capillary microscopy. Microvasc Res 1999;58:28-34.
709. Valensi P. Diabetic autonomic neuropathy: what are the risks? Diabet Metab 1998;24:66-72.
710. Mancia G, Paleari F, Parati G. Early diagnosis of diabetic autonomic neuropathy: present and future approaches. Diabetologia 1997;40:482-484.
711. Athyros VG, Didangelos TP, Karamitsos DT, et al. Long-term effect of converting enzyme inhibition on circadian sympathetic and parasympathetic modulation in patients with diabetic autonomic neuropathy. Acta Cardiol 1998;53:201-209.
712. Malmberg K, Norhammar A, Wedel H, Ryden L. Glycometabolic state at admission: important risk marker of mortality in conventionally treated patients with diabetes mellitus and acute myocardial infarction: long-term results from the Diabetes and Insulin-Glucose Infusion in Acute Myocardial Infarction (DIGAMI) study. Circulation 1999;99:2626-2632.
713. Kendall DM, Rooney DP, Smets YF, et al. Pancreas transplantation restores epinephrine response and symptom recognition during hypoglycemia in patients with long-standing type I diabetes and autonomic neuropathy. Diabetes 1997;46:249-257.
714. Burger AJ, Weinrauch LA, D'Elia JA, Aronson D. Effects of glycemic control on heart rate variability in type I diabetic patients with cardiac autonomic neuropathy. Am J Cardiol 1999;84:687-691.
715. Laederach-Hofmann K, Weidmann P, Ferrari P. Hypovolemia contributes to the pathogenesis of orthostatic hypotension in patients with diabetes mellitus. Am J Med 1999;106:50-58.
716. Denq JC, Opfer-Gehrking TL, Giuliani M, et al. Efficacy of compression of different capacitance beds in the amelioration of orthostatic hypotension. Clin Auton Res 1997;7:321-326.
717. Annese V, Bassotti G, Caruso N, et al. Gastrointestinal motor dysfunction, symptoms, and neuropathy in noninsulin-dependent (type 2) diabetes mellitus. J Clin Gastroenterol 1999;29:171-177.
718. Melga P, Mansi C, Ciuchi E, et al. Chronic administration of levosulpiride and glycemic control in IDDM patients with gastroparesis. Diabetes Care 1997;20:55-58.
719. Stacher G, Schernthaner G, Francesconi M, et al. Cisapride versus placebo for 8 weeks on glycemic control and gastric emptying in insulin-dependent diabetes: a double blind cross-over trial. J Clin Endocrinol Metab 1999;84:2357-2362.
720. Barone JA. Domperidone: a peripherally acting dopamine2-receptor antagonist. Ann Pharmacother 1999;33:429-440.
721. Silvers D, Kipnes M, Broadstone V, et al. Domperidone in the management of symptoms of diabetic gastroparesis: efficacy, tolerability, and quality-of-life outcomes in a multicenter controlled trial. DOM-USA-5 Study Group. Clin Ther 1998;20:438-453.
722. Erbas T, Varoglu E, Erbas B, et al. Comparison of metoclopramide and erythromycin in the treatment of diabetic gastroparesis. Diabetes Care 1993;16:1511-1514.
723. Vinik AI, Richardson D. Erectile dysfunction in diabetes. Diabetes Rev 1998;6:16-33.
724. Vinik AI, Richardson D. Erectile dysfunction in diabetes:pills for penile failure. Clinica Diabetes 1998;16:108-119.
725. Rendell MS, Rajfer J, Wicker PA, Smith MD. Sildenafil Diabetes Study Group. Sildenafil for treatment of erectile dysfunction in men with diabetes: a readomized controlled trial. JAMA 1999; 281:421-426.
726. Enzlin P, Mathieu C, Vanderschueren D, Demyttenaere K. Diabetes mellitus and female sexuality: a review of 25 years' research. Diabet Med 1998;15(10):809-815.
727. Shaw JE, Parker R, Hollis S, et al. Gustatory sweating in diabetes mellitus. Diabet Med 1996;13:1033-1037.
728. Shaw JE, Abbott CA, Tindle K, et al. A randomised controlled trial of topical glycopyrrolate, the first specific treatment for diabetic gustatory sweating. Diabetologia 1997;40:299-301.
729. Meyer C, Hering BJ, Grossmann R, et al. Improved glucose counterregulation and autonomic symptoms after intraportal islet transplants alone in patients with long-standing type I diabetes mellitus. Transplantation 1998;66:233-240.
730. Vinik A: Diagnosis and management of diabetic neuropathy. Clin Geriatr Med 1999;15:293-319.
731. Gu K, Cowie CC, Harris MI. Diabetes and decline in heart disease mortality in US adults. JAMA 1999;281:1291-1297.
732. Malmberg K, Yusuf S, Gerstein HC, et al. Impact of diabetes on long-term prognosis in patients with unstable angina and non–Q-wave myocardial infarction. Circulation 2000;102:1014-1019.
733. Mukamal KJ, Nesto RW, Cohen MC, et al. Impact of diabetes on long-term survival after acute myocardial infarction. Diabetes Care 2001;24:1422-1427.
734. Evans JM, Wang J, Morris AD. Comparison of cardiovascular risk between patients with type 2 diabetes and those who had a myocardial infarction: cross sectional and cohort studies. BMJ 2002;324:939-943.
735. Lee CD, Folsom AR, Pankow JS, et al. Cardiovascular events in diabetic and nondiabetic adults with or without a history of myocardial infarction. Circulation 2004;109:855-860.
736. Krolewski AS, Warram JH, Rand LI, et al. Epidemiologic approach to the etiology of type I diabetes mellitus and its complications. N Engl J Med 1987;317:1390-1398.
737. Orchard TJ, Olson JC, Erbey JR, et al. Insulin resistance-related factors, but not glycemia, predict coronary artery disease in type 1 diabetes. Diabetes Care 2003;26:1374-1379.
738. Soedamah-Muthu SS, Chaturvedi N, Toeller M, et al. EURODIAB Prospective Complications Study Group: Risk factors for coronary heart disease in type 1 diabetic patients in Europe: The EURODIAB Prospective Complications Study. Diabetes Care 2004;27: 530-537.
739. Pambianco G, Costacou T, Ellis D, et al. The 30-year natural history of type 1 diabetes complications: the Pittsburgh Epidemiology of Diabetes Complications Study experience. Diabetes 2006;55: 1463-1469.

740. Laing SP, Swerdlow AJ, Slater SD, et al. Mortality from heart disease in a cohort of 23,000 patients with insulin-treated diabetes. Diabetologia 2003;46:760-765.
741. Wilson PW, Kannel WB, Silbershatz H, et al. Clustering of metabolic factors and coronary heart disease. Arch Intern Med 1999;159:1104-1109.
742. Haffner SM, MykkanenL, Festa A, et al. Insulin-resistant prediabetic subjects hane more atherogenic risk factors than insulin-sensitive p[rediabetic subjects. Circulation 2000;101:975-980.
743. Festa A, Hanley AJG, Tracey RP, et al. Inflammation in the prediabetic state is related to increased insulin resistance rather that decreased insulin secretion. Ciruclation 2003;108:1822-1830.
744. Turner RC. The UK Prospective Diabetes Study: a review. Diabetes Care 1998;21(suppl 3):C35-C38.
745. Andersson DK, Svardsudd K. Long-term glycemic control relates to mortality in type II diabetes. Diabetes Care 1995;18:1534-1543.
746. Wei M, Gaskill SP, Haffner SM, et al. Effects of diabetes and level of glycemia on all-cause and cardiovascular mortality. The San Antonio Heart Study. Diabetes Care 1998;21:1167-1172.
748. Brunner EJ, Shipley MJ, Witte DR, et al. Relation between blood glucose and coronary mortality over 33 years in the Whitehall study. Diabetes Care 2006;29:26-31.
748. Tominaga M, Eguchi H, Manaka H, et al. Impaired glucose tolerance is a risk factor for cardiovascular disease but not impaired fasting glucose. Diabetes Care 1999;22:920-924.
749. DECODE study group. Glucose tolerance and mortality: comparison of WHO and American Diabetic Asociation diagnostic criteria. Lancet 1999;354:617-621.
750. Hu FB, Stampfner MJ, Haffner SM, et al. Elevated risk of cardiovascular disease prior to clinical diagnosis of type 2 diabetes. Diabetes Care 2002;25:1129-1134.
751. Klein R, Klein BE, Moss SE. The Wisconsin Epidemiologic Study of Diabetic Retinopathy: XVI. The relationship of C-peptide to the incidence and progression of diabetic retinopathy. Diabetes 1995;44:796-801.
752. Wingard DL, Barrett-Connor EL, Scheidt-Nave C, et al. Prevalence of cardiovascular and renal complications in older adults with normal or impaired glucose tolerance or NIDDM: a population-based study. Diabetes Care 1993;16:1022-1025.
753. Folsom AR, Eckfeldt JH, Weitzman S, et al. Relation of carotid artery wall thickness to diabetes mellitus, fasting glucose and insulin, body size, and physical activity. Atherosclerosis Risk in Communities (ARIC) Study Investigators. Stroke 1994;25: 66-73.
754. Temelkova-Kurktschiev TS, Koehler C, Leonhardt W, et al. Increased intimal-medial thickness in newly detected type 2 diabetes: risk factors. Diabetes Care 1999;22:333-338.
755. Hanefeld M, Koehler C, Schaper F, et al. Postprandial plasma glucose is an independent risk factor for increased carotid intima-media thickness in non-diabetic individuals. Atherosclerosis 1999;144:229-235.
756. National Cholesterol Education Program (NCEP) Expert Panel on the Detection, Evaluation, and Treatment of High Blood Cholesterol in Adults (Adult Treatment Panel III). Third report of the National Cholesterol Education Program (NCEP) Expert Panel on the Detection, Evaluation, and Treatment of High Blood Cholesterol in Adults (Adult Treatment Panel III). Final report. Circulation 2002;106:3143-3421.
757. Grundy SM, Brewer HB, Cleeman JI, et al. Definition of metabolic syndrome. Report of the National Heart, Lung, and Blood Institute/ American Heart Association Conference on Scientific Issues Related to Definition. Circulation 2004;109:433-438.
758. International Diabetes Foundation. The IDF worldwide definition of the metabolic syndrome. Available at http://www.idf.org/home/index.cfm?node=1429 (accessed March 21, 2007).
759. Ford ES, Giles WH, Dietz WH. Prevelence of the metabolic syndrome among US adults. Findings from the Third National Health and Nutrition Examination Survey. JAMA 2002;287:356-359.
760. Lakka, H-M, Laaksonen DE, Lakka TA, et al. The metabolic syndrome and total and cardiovascular disease mortality in middle-aged men. JAMA 2002;288:2709-2716.
761. Malik S, Wong ND, Franklin SS, et al. Impact of the metabolic syndrome on mortality from coronary heart disease, cardiovascular disease, and all causes in United States adults. Circulation 2004;110:1245-1250.
762. Sattar N, Gaw A, Scherbakova O, et al. Metabolic syndrome with and without C-reactive protein as a predictor of coronary heart disease and diabetes in the West of Scotland Coronary Prevention Study. Circulation 2003;108:414-419.
763. Ford ES. Risk for all-cause mortality, cardiovascular disease, and diabetes associated with the metabolic syndrome. Diabetes Care 2005;28:1769-1778.
764. Grundy SM, Cleeman JI, Daniels SR, et al. Diagnosis and management of the metabolic syndrome. An American Heart Association/National Heart, Lung, and Blood Institute scientific statement. Circulation 2005;112:2735-2752.
765. Deedwania PC. The deadly quartet revisited. Am J Med 1998; 105:1S-3S.
766. Howard G, O'Leary DH, Zaccaro D, et al. Insulin sensitivity and atherosclerosis. The Insulin Resistance Atherosclerosis Study (IRAS) Investigators. Circulation 1996;93:1809-1817.
767. Abraira C, Colwell J, Nuttall F, et al. Cardiovascular events and correlates in the Veterans Affairs Diabetes Feasibility Trial. Veterans Affairs Cooperative Study on Glycemic Control and Complications in Type II Diabetes. Arch Intern Med 1997;157:181-188.
768. Diabetes Control and Complications Trial/Epidemiology of Diabetes Interventions and Complications (DCCT/EDIC) Study Research Group. Intensive diabetes treatment and cardiovascular disease in patients with type 1 diabetes N Eng J Med 2005;353:2643-2653.
769. Dormandy JA, Charbonnel B, Eckland DJA, et al. Secondary prevention of macrovascular events in patients with type 2 diabetes in the PROactive Study (PROspective pioglitAzone Clinical Trial in macroVascular Events: a randomized controlled trial. Lancet 2005;366:1279-1289.
770. Gowri MS, Van der Westhuyzen DR, Bridges SR, et al. Decreased protection by HDL from poorly controlled type 2 diabetic subjects against LDL oxidation may be due to the abnormal composition of HDL. Arterioscler Thromb Vasc Biol 1999;19:2226-2233.
771. The Long-Term Intervention with Pravastatin in Ischemic Disease (LIPID) Study Group. Prevention of cardiovascular events and death in pravastatin patients with coronary heart disease and a broad range of initial cholesterol levels. N Engl J Med 1998; 339:1349-1357.
772. Haffner SM, Alexander CM, Cook TJ, et al. Reduced coronary events in simvastatin-treated patients with coronary heart disease and diabetes or impaired glucose levels. Arch Intern Med 1999;159:2661-2667.
773. Ballantyne CM, Olsson AG, Cook TJ, et al. Influence of low density high-density lipoprotein cholesterol and elevated triglyceride on coronary heart disease events and response to simvastatin therapy in 4S. Circulation 2001;104:3046-3051.
774. Deedwania P, Barter P, Carmena R, et al. Reduction of low-density lipoprotein cholesterol in patients with coronary heart disease and metabolic syndrome: analysis of the Treating to New Targets study. Lancet 2006;368:919-928.
775. Taylor AJ, Sullenberger LE, Lee HJ, et al. Arterial Biology for the Investigation of the Treatment Effects of Reducing Cholesterol (ARBITER 2): a double-blind, placebo-controlled study of extended-release niacin on atherosclerosis progression in secondary prevention patients treated with statins. Circulation 2004;110(23):3512-3517. Erratum in Circulation 2004;110(23):3615. Circulation 2005;111(24):e446.
776. Rubins HB, Robins SJ, Collins D, et al. Gemfibrozil for the secondary prevention of coronary heart disease in men with low levels of high-density lipoprotein cholesterol. Veterans Affairs High-Density Lipoprotein Cholesterol Intervention Trial Study Group. N Engl J Med 1999;341:410-418.
777. The FIELD Study Investigators. Effects of long-term fenofibrate therapy on cardiovascular events in 9795 people with type 2 diabetes mellitus (the FIELD study): randomized controlled trial. Lancet 2005;366:1849-1861.
778. Heart Protection Study Collaborative Group. MRC/BHF Heart protection Study of cholesterol lowering with simvastatin in 20,536 high-risk individuals: a randomized, placebo-controlled study. Lancet 2002;360:7-22.
779. Calhoun HM, Betteridge DJ, Durrington PN, et al. Primary prevention of cardiovascular disease with atorvastatin in type 2 diabetes in the Collaborative Atorvastatin Diabetes Study (CARDS): multicentre randomised placebo-controlled trial. Lancet 2004;364: 685-696.

780. Grundy SM, Cleeman JI, Merz MB, et al. Implications of recent clinical trials for the National Cholesterol Education Program Adult Treatment Panel III Guidelines. Circulation 2004;110: 227-239.
781. Chobanian AV, Bakris GL, Black HR, et al. The Seventh Report of the Joint National Committee on Prevention, Detection, Evaluation, and Treatment of High Blood Pressure (JNC VII). JAMA 2003;289:2560-2572.
782. Tuomilehto J, Rastenyte D, Birkenhager WH, et al. Effects of calcium-channel blockade in older patients with diabetes and systolic hypertension. Systolic Hypertension in Europe Trial Investigators. N Engl J Med 1999;340:677-684.
783. The Heart Outcomes Prevention Evaluation Study Investigators. Effects of an angiotensin-converting enzyme inhibitor, ramipril, on cardiovascular events in high-risk patients. N Engl J Med 2000;342: 145-153.
784. UK Prospective Diabetes Study Group. Efficacy of atenolol and captopril in reducing risk of macrovascular and microvascular complications in type 2 diabetes: UKPDS 39. BMJ 1998;317: 713-720.
785. Hansson L, Zanchetti A, Carruthers SG, et al. Effects of intensive blood pressure lowering and low-dose aspirin in patients with hypertension: principal results of the Hypertension Optimal Treatment (HOT) randomised trial. HOT Study Group. Lancet 1998;351:1755-1762.
786. Whelton PK, Barzilay J, Cushman WC, et al. Clinical outcomes in antihypertensive treatment of type 2 diabetes, impaired fasting glucose concentration, and normoglycemia. Arch Intern Med 2005;165:1401-1409.
787. Nesto RW, Zarich S. Acute myocardial infarction in diabetes mellitus: lessons learned from ACE inhibition. Circulation 1998;97: 12-15.
788. Jacoby RM, Nesto RW. Acute myocardial infarction in the diabetic patient: pathophysiology, clinical course and prognosis. J Am Coll Cardiol 1992;20:736-744.
789. Iwasaka T, Takahashi N, Nakamura S, et al. Residual left ventricular pump function after acute myocardial infarction in NIDDM patients. Diabetes Care 1992;15:1522-1526.
790. Bernardi L, Ricordi L, Lazzari P, et al. Impaired circadian modulation of sympathovagal activity in diabetes: a possible explanation for altered temporal onset of cardiovascular disease. Circulation 1992;86:1443-1452.
791. Zarich S, Waxman S, Freeman RT, et al. Effect of autonomic nervous system dysfunction on the circadian pattern of myocardial ischemia in diabetes mellitus. J Am Coll Cardiol 1994;24: 956-962.
792. Muller JE, Tofler GH, Stone PH. Circadian variation and triggers of onset of acute cardiovascular disease. Circulation 1989;79: 733-743.
793. Imperatore G, Riccardi G, Iovine C, et al. Plasma fibrinogen—a new factor of the metabolic syndrome: a population-based study. Diabetes Care 1998;21:649-654.
794. Sobel BE, Woodcock-Mitchell J, Schneider DJ, et al. Increased plasminogen activator inhibitor type 1 in coronary artery atherectomy specimens from type 2 diabetic compared with nondiabetic patients: a potential factor predisposing to thrombosis and its persistence. Circulation 1998;97:2213-2221.
795. Meigs JB, Mittleman MA, Nathan DM, et al. Hyperinsulinemia, hyperglycemia, and impaired hemostasis. The Framingham Offspring Study. JAMA 2000;283:221-228.
796. Woodfield SL, Lundergan CF, Reiner JS, et al. Angiographic findings and outcome in diabetic patients treated with thrombolytic therapy for acute myocardial infarction: the GUSTO-I experience. J Am Coll Cardiol 1996;28:1661-1669.
797. Mak KH, Moliterno DJ, Granger CB, et al. Influence of diabetes mellitus on clinical outcome in the thrombolytic era of acute myocardial infarction. GUSTO-I Investigators. Global Utilization of Streptokinase and Tissue Plasminogen Activator for Occluded Coronary Arteries. J Am Coll Cardiol 1997;30:171-179.
798. Sun D, Nguyen N, DeGrado T, et al. Ischemia-induced translocation of the insulin-responsive glucose transporter GLUT4 in the plasma membrane of cardiac myocytes. Circulation 1994;89: 793-798.
799. Oliver M, Opie H. Effects of glucose and fatty acids on myocardial ischaemia and arrhythmias. Lancet 1994;343:155-158.
800. Bellodi G, Manicardi V, Malavasi V, et al. Hyperglycemia and prognosis of acute myocardial infarction in patients without diabetes mellitus. Am J Cardiol 1989;64:885-888.
801. Oswald GA, Smith CC, Betteridge DJ, et al. Determinants and importance of stress hyperglycaemia in non-diabetic patients with myocardial infarction. BMJ 1986;293:917-922.
802. Fava S, Aquilina O, Azzopardi J, et al: The prognostic value of blood glucose in diabetic patients with acute myocardial infarction. Diabetes Med 1996;13:80-83.
803. Capes SE, Hunt D, Malmberg K, et al. Stress hyperglycemia and increased risk of death after myocardial infarction in patients with and without diabetes: a systematic overview. Lancet 2000;355: 773-778.
804. Malmberg K, Ryden L, Efendic S, et al. Randomized trial of insulin-glucose infusion followed by subcutaneous insulin treatment in diabetic patients with acute myocardial infarction (DIGAMI study): effects on mortality at 1 year. J Am Coll Cardiol 1995;26:57-65.
805. Malmberg K, Ryden L, Wedel H, et al. Intense metabolic control by means of insulin in patients with diabetes mellitus and acute myocardial infarction (DIGAMI 2): effects on mortality and morbidity. Eur Heart J 2005;26:650-661.
806. The CREATE-ECLA Trial Group Investigators. Effect of glucose-insulin-potassium infusion on mortality in patients with acute ST-segment elevation myocardial infarction. JAMA 2005; 293:437-446.
807. Garratt KN, Brady PA, Hassinger NL, et al. Sulfonylurea drugs increase early mortality in patients with diabetes mellitus after direct angioplasty for acute myocardial infarction. J Am Coll Cardiol 1999;33:119-124.
808. Cleveland JC Jr, Meldrum DR, Cain BS, et al. Oral sulfonylurea hypoglycemic agents prevent ischemic preconditioning in human myocardium: two paradoxes revisited. Circulation 1997;96:29-32.
809. Katsuda Y, Egashira K, Ueno H, et al. Glibenclamide, a selective inhibitor of ATP-sensitive K^+ channels, attenuates metabolic coronary vasodilatation induced by pacing tachycardia in dogs. Circulation 1995;92:511-517.
810. Davis CA III, Sherman AJ, Yaroshenko Y, et al. Coronary vascular responsiveness to adenosine is impaired additively by blockade of nitric oxide synthesis and a sulfonylurea. Am J Cardiol 1998;31:816-822.
811. O'Driscoll G, Green D, Maiorana A, et al. Improvement in endothelial function by angiotensin-converting enzyme inhibition in non-insulin-dependent diabetes mellitus. J Am Coll Cardiol 1999;33: 1506-1511.
812. Vaughan DE, Rouleau JL, Ridker PM, et al. Effects of ramipril on plasma fibrinolytic balance in patients with acute anterior myocardial infarction. HEART Study Investigators. Circulation 1997;96: 442-447.
813. Torlone E, Britta M, Rambotti AM, et al. Improved insulin action and glycemic control after long-term angiotensin-converting enzyme inhibition in subjects with arterial hypertension and type II diabetes. Diabetes Care 1993;16:1347-1355.
814. Zuanetti G, Latini R, Maggioni A, et al. Effect of the ACE-inhibitor lisinopril on mortality in diabetic patients with acute myocardial infarction: the data from the GISSI-3 study. Circulation 1997;96: 4239-4245.
815. Gustafsson I, Torp-Pedersen C, Kober L, et al. Effect of the angiotensin-converting enzyme inhibitor trandolapril on mortality and morbidity in diabetic patients with left ventricular dysfunction after acute myocardial infarction. Trace Study Group. J Am Coll Cardiol 1999;34:83-89.
816. Lakshman MR, Reda DJ, Materson BJ, et al. Diuretics and β-blockers do not have adverse effects at 1 year on plasma lipid and lipoprotein profiles in men with hypertension. Department of Veterans Affairs Cooperative Study Group on Antihypertensive Agents. Arch Intern Med 1999;159:551-558.
817. Shorr RI, Ray WA, Daugherty JR, et al. Antihypertensives and the risk of serious hypoglycemia in older persons using insulin or sulfonylureas. JAMA 1997;278:40-43.
818. Chen J, Marciniak TA, Radford MJ, et al. β-Blocker therapy for secondary prevention of myocardial infarction in elderly diabetic patients. Results from the National Cooperative Cardiovascular Project. J Am Coll Cardiol 1999;34:1388-1394.
819. Giugliano D, Acampora R, Marfella R. Metabolic and cardiovascular effects of carvedilol and atenolol in non–insulin-dependent

diabetes mellitus and hypertension. Ann Intern Med 1997;126: 955-959.
820. ETDRS Investigators. Aspirin effects on mortality and morbidity in patients with diabetes mellitus. Early Treatment Diabetic Retinopathy Study report 14. JAMA 1992;268:1292-1300.
821. American Diabetes Association. Aspirin therapy in diabetes. Diabetes Care 1997;20:772-1773.
822. Davi G, Catalano I, Averna M, et al. Thromboxane biosynthesis and platelet function in type II diabetes mellitus. N Engl J Med 1990; 322:1769-1774.
823. Hirsh J, Bhatt DL. Comparative benefits of clopidogrel and aspirin in high-risk patient populations. Lessons from the CAPRIE and CURE studies. Arch Intern Med 2004;164:2106-2110.
824. Platelet Receptor Inhibition in Ischemic Syndrome Management in Patients Limited by Unstable Signs and Symptoms (PRISM-PLUS) Study Investigators. Inhibition of the platelet glycoprotein IIb/IIIa receptor with tirofiban in unstable angina and non-Q-wave myocardial infarction. N Engl J Med 1998;338:1488-1497.
825. EPILOG Investigators. Platelet glycoprotein IIb/IIIa receptor blockade and low-dose heparin during percutaneous coronary revascularization. N Engl J Med 1997;336:1689-1696.
826. Lincoff AM, Califf RM, Moliterno DJ, et al. Complementary clinical benefits of coronary artery stenting and blockade of platelet glycoprotein IIb/IIIa receptors. Evaluation of Platelet IIb/IIIa Inhibition in Stenting Investigators. N Engl J Med 1999;341:319-327.
827. Bypass Angioplasty Revascularization Investigation (BARI) Investigators. Comparison of coronary bypass surgery with angioplasty in patients with multivessel disease. N Engl J Med 1996; 335:217-225.
828. Kannel WB, Hjortland M, Castelli WP. Role of diabetes in congestive heart failure. The Framingham study. Am J Cardiol 1974;34: 29-34.
829. Aronson D, Rayfield E, Cheseboro J. Mechanisms determining course and outcome of diabetic patients who have had acute myocardial infarction. Ann Intern Med 1997;126:296-306.
830. Cabin H, Roberts W. Quantitative comparison of extent of coronary narrowing and size of healed myocardial infarct in 33 necropsy patients with clinically recognized and in 28 with clinically unrecognized ("silent") previous acute myocardial infarction. Am J Cardiol 1982;50:677-681.
831. van Hoeven KH, Factor SM. A comparison of the pathological spectrum of hypertensive, diabetic, and hypertensive-diabetic heart disease. Circulation 1990;82:848-855.
832. Kawaguchi M, Techigawara M, Ishihata T, et al. A comparison of ultrastructural changes on endomyocardial biopsy specimens obtained from patients with diabetes mellitus with and without hypertension. Heart Vessels 1997;12:267-274.
833. Nahser P, Brown R, Oskarsson H, et al. Maximal coronary flow reserve and metabolic coronary vasodilation in patients with diabetes mellitus. Circulation 1995;91:635-640.
834. Depre C, Vanoverschelde JL, Taegtmeyer H. Glucose for the heart. Circulation 1999;99:578-588.
835. Azzarelli A, Dini F, Cristofani R, et al. NIDDM as unfavorable factor to the postinfarction ventricular function in the elderly: echocardiography study. Coron Artery Dis 1995;6:629-634.
836. Korup E, Dalsgaard D, Nyvad O, et al. Comparison of degrees of left ventricular dilation within three hours and up to six days after onset of first acute myocardial infarction. Am J Cardiol 1997;80:449-453.
837. Mayfield JA, Reiber GE, Maynard C, et al: Trends in lower limb amputation in the Veterans Health Administration, 1989-1998. J Rehabil Res Dev 2000;37:23-30.
838. Anichini R, de Bellis A, Cerretini I, et al. The number of amputations as a quality marker of diabetic foot therapy—results after 5 year implementation of a disease management project. Diabetologia; 2007 (in press).
839. Vileikyte L, Rubin RR, Leventhal H. Psychological aspects of diabetic neuropathy and its late sequalae. Diabet Metab Res Rev 2004;20(suppl 1):S13-S18.
840. Boulton, AJM, Cavanagh PR, Rayman G, eds. The Foot in Diabetes, 4th ed. Chichester, UK: John Wiley & Sons, 2006.
841. Bowker JH, Pfeifer MA, eds. Levin & O'Neal's The Diabetic Foot, 7th ed. St Louis: Mosby, 2006.
842. Boulton AJM, Vileikyte L, Kirsner RS. Neuropathic diabetic foot ulcers. N Engl J Med 2004;251:48-55.
843. Singh N, Armstrong DG, Lipsky BA. Preventing foot ulcers in patients with diabetes. JAMA 2005;293:217-228.
844. Abbott CA, Carrington AL, Ashe H et al: The North-West diabetes foot care study: incidence of, and risk factors for, new diabetic foot ulceration in a community-based cohort. Diabetic Med 2002;20:277-384.
845. Akbari CM, Pomposelli FB, Gibbons GW. Lower extremity revascularization in diabetes: late observations. Arch Surg 2000;135: 452-456.
846. Boulton AJM. The diabetic foot: from art to science. Diabetologia 2004;47:1343-1353.
847. Reiber GE, Vileikyte L, Boyko EJ, et al. Causal pathways for incident lower extremity ulcers in patients with diabetes from two settings. Diabetes Care 1999;22:157-162.
848. Boulton AJM. Why bother educating the multidisciplinary team and the patient? The example of prevention of lower extremity amputation in diabetes. Patient Educ Counsel 1995;26:183-188.
849. Armstrong DG, Lavery LA, Harkless LB. Validation of a diabetic wound classification system. Diabet Med 1998;14:855-859.
850. Oyibo S, Jude EB, Tarawneh I, et al. A comparision of two diabetic foot ulcer classification systems: the Wagner and the University of Texas wound classification systems. Diabetes Care 2001;24: 84-88.
851. Piaggesi A, Viacava P, Rizzo L et al. Semi-quantitative analysis of the histopathological features of the neuropathic foot ulcer—effects of pressure relief. Diabetes Care 2003;26:3123-3128.
852. Steed DL, Donohoe D, Webster MW, et al. Effect of extensive debridement and treatment on the healing of diabetic foot ulcers. J Am Coll Surg 1996;183:61-64.
853. Consensus statement on diabetic foot wound care. Diabetes Care 1999;22:1354-1360.
854. Armstrong DG, Nguyen HC, Lavery LA, et al: Off-loading the diabetic foot wound: a randomized clinical trial. Diabetes Care; 2001;24:1019-1022, 2001.
855. Katz I, Harlan A, Miranda-Palma B, et al. A randomized trial of two irremovable offloading devices in the treatment of plantar neuropathic diabetic foot ulcers. Diabetes Care 2005;28:555-559.
856. Lipsky BA. Intrnational consensus on diagnosing and treating the infected diabetic foot. Diabet Metab Res Rev 2004;20(suppl 1): S68-S77.
857. Smiell J, Wieman TJ, Steed DL, et al. Efficacy and safety of becaplermin in patients with non-healing lower extremity diabetic ulcers: a combined analysis of four randomised, controlled studies. Wound Rep Regen 1999;7:335-346.
858. Armstrong DG, Attinger C, Boulton AJM, et al. Guidelines regarding negative pressure wound therapy in the diabetic foot. Ostomy Wound Management 2004;50(suppl B):3S-27S.

CHAPTER 33

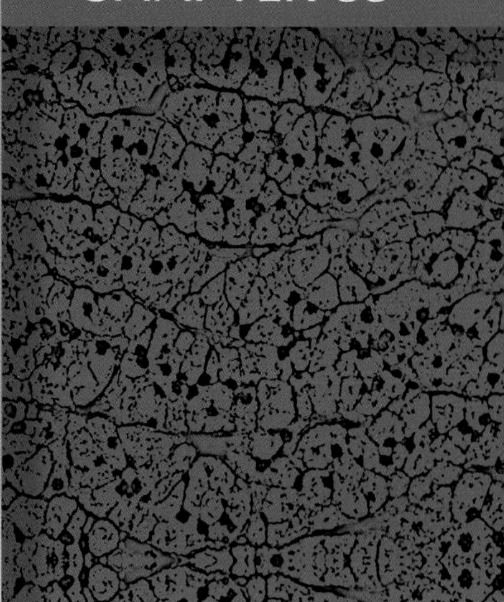

GLUCOSE HOMEOSTASIS AND HYPOGLYCEMIA

Philip E. Cryer

Glucose is an obligate metabolic fuel for the brain under physiologic conditions. In contrast, other organs oxidize fatty acids as well as glucose. Because of this unique dependence on glucose and because it cannot synthesize glucose or store more than a few minutes' supply as glycogen, the brain requires a continuous supply of glucose from the circulation. Facilitated diffusion of glucose from the blood to the brain is a direct function of the arterial plasma glucose concentration. At normal plasma glucose concentrations, the rate of blood-to-brain glucose transport exceeds the rate of brain glucose metabolism. However, as the plasma glucose concentration falls below the physiologic range, blood-to-brain glucose transport becomes limiting to brain energy metabolism and, thus, to survival. Given the immediate survival value of maintenance of the plasma glucose concentration, it is not surprising that physiologic mechanisms that prevent or rapidly correct hypoglycemia have evolved. Indeed, these mechanisms are so effective that hypoglycemia is an uncommon clinical event except in people who use drugs that lower glucose levels (e.g., insulin, sulfonylureas, or alcohol).

Insight into the physiology of glucose counterregulation—the mechanisms that normally prevent or rapidly correct hypoglycemia—and its pathophysiology in the context of clinical hypoglycemia, which have been reviewed in detail,[1-3] has improved the management of hypoglycemia. Nonetheless, major gaps in understanding remain. Both are discussed here.

Physiology of Systemic Glucose Regulation

This section summarizes glucose metabolism and systemic glucose balance and their regulation,[2] with emphasis on the aspects relevant to glucose counterregulation and the prevention of hypoglycemia.

Glucose Metabolism

Origins and Fates of Glucose

Glucose is derived from three sources: intestinal *absorption* that follows digestion of dietary carbohydrates; *glycogenolysis,* the breakdown of glycogen, which is the polymerized storage form of glucose; and *gluconeogenesis,* the formation of glucose from precursors including lactate (and pyruvate), amino acids (especially alanine and glutamine), and, to a lesser extent, glycerol (Fig. 33–1).

Although most tissues express the enzyme systems required to synthesize (glycogen synthase) and hydrolyze (phosphorylase) glycogen, only the liver and kidneys express glucose-6-phosphatase, the enzyme necessary for the release of glucose into the circulation, at levels sufficient to permit these organs to contribute to the systemic glucose pool. The liver and kidneys also express the enzymes necessary for gluconeogenesis (including the critical gluconeogenic enzymes pyruvate carboxylase, phosphoenolpyruvate carboxykinase, and fructose-1, 6-bisphosphatase).

There are multiple potential metabolic fates for glucose that is transported into cells; external losses are normally negligible (see Fig. 33–1). Glucose may be stored as glycogen, or it can undergo glycolysis to pyruvate, which can be reduced to lactate, transaminated to form alanine, or converted to acetyl coenzyme A (CoA), which in turn can be oxidized to carbon dioxide and water through the tricarboxylic acid cycle, converted to fatty acids (and stored as triglycerides), or used for ketone body (acetoacetate, β-hydroxybutyrate) or cholesterol synthesis. Finally, glucose may be released into the circulation. As

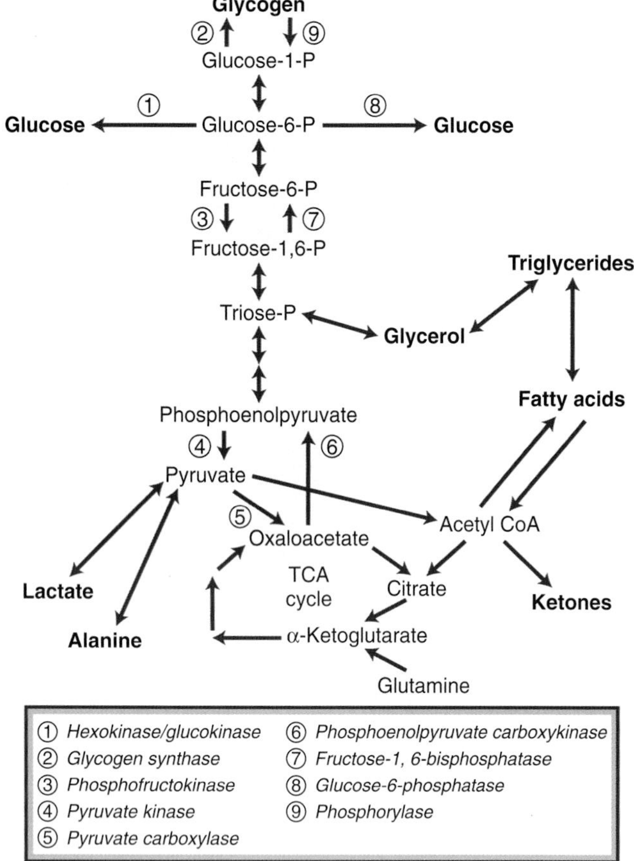

Figure 33–1 ▪ Schematic representation of glucose metabolism. CoA, coenzyme A; TCA, tricarboxylic acid.

summarized in the following paragraphs, these outcomes differ in different organs.

Hepatic (and Renal) Glucose Metabolism

The liver is remarkably flexible in its role in glucose homeostasis and is the major source of net endogenous glucose production (through glycogenolysis and gluconeogenesis).[4] Under conditions of high glucose output (e.g., fasting), the energy needs of the liver are largely provided by the beta oxidation of fatty acids. Conversely, the liver can also be an organ of net glucose uptake, with glucose stored as glycogen, oxidized for energy, or converted to fat that can either remain in the liver or be transported to other tissues as very-low-density lipoprotein (VLDL). The kidneys also produce (through gluconeogenesis) and use glucose.[5,6]

Glucose Utilization

Muscle can store glucose as glycogen or can metabolize glucose through glycolysis to pyruvate. The pyruvate is reduced to lactate or is transaminated to form alanine or is oxidized. Lactate (and pyruvate) released from muscle is transported to the liver, where it serves as a gluconeogenic precursor (the Cori or glucose-lactate cycle). However, to the extent that lactate and pyruvate carbons are derived from glucose, they cannot result in net new glucose formation. Alanine, glutamine, and other amino acids can also flow from muscle to liver, where they too serve as gluconeogenic precursors. Circulating alanine is also largely derived from glucose (glucose-alanine cycle). Glutamine is also a major precursor for new glucose formation, although it too is partially derived from glucose (glucose-glutamine cycle).

TABLE 33–1 SYSTEMIC GLUCOSE BALANCE

Glucose Influx into the Circulation	=	Glucose Efflux out of the Circulation
Exogenous glucose delivery		Ongoing brain glucose utilization
+		+
Endogenous glucose production In liver: glycogenolysis and gluconeogenesis[1,3,4] In kidneys: gluconeogenesis[1,4]		Variable glucose utilization by other tissues (e.g., muscle, fat, liver, kidneys etc.)[2,5]

[1]↓ by insulin; [2]↑ by insulin; [3]↑ by glucagon; [4]↑ by epinephrine; [5]↓ by epinephrine.

During a fast, muscle can reduce its glucose uptake virtually to zero, oxidize fatty acids for its energy needs, and, through proteolysis, mobilize amino acids for transport to the liver to serve as gluconeogenic precursors for net glucose formation.

Although quantitatively less important than muscle, adipose tissue can also use glucose for fatty acid synthesis or formation of glycerol-3-phosphate, which can then esterify fatty acids (derived largely from circulating VLDL) to form triglycerides. During a fast, adipocytes decrease their glucose utilization and satisfy energy needs from the beta oxidation of fatty acids. Other tissues, such as the formed elements of the blood and the renal medullae, do not have the capacity to decrease glucose utilization during fasting and therefore produce lactate at relatively fixed rates.

Glucose is the predominant metabolic fuel used by the brain under most conditions. Glucose undergoes terminal oxidation to carbon dioxide and water in the brain. The brain respiratory quotient is approximately 1.0. Although the adult brain constitutes only about 2.5% of body weight, its oxidative metabolism accounts for approximately 25% of the basal metabolic rate under physiologic conditions. However, when ketones are plentiful in the circulation, as during prolonged fasting, they can support the majority of the energy needs of the brain and thus reduce its glucose utilization.

Systemic Glucose Balance

Normally, rates of endogenous glucose influx into the circulation and those of glucose efflux out of the circulation into tissues other than the brain are coordinately regulated—largely by the plasma glucose–lowering (regulatory) hormone insulin and the plasma glucose–raising (counterregulatory) hormones glucagon and epinephrine—such that systemic glucose balance is maintained, hypoglycemia (as well as hyperglycemia) is prevented, and a continuous supply of glucose to the brain is ensured (Table 33–1). This is accomplished despite wide variations in exogenous glucose influx (e.g., after feeding versus during fasting) and in glucose efflux (e.g., during exercise versus during rest). Hypoglycemia occurs when rates of glucose appearance in the circulation (the sum of endogenous glucose production and of exogenous glucose delivery from ingested carbohydrates) fail to keep pace with rates of glucose disappearance from the circulation (the sum of ongoing brain glucose metabolism and of variable glucose utilization by tissues such as muscle and fat as well as the liver and kidneys, among others).

Fasting

The *postabsorptive state* is the interdigestive period that begins approximately 5 to 6 hours after a meal. However, the term is most commonly used to refer to data obtained after a 10- to 14-hour overnight fast. In healthy adults, the physiologic postabsorptive (fasting) plasma glucose concentration is approximately 4.0 to 6.0 mmol/L (72-108 mg/dL), with a mean of approximately 5.0 mmol/L (90 mg/dL). In the postabsorptive steady state, rates of glucose production and utilization are equal. They average 12 μmol/kg per minute (2.2 mg/kg per minute) and range from about 10 to 14 μmol/kg per minute (1.8-2.6 mg/kg per minute) in healthy adults after an overnight fast.[2] These rates are as much as threefold higher in infants, at least in part because of their greater brain mass relative to their body weight.

Approximately 60% of basal glucose utilization is accounted for by the brain. The remainder is used by glycolyzing tissues, such as the formed elements of the blood and the renal medullae and to some extent muscle and fat. Hepatic glucose production results from both glycogenolysis and gluconeogenesis even after an overnight fast.[5]

The liver is the predominant source of net endogenous glucose production after an overnight fast. The kidneys, which both use and produce glucose, contribute little to net glucose production. However, renal, like hepatic, glucose production is regulated.[5,6] It is suppressed by insulin and stimulated by epinephrine (but not by glucagon). Thus, net renal glucose production occurs under some conditions, including hypoglycemia.[6] Therefore, equating endogenous glucose production with hepatic glucose production is not precise.

The importance of gluconeogenesis in providing new glucose and supporting hepatic glycogen stores after an overnight fast becomes apparent when one considers the limited availability of preformed glucose. The glucose pool, namely free glucose in the extracellular fluid and in the cells of certain tissues (primarily in the liver but also small amounts in the kidneys, intestinal mucosa, pancreatic islet cells, brain, and blood cells), is about 83 to 111 mmol (15-20 g) in the normal adult. Glycogen that can be mobilized to provide circulating glucose (e.g., hepatic glycogen) contains approximately 390 mmol glucose (70 g), with a range of about 135 to 722 mmol (25-130 g). Thus, in an adult of average size, preformed glucose can provide as little as a 3-hour supply of glucose and less than an 8-hour supply on average, even at the diminished rate of glucose utilization that occurs in the postabsorptive state. Clearly, therefore, gluconeogenesis is important for maintenance of the plasma glucose concentration even during an overnight fast.[4]

If fasting is prolonged to 24 to 48 hours, the plasma glucose level declines and then stabilizes, hepatic glycogen content falls to less than 55 mmol (10 g), and gluconeogenesis becomes the sole source of glucose production.[4] Because amino acids are the main gluconeogenic precursors that result in net glucose formation, muscle protein is degraded. Glucose utilization by muscle and fat virtually ceases. As lipolysis and ketogenesis accelerate and circulating ketone levels rise, ketones become a major source of fuel for the brain. Thus, glucose utilization by the brain declines by about half, resulting in a decrease in the rate of gluconeogenesis required to maintain the plasma glucose concentration and hence in diminished protein wasting. After prolonged fasting (40 days), ketones provide an estimated 80% to 90% of the energy used by the brain, and renal gluconeogenesis provides up to half of the endogenous glucose production.[7]

Feeding

After a meal, glucose absorption into the circulation is more than twice the rate of postabsorptive endogenous glucose production, depending on the carbohydrate content of the meal and the rate of its digestion and absorption. As glucose is absorbed, endogenous glucose production is suppressed, and glucose utilization by liver, muscle, and fat accelerates. Thus, exogenous glucose is assimilated and the plasma glucose concentration returns to the postabsorptive level.

Exercise

Exercise increases glucose utilization (by muscle) to rates that can be several times greater than those of the postabsorptive state. Endogenous glucose production normally accelerates to match use so that the plasma glucose concentration is maintained.

From these examples, it is clear that the plasma glucose concentration is normally maintained within a narrow range despite wide variations in glucose flux, a homeostatic feat accomplished by hormonal, neural, and substrate glucoregulatory factors.[2] From a mechanistic perspective, hypoglycemia could result from decreased glucose production, increased glucose utilization, or both.

Glucoregulatory Factors

Hormonal Glucoregulatory Factors

Hormones are the most important glucoregulatory factors, and the regulation of their secretion is complex. Glucose, specifically the plasma glucose concentration, is the most important determinant of the secretion of glucoregulatory hormones, including insulin, glucagon, epinephrine, growth hormone, and cortisol.[2]

Insulin, the dominant glucose-lowering hormone, suppresses endogenous glucose production and stimulates glucose utilization by insulin-sensitive tissues, thereby lowering the plasma glucose concentration. Insulin is secreted from beta cells of the pancreatic islets into the hepatic portal circulation and acts on the liver and peripheral tissues. It inhibits hepatic glycogenolysis and gluconeogenesis and, in concert with other factors, converts the liver into an organ of net glucose uptake and fuel storage (glycogen and triglycerides). It also suppresses renal glucose production and stimulates glucose uptake, storage, and utilization by tissues such as muscle and fat. In the postabsorptive state, insulin regulates the plasma glucose concentration primarily by restraining hepatic glucose production. Higher levels, such as those that occur after meals, are required to stimulate glucose utilization. In addition to direct actions on hepatocytes, insulin reduces hepatic glucose production by suppressing circulating fatty acid, gluconeogenic precursor, and glucagon levels and by increasing vagal signaling, the latter through actions on the hypothalamus.[8,9]

Conversely, decreased insulin secretion causes increased hepatic and renal glucose production and decreased glucose utilization by insulin-sensitive tissues such as muscle and thus tends to raise the plasma glucose concentration. Insulin is therefore both a glucose-lowering (regulatory) and a glucose-raising (counterregulatory) hormone. The rate of insulin secretion is regulated by a number of factors,[2] the most important of which is glucose. A decrease in the plasma glucose concentration has an immediate inhibitory effect on insulin secretion, thereby limiting a further fall in the plasma glucose level. Insulin is a potent and critical hormone. Either profound insulin deficiency or marked insulin excess can be lethal. But it is not the only glucoregulatory hormone.

Glucose-raising or glucose counterregulatory hormones include glucagon, epinephrine, growth hormone, and cortisol.[2] In response to falling plasma glucose levels, glucagon is secreted from alpha cells of the pancreatic islets into the hepatic portal circulation and is believed to act exclusively on the liver under physiologic conditions. It activates glycogenolysis, and to some extent gluconeogenesis, and increases hepatic glucose production within minutes. This increase is transient. Despite ongoing hyperglucagonemia, glucose production returns toward basal

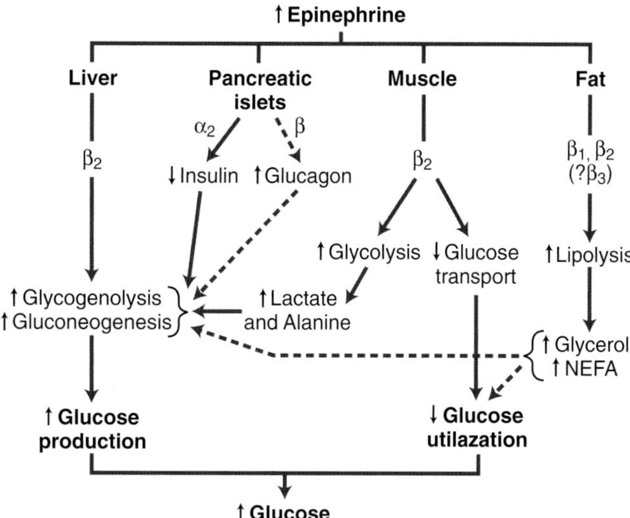

Figure 33–2 ▪ Schematic representation of the mechanisms of the hyperglycemic effect of epinephrine. NEFA, nonesterified fatty acids. (From Cryer PE. Catecholamines, pheochromocytoma and diabetes. Diabetes Rev 1993;1:309-317. Copyright 1993, American Diabetes Association, Alexandria, Va.)

rates over about 90 minutes, although the hormone continues to support glucose production. Glucagon-induced hyperglycemia is also transient because the glucagon-induced increase in glycogenolysis does not persist. The transient nature of the glycogenolytic response to sustained hyperglucagonemia is not the result of glycogen depletion because a further increase in glucagon causes a further increase in glucose release; instead, it is the result of glucose-induced insulin secretion and perhaps the autoregulatory effect of hyperglycemia (see later), although other factors may be involved. Because glucagon, unlike epinephrine, does not mobilize gluconeogenic precursors, glucagon alone has relatively little impact on gluconeogenesis.[10] Although glucagon is not thought to stimulate lipolysis under physiologic conditions, combined with low insulin levels glucagon favors hepatic ketogenesis.

The hyperglycemic effect of the adrenal hormone epinephrine (Fig. 33–2) is more complex.[2] Epinephrine is secreted from chromaffin cells of the adrenal medullae in response to falling plasma glucose levels and both stimulates hepatic (and renal) glucose production and limits glucose utilization. The actions of epinephrine are direct and indirect and are mediated through α-adrenergic and β-adrenergic receptors. α_2-Adrenergic limitation of insulin secretion is an important indirect hyperglycemic action of epinephrine. It allows the hyperglycemic response to occur. However, the increase in insulin secretion that occurs as plasma glucose rises limits the magnitude of the glycemic response. β-Adrenergic stimulation of glucagon secretion also occurs, but its contribution to the hyperglycemic effect of epinephrine appears to be minor under physiologic conditions.

Epinephrine acts directly (i.e., independent of changes in other hormones or substrates) to increase hepatic glycogenolysis and gluconeogenesis. In humans the hepatic effect is mediated predominantly through β_2-adrenergic mechanisms. Epinephrine also mobilizes gluconeogenic precursors (e.g., lactate, alanine, and glycerol) and fatty acids and, like glucagon, acts within minutes to produce a transient increase in glucose production and support basal rates of glucose production thereafter. In contrast to glucagon, however, epinephrine also limits glucose utilization (i.e., it reduces glucose clearance) by insulin-sensitive tissues such as skeletal muscle,[11] predominantly through direct β-adrenergic mechanisms. Because of the persistent effect on glucose utilization, sustained hyperepinephrinemia results in persistent hyperglycemia.

Long-term elevations of growth hormone and of cortisol limit glucose utilization and stimulate glucose production.[2] Initially, however, growth hormone has a plasma glucose–lowering (insulin-like) effect; its hyperglycemic effect does not appear for several hours. Similarly, cortisol causes an increase in the plasma glucose level after 2 to 3 hours. The hyperglycemic effect of the combination of glucagon, epinephrine, and cortisol is greater than the sum of the effects of the hormones individually.[12] Growth hormone and cortisol, like epinephrine, also stimulate lipolysis.

Neural Glucoregulatory Factors

The sympathetic neurotransmitter norepinephrine exerts hyperglycemic actions by mechanisms assumed to be similar to those of epinephrine, except that norepinephrine is released primarily from terminals of sympathetic postganglionic neurons.[2] These terminals are adjacent to adrenergic receptors on target cells within the innervated tissues. Sympathetic neural activation increases, and parasympathetic neural activation decreases, hepatic glucose production.[13,14] It is reasonable to anticipate that peptide neurotransmitters and neuromodulators also affect glucose metabolism.

Substrate Glucoregulatory Factors

Glucose per se shifts hepatic metabolism in favor of glycogen storage. Hepatic glucose autoregulation (namely hepatic glucose production as an inverse function of the plasma glucose concentration independent of hormonal and neural regulatory factors) may be a glucose counterregulatory factor.[2] Given the complexity of the direct and indirect effects of insulin to regulate glucose production,[8,9] it is difficult to document unequivocally that a change in glucose production associated with a change in plasma glucose concentrations is not the result of a change in a hormonal or neural glucoregulatory factor and thus to establish the contribution of glucose autoregulation. Fatty acids support glucose production (as an energy source) and limit glucose utilization.

Control of Glucoregulatory Factors

Hypoglycemia suppresses the secretion of insulin from pancreatic beta cells and stimulates the secretion of glucagon from pancreatic alpha cells, epinephrine from the adrenal medullae, cortisol from the adrenal cortices, and growth hormone from the pituitary gland, among other hormones.[2] It also stimulates the release of norepinephrine from sympathetic postganglionic neurons and acetylcholine from sympathetic and parasympathetic postganglionic neurons. An array of neuropeptides are also released from sympathetic, parasympathetic, and other neurons.[15]

Insulin secretion and glucagon secretion are regulated by substrate, neural, and hormonal signals[2] (see Chapter 29). Falling plasma glucose concentrations are sensed directly by pancreatic beta cells, resulting in decreased insulin secretion. During hypoglycemia, activated sympathetic neural and adrenomedullary systems further limit insulin secretion (by α-adrenergic mechanisms). Decreasing plasma glucose concentrations are also thought to be sensed directly by pancreatic alpha cells, but a decrease in intraislet insulin—secondary to a decrease in beta cell insulin secretion and resulting in decreased tonic alpha cell inhibition by insulin—is a signal critical to glucagon secretion.[16] Sympathoadrenal and parasympathetic activation also stimulates glucagon secretion.[17,18]

The autonomic (adrenomedullary, sympathetic, and parasympathetic), adrenocorticotropic hormone (ACTH)-mediated cortisol and growth hormone responses to hypoglycemia are mediated through the CNS.[2] Although sympathetic reflexes at the spinal cord level can be elicited by various stimuli in patients with spinal cord transections, sympathoadrenal responses to hypoglycemia do not occur in such persons.[19]

The ventromedial nucleus of the hypothalamus is an important site of glucose-sensing neurons that trigger CNS-mediated neuroendocrine responses to hypoglycemia.[20] However, there is evidence that there are widespread glucose-sensing sites within the brain[21] and in peripheral locations, including the portal vein.[22]

Glycemic Thresholds for Responses to Hypoglycemia

Falling plasma glucose concentrations normally elicit a typical sequence of responses.[2] Arterialized venous glycemic thresholds[23-25] for several of these are listed in Table 33–2 and illustrated in Figure 33–3. Insulin secretion decreases (favoring increased glucose production as well as decreased glucose utilization by tissues other than the brain) as plasma glucose levels decline within the physiologic range. Secretion of counterregulatory hormones including glucagon (which stimulates hepatic glycogenolysis and favors gluconeogenesis) and epinephrine (which stimulates hepatic glycogenolysis and, by mobilizing precursors, hepatic and renal gluconeogenesis and which limits glucose utilization by insulin-sensitive tissues) increases as plasma glucose levels fall just below the physiologic range. Lower plasma glucose concentrations cause symptoms and signs of hypoglycemia and, ultimately, brain dysfunction.

When the same methods are used, the glycemic thresholds for the various responses to falling plasma glucose concentrations in healthy subjects are quite reproducible from laboratory to laboratory (see Fig. 33–3).[23-25] Nonetheless, these thresholds are dynamic rather than static. As discussed later in this chapter, they shift to higher plasma glucose concentrations in people with poorly controlled diabetes (who often have symptoms of hypoglycemia at higher than normal glucose levels) and to lower plasma glucose concentrations in people who suffer recurrent hypoglycemia, such as those with well-controlled diabetes or with an insulinoma (who often tolerate subnormal glucose levels without symptoms).

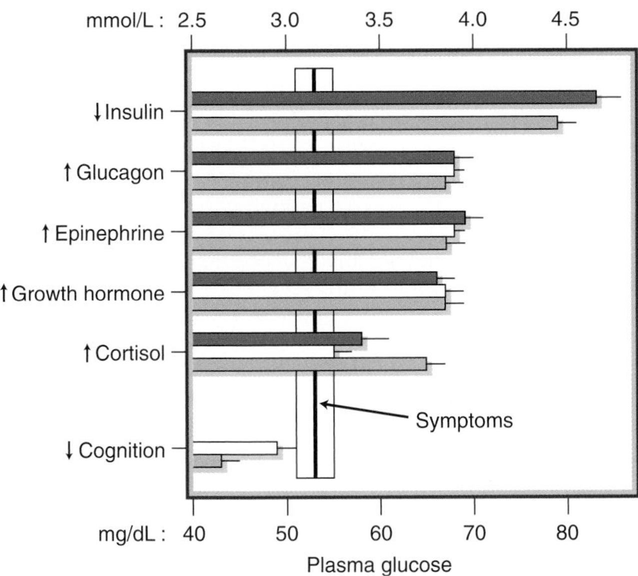

Figure 33–3 ▪ Mean (±SE) arterialized venous glycemic thresholds for decrements in insulin secretion (determined by measurement of C-peptide concentrations); increments in plasma glucagon, epinephrine, growth hormone, and cortisol concentrations; symptoms; and decrements in cognitive functions during decreasing plasma glucose concentrations in healthy humans in three different studies. (Data for *solid columns* from Schwartz NS, Clutter WE, Shah SD, et al. Glycemic thresholds for activation of glucose counterregulatory systems are higher than the threshold for symptoms. J Clin Invest 1987;79:777-781. Data for *open columns* from Mitrakou A, Ryan C, Veneman T, et al. Hierarchy of glycemic thresholds for counterregulatory hormone secretion, symptoms, and cerebral dysfunction. Am J Physiol 1991; 260:E67-E74. Data for *crosshatched* columns from Fanelli C, Pampanelli S, Epifano L, et al. Relative roles of insulin and hypoglycaemia on induction of neuroendocrine responses to, symptoms of, and deterioration of cognitive function in hypoglycaemia in male and female humans. Diabetologia 1994; 37:797-807. Reprinted from Cryer PE. Hypoglycemia. Pathophysiology, Diagnosis and Treatment. New York: Oxford University Press, 1997. Copyright 1997, Oxford University Press, New York.)

Glucose Counterregulation

The physiology of glucose counterregulation—the mechanisms that normally prevent or rapidly correct hypoglycemia[26-33]—has been reviewed in detail.[2] Early studies of the mechanisms of the correction of short-term insulin-induced hypoglycemia[26-29] and of more prolonged insulin-induced hypoglycemia[30-33] are summarized in Figures 33–4 and 33–5, respectively. These and

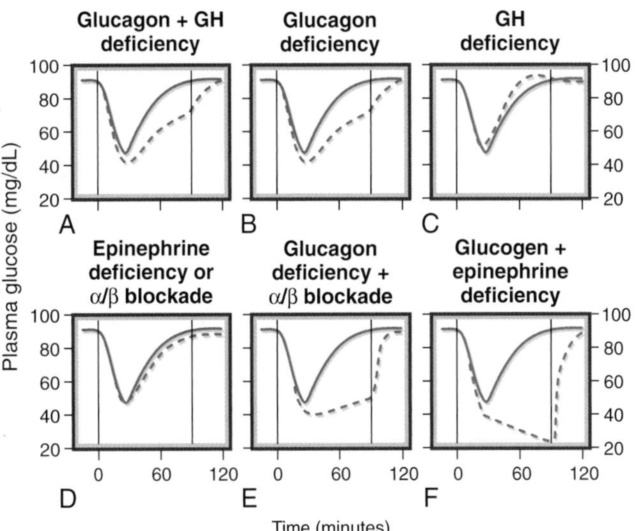

Figure 33–4 ▪ Summary of studies of the mechanisms of glucose recovery from short-term hypoglycemia in healthy humans. Insulin was injected intravenously at time 0 minutes. Interventions were started at time 0 minutes and stopped at time 90 minutes (i.e., between the vertical lines in each panel). Plasma glucose curves during control studies (*solid curves,* same in all six panels) and as modified *(dashed curves)* by the following: **A,** Somatostatin infusion (glucagon plus growth hormone [GH] deficiency. **B,** Somatostatin infusion plus growth hormone replacement (glucagon deficiency). **C,** Somatostatin infusion plus glucagon replacement (GH deficiency). **D,** Phentolamine and propranolol infusion (combined α-adrenergic and β-adrenergic blockade) or studies performed in bilaterally adrenalectomized persons (epinephrine deficiency). **E,** Somatostatin, phentolamine, and propranolol infusion (glucagon deficiency plus α-adrenergic and β-adrenergic blockade). **F,** Somatostatin infusion in bilaterally adrenalectomized persons (glucagon plus epinephrine deficiency). (*Curves* derived from data in Clarke WL, Santiago JV, Thomas L, et al. Adrenergic mechanisms in recovery from hypoglycemia in man: adrenergic blockade. Am J Physiol 1979;236: E147-E152; and Rizza RA, Cryer PE, Gerich JE. Role of glucagon, epinephrine and growth hormone in human glucose counterregulation: effects of somatostatin and adrenergic blockade on plasma glucose recovery and glucose flux rates following insulin induced hypoglycemia. J Clin Invest 1979;64:62-71. From Cryer PE. Glucose counterregulation in man. Diabetes 1981; 30:261-264. Copyright 1981, American Diabetes Association, Alexandria, VA.)

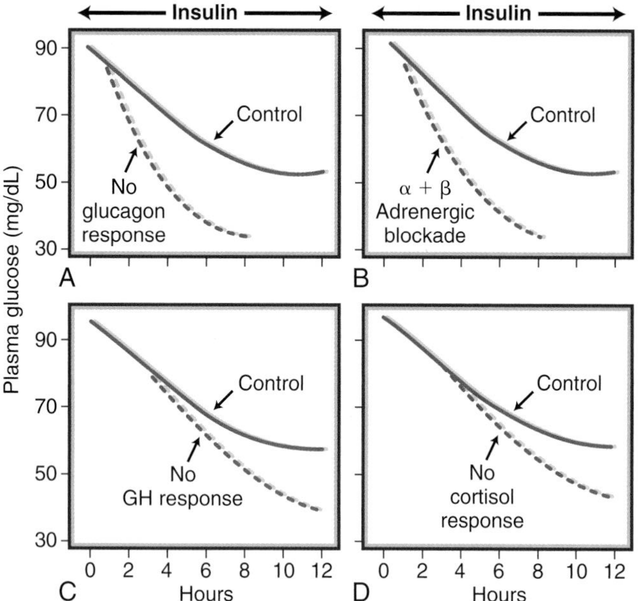

Figure 33–5 ▪ Summary of studies of the mechanisms of defense against prolonged hypoglycemia in healthy humans. Plasma glucose curves during control studies (*solid curves,* same in all panels) and as modified *(dashed curves)* by the following: **A,** Somatostatin infusion and metyrapone administration with cortisol and growth hormone (GH) replacement and endogenous epinephrine secretion (no glucagon response). **B,** Somatostatin infusion and metyrapone administration with glucagon, cortisol, and growth hormone replacement and endogenous epinephrine secretion and phentolamine and propranolol infusion (α-adrenergic + β-adrenergic blockade). **C,** Somatostatin infusion and metyrapone administration with glucagon and cortisol replacement and endogenous epinephrine secretion (no growth hormone response). **D,** Somatostatin infusion and metyrapone administration with glucagon and growth hormone replacement (no cortisol response). (Data from DeFeo P, Periello G, Torlone E, et al. Demonstration of a role for growth hormone in glucose counterregulation. Am J Physiol 1989;256:E835-E843; DeFeo P, Periello G, Torlone E, et al. Contribution of cortisol to glucose counterregulation. Am J Physiol 1989;257:E35-E42; DeFeo P, Perriello G, Torlone E, et al. Evidence against important catecholamine compensation for absent glucagon counterregulation. Am J Physiol 1991;260:E203-E212; DeFeo P, Perriello G, Torlone E, et al. Contribution of adrenergic mechanisms to glucose counterregulation in humans. Am J Physiol 1991;261:E725-E736. From Gerich JE. Glucose counterregulation and its impact on diabetes mellitus. Diabetes 1988; 37:1608-1617. Copyright 1988, American Diabetes Association, Alexandria, VA.)

studies of the prevention of hypoglycemia in the postabsorptive and postprandial states, during exercise, and during prolonged fasting are detailed elsewhere.[2]

The principles of glucose counterregulation are three.[2] First, the prevention and the correction of hypoglycemia involve both waning of insulin and activation of glucose counterregulatory factors. These are not due solely to waning of insulin. Second, although insulin is the dominant plasma glucose–lowering factor, there are redundant glucose counterregulatory factors including a decrease in insulin and increases in glucagon and epinephrine as well as growth hormone and cortisol. Thus, there is a fail-safe system that prevents failure of the counterregulatory process even when one, or perhaps more, of the components of the system fails. Third, there is a hierarchy among the counterregulatory factors. Some are more important than others.

The physiology of glucose counterregulation is also summarized in Table 33–2. The first defense against falling plasma glucose concentrations is decreased insulin secretion. Among the counterregulatory factors, increased glucagon secretion plays a primary role. Glucose recovery from hypoglycemia is impaired when glucagon secretion is deficient. Glucagon is the second defense against falling plasma glucose concentrations. Albeit demonstrably involved, increased epinephrine secretion is not normally critical. It becomes critical when glucagon is deficient. Epinephrine is the third defense against falling plasma glucose concentrations. Hypoglycemia develops or progresses when both glucagon and epinephrine are deficient and insulin is present despite the actions of the other glucose counterregulatory factors. Thus, insulin, glucagon, and epinephrine stand high in the hierarchy of redundant glucose counterregulatory factors.

Growth hormone and cortisol, both of which tend to increase plasma glucose concentrations after several hours, are involved in defense against prolonged hypoglycemia. However, neither is critical to recovery from even prolonged hypoglycemia or, at least in adults, to prevention of hypoglycemia after an overnight fast.[34]

There is some evidence that glucose autoregulation may be involved,[35] although only during severe hypoglycemia.[35,36] Other hormones, neurotransmitters, and substrates other than glucose (and fatty acids that mediate part of the effect of epinephrine) might also be involved. If so, they play relatively minor roles.

These principles apply to the correction of hypoglycemia and to its prevention when plasma glucose levels fall below the physiologic range in the postabsorptive and postprandial states and during exercise and prolonged fasting.[2] In contrast to acti-

TABLE 33–2 PHYSIOLOGIC RESPONSES TO DECREASING PLASMA GLUCOSE CONCENTRATIONS

Response	Glycemic Threshold* (mmol/L [mg/dL])	Physiologic Effects	Role in Prevention or Correction of Hypoglycemia (Glucose Counterregulation)
↓ Insulin	4.4-4.7 [80-85]	↑R_a (↓R_d)	Primary glucose regulatory factor, first defense against hypoglycemia
↑ Glucagon	3.6-3.9 [65-70]	↑R_a	Primary glucose counterregulatory factor, second defense against hypoglycemia
↑ Epinephrine	3.6-3.9 [65-70]	↑R_a, ↓R_d	Involved, critical when glucagon is deficient, third defense against hypoglycemia
↑ Cortisol and growth hormone	3.6-3.9 [65-70]	↑R_a, ↓R_d	Involved, not critical
Symptoms	2.8-3.1 [50-55]	↑Exogenous glucose	Prompt behavioral defense (food ingestion)
↓ Cognition	<2.8 [<50]	—	(Compromises behavioral defense)

*Arterialized venous, not venous, plasma glucose concentrations.

R_a, rate of glucose appearance, glucose production by the liver and kidneys; R_d, rate of glucose disappearance, glucose utilization by insulin-sensitive tissues such as skeletal muscle (no direct effect on central nervous system glucose utilization).

vation of glucose counterregulatory factors, insulin secretion responds to plasma glucose fluctuations within the physiologic range (Fig. 33–3, Table 33–2), and insulin is therefore the critical determinant of the normal postabsorptive plasma glucose concentration.[37]

Pathophysiology of Hypoglycemia

Clinical Manifestations of Hypoglycemia

Whipple's triad—symptoms consistent with hypoglycemia, a low plasma glucose concentration, and relief of those symptoms when the plasma glucose concentration is raised—provides compelling evidence of clinical hypoglycemia.

Symptoms of hypoglycemia can be divided into two categories, *neuroglycopenic* and *neurogenic* (autonomic) symptoms.[38-40] Neuroglycopenic symptoms are the direct result of CNS neuronal glucose deprivation. They include behavioral changes, confusion, fatigue or weakness, visual changes, seizure, loss of consciousness, and, if hypoglycemia is severe and prolonged, death. Neurogenic symptoms are the result of the perception of physiologic changes caused by the sympathoadrenal discharge triggered by hypoglycemia. They include adrenergic symptoms such as palpitations, tremor, and anxiety and cholinergic symptoms such as sweating, hunger, and paresthesias.[38] Adrenergic symptoms are mediated by norepinephrine released from sympathetic postganglionic neurons, the adrenal medullae, or both, and epinephrine released from the adrenal medullae. Cholinergic symptoms are mediated by acetylcholine released from sympathetic postganglionic neurons. Adrenergic and cholinergic symptoms are largely the result of sympathetic neural, rather than adrenomedullary, activation.[41]

Representative neurogenic and neuroglycopenic symptoms of hypoglycemia are listed in Figure 33–6, which also illustrates that awareness of hypoglycemia—the extent to which a person perceives that the blood sugar is low—is largely the result of the perception of neurogenic symptoms.[38] The autonomic response to hypoglycemia is initiated by glucose-sensitive neurons, including those in the ventromedial hypothalamus, that increase firing as extracellular glucose levels fall. Thus, although both neurogenic and neuroglycopenic symptoms could be viewed as fundamentally neuroglycopenic in origin, their mechanisms are different.

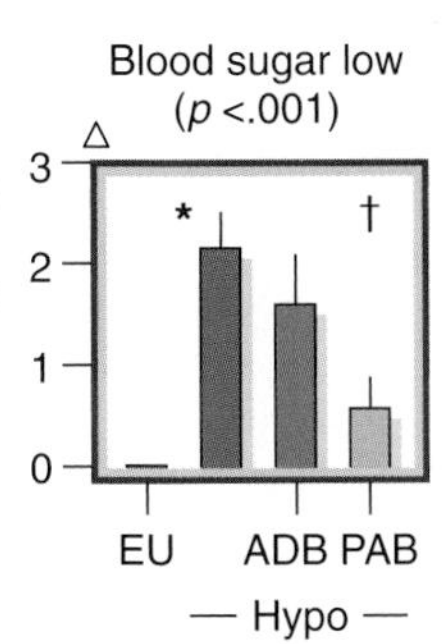

Figure 33–6 ▪ Neurogenic (autonomic) and neuroglycopenic symptoms of hypoglycemia in healthy humans. Among the neurogenic symptoms, "sweaty," "hungry," and "tingling" are cholinergic and "shaky/tremulous," "heart pounding," and "nervous/anxious" are adrenergic. See text for discussion. Mean (±SE) subject scores for awareness of hypoglycemia (low blood sugar) during clamped euglycemia (EU) and during hypoglycemia (Hypo) alone *(closed column)*, with combined α-adrenergic and β-adrenergic blockade with infused phentolamine and propranolol (ADB, *crosshatched column*), and with combined α-adrenergic and β-adrenergic blockade plus muscarinic cholinergic blockade with atropine, panautonomic blockade (PAB, *open column*), are also shown. (Data from Towler DA, Havlin CE, Craft S, Cryer PE. Mechanisms of awareness of hypoglycemia: perception of neurogenic [predominantly cholinergic] rather than neuroglycopenic symptoms. Diabetes 1993;42:1791-1798. Copyright 1994, American Diabetes Association, Alexandria, VA.)

Common signs of hypoglycemia include pallor and diaphoresis. Heart rate and systolic blood pressure are typically increased, but these findings might not be prominent. To the extent that they are observable, the neuroglycopenic manifestations are often valuable, albeit nonspecific, signs. Transient neurologic defects occur occasionally. Permanent neurologic damage is rare. (In monkeys, 5-6 hours of a blood glucose <1.1 mM/L [20 mg/dL] was required for the regular production of neurological damage.[42]) Brain damage is thought to be the result of the excitatory actions of increased glutamate release and involve activation of poly(ADP-ribose) polymerase, an enzyme normally involved in DNA repair, that leads to neuronal dysfunction and cell death.[43]

The magnitude of the responses to hypoglycemia is an inverse function of the nadir plasma glucose concentration rather than the rate of decrease in plasma glucose.[44,45] It was once thought that neurogenic symptoms are less prominent when hypoglycemia develops gradually. However, the relative paucity of symptoms at a given low plasma glucose concentration in persons with recurrent hypoglycemia, such as those with tightly controlled diabetes[46] or with an insulinoma,[47] is attributable to a shift in glycemic thresholds for sympathoadrenal responses to lower plasma glucose concentrations. Conversely, the thresholds shift to higher plasma glucose concentrations in patients with chronic hyperglycemia, resulting in symptoms of hypoglycemia at relatively high glucose levels.[46,48] The mechanism of these shifts in thresholds is unknown. Potential mechanisms are discussed later in this chapter.

Diagnosis of Hypoglycemia

The manifestations of hypoglycemia are nonspecific, vary among persons, and can change from time to time in the same person. They are also typically episodic. Thus, although the history is of fundamental importance in suggesting the possibility of hypoglycemia, the diagnosis cannot be made solely on the basis of symptoms and signs.

The diagnosis of hypoglycemia should also not be made solely on the basis of plasma glucose measurements unless they are unequivocally subnormal. It is not possible to define a plasma glucose concentration below which neuroglycopenia invariably occurs and above which neuroglycopenia never occurs. Although symptoms commonly occur with plasma glucose levels less than 3.0 mM/L (54 mg/dL),[23-25] they can occur at higher plasma glucose levels in poorly controlled diabetes[46,48] and only at lower glucose levels in well-controlled diabetes[46] or in other conditions that result in recurrent hypoglycemia, such as insulinoma.[47] In addition, venous plasma glucose concentrations substantially less than 3.0 mM/L (54 mg/dL) can occur in normal persons late after glucose ingestion (arterial glucose levels are higher) and in some women and children during fasting without producing recognizable symptoms. This is not to say that distinctly low plasma glucose measurements should be ignored. Some patients with endogenous hyperinsulinism[47] or intensively treated diabetes[46] tolerate glucose levels that are unequivocally subnormal, as mentioned earlier. Because these patients can have hypoglycemic symptoms at other times (presumably when glucose levels are even lower), it would be inappropriate to deny that they have hypoglycemia.

In general, venous plasma glucose concentrations greater than 3.9 mM/L (70 mg/dL) after an overnight fast are normal, those between 3.0 and 3.9 mM/L (54-70 mg/dL) suggest hypoglycemia, and those less than 3.0 mM/L (54 mg/dL) indicate postabsorptive hypoglycemia. Because substantial glucose extraction occurs across the forearm under hyperinsulinemic conditions, arterial glucose concentrations (those relevant to brain function) are as much as 30% higher than venous glucose concentrations after an oral glucose load. Artifactually low measured glucose levels can result from glycolysis in vitro (pseudohypoglycemia), particularly in the presence of leukocytosis or polycythemia, or both, or if separation of plasma from the formed elements of the blood is delayed. The diagnosis of hypoglycemia is most convincingly established when it is based on Whipple's triad: symptoms consistent with hypoglycemia, a low plasma glucose concentration, and relief of those symptoms when the plasma glucose concentration is increased to normal levels.

Postabsorptive versus Postprandial Hypoglycemia

Reproducible hypoglycemia in the postabsorptive state implies the presence of disease and requires diagnostic explanation and therapy. This condition is commonly referred to as *postabsorptive, or fasting, hypoglycemia.* However, it need not be apparent initially or exclusively during prolonged fasting or after an overnight fast; it might become symptomatic during the latter portion of any interdigestive period, especially with exercise. In contrast, *postprandial (reactive, stimulative) hypoglycemia* usually does not imply a serious underlying disorder. Thus, the distinction between postabsorptive and postprandial hypoglycemia is useful.

Mechanisms of Hypoglycemia

Hypoglycemia indicates that the rate of glucose efflux from the circulation exceeds that of glucose influx into the circulation. It can result from excessive glucose efflux (excessive utilization, external losses) or deficient glucose influx (deficient endogenous production in the absence of exogenous glucose delivery), or both. Conditions in which glucose utilization is increased include exercise, pregnancy, and sepsis; renal losses can occur at physiologic plasma glucose concentrations (e.g., renal glycosuria, pregnancy). However, because of the capacity of the normal liver (and kidneys) to increase glucose production several-fold, as discussed earlier, clinical hypoglycemia rarely results solely from excessive glucose efflux. Rather it is commonly the result of inappropriately low glucose production relative to the rate of glucose utilization.

Hypoglycemia can be caused by regulatory, enzymatic, or substrate defects. Glucoregulatory defects include excessive secretion of insulin or deficient secretion of glucose counterregulatory hormones. Enzymatic defects in glucose production may be primary or can result from hepatic disease. Substrate defects include failure to mobilize or utilize gluconeogenic substrates.

Clinical Classification of Hypoglycemia

Hypoglycemia can be classified on the basis of glucose kinetic patterns, pathogenic mechanisms, or disease groups. The last approach is used in this chapter (Table 33–3). Postabsorptive, or fasting, hypoglycemia can be the result of drugs, critical illnesses including hepatic or renal failure or sepsis, hormonal deficiencies, non–beta cell tumors, endogenous hyperinsulinism (including that caused by pancreatic beta cell tumors), or metabolic disorders of infancy and childhood. Postprandial, or reactive, hypoglycemia is rarely caused by endogenous hyperinsulinism or congenital enzyme defects but can follow gastric surgery and perhaps occurs rarely as an idiopathic disorder.

TABLE 33–3 CLINICAL CLASSIFICATION OF HYPOGLYCEMIA

POSTABSORPTIVE (FASTING) HYPOGLYCEMIA
Drugs
Especially insulin, sulfonylureas, alcohol
Also pentamidine, quinine
Rarely, salicylates, sulfonamides
Others
Critical Illnesses
Hepatic failure
Cardiac failure
Renal failure
Sepsis
Inanition
Hormonal Deficiencies
Cortisol or growth hormone, or both
Glucagon and epinephrine
Endogenous Hyperinsulinism
Pancreatic beta cell disorders
• Tumor (insulinoma)
• Nontumor
Beta cell secretagogue (e.g., sulfonylureas)
Autoimmune hypoglycemia
• Insulin antibodies
• Insulin receptor antibodies
• ? beta-cell antibodies
? Ectopic insulin secretion
Other
Non–beta-cell tumors
Hypoglycemias of infancy and childhood
POSTPRANDIAL (REACTIVE) HYPOGLYCEMIA
Endogenous Hyperinsulinism
Insulin antibodies
Noninsulinoma pancreatogenous hypoglycemia
Congenital Deficiencies of Enzymes of Carbohydrate Metabolism
Hereditary fructose intolerance
Galactosemia
Other
Alimentary hypoglycemia
Idiopathic (functional) postprandial hypoglycemia

Most episodes of hypoglycemia result from drugs, particularly insulin, sulfonylureas, or alcohol. In one series of patients treated in an emergency department for hypoglycemia, two thirds had diabetes mellitus and two thirds had been drinking alcohol.[49] Clearly, the combination of drug-treated diabetes and alcohol ingestion can be devastating. Nearly one fourth of the patients were septic, but diabetes or alcohol ingestion was common even in those patients. Drugs are also a common cause of hypoglycemia in inpatients.[50] In this case, however, critical illnesses such as renal or hepatic failure, sepsis, and inanition are common. Hypoglycemia resulting from hormonal deficiencies is uncommon but often treatable by hormone replacement. Hypoglycemia caused by non–beta cell tumors or by endogenous hyperinsulinism is rare.

Hypoglycemia in Diabetes Mellitus

Clinical Context

Iatrogenic hypoglycemia is the limiting factor in the glycemic management of diabetes.[3,51-53] It causes recurrent morbidity in most people with type 1 diabetes (T1DM) and many with type 2 diabetes (T2DM), and it is sometimes fatal. In addition, episodes of hypoglycemia, even asymptomatic episodes, impair defenses against subsequent hypoglycemia by causing hypoglycemia-associated autonomic failure—the clinical syndromes of defective glucose counterregulation and hypoglycemia unawareness—and thus a vicious cycle of recurrent hypoglycemia. Finally, the barrier of hypoglycemia precludes maintenance of euglycemia over a lifetime of diabetes and thus full realization of the well-established vascular benefits of glycemic control.[54-57]

In T1DM, aggressive attempts to achieve glycemic control increase the risk of severe, at least temporarily disabling, iatrogenic hypoglycemia (i.e., that requiring the assistance of another person) more than threefold (Fig. 33–7). That fact was documented in both of the controlled clinical trials with sample sizes large enough to demonstrate beneficial effects of intensive therapy on the long-term complications of diabetes, the Diabetes Control and Complications Trial (DCCT)[54,58,59] and the Stockholm Diabetes Intervention Study.[55,60] It was confirmed in a meta-analysis that also included 12 smaller controlled clinical trials of intensive therapy.[61] However, it is possible to reduce the risk of hypoglycemia during aggressive therapy of T1DM.[51] For example, the sixfold increased risk of severe hypoglycemia during intensive therapy in the feasibility phase of the DCCT[58] was reduced by half in the full-scale trial.[54]

It is not practical to detect all episodes of iatrogenic hypoglycemia. Asymptomatic episodes will be missed unless they are detected by routine glucose monitoring, and mild to moderate symptomatic episodes might not be recognized as such. Because of incomplete ascertainment, estimates of the incidence of hypoglycemia in a given patient group or under a given therapeutic condition are best considered minimum estimates. Because severe hypoglycemia is a dramatic event that is more likely to be recalled (by the patient or by associates), estimates of the incidence of severe hypoglycemia are more reliable although they represent only a small fraction of the total hypoglycemic experience.

Because of the interplay of therapeutic insulin excess and compromised physiologic and behavioral defenses against falling plasma glucose concentrations, as discussed later in this chapter, people with T1DM are at ongoing risk for episodes of hypoglycemia.[51] Those attempting to achieve glycemic control suffer untold numbers of episodes of asymptomatic hypoglycemia—plasma glucose levels may be lower than 2.8 mM/L (50 mg/dL) as much as 10% of the time—and an average of two episodes of symptomatic hypoglycemia per week. They suffer an episode of severe, at least temporarily disabling hypoglycemia, often with seizure or coma, every year on average (Table 33–4). Although seemingly complete recovery from even severe hypoglycemia is the rule, permanent neurologic deficits can result. It has been estimated that 2% to 4% of deaths of people with T1DM are caused by hypoglycemia.[51,62] In addition, hypoglycemia can cause recurrent or even persistent psychosocial morbidity. The reality of hypoglycemia, the rational fear of hypoglycemia, or both can be a barrier to glycemic control.

Iatrogenic hypoglycemia is generally less frequent in T2DM.[51] However, it occurs during treatment with sulfonylureas or other insulin secretagogues (and has been reported in patients treated with metformin[57,63]) or with insulin (Table 33–5; see Table 33–4). The frequency of hypoglycemia approaches that in T1DM in those who reach the insulin-deficient end of the spectrum of T2DM.[64] Indeed, in one series, the frequency of severe hypoglycemia was similar in patients with T2DM and T1DM matched for duration of insulin therapy.[65] The United Kingdom Prospective Diabetes Study (UKPDS) investigators concluded that over time, hypoglycemia becomes limiting in the treatment of T2DM just as it is in the treatment of T1DM.[64] Population-based data indicate that the event rates for severe hypoglycemia,[66] including that requiring emergency treatment,[67,68] approach those in T1DM in insulin-treated T2DM.

Given the now well-established long-term benefits of glycemic control and the short-term potentially devastating effects of iatrogenic hypoglycemia, it is clear that the goals of both reducing mean glycemia and minimizing hypoglycemia are important for people with diabetes.[51] Minimizing the risk of hypoglycemia in T1DM involves both application of the principles of aggressive therapy—education and empowerment of patients, frequent self-monitoring of blood glucose, flexible insulin (and other drug) regimens, individualized glycemic goals, and ongoing professional guidance and support—and implementation of hypoglycemia risk reduction. As discussed later in this chapter,

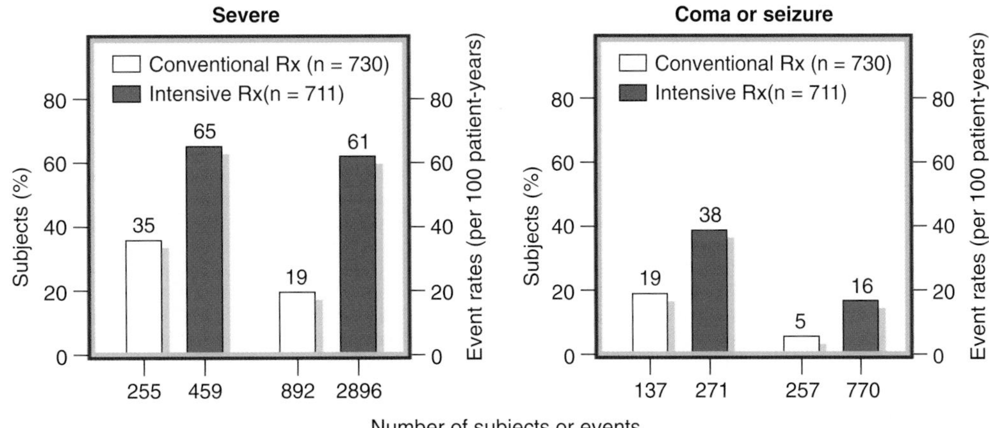

Figure 33–7 ▪ Fraction of patients affected and event rates for severe hypoglycemia *(left)* and severe hypoglycemia with coma or seizure *(right)* in the Diabetes Control and Complications Trial. Rx, therapy. (Data from The Diabetes Control and Complications Trial Research Group. Hypoglycemia in the Diabetes Control and Complications Trial. Diabetes 1997;46:271-286. From Cryer PE. Hypoglycemia. Pathophysiology, Diagnosis and Therapy. New York, Oxford University Press, 1997. Copyright 1997, Oxford University Press, New York.)

TABLE 33–4 SEVERE HYPOGLYCEMIA DURING AGGRESSIVE GLYCEMIC THERAPY OF DIABETES

Study	Reference	Episodes Per 100 Patient-Years
	TYPE 1 DIABETES	
Edinburgh	MacLeod et al (1993)	170
Utrecht	ter Braak et al (2000)	150
Danish-British Multicentre Survey	Pedersen-Bjergaard et al (2004)	130
Tayside	Donnelly et al (2005)	115
Stockholm Diabetes Intervention Study	Reichard & Pihl (1994)	110
Diabetes Control and Complications Trial	DCCT Research Group (1993)	62
	TYPE 2 DIABETES	
Edinburgh	MacLeod et al (1993)	73
Steno	Akram et al (2006)	44
Tayside	Donnelly et al (2005)	35
Veterans Affairs Pump Study*	Saudek et al (1996)	10
Veterans Affairs Cooperative Study	Abraira et al (1995)	3

*Multiple daily insulin injection subset.

Abraira C, Colwell JA, Nuttall FQ, et al. Veterans Affairs Cooperative Study on glycemic control and complications in type II diabetes (VA CSDM). Results of the feasibility trial. Veterans Affairs Cooperative Study in Type II Diabetes. Diabetes Care 1995;18(8):1113-1123.

Akram K, Pedersen-Bjergaard U, Carstensen B, et al. Frequency and risk factors of severe hypoglycaemia in insulin-treated type 2 diabetes: a cross-sectional survey. Diabet Med 2006;23(7):750-756.

Diabetes Control and Complications Trial (DCCT) Research Group. The effect of intensive treatment of diabetes on the development and progression of long-term complications in insulin-dependent diabetes mellitus. N Engl J Med 1993;329(14):977-986.

Donnelly LA, Morris AD, Frier BM, et al. Frequency and predictors of hypoglycaemia in type 1 and insulin-treated type 2 diabetes: a population-based study. Diabet Med 2005;22(6):749-755.

MacLeod KM, Hepburn DA, Frier BM. Frequency and morbidity of severe hypoglycaemia in insulin-treated diabetic patients. Diabet Med 1993;10(3):238-245.

Pedersen-Bjergaard U, Pramming S, Heller SR, et al. Severe hypoglycaemia in 1076 adult patients with type 1 diabetes: influence of risk markers and selection. Diabetes Metab Res Rev 2004;20(6):479-486.

Reichard P, Pihl M. Mortality and treatment side-effects during long-term intensified conventional insulin treatment in the Stockholm Diabetes Intervention Study. Diabetes 1994;43(2):313-317.

Saudek CD, Duckworth WC, Giobbie-Hurder A, et al. Implantable insulin pump vs multiple-dose insulin for non–insulin-dependent diabetes mellitus: a randomized clinical trial. Department of Veterans Affairs Implantable Insulin Pump Study Group. JAMA 1996;276(16):1322-1327.

ter Braak EW, Appelman AM, van de Laak M, et al. Clinical characteristics of type 1 diabetic patients with and without severe hypoglycemia. Diabetes Care 2000;23(10):1467-1471.

hypoglycemia risk reduction requires consideration of the roles of both therapeutic insulin excess and compromised physiologic and behavioral defenses against developing hypoglycemia.

Risk Factors

Insulin Excess

The conventional risk factors for iatrogenic hypoglycemia in T1DM[51] (Table 33–6) are based on the premise that relative or absolute therapeutic insulin excess, which must occur from time to time because of the pharmacokinetic imperfections of all current insulin replacement regimens, is the sole determinant of risk. Relative or absolute therapeutic insulin excess occurs when

- Insulin doses are excessive, ill-timed, or of the wrong type
- The influx of exogenous glucose is decreased (as during the overnight fast or after missed meals or snacks)
- Insulin-independent glucose utilization is increased (as during exercise)
- Endogenous glucose production is decreased (as after alcohol ingestion or administration or other drugs and with loss of renal parenchyma)
- Sensitivity to insulin is increased (as after exercise; in the middle of the night; with glycemic control; with increased fitness, weight loss, or both; or with administration of certain drugs)
- Insulin clearance is decreased (as in renal failure).

These are the issues with which people with diabetes and their health care providers deal routinely as they attempt to minimize iatrogenic hypoglycemia. However, it became clear early in the DCCT that these conventional risk factors explain only a minority of episodes of severe iatrogenic hypoglycemia.[58] Indeed, in a multivariate model none was found to be statistically significant. Clearly, we must look beyond these risk factors if we are to understand the majority of episodes of severe hypoglycemia in T1DM.

Interplay of Insulin Excess and Compromised Glucose Counterregulation

Iatrogenic hypoglycemia in T1DM is more appropriately viewed as the result of the interplay of relative or absolute therapeutic insulin excess (the conventional risk factors) and compromised glucose counterregulation (see Table 33–6).[3,51] Three clinically well-documented risk factors for iatrogenic hypoglycemia in T1DM are insulin deficiency[59,69-71]; a history of severe hypoglycemia, hypoglycemia unawareness, or both[59,70,71]; and aggressive glycemic therapy per se as evidenced by lower glycemic goals or lower hemoglobin (Hb) A_{1c} levels[59,70] (Table 33–6). (Obviously, iatrogenic hypoglycemia occurs in people with diabetes who are not severely insulin deficient, have no history of severe

TABLE 33–5 CUMULATIVE INCIDENCE OF HYPOGLYCEMIA (ANY, MAJOR) IN TYPE 2 DIABETES OVER 6 YEARS IN THE UNITED KINGDOM PROSPECTIVE DIABETES STUDY

Therapy*	*N*	HEMOGLOBIN A_{1C} (%)	PERCENTAGE WITH HYPOGLYCEMIA	
			Any	Major†
		GROUP 1		
Diet	379	8.0	3.0	0.2
Sulfonylurea	922	7.1	45.0	3.3
Insulin	689	7.1	76.0	11.2‡
		GROUP 2		
Diet	297	8.2	2.8	0.4
Metformin	251	7.4	17.6	2.4

*Taking assigned medication.
†Requiring medical assistance or admission to hospital.
‡Compared with severe hypoglycemia (that requiring the assistance of another individual) in 65% of intensively treated patients over 6.5 years in the Diabetes Control and Complications Trial.
From The United Kingdom Prospective Diabetes Study Research Group. Overview of 6 years of therapy of type II diabetes: a progressive disease. Diabetes 1995;44:1249-1258.

TABLE 33–6 COMPREHENSIVE RISK FACTORS FOR HYPOGLYCEMIA IN DIABETES

Premise: Iatrogenic hypoglycemia in type 1 diabetes and advanced type 2 diabetes is the result of the interplay of therapeutic insulin excess and compromised glucose counterregulation.

1. Absolute or relative therapeutic insulin excess (the conventional risk factors)
   a. Insulin doses excessive, ill-timed, wrong type
   b. Decreased food intake (e.g., missed meals, overnight fast)
   c. Increased glucose utilization (e.g., exercise)
   d. Decreased glucose production (e.g., alcohol)
   e. Increased sensitivity to insulin (e.g., after exercise, during the night, glycemic control, weight loss)
   f. Decreased insulin clearance (e.g., renal failure)
2. Compromised glucose counterregulation (hypoglycemia-associated autonomic failure)
   a. Insulin deficiency
      Beta cell dysfunction: No ↓ in insulin or ↑ in glucagon in response to ↓ glucose
   b. History of severe hypoglycemia, hypoglycemia unawareness, or both or aggressive therapy per se (lower glucose goals, lower hemoglobin A_{1C})

Episodes of hypoglycemia: Attenuated sympathoadrenal (including ↑ epinephrine) activation and symptoms in response to ↓ glucose (defective glucose counterregulation and hypoglycemia unawareness)

hypoglycemia, and are not practicing aggressive glycemic therapy. Nonetheless, these are associated with a substantially increased risk of hypoglycemia.) These three risk factors are clinical surrogates of compromised physiologic and behavioral defenses against falling plasma glucose concentrations: the clinical syndromes of defective glucose counterregulation and of hypoglycemia unawareness and the pathophysiologic concept of hypoglycemia-associated autonomic failure.

Pathophysiology of Glucose Counterregulation in Diabetes

Iatrogenic hypoglycemia is the result of the interplay of relative or absolute insulin excess and compromised physiologic and behavioral defenses against falling plasma glucose concentrations in patients with insulin deficient—T1DM and advanced T2DM—diabetes, as reviewed in detail elsewhere.[1,3,51-53] All three of the key physiologic defenses against hypoglycemia discussed earlier—decrements in insulin and increments in glucagon and epinephrine—are compromised. As plasma glucose concentrations fall, insulin levels do not decrease, glucagon levels do not increase,[72,73] and the increase in epinephrine levels is typically attenuated (Figure 33–8).[73,74] To the extent that endogenous insulin secretion is deficient, insulin levels are simply a function of the clearance of administered insulin. Loss of the glucagon response is plausibly attributed to insulin deficiency because, along with a decrease in glucose, a decrease in intraislet insulin is normally a signal to increase glucagon secretion.[16] The attenuated epinephrine response reflects a shift of the glycemic threshold for sympathoadrenal (sympathetic neural as well as adrenomedullary) responses to lower plasma glucose concentrations.[46,74] The latter is generally the result of recent antecedent hypoglycemia (Figure 33–9), although sleep and prior exercise have a similar effect.[3] The symptom responses are also reduced following antecedent hypoglycemia (Figure 33–10). In addition to the functional shift of the glycemic thresholds, there is likely an anatomic component of the reduced sympathoadrenal response to a given level of hypoglycemia in patients who also have classic diabetic autonomic neuropathy.[75,76] Nonetheless, the epinephrine response is typically reduced in patients with no clinical evidence of autonomic neuropathy (see Fig. 33–8).[74,75,76]

An attenuated adrenomedullary epinephrine response to falling plasma glucose concentrations, in the absence of insulin and glucagon responses, causes the clinical syndrome of *defective glucose counterregulation.*[1,3,51] Compared with persons who have normal epinephrine responses, affected patients are at 25-fold[77] or greater[78] increased risk for severe iatrogenic hypoglycemia during aggressive glycemic therapy. An attenuated sympathoadrenal response (largely an attenuated sympathetic neural response[41]) causes the clinical syndrome of *hypoglycemia unawareness* (loss of the warning, largely neurogenic, symptoms that previously allowed the patient to recognize a developing hypoglycemic episode and abort it by eating).[1,3,51] Affected patients are at about a sixfold increased risk for severe iatrogenic hypoglycemia.[79]

Based on the finding that hypoglycemia reduces the neuroendocrine and symptomatic responses to subsequent hypoglycemia,[80] the concept of *hypoglycemia-associated autonomic failure* (HAAF) in T1DM[74] and advanced T2DM[81] posits that recent antecedent iatrogenic hypoglycemia causes both defective glucose counterregulation and hypoglycemia unawareness and thus a vicious cycle of recurrent hypoglycemia.[1,3,51] The defective glucose counterregulation is caused by reducing epinephrine responses to a given level of subsequent hypoglycemia in the setting of absent decrements in insulin and absent increments in glucagon; the hypoglycemia unawareness is caused by reducing sympathoadrenal responses and the resulting neurogenic symptom responses to a given level of subsequent hypoglycemia. The HAAF concept has been extended to include sleep-related HAAF[3,82] and exercise-related HAAF.[3,83] The principles of HAAF are illustrated in Figure 33–11.

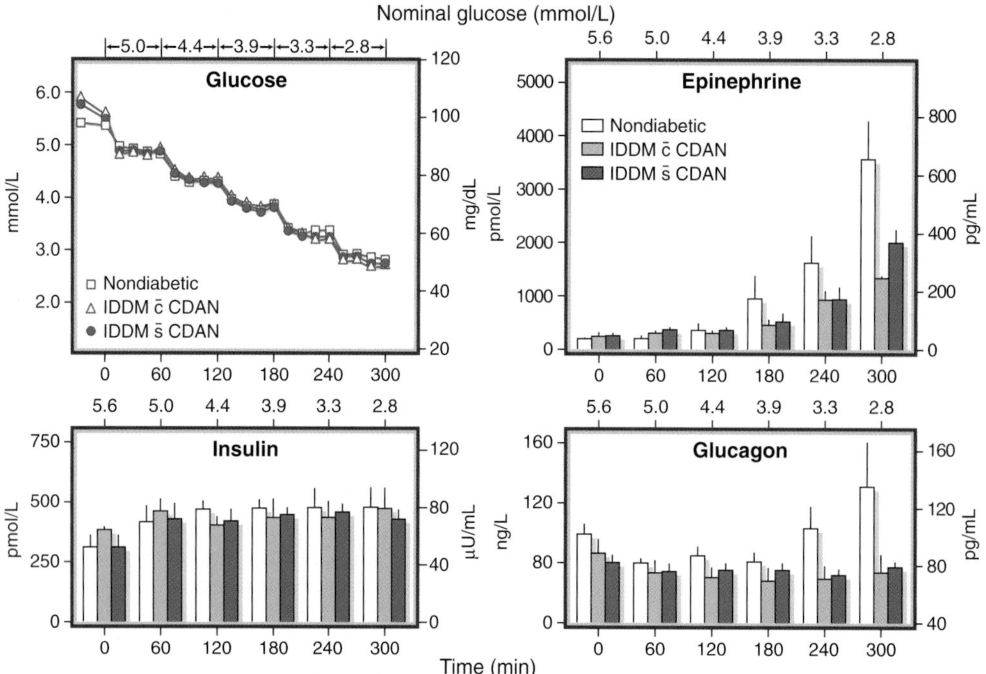

Figure 33–8 ▪ Mean (+SE) plasma glucose, insulin, epinephrine, and glucagon concentrations during hyperinsulinemic stepped hypoglycemic glucose clamps in nondiabetic subjects (*open squares* and *columns*), people with type 1 diabetes mellitus (IDDM, insulin-dependent diabetes mellitus) with classic diabetic autonomic neuropathy (CDAN, *open triangles* and *crosshatched columns*), and people with type 1 diabetes mellitus without CDAN (*closed circles* and *columns*). (From Dagogo-Jack SE, Craft S, Cryer PE. Hypoglycemia-associated autonomic failure in insulin dependent diabetes mellitus. J Clin Invest 1993;91:819-828. Copyright 1994, American Society for Clinical Investigation, New York.)

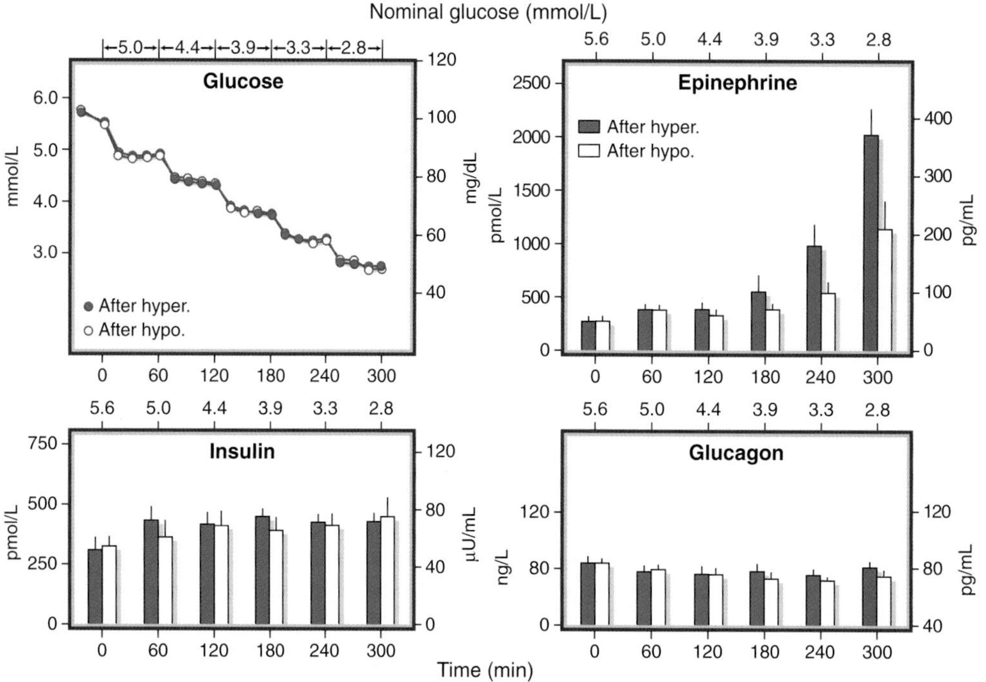

Figure 33–9 ▪ Mean (±SE) plasma glucose, insulin, epinephrine, and glucagon concentrations during hyperinsulinemic stepped hypoglycemic glucose clamps in patients with type 1 diabetes mellitus (IDDM, insulin-dependent diabetes mellitus) without classic diabetic autonomic neuropathy on mornings following afternoon hyperglycemia (Hyper., *closed circles* and *columns*) and on mornings following afternoon hypoglycemia (Hypo., *open circles* and *columns*). (From Dagogo-Jack SE, Craft S, Cryer PE. Hypoglycemia-associated autonomic failure in insulin dependent diabetes mellitus. J Clin Invest 1993;91:819-828. Copyright 1993, American Society for Clinical Investigation, New York.)

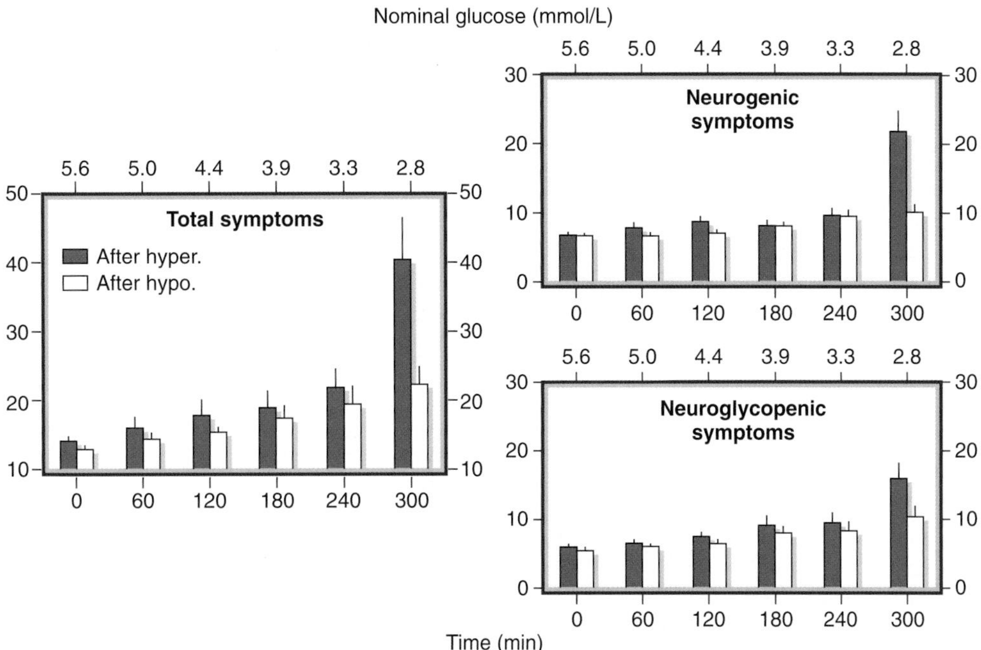

Figure 33–10 ▪ Mean (±SE) total, neurogenic, and neuroglycopenic symptom scores during hyperinsulinemic, stepped hypoglycemic glucose clamps in patients with type 1 diabetes mellitus (IDDM, insulin-dependent diabetes mellitus) without classic diabetic autonomic neuropathy on mornings following afternoon hyperglycemia (hyper., *closed columns*) and on mornings following afternoon hypoglycemia (hypo., *open columns*). (From Dagogo-Jack SE, Craft S, Cryer PE. Hypoglycemia-associated autonomic failure in insulin dependent diabetes mellitus. J Clin Invest 1993;91:819-828. Copyright 1993, American Society for Clinical Investigation, New York.[74])

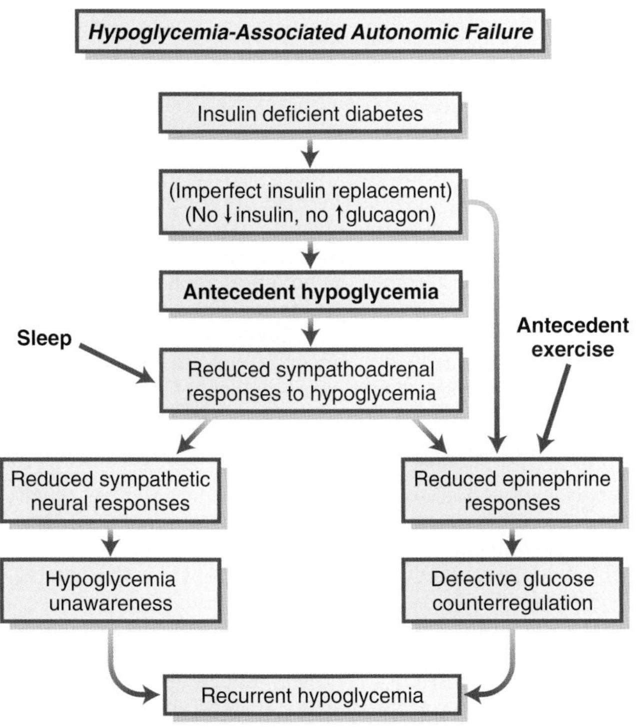

Figure 33–11 ▪ Schematic representation of the concept of hypoglycemia-associated autonomic failure in type 1 diabetes. See text for discussion. (Modified from Cryer PE. Diverse causes of hypoglycemia-associated autonomic failure in diabetes. N Engl J Med 2004;350:2272-2279. Copyright 2004, Massachusetts Medical Society, Boston, MA.)

The clinical impact of HAAF is well established in T1DM.[3,51,74,81,84-88] Recent antecedent hypoglycemia, even asymptomatic nocturnal hypoglycemia,[84] reduces sympathoadrenal epinephrine and neurogenic symptom responses[74,84,85] and cognitive dysfunction responses[84,85] to subsequent hypoglycemia. It also impairs glycemic defenses against hyperinsulinemia[74] and reduces detection of hypoglycemia in the clinical setting.[85] Perhaps the most compelling support for the concept of HAAF is the finding that as little as 2 to 3 weeks of scrupulous avoidance of hypoglycemia reverses hypoglycemia unawareness (Figure 33–12) and improves the reduced epinephrine component of defective glucose counterregulation in most affected patients.[86-88]

The clinical impact of HAAF is less well established in T2DM.[3,51,81] However, in people with advanced (insulin-deficient) T2DM, the glucagon response to hypoglycemia is lost, as it is in T1DM, and the glycemic thresholds for epinephrine and neurogenic symptom responses are shifted to lower plasma glucose concentrations by recent antecedent hypoglycemia in T2DM as they are in T1DM.[81] Thus, patients with advanced T2DM are also at risk for both components of HAAF.

In contrast to the clinical impact of HAAF, the mechanisms of HAAF, specifically the mechanisms of the key reduced sympathoadrenal responses, presumably occurring within the central nervous system, are largely unknown. Potential mechanisms have been reviewed.[53] The shift of the glycemic thresholds for sympathoadrenal responses to lower plasma glucose concentrations caused by antecedent hypoglycemia does not appear to be the result of release of a systemic mediator (e.g., cortisol or epinephrine) during antecedent hypoglycemia or of increased blood-to-brain glucose transport. Although the possibility of posthypoglycemic brain glycogen supercompensation

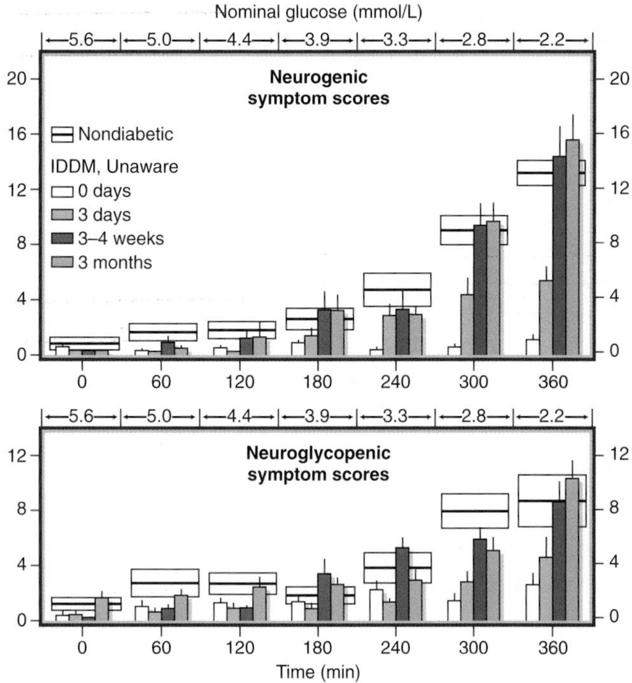

Figure 33–12 ▪ Mean (±SE) neurogenic (autonomic) and neuroglycopenic symptom scores during hyperinsulinemic stepped hypoglycemic glucose clamps in nondiabetic subjects *(rectangles)* and people with type 1 diabetes (IDDM, insulin-dependent diabetes mellitus) selected for hypoglycemia unawareness studied at baseline before (0 days, *open columns*), and after 3 days *(first set of cross-hatched columns)*, 3 to 4 weeks *(closed columns)*, and 3 months *(second set of crosshatched columns)* of scrupulous avoidance of iatrogenic hypoglycemia. (From Dagogo-Jack S, Rattarasarn C, Cryer PE. Reversal of hypoglycemia unawareness, but not defective glucose counterregulation, in IDDM. Diabetes 1994;43:1426-1434. Copyright 1994, American Diabetes Association, Alexandria, VA.)

has been proposed, it is likely the result of an as yet to be identified alteration of brain metabolism.

It is generally thought that hypoglycemia unawareness is due to reduced release of the sympathetic neural neurotransmitters norepinephrine and acetylcholine and perhaps that of adrenomedullary epinephrine.[41] However, there is some evidence of decreased β-adrenergic sensitivity, specifically reduced cardiac chronotropic sensitivity to isoproterenol,[89,90] in patients with unawareness. However, reduced symptomatic β-adrenergic sensitivity remains to be demonstrated in unaware patients, and one would also need to postulate reduced cholinergic sensitivity to explain reduced cholinergic symptoms such as sweating.

Definition and Classification of Hypoglycemia in Diabetes

The glycemic thresholds for activation of glucose counterregulatory systems, symptoms, and cognitive dysfunction are dynamic, as discussed earlier. They shift to lower plasma glucose concentrations in people with recurrent hypoglycemia such as those with tightly controlled diabetes[46] or an insulinoma.[47] They shift to higher plasma glucose concentrations in those with poorly controlled diabetes.[46,48]

Nonetheless, from a pragmatic perspective, the American Diabetes Association Workgroup on Hypoglycemia[52] recommended a plasma glucose concentration of less than 3.9 mM/L (70 mg/dL) as a conservative glucose level at which patients with diabetes should become concerned about developing hypoglycemia. A plasma glucose concentration of 3.9 mM/L approximates the lower limit of the postabsorptive physiologic range and the glycemic thresholds for activation of glucose counterregulatory systems in nondiabetic persons and the highest antecedent low plasma glucose levels that reduce responses to subsequent hypoglycemia.[91] This pragmatic action glucose level for people with diabetes should not be used to diagnose hypoglycemia in nondiabetic persons or hypoglycemia caused by mechanisms other than insulin or insulin-secretagogue treatment of diabetes. The Workgroup classified hypoglycemia in diabetes into five categories: severe, documented symptomatic, asymptomatic, probable symptomatic, and relative.

Severe Hypoglycemia

Severe hypoglycemia is an event requiring the assistance of another person to actively administer carbohydrate, glucagon, or other resuscitative actions. Plasma glucose measurements might not be available during such an event, but neurologic recovery attributable to the restoration of plasma glucose to normal is considered sufficient evidence that the event was induced by a low plasma glucose concentration.

Documented Symptomatic Hypoglycemia

Documented symptomatic hypoglycemia is an event during which typical symptoms of hypoglycemia are accompanied by a measured plasma glucose concentration less than 3.9 mM/L (70 mg/dL).

Asymptomatic Hypoglycemia

Asymptomatic hypoglycemia is an event not accompanied by typical symptoms of hypoglycemia but with a measured plasma glucose concentration less than 3.9 mM/L (70 mg/dL).

Probable Symptomatic Hypoglycemia

Probable symptomatic hypoglycemia is an event during which symptoms of hypoglycemia are not accompanied by a plasma glucose determination (but was presumably caused by a low plasma glucose level).

Relative Hypoglycemia

Relative hypoglycemia is an event during which the person with diabetes reports any of the typical symptoms of hypoglycemia and interprets those as indicating hypoglycemia, but with a measured plasma glucose concentration greater than 3.9 mM/L (70 mg/dL). This category reflects the fact that patients with poorly controlled diabetes can experience symptoms of hypoglycemia at plasma glucose concentrations greater than 3.9 mM/L as glucose levels decline toward that level.[46,48]

Hypoglycemia Risk Reduction in Diabetes

Clearly, every effort must be made to minimize the risk of iatrogenic hypoglycemia and eliminate the risk of severe hypoglycemia while pursuing the greatest degree of glycemic control that can be achieved safely in an individual person with diabetes.[51] Hypoglycemia risk reduction involves addressing the issue of hypoglycemia in every contact with the patient, applying the principles of aggressive glycemic therapy, and considering each of the comprehensive risk factors for hypoglycemia.

In addition to questioning the patient about episodes of symptomatic and biochemical hypoglycemia and looking for low values in the patient's self-monitoring of blood glucose (SMBG) log, it is important to assess the patient's awareness of hypoglycemia. A history of hypoglycemia unawareness identifies that clinical syndrome (and also implies defective glucose counterregulation). It is also important to determine the extent to which the patient is concerned about the reality or the possibility of hypoglycemia. Fear of hypoglycemia can be a barrier to glycemic control. If episodes of hypoglycemia are identified, their frequency, severity, timing, and clinical contexts need to be determined.

Once the problem of iatrogenic hypoglycemia is recognized, it is appropriate to review the treatment plan with respect to the principles of aggressive glycemic therapy. These include education and empowerment of the patient; frequent SMBG; flexible insulin (or other drug) regimens; rational, individualized glycemic goals; and ongoing professional guidance and support. Particularly in T1DM, but also in advanced T2DM, glycemic control is achieved safely by a well-informed, thoughtful person with diabetes who must make judgments about the management of his or her diabetes several times each day. The patient must be given the resources to make those judgments.

In the context of these therapeutic principles, hypoglycemia risk reduction requires consideration of both the conventional risk factors that lead to episodes of absolute or relative insulin excess—insulin (or other drug) dose, timing, and type; patterns of food ingestion and of exercise; interactions with alcohol or other drugs; and altered sensitivity to or clearance of insulin—and the risk factors for compromised glucose counterregulation that impair physiologic and behavioral defenses against developing hypoglycemia (see Table 33–6). The underlying principle is that iatrogenic hypoglycemia is the result of the interplay of insulin excess and compromised glucose counterregulation rather than insulin excess alone.

As discussed earlier, the clinical surrogates of risk attributable to compromised glucose counterregulation include insulin deficiency and a history of recurrent hypoglycemia or hypoglycemia unawareness or, absent that, aggressive glycemic therapy per se as evidenced by lower glycemic goals, lower hemoglobin A_{1c} levels, or both.[59,68-71] Insulin deficiency may be apparent from a history of ketosis-prone diabetes requiring insulin therapy from diagnosis, although it is now recognized that insulin deficiency can sometimes develop more gradually in late-onset T1DM or advanced T2DM.

Clinical hypoglycemia unawareness (which also suggests defective glucose counterregulation) implies recurrent antecedent iatrogenic hypoglycemia, whether that has or has not been documented. If such hypoglycemia is not apparent to the patient or to his or her family or in the SMBG log, it is probably occurring during the night. Indeed, hypoglycemia—including severe hypoglycemia—occurs most commonly during the night in people with T1DM.[54,58,59] That is typically the longest interdigestive period and time between SMBG and the time of maximal sensitivity to insulin.[92] In addition, sleep further reduces the sympathoadrenal responses to hypoglycemia and, probably because of their markedly reduced sympathoadrenal responses, people with T1DM are often not awakened by hypoglycemia.[82]

In addition to regimen adjustments, approaches to the problem of nocturnal hypoglycemia include use of insulin analogues and bedtime treatments. Substitution of a preprandial rapid-acting insulin analogue (e.g., lispro, aspart, or probably glulisine) for short-acting (regular) insulin during the day reduces the frequency of nocturnal hypoglycemia.[93] Substitution of a long-acting insulin analogue (e.g., glargine or detemir) for neutral protamine Hagedorn (NPH) insulin at bedtime also reduces the frequency of nocturnal hypoglycemia.[93] Bedtime treatments intended to reduce nocturnal hypoglycemia include bedtime snacks, although their efficacy has been questioned.[94] Experimental approaches include bedtime administration of uncooked cornstarch, of the glucagon-releasing amino acid alanine, or of the epinephrine-simulating β_2-adrenergic agonist terbutaline or administration of an α-glucosidase inhibitor with the evening meal (summarized in reference 94). Of these, bedtime terbutaline prevented nocturnal hypoglycemia in patients with aggressively treated T1DM.[94] However, in the dose used it also raised plasma glucose concentrations the following morning.

Obviously, with a history of recurrent hypoglycemia, one should determine when it occurs and adjust the treatment regimen appropriately. With a basal-bolus insulin analogue regimen, morning fasting hypoglycemia implicates the basal insulin and daytime hypoglycemia implicates the bolus insulin, all in the context of the other risk factors for insulin excess. In theory, because of its dosing flexibility, a continuous subcutaneous insulin infusion (CSII) regimen should minimize the risk of hypoglycemia. However, a clear advantage of a CSII over a basal-bolus regimen remains to be documented in rigorous trials.[95,96] For example, a crossover study of 100 patients with T1DM compared CSII with an insulin analogue to a basal-bolus regimen with insulin analogues. The CSII regimen reduced the frequency of nocturnal hypoglycemia but increased that of daytime hypoglycemia.[96]

A history of severe iatrogenic hypoglycemia—that requiring the assistance of another person—is a clinical red flag. Unless it was the result of an easily remediable factor, such as a missed meal after insulin administration or vigorous exercise without the appropriate regimen adjustment, a substantive change in the regimen must be made. If it is not, the risk of recurrent severe hypoglycemia is unacceptably high.[59,70]

In a patient with hypoglycemia unawareness, a 2- to 3-week period of scrupulous avoidance of iatrogenic hypoglycemia is advisable and can be assessed by return of awareness of hypoglycemia. This return of awareness has been accomplished without[86,87] or with minimal[88] compromise of glycemic control, but that required substantial involvement of health professionals. In practice, it can involve acceptance of somewhat higher glucose levels over the short term. However, with the return of symptoms of developing hypoglycemia, empirical approaches to better glycemic control can be tried.

Despite the promise of continuous or frequent glucose sensing, available subcutaneous or transcutaneous glucose sensors do not appear to detect hypoglycemia reliably in patients with T1DM, nor has their use been shown to improve glycemic control.[94,97,98]

It is possible to improve glycemic control and reduce the risk of hypoglycemia in many patients with diabetes.[51] Nonetheless, hypoglycemia continues to be a problem for many patients. Ultimately, the problem of hypoglycemia (and hyperglycemia) will likely be solved by methods that provide plasma glucose–regulated insulin replacement or secretion. Pending that, we need to learn to prevent, correct, or compensate for compromised glucose counterregulation in people with diabetes.

Treatment of Hypoglycemia in Diabetes

Most episodes of asymptomatic hypoglycemia (detected by SMBG) and mild to moderate symptomatic hypoglycemia are effectively self-treated by ingestion of glucose tablets or carbohydrate in the form of juices, soft drinks, milk, crackers, candy, or a meal.[99,100] A commonly recommended dose of glucose is 20 g (0.3 g/kg in children) (Figure 33–13). However, the glycemic response to oral glucose is transient, usually less than 2 hours in insulin-induced hypoglycemia in T1DM[100] (Fig. 33–13). Thus, ingestion of a more substantial mixed snack or meal shortly after the plasma glucose level is raised is generally advisable.

Parenteral treatment is necessary when a hypoglycemic patient is unable or unwilling (because of neuroglycopenia) to take carbohydrate orally. Glucagon is commonly injected sub-

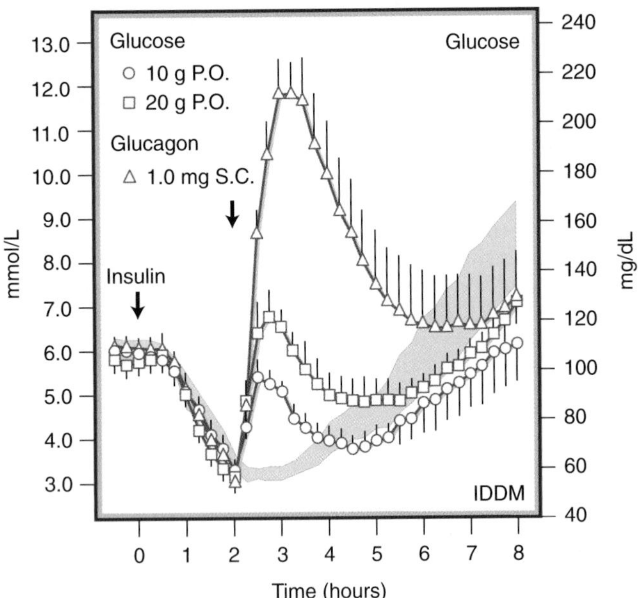

Figure 33–13 ▪ Mean (±SE) plasma glucose concentrations during hypoglycemia produced by subcutaneous insulin injection in people with type 1 diabetes in response to 10 g *(circles)* and 20 g *(squares)* of oral (P.O.) glucose and 1.0 mg of subcutaneous (S.C.) glucagon *(triangles)* compared with placebo *(shaded area)*. (From Wiethop BV, Cryer PE. Alanine and terbutaline in the treatment of hypoglycemia in IDDM. Diabetes Care 1993;16:1131-1136. Copyright 1993, American Diabetes Association, Alexandria, VA.)

cutaneously or intramuscularly by a spouse or family member.[101] The standard dose, 1 mg (15 μg/kg in children), can cause substantial but transient hyperglycemia[100] (see Fig. 33–13). It can also produce nausea and vomiting. Smaller doses (20 μg in children younger than 2 years and 10 μg/kg up to 150 μg), repeated if necessary, have been found to be effective without producing nausea in children with T1DM.[102] Because it stimulates insulin secretion, glucagon is less useful in T2DM than it is in T1DM. Although glucagon can be administered intravenously by medical personnel, intravenous glucose, 25 g initially, is the standard intravenous therapy. Because the glycemic response is transient, a subsequent glucose infusion is often needed and food should be provided orally as soon as the patient is able to take it safely.

The duration of a hypoglycemic episode is a function of the pharmacodynamic profile of the drug that induced it. A severe episode caused by a sulfonylurea overdose can be prolonged, and hospitalization for prolonged treatment and observation is often necessary.

Hypoglycemic Disorders

Hypoglycemia is most often caused by drugs, including those used to treat diabetes (just discussed) and alcohol.[1,49-51,103-105] Other causes of hypoglycemia (see Table 33–3) include several critical illnesses (hepatic, cardiac, and renal failure; sepsis; and inanition), endocrine deficiencies (cortisol, growth hormone, or both), non–beta cell tumors (non-islet cell tumor hypoglycemia), and endogenous, as well as exogenous, hyperinsulinemia (insulinoma among others). Some hypoglycemic disorders are unique to, or typically have their onset in, infancy and childhood. Clinical hypoglycemia in general[1] and that not resulting from the treatment of diabetes[103] have been reviewed in detail.

TABLE 33–7 ESTABLISHED AND PUTATIVE HYPOGLYCEMIA-CAUSING DRUGS

Drug	Disorder Treated
ESTABLISHED	
Insulin, sulfonylureas and other insulin secretagogues, metformin	Diabetes mellitus
Alcohol	—
Pentamidine, quinine, sulfonamides, quinolones (gatifloxacin, ciprofloxacin, levofloxacin)	Infections
Quinidine, disopyramide, cibenzoline	Arrhythmias
Acetylsalicylic acid	Pain
PUTATIVE	
Chloramphenicol, ketoconazole,, oxytetracycline, ethionamide isoniazid, *p*-aminosalicylic acid, *p*-aminobenzoate	Infection
Acetaminophen, indomethacin, propoxyphene, phenylbutazone	Pain
β-Adrenergic antagonists (nonselective > β_1-selective), angiotensin-converting enzyme inhibitors	Hypertension, heart disease
Furosemide, acetazolamide	Edema
Monoamine oxidase inhibitors, fluoxetine, imipramine	Depression
Haloperidol, chlorpromazine, perhexiline	Psychoses
Clofibrate, bezafibrate	Hyperlipidemia
Orphenadrine, diphenhydramine	Allergies
Cimetidine, ranitidine	Gastric hyperacidity
Colchicine, sulfinpyrazone	Gout
Phenytoin, gabapentin	Seizures
Enflurane, halothane	(Anesthetics)
Penicillamine	(Chelation)
Hypoglycins (in Jamaican akee fruit), thalidomide, selegiline, others	Miscellaneous

Fasting (Postabsorptive) Hypoglycemias

Drugs

Drugs are the most common cause of hypoglycemia.[1,49-51,104] Among these, insulin, sulfonylureas (and other insulin secretagogues), and perhaps metformin, used to treat diabetes, are the common offenders. Insulin and particularly sulfonylureas are possible causative agents even when there is no history of diabetes because these are sometimes taken surreptitiously, administered with criminal intent, or taken as the result of a pharmacy or other error.[105] Established and putative hypoglycemia-causing drugs are listed in Table 33–7.

Ethanol inhibits gluconeogenesis,[106] possibly because its metabolism to acetaldehyde and then acetate (by alcohol dehydrogenase and aldehyde dehydrogenase, respectively) depletes nicotinamide adenine dinucleotide (NAD^+), a cofactor critical to the entry of most precursors into the gluconeogenic pathway. It does not inhibit glycogenolysis. Ethanol also inhibits cortisol and growth hormone responses and can delay the epinephrine and glucagon responses to hypoglycemia.[106] In healthy humans, ethanol administration does not cause postabsorptive hypoglycemia or impair recovery from short-term hypoglycemia, presumably because of intact glucagon and epinephrine secretion and responsive hepatic glycogenolysis coupled with decreased sensitivity to insulin.[107,108] However, because gluconeogenesis becomes the dominant route of glucose production during prolonged hypoglycemia,[106] ethanol can contribute to the progression of hypoglycemia in patients with drug-treated diabetes. It can also cause postabsorptive hypoglycemia in states of glycogen depletion.[104]

Clinical alcohol-induced hypoglycemia typically follows (by 6 to 36 hours) a binge of moderate to heavy alcohol consumption during which the person eats little food (i.e., in the setting of glycogen depletion).[104] Hypoglycemia can be profound, and alcohol-induced hypoglycemia can be fatal. However, with restoration of normal glucose levels and supportive care, complete recovery is the rule. Ethanol is typically measurable in blood at the time of presentation, but its levels correlate poorly with glucose levels. On the other hand, hypoglycemia may be a late feature of alcoholic ketoacidosis, and ethanol might not be measurable in the blood at the time of presentation.[104]

Salicylates in relatively large doses (4 to 6 g/day) can produce hypoglycemia in children and, rarely, in adults.[104,109] Perhaps by inhibiting the serine kinase IKKβ, high-dose aspirin administration has been shown to reduce basal glucose production and plasma glucose concentrations and to increase sensitivity to insulin in people with T2DM.[110] Sulfonamides also rarely produce hypoglycemia by stimulating insulin secretion.[111]

Pentamidine is a beta cell toxin. Initially, it can cause hypoglycemia by causing insulin release. Ultimately, it can cause diabetes mellitus. In one series of immunocompromised patients with *Pneumocystis* pneumonia (PCP) treated with pentamidine, 7% experienced hypoglycemia, 14% experienced hypoglycemia followed by diabetes, and 18% experienced diabetes without detected hypoglycemia.[112] Risk factors for pentamidine-induced hypoglycemia include therapy of longer duration and increased doses, previous pentamidine therapy, and renal insufficiency.

Hypoglycemia occurs commonly in severe malaria. Although associated with relative hyperinsulinemia attributed to quinine-induced insulin release in some patients, hypoglycemia can occur in the absence of quinine therapy and in the absence of hyperinsulinemia in quinine-treated patients.[113] Nonetheless, quinine has been reported to cause hypoglycemia in persons not afflicted with malaria.[114] Quinolone antibiotics, particularly gatifloxacin and often in the setting of drug-treated diabetes, have also been reported to cause hypoglycemia.[115] Among antiarrhythmic drugs, quinidine, disopyramide,[116] and cibenzoline[117] have been reported to cause hypoglycemia.

Hypoglycemia has been attributed to many other drugs (see Table 33–7). In many cases, other potential causes of hypoglycemia have been present. For example, although hypoglycemia attributed to propranolol has been reported in healthy children,[118] most of the reported incidents occurred in insulin-treated diabetes. Although nonselective β-adrenergic antagonists such as propranolol would be expected to reduce symptoms of developing hypoglycemia and impair epinephrine-mediated glucose counterregulation,[119] compelling evidence that these drugs increase the frequency of clinical hypoglycemia in insulin-treated diabetes has not been forthcoming. Nonetheless, it would be reasonable to use a relatively selective β_1-adrenergic receptor antagonist (e.g., metoprolol or atenolol) in such patients.

Critical Illnesses

Among hospitalized patients, drugs, particularly insulin, are still the most common cause of hypoglycemia.[50] However, serious diseases—particularly renal failure but also hepatic or cardiac failure, sepsis, or inanition—are second only to drugs.

Hepatic Failure

In addition to appropriate glucoregulatory signals and a sufficient supply of gluconeogenic precursors, maintenance of the postabsorptive plasma glucose concentration requires a structurally and functionally intact liver. Renal glucose production notwithstanding, total hepatectomy results in hypoglycemia.[120] Extensive liver disease is required to produce hypoglycemia. Hepatogenous hypoglycemia occurs most commonly when destruction of the liver is rapid and massive (e.g., toxic hepatitis). It has been reported in fulminant viral hepatitis, in fatty liver attributed to alcohol ingestion, and in cholangitis and biliary obstruction. It is unusual in common forms of cirrhosis and hepatitis, although glucose metabolism is altered demonstrably (with lower postabsorptive plasma glucose concentrations, diminished glycemic responses to glucagon, and reduced hepatic glycogen contents) in uncomplicated viral hepatitis.[121] It is also unusual in metastatic liver disease despite extensive hepatic replacement.[122] Hypoglycemia can be caused by primary malignant tumors but is the result of a glucoregulatory abnormality, insulin-like growth factor II (IGF-II) overproduction (see "Non–Beta Cell Tumors").

Cardiac Failure

The pathogenesis of hypoglycemia in occasional patients with severe cardiac failure is unknown. Possibilities include hepatic congestion and hypoxia, inanition, and gluconeogenic precursor limitation. The finding of elevated blood lactate levels associated with hypoglycemia[123] raises the possibility of inhibited gluconeogenesis.

Renal Failure

Postabsorptive hypoglycemia occurs in some patients with renal failure,[124] and the finding of a high frequency of renal insufficiency among patients with low plasma glucose levels[50] suggests that compromised glucose counterregulation may be a feature of renal failure. However, the pathogenesis of hypoglycemia in such patients is not known; it might involve multiple mechanisms. It has been attributed to drugs, sepsis, or inanition.[50,124] Most patients with hypoglycemia attributed to renal failure are cachectic. One such patient had reduced glucose turnover, diminished gluconeogenesis from alanine, and reduced alanine turnover.[125] During fasting, plasma glucose levels fell, blood lactate levels did not increase, and blood alanine levels fell. Hypoglycemia was attributed to substrate limitation of gluconeogenesis. However, at least one patient did not respond to substrate (glycerol, alanine) administration.[126]

The kidneys are a major site of insulin clearance, and decreasing insulin requirements parallel decreasing renal function in patients with insulin-treated diabetes. In the absence of insulin or insulin secretagogue therapy, however, endogenous insulin secretion should decrease as glucose levels decline and hypoglycemia would, therefore, not be expected. The extent to which reduced renal glucose production contributes to hypoglycemia in end-stage renal disease is unknown. However, most people with end-stage renal disease and no functioning renal parenchyma do not suffer hypoglycemia, and renal transplantation does not correct postabsorptive hypoglycemia in patients with glucose-6-phosphatase deficiency.[127] Thus, one functioning kidney is not sufficient to provide normal endogenous glucose production in the virtual absence of hepatic glucose production.

Sepsis

Sepsis is a relatively common cause of hypoglycemia.[49,50,128] Increased glucose utilization (by skeletal muscle and by macrophage-rich tissues such as liver, spleen, and lung) and, initially, glucose production characterize experimental sepsis.[129] Hypoglycemia develops when hepatic glucose production decreases. The factors responsible for the increased glucose turnover and the ultimate failure of glucose production to keep pace in sepsis are not entirely clear. Proinflammatory cytokines such as tumor necrosis factor α (TNF-α) and interleukins, among others, are thought to increase glucose utilization.[130-132] The initial increase in glucose production is at least in part mediated by increased glucagon[133] and catecholamine[134,135] release, appropriate physiologic responses to accelerated glucose utilization. These can also be stimulated by cytokines. For example, in dogs, TNF-α infusion increases glucose production, an effect attributable to TNF-α-stimulated glucagon secretion.[131] The later decline in glucose production, which in the setting of persistently high rates of glucose utilization[129] results in hypoglycemia, is not the result of glucose counterregulatory failure. Rather, it is the result of decreased responsiveness to appropriate glucoregulatory stimuli, that is, low insulin and high glucagon and epinephrine levels.[136] This may be the result of cytokine-induced inhibition of gluconeogenesis and glucose release,[132] but hepatic and renal hypoperfusion is also a plausible mechanism.

Inanition

Hypoglycemia can be caused by inanition.[137] Because hypoglycemia can persist despite high rates of glucose infusion, such patients must have high rates of glucose utilization. Beyond this, the pathogenesis of hypoglycemia is unknown. An entirely speculative suggestion is that glucose becomes the sole oxidative fuel in the setting of total body fat depletion and that high rates of glucose utilization exceed the capacity to produce glucose because of limitation of substrates (e.g., amino acids). Postabsorptive hypoglycemia (with low blood alanine levels) has been reported in some patients with profound muscle atrophy[138,139]; hypoglycemia is presumably the result of substrate limitation of gluconeogenesis in such patients.

Hormonal Deficiencies

With the notable exception of defective glucose counterregulation in patients with established T1DM and advanced T2DM,[3,51,53] hormonal glucoregulatory abnormalities resulting in hypoglycemia are not common. These abnormalities include hyperinsulinism, discussed later, and deficiencies of glucose counterregulatory hormones.

Most adults with deficient secretion of cortisol, growth hormone, or both do not experience hypoglycemia. Indeed, plasma glucose concentrations (and endogenous glucose production) after an overnight fast are not distinguishable from normal in glucocorticoid-withdrawn patients with panhypopituitarism never treated with growth hormone.[34] Nonetheless, postabsorptive hypoglycemia can occur in patients with chronic deficiencies of these hormones, particularly in the neonatal period and in children younger than 5 years.[140]

Hypoglycemia in children with deficient secretion of cortisol, growth hormone, or both is generally preceded by a period of caloric deprivation. That is consistent with the observation that hypoglycemia can sometimes be provoked by 24 to 30 hours of fasting in children with hypopituitarism who do not exhibit hypoglycemia after an overnight fast.[141] This intolerance of fasting is largely corrected by glucocorticoid replacement, whereas growth hormone replacement has a lesser effect.[141,142] These findings suggest that a defect in gluconeogenesis causes hypoglycemia when hepatic glycogen stores are depleted.

Cortisol supports gluconeogenesis both by increasing gluconeogenic enzyme activities and by mobilizing gluconeogenic precursors to the liver (and the kidneys).[141,143] Postabsorptive hypoglycemia in hypopituitarism is associated with low levels of circulating gluconeogenic precursors.[141,144] However, oral alanine administration only partially reverses hypoglycemia.[144] Finally, because cortisol deficiency causes reduced epinephrine secretion[145]—presumably because of reduced induction of adrenomedullary phenylethanolamine *N*-methyltransferase by adrenocortical cortisol—epinephrine deficiency might contribute to the pathogenesis of hypoglycemia in this setting. Glucagon secretion is not reduced in such patients. Thus, given the key role of glucagon in glucose counterregulation, it is not surprising that glucose recovery, at least from short-term hypoglycemia, is generally normal in children with deficient secretion of cortisol, growth hormone, or both.[146] Adults with hypopituitarism occasionally suffer postabsorptive hypoglycemia, particularly when glucose utilization or loss is increased, as during exercise or in pregnancy, respectively,[147] or when gluconeogenesis is impaired, as after alcohol ingestion.[148] Again, these observations suggest that impaired gluconeogenesis becomes limiting to glucose production in the setting of glycogen depletion resulting from caloric deprivation.

As discussed earlier (see "Glucose Counterregulation"), hypoglycemia develops or progresses when both glucagon and epinephrine are deficient and insulin is present[2,3,51-53] (see Table 33–2). This combination occurs in patients with established T1DM. They must be treated with insulin, have no glucagon response to hypoglycemia, and typically have a reduced epinephrine response to hypoglycemia and are, as a result, at high risk for iatrogenic hypoglycemia[3,51,53] as discussed earlier (see "Hypoglycemia in Diabetes Mellitus"). It also occurs in advanced T2DM.[81]

Hypoglycemia is not a feature of the epinephrine-deficient state that results from bilateral adrenalectomy if glucocorticoid replacement is appropriate,[29,41] and hypoglycemia does not occur during pharmacologic blockade of catecholamine actions when other glucose counterregulatory systems are intact.[11,29,41,149] Hypoglycemia has been attributed to epinephrine deficiency in ketotic hypoglycemia of childhood,[150] and therapeutic responses to ephedrine, a catecholamine-releasing drug, have been reported in uncontrolled studies of such patients.[151,152] However, the latter does not document a causative role of epinephrine deficiency. Postabsorptive hypoglycemia has also been attributed to epinephrine deficiency in one member of each of three sets of twins.[153,154] However, the glucagon secretory responses were not evaluated, and the affected infants had inappropriately high insulin levels while they were hypoglycemic.[153] Finally, reduced epinephrine excretion in infants of diabetic mothers has been associated with the occurrence of neonatal hypoglycemia.[155]

Postabsorptive hypoglycemia has been reported in a glucagon-deficient adult, but cortisol secretion and growth hormone secretion were also deficient.[156] Neonatal hypoglycemia has also been attributed to glucagon deficiency.[157,158] However, plasma insulin levels were inappropriately high during hypoglycemia.

Elevated plasma levels of glucose counterregulatory hormones during hypoglycemia exclude deficiencies of these. Levels that are not elevated during a spontaneous episode of hypoglycemia provide a diagnostic clue that requires definitive testing. In a patient with postabsorptive hypoglycemia that is not readily explained, it is my practice to seek clinical clues of hypopituitarism or primary adrenocortical insufficiency—and often assess the plasma cortisol response to cosyntropin (synthetic ACTH)—and to pursue such clues with definitive testing (e.g., the responses to insulin-induced hypoglycemia). Given the evidence, just summarized, that isolated glucagon deficiency or isolated epinephrine deficiency rarely, if ever, causes postabsorptive hypoglycemia, these theoretical possibilities are generally not pursued.

Non–Beta Cell Tumors

Postabsorptive hypoglycemia is occasionally caused by non–beta cell tumors (non–islet cell tumor hypoglycemia).[159] The majority are large retroperitoneal, intra-abdominal, or intrathoracic mesenchymal tumors that are typically slow-growing albeit malignant. Epithelial tumors that can cause hypoglycemia include hepatomas, gastric or adrenocortical carcinomas, and carcinoid tumors. More common carcinomas and hematologic or lymphoid malignancies rarely cause hypoglycemia in the absence of cachexia. Affected patients often have relatively high rates of glucose utilization,[160] a pattern resembling that of hyperinsulinism. Reports of a few patients with hypoglycemia attributed to ectopic insulin secretion have been published,[161] but plasma insulin and C-peptide levels are suppressed appropriately during hypoglycemia in the vast majority of patients with non–beta cell tumor hypoglycemia.

Overproduction of IGF-II, specifically an incompletely processed form (big IGF-II) that does not complex normally with circulating binding proteins and thus more readily gains access to target tissues, is the cause of hypoglycemia in most patients.[162-165] The diagnosis is usually not difficult. The tumors are often apparent clinically, and plasma insulin, C-peptide, and proinsulin levels are low during hypoglycemia. Free IGF-II levels (and levels of pro-IGF-II [E1-21]) are elevated.[164,165] It should be noted, however, that both of these are often elevated in patients with renal failure. Presumably because of negative feedback mediated by IGF-II, growth hormone secretion is suppressed. Thus, serum IGF-I levels are low and the ratio of IGF-II to IGF-I is distinctly elevated. Curative surgery is seldom possible. Therapy with a glucocorticoid, growth hormone, or both has been reported to alleviate hypoglycemia.[165] A patient with hypoglycemia attributed to ectopic production of IGF-I has been reported.[166]

Endogenous Hyperinsulinemia

Hypoglycemia related to excessive endogenous insulin secretion[1,103,167,168] can be caused by a primary pancreatic islet beta cell disorder, typically a beta cell tumor (insulinoma), and sometimes multiple insulinomas. Especially in infants or young children but occasionally in adults, a functional beta cell disorder with beta cell hypertrophy or hyperplasia or without an anatomic correlate can cause endogenous hyperinsulinemia. It can also be caused by a beta cell secretagogue, often a sulfonylurea, theoretically a beta cell–stimulating autoantibody, or an antibody to insulin.

None of these is common. Endogenous hyperinsulinism is more likely in an overtly well person with postabsorptive hypoglycemia, that is, a person with no relevant drug history or critical illness and no clinical clues to hormone deficiencies or a non–beta cell tumor. In such an person, accidental, surreptitious, or even malicious administration of a sulfonylurea, another insulin-releasing drug, or insulin should also be considered.[105]

The critical pathophysiologic feature of endogenous hyperinsulinism is failure of insulin secretion, assessed by plasma insulin and C-peptide levels, to fall to very low rates during hypoglycemia.[1,103,167,168] The plasma insulin, C-peptide, proinsulin, sulfonylurea, and insulin antibody patterns in the various diagnostic categories (including exogenous as well as endogenous hyperinsulinism) are shown in Table 33–8.

Diagnosis

The diagnosis of hyperinsulinemic hypoglycemia, including that produced by an insulinoma, requires documentation of fasting hypoglycemia and documentation that insulin secretion is inappropriately high for a plasma glucose concentration less than 3.0 mM/L (54 mg/dL) with measurements of plasma insulin and C-peptide, and preferably proinsulin, concentrations.[1,103,167,168] Fasting hypoglycemia is documented by Whipple's triad: a plasma glucose concentration less than 3.0 mM/L (54 mg/dL), preferably less than 2.5 mM/L (45 mg/dL), with symptoms and relief of those symptoms after the glucose level is raised.

These criteria need not be fulfilled simultaneously, although that is often the case. The diagnostic plasma glucose concentration(s) must be measured with a precise analytical method, not with a glucose monitor. Because symptoms are important for documenting Whipple's triad, and for safety reasons, the patient must be observed by a medical professional. Because venous plasma glucose concentrations are usually measured, the patient should be in the postabsorptive state. Although the arteriovenous plasma glucose concentration difference is negligible in the postabsorptive state, high insulin levels in the postprandial state result in glucose extraction across the forearm and thus venous glucose levels as much as 30% lower than arterial glucose levels. It is, of course, arterial glucose levels that provide glucose to the brain. (See "The Postprandial Hypoglycemias," later, for exceptions.)

Many affected patients meet these criteria after an overnight fast, particularly if they are assessed on three separate occasions.[168] If the criteria are not demonstrable during an extended outpatient visit,[169] hospitalization for a prolonged diagnostic fast is necessary if clinical suspicion is high.[169,170] A negative prolonged fast makes a diagnosis of insulinoma highly unlikely (although it does not categorically exclude hyperinsulinemic hypoglycemia as discussed later). Traditionally, the failure to document hypoglycemia through 72 hours of fasting has been required to support the conclusion that the test is negative,[169] but it has been suggested that 48 hours is sufficient.[170] Two thirds of patients with proven insulinomas fulfill the diagnostic criteria by 24 hours of fasting,[169,170] and well over 90%,[169,170] perhaps 100%,[170] by 48 hours of fasting.

The adoption of highly specific, two-site assays of insulin, which unlike the earlier radioimmunoassays do not measure other species including proinsulin, has necessitated revised plasma insulin cut-off values for the diagnosis of hyperinsulinemic hypoglycemia. Plasma glucose concentrations in 33 healthy subjects declined to a median of 3.7 mmol/L, with a 5th to 95th percentile range of 3.0 to 4.4 mmol/L (67 mg/dL, range 54-79 mg/dL) during a 72-hour fast. In these subjects, immunofluorometric plasma insulin concentrations decreased to a median of 9 pmol/L, with a 5th to 95th percentile range of less

TABLE 33–8 BIOCHEMICAL PATTERNS IN PATIENTS WITH VARIOUS CAUSES OF HYPERINSULINEMIC HYPOGLYCEMIA

Insulin	C Peptide	Proinsulin	Sulfonylurea	Insulin Antibody	Diagnosis
↑	↓	↓	—	—	Exogenous insulin
↑	↑	↑	—	—	Insulinoma, CHI
↑	↑	↑	+	—	Sulfonylurea
↑	↑*	↑*	—	+	Insulin autoimmune
±↑	↓	↓	—	—	Insulin receptor autoimmune†

*Free C peptide and proinsulin ↓.
†Insulin receptor antibody+.
CHI, Congenital hyperinsulinism.

than 9 to 19 pmol/L (1.5 μU/mL, range <2-3 μU/mL).[171] Plasma C-peptide concentrations decreased to a median of 127 pmol/L, with a 5th to 95th percentile range of 74 to 295 pmol/L (0.38 ng/mL, range 0.22-0.89 ng/mL) and proinsulin concentrations decreased to a median of 3 pmol/L, with a 5th to 95th percentile range of 2 to 5 pmol/L.[171]

The criteria used at the Mayo Clinic to diagnose endogenous hyperinsulinemic hypoglycemia at a fasting plasma glucose concentration less than 2.5 mmol/L (45 mg/dL) are immunochemiluminometric plasma insulin concentrations greater than 18 pmol/L (3 μU/mL), C-peptide concentrations greater than 200 pmol/L (0.60 ng/mL), and proinsulin greater than 5 pmol/L.[103,172] In one series, immunoradiometric plasma insulin concentrations were less than 18 pmol/L (3 μU/mL) in 2 of 15 patients with insulinomas during fasting hypoglycemia.[173] Plasma C-peptide concentrations were greater than 200 pmol/L in all 15 patients. Many current insulin assays also have limited cross reactivity with insulin analogues (e.g., lispro, aspart, glargine), a potential problem in the documentation of hypoglycemia caused by exogenous insulin administration.[174]

In addition to plasma glucose, insulin, C-peptide, and proinsulin measurements, it is important to screen the serum for sulfonylureas and other insulin secretagogues (repaglinide, netaglinide) at the time of hypoglycemia. Because hyperinsulinemia suppresses lipolysis and ketogenesis, a substantial increase in blood β-hydroxybutyrate concentrations (e.g., to >2.7 mM/L) during a prolonged fast implies physiologic suppression of insulin secretion and thus predicts a negative fast. Circulating insulin antibodies should also be sought, but these need not be measured at the time of hypoglycemia.

Differential Diagnosis

With respect to the differential diagnosis of hyperinsulinemic hypoglycemia (Table 33–8), inappropriately high plasma insulin, C-peptide, and proinsulin concentrations occur in patients with insulinomas and other beta cell disorders including congenital hyperinsulinism. Sulfonylurea or other insulin secretagogue ingestion produces the same pattern, but the drug is measurable. Exogenous insulin administration produces high insulin levels with suppressed C-peptide and proinsulin levels.

Antibodies to insulin [175] typically cause hypoglycemia during the transition from the postprandial to the postabsorptive state as insulin—secreted in response to the earlier meal and bound to the antibodies—slowly dissociates from the antibodies and causes relative hyperinsulinism. Total and free plasma insulin concentrations are inappropriately high. Insulin secretion is suppressed appropriately and free plasma C-peptide (and proinsulin) levels are low, but total C-peptide (and proinsulin) levels may be high because of cross reactivity with antibody-bound proinsulin, including its C-peptide sequence.[176] Circulating antibodies to the insulin receptor are rare and often cause profound insulin resistance but sometimes are receptor agonists and cause fasting hypoglycemia.[177,178] During hypoglycemia, insulin secretion is suppressed and C-peptide levels are low, but insulin levels tend to be inappropriately high, presumably because receptor-bound antibodies impair the clearance of insulin.[177] Antibodies that stimulate beta cell insulin secretion in vitro have been described,[179,180] but a corresponding clinical syndrome has not been defined.

Ectopic insulin secretion has been reported.[161] Nonetheless, insulin arteriovenous differences across such tumors have not been reported.

An algorithm for the diagnostic approach for a patient with suspected hypoglycemia is shown in Figure 33–14.

Insulinomas

Insulinomas, the most common cause of hypoglycemia related to endogenous hyperinsulinism in adults,[103,167] are rare. The estimated incidence is one case per 250,000 patient-years.[181] However, because approximately 90% of insulinomas are benign, they are generally a treatable cause of potentially fatal hypoglycemia. Insulinomas can be sporadic or familial, a component of the autosomal dominant multiple endocrine neoplasia type 1 (MEN-1) syndrome (primary hyperparathyroidism, islet tumors including but not limited to insulinomas, and pituitary tumors).[182] Solitary insulinomas are the rule in adults with sporadic tumors; multiple insulinomas are common in MEN-1. In addition to insulin, these tumors can secrete other hormones including gastrin, chorionic gonadotropin, corticotropin, serotonin, glucagon, somatostatin, and pancreatic polypeptide. Indeed, somatostatin, glucagon, and insulin genes were expressed in four insulinomas in one report.[183] Overproduction of one hormone, such as insulin, can predominate at one time, and that of another can predominate later in the course of MEN-1.[183,184]

Insulinomas are almost invariably within the substance of the pancreas and are often small. Thus, they almost always come to clinical attention because of the hypoglycemia they cause rather than because of mass effects. Hyperinsulinism in the hepatic portal circulation (as well as the peripheral circulation) causes low rates of glucose production relative to glucose utilization (which need not be high in the absolute) and, thus, postabsorptive hypoglycemia.[185] Unusually low plasma glucose concentrations are required to produce symptoms of hypoglycemia in patients with an insulinoma because of the shift of glycemic thresholds to lower plasma glucose concentrations caused by recurrent hypoglycemia.[47] Although symptomatic hypoglycemia can occur after an overnight fast, it often follows exercise. Rarely, symptomatic hypoglycemia follows meals, but postabsorptive hypoglycemia is typically also demonstrable in such patients. Common symptoms in patients with an insulinoma[186] are listed in Table 33–9.

Given convincing clinical and biochemical evidence of an insulinoma, it is useful to localize the tumor.[187,188] However, insulinomas tend to be small—90% are less than 2.0 cm and 40% are less than 1.0 cm[189]—and negative imaging does not exclude the presence of the tumor. Computed tomography can detect approximately 70% to 80% of insulinomas, and magnetic resonance imaging can detect about 85%.[189] These generally detect metastases in the roughly 10% of patients with a malignant insulinoma. Transabdominal ultrasound identifies many insulinomas, and endoscopic ultrasound has a sensitivity of about 90%.[190,191] Somatostatin receptor scintigraphy is thought to detect insulinomas in about half of the patients,[192] but a sensitivity of 80% has been reported[193]; it, too, can identify metastases. Selective pancreatic arterial calcium injections, with the endpoint of a sharp increase (more than fivefold with specific insulin assays) in hepatic venous insulin levels, regionalizes insulinomas with high sensitivity,[194,195] but this invasive procedure is seldom necessary in the clinical setting.[196] The same is true of transhepatic

TABLE 33–9 SYMPTOMS OF HYPOGLYCEMIA IN PATIENTS WITH INSULINOMAS

Symptom	Incidence (%)
Various combinations of diplopia, blurred vision, sweating, palpitations, or weakness	85
Confusion or abnormal behavior	80
Unconsciousness or amnesia	53
Grand mal seizures	12

From Service FJ, Dale AJD, Elveback LR. Insulinoma: clinical and diagnostic features of 60 consecutive patients. Mayo Clin Proc 1976;51:417-429.[186]

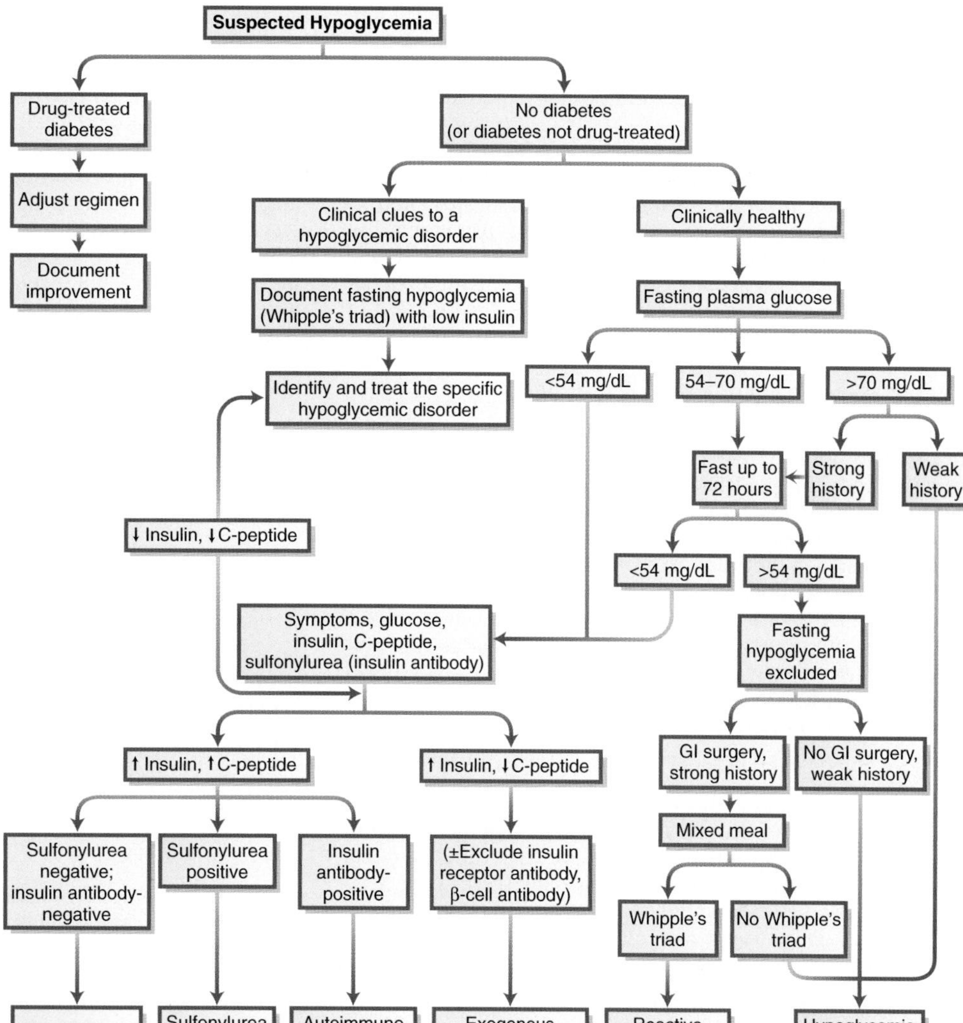

Figure 33–14 ▪ Diagnostic algorithm for suspected hypoglycemia. GI, gastrointestinal.

portal venous sampling.[197] The utility of positron emission tomography (PET) remains to be determined.[198] Intraoperative pancreatic ultrasonography almost invariably localizes insulinomas that are not readily palpable by the surgeon.

Surgical resection of solitary insulinomas is generally curative. Medical therapy of unresectable insulinomas includes administration of diazoxide[199]; the somatostatin analogue octreotide is sometimes effective.[200] The majority of infants and young children with hyperinsulinemic hypoglycemia do not have discrete insulinomas. Additional causes of hypoglycemia related to endogenous hyperinsulinism are discussed later in this chapter (see "Hypoglycemia in Infancy and Childhood").

Autoimmune Hypoglycemia

Autoimmune hypoglycemia is thought to be quite rare. The majority of the reported cases of hypoglycemia attributed to autoantibodies to insulin[175] have been from Japan. A history of other autoimmune disorders, particularly Graves' disease, and of treatment with sulfhydryl medications, particularly methimazole, is common. Whereas most autoantibodies against the insulin receptor are antagonists and cause (type B) insulin resistance, some are agonists and cause hypoglycemia.[178] Again, clinical or biochemical evidence of other autoimmune disorders, as well as the finding of acanthosis nigricans, are common.

Noninsulinoma Pancreatogenous Hypoglycemia Syndrome

Service and colleagues have recognized a novel syndrome of endogenous hyperinsulinemic hypoglycemia that they termed *noninsulinoma pancreatogenous hypoglycemia syndrome* (NIPHS).[201] The patients had postprandial symptoms and hyperinsulinemic hypoglycemia (albeit using criteria developed during prolonged fasts) but negative 72-hour fasts. (However, otherwise similar patients exhibited hyperinsulinemic hypoglycemia during 48-hour fasts.[202]) Evidence that the symptoms were, in fact, the result of endogenous hyperinsulinism included positive arterial calcium injection tests and amelioration of symptoms following partial pancreatic resection in nine of 10 patients. Histologic findings included beta cell hypertrophy with or without hyperplasia.

Subsequently, the same group[203] and others[204] recognized a similar syndrome following Roux-en-Y gastric bypass surgery for obesity. The post–gastric bypass patients also presented with postprandial symptoms; data from 72-hour fasts were not reported. Partial pancreatectomy ameliorated symptoms in three of six patients. The surgical specimens disclosed multiple insulinomas in one patient and beta cell hypertrophy and hyperplasia in the other five. The possibility that enhanced secretion of the incretin glucagon-like peptide 1 (GLP-1) might be involved in the pathogenesis of these beta cell changes has been raised[203,204] (see "Postprandial Hypoglycemia," later). Dietary and medical (diazoxide, octreotide, α-glucosidase inhibitor) therapies are sometimes useful, but partial pancreatectomy is often required.[204]

Further evidence that adults with endogenous hyperinsulinism do not necessarily have an insulinoma is the finding that 15 (4%) of 232 patients with fasting hypoglycemia attributed to endogenous hyperinsulinism did not have an insulinoma but rather histologic findings including pancreatic beta cell hypertrophy and, in some instances, hyperplasia.[205] Although the authors used the term *nesidioblastosis,* excessive budding of insulin-positive cells from pancreatic ducts was not found.[205]

Hypoglycemia in Infancy and Childhood

Causes of hypoglycemia unique to, or typically with their clinical onset in, infancy and childhood[206] (Table 33–10) include transient intolerance of fasting, hyperinsulinism, and enzymatic defects in carbohydrate, protein, or fat metabolism. Hypoglycemia in children can also be caused by the mechanisms discussed earlier (see Table 33–3). These include drugs and critical illnesses. For example, nine (18%) of 49 children receiving resuscitative care for altered consciousness, status epilepticus, respiratory failure, cardiac failure, or cardiopulmonary arrest were hypoglycemic, with plasma glucose levels ranging from 0.1 mM/L (2 mg/dL) to 1.8 mM/L (33 mg/dL).[207] Four of the nine were septic. Of the 10 who died, 5 were hypoglycemic.

Neonatal Hypoglycemia

In addition to changes in the level of consciousness (irritability, lethargy, stupor), tremor, seizures, and coma, signs consistent with hypoglycemia in infants include apnea, cyanotic spells, hypothermia, hypotonia, and poor feeding (especially after feeding well).[206] The definition of neonatal hypoglycemia is controversial. Plasma glucose concentrations ranging from 2.2 mmol/L (40 mg/dL) to 2.8 mmol/L (50 mg/dL) have been suggested. Plasma glucose levels less than 3.3 mmol/L (60 mg/dL) are unusual in healthy newborns after 24 hours of extrauterine life.

The fetus relies on a continuous supply of glucose from the maternal circulation. After birth, the neonate must make the transition to endogenous glucose production with only intermittent exogenous glucose delivery.[206] Probably because of their large brains relative to their body weights, infants have rates of glucose utilization approximately threefold higher than those of adults when expressed per unit of body weight.[208] Correspondingly high rates of endogenous glucose production are required to maintain systemic glucose balance. Because mobilizable glycogen stores are limited and feeding is intermittent, the newborn is largely dependent on gluconeogenesis for the first 4 to 6 hours after birth.

Therefore, appropriate glucoregulatory signals (particularly low insulin and high glucagon, epinephrine, and other glucose counterregulatory hormone levels), structural and enzymatic integrity of the liver (and kidneys), and availability of sufficient gluconeogenic precursors are essential. In the setting of relatively low plasma glucose concentrations, the combination of hypoinsulinemia and activated glucose counterregulatory systems also favors lipolysis. High nonesterified fatty acid levels provide an alternative fuel for tissues other than the brain and limit glucose utilization by muscle and fat. They also drive ketogenesis, thus providing an alternative fuel for the brain during neonatal life. These glucoregulatory signals also favor mobilization of gluconeogenic precursors. Impairment of any of these adaptations to extrauterine life can cause transient neonatal hypoglycemia. Persistent defects cause recurrent or persistent hypoglycemia.

TABLE 33–10 CAUSES OF HYPOGLYCEMIA UNIQUE TO, OR TYPICALLY WITH ONSET IN, INFANCY AND CHILDHOOD

TRANSIENT INTOLERANCE OF FASTING
Preterm or small-for-gestational age infants Hypopituitarism, adrenal hypoplasia, congenital adrenal hyperplasia Ketotic hypoglycemia of childhood
HYPERINSULINISM
Infant of a diabetic mother Maternal drugs (sulfonylurea, β_2-adrenergic agonist) Congenital hyperinsulinism, insulinoma Miscellaneous: Rh incompatibility, Beckwith-Wiedemann syndrome, exchange transfusions, perinatal stress
ENZYME DEFECTS
Carbohydrate metabolism: glycogen storage disease types I, III, and VI; glycogen synthase deficiency; fructose-1,6-bisphosphatase deficiency; fructose-1-phosphate aldolase deficiency; galactose-1-phosphate uridyltransferase deficiency Protein metabolism: branched-chain α-keto acid dehydrogenase complex deficiency Fat metabolism: fatty acid oxidation defects including deficiencies in the carnitine cycle, the beta oxidation spiral, the electron transport system, and the ketogenesis sequence

Intolerance of Fasting

Transient intolerance of fasting occurs in preterm or small-for-gestational age infants; in hypopituitarism, adrenal hypoplasia, or congenital adrenal hyperplasia; or, later, in ketotic hypoglycemia of childhood. At least in the absence of seizure or coma, neonatal hypoglycemia (that developing in the first 72 hours after birth) is usually transient. It is particularly common in preterm or small-for-gestational age infants and is thought to result from incomplete development of gluconeogenic mechanisms.[209] Deficiencies of cortisol, growth hormone, or both can be congenital and cause hypoglycemia through mechanisms discussed earlier.

In general, children tolerate fasting less well than adults. The syndrome of ketotic hypoglycemia of childhood, which typically has its onset between ages 2 and 5 years and remits spontaneously before age 10 years, might account for the fraction of children who are least tolerant of fasting. Hypoglycemia occurs when feeding is interrupted, typically during an intercurrent illness. The syndrome appears to involve diminished mobilization of gluconeogenic precursors including alanine.[210] Blood alanine levels are low during hypoglycemia, and alanine infusion increases plasma glucose levels. Glycogenolytic and gluconeogenic mechanisms appear to be intact and, aside from low epinephrine levels,[150] glucoregulatory signals are appropriate. Epinephrine deficiency per se does not cause hypoglycemia.

Hyperinsulinism

A common cause of transient hyperinsulinemic neonatal hypoglycemia is maternal diabetes.[206] Infants of diabetic mothers are hyperglycemic (in proportion to the mother's hyperglycemia) and correspondingly hyperinsulinemic. Presumably reflecting chronic stimulation of fetal insulin secretion in utero and its failure to become suppressed normally as glucose levels fall shortly after birth, transient neonatal hypoglycemia occurs. Transient hyperinsulinemia also underlies neonatal hypoglycemia in infants with Rh factor incompatibility or with the Beckwith-Wiedemann syndrome (macroglossia, omphalocele, and visceromegaly).[211] Hypoglycemia, resulting from hyperinsulinemia stimulated by glucose infusion during the procedure, can also follow exchange transfusion. Neonatal hypoglycemia can be caused by drugs given to the mother, including agents that stimulate fetal insulin secretion (e.g., a sulfonylurea) or that produce maternal and fetal hyperglycemia and thus fetal hyperinsulinemia (e.g., a β_2-adrenergic agonist used to delay labor). Accidental or malicious administration of a sulfonylurea or insulin is a rare cause of hyperinsulinemic hypoglycemia in children. Transient neonatal hyperinsulinemic hypoglycemia has also been attributed to perinatal stress such as asphyxia.[212]

Congenital Hyperinsulinism

In contrast to these causes of transient neonatal hyperinsulinemic hypoglycemia, congenital hyperinsulinism (or persistent hyperinsulinemic hypoglycemia of infancy) can persist from the neonatal period or become apparent clinically in the first year of life.[213,214] (Patients in that age range rarely have a discrete insulinoma, although insulinomas are found in children who develop hyperinsulinemic hypoglycemia after the first year.) Although partial pancreatectomy can become necessary, patients with congenital hyperinsulinism are treated medically initially—with glucose administration for stabilization; frequent feedings; and diazoxide (often with a thiazide), octreotide, and glucagon, often tried in that sequence—in the anticipation of amelioration of hypoglycemia over time because there is a high frequency of diabetes late after partial pancreatectomy.[213]

Congenital hyperinsulinism is the most common cause of nontransient neonatal hypoglycemia, although it occurs in only approximately 1 in 50,000 live births. It is often inherited as an autosomal recessive trait and the result of mutations of the genes that encode adenosine triphosphate (ATP)-sensitive potassium (K_{ATP}) channels, specifically the sulfonylurea receptor (SUR1) or, less commonly, the channel itself (Kir6.2).[213-215] Homozygous mutations result in diffuse beta cell hypersecretion; focal beta cell hypersecretion has been attributed to loss of maternal heterozygosity and expression of the paternal K_{ATP} mutation.[213,214] Loss of channel function leads to persistent beta cell membrane depolarization and thus insulin secretion despite low plasma glucose levels.[215]

In general, patients with K_{ATP} channel mutations suffer from severe neonatal hypoglycemia that is unresponsive to diazoxide which normally opens the channel and suppresses insulin secretion.[216] Successful treatment with the calcium channel antagonist nifedipine has been reported,[217] but partial pancreatectomy is often required. Resection of focal lesions can be curative; ^{18}F-dihydroxyphenylalanine positron emission tomography often identifies the focal lesion.[218]

Other causes of congenital hyperinsulinism[213-215]—which typically cause less marked hypoglycemia and are more likely to be responsive to diazoxide—include autosomal dominant activating mutations of the glutamate dehydrogenase gene (the hyperinsulinism-hyperammonemia syndrome) and of the glucokinase gene and homozygous mutations of the short-chain 3-hydroxylacyl-coenzyme A dehydrogenase (SCHAD) gene.[219] Gain-of-function glucokinase and glutamate dehydrogenase mutations can increase insulin secretion by increasing ATP synthesis.[215] The mechanism of hyperinsulinism with SCHAD mutations is unknown.[215] Hyperinsulinemic hypoglycemia has also been reported in infants with disorders of glycosylation[220] and with tyrosinemia type 1.[221]

Enzyme Defects

Hypoglycemia that develops in infancy or childhood, and persists into adulthood with effective therapy, can also be caused by enzymatic defects in carbohydrate metabolism (e.g., glycogen storage disease types I, III, and IV; glycogen synthase deficiency; fructose-1,6-bisphosphatase, phosphoenolpyruvate carboxykinase, or pyruvate kinase deficiency; fructose-1-phosphate aldolase deficiency; galactose-1-phosphate uridyltransferase deficiency; or glucose transporter defects),[222-231] in protein metabolism (e.g., branched-chain α-keto acid dehydrogenase complex deficiency),[232] or in fat metabolism (e.g., various defects in fatty acid oxidation).[233-236] All of these disorders cause postabsorptive hypoglycemia except for hereditary fructose intolerance caused by fructose-1-phosphate aldolase deficiency and galactosemia caused by galactose uridyltransferase deficiency, which cause postprandial hypoglycemia. Although clinical features and biochemical patterns suggest a subset of diagnostic possibilities and in some instances provide a specific diagnosis, definitive diagnosis often requires either documentation of deficient enzyme activity in affected tissues or, increasingly, identification of a mutation in the relevant gene.

As first documented by Cori and Cori[222] in 1952, deficient glucose-6-phosphatase activity causes glycogen storage disease type I (von Gierke's disease),[223] the prototype glycogen storage disease. Because hydrolysis of glucose-6-phosphate to glucose is the common pathway for systemic glucose production from both hepatic glycogenolysis and gluconeogenesis (and renal gluconeogenesis), glucose-6-phosphatase deficiency causes profound postabsorptive hypoglycemia with hypoinsulinemia; activated glucose counterregulatory systems with elevated lactate, alanine, nonesterified fatty acid, ketone body, and triglyceride levels; and metabolic acidosis with hyperuricemia. Hepatomegaly (caused by hepatocyte accumulation of fat as well as glycogen) is a universal finding. With the exception of hepatomegaly, the abnormalities can be reversed by the prevention of hypoglycemia with frequent feedings during waking hours and continuous intragastric glucose infusion during sleep or with bedtime administration of large doses of uncooked cornstarch. Liver transplantation corrects hypoglycemia and the associated metabolic abnormalities.[224] Hepatocyte transplantation may become an alternative.[225] Adults with (presumably inadequately treated) type I glycogen storage disease have a high incidence of hepatic adenomas and renal disease. Interestingly, renal transplantation does not correct hypoglycemia.[223] The mechanism by which these patients maintain some level of endogenous glucose production is unclear.[226]

The glucose-6-phosphatase system is complex. Most patients with type I glycogen storage disease have mutations of the gene encoding the catalytic subunit (type Ia). Others do not have such mutations; the defect has been attributed to mutations in the glucose-6-phosphate translocase gene (type Ib-Ic or non–type Ia). Hypoglycemia is less prominent in type III (amylo-1,6-glucosidase deficiency) and type IV (branching enzyme deficiency) and rare in types VI and IX (phosphorylase complex deficiency) glycogen storage diseases. Hypoglycemia can also be caused by glycogen synthase deficiency, which, unlike the glycogen storage diseases, does not cause hepatomegaly. Because it blocks gluconeogenesis, fructose-1,6-bisphosphatase deficiency causes profound postabsorptive hypoglycemia with lactic acidosis, ketosis, and elevated alanine levels. Hyperlipidemia, hyperuricemia, and hepatomegaly (related to fat accumulation) occur as in type I glycogen storage disease. Hypoglycemia has also been attributed to phosphoenolpyruvate carboxykinase and pyruvate carboxylase deficiencies.

Finally, with respect to postabsorptive hypoglycemia and defects in glucose metabolism, CNS glucopenia occurs in patients with mutations of the GLUT-1 glucose transporter gene.[228] Plasma glucose levels are normal, but cerebrospinal glucose levels are low because of reduced GLUT-1-mediated glucose transport across the blood-brain barrier. Treatment includes a ketogenic (low-carbohydrate) diet designed to raise ketone levels and thus provide an alternative fuel to the brain. Hypoglycemia has also been attributed to GLUT-2 deficiency in the Fanconi-Bickel syndrome.[228]

Postprandial, rather than postabsorptive, hypoglycemia can be a feature of hereditary fructose intolerance[229] and, rarely, galactosemia.[230] Fructose-1-phosphate aldolase deficiency, the enzymatic defect in hereditary fructose intolerance, causes vomiting and severe hypoglycemia after fructose ingestion. Fructose-1-phosphate accumulates and inhibits glycogenolysis (at the phosphorylase level) and gluconeogenesis (at the mutant aldolase level). The patients are well when fructose is omitted from the diet. Galactose uridyltransferase deficiency, one of the causes of galactosemia, can also cause postprandial hypoglycemia, which has been attributed to inhibition of glycogenolysis.[230,231]

Deficiencies of enzymes involved in protein metabolism that can cause postabsorptive hypoglycemia include that of the branched-chain keto acid dehydrogenase complex, the basis of branched-chain ketoaciduria (maple syrup urine disease).[232] The levels of leucine, isoleucine, and valine—particularly leucine—in plasma and urine are elevated. The pathogenesis of hypoglycemia is not entirely clear, although it results from defective gluconeogenesis.

Several defects that ultimately impair fatty acid oxidation result in postabsorptive hypoglycemia with *hypo*ketonemia.[233–236] Normally,[237] low-insulin, high-glucagon (and catecholamine) states such as fasting favor the mobilization of fatty acids from fat (lipolysis) and their transport to other tissues, including the liver and skeletal and cardiac muscle. These regulatory conditions also favor fatty acid oxidation (with ATP formation) and ketogenesis over triglyceride, phospholipid, and cholesterol ester synthesis and peroxisomal oxidation. Mitochondrial fatty acid oxidation and ketogenesis require transport of fatty acids across the plasma membrane, formation of fatty acyl-CoA derivatives, and transport of the derivatives into mitochondria. Because the inner mitochondrial membranes are not permeable to long-chain (as opposed to medium-chain and short-chain) fatty acyl-CoA esters, the long-chain fatty acyl-CoA esters are transesterified to fatty acylcarnitines at the outer surface of the membranes (by carnitine palmitoyltransferase I, CPT-I), transported across the membranes (by a translocase), and reconverted to the fatty acyl-CoA esters (by carnitine palmitoyltransferase II, CPT-II) at the inner surface of the membranes. Then they can be oxidized or converted to ketones.

Insulin decreases fat oxidation and ketogenesis by decreasing lipolysis and by increasing lipogenesis and the formation of malonyl-CoA, which inhibits CPT-I. Conversely, low insulin levels favor fatty acid oxidation and ketogenesis. High glucagon levels do so by decreasing malonyl-CoA. Catecholamines do so largely by stimulating lipolysis. Any defect in this sequence—defects in the carnitine cycle (carnitine transport defect, CPT-I deficiency, carnitine-acylcarnitine translocase deficiency, CPT-II deficiency), defects in the β-oxidation spiral (long-chain acyl-CoA dehydrogenase [LCAD] deficiency, long-chain L-3-hydroxylacyl-CoA dehydrogenase [LCHAD] deficiency, short-chain L-3-hydroxyacyl-CoA dehydrogenase [SCHAD] deficiency, 2,4-dienoyl-CoA reductase deficiency, medium-chain acyl-CoA dehydrogenase [MCAD] deficiency, short-chain acyl-CoA dehydrogenase [SCAD] deficiency), several defects of electron transfer or defects in ketogenesis (hydroxymethylglutaryl [HMG]-CoA lyase deficiency, HMG-CoA synthetase deficiency)—decreases fatty acid oxidation (and ketogenesis) and reciprocally increases glucose oxidation, resulting in hypoketonemic postabsorptive hypoglycemia. Reduced plasma carnitine levels (20% to 50% of normal) are the rule in these disorders, but extremely low carnitine levels characterize the carnitine transport defect, a true carnitine deficiency state that is responsive to carnitine supplementation.[233,234] CPT-I deficiency, a rare disorder, is treatable by administration of medium-chain triglycerides, which do not require the CPT system for oxidation, or by a high-carbohydrate, low-fat diet.[238] CPT-II deficiency, which is typically seen with episodes of muscle pain and myoglobinuria but can also cause hypoglycemia, is more common.[239]

The child affected with a disorder of fatty acid oxidation typically presents with hypoketonemic hypoglycemia; intravenous glucose causes prompt improvement. Some have presented with Reye's syndrome. All are at risk for sudden death, presumably from cardiac causes. Treatment includes provision of an adequate caloric intake, avoidance of fasting, and support of the plasma glucose concentration during intercurrent illnesses. The diagnosis of specific fatty acid oxidation defects is typically accomplished by blood acylcarnitine profiling,[240] although molecular diagnosis is increasingly possible. Interestingly, the presence of a defect in fatty acid oxidation in a fetus can have implications for the mother. While carrying a fetus with a specific mutation (Glu474Gln) causing long-chain 3-hydroxyacyl-CoA dehydrogenase deficiency, 15 (79%) of 19 mothers suffered fatty liver of pregnancy or the HELLP (hemolysis, elevated liver enzyme levels, and low platelet count) syndrome.[241]

Neonatal hypoglycemia with suppressed nonesterified fatty acid (NEFA) and ketone (e.g., β-hydroxybutyrate) levels suggests hyperinsulinism, and that with high NEFA but low ketone levels suggests a defect in fatty acid oxidation or ketogenesis. Hypoglycemia with high lactate levels suggests a defect in gluconeogenesis or glucose release. High NEFA and ketone levels suggest a defect in glucose production or release including deficiencies of cortisol, growth hormone, or both, although NEFA and ketone levels need not be elevated in patients with hypopituitarism.

Given the array of causes of hypoglycemia in infancy and childhood just summarized, it is reasonable to suggest an extensive biochemical assessment during a hypoglycemic episode when the hypoglycemic mechanism is obscure. In addition to the concurrent plasma glucose concentration, this might include plasma insulin, C peptide, sulfonylureas, growth hormone, and cortisol; plasma or blood lactate, amino acids (including alanine), nonesterified fatty acids, and β-hydroxybutyrate; serum liver enzymes; plasma acylcarnitine profile; and urine ketones and organic acid profile.

Postprandial (Reactive) Hypoglycemias

Postprandial (reactive, stimulative) hypoglycemia occurs exclusively after meals, typically within 4 hours after food ingestion. Some disorders that cause postabsorptive hypoglycemia can also result in hypoglycemia detected after a meal. However, the diagnostic and therapeutic approach is that of postabsorptive hypoglycemia in such a patient.

Postprandial hypoglycemia can occur in persons who have undergone gastric surgery that results in rapid movement of ingested food into the small intestine.[242] Termed *alimentary hypoglycemia,* this is thought to be the result of marked early hyperinsulinemia caused by rapid increments in plasma glucose and enhanced secretion of the gut incretin glucagon-like peptide-1 (GLP-1) coupled with suppression of glucagon secretion by GLP-1. Hypoglycemia occurs 1.5 to 3.0 hours after a meal. Symptoms of hypoglycemia need to be distinguished from those of the dumping syndrome—abdominal fullness, nausea, weakness—which occur less than an hour after ingestion. Administration of an α-glucosidase inhibitor (acarbose, miglitol) is a conceptually attractive treatment for alimentary hypoglycemia,[243] although controlled trials documenting its efficacy are lacking.

Some patients with an insulinoma have hypoglycemic episodes after a meal. Postprandial hypoglycemia occurs in patients with autoimmune hypoglycemia due to an antibody to insulin[175] or with noninsulinoma pancreatogenous hypoglycemia without[201,202] or with[203,204] previous gastric bypass surgery, as well as those with hereditary fructose intolerance[229] or galactosemia.[230] However, all of these disorders are rare.

Documentation of Whipple's triad—symptoms consistent with hypoglycemia, a low measured plasma glucose concentration, and relief of those symptoms after the glucose level is raised—is critical to a diagnosis of postprandial hypoglycemia. The recommended biochemical criteria are a plasma glucose concentration less than 3.0 mmol/L (54 mg/dL), an insulin concentration greater than 18 pmol/L (3.0 μU/mL), and a C-peptide concentration greater than 0.2 nmol/L (0.6 ng/mL).[201,203] It is conceivable that healthy persons might have a venous (as opposed to arterial) plasma glucose level less than 3.0 mmol/L and a corresponding insulin level greater than 18 pmol/L late after a meal given insulin-stimulated glucose extraction across the forearm and even with an insulin plasma half-time of 4 to 6 minutes. Given a plasma insulin half-time of 30 to 40 minutes, C-peptide levels would almost assuredly be greater than 0.2 nmol/L under those conditions. Thus, the C-peptide value would only serve as evidence against exogenous insulin administration.[203] It would not be appropriate to diagnose postprandial hypoglycemia in the absence of symptoms temporally related to the nadir plasma glucose concentration.

The frequency, and even the existence, of clinically relevant idiopathic (functional) postprandial hypoglycemia is a matter of debate.[244] Idiopathic postprandial hypoglycemia is often erroneously diagnosed by patients and by physicians. For example, only 16 of 118 patients suspected of having postprandial hypoglycemia in one series had both a plasma glucose concentration lower than the 10th percentile of asymptomatic control subjects and typical symptoms after an oral glucose load; only 5 of those 16 patients had similar symptoms after their regular meals.[245] Furthermore, most patients thought to have hypoglycemic symptoms and low glucose levels after glucose ingestion have normal glucose levels after a mixed meal. In one series in which blood glucose was measured during symptomatic episodes, only 5% of 132 episodes were associated with blood glucose levels of 2.8 mmol/L (50 mg/dL) or less.[246] Enhanced, presumably compensatory, plasma epinephrine responses have been reported in persons with sweating, tremor, and greater heart rates temporally related to the glucose nadir late after glucose ingestion.[247] In such persons, the postprandial syndrome may be the result of an appropriately enhanced sympathoadrenal response to falling plasma glucose concentrations rather than hypoglycemia per se.

A diagnosis of postprandial hypoglycemia should not be made on the basis of seemingly low plasma glucose concentrations during an oral glucose tolerance test. The lower limits of normal for venous plasma glucose concentrations late after glucose ingestion can be defined statistically. For example, in 650 subjects who remained asymptomatic after ingestion of 100 g of glucose, nadir glucose concentrations were lower 5th percentile, 2.4 mmol/L (43 mg/dL); lower 10th percentile, 2.6 mmol/L (47 mg/dL); and lower 25th percentile, 3.0 mmol/L (54 mg/dL).[248] (The absence of symptoms in response to such seemingly low plasma glucose concentrations is most plausibly explained by venous sampling.) Because the lowest glucose levels in these subjects cause no recognizable symptoms, have no known long-term ill effects, are self-limited, and do not imply the presence of disease, there is no reason to classify 2.5% or 5% of the population arbitrarily as abnormal. The diagnosis requires documentation of appropriate symptoms temporally related to a low plasma glucose concentration after a mixed meal and relief of those symptoms as the plasma glucose concentration rises (Whipple's triad).

Diets low in carbohydrate and high in protein are commonly recommended to patients thought to have postprandial hypoglycemia. Their efficacy has not been established by controlled clinical trials. Frequent feedings and avoidance of simple sugars are also advised. To the extent that an excessive initial increase in plasma glucose plays a role in the pathogenesis of alimentary hypoglycemia, administration of an α-glucosidase inhibitor to delay carbohydrate digestion is a conceptually attractive treatment.[241]

Treatment of Postabsorptive Hypoglycemia

In view of the vulnerability of the brain to prolonged hypoglycemia, the plasma glucose concentration must be raised at least to normal levels as rapidly as possible and recurrence of hypoglycemia must be prevented. Because it is self-limited, postprandial hypoglycemia rarely requires urgent treatment. In contrast, postabsorptive hypoglycemias are typically persistent or progressive and require short-term and long-term therapy.

The urgent treatment of iatrogenic hypoglycemia in persons with diabetes—with oral carbohydrate or glucose or with parenteral glucagon or glucose—was discussed earlier under "Hypoglycemia in Diabetes Mellitus." Clinical improvement should occur within about 15 to 20 minutes after the plasma glucose level is increased and maintained, provided that brain damage has not occurred. Whenever possible, the presence of hypoglycemia should be documented before therapy, and the response to therapy should be followed by frequent measurements of the plasma glucose level. If these are not available and there is no clinical response within 15 minutes, the initial therapy should be repeated and access to plasma glucose monitoring and intravenous glucose infusion should be obtained as soon as possible. Even if there is a response to initial therapy, glucose monitoring is essential to ensure maintenance of the plasma glucose concentration.

Although CNS function usually recovers promptly after restoration of the plasma glucose level, recovery may be delayed, perhaps because of cerebral edema. Unconsciousness lasting more than 30 minutes after the plasma glucose concentration has been raised to normal and maintained is referred to as posthypoglycemic coma.[249] It has been treated with intravenous mannitol (40 g as a 20% solution over 20 minutes) or glucocorticoids (e.g., dexamethasone,10 mg), or both,[249,250] along with maintenance of normal plasma glucose levels.

Definitive treatment of the postabsorptive hypoglycemias requires correction of the underlying defect whenever possible. When that is not possible, attempts must be made to increase exogenous delivery or endogenous glucose production and to limit glucose utilization by tissues other than the brain. Although the judicious use of snacks is sometimes a useful component of therapy for persons with diabetes, frequent feedings are less than ideal for the long-term treatment of chronic hypoglycemia. One problem is weight gain. However, frequent feedings, even overnight gastric infusions, are sometimes necessary when other measures are inadequate.

Hypoglycemia caused by drugs is limited to the duration of action of the offending drug. The management is straightforward: discontinuation of the drug (at least temporarily), maintenance of the plasma glucose level while drug action continues, and adjustment of subsequent drug regimens to avoid recurrent hypoglycemia if the causative drug is known. Therapy is more difficult if the drug is used surreptitiously or given accidentally or maliciously.

Postabsorptive hypoglycemia related to endogenous hyperinsulinism is often curable by the surgical removal of an insulinoma. If this is not possible because of multiple or metastatic tumors or the absence of a definable lesion, diazoxide is sometimes effective.[199,251] Diazoxide (100-800 mg/day in adults and 5-30 mg/kg/day in infants) raises the plasma glucose concentration by suppressing insulin secretion.[216] Diazoxide is bound tightly to albumin and has a plasma half-time of 20 to 30 hours.[250] When given by rapid intravenous injection, it is a potent hypotensive drug, but when given orally or by slow intravenous infusion, it has less hypotensive action. Nonetheless, hypotension is dose-limiting in the short-term; oral doses up to 6.0 mg/kg appear to be safe in this regard.[216] Although chemically related to the thiazide diuretics, diazoxide causes sodium retention. Coadministration of a thiazide diuretic both limits sodium retention and potentiates the hyperglycemic action of diazoxide.[199] Both edema formation and gastrointestinal side effects (anorexia, nausea, sometimes vomiting) are dose-related. Generalized growth of lanugo hair (hypertrichosis lanuginosa) can occur during prolonged therapy. Allergic reactions, including skin rashes and agranulocytosis, are rare. Other treatments include octreotide or calcium channel antagonists.[215]

The treatment of hypoglycemia associated with non–beta cell tumors involves short-term measures pending effective medical, surgical, or radiotherapeutic treatment of the tumor. Administration of a glucocorticoid or growth hormone sometimes alleviates hypoglycemia. The former, but not the latter, has been reported to reduce IGF-II levels.[166,252,253] Hypoglycemia resulting from glucocorticoid deficiency is corrected by replacement therapy. Hypoglycemia is rarely an indication for growth hormone replacement. Remissions of autoimmune hypoglycemias have been associated with immunosuppressive therapy, including glucocorticoids, but controlled trials are lacking. The treatment of hypoglycemia related to inanition, hepatic or renal disease, cardiac failure, or sepsis includes short-term measures and, when possible, treatment or management of the underlying disease process. The treatment of the hypoglycemias of infancy and childhood and that of postprandial hypoglycemia were discussed earlier.

TABLE 33–11 DIAGNOSTIC APPROACH TO AN ADULT WITH DOCUMENTED FASTING HYPOGLYCEMIA

1. Think of drugs, critical illness, endocrine deficiency, non–beta-cell tumor, and hyperinsulinism while supporting the plasma glucose concentration if necessary.
2. Search the history, physical examination, and available laboratory data for clinical clues to the hypoglycemic mechanism and pursue the plausible mechanism or mechanisms:
   a. For insulin-treated or sulfonylurea-treated diabetes: Adjust the therapeutic regimen
   b. For use of other drugs known or suspected to cause hypoglycemia: Discontinue the drug (substitute an alternative if necessary)
   c. For hepatic, renal, or cardiac failure, for sepsis, or for inanition: Treat the underlying disorder
   d. For anorexia, weight loss, change in skin pigmentation, known pituitary or adrenocortical disease, hypotension, hyponatremia, or hyperkalemia: Evaluate for adrenocortical insufficiency
   e. For known non-beta cell tumor, mass on examination or imaging studies: Measure free IGF-II and IGF-I
3. In the absence of clinical clues, consider medication error, endogenous hyperinsulinism, and surreptitious or malicious sulfonylurea or insulin administration.
4. A metabolic enzyme deficiency is rarely first detected in an adult.

IGF, insulin-like growth factor.

Approach to the Patient with Hypoglycemia

In addition to recognizing and documenting hypoglycemia and often giving urgent treatment, management of hypoglycemia requires diagnosing the hypoglycemic mechanism leading to treatment that prevents, or at least minimizes, recurrent hypoglycemia. The differential diagnosis of hypoglycemia, discussed earlier, is summarized in Table 33–3. A diagnostic algorithm is shown in Figure 33–14. The thought process is summarized in Table 33–11.

ACKNOWLEDGMENTS

The author acknowledges the substantive contributions of several colleagues and collaborators that shaped the views expressed in this chapter; the assistance of the nursing, dietary, laboratory, informatics, and biostatistical staffs of the Washington University General Clinical Research Center in performing the original work cited; and the help of Ms. Janet Dedeke in the preparation of the manuscript.

REFERENCES

1. Cryer PE. Hypoglycemia: Pathophysiology, Diagnosis and Treatment. New York: Oxford University Press, 1997.
2. Cryer PE. The prevention and correction of hypoglycemia. In Jefferson LS, Cherrington AD, eds. The Endocrine Pancreas and Regulation of Metabolism, vol II, The Endocrine System. Handbook of Physiology. New York: Oxford University Press, 2001: 1057-1092.
3. Cryer PE. Diverse causes of hypoglycemia-associated autonomic failure in diabetes. N Engl J Med 2004;350:2272-2279.
4. Boden G. Gluconeogenesis and glycogenolysis in health and disease. J Invest Med 2004;52:375-378.
5. Stumvoll M, Chintalapudi U, Perriello G, et al. Uptake and release of glucose by the human kidney. J Clin Invest 1995;96:2528-2533.
6. Woerle HJ, Meyer C, Popa EM, et al. Renal compensation for impaired hepatic glucose release during hypoglycemia in type 2 diabetes. Diabetes 2003;52:1386-1392.
7. Owen OE, Felig P, Morgan AP, et al. Liver and kidney metabolism during prolonged starvation. J Clin Invest 1969;48:574-583.
8. Cherrington AD. The role of hepatic insulin receptors in the regulation of glucose production. J Clin Invest 2005;45:1136-1139.
9. Pocai A, Lam TKT, Gutierrez-Juarez, et al. Hypothalamic K_{ATP} channels control hepatic glucose production. Nature 2005;434: 1026-1031.
10. Gustavson SM, Chu CA, Nishizawa M, et al. Glucagon's actions are modified by the combination of epinephrine and gluconeogenic precursor infusion. Am J Physiol 2003;285:E534-E544.
11. Laurent D, Petersen KF, Russell RR, et al. Effect of epinephrine on muscle glycogenolysis and insulin-stimulated muscle glycogen synthesis in humans. Am J Physiol 1998;274:E130-E138.
12. Shamoon H, Hendler R, Sherwin RS. Synergistic interactions among anti-insulin hormones in the pathogenesis of stress hyperglycemia in humans. J Clin Endocrinol Metab 1981;52:1235-1241.
13. Püschel GP. Control of hepatocyte metabolism by sympathetic and parasympathetic hepatic nerves. Anat Rec A Discov Mol Cell Evol Biol 2004;280A:854-867.
14. Boyle PJ, Liggett SB, Shah SD, et al. Direct muscarinic cholinergic inhibition of hepatic glucose production in humans. J Clin Invest 1988;82:445-449.
15. Ahrén B. Autonomic regulation of islet hormone secretion: implications for health and disease. Diabetologia 2000;43:393-410.
16. Raju B, Cryer PE. Loss of the decrement in intraislet insulin plausibly explains loss of the glucagon response to hypoglycemia in insulin-deficient diabetes. Diabetes 2005;54:757-764.
17. Coiro VM, Passeri M, Volpi R, et al. Effect of muscarinic and nicotinic cholinergic blockade on the glucagon response to insulin-induced hypoglycemia in normal man. Horm Metab Res 1989;21: 102-103.
18. Havel P, Ahrén B. Activation of autonomic nerves and the adrenal medulla contributes to increased glucagon secretion during

moderate insulin-induced hypoglycemia in women. Diabetes 1997;46:801-807.
19. Mathias CJ, Christensen NJ, Corbett JL, et al. Plasma catecholamines during paroxysmal neurogenic hypertension in quadriplegic man. Circ Res 1976;39:204-208.
20. Borg WP, Sherwin RS, During MJ, et al. Local ventromedial hypothalamus glucopenia triggers counterregulatory hormone release. Diabetes 1995;44:180-184.
21. Frizell RT, Jones EM, Davis SN, et al. Counterregulation during hypoglycemia is directed by widespread brain regions. Diabetes 1993;42:1253-1261.
22. Heavener AL, Bergman RN, Donovan CM. Portal vein afferents are critical for the sympathoadrenal response to hypoglycemia. Diabetes 2000;49:8-12.
23. Schwartz NS, Shah SD, Clutter WE, et al. Glycemic thresholds for activation of glucose counterregulatory systems are higher than the threshold for symptoms. J Clin Invest 1987;79:777-781.
24. Mitrakou A, Ryan C, Veneman T, et al. Hierarchy of glycemic thresholds for counterregulatory hormone secretion, symptoms and cerebral dysfunction. Am J Physiol 1991;260:E67-E74.
25. Fanelli C, Pampanelli S, Epifano L, et al. Relative roles of insulin and hypoglycaemia on induction of neuroendocrine responses to, symptoms of and deterioration of cognitive function in hypoglycemia in male and female humans. Diabetologia 1994;37:797-807.
26. Garber AJ, Cryer PE, Santiago JV, et al. The role of adrenergic mechanisms in the substrate and hormonal responses to hypoglycemia in man. J Clin Invest 1976;58:7-15.
27. Clarke WL, Santiago JV, Thomas L, et al. Adrenergic mechanisms in recovery from hypoglycemia in man: adrenergic blockade. Am J Physiol 1979;236:E147-E152.
28. Gerich JE, Davis J, Lorenzi M, et al. Hormonal mechanisms of recovery from insulin-induced hypoglycemia in man. Am J Physiol 1979;236:E380-E385.
29. Rizza RA, Cryer PE, Gerich JE. Role of glucagon, epinephrine and growth hormone in human glucose counterregulation: effects of somatostatin and adrenergic blockade on plasma glucose recovery and glucose flux rates following insulin induced hypoglycemia. J Clin Invest 1979;64:62-71.
30. DeFeo P, Periello G, Torlone E, et al. Demonstration of a role for growth hormone in glucose counterregulation. Am J Physiol 1989;256:E835-E843.
31. DeFeo P, Periello G, Torlone E, et al. Contribution of cortisol to glucose counterregulation. Am J Physiol 1989;257:E35-E42.
32. DeFeo P, Perriello G, Torlone E, et al. Evidence against important catecholamine compensation for absent glucagon counterregulation. Am J Physiol 1991;260:E203-E212.
33. DeFeo P, Perriello G, Torlone E, et al. Contribution of adrenergic mechanisms to glucose counterregulation in humans. Am J Physiol 1991;261:E725-E736.
34. Boyle PJ, Cryer PE. Growth hormone, cortisol, or both are involved in defense against, but are not critical to recovery from, prolonged hypoglycemia in humans. Am J Physiol 1991;260:E395-E402.
35. Bolli G, DeFeo P, Periello G, et al. Role of hepatic autoregulation in defense against hypoglycemia in humans. J Clin Invest 1985;75:1623-1631.
36. Camacho RC, Lacy DB, James FD, et al. Hepatic glucose autoregulation: responses to small, non–insulin-induced changes in arterial glucose. Am J Physiol 2004;287:E269-E274.
37. Raju B, Cryer PE. Maintenance of the postabsorptive plasma glucose concentration: insulin or insulin plus glucagon? Am J Physiol 2005;289:E181-E186.
38. Towler DA, Havlin CE, Craft S, Cryer PE. Mechanisms of awareness of hypoglycemia: perception of neurogenic (predominantly cholinergic) rather than neuroglycopenic symptoms. Diabetes 1993;42:1791-1798.
39. McAulay V, Deary IJ, Frier BM. Symptoms of hypoglycemia in people with diabetes. Diabetic Medicine 2001;18:690-705.
40. McCrimmon RJ, Deary IJ, Gold AE, et al. Symptoms reported during experimental hypoglycaemia: effect of method of induction of hypoglycaemia and diabetes per se. Diabetic Medicine 2003;20:507-509.
41. DeRosa MA, Cryer PE. Hypoglycemia and the sympathoadrenal system: neurogenic symptoms are largely the result of sympathetic neural, rather than adrenomedullary, activation. Am J Physiol 2004;287:E32-E41.
42. Kahn KJ, Myers RE. Insulin-induced hypoglycaemia in the non-human primate. I. Clinical consequences. In Brierley JB, Meldrum BS, eds. Brain Hypoxia. London: William Heinemann Medical Books, 1971:185-193.
43. Suh SW, Aoyama K, Chen Y, et al. Hypoglycemic neuronal death and cognitive impairment are prevented by poly(ADP-ribose) polymerase inhibitors administered after hypoglycemia. J Neurosci 2003;23:10681-10690.
44. Amiel SA, Simonson DC, Tamborlane WV, et al. Rate of glucose fall does not affect counterregulatory hormone responses to hypoglycemia in normal and diabetic humans. Diabetes 1987;36: 518-522.
45. Mitrakou A, Mokan M, Ryan C, et al. Influence of plasma glucose rate of decrease on hierarchy of responses to hypoglycemia. J Clin Endocrinol Metab 1993;76:462-465.
46. Amiel SA, Sherwin RS, Simonson DC, et al. Effect of intensive insulin therapy on glycemic thresholds for counterregulatory hormone release. Diabetes 1988;37:901-907.
47. Mitrakou A, Fanelli C, Veneman T, et al. Reversibility of hypoglycemia unawareness. N Engl J Med 1993;329:834-839.
48. Boyle PJ, Schwartz NS, Shah SD, et al. Plasma glucose concentrations at the onset of hypoglycemic symptoms in patients with poorly controlled diabetes and nondiabetics. N Engl J Med 1988;318:1487-1492.
49. Malouf R, Brust JCM. Hypoglycemia: causes, neurological manifestations, and outcome. Ann Neurol 1985;17:421-430.
50. Fischer KF, Lees JA, Newman JH. Hypoglycemia in hospitalized patients: causes and outcomes. N Engl J Med 1986;315:1245-1250.
51. Cryer PE, Davis SN, Shamoon H. Hypoglycemia in diabetes. Diabetes Care 2003;26:1902-1912.
52. American Diabetes Association Workgroup on Hypoglycemia. Defining and reporting hypoglycemia in diabetes. Diabetes Care 2005;28:1245-1249.
53. Cryer PE. Mechanisms of hypoglycemia-associated autonomic failure and its component syndromes in diabetes. Diabetes 2005;54:3592-3601.
54. The Diabetes Control and Complications Trial Research Group. The effect of intensive treatment of diabetes on the development and progression of long-term complications in insulin-dependent diabetes mellitus. N Engl J Med 1993;329:977-986.
55. Reichard P, Nilsson B-Y, Rosenqvist U. The effect of long-term intensified insulin treatment on the development of microvascular complications of diabetes mellitus. N Engl J Med 1993;329: 304-309.
56. The United Kingdom Prospective Diabetes Study Group. Intensive blood-glucose control with sulfonylureas or insulin compared with conventional treatment and risk of complications in patients with type 2 diabetes. Lancet 1998;352:837-853.
57. The United Kingdom Prospective Diabetes Study Group. Effect of intensive blood-glucose control with metformin on complications in overweight patients with type 2 diabetes. Lancet 1998;352: 854-865.
58. The Diabetes Control and Complications Trial Research Group. Epidemiology of severe hypoglycemia in the Diabetes Control and Complications Trial. Am J Med 1991;90:450-459.
59. The Diabetes Control and Complications Trial Research Group. Hypoglycemia in the Diabetes Control and Complications Trial. Diabetes 1997;46:271-286.
60. Reichard P, Berglund B, Britz A, et al. Intensified conventional insulin treatment retards the microvascular complications of insulin-dependent diabetes mellitus: the Stockholm Diabetes Intervention Study after 5 years. J Intern Med 1990;230:101-108.
61. Egger M, Davey Smith G, Stettler C, et al. Risk of adverse effects of intensified treatment in insulin-dependent diabetes mellitus: a meta-analysis. Diabet Med 1997;14:919-928.
62. Laing SP, Swerdlow AJ, Slater SD, et al. The British Diabetic Association Cohort Study. II. Cause-specific mortality in patients with insulin-treated diabetes mellitus. Diabet Med 1999;16: 466-471.
63. The United Kingdom Prospective Diabetes Study Research Group. Overview of 6 years of therapy of type II diabetes: a progressive disease. Diabetes 1995;44:1249-1258.
64. The United Kingdom Prospective Diabetes Study Group. A 6-year, randomized, controlled trial comparing sulfonylurea, insulin and metformin therapy in patients with newly diagnosed type 2 diabe-

tes that could not be controlled with diet therapy. Ann Intern Med 1998;128:165-175.
65. Hepburn DA, MacLeod KM, Pell ACH, et al. Frequency and symptoms of hypoglycemia experienced by patients with type 2 diabetes treated with insulin. Diabet Med 1993;10:231-237.
66. Donnelly LA, Morris AD, Frier BM, et al. Frequency and predictors of hypoglycaemia in type 1 and insulin-treated type 2 diabetes: a population based study. Diabet Med 2005;22:749-744.
67. Holstein A, Plaschke A, Egberts E-H. Clinical characteristics of severe hypoglycemia—a prospective population-based study. Exp Clin Endocrinol Diabetes 2003;111:364-369.
68. Leese GP, Wang J, Broomhall J, et al. Frequency of severe hypoglycemia requiring emergency treatment in type 1 and type 2 diabetes: a population based study of health service resource use. Diabetes Care 2003;26:1176-1180.
69. Fukuda M, Tanaka A, Tahara Y, et al. Correlation between minimal secretory capacity of pancreatic β-cells and stability of diabetic control. Diabetes 1988;37:81-88.
70. Mühlhauser I, Overmann H, Bender R, et al. Risk factors for severe hypoglycaemia in adult patients with type 1 diabetes: a prospective population based study. Diabetologia 1997;41:1274-1282.
71. Steffes MW, Sibley S, Jackson M, Thomas W. β-cell function and the development of diabetes-related complications in the Diabetes Control and Complications Trial. Diabetes Care 2003;26: 832-836.
72. Gerich JE, Langlois M, Noacco C, et al. Lack of glucagon response to hypoglycemia in diabetes: evidence for an intrinsic pancreatic alpha cell defect. Science 1973;182:171-173.
73. Bolli G, De Feo P, Compagnucci P, et al. Abnormal glucose counterregulation after subcutaneous insulin in insulin dependent diabetes mellitus: interaction of anti-insulin antibodies and impaired glucagon and epinephrine secretion. Diabetes 1983;32:134-141.
74. Dagogo-Jack SE, Craft S, Cryer PE. Hypoglycemia-associated autonomic failure in insulin dependent diabetes mellitus. J Clin Invest 1993;91:819-828.
75. Bottini P, Boschetti E, Pampanelli S, et al. Contribution of autonomic neuropathy to reduced plasma adrenaline responses to hypoglycemia in IDDM: evidence for a nonselective defect. Diabetes 1997;46:814-823.
76. Meyer C, Grobmann R, Mitrakou A, et al. Effects of autonomic neuropathy on counterregulation and awareness of hypoglycemia in type 1 diabetic patients. Diabetes Care 1998;21:1960-1966.
77. White NH, Skor D, Cryer PE, et al. Identification of type 1 diabetic patients at increased risk for hypoglycemia during intensive therapy. N Engl J Med 1983;308:485-491.
78. Bolli G, De Feo P, De Cosmo S, et al. A reliable and reproducible test for adequate glucose counterregulation in type I diabetes. Diabetes 1984;33:732-737.
79. Gold AE, MacLeod KM, Frier BM. Frequency of severe hypoglycemia in patients with type 1 diabetes with impaired awareness of hypoglycemia. Diabetes Care 1994;17:697-703.
80. Heller SR, Cryer PE. Reduced neuroendocrine and symptomatic responses to subsequent hypoglycemia after one episode of hypoglycemia in nondiabetic humans. Diabetes 1991;40:223-226.
81. Segel SA, Paramore DS, Cryer PE. Hypoglycemia-associated autonomic failure in advanced type 2 diabetes. Diabetes 2002;51: 724-733.
82. Banarer S, Cryer PE. Sleep-related hypoglycemia-associated autonomic failure in type 1 diabetes. Diabetes 2003;52:1195-1203.
83. Ertl AC, Davis SN. Evidence for a vicious cycle of exercise and hypoglycemia in type 1 diabetes mellitus. Diabetes Metab Res Rev 2004;20:124-130.
84. Fanelli CG, Paramore DS, Hershey T, et al. Impact of nocturnal hypoglycemia on hypoglycemic cognitive dysfunction in type 1 diabetes mellitus. Diabetes 1998;47:1920-1927.
85. Ovalle F, Fanelli CG, Paramore DS, et al. Brief twice weekly episodes of hypoglycemia reduce detection of clinical hypoglycemia in type 1 diabetes mellitus. Diabetes 1998;47:1472-1479.
86. Fanelli CG, Pampanelli S, Epifano L, et al. Long-term recovery from unawareness, deficient counterregulation and lack of cognitive dysfunction during hypoglycemia following institution of rational intensive therapy in IDDM. Diabetologia 1994;37:1265-1276.
87. Cranston I, Lomas J, Maran A, et al. Restoration of hypoglycemia unawareness in patients with long duration insulin-dependent diabetes mellitus. Lancet 1994;344:283-287.
88. Dagogo-Jack S, Rattarasarn C, Cryer PE. Reversal of hypoglycemia unawareness, but not defective glucose counterregulation, in IDDM. Diabetes 1994;43:1426-1434.
89. Berlin I, Grimaldi A, Payan C, et al. Hypoglycemic symptoms and decreased β-adrenergic sensitivity in insulin dependent diabetic patients. Diabetes Care 1987;10:742-747.
90. Fritsche A, Stefan N, Häring H, et al. Avoidance of hypoglycemia restores hypoglycemia awareness by increasing β-adrenergic sensitivity in type 1 diabetes. Ann Intern Med 2001;134:729-736.
91. Davis SN, Shavers C, Mosqueda-Garcia R, Costa F. Effects of differing antecedent hypoglycemia on subsequent counterregulation in normal humans. Diabetes 1997;46:1328-1335.
92. Perriello G, De Feo P, Torlone E, et al. The dawn phenomenon in type 1 (insulin dependent) diabetes mellitus: magnitude, frequency, variability, and dependence on glucose counterregulation and insulin sensitivity. Diabetes 1991;34:21-28.
93. Hirsh IB. Insulin analogues. N Engl J Med 2005;352:174-183.
94. Raju B, Arbelaez A, Breckenridge SM, Cryer PE. Nocturnal hypoglycemia in type 1 diabetes: an assessment of preventive bedtime treatments. J Clin Endocrinol Metab 2006;91:2087-2092.
95. DeVries JH. Will long acting insulin analogs influence the use of insulin pump therapy in type 1 diabetes? Curr Diabetes Rev 2005;1:23-26.
96. Hirsch IB, Bode BW, Garg S, et al. Continuous subcutaneous insulin infusion (CSII) of insulin aspart versus multiple daily injection of insulin aspart/insulin glargine in type 1 diabetic patients previously treated with CSII. Diabetes Care 2005;28: 533-538.
97. The Diabetes Research in Children (DirecNet) Study Group. Accuracy of the GlucoWatch G2 Biographer and the Continuous Glucose Monitoring System during hypoglycemia. Diabetes Care 2004;27: 722-726.
98. The Diabetes Research in Children (DirecNet) Study Group. A randomized multicenter trial comparing the GlucoWatch Biographer with standard glucose monitoring in children with type 1 diabetes. Diabetes Care 2005;28:1101-1106.
99. MacCuish AC. Treatment of hypoglycemia. In Frier BM, Fisher BM (eds). Diabetes and Hypoglycaemia. London: Edward Arnold, 1993:212-221.
100. Wiethop BV, Cryer PE. Alanine and terbutaline in the treatment of hypoglycemia in IDDM. Diabetes Care 1993;16:1131-1136.
101. Hvidberg AM, Jørgensen S, Hilsted J. The effect of genetically engineered glucagon on glucose recovery after hypoglycaemia in man. Br J Clin Pharmacol 1992;34:547-550.
102. Haymond MW, Schreiner B. Mini-dose glucagon rescue for hypoglycemia in children with type 1 diabetes. Diabetes Care 2001;24: 643-645.
103. Service FJ. Hypoglycemic disorders. Endocrinol Metab Clin North Am 1999;28:467-661.
104. Marks V, Teale JD. Drug-induced hypoglycemia. Endocrinol Metab Clin North Am 1999;28:555-578.
105. Marks V, Teale JD. Hypoglycemia: factitious and felonious. Endocrinol Metab Clin North Am 1999;28:579-601.
106. Lecavalier L, Bolli G, Cryer P, et al. Contributions of gluconeogenesis and glycogenolysis during glucose counterregulation in normal humans. Am J Physiol 1989;256:E844-E851.
107. Yki-Järvinen H, Koivisto VA, Ylikahri R, et al. Acute effects of ethanol and acetate on glucose kinetics in normal subjects. Am J Physiol 1988;254:E175-E180.
108. Avogaro A, Valerio A, Miola M, et al. Ethanol impairs insulin-mediated glucose uptake by an indirect mechanism. J Clin Endocrinol Metab 1996;81:2285-2290.
109. Raschke R, Arnold-Capell PA, Richeson R, et al. Refractory hypoglycemia secondary to topical salicylate intoxication. Arch Intern Med 1991;151:591-593.
110. Hundal RS, Petersen KF, Mayerson AB, et al. Mechanism by which high-dose aspirin improves glucose metabolism in type 2 diabetes. J Clin Invest 2002;109:1321-1326.
111. Poretsky L, Moses AC. Hypoglycemia associated with trimethoprim/sulfamethoxazole therapy. Diabetes Care 1984;7: 508-509.
112. Assan R, Perronne C, Assan D, et al. Pentamidine-induced derangements of glucose metabolism. Diabetes Care 1995;18:47-55.
113. Taylor TE, Molyneux ME, Wirima JJ, et al. Blood glucose levels in Malawian children before and during the administration of intra-

venous quinine for severe falciparum malaria. N Engl J Med 1988;319:1040-1047.
114. Limburg PJ, Katz H, Grant CS, et al. Quinine-induced hypoglycemia. Ann Intern Med 1993;119:218-219.
115. Park-Wyllie LY, Juurlink DN, Kopp A, et al. Outpatient gatifloxacin therapy and dysglycemia in older adults. N Engl J Med 2006; 354:1352-1361.
116. Cacoub P, Deray G, Baumelou A, et al. Disopyramide-induced hypoglycemia: case report and review of the literature. Fundam Clin Pharmacol 1989;3:527-535.
117. Moore N, Kreft-Jais C, Haramburu F, et al. Report of hypoglycaemia associated with use of ACE inhibitors and other drugs: a case/noncase study in French pharmacovigilance system database. Br J Pharmacol 1997;44:513-518.
118. Hesse B, Pedersen JT. Hypoglycemia after propranolol in children. Acta Med Scand 1973;193:551-552.
119. Hirsch IB, Boyle PJ, Craft S, et al. Higher glycemic thresholds for symptoms during β-adrenergic blockade in IDDM. Diabetes 1991;40:1177-1186.
120. Mann FC, Magath TB. Studies on the physiology of the liver. II: The effect of the removal of the liver on the blood sugar level. Arch Intern Med 1922;30:73-84.
121. Felig P, Brown WV, Levine RA, et al. Glucose homeostasis in viral hepatitis. N Engl J Med 1970;283:1436-1440.
122. Younus S, Soterakis J, Sosi AJ, et al. Hypoglycemia secondary to metastases to the liver. Gastroenterology 1977;72:334-337.
123. Medalle R, Webb R, Waterhouse C. Lactic acidosis and hypoglycemia. Arch Intern Med 1971;128:273-278.
124. Haviv YS, Sharkia M, Safadi R. Hypoglycemia in patients with renal failure. Ren Fail 2000;22:219-223.
125. Garber AJ, Bier DM, Cryer PE, et al. Hypoglycemia in compensated chronic renal insufficiency. Diabetes 1974;23:982-986.
126. Rutsky EA, McDaniel HG, Tarpe DL, et al. Spontaneous hypoglycemia in chronic renal failure. Arch Intern Med 1978;138: 1364-1368.
127. Chen YT, Burchell A. Glycogen storage diseases. In Scriver CR, Beaudetal AL, Sly WS, Valle D (eds). The Metabolic and Molecular Bases of Inherited Disease, 7th ed. New York: McGraw Hill, 1995:935-965.
128. Miller SI, Wallace RJ Jr, Musher DM, et al. Hypoglycemia as a manifestation of sepsis. Am J Med 1980;68:649-653.
129. Maitra SR, Wojnar MM, Lang CH. Alterations in tissue glucose uptake during the hyperglycemic and hypoglycemic phases of sepsis. Shock 2000;13:379-385.
130. Lee MD, Zentella A, Pekala PH, et al. Effect of endotoxin-induced monokines on glucose metabolism in the muscle cell line L6. Proc Natl Acad Sci U S A 1987;84:2590-2594.
131. Sakurai Y, Zhang X-J, Wolfe RR. TNF directly stimulates glucose uptake and leucine oxidation and inhibits FFA flux in conscious dogs. Am J Physiol 1996;270:E864-E872.
132. Metzger S, Nusair S, Planer D, et al. Inhibition of hepatic gluconeogenesis and enhanced glucose uptake contribute to the development of hypoglycemia in mice bearing interleukin-1β-secreting tumors. Endocrinology 2004;145:5150-5156.
133. Lang CH, Bagby GJ, Blakesley HL, et al. Importance of hyperglucagonemia in eliciting the sepsis-induced increase in glucose production. Circ Shock 1989;29:181-191.
134. McKechnie K, Dean HG, Furman BL, et al. Plasma catecholamines during endotoxin infusion in conscious unrestrained rats: effects of adrenal demedullation and/or guanethidine treatment. Circ Shock 1985;17:85-94.
135. Bagby GJ, Lang CH, Skrepnik N, et al. Attenuation of glucose metabolic changes resulting from TNF administration by adrenergic blockade. Am J Physiol 1992;262:R628-R635.
136. Hargrove DM, Lang CH, Bagby GJ, et al. Epinephrine-induced increase in glucose turnover is diminished during sepsis. Metabolism 1989;38:1070-1076.
137. Wharton B. Hypoglycemia in children with kwashiorkor. Lancet 1970;1:171-173.
138. Bruce AK, Jacobsen E, Dossing H, et al. Hypoglycaemia in spinal muscular atrophy. Lancet 1995;346:609-610.
139. Ørngreen MC, Zacho M, Hebert A, et al. Patients with severe muscle wasting are prone to develop hypoglycemia during fasting. Neurology 2003;61:997-1000.
140. Goodman HG, Grumbach MM, Kaplan SL. Growth and growth hormone. II: A comparison of isolated growth hormone deficiency and multiple pituitary hormone deficiencies in 35 patients with idiopathic hypopituitary dwarfism. N Engl J Med 1968;278:57-68.
141. Haymond MW, Karl I, Weldon VV, et al. The role of growth hormone and cortisone in glucose and gluconeogenic substrate regulation in fasted hypopituitary children. J Clin Endocrinol Metab 1976;42: 846-856.
142. Wolfsdorf JI, Sadeghi-Nejad A, Senior B. Hypoketonemia and age-related fasting hypoglycemia in growth hormone deficiency. Metabolism 1983;32:457-462.
143. Frizell RT, Campbell PJ, Cherrington AD. Gluconeogenesis and hypoglycemia. Diabetes Metab Rev 1988;4:51-70.
144. Aynsley-Green A, Moncrieff MW, Ratter S, et al. Isolated ACTH deficiency. Arch Dis Child 1978;53:499-502.
145. Rudman D, Moffitt SD, Fernhoff PM, et al. Epinephrine deficiency in hypocorticotropic hypopituitary children. J Clin Endocrinol Metab 1981;53:722-729.
146. Voorhees ML, Jakubowski AF, MacGillivray MH. The adrenomedullary and glucagon responses of hypopituitary children to insulin induced hypoglycemia. Pediatr Res 1981;15:912-915.
147. Smallridge RC, Corrigan DF, Thomason AM, et al. Hypoglycemia in pregnancy: occurrence due to adrenocorticotropic hormone and growth hormone deficiency. Arch Intern Med 1980;140: 564-565.
148. Steer P, Marnell R, Werk EE Jr. Clinical alcohol hypoglycemia and isolated adrenocorticotropic hormone deficiency. Ann Intern Med 1969;71:343-348.
149. Shah SD, Tse TF, Clutter WE, et al. The human sympathochromaffin system. Am J Physiol 1984;247:E380-E384.
150. Christensen NJ. Hypoadrenalinemia during insulin hypoglycemia in children with ketotic hypoglycemia. J Clin Endocrinol Metab 1974;38:107-112.
151. Rosenbloom AL, Tiwary CM. Ketotic (idiopathic glucagon unresponsive) hypoglycemia: catecholamine excretion and effects of ephedrine therapy. Arch Dis Child 1972;47:924-926.
152. Court JM, Dunlop ME, Boulton TJC. Effect of ephedrine in ketotic hypoglycemia. Arch Dis Child 1974;49:63-65.
153. Kerr DS, Brooke OG, Robinson HM. Fasting energy utilization in the smaller of twins with epinephrine-deficient hypoglycemia. Metabolism 1981;30:6-17.
154. Kerr DS, Picou DIM. Fasting glucose production in the smaller of twins with epinephrine-deficient hypoglycemia. Metabolism 1981;30:18-26.
155. Light IJ, Sutherland JM, Loggie JM, et al. Impaired epinephrine release in hypoglycemic infants of diabetic mothers. N Engl J Med 1967;277:394-398.
156. Starke AAR, Valverde I, Botazzo GF, et al. Glucagon deficiency associated with hypoglycaemia and the absence of islet cell antibodies in the polyglandular failure syndrome before the onset of insulin-dependent diabetes mellitus: a case report. Diabetologia 1983;25:336-339.
157. Vidnes J, Oyaseater S. Glucagon deficiency causing severe neonatal hypoglycemia in a patient with normal insulin secretion. Pediatr Res 1977;11:943-949.
158. Kollee LA, Monnens LA, Cejka V, et al. Persistent neonatal hypoglycemia due to glucagon deficiency. Arch Dis Child 1978;53: 422-424.
159. Fukuda I, Hizuka N, Ishikawa Y, et al. Clinical features of insulin-like growth factor-II producing non–islet-cell tumor hypoglycemia. Growth Hormone and IGF Research 2006;16:211-216.
160. Eastman RC, Carson RE, Orloff DG, et al. Glucose utilization in a patient with hepatoma and hypoglycemia. J Clin Invest 1992;89:1958-1963.
161. Seckl MJ, Mulholland PJ, Bishop AE, et al. Hypoglycemia due to an insulin-secreting small cell carcinoma of the cervix. N Engl J Med 1999;341:733-736.
162. Zapf J, Futo E, Peter M, et al. Can "big" insulin-like growth factor II in serum of tumor patients account for the development of extrapancreatic tumor hypoglycemia? J Clin Invest 1992;90:2574-2584.
163. Daughaday WH, Trivedi B, Baxter RC. Serum "big insulin-like growth factor II" from patients with tumor hypoglycemia lacks normal E-domain *O*-linked glycosylation, a possible determinant of normal propeptide processing. Proc Natl Acad Sci U S A 1993;90:5823-5827.

164. Daughaday WH. The pathophysiology of IGF-II hypersecretion in non–islet tumor hypoglycemia. Diabetes Rev 1995;3:62-72.
165. Bourcigaux N, Arnault-Quary G, Christol R, et al. Treatment of hypoglycemia using combined glucocorticoid and recombinant human growth hormone in a patient with metastatic non–islet cell tumor hypoglycemia. Clinical Therapeutics 2005;27:246-251.
166. Nauck MA, Reinecke M, Perren A, et al. Hypoglycemid due to paraneoplastic secretion of insulin-like growth factor-I in a patient with metastasizing large cell carcinoma of the lung. J Clin Endocrinol Metab 2007;92:1600-1605.
167. Marks V, Teale JD. Investigation of hypoglycaemia. Clin Endocrinol (Oxf) 1996;44:133-136.
168. Gama R, Teale JD, Marks V. Clinical and laboratory investigation of adult spontaneous hypoglycaemia. J Clin Path 2003;56: 641-646.
169. Service FJ, Natt N. The prolonged fast. J Clin Endocrinol Metab 2000;85:3973-3974.
170. Hirshberg B, Livi A, Bartlett DL, et al. Forty-eight-hour fast: the diagnostic test for insulinoma. J Clin Endocrinol Metab 2000;85: 3222-3226.
171. Højlund K, Wildner-Christensen M, Eshøj O, et al. Reference intervals for glucose, β-cell polypeptides, and counterregulatory factors during prolonged fasting. Am J Physiol 2001;280:E50-E58.
172. Thompson GB. Diagnosis and management of insulinoma. Endocr Pract 2002;8:385-386.
173. Vezzosi D, Bennet A, Fauvel J, et al. Insulin levels measured with an insulin-specific assay in patients with fasting hypoglycaemia related to endogenous hyperinsulinism. Eur J Endocrinol 2003;149:413-419.
174. Heald AH, Bhattacharya B, Cooper H, et al. Most commercial insulin assays fail to detect recombinant insulin analogues. Ann Clin Biochem 2006;43:306-308.
175. Basu A, Service FJ, Yu L, et al. Insulin autoimmunity and hypoglycemia in seven white patients. Endocr Pract 2005;11:97-103.
176. Goldman J, Baldwin D, Rubenstein AH, et al. Characterization of circulating insulin and proinsulin binding antibodies in autoimmune hypoglycemia. J Clin Invest 1979;63:1050-1059.
177. Kiyokawa H, Kono N, Hamaguchi T, et al. Hyperinsulinemia due to impaired insulin clearance associated with fasting hypoglycemia and postprandial hyperglycemia: an analysis of a patient with antiinsulin antibodies. J Clin Endocrinol Metab 1989;69: 616-621.
178. Arioglu E, Andewelt A, Diabo C, et al. Clinical course of the syndrome of autoantibodies to the insulin receptor (type B insulin resistance). Medicine (Baltimore) 2002;81:87-100.
179. Wilkin TJ, Hammonds P, Mirza JH, et al. Graves' disease of the β-cell: glucose dysregulation due to islet-cell stimulating antibodies. Lancet 1988;2:1155-1158.
180. Foggensteiner L, Bone AJ, Webster KA, et al. Increased preproinsulin mRNA in pancreatic islets incubated with islet cell–stimulating antibodies from serums of type I diabetic patients. Diabetes 1990;39:1165-1169.
181. Service FJ, McMahon MM, O'Brien PC, et al. Functioning insulinoma: incidence, recurrence, and long-term survival of patients. Mayo Clin Proc 1991;66:711-719.
182. Agarwal SK, Burns AL, Sukhodolets KE, et al. Molecular pathology of the *MEN1* gene. Ann N Y Acad Sci 2004;1014:189-198.
183. Philippe J, Powers AC, Mojsov S, et al. Expression of peptide hormone genes in human islet cell tumors. Diabetes 1988;37: 647-651.
184. D'Arcangues CM, Awoke S, Lawrence GD. Metastatic insulinoma with long survival and glucagonoma syndrome. Ann Intern Med 1984;100:233-235.
185. Rizza RA, Haymond MW, Verdonk CA, et al. Pathogenesis of hypoglycemia in insulinoma patients: suppression of hepatic glucose production by insulin. Diabetes 1981;30:377-381.
186. Service FJ, Dale AJD, Elveback LR, et al. Insulinoma: clinical and diagnostic features of 60 consecutive cases. Mayo Clin Proc 1976;51:417-429.
187. Kaltsas GA, Besser GM, Grossman AB. The diagnosis and medical management of neuroendocrine tumors. Endocr Rev 2004;25: 458-511.
188. Grossman AB, Reznek RH. Commentary: imaging of islet cell tumors. Best Pract Res Clin Endocrinol Metab 2005;19: 241-243.
189. Noone TC, Hosey J, Firat Z, Semelka RC. Imaging and localization of islet cell tumors of the pancreas on CT and MRI. Best Pract Res Clin Endocrinol Metab 2005;19:195-211.
190. Fritscher-Ravens A. Endoscopic ultrasound and neuroendocrine tumours of the pancreas. J Pancreas 2004;5:273-281.
191. McLean AM, Fairclough PD. Endoscopic ultrasound in the localization of pancreatic islet cell tumours. Best Pract Res Clin Endocrinol Metab 2005;19:177-193.
192. Virgolini I, Traub-Weidinger T, Decristoforo C. Nuclear medicine in the detection and management of pancreatic islet-cell tumors. Best Pract Res Clin Endocrinol Metab 2005;19:213-227.
193. Kumbasar B, Kamel IR, Tekes A, et al. Imaging of neuroendocrine tumors: accuracy of helical CT versus SRS. Abdom Imaging 2004;29:696-702.
194. Wiesli P, Brändle M, Schmid C, et al. Selective arterial calcium stimulation and hepatic venous sampling in the evaluation of hyperinsulinemic hypoglycemia: potential and limitations. J Vasc Interv Radiol 2004;15:1251-1256.
195. Jackson JE. Angiography and arterial stimulation venous sampling in the localization of pancreatic neuroendocrine tumours. Best Pract Res Clin Endocrinol Metab 2005;19:229-239.
196. Axelrod L. Insulinoma: cost-effective care in patients with rare disease. Ann Intern Med 1995;123:311-312.
197. Kinoshita Y, Nonaka H, Suzuki S, et al. Accurate localization of insulinomas using percutaneous transhepatic portal venous sampling: usefulness of simultaneous measurement of plasma insulin and glucagon levels. Clin Endocrinol (OxF) 1985;23:587-593.
198. Kauhanen S, Seppänenm, Minn H, et al. Flourine-18-L-dihydroxyphenylalanine (^{18}F-DOPA) positron emission tomography as a tool to localize an insulinoma or β-cell hyperplasid in adult patients. J Clin Endocrinol Metab 2007;92:1237-1244.
199. Marks V, Samols E. Diazoxide therapy of intractable hypoglycemia. Ann N Y Acad Sci 1968;150:442-454.
200. Hearn PR, Ahmed M, Woodhouse NJY. The use of SMS 201-995 (somatostatin analogue) in insulinomas. Horm Res 1988;29: 211-213.
201. Thompson GB, Service FJ, Andrews JC, et al. Noninsulinoma pancreatogenous hypoglycemia syndrome: an update in 10 surgically treated patients. Surgery 2000;128:937-945.
202. Starke A, Saddig C, Kirch B, et al. Islet hyperplasia in adults: challenge to preoperatively diagnose non-insulinoma pancreatogenic hypoglycemia syndrome. World J Surg 2006;30:670-679.
203. Service GJ, Thompson GB, Service FJ, et al. Hyperinsulinemic hypoglycemia with nesidioblastosis after gastric bypass surgery. N Engl J Med 2005;353:249-254.
204. Goldfine AB, Mun E, Patti ME. Hyperinsulinemic hypoglycemia following gastric bypass surgery for obesity. Curr Opin Endocrinol Diabetes 2006;13:419-424.
205. Anlauf M, Wieben D, Perren A, et al. Persistent hyperinsulinemic hypoglycemia in 15 adults with diffuse nesidioblastosis. Am J Surg Pathol 2005;29:524-533.
206. Sperling MA, Menon RK. Differential diagnosis and management of neonatal hypoglycemia. Pediatr Clin N Am 2004;51:703-723.
207. Losek J. Hypoglycemia and the ABC's (sugar) of pediatric resuscitation. Ann Emerg Med 2000;35:43-46.
208. Bier DM, Leake RD, Haymond MW, et al. Measurement of "true" glucose production rates with 6,6-dideuteroglucose. Diabetes 1977;26:1016-1023.
209. Haymond MW, Karl IE, Pagliara AS. Increased gluconeogenic substrates in small for gestational age infants. N Engl J Med 1974;291: 332-328.
210. Haymond MW, Karl IE, Pagliara AS. Ketotic hypoglycemia: an amino acid substrate limited disorder. J Clin Endocrinol Metab 1974;38:521-530.
211. Hussain K, Cosgrove KE, Shepherd RM, et al. Hyperinsulinemic hypoglycemia in Beckwith-Wiedemann syndrome due to defects in the function of pancreatic β-cell adenosine triphosphate–sensitive potassium channels. J Clin Endocrinol Metab 2005;90: 4376-4382.
212. Clark W, O'Donovan D. Transient hyperinsulinism in an asphyxiated newborn infant with hypoglycemia. Amer J Perinatol 2001;18:175-178.
213. Dunne MJ, Cosgrove KE, Shepherd RM, et al. Hyperinsulinism in infancy: from basic science to clinical disease. Physiol Rev 2004;84:239-275.

214. Giurgea I, Bellanné-Chantelot C, Ribeiro M, et al. Molecular mechanisms of neonatal hyperinsulinism. Horm Res 2006;66:289-296.
215. Ashcroft FM. ATP-sensitive potassium channelopathies: focus on insulin secretion. J Clin Invest 2005;115:2047-2058.
216. Raju B, Cryer PE. Mechanism, temporal patterns and magnitudes of the metabolic responses to the K_{ATP} channel agonist diazoxide. Am J Physiol 2005;288:E80-E85.
217. Bas F, Darendeliler F, Demirkol D, et al. Successful therapy with calcium channel blocker (nifedipine) in persistent neonatal hyperinsulinemic hypoglycemia of infancy. J Pediatr Endocrinol Metab 1999;12:873-878.
218. Mohnike K, Blankenstein O, Christesen HT, et al. Proposal for a standardized protocol for ^{18}F-DOPA-PET (PET/CT) in congenital hyperinsulinism. Horm Res 2006;66:40-42
219. Molven A, Matre GE, Duran M, et al. Familial hyperinsulinemic hypoglycemia caused by a defect in the SCHAD enzyme of mitochondrial fatty acid oxidation. Diabetes 2004;53:221-227.
220. Sun L, Eklund EA, Chung WK, et al. Congenital disorder of glycosylation ID presenting with hyperinsulinemic hypoglycemia and islet cell hyperplasia. J Clin Endocrinol Metab 2005;90:4371-4375.
221. Baumann U, Preece MA, Green A, et al. Hyperinsulinism in tyrosinaemia type I. J Inherit Metab Dis 2005;28:131-135.
222. Cori GT, Cori CF. Glucose-6-phosphatase of the liver in glycogen storage disease. J Biol Chem 1952;199:661-667.
223. Chen YT, Burchell A. Glycogen storage diseases. In Scriver CR, Beaudet AL, Sly WS, Valle D (eds). The Metabolic and Molecular Bases of Inherited Disease, 7th ed. New York: McGraw-Hill, 1995: 935-965.
224. Koestinger A, Gillet M, Chiol'ero R, et al. Effect of liver transplantation on hepatic glucose metabolism in a patient with type I glycogen storage disease. Transplantation 2000;69:2205-2207.
225. Muraca M, Gerunda G, Neri D, et al. Hepatocyte transplantation as a treatment for glycogen storage disease type 1a. Lancet 2002; 359:317-318.
226. Rother KI, Schwenk WF. Glucose production in glycogen storage disease I is not associated with increased cycling through hepatic glycogen. Am J Physiol 1995;269:E774-E778.
227. Van den Berghe G. Disorders of gluconeogenesis. J Inherit Metab Dis 1996;19:470-477.
228. Brown GK. Glucose transporters: structure, function and consequences of deficiency. J Inherit Metab Dis 2000;23:237-246.
229. Gitzelmann R, Steinmann B, van den Berghe G. Disorders of fructose metabolism. In Scriver CR, Beaudet AL, Sly WS, Valle D (eds). The Metabolic and Molecular Bases of Inherited Disease, 7th ed. New York: McGraw-Hill, 1995:905-934.
230. Segal S, Berry GT. Disorders of galactose metabolism. In Scriver CR, Beaudet AL, Sly WS, Valle D (eds). The Metabolic and Molecular Bases of Inherited Disease, 7th ed. New York: McGraw-Hill, 1995:967-1000.
231. Kaufman U, Froesch ER. Inhibition of phosphorylase-a by fructose-1-phosphate, α-glycerophosphate and fructose-1,6-diphosphate: explanation for fructose-induced hypoglycemia in hereditary fructose intolerance and fructose-1,6-diphosphatase deficiency. Eur J Clin Invest 1973;3:407-413.
232. Chuang DT, Shih VE. Disorders of branched chain amino acid and keto acid metabolism. In Scriver CR, Beaudet AL, Sly WS, Valle D (eds). The Metabolic and Molecular Bases of Inherited Disease, 7th ed. New York: McGraw-Hill, 1995:1239-1277.
233. Roe CR, Coates PM. Mitochondrial fatty acid oxidation disorders. In Scriver CR, Beaudet AL, Sly WS, Valle D (eds). The Metabolic and Molecular Bases of Inherited Disease, 7th ed. New York: McGraw-Hill, 1995:1501-1533.
234. Nezu J, Tamai I, Oku A, et al. Primary systemic carnitine deficiency is caused by mutations in a gene encoding sodium ion–dependent carnitine transporter. Nat Genet 1999;21:91-94.
235. Jist LI, Mandel H, Oostheim W, et al. Molecular basis of hepatic carnitine palmitoyltransferase I deficiency. J Clin Invest 1998;102:527-531.
236. Infante JP, Huszagh VA. Secondary carnitine deficiency and impaired docosahexaenoic (22:6n-3) acid synthesis: a common denominator in the pathophysiology of diseases of oxidative phosphorylation and β-oxidation. FEBS Lett 2000;468:1-5.
237. McGarry JD, Brown NF. The mitochondrial carnitine palmitoyltransferase system. Eur J Biochem 1997;244:1-14.
238. Bougnieres PF, Saudubray JM, Marsac C, et al. Fasting hypoglycemia resulting from hepatic carnitine palmitoyltransferase deficiency. J Pediatr 1981;98:742-746.
239. Yamamoto S, Abe H, Kohgo T, et al. Two novel gene mutations (Glu174 → Lys, Phe 383 → Tyr) causing the "hepatic" form of carnitine palmitoyltransferase II deficiency. Hum Genet 1996;98: 116-118.
240. Vianey-Saban C, Guffan N, Delolne F, et al. Diagnosis of inborn errors of metabolism by acylcarnitine profiling in blood using tandem mass spectrometry. J Inherit Metab Dis 1997;20:411-414.
241. Ibdah JA, Bennett MJ, Rinaldo P, et al. A fetal fatty-acid oxidation disorder as a cause of liver disease in pregnant women. N Engl J Med 1999;340:1723-1731.
242. Gebhard B, Holst JJ, Biegelmayer C, Miholic J. Postprandial GLP-1, norepinephrine and reactive hypoglycemia in dumping syndrome. Dig Dis Sci 2001;46:1915-1923.
243. Peter S. Acarbose and idiopathic reactive hypoglycemia. Horm Res 2003;60:166-167.
244. Service FJ. Hypoglycemic disorders. N Engl J Med 1995;332: 1144-1152.
245. Charles MA, Hofeldt F, Shackelford A, et al. Comparison of oral glucose tolerance tests and mixed meals in patients with apparent idiopathic postabsorptive hypoglycemia. Diabetes 1981;30: 465-470.
246. Palardy J, Havrankova J, Lepage R, et al. Blood glucose measurements during symptomatic episodes in patients with suspected postprandial hypoglycemia. N Engl J Med 1989;321:1421-1425.
247. Chalew SA, McLaughlin JV, Mersey J, et al. The use of the plasma epinephrine response in the diagnosis of idiopathic postprandial syndrome. JAMA 1984;251:612-615.
248. Lev-Ran A, Anderson RW. The diagnosis of postprandial hypoglycemia. Diabetes 1981;30:996-999.
249. Kay WW. The treatment of prolonged insulin coma. J Ment Sci 1961;107:194-238.
250. MacCuish AC, Munro JF, Duncan LJP. Treatment of hypoglycaemic coma with glucagon, intravenous dextrose, and mannitol infusion in a hundred diabetics. Lancet 1970;2:946-949.
251. Koch-Weser J. Diazoxide. N Engl J Med 1976;294:1271-1273.
252. Baxter RC, Holman SR, Corbould A, et al. Regulation of the insulin-like growth factors and their binding proteins by glucocorticoid and growth hormone in nonislet cell tumor hypoglycemia. J Clin Endocrinol Metab 1995;80:2700-2708.
253. Baxter RC. The role of insulin-like growth factors and their binding proteins in tumor hypoglycemia. Horm Res 1996;46:195-201.

Section IX

Body Fat and Lipid Metabolism

CHAPTER 34

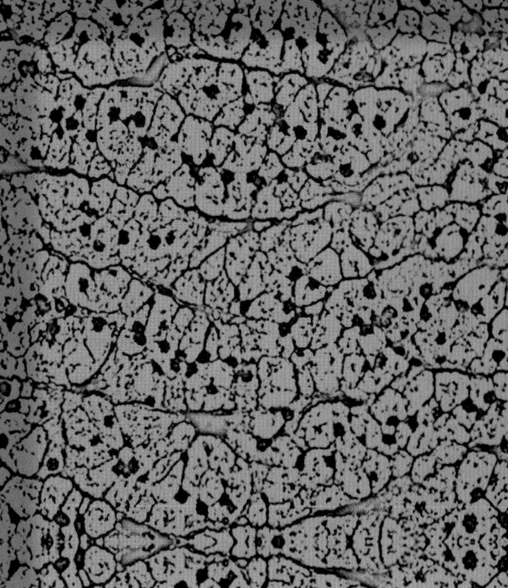

NEUROENDOCRINE CONTROL OF ENERGY STORES

Roger D. Cone and Joel K. Elmquist

INTRODUCTION AND HISTORICAL PERSPECTIVE

The increasing incidence of obesity and diabetes are major health issues facing society. Fortunately, in the past decade several key molecules including hormones and receptors controlling energy homeostasis have been identified. Indeed, we now have a rough central nervous system (CNS) roadmap through which key metabolic signals exert their effects. For example, it is established that key components of the central control of energy balance are located in the hypothalamus. In the twenty-first century it is taken for granted that the hypothalamus is required for coordinated control of food intake and energy homeostasis. The intimate interaction of the hypothalamus and the pituitary gland has been appreciated for some time. However, understanding the primary role of the hypothalamus in controlling long-term energy stores, and thus adipose mass, is relatively recent. For example, at the end of the nineteenth century, clinicians including Alfred Fröhlich described an adiposogenital dystrophic condition in patients with pituitary tumors. This condition became known as Fröhlich's syndrome and was characterized by pituitary tumors associated with excessive subcutaneous fat and hypogonadism.[1,2] However, whether the etiology of this syndrome was due to injury to the pituitary gland or to the overlying hypothalamus was extremely controversial. Several groups, including Cushing and his colleagues, argued that the syndrome was due to disruption of the pituitary gland.[3-5] However, Aschner demonstrated in dogs that mere removal of the pituitary gland without damage to the overlying hypothalamus did not result in obesity.[6] The most definitive evidence of the vital role of the hypothalamus was provided by Hetherington and Ranson when they demonstrated that destruction of the medial basal hypothalamus without damage to the pituitary gland could result in morbid obesity and neuroendocrine derangements in a very similar fashion to the patients reported by Fröhlich.[7] These and subsequent studies firmly established that an intact hypothalamus is required for normal energy and glucose homeostasis.

Following the discoveries that hypothalamic lesions could cause obesity, it also became apparent that lesions in other regions, such as the lateral hypothalamus, could cause leanness. Based on these results, it was suggested that a feeding center was located in the lateral hypothalamus and a satiety center in the ventromedial hypothalamus.[8] As a result of these and other studies, the importance of the hypothalamus as an integrator and effector of energy balance and neuroendocrine function was generally accepted. Humans and other mammals have a remarkable ability to match caloric intake and expenditure, leading to relative stability of body weight and adipose mass over long periods. Based on this observation, Kennedy[9] proposed a mechanism of body weight regulation in which a signal related to energy stores elicited compensatory changes in food intake and energy expenditure, with the result being maintenance of adipose mass at a presumed set point. This view was supported by studies in rodents showing that weight gain from forced overfeeding resulted in a compensatory decrease in voluntary food intake, increased energy expenditure, and eventual restoration of body weight to the previous level, while starvation or lipectomy stimulated feeding and decreased energy expenditure in order to restore body weight and adipose mass to a previous "set point."[10-12] However, the signals mediating the potential interaction between adipose tissue and the brain were not known for many years. Studies by Hervey[13-15] offered important insights into potential signals linking energy stores with energy homeostatic mechanisms. He showed that parabiosis between obese rats with ventromedial hypothalamic (VMH) lesions and normal (nonlesioned) rats led to starvation and weight loss in the latter. In contrast, the VMH-lesioned rats gained weight when parabiosed with lean rats or other VMH-lesioned rats. Results of these studies were thought to indicate that obese VMH-lesioned rats produced a circulating "satiety factor" leading to inhibition of feeding in nonlesioned parabiotic rats. In contrast, the lack of response in VMH-lesioned rats was consistent with the existence of a satiety center proposed in earlier studies.[8] This concept received further support following the discovery of recessive mutations in mice, *ob* and *db*, both of which led to hyperphagia, decreased energy expenditure, and morbid obesity.[16] Parabiosis of lean (wild-type) and *ob/ob* mice suppressed weight gain in *ob/ob* mice, while parabiosis of wild-type and *db/db* mice caused profound hypophagia and weight loss in the former.[17-19] These results were interpreted as meaning that the ob locus was necessary for or involved in the production of a circulating satiety factor, while the *db* locus encoded a component required for the response mechanism to the satiety factor. Predictions based on parabiosis studies were confirmed by the cloning of *ob* and *db* genes in the mid 1990s.[20-22] The hormone product of the *ob* gene was named "leptin" (from the Greek root *leptos*, meaning "thin"), because it potently inhibited feeding, body weight, and adipose mass when injected into leptin-deficient or normal mice.[23-26] In addition to the obese and diabetic mouse strains, the lethal yellow agouti *(A^Y)* mouse had long been known to express an obesity syndrome. Just as molecular cloning of the *ob* and *db* loci led to the discovery of the primary adipostatic factor and its receptor, cloning and characterization of the agouti gene[27-29] has led to characterization of one of the important CNS circuits involved in regulating energy homeostasis, the central melanocortin system.[30,31] These, and related discoveries over the past decade, have taken the understanding of energy homeostasis from the level of gross anatomy to the beginnings of a cellular and molecular basis for the neuroendocrine control of energy stores, the topic of this chapter (Fig. 34–1).

FEEDING AND SATIETY CIRCUITS

As noted, key circuits regulating energy homeostasis and food intake originate in the hypothalamus and brainstem (Fig. 34–2). The hypothalamus is an essential and evolutionarily highly conserved region of the mammalian brain and is the ultimate brain structure that allows mammals to maintain homeostasis. Destruction of the hypothalamus is not compatible with life.[32] Hypothalamic control of homeostasis stems from the ability of hypothalamic neurons to orchestrate behavioral, autonomic, and behavioral responses. This is due to the anatomic connections (both inputs and outputs) of the hypothalamus discussed briefly next.

The hypothalamus receives sensory inputs from the external environment (e.g., light) and information regarding the internal environment (e.g., blood glucose levels). In addition, several hormones known to be key in regulating food intake and metabolism (e.g., glucocorticoids, estrogen, leptin, ghrelin) directly act on neurons in the hypothalamus. The hypothalamus integrates all of this information and in turn provides motor outputs to key regulatory sites including the anterior pituitary gland, the posterior pituitary gland, the cerebral cortex, premotor and motor neurons in the brainstem and spinal cord, and autonomic (parasympathetic and sympathetic) preganglionic neurons. The patterned hypothalamic outputs to these effector sites ultimately result in coordinated endocrine, behavioral, and autonomic responses that maintain homeostasis in several physiologic systems, including energy balance. Within the hypothalamus, several hypothalamic sites are thought to be key in regulating energy homeostasis (see Fig. 34–1). The first group is comprised of groups located in the medial hypothalamus. These groups include arcuate nucleus, the ventral medial nucleus, the dorsal medial nucleus, and the paraventricular nucleus. In addition, the lateral hypothalamus (lateral hypothalamic area and perifornical hypothalamus) are key in regulating food intake and energy homeostasis.

In addition to the hypothalamus, it is now clear that circuits in the brain stem are involved in the coordinated control of food intake as well.[33] For example, in addition to the aforementioned inputs to the hypothalamus, the brain also receives a wide variety of signals from visceral organs including the gastrointestinal (GI) tract. This includes visceral sensory afferents that converge on the dorsal vagal complex. The dorsal vagal complex is comprised of the nucleus of the solitary tract, the dorsal motor nucleus of the vagus (vagal motor neurons), and the area postrema. Sensory afferent signals carried by the glossopharyngeal and vagus nerves include indications of taste, gastric stretch, and levels of glucose and lipids in the liver and portal vein. Nerve terminals carrying this information innervate the nucleus of the solitary tract. This information is relayed to the dorsal motor nucleus of the vagus. The vagal motor neurons in turn innervate the entire GI tract including the pancreas.

In addition, key sensory inputs to the nucleus of the solitary tract from the gastrointesital tract and taste information is directly relayed to the paraventricular, dorsomedial, and arcuate nuclei of the hypothalamus and the lateral hypothalamic area; the central nucleus of the amygdala and bed nucleus of the stria terminalis; and the parabrachial nucleus.[32,34] The parabrachial nucleus then projects to the thalamus, the cerebral cortex, the amygdala, and several hypothalamic sites.[32]

The area postrema is a circumventricular organ that lies directly above the nucleus of the solitary tract. Unlike the nucleus of the solitary tract, which lies inside the blood-brain barrier, and thus is not in direct contact with circulating factors and hormones, neurons in the area postrema sit outside the blood brain barrier.[35] Neurons in the area postrema may respond to circulating gut hormones (e.g., CCK, GLP-1) and relay those signals into the nucleus of the solitary tract and the parabrachial nucleus.[36-40]

The Arcuate Nucleus is a Key Node of Hypothalamic Control of Energy Balance

The arcuate nucleus is perhaps the best characterized hypothalamic nucleus involved in the control of energy balance. For example, the arcuate nucleus is thought to be critical in mediating the actions of metabolic signals such as leptin, insulin, and ghrelin. Specifically, pro-opiomelanocortin (POMC) and neuropeptide Y (NPY)/agouti-related protein (AgRP) neurons within the arcuate nucleus are required for regulating energy homeostasis, food intake, and glucose homeostasis. POMC is a multifunctional pro-peptide that is differentially processed into key peptides in different tissues[41] (Fig. 34–3). In the brain, melanocortin peptides like α-melanocyte stimulating hormone

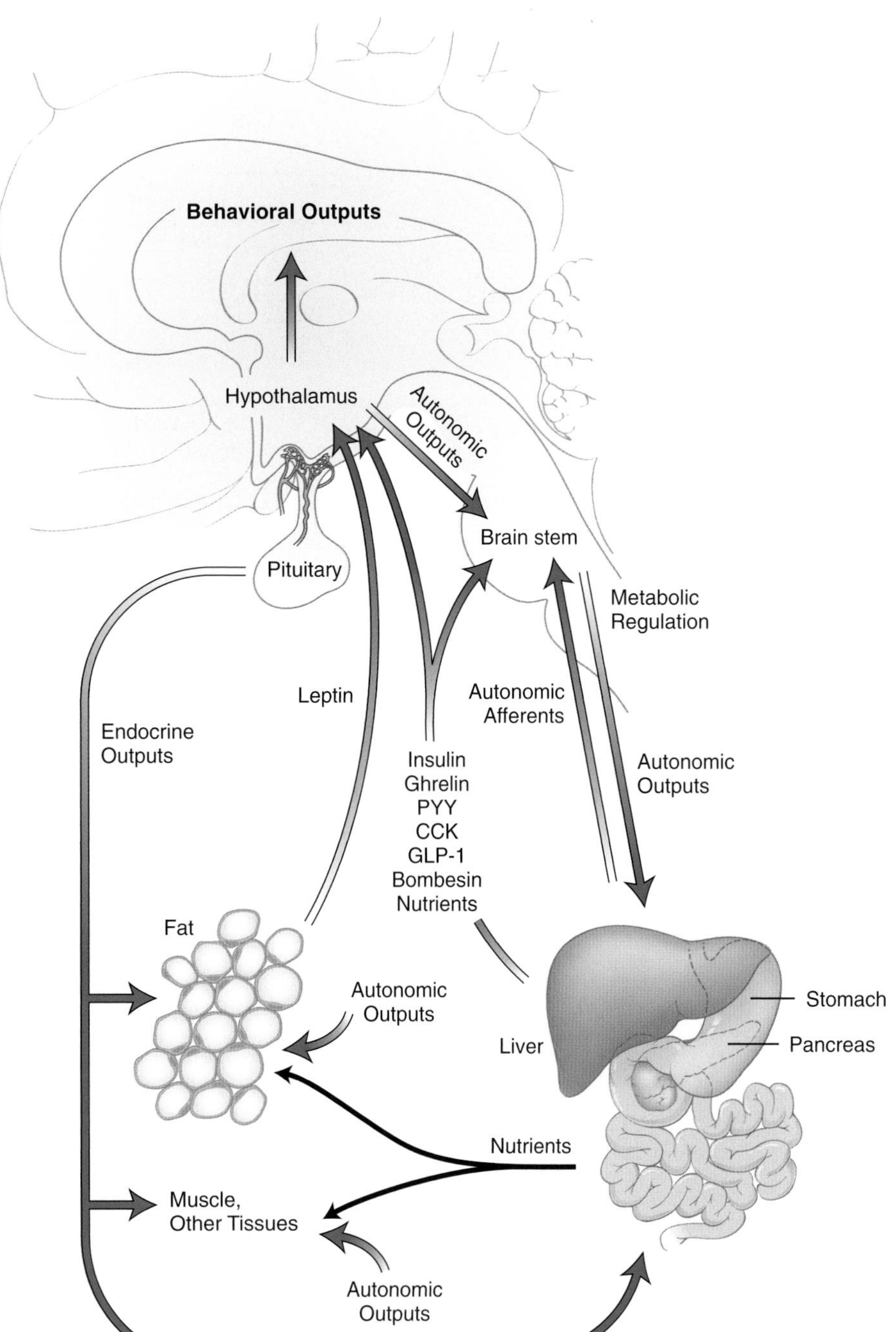

Figure 34–1 ▪ Regulation of energy homeostasis by the brain-gut-adipose axis. *CCK,* Cholecystokinin; *GLP-1,* glucagon-like peptide 1; *PYY,* peptide YY.

(α-MSH) are key products that regulate food intake and energy homeostasis. α-MSH is the agonist for the melanocortin-4 receptor (MC4-R), which is clearly established as key in regulating food intake, energy homeostasis, and glucose homeostasis in both mice and humans.[41,42] Uniquely, an endogenous MC4-R antagonist exists, agouti-related protein (AgRP), that is coexpressed with neuropeptide Y (NPY) in other neurons in the arcuate nucleus of the hypothalamus.

Supportive of a key role of the arcuate nucleus in regulating food intake and energy homeostasis, leptin deficiency (ob/ob mice), and fasting, which lowers leptin levels, results in decreased POMC expression and increased AgRP and NPY expression.[43,44] POMC and NPY/AgRP neurons are located in the arcuate nucleus (Figs. 34–4 and 34–5) and are directly regulated by leptin, ghrelin, glucose, and other metabolic signals. For example, leptin directly depolarizes (activates) POMC neurons and hyperpolarizes (inhibits) AgRP/NPY neurons,[45,46] and deletion of leptin receptors selectively in POMC neurons produces mild obesity.[47] However, leptin also has physiologically relevant actions outside the arcuate nucleus. For example, deletion of leptin receptors from neurons in the ventral medial nucleus produces obesity equal in magnitude to deletion from POMC neurons.[48,49]

In addition to leptin other key metabolic signals act directly on POMC and AgRP neurons in the arcuate nucleus. For example, ghrelin directly depolarizes AgRP/NPY neurons.[50] In addition, serotonin directly activates POMC neurons[51] and inhibitis NPY/AgRP neurons.[52] Moreover, the anorexic properties of

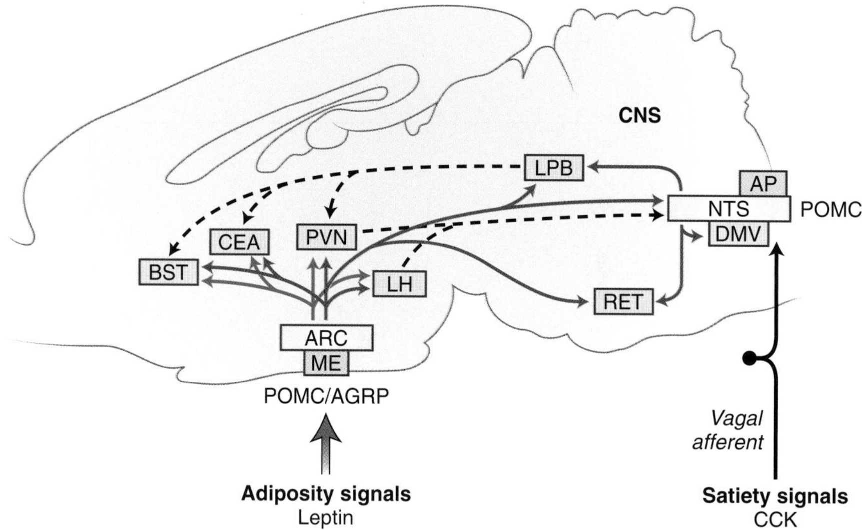

Figure 34–2 ▪ Brain structures involved in energy homeostasis. Receipt of long-term adipostatic signals and acute satiety signals by neurons in arcuate nucleus and brainstem, respectively. Blue: leptin-responsive neurons; yellow: nuclei containing MC4-R neurons that may serve to integrate adipostatic and satiety signals; pink: some circumventricular organs involved in energy homeostasis; red arrows: POMC projections; blue arrows: AgRP projections. *BST,* Bed nucleus of the stria terminalus; *CEA,* central nucleus of the amygdala; *PVN,* paraventricular nucleus of the hypothalamus; *LH,* lateral hypothalamic area; *LPB,* lateral parabrachial nucleus; *AP,* area postrema; *DMV,* dorsal motor nucleus of the vagus. (Adapted from Fan W, et al. Cholecystokinin-mediated suppression of feeding involves the brainstem melanocortin system. Nat Neurosci 2004;7:335-336.)

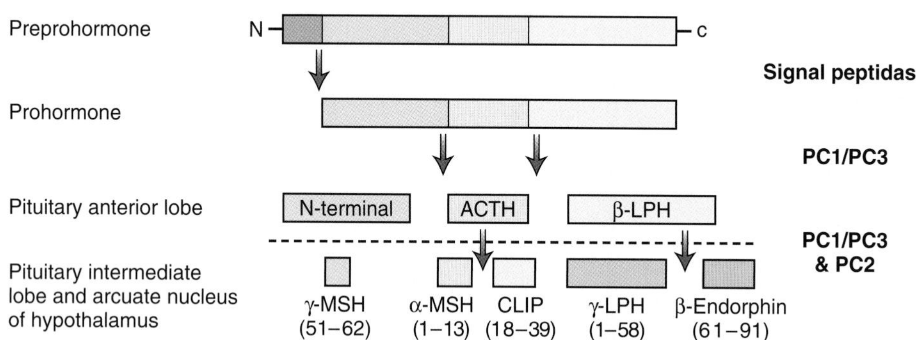

Figure 34–3 ▪ Organization of proopiomelanocortin (POMC), the precursor hormone of corticotropin (ACTH on figure), β-LPH, and related peptides. The precursor protein contains a leader sequence (signal peptide), followed by a long fragment that includes sequence 51-62 corresponding to γ-MSH. This fragment is cleaved at Lys-Arg bonds to form corticotropin 1-39, which in turn includes the sequences for α-MSH (corticotropin 1-13) and corticotropin-like intermediate lobe peptide (CLIP) (corticotropin 18-39), and a sequence corresponding to β-LPH (1-91) that includes γ-LPH 1-58), and β-endorphin (61-91). The β endorphin sequence also includes a sequence corresponding to met-enkephalin. The precursor molecule in the anterior lobe of the pituitary is processed predominantly to corticotropin and β-LPH. In the intermediate pituitary lobe (in the rat), corticotropin and β-LPH are further processed to α-MSH and a β-endorphin–like material. In all extrapituitary tissues, post-translational processing of the prohormone resembles that in the intermediate lobe. Hypothalamic processing is similar but not identical to that in the intermediate lobe. In the latter, β-endorphin and α-MSH are present predominantly in their acetylated forms. β-LPH, β-lipotropin; γ-MSH; γ-melanocyte-stimulating hormone; α-MSH, α-melanocyte-stimulating hormone; γ-LPH, γ-lipotropin. (Figure provided by Dr. Malcolm Low.)

fenfluramine depend in part on MC4-Rs.[52] This is interesting as fenfluramine was used in combination with phenteramine (Fen/Phen) to successfully reduce food intake and body weight in humans, before removal from the market as a result of heart valve disorders and pulmonary hypertension. Importantly, the NPY/AgRP neurons send dense projections to POMC neurons, and thus the orexigenic NPY/AgRP and anorexigenic POMC neurons of the arcuate are coordinately regulated by a wide variety of hormones, drugs, and perhaps nutrients (Fig. 34–6).

Melanocortin-4 Receptors Regulate Energy and Glucose Homeostasis

Several pieces of evidence definitively demonstrate the role for MC4-Rs in the regulation of energy homeostasis. For example, ectopic expression of MC4-R antagonists in the brain induces obesity and diabetes.[42,53] In addition, MC4-R deletion in mice produces obesity.[54] In addition, humans with MC4-R mutations display obesity.[55-58] Indeed, estimates suggest that 5% of cases of severe early onset obesity are the result of heterozygous MC4-R mutations.

MC4-Rs are widely expressed in the brain, many of which could play a role in regulating energy balance.[59-61] However, the sites in the brain that mediate the varied effects of MC4-R agonists are beginning to emerge. Evidence suggests that MC4-Rs expressed by hypothalamic neurons contribute to the effects of MC4-R agonists to regulate energy homeostasis.[62,63] For example, selective restoration of MC4-Rs in the paraventricular nucleus of the hypothalamus in mice lacking MC4-Rs everywhere else normalizes food intake and greatly reduces body weight.[63] However, evidence suggests that extrahypothalamic MC4-Rs contribute to melanocortin action to decrease adipose mass, food intake and

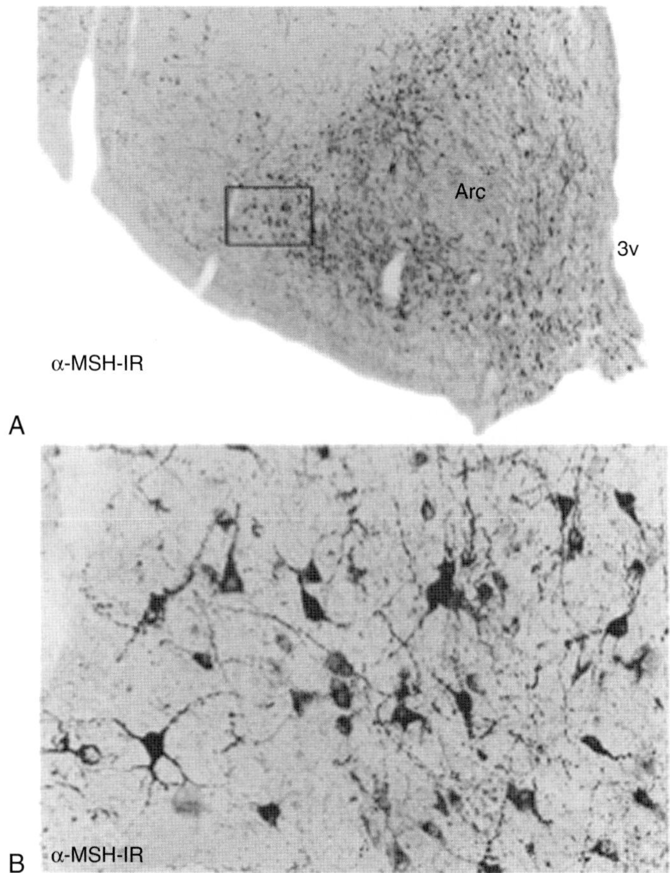

Figure 34–4 ▪ A series of photomicrographs demonstrate that α-melanocyte stimulating hormone-immunoreactive (α-MSH-IR) neurons are present in the human hypothalamus. The neurons are found in the arcuate nucleus of the hypothalamus (Arc; infundibular nucleus). *3v,* Third ventricle. (Modified from Elias CF, et al. Chemically defined projections linking the mediobasal hypothalamus and the lateral hypothalamic area. J Comp Neurol 1998;402:442-459.)

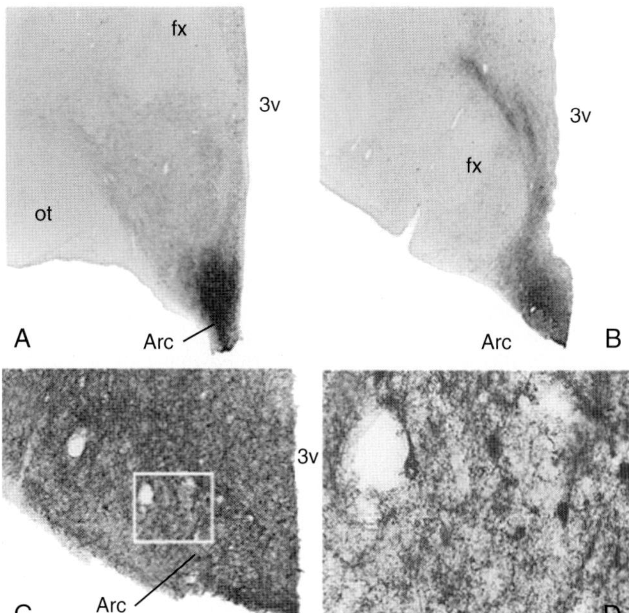

Figure 34–5 ▪ A series of photomicrographs demonstrate that agouti-related peptide-immunoreactive (AgRP-IR) neurons are present in the human hypothalamus. **A** and **B,** Two rostral to caudal low-power photomicrographs demonstrate that AgRP-IR neurons localize to the arcuate nucleus of the hypothalamus (Arc; infundibular nucleus). **B,** Immunoreactive fibers are also observed streaming dorsally out of the arcuate nucleus. **C** and **D,** AgRP-IR neurons are observed in the arcuate nucleus. **D** is a higher magnification of **C** (use box for orientation). *3v,* Third ventricle; *fx,* fornix. (Modified from Elias CF, et al. Chemically defined projections linking the mediobasal hypothalamus and the lateral hypothalamic area. J Comp Neurol 1998;402:442-459.)

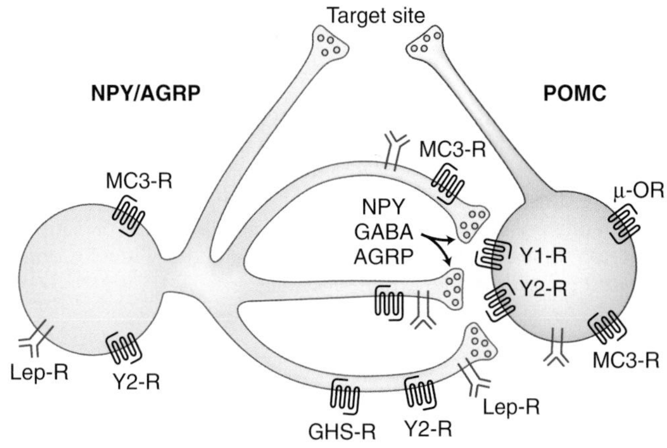

Figure 34–6 ▪ Regulation of the arcuate nucleus of the hypothalamus by various hormones and neuropeptides. NPY/AgRP and POMC neurons within the arcuate nucleus form a coordinately regulated network due to dense NPY/AgRP fibers projecting to POMC cell bodies. Some receptors for the large numbers of hormones and neuropeptides known to regulate the network are indicated. (Modified from Cowley MA, Smart JL, Rubinstein M, et al. Leptin activates anorexigenic POMC neurons through a neural network in the arcuate nucleus. Nature 2001; 411:480-484.)

increase energy expenditure. For example, MC4-R mRNA is densely expressed in the dorsal motor nucleus of the vagus (DMV)[64] including cholinergic parasympathetic preganglionic neurons.[60,61] In addition, injections of the MC4-R agonists into the fourth ventricle decreases food intake and similar injections of MC4-R antagonists dose dependently increases food intake.[65,66] Interestingly, injections of both MC4-R agonists and antagonists into the region of the DMV alter food intake. This is likely mediated by MC4-Rs in the brainstem as this occurs at doses that are ineffective when injected into the fourth ventricle. These findings suggest that extrahypothalamic MC4-Rs contribute to the effects of the MC4-R agonists to regulate food intake, insulin secretion, and energy expenditure. This includes the amplification of satiety signals emanating from the gut such as that mediated by the gut peptide cholecystokinin.[67]

The Lateral Hypothalamus Links Coordinated Food Intake Control and Arousal

The lateral hypothalamus includes the lateral hypothalamic area (LHA) and perifornical hypothalamus. This region of the brain has long been suggested to play a key role in the regulation of ingestive behavior since the early lesion studies of Anand and Brobeck.[68] In the past decade, two neuropeptides were discovered that are expressed by neurons in the lateral hypothalamus. These metabolically regulated peptides are melanin concentrating hormone (MCH) and the orexins (also known as hypocretins).[69-72] MCH and orexin are expressed by distinct subsets of intermingled neurons in the LHA.[73,74] However, both populations broadly innervate the entire neuraxis including monosynaptic projections to other hypothalamic sites, the cerberbral cortex, the amygdala, the brainstem, and the spinal cord.[69,75] The expression patterns of the receptors for both peptides are also widespread.[76-78]

Current data support the view that these LHA neuropeptides play a key role in regulating food intake, adipose mass, and glucose homeostasis. For example, injection of MCH into the brain increases food intake.[70] Mice lacking MCH (knockouts) are hypophagic and lean, and mice that overexpress MCH are obese and hyperleptinemic.[79,80] In addition, mice lacking MCH and leptin are leaner compared to mice that lack leptin but express MCH.[81] The role of orexins in regulating food intake is complex, but it is clear that orexins are required for normal energy balance.[82,83] For example, central injections of orexin peptides increase feeding behavior.[71,84] However, the best characterized role for orexins are in the regulation of state control and in the maintenance of wakefulness,[85,86] because it has been demonstrated that defective orexin signaling causes narcolepsy in mice, dogs, and humans. Other studies have recently demonstrated the ability of orexin neurons to sense changing levels of glucose (see section below).

The exact sites targeted by MCH and orexin neurons to induce feeding remain to be determined and represent an area of active investigation. However, both MCH and orexin neurons have very similar and widespread projection patterns that include the hypothalamus, the brainstem, the cerebral cortex, and the spinal cord. Targets in the brainstem include motor systems and cranial nerve motor nuclei that underlie behaviors like chewing, licking, and swallowing.[33,40] The MCH and orexin neurons also innervate the sympathetic and parasympathetic preganglionic nuclei in the medulla and the spinal cord suggesting that both may be key in regulating the autonomic nervous system. Finally, a key target for both MCH and orexin neurons in coordinating feeding behavior may be their reciprocal connections with the nucleus accumbens. The nucleus accumbens is known to be critical in mediating rewarding components of several stimuli including drugs of abuse, and potentially the rewarding aspects of feeding. Although still being investigated, it is likely that MCH and orexin neurons may be able to enhance the hedonic value of food.[40] Regardless of the specific sites that mediate these effects, it is clear that MCH and orexin neurons are ideally positioned to regulate complex behavior, endocrine function, and autonomic outflow, all of which are key for coordinated control of energy balance.

CENTRAL NERVOUS SYSTEM CONTROL OF THERMOGENESIS

Coordinated energy homeostasis necessarily includes a balance between energy intake and energy expenditure. Energy expenditure is often grouped into three categories: energy required for basal metabolism, energy required for voluntary and involuntary physical activity, and the thermic effect of food. The latter, often referred to as diet-induced thermogenesis (DIT) is estimated at 8% to 10% of total expenditure, and defined as the increased energy expenditure in response to energy intake.[87] This process is under the control of the sympathetic nervous system and the thyroid axis energy expenditure is increased by stimulation of β-adrenergic receptors, and/or elevation of thyroid hormone. In rodents, one tissue mediating this response is brown adipose tissue, which contains adipocytes with dense collections of mitochondria.[88] In addition, the brown adipocytes express uncoupling protein 1 (UCP-1), which uncouple mitochondrial respiration and thus induce energy expenditure and heat. In humans, the key tissue mediating energy expenditure in response to changing energy intake remains to be determined but likely includes skeletal muscle.[88] Regardless, it is clear that the sympathetic nervous system is required for coordinated control of energy expenditure and resistance to diet-induced obesity. For example, mice lacking β-adrenergic receptors (triple knockouts) develop severe obesity when placed on a high-fat diet.[89] Thus, coordinated control of the sympathetic nervous system is required for control of diet-induced thermogenesis.

As noted, the CNS integrates metabolic information into a coordinated set of endocrine, autonomic, and behavioral responses to maintain homeostasis.[32,90,91] Key mediators of these responses are parasympathetic and sympathetic preganglionic neurons (PGNs and SPNs) in the brainstem and spinal cord.[32,92] SPNs extend from the upper thoracic to the upper lumbar segments of the spinal cord and are found within the interomediolateral cell column (IML). Different rostral-caudal levels of the IML provide innervation to different target organs and thus, mediate distinct autonomic responses. For example, SPNs in the upper thoracic levels of the IML are thought to be important for control of the heart and cardiovascular system. Additionally, SPNs in the T6-T12 level of the IML provide innervation of the adrenal gland and endocrine pancreas.[90,93-97]

In addition to the autonomic preganglionic neurons themselves, a key component of the central autonomic control system is direct (monosynaptic) descending innervation from key regulatory groups in the hypothalamus and brainstem.[32,98,99] The projection to the SPNs in the spinal cord is composed of inputs from the arcuate nucleus/retrochiasmatic area, the paraventricular nucleus, and the lateral hypothalamus.[90,99-105] Major projection also arise from the brainstem and includes inputs from the raphe pallidus, catecholaminergic cells in the A5 group of the pons, and C1 cells in the rostral ventral lateral medulla that are critical in maintaining sympathetic tone in the cardiovascular system.[106-109] Thus, there is a relatively circumscribed distribution of neurons providing descending input to sympathetic preganglionic neurons that regulate the cardiovascular system, energy expenditure, adrenal catecholamine secretion, and the endocrine pancreas.

As noted, in rodents central melanocortins are known to regulate energy expenditure in addition to food intake. For example, it has been demonstrated that MC4-R blockade in mice prevents diet-induced thermogenesis[110] and blocks the upregulation of BAT activity,[111] for example, preventing upregulation of expression of uncoupling proteins normally seen when mice are placed on a high-fat diet.[112] The sites mediating the effects of MC4-R agonists on energy expenditure are still not definitively identified. However, a site of MC4-R action relevant to the control of energy expenditure may be the sympathetic preganglionic neurons themselves, which express MC4-Rs.[60] Notably, these neurons receive direct inputs from leptin-responsive POMC neurons.[113] Thus, MC4-Rs expressed by sympathetic preganglionic neurons in the spinal cord may contribute to melanocortin's effects on energy expenditure.

Recently, evidence has suggested that the effects on energy expenditure by MC4-R agonists are mediated by MC4-R-bearing neurons in the raphe pallidus (RPa) in the brainstem.[114,115] Neurons in the RPa innervate sympathetic preganglionic neurons in the IML.[116,117] In addition, RPa neurons are activated by "thermogenic" stimuli and have been shown to control brown adipose tissue thermogenesis.[118,119] Of note, injections of MC4-R agonists into the RPa increases sympathetic nerve activity to brown adipose tissue.[115] Thus, MC4-R expressing neurons in the raphe nucleus may be key in the ability of melanocortin receptor agonists to increase energy expenditure.

HORMONAL REGULATORS OF THE BRAIN-GUT-ADIPOSE AXIS

Adipostatic Factors

Leptin Is the Prototypical Regulator of Energy Homeostasis

In the past decade, the molecular basis for several obesity syndromes have been discovered; prominent among them are the hormone leptin[120] and its receptor[21]. Collectively, these observations have rapidly and dramatically increased our understanding of the pathophysiology of obesity and related disorders. Leptin, the product of the *ob* gene,[120] is produced by white adipose tissue and affects feeding behavior, thermogenesis, and neuroendocrine status. Leptin protein is highly conserved throughout evolution as demonstrated by mouse and human leptin being 84% homologous. Thus far, leptin has been found in birds, and has been tentatively identified in fish. This protein is 167 amino acids and 16 kd, and circulates in the blood at concentrations proportional to the amount of fat depots. Leptin circulates in the bloodstream both as a free protein but also bound to a soluble isoform of its receptor (Ob-Re). Leptin is secreted primarily from the adipocyte; however, minor levels of regulated leptin expression also occurs in other sites such as skeletal muscle, placenta, and stomach.[121,122]

Total lack of leptin or leptin signaling in rodents and humans causes morbid obesity that is accompanied by a wide array of neuroendocrine abnormalities. Replacement with exogenous leptin normalizes these abnormalities.[123-126] Starvation, a time of low energy stores, leads to a fall in serum leptin levels, and has profound effects on several neuroendocrine systems, including activation of the hypothalamic-pituitary-adrenal (HPA) axis, inhibition of the growth hormone and thyroid axes, and inhibition of reproductive function.[127-129] Therefore, lack of leptin has many physiologic responses that are also found in a state of starvation. Interestingly, many of these starvation-induced endocrine and autonomic changes are blocked or blunted by pretreatment with systemic leptin.[127] The dose needed to reverse these abnormalities is lower than needed to induce weight loss in normal rodents. These observations have led to the suggestion that circulating leptin may have evolved to signal the brain that energy stores are sufficient and that a lack of leptin may be responsible for multiple neuroendocrine abnormalities caused by starvation.[130,131] Soon after the discovery of leptin it was clear that most of the varied effects of leptin are mediated by the brain. Over the past few years, studies have begun to unravel some of the complex circuitry involved in leptin signaling.[49]

Distribution of Leptin Receptors

After its transport through the blood-brain barrier, leptin binds to specific receptors in the hypothalamus and brainstem. The "long form" leptin receptor (OB-Rb) is a member of the cytokine-receptor superfamily.[20,21,132] The leptin receptor binds janus kinases (JAK), tyrosine kinases involved in intracellular cytokine signaling. Activation of JAK leads to phosphorylation of members of the signal transduction and transcription (STAT) family of proteins. In turn, these STAT proteins activate transcription of leptin target genes.

The "long form" leptin receptor is required for normal energy homeostasis as mutations of this gene result in the obese phenotype of the *db/db* mouse and the Zucker rat.[20,133,134] Leptin receptors are highly expressed by several hypothalamic nuclei within the medial basal hypothalamus.[135-140] This includes the arcuate, dorsomedial, ventromedial, and ventral premamillary nuclei. Interestingly, leptin receptors are expressed in several extrahypothalamic sites including the nucleus of the solitary tract (where vagal afferents terminate), the substantia nigra, and the ventral tegmental area.

The role of extrahypothalamic leptin receptors is evolving, but evidence is accumulating that leptin has important sites of action within the brainstem. For example, leptin administration increased STAT-3 phosphorylation in several extrahypothalamic sites including the parabrachial nucleus, dorsal raphe, and nucleus of the solitary tract.[141] Moreover, administration of leptin into the fourth ventricle and into the dorsal vagal complex significantly reduced food intake.[33,142-145]

The Role of Insulin and Glucose in Regulating Energy Homeostasis

The concept that the CNS plays a primary role in the control of insulin action and glucose homeostasis is an old concept. This includes observations published in 1849 by Claude Bernard. He suggested that the CNS regulates blood glucose levels following his famous experiments that demonstrated that "piqure" of the floor of the fourth ventricle of rabbits produced increases in blood glucose that were measured by glucose levels in the urine.[4,146] Remarkably, he concluded that the effect was mediated by stimulation of the autonomic input to the liver. Later lesion studies of the hypothalamus also disassociated actions of insulin independent of food intake.[4] These early observations fit remarkably well with very recent findings that have predicted that similar to obesity, diabetes may be viewed as a disorder with underlying defects in the CNS.[147-151]

Insulin Action in the Brain

In addition to its well known role in increasing glucose uptake in tissues such as muscle and fat, insulin also has actions on the brain to regulate energy balance.[152] Insulin receptors are expressed in the brain and injections of insulin into the brain reduce food intake.[152,153] In addition, deletion of insulin receptors specifically from neurons results in mild obesity.[154] More recently, the role of insulin action in the CNS has been investigated in the context of regulation of glucose homeostasis. For example, down-regulation of insulin receptors affect glucose homeostasis, including glucose production by the liver.[150] Thus, insulin action in the brain may be key in coordinated physiological responses to changing levels of metabolic fuels. However, it should be noted that the physiologic significance and relative contributions of central vs peripheral actions of insulin in regulating glucose homeostasis, especially glucose production by the liver is still unclear.[155-157] Going forward a key area of diabetes and obesity research will be investigation of CNS control of glucose homeostasis including hepatic glucose production.

Glucose Levels Are Sensed by Neurons in the Brain

Changing levels of blood glucose are sensed by several distinct populations of neurons in the brain. This was first suggested by classic experiments[158] that demonstrated that some neurons are activated by rising concentrations of glucose while other classes of neurons are inhibited by rising glucose. This model has evolved such that several contemporary models predict that neurons that are activated by rising glucose respond and behave very similarly to β cells of the endocrine pancreas.[159-161] The chemical identity and location of these glucose sensing neurons is still to be determined. For example, several populations of glucose sensitive neurons have been described in the hypothalamus. However, it is clear neurons in the brainstem also sense glucose and are capable of inducing coordinated responses to falling levels of glucose.[162-164]

The cellular mechanisms underlying glucose mediated neuronal excitation likely involves a rise in ATP, resulting from an increase in glucose metabolism, promoting the closure of K_{ATP} channels.[161] In contrast, the mechanisms underlying the ability of neurons to be inhibited by rises in glucose (or conversely to be activated by falling glucose) are not as clearly defined, but may involve the TASK subfamily of two pore, potassium channels as mediating the glucose activated inhibitory current in orexin neurons.[165] Collectively, these observations have led to predictions that changes in glucose levels alter the electrical activity of specific neurons which in turn lead to changes in feeding behavior and glucose production. These models also predict that dysregulation of nutrient sensing in the CNS may contribute to the metabolic alterations characteristic of diabetes and obesity.

POMC Neurons Sense Changes in Glucose Concentration

Consistent with the demonstration that metabolic cues like leptin directly act on POMC neurons, a key role of the central melanocortin system in regulating glucose homeostasis has emerged over the past decade. For example, POMC neurons increase their activity in response to rising glucose.[161] In addition, mice lacking MC4-Rs are hyperinsulinemic before the onset of obesity.[54,148] Recent data has reinforced the concept that vagal input to the liver is a key regulator of hepatic glucose production, potentially including that mediated by melanocortin agonists.[166] The parasympathetic (cholinergic) innervation to the pancreas and liver is provided by the dorsal motor nucleus of the vagus.[97,167,168] The sympathetic innervation of the pancreas is from postganglionic neurons in the celiac ganglia[96,169] that are innervated by preganglionic neurons from mid-thoracic levels of the spinal cord.

In addition, central administration of MC4-R agonists decrease plasma insulin levels in lean and obese mice.[148] This effect was blocked by blockade of α-adrenergic receptors, suggesting that central MC4-R agonists inhibit insulin secretion by activating the sympathetic nervous system. Additionally, administration of MC4-R agonists increases glucose tolerance and lean MC4-R knockout mice are insulin resistant before the onset of obesity.[148] Moreover, MC4-R–deficient humans are hyperinsulinemic, more so than would be expected from their degree of obesity alone. Notably, subjects as young as 12 months old are hyperinsulinemic.[55,56] The sites in the CNS mediating these effects are to be determined, but MC4-Rs are expressed by both parasympathetic and sympathetic preganglionic neurons.[60,61] Thus, it is likely that MC4-R agonists exert a tonic inhibitory influence on insulin secretion by increasing the sympathetic input to the pancreas while simultaneously diminishing the parasympathetic input.[148]

As noted, the activity of orexin neurons of the lateral hypothalamus is altered by changing levels of blood glucose. Specifically, orexin neurons are activated by physiologically relevant decreases in glucose concentrations.[165,170-173] Though still evolving, orexin neurons may be key in coordinating endocrine and autonomic responses to falling glucose levels. It is also likely that orexin neurons may represent one of the populations of "glucose-inhibited" neurons in the lateral hypothalamus that respond to physiologic falls in glucose levels with an increase in activity.[160,174] Moreover, due to its unique anatomic and physiologic properties, the central orexin system may be required to link glucose sensing with wakefulness (i.e., hypoglycemic unawareness) and coordinated autonomic responses.

Satiety and Hunger Factors

Role of the Brain stem in Satiety/Hunger

The brain stem is classically understood as the center for detection and response to hunger/satiety signals. The nucleus of the solitary tract is the primary site for innervation by vagal afferents by the gut (for review, see reference 175; see also Fig. 34–2). The afferent branches deriving from different aspects of the GI tract map viscerotopically along the nucleus tractus solitarius (NTS), from its rostral to caudal aspect.[176] Rostrally, the NTS is a bilaterally symmetrical nucleus, which merges into a single medial body at its caudal extent, called the *commissural NTS*.[177] Vagal afferents deriving input from the upper GI tract are responsive to three basic stimuli, gastric and duodenal distention or contraction, chemical contents of the lumen, and gut peptides and neurotransmitters released from the stomach and duodenum in response to nutrients.[175] In the rat, vagal afferents responding to gastric and duodenal distention tend to map to the medial and commissural divisions of the NTS.[178,179] Vagal afferents responsive to the gut peptide cholecystokinin (CCK) also map to the caudal NTS.[180] The dorsal motor nucleus of the vagus, located just ventral to the NTS, is the primary site of motor efferents to the gut, and is densely innervated by NTS fibers. Together these cell groups, with the area postrema, a circumventricular organ, form the dorsal vagal complex (DVC), and serve as the neuroanatomic substrate for the vagovagal reflex.

Gut Peptides Involved in Satiety and Hunger

In addition to signals from gut distention, gut peptides stimulated by meal intake mediate satiety through centers in the brainstem. Signals received by the brainstem are then thought to interact primarily with long-term weight regulation centers via neural connections to the hypothalamus to regulate total daily intake by adjusting meal size, number, or both.

With the discovery of ghrelin, we now also must consider gut factors that stimulate food intake. Chapter 38 examines GI hormones in detail, focusing on their peripheral actions. Here we consider their central actions. As discussed below, newer data also suggest that a subset of these GI hormones may also act directly on hypothalamic control centers.

Cholecystokinin

Produced by the GI tract in response to meal ingestion, the diverse actions of CCK include stimulation of pancreatic enzyme secretion and intestinal motility, inhibition of gastric motility, and acute inhibition of feeding. Early experiments administering CCK peripherally supported a role for increased CCK levels in the early termination of a meal.[181,182] The finding that repeated injections of CCK lead to reduced meal size without a change in body weight, due to a compensatory increase in meal frequency, argued against CCK acting as a signal regulating long-term energy stores.[183,184]

Two subtypes of the CCK receptor belonging to the G-protein–coupled family of receptors have been described: CCKA and CCKB. Studies using CCK receptor specific antagonists as well as surgical or chemical vagotomy have demonstrated that the satiety effects of CCK are specifically mediated via CCKA receptors on afferent vagal nerves.[185-191]

This interaction between acute vagal input from CCKA receptors and meal termination involves activation of cells in the NTS and AP, modulated by neural connections from the hypothalamus receiving inputs from insulin and leptin. Peripheral administration of CCK potently activates large numbers of neurons in both the NTS and AP (Fig. 34–7). Furthermore, central admin-

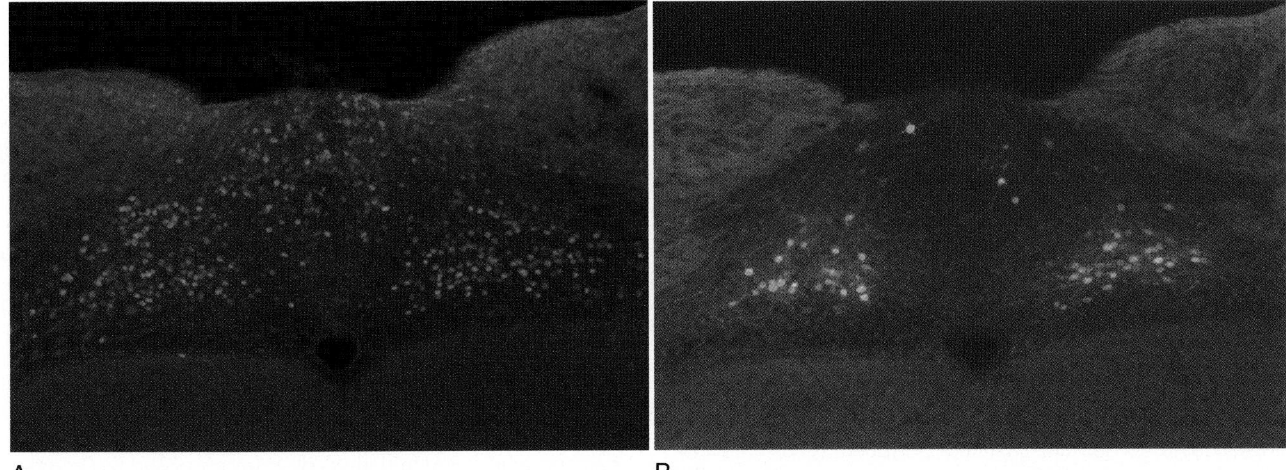

Figure 34–7 ▪ Brainstem neurons activated by satiety. Neurons activated by intraperitoneal administration of CCK (10 μg/kg) in the nucleus tractus solitarius (NTS) of the mouse **(A).** Neurons visualized by immunohistochemical reaction against C-fos, a marker of neuronal activation. Neurons in the NTS activated by CCK encompass a variety of different neurochemical subtypes, such as GLP-1 positive neurons, and the POMC-positive neurons **(B).** POMC neurons are visualized using immunohistochemical detection of green fluorescent protein in tissue from a transgenic mouse in which GFP is expressed under the control of the POMC promoter. (Reproduced from Cowley MA, Smart JL, Rubinstein M, et al. Leptin activates anorexigenic POMC neurons through a neural network in the arcuate nucleus. Nature 2001;411:480-484. Photos provided by Dr. Kate L.J. Ellacott.)

istration of insulin and leptin potentiates the satiety inducing effects of peripherally administered CCK[192-196] and leads to sustained weight loss with repeated injections that is greater than injection of the agents separately.[197] However, more remains to be learned regarding the neuroanatomical substrate underlying this convergence of long-term and short-term information. Whereas basomedial hypothalamic cell groups involved in leptin signaling are densely innervated by catecholaminergic neurons from the brainstem, a recent report demonstrates that norepinephrine is not required for CCK-induced reduction of feeding, in that the dopamine β-hydroxylase knockout mouse is still responsive to CCK-induced satiety.[198] The central melanocortin system may be one element of this integration of satiety with long-term energy homeostasis, because MC4 receptor blockade in the brainstem appears to inhibit the satiating activity of peripherally administered CCK.[67]

Besides inducing satiety through vagally mediated signaling, a small body of literature supports a central role for CCK action in regulation of feeding. Immunohistochemistry of the brain and spinal cord shows that the CCKA and CCKB receptors are widely distributed in the CNS, including in the arcuate nucleus[199] and other hypothalamic regions.[199,200] Intracerebroventricular administration of CCK to mice[201] inhibits food intake that is reversible by prior administration of a CCKA receptor antagonist. The significance of these hypothalamic-arcuate CCK receptors to weight regulation in the free feeding state is not known.

PYY

PYY, a peptide related to neuropeptide Y and pancreatic peptide (PP), is postprandially released by endocrine cells in the ileum and colon.[202] PYY is found in vivo in both a full length 36 amino acid and 34 amino acid form (PYY_{3-36}) in approximately a 2:1 to 1:1 molar ratio.[203] PYY is a potent agonist of both Y1 and Y2 receptors, while PYY_{3-36} is a Y2-specific agonist, with approximately a 1000 times greater affinity for the Y2 vs Y1 receptor.[204] Y1- and Y2-preferring binding sites are located in the area postrema and in the dorsal vagal complex (NTS and DMV). Peripheral administration of PYY (300 mg/kg) in the rat induces c-fos in the AP, as well as in the medial and commissural NTS, the latter being the same region of the NTS known to express POMC.[205] Infusion of PYY within the physiologic range has numerous effects, including inhibition of gastric emptying,[206] gastric acid secretion,[207] and pancreatic exocrine secretion.[207] Evidence shows that these actions of PYY appear to be mediated by PYY action directly on the dorsal vagal complex as well as on gastric mucosal enterochromaffin-like cells (for review, see reference 208). Both Y1 and Y2 receptors are found within the DVC.[209] For example, PYY appears to inhibit gastric acid secretion primarily through vagal innervation of the gastric fundus.[210] The ability of low-dose PYY and PYY_{3-36} to inhibit the activity of DMN efferents appears to be Y2-mediated, while Y1 agonists appear to stimulate these cells[208].

Peripheral administration of PYY_{3-36} in pharmacologic doses appears to have an anorexigenic effect in rodents as well as humans,[211-217] thus suggesting that the peptide also functions as a satiety factor. The mechanisms underlying the action of PYY_{3-36} in reduction of food intake have not been fully elucidated. Intraperitoneal (i.p.) administration of PYY_{3-36} was found to activate 12% to 13% of arcuate POMC neurons, as assayed by increase in expression of c-fos.[211,218] However, vagotomy also blocks PYY_{3-36}-induced inhibition of feeding.[219] A direct hypothalamic site of action has been challenged by several studies. Inhibition of feeding by PYY_{3-36} persists in the melanocortin-4 receptor (MC4-R) knockout mouse,[218] the proopiomelanocortin knockout mouse,[213] and in obese agouti mice.[220] Thus, release of melanocortin peptides derived from POMC and their subsequent activation of the MC4-R, a well-characterized anorexigenic pathway, does not appear to be required for the inhibition of feeding by PYY_{3-36}. Furthermore, PYY appears to induce conditioned taste aversion in rodents and nausea in some human studies, suggesting an aversive effect of the peptide likely to involve brainstem sites like the area postrema.

Despite the short-acting anorexic effects of the peptide in most experimental models, suggesting it may be a satiety factor like CCK, two knockout studies have demonstrated that removal of the gene encoding the peptide produces obese hyperinsulinemic mice,[221,222] these data suggest that the peptide may also play an important role in the regulation of long-term energy stores. One study suggests the peptide may be specifically involved in the satiating effects of protein in the diet.[221]

Ghrelin

Identified as an endogenous ligand for the growth-hormone secretagogue receptor (GHS-R),[223,224] ghrelin is an acylated 28 amino acid peptide predominantly secreted by the stomach, regulated by ingestion of nutrients[225-228] with potent effects on appetite.[227,228] Ghrelin levels are markedly reduced with meal ingestion in both rodents and humans but rebound to baseline before the next meal or increase after an overnight fast[226-228] (Fig. 34–8). In rodents, this was demonstrated to be a nutrient-specific effect in that a similar volume of saline infused into the stomach did not affect ghrelin levels.[227] GHS-R have been demonstrated on arcuate NPY containing neurons,[229] and pharmacologic doses of ghrelin injected peripherally or into the hypothalamus activate C-fos and Egrl solely in arcuate NPY neurons in rats,[230] and stimulate food intake and obesity, in part by stimulating NPY and AgRP expression,[231-236] which antagonize leptin's anorexic effect.[235]

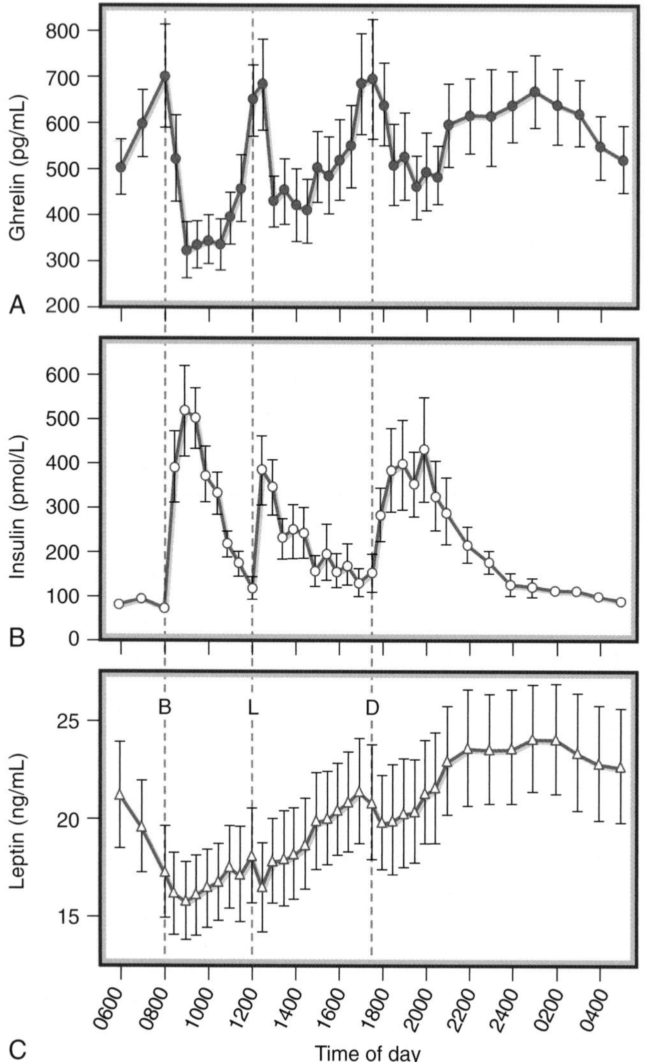

Figure 34–8 ▪ Average plasma ghrelin, insulin, and leptin concentrations during a 24-hour period in 10 human subjects consuming breakfast (B), lunch (L), and dinner (D) at the times indicated (0800, 1200, and 1730, respectively). (Reprinted from Cummings DE, et al. A preprandial rise in plasma ghrelin levels suggest a role in meal initiation in humans. Diabetes 2001;50:1714-1719.)

This orexigenic action occurs in rodents even with peripheral administration of ghrelin that matches fasting levels.[237] Stimulation of appetite and food intake during an infusion of ghrelin over 4.5 hours in humans has also been demonstrated.[238] Additionally, ghrelin may also effect gastric emptying. This study establishes that, similar to its action in rodents, ghrelin can stimulate appetite and food intake in humans when given in a supraphysiologic dose, but a role for physiologic changes in ghrelin levels or signaling in human energy homeostasis remains unknown.

Ghrelin's characteristics make it unique among the gut-derived signals. Unlike other enteropancreatic signals involved with energy homeostasis, ghrelin secretion is inhibited in response to meals; and instead of acting as a satiety signal (like CCK or PYY_{3-36}), ghrelin stimulates appetite, potentially through arcuate signaling. These properties strongly suggest that ghrelin is a candidate "meal initiating" signal as proposed by Cummings and colleagues.[228] In addition, fasting ghrelin levels have been shown to be inversely proportional to body weight[239] and to be higher in underweight subjects with anorexia nervosa and cardiac cachexia compared to controls.[225,240] Down-regulation of ghrelin in obese subjects suggests an adaptive response to the obese state while a rise in levels in weight-reduced subjects is compatible with a "counterregulatory" role to restore fat depots. These properties inversely parallel those of insulin, which is stimulated by meals, inhibits food intake when injected intracerebroventricularly (ICV), circulates in the fasting state in direct proportion to body weight, and whose secretion is decreased following weight loss.

Much work remains to establish the physiologic role of ghrelin in meal initiation and energy homeostasis and its mechanisms of action. With regard to mechanism of action, much evidence indicates the melanocortin system is central to ghrelin's effects on food intake. Stimulation of food intake by ghrelin administration is blocked by administration of NPY/Y1 and Y5 antagonists,[235] and reduced in the NPY −/− mouse . Administration of the melanocortin agonist MTII blocks further stimulation of weight gain by GHRP-2 in the NPY −/− mouse (Tschop, 2002).[240a] Finally, peripheral administration of ghrelin activates c-fos expression only in arcuate NPY/AgRP neurons, not in other hypothalamic or brainstem sites,[241] and ablation of the arcuate nucleus blocks the actions of ghrelin administration on feeding but not elevation of growth hormone.[242] Despite only activating c-fos in arcuate NPY neurons, peripheral ghrelin may access the arcuate via vagal afferents in that GHS receptor is expressed on vagal afferents, ghrelin suppresses firing of vagal nerves, and surgical or chemical vagotomy blocks stimulation of feeding *and* c-fos activation in the arcuate by peripheral but not central ghrelin administration.[243] Peripheral ghrelin may largely suppress brainstem satiety centers, thus explaining the lack of c-fos activation at these sites. The NTS sends dense catecholaminergic projections to the arcuate, so while a convergence of ascending vagal afferent information arrives at the arcuate from both brainstem and intermediate hypothalamic sites, it is possible that NTS neurons inhibited by ghrelin synapse directly with NPY arcuate neurons, thus explaining the absence of other hypothalamic neurons activated by peripheral ghrelin.

Recently, another peptide hormone derived from proghrelin, termed *obestatin,* was demonstrated to inhibit food intake when administered and was proposed to be the ligand for an orphan GPCR, termed *GPR39.*[244] However, most groups have been unable to repeat this finding, and even the identity of obestatin as a GPR39 ligand has been called into question.[245-247]

Preproglucagon-Derived Peptides

Current strategies for the treatment of type 2 diabetes mellitus are not optimally effective, and even multiple drug combinations often fail to normalize glycemia in a sustained manner in many subjects. Hence, there remains intense interest in new therapies that safely and effectively lower blood glucose in diabetic subjects. Recently, strategies mimicking the actions of incretin class of hormones is being used to treat type 2 diabetes and obesity.[248,249] Incretins are hormones that are released by oral ingestion of nutrients to increase insulin secretion. The prototypical incretin hormone is glucagon-like peptide 1 (GLP-1), which is derived from the proglucagon gene. The proglucagon-derived peptides are generated in the A cells of the pancreas (principally glucagon), the L cells of the intestine (GLP-1, GLP-2, and glicentin), and the brain (glucagon, GLP-1, GLP-2).[248,249]

As outlined in detail in Chapter 30, GLP-1 receptor agonists induce multiple desirable antidiabetic and antiobesity actions, and protease-resistant long-acting GLP-1 analogues are currently available for the treatment of type 2 diabetes.[248,249] The first of these drugs, Byetta (exenatide), is a potent GLP-1 receptor agonist and mimics the GLP-1 enhancement of glucose-dependent insulin secretion, slowing of gastric emptying, inhibiting gastric acid secretion, and reducing food intake. The latter effect may be due to action on circuits in the brain involved in the control of energy homeostasis (see below).

GLP-1 and GLP-1R Neurons in the Central Nervous System

Despite recent intense interest in GLP-1 and related peptides, it is much less appreciated that GLP-1 is an endogenous neuropeptide expressed by neurons in the CNS. The CNS actions are less well understood. Given the increasing likelihood that one or more GLP-1 analogues will be increasingly used to treat diabetic patients, understanding central actions of GLP-1 is quite relevant for predicting the biologic consequences of sustained GLP-1 administration.

Initial interest in the CNS actions of GLP-1 stemmed from the observation that GLP-1 inhibits food intake.[250-254] In humans, peripheral GLP-1 administration to normal and diabetic subjects induces satiety and reduces food intake in short-term studies.[255-258] Chronic continuous GLP-1 administration to human diabetic subjects was associated with modest weight loss.[259] The effects of GLP-1 on appetite may be mediated in part via inhibition of gastric emptying and may also reflect direct effects of GLP-1 on satiety and induction of taste aversion.[38,260-264]

The CNS expression of GLP-1 is very restricted and includes a population of neurons within the caudal NTS. Caudal NTS neurons receive and process viscerosensory information from thoracic and abdominal viscera. The NTS is reciprocally connected with various brain areas, including hypothalamic areas thought to regulate feeding.[177,265] Additionally, the NTS is located adjacent to a circumventricular organ, the area postrema (AP), and the NTS contains fenestrated capillaries potentially allowing circulating peptides access to the nucleus. Thus, neurons in the NTS (including GLP-1 cells) process information arising from a variety of neural and humoral sources. GLP-1 neurons are in a prime position to rapidly modify ingestive behavior in direct response to either transiently altered levels of metabolic cues such as leptin or glucose as well as neural modulators from other brain sites including pro-opiomelanocortin (POMC) neurons in the arcuate nucleus. For example, the adipocyte-derived hormone leptin communicates the status of energy stores to the brain. The vast majority of work investigating the neural circuits that mediate leptin action has focused on the hypothalamus. However, increasing evidence implicates a significant role for extrahypothalamic sites of leptin action.[33,142] For example, intravenous leptin increases neuronal activation (induces Fos-IR) in regions of the hindbrain including GLP-1 neurons in the NTS,[266] as well as POMC neurons in some cases.[267]

In addition to the varied inputs, GLP-1 neurons in the NTS also have a widespread projection pattern in the brain.[268] This includes direct innervations of several hypothalamic nuclei, including the paraventricular nucleus (PVH), lateral hypothalamic area (LHA), and arcuate nucleus. Accordingly, GLP-1 receptor mRNA has been found within the PVH, LHA, and arcuate.[269] The location of GLP-1 neurons in the NTS and their diffuse projection pattern suggest that GLP-1 neurons are ideally situated to integrate key signals and regulate complex physiologic processes.

Amylin

Amylin, or islet amyloid polypeptide (IAPP), is a 37 amino acid polypeptide that co-localizes with insulin in β cells in the pancreas. In humans, IAPP in the pancreas can form amyloid fibrils and is thought to play a role in the decline in islet cell function that accompanies type 2 diabetes (see reviews in references 270 and 271). In addition, amylin has been shown to impair gastric motility and have effects independent of insulin on energy homeostasis mediated through hypothalamic signaling.

Amylin is co-secreted with insulin in response to nutrient intake and insulin secretogogues.[272,273] Amylin readily enters the brain and high affinity amylin binding sites have been found in several brain regions including the hypothalamus and arcuate nucleus.[274,275] Both peripheral and ICV infusions of amylin inhibit food intake acutely and, during chronic infusion, leads to a sustained reduction in body weight.[274-279] This anorectic effect has been shown by Rushing and colleagues to be blocked by coadministration of the amylin antagonist AC187 centrally and for AC187 to result in a significant increase in body adiposity when infused ICV over 14 days compared to control animals.[279] Studies of coadminstration of amylin with other GI hormones has shown that the acute satiety effects of amylin are equipotent to CCK[280] and additive when peripherally coinjected with either CCK[281] or insulin.[282] The precise central neuroendocrine mechanism mediating amylin's anorexic effects has yet to be elucidated. The diverse CNS binding of amylin suggests that multiple sites may have roles in the anorectic effects of amylin, however the inhibition of appetite with ICV administration and demonstrated binding in the arcute suggests the hypothalamus may be an important site of amylin action.

Bariatric Surgery and the Role of the Gastrointestinal System in the Control of Energy Homeostasis

No pharmacologic treatment has yet been devised that is capable of resetting the adipostat—that is, allows significant long-term weight loss to be maintained. In contrast, certain types of bariatric surgery, such as the Roux-en-Y gastric bypass (described in Chapter 35; for reviews, see references 283 and 284) appear to not only cause significant weight loss, but also appear to allow this weight loss to be maintained for many years (Fig. 34–9). Furthermore, improvement in diabetes following these procedures is often seen before significant weight loss occurs, and this can now be modeled in rodents as well.[285] Both these findings imply that the procedures are having a profound impact on the central control of long-term energy stores, satiety, and glucose homeostasis. Conventional models have argued that GI hormones regulate satiety, but individually do not have significant impact on the control of long-term energy stores. For example, deletion or blockade of CCK increases meal size but not 24-hour food intake or body weight. The fact that bariatric surgery appears capable of creating a new stable weight set-point and the fact that PYY deletion causes obesity suggest that hormonal and/or vagal and nutritional signals from the gut may

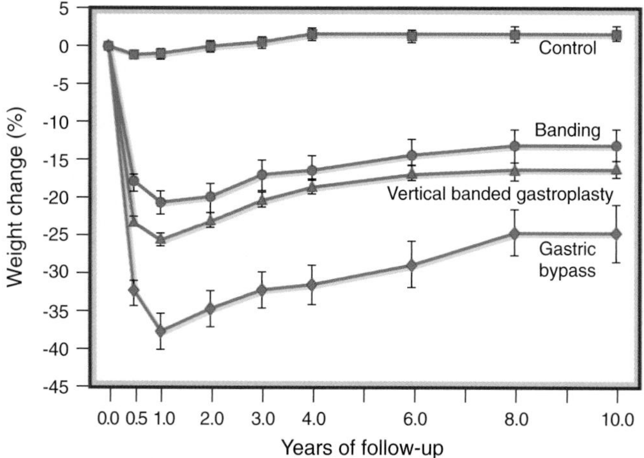

Figure 34–9 ▪ Apparent alteration of the adipostatic set point following bariatric surgery. (Modified from Sjostrom L, et al, and Swedish Obese Subjects Study Scientific Group. Lifestyle, diabetes, and cardiovascular risk factors 10 years after bariatric surgery. N Engl J Med 2004; 351:2683-2693.)

indeed have a more profound impact on long-term energy homeostasis than previously thought.

GLUCOCORTICOIDS AND GONADAL STEROIDS

Both glucocorticoids and gonadal steroids are known to act centrally on circuits involved in energy homeostasis. Orchiectomy decreases food intake in rodents, whereas ovariectomy has the opposite result (for review, see reference 286). Hormone replacement therapy with drugs such as tamoxifen has been demonstrated to reduce the weight gain seen with menopause.[287] Estrogen receptors appear to be expressed at significant levels in the arcuate nucleus of the hypothalamus. Recent data suggest that estrogen may act at both the POMC and NPY/AgRP neurons, perhaps explaining part of the cellular mechanism of the hormone's action in the CNS.[288,289] Furthermore, estrogen receptor α (ERα) knockout mice develop increased visceral adiposity, elevated insulin levels, and reduced glucose tolerance.[290] However, obesity in this knockout model does not appear to be due to hyperphagia. Furthermore, deletion of ERα exclusively in neurons of the ventromedial hypothalamus leads to a similar syndrome, obesity and metabolic syndrome, suggesting an important role for estrogen in the control of energy expenditure as well, and implicating the VMH in estrogen action.[291] The vagal nerve is also a site of estrogen action, where the hormone has been demonstrated to alter reposnsiveness to satiety factors, such as CCK.[286]

In contrast to estrogen, glucocorticoids stimulate food intake and weight gain. Excessive glucocorticoids are associated with the unusual deposition of excess adipose tissue seen, for example, in Cushing's disease (see Chapter 7). However, glucocorticoids have an enormous diversity of effects both in the periphery and in the CNS, and glucocorticoid receptor is extremely widely expressed throughout the CNS.[292] In the CNS, glucocorticoids have antiinflammatory effects, and they provide feedback inhibition to the HPA axis (see Chapter 7), both actions having secondary effects on energy homeostasis. Glucocorticoids also appear to be critical in determining the tone of adipostatic circuits (for review, see reference 286). For example, the ability of centrally administered NPY to produce obesity and the obesity resulting from leptin-deficiency are both dramatically reduced by adrenalectomy. ICV administration of dexamethasone to adrenalectomized rats also dose-dependently reduces leptin potency.

The complexity of the glucocorticoid action in energy homeostasis results from the broad number of tissues affected, the multiple physiologic systems involved, as well as action in a variety of time scales. Rapid actions of glucocorticoids in the hypothalamus, not mediated by the conventional glucocorticoid receptor, have also been linked in sites like the PVN to rapid synthesis and retrograde release of endocannabinoids, which suppress synaptic excitation through presynaptic CB1 receptors. In support of this newly identified pathway, leptin appears to block glucocorticoid-mediated endocannabinoid release.[293]

CYTOKINES AND ENERGY BALANCE

The profound effect of cytokines, largely derived from the immune system, on energy balance is most clearly evident in the case of disease wasting or cachexia. Cachexia describes a constellation of symptoms that occurs in multiple independent infectious and chronic diseases including some forms of cancer, heart failure, renal failure, and acquired immunodeficiency syndrome. These symptoms include anorexia, increased energy expenditure, and a loss of lean mass. Importantly, the normal response to anorexia and initial loss of adipose mass—a decrease in energy expenditure and neuroendocrine changes designed to save energy such as hypothyroidism—such as occur in anorexia nervosa do not occur in cachexia. Research in both rodents and humans demonstrate that cachexia results from the action of a variety of cytokines in the CNS and in particular the dysfunctional response of circuits involved in the central control of energy homeostasis

Neuroendocrine-Immune Interactions

Stimulation of the immune system by foreign pathogens leads to a stereotyped set of responses orchestrated by the CNS. These responses are the result of the complex interaction of the immune system and the CNS and are often referred to as the cerebral component of the acute phase reaction.[294] This constellation of stereotyped responses is adaptive and is mediated in large part by the hypothalamus and, just as in the normal control of energy homeostasis, includes coordinated autonomic, endocrine, and behavioral components. These responses include fever, alterations in the activity of nearly every neuroendocrine axis, changes in the sleep-wake cycle, anorexia, and inactivity. It is now clear that cytokines produced by white blood cells of the immune system mediate the CNS responses. Early evidence supporting this hypothesis was provided by the seminal observations that cytokines such as IL-1β can activate the HPA axis.[295-297] While it is established that cytokines modulate hypothalamic activity, it is also important to note that the immune system is modulated by the nervous system. This occurs largely via two routes: by endocrine mechanisms and by direct innervation. This innervation includes lymphoid organs such as the thymus and spleen, which receive direct inputs from the autonomic nervous system.[298,299] As noted earlier in Chapter 7, the hallmark of cytokine action on the hypothalamus is the activation of the HPA axis. The resultant glucocorticoid secretion acts as a classic negative feedback to the immune system to dampen down the immune response (Fig. 34–10). In general, glucocorticoids inhibit most limbs of the immune response, including lymphocyte proliferation, production of immunoglobulins, cytokines, and cytotoxicity. These inhibitory reactions form the basis of the antiinflammatory actions of glucocorticoids.

This section will address several of the hypothesized mechanisms by which cytokines engage neural pathways to mediate neuroendocrine and autonomic effects. It is also important to note that many nonlymphocyte cells including endocrine, adipose cells, and neurons also synthesize cytokines that exert effects independent of immunomodulation. Examples of cytokines secreted by adipocytes include leptin, and TNF-α, which have profound effects on metabolism.[300]

Mechanisms of Cytokine Signaling in the Central Nervous System

Cytokines made outside the CNS can alter the activity and function of populations of hypothalamic neurons. LPS administration is widely used as an experimental model and induces the secretion of several pyrogenic cytokines including interleukin-1β (IL-1β), tumor necrosis factor-α (TNF-α), and interleukin-6 (IL-6) that mimic the patterns of cytokine production seen in natural infections.[301-304] Many other studies have used systemic injections of cytokines such as IL-1β and TNF-α to stimulate the CNS. Using methodologies such as these, three models are discussed below to explain how immune system signals might act upon the CNS (Fig. 34–11).

Interaction of Cytokines with the Circumventricular Organs

The circumventricular organs (CVOs, described in detail above) are specialized regions along the margins of the ventricular system that have fenestrated capillaries and therefore no blood-brain barrier (BBB).[35] Many circulating hormones, such as angiotensin II, act on neurons in the CVOs, converting blood-borne signals into CNS responses.[294] Several models of fever production have hypothesized that cytokines may enter the CNS via the CVOs, particularly at the organum vasculosum of the

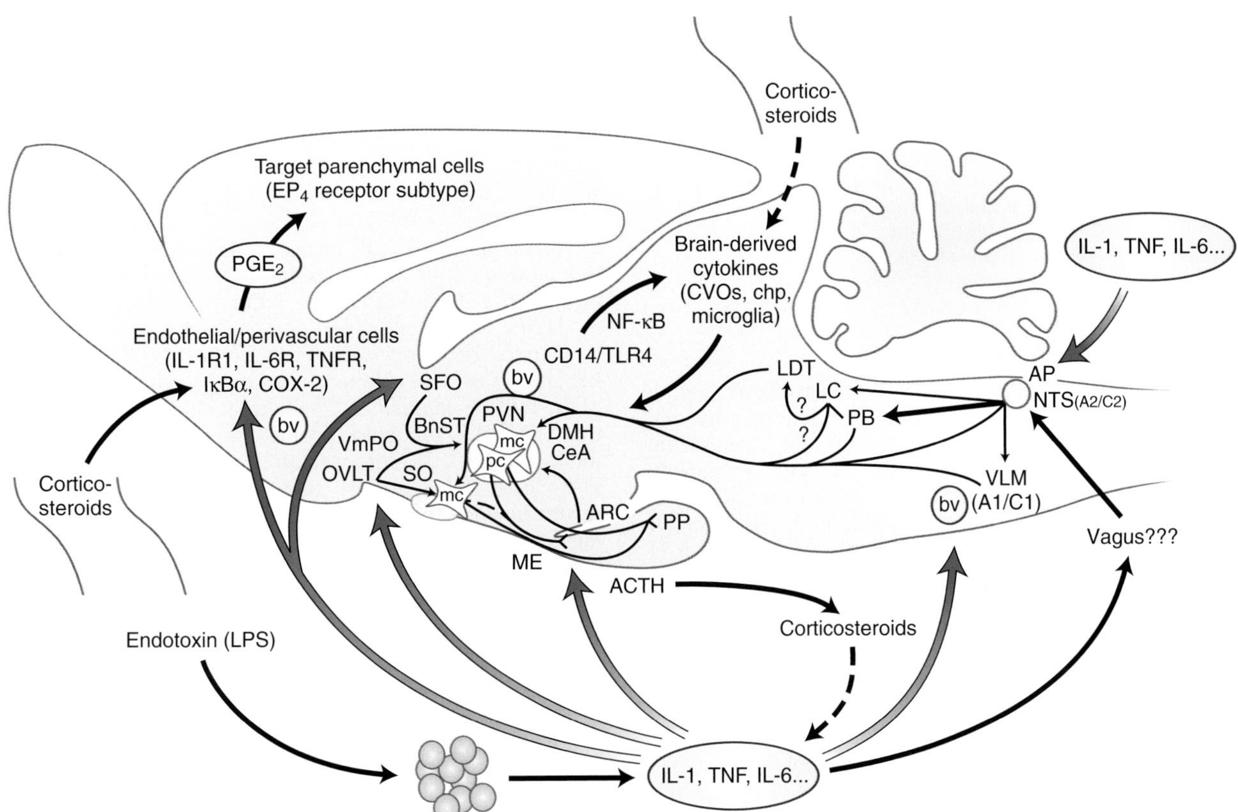

Figure 34–10 ▪ A model of the CNS circuitry activated by cytokines. Circumventricular organs (organs devoid of blood-brain barrier; CVOs) and the blood vessels (bv) are crucial target sites of cytokines of systemic origin produced during the acute-phase response. Among these integrative structures, the PVN is critical in coordinating autonomic and endocrine responses, including the activity of the HPA axis. For example, corticotropin-releasing factor (CRF) neurons of the parvocellular PVN confer HPA axis activation in endotoxin-treated animals. *ACTH,* Adrenocorticotropic hormone; *AP,* area postrema; *ARC,* arculate nucleus; *BnST,* bed nucleus of the stria terminalis; *bv,* blood vessels; *chp,* choroid plexus; *CeA,* central nucleus of the amygdala; *chp,* choroid plexus; *COX-2,* cyclooxygenase-2; *DMH,* dorsomedial nucleus of the hypothalamus; *EP,* prostaglandin E receptor; *IL-1β,* interleukin-1β; *IL-1R1,* IL-1 type 1 receptor; *IL-6,* interleukin-6; *IκBα,* NF-κB inhibitor; *LC,* locus coeruleus; *LDT,* laterodorsal tegmental nucleus; *LPS,* lipopolysaccharide; *LRNm,* lateral reticular nucleus medial; *ME,* median eminence; *MPOA,* medial preoptic area; *NF-κB;* nuclear factor-κB; *NTS,* nucleus of the solitary tract; *OVLT,* organum vasculosum of the lamina terminalis; *PGE2,* prostaglandin E2; *PB,* parabrachial nucleus; *PP,* posterior pituitary; *PVN,* paraventricular nucleus of the hypothalamus (parvocellular [pc] and magnocellular divisions [mc]); *SFO,* subfornical organ; *SON,* supraoptic nucleus; *TNF-α,* tumor necrosis factor-α; *VLM,* ventrolateral medulla. (Modified from Rivest, 2000.)

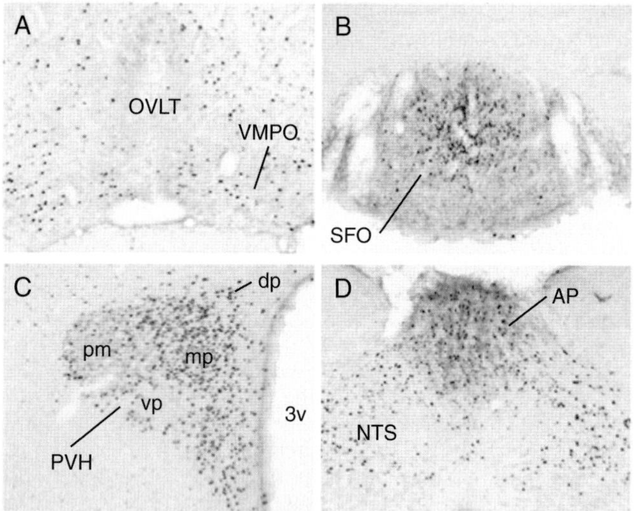

Figure 34–11 ▪ Immune stimulation activates key brain regions involved in energy homeostasis. A series of photomicrographs demonstrating the distribution of Fos-like immunoreactivity (Fos-IR) in the rat brain 2 hours following intravenous injections of lipopolysaccharide (LPS; 125 μg/kg). LPS administration is a commonly used model of immune stimulation and Fos-IR is a widely used marker of neuronal activation. LPS activates (induces Fos-IR) in the ventral medial preoptic area and organum vasculosum of the lamina terminalis (VMPO and OVLT; A), in the subfornical organ (SFO; B), in the paraventricular nucleus of the hypothalamus (PVH; C), and in the area postrema and nucleus of the solitary tract in the brainstem (AP, NTS; D). Note that prominent Fos-IR is seen throughout the subdivisions of the PVH including the dorsal (dp), ventral (vp), and medial (mp) parvocellular and posterior magnocellular (pm) divisions. Also note that LPS activates neurons in the circumventricular organs (OVLT, SFO, AP). *3v*, Third ventricle.

lamina terminalis (OVLT; see Fig. 34–10).[305-308] However, definitive evidence establishing this model as a predominant mechanism is still lacking. Large lesions of the preoptic area of the hypothalamus including the OVLT block fever, but they inevitably damage nearby regions that are critical for thermoregulation.[306] Small lesions of the OVLT do not block fever or corticotropin responses.[309] However, an inherent limitation of this type of study is that the lesion itself breaches the BBB, allowing entry of cytokines. Moreover, knife cuts just caudal to the OVLT, interrupting connections from the OVLT to the paraventricular nucleus of the hypothalamus, do not block activation of the HPA axis by IL-1.[310,311] Other studies have focused on the area postrema, a CVO located in the medulla oblongata lying along the surface of the nucleus of the solitary tract at the caudal end of the fourth ventricle (see Fig. 34–10). Lesions of the area postrema can block the IL-1-induced activation the HPA axis and the induction of c-fos mRNA in the paraventricular nucleus of the hypothalamus.[312] However, others have found that more circumscribed lesions, which do not injure the nucleus of the solitary tract, do not prevent CNS responses to intravenous (IV) IL-1.[313]

Interactions of Cytokines at the Barriers of the Brain: The Requirement of Prostaglandins

One of the hallmarks of CNS response to inflammation is that many of its components, including fever and activation of the HPA axis, can be prevented by blocking the production of prostaglandins. This is typically done by administration of nonsteroidal antiinflammatory drugs (NSAIDs) such as aspirin and indomethacin.[314-316] Indeed, decades ago, the work of Milton and Wendlandt demonstrated that central injections of prostaglandins increase body temperature.[317,318] Two isoforms of COX exist. COX-1 is the constitutive form of the enzyme and is not thought to be regulated by inflammatory stimuli. COX-2 is an inducible isoform and is increased in several cell types in response to immunologic stimuli.[319,320] In the normal brain, COX-2 mRNA and protein is found exclusively in neurons.[303,321-323] In contrast, immune stimulation by LPS or cytokines induces COX-2 mRNA and protein throughout the brain in nonneuronal cells associated with blood vessels, the meninges, and the choroid plexus. In addition, systemic administration of IL-1β induces the expression of prostaglandin E synthase mRNA.[324] This likely includes endothelial cells and perivascular microglial cells and meningeal macrophages.[325-327] Regardless of the cell type, it seems clear that circulating LPS or cytokines induce COX-2 in cells in the perivascular space, which in turn may produce PGs to stimulate nearby brain regions inside the BBB.

Prostaglandin E_2, the predominant endogenous isoform of PGE in the brain, is thought to be an essential mediator of cytokine modulation of hypothalamic function.[328] Evidence supporting this claim includes that microinjections of PGE receptor agonists into the brain of rats[308,329,330] and other species[331,332] produce fever. The preoptic area of the hypothalamus surrounding the OVLT is thought to be critical in the response to PGE. For example, microinjections of as little of 1 ng of PGE_2 into the anteroventral preoptic area of rats reliably produces fevers.[329] Conversely, a COX-2 inhibitor ketorolac attenuates LPS-induced fever with injections placed in this same region.[333] This PGE-sensitive zone is the same as the region containing the highest concentrations of PGE_2 binding sites.[334,335] The recent cloning of the prostaglandin E (EP) receptors will ultimately allow a more definitive analysis of the receptors in the hypothalamus that mediate the effects of PGEs on both fever and anorexia (see Fig. 34–11).

Four EP receptors have been identified: EP_1, EP_2, EP_3, and EP_4.[302,336,337] All four subtypes are expressed in the preoptic area of the hypothalamus.[302,338-342] Pharmacologic evidence suggests that EP_1 and EP_3 receptor agonist administration mimics PGE_2-induced fever.[343,344] Moreover, an EP_1 receptor antagonist blocks PGE_2 fever.[344] In contrast, targeted deletion of the EP_3 gene results in mice that do not show an early phase of fever after injection of LPS or PGE_2 (ICV).[337] EP_1 and EP_3 receptors do not individually appear to be essential for cancer-mediated anorexia in rodent models.[345] Interestingly, there is upregulation of EP_4 receptor expression in several areas of the brain, including the corticotropin-releasing hormone (CRH) neurons of the paraventricular nucleus, following immune challenge.[338,341] In addition, paraventricular neurons that express Fos after ICV PGE_2 also express EP_4 receptors.[341] Thus, production of PGE_2 is certainly an obligate step in the pathogenesis of the febrile response. Furthermore, knockout of the gene for enzyme microsomal prostaglandin E-synthase-1 (mPGES-1), essential for PGE_2 synthesis, blocks IL-1β induced anorexia.[346] However, LPS-induced anorexia remains intact in these animals, suggesting both PGE_2-dependent and -independent pathways are involved in the anorexic component of cachexia.[346]

Entry of Cytokines into the Brain

Circulating cytokines are proteins that cannot easily penetrate the BBB. The kinetics of entry of cytokines into the brain have been examined and evidence suggests that saturable transport of IL-1α, IL-1β, IL-6, and TNF-α into the brain occurs.[347-349] However, it is not clear if sufficient levels of cytokines are detectable in brain following acute IV administration to account for CNS responses to acute infection. Thus, the physiologic setting and significance of this mechanism remains to be established. Moreover, it is noteworthy that levels of circulating IL-1β do not rise significantly during immune challenges.[350,351] In contrast to IL-1β, large increases in circulating and brain IL-6 are found during fever. Although not completely understood, it appears that synthesis of IL-6 within the BBB and not peripheral IL-6 crossing the BBB is critical in the production of fever.[352] Moreover, several recent studies have demonstrated that cells located at the BBB and cells within the meninges respond to LPS stimulation with induction of IL-1β and TNF-α, the NF-κB inhibitor IκBα, and the LPS receptor CD14).[302,353-355] Cells with a similar morphology lining the blood vessels that penetrate the CNS and the meninges that cover it, also have IL-1 receptors, suggesting that they may respond to cytokines as well.[356] Hence, endothelial and perivascular cells at the blood-brain interface may have the ability to elaborate cytokines following an LPS or cytokine signal. The physiologic role of centrally produced cytokines in the response to peripheral immune cues has been recently reviewed in detail.[302,351]

Brain Regions Involved in the Cytokine Response

Many studies have used the immediate expression of early genes such as *c-fos* or its protein product Fos[357] as a marker of neuronal activity. This has allowed investigators to assess the involvement of extended neuronal systems during the complex physiologic responses following immune challenge. Mapping the patterns of activation in the CNS following either IL-1β or LPS administration, has allowed new insights into the functional neuroanatomy underlying the coordinated autonomic, endocrine, and behavioral responses during the febrile response.[311,314,358-369] Immune activation using moderate to high doses of LPS and IL-1β activates central autonomic and endocrine structures at nearly every level of the neuraxis, including several neuroendocrine regulator sites, such as central nucleus of the amygdala, paraventricular hypothalamic nucleus, arcuate nucleus of the hypothalamus, subfornical organ, OVLT, and ventral medial preoptic area. Brainstem sites engaged include the parabrachial nucleus, nucleus of the solitary tract, area postrema, and the rostral and caudal levels of the ventrolateral medulla.[311,314,358-369] In the paraventricular nucleus, LPS and cytokines activate parvicellular corticotropin releasing hormone neurons.

Although it is established that the hypothalamus is responsible for inducing a febrile response and anorexia, it is also important to note that hypothalamic systems also exist that attenuate rises in body temperature. These include arcuate POMC neurons (see Figs. 34–2 and 34–10) and arginine vasopressin neurons, both of which are thought to be endogenous antipyretic neuromodulators.[370-373] Thus, neuronal activation patterns elicited by LPS or cytokines likely include neurons engaged to limit rises in body temperature. Indeed, Tatro and colleagues have found that exogenous α-MSH administration can block LPS-induced fever.[375] The discovery that central melanocortin agonists could both inhibit food intake[30] and increase energy expenditure[374] suggested that stimulation of the central melanocortin system might be involved in mediating a component of cachexia. Direct experimental testing of this hypothesis demonstrated that the central melanocortin system does indeed contribute to anorexia during systemic illness.[375-377] In rodents, melanocortin-4 receptor blockade prevents illness-induced anorexia and cachexia associated with cancer and kidney failure.[378,379]

Recent experimental work has coupled neuroanatomic tract tracing with methods assessing immediate early gene expression to investigate the circuitry that is activated by peripheral immune signals. For example, IV administration of IL-1β induced Fos in C1 adrenergic neurons in the ventrolateral medulla that project to the PVH. The C1 adrenergic cell group targets the medial parvicellular subdivision of the PVH, the site of the CRH neurons 7-26).[311] Lesions interrupting the input from the C1 cells to the PVH prevent the HPA response to IL-1β. These studies suggest that the activation of C1 cells by locally produced prostaglandins[313] may play a critical role in activating the HPA axis in response to IL-1β.

Sympathetic preganglionic neurons in the intermediolateral cell column (IML), extending from the first thoracic through the upper lumbar segments of the spinal cord, also show Fos expression in response to LPS.[368] Preganglionic neurons in the upper thoracic (T1-4) levels mediate thermogenesis by brown adipose tissue,[380,381] which is a key mechanism used by rats to control heat production and body temperature.[382] Sympathetic preganglionic neurons in the T2-5 levels are important for control of the heart,[90,383] which is important as there are changes in cardiac output in the febrile state. Another important concept to keep in mind is that sympathetic preganglionic neurons receive direct, monosynaptic input from a series of well-defined nuclei in the brainstem and the hypothalamus (see Fig. 34–2). These cells provide another way in which the hypothalamus can contribute to the coordinated autonomic response to inflammatory signals. The major input to the sympathetic preganglionic column arises from neurons in the hypothalamus.[384] This innervation includes the paraventricular nucleus (dorsal, ventral, and lateral parvicellular subnuclei), the lateral hypothalamic area, and the arcuate nucleus and retrochiasmatic area.[100,177] Direct projections to the IML also arise in the brainstem from the A5 noradrenergic cell group in the ventral pons, the caudal part of the nucleus of the solitary tract, the ventromedial medulla including the medullary raphe nuclei, and the rostral ventrolateral medulla, including the C1 adrenergic cell group.[90,177,385]

Fos expression in hypothalamic and brainstem neurons projecting to the IML following LPS administration has been recently examined.[385] LPS-activated cells that innervate the IML are found in the rostral ventrolateral medulla (C1 adrenergic cell group) and the A5 noradrenergic cell group in the brainstem. Moreover, a prominent population of cells was found in the dorsal parvicellular division of the paraventricular nucleus in the hypothalamus. These results suggest that neurons in the parvicellular PVH specifically innervate sympathetic preganglionic neurons in the spinal cord that regulate LPS-induced fever. Furthermore, as noted above, activation of CRH neurons in the PVH is a signature of the CNS response to immune stimulation. Thus, the paraventricular hypothalamic nucleus is a key site for mediating both neuroendocrine and autonomic responses to immune stimulation.

INTERSECTION OF ENERGY BALANCE AND REWARD CIRCUITS

A relatively recent and novel concept to emerge is that food and drug rewards share some common neural substrates.[40,386] This is potentially quite important as it is logical to predict that if rational strategies to combat obesity are to be developed, then an increased understanding of the molecular mechanisms of the rewarding aspects of feeding behavior is required.[40] Motivation and reward have been studied in the context of drug addiction.[387-389] The nucleus accumbens (NAc) and its dopamine inputs have been strongly implicated in mediating several rewarding stimuli.[387,390]

Although dopamine is widely accepted to be involved in reward processes, it has become clear that the relationship between dopamine and reward is complex.[40] For example, lesions of the nucleus accumbens does reduce food intake[391] or the ability to display operant conditioning in response to food.[392] However, recent evidence has demonstrated a dopamine component of food reward. For example, mice lacking the ability to produce dopamine, which normally die of starvation, resume feeding after reintroduction of the dopamine into the striatum.[393,394]

Recent evidence has suggested that key metabolic cues act directly on dopamine neurons in the midbrain. For example, midbrain dopamine neurons express leptin and ghrelin receptors.[395-397] Interestingly, Fulton and colleagues demonstrated that leptin also affects brain self-stimulation,[398] suggesting that leptin has the ability to affect CNS circuits classically involved in reward. Taken together, these findings suggest that alterations of cues such as leptin and ghrelin may not only affect hypothalamic pathways, but may also act directly on midbrain dopamine neurons. While this field of study is still evolving, these findings lead to a model with potentially broad implications. These models could provide a mechanism for signals regulating food intake to intersect with brain circuitry critical in the regulation of motivated behaviors. Moreover, dysregulation of these pathways may be relevant to the pathophysiology of obesity as well as eating disorders such as anorexia nervosa.[399]

NEUROENDOCRINE DISORDERS OF ENERGY HOMEOSTASIS

A wide variety of disorders of hypothalamic and neuroendocrine function are known to produce obesity. For example, as discussed in the historical introduction to this chapter, insults to the function of the basal hypothalamus, including Fröelich's syndrome and craniopharyngioma are known to cause obesity. In the past 10 years there have been a number of important discoveries related to genetic syndromes underlying certain human obesity disorders; these are also reviewed briefly in Chapter 35, but two of the most informative monogenic disorders are discussed in detail below in the context of their effects on the neuroendocrine control of energy stores.

Leptin and Leptin Receptor Deficiency in Humans

Despite being extremely rare, leptin deficiency[400] and leptin receptor defects[401] in humans are illustrative of the physiologic importance of this hormone. For example, serum leptin levels in humans are generally proportional to adipose mass.[129,402] Thus, the vast majority of obese humans may be considered to be leptin-resistant rather than deficient in leptin.[42,128,403] Despite rapid increases in our understanding of obesity and leptin action, the molecular basis of leptin resistance remains poorly understood.

Clinical studies have now demonstrated that leptin treatment is safe and well-tolerated and clearly effective in individuals with congenital leptin deficiency[126] and in patients who are very low in adipose tissue.[404,405] For example, doses of methionyl-leptin were given to subjects with congenital deficiency that resulted in leptin levels 10% of that predicted based on body fat. Leptin in this study was well-tolerated and resulted in dramatic declines in appetite, body weight, and food intake.[126] In addition, administration of recombinant leptin to women with hypothalamic amenorrhea due to strenuous exercise training and very low body fat normalized several endocrine indices of reproductive function and bone density.[405] Unfortunately, in individuals with common obesity, leptin had only very modest effects on appetite and body weight.[406]

A recent concept that has emerged is that leptin has potent effects on whole body glucose and lipid homeostasis independent of its effects on body weight.[49,147] These studies of leptin action may be relevant to models linking diabetes and hypothalamic resistance to metabolic cues. Leptin deficiency, as seen in lipodystrophic mice and humans, induces severe insulin resistance. This extreme resistance is corrected by leptin replacement.[407-409] This can be explained by actions of leptin in the arcuate nucleus of the hypothalamus. Restoration of leptin receptors only in the arcuate nucleus in mice lacking leptin receptors everywhere had remarkably improved glucose homeostasis.[410,411] Thus, leptin action in the arcuate nucleus is sufficient to mediate the antidiabetic actions of leptin.

Obesity resulting from Defective Melanocortin Signaling

Evidence that the melanocortin obesity syndrome can occur in humans resulted from the astute recognition of an agouti-mouse like syndrome in two families, resulting from null mutations in the *POMC* gene[412] (Fig. 34–12). These patients have a rare syndrome that includes ACTH insufficiency, red hair, and obesity resulting from the lack of ACTH peptide in the serum, and a lack of melanocortin peptides in skin and brain respectively. These data demonstrated, for the first time, that the central melanocortin circuitry subserves energy homeostasis in humans as it does in the mouse. Shortly thereafter, heterozygous frameshift mutations in the human *MC4R* were reported, associated with nonsyndromic obesity in two separate families.[413,414] Additional reports[415-417] provide a clearer picture of the frequency and diversity of *MC4R* mutations and show that haploinsufficiency of the MC4-R in humans is the most common monogenic cause of severe obesity at the present time, accounting for up to 5% of

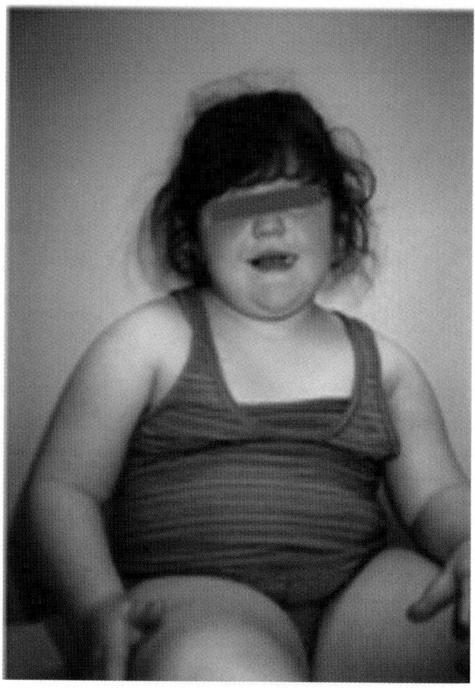

Figure 34–12 ▪ A monogenic neuroendocrine obesity syndrome of adrenocorticotropic hormone insufficiency, obesity, and red hair resulting from a null mutation in the pro-opiomelanocortin gene. (Photo provided by Dr. A. Gruters, Berlin.)

cases. Two recent reports provide a detailed clinical picture of the syndrome.[418,419] Remarkably, the syndrome is virtually identical to that reported for the mouse,[31,110,374] with increased adipose mass, increased linear growth and lean mass, hyperinsulinemia greater than that seen in matched obese controls, and severe hyperphagia.

REFERENCES

1. Bramwell B. Intracranial Tumours. Edinburgh: Pentland, 1888.
2. Fröhlich A. Ein fall von tumor der hypophysis cerebri ohne akromegalie. Wien Klin Rundsch, 1901;15:883.
3. Crowe SJ, Cushing H, Homans J. Bulletin Hopkins Hospital, 1910;21:127.
4. Stevenson JAF. Neural control of food and water intake. In Haymaker W, Anderson E, Nauta WJH, eds. The Hypothalamus. Springfield, IL: Charles C Thomas, 1969:524-621.
5. Elmquist JK, Elias CF, Saper CB. From lesions to leptin: hypothalamic control of food intake and body weight. Neuron 1999;22: 221-232.
6. Aschner B. Uber die funktion der hypophyse. Pflugers Arch Physiol 1912;146:1.
7. Hetherington AW, et al. Hypothalamic lesions and adiposity in the rat. Anat Rec 1940;78:149-172.
8. Stellar E. The physiology of motivation. Physiol Rev 1954;61:5-22.
9. Kennedy GC. The role of depot fat in the hypothalamic control of food intake in the rat. Proc R Soc Lond B Biol Sci 1953;140: 579-592.
10. Harris RB, Kasser TR, Martin RJ. Dynamics of recovery of body composition after overfeeding, food restriction or starvation of mature female rats. J Nutr 1986;116:2536-2546.
11. Harris RB. Role of set-point theory in regulation of body weight. Faseb J 1990;4:3310-3318.
12. Faust IM, Johnson PR, Hirsch J. Surgical removal of adipose tissue alters feeding behavior and the development of obesity in rats. Science 1977;197:393-396.
13. Hervey GR. The effects of lesions in the hypothalamus in parabiotic rats. J Physiol 1959;145:336-352.
14. Hervey GR. Physiological mechanisms for the regulation of energy balance. Proc Nutr Soc 1971;30:109-116.
15. Parameswaran SV, Steffens AB, Hervey GR, et al. Involvement of a humoral factor in regulation of body weight in parabiotic rats. Am J Physiol 1977;232:R150-R157.
16. Ingalls AM, Dickie MM, Snell GD. Obese, a new mutation in the house mouse. J Hered 1950;41:317-318.
17. Coleman DL, Hummel KP. Effects of parabiosis of normal with genetically diabetic mice. Am J Physiol 1969;217:1298-1304.
18. Coleman DL. Obese and diabetes: two mutant genes causing diabetes-obesity syndromes in mice. Diabetologia 1978;14: 141-148.
19. Coleman DL. Effects of parabiosis of obese with diabetes and normal mice. Diabetologia 1973;9:294-298.
20. Lee GH, Proenca R, Montez JM, et al. Abnormal splicing of the leptin receptor in diabetic mice. Nature 1996;379:632-635.
21. Tartaglia LA, Dembski M, Weng X, et al. Identification and expression cloning of a leptin receptor, OB-R. Cell, 1995;83:1263-1271.
22. Zhang Y, Proenca R, Maffei M, et al. Positional cloning of the mouse obese gene and its human homologue. Nature 1994;372: 425-432.
23. Campfield LA, Smith FJ, Guisez Y, et al. Recombinant mouse OB protein: evidence for a peripheral signal linking adiposity and central neural networks. Science 1995;269:546-549.
24. Halaas JL, Gajiwala KS, Maffei M, et al. Weight-reducing effects of the plasma protein encoded by the obese gene. Science 1995; 269:543-546.
25. Halaas JL, Boozer C, Blair-West J, et al. Physiological response to long-term peripheral and central leptin infusion in lean and obese mice. Proc Natl Acad Sci U S A 1997;94:8878-8883.
26. Pelleymounter MA, Cullen MJ, Baker MB, et al. Effects of the obese gene product on body weight regulation in ob/ob mice (see comments). Science 1995;269:540-543.
27. Miller MW, Duhl DM, Vrieling H, et al. Cloning of the mouse agouti gene predicts a novel secreted protein ubiquitously expressed in mice carrying the lethal yellow (A^y) mutation. Genes and Dev 1993;7:454-467.
28. Bultman SJ, Michaud EJ, Woychik RP. Molecular characterization of the mouse agouti locus. Cell 1992;71:1195-1204.
29. Lu D, Willard D, Patel IR, et al. Agouti protein is an antagonist of the melanocyte-stimulating hormone receptor. Nature 1994;371: 799-802.
30. Fan W, Boston BA, Kesterson RA, et al. Role of melanocortinergic neurons in feeding and the agouti obesity syndrome. Nature 1997;385:165-168.
31. Huszar D, Lynch CA, Fairchild-Huntress V, et al. Targeted disruption of the melanocortin-4 receptor results in obesity in mice. Cell 1997;88:131-141.
32. Saper CB. Central autonomic system. In Paxinos G, ed. The Rat Nervous System. San Diego: Academic Press, 1995:107-135.
33. Grill HJ, Kaplan JM. The neuroanatomical axis for control of energy balance. Front Neuroendocrinol 2002;23:2-40.
34. Herbert H, Moga MM, CB Saper. Connections of the parabrachial nucleus with the nucleus of the solitary tract and the medullary reticular formation in the rat. J Comp Neurol 1990;293:540-580.
35. Broadwell, RD and M.W. Brightman, Entry of peroxidase into neurons of the central and peripheral nervous systems from extracerebral and cerebral blood. J Comp Neurol 1976;166:257-283.
36. Herbert H, Saper CB. Cholecystokinin-, galanin-, and corticotropin-releasing factor-like immunoreactive projections from the nucleus of the solitary tract to the parabrachial nucleus in the rat. J Comp Neurol 1990;293:581-598.
37. Billig I, Yates BJ, Rinaman L. Plasma hormone levels and central c-Fos expression in ferrets after systemic administration of cholecystokinin. Am J Physiol Regul Integr Comp Physiol 2001;281: R1243-R1255.
38. Rinaman L. A functional role for central glucagon-like peptide-1 receptors in lithium chloride-induced anorexia. Am J Physiol 1999;277(5 Pt 2): R1537-R1540.
39. Yamamoto H, Kishi T, Lee CE, et al. Glucagon-like peptide-1 responsive catecholamine neurons in the area postrema link peripheral glucagon-like peptide-1 with central autonomic control sites. J Neurosci 2003;23:2939-2946.
40. Saper CB, Chou TC, Elmquist JK. The need to feed: homeostatic and hedonic control of eating. Neuron 2002;36:199-211.
41. Cone RD. Anatomy and regulation of the central melanocortin system. Nat Neurosci 2005;8:571-578.
42. Barsh GS, Farooqi IS, O'Rahilly S. Genetics of body-weight regulation. Nature 2000;404:644-651.
43. Schwartz MW, Seeley RJ, Woods SC, et al. Leptin increases hypothalamic pro-opiomelanocortin mRNA expression in the rostral arcuate nucleus. Diabetes 1997;46:2119-2123.
44. Stephens TW, Basinski M, Bristow PK, et al. The role of neuropeptide Y in the antiobesity action of the obese gene product. Nature 1995;377:530-532.
45. Cowley MA, Smart JL, Rubinstein M, et al. Leptin activates anorexigenic POMC neurons through a neural network in the arcuate nucleus. Nature 2001;411:480-484.
46. Spanswick D, Smith MA, Groppi VE, et al. Leptin inhibits hypothalamic neurons by activation of ATP-sensitive potassium channels. Nature 1997;390:521-525.
47. Balthasar N, Coppari R, McMinn J, et al. Leptin receptor signaling in POMC neurons is required for normal body weight homeostasis. Neuron 2004;42:983-991.
48. Dhillon H, Zigman JM, Ye C, et al. Leptin directly activates SF1 neurons in the VMH, and this action by leptin is required for normal body-weight homeostasis. Neuron 2006;49:191-203.
49. Elmquist JK, Coppari R, Balthasar N, et al. Identifying hypothalamic pathways controlling food intake, body weight, and glucose homeostasis. J Comp Neurol 2005;493:63-71.
50. Cowley MA, Smith RG, Diano S, et al. The distribution and mechanism of action of ghrelin in the CNS demonstrates a novel hypothalamic circuit regulating energy homeostasis. Neuron 2003;37: 649-661.
51. Heisler LK, Cowley MA, Tecott LH. Activation of central melanocortin pathways by fenfluramine. Science 2002;297:609-611.
52. Heisler LK, Jobst EE, Sutton GM, et al. Serotonin reciprocally regulates melanocortin neurons to modulate food intake. Neuron 2006;51:239-249.
53. Fan W, Boston BA, Kesterson RA, et al. Role of melanocortinergic neurons in feeding and the agouti obesity syndrome. Nature 1997;385:165-168.

54. Huszar D, Lynch CA, Fairchild-Huntress V. Targeted disruption of the melanocortin-4 receptor results in obesity in mice. Cell 1997;88:131-141.
55. Farooqi IS, Keogh JM, Yeo GS, et al. Clinical spectrum of obesity and mutations in the melanocortin 4 receptor gene. N Engl J Med 2003;348:1085-1095.
56. Farooqi IS, Yeo GS, Keogh JM, et al. Dominant and recessive inheritance of morbid obesity associated with melanocortin 4 receptor deficiency. J Clin Invest 2000;10:271-279.
57. Yeo GS, Farooqi IS, Aminian S, et al. A frameshift mutation in MC4R associated with dominantly inherited human obesity (letter). Nat Genet 1998;20:111-112.
58. Vaisse C, Clement K, Guy-Grand B, et al. A frameshift mutation in human MC4R is associated with a dominant form of obesity. Nat Genet 1998;20:113-114.
59. Mountjoy KG, Mortrud MT, Low MJ, et al. Localization of the melanocortin-4 receptor (MC4-R) in neuroendocrine and autonomic control circuits in the brain. Mol Endocrinol 1994;8:1298-1308.
60. Kishi T, Aschkenasi CJ, Lee CE, et al. Expression of melanocortin 4 receptor mRNA in the central nervous system of the rat. J Comp Neurol 2003;457:213-235.
61. Liu H, Kishi T, Roseberry AG, et al. Transgenic mice expressing green fluorescent protein under the control of the melanocortin-4 receptor promoter. J Neurosci 2003;23:7143-7154.
62. Cowley MA, Pronchuk N, Fan W, et al. Integration of NPY, AGRP, and melanocortin signals in the hypothalamic paraventricular nucleus: evidence of a cellular basis for the adipostat. Neuron 1999;24:155-163.
63. Balthasar N, Dalgaard LT, Lee CE, et al. Divergence of melanocortin pathways in the control of food intake and energy expenditure. Cell 2005;123:493-505.
64. Mountjoy KG, Mortrud MT, Low MJ, et al. Localization of the melanocortin-4 receptor (MC4-R) in neuroendocrine and autonomic control circuits in the brain. Mol Endocrinol 1994;8: 1298-1308.
65. Grill HJ, Ginsberg AB, Seeley RJ, et al. Brainstem application of melanocortin receptor ligands produces long- lasting effects on feeding and body weight. J Neurosci 1998;18:10128-10135.
66. Williams DL, Kaplan JM, Grill HJ. The role of the dorsal vagal complex and the vagus nerve in feeding effects of melanocortin-3/4 receptor stimulation. Endocrinology 2000;141:1332-1337.
67. Fan W, Ellacott KL, Halatchev IG, et al. Cholecystokinin-mediated suppression of feeding involves the brainstem melanocortin system. Nat Neurosci 2004;7:335-336.
68. Anand BK, Brobeck JR. Localization of a "feeding center" in the hypothalamus of the rat. Proc Soc Exp Biol Med 1951;77:323-324.
69. Bittencourt JC, Presse F, Arias C, et al. The melanin-concentrating hormone system of the rat brain: an immuno- and hybridization histochemical characterization. J Comp Neurol 1992;319:218-245.
70. Qu D, Ludwig DS, Gammeltoft S, et al. A role for melanin-concentrating hormone in the central regulation of feeding behaviour. Nature 1996;380:243-247.
71. Sakurai T, Amemiya A, Ishii M, et al. Orexins and orexin receptors: a family of hypothalamic neuropeptides and G protein-coupled receptors that regulate feeding behavior. Cell 1998;92:573-585.
72. de Lecea L, Kilduff TS, Peyron C, et al. The hypocretins: hypothalamus-specific peptides with neuroexcitatory activity. Proc Natl Acad Sci U S A 1998;95:322-327.
73. Elias CF, Saper CB, Maratos-Flier E, et al. Chemically defined projections linking the mediobasal hypothalamus and the lateral hypothalamic area. J Comp Neurol 1998;402:442-459.
74. Broberger C, De Lecea L, Sutcliffe JG, et al. Hypocretin/orexin- and melanin-concentrating hormone-expressing cells form distinct populations in the rodent lateral hypothalamus: relationship to the neuropeptide Y and agouti gene-related protein systems. J Comp Neurol 1998;402:460-474.
75. Peyron C, Tighe DK, van den Pol AN, et al. Neurons containing hypocretin (orexin) project to multiple neuronal systems. J Neurosci 1998;18:9996-10015.
76. Marcus JN, Aschkenasi CJ, Lee CE, et al. Differential expression of orexin receptors 1 and 2 in the rat brain. J Comp Neurol 2001; 435:6-25.
77. Saito Y, Cheng M, Leslie FM, et al. Expression of the melanin-concentrating hormone (MCH) receptor mRNA in the rat brain. J Comp Neurol 2001;435:26-40.
78. Kilduff TS, de Lecea L. Mapping of the mRNAs for the hypocretin/orexin and melanin-concentrating hormone receptors: networks of overlapping peptide systems. J Comp Neurol 2001;435:1-5.
79. Shimada M, Tritos NA, Lowell BB, et al. Mice lacking melanin-concentrating hormone are hypophagic and lean. Nature 1998;396: 670-674.
80. Ludwig DS, Tritos NA, Mastaitis JW, et al. Melanin-concentrating hormone overexpression in transgenic mice leads to obesity and insulin resistance. J Clin Invest 2001;107:379-386.
81. Segal-Lieberman G, Bradley RL, Kokkotou E, et al. Melanin-concentrating hormone is a critical mediator of the leptin-deficient phenotype. Proc Natl Acad Sci U S A 2003;100:10085-10090.
82. Willie JT, Chemelli RM, Sinton CM, et al. To eat or to sleep? Orexin in the regulation of feeding and wakefulness. Annu Rev Neurosci 2001;24:429-458.
83. Hara J, Beuckmann CT, Nambu T, et al. Genetic ablation of orexin neurons in mice results in narcolepsy, hypophagia, and obesity. Neuron 2001;30:345-354.
84. Clegg DJ, Air EL, Woods SC, et al. Eating elicited by orexin-a, but not melanin-concentrating hormone, is opioid mediated. Endocrinology 2002;143:2995-3000.
85. Chemelli RM, Willi JT, Sinton CM, et al. Narcolepsy in orexin knockout mice: molecular genetics of sleep regulation. Cell 1999;98:437-451.
86. Lin L, Faraco J, Li R, et al. The sleep disorder canine narcolepsy is caused by a mutation in the hypocretin (orexin) receptor 2 gene (see comments). Cell 1999;98:365-376.
87. Rothwell NJ. CNS regulation of thermogenesis. Crit Rev Neurobiol 1994;8:1-10.
88. Lowell BB, Bachman ES. Beta-adrenergic receptors, diet-induced thermogenesis, and obesity. J Biol Chem 2003;278:29385-29388.
89. Bachman ES, Dhillon H, Zhang CY, et al. betaAR signaling required for diet-induced thermogenesis and obesity resistance. Science 2002;297:843-845.
90. Jansen AS, Nguyen XV, Karpitskiy V, et al. Central command neurons of the sympathetic nervous system: basis of the fight-or-flight response. Science 1995;270:644-646.
91. Loewy AD. Forebrain nuclei involved in autonomic control. Prog Brain Res 1991;87:253-268.
92. Loewy AD, Spyer KM. Central regulation of autonomic functions. New York: Oxford University Press, 1990:xii, 390.
93. Strack AM, Sawyer WB, Platt KB, et al. CNS cell groups regulating the sympathetic outflow to adrenal gland as revealed by transneuronal cell body labeling with pseudorabies virus. Brain Res 1989;491:274-296.
94. Strack AM, Sawyer WB, Marubio LM, et al. Spinal origin of sympathetic preganglionic neurons in the rat. Brain Res 1988;455: 187-191.
95. Strack AM, Sawyer WB, Hughes GH, et al. A general pattern of CNS innervation of the sympathetic outflow demonstrated by transneuronal pseudorabies viral infections. Brain Res 1989;491:156-162.
96. Jansen AS, Hoffman JL, Loewy AD. CNS sites involved in sympathetic and parasympathetic control of the pancreas: a viral tracing study. Brain Res 1997;766:29-38.
97. Rinaman L, Miselis RR. The organization of vagal innervation of rat pancreas using cholera toxin-horseradish peroxidase conjugate. J Auton Nerv Syst 1987;21:109-125.
98. Saper CB, Loewy AD, Swanson LW, et al. Direct hypothalamo-autonomic connections. Brain Res 1976;117:305-312.
99. Loewy AD, McKellar S, Saper CB. Direct projections from the A5 catecholamine cell group to the intermediolateral cell column. Brain Res 1979;174:309-314.
100. Cechetto DF, Saper CB. Neurochemical organization of the hypothalamic projection to the spinal cord in the rat. J Comp Neurol 1988;272:579-604.
101. Loewy AD, Burton H. Nuclei of the solitary tract: efferent projections to the lower brain stem and spinal cord of the cat. J Comp Neurol 1978;181:421-449.
102. Loewy AD. Descending pathways to sympathetic and parasympathetic preganglionic neurons. J Auton Nerv Syst 1981;3:265-275.
103. Loewy AD. Descending pathways to the sympathetic preganglionic neurons. Prog Brain Res 1982;57:267-277.
104. Tucker DC, Saper CB. Specificity of spinal projections from hypothalamic and brainstem areas which innervate sympathetic preganglionic neurons. Brain Res 1985;360:159-164.

105. Tucker DC, Saper CB, Ruggiero DA, et al. Organization of central adrenergic pathways: I. Relationships of ventrolateral medullary projections to the hypothalamus and spinal cord. J Comp Neurol 1987;259:591-603.
106. Chan RK, Sawchenko PE. Spatially and temporally differentiated patterns of c-fos expression in brainstem catecholaminergic cell groups induced by cardiovascular challenges in the rat. J Comp Neurol 1994;348:433-460.
107. Morrison SF, Milner TA, Reis DJ. Reticulospinal vasomotor neurons of the rat rostral ventrolateral medulla: relationship to sympathetic nerve activity and the C1 adrenergic cell group. J Neurosci 1988;8:1286-1301.
108. Haselton JR, Guyenet PG. Electrophysiological characterization of putative C1 adrenergic neurons in the rat. Neuroscience 1989; 30:199-214.
109. Reis DJ, Ruggiero DA, Morrison SF. The C1 area of the rostral ventrolateral medulla oblongata. A critical brainstem region for control of resting and reflex integration of arterial pressure. Am J Hypertens 1989;2(12 Pt 2):363S-374S.
110. Butler AA, Marks DL, Fan W, et al. Melanocortin-4 receptor is required for acute homeostatic responses to increased dietary fat. Nat Neurosci 2001;4(6):605-611.
111. Yasuda T, Masaki T, Kakuma T, et al. Hypothalamic melanocortin system regulates sympathetic nerve activity in brown adipose tissue. Exp Biol Med (Maywood) 2004;229:235-239.
112. Voss-Andreae A, Murphy JG, Ellacott KL, et al. Role of the central melanocortin circuitry in adaptive thermogenesis of brown adipose tissue. Endocrinology 2007;148:1550-1560.
113. Elias CF, Lee C, Kelly J, et al. Leptin activates hypothalamic CART neurons projecting to the spinal cord. Neuron 1998;21: 1375-1385.
114. Morrison SF. Central pathways controlling brown adipose tissue thermogenesis. News Physiol Sci 2004;19:67-74.
115. Fan W, Voss-Andreae A, Cao WH, et al. Regulation of thermogenesis by the central melanocortin system. Peptides 2005;26: 1800-1813.
116. Loewy AD. Raphe pallidus and raphe obscurus projections to the intermediolateral cell column in the rat. Brain Res 1981;222: 129-133.
117. Bacon SJ, Zagon A, Smith AD. Electron microscopic evidence of a monosynaptic pathway between cells in the caudal raphe nuclei and sympathetic preganglionic neurons in the rat spinal cord. Exp Brain Res 1990;79:589-602.
118. Bamshad M, Song CK, Bartness TJ. CNS origins of the sympathetic nervous system outflow to brown adipose tissue. Am J Physiol 1999;276(6 Pt 2): R1569-R1578.
119. Morrison SF. Differential control of sympathetic outflow. Am J Physiol Regul Integr Comp Physiol 2001;281:R683-R698.
120. Zhang Y, Proenca R, Maffei R, et al. Positional cloning of the mouse obese gene and its human homologue. Nature 1994;372:425-432.
121. Wang J, Liu R, Hawkins M, Barzilai N, et al. A nutrient-sensing pathway regulates leptin gene expression in muscle and fat. Nature 1998;393:684-688.
122. Masuzaki H, Ogawa Y, Sagawa N, et al. Nonadipose tissue production of leptin: leptin as a novel placenta-derived hormone in humans. Nat Med 1997;3:1029-1033.
123. Pelleymounter MA, Cullen MJ, Baker MB, et al. Effects of the obese gene product on body weight regulation in ob/ob mice. Science 1995;269:540-543.
124. Campfield LA, Smith FJ, Guisez Y, et al. Recombinant mouse OB protein: evidence for a peripheral signal linking adiposity and central neural networks. Science 1995;269:546-549.
125. Halaas JL, Gajiwala KS, Maffei M, et al. Weight-reducing effects of the plasma protein encoded by the obese gene. Science 1995; 269:543-546.
126. Farooqi IS, Jebb SA, Langmack G, et al. Effects of recombinant leptin therapy in a child with congenital leptin deficiency. N Engl J Med 1999;341:879-884.
127. Ahima RS, Saper CB, Flier JS, et al. Role of leptin in the neuroendocrine response to fasting. Nature 1996;382:250-252.
128. Spiegelman BM, Flier JS. Obesity and the regulation of energy balance. Cell 2001;104:531-543.
129. Frederich RC, Hamann A, Anderson S, et al. Leptin levels reflect body lipid content in mice: evidence for diet- induced resistance to leptin action. Nat Med 1995;1:1311-1314.
130. Ahima RS, Saper CB, Flier JS, et al. Leptin regulation of neuroendocrine systems. Front Neuroendocrinol 2000;21:263-307.
131. Flier JS. Clinical review 94: what's in a name? In search of leptin's physiologic role. J Clin Endocrinol Metab 1998;83:1407-1413.
132. Tartaglia LA. The leptin receptor. J Biol Chem 1997;272: 6093-6096.
133. Chen H, Charlat O, Tartaglia LA, et al. Evidence that the diabetes gene encodes the leptin receptor: identification of a mutation in the leptin receptor gene in db/db mice. Cell 1996;84:491-495.
134. White DW, Wang DW, Chua SC Jr, et al. Constitutive and impaired signaling of leptin receptors containing the Gln –> Pro extracellular domain fatty mutation. Proc Natl Acad Sci U S A 1997;94: 10657-10662.
135. Mercer JG, Hoggard N, Williams LM, et al. Coexpression of leptin receptor and preproneuropeptide Y mRNA in arcuate nucleus of mouse hypothalamus. J Neuroendocrinol 1996;8:733-735.
136. Mercer JG, Hoggard N, Williams LM, et al. Localization of leptin receptor mRNA and the long form splice variant (Ob-Rb) in mouse hypothalamus and adjacent brain regions by in situ hybridization. FEBS Lett 1996;387:113-116.
137. Fei H, Okano HJ, Li C, et al. Anatomic localization of alternatively spliced leptin receptors (Ob-R) in mouse brain and other tissues. Proc Natl Acad Sci U S A 1997;94:7001-7005.
138. Schwartz MW, Seeley RJ, Campfield LA, et al. Identification of targets of leptin action in rat hypothalamus. J Clin Invest 1996;98: 1101-1106.
139. Elmquist JK, Bjorbaek C, Ahima RS, et al. Distributions of leptin receptor mRNA isoforms in the rat brain. J Comp Neurol 1998; 395:535-547.
140. Cheung CC, Clifton DK, Steiner RA. Proopiomelanocortin neurons are direct targets for leptin in the hypothalamus. Endocrinology 1997;138:4489-4492.
141. Hosoi T, Kawagishi T, Okuma Y, et al. Brain stem is a direct target for leptin's action in the central nervous system. Endocrinology 2002;143:3498-3504.
142. Grill HJ, Schwartz MW, Kaplan JM, et al. Evidence that the caudal brainstem is a target for the inhibitory effect of leptin on food intake. Endocrinology 2002;143:239-246.
143. Finn PD, Cunningham MJ, Rickard DG, et al. Serotonergic neurons are targets for leptin in the monkey. J Clin Endocrinol Metab 2001;86:422-426.
144. Mercer JG, Moar KM, Hoggard N. Localization of leptin receptor (Ob-R) messenger ribonucleic acid in the rodent hindbrain. Endocrinology 1998;139:29-34.
145. Mercer JG, Moar KM, Findlay PA, et al. Association of leptin receptor (OB-Rb), NPY and GLP-1 gene expression in the ovine and murine brainstem. Regul Pept 1998;75-76:271-278.
146. Bernard C. CR Soc Biol (Paris) Chiens rendus diabetiques. 1849;1:60.
147. Elmquist JK, Marcus JN. Rethinking the central causes of diabetes. Nat Med 2003;9:645-647.
148. Fan W, Dinulescu DM, Butler AA, et al. The central melanocortin system can directly regulate serum insulin levels. Endocrinology 2000;141:3072-3079.
149. Obici S, Feng Z, Arduini A, et al. Inhibition of hypothalamic carnitine palmitoyltransferase-1 decreases food intake and glucose production. Nat Med 2003;9:756-761.
150. Obici S, Feng Z, Karkanias G, et al. Decreasing hypothalamic insulin receptors causes hyperphagia and insulin resistance in rats. Nat Neurosci 2002;5(6):566-572.
151. Schwartz MW. Progress in the search for neuronal mechanisms coupling type 2 diabetes to obesity. J Clin Invest 2001;108: 963-964.
152. Schwartz MW, Woods SC, Porte D Jr, et al. Central nervous system control of food intake. Nature 2000;404:661-671.
153. Woods SC, Lotter EC, McKay LD, et al. Chronic intracerebroventricular infusion of insulin reduces food intake and body weight of baboons. Nature 1979;282:503-505.
154. Bruning JC, Gautam D, Burks DJ, et al. Role of brain insulin receptor in control of body weight and reproduction. Science 2000; 289:2122-2125.
155. Buettner C, Patel R, Muse ED, et al. Severe impairment in liver insulin signaling fails to alter hepatic insulin action in conscious mice. J Clin Invest 2005;115:1306-1313.

156. Okamoto H, Obici S, Accili D, et al. Restoration of liver insulin signaling in Insr knockout mice fails to normalize hepatic insulin action. J Clin Invest 2005;115:1314-1322.
157. Edgerton DS, Lautz M, Scott M, et al. Insulin's direct effects on the liver dominate the control of hepatic glucose production. J Clin Invest 2006;116:521-527.
158. Oomura Y, Ono T, Ooyama H, et al. Glucose and osmosensitive neurones of the rat hypothalamus. Nature 1969;222:282-284.
159. Levin BE. Metabolic sensing neurons and the control of energy homeostasis. Physiol Behav 2006;89:1107-1121.
160. Levin BE, Routh VH, Kang L, et al. Neuronal glucosensing: what do we know after 50 years? Diabetes 2004;53:2521-2528.
161. Ibrahim N, Bosch MA, Smart JL, et al. Hypothalamic proopiomelanocortin neurons are glucose responsive and express K(ATP) channels. Endocrinology 2003;144:1331-1340.
162. DiRocco RJ, Grill HJ. The forebrain is not essential for sympathoadrenal hyperglycemic response to glucoprivation. Science 1979;204:1112-1114.
163. Ritter S, Bugarith K, Dinh TT. Immunotoxic destruction of distinct catecholamine subgroups produces selective impairment of glucoregulatory responses and neuronal activation. J Comp Neurol 2001;432:197-216.
164. Ritter S, Dinh TT, Zhang Y. Localization of hindbrain glucoreceptive sites controlling food intake and blood glucose. Brain Res 2000;856:37-47.
165. Burdakov D, et al. Tandem-pore K+ channels mediate inhibition of orexin neurons by glucose. Neuron 2006;50:711-722.
166. Obici S, Feng Z, Tan J, et al. Central melanocortin receptors regulate insulin action. J Clin Invest 2001;108:1079-1085.
167. Fox EA, Powley TL. Tracer diffusion has exaggerated CNS maps of direct preganglionic innervation of pancreas. J Auton Nerv Syst 1986;15:55-69.
168. Loewy AD, Franklin MF, Haxhiu MA. CNS monoamine cell groups projecting to pancreatic vagal motor neurons: a transneuronal labeling study using pseudorabies virus. Brain Res 1994;638: 248-260.
169. Berthoud HR, Fox EA, Powley TL. Localization of vagal preganglionics that stimulate insulin and glucagon secretion. Am J Physiol 1990;258(1 Pt 2):R160-R168.
170. Cai XJ, Widdowson PS, Harrold J, et al. Hypothalamic orexin expression: modulation by blood glucose and feeding. Diabetes 1999;48:2132-2137.
171. Griffond B, Risold PY, Jacquemard C, et al. Insulin-induced hypoglycemia increases preprohypocretin (orexin) mRNA in the rat lateral hypothalamic area. Neurosci Lett 1999;262:77-80.
172. Moriguchi T, Sakurai T, Nambu T, et al. Neurons containing orexin in the lateral hypothalamic area of the adult rat brain are activated by insulin-induced acute hypoglycemia. Neurosci Lett 1999;264: 101-104.
173. Scott MM, Marcus JN, Elmquist JK. Orexin neurons and the TASK of glucosensing. Neuron 2006;50:665-667.
174. Oomura Y, Yoshimatsu H. Neural network of glucose monitoring system. J Auton Nerv Syst 1984;10:359-372.
175. Schwartz GJ. The role of gastrointestinal vagal afferents in the control of food intake: current prospects. Nutrition 2000;16: 866-873.
176. Altschuler SM, et al. Viscerotopic representation of the upper alimentary tract in the rat: sensory ganglia and nuclei of the solitary and spinal trigeminal tracts. J Comp Neurol 1989;283:248-268.
177. Saper CB. Central autonomic system. In Paxinos G, ed. The Rat Nervous System. San Diego: Academic Press, 1995:107-135.
178. Raybould HE, Gayton RJ, Dockray GJ. CNS effects of circulating CCK8: involvement of brainstem neurones responding to gastric distension. Brain Res 1985;342:187-190.
179. Zhang X, Fogel R, Renehan WE. Relationships between the morphology and function of gastric- and intestine-sensitive neurons in the nucleus of the solitary tract. J Comp Neurol 1995;363:37-52.
180. Rinaman L, et al. Distribution and neurochemical phenotypes of caudal medullary neurons activated to express cFos following peripheral administration of cholecystokinin. J Comp Neurol 1993;338:475-490.
181. Gibbs J, Falasco JD, McHugh PR. Cholecystokinin-decreased food intake in rhesus monkeys. Am J Physiol 1976;230:15-18.
182. Gibbs J, Young RC, Smith GP. Cholecystokinin decreases food intake in rats. J Comp Physiol Psych 1973;84:488-495.
183. Crawley JN, Beinfeld MC. Rapid development of tolerance to the behavioural actions of cholecystokinin. Nature 1983;302:703-706.
184. West D, Fey D, Woods S. Cholecystokinin persistently suppresses meal size but not food intake in free-feeding rats. Am J Physiol 1984;246:R776-R787.
185. Smith GP, et al. Abdominal vagotomy blocks the satiety effect of cholecystokinin in the rat. Science 1981;213:1036-1037.
186. South EH, Ritter RC. Capsaicin application to central or peripheral vagal fibers attenuates CCK satiety. Peptides 1988;9:601-612.
187. Hewson G, et al. The cholecystokinin receptor antagonist L364,718 increases food intake in the rat by attenuation of the action of endogenous cholecystokinin. Br J Pharmacol 1988;93:79-84.
188. Dourish CT, et al. Evidence that decreased feeding induced by systemic injection of cholecystokinin is mediated by CCK-A receptors. Eur J Pharmacol 1989;173:233-234.
189. Dourish C, Rycroft W, Iversen S. Postponement of satiety by blockade of brain cholecystokinin (CCKB) receptors. Science 1989;245: 1509-1511.
190. Reidelberger RD, O'Rourke MF. Potent cholecystokinin antagonist L 364718 stimulates food intake in rats. Am J Physiol 1989;257(6 Pt 2):R1512-R1518.
191. Gutzwiller JP, et al. Interaction between CCK and a preload on reduction of food intake is mediated by CCK-A receptors in humans. Am J Physiol Regul Integr Comp Physiol 2000;279: R189-R195.
192. Riedy CA, et al. Central insulin enhances sensitivity to cholecystokinin. Physiol Behav 1995;58:755-760.
193. Figlewicz DP, et al. Intraventricular insulin enhances the meal-suppressive efficacy of intraventricular cholecystokinin octapeptide in the baboon. Behav Neurosci 1995;109:567-569.
194. Matson CA, et al. Synergy between leptin and cholecystokinin (CCK) to control daily caloric intake. Peptides 1997;18:1275-1278.
195. Matson CA, Ritter RC. Long-term CCK-leptin synergy suggests a role for CCK in the regulation of body weight. Am J Physiol 1999;276:R1038.
196. Emond M, Schwartz GJ, Ladenheim EE, et al. Central leptin modulates behavioral and neural responsivity to CCK. Am J Physiol 1999;276(5 Pt 2):R1545-R1549.
197. Matson CA, et al. Cholecystokinin and leptin act synergistically to reduce body weight. Am J Physiol 2000;278:R882.
198. Cannon CM, Palmiter RD. Peptides that regulate food intake: norepinephrine is not required for reduction of feeding induced by cholecystokinin. Am J Physiol Regul Integr Comp Physiol 2003;284: R1384-R1388.
199. Lodge DJ, Lawrence AJ. Comparative analysis of the central CCK system in Fawn Hooded and Wistar Kyoto rats: extended localisation of CCK-A receptors throughout the rat brain using a novel radioligand. Regul Pept 2001;99:191-201.
200. Mercer LD, Beart PM. Histochemistry in rat brain and spinal cord with an antibody directed at the cholecystokininA receptor. Neurosci Lett 1997;225:97-100.
201. Hirosue Y, et al. Cholecystokinin octapeptide analogues suppress food intake via central CCK-A receptors in mice. Am J Physiol 1993;265(3 Pt 2):R481-R486.
202. Adrian TE, et al. Human distribution and release of a putative new gut hormone, peptide YY. Gastroenterology 1985;89:1070-1077.
203. Grandt D, et al. Two molecular forms of peptide YY (PYY) are abundant in human blood: characterization of a radioimmunoassay recognizing PYY 1-36 and PYY 3-36. Regul Pept 1994;51: 151-159.
204. Grandt D, et al. Characterization of two forms of peptide YY, PYY(1-36) and PYY(3-36), in the rabbit. Peptides 1994;15:815-820.
205. Bonaz B, Taylor I, Tache Y. Peripheral peptide YY induces c-fos-like immunoreactivity in the rat brain. Neurosci Lett 1993;163:77-80.
206. Allen JM, et al. Effects of peptide YY and neuropeptide Y on gastric emptying in man. Digestion 1984;30:255-262.
207. Adrian TE, et al. Effect of peptide YY on gastric, pancreatic, and biliary function in humans. Gastroenterology 1985;89:494-499.
208. Yang H. Central and peripheral regulation of gastric acid secretion by peptide YY. Peptides 2002;23:349-358.
209. Dumont Y, et al. Autoradiographic distribution of (125I)Leu31, Pro34)PYY and (125I)PYY3-36 binding sites in the rat brain evaluated with two newly developed Y1 and Y2 receptor radioligands. Synapse 1996;22:139-158.

210. Lloyd KC, et al. Candidate canine enterogastrones: acid inhibition before and after vagotomy. Am J Physiol 1997;272(5 Pt 1):G1236-G1242.
211. Batterham RL, et al. Gut hormone PYY(3-36) physiologically inhibits food intake. Nature 2002;418:650-654.
212. Adams SH, et al. Effects of peptide YY(3-36) on short-term food intake in mice are not affected by prevailing plasma ghrelin levels. Endocrinology 2004;145:4967-4975.
213. Challis BG, et al. Mice lacking pro-opiomelanocortin are sensitive to high-fat feeding but respond normally to the acute anorectic effects of peptide-YY(3-36). Proc Natl Acad Sci U S A 2004; 101:4695-4700.
214. Chelikani PK, Haver AC, Reidelberger RD. Intravenous infusion of peptide YY(3-36) potently inhibits food intake in rats. Endocrinology 2005;146:879-888.
215. Cox JE, Randich A. Enhancement of feeding suppression by PYY(3-36) in rats with area postrema ablations. Peptides 2004; 25:985-989.
216. Pittner RA, Moore CX, Bhavsar SP, et al. Effects of PYY(3-36) in rodent models of diabetes and obesity. Int J Obes Relat Metab Disord 2004;28:963-971.
217. Moran TH, et al. Peptide YY(3-36) inhibits gastric emptying and produces acute reductions in food intake in rhesus monkeys. Am J Physiol Regul Integr Comp Physiol 2005;288:R384-R388.
218. Halatchev IG, et al. Peptide YY3-36 inhibits food intake in mice through a melanocortin-4 receptor-independent mechanism. Endocrinology 2004;145:2585-2590.
219. Abbott CR, et al. The inhibitory effects of peripheral administration of peptide YY(3-36) and glucagon-like peptide-1 on food intake are attenuated by ablation of the vagal-brainstem-hypothalamic pathway. Brain Res 2005;1044:127-131.
220. Martin NM, et al. Pre-obese and obese agouti mice are sensitive to the anorectic effects of peptide YY(3-36) but resistant to ghrelin. Int J Obes Relat Metab Disord 2004;28:886-893.
221. Batterham RL, et al. Critical role for peptide YY in protein-mediated satiation and body-weight regulation. Cell Metab 2006;4: 223-233.
222. Boey D, et al. Peptide YY ablation in mice leads to the development of hyperinsulinaemia and obesity. Diabetologia 2006;49:1360-1370.
223. Kojima M, et al. Ghrelin is a growth-hormone-releasing acylated peptide from stomach. Nature 1999;402:656-660.
224. Kojima M, et al. Ghrelin: discovery of the natural endogenous ligand for the growth hormone secretagogue receptor. Trends Endocrinol Metab 2001;12:118-122.
225. Ariyasu H, et al. Stomach is a major source of circulating ghrelin, and feeding state determines plasma ghrelin-like immunoreactivity levels in humans. J Clin Endocrinol Metab 2001;86:4753-4758.
226. Tschop M, et al. Post-prandial decrease of circulating human ghrelin levels. J Endocrinol Invest 2001;24:RC19-RC21.
227. Tschop M, Smiley DL, Heiman ML. Ghrelin induces adiposity in rodents. Nature 2000;407:908-913.
228. Cummings DE, et al. A preprandial rise in plasma ghrelin levels suggest a role in meal initiation in humans. Diabetes 2001;50: 1714-1719.
229. Willesen M, Kristensen P, Romer J. Co-localization of growth hormone secretagogue receptor and NPY mRNA in the arcuate nucleus of the rat. Neuroendocrinol 1999;70:306-316.
230. Hewson AK, Dickson SL. Systemic administration of ghrelin induces Fos and Egr-1 proteins in the hypothalamic arcuate nucleus of fasted and fed rats. J Neuroendocrinol 2000;12: 1047-1049.
231. Kamegai J, et al. Central effect of ghrelin, an endogenous growth hormone secretagogue, on hypothalamic peptide gene expression. Endocrinology 2000;141:4797-4800.
232. Kamegai J, et al. Chronic central infusion of ghrelin increases hypothalamic neuropeptide Y and Agouti-related protein mRNA levels and body weight in rats. Diabetes 2001;50:2438-2443.
233. Asakawa A, et al. Ghrelin is an appetite-stimulatory signal from stomach with structural resemblance to motilin. Gastroenterology 2001;120:337-345.
234. Nakazato M, Murakami N, Date Y. A role for ghrelin in the central regulation of feeding. Nature 2001;409:194-198.
235. Shintani M, et al. Ghrelin, an endogenous growth hormone secretagogue, is a novel orexigenic peptide that antagonizes leptin action through the activation of hypothalamic neuropeptide Y/Y1 receptor pathway. Diabetes 2001;50:227-232.
236. Wren AM, et al. The novel hypothalamic peptide ghrelin stimulates food intake and growth hormone secretion. Endocrinology 2000;141:4325-4328.
237. Wren AM, et al. Ghrelin causes hyperphagia and obesity in rats. Diabetes 2001;50:2540-2547.
238. Wren AM, et al. Ghrelin enhances appetite and increases food intake in humans. J Clin Endocrinol Metab 2001;86:5992.
239. Tschop M, et al. Circulating ghrelin levels are decreased in human obesity. Diabetes 2001;50:707-709.
240. Nagaya N, et al. Chronic administration of ghrelin improves left ventricular dysfunction and attenuates development of cardiac cachexia in rats with heart failure. Circulation 2001;104: 1430-1435.
240a. Tschop M, et al. GH-releasing peptide-2 increases fat mass in mice lacking NPY: Indication for a crucial mediating role of hypothalamic agouti-related protein. Endocrinology 2002;143:558-568.
241. Wang L, Saint-Pierre DH, Tache Y. Peripheral ghrelin selectively increases Fos expression in neuropeptide Y—synthesizing neurons in mouse hypothalamic arcuate nucleus. Neurosci Lett 2002; 325:47-51.
242. Tamura H, et al. Ghrelin stimulates GH but not food intake in arcuate nucleus ablated rats. Endocrinology 2002;143:3268-3275.
243. Date Y, et al. The role of the gastric afferent vagal nerve in ghrelin-induced feeding and growth hormone secretion in rats. Gastroenterology 2002;123:1120-1128.
244. Zhang JV, et al. Obestatin, a peptide encoded by the ghrelin gene, opposes ghrelin's effects on food intake. Science 2005;310: 996-999.
245. Tremblay F, et al. Normal food intake and body weight in mice lacking the G protein-coupled receptor GPR39. Endocrinology 2007;148:501-506.
246. Lauwers E, et al. Obestatin does not activate orphan G protein-coupled receptor GPR39. Biochem Biophys Res Commun 2006; 351:21-25.
247. Nogueiras R, et al. Effects of obestatin on energy balance and growth hormone secretion in rodents. Endocrinology 2007;148: 21-26.
248. Drucker DJ. The biology of incretin hormones. Cell Metab 2006;3:153-165.
249. Drucker DJ, Nauck MA. The incretin system: glucagon-like peptide-1 receptor agonists and dipeptidyl peptidase-4 inhibitors in type 2 diabetes. Lancet 2006;368:1696-1705.
250. Thiele TE, et al. Central infusion of GLP-1, but not leptin, produces conditioned taste aversions in rats. Am J Physiol 1997;272(2 Pt 2): R726-R730.
251. Thiele TE, et al. Central infusion of glucagon-like peptide-1-(7-36) amide (GLP-1) receptor antagonist attenuates lithium chloride-induced c-Fos induction in rat brainstem. Brain Res 1998;801: 164-170.
252. Tang-Christensen M, et al. Central administration of GLP-1-(7-36) amide inhibits food and water intake in rats. J Physiol 1996;271: 848-856.
253. Turton MD, et al. A role for glucagon-like peptide-1 in the central regulation of feeding. Nature 1996;379:69-72.
254. McMahon LR, Wellman PJ. PVN infusion of GLP-1-(7-36) amide suppresses feeding but does not induce aversion or alter locomotion in rats. Am J Physiol 1998;274(1 Pt 2):R23-R29.
255. Flint A, et al. Glucagon-like peptide 1 promotes satiety and suppresses energy intake in humans. J Clin Invest 1998;101:515-520.
256. Gutzwiller JP, et al. Glucagon-like peptide-1 promotes satiety and reduces food intake in patients with diabetes mellitus type 2. Am J Physiol 1999;276(5 Pt 2):R1541-R1544.
257. Toft-Nielsen MB, Madsbad S, Holst JJ. Continuous subcutaneous infusion of glucagon-like peptide 1 lowers plasma glucose and reduces appetite in type 2 diabetic patients. Diabetes Care 1999; 22:1137-1143.
258. Verdich C, et al. A meta-analysis of the effect of glucagon-like peptide-1 (7-36) amide on ad libitum energy intake in humans. JCEM 2001;86:4382-4389.
259. Zander M, et al. Effect of 6-week course of glucagon-like peptide 1 on glycaemic control, insulin sensitivity, and beta-cell function in type 2 diabetes: a parallel-group study. Lancet 2002;359: 824-830.

260. Nakabayashi H, et al. Vagal hepatopancreatic reflex effect evoked by intraportal appearance of tGLP-1. Am J Physiol 1996;271(5 Pt 1):E808-E813.
261. Imeryuz N, et al. Glucagon-like peptide-1 inhibits gastric emptying via vagal afferent-mediated central mechanisms. Am J Physiol 1997;273(4 Pt 1):G920-G927.
262. Lachey JL, et al. The role of central glucagon-like peptide-1 in mediating the effects of visceral illness: differential effects in rats and mice. Endocrinology 2005;146:458-462.
263. Rinaman L. Interoceptive stress activates glucagon-like peptide-1 neurons that project to the hypothalamus. Am J Physiol 1999;277(2 Pt 2):R582-R590.
264. Rinaman L, RotheEE. GLP-1 receptor signaling contributes to anorexigenic effect of centrally administered oxytocin in rats. Am J Physiol Regul Integr Comp Physiol 2002;283:R99-R106.
265. Sawchenko PE, Swanson LW. The organization of forebrain afferents to the paraventricular and supraoptic nuclei of the rat. J Comp Neurol 1983;218:121-144.
266. Elias CF, et al. Chemical characterization of leptin-activated neurons in the rat brain. J Comp Neurol 2000;423:261-281.
267. Ellacott KL, Halatchev IG, Cone RD. Characterization of leptin-responsive neurons in the caudal brainstem. Endocrinology 2006;147:3190-3195.
268. Larsen PJ, et al. Distribution of glucagon-like peptide-1 and other preproglucagon-derived peptides in the rat hypothalamus and brainstem. Neuroscience 1997;77:257-270.
269. Merchenthaler I, Lane M, Shughrue P. Distribution of pre-pro-glucagon and glucagon-like peptide-1 receptor messenger RNAs in the rat central nervous system. J Comp Neurol 1999;403: 261-280.
270. Kahn SE, Andrikopoulos S, CB Verchere CB. Islet amyloid: a long-recognized but underappreciated pathological feature of type 2 diabetes. Diabetes 1999;48:241-253.
271. Hoppener JW, Ahren B, Lips CJ. Islet amyloid and type 2 diabetes mellitus. N Engl J Med 2000;343:411-419.
272. Hartter E, et al. Basal and stimulated plasma levels of pancreatic amylin indicate its co- secretion with insulin in humans. Diabetologia 1991;34:52-54.
273. Butler PC, Chou J, Carter WB, et al. Effects of meal ingestion on plasma amylin concentration in NIDDM and nondiabetic humans. Diabetes 1990;39:752-756.
274. Banks WA, et al. Permeability of the blood-brain barrier to amylin. Life Sci 1995;57:1993-2001.
275. Beaumont K, et al. High affinity amylin binding sites in rat brain. Mol Pharmacol 1993;44:493-497.
276. Morley, JE and JF Flood, Amylin decreases food intake in mice. Peptides 1991;12:865-869.
277. Arnelo U, et al. Effects of acute and chronic infusion of islet amyloid polypeptide on food intake in rats. Scand J Gastroenterol 1996;31:83-89.
278. Rushing PA, et al. Amylin: a novel action in the brain to reduce body weight. Endocrinology 2000;141:850-853.
279. Rushing PA, et al. Inhibition of central amylin signaling increases food intake and body adiposity in rats. Endocrinology 2001; 142:5035.
280. Reidelberger RD, et al. Comparative effects of amylin and cholecystokinin on food intake and gastric emptying in rats. Am J Physiol Regul Integr Comp Physiol 2001;280:R605-R611.
281. Bhavsar S, Watkins J, Young A. Synergy between amylin and cholecystokinin for inhibition of food intake in mice. Physiol Behav 1998;64:557-561.
282. Rushing PA, et al. Amylin and insulin interact to reduce food intake in rats. Horm Metab Res 2000;32:62-65.
283. Cummings DE, et al. Hormonal mechanisms of weight loss and diabetes resolution after bariatric surgery. Surg Obes Relat Dis 2005;1:358-368.
284. Sjostrom L, et al, and Swedish Obese Subjects Study Scientific Group. Lifestyle, diabetes, and cardiovascular risk factors 10 years after bariatric surgery. N Engl J Med 2004;351:2683-2693.
285. Rubino F, et al. The mechanism of diabetes control after gastrointestinal bypass surgery reveals a role of the proximal small intestine in the pathophysiology of type 2 diabetes. Ann Surg 2006;244:741-749.
286. Asarian L, Geary N. Modulation of appetite by gonadal steroid hormones. Philos Trans R Soc Lond B Biol Sci 2006;361: 1251-1263.
287. Lopez M, et al. Tamoxifen-induced anorexia is associated with fatty acid synthase inhibition in the ventromedial nucleus of the hypothalamus and accumulation of malonyl-CoA. Diabetes 2006;55:1327-1336.
288. Acosta-Martinez M, Horton T, Levine JE. Estrogen receptors in neuropeptide Y neurons: at the crossroads of feeding and reproduction. Trends Endocrinol Metab 2007;18:48-50.
289. Gao Q, et al. Anorectic estrogen mimics leptin's effect on the rewiring of melanocortin cells and Stat3 signaling in obese animals. Nat Med 2007;13:89-94.
290. Heine PA, et al. Increased adipose tissue in male and female estrogen receptor-alpha knockout mice. Proc Natl Acad Sci U S A 2000;97:12729-12734.
291. Musatov S, et al. Silencing of estrogen receptor (alpha) in the ventromedial nucleus of hypothalamus leads to metabolic syndrome. Proc Natl Acad Sci U S A 2007;104:2501-2506.
292. Aronsson M, et al. Localization of glucocorticoid receptor mRNA in the male rat brain by in situ hybridization. Proc Natl Acad Sci U S A 1988;85:9331-9335.
293. Tasker JG. Rapid glucocorticoid actions in the hypothalamus as a mechanism of homeostatic integration. Obesity (Silver Spring) 2006;14(suppl 5):259-265.
294. Saper C, Breder C. The neurologic basis of fever. N Engl J Med 1994;330:1880-1886.
295. Besedovsky H, et al. Immunoregulatory feedback between interleukin-1 and glucocorticoid hormones. Science 1986;233: 652-654.
296. Berkenbosch F, et al. Corticotropin-releasing factor-producing neurons in the rat activated by interleukin-1. Science 1987;238: 524-526.
297. Sapolsky R, et al. Interleukin-1 stimulates the secretion of hypothalamic corticotropin-releasing factor. Science 1987;238: 522-524.
298. Ader R, Cohen N, Felten D. Psychoneuroimmunology: interactions between the nervous system and the immune system. Lancet 1995;345:99-103.
299. Felten DL, et al. Noradrenergic and peptidergic innervation of lymphoid tissue. J Immunol 1985;135(suppl 2):755-765.
300. Spiegelman BM, Flier JS. Obesity and the regulation of energy balance. Cell 2001;104:531-543.
301. Chen TY, et al. Lipopolysaccharide receptors and signal transduction pathways in mononuclear phagocytes. Curr Top Microbiol Immunol 1992;181:169-188.
302. Rivest S, et al. How the blood talks to the brain parenchyma and the paraventricular nucleus of the hypothalamus during systemic inflammatory and infectious stimuli. Proc Soc Exp Biol Med 2000;223(1):22-38.
303. Elmquist, JK, Scammell TE, Saper CB. Mechanisms of CNS response to systemic immune challenge: the febrile response. Trends Neurosci 1997;20:565-570.
304. Reichlin S. Neuroendocrinology of infection and the innate immune system. Recent Prog Horm Res 1999;54:133-181.
305. Hellon R, Townsend Y. Mechanisms of fever. Pharmacol Ther 1982;19:211-244.
306. Blatteis CM. Role of the OVLT in the febrile response to circulating pyrogens. Prog Brain Res 1992;91:409-412.
307. Hunter WS, Sehic E, Blatteis CM. In Milton AS, ed. Temperature regulation: recent physiological and pharmacological advances. Basel: Birkhauser, 1994:75-85.
308. Stitt JT. Differential sensitivity in the sites of fever production by prostaglandin E1 within the hypothalamus of the rat. J Physiol (Lond) 1991;432:99-110.
309. Katsuura G, et al. Involvement of organum vasculosum of lamina terminalis and preoptic area in interleukin 1 beta-induced ACTH release. Am J Physiol 1990;258(1 Pt 1):E163-E171.
310. Kovacs KJ, Sawchenko PE. Mediation of osmoregulatory influences on neuroendocrine corticotropin-releasing factor expression by the ventral lamina terminalis. Proc Natl Acad Sci U S A 1993;90:7681-7685.
311. Ericsson A, Kovacs KJ, Sawchenko PE. A functional anatomical analysis of central pathways subserving the effects of interleukin-1 on stress-related neuroendocrine neurons. J Neurosci 1994;14: 897-913.
312. Lee HY, Whiteside MB, Herkenham M. Area postrema removal abolishes stimulatory effects of intravenous interleukin-1beta on hypothalamic-pituitary-adrenal axis activity and c- fos mRNA

in the hypothalamic paraventricular nucleus. Brain Res Bull 1998;46:495-503.
313. Ericsson A, Arias C, Sawchenko PE. Evidence for an intramedullary prostaglandin-dependent mechanism in the activation of stress-related neuroendocrine circuitry by intravenous interleukin-1. J Neurosci 1997;17:7166-7179.
314. Sagar SM, et al. Anatomic patterns of Fos immunostaining in rat brain following systemic endotoxin administration. Brain Res Bull 1995;36:381-392.
315. Vane JR. Inhibition of prostaglandin synthesis as a mechanism of action for aspirin-like drugs. Nature New Biol 1971;231:232-235.
316. Johnson RW, von Borell E. Lipopolysaccharide-induced sickness behavior in pigs is inhibited by pretreatment with indomethacin (published erratum appears in J Anim Sci 1994;72[3]:801). J Anim Sci 1994;72(2):309-314.
317. Milton AS, Wendlandt S. A possible role for prostaglandin El as a modulator for temperature regulation in the central nervous system of the cat. J Physiol (Lond) 1970;207:76P-77P.
318. Milton AS, Wendlandt S. Effects on body temperature of prostaglandins of the A, E and F series on injection into the third ventricle of unanaesthetized cats and rabbits. J Physiol (Lond) 1971; 218:325-336.
319. Goppelt-Struebe M. Regulation of prostaglandin endoperoxide synthase (cyclooxygenase) isozyme expression. Prostaglandins Leukot Essent Fatty Acids 1995;52:213-222.
320. Robertson RP. Molecular regulation of prostaglandin synthesis implications for endocrine systems. Trends Endocrinol Metab 1995;6:293-297.
321. Breder CD, Dewitt D, Kraig RP. Characterization of inducible cyclooxygenase in rat brain. J Comp Neurol 1995;355:296-315.
322. Breder CD, et al. Distribution and characterization of cyclooxygenase immunoreactivity in the ovine brain. J Comp Neurol 1992; 322:409-438.
323. Yamagata K, et al. Expression of a mitogen-inducible cyclooxygenase in brain neurons: regulation by synaptic activity and glucocorticoids. Neuron 1993;11:371-386.
324. Ek M, et al. Inflammatory response: pathway across the blood-brain barrier. Nature 2001;410:430-431.
325. Elmquist JK, et al. Intravenous lipopolysaccharide induces cyclooxygenase-II immunoreactivity in rat brain perivascular microglia. J Comp Neurol 1997;381:119-129.
326. Elmquist JK, et al. Leptin activates neurons in ventrobasal hypothalamus and brainstem. Endocrinology 1997;138:839-842.
327. Rivest S. What is the cellular source of prostaglandins in the brain in response to systemic inflammation? Facts and controversies. Mol Psychiatry 1999;4:500-507.
328. Blatteis CM, Sehic E. Cytokines and fever. Ann N Y Acad Sci 1998;840:608-618.
329. Scammell TE, et al. Ventromedial preoptic prostaglandin E2 activates fever-producing autonomic pathways. J Neurosci 1996; 16:6246-6254.
330. Williams JW, et al. An extensive exploration of the rat brain for sites mediating prostaglandin-induced hyperthermia. Brain Res 1977;120:251-262.
331. Feldberg W, Saxena PN. Further studies on prostaglandin E 1 fever in cats. J Physiol (Lond) 1971;219:739-745.
332. Morimoto A, et al. Pattern differences in experimental fevers induced by endotoxin, endogenous pyrogen, and prostaglandins. Am J Physiol 1988;254(4 Pt 2):R633-R640.
333. Scammell TE, et al. Microinjection of a cyclooxygenase inhibitor into the anteroventral preoptic region attenuates LPS fever. Am J Phys 1998;274:R783-789.
334. Watanabe Y, Watanabe Y, Hayaishi O. Quantitative autoradiographic localization of prostaglandin E2 binding sites in monkey diencephalon. J Neurosci 1988;8:2003-2010.
335. Matsumura K, et al. High density of prostaglandin E2 binding sites in the anterior wall of the 3rd ventricle: a possible site of its hyperthermic action. Brain Res 1990;533:147-151.
336. Coleman RA, et al. A novel inhibitory prostanoid receptor in piglet saphenous vein. Prostaglandins 1994;47:151-168.
337. Ushikubi F, et al. Impaired febrile response in mice lacking the prostaglandin E receptor subtype EP3. Nature 1998;395: 281-284.
338. Oka T, et al. Relationship of EP(1-4) prostaglandin receptors with rat hypothalamic cell groups involved in lipopolysaccharide fever responses. J Comp Neurol 2000;428:20-32.
339. Ek M, et al. Distribution of the EP3 prostaglandin E(2) receptor subtype in the rat brain: relationship to sites of interleukin-1-induced cellular responsiveness. J Comp Neurol 2000;428:5-20.
340. Sugimoto Y, et al. Distribution of the messenger RNA for the prostaglandin E receptor subtype EP3 in the mouse nervous system. Neuroscience 1994;62:919-928.
341. Zhang J, Rivest S. A functional analysis of EP4 receptor-expressing neurons in mediating the action of prostaglandin E2 within specific nuclei of the brain in response to circulating interleukin-1beta. J Neurochem 2000;74:2134-2145.
342. Nakamura K, et al. Immunocytochemical localization of prostaglandin EP3 receptor in the rat hypothalamus. Neurosci Lett 1999;260:117-120.
343. Oka T, Hori T. EP1-receptor mediation of prostaglandin E2-induced hyperthermia in rats. Am J Physiol 1994;267(1 Pt 2):R289-R294.
344. Oka K, Oka T, Hori T. PGE2 receptor subtype EP1 antagonist may inhibit central interleukin-1beta-induced fever in rats. Am J Physiol 1998;275(6 Pt 2):R1762-R1765.
345. Wang W, et al. Anorexia and cachexia in prostaglandin EP1 and EP3 subtype receptor knockout mice bearing a tumor with high intrinsic PGE2 production and prostaglandin related cachexia. J Exp Clin Cancer Res 2005;24:99-107.
346. Elander L, et al. IL-1(beta) and LPS induce anorexia by distinct mechanisms differentially dependent on microsomal prostaglandin E synthase-1. Am J Physiol Regul Integr Comp Physiol 2007;292: R258-267.
347. Banks WA, Kastin AJ, Durham DA. Bidirectional transport of interleukin-1 alpha across the blood-brain barrier. Brain Res Bull 1989;23:433-437.
348. Banks WA, et al. Human interleukin (IL) 1 alpha, murine IL-1 alpha and murine IL-1 beta are transported from blood to brain in the mouse by a shared saturable mechanism. J Pharmacol Exp Ther 1991;259:988-996.
349. Banks WA, Kastin AJ. Blood to brain transport of interleukin links the immune and central nervous systems. Life Sci 1991;48: PL117-PL1121.
350. Hopkins SJ, Rothwell NJ. Cytokines and the nervous system. I: Expression and recognition (see comments). Trends Neurosci 1995;18:83-88.
351. Rothwell NJ, Hopkins SJ. Cytokines and the nervous system II: actions and mechanisms of action (see comments). Trends Neurosci 1995;18:130-136.
352. Klir JJ, McClellan JL, Kluger MJ. Interleukin-1 beta causes the increase in anterior hypothalamic interleukin-6 during LPS-induced fever in rats. Am J Physiol 1994;266(6 Pt 2):R1845-1848.
353. Breder CD, et al. Regional induction of tumor necrosis factor alpha expression in the mouse brain after systemic lipopolysaccharide administration. Proc Natl Acad Sci U S A 1994;91:11393-11397.
354. Quan N, et al. Induction of inhibitory factor kappaBalpha mRNA in the central nervous system after peripheral lipopolysaccharide administration: an in situ hybridization histochemistry study in the rat. Proc Natl Acad Sci U S A 1997;94:10985-10990.
355. Laflamme N, Lacroix S, Rivest S. An essential role of interleukin-1beta in mediating NF-kappaB activity and COX-2 transcription in cells of the blood-brain barrier in response to a systemic and localized inflammation but not during endotoxemia. J Neurosci 1999;19:10923-10930.
356. Ericsson A, et al. Type 1 interleukin-1 receptor in the rat brain: distribution, regulation, and relationship to sites of IL-1-induced cellular activation. J Comp Neurol 1995;361:681-698.
357. Sagar SM, Sharp FR, Curran T. Expression of c-fos protein in brain: metabolic mapping at the cellular level. Science 1988;240: 1328-1331.
358. Elmquist JK, et al. Induction of Fos-like immunoreactivity in the rat brain following *Pasteurella multocida* endotoxin administration. Endocrinology 1993;133:3054-3057.
359. Elmquist JK, et al. Distribution of Fos-like immunoreactivity in the rat brain following intravenous lipopolysaccharide administration. J Comp Neurol 1996;371:85-103.
360. Elmquist JK, Saper CB. Activation of neurons projecting to the paraventricular hypothalamic nucleus by intravenous lipopolysaccharide. J Comp Neurol 1996;374:315-331.
361. Wan W, et al. Differential induction of c-fos immunoreactivity in hypothalamus and brain stem nuclei following central and peripheral administration of endotoxin. Brain Res Bull 1993;32: 581-587.

362. Wan W, et al. Neural and biochemical mediators of endotoxin and stress-induced c-fos expression in the rat brain. Brain Res Bull 1994;34:7-14.
363. Brady LS, et al. Systemic interleukin-1 induces early and late patterns of c-fos mRNA expression in brain. J Neurosci 1994;14: 4951-4964.
364. Chan RK, et al. A comparison of two immediate-early genes, c-fos and NGFI-B, as markers for functional activation in stress-related neuroendocrine circuitry. J Neurosci 1993;13: 5126-5138.
365. Hare AS, Clarke G, Tolchard S. Bacterial lipopolysaccharide-induced changes in FOS protein expression in the rat brain: correlation with thermoregulatory changes and plasma corticosterone. J Neuroendocrinol 1995;7:791-799.
366. Rivest S, Rivier C. Stress and interleukin-1 beta-induced activation of c-fos, NGFI-B and CRF gene expression in the hypothalamic PVN: comparison between Sprague-Dawley, Fisher-344 and Lewis rats. J Neuroendocrinol 1994;6:101-117.
367. Rivest S, Laflamme N. Neuronal activity and neuropeptide gene transcription in the brains of immune-challenged rats. J Neuroendocrinol 1995;7:501-525.
368. Tkacs NC, Strack AM. Systemic endotoxin induces Fos-like immunoreactivity in rat spinal sympathetic regions. J Auton Nerv Syst 1995;51:1-7.
369. Veening JG, et al. Intravenous administration of interleukin-1 beta induces Fos-like immunoreactivity in corticotropin-releasing hormone neurons in the paraventricular hypothalamic nucleus of the rat. J Chem Neuroanat 1993;6:391-397.
370. Huang QH, et al. Antipyretic role of endogenous melanocortins mediated by central mealanocortin receptors during endotoxin-induced fever. J Neurosci 1997;17:3343-3351.
371. Kasting NW, Cooper KE, Veale WL. Antipyresis following perfusion of brain sites with vasopressin. Experientia 1979;35:208-209.
372. Cooper KE, et al. Evidence supporting a role for endogenous vasopressin in natural suppression of fever in the sheep. J Physiol (Lond) 1979;295:33-45.
373. Shih ST, et al. Central administration of alpha-MSH antiserum augments fever in the rabbit. Am J Physiol 1986;250(5 Pt 2):R803-R806.
374. Fan W, et al. The central melanocortin system can directly regulate serum insulin levels. Endocrinology 2000;141:3072-3079.
375. Huang QH, Hruby VJ, Tatro JB. Role of central melanocortins in endotoxin-induced anorexia. Am J Physiol 1999;276(3 Pt 2): R864-R871.
376. Marks DL, Cone RD. Central melanocortins and the regulation of weight during acute and chronic disease. Recent Prog Horm Res 2001;56:359-375.
377. Marks DL, Ling N, Cone RD. Role of the central melanocortin system in cachexia. Cancer Res 2001;61:1432-1438.
378. Mak RH, et al. Orexigenic and anorexigenic mechanisms in the control of nutrition in chronic kidney disease. Pediatr Nephrol 2005;20:427-431.
379. Markison S, et al. The regulation of feeding and metabolic rate and the prevention of murine cancer cachexia with a small-molecule melanocortin-4 receptor antagonist. Endocrinology 2005;146: 2766-2773.
380. Bamshad M, et al. Central nervous system origins of the sympathetic nervous system outflow to white adipose tissue. Am J Physiol 1998;275(1 Pt 2):R291-R299.
381. Rothwell NJ, Stock MJ. Effects of denervating brown adipose tissue on the responses to cold, hyperphagia and noradrenaline treatment in the rat. J Physiol (Lond) 1984;355:457-463.
382. Lowell BB, Flier JS. Brown adipose tissue, beta 3-adrenergic receptors, and obesity. Annu Rev Med 1997;48:307-316.
383. Jansen AS, Wessendorf MW, Loewy AD. Transneuronal labeling of CNS neuropeptide and monoamine neurons after pseudorabies virus injections into the stellate ganglion. Brain Res 1995;683: 1-24.
384. Saper CB, et al. Direct hypothalamo-autonomic connections. Brain Res 1976;117: 305-312.
385. Zhang YH, et al. Lipopolysaccharide activates specific populations of hypothalamic and brainstem neurons that project to the spinal cord. J Neurosci 2000;20:6578-6586.
386. Kelley AE, et al. Opioid modulation of taste hedonics within the ventral striatum. Physiol Behav 2002;76:365-377.
387. Nestler EJ. Is there a common molecular pathway for addiction? Nat Neurosci 2005;8:1445-1449.
388. Berke JD, Hyman SE. Addiction, dopamine, and the molecular mechanisms of memory. Neuron 2000;25:515-532.
389. Laakso A, et al. Experimental genetic approaches to addiction. Neuron 2002;36:213-228.
390. Wise RA. Brain reward circuitry: insights from unsensed incentives. Neuron 2002;36:229-240.
391. Ikemoto S, Panksepp J. Dissociations between appetitive and consummatory responses by pharmacological manipulations of reward-relevant brain regions. Behav Neurosci 1996;110:331-345.
392. Balleine B, Killcross S. Effects of ibotenic acid lesions of the nucleus accumbens on instrumental action. Behav Brain Res 1994;65:181-193.
393. Szczypka MS, et al. Dopamine production in the caudate putamen restores feeding in dopamine-deficient mice. Neuron 2001;30: 819-828.
394. Szczypka MS, et al. Viral gene delivery selectively restores feeding and prevents lethality of dopamine-deficient mice. Neuron 1999; 22:167-178.
395. Figlewicz DP, et al. Expression of receptors for insulin and leptin in the ventral tegmental area/substantia nigra (VTA/SN) of the rat. Brain Res 2003;964:107-115.
396. Zigman JM, et al. Expression of ghrelin receptor mRNA in the rat and the mouse brain. J Comp Neurol 2006;494:528-548.
397. Figlewicz DP. Adiposity signals and food reward: expanding the CNS roles of insulin and leptin. Am J Physiol Regul Integr Comp Physiol 2003;284:R882-R892.
398. Fulton S, Woodside B, Shizgal P. Modulation of brain reward circuitry by leptin. Science 2000;287:125-128.
399. Zigman JM, Elmquist JK. Minireview: from anorexia to obesity—the yin and yang of body weight control. Endocrinology 2003; 144:3749-3756.
400. Montague CT, et al. Congenital leptin deficiency is associated with severe early-onset obesity in humans. Nature 1997;387: 903-908.
401. Clement K, et al. A mutation in the human leptin receptor gene causes obesity and pituitary dysfunction. Nature 1998;392: 398-401.
402. Considine RV, et al. Serum immunoreactive-leptin concentrations in normal-weight and obese humans. N Engl J Med 1996;334: 292-295.
403. Friedman JM. Leptin, leptin receptors, and the control of body weight. Nutr Rev 1998;56(2 Pt 2): s38-s46; discussion s54-s75.
404. Chan JL, Mantzoros CS. Role of leptin in energy-deprivation states: normal human physiology and clinical implications for hypothalamic amenorrhoea and anorexia nervosa. Lancet 2005;366: 74-85.
405. Welt CK, et al. Recombinant human leptin in women with hypothalamic amenorrhea. N Engl J Med 2004;351:987-997.
406. Heymsfield SB, et al. Recombinant leptin for weight loss in obese and lean adults: a randomized, controlled, dose-escalation trial. JAMA 1999;282:1568-1575.
407. Shimomura I, et al. Leptin reverses insulin resistance and diabetes mellitus in mice with congenital lipodystrophy. Nature 1999;401: 73-76.
408. Ebihara K, et al. Transgenic overexpression of leptin rescues insulin resistance and diabetes in a mouse model of lipoatrophic diabetes. Diabetes 2001;50:1440-1448.
409. Oral EA, Simha V, Ruiz E, et al. Leptin-replacement therapy for lipodystrophy. N Engl J Med 2002;346:570-578.
410. Coppari R, et al. The hypothalamic arcuate nucleus: a key site for mediating leptin's effects on glucose homeostasis and locomotor activity. Cell Metabolism 2005;1:63-72.
411. Morton GJ, et al. Leptin regulates insulin sensitivity via phosphatidylinositol-3-OH kinase signaling in mediobasal hypothalamic neurons. Cell Metab 2005;2:411-420.
412. Krude H, et al. Severe early-onset obesity, adrenal insufficiency and red hair pigmentation caused by POMC mutations in humans. Nat Genet 1998;19:155-157.
413. Vaisse C, et al. A frameshift mutation in human MC4R is associated with a dominant form of obesity. Nat Genet 1998;20:113-114.
414. Yeo GSH, et al. A frameshift mutation in MC4R associated with dominantly inherited human obesity. Nat Genet 1998;20: 111-112.

415. Hinney A, Schmidt A, Nottebom K, et al. Several mutations in the melanocortin-4 receptor gene including a nonsense and a frameshift mutation associated with dominantly inherited obesity in humans. J Clin Endocrinol Metab 1999;84:1483-1486.
416. Farooqi IS, Yeo GS, Keogh JM, et al. Dominant and recessive inheritance of morbid obesity associated with melanocortin 4 receptor deficiency. J Clin Invest 2000;106:271-279.
417. Vaisse C, Clement K, Durand E, et al. Melanocortin-4 receptor mutations are a frequent and heterogenous cause of morbid obesity. J Clin Invest 2000;106:253-262.
418. Farooqi IS, Keogh JM, Yeo GS, et al. Clinical spectrum of obesity and mutations in the melanocortin 4 receptor gene. N Engl J Med 2003;348:1160-1163.
419. Branson R, Potoczna N, Kral JG, et al. Binge eating as a major phenotype of melanocortin 4 receptor gene mutations. N Engl J Med 2003;348:1096-1103.

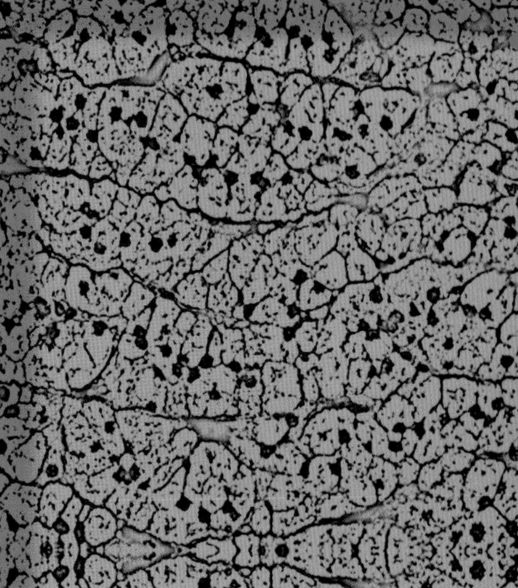

OBESITY

Samuel Klein and Johannes A. Romijn

Obesity is a chronic disease that is causally related to serious medical illnesses. In the United States alone, the consequences of obesity account for an estimated 300,000 deaths per year.[1] The medical expenses and cost of lost productivity due to obesity are greater than $100 billion per year.[2] This review addresses the important clinical and pathophysiologic issues in obesity.

Definition of Obesity

Body Mass Index

Body mass index (BMI) is calculated by dividing weight (in kilograms) by height (in meters squared) or weight (in pounds) multiplied by 704 and divided by height (in inches squared). There is a strong curvilinear relation between BMI and relative body fat mass.[3] However, the current practical definition of obesity is based on the relationship between BMI and health outcome rather than BMI and body composition.

Table 35–1 summarizes the guidelines for classifying weight status by BMI proposed by the major national and international health organizations.[4-7] Large epidemiologic studies[8,9] have established an inverse relationship between BMI and mortality above BMI values of 25.0 kg/m^2. Men and women with a BMI between 25.0 and 29.9 kg/m^2 are considered overweight, and those with a BMI greater than 30.0 kg/m^2 are considered obese. Obese persons are at higher risk for adverse health consequences than those who are overweight (Fig. 35–1). These criteria for overweight and obesity represent imposed cutoff values along a continuum between mortality rate and BMI. The prevalence of obesity-related diseases, such as diabetes, begins to increase at BMI values below 25.0 kg/m^2 (Fig. 35–2).

Factors Affecting Body Mass Index–Related Risk

As shown in Table 35–1, several factors influence BMI-related health risk. For example, obese persons with excess abdominal fat are at higher risk for diabetes, hypertension, dyslipidemia, and ischemic heart disease than obese persons whose fat is located predominantly in the lower body.[10] Waist circumference is highly correlated with abdominal fat mass and is, therefore, often used as a surrogate marker for abdominal (upper body) obesity (Table 35–2). Waist circumference values denoting increased risk for metabolic diseases have been proposed on the basis of epidemiologic data. For men, a waist circumference greater than 102 cm (40 in), and for women, a waist circumference greater than 88 cm (35 in) have been proposed as cutoff values for increased risk.[5] However, it should be realized that this proposal imposes arbitrary cutoff values on the continuous relationship between waist circumference and metabolic disease risk.

Another factor that modifies the risk of obesity-related complications is weight gain during adulthood. In both men and women, weight gain of 5 kg or more since the ages of 18 to 20

TABLE 35–1 WEIGHT CLASSIFICATION BY BODY MASS INDEX

Weight Classification	Obesity Class	BMI (kg/m²)	Risk of Disease
Underweight		<18.5	Increased
Normal		18.5-24.9	Normal
Overweight		25.0-29.9	Increased
Obesity	I	30.0-34.9	High
	II	35.0-39.9	Very High
Extreme Obesity	III	≥40.0	Extremely High

BMI, body mass index.
Adapted from the National Institutes of Health, National Heart, Lung, and Blood Institute. Clinical Guidelines on the Identification, Evaluation, and Treatment of Overweight and Obesity in Adults—The Evidence Report. Obes Res 1998;6(suppl 2):51S-209S.

TABLE 35–2 ADDITIONAL ADIPOSITY-RELATED RISK FACTORS

Risk Factor	Amount
Waist circumference	>40 inches in men >35 inches in women
Weight gain	≥5 kg since age 18-20 yr

Data from the National Institutes of Health, National Heart, Lung, and Blood Institute. Clinical Guidelines on the Identification, Evaluation, and Treatment of Overweight and Obesity in Adults—The Evidence Report. Obes Res 1998;6(suppl 2):51S-209S.

years increases the risk of developing diabetes, hypertension, and coronary heart disease, and the risk of disease increases with the amount of weight gained.[11-16]

Risks of developing obesity-associated diabetes or cardiovascular disease can also be modified by aerobic fitness. In a cohort of more than 8000 men who were followed for an average of 6 years, the incidences of diabetes[17] and cardiovascular mortality[18] were lower in those who were fit, as defined by maximal ability to consume oxygen during exercise, compared with those who were unfit across a range of body adiposity.

BMI-associated health risk is also influenced by ethnicity.[19] For example, when matched on BMI, the risk of diabetes is higher in Southeast Asian populations than in whites.

Physiology of Energy Homeostasis

A complex physiologic system regulates energy homeostasis by integrating signals from peripheral organs with central coordination in the brain. The hypothalamus functions as the main cerebral center in which these signals converge.[20] A balanced interaction between two sets of neurons occurs within the arcuate nucleus of the hypothalamus. Activation of neuropeptide Y (NPY)/Agouti related protein (AGRP) neurons promote food intake, whereas pro-opiomelanocortin (POMC)/cocaine and amphetamine related transcript (CART) neurons have an anorexigenic effect. The NPY/AGRP neurons also inhibit POMC/

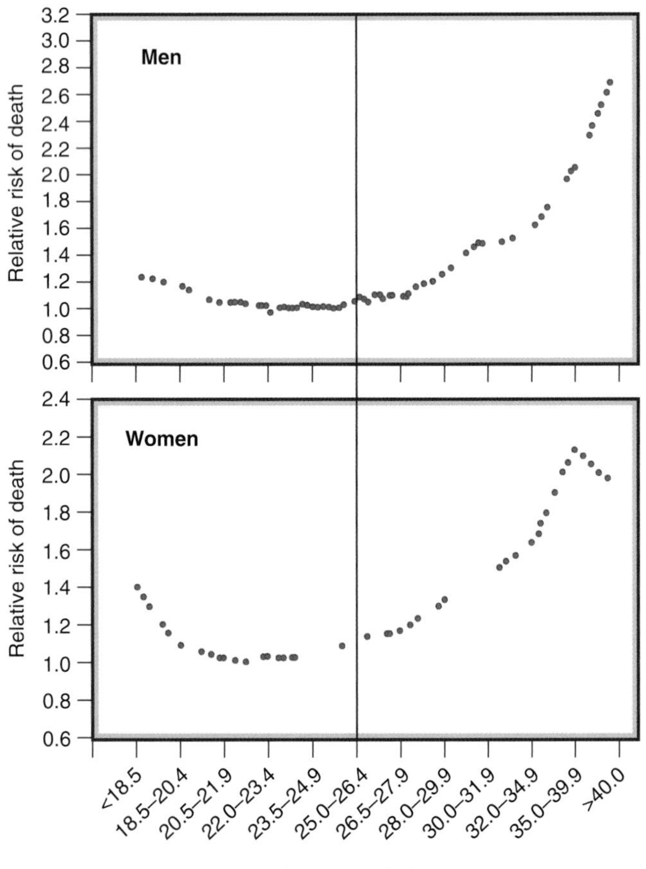

Figure 35–1 ▪ Relationship between body mass index and cardiovascular mortality in men and women in the United States who never smoked and had no preexisting illness. The vertical line separates underweight and lean subjects *(left side)* from overweight and obese subjects *(right side)*. (Adapted from Calle EE, Thun MJ, Petrelli JM, et al. CW. Body-mass index and mortality in a prospective cohort of U.S. adults. N Engl J Med 1999;341:1097-1105.)

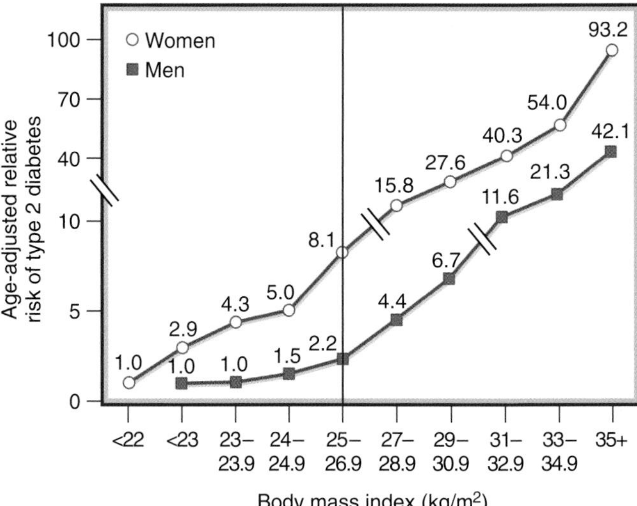

Figure 35–2 ▪ Relationship between body mass index and type 2 diabetes in men and women in the United States. The vertical line separates underweight and lean subjects *(left side)* from overweight and obese subjects *(right side)*. The data demonstrate that the risk of diabetes begins to increase at the upper end of the lean body mass index category. (Adapted from Colditz GA, Willett WC, Rotnitzky A, Manson JE. Weight gain as a risk factor for clinical diabetes mellitus in women. Ann Intern Med 1995;122:481-486; and Chan JM, Rimm EB, Colditz GA, et al. Obesity, fat distribution, and weight gain as risk factors for clinical diabetes in men. Diabetes Care 1994;17:961-969.)

CART neurons through γ-aminobutyric acid (GABA). The orexigenic and anorexigenic signals from the NPY/AGRP and POMC/CART neurons are sent to other brain nuclei, which ultimately results in alterations in food intake and energy expenditure.

The major peripheral organs participating in the regulation of food intake are the stomach, gut, pancreas, and adipose tissue.[20] The stomach and the duodenum secrete the orexigenic peptide ghrelin, which increases before eating and decreases after feeding. Insulin, secreted by the pancreas, has an anorexigenic effect through the arcuate nucleus. PYY 3-36 is secreted by the gastrointestinal tract after food ingestion and might have an anorexigenic effect.[21] Glucagon-like peptide–1 (GLP-1) is derived from pre-proglucagon and secreted upon food ingestion by the proximal gastrointestinal tract; it exerts pleiotropic effects, including slight anorexic effects.[22] Satiety is also mediated by other gut proteins, such as cholecystokinin (CCK). Leptin, secreted by the adipose tissue, also serves as an anorexigenic signal.

It has recently been shown that the endocannabinoid system, particularly the cannabinoid 1 (CB1) receptors and its endogenous ligands, anandamide and 2-arachidonoyl-glycerol, is involved in the regulation of food intake. Absence of CB1 receptors in mice with a disrupted CB1 gene causes hypophagia and leanness.[23] Administration of cannabinoids increases food intake and promotes body-weight gain. In addition, treatment with selective CB1 receptor antagonists decreases food intake and body weight.[24] Moreover, recent data from randomized, controlled trials (RCTs) conducted in obese subjects have shown that treatment with a CB1 receptor antagonist decreases body weight.[25,26] Therefore, the cannabinoid system has an important role in the regulation of ingestive behavior in animals and humans.[27]

Pathogenesis

Energy Balance

Obesity is caused by an excessive intake of calories in relation to energy expenditure over a long period of time. The gastrointestinal tract has the capacity to absorb large amounts of nutrients. Large increases in body fat can result from even minor, but chronic, differences between energy intake and energy expenditure. In 1 year, the ingestion of only 5% more calories than expended can promote the gain of approximately 5 kg in adipose tissue. Over 30 years, the ingestion of only 8 kcal/day more than expended can increase body weight by 10 kg. This represents the average amount of weight gained by Americans during the 30-year period between 25 and 55 years of age.[28]

Genes and Environment

Body size depends on the complex interaction between genetic background and environmental factors. In humans, genetic background explains only an estimated 40% of the variance in body mass.[29] The marked increase in the prevalence of obesity since the 1980s must have resulted largely from alterations in environmental factors that increase energy intake and reduce physical activity. For example, more meals are now eaten outside the home, there is greater availability of convenience and snack foods, serving sizes are larger, and daily physical activity has decreased because of sedentary lifestyle and work activities.

Environmental Effects in High-Risk Populations

Dramatic examples of the influence of environment on body weight have been reported globally. These examples illustrate that persons of certain genetic backgrounds are especially prone to gain weight and develop obesity-related diseases when exposed to a "modern" lifestyle.

Since the 1950s, striking changes in the lifestyle of Pima Indians living in Arizona have led to an epidemic of obesity and diabetes in this population.[30] The diet of these urbanized Pimas is much higher in fat (50% of energy as fat) than their traditional diet (15% of energy as fat). In addition, these urbanized Pimas are much more sedentary than the Pimas who remain in the Sierra Madre Mountains of Northern Mexico and are isolated from Western influences. These rural Pimas eat a traditional diet and are physically active as farmers and sawmill workers, and they have much lower incidences of obesity and diabetes than their Arizona kindred.

The Aborigines of northern Australia are another high-risk population whose weight and health status have been compromised by exposure to a modern environment. Urbanized Aborigines are heavier than their usually very lean (BMI <20.0 kg/m^2) hunter-gatherer kindred and have high prevalences of type 2 diabetes and hypertriglyceridemia.[31] The traditional hunter-gatherer lifestyle of the Aborigines involves a low-fat, low-calorie diet of wild game, fish, and plants and a high level of physical activity. Short-term (7 weeks) re-exposure to the traditional lifestyle has resulted in weight loss and significant improvements or normalization of glucose tolerance and fasting blood glucose, insulin, and triglyceride concentrations in urbanized Aborigines with type 2 diabetes and hypertriglyceridemia.[32]

Influences of Childhood and Parental Obesity

The risk of becoming an obese adult is influenced both by having been obese as a child and by having had at least one obese parent. The risk of adult obesity increases with increasing age and severity of obesity in childhood. For example, the risk of being obese at 21 to 29 years of age ranged from 8% for persons who were obese at 1 to 2 years of age and had nonobese parents to 79% for persons who were obese at 10 to 14 years of age and had at least one obese parent.[33] Although persons who were obese at 1 to 2 years of age and had lean parents did not have an increased risk of obesity in adulthood, persons who became obese after 6 years of age had more than a 50% chance of becoming obese adults.

Monogenic Causes of Obesity

Since the discovery of the adipose tissue protein leptin, much progress has been made in understanding the molecular basis of body-fat regulation. It has nonetheless been disappointing that a genetic cause of obesity has been identified in only a very few persons. Several rare, monogenic causes of obesity have been described in recent years.

Leptin Gene Mutations

The pathophysiologic relevance of leptin was established in two extremely obese cousins with hyperphagia who belonged to a consanguineous family of Pakistani origin.[34] These cousins were homozygous for a single nucleotide deletion at position 398 of the leptin gene. This mutation resulted in a frameshift of the leptin-coding region and a premature termination of leptin synthesis. The parents of the cousins were heterozygous for this mutation. Another mutation, this time involving a homozygous single-nucleotide transversion in the leptin gene that resulted in an Arg→Trp substitution in the mature peptide and low serum leptin levels, was discovered in three extremely obese persons. Two of these persons are adults. Both adults—a man and a woman—were hyperinsulinemic.[35] The man exhibited hypothalamic hypogonadism and dysfunction of the sympathetic nervous system, and the woman had primary amenorrhea.

Leptin treatment has successfully reversed the obesity of leptin-deficient patients. Treatment with recombinant human leptin resulted in a weight loss of 1 to 2 kg per month over a 12-month period. Loss of fat mass accounted for 95% of this weight loss.[36]

The possibility that leptin levels are reduced in obesity has been investigated in large groups of subjects. However, serum leptin levels increase exponentially with fat mass, suggesting that most obese persons are resistant or insensitive to body weight regulation by endogenous leptin.[37]

Leptin Receptor Mutation

Three extremely obese sisters from a consanguineous family were found to have markedly high serum leptin levels and were homozygous for a single-nucleotide substitution at the splice site of exon 16 of the leptin receptor gene.[38] This mutation resulted in a truncated protein, which lacked both the transmembrane and intracellular domains of the receptor. The sisters displayed hypogonadotropic hypogonadism, failure of pubertal development, growth delay, and secondary hypothyroidism. This finding confirms the endocrine abnormalities in leptin-deficient subjects and implies a role for the leptin–leptin receptor system in the central regulation of energy balance and hypothalamic endocrine functions in humans.

Prohormone Convertase 1 Gene Mutation

A mutation in the prohormone convertase 1 *(PC1)* gene was identified in a 43-year-old obese woman with a history of severe childhood obesity.[39] This woman had impaired glucose tolerance, postprandial hypoglycemia, low plasma cortisol levels, and hypogonadotropic hypogonadism. In addition, she had increased plasma concentrations of proinsulin and POMC but very low plasma insulin concentrations. She was a compound heterozygote for two mutations in the *PC1* gene, which resulted in loss of the autocatalytic cleavage ability of *PC1*.

A second patient was recently described.[40] Melanocortins, including α-melanocortin stimulating hormone (MSH), are formed through the processing of POMC by *PC1*. Therefore, reduced production of melanocortin might have been responsible for obesity in this patient.

Pro-opiomelanocortin Gene Mutation

A mutation in the pro-opiomelanocortin *(POMC)* gene was described in two obese children with hyperphagia.[41] The children also had red hair pigmentation and were deficient in adrenocorticotropic hormone (ACTH). The mutations resulted in complete loss of the ability to synthesize α-MSH and ACTH. The red hair pigmentation and obesity are believed to be due to deficiency of α-MSH.

Melanocortin 4 Receptor (MC4-R) Mutation

Although rare, melanocortin 4 receptor *(MC4-R)* mutations are the most common monogenic cause of obesity.[42] Moreover, *MC4-R* mutations are characterized by both dominant and recessive modes of inheritance, in contrast to the other monogenic forms of obesity, which have recessive modes of inheritance. In children with *MC4-R* mutations, the degree of obesity and hyperphagia correlates with the extent of impairment of *MC4-R* signaling. However, adult carriers of the mutations cannot be phenotypically distinguished from other obese subjects.[43]

TrkB

The survival and differentiation of neurons in the peripheral nervous system are dependent on neurotrophic factors, which are secreted by the target tissues. Neurotrophin signaling occurs through the specific activation of receptor tyrosine kinases of the Trk family. An 8-year-old boy has been described with a complex developmental syndrome and severe obesity. He was heterozygous for a de novo missense mutation resulting in a Y722C substitution in the neurotrophin receptor TrkB. This mutation markedly impaired receptor autophosphorylation and signaling to mitogen-activated protein (MAP) kinase. Mutation of the gene encoding for TrkB seems to result in a unique human syndrome of hyperphagic obesity.[44]

Obesity in Pleiotropic Syndromes

About 30 mendelian disorders have been described in which obesity is a clinical feature and is often associated with mental retardation, dysmorphic features, and organ-specific developmental abnormalities, the pleiotropic syndromes. Positional genetic techniques have led to the recent identification of different mutations underlying these syndromes. However, in most cases these genes encode for proteins with a yet-unresolved function.[45]

Obesity Syndromes due to Chromosomal Rearrangements

Prader-Willi Syndrome

The Prader-Willi syndrome is characterized by obesity, mental retardation, short stature, and secondary hypogonadism. It is the most common syndromal cause of obesity, occurring in 1:25,000 births.[46] In these patients, the paternal segment 15q11.2-q12 is absent. The omission can result from deletion of the paternal segment (75%) or the loss of the entire paternal chromosome 15, with the presence of two maternal homologs (uniparental maternal disomy). The role of the genes encoded by the paternal segment and the mechanisms by which they cause the obesity syndrome have not been resolved.[46]

SIM1 Gene Mutation

A de novo balanced translocation between chromosomes 1 and 6 was found in a severely obese girl who weighed 47 kg at 67 months of age.[47] The mutation caused a disruption in the *SIM1* gene, the human homolog of the *Drosophila* Single-minded (Sim) gene that regulates neurogenesis. The *SIM1* gene encodes a transcription factor involved in the formation of the paraventricular and supraoptic nuclei. It is likely that this abnormality altered energy balance by stimulating food intake because measured resting energy expenditure was normal.

Polygenic Causes of Obesity

In contrast to the small number of single gene mutations that clearly cause obesity, a large number of human genes have been identified that show variations in DNA sequences, which might also contribute to obesity. Overall, more than 600 genes, markers, and chromosomal regions have been associated or linked with human obesity phenotypes. The electronic version of the Obesity Gene Map, with links to useful publications and genomic and other relevant sites, can be found at http://obesitygene.pbrc.edu.[48] Some of these associations will undoubtedly prove to be more important than others. It remains a major challenge to identify genes that contribute to human obesity because of the potential interactions between multiple genes and the interaction between genes and environment that can lead to expression of an obesity phenotype.

Energy Metabolism

The components of daily total energy expenditure (TEE) are resting energy expenditure (REE), which accounts for approximately 70% of TEE; energy expended in physical activity, which accounts for approximately 20% of TEE; and the thermic effect of food (TEF), which accounts for approximately 10% of TEE. REE represents the energy expended for normal cellular and organ function under postabsorptive resting conditions. Energy expended in physical activity includes the energy costs of both volitional activity, such as exercise, and nonvolitional activity, such as spontaneous muscle contractions, maintaining posture, and fidgeting. The TEF represents the energy expended in digestion, absorption, and sympathetic nervous system activation after ingestion of a meal.

Cross-sectional studies have investigated whether alterations in energy metabolism are involved in obesity. Obese persons usually have greater rates of REE than lean persons of the same height because obese persons have greater lean and adipose tissue cell mass.[49]

Defects in REE or TEE have not been detected in "diet-resistant" patients who maintain their weight despite the claim of strict adherence to a low-calorie diet.[50,51] Instead, such patients appear to underestimate their food intake and actually consume twice as many calories as they record in food-intake diaries. Currently, it is not known whether obese persons expend less total energy in daily physical activity because they are less active than lean individuals. During non–weight bearing activity (e.g., cycling), obese persons expend the same amount of energy as lean persons to perform the same amount of work.[52] However, during weight-bearing activities, obese epersons expend more energy than lean ones because more work is required to carry their greater body weight.

Evidence from studies in obese and lean subjects, matched for either fat mass or lean body mass, suggests that obese subjects have a small (~75 kcal/day) but potentially important reduction in TEF. This reduction in TEF might arise from the insulin resistance and blunted sympathetic nervous system activity that occur in obesity.[53]

Although extensive research has failed to reveal significant defects in the energy metabolism of persons who are already obese, the possibility remains that inherent abnormalities in energy metabolism contribute to the development of obesity. However, currently available research technology has only a limited ability to detect small, but possibly clinically significant, chronic defects in energy metabolism. Moreover, it is difficult to establish a causal relationship between energy expenditure and the development of obesity because energy metabolism measurements capture only a brief point in time and therefore might not reveal abnormalities that emerge during specific life stages.

The majority of studies do not support the involvement of a defect in metabolic rate in the development of obesity. In one longitudinal study, daily TEE at 3 months of age was 21% lower in infants who later became overweight compared with those who maintained a normal weight.[54] However, larger subsequent studies (e.g., reference 55) have not confirmed this finding. In a longitudinal study of 126 Pima Indians, those in the lowest tertile of REE at baseline had the highest cumulative incidence of a 10-kg weight gain 1 to 4 years later.[56] In contrast, the Baltimore Longitudinal Study on Aging, which followed 775 men for an average of 10 years, did not detect a relationship between initial REE and weight change.[57]

When energy intake exceeds energy expenditure, weight gain usually occurs. However, genetic factors might influence the amount of weight gained with overfeeding. Bouchard and colleagues[58] observed variable weight gain among 12 monozygotic twin pairs who were chronically overfed 1000 kcal/day. However, members of a twin pair gained similar amounts of weight. In another study, the increase in body fat after 8 weeks of overfeeding was inversely related to changes in nonvolitional energy expenditure (e.g., fidgeting).[59] Therefore, in some persons, nonvolitional energy expenditure during periods of overingestion could be a mechanism that limits weight gain through the dissipation of excess ingested energy.

Diet-induced weight loss decreases REE, which promotes weight regain. This observation underlies the set-point theory, which posits that body weight is predetermined so that weight loss (or gain) promotes a decrease (or increase) in metabolic rate that acts to restore body weight to a preset level. In both lean and obese persons, hypocaloric feeding reduces REE by 15% to 30%. This reduction in REE cannot be completely accounted for by the accompanying decrease in body size or lean body mass and is considered a normal part of the physiologic adaptation to energy restriction.[60]

The reduction in REE that occurs during negative energy balance is transient and does not persist during maintenance of a lower body weight. As reported in several studies, long-term maintenance of weight loss is not associated with an abnormal decrease in REE or TEE when adjustments are made for changes in body composition.[61,62] In a meta-analysis of 15 studies, the REE of subjects who were formerly obese was found to be similar to that of subjects who were never obese.[63] Although the decrease in energy metabolism with weight loss is largely appropriate for the concomitant changes in body composition, this decrease might nonetheless promote weight regain.

Adipose Tissue and Triglyceride Metabolism

Triglycerides stored within adipose tissue constitute the body's major energy reserve (Table 35–3). Triglycerides are a much more compact fuel than glycogen because of the energy density and hydrophobic nature of fat. Triglycerides yield 9.3 kcal/g upon oxidation and are compactly stored as oil inside the fat

TABLE 35–3 ENDOGENOUS FUEL STORES IN A MAN WEIGHING 70 kg

Fuel Source	MASS Grams	Kcal
ADIPOSE TISSUE		
Triglyceride	13,000	120,000
LIVER		
Glycogen	100	400
Triglyceride	50	450
MUSCLE		
Glycogen	500	2,000
Triglyceride	300	2,700
BLOOD		
Glucose	15	60
Triglyceride	4	35
Free fatty acids	0.5	5

cell, accounting for 85% of adipocyte weight. Glycogen, in contrast, yields only 4.1 kcal/g upon oxidation and is stored intracellularly as a gel containing approximately 2 g of water for every 1 g of glycogen.

Adipose tissue is an effective storage mechanism for transportable fuel that allows mobility and survival when food is scarce. During starvation, the duration of survival is determined by the size of the adipose tissue mass. Lean persons die after only approximately 60 days of starvation when more than 35% of body weight is lost.[64] Obese persons, in contrast, have tolerated therapeutic fasts for more than a year without adverse effects. In the longest reported fast, a 207-kg man ingested only acaloric fluids, vitamins, and minerals for 382 days and lost 126 kg, or 61%, of his initial weight.[65]

Triglyceride Storage

The major function of adipocytes is the storage of triglycerides for future use as energy substrate. Lipogenesis from glucose makes only a limited contribution to triglyceride storage in the adipocyte.[66] Most of the triglyceride in adipocytes is derived from chylomicrons and very-low-density lipoprotein (VLDL) triglycerides that originate, respectively, from dietary and hepatic sources. These plasma triglycerides are hydrolyzed by lipoprotein lipase (LPL), a key regulator of fat cell triglyceride uptake from circulating triglycerides. Lipoprotein lipase is synthesized by adipocytes and transported to the endoluminal surface of endothelial cells. The interaction of LPL with chylomicrons and VLDL releases fatty acids from plasma triglycerides, which are then taken up by local adipocytes. Plasma free fatty acids themselves can also be taken up by adipose tissue, independent of LPL.

Insulin and cortisol are the principal hormones involved in regulation of LPL activity and expression.[67] The activity of LPL within individual tissues is a key factor in partitioning triglycerides among different body tissues. Insulin influences this partitioning through its stimulation of LPL activity in adipose tissue.[68] Insulin also promotes triglyceride storage in adipocytes through other mechanisms, including inhibition of lipolysis, stimulation of adipocyte differentiation, and escalation of glucose uptake. Cortisol's importance in fat distribution is supported by the clinical appearance of patients with Cushing's syndrome. The obesity-promoting effect of cortisol can involve a synergistic effect of cortisol and insulin on the induction of LPL in adipose tissue, as has been demonstrated in vitro. Testosterone, growth hormone, catecholamines, tumor necrosis factor (TNF), and other related cytokines inhibit lipoprotein lipase activity.[67]

Lipolysis

The balance between triglyceride storage and lipolysis is regulated by complex hormonal and neuronal mechanisms. To become available as energy substrate, triglycerides stored within adipocytes must be hydrolyzed by hormone sensitive lipase (HSL) into fatty acids. These fatty acids can be released from adipocytes into the circulation. The circulating half-life of plasma fatty acids is only 3 to 4 minutes. During resting conditions, fatty acid release by adipose tissue exceeds the rate of fatty acid oxidation.[69] The excess availability of fatty acids in plasma provides a ready supply of oxidizable substrate to respond to sudden changes in energy requirements, such as are induced by exercise. The plasma fatty acids that escape immediate oxidation are usually re-esterified to triglyceride in adipose tissue, muscle, or liver. These fatty acids are the major precursors of hepatic VLDL triglyceride synthesis.[70] In turn, VLDL triglycerides are secreted by the liver and redistributed throughout the body, depending on tissue-specific factors, such as the activity of LPL. These observations imply that there is continuous redistribution of triglycerides between adipose tissue and the rest of the body.

There is considerable variation in the rate of lipolysis and, consequently, plasma fatty acid level, both within and between subjects. Insulin and catecholamines are the major circulating hormones that influence lipolysis in adipocytes. Insulin inhibits lipolysis via its effect on HSL, whereas catecholamines stimulate lipolysis. Small changes in the plasma concentrations of insulin and catecholamines have major effects on lipolytic rate. Half-maximal suppression of lipolysis occurs at postabsorptive insulin levels, and maximal suppression of lipolysis occurs at insulin levels within the range observed after a regular meal.[71] Minor increases in resting catecholamine levels stimulate lipolysis. Other factors also modulate the rate of lipolysis. For example, growth hormone and cortisol stimulate lipolysis. In general, the effects of these other factors are less potent than the effects of insulin and catecholamines.

In contrast to the tight feedback regulation of insulin secretion by glucose levels, insulin and catecholamine concentrations are not regulated by lipolysis or fatty acid levels. Although free fatty acid levels affect glucose-stimulated insulin release, there is no feedback between insulin release and rate of lipolysis. The wide physiologic variations in plasma free fatty acid concentrations between individual persons can be explained, in part, by the finely tuned dose-response effects of insulin and catecholamines on lipolysis, in combination with the absence of tight feedback regulation of insulin and catecholamine levels by free fatty acids.

Basal plasma fatty acid concentrations are often increased in obese persons, particularly those with abdominal obesity. An increased rate of free fatty acid release into plasma because of an increased rate of lipolysis from upper-body subcutaneous fat is responsible for the higher levels of circulating fatty acids.[72,73] The excess free fatty acid availability in plasma might lead to increased hepatic free fatty acid uptake, VLDL triglyceride synthesis, intramuscular triglyceride formation, and insulin resistance.

Adipose Tissue as an Endocrine Organ

Traditionally, adipocytes have been viewed as energy depots that store triglycerides during feeding and release fatty acids during fasting to provide fuel for other tissues. However, adipose tissue secretes numerous proteins that have important physiologic functions (Table 35–4). These factors participate in autocrine and paracrine regulation within adipose tissue and can

TABLE 35–4 ADIPOCYTE-SECRETED PROTEINS

Category	Protein
Hormone	Leptin, resistin, angiotensinogen, ACRP 30, estrogens, visfatin
Cytokine	Interleukin-6, tumor necrosis factor-α
Extracellular matrix protein	Types I, III, IV, and VI collagen; fibronectin, osteonectin, laminin, entactin, MMP-2
Complement factor	Adipsin, complement C3, factor B
Enzyme	Cholester ester transfer protein, lipoprotein lipase
Acute phase response protein	α-1 Acid glycoprotein, haptoglobin
Other	Fatty acids, plasminogen activator inhibitor-1, prostacyclin

affect the functions of distant organs, such as muscle, the pancreas, the liver, and the central nervous system.

The function of adipose tissue as an endocrine organ has important implications for understanding the pathophysiologic relationship between excess body fat and pathologic states, such as insulin resistance and type 2 diabetes mellitus.[74,75] Not all products released by adipose tissue are produced by adipocytes. Other cells contained within the adipose tissue, including endothelial cells, macrophages, and adipocyte precursor cells, can also participate in endocrine functions. Select proteins produced by adipose tissue are reviewed next.

Leptin

Adipocytes produce leptin and secrete it into the bloodstream. Leptin has pleiotropic effects on food intake, hypothalamic neuroendocrine regulation, reproductive function, and energy expenditure.[76,77] There is a direct relationship between plasma leptin concentrations and BMI or body fat percentage.[78] However, there can be considerable variability in leptin concentrations among persons with the same BMI, suggesting that leptin production is also regulated by factors other than adipose tissue mass per se. Leptin levels decrease rapidly within 12 hours of the start of starvation. Conversely, leptin levels increase in response to overfeeding.[79] Therefore, plasma leptin concentrations reflect adipose tissue mass and are influenced by energy balance. In this perspective, leptin is a bidirectional signal that switches physiologic regulation between fed and starved states. Plasma leptin concentrations increase with increasing fat mass and decrease rapidly during early fasting. The relative importance of the central versus peripheral effects of leptin in body weight regulation in most obese persons is still unclear.[80]

Resistin

Resistin is another signaling polypeptide secreted by adipocytes.[81] Resistin levels are increased in mice with diet-induced and genetic forms of obesity and insulin resistance. Administration of recombinant resistin to normal mice impaired glucose tolerance and insulin action. Neutralization of resistin reduced hyperglycemia in obese, insulin-resistant mice, in part by improving insulin sensitivity. Resistin has, therefore, been proposed to be a hormone that links obesity to diabetes by inducing insulin resistance.

Adiponectin

Adiponectin is the most abundant secretory protein produced by adipocytes. In contrast to other secretory products of adipocytes, the plasma concentrations of adiponectin are decreased in obesity and insulin resistance. There is a close association between hypoadiponectinemia, insulin resistance, and hyperinsulinemia.[82] Conversely, adiponectin expression increases with improved insulin sensitivity and weight loss.[83] Interventions that improve insulin sensitivity, such as weight loss or treatment with thiazolidinediones, are associated with increased adipose tissue adiponectin gene expression and plasma concentrations.[84] Moreover, administration of recombinant adiponectin exerts glucose-lowering effects and ameliorates insulin resistance in mouse models of obesity or diabetes.[85] These data suggest that decreased plasma levels of adiponectin contribute to some of the metabolic complications associated with obesity.

Visfatin

Recently, a new adipocytokine was isolated and named visfatin.[86] The expression of this protein increases with the level of obesity. Visfatin corresponds with a protein previously known as pre–B cell colony-enhancing factor. Visfatin shares properties with insulin both in vitro and in vivo. It has insulin-like effects in cultured cells and lowers blood glucose levels in mice. Surprisingly, visfatin binds to and activates the insulin receptor, although in a manner distinct from insulin. At similar concentrations, visfatin and insulin have similar effects in activating insulin signaling. However, the plasma concentrations of visfatin are much lower (10%) than those of insulin. Additional studies are required to elucidate the potential physiologic and pathophysiologic roles of visfatin.

Estrogens

Adipose tissue has P450 aromatase activity. This enzyme is important for transforming androstenedione into estrone. Estrone is the second major circulating estrogen in premenopausal women and the most important estrogen in postmenopausal women.[75] The conversion rate of androstenedione into estrone increases with age and obesity, and is higher in lower-body obesity than in upper-body obesity. In addition to a role in endocrine regulation, the effects of P450 aromatase on estrogen metabolism might also have a role in autocrine and paracrine action because estrogen receptors are present in adipose tissue.

Tumor Necrosis Factor-α

Adipocytes secrete tumor necrosis factor-α (TNF-α, and TNF-α expression are increased in the enlarged adipocytes of obese subjects.[87] However, plasma TNF-α levels are generally at or below the detection limit of available assays, which suggests that the TNF-α produced in adipose tissue has paracrine, rather than endocrine, functions. The multiple effects of TNF-α on adipocytes include the impairment of insulin signaling. Therefore, it has been proposed that TNF-α might partially contribute to insulin resistance in obesity.[74]

Interleukin-6

Adipose tissue interleukin-6 (IL-6) secretion might account for 30% of circulating IL-6.[88,89] Obesity is associated with increased plasma IL-6 concentrations, which might contribute to systemic inflammation and insulin resistance. In fact, insulin sensitivity is inversely related to plasma IL-6 levels[90] and IL-6 directly impairs insulin signaling.[91] Administration of IL-6 to human subjects induces dose-dependent increases in fasting blood glucose, probably by stimulating glucagon release and other counterregulatory hormones or by inducing peripheral resistance to insulin action, or both.[92]

Adipocyte Biology

Obesity is associated with an increased number of adipocytes. A lean adult has about 35 billion adipocytes, each containing about 0.4 to 0.6 μg of triglyceride; an extremely obese adult can have four times as many adipocytes (125 billion), each containing twice as much lipid (0.8-1.2 μg of triglyceride).[93]

Our understanding of adipocyte differentiation is largely derived from studies conducted in preadipocytes in culture. The current concept is that adipocytes are derived from fibroblast precursor cells after the concerted actions of extracellular signals and intrinsic transcription factors and coactivators.

Many extranuclear factors and intracellular transduction pathways influence the adipogenic potential of cells in vitro and

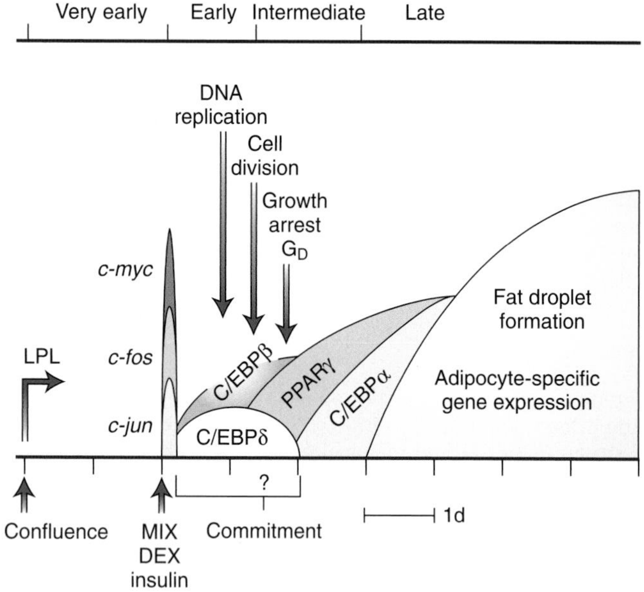

Figure 35–3 ▪ Progression of 3T3-L1 preadipocyte differentiation with subsequent changes in cellular characteristics. The distinct stages of differentiation (very early, early, intermediate, and late) are shown. C/EBP, CCAAT/enhancer binding protein; DEX, dexamethasone; LPL, lipoprotein lipase; MIX, methylisobutylxanthine; PPAR, peroxisome proliferator-activated receptor. (From Ntambi JM, Kim Y-C. Adipocyte differentiation and gene expression. J Nutr 2000;130:3122S-3126S.)

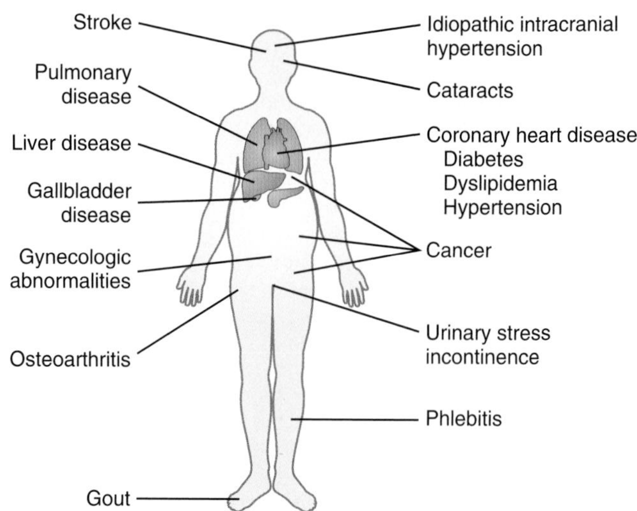

Figure 35–4 ▪ Medical complications associated with obesity.

in vivo (Fig. 35–3).[94] Although in the future it may be possible to regulate adipogenesis in vivo, decreasing adipogenesis without altering energy balance can result in the deposition of triglycerides in other tissues. Excessive amounts of triglycerides in nonadipose tissues can have deleterious effects, as suggested by the liver steatosis, dyslipidemia, and diabetes observed when adipogenesis was prevented in mice.[95]

The cornerstone of obesity therapy is to increase the use of endogenous fat stores as fuel by reducing energy intake below energy expenditure. With dieting, weight loss is composed of approximately 75% to 85% fat and 15% to 25% fat-free mass (FFM).[96] An energy deficit of approximately 3500 kcal is required to oxidize 1 lb of adipose tissue. However, because of the oxidation of lean tissue and associated water losses, a 3500-kcal energy deficit will reduce body weight by more than 1 lb.

The distribution of fat loss is characterized by regional heterogeneity.[97,98] Particularly in men and women with initially increased intraabdominal fat, there are greater relative losses of intraabdominal fat than total body fat mass. A decrease in the size (triglyceride content) of existing adipocytes accounts for most, if not all, of the fat loss.[99] In humans, there is also evidence that the number of adipocytes is reduced with large, long-term fat loss.[100] However, it is possible that this perception of decreased fat cell number is false because standard cell counting techniques might fail to detect adipocytes that have undergone marked shrinkage.

There are two possible mechanisms through which weight loss can eliminate fat cells: dedifferentiation, the morphologic and biochemical reversion of mature adipocytes to preadipocytes, and apoptosis. Adipocyte dedifferentiation has been observed in vitro, but there is no evidence that it occurs in vivo.[101] Adipocyte apoptosis has been induced in vitro,[102] and it has been demonstrated to occur in vivo in some patients with cancer.[103] To date, it is not known whether diet-mediated weight loss induces adipocyte apoptosis.

Prevalence of Obesity

The worldwide prevalence of obesity has increased dramatically over the last several decades. In the United States alone, about one third of adults aged 20 to 74 years are considered obese.[104] According to national population surveys conducted since 1960, the prevalence of obesity (BMI >30 kg/m^2) has more than doubled from 13% to 32%[104,105]; the prevalence of obesity increases progressively from 20 to 50 years of age, but it then declines after 60 to 70 years of age.

The prevalence of obesity has also risen in children and adolescents. As defined by a BMI greater than the 95th percentile for age and gender from the revised National Center for Health Statistics growth charts, 17% of 6- to 17-year-old children and adolescents in the United States are overweight.[104,106] These data indicate that overweight prevalence rates for children and adolescents, reported by earlier surveys, have doubled. Diseases commonly associated with obesity in adults, such as type 2 diabetes mellitus, hypertension, hyperlipidemia, gallbladder disease, nonalcoholic steatohepatitis (NASH), sleep apnea, and orthopedic complications, are now increasingly observed in children.[107]

Clinical Features and Complications of Obesity

Obesity causes many serious medical complications that impair quality of life and lead to increased morbidity and premature death[108] (Fig. 35–4). The complications associated with obesity have been reviewed in detail previously.[5]

Endocrine and Metabolic Diseases

The Metabolic or Insulin-Resistance Syndrome

In the metabolic or insulin-resistance syndrome, also known as syndrome X, the specific phenotype of upper-body, or abdominal, obesity is associated with a cluster of metabolic risk factors for coronary heart disease (CHD). Features of this syndrome include insulin resistance with associated hyperinsulinemia, impaired glucose tolerance, impaired insulin-mediated glucose disposal, and type 2 diabetes mellitus; dyslipidemia, characterized by hypertriglyceridemia and low serum HDL-cholesterol levels; and hypertension. Other metabolic risk factors, including increased serum levels of apolipoprotein B; small, dense LDL particles; and plasminogen activator inhibitor 1 (PAI-1) with impaired fibrinolysis have also been associated with abdominal obesity.[109,110] The metabolic syndrome usually occurs in persons with frank obesity, but it has also been reported in normal-weight persons who presumably have an increased amount of abdominal fat.[111]

The metabolic syndrome was originally identified and defined on the basis of epidemiologic associations. The underlying pathogenesis and the interrelationships between the individual features have not been completely elucidated. Insulin resistance has been hypothesized to be the common underlying pathogenic mechanism.[112] However, according to a factor analysis of data obtained from nondiabetic subjects in the Framingham Offspring Study, insulin resistance might not be the only precedent condition, and more than one independent physiologic process may be involved.[113]

Abdominal obesity is clearly associated with insulin resistance. However, it is unclear whether visceral (omental and mesenteric) or subcutaneous deposits of abdominal fat are more closely related to insulin resistance, because data from different studies are contradictory. In addition, it is difficult to define the relationship between abdominal and subcutaneous adipose tissue deposits and insulin resistance because the size of the deposits is closely correlated. Furthermore, it is not known whether visceral fat actually participates in the pathogenesis of the metabolic syndrome or merely serves as a marker of increased risk for the metabolic complications of obesity.[114]

There is increasing evidence that the ectopic distribution of triglycerides in nonadipose tissue may be involved in the complications of obesity. In cross-sectional studies, insulin resistance was highly correlated with the intramyocellular concentration of triglyceride.[115] It is not known whether triglycerides per se interfere with insulin action or whether triglycerides serve as surrogate markers for some other fatty acid–derived entity, from plasma or intracellular sources, that impairs insulin signaling.[116]

Type 2 Diabetes Mellitus

The marked increase in the prevalence of obesity has played an important role in the 25% increase in the prevalence of diabetes that has occurred in the United States over the last 20 years.[117] According to data from NHANES III, two thirds of the men and women in the United States with diagnosed type 2 diabetes have a BMI of 27.0 kg/m^2 or greater.[106] The risk of diabetes increases linearly with BMI: the prevalence of diabetes increased from 2% in those with a BMI of 25.0 to 29.9 kg/m^2, to 8% in those with a BMI of 30 to 34.9 kg/m^2, and to 13% in those with a BMI greater than 35 kg/m^2.[117] In the Nurses' Health Study, the risk of diabetes began to increase when BMI exceeded the "normal" value of 22 kg/m^2 (see Fig. 35–2).[13,118] In addition, the risk of diabetes increases with increases in abdominal fat mass, waist circumference, or waist-to-hip circumference ratio at any given BMI value.[119-121] The risk of diabetes also increases with weight gain during adulthood. Among men and women aged 35 to 60 years, the risk of diabetes was three times greater in those who gained 5 to 10 kg since the age of 18 to 20 years than in those who maintained their weight within 2 kg.[13,14]

Dyslipidemia

Obesity is associated with several serum lipid abnormalities including hypertriglyceridemia, reduced HDL cholesterol levels, and an increased fraction of small, dense LDL particles.[122,123] This association is especially strong in persons with abdominal obesity. In addition, most studies suggest that serum concentrations of total and LDL cholesterol are elevated in obesity. Data from NHANES III showed that in men, there was a progressive increase in the prevalence of hypercholesterolemia (total blood cholesterol >240 mg dL or 6.21 mmol/L) with increasing BMI.[124] In women, by contrast, the prevalence of hypercholesterolemia was highest at a BMI of 25.0 to 27.0 kg/m^2, and it did not increase further at higher BMI values. The serum lipid abnormalities associated with obesity are important risk factors for CHD.[125,126]

Cardiovascular Disease

Hypertension

There is a linear relationship between hypertension and BMI.[127,128] In NHANES III, the age-adjusted prevalence of hypertension (defined as systolic blood pressure >140 mm Hg, diastolic blood pressure >90 mm Hg, or use of antihypertensive medication) in obese men and women was 42% and 38%, respectively. These prevalence rates are more than twice as high as the prevalence rates of hypertension in lean men and women (~15% prevalence rate in both men and women).[124] The risk of hypertension also increases with weight gain. Among subjects followed in the Framingham Study, there was a 6.5-mm Hg increase in blood pressure with every 10% increase in body weight.[129]

Coronary Heart Disease

The risk of CHD is increased in obese persons, particularly in those with increased abdominal fat distribution and in those who gained weight during young adulthood. Moreover, CHD risk starts to increase at the "normal" BMI levels of 23.0 kg/m^2 in men and 22.0 kg/m^2 in women.[130] In the Nurses' Health Study, the risk of fatal and nonfatal myocardial infarctions was greater in women with the lowest BMI but highest waist-to-hip circumference ratio than in women with the highest BMI but lowest waist-to-hip circumference ratio.[131] At any BMI level, the risk of CHD increases with the presence of increased abdominal fat. The risk of fatal and nonfatal myocardial infarction also increases when 5 kg or more are gained after 18 years of age.[132]

Obesity-related CHD risk factors, particularly hypertension, dyslipidemia, impaired glucose tolerance, and diabetes, are largely responsible for the increase in CHD. However, even after adjusting for other known risk factors, several long-term epidemiologic studies still found that overweight and obesity increased the risk of CHD.[132] As a result, the American Heart Association recently classified obesity as a major preventable risk factor for CHD.[133,134]

Cerebrovascular and Thromboembolic Disease

The risk of fatal and nonfatal ischemic stroke is approximately twice as great in obese as in lean persons and increases progressively with increasing BMI.[135,136] The risks of venous stasis, deep vein thrombosis, and pulmonary embolism are also increased in obesity, particularly in persons with abdominal obesity.[137] Lower-extremity venous disease can result from increased intraabdominal pressure, impaired fibrinolysis, and the increase in inflammatory mediators.[138,139]

Pulmonary Disease

Restrictive Lung Disease

Obesity increases the pressure placed on the chest wall and thoracic cage, which restricts pulmonary function by decreasing respiratory compliance, increasing the work of breathing, restricting ventilation (measured as decreased total lung capacity, forced vital capacity, and maximal ventilatory ventilation), and limiting ventilation of lung bases.[140]

Obesity-Hypoventilation Syndrome

In obesity-hypoventilation syndrome, the PCO_2 is less than 50 mm Hg because of decreased ventilatory responsiveness to hypercapnea or hypoxia (or both) and an inability of respiratory muscles to meet the increased ventilatory demand imposed by the mechanical effects of obesity. There is reduced alveolar ventilation because of shallow and inefficient ventilation related to decreased tidal volume, inadequate inspiratory strength, and elevation of the diaphragm. Symptoms increase when patients are lying down because of increased abdominal pressure on the diaphragm. The resulting increase in intrathoracic pressure further compromises lung function and respiratory capacity.

The Pickwickian syndrome is a severe form of the obesity-hypoventilation syndrome. Named after an obese character in Charles Dickens' *The Pickwick Papers,* this syndrome involves extreme obesity, irregular breathing, somnolence, cyanosis, secondary polycythemia, and right ventricular dysfunction.

Obstructive Sleep Apnea

In obstructive sleep apnea, excessive episodes of apnea and hypopnea during sleep are caused by partial or complete upper airway obstruction, despite persistent respiratory efforts. Daytime sleepiness and cardiopulmonary dysfunction result from the interruption in nighttime sleep and arterial hypoxemia. In general, patients with sleep apnea are characterized by a BMI greater than 30.0 kg/m^2, excess abdominal fat, and a large neck girth (>17 inches in men and >16 inches in women).[141-143]

Musculoskeletal Disease

Gout

Hyperuricemia and gout are associated with obesity.[144,145]

Osteoarthritis

The risk of osteoarthritis of weight-bearing joints is increased in overweight and obese persons. The knees are most often involved because much more body weight is exerted across the knees than across the hips during weight-bearing activity.[146] There is a stronger relationship between body size and osteoarthritis in women than in men and, in women, even small increases in body weight can promote osteoarthritis. In a study of twins, symptomatic or asymptomatic lower extremity osteoarthritis was found in persons who were only 3 to 5 kg heavier than their twin sibling.[147]

Cancer

Overweight and obesity increase the risk of cancer. Based on data from a prospective study in more than 900,000 U.S. adults,[148] it was estimated that overweight and obesity could account for 14% of all deaths from cancer in men and 20% of deaths in women. In both men and women, BMI was also significantly associated with higher rates of death due to cancers of the esophagus, colon and rectum, liver, gallbladder, pancreas, and kidney; non-Hodgkin's lymphoma; and multiple myeloma. Significant trends of increasing risk with higher BMI values were observed for death from cancers of the stomach and prostate in men and for death from cancers of the breast, uterus, cervix, and ovary in women.[148] Most (e.g., references 148 and 149) but not all (e.g., reference 150) epidemiologic studies have found a direct relationship between BMI and colon cancer in both men and women. The risks of breast and endometrial cancer mortality increase with obesity and weight gain since age 18 years.[151] Specifically, the risk of breast cancer appears to increase with increasing BMI only in postmenopausal women; in premenopausal women, however, increased BMI may actually protect against breast cancer.[152]

Obesity is often correlated with ingestion of a high-fat, high-calorie diet, which is another risk factor for cancer. Therefore, it is difficult to distinguish how much of the relation between obesity and cancer is attributable to obesity per se and how much is attributable to dietary factors.

Genitourinary Disease in Women

Obese women are often affected by irregular menses, amenorrhea, and infertility.[153] Pregnant obese women are at increased risks for gestational diabetes and hypertension[154] and delivery complications,[155] and their babies are at increased risk for congenital malformations.[156] The risk of urinary incontinence is also increased in obese women.[157] In extremely obese patients, incontinence usually resolves after considerable weight loss, usually achieved by bariatric surgery.[158]

Neurologic Disease

Obesity increases the incidence of ischemic stroke. Obesity is also associated with idiopathic intracranial hypertension (IIH), also known as *pseudotumor cerebri.* This syndrome is manifested by headache, vision abnormalities, tinnitus, and sixth nerve paresis. Although the prevalence of IIH increases with increasing BMI, the risk of IIH is increased even in persons who are only 10% above ideal body weight.[159,160] The observation that weight loss in extremely obese patients with IIH decreases intracranial pressure and resolves most associated clinical signs and symptoms suggests there is a causal relationship between obesity and IIH.[161,162]

Cataracts

Overweight and obesity are associated with an increased prevalence of cataracts.[163] Moreover, persons with abdominal obesity are at greater risk than those with lower-body obesity, suggesting that insulin resistance may be involved in the pathogenesis of cataract formation.

Gastrointestinal Disease

Gastroesophageal Reflux Disease

The relationship between gastroesophageal reflux disease (GERD) and obesity is unclear because of conflicting data from different studies. A higher incidence of reflux symptoms in obese than in lean persons has been found in most,[164,165] but not all,[166] large epidemiologic studies. In addition, studies that evaluated gastroesophageal acid reflux by 24-hour pH monitoring have reported the presence of a significant relationship[167] and no relationship[168] between BMI and pathologic reflux, defined as the occurrence of esophageal pH of less than 4 more than 5% of the time.

Gallstones

The risk of symptomatic gallstones increases linearly with BMI.[16,169] The Nurses' Health Study found that the annual incidence of symptomatic gallstones was 1% in women with a BMI greater than 30.0 kg/m^2 and 2% in women with a BMI greater than 45.0 kg/m^2.[169] The risk of gallstones increases during weight loss, particularly when weight loss is rapid. This increased risk is related to increased bile cholesterol supersaturation, enhanced cholesterol crystal nucleation, and decreased gallbladder contractility.[170]

When the rate of weight loss exceeds 1.5 kg (~1.5% of body weight) per week, the risk of gallstone formation increases exponentially.[171] In obese patients who undergo rapid weight loss with a very-low-calorie (<600 kcal/day), low-fat (1-3 g/day) diet or gastric surgery, the respective incidence of new gallstones is approximately 25%[172,173] and 35%.[174] Gallstone formation is also promoted by the low fat content of very-low-calorie diets because more than 4 to 10 g of fat in a meal are needed to stimulate maximal gallbladder contractility.[175] Therefore, increasing the fat content of a very-low-calorie diet can prevent the development of new gallstones.[176] However, increasing dietary fat content might not be as important in preventing gallstones in patients consuming a low-calorie than in those consuming a very-low-calorie diet. Administration of ursodeoxycholic acid (600 mg/day) during weight loss markedly decreases gallstone formation.[177]

Pancreatitis

Obese patients would be expected to be at increased risk for gallstone pancreatitis because of their increased prevalence of gallstones. However, few studies have addressed this issue. Several studies show that overweight and obese patients with pancreatitis have a higher risk of local complications, severe pancreatitis, and death than lean patients.[178] It has been hypothesized that the increased deposition of fat in the peripancreatic and retroperitoneal spaces predisposes obese patients to develop peripancreatic fat necrosis and subsequent local and systemic complications.

Liver Disease

Obesity is associated with a spectrum of liver abnormalities, which are now referred to as *nonalcoholic steatohepatitis*.[179] These abnormalities include hepatomegaly, abnormal liver biochemistries, steatosis, steatohepatitis, fibrosis, and cirrhosis. Alanine aminotransferase (ALT) and aspartate aminotransferase (AST) are the most commonly elevated liver enzymes, but elevations of these enzymes generally do not exceed two times the upper limit of normal.[180] Moreover, enzyme levels often do not correlate with the severity of histologic abnormalities.[179] Most of the available data suggest that steatosis affects approximately 75%, steatohepatitis approximately 20%, and cirrhosis approximately 2% of obese patients.[180-182]

NASH is associated with abdominal obesity and the metabolic syndrome.[183,184] However, the factors underlying the development of NASH in obese persons are not clear. NASH has been hypothesized to result from two or more insults to the liver.[185] The first insult is steatosis, caused by obesity-induced alterations in lipid metabolism. One alteration is increased lipolysis of adipose tissue triglycerides, which increases the delivery of free fatty acids to the liver; another is increased de novo lipogenesis; a possible third alteration is inadequate hepatic fatty acid oxidation. The second insult might involve peroxidation of hepatic lipids and injury-related cytokines, which can promote direct cellular injury, inflammation, and fibrosis.[186]

Obese patients with NASH are usually advised to lose weight, but it is not known whether weight loss alters the progression of the disease. With a gradual weight loss of 10% or more, abnormalities in liver chemistries resolve and liver size, hepatic fat content, and features of steatohepatitis decrease.[185,187] The rapid weight loss that occurs with gastric surgery[181] or a very-low-calorie diet[188] also decreases hepatic fat content, but it can promote hepatic inflammation and worsen steatohepatitis.

Benefits of Intentional Weight Loss

Effect on Morbidity

Intentional weight loss improves many of the medical complications associated with obesity. Many of these beneficial effects have a dose-dependent relationship with the amount of weight lost, and they begin after only a modest weight loss of 5% of initial body weight.[5] In addition, weight loss can decrease the risk of developing new obesity-related diseases, such as diabetes.[189,190]

Type 2 Diabetes Mellitus

In obese patients with type 2 diabetes mellitus, weight loss improves insulin sensitivity and glycemic control. A 1-year study, conducted in obese patients with type 2 diabetes treated with oral hypoglycemic agents, showed that even a 5% weight loss decreased fasting blood glucose, insulin, and hemoglobin A_{1c} concentrations and the dosage of hypoglycemic medication.[191] All patients who lost 15% or more of their body weight decreased or eliminated the need for hypoglycemic medication. In patients with severe obesity who underwent gastric bypass surgery, the average loss of approximately 30% of initial body weight promoted marked long-term improvements in glucose homeostasis.[192] In this study, normal fasting blood glucose, insulin, and hemoglobin A_{1c} concentrations were achieved by 83% of the patients who had type 2 diabetes and by 99% of the patients who had impaired glucose tolerance. However, a subset of obese patients with severe diabetes might not experience improved glycemic control with weight loss.[193]

In obese patients with mild type 2 diabetes mellitus, both energy restriction and weight loss have important beneficial effects on insulin action and glycemic control. The initial negative energy balance associated with dieting acutely improves insulin sensitivity before there is a significant change in body weight. Subsequent weight and fat losses further improve glycemic control and insulin-mediated glucose uptake.[194,195]

Sustained weight loss can prevent the development of new cases of diabetes.[196,197] For example, the Swedish Obese Subjects (SOS) Study found that in severely obese patients (initial BMI 41 kg/m^2) who underwent gastric surgery, a 16% weight loss reduced the risk of diabetes fivefold over an 8-year period.[197] Data reported from the Finnish Diabetes Prevention Study demonstrated that changes in lifestyle that resulted in modest (~5%) weight loss decreased the 3-year incidence of diabetes by 58% in subjects with impaired glucose tolerance.[198]

Several studies have found that weight loss is more difficult in obese patients with type 2 diabetes than in those without diabetes.[199,200] Moreover, successful weight loss may be inversely related to the duration and severity of diabetes.[200] The reasons obese patients with diabetes are less responsive to weight-loss therapy are not known, but they might involve the energy-conserving effects of improved glycemic control (e.g., reduced glycosuria) and the tendency for weight gain associated with most drug treatments for diabetes.[201]

Dyslipidemia

Weight loss usually decreases serum triglyceride, total cholesterol, and LDL-cholesterol concentrations, and serum HDL-cholesterol concentrations increase.[5,202] Improvements in serum triglyceride, total cholesterol, and LDL-cholesterol concentrations are generally greatest during the first 4 to 8 weeks of a weight-loss program.[203] Serum HDL-cholesterol concentrations decrease during active weight loss but tend to increase once weight loss stabilizes.[202] A greater reduction in LDL cholesterol is observed when weight loss is induced by a program of diet plus exercise than with either treatment alone.[204]

Hypertension

Systolic and diastolic blood pressures decrease with weight loss, independent of sodium restriction.[205] In the Trials of Hypertension Prevention Phase II (TOHP II), which is one of the largest intervention studies to date, approximately 1200 overweight and obese patients were randomized to a dietary weight loss intervention or usual care.[206] This study showed a dose-response relationship between weight loss and change in blood pressure at 36 months. During the first 6 months, patients who successfully lost weight experienced a marked reduction in blood pressure. However, among patients who regained most or all of their lost weight, blood pressure steadily increased to near-baseline values.

The marked weight loss induced by gastric surgery improves or completely resolves hypertension in about two thirds of extremely obese hypertensive patients.[207] However, data recently compiled by the SOS Study indicate that the beneficial effect of weight loss on blood pressure might not persist.[208] Much of the improvement in blood pressure observed at 1 and 2 years after gastric surgery disappeared by 3 years. Over the next 5 years, both systolic and diastolic blood pressures gradually increased. These findings imply that current energy balance and the direction of weight change are also important in blood pressure control.

A decreased incidence of hypertension with weight loss has been reported by several large, prospective, epidemiologic and intervention studies. For example, TOHP II found that persons who maintained a weight loss of at least 4.5 kg at 36 months had a 65% decrease in the risk of hypertension compared with the control group participants who gained 1.8 kg.[206] The Nurses' Health Study observed a direct correlation between the risk of developing hypertension and changes in body weight among normotensive women who were followed for 12 to 15 years. With weight losses of 5.0 to 9.9 kg and 10 or more kg, the risk of developing hypertension decreased by 15% and 26%, respectively.[209]

Data from the SOS Study also question the ability of weight loss to prevent development of hypertension. In that study, the preventive effect of weight loss on the development of hypertension, which was observed 2 years after gastric surgery,[189] disappeared at 3 years.[208] In contrast, the SOS study found a marked effect of weight loss on the incidence of other obesity-related diseases. For example, the long-term maintenance of major weight loss after gastric surgery was associated with a marked and persistent reduction in the risk of diabetes.

Cardiovascular Disease

Modest weight loss can simultaneously affect the entire cluster of cardiovascular risk factors associated with obesity. In the Framingham Offspring Study, a weight loss of 5 lb (2.25 kg) or more over 16 years was associated with 48% (in men) and 40% (in women) reductions in the sum of risk factors (defined as the highest quintile of systolic blood pressure, serum triglyceride, serum total cholesterol, fasting blood glucose, and BMI and the lowest quintile of HDL cholesterol).[210] Improvements in cardiovascular structure and function associated with weight loss include reductions in blood volume and hemodynamic demands on the heart, left ventricular mass and chamber size, and septal wall thickness (e.g., reference 211). Such improvements in cardiac function may be responsible for the reduced frequency of chest pain and dyspnea reported by patients who lost weight after bariatric surgery.[212] Weight loss might also delay the progression of atherosclerosis. In one study, the progression of carotid artery intimal wall thickening over 4 years was three times higher in untreated obese subjects who did not lose weight than in obese subjects who lost weight after gastric surgery.[193]

Pulmonary Disease

Weight loss improves pulmonary function, obstructive sleep apnea, and the obesity-hypoventilation syndrome. Even modest weight loss reduces the severity of sleep apnea, improves sleep patterns, and decreases daytime hypersomnolence.[213,214] More marked weight loss, induced by bariatric surgery, has been shown to improve the obesity-hypoventilation syndrome by correcting resting room-air arterial blood gases, lung volume, and cardiac filling pressure.[215] Sustained weight loss maintains these improvements in sleep apnea and obesity hypoventilation; however, pulmonary symptoms recur with weight regain.

Reproductive and Urinary Tract Function in Women

Marked weight loss (>20% of initial body weight) has been shown to correct urinary overflow incontinence,[157] resolve amenorrhea, and improve fertility.

Effect on Mortality

To date, there is no conclusive evidence showing that weight loss in obese persons reduces mortality. In fact, most epidemiologic studies have indicated that weight loss or weight fluctuation increases mortality.[216] However, these studies did not distinguish between intentional and unintentional weight loss, so their results might have been confounded by unintentional weight loss caused by concomitant illness.

The effect of intentional weight loss on mortality has been addressed in three studies, which obtained baseline data between 1959 and 1960 and followed the participants for an average of 12 years.[217-219] The composite results of these studies suggest that intentional, and possibly transient, weight loss might increase survival among overweight and obese persons who have type 2 diabetes mellitus. However, these data are not conclusive because weight loss was self-reported and occurred at any time before the initial interview, and possible changes in weight that might have occurred during follow-up were not determined. Therefore, long-term, prospective trials are needed to determine the true relationship between intentional weight loss and survival in obese persons.

Obesity Therapy

Many obese persons can achieve short-term weight loss by dieting alone, but successful long-term weight maintenance is much more difficult to achieve. "Weight cycling" and "yo-yo dieting" are popular terms used to describe repetitive cycles of weight loss and subsequent regain.[220] Although some adverse consequences have been associated with weight cycling,[221] available data on the health effects of weight cycling are inconclusive and should not deter obese persons from attempting to lose weight.[220] Currently available weight-loss treatments include dietary intervention, increased physical activity, behavior modification, pharmacotherapy, and surgery.

Dietary Intervention

For most obese persons, negative energy balance is more readily achieved by decreasing food intake than by increasing physical activity. Therefore, dietary intervention is considered the cornerstone of weight-loss therapy. Weight-loss diets generally involve modifications of energy content and macronutrient composition. However, the degree of weight loss achieved primarily depends on the energy content, rather than the relative macronutrient composition, of the diet.

Energy Content

Weight-loss diets can be classified according to their energy content. A balanced-deficit diet of conventional foods usually contains less than 1500 kcal/day and an appropriate balance of macronutrients. Low-calorie diets (LCDs) contain 800 to 1500 kcal/day and are consumed as liquid formula, nutritional bars, conventional food, or a combination of these items. Very-low-calorie diets (VLCDs) contain less than 800 kcal/day and are generally high in protein (70-100 g/day) and low in fat (<15 g/day). Such diets may be consumed as a commercially prepared liquid formula and may include nutritional bars. VLCDs consumed as regular foods (mostly lean meat, fish, or fowl) are known as protein-sparing modified fasts.

According to the treatment guidelines recently issued by the U.S. National Institutes of Health (NIH),[5] persons who are overweight (BMI 25.0-29.9 kg/m^2) and have two or more cardiovascular disease risk factors and persons who have class I obesity (BMI 30.0-34.9 kg/m^2) should decrease their energy intake by approximately 500 kcal/day. This deficit in energy intake will generally promote weight loss of 1 lb (0.45 kg) per week and result in about a 10% reduction of initial weight at 6 months. The NIH guidelines recommend a more aggressive energy deficit of 500 to 1000 kcal/day for persons with more severe obesity (BMI ≥35.0 kg/m^2). In such persons, this energy deficit will generally produce weight loss of 1 to 2 lb/wk and result in a 10% weight loss at 6 months.

Total daily energy requirements can be estimated by using standard equations, such as the Harris-Benedict[222] or the World Health Organization equation,[223] which are based on the patient's size, age, sex, and activity level. However, the use of standard equations is cumbersome and may be unreliable in obese persons. The simple diet guidelines outlined in Tables 35–5 and 35–6 are suggested as an alternative to a specific energy-deficit diet based on the patient's daily energy requirements. Patients who follow these guidelines generally lose weight. Because many patients do not fully adhere to their prescribed diet, the energy content of the diet should be regularly adjusted according to the patient's weight loss response.

More than 30 prospective RCTs have investigated the effectiveness of LCDs for weight loss.[5] The composite results of these trials indicated that a 1000 to 1500 kcal/day LCD induces about an 8% weight loss after 16 to 26 weeks of treatment. However, these results might not be typical of the results obtained when an LCD is prescribed in routine clinical practice, because trial participants volunteered to enroll in a weight-loss study and most study protocols included some form of behavior modification therapy.

The use of VLCDs induces a weight loss of about 15% to 20% in 12 to 16 weeks of treatment, but this weight loss is not usually maintained.[224,225] In fact, several randomized trials have shown that weight regain is greater after VLCD than after LCD therapy.[226-229] Therefore, 1 year after treatment, weight loss with a VLCD is often similar to that obtained with a LCD. In addition, initial weight losses with a VLCD and an LCD are similar when the diets are consumed in the same manner. For example, the weight loss observed in patients given a liquid diet providing 420 kcal/day was not significantly greater than that observed in persons who consumed a liquid diet providing 800 kcal/day.[230] This suggests that patients treated with VLCDs are either less compliant with the diet or sustain a greater decline in energy expenditure than those treated with LCDs. With VLCDs, there is greater risk of the medical complications associated with dieting, such as hypokalemia, dehydration, and gallstone formation. Patients treated with a VLCD, therefore, require closer medical supervision than those treated with an LCD.

TABLE 35–5 SUGGESTED ENERGY COMPOSITION OF INITIAL REDUCED-CALORIE DIET

Body Weight (lbs)	Suggested Energy Intake (kcal/day)
150-199	1000
200-249	1200
250-299	1500
300-349	1800
≥350	2000

TABLE 35–6 SUGGESTED MACRONUTRIENT COMPOSITION OF INITIAL REDUCED-CALORIE DIET

Macronutrient	Suggested Amount
Fat	20%-30% of total calories
Saturated fatty acids	8%-10% of total calories
Monosaturated fatty acids	Up to 15% of total calories
Polyunsaturated fatty acids	Up to 10% of total calories
Cholesterol	<300 mg/day
Protein	15%-20% of total calories
Carbohydrate	55%-65% of total calories

Macronutrient Composition

Altering the macronutrient composition of the diet does not induce weight loss, unless total energy intake is reduced. Low-fat diets have traditionally been prescribed for weight loss because such diets facilitate energy restriction. Triglycerides, the principal component of dietary fat, increase the palatability and energy density of food. The results of epidemiologic and diet intervention studies suggest that increased dietary fat intake is associated with increases in total energy intake and body weight.[231] Conversely, data from a large number of studies suggest that decreasing fat intake is associated with spontaneous decreases in total energy intake and body weight, even when carbohydrate and protein intakes are not restricted.

A direct relationship between changes in dietary fat intake and body weight was found in a meta-analysis of 37 intervention studies involving the Step I or Step II low-fat (<30% kcal as fat) diet recommended by the National Cholesterol Education Program to lower cardiovascular risk.[232] Data from another meta-analysis suggest that the amount of weight loss induced by a low-fat diet is directly related to the severity of obesity.[233]

The weight-loss effects of a low-fat diet may be related to the effect of dietary fat on energy density. Energy density is defined as the energy (i.e., calories) present in a given weight (g) of food. Because the energy density of fat is so high, there is a high correlation between dietary fat content and diet energy density. According to short-term studies lasting up to 14 days, energy intake is regulated according to the weight of ingested food rather than its fat or energy content.[234] For example, the weight of food ingested was the same when lean and obese subjects were given either an ad libitum high-fat/high-energy-density (1.5 kcal/g) diet or a low-fat/low-energy-density (0.7 kcal/g) diet.[235] As a result, energy intake on the high-fat/high-energy-density diet (3000 kcal/day) was nearly double the intake on the low-fat/low-energy-density diet (1570 kcal/day). In other studies, the weight of food ingested also remained the same when subjects were given liquid diets that had the same energy density but varied in fat content (20% to 60%)[236] and when energy density was varied but fat content remained constant.[237] The results of these short-term studies show that dietary fat content itself does not affect total energy intake, apart from its effects on dietary energy density and food palatability. Whether diets of low energy density can help induce and maintain weight loss remains to be confirmed by long-term studies in obese subjects.

Low-carbohydrate diets have been evaluated as a potential therapy for obesity in RCTs. Several short-term (<12 wk) trials (e.g., reference 238) compared the effects of low-carbohydrate and high-carbohydrate diets on weight loss when energy intake was kept constant. These studies suggest that despite equal energy intakes, weight loss during the first 4 weeks may be greater with a low- than with a high-carbohydrate diet but that weight loss between 6 and 12 weeks was the same with either diet. The results of five of six RCTs conducted in adults[239-244] found that subjects randomized to a low-carbohydrate diet (approximately 25% to 40% carbohydrate) achieved greater short-term (6 months),[239-241] but not long-term (12 months),[239,243,244] weight loss than those randomized to a low-fat diet (approximately 25% to 30% fat, 55% to 60% carbohydrate). The data from these studies also found greater improvements in serum triglyceride and HDL-cholesterol concentrations, but not in serum LDL-cholesterol concentration, in the low-carbohydrate versus the low-fat group. The mechanism responsible for the decrease in body weight associated with a low-carbohydrate diet can be completely explained by a decrease in total energy intake.[245] However, the mechanism responsible for decreased energy consumption when dietary carbohydrates are restricted, despite an unlimited intake of fat and protein, is not known.

Physical Activity

Metabolic Rate

Although there is a profound increase in energy expenditure during an actual episode of exercise, the addition of regular exercise to a weight-loss program has negligible effects on REE. In a meta-analysis of prospective, controlled trials that randomized obese subjects to treatment with diet alone or diet plus exercise, the addition of exercise did circumvent the expected decline in REE, when REE was adjusted for body mass.[246]

Body Composition

The composition of weight loss can be influenced by the addition of exercise to a diet program. Pooled data from two meta-analyses found that exercise can reduce the loss of FFM that occurs with weight loss.[247] When diet-induced weight loss was approximately 10 kg, regular exercise of low or moderate intensity reduced the percentage of weight lost as FFM from approximately 25% to 12%. Although the difference in weight lost as FFM was large on a percentage basis, it nonetheless represented only a small (~1 kg) difference in the absolute amount of FFM lost. This preservation of FFM with exercise might not necessarily reflect preservation of muscle protein but might, instead, involve increased retention of body water and muscle glycogen. Indeed, nitrogen balance studies have not been able to detect any nitrogen sparing effect of exercise during diet-induced weight loss in women.[248] Whether there is a difference between the effects of endurance and resistance exercise on FFM conservation is not clear because the available data are limited and conflicting.

Diabetes and Coronary Heart Disease

Endurance exercise increases insulin sensitivity[249] and is associated with a decreased risk of developing diabetes[250,251] and dying from cardiovascular disease.[252]

Weight Loss

Increasing physical activity alone is not an effective strategy for promoting initial weight loss. Most studies have shown that moderate endurance exercise, such as brisk walking for 45 to 60 minutes, 4 times a week, for up to 1 year, usually induces only minor weight loss.[246] In obese persons, the energy deficit created by exercise is usually much less and requires more effort than the energy deficit created by a reduced-calorie diet. For example, to lose 1 lb of fat, an obese patient would have to walk or run approximately 4.5 miles/day for one week or to consume a 500-kcal/day-deficit diet for one week.

Although exercise alone is not an effective strategy for inducing initial weight loss, increasing physical activity might be an important component of successful long-term weight management. Several large-scale, cross-sectional case studies have shown that obese subjects who were successful in maintaining weight loss for 1 year or more engaged in regular exercise.[253,254] Retrospective analyses of data from prospective randomized studies found that subjects treated with diet-plus-exercise who continued to exercise sustained significantly larger long-term weight losses than subjects who stopped exercising or subjects treated with diet alone (e.g., reference 255). However, when data are analyzed on an intention-to-treat basis, most prospective randomized trials do not find that exercise has a statistically significant effect on the long-term maintenance of weight loss, presumably because adherence to the exercise program is often poor.[256]

The amount of exercise that is associated with weight-loss maintenance is considerable and requires expending approximately 2500 kcal/wk.[257,258] This level of energy expenditure can be accomplished through vigorous activity (aerobics, cycling, or jogging) for approximately 30 min/day or more moderate activity (brisk walking) for 60 to 75 min/day. Most obese persons cannot easily achieve this level of activity. Therefore, prescribed activity goals should be initially modest and increased gradually over time.

Behavior Modification

Principles

Behavior-modification therapy attempts to enable obese patients to recognize and subsequently alter eating and activity habits that promote their obesity. Behavior modification is derived from the classic conditioning principle that behavior is often triggered by an antecedent event. The association between the antecedent event, such as watching television, and the behavior, such as eating, is strengthened by repetition so that the more often the two are paired, the stronger becomes the association between them.

Behavior modification for the treatment of obesity usually involves multiple strategies to modify eating and activity habits. These strategies include: stimulus control (avoiding the cues that prompt eating), self-monitoring (keeping daily records of food intake and physical activity), problem-solving skills (developing a systematic manner of analyzing a problem and identifying possible solutions), cognitive restructuring (thinking in a positive manner), social support (cooperation from family members and friends in altering lifestyle behavior), and relapse prevention (methods to promote recovery from bouts of overeating or weight regain).

Effectiveness

Treatment by a comprehensive group behavior therapy approach generally results in about a 9% loss of initial weight in 20 to 26 weeks.[259] When treatment ends, weight regain is commonly observed. Although in the year following treatment, patients generally regain about 30% to 35% of their lost weight, most patients sustain clinically significant weight loss of more than 5% of initial body weight.[260] Increasing the duration of behavior therapy programs has only marginally improved total weight loss, but it probably prevents the weight regain that usually occurs when treatment is stopped.[261]

Pharmacotherapy

Overview

Conventional obesity therapy is associated with a high rate of recidivism. Therefore, the most important goal of pharmacotherapy is to maintain long-term weight loss. Pharmacotherapy should not be considered a short-term approach for weight loss because patients who lose weight with drug therapy usually regain weight when the therapy is discontinued.[262,263] Some obese patients do not respond to drug therapy, and long-term success is unlikely if weight loss does not occur within the first 4 weeks of drug treatment.[264]

Weight loss usually plateaus by 6 months of treatment and weight begins to increase after 1 year.[262,263] This observation implies that the efficacy of weight loss medications declines with time or obesity is a progressive disease, or both. Treatment outcome is less successful when pharmacotherapy is administered alone than when pharmacotherapy is administered as part of a comprehensive weight-loss program that includes diet, exercise, and behavior modification (Fig. 35–5).[256] The use of obesity pharmacotherapy alone exposes patients to the full risks of the drug without the full medical benefits of more comprehensive treatment.

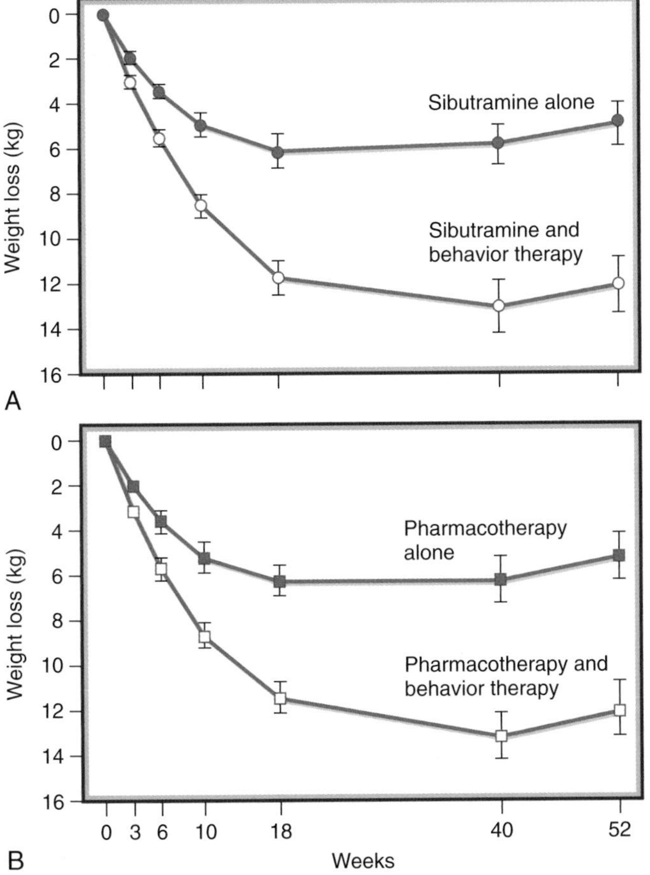

Figure 35–5 ▪ Weight loss in obese subjects treated with anorexiant medication (sibutramine) alone, group behavioral therapy alone, or medication plus group behavioral therapy. These data demonstrate that greater weight loss is achieved when antiobesity medications are used in conjunction with lifestyle modification than when they are used alone. (Adapted from Wadden TA, Berkowitz RI, Womble LG, et al. Randomized trial of lifestyle modification and pharmacotherapy for obesity. N Engl J Med 2005;353:2111-2120.)

Table 35–7 lists the drugs currently approved by the U.S. Food and Drug Administration for the treatment of obesity. All currently approved weight-loss drugs act as anorexiants, with the exception of orlistat, which inhibits the absorption of dietary fat. In the last several years, three anorexiant drugs were withdrawn from the market because of the increased incidence of either valvular heart disease (fenfluramine and dexfenfluramine)[265] or hemorrhagic stroke (phenylpropanolamine)[266] associated with their use.

All anorexiant drugs, except mazindol, are derived from β-phenylethylamine, the amphetamine precursor. The structures of these drugs have been chemically altered to reduce the potential for abuse. Anorexiant medications affect the monoamine (norepinephrine, serotonin, and dopamine) system in the hypothalamus and thereby enhance satiation (level of fullness during consumption of a meal, which influences the amount of food consumed), satiety (level of hunger after consumption of a meal, which influences the frequency of eating), or both.

Monoamine neurotransmitters are synthesized from tyrosine and stored in granules that release their contents from presynaptic nerve terminals into the interneuronal cleft between pre- and postsynaptic nerves. Only a small portion of the monoamines released into the interneuronal cleft actually bind to postsynaptic receptors and thus transmit a signal from one nerve to the other. Most of the released monoamines are taken back up into the presynaptic nerve terminal, where they are either degraded or repackaged into granules for future release.

Weight-loss pharmacotherapy is approved for patients who have no contraindications to therapy and who have a BMI greater than 30.0 kg/m^2, or a BMI between 27.0 and 29.9 kg/m^2 and an obesity-related medical condition. Since a comprehensive review of drug therapy for obesity has been published,[267] we will only review data from long-term (>6 months) prospective RCTs that investigated the weight-loss efficacy and safety of sibutramine and orlistat, the only drugs currently approved for long-term use in the management of obesity.

Sibutramine

Sibutramine inhibits the neuronal reuptake of norepinephrine, serotonin, and, to a lesser degree, dopamine. It enhances satiation, rather than satiety. In humans, sibutramine also appears to promote a small increase in metabolic rate several hours after its administration.[268] The currently recommended initial dose of sibutramine is 10 mg/day.[269] This daily dose can be decreased or increased by 5 mg if tolerance is poor or weight loss is inadequate. Administration of sibutramine at doses between 1 and

TABLE 35–7 DRUGS APPROVED BY THE U.S. FOOD AND DRUG ADMINISTRATION FOR THE TREATMENT OF OBESITY

Generic Name	Trade Name
Benzphetamine HCl	Didrex
Phendimetrazine tartrate	Bontril, Plegine, Prelu-2, X-Trozine
Phentermine	Ionamin, Adipex-P, Fastin, Oby-trim
Diethylpropion hydrochloride	Tenuate, Tenuate Dospan
Mazindol	Sanorex, Mazanor
Sibutramine HCl	Meridia
Orlistat	Xenical

30 mg/day for 24 weeks demonstrates a dose-dependent weight loss, ranging from 0.9% of initial body weight with placebo to 7.7% with 30 mg sibutramine/day.[270]

Results from two 1-year RCTs of the effectiveness of sibutramine treatment in producing and maintaining weight loss have been reported.[271,272] The results of one trial have only appeared in abstract form,[271] and the other trial involved only obese subjects with medication-controlled hypertension.[272] In both trials, all participants received minimal adjunctive weight-management therapy, and the placebo group lost less weight than usually observed in placebo groups from other trials. Compared with placebo-treated subjects, subjects treated with sibutramine (10-20 mg/day) lost more weight. In the first study, 39% of patients randomized to sibutramine therapy lost 10% or more of their initial body weight compared with 9% of patients randomized to receive placebo.[271] In the second study of hypertensive obese patients, 13% of patients randomized to sibutramine therapy lost 10% or more of their body weight compared with 4% of patients randomized to placebo.[272]

Results have also been reported from two prospective RCTs that evaluated the efficacy of sibutramine therapy in long-term weight management after a predetermined amount of weight was lost.[273,274] In the first trial, obese subjects who lost at least 6 kg after a 4-week VLCD resumed a regular diet with diet counseling and were randomly assigned to 1 year of treatment with placebo or sibutramine.[273] In the year after randomization, sibutramine-treated subjects lost an additional 5.2 kg and placebo-treated subjects gained 0.5 kg. Total study weight losses were 12.9 kg in sibutramine-treated subjects and 6.9 kg in subjects treated with placebo. The initial weight loss achieved with the VLCD was maintained or increased in 74% of sibutramine-treated subjects compared with only 41% of placebo-treated subjects.

In the second trial, obese subjects who lost more than 5% of initial weight after 6 months of treatment with sibutramine (10 mg/day) and a 600-kcal/day-deficit diet were randomized to treatment with either sibutramine (increased to 15 or 20 mg/day) or placebo.[274] All subjects received diet counseling. Nearly one half the subjects who entered the study failed to complete the 18-month treatment program. Among subjects who completed the study, 43% of those treated with sibutramine but only 16% of those treated with placebo maintained 80% or more of their original 6-month weight loss. On average, subjects who continued sibutramine maintained their weight loss for 1 year and then experienced a slight and progressive increase in weight, but subjects who were switched to placebo experienced a progressive increase in weight as soon as sibutramine therapy was stopped.

The most common side effects of sibutramine therapy are dry mouth, headache, constipation, and insomnia. Sibutramine also causes small increases in blood pressure (~2-4 mm Hg) and heart rate (~4-6 beats/min).[270] However, some patients experience much larger increases in blood pressure or heart rate and require dose reduction or discontinuation of therapy.

Orlistat

Orlistat is synthesized from lipstatin, a product of *Streptomyces toxytricini* mold, which inhibits most mammalian lipases.[275] Orlistat binds to lipases in the gastrointestinal tract and thereby blocks the digestion of dietary triglycerides. This inhibition of fat digestion reduces micelle formation and, subsequently, the absorption of long-chain fatty acids, cholesterol, and certain fat-soluble vitamins. The degree of fat malabsorption is directly related in a curvilinear fashion to the dose of orlistat administered.[276] Excretion of about 30% of ingested triglycerides, which is near the maximum plateau value, occurs at a dose of 360 mg/day (120 mg tid with meals). Orlistat has no effect on systemic lipases because less than 1% of the administered dose is absorbed.[277]

Many clinical trials of orlistat included treatment with low doses (30 and 60 mg tid) that were not effective, so only data obtained with the standard recommended dose of 120 mg tid are reviewed. The effectiveness of orlistat therapy (120 mg tid) in promoting and maintaining weight loss has been evaluated in several prospective RCTs that lasted longer than 1 year.[278-284] At 1 year, about one third more patients treated with orlistat than treated with placebo lost 5% or more of initial body weight; about twice as many patients treated with orlistat than treated with placebo lost 10% or more of initial weight. Subjects who were enrolled in a trial conducted in a primary care practice setting, which did not include behavior therapy or interaction with a dietitian,[272] did not do as well as those enrolled in trials that provided formal behavior modification and diet counseling.[278,279] Successful weight loss was also more difficult to achieve in patients with type 2 diabetes mellitus.[283]

The long-term efficacy of orlistat in maintaining initial weight loss after 1 year has been evaluated in several RCTs, including second-year extensions of the 1-year trials reviewed here (e.g., reference 278). During the second year of these trials, more liberal energy intake was allowed with a goal of preventing weight regain, rather than promoting additional weight loss. About one half of the initially randomized subjects completed the second year. After 1 year, both placebo- and orlistat-treated groups in all trials regained weight. However, at the end of 2 years, relative weight loss was greater with orlistat than placebo treatment.

The results of several RCTs suggest that orlistat administration is associated with a reduction of serum LDL-cholesterol concentrations that is independent of the effect of weight loss alone. Even after adjusting for percent weight loss, these studies found that subjects treated with orlistat sustained a greater reduction in serum LDL-cholesterol concentrations than those treated with placebo.[278,279] The mechanism responsible for this effect may be related to orlistat-induced inhibition of dietary cholesterol absorption.[285]

The most common side effects associated with orlistat therapy are gastrointestinal complaints. Approximately 70% to 80% of subjects treated with orlistat experienced one or more gastrointestinal events, compared with approximately 50% to 60% of those treated with placebo.[278-281,283] These gastrointestinal events were induced by fat malabsorption, usually occurred within the first 4 weeks of treatment, and were of mild or moderate intensity. Subjects rarely reported more than two episodes despite continued orlistat treatment. Orlistat treatment can also affect fat-soluble vitamin status and the absorption of some lipophilic medications.[278-280,286] Therefore, it is recommended that all patients treated with orlistat also receive a daily multivitamin supplement, and that orlistat not be taken for at least 2 hours before or after the ingestion of vitamin supplements or lipophilic drugs.

Surgical Therapy

Overview

Gastrointestinal surgery is the most effective approach for inducing major weight loss in extremely obese patients. In 1991, guidelines for the surgical treatment of obesity were established by an NIH Consensus Conference.[287] According to these guidelines, eligible candidates for surgery include patients with a BMI 40 kg/m^2 or more or those with a BMI of 35.0 to 39.9 kg/m^2 and one or more severe medical complications of obesity (e.g., hypertension, heart failure, type 2 diabetes mellitus, sleep apnea). Additional eligibility criteria are the inability to maintain weight loss with conventional therapy, acceptable operative

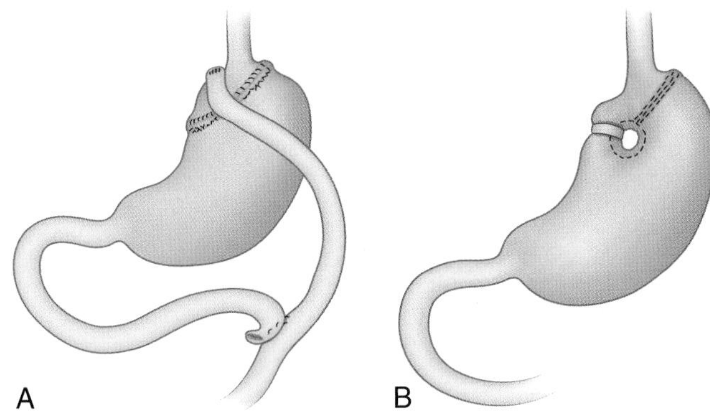

Figure 35–6 ■ Schematic diagram of the gastric bypass procedure **(A)** and vertical banded gastroplasty **(B)**. From Klein S, Wadden TA, Sugerman H. AGA technical review on obesity. Gastroenterology 2002; 123:882-932.

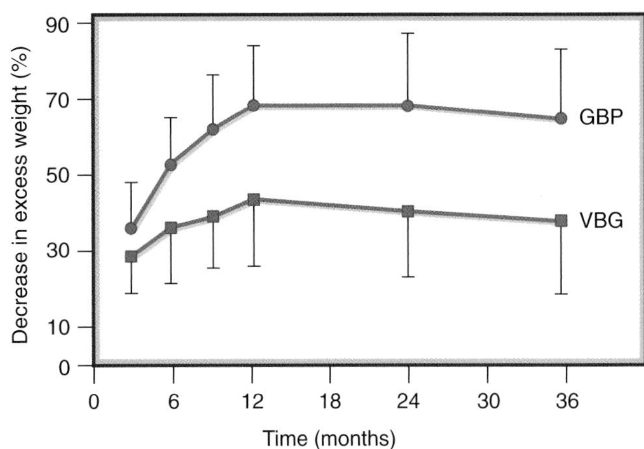

Figure 35–7 ■ Percentage of excess weight (mean ± SD) lost over 36 months after the gastric bypass procedure (GBP) and vertical banded gastroplasty (VBGP). Adapted from Sugerman HJ, Starkey JV, Birkenhauer R. A randomized prospective trial of gastric bypass versus vertical banded gastroplasty for morbid obesity and their effects on sweets versus non-sweets eaters. Ann Surg 1987;205:613-624.

risks, the absence of active substance abuse, and the ability to comply with the long-term treatment and follow-up required.

Current surgical procedures for obesity can be categorized as those that primarily cause gastric restriction and those that primarily cause nutrient maldigestion and malabsorption. All procedures have been performed laparoscopically, but the laparoscopic approach is technically challenging and usually requires more operating room time.

Gastric Bypass Procedure

The gastric bypass procedure, also known as Roux-en-Y gastric bypass, involves creating a small (10 mL to 30 mL) proximal gastric pouch that empties into a segment of jejunum that is anastomosed as a Roux-en-Y limb. The size of the patient determines the length of the Roux-en-Y limb (Fig. 35–6A). In patients with a BMI less than 50 kg/m^2, a 45- to 60-cm limb is generally used, but in patients with a BMI 50 kg/m^2 or more, a 150-cm limb (long-limb gastric bypass) promotes better weight loss without increasing the risk of nutrient deficiencies.[288] Although the gastric bypass is primarily a restrictive procedure, some malabsorption does occur as a result of the bypassed stomach, duodenum, and upper jejunum. Specific complications associated with the gastric bypass procedure include marginal ulcers, stomal stenosis, dilation of the bypassed stomach, staple line disruption, internal hernias, malabsorption of specific nutrients, and the dumping syndrome.

Gastroplasty

Vertical banded and Silastic ring gastroplasties, also known as gastric stapling, involve creating a small pouch from the gastroesophageal junction along the lesser curvature of the stomach, which has a stoma that is restricted by a 1-cm polypropylene or Silastic ring and empties into the rest of the stomach (see Fig. 35–6B).[289,290] Specific complications associated with gastroplasty include staple line disruption, stomal stenosis, and gastroesophageal reflux.

Gastric Bypass versus Gastroplasty

Data obtained from four prospective, randomized trials found that weight loss several years after surgery was consistently greater with the gastric bypass procedure (loss of ~65% of excess weight) than with gastroplasty (loss of ~40% of excess weight)[291-294] (Fig. 35–7). In addition, independent evaluations of each procedure suggest better long-term (10 to 14 years) results with the gastric bypass than with gastroplasty.[177,295] As a result of these findings, most centers now consider gastric bypass the gold standard for obesity surgery.

Gastric Banding

In the laparoscopically inserted adjustable silicone gastric banding (LASGB) procedure, a silicone band is placed around the upper stomach, just below the gastroesophageal junction. The band's circumference can be adjusted by inflating or deflating a balloon connected to a subcutaneously implanted port that is accessed percutaneously. This procedure is currently the most popular bariatric surgical procedure performed in Europe, and has recently been approved for use in the United States. The degree of weight loss achieved with LASBD has been similar to that achieved with vertical banded gastroplasty[296] and over time may equal that achieved by the GBP.[297]

Complications associated with LASGB include esophageal dilation, erosion of the band into the stomach, band slippage, band or port infections, and balloon or system leaks that lead to inadequate weight loss.[298,299] Esophageal dilation and dysphagia can result from the placement of the band at the gastroesophageal junction.[298] Although loosening the band usually relieves the dilation, removal of the band is sometimes necessary.[299] In some patients, the band erodes into the stomach and must be surgically removed. When the posterior stomach wall herniates through the band, the band slips. This can cause gastric obstruction and requires surgical revision.

Partial Biliopancreatic Bypass Procedures

The partial biliopancreatic bypass and the partial biliopancreatic bypass with duodenal switch result in gastric restriction, maldigestion, and malabsorption. Both procedures involve a partial gastrectomy and bypassing a considerable amount of small intestine from biliary and pancreatic secretions.[300,301] Partial biliopancreatic bypass induces malabsorption of protein, fat, fat-soluble vitamins, iron, calcium, and vitamin B_{12} and thus promotes more nutritional deficits than gastric restrictive procedures.[300,302] The incidence of protein deficiency is probably less common, and gastrointestinal side effects are not as severe, after partial biliopancreatic bypass with duodenal switch than after partial biliopancreatic bypass. Presumably these procedures cause greater weight loss (~75% of excess weight) than a standard gastric bypass, but the techniques have never been compared directly in a prospective randomized trial.

TABLE 35–8 SUGGESTED WEIGHT-LOSS TREATMENT OPTIONS BASED ON BMI AND RISK FACTORS

Treatment	BMI Category (kg/m²)				
	25.0-26.9	27.0-29.9	30.0-34.9	35.0-39.9	≥40.0
Diet, physical activity, and behavior therapy	With CHD risk factor or obesity-related disease	With CHD risk factor or obesity-related disease	Yes	Yes	Yes
Pharmacotherapy*		With obesity-related disease	Yes	Yes	Yes
Surgery†				With obesity-related disease	Yes

*Pharmacotherapy should only be considered in patients who are not able to achieve adequate weight loss by available conventional therapy (diet, physical activity, and behavior therapy) and who do not have any absolute contraindications for drug therapy.
†Bariatric surgery should only be considered in patients who are unable to lose weight with available conventional therapy and who do not have any absolute contraindications to surgery.
BMI, body mass index; CHD, coronary heart disease.

Jejunoileal Bypass

Jejunoileal bypass (JIB) was first described in 1969. This procedure was designed to bypass the major portion of the small intestine and thereby promote weight loss by inducing the malabsorption of ingested nutrients.[303,304] The JIB procedure is no longer performed because of an unacceptable incidence of serious side effects. The serious side effects of JIB result from protein-calorie malnutrition, bacterial overgrowth and translocation, and excess oxalate absorption (e.g., cirrhosis, interstitial nephritis, migratory arthritis, bypass enteritis, erythema nodosum, oxalate urolithiasis, hypocalcemia, and electrolyte imbalances) (e.g., references 305 to 309). Oral metronidazole is effective in treating the complications of JIB related to bacterial overgrowth (e.g., migratory arthritis, elevated liver enzymes, and bleeding from inflammation in the bypassed intestine).[308,309]

Inadequate Weight Loss after Surgery

About 15% of patients fail to lose more than 40% of their excess weight (10% to 15% of total weight) after a gastric bypass.[192,310] The percentage of patients who fail to lose this amount of weight after a gastroplasty procedure is even greater.[295] The major cause of inadequate weight loss after gastric bypass is the frequent ingestion of high-calorie soft foods and liquids (e.g., ice cream, cookies, milk shakes, and sodas) and high-fat snacks and fried foods (e.g., potato chips and fried potatoes). In patients who have undergone either a stapled gastroplasty or gastric bypass, increased food intake may be related to staple line disruption, particularly if the patient is able to eat much larger quantities of food at a time.

Perioperative Mortality

Perioperative mortality rate after bariatric surgery is less than 0.5% when the procedure is performed by experienced surgeons in experienced centers.[192,291] Approximately, three fourths of the deaths are due to anastamotic leaks and peritonitis and one fourth are due to pulmonary embolism.

Treatment Guidelines

Recently, a practical guide to the management of overweight and obesity was developed by the North American Association for the Study of Obesity in conjunction with the NIH.[269] An overview of these guidelines is shown in Table 35–8, which outlines a stepwise approach for weight loss. Certain kinds of behavior are common among patients who have achieved successful long-term weight loss without bariatric surgery.[311] Therefore, these four kinds of behavior should be a goal for all patients:

- Consume a diet that is low in calories (1300 to 1400 kcal/day) and fat (~25% kcal as fat)
- Engage in high levels of regular physical activity (expending ~2800 kcal/wk, which is equivalent to walking ~4 miles/day)
- Monitor food intake and physical activity
- Check weight regularly

Weight management is a key component in the treatment of overweight or obese patients with type 2 diabetes mellitus. Even a modest weight loss of 5% of initial body weight improves glycemic control and reduces the need for hypoglycemic medication. Moreover, modest weight loss also improves other diabetes-related risk factors for CHD. Unfortunately, successful weight management is more difficult to achieve in obese patients with type 2 diabetes than in those without diabetes.[199,200] In fact, treatment of diabetes itself is usually associated with an increase in body weight.[201] Therefore, the first principle of weight management in patients with diabetes is to use hypoglycemic therapy that is associated with the least amount of weight gain. Metformin is the preferred oral hypoglycemic agent because it produces minimal weight gain or slight weight loss.[312,313] In addition, providing long-acting insulin at night is associated with less weight gain than more frequent dosing.[314,315]

REFERENCES

1. Allison DB, Fontaine KR, Manson JE, et al. Annual deaths attributable to obesity in the United States. JAMA 1999;282:1530-1538.
2. Wolf AM, Colditz GA. Current estimates of the economic cost of obesity in the United States. Obesity Res 1998;6:97-106.
3. Gallagher D, Heymsfield SB, Heo M, et al. Health percentage body fat ranges: an approach for developing guidelines based on body mass index. Am J Clin Nutr 2000;72:694-701.
4. World Health Organization. Obesity: preventing and managing the global epidemic. Report of a WHO Consultation on Obesity. Geneva: World Health Organization, 1998.
5. National Institutes of Health, National Heart, Lung, and Blood Institute. Clinical Guidelines on the Identification, Evaluation, and Treatment of Overweight and Obesity in Adults—The Evidence Report. Obes Res 1998;6(suppl 2):51S-209S.
6. U.S. Department of Health and Human Services. Nutrition and overweight. In Healthy People 2010. Washington, D.C.: U.S. Government Printing Office, 2000.
7. U.S. Department of Agriculture and U.S. Department of Health and Human Services. Nutrition and your health: dietary guidelines for Americans. 5th ed. Washington, D.C.: U.S. Government Printing Office, 2000 (Home and Garden Bulletin no. 232).

8. Calle EE, Thun MJ, Petrelli JM, et al. CW. Body-mass index and mortality in a prospective cohort of U.S. adults. N Engl J Med 1999;341:1097-1105.
9. Flegal KM, Graubard BI, Williamson DF, Gail MH. Excess deaths associated with underweight, overweight, and obesity. JAMA 2005;293:1861-1867.
10. Kissebah AH, Videlingum N, Murray R, et al. Relation of body fat distribution to metabolic complications of obesity. J Clin Endocrinol Metab 1982;54:254-260.
11. Willett WC, Manson JE, Stampfer MJ, et al. Weight, weight change, and coronary heart disease in women: risk within the "normal" weight range. JAMA 1995;273:461-465.
12. Rimm EB, Stampfer MJ, Giovannucci E, et al. Body size and fat distribution as predictors of coronary heart disease among middle-aged and older U.S. men. Am J Epidemiol 1995;141:1117-1127.
13. Colditz GA, Willett WC, Rotnitzky A, Manson JE. Weight gain as a risk factor for clinical diabetes mellitus in women. Ann Intern Med 1995;122:481-486.
14. Chan JM, Rimm EB, Colditz GA, et al. Obesity, fat distribution, and weight gain as risk factors for clinical diabetes in men. Diabetes Care 1994;17:961-969.
15. Huang Z, Willett WC, Manson JE, et al. Body weight, weight change, and risk for hypertension in women. Ann Intern Med 1998;128:81-88.
16. Maclure KM, Hayes KC, Colditz GA, et al. Weight, diet, and risk of symptomatic gallstones in middle-aged women. N Engl J Med 1989;321:563-569.
17. Wei M, Gibbons L, Mitchell T, et al. The association between cardiorespiratory fitness and impaired fasting glucose and type 2 diabetes mellitus in men. Ann Intern Med 1999;130:89-96.
18. Lee CD, Blair SN, Jackson AS. Cardiorespiratory fitness, body composition, and all-cause and cardiovascular disease mortality in men. Am J Clin Nutr 1999;69:373-380.
19. McKeigue P, Shah B, Marmont MG. Relation of central obesity and insulin resistance with high diabetes prevalence and cardiovascular risk in South Asians. Lancet 1991;337: 382-386.
20. Badman MK, Flier JF. The gut and energy balance: visceral allies in the obesity wars. Science 2005;307:1909-1914.
21. McGowan BM, Bloom SR. Peptide YY and appetite control. Curr Opin Pharmacol 2004;4:583-588.
22. Deacon CF. Therapeutic strategies based on glucagon-like peptide 1. Diabetes 2004;53:2181-2189.
23. Cota D, Marsicano G, Tschöp M, et al. The endogenous cannabinoid system affects energy balance via central orexigenic drive and peripheral lipogenesis. J Clin Invest 2003;112:423-431.
24. Ravinet C, Arnone M, Delgorge C, et al. Anti-obesity effect of SR141716, a CB1 receptor antagonist, in diet-induced obese mice. Am J Physiol Regul Integr Comp Physiol 2003;284: R345-R353.
25. Pi-Sunyer FX, Aronne LJ, Heshmati HM, et al; RIO-North America Study Group. Effect of rimonabant, a cannabinoid-1 receptor blocker, on weight and cardiometabolic risk factors in overweight or obese patients: RIO-North America: a randomized controlled trial. JAMA 2006;295:761-775.
26. Despres JP, Golay A, Sjostrom L; Rimonabant in Obesity-Lipids Study Group. Effects of rimonabant on metabolic risk factors in overweight patients with dyslipidemia. N Engl J Med 2005;353: 2121-2134.
27. Vickers SP, Kennett GA. Cannabinoids and the regulation of ingestive behaviour. Curr Drug Targets 2005;6:215-223.
28. Rosenbaum M, Leibel RL, Hirsch J. Obesity. N Engl J Med 1997;337:396-408.
29. Bouchard C, Perusse L. Genetics of obesity. Annu Rev Nutr 1993;3:337-354.
30. Pratley RE. Gene-environment interactions in the pathogenesis of type 2 diabetes mellitus: lessons learned from the Pima Indians. Proc Nutr Soc 1998;57:175-181.
31. O'Dea K, White N, Sinclair A. An investigation of nutrition-related risk factors in an isolated Aboriginal community in Northern Australia: advantages of a traditionally-orientated life style. Med J Aust 1988;148:177-180.
32. O'Dea K. Marked improvement in carbohydrate and lipid metabolism in diabetic Australian Aborigines after temporary reversion to traditional lifestyle. Diabetes 1984;33:596-603.
33. Whitaker RC, Wright JA, Pepe MS, et al. Predicting obesity in young adulthood from childhood and parental obesity. N Engl J Med 1997;337:869-873.
34. Montague CT, Farooqi IS, Whitehead JP, et al. Congenital leptin deficiency is associated with severe early-onset obesity in humans. Nature 1997;387:903-908.
35. Strobel A, Issad T, Camoin L, et al. A leptin missense mutation associated with hypogonadism and morbid obesity. Nat Genet 1998;18:213-215.
36. Farooqi IS, Jebb SA, Langmack G, et al. Effects of recombinant leptin therapy in a child with congeital leptin deficiency. N Engl J Med 1999;341:879-884.
37. Consadine RV, Sinha MK, Heiman ML et al. Serum immunoreactive-leptin concentrations in normal-weight and obese humans. N Engl J Med 1996;334:292-295.
38. Clement K, Vaisse C, Lahlou N, et al. A mutation in the human leptin receptor gene causes obesity and pituitary dysfunction. Nature 1998;392:398-401.
39. Jackson RS, Creemers JW, Ohagi S, et al. Obesity and impaired prohormone processing associated with mutation of the human prohormone convertase 1 gene. Nat Genet 1997;16:218-220.
40. Jackson RS, Creemers JWM, Farooqi IS, et al. Small intestinal dysfunction accompanies the complex endocrinopathy of human proprotein convertase 1 deficiency. J Clin Invest 2003;112: 1550-1560.
41. Krude H, Biebermann H, Luck W, et al. Severe early-onset obesity, adrenal insufficiency and red hair pigmentation caused by POMC mutations in humans. Nat Genet 1998;19:155-157.
42. Farooqi IS, Yeo GS, Keogh JM, et al. Dominant and recessive inheritance of morbid obesity associated with melanocortin 4 receptor deficiency. J Clin Invest 2000;106:271-279.
43. Farooqi IS, Keogh JM, Giles SH, et al. Clinical spectrum of obesity and mutations in the melanocortin 4 receptor gene. New Engl J Med 2003;348:1085-1095.
44. Yeo GS, Connie Hung CC, Rochford J, et al. A de novo mutation affecting human TrkB associated with severe obesity and developmental delay. Nat Neurosci 2004;7:1187-1189.
45. Farooqi IS, O'Rahilly S. Monogentic obesity in humans. Annu Rev Med. 2005;56:443-458.
46. Goldstone AP. Prader-Willi syndrome: advances in genetics, pathophysiology and treatment. Trends Endocrinol Metab 2004;15: 12-20.
47. Holder JL Jr, Butte NF, Zinn AR. Profound obesity associated with a balanced translocation that disrupts the *SIM1* gene. Hum Mol Genet 2000;9:101-108.
48. Pérusse L, Rankinen T, Zuberi A, et al. The human obesity gene map: the 2004 update, Obes Res 2005;13:381-490.
49. Ravussin E, Burnand B, Schutz Y, Jequier E. Twenty-four-hour energy expenditure and resting metabolic rate in obese, moderately obese, and control subjects. Am J Clin Nutr 1982;35: 566-573.
50. Skov AR, Toubro S, Buemann B, Astrup A. Normal levels of energy expenditure in patients with reported "low metabolism." Clin Physiol 1997;17:279-285.
51. Lichtman SW, Pisarka K, Berman ER, et al. Discrepancy between self-reported and actual caloric intake and exercise in obese subjects. N Engl J Med 1992;327:1893-1898.
52. Segal KR, Presta E, Gutin B. Thermic effect of food during graded exercise in normal weight and obese men. Am J Clin Nutr 1984;40:95-100.
53. de Jonge L, Bray GA. The thermic effect of food and obesity: a critical review. Obesity Res 1997;5:622-631.
54. Roberts SB, Savage J, Coward WA, et al. Energy expenditure and intake from infants born to lean and overweight mothers. N Engl J Med 1988;318:461-466.
55. Stunkard AJ, Berkowitz RI, Stallings VA, Schoeller DA. Energy intake, not energy output, is a determinant of body size in infants. Am J Clin Nutr 1999;69:524-530.
56. Ravussin E, Stephen Lillioja MB, et al. Reduced rate of energy expenditure as a risk factor for body-weight gain. N Engl J Med 1988;318:467-472.
57. Seidell JC, Muller DC, Sorkin JD, Andres R. Fasting respiratory exchange ratio and resting metabolic rate as predictors of weight gain: the Baltimore Longitudinal Study on Aging. Int J Obes Relat Metab Disord 1992;16:667-674.

58. Bouchard C, Tremblay A, Despres JP, et al. The response to long-term overfeeding in identical twins. N Engl J Med 1990;322: 1477-1482.
59. Levine JA, Eberhardt NL, Jensen MD. Role of nonexercise activity thermogenesis in resistance to fat gain in humans. Science 1999;282:212-214.
60. Wadden TA, Foster GD, Letizia KA, Mullen JL. Long-term effects of dieting on resting metabolic rate in obese outpatients. JAMA 1990;264:707-711.
61. Amatruda JM, Statt MC, Welle SL. Total resting energy expenditure in obese women reduced to ideal body weight. J Clin Invest 1993;92:1236-1242.
62. Weinsier RL, Nagy TR, Hunter GR, et al. Do adaptive changes in metabolic rate favor weight regain in weight-reduced individuals? An examination of the set-point theory. Am J Clin Nutr 2000;72: 1088-1094.
63. Astrup A, Gotzsche PC, van de Werken K, et al. Meta-analysis of resting metabolic rate in formerly obese subjects. Am J Clin Nutr 1999;69:1117-122.
64. Leiter LA, Marliss EB. Survival during fasting may depend on fat as well as protein stores. JAMA 1982;248:2306-2307.
65. Stewart WK, Fleming LW. Features of a successful therapeutic fast of 382 days duration. Postgrad Med J 1973;49:203-209.
66. Angel A, Bray GA. Synthesis of fatty acids and cholesterol by the liver, adipose tissue and intestinal mucosa from obese and control subjects. Eur J Clin Invest 1979;9:355-362.
67. Ramsay TG. Fat cells. Endocrinol Metab Clin North Am 1996;25: 847-870.
68. Simsolo RB, Ong JM, Saffari B, et al. Effect of improved diabetes control on the expression of lipoprotein lipase in human adipose tissue. J Lipid Res 1992;33;89-95.
69. Heiling VJ, Miles JM, Jensen MD. How valid are isotopic measurements of fatty acid oxidation? Am J Physiol 1991;261:E572-E577.
70. Leweis GF. Fatty acid regulation of very low density lipoprotein production. Curr Opinion Lipidology 1997;8:146-153.
71. Jensen MD. Diet effects on fatty acid metabolism in lean and obese subjects. Am J Clin Nutr 1998;67:531S-534S.
72. Jensen MD, Haymond MW, Rizza RA, et al. Influence of body fat distribution on free fatty acid metabolism in obesity. J Clin Invest 1989;83:12168-12173.
73. Martin ML, Jensen MD. Effects of body fat distribution on regional lipolysis in obesity. J Clin Invest 1991;88:609-613.
74. Kahn BB, Flier JS. Obesity and insulin resistance. J Clin Invest 2000;106:473-481.
75. Wajchenberg BL. Subcutaneous and visceral adipose tissue: their relation to the metabolic syndrome. Endocr Rev 2000;21:697-738.
76. Friedman JM. Obesity in the new millenium. Nature 2000; 404:632-634.
77. Lee Y, Wang MY, Wang ZW, et al. Liporegulation in diet-induced obesity. The antisteatotic role of hyperleptinemia. J Biol Chem 2001;276:5629-5635.
78. Considine RV, Sinha MK, Heiman ML, et al. Serum immunoreactive leptin concentrations in normal weight and obese humans. N Engl J Med 1996;334:292-295.
79. Kolaczynsky JW, Ohammesian JP, Considine RV, et al. Response of leptin to short-term and prolonged overfeeding in humans. J Clin Endocrinol Metab 1996;81:4162-4165.
80. Flier JS. Clinical review 94: What's in a name? In search of leptin's physiologic role. J Clin Endocrinol Metab 1998;83:1407-1413.
81. Steppan CM, Bailey ST, Bhat S, et al. The hormone resistin links obesity to diabetes. Nature 2001;409:307-312.
82. Weyer C, Funahashi T, Tanaka S, et al. Hypoadiponectinemia in obesity and type 2 diabetes: close association with insulin resistance and hyperinsulinemia. J Clin Endocrinol Metab 2001;86: 1930-1935.
83. Yang WS, Lee WJ, Funahashi T, et al. Weight reduction increases plasma levels of an adipose-derived anti-inflammatory protein, adiponectin. J Clin Endocrinol Metab 2001;86:3815-3819.
84. Yu JG, Javorschi S, Hevener AL, et al. The effect of thiazolidinediones on plasma adiponectin levels in normal, obese, and type 2 diabetic subjects. Diabetes 2002;51:2968-2974.
85. Berg AH, Combs TP, Scherer PE. ACRP30/adiponectin: an adipokine regulating glucose and lipid metabolism. Trends Endocrinol Metab 2002;13:84-89.
86. Fukuhara A, Matsuda M, Segawa K, et al. Visfatin: a protein secreted by visceral fat that mimics the effects of insulin. Science 2005;307:426-430.
87. Peraldi P, Spiegelman B. TNF-α and insulin resistance: summary and future prospects. Mol Cell Biochem 1998;182:169-171.
88. Mohamed-Ali V, Pinkney JH, Coppack SW. Adipose tissue as an endocrine and paracrine organ. Int J Obes Relat Metab Disord 1998;22:1145-1158.
89. Bastard JP, Jardel C, Bruckert E, et al. Elevated levels of interleukin 6 are reduced in serum and subcutaneous adipose tissue of obese women after weight loss. J Clin Endocrinol Metab 2000;85: 3338-3342.
90. Bastard JP, Maachi M, Van Nhieu JT, et al. Adipose tissue IL-6 content correlates with resistance to insulin activation of glucose uptake both in vivo and in vitro. J Clin Endocrinol Metab 2002;87:2084-2089.
91. Senn JJ, Klover PJ, Nowak IA, Mooney RA. Interleukin-6 induces cellular insulin resistance in hepatocytes. Diabetes 2002;51: 3391-3399.
92. Tsigos C, Papanicolaou DA, Kyrou I, et al. Dose-dependent effects of recombinant human interleukin-6 on glucose regulation. J Clin Endocrinol Metab 1997;82:4167-4170.
93. Hirsch J, Knittle JL. Cellularity of obese and non-obese human adipose tissue. Fed Proc 1970;29:1516-1521.
94. Ntambi JM, Kim Y-C. Adipocyte differentiation and gene expression. J Nutr 2000;130:3122S-3126S.
95. Shimomura I, Hammer RE, Richardson JA, et al. Insulin resistance and diabetes mellitus in transgenic mice expressing nuclear SREBP-1c in adipose tissue: model for congenital generalized lipodystrophy. Genes Dev 1998;12:3182-3194.
96. Ballor DL, Poehlman ET. Exercise-training enhances fat-free mass preservation during diet-induced weight loss: a meta-analytical finding. Int J Obes Relat Metab Disord 1994;18:35-40.
97. Ross R, Rissanen J, Pedwell H, et al. Influence of diet and exercise on skeletal muscle and visceral adipose tissue in men. J Appl Physiol 1996;81: 2445-2455.
98. Smith SR, Zachwieja JJ. Visceral adipose tissue: a critical review of intervention strategies. Int J Obes Relat Metab Disord 1999; 23:329-335.
99. Knittle JL, Ginsberg-Fellner F. Effect of weight reduction on in vitro adipose tissue lipolysis and cellularity in obese adolescents and adults. Diabetes 1972;21:754-761.
100. Naslund I, Hallgren P, Sjostrom L. Fat cell weight and number before and after gastric surgery for morbid obesity in women. Int J Obes 1988;12:191-197.
101. Prins JB, O'Rahilly S. Regulation of adipose cell number in man. Clin Sci 1997;92:3-11.
102. Prins JB, Walker NL, Winterford CM, Cameron DP. Apoptosis of human adipocyte in vitro. Biochem Biophys Res Commun 1994;201:500-507.
103. Prins JB, Walker NL, Winterford CM, Cameron DP. Human adipocyte apoptosis occurs in malignancy. Biochem Biophys Res Commun 1994;205:625-630.
104. Ogden CL, Carroll MD, Curtin LR, et al. Prevalence of overweight and obesity in the United States, 1999-2004. JAMA 2006;295: 1549-1555.
105. Flegal KM, Carroll MD, Kuczmarski RJ, Johnson CL. Overweight and obesity in the United States: prevalence and trends, 1960-1994. Int J Obes Relat Metab Disord 1998;22:39-47.
106. Flegal KM, Troiano RP. Changes in the distribution of body mass index of adults and children in the U.S. population. Int J Obes Relat Metab Disord 2000;24:807-818.
107. Barlow SE, Dietz WH. Obesity evaluation and treatment: Expert Committee recommendations. The Maternal and Child Health Bureau, Health Resources and Services Administration and the Department of Health and Human Services. Pediatrics 1998;102: E29.
108. Flegal KM, Graubard BI, Williamson DF, Gail MH. Excess deaths associated with underweight, overweight, and obesity. JAMA 2005;293:1861-1867.
109. Landin K, Stigendal L, Eriksson E, et al. Abdominal obesity is associated with an impaired fibrinolytic activity and elevated plasminogen activator inhibitor-1. Metabolism 1990;39:1044-1048.
110. Lemieux I, Pascot A, Couillard C, et al. Hypertriglyceridemic waist: a marker of the atherogenic metabolic triad (hyperinsulinemia;

hyperapolipoprotein B; small, dense LDL) in men? Circulation 2000;102:179-184.
111. Ruderman N, Chisholm D, Pi-Sunyer X, Schneider S. The metabolically obese, normal-weight individual revisited. Diabetes 1998;47:699-713.
112. Reaven GM. Role of insulin resistance in human disease. Diabetes 1988;37:1595-1607.
113. Meigs JB, D'Agostino RB, Wilson WF, et al. Risk variable clustering in the insulin resistance syndrome. Diabetes 1997;46:1594-1600.
114. Frayn KN. Visceral fat and insulin resistance—causative or correlative? Brit J Nutr 2000;83(suppl 1):S71-S77.
115. Krssak M, Petersen KF, Dresner A, et al. Intramyocellular lipid concentrations are correlated with insulin sensitivity in humans: a ^{1}H NMR spectroscopy study. Diabeteologia 1999;42:113-116.
116. Dobbins RL, Szczepaniak LS, Bentley B, et al. Prolonged inhibition of muscle carnitine palmitoyltransferase I promotes intramyocellular lipid accumulation and insulin resistance in rats. Diabetes 2001;50:123-130.
117. Harris MI, Flegal KM, Cowie CC, et al. Prevalence of diabetes, impaired fasting glucose, and impaired glucose tolerance in U.S. adults. The Third National Health and Nutrition Examination Survey, 1988-1994. Diabetes Care 1998;21:518-524.
118. Colditz GA, Willett WC, Stampfer MJ, et al. Weight as a risk factor for clinical diabetes in women. Am J Epidemiol 1990;132:501-513.
119. Ohlson LO, Larsson B, Svardsudd K, et al. The influence of body fat distribution on the incidence of diabetes mellitus. Diabetes 1985;34:1055-1058.
120. Lundgren H, Bengtsson C, Blohme G, et al. Adiposity and adipose tissue distribution in relation to incidence of diabetes in women: results from a prospective population study in Gothenburg, Sweden. Int J Obes 1989;13:413-423.
121. Kaye SA, Folsom AR, Sprafka JM, et al. Increased incidence of diabetes mellitus in relation to abdominal adiposity in older women. J Clin Epidemiol 1991;44:329-334.
122. Reaven GM, Chen YDI, Jeppesen J, et al. Insulin resistance and hyperinsulinemia in individuals with small, dense, low density lipoprotein particles. J Clin Invest 1993;92:141-146.
123. Terry RB, Wood PD, Haskell WL, et al. Regional adiposity pattern in relation to lipids, lipoprotein cholesterol, and lipoprotein subfraction mass in men. J Clin Endocrinol Metab 1989;68:191-199.
124. Brown CD, Higgins M, Donato KA, et al. Body mass index and the prevalence of hypertension and dyslipidemia. Obes Res 2000;8:605-619.
125. Assmann G, Schulte H. Relation of high-density lipoprotein cholesterol and triglycerides to incidence of atherosclerotic coronary artery disease (the PROCAM Experience). Am J Cardiol 1992;70: 733-737.
126. Lamarche B, Lemieux I, Despres JP. The small, dense LDL phenotype and the risk of coronary heart disease: epidemiology, pathophysiology and therapeutic aspects. Diabetes Metab 1999;25: 199-211.
127. Hubert HB, Feinleib M, McNamara PM, Castelli WP. Obesity as an independent risk factor for cardiovascular disease: a 26-year follow-up of participants in the Framingham Heart Study. Circulation 1983;67:968-977.
128. Stamler R, Stamler J, Riedlinger WF, et al. Weight and blood pressure: findings in hypertension screening of 1 million Americans. JAMA 1978;240:1607-1609.
129. Kannel W, Brand N, Skinner J, et al. The relation of adiposity to blood pressure and development of hypertension. The Framingham study. Ann Intern Med 1967;67:48-59.
130. Stamler J, Wentworth D, Neaton JD. Is relationship between serum cholesterol and risk of premature death from coronary disease continuous or graded? Findings in 356,222 primary screenees of the Multiple Risk Factor Intervention Trial (MRFIT). JAMA 1986;256:2823-2828.
131. Rexrode KM, Carey VJ, Hennekens CH, et al. Abdominal adiposity and coronary heart disease in women. JAMA 1998;280: 1843-1848.
132. Manson JE, Willett WC, Stampfer MJ, et al. Body weight and mortality among women. N Engl J Med 1995;333:677-685.
133. Eckel RH, Krauss RM. American Heart Association call to action: obesity as a major risk factor for coronary heart disease. Circulation 1998;97:2099-2100.
134. Krause RM, Eckel RH, Howard B, et al. AHA Dietary guidelines revision 2000: a statement for healthcare professionals from the nutrition committee of the American Heart Association. Circulation 2000;102:2296-2311.
135. Walker SP, Rimm EB, Ascherio A, et al. Body size and fat distribution as predictors of stroke among U.S. men. Am J Epidemiol 1996;144:1143-1150.
136. Rexrode KM, Hennekens CH, Willett WC, et al. A prospective study of body mass index weight change, and risk of stroke in women. JAMA 1997;277:1539-1545.
137. Hansson PO, Eriksson H, Welin L, et al. Smoking and abdominal obesity: risk factors for venous thromboembolism among middle-aged men: "The study of men born in 1913." Arch Intern Med 1999;159:1886-1890.
138. Sugerman HJ, Windsor ACJ, Bessos MK, Wolfe L. Abdominal pressure, sagittal abdominal diameter and obesity co-morbidity. J Int Med 1997;241:71-79.
139. Visser M, Bouter LM, McQuillan GM, et al. Elevated C-reactive protein levels in overweight and obese adults. JAMA 1999;282: 2131-2135.
140. Strohl KP, Strobel RJ, Parisi RA. Obesity and pulmonary function. In Bray GA, Bouchard C, James WPT, eds. Handbook of Obesity. New York, NY: Marcel Dekker, 1998:725-739.
141. Vgontzas AN, Tan TL, Bixler EO, et al. Sleep apnea and sleep disruption in obese patients. Arch Intern Med 1994;154:1705-1711.
142. Davies RJ, Stradling JR. The relationship between neck circumference, radiographic pharyngeal anatomy, and the obstructive sleep apnoea syndrome. Eur Respir J 1990;3:509-514.
143. Katz I, Stradling J, Slutsky AS, et al. Do patients with obstructive sleep apnea have thick necks? Am Rev Respir Dis 1990;141: 1228-1231.
144. Roubenoff R, Klag MJ, Mead LA, et al. Incidence and risk factors for gout in white men. JAMA 1991;266:3004-3007.
145. Cigolini M, Targher G, Tonoli M, et al. Hyperuricaemia: relationships to body fat distribution and other components of the insulin resistance syndrome in 38-year-old healthy men and women. Int J Obes Relat Metab Disord 1995;19:92-96.
146. Felson DT, Anderson JJ, Naimark A, et al. Obesity and knee osteoarthritis. The Framingham Study. Ann Intern Med 1988;109:18-24.
147. Cicuttini FM, Baker JR, Spector TD. The association of obesity with osteoarthritis of the hand and knee in women: a twin study. J Rheumatol 1996;23:1221-1226.
148. Calle EE, Rodriguez C, Walker-Thurmond K, Thun MJ. Overweight, obesity and mortality from cancer in a prospectively studied cohort of U.S. adults. N Engl J Med 2003;348:1625-1638.
149. Giovannucci E, Ascherio A, Rimm EB, et al. Physical activity, obesity, and risk for colon cancer and adenoma in men. Ann Intern Med 1995;122:327-334.
150. Potter JD, Slattery ML, Bostick RM, Gapstur SM. Colon cancer: a review of the epidemiology. Epidemiol Rev 1993;15:499-545.
151. Huang Z, Hankinson SE, Colditz GA, et al. Dual effects of weight and weight gain on breast cancer risk. JAMA 1997;278:1407-1411.
152. Willett WC, Browne ML, Bain C, et al. Relative weight and risk of breast cancer among premenopausal women. Am J Epidemiol 1985;122:731-740.
153. Grodstein F, Goldman MB, Cramer DW. Body mass index and ovulatory infertility. Epidemiology 1994;5:247-250.
154. Johnson SR, Kolberg BH, Varner MW, Railsback LD. Maternal obesity and pregnancy. Surg Gynecol Obstet 1987;164:431-437.
155. Garbaciak JA Jr, Richter M, Miller S, Barton JJ. Maternal weight and pregnancy complications. Am J Obstet Gynecol 1985;152: 238-245.
156. Prentice A, Goldberg G. Maternal obesity increases congenital malformations. Nutr Rev 1996;54:146-152.
157. Dwyer PL, Lee ETC, Hay DM. Obesity and urinary incontinence in women. Br J Obstet Gynecol 1988;95:91-96.
158. Bump RC, Sugerman HJ, Fantl JA, McClish DK. Obesity and lower urinary tract function in women: effect of surgically induced weight loss. Am J Obstet Gynecol 1992;167:392-399.
159. Durcan FJ, Corbett JJ, Wall M. The incidence of pseudotumor cerebri: population studies in Iowa and Louisiana. Arch Neurol 1988;45:875-877.
160. Giuseffi V, Wall M, Siegel PZ, Rojas PB. Symptoms and disease associations in idiopathic intracranial hypertension (pseudotumor cerebri): a case-control study. Neurology 1991;41:239-244.

161. Sugerman HJ, Felton WL, Sismanis A, et al. Effects of surgically induced weight loss on pseudotumor cerebri in morbid obesity. Neurology 1995;45:1655-1659.
162. Sugerman HJ, Felton WL III, Sismanis A, et al. Gastric surgery for pseudotumor cerebri associated with severe obesity. Ann Surg 1999;229:634-642.
163. Glynn RJ, Christen WG, Manson JE, et al. Body mass index: an independent predictor of cataract. Arch Ophthalmol 1995;113:1131-1137.
164. Romero Y, Cameron AJ, Locke GR III, et al. Familial aggregation of gastroesophageal reflux in patients with Barrett's esophagus and esophageal adenocarcinoma. Gastroenterology 1997;113:1449-1456.
165. Locke GR, Talley NJ, Fett SL, et al. Risk factors associated with symptoms of gastroesophageal reflux. Am J Med 1999;106:642-649.
166. Lagergren J, Bergeström R, Nyrén O. No relation between body mass and gastro-oesophageal reflux symptoms in a Swedish population based study. Gut 2000;47:26-29.
167. Fisher BL, Pennathur A, Mutnick JLM, Little AG. Obesity correlates with gastroesophageal reflux. Dig Dis Sci 1999;44:2290-2294.
168. Lundell L, Ruth M, Sandberg N, Bove-Nielsen M. Does massive obesity promote abnormal gastroesophageal reflux? Dig Dis Sci 1995;40:1632-16350.
169. Stampfer MJ, Maclure KM, Colditz GA, et al. Risk of symptomatic gallstones in women. Am J Clin Nutr 1992;55:652-658.
170. Hay DW, Carey MC. Pathophysiology and pathogenesis of cholesterol gallstone formation. Semin Liver Dis 1990;10:159-170.
171. Weinsier RL, Wilson LJ, Lee J. Medically safe rate of weight loss for the treatment of obesity: a guideline based on risk of gallstone formation. Am J Med 1995;98:115-117.
172. Broomfield PH, Chopra R, Sheinbaum RC, et al. Effects of ursodeoxycholic acid and aspirin on the formation of lithogenic bile gallstones during loss of weight. N Engl J Med 1988;319:1567-1572.
173. Shiffman ML, Kaplan GD, Brinkman-Kaplan V, Vickers FF. Prophylaxis against gallstone formation with urosdeoxycholic acid in patients participating in a very-low-calorie diet program. Ann Intern Med 1995;122:899-905.
174. Wattchow DA, Hall JC, Whiting MJ, et al. Prevalence and treatment of gall stones after gastric bypass surgery for morbid obesity. Br Med J (Clin Res Ed) 1983;286:763.
175. Stone BG, Ansel HJ, Peterson FJ, Gebhard RL. Gallbladder emptying stimuli in obese and normal weight subjects. Hepatology 1990;12:795-798.
176. Festi D, Colecchia A, Orsini M, et al. Gallbladder motility and gallstone formation in obese patients following very low calorie diets. Use it (fat) to lose it (well). Int J Obes 1998;22:592-600.
177. Shoheiber O, Biskupiak JE, Nash DB. Estimation of the cost savings resulting from the use of ursodiol for the prevention of gallstones in obese patients undergoing rapid weight reduction. Int J Obes Relat Metab Disord 1997;21:1038-1045.
178. Funnell IC, Bornman PC, Weakley SP. Obesity: an important prognostic factor in acute pancreatitis. Br J Surg 1993;80:484-486.
179. Matteoni C, Younossi ZM, McCullough A. Nonalcoholic fatty liver disease: a spectrum of clinical pathological severity. Gastroenterology 1999;116:1413-1419.
180. Wanless IR, Lentz JS. Fatty liver hepatitis (steatohepatitis) and obesity: an autopsy study with analysis of risk factors. Hepatology 1990;12:1106-1110.
181. Luyckx FH, Desaive C, Thiry A, et al. Liver abnormalities in severely obese subjects: effect of a drastic weight loss after gastroplasty. Int J Obes Relat Metab Disord 1998;22:222-226.
182. Bellentani S, Saccocio G, Masutti F, et al. Prevalence of and risk factors for hepatic steatosis in Northern Italy. Ann Intern Med 2000;132:112-117.
183. Marchesini G, Brizi M, Morselli-Labate M, et al. Association of nonalcoholic fatty liver disease with insulin resistance. Am J Med 1999;107:450-455.
184. Cigolini M, Targher G, Agostino G, et al. Liver steatosis and its relation to plasma haemostatic factors in apparently healthy men. Role of the metabolic syndrome. Thromb Haemost 1996;76:69-73.
185. Day CO, James OFW. Steatohepatits: a tale of two "its." Gastroenterology 1998;114:842-845.
186. Tilg H, Diehl AM. Cytokines in alcoholic and nonalcoholic steatohepatitis. N Engl J Med 2000;343:1467-1476.
187. Palmer M, Schaffner F. Effect of weight reduction on hepatic abnormalities in overweight patients. Gastroenterology 1990;99:1408-1413.
188. Andersen T, Gluud C, Franzmann MB, Christoffersen P. Hepatic effects of dietary weight loss in morbidly obese subjects. J Hepatology 1991;12:224-226.
189. Sjostrom CD, Lissner L, Wedel H, Sjostrom L. Reduction in incidence of diabetes, hypertension and lipid disturbances after intentional weight loss induced by bariatric surgery: the SOS Intervention Study. Obes Res 1999;7:477-484.
190. Moore LL, Visioni AJ, Wilson PW, et al. Can sustained weight loss in overweight individuals reduce the risk of diabetes mellitus? Epidemiology 2000;11:269-273.
191. Wing RR, Koeske R, Epstein LH, et al. Long-term effects of modest weight loss in type II diabetic patients. Arch Intern Med 1987;147:1749-1753.
192. Pories WJ, Swanson MS, MacDonald KG, et al. Who would have thought it? An operation proves to be the most effective therapy for adult-onset diabetes mellitus. Ann Surg 1995;222:339-350.
193. Karason K, Wikstrand J, Sjostrom L, Wendelhag I. Weight loss and progression of early atherosclerosis in the carotid artery: a four-year controlled study of obese subjects. Int J Obes Relat Metab Disord 1999;23:948-956.
194. Hughes TA, Gwynne JT, Switzer BR, et al. Effects of caloric restriction and weight loss on glycemic control, insulin release and resistance, and atherosclerotic risk in obese subjects with type II diabetes mellitus. JAMA 1984;77:7-17.
195. Markovic TP, Jenkins AB, Campbell LV, et al. The determinants of glycemic responses to diet restriction and weight loss in obesity and NIDDM. Diabetes Care 1998;21:687-694.
196. Pan XR, Li GW, Hu YH, et al. Effects of diet and exercise in preventing NIDDM in people with impaired glucose tolerance. The Da Qing IGT and Diabetes Study. Diabetes Care 1997;20:537-544.
197. Sjostrom CD, Peltonen M, Wedel H, Sjostrom L. Differentiated long-term effects of intentional weight loss on diabetes and hypertension. Hypertension 2000;36:20-25.
198. Tuomilehto J, Lindstrom J, Eriksson JG, et al; Finnish Diabetes Prevention Study Group. Prevention of type 2 diabetes mellitus by changes in lifestyle among subjects with impaired glucose tolerance. N Engl J Med 2001;344:1343-1350.
199. Wing RR, Marcus MD, Epstein LH, Salata R. Type II diabetic subjects lose less weight than their overweight nondiabetic spouses. Diabetes Care 1987;10:563-566.
200. Khan MA, St Peter JV, Breen GA, et al. Diabetes disease stage predicts weight loss outcomes with long-term appetite suppressants. Obes Res 2000;8:43-48.
201. UK Prospective Diabetes Study (UKPDS) Group. Intensive blood-glucose control with sulphonylureas or insulin compared with conventional treatment and risk of complications in patients with type 2 diabetes (UKPDS 33). Lancet 1998;352:837-853.
202. Dattilo AM, Kris-Etherton PM. Effects of weight reduction on blood lipids and lipoproteins: a meta-analysis. Am J Clin Nutr 1992;56:320-328.
203. Wadden TA, Anderson DA, Foster GD. Two-year changes in lipids and lipoproteins associated with the maintenance of a 5% to 10% reduction in initial weight: some findings and some questions. Obes Res 1999;7:170-178.
204. Stefanick ML, Mackey S, Sheehan M, et al. Effects of diet and exercise in men and postmenopausal women with low levels of HDL cholesterol and high levels of LDL cholesterol. N Engl J Med 1998;339:12-20.
205. The Trials of Hypertension Prevention Collaborative Research Group. Effects of weight loss and sodium reduction intervention on blood pressure and hypertension incidence in overweight people with high-normal blood pressure. The Trials of Hypertension Prevention, phase II. Arch Intern Med 1997;157:657-667.
206. Stevens VJ, Obarzanek E, Cook NR, et al. Long-term weight loss and changes in blood pressure: results of the Trials of Hypertension Prevention, phase II. Ann Intern Med 2001;134:1-11.
207. Carson JL, Ruddy ME, Duff AE, et al. The effect of gastric bypass surgery on hypertension in morbidly obese patients. Arch Intern Med 1994;154:193-200.

208. Sjöström CD, Peltonen M, Wedel H, Sjöström L. Differentiated long-term effects of intentional weight loss on diabetes and hypertension. Hypertension 2000;36:20-25.
209. Huang Z, Willett WC, Manson JE, et al. Body weight, weight change, and risk for hypertension in women. Ann Intern Med 1998;128:81-88.
210. Wilson PW, Kannel WB, Silbershatz H, D'Agostino RB. Clustering of metabolic factors and coronary heart disease. Arch Intern Med 1999;159:1104-1109.
211. MacMahon SW, Wilcken D, MacDonald GJ. The effect of weight reduction on left ventricular mass. N Engl J Med 1986;314:334-339.
212. Karason K, Lindroos AK, Stenlof K, Sjostrom L. Relief of cardiorespiratory symptoms and increased physical activity after surgically induced weight loss: results from the Swedish Obese Subjects study. Arch Intern Med 2000;160:1797-1802.
213. Sugerman HJ, Fairman RP, Sood RK, et al. Long-term effects of gastric surgery for treating respiratory insufficiency of obesity. Am J Clin Nutr 1992;55:597S-601S.
214. Smith PL, Gold AR, Meyers DA, et al. Weight loss in mildly to moderately obese patients with obstructive sleep apnea. Ann Intern Med 1985;103:850-855.
215. Sugerman HJ, Baron PL, Fairman RP, et al. Hemodynamic dysfunction in obesity hypoventilation syndrome and the effects of treatment with surgically induced weight loss. Ann Surg 1988;207: 604-613.
216. Andres R, Muller DC, Sorkin JD. Long-term effects of change in body weight on all-cause mortality: a review. Ann Intern Med. 1993;119:737-743.
217. Williamson DF, Pamuk E, Thun M, et al. Prospective study of intentional weight loss and mortality in never-smoking overweight U.S. white women aged 40-64 years. Am J Epidemiol 1995;14: 1128-1141.
218. Williamson DF, Pamuk E, Thun M, et al. Prospective study of intentional weight loss and mortality in overweight weight white men aged 40-64 years. Am J Epidemiol 1999;149:491-503.
219. Williamson DF, Thompson TJ, Thun M, et al. Intentional weight loss and mortality among overweight individuals with diabetes. Diabetes Care 2000;23:1499-1504.
220. National Task Force on the Prevention and Treatment of Obesity. Weight cycling. JAMA 1994;272:1196-1202.
221. Lissner L, Odell PM, D'Agostino RB, et al. Variability of body weight and health outcomes in the Framingham population. N Eng J Med 1991;324:1839-1844.
222. Harris JA, Benedict FG. Standard basal metabolism constants for physiologists and clinicians. In A biometric study of basal metabolism in man. Publication 279, The Carnegie Institute of Washington. Philadelphia, JB Lippincott, 1919.
223. World Health Organization. WHO/FAO/UNO report: energy and protein requirements. WHO Technical Report Series, No. 724. Geneva: World Health Organization, 1985.
224. Wing RR, Marcus MD, Salata R, et al. Effects of a very-low-calorie diet on long-term glycemic control in obese type 2 diabetic subjects. Arch Intern Med 1991;151:1334-1340.
225. Torgerson JS, Lissner L, Lindross AK, et al. VLCD plus dietary and behavioral support versus support alone in the treatment of severe obesity: a randomised two-year clinical trial. Int J Obes Relat Metab Disord 1997;21:987-994.
226. Wadden TA, Foster GD, Letizia KA. One-year behavioral treatment of obesity: comparison of moderate and severe caloric restriction and the effects of weight maintenance therapy. J Consult Clin Psychol 1994;62:165-171.
227. Wadden TA, Stunkard AJ. A controlled trial of very-low-calorie diet, behavior therapy, and their combination in the treatment of obesity. J Consult Clin Psychol 1986;4:482-488.
228. Miura J, Arai K, Ohno M, Ikeda Y. The long term effectiveness of combined therapy by behavior modification and very low calorie diet: 2 year follow-up. Int J Obes 1989;13:73-77.
229. Ryttig KR, Flaten H, Rossner S. Long-term effects of a very low calorie diet (Nutrilett) in obesity treatment: a prospective, randomized, comparison between VLCD and a hypocaloric diet + behavior modification and their combination. Int J Obes Relat Metab Disord 1997;21:574-579.
230. Foster GD, Wadden TA, Peterson FJ, et al. A controlled comparison of three very-low-calorie diets: effects on weight, body composition, and symptoms. Am J Clin Nutr 1992;55:811-817.
231. Bray GA, Popkin BM. Dietary fat intake does affect obesity! Am J Clin Nutr 1998;68:1157-1173.
232. Yu-Poth S, Zhao G, Etherton T, et al. Effects of the National Cholesterol Education Program's Step I and Step II dietary intervention programs on cardiovascular disease risk factors: a meta-analysis. Am J Clin Nutr 1999;69:632-646.
233. Astrup A, Grunwald GK, Melanson EL, et al. The role of low-fat diets in body weight control: a meta-analysis of ad libitum dietary intervention studies. Int J Obes Relat Metab Disord 2000;24: 1545-1552.
234. Rolls BJ, Bell EA. Dietary approaches to the treatment of obesity. Med Clin North Am 2000;84:401-418.
235. Duncan KH, Bacon JA, Weinsier RL. The effects of high and low energy density diets on satiety, energy intake, and eating time of obese and nonobese subjects. Am J Clin Nutr 1983;37:763-767.
236. Stubbs RJ, Harbron CG, Murgatroyd PR, Prentice AM. Covert manipulation of dietary fat and energy density: effect on substrate flux and food intake in men eating ad libitum. Am J Clin Nutr 1995;62:316-329.
237. Bell EA, Castellanos VH, Pelkman CL, et al. Energy density of foods affects energy intake in normal-weight women. Am J Clin Nutr 1998;67:412-420.
238. Yang M-U, Van Itallie TB. Composition of weight lost during short-term weight reduction. J Clin Invest 1976;58:722-730.
239. Foster GD, Wyatt HR, Hill JO, et al. A randomized trial of a low-carbohydrate diet for obesity. N Engl J Med. 2003;348:2082-2090.
240. Samaha FF, Iqbal N, Seshadri P, et al. A low-carbohydrate as compared with a low-fat diet in severe obesity. N Engl J Med 2003;348:2074-2081.
241. Brehm BJ, Seeley RJ, Daniels SR, D'Alessio DA. A randomized trial comparing a very low carbohydrate diet and a calorie-restricted low fat diet on body weight and cardiovascular risk factors in healthy women. J Clin Endocrinol Metab 2003;88:1617-1623.
242. Yancy WS, Olsen MK, Guyton JR, et al. A low-carbohydrate, ketogenic diet versus a low-fat diet to treat obesity and hyperlipidemia. Ann Intern Med 2004;140:769-777.
243. Stern L, Iqbal N, Seshadri P, et al. The effects of low-carbohydrate versus conventional weight loss diets in severely obese adults: one-year follow up of a randomized trial. Ann Intern Med 2004;140:778-785.
244. Dansinger ML, Gleason JA, Griffith JL, et al. Comparison of the Atkins, Ornish, Weight Watchers, and Zone diets for weight loss and heart disease risk reduction: a randomized trial. JAMA 2005;293:43-53.
245. Boden G, Sargrad K, Homko C, et al. Effect of a low-carbohydrate diet on appetite, blood glucose levels, and insulin resistance in obese patients with type 2 diabetes. Ann Intern Med 2005;142: 403-411.
246. Ballor DL, Poehlman ET. A meta-analysis of the effects of exercise and/or dietary restriction on resting metabolic rate. Eur J Appl Physiol Occup Physiol 1995;71:535-542.
247. Garrow JS, Summerbell CD. Meta-analysis: effect of exercise, with or without dieting, on the body composition of overweight subjects. Eur J Clin Nutr 1995;49:1-10.
248. Warwick PM, Garrow JS. The effect of addition of exercise to a regime of dietary restriction on weight loss, nitrogen balance, resting metabolic rate and spontaneous physical activity in three obese women in a metabolic ward. Int J Obes Relat Metab Disord 1981;5:25-32.
249. Holloszy JO, Schultz J, Kusnierkiewicz J, et al. Effects of exercise on glucose tolerance and insulin resistance. Acta Med Scand 1986;711:55-65.
250. Helmrich SP, Ragland DR, Leung RW, Paffenbarger Jr RS. Physical activity and reduced occurrence of non–insulin-dependent diabetes mellitus. N Engl J Med 1991;325:147-152.
251. Wei M, Gibbons L, Mitchell T, et al. The association between cardiorespiratory fitness and impaired fasting glucose and type 2 diabetes mellitus in men. Ann Intern Med 1999;130:89-96.
252. Lee CD, Blair SN, Jackson AS. Cardiorespiratory fitness, body composition, and all-cause and cardiovascular disease mortality in men. Am J Clin Nutr 1999;69:373-380.
253. Klem ML, Wing RR, McGuire MT, et al. A descriptive study of individuals successful at long-term maintenance of substantial weight loss. Am J Clin Nutr 1997;66:239-246.

254. Kayman S, Bruvold W, Stern JS. Maintenance and relapse after weight loss in women: behavioral aspects. Am J Clin Nutr 1990;52:800-807.
255. Hill JO, Schlundt DG, Sbrocco T, et al. Evaluation of an alternating-calorie diet with and without exercise in the treatment of obesity. Am J Clin Nutr 1989;50:284-254.
256. Wadden TA, Berkowitz RI, Womble LG, et al. Randomized trial of lifestyle modification and pharmacotherapy for obesity. N Engl J Med 2005;353:2111-2120.
257. Schoeller DA, Shay K, Kushner RF. How much physical activity is needed to minimize weight gain in previously obese women? Am J Clin Nutr 1997;66:551-556.
258. Jakicic JM, Wing RR, Winters D. Effects of intermittent exercise and use of home exercise equipment on adherence, weight loss, and fitness in overweight women. JAMA 1999;282:1554-1560.
259. Wadden TA, Sarwer DB, Berkowitz RI. Behavioural treatment of the overweight patient. Bailliere's Clin Endocrin Metab 1999;13: 93-107.
260. Wadden TA, Foster GD. Behavioral treatment of obesity. Med Clin N Am 2000;84:441-461.
261. Perri MG, Nezu AM, Viegener BJ. Improving the Long-Term Management of Obesity: Theory Research and Clinical Guidelines. New York: John Wiley and Sons, 1992.
262. Sjostrom L, Rissanen A, Andersen T, et al. Randomised placebo-controlled trial of orlistat for weight loss and prevention of weight regain in obese patients. Lancet 1998;352:167-172.
263. Weintraub M, Sundaresan PR, Schuster B, et al. Long-term weight control study. V (weeks 190 to 210): follow-up of participants after cessation of medication. Clin Pharmacol Ther 1992;51:615-618.
264. Lean ME. Sibutramine—a review of clinical efficacy. Int J Obes Relat Metab Disord 1997;21(Suppl 1):S30-S36.
265. Khan MA, Herzog CA, St Peter JV, et al. The prevalence of cardiac valvular insufficiency assessed by transthoracic echocardiography in obese patients treated with appetite-suppressant drugs. N Engl J Med 1998;339:713-718.
266. Kernan WN, Viscoli CM, Brass LM, et al. Phenylpropanolamine and the risk of hemorrhagic stroke. N Engl J Med 2000;343: 1826-1832.
267. Bray GA, Greenway FL. Current and potential drugs for treatment of obesity. Endocrine Rev 1999;20:805-875.
268. Hansen DL, Toubro S, Stock MJ, et al. Thermogenic effects of sibutramine in humans. Am J Clin Nutr 1998;68:1180-1186.
269. National Institutes of Health; National Heart, Lung, and Blood Institute; North American Association for the Study of Obesity. Practical Guide to the Identification, Evaluation, and Treatment of Overweight and Obesity in Adults. NIH Publication Number 00-4084. Bethesda: National Institutes of Health, 2000.
270. Bray GA, Blackburn GL, Ferguson JM, et al. Sibutramine produces dose-related weight loss. Obes Res 1999;7:189-198.
271. Jones SP, Smith IG, Kelly F, Gray JA. Long-term weight loss with sibutramine [abstract]. Int J Obes Relat Metab Disord 1995;19:41.
272. McMahon FG, Fujioka K, Singh BN, et al. Efficacy and safety of sibutramine in obese white and African American patients with hypertension: a 1-year, double-blind, placebo-controlled, multicenter trial. Arch Intern Med 2000;160:2185-2191.
273. Apfelbaum M, Vague P, Ziegler O, et al. Long-term maintenance of weight loss after a very-low-calorie diet: a randomized blinded trial of the efficacy and tolerability of sibutramine. Am J Med 1999;106:179-184.
274. James WPT, Astrup A, Finer N, et al. Effect of sibutramine on weight maintenance after weight loss: a randomized trial. Lancet 2000;356:2119-2125.
275. Hadvary P, Lengsfield H, Wolfer H. Inhibition of pancreatic lipase in vitro by the covalent inhibitor tetrahydrolipstatin. Biochem J 1998;256:357-361.
276. Zhi J, Melia AT, Guerciolini R, et al. Retrospective population-based analysis of the dose-response (fecal fat excretion) relationship of orlistat in normal and obese volunteers. Clin Pharmacol Ther 1994;56:82-86.
277. Zhi J, Melia AT, Funk C, et al. Metabolic profiles of minimally absorbed orlistat in obese/overweight volunteers. J Clin Pharmacol 1996;36:1006-1011.
278. Sjöström L, Rissanen A, Andersen T, et al. Randomised placebo-controlled trial of orlistat for weight loss and prevention of weight regain in obese patients. Lancet 1998;352:167-172.
279. Davidson MH, Hauptman J, DiGirolamo M, et al. Weight control and risk factor reduction in obese subjects treated for 2 years with orlistat. JAMA 1999;281:235-242.
280. Rössner S, Sjöström L, Noack R, et al. Weight loss, weight maintenance, and improved cardiovascular risk factors after 2 years treatment with orlistat for obesity. Obes Res 2000;8:49-61.
281. Finer N, James WP, Kopelman PG, et al. One-year treatment of obesity: a randomized, double-blind, placebo-controlled, multicentre study of orlistat, a gastrointestinal lipase inhibitor. Int J Obes Relat Metab Disord 2000;24:306-313.
282. Hauptman J, Lucas C, Boldrin MN, et al. Orlistat in the long-term treatment of obesity in primary care settings. Arch Fam Med 2000;9:160-167.
283. Hollander PA, Elbein SC, Hirsch IB, et al. Role of orlistat in the treatment of obese patients with type 2 diabetes. Diabetes Care 1998;21:1288-1294.
284. Lindgarde F. The effect of orlistat on body weight and coronary heart disease risk profile in obese patients: the Swedish Multimorbidity Study. J Intern Med 2000;248:245-254.
285. Mittendorfer B, Ostlund R, Patterson BW, Klein S. Orlistat inhibits dietary cholesterol absorption. Obes Res 2001;9:599-604.
286. Colman E, Fossler M. Reduction in blood cyclosporin concentrations by orlistat. N Engl J Med 2000;342:1141-1142.
287. Consensus Development Conference Panel. NIH Conference: Gastrointestinal surgery for severe obesity. Ann Intern Med 1991; 115:956-961.
288. Brolin RE, Kenler HA, Gorman JH, Cody RP. Long-limb gastric bypass in the superobese: a prospective randomized study. Ann Surg 1992;215:387-395.
289. Mason EE. Vertical banded gastroplasty for obesity. Arch Surg 1982;117:701-706.
290. Eckhout GV, Willibanks OL, Moore JT. Vertical ring gastroplasty for morbid obesity: five year experience with 1,463 patients. Am J Surg 1986;152:713-716.
291. MacLean LD, Rhode BM, Sampalis J, Forse RA. Results of the surgical treatment of obesity. Am J Surg 1993;165:155-162.
292. Sugerman HJ, Starkey JV, Birkenhauer RA. A randomized prospective trial of gastric bypass versus vertical banded gastroplasty and their effects on sweets versus non-sweets eaters. Ann Surg 1987;205:613-624.
293. Hall JC, Watts JM, O'Brien PE, et al. Gastric surgery for morbid obesity. The Adelaide study. Ann Surg 1990;211:419-427.
294. Howard L, Malone M, Michalek A, et al. Gastric bypass and vertical banded gastroplasty: a prospective randomized comparison and 5-year follow-up. Obes Surg 1995;5:55-60.
295. Balsiger BM, Kelly KA, Poggio JL, et al. Long term prospective follow-up (>10 years) after vertical banded gastroplasty (VBG). Gastroenterology 2000;118;A1060.
296. Belachew M, Legrand M, Vincent V, et al. Laparoscopic adjustable gastric banding. World J Surg 1998;22:955-963.
297. DeMaria EJ, Sugerman HJ, Kellum JM, et al. High failure rate following laparoscopic adjustable silicone gastric banding for treatment of morbid obesity. Ann Surg 2001;233:809-818.
298. O'Brien PE, Dixon JB. Lap-band: outcomes and results. J Laparoendosc Adv Surg Tech A 2003;13:265-270.
299. Gustavsson S. Laparoscopic adjustable gastric banding—a caution. Surgery 2000;127:489-490.
300. Scopinaro N, Adami GF, Marinari GM, et al. Biliopancreatic diversion. World J Surg 1998;22:936-946.
301. Marceau P, Hould FS, Simard S, et al. Biliopancreatic diversion with duodenal switch. World J Surg 1998;22:947-954.
302. Clare MW. Reversals on 504 biliopancreatic surgeries over 12 years. Obes Surg 1993;3:169-173.
303. Payne JH, DeWind LT. Surgical treatment of obesity. Am J Surg 1969;118:141-147.
304. Scott HW Jr, Dean RH, Shull HJ, Gluck F. Results of jejunoileal bypass in two hundred patients with morbid obesity. Surg Gynecol Obstet 1977;145:661-673.
306. Hocking MP, Duerson MC, O'Leary JP, Woodward ER. Jejunoileal bypass for morbid obesity: late follow-up in 100 cases. N Engl J Med 1983;308:995-999.
306. Drenick EJ, Bassett LW, Stanley TM. Rheumatoid arthritis associated with jejunoileal bypass. Arthritis Rheum 1984;27:1300-1305.
307. Drenick EJ, Stanley TM, Wills CE. Renal damage after intestinal bypass. Int J Obes Relat Metab Disord 1981;5:501-508.

308. Drenick EJ, Fisler J, Johnson D. Hepatic steatosis after intestinal bypass—prevention and reversal with metronidazole, irrespective of protein-calorie malnutrition. Gastroenterolgy 1982;82:535-548.
309. Drenick EJ, Ament ME, Finegold SM, Passaro E Jr. Bypass enteropathy: an inflammatory process in the excluded segment with systemic complications. Am J Clin Nutr 1977;30:76-89.
310. Sugerman HJ, Kellum JM, Engle KM, et al. Gastric bypass for treating severe obesity. Am J Clin Nutr 1992:55:560S-566S.
311. Klem ML, Wing RR, McGuire MT, et al. A descriptive study of individuals successful at long-term maintenance of substantial weight loss. AmJ Clin Nutr 1997;66:239-246.
312. De Fronzo RA, Goodman AM. Efficacy of metformin in patients with non–insulin-dependent diabetes mellitus. N Engl J Med 1995;333:541-549.
313. Johansen K. Efficacy of metformin in the treatment of NIDDM: a meta-analysis. Diabetes Care 1999;22:33-37.
314. Yki-Jarvinen H, Kauppila M, Kujansuu E, et al. Comparison of insulin regimens in patients with non–insulin-dependent diabetes mellitus. N Engl J Med 1992;327:1426-1433.
315. Landstedt-Hallin L, Adamson U, Arner P, Bolinder J, Lins PE. Comparison of bedtime NPH or preprandial regular insulin combined with glibenclamide in secondary sulfonylurea failure. Diabetes Care 1995;18:1183-1186.

CHAPTER 36

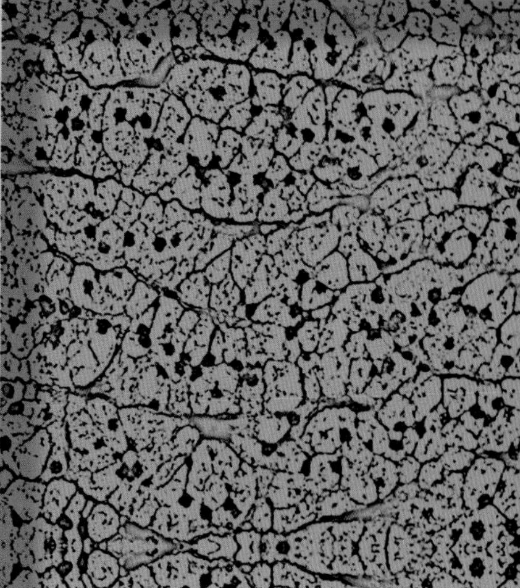

DISORDERS OF LIPID METABOLISM

Robert W. Mahley, Karl H. Weisgraber, and Thomas P. Bersot

Lipid Biochemistry and Cholesterol Metabolism

Lipids are hydrophobic molecules that are insoluble or minimally soluble in water. They are found in cell membranes, which maintain cellular integrity and allow the cytoplasm to be compartmentalized into specific organelles. Lipids function as a major form of stored nutrients (triglycerides), as precursors of adrenal and gonadal steroids and bile acids (cholesterol), and as extracellular and intracellular messengers (e.g., prostaglandins, phosphatidylinositol). Lipoproteins provide a vehicle for transporting the complex lipids in the blood as water-soluble complexes and deliver lipids to cells throughout the body.

Classes of Lipids. Structure and Function

Fatty Acids

Fatty acids vary in length and in the number and position of double bonds (Fig. 36–1). Saturated fatty acids lack double bonds (all carbon atoms have a full complement of hydrogen), and unsaturated fatty acids have one or more double bonds. Monounsaturated fatty acids have one double bond, and polyunsaturated fatty acids (PUFAs) have two or more. The major fatty acids and their sources in foods are listed in Table 36–1.

Cholesterol

Cholesterol is a four-ring hydrocarbon with an eight-carbon side chain (see Fig. 36–1). It plays a critical role as a major component of cell membranes and as a precursor of steroid hormones (adrenal and gonadal hormones). Cholesterol is also a precursor of bile acids, which are formed in the liver, stored in the gallbladder, and secreted in the intestine to participate in the absorption of fat. In the blood, about two thirds of the cholesterol is esterified (a fatty acid is esterified to the hydroxyl group at position 3).

Complex Lipids

Triglycerides (Triacylglycerol)

Triglycerides consist of three fatty acid molecules esterified to a glycerol molecule (see Fig. 36–1). Diglycerides (diacylglycerols) contain two fatty acids, and monoglycerides have only one fatty acid per glycerol molecule. Triglycerides store fatty acids and form large lipid droplets in adipose tissue. They are also transported as a component of certain lipoproteins. When triglycerides are hydrolyzed in adipocytes or on lipoprotein particles, free fatty acid (FFA) molecules are released to be used as a source of energy.

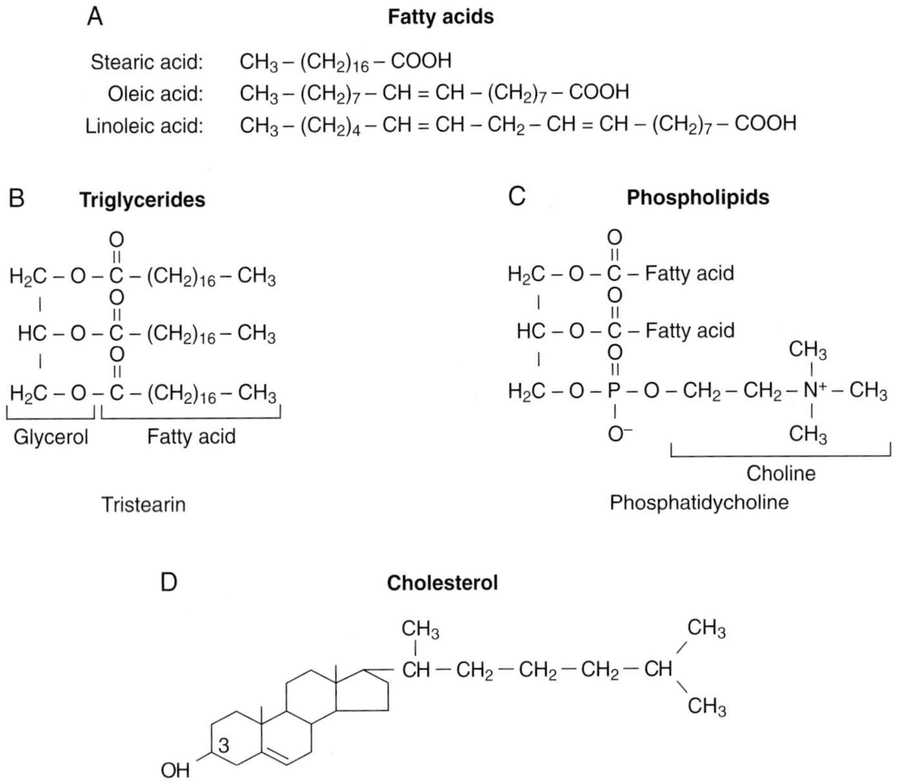

A **Fatty acids**

Stearic acid: $CH_3-(CH_2)_{16}-COOH$

Oleic acid: $CH_3-(CH_2)_7-CH=CH-(CH_2)_7-COOH$

Linoleic acid: $CH_3-(CH_2)_4-CH=CH-CH_2-CH=CH-(CH_2)_7-COOH$

B **Triglycerides**

$H_2C-O-C(=O)-(CH_2)_{16}-CH_3$

$HC-O-C(=O)-(CH_2)_{16}-CH_3$

$H_2C-O-C(=O)-(CH_2)_{16}-CH_3$

Glycerol Fatty acid

Tristearin

C **Phospholipids**

$H_2C-O-C(=O)-$ Fatty acid

$HC-O-C(=O)-$ Fatty acid

$H_2C-O-P(=O)(O^-)-O-CH_2-CH_2-N^+(CH_3)_2-CH_3$

Choline

Phosphatidycholine

D **Cholesterol**

CH3, CH – CH2 – CH2 – CH2 – CH, CH3, CH3

3

OH

Figure 36–1 ▪ Structures of the common lipids.

Phospholipids

Phospholipids have fatty acids esterified at two of the three hydroxyl groups of glycerol (see Fig. 36–1). The third hydroxyl group is esterified to phosphate (this complex lipid is referred to as phosphatidic acid). Typically, in mammalian tissue, the phosphatidic acid is esterified to the hydroxyl group of a hydrophilic molecule, such as choline, serine, or ethanolamine, to form phosphatidylcholine (commonly called lecithin), phosphatidylserine, or phosphatidylethanolamine, respectively.

TABLE 36–1 MAJOR FATTY ACIDS

Chemical Designation*	Common Name	Common Food
	SATURATED FATTY ACIDS (NO DOUBLE BONDS)	
C12:0	Lauric	Coconut oil
C14:0	Myristic	Coconut oil, butter fat
C16:0	Palmitic	Butter, cheese, meat
C18:0	Stearic	Beef, chocolate
	MONOUNSATURATED FATTY ACIDS (ONE DOUBLE BOND)	
C18:1 Δ^9	Oleic	Olive oil, canola oil
	POLYUNSATURATED FATTY ACIDS (TWO OR MORE DOUBLE BONDS)	
Omega-6 Fatty Acids		
C18:2ω6 Δ^9, Δ^{12}	Linoleic	Sunflower, corn, soybean, and safflower oils
C20:4ω6 Δ^5, Δ^8, Δ^{11}, Δ^{14}	Arachidonic	
Omega-3 Fatty Acids		
C18:3ω3	α-Linolenic	Canola, flaxseed, and soybean oils
C20:5ω3	Eicosapentaenoic (EPA)	Salmon, cod, mackerel, tuna
C22:6ω3	Docosahexaenoic (DHA)	Salmon, cod, mackerel, tuna

*The numeral after the C indicates the number of carbon atoms; the numeral after the colon indicates the number of double bonds. Carbon atom number 1 is the carboxylic acid carbon, and the ω carbon atom is the carbon atom most distant from the carboxyl group. The placement of the double bonds is shown by the Δ designations (e.g., Δ^9 indicates a double bond between carbons 9 and 10). In omega-6 fatty acids, the first double bond occurs after the sixth carbon atom from the ω carbon atom (indicated by ω6), and in omega-3 fatty acids it occurs after the third carbon atom from the ω carbon atom (ω3).

Lysolecithin is phosphatidylcholine from which one of the fatty acids has been removed. The combination of hydrophobic and hydrophilic regions in phospholipids enables them to be miscible at the water-lipid interface and makes them ideal components of membranes and of surface coats of lipoproteins. They are the most hydrophilic of the complex lipids.

Cholesterol Biosynthesis and the Low-Density Lipoprotein Receptor Pathway

Cholesterol is either absorbed from the diet or synthesized by cells in the body. All dietary cholesterol is of animal origin (from meats, dairy products, and eggs). Plants do not produce cholesterol; plant membranes contain sitosterol, which, except in a rare genetic disease, is not absorbed. Cholesterol is produced in many tissues (e.g., liver, skin, adrenals, gonads, brain, intestine). In most mammals, including humans, about 10% to 20% of cholesterol synthesis occurs in the liver.[1-4]

Cholesterol Biosynthesis

Cholesterol synthesis, illustrated schematically in Figure 36–2A, begins with acetate. Three molecules of acetate are condensed to form 3-hydroxy-3-methylglutaryl coenzyme A (HMG-CoA), which is then converted to mevalonic acid by the enzyme HMG-CoA reductase. Through a series of steps, mevalonic acid is converted to cholesterol. The key (rate-limiting) step in the regulation of cholesterol biosynthesis involves HMG-CoA reductase. Competitive inhibitors of this enzyme (the statins) reduce cholesterol biosynthesis and lower plasma cholesterol levels. Increased cholesterol content of cells feeds back on the HMG-CoA reductase and decreases its activity, thereby reducing cholesterol biosynthesis. Conversely, a deficiency of intracellular cholesterol increases reductase activity and increases cholesterol biosynthesis (see later discussion).[1-5]

Cholesterol cannot be eliminated by catabolism to carbon dioxide and water; it must be either excreted as free cholesterol in the bile or converted to bile acids and secreted into the intestine. About 50% of the cholesterol entering the intestine is reabsorbed and recirculates to the liver; the remainder is eliminated in the feces. Almost all of the secreted bile acids (97%) are reabsorbed from the intestine and transported back to the liver. This recirculation of cholesterol and bile acids from the intestine to the liver is called the *enterohepatic circulation* (see Fig. 36–2B). The reabsorbed cholesterol and bile acids regulate de novo cholesterol and bile acid synthesis in the liver. For example, if the amount of bile acids returning to the liver is decreased (as occurs in the intestine during treatment with bile acid–binding resins), bile acid synthesis is increased, enhancing the amount of cholesterol being converted to bile acids.

Cholesterol 7α-Hydroxylase

This enzyme of about 57 kd (503 amino acids), known as CYP7A (formerly $P450_{7\alpha}$), converts free cholesterol to 7α-hydroxycholesterol. This is the rate-limiting step in bile acid synthesis, and it is under feedback regulation by recirculated bile acids. The interruption of bile acid recirculation increases cholesterol 7α-hydroxylase activity. This enzyme and HMG-CoA reductase are closely coupled, and their activities usually change in parallel.[4,6,7] In this way, the intracellular cholesterol level for bile acid production remains rather constant.

Low-Density Lipoprotein Receptor

Cholesterol levels in the blood are controlled primarily through the low-density lipoprotein (LDL) receptor pathway.[4,5] This receptor is present on the surface of all cells throughout the body, including hepatocytes, and mediates the uptake of cholesterol-rich lipoproteins (e.g., LDL) from the blood. Specific proteins on the surface of certain lipoproteins (apolipoprotein [apo] B100 and apo-E) interact with the LDL receptor and facilitate lipoprotein internalization by cells. By this mechanism, cells that require cholesterol can obtain the preformed sterol. The LDL receptor also allows the liver (the principal site for LDL catabolism) to take up LDL and eliminate cholesterol from the body (discussed in "Lipoprotein Receptors Controlling Lipoprotein Metabolism").

The number of LDL receptors on the cell surface is tightly regulated.[4,5] If the cholesterol content of a cell is elevated, fewer receptors are synthesized (i.e., receptor expression is down-regulated). On the other hand, if a cell requires cholesterol, expression of LDL receptors is up-regulated and synthesis increases. This system keeps the intracellular cholesterol concentration relatively constant and prevents excessive and possibly toxic accumulation. Within the cell, cholesterol can be esterified by the enzyme acyl-CoA:cholesterol acyltransferase (ACAT).

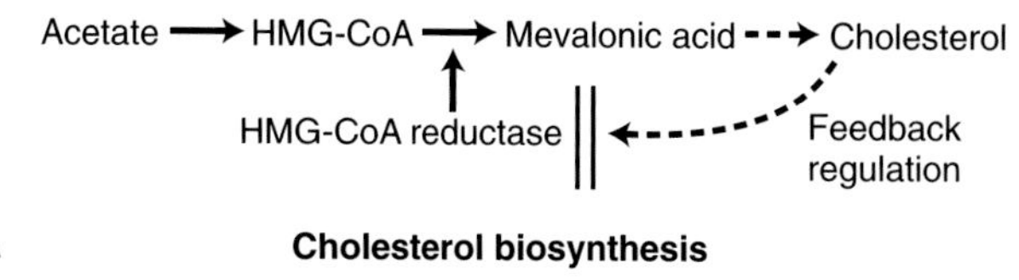

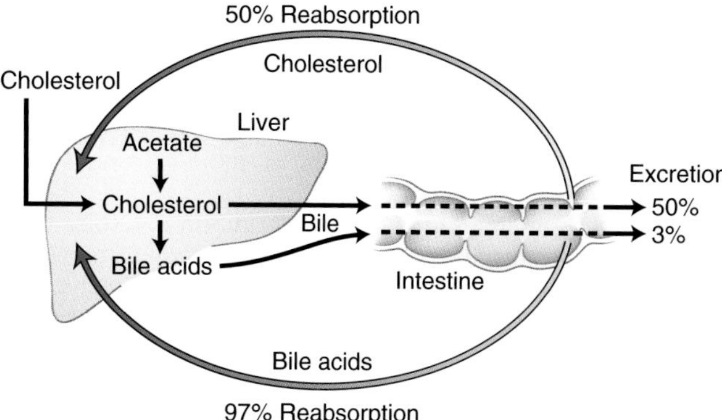

Figure 36–2 ▪ **A,** Cholesterol biosynthesis. 3-Hydroxy-3-methylglutaryl coenzyme A (HMG-CoA) reductase is a rate-limiting enzyme regulating cholesterol biosynthesis. The enzyme is down-regulated by excess cholesterol in the cell. **B,** Enterohepatic circulation of cholesterol and bile acids. About 50% of cholesterol and 97% of bile acids are reabsorbed from the intestine and recirculated to the liver. (**A** modified from Brown MS, Goldstein JL. A receptor-mediated pathway for cholesterol homeostasis. Science 1986;232:34-47.)

Acyl-Coenzyme A: Cholesterol Acyltransferase

ACAT is an enzyme of the endoplasmic reticulum (ER) (about 45 to 50 kd, 550 amino acids) that catalyzes the formation of cholesteryl esters from long-chain fatty acyl-CoA (e.g., oleoyl-CoA) and free cholesterol substrates.[8,9] When lipoproteins enter the cell by receptor-mediated endocytosis and are degraded within the lysosomes, the free cholesterol released can be transported to the ER, where it is esterified by ACAT. There are two ACAT enzymes. ACAT1 is present in macrophages, steroidogenic tissues, and sebaceous glands, and its action in macrophages has been implicated in foam cell formation and atherogenesis. ACAT2 is found in liver and intestine, where it plays a role in providing cholesteryl esters for assembly of apo-B–containing lipoproteins. In the intestine, ACAT2 promotes the absorption of dietary cholesterol. Agents that inhibit intestinal ACAT activity can provide a means to limit cholesterol absorption by the intestine.

Cholesteryl ester hydrolysis by cholesterol ester hydrolase generates free cholesterol, either for efflux from the cells or to serve as a biosynthetic substrate (e.g., for steroid hormones and cell membranes) within the cells. The pool of intracellular cholesterol and cholesteryl esters is dynamic.

Metabolism of Dietary Lipids

The digestion of dietary fats begins in the stomach and continues in the proximal small intestine.[10,11] Triglycerides are hydrolyzed to FFAs and small amounts of monoglycerides and diglycerides, cholesteryl esters are hydrolyzed to free cholesterol, and phospholipids are converted primarily to lysolecithin. Bile salt micelles disperse and partially solubilize water-insoluble lipids; this facilitates the intestinal transport and delivery of lipids to the unstirred water layer of intestinal epithelial cells, where they can be taken up by the cells. Bile acids also activate pancreatic lipase, which participates in the hydrolysis of triglycerides. Long-chain fatty acids are taken up primarily by the enterocytes of the duodenum and proximal jejunum, re-esterified into triglycerides, and used in the biosynthesis of intestinal lipoproteins (chylomicrons), which are delivered to the mesenteric lymph and enter the general circulation with the thoracic duct lymph. Medium-chain fatty acids (≤10 carbons) are absorbed into the portal blood without being esterified and are cleared directly from the blood by the liver. Bile acids are reabsorbed primarily from the ileum, enter the portal blood, and are taken up by the liver.

Triglyceride and Free Fatty Acid Metabolism

Storage and Use

Free fatty acids are released from triglycerides of chylomicrons and very-low-density lipoproteins (VLDLs) through the action of lipoprotein lipase (LPL). LPL is bound to the capillary endothelial cells adjacent to adipose, muscle, and breast tissue, where it liberates FFAs from lipoprotein triglyceride. The level of LPL in tissues differs under different physiologic circumstances so that FFAs are directed to tissues requiring them as substrates or energy sources.[12,13] During fasting, for example, LPL activity decreases in adipose tissue and increases in heart muscle. In the breast, LPL levels are low until parturition, when they increase 10-fold to promote milk formation.

In adipose tissue, high levels of glucose and insulin promote the conversion of FFAs to triglyceride for storage. Insulin stimulates LPL activity and fatty acid esterification through the formation of glycerol phosphate and decreases FFA release through the inhibition of hormone-sensitive lipase.[14] Insulin deficiency, as in diabetes mellitus, is associated with decreased LPL activity. Insulin and glucose also stimulate the biosynthesis of FFAs in the liver and, to a lesser degree, in adipocytes when dietary fat is replaced by carbohydrate. As a result, hepatic FFAs are converted to triglyceride and packaged into VLDL particles (discussed in the section on plasma lipoproteins).

Acyl-Coenzyme A:Diacylglycerol Acyltransferase

Triglyceride (triacylglycerol) synthesis is catalyzed by the enzyme acyl-CoA:diacylglycerol acyltransferase (DGAT)][15,16,17] (Fig. 36–3). A DGAT gene that is expressed in all tissues has been identified. Interestingly, the inactivation of this gene in mice has revealed that multiple pathways exist for triglyceride synthesis, including DGAT1 and DGAT2. The gene inactivation studies also reveal that DGAT plays an important role in energy metabolism.

Fatty Acid Release from Adipose Tissue

The net release of FFAs and glycerol from adipose triglyceride stores occurs during various physiologic conditions, including stress, exercise, fasting, and uncontrolled diabetes mellitus. This release occurs in response to hormones (Table 36–2), most of which act through cyclic adenosine monophosphate (cAMP) to activate a hormone receptor–coupled protein kinase, which in turn activates a hormone-sensitive lipase.[14] Unlike many hormones, insulin inhibits rather than stimulates hormone-sensitive lipase in adipose tissue. Growth hormone liberates FFAs by a different mechanism, which requires enhanced synthesis of hormone-sensitive lipase.

After triglyceride hydrolysis in adipose tissue, the released FFAs bind to albumin and circulate in the plasma. Released glycerol is taken up by the liver and kidney for triglyceride synthesis or for gluconeogenesis. The fate of the FFA–albumin complexes is determined in part by blood flow. With intense exercise

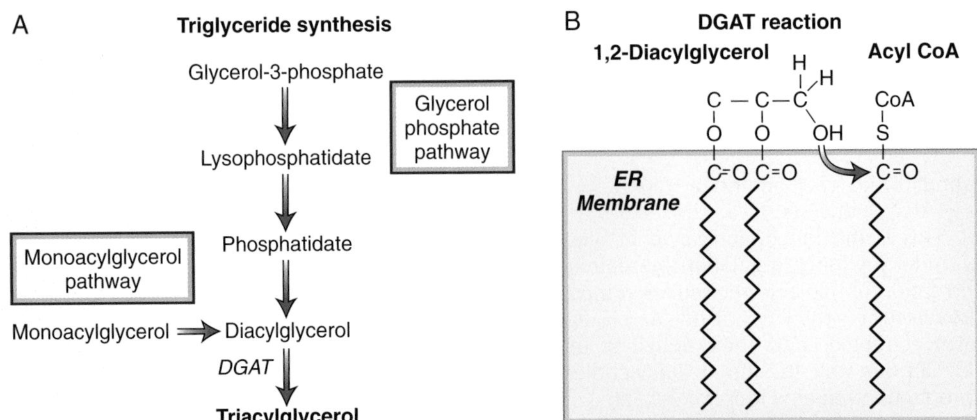

Figure 36–3 ▪ Triglyceride synthesis and the diacylglycerol acyltransferase (DGAT) reaction. **A,** Two major pathways of triglyceride synthesis have been described. the glycerol-phosphate pathway and the monoacylglycerol pathway, which is prominent in the small intestine. **B,** DGAT catalyzes a reaction in which 1,2-diacylglycerol and fatty acyl CoA react to form triacylglycerol at the surface of the endoplasmic reticulum. (From Farese RV Jr, Cases S, Smith SJ. Triglyceride synthesis. insights from the cloning of diacylglycerol acyltransferase. Curr Opin Lipidol 2000;11:229-234.)

TABLE 36–2 HORMONES THAT AFFECT LIPOLYSIS IN VITRO

RAPID STIMULATION
Catecholamines (β-1 agonists)
Corticotropin
Glucagon
Placental lactogen
Prolactin
Secretin
Thyrotropin
Vasoactive intestinal peptide
Vasopressin
SLOW STIMULATION
Glucocorticoids
Growth hormone
SUPPRESSION
Gastric inhibitory polypeptide
Insulin
Oxytocin
Prostaglandin
Somatomedins

Modified from Bierman EL, Glomset JA. Disorders of lipid metabolism. In Wilson JD, Foster DW (eds). Williams Textbook of Endocrinology, 8th ed. Philadelphia: WB Saunders, 1992:1367-1395.

and diminished blood flow to the splanchnic bed, FFAs are targeted to muscle. Depending on the metabolic state, FFAs taken up by the liver are reused for triglyceride or phospholipid synthesis (exported on VLDL), oxidized to carbon dioxide, or converted to ketone bodies.

Fatty Acid Oxidation and Ketogenesis

Oxidation and ketogenesis of fatty acids (except very-long-chain fatty acids) take place in the mitochondria; very-long-chain fatty acids (C-24 and C-26) are oxidized in peroxisomes. Because FFAs and their CoA derivatives can penetrate only the outer leaflet of the mitochondrial membrane, they are converted to carnitine derivatives within the mitochondrial membrane to allow transport across the inner membrane. Once inside the mitochondria, they are reconverted to CoA derivatives and undergo β-oxidation, which produces acetyl-CoA and the reduced forms of nicotinamide-adenine dinucleotide (NADH) and flavin-adenine dinucleotide (FADH).

With a normal flux of FFAs, the NADH and FADH enter the electron transport system, resulting in the formation of adenosine triphosphate (ATP) and water. The condensation of acetyl-CoA with oxaloacetic acid yields citrate, which can enter the citric acid cycle, where it is oxidized to carbon dioxide or is transported out of the mitochondria and converted again to FFAs. If FFA flux to the liver is massively increased, as in insulin-deficient states such as prolonged fasting or uncontrolled diabetes mellitus, the production of VLDL triglyceride from FFAs is limited. As a result, NADH, FADH, and acetyl-CoA accumulate in the mitochondria and give rise to the products of ketogenesis. acetoacetate, β-hydroxybutyrate, and acetone.

Ketogenesis occurs in several steps. Initially, acetyl-CoA condenses in two steps to form acetoacetyl-CoA and then HMG-CoA. The latter is cleaved to acetoacetate and acetyl-CoA, which leads to the liberation of CoA and its use in β-oxidation of FFAs. Acetoacetate can be reduced by NADH to form β-hydroxybutyrate; the NAD produced can be used for continued β-oxidation of fatty acids. Alternatively, the acetoacetate can decompose to form acetone. The ketones are released into the plasma and, if they accumulate, cause ketoacidosis.

Fatty Acid Biosynthesis

Under normal conditions, the diet supplies sufficient fatty acids through the ingestion of fat. However, increases in the ratio of carbohydrate to fat in the diet stimulate fatty acid synthesis by the liver and adipose tissue. Fatty acids are synthesized from two carbon units of acetyl-CoA. Because acetyl-CoA is produced in the mitochondria, it must first be converted to citrate by condensation with oxaloacetate and then transported into the cytosol, where it is reconverted to acetyl-CoA and oxaloacetate. Eight acetyl-CoA units are condensed to form palmitic acid (16 carbon atoms) in a series of reactions involving the enzymes fatty acid synthase and acetyl-CoA carboxylase. Longer fatty acids, such as stearic acid (18 carbon atoms) or oleic acid (18 carbon atoms with one double bond), are synthesized from palmitic acid by chain extension. In this way, fatty acid synthesis can meet most of the body's requirements.

Certain essential PUFAs cannot be synthesized in humans and must be supplied in the diet. These include linoleic acid (18 carbon atoms with two double bonds) and linolenic acid (18 carbon atoms with three double bonds). Essential fatty acids are required for a number of special functions, including prostaglandin synthesis.[18]

Plasma Lipoproteins. Apolipoproteins, Receptors, and Enzymes

General Structure and Major Classes of Lipoproteins

Lipoproteins function as vehicles to transport lipids in the blood in the form of soluble complexes of lipids and proteins. The lipids include triglycerides, cholesteryl esters, free cholesterol, and phospholipids. Twelve different protein moieties, called apolipoproteins, are associated with various lipoproteins and are given letter designations (Table 36–3).[19,20] Lipoproteins also transport fat-soluble vitamins (A, D, and E), drugs (e.g., probucol, cyclosporine), some viruses, and certain antioxidant enzymes (e.g., paraoxonase[21] and platelet-derived activating factor hydrolase[22]).

Lipoproteins are spherical particles with a core of mostly hydrophobic lipids (triglycerides and cholesteryl esters) and a surface layer of more hydrophilic constituents, namely protein, free cholesterol, and phospholipids (Figure 36–4). Six major classes of lipoproteins play different roles in lipid transport (Table 36–4), and the specific apolipoproteins on the surface determine the fate of the lipoproteins. To understand lipoprotein metabolism and the diseases associated with lipid abnormalities, it is necessary to consider the roles of the individual apolipoproteins in regulating lipid metabolism. Some of their physical properties are summarized in Table 36–4 and Figure 36–5.[19,20]

Major Apolipoproteins that Regulate Lipoprotein Metabolism

Apolipoprotein B

In human plasma, apo-B occurs in two forms, apo-B100 and apo-B48, which are derived from a single gene on the short arm of chromosome 2.[23] The human apo-B gene comprises 29 exons

TABLE 36–3 CHARACTERISTICS AND MAJOR FUNCTIONS OF HUMAN APOLIPOPROTEINS

Apolipoprotein	Average Plasma Concentration (mg/dL)	Chromosome	Molecular Weight (×1000)	Mature Protein (amino acids)	Major Sites of Synthesis	Major Functions
AI	130	11	~29	243	Liver, intestine	Structural protein/HDL Cofactor for LCAT Crucial role in reverse cholesterol transport. Ligand for ABCA1 and SR-BI
AII	40	1	~17 (dimer)	77	Liver	Inhibits apo-E binding to receptors (through the E-AII complex)
AIV	40	11	~45	376	Intestine	Might facilitate cholesterol efflux from cells Activator of LCAT Facilitates lipid secretion from the intestine
AV	<1	11	39	343	Liver	Activator of LPL-mediated lipolysis Maight inhibit hepatic VLDL synthesis
B100	85	2	~513	4536	Liver	Structural protein/VLDL and LDL Ligand for LDL receptor
B48	Variable		~241	2152	Intestine	Structural protein/chylomicrons
CI	6	19	~6.6	57	Liver	Modulates remnant binding to receptors. Activates LCAT
CII	3	19	8.9	79	Liver	Cofactor for LPL
CIII	12	11	8.8	79	Liver	Modulates remnant binding to receptors. Inhibitor of LPL
E	5	19	~34	299	Liver, brain, skin, testes, spleen	Ligand for LDL and remnant receptors. Local lipid redistribution Reverse cholesterol transport (HDL with apo-E)
apo(a)	Variable	6	~400-800	4000-6000	Liver	Modulates thrombosis/fibrinolysis
D	10	3	~20	169	Liver, intestine	Activator of LCAT (?)

ABCA1, ATP binding cassette transporter A1; apo, apolipoprotein; HDL, high-density lipoproteins; LCAT, lecithin:cholesterol acyltransferase; LDL, low-density lipoproteins; LPL, lipoprotein lipase; SR-BI, scavenger receptor BI; VLDL, very-low-density lipoproteins.

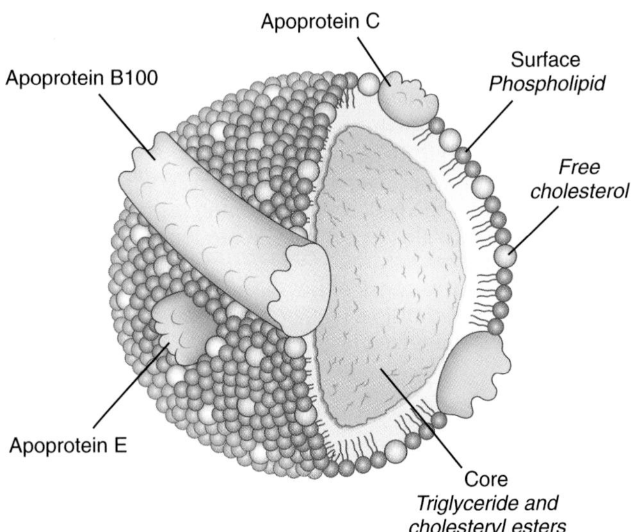

Figure 36–4 ▪ General structure of lipoproteins. Shown is a schematic representation of a very-low-density lipoprotein (VLDL) particle.

and 28 introns and is approximately 45 kb long. A unique RNA-editing mechanism (APOBEC1) is responsible for the synthesis of apo-B100 and apo-B48 from the apo-B mRNA (Fig. 36–6).[23,24,25] An editing protein (or proteins) interacts with the apo-B mRNA in the human intestine to change a single nucleotide, resulting in the synthesis of a truncated form of apo-B (apo-B48). In humans, this modification of the apo-B mRNA occurs only in the intestine and not in the liver; therefore, the liver produces the full-length apo-B100. Apo-B100 (but not apo-B48) is also expressed in the yolk sac of mammals.

Apo-B mRNA editing changes cytosine-6666 in the apo-B100 mRNA to a uracil. As a result, the codon CAA, which encodes a glutamine at amino acid residue 2153 in apo-B100, is changed to a UAA, a stop codon that terminates translation of the protein chain (see Fig. 36–6). Therefore, apo-B48 possesses only 2152 amino acids (apo-B100 has 4536). Apo-B100, a 513-kd protein, is synthesized in the liver; it serves as a structural protein of VLDL and of intermediate-density lipoproteins (IDLs) and is the exclusive protein constituent of LDL. Each VLDL, IDL, and LDL particle contains one molecule of apo-B100. The primary structure of apo-B contains many hydrophobic and amphipathic sequences, forming α-helices and β-strands, which occur

TABLE 36–4 MAJOR CLASSES OF PLASMA LIPOPROTEINS

Type	Density (g/mL)	Electrophoretic Mobility	Site of Origin	Major Lipids	Major Apolipoproteins
Chylomicrons	<0.95	Origin	Intestine	85% Triglyceride	B48, AI, AIV (E, CI, CII, CIII—by transfer from HDL)
Chylomicron remnants	<1.006	Origin	Intestine	60% Triglyceride, 20% cholesterol	B48, E
VLDL*	<1.006	Pre-β	Liver	55% Triglyceride, 20% cholesterol	B100, E, CI, CII, CIII
IDL*	1.006-1.019	β	Derived from VLDL	35% Cholesterol, 25% triglyceride	B100, E
LDL	1.019-1.063	β	Derived from IDL	60% Cholesterol, 5% triglyceride	B100
HDL	1.063-1.21	α	Liver, intestine, plasma	25% Phospholipid, 20% cholesterol, 5% triglyceride (50% protein)	AI, AII, CI, CII, CIII, E
HDL_2	1.063-1.125	α			
HDL_3	1.125-1.21	α			
Lp(a)	1.05-1.09	α	Liver	60% Cholesterol, 5% triglyceride	B100, apo(a)

*Small, partially lipolyzed VLDL and IDL are often called VLDL remnants.
IDL, intermediate-density lipoproteins; LDL, low-density lipoproteins; Lp(a), lipoprotein(a); VLDL, very-low-density lipoproteins.

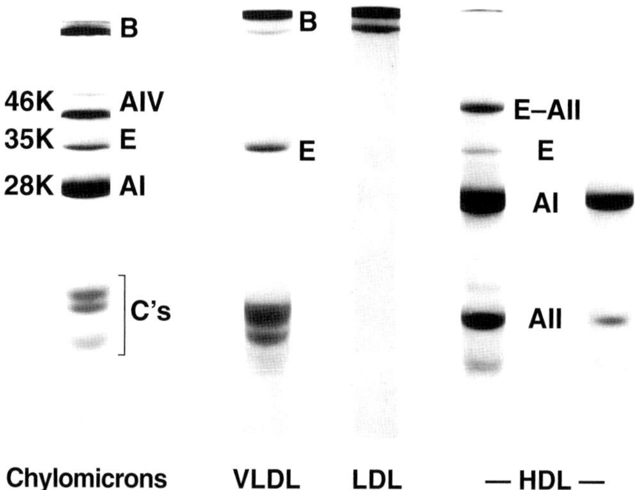

Figure 36–5 ▪ Polyacrylamide gel showing the various apolipoproteins characteristic of each type of plasma lipoprotein particle. HDL, high-density lipoprotein; LDL, low-density lipoprotein; VLDL, very-low-density lipoprotein. (Modified from Mahley RW, Innerarity TL. Lipoprotein receptors and cholesterol homeostasis. Biochim Biophys Acta 1983;737:197-222. With permission from Elsevier Science-NL, Sara Burgerhartstraat 25, 1055 KV Amsterdam, the Netherlands.)

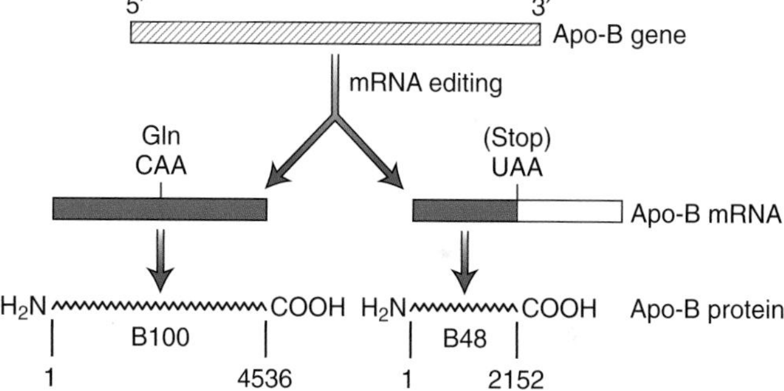

Figure 36–6 ▪ Synthesis of apolipoprotein B100 (apo-B100) and apo-B48 by a unique mRNA-editing mechanism. In the human intestine, a specific cytosine (C) is changed to a uracil (U) in the apo-B mRNA. This change results in a stop codon and the formation of apo-B48, which contains only the first 2152 amino acids of the full-length apo-B100 (4536 amino acids).

throughout the molecule and appear to function as lipid-binding domains. In addition to its structural role, apo-B100 is a ligand for the LDL receptor.

Apo-B48, a 241-kd protein, is a structural constituent of chylomicrons.[23] Each chylomicron appears to possess one or possibly two molecules of apo-B48. Because it lacks the carboxyl-terminal domain of apo-B100, apo-B48 cannot bind to the LDL receptor. The carboxyl-terminal domain of apo-B100 in the region of amino acids 3000 to 3700 is critical for the binding of apo-B100 to the LDL receptor (Fig. 36–7).[26-28] Selective chemical modification of the apo-B100 of LDL demonstrated that the positively charged (basic) amino acids arginine and lysine are important in the interaction of LDL with its receptor. When apo-B100 was sequenced, several regions enriched in arginines and lysines became candidates for receptor binding.[26-28] It is now apparent that the basic residues in the region of amino acids 3359 to 3369 are critical for receptor binding. However, it is also clear that the carboxyl-terminal region of apo-B100 in the vicinity of amino acid 3500 can modulate receptor-binding activity.[29] Patients expressing apo-B defective in binding have hypercholesterolemia and high LDL levels. This genetic disorder, familial defective apo-B100 (see later discussion), is caused by the substitution of glutamine for arginine at amino acid 3500 of apo-B100.[30]

Role of Apolipoprotein B in Lipid Metabolism

Apo-B100 and apo-B48 play critical roles in the biosynthesis of apo-B–containing lipoproteins.[20,31,32] In addition, the apo-B100 in LDL interacts with the LDL receptor. Although it is also a constituent of VLDL and IDL, apo-B100 does not play a major role in the binding of these lipoproteins to LDL receptors. Apo-E is responsible for most of the receptor-mediated clearance of VLDL and IDL[20,28]; presumably, the lipid or apolipoprotein

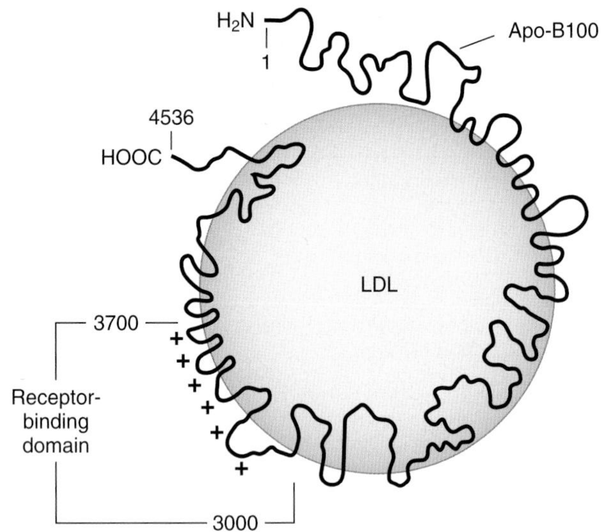

Figure 36–7 ▪ Schematic representation of apolipoprotein B100 (apo-B100) on the surface of a low-density lipoprotein (LDL) particle. The receptor-binding domain forms a cluster of positively charged arginine and lysine residues (a basic patch) capable of interacting with critical negatively charged glutamic and aspartic acid residues in the ligand-binding domain of the LDL receptor. (Adapted from Yang C-Y, Gu Z-W, Weng S-A, et al. Structure of apolipoprotein B-100 of human low density lipoproteins. Arteriosclerosis 1989;9:96-108.)

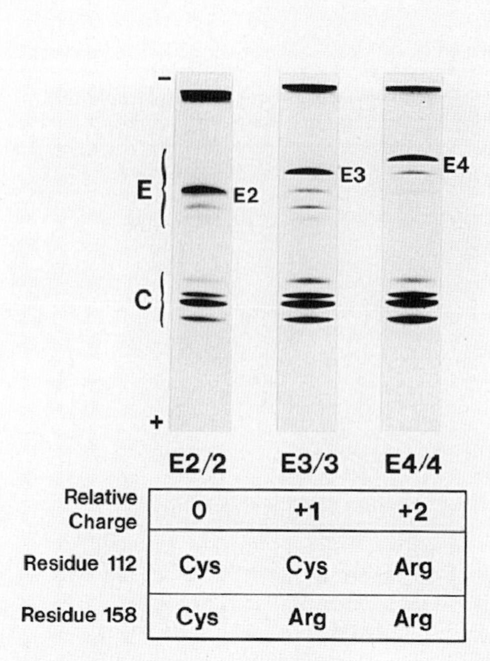

Figure 36–8 ▪ Isoelectric focusing gels of very-low-density lipoprotein (VLDL) apolipoproteins from three subjects homozygous for the common apo-E phenotypes. The relative charge differences among the different apo-E isoforms are accounted for by the specific amino acid substitutions that are responsible for the three isoforms. The minor, more acidic apo-E isoforms represent sialylated forms of the protein. (From Mahley RW, Rall SC Jr. Type III hyperlipoproteinemia (dysbetalipoproteinemia). the role of apolipoprotein E in normal and abnormal lipoprotein metabolism. In Scriver CR, Beaudet AL, Sly WS, et al [eds]. The Metabolic and Molecular Bases of Inherited Disease, 7th ed. New York. McGraw-Hill, 1995:1953-1980.)

content of the VLDL and IDL masks or alters the conformation of the receptor-binding domain of the apo-B100 on these particles. Apo-B100 is, however, the major (or exclusive) protein moiety of LDL and is responsible for directing the clearance of these lipoproteins through the LDL receptor pathway.

Overexpression of apo-B in transgenic mice increases the levels of LDL and other apo-B–containing lipoproteins,[33-35] resulting in increased susceptibility to diet-induced atherosclerosis.[34] Knockout of the apo-B gene in mice is embryonically lethal.[35,36] Production of apo-B in the yolk sac appears to play an essential role in the delivery of lipids to the developing mouse embryo; delivery of α-tocopherol may be particularly important to embryonic tissues.[37]

Apolipoprotein E

Apo-E mediates the interaction of apo-E–containing lipoproteins with the LDL receptor and with the chylomicron remnant receptor, the LDL receptor-related protein (LRP).[38-44] As a consequence, apo-E plays a critical role in determining the metabolic fate of several classes of lipoproteins and is of central importance in cholesterol metabolism. In addition, apo-E appears to participate in cholesterol transport to cells undergoing proliferation and repair and might modulate lymphocyte response and smooth muscle cell proliferation.[38,39,41]

Apo-E, a 34-kd protein composed of 299 amino acids, circulates in the plasma as a constituent of chylomicrons, chylomicron remnants, VLDL, and IDL and as a component of a minor subclass of high-density lipoproteins (HDLs), referred to as HDL with apo-E or HDL_1 (see Fig. 36–5).[38,41] Normal plasma apo-E levels range from 30 to 70 μg/mL, approximately half of which is associated with HDL and serves as a reservoir of apo-E for redistribution to chylomicrons and VLDLs as they enter the plasma. In lymph and interstitial fluid, apo-E is associated with lipid complexes (phospholipid-apo-E discs) or with HDL.

Approximately 75% of plasma apo-E is synthesized by hepatocytes, and the remainder is synthesized in a variety of tissues. Macrophages can synthesize and secrete apo-E, especially when they are loaded with cholesterol, and are responsible for a portion of the apo-E found in interstitial fluid. Apo-E is also synthesized by smooth muscle cells of arteries and keratinocytes in the skin (see Table 36–3). The tissue with the second highest level of apo-E mRNA (after the liver) is the brain, where apo-E is synthesized primarily by astrocytes and neurons. Cerebrospinal fluid contains apo-E derived from the brain (approximately 0.3 mg/dL, or 5% to 10% of plasma apo-E levels). Apo-E appears to play a key role in cholesterol transport in both the central and peripheral nervous systems and is involved in the pathogenesis of Alzheimer's disease.[38,41]

Located on chromosome 19, the apo-E gene is part of a gene cluster that includes the genes for apo-CI and apo-CII. The apo-E gene locus has multiple alleles that give rise to a common genetic protein polymorphism.[38-41] The three major forms of apo-E—apo-E2, apo-E3, and apo-E4—arise from three alleles, referred to as ε2, ε3, and ε4, that occur in several populations with a frequency of about 8%, 77%, and 15%, respectively (Fig. 36–8). There are three homozygous (E2/2, E3/3, and E4/4) and three heterozygous (E3/2, E4/2, and E4/3) phenotypes. About 60% of individuals are homozygous for apo-E3.

These genetic polymorphisms are caused by amino acid differences at two sites in the protein (see Fig. 36–8).[20,28,38,39,41] Apo-E3 has cysteine at position 112 and arginine at position 158, whereas apo-E2 has cysteine at both positions and apo-E4 has arginine. In addition, apo-E displays a second type of polymorphism, post-translational glycosylation. Carbohydrate attachment at threonine-194 and the presence of multiple sialic acid residues give rise to minor acidic isoforms.

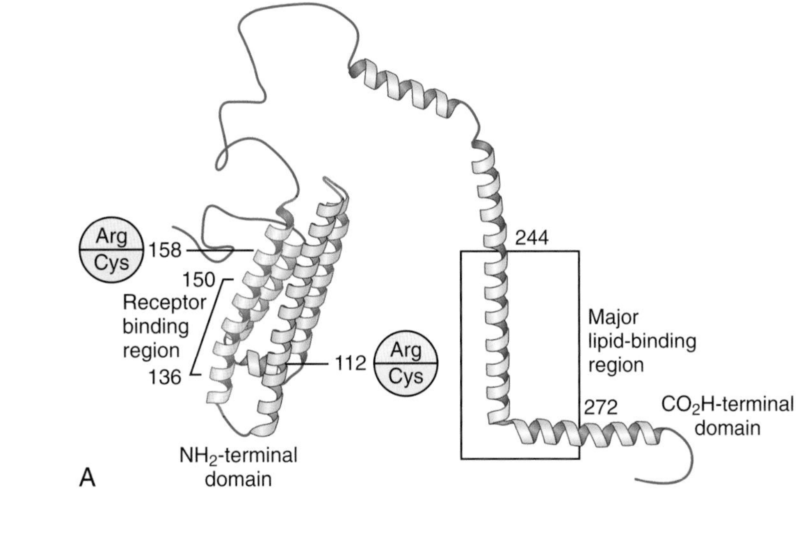

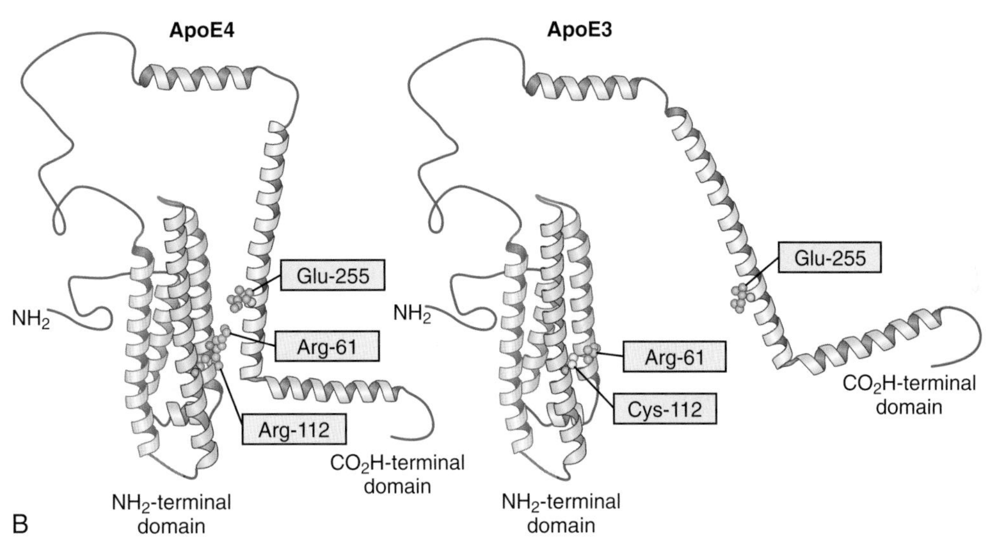

Figure 36–9 ▪ The amino-terminal domain of apo-E is composed of a four-helix bundle. A region of random structure encompassing residues 165 to 200 appears to form a connector or hinge region linked to the carboxyl-terminal domain. There are two major functional regions. residues 136 to 150 (yellow helix) encompass the receptor-binding region; residues 240 to 260 in the carboxyl domain encompass the lipid-binding region. Apo-E4 displays the unique property of domain interaction that distinguishes it from apo-E3 (Arg-61 in the amino-terminal domain interacts with Glu-255 in the carboxyl-terminal domain).

Apo-E functions in both receptor binding and lipid binding, and the different isoforms have different activities. Apo-E3 and apo-E4 are equally capable of interacting with LDL receptors, but the binding of apo-E2 to LDL receptors is impaired and is associated with the development of type III hyperlipoproteinemia under certain conditions.[44,45] Apo-E isoforms also interact differently with specific types of lipids and lipoproteins.[39,41] Apo-E4 binds preferentially to large, triglyceride-rich lipoproteins (e.g., VLDL), whereas apo-E3 and apo-E2 bind preferentially to smaller, phospholipid-rich HDL.

The apo-E primary translational product is a 317–amino acid protein; an 18–amino acid signal peptide is cleaved before the mature protein (299 amino acids, relative molecular mass ≈34 kd) is secreted into plasma. The molecule has two domains (Fig. 36–9A).[38,39,41] The amino-terminal domain (residues 1 to 191) contains the receptor-binding region. The amino acids of apo-E that mediate its binding to the LDL receptor are in the vicinity of residues 136 to 150 (see Fig. 36–9).[38,39,44,45] Positively charged arginines and lysines between amino acids 136 and 150 interact with the negatively charged glutamic and aspartic acids in the ligand-binding region of the LDL receptor. As shown by x-ray crystallography, the amino-terminal domain of apo-E (residues 1 to 191) forms a four-helix bundle.[46-48] The fourth helix encompasses residues 130 to 165, the area envisioned to contain the receptor-binding region. The basic residues in the vicinity of amino acids 134 to 150 are oriented away from the surface of the molecule and are probably involved in the direct interaction of apo-E with the LDL receptor.[47,48]

The carboxyl-terminal domain (residues 192 to 299) appears to have three amphipathic α-helices (one face being hydrophilic and the other hydrophobic) and is responsible for lipid binding. Residues 240 to 260 are key in the binding of apo-E to lipoproteins.[39,41] Paradoxically, the lipid-binding region of apo-E resides in the carboxyl-terminal domain, but the amino acid differences that distinguish the three major apo-E isoforms are in the amino-terminal domain (residues 112 and 158). The fact that the isoforms display different specificities for different types of lipoproteins (i.e., apo-E4 for VLDL and apo-E3 and apo-E2 for

HDL) suggests that the amino-terminal and carboxyl-terminal domains interact and that specific residues in the amino terminus alter the conformation and the specificity of the lipid-binding domain for certain types of lipoproteins. In fact, the amino-terminal and carboxyl-terminal domains of apo-E4, but not apo-E2 or apo-E3, interact. Crystallographic studies indicated that Arg-112 in apo-E4 causes the side chain of Arg-61 to extend away from the helical bundle. The Arg-61 in the amino terminus interacts with Glu-255 in the carboxyl terminus (see Fig. 36–9B). In apo-E2 and apo-E3, Arg-61 is tucked between helices 2 and 3 and is unavailable for interaction with other residues. Thus, domain interaction in apo-E4 modulates both its structure and function.[39,41,46]

The identification of naturally occurring mutants of apo-E that are defective in receptor binding has provided key insights into the specific residues involved (Fig. 36–10). The most common variant that is defective in binding is apo-E2 (Arg-158 → Cys). This substitution appears to impair receptor binding secondarily by altering the conformation of residues in the 136 to 150 region of apo-E.[41,48,49] Other variants that are defective in binding involve single amino acid substitutions. Arg-136 → Ser, Arg-142 → Cys, Arg-145 → Cys, and Lys-146 → Gln or Glu.

Site-directed mutagenesis showed that Arg-150 also plays a key role in receptor binding. A rare apo-E mutation, apo-E Leiden, involves a duplication of seven amino acids (residues 121 to 127) inserted in tandem at the junction between helices 3 and 4. This insertion probably disrupts receptor binding by altering the conformation of the 136 to 150 receptor-binding region.

Apo-E also binds to heparin and to heparan sulfate proteoglycans (HSPGs).[44,50] As discussed later, binding of apo-E to HSPG is important in the clearance of remnant lipoproteins by the LRP pathway. Residues in the 136 to 150 region of apo-E are responsible for the ionic interaction with the sulfate groups of heparin-like molecules and for binding to the LRP.

Roles of Apolipoprotein E in Lipid Metabolism

Apo-E functions in two aspects of lipid and cholesterol transport.[38,41,44,45,50] The first, involving chylomicron and VLDL metabolism, provides a global transport role for apo-E. The knockout of apo-E by gene targeting in mice results in marked hyperlipidemia and the development of severe atherosclerosis, confirming the importance of this protein in cholesterol homeostasis and lipid transport.[51,52] The second aspect involves the redistribution of lipids (including cholesterol) among cells within a tissue or organ. This local transport role redistributes lipids from cells with excess cholesterol to those requiring cholesterol, phospholipids, and other lipids for repair, proliferation, or other purposes. This pathway might involve lipid-laden HDL and apo-E that can acquire tissue lipids or apo-E–lipid complexes formed in the interstitial fluid. Apo-E is synthesized and secreted by a variety of cells and is available in interstitial fluid to transport lipids. Cells requiring cholesterol up-regulate their LDL receptors, and apo-E targets the apo-E–containing HDL or lipid complexes to cells deficient in necessary lipids. For example, the local transport pathway for apo-E is involved in lipid redistribution within a nerve after injury and during regeneration.[38,41,42]

Apolipoprotein AI

Apo-AI is a 29-kd protein encoded by a gene on the long arm of chromosome 11, part of a cluster that includes genes for apo-CIII, apo-AIV, and apo-AV.[19,53] The apo-AI gene is 1863 bp long, and its mRNA encodes a 267–amino acid protein that includes an 18–amino acid prepeptide and a 6–amino acid propeptide. The propeptide is cleaved extracellularly to yield the mature circulating protein of 243 amino acids (see Table 36–3).

Apo-AI is synthesized by the human intestine and liver and is a constituent of chylomicrons and HDL (see Fig. 36–5). It binds to lipids of these lipoproteins, mainly through a series of 22–amino acid amphipathic α-helices separated by helix-breaking proline residues.[54] The polar face of the amphipathic helix is exposed to the aqueous environment, whereas the nonpolar face binds to the lipid (primarily phospholipid) on the surface of the particle. There are eight complete 22–amino acid amphipathic helices and two 11–amino acid repeats in apo-AI.

In addition to its role as a structural protein in HDL, apo-AI activates lecithin:cholesterol acyltransferase (LCAT), which esterifies free cholesterol on HDL particles. It may facilitate the interaction of LCAT with phosphatidylcholine, the substrate of LCAT, and activate the enzyme. The specific regions of apo-AI involved in LCAT activation have been identified, including the amino acid residues responsible for enhanced catalytic activity.[54,55] Other apolipoproteins, such as apo-AIV and apo-CI, which have similar lipid-binding properties, can also activate LCAT (discussed in detail later).

Apo-AI-associated particles, either HDL or its phospholipid-rich precursor, pre-β HDL, serve as acceptors for cholesterol released from cells.[53,54] The efflux of cholesterol to HDL represents part of the *reverse cholesterol transport pathway* (discussed in "Metabolic Pathways Involving High-Density Lipoproteins").[53] Apo-AI serves as the recognition protein for the binding to the ATP binding cassette transporter A1 (ABCA1), ABCG1, and ABCG4, which mediate the efflux of cholesterol from cells (especially macrophages) and to the class B, type I scavenger

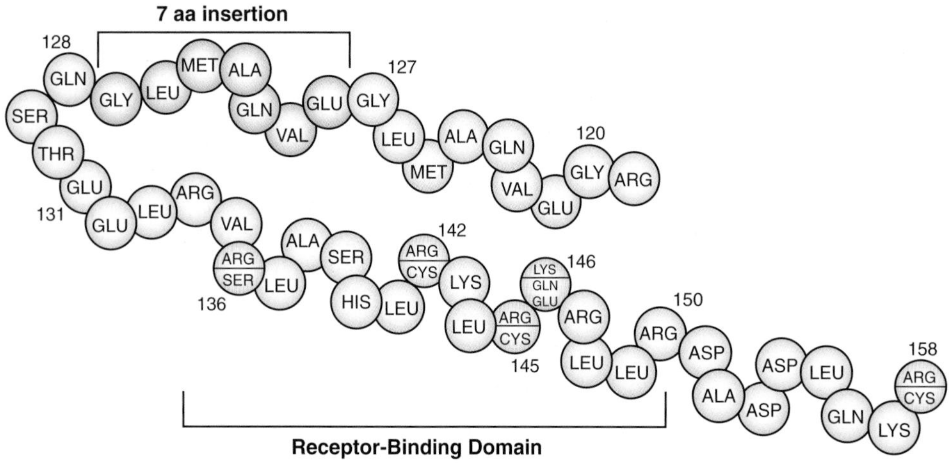

Figure 36–10 ▪ Schematic representation of the receptor-binding domain of apolipoprotein E, indicating the location and identity of naturally occurring amino acid substitutions that lead to type III hyperlipoproteinemia. In each substitution, the bottom amino acid represents the mutant.

receptor (SR-BI), which mediates cholesterol uptake by the liver.[53,54,56,57]

Mutations that give rise to apo-AI deficiency are characterized by absent or low levels of HDL (discussed in "Primary Disorders of High-Density Lipoprotein Metabolism").[54] Apo-AI synthesis is required for HDL production. Apo-AI deficiency causes a variety of manifestations. planar xanthomas, corneal clouding, and sometimes premature coronary heart disease (CHD). Apo-AI is often described as an antiatherogenic apolipoprotein. Although apo-E–deficient mice typically develop extensive atherosclerosis,[51,52] overexpression of human apo-AI in these mice causes an increase in HDL and a significant decrease in atherosclerosis.[58,59]

Apolipoprotein AII

The apo-AII gene is on the long arm of chromosome 1.[19,53,54] The mRNA encodes a 100–amino acid protein, but the mature circulating form of apo-AII is 77 amino acids in length. In the plasma, human apo-AII exists primarily as a homodimer (see Fig. 36–5). A cysteine at residue 6 of apo-AII forms a disulfide bond with a second apo-AII molecule. Heterodimers of apo-AII and apo-E occur only in persons with apo-E2 and apo-E3, which possess free cysteine residues. Heterodimer formation interferes with the ability of apo-E to bind to the LDL receptor.

Apo-AII is synthesized primarily in the liver.[19,53,54] It is found together with apo-AI on a subfraction of HDL referred to as LpAI/AII particles. Apo-AII might play a role in the activation of hepatic lipase and the inhibition of LCAT. The genetic absence of apo-AII in two sisters did not produce any obvious phenotypic effects and did not cause low HDL levels.[60]

Overexpression of apo-AII in mice increases susceptibility to atherosclerosis,[61] possibly because apo-AII displaces apo-AI from HDL. This could interfere with the normal ability of apo-AI–containing HDL to transport cellular cholesterol to the liver for excretion. Therefore, apo-AII is considered a proatherogenic apolipoprotein.

Apolipoprotein AV

Apo-AV is the newest member of the apo-AI/CIII/AIV gene cluster on chromosome 11 (see Table 36–3). It resides about 30 kb distal to the apo-AIV gene.[62,63] Apo-AV was not recognized for many years because of its very low concentration in the plasma (<0.1 mg/dL). Produced by the liver, apo-AV profoundly affects plasma triglyceride levels. Overexpression of apo-AV in transgenic mice decreases plasma triglyceride levels by half, whereas inactivation of the apo-AV gene increases triglyceride levels fourfold.[64]

Apo-AV is a potent activator of LPL-mediated lipolysis.[64] It might target triglyceride-rich lipoproteins to cell surface HSPG on vascular endothelial cells where LPL resides. On the other hand, apo-AV might inhibit hepatic VLDL production by interfering with assembly. Polymorphisms in the gene are associated with significant variability in triglyceride levels in humans across several populations. Interestingly, a nonsense mutation (Q139X), resulting in a truncated form of apo-AV, can cause hypertriglyceridemia and chylomicronemia.[65]

C Apolipoproteins

The genes for apo-CI and apo-CII reside on chromosome 19 near the gene that encodes apo-E, whereas the apo-CIII gene is part of the apo-AI and apo-AIV gene cluster on chromosome 11.[19,20] The C apolipoproteins (see Table 36–3 and Fig. 36–5) readily exchange among various lipoproteins and are synthesized primarily by the liver. (Apo-CI is also produced by macrophages and, in small amounts, by the intestine.) HDLs appear to serve as a reservoir for the C apolipoproteins, which can then be transferred to triglyceride-rich lipoproteins. The C apolipoproteins appear to regulate triglyceride metabolism and to influence the inverse relation between triglyceride levels and HDL cholesterol (HDL-C). Apo-CI (6.6 kd) modulates the uptake of triglyceride-rich lipoproteins (chylomicron remnants, VLDL, and IDL) by interfering with the ability of apo-E to mediate binding to lipoprotein receptor pathways. Similarly, apo-CIII (8.8 kd) can prevent the normal interaction of triglyceride-rich, apo-E–containing lipoproteins with receptors and cell-surface HSPG. Apo-CI and apo-CIII can displace apo-E from the particles. Apo-CII (8.9 kd) is a cofactor for LPL, and mutations in the apo-CII gene result in a marked hypertriglyceridemia (discussed later).

Overexpression of apo-CI, apo-CII, or apo-CIII in transgenic mice results in hypertriglyceridemia.[19] In the case of apo-CI and apo-CIII, the resulting hyperlipidemia appears to be caused by displacement of apo-E from triglyceride-rich particles, which results in impaired receptor-mediated uptake, and displacement of apo-CII, which impairs lipolytic processing. Mice lacking apo-CIII have low triglyceride levels resulting from more rapid clearance of postprandial lipoproteins. A polymorphism of the apo-CIII gene promoter region in mice is also associated with increased levels of apo-CIII and hypertriglyceridemia.

The hypertriglyceridemia that follows the overexpression of apo-CII was initially puzzling because apo-CII is a cofactor that activates LPL-mediated hydrolysis of triglycerides.[19] However, the triglyceride-rich lipoproteins that accumulate in the plasma are poor in apo-E and do not interact well enough with cell-surface HSPG to allow lipase activity to occur or with receptors in the proteoglycan-rich matrices of the hepatic cell surface to allow uptake. Therefore, either overproduction or underproduction of apo-CII can cause hypertriglyceridemia.

Lipoprotein Receptors Controlling Lipoprotein Metabolism

Low-Density Lipoprotein Receptor Gene Family

The LDL receptor family consists of seven members that are structurally closely related. the LDL receptor, the VLDL receptor, the apo-E receptor 2, the MEGF7, the LRP, the LRP1B, and the LRP2 (megalin, glycoprotein 330).[4,66-69] The common structural motifs that occur in the same repeating arrangement include ligand binding repeats (cysteine-rich containing ~40 amino acids each), a YWTD motif with a β-propeller domain, an epidermal growth factor precursor, a single membrane-spanning domain, and a short cytoplasmic tail containing one or more NPXY motifs, which are docking sites for a phosphotyrosine binding domain containing adapter proteins. The functions of this gene family extend beyond mediating lipid uptake by cells and include serving as transducers of extracellular signals involved in the normal development of the brain and the blood-brain barrier.[70]

Low-Density Lipoprotein Receptor

The LDL receptor, a glycoprotein with an apparent molecular weight of 160,000, is expressed on the surface of most cells and especially in the liver. It functions in the uptake of apo-B– and apo-E–containing lipoproteins, including LDL, chylomicron remnants, VLDL, VLDL remnants, IDL, and HDL_1.[20,28,38,41] Most HDL particles lack apo-E and do not interact with the LDL receptor. Cells can acquire cholesterol from the plasma by taking up these lipoproteins through the LDL receptor. The LDL receptor was first identified in 1973, and its gene was characterized in 1985 in the laboratory of Nobel laureates Joseph L. Goldstein and Michael S. Brown.[5,68] Two proteins on the lipoprotein surface, apo-B100 and apo-E, bind to the LDL receptor.

After the lipoprotein binds to the LDL receptor, the resulting complex becomes localized to a specialized area of the cell membrane called a coated pit. The coat contains a protein complex called clathrin, which clusters the receptors in a region of the cell membrane that can invaginate and form an intracellular vesicle to contain the lipoprotein. As these internalized vesicles, or endosomes, move into the cytoplasm, the internal environment becomes progressively more acidic, causing the receptor and the lipoprotein to dissociate. The lipoproteins are degraded in the lysosomes, and the unoccupied receptors recycle to the cell surface (Fig. 36–11).

The LDL receptor is synthesized in the ER as a protein of 839 amino acids with an apparent molecular weight of 120,000.[68] Glycosylation of the protein in the ER and in the Golgi apparatus increases its weight to about 160,000. The LDL receptor has five distinct structural and functional domains[68] (Fig. 36–12). Mutations within these domains disrupt the normal function of the receptor in lipoprotein metabolism and cause the genetic disorder familial hypercholesterolemia (FH) (discussed later).[68]

Ligand-Binding Domain

The ligand-binding domain of the LDL receptor consists of the 292 amino acids at the amino terminus (see Fig. 36–12). This region of the molecule is rich in cysteines and contains glutamic and aspartic acids that mediate the binding to apo-B and apo-E. It is composed of seven repeats of approximately 40 amino acids each. Each repeat contains six cysteines that form three intrarepeat disulfide bonds, resulting in a very stable structure. In addition, each repeat contains a Ser-Asp-Glu triplet that mediates the interaction of apo-B– and apo-E–containing lipoproteins with the LDL receptor. The ligand-receptor binding is an ionic interaction between positively charged arginines and lysines in apo-B100 and apo-E and negatively charged aspartic and glutamic acids in the ligand-binding domain of the LDL receptor.[38,41]

Site-directed mutagenesis and analysis of naturally occurring mutants of the LDL receptor associated with FH have provided insights into the roles of specific repeats and residues in ligand binding.[68] Ligand-binding domain repeat 1 does not play a major role in the binding of either apo-B–containing (LDL) or apo-E–containing (β-VLDL) lipoproteins. The deletion of repeats 2 through 7, however, markedly impairs the binding of LDL. The binding of β-VLDL is mediated by apo-E and is impaired only if repeat 5 is deleted. Therefore, the requirements for the binding of LDL are more stringent than those for the binding of β-VLDL.

Single amino acid substitutions of critical residues in the ligand-binding repeats also impair binding activity. For example, in patients with FH Puerto Rico, in which the serine of the ligand-binding triplet (Ser-Asp-Glu) in repeat 4 is changed to a leucine, the LDL fails to bind, although apo-E–containing β-VLDL binds with near-normal affinity. In FH Mexico, in which lysine is substituted for the glutamic acid of the ligand-binding triplet of repeat 5, neither LDL nor β-VLDL binds normally.

The defect in the Watanabe heritable hyperlipidemic (WHHL) rabbit with hypercholesterolemia and accelerated atherosclerosis involves a deletion of four amino acids in repeat 4. Although this defect is associated with a reduced number of receptors reaching the cell surface, those that do reach the surface retain the ability to bind β-VLDL (apo-E) but not LDL (apo-B).[68]

As demonstrated in the WHHL rabbit, mutations in the ligand-binding domain can also disrupt the normal transport of the LDL receptor to the cell surface. The decreased transport of the mutant receptor from the ER to the Golgi apparatus and to the cell surface is undoubtedly caused by improper folding of the molecule and increased intracellular degradation. For example, FH Afrikaner, which is caused by the presence of a glutamic acid rather than aspartic acid in the triplet of repeat 5, results in defective transport and lack of normal expression of the receptor on the cell surface.

Cytoplasmic Domain

The carboxyl-terminal region of the LDL receptor is composed of 50 amino acids and contains the sequence NPXY (N, asparagine; P, proline; X, any amino acid; Y, tyrosine), which is respon-

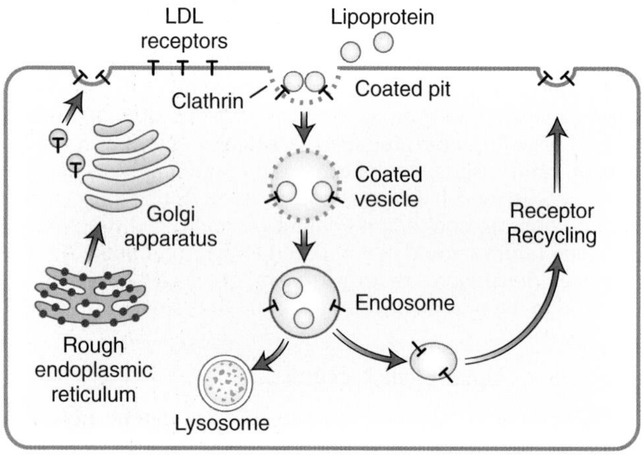

Figure 36–11 ▪ Low-density lipoprotein (LDL) receptor pathway. The LDLs interact with their receptors on the cell surface. The complex enters the coated pit and is internalized. The coated vesicle loses its clathrin coat and becomes an endosome, the site of lipoprotein and receptor dissociation. The receptors recycle to the cell surface, and the lipoproteins are degraded. Alternatively, new receptors are synthesized in the rough endoplasmic reticulum and transported to the cell surface. (Modified from Brown MS, Goldstein JL. A receptor-mediated pathway for cholesterol homeostasis. Science 1986;232:34-47; and Myant NB. Cholesterol Metabolism, LDL, and the LDL Receptor. San Diego. Academic Press, 1990.)

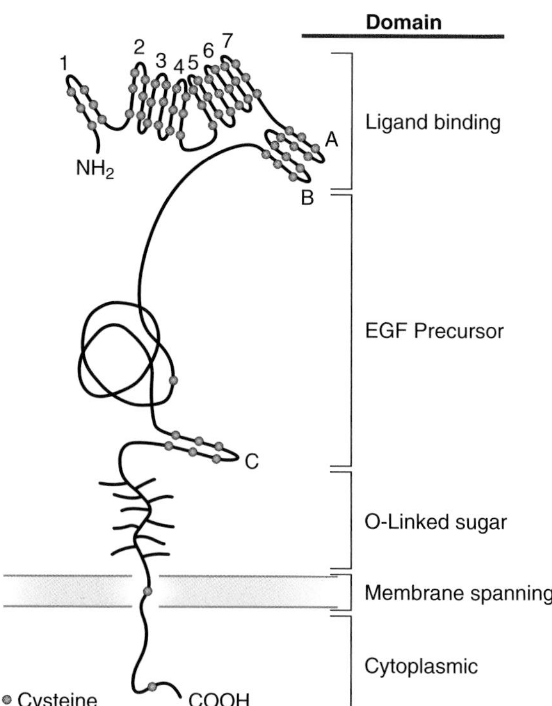

Figure 36–12 ▪ Functional domains of the low-density lipoprotein receptor. See text for complete description. EGF, epidermal growth factor. Numbers 1 to 7 indicate repeats.

sible for clustering the receptors in coated pits and mediating internalization of the receptors by the cells.[68] One of the early mutations associated with FH (J.D. allele, FH Bari) provided insights into the role of a critical residue for directing internalization. In the mutant form of the receptor, Tyr-807 is changed to a cysteine. Site-directed mutagenesis demonstrated that this position must be occupied by an aromatic amino acid (tyrosine, phenylalanine, or tryptophan) for normal internalization. The tetrameric sequence Asn-Pro-Val-Tyr, in which Tyr-807 occurs, is the signal directing the receptors to the coated pit.

Regulation of the Low-Density Lipoprotein Receptor Gene

The LDL receptor gene is 45 kb long and is located on the distal portion of the short arm of chromosome 19. Synthesis of the LDL receptor is regulated by DNA sequences in the 5′-flanking region of the LDL receptor gene (Fig. 36–13).[71-73] A sequence of approximately 10 bases in this region, called the sterol regulatory element (SRE), and two other repeats that bind the transcription factor Spl are necessary for the regulation of the LDL receptor mRNA levels. If intracellular sterol levels are high, LDL receptor mRNA is not transcribed. When the sterol content of the cells decreases, the expression of LDL receptors on the cell surface increases, causing increased uptake of apo-B– and apo-E–containing lipoproteins and increased delivery of cholesterol to the cells. The LDL receptor gene senses the sterol level of the cell and appropriately controls receptor mRNA production and protein biosynthesis to meet the needs of the cell.

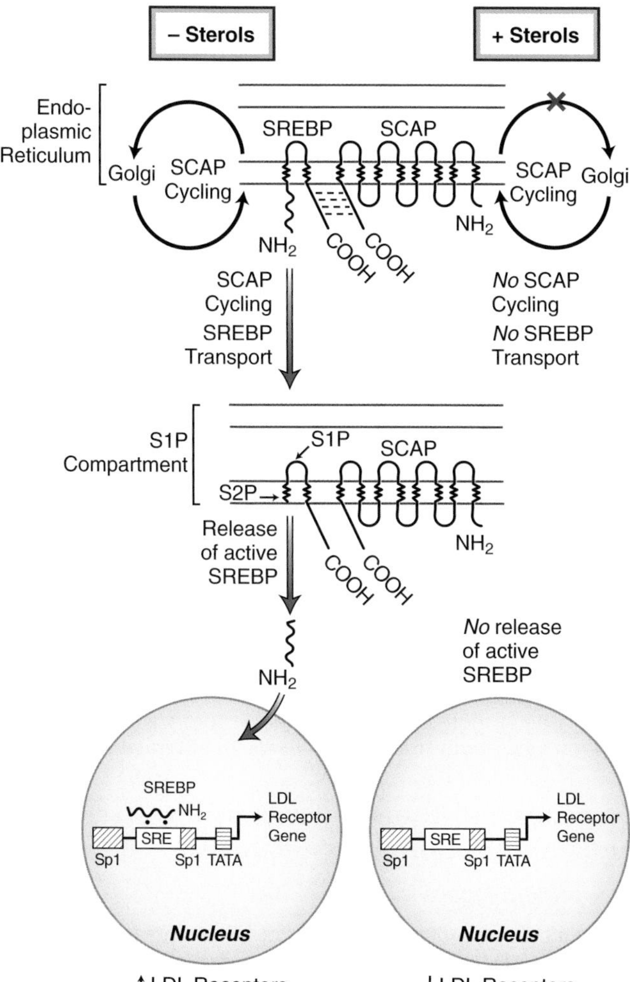

Figure 36–13 ▪ Low-density lipoprotein (LDL) receptor gene regulation. SREBP, sterol regulatory element–binding protein; SCAP, SREBP cleavage activating protein.

The control mechanism of LDL receptor expression has been elucidated in considerable detail.[71,72] Currently, there are three known structurally related transcription factors, SRE-binding proteins (SREBPs) la, lc, and 2, that regulate the level of LDL receptors and other genes encoding enzymes involved in the biosynthesis of cholesterol, unsaturated fatty acids, and triglycerides. SREBP-la and SREBP-lc arise from the same gene but use different promoters and have different first introns; SREBP-2 arises from a separate gene. The intact 125-kd SREBPs are three-domain integral membrane proteins containing two membrane-spanning regions (see Fig. 36–13). The amino-terminal domain of the SREBPs represents transcription factors of the loop-helix leucine zipper family and contains sequences that recognize the SREs on the genes that they control.

To become active transcription factors, the intact SREBPs must be cleaved in the correct order by two proteases in a post-ER compartment and then translocated to the nucleus to interact with the SREs. The first protease, designated site-l protease (SlP), cleaves the loop connecting the amino-terminal and carboxyl-terminal domains, both of which remain membrane bound after cleavage. The second protease, site-2 protease (S2P), further cleaves the amino-terminal domain just within the first membrane-spanning region, releasing the transcription factor to enter the nucleus and interact with the SREs (see Fig. 36–13).

Sterol control is exerted through a two-domain regulatory protein, SREBP cleavage-activating protein (SCAP), which is required for SlP cleavage of the SREBP. SCAP is membrane associated (eight transmembrane regions) and is tightly complexed to the SREBPs through its carboxyl-terminal domain. Five of the eight membrane-spanning segments serve as a sterol-sensing domain. It is not clear whether the sensing domain interacts directly or indirectly with sterols. What is known is that sterols regulate the ability of SCAP to transport SREBPs to the post-ER compartment where SlP is located.[74] SCAP cycles between the ER and Golgi apparatus, and whether SCAP transports the SREBPs to the SlP compartment depends on the processing of its N-linked carbohydrates by the Golgi apparatus. In sterol-depleted cells, SCAP cycles to the Golgi apparatus and its N-linked carbohydrates are modified; the modified SCAP returns to the ER to transport the SREBPs. Sterols block the movement of SCAP from the ER to the Golgi apparatus, preventing carbohydrate modification and the ability of SCAP to transport the SREBPs for SlP cleavage.

Low-Density Lipoprotein Receptor-Related Protein

The LRP is an integral membrane receptor composed of two components. a 515-kd amino-terminal extracellular domain and an 85-kd cytoplasmic and membrane-spanning domain (the precursor protein, composed of 4525 amino acids, is cleaved after synthesis).[66,67,75] This large protein is equivalent structurally to approximately four LDL receptors and possesses 31 ligand-binding domains. The LRP contains the four structural motifs characteristic of other members of the LDL receptor gene family. multiple ligand-binding repeats, EGF repeats and EGF precursor homology domains, a single membrane-spanning region, and two NPXY internalization signals. The LRP is expressed primarily in liver (parenchymal cells), brain (neurons), and placenta (syncytiotrophoblast cells). The LRP plays a key role in the brain.[67,70]

The LRP interacts with approximately 18 ligands and has several functions. With respect to lipoprotein metabolism, the LRP binds with high affinity to apo-E–enriched chylomicron remnants and VLDL remnants and internalizes them. Interaction of these lipoproteins with the LRP requires the addition of multiple apo-E molecules per particle, which serve as ligands. Initial binding of the lipoprotein to cell-surface HSPG is necessary to facilitate the interaction or transfer of the apo-E–enriched remnants to the LRP[50] (discussed further in "Chylomicron Remnant Receptors in Remnant Catabolism"). The LRP does not bind LDL.

The LRP can also interact with LPL[76] and hepatic lipase.[77] This interaction could mediate the hepatic binding and uptake of remnant lipoproteins possessing these enzymes on their surface. Other ligands for the LRP that are not directly related to lipid metabolism include α_2-macroglobulin, plasminogen activators and inhibitors, and bacterial toxins.[66,67] Knockout of the LRP in mice is lethal, demonstrating its critical importance.

A receptor-associated protein (RAP) of 39 kd can be isolated along with purified LRP and effectively competes with all the ligands for the LRP binding. This protein also binds to the gp330 and VLDL receptors (described later) and blocks ligand binding to these receptors as well. However, RAP does not appear to be secreted from the cells, and it may serve as an intracellular chaperone that occupies the ligand-binding sites for transport of the LRP to the cell surface. The knockout of RAP by gene targeting in mice markedly reduces LRP expression in both liver and brain, further suggesting an intracellular transport role for this protein. Alternatively, it may participate in the intracellular recycling of the receptors. Regardless of its physiologic role, RAP inhibits the interaction of LRP and its ligands both in cultured cells and in intact animals.

Glycoprotein 330

The gp330/megalin receptor, also referred to as the major Heymann nephritis antigen, is a large protein (about 600 kd) that possesses many of the structural motifs of the LDL receptor.[66,67] It is expressed in the proximal tubules of the kidney and the ependymal cells in the brain and is not present in liver. Although gp330 binds apo-E–containing lipoproteins and LDL, its role in lipoprotein metabolism is unknown. The knockout of gp330 by gene targeting does not have an obvious effect on lipoprotein metabolism, but it causes developmental abnormalities of the central nervous system (holoprosencephaly).[78]

Very-Low-Density Lipoprotein Receptor

The VLDL receptor closely resembles the LDL receptor except that it has an eighth ligand-binding repeat.[66,67] The VLDL receptor (about 130 kd) binds apo-E–containing lipoproteins and is present primarily in muscle, fat, and brain. In the nervous system, it is present in the choroid plexus and in some neurons. It is absent from liver, and its role in lipoprotein metabolism remains to be determined. It has been suggested, because the receptor is present in tissues that metabolize VLDL-derived fatty acids, that it might function to deliver triglyceride-rich lipoproteins to target tissues.

Apolipoprotein E Receptor 2

The apo-E receptor 2 (~106 kd) is expressed primarily in the brain and to a lesser extent in the placenta and can be expressed as various splice variants.[66,67] Although this receptor, like the LDL receptor, contains seven cysteine-rich repeats in the ligand-binding domain, the repeats are more closely related structurally to the VLDL receptor. Because the receptor is primarily expressed in the brain, it is likely to play a role in lipoprotein metabolism in the central nervous system. In addition to their roles in lipoprotein metabolism, the apo-E receptor 2 and the VLDL receptor have been implicated in normal brain development by transducing extracellular signals.[67]

Scavenger Receptors

Originally, it was thought that a single scavenger receptor existed on macrophages. Also known as the acetyl-LDL receptor, this receptor was characterized by its ability to interact with chemically modified LDL but not with native LDL. LDL particles that had been modified by acetylation, acetoacetylation, or malondialdehyde were taken up by high-affinity cell-surface receptors on macrophages, resulting in marked cholesterol accumulation. As a result of cloning efforts, it became apparent that the scavenger receptor actually represented a large family of receptors with specificities for a broad range of unrelated ligands and involvement in a spectrum of physiologic processes, including atherosclerosis, host defense, and central nervous system disorders.[79-82]

Currently, there are ten known subclasses (A to J) of the scavenger receptor family. Classes A, B, D, E, F, G, and H are expressed in atherosclerotic lesions and may be involved in foam cell formation. Class A receptors include types I, II, and III and MARCO. The type I and type II receptors are generated by alternative splicing of the mRNA encoded by a gene on chromosome 8.[80-82] The predicted structure is that of a trimer (~220 kd) composed of three identical subunits (each about 77 kd). The type I receptor contains six domains. a cytoplasmic amino-terminal domain (50 amino acids), a transmembrane domain (26 amino acids), a spacer (74 amino acids), an α-helical coiled-coil domain (121 amino acids), a collagen-like domain (72 amino acids with a Gly-X-Tyr repeat), and a cysteine-rich domain (110 amino acids). The type II scavenger receptor is identical to the type I receptor except that it lacks the carboxyl-terminal cysteine-rich domain; its collagen-like domain is responsible for ligand binding. Clusters of positively charged residues (lysines) appear to mediate the interaction with the chemically modified lipoproteins (see section on the LDL paradox and oxidized lipids for a discussion of the role of the scavenger receptor in atherogenesis). In addition to binding modified LDL, class A scavenger receptors bind anionic proteins, polynucleotides, and bacterial endotoxins (lipopolysaccharides). A deficiency of scavenger receptor A results in a decrease in foam cell formation.[81,82] Their main function appears to involve the clearance of microbial pathogens, senescent cells, and altered lipoproteins.

Class B scavenger receptors include CD36 and SR-BI (human homologue CLA-1).[81] These receptors possess two membrane-spanning regions and bind both oxidized and native lipoproteins. CD36 is expressed on the surface of platelets, capillary endothelial cells, adipose cells, circulating monocytes, macrophages, and other cell types. As discussed in the section "Transport Facilitated by a Cell-Surface Binding Protein," the SR-BI has a unique dual role. In the liver, it functions in the selective uptake of cholesteryl esters from HDL; in macrophages, however, it functions in the uptake of oxidized LDL and β-VLDL remnants, leading to foam cell formation.

There is much discussion as to whether the scavenger receptors are pro- or antiatherogenic. Removal of oxidized LDLs from the artery wall by macrophages may be beneficial because oxidized LDLs are toxic to cells. When macrophages are functioning normally, the excess lipid in the foam cells is effluxed by ABC transporters and delivered to the liver for excretion. Inhibitors of one or more of the scavenger receptors will shed further light on whether they are friend or foe in atherogenesis.[80-82]

Enzymes and Transfer Proteins Involved in Lipid and Lipoprotein Metabolism

Lipoprotein Lipase

Human LPL is a protein composed of 448 amino acids (approximately 50 kd). It is synthesized by adipocytes, by myocytes in skeletal and cardiac muscle, and by macrophages but is not produced by hepatocytes. After secretion from adipocytes and myocytes, LPL is transported to the surface of capillary endothelial cells of these tissues, where it attaches to HSPG and interacts with chylomicrons and VLDL in the circulation and mediates the hydrolysis of their triglycerides to release FFAs for use by the tissues. The fatty acids are stored as triglyceride in adipocytes and used as a source of energy in muscle and for triglyceride synthesis in the formation of hepatic VLDL.[13,83]

The active form of LPL is a dimer. Although its crystal structure is not known, LPL has a high degree of homology with another serine esterase, pancreatic lipase, whose structure is known. Based on similarities between LPL and pancreatic lipase, a model for LPL function has been suggested (Fig. 36–14), and five functional domains have been identified in LPL on the basis of structural and mutational studies.[13,83]

Heparin-Binding Site

The heparin-binding site mediates the interaction of LPL with HSPG on endothelial cells. Clusters of positively charged arginines and lysines on one face of LPL, particularly those in the carboxyl terminus, appear to mediate this interaction.

Lipid-Binding Site

The domain of the protein that allows the enzyme to interact with the surface of the chylomicron lies in the carboxyl terminus, particularly around residues 245 to 253.

Apolipoprotein CII-Binding Site

Apo-CII, an essential cofactor for LPL, binds to the carboxyl terminus at a site that has not been identified precisely.

Catalytic Site

This site mediates the hydrolysis of triglycerides, primarily to fatty acids and monoglyceride, and is thought to involve Ser-132, Asp-156, and His-241, which are at the bottom of a hydrophobic channel that is covered by a flap or catalytic lid. By assuming an open or closed conformation, the lid can mediate the interaction with the lipid substrate. LPL is a serine esterase with triglyceride hydrolase activity and, to a lesser extent, phospholipase activity.

LDL Receptor–Related Protein–Binding Site

The LRP-binding site is distinct from the heparin-binding site and involves the carboxyl-terminal domain. Through its interaction with the LRP, LPL can facilitate the binding and uptake of lipoproteins associated with the enzyme.

Hepatic Lipase

Hepatic lipase (about 53 kd, 477 amino acids) is primarily a phospholipase but also possesses triglyceride hydrolase activity.[19,50,84] It is synthesized by hepatocytes and is present primarily on liver endothelial cells and on HSPG in the space of Disse. Hepatic lipase is transported from the liver to the capillary endothelium of the adrenals, ovaries, and testes, where it functions in the release of lipids from lipoproteins for use in these organs. Its activity is increased by androgens and reduced by estrogens. Little is known about the structural domains of hepatic lipase except by analogy to similar domains within LPL, but the catalytic triad includes Ser-145, Asp-171, and His-256.

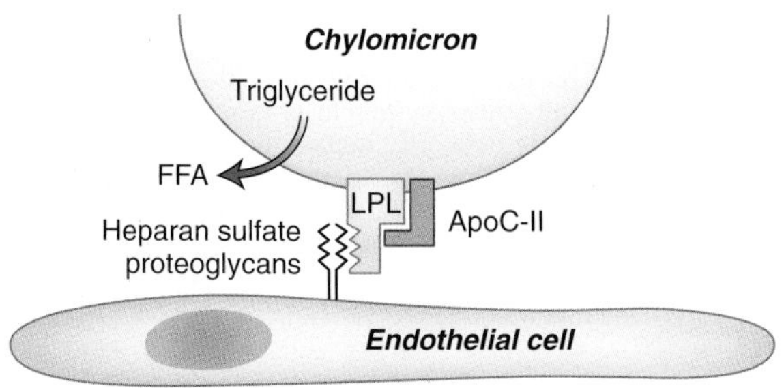

Figure 36–14 ■ Lipoprotein lipase (LPL), attached by interaction with glycosaminoglycans on the endothelial cells, interacts with chylomicrons to catalyze the hydrolysis of the chylomicron triglycerides (Tg) to form free fatty acids (FFA). Apolipoprotein (apo) CII on the lipoprotein serves as a cofactor for LPL.

Hepatic lipase has several roles in lipoprotein metabolism.[84,85] First, it hydrolyzes triglycerides and possibly excess surface phospholipids in the final processing of chylomicron remnants. This enzyme may be active in the space of Disse. It binds heparan sulfate and facilitates the interaction of remnant lipoproteins with the LRP, thereby delivering these lipoproteins to the receptor for internalization by hepatocytes. Second, it completes the processing of IDL to LDL (discussed in the section on IDL). Third, it participates in the conversion of HDL_2 to HDL_3 by the removal of triglyceride and phospholipid from HDL_2 (discussed in "Metabolic Pathways Involving High-Density Lipoproteins"). High levels of hepatic lipase activity decrease total HDL levels.

Contrasting Lipoprotein Lipase and Hepatic Lipase

LPL requires apo-CII as a cofactor to stimulate its catalytic activity, but apo-CII is not a cofactor for hepatic lipase.[84] In contrast, apo-E might facilitate both triglyceride and phospholipid hydrolysis by hepatic lipase and may be a cofactor for its enzymatic activity.[86] In other respects, the enzymes are similar. After intravenous injection of heparin, both enzymes are released from endothelial cells of the liver and peripheral tissues and are referred to as postheparin lipase. Therefore, measurements of total plasma lipolytic activity after heparin injection reflect the activities of both enzymes.

Mutations that impair or inactivate LPL cause hypertriglyceridemia[83] (discussed later). Likewise, deficiency of apo-CII prevents normal activation of LPL and also causes hypertriglyceridemia. Hepatic lipase deficiencies result in a variable and diverse pattern of lipoprotein changes, including the accumulation of remnant lipoproteins, IDL, and HDL_2. These changes are predictable on the basis of the functional roles of hepatic lipase. Knockout of the LPL gene in mice causes a particularly severe hypertriglyceridemia that becomes evident as soon as the newborns begin to suckle and causes death within the first 24 hours.[19] Knockout of the hepatic lipase gene causes less severe manifestations, including changes in HDL and increased plasma phospholipid levels.[87] In the mouse, LPL might take on some of the functions subserved by hepatic lipase in other species. Overexpression of human hepatic lipase in transgenic mice[88] and rabbits[89] markedly decreases HDL and IDL.

Lecithin: Cholesterol Acyltransferase

LCAT circulates in association with HDL in the plasma and functions to esterify free cholesterol.[90,91] In humans, most of the cholesteryl esters in plasma lipoproteins are formed by the action of LCAT. The major substrate for LCAT is the small HDL particle; to a lesser extent, LDL is also a substrate. The enzyme catalyzes the transfer of long-chain fatty acids from phosphatidylcholine (linoleic acid at position 2 of lecithin preferred) to the hydroxyl group at position 3 on cholesterol. The structure and function of LCAT are discussed more thoroughly later in the context of HDL metabolism.

Cholesteryl Ester Transfer Protein

The cholesteryl ester transfer protein (CETP) transfers cholesteryl esters from the larger HDL to VLDL, IDL, and remnant lipoproteins.[92,93] In return, triglyceride from these lipoproteins is transferred to HDL. LCAT and CETP function in concert in HDL metabolism, and the structure and function of CETP are discussed further in the section on HDL.

Plasma Lipoproteins. Structure, Function, and Metabolism

Chylomicrons

Characteristics

Chylomicrons (density *[d]* <0.95 g/mL) are the largest of the plasma lipoproteins (>1000 Å in diameter) and readily float after ultracentrifugation of plasma. They are composed of 98% to 99% lipid (85%-90% triglyceride) and 1% to 2% protein (see Table 36–4). Chylomicrons are present in postprandial plasma (but are absent after an overnight fast) and contain several apolipoproteins, including apo-B48, apo-AI, apo-AIV, apo-E, and the C apolipoproteins (see Fig. 36–5). The distinctive apolipoprotein is apo-B48, a form of apo-B that has an apparent molecular mass 48% that of apo-B100. Because it is the only form of apo-B synthesized by the intestine, apo-B48 is a marker for human lipoproteins produced by the intestinal epithelium.[20,28,32,94]

Origin

Chylomicrons are produced by the epithelial cells of the small intestine (duodenum and proximal jejunum) when dietary fat and cholesterol are presented to the brush border of the epithelial cell membranes as bile acid micelles. Free fatty acids and monoglycerides taken up by the intestinal epithelial cells are synthesized into triglycerides in the ER in the apical region of the intestinal cells. Triglycerides, phospholipids, and cholesterol (absorbed or synthesized by the intestinal cells) are used for chylomicron formation in the Golgi apparatus, where some of the apolipoproteins undergo final carbohydrate processing, and the chylomicrons are secreted into the space along the lateral borders of the intestinal cells. From there, they enter the mesenteric lymph and proceed through the thoracic duct lymph to the general circulation. Newly synthesized chylomicrons possess apo-B48, apo-AI, and apo-AIV (intestinally synthesized apolipoproteins); they acquire apo-E and C apolipoproteins in the lymph and blood, primarily from HDL.

Intestinal cholesterol absorption is mediated by the Niemann-Pick C1-like protein (NPC1L1), which appears to be the target for ezetimibe, which inhibits intestinal cholesterol absorption.[95] The dietary free cholesterol is esterified by the type 2 isozyme of ACAT before it is incorporated into the chylomicrons. ACAT2 in the intestine also regulates cholesterol absorption, and this may be a therapeutic target for lowering plasma cholesterol levels.[8,9] Triglyceride synthesis is regulated by DGAT. After their synthesis in the ER, the triglycerides are transferred to apo-B48 for assembly of the particles.

Metabolic Fate

In the circulation, LPL catalyzes the release of FFAs from chylomicron triglycerides and converts them into triglyceride-poor, cholesterol-enriched chylomicron remnants (Fig. 36–15). The FFAs are taken up by various tissues to be stored as triglyceride, oxidized as an energy source, or reutilized in hepatic lipoprotein-triglyceride synthesis. Hepatic lipase, acting primarily as a phospholipase and secondarily as a glyceride hydrolase, also plays a role in the final preparation of chylomicron remnants for uptake by hepatocytes. Chylomicron remnants are cleared rapidly from the plasma by the liver.[44,45,50,66,67] The metabolic pathways involved in their catabolism are discussed later.

The pathways responsible for chylomicron remnant clearance are understood (Fig. 36–16). The remnants rapidly appear in the liver in the space of Disse, which is bounded by endothelial cells lining the liver blood sinusoids and by liver cells covered with microvilli. Apo-E on the surface of chylomicron remnants and newly secreted by hepatocytes is critical for initiating plasma clearance of these lipoproteins, but both the plasma clearance and the catabolism of these particles are complex.[38,44,45,50]

Sequestration of chylomicron remnants within the space of Disse (see Fig. 36–16) appears to involve binding of the remnant lipoproteins to HSPG mediated by apo-E (or possibly LPL or hepatic lipase). The microvilli-covered surface of hepatocytes is coated with HSPG, which is abundant in the space of Disse. HSPGs bind apo-E by an ionic interaction between negatively charged sulfate groups of HSPG and basic amino acids within the 136 to 150 region of apo-E. The absence of proteoglycans on the cell surface impairs uptake of the particles.[50] Apo-E secreted by the hepatocytes appears to be bound to the cell-surface HSPG and further enhances the apo-E–mediated binding of remnant lipoproteins.

Chylomicron remnants may be *further processed* by lipases or other enzymes in the space of Disse. LPL is carried into the space of Disse on chylomicron remnants, and hepatic lipase produced by the liver may be localized there. These lipases

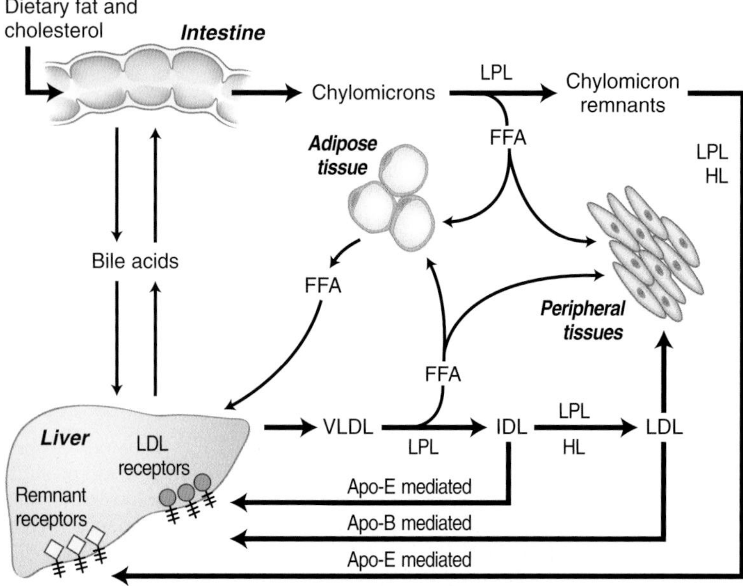

Figure 36–15 ■ General scheme summarizing the major pathways involved in the metabolism of chylomicrons synthesized by the intestine and very-low-density lipoprotein (VLDL) synthesized by the liver. Apo-E, apolipoprotein E; FFA, free fatty acid; HL, hepatic lipase; IDL, intermediate-density lipoprotein; LPL, lipoprotein lipase. (Modified from Mahley RW. Biochemistry and physiology of lipid and lipoprotein metabolism. In Becker KL [ed]. Principles and Practice of Endocrinology and Metabolism, 2nd ed. Philadelphia. JB Lippincott, 1995:1369-1378.)

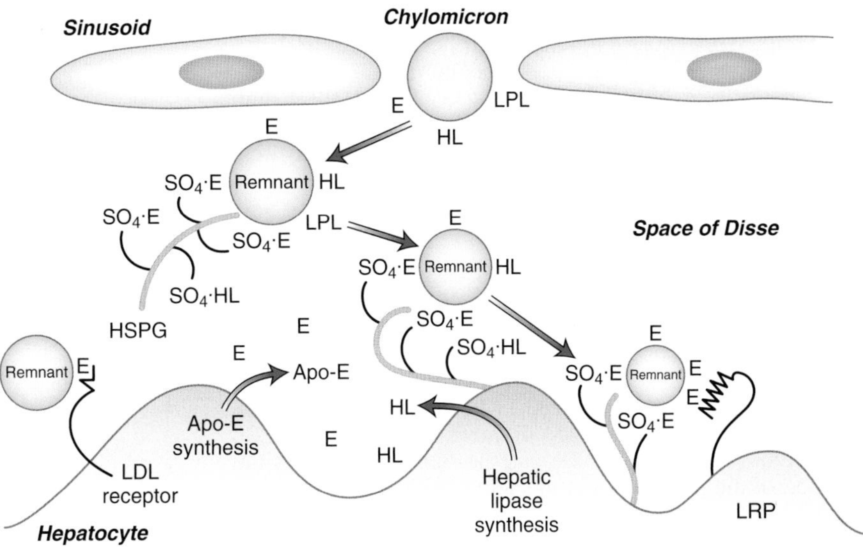

Figure 36–16 ■ Pathways involved in chylomicron remnant metabolism. In *sequestration,* chylomicron remnants are trapped in the space of Disse, through proteoglycan binding mediated by apolipoprotein E (E). In *processing,* enzymes, including lipases, can continue processing the remnants to smaller particles. In *uptake,* receptors involved in the uptake of the remnants appear to include the low-density lipoprotein (LDL) receptor and the LDL receptor–related protein (LRP). Apo-E, apolipoprotein E; HL, hepatic lipase; HSPG, heparan sulfate proteoglycans; LPL, lipoprotein lipase.

facilitate the binding and uptake of remnants by interacting with the LRP.

The actual uptake of the particles by hepatocytes can involve two or more receptors (see Fig. 36–16). the *LDL receptor,* which interacts with remnants containing apo-E, and a chylomicron remnant receptor, now known to be the LRP.[44,50,66,67]

Remnant particles with LPL or hepatic lipase on their surfaces can interact by means of these molecules with the HSPG in the space of Disse and facilitate binding and uptake by the LRP[76,77]; however, apo-E–mediated interactions with HSPG and the LRP or the LDL receptor are critical in remnant metabolism. Patients with apo-E mutations that prevent interaction with HSPG or lipoprotein receptors develop hyperlipidemia characterized by remnant lipoprotein accumulation despite having normal lipase activity.[45,50] In addition, knockout of apo-E by gene targeting in mice causes a massive accumulation of remnant lipoproteins.[51,52]

Role of the Low-Density Lipoprotein Receptor in Remnant Catabolism

The LDL receptor plays a key role in chylomicron remnant uptake by the liver.[50,66,67] The lack of accumulation of chylomicrons or chylomicron remnants in patients with absent or defective LDL receptors could reflect the fact that remnant clearance requires several steps, as described. For example, sequestration of the particles in the space of Disse (HSPG binding) is normal in patients with defective LDL receptors and could prevent the accumulation of remnants in plasma. Furthermore, the HSPG/LRP pathway can compensate for deficiency of LDL receptors. Both receptors probably function in the uptake of the remnants; if one is absent, the other continues to function.

Chylomicron Remnant Receptors in Remnant Catabolism

The LRP is the chylomicron remnant (apo-E) receptor, which belongs to the LDL receptor gene family (discussed previously).[66,67] The LRP binds with high affinity to apo-E–enriched lipoproteins but does not bind LDL to a significant extent. Apo-E must be added to remnant lipoproteins before they bind to the LRP with high affinity. Apo-E exists in the space of Disse in high concentration, probably because it is secreted by hepatocytes and binds to HSPG in the space of Disse. The HSPG might serve as a reservoir for apo-E, allowing enrichment of the remnants with this apolipoprotein (see Fig. 36–16).[45,50]

These and other observations have led to the hypothesis that apo-E functions in a process called *secretion-capture.*[50,96,97] It is envisioned that apo-E combines with lipids or lipoproteins and directs them to cells expressing LDL receptors or the LRP. In the liver, the LRP and apo-E could interact in this way to capture chylomicron remnants (see Fig. 36–16). The LRP is also present in other tissues, including brain, and might function locally in the uptake of lipids. The secretion-capture role of apo-E functions in peripheral nerve injury and repair and in the normal maintenance of neurons.[38,41]

As already stated, LRP-mediated uptake of remnants requires the initial interaction of apo-E–containing lipoproteins with cell-surface HSPG (see Fig. 36–16).[50] If HSPGs are hydrolyzed by treating cells with heparinase in vitro or by infusing heparinase into the portal vein of mice, apo-E–enriched remnants do not bind to the cell surface and do not interact with the LRP even though the receptor is present. After the lipoproteins interact with HSPG, the remnants may be transferred to the LRP for internalization by the cells, or the HSPG/LRP complex may be internalized. This two-step process involving cell-surface proteoglycans and receptors is referred to as the *HSPG/LRP pathway;* a similar two-step process has also been described for growth factors.[41,44,50] It is also possible that HSPG alone can mediate remnant uptake directly without the LRP.

Herz and colleagues demonstrated that the LRP is the chylomicron remnant (apo-E) receptor and documented its importance in remnant catabolism.[66,67] These studies used RAP, which blocks the interaction of all ligands with the LRP, to demonstrate the role of the LRP in remnant clearance in mice. Knockout of RAP in mice results in a loss of LRP expression in the liver. Double-knockout mice, in which both RAP and the LDL receptor are missing, develop hyperlipidemia characterized by the accumulation of remnant lipoproteins in the plasma.[98]

In summary, the catabolism of chylomicron remnants involves several steps and several components. sequestration, further lipolytic processing, and receptor-mediated endocytosis using both the LDL receptor pathway and the HSPG/LRP pathway.

Very-Low-Density Lipoproteins

Characteristics

VLDLs are particles 300 to 700 Å in diameter. Upon ultracentrifugation, they float at a density of less than 1.006 g/mL (see

Table 36–4). They are composed of 85% to 90% lipid (about 55% triglyceride, 20% cholesterol, and 15% phospholipid) and 10% to 15% protein. The distinctive apolipoprotein is apo-B100, the hepatic form of apo-B. VLDLs also contain apo-E and C apolipoproteins (see Fig. 36–5). VLDLs have pre-β or α_2-electrophoretic mobility and were previously called pre-β lipoproteins.[20,94]

Origin

VLDLs are synthesized by the liver, and their production is stimulated by increased delivery of FFAs to the hepatocytes, either from a high intake of dietary fat or from the mobilization of fatty acids from adipose tissue with fasting or uncontrolled diabetes mellitus. Triglycerides and phospholipids to be used in the formation of VLDL are synthesized in the liver, whereas VLDL cholesterol can be synthesized de novo or reused from LDL cholesterol (LDL-C). The VLDL particles are first visible at the junction of the rough ER and the smooth ER (transitional elements) before they enter the Golgi apparatus.[99] Several of the apolipoproteins undergo carbohydrate processing within the Golgi apparatus. Large Golgi secretory vesicles migrate to the brush border surface of the hepatocytes, fuse with the plasma membrane, and release the VLDL particles into the space of Disse, where they enter the plasma (Fig. 36–17). The major protein constituents of the newly synthesized VLDLs are apo-B100, apo-E, and small amounts of the C apolipoproteins. In plasma, VLDLs acquire additional C apolipoproteins and apo-E, primarily from HDL.

Although present in low concentration in the plasma, apo-AV is associated with plasma VLDL and modulates plasma triglyceride levels. Apo-AV appears to promote LPL-mediated lipolysis of VLDL.[62,63] Polymorphisms that decrease apo-AV are associated with hypertriglyceridemia.[64,65]

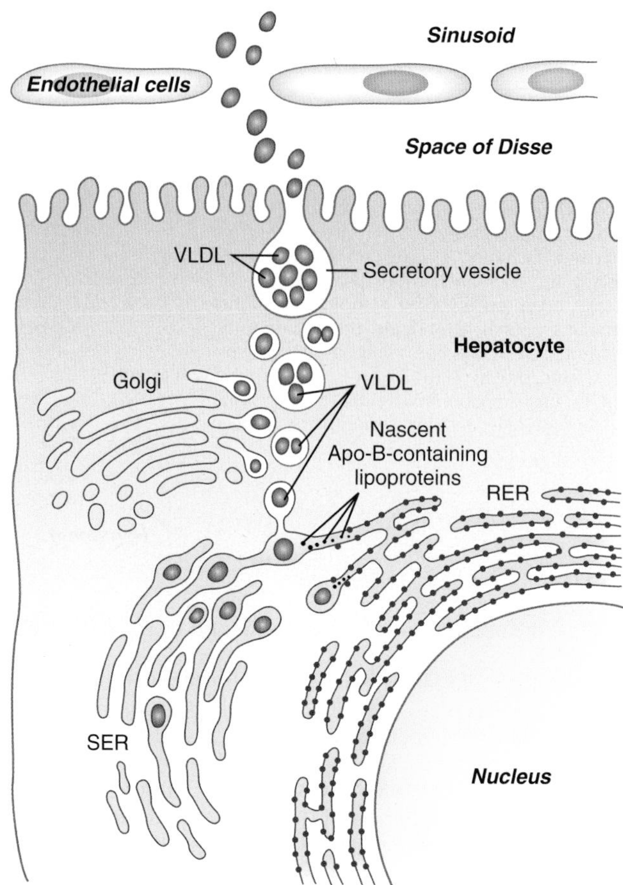

Figure 36–17 ▪ Very-low-density lipoprotein (VLDL) biosynthesis by hepatocytes. The nascent apolipoprotein B (apo-B)–containing apolipoproteins synthesized by the rough endoplasmic reticulum (RER) apparently combine with the lipids in the smooth endoplasmic reticulum (SER). The VLDLs are processed in the Golgi apparatus and accumulate in large secretory vesicles. They are then released into the space of Disse and enter the plasma. (Modified from Alexander CA, Hamilton RL, Havel RJ. Subcellular localization of B apoprotein of plasma lipoproteins in rat liver. J Cell Biol 1976;69:241-263; by copyright permission of The Rockefeller University Press.)

Control of Very-Low-Density Lipoprotein Secretion Rate

The quantity of VLDL secreted from the liver is not controlled by changes in apo-B100 mRNA levels. Apo-B100 is constitutively expressed and is not highly variable.[31,94,100,101] Newly synthesized apo-B100 is subject to two fates. It can be combined with lipid to form VLDL particles, or it can be degraded, in which case a VLDL particle is not secreted. If there is a stimulus for VLDL production, such as the delivery of FFAs to the liver, the balance is shifted away from apo-B100 degradation to the formation and secretion of apo-B100–containing VLDL.

Biosynthesis of Very-Low-Density Lipoproteins

Newly synthesized apo-B100 is translocated across the rough ER membrane. If not sufficiently lipidated as it is translocated, apo-B100 is destined to be degraded. If sufficient lipid is available, the apo-B100 binds the lipid as it enters the ER and forms triglyceride-rich particles. These particles can increase in size, enter the secretory pathway, and exit from the cell as mature VLDLs (see Fig. 36–17).[31,100,101] Apo-AV might promote VLDL assembly in the liver; however, the mechanism remains to be clearly defined (see Table 36–3).

The newly synthesized apo-B100 could associate with the inner leaflet of the ER and serve as a lipid nucleation site capable of accepting triglycerides to form a central core for the VLDL particles. Triglycerides and possibly cholesteryl esters and phospholipids are transferred into the particle by the microsomal triglyceride transfer protein (MTP),[102] and additional triglyceride, cholesterol, and phospholipid may be added as the VLDL precursor passes through the lumen of the rough ER. At the junction of the rough and smooth ER, lipid-rich particles lacking apo-B have been identified in rat liver, and these particles might fuse with the apo-B–containing VLDL precursors to form the mature particle. However, because rat liver synthesizes both apo-B100– and apo-B48–containing VLDLs, the fusion step might apply only to apo-B48 VLDL and may be more relevant to apo-B48–containing chylomicron synthesis by the intestine.

Microsomal Triglyceride Transfer Protein

MTP is produced in the liver at sites where apo-B100–containing VLDLs are synthesized and in the intestine at sites where apo-B48–containing chylomicrons are synthesized. MTP (97 kd) occurs as a heterodimer complex with the 58-kd protein disulfide isomerase, an association required for MTP activity. Protein disulfide isomerase reshuffles disulfide bonds of cysteine residues and therefore can play a role in altering the conformation of apo-B for lipidation. In addition to transferring triglycerides to these lipoprotein particles, MTP transfers cholesteryl esters and phospholipids.[102]

More than a dozen mutations of MTP interfere with its activity. Defective MTP is responsible for the lipid disorder abetalipoproteinemia, a condition in which patients essentially lack apo-B–containing lipoproteins in plasma.[102,103] Therefore, MTP is critical for the biosynthesis of both apo-B100 VLDLs in the liver and apo-B48 chylomicrons in the intestine.

The luminal surfaces of the hepatocytes express LDL receptors and the LRP, and VLDLs possess both apo-B100 and apo-E that can react with these receptors. How then do VLDLs traverse the space of Disse and enter the blood? First, lipids such as phosphatidylethanolamine on the surface of the newly secreted VLDLs can alter the reactivity of the lipoproteins with the receptors. Newly secreted VLDLs are rich in phosphatidylethanolamine, but VLDLs in the circulation are poor in phosphatidylethanolamine. This phospholipid can prevent the particle from interacting with the receptors (i.e., specific lipids can mask the receptor-binding domains of apo-B100 and apo-E).

Second, other apolipoproteins can mask the receptor-binding domains of the VLDL apo-B100 and apo-E. Although they are present in small amounts on newly secreted VLDLs, the C apolipoproteins can alter the conformation or availability of apolipoproteins that interact with lipoprotein receptors. Specifically, when VLDLs are formed in the liver and acquire apo-E, the C apolipoproteins may be positioned so as to mask the apo-E, blocking its ability to react with the receptor or with proteoglycans in the space of Disse. Alternatively, apo-E associated with the particles intracellularly might not be available to bind to the receptors; only newly acquired apo-E obtained from HDL might have the appropriate conformation for receptor binding.

Metabolic Fate

VLDL triglycerides are hydrolyzed by the actions of LPL and hepatic lipase. They are converted to smaller and smaller particles that become increasingly rich in cholesterol (see Fig. 36–14). The products of VLDL catabolism are IDLs (d = 1.006-1.019 g/mL). IDLs retain apo-B100 and apo-E but have lost most of the C apolipoproteins. IDLs are processed to LDLs (d = 1.019-1.063 g/mL) by LPL, with final processing by hepatic lipase. Approximately half of VLDLs are converted to LDLs, and the remainder are cleared directly by the liver as VLDL remnants (small VLDL) and IDLs (see Fig. 36–14). The uptake of VLDL remnants and IDLs by liver parenchymal cells is mediated by apo-E, and the uptake of LDL by the LDL receptor is mediated by apo-B100.[4,5,38,94]

Intermediate-Density Lipoproteins

IDLs (d = 1.006-1.019 g/mL) are normally present in low concentrations in the plasma and are intermediate in size and composition between VLDL and LDL (see Table 36–4). Their primary proteins are apo-B100 and apo-E.[4,94] The IDLs are precursors of LDLs and represent metabolic products of VLDL catabolism in the plasma by the action of lipases. As shown in Figure 36–15, IDLs may be further processed by hepatic lipase or removed from the plasma by the LDL receptor. IDLs are often considered to be VLDL remnants and to be atherogenic.

Low-Density Lipoproteins

Characteristics

LDLs (d = 1.019-1.063 g/mL), which are about 200 Å in diameter, are the major cholesterol-carrying lipoproteins in the plasma; about 70% of total plasma cholesterol is in LDL. LDLs are composed of approximately 75% lipid (about 35% cholesteryl ester, 10% free cholesterol, 10% triglyceride, and 20% phospholipid) and 25% protein (see Table 36–4). Apo-B100 is the principal protein in these particles, along with trace amounts of apo-E (see Fig. 36–5). LDLs have β-electrophoretic mobility and were previously referred to as β lipoproteins.[2,94]

Origin

LDLs are the end products of lipase-mediated hydrolysis of VLDLs (see Fig. 36–15). Moreover, as the triglyceride-rich core of the larger VLDL particles is removed, the surface lipids and proteins are remodeled and excess surface constituents are transferred to HDL, resulting in the formation of a small, cholesterol-rich LDL devoid of almost all apolipoproteins except apo-B100.

Metabolic Fate

About 75% of LDL is taken up by hepatocytes (see Fig. 36–15). Other tissues take up smaller amounts of LDL. Approximately two thirds of the uptake is mediated by the LDL receptor, and the remainder is mediated by a poorly defined process that does not involve receptors. LDLs are considered to be atherogenic.

Apolipoproteins B and E Determine Rate of Plasma Lipoprotein Clearance

The rate of clearance of lipoproteins from the plasma is determined by the apolipoprotein that mediates the interaction with the receptor and by the number of receptors expressed on the cell surface (primarily in the liver). VLDL and IDL are rapidly cleared from the plasma (their half-lives are measured in minutes to a few hours). Apo-E mediates their binding to the LDL receptors. Multiple apo-E molecules per lipoprotein can interact with more than one receptor or with multiple sites on a receptor. Multiple interactions enhance binding affinity and increase the clearance of these particles from the plasma. The clearance of LDL is mediated by apo-B100. The affinity of apo-B100 for the LDL receptor is lower than that of apo-E, and clearance of LDL is much slower (with a half-life of 2 to 3 days). Compared with apo-B100–containing LDLs, apo-E–containing lipoproteins have 20-fold greater affinity for the LDL receptor.[20,28,38]

This difference in affinity can affect the circulating levels of lipoproteins containing apo-B100 and apo-E. In the presence of high levels of apo-E associated with remnants, VLDL, and IDL, these lipoproteins compete effectively with LDL for binding to the LDL receptor, and LDL levels can rise. Conversely, in the presence of low levels of apo-E or of apo-E that is defective in receptor-binding activity (apo-E2 associated with type III hyperlipoproteinemia), these lipoproteins do not compete effectively with LDL for the LDL receptor; as a result, the LDL concentrations are lower. Thus, the difference in the affinities of apo-B100 and apo-E plays a role in plasma cholesterol homeostasis.

Role of Lipoprotein Cholesterol in Cellular Metabolism

All cells can synthesize cholesterol de novo.[1-4] However, LDL serves as a source of cholesterol for many cells. Cholesterol taken up by the liver has several fates. membrane biosynthesis, VLDL biosynthesis, excretion as cholesterol in the bile, and conversion to bile acids. Cholesterol is used as a precursor for steroid hormone production in the adrenals, ovaries, and testes. In other peripheral tissues, cholesterol is used in membrane biosynthesis for cell repair and proliferation.

Factors Affecting Low-Density Lipoprotein Levels in the Blood

Plasma LDL levels can be increased through two primary mechanisms. One is increased VLDL biosynthesis and secretion caused by increased flux of FFAs to the liver from dietary fats or from mobilization from adipose tissue, and the other is decreased LDL catabolism. Decreased catabolism can result from decreased LDL receptor levels in hepatic and extrahepatic tissues (LDL receptor expression is down-regulated when cells have enough cholesterol for their metabolic needs or when diets are high in saturated fat and cholesterol). Catabolism can also be decreased by increased numbers of high-affinity apo-E–containing lipoproteins that compete with LDL for receptor interaction, by defective LDL receptors incapable of normal interaction with apo-B100, or by defective apo-B100 incapable of normal interaction with LDL receptors.

High-Density Lipoproteins

Characteristics

HDLs are small particles (70-120 Å in diameter) that float at densities of 1.063 to 1.21 g/mL. They are somewhat arbitrarily divided into two major subclasses. HDL_2 (d = 1.063-1.125 g/mL) and HDL_3 (d = 1.125-1.21 g/mL). HDLs contain about 50% lipid (25% phospholipid, 15% cholesteryl ester, 5% free cholesterol, and 5% triglyceride) and 50% protein (see Table 36–4). Their major apolipoproteins are apo-AI (65%), apo-AII (25%), and smaller amounts of the C apolipoproteins and apo-E (see Fig. 36–5). Apo-E is a minor component of a subclass of HDL referred to as HDL_1, but about 50% of total plasma apo-E is in this HDL fraction. The major classes of HDLs lack apo-E and therefore do not interact with the LDL receptor. HDLs serve as a reservoir for apo-E and the C apolipoproteins to be distributed to other lipoproteins when they enter the plasma (e.g., chylomicrons, VLDLs). Subclasses of HDL can contain only apo-AI (called LpAI) or apo-AI and apo-AII (called LpAI/AII). Although LpAI and LpAI/AII do not correspond directly to the ultracentrifugal fractions, LpAI corresponds primarily to HDL_2 and LpAI/AII to HDL_3. The HDLs as a class have α-electrophoretic mobility and previously were referred to as α lipoproteins.[19,53,54,57,94,104]

Origin

HDLs originate from three major sources (Fig. 36–18). First, the liver secretes an apo-AI-phospholipid disc called *nascent* or *precursor HDL* (pre-β HDL). Second, the intestine directly synthesizes a small apo-AI–containing HDL particle. Third, HDLs are derived from surface material (primarily apo-AI and phospholipid) that comes from chylomicrons and VLDLs during lipolysis. As chylomicrons and VLDLs are acted on by LPL and the triglyceride-rich core is hydrolyzed, excess material is shed from the surface of the particle in combination with apo-AI to form small HDL discs. The phospholipid transfer protein facilitates the shedding of the surface material during lipolytic processing of triglyceride-rich lipoproteins to generate the HDL precursors.[105]

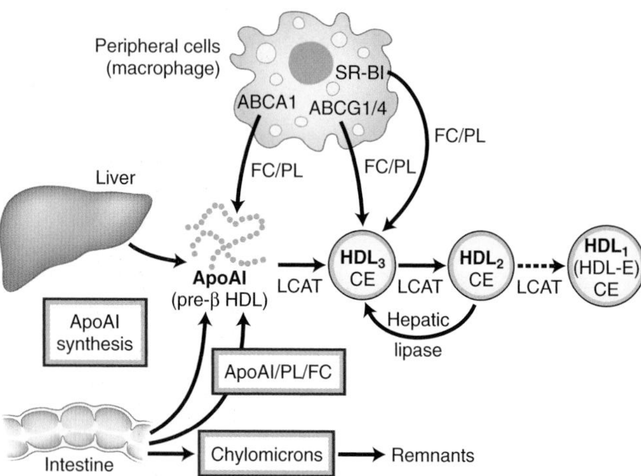

Figure 36–18 ▪ Origin of high-density lipoprotein (HDL) from liver, intestine, and surface material from chylomicrons and very-low-density lipoprotein (VLDL). ABCA, ATP binding cassette transporter; AI, apo-AI; CE, cholesteryl ester; FC, free cholesterol; HDL-E, HDL with apo-E; LCAT, lecithin:cholesterol acyltransferase; PL, phospholipid; SR-BI, class B, type I scavenger receptor; Tg, triglyceride.

Maturation of High-Density Lipoproteins

Apo-AI that is lipid-free or poorly lipidated can occur in the plasma and serve as a cholesterol and phospholipid acceptor (see Fig. 36–18). The nascent or precursor HDL particles exist as apo-AI-phospholipid discs. Designated pre-β_1, pre-β_2, and pre-β_3,[53,54,57,94,104] these discs are excellent acceptors of free cholesterol from cells with excess cholesterol or from other lipoproteins. The pre-β phospholipid discs can accommodate only a limited amount of free cholesterol. However, esterification of the cholesterol with a long-chain fatty acid increases its hydrophobicity, and the newly formed cholesteryl ester moves away from the surface of the disc, beginning the process of forming a cholesteryl ester–rich core and converting the disc to a sphere. The enzyme in plasma that converts free cholesterol to cholesteryl ester is LCAT.

The small, spherical, mature HDL particles (HDL_3) also serve as acceptors for free cholesterol; as more free cholesterol is acquired and esterified, the particles increase in size, forming HDL_2. These HDL subclasses can include LpAI, or they can be converted to LpAI/AII particles by the addition of apo-AII.

In some animals, and to a lesser extent in humans, HDL_2 can be further enriched in cholesteryl ester and at the same time acquire apo-E (Fig. 36–19). These apo-E–containing HDL_1 are a minor but metabolically active subclass of HDL.[20,28] The presence of apo-E targets the HDL_1 to cells expressing the LDL recep-

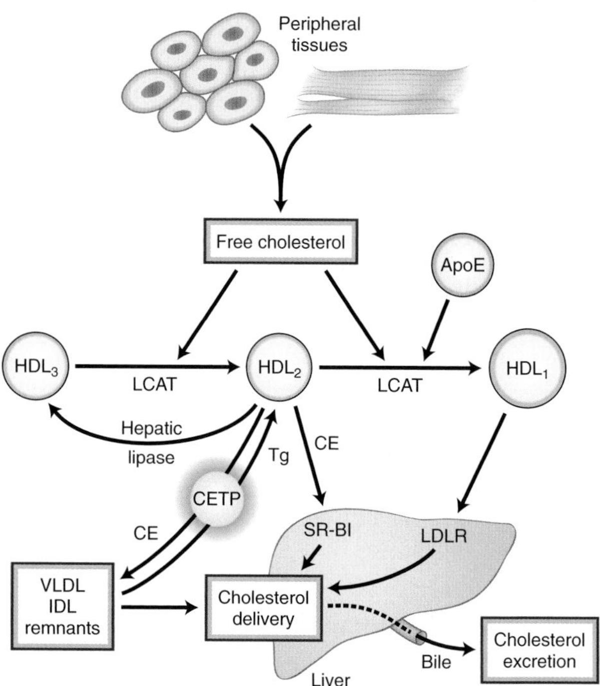

Figure 36–19 ▪ Role of high-density lipoprotein (HDL) in the redistribution of lipids from cells with excess cholesterol to cells requiring cholesterol or to the liver for excretion. The reverse cholesterol transport pathway is indicated by arrows (net transfer of cholesterol from cells → HDL → LDL → liver). CE, cholesteryl ester; CETP, cholesteryl ester transfer protein; FC, free cholesterol; HDL-E, HDL with apolipoprotein E; IDL, intermediate-density lipoprotein; LCAT, lecithin:cholesterol acyltransferase; LDL, low-density lipoprotein; LDLR, LDL receptor; PL, phospholipid; SR-BI, class B, type I scavenger receptor; Tg, triglyceride; VLDL, very-low-density lipoprotein.

tor. Typical HDLs lack apo-E and do not interact with the LDL receptor. The HDL_1 represent a major HDL class in many other species and in humans with abetalipoproteinemia or CETP deficiency.

HDL_1 can also arise from a precursor particle that displays γ-electrophoretic mobility and is called γLp-E.[106] This particle is approximately 80% protein and 20% lipid (primarily sphingomyelin and phosphatidylcholine, with some free cholesterol). The γLp-E is a good acceptor of free cholesterol from cells and appears to be converted to the larger HDL_1 by the action of LCAT. HDL_1 also contains apo-AI and sometimes apo-AII. It is difficult to fractionate these various subclasses of HDL.

Acquisition of Cholesterol by High-Density Lipoproteins

HDL, especially HDL_3, precursors of mature HDL, and lipid-poor apo-AI, can acquire cholesterol from cells by two mechanisms. aqueous transfer from cells and transport facilitated by a cell-surface binding protein (see Fig. 36–18).[53,54,57,104]

Aqueous Transfer from Cells

The HDLs come in close contact with cells having excess cholesterol and acquire free cholesterol (not cholesteryl ester) from the cell surface. Free cholesterol follows a physicochemical concentration gradient from the cell to the HDL particle, from a high concentration of free cholesterol in the membranes of cells with excess cholesterol to a low concentration at the surface of the HDL. This process is referred to as *passive desorption.*

Transport Facilitated by a Cell-Surface Binding Protein

At least four cell-surface proteins facilitate the efflux of free cholesterol from cells possessing excess cholesterol (see Fig. 36–18). The SR-BI binds HDL particles to the cell surface. This receptor can alter the organization of the cell membrane lipids, facilitating the efflux of free cholesterol from the membrane to the lipoprotein. The HDLs are not internalized by the cell and are released into the circulation when the particle is enriched in cholesterol.[53,54,57] The second receptor that participates in the efflux of cholesterol from cells is ABCA1. It appears to bind apo-AI or a pre-β HDL disc to the cell membrane and facilitate the transfer of free cholesterol and phospholipid from the cell to enrich the HDL precursors in these lipids.[53,104,107,108] Mutations in ABCA1 prevent the efflux of cholesterol from cells, resulting in absence of mature HDL and rapid catabolism of apo-AI and causing the lipid disorder called *Tangier disease.*[53,54,57,109] Two other ATP binding cassette transporters (ABCG1 and ABCG4) have been shown to mediate cholesterol efflux. However, they stimulate efflux to the mature HDL, including HDL_2 and HDL_3.[56]

Enzyme Involved in High-Density Lipoprotein Metabolism. Lecithin:Cholesterol Acyltransferase

LCAT (47 kd, 416 amino acids) is synthesized as a glycoprotein (25% of total mass is carbohydrate) primarily by the liver and to a lesser extent in the brain and testes.[90,91,94,110] In the plasma, it is associated primarily with LpAI or pre-β_3 and small mature HDL and to a lesser extent with LDL. Activated by apo-AI (and by apo-CI and apo-AIV), LCAT is responsible for the production of most cholesteryl esters in plasma lipoproteins in humans. Although HDLs are the preferred substrate for LCAT, a small fraction of free cholesterol is esterified on LDLs; LCAT has both α-LCAT activity (acting on HDL) and β-LCAT activity (acting on LDL). In the human disorder called *fish-eye disease,* a single amino acid substitution of threonine for isoleucine-123 blocks the ability of LCAT to esterify cholesterol in HDL, but the mutated protein still catalyzes the esterification of cholesterol on LDL. Therefore, this form of LCAT deficiency is less severe than complete LCAT deficiency.

LCAT has two different enzymatic activities. First, *lecithin cleavage (phospholipase activity)* involves the ester bond of the fatty acid in position 2 of lecithin, which is usually linoleic acid (C18:2), yielding lysolecithin and the fatty acid. The fatty acid becomes covalently linked to Ser-181 in the LCAT molecule. Second, *transesterification (transacylase activity)* involves the transfer of the fatty acid attached to LCAT to the 3β-hydroxyl position of cholesterol, forming a cholesteryl ester. The mechanism for the transfer of the fatty acid to cholesterol has not been well defined.

Much has been learned about the normal function of LCAT in lipoprotein metabolism by studying patients who have low or undetectable activity of this enzyme in plasma. LCAT deficiency can be caused by mutations that affect the structure of LCAT or of apo-AI. The disorder is manifested by low levels of cholesteryl esters, low levels of HDL, and clinical features ranging from mild symptoms such as corneal clouding (caused by accumulation of free cholesterol in the cornea) to severe disorders such as renal failure (see "Lecithin:Cholesterol Acyltransferase Deficiency").

Metabolic Pathways Involving High-Density Lipoproteins

HDLs function in the redistribution of lipids among lipoproteins and cells by a process called *reverse cholesterol transport.*[53,54,57] HDLs acquire cholesterol from cells and transport it to the liver for excretion or to other cells that require cholesterol. The scheme is shown in Figure 36–19.[54,90]

HDL_3 particles are converted to HDL_2 and then to HDL_1. Apo-E, which is associated with HDL_1, targets this minor HDL subclass to cells expressing LDL receptors.[20,28] In this way, cholesterol can be redistributed from cells that have excess cholesterol to cells that require cholesterol. This apo-E–mediated pathway can also deliver cholesterol to the liver for excretion. HDL_1 is a major transport pathway for cholesteryl ester delivery to the liver in some species (mice, rats, and dogs) but not in humans.

A second pathway of cholesterol redistribution involves CETP (see Fig. 36–19).[92,93,104,111] CETP transfers cholesteryl ester from HDL_2 to VLDL, IDL, LDL, and remnants. The cholesterol is thus delivered indirectly to the liver through VLDL and chylomicron remnant pathways. In exchange for transfer of the cholesteryl ester, CETP transfers triglyceride from VLDL, IDL, LDL, and remnants to HDL_2, which becomes enriched with triglycerides. The CETP pathway is the major route for the transport and delivery of cholesteryl esters from HDL to the liver in humans, nonhuman primates, and rabbits.

A third pathway involves SR-BI (see Fig. 36–19). Cholesteryl esters are removed from the particle by selective uptake and preferentially delivered to the liver, adrenal glands, and gonads.[108] The SR-BI can facilitate the transfer of cholesteryl esters from HDL to cells without the lipoprotein particle's entering the cell or being degraded. The SR-BI appears to function by transferring cholesteryl ester through a hydrophilic channel formed in the cell membrane.[108] Hepatic lipase may be involved in the selective uptake of cholesterol from the HDL by hydrolyzing the phospholipids on the particles and creating a chemical gradient that promotes the transfer of cholesterol from the particle to the cell. Recall that hepatic lipase is localized in the space of Disse of the liver and in the adrenal glands and ovaries.

HDL_2 Is Reconverted to HDL_3 to Regenerate These Cholesterol Acceptors

As stated previously, HDL_2 particles are partially depleted of cholesteryl esters and enriched in triglycerides by the action of

CETP. Hepatic lipase can then act on the large, triglyceride-enriched HDL_2 to hydrolyze the triglycerides (and possibly excess phospholipids), converting HDL_2 to HDL_3.[85] HDL_3 serves as an acceptor of free cholesterol, thus perpetuating the HDL_2-HDL_3 cycle (see Figs. 36–18 and 36–19).[112]

The mechanism of HDL catabolism is not entirely understood, but ultimately the particles are degraded in the liver. Although the HDL with apo-E represents a small fraction of total HDL, apo-E targets these particles to the liver, where they are taken up by the LDL receptors. In the kidneys, apo-AI is dissociated from the HDL, filtered, and degraded.

Selective Uptake of Cholesterol by Steroidogenic Cells

HDL is more efficient than LDL in delivering cholesterol to steroidogenic cells of the adrenal, ovary, and testis. In these organs, the lipoproteins concentrate on the surface of cells in microvillar channels.[108,113] The channels appear to represent flaps of cell-surface membrane that form a 150- to 250-Å-wide cleft in which the lipoproteins are trapped at least transiently. Within these channels, cholesteryl ester and free cholesterol can be extracted from the HDLs without endocytosis or degradation of the particles. Hepatic lipase is selectively localized to the same organs and is believed to modify HDL so as to facilitate the selective uptake of cholesterol. The SR-BI is highly expressed in steroidogenic cells, where it functions in the selective uptake of cholesteryl esters from HDL without internalization and degradation of the lipoproteins. The particles reenter the circulation after the cholesterol is extracted.[113]

The importance of HDL and specifically apo-AI–containing HDL for delivery of cholesterol to steroidogenic cells has been shown in apo-AI knockout mice.[108] In the adrenal glands, the reticularis and fasciculata cells are usually loaded with lipid droplets. In knockout mice, however, there is no lipid in these cells, lipoproteins are absent from the microvillar channels, and luteal cells of the ovary and Leydig's cells of the testis have markedly reduced levels of lipid. However, lipid and cell-surface lipoprotein particles are present in the adrenal gland, ovary, or testis of knockout mice lacking apo-AII or apo-E. Therefore, apo-AI appears to play an important role, possibly by targeting the particles to the channels or by providing particles with the proper composition to allow their entry into the channels for selective delivery of cholesterol to the cells. The importance of the apo-AI-HDL pathway in delivering cholesterol to the adrenal is further shown by the blunted synthesis and secretion of glucocorticoids in apo-AI knockout mice that are acutely stressed.

Cholesteryl Ester Transfer Protein

CETP facilitates the transfer of cholesteryl esters from HDL to the lower density, triglyceride-rich lipoproteins (primarily VLDL, IDL, and remnants).[92,93] CETP plays a pivotal role in lipid metabolism and can affect susceptibility or resistance to the development of atherosclerosis.[114] For example, humans, nonhuman primates, and rabbits have significant amounts of CETP activity in their plasma. As a consequence, they form only small amounts of HDL_1; they dispose of most of their HDL cholesteryl esters by delivering them to lower-density lipoproteins (see Fig. 36–19). Ultimately, most of the cholesteryl esters leave the plasma by the LDL pathway. These species are susceptible to atherosclerosis and tend to have higher levels of LDL. On the other hand, rats, mice, and dogs have no CETP activity, readily form HDL_1, and can deliver the cholesterol directly to the liver by the apo-E–mediated pathway. These animals have very low levels of LDL and are resistant to the development of atherosclerosis. These observations suggest that high levels of CETP activity accelerate atherogenesis and that inhibition of CETP may be beneficial in treating certain types of hyperlipidemia.

However, this concept has been brought into question by the observation that Japanese Americans with a deficiency of CETP have increased HDL but nevertheless develop CHD.[92,93] The HDL in these subjects tends to be the large HDL_1, and levels of the smaller HDL_3 are decreased. If these data concerning the atherogenicity of low CETP activity are confirmed, it might mean that low levels of HDL_3, which serves as the most potent acceptor of cellular cholesterol, are a major risk factor for CHD in these subjects; alternatively, high levels of the large apo-E–containing HDL_1 may be atherogenic.

Data obtained through overexpression of CETP in transgenic mice do not clarify whether high levels are protective or detrimental.[19,92,114] In one study, overexpression of CETP led to accelerated atherogenesis,[115] but in a study in which CETP was overexpressed in hypertriglyceridemic mice expressing high levels of apo-CIII, there was less atherosclerosis even though the mice were hyperlipidemic and had low HDL levels.[92] The potential therapeutic value of lowering CETP to retard atherogenesis must be questioned until these inconsistencies are sorted out.

High-Density Lipoproteins as Antiatherogenic Lipoproteins

Numerous studies have demonstrated that high levels of HDL-C are associated with a lower incidence of CHD. Conversely, low levels of HDL-C are associated with a higher incidence of CHD.[116] The protective mechanism involving HDL may be related to its role in reverse cholesterol transport, which results in redistribution of cholesterol away from the artery wall. Other potentially protective roles for HDL include inhibition of monocyte adhesion and antioxidative activity that could prevent LDL oxidation. HDLs contain paraoxonase and PAF-AH that possess antioxidative activity. HDL_3 appear to be the most potent inhibitors of LDL oxidation. It must be kept in mind that the HDLs are a heterogeneous group of molecules having different metabolic roles. Some may be protective (e.g., LpAI, HDL_2), and others may not be (e.g., LpAI/AII). As the complex nature of HDL is unraveled, it may be possible to define an antiatherogenic spectrum of HDL particles and determine the metabolic and therapeutic measures needed to alter these HDLs selectively.

Lipids and Atherosclerosis

Cholesterol and Cardiovascular Disease

Despite a very significant decrease in the incidence of vascular disease, CHD, cerebrovascular disease, and peripheral vascular disease remain the major causes of death in the United States (39% in 2001). The major risk factors are elevated LDL-C, reduced HDL-C, smoking, hypertension, insulin resistance with or without overt diabetes mellitus, age, and family history of premature CHD. Modifiable risk factors account for 85% of the excess CHD risk. Especially important is plasma cholesterol. Total cholesterol levels of less than 160 mg/dL markedly decrease CHD risk, even in the presence of other risk factors. Although a number of new risk factors have been proposed to increase the accuracy of predicting risk of CHD events, one of four conditions (dyslipidemia, hypertension, cigarette smoking, and diabetes) accounts for increased CHD risk in 90% of patients.[117,118]

The major role of hypercholesterolemia gave rise to the universally accepted cholesterol-diet-CHD hypothesis. This hypothesis states that increased plasma cholesterol concentrations increase the risk of CHD, that diets high in fat (especially saturated fat of animal origin) and cholesterol increase plasma cholesterol levels, and that lowering plasma cholesterol levels decreases the risk of CHD. Proof that cholesterol lowering prevented CHD required extensive epidemiologic studies and clinical trials.

Epidemiologic Evidence

Several epidemiologic studies have demonstrated a relation between the plasma cholesterol level and the risk of CHD. For example, the Multiple Risk Factor Intervention Trial (MRFIT) (Fig. 36–20) showed that there is increased risk at levels greater than 5.2 mM/L (200 mg/dL).[119] The Seven Countries Study also demonstrated a relation between an increased incidence of CHD and high plasma cholesterol levels.[120] The causal relationship between elevated plasma cholesterol levels and accelerated atherosclerosis is established. Epidemiologic studies have linked the intake of high levels of dietary fat, especially saturated fats, with increased plasma cholesterol levels.[10,11,120] Likewise, diets high in cholesterol also tend to increase plasma cholesterol levels.[10,11] Therefore, restriction of saturated fat and cholesterol is the cornerstone of dietary therapy to reduce elevated blood cholesterol levels.

Clinical Trials

Final compelling evidence supporting the cholesterol-diet-heart hypothesis comes from multiple human clinical trials examining the efficacy of several lipid-lowering drugs in reducing CHD (reviewed in the section on treatment of lipid disorders, clinical trials). In all groups examined, including patients with and without preexisting CHD over a range of initial plasma cholesterol levels, the results unequivocally demonstrated that sufficient lowering of plasma cholesterol levels reduces the risk of CHD regardless of baseline cholesterol levels (discussed later).

In summary, the current evidence overwhelmingly supports the cholesterol-diet-heart hypothesis and upholds the conclusion of the Cholesterol Consensus Conference on Lowering Blood Cholesterol to Prevent Coronary Heart Disease organized by the National Heart, Lung, and Blood Institute. that the cause-and-effect relation between cholesterol and CHD is clearly established.[121]

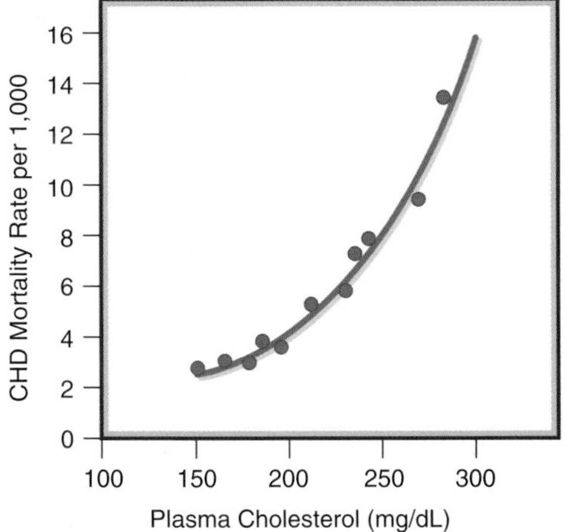

Figure 36–20 ■ Relation between plasma cholesterol levels and coronary heart disease (CHD) mortality in the Multiple Risk Factor Intervention Trial. (Modified from Stamler J, Wentworth D, Neaton JD. Is relationship between serum cholesterol and risk of premature death from coronary heart disease continuous and graded? Findings in 356,222 primary screenees of the Multiple Risk Factor Intervention Trial (MRFIT). JAMA 1986;256:2823-2828; Copyright © 1986, by the American Medical Association.)

Atherogenic Lipoproteins

In addition to LDL, almost all lipoproteins that contain apo-B100 (VLDL, β-VLDL, IDL, lipoprotein(a) [Lp(a)], and oxidized LDL) or apo-B48 (chylomicron remnants) are considered to be atherogenic. A common feature of these atherogenic lipoproteins is that they contain cholesteryl esters. In addition, Lp(a) contains apo(a), a protein that is disulfide-linked to apo-B and is homologous to plasminogen; apo(a) might contribute to atherogenesis by mechanisms related to thrombosis.[122] Finally, the atherogenic potential of LDL differs among the various LDL size and density subclasses, with the small, dense LDL subclass being the most atherogenic.[123]

Apo-B–containing remnant lipoproteins appear to be especially atherogenic[124,125] because β-VLDLs, which accumulate in the plasma of cholesterol-fed animals and in patients with type III hyperlipoproteinemia, are associated with accelerated formation of atherosclerotic lesions. These particles, representing chylomicron remnants and VLDL remnants (IDL), are taken up by macrophages, including, presumably, macrophages in the artery wall, in a nonsaturable manner. This uptake results in massive intracellular accumulation of cholesteryl esters in the form of lipid droplets. The lipid-engorged macrophages resemble the foam cells of the early fatty streak (discussed later).

Another related class of potentially atherogenic apo-B–containing lipoproteins is triglyceride-rich lipoproteins, which are associated with postprandial lipemia after ingestion of a fatty meal.[125] Whereas chylomicrons and large, triglyceride-rich VLDLs are not believed to be atherogenic, remnants derived from these particles are.

The Low-Density Lipoprotein Paradox and Oxidized Lipids

Because LDL-C levels are a strong predictor of CHD and atherosclerosis, it was expected that LDL would be taken up avidly by macrophages, leading to the formation of foam cells. However, in vitro experiments showed that only low levels of normal plasma LDL are taken up by macrophages. This low uptake presumably occurred because of the highly regulated LDL receptor pathway; the delivery of LDL-C to macrophages down-regulates LDL receptor expression, thereby protecting the cells from overaccumulation of LDL-C. These results led to the LDL paradox. How do LDLs contribute to atherosclerosis if only limited quantities are taken up by macrophages?[126] The explanation turned out to be that LDLs that have been modified are taken up by macrophages in an unregulated manner through receptors unrelated to the LDL receptor. These receptors are now commonly referred to as scavenger receptors (discussed in "Scavenger Receptors").[81,82]

In vitro experiments have demonstrated that a number of chemical modifications, including acetylation, acetoacetylation, and reaction with malondialdehyde, circumvent the LDL receptor pathway and cause massive amounts of modified LDL to enter macrophages by means of scavenger receptors. Furthermore, macrophages can alter LDL so that these particles can be taken up by macrophages in an unregulated manner. Other cells, including smooth muscle cells, can also modify LDL.[126]

The physiologically important LDL modification probably involves oxidation and results in lipid peroxidation. The oxidized-LDL hypothesis proposes that unsaturated lipids on the particle undergo oxidative modification, which subsequently leads to oxidation of apo-B, which alters the protein's affinity for cell-surface receptors. It appears that production of reactive oxygen species (i.e., free radicals) is an integral part of the modification and may be related to the general aging process, in which lipid peroxidation may be a component. Two products of lipid peroxidation, 4-hydroxynonenal and malondialdehyde, modify amino acids of apo-B100, resulting in its fragmentation. Modification is inhibited by antioxidants. Phospholipase and lipoxygenases have also been implicated in LDL modification. In addition to macrophage uptake, oxidized LDLs might participate directly in atherogenesis because they are cytotoxic, might serve as chemoattractants for circulating monocyte-macrophages, and are immunogenic.[81,82]

The role of oxidized LDL as a major contributor to atherosclerosis remains to be proved in vivo.[127] However, what appear to be oxidatively modified forms of LDL have been identified in atherosclerotic lesions and inflammatory fluid. Also, epitopes of malondialdehyde- and 4-hydroxynonenal-modified apo-B100 have been observed in lesions. Therefore, the formation of oxidized LDL, which can contribute to atherogenesis in a number of ways, is an attractive solution to the LDL paradox.

The most probable mechanism by which oxidized or modified LDLs are taken up by macrophages is by one or more of the scavenger receptors (see "Scavenger Receptors"). The roles of the various scavenger receptors and their relative importance in atherogenesis are still being clarified.[81,82,126] However, the receptor whose primary function is to take up oxidized or modified LDL within the artery wall and to contribute to the development and progression of atherosclerosis may well remain to be identified.

Overview of Atherogenesis

Atherogenesis involves several processes starting in the artery wall and ultimately leading to impaired blood flow to the cardiac muscle, brain, and peripheral organs, causing ischemia or infarction. One of the processes has been termed *response to injury,* in which endothelial cell dysfunction occurs in response to various injurious agents that damage the artery wall and initiate lesion formation.[128] Cholesterol-rich atherogenic lipoproteins can themselves injure the endothelium and can also contribute to the lipid accumulation in the intima of the artery.

The response-to-retention hypothesis envisions that the atherogenic lipoproteins are bound to arterial proteoglycans in the intima, where they undergo chemical modification.[129,130] Oxidation and other modifications of the retained lipoproteins target these lipoproteins for uptake by macrophages and initiate lesion formation.

It is now recognized that lesion formation involves a prominent inflammatory response in which monocytes become lipid-laden macrophage foam cells and lymphocytes and produce various inflammatory molecules and proteolytic enzymes that alter the nature of the lesion.[131] T-cells (predominantly $CD4^+$ lymphocytes) are always present in atherosclerotic lesions.[132] Antigens, such as oxidized LDL, are presented by macrophages to the type 1 helper T (Th1) cells, which then begin producing the macrophage-activating cytokine interferon-γ. This cytokine and others initiate the production of inflammatory and cytotoxic molecules from macrophages. These actions promote atherosclerosis. Inhibition of the Th1 pathway pharmacologically or genetically reduces atherogenesis in animals. The inflammatory cytokines from activated immune cells in the lesions induce the production of interleukin-6 (produced by various tissues), which enters the general circulation and stimulates the production of acute-phase reactants, such as C-reactive protein (CRP) from the liver. In certain patients, the serum level of CRP is useful as a clinical marker of inflammation caused by atherogenesis and of subsequent risk of sustaining a CHD event.

The atherogenic process occurs within the artery wall. Initially, it was thought that the lumen was progressively narrowed by the accumulation of macrophages, the proliferation of smooth muscle cells, and the deposition of cholesterol.[131,133] In fact, the truly dangerous lesion (the culprit lesion) may not cause marked luminal narrowing.[134] As atherosclerosis progresses, there is a compensatory expansion of the lumen that maintains lumen size rather constant. As the lesion develops within the intima, the complication of rupture of the overlying intima or endothelial erosion leads to exposure of the lesion content to platelets and initiates thrombosis. It is the acute thrombosis, not arterial lumen stenosis, that is responsible for infarctions in most cases. Rupture or erosion occurs where the fibrous cap is thin and where an active inflammatory process is occurring.[134,135]

The pattern of lesion formation does not occur randomly within the arterial tree but is focal in nature. Susceptible regions are more permeable to plasma components, and endothelial cell turnover is greater, although the endothelial surface appears to be intact. The focal nature of atherosclerosis suggests that local hemodynamic factors are involved.

Steps in Atherosclerotic Lesion Formation

Normally, the endothelium forms a relatively impermeable barrier. The endothelial cells and the relatively narrow region beneath them (subendothelial space), which contains an occasional smooth muscle cell, constitute the intima of the artery wall (Fig. 36–21A).[136] Beneath the intima is a layer of many smooth muscle cells, the media, which constitutes the bulk of the artery wall. The adventitia is the outermost layer of the artery wall and is composed of loose connective tissue.

A current model of atherogenesis is depicted in Figure 36–21B to E. The major cell types involved include endothelial cells, smooth muscle cells, and inflammatory mononuclear cells, such as macrophages and lymphocytes. One of the initial events is the focal attachment of circulating monocytes to the endothelial surface (see Fig. 36–21B). Oxidized or modified LDLs or other atherogenic lipoproteins retained in the subendothelium are probably a major initiating factor responsible for the adherence of monocytes; areas of microinjury might contribute as well. The monocytes modify the endothelial surface and induce the expression of leukocyte adhesion molecules such as vascular cell adhesion molecule (VCAM)-1.[137] Once adhered, the monocytes migrate between endothelial cells, enter the subendothelial space, and differentiate into macrophages (see Fig. 36–21B). In addition, LDLs and other atherogenic lipoproteins can enter this space, where they become entrapped in the matrix and undergo oxidation or further chemical modifications. The macrophages take up the oxidized or modified LDLs and begin to take on the appearance of foam cells as lipid accumulates. Lymphocyte infiltration is prominent. These initial steps set in motion a chain of events that includes the expression of growth factors (mediators of cell proliferation and chemotaxis) and cytokines (mediators involved in inflammation and immunity).

Monocyte chemoattractant protein 1 (MCP-1), produced by endothelial and smooth muscle cells, plays a role in further monocyte recruitment into lesions and may be induced by the presence of oxidized LDL. The role of MCP-1 in macrophage recruitment in the early stages of lesion development was established in MCP-1–deficient mice.[138] When the MCP-1–deficient mice were crossed with apo-E–deficient mice, a common mouse model of atherosclerosis, and fed a high-fat Western-type diet for 5 weeks, fewer macrophages were present in the aortas of the doubly transgenic mice than in the apo-E–deficient control mice. After 5 to 26 weeks of the diet, the doubly transgenic mice displayed significantly smaller lesions. These results establish a role for MCP-1 in the recruitment of macrophages into the artery wall at an early stage of lesion formation and establish MCP-1 as an important factor for atherogenesis.

Other growth factors that have been implicated in atherosclerosis include platelet-derived growth factor (PDGF), basic fibroblast growth factor (FGF), insulin-like growth factors (IGFs),

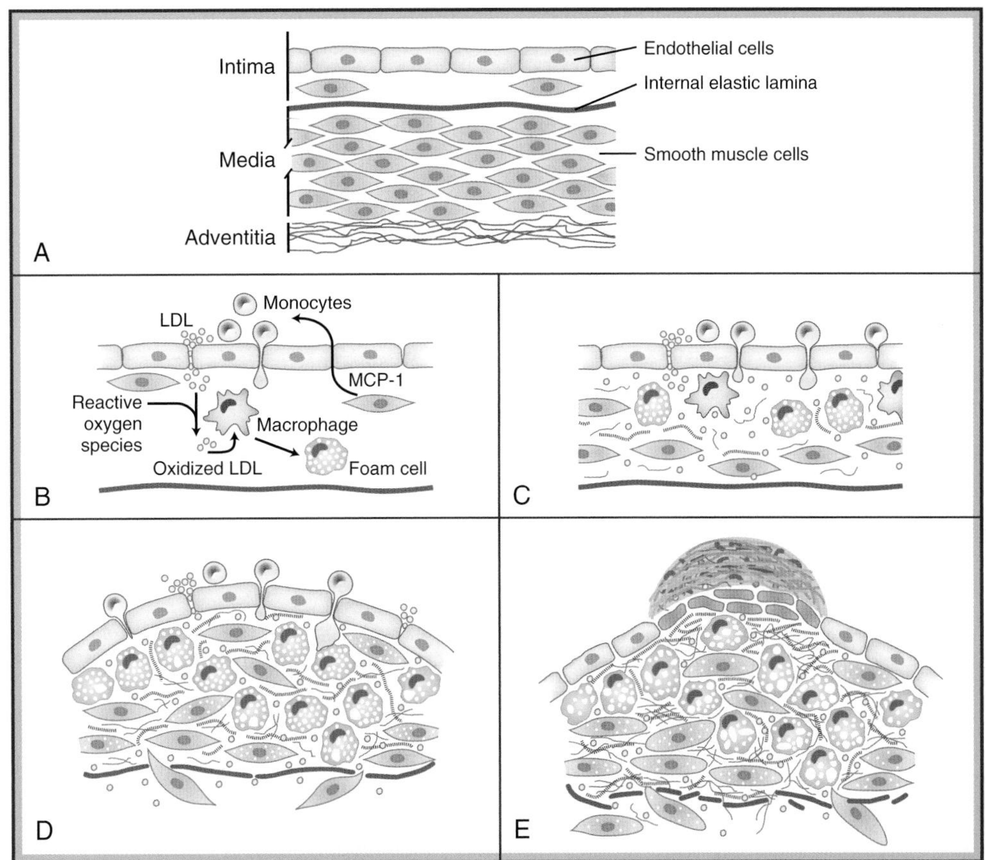

Figure 36–21 ■ Schematic representation of the progression of atherogenesis. ***A,*** Normal artery wall showing the three major regions of the vessel wall, intima, media, and adventitia. The thickness of the intima beneath the endothelial cell layer is exaggerated relative to the media to allow illustration of the changes that occur within the subendothelial intima. **B,** Initial events in lesion formation include the recruitment of monocyte-macrophages to the subendothelial space and the infiltration of plasma low-density lipoproteins (LDLs) *(small circles),* which are oxidized by unknown mechanisms that may include reactive oxygen species. Oxidized LDLs are taken up by macrophages, leading to the formation of foam cells. MCP-1, monocyte chemoattractant protein 1. **C,** Fatty streak lesion. Further recruitment of monocyte-macrophages from the plasma takes place along with smooth muscle cell proliferation and collagen synthesis (rows of vertical lines). Elastin fibers (thin curved lines) begin to accumulate. **D,** Proliferative or fibrous lesion. Atherogenesis continues as the lesion begins to extend into the vessel lumen. Necrosis of foam cells begins, and smooth muscle cells start to migrate from the media through the disrupted internal elastic lamina. Some smooth muscle cells accumulate lipid droplets. **E,** Complicated lesion. The endothelial cell layer covering the lesion is lost. As a result, the surface of the lesion becomes thrombogenic, inducing thrombus formation. Cellular debris increases. Calcification and appearance of cholesterol crystals can occur.

interleukin-1 (IL-1), tumor necrosis factor (TNF), and transforming growth factor β (TΓΦ-β).[131,133] These mitogenic factors, which can stimulate smooth muscle cell proliferation, are not expressed in the normal artery wall but are present in developing lesions. Several of these mitogens are also chemoattractants with the potential to attract smooth muscle cells or monocytes-macrophages into a developing lesion. Inflammatory response cytokines include IL-1, interferon (IFN)-γ, TNF-α, IL-2, and the colony-stimulating factors. Some of the cytokines produced in lesions enter the circulation and stimulate production of the CRP in the liver. Blood levels of CRP appear to predict the intensity of inflammation induced by atherosclerosis. In some patients, CRP measurement may be useful in assessing CHD risk.[139,140] It is unlikely that the various factors act in isolation from each other, but they probably act through a network of cellular interactions operating in a paracrine or autocrine manner.

The first grossly visible atherosclerotic lesion is referred to as a fatty streak (see Fig. 36–21C). Macrophages accumulate in abundance in the subendothelial space and are converted to foam cells, presumably through the uptake of oxidized LDLs or remnant lipoproteins. The recruitment of monocytes continues, and smooth muscle cells begin to migrate into the intima. Fatty streaks probably come and go, depending on the local stimuli present in the artery wall.

As the cycle of interactions continues, the fatty streak matures into a proliferative or fibrous plaque (see Fig. 36–21D). The foam cells begin to necrose, probably because of the cytotoxicity of the accumulated lipid; as the lesion progresses, cholesterol crystals develop. The death of foam cells leads to extracellular lipid deposition, accompanied by collagen synthesis and smooth muscle cell migration and proliferation. In the continued presence of factors that promote atherogenesis (e.g., high plasma concentrations of atherogenic lipoproteins), the plaque progresses to the complicated lesion stage (see Fig. 36–21E).

The surfaces of complicated lesions can become thrombogenic as endothelial cells are lost or the fibrous cap ruptures and the subendothelial space is exposed. Platelets can adhere to this exposed surface, promoting thrombus formation. In these unstable plaques, blood actually dissects into the artery wall, leading to the formation of a large thrombus. Calcification is also a feature of late lesions. Advanced lesions can weaken the elasticity and integrity of the artery wall, with the potential to lead to an aneurysm of the vessel. As clinical trial data have shown, removal or reduction of the atherogenic stimulus can result in plaque regression and stabilization, leaving a remnant devoid of lipid that resembles a wound scar and is less likely to serve as a nidus for thrombus formation.

Hyperlipidemia and Dyslipidemia. Definitions and Overview

Plasma lipid levels vary among individual members of different populations owing to genetic and dietary factors. For example, the age-adjusted mean plasma cholesterol concentration is 5.26 mM/L (202 mg/dL) in U.S. men[141] but 4.3 mM/L (165 mg/dL) in Chinese men.[142] For Western adults, cholesterol concentrations higher than 6.2 mM/L (240 mg/dL) or triglyceride concentrations higher than 1.7 mM/L (150 mg/dL) constitute high-risk hyperlipidemia. However, serum total cholesterol levels correlate with CHD risk over a broad range. In the Framingham study, the lowest risk was observed in subjects with total cholesterol levels less than 3.9 mM/L (150 mg/dL); one third of events occurred in those with cholesterol levels between 3.9 and 5.2 mM/L (150 to 200 mg/dL) and two thirds in those with total cholesterol levels greater than 5.2 mM/L (200 mg/dL).[143]

The guidelines from the 2001 National Cholesterol Education Program (NCEP) suggest that plasma cholesterol levels less than 5.2 mM/L (200 mg/dL) are desirable, that those between 5.2 and 6.2 mM/L (200 to 240 mg/dL) are borderline high, and that levels greater than 6.2 mM/L (240 mg/dL) are high.[144] Because plasma lipid levels increase with age,[144] cutoff values in children are lower. Total cholesterol between 4.4 and 5.2 mM/L (170 and 200 mg/dL) is borderline high and levels greater than 5.2 mM/L (200 mg/dL) are high. For triglycerides, the cutpoint is 1.7 mM/L (150 mg/dL).[145] These boundaries are arbitrary, and the designation of plasma cholesterol concentrations above 6.2 mM/L (240 mg/dL) as "high" and those between 5.2 and 6.2 mM/L (200-240 mg/dL) as "borderline high" detracts from the fact that risk increases continuously above values of 3.9 mM/L (150 mg/dL) (see Fig. 36–20).[146] The prevalence of CHD events in those with desirable cholesterol levels (3.9-5.2 mM/L [150-200 mg/dL]) is actually 20 out of 100 persons. Considering that 45% of the U.S. population has cholesterol levels in this range, there are 25 million persons at risk in the United States with desirable cholesterol levels. The challenge is how to identify the 20 out of 100 patients who are at risk so that they may be treated.[143] Patients with desirable total cholesterol levels who develop CHD commonly have low HDL-C levels and high triglyceride values. The term *dyslipidemia* is often applied to patients who are not hypercholesterolemic according to existing NCEP guidelines.

Hyperlipidemia is caused by increased concentrations of plasma lipoproteins. One or more classes of lipoproteins can accumulate in the bloodstream because of increased production or secretion into the circulation or because of decreased clearance or removal from the circulation; in some cases, both processes coexist. Alterations in metabolic processes are often related to alterations in the proteins involved in lipoprotein metabolism (see "Plasma Lipoproteins. Apolipoproteins, Receptors, and Enzymes"). Alterations resulting from genetic defects that directly affect lipoprotein metabolism are classified as *primary* disorders. Other disorders that alter lipoprotein metabolism indirectly, such as diabetes mellitus or hypothyroidism, lead to altered plasma lipoprotein concentrations; these are classified as *secondary* disorders of lipid metabolism. Often, hyperlipidemia results from mixed primary and secondary causes, as when diabetes mellitus occurs in a subject who has an inherited defect in one of the proteins involved in lipoprotein metabolism. In cases in which no known cause of hyperlipidemia can be identified, the disorder is classified as sporadic or possibly polygenic in origin.

When considering the causes of hyperlipidemia, it is possible to create a differential diagnosis on the basis of whether the concentration of plasma cholesterol or triglycerides (or both) is elevated. Table 36–5 illustrates such a diagnostic strategy. More extensive lists of primary and secondary disorders are given in Tables 36–6 and 36–7. Although it is often not essential to diagnose a genetic disorder in a hyperlipidemic subject for treatment purposes, the understanding of genetic causes can have important implications for family members. The recognition of secondary disorders is of great importance because therapy should be directed, at least in part, toward correcting the underlying disorder.

Primary Disorders of Hyperlipidemia

Familial Hypercholesterolemia

FH is a relatively common disorder caused by mutations in the LDL receptor gene that result in LDL receptor malfunction or absence in cells of the liver and peripheral tissues, leading to elevation of plasma LDL and total cholesterol concentrations (see Table 36–6).[4,5,68,168] Plasma cholesterol concentrations are typically elevated twofold to threefold above average in heterozygous subjects and threefold to sixfold in homozygous subjects.

TABLE 36–5 DIFFERENTIAL DIAGNOSIS OF HYPERLIPIDEMIA INCLUDING COMMON SECONDARY DISORDERS

Type of Disorder	MAJOR PLASMA LIPID ABNORMALITY		
	Increased Cholesterol	Increased Cholesterol and Triglyceride	Increased Triglyceride
Primary	Familial hypercholesterolemia Familial defective apo-B100 Polygenic hypercholesterolemia	Familial combined hyperlipidemia Type III hyperlipoproteinemia (dysbetalipoproteinemia)	Familial hypertriglyceridemia LPL deficiency Apo-CII deficiency Sporadic hypertriglyceridemia
Secondary	Hypothyroidism Nephrotic syndrome	Hypothyroidism Nephrotic syndrome Diabetes mellitus	Diabetes mellitus Alcoholic hyperlipidemia Estrogen therapy

Apo, apolipoprotein; LPL, lipoprotein lipase.

TABLE 36–6 MAJOR GENETIC HYPERLIPOPROTEINEMIAS RESULTING FROM SINGLE-GENE MUTATIONS

Disorder	Mutant Gene	Inheritance	Estimated Population Frequency	Elevated Plasma Lipoprotein	TYPICAL CLINICAL MANIFESTATIONS		
					Xanthomas	Pancreatitis	Premature Vascular Disease
Familial LPL deficiency	LPL	Autosomal recessive	1/10^6	Chylomicrons, VLDL	Eruptive	+	–
Familial apo-CII deficiency	Apo-CII	Autosomal recessive	1/10^6	Chylomicrons, VLDL	Eruptive (rarely)	+	–
Familial hypercholesterolemia	LDL receptor	Autosomal dominant	1/500 (heterozygous); 1/10^6 (homozygous)	LDL	Tendon; xanthelasma	–	+
Autosomal recessive hypercholesterolemia	ARH	Autosomal recessive	Very rare	LDL	Tendon	–	+
Familial defective apo-B100	Apo-B	Autosomal dominant	1/1000	LDL	Tendon	–	+
Familial type III hyperlipoproteinemia	Apo-E	Autosomal recessive (rarely dominant)	1/10000	Remnant lipoproteins (β-VLDL)	Palmar; tuberous	–	+
Familial combined hyperlipidemia	Unknown	Autosomal dominant	1/100	VLDL, LDL, or both	—	–	+
Familial hypertriglyceridemia	Unknown	Autosomal dominant	Uncertain	VLDL	—	–	Uncertain

Apo, apolipoprotein; ARH, autosomal recessive hypercholesterolemia; LDL, low-density lipoproteins; LPL, lipoprotein lipase; VLDL, very-low-density lipoproteins.

Clinical Features

Heterozygosity for FH occurs with an incidence of about 1 in 500 in the population and occurs in most ethnic groups, some with a much higher incidence than 1 in 500.[69] Typically, the plasma cholesterol concentration is higher than 7.8 mM/L (300 mg/dL), and the LDL-C concentration is higher than 6.5 mM/L (250 mg/dL). Plasma triglycerides are not elevated. The hyperlipidemia is present at birth, and the diagnosis can be suspected from elevated cholesterol concentrations in umbilical cord blood.

The characteristic physical finding in approximately 75% of affected patients is tendon xanthomas (Fig. 36–22C and D), usually on the Achilles tendons or extensor tendons of the hands. Xanthomas of the Achilles tendon can cause recurrent episodes of Achilles tendinitis.[169] These xanthomas may be subtle and apparent only as a thickening of the tendon (see Fig. 36–22C). Other common physical findings include xanthelasma (see Fig. 36–22A) and premature arcus corneae (i.e., in persons younger than 40 years).[170] Many affected subjects have no physical findings. Premature coronary artery disease is common; the age of onset of coronary disease is about 45 years in men and women who are heterozygous for FH. Affected subjects with other risk factors develop symptomatic vascular disease even earlier in life.[171]

Homozygosity for FH is rare, occurring at a frequency of about 1 in 10^6 in the population (i.e., ~250 persons in the U.S. population). These subjects come to clinical attention early in life because of the appearance of xanthomas younger than the age of 10, marked hypercholesterolemia apparent at birth, or premature CHD. Typical plasma cholesterol concentrations range from 15.5 mM/L (600 mg/dL) to 25.9 mM/L (1000 mg/dL), and LDL-C concentrations range from 14.2 mM/L (550 mg/dL) to 24.6 mM/L (950 mg/dL). In addition to the xanthelasma and tendon xanthomas found in heterozygotes, homozygous persons often have tuberous xanthomas (see Fig. 36–22E), which are almost unique to this disorder and almost always noticed by age 6 years. These xanthomas are cutaneous protuberances of cholesterol-filled macrophages that occur in the skin at areas of trauma, such as the elbows and knees. Symptomatic CHD can occur before age 10 years,[172] and, if not treated, these homozygous persons usually die from myocardial infarction by age 20 years. Myocardial infarction has been reported as early as age 18 months.[173] Homozygotes are also susceptible to both valvular and supravalvular aortic stenosis.[174]

Origin and Pathogenesis

FH is an autosomal dominant disorder caused by mutations in the LDL receptor gene.[4,5,68] Many different types of mutations have been described, including null mutations or nonsense mutations that affect the production of a functional protein, mutations that affect the ability of the receptor to bind its ligands on lipoproteins, and mutations in which receptors bind LDL normally but are unable to internalize the lipoprotein.[168] A milder phenotype occurs when the ability to bind LDL is impaired but not absent. Different LDL receptor mutations occur in different ethnic groups; for example, there is an increased prevalence (about 60%) of a large deletion mutation in French Canadians with heterozygous FH.[69] More than 900 mutations in the LDL receptor gene cause FH.[69]

The lack of LDL receptors impairs the clearance of lipoproteins that rely on the LDL receptor for this purpose; these include LDLs, in which apo-B100 is the ligand, and remnant lipoproteins (IDLs) that are cleared by apo-E. As a result, the plasma cholesterol concentration increases twofold to threefold in heterozygotes and threefold to sixfold in homozygotes. The high levels of LDL in the plasma are taken up by scavenger receptors on macrophages in a nonsaturable manner, possibly after the LDL undergoes oxidative modification,[79-82] leading to cholesteryl ester accumulation in tissue macrophages in the arterial wall and skin and pathologic processes in these tissues. In tendons,

TABLE 36–7 CLINICAL DISORDERS ASSOCIATED WITH SECONDARY HYPERLIPIDEMIA

Disorder	Elevated Plasma Lipoprotein	Proposed Mechanism	References*
		ENDOCRINE-METABOLIC	
Diabetes mellitus	VLDL, chylomicrons	Increased VLDL production; decreased VLDL catabolism	See text
Hypothyroidism	LDL (rarely β-VLDL)	Decreased LDL clearance	See text
Estrogen therapy	VLDL	Increased VLDL production (especially in genetically predisposed)	See text
Glucocorticoid therapy	VLDL, LDL	Increased VLDL production with conversion to LDL	147, 148
Hypopituitarism (ateliotic dwarfism)	LDL	Increased VLDL production with conversion to LDL	149
Acromegaly	Remnants, Lp(a)	Decreased lipoprotein lipase activity	150, 151
Anorexia nervosa	LDL	Decreased biliary excretion of cholesterol and bile acids	152
Lipodystrophy (congenital or acquired)	VLDL	Increased VLDL production associated with insulin resistance	153
Werner syndrome	LDL	Unknown	154
Acute intermittent porphyria	LDL	Unknown	155
Glycogen storage disease	VLDL	Increased VLDL production; decreased VLDL catabolism	156, 157
		NONENDOCRINE	
Alcohol	VLDL (rarely chylomicrons)	Increased VLDL production (especially in genetically predisposed)	See text
Nephrotic syndrome	VLDL, LDL	Increased VLDL production	See text
Uremia	VLDL	Decreased VLDL clearance, decreased HDL synthesis	158
Biliary obstruction/cholestasis	LP-X	Increased hepatic cholesterol synthesis	159, 160
Acute hepatitis	VLDL	Decreased LCAT	161
Paraproteinemia	Various	Antibodies (usually monoclonal) bindto lipoproteins or other proteins (e.g., receptors, enzymes) involved in lipoprotein metabolism; lipid levels may be increased or decreased; artifactual results of directly measured LDL-C and HDL-C occur	162-166
Protease inhibitors (antiretrovirals)	VLDL, chylomicrons	Insulin resistance	167

*References are given for disorders not discussed in the text. For a thorough review of the metabolism associated with many of the secondary hyperlipidemic disorders, see Havel RJ, Goldstein JL, Brown MS. Lipoproteins and lipid transport. In Bondy PK, Rosenberg LE (eds). Metabolic Control and Disease, 8th ed. Philadelphia: WB Saunders, 1980:393-494.

IDL, intermediate-density lipoproteins; LCAT, lecithin:cholesterol acyltransferase; LDL, low-density lipoproteins; Lp(a), lipoprotein(a); LPL, lipoprotein lipase; VLDL, very-low-density lipoproteins.

unesterified cholesterol accumulates extracellularly in association with collagen fibrils, whereas esterified cholesterol is found intracellularly in macrophages.[175]

Diagnosis

The diagnosis of heterozygous FH is suggested by the presence of high plasma levels of total cholesterol and LDL-C, normal plasma triglycerides, tendon xanthomas, and a family history of premature CHD. Up to 25% of subjects do not have xanthomas. Heterozygous FH should be suspected in any person with premature heart disease. In one study, heterozygous FH accounted for 4% of men who survived myocardial infarction before age 60 years.[176] The differential diagnosis includes familial defective apo-B100, which has many of the same phenotypic characteristics, including tendon xanthomas.[69] The pattern of isolated high LDL-C also occurs in the more common disorder of polygenic hypercholesterolemia, but tendon xanthomas are not usually a feature of the latter.

The diagnosis of FH is primarily a clinical diagnosis because tests to detect one of the many LDL receptor gene mutations or to demonstrate diminished LDL receptor function are performed only in specialized research laboratories. The clinical diagnosis of FH is important not only for proper treatment of the affected subject but also for identification of other family members who may be at high risk for developing CHD.

The diagnosis of homozygous FH should be suspected in any child with extremely high plasma cholesterol (typically >12.9 mM/L [500 mg/dL]) or the xanthomas characteristic of FH. Both parents are obligate heterozygotes and should manifest the phenotype of heterozygous FH.

Treatment

Because other risk factors modulate CHD risk of patients with heterozygous FH, the presence of additional risk factors should be sought, especially smoking and low levels of HDL-C.[171] Treatment of heterozygous FH consists of a diet low in total and saturated fat (approximately 20% and 6% of calories, respectively) and low in cholesterol (<2.6 mM/day [100 mg/day]) plus drug therapy.[177,178] Diet modifications usually result in only minor decreases in the plasma cholesterol levels (5% to 15%). With the development of more potent HMG-CoA reductase inhibitors, adequate cholesterol lowering in these patients can occasionally be achieved by a single therapeutic drug.[178] However, combinations of two or three drugs are often needed to reduce plasma cholesterol to desired levels.[179]

The first effective drug combinations developed usually included low doses of bile acid sequestrants together with HMG-CoA reductase inhibitors or niacin or all three agents combined.[177] Bile acid sequestrants and HMG-CoA reductase inhibitors deplete the hepatic cells of their cholesterol content

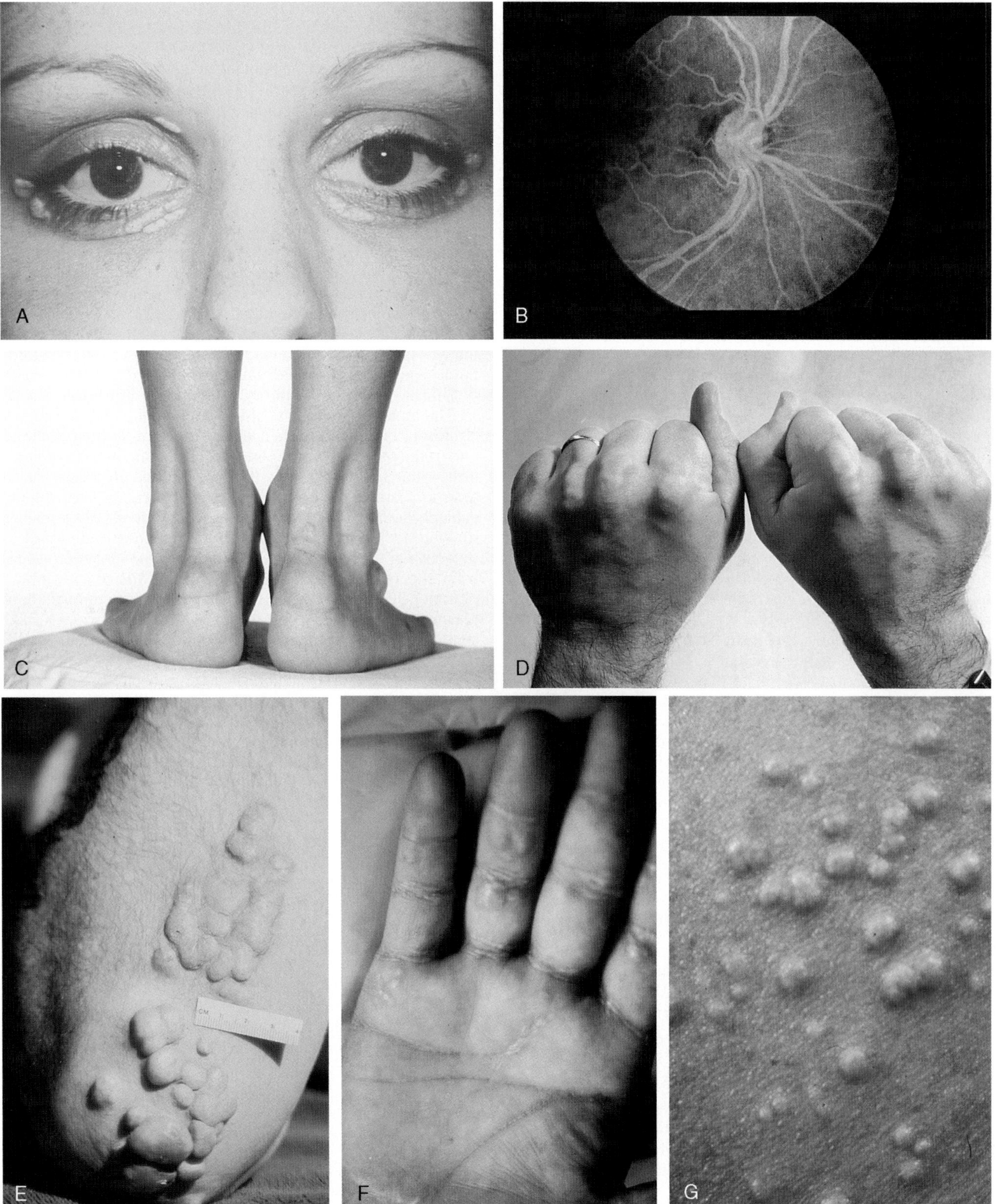

Figure 36–22 ■ Physical examination findings associated with hyperlipidemia. **A,** Xanthelasma. **B,** Lipemia retinalis. **C,** Achilles tendon xanthomas. Note the marked thickening of the tendons. **D,** Tendon xanthomas. **E,** Tuberous xanthomas. **F,** Palmar xanthomas. **G,** Eruptive xanthomas. (**A** and **B** courtesy of Dr. Mark Dresner and Hospital Practice [May 1990, p 15]. **C, D, E,** and **F** courtesy of Dr. Tom Bersot. **G** courtesy of Dr. Alan Chait.)

(see later discussion), thereby causing increased expression of functional LDL receptors (from the normal allele) on the surface of hepatocytes, which in turn lowers plasma cholesterol levels.[69] A more recent approach is to combine maximum-dose statin therapy with the intestinal cholesterol absorption inhibitor ezetimibe.[178,180] Ileal bypass surgery,[181] which, like bile acid sequestrants, causes decreased reabsorption of bile acids from the gut, may be considered in patients who cannot tolerate lipid-lowering drugs.

The age at which drug treatment should begin in heterozygous FH is somewhat controversial. On the one hand, development of atherosclerosis in these subjects is a long process that begins early in life, and one could argue that treatment should begin during the early stages of lesion development. Statins have been approved for the treatment of children with heterozygous FH who are 8 years of age.[178] On the other hand, CHD is usually not symptomatic until the fourth decade of life in men and women.[171] Because established CHD is reversible,[182,183] one could argue that medicines can be withheld until after age 25 years in men or age 35 years in women. A rational approach may be to use diet therapy and bile acid sequestrants, which do not cause systemic toxicity, in the early years and to add more potent drug combinations later. The presence of additional risk factors (e.g., low plasma HDL-C levels or smoking) in an affected patient is an indication for more aggressive treatment at a young age.

Unless there is some small percentage of residual LDL binding, drug therapy of FH homozygotes is usually ineffective for lowering plasma cholesterol. High doses (80 mg) of atorvastatin and simvastatin combined with ezetimibe can lower LDL-C levels by about 30%.[184] However, the most effective means of therapy in these patients is selective removal of LDL from the plasma or blood by extracorporeal apheresis combined with LDL adsorption performed every 1 to 3 weeks.[185,186] Experimental therapies include liver transplantation,[187] which provides functional LDL receptors but is accompanied by the usual complications associated with organ transplantation, as well as portacaval shunting[188,189] and gene therapy. Delivery of an LDL receptor transgene to the liver cells has been fraught with issues of efficacy and safety. Development of technology to deliver the complete LDL receptor genomic locus to cells in vitro results in regulated LDL receptor gene expression. Whole-animal experiments are in progress.[190]

Familial Defective Apolipoprotein B100

Familial defective apo-B100 is a relatively common disorder caused by a mutation in apo-B100, the ligand that binds LDL to the LDL receptor. It results in high plasma LDL and total cholesterol levels and increased susceptibility to CHD.[30] It is phenotypically similar to FH.

Clinical Features

This disorder occurs with a prevalence of 1 in 500 to 1 in 750 in white persons.[30,191] The prevalence of familial defective apo-B100 was 0.08% in an ethnically diverse, unselected population.[192,193] The clinical features of heterozygous familial defective apo-B100 overlap extensively with those of heterozygous FH and include isolated elevations of plasma LDL, tendon xanthomas, xanthelasmas, and premature CHD.[194]

Although there is extensive overlap, heterozygous familial defective apo-B100 is usually milder in its manifestations than homozygous FH.[30,194] Subjects who are homozygous for the familial defective apo-B100 mutation also appear to have a milder clinical phenotype than FH homozygotes. Total cholesterol and LDL-C levels are substantially lower in familial defective apo-B100 patients than in FH patients, and clinically evident atherosclerotic vascular disease does not appear until much later in life.[69] Presumably, the less severe phenotype is related to the fact that the binding of apo-B to LDL receptors is defective but not totally absent in familial defective apo-B100, whereas the apo-E–mediated clearance of remnant particles, which is impaired in FH, is normal in persons with familial defective apo-B100.

Origin and Pathogenesis

Familial defective apo-B100 is caused by a mutation in apo-B100 that impairs its ability to bind to the LDL receptor.[195,196] To date, a single mutation, the substitution of glutamine for arginine at amino acid 3500, accounts for almost all cases of familial defective apo-B100.[30] Apo-B allele haplotype analysis of DNA from affected subjects has indicated that almost all cases can be traced back to an original founder.[192] Only after extensive screening was this mutation detected in persons with a different apo-B haplotype for the allele carrying the mutation, one of whom was of Chinese ancestry[193] and one in a kindred from Germany.[197]

The mutation located at apo-B amino acid 3500 disrupts the conformation of the protein in the receptor-binding domain[198] and reduces receptor binding of LDL from heterozygotes to levels that are about one third of normal in tissue culture assays.[195] Isolation of the binding-defective LDL from affected subjects demonstrated that it binds with 4% to 9% of normal LDL binding activity to LDL receptors.[199] Decreased affinity of the defective apo-B100 for its receptor delays the clearance of LDL from the plasma (by about 50%) and leads to elevation of plasma LDL-C levels. Defective LDL particles accumulate in the plasma in increased proportions relative to normal LDL. A second mutation at amino acid 3500 (tryptophan for arginine) has been reported.[200]

Another mutation located near the receptor-binding region of the apo-B molecule (a substitution of cysteine for arginine at amino acid 3531) also impairs binding of apo-B to the LDL receptor.[201] This mutation decreases LDL binding to LDL receptors by 35% to 40% in tissue culture assays and is associated with moderate elevations in plasma LDL-C levels.

Diagnosis

As in heterozygous FH, the diagnosis of familial defective apo-B100 is suggested by the presence of increased plasma LDL-C and normal triglyceride levels, especially in a patient with tendon xanthomas and a family history of premature CHD. Without specialized testing, however, familial defective apo-B100 is clinically indistinguishable from FH. Because familial defective apo-B100 is caused primarily by one mutation, in contrast to the many mutations that cause FH,[69] it is possible to screen easily for the familial defective apo-B100 mutation using a polymerase chain reaction–based assay of genomic DNA isolated from blood.[69] This test is available only in specialized laboratories.

Treatment

Treatment of familial defective apo-B100 is similar to that of heterozygous FH and consists of a low-fat, low-cholesterol diet and a combination drug regimen.[178] Drugs that either decrease LDL production (e.g., niacin[202]) or increase the expression of LDL receptors to facilitate clearance of the normal apo-B100–containing particles effectively lower the plasma LDL-C level.[203] In two patients with homozygous familial defective apo-B100 whose LDL had receptor-binding affinities 10% to 20% of normal, treatment with HMG-CoA reductase inhibitors markedly reduced plasma cholesterol levels.[204] Family members at risk should also be screened for the dominant mutation.

Rare Mutations in Other Genes Associated with Elevated LDL Levels

Autosomal recessive hypercholesterolemia has been identified in families from Sardinia and Lebanon.[205] Affected patients have clinical features of homozygous FH, but the lipid levels of the parents are normal. The disorder is caused by mutations in *Arh*, the gene encoding ARH, a putative adaptor protein that is required for internalization of LDL bound by the LDL receptor on the surface of hepatocytes.[206] The mutation affects LDL receptor internalization by the liver and lymphocytes, not by skin fibroblasts.[205] As of 2003, eight mutations in *Arh* had been associated with autosomal recessive hypercholesterolemia, mostly in Italians (Sardinia) and Lebanese. In one case, treatment with high-dose statin therapy and ezetimibe reduced the LDL-C level well below 2.6 mM/L (100 mg/dL).[207]

Autosomal dominant hypercholesterolemia caused by a mutation in the gene encoding cholesterol 7α-hydroxylase has been reported in a single kindred.[208] Plasma cholesterol levels of homozygous patients vary between 7.8 and 10.4 mM/L (300-400 mg/dL), and cholelithiasis is a concomitant clinical feature. This is caused by a lack of synthesis of cholic acid from cholesterol due to the inability to synthesize 7α-hydroxycholesterol, a cholic acid precursor. Accumulation of cholesterol in hepatocytes associated with this mutation decreases the responsiveness to low-to-moderate dose statin therapy. Treatment requires combination therapy with maximum statin dosages and niacin.[208]

Another very rare cause of autosomal dominant hypercholesterolemia is a mutation of proprotein convertase subtilisin kexin 9 (PCSK9), which encodes neural apoptosis-regulated convertase-1 (NARC-1).[209] NARC-1 is highly expressed in the liver and is thought to play a role in LDL receptor catabolism, but its exact substrate has yet to be identified. Mutations in PCSK9 associated with hypercholesterolemia are thought to be gain-of-function mutations, because overexpression of PCSK9 in mice produces hypercholesterolemia.[210] Interestingly, loss-of-function mutations in PSCK9 are associated with low levels of total cholesterol and LDL-C. The prevalence of loss-of-function mutations is about 2% among African Americans, but less than 0.1% in white Americans.[210]

Familial Combined Hyperlipidemia

Originally described in 1973,[176,211,212] familial combined hyperlipidemia is a common disorder of unknown genetic cause associated with elevations of plasma cholesterol and triglyceride levels and increased susceptibility to CHD. It is inherited as an autosomal dominant trait. The phenotype of familial combined hyperlipidemia overlaps with and may be the same as that of familial hyperapobetalipoproteinemia,[213] in which subjects have elevations of total apo-B (>120 mg/dL, the 75th percentile value in North Americans) and small, dense LDL particles.[214] The phenotype of familial combined hyperlipidemia also is similar to that of patients with *syndrome X*, a disorder that includes documented insulin resistance, increased plasma levels of small, dense LDL, elevated plasma triglycerides, elevated apo-B levels, and low plasma HDL levels.[215]

Insulin resistance is thought to be the cornerstone of hyperapobetalipoproteinemia, syndrome X, and perhaps familial combined hyperlipidemia. Diagnosis of familial combined hyperlipidemia requires extensive study of the family members of suspected probands. Documentation of hyperapobetalipoproteinemia requires reliable measurements of apo-B levels, and a diagnosis of syndrome X requires measurement of insulin levels in the context of glucose tolerance testing, a procedure that is time consuming; moreover, insulin assays have problems with reliability and reproducibility. To help clinicians recognize patients at risk because of the constellation of risk factors associated with insulin resistance without resorting to specialized testing (glucose tolerance test, apolipoprotein measurements), the NCEP Adult Treatment Panel (ATP) III proposed a simple set of diagnostic criteria for a "metabolic syndrome."[216] The diagnostic criteria are based on readily available clinical tests. waist circumference, blood pressure, blood levels of triglycerides and HDL-C, and fasting glucose (see "Metabolic Syndrome").

Clinical Features

The features of familial combined hyperlipidemia include moderate elevations of plasma cholesterol or triglycerides, or both, within subjects of an affected kindred. The predominant lipid abnormality (hypertriglyceridemia, hypercholesterolemia, or both) can vary among affected family members or in a single person over time.[176] Variability in the type of dyslipidemia is a useful hint that the subject might have this disorder. Levels of HDL-C are often moderately decreased,[217] especially in the setting of increased plasma triglycerides.

Although it was originally thought that lipid abnormalities usually develop after puberty, it is now known that the phenotype can be detected in children.[176,218] Xanthomas are not a feature of familial combined hyperlipidemia. Associated metabolic disturbances include glucose intolerance, obesity, and hyperuricemia. Premature CHD in men younger than 50 years is a common feature; in one study of male survivors of myocardial infarction conducted in 1970 to 1971, familial combined hyperlipidemia was found in 11.3% of those younger than 60 years.[176]

Origin and Pathogenesis

The estimated prevalence originally described (0.5%-2.0%) is probably greater (~5%-7%) based on a more recent population-based study.[176,219] Neither its genetic cause nor its metabolic pathogenesis is clear. Given the dominant pattern of inheritance, it was initially presumed that familial combined hyperlipidemia is caused by a single gene defect.[176] Now it is believed that multiple genes may be involved, with specific alleles of the upstream stimulatory factor-1, hepatocyte nuclear factor 4a, and the APOA1/C3/A4/A5 gene cluster being implicated in the transmission of familial combined hyperlipidemia.[220] The phenotype of this disorder has also been mapped to loci on chromosomes 11, 16,[220] and 19.[221] Lifestyle choices and several additional loci might underlie the expression of the phenotype.[222-224] Other disorders such as heterozygous LPL deficiency, which aggravates hypertriglyceridemia, modulate the phenotypic expression of familial combined hyperlipidemia.[225] Assessment of the prevalence of the metabolic syndrome in patients affected by familial combined hyperlipidemia indicates that two thirds meet the diagnostic criteria defining the metabolic syndrome. Regression analysis of these patients with familial combined hyperlipidemia and CHD indicated that the metabolic syndrome accounted entirely for the increased CHD risk.[219]

A significant problem with mapping this disorder is the difficult task of assigning phenotypes to individual patients because of the fluctuating and indistinct clinical features. Familial hyperapobetalipoproteinemia, a disorder characterized by high plasma levels of apo-B and normal plasma cholesterol levels,[213] overlaps with the phenotype of familial combined hyperlipidemia. Both of these familial syndromes are characterized by small, dense LDL, as is syndrome X, which is defined by insulin resistance and other metabolic abnormalities.[226] The metabolic defect that leads to the hypercholesterolemia or hypertriglyceridemia, or both, is also unclear, but overproduction of apo-B may be a contributing factor[227,228]; apo-B overproduction can result in elevations in plasma VLDL, LDL, or both.[229] Similarly, the pathogenesis of the low HDL in this disorder remains unclear. Low HDL-C is commonly associated with hypertriglyceridemia. This finding could be related either to decreased substrate for HDL formation resulting from impaired catabolism of the apo-B–containing lipoproteins or to enhanced CETP-mediated cholesteryl ester transfer from HDL to the apo-B–containing lipoproteins.

Diagnosis

Familial combined hyperlipidemia should be suspected in subjects with moderate hypertriglyceridemia or moderate hypercholesterolemia, or both, especially in the setting of a family history of premature CHD. Xanthomas are not a feature of this disorder. Low plasma HDL-C, obesity, insulin resistance, and hyperuricemia are often present. Patients should also be assessed for the metabolic syndrome. The original diagnostic criteria are clinical ones; it requires demonstration of the clinical phenotype in the affected subject and family members and exclusion of other primary or secondary disorders. Recently, a phenotype of fasting hypertriglyceridemia (>1.5 mM/L [>133 mg/dL]) and apo-B greater than 125 mg/dL was shown to correctly identify patients affected by the original clinical criteria.[230] This has led to a proposal to redefine familial combined hyperlipidemia based only on triglyceride and apo-B levels using the cutpoints described.[231] Secondary disorders that produce a similar phenotype include diabetes mellitus, the nephrotic syndrome, and occasionally hypothyroidism.

Treatment

Weight reduction and dietary treatment can help correct metabolic abnormalities, such as obesity and insulin resistance, that contribute to the hyperlipidemia. Drug therapy should be directed at the predominant lipid abnormality. For example, plasma elevations of total cholesterol and LDL-C can be treated with HMG-CoA reductase inhibitors, niacin, ezetimibe, or bile acid sequestrants.[178] Of these, HMG-CoA reductase inhibitors may be preferable because niacin can cause or worsen glucose intolerance and hyperuricemia, and bile acid sequestrants can aggravate hypertriglyceridemia.[232] Fibrates can lower triglyceride and raise HDL-C levels, and they reduce the incidence of coronary events in insulin-resistant hypertriglyceridemic patients with low HDL-C levels.[233,234] Patients with low HDL-C levels should be treated with HMG-CoA reductase inhibitors. Addition of niacin, ezetimibe, and fibrates can further improve lipid profiles and reduce CHD risk.[178] Because familial combined hyperlipidemia is associated with premature CHD, affected family members should be identified.

Metabolic Syndrome

In 2001, the NCEP ATP III defined criteria for a metabolic syndrome to aid physicians in identifying patients at risk of developing CHD and type 2 diabetes mellitus due to a clustering of metabolic risk factors.[216] The metabolic risk factors include atherogenic dyslipidemia (a high triglyceride level, low HDL-C level, elevated apo-B level, and a preponderance of small LDL particles), elevated blood glucose, elevated blood pressure, a prothrombotic state, and a proinflammatory state. The clustering of these risk factors in some persons has been recognized for many years, and other names and definitions of these clustered risk factors have been proposed, including syndrome X, the insulin-resistance syndrome, the deadly quartet, and hypertriglyceridemic waist.

The NCEP ATP III proposed "the metabolic syndrome" because previous paradigms either failed to include all of the metabolic risk factors, failed to provide cutpoints defining risk factors, or required time-consuming testing (e.g., glucose tolerance testing) or research methodology (e.g., insulin clamp) to identify affected persons. The NCEP ATP III defines five easily measured criteria to identify those affected by the metabolic syndrome. These measurements are fasting levels of plasma triglycerides and glucose, HDL-C level, blood pressure, and abdominal waist circumference. The cutpoints defining the various risk factors are listed in Table 36–8. Persons affected by three of the five criteria proposed in Table 36–8 meet the criteria for the metabolic syndrome. However, with its aggregation of metabolic risk factors, this syndrome probably does not have a single underlying cause. Most importantly, this recently defined syndrome identifies people at high risk for developing atherosclerotic vascular disease and type 2 diabetes mellitus.

The prevalence of the metabolic syndrome in the United States, based on NHANES data collected between 1999 and 2002, is 34.5% of a population-based sample (N = 3601) of men and women 20 years or older.[235] This is an increase of about 10 percentage points (from ~25%) since the NHANES III study carried out between 1988 and 1994.[236] Prevalence increases with age. Among men and women older than 50 years, the prevalence (based on data of 1999-2002) was about 50%.[235] The prevalence varies by ethnic group and by gender in some ethnic groups.[235,236]

A diagnosis of the metabolic syndrome increases the relative risk of a subsequent cardiovascular disease event by 65% and increases the risk of developing type 2 diabetes mellitus threefold.[237] The data suggest that the metabolic syndrome accounts for 12% to 17% of atherosclerosis-induced vascular disease, 30% to 52% of type 2 diabetes mellitus, and 6% to 7% of all-cause mortality in the United States.

Pathogenesis

The pathogenetic basis of the metabolic syndrome has not been elucidated.[238] It remains to be determined if all the risk factors for the metabolic syndrome are due to a single cause or to multiple causes. It is clear that overweight and obesity are associated with the syndrome. The increasing prevalence of the metabolic syndrome since the 1970s is largely due to increasing weight. Weight gain probably modulates each of the metabolic risk factors, but there is evidence that expression of each risk factor is subject to its own genetic control. Some believe that insulin resistance is the single underlying factor responsible for the metabolic syndrome.[239] However, irrespective of the underlying cause, a diagnosis of the metabolic syndrome indicates increased risk of cardiovascular disease. The magnitude of the risk varies depending on which risk factors are present and their severity.[216]

Insulin resistance is common among persons with high triglycerides and low HDL-C levels, two of the most common risk factors among persons with a diagnosis of the metabolic syndrome.[236] However, impaired fasting glucose occurs in only about 12% of persons who meet the diagnostic criteria for the metabolic syndrome because it is the last of the risk factors to develop in metabolic syndrome patients. One of the objections to these criteria is the insensitivity of fasting glucose as an indicator of insulin resistance. In one study, insulin resistance indicated that only 46% of subjects with insulin resistance defined by the insulin clamp technique, the gold standard test, met the criteria for a diagnosis of the metabolic syndrome. Conversely, among those with a diagnosis of the metabolic syndrome, 24% were not found to be insulin resistant by the insulin clamp technique.[240] A simple indicator of insulin resistance in persons affected by the metabolic syndrome is to divide the fasting triglyceride concentration by the HDL-C level. A value of triglyceride/HDL-C = 3.5 mg/dL predicts insulin resistance as reliably as elevated fasting insulin levels.[241]

TABLE 36–8 CRITERIA FOR CLINICAL DIAGNOSIS OF THE METABOLIC SYNDROME

Measure*	Categorical Cutpoints	
Waist circumference†‡§	*Whites, African Americans, Latin Americans* Men: ≥102 cm (≥40 in) Women: ≥88 cm (≥35 in)	*Asians* Men: , ≥90 cm (≥35 in) Women: ≥80 cm (≥32 in)
Elevated triglycerides	≥1.7 mM/L (≥150 mg/dL) *or* On drug treatment for elevated triglycerides¶	
Reduced HDL-C	Men: <1.03 mM/L (<40 mg/dL) Women: <1.3 mM/L (<50 mg/dL) *or* On drug treatment for reduced HDL-C¶	
Elevated blood pressure	≥130 mm Hg systolic blood pressure *or* ≥85 mm Hg diastolic blood pressure *or* On antihypertensive drug treatment in a patient with a history of hypertension	
Elevated fasting glucose	≥5.6 mM/L (≥100 mg/dL) *or* On drug treatment for elevated glucose	

*Any three of five constitute diagnosis of the metabolic syndrome.
†To measure waist circumference, locate the top of the right iliac crest. Place a measuring tape in a horizontal plane around the abdomen at the level of the iliac crest. Before reading the tape measure, ensure that the tape is snug but does not compress the skin and is parallel to the floor. Measurement is made at the end of a normal expiration.
‡Overweight and obesity are associated with insulin resistance and the metabolic syndrome. However, the presence of abdominal obesity (indicated by elevated waist circumference) is as highly correlated with the metabolic risk factors as is an elevated body mass index. Therefore, the simple measurement of waist circumference is recommended to identify the body weight component of the metabolic syndrome.
§Some U.S. adults of non-Asian origin (e.g., white, black, Latin American) with marginally increased waist circumference (e.g., 97-101 cm [37-39 in] in men and 80-87 cm [31-34 in] in women) might have a strong genetic contribution to insulin resistance and should benefit from changes in lifestyle habits, similar to men with categorical increases in waist circumference.
¶Fibrates and nicotinic acid are the most commonly used drugs for elevated triglycerides and reduced HDL-C. Patients taking one of these drugs are presumed to have high triglycerides and low levels of HDL.
Adapted from Grundy SM, Cleeman JI, Daniels SR, et al. Diagnosis and management of the metabolic syndrome. An American Heart Association/National Heart, Lung, and Blood Institute scientific statement. Circulation 2005;112:2735-2752.
HDL-C, high-density lipoprotein cholesterol.

A detailed discussion of the pathogenesis of insulin resistance and its impact on lipid metabolism, glucose metabolism, and its relationship with obesity can be found in Chapter 39.

A second risk factor for the metabolic syndrome is abdominal obesity.[216] In fact, some diagnostic schemes for identifying the metabolic syndrome require the presence of abdominal obesity, which is assessed by measuring abdominal girth just above the superior iliac crest.[235] The absolute values of the cutpoints of abdominal girth defining abdominal obesity vary considerably by ethnic group (see Table 36–8 and reference 235 for definitions of abdominal obesity by ethnic group). The increasing prevalence of obesity, especially abdominal obesity, probably accounts for the increasing prevalence of the metabolic syndrome.[216]

Abdominal obesity contributes to increased insulin resistance, and with that comes increased flux of adipose-derived FFAs to the liver and worsening insulin resistance in muscle. Adipocyte expression of a specific retinal binding protein, RBP4, is increased in obese mice, and serum levels of RBP4 are increased in obese humans.[242] Animal studies indicate that RBP4 enhances skeletal muscle insulin resistance and that drugs reducing RBP4 levels also reduce insulin resistance. Although not enough data are available, RBP4 may be the compound produced in obesity that impairs insulin function in skeletal muscle, possibly by affecting insulin signaling.[242] Abdominal obesity is also associated with increased production of inflammatory cytokines (TNF-α, IL-6), macrophage accumulation in visceral fat, and production of plasminogen activator inhibitor 1.[243]

Diagnosis

As shown in Table 36–8, all patients older than 20 years should be assessed for the metabolic syndrome. In children, the metabolic syndrome can be assessed by using slightly different criteria. fasting triglycerides,100 mg/dL; HDL-C, less than 50 mg/dL (except for boys 15 to 19 years, <45 mg/dL); fasting glucose, 110 mg/dL; waist circumference, greater than 75th percentile for age and sex; and systolic blood pressure greater than 90th percentile for age, sex, and height.[244] Values of blood pressure and waist circumference for children by age are available.[245,246] Patients taking drugs that modify lipids, blood pressure, or glucose are considered to have the risk factor the drug is intended to treat. In patients with moderate increases in waist measurements (men 94-101 cm; women 80-87 cm), the metabolic syndrome may be considered to be present in those with a first-degree relative with type 2 diabetes mellitus before age 60, polycystic ovary disease, fatty liver, CRP greater than 3 mg/L, microalbuminuria, impaired glucose tolerance, or elevated total apo-B.[216]

Treatment

All patients with a diagnosis of the metabolic syndrome should be informed of their increased risk of developing cardiovascular disease and type 2 diabetes mellitus. Weight loss and increased physical activity are the best therapy and may be the only therapy that many metabolic syndrome patients require. All patients should be assessed according to existing guidelines for treating blood pressure, dyslipidemia, hypertension, and hyperglycemia.[216] Aspirin therapy is indicated because of the prothrombotic state.[216]

Type III Hyperlipoproteinemia (Familial Dysbetalipoproteinemia)

Type III hyperlipoproteinemia, or familial dysbetalipoproteinemia, is an uncommon disorder of lipoprotein metabolism characterized by moderate to severe hypertriglyceridemia and hypercholesterolemia caused by the accumulation of cholesterol-rich remnant particles in the plasma.[44,45] Premature peripheral vascular disease and coronary artery disease are common. The cause is mutations in the apo-E gene that result in defective binding of apo-E to lipoprotein receptors. The disorder is associated with the apo-E2 isoform (described previously) and in most instances is inherited as an autosomal recessive trait that requires a secondary exacerbating metabolic factor (either genetic or environmental) for expression of the phenotype.[38,41,44,45,50] Several rare apo-E mutations result in the dominant expression of the disorder.

Clinical Features

Type III hyperlipoproteinemia is usually diagnosed in adulthood and is rarely detected in persons younger than 20 years, with the exception of those with the rare autosomal dominant apo-E mutations.[45] The disorder is more common in men and is usually not manifested in women until after menopause. It is characterized by moderately severe elevations in plasma triglyceride and cholesterol levels; typically, these values range from 3.4 to 4.5 mM/L (300-400 mg/dL) and 7.8 to 10.3 mM/L (300-400 mg/dL), respectively. Concentrations of HDL-C are normal, and LDL-C is almost always reduced.

Xanthomas are present in more than half of affected subjects.[44,45] The presence of palmar xanthomas, which are planar xanthomas in the palmar creases (see Fig. 36–22F), is virtually pathognomonic for this disorder. Tuberous or tuboeruptive xanthomas (see Fig. 36–22E) are also common but are less specific for this disorder. Tendon xanthomas and xanthelasma occur in some patients. Premature vascular disease is common, and peripheral vascular disease occurs in addition to premature CHD.[45] Type III hyperlipoproteinemia accounts for 0.2% to 1.0% of lipid disorders associated with myocardial infarction in persons younger than 60 years. Coexisting metabolic conditions that exacerbate the phenotype of type III hyperlipoproteinemia, such as obesity, alcohol consumption, diabetes mellitus, and hypothyroidism, are often present.

Origin and Pathogenesis

Type III hyperlipoproteinemia is caused by the accumulation of cholesterol-rich remnants of VLDL, IDL, and chylomicron particles in the plasma.[44,45,50] The clearance defect is caused by mutant apo-E that binds defectively to remnant receptors, including LDL receptors (discussed in "Roles of Apolipoprotein E in Lipid Metabolism"). The remnants that accumulate have lost much of their triglyceride through LPL-mediated triglyceride hydrolysis and therefore are cholesterol rich. The predominant remnant particles, termed β-VLDL, can be isolated in the VLDL ultracentrifugation density range (<1.006 g/mL). In contrast to normal VLDLs, which migrate as pre-β particles, these remnants are characterized by β-migration on agarose gel electrophoresis.

Homozygosity for the ε2 allele encoding the apo-E2 isoform occurs at a frequency of about 1 in 100 in the general population. Despite this high prevalence, the type III hyperlipoproteinemia phenotype is relatively rare; the dyslipidemia develops in about 1% to 10% of apo-E2 homozygotes (overall prevalence of 1 in 10,000). Manifestation of the dyslipidemia appears to require a secondary factor, such as a metabolic condition that aggravates the impaired remnant clearance underlying the phenotype. Such conditions can be caused by lipoprotein overproduction syndromes, such as obesity, diabetes mellitus, or alcohol consumption, or by conditions that further impair lipoprotein clearance, such as hypothyroidism. In conditions characterized by VLDL overproduction, the increased generation of remnant particles through catabolism of VLDL overwhelms the ability to clear these remnants from the plasma. Because affected patients are so sensitive to conditions that increase hepatic lipoprotein production, lifestyle treatments directed at decreasing hepatic lipoprotein production, such as diet modifications, weight loss, and alcohol cessation, are extremely effective.

In addition to homozygosity for the apo-E2 isoform, six mutations in the apo-E gene are known to lead to the type III hyperlipoproteinemia phenotype in an autosomal dominant fashion.[44,45] In these dominantly inherited disorders, the phenotype is present at an early age and does not require a coexisting metabolic condition as an exacerbating factor. These rare dominant disorders are of great interest because they show that different mutations in a single protein can give rise to either recessively or dominantly inherited phenotypes.

How a given apo-E mutation interacts with the HSPG/LRP pathway is believed to determine whether the mutation gives rise to a dominant or recessive phenotype.[44,50] For example, in recessive expression of the disorder, as occurs with apo-E2 homozygosity, apo-E2 interacts poorly with the LDL receptor but almost normally with the HSPG/LRP pathway, so that in the absence of exacerbating secondary factors, remnant lipoproteins are cleared effectively. However, in the presence of a secondary factor that overwhelms or even slightly impairs the normal pathways, apo-E2 cannot mediate remnant clearance efficiently. In dominant expression of the disorder, apo-E interacts poorly with both the LDL receptor and the HSPG/LRP pathway, and remnant lipoprotein clearance is impaired even in the heterozygous state. Another contributing factor is the particular lipoprotein fraction with which the apo-E molecule preferentially associates[45] (discussed in "Roles of Apolipoprotein E in Lipid Metabolism").

The accumulation of cholesterol-rich remnant lipoproteins in the plasma leads to the deposition of cholesterol in tissue macrophages, which avidly bind and take up β-VLDL.[124,125] The deposition of β-VLDL-derived cholesterol in macrophages leads to foam cell formation and accumulation, manifested as skin xanthomas and as atherosclerotic vascular disease.[45] In addition to the frequent occurrence of CHD, β-VLDL hyperlipidemia appears to cause a disproportionately high incidence of peripheral vascular disease. Although hyperlipidemia typically does not develop until after about 20 years of age, the onset of premature CHD occurs at about 40 years of age in men and at about 50 years of age in women.[45] Developing clinically evident atherosclerosis after only 20 to 30 years of dyslipidemia indicates the potent atherogenicity of remnant lipoproteins.

Diagnosis

The diagnosis of type III hyperlipoproteinemia should be suspected in patients with moderately severe, nearly equal (based on values expressed as mg/dL) elevations in both plasma triglyceride and cholesterol concentrations.[45] Typically the cholesterol and triglyceride levels are in the range of 3.4 to 4.5 mM/L (300-400 mg/dL) and 7.8 to 10.3 mM/L (300-400 mg/dL), respectively. Because this disorder is most commonly recessive, there is often no family history of hyperlipidemia or premature CHD.

The presence of palmar or tuberous xanthomas makes the diagnosis highly likely.

In the absence of palmar or tuberous xanthomas, the specific diagnosis is more difficult and requires specialized testing. If available, a direct measurement of the VLDL cholesterol level allows detection of cholesterol-rich remnant particles. The directly measured VLDL cholesterol-to-plasma triglyceride ratio (lipid values in mg/dL) is a useful screen; in type III hyperlipoproteinemia, this ratio is usually greater than 0.3 (when hyperlipidemia is present). The normal VLDL cholesterol-to-triglyceride ratio is typically about 0.2 (i.e., the VLDL cholesterol concentration is about 20% of the plasma triglyceride level, a fact that is the basis for estimating VLDL cholesterol concentration using the Friedewald formula; see later). The ratio is elevated because β-VLDL remnants are rich in cholesterol and cause the VLDL fraction to be cholesterol rich. Electrophoresis of plasma samples on agarose gels typically demonstrates a broad band in the β-migrating lipoprotein region, hence the names *broad-β disease* and *dysbetalipoproteinemia* for type III hyperlipoproteinemia. Patients suspected of having type III hyperlipoproteinemia can be evaluated for apo-E2 homozygosity either by isoelectric focusing of plasma (see Fig. 36–8) or, more commonly, by apo-E genotyping of DNA obtained from leukocytes, a procedure that is available in many large clinical laboratories.[247] The other rare dominant mutations in apo-E can be diagnosed only in specialized laboratories.

Treatment

Because type III hyperlipoproteinemia is greatly influenced by coexisting metabolic conditions, a vigorous effort should be made to identify and treat obesity, diabetes mellitus, and hypothyroidism and to reduce alcohol consumption. If these efforts are successful, the lipid abnormalities can often be resolved and plasma lipids returned to normal without the use of drug therapies. Type III hyperlipoproteinemia associated with hypothyroidism, in particular, responds dramatically to thyroid hormone replacement therapy.[248] Diet therapy should be aimed at restricting total fat, saturated fat, and cholesterol (therapeutic lifestyle diet).[144] Caloric restriction to reduce weight is especially effective if a patient is overweight or obese. In postmenopausal women, treatment with estrogen may substantially improve the hyperlipidemia,[249] probably by stimulating LDL receptor-mediated remnant particle clearance. However, postmenopausal estrogen therapy enhances CHD risk in elderly women with established heart disease, so it is not usually recommended for these patients or for younger women.[250]

If diet therapy and treatment of coexisting metabolic conditions yield unsatisfactory results, drug therapy should be initiated using either niacin, fibric acid derivatives, or HMG-CoA reductase inhibitors, all of which are effective in the treatment of this disorder.[45,178] By decreasing VLDL synthesis and secretion, niacin lowers triglyceride and VLDL cholesterol levels by about 40% and LDL-C levels by 20% and can raise HDL-C concentrations by 20%.[251,252] The fibric acid derivatives, gemfibrozil, clofibrate, bezafibrate (not available in the United States), and fenofibrate can also lower triglyceride and VLDL cholesterol levels.[253,254] Through their ability to increase LDL receptor levels, the HMG-CoA reductase inhibitors can also lower the plasma cholesterol levels.[253,255] Cases that are refractory to treatment with individual drugs can be treated with combinations of fibric acid derivatives and HMG-CoA reductase inhibitors, although this combination should be used cautiously because of the risk of myopathy.[178,253,255] Fenofibrate is the safest fibrate to use in combination therapy with a statin.[178] Because the disorder is associated with premature vascular disease, first-degree relatives such as siblings (or offspring if the affected person's spouse has an apo-E2 allele) should be screened.

Lipoprotein Lipase Deficiency

LPL deficiency is a rare recessive disorder that results from mutations in the LPL gene.[83] These abnormalities cause LPL deficiency and severe hypertriglyceridemia by blocking the clearance of triglyceride-rich lipoproteins from the plasma. Massive accumulations of these lipoproteins in the plasma, known as the *chylomicronemia syndrome,*[256,257] can be accompanied by severe clinical manifestations, including pancreatitis.

Clinical Features

LPL deficiency is usually recognized in infancy or childhood as a chylomicronemia syndrome,[256,257] which consists of marked hypertriglyceridemia associated with recurrent abdominal pain or pancreatitis, which can be life-threatening. A syndrome of recurrent abdominal pain and severe hypertriglyceridemia but without overt pancreatitis or elevated serum amylase concentrations also exists.[256] The pain syndrome is associated with triglyceride levels of more than 22.6 mM/L (2000 mg/dL) and abates with triglyceride lowering. When plasma triglyceride levels exceed 22.6 mM/L (2000 mg/dL), the findings include eruptive xanthomas (see Fig. 36–22G) and lipemia retinalis (see Fig. 36–22B). The plasma may be visibly lipemic; plasma that has been refrigerated overnight might have a cream-like layer on the top, representing chylomicrons. If there is a turbid plasma infranatant, there is a high concentration of VLDL.

Chylomicrons can be assumed to be present if the fasting triglyceride concentration is greater than 11.3 mM/L (1000 mg/dL).[256] The degree of fasting chylomicronemia is determined by the dietary fat intake. Accumulation of triglycerides in tissue reticuloendothelial cells can lead to hepatomegaly and splenomegaly. Chylomicronemia can also cause neurologic manifestations[258-260] and dyspnea.[258] CHD is not a prominent feature, but recurrent episodes of pancreatitis can cause death prematurely. Massive triglyceride elevations can occupy significant plasma volume and lead to artifactually low measurements of serum electrolytes, such as sodium (pseudohyponatremia), if the serum is not cleared of triglyceride-rich lipoproteins by centrifugation before electrolyte measurements.

Subjects who are heterozygous for LPL mutations have reduced LPL activity and often have mild to moderate hypertriglyceridemia, increased VLDL cholesterol levels, and decreased HDL-C levels.[261] This phenotype is exacerbated by age and obesity.

Origin and Pathogenesis

Complete LPL deficiency results from homozygosity or compound heterozygosity for mutations in the LPL gene that lead to the absence or inactivation of the LPL protein.[83,257,262] A variety of mutations have been described. The combined frequency of homozygosity and compound heterozygosity is approximately 1 in 10^6 persons. Patients who are heterozygous for LPL deficiency have half-normal LPL activities,[261] and hypertriglyceridemia can develop in the presence of secondary factors.[261] Heterozygous LPL deficiency occurs at a frequency of 1 in 500 persons in the general population but as high as 1 in 40 in areas of Quebec.[263] In the absence of functional LPL,[257] triglyceride-rich lipoproteins accumulate in the plasma. Because of the impaired clearance of these lipoproteins, plasma triglyceride levels are especially sensitive to dietary fat intake. Chylomicrons are normally cleared from the plasma within 8 hours after eating, but in patients with this disorder, clearance can take days. The triglyceride-rich particles infiltrate organs, where they are taken up by reticuloendothelial cells. The accumulation of these lipoproteins in the plasma can cause pancreatitis, presumably resulting from chemical irritation by fatty acids and lysolecithin liberated by the action of pancreatic lipases.[256]

Diagnosis

LPL deficiency should be suspected in infants or children with pancreatitis or recurrent abdominal pain. Eruptive xanthomas are often present. Plasma triglyceride levels are usually higher than 11.3 mM/L (1000 mg/dL) and may be considerably higher, depending on the dietary fat intake. Eruptive xanthomas, lipemia retinalis, and pancreatitis are usually apparent only when triglyceride levels are greater than 22.6 mM/L (2000 mg/dL). Because LPL deficiency is a recessive disease, family history is usually uninformative except in siblings.

The definitive diagnosis is established by demonstrating the absence of lipase activity in plasma after heparin administration.[257] Heparin, when infused intravenously, displaces LPL from its binding sites on HSPG in capillary endothelium and releases it into plasma, which can be assayed for lipase activity. LPL deficiency must be distinguished from deficiency in the LPL cofactor apo-CII,[83] which is another cause of chylomicronemia. Because several different mutations can result in LPL deficiency, specific mutations can be identified only by specialized laboratories.

Treatment

During the initial stages of treatment of pancreatitis, a fat-free diet is provided until plasma triglycerides reach a safe level (e.g., <11.3 mM/L [1000 mg/dL]). After the acute pancreatitis syndrome has resolved, the mainstay of treatment is a diet that contains very small amounts of fat (e.g., <10% of calories or 20-25 g/day). Because medium-chain triglycerides, in contrast to long-chain triglycerides, are absorbed directly into the portal circulation and do not rely on chylomicron formation for hepatic uptake, they can provide a source of fat in the diet; however, these agents may cause hepatic toxicity.[264,265] Fat-soluble vitamin supplements should be administered. The goal of therapy is to maintain the plasma triglyceride level at less than 11.3 mM/L (1000 mg/dL), which prevents further episodes of pancreatitis.[256]

Drug therapy for primary LPL deficiency is largely ineffective; however, clofibrate, gemfibrozil, fenofibrate, or niacin can lower VLDL production and lessen the severity of the hypertriglyceridemia.[256] Orlistat lowers triglyceride levels significantly in some patients with severe hypertriglyceridemia.[266] Secondary causes of hypertriglyceridemia, such as diabetes mellitus or hypothyroidism, should be identified and treated if present (see "Treatment of the Chylomicronemia Syndrome").

Apolipoprotein CII Deficiency

Apo-CII deficiency is a rare autosomal recessive disorder that occurs in fewer than 1 in 10^6 persons and causes a chylomicronemia syndrome similar to that in LPL deficiency.[83,256,257] As in LPL deficiency, the features include pancreatitis or recurrent bouts of abdominal pain in children or young adults and, after a 12-hour fast, lipemic serum with chylomicrons that rise to the surface of serum that has stood undisturbed for 10 to 12 hours. Plasma triglyceride levels are usually severely elevated (>11.3 mM/L [1000 mg/dL]), reflecting the accumulation of chylomicrons, VLDL, or both lipoproteins in the plasma. This hyperlipoproteinemia results from the lack of apo-CII, an activating cofactor for LPL, which causes a functional LPL deficiency. More than 10 mutations are known to cause apo-CII deficiency.[257] The accumulation of triglyceride-rich particles results in a pathophysiologic process that is nearly identical to that described for LPL deficiency. Heterozygotes might have slightly elevated triglyceride concentrations, but they do not develop pancreatitis.

The diagnosis requires specialized testing to demonstrate that apo-CII is absent on electrophoresis of the plasma apolipoproteins or that the plasma is incapable of activating LPL in vitro.[83,257] The treatment of apo-CII deficiency is identical to that of primary LPL deficiency with the exception that severe hypertriglyceridemia in apo-CII-deficient patients with pancreatitis can be treated with transfusions of plasma, which contains apo-CII.

Familial Hypertriglyceridemia

Familial hypertriglyceridemia is characterized by increased plasma concentrations of triglyceride-rich VLDLs, which cause elevations of plasma triglycerides but not plasma cholesterol levels.

Clinical Features

Subjects with familial hypertriglyceridemia typically have plasma triglyceride levels in the range of 2.3 to 5.6 mM/L (200 to 500 mg/dL) and normal LDL-C levels. As the level of LDL-C considered to be normal has declined, the prevalence of persons with isolated elevations of plasma triglycerides has also diminished. The hypertriglyceridemia is often associated with low plasma HDL-C levels.[219,267] The elevated triglyceride levels are usually not evident until adulthood[176] and may be exacerbated by secondary factors, including hypothyroidism, estrogen therapy, or alcohol ingestion. Such exacerbations can be associated with severe elevations of triglycerides (>11.3 mM/L [1000 mg/dL]), placing subjects at risk for eruptive xanthomas and pancreatitis. However, xanthomas are usually not present. Obesity and insulin resistance are common.

Whether or not familial hypertriglyceridemia increases the risk of developing premature CHD has been uncertain.[176,268] Recent studies suggest that elevated triglyceride levels in patients with familial hypertriglyceridemia are associated with increased CHD risk.[219,269] Among patients with familial hypertriglyceridemia (or familial combined hyperlipidemia), CHD risk was substantially attenuated by accounting for the presence of the metabolic syndrome, diabetes mellitus, hypertension, and low HDL-C levels. More than 70% of patients with familial hypertriglyceridemia met the criteria for the metabolic syndrome.[219]

Origin and Pathogenesis

Familial hypertriglyceridemia appears to be caused by overproduction of VLDL triglycerides in the presence of near-normal apo-B production,[227,228] which leads to the secretion of large, triglyceride-rich VLDL. Secondary disorders (e.g., insulin resistance) that lead to VLDL overproduction can exacerbate the syndrome. The low plasma HDL levels commonly found in hypertriglyceridemia are associated with enhanced fractional catabolism of apo-AI.[270,271] Hepatic overproduction of bile acids in association with impaired intestinal absorption of bile acids has been demonstrated.[272,273] Increased expression of the ileal apical sodium bile acid transporter gene, SLC10A2, on chromosome 13 has been observed, but mutations in the coding and 5′ flanking region do not account for the observed decrease in intestinal bile acid transport.[273,274] Genetic loci on chromosome 15 are associated with triglyceride levels in familial combined hypertriglyceridemia kindreds.[275] Whether the large, triglyceride-rich VLDLs are atherogenic is unclear; an enhanced risk of premature CHD may be related to whether concomitant decreases in HDL-C occur.

Diagnosis

Familial hypertriglyceridemia should be suspected in patients with increased plasma triglyceride levels and normal plasma cholesterol levels. The disorder can be diagnosed only if hypertriglyceridemia is found in half of the first-degree relatives at risk, and it can be difficult to distinguish from familial combined hyperlipidemia, which can also occur as isolated hypertriglyceridemia related to increased plasma VLDL. Plasma lipid levels in children of affected parents have not been studied, so it is unknown if children in familial hypertriglyceridemia kindreds can be identified. Elevated VLDL levels impart a cloudy appearance to plasma after overnight refrigeration.

Treatment

In addition to dietary fat restriction, secondary disorders such as diabetes mellitus, estrogen administration, or alcohol intake should be screened for and treated. Drugs that lower triglyceride levels (e.g., niacin, gemfibrozil) may be useful. Because niacin can impair glucose tolerance, it should be used cautiously in patients with underlying insulin resistance.

Elevated Plasma Lipoprotein(a)

This disorder consists of elevations of modified LDL particles in the plasma, in which the apo-B protein of LDL is covalently bonded to apo(a).[276,277] Apo(a) is a protein of unknown function that shares high sequence homology with plasminogen but is not a catalytically active protease that degrades fibrin.[278] Some[217,279-281] but not all[282-286] studies suggest that elevated plasma Lp(a) concentrations are associated with an increased risk of CHD.

Clinical Features

There are no characteristic physical findings or lipoprotein patterns to suggest elevated plasma Lp(a) levels. Elevated Lp(a) may be suspected, however, in patients with symptomatic premature CHD. Plasma Lp(a) concentrations are influenced by heredity[287,288] and vary among different ethnic populations.[289] For example, African populations have higher levels.[290] Some data suggest that elevations of plasma Lp(a) may be associated with CHD events only in those with high concentrations of LDL or who are otherwise at high risk.[291-293] Thus, high Lp(a) levels may be viewed as a potent risk factor for CHD events in predisposed patients.[293]

Origin and Pathogenesis

Apo(a) is found only in humans, nonhuman primates, and hedgehogs.[290] Its function from an evolutionary perspective is unclear. Nevertheless, the presence of high plasma levels of apo(a) appears to have been selected for in certain populations.[289] Apo(a) is attached by a single disulfide bond to the apo-B protein of LDL.[294] Plasma Lp(a) levels in the absence of inflammation are in large part determined by heredity and appear to be related to the number of repeats of a kringle motif in the apo(a) protein.[287] The larger isoforms that contain more kringle repeats are found in lower concentrations in the plasma,[295] possibly related to impaired processing of these large forms for secretion by hepatocytes.

The factors that control the production and clearance of Lp(a) are largely unknown. Renal failure is associated with substantial elevations of Lp(a) levels, which revert to lower levels subsequent to renal transplantation. It is the higher molecular weight isoforms of apo(a) in Lp(a) that increase in concentration in renal failure and that revert to normal after transplantation.[296] An increased susceptibility to atherosclerosis modulated by Lp(a) particle size rather than Lp(a) concentrations has been suggested.[297] It is the smaller Lp(a) particles that are associated with higher risk. Lp(a) might promote atherosclerosis because of impaired fibrinolysis caused by competition for plasminogen receptors or inhibition of plasminogen activation,[298-300] effects on smooth muscle proliferation,[301] or unknown factors.

Diagnosis

The measurement of Lp(a) levels has been fraught with difficulties due to the genetically determined variability in apo(a) size, stability when samples are frozen, and the lack of suitable reference reagent.[302,303] Lp(a) levels should be reported in units of nmol/L of Lp(a) protein, with levels greater than 75 nmol/L as the definition of elevated.[302] Assays reporting values in mg/dL are not standardized, which precludes comparison of data from different laboratories. Conflicting effects of statins on Lp(a) levels have been reported.[302] Lp(a) is an acute phase protein that accounts for transient elevations of Lp(a) in patients with inflammatory disorders.[304] This should be kept in mind when blood samples are obtained to measure Lp(a) levels.

Treatment

Of the hypolipidemic drugs currently available, only niacin appears to lower plasma Lp(a) levels.[305] Treatment with niacin (4 g/day) lowers Lp(a) levels by 35% to 40%. In postmenopausal women, estrogen with or without a progestin lowers Lp(a) levels by 10% to 20%.[306] In a study of the effect of hormone replacement therapy in older women (mean age 66.7 years) with a history of CHD, those with the highest concentrations of Lp(a) had the greatest reductions in Lp(a) levels and in the incidence of nonfatal heart attacks or CHD death. Women with Lp(a) values in the normal range at baseline who received hormone replacement therapy experienced minimal change in Lp(a) levels and had a 50% increase in the risk of sustaining a primary endpoint event (nonfatal heart attack or CHD death) compared to women with the highest baseline Lp(a) values.[307] Scrupulous attention to management of the traditional risk factors can reduce the consequences of elevated Lp(a) levels.[292,293]

Polygenic Hypercholesterolemia

Hypercholesterolemia is defined as a cholesterol value that exceeds the 95th percentile for the population. A study by Goldstein and coworkers[176] suggested that about 10% of men sustaining a myocardial infarction before age 60 have familial combined hyperlipidemia and about 5% have FH. In another 5% of patients, the cause of the hypercholesterolemia appears to involve combinations of multiple genetic and environmental factors. Other genetic factors that contribute to hypercholesterolemia can involve physiologic processes that influence cholesterol absorption, bile acid metabolism, or intracellular cholesterol metabolism. Polygenic hypercholesterolemia is diagnosed by excluding other primary genetic causes, by the absence of tendon xanthomas, and by demonstrating that hypercholesterolemia is present in no more than 10% of first-degree relatives.[176] The hypercholesterolemia is treated according to NCEP ATP III guidelines (described later).

Sporadic Hypertriglyceridemia

As with high plasma cholesterol levels, unknown genetic and environmental factors can result in elevated plasma triglyceride levels.[176] This *sporadic hypertriglyceridemia* can be distinguished from familial syndromes by the absence of hypertriglyceridemia in relatives. The condition is evaluated and treated according to NCEP ATP III guidelines.

■ Primary Disorders of High-Density Lipoprotein Metabolism

Several genetic disorders can result in decreased or increased plasma levels of HDL-C (Table 36–9).

TABLE 36–9 GENETIC DISORDERS OF HIGH-DENSITY LIPOPROTEIN METABOLISM

Disorder	Mutant Gene	Mode of Inheritance	Population Frequency	Typical Plasma HDL-C (mM/L [mg/dL])	TYPICAL CLINICAL MANIFESTATIONS	
					Corneal Opacifications	Premature Vascular Disease
Familial hypoalphalipoproteinemia	Unknown	Autosomal dominant	~1/400	0.5-0.8 [20-30]	–	+
Familial apo-AI and apo-CIII deficiency	Apo-AI or apo-AI/apo-CIII	Autosomal recessive	Rare	<0.1 [5]	+	+
Apo-AI_{Milano}	Apo-AI	Autosomal dominant	Rare	~0.3 [10]	–	–
LCAT deficiency	LCAT	Autosomal recessive	Rare	<0.3 [10]	+	+
Fish-eye disease	LCAT	Autosomal recessive	Rare	<0.3 [10]	+	–
Tangier disease*	ABCA1	Autosomal recessive	Rare	<0.1 [5]	+	+
CETP deficiency	CETP	Autosomal recessive	Rare	>2.6 [100]	–	–

*Clinical manifestations also include orange tonsils.

ABCA1, ATP binding cassette transporter A1; apo, apolipoprotein; CETP, cholesteryl ester transfer protein; LCAT, lecithin:cholesterol acyltransferase.

TABLE 36–10 GUIDELINES BASED ON TC/HDL-C RATIO FOR TREATMENT OF LOW HDL-C POPULATIONS

Risk Category	GOALS			LIFESTYLE CHANGE INITIATED FOR			DRUG THERAPY INITIATED FOR		
	LDL-C (mg/dL)		TC/HDL-C	LDL-C (mg/dL)		TC/HDL-C	LDL-C (mg/dL)		TC/HDL-C
CHD or equivalent	<100	and	<3.5	≥100	or	≥3.5	≥100	or	≥3.5
2+ Risk factors	<130	and	<4.5	≥130	or	≥4.5	≥130	or	≥6.0
0-1 Risk factor	<160	and	<5.5	≥160	or	≥5.5	≥160	or	≥7.0

CHD, coronary heart disease; HDL-C, high-density lipoprotein cholesterol; LDL-C, low-density lipoprotein cholesterol; TC, total cholesterol.

Familial Hypoalphalipoproteinemia

The autosomal dominant disorder familial hypoalphalipoproteinemia is manifested by low plasma HDL-C levels, normal LDL-C and fasting triglyceride levels, and an increased risk of premature CHD.[217] The diagnosis is suggested by HDL-C levels that are less than the 10th percentile (<0.77 mM/L [30 mg/dL]) in men or the 15th percentile in women (1.04 mM/L [40 mg/dL]) based on a study of the distribution of HDL-C levels in the United States.[144] There are no characteristic physical findings, but there is often a family history of low HDL-C levels and premature CHD. The genetic and metabolic defects that lead to low plasma HDL levels are unknown, but it appears that up to 50% of low HDL-C levels can be linked to the hepatic lipase or apo-AI/apo-CIII/apo-AIV/apo-AV gene locus.[308] The lack of HDL in the plasma accelerates the development of atherosclerosis, presumably because reverse cholesterol transport or other protective effects of HDL are impaired.[309]

Drug therapy should be aimed at raising the plasma HDL concentration or lowering the plasma LDL concentration with statins (Table 36–10).[310] Fibrates (gemfibrozil, fenofibrate) raise HDL-C levels about 5% to 20%, similar to the effects of statins. Niacin is the most effective drug currently available to raise HDL-C levels. However, there is a paucity of data showing that fibrates and niacin as monotherapies reduce vascular disease events, and there is a plethora of data suggesting that statins prevent events in patients with low HDL-C levels. For this reason, statin therapy should be the first-line treatment; niacin or fibrate should be added (keeping in mind the risk of myopathy) if lipid goals cannot be reached with statin monotherapy.[178] Lifestyle and drug treatments can raise HDL levels. Lifestyle choices that raise HDL-C levels include exercise, smoking cessation, weight control, moderate alcohol use, and avoiding diets that are low in total fat and high in simple rather than complex carbohydrates.[311] Unfortunately these lifestyle choices are less effective in patients with low HDL-C levels than in those with normal levels.[312]

Low HDL levels have been found in certain ethnic groups. For example, persons from South and Southeast Asian, and specifically from the Indian subcontinent, have very low HDL levels in the context of insulin resistance.[313,314] In Turks, however, low HDL levels are associated with elevated hepatic lipase activity without insulin resistance.[315,316]

Apolipoprotein AI Mutations

Mutations in the apo-AI gene[54,317,318] can decrease HDL formation and result in low plasma HDL-C levels. Apo-AI deficiency can be caused by point mutations in the apo-AI gene or by deletions or gene rearrangements at the apo-AI/apo-CIII/apo-AIV/apo-AV gene locus.[317] Apo-AI deficiency typically results in plasma HDL-C levels less than 0.3 mM/L (10 mg/dL).[317] Mutations affecting residues 121 to 186 in the center of the apo-AI molecule are associated with low HDL-C levels. These apo-AI variants activate LCAT poorly. Mutations resulting in substitutions in amino-terminal residues 1 to 90 are not typically associated with low HDL-C levels but are associated with deposition of amyloid.[317,318] Manifestations include a predisposition to premature CHD, xanthomas, and corneal opacities.[318] The molecular diagnosis can be made only by specialized analysis, including electrophoresis of the plasma apolipoproteins and DNA analysis to identify the mutation. Inasmuch as it is difficult to raise the plasma apo-AI or HDL-C levels in these disorders, the treatment should be directed toward lowering the levels of plasma non-HDL-C (VLDL and LDL).

Other rare variants of apo-AI exist,[317] including apo-AI_{Milano},[319] which is caused by a substitution of cysteine for arginine at amino acid 173 and results in lower plasma HDL-C levels. This mutation is inherited as an autosomal dominant trait and has not been associated with premature CHD. Whether the mutation protects against the development of atherosclerosis or whether this kindred has mitigating genetic or environmental factors is not known. However, the results of a small trial in acute coronary syndrome patients infused weekly with apo-AI_{Milano} suggest that this treatment might reduce atheroma plaque volume.[320] Other apo-AI variants are associated with amyloidosis.[317]

Cholesteryl Ester Transfer Protein Deficiency

CETP deficiency is a hereditary syndrome in which plasma HDL-C levels are increased because of diminished activity of plasma CETP.[111,321] Once thought to be rare, the disorder is not uncommon in the Japanese population.[111] Its features include marked elevations of plasma HDL-C in homozygotes (usually >2.6 mM/L [100 mg/dL]); however, despite the elevated HDL-C levels, the effect on CHD risk of CETP gene mutations that reduce CETP activity is unclear.[111,321] Heterozygotes have moderately elevated HDL-C levels. The lower activity of CETP results in diminished transfer of cholesteryl esters from HDL to the apo-B–containing lipoproteins. As a result, more cholesteryl esters are found in HDL, and the ratio of total cholesterol to HDL-C is markedly reduced.

Studies in transgenic mice have confirmed a relation between CETP activity and atherosclerosis risk. Although mice normally do not have significant plasma CETP activity and have high plasma HDL-C levels, transgenic mice that express CETP have increased plasma LDL-C, decreased HDL-C, and increased susceptibility to atherosclerosis.[115] As discussed previously, subjects who are heterozygous for CETP deficiency experience CHD despite high plasma HDL,[111] and it remains to be determined if lowering CETP activity in humans would have therapeutic value. Inhibitors of CETP have been developed and are being studied in humans.[322] The molecular diagnosis of CETP deficiency requires the measurement of plasma CETP activity in vitro or identification of the DNA mutation. At present, there is no specific treatment.

Lecithin:Cholesterol Acyltransferase Deficiency

LCAT deficiency is a rare autosomal recessive disorder that causes corneal opacities,[170] normochromic anemia, and renal failure in young adults.[323] About 30 affected kindreds and a number of mutations have been described.[324] LCAT deficiency results in decreased esterification of cholesterol to cholesteryl esters on HDL particles.[325] As a result, free cholesterol accumulates on lipoprotein particles and in peripheral tissues such as the cornea, red blood cell membranes, and renal glomeruli, presumably because reverse cholesterol transport is impaired. Plasma cholesterol levels in LCAT deficiency are variable, HDL-C levels are reduced, and the ratio of free (unesterified) cholesterol to esterified cholesterol in the plasma is increased. Normally, free cholesterol accounts for about one third of the total cholesterol in the plasma; in LCAT deficiency, free cholesterol accounts for most of the plasma cholesterol. The accumulation of free cholesterol in vascular tissues can lead to premature CHD. A limited number of patients homozygous for LCAT mutations have been followed for 20 to 30 years. Despite their very low HDL levels they do not develop premature atherosclerosis. Paradoxically, those who are heterozygous have more pronounced atherosclerosis despite higher levels of HDL-C.[324,326] At present, there is no means to increase the plasma activity of LCAT; therefore, the treatment is preventive (by dietary fat restriction, statin therapy, or LDL apheresis)[318] and symptomatic (e.g., renal transplantation).

A variant of LCAT deficiency is called fish-eye disease.[327] Although this disorder is also caused by mutations of the LCAT gene,[324] the phenotype is less severe than that seen in complete LCAT deficiency. Fish-eye disease is characterized by low plasma HDL-C levels and corneal opacities; anemia and renal disease do not occur. Premature atherosclerosis, once thought not to be a feature of fish-eye disease, has been reported.[324] The phenotypic differences between LCAT deficiency and fish-eye disease have been attributed to whether mutations in the LCAT gene encode variants that fail to esterify cholesterol of both HDL and apo-B–containing lipoproteins (LCAT deficiency) or of HDL only (fish-eye disease)[328]; however, one subject with phenotypic fish-eye disease had normal HDL-associated LCAT activity.[323]

Tangier Disease

Tangier disease is a rare autosomal recessive disorder associated with hypolipidemia, including decreases in plasma HDL and LDL-C levels and orange tonsils.[329] Other features include corneal opacities,[170] hepatosplenomegaly, peripheral neuropathy, and premature CHD.[330] Metabolic studies have demonstrated that the disorder is associated with enhanced catabolism of plasma HDL.[331] Mutations in *ABCA1* have been causally linked to Tangier disease.[332-334] ABCA1 appears to promote cholesterol efflux from cells such as macrophages; the loss of this function apparently accounts for the impaired efflux of cholesterol from Tangier cells.[109] As a result, massive amounts of cholesteryl esters accumulate in macrophages of the reticuloendothelial system. The orange tonsils observed in this disorder are caused by cholesterol deposits. There is currently no specific treatment. Available data suggest that heterozygosity for *ABCA1* mutations occurs in about 10% of patients with inherited low-HDL–only syndromes.[335,336]

Primary Genetic Hypolipidemias

Familial Hypobetalipoproteinemia

Familial hypobetalipoproteinemia is defined as apo-B and LDL-C levels below the 5th percentile. The genetic bases of hypobetalipoproteinemia are poorly understood in the vast majority of cases.[337] One well-characterized type of familial hypobetalipoproteinemia is caused by mutations in the apo-B100 gene coding for truncated apo-B100 molecules. Reduced synthesis and enhanced clearance of VLDL containing truncated apo-B100 account for the reduced LDL levels. The disorder is inherited as an autosomal dominant trait.[338] A report describes hypobetalipoproteinemia associated with two nonsense mutations in *PCSK9*. Enhanced LDL receptor–mediated hepatic uptake of LDL accounts for the reduced LDL levels. The PCSK9 loss-of-function mutations might occur in as many as 2% of African Americans, but it is rare in persons of European descent.[210]

Clinical Features

The prevalence of heterozygous subjects with apo-B mutations causing low LDL-C levels is unknown, but it has been estimated to vary between 0.02% and 0.2%. Affected persons are usually asymptomatic but come to attention because of the detection of low plasma cholesterol levels. Typically, the total plasma cholesterol level is less than the 5th percentile, and it may be less than 2.6 mM/L (100 mg/dL). Plasma LDL-C levels are also reduced by one half or more, and HDL-C levels are normal or slightly increased.[338] Plasma triglyceride levels are reduced in some kindreds. Although heterozygotes are usually asymptomatic, fat malabsorption has been reported.[338,339] The syndrome is associated with longevity, probably the result of a low risk for CHD.[338]

Subjects who are homozygotes or compound heterozygotes for these apo-B mutations are rare, about 1 in 10^6 persons. Homozygotes may be detected at a young age because of fat malabsorption and decreased plasma cholesterol levels. Fat malabsorption is caused by inability to form chylomicrons in the intestine and subsequent failure to absorb fats and fat-soluble vitamins. Fat malabsorption may be accompanied by retinitis pigmentosa, erythrocyte acanthocytosis, and progressive neurologic degenerative disease resulting from vitamin E deficiency. The acanthocytosis is caused by alterations in red blood cell membrane lipids. Despite the low plasma cholesterol levels, steroidogenesis appears to be normal except when synthetic demands are quite high.[340] Homozygous subjects who produce enough of a truncated isoform of apo-B to facilitate some fat absorption might have a milder phenotype.

Origin and Pathogenesis

More than 30 mutations in the apo-B gene have been described; most are either nonsense or frameshift mutations that lead to the formation of truncated apo-B proteins.[338] Metabolic turnover studies indicate that these mutations impair the synthesis of apo-B–containing lipoproteins in some cases[341] and enhance their clearance from the plasma in others.[342] The decreased levels of apo-B–containing lipoproteins in the plasma cause low plasma cholesterol and triglyceride levels. Although many cases of hypobetalipoproteinemia involve apo-B mutations, additional undefined genetic factors can result in low cholesterol levels.[343,344]

In homozygous subjects, the absence of apo-B leads to impaired intestinal chylomicron formation, which in turn leads to impaired absorption of fats and fat-soluble vitamins. Cholesterol absorption is probably also impaired, as demonstrated in transgenic mice lacking intestinal apo-B expression and chylomicron formation.[345] As noted, vitamin E malabsorption results in low tissue stores of tocopherol and a degenerative neurologic disease. Retinal degeneration might also be related to deficiencies of fat-soluble vitamins.[346]

Diagnosis

The diagnosis of familial hypobetalipoproteinemia is suggested by low plasma total and LDL cholesterol levels inherited as an autosomal dominant trait. The homozygous condition is suggested by extremely low plasma cholesterol and triglyceride levels in an infant or child with fat malabsorption. The differential diagnosis of the homozygous state includes abetalipoproteinemia (see later discussion) and Anderson's disease (chylomicron retention disease).[347] The molecular diagnosis of hypobetalipoproteinemia caused by apo-B mutations can be performed only in specialized laboratories by gel electrophoresis of plasma apo-B or by DNA analysis to identify specific mutations.

Treatment and Prognosis

Because heterozygous subjects are almost always asymptomatic, no specific treatment is indicated, but dietary supplementation of fat-soluble vitamins (especially vitamin E) is reasonable. Heterozygotes should be informed that if their spouse also has a very low plasma cholesterol level, their children could have homozygous or compound heterozygous hypobetalipoproteinemia; in this scenario, subjects should be referred to a lipid clinic for genetic counseling.

Subjects with homozygous hypobetalipoproteinemia (phenotypic abetalipoproteinemia) should be treated with large doses of vitamin E orally (100 to 300 mg/kg/day), which can raise the tissue vitamin E concentrations and prevent the neurologic complications.[338] Administration of large doses of the other fat-soluble vitamins should be considered, because nearly fatal exsanguinating bleeding during childbirth occurred in a patient with severe vitamin K depletion.[338] It is imperative to make the diagnosis and begin treatment at an early age to prevent nutritional deficiencies. Fat should be provided in the diet up to a level that symptoms allow (usually 15% to 20% of calories). Supplementation with medium-chain triglycerides is probably contraindicated because of reports of liver toxicity.

Abetalipoproteinemia

Abetalipoproteinemia is a rare autosomal recessive disorder caused by a deficiency in MTP, which results in a virtual absence of apo-B–containing lipoproteins in the plasma.[103]

Clinical Features

Abetalipoproteinemia occurs in fewer than 1 in 10^6 persons and has the same phenotype as homozygous hypobetalipoproteinemia, including malabsorption of fat and fat-soluble vitamins from the intestine, which can lead to neurologic disease related to vitamin E deficiency. The disorder is usually detected in infancy because of fat malabsorption associated with marked decreases in plasma cholesterol and triglyceride levels.

Origin and Pathogenesis

Abetalipoproteinemia is caused by a deficiency of MTP,[103] a protein that transfers triglycerides or phospholipids onto nascent apo-B–containing lipoproteins during their formation in the ER. Insufficient lipidation of nascent particles impairs the synthesis and secretion of these particles by the intestine and the liver, and little if any apo-B is found in the plasma. At least 18 mutations in the MTP gene have been described.[103] The lack of MTP in the intestine leads to impaired chylomicron formation and malabsorption of fats and fat-soluble vitamins.

Diagnosis

The diagnosis is suggested by fat malabsorption associated with extremely low levels of plasma cholesterol (usually <1.3 mM/L [50 mg/dL]) and triglyceride in an infant or young child.[103] Cholesterol levels in the parents, who are obligate heterozygotes, are normal. The demonstration of the molecular defect requires a specialized laboratory for detection of low or absent MTP in intestinal biopsy specimens or DNA analysis to identify specific mutations. The differential diagnosis of abetalipoproteinemia includes homozygous hypobetalipoproteinemia, in which the obligate heterozygote parents have low plasma lipid levels, and Anderson's disease.[347] Also called *chylomicron retention syndrome,* Anderson's disease is a rare condition that is phenotypically similar to abetalipoproteinemia. Subjects with Anderson's disease cannot secrete chylomicrons from the intestine. Eight mutations in the SARA2 gene have been linked to Anderson's disease. This gene encodes Sar1b, a protein that is important in the transport of chylomicrons through the secretory pathway in enterocytes.[32,347]

Treatment

Abetalipoproteinemia caused by mutations in *MTP* or *SARA2* is treated in the same way as homozygous hypobetalipoproteinemia. Large doses of vitamin E are given by mouth to prevent the neurologic sequelae of vitamin E deficiency.

Other Rare Primary Lipid Disorders

Hepatic Lipase Deficiency

Hepatic lipase deficiency is a disorder associated with lack of heparin-releasable hepatic lipase activity in the plasma.[348] The disorder is inherited as an autosomal recessive trait, and five different missense mutations have been identified in the six known families with affected members.[349] Its features include combined hyperlipidemia, with elevated levels of plasma cholesterol (6.5-38.8 mM/L [250-1500 mg/dL]) and triglyceride (4.5-92.6 mM/L [395-8200 mg/dL]); palmar and tuboeruptive xanthomas; and premature arcus corneae. β-VLDL levels are increased because of impaired conversion of VLDL to IDL to LDL (however, the VLDL cholesterol-to-triglyceride ratio is <0.3, in contrast to type III hyperlipoproteinemia), and the LDL and HDL fractions are enriched threefold to fivefold in triglyceride. HDL-C levels are normal or slightly increased. Susceptibility to atherosclerosis is thought to be increased. The demonstration of hepatic lipase deficiency requires specialized in vitro assays of hepatic lipase activity in plasma or DNA analysis to identify mutations. Dietary restriction of fat and cholesterol can lower the plasma lipid levels. Fenofibrate normalizes plasma lipids primarily by enhancing the catabolism of VLDL and IDL, presumably by increasing the expression of LPL.[350]

Sitosterolemia

In this rare disorder, dietary sitosterol and other plant sterols, which are not normally absorbed in significant quantities in the intestine, are absorbed in large amounts, resulting in their accumulation in the plasma and in peripheral tissues.[351] Premature atherosclerosis can occur.[352] The molecular cause was identified as mutations in the genes encoding ABCG8 and ABCG5 on chromosome 2p21.[353,354] Clinically, affected subjects develop tendon xanthomas in childhood and have normal to high plasma levels of LDL-C; the differential diagnosis includes FH and cerebrotendinous xanthomatosis. The diagnosis can be confirmed by gas-liquid chromatography of plasma lipids to demonstrate the high levels of plant sterols. Treatment consists of restriction of plant sterols in the diet and treatment with ezetimibe, a drug that inhibits absorption of dietary sterols.[355]

Cerebrotendinous Xanthomatosis

Cerebrotendinous xanthomatosis[356] is a rare disorder of sterol metabolism associated with neurologic disease, tendon xanthomas, and cataracts in young adults. Neurologic manifestations include cerebellar ataxia, dementia, spinal cord paresis, and subnormal intelligence. Premature atherosclerosis is common. Osteoporosis has been reported and is presumably caused by alterations in vitamin D metabolism.[357] The disorder results from mutations that cause deficiencies of 27-hydroxylase, a key enzyme in cholesterol oxidation and bile acid synthesis.[356] As a result, high levels of cholesterol and cholestanol, a 5α-dihydro derivative of cholesterol, accumulate in the plasma, tendons, and tissues of the nervous system. Treatment is with chenodeoxycholic acid,[356] often in combination with an HMG-CoA reductase inhibitor, although there is concern that statin-induced enhanced cellular uptake of cholesterol might worsen the condition.[356,358,359]

Lysosomal Acid Lipase Deficiency

Lysosomal acid lipase deficiency is an autosomal recessive disorder that results in massive accumulation of cholesteryl esters and triglycerides in lysosomes.[360-362] In the variant called *Wolman's disease,* which is usually fatal in the first year of life, there is a complete deficiency of the lysosomal lipase. Cholesteryl ester storage disease is a milder variant in which there is less accumulation of triglycerides than in Wolman's disease, possibly because of some residual enzyme activity; affected subjects can survive past childhood but can develop premature CHD.

Familial Isolated Vitamin E Deficiency

Familial isolated vitamin E deficiency is a rare disorder characterized by low plasma levels of vitamin E in association with progressive degenerative neurologic disease.[363,364] It is caused by lack of hepatic α-tocopherol transfer protein,[365] which is thought to facilitate the incorporation of α-tocopherol onto nascent VLDLs during their formation in the liver. In the absence of the protein, there is a lack of vitamin E on VLDL, which is a major transport mechanism for delivery of vitamin E to peripheral tissues. Treatment consists of daily supplementation with large doses of oral vitamin E.

Secondary Disorders of Lipid Metabolism

A number of metabolic diseases and drug therapies influence plasma lipid levels.[366] The secondary disorders of hyperlipidemia are listed in Table 36–7. Factors that affect HDL levels are listed in Table 36–11.

Diabetes Mellitus

Of the common diseases, diabetes mellitus exerts some of the most profound effects on plasma lipid metabolism.[367-369] Hyper-

TABLE 36–11 FACTORS AFFECTING PLASMA HIGH-DENSITY LIPOPROTEIN LEVELS

FACTORS THAT INCREASE HDL
Alcohol Drugs: Nicotinic acid, fibrates, HMG-CoA reductase inhibitors Estrogens Exercise
FACTORS THAT DECREASE HDL
Androgens Cigarette smoking Drugs: β-blockers, anabolic steroids Low-fat diet Obesity Progestogens

HDL, high-density lipoproteins; HMG-CoA, 3-hydroxy-3-methylglutaryl coenzyme A.

triglyceridemia is found in up to one third of all diabetic patients and is related to the critical role of insulin in the production and clearance of triglyceride-rich lipoproteins from the plasma.[367] In addition, diabetic patients often have high plasma levels of atherogenic lipoproteins and low plasma HDL, predisposing them to premature CHD, a leading cause of death in diabetes.

In type 1 diabetes, insulin deficiency and poor glycemic control lead to increases in the plasma levels of triglycerides and apo-B–containing lipoproteins because of effects on plasma lipid metabolism in peripheral tissues and the liver. In peripheral tissues, insulin deficiency results in impaired LPL activity and diminished clearance of triglyceride-rich particles.[370] Insulin deficiency also enhances lipolysis, which increases FFA flux to the liver. In the liver, increased FFA flux drives triglyceride synthesis and VLDL triglyceride synthesis and secretion. Plasma LDL-C levels may also be increased, possibly because insulin stimulates LDL receptor–mediated degradation of LDL,[371] and this is diminished in type 1 diabetes.

In its most severe form, insulin deficiency can cause a chylomicronemia syndrome known as *diabetic lipemia*.[370,372] In this disorder, massive increases in plasma triglyceride levels (>22.6 mM/L [2000 mg/dL]) can result in lipemia retinalis, eruptive xanthomas, fatty liver, and pancreatitis. This disorder arises from an acquired LPL deficiency[370] and is relatively rare in the modern era of insulin therapy. The acquired lack of LPL activity results in accumulation of chylomicrons in the plasma, similar to that seen in primary genetic LPL deficiency. The disorder might result from diabetes mellitus in combination with an underlying disorder of triglyceride metabolism.[373] The hyperlipidemia related to insulin deficiency and type 1 diabetes is reversible with insulin therapy. Persistent lipid abnormalities in patients with type 1 diabetes with excellent glycemic control suggest that another disorder of lipid metabolism is present.

In type 2 diabetes, which accounts for more than 90% of cases, the metabolic defect is related to insulin resistance and relative insulin deficiency. The insulin resistance appears to be caused by both genetic and acquired factors; metabolic abnormalities that accompany the insulin resistance include obesity, hyperglycemia, hypertension, plasma lipid abnormalities, and hyperuricemia, which are referred to as *syndrome X* or the *metabolic syndrome*.[215,216] One of the most common lipid abnormalities in type 2 diabetes is a moderate hyperlipidemia characterized by an increase in VLDL, which may be accompanied by chylomicronemia, depending on how well blood glucose levels are regulated and on the dietary fat intake. This disorder is characterized by the accumulation of apo-B–containing lipoproteins, which are proatherogenic, in the plasma. The fasting plasma triglyceride and cholesterol levels are often moderately elevated, the HDL-C concentration is usually low, and remnants of VLDL and chylomicrons, which are atherogenic, are also often increased. Plasma levels of LDL are increased in some but not all subjects. However, the hyperlipidemia in type 2 diabetes is often characterized by an increase in small, dense LDLs (LDL subclass pattern B),[215] which are particularly atherogenic; this increase occurs even in the absence of elevated total cholesterol levels.[215] In addition, a portion of the plasma LDL undergoes glycosylation, which can increase binding to arterial wall proteoglycans and susceptibility to oxidation.[374,375] Xanthomas are usually absent in this disorder.

Factors that contribute to the lipoprotein abnormalities in type 2 diabetes include decreased LPL activity in muscle and adipose tissue and increased FFA flux to the liver from peripheral adipose tissue stores.[215] Combined with hepatic overproduction of apo-B, which occurs in insulin resistance,[376] the FFA flux drives triglyceride synthesis and VLDL production in the liver.[215] The lipid abnormalities associated with VLDL overproduction may be exacerbated by a primary genetic disorder of lipid metabolism.[373,377]

A cornerstone of therapy for patients with type 2 diabetes with hyperlipidemia is glycemic control through regular exercise, diet, oral hypoglycemic agents, or insulin therapy. Periodic monitoring of the glycosylated hemoglobin is helpful in assessing the glycemic control. However, in contrast to the situation in type 1 diabetes, the hyperlipidemia in type 2 diabetes cannot be eradicated even with excellent glycemic control because these subjects have accompanying genetic and acquired metabolic abnormalities that are not resolved by returning blood sugar levels to normal. Decreasing insulin resistance through weight loss and exercise can, however, have dramatic effects on both the hyperglycemia and the hyperlipidemia.[378] Metformin, a hypoglycemic agent, may lower plasma glucose levels and produce a modest lowering of plasma lipid levels.[379] In addition to glycemic control, drugs for diabetic hyperlipidemia include HMG-CoA reductase inhibitors, a mandated therapy for all type 2 diabetes patients, and, in certain cases, addition of fibrate or niacin therapy may be beneficial. Niacin should be used with caution because it can impair or worsen glucose tolerance. Treatment with insulin can lower plasma LDL-C levels in both type 1[380] and type 2[381] diabetes mellitus.

Hypothyroidism

Alterations in thyroid function can have profound effects on plasma lipids,[382,383] and all patients with significant hyperlipidemia should be screened for hypothyroidism. The classic manifestation of hypothyroidism is an elevation of the plasma LDL-C level (6.5 to 15.5 mM/L [250 to 600 mg/dL]), but this disorder can also be associated with high plasma triglyceride levels.[383] Levels of HDL-C are usually unchanged or slightly lower in hypothyroidism and may be reduced in hyperthyroidism[384]; the latter effect may be related to alterations in hepatic lipase activity.[384] The elevations of plasma LDL-C in hypothyroidism are associated with impaired clearance of LDL,[385] probably reflecting decreased LDL receptor expression.[386] The high LDL-C levels in hypothyroidism are associated with an increased risk of atherosclerosis,[387] but risk of myocardial infarction is not necessarily increased,[387,388] perhaps because hypothyroidism decreases myocardial oxygen demand. Subclinical hypothyroidism, in which metabolic abnormalities are present without symptoms, can also cause hypercholesterolemia that responds to treatment with thyroid hormone. Hypothyroidism is also associated with low LPL activity,[383] predisposing to increased plasma triglyceride levels. Hyperlipidemia with hypothyroidism may be more marked in those with an underlying genetic susceptibility,[248,389] but it responds dramatically to thyroid hormone replacement. In elderly patients with CHD or significant risk factors, thyroid hormone should be replaced cautiously to avoid precipitating ischemic heart disease clinical events.

Estrogen Therapy

Although once thought to reduce CHD risk, estrogen therapy in postmenopausal women is now known to increase CHD event risk in older women with a history of myocardial infarction.[390] Estrogen therapy increases plasma triglyceride levels[391] and can occasionally cause marked hypertriglyceridemia, especially in predisposed persons.[392] The hypertriglyceridemia appears to be dose-related.[393] Although most women taking either oral contraceptives or oral postmenopausal estrogens maintain triglyceride levels in the normal range, massive hypertriglyceridemia can on occasion cause pancreatitis.[392] For this reason, triglyceride levels should be measured in women before estrogen therapy is initiated. Women who develop hypertriglyceridemia after initiating oral estrogen therapy experience significant reductions in triglyceride levels after changing to transdermal estrogen administration.[394] Estrogens appear to cause hypertriglyceridemia through increased production of VLDL.[395] LPL activity in adipose tissue is not altered. Tamoxifen, a selective estrogen receptor modulator used in breast cancer patients, can also cause severe hypertriglyceridemia and pancreatitis.[392] Raloxifene, another selective estrogen receptor modulator, does not raise triglycerides.[396]

Estrogen therapy also enhances the clearance of LDL from the circulation[391] and lowers plasma LDL-C. Enhanced LDL clearance probably results from increased hepatic LDL receptor expression.[397] Treatment of postmenopausal women with estrogen can lower LDL-C by 15%.[391] Estrogens can also reduce the hyperlipidemia of type III hyperlipoproteinemia.[249]

Estrogens have significant effects on HDL metabolism, increasing HDL-C in postmenopausal women by more than 15%,[391] primarily by increasing the HDL_2 subfraction. Women have higher HDL-C levels than men at all ages after puberty. This is presumably a result of the effects of androgens because HDL-C levels decrease at puberty in men but remain constant in women.[398] The mechanism by which gonadal hormones alter the HDL-C levels in men, but not women, is uncertain but might involve an androgen-mediated increase in hepatic lipase activity that does not occur with estrogen.[399] However, oral androgen administration to men with genetic hepatic lipase deficiency significantly lowered HDL-C and apo-AI levels without stimulating hepatic lipase activity.[400] This suggests than androgens affect HDL metabolism independently of their effects on hepatic lipase. The effects of exogenously administered estrogen, which raises HDL and lowers LDL-C levels, can be diminished if estrogens are combined with progestational agents, which lower HDL and raise LDL-C levels.[391]

Alcohol Consumption

The regular consumption of large amounts of alcohol can significantly affect plasma triglyceride metabolism.[401] Alcohol metabolism results in increased NADH levels, which inhibit fatty acid oxidation in the liver. This inhibition leads to increased triglyceride synthesis, fatty liver, and enhanced VLDL production.[401] The enhanced VLDL production raises plasma triglycerides and occasionally causes massive hypertriglyceridemia and pancreatitis, especially in persons with underlying hypertriglyceridemia. VLDL accumulates in the plasma, and occasionally chylomicronemia occurs, as these particles of hepatic and intestinal origin compete for saturable clearance mechanisms.[256] Subjects with type III hyperlipoproteinemia are particularly sensitive to the effects of alcohol consumption because the alcohol-induced overproduction of VLDL and associated remnant particles occurs in the setting of impaired remnant clearance.

Alcohol consumption is also associated with higher plasma levels of HDL-C, which in turn might explain why moderate alcohol consumption may protect against CHD. Indeed, moderate consumption of alcohol is inversely correlated with CHD mortality.[402]

Nephrotic Syndrome

Hyperlipidemia almost always accompanies the nephrotic syndrome. Total cholesterol, VLDL, LDL-C, total triglycerides, and plasma apo-B are all elevated.[403] The ratio of total cholesterol to HDL-C is increased, consistent with an atherogenic phenotype. Plasma Lp(a) levels can also be elevated.[404] The pathogenesis of the hyperlipidemia appears to be related to increased rates of production of LDL or VLDL, or both.[404,405] The cause of VLDL overproduction is unclear, but it may be related to a generalized hypersecretion phenomenon in the liver. Because myocardial infarction ranks second only to renal failure as the cause of death in subjects with the nephrotic syndrome, the hyperlipidemia should be treated vigorously. HMG-CoA reductase inhibitors appear to be particularly effective.[404]

Protease Inhibitor Use in Human Immunodeficiency Virus Infection

Therapy with protease inhibitors for human immunodeficiency virus infection has been associated with metabolic changes, including hyperlipidemia, lipodystrophy, and insulin resistance, in many patients.[167] The cause of this syndrome is thought to be associated with antagonism of insulin-mediated glucose transport by protease inhibitors. With the improved life expectancy in patients receiving protease inhibitor regimens, there is increased concern about the risk of CHD related to HIV infection directly and the metabolic side effects of anti-HIV drugs. Although definitive data are lacking, some evidence suggests increased risk of CHD.[406] Many affected subjects are currently treated with regimens similar to those used in patients with insulin resistance or diabetes not associated with HIV infection. The advent of atazanavir, a protease inhibitor that is not associated with the dysmetabolic effects of earlier protease inhibitors, opens a new chapter in the management of HIV-positive patients.[407] Guidelines for managing dyslipidemia in HIV patients have been published.[408]

Other Drugs

In addition to estrogens, other therapeutic agents can cause hyperlipidemia. These agents include glucocorticoids[147,148,409] and antihypertensive agents such as thiazide diuretics and β-adrenergic blockers.[410-412] Exogenous androgens can reduce HDL-C levels.[413,414]

Treatment of Lipid Disorders

Clinical Trials Providing Rationale for Treating Hyperlipidemia

It is clear that optimal management of patients to control risk factors substantially reduces the risk of sustaining clinical events caused by atherosclerosis. However, current "optimal" treatment of patients with clinical manifestations of atherosclerosis is still associated with a very high residual risk of death. Data from the Framingham Heart Study and other studies suggest that 10-year mortality (as of 2003) after myocardial infarction or acute coronary syndrome is about 40% to 60% depending on the degree of compliance with guidelines established 10 years earlier.[415-417]

The benefit of lipid-lowering therapies in clinical trials of post–myocardial infarction patients is presented in Figure 36–23. For comparison of outcomes between the trials, a common end point of fatal and nonfatal CHD events was chosen, although it was not the primary end point in several studies (for a review of clinical trials, see references 178, 418). Five trials—the Heart Protection Study (HPS), the Scandinavian Simvastatin Survival Study (4S), Cholesterol and Recurrent Events (CARE), Long-term Intervention with Pravastatin in Ischemic Disease (LIPID), and Veterans Affairs High Density Lipoprotein Intervention Trial (VA HIT)—compared a lipid-lowering agent versus placebo. Three trials—Pravastatin or Atorvastatin Evaluation and Infection Therapy (PROVE-IT), Treating to New Targets (TNT), and Incremental Decrease in End Points Through Aggressive Lipid Lowering (IDEAL)—compared the effect of more efficacious lipid-lowering versus less efficacious lipid-lowering (PROVE-IT, 80 mg atorvastatin vs 40 mg pravastatin; TNT, 80 vs 10 mg atorvastatin; IDEAL, 80 mg atorvastatin vs 20 or

40 mg simvastatin). In all of the trials except PROVE-IT, eligible patients were 3 to 6 months post–myocardial infarction. In PROVE-IT, the patients were hospitalized acute coronary syndrome patients, and the mean duration of participation in the trial was 2 years. In all of the other trials the mean or median duration was about 5 years.

The relative risk reduction of sustaining a fatal or nonfatal CHD event was 22% to 34% in the trials in which drug treatment was compared to placebo. In trials that compared less efficacious versus more efficacious LDL-C lowering (PROVE-IT, TNT, and IDEAL), the relative risk reduction was 11% to 20%. These relative risk reductions and the low number of subjects requiring treatment to prevent one event (<25 in all of the trials) provide evidence that lipid-lowering therapy reduces the risk of sustaining an event in a cost-effective manner. However, a closer look at the data indicates that patients remain at high risk despite aggressive lipid-lowering therapy. Between 6% and 10% of patients with LDL-C levels of 77 to 97 mg/dL had fatal or nonfatal CHD events over 5 years of treatment in HPS, CARE, LIPID, TNT, and IDEAL. In PROVE-IT, a trial only 2 years long, 8.3% of patients had a fatal or nonfatal myocardial infarction despite a mean on-treatment LDL-C value of 62 mg/dL. The 5-year risk would be much higher in these acute coronary syndrome patients, and the 10-year risk of the most aggressively managed patients in all of these trials approaches 20%. A high percentage of subjects in PROVE-IT, TNT, and IDEAL also received other current treatments (aspirin, β-blockers, angiotensin-converting enzyme inhibitors).[419] Meta-analyses of the effects of treatment with contemporary lipid-lowering agents support the concept that residual risk of CHD events after a myocardial infarction is about 50% over 8 to 10 years[417,418,420] and that an average of 14.2 years of life are lost.

The results of these clinical trials support the use of lipid-lowering therapy to reduce the risk of CHD events in patients who have had an atherosclerosis-induced ischemic event.[178] Furthermore, the trials provide definitive evidence that treatment with statins is safe. Cancer is not associated with statin therapy.[418] Although real, the risk of death from statin-induced myopathy or liver failure is remote. about one person per million person years of use.[420] In clinical trials involving nearly 40,000 persons each in placebo and active statin therapy groups, the incidence of rhabdomyolysis was extremely low in both groups ($N = 9$ vs 14), and the difference was not statistically significant.[418]

Given the high risk of patients who have had a myocardial infarction despite current best practices, it is obvious that prevention of first heart attacks provides the greatest opportunity to prevent death and morbidity. In the Framingham Heart Study, morbidity and mortality were lowest in those who had LDL-C less than 130 mg/dL, blood pressure (without treatment) less than 120/80 mm Hg, and HDL-C greater than 60 mg/dL and who did not smoke or have diabetes mellitus. In this group, the lifetime risk of developing CHD was 8% compared to the United States average of 50% of men and 35% of women.[421] This risk factor profile can be attained by lifestyle measures in 80% to 90% of the population. Unfortunately, only about 5% of adults in the United States maintain a lifestyle compatible with maintaining such a low-risk status.[421]

Treatment of high-risk primary prevention patients is cost effective. Moderate doses of statins lower LDL-C about 25% to 35%. Patients so treated who are at risk because of age (>40 years) and who have very high LDL-C levels, low HDL-C levels, or multiple risk factors have 30% to 40% reductions in the risk of having a vascular disease event.[422-424]

Approach to the Hyperlipidemic Patient

Evaluation for a lipid disorder is prompted by the presence of atherosclerotic vascular disease, pancreatitis, or xanthomas or because a high plasma cholesterol or triglyceride level or a low HDL-C level has been detected. The initial evaluation of these patients includes a history and physical examination, including assessment of CHD risk factors (Table 36–12) and measurement of plasma lipids (Table 36–13). Exclusion of disorders causing secondary lipid abnormalities (see Table 36–7) by appropriate history, physical examination, and laboratory measures is important.

Risk Factors

The initial examination should include an assessment of risk factors (see Table 36–12) for atherosclerotic vascular disease.[144] Obesity is an independent risk factor for CHD not included in the formal list of NCEP risk factors.[425] Obesity aggravates hypertension and insulin resistance and is a target of therapy irrespective of the severity of traditional CHD risk factors. Particular emphasis should be placed on obtaining a detailed history of all first-degree relatives to identify cholesterol disorders or premature CHD.

Physical Examination

A thorough physical examination should be performed with emphasis on the cardiovascular system, the manifestations of hyperlipidemia, and disorders causing secondary lipid abnormalities. Plasma lipids (cholesterol or triglycerides) can accumulate in macrophage reticuloendothelial cells in many tissues, but only those affecting the skin, eye, liver, and spleen can be observed by physical examination. Deposits in tendons are a result of physical interaction between collagen fibrils and cholesterol. In almost all cases, these tissue lipid deposits are reversible with lipid-lowering therapy. Several of the clinical findings are illustrated in Figure 36–22.

Xanthelasmas (see Fig. 36–22A), a type of xanthoma, are small, raised, yellowish macules that typically appear around the medial canthus. Involvement can extend to the eyelids or skin immediately below the eye. They occur in patients with FH, familial defective apo-B100, and type III hyperlipoproteinemia. Xanthelasmas occasionally occur in patients with normal

TABLE 36–12 MAJOR RISK FACTORS FOR CORONARY HEART DISEASE

POSITIVE
Age (men ≥45 yr; women ≥55 yr)
Current cigarette smoking (smoking within the 30 days prior to evaluation)
Diabetes mellitus*
Family history of premature CHD (male parent or sibling <55 yr, female parent or sibling <65 yr, or grandparents)
Hypertension (blood pressure ≥140 systolic or 90 diastolic mm Hg or on antihypertensive medication)
Low HDL-C (<1.0 mM/L [<40 mg/dL])
NEGATIVE
High HDL-C (≥1.6 mM/L [≥60 mg/dL])

*Diabetes mellitus or any clinical manifestation of atherosclerosis (claudication, stroke, abdominal aortic aneurysm) is regarded as a CHD-equivalent, that is, >20% risk of a CHD event within 10 years.

Adapted from The Expert Panel. Third Report of the National Cholesterol Education Program (NCEP) Expert Panel on Detection, Evaluation, and Treatment of High Blood Cholesterol in Adults (Adult Treatment Panel III). Final report. Circulation 2002;106:3143-3421.

CHD, coronary heart disease; HDL-C, high-density lipoprotein cholesterol.

TABLE 36–13 CLASSIFICATION OF PLASMA LIPID LEVELS

Level	Classification
	TOTAL CHOLESTEROL
<200 mg/dL	Desirable
200-239 mg/dL	Borderline high
≥240 mg/dL	High
	HDL-C
<40 mg/dL	Low (consider <50 mg/dL low for women)
>60 mg/dL	High
	LDL-C
<70 mg/dL	
<100 mg/dL	Optimal
100-129 mg/dL	Near optimal
130-159 mg/dL	Borderline high
160-189 mg/dL	High
≥190 mg/dL	Very high
	TRIGLYCERIDES
<150 mg/dL	Normal
150-199 mg/dL	Borderline high
200-499 mg/dL	High
≥500 mg/dL	Very high

HDL-C, high-density lipoprotein cholesterol; LDL-C, low-density lipoprotein cholesterol.
Adapted from The Expert Panel. Third Report of the National Cholesterol Education Program (NCEP) Expert Panel on Detection, Evaluation, and Treatment of High Blood Cholesterol in Adults (Adult Treatment Panel III). Final report. Circulation 2002;106:3143-3421; and Grundy SM, Cleeman JI, Merz CNB, et al. Implications of recent clinical trials for the National Cholesterol Education Program Adult Treatment Panel III guidelines. Circulation 2004;110:227-239.

plasma cholesterol levels, possibly as the result of enhanced uptake of oxidized or modified lipoproteins by tissue macrophages. Xanthelasmas typically regress with cholesterol lowering and may be treated effectively in the setting of normal cholesterol levels with cholesterol-lowering drugs.

Lipemia retinalis (see Fig. 36–22B), a condition in which lipemic blood causes opalescence of retinal arterioles, can be observed upon funduscopic examination. It is typically seen only when the triglyceride levels are 22.6 mM/L (2000 mg/dL) or higher.

Tendon xanthomas (see Fig. 36–22C and D) are nodular deposits of cholesterol that accumulate in tissue macrophages in the Achilles and other tendons, including the extensor tendons in the hands, knees, and elbows. Tendon xanthomas are often present in FH (approximately 75% of subjects), in familial defective apo-B100, and sometimes in type III hyperlipoproteinemia. Small tendon xanthomas can be easily overlooked. The examination of the Achilles tendon should include an assessment of thickness and for irregularities of contour (see Fig. 36–22C).

Tuberous or *tuboeruptive xanthomas* (see Fig. 36–22E) are subcutaneous nodules that develop in the skin over areas susceptible to trauma such as the elbows and knees. They may be single or multiple and can range from pea-sized to lemon-sized. Tuberous xanthomas are most often seen in type III hyperlipoproteinemia and also occur in FH.

Palmar xanthomas (see Fig. 36–22F) are cutaneous deposits in the palmar and digital creases of the hands. This type of xanthoma is almost pathognomonic for high plasma levels of β-VLDL and type III hyperlipoproteinemia.

Eruptive xanthomas (see Fig. 36–22G) are cutaneous xanthomas that appear as small, yellowish, round papules that contain a pale center and an erythematous base. They can be mistaken for acne. The distribution of eruptive xanthomas includes the abdominal wall, the back, the buttocks, and other pressure contact areas. They are caused by accumulation of triglyceride in dermal histiocytes and generally occur when the plasma triglyceride level is 11.3 to 22.6 mM/L (1000 to 2000 mg/dL) or more. They can disappear rapidly with lowering of the plasma triglyceride level.

Screening for Secondary Disorders

The history and physical examination should be directed toward uncovering secondary disorders of lipid metabolism (e.g., diabetes mellitus, hypothyroidism, or the nephrotic syndrome) and identifying agents that could cause hyperlipidemia (e.g., estrogens, alcohol, or β-adrenergic blockers) (see Table 36–7). Laboratory studies should be performed to measure fasting blood sugar or glycosylated hemoglobin, or both, and to assess renal and hepatic function and urinary protein. To screen for hypothyroidism, the plasma thyroid-stimulating hormone (thyrotropin) level should be assessed because the prevalence of hypothyroidism is increased in dyslipidemic subjects.[426]

Measurement of Plasma Lipids

Ideally, plasma lipids should be measured at least twice under fasting steady-state conditions before therapeutic decisions are made (see Table 36–13). Plasma lipids are usually measured after a 12-hour fast to preclude detection of significant elevations in atherogenic remnant lipoproteins. Because cholesterol is a minor component of chylomicrons, total plasma cholesterol can be measured in either the fasting or nonfasting state. Plasma lipids can be decreased in the setting of acute myocardial infarction,[427] and follow-up measurements are essential in these patients.

Most clinical laboratories measure plasma levels of total triglycerides, total cholesterol, and HDL-C; the last analysis is performed after apo-B–containing lipoproteins are removed from the plasma or complexed with one of a number of polyanionic agents.[428] The plasma LDL-C concentration is then calculated from these measurements by the Friedewald formula[429]:

$$\text{LDL cholesterol} = \text{total cholesterol} - \text{HDL} - \text{VLDL} - (\text{triglycerides}/5).$$

This formula relies on an estimate of the VLDL cholesterol that assumes that the cholesterol content of VLDL is about 20% of the fasting plasma triglyceride level. It is reliable only when triglyceride levels are 4.5 mM/L (400 mg/dL) or less. Plasma LDL concentrations calculated by this formula may be inaccurate in the setting of severe hypertriglyceridemia or when the triglyceride-to-cholesterol ratio of VLDL differs from the usual 5:1 ratio (as occurs in the presence of high concentrations of remnant lipoproteins). Specialized lipid laboratories separate the plasma into different density fractions (e.g., VLDL, LDL, and HDL) by sequential ultracentrifugation of the plasma and then measure the lipid concentrations in each fraction. The main advantage of the latter technique is that VLDL cholesterol, which can reflect atherogenic remnant lipoproteins, is measured directly. Direct measurement of LDL-C not requiring ultracentrifugation is also available in many clinical laboratories.

Because the plasma lipids can be divided roughly into the proatherogenic apo-B–containing lipoproteins and the antiatherogenic HDL, assessment of the relative proportions of cholesterol in these two fractions can be valuable in the individual lipid profile. One method is to assess absolute levels of HDL and non-HDL cholesterol.[144] Another method is to determine the ratio of total cholesterol to HDL-C[430,431]; the optimal ratio is about 3.5 or lower (i.e., at least 30% of the plasma cholesterol is in the HDL fraction). Both methods allow incorporation of the potentially atherogenic apo-B–containing lipoproteins in the assessment of cardiovascular risk from hyperlipidemia by including VLDL cholesterol levels in the assessment.

Several caveats for interpreting the plasma triglyceride level deserve mention. First, a triglyceride level higher than 11.3 mM/L (1000 mg/dL) usually signifies the presence of two or more abnormalities of lipid metabolism (e.g., estrogen therapy in the presence of underlying familial hypertriglyceridemia).[256] Second, elevated plasma triglyceride levels can fluctuate markedly in a single person over short periods. The fluctuation occurs because the LPL-mediated clearance mechanisms for triglyceride-rich particles become saturated at plasma triglyceride concentrations of approximately 5.6 mM/L (500 mg/dL), and above this level plasma triglyceride levels largely reflect dietary fat intake. In this range, the plasma triglyceride levels can rise precipitously as dietary fat intake increases and can fall rapidly with dietary fat restriction.[256]

In some instances, visual inspection of plasma after it has been refrigerated overnight can be helpful in understanding a disorder of lipoprotein metabolism. To accomplish this, plasma should be collected in a tube containing ethylenediaminetetraacetic acid (EDTA) and refrigerated overnight. A cream-like layer on the top signifies the presence of chylomicrons, which are less dense than plasma and float to the surface. A turbid plasma infranatant signifies high levels of VLDL. The combination of a cream-like top layer and turbid plasma indicates the presence of both chylomicrons and VLDL.

Other tests used to assess CHD risk and guide the therapy of patients with plasma lipid disorders include measurements of plasma Lp(a) levels, measurements of plasma apolipoproteins AI and B, and screening of genomic DNA for mutations (see "Apolipoprotein CII Deficiency. Diagnosis" for a discussion of the measurement of plasma Lp(a) levels by standardized assays). The Lp(a) assay must distinguish the apo(a) protein from plasminogen, which is highly homologous. Plasma Lp(a) measurement is occasionally helpful in assessing CHD risk, and high levels of Lp(a) can suggest the use of niacin as a therapeutic agent.[305] Plasma apo-B and apo-AI levels may be of great value in predicting CHD risk[432]; however, it is controversial if assays of these apolipoproteins add to the risk assessment obtained from plasma cholesterol measurements. Specialized tests such as in vitro assays for enzyme activities (e.g., LPL, CETP) or DNA screening for mutations (e.g., the familial defective apo-B100 mutation) are currently performed in specialized laboratories.

Selection of Patients for Plasma Lipid Measurements

Guidelines developed by the NCEP in 2001 recommend that a complete plasma lipid profile (total cholesterol, LDL-C, HDL-C, and triglycerides) be measured in all adults 20 years of age and older at least once every 5 years.[216] The classification of plasma lipid levels is shown in Table 36–13. An analysis of large, long-term observational cohort studies has provided evidence that young men with hypercholesterolemia are at substantially increased risk for morbidity from CHD.[433]

The widespread focus on assessing 10-year risk and treating only those with very high cholesterol levels or with several risk factors results in therapy being recommended for those who are middle-aged or older. This approach actually supports the concept of delaying screening until age 40 to 50 years. Less well known is the concept of lifetime risk.[144,434]

The lifetime risk of developing CHD in the United States is 50% for men and 33% for women. Among persons younger than 65 years, mortality 8 years after a myocardial infarction is about 50%, despite optimal therapy.[417] In addition, sudden death is the first sign of CHD in about 15% of patients who die of CHD. Given the high prevalence of CHD and the treatment outcomes of heart attack survivors, waiting to evaluate and treat patients until middle age makes little sense. Young adults should be apprised of the high prevalence of CHD in our population and advised about lifestyle choices that reduce CHD risk. The optimal risk factor profile associated with the lowest risk of developing CHD (<10% lifetime risk) is LDL-C lower than 130 mg/dL, blood pressure lower than 120/80 mm Hg, no smoking, HDL-C higher than 60 mg/dL, and no diabetes mellitus.[421] Everyone should be instructed to strive to attain this profile.

Plasma triglycerides should be measured in all patients with pancreatitis.

Selection of Patients for Treatment

The 2001 NCEP treatment guidelines as modified in 2004[435] are based on measurements of plasma cholesterol levels and assessment of risk factors.[216] The first step in risk assessment is to determine whether CHD or a CHD equivalent (e.g., diabetes mellitus, symptomatic cerebrovascular disease, peripheral arterial disease, abdominal aortic aneurysm) is present, because these disorders confer more than 20% risk of a subsequent CHD event within 10 years. In all others the presence or absence of the risk factors listed in Table 36–12 should be determined. Patients with two or more risk factors should have the 10-year risk of a future CHD event calculated according to the Framingham Risk Tables (Table 36–14).[216] Subjects with multiple risk factors and scores conferring a 10-year risk of more than 20% are also classified as high-risk, CHD-equivalent patients. Treatment options, based on risk stratification, are discussed below. Guidelines for managing dyslipidemia based on risk assessment were also published by the European Atherosclerosis Society in 1998.[436]

Treatment decisions can be divided into two major categories. treatment of hyperlipidemia in patients with established CHD (sometimes referred to as *secondary-prevention patients*) and treatment of patients who do not have CHD *(primary-prevention patients)*.[178] Subjects with hyperlipidemia and established CHD should be aggressively treated to lower plasma cholesterol to NCEP treatment guideline levels. The rationale for this recommendation is that lowering of plasma cholesterol in patients with established CHD decreases subsequent risk of cardiac events[181,182,418,420] and decreases mortality from cardiac events. Studies also have demonstrated a reduction in overall mortality in treated patients.[418,420] In subjects with established CHD, lipid-lowering therapy causes atherosclerotic lesions to stabilize or regress.[181-183,437-439] However, despite the overwhelming evidence demonstrating the benefits of lipid-lowering treatment, many people with hypercholesterolemia and CHD remain inadequately treated.[440]

When to initiate lipid-lowering therapy in subjects with dyslipidemia and no known CHD (i.e., therapy for primary prevention) is an evolving issue.[441] This issue arises in part because there is no reliable noninvasive test for assessing the degree of atherosclerosis in arteries or predicting when a person will have a clinical event caused by atherosclerosis. Treatment recommendations for asymptomatic persons have been based largely on studies of high-risk groups of primary-prevention patients. Trials have shown that lipid lowering reduces risk in middle-aged or older patients who have high total cholesterol and LDL-C levels and low HDL-C levels and in patients who have three or more risk factors and LDL-C levels greater than 100 mg/dL.[418,420,435] No trial of lipid lowering has shown a statistically

TABLE 36–14 FRAMINGHAM RISK SCORING TABLES

ESTIMATE OF 10-YEAR RISK FOR MEN

Age (yr)	Points
20-34	−9
35-39	−4
40-44	0
45-49	3
50-54	6
55-59	8
60-64	10
65-69	11
70-74	12
75-79	13

Points

Total Cholesterol (mg/dL)	Age 20-39 yr	Age 40-49 yr	Age 50-59 yr	Age 60-69 yr	Age 70-79 yr
<160	0	0	0	0	0
160-199	4	3	2	1	0
200-239	7	5	3	1	0
240-279	9	6	4	2	1
≥280	11	8	5	3	1

Points

	Age 20-39 yr	Age 40-49 yr	Age 50-59 yr	Age 60-69 yr	Age 70-79 yr
Nonsmoker	0	0	0	0	0
Smoker	8	5	3	1	1

HDL (mg/dL)	Points
≥60	−1
50-59	0
40-49	1
<40	2

Systolic BP (mm Hg)	If Untreated	If Treated
<120	0	0
120-129	0	1
130-139	1	2
140-159	1	2
≥160	2	3

Point Total	10-yr Risk (%)
<0	<1
0	1
1	1
2	1
3	1
4	1
5	2
6	2
7	3
8	4
9	5
10	6
11	8
12	10
13	12
14	16
15	20
16	25
≥17	≥30

ESTIMATE OF 10-YEAR RISK FOR WOMEN

Age (yr)	Points
20-34	−7
35-39	−3
40-44	0
45-49	3
50-54	6
55-59	8
60-64	10
65-69	12
70-74	14
75-79	16

Points

Total Cholesterol (mg/dL)	Age 20-39 yr	Age 40-49 yr	Age 50-59 r	Age 60-69 yr	Age 70-79 yr
<160	0	0	0	0	0
60-199	4	3	2	1	1
200-239	8	6	4	2	1
240-279	11	8	5	3	2
≥280	13	10	7	4	2

Points

	Age 20-39 yr	Age 40-49 yr	Age 50-59 yr	Age 60-69 yr	Age 70-79 yr
Nonsmoker	0	0	0	0	0
Smoker	9	7	4	2	1

HDL (mg/dL)	Points
≥60	−1
50-59	0
40-49	1
<40	2

Systolic BP (mm Hg)	If Untreated	If Treated
<120	0	0
120-129	1	3
130-139	2	4
140-159	3	5
≥160	4	6

Point Total	10-yr Risk (%)
<9	<1
9	1
10	1
11	1
12	1
13	2
14	2
15	3
16	4
17	5
18	6
19	8
20	11
21	14
22	17
23	22
24	27
≥25	≥30

BP, blood pressure; HDL, high-density lipoprotein.

Adapted from The Expert Panel. Third Report of the National Cholesterol Education Program (NCEP) Expert Panel on Detection, Evaluation, and Treatment of High Blood Cholesterol in Adults (Adult Treatment Panel III). Final report. Circulation 2002;106:3143-3421.

significant reduction in total mortality, although one trial that was stopped after 3 years instead of the planned 5 years demonstrated a 13% reduction in total mortality that was not statistically significant (P = 0.16). Current guidelines for managing dyslipidemia in primary prevention match the intensity of treatment to the calculated risk of having a CHD event within 10 years of the risk assessment.[144,435]

A benefit from treating hypercholesterolemia in persons older than 85 years has yet to be documented, because no prospective studies have addressed the benefits of treatment in this population. Nevertheless, CHD accounts for a high percentage of deaths in this age group, and several trials have demonstrated the survival benefits of treatment in elderly patients up to the age of 85 years and who have established CHD.[418,435]

Patients with type 2 diabetes mellitus have at least a twofold increase in the risk for CHD,[442] and diabetics without diagnosed CHD have the same risk as nondiabetics with established CHD.[443] In the HPS, diabetic patients were a prespecified subgroup. Treatment with simvastatin, 40 mg daily, reduced their risk of having a fatal or nonfatal CHD event by 27%.[444] The American Diabetes Association recommends that all patients with type 2 diabetes mellitus who are older than 40 years be treated to reduce LDL-C by at least 30%.[445] In post hoc analyses, every clinical trial using statins to lower LDL-C levels demonstrated 20% to 55% reductions in CHD events in diabetic patients.[418] For these reasons, the American Heart Association and the American Diabetes Association have recommended that guidelines for treating hyperlipidemia in diabetics be the same as for patients with CHD.[144,445] Accordingly, the latest NCEP guidelines define diabetes mellitus as a CHD equivalent, and treatment goals for lipids in diabetic patients are the same as for established CHD patients, irrespective of whether a diabetic patient has a history of a prior CHD event. HMG-CoA reductase inhibitors have been recommended as a first-line treatment.

Severe hypertriglyceridemia (>11.3 mM/L [1000 mg/dL]) should be treated aggressively because it is associated with a high risk of pancreatitis, a potentially fatal disease.[256]

Treatment Goals

The treatment goals of the 2001 NCEP guidelines as modified in 2004, based on LDL-C and risk assessment, are summarized in Table 36–15.[144,435] For patients with clinical CHD, the treatment goal for LDL-C should be a level less than 2.6 mM/L (100 mg/dL). In some very high risk patients, a goal of less than 1.8 mM/L (<70 mg/dL) has been proposed.[435] A useful rule is to lower total cholesterol to roughly 4.1 mM/L (160 mg/dL) and LDL-C to 2.6 mM/L (100 mg/dL). These values are similar to the average cholesterol levels in populations in which CHD is much less prevalent. Based on short-term (10-year) risk assessment, the NCEP ATP III guidelines suggest LDL-C levels should be lowered to less than 4.1 mM/L (160 mg/dL) for patients with minimal risk (10-year risk <10%) and to less than 3.4 mM/L (130 mg/dL) in those with moderate risk (10-year risk 10% to 20%). Because the Framingham risk score can underestimate risk in primary prevention patients with two or more risk factors and 10% to 20% 10-year risk scores, consideration of an LDL-C goal less than 100 mg/dL related to a variety of indicators has been proposed (see Table 38-15).[435] It is also useful to monitor the ratio of total cholesterol to HDL-C, which should be 4.5 or less. However, to reduce lifetime risk of developing CHD (50% risk for men; 33% risk for women) *all* patients should be told to maintain LDL less than 130 mg/dL irrespective of their 10-year short-term risk.

In patients with severe hypertriglyceridemia, the goal is to lower the plasma triglyceride level to less than 4.5 mM/L (400 mg/dL), which markedly reduces the risk of developing pancreatitis. The 2001 NCEP guidelines[144] reflect the fact that even moderate hypertriglyceridemia (>1.7 mM/L, or 150 mg/dL) is associated with increased CHD risk. If plasma triglycerides remain higher 2.3 mM/L (200 mg/dL) after the LDL-C goal is reached, further reduction may be achieved by increasing the drug therapy.

Treatment of Hyperlipidemia

The treatment of hyperlipidemia is directed primarily at lowering plasma cholesterol levels to prevent morbidity and mortality from CHD.[178] The rationale and the use of diet or drugs for this purpose have been reviewed.[446,447] Treatment modalities recommended by the NCEP are therapeutic lifestyle changes, which include diet, weight management, and physical activity recommendations, and drug therapy.[144] A major goal in the treatment of severe hypertriglyceridemia is to prevent pancreatitis. Patients with CHD or a CHD-equivalent diagnosis should immediately

TABLE 36–15 LDL-C GOALS AND CUTPOINTS FOR THERAPEUTIC LIFESTYLE CHANGES AND DRUG THERAPY IN DIFFERENT RISK CATEGORIES

Risk Category	LDL Goal, mM/L (mg/dL)	LDL Level at Which to Initiate Therapeutic Lifestyle Changes,* mM/L (mg/dL)	LDL-C Level at Which to Consider Drug Therapy, mM/L (mg/dL)
CHD or CHD risk equivalents (10-year risk >20%)	<2.6 (100) <1.8 (70)†	No threshold	No threshold
2+ Risk factors (10-year risk ≤20%)	<3.4 (130) <2.6 (100)*	≥3.4 (130) ≥2.6 (100)	10-year risk 10%-20%: ≥3.4 (130) 10-year risk <10%: ≥4.1 (160)
0-1 Risk factor‡	<4.1 (160)	>4.1 (160)	>4.9 (190) (4.1-4.9 [160-189]: LDL-lowering drug optional)

*For patients with 2+ risk factors, 10% to 20% 10-year risk, *and* any of items 2-5 in footnote † *or* any of the following: age >50 years, high-density lipoprotein cholesterol ≤40 mg/dL, C-reactive protein level >3 mg/L, coronary artery calcium score >75th percentile.

†LDL <1.8 mM/L (70 mg/dL) *only* for patients with a CHD event, stroke, TIA (SPELL), peripheral vascular disease, *and one of the following:* acute coronary syndrome, type 2 diabetes mellitus, the metabolic syndrome, a *single poorly controlled* risk factor, three risk factors irrespective of how well controlled.

‡Almost all people with 0-1 risk factor have a 10-year risk <10%; thus 10-year risk assessment in people with 0-1 risk factor is not necessary.

CHD, coronary heart disease, LDL-C, low-density lipoprotein cholesterol; TIA, transient ischemic attack.

Adapted from The Expert Panel. Third Report of the National Cholesterol Education Program (NCEP) Expert Panel on Detection, Evaluation, and Treatment of High Blood Cholesterol in Adults (Adult Treatment Panel III). Final report. Circulation 2002;106:3143-3421; and Grundy SM, Cleeman JI, Merz CNB, et al. Implications of recent clinical trials for the National Cholesterol Education Program Adult Treatment Panel III guidelines. Circulation 2004;110:227-239.

start appropriate lipid-lowering therapy and lifestyle change advice (diet and exercise). Patients without CHD or a CHD-equivalent diagnosis should be encouraged to alter lifestyle behavior for 3 to 6 months before starting drug therapy.

The NCEP guidelines recognize the increased risk of developing diabetes mellitus associated with the metabolic syndrome, which is characterized by the presence of at least three of five metabolic risk factors (see Table 36–8).[144,216] Because these risk factors are also associated with increased CHD risk, each risk factor should be managed according to existing guidelines specific to each risk factor.[216,448]In addition to treating increased LDL-C levels, treatment for these patients should focus on weight loss and increased physical activity, because obesity appears to exacerbate these metabolic abnormalities.

Lifestyle Treatment

All patients should receive instruction about restriction of dietary saturated fat and cholesterol. On average, diets consumed in countries with a high prevalence of CHD contain 35% to 40% of calories as fat (about 15% to 20% saturated fat, 10% polyunsaturated fat, and 10% monounsaturated fat) and approximately 380 mg of cholesterol per day. In the past, the average diet in many underdeveloped countries contained closer to 10% of calories as fat. This has changed since the 1990s because dietary fat has become less expensive. At this time, about 80% of CHD deaths occur in low-income and middle-income countries.[449] The American Heart Association has recommended a single diet (formerly termed *step 1 dietary therapy* by the NCEP) for all persons older than 2 years.[450] The diet consists of 50% of calories in the form of carbohydrate (complex carbohydrates preferred), 20% as protein, and no more than 30% as fat. Saturated fat plus *trans* fat should constitute less than 10% of total calories, monounsaturated fat 10% to 15% of calories, and polyunsaturated fat up to 10% of total calories. Cholesterol intake should be limited to 300 mg/day or less. A more stringent restriction of saturated fat plus *trans* fat (<7% of calories) and cholesterol (≤200 mg/day) intake (therapeutic lifestyle diet) is recommended for patients with elevated LDL-C levels or with established coronary artery disease.[144] The composition of this therapeutic lifestyle change, as it is termed by the NCEP, is shown in Table 36–16. In patients with established CHD, drug therapy should be instituted concomitantly with diet therapy.

Changing from a typical high-saturated-fat, high-cholesterol diet to the diet recommended for the general population lowers plasma cholesterol levels by 5% to 10%, an effect that would decrease CHD events by 10% to 20%.[451,452] The adoption of a therapeutic lifestyle diet (25% of calories as fat) has produced mixed results in two types of studies. In one study, restricting fat intake to 25% of calories lowered cholesterol levels by only 5%; however, in this outpatient study, it was not clear that the diets were strictly adhered to, as evidenced by comparison of the expected and the actual weight loss in participants.[453] In two metabolic ward studies, reducing fat intake to 25% of calories lowered total cholesterol levels by 15% to 20% and LDL-C levels by 18% to 23%.[454,455] Even more stringent limitation of fat intake (e.g., 10% of calories) can further lower plasma lipids. In conjunction with modifications of other lifestyle factors, this diet achieved a reduction of about 25% in total plasma cholesterol levels, an average weight loss of 10 kg, and angiographic regression of coronary artery disease.[438] The latter studies suggest that dietary restriction of fat intake can lower plasma cholesterol levels provided the diet is followed.

The effects of various types of fat in the diet have been studied extensively.[456] Current recommendations are that dietary fat intake be lowered, primarily by restricting saturated fat intake because saturated fats appear to have the greatest propensity to elevate plasma cholesterol levels.[11] The mechanism of this effect appears to involve decreased receptor-mediated clearance of LDL from the plasma.[457] Similarly, high levels of cholesterol intake raise plasma cholesterol by reducing receptor-mediated catabolism of LDL and by increasing LDL synthesis.[73]

PUFAs, such as linoleic acid, which are chiefly found in vegetable oils, have less deleterious effects on plasma cholesterol levels than saturated fats do.[11,458] However, because the long-term effects of consumption of large amounts of PUFAs are unknown, current recommendations are that polyunsaturated fat constitute no more than 10% of total calories.[144] PUFAs that have been hardened by hydrogenation (e.g., in margarines) result in the conversion of some double bonds in the fatty acid from the *cis* to the *trans* configuration; these *trans* fatty acids exert effects on LDL-C levels that are comparable to those of saturated fatty acids, but they also reduce HDL-C levels.[459]

Fish oils are rich in a particular subset of long-chain PUFAs containing double bonds at the n-3 or ω-3 position, such as eicosapentaenoic acid (C-20) (EPA) or docosahexaenoic acid (C-22) (DHA). Because the incidence of CHD is decreased in populations that consume relatively large amounts of fish oils,[460] these PUFAs have been evaluated for the treatment of hyperlipidemia and the prevention of CHD.[460] Daily doses of 4 g of EPA plus DHA lower VLDL levels and are effective for treating hypertriglyceridemia. LDL levels in many patients with hypertriglyceridemia are increased, but non-HDL-C (sum of VLDL cholesterol and LDL-C) is decreased by about 15%.[461] However, as little as 1 g of EPA plus DHA daily reduces sudden death risk in post–myocardial infarction patients by 30% to 50%. This effect is thought to be due to prevention of ventricular arrhythmias.[462] Based on the results of studies of both primary- and secondary-prevention patients, it is recommended that persons free of CHD consume two fish meals weekly and that secondary-prevention patients take fish oil capsules providing about 1 g/day of EPA plus DHA.[460] Large doses of fish oil supplements can worsen glycemic control in persons with type 2 diabetes.[463]

Of all the types of fatty acids, monounsaturated fats might have the least deleterious effects on plasma lipoprotein metabolism.[11,464] Monounsaturated fats, such as oleic acid, are found in high quantities in olive oil and canola oil. When substituted for saturated fats, monounsaturated fats lowered total plasma cho-

TABLE 36–16 NATIONAL CHOLESTEROL EDUCATION PROGRAM: THERAPEUTIC LIFESTYLE CHANGES FOR REDUCING CORONARY HEART DISEASE RISK

Therapeutic lifestyle changes diet:
- Saturated fat (and *trans*-esterified fatty acids) less than 7% of total calories
- Polyunsaturated fat up to 10% of total calories
- Monounsaturated fat up to 20% of total calories
- Total fat 25%-35% of total calories
- Carbohydrates (predominantly complex) 50%-60% of total calories
- Fiber 20-30 g/d*
- Protein ~15% of total calories
- Cholesterol <5.2 mM/L (200 mg/dL)
- Consider plant stanols/sterols (2 g/d) to enhance LDL-C lowering

Weight reduction

Increased physical activity

LDL-C, low-density lipoprotein cholesterol.

*Adapted from National Cholesterol Education Program Expert Panel. Executive summary of the third report of the National Cholesterol Education Program (NCEP) Expert Panel on Detection, Evaluation, and Treatment of High Blood Cholesterol in Adults (Adult Treatment Panel III). JAMA 2001;285:2486-2497.

lesterol levels without lowering plasma HDL-C levels.[464] There is some evidence suggesting that α-linolenic acid consumption can reduce CHD mortality.[460,465] Canola oil is the most readily available source of α-linolenic acid, and it should be recommended when margarine or cooking oil is necessary.

Other dietary components can influence plasma lipid levels. For example, soluble fibers such as psyllium or oat bran, which can bind bile acids in the gut and promote net cholesterol excretion, can result in modest (<10%) decreases in LDL-C levels.[466-468] Margarine containing sitostanol, a nonabsorbed plant sterol that inhibits cholesterol absorption, reduces serum cholesterol by about 10%.[469] Garlic[470] and walnuts[471] are reported to result in modest decreases in plasma cholesterol levels. Combination of these minor nutrients, along with restriction of saturated fat and cholesterol, reduces LDL-C levels by about 30%.[472]

Making diet changes is difficult, and given the increasing prevalence of overweight and obesity in many countries (including the United States), the approach to helping patients change eating behavior needs to be changed. Almost all physicians, most nurses, and most pharmacists have insufficient knowledge about the suitability of many kinds of foods for patients attempting to change lifelong dietary habits. A collaborative approach including experienced nutritionists and dieticians working with other providers holds promise of better patient outcomes. Recommendations for managing patients in such a collaborative fashion have been developed.[473]

Drug Treatment

Categories of drugs for treatment of lipid abnormalities[144,178] are listed in Table 36–17. These include drugs that interfere with bile acid absorption from the gut (e.g., bile acid sequestrants), with cholesterol biosynthesis in cells (e.g., HMG-CoA reductase inhibitors), or with cholesterol absorption from the gut (i.e., ezetimibe). These agents reduce cholesterol levels and increase LDL receptor expression primarily in hepatocytes, thereby lowering plasma LDL concentrations. Other agents, including niacin, fibrates, and ω-3 fatty acids, either inhibit VLDL synthesis and secretion or enhance the clearance of triglyceride-rich particles by enhancing LPL-mediated catabolism of triglyceride-rich lipoproteins. The choice of drug for treating hyperlipidemia depends primarily on which lipids are abnormal (Table 36–18) and on the side effects of each drug. In cases of severe hypercholesterolemia (e.g., FH) or to attain very low LDL-C goals (<1.8 mM/L [70 mg/dL]), combinations of agents might be required to reduce plasma cholesterol concentrations sufficiently.

HMG-CoA Reductase Inhibitors

Six potent inhibitors of HMG-CoA reductase, the enzyme that catalyzes the rate-limiting step in cholesterol biosynthesis, are available (Table 36–19).[178] Inhibition of cholesterol biosynthesis up-regulates cellular LDL receptors and enhances clearance of LDL from the plasma into cells.[69] About two thirds of the body's LDL receptors are on the surface of hepatocytes. The structural differences of the inhibitors account for the differences in LDL-lowering efficacy.[178] Lovastatin and simvastatin are administered as lactone prodrugs that are converted in the liver to hydroxy acids capable of inhibiting HMG-CoA reductase. The other four inhibitors are administered as hydroxy acids. The relative water insolubility of lovastatin and simvastatin compared to the other drugs is of no clinical consequence.

TABLE 36–17 DRUGS COMMONLY USED FOR TREATING HYPERLIPIDEMIA

Class	Drugs Available	Dosage	Major Lipoprotein Decreased	Mechanism	Side Effects
Bile acid sequestrants	Cholestyramine Colestipol	4-12 g bid 5-15 g bid	LDL	Increase sterol excretion; increase LDL receptor-mediated removal of LDL	Gastrointestinal symptoms; can increase triglycerides; binds other drugs
Nicotinic acid	Colesevelam Niacin (crystalline)	3.75-4.375 g qd 1-2 g tid	VLDL (LDL)	Decrease VLDL production	Flushing; hyperglycemia; hepatic dysfunction; gout
Fibric acid derivatives	Gemfibrozil Clofibrate Fenofibrate*	600 mg bid 1 g bid 48-200 mg qd	VLDL (LDL)	Decrease VLDL production; enhance LPL action	Gallstones; myopathy
HMG-CoA reductase inhibitors	Lovastatin Pravastatin Simvastatin Fluvastatin Atorvastatin Rosuvastatin	10-80 mg qd 10-40 mg qd 5-80 mg qd 20-80 mg qd 10-80 mg qd 5-40 mg qd	LDL	Decrease cholesterol synthesis; increase LDL receptor-mediated removal of LDL	Hepatic dysfunction; myopathy
Intestinal cholesterol absorption inhibitor	Ezetimibe	10 mg qd	LDL (also reduces chylomicron cholesterol content	Inhibits cholesterol absorption	None known
Omega-3 fatty acids	Omacor (1-g capsule contains EPA, 465 mg, and DHA, 375 mg)	4 g qd	VLDL	Inhibition of hepatic triglyceride synthesis and increased fatty acid oxidation in the liver (reduces VLDL production)	Potential for bleeding associated with anticoagulant therapy

*There are several different preparations of fenofibrate that are dosed differently. Prescribing information for each preparation should be read before issuing prescriptions to patients.

EPA, highly concentrated ethyl esters of eicosapentaenoic acid; DHA, docosahexaenoic acid; HMG-CoA, 3-hydroxy-3-methylglutaryl coenzyme A; LDL, low-density lipoproteins; VLDL, very-low-density lipoproteins.

Therapeutic doses of these agents reduce total cholesterol and LDL-C levels by 20% to 55% (see Table 36–19). Plasma triglyceride levels greater than 250 mg/dL are reduced by amounts that are comparable to the reductions in LDL-C.[474] Atorvastatin or simvastatin at 80-mg doses, and rosuvastatin at 40-mg doses, reduce triglyceride levels by 35% to 40%. In patients with triglyceride levels less than 250 mg/dL, statins reduce triglyceride levels by less than 25%.[474] Statins also increase plasma HDL-C levels by 5% to 10%. In addition, a multitude of potentially cardioprotective non–lipid-lowering effects are being ascribed to statins, including improved endothelial function, increased plaque stability, decreased inflammation, decreased lipoprotein oxidation, and improved circulation.[178,475]

The reductase inhibitors are well tolerated and cause few side effects.[178] The most serious potential side effect is myopathy. Myopathy is defined as creatine kinase (CK) values exceeding 10 times the upper limit of normal, which occurs in approximately 0.01% of persons taking statins and can cause myoglobinuria and renal failure.[476] Patients taking HMG-CoA reductase inhibitors in whom myalgias develop should have serum CK measured immediately, and consideration should be given to stopping the drug if CK values are increased more than fivefold above the normal range. The risk of myopathy increases in proportion to plasma concentrations of HMG-CoA reductase inhibitors. Consequently, inhibition of statin catabolism is associated with increased myopathy risk. This problem tends to occur more often in persons older than 80 years, in patients with hepatic or renal dysfunction, during perioperative periods, in patients with multisystem disease, in persons with small body size, and in patients with untreated hypothyroidism.[477,478] Use of other drugs that reduce statin catabolism is associated with myopathy in 50% to 60% of cases.[478] As a fraction of 3339 cases reported to the FDA between 1990 and 2002, the most common interactions associated with rhabdomyolysis were statin with fibrates (38%), cyclosporine (4%), digoxin (5%), warfarin (4%), macrolide antibiotics (3%), mibefradil (2%), and azole antifungals (1%). Other drugs that increase myopathy risk are niacin (rare), amiodarone, nefazodone, and HIV protease inhibitors.[477,478]

TABLE 36–18 DRUG SELECTION BASED ON MAJOR LIPID ABNORMALITY

Major Elevated Plasma Lipid(s)	Drugs
Total cholesterol	HMG-CoA reductase inhibitor Niacin Bile acid sequestrants Ezetimibe
Total cholesterol and fasting triglycerides	Niacin Fibric acid derivative HMG-CoA reductase inhibitor Ezetimibe
Fasting triglycerides	Niacin Fibric acid derivative Omega-3 fatty acids HMG-CoA reductase inhibitor
Lp(a)	Niacin

HMG-CoA, 3-hydroxy-3-methylglutaryl coenzyme A; Lp(a), lipoprotein(a).

To minimize the risk of myopathy, these drug combinations should be avoided. However, statins may be used with a predisposing drug without increasing myopathy risk if the statin is administered at no more than 25% of its maximum dose.[178] If such combinations are used, it is important to be aware that myopathy can occur several years after starting therapy. There is usually no antecedent CK elevation before the onset of rhabdomyolysis, which negates the value of serial CK measurements. Serum transaminase elevations (greater than three times normal) occur in 1% to 2% of patients. The long-term side effects of HMG-CoA reductase inhibitor therapy are not known, but no significant long-term toxicities have been observed with lovastatin, which has now been in use for more than two decades. Serious hepatoxicity is extremely rare (liver failure rate of 1 case per million person-years of use).[420] Patients taking statins should have serum ALT measured at baseline and at 3 months after starting treatment. If the values are normal, ALT should then be measured only if clinically indicated.[420]

Bile Acid Sequestrants

Bile acid sequestrants are anion-exchange resins that exchange chloride for negatively charged bile acids.[178] The bound bile acids are then excreted in the feces.[479] The increased excretion of bile acids causes increased oxidation of cholesterol to form bile acids in hepatocytes, and the resultant up-regulation of hepatic LDL receptors in turn lowers plasma LDL concentrations.[480] Because bile acid sequestrants act in the intestine, the side effects are limited to local effects in the gastrointestinal system (e.g., bloating, gas, constipation). At therapeutic doses, these agents can lower plasma cholesterol levels by 15% to 25%. However, they can increase plasma triglyceride levels[481] and must be used with caution in patients predisposed to hypertriglyceridemia. In addition, because they bind negatively charged molecules in the intestine, these agents can interfere with the absorption of other medications, including levothyroxine, digoxin, warfarin, and thiazide diuretics. Therefore, resins are given at least 4 hours before or 1 hour after other medications. Colesevelam does not bind other drugs to the same extent as the resins cholestyramine and colestipol.

Niacin

The most inexpensive drug for treating hyperlipidemia is the B vitamin niacin.[178] Therapeutic doses of crystalline niacin (typically 2.0 to 6.0 g/day) lower both total and LDL cholesterol by

TABLE 36–19 PERCENTAGE REDUCTIONS IN LOW-DENSITY LIPOPROTEIN CHOLESTEROL FROM BASELINE

Reduction from Baseline (%)	DOSE (mg)					
	Atorvastatin	Fluvastatin	Lovastatin	Pravastatin	Simvastatin	Rosuvastatin
20-25	—	20	10	10	—	—
26-30	—	40	20	20	10	—
31-35	10	80	40	40	20	—
36-40	20		80		40	5
41-50	40				80	10
51-55	80					20, 40

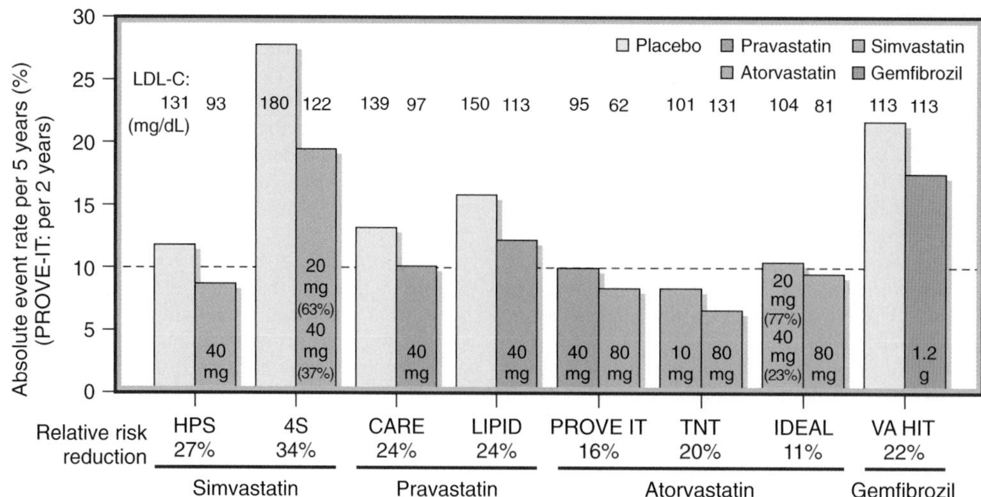

Figure 36–23 ▪ Rates of fatal and nonfatal myocardial infarction in recent major lipid-lowering trials conducted in patients with CHD or CHD-equivalent disorders. In all trials, lower LDL-C levels were associated with lower event rates. The relative risk reductions were 11% to 34%. Absolute event rates approached 10% per 5 years (2% per year) for all patients in all trials irrespective of treatment. In PROVE-IT (Pravastatin or Atorvastatin Evaluation and Infection Therapy), the only trial of patients with acute coronary syndrome, the 2-year event rate was 8.3% despite average on-treatment LDL-C = 1.61 mM/L (62 mg/dL). 4S, Scandinavian simvastatin survival study; CARE, cholesterol and recurrent events; IDEAL, incremental decrease in endpoints through aggressive lipid lowering; LIPID, long-term intervention with pravastatin in ischemic disease; TNT, treating to new targets; VA-HIT, Veterans Administration HDL intervention trial.

15% to 30%, lower triglyceride levels by 30% to 40%, and raise HDL-C levels by 15% to 25%.[178] Maximum HDL increases usually occur with therapeutic doses of 1.5 to 2.0 g/day. Niacin also lowers plasma Lp(a) concentrations by up to 40%.[305,482] The preparation must be niacin and not niacinamide, which has no efficacy. The mechanism whereby niacin affects plasma lipids is unclear, but it seems to be associated with decreased hepatic VLDL production.

The most troublesome side effect of niacin therapy is a flushing syndrome that occurs shortly after taking the medicine. Flushing can be minimized by initiating therapy with small doses (e.g., 100 mg) and gradually increasing the dosage to the therapeutic range over weeks to months. Repeated dosing is associated with a gradual tolerance to the flushing syndrome. In addition, taking an aspirin about 1 hour before the niacin can diminish the flushing, possibly by inhibiting prostaglandin-mediated side effects.

The most serious complication of niacin therapy is hepatotoxicity, and therapy should be accompanied by monitoring of serum liver function tests. Mild increases in serum transaminases are common when doses are increased rapidly; however, therapy should be discontinued if transaminases reach highly elevated levels (e.g., >3 times normal). Because hepatotoxicity appears to be more common with sustained-release preparations of niacin,[483] the immediate-release crystalline form is preferred. Other side effects of niacin therapy include impairment or worsening of glucose tolerance and hyperuricemia. Data suggest that niacin can be used safely in patients with glucose intolerance or diabetes mellitus,[484] but the drug should be used with great caution in patients with a history of gout and is contraindicated in patients with active peptic ulcer disease. A prescription formulation of niacin, Niaspan, is characterized as extended-release as opposed to sustained-release. Diminished hepatotoxicity is reported for this drug, but careful monitoring of hepatic transaminase (ALT) is still required. Niaspan should be taken at bedtime in amounts of 500 to 2000 mg daily.

Fibric Acid Derivatives

The fibric acid derivatives—clofibrate, gemfibrozil, and fenofibrate—lower plasma triglycerides by about 40% and increase HDL-C levels by about 10%[233] but have only minor effects on LDL-C.[178] These agents act by activating the peroxisome proliferator-activated receptor (PPAR) α, a nuclear hormone receptor that is expressed in the liver and other tissues.[485] This results in increased fatty acid oxidation, increased LPL synthesis, and reduced expression of apo-CIII, all of which contribute to lowering plasma triglycerides.[485] The physiologic results are a decrease in VLDL triglyceride production and an increase in LPL-mediated catabolism of triglyceride-rich lipoproteins.[486] This receptor also stimulates the expression of apo-AI and apo-AII, leading to increased HDL levels. Fenofibrate may be taken once daily. The other two agents are given twice a day.

Side effects include gastrointestinal discomfort and possibly an increased incidence of cholesterol gallstones (documented for clofibrate). Fibric acid derivatives should be used with great caution in the setting of renal insufficiency because these drugs are excreted into the urine. Patients with this condition have an increased risk of myopathy.[487] Fenofibrate, which does not interfere with statin metabolism and has a much lower risk of causing myopathy, is the preferred fibrate to use in combination with a statin.[488-492] However, the fenofibrate dose needs to be reduced in patients with renal insufficiency.

Clofibrate received adverse publicity because of a large clinical trial in which slightly more cancer deaths were noted in the clofibrate-treated group.[493] However, a later analysis did not substantiate this finding,[494] and there is no firm evidence that the drug is carcinogenic in humans. In two subsequent trials, the Helsinki Heart Study (primary prevention) and the VA HIT (secondary prevention), gemfibrozil treatment reduced fatal and nonfatal CHD events without changes in mortality rates or increased mortality from noncardiac causes.[233,234]

Ezetimibe, an Inhibitor of Intestinal Cholesterol Absorption

Ezetimibe is the first drug that inhibits cholesterol absorption by enterocytes in the intestine.[495] As monotherapy, the 10-mg standard dose lowers LDL-C by 15% to 20%. It is rarely used except in combination with statins. Ezetimibe lowers LDL-C by an additional 15% to 20% when it is combined with any statin at any dose. Increasing statin doses from 20 to 80 mg provides only an additional 12% reduction in LDL-C, whereas adding ezetimibe, 10 mg daily, to 20 mg of a statin will reduce LDL-C by an additional 15% to 20%.[496-498] Outcome studies employing ezetimibe administered in combination with a statin are in progress.

Omega-3 Fatty Acids

Fish-derived ω-3 fatty acids (eicosapentaenoic acid, C20:5n-3; or EPA and docosahexaenoic acid, C22:6n-3; or DHA) have a number of effects upon plasma lipid levels and antiarrhythmic effects that reduce the risk of sudden death.[460] In the United States, the FDA has approved a preparation, Omacor, for the sole indication of lowering triglyceride levels in persons with fasting triglyceride levels greater than 5.6 mM/L (500 mg/dL). Omacor is prepared in capsule form containing a gram of oil, which includes 900 mg of the ethyl esters of ω-3 fatty acids. Each capsule contains about 465 mg of EPA and 375 mg of DHA, or a total of 840 mg of EPA plus DHA. At the recommended dosage of four capsules daily given to patients who have triglycerides of 5.7-22.6 mM/L (500-2000 mg/dL), Omacor lowers triglycerides by about 50%, raises HDL-C by about 10%, lowers VLDL-C by about 40%, and raises LDL-C by about 50%. Overall the total cholesterol-to-HDL-C ratio is reduced by about 20% and the non-HDL-C is lowered by about 10%.[461,499] As with fibrates, the distribution of LDL particles shifts to one with higher concentrations of buoyant LDL and lower concentrations of smaller, denser LDL particles.[500] Unlike fibrates, however, EPA and DHA have no effect on statin metabolism, and there is virtually no increase in the risk of myopathy when Omacor is used in combination with statins.

Combination Therapy

For patients with severe elevations of plasma cholesterol (e.g., >7.8 mM/L [300 mg/dL]) or in whom treatment goals are to reduce the plasma cholesterol and LDL-C levels by 50% or more, combination drug therapy is usually required.[178] Often goals can be achieved with drug combinations that employ lower doses than needed when these agents are used singly. For example, combined therapy with an HMG-CoA reductase inhibitor and either ezetimibe,[501] niacin,[502,503] or a bile acid sequestrant[504] can lower plasma cholesterol levels by more than 50%.[501] Vytorin, a preparation of simvastatin (10 mg, 20 mg, 40 mg, or 80 mg) plus ezetimibe (10 mg), can lower LDL-C by 60%. Alternatively, combinations that include an HMG-CoA reductase inhibitor, niacin, and a bile acid sequestrant can achieve the desired lipid-lowering effect.[505] Patients with diabetes mellitus who have high plasma levels of triglyceride and VLDL-C may benefit from combination therapy with a low dose of an HMG-CoA reductase inhibitor and gemfibrozil or fenofibrate. Because the use of HMG-CoA reductase inhibitors with niacin or gemfibrozil is associated with a higher risk of myopathy, such combinations must be used with caution. Fenofibrate is preferable because it is less likely to cause myopathy. Statin doses should be limited to approximately 25% of maximum dosages in most patients. It is not advisable to give gemfibrozil with rosuvastatin at doses greater than 10 mg of rosuvastatin.

Drugs on the Horizon

A number of strategies to improve the treatment of dyslipidemia are under development.[178] For example, more potent statins capable of lowering LDL-C levels by more than 65% are being developed.[506] Inhibitors of MTP represent another strategy.[507] These agents have the potential to lower both plasma triglyceride and cholesterol levels by inhibiting hepatic VLDL production. An ACAT2 inhibitor[508] might offer an alternative to ezetimibe for lowering plasma cholesterol levels by inhibiting intestinal cholesterol absorption. CETP inhibitors raise HDL levels by 100% and might prevent clinical events caused by complications of atherosclerosis. Clinical trials of two CETP inhibitors, JTT705 and torcetrapib, are under way.[509]

There has been intense interest in the use of antioxidants to treat or prevent atherosclerosis. Apo-AI administration or administration of mutant isoforms of apo-AI may slow the progression of atherosclerosis.[320,510] Apo-AI mimetic peptides synthesized from D-amino acids rather than L-amino acids hold promise for oral therapies that will enhance reverse cholesterol transport.[511]

Surgical Treatment

Partial ileal bypass surgery has been used to reduce lipid levels in patients with severe hypercholesterolemia who cannot tolerate lipid-lowering drugs. This surgical therapy can reduce total cholesterol levels by 20% to 25% and cause regression of angiographically measured atherosclerotic lesions.[181] In addition, liver transplantation[187] and portacaval shunting[188,189] have been used as experimental therapies for homozygous FH (see previous discussion).

Treatment of Patients with Low Levels of High-Density Lipoprotein Cholesterol

Patients with familial hypoalphalipoproteinemia can have normal or modestly increased plasma cholesterol levels but have very low HDL-C levels, resulting in a predisposition to CHD. Such patients can have high ratios of total cholesterol to HDL-C (e.g., >10) despite having a normal plasma cholesterol level. At present, there are no highly effective therapies to raise HDL-C levels.[512] Exercise in sustained amounts only modestly increases HDL-C levels in persons with low HDL-C levels.[513] In a study of recreational runners, HDL-C levels increased by approximately 2 mg/dL for every 10 miles run per week.[514] Alcohol, when consumed in modest quantities, can also increase HDL-C levels.[401] Of the available drug therapies, niacin results in the largest increase in HDL-C levels (about 15% to 25%)[515]; fibrates and HMG-CoA reductase inhibitors increase HDL-C by about 10%. However, the potent ability of HMG-CoA reductase inhibitors to lower LDL-C and total cholesterol is the most efficacious way to lower the total cholesterol/HDL-C ratio,[516] and statins reduce the risk of clinical events without significantly raising HDL-C levels.[517]

Management of patients with low HDL levels is best accomplished by employing treatment goals for both LDL-C and for the total cholesterol-to-HDL-C ratio, because LDL-C targets of therapy need to be lower for patients who have low HDL-C levels than for those who don't. Table 36–10 provides guidance for this approach.[310] An alternative approach is used in the current NCEP ATP III guidelines, which advise additional treatment of low HDL-C patients if they are at their goal for LDL-C and if they have triglyceride levels greater than 2.25 mM/L (200 mg/dL). In such patients, a secondary goal for non–HDL-C is calculated as total cholesterol minus HDL-C. The non-HDL-C goal is the same as a patient's LDL-C goal plus 0.8 mM/L (30 mg/dL).[216]

Treatment of the Chylomicronemia Syndrome

Patients with the chylomicronemia syndrome often present with acute pancreatitis and severe hypertriglyceridemia (triglycerides >22.6 mM/L [2000 mg/dL]).[256] These patients should be treated with total fat restriction until the triglyceride level falls to a safe range (e.g., <11.3 mM/L [1000 mg/dL]), at which time a fat-restricted diet (e.g., <10% of calories) can be instituted and the plasma triglyceride level further monitored. The goal is to maintain the triglyceride level at less than 11.3 mM/L (1000 mg/dL) and preferably less than 4.5 mM/L (400 mg/dL). Often this can be accomplished by modifying the diet and eliminating or modifying secondary causes of hyperlipidemia such as drugs, glucose intolerance, or alcohol consumption. However, such patients often require a triglyceride-lowering drug, such as a fibrate or niacin, to maintain the plasma triglyceride level in a range that prevents subsequent episodes of pancreatitis. Recommendations for the management of the hypertriglyceridemia associated with pregnancy have been described.[518] In some patients who hvae severe hypertriglyceridemia despite use of highly restricted dietary fat intake, therapy with orlistat has been beneficial.[266]

REFERENCES

1. Goldstein JL, Brown MS. Regulation of the mevalonate pathway. Nature 1990;343:425-430.
2. Myant NB. Cholesterol Metabolism, LDL, and the LDL Receptor. San Diego. Academic Press, 1990.
3. Dietschy JM, Turley SD, Spady DK. Role of liver in the maintenance of cholesterol and low density lipoprotein homeostasis in different animal species, including humans. J Lipid Res 1993;34:1637-1659.
4. Rader DJ, Hobbs HH. Disorders of lipoprotein metabolism. In Kasper DL, Braunwald E, Fauci AS (eds). Harrison's Principles of Internal Medicine, 16th ed. New York. McGraw-Hill, 2005: 2286-2298.
5. Brown MS, Goldstein JL. A receptor-mediated pathway for cholesterol homeostasis. Science 1986;232:34-47.
6. Björkhem I, Eggertsen G. Genes involved in initial steps of bile acid synthesis. Curr Opin Lipidol 2001;12:97-103.
7. Russell DW. The enzymes, regulation, and genetics of bile acid synthesis. Annu Rev Biochem 2003;72:137-174.
8. Buhman KF, Accad M, Farese RV Jr. Mammalian acyl-CoA: cholesterol acyltransferases. Biochim Biophys Acta 2000;1529:142-154.
9. Buhman KK, Chen HC, Farese RV Jr. The enzymes of neutral lipid synthesis. J Biol Chem 2001;276:40369-40372.
10. Gotto AM. Cholesterol intake and serum cholesterol level. N Engl J Med 1991;324:912-913.
11. Grundy SM, Denke MA. Dietary influences on serum lipids and lipoproteins. J Lipid Res 1990;31:1149-1172.
12. Kuwajima M, Foster DW, McGarry JD. Regulation of lipoprotein lipase in different rat tissues. Metabolism 1988;37:597-601.
13. Stein Y, Stein O. Lipoprotein lipase and atherosclerosis. Atherosclerosis 2003;170:1-9.
14. Strålfors P, Olsson H, Belfrage P. Hormone-sensitive lipase. In Boyer PD, Krebs EG (eds). The Enzymes, 3rd ed, vol 18. Orlando. Academic Press, 1987:147-177.
15. Chen HC, Farese RV Jr. DGAT and triglyceride synthesis. a new target for obesity treatment? Trends Cardiovasc Med 2000;10: 188-192.
16. Cases S, Stone SJ, Zhou P, et al. Cloning of *DGAT2*, a second mammalian diacylglycerol acyltransferase, and related family members. J Biol Chem 2001;276:38870-38876.
17. Chen HC, Farese RV Jr. Inhibition of triglyceride synthesis as a treatment strategy for obesity. Lessons from DGAT1-deficient mice. Arterioscler Thromb Vasc Biol 2005;25:482-486.
18. Needleman P, Turk J, Jakschik BA, et al. Arachidonic acid metabolism. Annu Rev Biochem 1986;55:69-102.
19. Breslow JL. Insights into lipoprotein metabolism from studies in transgenic mice. Annu Rev Physiol 1994;56:797-810.
20. Mahley RW, Innerarity TL, Rall SC Jr, Weisgraber KH. Plasma lipoproteins. apolipoprotein structure and function. J Lipid Res 1984;25:1277-1294.
21. Mackness MI, Durrington PN. HDL, its enzymes and its potential to influence lipid peroxidation. Atherosclerosis 1995;115:243-253.
22. Tjoelker LW, Wilder C, Eberhardt C, et al. Anti-inflammatory properties of a platelet-activating factor acetylhydrolase. Nature 1995;374:549-553.
23. Innerarity TL, Borén J, Yamanaka S, Olofsson S-O. Biosynthesis of apolipoprotein B48–containing lipoproteins. Regulation by novel post-transcriptional mechanisms. J Biol Chem 1996;271: 2353-2356.
24. Anant S, Davidson NO. Molecular mechanisms of apolipoprotein B mRNA editing. Curr Opin Lipidol 2001;12:159-165.
25. Anant S, Davidson NO. Identification and regulation of protein components of the apolipoprotein B mRNA editing enzyme. A complex event. Trends Cardiovasc Med 2002;12:311-317.
26. Knott TJ, Pease RJ, Powell LM, et al. Complete protein sequence and identification of structural domains of human apolipoprotein B. Nature 1986;323:734-738.
27. Yang C-Y, Gu Z-W, Weng S-A, et al. Structure of apolipoprotein B-100 of human low density lipoproteins. Arteriosclerosis 1989;9: 96-108.
28. Mahley RW, Innerarity TL. Lipoprotein receptors and cholesterol homeostasis. Biochim Biophys Acta 1983;737:197-222.
29. Borén J, Lee I, Zhu W, et al. Identification of the low density lipoprotein receptor–binding site in apolipoprotein B100 and the modulation of its binding activity by the carboxyl terminus in familial defective apo-B100. J Clin Invest 1998;101:1084-1093.
30. Innerarity TL, Mahley RW, Weisgraber KH, et al. Familial defective apolipoprotein B100. a mutation of apolipoprotein B that causes hypercholesterolemia. J Lipid Res 1990;31:1337-1349.
31. Shelness GS, Ledford AS. Evolution and mechanism of apolipoprotein B–containing lipoprotein assembly. Curr Opin Lipidol 2005;16:325-332.
32. Hussain MM, Fatma S, Pan X, Iqbal J. Intestinal lipoprotein assembly. Curr Opin Lipidol 2005;16:281-285.
33. Young SG, Farese RV Jr, Pierotti VR, et al. Transgenic mice expressing human $apoB_{100}$ and $apoB_{48}$. Curr Opin Lipidol 1994;5: 94-101.
34. Purcell-Huynh DA, Farese RV Jr, Johnson DF, et al. Transgenic mice expressing high levels of human apolipoprotein B develop severe atherosclerotic lesions in response to a high-fat diet. J Clin Invest 1995;95:2246-2257.
35. Farese RV Jr, Ruland SL, Flynn LM, et al. Knockout of the mouse apolipoprotein B gene results in embryonic lethality in homozygotes and protection against diet-induced hypercholesterolemia in heterozygotes. Proc Natl Acad Sci U S A 1995;92:1774-1778.
36. Huang L-S, Voyiaziakis E, Markenson DF, et al. Apo B gene knockout in mice results in embryonic lethality in homozygotes and neural tube defects, male infertility, and reduced HDL cholesterol ester and apo A-I transport rates in heterozygotes. J Clin Invest 1995;96:2152-2161.
37. Farese RV Jr, Cases S, Ruland SL, et al. A novel function for apolipoprotein B. lipoprotein synthesis in the yolk sac is critical for maternal-fetal lipid transport in mice. J Lipid Res 1996;37: 347-360.
38. Mahley RW. Apolipoprotein E. cholesterol transport protein with expanding role in cell biology. Science 1988;240:622-630.
39. Weisgraber KH. Apolipoprotein E. structure-function relationships. Adv Protein Chem 1994;45:249-302.
40. Davignon J, Gregg RE, Sing CF. Apolipoprotein E polymorphism and atherosclerosis. Arteriosclerosis 1988;8:1-21.
41. Mahley RW, Rall SC Jr. Apolipoprotein E. Far more than a lipid transport protein. Annu Rev Genomics Hum Genet 2000;1: 507-537.
42. Mahley RW, Huang Y. Apolipoprotein E. structure and function in lipid metabolism and neurobiology. In Rosenberg RN, Prusiner SB, DiMauro S (eds). The Molecular and Genetic Basis of Neurologic and Psychiatric Disease, 3rd ed. Philadelphia. Butterworth Heinemann, 2003:565-573.
43. Mahley RW, Huang Y. Apolipoprotein E. from atherosclerosis to Alzheimer's disease and beyond. Curr Opin Lipidol 1999;10: 207-217.
44. Mahley RW, Huang Y, Rall SC Jr. Pathogenesis of type III hyperlipoproteinemia (dysbetalipoproteinemia). questions, quandaries, and paradoxes. J Lipid Res 1999;40:1933-1949.
45. Mahley RW, Rall SC Jr. Type III hyperlipoproteinemia (dysbetalipoproteinemia). The role of apolipoprotein E in normal and abnormal lipoprotein metabolism. In Scriver CR, Beaudet AL, Sly WS

(eds). The Metabolic and Molecular Bases of Inherited Disease, 8th ed, vol 2. New York. McGraw-Hill, 2001:2835-2862.
46. Dong L-M, Wilson C, Wardell MR, et al. Human apolipoprotein E. Role of arginine 61 in mediating the lipoprotein preferences of the E3 and E4 isoforms. J Biol Chem 1994;269:22358-22365.
47. Wilson C, Wardell MR, Weisgraber KH, et al. Three-dimensional structure of the LDL receptor-binding domain of human apolipoprotein E. Science 1991;252:1817-1822.
48. Wilson C, Mau T, Weisgraber KH, et al. Salt bridge relay triggers defective LDL receptor binding by a mutant apolipoprotein. Structure 1994;2:713-718.
49. Dong L-M, Parkin S, Trakhanov SD, et al. Novel mechanism for defective receptor binding of apolipoprotein E2 in type III hyperlipoproteinemia. Nat Struct Biol 1996;3:718-722.
50. Mahley RW, Ji Z-S. Remnant lipoprotein metabolism. Key pathways involving cell-surface heparan sulfate proteoglycans and apolipoprotein E. J Lipid Res 1999;40:1-16.
51. Zhang SH, Reddick RL, Piedrahita JA, Maeda N. Spontaneous hypercholesterolemia and arterial lesions in mice lacking apolipoprotein E. Science 1992;258:468-471.
52. Plump AS, Smith JD, Hayek T, et al. Severe hypercholesterolemia and atherosclerosis in apolipoprotein E-deficient mice created by homologous recombination in ES cells. Cell 1992;71:343-353.
53. Linsel-Nitschke P, Tall AR. HDL as a target in the treatment of atherosclerotic cardiovascular disease. Nat Rev Drug Discov 2005; 4:193-205.
54. Tall AR, Breslow JL, Rubin EM. Genetic disorders affecting plasma high-density lipoproteins. In Scriver CR, Beaudet AL, Sly WS (eds). The Metabolic and Molecular Bases of Inherited Disease, 8th ed, vol 2. New York. McGraw-Hill, 2001:2915-2936.
55. Cho K-H, Durbin DM, Jonas A. Role of individual amino acids of apolipoprotein A-I in the activation of lecithin:cholesterol acyltransferase and in HDL rearrangements. J Lipid Res 2001;42: 379-389.
56. Wang N, Lan D, Chen W, et al. ATP-binding cassette transporters G1 and G4 mediate cellular cholesterol efflux to high-density lipoproteins. Proc Natl Acad Sci U S A 2004;101:9774-9779.
57. Yokoyama S. Assembly of high density lipoprotein by the ABCA1/ apolipoprotein pathway. Curr Opin Lipidol 2005;16:269-279.
58. Plump AS, Scott CJ, Breslow JL. Human apolipoprotein A-I gene expression increases high density lipoprotein and suppresses atherosclerosis in the apolipoprotein E–deficient mouse. Proc Natl Acad Sci U S A 1994;91:9607-9611.
59. Pászty C, Maeda N, Verstuyft J, Rubin EM. Apolipoprotein AI transgene corrects apolipoprotein E deficiency-induced atherosclerosis in mice. J Clin Invest 1994;94:899-903.
60. Deeb SS, Takata K, Peng R, et al. A splice-junction mutation responsible for familial apolipoprotein A-II deficiency. Am J Hum Genet 1990;46:822-827.
61. Warden CH, Hedrick CC, Qiao J-H, et al. Atherosclerosis in transgenic mice overexpressing apolipoprotein A-II. Science 1993; 261:469-472.
62. Pennacchio LA, Olivier M, Hubacek JA, et al. An apolipoprotein influencing triglycerides in humans and mice revealed by comparative sequencing. Science 2001;294:169-173.
63. Pennacchio LA, Olivier M, Hubacek JA, et al. Two independent apolipoprotein A5 haplotypes influence human plasma triglyceride levels. Hum Mol Genet 2002;11:3031-3038.
64. Merkel M, Heeren J. Give me A5 for lipoprotein hydrolysis! J Clin Invest 2005;115:2694-2696.
65. Marçais C, Verges B, Charrière S, et al. Apoa5 Q139X truncation predisposes to late-onset hyperchylomicronemia due to lipoprotein lipase impairment. J Clin Invest 2005;115:2862-2869.
66. Willnow TE. The low-density lipoprotein receptor gene family. Multiple roles in lipid metabolism. J Mol Med 1999;77:306-315.
67. Willnow TE, Nykjaer A, Herz J. Lipoprotein receptors. New roles for ancient proteins. Nat Cell Biol 1999;1:E157-E162.
68. Goldstein JL, Hobbs HH, Brown MS. Familial hypercholesterolemia. In Scriver CR, Beaudet AL, Sly WS (eds). The Metabolic and Molecular Bases of Inherited Disease, 8th ed, vol 2. New York. McGraw-Hill, 2001:2863-2913.
69. Rader DJ, Cohen J, Hobbs HH. Monogenic hypercholesterolemia. New insights in pathogenesis and treatment. J Clin Invest 2003;111:1795-1803.
70. Herz J. LRP. A bright beacon at the blood-brain barrier. J Clin Invest 2003;112:1483-1485.
71. Brown MS, Goldstein JL. Sterol regulatory element binding proteins (SREBPs). controllers of lipid synthesis and cellular uptake. Nutr Rev 1998;56:S1-S3.
72. Goldstein JL, DeBose-Boyd RA, Brown MS. Protein sensors for membrane sterols. Cell 2006;124:35-46.
73. Horton JD, Goldstein JL, Brown MS. SREBPs. Activators of the complete program of cholesterol and fatty acid synthesis in the liver. J Clin Invest 2002;109:1125-1131.
74. Nohturfft A, DeBose-Boyd RA, Scheek S, et al. Sterols regulate cycling of SREBP cleavage-activating protein (SCAP) between endoplasmic reticulum and Golgi. Proc Natl Acad Sci U S A 1999;96:11235-11240.
75. Herz J, Strickland DK. LRP. a multifunctional scavenger and signaling receptor. J Clin Invest 2001;108:779-784.
76. Beisiegel U, Weber W, Bengtsson-Olivecrona G. Lipoprotein lipase enhances the binding of chylomicrons to low density lipoprotein receptor–related protein. Proc Natl Acad Sci U S A 1991;88: 8342-8346.
77. Ji Z-S, Lauer SJ, Fazio S, et al. Enhanced binding and uptake of remnant lipoproteins by hepatic lipase-secreting hepatoma cells in culture. J Biol Chem 1994;269:13429-13436.
78. Willnow TE, Hilpert J, Armstrong SA, et al. Defective forebrain development in mice lacking gp330/megalin. Proc Natl Acad Sci U S A 1996;93:8460-8464.
79. Witztum JL, Steinberg D. The oxidative modification hypothesis of atherosclerosis. Does it hold for humans? Trends Cardiovasc Med 2001;11:93-102.
80. Trigatti BL, Krieger M, Rigotti A. Influence of the HDL receptor SR-BI on lipoprotein metabolism and atherosclerosis. Arterioscler Thromb Vasc Biol 2003;23:1732-1738.
81. Witztum JL. You are right too! J Clin Invest 2005;115:2072-2075.
82. van Berkel TJC, Out R, Hoekstra M, et al. Scavenger receptors. Friend or foe in atherosclerosis? Curr Opin Lipidol 2005;16: 525-535.
83. Brunzell JD, Deeb SS. Familial lipoprotein lipase deficiency, apo C-II deficiency, and hepatic lipase deficiency. In Scriver CR, Beaudet AL, Sly WS (eds). The Metabolic and Molecular Bases of Inherited Disease, 8th ed, vol 2. New York. McGraw-Hill, 2001: 2789-2816.
84. Kern PA. Lipoprotein lipase and hepatic lipase. Curr Opin Lipidol 1991;2:162-169.
85. Cohen JC, Vega GL, Grundy SM. Hepatic lipase. new insights from genetic and metabolic studies. Curr Opin Lipidol 1999;10: 259-267.
86. Thuren T, Weisgraber KH, Sisson P, Waite M. Role of apolipoprotein E in hepatic lipase catalyzed hydrolysis of phospholipid in high-density lipoproteins. Biochemistry 1992;31:2332-2338.
87. Homanics GE, de Silva HV, Osada J, et al. Mild dyslipidemia in mice following targeted inactivation of the hepatic lipase gene. J Biol Chem 1995;270:2974-2980.
88. Busch SJ, Barnhart RL, Martin GA, et al. Human hepatic triglyceride lipase expression reduces high density lipoprotein and aortic cholesterol in cholesterol-fed transgenic mice. J Biol Chem 1994;269:16376-16382.
89. Fan J, Wang J, Bensadoun A, et al. Overexpression of hepatic lipase in transgenic rabbits leads to a marked reduction of plasma high density lipoproteins and intermediate density lipoproteins. Proc Natl Acad Sci U S A 1994;91:8724-8728.
90. Glomset JA, Assmann G, Gjone E, Norum KR:.Lecithin:cholesterol acyltransferase deficiency and fish eye disease. In Scriver CR, Beaudet AL, Sly WS, Valle D (eds). The Metabolic and Molecular Bases of Inherited Disease, 7th ed, vol 2. New York. McGraw-Hill, 1995:1933-1951.
91. Stein O, Stein Y. Lipid transfer proteins (LTP) and atherosclerosis. Atherosclerosis 2005;178:217-230.
92. Tall A. Plasma lipid transfer proteins. Annu Rev Biochem 1995;64: 235-257.
93. Barter PJ, Brewer HB Jr, Chapman MJ, et al. Cholesteryl ester transfer protein. A novel target for raising HDL and inhibiting atherosclerosis. Arterioscler Thromb Vasc Biol 2003;23:160-167.
94. Havel RJ, Kane JP. Introduction. Structure and metabolism of plasma lipoproteins. In Scriver CR, Beaudet AL, Sly WS (eds). The

Metabolic and Molecular Bases of Inherited Disease, 8th ed, vol 2. New York. McGraw-Hill, 2001:2705-2716.

95. Altmann SW, Davis HR Jr, Zhu L-J, et al. Niemann-Pick C1 like 1 protein is critical for intestinal cholesterol absorption. Science 2004;303:1201-1204.
96. Brown MS, Herz J, Kowal RC, Goldstein JL. The low-density lipoprotein receptor-related protein. Double agent or decoy? Curr Opin Lipidol 1991;2:65-72.
97. Ji Z-S, Fazio S, Lee Y-L, Mahley RW. Secretion-capture role for apolipoprotein E in remnant lipoprotein metabolism involving cell surface heparan sulfate proteoglycans. J Biol Chem 1994;269: 2764-2772.
98. Willnow TE, Armstrong SA, Hammer RE, Herz J. Functional expression of low density lipoprotein receptor–related protein is controlled by receptor-associated protein in vivo. Proc Natl Acad Sci U S A 1995;92:4537-4541.
99. Alexander CA, Hamilton RL, Havel RJ. Subcellular localization of B apoprotein of plasma lipoproteins in rat liver. J Cell Biol 1976;69:241-263.
100. Olofsson S-O, Asp L, Borén J. The assembly and secretion of apolipoprotein B–containing lipoproteins. Curr Opin Lipidol 1999;10: 341-346.
101. Fisher EA, Ginsberg HN. Complexity in the secretory pathway. the assembly and secretion of apolipoprotein B–containing lipoproteins. J Biol Chem 2002;277:17377-17380.
102. Gregg RE, Wetterau JR. The molecular basis of abetalipoproteinemia. Curr Opin Lipidol 1994;5:81-86.
103. Berriot-Varoqueaux N, Aggerbeck LP, Samson-Bouma M-E, Wetterau JR. The role of the microsomal triglyceride transfer protein in abetalipoproteinemia. Annu Rev Nutr 2000;20:663-697.
104. Lewis GF, Rader DJ. New insights into the regulation of HDL metabolism and reverse cholesterol transport. Circ Res 2005;96: 1221-1232.
105. Jiang X-C, Bruce C, Mar J, et al. Targeted mutation of plasma phospholipid transfer protein gene markedly reduces high-density lipoprotein levels. J Clin Invest 1999;103:907-914.
106. Huang Y, von Eckardstein A, Wu S, et al. A plasma lipoprotein containing only apolipoprotein E and with G mobility on electrophoresis releases cholesterol from cells. Proc Natl Acad Sci U S A 1994;91:1834-1838.
107. Krieger M. Charting the fate of the "good cholesterol". Identification and characterization of the high-density lipoprotein receptor SR-BI. Annu Rev Biochem 1999;68:523-558.
108. Williams DL, Connelly MA, Temel RE, et al. Scavenger receptor BI and cholesterol trafficking. Curr Opin Lipidol 1999;10:329-339.
109. Oram JF. Tangier disease and ABCA1. Biochim Biophys Acta 2000;1529:321-330.
110. Jonas A. Lecithin cholesterol acyltransferase. Biochim Biophys Acta 2000;1529:245-256.
111. Yamashita S, Hirano K-I, Sakai N, Matsuzawa Y. Molecular biology and pathophysiological aspects of plasma cholesteryl ester transfer protein. Biochim Biophys Acta 2000;1529:257-275.
112. Tall AR, Jiang X-C, Luo Y, Silver D. 1999 George Lyman Duff Memorial Lecture. Lipid transfer proteins, HDL metabolism, and atherogenesis. Arterioscler Thromb Vasc Biol 2000;20:1185-1188.
113. Rigotti A, Miettinen HE, Krieger M. The role of the high-density lipoprotein receptor SR-BI in the lipid metabolism of endocrine and other tissues. Endocr Rev 2003;24:357-387.
114. Morton RE. Cholesteryl ester transfer protein and its plasma regulator. Lipid transfer inhibitor protein. Curr Opin Lipidol 1999;10: 321-327.
115. Marotti KR, Castle CK, Boyle TP, et al. Severe atherosclerosis in transgenic mice expressing simian cholesteryl ester transfer protein. Nature 1993;364:73-75.
116. Genest JJ, McNamara JR, Salem DN, Schaefer EJ. Prevalence of risk factors in men with premature coronary artery disease. Am J Cardiol 1991;67:1185-1189.
117. Greenland P, Knoll MD, Stamler J, et al. Major risk factors as antecedents of fatal and nonfatal coronary heart disease events. JAMA 2003;290:891-897.
118. Khot UN, Khot MB, Bajzer CT, et al. Prevalence of conventional risk factors in patients with coronary heart disease. JAMA 2003;290: 898-904.
119. The Multiple Risk Factor Intervention Trial Research Group. Mortality rates after 10.5 years for participants in the Multiple Risk Factor Intervention Trial. Findings related to a priori hypotheses of the trial. JAMA 1990;263:1795-1801.
120. Keys A. Coronary heart disease—the global picture. Atherosclerosis 1975;22:149-192.
121. Consensus conference. Lowering blood cholesterol to prevent heart disease. JAMA 1985;253:2080-2086.
122. Berg K. Lp(a) lipoprotein. An overview. Chem Phys Lipids 1994; 67/68:9-16.
123. Krauss RM. Low-density lipoprotein subclasses and risk of coronary artery disease. Curr Opin Lipidol 1991;2:248-252.
124. Mahley RW. Atherogenic lipoproteins and coronary artery disease. concepts derived from recent advances in cellular and molecular biology. Circulation 1985;72:943-948.
125. Mahley RW, Weisgraber KH, Innerarity TL, Rall SC Jr. Genetic defects in lipoprotein metabolism. Elevation of atherogenic lipoproteins caused by impaired catabolism. JAMA 1991;265: 78-83.
126. Steinberg D. Lipoproteins and the pathogenesis of atherosclerosis. Circulation 1987;76:508-514.
127. Steinberg D. Is there a potential therapeutic role for vitamin E or other antioxidants in atherosclerosis? Curr Opin Lipidol 2000;11:603-607.
128. Ross R. Atherosclerosis—an inflammatory disease. N Engl J Med 1999;340:115-126.
129. Williams KJ, Tabas I. The response-to-retention hypothesis of early atherogenesis. Arterioscler Thromb Vasc Biol 1995;15:551-561.
130. Williams KJ, Tabas I. Lipoprotein retention—and clues for atheroma regression. Arterioscler Thromb Vasc Biol 2005;25: 1536–1540.
131. Hansson GK. Inflammation, atherosclerosis, and coronary artery disease. N Engl J Med 2005;352:1685-1695.
132. Mallat Z, Ait-Qufella H, Tedgui A. Regulatory T cell responses. potential role in the control of atherosclerosis. Curr Opin Lipidol 2005;16:518-524.
133. Libby P. Changing concepts of atherogenesis. J Intern Med 2000;247:349-358.
134. Virmani R, Kolodgie FD, Burke AP, et al. Lessons from sudden coronary death. A comprehensive morphological classification scheme for atherosclerotic lesions. Arterioscler Thromb Vasc Biol 2000;20:1262-1275.
135. Davies MJ. Stability and instability. two faces of coronary atherosclerosis. The Paul Dudley White Lecture 1995. Circulation 1996;94:2013-2020.
136. Stary HC. The sequence of cell and matrix changes in atherosclerotic lesions of coronary arteries in the first forty years of life. Eur Heart J 1990;11(suppl E):3-19.
137. Cybulsky MI, Gimbrone MA Jr. Endothelial expression of a mononuclear leukocyte adhesion molecule during atherogenesis. Science 1991;251:788-791.
138. Peters W, Charo IF. Involvement of chemokine receptor 2 and its ligand, monocyte chemoattractant protein-1, in the development of atherosclerosis. Lessons from knockout mice. Curr Opin Lipidol 2001;12:175-180.
139. Smith SC Jr, Anderson JL, Cannon III RO, et al. CDC/AHA Workshop on Markers of Inflammation and Cardiovascular Disease. Application to Clinical and Public Health Practice. Report from the Clinical Practice Discussion Group. Circulation 2004;110: e550-e553.
140. Koenig W. Predicting risk and treatment benefit in atherosclerosis. the role of C-reactive protein. Int J Cardiol 2005;98:199-206.
141. Carroll MD, Lacher DA, Sorlie PD, et al. Trends in serum lipids and lipoproteins of adults, 1960-2002. JAMA 2005;294:1773-1781.
142. Wu Z, Yao C, Zhao D, et al. Cardiovascular disease risk factor levels and their relations to CVD rates in China—results of Sino-MONICA project. Eur J Cardiovasc Prev Rehabil 2004;11:275-283.
143. Castelli WP. Making practical sense of clinical trial data in decreasing cardiovascular risk. Am J Cardiol 2001;88(suppl):16F-20F.
144. The Expert Panel. Third Report of the National Cholesterol Education Program (NCEP) Expert Panel on Detection, Evaluation, and Treatment of High Blood Cholesterol in Adults (Adult Treatment Panel III). Final report. Circulation 2002;106:3143-3421.
145. Kavey R-EW, Daniels SR, Lauer RM, et al. American Heart Association guidelines for primary prevention of atherosclerotic cardiovascular disease beginning in childhood. Circulation 2003; 107:1562-1566.

146. Martin MJ, Hulley SB, Browner WS, et al. Serum cholesterol, blood pressure, and mortality. implications from a cohort of 361,662 men. Lancet 1986;2:933-936.
147. Taskinen M-R, Nikkilä EA, Pelkonen R, Sane T. Plasma lipoproteins, lipolytic enzymes, and very low density lipoprotein triglyceride turnover in Cushing's syndrome. J Clin Endocrinol Metab 1983;57:619-626.
148. Ettinger WH Jr, Hazzard WR. Prednisone increases very low density lipoprotein and high density lipoprotein in healthy men. Metabolism 1988;37:1055-1058.
149. Maison P, Griffin S, Nicoue-Beglah M, et al. Impact of growth hormone (GH) treatment on cardiovascular risk factors in GH-deficient adults. a metaanalysis of blinded, randomized, placebo-controlled trials. J Clin Endocrinol Metab 2004;89: 2192-2199.
150. Maldonado Castro GF, Escobar-Morreale HF, Ortega H, et al. Effects of normalization of GH hypersecretion on lipoprotein(a) and other lipoprotein serum levels in acromegaly. Clin Endocrinol 2000;53:313-319.
151. Twickler TB, Dallinga-Thie GM, Zelissen PMJ, et al. The atherogenic plasma remnant-like particle cholesterol concentration is increased in the fasting and postprandial state in active acromegalic patients. Clin Endocrinol 2001;55:69-75.
152. Weinbrenner T, Züger M, Jacoby GE, et al. Lipoprotein metabolism in patients with anorexia nervosa. a case-control study investigating the mechanisms leading to hypercholesterolaemia. Br J Nutr 2004;91:959-969.
153. Garg A. Gender differences in the prevalence of metabolic complications in familial partial lipodystrophy (Dunnigan variety). J Clin Endocrinol Metab 2000;85:1776-1782.
154. Epstein CJ, Martin GM, Schultz AL, Motulsky AG. Werner's syndrome. A review of its symptomatology, natural history, pathologic features, genetics and relationship to the natural aging process. Medicine (Baltimore) 1966;45:177-221.
155. Lees RS, Song CS, Levere RD, Kappas A. Hyperbeta-lipoproteinemia in acute intermittent porphyria. N Engl J Med 1970;282: 432-433.
156. Hülsmann WC, Eijkenboom WHM, Koster JF, Fernandes J. Glucose-6-phosphatase deficiency and hyperlipaemia. Clin Chim Acta 1970;30:775-778.
157. Jakovcic S, Khachadurian AK, Hsia DY-Y. The hyperlipidemia in glycogen storage disease. J Lab Clin Med 1966;68:769-779.
158. Moestrup SK, Nielsen LB. The role of the kidney in lipid metabolism. Curr Opin Lipidol 2005;16:301-306.
159. Bertolotti M, Carulli L, Concari M, et al. Suppression of bile acid synthesis, but not of hepatic cholesterol 7α-hydroxylase expression, by obstructive cholestasis in humans. Hepatology 2001;34: 234-242.
160. Campbell KM, Sabla GE, Bezerra JA. Transcriptional reprogramming in murine liver defines the physiologic consequences of biliary obstruction. J Hepatol 2004;40:14-23.
161. Miller JP. Dyslipoproteinaemia of liver disease. Baillieres Clin Endocrinol Metab 1990;4:807-832.
162. Taylor JS, Lewis LA, Battle JD Jr, et al. Plane xanthoma and multiple myeloma with lipoprotein-paraprotein complexing. Arch Dermatol 1978;114:425-431.
163. Tsai L-Y, Tsai S-M, Lee S-C, Liu S-F. Falsely low LDL-cholesterol concentrations and artifactual undetectable HDL-cholesterol measured by direct methods in a patient with monoclonal paraprotein. Clin Chim Acta 2005;358:192-195.
164. Kihara S, Matsuzawa Y, Kubo M, et al. Autoimmune hyperchylomicronemia. N Engl J Med 1989;320:1255-1259.
165. Corsini A, Roma P, Sommariva D, et al. Autoantibodies to the low density lipoprotein receptor in a subject affected by severe hypercholesterolemia. J Clin Invest 1986;78:940-946.
166. Nozaki S, Ito Y, Nakagawa T, et al. Autoimmune hyperlipidemia with inhibitory monoclonal antibodies against low density lipoprotein binding to fibroblasts in a case with multiple myeloma. Intern Med 1997;36:920-925.
167. Lee GA, Rao MN, Grunfeld C. The effects of HIV protease inhibitors on carbohydrate and lipid metabolism. Curr HIV/AIDS Rep 2005;2:39-50.
168. Hobbs HH, Brown MS, Goldstein JL. Molecular genetics of the LDL receptor gene in familial hypercholesterolemia. Hum Mutat 1992;1:445-466.
169. Shapiro JR, Fallat RW, Tsang RC, Glueck CJ. Achilles tendinitis and tenosynovitis. A diagnostic manifestation of familial type II hyperlipoproteinemia in children. Am J Dis Child 1974;128:486-490.
170. Barchiesi BJ, Eckel RH, Ellis PP. The cornea and disorders of lipid metabolism. Surv Ophthalmol 1991;36:1-22.
171. Neil HAW, Seagroatt V, Betteridge DJ, et al. Established and emerging coronary risk factors in patients with heterozygous familial hypercholesterolaemia. Heart 2004;90:1431-1437.
172. Sprecher DL, Schaefer EJ, Kent KM, et al. Cardiovascular features of homozygous familial hypercholesterolemia. Analysis of 16 patients. Am J Cardiol 1984;54:20-30.
173. Coetzee GA, van der Westhuyzen DR, Berger GMB, et al. Low density lipoprotein metabolism in cultured fibroblasts from a new group of patients presenting clinically with homozygous familial hypercholesterolemia. Arteriosclerosis 1982;2:303-311.
174. Allen JM, Thompson GR, Myant NB, et al. Cardiovascular complications of homozygous familial hypercholesterolaemia. Br Heart J 1980;44:361-368.
175. Tsouli SG, Kiortsis DN, Argyropoulou MI, et al. Pathogenesis, detection and treatment of Achilles tendon xanthomas. Eur J Clin Invest 2005;35:236–244.
176. Goldstein JL, Schrott HG, Hazzard WR, et al. Hyperlipidemia in coronary heart disease. II. Genetic analysis of lipid levels in 176 families and delineation of a new inherited disorder, combined hyperlipidemia. J Clin Invest 197352:1544-1568.
177. Hopkins PN. Familial hypercholesterolemia-improving treatment and meeting guidelines. Int J Cardiol 2003;89:13-23.
178. Mahley RW, Bersot TP. Drug therapy for hypercholesterolemia and dyslipidemia. In Brunton LL, Lazo JS, Parker KL (eds). Goodman & Gilman's The Pharmacological Basis of Therapeutics, 11th ed. New York: McGraw-Hill, 2006:933-966.
179. Illingworth DR. Management of hypercholesterolemia. Med Clin North Am 2000;84:23-42.
180. Stein E, Stender S, Mata P, et al. Achieving lipoprotein goals in patients at high risk with severe hypercholesterolemia. Efficacy and safety of ezetimibe co-administered with atorvastatin. Am Heart J 2004;148:447-455.
181. Buchwald H, Varco RL, Matts JP, et al. Effect of partial ileal bypass surgery on mortality and morbidity from coronary heart disease in patients with hypercholesterolemia. Report of the Program on the Surgical Control of the Hyperlipidemias (POSCH). N Engl J Med 1990;323:946-955.
182. Brown G, Albers JJ, Fisher LD, et al. Regression of coronary artery disease as a result of intensive lipid-lowering therapy in men with high levels of apolipoprotein B. N Engl J Med 1990;323: 1289-1298.
183. Kane JP, Malloy MJ, Ports TA, et al. Regression of coronary atherosclerosis during treatment of familial hypercholesterolemia with combined drug regimens. JAMA 1990;264:3007-3012.
184. Gagné C, Gaudet D, Bruckert E. Efficacy and safety of ezetimibe coadministered with atorvastatin or simvastatin in patients with homozygous familial hypercholesterolemia. Circulation 2002;105: 2469-2475.
185. Ziajka P. Role of low-density lipoprotein apheresis. Am J Cardiol 2005;96:67E-69E.
186. Bosch T. Practical aspects of direct adsorption of lipoproteins from whole blood by DALI LDL-apheresis. Transfus Apheresis Sci 2004;31:83-88.
187. Bilheimer DW, Goldstein JL, Grundy SM, et al. Liver transplantation to provide low-density-lipoprotein receptors and lower plasma cholesterol in a child with homozygous familial hypercholesterolemia. N Engl J Med 1984;311:1658-1664.
188. Forman MB, Baker SG, Mieny CJ, et al. Treatment of homozygous familial hypercholesterolaemia with portacaval shunt. Atherosclerosis 1982;41:349-361.
189. McNamara DJ, Ahrens EH Jr, Kolb R, et al. Treatment of familial hypercholesterolemia by portacaval anastomosis. Effect on cholesterol metabolism and pool sizes. Proc Natl Acad Sci U S A 1983;80:564-568.
190. Wade-Martins R, Saeki Y, Chiocca EA. Infectious delivery of a 135-kb *LDLR* genomic locus leads to regulated complementation of low-density lipoprotein receptor deficiency in human cells. Mol Ther 2003;7:604-612.
191. Tybjærg-Hansen A, Gallagher J, Vincent J, et al. Familial defective apolipoprotein B-100. Detection in the United Kingdom and

Scandinavia, and clinical characteristics of ten cases. Atherosclerosis 1990;80:235-242.
192. Ludwig EH, McCarthy BJ. Haplotype analysis of the human apolipoprotein B mutation associated with familial defective apolipoprotein B100. Am J Hum Genet 1990;47:712-720.
193. Bersot TP, Russell SJ, Thatcher SR, et al. A unique haplotype of the apolipoprotein B-100 allele associated with familial defective apolipoprotein B-100 in a Chinese man discovered during a study of the prevalence of this disorder. J Lipid Res 1993;34:1149-1154.
194. Miserez AR, Keller U. Differences in the phenotypic characteristics of subjects with familial defective apolipoprotein B-100 and familial hypercholesterolemia. Arterioscler Thromb Vasc Biol 1995; 15:1719-1729.
195. Innerarity TL, Weisgraber KH, Arnold KS, et al. Familial defective apolipoprotein B-100. Low density lipoproteins with abnormal receptor binding. Proc Natl Acad Sci U S A 1987;84:6919-6923.
196. Soria LF, Ludwig EH, Clarke HRG, et al. Association between a specific apolipoprotein B mutation and familial defective apolipoprotein B-100. Proc Natl Acad Sci U S A 1989;86:587-591.
197. Rauh G, Schuster H, Schewe CK, et al. Independent mutation of arginine(3500) $\rightarrow$ glutamine associated with familial defective apolipoprotein B-100. J Lipid Res 1993;34:799-805.
198. Lund-Katz S, Innerarity TL, Arnold KS, et al. ^{13}C NMR evidence that substitution of glutamine for arginine 3500 in familial defective apolipoprotein B-100 disrupts the conformation of the receptor-binding domain. J Biol Chem 1991;266:2701-2704.
199. Arnold KS, Balestra ME, Krauss RM, et al. Isolation of allele-specific, receptor-binding-defective low density lipoproteins from familial defective apolipoprotein B-100 subjects. J Lipid Res 1994;35:1469-1476.
200. Gaffney D, Reid JM, Cameron IM, et al. Independent mutations at codon 3500 of the apolipoprotein B gene are associated with hyperlipidemia. Arterioscler Thromb Vasc Biol 1995;15: 1025-1029.
201. Pullinger CR, Hennessy LK, Chatterton JE, et al. Familial ligand-defective apolipoprotein B. Identification of a new mutation that decreases LDL receptor binding affinity. J Clin Invest 1995;95: 1225-1234.
202. Schmidt EB, Illingworth DR, Bacon S, et al. Hypolipidemic effects of nicotinic acid in patients with familial defective apolipoprotein B-100. Metabolism 1993;42:137-139.
203. Schmidt EB, Illingworth DR, Bacon S, et al. Hypocholesterolemic effects of cholestyramine and colestipol in patients with familial defective apolipoprotein B-100. Atherosclerosis 1993;98:213-217.
204. Gallagher JJ, Myant NB. The affinity of low-density lipoproteins and of very-low-density lipoprotein remnants for the low-density lipoprotein receptor in homozygous familial defective apolipoprotein B-100. Atherosclerosis 1995;115:263-272.
205. Cohen JC, Kimmel M, Polanski A, Hobbs HH. Molecular mechanisms of autosomal recessive hypercholesterolemia. Curr Opin Lipidol 2003;14:121-127.
206. Garuti R, Jones C, Li W-P, et al. The modular adaptor protein autosomal recessive hypercholesterolemia (ARH) promotes low density lipoprotein receptor clustering into clathrin-coated pits. J Biol Chem 2005;280:40996-41004.
207. Lind S, Olsson AG, Eriksson M, et al. Autosomal recessive hypercholesterolaemia. Normalization of plasma LDL cholesterol by ezetimibe in combination with statin treatment. J Intern Med 2004;256:406-412.
208. Pullinger CR, Eng C, Salen G, et al. Human cholesterol 7α-hydroxylase (CYP7A1) deficiency has a hypercholesterolemic phenotype. J Clin Invest 2002;110:109-117.
209. Maxwell KN, Breslow JL. Proprotein convertase subtilisin kexin 9. The third locus implicated in autosomal dominant hypercholesterolemia. Curr Opin Lipidol 2005;16:167-172.
210. Cohen J, Pertsemlidis A, Kotowski IK, et al. Low LDL cholesterol in individuals of African descent resulting from frequent nonsense mutations in *PCSK9*. Nat Genet 2005;37:161-165.
211. Rose HG, Kranz P, Weinstock M, et al. Inheritance of combined hyperlipoproteinemia. Evidence for a new lipoprotein phenotype. Am J Med 1973;54:148-160.
212. Nikkilä EA, Aro A. Family study of serum lipids and lipoproteins in coronary heart-disease. Lancet 19731:954-959.
213. Sniderman A, Shapiro S, Marpole D, et al. Association of coronary atherosclerosis with hyper*apo*betalipoproteinemia (increased protein but normal cholesterol levels in human plasma low density (b) lipoproteins). Proc Natl Acad Sci U S A 1980;77:604-608.
214. Sniderman AD. Applying apoB to the diagnosis and therapy of the atherogenic dyslipoproteinemias. A clinical diagnostic algorithm. Curr Opin Lipidol 2004;15:433-438.
215. Reaven GM. Compensatory hyperinsulinemia and the development of an atherogenic lipoprotein profile. The price paid to maintain glucose homeostasis in insulin-resistant individuals. Endocrinol Metab Clin North Am 2005;34:49-62.
216. Grundy SM, Cleeman JI, Daniels SR, et al. Diagnosis and management of the metabolic syndrome. An American Heart Association/National Heart, Lung, and Blood Institute scientific statement. Circulation 2005;112:2735-2752.
217. Genest JJ Jr, Martin-Munley SS, McNamara JR, et al. Familial lipoprotein disorders in patients with premature coronary artery disease. Circulation 1992;85:2025-2033.
218. Cortner JA, Coates PM, Gallagher PR. Prevalence and expression of familial combined hyperlipidemia in childhood. J Pediatr 1990;116:514-519.
219. Hopkins PN, Heiss G, Ellison RC, et al. Coronary artery disease risk in familial combined hyperlipidemia and familial hypertriglyceridemia. A case-control comparison from the National Heart, Lung, and Blood Institute Family Heart Study. Circulation 2003;108: 519-523.
220. Shoulders CC, Naoumova RP. USF1 implicated in the aetiology of familial combined hyperlipidaemia and the metabolic syndrome. Trends Mol Med 2004;10:362-365.
221. Nishina PM, Johnson JP, Naggert JK, Krauss RM. Linkage of atherogenic lipoprotein phenotype to the low density lipoprotein receptor locus on the short arm of chromosome 19. Proc Natl Acad Sci U S A 1992;89:708-712.
222. Rotter JI, Bu X, Cantor R, et al. Multilocus genetic determination of LDL particle size in coronary artery disease families [abstract]. Clin Res 1994;42:16A.
223. Pajukanta P, Terwilliger JD, Perola M, et al. Genomewide scan for familial combined hyperlipidemia genes in Finnish families, suggesting multiple susceptibility loci influencing triglyceride, cholesterol, and apolipoprotein B levels. Am J Hum Genet 1999; 64:1453-1463.
224. Aouizerat BE, Allayee H, Bodnar J, et al. Novel genes for familial combined hyperlipidemia. Curr Opin Lipidol 1999;10:113-122.
225. Babirak SP, Brown BG, Brunzell JD. Familial combined hyperlipidemia and abnormal lipoprotein lipase. Arterioscler Thromb 1992;12:1176-1183.
226. Reaven GM. Pathophysiology of insulin resistance in human disease. Physiol Rev 1995;75:473-486.
227. Chait A, Albers JJ, Brunzell JD. Very low density lipoprotein overproduction in genetic forms of hypertriglyceridaemia. Eur J Clin Invest 1980;10:17-22.
228. Janus ED, Nicoll AM, Turner PR, et al. Kinetic bases of the primary hyperlipidaemias. Studies of apolipoprotein B turnover in genetically defined subjects. Eur J Clin Invest 1980;10:161-172.
229. Brunzell JD, Albers JJ, Chait A, et al. Plasma lipoproteins in familial combined hyperlipidemia and monogenic familial hypertriglyceridemia. J Lipid Res 1983;24:147-155.
230. Demacker PNM, Veerkamp MJ, Bredie SJH, et al. Comparison of the measurement of lipids and lipoproteins versus assay of apolipoprotein B for estimation of coronary heart disease risk. A study in familial combined hyperlipidemia. Atherosclerosis 2000;153: 483-490.
231. Sniderman AD, Castro Cabezas M, Ribalta J, et al. A proposal to redefine familial combined hyperlipidaemia. Third workshop on FCHL held in Barcelona from 3 to 5 May 2001, during the Scientific Sessions of the European Society for Clinical Investigation. Eur J Clin Invest 2002;32:71-73.
232. Crouse III JR. Hypertriglyceridemia. A contraindication to the use of bile acid binding resins. Am J Med 1987;83:243-248.
233. Frick MH, Elo O, Haapa K, et al. Helsinki Heart Study. Primary-prevention trial with gemfibrozil in middle-aged men with dyslipidemia. Safety of treatment, changes in risk factors, and incidence of coronary heart disease. N Engl J Med 1987;317:1237-1245.
234. Rubins HB, Robins SJ, Collins D, et al. Gemfibrozil for the secondary prevention of coronary heart disease in men with low levels of high-density lipoprotein cholesterol. N Engl J Med 1999;341: 410-418.

235. Ford ES. Prevalence of the metabolic syndrome defined by the International Diabetes Federation among adults in the U.S. Diabetes Care 2005;28:2745-2749.
236. Ford ES, Giles WH, Dietz WH. Prevalence of the metabolic syndrome among US adults. Findings from the Third National Health and Nutrition Examination Survey. JAMA 2002;287:356-359.
237. Ford ES. Risks for all-cause mortality, cardiovascular disease, and diabetes associated with the metabolic syndrome. A summary of the evidence. Diabetes Care 2005;28:1769-1778.
238. Special Feature. Metabolic syndrome. Nat Med 2006;12:26-61.
239. Reaven G. The metabolic syndrome or the insulin resistance syndrome? Different names, different concepts, and different goals. Endocrinol Metab Clin North Am 2004;33:283-303.
240. Cheal KL, Abbasi F, Lamendola C, et al. Relationship to insulin resistance of the Adult Treatment Panel III diagnostic criteria for identification of the metabolic syndrome. Diabetes 2004;53: 1195-1200.
241. McLaughlin T, Reaven G, Abbasi F, et al. Is there a simple way to identify insulin-resistant individuals at increased risk of cardiovascular disease? Am J Cardiol 2005;96:399-404.
242. Yang Q, Graham TE, Mody N, et al. Serum retinol binding protein 4 contributes to insulin resistance in obesity and type 2 diabetes. Nature 2005;436:356-362.
243. Ruan H, Lodish HF. Regulation of insulin sensitivity by adipose tissue–derived hormones and inflammatory cytokines. Curr Opin Lipidol 2004;15:297-302.
244. de Ferranti SD, Gauvreau K, Ludwig DS, et al. Prevalence of the metabolic syndrome in American adolescents. Findings from the Third National Health and Nutrition Examination Survey. Circulation 2004;110:2494-2497.
245. National High Blood Pressure Education Program Working Group on Hypertension Control in Children and Adolescents. Update on the 1987 Task Force Report on High Blood Pressure in Children and Adolescents. A working group report from the National High Blood Pressure Education Program. Pediatrics 1996;98:649-658.
246. Zhu S, Wang Z, Heshka S, et al. Waist circumference and obesity-associated risk factors among whites in the third National Health and Nutrition Examination Survey. Clinical action thresholds. Am J Clin Nutr 2002;76:743-749.
247. Hixson JE, Vernier DT. Restriction isotyping of human apolipoprotein E by gene amplification and cleavage with *HhaI*. J Lipid Res 1990;31:545-548.
248. Hazzard WR, Bierman EL. Aggravation of broad-b disease (type 3 hyperlipoproteinemia) by hypothyroidism. Arch Intern Med 1972;130:822-828.
249. Kushwaha RS, Hazzard WR, Gagne C, et al. Type III hyperlipoproteinemia. Paradoxical hypolipidemic response to estrogen. Ann Intern Med 1977;87:517-525.
250. Grodstein F, Clarkson TB, Manson JE. Understanding the divergent data on postmenopausal hormone therapy. N Engl J Med 2003;348:645-650.
251. Hoogwerf BJ, Bantle JP, Kuba K, et al. Treatment of type III hyperlipoproteinemia with four different treatment regimens. Atherosclerosis 1984;51:251-259.
252. Schaefer EJ, (discussant). Type III hyperlipoproteinemia. Diagnosis, molecular defects, pathology, and treatment. Dietary and drug treatment. Ann Intern Med 1983;98:633-640.
253. Feussner G, Eichinger M, Ziegler R. The influence of simvastatin alone or in combination with gemfibrozil on plasma lipids and lipoproteins in patients with type III hyperlipoproteinemia. Clin Investig 1992;70:1027-1035.
254. Feussner G, Kurth B, Lohrmann J. Comparative effects of bezafibrate and micronised fenofibrate in patients with type III hyperlipoproteinemia. Eur J Med Res 1997;2:165-168,.
255. Illingworth DR, O'Malley JP. The hypolipidemic effects of lovastatin and clofibrate alone and in combination in patients with type III hyperlipoproteinemia. Metabolism 1990;39:403-409.
256. Chait A, Brunzell JD. Chylomicronemia syndrome. Adv Intern Med 1991;37:249-273.
257. Santamarina-Fojo S. The familial chylomicronemia syndrome. Endocrinol Metab Clin North Am 1998;27:551-567.
258. Chait A, Robertson HT, Brunzell JD. Chylomicronemia syndrome in diabetes mellitus. Diabetes Care 1981;4:343-348.
259. Heilman KM, Fisher WR. Hyperlipidemic dementia. Arch Neurol 1974;31:67-68.
260. Mathew NT, Meyer JS, Achari AN, Dodson RF. Hyperlipidemic neuropathy and dementia. Eur Neurol 1976;14:370-382.
261. Babirak SP, Iverius P-H, Fujimoto WY, Brunzell JD. Detection and characterization of the heterozygote state for lipoprotein lipase deficiency. Arteriosclerosis 1989;9:326-334.
262. Hayden MR, Ma Y, Brunzell J, Henderson HE. Genetic variants affecting human lipoprotein and hepatic lipases. Curr Opin Lipidol 1991;2:104-109.
263. Gagné C, Brun L-D, Julien P, et al. Primary lipoprotein-lipase-activity deficiency. Clinical investigation of a French Canadian population. Can Med Assoc J 1989;140:405-411.
264. Illingworth DR, Connor WE, Miller RG. Abetalipoproteinemia. Report of two cases and review of therapy. Arch Neurol 1980; 37:659-662.
265. Partin JS, Partin JC, Schubert WK, McAdams AJ. Liver ultrastructure in abetalipoproteinemia. Evolution of micronodular cirrhosis. Gastroenterology 1974;67:107-118.
266. Wierzbicki AS, Reynolds TM, Crook MA. Usefulness of orlistat in the treatment of severe hypertriglyceridemia. Am J Cardiol 2002;89:229-231.
267. Schaefer EJ. Familial lipoprotein disorders and premature coronary artery disease. Med Clin North Am 1994;78:21-39.
268. Brunzell JD, Schrott HG, Motulsky AG, Bierman EL. Myocardial infarction in the familial forms of hypertriglyceridemia. Metabolism 1976;25:313-320.
269. Austin MA, McKnight B, Edwards KL, et al. Cardiovascular disease mortality in familial forms of hypertriglyceridemia. A 20-year prospective study. Circulation 2000;101:2777-2782.
270. Schaefer EJ, Zech LA, Jenkins LL, et al. Human apolipoprotein A-I and A-II metabolism. J Lipid Res 1982;23:850-862.
271. Brinton EA, Eisenberg S, Breslow JL. Increased apo A-I and apo A-II fractional catabolic rate in patients with low high density lipoprotein-cholesterol levels with or without hypertriglyceridemia. J Clin Invest 1991;87:536–544.
272. Angelin B, Hershon KS, Brunzell JD. Bile acid metabolism in hereditary forms of hypertriglyceridemia. Evidence for an increased synthesis rate in monogenic familial hypertriglyceridemia. Proc Natl Acad Sci U S A 1987;84:5434-5438.
273. Duane WC, Hartich LA, Bartman AE, Ho SB. Diminished gene expression of ileal apical sodium bile acid transporter explains impaired absorption of bile acid in patients with hypertriglyceridemia. J Lipid Res 2000;41:1384-1389.
274. Love MW, Craddock AL, Angelin B, et al. Analysis of the ileal bile acid transporter gene, *SLC10A2,* in subjects with familial hypertriglyceridemia. Arterioscler Thromb Vasc Biol 2001;21:2039-2045.
275. Austin MA, Edwards KL, Monks SA, et al. Genome-wide scan for quantitative trait loci influencing LDL size and plasma triglyceride in familial hypertriglyceridemia. J Lipid Res 2003;44:2161-2168.
276. Scanu AM, Fless GM. Lipoprotein(a). Heterogeneity and biological relevance. J Clin Invest 1990;85:1709-1715.
277. Gaw A, Hobbs HH. Molecular genetics of lipoprotein(a). New pieces to the puzzle. Curr Opin Lipidol 1994;5:149-155.
278. McLean JW, Tomlinson JE, Kuang W-J, et al. cDNA sequence of human apolipoprotein(a) is homologous to plasminogen. Nature 1987;330:132-137.
279. Dahlen GH, Guyton JR, Attar M, et al. Association of levels of lipoprotein Lp(a), plasma lipids, and other lipoproteins with coronary artery disease documented by angiography. Circulation 1986; 74:758-765.
280. Sandkamp M, Funke H, Schulte H, et al. Lipoprotein(a) is an independent risk factor for myocardial infarction at a young age. Clin Chem 1990;36:20-23.
281. Genest J Jr, Jenner JL, McNamara JR, et al. Prevalence of lipoprotein(a) [Lp(a)] excess in coronary artery disease. Am J Cardiol 1991;67:1039-1045.
282. Gurewich V, Mittleman M. Lipoprotein(a) in coronary heart disease. Is it a risk factor after all? JAMA 1994;271:1025-1026.
283. Ridker PM, Hennekens CH, Stampfer MJ. A prospective study of lipoprotein(a) and the risk of myocardial infarction. JAMA 1993;270:2195-2199.
284. Jauhiainen M, Koskinen P, Ehnholm C, et al. Lipoprotein(a) and coronary heart disease risk. A nested case-control study of the Helsinki Heart Study participants. Atherosclerosis 1991;89:59-67.
285. Schaefer EJ, Lamon-Fava S, Jenner JL, et al. Lipoprotein(a) levels and risk of coronary heart disease in men. The Lipid Research

Clinics Coronary Primary Prevention Trial. JAMA 1994;271: 999-1003.
286. Rosengren A, Wilhelmsen L, Eriksson E, et al. Lipoprotein(a) and coronary heart disease. A prospective case-control study in a general population sample of middle aged men. Br Med J 1990;301:1248-1251.
287. Boerwinkle E, Leffert CC, Lin J, et al. Apolipoprotein(a) gene accounts for greater than 90% of the variation in plasma lipoprotein(a) concentrations. J Clin Invest 1992;90:52-60.
288. Lamon-Fava S, Jimenez D, Christian JC, et al. The NHLBI Twin Study. Heritability of apolipoprotein A-I, B, and low density lipoprotein subclasses and concordance for lipoprotein(a). Atherosclerosis 1991;91:97-106.
289. Sandholzer C, Hallman DM, Saha N, et al. Effects of the apolipoprotein(a) size polymorphism on the lipoprotein(a) concentration in 7 ethnic groups. Hum Genet 1991;86:607-614.
290. Utermann G. The mysteries of lipoprotein(a). Science 1989;246: 904-910.
291. Sandholzer C, Saha N, Kark JD, et al. Apo(a) isoforms predict risk for coronary heart disease. A study in six populations. Arterioscler Thromb 1992;12:1214-1226.
292. Maher VMG, Brown BG, Marcovina SM, et al. Effects of lowering elevated LDL cholesterol on the cardiovascular risk of lipoprotein(a). JAMA 1995;274:1771-1774.
293. von Eckardstein A, Schulte H, Cullen P, Assmann G. Lipoprotein(a) further increases the risk of coronary events in men with high global cardiovascular risk. J Am Coll Cardiol 2001;37:434-439.
294. McCormick SPA, Ng JK, Taylor S, et al. Mutagenesis of the human apolipoprotein B gene in a yeast artificial chromosome reveals the site of attachment for apolipoprotein(a). Proc Natl Acad Sci U S A 1995;92:10147-10151.
295. Gavish D, Azrolan N, Breslow JL. Plasma Lp(a) concentration is inversely correlated with the ratio of Kringle IV/Kringle V encoding domains in the apo(a) gene. J Clin Invest 1989;84:2021-2027.
296. Kronenberg F, Lhotta K, König P, et al. Apolipoprotein(a) isoform-specific changes of lipoprotein(a) after kidney transplantation. Eur J Hum Genet 2003;11:693-699.
297. Holmer SR, Hengstenberg C, Kraft H-G, et al. Association of polymorphisms of the apolipoprotein(a) gene with lipoprotein(a) levels and myocardial infarction. Circulation 2003;107:696-701.
298. Buechler C, Ullrich H, Ritter M, et al. Lipoprotein (a) up-regulates the expression of the plasminogen activator inhibitor 2 in human blood monocytes. Blood 2001;97:981-986.
299. Hajjar KA, Gavish D, Breslow JL, Nachman RL. Lipoprotein(a) modulation of endothelial cell surface fibrinolysis and its potential role in atherosclerosis. Nature 1989;339:303-305.
300. Miles LA, Fless GM, Levin EG, et al. A potential basis for the thrombotic risks associated with lipoprotein(a). Nature 1989;339: 301-303.
301. Grainger DJ, Kirschenlohr HL, Metcalfe JC, et al. Proliferation of human smooth muscle cells promoted by lipoprotein(a). Science 1993;260:1655-1658.
302. Marcovina SM, Koschinsky ML, Albers JJ, Skarlatos S. Report of the National Heart, Lung, and Blood Institute workshop on lipoprotein(a) and cardiovascular disease. Recent advances and future directions. Clin Chem 2003;49:1785-1796.
303. Dati F, Tate JR, Marcovina SM, Steinmetz A. First WHO/IFCC International Reference Reagent for Lipoprotein(a) for Immunoassay—Lp(a) SRM 2B. Clin Chem Lab Med 2004;42:670-676.
304. Min W-K, Lee JO, Huh JW. Relation between lipoprotein(a) concentrations in patients with acute-phase response and risk analysis for coronary heart disease. Clin Chem 1997;43:1891-1895.
305. Carlson LA, Hamsten A, Asplund A. Pronounced lowering of serum levels of lipoprotein Lp(a) in hyperlipidaemic subjects treated with nicotinic acid. J Intern Med 1989;226:271-276.
306. Espeland MA, Marcovina SM, Miller V, et al. Effect of postmenopausal hormone therapy on lipoprotein(a) concentration. Circulation 1998;97:979-986.
307. Shlipak MG, Simon JA, Vittinghoff E, et al. Estrogen and progestin, lipoprotein(a), and the risk of recurrent coronary heart disease events after menopause. JAMA 2000;283:1845-1852.
308. Cohen JC, Wang Z, Grundy SM, et al. Variation at the hepatic lipase and apolipoprotein AI/CIII/AIV loci is a major cause of genetically determined variation in plasma HDL cholesterol levels. J Clin Invest 1994;94:2377-2384.
309. Ansell BJ, Watson KE, Fogelman AM, et al. High-density lipoprotein function. Recent advances. J Am Coll Cardiol 2005;46: 1792-1798.
310. Bersot TP, Pépin GM, Mahley RW. Risk determination of dyslipidemia in populations characterized by low levels of high-density lipoprotein cholesterol. Am Heart J 2003;146:1052-1060.
311. Ashen MD, Blumenthal RS. Low HDL cholesterol levels. N Engl J Med 2005;353:1252-1260.
312. Williams PT. The relationships of vigorous exercise, alcohol, and adiposity to low and high high-density lipoprotein-cholesterol levels. Metabolism 2004;53:700-709.
313. Dhawan J. Coronary heart disease risks in Asian Indians. Curr Opin Lipidol 1996;7:196-198.
314. Tai E-S, Emmanuel SC, Chew S-K, et al. Isolated low HDL cholesterol. An insulin-resistant state only in the presence of fasting hypertriglyceridemia. Diabetes 1999;48:1088-1092.
315. Mahley RW, Palaoglu KE, Atak Z, et al. Turkish Heart Study. Lipids, lipoproteins, and apolipoproteins. J Lipid Res 1995;36: 839-859.
316. Bersot TP, Vega GL, Grundy SM, et al. Elevated hepatic lipase activity and low levels of high density lipoprotein in a normotriglyceridemic, nonobese Turkish population. J Lipid Res 1999;40: 432-438.
317. Sorci-Thomas MG, Thomas MJ. The effects of altered apolipoprotein A-I structure on plasma HDL concentration. Trends Cardiovasc Med 2002;12:121-128.
318. von Eckardstein A. Differential diagnosis of familial high density lipoprotein deficiency syndromes. Atherosclerosis (in press).
319. Franceschini G, Sirtori CR, Capurso A, et al. A-I_{Milano} apoprotein. Decreased high density lipoprotein cholesterol levels with significant lipoprotein modifications and without clinical atherosclerosis in an Italian family. J Clin Invest 1980;66:892-900.
320. Nissen SE, Tsunoda T, Tuzcu EM, et al. Effect of recombinant apoA-I Milano on coronary atheroclerosis in patients with acute coronary syndromes. A randomized controlled trial. JAMA 2003;290: 2292-2300.
321. Boekholdt SM, Kuivenhoven J-A, Hovingh GK, et al. CETP gene variation. Relation to lipid parameters and cardiovascular risk. Curr Opin Lipidol 2004;15:393-398.
322. de Grooth GJ, Klerkx AH, Stroes ES, et al. A review of CETP and its relation to atherosclerosis. J Lipid Res 2004;45:1967-1974.
323. Santamarina-Fojo S, Hoeg JM, Assmann G, Brewer HB Jr. Lecithin cholesterol acyltransferase deficiency and fish eye disease. In Scriver CR, Beaudet AL, Sly WS (eds). The Metabolic and Molecular Bases of Inherited Disease, 8th ed, vol 2. New York: McGraw-Hill, 2001:2817-2833.
324. Kuivenhoven JA, Pritchard H, Hill J, et al. The molecular pathology of lecithin:cholesterol acyltransferase (LCAT) deficiency syndromes. J Lipid Res 1997;38:191-205.
325. Glomset JA. The plasma lecithin:cholesterol acyltransferase reaction. J Lipid Res 1968;9:155-167.
326. Ayyobi AF, McGladdery SH, Chan S, et al. Lecithin:cholesterol acyltransferase (LCAT) deficiency and risk of vascular disease. 25 year follow-up. Atherosclerosis 2004;177:361-366.
327. Carlson LA, Philipson B. Fish-eye disease. A new familial condition with massive corneal opacities and dyslipoproteinæmia. Lancet 1979;2:921-924.
328. Carlson LA, Holmquist L. Evidence for the presence in human plasma of lecithin:cholesterol acyltransferase activity (b-LCAT) specifically esterifying free cholesterol of combined pre-b- and b-lipoproteins. Studies of fish eye disease patients and control subjects. Acta Med Scand 1985;218:197-205.
329. Assmann G, von Eckardstein A, Brewer HB, Jr. Familial analphalipoproteinemia. Tangier disease. In Scriver CR, Beaudet AL, Sly WS (eds). The Metabolic and Molecular Bases of Inherited Disease, 8th ed, vol 2. New York. McGraw-Hill, 2001:2937-2960.
330. Serfaty-Lacrosniere C, Civeira F, Lanzberg A, et al. Homozygous Tangier disease and cardiovascular disease. Atherosclerosis 1994;107:85-98.
331. Bojanovski D, Gregg RE, Zech LA, et al. In vivo metabolism of proapolipoprotein A-I in Tangier disease. J Clin Invest 1987;80: 1742-1747.
332. Bodzioch M, Orsó E, Klucken J, et al. The gene encoding ATP-binding cassette transporter 1 is mutated in Tangier disease. Nat Genet 1999;22:347-351.

333. Brooks-Wilson A, Marcil M, Clee SM, et al. Mutations in *ABC1* in Tangier disease and familial high-density lipoprotein deficiency. Nat Genet 1999;22:336–345.
334. Rust S, Rosier M, Funke H, et al. Tangier disease is caused by mutations in the gene encoding ATP-binding cassette transporter 1. Nat Genet 1999;22:352-355.
335. Frikke-Schmidt R, Nordestgaard BG, Jensen GB, Tybjærg-Hansen A. Genetic variation in ABC transporter A1 contributes to HDL cholesterol in the general population. J Clin Invest 2004;114: 1343-1353.
336. Cohen JC, Kiss RS, Pertsemlidis A, et al. Multiple rare alleles contribute to low plasma levels of HDL cholesterol. Science 2004; 305:869-872.
337. Wu J, Kim J, Li Q, et al. Known mutations of apoB account for only a small minority of hypobetalipoproteinemia. J Lipid Res 1999;40:955-959.
338. Linton MF, Farese RV Jr, Young SG. Familial hypobetalipoproteinemia. J Lipid Res 1993;34:521-541.
339. Levy E, Roy CC, Thibault L, et al. Variable expression of familial heterozygous hypobetalipoproteinemia. Transient malabsorption during infancy. J Lipid Res 1994;35:2170-2177.
340. Illingworth DR, Kenny TA, Orwoll ES. Adrenal function in heterozygous and homozygous hypobetalipoproteinemia. J Clin Endocrinol Metab 1982;54:27-33.
341. Aguilar-Salinas CA, Barrett PHR, Parhofer KG, et al. Apoprotein B-100 production is decreased in subjects heterozygous for truncations of apoprotein B. Arterioscler Thromb Vasc Biol 1995;15: 71-80.
342. Parhofer KG, Daugherty A, Kinoshita M, Schonfeld G. Enhanced clearance from plasma of low density lipoproteins containing a truncated apolipoprotein, apoB-89. J Lipid Res 1990;31: 2001-2007.
343. Vega GL, von Bergmann K, Grundy SM, et al. Increased catabolism of VLDL-apolipoprotein B and synthesis of bile acids in a case of hypobetalipoproteinemia. Metabolism 1987;36:262-269.
344. Cohen JC, Pertsemlidis A, Fahmi S, et al. Multiple rare variants in *NPC1L1* associated with reduced sterol absorption and plasma low-density lipoprotein levels. Proc Natl Acad Sci U S A 2006; 103:1810-1815.
345. Young SG, Cham CM, Pitas RE, et al. A genetic model for absent chylomicron formation. Mice producing apolipoprotein B in the liver, but not in the intestine. J Clin Invest 1995;96: 2932-2946.
346. Runge P, Muller DPR, McAllister J, et al. Oral vitamin E supplements can prevent the retinopathy of abetalipoproteinaemia. Br J Ophthalmol 1986;70:166-173.
347. Jones B, Jones EL, Bonney SA, et al. Mutations in a Sar1 GTPase of COPII vesicles are associated with lipid absorption disorders. Nat Genet 2003;34:29-31.
348. Breckenridge WC, Little JA, Alaupovic P, et al. Lipoprotein abnormalities associated with a familial deficiency of hepatic lipase. Atherosclerosis 1982;45:161-179.
349. Ruel IL, Couture P, Gagné C, et al. Characterization of a novel mutation causing hepatic lipase deficiency among French Canadians. J Lipid Res 2003;44:1508-1514.
350. Ruel IL, Lamarche B, Mauger J-F, et al. Effect of fenofibrate on plasma lipoprotein composition and kinetics in patients with complete hepatic lipase deficiency. Arterioscler Thromb Vasc Biol 2005;25:2600-2607.
351. Björkhem I, Boberg KM, Leitersdorf E. Inborn errors in bile acid biosynthesis and storage of sterols other than cholesterol. In Scriver CR, Beaudet AL, Sly WS (eds). The Metabolic and Molecular Bases of Inherited Disease, 8th ed, vol 2. New York. McGraw-Hill, 2001:2961-2988.
352. Salen G, Shefer S, Nguyen L, et al. Sitosterolemia. J Lipid Res 1992;33:945-955.
353. Berge KE, Tian H, Graf GA, et al. Accumulation of dietary cholesterol in sitosterolemia caused by mutations in adjacent ABC transporters. Science 2000;290:1771-1775.
354. Lee M-H, Lu K, Hazard S, et al. Identification of a gene, *ABCG5,* important in the regulation of dietary cholesterol absorption. Nat Genet 2001;27:79-83.
355. Salen G, von Bergmann K, Lütjohann D, et al. Ezetimibe effectively reduces plasma plant sterols in patients with sitosterolemia. Circulation 2004;109:966-971.
356. Moghadasian MH. Cerebrotendinous xanthomatosis. Clinical course, genotypes and metabolic backgrounds. Clin Invest Med 2004;27:42-50.
357. Berginer VM, Shany S, Alkalay D, et al. Osteoporosis and increased bone fractures in cerebrotendinous xanthomatosis. Metabolism 1993;42:69-74.
358. Nakamura T, Matsuzawa Y, Takemura K, et al. Combined treatment with chenodeoxycholic acid and pravastatin improves plasma cholestanol levels associated with marked regression of tendon xanthomas in cerebrotendinous xanthomatosis. Metabolism 1991;40:741-746.
359. Peynet J, Laurent A, De Liege P, et al. Cerebrotendinous xanthomatosis. Treatments with simvastatin, lovastatin, and chenodeoxycholic acid in 3 siblings. Neurology 1991;41:434-436.
360. Klima H, Ullrich K, Aslanidis C, et al. A splice junction mutation causes deletion of a 72-base exon from the mRNA for lysosomal acid lipase in a patient with cholesteryl ester storage disease. J Clin Invest 1993;92:2713-2718.
361. Schmitz G, Assmann G. Acid lipase deficiency. Wolman disease and cholesteryl ester storage disease. In Scriver CR, Beaudet AL, Sly WS, Valle D (eds). The Metabolic Basis of Inherited Disease, 6th ed, vol 2. New York. McGraw-Hill, 1989:1623-1644.
362. Anderson RA, Byrum RS, Coates PM, Sando GN. Mutations at the lysosomal acid cholesteryl ester hydrolase gene locus in Wolman disease. Proc Natl Acad Sci U S A 1994;91:2718-2722.
363. Sokol RJ, Kayden HJ, Bettis DB, et al. Isolated vitamin E deficiency in the absence of fat malabsorption—familial and sporadic cases. Characterization and investigation of causes. J Lab Clin Med 1988;111:548-559.
364. Kayden HJ. The neurologic syndrome of vitamin E deficiency. A significant cause of ataxia. Neurology 1993;43:2167-2169.
365. Cavalier L, Ouahchi K, Kayden HJ, et al. Ataxia with isolated vitamin E deficiency. Heterogeneity of mutations and phenotypic variability in a large number of families. Am J Hum Genet 1998;62:301-310.
366. Stone NJ. Secondary causes of hyperlipidemia. Med Clin North Am 1994;78:117-141.
367. Bierman EL. Insulin and hypertriglyceridemia. Isr J Med Sci 1972;8:303-308.
368. Reaven GM, Greenfield MS. Diabetic hypertriglyceridemia. Evidence for three clinical syndromes. Diabetes 1981;30(suppl 2):66-75.
369. Tomkin GH, Owens D. Insulin and lipoprotein metabolism with special reference to the diabetic state. Diabetes Metab Rev 1994;10:225-252.
370. Bagdade JD, Porte D Jr, Bierman EL. Acute insulin withdrawal and the regulation of plasma triglyceride removal in diabetic subjects. Diabetes 1968;17:127-132.
371. Chait A, Bierman EL, Albers JJ. Low-density lipoprotein receptor activity in cultured human skin fibroblasts. Mechanism of insulin-induced stimulation. J Clin Invest 1979;64:1309-1319.
372. Bagdade JD, Porte D Jr, Bierman EL. Diabetic lipemia. A form of acquired fat-induced lipemia. N Engl J Med 1967;276:427-433.
373. Brunzell JD, Hazzard WR, Motulsky AG, Bierman EL. Evidence for diabetes mellitus and genetic forms of hypertriglyceridemia as independent entities. Metabolism 1975;24:1115-1121.
374. Bowie A, Owens D, Collins P, et al. Glycosylated low density lipoprotein is more sensitive to oxidation. Implications for the diabetic patient? Atherosclerosis 1993;102:63-67.
375. Edwards IJ, Terry JG, Bell-Farrow AD, Cefalu WT. Improved glucose control decreases the interaction of plasma low-density lipoproteins with arterial proteoglycans. Metabolism 2002;51: 1223-1229.
376. Sparks JD, Sparks CE. Insulin modulation of hepatic synthesis and secretion of apolipoprotein B by rat hepatocytes. J Biol Chem 1990;265:8854-8862.
377. Eto M, Watanabe K, Sato T, Makino I. Apolipoprotein-E2 and hyperlipoproteinemia in noninsulin-dependent diabetes mellitus. J Clin Endocrinol Metab 1989;69:1207-1212.
378. Bogardus C, Lillioja S, Mott DM, et al. Relationship between degree of obesity and in vivo insulin action in man. Am J Physiol 1985;248: E286-E291.
379. DeFronzo RA, Goodman AM, the Multicenter Metformin Study Group. Efficacy of metformin in patients with non–insulin-dependent diabetes mellitus. N Engl J Med 1995;333:541-549.

380. Rosenstock J, Vega GL, Raskin P. Effect of intensive diabetes treatment on low-density lipoprotein apolipoprotein B kinetics in type I diabetes. Diabetes 1988;37:393-397.
381. Taskinen M-R, Kuusi T, Helve E, et al. Insulin therapy induces antiatherogenic changes of serum lipoproteins in noninsulin-dependent diabetes. Arteriosclerosis 1988;8:168-177.
382. Koppers LE, Palumbo PJ. Lipid disturbances in endocrine disorders. Med Clin North Am 1972;56:1013-1020.
383. Valdemarsson S, Hansson P, Hedner P, Nilsson-Ehle P. Relations between thyroid function, hepatic and lipoprotein lipase activities, and plasma lipoprotein concentrations. Acta Endocrinol 1983;104:50-56.
384. Hansson P, Valdemarsson S, Nilsson-Ehle P. Experimental hyperthyroidism in man. Effects on plasma lipoproteins, lipoprotein lipase and hepatic lipase. Horm Metab Res 1983;15:449-452.
385. Thompson GR, Soutar AK, Spengel FA, et al. Defects of receptor-mediated low density lipoprotein catabolism in homozygous familial hypercholesterolemia and hypothyroidism in vivo. Proc Natl Acad Sci U S A 1981;78:2591-2595.
386. Chait A, Bierman EL, Albers JJ. Regulatory role of triiodothyronine in the degradation of low density lipoprotein by cultured human skin fibroblasts. J Clin Endocrinol Metab 1979;48:887-889.
387. Vanhaelst L, Neve P, Chailly P, Bastenie PA. Coronary-artery disease in hypothyroidism. Observations in clinical myxœdema. Lancet 1967;2:800-802.
388. Steinberg AD. Myxedema and coronary artery disease—a comparative autopsy study. Ann Intern Med 1968;68:338-344.
389. Tanis BC, Westendorp RGJ, Smelt AHM. Effect of thyroid substitution on hypercholesterolaemia in patients with subclinical hypothyroidism. A reanalysis of intervention studies. Clin Endocrinol 1996;44:643-649.
390. Hulley S, Grady D, Bush T, et al. Randomized trial of estrogen plus progestin for secondary prevention of coronary heart disease in postmenopausal women. JAMA 1998;280:605-613.
391. Barrett-Connor E, Slone S, Greendale G, et al. The postmenopausal estrogen/progestin interventions study. Primary outcomes in adherent women. Maturitas 1997;27:261-274.
392. Glueck CJ, Lang J, Hamer T, Tracy T. Severe hypertriglyceridemia and pancreatitis when estrogen replacement therapy is given to hypertriglyceridemic women. J Lab Clin Med 1994;123:59-64.
393. Knopp RH, Walden CE, Wahl PW, et al. Oral contraceptive and postmenopausal estrogen effects on lipoprotein triglyceride and cholesterol in an adult female population. Relationships to estrogen and progestin potency. J Clin Endocrinol Metab 1981;53: 1123-1132.
394. Sanada M, Tsuda M, Kodama I, et al. Substitution of transdermal estradiol during oral estrogen-progestin therapy in postmenopausal women. Effects on hypertriglyceridemia. Menopause 2004;11:331-336.
395. Glueck CJ, Fallat RW, Scheel D. Effects of estrogenic compounds on triglyceride kinetics. Metabolism 1975;24:537-545.
396. Mosca L, Harper K, Sarkar S, et al. Effect of raloxifene on serum triglycerides in postmenopausal women. Influence of predisposing factors for hypertriglyceridemia. Clin Ther 2001;23:1552-1565.
397. Windler EET, Kovanen PT, Chao Y-S, et al. The estradiol-stimulated lipoprotein receptor of rat liver. A binding site that mediates the uptake of rat lipoproteins containing apoproteins B and E. J Biol Chem 1980;255:10464-10471.
398. Heiss G, Tamir I, Davis CE, et al. Lipoprotein-cholesterol distributions in selected North American populations. The Lipid Research Clinics Program Prevalence Study. Circulation 1980;61:302-315.
399. Herbst KL, Amory JK, Brunzell JD, et al. Testosterone administration to men increases hepatic lipase activity and decreases HDL and LDL size in 3 wk. Am J Physiol Endocrinol Metab 2003;284: E1112-E1118.
400. Bausserman LL, Saritelli AL, Herbert PN. Effects of short-term stanozolol administration on serum lipoproteins in hepatic lipase deficiency. Metabolism 1997;46:992-996.
401. Steinberg D, Pearson TA, Kuller LH. Alcohol and atherosclerosis. Ann Intern Med 1991;114:967-976.
402. Hill JA. In vino veritas. Alcohol and heart disease. Am J Med Sci 2005;329:124-135.
403. Joven J, Villabona C, Vilella E, et al. Abnormalities of lipoprotein metabolism in patients with the nephrotic syndrome. N Engl J Med 1990;323:579-584.
404. Saland JM, Ginsberg H, Fisher EA. Dyslipidemia in pediatric renal disease. Epidemiology, pathophysiology, and management. Curr Opin Pediatr 2002;14:197-204.
405. Warwick GL, Caslake MJ, Boulton-Jones JM, et al. Low-density lipoprotein metabolism in the nephrotic syndrome. Metabolism 1990;39:187-192.
406. Sani MU, Okeahialam BN, Aliyu SH, Enoch DA. Human immunodeficiency virus (HIV) related heart disease. A review. Wien Klin Wochenschr 2005;117:73-81.
407. Cahn PE, Gatell JM, Squires K, et al. Atazanaviræa once-daily HIV protease inhibitor that does not cause dyslipidemia in newly treated patients. Results from two randomized clinical trials. J Int Assoc Physicians AIDS Care 2004;3:92-98.
408. Dubé MP, Stein JH, Aberg JA, et al. Guidelines for the evaluation and management of dyslipidemia in human immunodeficiency virus (HIV)-infected adults receiving antiretroviral therapy. Recommendations of the HIV Medicine Association of the Infectious Disease Society of America and the Adult AIDS Clinical Trials Group. Clin Infect Dis 2003;37:613-627.
409. Bagdade JD, Porte D Jr, Bierman EL. Steroid-induced lipemia. A complication of high-dosage corticosteroid therapy. Arch Intern Med 1970;125:129-134.
410. Lardinois CK, Neuman SL. The effects of antihypertensive agents on serum lipids and lipoproteins. Arch Intern Med 1988;148: 1280-1288.
411. Pollare T, Lithell H, Berne C. A comparison of the effects of hydrochlorothiazide and captopril on glucose and lipid metabolism in patients with hypertension. N Engl J Med 1989;321:868-873.
412. Rohlfing JJ, Brunzell JD. The effects of diuretics and adrenergic-blocking agents on plasma lipids. West J Med 1986;145:210-218.
413. Haffner SM, Kushwaha RS, Foster DM, et al. Studies on the metabolic mechanism of reduced high density lipoproteins during anabolic steroid therapy. Metabolism 1983;32:413-420.
414. Webb OL, Laskarzewski PM, Glueck CJ. Severe depression of high-density lipoprotein cholesterol levels in weight lifters and body builders by self-administered exogenous testosterone and anabolic-androgenic steroids. Metabolism 1984;33:971-975.
415. Allen LA, O'Donnell CJ, Giugliano RP, et al. Care concordant with guidelines predicts decreased long-term mortality in patients with unstable angina pectoris and non–ST-elevation myocardial infarction. Am J Cardiol 2004;93:1218-1222.
416. Lloyd-Jones DM, Camargo CA, Allen LA, et al. Predictors of long-term mortality after hospitalization for primary unstable angina pectoris and non–ST-elevation myocardial infarction. Am J Cardiol 2003;92:1155-1159.
417. American Heart Association. Heart Disease and Stroke Statistics—2006 Update. Dallas. American Heart Association, 2006.
418. Cholesterol Treatment Trialists' Collaborators. Efficacy and safety of cholesterol-lowering treatment. Prospective meta-analysis of data from 90,056 participants in 14 randomised trials of statins. Lancet 2005;366:1267-1278.
419. Antman EM, Anbe DT, Armstrong PW, et al. ACC/AHA guidelines for the management of patients with ST-elevation myocardial infarction. A report of the American College of Cardiology/American Heart Association Task Force on Practice Guidelines (Committee to Revise the 1999 Guidelines for the Management of Patients With Acute Myocardial Infarction). Circulation 2004;110: e82-e293.
420. Law MR, Wald NJ, Rudnicka AR. Quantifying effect of statins on low density lipoprotein cholesterol, ischaemic heart disease, and stroke. Systematic review and meta-analysis. Br Med J 2003; 326:1423.
421. Wilson PWF, D'Agostino RB, Levy D, et al. Prediction of coronary heart disease using risk factor categories. Circulation 1998;97: 1837-1847.
422. Shepherd J, Cobbe SM, Ford I, et al. Prevention of coronary heart disease with pravastatin in men with hypercholesterolemia. N Engl J Med 1995;333:1301-1307.
423. Sacks FM, Pfeffer MA, Moye LA, et al. The effect of pravastatin on coronary events after myocardial infarction in patients with average cholesterol levels. N Engl J Med 1996;335:1001-1009.
424. Sever PS, Dahlöf B, Poulter NR, et al. Prevention of coronary and stroke events with atorvastatin in hypertensive patients who have average or lower-than-average cholesterol concentrations, in the Anglo-Scandinavian Cardiac Outcomes Trial-Lipid Lowering Arm

(ASCOT-LLA). A multicentre randomised controlled trial. Lancet 2003;361:1149-1158.

425. Pi-Sunyer FX, Becker DM, Bouchard C, et al. Clinical Guidelines on the Identification, Evaluation, and Treatment of Overweight and Obesity in Adults. The Evidence Report. Bethesda, MD. U.S. Department of Health and Human Services, Public Health Service, National Institutes of Health (NIH Publ. No. 98-4083), 1998:58-59.
426. Diekman T, Lansberg PJ, Kastelein JJP, Wiersinga WM. Prevalence and correction of hypothyroidism in a large cohort of patients referred for dyslipidemia. Arch Intern Med 1995;155:1490-1495.
427. Watson WC, Buchanan KD, Dickson C. Serum cholesterol levels after myocardial infarction. Br Med J 1963;2:709-712.
428. Warnick GR, Nauck M, Rifai N. Evolution of methods for measurement of HDL-cholesterol. From ultracentrifugation to homogeneous assays. Clin Chem 2001;47:1579-1596.
429. Friedewald WT, Levy RI, Fredrickson DS. Estimation of the concentration of low-density lipoprotein cholesterol in plasma, without use of the preparative ultracentrifuge. Clin Chem 1972;18: 499-502.
430. Castelli WP, Garrison RJ, Wilson PWF, et al. Incidence of coronary heart disease and lipoprotein cholesterol levels. The Framingham Study. JAMA 1986;256:2835-2838.
431. Castelli WP, Abbott RD, McNamara PM. Summary estimates of cholesterol used to predict coronary heart disease. Circulation 1983;67:730-734.
432. Stampfer MJ, Sacks FM, Salvini S, et al. A prospective study of cholesterol, apolipoproteins, and the risk of myocardial infarction. N Engl J Med 1991;325:373-381.
433. Stamler J, Daviglus ML, Garside DB, et al. Relationship of baseline serum cholesterol levels in 3 large cohorts of younger men to long-term coronary, cardiovascular, and all-cause mortality and to longevity. JAMA 2000;284:311-318.
434. Lloyd-Jones DM, Leip EP, Larson MG, et al. Prediction of lifetime risk for cardiovascular disease by risk factor burden at 50 years of age. Circulation 2006;113:791-798.
435. Grundy SM, Cleeman JI, Merz CNB, et al. Implications of recent clinical trials for the National Cholesterol Education Program Adult Treatment Panel III guidelines. Circulation 2004;110: 227-239.
436. Wood D, De Backer G, Faergeman O, et al. Prevention of coronary heart disease in clinical practice. Recommendations of the Second Joint Task Force of European and Other Societies on Coronary Prevention. Summary of recommendations. Eur Heart J 1998; 19:1434-1503.
437. Blankenhorn DH, Nessim SA, Johnson RL, et al. Beneficial effects of combined colestipol-niacin therapy on coronary atherosclerosis and coronary venous bypass grafts. JAMA 1987;257:3233-3240.
438. Ornish D, Brown SE, Scherwitz LW, et al. Can lifestyle changes reverse coronary heart disease? The Lifestyle Heart Trial. Lancet 1990;336:129-133.
439. Brown BG, Zhao X-Q, Sacco DE, Albers JJ. Lipid lowering and plaque regression. New insights into prevention of plaque disruption and clinical events in coronary disease. Circulation 1993;87: 1781-1791.
440. Foley KA, Simpson RJ Jr, Crouse III JR, et al. Effectiveness of statin titration on low-density lipoprotein cholesterol goal attainment in patients at high risk of atherogenic events. Am J Cardiol 2003;92:79-81.
441. Criqui MH. Cholesterol, primary and secondary prevention, and all-cause mortality. Ann Intern Med 1991;115:973-976.
442. Grundy SM, Benjamin IJ, Burke GL, et al. Diabetes and cardiovascular disease. A statement for healthcare professionals from the American Heart Association. Circulation 1999;100:1134-1146.
443. Haffner SM, Lehto S, Rönnemaa T, et al. Mortality from coronary heart disease in subjects with type 2 diabetes and in nondiabetic subjects with and without prior myocardial infarction. N Engl J Med 1998;339:229-234.
444. Heart Protection Study Collaborative Group. MRC/BHF Heart Protection Study of cholesterol-lowering with simvastatin in 5963 people with diabetes. A randomised placebo-controlled trial. Lancet 2003;361:2005-2016.
445. American Diabetes Association. Dyslipidemia management in adults with diabetes. Diabetes Care 2004;27(suppl 1):S68-S71.
446. The Expert Panel. Summary of the second report of the National Cholesterol Education Program (NCEP) Expert Panel on Detection, Evaluation, and Treatment of High Blood Cholesterol in Adults (Adult Treatment Panel II). JAMA 1993;269:3015-3023.
447. Connor WE, Connor SL. The dietary treatment of hyperlipidemia. Rationale, technique and efficacy. Med Clin North Am 1982; 66:485-518.
448. Kohli P, Greenland P. Role of the metabolic syndrome in risk assessment for coronary heart disease. JAMA 2006;295:819-821.
449. Strong K, Mathers C, Leeder S, Beaglehole R. Preventing chronic diseases. How many lives can we save? Lancet 2005;366: 1578-1582.
450. Krauss RM, Eckel RH, Howard B, et al. AHA dietary guidelines. Revision 2000. A statement for healthcare professionals from the Nutrition Committee of the American Heart Association. Circulation 2000;102:2284-2299.
451. Denke MA, Grundy SM. Individual responses to a cholesterol-lowering diet in 50 men with moderate hypercholesterolemia. Arch Intern Med 1994;154:317-325.
452. Ginsberg HN, Barr SL, Gilbert A, et al. Reduction of plasma cholesterol levels in normal men on an American Heart Association Step 1 diet or a Step 1 diet with added monounsaturated fat. N Engl J Med 1990;322:574-579.
453. Hunninghake DB, Stein EA, Dujovne CA, et al. The efficacy of intensive dietary therapy alone or combined with lovastatin in outpatients with hypercholesterolemia. N Engl J Med 1993; 328:1213-1219.
454. Cobb MM, Teitelbaum HS, Breslow JL. Lovastatin efficacy in reducing low-density lipoprotein cholesterol levels on high- vs low-fat diets. JAMA 1991;265:997-1001.
455. Schaefer EJ, Lichtenstein AH, Lamon-Fava S, et al. Efficacy of a National Cholesterol Education Program Step 2 diet in normolipidemic and hypercholesterolemic middle-aged and elderly men and women. Arterioscler Thromb Vasc Biol 1995;15:1079-1085.
456. Willett WC. Diet and health. What should we eat? Science 1994; 264:532-537.
457. Horton JD, Cuthbert JA, Spady DK. Dietary fatty acids regulate hepatic low density lipoprotein (LDL) transport by altering LDL receptor protein and mRNA levels. J Clin Invest 1993;92:743-749.
458. Mensink RP, Katan MB. Effect of a diet enriched with monounsaturated or polyunsaturated fatty acids on levels of low-density and high-density lipoprotein cholesterol in healthy women and men. N Engl J Med 1989;321:436–441.
459. Katan MB, Zock PL, Mensink RP. *Trans* fatty acids and their effects on lipoproteins in humans. Annu Rev Nutr 1995;15:473-493.
460. Kris-Etherton PM, Harris WS, Appel LJ. Fish consumption, fish oil, omega-3 fatty acids, and cardiovascular disease. Circulation 2002;106:2747-2757.
461. Harris WS, Ginsberg HN, Arunakul N, et al. Safety and efficacy of Omacor in severe hypertriglyceridemia. J Cardiovasc Risk 1997;4: 385-391.
462. Leaf A, Xiao Y-F, Kang JX, Billman GE. Prevention of sudden cardiac death by n-3 polyunsaturated fatty acids. Pharmacol Ther 2003;98:355-377.
463. Friday KE, Childs MT, Tsunehara CH, et al. Elevated plasma glucose and lowered triglyceride levels from omega-3 fatty acid supplementation in type II diabetes. Diabetes Care 1989;12:276-281.
464. Grundy SM. Comparison of monounsaturated fatty acids and carbohydrates for lowering plasma cholesterol. N Engl J Med 1986;314:745-748.
465. Sacks FM, Katan M. Randomized clinical trials on the effects of dietary fat and carbohydrate on plasma lipoproteins and cardiovascular disease. Am J Med 2002;113:13S-24S.
466. Connor WE. Dietary fiber—nostrum or critical nutrient? N Engl J Med 1990;322:193-195.
467. Jenkins DJA, Wolever TMS, Rao AV, et al. Effect on blood lipids of very high intakes of fiber in diets low in saturated fat and cholesterol. N Engl J Med 1993;329:21-26.
468. Sprecher DL, Harris BV, Goldberg AC, et al. Efficacy of psyllium in reducing serum cholesterol levels in hypercholesterolemic patients on high- or low-fat diets. Ann Intern Med 1993;119: 545-554.
469. Miettinen TA, Puska P, Gylling H, et al. Reduction of serum cholesterol with sitostanol-ester margarine in a mildly hypercholesterolemic population. N Engl J Med 1995;333:1308-1312.
470. Warshafsky S, Kamer RS, Sivak SL. Effect of garlic on total serum cholesterol. A meta-analysis. Ann Intern Med 1993;119:599-605.

471. Sabaté J, Fraser GE, Burke K, et al. Effects of walnuts on serum lipid levels and blood pressure in normal men. N Engl J Med 1993;328:603-607.
472. Jenkins DJA, Kendall CWC, Marchie A, et al. Effects of a dietary portfolio of cholesterol-lowering foods vs lovastatin on serum lipids and C-reactive protein. JAMA 2003;290:502-510.
473. Fletcher B, Berra K, Ades P, et al. Managing abnormal blood lipids. A collaborative approach. Circulation 2005;112:3184-3209.
474. Stein EA, Lane M, Laskarzewski P. Comparison of statins in hypertriglyceridemia. Am J Cardiol 1998;81:66B-69B.
475. Liao JK. Effects of statins on 3-hydroxy-3-methylglutaryl coenzyme A reductase inhibition beyond low-density lipoprotein cholesterol. Am J Cardiol 2005;96(suppl):24F-33F.
476. Omar MA, Wilson JP, Cox TS. Rhabdomyolysis and HMG-CoA reductase inhibitors. Ann Pharmacother 2001;35:1096-1107.
477. Pasternak RC, Smith SC Jr, Bairey-Merz CN, et al. ACC/AHA/NHLBI Clinical Advisory on the Use and Safety of Statins. Circulation 2002;106:1024-1028.
478. Thompson PD, Clarkson P, Karas RH. Statin-associated myopathy. JAMA 2003;289:1681-1690.
479. Ast M, Frishman WH. Bile acid sequestrants. J Clin Pharmacol 1990;30:99-106.
480. Shepherd J, Packard CJ, Bicker S, et al. Cholestyramine promotes receptor-mediated low-density-lipoprotein catabolism. N Engl J Med 1980;302:1219-1222.
481. Beil U, Crouse JR, Einarsson K, Grundy SM. Effects of interruption of the enterohepatic circulation of bile acids on the transport of very low density-lipoprotein triglycerides. Metabolism 1982;31: 438-444.
482. Gurakar A, Hoeg JM, Kostner G, et al. Levels of lipoprotein Lp(a) decline with neomycin and niacin treatment. Atherosclerosis 1985;57:293-301.
483. McKenney JM, Proctor JD, Harris S, Chinchili VM. A comparison of the efficacy and toxic effects of sustained- vs immediate-release niacin in hypercholesterolemic patients. JAMA 1994;271: 672-677.
484. Elam MB, Hunninghake DB, Davis KB, et al. Effect of niacin on lipid and lipoprotein levels and glycemic control in patients with diabetes and peripheral arterial disease. The ADMIT study. A randomized trial. JAMA 2000;284:1263-1270.
485. Kersten S, Desvergne B, Wahli W. Roles of PPARs in health and disease. Nature 2000;405:421-424.
486. Kissebah AH, Adams PW, Harrigan P, Wynn V. The mechanism of action of clofibrate and tetranicotinoylfructose (bradilan) on the kinetics of plasma free fatty acid and triglyceride transport in Type IV and Type V hypertriglyceridaemia. Eur J Clin Invest 1974;4: 163-174.
487. Pierides AM, Alvarez-Ude F, Kerr DNS, Skillen AW. Clofibrate-induced muscle damage in patients with chronic renal failure. Lancet 1975;2:1279-1282.
488. Prueksaritanont T, Subramanian R, Fang X, et al. Glucuronidation of statins in animals and humans. A novel mechanism of statin lactonization. Drug Metab Disp 2002;30:505-512.
489. Prueksaritanont T, Tang C, Qiu Y, et al. Effects of fibrates on metabolism of statins in human hepatocytes. Drug Metab Disp 2002; 30:1280-1287.
490. Prueksaritanont T, Zhao JJ, Ma B, et al. Mechanistic studies on metabolic interactions between gemfibrozil and statins. J Pharmacol Exp Ther 2002;301:1042-1051.
491. Bergman AJ, Murphy G, Burke J, et al. Simvastatin does not have a clinically significant pharmacokinetic interaction with fenofibrate in humans. J Clin Pharmacol 2004;44:1054-1062.
492. Martin PD, Dane AL, Schneck DW, Warwick MJ. An open-label, randomized, three-way crossover trial of the effects of coadministration of rosuvastatin and fenofibrate on the pharmacokinetic properties of rosuvastatin and fenofibric acid in healthy male volunteers. Clin Ther 2003;25:459-471.
493. Committee of Principal Investigators. A co-operative trial in the primary prevention of ischaemic heart disease using clofibrate. Report from the Committee of Principal Investigators. Br Heart J 1978;40:1069-1118.
494. Heady JA, Morris JN, Oliver MF. WHO clofibrate/cholesterol trial. Clarifications. Lancet 1992;340:1405-1406.
495. van Heek M, Farley C, Compton DS, et al. Comparison of the activity and disposition of the novel cholesterol absorption inhibitor, SCH58235, and its glucuronide, SCH60663. Br J Pharmacol 2000; 129:1748-1754.
496. Ballantyne CM, Houri J, Notarbartolo A, et al. Effect of ezetimibe coadministered with atorvastatin in 628 patients with primary hypercholesterolemia. A prospective, randomized, double-blind trial. Circulation 2003;107:2409-2415.
497. Melani L, Mills R, Hassman D, et al. Efficacy and safety of ezetimibe coadministered with pravastatin in patients with primary hypercholesterolemia. A prospective, randomized, double-blind trial. Eur Heart J 2003;24:717-728.
498. Ballantyne CM, Blazing MA, King TR, et al. Efficacy and safety of ezetimibe co-administered with simvastatin compared with atorvastatin in adults with hypercholesterolemia. Am J Cardiol 2004;93:1487-1494.
499. Pownall HJ, Brauchi D, Kilinç C, et al. Correlation of serum triglyceride and its reduction by w-3 fatty acids with lipid transfer activity and the neutral lipid compositions of high-density and low-density lipoproteins. Atherosclerosis 1999;143:285-297.
500. Stalenhoef AFH, de Graaf J, Wittekoek ME, et al. The effect of concentrated n-3 fatty acids versus gemfibrozil on plasma lipoproteins, low density lipoprotein heterogeneity and oxidizability in patients with hypertriglyceridemia. Atherosclerosis 2000;153: 129-138.
501. Feldman T, Koren M, Insull W Jr, et al. Treatment of high-risk patients with ezetimibe plus simvastatin co-administration versus simvastatin alone to attain National Cholesterol Education Program Adult Treatment Panel III low-density lipoprotein cholesterol goals. Am J Cardiol 2004;93:1481-1486.
502. Kane JP, Malloy MJ, Tun P, et al. Normalization of low-density-lipoprotein levels in heterozygous familial hypercholesterolemia with a combined drug regimen. N Engl J Med 1981;304: 251-258.
503. Illingworth DR, Phillipson BE, Rapp JH, Connor WE. Colestipol plus nicotinic acid in treatment of heterozygous familial hypercholesterolaemia. Lancet 1981;1:296-298.
504. Mabuchi H, Sakai T, Sakai Y, et al. Reduction of serum cholesterol in heterozygous patients with familial hypercholesterolemia. Additive effects of compactin and cholestyramine. N Engl J Med 1983;308:609-613.
505. Malloy MJ, Kane JP, Kunitake ST, Tun P. Complementarity of colestipol, niacin, and lovastatin in treatment of severe familial hypercholesterolemia. Ann Intern Med 1987;107:616-623.
506. Olsson AG, Pears JS, McKellar J, et al. Pharmacodynamics of new HMG-CoA reductase inhibitor ZD4522 in patients with primary hypercholesterolaemia [abstract]. Atherosclerosis 2000; 151:39.
507. Wetterau JR, Gregg RE, Harrity TW, et al. An MTP inhibitor that normalizes atherogenic lipoprotein levels in WHHL rabbits. Science 1998;282:751-754.
508. Buhman KK, Accad M, Novak S, et al. Resistance to diet-induced hypercholesterolemia and gallstone formation in ACAT2-deficient mice. Nat Med 2000;6:1341-1347.
509. van der Steeg WA, Kuivenhoven JA, Klerkx AH, et al. Role of CETP inhibitors in the treatment of dyslipidemia. Curr Opin Lipidol 2004;15:631-636.
510. Rader DJ. High-density lipoproteins as an emerging therapeutic target for atherosclerosis. JAMA 2003;290:2322-2324.
511. Navab M, Anantharamaiah GM, Reddy ST, et al. Apolipoprotein A-I mimetic peptides. Arterioscler Thromb Vasc Biol 2005;25: 1325-1331.
512. Rosenson RS. Low levels of high-density lipoprotein cholesterol (hypoalphalipoproteinemia). An approach to management. Arch Intern Med 1993;153:1528-1538.
513. Gordon DJ, Witztum JL, Hunninghake D, et al. Habitual physical activity and high-density lipoprotein cholesterol in men with primary hypercholesterolemia. The Lipid Research Clinics Coronary Primary Prevention Trial. Circulation 1983;67:512-520.
514. Williams PT. High-density lipoprotein cholesterol and other risk factors for coronary heart disease in female runners. N Engl J Med 1996;334:1298-1303.
515. Packard CJ, Stewart JM, Third JLHC, et al. Effects of nicotinic acid therapy on high-density lipoprotein metabolism in type II and

type IV hyperlipoproteinaemia. Biochim Biophys Acta 1980;618: 53-62.
516. Vega GL, Grundy SM. Lipoprotein responses to treatment with lovastatin, gemfibrozil, and nicotinic acid in normolipidemic patients with hypoalphalipoproteinemia. Arch Intern Med 1994; 154:73-82.
517. Heart Protection Study Collaborative Group. MRC/BHF Heart Protection Study of cholesterol lowering with simvastatin in 20 536 high-risk individuals. a randomised placebo-controlled trial. Lancet 2002;360:7-22.
518. Sanderson SL, Iverius P-H, Wilson DE. Successful hyperlipemic pregnancy. JAMA 1991;265:1858-1860.

CHAPTER 37

ENDOCRINOLOGY OF HIV AND AIDS

Steven K. Grinspoon

Human immunodeficiency virus (HIV) disease affects up to 44 million patients worldwide and more than 1 million in the United States. In many parts of the world, for example in sub-Saharan Africa, HIV remains epidemic; an estimated 25 million people are infected, and the adult infection rate is 7.5%.[1] In addition, the number of patients with HIV infection and acquired immunodeficiency syndrome (AIDS) is growing rapidly in Asia and other parts of the world.

Endocrine dysfunction is common among HIV-infected patients. Adrenal, gonadal, thyroid, bone, and metabolic abnormalities have all been reported. HIV itself, related infectious organisms, cytokines, and antiretroviral medications can all affect endocrine function. Endocrine disorders in HIV disease, for example hypogonadism, adrenal insufficiency, diabetes and bone loss, can cause significant morbidity and are thus important to diagnose. Furthermore, treatment can improve quality of life and long-term mortality through effects on critical metabolic and body composition parameters, including loss of muscle mass (sarcopenia) in AIDS wasting and fat redistribution (central adiposity) in HIV lipodystrophy that may affect long-term mortality. However, diagnosis and treatment may be difficult due to varying nutritional conditions and effects of the varied medications used to treat HIV disease. In addition, specific endocrine disorders can provide a clue to local or disseminated infections that are also critical to diagnose and treat.

As HIV patients live longer due to the success of antiretroviral medications, adverse effects resulting from these very medications have resulted in increased cardiovascular risk and metabolic changes that require intervention and long-term management by the endocrine specialist (Fig. 37–1). This chapter reviews the prevalence, mechanisms, and optimal treatment strategies for endocrine abnormalities in HIV-infected patients.

Adrenal Function

Adrenal dysfunction may be suspected in the patient with advanced HIV disease because of fatigue, hyponatremia, and other features of adrenal insufficiency. Although clinical adrenal dysfunction is rare among patients with AIDS, recent data suggest that subtle impairments in adrenal reserve are common in this population. Adrenal dysfunction most often is caused by destruction of adrenal tissue by cytomegalovirus (CMV) in patients with advanced HIV disease, but adrenal dysfunction might also be caused by medications, hypothalamic or pituitary disease from opportunistic infections, idiopathic inflammation or tissue destruction, or, in rare cases, cortisol resistance. Excess cortisol production may be seen in association with severe stress. In addition, some features of Cushing's syndrome may be seen among patients with lipodystrophy, but true Cushing's syndrome is rare.

Adrenal Insufficiency

Biochemical evidence of adrenal insufficiency is relatively common among hospitalized AIDS patients; 17% of 74 hospitalized AIDS patients screened by cosyntropin test demonstrated

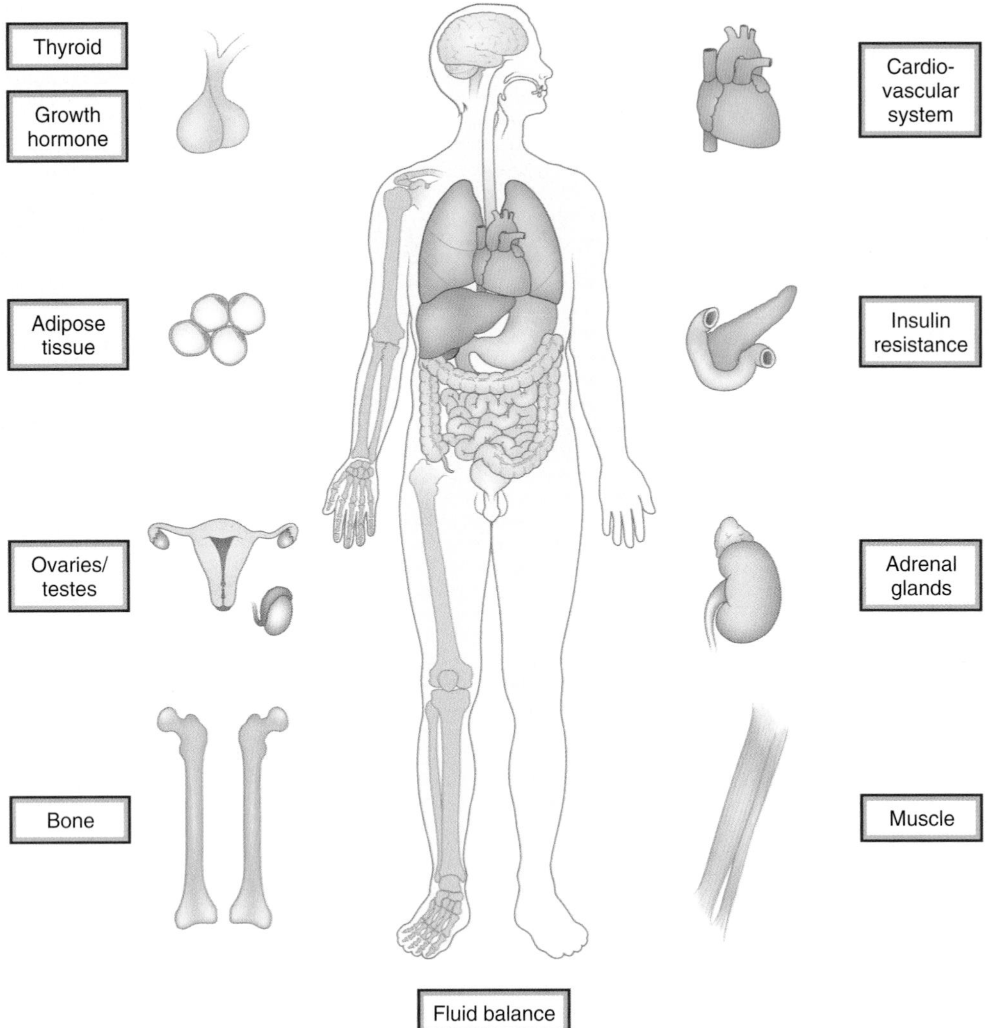

Figure 37–1 ▪ Potential areas of endocrine involvement in HIV disease.

inadequate adrenal stimulation (1 h cortisol <18 μg/dL) in an early study. In contrast, fewer patients (4%) demonstrate clinical symptoms of adrenal insufficiency.[2] Among patients with clinical symptoms and signs of adrenal insufficiency, including hyponatremia, a higher percentage (up to 30%) demonstrate inadequate testing using cosyntropin.[3]

Adrenal insufficiency occurring in the context of advanced HIV disease is most often caused by tissue destruction of the adrenal glands from opportunistic infections. CMV adrenalitis is the most common etiology, seen in approximately 40% to 90% of patients with CMV infections at autopsy (Fig. 37–2). However, adrenocortical destruction caused by CMV is usually less than 50% and therefore unlikely to cause adrenal insufficiency,[4] and CMV disease is rare with well-preserved immune function in patients on newer potent antiretroviral therapies. Other organisms and processes that have been associated with adrenal destruction in HIV disease include *Mycobacterium tuberculosis, Mycobacterium avium-intracellulare* (MAI), *Cryptococcus,* and hemorrhage. Additionally, pituitary and hypothalamic destruction resulting in secondary adrenal insufficiency may be caused in rare instances by opportunistic infection (e.g. toxoplasmosis, cryptococcosis, and CMV). Idiopathic adenohypophyseal necrosis is also observed in a minority of patients, approximately 10% at autopsy, and may be related to a direct effect of HIV.[5]

Impaired Adrenal Reserve

Longitudinal evaluation of adrenal function in HIV-infected patients suggests that impaired adrenal reserve may be common. In one study, normal cortisol, but reduced aldosterone and dehydroepiandrosterone (DHEA) responses to adrenocorticotropic hormone (ACTH) were seen, particularly among patients with advanced HIV disease. Over time, ACTH levels increased, suggesting impaired adrenal reserve and subclinical adrenal dysfunction.[6] However, the usefulness of glucocorticoid treatment in such patients with slightly increased ACTH levels but normal cortisol response to cosyntropin testing has not been demonstrated.

Glucocorticoid Excess

Increased cortisol levels may also be seen in HIV-infected patients. More commonly, increased cortisol levels are seen as a stress response, in association with low weight or increasing degree of illness. Intraadrenal shunting toward cortisol synthesis, potentially as a result of 17,20 lyase dysfunction, has been suggested by studies demonstrating a reduced DHEA-to-cortisol ratio on cosyntropin testing (Fig. 37–3).[7]

Cytokine modulation of the hypothalamic-pituitary-adrenal axis might also contribute to increased cortisol levels. Interleu-

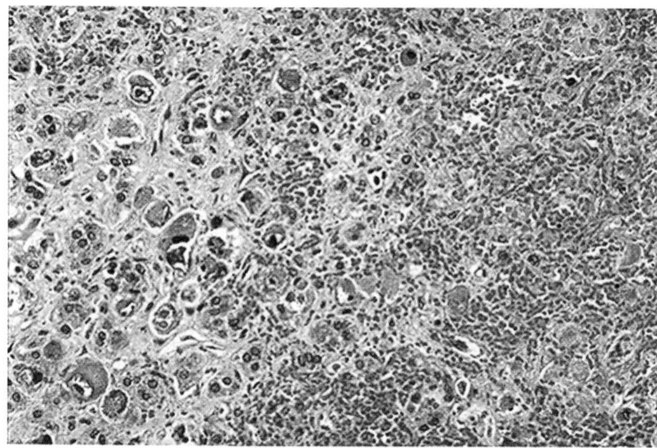

Figure 37–2 ■ Cytomegalovirus adrenalitis associated with HIV infection. (Reprinted from WebPath [Edward Klatt, MD; http://library.med.utah.edu/WebPath/webpath.html] with permission.)

kin-1 (IL-1), produced in the median eminence, has been shown to increase corticotropin-releasing hormone and ACTH secretion in vitro and in animal studies. Increased IL-1 secretion from infected monocytes in the median eminence is thus another possible cause of increased cortisol secretion in HIV-infected patients.

Glucocorticoid resistance has also been shown in rare patients with advanced HIV disease, who demonstrate addisonian symptoms, including hyperpigmentation, in the setting of hypercortisolism and increased ACTH. Abnormalities of glucocorticoid receptor function have been shown in association with increased interferon-α (IFN-α) in such patients.[8] Monocytes from such patients are resistant to dexamethasone and exhibit increased concentration of glucocorticoid receptors with decreased apparent affinity for dexamethasone, in contrast to patients with primary glucocorticoid resistance.

Medication Effects

Medications can contribute to adrenal insufficiency in HIV patients (Table 37–1). Ketoconazole, an antifungal agent, inhibits side chain cleavage enzyme and 11-hydroxylase. These effects are not generally seen with fluconazole, itraconazole, and the more recently introduced imidazole derivatives. Phenytoin, opiates, and rifampin, among other drugs, affect cortisol metabolism. For example, adrenal insufficiency may be precipitated by the use of rifampin for treatment of tuberculosis in patients with reduced adrenal reserve.

Megestrol acetate, a potent synthetic progestational derivative, has glucocorticoid properties and decreases ACTH. Abrupt withdrawal of megestrol acetate can precipitate adrenal insufficiency, and such patients should be tested before megestrol acetate is administered and receive physiologic glucocorticoid administration as needed after megestrol acetate is withdrawn. In addition, megestrol acetate can decrease gonadal function, which should also be monitored during and after therapy.

Clinical Assessment

HIV-infected patients with symptoms of adrenal insufficiency and particularly those with hyponatremia and risk factors for adrenal insufficiency (e.g., known disseminated CMV or recent use of megestrol acetate) should be evaluated. Evaluation of the cortisol axis should proceed as in other patients with suspected adrenal dysfunction. Cosyntropin testing is usually an adequate first step, except in patients in whom hypothalamic or pituitary insufficiency of recent onset is suspected. In such patients, use

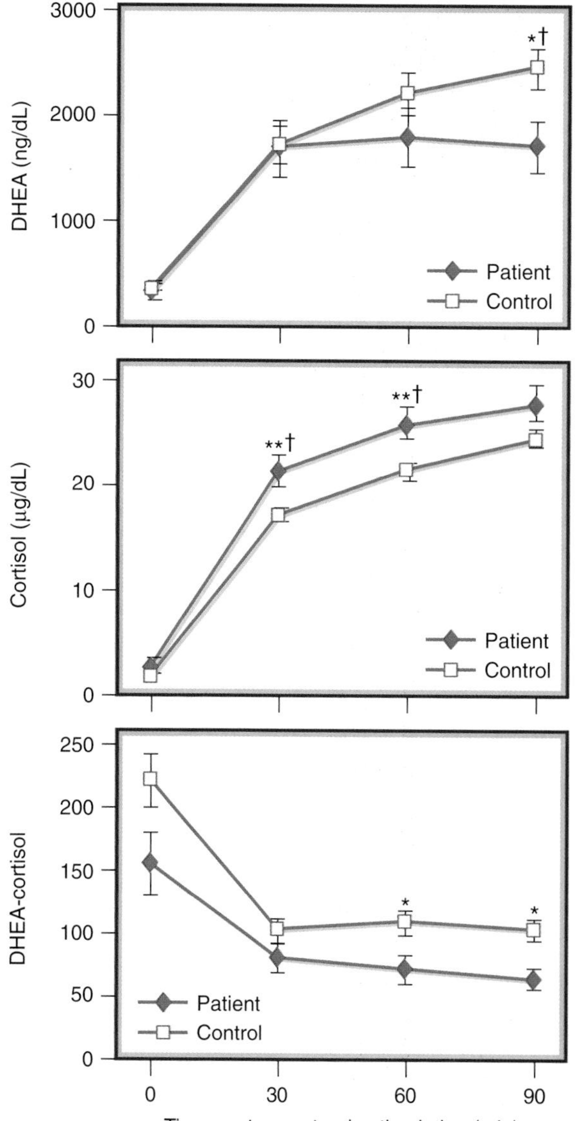

Figure 37–3 ■ Dehydroepiandrosterone (DHEA) and cortisol response to cosyntropin stimulation in HIV-infected women with the wasting syndrome *(closed diamonds)* and normal controls *(open squares)*. $^*P<0.05$ vs. controls, $^{**}P<0.01$ vs. controls, $^{\dagger}P<0.05$ and $^{\dagger\dagger}P<0.01$ (†,†† for comparison of change from baseline at each time point, HIV-infected vs. control subjects). (Data from Grinspoon S, Corcoran C, Stanley T, et al. Mechanisms of androgen deficiency in human immunodeficiency virus–infected women with the wasting syndrome. J Clin Endocrinol Metab 2001;86[9]:4120-4126, with permission.)

of morning cortisol levels, metyrapone, or insulin tolerance testing may be necessary if there are no contraindications. After adrenal insufficiency is documented, ACTH testing and appropriate imaging are used to localize the defect. In patients with clinical symptoms of adrenal insufficiency and elevated cortisol levels, cortisol resistance may be present and the diagnosis may be made by glucocorticoid receptor studies in blood monocytes.

Gonadal Function

Male

Gonadal dysfunction is common among HIV-infected men. Initial studies indicated biochemical hypogonadism in

TABLE 37–1 ENDOCRINE EFFECTS OF THE 21 APPROVED ANTIRETROVIRALS AND OTHER MEDICATIONS USED IN HIV CARE

Medication	Relevant Endocrine Effects	Site of Metabolism	Method of Metabolism
PROTEASE INHIBITORS			
Amprenavir	Hypertriglyceridemia, hyperglycemia, fat redistribution	Liver	CYP3A4
Atazanavir	Only minimal effects on glucose and lipid levels	Liver	CYP3A
Fosamprenavir	Diabetes mellitus, hyperkalemia, hyponatremia, fat redistribution, hypertriglyceridemia	Liver	CYP3A4
Indinavir	Hyperglycemia, hyperlipidemia, fat redistribution	Liver	CYP3A4
Lopinavir/Ritonavir	Fat redistribution, diabetes mellitus, hyperlipidemia	Liver	CYP3A4
Nelfinavir	Fat redistribution, diabetes mellitus, dyslipidemia	Liver	CYP3A4, CYP2C19, CYP2C9 and CYP2D6
Ritonavir	Diabetes mellitus, hyperlipidemia	Liver	CYP3A4 and CYP2D6
Saquinavir	Diabetes mellitus, hyperlipidemia, gynecomastia	Liver	CYP3A4
Tipranavir	Hyperglycemia, hyperlipidemia	Liver	CYP3A4
NUCLEOSIDE REVERSET RANSCRIPTASE INHIBITORS			
Abacavir	Hyperglycemia, fat redistribution	Liver	Alcohol dehydrogenase and glucuronyl transferase
Didanosine	Abnormal glucose, hypertriglyceridemia Hypocalcemia, hypomagnesemia, hypokalemia, gynecomastia, fat redistribution		Purine metabolism pathway
Emtricitabine	None	Liver	Sulfoxide and glucuronide metabolites
Lamivudine	Fat redistribution, hyperglycemia	Kidney	*trans*-Sulfoxide metabolite
Stavudine	Fat redistribution; possibly gynecomastia	Liver and Kidney	Unknown
Zalcitabine	Hypophosphatemia, hypomagnesemia, hypocalcemia Abnormal glucose, triglycerides, and sodium Weight loss, appetite loss, fat redistribution	Liver	Insignificant
Zidovudine	Gynecomastia, fat redistribution	Liver	Metabolized to GZDV
NUCLEOTIDE REVERSET RANSCRIPTASE INHIBITORS			
Disoproxil	Fat redistribution, hypophosphatemia	Plasma	Esterases
Fumarate	Fat redistribution, hypophosphatemia	Plasma	Esterases
Tenofovir	Fat redistribution, hypophosphatemia	Plasma	Esterases
NON-NUCLEOSIDE REVERSET RANSCRIPTASE INHIBITORS			
Delavirdine	Fat redistribution	Liver	CYP3A, CYP2D6, CYP2C9, and CYP2C19
Efavirenz	Fat redistribution, hyperlipidemia	Liver	CYP3A4 and CYP2B6
Nevirapine	Fat redistribution, hyperlipidemia	Liver	CYP3A4 and CYP2B6
ENTRY INHIBITOR			
Enfuvirtide	Hyperglycemia, hyperlipidemia, fat redistribution	Liver	Hydrolysis
ADDITIONAL MEDICATIONS			
Foscarnet	Hyperphosphatemia, hypocalcemia, hypokalemia	None	None
Ketoconazole	Gynecomastia, hypogonadism, vitamin D deficiency, adrenal insufficiency, hypertriglyceridemia	Liver	Oxidation, dealkylation, and hydroxylation
Megestrol acetate	Cushingoid features, weight gain; hyperglycemia, hypogonadism, adrenal insufficiency on withdrawal	Liver	Inactivation
Pentamidine	Pancreatitis, hypocalcemia, hyperkalemia, hypomagnesemia, abnormal glucose	None	None
Phenytoin	Vitamin D deficiency, gynecomastia, hyperglycemia, hyperprolactinemia	Liver	Hydroxylation
Rifampicin	Hyperglycemia, adrenal insufficiency	Liver	Deacetylation
Trimethoprim	Hyperkalemia, hyponatremia, decreased uric acid	Liver	Oxidation, hydroxylation, demethylation, carbonylation, and conjugation

Note: For a complete list of side effects and methods of metabolism, consult the *Physician's Desk Reference.*
Data from 2005 Physician's Desk Reference. Montvale, NJ: Thomson Healthcare, 2004.

approximately 50% of men with AIDS[9] in association with increased disease severity. More recent studies suggest a prevalence of up to 20% among men in the current era of potent antiretroviral treatment.[10] The mechanisms of hypogonadism in HIV-infected patients might relate to severe illness or effects of undernutrition on gonadotropin secretion, medication effects or, more rarely, tissue destruction from opportunistic infections. Most often, hypogonadism is secondary, with low or inappropriately normal gonadotropin levels. Primary hypogonadism is seen less often and may be caused by cytokine effects on the testes, including effects of TNF to inhibit steroidogenesis via effects on the side chain cleavage enzyme and of IL-I to inhibit Leydig cell steroidogenesis and LH binding to the Leydig cell.[11-13] In addition, opportunistic infections of the testes have rarely been reported, and up to 25% of HIV-infected patients with AIDS demonstrate testicular involvement of widespread opportunistic infection or systemic neoplasms, including CMV, toxoplasmosis, Kaposi's sarcoma, and testicular lymphoma.[14]

In addition, a number of medications can affect the HPG axis. Ketoconazole inhibits side chain cleavage enzyme and other critical enzymes in testicular steroidogenesis. Megestrol acetate suppresses gonadotropin secretion. Opiate therapy affects GnRH secretion and can result in hypogonadotropic hypogonadism (see Table 37–1).

Increased prolactin levels and gynecomastia have been demonstrated among HIV-infected patients. In a case-control study, gynecomastia was seen in 1.8% of 2275 consecutively screened HIV-infected patients and was associated with hypogonadism, hepatitis C, and degree of lipoatrophy (subcutaneous fat loss associated with potent antiretroviral therapy). Thyroid-stimulating hormone (TSH) levels were increased, although the percentage with hypothyroidism was not different.[15] Hyperprolactinemia was reported in 21% of HIV-infected men with stable HIV disease and was significantly associated with opioid use and increased CD4 count but not with changes in body composition or gynecomastia.[16] Evidence suggests increased bioactivity of prolactin in HIV-infected patients that can arise from reduced dopaminergic tone.[17] Increased prolactin levels in association with galactorrhea have also been described among patients treated with protease inhibitors (PIs). The mechanism of this effect is unclear and might relate to a direct stimulation of prolactin secretion by specific PIs or effects on the P450 system to potentiate the dopamine antagonistic effect of other drugs.[18] Dopamine agonists should be used cautiously among HIV-infected men receiving PIs because of the potential for interactions.

Sex-hormone binding levels are increased in 30% to 55% of HIV-infected patients. Therefore, use of bioavailable or free testosterone assays is recommended to diagnose hypogonadism, because total testosterone assays can underestimate the prevalence of true hypogonadism in this population. For example, hypogonadism was diagnosed by low levels of free testosterone in 49% of patients compared with diagnosis in 26% by low levels of total testosterone in an early study of HIV-infected men with weight loss.[19]

Decreased gonadal function is associated with sarcopenia and reduced strength in HIV-infected men.[19] Treatment with physiologic testosterone replacement results in increased lean body mass, improved quality of life, and reduction in indices of depression in HIV-infected men with hypogonadism (Table 37–2, Fig. 37–4). Sustained increases in lean body mass of almost 8% (~3.7 kg) have been shown with 1 year of intramuscular testosterone treatment.[20] In addition, a number of studies have investigated anabolic steroids such as nandrolone and oxandrolone as well as pharmacologic doses of testosterone

TABLE 37–2 SELECT STUDIES* OF TESTOSTERONE REPLACEMENT IN HIV-INFECTED PERSONS

Study	N	Duration	Route	Dose	Primary End-point	Result
				STUDIES IN MEN		
Berger[91]	63	16 wk	PO	15 mg/day†	Weight, muscle strength, and well-being	Weight and well-being improved; no change in muscle strength
Bhasin[101]	61	16 wk	IM	100 mg/wk	Muscle strength	Muscle strength improved 18%-30%
Bhasin[177]	41	12 wk	Transdermal patch	5 mg/day	LBM	LBM increased
Dobs[178]	133	12 wk	Transscrotal patch	6 mg/day	BCM and DHEA	DHEA levels improved, no change in BCM
Grinspoon[176,89]	51	6 mo	IM	300 mg every 3 wk	LBM	Gained 2 kg fat-free mass
Piketty[179]	32	16 wk	PO	50 mg/day‡	QOL	Mental health and health distress improved
Strawford[102]	24	8 wk	PO	20 mg/day†	LBM and strength	LBM and strength increased
				STUDIES IN WOMEN		
Choi[24]	52	24 wk	Transdermal patch	300 μg biw	Fat-free mass, muscle strength, weight	No significant change in body composition compared with placebo
Dolan[90]	57	6 mo	Transdermal patch	150 μg biw	Muscle strength	Muscle strength improved
Miller[180]	53	12 wk	Transdermal patch	150 and 300 μg biw	Change in free testosterone	Free testosterone and weight increased significantly

*All studies are randomized, doubles-blind, and placebo-controlled trials.
†Oxandrolone
‡DHEA
BCM, body cell mass; DHEA, dehydroepiandrosterone; LBM, lean body mass; QOL, quality of life.

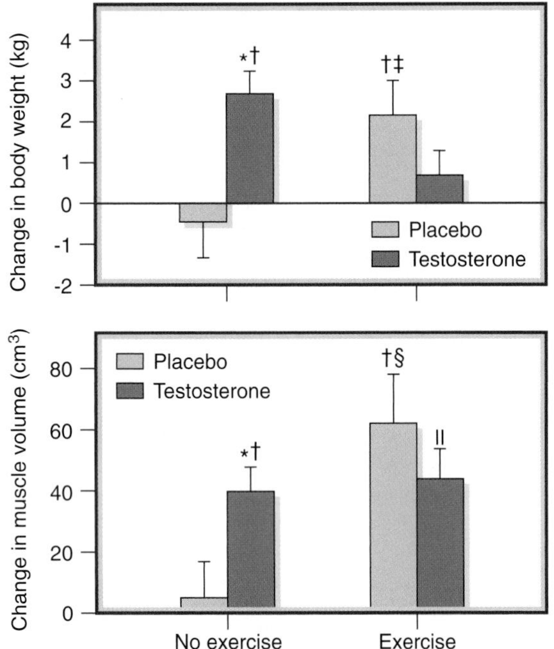

Figure 37–4 ▪ Effects of testosterone replacement and resistance exercise on changes in body weight and muscle volume in HIV-infected men with low testosterone levels. *$P<0.001$ vs. zero change; †$P<0.01$ vs. placebo and no exercise; ††$P=0.02$ vs. zero change; §$P=0.003$ vs. zero change; ||$P=0.001$. (Data from Bhasin S, Storer TW, Javanbakht M, et al. Testosterone replacement and resistance exercise in HIV-infected men with weight loss and low testosterone levels. JAMA 2000;283:763-770, with permission.)

alone or in combination with progressive resistance training (see Table 37–2). Oral anabolic steroids are associated with liver dysfunction and should be avoided. Pharmacologic doses of testosterone, although effective in increasing lean body mass without causing liver dysfunction, result in decreased high-density lipoprotein (HDL) and are likely to result in suppression of the hypothalamic-pituitary-gonadal axis. Progressive resistance training also increases lean body mass in men with AIDS wasting and is associated with increased HDL.[21]

Appropriate use of physiologic testosterone replacement in HIV-infected men is unlikely to suppress endogenous gonadal function. Safety assessment should include monitoring of prostate-specific antigen (PSA), as is generally recommended for older men receiving testosterone. In patients with resolution of acute or chronic illness, retesting of gonadal function by measuring an early morning bioavailable testosterone level is recommended, because endogenous function can return with improved health. No clear benefit has been demonstrated for the combined use of testosterone and anabolic steroids.

Female

Amenorrhea is seen in approximately 25% of HIV-infected women[22] and may be caused by the reduction of gonadotropin production associated with the stress of illness. In contrast, anovulation may be seen in up to 50% of HIV-infected women in association with reduced CD4 counts. Among anovulatory HIV-infected women, changes in menstrual function are three times as likely compared with normally ovulating patients. Early menopause has been reported in up to 8% of HIV-infected women.[23]

Androgen levels are often reduced in HIV-infected women. In one study, androgen levels, assessed with the use of a free testosterone assay, were reduced below the level seen in age-matched healthy women in more than 50% of HIV-infected women with significant weight loss and in more than one third of HIV-infected women without weight loss.[22] The mechanisms of androgen deficiency in HIV disease may be caused in part by intraadrenal shunting toward cortisol production and away from androgen production, particularly in women with significant weight loss (see Fig. 37–3, see the discussion of adrenal function, earlier).[7] In contrast, hCG testing showed ovarian androgen production to be intact.

Two studies have investigated testosterone administration to HIV-infected women using a transdermal patch designed to deliver a low, physiologic dose of 150 μg/day (see Table 37–2). In the longer of the two studies, functional capacity and strength significantly improved, and there was a trend toward increased lean body mass. Hirsutism was not seen and virilization did not occur. In contrast, studies using nandrolone and other anabolic steroids have demonstrated significant increases in lean body mass but reductions in HDL and other side effects. Physiologic testosterone replacement appears to be useful to increase physical function in HIV-infected women, but such doses may be too low to significantly increase lean body mass. A more recent study using a larger dose of 300 μg/day by transdermal administration among normal-weight HIV-infected women did not show an increase in weight or lean body mass, but testosterone was well tolerated.[24]

Thyroid Function

Altered thyroid function test (TFT) results are common in HIV-infected patients. Thyroid-binding globulin (TBG) levels are increased in HIV-infected patients and correlate inversely with CD4 counts. For example, Bourdoux and colleagues demonstrated that TBG levels were increased in 16 of 54 HIV-infected patients.[25] Abnormal thyroid function test results may be caused by the stress of illness in patients with advanced disease or concomitant morbidities, as found in other patients with euthyroid sick syndrome. However, among adults, some studies have shown that reverse triiodothyronine (T_3) (rT_3) levels do not rise in association with decreasing T_3 levels, as one would expect in nonthyroid illness.[3] Patients with progressive HIV disease therefore exhibit decreased T_3 levels, increased TBG, and decreased rT_3 levels with increasing illness.

In addition to the euthyroid sick syndrome, recent large screening studies have demonstrated an increased prevalence of primary hypothyroidism in HIV-infected patients. Among 350 patients studied in France, 2.6% had clinically evident hypothyroidism, 6.6% had subclinical hypothyroidism based on increased TSH levels but normal free T_4 levels, and 6.8% demonstrated a low free T_4 level. The prevalence of subclinical hypothyroidism was higher in men. Use of stavudine and low CD4 were predictive of thyroid disease in multivariate modeling.[26] In a Spanish cohort, free T_4 was found to be below normal in only 1.3% of patients, and low free T_4 was shown to correlate with low CD4 count. Increased TSH levels and normal free T_4 were found in 3.5% of patients, but no relationship with specific antiviral drugs was found.[27] Subclinical hypothyroidism is not uncommon among adult HIV-infected patients and is seen most often in the context of low CD4 count. Hypothyroidism in HIV-infected patients is not often seen in association with antithyroid antibodies, and the etiology remains unclear.[28,29]

Among children, increased TSH was seen in 8 of 11 children with an average age of 1.5 years and failure to thrive. T_4 levels were normal, but thyrotropin-releasing hormone (TRH) testing showed exaggerated TSH responses, and growth rates increased in response to thyroid hormone.[30] Fundaro and colleagues demonstrated increased antithyroglobulin antibodies in 34% of symptomatic HIV-infected children.[31] Increased TSH levels were found in 28% of HIV-infected children, particularly those with severe immunosuppression. In contrast, a larger study in perinatally infected children demonstrated reduced total T_3, total T_4, and free T_4 and increased rT_3, TBG, and TSH, with negative autoantibodies, suggesting a euthyroid sick syndrome pattern, particularly in those with severe immunosuppression. HIV-infected children with failure to thrive should be screened for true hypothyroidism, but more often the TFTs reflect nonthyroid illness and the severity of immune compromise.[32]

Recently, thyroid dysfunction has been described with an immune reconstitution syndrome, in which autoimmune thyroid disease occurs in association with potent antiretroviral therapy and improved immune function. Graves' disease is most often reported in this context. The estimated prevalence for immune reconstitution thyroid disease with initiation of highly active antiretroviral therapy (HAART) was 3% for women and 0.2% for men.[33] Graves' disease has also been described after IL-2 therapy in HIV-infected patients.[34]

In addition to autoimmune etiologies, thyroid disease related to anatomic replacement and infection of the thyroid has been reported in HIV-infected patients. *Pneumocystis* thyroiditis has been reported to cause a painful thyroiditis-like picture, with hyperthyroidism followed by hypothyroidism, decreased uptake on scanning, and a firm, tender gland.[35] *Pneumocystis* thyroiditis might result from the increased use of inhaled pentamidine, which is associated with extrapulmonary *Pneumocystis* infections.

CMV, MAI, *Cryptococcus*, and Kaposi's sarcoma have been demonstrated in the thyroid at autopsy but have not been related to clinical thyroid disease among patients with AIDS. Clinically apparent thyroidal abscesses from *Aspergillus* and *Rhodococcus equi* have been reported. Hypothalamic or pituitary replacement from opportunistic infections, such as toxoplasmosis and CMV, has also been reported to cause secondary hypothyroidism.

Medications can affect thyroid function. Rifampin influences hepatic clearance of thyroxine, and interferon is associated with an increased incidence of autoimmune hypothyroidism.

Fluid Balance and Electrolytes

Disorders of fluid balance and electrolytes are common among patients with AIDS. Hyponatremia may be seen in upward of 50% of patients and is most often related to the secretion of inappropriate antidiuretic hormone (SIADH). Hyperkalemia is also frequently reported and may be seen in association with various drugs, such as trimethoprim (Bactrim). More rarely, hyperkalemia may be associated with adrenal insufficiency.

Sodium

Hyponatremia (Na<130 mM/L) is seen in 40% to 60% of hospitalized patients with AIDS and 20% of outpatients. SIADH (volume-replete patients with low levels of serum sodium and inappropriately elevated urine osmolarity) is seen in 23% to 47% of hyponatremic patients. SIADH may be caused by various infections and tumors and is treated with fluid restriction and hypertonic saline if it is severe.

Adrenal insufficiency is documented in 30% of volume-deplete, hyponatremic HIV-infected patients.[36] Volume depletion (diarrhea, vomiting) with excessive free water and impaired water clearance (HIV nephropathy) can cause hyponatremia among ill HIV-infected patients, especially those in the hospital. Volume repletion is the treatment. Hyporeninemic hypoaldosteronism,[37] more typically associated with hyperkalemia, may be another cause of hyponatremia. Treatment is with mineralocorticoids. Medications such as vidarabine, miconazole, and pentamidine are associated with hyponatremia of unknown etiology. Hypernatremia may be caused by foscarnet-induced nephrogenic diabetes insipidus.

Potassium

Hyperkalemia occurs in 20% to 53% of AIDS patients taking trimethoprim because trimethoprim is structurally similar to amiloride and because it inhibits tubular potassium excretion.[38] Other potential etiologies include pentamidine-associated tubular nephropathy, HIV-nephropathy (glomerular sclerosis), primary adrenal insufficiency and rarely, hyporeninemic hypoaldosteronism. Physiologic studies investigating potassium balance in HIV-infected patients also suggest an inadequate aldosterone response to hyperkalemia in HIV-infected patients.[39]

Bone

Bone Loss

Reduced bone density is common among HIV-infected patients. Fairfield and colleagues demonstrated reduced bone density in the hip and spine among men with AIDS and weight loss.[40] Studies during the era of HAART, in patients without significant weight loss, also demonstrated reduced bone density. Tebas and colleagues demonstrated a significant reduction in lumbar spine bone density, as determined by dual-energy x-ray absorptiometry (DEXA), among HIV-infected men receiving combined antiretroviral therapy.[41] Osteoporosis or osteopenia, or both, were seen in 73% of HIV-infected versus 30% of HIV-negative patients of similar age. The study suggested that PI therapy was associated with reduced bone density. Men receiving PI therapy had an increased incidence of osteopenia and osteoporosis (relative risk [RR], 2.19; $P=0.02$) compared with HIV-infected men not receiving PI therapy and with non–HIV-infected men. In contrast, Mondy and coworkers showed a 46% prevalence of osteopenia or osteoporosis in a primarily (86%) male population, in whom traditional risk factors including low weight, smoking, and steroid use were associated with bone loss.[42] Duration of HAART, but not use of specific PIs, was associated with bone loss.[42] Likewise, Amiel and colleagues demonstrated a prevalence of osteoporosis of 16% in HIV-positive men compared with 4% in the control population. Age-adjusted bone density was reduced in association with HIV infection but was not affected by HIV treatment.[43]

Osteopenia was demonstrated in more than 50% of consecutively screened outpatients in either the hip or the spine and was 2.4 times as likely in HIV-infected women compared with age- and BMI-matched control subjects. Low bone density was associated with low weight and other nutritional factors[44] but not menstrual function or estrogen levels, arguing against an effect of simple estrogen deficiency. Markers of bone resorption were increased, but there was no association with specific PI use. In contrast, histomorphometric studies performed before the current era of potent antiretroviral therapy showed reduced bone turnover in association with increased disease severity.[45] Reduced vertebral bone density has also been associated with increased visceral adiposity among HIV-infected patients.[46] Researchers debate whether HIV can directly infect osteocytes, but preliminary data suggest that HIV is unlikely to affect osteoblasts and that these cells are unlikely to serve as a reservoir for HIV disease.[47]

Other studies in HIV-infected patients receiving HAART have investigated markers of bone resorption and formation and found evidence of increased bone turnover.[48] Tebas and colleagues evaluated serum and urine bone markers in 73 HIV-positive patients receiving PI therapy.[41] Increased serum bone alkaline phosphatase and urine *N*-telopeptides (NTXs) were found to be inversely correlated with bone mineral density T- and Z-scores measured by DEXA, suggesting an increased rate of bone turnover among HIV-infected patients receiving PI therapy.[41] Despite the evidence demonstrating reduced bone density and increased bone turnover, formal, longitudinal studies of fracture risk have not been performed in patients with HIV disease.

Reduced bone density has also been reported in HIV-infected children. O'Brien's group demonstrated reduced total body bone density in perinatally infected girls at age 9 years in association with increased NTX and parathyroid hormone (PTH) levels.[49] Bone density is reduced among children receiving HAART, and it is lowest among those with lipodystrophy.[50] Arpadi and coworkers demonstrated persistent reduction after controlling for height and weight, but the degree of bone loss increased with age.[51] In contrast to increased markers of resorption, reduced osteocalcin levels have been reported in HIV-infected children, suggesting reduced bone formation and a relative discrepancy between increased resorption and reduced formation in this group.[52] Similar to data in adults, bone density is related to insulin-like growth factor (IGF)-I in HIV-infected children, suggesting a potential effect of low growth hormone (GH) on bone.[53] Mora's group followed bone density longitudinally over 1 year to compare changes in HIV-infected children and control subjects. They demonstrated relative reductions in total body bone density accrual but not spinal bone density accrual, as well as relative increases in bone turnover.[50] Additional studies controlling for potential differences in bone size are necessary to assess changes in bone density among HIV-infected children.

A number of endocrine factors can contribute to reduced bone density in HIV-infected patients, including hypogonadism and relative GH deficiency associated with excess visceral adiposity. GH pulse area determined from overnight frequent sampling of GH was reduced in patients with central fat accumulation and correlated significantly with vertebral bone density.[46] PIs might also inhibit 1α-hydroxylase and result in vitamin D deficiency.[54]

Limited data are available on treatment strategies for bone loss in AIDS patients. Among patients with idiopathic bone loss and high bone turnover, recent studies suggest that alendronate is effective in increasing bone density, resulting in a 5.2% increase in spinal bone density over 48 weeks.[55] Among men with AIDS wasting, testosterone at high doses (200 mg/week) has been shown to increase bone density.[40]

Avascular Necrosis

Miller and colleagues demonstrated a 4.4% prevalence of avascular necrosis (AVN) among 339 asymptomatic HIV-infected patients.[56] A significant relationship was reported between AVN and prior use of systemic corticosteroids ($P=0.02$). Other potential factors significantly associated with an increased risk of AVN included the presence of anticardiolipin antibodies, as well as routine bodybuilding and its associated mechanical stress. The relationship between AVN and HAART is unclear. Gutierrez demonstrated an increased prevalence of AVN from 1.6 per 1000 patients during the early 1990s to 14 per 1000 patients in the late 1990s.[57] Ninety-one percent of patients had prior exposure to HAART and 70% had been given HAART before developing AVN.[57]

Calcium Homeostasis

Hypocalcemia is common in HIV-infected patients. Hypocalcemia determined from albumin-adjusted total calcium levels was demonstrated in 6.5% of a large cohort of patients with AIDS. Calcium decreased progressively with stage of disease. Among patients with hypocalcemia, 48% were vitamin D deficient, and the expected increase in PTH levels was lacking in the majority.[58] Jaeger and colleagues also demonstrated decreased PTH secretion in severely immunocompromised patients with AIDS, but the mechanism of PTH decrease is unknown.[59] In addition, decreased PTH can occur in the setting of hypomagnesemia during severe illness or in association with renal magnesium wasting. Vitamin D deficiency may be caused by malabsorption from AIDS enteropathy or by specific effects of antiretroviral drugs, such as an effect of PIs to inhibit 1α-hydroxylation of 25(OH)D_3 (25-hydroxyvitamin D_3).[54] Severe vitamin D deficiency of nutritional origin has also been described in HIV-infected children.[60] Recently, Earle and coworkers described three cases of Fanconi's syndrome in HIV-infected adults, characterized by excess phosphate excretion and osteomalacia in the context of tenofovir and cedofovir administration.[61] In addition, hypocalcemia related to severe illness may be caused by abnormal calcium-binding proteins or increased free fatty acid (FFA) levels.

A number of drugs can affect calcium homeostasis (see Table 37–1). Foscarnet complexes with calcium to decrease ionized calcium levels and can also induce severe hypomagnesemia. Pentamidine therapy has been associated with renal magnesium wasting and severe hypomagnesemia, which can cause hypocalcemia through decreased PTH release and resistance to circulating PTH. Ketoconazole inhibits 1,25$(OH)_2D_3$ (1,25-dihydroxyvitamin D_3) synthesis. Among patients with HIV disease, hypercalcemia can be caused by excessive 1,25$(OH)_2D_3$ production in the setting of granulomatous disease (tuberculosis) or lymphoma, by local osteoclastic bone resorption from disseminated CMV,[62] or by human T-lymphotropic virus 1 (HTLV-1)–related activation of PTH-related protein (PTHrP).

Growth Hormone

Significant abnormalities in the GH–IGF-1 axis occur in HIV-infected patients. Among patients with AIDS wasting and significant weight loss, GH levels are increased in association with reduced IGF-1 levels,[19] a pattern typical of GH resistance seen with malnutrition.[63] In contrast, in patients with HIV lipodystrophy and visceral fat accumulation, frequent sampling of GH levels over 24 hours has suggested a different pattern.[64] Mean overnight GH levels and GH pulse amplitude were decreased in this setting, whereas pulse frequency was not different compared with age- and BMI-matched nonlipodystrophic HIV and non–HIV-infected patients. Reduced GH levels were strongly predicted by increased visceral fat in the patients.

In subsequent studies, the percentage of patients failing a GHRH-arginine stimulation test using a highly stringent cutoff of 3.3 ng/mL was 18% in patients with lipodystrophy compared with 0% for age- and BMI-matched healthy control subjects. The prevalence of GH deficiency increased to 30% using a cutoff of 5 ng/mL. GH responses to GHRH-arginine were highly inversely correlated with visceral adiposity as well as with circulating FFA levels.[65] Using a subtraction algorithm, physiologic testing comparing stimulation with GHRH alone or GHRH-arginine demonstrated a significantly greater increase with the addition of arginine compared with control subjects, suggesting increased somatostatin tone in such patients.[66] Furthermore, levels of ghrelin, a stimulator of GH release, were reduced in patients with lipodystrophy and were associated with the peak GH response to GHRH.

A role for suppression of GH release by FFAs was suggested by experiments in which acipimox, a nicotinic acid derivative that blocks peripheral tissue lipolysis and lowers FFA levels was administered. Peak GH response to GHRH was increased in response to acipimox, in inverse association to the change in FFA.[66] In patients with AIDS wasting, GH levels are increased in association with GH resistance; in contrast, physiologic studies of GH in HIV-infected patients suggest a schema whereby increased somatostatin tone, reduced ghrelin, and increased lipolysis contribute to reduced GH secretion in viscerally obese HIV-infected patients with lipodystrophy.

GH and GH secretagogues have been used in HIV-infected patients both to increase lean body mass in sarcopenic patients with AIDS wasting and to reduce visceral adiposity in HIV-infected patients with the lipodystrophy syndrome. Among patients with AIDS wasting, Schambelan and coworkers investigated the effects of high-dose supraphysiologic GH (0.1 mg/kg per day). Relatively small but significant effects on weight (1.6 kg) were seen over 3 months in a placebo-controlled study.[67] Larger effects on lean body mass (3.0 kg) were achieved over 3 months but a portion of this gain was attributed to increased total body water (Fig. 37–5).[67] GH administration at 0.1 mg/kg has also been shown to increase work output during treadmill exercise[67] and quality of life, as well as peripheral muscle oxygen extraction and utilization in patients with AIDS wasting.[68]

Other studies have investigated combination GH and IGF-1 therapy in AIDS wasting. However, use of a lower GH dose (0.68 mg/day) and IGF-1 (10 mg/day) was only marginally effective at increasing lean body mass, although it resulted in significant fat loss,[69] suggesting that large doses of GH may be necessary to significantly increase lean mass in patients with AIDS wasting and nutritionally mediated resistance to GH. Furthermore, responsiveness of muscle protein synthesis to GH has been shown to decline with diseased severity.[70]

Short-term high-dose GH (6 mg/day) has also been used successfully to increase lean body mass at the time of acute opportunistic infection. However, high-dose GH is associated with side effects including hyperglycemia and fluid retention[71] and is not well tolerated in the long term. GH has not been shown to worsen viral load among patients with HIV disease, and it was shown to increase thymic mass and circulating CD4 cells in one study.[72]

Growth hormone has also been used to reduce visceral fat in patients with the HIV lipodystrophy syndrome. Use of high-dose GH (6 mg/day) over 12 weeks significantly decreased visceral fat and cholesterol, but it also reduced subcutaneous fat and was associated with joint pain and hyperglycemia. In a large randomized, placebo-controlled study, Kotler and colleagues investigated 4 mg of daily GH compared with treatment on alternate days with GH and placebo.[73] The 4-mg daily dose was associated with an −18.8% reduction in visceral adipose tissue over 12 weeks, whereas the alternating dose reduced visceral adipose tissue by −16.8%. Both doses reduced total and non-HDL cholesterol levels but also increased glucose levels.[73] Lower doses of GH at 1 mg/day did not decrease visceral adipose tissue.[74]

In contrast, GH secretagogues have been used to successfully increase lean body mass and reduce visceral and truncal fat, without significant effects on glucose. Subcutaneous GHRH1-29 at a dose of 1 mg twice a day reduced visceral and truncal fat and increased extremity fat, thereby improving the ratio of truncal to extremity fat (Fig. 37–6).[75] A synthetically modified form of GHRH1-44 also reduced truncal fat without decreasing extremity fat over 12 weeks.[76] Use of GH secretagogues was associated with physiologic increases in IGF-1 levels and was not associated with increased glucose levels. In addition, GHRH was shown to increase bone turnover in HIV-infected patients.[46]

Currently, GH and GH secretagogue treatment remains investigational for HIV lipodystrophy, but large phase III trials are under way to establish the long-term clinical benefits of this therapeutic strategy to reduce visceral adiposity. In contrast, GH

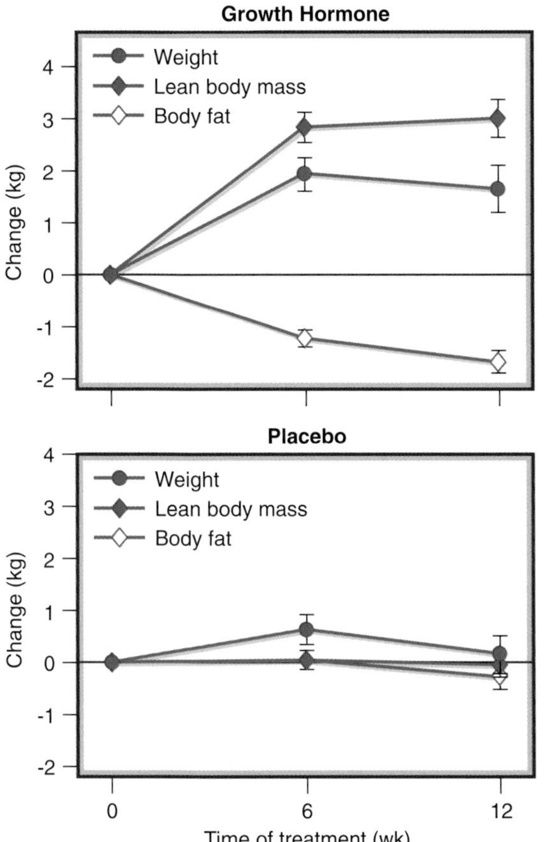

Figure 37–5 ▪ Effects of 3 months of treatment with growth hormone *(left panel)* or placebo *(right panel)* on change in weight *(closed circles)*, lean body mass *(closed diamonds)*, and body fat *(open diamonds)* in subjects with HIV wasting. (Data from Schambelan M, Mulligan K, Grunfeld C, et al. Recombinant human growth hormone in patients with HIV-associated wasting: a randomized, placebo-controlled trial. Serostim Study Group. Ann Intern Med 1996;125[11]:873-882, with permission.)

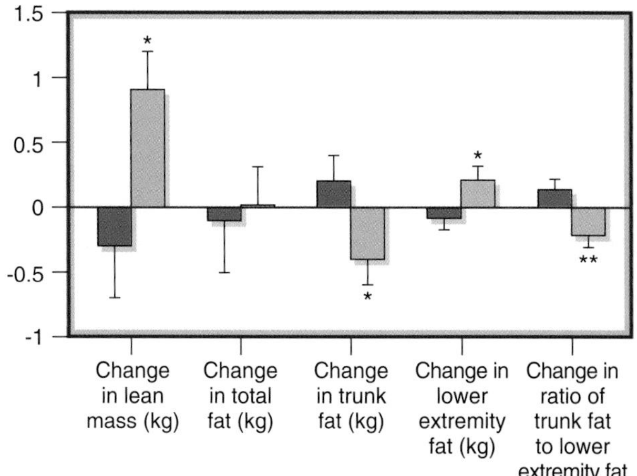

Figure 37–6 ▪ Effects of 3 months of treatment with growth hormone–releasing hormone *(purple)* vs. placebo *(blue)* on body composition in HIV-lipodystrophic men. *P=0.05, **P=0.01. (Data modified from Koutkia P, Canavan B, Breu J, et al. Growth hormone–releasing hormone in HIV-infected men with lipodystrophy: a randomized, controlled trial. JAMA 2004;292:210-218, with permission.)

is approved by the U.S. Food and Drug Administration (FDA) to treat severe loss of muscle mass in the AIDS wasting syndrome (see later).

GH deficiency is a potential cause of growth failure in HIV-infected children,[77] and treatment with GH results in improved auxologic parameters in such children.[78] Increased IGF binding protein 3 (IGFBP3) proteolysis and reduced IGF-1, IGFBP3, and acid labile subunit of the IGFBP3 ternary complex are demonstrated among HIV-infected children with failure to thrive.[79] IGF-I and IGFBP3 responses to GH may be impaired in HIV-infected children,[80] suggesting a degree of GH insensitivity in this population, which might improve with weight and improved immune function in response to HAART.[81] GH deficiency can also disrupt the normal thymic development in HIV-infected children.[82] GH has been used to increase height in HIV-infected children with normal GH responses to stimulatory testing.[78] Among HIV-infected children with lipodystrophy, reduced GH secretion is associated with excess visceral adiposity.[83]

Glucose Homeostasis and Pancreatic Function

Disorders of glucose homeostasis were relatively infrequent prior to the institution of potent antiretroviral therapy, but they are common in association with dyslipidemia and fat redistribution in the HIV lipodystrophy syndrome (see the discussion under "HIV Lipodystrophy Syndrome," later). The pancreas is a frequent target of opportunistic infections and malignancies in patients with HIV disease. However, clinical endocrine dysfunction rarely results, except in cases of massive pancreatic replacement from lymphoma or Kaposi's sarcoma. For example, opportunistic infections of the pancreas are seen on postmortem examination but are rarely clinically relevant.

More commonly, pancreatitis and hypoglycemia follow the use of certain drugs, such as pentamidine, didanosine, or zalcitabine. Hypoglycemia can result from pentamidine administration secondary to islet cell inflammation and insulin release, especially in the context of high dose therapy and azotemia. Subsequently, chronic hyperglycemia from pancreatic beta cell destruction can follow pentamidine use. Megestrol acetate use has been associated with new-onset diabetes mellitus because of its potent glucocorticoid action. Pancreatitis is common among patients with HIV and most often related to a drug effect, especially from pentamidine, trimethoprim, didanosine, or zalcitabine. Amylase levels might also be elevated in HIV-infected patients secondary to macroamylasemia and salivary amylase.

AIDS Wasting Syndrome

Wasting is a common feature of progressive HIV disease, known originally as "slim disease." The AIDS wasting syndrome is currently defined by body weight less than 90% of ideal or weight loss greater than 10% of body weight over 3 months. It is characterized by a disproportionate loss of lean body mass, with a relative sparing of body fat, particularly in men. In women, fat mass may be lost disproportionately with disease progression.[22] The loss of lean body mass occurs early and can antedate weight loss.[84] Muscle wasting, weakness, increased resting energy expenditure (8% to 9% at baseline), and increased triglyceride levels are also features of this disease. Macallan and colleagues demonstrated that energy expenditure fell during periods of rapid weight loss, but less than the decrease in caloric intake.[85]

Cytokines associated with severe illness can increase energy expenditure and decrease appetite. In addition, chronic weight loss may be associated with gastrointestinal disease, including malabsorption.[86] Weight loss is a significant predictor of mortality in HIV infection: BMI of less than 18.4 kg/m^2 is associated with a 2.2-fold increase in mortality, and BMI of less than 16.0 kg/m^2 is associated with a 4.4-fold increase in mortality.[87] Wasting remains common in the era of HAART, estimated at 34% in a longitudinal cohort study.[88]

One potential endocrine mechanism that might predispose to a disproportionate loss of lean body mass is hypogonadism. Hypogonadism, most usually central in etiology, is observed in 30% to 50% of men with AIDS wasting and is associated with decreased lean body mass, decreased muscle mass, and decreased exercise functional capacity.[19] Testosterone has been successfully used to increase lean body mass in men with AIDS wasting (see Table 37–2). Route of administration can be either intramuscular (testosterone enanthate or cypionate) or transdermal (scrotal, nonscrotal, or newer gel preparations). Skin reaction is reported in up to 30% with the nonscrotal skin patches. Randomized studies of IM testosterone for hypogonadal men with AIDS wasting suggest a beneficial effect of testosterone administration on lean body mass (2.0 kg over 6 months) and improved quality of life.[89] Testosterone in women with AIDS wasting has also recently been shown to be safe and well tolerated and to increase physical function over 6 months.[90]

Although a limited number of studies (see Table 37–2) have shown a benefit of anabolic steroids in HIV-infected patients with wasting, these agents potently suppress endogenous gonadal function and can thus cause hypogonadism. Methyltestosterone and anabolic steroids can cause problems with the liver including peliosis hepatitis, worsening liver function, and, potentially, malignancy. Oxandrolone, an oral anabolic steroid, was shown to be safe but ineffective for AIDS wasting at low doses.[91] Doses higher than 20 mg/day may be associated with liver dysfunction. Recently, nandrolone (100 mg IM every other week) was shown to be effective in increasing weight and lean body mass in HIV-infected women with weight loss.[92] Anabolic steroids are associated with decreased HDL and other side effects, though, and hold no advantage over natural testosterone in treating hypogonadism associated with AIDS-related weight loss. Short-term use of anabolic steroids may be considered in eugonadal patients with severe wasting, but may be associated with adverse effects.

Megestrol acetate (Megace) is a synthetic progestational agent with glucocorticoid-like properties. Two randomized studies, one by Von Roenns' group[93] and one by Oster's group,[94] show that megestrol acetate increases weight 3 to 4 kg over 12 weeks with an increase in caloric intake (+688 kcal/day). However, the weight increase is almost entirely fat mass without an increase in lean body mass. In addition, megestrol acetate, because of its glucocorticoid-like properties, is associated with a number of side effects, including hypogonadism and hyperglycemia, and abrupt withdrawal can precipitate adrenal crisis. In children, megestrol acetate promotes weight gain without improving linear growth.[95]

A number of other agents have been used in the setting of AIDS wasting. Thalidomide blocks the action of TNF-α and decreases esophageal ulcers in AIDS patients.[96] Clinical studies demonstrate a modest beneficial short-term effect of thalidomide on weight indices, but there are also significant associated adverse effects, including rash and fever. Human chorionic gonadotropin (hCG) results in increased testosterone levels and might have independent effects that inhibit Kaposi's sarcoma.[97] No data are available from randomized, controlled studies to determine the effects on wasting in humans. Small short-term studies have also shown benefits of an amino acid mixture of glutamine and arginine to increase lean body mass.[98] In contrast, no effects of omega-3 fatty acids[99] or pentoxyfiline[100] on weight indices have been shown.

Progressive resistance training has been shown to increase lean body mass by 2.3 kg over 12 weeks in men with AIDS wasting. Resistance training may be even more effective when combined with anabolic therapies, such as testosterone,[101] oxandrolone,[101] or nandrolone.[103]

In addition, patients with AIDS wasting can demonstrate a typical pattern of nutrition-related GH resistance. These patients exhibit elevated GH levels but decreased IGF-1, the primary hormone mediating the action of GH on muscle, suggesting GH resistance.[104,105] GH resistance is likely a secondary phenomenon in AIDS wasting, but the HIV envelope protein gp120 has been shown to decrease GH release in vitro and in animal studies,[106] potentially leading to a relative reduction in GH secretion. GH at supraphysiologic doses has been shown to increase lean body mass in AIDS wasting and is FDA approved for this purpose at a dose of 6 mg/day. However, caution should be used in the long-term treatment of HIV patients with this dose, which can cause acute and chronic side effects of GH excess.

Taken together, the data suggest a systematic multidisciplinary approach to the AIDS wasting syndrome. Optimization of antiretroviral therapy is paramount in conjunction with provision of adequate nutrition and protein intake. However, even in this context, weight and muscle loss can occur due to the highly catabolic nature of the disease. In such cases, endocrine evaluation should include assessment of gonadal function, which is often reduced. Testosterone administration can prove useful to increase lean body mass in this context, and it may be used in conjunction with resistance training in appropriate patients to optimally increase muscle mass. Growth hormone levels are increased in AIDS wasting, but supraphysiologic administration, as approved by the FDA, can further increase lean body mass. This strategy is best reserved for severe wasting refractory to other treatments. Other therapeutic strategies that increase weight by stimulating appetite, including megestrol acetate, are not associated with gain in lean body mass and may be associated with side effects.

HIV Lipodystrophy Syndrome

The HIV lipodystrophy syndrome is characterized by changes in body composition such as buffalo hump, truncal obesity, facial and peripheral fat atrophy, and breast enlargement in women. In addition, this syndrome is characterized by insulin resistance and hyperglycemia, as well as hypertriglyceridemia. Not all components of the syndrome are present in all patients, so there is significant variability and heterogeneity in the presentation.

Prevalence

The HIV lipodystrophy syndrome is observed in approximately 40% to 50% of ambulatory HIV-infected patients,[107] with a higher proportion in patients receiving HAART. However, the prevalence of HIV lipodystrophy varies greatly across populations and also among studies, in part due to differences in body composition characteristics used to define the syndrome. In an early study, Carr and coworkers investigated body composition by DEXA, clinical examination, and patient self-report. The lipodystrophy syndrome was noted in 63% of protease inhibitor–treated patients.[108] Among women, Dong and colleagues noted a prevalence of 16% by self-report.[109] Among the affected patients, 71% noted breast enlargement. HIV lipodystrophy has been most widely recognized since the introduction of HAART, but characteristics of the syndrome, including abnormal fat distribution, can be seen in antiretroviral-naïve patients.

Etiology

Most studies indicate that the HIV lipodystrophy syndrome is associated with the use of PPIs. However, a number of studies have documented cases of the lipodystrophy syndrome occurring among patients who are not receiving PIs.[110] These studies raise the question of whether the syndrome is due to PI therapy alone, other agents, or improved immune function due to HAART.

In patients with improved immune function and weight gain, abnormal repartitioning of energy substrate can occur. To support this argument, Kotler and colleagues have analyzed data from patients prior to the era of PI therapy, noting an increased waist-to-hip ratio. PIs might have direct effects on adipogenesis (via inhibition of nuclear localization of sterol regulatory element–binding protein 1 [SREBP1] and reduction in peroxisome proliferator-activated receptor γ [PPARγ] expression),[111] and nucleoside reverse transcriptase inhibitors (NRTIs) might have direct effects on lipolysis,[112] contributing to fat redistribution and further insulin resistance.

An effect of NRTIs to impair mitochondrial polymerase γ and alter mitochondrial function has been observed in the subcutaneous fat of lipoatrophic patients[113] and might also contribute to subcutaneous fat loss. Reduced mitochondrial DNA is most often associated with the use of specific NRTIs, including stavudine.[114] The etiology for central adiposity among HIV-infected patients receiving HAART is unknown, but the syndrome might result from nutrient partitioning to relatively preserved central adipose stores less affected by NRTI administration and mitochondrial toxicity. Alternatively, fat redistribution might result in part from altered cytokines, including increased IL-6 and TNF,[115] or altered steroid milieu (Fig. 37–7).

The lipodystrophy syndrome bears some similarities to Cushing's syndrome, with dorsocervical fat accumulation and centripetal fat distribution, but it is not associated with more specific stigmata of true Cushing's syndrome, including proximal muscle weakness, facial plethora, thin skin, bruising, or violaceous striae, and it has therefore been termed a pseudo-Cushing's syndrome.[110] Miller and colleagues observed normal cortisol levels and adequate suppression in response to dexamethasone among HIV-infected patients with cushingoid features.[110]

Yanovski and colleagues compared HIV-infected patients who had PI-associated lipodystrophic changes in fat with control patients and those with true Cushing's syndrome.[116] In contrast to patients with true Cushing's syndrome, patients with PI-associated lipodystrophy demonstrated normal diurnal variation in cortisol levels. Their 24-hour urine free cortisol levels were reduced and 17-hydroxysteroid levels were increased compared with those of controls. ACTH levels were somewhat increased after corticotropin-releasing hormone testing, but these changes did not appear to be related to changes in abdominal adiposity and did not suggest pathologic activation of the cortisol axis as an etiology of lipodystrophic changes in fat distribution.

In contrast, stress activation of the adrenal axis can contribute to increased cortisol production. Evidence of shunting toward cortisol production and away from androgen production in the adrenal glands has been demonstrated in association with weight loss, disease severity, and immune compromise in HIV-infected patients (see Fig. 37–3).[7,117] Among patients with HIV lipodystrophy, increased 11β-hydroxysteroid dehydrogenase expression in subcutaneous adipose tissue has been demonstrated in association with an increased ratio of urinary cortisol to cortisone metabolites and might also contribute to increased cortisol production.[118]

Other abnormalities of steroid metabolism have been noted in lipodystrophy. In a longitudinal evaluation, the development of lipodystrophy was associated with reduced DHEA, increased cortisol-to-DHEA ratio, and increased IFN-α.[119] Increased

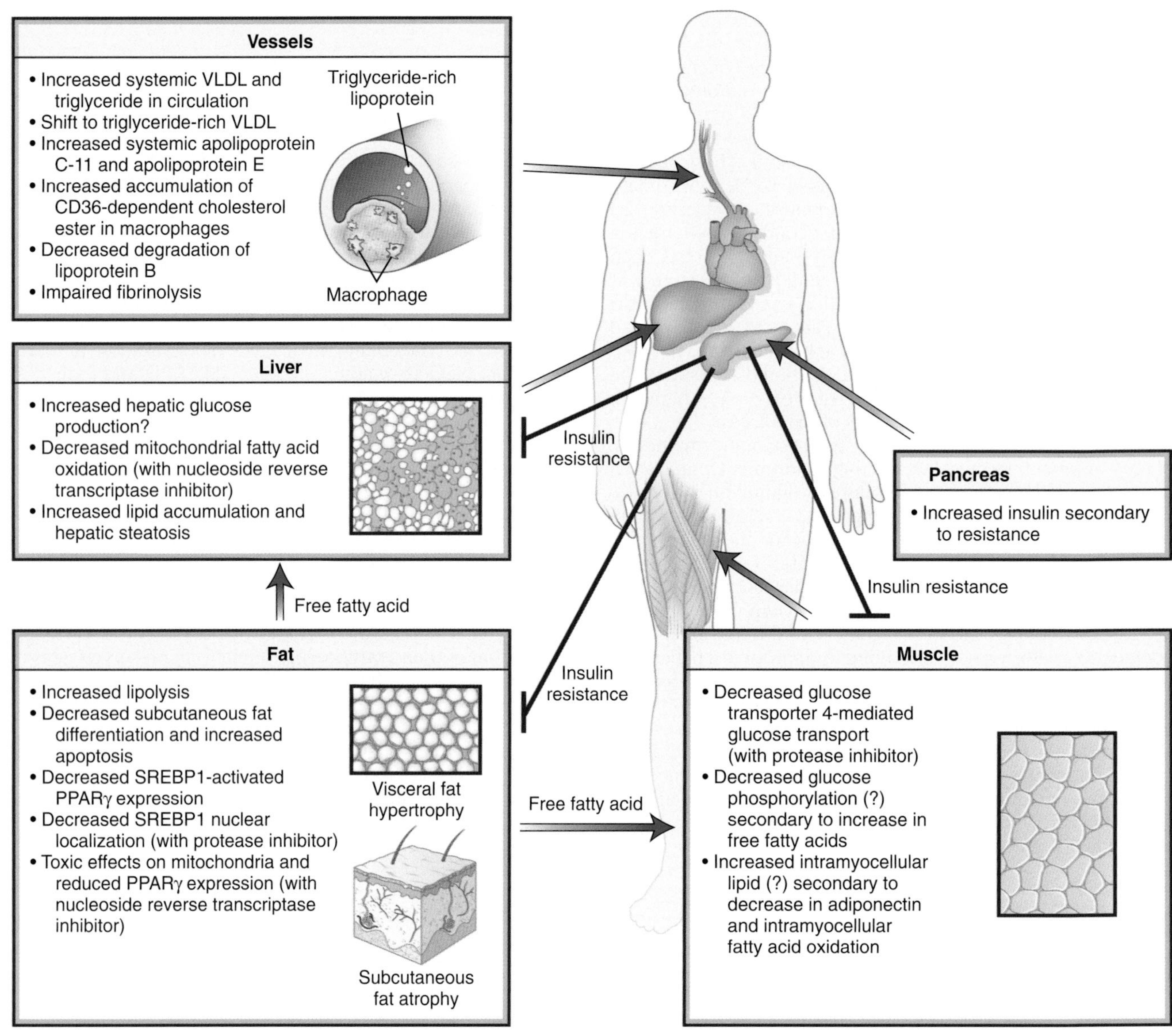

Figure 37–7 ▪ Potential mechanisms underlying HIV-related metabolic abnormalities. PPAR, peroxisome proliferator–activated receptor; SREBP, sterol regulatory element–binding protein; VLDL, very-low-density lipoprotein. (From Grinspoon S, Carr A. Cardiovascular risk and body fat abnormalities in HIV-infected adults. N Engl J Med 2005;352[1]:48-62, with permission.)

cortisol regeneration from affected fat depots might contribute to insulin resistance and further fat redistribution.

Lipid Abnormalities

Lipid abnormalities are highly prevalent among HIV-infected patients, particularly those with changes in fat distribution. Hypertriglyceridemia has long been associated with HIV infection and was observed before the introduction of potent antiretroviral therapy. It is related in part to increased very-low-density lipoprotein (VLDL) secretion and decreased clearance.[120] The etiology of these changes is not known but might relate to the effects of viral infection itself, altered cytokines, including IFN-α,[121] or increased apolipoprotein E.[122] In longitudinal studies, reductions in HDL, total, and low-density lipoprotein (LDL) cholesterol are observed with seroconversion. With antiretroviral treatment, total cholesterol and LDL rise to preinfection levels, but low HDL levels persist.[123]

Among HIV-infected patients receiving combination antiretroviral therapy including a PI, hypercholesterolemia (>240 mg/dL), hypertriglyceridemia (>200 mg/dL), and low HDL (<35 mg/dL) were reported in 27%, 40%, and 27% respectively, compared with corresponding percentages of 8%, 15%, and 26% in previously untreated patients.[124] Among patients with changes in fat distribution, 57% demonstrated hypertriglyceridemia and 46% low HDL in comparison with an age- and BMI-matched cohort from the Framingham Offspring Study (Fig. 37–8).[125] Severe dyslipidemia among HIV-infected patients might result from the effects of antiretroviral drugs, including specific PIs, such as ritonavir, which have been shown to increase triglyceride levels.[126] PIs might also be associated with an atherogenic dyslipidemia and an increase in small dense LDL2,[127] increased

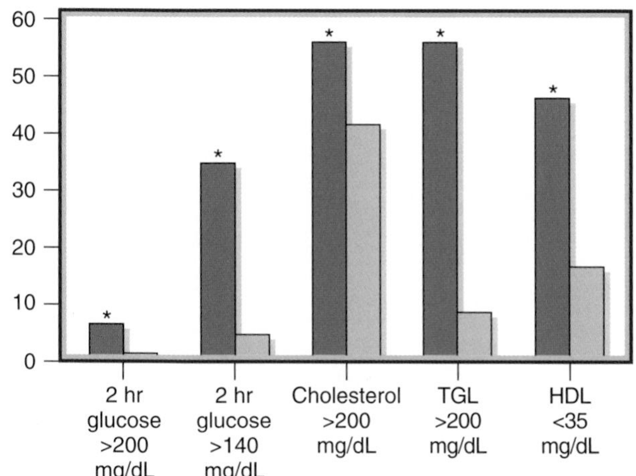

Figure 37–8 ■ Percentage of HIV-infected subjects with lipodystrophy *(blue bars)* compared with age- and BMI-matched controls *(purple bars)* from the Framingham cohort. The readings for the metabolic profile are the glucose readings 2 hours after the oral glucose tolerance test. *P=0.05. Chol, cholesterol; HDL, high-density lipoprotein; TGL, triglyceride lipoprotein. (Data modified from Hadigan C, Meigs JB, Corcoran C, et al. Metabolic abnormalities and cardiovascular disease risk factors in adults with human immunodeficiency virus infection and lipodystrophy. Clin Infect Dis 2001;32[1]:130-139, with permission.)

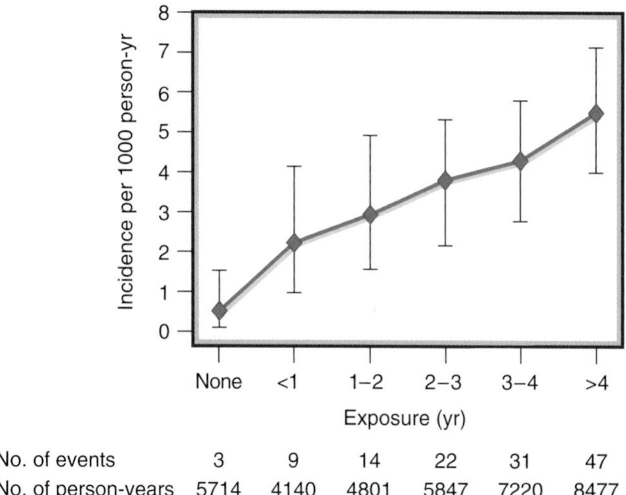

No. of events	3	9	14	22	31	47
No. of person-years	5714	4140	4801	5847	7220	8477

Figure 37–9 ■ Incidence of myocardial infarction stratified by time of exposure to highly active antiretroviral therapy (the DAD study). (Data from Friis-Moller N, Sabin CA, Weber R, et al. Combination antiretroviral therapy and the risk of myocardial infarction. N Engl J Med 2003;349[21]:1993-2003, with permission.)

apolipoprotein C-III and apolipoprotein E and decreased proteosomal degradation of apolipoprotein B.[128,129]

Hyperglycemia and Insulin Resistance

Insulin resistance and diabetes mellitus are increasingly common among HIV-infected patients with the lipodystrophy syndrome. In a longitudinal study, diabetes mellitus was 3.1 times more likely to develop in HIV-infected patients receiving combination antiretroviral therapy than in control subjects.[130] Among HIV-infected patients with changes in fat distribution, including visceral adiposity and loss of subcutaneous fat, impaired glucose tolerance is seen in approximately 35% of patients (see Fig. 37–8).[125] Hyperinsulinemia in such patients is consistent with insulin resistance as the primary mechanism for impaired glucose tolerance and diabetes. Insulin resistance among HIV-infected women is not associated with the typical features, such as polycystic ovary syndrome, that are common in the general population with insulin resistance.[131]

The mechanisms of insulin resistance among HIV-infected patients may be caused by the abnormal fat distribution itself, such as increased central adiposity,[132] loss of peripheral subcutaneous fat,[133] altered cytokines (e.g., low adiponectin[134] or elevated TNF[133]), or other factors, including increased lipolysis,[135] and increased accumulation of fat in the muscle[136] and liver.[137] In addition, significant evidence suggests direct effects of specific antiretroviral drugs to reduce insulin sensitivity. PIs have now been shown to decrease glucose uptake by inhibiting the transport function of GLUT-4 in vitro,[138] and they have been shown to reduce insulin sensitivity in vivo.[139] NRTIs are associated with insulin resistance, which may be a direct effect, potentially related to mitochondrial toxicity[139a] or through effects on subcutaneous fat.[140]

Cardiovascular Risk in HIV Lipodystrophy

Cardiovascular disease is increased among HIV-infected patients treated with HAART. The Framingham equation predicts increased myocardial infarction (MI) rates among HIV-infected patients with fat redistribution.[141] More than 40% of such subjects meet the definition of the metabolic syndrome, and predicted MI rates are most increased in this subgroup.[141] Risk factors for cardiovascular disease include insulin resistance, atherogenic dyslipidemia,[142] truncal adiposity, hypertension,[143] impaired fibrinolysis, and increased plasminogen activator inhibitor 1 (PAI-1) and tissue plasminogen activator (tPA) levels,[144] as well as increased C-reactive protein (CRP) and reduced adiponectin.[145] Surrogate markers, including carotid intima-medial thickness and endothelial function suggest increased cardiovascular disease in HIV-infected patients. Hsue and coworkers demonstrated increased carotid intima-medial thickness in HIV-infected patients in association with cigarette smoking, increased LDL, and hypertension.[146] Progression rates were also greater in HIV-infected patients during longitudinal follow-up.

Endothelial dysfunction, as determined by impaired flow-mediated dilation, is seen among HIV-infected adults receiving PIs.[142] Abnormal endothelial function correlated with dyslipidemia, including increased chylomicrons, VLDL, and IDL and reduced HDL. Protease inhibitors might also directly affect endothelial function through an effect on endothelial nitric oxide synthase (eNOS).[147] Pravastatin improves lipid parameters and tends to improve endothelial function in HIV-infected patients receiving a PI.[148] In addition, evidence suggests increased intima-medial thickness and reduced flow-mediated dilation in children receiving PIs.[149]

Krause and coworkers demonstrated a relative hazard ratio of 2.6 for increased MIs in HIV-infected patients receiving a PI for 18 months or more in a French cohort.[150] In contrast, data from a U.S. retrospective cohort study demonstrated an increased MI rate among HIV-infected patients but did not suggest an independent effect of PIs.[151] In retrospective studies, the risk of coronary heart disease related to antiretroviral therapy use may be most pronounced among younger HIV-infected patients.[152] In a large prospective study of 23,468 patients, the covariate-adjusted risk was 1.26 per each additional year of antiretroviral exposure (Fig. 37–9). Other risk factors included male gender, diabetes, age, previous MI, hypertension, and dyslipidemia.[153] Controlling for dyslipidemia significantly reduced the effects of HAART exposure, suggesting that dyslipidemia is a significant mechanism by which HAART contributes to excess coronary artery disease in HIV-infected patients.

Women represent an increasing percentage of patients with clinical lipodystrophy and are at risk for increased cardiovascular disease. Increased waist-to-hip ratio, visceral adiposity, triglyceride, and LDL and reduced HDL have been demonstrated in HIV-infected women compared with age- and BMI-matched control subjects. In addition to traditional risk factors, CRP and IL-6 are increased and adiponectin is reduced. Central adiposity, more than other factors, was significantly predictive of abnormal cardiovascular disease risk indices, including newer inflammatory indices.[145] In contrast, HIV status and viral load were not predictive, suggesting that central adiposity and changes in fat distribution are primarily responsible for increased cardiovascular disease risk in HIV-infected women.

Treatment

There are a number of options available for the treatment of body composition and metabolic abnormalities in HIV-infected patients. Switching to less toxic NRTIs or PIs may be useful for improving changes in fat distribution and hyperlipidemia.[154] Exercise and lifestyle modification can improve lipid levels and visceral adiposity associated with the lipodystrophy syndrome.[155] Progressive resistance training may also confer significant benefits on glucose homeostasis in HIV-infected patients with the lipodystrophy syndrome through a reduction in muscle adiposity.[156] However, resistance training is unlikely to improve the often debilitating loss of subcutaneous fat associated with the lipodystrophy syndrome.

Testosterone and Anabolic Steroids

Testosterone reduces fat and builds muscle mass in hypogonadal HIV-infected men,[89] as in non–HIV-infected men, and reduces total fat but not visceral fat the lipodystrophy syndrome.[156b] Among HIV-infected patients without clinically defined lipodystrophy, nandrolone results in reduced HDL with no effect on LDL particle size.[157] Effects of high-dose testosterone and anabolic steroids on lipid parameters can limit the usefulness of this class of drugs to reduce visceral fat in the HIV lipodystrophy syndrome.

Insulin-Sensitizing Agents

Significant insulin resistance occurs among HIV-infected patients with the lipodystrophy syndrome receiving HAART. Among non–HIV-infected persons, numerous studies have documented that hyperinsulinemia and truncal obesity are strong independent risk factors contributing to coronary artery disease with significant associated morbidity and mortality. In non–HIV-infected insulin-resistant but nondiabetic populations, such as patients with polycystic ovary disease, the use of insulin-sensitizing agents has resulted in successful reduction of fasting hyperinsulinemia and weight loss. Metformin is particularly appropriate for use in patents with significant truncal adiposity and increased FFA concentrations, in whom insulin resistance is in part attributable to increased hepatic glucose production. In addition, metformin has a modest favorable effect on lipids. In patients with hyperlipidemia, metformin has been demonstrated to decrease triglyceride and LDL levels without adversely affecting other parameters. The modest 10% to 20% reduction in plasma triglyceride levels is believed to be caused by decreased hepatic VLDL production.

The effects of metformin were recently reported in HIV-infected patients with the lipodystrophy syndrome, using oral metformin 500 mg twice a day in a randomized 12-week study.[158] Hadigan's and colleagues demonstrated that low-dose metformin used over 12 weeks significantly reduced insulin resistance, waist circumference, diastolic blood pressure, and tPA and PAI concentrations, thus improving the cardiovascular risk profiles of such patients (Fig. 37–10).[144,158] The effects of metformin were sustained over 9 months.[159] These data also suggest the need for further studies to assess the long-term efficacy of metformin in terms of fat redistribution and cardiovascular risk. In a randomized trial, the effects of metformin and progressive resistance training were compared with metformin alone, and the addition of progressive resistance training further significantly improved central adiposity, blood pressure, and insulin resistance.[160]

The loss of subcutaneous fat in patients with the HIV lipodystrophy syndrome might further contribute to insulin resistance by limiting peripheral glucose and triglyceride uptake. Therefore, attention has focused on insulin-sensitizing strategies that

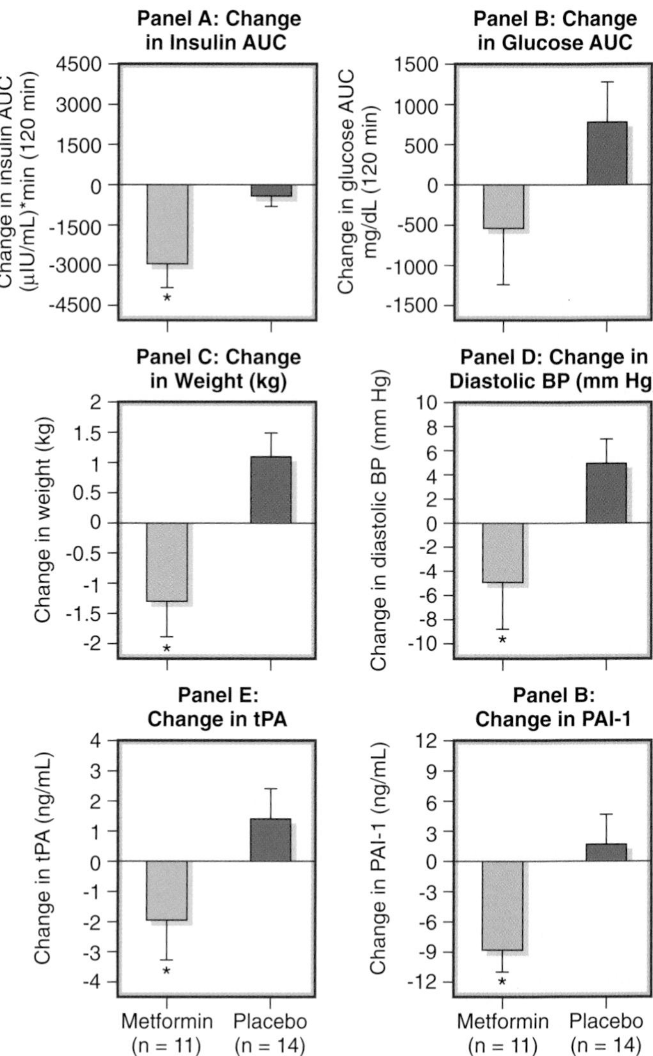

Figure 37–10 ▪ Effects of 3 months of treatment with metformin *(purple)* vs. placebo *(blue)* on insulin and glucose response to oral glucose tolerance test, weight, blood pressure, tPA, and PAI-1 in 26 HIV-lipodystrophic subjects. **P*=0.05. AUC, area under the curve; BP, blood pressure; PAI, plasminogen activator inhibitor; tPA, tissue plasminogen activator. (Data modified from Hadigan C, Meigs JB, Rabe J, et al. Increased PAI-1 and tPA antigen levels are reduced with metformin therapy in HIV-infected patients with fat redistribution and insulin resistance. J Clin Endocrinol Metab 2001;86[2]:939-943; and Hadigan C, Corcoran C, Basgoz N, et al. Metformin in the treatment of HIV lipodystrophy syndrome: a randomized controlled trial. JAMA 2000;284[4]:472-477; with permission.)

might act to increase subcutaneous adipogenesis. Metformin, although a potent insulin-sensitizing agent, is not expected to restore peripheral adipogenesis but rather to act primarily via a reduction of hepatic insulin resistance. In contrast, a novel class of therapeutic agents, the thiazolidinediones (TZDs) have been shown to promote adipogenesis, primarily through activation of PPARγ. Although the TZDs have effects on both hepatic and peripheral insulin resistance, the dominant effect is to improve peripheral glucose uptake. For example, troglitazone was shown to significantly increase peripheral glucose uptake with only modest effects on hepatic insulin sensitivity in a recently completed study of patients with type 2 diabetes (T2DM). TZDs have potent effects on muscle glucose uptake.

The therapeutic efficacy of the TZDs has been well established among patients with T2DM. Short-term studies have demonstrated an effect on HbA_{1c} and fasting glucose after 12 weeks. The TZDs also reduce plasma triglyceride levels by 10% to 20% and increase HDL by 5% to 10% in diabetic patients. Weight has been reported to increase in response to TZDs, in contrast to metformin, which is associated with weight loss. Hepatic toxicity has been reported among patients receiving troglitazone, but not in patients receiving rosiglitazone. In a series of clinical trials, rosiglitazone was efficacious in reducing HbA_{1c} and fasting glucose in non–HIV-infected patients with diabetes, and it was safe, with no liver toxicity. Based on the clinical experience to date with rosiglitazone and its known effects to stimulate insulin sensitivity through PPARγ and promote adipogenesis, rosiglitazone might be appropriate to reverse insulin resistance and promote adipogenesis in patients with HIV lipodystrophy, in whom subcutaneous fat cell loss has been shown to correlate inversely with insulin resistance.

Gelato and colleagues demonstrated that TZDs increase fat mass and improve insulin resistance in an open-label study.[161] In a 3-month randomized, placebo-controlled study involving 28 patients selected based on insulin resistance, rosiglitazone was shown to improve insulin sensitivity, adiponectin, FFA, and subcutaneous fat mass.[162] In contrast, an effect of rosiglitazone on subcutaneous fat was not shown over 48 weeks in patients with lipoatrophy, who were selected for fat loss but not for insulin resistance.[163] Adiponectin significantly increased and resistin levels decreased in response to rosiglitazone in HIV lipodystrophy, changes that might contribute to improved insulin sensitivity.[162,164] Rosiglitazone and other such TZDs may be effective in selective subpopulations of HIV-infected patients, particularly those with insulin resistance.[165] Slight but significant adverse effects on lipid levels suggest that other agents, including pioglitazone, should be investigated to optimize effects on lipid levels. In addition, the thiazolidinediones are not appropriate for severely overweight patients with HIV lipodystrophy but rather are best reserved for patients with lipoatrophy and insulin resistance.

Lipid Management

Lipid abnormalities are common among HIV-infected patients in general, and particularly those with the HIV lipodystrophy syndrome. Hypertriglyceridemia is more common than hypercholesterolemia and is associated with HIV infection and increased VLDL secretion. In addition to the effects of HIV itself, specific antiviral drugs contribute significantly to hypertriglyceridemia. Mulligan and colleagues demonstrated that changes in lipid levels occur within 3 months of PI therapy,[166] and Purnell's group recently confirmed significant increases in triglyceride levels among HIV-negative patients receiving a short course of ritonavir after 2 weeks.[126] Hypertriglyceridemia is most severe among patients treated with ritonavir or a ritonavir-saquinavir combination. Nelfinavir and indinavir are less often associated with abnormalities in triglyceride levels. Among the currently approved PIs, atazanavir is least often associated with hyperlipidemia.[167]

Treatment for hyperlipidemia among HIV-infected patients is indicated to reduce cardiovascular risk and should proceed according to standard National Cholesterol Education Program (NCEP) guidelines. Severe hypertriglyceridemia should be treated to reduce the risk of pancreatitis. Triglyceride levels greater than 1000 mg/dL are highly associated with pancreatitis, but lesser elevations are often asymptomatic and of unknown risk. If triglyceride levels increase substantially (>750 mg/dL), lipid-lowering therapy should be considered. An initial option in patients with severe elevations in triglyceride levels is to switch treatment to a PI less likely to cause dyslipidemia.

Triglyceride levels are reduced approximately 20% by diet[168] and 30% by exercise[169] in HIV-infected patients. Neither diet nor exercise is likely to normalize triglyceride levels in the HIV-infected population with severe dyslipidemia.

Fenofibrate resulted in a 40% reduction in triglyceride levels and a 14% reduction in total cholesterol levels over 3 months in HIV-infected patients with hypertriglyceridemia.[170] Lesser but nonetheless beneficial effects may be seen with gemfibrozil or other fibrate derivatives.[171,172] Niacin also significantly reduces triglyceride level but might aggravate glucose tolerance in HIV-infected patients.[173] In addition, niacin may be difficult to use because of its associated flushing and potential liver abnormalities. Fish oil may also be useful to improve lipid levels in HIV-infected patients.[173b]

3-Hydroxy-3-methylglutaryl-coenzyme A (HMG-CoA) reductase inhibitors are most useful for lowering cholesterol levels in HIV-infected patients, but they are less effective in lowering triglyceride levels. For example, pravastatin combined with diet advice reduced total cholesterol levels by 17% over 24 weeks, without effects on triglyceride levels.[174] In addition, pravastatin reduced the number of small LDL particles by 27%.[148] The combination of gemfibrozil and atorvastatin resulted in a 30% reduction in cholesterol and 60% reduction in triglycerides in HIV-infected patients,[168] and it may be useful in HIV-infected patients with combined hyperlipidemia. When using the combination of HMG-CoA reductase inhibitors and fibric acid derivatives, the risk of rhabdomyolysis increases. In addition, recent data suggest that the PIs can themselves affect metabolism of the HMG-CoA reductase inhibitors. In this regard, ritonavir was shown to increase simvastatin levels by 2600% and atorvastatin levels by 74%.[175] Simvastatin should be avoided in patients receiving PI therapy.

The lipodystrophy syndrome is associated with metabolic derangements that increase cardiovascular risk in HIV-infected patients and is therefore important to identify and treat. In particular, dyslipidemia and diabetes are increasingly common among patients treated with HAART, and they may be caused by direct effects of the antiretroviral medications or the inflammation and fat redistribution associated with the syndrome. Treatment of dyslipidemia should be based on standard NCEP guidelines, but it can involve adjusting antiretroviral medications if lipid levels are severely increased. As triglyceride levels are most often severely affected, treatment often begins with fibric acid inhibitors, but it can involve other agents as needed. Treatment of diabetes should also follow standardized guidelines. However, recognition of severe underlying insulin resistance is critical, and use of insulin-sensitizing agents can have multiple beneficial effects, including reduction of visceral fat (e.g., with metformin) and potential improvement of subcutaneous fat loss (e.g., with thiazolidinediones).

REFERENCES

1. AVERT. Worldwide HIV and AIDS statistics. Available at http://www.avert.org/worldstats.htm (accessed January 9, 2007).

2. Membreno L, Irony I, Dere W, et al. Adrenocortical function in acquired immune deficiency syndrome. J Clin Endocrinol Metab 1987;65:482-487.
3. Grinspoon SK, Bilezikian JB. HIV disease and the endocrine system. N Engl J Med 1992;327:1360-1365.
4. Glasgow BJ, Steinsapir KD, Anders K, Layfield LJ. Adrenal pathology in the acquired immune deficiency syndrome. Am J Clin Path 1985;84:594-597.
5. Ferreiro J, Vinters HV. Pathology of the pituitary gland in patients with the acquired immune deficiency syndrome (AIDS). Pathology 1988;20:211-215.
6. Findling JW, Buggy BP, Gilson IH, et al. Longitudinal evaluation of adrenocortical function in patients with the human immunodeficiency virus. J Clin Endocrinol Metab 1994;79:1091-1096.
7. Grinspoon S, Corcoran C, Stanley T, et al. Mechanisms of androgen deficiency in human immunodeficiency virus–infected women with the wasting syndrome. J Clin Endocrinol Metab 2001;86(9): 4120-4126.
8. Norbiato G, Bevilacqua M, Vago T, Clerici M. Glucocorticoids and interferon-alpha in the acquired immunodeficiency syndrome. J Clin Endocrinol Metab 1996;81(7):2601-2606.
9. Dobs AS, Dempsey MA, Ladenson PW, Polk BF. Endocrine disorders in men infected with human immunodeficiency virus. Am J Med 1988;84(3 Pt 2):611-616.
10. Rietschel P, Corcoran C, Stanley T, et al. Prevalence of hypogonadism among men with weight loss related to human immunodeficiency virus infection who were receiving highly active antiretroviral therapy. Clin Infect Dis 2000;31(5):1240-1244.
11. Xiong Y, Hales DB. The role of tumor necrosis factor-alpha in the regulation of mouse Leydig cell steroidogenesis. Endocrinology 1993;132(6):2438-2444.
12. Hales DB. Interleukin-1 inhibits Leydig cell steroidogenesis primarily by decreasing 17α-hydroxylase/C17-20 lyase cytochrome P450 expression. Endocrinology 1992;131(5):2165-2172.
13. Calkins JH, Siegel MM, Nankin HR, Lin T. Interleukin-l inhibits leydig cell steroidogenesis in primary cell culture. J Clin Endocrinol Metab 1988;123:1605-1610.
14. Chabon AB, Stenger RJ, Grabstald H. Histopathology of testis in acquired immune deficiency syndrome. Urology 1987;29(6):658-663.
15. Biglia A, Blanco JL, Martinez E, et al. Gynecomastia among HIV-infected patients is associated with hypogonadism: a case-control study. Clin Infect Dis 2004;39(10):1514-1519.
16. Collazos J, Ibarra S, Martinez E, Mayo J. Serum prolactin concentrations in patients infected with human immunodeficiency virus. HIV Clin Trials 2002;3(2):133-138.
17. Parra A, Ramirez-Peredo J, Larrea F, et al. Decreased dopaminergic tone and increased basal bioactive prolactin in men with human immunodeficiency virus infection. Clin Endocrinol (Oxf) 2001;54(6):731-738.
18. Hutchinson J, Murphy M, Harries R, Skinner CJ. Galactorrhoea and hyperprolactinaemia associated with protease-inhibitors. Lancet 2000;356(9234):1003-1004.
19. Grinspoon S, Corcoran C, Lee K, et al. Loss of lean body and muscle mass correlates with androgen levels in hypogonadal men with acquired immunodeficiency syndrome and wasting. J Clin Endocrinol Metab 1996;81(11):4051-4058.
20. Grinspoon S, Corcoran C, Anderson E, et al. Sustained anabolic effects of long-term androgen administration in men with AIDS wasting. Clin Infect Dis 1999;28(3):634-636.
21. Grinspoon S, Corcoran C, Parlman K, et al. Effects of testosterone and progressive resistance training in eugonadal men with AIDS wasting. Ann Int Med 2000;133:348-355.
22. Grinspoon S, Corcoran C, Miller K, et al. Body composition and endocrine function in women with acquired immunodeficiency syndrome wasting [published erratum appears in J Clin Endocrinol Metab 1997;82(10):3360]. J Clin Endocrinol Metab 1997;82(5): 1332-1337.
23. Clark RA, Mulligan K, Stamenovic E, et al. Frequency of anovulation and early menopause among women enrolled in selected adult AIDS clinical trials group studies. J Infect Dis 2001;184(10): 1325-1327.
24. Choi HH, Gray PB, Storer TW, et al. Effects of testosterone replacement in human immunodeficiency virus–infected women with weight loss. J Clin Endocrinol Metab 2005;90(3):1531-1541.
25. Bourdoux PP, De Wit SA, Servais GM, et al. Biochemical thyroid profile in patients infected with the human immunodeficiency virus. Thyroid 1991;1(2):147-149.
26. Beltran S, Lescure FX, Desailloud R, et al. Increased prevalence of hypothyroidism among human immunodeficiency virus–infected patients: a need for screening. Clin Infect Dis 2003;37(4):579-583.
27. Collazos J, Ibarra S, Mayo J. Thyroid hormones in HIV-infected patients in the highly active antiretroviral therapy era: evidence of an interrelation between the thyroid axis and the immune system. AIDS 2003;17(5):763-765.
28. Calza L, Manfredi R, Chiodo F. Subclinical hypothyroidism in HIV-infected patients receiving highly active antiretroviral therapy. J Acquir Immune Defic Syndr 2002;31(3):361-363.
29. Quirino T, Bongiovanni M, Ricci E, et al. Hypothyroidism in HIV-infected patients who have or have not received HAART. Clin Infect Dis 2004;38(4):596-597.
30. Rana S, Nunlee-Bland G, Valyasevi R, Iqbal M. Thyroid dysfunction in HIV-infected children: is L-thyroxine therapy beneficial? Pediatr AIDS HIV Infect 1996;7(6):424-428.
31. Fundaro C, Olivieri A, Rendeli C, et al. Occurrence of anti-thyroid autoantibodies in children vertically infected with HIV-1. J Pediatr Endocrinol Metab 1998;11(6):745-750.
32. Chiarelli F, Galli L, Verrotti A, et al. Thyroid function in children with perinatal human immunodeficiency virus type 1 infection. Thyroid 2000;10(6):499-505.
33. Chen F, Day SL, Metcalfe RA, et al. Characteristics of autoimmune thyroid disease occurring as a late complication of immune reconstitution in patients with advanced human immunodeficiency virus (HIV) disease. Medicine (Baltimore) 2005;84(2):98-106.
34. Jimenez C, Moran SA, Sereti I, et al. Graves' disease after interleukin-2 therapy in a patient with human immunodeficiency virus infection. Thyroid 2004;14(12):1097-1102.
35. Drucker DJ, Bailey D, Rotstein L. Thyroiditis as the presenting manifestation of disseminated extrapulmonary *Pneumocystis carinii* infection. J Clin Endocrinol Metab 1990;71(6):1663-1665.
36. Tang WW, Kaptein E, Feinstein EI, Massry SG. Hyponatremia in hospitalized patients with the acquired immunodeficiency syndrome (AIDS) and the AIDS-related complex. Am J Med 1993;94:169-174.
37. Kalin MF, Poretsky L, Seres DS, Zumoff B. Hyporeninemic hypoaldosteronism associated with acquired immune deficiency syndrome. Am J Med 1987;82:1035-1038.
38. Choi MJ, Fernandez PC, Patnaik A, et al. Brief report: trimethoprim-induced hyperkalemia in a patient with AIDS. Ann Int Med 1993;328:703-706.
39. Caramelo C, Bello E, Ruiz E, et al. Hyperkalemia in patients infected with the human immunodeficiency virus: involvement of a systemic mechanism. Kidney Int 1999;56(1):198-205.
40. Fairfield WP, Finkelstein JS, Klibanski A, Grinspoon SK. Osteopenia in eugonadal men with acquired immune deficiency syndrome wasting syndrome. J Clin Endocrinol Metab 2001;86(5): 2020-2026.
41. Tebas P, Powderly WG, Claxton S, et al. Accelerated bone mineral loss in HIV-infected patients receiving potent antiretroviral therapy. AIDS 2000;14(4):F63-67.
42. Mondy K, Yarasheski K, Powderly WG, et al. Longitudinal evolution of bone mineral density and bone markers in human immunodeficiency virus–infected individuals. Clin Inf Dis 2003;36:482-490.
43. Amiel C, Ostertag A, Slama L, et al. BMD is reduced in HIV-infected men irrespective of treatment. J Bone Miner Res 2004;19(3): 402-409.
44. Dolan SE, Huang JS, Killilea KM, et al. Reduced bone density in HIV-infected women. AIDS 2004;18(3):475-483.
45. Serrano S, Marinoso ML, Soriano JC, et al. Bone remodelling in human immunodeficiency virus-l-infected patients: a histomorphometric study. Bone 1995;16(2):185-191.
46. Koutkia P, Canavan B, Breu J, Grinspoon S. Effects of growth hormone–releasing hormone on bone turnover in human immunodeficiency virus–infected men with fat accumulation. J Clin Endocrinol Metab 2005;90(4):2154-2160.
47. Nacher M, Serrano S, Gonzalez A, et al. Osteoblasts in HIV-infected patients: HIV-1 infection and cell function. AIDS 2001;15(17): 2239-2243.
48. Aukrust P, Haug CJ, Ueland T, et al. Decreased bone formative and enhanced resorptive markers in human immunodeficiency virus

infection: indication of normalization of the bone-remodeling process during highly active antiretroviral therapy. J Clin Endocrinol Metab 1999;84(1):145-150.
49. O'Brien KO, Razavi M, Henderson RA, et al. Bone mineral content in girls perinatally infected with HIV. Am J Clin Nutr 2001;73(4): 821-826.
50. Mora S, Zamproni I, Beccio S, et al. Longitudinal changes of bone mineral density and metabolism in antiretroviral-treated human immunodeficiency virus–infected children. J Clin Endocrinol Metab 2004;89(1):24-28.
51. Arpadi SM, Horlick M, Thornton J, et al. Bone mineral content is lower in prepubertal HIV-infected children. J Acquir Immune Defic Syndr 2002;29(5):450-454.
52. Zamboni G, Antoniazzi F, Bertoldo F, et al. Altered bone metabolism in children infected with human immunodeficiency virus. Acta Paediatr 2003;92(1):12-16.
53. Stagi S, Bindi G, Galluzzi F, et al. Changed bone status in human immunodeficiency virus type 1 (HIV-1) perinatally infected children is related to low serum free IGF-I. Clin Endocrinol (Oxf) 2004;61(6):692-699.
54. Cozzolino M, Vidal M, Arcidiacono MV, et al. HIV-protease inhibitors impair vitamin D bioactivation to 1,25-dihydroxyvitamin D. AIDS 2003;17(4):513-520.
55. Mondy K, Powderly WG, Claxton SA, et al. Alendronate, vitamin D, and calcium for the treatment of osteopenia/osteoporosis associated with HIV infection. J Acquir Immune Defic Syndr 2005; 38(4):426-431.
56. Miller KD, Masur H, Jones EC, et al. High prevalence of osteonecrosis of the femoral head in HIV-infected adults. Ann Intern Med 2002;137(1):17-25.
57. Gutierrez F, Padilla S, Ortega E, et al. Avascular necrosis of the bone in HIV-infected patients: incidence and associated factors. AIDS 2002;16(3):481-483.
58. Kuehn EW, Anders HJ, Bogner JR, et al. Hypocalcaemia in HIV infection and AIDS. J Intern Med 1999;245(1):69-73.
59. Jaeger P, Otto S, Speck RF, et al. Altered parathyroid gland function in severely immunocompromised patients infected with human immunodeficiency virus. J Clin Endocrinol Metab 1994;79:1701-1705.
60. Chao D, Rutstein RM, Steenhoff AP, et al. Two cases of hypocalcemia secondary to vitamin D deficiency in an urban HIV-positive pediatric population. AIDS 2003;17(16):2401-2403.
61. Earle KE, Seneviratne T, Shaker J, Shoback D. Fanconi's syndrome in HIV$^+$ adults: report of three cases and literature review. J Bone Miner Res 2004;19(5):714-721.
62. Zaloga GP, Chernow B, Eil C. Hypercalcemia and disseminated cytomegalovirus infection in the acquired immunodeficiency syndrome. Ann Int Med 1985;102:331-333.
63. Grinspoon S, Baum H, Lee K, et al. Effects of short-term recombinant human insulin-like growth factor-I administration on bone turnover in osteopenic women with anorexia nervosa. J Clin Endocrinol Metab 1996;81:3864-3870.
64. Rietschel P, Hadigan C, Corcoran C, et al. Assessment of growth hormone dynamics in human immunodeficiency virus–related lipodystrophy. J Clin Endocrinol Metab 2001;86(2): 504-510.
65. Koutkia P, Canavan B, Breu J, Grinspoon S. Growth hormone (GH) responses to GH-releasing hormone–arginine testing in human immunodeficiency virus lipodystrophy. J Clin Endocrinol Metab 2005;90(1):32-38.
66. Koutkia P, Meininger G, Canavan B, et al. Metabolic regulation of growth hormone by free fatty acids, somatostatin, and ghrelin in HIV-lipodystrophy. Am J Physiol Endocrinol Metab 2004;286(2): E296-303.
67. Schambelan M, Mulligan K, Grunfeld C, et al. Recombinant human growth hormone in patients with HIV-associated wasting. A randomized, placebo-controlled trial. Serostim Study Group. Ann Intern Med 1996;125(11):873-882.
68. Esposito JG, Thomas SG, Kingdon L, Ezzat S. Growth hormone treatment improves peripheral muscle oxygen extraction-utilization during exercise in patients with human immunodeficiency virus–associated wasting: a randomized controlled trial. J Clin Endocrinol Metab 2004;89(10):5124-5131.
69. Ellis KJ, Lee PD, Pivarnik JM, et al. Changes in body composition of human immunodeficiency virus–infected males receiving insulin-like growth factor I and growth hormone. J Clin Endocrinol Metab 1996;81(8):3033-3038.
70. McNurlan MA, Garlick PJ, Steigbigel RT, et al. Responsiveness of muscle protein synthesis to growth hormone administration in HIV-infected individuals declines with severity of disease. J Clin Invest 1997;100(8):2125-2132.
71. Moyle GJ, Daar ES, Gertner JM, et al. Growth hormone improves lean body mass, physical performance, and quality of life in subjects with HIV-associated weight loss or wasting on highly active antiretroviral therapy. J Acquir Immune Defic Syndr 2004;35(4): 367-375.
72. Napolitano LA, Lo JC, Gotway MB, et al. Increased thymic mass and circulating naive CD4 T cells in HIV-1-infected adults treated with growth hormone. AIDS 2002;16(8):1103-1111.
73. Kotler DP, Muurahainen N, Grunfeld C, et al. Effects of growth hormone on abnormal visceral adipose tissue accumulation and dyslipidemia in HIV-infected patients. J Acquir Immune Def Syndr 2004;35:239-252.
74. Lo JC, Mulligan K, Noor MA, et al. The effects of low-dose growth hormone in HIV-infected men with fat accumulation: a pilot study. Clin Infect Dis 2004;39(5):732-735.
75. Koutkia P, Canavan B, Breu J, et al. Growth hormone–releasing hormone in HIV-infected men with lipodystrophy: a randomized, controlled trial. JAMA 2004;292:210-218.
76. Falutz J, Allas S, Kotler D, et al. A placebo-controlled, dose-ranging study of a growth hormone releasing factor in HIV-infected patients with abdominal fat accumulation. AIDS 2005;19(12):1279-1287.
77. Ratner Kaufman F, Gertner JM, et al. Growth hormone secretion in HIV-positive versus HIV-negative hemophilic males with abnormal growth and pubertal development. The Hemophilia Growth and Development Study. J Acquir Immune Defic Syndr Hum Retrovirol 1997;15(2):137-144.
78. Pinto G, Blanche S, Thiriet I, et al. Growth hormone treatment of children with human immunodeficiency virus-associated growth failure. Eur J Pediatr 2000;159(12):937-938.
79. Frost RA, Nachman SA, Lang CH, Gelato MC. Proteolysis of insulin-like growth factor–binding protein–3 in human immunodeficiency virus–positive children who fail to thrive. J Clin Endocrinol Metab 1996;81(8):2957-2962.
80. Rondanelli M, Caselli D, Arico M, et al. Insulin-like growth factor I (IGF-I) and IGF-binding protein 3 response to growth hormone is impaired in HIV-infected children. AIDS Res Hum Retroviruses 2002;18(5):331-339.
81. Van Rossum AM, Gaakeer MI, Verweel S, et al. Endocrinologic and immunologic factors associated with recovery of growth in children with human immunodeficiency virus type 1 infection treated with protease inhibitors. Pediatr Infect Dis J 2003;22(1): 70-76.
82. Vigano A, Saresella M, Trabattoni D, et al. Growth hormone in T-lymphocyte thymic and postthymic development: a study in HIV-infected children. J Pediatr 2004;145(4):542-548.
83. Vigano A, Mora S, Brambilla P, et al. Impaired growth hormone secretion correlates with visceral adiposity in highly active antiretroviral treated HIV-infected adolescents. AIDS 2003;17(10): 1435-1441.
84. Ott M, Lembcke B, Fischer H, et al. Early changes of body composition in human immunodeficiency virus–infected patients: tetrapolar body impedance analysis indicates significant malnutrition. Am J Clin Nutr 1993;57(1):15-19.
85. Macallan DE, Noble C, Baldwin C, et al. Energy expenditure and wasting in human immunodeficiency virus infection. N Engl J Med 1995;333:83-88.
86. Macallan DC, Noble C, Baldwin C, et al. Prospective analysis of patterns of weight change in stage IV human immunodeficiency virus infection. Am J Clin Nutr 1993;58(3):417-424.
87. Thiebaut R, Malvy D, Marimoutou C, Davis F. Anthropometric indices as predictors of survival in AIDS adults. Aquitaine Cohort, France, 1985-1997. Groupe d'Epidemiologie Clinique du Sida en Aquitaine (GECSA). Eur J Epidemiol 2000;16(7):633-639.
88. Wanke C, Silva M, Knox T, et al. Weight loss and wasting remain common complications in individuals infected with HIV in the era of highly active antiretroviral therapy. Clin Inf Dis 2000;31: 803-805.
89. Grinspoon S, Corcoran C, Askari H, et al. Effects of androgen administration in men with the AIDS wasting syndrome: a random-

ized, double-blind, placebo-controlled trial. Ann Intern Med 1998;129(1):18-26.
90. Dolan S, Wilkie S, Aliabadi N, et al. Effects of testosterone administration in human immunodeficiency virus–infected women with low weight: a randomized, placebo-controlled study. Arch Intern Med 2004;164:897-904.
91. Berger JR, Pall L, Hall CD, et al. Oxandrolone in AIDS wasting myopathy. AIDS 1996;1996:1657-1662.
92. Mulligan K, Zackin R, Clark RA, et al. Effect of nandrolone decanoate therapy on weight and lean body mass in HIV-infected women with weight loss: a randomized, double-blind, placebo-controlled, multicenter trial. Arch Intern Med 2005;165(5):578-585.
93. Von Roenn JH, Armstron D, Kotler DP, et al. Megesterol acetate in patients with AIDS-related cachexia. Ann Int Med 1994;121: 393-399.
94. Oster MH, Enders SR, Samuels SJ, et al. Megesterol acetate in patients with AIDS and cachexia. Ann Int Med 1994;121:400-408.
95. Clarick RH, Hanekom WA, Yogev R, Chadwick EG. Megestrol acetate treatment of growth failure in children infected with human immunodeficiency virus. Pediatrics 1997;99(3):354-357.
96. Makonkawkeyoon S, Limson-Pobre RNR, Moreira AL, et al. Thalidomide inhibits the replication of human immunodeficiency virus type 1. Proc Natl Acad Sci U S A 1993;90:5974-5978.
97. Lunardi-Iskandar Y, Bryant JL, Zeman RA, et al. Tumorigenesis and metastasis of neoplastic Kaposi's sarcoma cell line in immunodeficient mice blocked by a human pregnancy hormone. Nature 1995;375(6526):64-68.
98. Clark RH, Feleke G, Din M, et al. Nutritional treatment for acquired immunodeficiency virus-associated wasting using β-hydroxy β-methylbutyrate, glutamine, and arginine: a randomized, double-blind, placebo-controlled study. JPEN J Parenter Enteral Nutr 2000;24(3):133-139.
99. Hellerstein MK, Wu K, McGrath M, et al. Effects of dietary omega-3 fatty acid supplementation in men with weight loss associated with the acquired immune deficiency syndrome: relation to indices of cytokine production. J Acquir Immune Defic Syndr Hum Retrovirol 1996;11(3):258-270.
100. Landman D, Sarai A, Sathe SS. Use of pentoxifylline therapy for patients with AIDS-related wasting: pilot study. Clin Infect Dis 1994;18(1):97-99.
101. Bhasin S, Storer TW, Javanbakht M, et al. Testosterone replacement and resistance exercise in HIV-infected men with weight loss and low testosterone levels. JAMA 2000;283:763-770.
102. Strawford A, Barbieri T, Van Loan M, et al. Resistance exercise and supraphysiologic androgen therapy in eugonadal men with HIV-related weight loss. JAMA 1999;281:1282-1290.
103. Sattler FR, Jaque SV, Schroeder ET, et al. Effects of pharmacological doses of nandrolone decanoate and progressive resistance training in immunodeficienct patients infected with human immunodeficiency virus. J Clin Endocrinol Metab 1999;84:1268-1276.
104. Grinspoon S, Corcoran C, Stanley T, et al. Effects of androgen administration on the growth hormone–insulin-like growth factor I axis in men with acquired immunodeficiency syndrome wasting. J Clin Endocrinol Metab 1998;83(12):4251-4256.
105. Frost RA, Fuhrer J, Steigbigel R, et al. Wasting in the acquired immune deficiency syndrome is associated with multiple defects in the serum insulin-like growth factor system. Clin Endocrinol (Oxf) 1996;44(5):501-514.
106. Mulroney SE, McDonnell KJ, Pert CB, et al. HIV gp120 inhibits the somatotropic axis: a possible GH-releasing hormone receptor mechanism for the pathogenesis of AIDS wasting. Proc Natl Acad Sci U S A 1998;95(4):1927-1932.
107. Lichtenstein KA, Ward DJ, Moorman AC, et al. Clinical assessment of HIV-associated lipodystrophy in an ambulatory population. AIDS 2001;15(11):1389-1398.
108. Carr A, Samaras K, Thorisdottir A, et al. Diagnosis, prediction, and natural course of HIV-1 protease-inhibitor–associated lipodystrophy, hyperlipidaemia, and diabetes mellitus: a cohort study. Lancet 1999;353(9170):2093-2099.
109. Dong KL, Bausserman LL, Flynn MM, et al. Changes in body habitus and serum lipid abnormalities in HIV-positive women on highly active antiretroviral therapy (HAART). J Acquir Immune Defic Syndr 1999;21(2):107-113.
110. Miller KK, Daly PA, Sentochnik D, et al. Pseudo-Cushing's syndrome in human immunodeficiency virus–infected patients. Clin Infect Dis 1998;27(1):68-72.
111. Caron M, Auclair M, Vigouroux C, et al. The HIV protease inhibitor indinavir impairs sterol regulatory element–binding protein-1 intranuclear localization, inhibits preadipocyte differentiation, and induces insulin resistance. Diabetes 2001;50(6):1378-1388.
112. Hadigan C, Borgonha S, Rabe J, et al. Increased rates of lipolysis among HIV-infected men receiving highly active antiretroviral therapy. Metabolism 2002;51:1143-1147.
113. Shikuma CM, Hu N, Milne C, et al. Mitochondrial DNA decrease in subcutaneous adipose tissue of HIV-infected individuals with peripheral lipoatrophy. AIDS 2001;15(14):1801-1809.
114. Buffet M, Schwarzinger M, Amellal B, et al. Mitochondrial DNA depletion in adipose tissue of HIV-infected patients with peripheral lipoatrophy. J Clin Virol 2005;33(1):60-64.
115. Johnson JA, Albu JB, Engelson ES, et al. Increased systemic and adipose tissue cytokines in patients with HIV-associated lipodystrophy. Am J Physiol Endocrinol Metab 2004;286(2):E261-271.
116. Yanovski JA, Miller KD, Kino T, et al. Endocrine and metabolic evaluation of human immunodeficiency virus–infected patients with evidence of protease inhibitor–associated lipodystrophy. J Clin Endocrinol Metab 1999;84(6):1925-1931.
117. Christeff N, Nunez EA, Gougeon ML. Changes in cortisol/DHEA ratio in HIV-infected men are related to immunological and metabolic perturbations leading to malnutrition and lipodystrophy. Ann N Y Acad Sci 2000;917:962-970.
118. Sutinen J, Kannisto K, Korsheninnikova E, et al. In the lipodystrophy associated with highly active antiretroviral therapy, pseudo-Cushing's syndrome is associated with increased regeneration of cortisol by 11β-hydroxysteroid dehydrogenase type 1 in adipose tissue. Diabetologia 2004;47(10):1668-1671.
119. Christeff N, De Truchis P, Melchior JC, et al. Longitudinal evolution of HIV-1-associated lipodystrophy is correlated to serum cortisol: DHEA ratio and IFN-α. Eur J Clin Invest 2002;32(10):775-784.
120. Hellerstein MK, Grunfeld C, Wu K, et al. Increased de novo hepatic lipogenesis in human immunodeficiency virus infection. J Clin Endocrinol Metab 1993;76(3):559-565.
121. Grunfeld C, Pang M, Doerrler W, et al. Lipids, lipoproteins, triglyceride clearance, and cytokines in human immunodeficiency virus infection and the acquired immunodeficiency syndrome. J Clin Endocrinol Metab 1992;74(5):1045-1052.
122. Grunfeld C, Doerrler W, Pang M, et al. Abnormalities of apolipoprotein E in the acquired immunodeficiency syndrome. J Clin Endocrinol Metab 1997;82(11):3734-3740.
123. Riddler SA, Smit E, Cole SR, et al. Impact of HIV infection and HAART on serum lipids in men. JAMA 2003;289(22):2978-2982.
124. Friis-Moller N, Weber R, Reiss P, et al. Cardiovascular disease risk factors in HIV patients—association with antiretroviral therapy. Results from the DAD study. AIDS 2003;17(8):1179-1193.
125. Hadigan C, Meigs JB, Corcoran C, et al. Metabolic abnormalities and cardiovascular disease risk factors in adults with human immunodeficiency virus infection and lipodystrophy. Clin Infect Dis 2001;32(1):130-139.
126. Purnell JQ, Zambon A, Knopp RH, et al. Effect of ritonavir on lipids and post-heparin lipase activities in normal subjects. AIDS 2000;14(1):51-57.
127. Schmitz M, Michl GM, Walli R, et al. Alterations of apolipoprotein B metabolism in HIV-infected patients with antiretroviral combination therapy. J Acquir Immune Defic Syndr 2001;26(3):225-235.
128. Bonnet E, Ruidavets JB, Tuech J, et al. Apoprotein C-III and E-containing lipoparticles are markedly increased in HIV-infected patients treated with protease inhibitors: association with the development of lipodystrophy. J Clin Endocrinol Metab 2001; 86(1):296-302.
129. Liang JS, Distler O, Cooper DA, et al. HIV protease inhibitors protect apolipoprotein B from degradation by the proteasome: a potential mechanism for protease inhibitor-induced hyperlipidemia. Nat Med 2001;7(12):1327-1331.
130. Brown TT, Cole SR, Li X, et al. Antiretroviral therapy and the prevalence and incidence of diabetes mellitus in the multicenter AIDS cohort study. Arch Intern Med 2005;165(10):1179-1184.
131. Johnsen S, Dolan SE, Fitch KV, et al. Absence of polycystic ovary syndrome features in human immunodeficiency virus–infected

women despite significant hyperinsulinemia and truncal adiposity. J Clin Endocrinol Metab 2005;90(10):5596-5604.
132. Meininger G, Hadigan C, Rietschel P, Grinspoon S. Body-composition measurements as predictors of glucose and insulin abnormalities in HIV-positive men. Am J Clin Nutr 2002;76(2): 460-465.
133. Mynarcik DC, McNurlan MA, Steigbigel RT, et al. Association of severe insulin resistance with both loss of limb fat and elevated serum tumor necrosis factor receptor levels in HIV lipodystrophy. J Acquir Immune Defic Syndr 2000;25(4):312-321.
134. Tong Q, Sankale JL, Hadigan CM, et al. Regulation of adiponectin in human immunodeficiency virus–infected patients: relationship to body composition and metabolic indices. J Clin Endocrinol Metab 2003;88(4):1559-1564.
135. Hadigan C, Rabe J, Meininger G, et al. Inhibition of lipolysis improves insulin sensitivity in protease inhibitor–treated HIV-infected men with fat redistribution. Am J Clin Nutr 2003;77: 490-494.
136. Gan SK, Samaras K, Thompson CH, et al. Altered myocellular and abdominal fat partitioning predict disturbance in insulin action in HIV protease inhibitor-related lipodystrophy. Diabetes 2002; 51(11):3163-3169.
137. Sutinen J, Hakkinen AM, Westerbacka J, et al. Increased fat accumulation in the liver in HIV-infected patients with antiretroviral therapy–associated lipodystrophy. AIDS 2002;16(16):2183-2193.
138. Murata H, Hruz PW, Mueckler M. The mechanism of insulin resistance caused by HIV protease inhibitor therapy. J Biol Chem 2000;275(27):20251-20254.
139. Noor MA, Seneviratne T, Aweeka FT, et al. Indinavir acutely inhibits insulin-stimulated glucose disposal in humans: a randomized, placebo-controlled study. AIDS 2002;16(5):F1-8.
139b. Fleischman A, Johnsen S, Systrom DM, et al: Effects of a nucleoside reverse transcriptase inhibitor, stavudine, on glucose disposal and mitochondrial function in muscle of healthy adults. J Am Physiol Endocrinol Metab. 2007; [pub ahead of print].
140. Mallon PW, Unemori P, Sedwell R, et al. In vivo, nucleoside reverse-transcriptase inhibitors alter expression of both mitochondrial and lipid metabolism genes in the absence of depletion of mitochondrial DNA. J Infect Dis 2005;191(10):1686-1696.
141. Hadigan C, Meigs JB, Wilson PW, et al. Prediction of coronary heart disease risk in HIV-infected patients with fat redistribution. Clin Infect Dis 2003;36(7):909-916.
142. Stein JH, Klein MA, Bellehumeur JL, et al. Use of human immunodeficiency virus-1 protease inhibitors is associated with atherogenic lipoprotein changes and endothelial dysfunction. Circulation 2001;104(3):257-262.
143. Sattler FR, Qian D, Louie S, et al. Elevated blood pressure in subjects with lipodystrophy. AIDS 2001;15(15):2001-2010.
144. Hadigan C, Meigs JB, Rabe J, et al. Increased PAI-1 and tPA antigen levels are reduced with metformin therapy in HIV-infected patients with fat redistribution and insulin resistance. J Clin Endocrinol Metab 2001;86(2):939-943.
145. Dolan SE, Hadigan C, Killilea KM, et al. Increased cardiovascular disease risk indices in HIV-infected women. J Acquir Immune Defic Syndr 2005;39(1):44-54.
146. Hsue PY, Lo JC, Franklin A, et al. Progression of atherosclerosis as assessed by carotid intima-media thickness in patients with HIV infection. Circulation 2004;109:1603-1608.
147. Fu W, Chai H, Yao Q, Chen C. Effects of HIV protease inhibitor ritonavir on vasomotor function and endothelial nitric oxide synthase expression. J Acquir Immune Defic Syndr 2005;39(2): 152-158.
148. Stein JH, Merwood MA, Bellehumeur JL, et al. Effects of pravastatin on lipoproteins and endothelial function in patients receiving human immunodeficiency virus protease inhibitors. Am Heart J 2004;147(4):E18.
149. Charakida M, Donald AE, Green H, et al. Early structural and functional changes of the vasculature in HIV-infected children: impact of disease and antiretroviral therapy. Circulation 2005; 112(1):103-109.
150. Mary-Krause M, Cotte L, Simon A, et al. Increased risk of myocardial infarction with duration of protease inhibitor therapy in HIV-infected men. AIDS 2003;17(17):2479-2486.
151. Klein D, Hurley LB, Quesenberry CP Jr, Sidney S. Do protease inhibitors increase the risk for coronary heart disease in patients with HIV-1 infection? J Acquir Immune Defic Syndr 2002;30(5): 471-477.
152. Currier JS, Taylor A, Boyd F, et al. Coronary heart disease in HIV-infected individuals. J Acquir Immune Defic Syndr 2003;33(4): 506-512.
153. Friis-Moller N, Sabin CA, Weber R, et al. Combination antiretroviral therapy and the risk of myocardial infarction. N Engl J Med 2003;349(21):1993-2003.
154. Carr A, Workman C, Smith DE, et al. Abacavir substitution for nucleoside analogs in patients with HIV lipoatrophy: a randomized trial. JAMA 2002;288(2):207-215.
155. Jones SP, Doran DA, Leatt PB, et al. Short-term exercise training improves body composition and hyperlipidaemia in HIV-positive individuals with lipodystrophy. AIDS 2001;15(15):2049-2051.
156. Driscoll SD, Meininger GE, Ljunquist K, et al. Differential effects of metformin and exercise on muscle adiposity and metabolic indices in human immunodeficiecy virus–infected patients. J Clin Endocrinol Metab 2004;89(5):2171-2178.
156b. Bhasin S, Parker RA, Sattler F, et al: Effects of testosterone supplementation on whole body and regional fat mass and distribution in human immunodeficiency virus-infected men with abdominal obesity. J Clin Endocrinol Metab 2007;92:1049-1057.
157. Sattler FR, Schroeder ET, Dube MP, et al. Metabolic effects of nandrolone decanoate and resistance training in men with HIV. Am J Physiol Endocrinol Metab 2002;283(6):E1214-E1222.
158. Hadigan C, Corcoran C, Basgoz N, et al. Metformin in the treatment of HIV lipodystrophy syndrome: a randomized controlled trial. JAMA 2000;284(4):472-477.
159. Hadigan C, Rabe J, Grinspoon S. Sustained benefits of metformin therapy on markers of cardiovascular risk in human immunodeficiency virus–infected patients with fat redistribution and insulin resistance. J Clin Endocrinol Metab 2002;87:4611-4615.
160. Driscoll SD, Meininger GE, Lareau MT, et al. Effects of exercise training and metformin on body composition and cardiovascular indices in HIV infected patients. AIDS 2004;18(3):465-473.
161. Gelato MC, Mynarcik DC, Quick JL, et al. Improved insulin sensitivity and body fat distribution in HIV-infected patients treated with rosiglitazone: a pilot study. J Acquir Immune Defic Syndr 2002; 31(2):163-170.
162. Hadigan C, Yawetz S, Thomas A, et al. Metabolic effects of rosiglitazone in HIV lipodystrophy: a randomized controlled trial. Ann Intern Med 2004;140(10):786-794.
163. Carr A, Workman C, Carey D, et al. No effect of rosiglitazone for treatment of HIV-1 lipoatrophy: randomized, double-blind, placebo-controlled trial. Lancet 2004;363(9407):429-438.
164. Kamin D, Hadigan C, Lehrke M, et al. Resistin levels in human immunodeficiency virus–infected patients with lipoatrophy decrease in response to rosiglitazone. J Clin Endocrinol Metab 2005;90(6):3423-3426.
165. van Wijk JP, de Koning EJ, Cabezas MC, et al. Comparison of rosiglitazone and metformin for treating HIV lipodystrophy: a randomized trial. Ann Intern Med 2005;143(5):337-346.
166. Mulligan K, Tai VW, Algren H, et al. Altered fat distribution in HIV-positive men on nucleoside analog reverse transcriptase inhibitor therapy. J Acquir Immune Defic Syndr 2001;26(5):443-448.
167. Wood R, Phanuphak P, Cahn P, et al. Long-term efficacy and safety of atazanavir with stavudine and lamivudine in patients previously treated with nelfinavir or atazanavir. J Acquir Immune Defic Syndr 2004;36(2):684-692.
168. Henry K, Melroe H, Huebesch J, et al. Atorvastatin and gemfibrozil for protease-inhibitor-related lipid abnormalities. Lancet 1998; 352(9133):1031-1032.
169. Yarasheski KE, Tebas P, Stanerson B, et al. Resistance exercise training reduces hypertriglyceridemia in HIV-infected men treated with antiviral therapy. J Appl Physiol 2001;90(1):133-138.
170. Badiou S, De Boever M, Dupuy AM, et al. Fenofibrate improves the atherogenic lipid profile and enhances LDL resistance to oxidation in HIV-positive adults. Atherosclerosis 2004;172:273-279.
171. Miller J, Brown D, Amin J, et al. A randomized, double-blind study of gemfibrozil for the treatment of protease inhibitor–associated hypertriglyceridaemia. AIDS 2002;16(16):2195-2200.
172. Calza L, Manfredi R, Chiodo F. Statins and fibrates for the treatment of hyperlipidaemia in HIV-infected patients receiving HAART. AIDS 2003;17(6):851-859.

173. Gerber MT, Mondy KE, Yarasheski KE, et al. Niacin in HIV-infected individuals with hyperlipidemia receiving potent antiretroviral therapy. Clin Infect Dis 2004;39(3):419-425.
173b. De Truchis P, Kirstetter M, Perier A, et al: Reduction in triglyceride level with N-3 polyunsaturated fatty acids in HIV-infected patients taking potent antiretroviral therapy: a randomized prospective study. J Acquir Immune Defic Syndr 2007;44:278-85.
174. Moyle GJ, Lloyd M, Reynolds B, et al. Dietary advice with or without pravastatin for the management of hypercholesterolaemia associated with protease inhibitor therapy. AIDS 2001;15(12):1503-1508.
175. Fichtenbaum CJ, Gerber JG. Interactions between antiretroviral drugs and drugs used for the therapy of the metabolic complications encountered during HIV infection. Clin Pharmacokinet 2002;41(14):1195-1211.
176. Grinspoon S, Carr A. Cardiovascular risk and body fat abnormalities in HIV-infected adults. N Engl J Med 2005;352(1):48-62.
177. Bhasin S, Storer TW, Asbel-Sethi N, et al: Effects of testosterone replacement with a nongenital transdermal system, Androderm, in human immunodeficiency virus-infected men with low testosterone levels. J Clin Endocrinol Metab 1998;83:3155-3162.
178. Dobs AS, Cofrancesco J, Nolten WE, et al. The use of a transcrotal testosterone delivery system in the treatment of patients with weight loss related to human immunodeficiency virus. Am J Med 1999;107:126-132.
179. Piketty C, Jayle D, Leplege A, et al. Double-blind placebo-controlled trial of oral dehydroepiandrosterone in patients with advanced HIV disease. Clin Endocrinol (Oxf) 2001;55(3):325-330.
180. Miller K, Corcoran C, Armstrong C, et al. Transdermal testosterone administration in women with acquired immunodeficiency syndrome wasting: a pilot study. J Clin Endocrinol Metab 1998;83(8):2717-2725.

CHAPTER 38

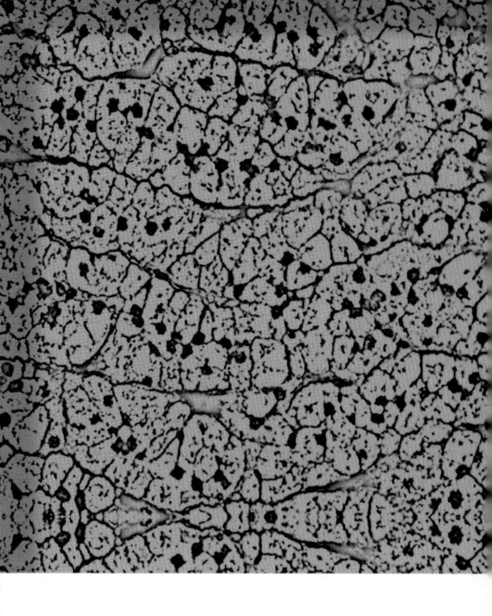

GASTROINTESTINAL HORMONES AND GUT ENDOCRINE TUMORS

Daniel J. Drucker

Endocrine tumors originating from islet or enteroendocrine cells can manifest with unique clinical symptoms that reflect the biological actions of secreted peptide hormones. In this chapter, we discuss how endocrine cell lineages develop during organogenesis in the endocrine pancreas and intestine, and we review the biological actions of peptide hormones produced in pancreatic and intestinal endocrine cells and enteric nerves. Although numerous physiologic actions of these peptides are still poorly understood and under active investigation, excessive production of one or more of these peptides often accounts for the clinical symptoms attributable to endocrine tumors arising from the gastrointestinal tract and pancreas.

Endocrine Cell Development in the Pancreas

The endocrine and exocrine pancreas develops from the primitive foregut endoderm. Pancreatic morphogenesis is a complex process that begins with the evagination of the embryonic foregut into ventral and dorsal buds at 28 days' gestation in humans and at embryonic day 8 day in mice. Rotation of the stomach and duodenum during development results in simultaneous rotation of the ventral bud that undergoes fusion with the dorsal bud to give rise to the primitive pancreas. The ventral bud develops into the posterior portion of the pancreatic head, including the uncinate process, and the remaining pancreas is derived from the dorsal bud. In mice, a complex treelike epithelial-lined ductal system develops within the pancreatic diverticula with glucagon immunoreactive cells detected as early as embryonic day 9.5 (E9.5), followed by detection of cells containing insulin at E10.5. Stem cells that give rise to both terminally differentiated endocrine and exocrine acinar cells are believed to reside in the ductal epithelium.

In humans, islet formation begins at gestational week 12 with the aggregation of polyclonal endocrine cells. Between gestational weeks 13 and 16, small aggregates of endocrine cells arise from the pancreatic duct and develop their own blood supply. At gestational weeks 17 to 20, fewer islets are observed in contact with the ducts and a mantle of nonbeta endocrine cells forms around the beta cells. Between gestational weeks 21 and 26, a continual increase in the portion of islet tissue and in the average size of the islets is observed, with occasional nonbeta cells in the center of the islet, a morphologic appearance that is characteristic of the postnatal islet. At birth, the endocrine pancreas accounts for 1% to 2% of the entire pancreatic cell mass.

Although genetic studies in mice have yielded valuable insights into the ontogeny of islet development, the relative order of appearance of unique populations of hormone-producing islet endocrine cells differs in humans and mice. Somatostatin and pancreatic polypeptide (PP)–positive cells are detected at 7 weeks' gestation in the human pancreas, scattered among ductal cells. One week later, glucagon cells appear, and by 9 to 10 weeks' gestation, insulin-producing cells are detectable. In mice, both insulin-expressing and glucagon-expressing cells are first detected between E9.5 and E10.5, and somatostatin and PP are expressed by E15.5. Although cells coexpressing insulin and glucagon are detected during early islet development, cell lineage studies employing specific transgenes that mark or ablate islet cell precursors suggest that the alpha and beta cell lineages arise independently during ontogeny in the mouse.[1] Peptide YY (PYY) colocalizes with each of the four main islet hormones in the developing pancreas; however, genetic evidence for an essential role of a PYY-producing precursor cell in pancreatic endocrine development has not been forthcoming.

Delineation of the genetic determinants that regulate the developmental formation and organization of pancreatic endocrine cell populations has been facilitated by studies of mice with disruption of candidate regulatory genes, principally islet transcription factors (Table 38–1). The homeobox transcription factor Pdx-1 is required for insulin gene transcription in the adult beta cell and for developmental formation of the entire pancreas. Similarly, the homeodomain transcription factor Prox1 controls pancreatic morphogenesis and formation of islet cell precursors after E13.5. Mice homozygous for a null mutation in Pdx-1 fail to develop a pancreas, whereas restricted inactivation of Pdx-1 in the murine beta cell produces insulin deficiency and diabetes. Similarly, pancreatic agenesis has also been reported in human subjects homozygous for a loss of function Pdx-1 mutation,[2] whereas subjects heterozygous for Pdx-1 develop a form of maturity-onset diabetes of the young (MODY4).

Targeted disruption of the LIM domain *Isl-1* gene in mice results in abnormal development of the dorsal pancreatic mesenchyme and abnormal differentiation of islet cells, whereas a heterozygous human *ISL-1* mutation has been reported in a single patient with type 2 diabetes. Although mutations in the *pax4* and *pax6* genes produce profound abnormalities in developmental formation of murine pancreatic endocrine cells,[3] islet function has not been extensively studied in human subjects with *PAX* mutations. Nevertheless, binding sites for the MODY genes *Pdx-1, HNF1α,* and *HNF4α* have been identified in the pax4 promoter, suggesting that MODY genes may be upstream regulators of genes critical for islet cell formation and islet function in the pancreas.

Genes encoding members of the Notch receptor family, and their ligands and downstream targets, are essential for developmental formation of the endocrine pancreas (see Table 38–1). Targeted inactivation of genes in the Notch signaling pathway markedly perturbs the normal development and differentiation of pancreatic endocrine cells. Mice lacking neurogenin 3 (ngn 3), a basic helix-loop-helix (bHLH) transcription factor, fail to develop pancreatic endocrine cells and die from diabetes postnatally, whereas overexpression of ngn 3 produces accelerated differentiation of pancreatic endocrine cells. These findings, together with the loss of *Isl-1, Pax4, Pax6,* and *NeuroD* expression in $ngn3^{-/-}$ mice, implicate *ngn3* as a key upstream regulator of pancreatic endocrine cell development.[4]

The transcription factor Arx is expressed in a *ngn3*-dependent manner, and targeted inactivation of the *Arx* gene results in hypoglycemia and neonatal lethality, with a failure to develop islet alpha cells.[5] Similarly, the NKX transcription factor family appears essential for the formation of both beta and alpha cell lineages in the mouse.[6] Intriguingly, targeted deletion of the *Nkx2.2* gene produces murine islets expressing ghrelin,[7] and studies have demonstrated that ghrelin is produced in a subset of normal islet alpha cells and in a small portion of newly identified ghrelin-producing epsilon cells.[7]

Research into the identification of upstream control mechanisms and downstream targets that promote islet cell formation, growth, and differentiation is likely to proceed rapidly in the next few years, providing scientists and clinicians with an enhanced understanding of the genetic determinants regulating the growth of normal and neoplastic endocrine cells. A summary of genetic mutations associated with abnormal formation of pancreatic endocrine cells is provided in Table 38–1.

TABLE 38–1 EFFECTS OF DISRUPTING GENES IMPORTANT FOR PANCREATIC ENDOCRINE CELL DEVELOPMENT

Gene	Phenotype in Homozygous (–/–) Mutant Mice
Arx	Failure to develop glucagon$^+$ alpha cells
Hes-1	Increased glucagon$^+$ alpha cells, pancreatic hypoplasia
Hlxb-9	Dorsal lobe agenesis, small islets, reduced beta cells
Isl-1	Loss of differentiated islet cells
NeuroD	Reduced beta cells, arrested islet morphogenesis
Nkx-2.2	Absent mature beta cells, reduced alpha and PP cells
Nkx-6.1	Reduced beta cell precursors
Ngn3	Absent islet cells and defective enteroendocrine cell formation
Pax4	Absent islet beta and alpha cells
Pax6	Absent islet alpha cells
Pbx1	Marked reductions in islet alpha and beta cells
Pdx-1	Pancreatic agenesis

Endocrine Cell Development in the Intestine

Stem cells associated with the intestinal epithelium differentiate into four different cell lineages: enterocytes, Paneth cells, goblet cells, and enteroendocrine cells. The bHLH gene *Math1* is a critical regulator of intestinal secretory cell lineages; deletion of *Math1* results in failure to develop goblet, Paneth, or enteroendocrine cell lineages.[8] The enteroendocrine cell population forms less than 1% of all intestinal epithelial cells but represents the largest mass of endocrine cells in the body.

Compared with studies of pancreatic endocrine cell development, much less is known about the molecular control of enteroendocrine cell formation and differentiation. Numerous enteroendocrine cell types have been identified that can be classified based on morphologic criteria and expression of one or more secretory products. In the stomach, gastrin cells first appear in the duodenum and then are localized to the antrum and pylorus in adult gastric mucosa. In the small bowel, a secretin-precursor cell appears important for enteroendocrine cell lineage formation. In the murine colon, PYY is the first detectable hormone marking appearance of enteroendocrine cells and is coexpressed in most endocrine cells in the large intestine as they first differentiate.

The Notch signaling pathway is essential for developmental formation of enteroendocrine bHLH cells. Activation of Notch results in increased expression of the transcriptional repressor Hes1 that functionally antagonizes bHLH genes that regulate cellular differentiation. Mice deficient in Hes1 demonstrate premature cellular differentiation and severe pancreatic hypoplasia due to depletion of pancreatic epithelial precursors.[9] These mice also demonstrate excessive differentiation of multiple endocrine cell types in the developing stomach and gut, suggesting that Hes1 is a negative regulator of endodermal endocrine differentiation. Ngn3 is expressed at early time points during gut development and is essential for development of enteroendocrine cells in the small intestine[10] and in the stomach.[11] Both Notch1 and Neurogenin3 act upstream of BETA2/NeuroD, a bHLH protein important for differentiation of endocrine cells in both the pancreas and intestine[12] (Table 38–2).

Mice homozygous for a null mutation in the *Pdx-1* gene demonstrate poorly differentiated duodenal intestinal epithelium, with absence of Brunner's glands and a deficiency of gastrin cells in the stomach. Just distal to the abnormal epithelium, a reduction in the number of enteroendocrine cells is observed. In contrast, expression of Pdx-1 in gut epithelial cells redirects cell lineage toward an enteroendocrine phenotype. Inactivation of BETA2/NeuroD in mice results in absence of secretin-producing and cholecystokinin (CCK)-producing enteroendocrine cells.[12] The complexity of lineage relationships between gut endocrine cell populations is further illustrated by studies in mice with targeted ablation of secretin-producing cells. These mice exhibit nearly complete elimination of enteroendocrine cell populations producing CCK and PYY/glucagon and a reduction in cells producing gastric inhibitory polypeptide (GIP), somatostatin, and serotonin.[13]

Members of the Pax gene family are also essential for the formation of enteroendocrine cells (see Table 38–2). Targeted disruption of *Pax4* markedly reduces the number of murine duodenal cells immunopositive for serotonin, secretin, GIP, PYY, and CCK and decreases the number of somatostatin- and serotonin-positive cells in the stomach. Complete disruption of the *Pax6* locus more selectively reduces the number of duodenal cells expressing GIP and CCK[14] and decreases the number of gastrin and somatostatin-immunopositive cells in the stomach. However, SEY^{NEU} mice that express a dominant negative mutant *Pax6* allele demonstrate markedly reduced levels of proglucagon mRNA transcripts in both the small and large intestine, with almost complete depletion of enteroendocrine cells exhibiting glucagon-like peptide 1 (GLP-1) and GLP-2 immunoreactivity (Fig. 38–1).[15]

At present, the classification of enteroendocrine cells is based principally on the phenotype ascribed to the production of one or more peptide hormones. Nevertheless, it seems likely that additional enteroendocrine cell subpopulations will be described in different regions of the gut that exhibit considerable biologic complexity beyond what is currently appreciated.

TABLE 38–2 CONSEQUENCES OF DISRUPTING GENES IMPORTANT FOR DEVELOPMENT OF ENTEROENDOCRINE CELLS

Gene	Phenotype in homozygous (–/–) mutant mice
Hes-1	Enhanced numbers of enteroendocrine cells
NeuroD	Absent secretin and CCK lineages
Ngn3	Absent enteroendocrine cell development in the small intestine
Pax4	Reduced endocrine cell lineages in duodenum and stomach
Pax6	Reduced number of GIP$^+$ K cells, antral gastrin and somatostatin cells, and L cells
Pdx-1	Reduced enteroendocrine cells in stomach and duodenum
Ihh	Reduced enteroendocrine cells in duodenum

CCK, cholecystokinin; GIP, gastric inhibitory polypeptide.

Pancreatic and Gut Hormones

Amylin

Amylin, also known as islet amyloid associated peptide (IAPP), is a 37–amino acid hormone produced in islet beta cells and in scattered endocrine cells in the stomach and in the proximal small intestine. Exogenous administration of amylin inhibits gastric emptying and glucagon secretion in rodents and humans. Excess amylin secretion and deposition in the endocrine pancreas has been implicated as a potential pathogenic feature in some subjects with type 2 diabetes, and transgenic mice engineered to overexpress human amylin develop islet amyloid and impaired insulin secretion following high-fat feeding.[16]

Amylin exerts its physiologic actions through interaction with the calcitonin receptor in the presence of a receptor activity–modifying protein (RAMP). Mice deficient in amylin display modest perturbations in islet function and enhanced glucose clearance following glucose challenge. The role of gut-derived amylin in human physiology has not been clearly established; however, the amylin analogue pramlintide has been approved for treatment of type 1 and type 2 diabetes as adjunctive therapy to concomitant insulin administration.[17] Although amylin expression has been detected in both pancreatic and gut endocrine tumors, a specific syndrome attributable to amylin overexpression has not been delineated.

Apelin

Apelin is a 36–amino acid peptide originally purified from bovine stomach extracts. It is the endogenous ligand for the orphan APJ G protein–coupled receptor (GPCR).[18] Apelin and its receptor are widely expressed in peripheral tissues such as the lungs, heart, and mammary gland and in the CNS. In the gastrointestinal tract, apelin is most abundant in the stomach.[19] Apelin produces vasodilator and inotropic actions in the cardiovascular system.[20] The Apelin receptor functions as a coreceptor for HIV in vitro, and apelin-related peptides act as antagonists of HIV infection in vitro.[20]

Calcitonin Gene–Related Peptide

Calcitonin gene–related peptide (CGRP) is a member of a larger family of peptides that includes calcitonin, amylin, and adrenomedullin. In humans, distinct genes *CALC-A* and *CALC-B* encode for both calcitonin and CGRP and give rise to two 37–amino acid C-terminal amidated neuropeptides designated α-CGRP and β-CGRP. These neuropeptides share considerable amino acid

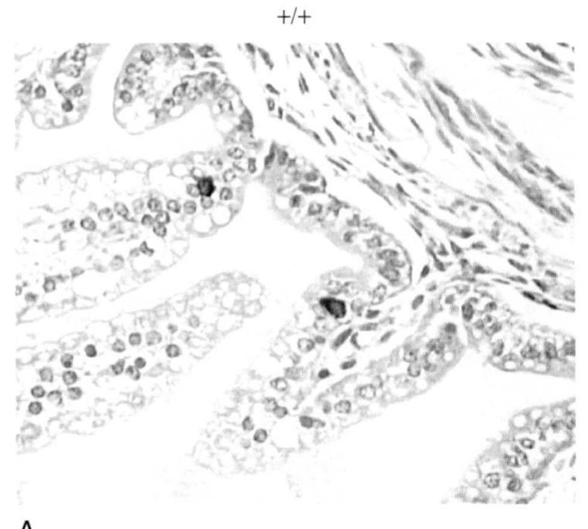

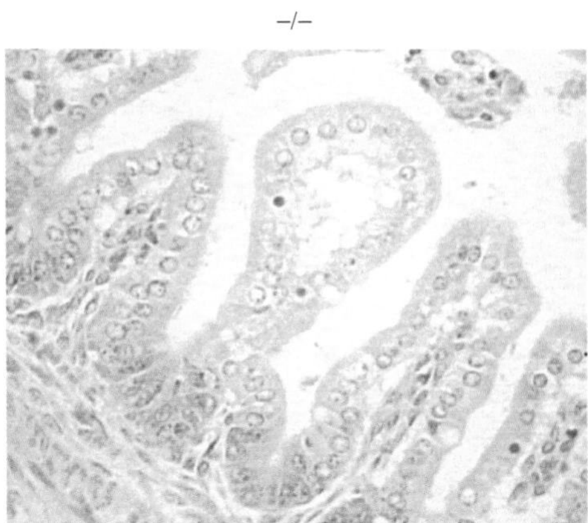

Figure 38–1 ■ Essential requirement for *Pax6* for glucagon$^+$ enteroendocrine cell formation in the murine intestine. *Pax6* SEY^{NEU} mutant mice (–/–) exhibit markedly reduced numbers of glucagon-immunopositive cells in the small and large intestine.

sequence homology, differing by only three amino acids in humans. α-CGRP is expressed predominantly in primary afferent sensory neurons arising from the spinal cord, and β-CGRP is expressed in enteric neurons. Two calcitonin-CGRP seven-transmembrane domain GPCRs[21] both interact with a family of RAMPs; coexpression of calcitonin receptor–like receptor with RAMP1 results in ligand specificity for CGRP, and expression of the same receptor with RAMP2 results in specificity for adrenomedullin.[22]

CGRP immunoreactivity has been localized to enteroendocrine cells of the human rectum and to endocrine cells and neurons in the small intestine. Intestinal CGRP is released in response to glucose and by gastric acid secretion. CGRP produces marked vasodilation in the stomach, splanchnic, and peripheral circulation through stimulating nitric oxide (NO) release. CGRP also inhibits gastric acid and pancreatic exocrine secretion, likely through stimulating somatostatin release. Although focal CGRP positivity has been detected in some human carcinoid and pancreatic endocrine tumors, its usefulness as a tumor marker has not been firmly established.

Cholecystokinin

CCK was first characterized as a factor that stimulates gallbladder contraction. The CCK gene is expressed in open-type enteroendocrine I-cells in the proximal small intestine (Table 38–3) and in nerve fibers branching to the gastric and colonic myenteric plexus and submucosal plexus, where CCK acts as a neurotransmitter. CCK-immunoreactive peptides are found in the cerebral cortex and limbic system and in pituitary corticotrophs, C-cells of the thyroid, adrenal medulla, and the acrosome of the developing and mature spermatozoa. The CCK gene encodes a 94–amino acid prohormone that is posttranslationally processed in a tissue-specific fashion into multiple molecular forms of CCK-83, 58, 39, 33, 22, 8, and 5, all sharing a common C-terminus. The major active form, CCK-8, is an octapeptide containing a sulfated tyrosine residue and an amidated C-terminal phenylalanine residue. CCK-33 appears to be the predominant circular form in human plasma.[23]

CCK binds with high affinity to the CCK-A receptor, a seven-transmembrane domain GPCR expressed in pancreatic acinar cells, gallbladder, smooth muscle, chief and D cells of the gastric mucosa, and the central and peripheral nervous system. In the stomach, CCK inhibits proximal gastric motility while increasing the force of antral and pyloric contractions. CCK also regulates meal-stimulated pancreatic enzyme secretion and gallbladder contraction.

CCK exhibits tropic effects on pancreatic acini in rats. Experimental manipulations that increase levels of circulating CCK, such as treatment with soybean trypsin inhibitor or long-term pancreatobiliary diversion, result in pancreatic growth and premalignant changes. Elevated circulating levels of CCK also enhance the development of preneoplastic acinar lesions induced by azaserine, a pancreatic carcinogen in rats. In contrast, the Otsuka Long-Evans Tokushima fatty (OLETF) rat fails to express a functional CCK-A receptor and demonstrates reduced pancreatic size.[24]

Exogenous administration of CCK decreases the size of spontaneously ingested meals, and CCK-A–receptor antagonists increase appetite and delay gastric emptying in humans. A human subject with polyglandular syndrome type 1 exhibited severe diarrhea and malabsorption, in association with reduced numbers of enteroendocrine cells and CCK deficiency.[25] Thus, CCK secretion in response to oral nutrient ingestion likely regulates nutrient absorption and postprandial satiety. Nevertheless, CCK receptors do not appear essential for weight regulation in vivo, because mice with targeted disruption of the CCK-A and CCK-B receptors exhibit normal food intake and weight gain well into adult life. Emerging evidence suggests that CCK might represent an important growth factor for adaptive islet growth in rodents.

TABLE 38–3 LOCATION OF ENTEROENDOCRINE CELLS AND THEIR ASSOCIATED PEPTIDE HORMONES IN THE GASTROINTESTINAL TRACT

Hormones	Enteroendocrine Cell	Location
Somatostatin	D cells	Stomach, duodenum, small intestine, colon
Gastrin, TRH	G cells	Stomach and duodenum
CCK	I cells	Duodenum and jejunum
GIP	K cells	Duodenum and proximal jejunum
GLP-1, GLP-2, PYY	L cells	Ileum, colon, and rectum
Motilin	M cells	Duodenum and proximal jejunum
Neurotensin	N cells	Small intestine especially ileum
Secretin	S cells	Duodenum and proximal jejunum

CCK, cholecystokinin; GIP, gastric inhibitory polypeptide; GLP, glucagon-like peptide; TRH, thyrotropin-releasing hormone.

Galanin

Galanin was initially isolated from porcine intestine as a 29–amino acid C-terminally amidated neuropeptide. Humans have two molecular forms of galanin, which are 19 and 30 amino acids in length. Galanin is expressed in the central and peripheral nervous systems, in the pituitary, and in neural structures of the gut, pancreas, thyroid, and adrenal gland. In the intestine, galanin immunoreactivity is detected predominantly in enteric neurons located in the myenteric and submucosal plexus that innervate the mucosa and the circular and longitudinal smooth muscle layer. Galanin is released by enteric neurons in response to intestinal distention, chemical stimulation of the mucosa, electrical stimulation of periarterial nerves, and extrinsic sympathetic neurons.

At least three different galanin receptor subtypes have been identified: GalR1, GalR2, and GalR3. These are widely expressed in gastric and intestinal smooth muscle cells, pancreas, and the CNS.[26] The actions of galanin include regulation of food intake, memory and cognition, antinociception, and modulation of multiple neuroendocrine systems in the pituitary, pancreas, and gut.

Galanin exhibits potent anticonvulsant activity in experimental rodent models of seizure disorders,[27] likely via modulation of glutamate release. Galanin might also act as a neuroprotective factor, and galanin knockout mice exhibit enhanced sensitivity to neuronal injury.[28] Although $GalR1^{-/-}$ mice exhibit increased anxiety and abnormal nociceptive sensitivity, mice with inactivation of the GalR2 receptor are normal and do not exhibit defects in classic phenotypes ascribed to galanin. The importance of galanin for pituitary lactotroph biology is exemplified by studies of galanin knockout mice that exhibit normal growth rates but reduced levels of prolactin and complete failure of lactation.[29]

Although galanin can inhibit GIP-induced and GLP-1–induced proinsulin gene transcription and insulin secretion, infusion of galanin in humans has no effect on levels of plasma insulin. Galanin also inhibits both pancreatic exocrine secretion and intestinal ion transport and induces both the contraction and relaxation of intestinal smooth muscle. In humans, intravenous administration of galanin delays gastric emptying and prolongs colonic transit times. Although galanin expression has been detected in hypothalamic, pituitary, and adrenal tumors, galanin-immunopositivity in pancreatic or gut endocrine tumor cells is rare.

Gastric Inhibitory Polypeptide

Gastric inhibitory polypeptide (GIP; also called glucose-dependent insulinotropic polypeptide) is a 42–amino acid peptide secreted by enteroendocrine K-cells located in the duodenum and proximal jejunum. GIP levels rise immediately following nutrient ingestion, leading to modest inhibitory effects on gastric acid secretion and gastrointestinal motility. The precise role of GIP as an enterogastrone remains controversial, because supraphysiologic concentrations of GIP are required to inhibit both gastric acid secretion and gastric emptying in humans.

The actions of GIP on the pancreatic beta cell are primarily those of an incretin, a gut-derived peptide that stimulates insulin secretion in the setting of raised plasma glucose levels following oral nutrient ingestion. GIP-receptor knockout mice are viable but exhibit impaired oral glucose tolerance and enhanced susceptibility to diabetes following high-fat feeding.[30] Intriguingly, GIP receptors are expressed on adipocytes, where they modulate lipid accumulation. Transient blockade of GIP receptor signaling with GIP peptide antagonists or genetic elimination of the GIP receptor in mice reduces fat storage in adipocytes and might contribute to improved insulin sensitivity via reduction of adipokine expression.[31]

GIP is an essential determinant of bone resorption in rodents; however, the role of GIP in the control of bone turnover in human subjects remains uncertain. GIP is a potent stimulator of glucose-dependent insulin secretion in normal rodents and human subjects, and experimental or clinical diabetes is associated with defective GIP action and reduced insulinotropic activity of exogenous GIP. GIP-secreting endocrine tumors are rare; however, gut-derived GIP might contribute to the development of food-induced Cushing's syndrome in a subset of patients with adrenal adenomas that express the GIP receptor.[32]

Gastrin

A single mRNA transcript encodes a pre-progastrin precursor of 101 amino acids that undergoes posttranslational processing into multiple biologically active molecular forms of circulating gastrin including G34, G17, and G14. Gastrin is produced predominantly in G cells located in the gastric antrum and duodenal bulb. However, gastrin immunoreactivity has also been detected in the central and peripheral nervous systems, pituitary, adrenal gland, genital tract, respiratory tract, and tumors.

The fetal endocrine pancreas produces large amounts of amidated gastrin, suggesting a possible role of gastrin in pancreatic development. However, gastrin-deficient mice do not demonstrate overt abnormalities in pancreatic islet morphology. A possible role for gastrin in human islet biology derives from studies of the CCK-2 receptor on pancreatic A cells, which secrete glucagon in response to gastrin in vitro. Gastrin$^{-/-}$ mice, however, exhibit modest fasting hypoglycemia and defective glucagon secretion in response to hypoglycemia.[33]

G cells are open type endocrine cells subject to regulation by luminal contents in addition to humoral and neural influences. The effects of gastrin on acid secretion are mediated by the fully processed amidated forms of gastrin (G-17 and G-34) at the CCK-2 receptor (formerly known as the CCK-B/gastrin receptor) located on the enterochromaffin-like (ECL) cells of the oxyntic mucosa. Gastrin stimulates histamine synthesis and release from ECL cells, which then induce acid secretion by binding to the H_2 receptor located on the basolateral aspect of the parietal cell. Gastrin also stimulates acid secretion from parietal cells via the CCK-2 receptor.

The physiologic roles of progastrin and glycine-extended gastrin (G-Gly) are less completely defined but might involve regulation of the growth and differentiation of the gastrointestinal tract. Amidated gastrin is tropic to the oxyntic mucosa of the stomach, where it stimulates proliferation of gastric stem cells and ECL cells, resulting in increased parietal and ECL mass. G-Gly exerts tropic effects on the colonic mucosa and stimulates growth of a diverse number of human cancers. Transgenic mice expressing progastrin or G-Gly exhibit increased colonic proliferation and mucosal thickness and are more prone to formation of aberrant crypt foci following treatment with azoxymethane, whereas inactivation of the gastrin gene results in reduced basal rates of colonic proliferation.[34]

Gastrin has been reported to induce proliferation of colon cancer cell lines expressing the CCK-2 receptor; however, most colon cancers and normal colonic epithelium do not normally express the CCK-2 receptor. A truncated gastrin-binding receptor has been described in some colon cancer cell lines and in a constitutively active CCK-2 receptor mutant, CCK2i4svR, that confers ligand-independent growth to transfected cells and has been identified in human colorectal and pancreatic cancers.[35,36] Both the CCK-1 and CCK-2 receptors can form homo- and heterodimers, and heterodimerization appears to modulate the sensitivity to agonist-induced cell growth.[37]

The tropic effects of gastrin have led to studies of gastrin-neutralizing antisera for the potential treatment of intestinal neoplasia.[38] Conversely, gastrin-17 has also been shown to reduce cell proliferation and induce apoptosis in human colon cancer cells expressing the CCK-2 receptor.[39] Gastrin is also mitogenic for rodent and human pancreatic islet and ductal cells cultured in vitro or propagated in immunodeficient nonobese diabetic–severe combined immune deficiency mice.[40] Treatment of NOD (nonobese diabetic) mice with gastrin and EGF induces regeneration of beta cell mass and reverses experimental type 1 diabetes.[41] These findings implicate a role for gastrin or EGF, or both, in the modulation of the immune response that initiates the development of type 1 diabetes in the NOD mouse.

Gastrin-Releasing Peptide and Related Peptides

The bombesin family of peptides was originally isolated from frog skin and includes bombesin, gastrin-releasing peptide (GRP, the mammalian homolog of bombesin), neuromedin B (NMB), and neuromedin C (NMC). GRP is a 27–amino acid peptide, and NMB and NMC are decapeptides. These peptides share an identical C-terminal α-amidated heptapeptide sequence that is essential for biologic activity. GRP is expressed in the central, peripheral, and enteric nervous system, reproductive tract, and lung, where it acts as a neurotransmitter. NMB is expressed predominantly in the brain and GI tract. In the intestine, GRP and NMB are localized to neurons in the submucosal and myenteric plexus of the stomach, small intestine, and colon. GRP-containing neurons are also distributed throughout the human pancreas. Bombesin and GRP stimulate smooth muscle cell contraction in the stomach, intestine, and gallbladder. GRP stimulates the release of CCK, gastrin, GIP, glucagon, GLP-1 and GLP-2, motilin, PP, PYY, and somatostatin in some but not all species.

Three GRP receptor subtypes have been cloned that are seven transmembrane domain GPCRs that bind bombesin-like peptides. The subtypes include a GRP-preferring subtype (expressed throughout the intestine), an NMB-preferring subtype (expressed in the esophageal and intestinal muscularis), and a third subtype designated *bombesin receptor subtype 3* (BRS-3), which preferentially binds GRP over NMB and is expressed in testes and small cell lung cancer. GRP regulates appetite, memory, and thermoregulation and suppresses appetite following intracerebroventricular or systemic administration. GRP-preferring (GRP-R) knockout mice exhibit defective control of food intake and increased body weight gain.[42] GRP stimulates pancreatic growth in part via a CCK-dependent mechanism. The expression of GRP in human tumors with neuroendocrine properties, such as small cell lung carcinoma and medullary thyroid carcinoma, together with its autocrine and endocrine effects on cell growth, suggest that GRP contributes to regulation of tumor cell growth.[43] GRP also exhibits angiogenic properties, and GRP antagonists reduce tumor growth and angiogenesis in vivo.[44]

Ghrelin

Ghrelin, a motilin-related peptide, is a 28–amino acid growth hormone–releasing factor originally purified from rat stomach that stimulates growth hormone release via the growth hormone secretagogue receptor (GHS-R). Fasting increases gastric ghrelin gene expression, and ghrelin exhibits gastric prokinetic activity and orexigenic activity following intracerebroventricular and peripheral administration via the ghrelin receptor expressed in hypothalamic nuclei. Ghrelin expression is also induced by stressors, and ghrelin might play a role in the anxiogenic stress response in a CRF-dependent manner in mice. The majority of rat and human gut endocrine cells that express ghrelin are localized to the stomach, and a small number of ghrelin-positive cells have been identified in the small and large intestine.[45] The GHS-R is also expressed in the gut; however, the function of the intestinal ghrelin-GHS-R axis remains poorly understood. Bioactive ghrelin is acylated, and circulating immunoreactive ghrelin represents a mixture of the free acylated form as well as molecules bound to higher molecular weight proteins.[45]

Circulating levels of ghrelin in human subjects increase and fall before and after food ingestion, consistent with a role for ghrelin in appetite regulation. The effects of ghrelin on stimulation of appetite, but not on growth hormone secretion, require an intact vagus nerve.[46] A large number of hormonal mediators regulate plasma levels of ghrelin, including PYY3-36, which suppresses appetite in association with a reduction in circulating ghrelin. Diet-induced weight loss is associated with a compensatory increase in circulating ghrelin, whereas some patients with weight loss following gastric bypass surgery fail to up-regulate plasma levels of ghrelin.[47] Ghrelin exhibits a number of actions beyond control of appetite, including regulation of insulin sensitivity and hepatic glucose output and regulation of immature Leydig cell proliferation. Ghrelin is expressed in pancreatic islet alpha cells and might regulate glucose-induced insulin secretion. Ghrelin also exhibits effects on cardiovascular function including vasodilation, inhibition of a proinflammatory response in endothelial cells, and improvement of left ventricular contractility, and exercise capacity in human subjects with left ventricular failure.[48]

Glucagon, Glucagon-like Peptide-1, and Glucagon-like Peptide-2

The proglucagon gene is expressed in the pancreatic A cell, intestinal L cell, and specialized regions of the brain, primarily neurons in the brain stem and, to a lesser extent, the hypothalamus. In mammals, a single proglucagon precursor is differentially processed to yield multiple proglucagon-derived peptides (PGDPs) including glucagon in the islet A cell, and glicentin, oxyntomodulin, GLP-1, GLP-2, and several spacer or intervening peptides in the gut enteroendocrine L cell.

Pancreatic glucagon is a 29–amino acid peptide that regulates plasma glucose levels via effects on gluconeogenesis and glycogenolysis. Glucagon excess represents one of the hallmark metabolic derangements that contribute to the development of hyperglycemia in both type 1 and type 2 diabetes. Conversely, appropriately increased glucagon secretion functions as the primary counterregulatory mechanism to restore normal levels of plasma glucose in hypoglycemia, and patients prone to frequent episodes of hypoglycemia may use glucagon injections for emergency management of severe hypoglycemia.

The physiologic importance of glucagon action has been examined using genetic or transient interruption of glucagon receptor expression. Glucagon receptor knockout mice exhibit modest fasting hypoglycemia, pancreatic alpha cell hyperplasia, and markedly elevated levels of circulating glucagon.[49] Similarly, transient reduction of glucagon receptor mRNA transcripts in rodents markedly lowers blood glucose, improves insulin secretion, and increases levels of circulating GLP-1 in rodents with experimental diabetes.

GLP-1 secreted from the gut endocrine cell enhances glucose disposal following nutrient ingestion by inhibition of gastric emptying, stimulation of insulin secretion, and inhibition of glucagon secretion.[50] Pharmacologic levels of GLP-1 also inhibit food intake, stimulate pancreatic islet neogenesis and proliferation, and inhibit beta cell apoptosis (Fig. 38–2), biologic actions that facilitate long-term control of nutrient homeostasis. The physiologic importance of endogenous GLP-1 has been studied using the GLP-1 receptor antagonist exendin9-39 and GLP-1R$^{-/-}$ mice. Exendin9-39 deteriorates glycemic control, increases insulin and decreases glucagon, and increases gastric emptying, illustrating the essential importance of endogenous GLP-1 in the control of islet hormone secretion and gut motility. Similarly, GLP-1R$^{-/-}$ mice exhibit defective glucose-stimulated insulin secretion, glucose intolerance, and enhanced susceptibility to islet injury.[51] In contrast, interruption or elimination of GLP-1 action does not have a significant effect on food intake or long-term control of body weight.

A GLP-1R agonist, exendin-4 (exenatide), has been used to treat patients whose type 2 diabetes was previously subopti-

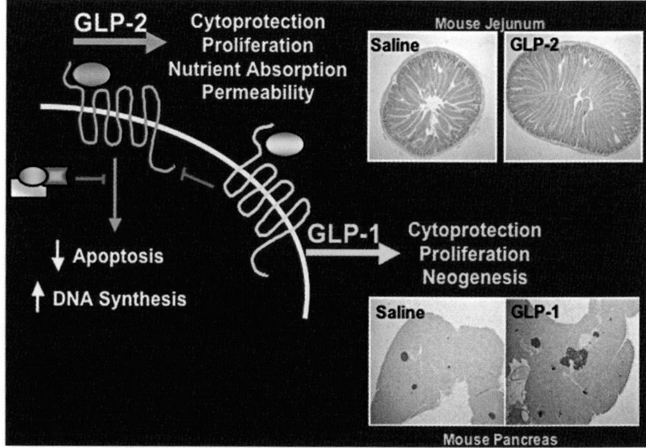

Figure 38–2 ▪ Molecular mechanisms of glucagon-like peptide (GLP) action. The GLP-1 receptor expressed on islet beta cells promotes growth and cytoprotection, leading to expansion of beta cell mass. The GLP-2 receptor, expressed on human gut endocrine cells, enteric neurons, and myofibroblasts, indirectly activates pathways coupled to control of mucosal permeability, cell proliferation, and apoptosis, leading to expansion of the surface area of the small bowel mucosal epithelium.

mally controlled on one or two oral hypoglycemic agents. Twice-daily administration of exenatide reduced hemoglobin A_{1c} (HbA_{1c}) and prevented weight gain in 6-month randomized clinical trials.[52-54] The principal side effects associated with exenatide use were gastrointestinal, predominantly nausea. Antibodies against exenatide were detected in about 40% of treated patients, but they did not seem to correlate with therapeutic outcome. Exenatide was approved for the treatment of type 2 diabetes in the United States in April 2005.

GLP-2 is a 33–amino acid peptide that is cosecreted with GLP-1, oxyntomodulin, and glicentin from enteroendocrine cells in a nutrient-dependent manner. GLP-2 inhibits both centrally induced antral motility and meal-stimulated gastric acid secretion. GLP-2 exhibits tropic actions in the small intestine and colon, via stimulation of crypt cell proliferation and reduction of apoptosis within the crypt and villus compartments (see Fig. 38–02).[55] GLP-2 also exerts actions independent of intestinal growth, including enhancement of intestinal epithelial barrier function and stimulation of intestinal hexose transport.[56] The beneficial therapeutic actions of GLP-2 in experimental models of intestinal injury and in human subjects with short bowel syndrome suggest that GLP-2 may be useful for preventing injury and enhancing repair and regeneration in the gastrointestinal epithelium.[56,57]

The actions of GLP-1 and GLP-2 are transduced via distinct GLP-1 and GLP-2 receptors; however, both GLP-1 and GLP-2 are rapidly inactivated by the same enzyme, dipeptidyl peptidase-4 (DPP-4). Genetic elimination of DPP-4 action in rodents increases the levels of GIP and GLP-1, enhances glucose-stimulated insulin secretion, and lowers blood glucose.[58] Conversely, chemical inhibitors of DPP-4 lower glucose and HbA_{1c} in preclinical models as well as in human subjects with type 2 diabetes.[59] DPP-4 inhibitors are in late-stage clinical testing and sitaglptin has been approved for the treatment of type 2 diabetes in 2006.

In contrast to GLP-1 and GLP-2, the biologic actions of the PGDPs glicentin and oxyntomodulin are less well established. Glicentin appears tropic for the gut mucosal epithelium, whereas oxyntomodulin inhibits short-term food intake and pentagastrin-stimulated gastric acid secretion both in vitro and in vivo. Oxyntomodulin administered three times daily for 4 weeks reduced body weight in overweight and obese human subjects.[60] Although distinct GPCRs for glucagon, GLP-1, and GLP-2 have been characterized, separate receptors that mediate the actions of glicentin and oxyntomodulin have not yet been identified, and the anorectic action of oxyntomodulin requires a functional GLP-1 receptor.[61]

Motilin

Motilin is a 22–amino acid peptide originally isolated from porcine intestine. Motilin immunoreactivity has been detected in open-type enteroendocrine epithelial M cells located predominantly in the duodenum and proximal jejunum. Secretion of motilin occurs in a cyclic manner during the interdigestive state between meals. The presence of nutrients in the duodenum suppresses the endogenous release of motilin in dogs and humans. Duodenal alkalinization, sham feeding, gastric distension, and the administration of opioid agonists promote motilin secretion.

A putative motilin receptor has been cloned that exhibits 52% amino acid identity with the human receptor for growth hormone secretagogues. The motilin receptor also binds erythromycin and is expressed in multiple regions of the GI tract, predominantly in smooth muscle and enteric neurons.[62]

Motilin induces phase III contractions in the stomach, an effect that can be abolished by food ingestion, duodenal acidification, somatostatin, pentagastrin, and CCK. Atropine and 5-hydroxytryptamine (serotonin) antagonists also abolish phase III contractions, emphasizing the importance of the cholinergic and serotoninergic neuronal pathways. Motilin stimulates gastric and pancreatic enzyme secretion and induces contraction of the gallbladder, sphincter of Oddi, and lower esophageal sphincter. Administration of motilin induces nausea and inhibits gastric emptying in human subjects.

Neuropeptide Y (NPY)

NPY is primarily synthesized and secreted by neurons in the central and peripheral nervous system. In the brain, NPY is expressed not only in the hypothalamus, where it exhibits extremely potent effects on nutrient intake, but also in the cortex, hippocampus, basal forebrain striation, limbic structures, amygdala, and brain stem. In the peripheral nervous system, NPY expression occurs predominantly in sympathetic neurons and in the myenteric and submucous plexuses of the enteric nervous system. NPY and vasoactive intestinal peptide (VIP) are often coexpressed in enteric neurons. NPY is synthesized in and released from pancreatic islet cells and inhibits glucose-stimulated insulin secretion via the Y1 receptor. Elevated circulating NPY levels are observed following sympathetic nervous system activation and in patients with pancreatic endocrine tumors and carcinoid tumors and with neurogenic tumors including neuroblastomas and pheochromocytomas.

NPY exerts its actions via at least four receptor subtypes including, the Y1 and Y2 receptors (which bind NPY and PYY with similar affinities) and the Y3 receptor (which exhibits a preference for NPY over PYY). Increased hypothalamic NPY is a potent stimulator of food intake in rodents; however, NPY antagonists have not yet proved useful for treating human obesity. NPY actions in the cardiovascular system include stimulation of vascular smooth muscle cell growth and neointima formation via Y1 and Y1 receptors, whereas angiogenic effects are mediated via Y2 and Y5 receptor activation.[63] NPY and PYY are targets for N-terminal degradation by the enzyme dipeptidyl peptidase IV (DP IV), leading to the generation of NPY3-36 and PYY3-36 peptides, which exhibit preferential binding to the Y2 receptor. In the gastrointestinal tract, NPY reduces fluid and electrolyte secretion and inhibits both gastric and small intestinal motility. Intravascular administration of NPY is associated with marked vasoconstriction of the splanchnic circulation, an effect that is not effected by α- or β-adrenergic blockade.

Neurotensin

Neurotensin (NT) is a 13–amino acid peptide originally detected in the bovine hypothalamus. NT-related peptides include neuromedin N, a 6–amino acid neurotensin-like peptide coencoded in proneurotensin, as well as xenin and xenopsin. In the gastrointestinal tract, NT processing favors the generation of NT in N cells of the ileum and in enteric neurons. NT is also produced in the central and peripheral nervous system, heart, adrenal gland, pancreas, and respiratory tract. NT secretion is stimulated by luminal nutrients, especially lipids but not amino acids or carbohydrates. GRP also stimulates NT release, and somatostatin exerts an inhibitory effect.

At least three different NT receptor/binding proteins (NTS1-3) have been identified. NTS1-2 belong to the GPCR family, and NTS3 represents a structurally unrelated protein with neurotensin-binding properties.[64] NTS1 is expressed in the brain and intestine, and NTS2-3 is expressed exclusively in the brain. Neurotensin administration to rats augments the adaptive response to small bowel resection in the intestinal remnant, and NT stimulates growth of the colonic epithelium in vivo. NT also inhibits postprandial gastric acid secretion and pancreatic exocrine secretion, stimulates colonic motility, and inhibits gastric and small intestinal motility. NT facilitates fatty acid uptake in the proximal small intestine and induces histamine release from mast cells.

NT receptor expression has been detected in a subset of human colon and pancreatic ductal cancers, and NT is tropic for some pancreatic and colon cancer cells in vitro. Experiments using NT antagonists or knockout mice implicate a role for neurotensin in pain perception or nociception.

Pituitary Adenylate Cyclase–Activating Peptide

Pituitary adenylate cyclase–activating peptide (PACAP), VIP, and GRF are structurally related members of the glucagon-secretin superfamily.[65] PACAP-immunoreactive nerve fibers are distributed along the gastrointestinal tract from the esophagus to the colon. PACAP1-38 and PACAP1-27 are detected in many tissues, but is generally the predominant peptide. PACAP stimulates histamine release from the stomach; increases the secretion of pancreatic fluid, protein, and bicarbonate; and stimulates insulin secretion and catecholamine release. PACAP signaling in gastric ECL cells might also constitute an important component of the neural regulation of gastric acid secretion.

PACAP exerts neuroprotective agents in the peripheral and central nervous systems likely related to stimulation of cyclic adenosine monophosphate (cAMP) accumulation. PACAP might also play a role in the central control of ventilation, because PACAP-deficient mice experience prolonged apneas, atrioventricular block, and an increased incidence of sudden death. Intriguingly, PACAP modulates platelet function, and PACAP overexpression may be associated with increased platelet cAMP accumulation and effective platelet aggregation.[66] Three PACAP receptors, designated PAC1, VPAC1, and VPAC2, have been cloned and bind PACAP and VIP with varying affinities. Consistent with the putative importance of PACAP for islet function, PAC1-receptor knockout mice exhibit defective glucose-stimulated insulin secretion. Furthermore, PACAP exhibits vasodilative effects in the pulmonary vasculature, whereas PAC1-receptor–deficient mice exhibit pulmonary artery hypertension and right ventricular failure.[67] PACAP1-38 is also a substrate for DPP-4, hence DPP-4 inhibition potentially modulates the clearance of PACAP in vivo.

Peptide YY

PYY, together with NPY and PP, are members of the pancreatic polypeptide family. These peptides consist of 36 amino acids, contain several tyrosine residues, and share considerable amino acid identity with amidated C-terminal ends. Although these peptides likely share a common ancestry, they exhibit unique actions and patterns of tissue-specific expression. PYY and PP act as hormones, and NPY acts primarily as a neurotransmitter.

PYY is expressed in the fetal and adult gastrointestinal tract in enteroendocrine cells. Distinct enteroendocrine subpopulations have been identified that express PYY alone, or both PYY and GLP-1, in the ileum, colon, and rectum. Immunoreactive PYY has also been detected in the developing endocrine pancreas and in a subpopulation of glucagon-producing alpha cells in mature islets. PYY is secreted as a 36–amino acid peptide and circulates as two molecular forms, PYY1-36 and an N-terminally truncated form, PYY3-36. Luminal nutrients, CCK, GRP, and vagal tone regulate PYY secretion.

PYY exerts its actions in part through the NPY Y1 and Y2 receptors. PYY1-36 binds both Y1 and Y2 receptors, but PYY3-36 is selective for the Y2 receptor. PYY demonstrates inhibitory effects on gastrointestinal secretion, motility, and blood flow. In the stomach, PYY functions as enterogastrone, inhibiting both gastric acid secretion and gastric emptying. PYY also increases intestinal transit times by inhibiting motility of the small and large intestines. The role of PYY as an intestinal epithelial growth factor remains unclear, because some but not all studies demonstrate an intestine tropic effect of PYY in rodents. In the pancreas, both PYY1-36 and PYY3-36 inhibit pancreatic exocrine secretion.

Administration of PYY3-36 to rodents and to normal and obese humans potently inhibits food intake in short-term studies.[68] PYY3-36 produces a conditioned taste aversion in some but not all studies in rodents. Obese human subjects exhibit attenuated release of PYY3-36 and reduced satiety in response to meal ingestion. Whether prolonged PYY3-36 administration will produce weight loss in obese human subjects has not yet been determined. In contrast, endogenous PYY does not seem to be essential for food intake and body weight homeostasis in mice, as exemplified by the normal ingestive behavior and body weight of $PYY^{-/-}$ mice.[69]

Pancreatic Polypeptide

Pancreatic polypeptide (PP) was isolated from chicken pancreatic extracts as a by-product of insulin purification. Most PP is expressed in pancreatic endocrine cells located predominantly in the periphery of islets in the pancreatic head and uncinate process. Elevated plasma levels of PP have been detected in patients with gastrointestinal endocrine tumors; hence, PP may be used as a tumor marker in appropriate clinical scenarios. Nutrients, hormones, neurotransmitters, gastric distension, insulin-induced hypoglycemia, and direct vagal nerve stimulation regulate PP secretion, and hyperglycemia, bombesin, and somatostatin inhibit PP secretion.

The actions of PP are mediated by the Y4 receptor, a GPCR coupled to inhibition of cAMP accumulation.[70] The human Y4 receptor is expressed in the stomach, small intestine, colon, pancreas, prostate, the enteric nervous system, and select CNS neurons. Exogenous administration of PP reduces CCK-induced gastric acid secretion and increases intestinal transit times by reducing gastric emptying and upper intestinal motility. PP also inhibits postprandial exocrine pancreas secretion via a vagal-dependent pathway. Transgenic mice that overexpress PP exhibit reduced weight gain and rate of gastric emptying and decreased fat mass. The biologic actions of PP in the gastrointestinal tract and pancreas are in part centrally mediated: Intracisternal injections of PP cause an increase in gastric acid secretion and gastric motility, and a reduction in pancreatic secretion. Administration of PP inhibits gastric emptying and reduces food intake in human subjects over a 24-hour study period.[71]

Secretin

Secretin is a 27–amino acid peptide synthesized predominantly in the brain and gastrointestinal tract. In the gut, secretin is produced by the enteroendocrine S-cell in the duodenum and proximal jejunum. Gastric acid, bile salts and luminal nutrients stimulate and somatostatin inhibits the release of secretin. Secretin stimulates pancreatic and biliary bicarbonate and water secretion, and it might regulate pancreatic enzyme secretion. Secretin also stimulates gastric secretion of pepsinogen and inhibits lower esophageal sphincter tone, postprandial gastric emptying, gastrin release, and gastric acid secretion. Although secretin is expressed in the fetal endocrine pancreas, its function in islet biology remains uncertain. To date, only a single secretin receptor has been isolated and characterized. Secretin has been proposed as a treatment for autism; however, clinical trial results examining this issue have not been consistently positive.[72]

Somatostatin

Somatostatin, originally isolated as a hypothalamic growth hormone release–inhibiting factor, is also expressed in the intestine and pancreas. Posttranslational processing of prosomatostatin results in the generation of SS-14 and SS-28, biologically active peptides corresponding to the C-terminal 14 and 28 amino acids of prosomatostatin. SS-28 is the predominant molecular form liberated by enteroendocrine D cells, and SS-14 is the predominant species liberated by D cells in the stomach and pancreas.

Five somatostatin (SMS) receptor subtypes (SST1-5) have been identified that are expressed in a tissue-specific manner.[73] Somatostatin actions are generally inhibitory; SMS inhibits the secretion of growth hormone and thyrotropin in the pituitary, and insulin, glucagon, and pancreatic polypeptide in the endocrine pancreas. In the gastrointestinal tract, somatostatin inhibits the secretion of a broad range of gut peptides. Somatostatin inhibits pancreatic exocrine secretion and also acts in a paracrine manner on G cells, ECL cells, and parietal cells to inhibit gastric acid secretion. In the brain, somatostatin regulates metabolism of amyloid beta peptide, a primary pathogenic agent of Alzheimer's disease, through modulating proteolytic degradation catalyzed by neprilysin.[74]

The inhibitory properties of somatostatin make it suitable for the treatment of conditions characterized by excess hormone secretion. Although the circulating half-life of native somatostatin is short, longer-acting synthetic somatostatin analogues such as octreotide and lanreotide are useful in treating neuroendocrine tumors, acromegaly, and portal hypertension.[75] Octreotide and lanreotide are octapeptides that bind the SST2 and SST5 somatostatin receptor subtypes, receptors commonly expressed in neuroendocrine tumors. A meta-analysis of clinical trials using these analogues for therapy of acromegaly demonstrated that the efficacy of octreotide LAR is greater than lanreotide SR among subjects unselected for prior somatostatin analogue responsiveness.[76] Somatostatin analogues are also employed for treating portal hypertension and gastrointestinal bleeding. Tumor-associated somatostatin receptor expression forms the basis for the radiolabeled octreotide scan, a test that appears useful for detecting a broad spectrum of human neoplasms.[77] Somatostatin-deficient mice exhibit normal growth but defects in sexually dimorphic hepatic gene expression.

Tachykinins

The family of tachykinins includes substance P (SP), neurokinin A (NKA), and neurokinin B (NKB), all of which share a common C-terminal pentapeptide sequence essential for biologic action. Two genes encode the tachykinins (TKs): a pre-protachykinin (PPT)-A gene that encodes SP and NKA and a PPT-B gene that encodes NKB. Tachykinins are synthesized in neurons localized to the submucous and myenteric plexuses, extrinsic sensory fibers, and enterochromaffin cells in the gut epithelium. Tachykinins are also widely distributed throughout the central and peripheral nervous systems; the respiratory tract, skin, sensory organs; and the urogenital tract.

Four different TK receptors have been cloned and designated NK1-4. They bind tachykinin peptides with different affinities. NK1 receptors preferentially bind SP, NK2 preferentially binds NKA, and NK3 and NK4 preferentially bind NKB.[78] The tachykinins regulate vasomotor and gastrointestinal motor activity, and the ability of tachykinins to induce vasodilation or vasoconstriction appears to be specific to the species and the vascular bed.

Tachykinins exhibit both direct and indirect effects on intestinal smooth muscle contractile activity. Activation of NK1 receptors on the interstitial cells of Cajal and NK2 receptors on intestinal smooth muscle cells directly promotes peristalsis, and activation of NK3 receptors on enteric neurons exerts a prokinetic effect that is indirectly mediated through cholinergic stimulation of enteric smooth muscle cells. The NK1 and NK3 receptors can exhibit inhibitory effects on intestinal motility by inducing the release of inhibitory molecules such as NO and VIP from inhibitory neurons. NK2 receptors can also inhibit intestinal motility either by stimulation of sympathetic ganglia or activation of nonadrenergic inhibitory mechanisms.

NK2 receptor antagonists reduce or prevent trinitrobenzenesulfonic acid (TNBS)-induced weight loss and intestinal injury, and an NK1 receptor antagonist exhibits protective effects in acetic acid–induced colitis. TKs are commonly produced by gut carcinoids and may be responsible for mediating some of the clinical manifestations associated with these tumors. There is considerable interest in determining whether blockade of NK1 and NK2 receptors represent a therapeutic approach for the treatment of asthma. Similarly, the NK1 and NK3 receptors are targets for the development of therapeutic agents that modulate gut motility and pain, potentially in the setting of irritable bowel syndrome.

Thyrotropin-Releasing Hormone

Originally isolated as a hypothalamic regulatory peptide, thyrotropin-releasing hormone (TRH) is expressed throughout the gastrointestinal tract including the stomach, colon, and pancreas. In the pancreas, TRH is most abundantly expressed during perinatal development. Pre-pro-TRH is synthesized by islet beta cells, G cells in the stomach, and neurons composing the myenteric plexus of the esophagus, stomach, and intestine. In the stomach, histamine and serotonin stimulate and endogenous opioids inhibit TRH release.

TRH acts via two related GPCRs, TRHR1, and TRHR2. TRH suppresses pentagastrin-stimulated gastric acid secretion, and chronic administration of TRH induces pancreatic hyperplasia and inhibits amylase release. Centrally administered TRH modulates pancreatic blood flow and gastric mucosal permeability. TRH also attenuates CCK-induced gallbladder smooth muscle contraction and inhibits cholesterol synthesis in the intestinal mucosa.

Vasoactive Intestinal Peptide

VIP is a 28–amino acid member of a peptide superfamily that includes pituitary adenylate cyclase–activating peptide (PACAP), peptide histidine isoleucine (PHI), and peptide histidine methionine (PHM), all neurotransmitters and neuromodulators of the enteric nervous system. The VIP gene is widely expressed in the central and peripheral nervous system. Receptors for VIP and PACAP belong to the same family of GPCRs. The PAC1 receptor binds both PACAP 1-27 and PACAP1-38 with the same affinity, but it is unable to bind VIP. The VPAC1 and VPAC2 receptors recognize both VIP and PACAP.[65]

In the digestive tract, VIP functions as an inhibitory neurotransmitter that induces relaxation of vascular and nonvascular smooth muscle. VIP mediates the relaxation of the lower esophageal sphincter, the sphincter of Oddi, and the anal sphincter. VIP also regulates relaxation associated with gut contraction and may be involved in reflex vasodilation in the small intestine, in part through a nitric oxide (NO)-dependent mechanism. In humans, VIP and PACAP may be colocalized to some neuronal subpopulations and are coreleased as neurotransmitters leading to NO regeneration. VIP inhibits gastric acid secretion but stimulates biliary water and bicarbonate, pancreatic enzymes, and intestinal chloride secretion. VIP might also regulate pancreatic release of insulin and glucagon.

VIP exerts either tropic or growth-inhibitory effects on normal and neoplastic cells.[79] In the lung, VIP functions as a bronchodilator via the VPAC2 receptor. Consistent with the importance of the PAC1 receptor for control of pulmonary artery pressure,[67] VIP reduced mean pulmonary artery pressure, increased cardiac output, and mixed venous oxygen saturation in eight human subjects with pulmonary hypertension.[80]

Miscellaneous Gut Endocrine Peptides

In addition to the peptide hormones just outlined and summarized in Table 38–4, several other gut endocrine peptides exist. Chromogranins and secretogranins are a family of secretory proteins that are found in secretory vesicles of endocrine cells and neurons. Chromogranin A (CgA) is a protein belonging to this family of peptides and is secreted into the circulation by several neuroendocrine tumors, especially small gastrinomas and pheochromocytomas.[81] There is a direct correlation between circulating levels of CgA and tumor burden, making this a well-suited marker for assessing treatment response. A role for chromogranin A in the regulation of blood pressure control is suggested by studies demonstrating that elimination of CgA expression in a knockout mouse led to decreased size and number of chromaffin granules and hypertension, whereas transgenic expression of human CgA or exogenous injection of human catestatin, a CgA-derived cholinergic antagonist, restored normal blood pressure in CgA knockout mice.[82]

Opioid peptides regulate intestinal motility and inhibit gastric acid secretion. Neuromedin B and its receptor are both expressed in the gut, where they activate pathways coupled to epithelial mitogenesis. Neuromedin U is a neurotransmitter that is expressed in the enteric nervous system, where it regulates intestinal motility and ion secretion.

A number of hormones are secreted by the gastrointestinal tract directly into the lumen, where they modulate secretion and the release of other hormones. Guanylin and uroguanylin stimulate water, bicarbonate, and chloride secretion by the intestine and kidney while inhibiting sodium reabsorption.[83] Guanylin might also regulate cell proliferation in the colon; guanylin$^{-/-}$ mice exhibit increased epithelial cell migration and colonocyte proliferation. Other luminally secreted peptides include sorbin, a 153–amino acid peptide involved with monitoring fluid and sodium fluxes in the duodenum, and monitor peptide, which is a 61–amino acid peptide that stimulates CCK release.

Pancreatic and Gut Endocrine Tumors

Understanding the ontogeny of pancreatic and gut endocrine cell development provides some insight into the molecular pathophysiology of pancreatic endocrine tumors (PETs). Although gastrin is not normally produced in human adult islets of Langerhans, the finding of gastrinomas arising from the adult endocrine pancreas might reflect the dedifferentiation of neoplastic endocrine tumor cells that recapitulates in part, patterns of islet gene expression observed during embryonic development. Similarly, the observation that pancreatic and gut endocrine tumors are often plurihormonal is consistent with studies demonstrating colocalization of peptide hormones in fetal and adult endocrine cells in the pancreas and gut.

Pancreatic endocrine tumors can occur in isolation or as part of a genetic syndrome. Examples include multiple endocrine neoplasia type 1 (MEN-1); the phakomatoses of von Hippel-Lindau disease, von Recklinghausen's disease, or neurofibromatosis type 1; and tuberous sclerosis. Defects in distinct tumor suppressor genes account for the phenotypic manifestations and development of tumors in these syndromes (Table 38–5). Loss of heterozygosity at 10q has been detected in several sporadic pancreatic endocrine tumors, with cellular rather than nuclear localization of PTEN (phosphatase and tensin homolog deleted on chromosome 10) detected in a substantial proportion of malignant PETs.[84] Similarly, loss of heterozygosity at the 11q13 MEN-1 locus has also been detected in a few sporadic PETs.

Genetic mutations in the menin gene give rise to the MEN-1 syndrome associated with an increased incidence of endocrine tumors in many organs, including the pancreas and gut carcinoids in the stomach.[85] The MEN-1 gene encodes a 610–amino acid nuclear protein that interacts with the N-terminus of the JunD transcription factor, presumably resulting in de-repressed cell growth. Menin regulates cell growth via control of histone methylation and regulation of cyclin-dependent kinase (CDK) inhibitors. About 10% of all MEN-1 germline mutations arise de novo. The current usefulness of genetic testing for all suspected patients with the MEN-1 remains unclear due to the large number of heterogeneous mutations identified in the menin gene. The likelihood of detecting MEN-1 mutations correlates directly with the number of MEN-1–related tumors in the index case at presentation.[86] Potentially affected family members might find usefulness in ruling out the diagnosis with genetic testing, thereby precluding years of biochemical testing and imaging studies.

A search for clinical manifestations of diseases associated with these genetic syndromes is an important component in the initial diagnosis and ongoing management of patients with PETs. More careful clinical phenotype-genotype analyses have ascertained that facial angiofibromas, collagenomas, lipomas, leiomyomas, and adrenocortical tumors may be seen with increased frequency in patients with MEN-1.[87] Moreover, somatic mutations of the menin gene have been described in isolated cases of gastrinomas, insulinomas, and gut endocrine tumors.[87]

The secretion of one or more peptide hormones resulting in the production of symptoms attributable to hormone excess, such as hypoglycemia, gastric ulceration, or profuse watery diarrhea in patients with insulinoma, gastrinoma, or VIPoma, respectively, clearly facilitates the diagnosis of a hormone-secreting endocrine tumor. In some instances, pancreatic or gut endocrine tumors are not associated with clinically or biochemically detectable hormone excess, and the development of a recognizable syndrome and analysis of the tumor might fail to reveal evidence for peptide hormone biosynthesis. Nonfunctioning pancreatic endocrine tumors are more common, often larger, and more commonly malignant at the time of diagnosis. The term "nonfunctioning" may be a misnomer, because these tumors can produce peptide hormones (Fig. 38–3) whose biologic actions are less clinically apparent. In some instances, tumor-associated defects in posttranslational processing can preclude the efficient synthesis and secretion of peptide hormones. Factors affecting prognosis include liver metastases, incomplete resection of the primary tumor, and poorly differentiated tumor cells.

Somatostatin receptor scintigraphy (SRS) and measurement of gene products commonly expressed in endocrine cells such as chromogranin, pancreatic polypeptide, neuron-specific enolase, or glycoprotein hormone subunits, may be useful as an adjunct for monitoring the tumor response to therapy. The widespread expression of receptors for somatostatin and multiple peptide hormone GPCRs has stimulated efforts directed at developing novel radiolabeled peptide ligands for localizing and treating endocrine and nonendocrine neoplasms.

Despite the large number and complexity of endocrine cell populations in the human small bowel, gut endocrine tumors,

TABLE 38–4 SUMMARY OF GASTROINTESTINAL-DERIVED HORMONES

Hormone	Cell or Tissue of Origin	Related Peptides	Actions	Secretory Stimuli
Amylin	Pancreatic beta cell, endocrine cells of stomach and small intestine	Calcitonin, CGRP, adrenomedulin	Inhibits gastric emptying Inhibits arginine-stimulated and postprandial glucagon secretion Inhibits insulin secretion Satiety factor	Cosecreted with insulin in response to oral nutrient ingestion
CGRP	α-CGRP is expressed predominantly in afferent sensory nerves from the spinal cord β-CGRP is expressed in enteric neurons and enteroendocrine cells of the rectum	Calcitonin, amylin, adrenomedulin	Produces marked vasodilation in the splanchnic and peripheral circulation by stimulating nitric oxide release Inhibits gastric acid and pancreatic exocrine secretion Induces intestinal smooth muscle relaxation	Glucose and gastric acid secretion
CCK	Enteroendocrine I cells and enteric nerves, CNS, pituitary corticotrophs, C cells of the thyroid, adrenal medulla, and the acrosome of developing and mature spermatozoa		Inhibits proximal gastric motility while increasing antral and pyloric contractions Regulates meal-stimulated pancreatic enzyme secretion and gallbladder contraction Trophic effects on pancreatic acini in rats Postprandial satiety In the brain, CCK affects memory, sleep, sexual behavior, and anxiety	Oral nutrient ingestion Several intestine-derived hormones, including GRP and bombesin Activation of β-adrenergic receptors
Galanin	Central and peripheral nervous systems, pituitary, neural structures of the gut, pancreas, thyroid, and adrenal gland		In the brain, regulation of food intake, memory and cognition, and antinociception Inhibits pancreatic exocrine secretion and intestinal ion transport Induces both contraction and relaxation of intestinal smooth muscle, depending on the species examined Delays gastric emptying and prolongs colonic transit times Inhibits secretion of insulin, PYY, gastrin, somatostatin, enteroglucagon, neurotensin, and PP	Intestinal distention Chemical stimulation of the intestinal mucosa Electrical stimulating of periarterial nerves Extrinsic sympathetic neurons
GIP	Neuroendocrine K cells in the duodenum and proximal jejunum		Inhibits gastric acid secretion and GI motility Increases insulin release and regulates glucose and lipid metabolism Exerts anabolic actions in bone	Oral nutrient ingestion, especially long-chain fatty acids
Gastrin	Predominantly enteroendocrine G cells of the stomach and duodenal bulb, CNS and PNS, pituitary, adrenal gland, genital tract, respiratory tract, fetal pancreas		Induces gastric acid secretion Amidated gastrins are trophic to the oxyntic mucosa of the stomach Progastrin and glycine-extended gastrin induce colonic epithelial proliferation	Luminal contents, especially partially digested aromatic amino acids, small peptides, calcium, coffee, and ethanol Humoral and neural influences, including the vagus nerve, β-adrenergic and GABA neurons, and GRP
GRP and related peptides	CNS, enteric nervous system; reproductive tract, and the lungs, where it acts as a neurotransmitter; GRP neurons also distributed through the human pancreas	Bombesin, neuromedin B, neuromedin C	Stimulates smooth muscle contraction in the stomach, intestine, and gallbladder Stimulates release of CCK, gastrin, GIP, glucagon, GLP-1, GLP-2, motilin, PP, PYY, and somatostatin Stimulates gastric acid secretion via direct effect on G cells In the brain, regulates appetite, memory, thermogenesis, and cardiac function Stimulates pancreatic growth In the lungs, growth factor for normal and neoplastic tissue	Cholinergic stimulation

Table continued on following page

TABLE 38–4 SUMMARY OF GASTROINTESTINAL-DERIVED HORMONES (Continued)

Hormone	Cell or Tissue of Origin	Related Peptides	Actions	Secretory Stimuli
Ghrelin	CNS, stomach, small intestine, colon	Motilin	Stimulates GH release Stimulates gastric kinetic activity Orexigenic activity Stimulates energy production and signals hypothalamic regulatory nuclei that control energy homeostasis	Fasting
Glucagon	Pancreatic alpha cell, CNS		Primary counterregulatory mechanism to restore plasma glucose levels in hypoglycemia by increasing gluconeogenesis, glycogenolysis, and protein-lipid flux in the liver and periphery GI smooth muscle relaxation	Neural and humoral factors released in response to hypoglycemia
GLP-1	Enteroendocrine L cells located in the ileum and colon, CNS		Enhances glucose disposal following nutrient ingestion by inhibiting gastric emptying, stimulating insulin secretion, and inhibiting glucagon secretion Inhibits food intake Stimulates pancreatic islet neogenesis and proliferation Inhibits sham feeding–induced gastric acid secretion	Oral nutrient ingestion, especially carbohydrates and fat-rich meals Vagal nerve, GRP, and GIP ACh and neuromedin C Somatostatin inhibits secretion
GLP-2	Enteroendocrine L cells located in the ileum and colon, CNS		Induces small intestinal and colonic mucosal growth by stimulating crypt cell proliferation and inhibiting apoptosis Inhibits centrally induced antral motility and meal-stimulated gastric acid secretion Enhances intestinal epithelial barrier function Stimulates intestinal hexose transport Inhibits short-term control of food intake	Oral nutrient ingestion, especially carbohydrates and fat-rich meals Vagus nerve, GRP, and GIP ACh and neuromedin C Somatostatin inhibits secretion
Motilin	Brain, bronchoepithelial cells, and enteroendocrine M cells located in the duodenum and proximal jejunum	Ghrelin	Induces phase III contractions in the stomach Stimulates gastric and pancreatic enzyme secretion Induces contraction of the gallbladder, sphincter of Oddi, and LES	Duodenal alkalinization, sham feeding, gastric distention, opioid agonists promote secretion Unlike most GI hormones, secretin is suppressed in the presence of duodenal nutrients
NPY	CNS and PNS, pancreatic islet cells	PYY and PP	Potent stimulator of oral nutrient intake Inhibits glucose-stimulated insulin secretion Reduces GI fluid and electrolyte secretion Inhibits gastric and small intestinal motility Induces marked vasoconstriction of the splanchnic circulation	Oral nutrient ingestion Activation of the sympathetic nervous system
NT	N cells located in the small intestinal mucosa, especially the ileum; CNS and PNS, including the enteric nervous system; heart, adrenal gland, pancreas, and respiratory tract	Neuromedin N, xenin, and xenopsin	Stimulates growth of the colonic epithelium Inhibits postprandial gastric acid secretion and pancreatic exocrine secretion Stimulates colonic motility but inhibits gastric and small intestinal motility Facilitates fatty acid uptake in the proximal and small intestine and induces histamine release from mast cells Trophic in some pancreatic and colon cancer cells lines in vitro	Luminal nutrients, especially lipids, but not amino acids or carbohydrates GRP and bombesin Somatostatin inhibits secretion

Table continued on following page

TABLE 38–4 SUMMARY OF GASTROINTESTINAL-DERIVED HORMONES (Continued)

Hormone	Cell or Tissue of Origin	Related Peptides	Actions	Secretory Stimuli
PP	Major site of expression is pancreatic endocrine cells located in periphery of islets in pancreatic head and uncinate process	NPY and PYY	Reduces CCK-induced gastric acid secretion Increases intestinal transit times by reducing gastric emptying and upper intestinal motility Inhibits postprandial exocrine pancreas secretion via vagal-dependent pathway	Stimulated by nutrients, hormones, neurotransmitters, gastric distention, insulin-induced hpoglycemia, and direct vagal nerve stimulation Hyperglycemia, bombesin, and somatostatin inhibit secretion
PYY	Enteroendocrine cells, developing endocrine pancreas, subpopulation of pancreatic alpha cells in mature islets	NPY and PP	Enterogastrone inhibits gastric acid secretion and gastric motility Increases intestinal transit time by reducing intestinal motility Inhibits pancreatic exocrine secretion Role as an intestinal epithelial growth factor remains controversial Peripheral vasoconstriction and reduced mesenteric and pancreatic vascular blood flow	Following oral nutrient ingestion, early secretion is mediated by the vagus nerve and hormonal influences; subsequently, secretion occurs as a result of direct L-cell stimulation Bile acids and fatty acids Amino acids administered intracolonically
PACAP	Brain, respiratory tract, and enteric nervous system	VIP, PHI, and PHM	Stimulates histamine release from the stomach Increases secretion of pancreatic fluid, protein, and bicarbonate Stimulates insulin and catecholamine release Neural regulation of gastric acid secretion	Activation of CNS
Secretin	CNS, fetal endocrine pancreas, and enteroendocrine S cells located in the duodenum and proximal jejunum		Principal hormonal stimulant of pancreatic and biliary bicarbonate and water secretion Regulates pancreatic enzyme secretion Stimulates gastric secretion of pepsinogen Inhibits LES tone, postprandial gastric emptying, gastrin release, and gastric acid secretion	Gastric acid, bile salts, and luminal nutrients, especially fatty acids, peptides, and ethanol Somatostatin inhibits secretion
Somatostatin	CNS, pancreatic delta cells, enteroendocrine D cells		Inhibits secretion of islet hormones, including insulin, glucagon, and PP Inhibits secretion of gut peptides, including gastrin, secretin, VIP, CCK, GLP-1, GLP-2 Inhibits pancreatic exocrine secretion Acts in a paracrine manner on G cells, enterochromaffin-like cells, and parietal cells to inhibit gastric acid secretion Reduces splanchnic blood flow, intestinal motility, and carbohydrate absorption while increasing water and electrolyte absorption	Luminal nutrients Gastrin, CCK, bombesin, GLP-1, and GIP Neural influences, including PACAP, VIP, and β-adrenergic agonists stimulate while ACh inhibits secretion
Tachykinins	Throughout the CNS and PNS, including the respiratory tract, skin, sensory organs, and urogenital tract; in the GI tract, neurons localized in teh submucous and myenteric plexuses, extrinsic sensory fibers, and enterochromaffin cells in the gut epithelium	Substance P, neurokinin A, and neurokinin B	Regulate vasomotor and GI smooth muscle contractility Chemotaxis and activation of immune cells, mucus secretion, water absorption and secretion Role in visceral inflammation, hyperreflexia, and hyperalgesia	Direct and/or indirect activation of neurons

Table continued on following page

TABLE 38–4 SUMMARY OF GASTROINTESTINAL-DERIVED HORMONES (Continued)

Hormone	Cell or Tissue of Origin	Related Peptides	Actions	Secretory Stimuli
TRH	CNS and enteric nervous system, colon, G cells of the stomach, pancreatic islet beta cells		Suppresses pentagastrin-stimulated gastric acid secretion Chronic administration induces pancreatic hyperplasia and inhibits amylase release Attenuates CCK-induced gallbladder smooth muscle contraction Inhibits cholesterol synthesis within the intestinal mucosa	In the stomach, histamine and serotonin stimulate and endogenous opioids inhibit secretion
VIP	Widely expressed in the CNS and PNS (including the enteric nervous system)	PACAP, PHI, and PHM	Induces relaxation of vascular and nonvascular smooth muscle Mediates relaxation of the LES, sphincter of Oddi, and anal sphincter Regulates relaxation-associated gut contraction and may be involved with reflex vasodilation in the small intestine Inhibits gastric acid secretion Stimulates biliary water, bicarbonate, pancreatic enzyme, and intestinal chloride secretion	Mechanical stimulation Activation of the central and peripheral nervous systems

ACh, acetylcholine; CCK, cholecystokinin; CGRP, calcitonin gene–related peptide; CNS, central nervous system; GABA, γ-aminobutyric acid; GH, growth hormones; GI, gastrointestinal; GIP, gastric inhibitory polypeptide; GLP, glucagon-like peptide; GRP, gastrin-releasing peptide; LES, lower esophageal sphincter; NPY, neuropeptide Y; NT, neurotensin; PACAP, pituitary adenylate cyclase–activating peptide; PHI, peptide histidine isoleucine; PHM, peptide histidine methionine; PNS, peripheral nervous system; PP, pancreatic polypeptide; PYY, peptide YY; TRH, thyrotropin-releasing hormone; VIP, vasoactive intestinal peptide.

TABLE 38–5 GENETIC DISEASES ASSOCIATED WITH DEVELOPMENT OF PANCREATIC OR GUT ENDOCRINE TUMORS

Gene	Disease	Phenotype
Menin	MEN-1	Parathyroid, pituitary, and pancreatic endocrine tumors
VHL	von Hippel-Lindau	Pancreatic endocrine tumors, hemangiomas, and multiple neoplasms
NF-1	Neurofibromatosis	Neurofibroma, pheochromocytoma
TSC1/2	Tuberous sclerosis	Pancreatic endocrine tumors, hamartoma

including ileal carcinoids, are comparatively rare. Similarly, although human colon cancer remains a major cause of cancer-associated morbidity and mortality, peptide hormone–secreting carcinoid tumors arising from the colon are comparatively much less common than colonic adenocarcinomas. The molecular basis for the infrequent malignant transformation of human gut endocrine cells remains incompletely understood. Mutations in the *reg I alpha* gene have been identified in a subset of patients with ECL tumors and associated hypergastrinemia; however, the contribution of this genetic mutation to transformation of ECL cells remains unclear.

The clinical presentation, diagnosis, and treatment of several more common pancreatic and gut endocrine tumors are reviewed next, and both medical and surgical perspectives to treatment have been reviewed.[88,89] Surgical resection remains the principal therapeutic strategy, with chemotherapeutic regimens exhibiting only modest degrees of success in patients with malignant tumors.

Gastrinoma

In 1955, Zollinger and Ellison described two patients with intractable peptic ulcer disease and pancreatic islet cell tumors.[90] Subsequent studies demonstrated elevated levels of circulating gastrin associated with gastric acid hypersecretion in patients with Zollinger-Ellison syndrome (ZES). Although the gastrin gene is not normally expressed in the adult pancreas, gastrinomas commonly arise from within the pancreas and manifest as endocrine carcinomas, solitary adenomas, microadenomas, or endocrine cell hyperplasia. Gastrinomas and insulinomas represent the two most common pancreatic endocrine tumors. A smaller fraction of gastrin-secreting tumors, 20% to 40%, arise from the duodenum. Most (75%) gastrinomas occur sporadically, but about 25% are associated with the MEN-1 syndrome.

Duodenal gastrinomas in patients with sporadic ZES are usually small, most commonly located in the proximal duodenum, and associated with regional lymph node metastases in 60%.[91] Patients presenting with gastrinoma as a component of the MEN-1 syndrome often develop pituitary (60%) and adrenal (45%) disease and carcinoid tumors (30%).[92] A substantial percentage of MEN-1 patients also present with benign skin lesions such as angiofibromas and collagenomas.[93] Patients with MEN-1–related duodenal gastrinomas also commonly exhibit proliferative hyperplastic foci of gastrin-immunopositive cells in the adjacent nontumorous duodenal tissue. Sporadic gastrinomas may also contain menin gene mutations. MEN-1 patients tend to exhibit a younger age at onset at the time of diagnosis.

Sporadic tumors are most often solitary and malignant; MEN-1–associated tumors are usually multiple but may be more localized at the time of diagnosis. It is estimated that 50% to 60% of gastrinomas are malignant, based on the presence of metasta-

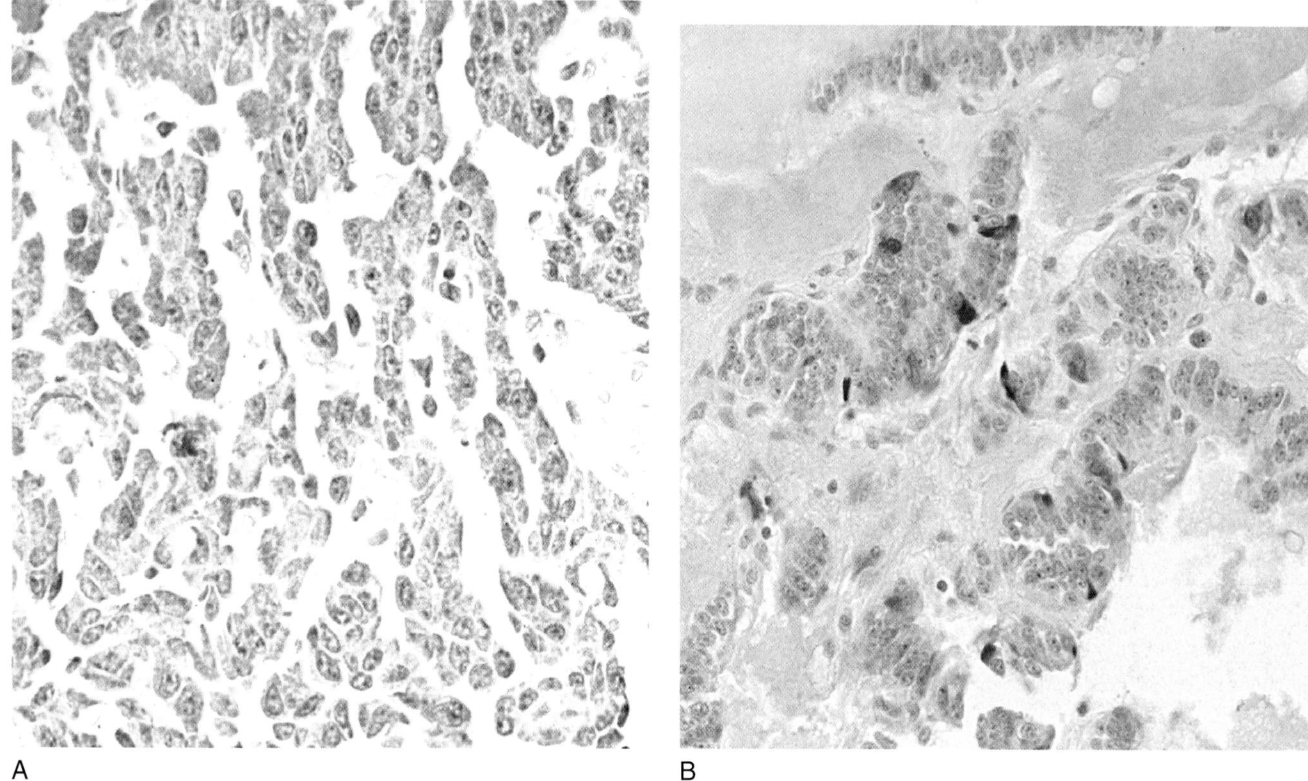

Figure 38–3 ▪ Clinically nonfunctioning tumors are often found to express one or more peptide hormones following immunocytochemical analyses. **A** and **B,** Histologic sections from a nonfunctioning human pancreatic endocrine tumor. **A,** Section of tumor exhibiting immunopositivity for glucagon. **B,** Section of tumor exhibiting pancreatic polypeptide.

ses at the time of diagnosis, perhaps partly because of the long delay between initial clinical presentation and diagnosis of ZES. Nevertheless, gastrin-secreting tumors are often slow growing and associated with prolonged survival despite complications arising from intestinal ulceration. Loss of heterozygosity at 1q or on the X chromosome may be associated with a more aggressive clinical presentation.

Clinical manifestations of gastrinomas are usually related to excessive gastric acid secretion resulting in severe refractory peptic ulceration complicated by hemorrhage, perforation, and stricture. Many patients report symptoms for 5 to 6 years before the diagnosis of ZES is established.[92] Abdominal pain, diarrhea, and heartburn are common manifesting symptoms, with diarrhea and pain observed in more than 70% of ZES patients.[94] The diarrhea results in part from fat malabsorption due to pancreatic lipase degradation by excess gastric acid. Small bowel inflammation and impaired nutrient absorption can also arise from excess gastric acid. Antisecretory therapy usually abolishes the diarrhea and diminishes many clinical features of the ZES.[94]

The diagnosis of gastrinoma is based on the detection of elevated fasting circulating gastrin levels (>200 pg/mL) and gastric acid hypersecretion (basal acid output >15 mEq/h with an intact stomach or >5 mEq/h after ulcer surgery) in patients off all acid antisecretory medication (14 days for H^+/K^+-ATPase inhibitors and 3 days for H_2-receptor antagonists).[94] Although many patients with ZES have serum gastrin values that exceed 500 pg/mL, a secretin stimulation test may be performed when the serum gastrin levels are in the range of 200 to 500 pg/mL to confirm the diagnosis. Provocative testing requires overnight fasting and intravenous administration of secretin (2 U/kg bolus) followed by serial measurements of circulating gastrin levels at 2, 5, 10, 15, and 20 minutes. A rise in the serum gastrin level of more than 200 pg/mL within 15 minutes or a doubling of the fasting gastrin levels strongly suggests the presence of a gastrinoma. Provocative testing may be useful in distinguishing gastrinomas from other causes of ulcerogenic hypergastrinemia such as gastric outlet obstruction, retained antrum after a Billroth II gastrectomy, antral G-cell hyperplasia, and *Helicobacter pylori* infection, which demonstrate a flat gastrin response to secretin. Difficulty in obtaining clinical supplies of secretin can preclude the routine use of the secretin test, and intravenous calcium administration has been successfully used to stimulate gastrin secretion in several cases. More than 90% of patients exhibit prominent gastric folds at the time of endoscopy, consistent with the tropic effect of gastrin on the stomach mucosa.[94] Serum calcium and PTH, along with baseline pituitary function and imaging studies, should also be considered to rule out the presence of the MEN-1 syndrome.

Localization of small primary tumors or endocrine hyperplasia can be difficult. Conventional endoscopy or an upper gastrointestinal series can occasionally be used to directly visualize duodenal lesions; however, tumors are often confined to the submucosa, making detection and biopsy challenging. Radiolabeled octreotide scanning can be useful for detecting the primary tumor and metastases. Magnetic resonance imaging (MRI) or computed tomography (CT) scans can also be informative; however, the primary tumor might not be detected with these modalities alone. Endoscopic ultrasound has been used for tumor localization with increasing success, and, less commonly, angiography with selective venous sampling may be helpful in localizing occult tumors. Primary tumors might also be localized to lymph nodes, and ectopic gastrinomas in sites such as the ovary have also been reported.

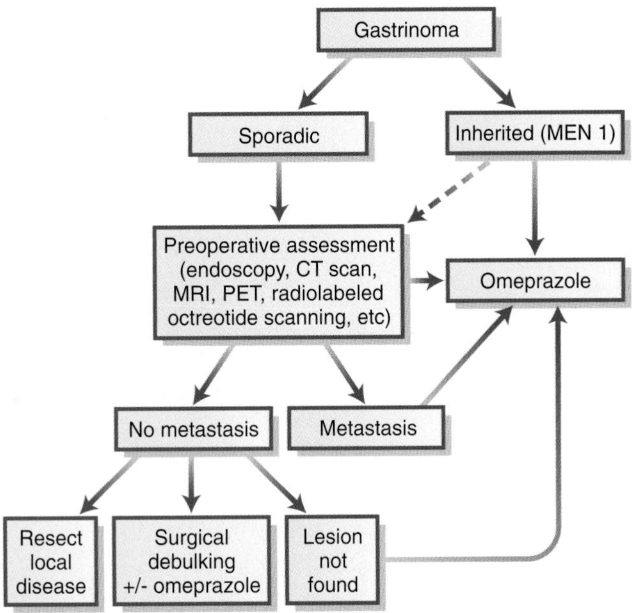

Figure 38–4 ▪ Treatment algorithm for management of a patient with gastrinoma. The *dotted line* indicates that in some circumstances, patients with familial gastrinoma might also be candidates for surgical resection if disease is very limited. CT, computed tomography; MEN, multiple endocrine neoplasia; MRI, magnetic resonance imaging; PET, positron-emission tomography.

Initial treatment of patients with gastrinoma is directed at pharmacologic reduction of gastric acid secretion. Although H_2 blockers have been used with some success, H^+/K^+-ATPase inhibitors such as omeprazole have become the drugs of choice due to their longer duration of action. Doses should be titrated to keep the H^+ ion output to less than 10 mEq/hour (5 mEq/hour in patients with previous acid-reducing surgery) for the hour before receiving the next dose of the drug.

As outlined in Figure 38–4, in the absence of unresectable disease, all patients with sporadic gastrinoma should undergo surgical exploration with the intent of curative surgical resection. Exploration should include a combination of duodenal palpation, endoscopic transillumination, intraoperative ultrasound, and duodenotomy. In up to 20% of patients undergoing surgical exploration, the primary tumor remains undetected at laparotomy despite meticulous exploration of the abdominal cavity. Total gastrectomy should be performed only under rare circumstances in patients with severe ulcer disease refractory to medical therapy in which the primary tumor cannot be resected. Surgery is generally not indicated in patients with gastrinoma and MEN-1 syndrome because these patients often have multiple small pancreatic tumors that are not all amenable to surgical resection.

Glucagonomas

The vast majority of glucagonomas are pancreatic in origin. Approximately 80% of tumors occur sporadically, and the remainder are associated with the MEN-1 syndrome. Most glucagonomas (~75%) are malignant and have metastasized by the time of diagnosis. The clinical presentation reflects the various actions of the PGDPs and can vary depending on the profile of PGDPs liberated due to tumor-specific differences in the posttranslational processing of proglucagon. A hallmark of this syndrome is necrolytic migratory erythema (NME), a skin rash that usually begins in the groin and perineum as a raised erythematous patch with occasional bullae that can also involve the lower extremities and perioral area. The exact etiology of the skin rash remains unknown, and elevated plasma glucagon levels, as well as deficiencies of zinc, amino acids, and fatty acids, might represent contributing factors.

Patients with glucagonomas can exhibit weight loss, abdominal pain, diabetes, stomatitis, glossitis, cheilitis, nail dystrophy, thromboembolic events, anemia, hypoaminoacidemia, and neuropsychiatric symptoms. The triad of hyperglucagonemia, NME, and a pancreatic tumor is seen in a minority of cases. Intestinal obstructive symptoms and increased intestinal transit times have also been reported and may reflect tumor-specific liberation of GLP-1 and GLP-2, peptides with antimotility and intestinotrophic properties, respectively.[95]

The diagnosis may be confirmed by demonstrating significantly elevated levels of plasma glucagon in association with a pancreatic mass. Extremely high levels of glucagon are more often seen with the classic glucagonoma syndrome, whereas more modest elevations of glucagon are detected in the setting of plurihormonal tumors. In contrast to insulinomas, glucagonomas are often large and more easily localized with imaging modalities. SRS is effective in detecting metastatic disease that most commonly involves the liver, lymph nodes, adrenal glands, or vertebrae.

Therapy with a somatostatin analogue may be useful in the setting of metastatic disease by reducing levels of circulating glucagon via the SST2 receptor, improving the skin rash, and promoting weight gain. The skin rash might also respond to selective nutrient supplementation. Whereas somatostatin analogues can reduce glucagon secretion and tumor-associated symptoms, effects on tumor growth are often modest. Patients with nonresectable or recurrent disease can be treated with chemotherapeutic agents such as streptozotocin and decarbazine (DTIC), interferon, or the selective use of arterial embolization.

Somatostatinoma

Somatostatinomas are extremely rare tumors that arise in the pancreas and the duodenum. Most clinical symptoms observed in the originally described somatostatinoma syndrome reflect the inhibitory properties of somatostatin on most digestive organs. A classic triad involving mild diabetes mellitus, steatorrhea, and cholelithiasis is observed in a minority of patients due to reduced insulin secretion, reduced biliary and pancreatic secretions, and inhibition of gallbladder motility. More prominent symptoms seen with duodenal tumors include weight loss, postprandial fullness and abdominal pain, cholelithiasis, anemia, and hypochlorhydria. Many patients do not present with the classic triad and exhibit only nonspecific symptoms. As a result, somatostatinomas are often malignant with extensive metastasis to the liver by the time of diagnosis.

Duodenal tumors (Fig. 38–5) are more commonly seen in association with neurofibromatosis type 1 or, less commonly, von Hippel-Lindau syndrome, and they therefore may be associated with pheochromocytomas. Most duodenal tumors are not associated with symptoms of classic somatostatinoma syndrome and can manifest with local obstruction and abdominal pain. Pancreatic tumors usually occur sporadically or as part of the MEN-1 syndrome and are most commonly located in the head of the pancreas. The diagnosis is confirmed by the presence of markedly elevated levels of plasma somatostatin. CT scan and both conventional and endoscopic ultrasounds can localize the duodenal tumors. In the small fraction of patients with localized disease, surgical resection can be curative. Patients with incurable or recurrent disease can be treated with the chemotherapeutic agents streptozotocin and decarbazine (DTIC).

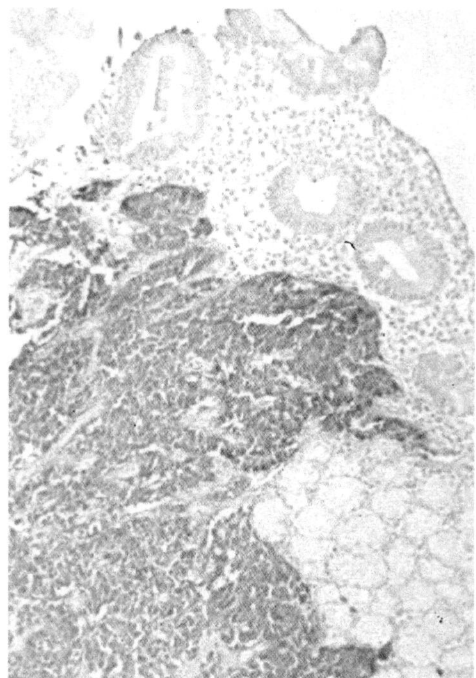

Figure 38–5 ▪ Somatostatin immunoreactivity in a human duodenal D cell tumor. This low-power micrograph illustrates the diffuse somatostatin immunoreactivity. Note the Brunner's glands *(lower right)* and the partly eroded mucosa *(upper right)* of the immunopositive endocrine tumor.

VIP-Secreting Tumors

The VIPoma syndrome is also known as pancreatic cholera, the Verner-Morrison syndrome, or the WDHA (watery diarrhea, hypokalemia, and achlorhydria) syndrome. Approximately 90% of patients with a VIPoma present with a pancreatic endocrine tumor that secretes VIP and, often, prostaglandins. The remaining tumors are extrapancreatic, usually involving the sympathetic chain or adrenal medulla. VIPomas can manifest as sporadic tumors or as part of the MEN-1 syndrome.

Clinical manifestations include intermittent severe watery diarrhea that contains large quantities of potassium, bicarbonate, and chloride. As a result, patients can exhibit signs and symptoms of hypokalemia, metabolic acidosis, and dehydration. Hypotension can occur due to dehydration and the vasodilator effects of VIP. Diarrhea is secretory and does not respond to antidiarrheal medications. Gastric analysis usually reveals hypochlorhydria or achlorhydria, although an appropriate increase in acid secretion is observed in response to a pentagastrin challenge. Glucose intolerance may be present due to hypokalemia and altered insulin sensitivity. Cutaneous flushing of the head and trunk may be observed in 15% of patients, usually during a bout of diarrhea, and may be associated with a patchy erythematous rash.

The diagnosis of VIPoma may be challenging because the symptoms are intermittent. A history of recurrent severe diarrhea together with elevated fasting levels of plasma VIP (>200 pg/mL), should prompt a search for a pancreatic tumor. Increased circulating levels of peptide histidine methionine (PHM), PP, NT, and prostaglandins have also been detected in patients with VIP-producing tumors. VIPomas can be localized by ultrasound, CT scan, and SRS imaging. Exploratory laparotomy with intraoperative ultrasound may also be used to identify the tumor.

Initial treatment of patients with the VIPoma syndrome involves aggressive fluid and electrolyte replacement. Somatostatin analogues may be used preoperatively to control the diarrhea by lowering circulating VIP and directly inhibiting intestinal secretion. Definitive treatment requires surgical resection of the tumor, which is commonly located in the body or tail of the pancreas. Although tumors are usually solitary, 60% are malignant at the time of diagnosis, and 75% metastasize to the liver and regional lymph nodes and less commonly to the lungs, mediastinum, stomach, and kidney. If a pancreatic tumor cannot be identified, exploration of the retroperitoneum, including the adrenal glands and sympathetic chains, is indicated. If no pancreatic tumor is identified, some patients elect to be closely monitored and others opt for an 80% distal pancreatectomy. This latter strategy may be beneficial for the 10% to 20% of symptomatic patients with diffuse islet cell hyperplasia. In patients with an inoperable or metastatic tumor, a combination 5-fluorouracil and streptozotocin may be effective.

Miscellaneous Gut Hormone–Producing Tumors

Pancreatic endocrine tumors can secrete PTH, GHRH, and ACTH, although this is rare. Secretion of these hormones leads to the development of hypercalcemia, acromegaly, and Cushing's syndrome, respectively. A large number of peptide hormones may be produced by pancreatic endocrine tumor cells, including PYY, calcitonin, neurotensin, melanocyte-stimulating hormone (MSH), corticotropin-releasing hormone (CRH), NPY, NMB, CGRP, GRP, and motilin. In some cases, the hormone precursors may be produced, but the correctly processed intact hormone might not be secreted by the tumor. Accordingly, excessive production of many of these hormones might not always be associated with characteristic signs and symptoms. Similarly, carcinoid tumors of the gastrointestinal tract often exhibit immunopositivity for multiple peptide hormones in the absence of a recognizable clinical syndrome.

Summary

A large number of peptides are synthesized in and secreted by endocrine cells of the pancreas and gastrointestinal tract. Many of these peptides circulate as hormones, but they also function as paracrine modulators or neurotransmitters, not only in the gut but also in the central and peripheral nervous system. Although some biologic actions for many of these peptides have been delineated, it seems likely that new peptides, new receptors, and novel biologic functions will continue to be discovered, which might provide new opportunities for understanding the pathophysiology, diagnosis, and treatment of endocrine disease.

REFERENCES

1. Herrera PL. Adult insulin- and glucagon-producing cells differentiate from two independent cell lineages. Development 2000;127:2317-2322.
2. Stoffers DA, Zinkin NT, Stanojevic V, et al. Pancreatic agenesis attributable to a single nucleotide deletion in the human IPF-1 gene coding sequence. Nat Genet 1997;15:106-110.
3. Dohrmann C, Gruss P Lemaire L. Pax genes and the differentiation of hormone-producing endocrine cells in the pancreas. Mech Dev 2000;92:47-54.
4. Apelqvist A, Li H, Sommer L, et al. Notch signaling controls pancreatic cell differentiation. Nature 1999;400:877-881.
5. Collombat P, Mansouri A, Hecksher-Sorensen J, et al. Opposing actions of Arx and Pax4 in endocrine pancreas development. Genes Dev 2003;17:2591-2603.
6. Henseleit KD, Nelson SB, Kuhlbrodt K, et al. NKX6 transcription factor activity is required for alpha- and beta-cell development in the pancreas. Development 2005;132:3139-3149.

7. Prado CL, Pugh-Bernard AE, Elghazi L, et al. Ghrelin cells replace insulin-producing beta cells in two mouse models of pancreas development. Proc Natl Acad Sci U S A 2004;101:2924-2929.
8. Yang Q, Bermingham NA, Finegold MJ, et al. Requirement of Math1 for secretory cell lineage commitment in the mouse intestine. Science 2001;294:2155-2158.
9. Jensen J, Pedersen EE, Galante P, et al. Control of endodermal endocrine development by Hes-1. Nat Genet 2000;24:36-44.
10. Jenny M, Uhl C, Roche C, et al. Neurogenin 3 is differentially required for endocrine cell fate specification in the intestinal and gastric epithelium. Embo J 2002;21:6338-6347.
11. Lee CS, Perreault N, Brestelli JE, et al. Neurogenin 3 is essential for the proper specification of gastric enteroendocrine cells and the maintenance of gastric epithelial cell identity. Genes Dev 2002; 16:1488-1497.
12. Naya FJ, Huang H, Qiu Y, et al. Diabetes, defective pancreatic morphogenesis, and abnormal enteroendocrine differentiation in BETA2/NeuroD-deficient mice. Genes Dev 1997;11:2323-2334.
13. Rindi G, Ratineau C, Ronco A, et al. Targeted ablation of secretin-producing cells in transgenic mice reveals a common differentiation pathway with multiple enteroendocrine cell lineages in the small intestine. Development 1999;126:4149-4156.
14. Larsson LI, St-Onge L, Hougaard DM, et al. Pax 4 and 6 regulate gastrointestinal endocrine cell development. Mech Dev 1998;79: 153-159.
15. Hill ME, Asa SL Drucker DJ. Essential requirement for Pax6 in control of enteroendocrine proglucagon gene transcription. Mol Endocrinol 1999;13:1474-1486.
16. Hull RL, Andrikopoulos S, Verchere CB, et al. Increased dietary fat promotes islet amyloid formation and beta-cell secretory dysfunction in a transgenic mouse model of islet amyloid. Diabetes 2003; 52:372-379.
17. Schmitz O, Brock B Rungby J. Amylin agonists: a novel approach in the treatment of diabetes. Diabetes 2004;53(Suppl 3):S233-S238.
18. Tatemoto K, Hosoya M, Habata Y, et al. Isolation and characterization of a novel endogenous peptide ligand for the human APJ receptor. Biochem Biophys Res Commun 1998;251:471-476.
19. Wang G, Anini Y, Wei W, et al. Apelin, a new enteric peptide: localization in the gastrointestinal tract, ontogeny, and stimulation of gastric cell proliferation and of cholecystokinin secretion. Endocrinology 2004;145:1342-1348.
20. Kleinz MJ Davenport AP. Emerging roles of apelin in biology and medicine. Pharmacol Ther 2005;107:198-211.
21. Wimalawansa SJ. Calcitonin gene–related peptide and its receptors: molecular genetics, physiology, pathophysiology, and therapeutic potentials. Endocr Rev 1996;17:533-585.
22. McLatchie LM, Fraser NJ, Main MJ, et al. RAMPs regulate the transport and ligand specificity of the calcitonin-receptor–like receptor. Nature 1998;393:333-339.
23. Rehfeld JF, Sun G, Christensen T, et al. The predominant cholecystokinin in human plasma and intestine is cholecystokinin-33. J Clin Endocrinol Metab 2001;86:251-258.
24. Moran TH, Katz LF, Plata-Salaman CR, et al. Disordered food intake and obesity in rats lacking cholecystokinin A receptors. Am J Physiol 1998;274:R618-625.
25. Hogenauer C, Meyer RL, Netto GJ, et al. Malabsorption due to cholecystokinin deficiency in a patient with autoimmune polyglandular syndrome type I. N Engl J Med 2001;344:270-274.
26. Branchek TA, Smith KE, Gerald C, et al. Galanin receptor subtypes. Trends Pharmacol Sci 2000;21:109-117.
27. Haberman RP, Samulski RJ McCown TJ. Attenuation of seizures and neuronal death by adeno-associated virus vector galanin expression and secretion. Nat Med 2003;9:1076-1080.
28. Elliott-Hunt CR, Marsh B, Bacon A, et al. Galanin acts as a neuroprotective factor to the hippocampus. Proc Natl Acad Sci U S A 2004;101:5105-5110.
29. Wynick D, Small CJ, Bacon A, et al. Galanin regulates prolactin release and lactotroph proliferation. Proc Natl Acad Sci U S A 1998;95:12671-12676.
30. Miyawaki K, Yamada Y, Yano H, et al. Glucose intolerance caused by a defect in the entero-insular axis: a study in gastric inhibitory polypeptide receptor knockout mice. Proc Natl Acad Sci U S A 1999;96:14843-14847.
31. Miyawaki K, Yamada Y, Ban N, et al. Inhibition of gastric inhibitory polypeptide signaling prevents obesity. Nat Med 2002;8:738-742.
32. Lacroix A, Ndiaye N, Tremblay J, et al. Ectopic and abnormal hormone receptors in adrenal Cushing's syndrome. Endocr Rev 2001;22:75-110.
33. Boushey RP, Abadir A, Flamez D, et al. Hypoglycemia, defective islet glucagon secretion, but normal islet mass in mice with a disruption of the gastrin gene. Gastroenterology 2003;125:1164-1174.
34. Dockray GJ, Varro A, Dimaline R, et al. The gastrins: their production and biological activities. Annu Rev Physiol 2001;63:119-139.
35. Hellmich MR, Rui XL, Hellmich HL, et al. Human colorectal cancers express a constitutively active cholecystokinin-B/gastrin receptor that stimulates cell growth. J Biol Chem 2000;275:32122-32128.
36. Olszewska-Pazdrak B, Townsend CM Jr, Hellmich MR. Agonist-independent activation of Src tyrosine kinase by a cholecystokinin-2 (CCK2) receptor splice variant. J Biol Chem 2004;279:40400-40404.
37. Cheng ZJ, Harikumar KG, Holicky EL, et al. Heterodimerization of type A and B cholecystokinin receptors enhance signaling and promote cell growth. J Biol Chem 2003;278:52972-52979.
38. Ferrand A, Wang TC. Gastrin and cancer: a review. Cancer Lett 2006;238(1):15-29.
39. Muerkoster S, Isberner A, Arlt A, et al. Gastrin suppresses growth of CCK2 receptor expressing colon cancer cells by inducing apoptosis in vitro and in vivo. Gastroenterology 2005;129:952-968.
40. Suarez-Pinzon WL, Lakey JR, Brand SJ, Rabinovitch A. Combination therapy with epidermal growth factor and gastrin induces neogenesis of human islet β-cells from pancreatic duct cells and an increase in functional β-cell mass. J Clin Endocrinol Metab 2005; 90:3401-3409.
41. Suarez-Pinzon WL, Yan Y, Power R, et al. Combination therapy with epidermal growth factor and gastrin increases beta-cell mass and reverses hyperglycemia in diabetic NOD mice. Diabetes 2005;54: 2596-2601.
42. Ladenheim EE, Hampton LL, Whitney AC, et al. Disruptions in feeding and body weight control in gastrin-releasing peptide receptor deficient mice. J Endocrinol 2002;174:273-281.
43. Zhou J, Chen J, Mokotoff M, et al. Targeting gastrin-releasing peptide receptors for cancer treatment. Anticancer Drugs 2004;15:921-927.
44. Martinez A, Zudaire E, Julian M, et al. Gastrin-releasing peptide (GRP) induces angiogenesis and the specific GRP blocker 77427 inhibits tumor growth in vitro and in vivo. Oncogene 2005;24: 4106-4113.
45. Kojima M Kangawa K: Ghrelin: structure and function. Physiol Rev 2005;85:495-522.
46. le Roux CW, Neary NM, Halsey TJ, et al. Ghrelin does not stimulate food intake in patients with surgical procedures involving vagotomy. J Clin Endocrinol Metab 2005;90:4521-4524.
47. Cummings DE, Weigle DS, Frayo RS, et al. Plasma ghrelin levels after diet-induced weight loss or gastric bypass surgery. N Engl J Med 2002;346:1623-1630.
48. Nagaya N, Moriya J, Yasumura Y, et al. Effects of ghrelin administration on left ventricular function, exercise capacity, and muscle wasting in patients with chronic heart failure. Circulation 2004;110: 3674-3679.
49. Gelling RW, Du XQ, Dichmann DS, et al. Lower blood glucose, hyperglucagonemia, and pancreatic alpha cell hyperplasia in glucagon receptor knockout mice. Proc Natl Acad Sci U S A 2003; 100:1438-1443.
50. Drucker DJ. Enhancing incretin action for the treatment of type 2 diabetes. Diabetes Care 2003;26:2929-2940.
51. Hansotia T Drucker DJ: GIP and GLP-1 as incretin hormones: lessons from single and double incretin receptor knockout mice. Regul Pept 2005;128:125-134.
52. Buse JB, Henry RR, Han J, et al. Effects of exenatide (exendin-4) on glycemic control over 30 weeks in sulfonylurea-treated patients with type 2 diabetes. Diabetes Care 2004;27:2628-2635.
53. Kendall DM, Riddle MC, Rosenstock J, et al. Effects of exenatide (exendin-4) on glycemic control over 30 weeks in patients with type 2 diabetes treated with metformin and a sulfonylurea. Diabetes Care 2005;28:1083-1091.
54. DeFronzo RA, Ratner RE, Han J, et al. Effects of exenatide (exendin-4) on glycemic control and weight over 30 weeks in metformin-treated patients with type 2 diabetes. Diabetes Care 2005;28: 1092-1100.

55. Drucker DJ, Ehrlich P, Asa SL, et al. Induction of intestinal epithelial proliferation by glucagon-like peptide 2. Proc Natl Acad Sci U S A 1996;93:7911-7916.
56. Estall JL Drucker DJ. Tales beyond the crypt: glucagon-like peptide–2 and cytoprotection in the intestinal mucosa. Endocrinology 2005;146:19-21.
57. Jeppesen PB, Sanguinetti EL, Buchman A, et al. Teduglutide (ALX-0600), a dipeptidyl peptidase IV resistant glucagon-like peptide 2 analogue, improves intestinal function in short bowel syndrome patients. Gut 2005;54:1224-1231.
58. Marguet D, Baggio L, Kobayashi T, et al. Enhanced insulin secretion and improved glucose tolerance in mice lacking CD26. Proc Natl Acad Sci U S A 2000;97:6874-6879.
59. Deacon CF. Therapeutic strategies based on glucagon-like peptide 1. Diabetes 2004;53:2181-2189.
60. Wynne K, Park AJ, Small CJ, et al. Subcutaneous oxyntomodulin reduces body weight in overweight and obese subjects: a double-blind, randomized, controlled trial. Diabetes 2005;54:2390-2395.
61. Baggio LL, Huang Q, Brown TJ, et al. Oxyntomodulin and glucagon-like peptide–1 differentially regulate murine food intake and energy expenditure. Gastroenterology 2004;127:546-558.
62. Feighner SD, Tan CP, McKee KK, et al. Receptor for motilin identified in the human gastrointestinal system. Science 1999;284:2184-2188.
63. Pons J, Lee EW, Li L, et al. Neuropeptide Y: multiple receptors and multiple roles in cardiovascular diseases. Curr Opin Investig Drugs 2004;5:957-962.
64. Vincent JP, Mazella J Kitabgi P: Neurotensin and neurotensin receptors. Trends Pharmacol Sci 1999;20:302-309.
65. Vaudry D, Gonzalez BJ, Basille M, et al. Pituitary adenylate cyclase–activating polypeptide and its receptors: from structure to functions. Pharmacol Rev 2000;52:269-324.
66. Freson K, Hashimoto H, Thys C, et al. The pituitary adenylate cyclase–activating polypeptide is a physiological inhibitor of platelet activation. J Clin Invest 2004;113:905-912.
67. Otto C, Hein L, Brede M, et al. Pulmonary hypertension and right heart failure in pituitary adenylate cyclase–activating polypeptide type I receptor–deficient mice. Circulation 2004;110:3245-3251.
68. Batterham RL, Cohen MA, Ellis SM, et al. Inhibition of food intake in obese subjects by peptide YY3-36. N Engl J Med 2003;349: 941-948.
69. Schonhoff S, Baggio L, Ratineau C, et al. Energy homeostasis and gastrointestinal endocrine differentiation do not require the anorectic hormone peptide YY. Mol Cell Biol 2005;25:4189-4199.
70. Michel MC, Beck-Sickinger A, Cox H, et al. XVI. International Union of Pharmacology recommendations for the nomenclature of neuropeptide Y, peptide YY, and pancreatic polypeptide receptors. Pharmacol Rev 1998;50:143-150.
71. Batterham RL, Le Roux CW, Cohen MA, et al. Pancreatic polypeptide reduces appetite and food intake in humans. J Clin Endocrinol Metab 2003;88:3989-3992.
72. Unis AS, Munson JA, Rogers SJ, et al. A randomized, double-blind, placebo-controlled trial of porcine versus synthetic secretin for reducing symptoms of autism. J Am Acad Child Adolesc Psychiatry 2002;41:1315-1321.
73. Low MJ: Clinical endocrinology and metabolism: the somatostatin neuroendocrine system: physiology and clinical relevance in gastrointestinal and pancreatic disorders. Best Pract Res Clin Endocrinol Metab 2004;18:607-622.
74. Saito T, Iwata N, Tsubuki S, et al. Somatostatin regulates brain amyloid beta peptide Abeta42 through modulation of proteolytic degradation. Nat Med 2005;11:434-439.
75. van der Hoek J, Hofland LJ Lamberts SW: Novel subtype specific and universal somatostatin analogues: clinical potential and pitfalls. Curr Pharm Des 2005;11:1573-1592.
76. Freda PU, Katznelson L, van der Lely AJ, et al. Long-acting somatostatin analog therapy of acromegaly: a meta-analysis. J Clin Endocrinol Metab 2005;90:4465-4473.
77. Gibril F Jensen RT. Diagnostic uses of radiolabelled somatostatin receptor analogues in gastroenteropancreatic endocrine tumours. Dig Liver Dis 2004;36(Suppl 1):S106-120.
78. Page NM. New challenges in the study of the mammalian tachykinins. Peptides 2005;26:1356-1368.
79. Gozes I Furman S. Clinical endocrinology and metabolism: potential clinical applications of vasoactive intestinal peptide: a selected update. Best Pract Res Clin Endocrinol Metab 2004;18:623-640.
80. Petkov V, Mosgoeller W, Ziesche R, et al. Vasoactive intestinal peptide as a new drug for treatment of primary pulmonary hypertension. J Clin Invest 2003;111:1339-1346.
81. Taupenot L, Harper KL O'Connor DT: The chromogranin-secretogranin family. N Engl J Med 2003;348:1134-1149.
82. Mahapatra NR, O'Connor DT, Vaingankar SM, et al. Hypertension from targeted ablation of chromogranin A can be rescued by the human ortholog. J Clin Invest 2005;115:1942-1952.
83. Forte LR Jr. Uroguanylin and guanylin peptides: pharmacology and experimental therapeutics. Pharmacol Ther 2004;104:137-162.
84. Perren A, Komminoth P, Saremaslani P, et al. Mutation and expression analyses reveal differential subcellular compartmentalization of PTEN in endocrine pancreatic tumors compared to normal islet cells. Am J Pathol 2000;157:1097-1103.
85. Chandrasekharappa SC, Guru SC, Manickam P, et al. Positional cloning of the gene for multiple endocrine neoplasia–type 1. Science 1997;276:404-407.
86. Ellard S, Hattersley AT, Brewer CM, et al. Detection of an MEN1 gene mutation depends on clinical features and supports current referral criteria for diagnostic molecular genetic testing. Clin Endocrinol (Oxf) 2005;62:169-175.
87. Schussheim DH, Skarulis MC, Agarwal SK, et al. Multiple endocrine neoplasia type 1: new clinical and basic findings. Trends Endocrinol Metab 2001;12:173-178.
88. Warner RR. Enteroendocrine tumors other than carcinoid: a review of clinically significant advances. Gastroenterology 2005;128: 1668-1684.
89. de Herder WW Lamberts SW. Clinical endocrinology and metabolism. Gut endocrine tumours. Best Pract Res Clin Endocrinol Metab 2004;18:477-495.
90. Zollinger RM Ellison EH. Primary peptic ulcerations of the jejunum associated with islet cell tumors of the pancreas. Ann Surg 1955;142:709-723; discussion, 724-708.
91. Zogakis TG, Gibril F, Libutti SK, et al. Management and outcome of patients with sporadic gastrinoma arising in the duodenum. Ann Surg 2003;238:42-48.
92. Gibril F, Schumann M, Pace A, et al. Multiple endocrine neoplasia type 1 and Zollinger-Ellison syndrome: a prospective study of 107 cases and comparison with 1009 cases from the literature. Medicine (Baltimore) 2004;83:43-83.
93. Asgharian B, Turner ML, Gibril F, et al. Cutaneous tumors in patients with multiple endocrine neoplasm type 1 (MEN1) and gastrinomas: prospective study of frequency and development of criteria with high sensitivity and specificity for MEN1. J Clin Endocrinol Metab 2004;89:5328-5336.
94. Roy PK, Venzon DJ, Shojamanesh H, et al. Zollinger-Ellison syndrome: clinical presentation in 261 patients. Medicine (Baltimore) 2000;79:379-411.
95. Brubaker PL, Drucker DJ, Asa SL, et al. Prolonged gastrointestinal transit in a patient with a glucagon-like peptide (GLP)-1– and -2–producing neuroendocrine tumor. J Clin Endocrinol Metab 2002; 87:3078-3083.

SECTION X

Polyendocrine Disorders

CHAPTER 39

PATHOGENESIS OF ENDOCRINE TUMORS

Andrew Arnold

A great deal is now known about the mechanisms underlying human tumorigenesis in general and about neoplasia of the endocrine glands in particular. The application of general principles of neoplasia to endocrine tumors has been a productive area of research and is now being translated into clinical applications. Endocrine tumorigenesis also involves some special, if not unique, features that must be considered in understanding the pathogenesis of endocrine tumors. The aim of this chapter is to present the general principles of neoplasia as a framework through which current knowledge about and future advances in endocrine tumorigenesis can be understood.

Molecular Tumor Biology

Both inherited tumor predisposition syndromes and the more common noninherited *(sporadic)* forms of neoplasia are genetic diseases in the sense that tumors develop when specific damage to genes leads to deregulated cell growth. As a general rule, damage to one such gene controlling cell growth is not sufficient to confer a neoplastic phenotype on a cell; instead, mutations in multiple genes accumulate over time. Inherited tumor syndromes constitute a special case in which mutation of one key gene is already present in each somatic cell at birth.

Clonality

Concepts of Clonality and Clonal Evolution

All cancers and many benign hypercellular expansions are *monoclonal;* that is, they are composed of cells that are the descendants of a single clonal progenitor cell in which the accumulation of a sufficient number of DNA alterations (and, perhaps, other epigenetic damage that does not actually change the nucleotide sequence) caused a selective advantage. Over time, this selective advantage, manifested as an increase in proliferative capacity, a decrease in the normal cell death rate, or both, leads to the development of a neoplasm.

The monoclonality of tumors implies that the necessary accumulation of mutations occurs only rarely in the large population of cells in a tissue. Viewed in another way, the identification of a specific monoclonal (also called *clonal*) change in DNA, found in all or most of the cells of a neoplasm but not in that person's constitutional DNA (e.g., obtained from adjacent normal tissue or leukocytes), indicates that this DNA alteration had been advantageous in the accelerated evolutionary process that is oncogenesis. Such a DNA lesion, especially if it recurs in other tumors of the same type, is therefore highly likely to contribute to tumor development[1] (although this conclusion must be drawn more cautiously in rare circumstances, such as an inherited DNA mismatch repair deficiency, in which the underlying global mutation rate is exceedingly high). In fact, one of the strongest types of evidence to implicate a given gene as a driving force in tumorigenesis is the recurrent demonstration of clonal DNA changes in or near that gene.

This situation contrasts with the one in which an increase or a decrease in the expression (RNA or protein levels) of a particular gene occurs in a tumor; such changes can be secondary consequences of tumor-related processes and might or might not themselves drive or contribute to the neoplastic phenotype. This caveat is especially important to bear in mind, given that the Human Genome Project and modern microarray technology have made it possible to examine expression changes in a huge number of genes in a tissue or tumor simultaneously.

An original clonal progenitor or transformed cell does not necessarily contain all the genetic lesions that are ultimately present in the mature, clinically apparent tumor. A continuing process of *clonal evolution* can result in the development of additional DNA damage that provides an incremental selective advantage to the single tumor cell in which it occurs. Over time, the progeny of this cell might become the dominant clonal population. The percentage of neoplastic cells in the final tumor that contain such a later mutation can vary markedly and depends on factors such as the duration of the mutation's existence and the relative rates of proliferation and death of the various cell populations.

Endocrine tumors are often sufficiently differentiated to express the hormonal activity characteristic of the corresponding normal cell type, but the hormonal function of the tumor is typically regulated in an abnormal fashion. It is important to understand that the genes that cause tumors of endocrine tissues do so only because of their effects on cell proliferation and accumulation. Such genes need not influence hormonal function. Furthermore, a mutant gene that alters hormonal function but confers no selective growth advantage is not tumorigenic. Nevertheless, the frequent coexistence of growth deregulation and hormonal hyperfunction in endocrine tumors does indicate that the tumor-causing genes can directly or indirectly alter hormone control pathways.

In certain instances, such as a mutation affecting the α subunit of stimulatory G protein ($G_{s\alpha}$) in growth hormone–producing and thyroid adenomas, a single mutant gene can directly contribute to both cell proliferation and hormonal hyperfunction. In general, however, the relation between hypercellularity caused by clonally selected mutant genes and hormonal hyperfunction is poorly understood.

Hyperplasia versus Neoplasia

Not all hypercellular expansions are monoclonal. For instance, the generalized proliferative response of all cells of a tissue to an extrinsic stimulus yields a polyclonal expansion, examples of which include the hyperthyroidism of Graves' disease and the early, reversible secondary hyperparathyroidism in states of chronic hypocalcemia. Such polyclonal expansions represent biologic hyperplasia, whereas any monoclonal growth (benign or malignant) is a true neoplasm. Analyses of tumor clonality have been used to distinguish between these types of tumorigenic mechanisms. Nevertheless, the genesis of some tumors can involve both types of processes. For example, a generalized stimulus to polyclonal hyperplasia can, by increasing the chances of mitosis-related DNA damage in one cell, foster the emergence of a monoclonal population capable of eventually overwhelming or replacing its hyperplastic neighbors.

The clinical and histopathologic use of the term *hyperplasia* does not necessarily correspond to the biologic meaning described earlier, a situation that has engendered much confusion. For example, the usual tumors responsible for primary hyperparathyroidism have been clinicopathologically classified as adenomas when a single gland is abnormal and as hyperplasia when the individual patient has multiple hypercellular glands. No histopathologic criteria can reliably predict whether a single or multiple glands are involved on the basis of analysis of only one such gland. Not only are clinical adenomas monoclonal neoplasms,[2] but also many parathyroid glands from patients with multigland "hyperplasia" are also monoclonal.[3] It is therefore important to ensure that the terms used in the description of endocrine tumorigenesis are clearly defined.

Insights into Tumor Pathogenesis

The clonal status of a cellular proliferation is of fundamental importance in deciphering its pathogenesis; thus, endocrine tumors have been studied to determine whether the expansion is monoclonal or polyclonal. One way of determining that a tumor is monoclonal is to identify a DNA or chromosomal lesion that, because of its tumor specificity and presence in all or most of the neoplastic cells, directly defines the expansion as monoclonal. Examples of cytogenetically defined clonal abnormalities are chromosome translocations such as the t(9;22) Philadelphia translocation in chronic myelogenous leukemia and the t(14;18) translocation in follicular lymphoma.

The use of classic cytogenetics is technically more difficult in solid tumors than in hematopoietic tumors because hematopoietic cells divide in culture much more readily and yield excellent metaphase chromosomal spreads. Specimens of endocrine tumors are difficult to obtain for culture and to analyze cytogenetically. Fortunately, improved methods for the cytogenetic and molecular cytogenetic study of tumors, including fluorescence in situ hybridization (FISH), comparative genomic hybridization, and chromosome painting, have opened up new avenues for detecting clonal chromosomal lesions in endocrine tumors.[4,5]

Examples of monoclonal abnormalities defined by molecular methods in endocrine neoplasia include $G_{s\alpha}$ gene mutations in growth hormone–producing pituitary tumors,[6] thyrotropin (TSH) receptor gene mutations in thyroid tumors,[7] and cyclin D1 or *PRAD1* gene rearrangements in parathyroid adenomas.[8,9] Identification of tumor-specific changes, such as deletions of DNA markers in particular regions of the tumor genome, also serves as evidence of monoclonality, even though the specific genes affected by such deletions might not be known.[4,10]

Indirect methods can determine the clonal status of tumors without the necessity of identifying the specific genes or chromosomal regions that are clonally mutated and involved in tumorigenesis. These methods have generally exploited the phenomenon of random X chromosome inactivation (the *Lyon phenomenon*) in women.[11] Random X chromosome inactivation occurs early in female embryonic development in all somatic cells. In any cell, the choice of which X chromosome is inactivated is random; once that choice is made, however, the decision is faithfully transmitted to all progeny of that cell. Usually, therefore, the maternally derived X chromosome is inactive in about 50% of the cells in a normal tissue, and the paternally derived X chromosome is inactive in about 50%.

Polyclonal growth, representing a generalized expansion of many or all original cells within a tissue, maintains the relatively even mix of active maternal and paternal X chromosomes characteristic of the normal tissues. In contrast, the neoplastic cells in a monoclonal tumor are derived from a single progenitor, and all should reflect an identical X chromosome pattern, with either the maternal or the paternal X chromosome uniformly inactivated.

A unifying feature of methods based on the analysis of X chromosome inactivation to determine the clonal status of a tumor is the use of a normally occurring variant, or *polymorphism,* at the genetic or protein level to distinguish between a woman's two X chromosomes. The other step involves assaying some property that reflects the state of X chromosome inactivation imposed on the tumor cell chromosomes at the polymorphic site. Assays to reflect X chromosome inactivation status include assessment of gene expression (RNA or protein levels) or regional DNA methylation.

A polymorphism in glucose-6-phosphate dehydrogenase (G6PD) was the first to be used in X chromosome inactivational analyses of tumor clonality.[12] A disadvantage of the G6PD system is that only a small minority of women are heterozygous for electrophoretically distinguishable isoforms of this X chromosome–encoded enzyme. Thus, most tumors have been unsuitable for clonal analysis. Furthermore, the method fails to detect the monoclonality of certain tumors,[2,13,14] perhaps because of differences in the level of G6PD expression in tumor cells compared with contaminating admixed normal cells within the analyzed samples.

DNA polymorphisms are now preferred for clonal analyses to distinguish between the two X chromosomes. High rates of heterozygosity make it possible to analyze most tumors. Some multiallelic polymorphisms, based on differences in the number of highly repeated sequence units in a genomic location, are heterozygous in more than 90% of women, and a large number of DNA polymorphisms have been described on the X chromosome (and on all chromosomes). Most, however, cannot be used in clonality studies because they have not been characterized for detectable changes that correlate with the state of activity of the X chromosome on which an allele resides. Some of the X-linked polymorphisms that have been valuable in clonal analyses of human tumors include restriction fragment length polymorphisms in the *HPRT* and *PGK* gene regions,[15] a minisatellite repeat (>10 nucleotide core repeated unit) region called M27 or DXS255,[3] and a microsatellite repeat (<10 nucleotide core repeated unit) locus in the androgen receptor gene.[16]

Changes in DNA methylation in the vicinity of certain polymorphic sites on the X chromosome correlate with the activity of that X chromosome and are useful in clonal analyses. Methylation of specific cytosine nucleotides is an epigenetic process that is faithfully replicated from a given cell to its progeny, and this process may have a role in maintaining the activity status of the particular X chromosome. Methylation at certain specific sites may be easily detected through the action of methylation-sensitive restriction endonucleases, which cleave when their target sites are unmethylated but cannot do so when a methyl group is present.

One cannot predict how or whether X chromosome inactivation will affect the methylation of a particular nucleotide in or near a gene; correlations must be established separately for individual genomic sites. For example, a useful restriction site in the *HPRT* region is consistently methylated when on the active X chromosome and unmethylated when on the inactive X chromosome; the opposite pattern is observed for an informative site in the *PGK* region. Despite the need for such empiric validation, the use of DNA methylation as a surrogate marker for the status of X chromosome activity has major advantages in clonality studies and eliminates the vulnerability of the assay to the vagaries of gene expression in tumor cells.

The analysis of clonality in endocrine tumors has yielded important insights. For example, most corticotropin-producing pituitary tumors are monoclonal, which shows that Cushing's disease is not explained solely by a generalized hypothalamic stimulation of corticotrophs.[17,18] Typical parathyroid adenomas are also monoclonal outgrowths[2,10] and are not, as previously suggested, asymmetric forms of multiglandular hyperplasia.[13,14] In patients with multifocal papillary thyroid cancer, clonal analysis of physically distinct individual tumors showed these foci are often clonally unrelated and, therefore, of independent origins,[16] suggesting an underlying predisposition to thyroid tumorigenesis in such patients (Fig. 39–1).

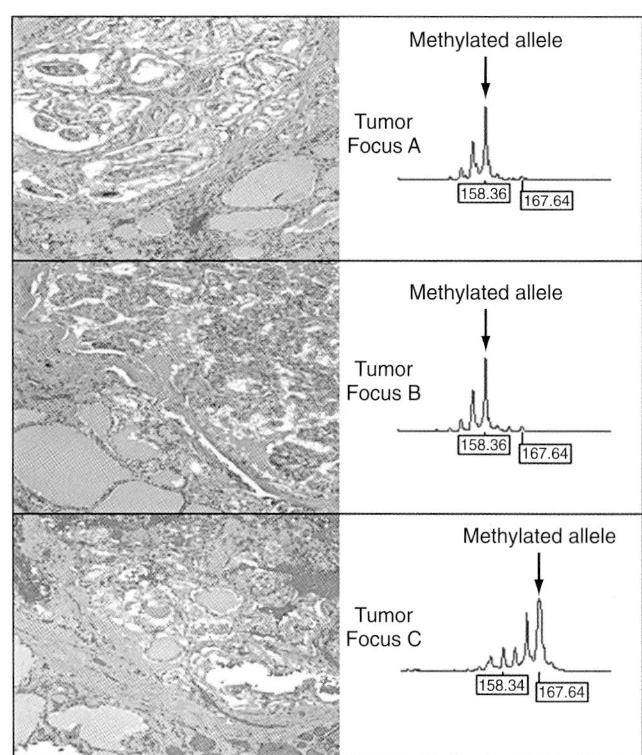

Figure 39–1 ▪ Example of discordant X-inactivation clonality patterns in distinct tumor foci from one patient with multifocal papillary thyroid carcinomas. Shown in the left panels are photomicrographs (stained with hematoxylin and eosin, ×40) of a single patient's three tumor foci, labeled A, B, and C. Even though the three discrete carcinomas have a similar microscopic appearance, they do not share an identical X-inactivation pattern. For each tumor, the corresponding plot to the right shows the size and amount of fluorescent polymerase chain reaction (PCR) products amplified from tumor DNA when analyzed on an automated sequencer. Products are plotted from left to right from smaller to larger alleles, differing at a polymorphic site in the androgen-receptor gene on the X-chromosome. Height of the peaks corresponds to the amount of product present. Methylation-sensitive PCR of tumor foci A and B shows that in each focus the smaller allele is methylated and therefore inactivated, and the larger allele is unmethylated. Tumor focus C, from the same patient, shows the opposite pattern, with the larger allele methyated and the smaller allele unmethylated. The number in the box under the peaks indicates the estimated allele size in base pairs. The discordant X-inactivation patterns indicate that tumor focus C originated independently from A and from B. Foci A and B might also have separate origins from each other and share an X-inactivation pattern by chance (such concordance expected in 50% of independently originating tumors), or they could be clonally related. (Modified from Shattuck TM, Shattuck TM, Westra WH, et al. Independent clonal origins of distinct tumor foci in multifocal papillary thyroid carcinoma. N Engl J Med 2005; 352:2406-2412. Copyright © Massachusetts Medical Society.)

In severe secondary (or tertiary) hyperparathyroidism in patients with uremia, the typical finding of multigland involvement had led to the assumption that this disease predominantly involves polyclonal (nonneoplastic) cellular proliferations. However, examination of clonality using X-inactivation showed that 64% of informative patients with renal failure undergoing hemodialysis and with refractory hyperparathyroidism harbored at least one monoclonal parathyroid tumor, and 63% of all tumors examined had monoclonal X inactivation patterns.[3] One often overlooked pitfall in the interpretation of any X inactivation analysis must be emphasized: Polyclonal patterns cannot be interpreted definitively. For example, admixed normal cells or tumor-specific aberrations in DNA methylation can obscure the detection of a monoclonal cell population. Thus, the true extent of monoclonality in severe secondary or tertiary hyperparathyroidism might be even higher (but not lower) than demonstrated. These unexpected results indicate that monoclonal parathyroid neoplasms are common in uremic refractory hyperparathyroidism and suggest that autonomous parathyroid function in this disorder is due to the outgrowth of true neoplasms, presumably on a background of preexisting (and more reversible) polyclonal parathyroid hyperplasia.

Predisposing Influences

Both environmental and genetic factors can contribute to the risk of a particular type of tumor development over a lifetime. In highly penetrant inherited syndromes, the genetic predisposition is overriding; in most instances, however, the intimate relation between environmental and (often multiple) genetic factors makes the traditional nature versus nurture question difficult to assess.

A commonly overlooked genetic component of tumor predisposition is gender; however, the specific mechanisms by which gender influences the risk of endocrine tumors such as thyroid cancer and parathyroid adenoma are not well understood. Additional genetic variables, which may be common in the population, also influence the chance of tumor development. To date, however, it has been notoriously difficult to isolate these specific genetic variations, each of which might confer only a small degree of risk or might increase risk only when present in particular combinations with other DNA polymorphisms.

An important environmental factor in endocrine tumorigenesis is ionizing radiation. Both thyroid and parathyroid tumors have been linked to prior head and neck irradiation in a dose-dependent fashion.[19,20] Whereas the latency period for tumor development after radiation exposure in the United States is quite long, childhood thyroid cancer has been observed with markedly increased frequency in the aftermath of the 1986 Chernobyl nuclear accident.[21] This heightened susceptibility might not be solely a function of age and amount of exposure, but it might be modified by other factors such as iodine deficiency in the region,[21] highlighting the point that tumor predisposition and development can be influenced by complex interacting factors.

Oncogenes and Tumor Suppressor Genes

Two broad categories of genes are implicated in the excessive cell proliferation and other properties that result in the outgrowth and evolution of a neoplastic clone. An *oncogene* carries a gain-of-function mutation in its regulatory or coding region that results in dysregulation of its normal product or in the formation of an abnormal protein product. Typically, only one mutated allele need be present for an oncogene to exert its tumorigenic action. The normal, unmutated version of an oncogene is called a *proto-oncogene.* Proto-oncogenes may be converted to oncogenes by various molecular genetic mechanisms, such as fusion of part of its coding region with that of another gene, chromosomal translocations or inversions that alter its regulatory environment, or point mutations.

A *tumor suppressor gene,* in contrast, normally acts to restrain cell proliferation or other potential aspects of the malignant phenotype. This restraint can directly control proliferation, for example, by regulating the cell cycle, or affect proliferation indirectly, for example, by maintaining genomic stability. Thus, the definition of a tumor suppressor gene is not restrictive concerning its specific cellular function.[22] Tumors are provoked or fostered by inactivating or loss-of-function mutations in such genes; common inactivating mechanisms are gene deletion, point mutations, and microdeletions or small base insertions that cause a frameshift. Both alleles of a classic tumor suppressor gene must be inactivated to eliminate the functional protein product and to contribute to tumorigenesis.

The existence of a critical tumor suppressor gene is often inferred from the finding that a particular subchromosomal stretch of DNA is recurrently and nonrandomly lost in a particular tumor type. The loss typically involves only one of a gene's two alleles. Because these regions of loss of heterozygosity are often large and can encompass many innocent bystander genes, the case that the correct tumor suppressor gene has been found can be made most convincingly when the remaining allele of the gene is shown to harbor another, more specific, clonal inactivating lesion, such as an intragenic coding region mutation or microdeletion. It is also possible (albeit unproved in human neoplasia) that certain nonclassic tumor suppressors might exist, contributing to neoplasia through acquired haploinsufficiency, in which somatic inactivation of only one allele provides the relevant selective advantage.[23]

Although there has been some evolution in, and even controversy about, the best definition of a tumor suppressor gene, "the simplest, most inclusive, and cleanest genetic definition" is that favored by Haber and Harlow,[22] namely "genes that sustain loss-of-function mutations in the development of neoplasia." This definition, although unrestricted concerning the function of the tumor suppressor, "does have an essential component—the unequivocal demonstration of inactivating mutations."[22] Thus, evidence for reduced or absent expression of a gene in a particular tumor, or even the ability of a gene to inhibit cell proliferation, should not be accepted as sufficient to award it designation as a tumor suppressor if it is not accompanied by clear and recurrent evidence of clonal mutation.

Some oncogenes or tumor suppressor genes contribute to tumors of only one or a few cell types, whereas other genes are involved in many different types of tumors. It is rare for any one particular gene to be invariably involved in the development of a given type of tumor, and different combinations of mutated genes can have similar cellular and clinical consequences (genetic heterogeneity).

Finally, genetic hits affecting multiple oncogenes and tumor suppressor genes in a single cell appear to be required if that cell is to become neoplastic. Thus, in most instances, no single activated oncogene or inactivated tumor suppressor gene is sufficient for the development of tumors.

Mutational Mechanisms and the Primary Role of Selection in Tumorigenesis

Tumors can acquire mutations that in themselves increase the rate at which new mutations develop at other sites in the genome. Many tumor biologists have commented on the apparently excessive number of genetic changes observed in individual cancers compared with measured rates of mutation in normal cells. Genetic changes are usually considered to occur or to be fixed during DNA replication or mitosis.[24,25] However, some mutations may be time-dependent rather than replication-dependent, meaning that they can arise even in the absence of cell proliferation.[24,26]

One mechanism by which somatic mutations might occur would be a defect in post-replication mismatch repair, the pathway responsible for removing and correcting mismatched base pairs in DNA.[26] At least one form of inherited genetic instability can result from inactivation of mutator genes in the mismatch repair system, *hMSH2* or *hMLH1,* for example.[27] Although such mutational mechanisms might in theory be quite important in benign or slow-growing endocrine tumors that derive from slowly proliferating normal tissues, to date little direct evidence supports this hypothesis. Furthermore, some investigators have drawn conclusions about the extent of genomic instability in endocrine tumors based on the number of observed chromosomal abnormalities. Such conclusions cloud the distinction between state and rate.[28] One must note that the presence of genetic alterations in a tumor, even in large numbers, does not necessarily imply that the tumor is genetically unstable. True instability is defined as an abnormal rate, and the snapshot of a mature tumor's complement of mutations (state) does not provide information about their rate of occurrence.

As noted by Lengauer and colleagues,[28] several factors in addition to true instability might explain the greater frequency of observed mutations in tumors than in nonneoplastic tissues. These include potentially crucial differences in the selective conditions of the tumor versus normal cell context, differences that involve humoral and intercellular interactions.[29] Thus, a given mutation might confer an important selective advantage and lead to clonal expansion only when it occurs in a tumor cell environment, whereas the same mutation (occurring at the same rate) in a normal cell environment would not lead to clonal expansion, might even cause apoptosis, and would thus avoid detection. In most instances it does not appear to be necessary to invoke an increased mutation rate in explaining the evolutionary process of tumor outgrowth, and often an increased mutation rate might well confer a disadvantage on the cell.[1,30]

In summary, selection is the driving force for tumor growth; this key principle is as applicable to slow-growing and benign endocrine tumors as it is to aggressive cancers.

Genetic Alterations in Endocrine Tumors: Examples

Neoplasia is, in large part, a genetic disease in which most of the critical DNA damage occurs somatically rather than through inheritance (germline mutations). Somatic alterations of proto-oncogenes and tumor suppressor genes are implicated in endocrine tumorigenesis; in other words, such mutations can be of either the gain-of-function or the loss-of-function type. Germline mutations that predispose to endocrine neoplasia can also occur in either proto-oncogenes or tumor suppressor genes. Germline mutations in *RET,* causing multiple endocrine neoplasia types 2A (MEN2A) and 2B (MEN2B), and familial medullary thyroid cancer (FMTC), are prominent examples of the former and are discussed in Chapter 40. However, most germline mutations identified to date are inactivating mutations, thus identifying the affected genes as tumor suppressors by definition.

Patients in whom a particular tumor develops on the basis of a strong inherited predisposition typically constitute only a minority of patients with that tumor. Nonetheless, the lessons learned from identifying the molecular basis of inherited tumor predisposition are important, both clinically and from a fundamental biologic perspective. In addition, some genes found to cause rare genetic syndromes through germline mutations have subsequently been found to be somatically mutated in the more common, sporadic occurrences of the same tumors. Two examples, *MEN1* and *HRPT2,* illustrate this point.

Thyrotropin Receptor and $G_{\alpha S}$ in Toxic Thyroid Adenomas

The fact that solitary toxic thyroid adenomas often contain somatic mutations in different genes whose products are functionally interrelated highlights the point that heterogeneous genetic lesions can converge on common pathways to predispose to neoplasia. Solitary toxic thyroid adenomas are characterized by autonomous *(TSH-independent)* hyperfunction and growth. Because TSH is normally a stimulus to both functional activity and growth of thyroid cells, toxic adenomas chronically and inappropriately behave as though they are stimulated by TSH. Somatic mutations in the TSH receptor itself can lead to TSH-independent *(constitutive)* activation of the receptor and cause both clonal expansion and hyperthyroidism in a subset of toxic adenomas.[31] Thus, the TSH receptor is a proto-oncogene that can be activated by a variety of point mutations. Analysis of how these point mutations mimic the effects of TSH binding has provided insight into the mechanism of activation of G protein–coupled receptors.

The TSH receptor is a member of the large family of G protein–coupled receptors, and its major actions on thyrocyte proliferation and differentiated function are mediated through the cyclic adenosine monophosphate (cAMP) signaling pathway. The predominant G protein involved in transducing the stimulatory effect of the receptor on adenylyl cyclase is $G_{s\alpha}$. $G_{s\alpha}$ is also a proto-oncogene and has undergone clonally selected activating point mutation in a subset of toxic thyroid adenomas.[32] $G_{s\alpha}$ genes bearing such gain-of-function mutations have been termed *gsp* oncogenes and are also present in some growth hormone–secreting pituitary tumors. Not surprisingly, these pituitary tumors demonstrate constitutive activation of the cAMP pathway, a prime mediator of proliferation and hormonal function in the somatotroph.

In this context, it is instructive to raise the example of McCune-Albright syndrome (see Chapter 24), in which activating $G_{s\alpha}$ mutations are present in multiple tissues of a given patient owing to mutation early in embryonic development and subsequent genetic mosaicism. Hyperthyroidism and acromegaly are among the characteristic components of this syndrome. Another gene encoding an element in the cAMP signaling pathway, the protein kinase A type I-α regulatory subunit gene *PPKAR1A,* has been implicated in the familial syndrome termed *Carney's complex,* which includes corticotropin-independent Cushing's syndrome related to autonomously functioning adrenocortical nodules, growth hormone–secreting pituitary tumors, and male precocious puberty caused by hormonally active testicular tumors.[33,34]

Cyclin D1 (PRAD1) in Hyperparathyroidism and General Oncology

Another illustrative example is that of the cyclin D1, or *PRAD1,* oncogene. Unlike many endocrine tumor–associated oncogenes, cyclin D1 is also commonly involved in nonendocrine tumors. Interestingly, this gene, now appreciated to be of central importance to molecular oncology and to normal cellular physiology, was discovered in the molecular dissection of an endocrine tumor.

Many human oncogenes were discovered because they are adjacent to nonrandom chromosome breakpoints in tumors. Chromosome breaks and rearrangements probably occur often in normal cells but are recognized only when they result in deregulation of the expression of a growth-related gene and confer a selective advantage on the cell. Cyclin D1 or *PRAD1* was identified as the putative oncogene adjacent to one such breakpoint on chromosome 11 in a subset of parathyroid adenomas (Fig. 39–2).[8,35,36] On the 11q13 side of the inversion breakpoint, the promoter and coding exons of the cyclin D1 gene remain in contiguity with each other. Across the breakpoint are regulatory sequences from the upstream region of the parathyroid hormone *(PTH)* gene on 11p15 that normally function to enhance *PTH* gene transcription in the presence of parathyroid

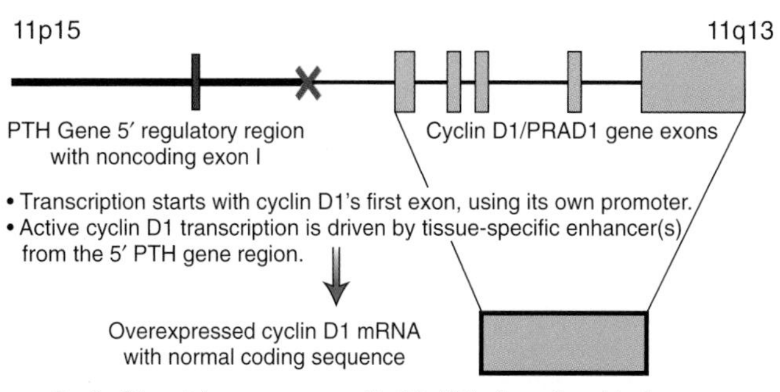
11p15
11q13
PTH Gene 5′ regulatory region
with noncoding exon I
Cyclin D1/PRAD1 gene exons
• Transcription starts with cyclin D1's first exon, using its own promoter.
• Active cyclin D1 transcription is driven by tissue-specific enhancer(s)
from the 5′ PTH gene region.
Overexpressed cyclin D1 mRNA
with normal coding sequence
Cyclin D1 protein overexpressed in 20–40% of parathyroid adenomas
by rearrangement/other mechanisms

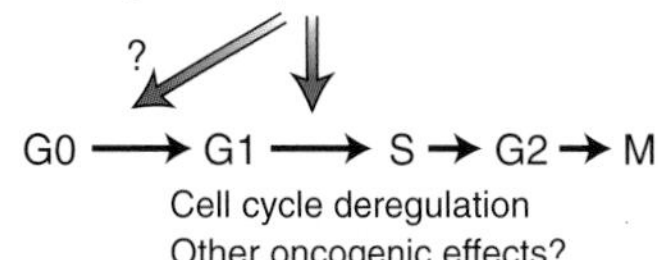
?
G0 → G1 → S → G2 → M
Cell cycle deregulation
Other oncogenic effects?

Figure 39–2 ■ Diagram of the molecular structure of the parathyroid hormone–cyclin D1 DNA rearrangement in a subset of parathyroid adenomas and its functional consequences. The dark X represents the chromosome breakpoint between the *PTH* gene regulatory region, plus *PTH* noncoding exon 1 *(solid light vertical bar)* and part of its first intron, from 11p15 *(left),* and the intact promoter and five exons of the cyclin D1 gene from 11q13. Cyclin D1 gene transcription proceeds in a left-to-right direction, as drawn. (Modified from Arnold A. Genetic basis of endocrine disease: 5. Molecular genetics of parathyroid gland neoplasia. J Clin Endocrinol Metab 1993; 77:1108-1112. Copyright © 1993, The Endocrine Society.)

tissue–specific signals (likely to be DNA-binding proteins found in the nucleus). Such transcriptional enhancer sequences can act over distances of many kilobases to enhance transcription, and cyclin D1 transcription is increased in these tumors. Although the true incidence of such rearrangements has not yet been determined because of variability in breakpoint sites, cyclin D1 protein levels are elevated in 20% to 40% of parathyroid adenomas.[9]

In a broader context, the tissue-specific enhancer-driven expression of cyclin D1 in parathyroid tumors is analogous to the activation of oncogenes such as *BCL2* or *MYC* in B-cell lymphomas. In these tumors, chromosomal rearrangements lead to a juxtaposition of immunoglobulin gene enhancer elements and the oncogene, which is thereby inappropriately activated.

The *PRAD1* gene product was initially recognized as a cyclin by virtue of its structural relation to the cyclin family of proteins, known to be involved in controlling the cell cycle. However, before discovery of *PRAD1* (cyclin D1), no mammalian cyclins were known to participate in the control of the critical transition from G_1 to S phase; this checkpoint would be an appropriate site for attack by an oncogenic protein because movement into S phase commits a cell to the remainder of the cycle and another mitosis. It is now widely accepted that cyclin D1 is a G_1 cyclin that functions to push the cell toward or through this key juncture.[37]

One cautionary note: This functional assignment for cyclin D1 as a G_1 cyclin is overwhelmingly derived from cultured cell systems, which might not fully reflect the true in vivo roles of this key oncoprotein. Thus, the detailed mechanism of action of cyclin D1, both normally and especially when dysregulated in tumorigenesis, deserves further exploration.[36]

Cyclins are regulatory subunits of holoenzymes whose catalytic subunits are cyclin-dependent kinases (CDKs). The major kinase partner for cyclin D1 appears to be CDK4 or, in some cell types, CDK6. The protein product of the retinoblastoma tumor suppressor gene, *pRB,* has been recognized as one substrate for phosphorylation by cyclin D–cdk complexes. Natural inhibitors of CDK function also exist, and $p16^{INK4a}$ is recognized as a key inhibitor of cyclin D–CDK4/6 complexes. Thus, inactivation of *p16* might be expected to be as oncogenic as cyclin D1 overexpression, and *p16* is, indeed, a tumor suppressor gene in familial melanoma and several types of sporadic human tumors. Interestingly, inactivating mutations of *p16* are uncommon, if they occur at all, in parathyroid adenomas.[38] Hence, the cellular consequences of *p16* loss and cyclin D1 activation might not precisely overlap. Consistent with this observation, increasing evidence exists for possible non-CDK-dependent actions of cyclin D1.[36]

The significance of cyclin D1 in human neoplasia extends far beyond its involvement in endocrine tumors. For example, it is the long-sought *BCL1* oncogene that is deregulated by the characteristic t(11;14) translocation in mantle cell or centrocytic B-cell lymphomas. Thus, assessment of cyclin D1 gene rearrangement or expression is clinically useful in the molecular diagnosis of B-cell neoplasia. In addition, cyclin D1 is a key oncogene in breast cancer, myeloma, squamous cell cancers of the head and neck, esophageal cancer, and a variety of other tumors.[36] Cyclin D1 and other members of its oncogenic pathway or pathways might serve as targets for development of antineoplastic therapies.

MEN1 Tumor Suppressor Gene

Multiple endocrine neoplasia type 1 (MEN1) is a familial predisposition to tumors of the parathyroid glands, anterior pituitary, pancreatic islets, and duodenum. Other tumors, including carcinoid tumors, lipomas, and angiofibromas, also occur with increased frequency in this disorder (see Chapter 40).

MEN1 is inherited in an autosomal dominant pattern with high penetrance, indicating that a single mutant gene is responsible for transmitting the tumor predisposition. *MEN1,* the normal gene whose mutant form causes MEN1, was identified by positional cloning.[39] *MEN1* germline mutations have been detected in most MEN1 families and in clinically sporadic MEN1, that is, in MEN1 patients with a negative family history. Many of these mutations would clearly be expected to truncate the translated product severely and can safely be categorized as *inactivating* mutations. It can be reasonably anticipated that when definitive functional testing is available, other reported mutations, especially in the missense category, will prove to be inactivating lesions as well.

The identification of *MEN1* also opened up the potential for direct presymptomatic molecular diagnosis in established or suspected MEN1 kindreds or individual patients. However, the benefits of such DNA testing with respect to prophylactic interventions are more restricted, and improvements in morbidity or mortality are less well established, than, for example, in *RET* testing for MEN2.[40] Furthermore, because the gene is large, with many introns, and because inactivating mutations can occur throughout the gene, a substantial fraction of mutations cannot be identified in MEN1 patients when exons are sequenced in research or commercial laboratories. Thus, a negative genetic test does not eliminate the diagnosis of MEN1 in a new patient.

The *MEN1* gene encodes a 610–amino acid protein termed *menin.* The structure of menin has yielded few clues to menin's normal function except for its nuclear localization signals. Menin might play a role in regulation of gene transcription; this role has been suggested by the finding that it can bind a member of the activator protein 1 (AP-1) transcription factor family, JunD, and inhibit the ability of JunD to activate transcription.[41] Tissue surveys have shown *MEN1* expression to be nearly ubiquitous.

The molecular pathology of *MEN1* strongly suggests that it functions as a classic tumor suppressor gene, requiring biallelic inactivation in order to drive the emergence of a clinically significant tumor. In a patient with MEN1, after somatic deletion on 11q13 has occurred in a particular parathyroid or islet cell, for example, that cell would be devoid of the normal tumor suppressor function of the *MEN1* gene product and would thereby acquire an actual or potential selective advantage over its neighbors. The high incidence of endocrine tumors in MEN1 (which demonstrates almost 100% penetrance) implies that this somatic inactivation of the remaining normal gene copy (second hit) is a common development in the context of the patient's entire endocrine tissue complement. Cells in tissues not affected in MEN1 probably sustain second hits as well but are able to tolerate the menin loss without fostering tumorigenesis,[42] indicating the crucial importance of cell and tissue context in endocrine tumor specificity in this disorder and others. Also, one should not assume that loss of function in both *MEN1* alleles is *sufficient* for tumorigenesis in susceptible tissues, and additional cooperating oncogenic lesions are likely needed.[43]

Allelic losses of DNA markers on 11q13, including the *MEN1* region, are found in some of the more common, sporadically occurring versions of the tumors associated with familial MEN1. They include a frequency of 25% to 40% for 11q13 allelic loss in sporadic parathyroid adenomas, for example. However, most studies have found putatively inactivating mutations of the nondeleted *MEN1* allele in only 12% to 17% of parathyroid adenomas. This gap, which is larger than expected from comparisons with other established tumor suppressors, suggests that another tumor suppressor on 11q might exist, serving as the target for specific acquired mutation in many of the tumors with 11q allelic loss but with an apparently intact remaining *MEN1* allele. However, the possibility remains that *MEN1* is the only 11q tumor suppressor relevant in these tumors and that epigenetic or noncoding alterations are disproportionately frequent mechanisms of somatic (but not germline) inactivation of *MEN1*.

HRPT2 Tumor Suppressor Gene

The hereditary hyperparathyroidism–jaw tumor syndrome (HPT-JT) is a rare autosomal dominant predisposition to parathyroid gland neoplasms, ossifying fibromas of the mandible and maxilla, renal abnormalities including cystic lesions and hamartomas, and possibly uterine tumors.[44,45] Using genetic linkage and positional cloning approaches, the *HRPT2* gene was identified as the source of predisposing germline mutations in the majority of HPT-JT kindreds examined.[46] The remaining 30% to 40% of kindreds most likely also have *HRPT2* mutations that are located outside the sequenced coding region and thereby evade detection. Similar germline mutations occur in a subset of kindreds with familial isolated hyperparathyroidism (FIHP).[47] Mutations of *HRPT2* are predicted to inactivate or eliminate its protein product, parafibromin, again consistent with a tumor suppressor mechanism. Parafibromin's normal cellular function appears to involve regulation of gene expression and chromatin modification as part of the human Paf complex,[48] and interestingly its regulatory targets might include cyclin D1.[49]

Hyperparathyroidism is the most penetrant component of HPT-JT, and it can develop as early as the first or second decade of life. Although the inherited mutation puts all the parathyroid glands at increased risk for tumor development over a patient's lifetime, the tumors can develop asynchronously, and only a solitary parathyroid tumor may be present at the time of initial diagnosis and surgical exploration. Furthermore, whereas most such parathyroid tumors are classified as adenomas, parathyroid carcinoma is found in an impressively high proportion (15%) relative to its less than 1% incidence among parathyroid tumors in the general population. The latter observation led investigators to consider *HRPT2* as a possible target for *somatic* mutations in nonfamilial sporadic cases of parathyroid carcinoma and indeed, somatic inactivating *HRPT2* mutations were discovered in the majority of sporadic parathyroid carcinomas.[50] Even the impressive combined prevalence of over 75% in this and subsequent studies is likely to underestimate the true role of *HRPT2* mutation in sporadic parathyroid cancer because noncoding mutations equally capable of inactivating the gene would have escaped detection. Thus, *HRPT2* mutation is central to the pathogenesis of most, and perhaps virtually all, sporadic parathyroid carcinomas. In contrast, although *HRPT2* was an equally plausible candidate for involvement in benign parathyroid neoplasia, somatic *HRPT2* mutations are rarely if ever present in unselected series of typical sporadic parathyroid adenomas.[51]

Importantly and unexpectedly, Shattuck and colleagues also found that some patients with *sporadic* presentations of parathyroid carcinoma harbor *germline* mutations in *HRPT2*.[50] Whether such patients represent newly recognized classic HPT-JT or have a distinct syndrome (akin to MEN2A and familial isolated medullary thyroid cancer being alternative expressions of the same *RET* mutation) is unknown, but in either case this molecular genetic insight has yielded a new clinical indication for DNA-based carrier identification in family members of patients with parathyroid cancer, aimed at preventing parathyroid malignancy.

Genetic paradigms that have originated in the study of malignant neoplasia are useful in the molecular dissection of endocrine tumors, including common benign endocrine tumors. Identification of clonally selected mutations in oncogenes and tumor suppressor genes has opened the door to understanding the control of growth in endocrine tissues and has already resulted in important advances in clinical diagnosis and management. Furthermore, the fact that these genetic alterations can affect endocrine cell function as well as cell number may be exploited in devising medical therapies in the future.

REFERENCES

1. Wang TL, Rago C, Silliman N, et al. Prevalence of somatic alterations in the colorectal cancer cell genome. Proc Natl Acad Sci U S A 2002;99:3076-3080.
2. Arnold A, Staunton CE, Kim HG, et al. Monoclonality and abnormal parathyroid hormone genes in parathyroid adenomas. N Engl J Med 1988;318:658-662.
3. Arnold A, Brown MF, Urena P, et al. Monoclonality of parathyroid tumors in chronic renal failure and in primary parathyroid hyperplasia. J Clin Invest 1995;95:2047-2053.
4. Weir B, Zhao X, Meyerson M. Somatic alterations in the human cancer genome. Cancer Cell 2004;6:433-438.
5. Kroll TG, Sarraf P, Pecciarini L, et al. *PAX8-PPARγ1* fusion oncogene in human thyroid carcinoma. Science 2000;289:1357-1360.
6. Levy A, Lightman S. Molecular defects in the pathogenesis of pituitary tumours. Front Neuroendocrinol 2003;24:94-127.
7. van Sande J, Parma J, Tonacchera M, et al. Genetic basis of endocrine disease: somatic and germline mutations of the TSH receptor gene in thyroid diseases. J Clin Endocrinol Metab 1995;80:2577-2585.
8. Arnold A. Genetic basis of endocrine disease 5: molecular genetics of parathyroid gland neoplasia. J Clin Endocrinol Metab 1993;77:1108-1112.
9. Arnold A. Molecular basis of primary hyperparathyroidism. In Bilezikian JP, Marcus R, Levine MA, eds. The Parathyroids, 2nd ed. San Diego: Academic Press, 2001:331-347.
10. Palanisamy N, Imanishi Y, Rao P, et al. Novel chromosomal abnormalities identified by comparative genomic hybridization in parathyroid adenomas. J Clin Endocrinol Metab 1998;83:1766-1770.
11. Lyon M. Gene action in the X-chromosome of the mouse. Nature 1961;190:372-373.
12. Fialkow PJ. Clonal origin of human tumors. Biochim Biophys Acta 1976;458:283-321.
13. Fialkow PJ, Jackson CE, Block MA, et al. Multicellular origin of parathyroid "adenomas." N Engl J Med 1977;297:696-698.
14. Jackson CE, Cerny JC, Block MA, et al. Probable clonal origin of aldosteronomas versus multicellular origin of parathyroid "adenomas." Surgery 1982;92:875-879.
15. Vogelstein B, Fearon ER, Hamilton SR, et al. Clonal analysis using recombinant DNA probes from the X-chromosome. Cancer Res 1987;47:4806-4813.
16. Shattuck TM, Shattuck TM, Westra WH, et al. Independent clonal origins of distinct tumor foci in multifocal papillary thyroid carcinoma. N Engl J Med 2005;352:2406-2412.
17. Biller BMK, Alexander JM, Zervas NT, et al. Clonal origins of adrenocorticotropin-secreting pituitary tissue in Cushing's disease. J Clin Endocrinol Metab 1992;75:1303-1309.
18. Gicquel C, Le Bouc Y, Luton J-P, et al. Monoclonality of corticotroph macroadenomas in Cushing's disease. J Clin Endocrinol Metab 1992;75:472-475.
19. Mihailescu D, Shore-Freedman E, Mukani S, et al. Multiple neoplasms in an irradiated cohort: pattern of occurrence and relationship to thyroid cancer outcome. J Clin Endocrinol Metab 2002;87:3236-3241.
20. Schneider AB, Ron E, Lubin J, et al. Dose-response relationships for radiation-induced thyroid cancer and thyroid nodules: evidence for the prolonged effects of radiation on the thyroid. J Clin Endocrinol Metab 1993;77:362-369.
21. Cardis E, Kesminiene A, Ivanov V, et al. Risk of thyroid cancer after exposure to ^{131}I in childhood. J Natl Cancer Inst 2005;97:724-732.
22. Haber D, Harlow E. Tumour-suppressor genes: evolving definitions in the genomic age. Nat Genet 1997;16:320-322.
23. Payne SR, Kemp CJ. Tumor suppressor genetics. Carcinogenesis 2005;26:2031-2045.
24. Strauss B. The origin of point mutation in human tumor cells. Cancer Res 1992;52:249-253.
25. O'Neill JP. DNA damage, DNA repair, cell proliferation, and DNA replication: how do gene mutations result? Proc Natl Acad Sci USA 2000;97:11137-11139.

26. MacPhee D. Mismatch repair, somatic mutations, and the origins of cancer. Cancer Res 1995;55:5489-5492.
27. Loeb L. Microsatellite instability: marker of a mutator phenotype in cancer. Cancer Res 1994;54:5059-5063.
28. Lengauer C, Kinzler KW, Vogelstein B. Genetic instabilities in human cancers. Nature 1998;396:643-649.
29. Rubin H. The role of selection in progressive neoplastic transformation. Adv Cancer Res 2001;83:159-207.
30. Tomlinson I, Bodmer W. Selection, the mutation rate and cancer: ensuring that the tail does not wag the dog. Nat Med 1999;5:11-12.
31. Russo D, Arturi F, Suarez HG, et al. Thyrotropin receptor gene alterations in thyroid hyperfunctioning adenomas. J Clin Endocrinol Metab 1996;81:1548-1551.
32. Lyons J, Landis C, Harsh G, et al. Two G protein oncogenes in human endocrine tumors. Science 1990;249:655-659.
33. Wilkes D, McDermott DA, Basson CT. Clinical phenotypes and molecular genetic mechanisms of Carney complex. Lancet Oncol 2005;6:501-8.
34. Bossis I, Stratakis CA. Minireview: PRKAR1A: normal and abnormal functions. Endocrinology 2004;145:545.
35. Motokura T, Bloom T, Kim HG, et al. A novel cyclin encoded by a *bcl1*-linked candidate oncogene. Nature 1991;350:512-515.
36. Arnold A, Papanikolaou A. Biology of neoplasia—cyclin D1 in breast cancer pathogenesis. J Clin Oncol 2005;23:4215-4224.
37. Sherr CJ. Cancer cell cycles. Science 1996;274:1672-1677.
38. Tahara H, Smith A, Gaz R, Arnold A. Loss of chromosome arm 9p DNA and analysis of the p16 and p15 cyclin-dependent kinase inhibitor genes in human parathyroid adenomas. J Clin Endocrinol Metab 1996;81:3663-3667.
39. Chandrasekharappa S, Guru S, Manickam P, et al. Positional cloning of the gene for multiple endocrine neoplasia type 1. Science 1997;276:404-407.
40. Brandi ML, Gagel RF, Angeli A, et al. Guidelines for diagnosis and therapy of MEN type 1 and type 2. J Clin Endocrinol Metab 2001;86:5658-5671.
41. Agarwal SK, Kennedy PA, Scacheri PC, et al. Menin molecular interactions: insights into normal functions and tumorigenesis. Horm Metab Res 2005;37:369-374.
42. Scacheri PC, Crabtree JS, Kennedy AL, et al. Homozygous loss of menin is well tolerated in liver, a tissue not affected in MEN1. Mamm Genome 2004;15:872-877.
43. Crabtree JS, Scacheri PC, Ward JM, et al. Of mice and MEN1: insulinomas in a conditional mouse knockout. Mol Cell Biol. 2003;23: 6075-6085.
44. Szabo J, Heath B, Hill VM, et al. Hereditary hyperparathyroidism–jaw tumor syndrome: the endocrine tumor gene *HRPT2* maps to chromosome 1q21-q31. Am J Hum Genet 1995;56:944-950.
45. Bradley KJ, Hobbs MR, Buley ID, et al. Uterine tumours are a phenotypic manifestation of the hyperparathyroidism–jaw tumour syndrome. J Intern Med 2005;257:18-22.
46. Carpten JD, Robbins CM, Villablanca A, et al. *HRPT2,* encoding parafibromin, is mutated in hyperparathyroidism–jaw tumor syndrome. Nat Genet 2002;32:676-680.
47. Simonds WF, Robbins CM, Agarwal SK, et al. Familial isolated hyperparathyroidism is rarely caused by germline mutation in *HRPT2,* the gene for the hyperparathyroidism–jaw tumor syndrome. J Clin Endocrinol Metab 2004;89:96-102.
48. Rozenblatt-Rosen O, Hughes CM, Nannepaga SJ, et al. The parafibromin tumor suppressor protein is part of a human Paf1 complex. Mol Cell Biol 2005;25:612-620.
49. Woodard GE, Lin L, Zhang JH, et al. Parafibromin, product of the hyperparathyroidism–jaw tumor syndrome gene *HRPT2,* regulates cyclin D1/PRAD1 expression. Oncogene 2005;24:1272-1276.
50. Shattuck TM, Valimaki S, Obara T, et al. Somatic and germ-line mutations of the *HRPT2* gene in sporadic parathyroid carcinoma. N Engl J Med 2003;349:1722-1729.
51. Krebs LJ, Shattuck TM, Arnold A. *HRPT2* mutational analysis of typical sporadic parathyroid adenomas. J Clin Endocrinol Metab 2005;90:5015-5017.

CHAPTER 40

MULTIPLE ENDOCRINE NEOPLASIA

Robert F. Gagel and Stephen J. Marx

Overview of Multiple Endocrine Neoplasia Syndromes

The multiple endocrine neoplasia (MEN) syndromes were described in the early part of the 20th century[1] and subsequently classified into two principal categories, MEN type 1 (MEN-1) and MEN type 2 (MEN-2). They were named *multiple endocrine neoplasia* or *multiple endocrine adenomatosis* syndromes because they affect multiple types of hormone-secreting organs and produce multiple hormonal syndromes. Although there were individual case reports of multiple endocrine neoplasms distributed throughout the literature, there was no clarity regarding the nature of these syndromes and their familial transmission during the first 50 years.

During the period 1950 to 1980, the development of techniques to measure steroid and peptide hormones, improvements in imaging and histopathology, and the recognition of the importance of genetic disease led to a more careful delineation of these syndromes and the development of strategies to diagnose and treat. The convergence of these technologies led to the recognition that a specific spectrum of endocrine tumors occurred in certain families with regularity. It was also recognized that unique sets of hormones were associated with specific tumor types and cell types and caused specific clinical syndromes. Among the earliest examples was the recognition that growth hormone or prolactin production by pituitary tumors or gastrin production by islet cell tumors caused specific clinical syndromes.

It was also during this period that investigators first proposed the concept of using hormone measurement to identify specific neoplastic components of these syndromes with the hope that earlier recognition would modify the course of the syndrome. Prominent among these are the use of measurements of prolactin to identify microadenomas of the pituitary, gastrin and insulin to identify enteropancreatic tumors, catecholamines or their metabolites to identify adrenal medullary tumors, and calcitonin to identify medullary thyroid carcinoma (MTC). In these and other examples, development of radioimmunoassay technology facilitated early and correct diagnosis and, in some cases, led to curative surgical removal of the affected organ.

During this same period, awareness developed that there were at least six multiple endocrine neoplasia syndromes with several subvariants: MEN-1, MEN-2, von Hippel-Lindau (VHL) disease, neurofibromatosis type 1 (NF-1), Carney's complex (CNC), and McCune-Albright syndrome (MAS) (Table 40–1).[2-8] The first five of these are transmitted in the germline with autosomal dominant transmission; the sixth, McCune-Albright syndrome, develops as a result of very early somatic mutations leading to involvement of multiple endocrine and nonendocrine cell types. Each of these syndromes meets the definition established earlier of multiple endocrine organ involvement with potential production of multiple hormones. What was not completely recognized at the time of their description or categorization is that each of these syndromes affects nonendocrine tissues and, in some cases, the nonendocrine manifestations provide the most problematic management issues.

Although this chapter will not provide an in-depth review of the management of nonendocrine manifestations, we will provide appropriate references. This chapter will also not address other genetic endocrine syndromes associated with single hormone or endocrine tumor involvement. For example, the hereditary paraganglioma syndromes can affect multiple sympathetic or parasympathetic ganglia or the adrenal medullae, but the cell types involved represent a single cell or organ type and the hormones secreted belong to a single class or category,[9] failing to meet the overall criteria of *multiplicity* in type of gland involved.

The current phase in our understanding of these syndromes, the elucidation of the genetic causes, began in the 1980s and continues today. The genes for five of the six syndromes (MEN-1, MEN-2, VHL, NF1, and CNC) were identified by classic linkage techniques. The prominent clinical syndromes associated with these syndromes led to the identification of large and well-defined kindreds and made them tempting targets for application of newly resurrected genetic linkage techniques in the late 1980s. During the period from 1987 through 1993, the causative genes for each of these disorders were mapped and cloned. The

TABLE 40–1 FEATURES OF MULTIPLE ENDOCRINE NEOPLASIA TYPE 1 IN ADULTS

ENDOCRINE FEATURES (ESTIMATED AVERAGE PENETRANCE)
Parathyroid adenoma (95%)
Enteropancreatic
Gastrinoma (40%)
Insulinoma (10%)
Nonfunctioning,* including pancreatic polypeptide-oma† (20%)
Other: glucagonoma, VIPoma, somatostatinoma, etc. (each <2%)
Foregut Carcinoid
Thymic carcinoid nonfunctioning (2%)
Bronchial carcinoid nonfunctioning (4%)
Gastric enterochromaffin-like tumor nonfunctioning (10%)
Anterior Pituitary
Prolactinoma (25%)
Other: nonfunctioning (10%), growth hormone + prolactin, growth hormone (5%), ACTH (2%), thyrotropin (5%)
Adrenal
Cortex: Nonfunctioning (30%); functioning or cancer (2%)
Medulla: Pheochromocytoma (<1%)
NONENDOCRINE FEATURES (ESTIMATED AVERAGE PENETRANCE)
Facial angiofibroma (85%)
Collagenoma (70%)
Lipoma (30%)
Leiomyoma (5%)
Meningioma (5%)

Italics indicate tumor type with substantial (>20% of cases) malignant potential.
*Many nonfunctioning MEN-1 tumors synthesize a peptide hormone or other factors (such as small amine) but do not oversecrete enough to produce a hormonal expression.
†Omits nearly 100% prevalence of nonfunctioning and clinically silent tumors, some of which are detected incidental to enteropancreatic surgery in MEN-1.
ACTH, adrenocorticotropic hormone; MEN, multiple endocrine neoplasia; VIP, vasoactive intestinal peptide.

elucidation of the genetic disorder in McCune-Albright syndrome derived from earlier observations that G-protein-coupled signaling was activated in endocrine tissues expressing the mutant gene, leading to the identification of mutations of the guanine nucleotide-binding protein, α-stimulating activity polypeptide (GNAS, $G_s\alpha$). Although it should be considered a part of the multiple endocrine neoplasia, it is discussed in Chapter 24 and will not be discussed further here.

The elucidation of the genetic basis for each of these syndromes has clarified some important questions. It has provided molecular evidence that most of the clinical variants of each syndrome are in fact initiated by mutations of a single gene. The only exceptions to this at present are MEN-1 and CNC, where a second gene at a different chromosomal locus remains to be identified or explored. In two of these syndromes, VHL and MEN-2, specific mutations of the causative genes define unique clinical variants, making genetic information useful for determining the phenotype. In at least one of these syndromes, MEN-2, the identification of the molecular defect has led to the development of pharmacologic agents that may blunt the signal transduction abnormalities and has led to human clinical trials to reverse malignant tumor growth. Finally, for most of these disorders, mutations of the same gene have been found in sporadic tumors of the same type, indicating a broader importance for these genes in endocrine and nonendocrine neoplasia. Examples include the identification of a somatic mutations of MEN-1 in a high percentage of pancreatic islet tumors, VHL mutations in sporadic renal cell carcinoma, and somatic mutations of *RET* in sporadic MTCs, each of which will be discussed later in this chapter.

The molecular abnormalities in these tumor syndromes are representative of the oncogene abnormalities found in human neoplasia: MEN-1, VHL, CNC, and NF1 are caused by inactivating mutations, and MAS and MEN-2 are caused by activating mutations. Although progress has been rapid, a number of important and unanswered questions remain: How do the molecular defects cause transformation? What is the mechanism of cell or tissue specificity? Are there signaling events that can be used as therapeutic targets? For each of these disorders the relevant signal transduction pathways are being defined and studied. Progress toward answers to these questions will be described in relevant sections of this chapter.

Multiple Endocrine Neoplasia Type 1

The association of parathyroid, enteropancreatic endocrine, and pituitary neoplasia is called *multiple endocrine neoplasia type 1.* Although there were earlier descriptions,[1] the syndrome was recognized as a clinical and familial syndrome by Moldawer and colleagues[3] and Wermer[4] in 1954 (thus the eponym Wermer syndrome). MEN-2 was recognized and classified as distinct from it in 1968.[7] In previous years, MEN-1 patients presented with advanced manifestations of parathyroid, pancreatic islet, or pituitary neoplasia (or some combination of these) in the third and fourth decades of life. However, improved carrier ascertainment and improved tumor surveillance have now resulted in earlier identification and earlier treatment of its hormonal syndromes.

The most common mode of presentation for MEN-1 is currently within the context of a previously identified kindred; less often, a patient with newly diagnosed advanced disease may be the propositus of a new kindred or an example of a sporadic case. MEN-1 remains the most challenging of the MEN syndromes. The many affected tissues cause complexity and expense in diagnosis and treatment. Each affected patient can be expected to undergo at least two surgical procedures. It is important for the clinician to recognize the high probability of recurrent or new neoplasms in many affected organ systems and to balance this likelihood against the potential effects of a deficiency syndrome associated with complete organ removal. Furthermore, even with satisfactory control of symptoms from hormone excess, patients have a high likelihood of eventual MEN-1–related cancer.

Hyperparathyroidism in Multiple Endocrine Neoplasia Type 1

MEN-1 is uncommon. The population prevalence is about 1 in 30,000, and it accounts for only about 1% to 3% of cases of primary hyperparathyroidism.[10] Hyperparathyroidism is the most common hormonal manifestation of MEN-1 (see Table 40–1).[6,10-14] Prospective tumor surveillance in members of MEN-1 families has shown hyperparathyroidism as early as age 8 years[11,12,15-19]; by age 40 years, about 95% of MEN-1 carriers have been hypercalcemic.[11,13,20]

Expressions of Hyperparathyroidism

Hyperparathyroidism in MEN-1 is most commonly asymptomatic; expressions include hypercalcemia, urolithiasis, parathyroid hormone (PTH)-induced bone abnormalities, musculoskeletal complaints, weakness, and alterations of mental status. These features are similar to those associated with other forms of hyperparathyroidism (see Chapter 27).

Hyperparathyroidism in MEN-1 differs in some ways from that caused by a sporadic adenoma. The first way is a difference in epidemiology. Hyperparathyroidism in MEN-1 has an earlier age of onset (typically 25 years versus 55 years)[13,14] (Fig. 40–1) and lack of gender imbalance (1 : 1 vs. 3 : 1 female-to-male ratio). Earlier onset implies that it can last longer. In particular, bone undermineralization among women with MEN-1–related hyperparathyroidism seems increased by their 20s and 30s.[21] Second is a different parathyroid pathology; enlargement, albeit highly asymmetric, of multiple parathyroid glands is usually present at the time of parathyroid exploration in MEN-1 (Fig. 40–2).[22,23] Third, the distributions of outcomes of parathyroid surgery differ. The presence of multiglandular disease and the resulting need to examine each gland during an initial surgical procedure inevitably result in a higher postoperative rate of hypoparathyroidism and a lower rate of euparathyroidism.[22,24] Successful subtotal parathyroidectomy is also followed within 10 years by recurrent hyperparathyroidism in half of MEN-1 cases.[22,24] In fact, true recurrent hyperparathyroidism in sporadic hyperparathyroidism is unusual, and recurrence should suggest the possibility of unrecognized MEN-1. True recurrent hyperparathyroidism, as with other tumor recurrences in MEN-1, could arise theoretically from a small remnant of tumor tissue or from a new mutation (second hit) in residual normal tissue. Fourth, hyperparathyroidism in MEN-1 almost never progresses to parathyroid cancer, although untreated hyperparathyroidism lasts longer in MEN-1 than in sporadic cases.[25]

There are several characteristics of hyperfunctioning parathyroid cells in MEN-1 that can have mechanistic implications. First, most or all parathyroid glands have been overgrown by one or a few neoplastic clones by the time of parathyroid surgery in MEN-1 (Fig. 40–3, *top*).[26] Second, a circulating growth factor is specific to the plasma of MEN-1 patients and mitogenic toward normal parathyroid cells in vitro (see later).[27] Third, a phenomenon observed in sporadic parathyroid adenomas, an abnormal rightward shift in the set-point for calcium suppression of PTH secretion, occurs to a lesser extent in MEN-1 parathyroid tumors (see Chapter 27).[28] This set-point abnormality may be caused by secondary decrease in the amount of the calcium-sensing receptor on the parathyroid cell surface.[29]

Hyperparathyroidism Management

Decision for Surgery

Surgery is the treatment of choice for hyperparathyroidism in MEN-1, although the timing and the type of operation remain controversial. Parathyroid surgery is definitely indicated in a MEN-1 patient with a moderately elevated PTH and other moderately advanced features, such as an albumin-adjusted serum calcium level higher than 3.0 mM/L (12.0 mg/dL), kidney stones, or PTH-induced bone disease.

Prospective surveillance for hyperparathyroidism in MEN-1 families has led to systematic identification of members, including some at ages 10 to 15 years, with minimal elevations of serum calcium and PTH concentration. The optimal management of such patients is not clear.

Early parathyroid surgery in MEN-1 has been advocated by some on the basis of the philosophy that hyperparathyroidism should always be treated as early as possible or the speculation that normalization of the serum calcium concentration might lead to a reduction of gastrin secretion and, possibly, lowered pancreatic islet cell growth or transformation, or both.[10] Although parathyroidectomy can decrease gastrin secretion by gastrinoma in MEN-1 (Fig. 40–4), there is no evidence that this intervention prevents or slows gastrin-cell transformation.[30] For this reason, and because drug control of gastric acid oversecretion is excellent, the coexistence of a gastrinoma is not a sufficient indication for parathyroidectomy in MEN-1, except in the rare case in which medical control of Zollinger-Ellison syndrome (ZES) is difficult.

Preoperative and Intraoperative Assessment of Tumors

Preoperative noninvasive imaging (ultrasonography, technetium 99m sestamibi, high-resolution CT scan, or all three) for parathyroid surgery is being performed with increasing

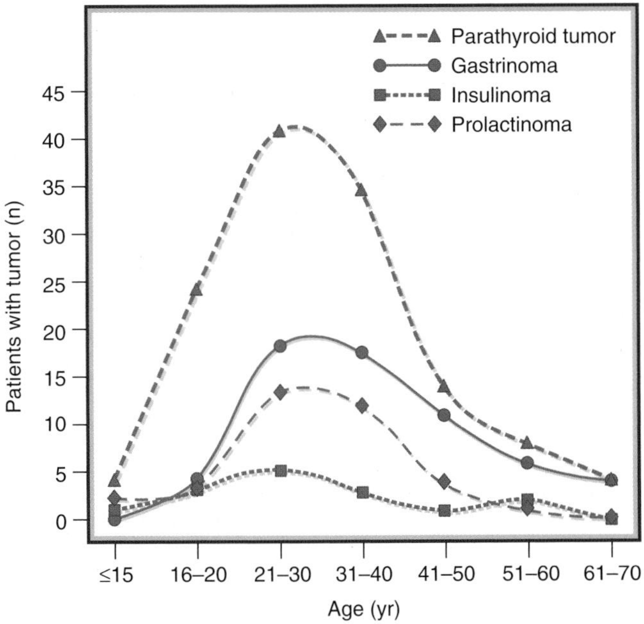

Figure 40–1 ▪ Age at onset for endocrine tumor expressions in multiple endocrine neoplasia type 1 (MEN-1). Data from retrospective analysis of multiple tumor expressions in 130 inpatients with MEN-1 during 15 years. Age of tumor onset was defined as the earlier of age at first symptom and age at first abnormal test result. (Modified from Marx S, Spiegel AM, Skarulis MC, et al. Multiple endocrine neoplasia type 1: clinical and genetic topics. Ann Intern Med 1998;129:484-494.)

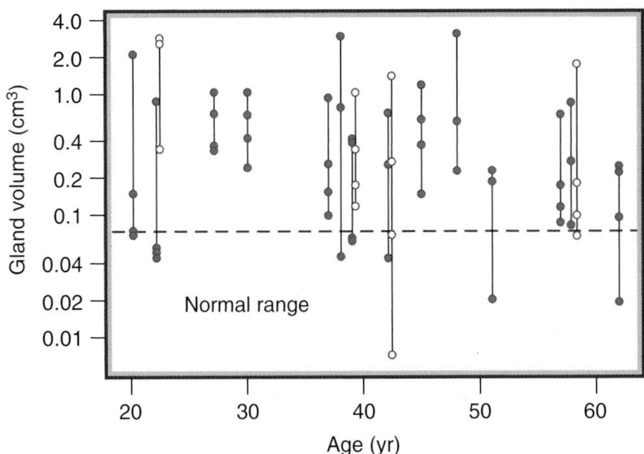

Figure 40–2 ▪ Parathyroid gland sizes at initial parathyroidectomy for 18 cases with familial multiple endocrine neoplasia type 1. The mean ratio of largest vs smallest turmor at an operation is 9:1 Volumes of all glands at one operation are connected by a *vertical line.* Adjacent symbols are highlighted by open circles. *Dashed horizontal line* is upper limit of normal gland volume (0.075 cm^3, equivalent to 75 mg mass). (Modified from Marx SJ, Menczel J, Campbell G, et al. Heterogeneous size of the parathyroid glands in familial multiple endocrine neoplasia type 1. Clin Endocrinol [Oxf] 1991;35:521-526.)

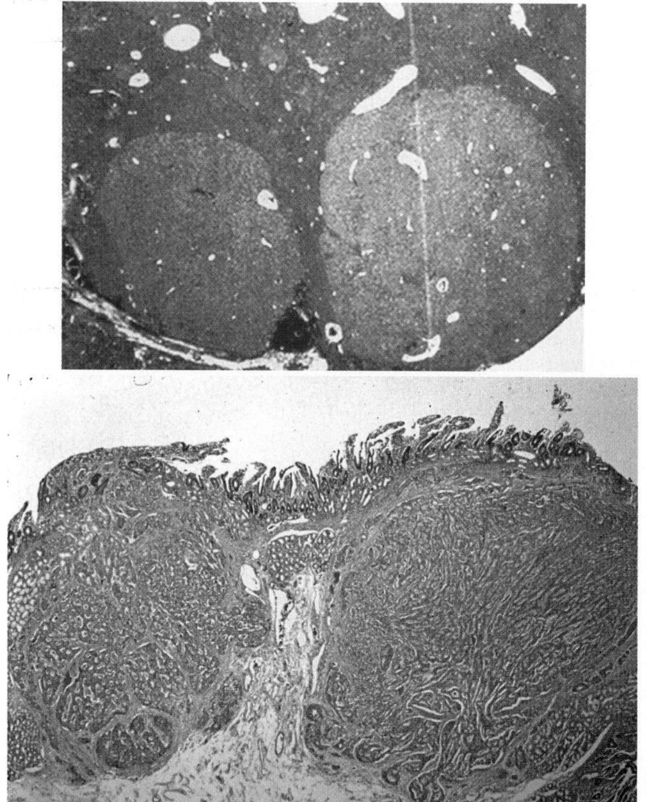

Figure 40–3 ▪ Tumor multiplicity within a tissue in multiple endocrine neoplasia type 1 (MEN-1). *Top,* Hypercellular parathyroid gland from patient with MEN-1. The gland is totally replaced by diffuse sheets of chief cells and two discrete nodules of chief cells. It suggests three or more abnormal parathyroid clones. This image could reflect three or more second hits to the normal copy of the *MEN1* gene in three different clone precursor cells and thus growth of three or more independent clones. An alternative pathogenesis could be stepwise evolution from one clone, that is, third hits to genes other than *MEN1. Bottom,* Duodenal mucosa from a second MEN-1 patient, showing two large submucosal microgastrinomas. Each tumor was positive for gastrin immunostain and negative for other peptide hormones. Possible development of these two adjacent tumors could have followed mechanisms suggested for the two parathyroid nodules at the top. (Both panels from I. Lubensky, National Institutes of Health, Bethesda, MD.)

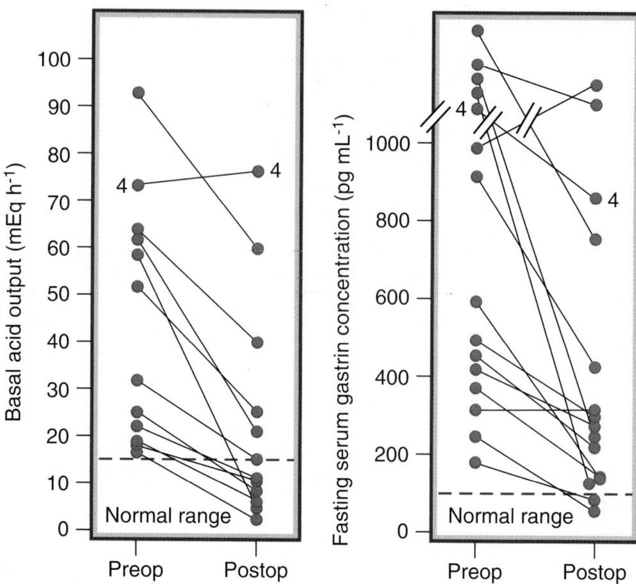

Figure 40–4 ▪ Effect of parathyroidectomy in patients with both multiple endocrine neoplasia type 1 and Zollinger-Ellison syndrome. Basal acid output and fasting serum gastrin are shown. All patients became normocalcemic except for one (case 4), who remained hypercalcemic. (From Jensen RT. Management of the Zollinger-Ellison syndrome in patients with multiple endocrine neoplasia type 1. J Intern Med 1998;243:477-488.)

frequency.[31] The major justification for the added costs of these procedures in sporadic hyperparathyroidism is to perform a unilateral or even more limited neck exploration, thereby reducing operative morbidity, time, and cost.[32] In MEN-1 the likely presence of multiple parathyroid tumors makes it necessary to perform an exploration of four or more glands at initial surgery, thereby eliminating one major rationale for preoperative imaging procedures.[10] A separate, and less frequent, concern is that if four glands are overactive, there is a fourfold greater possibility that one tumor has an abnormal location. A much stronger case can be made for the use of noninvasive and carefully selected invasive procedures (ultrasound-guided fine-needle aspiration for PTH assay, high resolation computerized tomography, selective arteriography, and selective venous sampling for PTH, when indicated) in MEN-1 patients undergoing reoperation.[33,34]

Several intraoperative tools can increase the likelihood of successful parathyroid surgery. Rapid on-line assay of PTH can be done at 5-minute intervals, with a turnaround time of 10 minutes for each result.[35-37] A substantial PTH fall from baseline predicts that no hyperfunctioning parathyroid tissue remains (Fig. 40–5). Sensitive ultrasound transducers routinely image parathyroid tumors intraoperatively in difficult locations, such as within the thyroid gland and within scar from prior surgery.[31] Availability of intraoperative PTH assay and ultrasonography may be useful as a backup option at initial parathyroid surgery, particularly in any patient expected to have multiple parathyroid tumors (as in MEN-1). These tests are even more likely to be helpful during parathyroid reoperations in MEN-1, because the number and locations of tumors during a second operative procedure are particularly hard to predict.

Surgical Objectives

The standard surgical approach for initial parathyroidectomy in MEN-1 is removal of 3.5 glands and conservation of approximately 50 mg of the most normal-appearing gland, attached to its vascular pedicle. Because eventual parathyroid reoperation in MEN-1 is likely, the recording of careful operative notes and diagrams and the marking of remaining tissue with nonresorbable materials enhance the likelihood of success in subsequent operations.

An alternative is attempted complete removal of parathyroid tissue from the neck and immediate autotransplantation of small fragments to pockets in the nondominant forearm.[38] Use of this strategy is dependent on the likelihood of achieving a high rate of graft success. This technique does not prevent recurrent hyperparathyroidism but can simplify its management. For example, a PTH concentration in the venous effluent of the graft greater than in the effluent from the contralateral arm confirms graft function (this does not exclude other parathyroid tissue in the neck or chest). Lastly, surgical removal of parathyroid tissue from the forearm graft bed during the likely second or third operation is technically easier than a neck reexploration. Cryopreservation of parathyroid tumor fragments is a useful option

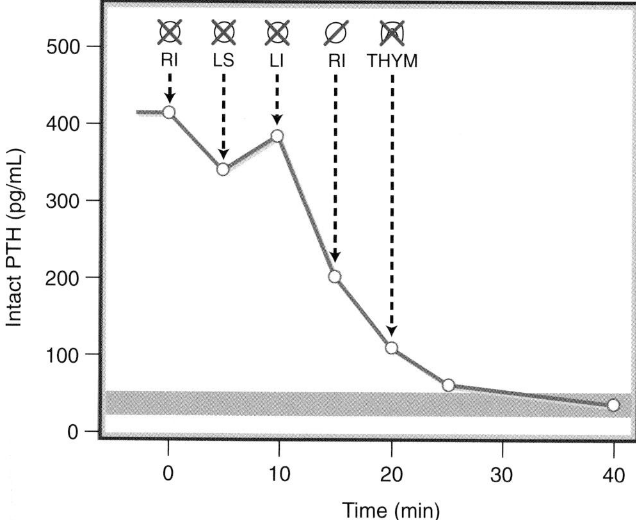

Figure 40–5 ▪ Intact parathyroid hormone (PTH) by rapid assay during parathyroid surgery. Normal range is indicated by *shading*. The patient had multiple endocrine neoplasia type 1 and primary hyperparathyroidism without prior parathyroidectomy. Three and one half similarly enlarged parathyroid glands (0.8-1.6 g; normal is <0.08 g) and the accessible portions of the thymus were removed at the times indicated; the thymus contained no identified parathyroid tumor. A rapid fall of PTH below a cutoff criterion indicates that little or no hyperfunctioning parathyroid tumor remains. Removal of the first two parathyroid tumors was not followed by a fall in PTH. The PTH assay result for each time point was available within several minutes to help establish the time at which no hyperfunctioning parathyroid tumor remained and thereby contribute to serial decisions about extending or ending the operation. (From S. K. Libutti, H. R. Alexander, and A. Remaley, National Institutes of Health, Bethesda, MD.)

in MEN-1, given the high rate of postoperative hypoparathyroidism in MEN-1. Cryopreservation permits a late parathyroid autograft.[38]

At initial parathyroid operation in MEN-1, partial thymectomy should be done through the cervical incision. This procedure not only results in removal of intrathymic parathyroid tissue but also can remove thymic carcinoid tissue, an issue discussed later in this chapter. It is important to do this during the initial operation because scar tissue can prevent a simple transcervical thymectomy at parathyroid reoperation.

Parathyroid surgery in the patient with MEN-1 requires judgment, familiarity with neck anatomy, and experience. The probability of an excellent outcome is improved substantially when initial or reoperative procedures are performed by an experienced endocrine surgery team.

Enteropancreatic Neuroendocrine Tumors

Neoplasia of the enteropancreatic neuroendocrine cells is the second most common endocrine manifestation of MEN-1 and eventually occurs in about 60% or more of MEN-1 patients (see Table 40–1). Also, multiple clinically silent enteropancreatic macroadenomas may be recognized at surgery or autopsy in nearly 100% of MEN-1 patients older than 40 years.[39,40] Gastric carcinoid tumors are described in a separate section (see "Foregut Carcinoid Tumors"). The enteropancreatic tumors are multiple, can oversecrete various hormones, and can become malignant. Approximately one third of MEN-1 patients die from MEN-1–related cancer, particularly gastrinoma; among these fatal cancers, the ratio of enteropancreatic neuroendocrine cancer to malignant carcinoid is 2 : 1.[41,42] It is similarly notable that in this era of excellent pharmacotherapy for gastric hyperacidity, about one sixth of MEN-1 patients with gastrinoma can die from metastatic gastrinoma but rarely from hypergastrinemia-induced metabolic complications.[43]

Although the MEN-1 patient can show symptoms or signs caused by one enteropancreatic hormone, there are often several associated and asymptomatic tumors with production of the same or other hormones.[44,45] The frequency of peptide immunostaining in MEN-1 pancreatic islet tumors is glucagon 35%, insulin 25%, pancreatic polypeptide 25%, and no hormone 10%; limited data are available for immunostaining of commonly observed duodenal gastrinomas.[44-46]

Interpretation of pancreatic islet histology in MEN-1 has changed over the decades. Early studies emphasized hyperplastic processes and budding of islet cells from ducts (nesidioblastosis).[47] Such features have now been reinterpreted as nonspecific. The overriding and important islet lesion in MEN-1, now termed *multifocal microadenoma,*[44] is a monoclonal or oligoclonal process (see Fig. 40–3, *legend*).[48,49] Molecular evidence for a hyperplastic precursor stage to tumor is accumulating. Hyperplastic foci of gastrin cells are seen by light microscopy in the duodenum of gastrinoma specimens from MEN-1 but not from sporadic gastrinoma.[50] Furthermore, heterozygous knockout of the *MEN1* gene in the mouse provides a good model of human *MEN1;* multiple giant hyperplastic islets are striking and precede insulinoma in this model, suggesting that subtle islet hyperplasia is an undetected tumor precursor lesion also in MEN-1 of humans.[51]

Rarely, enteropancreatic neuroendocrine tumors occur in several members of a family without other features of MEN-1; these have been insulinomas.[52] Nonfunctioning pancreatic islet tumors and pheochromocytoma can also appear uncommonly in a familial setting as expressions of VHL syndrome.[53]

Gastrinoma

Expressions of Gastrinomas

Gastrinoma is the second commonest endocrine tumor and the commonest cause of severe symptoms and signs in MEN-1. The symptoms and signs reflect two processes, malignancy and gastrin induction of excessive acid secretion by the stomach. Gastrinomas are found in about 40% of adults with MEN-1 (see Table 40–1).[10,13,30] ZES is defined here as symptoms or signs of gastric acid hypersecretion caused by a gastrin-secreting enteropancreatic neuroendocrine tumor or tumors. Among all patients with ZES, MEN-1 is found often, on the order of 25% in large series.[54] MEN-1 in most of these patients is readily recognizable from personal and family history. In contrast, among carefully defined sporadic ZES cases without obvious MEN-1, occult MEN-1 is much less frequent, a conclusion based on lack of family history, long-term follow-up, and mutational analysis of the *MEN1* gene.[55]

Symptoms of ZES include diarrhea, esophageal reflux, and those associated with peptic ulceration. Prospective tumor surveillance studies have more clearly defined the range of presenting features. Symptoms can antedate recognition of fasting hypergastrinemia. At one extreme, ulcer perforation can be caused infrequently by hypergastrinemia, even without prior symptoms.[56] The laboratory diagnosis of gastrinoma is established mainly by finding an elevated serum gastrin level. Other causes of elevated gastrin (false-positive results) that must be differentiated from gastrinoma include hypochlorhydria, including that resulting from autoimmunity or from pharmacologic agents that inhibit peptic acid secretion.[57] Hyperparathyroidism in MEN-1 can exacerbate hypergastrinemia (see earlier) (see Fig. 40–4).

Recognition of elevated gastrin or acid-related symptoms should be followed by assessment of the gastric acid secretion rate without acid-blocking drugs; the normal rate is less than 15 mEq/hr (or less than 5 mEq/hr after acid-reducing surgery).[57]

The diagnosis of gastrinoma can also be confirmed by measuring the serum gastrin response to intravenous synthetic secretin. A gastrin increase of more than 114 pM/L (200 pg/mL) diagnoses gastrinoma. This test differentiates gastrinoma from other hypergastrinemic states, such as retained gastric antrum, massive small bowel resection, or gastric outlet obstruction. Gastric endoscopy and ultrasound are advisable at the initial evaluation for ZES in MEN-1 and allow assessment of peptic ulcerations and duodenal gastrinomas. Imaging should also be used to search for gastric carcinoids, which are common in MEN-1 (see later).[58]

Like parathyroid adenomas, gastrinomas have two features that are relatively specific for MEN-1. One is earlier age of onset than sporadic tumors: On the average, gastrinoma begins 10 years earlier with MEN-1 than without it, a lesser age differential than 30 years for hyperparathyroidism.[59] The second is multifocal tumor: The gastrinomas in MEN-1 are often small, multiple, and intraduodenal (see Fig. 40–3, *bottom*).[46] The duodenal predominance differs only modestly from that in sporadic gastrinoma.[39,60] Because the gastrin cell or D cell is not normally found in the duodenum or pancreas, a gastrinoma in these locations may be judged ectopic and malignant, independent of its histologic grade. Gastrinomas in MEN-1 have a high propensity to metastasize to local nodes.[30] High-grade aggressive behavior, including distant spread to the liver and occasionally other tissues, also occurs in about 20% of cases.[61] Diffuse hepatic metastases are particularly ominous, predicting a 5-year survival of only 50%.[43] The prognosis of gastrinoma in MEN-1 is similar to that in sporadic cases.[43] No early features have allowed reliable prediction of which gastrinomas will behave aggressively.

Therapy of Gastrinoma

Most centers have reported virtually zero success rate for cure of gastrinoma in MEN-1 by surgery, even though one third of gastrinoma patients without MEN-1 are cured by surgery.[60,62] Unique characteristics of gastrinoma in MEN-1 that contribute to the low rate of curative resection are the multiplicity of small tumors and the frequency of local metastases. The largest tumor was not a gastrinoma in 40% of operations. Extreme approaches including total pancreatectomy have been suggested,[63] but long-term benefit is unproven and the associated surgical morbidity seems unacceptable. Only two groups have reported (without full details) frequent surgical cure of gastrinoma in MEN-1.[64,65] Other groups have not reported similar success rates despite the use of similar approaches.[60] Differences in criteria for cure and in selection of patients, such as age, can contribute to the difference in outcome.

The development of H_2 histamine receptor antagonists (cimetidine and ranitidine) and proton pump inhibitors (PPIs; omeprazole and other members of this class) makes it possible to perform a pharmacologic gastrectomy for ZES.[57,66] The PPIs are even more effective than the H_2 receptor antagonists. If compliance is good, the need for total gastrectomy is eliminated.[67,68] Side effects, including those from achlorhydria, are mild. Gastric carcinoids develop in rats given large doses of PPIs.[69] Gastric carcinoids are also seen in MEN-1[70]; however, the PPIs do not seem to exacerbate them in MEN-1. There remains disagreement about whether the PPIs worsen enterochromaffin-like cell hyperplasia in sporadic ZES.[65,71,72] The somatostatin analogue octreotide inhibits the secretion of both gastrin and gastric acid,[73] and it is under evaluation for a role in malignant gastrinoma.[74] In addition, the gastrin-lowering effect of somatostatin analogues might account for their effective suppression of gastric carcinoid mass in MEN-1.[75]

Although medical therapy for ZES in MEN-1 is effective and preferred, the need for lifetime medical therapy, the recognition that small duodenal gastrinomas cause a high percentage of cases, and the poor outcome (50% 5-year survival) in patients with hepatic metastasis lead to frequent reexamination of treatment choices.

Insulinoma

Insulinoma is the second most common hormone-secreting enteropancreatic neuroendocrine tumor in MEN-1, with an overall lifetime prevalence of 10% among adults with MEN-1 (see Table 40–1).[13,14] By coincidence, MEN-1 also accounts for approximately 10% of all patients with insulinoma.[14] The clinical features and diagnostic criteria are the same in MEN-1 and sporadic cases: glucopenic symptoms and fasting hypoglycemia with high insulin, C peptide, or proinsulin (see Chapter 33). Insulinoma syndrome in MEN-1 is usually caused by a single dominant and benign pancreatic islet tumor, although simultaneous non-hypersecreting islet tumors that stain for insulin or another gut hormone are common in MEN-1. The main insulinoma is generally 2 to 3 cm in diameter and located anywhere in the pancreas. Removal of the main insulinoma is usually curative.[14] Rarely, more than one tumor causes the insulinoma syndrome in MEN-1 at one time or sequentially. The postoperative recurrence rate of insulinoma may be higher in MEN-1 than in sporadic cases. As is the case with recurrent hyperparathyroidism in MEN-1, recurrent insulinoma in MEN-1 might, in theory, have arisen from residual tumor or a new clone.

Preferred treatment is surgical removal of the insulinoma. Other incidental pancreatic islet macroadenomas should also be removed because of the possibility that one may be a hypersecreting insulinoma and also because it might become malignant. Somatostatin receptor scintigraphy (SRS) can give 30% to 60% true-positive images.[76] When surgery is performed with guidance only by intraoperative ultrasonography,[77,78] the success rate should be satisfactory, although no large series has yet documented this in insulinoma of MEN-1. In some centers, routine distal pancreatectomy is performed as an adjunct in MEN-1 for prevention of other tumors.

Several techniques, based on insulin radioimmunoassay, can be useful for localization of an insulinoma in patients with MEN-1. These include infusion of calcium into selectively catheterized pancreatic arteries with measurement of insulin in right or left hepatic venous effluent.[79] Identification of an insulin peak after an intra-arterial calcium infusion localizes the insulinoma to the distribution of the artery. Other tests that have been useful include rapid intraoperative insulin and glucose levels in serum[80] or intraoperative insulin levels in fine-needle aspirates of a pancreatic tumor (S. K. Libutti, et al., National Institutes of Health, Bethesda, MD, unpublished observation).

Metastatic insulinoma causing hypoglycemia should be treated surgically for palliation, but operative strategies are not likely to be curative.[81,82] Hypoglycemia caused by unlocated or metastatic insulinoma can be controlled with diazoxide[81]; somatostatin analogues are less effective.[83]

Tumors Secreting Glucagon, Vasoactive Intestinal Peptide, or Other Hormones

Glucagonoma Syndrome

This syndrome consists of hyperglycemia, anorexia, glossitis, anemia, diarrhea, venous thrombosis, and a characteristic skin rash termed *necrolytic migratory erythema* (see Chapter 38). Glucagonoma syndrome is rare in MEN-1,[84] although one third of MEN-1 enteropancreatic neuroendocrine tumors immunostain for glucagon.[45] Glucagonoma is usually large and metastatic at presentation. Palliation is often possible with surgery or another ablative procedure (see later). Some patients have responded to the somatostatin analogue octreotide, although an initial response has not predicted a long-term response.[85]

Watery Diarrhea, Hypokalemia, Hypochlorhydria, and Acidosis

Although the most common cause of diarrhea in MEN-1 is gastrinoma, a separate syndrome is caused by oversecretion of vasoactive intestinal peptide (VIP) and is thus termed *WDHA* (watery diarrhea, hypokalemia, and achlorhydria) or *VIPoma* syndrome[86] (see Chapter 38). In MEN-1 it is rare and can occur with an enteropancreatic neuroendocrine tumor.[84] Half of such tumors also cause hypercalcemia, perhaps by cosecreting PTH-related peptide[87]; of course, coexistent primary hyperparathyroidism is similarly common in patients with MEN-1. The tumor is usually malignant, large, and metastatic at presentation. Treatment considerations are the same as with glucagonoma (see later).

Growth Hormone–Releasing Hormone Oversecretion

Oversecretion of growth hormone–releasing hormone (GHRH) is a rare manifestation of an enteropancreatic neuroendocrine tumor; however, half of such cases are found with MEN-1 (see later).[88] GHRH oversecretion can also occur with bronchial carcinoid in MEN-1.[89]

Other Ectopic Hormones

Other peptides that are oversecreted by enteropancreatic neuroendocrine tumors in MEN-1 include adrenocorticotropic hormone (ACTH), PTH-related peptide,[87] somatostatin,[90] and calcitonin.[91] The last can cause confusion with thyroidal C-cell cancer, but serum calcitonin levels are generally higher in C-cell cancer than in MEN-1 cancers.

Pancreatic Polypeptide–Secreting and Other Nonfunctional Tumors

One third of enteropancreatic neuroendocrine tumors in MEN-1 immunostain mainly for pancreatic polypeptide, similar to the percentages that immunostain mainly for insulin or for glucagon.[44,45] Enteropancreatic neuroendocrine tumors in MEN-1 commonly also oversecrete pancreatic polypeptide. [92,93] Production of this peptide is not associated with any identifiable hormonal syndrome. Like other nonfunctional enteropancreatic neuroendocrine tumors in MEN-1, these are often large, malignant, and metastatic at presentation.[84]

Nonfunctional tumor is an abused but convenient term. In the context of MEN-1, it is applied to enteropancreatic neuroendocrine tumors, anterior pituitary tumors, or foregut carcinoids that do not immunostain for the common hormones of that tissue or that immunostain for one or more hormones but do not hypersecrete the hormone. Most enteropancreatic tumors in MEN-1 fit this definition,[40] and most never become a clinical problem. Of course, one oversecreting tumor is sufficient to dominate the clinical features. If a nonfunctioning tumor becomes malignant, its lack of symptomatic hormone hypersecretion can allow progression to an advanced stage before recognition.

Staging of Enteropancreatic Neuroendocrine Tumors

Appropriate management of enteropancreatic neuroendocrine tumor or tumors in MEN-1 is challenging because of the multicentric nature of the tumors and the need to decide between surgical and other approaches. An enteropancreatic tumor causing a hormone excess state in MEN-1 is likely to be accompanied by nonfunctional tumor(s). Much of the experience acquired with imaging of sporadic tumors of the same types cannot be generalized to MEN-1 tumors. Accurate localization of tumor and, in particular, identification of metastatic disease is critical for preoperative decision making. The multicentricity and variable size of these tumors stretch the limitations of radiologic techniques that have difficulty imaging tumors smaller than 1 cm in diameter. And their rarity has prevented organization of controlled trials. Despite these challenges, there has been considerable progress since the 1990s.

Somatostatin receptor scintigraphy (SRS) (^{111}In-octreotide scan) is a generally useful method for imaging enteropancreatic neuroendocrine and foregut neuroendocrine tumors.[60,94] It can image primary tumor and local or distant metastases.[95,96] It is particularly useful for gastrinomas in MEN-1,[97,98] and it has replaced most angiographic procedures in MEN-1–associated gastrinoma.[60,99,100] Although it is the single most powerful imaging test, SRS still fails to image one third of lesions identified at surgery even in sporadic gastrinoma.[100] The yield of SRS with sporadic insulinoma is somewhat lower than with other pancreatic islet tumors, with 30% to 60% true positives.[76] Abdominal imaging by computed tomography (CT), particularly helical CAT,[101,102] combined with early-phase images after contrast injection or magnetic resonance imaging (MRI) provides enhanced sensitivity for detection of small lesions and is complementary to SRS.[60,103] ^{11}C-5-Hydroxytryptophan PET scanning is a relatively new method restricted to one center; it is generally more sensitive than SRS but has not been explored in MEN-1.[104]

No imaging technique used for evaluation of MEN-1 enteropancreatic tumors is completely satisfactory. Endoscopic ultrasonography with or without needle aspiration of a pancreatic mass is useful for characterizing enteropancreatic abnormalities but is a technically demanding and expensive option for the foreseeable future.[105,106] With the exception of endoscopic ultrasonography, the current preoperative imaging methods are not able to image tumors confined to the pancreas and smaller than 1.5 cm in diameter. They also fail to identify metastases in 25% of cases and the extent of tumor multiplicity in MEN-1 cases.[94] In contrast, intraoperative ultrasonography is a useful tool for localizing small tumors not detectable by the eye or fingers of the surgeon. This technique has become the primary approach for diagnosis of small insulinomas in most medical centers, although experience has been limited to sporadic tumors.[77,107]

Functional (i.e., insulin-specific) testing can be useful to assess insulinoma because, unlike other enteropancreatic neuroendocrine tumors in MEN-1, insulinoma may be symptomatic when it is small and solitary (see earlier).

Serum markers in MEN-1, mainly chromogranin-A, provide useful diagnostic tools in monitoring mass of an enteropancreatic tumor.[108] Chromogranin-A has not been helpful in insulinoma, perhaps because of the small tumor mass.[109] An example of the usefulness of hormonal markers is the relationship between glucose and insulin, C peptide, and proinsulin in the diagnosis of quite small insulinomas. In contrast, chromogranin-A and gastrin as possible tumor markers have not been reliable indices of gastrinoma extent or progression.[110]

Treatment of Enteropancreatic Neuroendocrine Tumors

Aspects of treatment specific to gastrinomas and insulinoma in MEN-1 have already been described. Treatment of these and other enteropancreatic neuroendocrine tumors in MEN-1 is controversial and guided in part by staging procedures and local preferences. The main controversies are highlighted.

Is Tumor Size Important?

Metastasis has been associated with gastrinomas more than 3 cm in diameter. This association has led some to recommend resection for all enteropancreatic tumors larger than 2.5 to 3 cm.[111] Another analysis of this strategy suggested a failure to prevent later emergence of hepatic metastases.[112] Some others have not found a relation of tumor size and metastasis and do not use a size criterion.[113]

Should All Enteropancreatic Neuroendocrine Tumors in MEN-1 Be Removed?

There is no consensus on this point. A reality confronted in MEN-1 is that for every identifiable pancreatic tumor there are likely to be several smaller unidentified tumors (clones) that coexist or emerge at a later date. Improvements in pancreatic surgical technique, however, have made it possible to excise smaller lesions surgically, although the rationale for doing this is less clear. Certainly there is no compelling evidence to suggest that surgical removal of small tumors, unless they produce a hormonal syndrome, improves overall outcome. Some urge removal of all detectable macroadenomas if removal would not be dangerous.[114] Others urge a large size cutoff (2.5-3 cm in diameter) for removal.

Should Metastatic Enteropancreatic Cancer Be Debulked?

Total pancreatectomy with a high rate of complications has been used for very large tumors.[115] Many methods are under exploration for resecting or otherwise ablating enteropancreatic neuroendocrine cancer.[116,117] Results are too preliminary to justify endorsing any of these.

Should Medications Be Used to Control Tumor Progression?

Enteropancreatic neuroendocrine tumors are generally differentiated and quite resistant to chemotherapy. Several regimens have been tried including streptozotocin, doxorubicin, or interferon, but there is no proof of long-term efficacy.[118-121] Octreotide has been effective in inhibiting hormone secretion by benign and malignant enteropancreatic neuroendocrine tumors[83,122-124]; however, it has not been effective by itself in blocking growth of these tumors except to a small degree for malignant gastrinoma.[74,125] Its use in multidrug regimens needs further evaluation.

Pituitary Adenoma

Anterior pituitary tumor occurs in about one third of MEN-1 patients.[13,14,126] The frequency of MEN-1 in cases of apparently sporadic pituitary tumor is probably less than 5%, although estimates vary widely to as high as 15% with prolactinoma.[127,128] The overall frequency of hormones hypersecreted is similar to those in non–MEN-1 pituitary tumors: oversecretion of prolactin 60%, oversecretion of growth hormone with or without prolactin 15%, nonsecreting 25%, and oversecretion of ACTH 5%; excessive secretion of thyrotropin or gonadotropins is rare.[13,14,126] Pituitary mass effects can be the principal problem.[129] In fact, pituitary tumors in MEN-1 have been larger and less responsive to treatment than those without MEN-1.[126] Pituitary tumor can occur early in MEN-1 and is occasionally the first recognized feature.[126,129,130] Rarely, two independent pituitary tumors have been suggested.[131]

Prolactinoma

Prolactinoma is the most common pituitary tumor in MEN-1 and the third most common endocrine tumor in MEN-1 after parathyroid tumors and gastrinomas (see Table 40–1). The general properties are similar to those of sporadic prolactinoma (see Chapter 8); MEN-1 prolactinoma may be larger.[126,132] Dopamine agonists (e.g., cabergoline, bromocriptine, quinagolide) are the preferred treatment.[133,134] A reduction in side effects and greater potency make cabergoline the current treatment of choice and have improved patients' compliance. In patients who escape the growth-inhibitory effects of these dopamine agonists or who are noncompliant, transsphenoidal surgery combined with radiation therapy is usually effective.

Tumors that Produce Growth Hormone or Growth Hormone–Releasing Hormone

The clinical features of growth hormone excess are similar in cases with and without MEN-1. There are two different etiologic mechanisms with different treatment implications. The majority of MEN-1 pituitary adenomas arise clonally from inactivation of both alleles of the *MEN1* gene in a tumor precursor cell.[135] Additional genes such as AIP or GNAS (encodes the α subunit of the stimulatory G protein) may be implicated, in this case by activating mutation of Gsp.[136] The second mechanism of pituitary GH tumorigenesis is overproduction of GHRH by pancreatic islet or carcinoid tumor.[89,137-139] The resulting secondary pituitary tumor is a polyclonal or hyperplastic process, which responds poorly to therapy directed only at the pituitary; removal of the primary GHRH-producing tumor is essential. Although acromegaly secondary to GHRH is rare in sporadic or MEN-1 cases,[137] a disproportionate fraction of such patients have had MEN-1. Thus, measurement of serum GHRH in MEN-1 acromegalic patients seems worthwhile. GH-producing pituitary tumors also produce GHRH locally, but this has not interfered with the interpretation of serum GHRH levels.[138,140]

Treatment for acromegaly with MEN-1 is the same as without MEN-1 (see Chapter 8). Surgery is usually the first choice, but the development of other pharmacologic therapies including long-acting somatostatin receptor antagonists and growth hormone receptor antagonists can provide effective, albeit expensive, control.[141,142] In patients with large tumors causing mass effects or those in whom GH effects are not controlled by surgery or pharmacologic therapy, radiation using an external beam, gamma knife, or proton beam is an alternative (see Chapter 8).

Corticotropin Hypersecretion or Primary Adrenocortical Hyperfunction

Cushing's syndrome in MEN-1 can be caused by a pituitary tumor producing corticotropin (ACTH),[143,144] or uncommonly by ectopic production of ACTH from a carcinoid or an islet tumor, or by ectopic production of ACTH-releasing hormone (CRH). Therapy should be directed initially to treat the ACTH- or CRH-producing primary tumor. When therapy directed toward the primary source is not successful, corticosteroid production can be controlled by bilateral adrenalectomy or medical therapy (see Chapters 8 and 14).

One or both adrenal glands are enlarged in up to 40% of MEN-1 patients.[145] This enlargement, most often discovered during pancreatic imaging, is generally clinically silent and rarely requires treatment. The silent enlargement represents a presumably polyclonal or hyperplastic process of unknown etiology,[145] and it rarely behaves as a neoplasm. Rare MEN-1 cases have been identified with primary hypercortisolism, hyperaldosteronism, or adrenocortical cancer[145,146]; these have not been proved to be intrinsic features of MEN-1.

Foregut Carcinoid Tumors

Carcinoid tumor is recognized in 5% to 15% of MEN-1 patients.[14,126] Although sporadic carcinoid is derived mainly from midgut and hindgut, MEN-1 carcinoid is primarily found in derivatives of the foregut (thymus, bronchus, stomach, etc.). Certain carcinoid tumors, unlike any other manifestation of MEN-1, have a sex-specific distribution. Thymic carcinoid is found mainly in male patients, and bronchial carcinoid is found mainly in female patients.[147-149] The average age of carcinoid recognition in MEN-1 is 45 years,[150] later than that of other MEN-1 tumors. This later age might reflect their lack of compression-induced symptoms and the lack of a hormone oversecretion syndrome as with most MEN-1 carcinoids.

Thymic carcinoid in MEN-1 is usually found at an already advanced stage as a large invasive mass. Less commonly it is recognized during chest imaging or during thymectomy adjunctive to parathyroidectomy. Thymic carcinoid is more often malignant (about 70%) than bronchial carcinoid (about 20%) in MEN-1.[148,149,151,152] MEN-1 thymic or bronchial carcinoids rarely oversecrete ACTH, calcitonin, or GHRH; similarly, they rarely oversecrete serotonin or histamine and rarely cause the carcinoid syndrome. Most can thus be considered clinically nonfunctioning. Mediastinal or bronchial carcinoids are best imaged by CT; however, SRS is often positive and therefore useful.[153]

Gastric carcinoid has been recognized more recently and is less well characterized in MEN-1. It is a tumor of enterochromaffin-like cells. Large gastric carcinoids can cause a hormonal syndrome from serotonin and histamine in MEN-1.[154] In up to 15% of MEN-1 patients, they have been recognized incidentally during endoscopy.[58] The overall malignancy rate seems low, but there are exceptions.[154,155] At early stages they can regress after treatment with somatostatin analogues.[75]

Carcinoid occurs occasionally in several members of a small family without other manifestations of MEN-1.[156,157] The etiology of these associations is not known.[158-160]

Miscellaneous Features of Multiple Endocrine Neoplasia Type 1

Miscellaneous Endocrine Tumors in Multiple Endocrine Neoplasia Type 1

Pheochromocytoma

Pheochromocytoma is a rare feature in MEN-1. There have been fewer than 10 reported cases.[10] Most have been unilateral and chemically silent; one was malignant.[129] In two tumors, 11q13 loss of heterozygosity (LOH) was documented,[161] making it likely that all or most of these rare pheochromocytomas in MEN-1 are true clonal expressions from biallelic *MEN1* gene inactivation. This is supported by more frequent pheochromocytoma in a mouse model of MEN-1.[51]

Thyroid Follicular Neoplasm

Thyroid follicular neoplasm has been associated with MEN-1 since the earliest reviews. This association is likely related to the high incidence of thyroid follicular neoplasms in the general population (unrelated to MEN-1) that are uncovered during the inevitable neck exploration for parathyroid disease in MEN-1.[6] Further support for a coincidental association is the failure to identify *MEN1* gene mutations in sporadic thyroid follicular tumors.[162]

Miscellaneous Nonendocrine Tumors

MEN-1 has nonendocrine features that vary from rare to common, with some offering possible use in the diagnosis of MEN-1.

Lipoma

Lipoma has been associated with MEN-1 since the 1960s.[6] MEN-1 lipomas are generally dermal, small, and sometimes multiple. Their frequency in MEN-1 is about 30% versus 5% in control subjects without MEN-1.[163] The frequency of lipomas in normal subjects has limited their use for MEN-1 carrier ascertainment.

Multiple Facial Angiofibromas

Multiple facial angiofibromas have been found in 85% of MEN-1 patients but not in control subjects.[163,164] Half of MEN-1 patients have five or more. They are acneiform papules that do not regress and that can extend across the vermilion border of the lips (Fig. 40–6).

Collagenoma

Collagenoma was also observed in 70% of MEN-1 patients but not in control subjects.[163,164] Collagenomas are whitish macular lesions about the trunk, sparing the face and neck. The MEN-1 lipomas, angiofibromas, and collagenomas show loss of one copy of 11q13.[165] Thus, it is likely that these are clonal neoplasms and caused by inactivation of the (first and then) second copy of the *MEN1* gene.

Spinal Cerebellar Ependymoma

Spinal cerebellar ependymoma has been seen in four MEN-1 patients.[10,166] There are no studies to determine whether 11q13 LOH or other *MEN1* gene abnormalities are causative.

Malignant Melanoma

Malignant melanoma has occurred in at least seven MEN-1 patients, but direct involvement of the *MEN1* gene has not been tested.[167]

Leiomyoma (of Esophagus, Lung, Rectum, or Uterus)

Leiomyoma has been reported in several MEN-1 patients.[6,168,169] Analyses of 11q13 LOH established that esophageal and uterine leiomyoma are specific to MEN-1 patients.[170] Similar *MEN1*

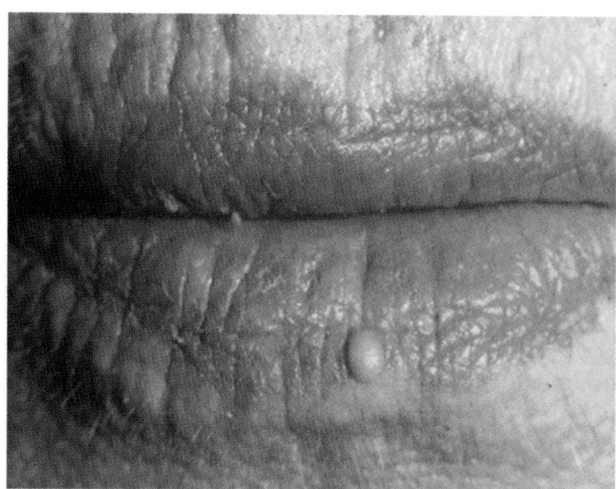

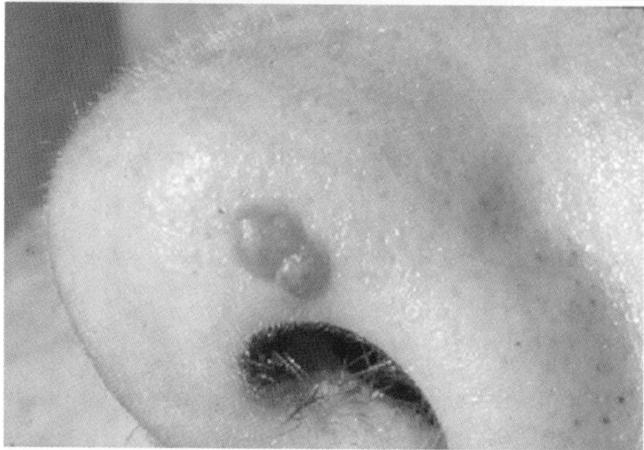

Figure 40–6 ▪ Facial angiofibroma in patients with multiple endocrine neoplasia type 1. A small, light pink lesion on the vermilion border of the lip *(top)* and a large, reddish angiofibroma on the nose *(bottom)* are shown. Typical lesions are smaller and multiple and might require biopsy for confirmation. (From T. Darling and M. Turner, National Institutes of Health, Bethesda, MD.)

inactivation was not implicated in sporadic uterine leiomyoma.[170] It is not known if uterine leiomyoma differs clinically between these two settings.

Meningioma (Cranial)

A large prospective series reported meningioma in 8% of MEN-1 patients. These tumors are mostly small and would not be recognized without imaging.[171] A large and locally aggressive meningioma was seen in one MEN-1 patient who had prior radiation to a pituitary tumor (SJM, personal observation). This tumor showed biallelic inactivation of MEN-1.[171]

Varying Penetrance of Tumors by Tissue or by Age

MEN-1 is perhaps the most heterogeneous of all multiple neoplasia syndromes.[172] The many tumors of MEN-1 have a wide range of penetrance (see Table 40–1). If the organ is paired and the penetrance is high, the tumors are generally bilateral (e.g., parathyroid adenomas); if the tumor is rare in MEN-1, its random occurrence is generally unilateral even in a paired organ (e.g., pheochromocytoma). Naturally, the apparent penetrance of any tumor type is heavily dependent upon the scrutiny that the organ is given. Thus, the frequent facial angiofibromas of MEN-1 were not recognized until 1997.[163] When symptoms alone are the main basis for disease recognition, the first feature of MEN-1 in adolescents is not hyperparathyroidism but rather prolactinoma or insulinoma.[173]

For each tumor type, penetrance necessarily increases with age (see Fig. 40–1). Overall, the penetrance for MEN-1 (usually includes parathyroid adenomas) reaches nearly 100% by age 50 years,[13] but occasional obligate *MEN1* mutation carriers have not shown any tumor beyond age 70 years.[166] Earliest penetrance and earliest preventable morbidity must be evaluated in decisions about when to begin tumor surveillance in a likely carrier. The earliest ages for identification of specific tumor expression in MEN-1 have been as follows: prolactinoma at age 5 years,[130] insulinoma at age 6 years,[174] hyperparathyroidism at age 8 years,[13] and gastrinoma at age 12 years (R. Jensen, personal communication). The information about morbidity for most of these young patients is incomplete; thus, more information is needed before it is possible to improve the consensus recommendations regarding the correct age at which to begin tumor surveillance and possibly intervention.

Phenotypes or Varying Tumor Penetrance by Family

Clustering of clinical subvariants of MEN-1, similar to that seen for MEN-2 (see later), has been evaluated. Preliminary analyses in small MEN-1 families suggested clusters of ACTH-producing pituitary tumors,[172] insulinomas[175,176] intestinal carcinoids,[149] and aggressive gastrinomas.[151] Identification of a specific MEN-1 mutation that correlates with a specific clinical variant in multiple kindreds would be most meaningful. Although subsequent analysis has failed to identify such a relationship (see later), increasing the likelihood of random clustering in most of these families, it is important to continue evaluating such subvariants because some may be united by an as yet undiscovered genetic basis.

Prolactinoma Variant of MEN-1

The prolactinoma variant of MEN-1 is defined in a family with high penetrance for hyperparathyroidism and prolactinoma but low penetrance for gastrinoma (typically 90%, 50%, and 5%, respectively among adults). Three such families have been reported, each with eight or more affected members.[177] The largest has more than 100 affected members. Because their ancestors colonized the Burin Peninsula of Newfoundland, Canada, their trait has been termed MEN-1_{Burin}. Several smaller families seem similar. Foregut carcinoid tumors were prominent in MEN-1_{Burin}.

Hyperparathyroidism Variant

Hyperparathyroidism is the most common clinical feature of MEN-1 and often occurs at a relatively young age. It would therefore not be surprising to identify isolated hyperparathyroidism in small families with early or occult MEN-1, particularly those with a disproportionate number of young members. Larger families (four, five, or more affected members) have been identified with familial isolated hyperparathyroidism (FIH) and an identifiable *MEN1* mutation but still could represent a random part of the normal spectrum of MEN-1 expression.[178] Eventually, most would probably develop other clinical features of MEN-1.[179] Two FIH families with *MEN1* mutation have been particularly large, with 11 and 14 hyperparathyroid members, raising the likelihood that in some families, isolated hyperparathyroidism can exist and continue as the only manifestation of *MEN1* mutation.[178,180] Though these patients have *MEN1* mutation, *MEN1* mutation is rare among all of the families with FIH (see later).[181]

Phenocopies and Differential Diagnoses of Multiple Endocrine Neoplasia Type 1

When MEN-1 occurs in its typical forms, it is easily diagnosed. Presentation as a single sporadic tumor, as FIH, or as familial isolated pituitary tumor (see earlier) not only is rare but also presents the clinician with a difficult diagnostic challenge.

Sporadic Tumor or Tumors

MEN-1 can occur without a recognized or even recognizable family history of MEN-1. When sporadic patients present with two or more typical tumors, some meet the definition criteria for MEN-1[182]; for others, the suspicion of MEN-1 is high. The prevalence of *MEN1* mutation is 10% to 90%, depending on the specific tumors (see later). When the sporadic case manifests with tumor in only one tissue, the suspicion and the true frequency of *MEN1* mutation are low. The frequency of occult MEN-1 with sporadic tumor can be estimated as follows: hyperparathyroidism, 2%[10,183]; gastrinoma, 5%[55]; prolactinoma, 5%.[128,184,185] Factors that increase the likelihood of MEN-1 in these settings are earlier onset and tumor multiplicity in the same organ.

Familial Isolated Hyperparathyroidism

When hyperparathyroidism is familial and isolated, the main possibilities include occult MEN-1 (see earlier), familial hypocalciuric hypercalcemia (FHH), hyperparathyroidism–jaw tumor syndrome (HPT-JT), MEN-2A, and so-called true FIH[181] (see Chapter 27). FHH, with a frequency similar to that of MEN-1, is an autosomal dominant disorder characterized by lifelong hypercalcemia with normal urine calcium excretion.[186,187] PTH levels and parathyroid gland mass are normal or minimally increased.[188,189] After subtotal parathyroidectomy, the residual parathyroid tissue directs persistent hypercalcemia. The parathyroid dysfunction is not monoclonal but polyclonal.[190] A remarkably high rate of persistence after subtotal parathyroidectomy and a low morbidity without surgery justify efforts to avoid parathyroid surgery in FHH. Useful diagnostic features of FHH are the low ratio of renal calcium clearance to creatinine clearance (in the presence of hypercalcemia), normal PTH level despite hypercalcemia, and the onset of hypercalcemia in relatives typically before age 1 year.

Two thirds of FHH index cases have an inactivating mutation of the calcium-sensing receptor gene *(CASR)*.[28] Most of the rest are believed to have an undetected mutation of *CASR*, suggested by genetic linkage to chromosome 3q; occasional families have the FHH syndrome with mutation in unknown genes at 19p or 19q.[192,193] One family with a missense mutation of *CASR* had features intermediate between FHH and typical hyperparathyroidism.[194] Two large prospective studies of FIH found unexpected germline mutation of *CASR* in 15% of families. These families were small (mainly with 2 or 3 affected members), and no family had typical clinical features of FHH.[181,195]

HPT-JT is a syndrome of hyperparathyroidism, jaw tumors, and renal lesions.[196] Transmission is autosomal dominant. The commonest and sometimes the only feature is hyperparathyroidism.[197] The hyperparathyroidism typically involves one parathyroid gland at a time, and there is a uniquely high malignant potential in the parathyroid tumor; 15% of patients have had parathyroid cancer.[181,198] Germline *HRPT2* mutation is found in most sporadic parathyroid cancers, suggesting an occult familial component.[199] The associated jaw tumors (in 25%) are ossifying or cementifying fibromas.[200] Unlike the jaw tumors of hyperparathyroidism, they are not influenced by the parathyroid status. The associated renal lesions (in 5%) are multiple renal cysts, hamartomas, or Wilms' tumor.[201] Uterine tumors are common and can impair fertility of the women.[202] *HRPT2* mutation has been found in 5% to 10% of kindreds with FIH.[181,203,204] Occult MEN-2A, theoretically another cause of FIH, has not been identified in the form of FIH.[205,206]

Many small kindreds with two or three affected members receive a diagnosis of FIH.[181,207,208] For years FIH was not pursued as a syndrome because of its bland features and the belief that most kindreds had occult MEN-1. Analyses of many kindreds with FIH have recently found occult MEN-1, FHH, or HPT-JT in the minority.[181] Probably mutation in undiscovered genes will account for these kindreds with FIH. One such gene seems to be on chromosome 2 by genetic linkage analysis.[194]

Familial Isolated Pituitary Tumor

Familial isolated tumor of the anterior pituitary has been recognized in several small and a few large families.[209] The tumors are usually somatotropinomas, occasionally prolactinomas. In theory, familial isolated tumor of the anterior pituitary could be an expression of occult MEN-1. To date, however, no family with familial isolated somatotropinoma has had a *MEN1* mutation (see later). It is more likely that most of these families harbor mutations of another unknown gene or genes, in particular the *AIP* gene.[210]

The *MEN1* Gene: Normal or Mutated

The Normal MEN-1 *Gene and Normal Menin*

Larsson and colleagues[211] showed in 1988 that the *MEN1* gene mapped to chromosome 11q13 and that it was probably a tumor suppressor gene (see the following).[212,213] However, almost a full decade passed before the *MEN1* gene was identified by positional cloning.[214] This strategy involved a progressive narrowing of the candidate gene interval,[215] cloning all the DNA in the narrowed interval,[216] and identifying all or most genes therein.[216] The final step required sequence analysis of each of these genes in a panel of DNA from familial MEN-1 index cases, a systematic process that led to the identification of the one gene that carried the defining mutations.[211,217,218]

The *MEN1* gene is 10 kb and encodes transcripts of 2.7 and 3.1 kb.[219] The transcripts are expressed in all or most tissues and with little cell cycle dependence.[220] They encode a 610-amino-acid protein termed menin. Rat, mouse, zebra fish, snail, *Drosophila*, and human menins are highly homologous.[221]

Menin has two nuclear localization signals near the carboxyl terminus that are likely to be responsible for its predominantly nuclear compartmentalization.[220] The first interacting protein partner identified for menin was selectively junD but not other members of the activator protein-1 (AP1) transcription factor family including fos, fra, or other jun proteins.[222,223] The menin-junD interaction can confer upon junD unique effects by which junD differs from other members of the AP1 transcription family. For example, junD has several actions opposite to those of C-jun, and in the absence of menin binding to it, junD behaves more like C-jun.[224] The importance of the menin-junD interaction for the development of MEN-1 is unclear. Homozygous knockout of junD in the mouse resulted in no identifiable abnormality of tissues involved in MEN-1.[225] Other studies have identified an MLL-containing complex, SMAD3, PEM, NM23, nuclear factor κB, and several other proteins that potentially interact with menin. Each interaction has unknown importance.[226]

Tumorigenesis: Sequential Two-Step Inactivation of the MEN-1 *Gene*

The first DNA-based discoveries in MEN-1 suggested that the *MEN1* gene was a tumor suppressor[211-213] (see Chapter 39), observations supported by subsequent studies (see later). Complete inactivation of a gene's function requires, in addition to the inherited or somatically acquired first hit (inactivating mutation), a second hit at the same genetic locus that finishes the inactivation of both copies of the *MEN1* gene. Inactivation of the second allele can be by mutation or other (epigenetic) means such as promoter methylation, though the latter has not been found for MEN-1.[227] A two-hit model for tumorigenesis was developed by Alfred Knudson[212,213] to account for epidemiologic observations in retinoblastoma: In comparison with sporadic cases, some hereditary tumors occurred earlier and in multiple sites. This can now be generalized to say that in a hereditary tumor, the germline mutation is obligatorily present in every cell. Thus, the earliest step seen in sporadic tumorigenesis caused by the *MEN1* gene is bypassed. Multiple independent cells in susceptible organs are thus primed for somatic mutations at the second and still normal copy to cause early and multiple tumors. Surprisingly, this model can be extended to stepwise tumorigenesis by an oncogene such as *RET* (see later).

Somatic Point Mutations (First Hits) of the MEN1 Gene in Sporadic Tumors

MEN1 is one of the most commonly mutated genes in sporadic endocrine tumors. The frequency of *MEN1* mutation is 10% to 20% in parathyroid adenomas,[228-231] 25% in gastrinomas,[232-234] 10% to 20% in insulinomas,[232,235] 50% in VIPomas,[232,235] and 25% to 35% in bronchial carcinoids.[232,235] Some other sporadic endocrine tumors show a lower frequency of *MEN1* somatic mutation: 0% to 5% in anterior pituitary tumor,[237-241] 0% in thyroid tumor,[162] 0% in benign or malignant adrenocortical neoplasm,[242,243] 0% in uremic secondary hyperparathyroidism,[242,244] and 0% in parathyroid cancer.[245] Sporadic nonendocrine tumors have undergone little evaluation; the *MEN1* mutation frequency was 2 in 19 in angiofibromas,[246] 1 in 6 in lipomas,[247] 0% in lung cancer other than carcinoid,[248] 1% in malignant melanoma,[167,249] and 0% in leukemia.[250]

The First Step (First Hit) Can Be in Germline or in Somatic Tissue

Virtually all germline or somatic first hits at the *MEN1* gene have been small mutations, involving one or several bases.[251,252] The mutations are broadly distributed across the *MEN1* open reading frame, so much so that half of newly ascertained index cases are found to have a novel mutation. At the same time, the other half shows a recurring mutation. These are equally distributed between cause by common ancestry (founder effect)[251,253-257] and cause by a hot spot for new mutation.[251]

Accumulated patterns of germline and somatic first-hit *MEN1* mutations have further supported the two-hit gene inactivation hypothesis for the *MEN1* gene (Fig. 40–7). Three fourths of *MEN1* first-hit mutations predict premature truncation of the menin protein. Although the biologic functions of menin are not established, such truncation mutations would probably cause menin inactivation or even absence. For example, all truncation-type *MEN1* mutations cause loss of the most carboxyl-terminal nuclear localization signal (see Fig. 40–7) and could thus compromise the nuclear localization of menin.[220] The remainder predict missense or replacement of one to three amino acids. The functional consequences of any one missense mutation are uncertain and even hard to distinguish from a rare benign polymorphism; however, their frequent occurrence specifically in MEN-1 establishes that all or most are deleterious mutations. Loss of menin function in the junD-mediated transcription assay occurs even with many missense (amino acid–changing) *MEN1* mutations;[222] this result also predicts menin inactivation.

The Second Hit in MEN-1 Tumorigenesis

The second hit is usually a large chromosomal or subchromosomal rearrangement (mutation), causing a deletion that includes the remaining normal *MEN1* gene. Another mechanism for creating a mutant second copy is deletion of the normal copy and then duplication of the DNA from the mutant chromosome 11, called *gene conversion.* In either case, the result is that neither copy of the *MEN1* gene remains normal. LOH or loss of alleles at the affected locus is usually inherent in this process and can provide evidence that gene inactivation has occurred in that chromosomal segment. Less common mechanisms for the second hit include small mutations (one to three bases) or promoter methylation.[227] The second hit is delayed after the first hit. It is always in somatic tissue and usually occurs postnatally.

Loss of Heterozygosity about Chromosome 11q13 as a Research Tool

LOH about 11q13 has been used mainly to deduce loss of the normal copy of the *MEN1* gene. In MEN-1, 11q13 LOH was found for almost 100% of parathyroid tumors,[26,258] gastrinoma and other pancreatic islet tumors,[48,49] gastric carcinoid,[259] anterior pituitary tumors,[135] and mesenchymal tumors (lipoma, angiofibroma, collagenoma, and leiomyoma).[165,168,170] Surprisingly, thymic carcinoid tumor and adrenocortical tumor in MEN-1 have not shown 11q13 LOH.[145,150,260] This has led to speculation that the normal *MEN1* copy can be inactivated by other mechanisms, such as promoter methylation.

Among sporadic endocrine tumors of the type found in MEN-1, some but not all have frequent 11q13 LOH. The frequencies of 11q13 LOH in these tumors have been as follows: sporadic parathyroid 30% to 40%,[228-230,261] uremic parathyroid 0% to 5%,[244,262-265] parathyroid cancer 0%,[245] gastrinoma 25% to 70%,[49,232] insulinoma 30%,[49] bronchial and other carcinoid 40% to 70%,[236,266] and

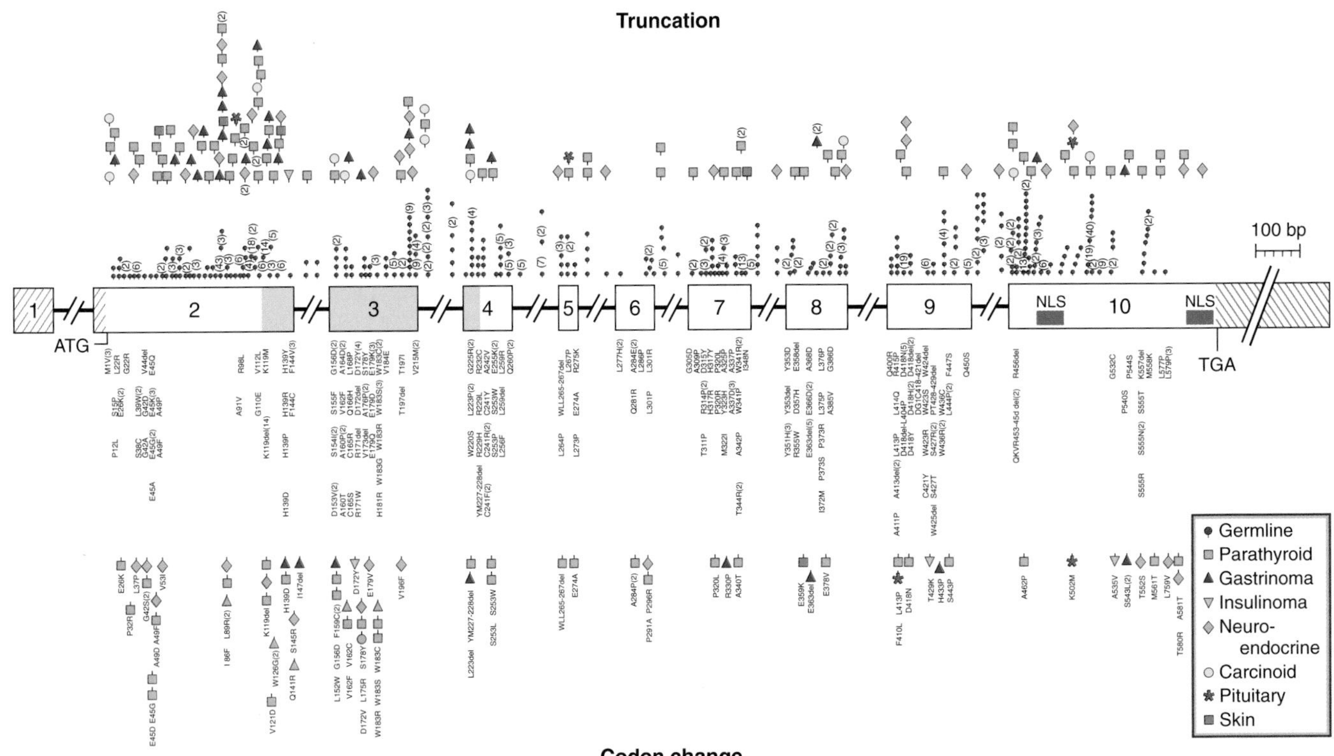

Figure 40–7 ▪ Germline and somatic mutations of the *MEN1* gene. Unique germline *MEN1* mutations in families, sporadic cases, and nonhereditary tumors. Figure shows 670 unique mutations as of 2006. Germline mutations are shown as black lollipops or as code about the mRNA. Somatic *MEN1* mutations in diverse tumors are shown separately as flags along the upper and lower border and as code. *MEN1* mRNA is diagrammed with exons numbered; untranslated regions are *crosshatched.* Truncating mutations (frameshift mutations, splice error, and nonsense [stop codon] mutations) are shown above the mRNA. Codon change mutations (missense mutations or small in-frame deletions) are shown below with their three-letter amino acid code. Repeating mutations within the germline or somatic category are shown only once, with a small number in parentheses to indicate total occurrences. *Stippling* about exon 3 represents the main zone of menin interaction with junD. Several large deletions, probably of the entire *MEN1* gene, are not shown.[252] NLS, nuclear localization sequence.

anterior pituitary 5% to 10%.[136,236-241] In the adrenal cortex, 11q13 LOH was less common in benign than in malignant tumors (20% and 80%, respectively).[242,243] Assessment of 11q13 LOH is not useful in clinical practice; however, it has been used in research as an indicator of an underlying first hit in a tumor suppressor gene at that locus. Thus, in sporadic MEN-1–like tumors, the underlying mutation at 11q13 has been traced to the *MEN1* gene in only about one half of tumors with 11q13 LOH.

11q13 LOH has also been used as an indicator of tissue monoclonality or oligoclonality. Because 11q13 LOH is a DNA rearrangement, it can be detected only if it is present in the DNA of most or a substantial minority of cells in a specimen. Thus, the nuclei are deduced to be monoclonal or oligoclonal descendants from one or a few precursor cells with that rearrangement or mutation. Early studies of MEN-1 parathyroid glands by light microscopy suggested oncogenesis through a polyclonal hyperplastic process, an observation supported by the finding in MEN-1 plasma of a factor mitogenic for parathyroid cells.[27] The subsequent finding of nearly universal 11q13 LOH in MEN-1 parathyroids[26,215,222,258] established that clonal growth was predominant, that tumorigenesis was by gene inactivation, and that a MEN-1 growth factor for parathyroid glands in MEN-1 could not represent the immediate product of the *MEN1* gene.

Tumorigenesis: Steps Distal to MEN1 Inactivation

Other unknown genes can be implicated in MEN-1 tumor evolution through gene loss of function (tumor suppressor gene) or gene gain of function (oncogene).[267,268] Inactivation of certain other tumor suppressor genes, alone or in combination, can cause specific endocrine tumors in mice. In particular, mice with homozygous knockout of both *p18INK4c* and *p27KIP1* develop at least eight types of proliferative tissue, including tumors of parathyroid, pituitary, pancreas islet, and duodenum (as in MEN-1); in addition, they develop C-cell cancers and pheochromocytoma (as in MEN-2).[269] The knocked out genes encode members of the two cyclin-dependent kinase inhibitor families that participate in the cell cycling pathway, which also includes retinoblastoma and cyclin D1.[270] This syndromic resemblance to MEN-1 and MEN-2 raises the possibility that the tumorigenic pathways of MEN-1 or MEN-2, or both, overlap and interact with the cell cycling pathway.

The earliest tissue-level effects toward tumorigenesis in MEN-1 are not well defined. Although a widespread role for hyperplasia prior to neoplasia has been seen in MEN-2, hyperplasia has been subtle or absent in MEN-1 tissues. However, the mouse *MEN1* knockout model for MEN-1 has striking giant hyperplastic islets as a precursor for insulinoma,[51] suggesting that more subtle hyperplasia might have gone unrecognized in human MEN-1. If there is a role for hyperplasia, it would still be uncertain whether this is an expression of inactivation of one *MEN1* allele or further processes.

Genome instability has been suggested in studies of MEN-1 lymphocytes and fibroblasts.[271,272] MEN-1 leukocytes show a subtle deficiency in repair of DNA damage.[273] Clonal cell proliferation has been identified in mesenchymal perivascular tissues about MEN-1 angiofibromas[274]; this could represent a precursor stage of that tumor.[275] MEN-1 plasma contains a growth factor that promotes mitogenesis in normal parathyroid cells.[27,276] Considering the overriding roles of *MEN1* gene inactivation and of clonal growth, it is not certain whether the growth factor is a contributor to or a consequence of oncogenesis in MEN-1.

Germline MEN1 Mutations: Multiple Endocrine Neoplasia Type 1 Phenotypes and Phenocopies

There have been no clear relations of *MEN1* genotype with phenotype, unlike the situation in MEN-2 (see later). The truncating *MEN1* mutations have the same diverse types of tumor expression as the missense mutations, and phenotypic expression does not differ between amino-terminal and carboxyl-terminal mutations. The distribution of somatic mutations about the open reading frame is similar to that of germline mutations (see Fig. 40–7) and seems not entirely random. In particular, there appears to be a deficiency of missense mutations near the carboxyl terminus and a cluster of missense mutations between amino acids 100 and 200. Otherwise, there is no clear clustering of missense mutations that could point to a zone of menin protein susceptible to change of function.

The prolactinoma variant of MEN-1, one of the clinical variants described before in four unrelated kindreds, was associated with three or four different *MEN1* mutations.[277] *MEN1* mutation has been found in 20% or less of tested families with isolated hyperparathyroidism (FIH).[178,181] Two of the largest *MEN1* mutation-positive families with isolated hyperparathyroidism had similarly located missense mutations (E255K and Q260P).[178,278] However, *MEN1* mutations in 14 other kindreds with FIH show no patterns of similarity.[181] Thus, FIH and the prolactinoma variant can be MEN-1 phenotypes without specific genotypes.

A *MEN1* mutation has not been found with familial isolated anterior pituitary tumor, although more than 100 such families have been evaluated.[174,240,253,254,280] Thus, most kindreds with isolated pituitary tumor, like most with FIH, represent MEN-1 phenocopies, that is, probably caused by mutation in genes (such as the *AIP* gene[210]) other than *MEN1*. There has also been no relationship between a specific somatic *MEN1* mutation and tumor type. Furthermore, tumor testing for somatic *MEN1* mutation has not shown prognostic or staging value when evaluated in sporadic gastrinomas of varying aggressiveness.[234]

Germline mutation of the *p27*^{KIP1} gene *(CDKN1B)* was identified in a rat strain with overlapping features of MEN-1 and MEN-2. One human family with MEN-1 (parathyroid tumors, somatotropinomas, renal angiomyolipoma, and other tumors) was then shown to have p27 mutation as the apparent cause of their MEN-1, thus representing an uncommon MEN-1 genotype.[279]

Testing for Carrier State and for Tumor Emergence in Multiple Endocrine Neoplasia Type 1

Screening and Counseling for Multiple Endocrine Neoplasia Type 1

A screening program for MEN-1 patients should routinely meet three main objectives: identify MEN-1 carriers, identify MEN-1 tumors particularly at a treatable stage, and be cost-effective (Fig. 40–8). [212] The term *screening* has been applied to several processes in the setting of MEN1. Herein, a distinction is made between testing for carrier ascertainment and testing for periodic surveillance of tumors. Note that when carrier testing with DNA (mutation or haplotype test) is not possible, streamlined and periodic tumor surveillance becomes the preferred method for carrier ascertainment.

Encounters for carrier ascertainment often involve counseling patients. In addition to standard genetics topics, counseling in MEN-1 addresses two different faces of MEN-1: an endocrinopathy with good but complex management options and a cancer syndrome with limited management options. A MEN-1 information Web page can help in orientation.[281] Experience with tumor surveillance in MEN-1 families has shown that compliance with a simple and regular surveillance protocol is high (Table 40–2); complicated, expensive, and erratic efforts are associated with lower compliance.

TABLE 40–2 REPRESENTATIVE PROTOCOL OF TESTS AND SCHEDULES TO SURVEY FOR TUMOR EXPRESSION IN A HIGHLY LIKELY CARRIER OF MULTIPLE ENDOCRINE NEOPLASIA TYPE 1

Tumor	Age to Begin Testing (yr)	Biochemical Tests Annually	Imaging Tests Every 3-5 yr
Anterior pituitary	5	Prolactin; IGF-I	MRI
Foregut carcinoid[‡]	20		CAT
Gastrinoma	20	Gastrin*	None
Insulinoma	5	Fasting glucose	None
Other enteropancreatic	20		^{111}In-DTPA octreotide[†]; CAT or MRI
Parathyroid adenoma	8	Calcium (especially Ca^{2+}), PTH	None

*Gastric acid output measured if gastrin is high; secretin-stimulated gastrin measured if gastrin is high or if gastric acid output is high.
[†]Stomach best evaluated for carcinoids (ECLomas) incidental to gastric endoscopy. Thymus removed partially at parathyroidectomy in MEN-1.

CT, computed tomography; DTPA, diethylenetriaminepentaacetic acid; ECL, enterochromaffin-like; IGF-I, insulin-like growth factor I; MRI, magnetic resonance imaging; PTH, parathyroid hormone.

Modified from Brandi ML, Gagel RF, Angeli A, et al. Guidelines for diagnosis and therapy of MEN type 1 and type 2. J Clin Endocrinol Metab 2001;86:5658-5671.

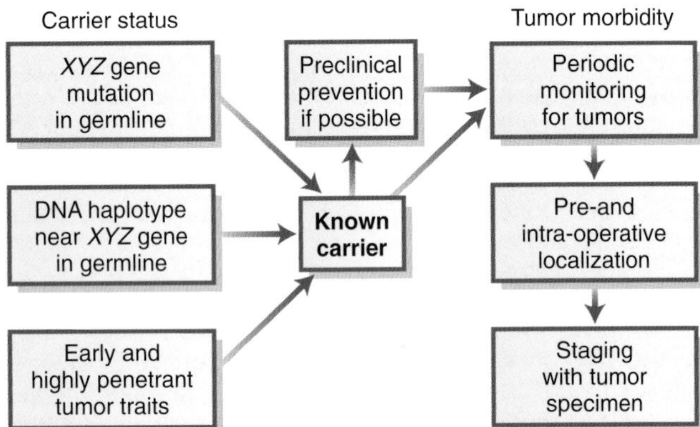

Figure 40–8 ▪ Test categories and test methods in a hereditary tumor syndrome. Tests of the germline carrier status *(left)* are largely distinguished from tests of tumor status *(right)*. When DNA testing is not informative, carrier status can be tested by streamlined surveillance of tumors (lower left).

Benefits and Limitations of Carrier Ascertainment

The benefits of this type of analysis are several. First is the secure proof of the MEN-1 carrier state in a person with a mutation and, equally important, the potential to exclude the MEN-1 carrier state by a normal sequence analysis when an affected member of the kindred has an identified mutant *MEN1* gene sequence.[182] This type of information can assist in decisions about family planning, future medical needs, and so forth. Second, the information from an index case, if shared, can be helpful to relatives unaware of their status. In particular, after a germline *MEN1* mutation is first identified, the information may be shared with a laboratory and with relatives, and DNA-based information may be used to develop an accurate shortcut test for that mutation in relatives (see later). Third, the information is useful to the physician. It assists in further plans about counseling and tumor surveillance. Occasionally, it is important in a decision about surgery, as in a case of apparently sporadic gastrinoma.

What the MEN-1 carrier ascertainment test does not do is also important. MEN-1 carrier ascertainment, unlike similar testing for MEN-2, does not routinely lead to a recommendation for medical or surgical intervention. MEN-1 cancers, in contrast to MTC in the thyroid, arise in tissues that cannot easily be ablated. This lack of mutation-guided intervention makes mutation testing at early ages in MEN-1 less urgent than in MEN-2. One approach is to recommend DNA testing in children of gene carriers at age 5 years, the youngest age at which a morbid and possibly treatable MEN-1–related tumor (prolactinoma) has been identified.[130] An alternative, based on the fact that MEN-1 morbidity is rare before the age of 20 years, is to delay carrier ascertainment until the child can make a mature decision about a test that could affect availability of insurance or job opportunities.

No identifiable *MEN1* mutation is found in up to 40% of typical MEN-1 kindreds, although most are believed to harbor MEN1 mutations not detected by the most common DNA sequencing strategies. Carrier ascertainment in such kindreds can be established by 11q13 haplotype analysis or by streamlined tumor surveillance (see later) (see Fig. 40–8). The potential for benefit from the *MEN1* mutation test is generally proportional to the likelihood of finding a *MEN1* mutation. Thus, obvious benefit is possible for an index case with familial or sporadic MEN-1 or with a state that resembles MEN-1 but does not quite meet the usual definitions. For example, a *MEN1* germline mutation was found in each of four patients with sporadic hyperparathyroidism and carcinoid tumor.[183] The likelihood of benefit in a case of atypical MEN-1 is generally much lower and varies greatly with the specific tumor identified. For example, the likelihood of finding a *MEN1* germline mutation in a case of sporadic hyperparathyroidism is probably less than 3%.[183] The mutation yield in apparently sporadic gastrinoma would probably be much higher, and gene testing is further justified by the independent impact that *MEN1* mutation status would have on a decision regarding gastrinoma surgery.

Germline DNA: Mutation or Haplotype Ascertainment

The following sections cover carrier ascertainment by mutation testing, haplotype testing, and tumor surveillance. The general principles of alternative ascertainment methods, with slight modification, are applicable to MEN-2 and to many hereditary syndromes (see Fig. 40–8).

Germline DNA mutation analysis can identify or rule out most *MEN1* mutation carriers by a test applied only one time during the life span. This test is available through several commercial and academic laboratories.[282] The usual tissue surrogate for germline DNA is blood leukocytes; MEN-1–associated tumor is less satisfactory because any identified mutation could have occurred somatically. The *MEN1* mutation test is based on polymerase chain reaction amplification of the nine translated exons (the open reading frame) and the intron-exon boundaries. Laboratories use modestly differing protocols.

MEN1 germline mutations have been detected in 60% to 100% of well-defined MEN-1 families.[277,283-285] The wide variability in mutation detection is explained partly by family selection but more likely by differences in laboratory detection methods. Genetic linkage analysis previously mapped all well-characterized MEN-1 kindreds to 11q13, making it likely that mutation of the *MEN1* gene causes almost all familial MEN-1.[280,286] Three atypical MEN-1 families have not been linked to 11q13.[174,279,287] Failure to identify a *MEN1* mutation could be explained by the presence of mutations involving 5′ or 3′ untranslated or central intronic regions, sequences that are not normally examined, or by a large *MEN1* deletion that results in no abnormal polymerase chain reaction product.[252]

The *MEN1* mutation detection rate has been lower (10% to 80%) in sporadic than in familial MEN-1,[169,174,253,254,277,283,285] probably because of differences in selection of patients. The *MEN1* germline mutation rate has been high (about 75%) in sporadic cases with hyperparathyroidism and ZES,[277] but it is far lower (about 10%) in sporadic cases with hyperparathyroidism and acromegaly.[288] For the same reason, the *MEN1* mutation detection rate has also been low (0% to 30%) in sporadic cases with atypical MEN-1, a truly broad category without a consensus definition.[169,174,277,289] Most *MEN1* mutations are familial, but about 10% arise de novo.[289]

When *MEN1* mutation cannot be detected in the germline DNA of a MEN-1 index case, ascertainment of the carrier state in relatives is more difficult. Carrier ascertainment can still be based on streamlined periodic tumor surveillance in a relative (see later) or on haplotype analysis (similar to genetic linkage analysis) in a kindred (see Fig. 40–8). Haplotype or linkage analysis for the MEN-1 trait can be done with high degrees of confidence[290]; however, few laboratories are doing these analyses.

Multiple Endocrine Neoplasia Type 1 Carrier Ascertainment by Streamlined Surveillance for Tumors: An Alternative to DNA Testing

In kindreds with no identifiable *MEN1* mutation or possibility of 11q13 haplotype analysis, it is necessary to base assignment of carrier status on the clinical identification of one of the major tumors of MEN-1 (see Fig. 40–8). Streamlined periodic surveillance for tumors by biochemical tests should be offered every 3 to 5 years. Hyperparathyroidism is the most common and usually the earliest manifestation of MEN-1, and therefore its recognition is central to this carrier-ascertainment strategy. The preferred parathyroid tumor surveillance test is the ionized calcium test, beginning at the age of 8 years or later. If the ionized calcium test is unavailable, an albumin-adjusted calcium test is suitable and is preferable to measuring total serum calcium.[11] A serum PTH assay should be performed at the same time.

Five years is a suggested starting age for prolactinoma surveillance, based on the occurrence of a macroprolactinoma in a child of that age with MEN-1.[130] Because serum prolactin rises with stress, avoidance of phlebotomy stress in a child can require an indwelling venous catheter and three blood samples at 20-minute intervals.[291] Gastrinoma surveillance can be introduced during adulthood because of the generally later age of onset of ZES in MEN-1 (see Fig. 40–1). Only rarely is gastrinoma the first clinical tumor to occur in MEN-1.[292] Surveillance for cutaneous manifestations of MEN-1, collagenomas or facial angiofibromas, may be promising but has not yet been explored in children.[163] False-positive test results are often found in MEN-1 tumor surveillance through the assays of prolactin (stress, pregnancy, or psychotropic medications) or gastrin (mainly hypochlorhydria, including that resulting from inhibitors of gastric acid secretion). Rarely, a sporadic but common endocrine tumor (such as parathyroid adenoma or pituitary tumor) occurs in a family member who is not a MEN-1 carrier.[293]

Periodic Surveillance for Tumors after Proving the Multiple Endocrine Neoplasia Type 1 Carrier State

When the MEN-1 carrier status has been identified by any method, it is appropriate to focus continued and increased attention on the patient with the goal of identifying and treating neoplastic manifestations at an appropriate stage (see Table 40–2). Surveillance for parathyroid tumor, prolactinoma, and insulinoma can begin in proven carriers at age 5 to 8 years; surveillance for gastrinoma, other islet tumors, and foregut carcinoids should be delayed until after the age of 20 years. Cost-effective surveillance combines a carefully obtained history focused on clinical symptoms associated with these tumors, limited hormonal and serum chemistry analysis, and carefully defined (i.e., selective and less frequent) use of imaging (see Table 40–2).[182]

Some have recommended more extensive surveillance measures that include measurement of pancreatic polypeptide,[93,94] insulin, proinsulin, or cortisol.[294] Furthermore, a meal-stimulated test was developed in the hope of increasing the MEN-1–related diagnostic information from pancreatic polypeptide and other markers.[92,108] Although a case can be made that these tests can result in earlier tumor recognition, it is unclear whether such detection results in benefit to the patient.

Multiple Endocrine Neoplasia Type 2

Multiple Endocrine Neoplasia Type 2A

In 1959, John Sipple was asked to see a hypertensive patient who subsequently died. At autopsy, Sipple "was amazed when [he] saw large, bilateral pheochromocytomas and a 2-cm pale tan mass in each lobe of the thyroid gland and nodular enlargement of the only parathyroid gland [he] could find."[295] He reported this case and reviewed five others from the literature[5]; subsequently, the familial nature of the syndrome[7,296] and the recognition of the thyroid tumor as medullary thyroid carcinoma were clarified by others.[297] Williams[298] reasoned that because MTC was a malignancy of the C cells it might produce calcitonin, a concept that led to the use of serum calcitonin measurements for early diagnosis of MTC and of MEN-2.[8,299-301]

The clinical syndrome of MEN-2A, as described by Sipple[5] and others,[7] consists of bilateral and multicentric MTC, unilateral or bilateral pheochromocytoma, and, less commonly, parathyroid hyperplasia or adenomas. In the decade after Sipple's description, patients with this syndrome commonly presented with manifestations of a pheochromocytoma, a thyroid nodule, hypercalcemia, or some combination of the three. Such clinical presentations are still observed, but MEN-2 syndrome identification and routine carrier ascertainment in affected families now make early thyroid C-cell hyperplasia or microscopic MTC without metastasis the most common initial presentation.[302-306] Pheochromocytomas are subsequently identified in about half of patients, and parathyroid abnormalities occur in 10% to 35%.[7,8,307]

MEN-2 differs from MEN-1 in several important ways. The first is the clinical spectrum of organ involvement; the only overlap feature is hyperparathyroidism and the rare occurrence of a pheochromocytoma in MEN-1. The second is the clear finding of hyperplasia that precedes development of a tumor, benign or malignant. There is only a weaker precedent for this in MEN-1. The third is the causation of this syndrome by a germline activating mutation of a tyrosine kinase receptor, unlike the inactivating mutations that cause a dysfunctional or nonfunctioning menin seen in MEN-1. This last criterion has provided a specific target for pharmacologic agents in MEN-2 to reverse the activation, a strategy that is in its preliminary stages but has generated much excitement.

Medullary Thyroid Carcinoma in Multiple Endocrine Neoplasia Type 2

Evolution of C-Cell Abnormalities

MTC in all variants of MEN-2 is a multicentric neoplasm of the parafollicular or C cell of the thyroid gland (Fig. 40–9). The earliest demonstrable abnormality in the thyroid gland of patients with this syndrome is hyperplasia of C cells,[308] followed by progression to nodular hyperplasia, microscopic MTC, and finally frank MTC (Fig. 40–10). These changes are multicentric, with the frequent occurrence of more than one type of histologic lesion in one or both lobes of the thyroid.[309] The time required for progression through these several histologic stages is not known, but malignant changes have been noted as early as 3 years of age in MEN-2A and during the first month of life in MEN-2B.[310,311] It is also not known with certainty at which earliest histologic stage metastasis occurs, but local lymph node metastasis occurs in 80% or more when the tumor diameter is larger than 1 cm, [312] whereas lymph node metastasis is rare in thyroid glands with only C-cell hyperplasia.[304,313,314] Occasionally, foci of MTC occur in extrathyroid locations such as the thymus gland. Whether these lesions are primary or metastatic has not been determined with certainty.

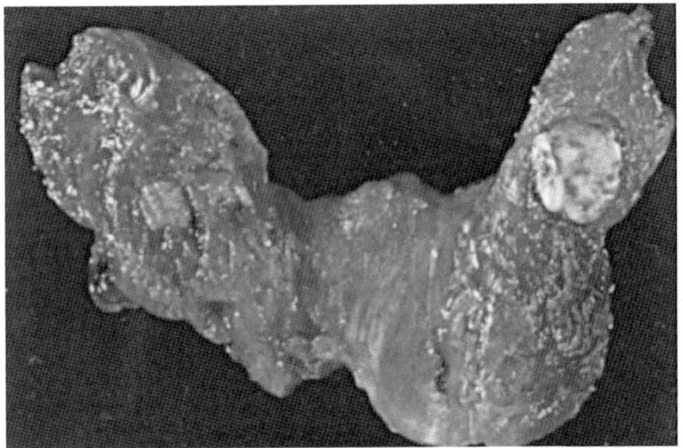

Figure 40–9 ▪ Bilateral medullary thyroid carcinoma in multiple endocrine neoplasia type 2A. Large bilateral foci of medullary thyroid carcinoma are located in each lobe of the thyroid gland.

Tumor Markers Associated with Medullary Thyroid Carcinoma

Potential tumor markers expressed by the normal C cell and by MTC include calcitonin, calcitonin gene–related peptide,[315] somatostatin,[316] dihydroxyphenylalanine decarboxylase,[317] and chromogranin-A.[318] Proteins that are not normally expressed in the C cell but that are expressed by MTC include proopiomelanocortin, thyrotropin-releasing hormone,[319] gastrin-releasing peptide,[320] VIP, neurotensin, substance P, carcinoembryonic antigen (CEA), histaminase,[321] and others.[322] The only reported clinical syndrome associated with ectopic hormone production is the ectopic ACTH syndrome in less than 5% of patients with extensive MTC (see Chapter 8). Diarrhea associated with advanced MTC is probably caused by a secretory product of the transformed C cell, although the specific causative agent has not been identified. With the exception of calcitonin and CEA, tumor markers are not generally used for recognition of a tumor in MEN-2 and are rarely used for monitoring a tumor.

Treatment of Visible Hereditary Medullary Thyroid Carcinoma

There has been an evolution in thinking about surgical management of hereditary MTC. The ready availability of genetic testing (see later discussion of genetic testing) has led to the routine genetic screening of kindreds with known hereditary MTC. Management of these patients, now most often children, is discussed in detail in the section focused on the use of genetic information in the management of MEN-2. Less commonly, a person with hereditary MTC comes to attention as a result of delayed genetic testing or identification of hereditary disease in a relative with

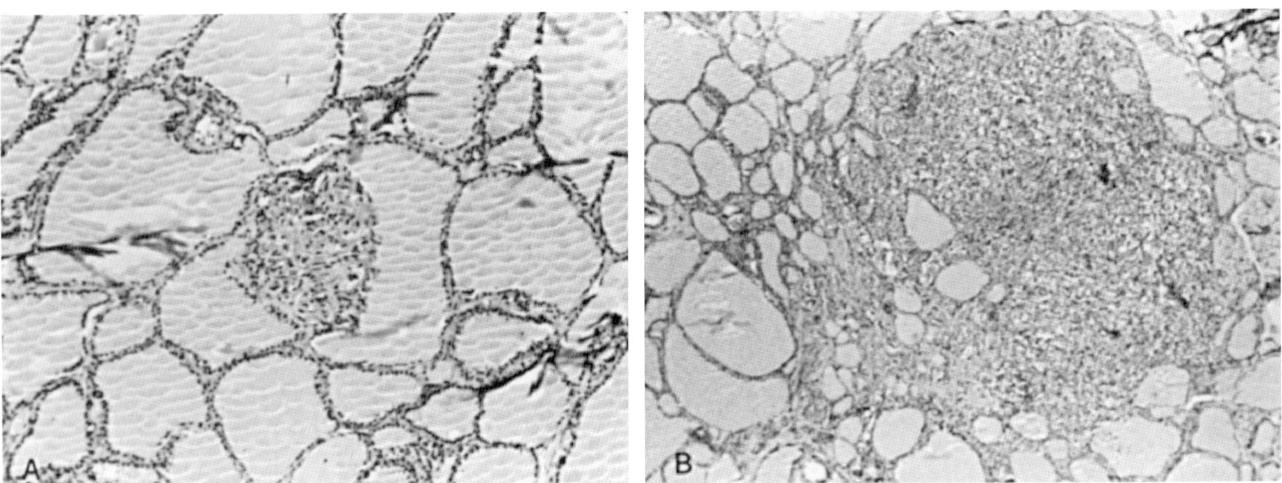

Figure 40–10 ▪ Progression of histologic changes from C-cell hyperplasia to medullary thyroid carcinoma. These sections were taken from a single thyroid lobe of a patient with hereditary medullary thyroid carcinoma and demonstrate the multicentric nature of this tumor. **A,** Nodular hyperplasia with containment of C cells within a thyroid follicle. Magnification ×250. **B,** Microscopic medullary thyroid carcinoma that is locally invasive. Magnification ×100.

apparent sporadic MTC who was determined to have hereditary MTC by genetic testing. In most cases these patients have palpable MTC. Primary therapy for these patients is total thyroidectomy.

The identification of lymph node metastasis in more than 80% of patients with an MTC larger than 1 cm[312] and a literature that indicates some small percentage (5%-15%) of these patients can be cured by extensive but not disfiguring lymph node dissection has led some to recommend bilateral dissection of level II to VI nodes at the time of primary surgery.[312,323,324] The complications of such a surgical procedure, hypoparathyroidism and XIth nerve injury, and the fact that one in 10 will be definitively cured have led some to question the routine application of extensive neck dissection. In practice, younger patients with an entire life in front of them are most likely to consider extensive and potentially curative surgery.

All patients with hereditary MTC should have studies performed to exclude hyperparathyroidism and pheochromocytoma prior to surgery. Pheochromocytomas should be removed before thyroid surgery.

Monitoring after Surgery for Medullary Thyroid Carcinoma

At 3 to 6 months following thyroidectomy, patients should be reevaluated by measurement of serum calcitonin and an ultrasound examination of the neck. Earlier postoperative measurement of serum calcitonin is discouraged because serum calcitonin values can remain elevated for 3 to 6 months after thyroid surgery and become normal later.[302,325] Elevation of the serum calcitonin in the immediate postoperative period is presumed to be related to the generalized rise in serum calcitonin that occurs during inflammation or sepsis.[326,327] Equally important, the fact that calcitonin gene expression can be activated in inflamed or infected tissue unrelated to the C cell suggests that one should be careful about overinterpreting the significance of a minimal or transient rise in the serum calcitonin value. Stimuli as nonspecific as exercise can cause a serum calcitonin rise.[328]

Calcitonin should be measured after calcium or pentagastrin stimulation at 6 to 12 months if basal serum calcitonin values are undetectable. Provocative testing with pentagastrin (not currently available in the United States) or calcium should be performed only if the result would direct a specific clinical action (discussed later). Serial measurement of the basal serum calcitonin or CEA is a useful indicator of long-term disease progression and helps define the aggressiveness of MTC in a patient with metastatic disease. Measurement of serum calcitonin and CEA and plotting biannual measurements over 5 to 10 years provides an indication of the growth rate of the MTC. Doubling times of less than 2 years indicate aggressive MTC. This type of information may be useful for making decisions regarding intervention with chemotherapy, reoperation, or prognostication.

Calcitonin is a secretory peptide, and there is considerable variability of the serum concentration. It can vary by as much as 50% or more from measurement to measurement without evidence of progression of disease. It is important to advise patients of this variability to provide them with a framework of how this information will be used over an extended period. There is frequent divergence between the rate of rise of calcitonin and CEA, presumably reflecting the impact of the transformation process on the expression of these two genes.

Reoperation for Locally Metastatic Medullary Thyroid Carcinoma

There has been an evolution in thought processes regarding reoperation for presumed locally metastatic MTC. Initial reoperative efforts were largely unsuccessful.[329-331] Improvement of surgical techniques led to a reexamination of this question in the 1980s; initial reports described normalization of the serum calcitonin values in approximately one third of reoperated patients.[332] This experience has led others to examine the usefulness of reoperation, and a larger experience suggests that approximately 5% to 15% of carefully selected patients (patients with no evidence of pulmonary, hepatic, or bone metastasis) have normal or nondetectable calcitonin values after reoperation.[324,332-334]

Several lines of evidence suggest that nondetectable basal and calcium- or pentagastrin-stimulated calcitonin after surgery is likely to indicate a cure. These include promising results after the short-term follow-up (5 to 10 years) of reoperated patients[324,332,335,336] and the generally favorable long-term outcome in patients with MTC and local nodal metastasis who had nondetectable calcitonin values after primary surgery.[325,329,337] Whether a 5% to 15% cure rate justifies the extensive repeat operative procedure is debated, but the generally poor outcomes of reoperative strategies suggested by earlier reports should be reconsidered in selected cases.

Pheochromocytoma in Multiple Endocrine Neoplasia Type 2

Evolution of Pheochromocytoma

Adrenal chromaffin tissue in patients with MEN-2A undergoes the same type of histologic progression as observed for the C cell, including hyperplasia, diffuse expansion of the adrenal medulla, and pheochromocytoma. The usual finding is single or multiple pheochromocytomas, with a background of hyperplastic chromaffin tissue (Fig. 40–11).[338-340] The pheochromocytomas may be unilateral or bilateral. If a tumor is present in one adrenal gland, hyperplastic changes are likely in the contralateral gland.[325,338] Invasion of the adrenal capsule by chromaffin cells is observed, but it is rare for these tumors to metastasize.[309,339] Pheochromocytomas in MEN-2B do not differ substantially from those identified in MEN-2A.[341]

Most of the pheochromocytomas in MEN-2 are intra-adrenal. There are rare examples of pheochromocytomas that develop in adrenal rest tissue, including one with multiple adrenal rests.[342] Other series have described extra-adrenal pheochromocytomas,[343] although it is difficult to determine whether these pheochromocytomas occurred in adrenal rest tissue or along the sympathetic chain. Recurrences are observed in a small percentage of patients, predominantly in the surgical bed.[343] It is unclear whether these recurrences represent additional pheochromocytomas that have developed in adrenal rest tissue or result from residual tissue or seeding. In most cases, they can be easily resected during a second procedure.

Malignant pheochromocytoma occurs rarely in MEN-2, and most of the described cases occurred in older series and were associated with larger pheochromocytomas.[344-347] Reports of malignant pheochromocytoma in MEN-2 have become uncommon,[348-351] suggesting that resection of smaller pheochromocytomas can eliminate not only cardiovascular risk but also the potential for malignant transformation. Malignant pheochromocytoma has been observed in the context of MEN-2B.[352] The identification of malignant pheochromocytoma in some families has led to the performance of bilateral prophylactic adrenalectomy in some kindreds,[338] although this approach should be considered only if there is a proven pattern of adrenal medullary malignancy within a family.

The clinical syndrome caused by adrenomedullary disease has changed since the 1980s. Before prospective tumor surveillance, patients commonly presented with hypertension, headaches, cardiac arrhythmias, and large pheochromocytomas. Death caused by a cardiac arrest or stroke was as likely as death from metastatic MTC.[8] Routine surveillance and detection of

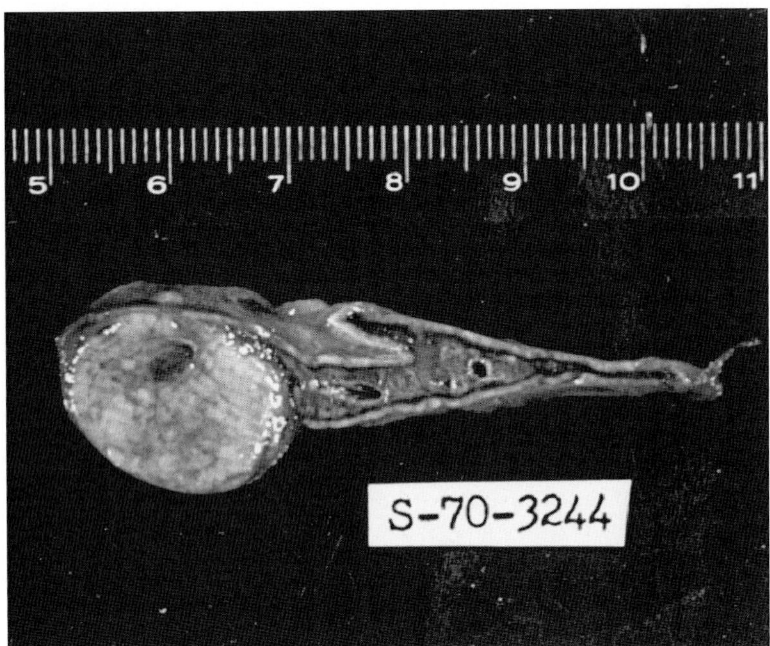

Figure 40–11 ■ A pheochromocytoma set on a background of diffuse adrenomedullary hyperplasia in multiple endocrine neoplasia type 2A. In the normal adrenal gland, the adrenal cortices are separated by a thin (less than 1 mm) band of adrenal medulla (not shown). Near to this pheochromocytoma there is diffuse expansion of the adrenal medulla.

pheochromocytomas coupled with α-adrenergic and β-adrenergic antagonist use and improved surgical management have resulted in improved outcomes. Early adrenomedullary abnormalities can cause intermittent headaches, palpitations, and nervousness; hypertension is uncommon.[325] Death caused by pheochromocytoma is uncommon, and the reported deaths since the 1990s have occurred largely in patients in whom prospective surveillance was not performed because of either an unrecognized gene carrier or noncompliance with routine surveillance.

Clinicians should be particularly vigilant with women of childbearing age or during pregnancy because of deaths during labor and delivery.[353,354] If a pheochromocytoma is identified during pregnancy, the conventional practice is to resect the tumor during pregnancy (under the coverage of adrenergic blockade). However, through an unusual set of circumstances, one of us (RFG) has managed a patient through a successful pregnancy and delivery. She received adrenergic antagonists throughout her pregnancy and underwent postpartum surgery for the pheochromocytoma.

Biochemical and Imaging Tests: Diagnosis and Localization of Pheochromocytoma

Adrenomedullary abnormalities associated with MEN-2A produce distinctive biochemical features. Increased urinary excretion of epinephrine and elevations of serum metanephrine are the most sensitive indicators of abnormality (Fig. 40–12).[325,355] Later in the course of the disease or with larger pheochromocytomas, the 24-hour excretion of epinephrine, norepinephrine, metanephrine, and normetanephrine metabolites is usually increased. Urinary vanillylmandelic acid excretion is usually normal early in the course of disease and is not useful for prospective tumor surveillance. Provocative testing (with glucagon or histamine) is rarely required and carries some risk (see Chapter 15).

The diagnosis of pheochromocytoma is confirmed by CT or MRI scanning of the abdomen in the context of abnormal catecholamines. In most cases, CT scanning provides greater anatomic resolution, is less expensive, and is adequate for patients whose catecholamines are abnormal. Other techniques may be useful for specific purposes. MRI provides greater specificity (bright image on T2-weighted images) and may be useful for differentiating between a small pheochromocytoma and an adrenal cortical adenoma. Scanning with ^{131}I metaiodobenzylguanidine (MIBG), a catecholamine analogue that is selectively concentrated in adrenal chromaffin tissue, is useful for confirming the presence of functioning intra-adrenal chromaffin tissue and excluding the rare extra-adrenal pheochromocytoma.[344,356] It is generally not useful for distinguishing between adrenal medullary hyperplasia and pheochromocytoma because it can be positive in either.[357] Octreotide scanning, although useful for identifying extra-adrenal sporadic pheochromocytomas, has little utility in the management of pheochromocytomas associated with MEN-2 (see Chapter 15).

Therapy

There has been an evolution of thought regarding management of pheochromocytoma in MEN-2A or MEN-2B, influenced by several factors. The first is the recognition that death from pheochromocytoma in this syndrome is now uncommon. Combined early detection and early therapy with α- and β-adrenergic antagonists have lessened the risk of cardiovascular death. Second, death caused by adrenal insufficiency in patients who have undergone bilateral adrenalectomy might in fact now be more common in MEN-2 than death from pheochromocytoma. Third, there have been dramatic improvements in imaging and laparoscopic surgical technology over the past decade that have simplified management of pheochromocytoma.

Radiographic evaluation is generally considered equivalent or superior to direct visualization of the adrenal gland by the surgeon. Laparoscopic adrenalectomy, particularly for small pheochromocytomas, has largely replaced other operative techniques. Current management approaches focus on the identification and treatment of adrenal medullary abnormalities *before* they become life threatening. The following discussion focuses on the range of approaches for specific clinical presentations.

Multiple Endocrine Neoplasia Type 2A Family Member with Symptoms of a Pheochromocytoma but No Catecholamine Abnormality

Occasionally, a patient with known MEN-2A or 2B presents with symptoms suggesting a pheochromocytoma and no identifiable catecholamine or radiographic abnormality. In these cases clinical judgment is required to separate anxiety from intermittent,

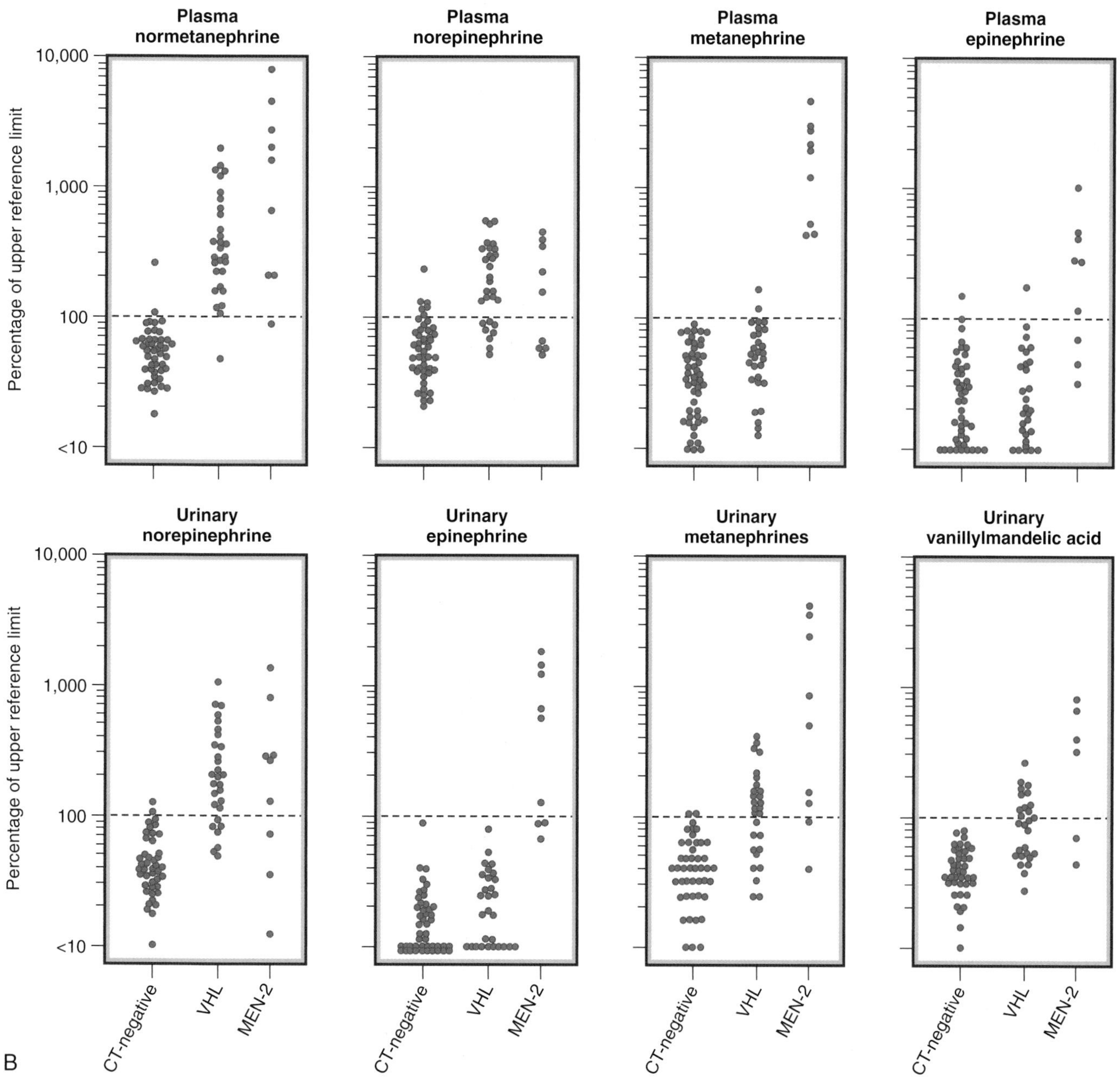

Figure 40–12 ▪ Surveillance for pheochromocytoma in multiple endocrine neoplasia type 2 (MEN-2) using catecholamines and their metabolites. Plasma concentrations of normetanephrine, norepinephrine, metanephrine, and epinephrine *(top)* and urinary excretion of norepinephrine, epinephrine, metanephrines, and vanillylmandelic acid *(bottom)*. The values are expressed as percentages of the upper reference limit for each test. Data on individual patients are shown for three groups of patients with von Hippel-Lindau (VHL) disease and MEN-2 as follows: patients with VHL disease or MEN-2 in whom a pheochromocytoma was ruled out on the basis of normal computed tomography (CT-negative), patients with VHL disease who had histologically verified pheochromocytomas (VHL), and patients with MEN-2 who had histologically verified pheochromocytomas (MEN-2). The values for patients with pheochromocytoma were determined when the tumors were first identified by CT. The dotted *horizontal line* represents the upper reference limit for each test. The scales are logarithmic. (Data from Eisenhofer G, Lenders JWM, Linehan WM, et al. Plasma normetanephrine and metanephrine for detecting pheochromocytoma in von Hippel-Lindau disease and multiple endocrine neoplasia type 2. N Engl J Med 1999;340:1872-1879.)

abnormal secretion of catecholamines by a hyperplastic adrenal gland. If the symptoms are persistent, are not improved by antianxiety agents, and become disabling or alarming to the patient, pressure to take some action builds. In this situation, a trial of β-adrenergic antagonists might, over time, make it possible to separate anxiety from symptoms caused by intermittent catecholamine production. Such an approach, if effective, might also provide a therapeutic option, thereby delaying a surgical procedure until there is a clearly defined radiographic abnormality.

Although there is no literature regarding the usefulness of MIBG or octreotide scanning in this situation, if a unilateral abnormality were defined, such information might be helpful. A decision to proceed with a blind exploration (with no imageable abnormality) should be made on a case-by-case basis and is generally discouraged. Direct visualization of the adrenal glands through an abdominal approach rarely provides greater information than imaging studies, and it is preferable to wait until a radiographic abnormality is detected.

Unilateral Pheochromocytoma

Unilateral pheochromocytomas may be identified by the development of adrenergic symptoms, by abnormal urine or plasma catecholamines, or by an imaging procedure. The unilateral adrenal nodule in MEN-2A or 2B is most often a pheochromocytoma, although metastatic MTC or benign adrenal cortical nodules have occasionally been identified. It is difficult and time consuming to differentiate among pheochromocytoma, metastatic MTC, or a benign cortical nodule in this situation. If catecholamines or metanephrine measurements are abnormal, it is appropriate to perform adrenal surgery. CT-guided fine-needle aspiration or selective adrenal vein sampling is generally discouraged.

Two different approaches have been employed to treat unilateral pheochromocytomas. The first is unilateral laparoscopic adrenalectomy. Reports of several deaths caused by adrenocortical insufficiency since the 1980s[358,359] raise the distinct possibility that at present, corticoid deficiency is a greater threat to life in MEN-2 than a pheochromocytoma, and therefore the contralateral normal adrenal should remain untouched if it is radiographically normal. A second approach, developed to maintain adrenocortical function, is cortical sparing adrenalectomy. This is an old technique that has gained increasing favor as the risks of death from adrenocortical insufficiency associated with bilateral adrenalectomy have become apparent. This approach has been applied to small groups of patients with MEN-2–related pheochromocytomas with retention of adrenal function in approximately 80% of treated patients.[347,360-362]

Resection of an intra-adrenal pheochromocytoma using the cortical sparing approach raises the inevitable possibility of late recurrence of pheochromocytoma caused by adrenal chromaffin tissue at the corticomedullary interface that develops into a tumor at a later time in approximately 20% of patients.[347] If retention of adrenocortical function is considered essential (e.g., for employment purposes),[363] consideration should be given to performance of a cortical-sparing adrenalectomy on the first identified pheochromocytoma, thereby providing an opportunity for a successful procedure on the contralateral adrenal gland if the first procedure fails. It is also difficult to know whether the first procedure is successful without detailed studies of corticoid secretory function that involve venous catheterization with selective sampling.[364] Cortical sparing adrenalectomy is generally performed through a flank incision; although it is technically feasible to perform this procedure by a laparoscopic approach, only a few of these have been performed.[365]

Bilateral Pheochromocytoma

Bilateral pheochromocytomas eventually develop in approximately one half of MEN-2A or MEN-2B gene carriers, although there has been a change in the clinical presentation. In the 1970s, pheochromocytomas were generally detected at a much later stage in the clinical course of the disease and, therefore, a higher percentage of patients had bilateral pheochromocytomas at presentation. Measurement of catecholamines and metanephrines, now routinely employed, has led to routine identification of pheochromocytoma at an earlier stage, yielding a higher percentage of unilateral pheochromocytomas at initial presentation. Of those who initially present with a unilateral pheochromocytoma, in 50% a pheochromocytoma develops in the contralateral adrenal gland over a period of 8 to 10 years.[325] Thus, the mode of clinical evolution has changed, but eventually approximately one half of MEN-2A or 2B patients experience pheochromocytoma.

The management for patients with bilateral pheochromocytomas follows a paradigm similar to that described for a unilateral pheochromocytoma. Because bilateral tumors are more likely to produce catecholaminergic signs and symptoms, adrenergic antagonists and inhibition of catecholamine synthesis with α-methyltyrosine become doubly important (see Chapter 15). Bilateral laparoscopic adrenalectomy or cortical sparing adrenalectomy should be performed. In patients with very large pheochromocytomas, laparoscopic adrenalectomy might not be possible, necessitating bilateral flank approaches or the less-preferred anterior abdominal approach.

Hyperparathyroidism

Reports from the 1960s and early 1970s described hyperparathyroidism in 10% to 35% of persons with MEN-2A.[7,8] These reports described the presence of either parathyroid hyperplasia or multiple parathyroid adenomas in association with hypercalcemia, urolithiasis, or osteitis fibrosa cystica. A careful review of the histology of these tumors has demonstrated occasional adenomatous formation with a background of parathyroid hyperplasia,[366] a finding that is analogous to that observed for C-cell hyperplasia in the thyroid gland and chromaffin cell hyperplasia in the adrenal medulla.

Simultaneous hyperparathyroidism is almost never seen in patients whose thyroids have been removed for early C-cell abnormalities, although histologic findings consistent with parathyroid hyperplasia have been observed.[325] Partly for this reason, most surgeons attempt to preserve parathyroid tissue, particularly in children who have a prophylactic total thyroidectomy. Whether patients who have had a prophylactic thyroidectomy for MTC eventually experience hyperparathyroidism is unknown. Surgical management of hyperparathyroidism is similar to that described for MEN-1, although recurrent hyperparathyroidism is a less common occurrence in MEN-2.

One concern related to thyroid surgery is the potential for development of hypoparathyroidism after aggressive thyroidectomy. A careful review of most series documents an incidence of hypoparathyroidism that is comparable to or higher than that for other thyroid surgical indications. To address this issue, some surgeons routinely perform a total thyroidectomy and autograft parathyroid tissue into the nondominant arm.[313,367]

Variants of Multiple Endocrine Neoplasia Type 2A

A number of MEN-2A variants have been described (Table 40–3). The most common is familial medullary thyroid carcinoma (FMTC) without pheochromocytoma or parathyroid disease.[368] Kindreds with this syndrome account for approximately 10% to 15% of all those with hereditary MTC. Familial MTC is most likely to be confused with sporadic MTC because of the absence of dramatic symptomatology associated with pheochromocytomas that is found in MEN-2A. Because the penetrance of pheochromocytoma in MEN-2A is much lower than that for MTC, it is possible to designate small kindreds with MEN-2A incorrectly as having FMTC. The concern, of course, is that there will be a failure to screen for and diagnose pheochromocytomas in such kindreds.

At least 15 families have been identified with the MEN-2A cutaneous lichen amyloidosis variant.[369,370] In these families, affected persons had a pruritic skin lesion over the scapular region of the upper back consisting of multiple infiltrated papules overlying a well-demarcated plaque (Fig. 40–13A). The histology is that of cutaneous lichen amyloidosis (deposition of amyloid at the juncture of the epidermis and dermis) in patients with the fully formed skin lesion. In most patients, intense pruritus precedes the development of the skin lesion by 3 to 5 years,

TABLE 40–3 MULTIPLE ENDOCRINE NEOPLASIA TYPE 2

MULTIPLE ENDOCRINE NEOPLASIA TYPE 2A (MEN-2A)
Medullary thyroid carcinoma (100%) Pheochromocytoma (50%) Parathyroid neoplasia (10%-35%)
VARIANTS OF MEN-2A
MEN-2A with cutaneous lichen amyloidosis (MEN-2A/CLA) MEN-2A or FMTC with Hirschsprung's disease FMTC
MULTIPLE ENDOCRINE NEOPLASIA TYPE 2B (MEN-2B)
Medullary thyroid carcinoma (100%) Pheochromocytoma (50%) Absence of parathyroid disease Marfanoid habitus (>95%) Intestinal ganglioneuromatosis and mucosal neuromas (>98%)

FMTC, familial medullary thyroid carcinoma.

suggesting that the primary defect may be a sensory abnormality in the C6-T6 dermatomes, leading to chronic irritation and friction amyloidosis.[371,372] In support of this hypothesis, there is RET expression in the normal dorsal root ganglion, the site at which the sensory nerve cells for this region are located.[373] Neurologic and electromyographic abnormalities have been observed in some of these patients.[374]

A third variant is MEN-2A associated with Hirschsprung's disease,[375] which can be differentiated by rectal biopsy from the ganglioneuromatosis identified in MEN-2B. Although this variant was considered uncommon in the 1990s, the increasing focus on the role of the *RET* proto-oncogene in the development of the enteric nervous system has led to more frequent identification of this variant.[376-379]

Multiple Endocrine Neoplasia Type 2B

The association of MTC and pheochromocytoma with multiple mucosal neuromas is termed *MEN-2B* (formerly MEN-3).[298,380,381] The hallmark of this syndrome is the presence of characteristic mucosal neuromas on the distal portion of the tongue (see Fig. 40–13B and C), on the lips and subconjunctival areas, and throughout the gastrointestinal tract.[380,382] Thickened corneal nerves may be identified by slit lamp examination, and enlarged nerves are often noted during neck or abdominal surgery. Ganglioneuromatosis of the gastrointestinal tract can cause obstruction, dilation of the colon, or a colic-like childhood syndrome with associated diarrhea[383,384] and may be the first clinical manifestation of MEN-2B. Other features associated with this syndrome include a marfanoid habitus, pectus excavatum, slipped femoral epiphysis, and long, thin extremities.[380-382]

The mucosal neuroma phenotype is associated, in all reported cases, with bilateral and multicentric C-cell hyperplasia or MTC, or both. The MTC in this syndrome is more aggressive than that in MEN-2A. Metastatic C-cell disease can occur in children younger than 1 year,[385-387] and there is a shorter average survival time in patients with metastatic disease.[388] However, the presence of multigenerational families and a more extensive compilation of outcomes suggest that long-term survival is more common than indicated by earlier reports.[389,390] MEN-2B is transmitted as an autosomal dominant trait, but a large percentage of cases appear to represent new mutations.[391] Unilateral or bilateral pheochromocytoma occurs in approximately half of the patients with this disorder,[392,393] occurs at similar ages,[341] and is histologically similar to that seen in MEN-2A.

The identification of the mucosal neuroma phenotype in a child should alert the physician to the diagnosis of MTC. It is important to confirm the diagnosis of MEN-2B by DNA testing (discussed later) because there are rare examples of mucosal neuromas without other features of MEN-2B or a *RET* mutation.[394-396] In most cases, a *RET* mutation is identified; in those who do not have a codon 918, 883, or 922 mutation, calcitonin testing would be appropriate. In children with MEN-2B, total thyroidectomy should be performed during the first month of life. It is not known whether such treatment is curative because experience is limited. The expressivity of the mucosal neuroma phenotype may be less than 100%. A case report in which a mother and one child had mucosal neuromas and MTC and a second child had MTC but no evidence of the mucosal neuroma syndrome suggests this possibility.[397] We are aware of other anecdotal examples of a mild MEN-2B phenotype. Therefore, all children born to a parent expressing the phenotype, whether or not clinical evidence of ganglioneuromatosis is present, should have carrier analysis for MEN-2B as discussed subsequently. Hyperparathyroidism is rare in MEN-2B.[392]

RET Proto-Oncogene: Normal or Mutated

Linkage analysis led to the mapping of all variants of MEN-2 to proximal chromosome 10,[398,399] and in 1993 mutations of the *RET* proto-oncogene were identified in MEN-2A and FMTC.[400,401] Subsequent workers confirmed these observations[376] and identified point mutations of the *RET* proto-oncogene in MEN-2B,[391,402,403] MEN-2A Hirschsprung's disease variant,[404-406] MEN-2A cutaneous lichen amyloidosis,[376,407] and Hirschsprung's disease (Table 40–4).[408-410] Later reports identified somatic (present only in the tumor) *RET* proto-oncogene point mutations in at least 25% of sporadic MTCs (Fig. 40–14, and see Table 40–4).[406,411-413]

To understand better how and why small DNA changes within the RET tyrosine kinase receptor cause the unique clinical syndromes associated with MEN-2, it is important to review current understanding of the RET receptor complex and the expression of its components and gain insight into its physiologic function. A brief synopsis is presented next.

The Discovery of RET *and Elucidation of Its Transforming Effects*

The *RET* proto-oncogene was discovered in 1985 by Takahashi and colleagues[414] as a result of a chance rearrangement of this gene during DNA extraction. This rearranged form was shown to cause transformation (RET = *re*arranged during *t*ransfection). The *RET* gene has 21 exons covering more than 60 kb of genomic DNA. It encodes a tyrosine kinase receptor composed of a large extracellular domain, a single transmembrane region, and an intracellular tyrosine kinase domain.[415] The extracellular domain includes a cadherin ligand-binding site that may be important for cell-cell signaling and a cysteine-rich extracellular region that is important for receptor dimerization. A number of variants of RET with different molecular weights have been identified, most of which result from alternative RNA processing events.

The *RET* gene was first shown to be a naturally occurring oncogene with the discovery of the papillary thyroid carcinoma oncogene (*RET-PTC* oncogene) 5 years later.[416,417] More than eight different rearrangements (three account for most of the identified forms) have been identified in 25% to 35% of papillary thyroid carcinomas.[418-420] The rearrangements permanently fuse two different genes, appear to result from physical adjacency of *RET* and other genes,[421] and appear to be triggered randomly by insults such as radiation.[422] The net effect of these

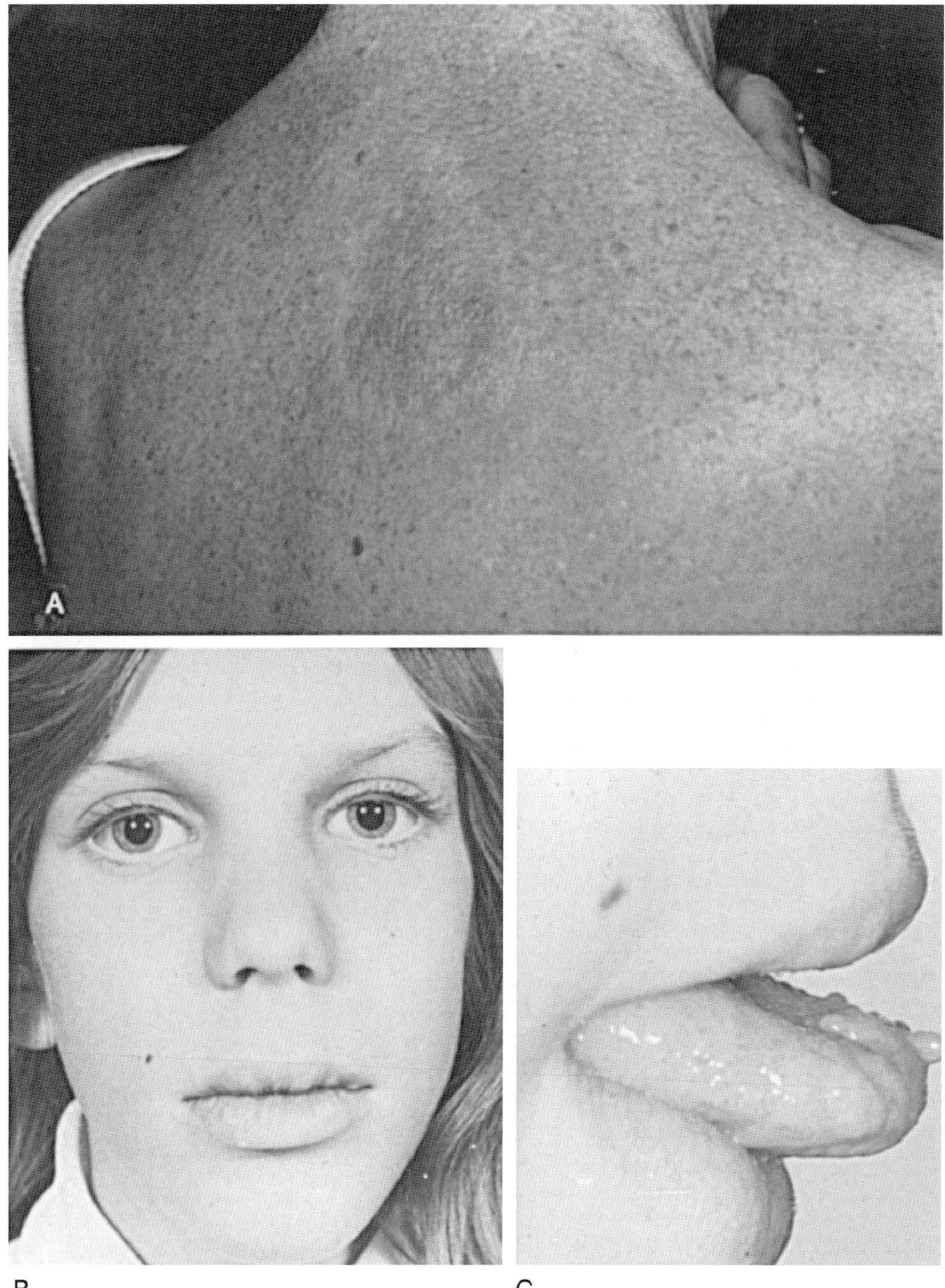

Figure 40–13 ■ Cutaneous and oral manifestations in multiple endocrine neoplasia type 2 (MEN-2) variants. **A,** The characteristic clinical picture of cutaneous lichen amyloidosis associated with MEN-2A. The pruritic skin lesion can cover a small area or the entire right or left upper back, as shown in this patient. **B** and **C,** Patient with MEN-2B demonstrating thick bumpy lips and eversion of upper eyelids **(B)** and neuromas on the anterior third of the tongue **(C).** (**A** from Gagel RF, Levy ML, Donovan DT, et al. Multiple endocrine neoplasia type 2A associated with cutaneous lichen amyloidosis. Ann Intern Med 1989;111:802-806; **B** and **C** from Brown RS, Colle E, Tashjian AH Jr. The syndrome of multiple mucosal neuromas and medullary thyroid carcinoma in childhood. Importance of recognition of the phenotype for the early detection of malignancy. J Pediatr 1975;86:77-83.)

rearrangements is that the tyrosine kinase of RET is expressed in a cell type (the thyroid follicular cell) that does not normally express this gene. These rearrangements involve two different genes and differ substantially from the single nucleotide changes most commonly associated with MEN-2, discussed later. These gene rearrangements lead to expression of a structurally normal RET kinase domain fused to one of several proteins expressed in thyroid follicular cells. Other than a few reports of rearrangement of *RET* in lymphoma and Hürthle cell neoplasms,[423] activated forms of the *RET* gene are often involved only in the pathogenesis of two malignant neoplasms, papillary thyroid carcinoma and the several neoplasms found in MEN-2.[420]

TABLE 40–4 GERMLINE MUTATIONS OF THE *RET* PROTO-ONCOGENE IN MULTIPLE ENDOCRINE NEOPLASIA TYPE 2

Affected Codon	Exon	Amino Acid Change Normal → Mutant	Nucleotide Change Normal → Mutant	Clinical Syndrome	Percentage of All MEN-2 Mutations
609	10	Cys → Arg	TGC → CGC	MEN-2A/FMTC	0-1
		Cys → Tyr	TGC → TAC*		
611	10	Cys → Tyr	TGC → TAC	MEN-2A/FMTC	2-3
		Cys → Trp	TGC → TGG	FMTC	
		Cys → Gly	TGC → GGC		
618	10	Cys → Ser	TGC → AGC†	MEN-2A/FMTC	3-5
		Cys → Gly	TGC → GGC		
		Cys → Arg	TGC → CGC		
		Cys → Phe	TGC → TTC		
		Cys → Ser	TGC → TCC		
		Cys → Tyr	TGC → TAC		
		Cys → End	TGC → TGA		
620	10	Cys → Arg	TGC → CGC*	MEN-2A/FMTC	6-8
		Cys → Tyr	TGC → TAC†		
		Cys → Phe	TGC → TTC		
		Cys → Ser	TGC → TCC		
		Cys → Gly	TGC → GGC		
630	11	Cys → Phe	TGC → TTC	FMTC	<0.1
634	11	Cys → Ser	TGC → AGC	MEN-2A‡	80-90
		Cys → Gly	TGC → GGC		
		Cys → Arg	TGC → CGC		
		Cys → Tyr	TGC → TAC		
		Cys → Phe	TGC → TTC		
		Cys → Ser	TGC → TCC		
		Cys → Trp	TGC → TGG		
768	13	Glu → Asp	GAG → GAC	FMTC	0-1
790	13	Leu → Phe	TTG → TTT	MEN-2A/FMTC	<0.1
791	13	Tyr → Phe	TAT → TTT	FMTC	<0.1
804	14	Val → Met	GTG → ATG	FMTC	0-1
		Val → Leu	GTG → TTG		
883	15	Ala → Phe	GCT → TTT	MEN-2B	—
891	15	Ser → Ala	TCG → GCG	FMTC	0-1
918	16	Met → Thr	ATG → ACG	MEN-2B	10-20

This table describes *RET* mutations identified in most germline carriers of MEN-2. A more complete listing of rare mutations can be found in the Human Gene Mutation Database (http://www.hgmd.cf.ac.uk/ac/index.php) and Online Mendelian Inheritance in Man (http://www.ncbi.nlm.nih.gov/entrez/query.fcgi?db=OMIM). In addition, there are rare mutations that have been identified in individual patients or in sporadic tumors. In some cases, the physical location of these rare coding changes is adjacent to a sequence known to be mutated, which gives credibility to the role of the mutant sequence; in others the relevance is unclear. Further clarification of their relevance awaits examination of their transforming abilities or additional genotype-phenotype correlation.

*Mutations of these two codons have been reported in Hirschsprung's disease.

†Reported cases of MEN-2A/Hirschsprung's disease variants have these mutations.

‡A codon 634 Cys → Arg (TGC → CGC) mutation accounts for approximately 50% of all mutations associated with MEN-2A.

FMTC, familial medullary thyroid carcinoma; MEN-2, multiple endocrine neoplasia type 2.

Normal Physiologic Functions of RET Protein

RET and a second extracellular protein, GFRα-1, together form an extracellular receptor for glial cell–derived neurotrophic factor (GDNF), a secretory peptide. A fascinating series of experiments led investigators to piece together the components of this signaling system.[418,420] Investigators seeking to understand the roles of RET and GDNF created transgenic knockout mouse models for these two genes and independently discovered a nearly identical phenotype in both.[424-428] In a parallel search for a GDNF receptor, a 468–amino acid protein that bound GDNF was isolated from an embryonic rat midbrain complementary DNA library.[429] This protein was designated GDNFRα-1/GDNF receptor α, now GFRα-1. GFRα-1 is a glycosyl-phosphatidylinositol–linked cell-surface protein that lacks cytoplasmic and transmembrane domains. It is expressed in GDNF-responsive cells and binds GDNF with high affinity.[429] GFRα-1 is required for GDNF to bind and activate the RET receptor, forming a multisubunit receptor system in which GFRα-1 is a ligand-binding component and RET is the signaling component (Fig. 40–15).[430,431] Subsequent experiments showed that targeted disruption of GFRα-1 produced the same phenotype as disruption of RET or GDNF.[432] Since the turn of the 21st century, a family of GFR proteins (GFRα-2, GFRα-3) and GDNF-related ligands (artemin, persephin, and neurturin) has been identified. Each of these is likely to have an important developmental role, but there is currently no evidence for their involvement in MEN-2.

One important and well-defined function of the RET receptor complex is to direct normal migration of several cell types during embryologic development. The targeting occurs through an interaction of the RET receptor system (RET and GFRα-1) with GDNF. RET is expressed in several tissues of neural crest derivation including the C cells of the thyroid gland,[433] the adrenal medulla,[434] and the parasympathetic, sympathetic, and enteric ganglia.[435,436] It is also expressed in parathyroid cells derived from the branchial arches[437] and in the ureteric bud.[438] The most well-characterized description of the role played by the RET/GFRα-1/GDNF receptor system is in the developing

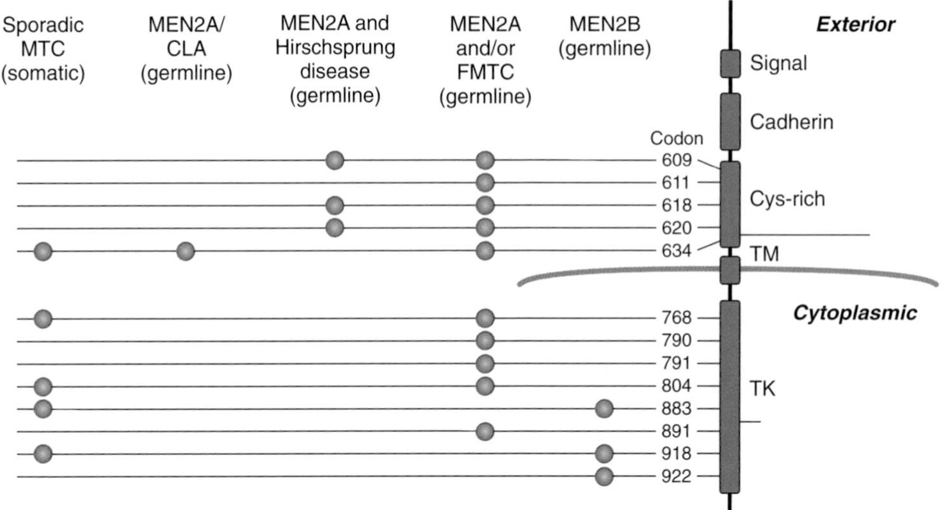

Figure 40–14 ▪ Molecular abnormalities of the *RET* proto-oncogene in multiple endocrine neoplasia type 2 (MEN-2). Mutations of the *RET* proto-oncogene have been identified in MEN-2A, familial medullary thyroid carcinoma (FMTC), MEN-2A associated with Hirschsprung's disease, MEN-2A associated with cutaneous lichen amyloidosis (CLA), and as somatic mutations in sporadic medullary thyroid carcinoma (MTC). Two regions of the RET tyrosine kinase are affected. The first is a cysteine-rich extracellular domain (Cys-Rich) important for dimerization of the ret receptor (codons 609, 611, 618, 620, 634). Mutations of individual cysteines at these codons cause RET dimerization, activation, autophosphorylation, and transformation. Mutations of the second region, the intracellular tyrosine kinase (TK) domain involving codons 768, 790, 791, 804, 883, 891, 918, and 922, cause activation, autophosphorylation, and transformation. A role for the cadherin-like region (Cadherin) has not been defined, although it may be involved in an interaction with the glial cell line–derived neurotrophic factor receptor. The most common germline mutation is a codon 634 mutation that converts a cysteine to an arginine and accounts for 50% or more of all MEN-2 mutations. Somatic mutations of codons 768, 804, and 918 have been identified as somatic mutations in sporadic MTC. Codon 768 and 804 mutations are rare; a somatic codon 918 mutation is identified in approximately 25% of sporadic MTCs. TM, transmembrane domain.

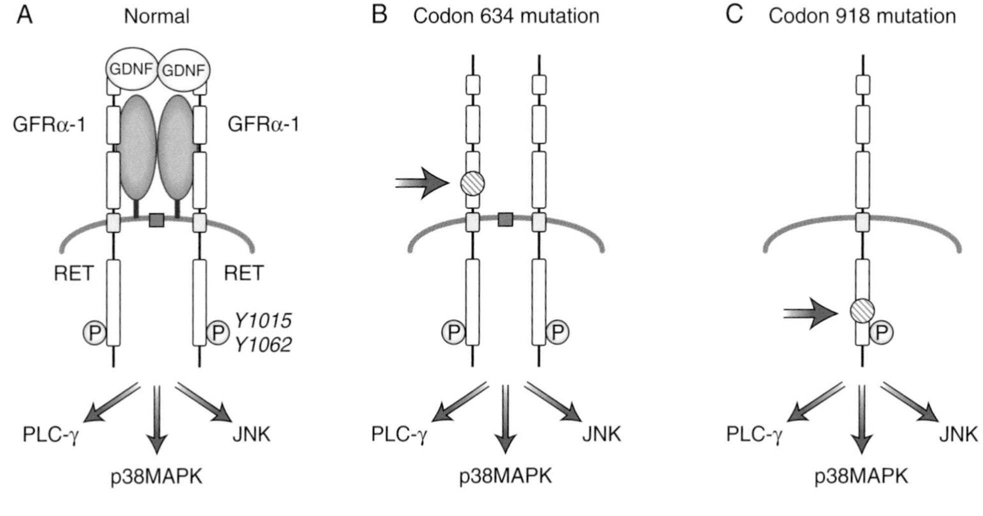

Figure 40–15 ▪ The RET tyrosine kinase and glial cell line–derived neurotrophic factor receptor signaling system. **A,** The RET receptor is a tyrosine kinase receptor that couples with the glial cell line–derived neurotrophic factor receptor (GFRα-1) to form a receptor for glial cell line–derived neurotrophic factor (GDNF). In the absence of GDNF, RET and GFRα-1 exist in an undimerized form. Addition of ligand results in activation of the receptor system, autophosphorylation (P), and activation of downstream signaling pathways (phospholipase Cγ [PLCγ], p38MAPK, and JNK pathways). **B,** Mutations of the extracellular cysteine-rich domain (codon 634) cause dimerization, autophosphorylation of the RET receptor complex, and activation of downstream signaling pathways. **C,** Mutations of the intracellular tyrosine kinase (codon 918) cause autophosphorylation and activation of the kinase domain in the absence of dimerization. MAPK, mitogen-activated protein kinase; JNK, c-Jun N-terminal terminal.

kidney. Normally, the developing ureteric bud invades the mesonephros, developing into the kidney collecting system by branching during growth into the kidney. RET and GFRα-1 are expressed in the ureteric bud; GDNF is expressed in the mesonephros. Targeted disruption of any of the *RET*, GFRα-1, or GDNF genes in mice causes renal agenesis. In the case of the GDNF knockout, the knockout phenotype can be rescued by implantation of pellets containing GDNF into the developing kidneys.[427] Thus, it appears that GDNF expression in the mesoderm entices the RET/GFRα-1-expressing ureteric bud to grow into the developing kidney, creating the ureteral collecting system.

There is a similar relationship in the gastrointestinal tract. RET/GFRα-1–expressing neurons from the neural crest migrate into the developing gastrointestinal tract, presumably enticed by GDNF-expressing cells.[427] Predictably, disruption of any component of this system leads to a disordered migration of neurons into the gastrointestinal tract and a Hirschsprung-like phenotype. These observations are clinically relevant to both the development of mucosal neuromas (derived from the enteric nervous system) in MEN-2B and disordered neural ganglia found in Hirschsprung's disease. The *RET* mutations found in MEN-2B are activating,[402,403] whereas about 50% of hereditary Hirschsprung's disease is attributable to inactivating mutations of *RET*.[439] There is an unresolved and interesting paradox of hereditary Hirschsprung's disease arising from either activating or inactivating mutation of *RET*.

Mutations of the RET *Proto-oncogene: Correlations with Multiple Endocrine Neoplasia Type 2 Variant or with Tumor Phenotype*

RET can undergo gain of function by two types of mutation. The first, discussed earlier, is a rearrangement in which genomic DNA from the *RET* kinase region is fused to a promoter sequence of another gene, creating the *RET-PTC* oncogene. The mutations of *RET* found in MEN-2 are missense (amino acid or codon change) mutations. *RET* missense mutations in MEN-2 fall into two broad categories: those that affect a group of highly conserved extracellular cysteine residues and a second group of intracellular mutations.

Germline RET Mutations

The most common mutations in MEN-2 affect codons 609, 611, 618, 620, 630, and 634, all encoding extracellular cysteine residues (see Fig. 40–14).[376,402] Mutations at codon 634 account for more than 80% of mutations in MEN-2, and a single coding change, cysteine to arginine at codon 634, is found in approximately 50% of cases.[376] In contrast to MEN-1, in which there is no relationship between a specific mutation and clinical phenotype, in MEN-2 there is a high degree of correlation. Kindreds with any substitution at codon 634 invariably have MEN-2A or one of its variants (see Table 40–3), and all reported patients with the MEN-2A cutaneous lichen amyloidosis variant have a mutation at the same codon. Mutations of codons 609, 618, and 620 have been identified in the MEN-2A Hirschsprung's variant of MEN-2.[406,440] Other less common extracellular mutations are listed in Table 40–4.

Mutations of the intracellular domain of RET predominantly affect codons 666, 768, 790, 791, 804, 883, 891, 918, and 922. Most cases of MEN-2B have a codon 918 mutation, although there are rare examples of codon 883 and 922 mutations. Codon 883, 918, and 922 mutations account for approximately 5% of all mutations in hereditary MTC. The other intracellular domain mutations (codons 768, 790, 791, 804, and 891) are uncommon and account for 2% to 3% of all mutations.[441] They are, however, important because mutations at these codons are most commonly associated with FMTC and are the most likely to be confused with sporadic MTC.

Familial MTC has been identified in kindreds with codon 609, 611, 618, 620, 768, V804M, and 891 mutations,[401,442-448] making the genotype-phenotype correlation for this clinical syndrome the least specific of the MEN-2 variants. Indeed, there is overlap between FMTC and MEN-2A for codon 609, 611, 618, 620, and 891 mutations. In a large French series, 60% of 148 patients with FMTC in 47 kindreds had intracellular noncysteine mutations (codons 768, 790, 804, 891); the remaining 40% had extracellular cysteine mutations at codons 611, 618, and 620.[441] One experimentally based hypothesis to explain this overlap is that mutations of codons 609, 611, 618, 620, 768, 804, and 891, relative to codon 634 or 918 mutations, have a lower in vitro transforming efficiency.[449] Because MTC is most often the earliest manifestation of MEN-2A, it is possible that kindreds with these *RET* mutations would develop other manifestations of MEN-2A if they lived long enough. Alternatively, other potential explanations such as small population-based polymorphisms of the *RET* gene or GFRα-1 or GDNF causing differential activity of this receptor system could be invoked.

The *RET* genotype-phenotype correlation is remarkable. Not only is it possible to predict the clinical phenotype with reasonable certainty (see Fig. 40–14), it is also possible to predict, albeit with considerably less certainty, the aggressiveness of MTC associated with a particular germline mutation.[449,450] Although it is difficult at present to predict clinical behavior based solely on the identification of a specific mutation, within a given family, specific mutations appear to behave in a more predictable manner. For example, in some kindreds with intracellular domain mutations with FMTC, there has never been a death caused by MTC, although the same mutations in other kindreds can be associated with more aggressive disease. These findings suggest that genetic differences of the *RET* gene or other components of the RET signaling system (GDNF, GFRα-1, or downstream effectors in the kinase signaling cascade) can modify the impact of a particular mutation. Recent reports in rodents document that the genetic background in which a mutant RET is expressed modify the growth rate and metastatic potential of medullary thyroid carcinoma substantially.[451]

Germline mutations of the *RET* proto-oncogene have also been identified in Hirschsprung's disease. Most of these are *inactivating* mutations,[408-410,452,453] although the association of Hirschsprung's disease alone, or the MEN-2A/Hirschsprung's disease variant, with apparent *activating* mutations at codons 609, 618, and 620 (see Table 40–4) suggests that disordered expression can also lead to this phenotype.[410]

Sporadic (Nonhereditary) RET Mutations

Somatic mutation of the *MEN1* gene contributes to the causation of certain sporadic tumors, with a spectrum similar to that of the tumors seen in MEN-1. A similar phenomenon is seen for somatic *RET* mutations in sporadic MTC and, to a much lesser extent, pheochromocytoma. Twenty-five percent of sporadic MTCs have a *somatic RET* mutation (60 of 236 reported cases).[403,443,454-466] The most common is a somatic codon 918 mutation identical to that found in the germline in MEN-2B, but other codons (609, 611, 618, 620, 631, 634, 768, 804, 883, and 891) are also mutated somatically. The presence of a codon 918 somatic mutation in an MTC is associated with a greater frequency of distant metastasis[412] and shorter survival.[462] In this respect, the behavior of the sporadic tumor with a somatic mutation parallels the aggressive behavior of MTC in the context of MEN-2B caused by a germline codon 918 mutation.[182]

Somatic RET mutations are considerably less common in sporadic pheochromocytomas than in sporadic MTC. Somatic *RET* mutations were identified in 2 of 35,[467] 2 to 4 of 48,[468] and 0 of 17[469] sporadic pheochromocytomas, for a total of 4 to 6 of 100 (4% to 6%). These results indicate that somatic *RET* mutation is an infrequent cause of sporadic pheochromocytoma. Similarly, in an examination for the presence of somatic *RET* mutations in sporadic parathyroid tumors, none of 35 tumors examined had codon 609, 611, 618, 620, 630, 634, or 918 mutations, making it unlikely that somatic *RET* mutations play any significant role in sporadic hyperparathyroidism.[437]

Tumorigenesis: Mechanism of RET-Induced Transformation

The *RET* gene is normally expressed in the several cell types involved in MEN-2, including the C cell, the parathyroid cell, and the adrenal medullary cell. Studies demonstrating tumorigenic mechanisms were performed in an in vitro transformation assay (the NIH3T3 cell culture system), using a cell type that does not usually express RET (hence only the mutant RET was expressed) and is readily transformed. These studies, from several different laboratories,[470-472] provide evidence for two different mechanisms of transformation in MEN-2.

The first mechanism is applicable to extracellular cysteine mutations (prototype was mutant codon 634). The cysteine-rich region has been shown to be important for normal RET receptor dimerization. Homozygous expression of a mutant RET receptor in NIH3T3 cells resulted in dimerization in the absence of either ligand or GFRα-1 and activation of downstream signaling pathways.[476,477] There is evidence that GDNF is not required for activation of the dimerized RET and, indeed, does not further activate the tyrosine kinase.[473] A second mechanism has been demonstrated for a mutation of the tyrosine kinase domain at codon 918. This mutation causes autophosphorylation of the kinase domain and phosphorylation of downstream substrates (in the absence of RET dimerization or interaction with either GFRα-1 or GDNF).

Activation of RET by GDNF or by intragenic activating mutations leads to autophosphorylation of the tyrosine at codons 1015 and 1062 (see Fig. 40–15).[474] There is considerable evidence that autophosphorylation of tyrosine 1062 is required for activation of downstream effector pathways and transformation.[475,476]

Tumorigenesis: Steps Distal to RET

At least three different pathways, JNK,[477] p38MAPK,[478] and phospholipase C gamma,[418,479] are activated through shc-grb2-src proteins linked to ret.[480,481] There is also evidence that nuclear factor κB is activated by mutant *RET* and depends on activation of raf and MEKK1.[482] It appears that additional genetic events are involved in the development or progression of the transformed phenotype. Multiple studies have demonstrated a consistent LOH of chromosome 1p, 3p, and 22q in MEN-2–related MTC[483-485] and pheochromocytoma.[483-488]

Loss of the normal *RET* allele or amplification of the mutant *RET* allele is found in a significant number of MEN-2 tumors.[489,490] These studies demonstrate somatic amplification of the mutant *RET* allele by at least two different mechanisms: trisomy of chromosome 10 and duplication of the mutant *RET* allele.[490,491] Alternatively, in a small percentage of tumors there is loss of the normal *RET* allele. These mutational rearrangements are formally analogous to the second hit at a tumor suppressor gene (see earlier). They help explain why germline gain-of-function tumorigenesis as in MEN-2 shares major properties with germline loss-of-function tumorigenesis as in MEN-1; specifically, both processes have early onset and tumor multiplicity.

Researchers hypothesize that the effect of amplification of the mutant *RET* allele or loss of the normal copy results in predominant expression of a mutant RET receptor, a model analogous to that demonstrated for *KRAS*[492] and *MET*.[493] In these examples, the normal oncogene moderates the impact of the mutant version. Several mechanisms could be envisioned to explain this mechanism for RET that are directly related to dimerization of the receptor, interaction of the receptor variants with GDNF or linker molecules, or differential activation of downstream mediators by the two different variants. None of these has been proved.

Studies have also implicated loss of function of p27 (chromosome 1p) in the progression of MTC. The evidence for this is indirect at present. Mapping studies have shown that the region of chromosome 1p lost in most MTCs contains p27. In addition, p27 has been found to be expressed at higher levels in cells in which RET is overexpressed, arguing for a role for this cell-cycle regulator.[494]

Testing for Carrier State and for Tumor Emergence In Multiple Endocrine Neoplasia Type 2

The identification of *RET* proto-oncogene mutations causing MEN-2 and FMTC has simplified carrier ascertainment and MTC surveillance in families with identifiable mutations (see Table 40–4).[304,305,495] Several different analytic techniques have been applied to the identification of mutations,[496] although direct DNA sequencing remains the most widely used. These analytic tests are readily available throughout North America and Europe at modest cost from several commercial sources. In the time since the discovery of *RET* mutations in MEN-2, DNA-based diagnosis has replaced measurement of calcitonin after pentagastrin or calcium stimulation for carrier ascertainment. During this period, additional mutations have been described with some regularity, and there are now few kindreds with hereditary MTC that do not have an identifiable mutation. In the rare kindred in which a mutation is not identified, continued calcitonin stimulation testing with calcium or pentagastrin (pentagastrin is not currently available in the United States but is available in other countries) is required. It might also be prudent to consider sequencing the entire *RET* gene in a single affected kindred member to identify a previously unrecognized mutation. A listing of available commercial testing sources is available.[282]

Calcitonin Measurement for Carrier Ascertainment and for Tumor Surveillance

The pentagastrin test is performed by measuring the serum calcitonin level before and 2, 5, and 10 minutes after the intravenous injection of pentagastrin (0.5 μg/kg body weight).[299,497] Administration of calcium immediately before the pentagastrin injection enhances the sensitivity of the test. A short calcium infusion (15 minutes) can also be used to stimulate calcitonin release.[498] Calcium is the only potent calcitonin secretagogue currently available in the United States.

A positive test is one in which either the basal serum calcitonin concentration is elevated and is further increased by the administration of pentagastrin or calcium or one in which the basal value is normal but increases into the abnormal range after the administration of pentagastrin or calcium. It is important that the samples be analyzed with the most sensitive assay available and with proper control samples; it is now possible to measure normal serum calcitonin levels (0.15 to 3 pM/L [0.5 to 10 pg/mL]) using two-site assays available from several commercial laboratories. Criteria that are useful for separation of normal from abnormal kindred members include a parent known to be affected and a consistently abnormal test result (two or more nonconsecutive test results that are abnormal).[302,325] Use of the pentagastrin or calcium stimulation test is currently limited to the rare kindred in whom a *RET* mutation is not identified.

However, there is considerable overlap between the normal range of serum calcitonin after a provocative test and that observed in patients with early abnormalities of the C cell, a finding that was not fully recognized until *RET* mutation testing became available in 1993. In nearly every large kindred in which calcitonin abnormalities were used to determine carrier status, there are examples of false-positive calcitonin tests that in some kindreds approached 15% of the total number of carriers. In retrospect, the use of calcitonin testing was less of a gold standard than thought at the time.

False-positive calcitonin test results have become much less common in an era of two-site immunologic assays for calcitonin, but the clinician should be aware that stimuli such as exercise or alcohol can raise serum calcitonin values. In addition, production of calcitonin by a tumor other than MTC (lung carcinoma, hepatoma, pheochromocytoma, pancreatic islet cell tumor, or benign liver disease) can cause further confusion. Establishment of ectopic production of calcitonin by a tumor other than MTC can be difficult, but it should be pursued when the pieces of the diagnostic schema for MTC do not fit together.

Method of RET *Sequence Testing in DNA*

DNA diagnostic techniques currently in use to identify MEN-2 gene carriers are based on the use of polymerase chain reaction techniques to amplify selected portions of the *RET* proto-oncogene known to be mutated in MEN-2. All laboratories analyze for mutations in exons 10, 11, and 16 (codons 609, 611, 618, 620, 630, 634, and 918), those most commonly found in MEN-2. If a mutation is not identified in one of these codons, some but not all laboratories analyze for mutations in exons 13, 14, and 15 (codons 768, 790, 791, 804, 883, and 891). If a mutation is not identified in exon 10, 11, or 16, it is important to identify a laboratory that will examine the other exons before concluding that no mutation is present. This is particularly true for kindreds with FMTC, a disproportionate number of which have an exon 13, 14, or 15 mutation.[441] Although there is a potential for several types of errors in mutational analysis,[314,499] a repeated analysis of each positive or negative test result in a separate testing facility with an independently obtained DNA sample provides nearly 100% certainty that an individual test result is accurate.

Germline RET *Mutation: Three Categories of Risk*

There is now consensus that all patients with a *RET* mutation should be offered a total thyroidectomy. Since the identification of these mutations, greater awareness of the relationship between mutation at a specific *RET* codon and the clinical aggressiveness of the MTC has developed. A consensus has developed within the field that these differences should be considered in the decision-making process regarding early thyroidectomy. The consensus guidelines have divided hereditary MTC into three different risk categories.[182]

Category 1: Highest Risk

In the highest risk category are those with MEN-2B and a codon 883, 918, or 922 *RET* mutation. In these children, MTC with metastasis can occur during the first year of life,[386,387] prompting a recommendation for total thyroidectomy and central lymph node dissection in such children during the first 6 months of life. During this procedure, other level II to V lymph nodes should be sampled, and more extensive lymph node dissection should be performed if metastatic disease is identified.

Category 2: High Risk

Patients with *RET* mutations of codons 609, 611, 618, 620, or 634 are classified as having high risk. They should have a total thyroidectomy, including removal of the posterior capsule, before the age of 5 years. This recommendation is based on the finding of microscopic MTC in two children with a codon 634 mutation at age 2 years[500,501] and nodal metastasis in children at ages 5[311,386] and 6[501] years. There is less consensus regarding the need for central node dissection, although a majority of surgeons perform this dissection during the primary surgery so that they do not need to reoperate in the central compartment if primary surgery is not curative.[183,313,334]

Category 3: Intermediate Risk

Patients with codon 768, 790, 791, 804, or 891 mutations are classified as having intermediate risk. The biologic behavior and clinical aggressiveness of MTC in patients with such mutations vary, but the MTC tends to be less aggressive. Lymph node metastasis and death related to MTC have been identified with all these mutations, but it is uncommon for most. There is no consensus regarding the age of total thyroidectomy in such children. Several approaches are used. Some classify these patients with the high-risk category and perform a total thyroidectomy by the age of 5 years. Some recommend thyroidectomy by the age of 10 years. Others observe patients with these mutations with periodic provocative tests for calcitonin and perform a total thyroidectomy when calcitonin levels become clearly abnormal. There is consensus, however, that these patients should be followed up especially carefully if an early thyroidectomy is not performed. There are large kindreds with some of these mutations in which there has never been a death caused by MTC, making it difficult to convince family members that early thyroidectomy is indicated.

Multiple Endocrine Neoplasia Type 2 Kindred with Known RET *Mutation*

A normal *RET* analysis in a kindred with a known *RET* mutation excludes the carrier state with nearly 100% certainty. A person with two independently obtained negative DNA test results in the context of a family with an identified missense mutation can be excluded from further carrier ascertainment. Pentagastrin testing in this situation adds nothing to the diagnostic accuracy and can actually confuse the clinical assessment because of a high incidence of false-positive results.[314]

Occult Phenotypes

Should *RET* germline be tested in a patient with an apparently sporadic tumor in the spectrum of MEN-2?

Germline Mutations in Sporadic Medullary Thyroid Carcinoma

A compilation of more than 200 patients with apparent sporadic MTC who were examined for *germline RET* mutations (codons 609, 611, 618, 620, 630, and in some cases 768) has identified mutations in approximately 6% of the total (this contrasts with data presented later showing that approximately 25% of sporadic MTCs have a *somatic RET* mutation without a corresponding germline abnormality).[406,456,466,502] Subsequent investigation of the subjects in these studies with germline *RET* mutations has demonstrated that the majority were members of previously unidentified kindreds or descendants of gene carriers who were separated from their families without knowledge of MEN-2 in the family. There have been at least eight examples of *de novo* germline mutations in which the affected person carries a *RET* proto-oncogene mutation but neither parent is affected.[406,466,503,504] In four of these cases in which it was tested and in most new MEN-2B probands,[391] the newly mutated allele is derived from the unaffected father, suggesting acquisition of the mutation during spermatogenesis.

The finding that 6% of patients with apparent sporadic MTC carry germline *RET* mutations suggests that all patients with MTC should have a *RET* germline analysis performed. This is especially important because identification of one hereditary case can have a multiplier effect, leading to the diagnosis of unsuspected cases in the family and effective early treatment.[406] Negative family history, although useful, clearly does not exclude hereditary disease. A second reason for performing a *RET* germline analysis is to reassure the patient and family members that there is no hereditary component. If the *RET* analysis is negative, hereditary disease can be excluded with greater than 99% certainty.[406] Most families of patients with sporadic MTC are assured by a less than 1% probability of hereditary disease; for those who want hereditary MTC excluded with 100% certainty, continued provocative calcitonin testing in relatives is required.

Germline Mutations in Sporadic Pheochromocytoma

The situation is less clear for apparently sporadic pheochromocytoma. Three genetic syndromes—MEN-2, VHL, and hereditary pheochromocytoma or paraganglioma syndrome—can manifest as a sporadic pheochromocytoma. This presentation is unlikely for type 1 neurofibromatosis. Estimates of frequency of heredity for pheochromocytoma in the general population have ranged from 9%[301] to as high as 24%[505] in some series. It is important to recognize that these estimates came from tertiary care centers, where there is a high incidence of genetic pheochromocytoma, raising the question of whether these percentages are relevant to the general population.[505] Based on a summary of all reports, a reasonable estimate is 17%.[506] Genetic testing should be pursued in patients considered to be at high risk for hereditary pheochromocytoma: those younger than 20 years, those with a positive family history, and persons with sympathetic paragangliomas.[506]

Germline mutation of GDNF has been identified in 1 of 50 sporadic pheochromocytomas.[507,508] The significance of this single mutation is unclear. Similarly, germline VHL mutations in apparent sporadic pheochromocytoma are uncommon, being found in only nine of 173 sporadic pheochromocytomas (5.2%) in four series.[475,509-511] Finally, there are at least four different familial pheochromocytoma-paraganglionoma syndromes that have been mapped (PGL1, PGL2, PGL3, and familial pheochromocytoma-paraganglioma syndrome). Mutations of components of the succinate dehydrogenase complex gene, putative tumor suppressor genes because each of the mutations appears to be inactivating, have been identified in three of the four variants.[512-518]

Periodic Tumor Surveillance in a Known Carrier

Should evaluation for tumors other than medullary thyroid carcinoma be performed in kindreds with familial medullary thyroid carcinoma?

Mutations at codons 768, 791, V804M, and 891 have been associated exclusively with FMTC; nonetheless, it would be prudent to consider a screening urine catecholamine or metanephrine test for pheochromocytoma at the time of diagnosis and perhaps at 5-year intervals. Codon 609, 611, 618, 620, or 630 mutations have been associated with either FMTC or MEN-2A. Unless there is a several-generation pattern of FMTC in more than 10 affected family members, it would be prudent to screen every 1 to 3 years for pheochromocytoma. The molecular basis for the phenotypic variability (FMTC or MEN-2A) with codon 609, 611, 618, 620, or 630 mutations is unknown at present.

Management of an Established Multiple Endocrine Neoplasia Type 2 Kindred

Counseling

Family education is an important component in the management of MEN-2. Although a physician's legal responsibility might end after immediate family members have been notified of the genetic nature of the disease, it is prudent to encourage patients to make even family members at distant risk aware of the nature of the disease. The fact that the disease appears to be benign in one generation should not deter carrier ascertainment and tumor surveillance efforts because the disease can assume a more virulent expression in a subsequent generation.[518] This notification can be done by giving pamphlets describing the syndrome to immediate family members for distribution to more distant relatives.[519]

Prospects for Surgical Cure of Medullary Thyroid Carcinoma in Multiple Endocrine Neoplasia Type 2

Widespread prospective carrier ascertainment and tumor surveillance have had an impact on the natural history of the syndrome. The age at carrier ascertainment has progressively fallen from a mean of 33 years when prospective carrier ascertainment through tumor surveillance first began in 1969 to a mean less than 13 years in 1988.[520,521] The current mean age with widespread DNA testing is likely to be earlier than age 5 years. Testing for *RET* mutations now makes it possible to identify carrier status at birth or in utero.

Whether prospective DNA-based ascertainment and early thyroidectomy are curative for the thyroid neoplasm is less clear. Follow-up data from several groups indicate that approximately 85% to 90% but not 100% of kindred members who received thyroidectomy for early disease on the basis of pentagastrin testing have normal calcitonin values at mean follow-up periods ranging from 1 to 15 years.[325,337,522] It can be anticipated that earlier DNA-based ascertainment and treatment are likely to improve the outcome in gene carriers. None of the patients with MEN-2A or FMTC identified by DNA-based carrier ascertainment and treated surgically before the age of 5 years have had identifiable metastasis,[304,313,314,500,501,523-528] although there was considerable variability in these small series in the numbers of nodes sampled. A 5-year follow-up of patients receiving thyroidectomy for hereditary MTC showed that 24 children operated on before the age of 8 years had no detectable calcitonin basally or after pentagastrin stimulation.[305] These data are encouraging, but longer-term data are required to demonstrate with certainty the impact of earlier treatment in this syndrome.

Therapies Based on Reversal of *RET* Activation

Activating mutations of tyrosine kinase receptors cause phosphorylation of the receptor and downstream signaling molecules, thereby initiating cellular processes that cause transformation. This recognition led to the development of small molecules that block phosphorylation by binding preferentially to the intracellular ATP binding pocket of the receptor. Reports since the turn of the 21st century have documented the effectiveness of several tyrosine kinase inhibitors in disorders caused by activating mutations of tyrosine kinases including chronic myelogenous leukemia, gastrointestinal stromal tumors, and lung and renal cancer, among others.[529]

In each of these examples, a cytoplasmic or receptor tyrosine kinase mutation initiated or maintained transformation. A number of these tyrosine kinase inhibitors, particularly those directed against the vascular endothelial growth factor family of receptors, are now known to also inhibit phosphorylation of the *RET* proto-oncogene.[530,531] Three of these agents, vandetanib (ZD 6474), AMG 706, and sorafenib (BAY 43-9006) are in phase II trials for treatment of medullary thyroid carcinoma.[532] A preliminary analysis of the use of ZD 6474 in MEN-2–associated medullary thyroid carcinoma has show objective evidence of regression in approximately 20% of treated patients.[533] A phase III trial of this agent is under way, and results of a phase II trial of AMG 706 are expected. At least two other agents (XL184 and

AG-013736) have preliminarily shown activity in phase I studies. Although it is not clear whether any of these agents will have long-term efficacy and will be approved for treatment, preliminary results are encouraging and have already provided proof of the concept that inactivation of *RET* will have therapeutic efficacy.

Multiple Endocrine Neoplasia of Mixed Type

Overlap Syndromes

Overlap syndromes in single patients include gastrinoma in a MEN-2 patient,[534] adenomatous polyposis coli with MEN-1 or MEN-2B,[535,536] posterior pituitary tumor and MEN-1,[537] prolactinoma in a patient with MEN-2A,[538] and pheochromocytomas in MEN-1 (see earlier). There is a single case report of an ovarian strumal carcinoid tumor, a variant of an ovarian teratoma, in a patient with MEN-2A. The tumor was composed of neuroendocrine cells with thyroid-like follicles that stained positive for thyroglobulin.[539]

Most cases of overlap of MEN-1 and MEN-2 were published before the era of discovery of syndrome-causing genes. Currently, most can be understood as follows:

- Unusual expressions of a syndrome. VHL can cause pheochromocytoma and islet tumor (see later), neurofibromatosis type 1 (NF1) can cause pheochromocytoma and duodenal somatostatinoma (see later), and MEN-1 can cause pheochromocytoma with any other feature of MEN-1 (see earlier).
- Coexistence of two rare disorders.
- Rare syndromes that have not yet been characterized sufficiently.
- Few cases of unexplained overlap. In this regard, a rat strain[279] and a mouse model (see earlier) have many features of both MEN-1 and MEN-2, suggesting a single pathway to both syndromes or an overlap.[269]

Familial Occurrence of Two or More Endocrine Neoplastic Disorders

MEN-1 and MEN-2 are the only multiple neoplasia syndromes in which the two most prominent features are hormone-secreting tumors. In other MEN syndromes, nonhormonal tumors are more urgent. For example, the McCune-Albright syndrome (which is not hereditary) features fibrous dysplasia of bone and café-au-lait spots of skin (Chapter 27), and VHL syndrome features papillary renal cancer and central nervous system hemangioblastomas.

Von Hippel-Lindau Disease

VHL syndrome is an autosomal dominant neoplastic syndrome characterized by hemangioblastomas of the central nervous system, retinal angiomas, renal cell carcinomas, visceral cysts, pheochromocytoma, and islet cell tumors.[540,541] More than 90% of gene carriers express one or more of the manifestations of this disorder by the age of 60 years. More than 70% of gene carriers have one or more central nervous system tumors.[542] Of particular relevance to endocrinologists is the observation that 25% to 35% of these patients have unilateral or bilateral pheochromocytomas and 15% to 20% have islet cell tumors.[540,543] Although the islet cell tumors might immunostain weakly for insulin, they virtually never hypersecrete it.[54]

The *VHL* gene was mapped to chromosome 3p25.3[544] and identified by positional cloning.[545] This gene is a tumor suppressor gene, implying that loss of function or inactivating mutations of both alleles or copies of this gene are associated with tumor formation. Studies have described an inhibitory effect of the *VHL*-encoded protein on transcription elongation through its binding to an elongin B/C complex. Mutation of the *VHL* gene, particularly in the region of codons 150 to 170, interferes with this interaction, resulting in an accelerated rate of transcription elongation.[546-548] Another mechanism might explain many of the properties of the *VHL* protein and disease. The action of the VHL protein to facilitate the proteasome-mediated degradation of the hypoxia-inducible factor 1 (HIF-1) protein and other proteins can prove central to many manifestations of *VHL* gene alteration.[549] Mutation of codon 238 was identified in more than 40% of VHL families with pheochromocytoma, suggesting that families with a mutation in this codon should be surveyed routinely for pheochromocytoma.[550] As with other recessive oncogenes, a large number of inactivating mutations have been described for *VHL*.

Clinical management for patients with VHL syndrome is often complicated by the presence of renal or central nervous system tumors. Pheochromocytomas or islet cell tumors associated with hypertension, cardiac arrhythmias, hypoglycemia, watery diarrhea, carcinoid, or a glucagonoma-like picture should be surgically excised. Judgment is required in the management of other malignant features associated with VHL. For example, a less aggressive approach to the management of pheochromocytoma or islet cell tumor may be indicated in a patient with VHL and a renal cell carcinoma with metastasis. An adrenal cortical–sparing operation may be appropriate for pheochromocytoma in such a patient.[347]

The association of pheochromocytoma and islet cell tumors can occur in familial[551-553] or nonfamilial[554-556] patterns. There is little information about the molecular genetics of these rare disorders, although it is possible that abnormalities of the *VHL* gene are involved.

Neurofibromatosis Type 1

The main features of NF1 are neurofibromas and dermal café-au-lait spots. NF1 has been associated with a variety of endocrine neoplasms including pheochromocytoma,[557] hyperparathyroidism,[558] somatostatin-producing carcinoid tumors of the duodenal wall,[559,560] MTC,[561] and hypothalamic or optic nerve tumors that cause precocious puberty.[562] The causative gene for NF1 encodes a ras guanosine triphosphatase (GTPase)-activating protein (GAP) of 2818 amino acids, named *neurofibromin*, which accelerates GTP hydrolysis on p21 ras. Loss of the GTPase-activating function of neurofibromin (through mutation or allelic loss) leads to p21 *ras* activation.[563] More specific evidence for a role of this protein in endocrine tumors is suggested by allelic loss of this gene in NF1-associated[564] or sporadic[565] pheochromocytomas. Targeted disruption of the mouse *NF1* gene resulted in sympathetic ganglia hyperplasia, providing additional evidence for a potential role of this gene in the genesis of endocrine tumors derived from neural crest tissue.[566]

Carney's Complex

Carney's complex includes myxomas of the heart, skin, and breast; spotty skin pigmentation; testicular, adrenal cortical, and growth hormone–secreting pituitary tumors; and peripheral nerve schwannomas.[567-569] Linkage analysis has identified a locus at 2p in half of the families and another locus at 17q in most others.[570] The gene at 17q has been identified as encoding the regulatory subunit (type IA) of protein kinase A *(PRKA1A)*, and it has tumor suppressor properties.[571] Several small kindreds with only bilateral adrenal hyperplasia have mutation of a phosphodiesterase (PDE11A) at chromosome 2p.[572] The activating *GNAS* mutations in McCune-Albright syndrome and the inactivating *PRKA1A* mutations in Carney's complex are likely to cause tumors in selected tissues with a similar tissue spectrum by raising cyclic adenosine monophosphate.

REFERENCES

1. Erdheim J. Zur normalen und pathologischen Histologie der Glandula Thyreoidea, Parathyreoidea und Hypophysis. Beitr Pathol Anat 1903;33:158-236.
2. Underdahl LO, Woolner LB, Black BM. Multiple endocrine adenomas: report of 8 cases in which the parathyroids, pituitary and pancreatic islets were involved. J Clin Endocrinol 1953;13:20-47.
3. Moldawer MP, Nardi GL, Raker JW. Concomitance of multiple adenomas of parathyroids and pancreatic islets with tumor of pituitary: syndrome with familial incidence. Am J Med Sci 1954; 228:190-206.
4. Wermer P. Genetic aspects of adenomatosis of endocrine glands. Am J Med 1954;16:363-371.
5. Sipple JH. The association of pheochromocytoma with carcinoma of the thyroid gland. Am J Med 1961;31:163-166.
6. Ballard HS, Frame B, Hartsock RJ. Familial multiple endocrine adenoma–peptic ulcer complex. Medicine 1964;43:481-516.
7. Steiner AL, Goodman AD, Powers SR. Study of a kindred with pheochromocytoma, medullary carcinoma, hyperparathyroidism and Cushing's disease: multiple endocrine neoplasia, type 2. Medicine 1968;47:371-409.
8. Melvin KEW, Tashjian AH Jr, Miller HH. Studies in familial (medullary) thyroid carcinoma. Recent Prog Horm Res 1972;28:399-470.
9. Baysal BE. Genetics of familial paragangliomas: past, present, and future. Otolaryngol Clin North Am 2001;34:863-879, vi.
10. Marx S. Multiple endocrine neoplasia type 1. In Bilezekian JP, Marcus R, Levine MA (eds). The Parathyroids: Basic and Clinical Concepts, 2nd ed. San Diego: Academic Press, 2001:535-584.
11. Marx SJ, Vinik AI, Santen RJ, et al. Multiple endocrine neoplasia type I: assessment of laboratory tests to screen for the gene in a large kindred. Medicine (Baltimore) 1986;65:226-241.
12. Benson L, Ljunghall S, Akerstrom G, Oberg K. Hyperparathyroidism presenting as the first lesion in multiple endocrine neoplasia type 1. Am J Med 1987;82:731-737.
13. Trump D, Farren B, Wooding C, et al. Clinical studies of multiple endocrine neoplasia type 1 (MEN1). Q J Med 1996;89:653-669.
14. Marx S, Spiegel AM, Skarulis MC, et al. Multiple endocrine neoplasia type 1: clinical and genetic topics. Ann Intern Med 1998;129: 484-494.
15. Jackson CE, Boonstra CE. The relationship of hereditary hyperparathyroidism to endocrine adenomatosis. Am J Med 1967; 43:727-734.
16. Johnson GJ, Summerskill WH, Anderson VE, Keating FR Jr. Clinical and genetic investigation of a large kindred with multiple endocrine adenomatosis. N Engl J Med 1967;277:1379-1385.
17. Craven DE, Goodman D, Carter JH. Familial multiple endocrine adenomatosis. Multiple endocrine neoplasia, type I. Arch Intern Med 1972;129:567-569.
18. Snyder N, III, Scurry MT, Deiss WP. Five families with multiple endocrine adenomatosis. Ann Intern Med 1972;76:53-58.
19. Jung RT, Grant AM, Davie M, et al. Multiple endocrine adenomatosis (type I) and familial hyperparathyroidism. Postgrad Med 1978;54:92-94.
20. Eberle F, Grun R. Multiple endocrine neoplasia, type I (MEN I). Ergeb Inn Med Kinderheilkd 1981;46:76-149.
21. Burgess JR, David R, Greenaway TM, et al. Osteoporosis in multiple endocrine neoplasia type 1: severity, clinical significance, relationship to primary hyperparathyroidism, and response to parathyroidectomy. Arch Surg 1999;134:1119-1123.
22. Rizzoli R, Green J, III, Marx SJ. Primary hyperparathyroidism in familial multiple endocrine neoplasia type I. Long-term follow-up of serum calcium levels after parathyroidectomy. Am J Med 1985;78:467-474.
23. Marx SJ, Menczel J, Campbell G, et al. Heterogeneous size of the parathyroid glands in familial multiple endocrine neoplasia type 1. Clin Endocrinol (Oxf) 1991;35:521-526.
24. Hellman P, Skogseid B, Oberg K, et al. Primary and reoperative parathyroid operations in hyperparathyroidism of multiple endocrine neoplasia type 1. Surgery 1998;124:993-999.
25. Sato M, Miyauchi A, Namihira H, et al. A newly recognized germline mutation of MEN1 gene identified in a patient with parathyroid adenoma and carcinoma. Endocrine 2000;12:223-226.
26. Friedman E, Sakaguchi K, Bale AE, et al. Clonality of parathyroid tumors in familial multiple endocrine neoplasia type 1. N Engl J Med 1989;321:213-218.
27. Brandi ML, Aurbach GD, Fitzpatrick LA, et al. Parathyroid mitogenic activity in plasma from patients with familial multiple endocrine neoplasia type 1. N Engl J Med 1986;314:1287-1293.
28. Brown EM, Pollak M, Hebert SC. The extracellular calcium-sensing receptor: its role in health and disease. Annu Rev Med 1998; 49:15-29.
29. Kifor O, Moore FD Jr, Wang P, et al. Reduced immunostaining for the extracellular Ca^{2+}-sensing receptor in primary and uremic secondary hyperparathyroidism. J Clin Endocrinol Metab 1996;81: 1598-1606.
30. Jensen RT. Management of the Zollinger-Ellison syndrome in patients with multiple endocrine neoplasia type 1. J Intern Med 1998;243:477-488.
31. Shawker TH, Avila N, Premkumar A, et al. Ultrasound evaluation of primary hyperparathyroidism. Ultrasound Quart 2000;16: 73-87.
32. Norman J, Chheda H, Farrell C. Minimally invasive parathyroidectomy for primary hyperparathyroidism: decreasing operative time and potential complications while improving cosmetic results. Am Surg 1998;64:391-395; discussion 395-396.
33. Thompson GB, Grant CS, Perrier ND, et al. Reoperative parathyroid surgery in the era of sestamibi scanning and intraoperative parathyroid hormone monitoring. Arch Surg 1999;134:699-704; discussion 704-695.
34. Jaskowiak N, Norton JA, Alexander HR, et al. A prospective trial evaluating a standard approach to reoperation for missed parathyroid adenoma. Ann Surg 1996;224:308-320; discussion 320-301.
35. Irvin GL 3rd, Molinari AS, Figueroa C, Carneiro DM. Improved success rate in reoperative parathyroidectomy with intraoperative PTH assay. Ann Surg 1999;229:874-878; discussion 878-879.
36. Tonelli F, Spini S, Tommasi M. Intraoperative PTH measurement in patients with MEN1 syndrome and hyperparathyroidism. World J Surg 1999;24:556-563.
37. Libutti SK, Alexander HR, Bartlett DL, et al. Kinetic analysis of the rapid intraoperative parathyroid hormone assay in patients during operation for hyperparathyroidism. Surgery 1999;126:1145-1150; discussion 1150-1141.
38. Feldman AL, Sharaf RN, Skarulis MC, et al. Results of heterotopic parathyroid autotransplantation: a 13-year experience. Surgery 1999;126:1042-1048.
39. Majewski JT, Wilson SD. The MEA-I syndrome: an all or none phenomenon? Surgery 1979;86:475-484.
40. Skogseid B, Oberg K, Eriksson B, et al. Surgery for asymptomatic pancreatic lesion in multiple endocrine neoplasia type I. World J Surg 1996;20:872-876; discussion 877.
41. Wilkinson S, Teh BT, Davey KR, et al. Cause of death in multiple endocrine neoplasia type 1. Arch Surg 1993;128:683-690.
42. Doherty GM, Olson JA, Frisella MM, et al. Lethality of multiple endocrine neoplasia type I. World J Surg 1998;22:581-586; discussion 586-587.
43. Yu F, Venzon DJ, Serrano J, et al. Prospective study of the clinical course, prognostic factors, causes of death, and survival in patients with long-standing Zollinger-Ellison syndrome. J Clin Oncol 1999;17:615-630.
44. Kloppel G, Willemer S, Stamm B, et al. Pancreatic lesions and hormonal profile of pancreatic tumors in multiple endocrine neoplasia type I. An immunocytochemical study of nine patients. Cancer 1986;57:1824-1832.
45. Le Bodic MF, Heymann MF, Lecomte M, et al. Immunohistochemical study of 100 pancreatic tumors in 28 patients with multiple endocrine neoplasia, type I. Am J Surg Pathol 1996;20:1378-1384.
46. Pipeleers-Marichal M, Somers G, Willems G, et al. Gastrinomas in the duodenums of patients with multiple endocrine neoplasia type 1 and the Zollinger-Ellison syndrome. N Engl J Med 1990;322: 723-727.
47. Ariel I, Kerem E, Schwartz-Arad D, et al. Nesidiodysplasia—a histologic entity? Hum Pathol 1988;19:1215-1218.

48. Lubensky IA, Debelenko LV, Zhuang Z, et al. Allelic deletions on chromosome 11q13 in multiple tumors from individual MEN1 patients. Cancer Res 1996;56:5272-5278.
49. Debelenko LV, Zhuang Z, Emmert-Buck MR, et al. Allelic deletions on chromosome 11q13 in multiple endocrine neoplasia type 1–associated and sporadic gastrinomas and pancreatic endocrine tumors. Cancer Res 1997;57:2238-2243.
50. Anlauf M, Perren A, Meyer CL, et al. Precursor lesions in patients with multiple endocrine neoplasia type 1–associated duodenal gastrinomas. Gastroenterol 2006;128:1187-1198.
51. Crabtree JS, Scacheri PC, Ward JM, et al. A mouse model of multiple endocrine neoplasia, type 1, develops multiple endocrine tumors. Proc Natl Acad Sci U S A 2001;98:1118-1123.
52. Maioli M, Ciccarese M, Pacifico A, et al. Familial insulinoma: description of two cases. Acta Diabetol 1992;29:38-40.
53. Lubensky IA, Pack S, Ault D, et al. Multiple neuroendocrine tumors of the pancreas in von Hippel-Lindau disease patients: histopathological and molecular genetic analysis. Am J Pathol 1998;153: 223-231.
54. Farley DR, van Heerden JA, Grant CS, et al. The Zollinger-Ellison syndrome. A collective surgical experience. Ann Surg 1992;215:561-569; discussion 569-570.
55. Serrano J, Goebel SU, Heppner C, et al. Occurrence of multiple endocrine neoplasia type 1 *(MEN1)* gene mutations in Zollinger Ellison syndrome (ZES) [abstract]. Gastroenterol 1998;114: G2022.
56. Waxman I, Gardner JD, Jensen RT, Maton PN. Peptic ulcer perforation as the presentation of Zollinger-Ellison syndrome. Dig Dis Sci 1991;36:19-24.
57. Metz DC, Jensen RT, Bale AE, et al. Multiple endocrine neoplasia type 1: clinical features and management. In Bilezekian JP, Levine MA, Marx SJ, eds. The Parathyroids, ed 1. New York: Raven Press, 1994:591-646.
58. Benya RV, Metz DC, Hijazi YJ, et al. Fine needle aspiration cytology of submucosal nodules in patients with Zollinger-Ellison syndrome. Am J Gastroenterol 1993;88:258-265.
59. Roy PK, Venzon DJ, Shojamanesh H, et al. Zollinger-Ellison syndrome. Clinical presentation in 261 patients. Medicine (Baltimore) 2000;79:379-411.
60. Norton JA, Fraker DL, Alexander HR, et al. Surgery to cure the Zollinger-Ellison syndrome. N Engl J Med 1999;341:635-644.
61. Gibril F, Venzon DJ, Ojeaburu JV, et al. Prospective study of the natural history of gastrinoma in patients with MEN1: definition of an aggressive and a nonaggressive form. J Clin Endocrinol Metab 2001;86:5282-5293.
62. Ruszniewski P, Podevin P, Cadiot G, et al. Clinical, anatomical, and evolutive features of patients with the Zollinger-Ellison syndrome combined with type I multiple endocrine neoplasia. Pancreas 1993;8:295-304.
63. Stadil F, Bardram L, Gustafsen J, Efsen F. Surgical treatment of the Zollinger-Ellison syndrome. World J Surg 1993;17:463-467.
64. Thompson NW. Current concepts in the surgical management of multiple endocrine neoplasia type 1 pancreatic-duodenal disease. Results in the treatment of 40 patients with Zollinger-Ellison syndrome, hypoglycaemia or both. J Intern Med 1998;243:495-500.
65. Tonelli F, Fratini G, Nesi G, et al. Pancreatectomy in multiple endocrine neoplasia type 1–related gastrinomas and pancreatic endocrine neoplasias. Ann Surg 2006;244:61-70.
66. Frucht H, Maton PN, Jensen RT. Use of omeprazole in patients with Zollinger-Ellison syndrome. Dig Dis Sci 1991;36:394-404.
67. Maton PN. Review article: the management of Zollinger-Ellison syndrome. Aliment Pharmacol Ther 1993;7:467-475.
68. Maton PN. Omeprazole. N Engl J Med 1991;324:965-975.
69. Jensen RT. Gastrinoma as a model for prolonged hypergastrinemia. In Walsh JH, ed. Gastrin. New York: Raven Press, 1993: 373-393.
70. Solcia E, Capella C, Fiocca R, et al. Gastric argyrophil carcinoidosis in patients with Zollinger-Ellison syndrome due to type 1 multiple endocrine neoplasia. A newly recognized association. Am J Surg Pathol 1990;14:503-513.
71. Maton PN, Lack EE, Collen MJ, et al. The effect of Zollinger-Ellison syndrome and omeprazole therapy on gastric oxyntic endocrine cells. Gastroenterology 1990;99:943-950.
72. Cadiot G, Lehy T, Ruszniewski P, et al. Gastric endocrine cell evolution in patients with Zollinger-Ellison syndrome. Influence of gastrinoma growth and long-term omeprazole treatment. Dig Dis Sci 1993;38:1307-1317.
73. Gyr K, Whitehouse I, Beglinger C, et al. Human pharmacological effects of SMS 201-995 on gastric secretion. Scan J Gastroenterol 1986;21(suppl 119):96-102.
74. Shojamanesh H, Gibril F, Louie A, et al. Prospective study of the antitumor efficacy of long-term octreotide treatment in patients with progressive metastatic gastrinoma. Cancer Res 2002;94: 331-343.
75. Tomassetti P, Migliori M, Caletti GC, et al. Treatment of type II gastric carcinoid tumors with somatostatin analogues. N Engl J Med 2000;343:551-554.
76. Proye C, Malvaux P, Pattou F, et al. Noninvasive imaging of insulinomas and gastrinomas with endoscopic ultrasonography and somatostatin receptor scintigraphy. Surgery 1998;124:1134-1143; discussion 1143-1134.
77. Norton JA. Intra-operative procedures to localize endocrine tumours of the pancreas and duodenum. Ital J Gastroenterol Hepatol 1999;31 Suppl 2:S195-S197.
78. Boukhman MP, Karam JM, Shaver J, et al. Localization of insulinomas. Arch Surg 1999;134:818-822; discussion 822-813.
79. Doppman JL, Chang R, Fraker DL, et al. Localization of insulinomas to regions of the pancreas by intra-arterial stimulation with calcium. Ann Intern Med 1995;123:269-273.
80. Proye C, Pattou F, Carnaille B, et al. Intraoperative insulin measurement during surgical management of insulinomas. World J Surg 1998;22:1218-1224.
81. Stefanini P, Carboni M, Patrassi N, et al. Beta-islet cell tumors of the pancreas: results of a study on 1,067 cases. 1974;75:597-609.
82. Goode PN, Farndon JR, Anderson J, et al. Diazoxide in the management of patients with insulinoma. World J Surg 1986;10: 586-592.
83. Lamberts SW, Pieters GF, Metselaar HJ, et al. Development of resistance to a long-acting somatostatin analogue during treatment of two patients with metastatic endocrine pancreatic tumours. Acta Endocrinol (Copenh) 1988;119:561-566.
84. Levy-Bohbot N, Merle C, Goudet P, et al. Prevalence, characteristics and prognosis of MEN 1–associated glucagonomas, VIPomas, and somatostatinomas: study from the GTE (Groupe des Tumeurs Endocrines) registry. Gastroenterol Clin Biol 2004;28:1075-1081.
85. Gorden P, Comi RJ, Maton PN, Go VLW. Somatostatin and somatostatin analogue (SMS 201-995) in treatment of hormone-secreting tumors of the pituitary and gastrointestinal tract and non-neoplastic diseases of the gut. Ann Intern Med 1989; 110:35-50.
86. Park SK, O'Dorisio MS, O'Dorisio TM. Vasoactive intestinal polypeptide–secreting tumours: biology and therapy. Baillieres Clin Gastroenterol 1996;10:673-696.
87. Wu TJ, Lin CL, Taylor RL, et al. Increased parathyroid hormone–related peptide in patients with hypercalcemia associated with islet cell carcinoma. Mayo Clin Proc 1997;72:1111-1115.
88. Liu SW, van de Velde CJ, Heslinga JM, et al. Acromegaly caused by growth hormone-relating hormone in a patient with multiple endocrine neoplasia type I. Jpn J Clin Oncol 1996;26:49-52.
89. Ezzat S, Asa SL, Stefaneanu L, et al. Somatotroph hyperplasia without pituitary adenoma associated with a long standing growth hormone–releasing hormone–producing bronchial carcinoid. J Clin Endocrinol Metab 1994;78:555-560.
90. Pedrazzoli S, Pasquali C, Sperti C, et al. Clinically silent pancreatic "somatostatinoma" in MEN-1 syndrome, and literature review. GI Cancer 1996;1:191-206.
91. Fleury A, Flejou JF, Sauvanet A, et al. Calcitonin-secreting tumors of the pancreas: about six cases. Pancreas 1998;16:545-550.
92. Skogseid B, Oberg K, Benson L, et al. A standardized meal stimulation test of the endocrine pancreas for early detection of pancreatic endocrine tumors in multiple endocrine neoplasia type 1 syndrome: five years experience. J Clin Endocrinol Metab 1987;64:1233-1240.
93. Mutch MG, Frisella MM, DeBenedetti MK, et al. Pancreatic polypeptide is a useful plasma marker for radiographically evident pancreatic islet cell tumors in patients with multiple endocrine neoplasia type 1. Surgery 1997;122:1012-1019; discussion 1019-1020.
94. Skogseid B, Oberg K, Akerstrom G, et al. Limited tumor involvement found at multiple endocrine neoplasia type I pancreatic

exploration: can it be predicted by preoperative tumor localization? World J Surg 1998;22:673-677; discussion 667-678.

95. Pisegna JR, Doppman JL, Norton JA, et al. Prospective comparative study of ability of MR imaging and other imaging modalities to localize tumors in patients with Zollinger-Ellison syndrome. Dig Dis Sci 1993;38:1318-1328.
96. Frilling A, Malago M, Martin H, Broelsch CE. Use of somatostatin receptor scintigraphy to image extrahepatic metastases of neuroendocrine tumors. Surgery 1998;124:1000-1004.
97. Yim JH, Siegel BA, DeBenedetti MK, et al. Prospective study of the utility of somatostatin-receptor scintigraphy in the evaluation of patients with multiple endocrine neoplasia type 1. Surgery 1998;124:1037-1042.
98. Cadiot G, Bonnaud G, Lebtahi R, et al. Usefulness of somatostatin receptor scintigraphy in the management of patients with Zollinger-Ellison syndrome. Groupe de Recherche et d'Etude du Syndrome de Zollinger-Ellison (GRESZE). Gut 1997;41:107-114.
99. Doppman JL, Miller DL, Chang R, et al. Gastrinomas: localization by means of selective intraarterial injection of secretin. Radiology 1990;174:25-29.
100. Alexander HR, Fraker DL, Norton JA, et al. Prospective study of somatostatin receptor scintigraphy and its effect on operative outcome in patients with Zollinger-Ellison syndrome. Ann Surg 1998;228:228-238.
101. Legmann P, Vignaux O, Dousset B, et al. Pancreatic tumors: comparison of dual-phase helical CT and endoscopic sonography. AJR Am J Roentgenol 1998;170:1315-1322.
102. Sheridan MB, Ward J, Guthrie JA, et al. Dynamic contrast-enhanced MR imaging and dual-phase helical CT in the preoperative assessment of suspected pancreatic cancer: a comparative study with receiver operating characteristic analysis. AJR Am J Roentgenol 1999;173:583-590.
103. Ichikawa T, Peterson MS, Federle MP, et al. Islet cell tumor of the pancreas: biphasic CT versus MR imaging in tumor detection. Radiology 2000;216:163-171.
104. Orlefors H, Sundin A, Garske U, et al. Whole-body ^{11}C-5-hydroxytryptophan positron emission tomography as a universal imaging technique for neuroendocrine tumors: comparison with somatostatin receptor scintigraphy and computed tomography. J Clin Endocrinol Metab 2005;90:3392-3400.
105. Bansal R, Tierney W, Carpenter S, et al. Cost effectiveness of EUS for preoperative localization of pancreatic endocrine tumors. Gastrointest Endosc 1999;49:19-25.
106. Suits J, Frazee R, Erickson RA. Endoscopic ultrasound and fine needle aspiration for the evaluation of pancreatic masses. Arch Surg 1999;134:639-642; discussion 642-633.
107. Hiramoto JS, Feldstein VA, LaBerge JM, Norton JA. Intraoperative ultrasound and preoperative localization detects all occult insulinomas. Arch Surg 2001;136:1020-1025.
108. Granberg D, Stridsberg M, Seensalu R, et al. Plasma chromogranin A in patients with multiple endocrine neoplasia type 1. J Clin Endocrinol Metab 1999;84:2712-2717.
109. Nobels FR, Kwekkeboom DJ, Coopmans W, et al. Chromogranin A as serum marker for neuroendocrine neoplasia: comparison with neuron-specific enolase and the α-subunit of glycoprotein hormones. J Clin Endocrinol Metab 1997;82:2622-2628.
110. Goebel SU, Serrano J, Yu F, et al. Prospective study of the value of serum chromogranin A or serum gastrin levels in the assessment of the presence, extent, or growth of gastrinomas. Cancer 1999; 85:1470-1483.
111. Weber HC, Venzon DJ, Lin JT, et al. Determinants of metastatic rate and survival in patients with Zollinger-Ellison syndrome: a prospective long-term study. Gastroenterology 1995;108:1637-1649.
112. Cadiot G, Vuagnat A, Doukhan I, et al. Prognostic factors in patients with Zollinger-Ellison syndrome and multiple endocrine neoplasia type 1. Groupe d'Etude des Neoplasies Endocriniennes Multiples (GENEM) and Groupe de Recherche et d'Etude du Syndrome de Zollinger-Ellison (GRESZE). Gastroenterology 1999;116:286-293.
113. Lowney JK, Frisella MM, Lairmore TC, Doherty GM. Pancreatic islet cell tumor metastasis in multiple endocrine neoplasia type 1: correlation with primary tumor size. Surgery 1998;124:1043-1048, discussion 1048-1049.
114. Wiedenmann B, Jensen RT, Mignon M, et al. Preoperative diagnosis and surgical management of neuroendocrine gastroenteropancreatic tumors: general recommendations by a consensus workshop. World J Surg 1998;22:309-318.
115. Lairmore TC, Chen VY, DeBenedetti MK, et al. Duodenopancreatic resections in patients with multiple endocrine neoplasia type 1. Ann Surg 2000;231:909-918.
116. Carty SE, Jensen RT, Norton JA. Prospective study of aggressive resection of metastatic pancreatic endocrine tumors. Surgery 1992;112:1024-1031; discussion 1031-1022.
117. Kim YH, Ajani JA, Carrasco CH, et al. Selective hepatic arterial chemoembolization for liver metastases in patients with carcinoid tumor or islet cell carcinoma. Cancer Invest 1999;17:474-478.
118. Eriksson B, Oberg K, Alm G, et al. Treatment of malignant endocrine pancreatic tumours with human leucocyte interferon. Lancet 1986;2:1307-1309.
119. Moertel CG, Lefkopoulo M, Lipsitz S, et al. Streptozocin-doxorubicin, streptozocin-fluorouracil or chlorozotocin in the treatment of advanced islet-cell carcinoma. N Engl J Med 1992;326:519-523.
120. Pisegna JR, Slimak GG, Doppman JL, et al. An evaluation of human recombinant α-interferon in patients with metastatic gastrinoma. Gastroenterology 1993;105:1179-1183.
121. Frank M, Klose KJ, Wied M, et al. Combination therapy with octreotide and α-interferon: effect on tumor growth in metastatic endocrine gastroenteropancreatic tumors. Am J Gastroenterol 1999;94: 1381-1387.
122. Tomassetti P, Migliori M, Corinaldesi R, Gullo L. Treatment of gastroenteropancreatic neuroendocrine tumours with octreotide LAR. Aliment Pharmacol Ther 2000;14:557-560.
123. Maton PN, Gardner JD, Jensen RT. Use of long-acting somatostatin analog SMS 201-995 in patients with pancreatic islet cell tumors. Dig Dis Sci 1989;34:28S-39S.
124. Wymenga AN, Eriksson B, Salmela PI, et al. Efficacy and safety of prolonged-release lanreotide in patients with gastrointestinal neuroendocrine tumors and hormone-related symptoms. J Clin Oncol 1999;17:1111.
125. di Bartolomeo M, Bajetta E, Buzzoni R, et al. Clinical efficacy of octreotide in the treatment of metastatic neuroendocrine tumors. A study by the Italian Trials in Medical Oncology Group. Cancer 1996;77:402-408.
126. Verges B, Boureille F, Goudet P, et al. Pituitary disease in MEN type 1 (MEN1): data from the France-Belgium MEN1 multicenter study. J Clin Endocrinol Metab 2002;87:457-465.
127. Corbetta S, Pizzocaro A, Peracchi M, et al. Multiple endocrine neoplasia type 1 in patients with recognized pituitary tumours of different types [see comments]. Clin Endocrinol 1997;47:507-512.
128. Tortosa F, Chico A, Rodriguez-Espinosa J, et al. Prevalence of MEN 1 in patients with prolactinoma. MEN1 Study Group of the Hospital de la Santa Creu i Sant Pau of Barcelona. Clin Endocrinol (Oxf) 1999;50:272.
129. Carty SE, Helm AK, Amico JA, et al. The variable penetrance and spectrum of manifestations of multiple endocrine neoplasia type 1. Surgery 1998;124:1106-1113; discussion 1113-1104.
130. Stratakis CA, Schussheim DH, Freedman SM, et al. Pituitary macroadenoma in a 5-year-old: an early expression of multiple endocrine neoplasia type 1. J Clin Endocrinol Metab 2000;85: 4776-4780.
131. Sahdev A, Jager R. Bilateral pituitary adenomas occurring with multiple endocrine neoplasia type one. AJNR Am J Neuroradiol 2000;21:1067-1069.
132. O'Brien T, O'Riordan DS, Gharib H, et al. Results of treatment of pituitary disease in multiple endocrine neoplasia, type I. Neurosurgery 1996;39:273-278; discussion 278-279.
133. Weil C. The safety of bromocriptine in long-term use: a review of the literature. Curr Med Res Opin 1986;10:25-51.
134. Bevan JS, Webster J, Burke CW, Scanlon MF. Dopamine agonists and pituitary tumor shrinkage. Endocr Rev 1992;13:220-240.
135. Weil RJ, Vortmeyer AO, Huang S, et al. 11q13 allelic loss in pituitary tumors in patients with multiple endocrine neoplasia syndrome type 1. Clin Cancer Res 1998;4:1673-1678.
136. Thakker RV, Pook MA, Wooding C, et al. Association of somatotrophinomas with loss of alleles on chromosome 11 and with Gsp mutations. J Clin Invest 1993;91:2815-2821.
137. Thorner MO, Frohman LA, Leong DA, et al. Extrahypothalamic growth-hormone-releasing factor (GRF) secretion is a rare cause of acromegaly: plasma GRF levels in 177 acromegalic patients. J Clin Endocrinol Metab 1984;59:846-849.

138. Sano T, Yamasaki R, Saito H, et al. Growth hormone–releasing hormone (GHRH)-secreting pancreatic tumor in a patient with multiple endocrine neoplasia type I. Am J Surg Pathol 1987;11:810-819.
139. Asa SL, Singer W, Kovacs K, et al. Pancreatic endocrine tumour producing growth hormone–releasing hormone associated with multiple endocrine neoplasia type I syndrome. Acta Endocrinol (Copenh) 1987;115:331-337.
140. Oka H, Kameya T, Sato Y, et al. Significance of growth hormone–releasing hormone receptor mRNA in non-neoplastic pituitary and pituitary adenomas: a study by RT-PCR and in situ hybridization. J Neurooncol 1999;41:197-204.
141. Newman CB, Melmed S, Snyder PJ, et al. Safety and efficacy of long-term octreotide therapy of acromegaly: results of a multicenter trial in 103 patients—a clinical research center study. J Clin Endocrinol Metab 1995;80:2768-2775.
142. Trainer PJ, Drake WM, Katznelson L, et al. Treatment of acromegaly with the growth hormone–receptor antagonist pegvisomant. N Engl J Med 2000;342:1171-1177.
143. Lamers CB, Froeling PG. Clinical significance of hyperparathyroidism in familial multiple endocrine adenomatosis type I (MEA I). Am J Med 1979;66:422-424.
144. Stewart PM. Current therapy for acromegaly. Trends Endocrinol Metab 2000;11:128-132.
145. Skogseid B, Larsson C, Lindgren PG, et al. Clinical and genetic features of adrenocortical lesions in multiple endocrine neoplasia type 1. J Clin Endocrinol Metab 1992;75:76-81.
146. Houdelette P, Chagnon A, Dumotier J, Marthan E. [Malignant adrenocortical tumor as a part of Wermer's syndrome. Apropos of a case]. J Chir (Paris) 1989;126:385-387.
147. Abe T, Yoshimoto K, Taniyama M, et al. An unusual kindred of the multiple endocrine neoplasia type 1 (MEN1) in Japanese. J Clin Endocrinol Metab 2000;85:1327-1330.
148. Harpole DH Jr, Feldman JM, Buchanan S, et al. Bronchial carcinoid tumors: a retrospective analysis of 126 patients. Ann Thorac Surg 1992;54:50-54; discussion 54-55.
149. Teh BT. Thymic carcinoids in multiple endocrine neoplasia type 1. J Intern Med 1998;243:501-504.
150. Teh BT, Zedenius J, Kytola S, et al. Thymic carcinoids in multiple endocrine neoplasia type 1. Ann Surg 1998;228:99-105.
151. Burgess JR, Greenaway TM, Parameswaran V, et al. Enteropancreatic malignancy associated with multiple endocrine neoplasia type 1: risk factors and pathogenesis. Cancer 1998;83:428-434.
152. Gould PM, Bonner JA, Sawyer TE, et al. Bronchial carcinoid tumors: importance of prognostic factors that influence patterns of recurrence and overall survival. Radiology 1998;208:181-185.
153. Musi M, Carbone RG, Bertocchi C, et al. Bronchial carcinoid tumours: a study on clinicopathological features and role of octreotide scintigraphy. Lung Cancer 1998;22:97-102.
154. Norton JA, Melcher ML, Gibril F, Jensen RT. Gastric carcinoid tumors in multiple endocrine neoplasia-1 patients with Zollinger-Ellison syndrome can be symptomatic, demonstrate aggressive growth, and require surgical treatment. Surgery 2004;136:1267-1274.
155. Bordi C, Falchetti A, Azzoni C, et al. Aggressive forms of gastric neuroendocrine tumors in multiple endocrine neoplasia type I. Am J Surg Pathol 1997;21:1075-1082.
156. Anderson RE. A familial instance of appendiceal carcinoid. Am J Surg 1966;111:738-740.
157. Yeatman TJ, Sharp JV, Kimura AK. Can susceptibility to carcinoid tumors be inherited? Cancer 1989;63:390-393.
158. Oliveira AM, Tazelaar HD, Wentzlaff KA, et al. Familial pulmonary carcinoid tumors. Cancer 2001;91:2104-2109.
159. Babovic-Vuksanovic D, Constantinou CL, Rubin J, et al. Familial occurrence of carcinoid tumors and association with other malignant neoplasms. Cancer Epidemiol Biomarkers Prev 1999;8:715-719.
160. Hemminki K, Li X. Familial carcinoid tumors and subsequent cancers: a nation-wide epidemiologic study from Sweden. Int J Cancer 2001;94:444-448.
161. Cote GJ, Lee JE, Evans DB, Gagel RF. The spectrum of mutations in the MEN1 variant syndromes. Program of the Annual Meeting of the Endocrine Society 1998:106.
162. Nord B, Larsson C, Wong FK, et al. Sporadic follicular thyroid tumors show loss of a 200-kb region in 11q13 without evidence for mutations in the MEN1 gene. Genes Chromosomes Cancer 1999;26:35-39.
163. Darling TN, Skarulis MC, Steinberg SM, et al. Multiple facial angiofibromas and collagenomas in patients with multiple endocrine neoplasia type 1. Arch Dermatol 1997;133:853-857.
164. Asgharian B, Turner ML, Gibril F, et al. Cutaneous tumors in patients with multiple endocrine neoplasm type 1 (MEN1) and gastrinomas: prospective study of frequency and development of criteria with high sensitivity and specificity for MEN1. J Clin Endocrinol Metab 2004;89:5328-5336.
165. Pack S, Turner ML, Zhuang Z, et al. Cutaneous tumors in patients with multiple endocrine neoplasia type 1 show allelic deletion of the MEN1 gene. J Invest Dermatol 1998;110:438-440.
166. Giraud S, Choplin H, Teh BT, et al. A large multiple endocrine neoplasia type 1 family with clinical expression suggestive of anticipation. J Clin Endocrinol Metab 1997;82:3487-3492.
167. Nord B, Platz A, Smoczynski K, et al. Malignant melanoma in patients with multiple endocrine neoplasia type 1 and involvement of the MEN1 gene in sporadic melanoma. Int J Cancer 2000;87:463-467.
168. Vortmeyer AO, Lubensky IA, Skarulis M, et al. Multiple endocrine neoplasia type 1: atypical presentation, clinical course, and genetic analysis of multiple tumors. Mod Pathol 1999;12:919-924.
169. Dackiw AP, Cote GJ, Fleming JB, et al. Screening for MEN1 mutations in patients with atypical endocrine neoplasia. Surgery 1999;126:1097-1103; discussion 1103-1094.
170. McKeeby JL, Li X, Zhuang Z, et al. Multiple leiomyomas of the esophagus, lung, and uterus in multiple endocrine neoplasia type 1. Am J Pathol 2001;159:1121-1127.
171. Asgharian B, Chen YJ, Patronas NJ, et al. Meningiomas may be a component tumor of multiple endocrine neoplasia type 1. Clin Cancer Res 2004;10:869-880.
172. Fearon ER. Human cancer syndromes: clues to the origin and nature of cancer. Science 1997;278:1043-1050.
173. Shepherd JJ. The natural history of multiple endocrine neoplasia type 1. Highly uncommon or highly unrecognized? Arch Surg 1991;126:935-952.
174. Giraud S, Zhang CX, Serova-Sinilnikova O, et al. Germ-line mutation analysis in patients with multiple endocrine neoplasia type 1 and related disorders. Am J Hum Genet 1998;63:455-467.
175. Skogseid B, Eriksson B, Lundqvist G, et al. Multiple endocrine neoplasia type 1: a 10-year prospective screening study in four kindreds. J Clin Endocrinol Metab 1991;73:281-287.
176. Gaitan D, Loosen PT, Orth DN. Two patients with Cushing's disease in a kindred with multiple endocrine neoplasia type I. J Clin Endocrinol Metab 1993;76:1580-1582.
177. Hao W, Skarulis MC, Simonds WF, et al. Multiple endocrine neoplasia type 1 variant with frequent prolactinoma and rare gastrinoma. J Clin Endocrinol Metab 2004;89:3776-3784.
178. Kassem M, Kruse TA, Wong FK, et al. Familial isolated hyperparathyroidism as a variant of multiple endocrine neoplasia type 1 in a large Danish pedigree. J Clin Endocrinol Metab 2000;85:165-167.
179. Marx SJ, Spiegel AM, Levine MA, et al. Familial hypocalciuric hypercalcemia: the relation to primary parathyroid hyperplasia. N Engl J Med 1982;307:416-426.
180. Carrasco CA, Gonzalez AA, Carvajal CA, et al. Novel intronic mutation of MEN1 gene causing familial isolated primary hyperparathyroidism. J Clin Endocrinol Metab 2004;89:4124-4129.
181. Simonds WF, James-Newton LA, Agarwal SK, et al. Familial isolated hyperparathyroidism: clinical and genetic characteristics of 36 kindreds. Medicine (Baltimore) 2002;81:1-26.
182. Brandi ML, Gagel RF, Angeli A, et al. Guidelines for diagnosis and therapy of MEN type 1 and type 2. J Clin Endocrinol Metab 2001;86:5658-5671.
183. Uchino S, Noguchi S, Sato M, et al. Screening of the *Men1* gene and discovery of germ-line and somatic mutations in apparently sporadic parathyroid tumors. Cancer Res 2000;60:5553-5557.
184. Andersen HO, Jorgensen PE, Bardram L, Hilsted L. Screening for multiple endocrine neoplasia type 1 in patients with recognized pituitary adenoma. Clin Endocrinol (Oxf) 1990;33:771-775.
185. Corbetta S, Pizzocaro A, Peracchi M, et al. Multiple endocrine neoplasia type 1 in patients with recognized pituitary tumours of different types. Clin Endocrinol (Oxf) 1997;47:507-512.

186. Marx SJ, Attie MF, Levine MA, et al. The hypocalciuric or benign variant of familial hypercalcemia: clinical and biochemical features in fifteen kindreds. Medicine (Baltimore) 1981;60:397-412.
187. Law WM Jr, Heath H III. Familial benign hypercalcemia (hypocalciuric hypercalcemia). Clinical and pathogenetic studies in 21 families. Ann Intern Med 1985;102:511-519.
188. Firek AF, Kao PC, Heath H 3rd. Plasma intact parathyroid hormone (PTH) and PTH-related peptide in familial benign hypercalcemia: greater responsiveness to endogenous PTH than in primary hyperparathyroidism. J Clin Endocrinol Metab 1991;72:541-546.
189. Thorgeirsson U, Costa J, Marx SJ. The parathyroid glands in familial hypocalciuric hypercalcemia. Hum Pathol 1981;12:229-237.
190. Marx SJ. Clinical review 109: Contrasting paradigms for hereditary hyperfunction of endocrine cells. J Clin Endocrinol Metab 1999;84:3001-3009.
191. Heath H 3rd, Jackson CE, Otterud B, Leppert MF. Genetic linkage analysis in familial benign (hypocalciuric) hypercalcemia: evidence for locus heterogeneity. Am J Hum Genet 1993;53:193-200.
192. Lloyd SE, Pannett AA, Dixon PH, et al. Localization of familial benign hypercalcemia, Oklahoma variant (FBHOk), to chromosome 19q13. Am J Hum Genet 1999;64:189-195.
193. Carling T, Szabo E, Bai M, et al. Familial hypercalcemia and hypercalciuria caused by a novel mutation in the cytoplasmic tail of the calcium receptor. J Clin Endocrinol Metab 2000;85: 2042-2047.
194. Warner JV, Nyholt DR, Busfield F, et al. Familial isolated hyperparathyroidism is linked to a 1.7 Mb region on chromosome 2p13.3-14. J Med Genet 2006;43:e12.
195. Warner J, Epstein M, Sweet A, et al. Genetic testing in familial isolated hyperparathyroidism: unexpected results and their implications. J Med Genet 2004;41:155-160.
196. Jackson CE, Norum RA, Boyd SB, et al. Hereditary hyperparathyroidism and multiple ossifying jaw fibromas: a clinically and genetically distinct syndrome. Surgery 1990;108:1006-1012.
197. Teh BT, Farnebo F, Twigg S, et al. Familial isolated hyperparathyroidism maps to the hyperparathyroidism–jaw tumor locus in 1q21-q32 in a subset of families. J Clin Endocrinol Metab 1998;83: 2114-2120.
198. Streeten EA, Weinstein LS, Norton JA, et al. Studies in a kindred with parathyroid carcinoma. J Clin Endocrinol Metab 1992;75: 362-366.
199. Shattuck TM, Valimaki S, Obara T, et al. Somatic and germ-line mutations of the HRPT2 gene in sporadic parathyroid carcinoma. N Engl J Med 2003;349:1722-1729.
200. Szabo J, Heath B, Hill VM, et al. Hereditary hyperparathyroidism–jaw tumor syndrome: the endocrine tumor gene *HRPT2* maps to chromosome 1q21-q31. Am J Hum Genet 1995;56:944-950.
201. Teh BT, Farnebo F, Kristoffersson U, et al. Autosomal dominant primary hyperparathyroidism and jaw tumor syndrome associated with renal hamartomas and cystic kidney disease: linkage to 1q21-q32 and loss of the wild type allele in renal hamartomas. J Clin Endocrinol Metab 1996;81:4204-4211.
202. Bradley KJ, Hobbs MR, Buley ID, et al. Uterine tumours are a phenotypic manifestation of the hyperparathyroidism–jaw tumour syndrome. J Intern Med 2005;257:18-26.
203. Warner J, Epstein M, Sweet A, et al. Genetic testing in familial isolated hyperparathyroidism: unexpected results and their implications. J Med Genet 2004;41:155-160.
204. Simonds WF, Robbins CM, Agarwal SK, et al. Familial isolated hyperparathyroidism is rarely caused by germline mutation in *HRPT2*, the gene for the hyperparathyroidism–jaw tumor syndrome. J Clin Endocrinol Metab 2004;89:96-102.
205. Keiser HR, Beaven MA, Doppman J, et al. Sipple's syndrome: medullary thyroid carcinoma, pheochromocytoma, and parathyroid disease. Ann Intern Med 1973;78:561-579.
206. Schuffenecker I, Virally-Monod M, Brohet R, et al. Risk and penetrance of primary hyperparathyroidism in multiple endocrine neoplasia type 2A families with mutations at codon 634 of the RET proto-oncogene. Groupe D'etude des Tumeurs a Calcitonine. J Clin Endocrinol Metab 1998;83:487-491.
207. Huang SM, Duh QY, Shaver J, et al. Familial hyperparathyroidism without multiple endocrine neoplasia. World J Surg 1997;21:22-28; discussion 29.
208. Watanabe T, Tsukamoto F, Shimizu T, et al. Familial isolated hyperparathyroidism caused by single adenoma: a distinct entity different from multiple endocrine neoplasia. Endocr J 1998;45: 637-646.
209. Berezin M, Karasik A. Familial prolactinoma. Clin Endocrinol (Oxf) 1995;42:483-486.
210. Vierimaa O, Georgitsi M, Lehtonen R, et al. Pituitary adenoma. predisposition caused by germline mutations in the AIP gene. Science 2006; 312:1228-1230.
211. Larsson C, Skogseid B, Oberg K, et al. Multiple endocrine neoplasia type 1 gene maps to chromosome 11 and is lost in insulinoma. Nature 1988;332:85-87.
212. Knudson AG Jr. Mutation and cancer: Statistical study of retinoblastoma. Proc Natl Acad Sci USA 1971;68:820-823.
213. Knudson AG. Hereditary cancer: two hits revisited. J Cancer Res Clin Oncol 1996;122:135-140.
214. Chandrasekharappa SC, Guru SC, Manickam P, et al. Positional cloning of the gene for multiple endocrine neoplasiatype 1. Science 1997;276:404-407.
215. Emmert-Buck MR, Lubensky IA, Dong Q, et al. Localization of the multiple endocrine neoplasia type I (MEN1) gene based on tumor loss of heterozygosity analysis. Cancer Res 1997;57:1855-1858.
216. Guru SC, Agarwal SK, Manickam P, et al. A transcript map for the 2.8-Mb region containing the multiple endocrine neoplasia type 1 locus [letter]. Genome Research 1997;7:725-735.
217. Lemmens I, Van de Ven WJ, Kas K, et al. Identification of the multiple endocrine neoplasia type 1 (MEN1) gene. The European Consortium on MEN1. Human Molecular Genetics 1997;6: 1177-1183.
218. Mayr B, Brabant G, von zur Muhlen A. Menin mutations in MEN1 patients [letter; comment]. J Clin Endocrinol Metab 1998;83: 3004-3005.
219. Guru SC, Olufemi SE, Manickam P, et al. A 2.8-Mb clone contig of the multiple endocrine neoplasia type 1 (MEN1) region at 11q13. Genomics 1997;42:436-445.
220. Guru SC, Goldsmith PK, Burns AL, et al. Menin, the product of the *MEN1* gene, is a nuclear protein. Proc Natl Acad Sci U S A 1998;95:1630-1634.
221. Manickam P, Vogel AM, Agarwal SK, et al. Isolation, characterization, expression and functional analysis of the zebrafish ortholog of *MEN1*. Mamm Genome 2000;11:448-454.
222. Agarwal SK, Guru SC, Heppner C, et al. Menin interacts with the AP1 transcription factor JunD and represses JunD-activated transcription. Cell 1999;96:143-152.
223. Gobl AE, Berg M, Lopez-Egido JR, et al. Menin represses JunD-activated transcription by a histone deacetylase-dependent mechanism. Biochim Biophys Acta 1999;1447:51-56.
224. Knapp JI, Heppner C, Hickman AB, et al. Identification and characterization of JunD missense mutants that lack menin binding. Oncogene 2000;19:4706-4712.
225. Thepot D, Weitzman JB, Barra J, et al. Targeted disruption of the murine junD gene results in multiple defects in male reproductive function. Development 2000;127:143-153.
226. Agarwal SK, Scacheri PC, Rice TS et al. MEN1 gene: mutation and pathophysiology. Ann d'Endocrinol 67 Suppl 4: IS12-IS13, 2006.
227. Herman JG, Latif F, Weng Y, et al. Silencing of the VHL tumor-suppressor gene by DNA methylation in renal carcinoma. Proc Natl Acad Sci U S A 1994;91:9700-9704.
228. Heppner C, Kester MB, Agarwal SK, et al. Somatic mutation of the *MEN1* gene in parathyroid tumours. Nature Genet 1997;16: 375-378.
229. Farnebo F, Teh BT, Kytola S, et al. Alterations of the *MEN1* gene in sporadic parathyroid tumors [see comments]. J Clin Endocrinol Metab 1998;83:2627-2630.
230. Carling T, Correa P, Hessman O, et al. Parathyroid *MEN1* gene mutations in relation to clinical characteristics of nonfamilial primary hyperparathyroidism [see comments]. J Clin Endocrinol Metab 1998;83:2960-2963.
231. Farnebo F, Kytola S, Teh BT, et al. Alternative genetic pathways in parathyroid tumorigenesis. J Clin Endocrinol Metab 1999;84: 3775-3780.
232. Zhuang Z, Vortmeyer AO, Pack S, et al. Somatic mutations of the MEN1 tumor suppressor gene in sporadic gastrinomas and insulinomas. Cancer Res 1997;57:4682-4686.
233. Wang EH, Ebrahimi SA, Wu AY, et al. Mutation of the *MENIN* gene in sporadic pancreatic endocrine tumors. Cancer Research 1998;58:4417-4420.

234. Goebel SU, Heppner C, Burns AL, et al. Genotype/phenotype correlation of multiple endocrine neoplasia type 1 gene mutations in sporadic gastrinomas. J Clin Endocrinol Metab 2000;85: 116-123.
235. Gortz B, Roth J, Krahenmann A, et al. Mutations and allelic deletions of the *MEN1* gene are associated with a subset of sporadic endocrine pancreatic and neuroendocrine tumors and not restricted to foregut neoplasms. Am J Pathol 1999;154:429-436.
236. Debelenko LV, Brambilla E, Agarwal SK, et al. Identification of *MEN1* gene mutations in sporadic carcinoid tumors of the lung. Hum Mol Genet 1997;6:2285-2290.
237. Zhuang Z, Ezzat SZ, Vortmeyer AO, et al. Mutations of the MEN1 tumor suppressor gene in pituitary tumors. Cancer Research 1997;57:5446-5451.
238. Tanaka C, Kimura T, Yang P, et al. Analysis of loss of heterozygosity on chromosome 11 and infrequent inactivation of the *MEN1* gene in sporadic pituitary adenomas. J Clin Endocrinol Metab 1998;83: 2631-2634.
239. Prezant TR, Levine J, Melmed S. Molecular characterization of the men1 tumor suppressor gene in sporadic pituitary tumors. J Clin Endocrinol Metab 1998;83:1388-1391.
240. Tanaka C, Yoshimoto K, Yamada S, et al. Absence of germ-line mutations of the multiple endocrine neoplasia type 1 (MEN1) gene in familial pituitary adenoma in contrast to MEN1 in Japanese [see comments]. J Clin Endocrinol Metab 1998;83:960-965.
241. Schmidt MC, Henke RT, Stangl AP, et al. Analysis of the MEN1 gene in sporadic pituitary adenomas. J Pathol 1999;188:168-173.
242. Gortz B, Roth J, Speel EJ, et al. *MEN1* gene mutation analysis of sporadic adrenocortical lesions. Int J Cancer 1999;80:373-379.
243. Heppner C, Reincke M, Agarwal SK, et al. *MEN1* gene analysis in sporadic adrenocortical neoplasms. J Clin Endocrinol Metab 1999;84:216-219.
244. Tahara H, Imanishi Y, Yamada T, et al. Rare somatic inactivation of the multiple endocrine neoplasia type 1 gene in secondary hyperparathyroidism of uremia. J Clin Endocrinol Metab 2000; 85:4113-4117.
245. Imanishi Y, Palanisamy N, Tahara H, et al. Molecular pathogenetic analysis of parathyroid carcinoma [abstract]. J Bone Miner Res 1999;14(suppl 1):S421.
246. Boni R, Vortmeyer AO, Pack S, et al. Somatic mutations of the MEN1 tumor suppressor gene detected in sporadic angiofibromas [letter]. J Invest Dermatol 1998;111:539-540.
247. Vortmeyer AO, Boni R, Pak E, et al. Multiple endocrine neoplasia 1 gene alterations in MEN1-associated and sporadic lipomas [letter]. J Natl Cancer Inst 1998;90:398-399.
248. Debelenko LV, Swalwell JI, Kelley MJ, et al. MEN1 gene mutation analysis of high-grade neuroendocrine lung carcinoma. Genes Chromosomes Cancer 2000;28:58-65.
249. Boni R, Vortmeyer AO, Huang S, et al. Mutation analysis of the MEN1 tumour suppressor gene in malignant melanoma. Melanoma Res 1999;9:249-252.
250. Thieblemont C, Pack S, Sakai A, et al. Allelic loss of 11q13 as detected by MEN1-FISH is not associated with mutation of the *MEN1* gene in lymphoid neoplasms. Leukemia 1999;13: 85-91.
251. Agarwal SK, Debelenko LV, Kester MB, et al. Analysis of recurrent germline mutations in the *MEN1* gene encountered in apparently unrelated families. Hum Mutat 1998;12:75-82.
252. Kishi M, Tsukada T, Shimizu S, et al. A large germline deletion of the *MEN1* gene in a family with multiple endocrine neoplasia type 1. Jpn J Cancer Res 1998;89:1-5.
253. Teh BT, Kytola S, Farnebo F, et al. Mutation analysis of the *MEN1* gene in multiple endocrine neoplasia type 1, familial acromegaly and familial isolated hyperparathyroidism. J Clin Endocrinol Metab 1998;83:2621-2626.
254. Poncin J, Abs R, Velkeniers B, et al. Mutation analysis of the *MEN1* gene in Belgian patients with multiple endocrine neoplasia type 1 and related diseases. Hum Mutat 1999;13:54-60.
255. Mutch MG, Dilley WG, Sanjurjo F, et al. Germline mutations in the multiple endocrine neoplasia type 1 gene: evidence for frequent splicing defects. Hum Mutat 1999;13:175-185.
256. Mayer K, Ballhausen W, Rott HD. Mutation screening of the entire coding regions of the *TSC1* and the *TSC2* gene with the protein truncation test (PTT) identifies frequent splicing defects. Hum Mutat 1999;14:401-411.
257. Olufemi SE, Green JS, Manickam P, et al. Common ancestral mutation in the *MEN1* gene is likely responsible for the prolactinoma variant of MEN1 (MEN1Burin) in four kindreds from Newfoundland. Hum Mutat 1998;11:264-269.
258. Thakker RV, Bouloux P, Wooding C, et al. Association of parathyroid tumors in multiple endocrine neoplasia type 1 with loss of alleles on chromosome 11. N Engl J Med 1989;321: 218-224.
259. Debelenko LV, Emmert-Buck MR, Zhuang Z, et al. The multiple endocrine neoplasia type I gene locus is involved in the pathogenesis of type II gastric carcinoids. Gastroenterology 1997;113: 773-781.
260. Teh BT, McArdle J, Chan SP, et al. Clinicopathologic studies of thymic carcinoids in multiple endocrine neoplasia type 1. Medicine (Baltimore) 1997;76:21-29.
261. Tahara H, Smith AP, Gas RD, et al. Genomic localization of novel candidate tumor suppressor gene loci in human parathyroid adenomas. Cancer Res 1996;56:599-605.
262. Shan L, Nakamura Y, Murakami M, et al. Clonal emergence in uremic parathyroid hyperplasia is not related to MEN1 gene abnormality. Jpn J Cancer Res 1999;90:965-969.
263. Arnold A, Brown MF, Urena P, et al. Monoclonality of parathyroid tumors in chronic renal failure and in primary parathyroid hyperplasia. J Clin Invest 1995;95:2047-2053.
264. Falchetti A, Bale AE, Amorosi A, et al. Progression of uremic hyperparathyroidism involves allelic loss on chromosome 11. J Clin Endocrinol Metab 1993;76:139-144.
265. Farnebo F, Farnebo LO, Nordenstrom J, Larsson C. Allelic loss on chromosome 11 is uncommon in parathyroid glands of patients with hypercalcaemic secondary hyperparathyroidism. Eur J Surg 1997;163:331-337.
266. Jakobovitz O, Nass D, DeMarco L, et al. Carcinoid tumors frequently display genetic abnormalities involving chromosome 11. J Clin Endocrinol Metab 1996;81:3164-3167.
267. Williamson C, Pannett A, Pang JT, et al. Localisation of a tumour suppressor gene causing endocrine tumours to a four centimorgan region on chromosome 1. Program of the Annual Meeting of the Endocrine Society 1996;Abstract.
268. Kytola S, Makinen MJ, Kahkonen M, et al. Comparative genomic hybridization studies in tumours from a patient with multiple endocrine neoplasia type 1. Eur J Endocrinol 1998;139:202-206.
269. Franklin DS, Godfrey VL, O'Brien DA, et al. Functional collaboration between different cyclin-dependent kinase inhibitors suppresses tumor growth with distinct tissue specificity. Mol Cell Biol 2000;20:6147-6158.
270. Pestell RG, Albanese C, Reutens AT, et al. The cyclins and cyclin-dependent kinase inhibitors in hormonal regulation of proliferation and differentiation. Endocr Rev 1999;20:501-534.
271. Scappaticci S, Fossati GS, Valenti L, et al. A search for double minute chromosomes in cultured lymphocytes from different types of tumors. Cancer Genet Cytogenet 1995;82:50-53.
272. Sakurai A, Katai M, Itakura Y, et al. Premature centromere division in patients with multiple endocrine neoplasia type 1. Cancer Genet Cytogenet 1999;109:138-140.
273. Ikeo Y, Sakurai A, Suzuki R, et al. Proliferation-associated expression of the MEN1 gene as revealed by in situ hybridization: possible role of the menin as a negative regulator of cell proliferation under DNA damage. Lab Invest 2000;80:797-804.
274. Vortmeyer AO, Boni R, Pack SD, et al. Perivascular cells harboring multiple endocrine neoplasia type 1 alterations are neoplastic cells in angiofibromas. Cancer Res 1999;59:274-278.
275. Deng G, Lu Y, Zlotnikov G, et al. Loss of heterozygosity in normal tissue adjacent to breast carcinomas. Science 1996;274: 2057-2059.
276. Zimering MB, Katsumata N, Sato Y, et al. Increased basic fibroblast growth factor in plasma from multiple endocrine neoplasia type 1: relation to pituitary tumor. J Clin Endocrinol Metab 1993;76: 1182-1187.
277. Agarwal SK, Kester MB, Debelenko LV, et al. Germline mutations of the *MEN1* gene in familial multiple endocrine neoplasia type 1 and related states. Hum Mol Genet 1997;6:1169-1175.
278. Teh BT, Esapa CT, Houlston R, et al. A family with isolated hyperparathyroidism segregating a missense *MEN1* mutation and

showing loss of the wild-type alleles in the parathyroid tumors. Am J Hum Genet 1998;63:1544-1549.

279. Pellegata NS, Quintanilla-Martinez L, Siggelkow H, et al 2006 Germ-line mutations in p27Kip1 cause a multiple endocrine neoplasia syndrome in rats and humans. Proc Natl Acad Sci U S A 103: 15558-15563; erratum in Proc Nat Acad Sci U S A 2006;103: 19213.
280. Larsson C, Calender A, Grimmond S, et al. Molecular tools for presymptomatic testing in multiple endocrine neoplasia type 1. J Intern Med 1995;238:239-244.
281. National Institute of Diabetes and Digestive and Kidney Dieseasess. Multiple Endocrine Neoplasia Type 1. Available at http://www.niddk.nih.gov/health/endo/pubs/fMEN1/fMEN1.htm (accessed March 7, 2007).
282. GeneTests. Laboratory directory. Available at http://www.genetests.org/servlet/access?id=8888891&key=Zf69pk1FekTOW&fcn=y&fw=8Cni&filename=/about/content/lab.html (accessed March 7, 2007).
283. Roijers JF, de Wit MJ, van der Luijt RB, et al. Criteria for mutation analysis in MEN 1-suspected patients: MEN 1 case-finding. Eur J Clin Invest 2000;30:487-492.
284. Hai N, Aoki N, Matsuda A, et al. Germline *MEN1* mutations in sixteen Japanese families with multiple endocrine neoplasia type 1 (MEN1). Eur J Endocrinol 1999;141:475-480.
285. Morelli A, Falchetti A, Martineti V, et al. *MEN1* gene mutation analysis in Italian patients with multiple endocrine neoplasia type 1. Eur J Endocrinol 2000;142:131-137.
286. Courseaux A, Grosgeorge J, Gaudray P, et al. Definition of the minimal *MEN1* candidate area based on a 5-Mb integrated map of proximal 11q13. The European Consortium on Men1, (GENEM 1; Groupe d'Etude des Neoplasies Endocriniennes Multiples de type 1). Genomics 1996;37:354-365.
287. Stock JL, Warth MR, Teh BT, et al. A kindred with a variant of multiple endocrine neoplasia type 1 demonstrating frequent expression of pituitary tumors but not linked to the multiple endocrine neoplasia type 1 locus at chromosome region 11q13. J Clin Endocrinol Metab 1997;82:486-492.
288. Hai N, Aoki N, Shimatsu A, et al. Clinical features of multiple endocrine neoplasia type 1 (MEN1) phenocopy without germline *MEN1* gene mutations: analysis of 20 Japanese sporadic cases with MEN1. Clin Endocrinol (Oxf) 2000;52:509-518.
289. Bassett JH, Forbes SA, Pannett AA, et al. Characterization of mutations in patients with multiple endocrine neoplasia type 1. Am J Hum Genet 1998;62:232-244.
290. Waterlot C, Porchet N, Bauters C, et al. Type 1 multiple endocrine neoplasia (MEN1): contribution of genetic analysis to the screening and follow-up of a large French kindred. Clin Endocrinol (Oxf) 1999;51:101-107.
291. Grayson RH, Halperin JM, Sharma V, et al. Changes in plasma prolactin and catecholamine metabolite levels following acute needle stick in children. Psychiatry Res 1997;69:27-32.
292. Benya RV, Metz DC, Venzon DJ, et al. Zollinger-Ellison syndrome can be the initial endocrine manifestation in patients with multiple endocrine neoplasia type I. Am J Med 1994;97:436-444.
293. Burgess JR, Nord B, David R, et al. Phenotype and phenocopy: the relationship between genotype and clinical phenotype in a single large family with multiple endocrine neoplasia type 1 (MEN 1). Clin Endocrinol (Oxf) 2000;53:205-211.
294. Oberg K, Skogseid B. The ultimate biochemical diagnosis of endocrine pancreatic tumours in MEN-1. J Intern Med 1998;243: 471-476.
295. Sipple JH. Multiple endocrine neoplasia type 2 syndromes: historical perspectives. Henry Ford Hosp Med J 1984;32:219-221.
296. Cushman P Jr. Familial endocrine tumors: report of two unrelated kindred affected with pheochromocytomas, one also with multiple thyroid carcinomas. Am J Med 1962;32:352-360.
297. Hazard JB, Hawk WA, Crile G Jr. Medullary (solid) carcinoma of the thyroid: A clinicopathologic entity. J Clin Endocrinol Metab 1959;19:152-161.
298. Williams ED. A review of 17 cases of carcinoma of the thyroid and phaeochromocytoma. J Clin Pathol 1965;18:288-292.
299. Wells SA Jr, Ontjes DA, Cooper CW, et al. The early diagnosis of medullary carcinoma of the thyroid gland in patients with multiple endocrine neoplasia type II. Ann Surg 1975;182:362-370.
300. Melvin KEW, Miller HH, Tashjian AH Jr. Early diagnosis of medullary carcinoma of the thyroid gland by means of calcitonin assay. N Engl J Med 1971;285:1115-1120.
301. Sizemore GW, Carney JA, Heath H III,. Epidemiology of medullary carcinoma of the thyroid gland: a 5 year experience. Surg Clin North Am 1977;57:633-645.
302. Graze K, Spiler IJ, Tashjian AH Jr, et al. Natural history of familial medullary thyroid carcinoma: effect of a program for early diagnosis. N Engl J Med 1978;299:980-985.
303. Gagel RF, Tashjian AH Jr, Cummings T, et al. Impact of prospective screening for multiple endocrine neoplasia type 2. Henry Ford Hosp Med J 1987;35:94-98.
304. Lips CJ, Landsvater RM, Hoppener JW, et al. Clinical screening as compared with DNA analysis in families with multiple endocrine neoplasia type 2A. N Engl J Med 1994;331:828-835.
305. Skinner MA, Moley JA, Dilley WG, et al. Prophylactic thyroidectomy in multiple endocrine neoplasia type 2A. N Engl J Med 2005;353:1105-1113.
306. Machens A, Niccoli-Sire P, Hoegel J, et al. Early malignant progression of hereditary medullary thyroid cancer. N Engl J Med 2003;349:1517-1525.
307. Heath H III, Sizemore GW, Carney JA. Preoperative diagnosis of occult parathyroid hyperplasia by calcium infusion in patients with multiple endocrine neoplasia, type 2a. J Clin Endocrinol Metab 1976;43:428-435.
308. Wolfe HJ, Melvin KEW, Cervi-Skinner SJ, et al. C-cell hyperplasia preceding medullary thyroid carcinoma. N Engl J Med 1973;289: 437-441.
309. Wolfe HJ, DeLellis RA. Familial medullary thyroid carcinoma and C-cell hyperplasia. Clin Endocrinol Metab 1981;10:351-365.
310. Samaan NA, Draznin MB, Halpin RE, et al. Multiple endocrine syndrome type IIb in early childhood. Cancer 1991;68:1832-1834.
311. Graham SM, Genel M, Touloukian RJ, et al. Provocative testing for occult medullary carcinoma of the thyroid: findings in seven children with multiple endocrine neoplasia type IIa. J Pediatr Surg 1987;22:501-503.
312. Moley JF, DeBenedetti MK. Patterns of nodal metastases in palpable medullary thyroid carcinoma: recommendations for extent of node dissection. Ann Surg 1999;229:880-887; discussion 887-888.
313. Wells SA Jr, Chi DD, Toshima K, et al. Predictive DNA testing and prophylactic thyroidectomy in patients at risk for multiple endocrine neoplasia type 2A. Ann Surg 1994;220:237-247; discussion 247-250.
314. Gagel RF, Cote GJ, Martins Bugalho MJ, et al. Clinical use of molecular information in the management of multiple endocrine neoplasia type 2A. J Intern Med 1995;238:333-341.
315. Cote GJ, Gould JA, Huang SC, Gagel RF. Studies of short-term secretion of peptides produced by alternative RNA processing. Mol Cell Endocrinol 1987;53:211-219.
316. Gagel RF, Palmer WN, Leonhart K, et al. Somatostatin production by a human medullary thyroid carcinoma cell line. Endocrinology 1986;118:1643-1651.
317. Atkins FL, Beaven MA, Keiser HR. Dopa decarboxylase in medullary carcinoma of the thyroid. N Engl J Med 1973;289: 545-548.
318. O'Connor DT, Deftos LJ. Secretion of chromogranin A by peptide-producing endocrine neoplasms. N Engl J Med 1986;314: 1145-1151.
319. Sevarino KA, Wu P, Jackson IMD, et al. Biosynthesis of thyrotropin releasing hormone by a rat medullary thyroid carcinoma cell line. J Biol Chem 1988;263:620-623.
320. Yamaguchi K, Abe K, Adachi I, et al. Concomitant production of immunoreactive gastrin-releasing peptide and calcitonin in medullary carcinoma of the thyroid. Metabolism 1984;33:724-727.
321. Baylin SB, Beaven MA, Buja LM, et al. Histaminase activity: a biochemical marker for medullary carcinoma of the thyroid. Am J Med 1972;53:723-733.
322. Gagel R. Tumor markers of medullary thyroid carcinoma. In Fishman W, ed. Oncodevelopmental Markers: Biologic, Diagnostic and Monitoring Aspects. New York: Academic Press, 1983: 222-239.
323. Guillem JG, Wood WC, Moley JF, et al. ASCO/SSO review of current role of risk-reducing surgery in common hereditary cancer syndromes. J Clin Oncol 2006;24:4642-4660.

324. Fleming JB, Lee JE, Bouvet M, et al. Surgical strategy for the treatment of medullary thyroid carcinoma. Ann Surg 1999;230: 697-707.
325. Gagel RF, Tashjian AH Jr, Cummings T, et al. The clinical outcome of prospective screening for multiple endocrine neoplasia type 2a: an 18-year experience. N Engl J Med 1988;318:478-484.
326. Becker KL, Walton-Moss BJ. Young woman with recurrent yeast infections. Lippincotts Prim Care Pract 2000;4:125-131.
327. Muller B, Becker KL, Schachinger H, et al. Calcitonin precursors are reliable markers of sepsis in a medical intensive care unit. Crit Care Med 2000;28:977-983.
328. Aloia JF, Rasulo P, Deftos LJ, et al. Exercise-induced hypercalcemia and the calciotropic hormones. J Lab Clin Med 1985;106: 229-232.
329. Samaan NA, Schultz PN, Hickey RC. Medullary thyroid carcinoma: prognosis of familial versus sporadic disease and the role of radiotherapy. J Clin Endocrinol Metab 1988;67:801-805.
330. Jackson CE, Talpos GB, Kambouris A, et al. The clinical course after definitive operation for medullary thyroid carcinoma. Surgery 1983;94:995-1001.
331. van Heerden JA, Grant CS, Gharib H, et al. Long-term course of patients with persistent hypercalcitoninemia after apparent curative primary surgery for medullary thyroid carcinoma. Ann Surg 1990;212:395-400.
332. Tisell L, Hansson G, Jansson S, Salander H. Reoperation in the treatment of asymptomatic metastasizing medullary thyroid carcinoma. Surgery 1986;99:60-66.
333. Moley JF, Dilley WG, DeBenedetti MK. Improved results of cervical reoperation for medullary thyroid carcinoma. Ann Surg 1997;225: 734-740.
334. Evans DB, Fleming JB, Lee JE, et al. The surgical treatment of medullary thyroid carcinoma. Semin Surg Oncol 1999;16:50-63.
335. Buhr HJ, Kallinowski F, Raue F, et al. Microsurgical neck dissection for metastasizing medullary thyroid carcinoma. Eur J Surg Oncol 1995;21:195-197.
336. Moley JF, Wells SA, Dilley WG, Tisell LE. Reoperation for recurrent or persistent medullary thyroid carcinoma. Surgery 1993;114: 1090-1096.
337. Wells SA Jr, Baylin SB, Leight GS, et al. The importance of early diagnosis in patients with hereditary medullary thyroid carcinoma. Ann Surg 1982;195:595-599.
338. Carney JA, Sizemore GW, Tyce GM. Bilateral adrenal medullary hyperplasia in multiple endocrine neoplasia, type 2: the precursor of bilateral pheochromocytoma. Mayo Clin Proc 1975;50:3-10.
339. Carney JA, Sizemore GW, Sheps SG. Adrenal medullary disease in multiple endocrine neoplasia, type 2: pheochromocytoma and its precursors. Am J Clin Pathol 1976;66:279-290.
340. DeLellis RA, Wolfe HJ, Gagel RF, et al. Adrenal medullary hyperplasia. A morphometric analysis in patients with familial medullary thyroid carcinoma. Am J Pathol 1976;83:177-196.
341. Carney JA, Sizemore GW, Hayles AB. Multiple endocrine neoplasia, type 2b. Pathobiol Annu 1978;8:105-153.
342. Lips KJ, Van der Sluys Veer J, Struyvenberg A, et al. Bilateral occurrence of pheochromocytoma in patients with the multiple endocrine neoplasia syndrome type 2A (Sipple's syndrome). Am J Med 1981;70:1051-1060.
343. Modigliani E, Vasen H, Raue K, et al. Pheochromocytoma in multiple endocrine neoplasia type 2: European study. J Int Med 1995;238:363-367.
344. Sisson JC, Shapiro B, Beierwaltes WH. Scintigraphy with I-131 MIBG as an aid to the treatment of pheochromocytomas in patients with the multiple endocrine neoplasia type 2 syndromes. Henry Ford Hosp Med J 1984;32:254-261.
345. Casanova S, Rosenberg-Bourgin M, Farkas D, et al. Phaeochromocytoma in multiple endocrine neoplasia type 2 A: survey of 100 cases. Clin Endocrinol (Oxf) 1993;38:531-537.
346. Westfried M, Mandel D, Alderete MN, et al. Sipple's syndrome with a malignant pheochromocytoma presenting as a pericardial effusion. Cardiology 1978;63:305-311.
347. Lee JE, Curley SA, Gagel RF, et al. Cortical-sparing adrenalectomy for patients with bilateral pheochromocytoma. Surgery 1996; 120:1064-1070.
348. Chevinsky AH, Minton JP, Falko JM. Metastatic pheochromocytoma associated with multiple endocrine neoplasia syndrome type II. Arch Surg 1990;125:935-938.
349. Namba H, Kondo H, Yamashita S, et al. Multiple endocrine neoplasia type 2 with malignant pheochromocytoma—long term follow-up of a case by ^{131}I-meta-iodobenzylguanidine scintigraphy. Ann Nucl Med 1992;6:111-115.
350. Hinze R, Machens A, Schneider U, et al. Simultaneously occurring liver metastases of pheochromocytoma and medullary thyroid carcinoma—a diagnostic pitfall with clinical implications for patients with multiple endocrine neoplasia type 2a. Pathol Res Pract 2000;196:477-481.
351. Gentile S, Rainero I, Savi L, et al. Brain metastasis from pheochromocytoma in a patient with multiple endocrine neoplasia type 2A. Panminerva Med 2001;43:305-306.
352. Scopsi L, Castellani MR, Gullo M, et al. Malignant pheochromocytoma in multiple endocrine neoplasia type 2B syndrome. Case report and review of the literature. Tumori 1996;82:480-484.
353. Chodankar CM, Abhyankar SC, Deodhar KP, Shanbhag AM. Sipple's syndrome (multiple endocrine neoplasia) in pregnancy—case report. Aust N Z J Obstet Gynaecol 1982;22:243-244.
354. Moraca Kvapilova L, Op de Coul AA, Merkus JM. Cerebral haemorrhage in a pregnant woman with a multiple endocrine neoplasia syndrome (type 2A or Sipple's syndrome). Eur J Obstet Gynecol Reprod Biol 1985;20:257-263.
355. Eisenhofer G, Lenders JW, Linehan WM, et al. Plasma normetanephrine and metanephrine for detecting pheochromocytoma in von Hippel-Lindau disease and multiple endocrine neoplasia type 2. N Engl J Med 1999;340:1872-1879.
356. Valk TW, Frager MS, Gross MD, et al. Spectrum of pheochromocytoma in multiple endocrine neoplasia. A scintigraphic portrayal using ^{131}I-metaiodobenzylguanidine. Ann Intern Med 1981;94: 762-767.
357. Yobbagy JJ, Levatter R, Sisson JC, et al. Scintigraphic portrayal of the syndrome of multiple endocrine neoplasia type-2B. Clin Nucl Med 1988;13:433-437.
358. Lairmore TC, Ball DW, Baylin SB, Wells SA Jr. Management of pheochromocytomas in patients with multiple endocrine neoplasia type 2 syndromes. Ann Surg 1993;217:595-601.
359. Telenius-Berg M, Ponder MA, Berg B, et al. Quality of life after bilateral adrenalectomy in MEN 2. Henry Ford Hosp Med J 1989;37:160-163.
360. Jansson S, Khorram-Manesh A, Nilsson O, et al. Treatment of bilateral pheochromocytoma and adrenal medullary hyperplasia. Ann N Y Acad Sci 2006;1073:429-435.
361. Diner EK, Franks ME, Behari A, et al. Partial adrenalectomy: the National Cancer Institute experience. Urology 2005;66:19-23.
362. Yip L, Lee JE, Shapiro SE, et al. Surgical management of hereditary pheochromocytoma. J Am Coll Surg 2004;198:525-534.
363. van Heerden JA, Sizemore GW, Carney JA, et al. Bilateral subtotal adrenal resection for bilateral pheochromocytomas in multiple endocrine neoplasia, type IIa: a case report. Surgery 1985;98: 363-366.
364. Evans DB, Lee JE, Merrell RC, Hickey RC. Adrenal medullary disease in multiple endocrine neoplasia type 2. Appropriate management. Endocrinol Metab Clin North Am 1994;23:167-176.
365. Ikeda Y, Takami H, Tajima G, et al. Laparoscopic partial adrenalectomy. Biomed Pharmacother 2002;56 Suppl 1:126s-131s.
366. Carney JA, Roth SI, Heath H, III, et al. The parathyroid glands in multiple endocrine neoplasia type 2b. Am J Pathol 1980; 99:387-398.
367. Skinner MA, Norton JA, Moley JF, et al. Heterotopic autotransplantation of parathyroid tissue in children undergoing total thyroidectomy. J Pediatr Surg 1997;32:510-513.
368. Farndon JR, Leight GS, Dilley WG, et al. Familial medullary thyroid carcinoma without associated endocrinopathies: a distinct clinical entity. Br J Surg 1986;73:278-281.
369. Gagel RF, Levy ML, Donovan DT, et al. Multiple endocrine neoplasia type 2a associated with cutaneous lichen amyloidosis. Ann Intern Med 1989;111:802-806.
370. Nunziata V, di Giovanni G, Lettera AM, et al. Cutaneous lichen amyloidosis associated with multiple endocrine neoplasia type 2A. Henry Ford Hosp J 1989;37:144-146.
371. Chabre O, Labat F, Pinel N, et al. Cutaneous lesion associated with multiple endocrine neoplasia type 2A: lichen amyloidosis or notalgia paresthetica. Henry Ford Hosp J 1992;40:245-248.
372. Wong C-K, Lin C-S. Friction amyloidosis. Int J Dermatol 1988;27: 302-307.

373. Durbec PL, Larsson-Blomberg LB, Schuchardt A, et al. Common origin and developmental dependence on c-ret of subsets of enteric and sympathetic neuroblasts. Development 1996;122: 349-358.
374. Gagel RF. When "The 7-year itch" is indicative of an endocrine malignant condition. Endocr Pract 2002;8:72-74.
375. Verdy MB, Cadotte M, Schurch W, et al. A French Canadian family with multiple endocrine neoplasia type 2 syndromes. Henry Ford Hosp Med J 1984;32:251-253.
376. Eng C, Clayton D, Schuffenecker I, et al. The relationship between specific RET proto-oncogene mutations and disease phenotype in multiple endocrine neoplasia type 2. International RET mutation consortium analysis. JAMA 1996;276:1575-1579.
377. Inoue K, Shimotake T, Tokiwa K, Iwai N. Mutational analysis of the RET proto-oncogene in a kindred with multiple endocrine neoplasia type 2A and Hirschsprung's disease. J Pediatr Surg 1999;34: 1552-1554.
378. Ito S, Iwashita T, Asai N, et al. Biological properties of Ret with cysteine mutations correlate with multiple endocrine neoplasia type 2A, familial medullary thyroid carcinoma, and Hirschsprung's disease phenotype. Cancer Res 1997;57:2870-2872.
379. Sasaki Y, Shimotake T, Go S, Iwai N. Total thyroidectomy for hereditary medullary thyroid carcinoma 12 years after correction of Hirschsprung's disease. Eur J Surg 2001;167:467-469.
380. Williams ED, Pollock DJ. Multiple mucosal neuromata with endocrine tumours: a syndrome allied to Von Recklinghausen's disease. J Pathol Bacteriol 1966;91:71-80.
381. Rashid M, Khairi MR, Dexter RN, et al. Mucosal neuroma, pheochromocytoma and medullary thyroid carcinoma: multiple endocrine neoplasia type 3. Medicine (Baltimore) 1975;54:89-112.
382. Carney JA, Sizemore GW, Hayles AB. C-cell disease of the thyroid gland in multiple endocrine neoplasia, type 2b. Cancer 1979; 44:2173-2183.
383. Carney JA, Go VL, Sizemore GW, Hayles AB. Alimentary-tract ganglioneuromatosis. A major component of the syndrome of multiple endocrine neoplasia, type 2b. N Engl J Med 1976;295: 1287-1291.
384. Khan AH, Desjardins JG, Youssef S, et al. Gastrointestinal manifestations of Sipple syndrome in children. J Pediatr Surg 1987; 22:719-723.
385. Stjernholm MR, Freudenbourg JC, Mooney HS, et al. Medullary carcinoma of the thyroid before age 2 years. J Clin Endocrinol Metab 1980;51:252-253.
386. Gill JR, Reyes-Mugica M, Iyengar S, et al. Early presentation of metastatic medullary carcinoma in multiple endocrine neoplasia, type IIA: implications for therapy. J Pediatr 1996;129:459-464.
387. Smith VV, Eng C, Milla PJ. Intestinal ganglioneuromatosis and multiple endocrine neoplasia type 2B: implications for treatment. Gut 1999;45:143-146.
388. Kakudo K, Carney JA, Sizemore GW. Medullary carcinoma of thyroid. Biologic behavior of the sporadic and familial neoplasm. Cancer 1985;55:2818-2821.
389. Sizemore GW, Carney JA, Gharib H, Capen CC. Multiple endocrine neoplasia type 2B: eighteen-year follow-up of a four-generation family. Henry Ford Hosp J 1992;40:236-244.
390. Vasen HFA, van der Feltz M, Raue F, et al. The natural course of multiple endocrine neoplasia type IIb: a study of 18 cases. Arch Intern Med 1992;152:1250-1252.
391. Carlson KM, Bracamontes J, Jackson CE, et al. Parent-of-origin effects in multiple endocrine neoplasia type 2B. Am J Hum Genet 1994;55:1076-1082.
392. Dyck PJ, Carney JA, Sizemore GW, et al. Multiple endocrine neoplasia, type 2b: phenotype recognition, neurological features and their pathological basis. Ann Neurol 1979;6:302-314.
393. Hubner A, Holschneider AM. Multiple endocrine neoplasias in 3 generations. Langenbecks Arch Chir 1987;372:747-750.
394. Pujol RM, Matias-Guiu X, Miralles J, et al. Multiple idiopathic mucosal neuromas: a minor form of multiple endocrine neoplasia type 2B or a new entity? J Am Acad Dermatol 1997;37:349-352.
395. Gomez JM, Biarnes J, Volpini V, Marti T. Neuromas and prominent corneal nerves without MEN 2B. Ann Endocrinol 1998;59: 492-494.
396. Valentines J, Marigo M, Quintana M, Gomez JM. Familial mucosal neuromatosis: a minor form of the MEN-2b syndrome. J Fr Ophtalmol 1984;7:479-484.
397. Sciubba JJ, D'Amico E, Attie JN. The occurrence of multiple endocrine neoplasia type IIb, in two children of an affected mother. J Oral Pathol 1987;16:310-316.
398. Mathew CG, Chin KS, Easton DF, et al. A linked genetic marker for multiple endocrine neoplasia type 2A on chromosome 10. Nature 1987;328:527-528.
399. Simpson NE, Kidd KK, Goodfellow PJ, et al. Assignment of multiple endocrine neoplasia type 2A to chromosome 10 by linkage. Nature 1987;328:528-530.
400. Mulligan LM, Kwok JB, Healey CS, et al. Germ-line mutations of the RET proto-oncogene in multiple endocrine neoplasia type 2A. Nature 1993;363:458-460.
401. Donis-Keller H, Dou S, Chi D, et al. Mutations in the RET proto-oncogene are associated with MEN 2A and FMTC. Hum Mol Genet 1993;2:851-856.
402. Carlson KM, Dou S, Chi D, et al. Single missense mutation in the tyrosine kinase catalytic domain of the RET protoncogene is associated with multiple endocrine neoplasia type 2B. Proc Natl Acad Sci USA 1994;91:1579-1583.
403. Hofstra RM, Landsvater RM, Ceccherini I, et al. A mutation in the RET proto-oncogene associated with multiple endocrine neoplasia type 2B and sporadic medullary thyroid carcinoma. Nature 1994;367:375-376.
404. Lacroix A, Blanchard L, Villeneuve L, et al. Cosegregation of Hirschsprung's disease (HSCR) with chromosome 10 markers and a ret mutation in a French Canadian family with MEN 2A. Presented as abstract at the V International Workshop on Multiple Endocrine Neoplasia, Stockholm, Sweden, ·· ··-··, 1994.
405. Borst MJ, Van Camp JM, Peacock ML, Decker RA. Mutational analysis of multiple endocrine neoplasia type 2A associated with Hirschsprung's disease. Surgery 1995;117:386-391.
406. Wohllk N, Cote GJ, Bugalho MMJ, et al. Relevance of RET proto-oncogene mutations in sporadic medullary thyroid carcinoma. J Clin Endocrinol Metab 1996;81:3740–3745.
407. Ceccherini I, Romei C, Barone V, et al. Identification of the cys 634-to-tyr mutation of the RET proto-oncogene in a pedigree with mutliple endocrine neoplasia type 2A and localized cutaneous lichen amyloidosis. J Endocr Invest 1994;17:201-204.
408. Edery P, Lyonnet S, Mulligan LM, et al. Mutations of the RET proto-oncogene in Hirschsprung's disease. Nature 1994;367: 378-380.
409. Romeo G, Ronchetto P, Luo Y, et al. Point mutations affecting the tyrosine kinase domain of the RET proto-oncogene in Hirschsprung's disease. Nature 1994;367:377-378.
410. Angrist M, Bolk S, Thiel B, et al. Mutation analysis of the RET receptor tyrosine kinase in Hirschsprung disease. Hum Mol Genet 1995;4:821-830.
411. Eng C, Mulligan LM, Smith DP, et al. Low frequency of germline mutations in the RET proto-oncogene in patients with apparently sporadic medullary thyroid carcinoma. Clin Endocrinol 1995;43: 123-127.
412. Zedenius J, Larsson C, Bergholm U, et al. Mutations of codon 918 in the RET proto-oncogene correlate to poor prognosis in sporadic medullary thyroid carcinomas. J Clin Endocrinol Metab 1995;80: 3088-3090.
413. Komminoth P, Kunz E, Hiort O, et al. Detection of RET proto-oncogene point mutations in paraffin-embedded pheochromocytoma specimens by nonradioactive single-strand conformation polymorphism analysis and direct sequencing. Am J Pathol 1994; 145:922-929.
414. Takahashi M, Ritz J, Cooper GM. Activation of a novel human transforming gene, ret, by DNA rearrangement. Cell 1985;42: 581-588.
415. Takahashi M, Buma Y, Iwamoto T, et al. Cloning and expression of the ret proto-oncogene encoding a tyrosine kinase with two potential transmembrane domains. Oncogene 1988;3:571-578.
416. Donghi R, Sozzi G, Pierotti MA, et al. The oncogene associated with human papillary thyroid carcinoma (PTC) is assigned to chromosome 10 q11-q12 in the same region as multiple endocrine neoplasia type 2A (MEN2A). Oncogene 1989;4:521-523.
417. Bongarzone I, Pierotti MA, Monzini N, et al. High frequency of activation of tyrosine kinase oncogenes in human papillary thyroid carcinoma. Oncogene 1989;4:1457-1462.
418. Takahashi M. The GDNF/RET signaling pathway and human diseases. Cytokine Growth Factor Rev 2001;12:361-373.

419. Vecchio G, Santoro M. Oncogenes and thyroid cancer. Clin Chem Lab Med 2000;38:113-116.
420. Hoff AO, Cote GJ, Gagel RF. Multiple endocrine neoplasias. Annu Rev Physiol 2000;62:377-411.
421. Nikiforova MN, Stringer JR, Blough R, et al. Proximity of chromosomal loci that participate in radiation-induced rearrangements in human cells. Science 2000;290:138-141.
422. Nikiforov YE, Rowland JM, Bove KE, et al. Distinct pattern of ret oncogene rearrangements in morphological variants of radiation-induced and sporadic thyroid papillary carcinomas in children. Cancer Res 1997;57:1690-1694.
423. Chiappetta G, Toti P, Cetta F, et al. The *RET/PTC* oncogene is frequently activated in oncocytic thyroid tumors (Hürthle cell adenomas and carcinomas), but not in oncocytic hyperplastic lesions. J Clin Endocrinol Metab 2002;87:364-369.
424. Sanchez M, Silos-Santiago I, Frisen J, et al. Newborn mice lacking GDNF display renal agenesis and absence of enteric neurons, but no deficits in midbrain dopaminergic neurons. Nature 1996;382: 70-73.
425. Robbins J, Gulick J, Sanchez A, et al. Mouse embryonic stem cells express the cardiac myosin heavy chain genes during development in vitro. J Biol Chem 1990;265:11905-11909.
426. Moore MW, Klein RD, Farinas I, et al. Renal and neuronal abnormalities in mice lacking GDNF. Nature 1996;382:76-79.
427. Pichel JG, Shen L, Sheng HZ, et al. Defects in enteric innervation and kidney development in mice lacking GDNF. Nature 1996; 382:73-76.
428. Schuchardt A, D'Agati V, Larsson-Blomberg L, et al. Defects in the kidney and enteric nervous system of mice lacking the tyrosine kinase receptor Ret. Nature 1994;367:380-383.
429. Jing S, Wen D, Yu Y, et al. GDNF-induced activation of the Ret protein tyrosine kinase is mediated by GDNFR-α, a novel receptor for GDNF. Cell 1996;85:1113-1124.
430. Durbec P, Marcos-Gutierrez CV, Kilkenny C, et al. GDNF signalling through the Ret receptor tyrosine kinase [see comments]. Nature 1996;381:789-793.
431. Treanor JJ, Goodman L, de Sauvage F, et al. Characterization of a multicomponent receptor for GDNF [see comments]. Nature 1996;382:80-83.
432. Cacalano G, Farinas I, Wang LC, et al. GFRα1 is an essential receptor component for GDNF in the developing nervous system and kidney. Neuron 1998;21:53-62.
433. Santoro M, Rosati R, Grieco M, et al. The *ret* proto-oncogene is consistently expressed in human pheochromocytomas and thyroid medullary carcinomas. Oncogene 1990;5:1595-1598.
434. Edstrom E, Frisk T, Farnebo F, et al. Expression analysis of RET and the GDNF/GFRα-1 and NTN/GFRα-2 ligand complexes in pheochromocytomas and paragangliomas. Int J Mol Med 2000; 6:469-474.
435. Pachnis V, Mankoo B, Costantini F. Expresssion of the *c-ret* proto-oncogene during mouse embryogenesis 1993;119:1005-1017.
436. Tsuzuki T, Takahashi M, Asai N, et al. Spatial and temporal expression of the *ret* proto-oncogene product in embryonic, infant and adult rat tissues. Oncogene 1995;10:191-198.
437. Pausova Z, Soliman E, Amizuka N, et al. Role of the *RET* proto-oncogene in sporadic hyperparathyroidism and in hyperparathyroidism of multiple endocrine neoplasia type 2. J Clin Endocrinol Metab 1996;81:2711-2718.
438. Attie-Bitach T, Abitbol M, Gerard M, et al. Expression of the *RET* proto-oncogene in human embryos. Am J Med Genet 1998;80: 481-486.
439. Attie T, Pelet A, Edery P, et al. Diversity of *RET* proto-oncogene mutations in familial and sporadic Hirschsprung disease. Hum Mol Genet 1995;4:1381-1386.
440. Borst M, Peacock BA, Minth C, Decker R. Mutational analysis of Hirschsprung's disease associated with multiple endocrine neoplasia type 2A. Presented at the Fifth International Workshop on Multiple Endocrine Neoplasia, Stockholm, Sweden, 6/29-7/2, 1994.
441. Niccoli-Sire P, Murat A, Rohmer V, et al. Familial medullary thyroid carcinoma with noncysteine ret mutations: phenotype-genotype relationship in a large series of patients. J Clin Endocrinol Metab 2001;86:3746-3753.
442. Kitamura Y, Goodfellow PJ, Shimizu K, et al. Novel germline *RET* proto-oncogene mutations associated with medullary thyroid carcinoma (MTC): mutation analysis in Japanese patients with MTC. Oncogene 1997;14:3103-3106.
443. Eng C, Smith DP, Mulligan LM, et al. A novel point mutation in the tyrosine kinase domain of the *RET* proto-oncogene in sporadic medullary thyroid carcinoma and in a family with FMTC. Oncogene 1995;10:509-513.
444. Bolino A, Schuffenecker I, Luo Y, et al. *RET* mutations in exons 13 and 14 of FMTC patients. Oncogene 1995;10:2415-2419.
445. Moers AM, Landsvater RM, Schaap C, et al. Familial medullary thyroid carcinoma: not a distinct entity? Genotype-phenotype correlation in a large family. Am J Med 1996;101:635-641.
446. Berndt I, Reuter M, Saller B, et al. A new hot spot for mutations in the *ret* protooncogene causing familial medullary thyroid carcinoma and multiple endocrine neoplasia type 2A. J Clin Endocrinol Metab 1998;83:770-774.
447. Hofstra RM, Fattoruso O, Quadro L, et al. A novel point mutation in the intracellular domain of the *ret* protooncogene in a family with medullary thyroid carcinoma. J Clin Endocrinol Metab 1997;82:4176-4178.
448. Dang GT, Cote GJ, Schultz PN, et al. A codon 891 exon 15 *RET* proto-oncogene mutation in familial medullary thyroid carcinoma: a detection strategy. Mol Cell Probes 1999;13:77-79.
449. Iwashita T, Kato M, Murakami H, et al. Biological and biochemical properties of *Ret* with kinase domain mutations identified in multiple endocrine neoplasia type 2B and familial medullary thyroid carcinoma. Oncogene 1999;18:3919-3922.
450. Carlomagno F, Salvatore G, Cirafici AM, et al. The different *RET*-activating capability of mutations of cysteine 620 or cysteine 634 correlates with the multiple endocrine neoplasia type 2 disease phenotype. Cancer Research 1997;57:391-395.
451. Cranston AN, Ponder BA. Modulation of medullary thyroid carcinoma penetrance suggests the presence of modifier genes in a *RET* transgenic mouse model. Cancer Res 2003;63:4777-4780.
452. Edery P, Pelet A, Mulligan LM, et al. Long segment and short segment familial Hirschsprung's disease: variable clinical expression at the *RET* locus. J Med Genet 1994;31:602-606.
453. Lyonnet S, Edery P, Mulligan LM, et al. [Mutations of *RET* proto-oncogene in Hirschsprung disease]. C R Acad Sci III 1994;317: 358-362.
454. Alemi M, Lucas SD, Sallstrom JF, et al. A complex nine base pair deletion in *RET* exon 11 common in sporadic medullary thyroid carcinoma. Oncogene 1997;14:2041-2045.
455. Chiefari E, Russo D, Giuffrida D, et al. Analysis of *RET* proto-oncogene abnormalities in patients with MEN 2A, MEN 2B, familial or sporadic medullary thyroid carcinoma. J Endocrinol Invest 1998;21:358-364.
456. Eng C, Mulligan LM, Smith DP, et al. Mutation of the *RET* protooncogene in sporadic medullary thyroid carcinoma. Genes Chromosomes Cancer 1995;12:209-212.
457. Frilling A, Bockhorn M, Kalinin V, et al. [Somatic *ret* proto-oncogene mutations in sporadic C-cell carcinoma of the thyroid gland]. Chirurg 1997;68:789-793.
458. Huang CN, Wu SL, Chang TC, et al. *RET* protooncogene mutations in patients with apparently sporadic medullary thyroid carcinoma. J Formos Med Assoc 1998;97:541-546.
459. Maeda S, Namba H, Takamura N, et al. A single missense mutation in codon 918 of the *RET* proto-oncogene in sporadic medullary thyroid carcinomas. Endocr J 1995;42:245-250.
460. Marsh DJ, Learoyd DL, Andrew SD, et al. Somatic mutations in the *RET* proto-oncogene in sporadic medullary thyroid carcinoma. Clin Endocrinol 1996;44:249-257.
461. Eng C, Mulligan LM, Healey CS, et al. Heterogeneous mutation of the *RET* proto-oncogene in subpopulations of medullary thyroid carcinoma. Cancer Research 1996;56:2167-2170.
462. Schilling T, Burck J, Sinn HP, et al. Prognostic value of codon 918 (ATG → ACG) *RET* proto-oncogene mutations in sporadic medullary thyroid carcinoma. Int J Cancer 2001;95:62-66.
463. Scurini C, Quadro L, Fattoruso O, et al. Germline and somatic mutations of the *RET* proto-oncogene in apparently sporadic medullary thyroid carcinomas. Mol Cell Endocrinol 1998;137:51-57.
464. Takano T, Miyauchi A, Yoshida H, et al. Large-scale analysis of mutations in *RET* exon 16 in sporadic medullary thyroid carcinomas in Japan. Jpn J Cancer Res 2001;92:645-648.
465. Uchino S, Noguchi S, Yamashita H, et al. Somatic mutations in *RET* exons 12 and 15 in sporadic medullary thyroid carcinomas: differ-

ent spectrum of mutations in sporadic type from hereditary type. Jpn J Cancer Res 1999;90:1231-1237.
466. Zedenius J, Wallin G, Hamberger B, et al. Somatic and MEN 2A de novo mutations identified in the *RET* proto-oncogene by screening of sporadic MTCs. Hum Molec Genet 1994;3:1259-1262.
467. Rodien P, Jeunemaitre X, Dumont C, et al. Genetic alterations of the *RET* proto-oncogene in familial and sporadic pheochromocytomas. Hormone Research 1997;47:263-268.
468. Eng C, Crossey PA, Mulligan LM, et al. Mutations in the *RET* proto-oncogene and the von Hippel-Lindau disease tumour suppressor gene in sporadic and syndromic phaeochromocytomas. J Med Genet 1995;32:934-937.
469. Bender BU, Gutsche M, Glasker S, et al. Differential genetic alterations in von Hippel-Lindau syndrome–associated and sporadic pheochromocytomas. J Clin Endocrinol Metab 2000;85:4568-4574.
470. Asai N, Iwashita T, Matsuyama M, Takahashi M. Mechanism of activation of the *ret* proto-oncogene by multiple endocrine neoplasia 2A mutations. Mol Cell Biol 1995;15:1613-1619.
471. Santoro M, Carlomagno F, Romano A, et al. Activation of *RET* as a dominant transforming gene by germline mutations of MEN 2A and MEN 2B. Science 1995;267:381-383.
472. Xing S, Smanik PA, Oglesbee MJ, et al. Characterization of *ret* oncogenic activation in MEN2 inherited cancer syndromes. Endocrinology 1996;137:1512-1519.
473. Carlomagno F, Melillo RM, Visconti R, et al. Glial cell line–derived neurotrophic factor differentially stimulates *ret* mutants associated with the multiple endocrine neoplasia type 2 syndromes and Hirschsprung's disease. Endocrinology 1998;139:3613-3619.
474. Salvatore D, Barone MV, Salvatore G, et al. Tyrosines 1015 and 1062 are in vivo autophosphorylation sites in *ret* and *ret*-derived oncoproteins. J Clin Endocrinol Metab 2000;85:3898-3907.
475. Ishiguro Y, Iwashita T, Murakami H, et al. The role of amino acids surrounding tyrosine 1062 in *ret* in specific binding of the shc phosphotyrosine-binding domain. Endocrinology 1999;140:3992-3998.
476. Hayashi Y, Iwashita T, Murakamai H, et al. Activation of BMK1 via tyrosine 1062 in *RET* by *GDNF* and *MEN2A* mutation. Biochem Biophys Res Commun 2001;281:682-689.
477. Chiariello M, Visconti R, Carlomagno F, et al. Signalling of *RET* receptor tyrosine kinase through the C-Jun NH2-terminal protein kinases (JNKS)—evidence for a divergence of the erks and jnks pathways induced by *RET.* Oncogene 1998;16:2435-2445.
478. De Vita G, Melillo RM, Carlomagno F, et al. Tyrosine 1062 of *RET-MEN2A* mediates activation of Akt (protein kinase B) and mitogen-activated protein kinase pathways leading to PC12 cell survival. Cancer Res 2000;60:3727-3731.
479. Hayashi H, Ichihara M, Iwashita T, et al. Characterization of intracellular signals via tyrosine 1062 in *RET* activated by glial cell line–derived neurotrophic factor. Oncogene 2000;19:4469-4475.
480. Ohiwa M, Murakami H, Iwashita T, et al. Characterization of Ret-Shc-Grb2 complex induced by GDNF, MEN 2A, and MEN 2B mutations. Biochem Biophys Res Comm 1997;237:747-751.
481. Melillo RM, Barone MV, Lupoli G, et al. *Ret*-mediated mitogenesis requires *Src* kinase activity. Cancer Res 1999;59:1120-1126.
482. Ludwig L, Kessler H, Wagner M, et al. Nuclear factor-κB is constitutively active in C-cell carcinoma and required for *RET*-induced transformation. Cancer Res 2001;61:4526-4535.
483. Khosla S, Patel VM, Hay ID, et al. Loss of heterozygosity suggests multiple genetic alterations in pheochromocytmoas and medullary thyroid carcinomas. J Clin Invest 1991;87:1691-1699.
484. Yang KP, Nguyen CV, Castillo SG, Samaan NA. Deletion mapping on the distal third region of chromosome 1p in multiple endocrine neoplasia type IIA. Anticancer Res 1990;10:527-533.
485. Takai S, Tateishi H, Nishisho I, et al. Loss of genes on chromosome 22 in medullary thyroid carcinoma and pheochromocytoma. Jpn J Cancer Res 1987;78:894-898.
486. Benn DE, Dwight T, Richardson AL, et al. Sporadic and familial pheochromocytomas are associated with loss of at least two discrete intervals on chromosome 1p. Cancer Res 2000;60:7048-7051.
487. Moley JF, Brother MB, Fong CT, et al. Consistent association of 1p loss of heterozygosity with pheochromocytomas from patients with multiple endocrine neoplasia type 2 syndromes. Cancer Res 1992;52:770-774.
488. Shin E, Fujita S, Takami K, et al. Deletion mapping of chromosome 1p and 22q in pheochromocytoma. Jpn J Cancer Res 1993;84:402-408.
489. Uchino S, Noguchi S, Adachi M, et al. Novel point mutations and allele loss at the *RET* locus in sporadic medullary thyroid carcinomas. Jpn J Cancer Res 1998;89:411-418.
490. Huang SC, Koch CA, Vortmeyer AO, et al. Duplication of the mutant *RET* allele in trisomy 10 or loss of the wild- type allele in multiple endocrine neoplasia type 2–associated pheochromocytomas. Cancer Res 2000;60:6223-6226.
491. Koch CA, Huang SC, Moley JF, et al. Allelic imbalance of the mutant and wild-type *RET* allele in MEN 2A–associated medullary thyroid carcinoma. Oncogene 2001;20:7809-7811.
492. Zhang Z, Wang Y, Vikis HG, et al. Wildtype *Kras2* can inhibit lung carcinogenesis in mice. Nat Genet 2001;29:25-33.
493. Zhuang Z, Park WS, Pack S, et al. Trisomy 7–harbouring non-random duplication of the mutant *MET* allele in hereditary papillary renal carcinomas. Nat Genet 1998;20:66-69.
494. Drosten M, Hilken G, Bockmann M, et al. Role of MEN2A-derived *RET* in maintenance and proliferation of medullary thyroid carcinoma. J Natl Cancer Inst 2004;96:1231-1239.
495. Machens A. Early malignant progression of hereditary medullary thyroid cancer. N Engl J Med 2004;350:943.
496. Cote GJ, Wohllk N, Evans D, et al. *RET* proto-oncogene mutations in multiple endocrine neoplasia type 2 and medullary thyroid carcinoma. Bailliere Clin Endocrinol Metab 1995;9:609-630.
497. Wells SA Jr, Baylin SB, Linehan WM, et al. Provocative agents and the diagnosis of medullary carcinoma of the thyroid gland. Ann Surg 1978;188:139-1341.
498. Parthemore JG, Bronzert D, Roberts G, Deftos LJ. A short calcium infusion in the diagnosis of medullary thyroid carcinoma. J Clin Endocrinol Metab 1974;39:108-111.
499. Wohllk N, Cote GJ, Evans D, et al. Application of genetic screening information to the management of medullary thyroid carcinoma and multiple endocrine neoplasia. Endocrine Metab Clin North Am 1996;25:1-25.
500. van Heurn LW, Schaap C, Sie G, et al. Predictive DNA testing for multiple endocrine neoplasia 2: a therapeutic challenge of prophylactic thyroidectomy in very young children. J Pediatr Surg 1999;34:568-571.
501. Arts CH, Bax NM, Jansen M, et al. [Prophylactic total thyroidectomy in childhood for multiple endocrine neoplasia type 2A: preliminary results]. Ned Tijdschr Geneeskd 1999;143:98-104.
502. Komminoth P, Kunz EK, Matias-Guiu X, et al. Analysis of *RET* proto-oncogene point mutations distinguishes heritable from nonheritable medullary thyroid carcinomas. Cancer 1995;76:479-489.
503. Shirahama S, Ogura K, Takami H, et al. Mutational analysis of the *RET* proto-oncogene in 71 Japanese patients with medullary thyroid carcinoma. J Hum Genet 1998;43:101-106.
504. Mulligan LM, Eng C, Healey CS, et al. A de novo mutation of the *RET* proto-oncogene in a patient with MEN 2A. Hum Mol Genet 1994;3:1007-1008.
505. Neumann HP, Bausch B, McWhinney SR, et al. Germ-line mutations in nonsyndromic pheochromocytoma. N Engl J Med 2002;346:1459-1466.
506. Jimenez C, Cote G, Arnold A, Gagel RF. Review: Should patients with apparently sporadic pheochromocytomas or paragangliomas be screened for hereditary syndromes? J Clin Endocrinol Metab 2006;91:2851-2858.
507. Woodward ER, Eng C, McMahon R, et al. Genetic predisposition to phaeochromocytoma: analysis of candidate genes *GDNF, RET* and *VHL.* Hum Mol Genet 1997;6:1051-1056.
508. Dahia PL, Toledo SP, Mulligan LM, et al. Mutation analysis of glial cell line–derived neurotrophic factor (GDNF), a ligand for the *RET/GDNF* receptor α complex, in sporadic phaeochromocytomas. Cancer Res 1997;57:310-313.
509. Brauch H, Hoeppner W, Jahnig H, et al. Sporadic pheochromocytomas are rarely associated with germline mutations in the *vhl* tumor suppressor gene or the *ret* protooncogene. J Clin Endocrinol Metab 1997;82:4101-4104.
510. van der Harst E, de Krijger RR, Dinjens WN, et al. Germline mutations in the *vhl* gene in patients presenting with phaeochromocytomas. Int J Cancer 1998;77:337-340.

511. Bar M, Friedman E, Jakobovitz O, et al. Sporadic phaeochromocytomas are rarely associated with germline mutations in the von Hippel-Lindau and *RET* genes. Clin Endocrinol 1997;47:707-712.
512. Astuti D, Douglas F, Lennard TW, et al. Germline *SDHD* mutation in familial phaeochromocytoma. Lancet 2001;357:1181-1182.
513. Niemann S, Muller U. Mutations in *SDHC* cause autosomal dominant paraganglioma, type 3. Nat Genet 2000;26:268-270.
514. Astuti D, Latif F, Dallol A, et al. Gene mutations in the succinate dehydrogenase subunit SDHB cause susceptibility to familial pheochromocytoma and to familial paraganglioma. Am J Hum Genet 2001;69:49-54.
515. Gimenez-Roqueplo AP, Favier J, Rustin P, et al. The R22X mutation of the *SDHD* gene in hereditary paraganglioma abolishes the enzymatic activity of complex II in the mitochondrial respiratory chain and activates the hypoxia pathway. Am J Hum Genet 2001;69: 1186-1197.
516. Gimm O, Armanios M, Dziema H, et al. Somatic and occult germline mutations in *SDHD,* a mitochondrial complex II gene, in nonfamilial pheochromocytoma. Cancer Res 2000;60:6822-6825.
517. Chew SL. Paraganglioma genes. Clin Endocrinol (Oxf) 2001;54: 573-574.
518. Ponder BA, Ponder MA, Coffey R, et al. Risk estimation and screening in families of patients with medullary thyroid carcinoma. Lancet 1988;1:397-401.
519. MD Anderson Cancer Center. Endocrine neoplasia and hormonal disorders. Patient education materials. Available at http://www.mdanderson.org/departments/endocrinology (accessed March 7, 2007).
520. Gagel RF, Jackson CE, Block MA, et al. Age-related probability of development of hereditary medullary thyroid carcinoma. J Pediatr 1982;101:941-946.
521. Easton DF, Ponder MA, Cummings T, et al. The clinical and screening age-at-onset distribution for the MEN-2 syndrome. Am J Hum Genet 1989;44:208-215.
522. Telander RL, Zimmerman D, van Heerden JA, Sizemore GW. Results of early thyroidectomy for medullary thyroid carcinoma in children with multiple endocrine neoplasia type 2. J Pediatr Surg 1986;21:1190-1194.
523. Machens A, Gimm O, Hinze R, et al. Genotype-phenotype correlations in hereditary medullary thyroid carcinoma: oncological features and biochemical properties. J Clin Endocrinol Metab 2001;86:1104-1109.
524. Niccoli-Sire P, Murat A, Baudin E, et al. Early or prophylactic thyroidectomy in MEN 2/FMTC gene carriers: results in 71 thyroidectomized patients. The French Calcitonin Tumours Study Group (GETC). Eur J Endocrinol 1999;141:468-474.
525. Sanso G, Domene HM, Iorcansky S, Barontini M. [Early diagnosis of multiple endocrine neoplasia type 2 (MEN 2) by detection of mutated *RET* proto-oncogene carriers]. Medicina 1998;58: 179-184.
526. Lallier M, St-Vil D, Giroux M, et al. Prophylactic thyroidectomy for medullary thyroid carcinoma in gene carriers of MEN2 syndrome. J Pediatr Surg 1998;33:846-848.
527. Dralle H, Gimm O, Simon D, et al. Prophylactic thyroidectomy in 75 children and adolescents with hereditary medullary thyroid carcinoma: German and Austrian experience. World J Surg 1998;22:744-750.
528. Frank-Raue K, Hoppner W, Buhr H, et al. Results and follow-up in eleven MEN 2A gene carriers after prophylactic thyroidectomy. Exp Clin Endocrinol Diabetes 1997;105:76-78.
529. Krause DS, Van Etten RA. Tyrosine kinases as targets for cancer therapy. N Engl J Med 2005;353:172-187.
530. Carlomagno F, Vitagliano D, Guida T, et al. ZD6474, an orally available inhibitor of KDR tyrosine kinase activity, efficiently blocks oncogenic *RET* kinases. Cancer Res 2002;62:7284-7290.
531. Carlomagno F, Anaganti S, Guida T, et al. BAY 43-9006 inhibition of oncogenic *RET* mutants. J Natl Cancer Inst 2006;98:326-334.
532. American Thyroid Association. Thyroid Clinical Trials. Available at http://www.thyroidtrials.org (accessed March 7, 2007).
533. Wells SA, Gosnell J, Gagel RF, et al. Vandetanib in metastatic hereditary medullary thyroid cancer: follow-up results of an open label phase II trial. Am Soc Clin Oncol 2007.
534. Cameron D, Spiro HM, Landsberg L. Zollinger-Ellison syndrome with multiple endocrine adenomatosis type II [letter]. N Engl J Med 1978;299:152-153.
535. Sakai Y, Koizumi K, Sugitani I, et al. Familial adenomatous polyposis associated with multiple endocrine neoplasia type 1–related tumors and thyroid carcinoma: a case report with clinicopathologic and molecular analyses. Am J Surg Pathol 2002;26:103-110.
536. Perkins JT, Blackstone MO, Riddell RH. Adenomatous polyposis coli and multiple endocrine neoplasia type 2b. A pathogenetic relationship. Cancer 1985;55:375-381.
537. Tuch BE, Carter JN, Armellin GM, Newland RC. The association of a tumour of the posterior pituitary gland with multiple endocrine neoplasia type 1. Aust N Z J Med 1982;12:179-181.
538. Bertrand JH, Ritz P, Reznik Y, et al. Sipple's syndrome associated with a large prolactinoma. Clin Endocrinol (Oxf) 1987;27: 607-614.
539. Tamsen A, Mazur MT. Ovarian strumal carcinoid in association with multiple endocrine neoplasia, type IIA. Arch Pathol Lab Med 1992;116:200-203.
540. Binkovitz LA, Johnson CD, Stephens DH. Islet cell tumors in von Hippel-Lindau disease: increased prevalence and relationship to the multiple endocrine neoplasias. AJR Am J Roentgenol 1990;155:501-505.
541. Hough DM, Stephens DH, Johnson CD, Binkovitz LA. Pancreatic lesions in von Hippel-Lindau disease: prevalence, clinical significance, and CT findings. AJR Am J Roentgenol 1994;162: 1091-1094.
542. Filling-Katz MR, Choyke PL, Oldfield E, et al. Central nervous system involvement in von Hippel-Lindau disease. Neurology 1991;41:41-46.
543. Neumann HP, Dinkel E, Brambs H, et al. Pancreatic lesions in the von Hippel-Lindau syndrome. Gastroenterology 1991;101: 465-471.
544. La Forgia S, Lasota J, Latif F, et al. Detailed genetic and physical map of the 3p chromosome region surrounding the familial renal cell carcinoma chromosome translocation, t(3; 8)(p14.2; q24.1). Cancer Res 1993;53:3118-3124.
545. Latif F, Kalman T, Gnarra J, et al. Identification of the von Hippel-Lindau disease tumor suppressor gene. Science 1993;260: 1317-1320.
546. Aso T, Lane WS, Conaway JW, Conaway RC. Elongin (SIII): a multisubunit regulator of elongation by RNA polymerase II. Science 1995;269:1439-1443.
547. Duan DR, Pause A, Burgess WH, et al. Inhibition of transcription elongation by the VHL tumor suppressor protein. Science 1995; 269:1402-1406.
548. Kibel A, Iliopoulos O, De Caprio JA, Kaelin WG Jr. Binding of the von Hippel-Lindau tumor suppressor protein to elongin B and C. Science 1995;269:1444-1446.
549. Maxwell PH, Wiesener MS, Chang GW, et al. The tumour suppressor protein VHL targets hypoxia-inducible factors for oxygen-dependent proteolysis. Nature 1999;399:271-275.
550. Chen F, Kishida T, Yao M, et al. Germline mutations in the von Hippel-Lindau disease tumor suppressor gene: correlations with phenotype. Hum Mutat 1995;5:66-75.
551. Janson KL, Roberts JA, Varela M. Multiple endocrine adenomatosis: in support of the common origin theories. J Urol 1978;119: 161-165.
552. Hull MT, Warfel KA, Muller J, Higgins JT. Familial islet cell tumors in Von Hippel-Lindau's disease. Cancer 1979;44:1523-1526.
553. Carney JA, Go VLW, Gordon H, et al. Familial pheochromocytoma and islet cell tumor of the pancreas. Am. J Med 1980;68:515-521.
554. Mori Y, Kiyohara H, Miki T, et al. Pheochromocytoma with prominent calcification and associated pancreatic islet cell tumor. J Urol 1977;118:843-844.
555. Nathan DM, Daniels GH, Ridgway EC. Gastrinoma and phaeochromocytoma: is there a mixed multiple endocrine adenoma syndrome. Acta Endocrinol 1980;93:91-93.
556. Zeller JR, Kauffman HM, Komorowski RA, Itskovitz HD. Bilateral pheochromocytoma and islet cell adenoma of the pancreas. Arch Surg 1982;117:827-830.
557. Cantor AM, Rigby CC, Beck PR, et al. Neurofibromatosis, phaeochromocytoma, and somatostatinoma. BMJ 1982;285:1618-1619.
558. Chakrabarti S, Murugesan A, Arida EJ. The association of neurofibromatosis and hyperparathyroidism. Am J Surg 1979;137: 417-420.
559. Saurenmann P, Binswanger R, Maurer R, et al. [Somatostatin-producing endocrine pancreatic tumor in Recklinghausen's neurofi-

bromatosis. Case report and literature review]. Schweiz Med Wochenschr 1987;117:1134-1139.

560. Chen CH, Lin JT, Lee WY, et al. Somatostatin-containing carcinoid tumor of the duodenum in neurofibromatosis: report of a case. J Formos Med Assoc 1993;92:900-903.
561. Hansen OP, Hansen M, Hansen HH, Rose B. Multiple endocrine adenomatosis of mixed type. Acta Med Scand 1976;200:327-331.
562. Habiby R, Silverman B, Listernick R, Charrow J. Precocious puberty in children with neurofibromatosis type 1. J Pediatr 1995;126:364-367.
563. Nur-E-Kamal MS, Varga M, Maruta H. The GTPase-activating NF1 fragment of 91 amino acids reverses v-Ha-Ras-induced malignant phenotype. J Biol Chem 1993;268:22331-22337.
564. Gutmann DH, Cole JL, Stone WJ, et al. Loss of neurofibromin in adrenal gland tumors from patients with neurofibromatosis type I. Genes Chromosom Cancer 1994;10:55-58.
565. Gutmann DH, Cole JL, Collins FS. Expression of the neurofibromatosis type 1 (NF1) gene during mouse embryonic development. Prog Brain Res 1995;105:327-335.
566. Brannan CI, Perkins AS, Vogel KS, et al. Targeted disruption of the neurofibromatosis type-1 gene leads to developmental abnormalities in heart and various neural crest–derived tissues. Genes Dev 1994;8:1019-1029.
567. Carney JA, Gordon H, Carpenter PC, et al. The complex of myxomas, spotty pigmentation, and endocrine overactivity. Medicine (Baltimore) 1985;64:270-283.
568. Carney JA. The Carney complex (myxomas, spotty pigmentation, endocrine overactivity, and schwannomas). Dermatol Clin 1995;13:19-26.
569. Stratakis CA, Kirschner LS, Carney JA. Clinical and molecular features of the Carney complex: diagnostic criteria and recommendations for patient evaluation. J Clin Endocrinol Metab 2001;86:4041-4046.
570. Stratakis CA. Genetics of Peutz-Jeghers syndrome, Carney complex and other familial lentiginoses. Horm Res 2000;54:334-343.
571. Kirschner LS, Carney JA, Pack SD, et al. Mutations of the gene encoding the protein kinase A type I-α regulatory subunit in patients with the Carney complex. Nat Genet 2000;26:89-92.
572. Horvath A, Boikos S, Giatzakis C, et al. A genome-wide scan identifies mutations in the gene encoding phosphodiesterase 11A4 (PDE11A) in individuals with adrenocortical hyperplasia. Nature Genet 2006;38:794-800.

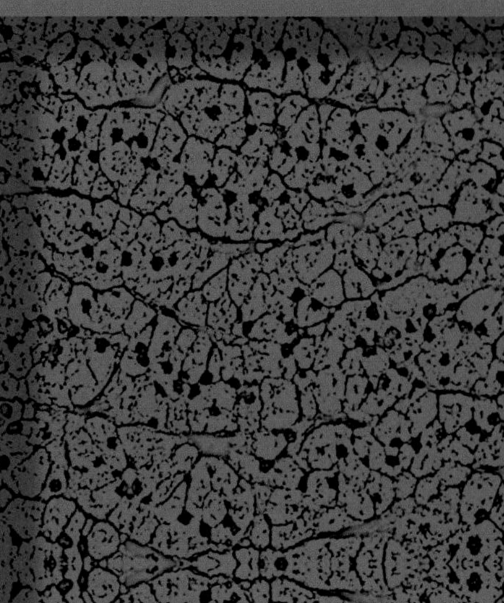

CHAPTER 41

THE IMMUNOENDOCRINOPATHY SYNDROMES

Jennifer M. Barker, Peter A. Gottlieb, and George S. Eisenbarth

What we now recognize as the immunoendocrinopathy syndromes has contributed to our understanding of endocrinology and immunology for more than 100 years. An illustration from Addison's initial description of primary adrenal insufficiency shows a patient with two autoimmune diseases: vitiligo and the hyperpigmentation of Addison's disease (Fig. 41–1). Geneticists, immunologists, and endocrinologists have generated a wealth of new information concerning the pathogenesis of the polyendocrine autoimmune syndromes and their component disorders. In particular, the genetic loci underlying disease susceptibility and organ-specific autoantigens targeted by the immune system are being defined. Multiple distinct molecules are often the targets of autoimmunity for a single organ-specific autoimmune disorder. In polyendocrine autoimmunity, multiple molecules of multiple organs are usually targeted.

Most autoimmune endocrine disorders occur in isolation (e.g., type 1 diabetes, autoimmune thyroid disease). Two distinct autoimmune polyendocrine syndromes with characteristic groupings of manifestations are readily recognized. *Autoimmune polyendocrine syndrome type I* (APS-I) is a rare disorder with autosomal recessive inheritance that is caused by defects in the autoimmune regulator *(AIRE)* gene on chromosome 21. In contrast, the most common syndrome discussed in this chapter, *autoimmune polyendocrine syndrome type II* (APS-II), is less well defined and includes overlapping groups of disorders. A unifying characteristic within APS-II is the strong association with polymorphic genes of the human leukocyte antigen (HLA) region located on the short arm of chromosome 6 (band 6p21.3). In addition to HLA, many other genetic loci are likely to contribute to susceptibility to APS-II. In this chapter, *APS-II* encompasses what some clinicians divide into APS-II (Addison's disease plus type 1 diabetes or thyroid autoimmunity), APS-III (thyroid autoimmunity plus other autoimmune diseases, not Addison's or type 1 diabetes), and APS-IV (two or more other organ-specific autoimmune disorders).

APS-II has also been known by various other names: Schmidt's syndrome, polyglandular autoimmune disease, polyglandular failure syndrome, organ-specific autoimmune disease, and polyendocrinopathy diabetes. Such diverse names reflect the large number of studies and case reports of this syndrome and its historical importance. Studies of patients with APS-II were instrumental in identifying the autoimmune basis of several diseases and developing autoantibody assays (e.g., type 1 diabetes and cytoplasmic islet cell antibodies). Each of these other names has some shortcomings, such as failure to include the fact that both hyperfunction and hypofunction of endocrine glands can occur or failure to recognize that nonendocrine disorders such as pernicious anemia and celiac disease are parts of the syndrome.

Other rare autoimmune endocrine disorders have contributed to our understanding of the development of autoimmunity. For example, the rare disorder immunodysregulation polyendocrinopathy enteropathy X linked syndrome (IPEX) is caused by a mutation of the *FOXp3* gene. *FOXp3* plays a role in the development of regulatory $CD4^+/CD25^+$ T cells that function to maintain tolerance to self. The influence of these cells on the development of autoimmunity is an area of active investigation. A thorough understanding of these rare and often genetically simple disorders provides insight into the development of disorders that are characterized by polygenic inheritance and that affect a larger group of patients.

Autoimmunity Primer

T lymphocytes and autoantibodies produced by B lymphocytes are major determinants of autoimmune endocrine diseases (Fig. 41–2). These two arms of the immune system differ fundamentally in their recognition of target antigens. Autoantibodies react with intact molecules (including both soluble and cell-surface molecules) and usually interact with conformational determinants of the autoantigen. In contrast, T lymphocytes recognize peptide fragments of autoantigens, often 8 to 12 amino acids in length presented on the surface of another cell by major histocompatibility molecules. $CD4^+$ (helper) T cells typically react with peptides that are derived from the extracellular fluid and bound by class II histocompatibility molecules (HLA-DP, HLA-DQ, or HLA-DR in humans). Effective presentation requires specialized antigen-presenting cells (APCs) such as macrophages, dendritic cells, and B lymphocytes. $CD8^+$ (cytotoxic) T cells react with peptides bound by class I histocompatibility molecules (HLA-A, HLA-B, and HLA-C). Class I molecules are present on the surface of nearly all nucleated cells. The antigen peptide in this case is derived from the presenting cell. Recognition of the antigenic peptide by $CD8^+$ T cells typically leads to the release of cytotoxic chemicals that kill the cell.

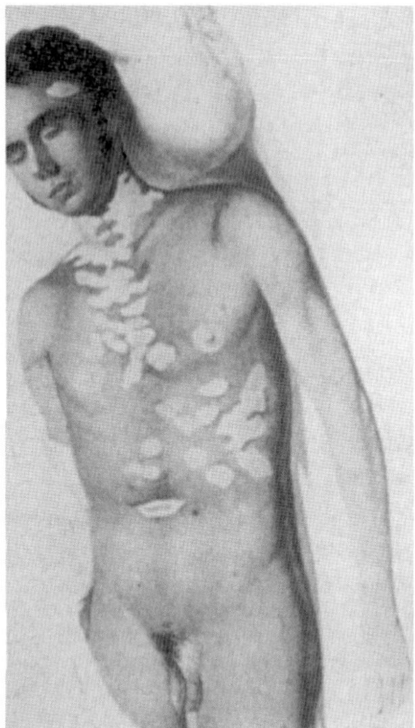

Figure 41–1 ■ Reproduction of an illustration from Addison's initial description of primary adrenal insufficiency (Addison's disease). (From Addison T. On the Constitutional and Local Effects of Disease of the Supra-renal Capsules. London, Samuel Highley, 1855.)

The crystal structure of histocompatibility molecules has been elucidated, and these molecules resemble a hot dog in a bun, with the antigenic peptide (the hot dog) bound in the groove of the histocompatibility molecule (the bun). Histocompatibility molecules are extremely polymorphic, with different amino acids lining the peptide-binding groove. These variable amino acids determine which peptides are bound and presented to T lymphocytes.

The T-cell response depends on the context in which the antigen is presented. The simple expression of histocompatibility molecules and recognition of antigen by a T cell are not sufficient for T-cell activation. This context is at least partially determined by the interaction of cell surface molecules on both the T cell and the APC. The interaction of major histocompatibility complex (MHC), peptide, and T-cell receptor (called signal one) is critical to the activation process, and other molecules help to define the nature of the immune response (signal two). For example, the cell-surface molecule B7 engages the CD80 receptor on the T cell and amplifies signal one, which leads to T-cell activation. When a T cell recognizes an antigen in the context of the MHC and does not receive the appropriate second

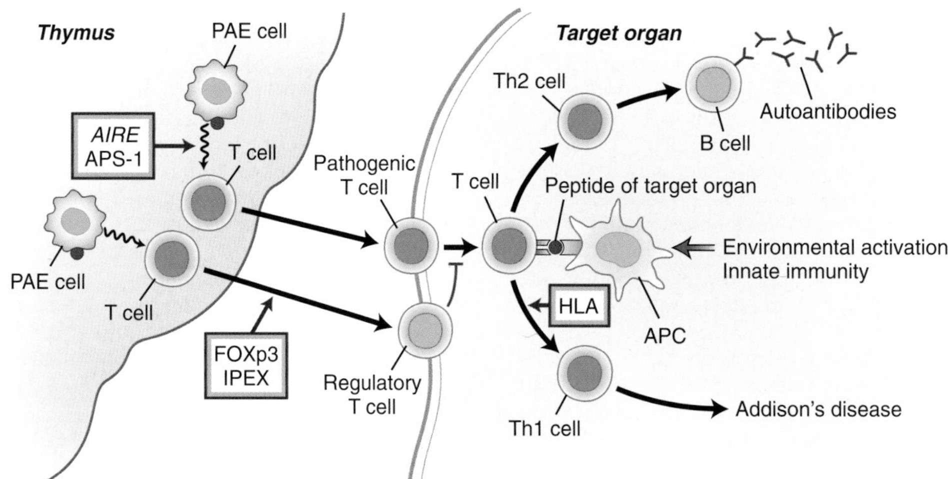

Figure 41–2 ■ Model of the pathogenesis of autoimmunity in polyendocrine disorders. The development of autoimmune disease is determined by a group of T cells that recognize one or more organ-specific epitomes. Peptides are presented in the HLA molecule and are recognized by the T-cell receptor (TCR). Recognition of self molecules depends on the maturation of the T cell, a process that begins in the thymus and continues in the periphery. FOXp3 stimulates the development of $CD4^+$ $CD25^+$ regulatory T cells. B cells produce autoantibodies under the stimulation of T cells. AIRE, autoimmune regulator; APS-I, autoimmune polyendocrine syndrome I; HLA, human leukocyte antigen; IPEX, immune dysregulation, polyendocrinopathy, enteropathy, X-linked; PAE, peripheral antigen-expressing cell; Th1, type 1 helper T cell; Th2, type 2 helper T cell. (Reproduced from Eisenbarth GS, Gottlieb PA. Autoimmune polyendocrine syndromes. NEJM 2004;350: 2068-2079.)

signal, anergy results. Cell surface molecules and receptors such as PD-1 and cytokine and chemokine signals can modulate the signal delivered to the T cell and lead to apoptosis or even to the generation of different types of regulatory T cells.

Autoimmunity results from the loss of tolerance, or the ability to differentiate between self and nonself. Tolerance induction is a staged process that initiates in the thymus during T-cell maturation. This process depends in part on the presence of *peripheral antigens* in the thymus. Peripheral antigens are antigens normally expressed in tissues outside of the immune system (e.g. insulin), which are expressed at low levels in the thymus. T cells that react strongly to these peripheral molecules in the context of the MHC are deleted in the thymus. T cells that react with peripheral antigens that are not expressed in the thymus have a greater opportunity to escape tolerance. Study of *AIRE* gene knockout mice has supported the importance of these phenomena in the development of autoimmunity. These mice have low levels of expression of peripheral antigens in the thymus and develop lymphocytic infiltrates in multiple organs.[1,2]

Peripheral tolerance is an important mechanism for tolerance induction after T cells have matured in the thymus. Anergic and regulatory T cells are integral in the development of tolerance for naïve T cells. A major population of T-regulatory cells carries the cell surface markers CD4, CD25, and GITR. The function of the population of $CD4^+/CD25^+$ cells continues to be elucidated. Maturation of these cells in the thymus depends on the transcription factor FOXp3. Deletion of this transcription factor leads to fulminant autoimmunity in neonates (e.g., neonatal type 1 diabetes and enteropathy), often resulting in death within the first year of life (the IPEX syndrome).

$CD4^+$ T cells activate B cells to produce the humoral immune response. This occurs after the $CD4^+$ T cell engages an antigen in the context of the MHC on the cell surface of a B cell. The cytokines (interleukin [IL]-4, IL-5, and IL-6) produced by the $CD4^+$ T cells induce the maturation of a B cell. Depending on the cytokine milieu, the B cell will switch from producing immuloglobulin M (IgM) to IgG, IgE, or IgA. The $CD4^+$ T cell and the B cell recognize the same antigen, which has initially bound the immunoglobulin receptor on the surface of the B cell and been internalized and processed for presentation by the MHC class II molecules. This is a process termed *linked recognition.* The development of B-cell tolerance is partially dependent on this linked recognition such that autoreactive B cells clones that do not have a $CD4^+$ T cell that will bind with the antigen in its MHC groove will not normally be activated.

Natural History of Autoimmune Disorders

The natural history of autoimmune disorders can be divided into a series of stages beginning with genetic susceptibility, followed by triggering of autoimmunity (e.g., dietary gliadin exposure in celiac disease), active autoimmunity preceding clinical manifestations (e.g., progressive glandular destruction), and, finally, overt disease.

Genetic Associations

Although there is familial aggregation of APS-II and its component disorders, there is no simple pattern of inheritance (Table 41–1). Susceptibility is probably determined by multiple genetic loci (with HLA having the strongest effect) interacting with environmental factors. For type 1 diabetes, the overall concordance of identical twins is approximately 50%, suggesting a possible role for environmental or other nongenetic factors, such as somatic mutation or the random rearrangement of T-cell receptors that occurs during the development of the immune system. We found that diabetes developed in identical twins much more often if it arose in the proband before 25 years of age but that

TABLE 41–1 GENETIC ASSOCIATIONS WITH AUTOIMMUNE DISEASE

Gene	Proposed Mechanism of Action	Polymorphism/Mutation	Disease	Inheritance
HLA	Antigen presentation	DR3-DQ2/DR4-DQ8	Type 1 diabetes	Multigenic
		DR3-DQ2	Celiac disease	
		DR3-DQ2/DRB1*0404-DQ8	Addison's disease	
		DR3-DQ2/DR4-DQ8	Graves' disease	
		DR3 DR5	Hypothyroidism	
MIC-A	Priming of naïve T cells	5, 5.1	Type 1 diabetes	Multigenic
		4, 5.1	Celiac disease	
		5.1	Addison's disease	
PTPN22	T-cell receptor signaling pathway through interaction with regulatory kinases	Tryptophan substitution for arginine at position 620	Type 1 diabetes SLE RA Graves' disease Hypothyroidism Vitiligo	Multigenic
CTLA-4	Receptor on activated $CD4^+$ and $CD8^+$ T cells; decreases T-cell activation	CT60	Type 1 diabetes	Multigenic
		CT60; +49A/G	Graves' disease	
		CT60; +49A/G	Hypothyroidism	
		+49A/G	Celiac disease	
		+49A/G	Addison's disease	
AIRE	"Peripheral" antigen presentation in the thymus	Multiple reported mutations	APS-I	Autosomal recessive
FOXp3	Transcription factor important for maturation of $CD4^+/CD25^+$ regulatory T cells	Multiple reported mutations	IPEX	X-linked

APS, autoimmune polyendocrine syndrome; IPEX, immunodysregulation polyendocrinopathy enteropathy X-linked syndrome; RA, rheumatoid arthritis; SLE, systemic lupus erythematosus.

initially discordant twins can become diabetic even after a prolonged period of discordance.[3] Furthermore, approximately 40% of long-term discordant twins (>7 years) have persistent autoantibodies or loss of first-phase insulin release, or both. Identical twins can also be discordant for other autoimmune diseases such as Addison's disease, Graves' disease, and celiac disease.

Autoimmune diseases share common genetic risk factors including HLA, the major histocompatibility complex class I–related gene A (*MIC-A*), the gene for lymphoid tyrosine phosphatase *(PTPN22),* and the cytotoxic T-lymphocyte associated antigen 4 (CTLA-4). In addition, genetic susceptibility for some autoimmune diseases has been linked to polymorphisms that are organ specific; for example, polymorphisms in the variable nucleotide tandem repeat (VNTR) upstream from the insulin gene have been associated with risk for type 1 diabetes.[4]

Molecular HLA genotyping has revealed many subtypes of the older serologically defined alleles, and the unique genetic sequence encoding each polymorphic chain of the histocompatibility molecules is now given a unique identifying number. Thus, for the DQ molecule, which is the histocompatibility molecule most strongly associated with endocrine autoimmunity, a number is given for each unique alpha and beta chain sequence. Examples are DQA1*0501 for the alpha chain and DQB1*0201 for the beta chain of the DQ molecule (also termed DQ2) commonly encoded on DR3 (DRB1*0301) haplotypes. A haplotype consists of a series of alleles of different genes on a contiguous region of a chromosome (e.g., DQA1 and DQB1 alleles) that are inherited together. A genotype is the combination of the haplotypes of both chromosomes. For example, the highest-risk HLA genotype for type 1 diabetes is DR3-DQ2, DR4-DQ8 (DQ8 = DQA1*0301-DQB1*0302). A specific DR4 subtype, DRB1*0404, of this gene shows a strong association with Addison's disease.[5,6] The DR3-DQ2 haplotype is associated with celiac disease both in the presence[7] and absence[8] of type 1 diabetes. This haplotype has been associated with autoimmune thyroid disease,[9] although conflicting reports exist.[10] Many of the disorders of APS-II are associated with an HLA extended haplotype formed by HLA-A1, B8, DR3, DQA1*0501, DQB1*0201[11] and HLA-DR4, DQA1*0301, DQB1*0302.[5] These include Graves' disease, atrophic thyroiditis, type 1A diabetes (also DR4-associated), Addison's disease (also DR4-associated), myasthenia gravis, and celiac disease.

Whereas some HLA alleles increase disease risk, others are associated with protection from disease. For example, the DQ alleles DQA1*0102-DQB1*0602 (usually associated with DR2) confer strong protection from type 1A diabetes in a dominant fashion[12] but confer susceptibility to another autoimmune disorder, multiple sclerosis. Furthermore, this protection is not general to endocrine autoimmunity because no protection from Addison's disease is afforded by DQB1*0602.

The major histocompatibility complex class I–related gene A *(MIC-A)* produces a gene that is expressed in the thymus and in naïve CD8$^+$ T cells. Polymorphisms of *MIC-A* have been associated with type 1 diabetes,[13] celiac disease,[14] and Addison's disease.[15] In a series of in vitro experiments on intestinal epithelium from patients with celiac disease, it has been shown that *MIC-A* is expressed on intestinal epithelial cells[16] and its expression is induced by gliadin.[17,18] This suggests a link between the genetic association and pathophysiologic role of this polymorphism in the development of autoimmunity.

The *PTPN22* gene encodes lymphoid tyrosine phosphatase (LYP) protein. LYP, through interactions with regulatory kinases such as Csk, appears to act as an inhibitor of the signal cascade downstream from the T-cell receptor. A specific polymorphism associated with a tryptophan substitution for arginine at position 620 (R620W) blocks LYP's interaction with Csk.[19] This polymorphism has been associated with type 1 diabetes,[19] rheumatoid arthritis,[20] systemic lupus erythematosus (SLE),[21] Graves' disease,[22] vitiligo,[23] and weakly associated with Addison's disease.[22] This polymorphism has also been associated with SLE, rheumatoid arthritis, type 1 diabetes, and autoimmune hypothyroidism in families with several members affected by more than one autoimmune disease.[24]

Cytotoxic T lymphocyte–associated antigen-4 (CTLA-4) is expressed on activated CD4$^+$ and CD8$^+$ T cells where it is hypothesized to act as a negative regulator.[25] Several polymorphisms within the CTLA-4 gene have been associated with autoimmune diseases. One polymorphism associated with AT repeats has been shown to reduce the inhibitory function of CTLA-4 in subjects with Graves' disease.[26] A single nucleotide polymorphism in the 3′ untranslated region denoted CT60 has been associated with Graves' disease[27] and autoimmune hypothyroidism.[28] An additional polymorphism denoted $^+$49A/G has been associated with celiac disease in the Dutch population,[29] autoimmune thyroid disease,[30] and Addison's disease.[31]

Organ-specific genetic polymorphisms have been associated with the development of specific autoimmune diseases. For example, polymorphisms of the variable number of tandem repeats (VNTR) upstream of the insulin gene have been associated with the development of type 1 diabetes. Higher numbers of tandem repeats are associated with increased production of insulin in the thymus and protection from type 1 diabetes.[4] Similarly, polymorphisms of the thyroglobulin gene are associated with autoimmune thyroid disease.[32]

Single gene defects such as *AIRE* and *FOXp3* cause multiorgan autoimmunity and are discussed in sections devoted to the topic. Analysis of mutations of the *AIRE* gene indicates that it does not play a role in APS-II or sporadic Addison's disease, with 1 of 90 (1.1%) patients with Addison's disease (non-APS-I) and 1 of 576 (0.2%) control subjects having *AIRE* mutations.[31]

Environmental Triggers

Although genetics is known to play an important role in the development of autoimmunity, it does not tell the whole story. For example, the highest risk HLA genotype for type 1 diabetes (DR3-DQ2, DR4-DQ8) is associated with a risk of 1 in 20 for the development of diabetes.[33] Although this is greater than the general population prevalence rates of 1 in 200 by the age of 20 years, it is not nearly a 100% risk. Therefore, other factors (genetic and environmental) must be involved in the initiation of autoimmunity. Some theorize that these factors may be environmental triggers. For one disease, celiac disease, the underlying environmental trigger has been identified: gluten. In addition, through studies such as the Diabetes Autoimmunity Study in the Young (DAISY), BabyDiab, and Celiac Disease Autoimmunity Research (CEDAR), the timing of first exposure to cereal has been identified as a risk factor for the development of diabetes and celiac disease autoimmunity. Infants exposed at a very young age to cereal developed diabetes and celiac-associated autoimmunity at a greater rate than those who had cereal introduced at a later date.[34,35,36] Further investigation might identify additional environmental associations.

Immunologic therapies, especially in patients with an autoimmune disease, can induce autoimmunity. A remarkable example is the treatment of patients with multiple sclerosis with an anti-CD52 monoclonal antibody. One third of 27 patients given the monoclonal antibody developed antithyrotropin receptor autoantibodies and hyperthyroidism.[37] Interferon-α (IFN-α) therapy for hepatitis has been associated with thyroid autoimmunity[38] and potentially type 1 diabetes.[39] Severe hypoglycemia associated with insulin autoantibodies in the absence of insulin administration, termed *Hirata's disease,* is associated with methimazole treatment of Graves' disease. The development of Hirata's disease in these patients is associated with HLA-Bw62/Cw4/DR4 with a specific DRB1 allele (DRB1*0406).[40]

Development of Organ-Specific Autoimmunity and Dysfunction

Autoantibodies highly specific for a given disorder are present before disease onset, such as anti-islet antibodies in type 1 diabetes and 21-hydroxylase autoantibodies in Addison's disease. Anti-islet antibodies include antibodies to GAD, islet cell antibody (ICA) 512 (also termed *insulinoma antigen-2* [IA-2]), and insulin. Each specific autoantibody reacts with only a single autoantigen, although autoantigens may be present in multiple tissues. For example, 17α-hydroxylase is present in the adrenal glands and the gonads. The very strong coincidence of Graves' hyperthyroidism and Graves' ophthalmopathy implies a specific shared immune target. For the most part, however, the targets of autoantibodies appear to be unrelated except that for organ-specific autoimmunity they are usually expressed in specific cells and cellular sites.

In contrast, less is known concerning the specificity of pathogenic T cells. Given the observation that cross-reactive recognition by pathogenic T-cell clones may be determined by as few as four properly spaced amino acids of a nonapeptide and the estimate that each T-cell receptor might react with a million different peptides, there is considerable potential for patterns of autoimmunity to be determined by cross-reactive T cells. An important development has been the discovery in the thymus and other lymphoid tissues of peripheral antigen-expressing cells that express autoantigens such as insulin. Minute quantities of such molecules in the thymus can contribute to tolerance. Insulin messenger RNA (mRNA) in the thymus is regulated by genetic polymorphisms of the insulin gene associated with diabetes risk.[4] There is also evidence that lymphoid cells (CD11c$^+$) in the spleen, lymph nodes, and circulation express multiple similar antigens.[41]

Organ-specific autoantibodies (with appropriate assays) are rarely present (approximately 1/100) in the general population and identify a subset of the population that is at greater risk for clinical disease. These autoantibodies may be expressed for years before the disease develops, and development of autoantibodies can continue over time. The pace at which disease develops is highly variable. For example, children as young as 1 year can present with type 1 diabetes. In contrast, a subset of subjects (5% to 10%) with type 2 diabetes diagnosed in adulthood has autoimmunity as the underlying cause. This may be in part due to genetics, because subjects who develop autoimmune diabetes at an older age have a higher proportion of the protective diabetes allele DQB1*0602, though even in adults DQB1*0602 provides dramatic protection.[42] Organ dysfunction develops over time and can include a period of intermediate function that may be characterized by increased levels of the stimulatory hormones (e.g. TSH, ACTH) with normal levels of the hormones (T_3, T_4, and cortisol). Once a significant portion of the gland has been destroyed, overt disease is present.

Autoimmune Polyendocrine Syndrome Type I

Clinical Features

Table 41–2 compares the features of APS-I with those of APS-II. Table 41–3 shows the clinical features and recommended follow-up of patients with APS-I.

Autoimmune polyendocrine syndrome type I (APS-I) (MIM 240300), also known as *autoimmune polyendocrinopathy-candidiasis-ectodermal dystrophy* (APECED), is characterized by the classic triad of mucocutaneous candidiasis, autoimmune hypoparathyroidism, and Addison's disease, which form three of the most common components of the disorder. Patients with APS-I are at risk for developing autoimmune diseases affecting almost every organ. More than 140 patients have been reported, including subjects in two large series from Finland[43,44,45] and the United States.[46] Of note "100%" of patients have anti-interferon antibodies.[47a]

In a series of 89 Finnish patients described by Perheentupa, all had chronic candidiasis at some time, 86% had hypoparathyroidism, and 79% had Addison's disease. Gonadal failure (72% in women, 26% in men) and hypoplasia of the dental enamel (77%) were also frequent findings. Other manifestations that occurred less often included alopecia (40%), vitiligo (26%), intestinal malabsorption (18%), type 1 diabetes (23%), pernicious anemia (31%), chronic active hepatitis (17%), and hypothyroidism (18%).[43] The incidence rates for many of these disorders peak in the first or second decade of life, and the disease continues to develop over decades (Fig. 41–3). Thus, reported prevalence rates of component disorders are highly dependent on the age at which follow-up ended.

APS-I is characteristically recognized in early childhood. Infants can present with chronic or recurrent mucocutaneous candidiasis in the first year of life that is then followed by hypoparathyroidism and Addison's disease, but new components can develop at any age. Decades can elapse between the diagnosis of one disorder and the onset of another in the same patient. Consequently, lifelong follow-up is important to allow early detection of additional components.

TABLE 41–2 CONTRASTING FEATURES OF AUTOIMMUNE POLYENDOCRINE SYNDROME

Feature	APS-I	APS-II
Inheritance pattern	Autosomal recessive (only siblings affected)	Polygenic (multiple generations affected)
Associated gene	*AIRE* gene mutation	*HLA-DR3* and *DR-4* associated
Gender association	Equal gender incidence	Female preponderance
Age at onset	Onset in infancy	Peak onset 20 to 60 years
Clinical features	Mucocutaneous candidiasis Hypoparathyroidism Addison's disease	Type 1 diabetes Autoimmune thyroid disease Addison's disease
"Diagnostic" Antibodies	Anti-Interferon	

APS, autoimmune polyendocrine syndrome.

TABLE 41–3 CLINICAL FEATURES AND RECOMMENDED FOLLOW-UP FOR APS-I AND APS-II

Component Disease	Frequency*	Recommended Evaluation
		AUTOIMMUNE POLYENDOCRINE SYNDROME TYPE I
Addison's disease	79%	Sodium, potassium, ACTH, cortisol, plasma renin activity, 21-hydroxylase autoantibodies
Diarrhea	18%	History
Ectodermal dysplasia	50%-75%	Physical examination
Hypoparathyroidism	86%	Serum calcium, phosphate, PTH
Hepatitis	17%	Liver function test
Hypothyroidism	18%	TSH; thyroid peroxidase and/or thyroglobulin autoantibodies
Male hypogonadism	26%	FSH/LH
Mucocutaneous candidiasis	100%	Physical examination
Obstipation	21%	History
Ovarian failure	72%	FSH/LH
Pernicious anemia	31%	CBC, vitamin B_{12} levels
Splenic atrophy	15%	Blood smear for Howell Jolly bodies; platelet count Ultrasound if positive
Type 1 diabetes	23%	Glucose, hemoglobin A_{1c}, diabetes-associated autoantibodies (insulin, GAD65, IA-2)
		AUTOIMMUNE POLYENDOCRINE SYNDROME TYPE II†
Addison's disease	0.5%	21-hydroxylase autoantibodies ACTH stimulation testing if positive
Alopecia		Physical examination
Autoimmune hypothyroidism	15%-30%	TSH; thyroid peroxidase and/or thyroglobulin autoantibodies
Celiac disease	5%-10%	Transglutaminase autoantibodies Small intestine biopsy if positive
Cerebellar ataxia	Rare‡	Dictated by signs and symptoms of disease
Chronic inflammatory demyelinating polyneuropathy	Rare‡	Dictated by signs and symptoms of disease
Hypophysitis	Rare‡	Dictated by signs and symptoms of disease
Idiopathic heart block	Rare‡	Dictated by signs and symptoms of disease
IgA deficiency	0.5%	IgA level
Myasthenia gravis	Rare‡	Dictated by signs and symptoms of disease
Myocarditis	Rare‡	Dictated by signs and symptoms of disease
Pernicious anemia	0.5%-5%	Antiparietal cell autoantibodies CBC, vitamin B_{12} levels if positive
Serositis	Rare‡	Dictated by signs and symptoms of disease
Stiff-man syndrome	Rare‡	Dictated by signs and symptoms of disease
Vitiligo	1%-9%	Physical examination

*At age 40.
†In the population with type 1 diabetes.
‡Rare reported disorders in subjects with APS-II.
ACTH, adrenocorticotropic hormone; APS, autoimmune polyendocrine syndrome; CBC, complete blood count; FSH, follicle-stimulating hormone; GAD, glutamic acid carboxylase; IgA, immunoglobulin A; LH, luteinizing hormone; PTH, parathyroid hormone; TSH, thyroid-stimulating hormone.

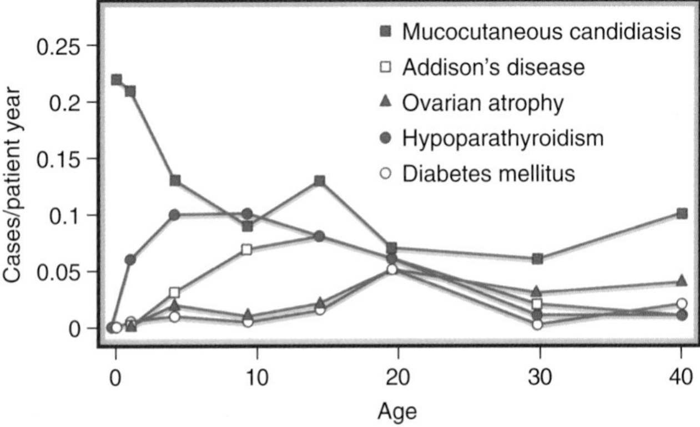

Figure 41–3 ▪ Incidence of disease development by age in patients with autoimmune polyendocrine syndrome type I (APS-I). (Reproduced from Perheentupa J. APS-I/APECED: the clinical disease and therapy. Endocrinol Metab Clin N Am 2002;31:295-320.)

Recurrent candidiasis commonly affects the mouth and nails and, less frequently, the skin and esophagus.[43] Chronic oral candidiasis can result in atrophic disease with areas suggestive of leukoplakia. If this develops, the patient is at significant risk for developing carcinoma of the oral mucosa (with its high mortality).

Ectodermal dystrophy is another component of the syndrome (manifested by pitted nails, keratopathy, and enamel hypoplasia) and cannot be attributed to hypoparathyroidism. Enamel hypoplasia can precede the onset of hypoparathyroidism and, despite adequate replacement therapy, can also affect teeth forming after the onset of hypoparathyroidism.[47]

Friedman and colleagues[48] reported the frequent occurrence of asplenism and cholelithiasis as additional features of APS-I. Splenic atrophy may also cause immune deficiency. Although the etiology of this disorder is unknown, it is relatively common: up to 15% of patients are asplenic.[43] Evidence of asplenia can be identified by the presence of Howell-Jolly bodies on peripheral smear. If asplenia is identified, immunization with polyvalent pneumococcal vaccine should be administered and follow-up antibody titers should be obtained. If an adequate response is not produced, daily prophylactic antibiotics may be necessary.

Malabsorption with steatorrhea is of uncertain origin, is usually intermittent, and may be exacerbated by hypocalcemia. Bereket and associates[49] reported a case with patchy intestinal lymphangiectasia discovered by endoscopically directed biopsy. Pancreatic insufficiency has been treated with cyclosporine.[50] Autoantibodies (e.g., tryptophan hydroxylase and histidine decarboxylase) reacting with intestinal endocrine cells (enterochromaffin, cholecystokinin, and enterochromaffin-like) occur and are associated with loss of endocrine cells on biopsy and with gastrointestinal dysfunction.[51,52]

Antiparathyroid and antiadrenal antibodies have been reported.[53] Cross-reactive autoantibodies might play a role in the multiorgan involvement of these disorders, as noted in several case reports. A target antigen for the autoantibodies found in autoimmune hypoparathyroidism was described by Li and colleagues,[54] who showed that 56% of 25 patients, 17 with APS-I, reacted to the extracellular domain of a membrane-associated antigen of 120 to 140 kd, which was identified as the calcium-sensing receptor. This is a controversial finding not confirmed in a population of 72 patients with APS-I and hypoparathyroidism.[55] Whereas 21-hydroxylase appears to be the major autoantigen in isolated Addison's disease and in Addison's disease associated with APS-II, autoantibodies against 17α-hydroxylase and cytochrome P450 side-chain cleavage enzyme (CYP11A1) have also been reported in Addison's disease associated with APS-I.[56]

Other autoantibodies that may be involved in other components of this disorder have been reported. These include antibodies to tryptophan hydroxylase in intestinal disease, tyrosine hydroxylase in alopecia areata, L-amino acid decarboxylase in hepatitis and vitiligo, and phenylalanine hydroxylase[57,58] and antibodies reacting with hair follicles.[59]

Tuomi and coworkers originally observed that many more APS-I patients (41%) express anti-GAD65 autoantibodies than become diabetic.[60] Among patients with APS-I in this study in whom diabetes developed, GAD65 autoantibodies could be detected up to 8 years before the onset of overt diabetes. They subsequently noted that many of the antibody-negative patients demonstrated T-cell responses to GAD65. Nearly 76% of all tested subjects showed either autoantibody or T-cell responses to GAD65 but only 18% had diabetes (8 of 44 subjects),[61] again suggesting that reactivity to this single autoantigen has low predictive value.

Genetics

APS-I is unique among autoimmune endocrine disorders in that the syndrome is not associated with high-risk class II HLA alleles, although the protective allele DQB1*0602 might protect against type 1 diabetes and DR3 is associated with diabetes risk.[60] APS-I shows an autosomal recessive pattern of inheritance, with a 25% recurrence risk for siblings of affected persons. The disorder has a high prevalence in Sardinia and Finland and in consanguineous Iranian Jewish families.

The etiologic gene was localized to the short arm of chromosome 21 (near markers D21s49 and D21s171 on 21p22.3) by Aaltonen and coworkers[62] and identified as the autoimmune regulator gene *AIRE*. The gene encodes a putative DNA-binding protein of unknown function expressed in the thymus and in lymphoid and other tissues. It has been localized to the nucleus, and mutations have been demonstrated to be associated with decreased transcription of reporter products.[63,64] *AIRE* gene knockout mice have decreased production of peripheral antigens within the thymus.[1,2] Reserchers hypothesize that *AIRE* acts as a transcriptional factor in cells of the thymus and that it promotes the expression of peripheral antigens in these APCs. Mutations in the *AIRE* gene are hypothesized to decrease central tolerance.

Multiple mutations of the AIRE gene have been identified in subjects with APS-I. The frequency of specific mutations varies in different populations. For example, in Sardinia, a deletion of amino acid 257 is present in 90% of mutated alleles. A 136-bp deletion in exon 8 is present in 71% of British alleles and 56% of alleles in the United States. Analysis of haplotypes indicates that this deletion has arisen on many occasions.

Diagnosis

The diagnosis of APS-I is highly likely when two or more of the primary component disorders are present (mucocutaneous candidiasis, hypoparathyroidism, and Addison's disease). Siblings of an affected patient should be considered affected with only one of the affected disorders. Analysis of the *AIRE* gene for the common mutations may be helpful in identifying subjects with APS-I. However, because multiple mutations have been discovered, the absence of a common mutation does not exclude APS-I. Any patient with any of the component disorders deserves careful follow-up to watch for development of additional disease.

Therapy

The treatment of adrenal insufficiency and hypoparathyroidism is the same as that discussed in other chapters with the caveat that malabsorption can complicate treatment. The therapy for mucocutaneous candidiasis has been improved with orally active antifungal drugs such as fluconazole and ketoconazole. Infection often recurs when the drug is discontinued or when the dosage is decreased. Patients must be monitored carefully because ketoconazole can inhibit adrenal and gonadal steroid synthesis and can precipitate adrenal failure. It is also associated with transient elevation of liver enzyme levels and, occasionally, hepatitis. Fluconazole is associated with a lower frequency of hepatitis and does not inhibit steroidogenesis when given in the recommended doses.

Screening to allow the early detection of new disorders before overt symptoms and signs develop is recommended, including autoantibody studies, electrolytes, calcium and phosphorus levels, thyroid and liver function tests, blood smear, and plasma vitamin B_{12}. Patients at risk for adrenal failure can be screened by measurement of basal ACTH and supine plasma renin activity (PRA) levels, followed by dynamic testing as appropriate. Evaluation for asplenism[48] with abdominal ultrasonography and blood smear examination for Howell-Jolly bodies is warranted, with pneumococcal vaccination and appropriate antibiotic coverage for affected patients.

Hypocalcemia has been associated with the intermittent steatorrhea characteristic of APS-I, and therapies that restore calcium levels have been beneficial. Treatment includes magnesium replacement for hypomagnesemia. Nevertheless, in individual patients, specific etiologic factors for intestinal dysfunction have been implicated, including pancreatic insufficiency, *Giardia lamblia* infection, and lymphangiectasia, and individualized therapy is required for these potentially diverse causes.

There are case reports of severely affected patients who have benefited from immunosuppressive therapy. For example, Ward and colleagues[50] treated a 13-year-old patient who had keratoconjunctivitis, hepatitis, and severe pancreatic insufficiency. Treatment with cyclosporine was associated with normalization of stool fat (from 31.5 g/day to 2.5 g/day).

Autoimmune Polyendocrine Syndrome Type II

Clinical Features

Autoimmune polyendocrine syndrome type II (APS-II) (MIM 269200) is more common than APS-I. It occurs more often in female than in male patients, often has its onset in adulthood, and exhibits familial aggregation (see Table 41–2). APS-II is usually defined by the occurrence in the same patient of two or more of the following: primary adrenal insufficiency (Addison's disease), Graves' disease, autoimmune thyroiditis, type 1A diabetes mellitus, primary hypogonadism, myasthenia gravis, or celiac disease. Vitiligo, alopecia, serositis, and pernicious anemia also occur with increased frequency in patients with this syndrome and their family members (see Table 41–3). Rare autoimmune disorders can also occur. For example, a case has been reported of autoimmune hyperparathyroidism in association with autoantibodies to the calcium receptor in a woman affected by multiple autoimmune diseases including autoimmune hypophysitis.[65]

When one of the component disorders is present, an associated disorder occurs more commonly than in the general population. Furthermore, circulating organ-specific autoantibodies are often present even in the absence of overt clinical disease. For example, in subjects with type 1 diabetes, there is a 15% to 20% risk of hypothyroidism, a 5% to 10% risk of celiac-related autoimmunity, and a 1.5% risk of adrenal autoimmunity. The risk of autoimmunity is greater in relatives of patients with APS-II. In our assessment of APS-II families with Addison's disease, we have noted that up to 15% of relatives have 21-hydroxylase autoantibodies (Addison's disease–associated autoantibodies), anti-islet autoantibodies, or transglutaminase (tTG) autoantibodies (celiac disease–associated autoantibodies). The initial lesion and precipitating events that result in the syndrome are unknown, but immunogenetic and immunologic similarities are present with regard to both the time course and the pathogenesis of each of the component disorders.

Because of the chronic development of organ-specific autoimmunity, patients with the syndrome and their families should have endocrinologic evaluations over time. In a family in which the syndrome has been documented, relatives should be advised of the early symptoms and signs of the principal component diseases. A list is available at www.barbaradaviscenter.org. Relatives of patients with multiple disorders should have a medical history, physical examination, and screening every 3 to 5 years, with measurement of anti-islet autoantibodies, a sensitive thyrotropin assay, and measurement of serum vitamin B_{12} levels. If there are any symptoms or signs or 21-hydroxylase autoantibodies, the patient should have annual assays of basal corticotropin and corticotropin-stimulated cortisol levels with cortrosyn stimulation testing.

Among 224 patients with Addison's disease and APS-II reported by Neufeld and colleagues,[46] type 1 diabetes (52%) and autoimmune thyroid disease (69%) were the most common coexisting conditions. Other components were less common, including vitiligo (5%) and gonadal failure (4%).

Among patients with type 1A diabetes, thyroid autoimmunity and celiac disease coexist with sufficient frequency to justify screening. Thyroid peroxidase autoantibodies are present in 10% to 20% of children with type 1 diabetes; this incidence is higher in female patients and increases in all patients with age and with diabetes duration. A significant fraction of patients with type 1 diabetes and thyroid peroxidase autoantibodies develops thyroid disease. One study showed that after follow-up for more than 15 years, 80% of patients with thyroid peroxidase autoantibodies and type 1 diabetes became hypothyroid.[66] However, several studies have shown that a subset of patients with negative autoantibodies develops thyroid disease. Thus, patients with type 1 diabetes should be screened annually for thyrotropin levels, which is a cost-effective approach.

With the identification of transglutominase as the major endomysial autoantigen of celiac disease, radioimmunoassays were developed and demonstrated that 10% to 12% of patients with type 1 diabetes have tTG autoantibodies.[7] The prevalence of tTG autoantibodies was higher in diabetic patients with HLA-DQ2; one third of DQ2-homozygous subjects were found to express anti-tTG antibody. Seventy percent of those with high-titer antibody who underwent biopsy were subsequently found to have the disease.[67] Therefore, screening with anti-tTG antibody can be carried out; if the results are positive and are confirmed on repeat assay, small bowel biopsy to document celiac disease is warranted, with institution of a gluten-free diet if the disease is present. Many patients have asymptomatic celiac disease that is nevertheless associated with osteopenia and impaired growth. Untreated, symptomatic celiac disease is also associated with an increased risk of gastrointestinal malignancy, especially lymphoma.

Hypoparathyroidism often occurs in APS-I but is rare in APS-II. If hypocalcemia occurs in a patient with the type II syndrome, celiac disease may be a more likely diagnosis than primary hypoparathyroidism. Nevertheless, we have described several elderly patients with APS-II who had a distinct form of hypoparathyroidism that, on the basis of a small series of patients, may be termed *geriatric hypoparathyroidism*. These patients form a distinct group because they have antibodies to the surface of parathyroid cells capable of suppressing parathyroid function and have a self-limited course of antibody presence and hypoparathyroidism.

Diagnosis

Improved assays for several organ-specific autoantibodies have been developed with the cloning of specific autoantigens and the development of assays that use recombinant antigens. These radioimmunoassays are superior to assays based on immunofluorescence with tissue sections, such as ICA testing. The most notable finding is the identification of a large number of different autoantigens that are targeted even in single autoimmune disorders. Most of the endocrine autoantigens are hormones (such as insulin) or enzymes associated with differentiated endocrine function: thyroid peroxidase in thyroiditis; glutamic acid decarboxylase, carboxypeptidase H, and ICA512/IA-2 in type 1 diabetes; 17α-hydroxylase and 21-hydroxylase in Addison's disease; and the parietal cell enzyme H^+/K^+-adenosine triphosphatase in pernicious anemia.

In type 1 diabetes, the four most informative assays currently available determine autoantibodies that react with insulin, GAD65 (glutamic acid decarboxylase), ICA512/IA-2, and ICA512β/IA-2β. In a similar manner, a radioassay format for the detection of autoantibodies that react with the enzyme 21-hydroxylase in Addison's disease has been developed and provides excellent disease specificity and sensitivity. Adrenal autoantibodies reacting with recombinant 21-hydroxylase usually precede the development of Addison's disease. However, as with thyroid autoantibodies, there may be patients who present with antibodies but who have normal production of cortisol in response to ACTH. Continued endocrine testing every year initially and then every other year are indicated in this situation.

In contrast to the autoimmune polyendocrine disorders with T cell–mediated glandular destruction, autoantibodies may also be pathogenic. A hallmark of pathogenic autoantibodies is the existence of a neonatal form of the disorder, secondary to transplacental passage of the autoantibody. Examples include neonatal Graves' disease (anti-thyrotropin–receptor autoantibodies) and neonatal myasthenia gravis (anti–acetyl choline–receptor autoantibodies).

Therapy

Treatment of the individual diseases of the polyendocrine autoimmune syndrome is discussed in other chapters. Therapeutic considerations related specifically to APS-II are discussed here.

Many of the component disorders of the syndrome have a long prodromal phase and are associated with the expression of autoantibodies before overt disease. The way the disorders develop allows the consideration of disease prediction and of clinical trials for prevention. This is particularly important for type 1A diabetes but is also likely to apply to Addison's disease and hypogonadism.

Because of the autoimmune nature of these disorders, several studies have evaluated immunosuppressive drugs. Drugs such as cyclosporine have preserved some residual insulin secretion. However, because cyclosporine is nephrotoxic and potentially oncogenic, its more generalized use is precluded. Newer immunosuppressive agents (mycophenolate mofetil or sirolimus) and biologics such as anti-IL-2 receptor (daclizumab) or nonmitogenic CD3 antibodies have been shown to prolong C-peptide production and result in a decreased insulin dose through the first year of diabetes compared with control subjects.[68]

Mucosal administration of antigens is commonly associated with bystander immunosuppression, in which T cells specific to the antigen are apparently induced to produce suppressive T_H2-like or T_H3-like cytokines (e.g., IL-4, IL-10, and transforming growth factor-β). In addition, subcutaneous administration of insulin prevents diabetes and insulitis in animal models, and subcutaneous administration of insulin peptides in adjuvants can prevent diabetes but not insulitis. A large National Institutes of Health (NIH) trial, the Diabetes Prevention Trial—Type 1 (DPT-1), directly tested oral and parenteral insulin for prevention of diabetes. DPT-1 had two arms: intravenous-subcutaneous for those at high risk (risk of diabetes more than 50% within 5 years) and oral insulin for those at moderate risk (risk of diabetes 25% to 50% within 5 years). Neither parenteral[69] nor oral[70] insulin slowed progression to diabetes. However, in a subgroup analysis of subjects in the DPT-1 oral trial, a treatment effect was noted for subjects who had the higher insulin autoantibody levels at diagnosis,[70] and further trials are underway. In preclinical Addison's disease, a short course of glucocorticoids appeared to suppress the expression of adrenal autoantibodies and prevent progressive adrenal destruction.[71]

There are several life-threatening autoimmune disorders including myocarditis that have been reported in patients with APS syndromes. This has been modeled in nonobese diabetic (NOD) mice, in which fatal myocarditis occurs in mice where the human DQ8 diabetes allele has been introduced.[72] For such patients, aggressive immunotherapies are considered, and because the disease is rare, there is a lack of clinical trials to guide therapies. Novel agents are being considered, such as monoclonal antibodies that react with the IL2-receptor followed by mycophenolate mofetil (current new-onset diabetes TrialNet study) and anti-B cell (ant-CD20) monoclonal antibodies. It would appear counterintuitive to use a monoclonal antibody to the IL-2 receptor (e.g., CD25) because $CD4^+/CD25^+$ T cells are important regulatory cells, but such antibodies have dramatic effects in uveitis and multiple sclerosis. The anti-CD20 antibody, though targeting B lymphocytes, has had apparent beneficial effects in rheumatoid arthritis, and trials in diabetes are planned. The anti-CD20 monoclonal antibodies might work in predominantly T cell–mediated disorders by effects on B-lymphocyte presentation of antigen to T cells.

Thyroxine therapy can precipitate a life-threatening addisonian crisis in a patient with untreated adrenal insufficiency and hypothyroidism. Thus, it is necessary to evaluate adrenal function in all hypothyroid patients in whom the syndrome is suspected before instituting such therapy. A decreasing insulin requirement in a patient with insulin-dependent diabetes mellitus can be one of the earliest indications of adrenal insufficiency, occurring before the development of hyperpigmentation or electrolyte abnormalities.

Other Polyendocrine Deficiency Autoimmune Syndromes

Rare polyendocrine syndromes are listed in Table 41–4.

Anti-Insulin–Receptor Autoantibodies

In this rarely reported disorder (~25 patients), also known as type B insulin resistance and acanthosis nigricans, insulin resistance is due to the presence of anti-insulin–receptor antibodies.[73] Approximately one third of patients with these antibodies have an associated autoimmune illness such as SLE or Sjögren's syndrome. Arthralgia, vitiligo, alopecia, and secondary amenorrhea have also been reported. One patient had a daughter with hyperthyroidism and a granddaughter with SLE. Autoimmune thyroid disease has been described in two such patients, one with hypothyroidism and the other with antithyroid antibodies. Antinuclear antibodies and an elevated erythrocyte sedimentation rate, hyperglobulinemia, leukopenia, and hypocomplementemia are common.[74]

The major clinical manifestations are related to the anti-insulin–receptor antibodies. Insulin resistance is profound, and up to 175,000 U of insulin given intravenously per day may be ineffective in lowering the elevated glucose. Despite hyperglycemia and marked insulin resistance, ketoacidosis is uncommon. The course of the diabetes is variable, and several patients have had spontaneous remissions. Other patients have had severe hypoglycemia (perhaps related to the insulin-like effects of anti-insulin–receptor antibodies demonstrable in vitro).[74] The acanthosis nigricans, which is due to hypertrophy and folding of otherwise histologically normal skin, appears to be related to the insulin-resistant state. Other forms of marked insulin resistance in the absence of antireceptor antibodies are also associated with acanthosis nigricans.

POEMS Syndrome

The components of the multisystem disorder POEMS (*p*lasma cell dyscrasia with polyneuropathy, *o*rganomegaly, *e*ndocrinopathy, *M* protein, and *s*kin changes, aka Crow-Fukase syndrome; MIM 192240) consist of diabetes mellitus (20%-50% of patients), primary gonadal failure (55%-70% of patients), plasma cell dyscrasia, sclerotic bone lesions, and neuropathy.[75] Patients usually present with severe progressive sensorimotor polyneuropathy, hepatosplenomegaly, lymphadenopathy, and hyperpigmentation. On evaluation, they are found to have plasma cell dyscrasia and sclerotic bone lesions. Patients present in the fifth to sixth decade of life and have a median survival after diagnosis of less than 3 years.[75]

POEMS is assumed to be secondary to circulating immunoglobulins, but binding of antibody directly to involved tissues has not been demonstrated. There is evidence implicating cytokines such as IL-1a, IL-6, and tumor necrosis factor α in addition to the M protein in the pathogenesis of this disorder. Several studies have also demonstrated that elevated levels of vascular endothelial growth factor (VEGF) correlate with the disease

TABLE 41–4 RARE POLYENDOCRINE DISORDERS

Disorder	Clinical Features	Cause
Hirata's disease (insulin resistance syndrome)	Hypoglycemia	Insulin autoantibodies Associated with methimazole
IPEX	Type 1 diabetes Enteropathy	Mutations of *FOXp3* gene
Kearns-Sayre syndrome	Hypoparathyroidism Primary gonadal failure Nonautoimmune diabetes Hypopituitarism	Deletions of mitochondrial DNA
POEMS	Polyneuropathy Organomegaly Diabetes Primary gonadal failure	Plasma cell dyscrasia with production of M protein and cytokines
Thymic tumors	Myasthenia gravis Red blood cell hypoglobulinemia Autoimmune thyroid disease Adrenal insufficiency	Thymomas
Type B insulin resistance	Severe insulin resistance	Insulin receptor autoantibodies
Wolfram's syndrome	Diabetes insipidus Nonautoimmune diabetes Bilateral optic atrophy Sensorineural deafness	Mutations of *WSF1* gene, which encodes wolframin gene

IPEX, immunodysregulation polyendocrinopathy enteropathy X-linked syndrome; POEMS, plasma cell dyscrasia with *p*olyneuropathy, *o*rganomegaly, *e*ndocrinopathy, *M* protein, and *s*kin changes.

state and that treatment with immunosuppressive agents reduced the symptoms of the disease and the levels of VEGF, suggesting that this growth factor plays a role in the disease.[76,77] A case report of the use of ticlopidine, which has been shown to decrease VEGF in experimental rats, showed decrease of VEGF with resolution of ascites, edema, and pleural effusions and no change in the remainder of clinical disease.[78] A therapeutic trial of an anti-VEGF antibody would provide more definitive evidence for this hypothesis.

The diabetes mellitus responds to small subcutaneous doses of insulin. The hypogonadism is associated with elevated plasma levels of follicle-stimulating hormone and luteinizing hormone. Temporary resolution of disease, including a return of the blood glucose level to normal, might occur after radiotherapy for localized plasma cell lesions of bone. Peripheral blood stem cell transplantation has been performed and shows promise with stabilization or improvement of the components of POEMS in transplanted patients. However, transplantation is not without risks, including death and respiratory failure.[79,80]

Kearns-Sayre Syndrome

The rare Kearns-Sayre syndrome (MIM 530000), also known as oculocraniosomatic disease or oculocraniosomatic neuromuscular disease with ragged red fibers, is characterized by myopathic abnormalities leading to ophthalmoplegia and progressive weakness in association with several endocrine abnormalities, including hypoparathyroidism, primary gonadal failure, diabetes mellitus, and hypopituitarism.[81] Crystalline mitochondrial inclusions are found in muscle biopsy specimens, and such inclusions have also been observed in the cerebellum. The relation between the mitochondrial disorders and endocrinologic abnormalities is not known. Antiparathyroid antibodies have not been described; however, antibodies to the anterior pituitary gland and striated muscle have been found, and the disease may have autoimmune components. Other abnormalities include retinitis pigmentosa and heart block. Deletions in mitochondrial DNA have been associated with Kearns-Sayre syndrome.[82] The mutations generally occur sporadically and are therefore not associated with a familial syndrome.

Thymic Tumors

The thymus is a complex tissue with a specialized endocrine epithelium that synthesizes a variety of biologically active peptides involved in the control of T-cell maturation. This epithelium is derived from the neural crest and contains complex gangliosides that react with monoclonal antibody (A2B5) and tetanus toxin in a manner similar to that of pancreatic islets.

The illnesses associated with thymomas are similar to those in APS-II,[83] although the incidence of specific disorders is different. In one review of patients with thymoma, myasthenia gravis occurred in 44% of the patients, red blood cell aplasia in approximately 20%, hypoglobulinemia in 6%, autoimmune thyroid disease in 2%, and adrenal insufficiency in 1 of 423 patients (0.0024%). The incidence of autoimmune thyroid disease reported in patients with thymoma is probably an underestimate, given the incidence of unsuspected thyroid disease in patients with myasthenia gravis. Mucocutaneous candidiasis in adults is also associated with thymomas. In most patients, the thymomas are malignant, although temporary remissions of the autoimmune disease can occur with resection of the tumor.

Trisomy 21

Down syndrome, or trisomy 21 (MIM 190685), is associated with the development of type 1 diabetes mellitus and thyroiditis. We have observed one patient with a partial distal translocation "leading" to trisomy 21 and "associated" with adrenal insufficiency, celiac disease, hypothyroidism, and diabetes. Patients with trisomy 21 also have T cell abnormalities, including increased Ia-positive T cells and a premature increase in the 3G5 age-related T cell subset.[84] It is not known whether the observed chromosomal abnormality influences the development of autoimmunity or whether part of the susceptibility to autoimmunity is associated with chromosomal disorders.[85] Organ-specific autoimmunity also occurs with gonadal dysgenesis.[86]

Congenital Rubella

Patients with congenital rubella have an almost 20% risk of acquiring diabetes mellitus and a higher than normal risk of acquiring thyroiditis and hypothyroidism.[87,88] Those at highest risk for diabetes express diabetes-associated HLA-DR3 and HLA-DR4 alleles.[89] Rubella appears to be associated with diabetes primarily after fetal infection, and it is not known if the virus increases the probability of subsequent autoimmunity because it has permanent effects on the developing immune system.[90] Due to the intensive effort to immunize against the rubella virus, recent reports from the Centers from Disease Control and Prevention (CDC) indicate that rubella is no longer endemic in the United States.[91]

Wolfram's Syndrome

Wolfram's syndrome (MIM 222300, chromosome 4; 598500, mitochondrial) is a rare autosomal recessive disease that is also called DIDMOAD (*d*iabetes *i*nsipidus, *d*iabetes *m*ellitus, progressive bilateral *o*ptic *a*trophy, and sensorineural *d*eafness). In addition, neurologic and psychiatric disturbances are prominent in most patients and can cause severe disability. Atrophic changes in the brain have been found with magnetic resonance imaging.[92] Segregation analysis of the mutations found in familial and sporadic cases of Wolfram's syndrome led to the identification of wolframin, encoded by the gene *WFS1*, a 100-kd transmembrane protein encoded by a gene located at 4p16.1.116. Genotype and phenotype analyses have identified the severe phenotype (defined as the development of neurologic disease within the first decade) in truncated proteins and with mutations on the C-terminal of the protein and deafness.[93]

Wolframin has been localized to the endoplasmic reticulum[94] and found in neuronal and neuroendocrine tissue.[95] Its expression induces ion channel activity with the resultant increase in intracellular calcium and might play an important role in intracellular calcium homeostasis.[96] Functional studies of *WFS1* mutations have shown that reported mutations lead to decreased stability of the protein wolframin.[95] Linkage to other loci in addition to *WFS1* might explain the variability in phenotype seen in this disorder.

Wolfram's syndrome appears to be a slowly progressive neurodegenerative process, and there is also (nonautoimmune) selective destruction of the pancreatic beta cells. This association is likely due to the expression pattern of *WFS1*. Diabetes mellitus with an onset in childhood is usually the first manifestation. Diabetes mellitus and optic atrophy are present in all reported cases, but expression of the other features is variable. Duration of diabetes is linked to the development of microvascular complications.[97] Additional endocrinologic diseases such as ACTH deficiency and growth hormone deficiency have been reported.[97] In one case report, two related children with Wolfram's syndrome had megaloblastic and sideroblastic anemia that responded to treatment with thiamine. Furthermore, thiamine treatment was associated with a marked decrease in insulin requirements.[98]

Immunodysregulation Polyendocrinopathy Enteropathy X-Linked Syndrome

IPEX (MIM 340790, MIM 300292), first described in 1982, is a rare X-linked recessive disorder characterized by immune dysregulation and resulting in multiple autoimmune diseases and early death (Fig. 41–4). Its clinical features include early type 1 diabetes and severe enteropathy resulting in failure to thrive. Other reported abnormalities include eczema or atopy, thrombocytopenia, hemolytic anemia, hypothyroidism and lymphadenopathy.[99]

Characteristics of the scurfy mouse gene *(sf)* bear a number of similarities to this syndrome, and abnormalities in the *sf* gene lead to abnormalities in the amount and function of scurfin, a DNA-binding protein in these mice.[100] Implanting thymus from scurfy mouse into immunoincompetent mice transfers disease, but transplanting thymus into immunocompetent mice does not transfer disease, and injections of normal T cells could rescue the phenotype. These observations suggest that a regulatory cell was involved in the pathogenesis of this disorder.

Linkage analysis demonstrated that a 17-cM stretch of the X chromosome (Xp11.1-q13.3) is associated with IPEX, and mutations within the *FOXp3* gene have been identified in the majority of families studied thus far.[101] The *FOXp3* gene encodes a protein called scurfin and belongs to the forkhead class of winged helix transcription factors. It is hypothesized to function as a transcription factor. *FOXp3* has been shown to be expressed in $CD4^+/CD25^+$ regulatory T cells.[102] These T cells can suppress activation of other T cells[102] (see Fig. 41–4). Thus, mutations in FOXp3 result in the inability to generate regulatory T cells and the development of IPEX.

Therapy has been targeted to the component disorders. Bone marrow transplantation (BMT) has been attempted with mixed success, and there is evidence for disease regression in most subjects.[103] Use of immunosuppressive therapy with sirolimus has been reported to have beneficial effects in three patients with IPEX.[104]

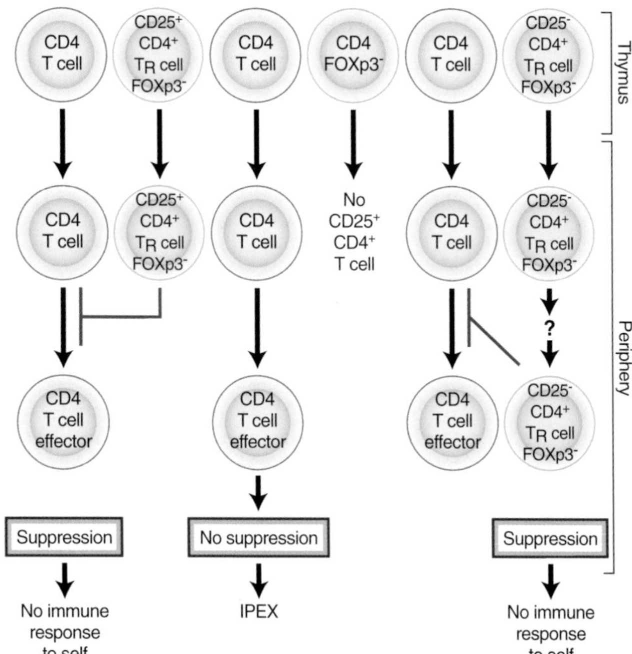

Figure 41–4 ▪ The development of $CD4^+/CD25^+$ regulatory T cells in the thymus is dependent on FOXp3 expression. The lack of FOXp3 in immune dysregulation, polyendocrinopathy, enteropathy, X-linked (IPEX) syndrome prevents the development of these regulatory T cells and promotes the development of autoimmunity. (Reproduced from Sakaguchi S. The origin of FOXp3-expression regulatory T-cells: thymus or periphery. J Clin Invest 2003;112:1310-1312.)

Omenn's Syndrome

Omenn's syndrome (MIM 603554) is a primary immunodeficiency syndrome with autoimmune manifestations primarily affecting the skin and gastrointestinal tract. Mutations associated with decreased recombination of the T-cell receptor have been described. A recent report has shown that the levels of *AIRE* gene expression are decreased in the thymus of two affected patients and that was associated with decreased expression of peripheral antigens compared with controls.[105]

Conclusion

Through the understanding of rare disorders such as APS-I and IPEX, the processes of thymic expression of peripheral antigens and the development of regulatory T cells are beginning to be defined. This understanding provides invaluable insight into the development of the normal immune system and mistakes that can occur and lead to autoimmunity. Lessons learned from these rare diseases will help to better define the pathophysiology of more common autoimmune endocrine disorders, hopefully leading to the development of immunologic methods for preventing and treating these disorders.

REFERENCES

1. Ramsey C, Winqvist O, Puhakka L, et al. AIRE deficient mice develop multiple features of APECED phenotype and show altered immune response. Hum Mol Genet 2002;11:397-409.
2. Anderson MS, Venanzi ES, Klein L, et al. Projection of an immunological self shadow within the thymus by the AIRE protein. Science 2002;298:1395-1401.
3. Redondo MJ, Yu L, Hawa M, et al. Heterogenity of type 1 diabetes: analysis of monozygotic twins in Great Britain and the United States. Diabetologia 2001;44:354-362.
4. Pugliese A, Zeller M, Fernandez A, et al. The insulin gene is transcribed in the human thymus and transcription levels correlate with allelic variation at the INS VNTR-IDDM2 susceptibility locus for type I diabetes. Nat Genet 1997;15:293-297.
5. Yu L, Brewer KW, Gates S, et al. DRB1*04 and DQ alleles: expression of 21-hydroxylase autoantibodies and risk of progression to Addison's disease. J Clin Endocrinol Metab 1999;84:328-335.
6. Myhre AG, Undlien DE, Lovas K, et al. Autoimmune adrenocortical failure in Norway: autoantibodies and HLA class II associations related to clinical features. J Clin Endocrinol Metab 2002; 87:618-623.
7. Bao F, Yu L, Babu S, et al. One third of HLA DQ2 homozygous patients with type 1 diabetes express celiac disease associated transglutaminase autoantibodies. J Autoimmunity 1999;13:143-148.
8. Hoffenberg EJ, McKenzie TL, Barriga KJ, et al. A prospective study of the incidence of childhood celiac disease. J Paediatr 2003; 143:308-314.
9. Levin L, Ban Y, Concepcion E, et al. Analysis of HLA genes in families with autoimmune diabetes and thyroiditis. Hum Immunol 2004;65:640-647.
10. Ban Y, Davies TF, Greenberg DA, et al.: The influence of human leucocyte antigen (HLA) genes on autoimmune thyroid disease (AITD): results of studies in HLA-DR3 positive AITD families. Clin Endocrinol (Oxf) 2002;57:81-88.
11. Huang W, Connor E, Rosa TD, et al.: Although DR3-DQB1*0201 may be associated with multiple component diseases of the autoimmune polyglandular syndromes, the human leukocyte antigen DR4-DQB1*0302 haplotype is implicated only in beta-cell autoimmunity. J Clin Endocrinol Metab 1996;81:2559-2563.
12. Baisch JM, Weeks T, Giles R, et al. Analysis of HLA-DQ genotypes and susceptibility in insulin-dependent diabetes mellitus. N Engl J Med 1990;322:1836-1841.
13. Zake LN, Ghaderi M, Park YS, et al. MHC class I chain-related gene alleles 5 and 5.1 are transmitted more frequently to type 1 diabetes offspring in HBDI families. Ann N Y Acad Sci 2002;958:309-311.
14. Bilbao JR, Martin-Pagola A, Vitoria JC, et al. HLA-DRB1 and MHC class 1 chain-related A haplotypes in Basque families with celiac disease. Tissue Antigens 2002;60:71-76.
15. Park YS, Sanjeevi CB, Robles D, et al. Additional association of intra-MHC genes, MICA and D6S273, with Addison's disease. Tissue Antigens 2002;60:155-163.
16. Martin-Pagola A, Ortiz L, Perez dN, et al. Analysis of the expression of MICA in small intestinal mucosa of patients with celiac disease. J Clin Immunol 2003;23:498-503.
17. Hue S, Mention JJ, Monteiro RC, et al. A direct role for NKG2D/MICA interaction in villous atrophy during celiac disease. Immunity 2004;21:367-377.
18. Martin-Pagola A, Perez-Nanclares G, Ortiz L, et al. MICA response to gliadin in intestinal mucosa from celiac patients. Immunogenetics 2004;56:549-554.
19. Bottini N, Muscumeci L, Alonso A, et al. A functional variant of lymphoid tyrosine phosphatase is associated with type I diabetes. Nature Genet 2004;36:337-338.
20. van Oene M, Wintle RF, Liu X, et al. Association of the lymphoid tyrosine phosphatase R620W variant with rheumatoid arthritis, but not Crohn's disease, in Canadian populations. Arthritis Rheum 2005;52:1993-1998.
21. Orozco G, Sanchez E, Gonzalez-Gay MA, et al. Association of a functional single-nucleotide polymorphism of PTPN22, encoding lymphoid protein phosphatase, with rheumatoid arthritis and systemic lupus erythematosus. Arthritis Rheum 2005;52:219-224.
22. Velaga MR, Wilson V, Jennings CE, et al. The codon 620 tryptophan allele of the lymphoid tyrosine phosphatase (LYP) gene is a major determinant of Graves' disease. J Clin Endocrinol Metab 2004; 89:5862-5865.
23. Canton I, Akhtar S, Gavalas NG, et al. A single-nucleotide polymorphism in the gene encoding lymphoid protein tyrosine phosphatase (PTPN22) confers susceptibility to generalised vitiligo. Genes Immun 2005;6:584-587.
24. Criswell LA, Pfeiffer KA, Lum RF, et al. Analysis of families in the multiple autoimmune disease genetics consortium (MADGC) collection: the PTPN22 620W allele associates with multiple autoimmune phenotypes. Am J Hum Genet 2005;76:561-571.
25. Vaidya B, Pearce S. The emerging role of the CTLA-4 gene in autoimmune endocrinopathies. Eur J Endocrinol 2004;150: 619-626.
26. Takara M, Kouki T, DeGroot LJ. CTLA-4 AT-repeat polymorphism reduces the inhibitory function of CTLA-4 in Graves' disease. Thyroid 2003;13:1083-1089.
27. Ban Y, Concepcion ES, Villanueva R, et al. Analysis of immune regulatory genes in familial and sporadic Graves' disease. J Clin Endocrinol Metab 2004;89:4562-4568.
28. Ban Y, Tozaki T, Taniyama M, et al. Association of a CTLA-4 3′ untranslated region (CT60) single nucleotide polymorphism with autoimmune thyroid disease in the Japanese population. Autoimmunity 2005;38:151-153.
29. Van Belzen MJ, Mulder CJ, Zhernakova A, et al. CTLA4 +49 A/G and CT60 polymorphisms in Dutch coeliac disease patients. Eur J Hum Genet 2004;12:782-785.
30. Ban Y, Davies TF, Greenberg DA, et al. Analysis of the CTLA-4, CD28, and inducible costimulator (ICOS) genes in autoimmune thyroid disease. Genes Immun 2003;4:586-593.
31. Vaidya B, Imrie H, Geatch DR, et al.: Association analysis of the cytotoxic T lymphocyte antigen–4 (CTLA-4) and autoimmune regulator–1 (AIRE-1) genes in sporadic autoimmune Addison's disease. J Clin Endocrinol Metab 2000;85:688-691.
32. Tomer Y, Greenberg DA, Concepcion E, et al. Thyroglobulin is a thyroid specific gene for the familial autoimmune thyroid diseases. J Clin Endocrinol Metab 2002;87:404-407.
33. Lambert AP, Gillespie KM, Thomson G, et al. Absolute risk of childhood-onset type 1 diabetes defined by human leukocyte antigen class ii genotype: a population-based study in the United Kingdom. J Clin Endocrinol Metab 2004;89:4037-4043.
34. Norris JM, Barriga K, Hoffenberg EJ, et al. Risk of celiac disease autoimmunity and timing of gluten introduction in the diet of infants at increased risk of disease. JAMA 2005;293:2343-2351.
35. Norris JM, Barriga K, Klingensmith G, et al. Timing of cereal exposure in infancy and risk of islet autoimmunity. The Diabetes Autoimmunity Study in the Young (DAISY). JAMA 2003;290:1713-1720.

36. Ziegler AG, Schmid S, Huber D, et al. Early infant feeding and risk of developing type 1 diabetes–associated autoantibodies. JAMA 2003;290:1721-1728.
37. Coles AJ, Wing M, Smith S, et al. Pulsed monoclonal antibody treatment and autoimmune thyroid disease in multiple sclerosis. Lancet 1999;354:1691-1695.
38. Gisslinger H, Gilly B, Woloszczuk W, et al.: Thyroid autoimmunity and hypothyroidism during long-term treatment with recombinant interferon-alpha. Clin Exp Immunol 1992;90:363-367.
39. Bosi E, Minelli R, Bazzigaluppi E, et al. Fulminant autoimmune type 1 diabetes during interferon-alpha therapy: a case of Th1-mediated disease? Diabet Med 2001;18:329-332.
40. Uchigata Y, Kuwata S, Tsushima T, et al. Patients with Graves' disease who developed insulin autoimmune syndrome (Hirata disease) possess HLA-Bw62/Cw4/DR4 carrying DRB1*0406. J Clin Endocrinol Metab 1993;77:249-254.
41. Pugliese A, Brown D, Garza D, et al. Self-antigen presenting cells expressing islet cell molecules in human thymus and peripheral lymphoid organs: phenotypic characterization and implications for immunological tolerance and type 1 diabetes. J Clin Invest 2001;107:555-564.
42. Lohmann T, Sessler J, Verlohren HJ, et al. Distinct genetic and immunological features in patients with onset of IDDM before and after age 40. Diabetes Care 1997;20:524-529.
43. Perheentupa J. APS-I/APECED: The clinical disease and therapy. Endocrinol Metab Clinic North Am 2002;31:295-320.
44. Ahonen P, Myllarniemi S, Sipila I, et al. Clinical variation of autoimmune polyendocrinopathy—candidiasis—ectodermal dystrophy (APECED) in a series of 68 patients. N Engl J Med 1990; 322:1829-1836.
45. Perheentupa J, Miettinen A. Autoimmune polyendocrinopathy-candidiasis-ectodermal dystrophy. In Eisenbarth GS, ed. Endocrine and Organ Specific Autoimmunity. Austin, TX: RG Landes, 1999:19-40.
46. Neufeld M, Maclaren NK, Blizzard RM. Two types of autoimmune Addison's disease associated with different polyglandular autoimmune (PGA) syndromes. Medicine (Baltimore) 1981;60:355-362.
47. Walls AWG, Soames JV. Dental manifestations of autoimmune hypoparathyroidism. Oral Surg Oral Med Oral Pathol 1993; 75:452-454.
47a. Meager A, Visvalingam K, Peterson P, et al. Anti-interferon Antibodies in Autoimmune Polyendocrine Syndrome Type 1. PloS Medicine 3:e289, 2006.
48. Friedman TC, Thomas PM, Fleisher TA, et al. Frequent occurrence of asplenism and cholelithiasis in patients with autoimmune polyglandular disease type I. Am J Med 1991;91:625-630.
49. Bereket A, Lowenheim M, Blethen SL, et al. Intestinal lymphangiectasia in a patient with autoimmune polyglandular disease type I and steatorrhea. J Clin Endocrinol Metab 1995;80:933-955.
50. Ward L, Paquette J, Seidman E, et al. Severe autoimmune polyendocrinopathy-candidiasis-ectodermal dystrophy in an adolescent girl with a novel AIRE mutation: response to immunosuppressive therapy. J Clin Endocrinol Metab 1999;84:844-852.
51. Gianani R, Eisenbarth GS. Autoimmunity to gastrointestinal endocrine cells in autoimmune polyendocrine syndrome type I. J Clin Endocrinol Metab 2003;88:1442-1444.
52. Hogenauer C, Meyer RL, Netto GJ, et al. Malabsorption due to cholecystokinin deficiency in a patient with autoimmune polyglandular syndrome type I. N Engl J Med 2001;344:270-274.
53. Blizzard RM, Chee D, Davis W. The incidence of parathyroid and other antibodies in the sera of patients with idiopathic hypoparathyroidism. Clin Exp Immunol 1966;1:119-128.
54. Li Y, Song Y-H, Rais N, et al. Autoantibodies to the extracellular domain of the calcium sensing receptor in patients with acquired hypoparathyroidism. J Clin Invest 1996;97:910-914.
55. Soderbergh A, Myhre AG, Ekwall O, et al. Prevalence and clinical associations of 10 defined autoantibodies in autoimmune polyendocrine syndrome type I. J Clin Endocrinol Metab 2004;89: 557-562.
56. Uibo R, Aavik E, Peterson P, et al. Autoantibodies to cytochrome P450 enzymes P450scc, P450c17, and P450c21 in autoimmune polyglandular disease types I and II and in isolated Addison's disease. J Clin Endocrinol Metab 1994;78:323-328.
57. Ekwall O, Hedstrand H, Haavik J, et al. Pteridin-dependent hydroxylases as autoantigens in autoimmune polyendocrine syndrome type I. J Clin Endocrinol Metab 2000;85:2944-2950.
58. Husebye ES, Boe AS, Rorsman F, et al. Inhibition of aromatic L-amino acid decarboxylase activity by human autoantibodies. Clin Exp Immunol 2000;120:420-423.
59. Hedstrand H, Perheentupa J, Ekwall O, et al. Antibodies against hair follicles are associated with alopecia totalis in autoimmune polyendocrine syndrome type I. J Invest Dermatol 1999;113: 1054-1058.
60. Tuomi T, Björses P, Falorni A, et al. Antibodies to glutamic acid decarboxylase and insulin-dependent diabetes in patients with autoimmune polyendocrine syndrome type I. J Clin Endocrinol Metab 1996;81:1488-1494.
61. Klemetti P, Bjorses P, Tuomi T, et al. Autoimmunity to glutamic acid decarboxylase in patients with autoimmune polyendocrinopathy-candidiasis-ectodermal dystrophy (APECED). Clin Exp Immunol 2000;119:419-425.
62. Aaltonen J, Bjorses P, Sandkuijl L, et al. An autosomal locus causing autoimmune disease: autoimmune polyglandular disease type I assigned to chromosome 21. Nat Genet 1994;8:83-87.
63. Bjorses P, Halonen M, Palvimo JJ, et al. Mutations in the AIRE gene: effects on subcellular location and transactivation function of the autoimmune polyendocrinopathy-candidiasis-ectodermal dystrophy protein. Am J Hum Genet 2000;66:378-392.
64. Halonen M, Kangas H, Ruppell T, et al. APECED-causing mutations in AIRE reveal the functional domains of the protein. Hum Mutat 2004;23:245-257.
65. Pallais JC, Kifor O, Chen YB, et al. Acquired hypocalciuric hypercalcemia due to autoantibodies against the calcium-sensing receptor. N Engl J Med 2004;351:362-369.
66. Umpierrez GE, Latif KA, Murphy MB, et al. Thyroid dysfunction in patients with type 1 diabetes: a longitudinal study. Diabetes Care 2003;26:1181-1185.
67. Hoffenberg EJ, Bao F, Eisenbarth GS, et al. Transglutaminase antibodies in children with a genetic risk for celiac disease. J Pediatr 2000;137:356-360.
68. Herold KC, Gitelman SE, Masharani U, et al. A single course of anti-CD3 monoclonal antibody hOKT3γ1(Ala-Ala) results in improvement in C-peptide responses and clinical parameters for at least 2 years after onset of type 1 diabetes. Diabetes 2005;54:1763-1769.
69. Diabetes Prevention Trial Type 1. Effects of insulin in relatives of patients with type 1 diabetes mellitus. N Engl J Med 2002; 346:1685-1691.
70. Diabetes Prevention Trial Type 1. Effects of oral insulin in relatives of patients with type 1 diabetes: The Diabetes Prevention Trial—Type 1. Diabetes Care 2005;28:1068-1076.
71. De Bellis A, Bizzarro A, Rossi R, et al. Remission of subclinical adrenocortical failure in subjects with adrenal autoantibodies. J Clin Endocrinol Metab 1993;76:1002-1007.
72. Elliott JF, Liu J, Yuan ZN, et al. Autoimmune cardiomyopathy and heart block develop spontaneously in HLA-DQ8 transgenic IAβ knockout NOD mice. Proc Natl Acad Sci U S A 2003;100: 13447-13452.
73. Kahn CR, Flier JS, Bar RS, et al. The syndromes of insulin resistance and acanthosis nigricans: insulin-receptor disorders in man. N Engl J Med 1976;294:739-745.
74. Flier JS, Bar RS, Muggeo M, et al. The evolving clinical course of patients with insulin receptor autoantibodies: spontaneous remission or receptor proliferation with hypoglycemia. J Clin Endocrinol Metab 1978;47:985-995.
75. Dispenzieri A, Kyle RA, Lacy MQ, et al. POEMS syndrome: definitions and long-term outcome. Blood 2003;101:2496-2506.
76. Soubrier M, Dubost JJ, Serre AF, et al. Growth factors in POEMS syndrome: evidence for a marked increase in circulating vascular endothelial growth factor. Arthritis Rheum 1997;40:786-787.
77. Watanabe O, Maruyama I, Arimura K, et al. Overproduction of vascular endothelial growth factor/vascular permeability factor is causative in Crow-Fukase (POEMS) syndrome. Muscle Nerve 1998;21:1390-1397.
78. Matsui H, Udaka F, Kubori T, et al. POEMS syndrome demonstrating VEGF decrease by ticlopidine. Intern Med 2004;43:1082-1083.
79. Dispenzieri A, Moreno-Aspitia A, Suarez GA, et al. Peripheral blood stem cell transplantation in 16 patients with POEMS

syndrome, and a review of the literature. Blood 2004;104:3400-3407.

80. Hogan WJ, Lacy MQ, Wiseman GA, et al. Successful treatment of POEMS syndrome with autologous hematopoietic progenitor cell transplantation. Bone Marrow Transplant 2001;28:305-309.
81. Harvey JN, Barnett D. Endocrine dysfunction in Kearns-Sayre syndrome. Clin Endocrinol 1992;37:97-104.
82. De Block CE, De Leeuw IH, Maassen JA, et al. A novel 7301-bp deletion in mitochondrial DNA in a patient with Kearns-Sayre syndrome, diabetes mellitus, and primary amenorrhoea. Exp Clin Endocrinol Diabetes 2004;112:80-83.
83. Combs RM. Malignant thymoma, hyperthyroidism and immune disorder. South Med J 1968;61:337-341.
84. Rabinowe SL, Rubin IL, George KL, et al. Trisomy 21 (Down's syndrome): autoimmunity, aging and monoclonal-antibody defined T-cell abnormalities. J Autoimmun 1989;2:25-30.
85. Fialkow PJ, Thuline HC, Hecht F, et al. Familial predisposition to thyroid disease in Down's syndrome: controlled immunoclinical studies. Am J Hum Genet 1971;23:67-86.
86. Fleming S, Cowell C, Bailey J, et al. Hashimoto's disease in Turner's syndrome. Clin Invest Med 1988;11:243-246.
87. Menser MA, Forrest JM, Bransby RD. Rubella infection and diabetes mellitus. Lancet 1978;1:57-60.
88. Clarke WL, Shaver KA, Bright GM, et al. Autoimmunity in congenital rubella syndrome. J Pediatr 1984;104:370-373.
89. Rubenstein P. The HLA system in congenital rubella patients with and without diabetes. Diabetes 1982;31:1088-1091.
90. Rabinowe SL, George KL, Loughlin R, et al. Congenital rubella: monoclonal antibody–defined T cell abnormalities in young adults. Am J Med 1986;81:779-782.
91. Centers for Disease Control and Prevention. Elimination of rubella and congenital rubella syndrome—United States, 1969-2004. MMWR Morb Mortal Wkly Rep 2005;54:279-282.
92. Rando TA, Horton JC, Layzer RB. Wolfram syndrome: evidence of a diffuse neurodegenerative disease by magnetic resonance imaging. Semin Neurol 1992;42:1220-1224.
93. Smith CJ, Crock PA, King BR, et al. Phenotype-genotype correlations in a series of Wolfram syndrome families. Diabetes Care 2004;27:2003-2009.
94. Takeda K, Inoue H, Tanizawa Y, et al. WFS1 (Wolfram syndrome 1) gene product: predominant subcellular localization to endoplasmic reticulum in cultured cells and neuronal expression in rat brain. Hum Mol Genet 2001;10:477-484.
95. Hofmann S, Philbrook C, Gerbitz KD, et al. Wolfram syndrome: structural and functional analyses of mutant and wild-type wolframin, the WFS1 gene product. Hum Mol Genet 2003;12:2003-2012.
96. Osman AA, Saito M, Makepeace C, et al. Wolframin expression induces novel ion channel activity in endoplasmic reticulum membranes and increases intracellular calcium. J Biol Chem 2003;278:52755-52762.
97. Medlej R, Wasson J, Baz P, et al. Diabetes mellitus and optic atrophy: a study of Wolfram syndrome in the Lebanese population. J Clin Endocrinol Metab 2004;89:1656-1661.
98. Borgna-Pignatti C, Marradi P, Pinelli L, et al. Thiamine-responsive anemia in DIDMOAD syndrome. J Pediatr 1989;114:405-410.
99. Powell BR, Buist NR, Stenzel P. An X-linked syndrome of diarrhea, polyendocrinopathy, and fatal infection in infancy. J Pediatr 1982;100:731-737.
100. Godfrey VL, Wilkinson JE, Russell LB. X-linked lymphoreticular disease in the scurfy (sf) mutant mouse. Am J Pathol 1991;138: 1379-1387.
101. Chatila TA, Blaeser F, Ho N, et al. JM2, encoding a fork head-related protein, is mutated in X-linked autoimmunity-allergic disregulation syndrome. J Clin Invest 2000;106:R75-R81.
102. Walker MR, Kasprowicz DJ, Gersuk VH, et al. Induction of FoxP3 and acquisition of T regulatory activity by stimulated human $CD4^+$ $CD25^-$ T cells. J Clin Invest 2003;112:1437-1443.
103. Baud O, Goulet O, Canioni D, et al. Treatment of the immune dysregulation, polyendocrinopathy, enteropathy, X-linked syndrome (IPEX) by allogeneic bone marrow transplantation. N Engl J Med 2001;344:1758-1762.
104. Bindl L, Torgerson T, Perroni L, et al. Successful use of the new immune-suppressor sirolimus in IPEX (immune dysregulation, polyendocrinopathy, enteropathy, X-linked syndrome). J Pediatr 2005;147:256-259.
105. Cavadini P, Vermi W, Facchetti F, et al. AIRE deficiency in thymus of 2 patients with Omenn syndrome. J Clin Invest 2005;115: 728-732.

SECTION XI

Paraendocrine and Neoplastic Syndromes

CHAPTER 42

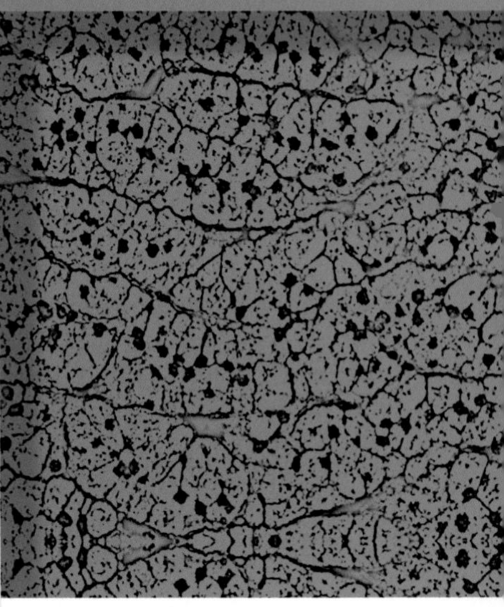

ENDOCRINE-RESPONSIVE CANCER

Richard Santen

BREAST CANCER

Etiology

A variety of data suggest that estrogens contribute to the development of breast cancer. Administration of exogenous estrogens to various animal species results in breast cancer. Spontaneous development of breast cancer in aging rats can be prevented by oophorectomy or administration of aromatase inhibitors (AIs) to block estrogen production. Oophorectomy before the age of 35 years in women lowers the risk of breast cancer by 75% over a 25-year period. Administration of antiestrogens to women at high risk for developing breast cancer results in a 50% reduction in tumor development. These observations and other data have led to the classification of estrogen as a carcinogen.[1]

Sources of Estrogen

The estradiol present in breast tissue is synthesized in three sites: the ovary, extraglandular tissues, and the breast itself. Direct glandular secretion by the ovary results in delivery of estradiol to the breast through an endocrine mechanism in premenopausal women. After the menopause, extraglandular production of estrogen from ovarian and adrenal androgens in fat and muscle provides the second source of estradiol. Third, the breast itself can synthesize estradiol via aromatization of androgens to estrogens or cleavage of estrone sulfate to estrone via the enzyme sulfatase. Estradiol acts through paracrine, autocrine, and intracrine mechanisms on cells in the breast. Several factors regulate in situ estradiol synthesis but the most important is the degree of obesity, which increases the amount of aromatase in breast and, consequently, estradiol production.

Estrogen-Induced Carcinogenesis

Mutations of key genes involved in cell proliferation, DNA repair, vasculogenesis, or apoptosis must accumulate to produce cancer.[2] It is likely that mitogenic as well as mutagenic effects of estradiol act in concert to initiate and promote the development of breast cancer.[3,4] As a general rule, the frequency of mutations increases in parallel with the number of mitotic divisions in a proliferating tissue. Accordingly, estrogens can *initiate* mutations leading to neoplastic transformation by increasing the rate of cell proliferation. As cells divide more rapidly, less time is available for DNA repair. Estrogens also enhance tumor *promotion* by increasing the rate of cell division with propagation of the mutations already present.

Metabolites of estradiol may be directly mutagenic through a pathway involving the 1B1 cytochrome P450 enzyme.[3] This catalyzes conversion of estradiol to the catechol estrogen 4-OH estradiol, which is then further metabolized to 3,4-estradiol quinone. This highly reactive species binds covalently to guanine or adenine molecules in the DNA helix and forms an unstable complex, which results in depurination. Error-prone or replicative repair of the depurinated sites leads to point mutations.[3] The direct mutagenic hypothesis is supported experimentally by studies demonstrating the mutagenic potential of estradiol on MCF-10 benign breast cells in vitro and the transformation of these cells to cancer in vivo.[5]

Estradiol is not the sole factor mediating the development of breast cancer. A number of specific genetic mutations are associated with a high incidence of breast cancer (Fig. 42–1).[6] Studies in twins suggest that approximately 27% of breast cancers arise because of genetic factors.[7] The most common mutations involve the *BRCA1* and *BRCA2* genes, which cause approximately 5% of breast cancer cases. Rarer genetic syndromes include mutations of the *p53* gene in the Li-Fraumeni syndrome, impaired cell-cycle checkpoint surveillance in the ataxia-telangiectasia syndrome, mutations in the *PTEN* gene in the Cowden syndrome, the *MLH1/MSH2* genes in the Muir-Torre syndrome, an *STK11* mutation in the Peutz-Jeghers syndrome, and *Chek 2* mutations.[6]

Dietary and environmental factors play a key role in breast cancer etiology and contribute to the fourfold differences in incidence between Japan, where the rate is 23 women per 100,000 woman-years, and the United States, where the rate is 90 women per 100,000 woman-years. Epidemiologic observations suggest a role for high-fat diet and resultant obesity in the genesis of breast cancer. In Japan, the rate of breast cancer peaks at the age of menopause, but in the United States, incidence continues to increase until age 90 years. The difference in postmenopausal patterns might result from the increase in obesity and associated aromatase increments in women in the United States compared to women in Japan. This different postmenopausal rate does not appear genetic, because Japanese women who move to the United States experience an increased rate of breast cancer that later approaches that of U.S. women.

Hormonal Risk Factors for Breast Cancer

The majority of risk factors for breast cancer relate to the duration or intensity of a woman's exposure to endogenous or exogenous estrogens (Fig. 42–2). Early menarche, late menopause, or both increase breast cancer risk.[8] Elevations in circulating estradiol levels predict the risk of developing breast cancer over the ensuing years in postmenopausal women (Figs. 42–2, 42–3).[9] A recent analysis concluded that estrogen levels provide information independent of other known risk factors.[10] An estradiol in the top quintile increases the relative risk of breast cancer by as much as fivefold.[9]

Putative markers of long-term estrogen exposure such as bone density are also predictive. Women in the top quartile of bone density have a threefold increased risk of breast cancer; a history of fracture or height loss lowers the risk.[11,12] Late first birth increases the risk 2.8-fold and is believed to relate to the lack of the differentiating effect of pregnancy on type of breast lobule present. Gain of at least 20 kg as an adult increases breast cancer risk twofold.[13] This effect was only observed in women who did not use MHT (menopausal hormone therapy). Increased waist-to-hip ratio exerts a similar increase in risk. Several but not all studies suggest that alcohol intake can increase the risk of breast cancer, perhaps by decreasing the clearance of estradiol. Increased exposure to estradiol in utero, as shown by twin studies, might increase risk of breast cancer by as much as twofold. Early pregnancy and prolonged duration of breastfeeding diminish the risk. More dramatic is the 75% reduction in risk caused by bilateral oophorectomy before age 35 years.[14]

Mammography density represents the most powerful risk factor for breast cancer (Fig. 42–4).[15] Increased breast density probably reflects either an increase in exposure to estrogen or sensitivity to it. Exogenous estrogens increase and antiestrogens reduce breast density. Because of these effects, MHT alters the sensitivity and specificity of reading standard film screen mammograms.[16] Increase in breast cancer risk from lowest to highest breast density category is on the order of fivefold, depending upon the age of the patient (see Fig. 42–4), with greater relative risk in older women.

Gene	Freq.	RR <50	RR 50–69	Abs. risk
BRCA1	0.1%	33	15	~65%
BRCA2	0.13%	12	12	~45%
TP53	0.01%	NA	NA	90%
PTEN	<0.01%	NA	NA	30%
ATM	0.5%	5	1.5	15%
CHEK2	0.5%	3	2	10%

Figure 42–1 ▪ Genetic mutations associated with development of breast cancer. Abs, absolute; Freq, frequency; RR, relative risk, NA, not available. (From Thompson D, Easton D. The genetic epidemiology of breast cancer genes. J Mammary Gland Biol Neoplasia 2004; 9[3]:221-236.)

Exogenous Estrogens and Breast Cancer Risk

In premenopausal women, use of oral contraceptives for 10 or more years increases the relative risk of breast cancer by approximately 10%.[17] However, this increase in relative risk affects very few women because the age-related incidence of breast cancer is quite low in women taking oral contraceptives.

Controversy previously surrounded the concept that MHT in postmenopausal women increases the risk of breast cancer. More than 50 observational studies have examined this question but reported conflicting results.[18,18] However, several recent key

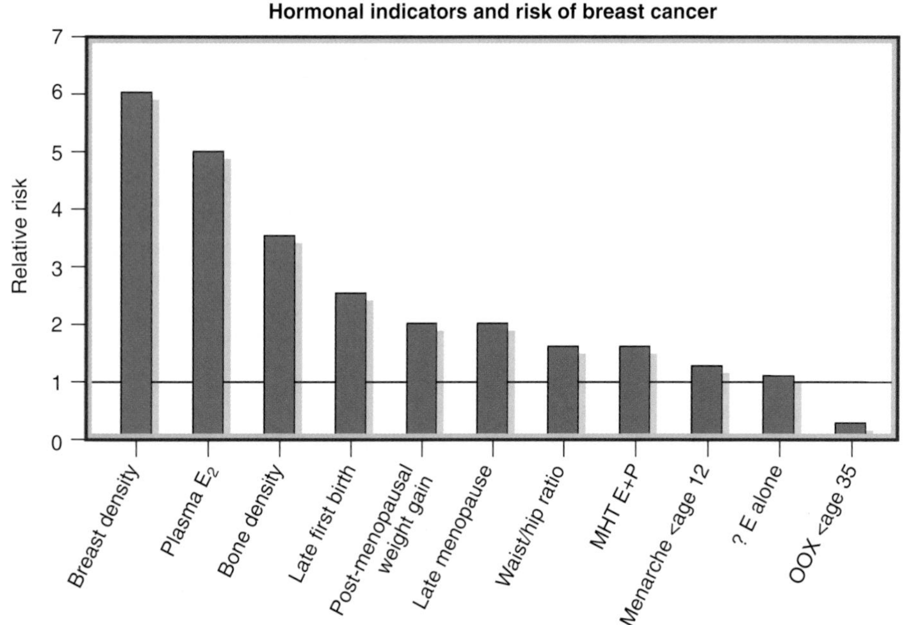

Figure 42–2 ▪ Relative risk of breast cancer as a function of several factors that relate to long-term exposure to estradiol (E_2). E, estrogen; HT, hormone therapy; OOX, oophorectomy; P, progesterone.

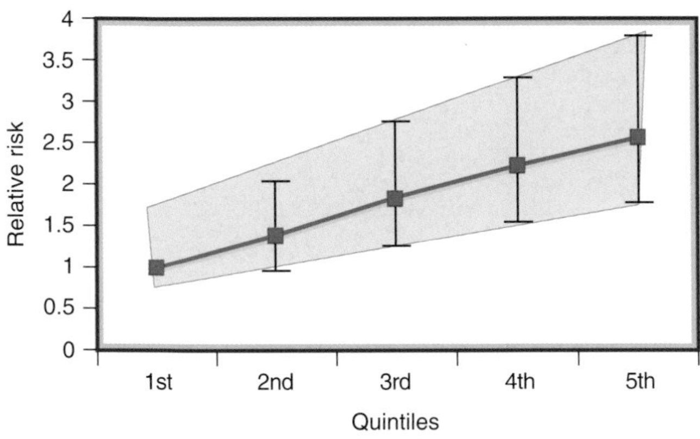

Figure 42–3 ▪ Risk of breast cancer related to endogenous levels of plasma estradiol in postmenopausal women. (From Key T, Appleby P, Barnes I, Reeves G, and Endogenous Hormones and Breast Cancer Collaborative Group. Endogenous sex hormones and breast cancer in postmenopausal women: reanalysis of nine prospective studies. J Natl Cancer Inst 2002;94[8]:606-616.)

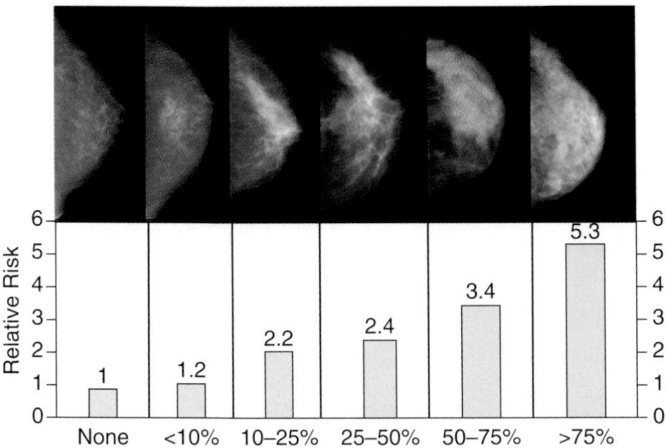

Figure 42–4 ▪ Relative risk of breast cancer as a function of the degree of mammographic density. (From Boyd NF, Byng JW, Jong RA, et al. Quantitative classification of mammographic densities and breast cancer risk: results from the Canadian National Breast Screening Study. J Natl Cancer Inst 1995;87:670-675.)

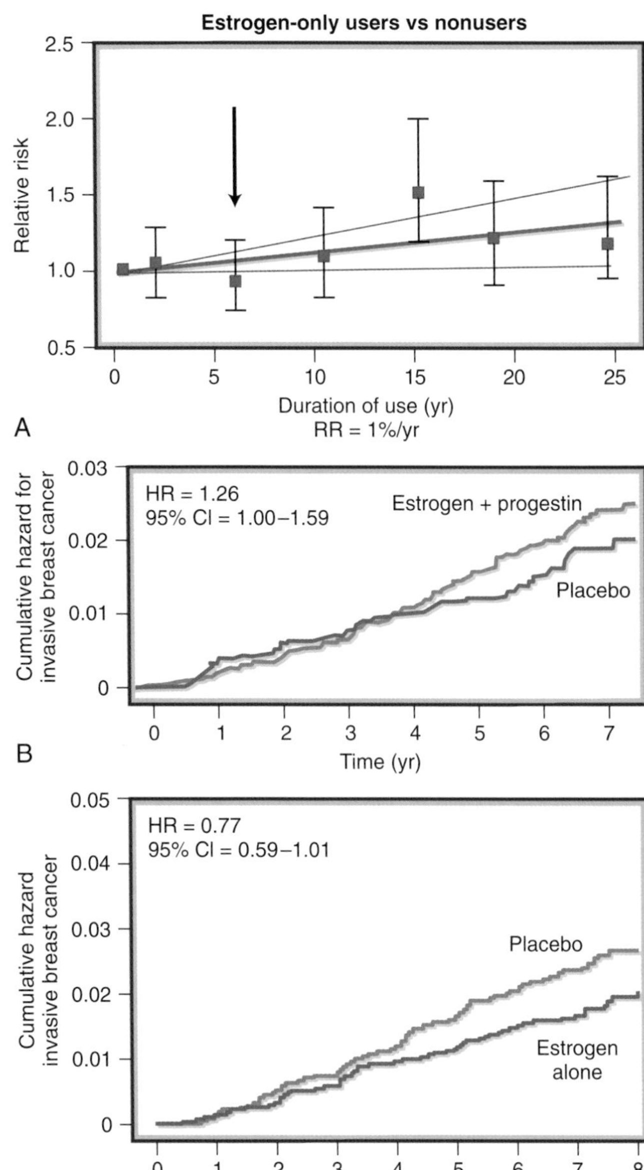

Figure 42–5 ▪ **A,** Observational data on the risk of breast cancer in women taking estrogen alone. **B,** Data from the Women's Health Initiative relating risk of breast cancer to use of conjugated equine estrogen plus medroxyprogesterone acetate. **C,** Randomized, controlled trial data from the Women's Health Initiative relating risk of breast cancer to use of estrogen alone. CI, confidence interval; HR, hazard ratio; RR, relative risk. (**A** from Schairer C, Lubin J, Troisi R, et al. Menopausal estrogen and estrogen-progestin replacement therapy and breast cancer risk. JAMA 2000;283:485-491; **B** from Rossouw JE, Anderson GL, Prentice RL, et al. Risks and benefits of estrogen plus progestin in healthy postmenopausal women: principal results From the Women's Health Initiative randomized controlled trial. JAMA 2002;288:321-333.) (**C** from Anderson GL, Limacher M, Assaf AR, et al. Effects of conjugated equine estrogen in postmenopausal women with hysterectomy: the Women's Health Initiative randomized, controlled study. JAMA 2004; 291:1701–1712.)

studies clarified the factors responsible for the differing conclusions among the various observational reports. One study, the meta-analysis from the Collaborative Group on Hormonal Factors in Breast Cancer (CGHFBC),[18,18] examined data from 52,705 women with breast cancer and 108,411 without. Five objective factors that confounded interpretation of prior studies were identified.

- The relative risk of breast cancer from MHT appears to be quite small, and large studies with a long duration of follow-up are required to minimize type I and type II statistical errors.
- The risk of breast cancer appears to increase linearly with duration of MHT use. Accordingly, comparisons of ever users with never users are invalid because duration of estrogen use is not considered.
- The increased risk of breast cancer *imparted by MHT* appears to dissipate within 4 years of cessation of therapy. Therefore, only women using MHT within 4 years of study might be found to be at increased risk.
- Breast cancer risk diminishes over a 4-year period *following the menopause*, presumably as a reflection of decreased estrogen levels. As a result, analyses of observational studies need to match users and nonusers for time following menopause.
- The increased risk of breast cancer appears to be limited to nonobese women (body mass index [BMI] <25 kg/m^2). Inclusion of a large percentage of obese women in a single study might then obscure an association between MHT use and breast cancer risk.

Taking into account these five factors, the CGHFBC meta-analysis concluded that the relative risk of breast cancer increases linearly by 2.3% per year of MHT for up to 25 years.[18,18] The slope of the line correlating relative risk with duration of use of MHT was statistically significant, indicating an effect of duration of MHT use. The overall risk of breast cancer among MHT users, regardless of duration of use, was also highly statistically significant. This study detected no increased risk of breast cancer with MHT use in obese women (BMI >25 kg/m^2). A hypothetical explanation for the differences between obese and thin women relates to the degree of in situ estrogen production. Obese women might have an increase in breast tissue estrogen as a result of increased aromatase activity, whereas lean women would have lower levels. Exogenous estrogen might then produce a greater percentage increase in breast tissue estradiol levels in thin than in obese women.

Another large observational database, the Million Women Study, supported the CGHFBC findings and extended them by comparing the use of estrogen alone to estrogen plus a progestin.[19] The relative risk of breast cancer from estrogen alone used for more than 10 years was increased (relative risk [RR], 1.37; 95% confidence interval [CI], 1.22-1.54), but use of estrogen plus a progestin for longer than 10 years was associated with an even greater relative risk (RR, 2.31; 95% CI, 2.08-2.56). Other observational studies report a linear increase in risk of breast cancer first appearing after 10 years of use and continuing to increase in a linear fashion for up to 25 years of use (Fig. 42–5A).[20]

Until recently, only observational studies were available to assess breast cancer risk, and unidentified biases could have confounded data interpretation. However, the large prospective, randomized Women's Health Initiative (WHI) trial in postmenopausal women provided compelling evidence for an adverse effect of an estrogen-progestin combination on breast cancer incidence.[21] Nearly 16,000 postmenopausal women with an average age of 63 years enrolled in the estrogen-plus-progestin arm of the WHI study and received either placebo or conjugated estrogens (0.625 mg) plus medroxyprogesterone acetate (2.5 mg) for 5 years. The study was terminated early because of an increased incidence of breast cancer in the MHT group, with a relative risk of 1.26 and a 95% confidence interval of 1.00-1.59. (see Fig. 42–5B). The absolute excess of cases was small, with only four more invasive breast cancers per 1000 women over 5 years of therapy in the MHT group. Nonetheless, these data confirm the prior observational studies and indicate a relative risk increase of 5.5% per year in those receiving MHT. This is similar to the 8% per year reported in the observational studies.

Another arm of the WHI study compared placebo with conjugated equine estrogen alone in women who had previously undergone a total abdominal hysterectomy.[22] This study did not demonstrate an increased risk of breast cancer after 5 years of hormonal therapy. Surprisingly, the risk of invasive breast cancer (hazard ratio [HR], 0.77) was reduced—although not statistically significantly (95% confidence interval (CI), 0.59-1.01)—at 5 years in those in the hormonal arm (see Fig. 42–5C). A post hoc subset analysis reported a statistically significant reduction in risk in three subgroups: those with localized tumors (HR, 0.69; 95% CI, 0.51-0.95), those with invasive ductal carcinoma (HR, 0.71; 95% CI, 0.52-0.99), and women adherent to the study protocol and not dropping out (HR, 0.67; 95% CI, 0.47-0.97).[22] The Nurses Health Observational Study reported a similar, statistically significant reduction in risk in women with a BMI greater than 25 who took estrogen alone for 5 to 9 years (HR, 0.74; 95% CI, 0.55-1.00).[23] The reduction in risk at 5 years in the observational study of Shairer's group also supports a potential beneficial effect of short-term estrogen (Fig. 42–5A: see arrow at 5 years).[20] Observational data regarding long-term use of estrogen alone reports the opposite effect, namely a 41% to 77%

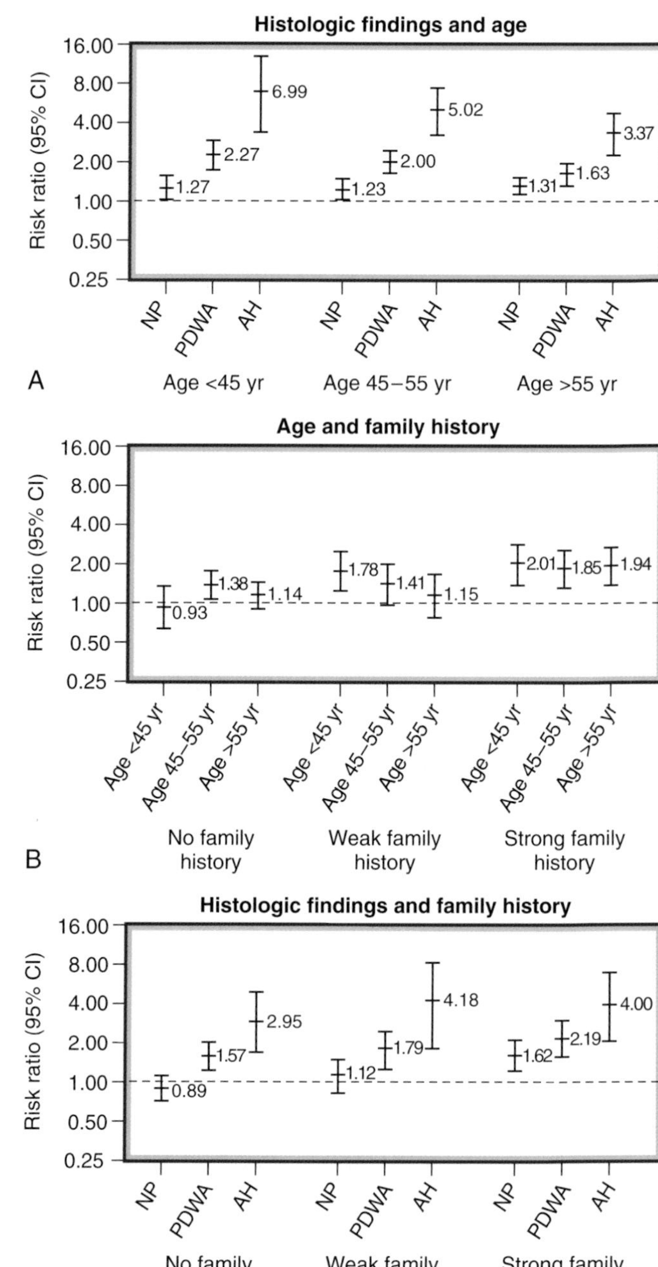

Figure 42–6 ▪ Risk of breast cancer related to various benign breast lesions and family history of breast cancer. AH, atypical hyperplasia; CI, confidence interval; NP, nonproliferative disease; PDWA, proliferative disease without atypia. (From Hartmann LC, Sellers TA, Frost MH, et al. Benign breast disease and the risk of breast cancer. N Engl J Med 2005;353:229-237.)

increase in relative risk of breast cancer at 25 years as observed in both the Schairer and Nurses Health studies.[23]

Comparison of short-term estrogen use, which might decrease breast cancer risk by 30%, with long-term administration, which appears to increase risk by 41% to 77%, suggests an estrogen paradox.[23a] One potential explanation for the estrogen paradox is that estradiol can exert two separate mechanistic effects: estradiol-induced apoptosis and initiation or promotion of new cancers. Recent studies demonstrate that estradiol can induce apoptosis in breast tumors that have been deprived of estradiol long term.[24] At entry to the WHI estrogen alone study, the average age of the women was 63 years, 12 years beyond the average age of menopause. Accordingly, women who never previously took hormone therapy were in a state of long-term estradiol deprivation for 12 years on average. A review of 10 studies[23a] that examined 1787 breasts at autopsy revealed a 5.9% prevalence of undiagnosed ductal carcinoma in situ. Two of the more recent studies describe the meticulous methodology needed to detect all occult tumors.[25,26] What effect would estrogen have on those small undiagnosed lesions? A proapoptotic effect of estradiol would be expected to reduce the size of those tumors such that they would not be detected over the 5 years of follow-up. This could explain the significant reductions of breast cancer in subgroups of women in the WHI and Nurses health studies. This short-term estrogen effect might then be superseded by a pro-carcinogenic effect of estradiol if the patients received this hormone over a prolonged period of up to 25 years (see Fig. 42–5A).[23,20]

The estrogen paradox hypothesis is speculative and will require prospective randomized, controlled trials over a longer period for confirmation. At present, only observational studies with long-term follow-up are available, and these suggest a 1% increase in relative risk of breast cancer with estrogen alone, which is only apparent after 10 to 15 years of exposure (see Fig. 42–5A).[23,20]

Critical review of the WHI data suggest that the adverse effects on breast cancer risk over the 5-year period resulted from the addition of a progestin to the administered estrogen. It is unclear if this is a progestin class effect or unique to the progestin used, medroxyprogesterone acetate. Several observational studies examined the effects of various types of progestin as well as differences between combined continuous and sequential regimens.[19,21] The Million Women Study suggested that all types of progestin are associated with an increased risk of breast cancer and that a class effect of progestins is responsible. Another large observational study, the Etude Epidémiologique de Femmes de la Mutuelle Général de l'Education Nationale (E3N) European Prospective Investigation into Cancer (EPIC) study, on the other hand, reported no increased risk of breast cancer from use of crystalline progesterone, but it found increased risks similar to those in the Million Women Study with other types of progestin.[27] More data are necessary to confirm this finding regarding crystalline progesterone, which, if valid, has major implications regarding which progestin should be used clinically.

An understanding of the physiologic basis for the association of progestins with breast cancer rests on data indicating that progestins are mitogenic on breast tissue, in contrast to their antimitogenic effects on the uterus.[28] Although data from cell cultures or animal studies are conflicting, the weight of evidence from patients suggests that progestins are mitogenic in breast tissue. Mammographic studies demonstrate that estrogen-progestin combinations increase breast density to a greater extent than estrogen alone or placebo.[29] Histologic examination demonstrates enhanced cell proliferation and percentage of the breast containing glandular tissue as a function of duration of progestin use.[28] Increased proliferation would be expected to increase both *initiation* and *promotion* of breast cancer in a manner similar to that thought to occur with estrogens.[3]

Relative, Absolute, and Attributable Risks from Menopausal Hormone Therapy

A full understanding of the magnitude of risk from MHT requires knowledge of the precise meaning of statistical terms. Epidemiologists use relative risk analysis as a tool that provides substantial power to determine the statistical significance of differences between groups. However, the term "relative risk" is misleading to patients, because absolute or actual risk may be quite small when relative risk is high. The lay press, patients, and many physicians confuse the terms relative, absolute, and attributable risk.

Relative risk is defined as the ratio of risk under one condition compared to another and does not take into account the frequency of occurrence of that condition. *Absolute risk* is determined by multiplying the relative risk by the underlying incidence rate in the group being considered. For example, an average 50-year-old woman in the United States has an absolute risk of developing breast cancer of 1.26 per 100 women over a 5-year period. A 35% increase in relative risk resulting from an estrogen-progestin combination increases her absolute chances of getting a breast cancer to 1.70 per 100 women. *Attributable* risk (alternatively called "excess risk") is defined as the number of women who would develop a breast cancer that would not have otherwise occurred unless they had used estrogen-progestin therapy. Using the previous example, the difference between breast cancer risk of 1.26 per 100 and 1.70 per 100 represents the increased (or excess) risk *attributable* to estrogen, or 0.44 per 100 women (or 4.4 per 1000 women). This increase is interpreted by patients to be less than that conveyed by an increase in relative risk of 26%.

Benign Breast Disease and Risk of Breast Cancer

A large recent study from the Mayo clinic confirmed prior observations that benign breast lesions with an enhanced rate of proliferation predict an increased incidence of breast cancer over time (Fig. 42–6).[30] Hyperplastic ductal lesions are often multicentric, suggesting that some type of underlying abnormality is present that predisposes to such lesions. This has been called a "field defect" or, more recently, a "mutator phenotype."[31] The multifocal nature of the associated benign hyperplastic lesions is most apparent in breast tissue from women with cancer. Examination of tissue adjacent to an invasive breast cancer or in the contralateral breast reveals one or more additional hyperplastic lesions in approximately 40% of patients.[32]

The nature of the *field defect* or mutator phenotype has not been specifically identified but hypothetically could represent a single mutation of a gene controlling local estrogen production, cellular proliferation, DNA repair, metabolism of procarcinogens to carcinogens, or other cellular events. Preliminary data suggest progression from adenomas to frank neoplasms. Eighty percent to 90% of hyperplastic lesions contain DNA mutations similar to those in the contiguous tumors. Extensive molecular genetic studies have now described progression of abnormalities in the spectrum of breast lesions.[31]

A major consideration for women who present with breast problems is whether they have a higher than normal risk of developing breast cancer. Certain breast lesions, such as fibrocystic changes, are associated with no increased risk of subsequent breast cancer (Fig. 42–7) unless a strong family history is present. Other lesions, characterized by the presence of increased cellular proliferation, impart an increased risk.[31] The relative risk of development of invasive cancer is increased 10- to 12-fold when ductal carcinoma in situ (DCIS) and lobular carcinoma in situ (LCIS) are present. Proliferative lesions can progress to invasive cancer as evidenced by the increase in ipsilateral breast cancer in women harboring these lesions. However, the presence of proliferative lesions also reflects a "field defect" or "mutator phenotype" because risk of contralateral breast cancer is also increased when the period of observation extends over more than 10 years. The Mayo Clinic study of nearly 15,000 women confirmed the concept that only lesions with increased proliferation impart an increased risk of breast cancer unless a strong family history is present.[30] This clarified a prior study that did not distinguish proliferative from non-

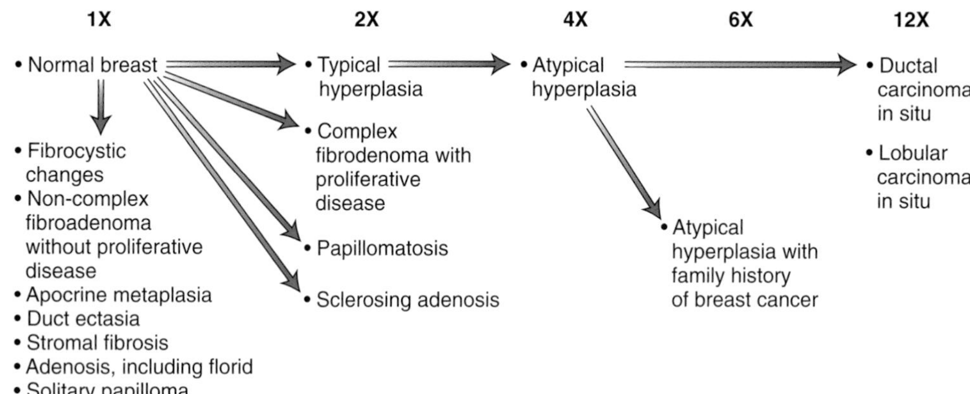

Figure 42–7 ▪ The relative risk of breast cancer (1X-12X) related to several benign breast lesions in women followed long term.

proliferative and concluded that low-category breast disease, including fibrocystic changes, conveys an increased risk.[33]

Estimating Breast Cancer Risk

To aid in assessing breast cancer risk, a questionnaire developed by Gail, uses answers to seven questions to calculate the 5-year and lifetime risk of developing breast cancer.[34] This model has recognized deficiencies in that it does not consider breast density, plasma estradiol levels, bone density, BMI, weight gain in adulthood, second-degree relatives with breast cancer, proliferative lesions of breast other than ADH, alcohol intake, or birth control pill and MHT use. Nonetheless, two major prospective studies validated the Gail model in a high-risk (National Surgical Adjuvant Breast and Bowel Project [NSABP] prevention study) and in an average-risk population of women (The Nurses' Health Study). The ratio of observed to expected cancers using this tool was 1.03 (95% CI 0.88-1.21) in the high-risk patients and 0.94 (95% CI 0.89-0.99) in average-risk women, and both were highly statistically significant. This risk tool is available as the RISK DISK from the National Cancer Institute. When second-degree relatives with breast cancer predominate to increase risk, the Claus model provides a more valid risk-assessment tool.

Newer models are being developed to enhance the power of risk prediction. Although only validated in one prospective study, the Tyrer-Cuzick model appeared to outperform the Gail and Claus models in a population with a high familial breast cancer component.[35] This new model combines the factors used in the Claus and Gail models as well as a history of MHT use, and it appears quite promising as a new risk-prediction tool.

Breast Cancer Risk and Clinical Decisions

Knowledge about underlying breast cancer risk influences advice given by health care providers and choices made by patients. Women known to be at high risk for breast cancer often choose a surrogate for MHT (see later) to treat menopausal symptoms. Those at low risk usually chose estrogen or an estrogen-progestin combination to relieve symptoms of estrogen deficiency. Those at intermediate risk of breast cancer have several options including use of a selective estrogen-receptor modulator (SERM), other alternatives to estrogen, watchful waiting, or MHT.

As a working guide, we arbitrarily define risk categories based upon use of risk prediction models: high risk is more than a 3% chance of breast cancer in 5 years; intermediate risk is a 1.5 to 3% chance, and low risk is less than 1.5%. Those classified as high risk include patients with a strong family history of breast cancer (particularly if it is associated with ovarian cancer), prior history of ADH or lobular carcinoma in situ, and age older than 60 years when combined with early menarche, late menopause, or first live birth. Intermediate-risk patients have some risk factors but not others. Low-risk patients are younger than 60 years; have a late onset of menarche, early menopause, early age of first live birth, and no family history of breast cancer; and lack predisposing breast lesions. Because no formal risk tool incorporates breast density, bone density, nor plasma estradiol levels into its assessment, a physician must take these factors into account in advising patients.

Prevention

Selective Estrogen-Receptor Modulators

Depending upon risk category, women may wish to take tamoxifen or raloxifene to prevent breast cancer. Only the antiestrogen tamoxifen is approved for this use in the United States. Evidence supporting antiestrogens for prevention is substantial. A meta-analysis of the five large prevention trials demonstrated a 50% reduction in breast cancer risk with tamoxifen when compared to placebo.[36] The most definitive trial, the first NSABP prevention trial (NSABP P-1), involved 13,388 women randomized to receive either placebo or 20 mg of tamoxifen daily.[37] Eligibility for the study required an intermediate or high risk of developing breast cancer, defined in the study as a 1.67% or greater chance of developing a new breast cancer over a 5-year period.

The rate of breast cancers in the placebo group was 9.4 per 1000 woman-years versus 4.7 in the tamoxifen group, a relative risk reduction of 50% (RR 0.50) (Fig. 42–8A). Considered separately, the risk of invasive breast cancer was reduced by 49% and noninvasive breast cancer by 50%. This effect occurred in women of all ages studied (younger than 49, 50-59, 60-69, and older than 70 years) and in those with LCIS, ADH, and a family history of breast cancer. The benefits of tamoxifen related to the underlying risk of breast cancer and the specific risk factor present (see Fig. 42–8B) These results led a panel of experts commissioned by the American Society of Clinical Oncology (ASCO) to conclude that tamoxifen does reduce the incidence of newly diagnosed breast cancer in high-risk women.[38]

Tamoxifen

Tamoxifen for treatment of breast cancer is considered well tolerated and safe. However, for use in otherwise normal women, infrequent side effects and toxicity become more important. Up to 40% of women starting on tamoxifen do not continue it

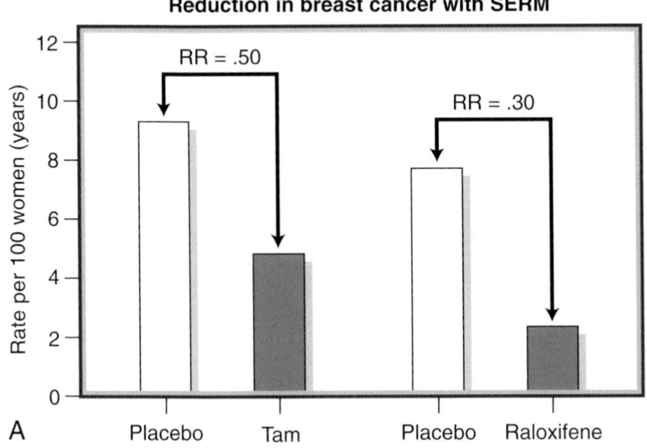

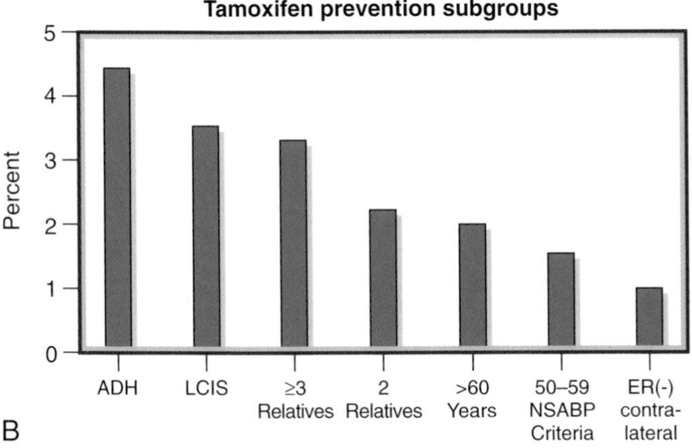

Figure 42–8 ▪ **A,** Reduction in risk of breast cancer in response to the administration of tamoxifen or to raloxifene for a mean duration of 4 years. **B,** Absolute benefit from tamoxifen expressed as a percentage of women whose breast cancer was prevented as a function of the underlying risk factor present. ADH, atypical ductal hyperplasia; ER, estrogen receptor; LCIS, lobular carcinoma in situ; NSABP, National Surgical Adjuvant Breast and Bowel Project; RR, relative risk; Tam, tamoxifen. (**A** from Fisher B, Costantino JP, Wickerham DL, et al. Tamoxifen for prevention of breast cancer: report of the National Surgical Adjuvant Breast and Bowel Project P-1 Study. J Natl Cancer Inst 1998;90:1371-1388; Cummings SR, Eckert S, Krueger KA, et al. The effect of raloxifene on risk of breast cancer in postmenopausal women: results from the MORE randomized trial. Multiple Outcomes of Raloxifene Evaluation. JAMA 1999;281:2189-2197.)

because of perceived side effects including depression and mood changes. Tamoxifen is one of the SERMS. Agents in this class exert antiestrogenic effects on tissues such as breast but estrogenic effects on others such as uterus and liver. These various actions of the SERMs must be factored in when estimating risks and benefits in the setting of breast cancer prevention.

To compare risks and benefits in a meaningful way, the NSABP data are expressed as the number of women per 100 with a specific benefit or adverse event after 5 years of study. With respect to benefits, new invasive breast cancers were prevented in 1.7 of 100 women, noninvasive cancers in 0.67, and bone fractures in 0.50 for a total of 2.87 in 100 women benefiting after 5 years. Risks of tamoxifen are primarily related to its estrogenic effects on the uterus, a prothrombotic effect, and adverse effects on the lens of the eye. To validly estimate actual risks to a patient, one must correct for the underlying risks in the population under study. For that reason, analysis of adverse events includes determination of *attributable risk* and involves subtracting the underlying rate from the total observed on tamoxifen. This indicates an excess of 1.5 per 100 women who developed cataracts, 0.69 with endometrial cancer (nearly exclusively in postmenopausal women), 0.27 with cerebrovascular accident (CVA), 0.25 with deep venous thrombosis (DVT), and 0.23 with pulmonary embolus, for a total of 2.94 per 100.[39] The new endometrial cancers were predominantly stage I and pulmonary emboli were nonfatal. Neither risk nor benefit was observed regarding cardiovascular effects, but the number of patients was not sufficient for statistical significance.

The increased incidence of uterine cancer in patients on tamoxifen presents a clinical management problem. Substantial study has examined how best to detect this cancer early.[40] Transvaginal ultrasound was initially proposed as a means of assessing both endometrial hyperplasia, as a precursor lesion, and early cancer. A prospective study demonstrated a mean increase in endometrial thickness from 3.5 ± 1.1 to 9.2 ± 5.1 mm in response to 5 years of tamoxifen. In 20% of women, endometrial thickness exceeded 10 mm or appeared suspicious for neoplasm. In this subset of women, biopsies revealed atrophy in 73%, polyps in 17%, hyperplasia in 7.7%, but endometrial cancer in only one patient.[41] This and other studies conclude that endometrial thickness does not usually indicate hyperplasia but rather the presence of edema and dilated myometrial glands. It should be noted that nonprospective studies report a higher prevalence of benign polyps (5%-55%) and hyperplasia (8%-16%),[42,43] but these are likely to be overestimates from selection bias. Based upon these studies, recommendations for screening include yearly gynecologic exam and endometrial sampling and ultrasound for only those with signs of abnormal vaginal bleeding.[40,41]

Raloxifene

Another SERM, raloxifene, appears to prevent breast cancer without increasing the risk of endometrial cancer. The MORE trial and its follow-on extension, the Core Trial, compared raloxifene with placebo in osteoporotic women and demonstrated a 75% reduction in breast cancer risk over an 8-year period in women with an average or reduced risk of breast cancer (see Fig. 42–8A).

The STAR (Study of Tamoxifen and Raloxifene) trial then compared raloxifene with tamoxifen in a head-to-head prevention trial in 18,000 postmenopausal women with a predicted risk of more than 1.67% at 5 years. Both agents prevented invasive breast cancer similarly (by an estimated 50%), but raloxifene exhibited a superior toxicity profile, with 30% fewer thromboembolic events ($P = 0.01$), 38% fewer endometrial cancers ($P = 0.07$), 21% fewer cataracts ($P = 0.002$), an 84% reduction in uterine hyperplasia ($P < 0.01$), and 55% fewer unplanned hysterectomies. No differences between agents were observed in cardiovascular events, strokes, or fracture rates. A surprising finding was that raloxifene did not appear to prevent noninvasive breast cancer, whereas tamoxifen has previously been shown to do so.[44] These effects of raloxifene were confirmed in a randomized comparison to placebo in the RUTH (Raloxifene Use for The Heart) trial.[45]

Although raloxifene is not yet approved for breast cancer prevention, the STAR and RUTH trials would suggest that this agent provides a reasonable preventive option for postmenopausal women at increased risk of breast cancer, particularly if they have low bone density or an intact uterus, or both.

Guidelines for Breast Cancer Prevention

Premenopausal women with a 5-year risk of breast cancer greater than 1.67% over 5 years are candidates for tamoxifen unless they are at increased risk for DVT or pulmonary emboli.

Postmenopausal women with similar breast cancer risk are candidates for tamoxifen if they no longer have a uterus and lack a predisposing risk for DVT or pulmonary emboli. Raloxifene may be preferred over tamoxifen in women with a uterus. The decision to take tamoxifen or raloxifene should be made by the patient in partnership with her health care provider and based upon a full discussion of individual risks and benefits expressed in absolute and not relative terms.[38] Prevention strategies for women carrying *BRCA1* or *BRCA2* mutations often involve more aggressive steps such as bilateral oophorectomy or mastectomy, but tamoxifen may also be effective in these patients.[46]

Critical Assessment of Breast Cancer Prevention Strategies

Estimates indicate that between 20 and 100 women (depending upon underlying risk) need to be treated to prevent one breast cancer. Clinical decisions depend upon analysis of risk-to-benefit ratios and should be made after full discussion between health care provider and patient. Regarding efficacy, available data demonstrate only a reduction in newly diagnosed breast cancers, but effects on overall survival are not yet known. Whether tamoxifen actually prevents breast cancer, cures some preexisting subclinical cancers, or delays the onset of diagnosis of small tumors remains to be determined. Mathematical modeling techniques suggest that the preventive effects of tamoxifen are equally divided between blockade of growth of occult tumors and prevention of new ones.[47] Tumors whose growth was blocked by tamoxifen during its 5 years of administration might be expected to regrow later. For this reason, long-term data on overall survival (from the ongoing first International Breast Cancer Intervention Study [IBIS 1]) will be critically important, but at present no survival benefit is evident.[36,36a]

Future studies will need to use additional factors to select women at higher risk of developing breast cancer. A study of raloxifene examined women with factors suggesting long-term high exposure to estrogen (increased bone mineral density, high BMI, and high plasma estradiol levels). Results indicated that raloxifene was more effective in preventing breast cancer in women with high than with low long-term estrogen exposure. For example, for those with high versus low bone mineral density, the prevention rates were 94% versus 56%; for the high versus low BMI groups, 82% versus 64%; and for the high versus low plasma estradiol groups, 77% versus 55% ($P < 0.005$).[48] A critical need at present is to develop a more powerful breast cancer risk model that incorporates breast density, plasma estrogen levels, history of fracture, waist-to-hip ratio, and obesity as well as the factors used in the Gail and Claus risk-prediction models.[48a]

Trials of the AIs in the adjuvant setting uniformly demonstrate a greater reduction of contralateral cancers with the AIs than with tamoxifen.[49,50,51,52] The crossover study from tamoxifen to letrozole or placebo at 5 years also demonstrated a reduction of contralateral breast cancer incidence with the AI.[53] These data provide strong indirect evidence that AIs will be more effective than tamoxifen in breast cancer prevention. Two trials (IBIS II and MAP 3 [Treatment with Examestane, an Aromatase Inhibitor, versus Placebo, for Postmenopausal Women at High Risk for Developing Breast Cancer]) have been initiated to examine this issue, and data should be forthcoming by 2010.

■ Treatment of Established Breast Cancers

The American Cancer Society estimates that 178,400 new cases of breast cancer will be diagnosed in the United States in 2007 and 40,460 will die of this disease. Use of digital mammography and MRI have increased the sensitivity of detecting early disease.[54] The death rate from breast cancer has declined by 12% since the mid-1990s in the United States and in Western Europe. This has probably resulted from early screening and use of adjuvant therapy.

The mechanisms whereby estradiol stimulates breast cancer growth are complex and involve direct regulation of genes involved in control of proliferation and apoptosis, induction of growth factors through secondary actions, and cross-talk between growth factor and estrogen pathways at both upstream and downstream levels.[55] Membrane-initiated (extranuclear) effects of estradiol on growth factor–mediated mitogenic pathways might also be involved. Treatment strategies use agents that abrogate the effects of estrogen on these pathways and thus inhibit growth and induce apoptosis. Emerging evidence suggests that tumor stem cells are the most important target for therapy.

Common approaches involve antiestrogens or blockade of estrogen synthesis with AIs or GnRH superagonist analogues.[56] Patients who initially respond to hormonal therapy eventually relapse. A standard strategy is that responders to first-line treatment benefit from secondary and tertiary hormonal therapies upon relapse. The sequential responses to hormonal therapies suggest an adaptive process whereby tumors do not become totally resistant to hormonal therapy but develop a transitional state during which alternative means of blocking hormonal pathways causes tumor regression. Patients relapsing following oophorectomy or tamoxifen treatment commonly respond secondarily to inhibitors of estrogen production (AIs) or rarely to withdrawal of tamoxifen.[56]

Development of Hormonal Resistance

Women respond to each hormonal therapy on average for 12 to 18 months and then relapse.[56] At some time in the course of treatment, tumors become totally resistant to further hormonal therapy. Several explanations for development of secondary resistance have been suggested, including:

- Changes in metabolism of tamoxifen with production of estrogenic metabolites
- A constitutive increase in growth factor production as a result of additional oncogene mutations
- Enhanced growth factor receptor functionality
- Increased use of extranuclear estrogen receptor (ER) pathways
- Down-regulation of transcriptional corepressors
- Outgrowth or selection of hormone-resistant clones of tumor cells
- Up-regulation of nuclear receptor coactivators
- Other adaptive mechanisms

An additional hypothesis to explain resistance is that tumors adapting to hormonal therapy become hypersensitive to lower amounts of circulating estrogen or to the estrogen-agonist properties of tamoxifen.[57] Experimental support for this concept emanates from observations in xenograft models and in vitro studies. Breast tumor xenografts adapt to long-term exposure to tamoxifen by responding to it as an estrogen, rather than as an antiestrogen. Under these circumstances, the pure antiestrogen fulvestrant blocks the stimulatory effect of tamoxifen, causing tumor regression. In cell culture systems, long-term deprivation of estradiol renders breast cancer cells hypersensitive to the proliferative effects of this sex steroid.[58] This adaptive process is associated with increments in mitogen-activated protein (MAP) kinase, an enzyme that stimulates cell proliferation and in growth factor pathways involving phosphatidylinositol 3 (PI3) kinase and mammalian target of rapamycin (mTOR). The hypersensitivity concept could explain secondary responses to AIs in patients relapsing after oophorectomy or tamoxifen and secondary responses to the pure antiestrogen fulvestrant.

Data from several laboratories have demonstrated several events that occur commonly in vitro in cells exposed long term to estrogen deprivation or tamoxifen. These include up-regulation of the MAP kinase pathway, increased phosphorylation of AKT, enhancement of mTOR, increased activation of the insulin-like growth factor (IGF)-1, epidermal growth factor (EGF), and *HER2/Neu* receptors, up-regulation of adaptor proteins such as CAS (Crk-associated protein) 130, and increased activation of ER-mediated transcription.[55] One theory is that the growth factor–activated kinases phosphorylate the ER to render it transcriptionally more active and at the same time phosphorylate coactivators such as AIB1 (activated in breast cancer 1). Another is that cells adapt to the pressure exerted by hormonal therapy to enhance utilization of membrane-initiated signaling pathways involving the ER.[55,59] Under these circumstances, tamoxifen becomes an estrogen agonist at the level of the cell membrane, and cells grow in its presence. Clinical data support these concepts in that tumors that overexpress *HER2/Neu* and AIB1 exhibit resistance to tamoxifen.[55] Secondary responses to AIs in patients resistant to tamoxifen might also reflect hypersensitivity to estrogen, because the third-generation AIs lower estradiol levels by more than 99%. De novo or primary resistance to endocrine therapy might also involve many of the mechanisms occurring during development of secondary resistance. As an example, primary tumors overexpressing *HER2/Neu* appear to be relatively resistant to tamoxifen therapy.

Prognostic Factors

Clinical decision making requires knowledge of the degree of aggressiveness and natural history of the type of breast cancer present. Much attention has been directed toward multivariate and neural network analysis to calculate the precise prognosis in individual women. Investigators previously developed means of pooling various risk factors in order to improve prognostication. The Nottingham index is an example of a method that integrates the findings of tumor size, nodal status, and histologic grade of the tumor. In general, these methods have not been particularly useful in practical decision making, and individual factors are used in treatment algorithms. However, a recently developed Web-based tool (adjuvantonline.com) has been very useful to calculate prognosis in individual women and to guide patients and their physicians in the choice of various therapeutic options.

Figure 42–9 illustrates the prognostic power of various biologic factors by comparing the effects of individual parameters on 5-year survival. The most powerful clinical and pathologically based prognostic parameters include nodal status, tumor grade and size, proliferative indices, and ER status. Other prognostic characteristics include *HER2/Neu* positivity by fluorescent in situ hybridization (FISH) analysis, degree of aneuploidy, and overexpression of certain oncogenes or co-activators (e.g., D-cyclin, A1B1, MAP kinase, Ras, HER III and IV, heregulin, c-Src, and ODC levels).[60] Finally, based upon data from the WHI study, tumors diagnosed in postmenopausal women while they were receiving conjugated equine estrogen plus medroxyprogesterone acetate are associated with larger size and more commonly involved lymph nodes.[21] These new findings contradict conclusions from observational studies that such tumors have lower histologic grade and a 10% better prognosis than those in women not receiving MHT.

Studies have detected circulating tumor cells in the blood of patients with breast cancer as well as micrometastases in lymph nodes and bone marrow.[60,61] This information clearly provides prognostic information, but no data are yet available on how these findings should be used to influence therapeutic decisions.[62]

cDNA Array–Derived Biologic Subtypes

A major recent advance is the performance of cDNA array analysis to assess the effect of a particular tumor signature on prognosis.[63] This type of analysis has allowed a new biologic

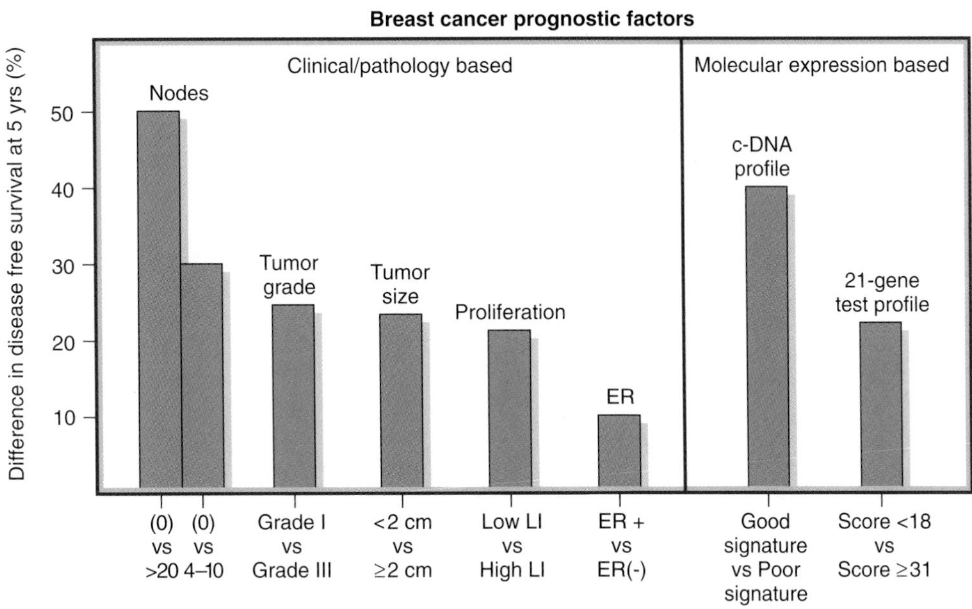

Figure 42–9 ▪ The prognostic value of several parameters related to patients with an initial diagnosis of breast cancer. All values are presented as the percentage difference (i.e., improvement) in disease-free survival at the 5-year interval. This method of presentation allows one to determine the increased number of women per 100 who would be free of disease at 5 years if they have a favorable prognostic factor compared with those with an unfavorable factor. ER, estrogen receptor; LI, labeling index.

classification of breast cancer based upon the degree of expression of key discriminant genes. Five subtypes of breast cancer are defined: luminal A, luminal B, basal epithelial, *ERB-B2*⁺, and normal breast tissue–like subtype.[63] As shown in Figure 42–10, each subtype has a different prognosis. All *BRCA1*-positive tumors fell into the basal subtype category.[63] Further validation of these techniques in subsets of patients categorized by tumor size, nodal status, tumor grade, age, and type of treatment will be necessary before common clinical application of this methodology is implemented.

Predictive Factors

Other biologic parameters allow assessment of the potential effectiveness of certain therapies. Older age, long disease-free survival, high degree of tumor differentiation, and prior response to endocrine therapy predict a higher likelihood of response to hormonal therapy.[56] The ability to measure receptors markedly improves the process of selection of patients for hormonal therapy. Absence of ER in the tumor predicts that less than 5% to 10% of women will respond to hormonal therapy. If both ER and PR are negative, an even lower percentage will respond. Patients with ER^+ or PR^+ tumors respond to hormonal therapy 50% to 75% of the time, and 30% to 50% of ER^+ but PgR^- tumors are responsive.[56,64] Emerging data suggest that patients with ER^+ and PR^+ tumors respond to tamoxifen therapy less often if

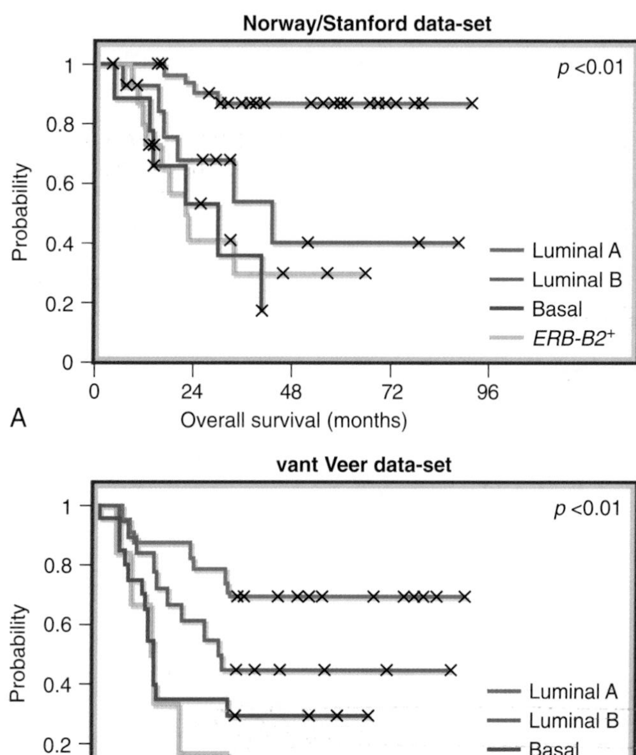

Figure 42–10 ▪ cDNA analysis of breast cancer tissues with categorization into Luminal A, Luminal B, Basal, and ERBP2 and the probability of overall survival and time to distant metastasis. The "x" symbols represent censored patients. The normal subtype is not shown. (Data reproduced from Sotiriou C, Neo SY, McShane LM, et al. Breast cancer classification and prognosis based on gene expression profiles from a population-based study. Proc Nat Acad Sci U S A 2003;100:10393-10398, with the permission of the authors and publisher.

HER2/Neu is positive.[65] However, *HER2/Neu*-positive tumors and *HER2/Neu*-negative tumors respond similarly to AIs. New data confirm the old observations of Lippmann and Allegra that low ER levels, in addition to predicting nonresponsiveness to hormonal therapy, predict a high likelihood of responding to chemotherapy.[66,67]

Receptor measurements are commonly performed by immunocytochemical analysis that correlates well with the ligand-binding assays. An increasing trend is to semiquantitate the level of ER positivity in tumors using the Allred scoring system, which classifies tumors on the basis of fraction of cells positive and intensity of staining with a scale of 0 to 8.[68] With routinely used immunocytochemical techniques, only ERα is measured, but half of breast tumors also contain ERβ. One study suggests that low levels of ERβ predict resistance to tamoxifen therapy.[69] However, current data are insufficient to show the precise clinical value of ERβ measurements. Some data suggest that certain tumors make ERβ variant proteins that can heterodimerize with full-length ERα or ERβ and exert dominant negative effects.[70] This concept suggests that further refinement of receptor assays could improve their predictive value.

An assay using quantitative PCR of selected genes has been validated in a prospective study to determine which patients with node-negative, ER^+ disease will experience distant disease recurrence while on tamoxifen.[71,72] This assay, the Oncotype DX assay, measures 16 informative genes and five housekeeping genes as controls. On this basis, women with node negative, ER^+ breast cancers are categorized into groups with low, intermediate, or high risk of recurrence. The low risk group had a 6.8% recurrence at 10 years versus a rate of 30.5% in the high-risk group. When patient age and tumor size were added to the model, only the cDNA score remained statistically significant upon multivariate analysis. These data provide prognostic information as well as predictive information about the treatment of women with ER^+, node-negative disease. Emerging data from the Oncotype DX assay suggests that the absolute level of ER mRNA, which varies by more than a 300-fold range, may be a better predictor of responses to hormonal therapy than qualitative immunohistochemistry assessment of ER protein content. Although it is not currently used routinely, cDNA array or quantitative PCR technology will probably be used commonly in the clinic within the next few years.

New Prognostic and Predictive Classification System

Investigators at the 2005 St. Gallen meeting devised a new, logical method to be used for both prognostic and predictive use.[62] This provides a practical means of choosing specific therapies. The first level of categorization places patients into one of three predictive groups: endocrine responsive (high receptor content), endocrine response uncertain (low receptor content), and endocrine nonresponsive (no receptor present). The second level of categorization places patients into prognostic groups including high risk, intermediate risk, and low risk as defined in Table 42–1.

Hormonal Therapies

Basic Mechanistic Principles

Surgical Ablative Therapies

Historically, the initial approach to hormonal therapy involved surgical removal of endocrine glands responsible for synthesis of estrogen or its precursors. Beatson in 1896 first demonstrated that oophorectomy caused regression of breast cancer in premenopausal women, and comprehensive studies later docu-

TABLE 42–1 DEFINITION OF RISK CATEGORIES FOR PATIENTS WITH POSTOPERATIVE BREAST CANCER

RISK CATEGORY
Low Risk
Node negative *and* all of the following features: pT ≤2 cm Grade 1 Absence of peritumoral vascular invasion HER2/*Neu* gene neither overexpressed nor amplified Age ≥35 years
Intermediate Risk
Node negative *and* at least one of the following features: pT >2 cm, Grade 2-3 Presence of peritumoral vascular invasion HER2/*Neu* gene overexpressed or amplified Age <35 years *or* Node positive (1-3 involved nodes) *and* HER2/*Neu* gene neither overexpressed nor amplified
High Risk
Node positive (1-3 involved nodes) *and* HER2/*Neu* gene overexpressed or amplified *or* Node positive (4 or more involved nodes)
ENDOCRINE RESPONSE CATEGORY
Endocrine Responsive
Cells express steroid hormone receptors at adequate levels (i.e. >10% of cells positive on IHC)
Endocrine Response Uncertain
Quantitatively low receptor level (i.e. receptor$^+$ but <10% of cells +PgR negative) PgR negative *HER2/Neu* overexpressed or amplified
Endocrine Nonresponsive
Cells have no detectable expression of steroid receptors

mented responses in one third of patients not selected with ER measurements.[56] The availability of glucocorticoid replacement therapy in the 1940s enabled the use of adrenalectomy or hypophysectomy. More recently, development of medical means to block hormone synthesis or action has replaced adrenalectomy and hypophysectomy while surgical oophorectomy is still used.[56]

Hormone-Additive Therapies

Clinicians learned from empirical observations that high doses of estrogen, androgen, or progestins caused tumor regression.[56,73] High-dose estrogen therapy is most effective in women who had experienced menopause several years previously. A series of recent studies suggests a possible mechanism to explain this paradoxical effect: estrogen-induced apoptotic cell death.[24] With prolonged deprivation of estradiol, tumors up-regulate the estrogen-responsive Fas/Fas ligand death-receptor system and down-regulate the antiapoptotic factor nuclear factor kappa B (NFκB). With respect to androgens, a variety of observations suggest that an increased ratio of androgens to estrogens exerts an antagonistic effect on breast tissue. Progestins exert glucocorticoid actions, which suppress circulating estrogen levels and could also act via progestational mechanisms.

Medical Ablative Therapies

Gonadotropin Receptor Hormone Agonist Analogues

Medical means of ablating hormone secretion or action avoid major surgery and can effectively replicate the hormonal and clinical effects of these procedures. High doses of GnRH agonist analogues suppress ovarian function to the same extent as surgical oophorectomy. This strategy is referred to as *medical oophorectomy* in this chapter. The pituitary requires pulsatile exposure to GnRH to maintain gonadotropin secretion. GnRH agonists suppress LH and FSH by exposing the pituitary to a continuous GnRH stimulus, which causes a paradoxical gonadotropin inhibition. Preparations lasting 3 to 6 months can be given by IM injection. For the first several days after initiation of therapy, an increase in LH, FSH, and estradiol occurs, but thereafter, suppression ensues.

Selective Estrogen-Receptor Modulators

Blockade of estrogen action rather than synthesis provides an additional strategy. In premenopausal women, these agents exert effects similar to those of surgical oophorectomy, and in postmenopausal women the effects are similar to those of hypophysectomy or adrenalectomy. Tamoxifen, the initial antiestrogen of this type, was introduced for use in the United States in the mid 1970s.[56] Early clinical observations noted that this drug is an antiestrogen on breast tissue but an estrogen agonist on uterus, vagina, bone, pituitary, and liver.[56]

Attempts to determine the divergent actions of tamoxifen led to an understanding of the complexity of ER-mediated transcriptional regulation and actions of the antiestrogens (reviewed briefly here and covered in detail in Chapter 16.) Tamoxifen binds to both ERα and ERβ in the ligand binding domain (AF2) of the receptor, which then facilitates the binding of the antiestrogen-ER complex to specific estrogen response elements on DNA (EREs). Conformational changes in the ER-binding pocket at helix 12 induced by antiestrogens do not allow binding of coactivators to the ER but rather facilitate binding of corepressors. The continued presence of corepressor in the complex is thought to explain the antiestrogenic properties of tamoxifen. The relative amounts of corepressor and coactivator in certain tissues and the presence of other unknown factors regulate whether tamoxifen acts as an agonist or antagonist. As one example, up-regulation of *HER2/Neu* and AIB1 appear to enhance the estrogen-agonistic properties of tamoxifen.[74] Additional estrogenic effects are mediated by membrane initiated (extranuclear) actions at the cell membrane as well as by protein-protein interactions between ER and binding sites on c-Jun, SP-1, IGF-R, PI3 kinase, *HER2/Neu*, c-Src, and potentially other factors.[75]

Based upon the SERM concept, other agents have been introduced or are being developed to enhance breast-antagonistic and bone-agonistic properties. One of these, toremiphene, is quite similar to tamoxifen, albeit slightly less effective as an agonist on bone. Raloxifene, on the other hand, appears not to stimulate uterus or cause endometrial cancer, and yet it is an antiestrogen on breast. The STAR and RUTH trials[44,45] established the efficacy of raloxifene as a breast cancer preventive drug, but minimal data are available regarding its efficacy for treatment. Preliminary results from other agents have been reported.

Pure Antagonist Antiestrogens

Clinical and experimental data suggest that long-term exposure to tamoxifen might induce tumors to undergo adaptive mechanisms to cause the agonistic properties of this SERM to predominate.[74] Based upon these observations, antiestrogens were developed that were devoid of agonist properties. Fulvestrant, the U.S. Food and Drug Administration (FDA)-approved drug in this class, increases the rate of degradation of the ER and also inhibits E2-mediated transcription by favoring binding of corepressors to the ER complex.[76] Because of its effect to reduce the concentration of the ER, fulvestrant has been termed an *estrogen-receptor down-regulator* (SERD).

Inhibitors of Estradiol Synthesis

Aromatase catalyzes the rate-limiting step in the conversion of androgens to estrogens.[77] Aromatase has been a key target for development of inhibitors since 1980. The first-generation inhibitor, aminoglutethimide, inhibited aromatase by 90% in postmenopausal women and was as effective as tamoxifen in causing breast tumor regressions. The greater side effect profile of aminoglutethimide served as an impetus to develop second- and third-generation inhibitors.[56]

Three third-generation agents (anastrozole, letrozole, and exemestane) are now approved drugs in the United States and Europe. These agents are 100-fold to 10,000-fold more potent than aminoglutethimide and are called selective aromatase inhibitors (SAIs) because they do not inhibit other enzymatic steps. The two major subclasses include nonsteroidal competitive inhibitors and steroidal enzyme inactivators.[77] The competitive inhibitors bind to the active site of the enzyme with high affinity and compete with substrate. Aromatase inactivators bind covalently to the enzyme and permanently destroy its activity. Theoretically, the inactivators could have advantages over the competitive AIs because inhibition might continue if a patient missed one or more doses of medication. However, no experimental proof of this advantage is as yet available in patients.

Both subclasses of inhibitor reduce aromatase to 1% to 2.5% of baseline activity,[78] substantially reduce plasma estradiolt levels, and suppress tissue concentrations of this steroid in breast tumors (Fig. 42–11). The greater degree of suppression with the third-generation than with first-generation inhibitors might explain their enhanced efficacy in causing tumor regression. Because the AIs are devoid of estrogen agonistic properties, these agents do not increase the incidence of endometrial cancer, as occurs with tamoxifen. However, as expected from the known effects of estrogen deprivation on bone, the AIs do accelerate the rate of bone loss and increase fracture incidence.[79] Although a trend toward an increased incidence of cardiac events has been reported, these adverse findings are inconsistent among studies and not yet statistically significant.[53] Preliminary data show no adverse effects on lipid concentrations, but more systematic data are needed.

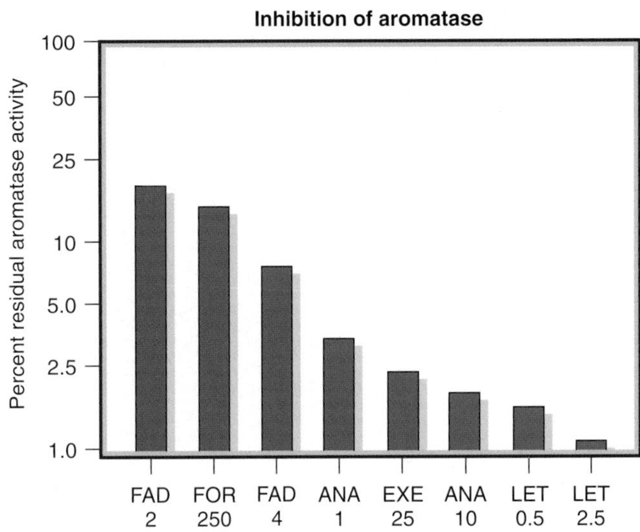

Figure 42–11 ▪ Aromatase activity remaining during the administration of first-, second-, and third-generation aromatase inhibitors and inactivators (mg/day). Data are expressed on a log scale to emphasize the expected log dose response characteristics of hormone actions. With the most potent inhibitor, only 1% of aromatase activity persists during therapy. Degree of aromatase suppression was determined by an isotopic kinetic method using ^{3}H-androstenedione and ^{14}C-estrone to assess the rho value before and during therapy. The Rho value represents the percentage conversion of androgens to estrogens under equilibrium conditions. ANA, anastrozole; EXE, exemestane; FAD, fadrozole; FOR, formestane; LET, letrozole. (From Geisler J, Lonning PE. Endocrine effects of aromatase inhibitors and inactivators in vivo: review of data and method limitations. J Steroid Biochem Mol Biol 2005;95[1-5]: 75-81.)

Chemical Castration

Chemotherapeutic agents destroy granulosa cells in the ovary and can result in transient or permanent amenorrhea in premenopausal women.[80] Accordingly, practical clinical issues of infertility and menopausal symptoms ensue. Complete ovarian destruction, as evidenced by the onset of amenorrhea, is more common in women older than 40 years as opposed to those younger (Fig. 42–12). Menses returns in up to 20% of women older than 40 years when an AI is started.[81] Incomplete information is available regarding estradiol levels under these circumstances. The effect of chemical castration was not initially felt to be clinically important. However, recent data suggest that adjuvant chemotherapy in premenopausal women exerts its antitumnor effects on neoplasms with high ER levels through an ovarian ablative effect to a substantial degree.[82]

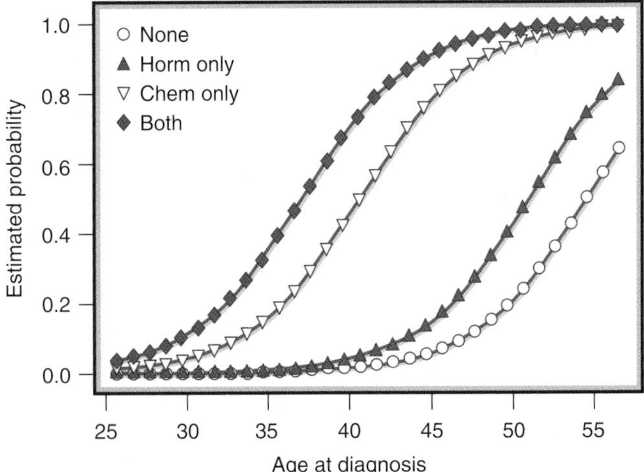

Figure 42–12 ▪ Cumulative frequency analysis of development of amenorrhea as a function of age in response to chemotherapy (Chem), hormonal therapy (Horm), or both in women with breast cancer in comparison with no treatment. The effect of chemotherapy on ovarian function reduces the age of menopause by an average of nearly 20 years. (Taken from the data of Goodwin PJ., Ennis M, Pritchard KI, et al. Risk of menopause during the first year after breast cancer diagnosis. J Clin Oncol 1999;17:2365-2370.)

Radiation Castration

Radiation treatment (RT) of the ovaries in premenopausal women has been used as adjuvant treatment of breast cancer for many years, but the majority of studies do not adequately document the degree of suppression of estradiol levels. An

Eastern Cooperative Oncology Group study examined 22 women receiving RT to induce ovarian ablation. Only 75% experienced complete ablation based upon estradiol or FSH levels. In one quarter of patients, the effect was delayed until 7 to 28 months after RT was completed. These data suggest that surgical or medical oophorectomy with GnRH agonists should be used in preference to RT to induce ovarian ablation.[83]

Complete versus Partial Estradiol Ablation

The concept of complete versus partial medical ablation arose from observations in men with prostate cancer (see later). Removal of the testes reduces androgen secretion only partially because precursor steroids from the adrenal can be enzymatically converted into potent androgens in prostate tissue. Partial androgen-deprivation therapy consists of reduction of testicular androgens, whereas addition of an antiandrogen or adrenal inhibitor accomplishes complete androgen blockade.

By analogy, removal of the ovaries causes a marked decrease in estradiol production, but adrenal precursors remain to be aromatized to estrogens in peripheral tissues or in the breast cancer itself. Accordingly, partial estrogen deprivation involves surgical or medical oophorectomy, and complete deprivation consists of addition of either tamoxifen or an AI to the oophorectomy regimen. A major focus of investigation currently is to determine if complete estrogen deprivation is superior to partial deprivation and if AIs are superior to tamoxifen to produce complete estrogen deprivation.

Overview of Clinical Efficacy

Background

Nearly all patients with breast cancer undergo lumpectomy or mastectomy and, if warranted, radiation therapy. Most patients then receive adjuvant therapy to destroy occult cancer cells at locoregional and distant metastatic sites. Upon tumor recurrence, first-, second-, and third-line hormonal or chemotherapies are then used in sequence for advanced disease. A recently introduced approach, called *neoadjuvant hormonal therapy*, involves use of hormonal therapy for 3 to 4 months before surgery for patients with large tumors.[84] The goal is to reduce the size of the lesion so as to make lumpectomy a feasible alternative to mastectomy.

Selective Estrogen-Receptor Modulators

Tamoxifen was the first antiestrogen approved for treatment of breast cancer. Until recently, the overall benefit of tamoxifen was usually reported as the relative improvement in frequency of defined events such as tumor recurrence or survival. In the neoadjuvant, adjuvant, and advanced disease settings, tamoxifen results in a *relative benefit* of approximately 50%. However, a more useful parameter, the absolute benefit rate, has now been widely accepted. This is defined as the number of women per hundred treated who benefit from taking tamoxifen. As illustrated in Figure 42–13, the absolute benefit increases as the event becomes more common, even though the relative percentage benefit remains approximately 50%.

Adjuvant Therapy

When tamoxifen is used as adjuvant therapy, pre- or postmenopausal women with positive lymph nodes at the time of diagnosis experience approximately a 17% absolute increase of recurrence-free survival at 5 years, and women with negative nodes experience approximately a 12% absolute increase (Fig. 42–14).[85] Tamoxifen causes an absolute reduction of contralateral breast cancers of 1% to 5% at 5 years depending on underlying risk factors. Tamoxifen is active in both pre- and postmenopausal women with breast cancer but only in those whose tumors are ER^+ or PR^+, or both.

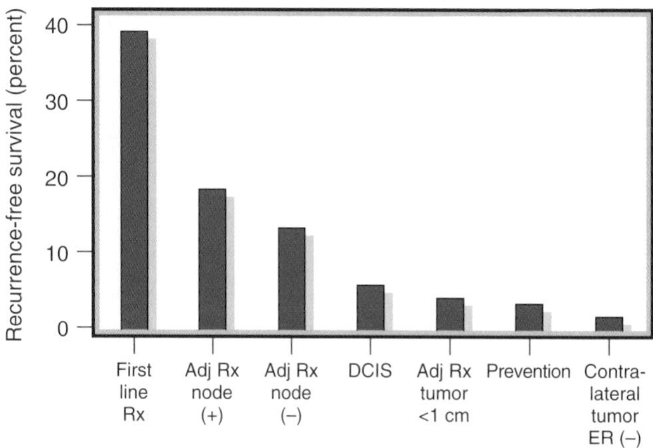

Figure 42–13 ▪ Absolute benefit from tamoxifen in the treatment and prevention setting. Absolute benefit is defined as the number of women per 100 who will benefit from the use of tamoxifen. In the adjuvant or treatment settings, tamoxifen was used for a period of 5 years. Adj Rx, adjuvant therapy; DCIS, ductal carcinoma in situ; ER, estrogen receptor.

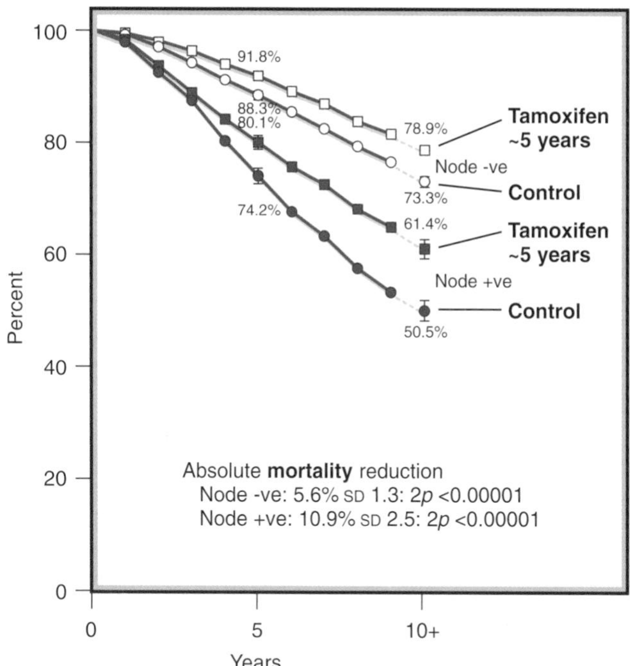

Figure 42–14 ▪ Disease specific survival in percent in women receiving tamoxifen or a placebo as adjuvant therapy for breast cancer. –ve, negative; +ve, positive. (Data taken from Early Breast Cancer Trialists' Collaborative Group. Tamoxifen for early breast cancer: an overview of the randomised trials. Lancet 1998;351[9114]:1451-1467.)

The optimal duration of use is 5 years. Direct comparative studies indicate superiority of 5 years versus 1 or 2 years of tamoxifen therapy, whereas 10 years of therapy provides no additional benefit over 5 years.[86] In two studies, tamoxifen for 10 as opposed to 5 years slightly reduced disease-free and overall survival.[87,88] This finding might be explained by tumor adaptation and emergence of a predominant estrogen-agonistic effect of tamoxifen, as initially suggested in animal studies.[89] Although tamoxifen is only administered for 5 years, benefit persists long term (carryover effect) because disease-specific survival increases from approximately 6% at 5 years to 10% at 10 years in node-positive patients.[85]

In premenopausal women, tamoxifen is used as the preferred hormonal agent either alone in low-risk patients or after chemotherapy in those at high risk. In postmenopausal women, the role of tamoxifen is undergoing reconsideration in light of the greater efficacy of AIs in this setting.[90]

Advanced Disease

Approximately 40% of women with advanced disease benefit from tamoxifen. Responses last 12 to 18 months on average before relapse.[56] Efficacy is limited to those with ER^+ or PR^+ tumors.[85] The presence of *HER2/Neu* appears to be associated with a decreased response to tamoxifen.[65,91] One large study, ATAC (Anastrazole and Tamoxifen Alone and in Combination), also suggested that ER^+/PR^- tumors respond less well to tamoxifen, but another, BIG FEMTA (Femara-Tamoxifen Breast International Group), did not confirm this observation.[49,50] Women with disease in soft tissue, bone, or viscera are the best candidates for tamoxifen, whereas chemotherapy is indicated when extensive liver metastases, brain metastases, or lymphangitic spread to lung is present.[56] The other SERM, toremifene, appears to exert clinical effects similar to those of tamoxifen.

Pure Antagonistic Antiestrogens

Fulvestrant is an agent that exhibits primarily antiestrogenic effects and acts both by down-regulating the ER molecule itself and by interfering with estradiol-induced transcription. A comparative study in 458 women with advanced disease demonstrated similar efficacy in patients treated with fulvestrant as with the AI anastrozole in patients progressing after prior endocrine treatment. Clinical benefit (complete objective response, partial objective response, or stable disease for 6 months) occurred in 44.5% receiving fulvestrant versus 45% receiving the aromatase inhibitor anastrozole. Another study compared tamoxifen with fulvestrant as first-line therapy of advanced breast cancer and found similar efficacy with respect to all parameters examined.[92] Finally, patients who were initially treated with fulvestrant and who relapsed continue to maintain responsiveness to AIs or to tamoxifen. Based upon these data, the appropriate role of fulvestrant in the clinical armamentarium remains to be fully defined.

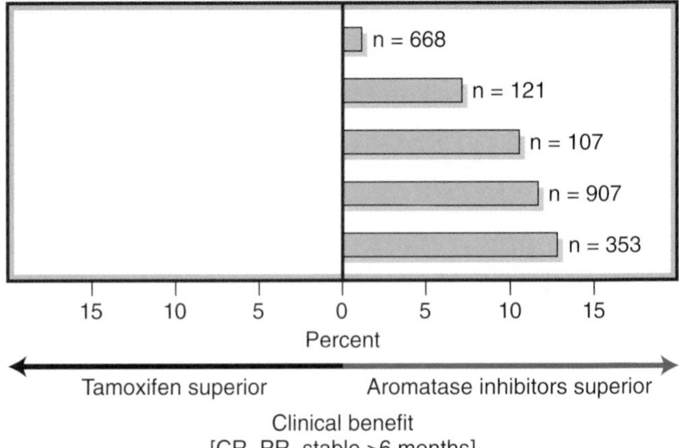

Figure 42–15 ▪ Comparison of tamoxifen versus aromatase inhibitors in five randomized, controlled studies in advanced disease. CR, complete objective response; PR, partial objective response. (Data taken from Bonneterre J, Thurlimann B, Robertson JF, et al. Anastrozole versus tamoxifen as first-line therapy for advanced breast cancer in 668 postmenopausal women: results of the Tamoxifen or Arimidex Randomized Group Efficacy and Tolerability study. J Clin Oncol 2000;18[22]:3748-3757; Nabholtz JM, Buzdar A, Pollak M, et al. Anastrozole is superior to tamoxifen as first-line therapy for advanced breast cancer in postmenopausal women: results of a North American multicenter randomized trial. Arimidex Study Group. J Clin Oncol 2000;18[22]:3758-3767.; Mouridsen H, Gershanovich M, Sun Y, et al. Phase III study of letrozole versus tamoxifen as first-line therapy of advanced breast cancer in postmenopausal women: analysis of survival and update of efficacy from the International Letrozole Breast Cancer Group. J Clin Oncol 2003;21[11]:2101-2109; Milla-Santos A, Milla L, Portella J, et al. Anastrozole versus tamoxifen as first-line therapy in postmenopausal patients with hormone-dependent advanced breast cancer: a prospective, randomized, phase III study. Am J Clin Oncol 2003;26[3]:317-322; Smith R, Sun Y, Garin A, et al, and the Letrozole International Breast Cancer Study Group. Femara (letrozole) showed significant improvement in efficacy over tamoxifen as first-line treatment in postmenopausal women with advanced breast cancer. Breast Cancer Res Treat 2000;64[1]:27.)

Aromatase Inhibitors

Only postmenopausal patients benefit from AIs because interruption of estradiol negative feedback results in override of aromatase blockade in premenopausal women. Until recently, tamoxifen was considered the preferred agent for the initial treatment of breast cancer in both the adjuvant and advanced disease settings. However, the third-generation AIs anastrozole, letrozole, and exemestane have now been proved superior to tamoxifen in direct head-to-head trials.[49,50]

Advanced Disease

Five large, multicenter, multinational, randomized trials directly compared the AIs with tamoxifen (Fig. 42–15).[93,94,94-98,99] All followed similar trial designs and included postmenopausal patients with locally advanced or metastatic breast cancer. No women had received adjuvant tamoxifen within 12 months and none were known to be ER negative. All trials demonstrated the superiority of the AIs in clinical efficacy, with incremental responses ranging from 2% to 13% (Fig. 42–15). The differences were statistically significant in all but one trial, in which the receptor status was unknown in 55% of patients.[93]

Pooled data indicate that tamoxifen was associated with DVT and pulmonary emboli (7.6% vs. 4.5%) significantly more often than the AI anastrozole.[97,99,100] If one combines observations from all trials, it appears that nausea, hot flushes, and GI distress were comparable with tamoxifen or an AI. Comparisons of AIs with placebo (or with tamoxifen) reveal an increase in hot flushes, arthritis, osteoporosis, arthralgia, and myalgia with AIs. Surprisingly, women receiving placebo or tamoxifen also experience these same side effects quite commonly (Table 42–2).

Taken together, these trials provide evidence that the third-generation AIs are superior in efficacy and toxicity to tamoxifen in the advanced disease setting. Letrozole, anastrozole, and exemestane have now been approved in the United States and Europe as first-line therapy for advanced breast cancer. These trials showed for the first time that one endocrine therapy could be superior to another. Prior to these studies, dogma held that each available endocrine therapy produced similar rates of response and could be distinguished only on the basis of side effects and cost.

Comprehensive, direct head-to-head comparisons of the three approved AIs (letrozole, anastrozole, and exemestane) are now needed to determine if one agent is superior to the other. This is particularly important because hormonal data suggest that letrozole may be more potent as an AI than anastrozole.[101] At present, only one such direct comparison is available in which anastrozole and letrozole were used in 713 women with advanced breast cancer. Letrozole was superior with respect to objective response rate (19.1% vs. 12.3%, $P = 0.013$)

TABLE 42–2 SIDE EFFECTS FROM AROMATASE INHIBITORS VERSUS TAMOXIFEN OR PLACEBO

Side Effect	Exemestane (%)	Letrozole (%)	PLACEBO		TAMOXIFEN	
			%	Probability	%	Probability
Arthralgia	5.4	21.3	16.6	$P < .001$	3.6	$P = 0.01$
Arthritis	—	5.6	3.5	$P < .001$	—	
Hot flushes	42.0	47.2	40.5	$P < .001$	39.6	$P = .28$
Myalgia	—	11.8	9.5	$P = 0.02$	—	
Osteoporosis	7.4	5.8	4.5	$P = 0.07$	5.7	$P = 0.05$

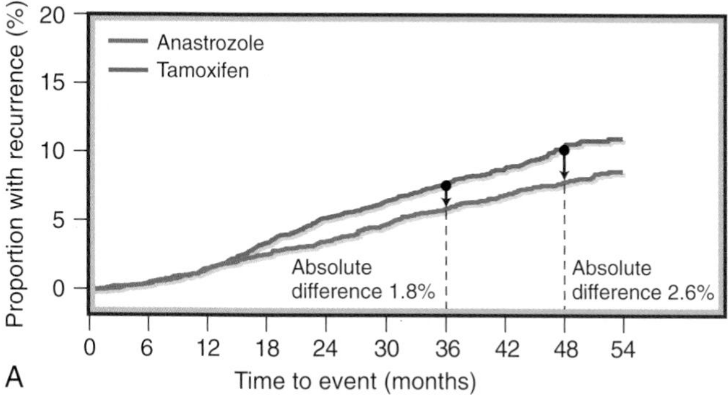

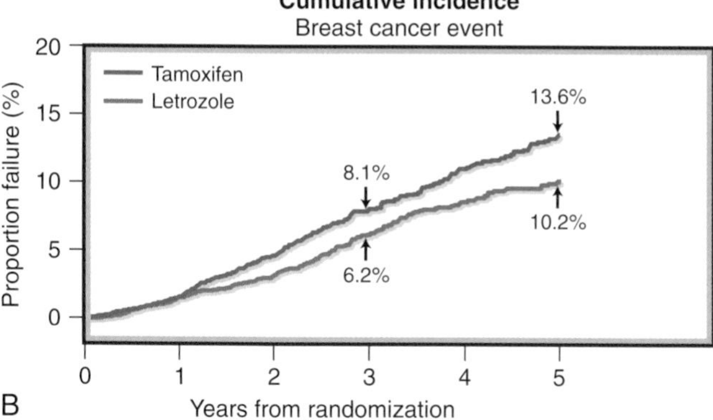

Figure 42–16 ▪ **A,** Comparison of tamoxifen with anastrozole in the ATAC trial of breast cancer treatment in the adjuvant setting. **B,** Comparison of tamoxifen with letrozole in the BIG FEMTA trial of breast cancer treatment in the adjuvant setting. (**A** from The ATAC Trialists' Group. Anastrozole alone or in combination with tamoxifen versus tamoxifen alone for adjuvant treatment of postmenopausal women with early breast cancer: first results of the ATAC randomised trial. Lancet 2002;359:2131-2139; Howell A, Cuzick J, Baum M, et al. Results of the ATAC (Arimidex, Tamoxifen, Alone or in Combination) trial after completion of 5 years' adjuvant treatment for breast cancer. Lancet 2005;365(9453):60-62; Coates AS, Keshaviah A, Thurlimann B et al: Five years of letrozole compared to tamoxifen as initial adjuvant therapy for postmenopausal women with endocrine-responsive early breast cancer: update of study BIG 1-98. J Clin Oncol 2007;25:486–492.

but no differences in time to progression, time to treatment failure, or duration of response were observed. Additional studies are considered necessary before clinical decisions can be made regarding equivalency or superiority of one agent over the other.

The choice of AIs over tamoxifen as first-line therapy for advanced disease at present is considered reasonable[90] but based upon incomplete data. Prior comparisons of tamoxifen with the first-generation AI aminoglutethimide demonstrated equal efficacy but a different pattern of cross resistance.[56] The AIs were efficacious if used after tamoxifen, but tamoxifen appeared less effective when used after the AIs. If this were true for the third-generation AIs, tamoxifen might remain the first-line agent. However, preliminary data suggest that tamoxifen is effective after crossover from the AI anastrozole. In a crossover comparison, 48.7% of 119 patients experienced clinical benefit from tamoxifen when used as a second-line agent after initial use of letrozole. By comparison, second-line letrozole following initial tamoxifen produced clinical benefit in 56.8%% of 95 patients.[102] The issue of choosing the proper sequence between the AIs and tamoxifen is currently being tested in a four-arm study, the BIG FEMTA trial.

Adjuvant Therapy

AIs provide a means to block estrogen effectively without the emergence of estrogen agonistic effects in the adjuvant setting. On the other hand, detrimental effects could result from deprivation of estradiol on vaginal mucosa, bone density, and cholesterol levels. Two similar large trials, the ATAC and the BIG FEMTA trial, compared the effects of either agent on time to progression of disease, time to treatment failure, and on overall survival.[49,50] At 5 years of follow-up, both trials demonstrated an absolute superiority of the AI of approximately 3% (Fig. 42–16A and B). Overall survival with either therapy was similar. In this setting, tamoxifen caused an increase in endometrial cancer and in venothrombotic episodes (VTEs). AIs were associated with accelerated bone loss, symptoms of urogenital atrophy, and arthralgias. Lipid parameters do not appear to deteriorate significantly with the AIs, but there is a trend toward a higher incidence of cardiovascular disease.[50] On the basis of these data, the AIs have now been approved in the Untied States for use in the adjuvant setting. Published guidelines still suggest initial use of tamoxifen unless patients are at risk for VTEs.[62,90] Use of an AI should be also considered in patients with *HER2/Neu* or ER^+/PR^- tumors (who in one trial appeared to respond less well to tamoxifen)[49] or in high-risk patients.

Recent data suggest a hypothesis why the AIs might be superior to tamoxifen. The enzyme cytochrome p4502D6 (CYP2D6). is required to convert tamoxifen to its active metabolite, endoxifen. Six percent to 8% of women taking tamoxifen harbor relatively inactive alleles of this enzyme, and SSRIs such as paroxetine, fluoxetine, sertraline, and citalopram can inhibit CYP2D6. Patients with reduced activity of 2D6 on a genetic or drug-drug interaction basis exhibit lower plasma levels of endoxifen. In a large study, women with defective 2D6 experienced a shortened disease-free and overall survival compared to those with normal function.[103] Accordingly, the lack of activating metabolism of tamoxifen to endoxifen might at least partially explain the inferiority of tamoxifen to the AIs.[104]

Several studies are currently comparing the sequential use of AIs after initial adjuvant therapy with tamoxifen (Fig. 42–17A and B). The MA.17 trial compared placebo to tamoxifen in women who had received tamoxifen for 5 years.[53] The results demonstrate a 35% greater relative reduction in new events and

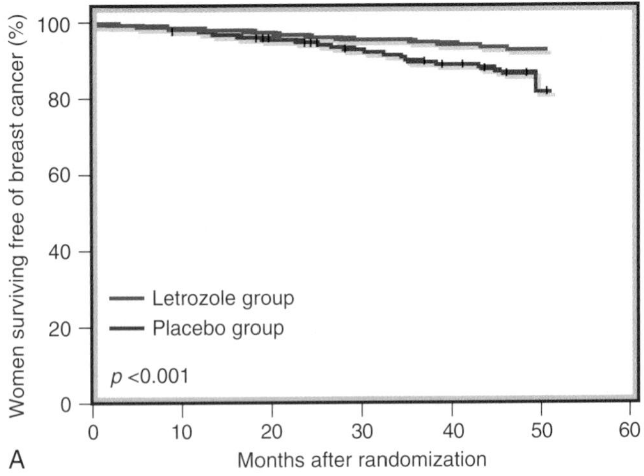

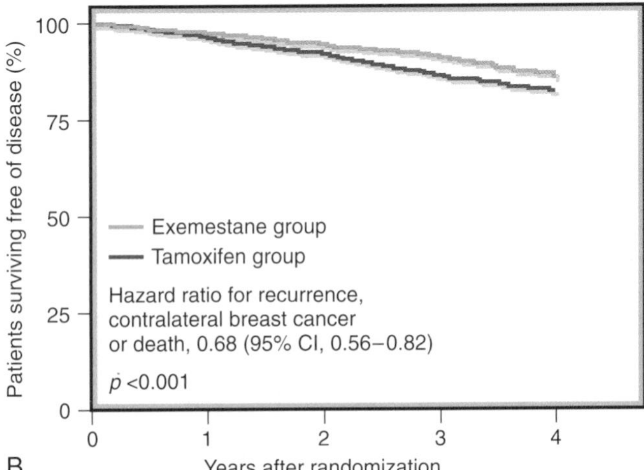

Figure 42–17 ▪ **A,** Comparison of placebo with letrozole in patients with breast cancer treated initially with tamoxifen in the adjuvant setting and randomized to receive letrozole or placebo with therapy after 5 years of tamoxifen. **B,** Comparison of tamoxifen with exemestane in patients with breast cancer treated initially with tamoxifen and then randomized to exemestane or continued tamoxifen after 2-3 years of tamoxifen. CI, confidence interval. (**A** from Goss PE, Ingle JN, Martino S, et al. A randomized trial of letrozole in postmenopausal women after five years of tamoxifen therapy for early-stage breast cancer. N Engl J Med 2003;349[19]:1793-1802. **B** from Coombes RC, Hall E, Gibson LJ, et al. A randomized trial of exemestane after two to three years of tamoxifen therapy in postmenopausal women with primary breast cancer. N Engl J Med 2004;350[11]:1081-192.)

an absolute reduction of 4% in women receiving the AI (see Fig. 42–17A). Overall survival was improved only in the node-positive group. As shown in Table 42–2, the AI was associated with an increase in hot flushes, bone loss, and arthralgia. The increase in arthralgia attributable to the AI was less than expected because of the high rate in the placebo group (16.6% placebo, 21.3% letrozole). The IES study (International Exemestane Study) compared the effect of 5 years of tamoxifen with 2 to 3 years of tamoxifen, with crossover to exemestane at 2 to 3 years (see Fig. 42–17B).[52] This study also showed a reduction in new cancer events in the AI compared to the tamoxifen group. The ABCSG/ARNO trial (Austrian Breast Cancer Study Group and German Adjuvant Breast Cancer Group) was similar but used anastrozole rather than exemestane. Switch to the AI resulted in a 3% improvement in event-free survival.[105] These crossover data demonstrate that women with breast cancer can

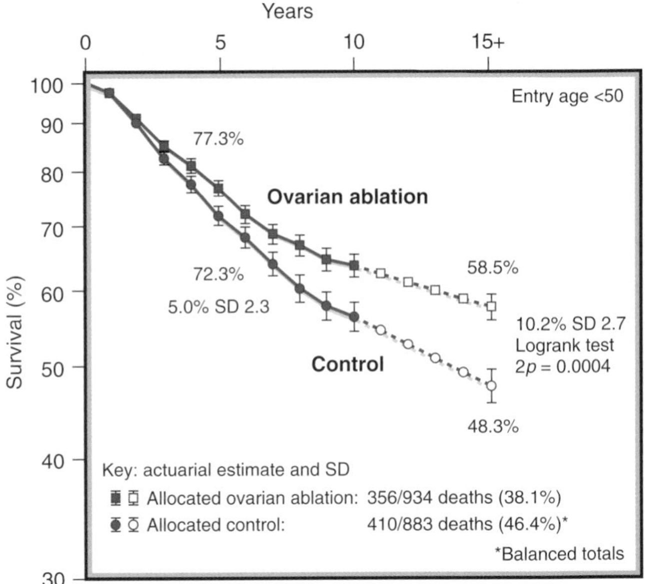

Figure 42–18 ▪ Survival data in patients undergoing a prophylactic oophorectomy in comparison with a group of women not receiving this therapy. SD, standard deviation. (From Early Breast Cancer Trialists' Collaborative Group. Ovarian ablation in early breast cancer: overview of the randomised trials. Lancet 1996;348[9036]:1189-1196.)

experience additional benefit by the sequential addition of an AI after tamoxifen. Based upon these three studies, the American Society of Clinical Oncology (ASCO) guidelines recommend that appropriate therapy is now to use an AI somewhere in the course of adjuvant therapy.[90]

Hormone Additive Therapy

Androgens or estrogens are generally considered inferior to use of tamoxifen and AIs.[56] Until recently, high-dose estrogen had been used sparingly because of the increased side-effect profile versus tamoxifen. However, a 20-year follow-up of a randomized comparison of tamoxifen with diethylstilbestrol (DES) reported a significant survival advantage in patients receiving the estrogen and lack of cross-resistance between these two therapeutic approaches.[73] This surprising study suggests reconsideration of use of high-dose estrogen in selected patients.[106]

A series of preclinical studies demonstrated the likely mechanism for the beneficial effects of estradiol, namely the stimulation of apoptotic tumor cell death by estrogens.[24,107] A recent review reports a 30% response to use of high-dose estrogen in women refractory to multiple hormonal agents.[106] Clinical trials to assess its place in the therapeutic armamentarium are under way (VC Jordan, M Ellis, personal communications).

Surgical Oophorectomy

Prophylactic oophorectomy represented the first adjuvant endocrine therapy for breast cancer. Although initially thought to be ineffective, recent meta-analyses demonstrate clear benefit, with a 6% absolute survival advantage at 15 years for patients younger than 50 years who are lymph-node negative and a 12.5% survival advantage for node-positive patients (Fig. 42–18).[108] Because receptor status was unknown in patients in these trials, a large fraction of receptor-negative patients were likely included. Accordingly, one would have expected even better results if hormone receptor–positive patients only were so treated.[108] In the advanced disease setting, surgical oophorectomy induces clinical benefit in approximately 50% of ER^+ or PR^+ patients.[56]

Medical Oophorectomy

Emerging data support the use of GnRH-induced medical oophorectomy in the adjuvant setting, and recent research emphasis has focused upon this strategy.[109] In the opinion of some experts, this approach might soon replace surgical oophorectomy, but others believe that laparoscopic oophorectomy might still be a more attractive approach. Demonstration of the effectiveness of prophylactic oophorectomy (see Fig. 42–18) was surprising to the medical community and led to a reconsideration of this approach, albeit with use of GnRH agonists rather than surgery. The goal of these studies was to determine the efficacy of medical oophorectomy in patients who are exclusively ER$^+$. Two studies in the advanced setting indicate that the GnRH analogues produce clinical effects similar to those induced by surgical oophorectomy.[110,111] No data are available to compare medical oophorectomy alone versus no treatment or versus surgical oophorectomy in the adjuvant setting.

Rather than comparing medical oophorectomy to no treatment, studies examined the effects of chemotherapy versus medical oophorectomy in the adjuvant setting. The Zoladex Early Breast Cancer Research Association (ZEBRA) study demonstrated equivalence of goserelin to standard CMF (cytoxan, methotrexate, 5-fluorouracil) chemotherapy on overall survival but only in ER$^+$ patients.[112] This study has been criticized on the basis that CMF is not as effective as anthracycline-based regimens such as FAC (5-fluorouracil, adriamycin, and cytoxan), and FAC might be more effective than medical oophorectomy. Tamoxifen can also be considered a form of medical oophorectomy, and studies demonstrate similar efficacy of this approach when compared with surgical oophorectomy.

Complete Estrogen Blockade

Recent trials have compared medical oophorectomy alone (partial estrogen deprivation) versus medical oophorectomy plus tamoxifen or an AI in the advanced disease setting. Complete estrogen blockade (medical oophorectomy plus tamoxifen) appeared superior to tamoxifen alone in a single large trial and in a meta-analysis of four similar studies.[113] The combined approach resulted in more frequent objective response rates and improved progression-free and overall patient survival. In the adjuvant setting, use of medical oophorectomy plus an AI or tamoxifen is the subject of the ongoing SOFT (Suppression of Ovarian Function Trial), TEXT (Tamoxifen and Exemestane Trial), and PERCHE (Premenopausal Endocrine-Responsive Chemotherapy) studies.[62]

Chemical Castration

Chemotherapy generally causes permanent amenorrhea in women older than 40 years and temporary cessation of menses in younger women (see Fig. 42–12).[80] Studies are ongoing to determine whether chemotherapy exerts some if its actions via suppression of estrogen production in premenopausal women. At least three possibilities for tumor regression exist:

- Hormonal effects resulting from chemotherapeutic destruction of the ovary
- Direct cytotoxic effects on the tumor
- A combination of these two effects.

Several trials have compared adjuvant chemotherapy to medical oophorectomy with and without tamoxifen in premenopausal women.[114-116] The chemotherapy and hormonal therapies appear to produce comparable antitumor effects in women with moderate or high levels of estrogen receptor (ZEBRA trial).[114] The International Breast Cancer Study Group (IBCSG) trial VII compared CMF with goserelin as adjuvant therapy in premenopausal women. In those with ER$^+$ tumors, disease-free survival was 81% in both groups at 5 years.[117] However, trends suggest that in ER$^-$ patents, chemotherapy is more effective than medical oophorectomy.[62,114] These results suggest that at least part of the benefit of chemotherapy in premenopausal women results from chemical castration.

Further support of the chemotherapy castration hypothesis comes from studies showing that chemotherapy is less effective in patients without complete cessation of menses[118,119] and that addition of medical oophorectomy is this setting provides improved responses.[118] Although effects of varying chemotherapeutic regimens on ovarian function differ, nearly 100% of women older than 40 years develop permanent amenorrhea following adjuvant chemotherapy (see Fig. 42–12). However, it was recently observed that use of AIs in this setting can induce return of menses, a potentially problematic phenomenon, and careful monitoring according to written guidelines followed.[81]

It would appear then, that in women younger than 40 years, addition of medical oophorectomy to chemotherapy would be beneficial. On the other hand, addition of medical oophorectomy to chemotherapy in women older than 40 years with ER$^+$ tumors might not be beneficial because chemical castration will be complete. In younger women at high risk for recurrence, chemotherapy followed by hormonal therapy is more efficacious than chemotherapy alone. These and other observations suggest that effects of chemotherapy are partially due to a reduction of hormone secretion and partially to cytotoxic effects.

Hormonal Therapy Alone in Premenopausal Women

Nearly all premenopausal women are treated with chemotherapy in the adjuvant setting, and the evidence for this in women in high-risk groups is substantial. However, for patients in the low- or intermediate-risk, endocrine-responsive categories, current data support equivalent efficacy of hormone therapy and chemotherapy. On this basis, the new St. Gallen guidelines favor the use of hormone therapy without chemotherapy in low-risk and intermediate-risk, hormone-responsive premenopausal patients (Fig. 42–19A and B).[62]

Chemotherapy Followed by Hormonal Therapy

Based upon a meta-analysis, the combination of surgical or medical oophorectomy (GnRH agonists or tamoxifen) plus chemotherapy provides additional benefit over chemotherapy alone in the adjuvant setting in premenopausal women.[120] The addition of the GnRH agonists might be particularly important for women younger than 40 years in whom estradiol remained in the premenopausal range after chemotherapy, as suggested by a recent trial.[109,121] In postmenopausal women, addition of tamoxifen after six courses of cytoxan, doxorubicin, fluorouracil (CAF) chemotherapy improved disease-free survival compared to tamoxifen alone,[122] but the chemotherapy provided little benefit in the subgroup with very high ER levels.[123] Recent data indicate that chemotherapy should be given first followed by endocrine therapy later to allow maximal effectiveness of the chemotherapy.

Chemotherapy Followed by Complete Estrogen Deprivation

Ongoing studies are addressing two questions. The first is whether chemotherapy followed by complete ovarian deprivation is superior to chemotherapy followed by partial ovarian deprivation. Davidson et al showed the superiority of CAF followed by medical oophorectomy plus tamoxifen versus CAF alone or CAF plus medical oophorectomy.[109] The complete estrogen blockade strategy (medical oophorectomy plus tamoxifen) improved time to treatment failure and disease-free

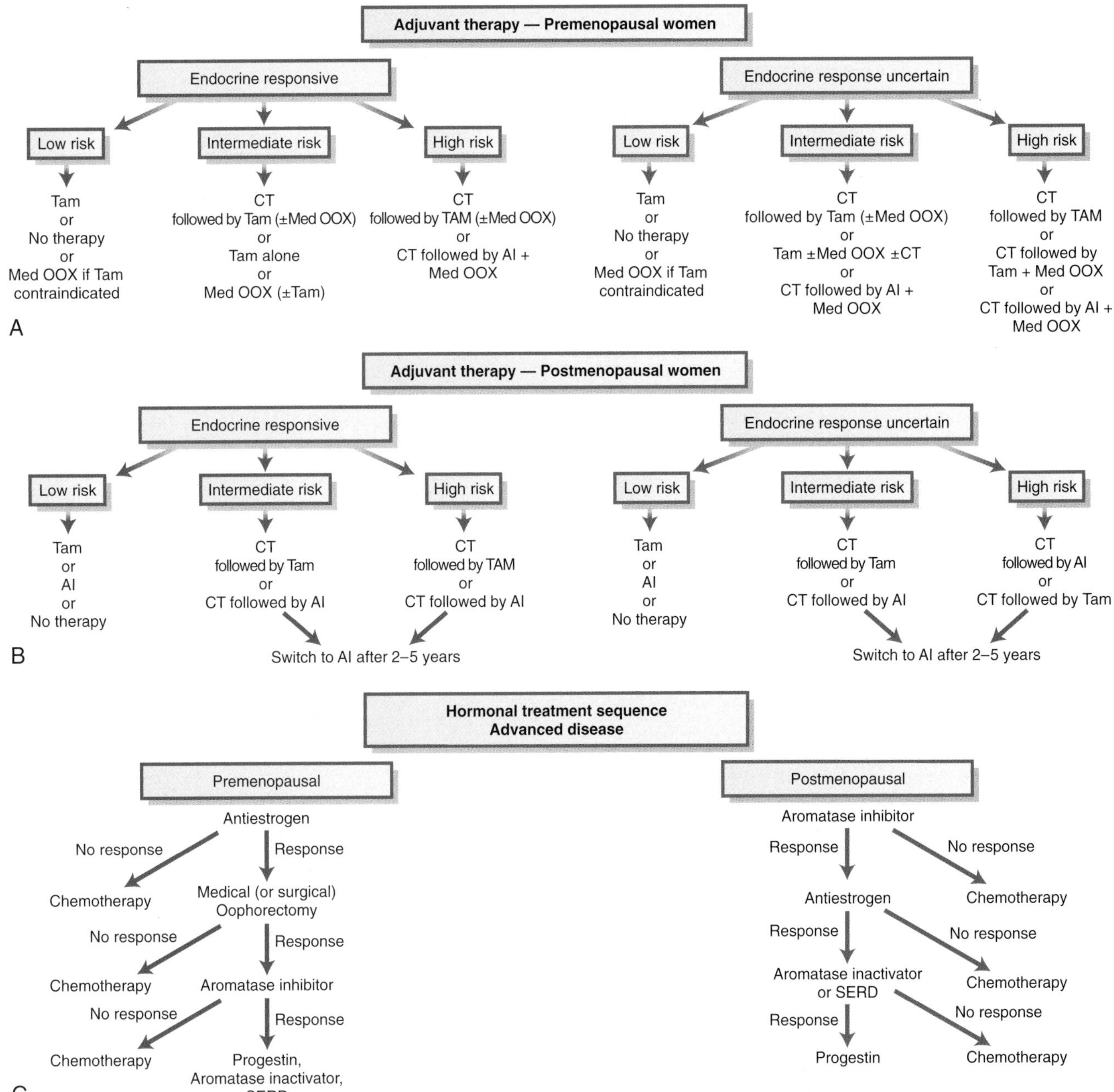

Figure 42–19 ■ Decisionmaking algorithm for breast cancer. **A** and **B,** The approach to adjuvant hormonal therapy in premenopausal women **(A)** and postmenopausal women **(B)** is based on guidelines from the 2005 St. Gallen conference, which divides women into endocrine responsive and endocrine response uncertain categories and into low, intermediate, and high risk.[62] Tamoxifen (Tam) is considered the preferred endocrine therapy based upon level I evidence. Medical oophorectomy (Med OOX) is preferred if tamoxifen is contraindicated. Sequences using combinations of tamoxifen and medical oophorectomy or medical oophorectomy plus an aromatase inhibitor (AI) are currently undergoing study and are considered acceptable alternatives. Chemotherapy (CT) is often recommended prior to endocrine therapy, and the various types of CT are outlined in the National Comprehensive Cancer Network guidelines.[129] **C,** The sequence of therapies for advanced disease in women still considered to be antiestrogen responsive (see text). This algorithm is applicable for patients who have never received an antiestrogen or who have taken this therapy but have been off it for at least 1 year. In patients thought to have very aggressive disease, chemotherapy may be chosen prior to hormonal therapy. SERD, selective estrogen receptor down-regulator (fulvestrant). (**A** and **B** adapted from Goldhirsch A, Glick JH, Gelber RD, et al. Meeting highlights: international expert consensus on the primary therapy of early breast cancer. Ann Oncol 2005;16[10]:1569-1583. **C** from Guidelines Committee. National comprehensive Cancer Center Network Practice Guidelines, Brenst Cancer 2007. Available at http://nccn.org/professionals/physician_gls/PDF/breast.pdf (accessed August 24, 2007).

survival but not overall survival when compared to medical oophorectomy without tamoxifen. One component of the SOFT trial is also addressing this point by comparing tamoxifen alone, versus medical oophorectomy plus tamoxifen, versus medical oophorectomy plus an AI in patients who had received standard chemotherapy.[114]

The second question addresses whether AIs are superior to tamoxifen for complete ovarian deprivation when given following chemotherapy and medical oophorectomy. The TEXT trial is addressing this issue by comparing medical oophorectomy plus tamoxifen with medical oophorectomy plus exemestane. Finally, to determine if chemotherapy is required at all when using complete estrogen deprivation, the PERCHE study will compare a chemotherapy plus complete estrogen-deprivation arm with one using only complete estrogen deprivation. Complete analyses of these various approaches and trials can be found in a review.[114,124] Very young patients with cancer have a worse prognosis than older premenopausal women. The ongoing trials (SOFT, TEXT, PERCHE) that examine the individual roles of medical oophorectomy, an AI, chemotherapy, and the combination of these agents should provide information regarding this subset of patients.

Emerging Therapies

Neoadjuvant therapy represents the use of an antitumor agent before surgery in an attempt to shrink the tumor sufficiently to allow lumpectomy rather than mastectomy.[84] The concept of neoadjuvant chemotherapy has been adopted into clinical practice, whereas neoadjuvant hormonal therapy is now undergoing clinical trial. A nonrandomized trial demonstrated an 81% reduction in tumor volume with letrozole versus 75% with anastrozole and 48% with tamoxifen.[125] More recently, a randomized trial involving 324 patients compared letrozole 2.5 mg daily with tamoxifen 20 mg daily in women with ER^+ tumors of greater than 2 cm.[126] Letrozole caused a 55% rate of objective response (CR and PR) versus 36% for tamoxifen ($P < 0.001$). Breast-conserving surgery was chosen in 45% of patients receiving letrozole and 35% receiving tamoxifen ($P < 0.001$). Approximately 50% of women had a sufficient reduction in size of tumor to allow lumpectomy. *HER2/Neu*$^+$ tumors responded better to the AI (88% response) than to tamoxifen (21%).[65]

A similar trial (Immediate Preoperative Anastrozole Tamoxifen or Combined with Tamoxifen [IMPACT]) confirmed the greater ability to perform lumpectomy in women receiving the AI (46% vs. 22%, $P = 0.03$), but objective tumor responses in the AI and tamoxifen arms were similar.[127] Current guidelines consider neoadjuvant endocrine therapy still to be experimental, but this approach is becoming more widely used with emergence of these two studies. Nonetheless, comparison of groups of patients treated conventionally and with neoadjuvant endocrine therapy with analysis of survival will be required to confirm the major utility of this approach.

Preclinical data suggest that tumors exposed to tamoxifen or to AIs adapt by up-regulating growth factor pathways. A compelling hypothesis is to administer growth factor pathway inhibitors concomitantly with endocrine therapies to inhibit the development of resistance. Several studies in xenograft models have proved the principle that this strategy can work and several clinical trials of this concept are under way.

Use of the monoclonal antibody against *HER2/Neu* (trastuzumab) in combination with or after adjuvant chemotherapy in women with breast cancer has been highly successful in delaying recurrence and perhaps implementing cure.[128] Pertinent studies included women with receptor-positive tumors but did not examine the interactions of trastuzumab and endocrine therapy. It is expected that such studies will be forthcoming in the near future with the possibility that use of all three approaches will add to the efficacy of current regimens.

Recommended Approaches

Several highly specific guidelines are available that base recommendations on nine subgroups of patients categorized as to low-, intermediate-, and high-risk prognostic categories and endocrine-responsive, nonresponsive, and uncertain predictive categories (see Fig. 42–19 A-C).[62] Level I evidence supports the use of tamoxifen as adjuvant hormonal therapy for both pre- and postmenopausal women. Medical oophorectomy provides an acceptable alternative for women in whom tamoxifen is contraindicated. Conclusive data regarding the superior efficacy of complete estrogen deprivation with medical oophorectomy plus tamoxifen or an AI are lacking and the subject of ongoing study. Nonetheless, the St. Gallen panel accepted the concept of complete estrogen suppression as reasonable for very young patients, especially in the intermediate-risk and high-risk groups. This approach was also considered appropriate alternative therapy for premenopausal women at any age at high risk, especially if chemotherapy did not induce complete ovarian failure. The Panel did not recommend GnRH analogues plus AIs outside of clinical trials. The St. Gallen guidelines are more specific than those of the National Comprehensive Cancer Center Network, but in general the two sets of guidelines do not substantially conflict.[62,129]

Adjuvant Therapy

Premenopausal Women

Current opinion recommends initial chemotherapy for most premenopausal women with ER^+ tumors larger than 1 cm in diameter followed by the addition of tamoxifen for 5 years after completion of chemotherapy (see Fig. 42–19). Those considered to have low-risk disease might benefit from tamoxifen alone. Evidence regarding combined therapy comes from a meta-analysis that demonstrated statistically significant prolongation of survival with a combination of tamoxifen plus chemotherapy versus chemotherapy alone.[120] Clinical data have established that the chemotherapy must be given first and completed before initiating tamoxifen. Medical oophorectomy with tamoxifen could be considered as an alternative for women averse to chemotherapy, particularly those at low risk of recurrence and with a high level of ER.[62] The use of medical oophorectomy and an AI is suggested only if tamoxifen is contraindicated.

Current recommendations suggest tamoxifen after chemotherapy, but medical oophorectomy in combination with an AI might later be proved to be superior to tamoxifen alone in young women with aggressive disease. This is the subject of the ongoing studies in the TEXT and PERCHE trials.[114] Some women who develop amenorrhea after chemotherapy may be candidates for AIs. However, medical oophorectomy is considered necessary in women younger than 40 years whose amenorrhea may only be temporary following chemotherapy and in women older than 40 years with return of menses.[81] The use of AIs in women older than 40 years who are rendered amenorrheic after chemotherapy might pose an unexpected problem regarding return of menses. This clinical scenario is being encountered by oncologists and requires hormonal monitoring.[81] By interrupting estradiol negative feedback, the AI might trigger return of ovulation and overcome the AI effects.

Postmenopausal Women

Tamoxifen is the preferred initial adjuvant therapy for postmenopausal women with ER^+ or PR^+ tumors larger than 1 cm unless there are contraindications. If the tumor is *HER2/Neu*$^+$ or ER^+/PR^-,[62] an AI would generally be considered preferable according to recent guidelines. Crossover to an AI after either 2 to 3 years or 5 years of tamoxifen is now recommended in responding patients.[90,120] Several trials have now shown that crossover to an

AI after 2 to 5 years of tamoxifen results in prolongation of disease-free survival (see Fig. 42–17A and B).[52,53,130] Only in the MA.17 trial was overall survival improved. and this only in the node-positive subgroup.[53] A more recent study with exemestane reported prolonged survival in both node-positive and node-negative patients whose tumors contained estrogen receptors.[53a] In women considered to have aggressive disease, particularly those who are younger, chemotherapy followed by tamoxifen may be chosen.[131] Information obtained from meta-analyses suggests that chemotherapy followed by tamoxifen may be preferable to use of tamoxifen alone in postmenopausal women.

Recommendations regarding the initial use of an AI rather than tamoxifen are rapidly evolving. The most recent ASCO guidelines stated that "optimal hormonal therapy for postmenopausal women with ER+ breast cancer should include an AI."[90] Whether an AI should be used initially (replacing tamoxifen) or at some time after (either 2 to 3 years or 5 years) remains uncertain and should be resolved by the upcoming results of the BIG FEMTA trial.[50] For patients at low risk for relapse or with comorbidity raising concern about the safety of an AI, adjuvant tamoxifen alone remains a reasonable alternative and may be the only economically viable option in many situations.

The major problems with the AIs in the extended adjuvant setting may be an increased risk of cardiovascular and cerebrovascular events, although this has not yet been shown to be statistically significant in randomized trials.[52] An increased rate of fracture has been demonstrated, but this can be prevented by concomitant use of a bisphosphonate.[79] Quality of life may be affected in the AI-treated patients with respect to an increase in arthralgia, vaginal dryness, dyspareunia, decreased libido, and an increase in hot flushes. On the other hand, the major problems with tamoxifen are the increased risk of VTEs and the increased incidence of endometrial carcinoma.

Small Tumors in Pre- and Postmenopausal Women

No randomized trial has examined use of tamoxifen in women with tumors of 1 cm or less. However, pooled data from four NSABP trials indicates a 4% absolute benefit regarding disease-free recurrence and 5% survival benefit for this group of women when given tamoxifen.[132] Individual decisions are made based upon risk-to-benefit analysis, and not all women are offered this therapy. With availability of the Oncotype DX test, one can stratify risk and offer tamoxifen to those at high or intermediate risk for recurrence.[71,72]

Ductal Carcinoma in Situ

Tamoxifen appears to provide benefit for women with DCIS[133] if the tumor is ER$^+$. In a large NSABP clinical trial, 13% of women treated with lumpectomy, irradiation, and placebo experienced a new tumor event over 5 years.[133] One third of these new events involved appearance of a contralateral breast cancer, one third involved a new ipsilateral tumor, and one third involved local recurrence of the original tumor. Tamoxifen reduced these events in absolute terms by 5% with equal benefit in reducing new contralateral, ipsilateral, and original tumor events. A later post hoc analysis reported that only women with ER$^+$ tumors benefited from this approach.[134] Risk-to-benefit analysis for tamoxifen is required to advise patients appropriately.

Decision Making

An overview of these data suggest that all women with ER$^+$ or PR$^+$ tumors are potential candidates for tamoxifen as adjuvant therapy with crossover to an AI later in postmenopausal women. In order to guide informed decision making, one must determine whether the benefits of tamoxifen outweigh the risks in individual patients (see Fig. 42–19). From the NSABP prevention trial, the absolute risks of tamoxifen are known and include uterine cancer, cataracts, DVT, pulmonary emboli, and CVA.[39] Presence of a uterus, past history of DVT or pulmonary embolus, or existent cataract would enhance these risks. Presence of larger or invasive tumors would enhance the absolute benefits of tamoxifen. In general, most women with invasive tumors larger than 1 cm should be advised to take tamoxifen. Those with small or noninvasive tumors should be counseled based upon risk-to-benefit ratios. Those without prior history of thromboembolic event or cataract and with prior hysterectomy might be advised to take tamoxifen, particularly if they also have osteopenia. Raloxifene has not been used in the adjuvant setting and would not be advised for the patients discussed here.

With the demonstrated superiority of the AIs in postmenopausal women in this setting, the risks and benefits of these agents versus tamoxifen should be considered. Regarding the AIs, risk of development of osteoporosis and heart disease should be weighed against the risks associated with tamoxifen. Based upon current guidelines, all postmenopausal women with lesions larger than 1 cm should receive an AI at some point in the adjuvant treatment sequence.

Treatment of Advanced Disease

Most women who develop advanced disease had previously received tamoxifen as adjuvant therapy. Those experiencing tumor recurrence while receiving tamoxifen or within 1 year of its cessation are considered resistant to this antiestrogen. For them, other hormonal therapies are chosen. Women whose tumors recur more than 1 year after stopping tamoxifen are candidates for an additional course of tamoxifen. An algorithm can then be used to choose hormonal therapy in women considered candidates for tamoxifen (see Fig. 42–19 C). In those resistant to tamoxifen, the next therapy in the sequential approach can be used.

Premenopausal Women

Initial therapy would usually consist of a course of chemotherapy followed later by hormonal therapy. It should be emphasized that AIs do not effectively inhibit ovarian estrogen production in premenopausal women who have not experienced amenorrhea from chemotherapy. In women younger than 40 years with chemotherapy-induced amenorrhea, tamoxifen (or toremifene) is usually considered first-line therapy for recurrent tumors. Based upon current data, this might be combined with a GnRH analogue to induce a medical oophorectomy in high-risk patients. If the initial therapy is tamoxifen alone, medical oophorectomy with use of a GnRH agonist analogue as second-line therapy would be recommended. Surgical oophorectomy could be substituted for the GnRH analogue.[62] AIs could then be used if the GnRH analogue is continued. Megestrol acetate is then advised as additional therapy.

Postmenopausal Women

Data from trials comparing AIs with tamoxifen as first-line therapy for advanced disease suggest that AIs be considered the first choice of endocrine therapy.[93,98,100,135] Responders would then be treated with tamoxifen as second-line therapy upon relapse, and nonresponders would be treated with chemotherapy. Third-line therapy would be megestrol acetate. After this, high-dose estrogen or androgens might be chosen. The use of the pure antiestrogen fulvestrant could be substituted for tamoxifen. If the patient develops rapidly progressive disease at any time in this sequence, chemotherapy may be chosen instead of the next endocrine therapy.

Chemotherapy

Discussion of the current choices of chemotherapy is beyond the scope of this chapter. The interested reader is referred to the book on management of breast diseases by Lippmann, Harris, Morrow, et al.[136]

Long-Term Quality of Life in Breast Cancer Survivors

With earlier diagnosis of breast cancer, an increasing percentage of women survive breast cancer long term. Two thirds of these women are menopausal at the time of diagnosis, and half of the premenopausal women undergo permanent ovarian failure as a result of chemotherapy. MHT is generally thought to be contraindicated in these women because estrogens might cause regrowth of residual tumor tissue after surgery or cause a second primary.[137,138] Data from observational studies, however, do not provide evidence of a deleterious effect. Prospective studies of the safety of MHT in this setting are conflicting: the Habits trial[139] reports an increase in risk of recurrent breast cancer with MHT, but the Stockholm trial does not.[140] The differences in results might relate to the increased use of tamoxifen (51%) in the Stockholm trial versus the Habits trial (22%), but this conclusion requires experimental confirmation. Until this issue is more definitively resolved, it is prudent to avoid estrogens in breast cancer survivors if alternatives to estrogen are effective.[137]

Effective agents are available to substitute for estrogen. These include bisphosphonates to prevent or treat osteoporosis, statins to prevent heart disease, venlafaxine (see earlier regarding CYP2D6 and tamoxifen) and gabapentin[141,142] to diminish the number and severity of hot flushes, low-dose vaginal estrogen for symptoms of urogenital atrophy, and SSRIs for depression thought to be related to estrogen deficiency. This approach does not protect against Alzheimer's disease or improve cognitive function, but the recent WHI study demonstrated that MHT increased rather than decreased the risk of dementia.[143] If alternatives to estrogen are not satisfactory, women might choose to receive MHT after a full discussion of the risks and benefits and with informed consent.

Breast Cancer in Men

The incidence of breast cancer in men is 100-fold lower than in women, with 1450 new cases in 2004 and 470 deaths. The incidence of male breast cancer increased since 1980 from 0.86 per 100,000 population to 1.08. Known risk factors include clinical disorders associated with reduced testosterone production or estrogen excess, such as orchitis, orchiectomy, undescended testes, testicular injury, Klinefelter's syndrome, radiation exposure, *BRCA2* carrier, family history, obesity, and exogenous estrogen.[144] Suggestive risk factors include Cowden's syndrome and cirrhosis. Inconclusive factors reported in the literature to be possibly associated include mutations of the androgen receptor gene, the *Chek 2* gene, prostate cancer, gynecomastia, occupational exposures, electromagnetic frequency exposure, high temperatures, diet, and alcohol.[144]

At presentation with breast cancer, 37.5% of men have regional lymph node involvement versus only 29.2% of women with this disease. Tumors are larger at diagnosis in men than in women, and 41.7% of men have tumors localized to their breast versus 50.5% of women. The percent ER$^+$ and PR$^+$ is higher in men (90.6% and 81.2%, respectively) than in women (76% and 66.7%, respectively). The 5-year survival rate is 63% and the 10-year survival rate is 41%.

Breast cancer is suspected when a subareolar or upper outer quadrant firm, painless lesion is palpated. Diagnosis is made by mammography and biopsy of the lesion. Most patients are then treated by mastectomy and adjuvant tamoxifen. Later therapy could include orchiectomy followed by AIs or progestins and chemotherapy upon relapse. No randomized, controlled trials are available to accurately assess relative efficacies of various therapies.

ENDOMETRIAL CANCER

Etiology

Approximately 40,800 new cases of endometrial cancer occur annually in the United States, and 3710 women die of this disease every year. Genetic factors such as those underlying the HNPCC (hereditary nonpolyposis colorectal cancer) syndrome, probably related to one or more polymorphic alleleles, are related to uterine cancer.[145] Exogenous factors include estrogen-only hormonal therapy and obesity.

Hormonal risk factors relate to conditions causing overexposure to endogenous or exogenous estrogen. Enhanced tumor initiation and promotion mediated by the proliferative effects of estrogen occur as with breast cancer.[146] Progestins are antimitogenic on the endometrium as opposed to breast tissue and result in a decreased rate of cell proliferation. Thus, unopposed estrogen increases the risk of endometrial cancer and progestins reduce that risk.[147,148] Continued stimulation of the endometrium without progestin induced endometrial shedding causes an increase in cell proliferation rate and a concomitant increase in genetic mutations. Mutations that are not repaired accumulate and ultimately result in neoplastic growth. With prolonged stimulation of the endometrial lining, typical hyperplasia occurs first, followed by atypical adenomatous hyperplasia, a premalignant lesion. It is thought that 30% of such lesions later progress to frank cancer.

Clinical Conditions

Several clinical conditions are characterized by increased estradiol production and anovulation, a state in which the proliferative effects of estrogen are not opposed by the antimitotic effects of progesterone.

One of these involves exogenous obesity. As the number of adipocytes increases, the amount of aromatase enzyme increases proportionately. With a normal amount of androgenic substrate, estradiol production increases as a function of the amount of enzyme present and in proportion to the degree of obesity.

The polycystic ovarian syndrome is associated with increases in estrone levels and lack of cyclic increments in progesterone as a result of absence of the luteal phase of the cycle. It is also associated with decreased sex steroid binding globulin (SHBG) and presumably an increase in the free fraction of estradiol and an increased rate of conversion of androgens to estrogens (aromatase excess).

Estrogen-producing ovarian and adrenal tumors are also conditions of unopposed estrogen and increased incidence of endometrial cancer. Other risk factors for endometrial cancer include nulliparity, late menopause, increasing age, the metabolic syndrome, history of breast cancer, long-term use of tamoxifen, HNPCC family syndrome, first-degree relative with endometrial cancer, radiation to the pelvis, diabetes, and hypertension.[149]

Menopausal Hormone Therapy

A large body of observational data reported the risks of endometrial carcinoma in women receiving MHT.[150] Estrogen unopposed by a progestin increases the relative risk of endometrial cancer by twofold to fourfold, depending upon duration of use.[147,148,151] This risk increases over time, with a relative risk of 1.30 for 2 years of use of unopposed estrogen, 2.22 for 2 to 5 years, and 4.49 for 5 to 10 years.[152] Progestins reduce this risk by opposing the mitogenic effects of estrogen on the endometrium and reducing the proliferative stimulus.

Four estrogen-progestin regimens commonly used include:

- Combined continuous estrogen plus progestin
- Sequential addition of a progestin to an estrogen for 10 or more days each month
- Sequential addition of a progestin to an estrogen for less than 10 days, usually 5 to 7 days
- The so-called long cycle, with progestin added to an estrogen for 14 days every 3 to 4 months.

The combined continuous regimen reduces endometrial cancer risk substantially, if not completely. Pike and colleagues[152] report a relative risk of 1.07 (95% CI 0.80-1.43) for combined continuous estrogen plus progesterone but a nonsignificant trend of increased risk for more than 5 years of use (RR 1.34; no CI given.) The large randomized, controlled WHI study now provides level I evidence regarding MHT use and risk of endometrial cancer. This study compared women receiving continuous conjugated equine estrogen plus medroxyprogesterone acetate with women taking placebo. After an average follow-up of 5.6 years, the hazard ratio for endometrial cancer was 0.81 (95% CI 0.48-1.36). There were no differences in tumor histology, stage, or grade between the women receiving MHT or placebo.

For sequential use of a progestin for 10 or more days each month and use for less than 5 years, there is no increase in endometrial cancer (Pike and colleagues[152]: RR 1.07, 95% CI 0.82-1.41; Beresford and colleagues[148]: 0.7, 95% CI 0.4-1.4). There was a trend, however, for an increase in endometrial cancer with longer-term use of this continuous regimen. Beresford and colleagues[148] report a relative risk of 2.7 (95% CI 1.2-6.0) for current users of this regimen for more than 5 years, whereas Pike and colleagues report a relative risk of 1.09 (nonsignificant).[152] Caution should then be advised for long-term use of such regimens.

Sequential regimens that administer a progestin for less than 10 days are associated with an increase in risk of endometrial cancer. Pike and colleagues report an increase in relative risk of 1.87 per 5 years of use (95% CI 1.33-2.65)[152] and Beresford 2.2 (0.9-5.2)[148] for less than 5 years of use and 4.8 (95% CI 2.0-11.0) for more than 5 years of use. Use of the long cycle approach also may not be not associated with an increased risk of endometrial cancer but additional data are needed for confirmation.[153]

Taken together, these data suggest that progestins protect against estrogen-induced endometrial cancer when taken continuously with an estrogen. In premenopausal women, oral contraceptives containing both estrogen and a progestin decrease the risk of endometrial cancer. Multiple pregnancies also increase the duration of exposure to large amounts of progesterone and decrease the risk.

Tibolone is a hormonal agent used in Europe for more than 2 decades for treatment of menopausal symptoms. The relative risk of endometrial cancer in women using this agent was reported as 1.79 in the Million Women Study (95% CI 1.43-2.25).[150] Although the overall data analysis in the Million Women study has been criticized, the other results reported regarding use of estrogen alone and cyclic progestin with estrogen appear to confirm other reports regarding MHT and breast cancer risk. Data from prospective trials regarding endometrial cancer are now needed before a clear conclusion regarding tibolone can be drawn.

Tamoxifen

Use of tamoxifen as adjuvant therapy for breast cancer or prevention is associated with an increased risk of endometrial cancer as well as hyperplasia and polyps (see earlier). However, raloxifene, another SERM, did not cause an increase in endometrial cancer in a large study monitoring this as a safety parameter.[154] Animal studies with raloxifene suggest that this SERM does not exert estrogen agonistic effects on uterus, whereas tamoxifen does.

Endocrinology

Endometrial carcinoma is divided into two general types: endometrioid (type I: low-grade lesions, 90% of endometrial cancers) and nonendometrioid (type II: high-grade lesions).Nonendometrioid tumors are not estrogen driven, and most are associated with endometrial atrophy. Serous carcinoma is the most aggressive type of nonendometroid tumor. Only the type I lesions retain some degree of hormonal responsiveness.

Most endometrial cancers contain appreciable levels of estrogen receptor, but only differentiated ones generally have progesterone receptors.[155] Tumors resulting from estrogen replacement therapy are generally well differentiated, have estrogen and progesterone receptors, and are of low grade and stage. The diagnosis is suspected when unexplained vaginal bleeding is detected. Instillation of saline into the uterine cavity followed by ultrasound can reveal an area of focal thickening that biopsy proves is cancer. An associated finding is generalized thickening of the endometrial stripe to greater than 6 mm as a sign of concomitant endometrial hyperplasia. Any unexplained vaginal bleeding in a postmenopausal women requires such evaluation to rule out endometrial cancer.

Treatment

Treatment requires initial hysterectomy and bilateral oophorectomy in all patients. The use of preoperative radiation therapy has been abandoned because it interferes with adequate surgical staging and there is no proven benefit over postoperative radiation therapy. Those with a poor prognosis (approximately 25% of patients) are treated postoperatively with external beam radiation therapy or with implants. Upon recurrence, one may use high doses of systemic progestagens. Response to therapy is independent of age, site of metastasis, or previous or concurrent therapy.

Two large Gynecologic-Oncology Group studies reported that objective responses to a progestin occurred in 24% to 25% of patients.[156,157] The exact mechanism causing tumor regression is unknown but could involve direct effects on tumor cells; stimulation of the inactivating 17β-hydroxysteroid dehydrogenase type I enzyme, which converts estradiol to estrone; inhibition of the production by the adrenals of androgenic estrogen precursors; down-regulation of estrogen receptors by progestagen; or suppression of gonadotropin production in premenopausal women. Experimental trials are ongoing to test the efficacy of AIs, antiestrogens, GnRH analogues, and combinations of these agents. Various chemotherapeutic regimens are also available for such patients.

Endometrial cancer survivors with an excellent prognosis and disease-free survival for at least 1 year may be treated with MHT to relieve menopausal symptoms. This recommendation is based upon several nonrandomized studies as well as a large randomized Gynecologic-Oncology Group study.[158]

PROSTATE CANCER

Incidence

In the United States, 218,00 new cases of prostate cancer are predicted for 2007 and 27,050 deaths. African American men have an age-adjusted relative risk of 1.73 (95% CI 1.23-2.45) compared to white men. The mortality of African American men compared to white men is nearly double. Introduction of PSA screening in the mid 1980s resulted in a tripling of prostate cancer detection rates between 1985 and 1997 from 96,000 per year to 334,500. However, estimated case detection rates then gradually declined to 198,000 in 2001 as the pool of previously undiagnosed cases diminished. Since the turn of the 21st century, incidence rates have again been on the rise in the United States. Currently, prostate cancer will be diagnosed in one in 6.25 men during their lifetimes in the United States. As a result of PSA screening, the percentage of patients with low-risk disease at diagnosis has increased. According to one set of criteria, low-risk disease is defined as PSA 10ng/mL or less, Gleason score less than 7, no Gleason 4 or 5 disease on biopsy, and clinical stage T1c or T2a. In 1989, 31% of men at diagnosis met these criteria, whereas in 2002, 47% were in the low-risk category.[159]

Etiology

Genetic Factors

Genetic factors play a major role in prostate cancer etiology as evidenced by epidemiologic data.[160] Twin studies suggest a genetic component in 42% (95% CI 29%-50%) of patients with prostate cancer.[7] Men with prostate cancer report a family history of this tumor 3.1 to 4.3 times more commonly than healthy men. The relative risk of prostate cancer is increased approximately twofold in men with one first-degree relative with prostate cancer.

Specific genetic lesions resulting in prostate cancer are uncommon, and incontrovertible evidence regarding causality is lacking. Candidate genes based on linkage analysis include RNASEL (an endoribonuclease), MSR1 (a macrophage scavenger receptor 1 gene), AR (the androgen receptor), CYP 17 (a cytochrome P450 responsible for the 17-hydroxylation of steroids), and SRD5A2 (the predominant form of 5α-reductase in the prostate).[161] Several genetic epidemiologic studies have shown a correlation between the number of polyglutamine repeats (CAG) on the androgen receptor and incidence of prostate cancer, but other studies have not confirmed this finding.[161] Recent data from the Utah pedigrees identified another high-risk gene on chromosome 17P called *ELAC/HPC2* in exon 1 of the androgen receptor gene. *BRCA2,* but not *BRCA1,* was associated with prostate cancer in Ashkenazi Jews, whereas most series in unselected populations do not show this association.[162] A recent preliminary finding suggested that fusions between two genes could activate carcinogenic pathways, a concept analogous to the fusion of the *BCR-ABL* genes in leukemia. Based upon outlier cDNA studies, fusions between the *TMPRSS2* and the ETS genes *EGR* and *ETV1* were commonly found in prostate cancer (in >90% of the 57% of tumors that overexpress *EGR* or *ETV1*) and might play an etiologic role.[163]

Diet and Environmental Factors

Age-standardized global incidence figures vary widely, from 1.9 per 100,000 person-years in Tianjin, China, to 100.8 per 100,000 person-years in the United States in white men and 137.0 per 100,000 person-years in black men.[164] Dietary or environmental explanations for this wide variance are likely. As evidence for this, Japanese living in Japan have an incidence of 10.8 per 100,000 person years, but this increases to 47.2 per 100,000 person-years in Japanese men who have moved to the United States.[164]

Variations in ingestion of high-fat diets, red meat, green tea, or soy products provide potential explanations for the divergent rates of prostate cancer among different populations.[164165,166] One hypothesis is that cooking meats at high temperature or on charcoal grills produces carcinogens such as heterocyclic aromatic amines and polycyclic aromatic hydrocarbons. Others suggest that components of vegetables such as lycopene or antioxidants such as vitamin E and selenium might reduce the risk of prostate cancer.

The incidence of premalignant prostate lesions and latent prostate cancer[167,168] is the same in Japan and China as in the United States, whereas the rates of invasive cancer differ markedly.[169] The additional mutations or promotional factors necessary to convert latent to invasive cancer apparently occur less commonly in the Japanese and Chinese living in Asia. In contrast, the initial mutation or mutations leading to latent cancer occur at the same rate. This observation suggests that environmental or dietary factors might influence later steps in the mutational process or events influencing promotion more specifically.

Inflammation and Oxidative Stress

Chronic or recurrent inflammation might play a role in the development of prostate cancer. Prostatitis, diagnosed by symptoms, occurs in 9% of men between 40 and 79 years of age.[161] Inflammatory cells release oxidants that could result in DNA damage and act as initiators of prostate cancer. A lesion called *proliferative inflammatory atrophy* has been proposed as a precursor to prostatic intraepithelial neoplasia (PIN) and prostate cancer. Chronic inflammation is associated with proliferative inflammatory atrophy and signs of molecular stress such as high levels of glutathione S transferase A1 and cyclooxygenase-2 (COX-2). On the basis of these concepts, it has been suggested that inflammation increases oxidative stress, which in turn causes DNA adducts that could contribute to the development of prostate cancer.[161]

Hormonal Factors

Hormonal factors, and particularly circulating androgens, probably play a role in the initiation and promotion of prostatic cancer. Men surgically orchiectomized before the age of 30 years are said to develop prostate cancer rarely, although this has been difficult to document in the published literature (Peter Gann, personal communication. Ross and colleagues suggested that the lower incidence of prostate cancer in Japanese and Chinese populations might relate to a lower level of 5αreductase activity than in their white counterparts, perhaps on a genetic basis. This could lead to lower levels of dihydrotestosterone (DHT) in prostatic tissue and less androgen-induced proliferation. However, direct isotopic kinetic measurements of 5α-reductase activity in Chinese versus white men demonstrated no differences in the levels of this enzyme, at least in peripheral tissues.[170]

Clinical Approach

Prostate Cancer Prevention

A large randomized, controlled trial tested the hypothesis that reduction of DHT formation with the type 2 5α-reductase inhibitor finasteride would reduce the incidence of prostate cancer.[171] At the time of final analysis, after 7 years of therapy, 4368 men receiving finasteride and 4692 receiving placebo were available for analysis. The finasteride group experienced a 24.8% reduction in prostate cancer diagnosis (803 in the finasteride group and 1147 in the placebo group, 95% CI 18.6-30.6%, $P < 0.001$). However, tumors of Gleason grade 7, 8, 9, or 10 occurred in a higher percentage of the men receiving finasteride (280 of 757 tumors or 37%) than in the placebo group (237 of 1068 tumors or 22.2%, $P < 0.001$). High-grade disease occurred in 6.4% of the finasteride group and 5.1% of the placebo group. Five deaths due to prostate cancer occurred in each study arm. Side effects in the finasteride group included reduced volume of ejaculate, erectile dysfunction, loss of libido, and gynecomastia ($P < 0.001$ vs placebo), but attributable risks of these side effects ranged only from 1% to 13%. A debate continues whether the increased prevalence of higher grade tumors was real, based upon plausible biologic principles or whether it was artifactual based upon effects of finasteride on histologic evaluation. Analysis of the lifetime implications and cost effectiveness of using finasteride for prostate cancer prevention does not support its routine use. The REDUCE (Reduction by Dutasteride of Prostate Cancer Events) trial is testing an agent that blocks both the type I and type II 5α-reductase enzymes to prevent prostate cancer.

With respect to other approaches, epidemiologic and secondary endpoint data support the possibility that selenium, vitamin E, and lycopene might be active for prevention of prostate cancer. The SELECT trial (Selenium and Vitamin E Cancer Prevention Trial) is examining the effects of selenium and vitamin E alone and in combination.

Early Case Detection

Until introduction of PSA measurements, digital rectal examination (DRE) followed by biopsy represented the standard screening procedures. Currently, PSA measurements detect cancers at a time when most are not palpable by DRE. The principle behind PSA screening is that tumors release more PSA into the bloodstream per gram of tissue than does BPH or normal tissue. PSA may be transiently increased by prostatitis, after endoscopic urethral manipulation, after prostatic biopsy, or to a lesser extent by ejaculation. Routine DRE has minimal effect on PSA levels, but most physicians defer PSA testing until several days after this examination.

The sensitivity of case detection with PSA is high but specificity is low, and routine PSA screening has been controversial.[172] In addition, there may be no advantage in detecting latent prostate cancers. Several attempts to increase specificity include use of age-related PSA normal ranges, PSA density (PSA divided by ultrasound-determined prostate volume), PSA velocity (rate of increase in PSA over time), and percentage of free PSA.[173] The free PSA measurement might provide the most useful information. A higher fraction of free PSA is present in men without prostate cancer. When used in patients with borderline PSA values of 4.0 to 10.0 ng/mL and normal DRE, the rate of biopsy-proven prostate cancer increases from 8% to 20% to 56% with free PSA fractions of greater than 25%, 15% to 20%, and 0 to 10%, respectively.[174]

Various professional societies have provided guidelines for PSA screening, both for and against, but no general agreement exists.[172] Randomized trials to determine whether screening improves survival are not yet conclusive. A common sense approach suggests screening only when test results would dictate diagnostic and therapeutic decisions. The patient needs to understand the consequences of a positive test and be willing to proceed with further diagnostic and therapeutic measures if the PSA is positive. Accordingly, patients selected for screening should be those in whom definitive treatment or hormonal manipulations and not watchful waiting would be the likely choice if cancer were detected. Based upon this reasoning, informed consent of the patient is required before embarking on screening with PSA.

Men with borderline PSA values (2.6-4.0 ng/mL) often undergo prostate biopsy under ultrasound, and in 75% of them, the biopsy reveals no evidence of prostate cancer. When to rebiopsy these patients is an unresolved but important clinical question. One study analyzed the records of 24,893 men being followed as part of a community-based screening study and identified 1011 with subsequent prostate cancer. Based upon these data, the authors recommended repeat biopsy in men with a PSA of 2.6 to 4.0 ng/mL if they had high-grade prostatic intraepithelial neoplasia (HGPIN), initial PSA of 3.6 to 4.0 ng/mL, abnormal DRE, a family history of prostate cancer, or a PSA velocity of 0 ng/mL or greater.[175] The complication rate of ultrasound-guided biopsy is reasonably low and increases slightly when 10 or 15 cores are taken rather than six.

Evaluation of Abnormal PSA or DRE

If the PSA is elevated to greater than 10 ng/mL or the DRE is abnormal, transrectal ultrasound (TRUS)-guided biopsy is indicated.[176] An algorithm for those with PSA values between 4 and 10 ng/mL has been described.[177] Common practice involves obtaining biopsies of ultrasound-detected hypoechoic lesions as well as blind biopsies.

Clinical Staging

Clinical staging of prostate cancer provides a means of determining prognosis and is used for making treatment decisions. Two analogous systems have been used in the past (Fig. 42–20), but the TMN classification is now preferred.

Endocrinology of Prostatic Cancer Growth

Dihydrotestosterone (DHT), the 5α-reduced product of testosterone, binds to androgen receptors with 2.5-fold higher affinity than testosterone itself and serves as the major regulator of prostatic tumor growth. Direct effects of androgen itself, indirect effects induced by stimulation of growth factors, or a combination of these two mechanisms can mediate androgen-induced proliferation.[178] Approximately 7000 μg of testosterone is secreted daily by the testes, of which 500 μg is converted into DHT in various peripheral tissues. The adrenal gland provides an additional 5% of the androgen produced in adults. Testosterone as well as preandrogens such as androstenedione, dehydroepiandrosterone (DHEA), and DHEA sulfate originate in the adrenal and are also converted in peripheral tissues into DHT. In addition to peripheral conversion, a large fraction of the DHT present in benign and malignant prostatic tissue is produced locally in the prostate gland from circulating precursors. Approximately 40% of prostatic DHT originates from steroids of adrenal origin.

Prostate cancer cells contain androgen receptors that bind DHT and transmit proliferative signals in androgen-dependent prostate cancer. As opposed to the use of receptor assays in breast cancer, measurement of the androgen receptor does not provide predictive information regarding hormone responsiveness. Mutations of the androgen receptor occur, but the frequency in primary prostate cancer is controversial. An early study found a 30% incidence of androgen receptor mutations in primary prostate cancers. Others have found a much lower incidence (0%-5%). All investigators find mutations in metastatic disease ranging from 10% to 50%.[179]

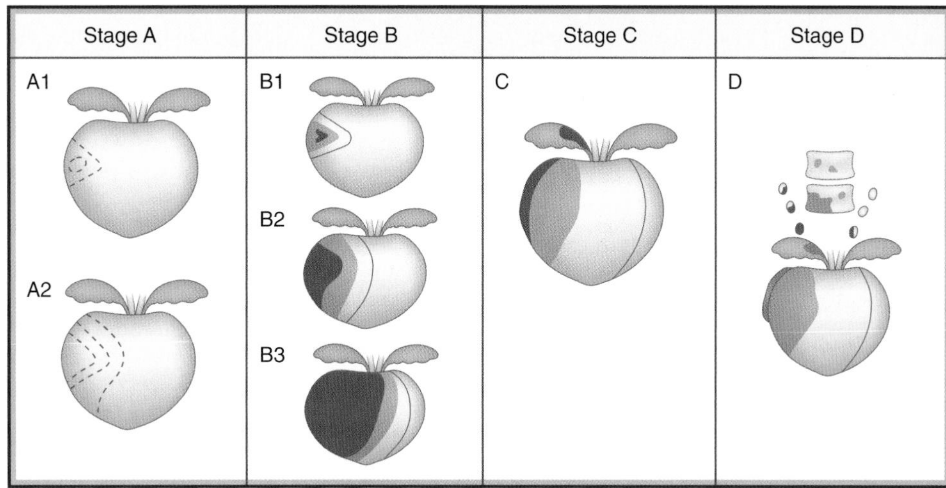

TNM classification

T1, N0 M0	T2, N0 M0	T3, N0 M0	T2–4, Nx Mx
T1a – incidental tumor ≤5% T1b – incidental tumor >5% T1c – identified by biopsy-PSA screening N0, M0	T2a – palpable or seen on TRUS-one lobe T2b – palpable or seen on TRUS-2 lobes N0, M0	T3a – extracapsular extension T3b – seminal vesicle involvement N0, M0	T4 – bladder neck, external sphincter, rectal levator muscles, or pelvic wall involvement N0 – no regional nodes or N1 – regional nodes M1 – nonregional nodes M1b – bone M1c – other sites

Figure 42–20 ■ Two analogous systems for classifying prostate cancer. The TNM system is generally used for a wide range of neoplasms and involves an estimate of tumor size, lymph nodes containing tumor, and presence of distant metastases. The Jewitt classification integrates these factors into stages A-D, which indicate progressively more severe disease. Because both are used by various authors, this figure demonstrates the parallels between the two systems.

The frequency and type of mutation appears to be influenced by the selective pressure exerted by antiandrogens. For example, in men receiving flutamide,[180] 5 of 16 treated patients had mutations versus 1 of 17 in those not receiving flutamide. The majority of these mutations involve a mutation at AA 877, the site involved in human lymph node prostate cancer (LNCaP) cells, which allows flutamide to become an androgen agonist. This finding could explain the occurrence of flutamide withdrawal responses observed in men with prostatic cancer (see later).[181-183]

Development of Androgen Resistance

Men with prostate cancer respond to deprivation of androgens for a variable length of time. After initial responses to blockade of androgen secretion or action, tumors regrow. Secondary responses to blockade of adrenal androgens occur, as evidenced by a 50% or greater decrease in PSA levels and often by pain reduction and improvement of fatigue but rarely by objective regression of tumor mass or healing of bone lesions.

Several theories might explain secondary hormonal responses and evolution into completely androgen-independent growth, but none are definitively proven. A concept that underlies all of the proposed theories is that growth factor pathways become up-regulated and that cross-talk between androgen receptor–mediated and growth factor–signaling molecules occurs. Non-mutually exclusive mechanistic theories include development of hypersensitivity to residual androgens, enhancement of androgen receptor action by phosphoryation of key sites in the receptor, and ligand independent activation of the receptor via growth factors or mutations.

An appealing theory is that tumors escape androgenic regulation of growth and co-opt mechanisms using ligand-independent activation of androgen receptors, up-regulation of growth factor pathways, or a combination of these mechanisms. Considerable experimental support for these concepts derives from demonstration of increased activated MAP kinase activity (a protein that mediates mitogenesis) and enhanced phosphorylation of the androgen receptor, a marker of ligand-independent receptor activation.

Another signaling pathway activated in androgen-resistant tumors involves PI3 kinase, AKT, and its downstream targets mTOR, p70 S6 kinase, and 4 E-BP1.[184] Mutations or inactivation of PTEN are found commonly in advanced prostate cancer. PTEN is a phosphatase that dephosphorylates and inactivates PI3 kinase. With mutational inactivation of PTEN, an associated up-regulation of phosphorylated, activated AKT occurs, as well as downstream activation of mTOR. Antibody-based approaches to demonstrate activation of this pathway demonstrate that loss of PTEN is highly correlated with activation of AKT and with phosphorylation and activation of S6, a substrate of p70S6 kinase. For this reason, use of agents to block mTOR, such as

CCI-779, are being examined in prostate cancer. COX-2 and matrix metalloproteinase (MMP)-9 are also up-regulated in the process of development of resistance and could serve as additional targets for therapy.

Treatment

Risk Stratification

Logical choices among various therapeutic options require assessment of the likelihood that complications and death from prostate cancer will ensue. Several algorithms provide a means to assess risk; the most widely used is called PROS-A.[185] The National Comprehensive Cancer Network (NCCN) has devised another practical risk stratification system (Table 42–3) that initially divides patients into clinically localized, locally advanced, and metastatic disease; then into low, intermediate, and high-risk subgroups; and finally according to expected survival of less than 10 years or 10 years or longer. The NCCN guidelines use this method as a means to choose appropriate therapies.[186]

One underlying principle in assessing risk is that prostate cancers exhibit a spectrum of biologic aggressiveness. At one end of the spectrum are *latent prostate cancers*, a term that has been applied to lesions less than 0.5 g that do not progress and do not result in cause-specific death. On the other end of the spectrum are large bulky tumors with high Gleason grade, which can progress rapidly. A key consideration is that older men often die of other existing medical conditions and not prostate cancer (Fig. 42–21). In men with a limited life expectancy as a result of other medical conditions, the risks of definitive therapy for prostate cancer might outweigh the benefits.

TABLE 42–3 RISK STRATIFICATION FOR PROSTATE CANCER

CLINICALLY LOCALIZED
Low Risk T1-2 Gleason score 2-6 PSA <10 mg/mL
Intermediate Risk T2b to Tc *or* Gleason score 7 *or* PSA 10-20
High Risk T3a *or* Gleason score 8-10 *or* PSA >20 mg/mL
LOCALLY ADVANCED
T3b-T4
METASTATIC
Lower Risk Any T, N1
Higher Risk Any T, any N, M1

Definitive Strategies in Localized Disease

Three competing strategies are recommended for management of localized prostate cancer: watchful waiting, radical prostatectomy, and radiation therapy. A key question is whether radical prostatectomy prolongs disease-free and overall survival when compared to watchful waiting. This issue has recently been examined in a randomized, controlled clinical trial comparing watchful waiting to radical prostatectomy in men with clinically localized disease.[187] A group of 695 men with localized prostate cancer, a life expectancy of greater than 10 years, and a mean age of 64.7 years were randomized and followed for a median of 8.2 years. Eighty-three men in the surgery group and 106 in the watchful waiting group died of all causes ($P = 0.04$) (Fig. 42–22). Death was due to prostate cancer in 8.6% of the surgical group and 14.5% of the watchful waiting group. The difference in death rates became greater at the 10-year time period (5.3 percentage points) than at the 5-year time period (2.0 percentage points). The risk of distant metastases was reduced from 10.2% to 1.7% by surgery and the rate of local progression from 25.1% to 19.1%. This study demonstrated that radical prostatectomy statistically significantly reduces disease-specific mortality and overall mortality after 8 years but this effect is numerically small. On the other hand, the decrease in incidence of metastases and local tumor progression is substantial.[187]

Observational studies over several decades demonstrated the efficacy of radiation therapy (both delivered in the conventional external beam format and as brachytherapy) as definitive therapy in men with prostate cancer and as an alternative to surgical prostatectomy. Studies have addressed whether neoadjuvant or adjuvant androgen deprivation therapy enhances the overall efficacy of therapy in men with aggressive disease. Radiation Therapy Oncology Group (RTOG) trial 86-10 examined the role of neoadjuvant endocrine therapy prior to radiation. The incidence of local progression at 5 years was 46% for patients with T2-4 tumors receiving adjuvant hormonal therapy and 71% for those receiving radiation alone ($P = 0.001$), but no difference in overall survival was noted.

Radiation therapy with concomitant (adjuvant) androgen-deprivation therapy has been the subject of two randomized trials.[188,189] An RTOG study[190] involved patients with T3 and T4 disease given radiation therapy followed by medical castration with goserelin starting at the last week of irradiation. Disease-free survival at 5 years was 60% for the goserelin arm and 44% for radiation alone ($P < 0.0001$). Only the subset of men with Gleason grade 8 to 10 tumors experienced a survival benefit from 66% to 55% ($P = 0.03$). However, the 10-year follow-up demonstrated a survival benefit for all patients treated with adjuvant hormonal therapy (HR 1.3, $P < 0.001$ in the multivariate analysis). The disease-free survival was also improved (HR 2.2, $P < 0.0003$).[190] In a similar European Organization for Research and Treatment of Cancer (EORTC) trial, the 5-year disease-free survival was 85% in the adjuvant hormone–treated group (goserelin) versus 48% in the radiation alone ($P < 0.001$) group. Importantly, overall survival was 79% for the adjuvant hormonal group versus 62% for the radiation-alone group, and this difference was statistically significant ($P = 0.001$).

The majority of data favor the use of adjuvant hormonal therapy in patients undergoing radiation therapy as definitive treatment for prostate cancer but only for high-risk localized or locally advanced disease.[186,191,192] An analysis of pooled data from the RTOG neoadjuvant and adjuvant trials concluded that the key consideration may be the necessity for long-term rather than short-term hormonal therapy in either neoadjuvant or adjuvant therapy approaches.[192] In men receiving short-term hormonal therapy (goserelin and flutamide for 2 months before and 2 months after radiation therapy) statistically significant improvements were observed for two endpoints, distant metastasis-free

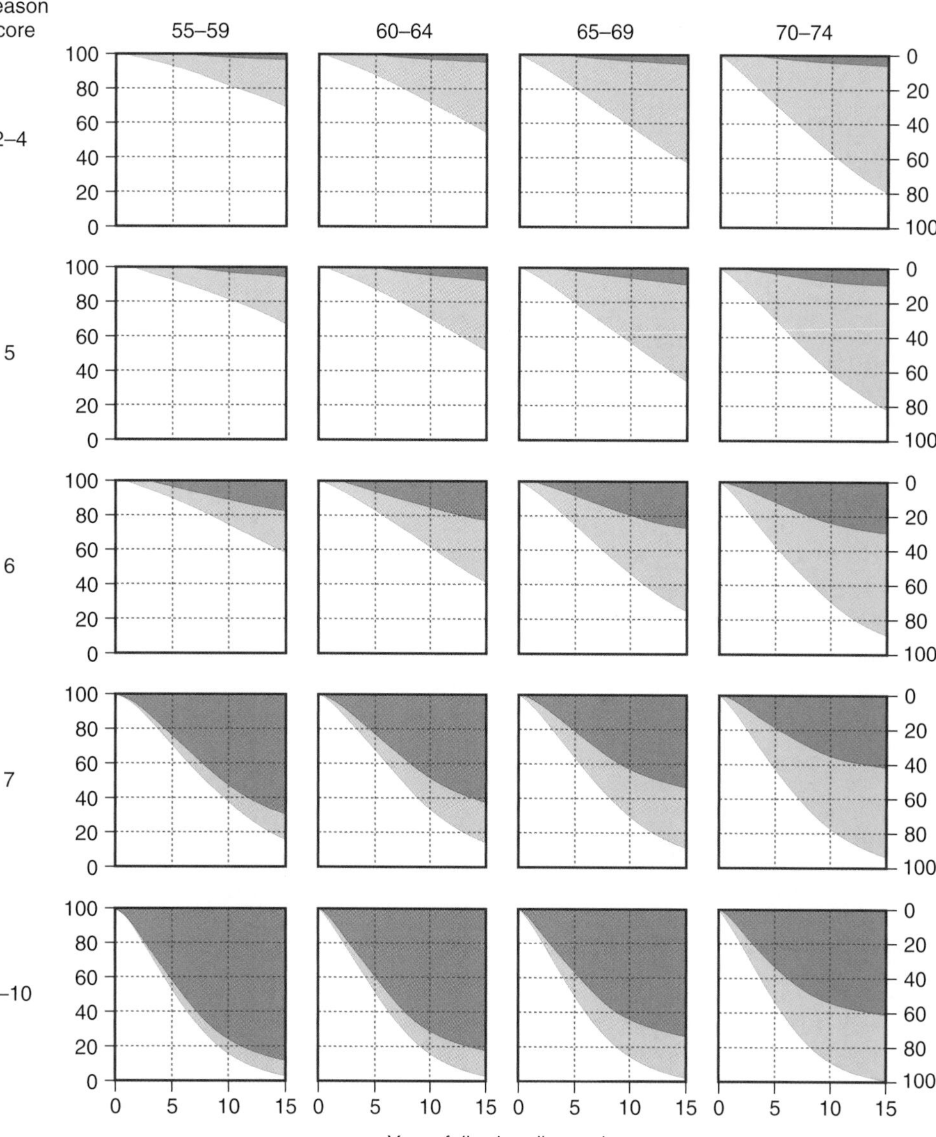

Figure 42–21 ▪ Illustration of death rates in men of various ages with prostate cancer. The *heavily shaded areas* represent death from all causes, and the *lightly shaded areas* indicate prostate cancer–related death rates. (From Albertsen, PC, Hanley JA, Gleason DF, Barry MJ. Competing risk analysis of men aged 55 to 74 years at diagnosis managed conservatively for clinically localized prostate cancer. JAMA 1998;280[11]:975-880. Reprinted with the permission of the American Medical Association.)

intervals and no evaluable disease (NED) free intervals but not for overall survival. Only long-term adjuvant therapy improved overall survival and only in the subset of men with Gleason grade 7 to 10 tumors. These conclusions on long-term versus short-term adjuvant hormonal therapy were supported by a nonrandomized Canadian trial.[193]

Brachytherapy, conformal radiation therapy, and intensity-modulated radiation therapy (IMRT) provide approaches that minimize side effects and allow higher radiation doses to the cancer tissue.[194-196] Current guidelines suggest the use of conformal or IMRT in preference to standard dosimetry methods. IMRT allows dose intensification, which might or might not eliminate the need for adjuvant hormonal therapy. Brachytherapy with implanted seeds provides another useful alternative.

Therapy for Locally Advanced or Metastatic Disease

Androgen deprivation represents the earliest form of systemic therapy for locally advanced and metastatic prostate cancer, and observational studies demonstrated its efficacy. Three methods have been used: surgical castration, high-dose estrogen, and GnRH analogues. Surgical castration and high-dose estrogen in the form of DES have been used as treatment of prostatic cancer since the 1940s. In the VACURG studies, 5 mg of DES decreased the rate of recurrence of prostate cancer but increased the cardiovascular death rate. Following this observation, careful dose-response studies indicated that 3 mg of DES daily minimizes the risk of cardiovascular disease acceleration and maximizes the beneficial effects on prostate cancer. Gynecomastia and impotence are the major side effects. However, DES is no longer available in the United States.

GnRH superagonist analogues or antagonists are now available that suppress testosterone to castrate levels and cause tumor responses equivalent to those induced by castration. Comparison of the various monotherapies was the subject of a meta-analysis involving 10 separate trials, which concluded that orchiectomy, GnRH agonist analogues, and DES produced equivalent survival in men and that no differences existed among the various GnRH analogues available.[197]

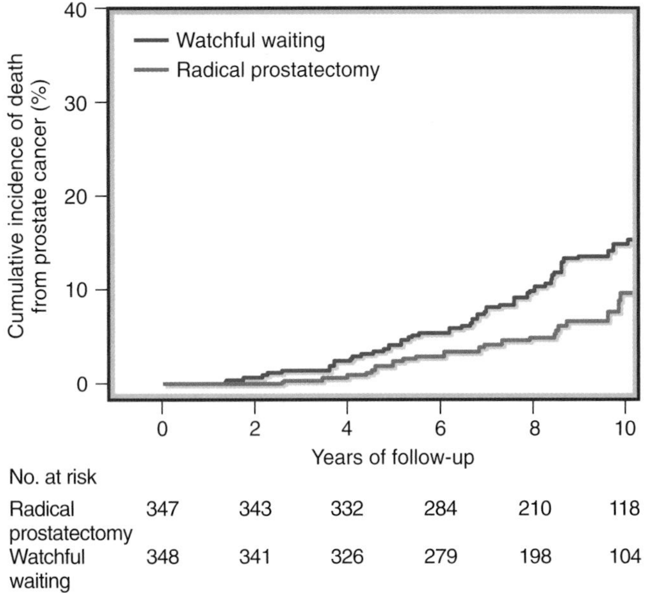

Figure 42–22 ▪ Death rates in men with prostate cancer randomized to radical prostatectomy or watchful waiting. (From Bill-Axelson A, Holmberg L, Ruutu M, et al. Radical prostatectomy versus watchful waiting in early prostate cancer. N Engl J Med 2005;352[19]:1977-1984. Data reproduced with permission of authors and publisher from the New England Journal of Medicine.)

Whether to recommend surgical castration or GnRH analogues represents a major question. Surgical orchiectomy produces a rapid decrease in serum androgen levels, does not require patient compliance long term, and is effective in inducing tumor regression in nearly 90% of patients. The clinician can be assured that testicular androgens are completely suppressed. However, more than half of men in the United States prefer medical castration as a means to avoid surgery.

Highly potent agonist analogues of GnRH have been approved for use in prostate cancer and effectively produce a medical orchiectomy. These compounds paradoxically inhibit LH secretion by the pituitary and thereby suppress testicular testosterone production. Clinically, the GnRH analogues stimulate LH three- to fourfold and testosterone twofold for 1 to 2 weeks upon initiation of therapy. Thereafter, LH is profoundly suppressed and plasma testosterone levels fall from approximately 500 ng/dL to castrate levels of 15 ng/dL. No escape from hormonal inhibition occurs for up to 2 years of continuous therapy. The initial rise in testosterone causes a transient disease flare in 5% to 10% of patients. This produces an objective increase in tumor size in approximately 3% of patients and a subjective increase in bone pain in the remainder. Although tumor flare is usually transient, severe reactions with spinal cord compression or death have been observed in occasional patients. For this reason, it is necessary to administer an antiandrogen during the first month of GnRH analogue therapy. A GnRH antagonist (abarelix) as a means to abrogate the flare phenomenon and its concomitant clinical problems has now been approved by the FDA.

The rationale for using GnRH analogues is to induce a medical castration selectively. Testosterone and DHT levels in patients treated with GnRH analogues and with surgical orchiectomy fall to a similar extent. Hormonal effects with the GnRH analogues are selective, with no alterations of adrenal, thyroid, parathyroid, or pancreatic function. Objective regressions occur as often as with orchiectomy. A meta-analysis (10 randomized, controlled trials, 1908 patients) provided evidence that medical castration and surgical castration exert equal clinical effects.[198]

Initially, a major problem with GnRH analogue therapy was the requirement for daily subcutaneous administration, with the possibility of noncompliance with daily injections and incomplete androgen suppression. Third-generation formulations are now available that allow injections at 3- to 6-month intervals or implants yearly. These biodegradable preparations appear highly effective, well tolerated, and acceptable to patients. Because some androgen-responsive cells remain in prostate tumors after relapse on the GnRH agonists, continued GnRH analogue treatment is advocated upon disease relapse and preferably for the remainder of the patient's life.

Immediate Versus Delayed Hormonal Therapy

Approximately 25% of men now present with either metastatic (M^+ or stage D) disease or with local spread into lymph nodes (N^+). Whether to initiate hormonal treatment immediately in these patients or to defer until they are symptomatic is a major question. Because cure with hormones is not possible, the two goals of treatment are to increase life expectancy and to relieve symptoms. If treatment were to be advocated in asymptomatic patients, the therapy should improve the length of patient survival.

Rigorously controlled series from the Veterans Administration Cooperative Urological Research Group (VACURG) trials during the 1960s indicated no clear survival benefit from endocrine therapy in patients with stage C or D disease at the time of diagnosis. Based upon these findings, standard practice until recently usually involved withholding hormonal therapy until symptomatic metastatic (stage D) disease was present. However, two recent studies provide evidence favoring therapy immediately upon detection of metastatic disease.

Messing and colleagues studied men with prostate cancer found to have positive pelvic lymph nodes at the time of radical prostatectomy.[199] They randomized these men into an immediate therapy group (medical or surgical orchiectomy) and into a group who were observed until an indication occurred. Death due to prostate cancer occurred in 3 of 47 men in the immediate-treatment group and 16 of 51 in the deferred group ($P < 0.01$).

In another study, 934 men with locally advanced prostate cancer or with asymptomatic metastatic disease were randomized to immediate versus deferred hormonal therapy. An initial report concluded that there was an overall survival benefit from immediate therapy. Overall, 203 men died from prostate cancer in the immediate therapy arm and 257 in the deferred group ($P = 0.02$).[200] However, on extended follow-up, the overall survival benefit was no longer statistically significant. Nonetheless, deaths due to prostate cancer were reduced to 241 in the immediate therapy arm versus 287 in the deferred arm ($P = 0.0019$).[201] In this group of elderly men, deaths from other causes occurred commonly and were not influenced by immediate hormonal therapy. Nonetheless, there were fewer cases of cord compression (10 vs. 24), pathologic fracture (14 vs. 22), extraskeletal metastases (47 vs. 62), and ureteral obstruction (49 vs. 64) in the immediate treatment group.[201]

A more recent study randomized men not accepting radical prostatectomy to immediate or deferred androgen therapy[202] and found no differences in overall pain-free time and performance status. Cancer-free survival tended to be longer in the immediate group ($P = 0.09$), but overall survival was identical ($P = 0.96$).

Other evidence of efficacy of early therapy comes from nonrandomized studies from the Mayo clinic. These studies demonstrated a statistically significant survival advantage for early endocrine therapy (castration) in men with stage D1 (T0-3, N1-2, M0) disease.[203] Seventy-three patients underwent either radical retropubic prostatectomy or radical prostatectomy plus orchiectomy. An advantage for immediate adjuvant therapy was demonstrated: 5-year survival rates were 93% in the immediate orchiectomy group and 80% in the deferred orchiectomy group. In another study, they demonstrated that benefit was only seen in patients with diploid and not in those with tetraploid or aneuploid tumors.[204] Finally, a subset analysis of men in the RTOG 85-31 study examined a group of 139 men with capsular penetration or seminal vesicle involvement. Seventy-one men received RT plus luteinizing hormone–releasing hormone (LHRH) agonist therapy, and 68 received RT alone. Statistically significant improvement in progression-free survival and freedom from biochemical relapse (rising PSA), was observed in the LHRH group. Overall survival was not statistically significantly different in this relatively small subset of men followed for a median of 5 years only.

A systematic review concluded that early androgen-deprivation therapy resulted in significant reductions in both disease-free progression and complications due to progression.[205] Progression-free survival was significantly higher at years I, 2, 5, and 10 (OR 3.99, 4.79, 3.15, and 3.49, respectively) in men treated with early androgen deprivation. Overall survival at 10 years was also improved (OR = 1.5; 95% CI 1.04-2.16). Taken together, these data suggest, but do not prove, that immediate hormonal therapy may be efficacious for asymptomatic men presenting with lymph node spread. In elderly men with increased risk of dying of nonprostate cancer causes, deferred therapy appears to be a reasonable choice.

The American Society of Clinical Oncology (ASCO) critically analyzed these data and commented that all of the trials just cited were conducted before the routine use of PSA testing. The ASCO review was considered to be limited by the variability in the interventions as well as in the stages of the cancers of the patients enrolled. From this analysis, the guidelines concluded that data at present do not provide definitive evidence that early endocrine therapy is beneficial regarding improved survival of patients presenting with metastatic (M^+) disease. Longer follow-up and additional studies sufficiently powered to detect an increase in overall survival are needed before definitive conclusions are warranted.[201,206]

Men who experience a rising PSA (biochemical failure) after an initial fall to undetectable levels after radical prostatectomy might also benefit from hormonal therapy. Data indicate that a rapid rise in PSA suggests the presence of metastatic disease, whereas a slow rise suggests local recurrence. In a single small study, 68% of men progressed to detectable clinical disease upon observation for a median of 19 months. With adjuvant hormonal therapy or radiation therapy, the rate of progression to clinically detectable disease decreased to 21%.[207] Use of the ProstaScint radiation isotopic scan has been advocated to identify patients with disseminated disease. Such patients would not be considered candidates for salvage radiation therapy to the pelvis.

Adverse Effects of Androgen-Deprivation Therapy

Medical or surgical orchiectomy causes an abrupt reduction of androgen levels. This results in hot flushes in up to 80% of patients, and up to 27% report this as the most troublesome adverse event. Bone density falls in men in response to declines in androgens and their aromatized estrogen metabolites. The risk of fracture increases starting 1 year after initiation of therapy. Either pamidronate or zoledronic acid, both potent intravenous bisphosphonates, can completely abrogate the effects of androgen deprivation on bone. Complete cessation of erectile function occurred in 78.6% of men after orchiectomy and in 73.3% during GnRH analogue therapy.[208] Other metabolic effects occur, such as decrease in hemoglobin and lean body mass, increase in total body fat mass, and rises in total cholesterol and triglyceride. Fatigue and psychological distress occurred more commonly in men receiving androgen-deprivation therapy than in those choosing to defer this treatment. Gynecomastia occurred in 1% to 16% of men treated with androgen-deprivation therapy.

Secondary Hormonal Therapies for Recurrent Disease

Men whose prostate cancer recurs following medical or surgical orchiectomy are treated with secondary hormonal therapies. Prior to PSA measurements, the clinician had to rely on bone x-rays and soft tissue changes to document responses, and these were rarely observed. Consequently, the efficacy of secondary hormonal therapies was controversial. More recently, clinicians have accepted a 50% decline in PSA as reflecting an objective response to therapy. Studies have shown that this PSA endpoint predicts a significantly prolonged median overall survival, objective progression-free survival, and time to pain progression. Using PSA measurements, it has now been possible to demonstrate efficacy of a number of secondary hormonal therapies. Responses to antiandrogens, ketoconazole, flutamide, bicalutamide, aminoglutethimide, DES, and glucocorticoids alone range from 14% to 60% (Table 42–4). Head-to-head comparisons are unavailable for these agents, and relative efficacy cannot be compared.[209]

Antiandrogen Withdrawal

Experimental studies with LNCaP cells in vitro detected a mutation in the androgen receptor in this cell line that caused it to respond to flutamide with increased proliferation. As a result of this observation, clinical studies examined whether tumors in some patients might adapt to flutamide by developing mutations allowing flutamide to behave as an androgen agonist. In support of this possibility, approximately 40% of men on flutamide experienced tumor regression after withdrawal (withdrawal responses). These data suggest that a first step in patients receiving flutamide, either as part of a complete androgen blockade regimen (see later) or as secondary hormonal therapy, is to stop flutamide. These withdrawal responses occur with bicalutamide as well, but less commonly.[210]

Other Secondary Hormonal Therapies

Prior to the PSA era, objective regression, stabilization, or symptomatic relief were reported with several agents. These included a high-dose formulation of DES (stilphostrol) and tamoxifen (20 mg daily). A more recent study using high-dose tamoxifen (160 mg/m^2/per day) observed only a 3.3% rate of objective response based upon PSA in heavily pretreated men with prostate cancer.[211] Each of these agents could be considered for patients relapsing slowly after castration.

Other Nonhormonal Treatment Measures

Potent bisphosphonates effectively reduce the incidence of skeletal-related events in men with hormone-refractory prostate cancer. A large randomized phase III trial demonstrated that zoledronic acid significantly reduced the incidence of pathologic fractures, spinal cord compression, the need to treat with radiation therapy for bone, and bone pain in men with prostate cancer. The dose used was 4 mg every 3 weeks for 24 months. The number of subjects with an SRE (skeletal-related event) decreased from 49% for placebo to 38% with zoledronic acid ($P = 0.28$).[212] A recent set of guidelines suggested that zoledronic acid be used routinely in patients who have hormone-refractory prostate cancer and at least one bone metastasis. In patients with no lesions, routine bone scans should be used to detect new lesions and zoledronic acid started when an initial lesion is found.

TABLE 42–4 SECONDARY HORMONAL THERAPIES FOR PROSTATE CANCER

Modality	Responders	Total Patients	Response	Clinical Setting	References
Flutamide	23	100	23%	First relapse after medical or surgical orchiectomy	Fossa et al
Prednisone	21	101	21%	First relapse after medical or surgical orchiectomy	Fossa et al
Flutamide withdrawal	29	138	21%	Relapse after combined androgen blockade or flutamide monotherapy	Scher & Kelly Small & Srinivas
AG/HC	14	29	49%	After antiandrogen withdrawal	Sartor & Cooper
HC	16	82	20%	After antiandrogen withdrawal	Dawson et al (1995)
Ketoconazole/HC	43	72	60%	After antiandrogen withdrawal	Small et al
Megestrol acetate	17	119	14%	After antiandrogen withdrawal	Dawson et al (2000)
DES	71	243	29%	After antiandrogen withdrawal	Berman et al

AG, aminoglutethimide; DES, diethylstilbestrol; HC, hydrocortisone.

Berman C, Glode LM, Crawford ED, Wilroy S. Vitamin D, dexamethasone and carboplatin for hormone refractory prostate cancer, a phase II study. Proc Am Soc Clin Oncol 2002;21:abstr 2455.

Dawson NA, Conaway M, Halabi S, et al. A randomized study comparing standard versus moderately high dose megestrol acetate for patients with advanced prostate carcinoma: cancer and leukemia group B study 9181. Cancer 2000;88:825-834.

Dawson NA, Cooper MR, Figg WD, et al. Antitumor activity of suramin in hormone-refractory prostate cancer controlling for hydrocortisone treatment and flutamide withdrawal as potentially confounding variables. Cancer 1995;76(3):453-462.

Fossa SD, Slee PH, Brausi M, et al. Flutamide versus prednisone in patients with prostate cancer symptomatically progressing after androgen-ablative therapy: a phase III study of the European organization for research and treatment of cancer genitourinary group. J Clin Oncol 2001;19(1):62-71.

Sartor O, Cooper M, Weinberger M, et al. Surprising activity of flutamide withdrawal, when combined with aminoglutethimide, in treatment of "hormone-refractory" prostate cancer. J Natl Cancer Inst 1994;86(3):222-227. Erratum in: J Natl Cancer Inst 1994;86(6):463.

Scher HI, Kelly WK. Flutamide withdrawal syndrome: its impact on clinical trials in hormone-refractory prostate cancer. J Clin Oncol 1993;11(8):1566-1572.

Small EJ, Baron AD, Fippin L, Apodaca D. Ketoconazole retains activity in advanced prostate cancer patients with progression despite flutamide withdrawal. J Urol 1997;157:1204-1207.

Small EJ, Srinivas S. The antiandrogen withdrawal syndrome. Experience in a large cohort of unselected patients with advanced prostate cancer. Cancer 1995;76(8):1428-1434.

Treatment of Hormone-Refractory Recurrent Disease

At some point in the patient's course, the tumor becomes completely refractory to hormonally based therapies. No diagnostic test is available to make the distinction between hormone dependence and independence. Men with a rapid downhill course with widespread systemic metastases should probably receive chemotherapy. Others will have already been treated with all available options of endocrine therapy. Chemotherapy or combination chemo-hormonal therapy is chosen at that point. The interested reader is referred to a comprehensive treatise.[213]

Alternative Approaches to Prostate Cancer Therapy

Monotherapy with antiandrogens, either steroidal or nonsteroidal, provides an alternative to surgical or medical castration. The nonsteroidal agents, flutamide and bicalutamide, bind to androgen receptors and block the cellular effects of circulating testosterone and DHT on cell proliferation. Interruption of the androgen negative-feedback system results in reflex increments in serum LH, testosterone, and DHT levels. Prior studies with antiandrogens suggested that these agents partially preserve erectile function. More recent data suggest that only 20% of all treated men maintain morning erections and sexual activity with antiandrogen therapy. When only men capable of sexual function before treatment are considered, 18% reported a reduction in sexual function score on bicalutamide and 37% after castration.[214] Side effects occur in 4% to 10% of patients[206] and include hot flushes, gynecomastia, hepatotoxicity, nonspecific ophthalmologic changes, and diarrhea (particularly for flutamide). Bone density improves in men receiving bicalutamide, probably because of the 146% increase in estradiol and because estradiol is the major mediator of bone density in men.[215]

Randomized trials have compared antiandrogens as monotherapy with medical or surgical castration. Initial studies showed that 50 mg of bicalutamide is not as effective as orchiectomy. Later studies used 150 mg of bicalutamide and compared medical or surgical castration with 150 mg of bicalutamide in patients with locally advanced (T1-4, N^+, M0) and metastatic (T-1-4, Nx, M0) disease. Bicalutamide was equivalent to medical or surgical castration for locally advanced[214] but not metastatic disease (HR for survival, 1.3). Pooled mature data from these studies suggest no survival difference between bicalutamide 150 mg daily and surgical castration. Other available data suggest that bicalutamide is not as effective as castration.[216]

Meta-analyses of studies involving 2717 patients comparing monotherapy with various antiandrogens suggested that the hazard ratio for recurrence was greater with antiandrogen monotherapy than with medical or surgical castration, but statistical significance was approached but not reached (HR 1.22, 95% CI 0.99-1.50).[217] Even though antiandrogen monotherapy appears less effective than castration, some men choose this therapy in preference to watchful waiting.[218] The ASCO guideline indicated that monotherapy with a nonsteroidal antiandrogen may be discussed as an alternative to surgical castration or GNRH analogues. This recommendation was based upon the data indicating less toxicity with respect to libido and physical capacity but inferior time to progression of disease compared to the LHRH agonists.[206]

Neoadjuvant Hormonal Therapy Prior to Radical Prostatectomy

Neoadjuvant hormonal therapy before radical prostatectomy involves medical castration with GnRH analogues, steroidal or nonsteroidal antiandrogens, or a combination of these agents prior to prostatectomy. Neoadjuvant strategies used for 3 to 6 months before radical prostatectomy result in an increase in organ-confined cancers and a decrease in positive surgical margins.[219] However, no differences in PSA detectable relapse rates have yet been observed in several trials. Data are not yet sufficiently mature to assess overall survival rates. A large ongoing study is randomizing men to placebo or 150 mg of bicalutamide daily following radical prostatectomy or radiation therapy or during watchful waiting. A total of 8055 patients have been entered. Bicalutamide significantly reduced the incidence of disease progression by 42% (HR 0.58, 95% CI 0.51 to 0.66, $P < 0.0001$). A recent analysis reported no increase in overall survival with these approaches.[220] However, the jury is still out on the efficacy of this maneuver because longer follow-up is needed before definitive conclusions regarding overall survival can be reached.

Complete Androgen Blockade

A more comprehensive strategy for the endocrine treatment of prostate cancer, called *complete or maximum androgen blockade,* has been proposed. The rationale rests upon three considerations:

- The adrenal glands contribute 5% of the total androgen pool.
- The concentrations of DHT in prostate cancer tissue of patients fall by only 50% to 80% after surgical orchiectomy, and DHT levels in that tissue after castration still are higher than in nonandrogen-target tissues.
- *In vitro* systems demonstrate that some tumor cells clones are hypersensitive to the proliferative effects of androgen.

Based upon these considerations, it was thought that inhibition of both testicular and adrenal androgens (maximum androgen blockade, MAB) might be more effective than inhibition of testicular secretion alone (testicular androgen suppression, TAS). Thirty-six studies have examined the concept of MAB as initial endocrine therapy for advanced disease (Stage D or Tx, Nx, M^+ disease) in randomized trials, but the results and conclusions drawn from them conflict. However, three systematic reviews (two with meta-analysis of the literature), one meta-analysis of individualized patient data, one large randomized trial, and one Markov model critically examined this issue.[217,221-223] These studies, involving nearly 90% of men treated worldwide, provided several definitive conclusions regarding this strategy. The benefits of complete androgen blockade are minimal and range from 1% to 5% improvement in overall survival. Figure 42–23 demonstrates the results of one meta-analysis. The additional cost of complete androgen blockade as opposed to testicular androgen suppression (TAS) approximates $1,110,000 per quality-adjusted life year, and the number needed to treat (NNT) to benefit one patient is estimated to be between 20 and 100.

These meta-analyses provide reasons for discrepancies among prior results. First, MAB regimens using nonsteroidal antiandrogens provide only a 1% to 5% improvement in overall survival. An example of data from one of the meta-analyses is presented in Figure 42–23.[221] This difference is statistically significant ($P = 0.005$) but of marginal significance clinically. Second, MAB regimens using the steroidal antiandrogen cyproterone acetate produce adverse survival effects compared to TAS. Third, analysis of studies of MAB that pool patients treated either with cyproterone acetate or nonsteroidal antiandrogens demonstrate no survival benefit produced by MAB over TAS. Fourth, men with disease limited to the axial skeleton did not gain more benefit from MAB than those with metastases to the appendicular skeleton. A large prior study had reported this to be the case. Fifth, results were similar when subsets of men treated with surgical or medical castration or with flutamide or nilutamide were examined.

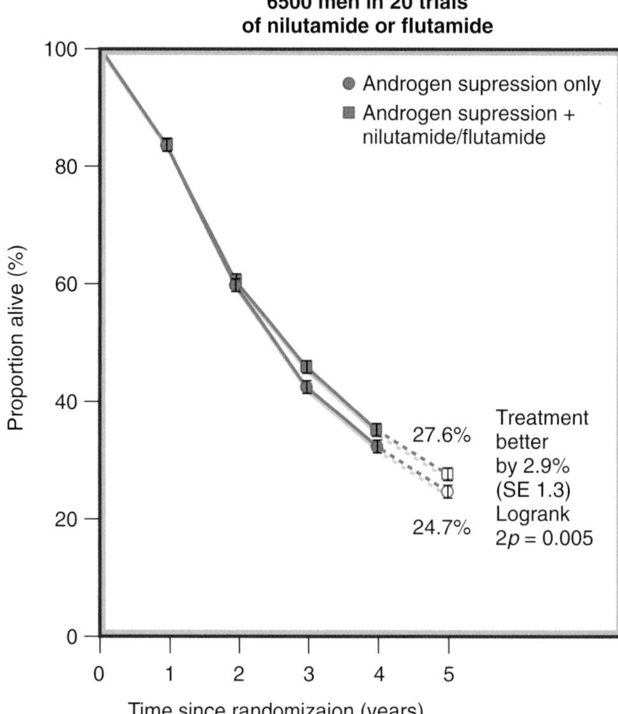

Figure 42–23 ▪ Results of complete versus partial androgen blockade in men with prostate cancer. Survival curves represent pooled data from a meta-analysis of multiple studies. SE, standard error. (From Prostate Cancer Trialists' Collaborative Group. Maximum androgen blockade in advanced prostate cancer: an overview of the randomised trials. Lancet 2000;355[9214]:1491-1498.)

Past controversies about MAB can be explained by fact that some trials used cyproterone acetate, an antiandrogen that shortens survival in these patients.[221] Other trials did not use short-term antiandrogen in the medical castration group, and the disease flare might have compromised overall efficacy. Finally, early trials used daily GnRH injections, which might not have induced effective medical castration because of the need for compliance with daily injections for 5 years.

No properly designed study has compared MAB to sequential androgen blockade (SAB, defined as initial castration followed by antiandrogen upon relapse). In the largest study of MAB,[222] use of antiandrogen upon relapse in the placebo group was left to the investigator's discretion, and only 50% of men in the placebo arm later took an antiandrogen. For this reason, no information is available whether antiandrogen therapy given at the time of relapse after medical or surgical orchiectomy (SAB) is as effective MAB. This is an important issue because flutamide given upon relapse after castration (sequential androgen blockade) causes objective benefit in 23% of patients.

Based on the data presented and the additional considerations discussed, the ASCO guidelines favor the SAB strategy and use of antiandrogens only after relapse from medical or surgical orchiectomy.[206] However, if GnRH agonists are used to produce a medical orchiectomy, short-term use of an antiandrogen to prevent disease flare is necessary. In patients with metastatic disease, GnRH analogues should not be used in men at risk for neurological compromise due to metastasis, ureteral or bladder outlet obstruction due to local encroachment, or severe bone pain persisting with narcotic analgesic use.

Experimental Hormonal Approaches

Experimental data from Shionogi tumors in mice suggest that intermittent androgen withdrawal might control tumor growth and delay development of hormonal resistance. Several pilot reports suggest the feasibility of this approach,[224] and observations are ongoing. This strategy cannot be recommended until sufficient data are available to support its efficacy.[206] Both type I and II GnRH receptors are present on prostate cancer cells, and preclinical studies are examining the effects of agents that bind to these proteins as a means of inhibiting prostate cancer growth.

Algorithm for Treatment of Prostate Cancer

No standard approach to the treatment of prostatic cancer has been universally agreed upon. To outline the options available, the algorithm in Figure 42–24 details decision branch points. Specific accepted options for each risk group are included in the National Comprehensive Cancer guidelines and detailed in Table 42–5.[186]

Considerations Regarding Initial Treatment of Clinically Localized Prostate Cancer

No consensus exists regarding selection of radical prostatectomy, radiation therapy, or watchful waiting.[225] Individual considerations including age, risk factors for recurrence, overall health of the patient, and life expectancy influence these decisions, which are often based on personal choices. In general, the younger and healthier the patient, the more likely is a choice of radical prostatectomy. The older and more debilitated, the more likely is the choice of watchful waiting.

In men with T3 disease, radiation therapy plus hormonal therapy is generally preferred over radical prostatectomy except in a few T3 cases with low-volume disease. Radiation therapy is often selected for patients falling at neither extreme. Adjuvant hormonal therapy to be used with radiation therapy should be limited to patients with high-risk disease. The likelihood of recurrence with low- or intermediate-risk disease may be too small to warrant the associated symptoms, bone loss, anemia, and other problems associated with androgen deprivation.

Considerations Regarding Initial Therapy in Men with Metastatic Disease at Time of Diagnosis

Men with metastatic disease (T1-4, N^+, M^+) at presentation are not treated definitively with radical prostatectomy or irradiation but often are offered hormonal therapy before symptomatic disease develops. This decision is based upon incomplete data suggesting superior efficacy of early rather than late hormonal therapy in locally advanced disease. Randomized trials with a large number of patients will be required before definitive advice can be given regarding management of patients with PSA relapses.

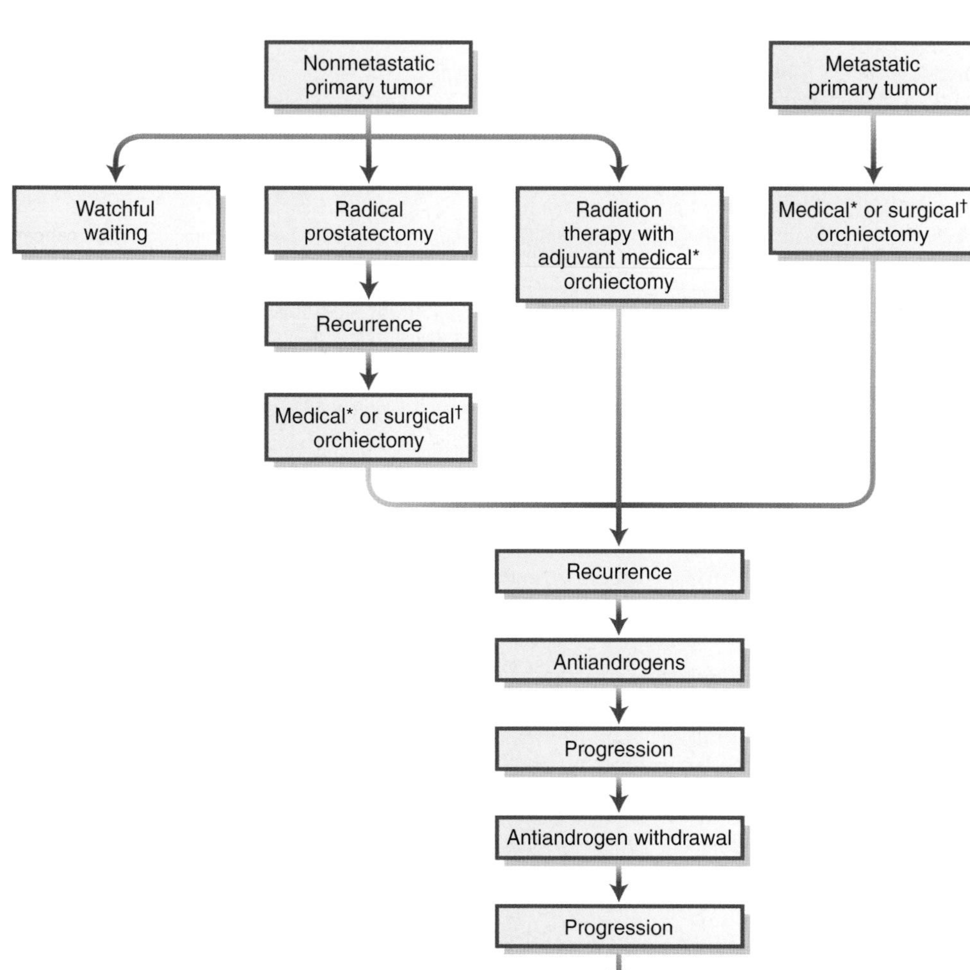

Figure 42–24 ▪ Algorithm of preferred treatment strategies for localized and advanced prostate cancer. *Medical orchiectomy refers to use of a GnRH analogue to suppress testicular function. †Surgical orchiectomy refers to removal of both testes surgically.

TABLE 42–5 INITIAL TREATMENT OF LOCALIZED DISEASE

LOW RISK
<10-yr life expectancy: Watchful waiting or radiation therapy >10-yr life expectancy: Watchful waiting or radiation therapy or radical prostatectomy
INTERMEDIATE RISK
<10-y-r life expectancy: Watchful waiting or radiation therapy or radical prostatectomy >10-y-r life expectancy: Radical prostatectomy or radiation therapy
HIGH RISK
Androgen ablation (2-3 yr) plus radiation therapy or radiation therapy and short-term androgen ablation or radical prostatectomy (if low volume and no fixation)
Initial Treatment of Locally Advanced Disease
androgen ablation for 2-3 yr or RT and androgen ablation
Initial Treatment of Metastatic Disease
Any T, N1: Androgen ablation or RT and androgen ablation Any T, any N, M1: Androgen ablation

Which hormonal therapy to use is a matter of choice. Meta-analyses of several trials suggests that medical castration, surgical castration, and DES all have equal efficacy,[198,206] but individual trials indicate that antiandrogens are less effective. In my opinion, surgical orchiectomy appears preferable for the initial treatment of these patients. The operation is relatively minor, it can be performed under local anesthesia, if desired, and it is cost effective. Rapid and complete cessation of testicular androgen secretion ensues, and patient compliance after surgery is not a factor. Unwarranted cardiovascular or other toxic side effects such as occur with DES are unknown. The incidence of impotence and loss of libido is the same as with other available therapies with the exception of the antiandrogens.

In actual practice, nearly half of patients in the United States prefer a form of medical castration for psychological or other reasons. The greater safety of the GnRH analogues favor their use over DES, and for this reason, DES is no longer available in the United States. To prevent tumor flare, antiandrogens should be used for at least 1 month during and after initiation of GnRH therapy. Maximum androgen blockade in the long term is not recommended based upon the individual studies and meta-analysis reviewed earlier but should be discussed with the patient.[206] Some patients choose to continue the antiandrogens long term to gain the slight (1% to 5%) maximal benefit from MAB. An antiandrogen alone could be chosen as an alternative but is not preferred, and DES is no longer available in the United States.

At present, medical castration with GnRH agonists can be achieved with 3 to 6 monthly injections or with yearly implants, which are well tolerated and should not be associated with cardiovascular complications. Cost is the limiting factor. When concern regarding erectile dysfunction is a major issue, the persistence of libido and erectile function in a subset of patients treated with antiandrogens as primary therapy may be a decisive factor. Under these circumstances, some men choose monotherapy with antiandrogens, even though this approach is not as effective as medical or surgical castration. This decision represents a quality of life issue, which is an increasingly important consideration in prostate cancer therapy.

Considerations Regarding Disease Recurrence

Upon first recurrence, men treated with radiation therapy or radical prostatectomy are then treated with either medical or surgical orchiectomy. Antiandrogen monotherapy can be offered but is not preferred. Antiandrogen therapy provides a reasonable next option after medical or surgical castration unless previously given as part of a maximum androgen blockade regimen. Those receiving an antiandrogen as part of a complete androgen blockade regimen are observed for an antiandrogen withdrawal response. Regarding choice of antiandrogen, bicalutamide is preferred to flutamide because of its better side effect profile and potentially superior efficacy. Upon relapse, men are observed for antiandrogen withdrawal response and only treated further when progressive disease is documented.

A variety of therapies are available for men relapsing after antiandrogen withdrawal. One group[183] prefers ketoconazole and hydrocortisone because of its lack of toxicity and observed efficacy (60% PSA response rate). Each of the other agents listed in Table 42–4 could be used as alternatives or as third-line therapies. Further choices of chemotherapy alone or chemotherapy in combination with hormonal agents are a matter of individual preference.

REFERENCES

1. International Agency for Research on Cancer (IARC). Hormonal contraception and postmenopausal hormone therapy. IARC Monographs on the Evaluation of Carcinogenic Risks to Humans, vol 72. Lyon, France, IARC, 1999.
2. Hahn WC, Weinberg RA. Rules for making human tumor cells. N Engl J Med 2002;347(20):1593-1603.
3. Yager JD, Davidson NE. Estrogen carcinogenesis in breast cancer. N Engl J Med 2006;354(3):270-282.
4. Preston-Martin S, Pike MC, Ross RK, Henderson BE. Epidemiologic evidence for the increased cell proliferation model of carcinogenesis. Environ Health Perspect 1993;101(suppl 5):137-138.
5. Cavalieri E, Chakravarti D, Guttenplan J, et al. Catechol estrogen quinones as initiators of breast and other human cancers: implications for biomarkers of susceptibility and cancer prevention. Biochim Biophys Acta 2006;1766(1):63-78.
6. Thompson D, Easton D. The genetic epidemiology of breast cancer genes. J Mammary Gland Biol Neoplasia 2004;9(3):221-236.
7. Lichtenstein P, Holm NV, Verkasalo PK, et al. Environmental and heritable factors in the causation of cancer—analyses of cohorts of twins from Sweden, Denmark, and Finland. N Engl J Med 2000;343(2):78-85.
8. Hulka BS. Epidemiologic analysis of breast and gynecologic cancers. Prog Clin Biol Res 1997;396:17-29.
9. Key T, Appleby P, Barnes I, Reeves G, and Endogenous Hormones and Breast Cancer Collaborative Group. Endogenous sex hormones and breast cancer in postmenopausal women: reanalysis of nine prospective studies. J Natl Cancer Inst 2002;94(8):606-616.
10. Eliassen AH, Missmer SA, Tworoger SS, and Hankinson SE. Endogenous steroid hormone concentrations and risk of breast cancer: does the association vary by a woman's predicted breast cancer risk? J Clin Oncol 2006;24(12):1823-1830.
11. Kuller LH, Cauley JA, Lucas L, et al. Sex steroid hormones, bone mineral density, and risk of breast cancer. Environ Health Perspect 1997;105(suppl 3):593-599.
12. Newcomb PA, Trentham-Dietz A, Egan KM, et al. Fracture history and risk of breast and endometrial cancer. Am J Epidemiol 2001;153(11):1071-1078.
13. Feigelson HS, Patel AV, Teras LR, et al. Adult weight gain and histopathologic characteristics of breast cancer among postmenopausal women. Cancer 2006;107(1):12-21.

14. Feinleib M. Breast cancer and artificial menopause: a cohort study. J Natl Cancer Inst 1968;41(2):315-329.
15. Boyd NF, Byng JW, Jong RA, et al. Quantitative classification of mammographic densities and breast cancer risk: results from the Canadian National Breast Screening Study. J Natl Cancer Inst 1995;87(9):670-675.
16. Harvey JA, Bovbjerg VE. Quantitative assessment of mammographic breast density: relationship with breast cancer risk.Radiology 2004;230(1):29-41.
17. Ursin G, Ross RK, Sullivan-Halley J, et al. Use of oral contraceptives and risk of breast cancer in young women. Breast Cancer Res Treat 1998;50(2):175-184.
18. Collaborative Group on Hormonal Factors in Breast Cancer. Breast cancer and hormone replacement therapy: collaborative reanalysis of data from 51 epidemiological studies of 52,705 women with breast cancer and 108,411 women without breast cancer. Lancet 1997;350(9084):1047-1059.
19. Beral V; Million Women Study Collaborators. Breast cancer and hormone-replacement therapy in the Million Women Study. Lancet 2003;362(9382):419-427.
20. Schairer C, Lubin J, Troisi R, et al. Menopausal estrogen and estrogen-progestin replacement therapy and breast cancer risk. JAMA 2000;283(4):485-491.
21. Rossouw JE, Anderson GL, Prentice RL, et al. Risks and benefits of estrogen plus progestin in healthy postmenopausal women: principal results From the Women's Health Initiative randomized controlled trial. JAMA 2002;288(3):321-333.
22. Stefanick ML, Anderson GL, Margolis KL, et al. Effects of conjugated equine estrogens on breast cancer and mammography screening in postmenopausal women with hysterectomy. JAMA 2006;295(14):1647-1657.
23. Chen WY, Manson JE, Hankinson SE, et al. Unopposed estrogen therapy and the risk of invasive breast cancer. Arch Intern Med 2006;166(9):1027-1032.
23a. Santen RJ, Allred DC. The estrogen paradox 2007. Nat Clin Prac Endocrinol Metab 2007;3:426-497.
24. Song RX, ZhangZ, Mor G, Santen RJ. Down-regulation of Bcl-2 enhances estrogen apoptotic action in long-term estradiol-depleted ER+ breast cancer cells. Apoptosis 2005;10(3):667-678.
25. Khurana KK, Loosmann A, Numann PJ, Khan SA. Prophylactic mastectomy: pathologic findings in high-risk patients. Arch Pathol Lab Med 2000;124(3):378-381.
26. Nielsen M, Thomsen JL, Primdahl S, et al. Breast cancer and atypia among young and middle-aged women: a study of 110 medicolegal autopsies. Br J Cancer 1987;56(6):814-819.
27. Fournier A, Berrino F, Riboli E, et al. Breast cancer risk in relation to different types of hormone replacement therapy in the E3N-EPIC cohort. Int J Cancer 2005;114(3):448-454.
28. Hofseth LJ, Raafat AM, Osuch JR, et al. Hormone replacement therapy with estrogen or estrogen plus medroxyprogesterone acetate is associated with increased epithelial proliferation in the normal postmenopausal breast. J Clin Endocrinol Metab 1999; 84(12):4559-4565.
29. Greendale GA, Reboussin BA, Sie A, et al. Effects of estrogen and estrogen-progestin on mammographic parenchymal density. Postmenopausal Estrogen/Progestin Interventions (PEPI) Investigators. Ann Intern Med 1999;130(4 Pt 1):262-269.
30. Hartmann LC, Sellers TA, Frost MH, et al. Benign breast disease and the risk of breast cancer. N Engl J Med 2005;353(3):229-237.
31. Santen RJ, Mansel R. Benign breast disorders. N Engl J Med 2005;353(3):275-285.
32. O'Connell P, Pekkel V, Fuqua SA, et al. Analysis of loss of heterozygosity in 399 premalignant breast lesions at 15 genetic loci. J Natl Cancer Inst 1998;90(9):697-703.
33. Wang J, Costantino JP, Tan-Chiu E, et al. Lower-category benign breast disease and the risk of invasive breast cancer. J Natl Cancer Inst 2004;96(8):616-620.
34. Rockhill B, Spiegelman D, Byrne C, et al. Validation of the Gail et al. model of breast cancer risk prediction and implications for chemoprevention. J Natl Cancer Inst 2001;93(5):358-366.
35. Tyrer J, Duffy SW, Cuzick J. A breast cancer prediction model incorporating familial and personal risk factors. Stat Med 2004; 23(7):1111-1130.
36. Cuzick J; and International Breast Cancer Intervention Study. A brief review of the International Breast Cancer Intervention Study (IBIS), the other current breast cancer prevention trials, and proposals for future trials. Ann N Y Acad Sci 2001;949: 123-133.
36a. Cuzick J, Forbes JF, Sestak I, et al. Long-term results of tamoxifen prophylaxis for breast cancer—96-month follow-up of the randomized IBIS-I trial. J Natl Cancer Inst 2007;99:272–282.
37. Fisher B, Costantino JP, Wickerham DL, et al. Tamoxifen for the prevention of breast cancer: current status of the National Surgical Adjuvant Breast and Bowel Project P-1 study. J Natl Cancer Inst 2005;97(22):1652-1662.
38. Chlebowski R T, Collyar DE, Somerfield MR, and Pfister DG. American Society of Clinical Oncology technology assessment on breast cancer risk reduction strategies: tamoxifen and raloxifene. J Clin Oncol 1999;17(6):1939-1955.
39. Fisher B, Costantino JP, Wickerham DL, et al. Tamoxifen for prevention of breast cancer: report of the National Surgical Adjuvant Breast and Bowel Project P-1 Study. J Natl Cancer Inst 1998; 90(18):1371-1388.
40. Barakat RR. Screening for endometrial cancer in the patient receiving tamoxifen for breast cancer. J Clin Oncol 1999;17(7): 1967-1968.
41. Gerber B, Krause A, Muller H, et al. Effects of adjuvant tamoxifen on the endometrium in postmenopausal women with breast cancer: a prospective long-term study using transvaginal ultrasound. J Clin Oncol 2000;18(20):3464-3470.
42. Mourits MJ, Van der Zee AG, Willemse PH, et al. Discrepancy between ultrasonography and hysteroscopy and histology of endometrium in postmenopausal breast cancer patients using tamoxifen. Gynecol Oncol 1999;73(1):21-26.
43. Ozsener S, Ozaran A, Itil I, Dikmen Y. Endometrial pathology of 104 postmenopausal breast cancer patients treated with tamoxifen. Eur J Gynaecol Oncol 1998;19(6):580-583.
44. Vogel VG, CostantinoJP, Wickerham DL, et al. Effects of tamoxifen vs raloxifene on the risk of developing invasive breast cancer and other disease outcomes: the NSABP Study of Tamoxifen and Raloxifene (STAR) P-2 trial. JAMA 2006;295(23):2727-2741.
45. Barrett-Connor E, Mosca L, Collins P, et al, and Raloxifene Use for The Heart (RUTH) Trial Investigators. Effects of raloxifene on cardiovascular events and breast cancer in postmenopausal women. N Engl J Med 2006;355(2):125-137.
46. Narod SA, Offit K. Prevention and management of hereditary breast cancer. J Clin Oncol 2005;23(8):1656-1663.
47. Radmacher MD, Simon R. Estimation of tamoxifen's efficacy for preventing the formation and growth of breast tumors. J Natl Cancer Inst 2000;92(1):48-53.
48. Lippman ME, Krueger KA, Eckert S, et al. Indicators of lifetime estrogen exposure: effect on breast cancer incidence and interaction with raloxifene therapy in the multiple outcomes of raloxifene evaluation study participants. J Clin Oncol 2001; 19(12):3111-3116.
48a. Santen RJ, Boyd NF, Chlebowski RT, et al. Critical assessment of new risk factors for breast cancer: considerations for development of an improved risk prediction model. Endocr Relat Cancer 2007;14:169-187.
49. Howell A, Cuzick J, Baum M, et al. Results of the ATAC (Arimidex, Tamoxifen, Alone or in Combination) trial after completion of 5 years' adjuvant treatment for breast cancer. Lancet 2005;365(9453): 60-62.
50. Coates AS, Keshaviah A, Thürliman B, et al: Five years of letrozole compared with tamoxifen as initial adjuvant therapy for postmenopausal women with endocrine-responsive early breast cancer: update of study BIG 1-98. J Clin Oncol 2007;25:486-492.
51. Jakesz R, Kaufmann M, Gnant M, et al. Benefits of switching postmenopausal women with hormone-sensitive early breast cancer to anastrozole after 2 years adjuvant tamoxifen: Combined results from 3,123 women enrolled in the ABCSG Trial 8 and the ARNO 95 trial. Breast Cancer Res Treat 2004;88(suppl 1):S7.
52. Coombes RC, Hall E, Gibson LJ, et al. A randomized trial of exemestane after two to three years of tamoxifen therapy in postmenopausal women with primary breast cancer. N Engl J Med 2004;350(11):1081-192.
53. Goss PE, Ingle JN, Martino S, et al. A randomized trial of letrozole in postmenopausal women after five years of tamoxifen therapy for early-stage breast cancer. N Engl J Med 2003;349(19): 1793-1802.

53a. Coombes RC, Kilburn LS, Snowdon CF, et al. Survival and safety of exemestane versus tamoxifen after 2-3 years tamoxifen treatment. Lancet 2007;369:559-570.
54. Pisano ED, Gatsonis C, Hendrick E. Digital Mammographic Imaging Screening Trial (DMIST) Investigators Group. Diagnostic performance of digital versus film mammography for breast-cancer screening. N Engl J Med 2005;353(17):1773-1783.
55. Osborne CK, Shou J, Massarweh S, Schiff R. Crosstalk between estrogen receptor and growth factor receptor pathways as a cause for endocrine therapy resistance in breast cancer. Clin Cancer Res 2005;11(2 Pt 2):865S-870S.
56. Santen RJ, Manni A, Harvey H, Redmond C. Endocrine treatment of breast cancer in women. Endocr Rev 1990;11(2): 221-265.
57. Shim WS, Conaway M, Masamura S, et al. Estradiol hypersensitivity and mitogen-activated protein kinase expression in long-term estrogen deprived human breast cancer cells in vivo. Endocrinology 2000;141(1):396-405.
58. Chan CM, Martin LA, Johnston SR, et al. Molecular changes associated with the acquisition of oestrogen hypersensitivity in MCF-7 breast cancer cells on long-term oestrogen deprivation. J Steroid Biochem Mol Biol 2002;81(4-5):333-3341.
59. Santen RJ, Song RX, Zhang Z, et al. Adaptive hypersensitivity to estrogen: mechanism for sequential responses to hormonal therapy in breast cancer. Clin Cancer Res 2004;10(1 Pt 2): 337S-345S.
60. Hayes DF. Prognostic and predictive factors for breast cancer: translating technology to oncology. J Clin Oncol 2005;23(8): 1596-1597.
61. Cristofanilli M, Hayes DF, Budd GT, et al. Circulating tumor cells: a novel prognostic factor for newly diagnosed metastatic breast cancer. J Clin Oncol 2005;23(7):1420-1430.
62. Goldhirsch A, Glick JH, Gelber RD, et al. Meeting highlights: international expert consensus on the primary therapy of early breast cancer. Ann Oncol 2005;16(10):1569-1583.
63. Sorlie T. Molecular portraits of breast cancer: tumour subtypes as distinct disease entities. Eur J Cancer 2004;40(18):2667-2675.
64. Ellis MJ, Hayes DF, Lippman M. Treatment of metastatic breast cancer. In Harris JR, Lippman M, Morrow M, Osborne CK (eds). Diseases of the Breast. Philadelphia: Lippincott Williams & Wilkins, 2000:749-797.
65. Ellis MJ, Coop A, Singh B, et al. Letrozole is more effective neoadjuvant endocrine therapy than tamoxifen for ErbB-1- and/or ErbB-2-positive, estrogen receptor–positive primary breast cancer: evidence from a phase III randomized trial. J Clin Oncol 2001; 19(18):3808-3816.
66. Colleoni M, Viale G, Zahrieh D, et al. Chemotherapy is more effective in patients with breast cancer not expressing steroid hormone receptors: a study of preoperative treatment. Clin Cancer Res 2004;10(19):6622-6628.
67. Lippman ME, Allegra JC, Thompson EB, et al. The relation between estrogen receptors and response rate to cytotoxic chemotherapy in metastatic breast cancer. N Engl J Med 1978;298(22): 1223-1228.
68. Harvey JM, Clark GM, Osborne CK, Allred DC. Estrogen receptor status by immunohistochemistry is superior to the ligand-binding assay for predicting response to adjuvant endocrine therapy in breast cancer. J Clin Oncol 1999;17(5):1474-1481.
69. Hopp TA, Weiss HL, Parra IS, et al. Low levels of estrogen receptor beta protein predict resistance to tamoxifen therapy in breast cancer. Clin Cancer Res 2004;10(22):7490-7499.
70. Pettersson K, Gustafsson JA. Role of estrogen receptor beta in estrogen action. Annu Rev Physiol 2001;63:165-192.
71. Paik S, Shak S, Tang G, et al. A multigene assay to predict recurrence of tamoxifen-treated, node-negative breast cancer. N Engl J Med 2004;351:2817-2826.
72. Paik S, Shak S, Tang G, et al. A multigene assay to predict recurrence of tamoxifen-treated, node-negative breast cancer. N Engl J Med 2004;351(27):2817-2826.
73. Peethambaram PP, Ingle JN, Suman VJ, et al. Randomized trial of diethylstilbestrol vs. tamoxifen in postmenopausal women with metastatic breast cancer. An updated analysis. Breast Cancer Res Treat 1999;54(2):117-122.
74. Shou J, Massarweh S, Osborne CK, et al. Mechanisms of tamoxifen resistance: increased estrogen receptor-*HER2/Neu* cross-talk in ER/*HER2*-positive breast cancer. J Natl Cancer Inst 2004;96(12): 926-935.
75. Shupnik MA. Crosstalk between steroid receptors and the c-Src-receptor tyrosine kinase pathways: implications for cell proliferation. Oncogene. 2004;23(48):7979-7989.
76. Bundred N. Preclinical and clinical experience with fulvestrant (Faslodex) in postmenopausal women with hormone receptor-positive advanced breast cancer. Cancer Invest 2005;23(2): 173-181.
77. Brueggemeier RW, Hackett JC, Diaz-Cruz ES. Aromatase inhibitors in the treatment of breast cancer. Endocr Rev 2005;26(3): 331-345.
78. Geisler J, Lonning PE. Endocrine effects of aromatase inhibitors and inactivators in vivo: review of data and method limitations. J Steroid Biochem Mol Biol 2005;95(1-5):75-81.
79. Eastell R, Hannon R. Long-term effects of aromatase inhibitors on bone. J Steroid Biochem Mol Biol 2005;95(1-5):151-154.
80. Goodwin PJ., Ennis M, Pritchard KI, et al. Risk of menopause during the first year after breast cancer diagnosis. J Clin Oncol 1999;17(8):2365-2370.
81. Smith I E, Dowsett M, Yap YS, et al. Adjuvant aromatase inhibitors for early breast cancer after chemotherapy-induced amenorrhoea: caution and suggested guidelines. J Clin Oncol 2006;24(16): 2444-2447.
82. Rutqvist LE. Adjuvant endocrine therapy. Baillieres Best Pract Res Clin Endocrinol Metab 2004;18(1):81-95.
83. Hughes LL, Gray RJ, Solin LJ; Eastern Cooperative Oncology Group, Southwest Oncology Group, et al. Efficacy of radiotherapy for ovarian ablation: results of a breast intergroup study. Cancer. 2004;101(5):969-972.
84. Ellis MJ. Neoadjuvant endocrine therapy for breast cancer: more questions than answers. J Clin Oncol 2005;23(22):4842-4844.
85. Early Breast Cancer Trialists' Collaborative Group. Tamoxifen for early breast cancer: an overview of the randomised trials. Lancet 1998;351(9114):1451-1467.
86. Ferno M, Stal O, Baldetorp B, et al. Results of two or five years of adjuvant tamoxifen correlated to steroid receptor and S-phase levels. South Sweden Breast Cancer Group, and South-East Sweden Breast Cancer Group. Breast Cancer Res Treat 2000;59(1):69-76.
87. Fisher B, Dignam J, Bryant J, et al. 1996. Five versus more than five years of tamoxifen therapy for breast cancer patients with negative lymph nodes and estrogen receptor–positive tumors. J Natl Cancer Inst 88(21):1529-1542.
88. Stewart HJ, Prescott RJ, Forrest AP. Scottish adjuvant tamoxifen trial: a randomized study updated to 15 years. J Natl Cancer Inst 2001;93(6):456-462.
89. Santen RJ. Long-term tamoxifen therapy: can an antagonist become an agonist? J Clin Endocrinol Metab 1996;81(6): 2027-2029.
90. Winer EP, Hudis C, Burstein HJ, et al. American Society of Clinical Oncology technology assessment on the use of aromatase inhibitors as adjuvant therapy for postmenopausal women with hormone receptor–positive breast cancer: status report J Clin Oncol 2005;23(3):619-629.
91. Gutierrez MC, Detre S, Johnston S, et al. Molecular changes in tamoxifen-resistant breast cancer: relationship between estrogen receptor, HER-2, and p38 mitogen–activated protein kinase. J Clin Oncol 2005;23(11):2469-2476.
92. Howell A, Robertson JF, Abram P, et al. Comparison of fulvestrant versus tamoxifen for the treatment of advanced breast cancer in postmenopausal women previously untreated with endocrine therapy: a multinational, double-blind, randomized trial. J Clin Oncol 2004;22(9):1605-1613.
93. Bonneterre J, Thurlimann B, Robertson JF, et al. Anastrozole versus tamoxifen as first-line therapy for advanced breast cancer in 668 postmenopausal women: results of the Tamoxifen or Arimidex Randomized Group Efficacy and Tolerability study. J Clin Oncol 2000;18(22):3748-3757.
94. Nabholtz JM, Buzdar A, Pollak M, et al. Anastrozole is superior to tamoxifen as first-line therapy for advanced breast cancer in postmenopausal women: results of a North American multicenter randomized trial. Arimidex Study Group. J Clin Oncol 2000;18(22): 3758-3767.
95. Mouridsen H, Gershanovich M, Sun Y, et al. Phase III study of letrozole versus tamoxifen as first-line therapy of advanced breast

cancer in postmenopausal women: analysis of survival and update of efficacy from the International Letrozole Breast Cancer Group. J Clin Oncol 2003;21(11):2101-2109.

96. Cuzick J, Buzdar A, Baum M, et al. Adjuvant use of anastrozole in breast cancer. J Clin Oncol 2004;22(8):1524-1525.
97. Buzdar AU. Phase III study of letrozole versus tamoxifen as first-line therapy of advanced breast cancer in postmenopausal women: analysis of survival and update of efficacy from the international letrozole breast cancer group. J Clin Oncol 2004;22(15):3199-200.
98. Milla-Santos A, Milla L, Portella J, et al. Anastrozole versus tamoxifen as first-line therapy in postmenopausal patients with hormone-dependent advanced breast cancer: a prospective, randomized, phase III study. Am J Clin Oncol 2003;26(3):317-322.
99. Nabholtz JM, Bonneterre J, Buzdar A, et al. Anastrozole (Arimidex) versus tamoxifen as first-line therapy for advanced breast cancer in postmenopausal women: survival analysis and updated safety results. Eur J Cancer 2003;39(12):1684-1689.
100. Bonneterre J, Buzdar A, Nabholtz JM, et al. Anastrozole is superior to tamoxifen as first-line therapy in hormone receptor positive advanced breast carcinoma. Cancer 2001;92(9):2247-2258.
101. Geisler J, Haynes B, Anker G, et al. Influence of letrozole and anastrozole on total body aromatization and plasma estrogen levels in postmenopausal breast cancer patients evaluated in a randomized, cross-over study. J Clin Oncol 2002;20:751-757.
102. Thurlimann B, Robertson JF, Nabholtz JM, and Arimidex Study Group. Efficacy of tamoxifen following anastrozole (Arimidex) compared with anastrozole following tamoxifen as first-line treatment for advanced breast cancer in postmenopausal women. Eur J Cancer 2003;39(16):2310-2317.
103. Goetz MP, Knox SK, Suman V, et al. The impact of cytochrome P450 2D6 metabolism in women receiving adjuvant tamoxifen. Breast Cancer Res Treat 2007;101:113-121.
104. Jin Y, Desta Z, Stearns V, et al. CYP2D6 genotype, antidepressant use, and tamoxifen metabolism during adjuvant breast cancer treatment. J Natl Cancer Inst 2005;97(1):30-39.
105. Jakesz R, Jonat W, Gnant M, et al. Switching of postmenopausal women with endocrine-responsive early breast cancer to anastrozole after 2 years' adjuvant tamoxifen: combined results of ABCSG trial 8 and ARNO 95 trial. Lancet 2005;366(9484):455-462.
106. Lonning PE, Taylor PD, Anker G, et al. High-dose estrogen treatment in postmenopausal breast cancer patients heavily exposed to endocrine therapy. Breast Cancer Res Treat 2001;67(2):111-116.
107. Lewis JS, Osipo C, Meeke K, and Jordan VC. Estrogen-induced apoptosis in a breast cancer model resistant to long-term estrogen withdrawal. J Steroid Biochem Mol Biol 2005;94(1-3):131-141.
108. Early Breast Cancer Trialists' Collaborative Group. Ovarian ablation in early breast cancer: overview of the randomised trials. Lancet 1996;348(9036):1189-1196.
109. Davidson NE, O'Neill AM, Vukov AM, et al. Chemoendocrine therapy for premenopausal women with axillary lymph node-positive, steroid hormone receptor-positive breast cancer: results from INT 0101 (E5188). J Clin Oncol 2005;23(25):5973-5982.
110. Taylor CW, Green S, Dalton WS, et al. Multicenter randomized clinical trial of goserelin versus surgical ovariectomy in premenopausal patients with receptor-positive metastatic breast cancer: an intergroup study. J Clin Oncol 1998;16(3):994-999.
111. Boccardo F, Rubagotti A, Perrotta A, et al. Ovarian ablation versus goserelin with or without tamoxifen in preperimenopausal patients with advanced breast cancer: results of a multicentric Italian study. Ann Oncol 1994;5(4):337-342.
112. Kaufmann M, Jonat W, Blamey R, and Zoladex Early Breast Cancer Research Association (ZEBRA) Trialists' Group. Survival analyses from the ZEBRA study. Goserelin (Zoladex) versus CMF in premenopausal women with node-positive breast cancer. Eur J Cancer 2003;39(12):1711-1717.
113. Klijn JG, Blamey RW, Boccardo F, and Combined Hormone Agents Trialists' Group and the European Organization for Research and Treatment of Cancer. Combined tamoxifen and luteinizing hormone–releasing hormone (LHRH) agonist versus LHRH agonist alone in premenopausal advanced breast cancer: a meta-analysis of four randomized trials. J Clin Oncol 2001;19:343-353.
114. Dellapasqua S, Colleoni M, Gelber RD, Goldhirsch A. Adjuvant endocrine therapy for premenopausal women with early breast cancer. J Clin Oncol 2005;23(8):1736-1750.
115. Robertson JF, Blamey RW. The use of gonadotrophin-releasing hormone (GnRH) agonists in early and advanced breast cancer in pre- and perimenopausal women. Eur J Cancer 2003;39(7):861-869.
116. Boccardo F, Rubagotti A, Amoroso D, et al. Cyclophosphamide, methotrexate, and fluorouracil versus tamoxifen plus ovarian suppression as adjuvant treatment of estrogen receptor-positive pre-/perimenopausal breast cancer patients: results of the Italian Breast Cancer Adjuvant Study Group 02 randomized trial. J Clin Oncol 2000;18(14):2718-2727.
117. Castiglione-Gertsch M, O'Neill A, Price KN, and International Breast Cancer Study Group. Adjuvant chemotherapy followed by goserelin versus either modality alone for premenopausal lymph node-negative breast cancer: a randomized trial. J Natl Cancer Inst 2003;95(24):1833-1846.
118. Pagani O, O'Neill A, Castiglione M, et al. Prognostic impact of amenorrhoea after adjuvant chemotherapy in premenopausal breast cancer patients with axillary node involvement: results of the International Breast Cancer Study Group (IBCSG) Trial VI. Eur J Cancer 1998;34(5):632-640.
119. Bianco AR, Del Mastro L, Gallo C, et al. Prognostic role of amenorrhea induced by adjuvant chemotherapy in premenopausal patients with early breast cancer. Br J Cancer 1991;63(5):799-803.
120. Early Breast Cancer Trialists' Collaborative Group. Effects of chemotherapy and hormonal therapy for early breast cancer on recurrence and 15-year survival: an overview of the randomised trials. Lancet 2005;365(9472):1687-1717.
121. Albain KS, Green SJ, Ravdin PM, et al. Adjuvant chemohormonal therapy for primary breast cancer should be sequential instead of concurrent. Proc Am Soc Clin Oncol 2002;21: (abstr 143).
122. Albain K, Barlow W, O'Malley F, et al.: Concurrent (CAFT) versus sequential (CAF-T) chemohormonal therapy (cyclophosphamide, doxorubicin, 5-fluorouracil, tamoxifen) versus T alone for postmenopausal, node-positive, estrogen (ER) and/or progesterone (PgR) receptor-positive breast cancer: mature outcomes and new biologic correlates on phase III intergroup trial 0100 (SWOG-8814). [Abstract] Breast Cancer Res Treat 88(Suppl 1):A-37, 2004.
123. Albain KS. Do all patients with endocrine-responsive early breast cancer need adjuvant chemotherapy before endocrine treatment? Breast 2005;14(suppl):S9-S10.
124. Goldhirsch A, Glick JH, Gelber RD, et al. Meeting highlights: International Consensus Panel on the Treatment of Primary Breast Cancer. Seventh International Conference on Adjuvant Therapy of Primary Breast Cancer. J Clin Oncol 2001;19:3817-3827.
125. Dixon JM, Renshaw L, Bellamy C, et al. The effects of neoadjuvant anastrozole (Arimidex) on tumor volume in postmenopausal women with breast cancer: a randomized, double-blind, single-center study. Clin Cancer Res 2000;6(6):2229-2235.
126. Eiermann W, Paepke S, Appfelstaedt J, et al. Preoperative treatment of postmenopausal breast cancer patients with letrozole: a randomized double-blind multicenter study. Ann Oncol 2001;12(11):1527-1532.
127. Smith IE, Dowsett M, Ebbs SR, et al. Neoadjuvant treatment of postmenopausal breast cancer with anastrozole, tamoxifen, or both in combination: the Immediate Preoperative Anastrozole, Tamoxifen, or Combined with Tamoxifen (IMPACT) multicenter double-blind randomized trial. J Clin Oncol 2005;23(22):5108-5116.
128. Romond EH, Perez EA, Bryant J, et al. Trastuzumab plus adjuvant chemotherapy for operable *HER2*-positive breast cancer. N Engl J Med 2005;353(16):1673-1684.
129. Guidelines Committee. National Comprehensive Cancer Center Network Practice Guidelines, Breast Cancer 2007. Available at http://nccn.org/professionals/physician_gls/PDF/breast.pdf (accessed August 24, 2007).
130. Boccardo F, Rubagotti A, Amoroso D, et al. Sequential tamoxifen and aminoglutethimide versus tamoxifen alone in the adjuvant treatment of postmenopausal breast cancer patients: results of an Italian cooperative study. J Clin Oncol 2001;19:4209-4215.
131. Fisher B, Jeong JH, Bryant J, et al. Treatment of lymph-node-negative, oestrogen-receptor-positive breast cancer: long-term findings from National Surgical Adjuvant Breast and Bowel Project randomised clinical trials. Lancet 2004;364(9437):858-868.

132. Fisher B, Dignam J, Tan-Chiu E, et al. Prognosis and treatment of patients with breast tumors of one centimeter or less and negative axillary lymph nodes. J Natl Cancer Inst 2001;93(2):112-120.
133. Fisher B, Dignam J, Wolmark N, et al. Tamoxifen in treatment of intraductal breast cancer: National Surgical Adjuvant Breast and Bowel Project B-24 randomised controlled trial. Lancet 1999;353(9169):1993-2000.
134. Allred DC, Bryant J, Land S, et al. Estrogen receptor expression as a predictive marker of the effectiveness of tamoxifen in the treatment of DCIS: findings from NSABP Protocol B-24. Breast Cancer Res Treat 2002;76(1):S36.
135. Mouridsen H, Gershanovich M, Sun Y, et al. Superior efficacy of letrozole versus tamoxifen as first-line therapy for postmenopausal women with advanced breast cancer: results of a phase III study of the International Letrozole Breast Cancer Group. J Clin Oncol 2001;19:2596-2606.
136. Harris JR, Lippman ME, Morrow M, Osborne CK. Diseases of the Breast, ed 3. Philadelphia: Lippincott Williams & Wilkins, 2004.
137. Santen R, Pritchard K, Burger H. The consensus conference on treatment of estrogen deficiency symptoms in women surviving breast cancer. Obstet Gynecol Surv 1998;53(10 suppl):S1-S83.
138. The Hormone Foundation, Canadian Breast Cancer Research Initiative, National Cancer Institute of Canada, Endocrine Society, and the University of Virginia Cancer Center and Woman's Place. Treatment of estrogen deficiency symptoms in women surviving breast cancer. J Clin Endocrinol Metab 1998;83(6):1993-2000.
139. Holmberg L, Anderson H, and HABITS Steering and Data Monitoring committees. HABITS (hormonal replacement therapy after breast cancer—is it safe?), a randomised comparison: trial stopped. Lancet 2004;363(9407):453-455.
140. von Schoultz E, Rutqvist LE, and Stockholm Breast Cancer Study Group. Menopausal hormone therapy after breast cancer: the Stockholm randomized trial. J Natl Cancer Inst 2005;97(7): 533-535.
141. Loprinzi CL, Kugler JW, Sloan, JA. Randomized phase III controlled trial of venlafaxine in the management of hot flashes. Lancet 2000;356:2059-2063.
142. Pandya KJ, Morrow GR, Roscoe JA, et al. Gabapentin for hot flashes in 420 women with breast cancer: a randomised double-blind placebo-controlled trial. Lancet 2005;366(9488): 818-824.
143. Shumaker SA, Legault C, Kuller L, et al. Conjugated equine estrogens and incidence of probable dementia and mild cognitive impairment in postmenopausal women: Women's Health Initiative Memory Study. JAMA 2004;291(24):2947-2958.
144. Weiss JR, Moysich KB, Swede H. Epidemiology of male breast cancer. Cancer Epidemiol Biomarkers Prev 2005;14(1):20-26.
145. Boyd,J. Genetic basis of familial endometrial cancer: is there more to learn? J Clin Oncol 2005;23(21):4570-4573.
146. Liehr JG. Is estradiol a genotoxic mutagenic carcinogen? Endocr Rev 2000;21(1):40-54.
147. Pike MC, Ross RK. Progestins and menopause: epidemiological studies of risks of endometrial and breast cancer. Steroids.2000; 65(10-11):659-664.
148. Beresford SA, Weiss NS, Voigt LF, McKnight B. Risk of endometrial cancer in relation to use of oestrogen combined with cyclic progestagen therapy in postmenopausal women. Lancet 1997; 349(9050):458-461.
149. Amant F, Moerman P, Neven P, et al. Endometrial cancer. Lancet 2005;366(9484):491-505.
150. Beral V, Bull D, Reeves G, Million Women Study Collaborators. Endometrial cancer and hormone-replacement therapy in the Million Women Study. Lancet 2005;365(9470):1543-1551.
151. Anderson GL, Judd HL, Kaunitz AM, et al, and Women's Health Initiative Investigators. Effects of estrogen plus progestin on gynecologic cancers and associated diagnostic procedures: the Women's Health Initiative randomized trial. JAMA 2003;290(13): 1739-1748.
152. Pike MC, Peters RK, Cozen W, et al. Estrogen-progestin replacement therapy and endometrial cancer. J Natl Cancer Inst 1997;89(15):1110-1116.
153. Erkkola R, Kumento U, Lehmuskoski S, et al. No increased risk of endometrial hyperplasia with fixed long-cycle oestrogen-progestogen therapy after five years. J Br Menopause Soc 2004;10(1): 9-13.
154. Martino S, Cauley JA, Barrett-Connor E, and CORE Investigators. Continuing Outcomes Relevant to Evista: breast cancer incidence in postmenopausal osteoporotic women in a randomized trial of raloxifene. J Natl Cancer Inst 2004;96(23):1751-1761.
155. Ehrlich CE, Young PC, Stehman FB, et al. Steroid receptors and clinical outcome in patients with adenocarcinoma of the endometrium. Am J Obstet Gynecol 1988;158(4):796-807.
156. Lentz SS, Brady MF, Major FJ, et al. High-dose megestrol acetate in advanced or recurrent endometrial carcinoma: a Gynecologic Oncology Group Study. J Clin Oncol 1996;14(2):357-361.
157. Thigpen JT, Brady MF, Alvarez RD, et al. Oral medroxyprogesterone acetate in the treatment of advanced or recurrent endometrial carcinoma: a dose-response study by the Gynecologic Oncology Group. J Clin Oncol 1999;17(6):1736-1744.
158. Barakat RR, Bundy BN Spirtos NM et al. A prospective randomized double blind trial of estrogen replacement therapy vs. placebo in women with stage I or II endometrial cancer: a Gynecologic Oncology Group study. Proceedings of the 35th Annual meeting of the Society of Gynecol Oncol. J Clin Oncol 2006;24:587-592.
159. Cooperberg MR, Broering JM, Litwin MS, et al, and CaPSURE Investigators. The contemporary management of prostate cancer in the United States: lessons from the cancer of the prostate strategic urologic research endeavor (CapSURE), a national disease registry. J Urol 2004;171(4):1393-1401.
160. McLellan DL, Norman RW. Hereditary aspects of prostate cancer. CMAJ 1995;153(7):895-900.
161. Nelson WG, De Marzo AM, Isaacs WB. Prostate cancer. N Engl J Med 2003;349(4):366-381.
162. Kirchhoff T, Kauff ND, Mitra N, et al. *BRCA* mutations and risk of prostate cancer in Ashkenazi Jews. Clin Cancer Res 2004;10(9): 2918-2921.
163. Tomlins SA, Rhodes DR, Perner S, et al. Recurrent fusion of TMPRSS2 and ETS transcription factor genes in prostate cancer. Science 2005;310(5748):644-648.
164. Gronberg H. Prostate cancer epidemiology. Lancet 2003;361(9360): 859-864.
165. Griffiths K, Morton MS, Denis L. Certain aspects of molecular endocrinology that relate to the influence of dietary factors on the pathogenesis of prostate cancer. Eur Urol 1999;35(5-6): 443-455.
166. Chan JM, Stampfer MJ, Giovannucci EL. What causes prostate cancer? A brief summary of the epidemiology. Semin Cancer Biol 1998;8(4):263-273.
167. Yang CR, Ou YC, Ho HC. Unsuspected prostate carcinoma and prostatic intraepithelial neoplasm in Taiwanese patients undergoing cystoprastatectomy. Mol Urol 1999;3:33-39.
168. Shin M, Takayama H, Nonomura N, et al. Extent and zonal distribution of prostatic intraepithelial neoplasia in patients with prostatic carcinoma in Japan: analysis of whole-mounted prostatectomy specimens. Prostate 2000;42(2):81-87.
169. de la Torre M, Haggman M, Brandstedt S, Busch C. Prostatic intraepithelial neoplasia and invasive carcinoma in total prostatectomy specimens: distribution, volumes and DNA ploidy. Br J Urol 1993;72(2):207-213.
170. Santner SJ, Albertson B, Zhang GY, et al. Comparative rates of androgen production and metabolism in caucasian and Chinese subjects. J Clin Endocrinol Metab 1998;83(6):2104-2109.
171. Thompson IM, Goodman PJ, Tangen CM, et al. The influence of finasteride on the development of prostate cancer. N Engl J Med 2003;349(3):215-224.
172. Frankel S, Smith GD, Donovan J, Neal D. Screening for prostate cancer. Lancet 2003;361(9363):1122-1128.
173. Carter HB, Pearson JD. Prostate-specific antigen velocity and repeated measures of prostate-specific antigen. Urol Clin North Am 1997;24(2):333-338.
174. Catalona WJ, Smith DS, Wolfert RL, et al. Evaluation of percentage of free serum prostate-specific antigen to improve specificity of prostate cancer screening. JAMA 1995;274(15):1214-1220.
175. Eggener SE, Roehl KA, Catalona WJ. Predictors of subsequent prostate cancer in men with a prostate specific antigen of 2.6 to 4.0 ng/mL and an initially negative biopsy. J Urol 2005;174(2): 500-504.
176. Chang JJ, Shinohara K, Hovey RM, et al. Prospective evaluation of systematic sextant transition zone biopsies in large prostates for cancer detection. Urology 1998;52(1):89-93.

177. Carroll PR, Lee KL, Fuks Z, Kantoff P. Cancer of the prostate. In DeVita VT, Hellman S, Rosenberg SA (eds). Cancer: Principles and Practice of Oncology. Philadelphia: Lippincott Williams & Wilkins, 2001:1418-1479.
178. Denis LJ, Griffiths K. Endocrine treatment in prostate cancer. Semin Surg Oncol 2000;18(1):52-74.
179. Taplin ME, Rajeshkumar B, Halabi S, et al. Androgen receptor mutations in androgen-independent prostate cancer: Cancer and Leukemia Group B Study 9663. J Clin Oncol 2003;21(14): 2673-2678.
180. Taplin ME, Bubley GJ, Ko YJ, et al. Selection for androgen receptor mutations in prostate cancers treated with androgen antagonist. Cancer Res 1999;59(11):2511-2515.
181. Richie JP. Anti-androgens and other hormonal therapies for prostate cancer. Urology 1999;54(6A Suppl):15-18.
182. Small EJ, Srinivas S. The antiandrogen withdrawal syndrome. Experience in a large cohort of unselected patients with advanced prostate cancer. Cancer 1995;76:1428-1434.
183. Small EJ, Vogelzang NJ. Second-line hormonal therapy for advanced prostate cancer: a shifting paradigm. J Clin Oncol 1997; 15(1):382-388.
184. Miyamoto H, Altuwaijri S, Cai Y, et al. Inhibition of the Akt, cyclooxygenase-2, and matrix metalloproteinase-9 pathways in combination with androgen deprivation therapy: potential therapeutic approaches for prostate cancer. Mol Carcinog 2005; 44(1):1-10.
185. Partin AW, Mangold LA, Lamm DM, et al. Contemporary update of prostate cancer staging nomograms (Partin Tables) for the new millennium. Urology 2001;58(6):843-848.
186. Guideline Panel. Practice Guidelines in Oncology: Prostate Cancer, 2005. PDF available at http://www.nccn.org/professionals/physician_gls/PDF/prostate.pdf (accessed March 1, 2007).
187. Bill-Axelson A, Holmberg L, Ruutu M, et al. Radical prostatectomy versus watchful waiting in early prostate cancer. N Engl J Med 2005;352(19):1977-1984.
188. Zagars GK, Pollack A, Smith LG. Conventional external-beam radiation therapy alone or with androgen ablation for clinical stage III (T3, NX/N0, M0) adenocarcinoma of the prostate. Int J Radiat Oncol Biol Phys 1999;44(4):809-819.
189. Laverdiere J, Gomez JL, Cusan L, et al. Beneficial effect of combination hormonal therapy administered prior and following external beam radiation therapy in localized prostate cancer. Int J Radiat Oncol Biol Phys 1997;37(2):247-252.
190. Pilepich MV, Winter K, Lawton CA, et al. Androgen suppression adjuvant to definitive radiotherapy in prostate carcinoma—long-term results of phase III RTOG 85-31. Int J Radiat Oncol Biol Phys 2005;61(5):1285-1290.
191. Pollack A, Zagars GK. Androgen ablation in addition to radiation therapy for prostate cancer: is there true benefit? Semin Radiat Oncol 1998;8(2):95-106.
192. Horwitz EM, Winter K, Hanks GE, et al. Subset analysis of RTOG 85-31 and 86-10 indicates an advantage for long-term vs. short-term adjuvant hormones for patients with locally advanced nonmetastatic prostate cancer treated with radiation therapy. Int J Radiat Oncol Biol Phys 2001;49(4):947-956.
193. Ludgate CM, Lim JT, Wilson AG, et al. Neoadjuvant hormone therapy and external beam radiation for localized prostate cancer: Vancouver Island Cancer Centre experience. Can J Urol 2000;7(1):937-943.
194. Horwitz EM, Hanlon AL, Hanks GE. Update on the treatment of prostate cancer with external beam irradiation. Prostate 1998;37(3):195-206.
195. Shipley WU, Thames HD, Sandler HM, et al. Radiation therapy for clinically localized prostate cancer: a multi-institutional pooled analysis. JAMA 1999;281(17):1598-1604.
196. Zelefsky MJ, Leibel SA, Gaudin PB, et al. Dose escalation with three-dimensional conformal radiation therapy affects the outcome in prostate cancer. Int J Radiat Oncol Biol Phys 1998;41(3):491-500.
197. Seidenfeld J, Samson J, Aronson N, et al. Relative effectiveness and cost-effectiveness of methods of androgen suppression in the treatment of advanced prostate cancer. Evid Rep Technol Assess (Summ) 1999;(4):i-x, 1-246, 11-36, passim.
198. Seidenfeld J, Samson DJ, Hasselblad V, et al. Single-therapy androgen suppression in men with advanced prostate cancer: a systematic review and meta-analysis. Ann Intern Med.2000;132(7): 566-77.
199. Messing EM, Manola J, Sarosdy M, et al. Immediate hormonal therapy compared with observation after radical prostatectomy and pelvic lymphadenectomy in men with node-positive prostate cancer. N Engl J Med 1999;341(24):1781-1788.
200. The Medical Research Council Prostate Cancer Working Party Investigators Group. Immediate versus deferred treatment for advanced prostatic cancer: initial results of the Medical Research Council Trial. Br J Urol 1997;79(2):235-246.
201. Kirk D. Timing and choice of androgen ablation. Prostate Cancer Prostatic Dis 2004;7(3):217-22.
202. Studer UE, Hauri D, Hanselmann S, et al. Immediate versus deferred hormonal treatment for patients with prostate cancer who are not suitable for curative local treatment: results of the randomized trial SAKK 08/88.[erratum appears in J Clin Oncol 2005;23(4):936]. J Clin Oncol 2004;22(20):4109-4118.
203. Zincke H, Bergstralh EJ, Larson-Keller JJ, et al. Stage D1 prostate cancer treated by radical prostatectomy and adjuvant hormonal treatment. Evidence for favorable survival in patients with DNA diploid tumors. Cancer. 1992;70(1 Suppl):311-323.
204. Seay TM, Blute ML, Zincke H. Long-term outcome in patients with pTxN$^+$ adenocarcinoma of prostate treated with radical prostatectomy and early androgen ablation. J Urol 1998;159(2): 357-364.
205. Wilt T, Nair B, MacDonald R, Rutks I. Early versus deferred androgen suppression in the tratment of advanced prostate cancer. Cochrane Database Syst Rev 2002;(1):CD))3506
206. Loblaw DA, Mendelson DS, Talcott JA, et al. American Society of Clinical Oncology recommendations for the initial hormonal management of androgen-sensitive metastatic, recurrent, or progressive prostate cancer.[erratum appears in J Clin Oncol. 2004; 22(21):4435]. J Clin Oncol 2004;22(14):2927-2941.
207. Kupelian PA, Katcher J, Levin HS, Klein EA. Stage T1-2 prostate cancer: a multivariate analysis of factors affecting biochemical and clinical failures after radical prostatectomy. Int J Radiat Oncol Biol Phys 1997;37(5):1043-1052.
208. Sharifi N, Gulley JL, Dahut WL. Androgen deprivation therapy for prostate cancer. JAMA 2005;294(2):238-244.
209. Scher HI. Prostate carcinoma: defining therapeutic objectives and improving overall outcomes. Cancer 2003;97(3 suppl):758-771.
210. Nieh PT. Withdrawal phenomenon with the antiandrogen casodex. J Urol 1995;153(3 Pt 2):1070-1072; discussion 1072-1073.
211. Bergan RC, Reed E, Myers CE, et al. A Phase II study of high-dose tamoxifen in patients with hormone-refractory prostate cancer. Clin Cancer Res 1999;5(9):2366-2373.
212. Saad F, Karakiewicz P, Perrotte P. The role of bisphosphonates in hormone-refractory prostate cancer. World J Urol 2005;23(1): 14-18.
213. Pienta KJ, Smith DC. Advances in prostate cancer chemotherapy: a new era begins. CA Cancer J Clin 2005;55(5):300-318.
214. Iversen P, Tyrrell CJ, Kaisary AV, et al. Bicalutamide monotherapy compared with castration in patients with nonmetastatic locally advanced prostate cancer: 6.3 years of followup. J Urol 2000; 164(5):1579-582.
215. Bilezikian JP. The role of estrogens in male skeletal development. Reprod Fertil Devel 2001;13(4):253-259.
216. Iversen P, Tveter K, Varenhorst E. Randomised study of Casodex 50 MG monotherapy vs orchidectomy in the treatment of metastatic prostate cancer. The Scandinavian Casodex Cooperative Group. Scand J Urol Nephrol 1996;30(2):93-98.
217. Samson D., Seidenfeld J, Schmitt B, et al. Systematic review and meta-analysis of monotherapy compared with combined androgen blockade for patients with advanced prostate carcinoma. Cancer 2002;95(2):361-376.
218. Tyrrell CJ, Kaisary AV, Iversen P, et al. A randomised comparison of 'Casodex' (bicalutamide) 150 mg monotherapy versus castration in the treatment of metastatic and locally advanced prostate cancer. Eur Urol 1998;33(5):447-456.
219. Fair WR, Rabbani F, Bastar A. Neoadjuvant hormone therapy before radical prostatectomy: update on the Memorial Sloan-Kettering Cancer Center trials. Molec Urol 1999;3, 253-260.
220. Wirth M, Tyrrell C, Delaere K, et al. Bicalutamide ('Casodex') 150 mg in addition to standard care in patients with nonmetastatic prostate cancer: updated results from a randomised double-blind

phase III study (median follow-up 5.1 y) in the early prostate cancer programme. Prostate Cancer Prostatic Dis 2005;8(2): 194-200.
221. Prostate Cancer Trialists' Collaborative Group. Maximum androgen blockade in advanced prostate cancer: an overview of the randomised trials. Lancet 2000;355(9214):1491-1498.
222. Eisenberger MA, Blumenstein BA, Crawford ED, et al. Bilateral orchiectomy with or without flutamide for metastatic prostate cancer. N Engl J Med 1998;339(15):1036-1042.
223. Bayoumi AM, Brown AD, Garber AM. Cost-effectiveness of androgen suppression therapies in advanced prostate cancer. J Natl Cancer Inst 2000;92(21):1731-1739.
224. Bruchovsky N, Klotz LH, Sadar M, et al. Intermittent androgen suppression for prostate cancer: Canadian Prospective Trial and related observations. Molec Urol 2000;4(3):191-199.
225. Carroll PR, Altwein J, Brawley O, et al: Management of disseminated prostate cancer. In Denis L, Bartsch G, Khoury S et al (eds). Prostate Cancer: 3rd International Consultation on Prostate Cancer—Paris. Paris: Health Publications, 2003:249–284.
226. Cummings SR, Eckert S, Krueger KA, et al. The effect of raloxifene on risk of breast cancer in postmenopausal women: results from the MORE randomized trial. Multiple Outcomes of Raloxifene Evaluation. [erratum appears in JAMA 1999;282(22):2124]. JAMA 1999;281(23):2189-2197.
227. Sotiriou C, Neo SY, McShane LM, et al. Breast cancer classification and prognosis based on gene expression profiles from a population-based study. Proc Nat Acad Sci U S A 2003;100(18): 10393-10398.
228. Smith R, Sun Y, Garin A, et al, and the Letrozole International Breast Cancer Study Group. Femara (letrozole) showed significant improvement in efficacy over tamoxifen as first-line treatment in postmenopausal women with advanced breast cancer. Breast Cancer Res Treat 2000;64(1):27.
229. The ATAC Trialists' Group. Anastrozole alone or in combination with tamoxifen versus tamoxifen alone for adjuvant treatment of postmenopausal women with early breast cancer: first results of the ATAC randomised trial. Lancet 2002;359:2131-2139.
230. Goss PE, Strasser K. Aromatase inhibitors in the treatment and prevention of breast cancer. J Clin Oncol 2001;19:881-894.
231. Albertsen, PC, Hanley JA, Gleason DF, Barry MJ. Competing risk analysis of men aged 55 to 74 years at diagnosis managed conservatively for clinically localized prostate cancer. JAMA 1998;280(11): 975-880.

CHAPTER 43

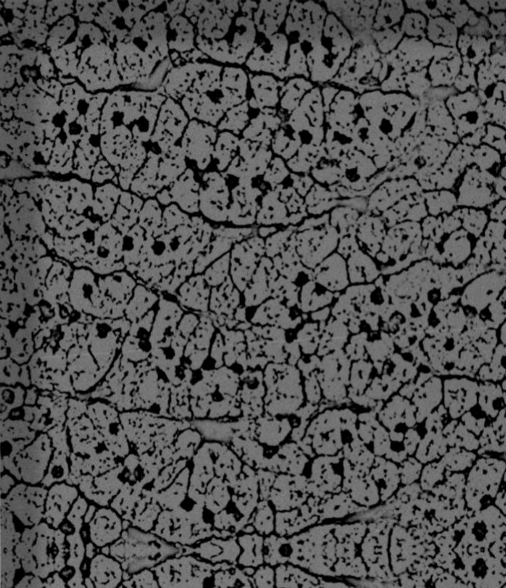

HUMORAL MANIFESTATIONS OF MALIGNANCY

Gordon J. Strewler

The syndrome of ectopic secretion of corticotropin (adrenocorticotropic hormone, ACTH) was first described by Brown in 1928 in a woman with bronchogenic carcinoma,[1] 4 years before Cushing's description of the clinical syndrome of corticotropin excess and before the relationship between the hormone and the clinical syndrome was recognized. In 1941, Albright proposed the idea that tumors can cause endocrine syndromes by secreting hormones inappropriately; he suggested that hypercalcemia in a patient with renal carcinoma might be due to production of parathyroid hormone (PTH) by the tumor.[2] Albright was led to this conclusion by the coexistence of hypercalcemia with hypophosphatemia (biochemical features of primary hyperparathyroidism) in a patient with a single bone metastasis.

In 1956, cases were reported in which hypercalcemia was cured by resection of the primary tumor,[3,4] supporting Albright's hypothesis that the neoplasm produced humoral hypercalcemia. Subsequently, Schwartz and colleagues[5] described the syndrome secretion of inappropriate vasopressin (antidiuretic hormone, ADH) in bronchogenic carcinoma. Meador and coworkers[6] described the ectopic corticotropin syndrome in lung carcinoma, and Liddle and colleagues[7] coined the term *ectopic hormone syndrome* to describe such situations.

Inappropriate Hormone Secretion in Malignancy

Common Features

Inappropriate secretion of peptide hormones is probably the most common cause of paraneoplastic syndromes. Although the manifestations vary widely, paraneoplastic hormonal syndromes have features that distinguish them from overproduction of hormones by endocrine glands (Table 43–1).

First, the secretion of hormones by extraglandular tumors is rarely suppressible. Tumor cells that secrete hormones typically do not possess the cellular machinery that allows regulation of hormone secretion. The most notable exception to this general rule is the secretion of corticotropin by carcinoid tumors of the lung or thymus. Corticotropin secretion by these tumors is often suppressible by glucocorticoids, with secretory dynamics that can be difficult to distinguish from those of corticotropic adenomas of the pituitary.

Second, because extraglandular tumors produce hormones relatively inefficiently, clinical syndromes of hormone excess become evident only in patients with advanced malignancies.

TABLE 43–1 GENERAL CHARACTERISTICS OF PARANEOPLASTIC HORMONAL SYNDROMES

- Secretion of hormones is rarely suppressible.
- Clinical syndromes are usually associated with advanced malignancies.
- Hormones are not useful as tumor markers for nonendocrine tumors.
- Tumors can mimic syndromes of hormone excess by secreting a related peptide (e.g., insulin-like growth factor II, causing hypoglycemia).

TABLE 43–2 HORMONES PRODUCED BY TUMORS

Atrial natriuretic peptide
Calcitonin
Corticotropin (ACTH)
Corticotropin-releasing hormone
Endothelin
Erythropoietin
FGF23 (phosphatonin)
Growth hormone
Growth hormone–releasing hormone
Human chorionic gonadotropin (hCG)
Human placental lactogen (hPL)
Hypercalcemia factors
- 1,25-Dihydroxycholecalciferol (1,25(OH)$_2$D$_3$)
- Parathyroid hormone (PTH)
- PTH-related protein (PTHrP)
- Prostaglandins
- Tumor necrosis factor

Insulin
Insulin-like growth factor II (IGF-II)
Luteinizing hormone (LH)
Renin
Vasopressin
Other gut hormones
- Gastrin-releasing peptide
- Glucose-dependent insulinotropic peptide (gastrin inhibitory peptide)
- Motilin
- Pancreatic polypeptide
- Somatostatin
- Substance P
- Vasoactive intestinal peptide (VIP)

It is probably for this reason that hormones are disappointing as tumor markers.

Third, tumors often lack the ability to process peptide hormones normally and secrete large, incompletely processed forms of hormones with reduced biologic activity.

Finally, some malignant tumors mimic syndromes of hormone excess not by secreting the expected hormone but by secreting related hormones that mimic the biologic actions of the expected hormone. For example, non–islet cell tumors can cause hypoglycemia not by secreting insulin but by secreting the related peptide insulin-like growth factor II (IGF-II).[8] IGF-II does not ordinarily play a major role in glucose metabolism, but it has insulin-like activity and in large amounts causes hypoglycemia. Similarly, hypercalcemia in malignancy is a manifestation not of PTH excess but of an excess of parathyroid hormone–related protein (PTHrP). PTHrP resembles PTH and in most circumstances is a local regulator, but it acts as a hormone when it is released into the circulation by malignant tumors.

Ectopic versus Eutopic Secretion

The term *ectopic hormone secretion* is a misnomer. Ectopic means "out of place," implying secretion of a hormone by tissues that do not ordinarily do so, whereas hormones that are secreted by tumors are usually present in the nonmalignant precursor cells, albeit often in small amounts. For example, many of the hormones typically secreted by small cell lung carcinoma—vasopressin, calcitonin, and gastrin-releasing peptide (GRP)—are thought to be present in the neuroendocrine cells in the normal bronchial mucosa that are the probable precursors of the tumor. PTHrP is a normal product of the keratinocyte, the cell of origin of squamous carcinomas that cause humoral hypercalcemia by secreting PTHrP. Human chorionic gonadotropin (hCG), usually considered a placental hormone, is not under tight transcriptional control, and low levels of the hormone are detectable in a variety of other normal tissues, a finding that is in keeping with the occurrence of hCG secretion by many tumor types.[9]

Thus, most endocrine manifestations of malignancy are caused by eutopic secretion of hormones by cells that were previously programmed to secrete them. This feature has implications for the pathogenesis of the humoral manifestations of malignancy that are discussed later. As for nosology, the term *ectopic* is firmly ingrained and will not soon be abandoned, even though true ectopic secretion of hormones is rare.

Peptide versus Nonpeptide Hormones

Nonendocrine malignant tumors are capable of secreting most peptide hormones (Table 43–2), with some exceptions. Biologically active glycoprotein hormones—follicle-stimulating hormone (FSH), luteinizing hormone (LH), and thyrotropin (TSH)—are rarely produced by extrapituitary tumors. Although doing so necessitates expressing the genes for two subunits, glycosylating the subunits appropriately, and assembling the complete dimer to produce a biologically active hormone, the glycoprotein hormone hCG is commonly secreted by nontrophoblastic tumors, illustrating that the requisite machinery is present in nonpituitary cells.

Pituitary glycoprotein hormone synthesis is tightly controlled by a series of pituitary-specific transcription factors, whereas hCG is normally expressed at low levels in a variety of nontrophoblastic cells. In the same vein, extrapancreatic secretion of insulin is rare.[10,11] Although a few copies per cell of insulin messenger ribonucleic acid (mRNA) can be detected in many cells by sensitive polymerase chain reaction (PCR) methods, physiologic expression of the insulin gene is driven by transcription factors that are specific to the pancreatic beta cell, and these factors are rarely, if ever, expressed in other cell types. Thus, the propensity of a peptide hormone for secretion by extraglandular tumors may be a function of the tightness of its transcriptional suppression in normal extraglandular tissues.

Steroid and thyroid hormones are not secreted by extraglandular tumors, although they are occasionally produced by teratomas that contain glandular elements. Their synthesis requires an extended series of enzymatic steps that are not present in nonsteroidogenic tissues. In contrast, 1,25-dihydroxycholecalciferol (1,25(OH)$_2$D$_3$, also called 1,25-dihydroxyvitamin D$_3$) is secreted by lymphomas as well as macrophages resident in granulomas of sarcoidosis and other granulomatous disorders. In these tissues, the synthesis of 1,25(OH)$_2$D$_3$ requires a single enzymatic step, the 1α-hydroxylation of the circulating precursor, 25-hydroxycholecalciferol.

Cellular Basis of Ectopic Hormone Secretion

Why is the secretion of hormones by malignant neoplasms so commonplace? Random sets of genes could be de-repressed in the cancer cell, including genes that code for hormones. However, the association of tumors and hormone secretion is nonrandom, with certain tumors (e.g., lung carcinoma) characteristically secreting certain hormones (e.g., corticotropin or vasopressin). The *dedifferentiation hypothesis* posits a retrograde movement of tumor cells along the pathway of differentiation, leading to the expression of fetal proteins (e.g., α-fetoprotein and carcinoembryonic antigen [CEA]) or hormones that are normally formed in immature cells. This hypothesis would account for both the nonrandom nature of ectopic hormone secretion and the propensity for secretion of hormones that play a critical role in development, for example, IGF-II, PTHrP, and possibly GRP and other peptides of neuroendocrine cells. In addition, tumors often secrete other fetal proteins (carcinoembryonic antigen, α-fetoprotein). However, there is no compelling evidence for a generalized pattern of expression of primitive genes in tumor cells.

The *dysdifferentiation hypothesis* of Baylin and Mendelsohn[12] holds that epithelial malignancy is the result of clonal expansion of a particular cell type that occurs along a complex pathway of epithelial differentiation. This process might give rise to overexpression of a hormone either because of expansion of a normally rare population of committed cells or clonal expansion of a primitive cell type not normally present in the mature epithelium. It is now thought that tumors are often derived from tumor stem cells, which can give rise to heterogeneous populations of tumor cells because of epigenetic as well as genetic events.[13,14] In this view, dysdifferentiation is fundamental to the origins of cancer as well as inappropriate secretion of hormones.

In a few instances, an oncogenic event directly activates transcription of a hormone gene. Loss of the von Hippel-Lindau tumor suppressor gene *VHL,* normally involved in gene regulation by hypoxia, is associated with the development of cerebellar hemangioblastoma and renal carcinoma. Expression of the erythropoietin gene, a classic target for up-regulation by hypoxia, is directly activated by this oncogenic event.[15,16]

Secretion of a hormone might stimulate the growth of tumor cells by an autocrine or a paracrine mechanism, so that hormone secretion provides a growth advantage, leading to selective outgrowth of cells that secrete high levels of the hormone. One of the characteristic products of small cell lung carcinoma (SCLC) is GRP, the mammalian counterpart of the amphibian hormone bombesin. GRP fulfills criteria for being an autocrine growth factor in SCLC: It is secreted by tumor cells and can stimulate replication of the cells via specific receptors, and blockade of its action by neutralizing antibodies to GRP or peptide antagonists inhibits cell replication in vitro and tumor formation in vivo.[17,18] Endothelin-1 and its receptor are often coexpressed on tumor cells, and endothelin-1 is reported to have paracrine effects on tumor cell growth and angiogenesis; antagonists of the endothelin receptor are in clinical trials.[19] Prolactin and its receptor are expressed by breast cancer cells, although rarely, if ever, at high enough levels to raise serum prolactin levels, and an autocrine pathway has been described in which prolactin induces constitutive phosphorylation of *erbB-2* (Her/Neu), an oncogene that is important in growth of breast cancer.[20] IGF-II, the factor that is believed to cause hypoglycemia in non–islet cell tumors, is also a growth factor. However, there is no direct evidence for a role of IGF-II in the growth of these neoplasms.

Epigenetic events associated with tumorigenesis might activate the transcription of hormone genes. Demethylation of the proopiomelanocortin (POMC) promoter might also be involved in expression of corticotropin in neuroendocrine tumor cells.[21,22] Altered methylation of CpG islands appears to play a role in the expression of PTHrP in renal carcinoma, with undermethylation of the PTHrP promoter in tumors that express the gene.[23]

Thus, ectopic hormone production can be partly understood in the context of the determinants of tumor cell behavior generally. Nevertheless, why specific tumor types overexpress particular hormone genes and why overexpression occurs in some tumors of a given type (e.g., SCLC) and not others are questions that remain largely unanswered.

Neuroendocrine Cells and Hormone Secretion

Tumors that secrete corticotropin, vasopressin, calcitonin, gut peptides (GRP, somatostatin, vasoactive intestinal peptide [VIP]), and biogenic amines such as 5-hydroxytryptamine (5-HT) are characteristically of neuroendocrine cell origin. Neuroendocrine cells specialized for the production of peptide hormones and biogenic amines possess pathways for the rapid release of peptides or neurotransmitters in response to stimuli; such regulated pathways for protein secretion are distinct from the mechanism of constitutive secretion, which is ubiquitous in eukaryotic cells.

The most readily recognizable feature of the regulated pathway is the dense neurosecretory granule, which secretes peptides and amines.[24,25] The neurosecretory granule, which is involved in both the storage of hormones in concentrated form and the rapid release of these stores in response to stimulation, is recognizable histologically because it is electron dense and intensely argyrophilic, reflecting the dense, nearly crystalline packing of its contents.

The neurosecretory granule buds from the trans-Golgi network after it is packed with its peptide or neurotransmitter contents. Proteins on the surface of the neurosecretory granule, in the vesicular compartments from which the granule buds, and on the plasma membrane of neurosecretory cells collectively determine the properties of the regulated pathway of hormone secretion.[25] They are probably important in ectopic hormone secretion. In addition to stored hormones, the neuroendocrine granule contains one or more acidic proteins called *chromogranins,* which are released together with stored hormone and serve as additional neuroendocrine tumor markers, both in immunohistology and in the circulation. The chromogranins are highly conserved in evolution and play a role in the assembly of neurosecretory granules.[26]

The neurosecretory granules contain serine proteases called *prohormone convertases* (PCs), which process precursor proteins to their mature forms.[27] The prohormone convertase family is widely distributed in evolution, and several members of the family, such as furin, are localized in the trans-Golgi network and process a wide variety of proteins in the constitutive pathway. The two members of the family that occur mainly in neurosecretory granules, PC2 (subtilisin-like PC2 [SPC2]) and PC1/PC3 (subtilisin-like PC2 [SPC3]), have acidic pH optima and are dependent on calcium, suiting them for the environment of the neurosecretory granule. Both enzymes cleave their substrate peptides on the carboxyl-terminal side of polybasic residues, but they have slightly different specificities, and their different distribution in the pituitary accounts for the differences in processing of POMC in the anterior and intermediate pituitary lobes.

The prohormone convertases are important for our understanding of ectopic hormone secretion. Their levels in tumor cells account for the efficiency of precursor processing to mature and biologically active versions of peptide hormones, thus determining whether a given tumor produces a clinical syndrome of hormone excess. Further, they determine the pattern of peptides produced (e.g., from the polyhormone precursor POMC) and thus the nature of the clinical syndrome.

Neuroendocrine cells are scattered through the bronchial mucosa of the developing and mature lung and might function in development, in sensing hypoxia, and in the immune response.[28] They occur singly and in distinct innervated corpuscles referred to as neuroepithelial bodies. Subpopulations of the cells contain the peptides calcitonin, GRP, vasopressin, and leu-enkephalin, and some might also contain somatostatin, motilin, or pancreatic polypeptide. Neuroendocrine (enterochromaffin) cells are also scattered through the gastrointestinal mucosa and are found in other organs, such as the ovaries and the prostate gland. Some years ago, Pearce suggested that neuroendocrine cells, which he called *APUD cells* (*a*mine *p*recursor *u*ptake and *d*ecarboxylation), although widely scattered in many tissues, have a common origin in the neural crest and represent a *diffuse neuroendocrine system*, a third branch of the nervous system. Not all APUD cells are of neural crest origin, however; some arise from primitive endoderm.

Neuroendocrine tumors are typically deficient in the tumor suppressor genes *Rb1* and *Trp53* (which encodes p53); removal of these genes from lung epithelium generates SCLC.[29] Genetic experiments indicate that the Rb family inhibits neuroendocrine differentiation in normal lung epithelium.[30] Neuroendocrine cells in the gut and lung are specified by a set of basic helix-loop-helix (bHLH) transcription factors that are involved in determining neuronal fate in mammals and *Drosophila*.[31] Transient expression of the mouse achaete-scute homologue-1 *(mASH1)* is required for neurogenesis of autonomic and enteric neurons and adrenal chromaffin cells. Pulmonary neuroendocrine cells do not develop in mice deficient in mASH1, and forced expression of mASH1 induces metaplasia and cooperates with simian virus 40 (SV40) T antigen in tumorigenesis.[32] Neuroendocrine tumor cells such as SCLC cells express the human orthologue hASH1.[33]

Disruption of an inhibitory pathway might also lead to neuroendocrine cell expansion. *Drosophila* and vertebrate neurogenesis is characterized by lateral inhibition, a cell-cell interaction in which differentiating neuronal cells inhibit neuronal differentiation of their neighbors through actions of a transmembrane receptor, Notch, and the ligand Delta.[34] One of the chief targets of the inhibitory pathway is hairy-enhancer-of-split-1 (Hes-1), which inhibits the proneural genes neurogenin, neuroD, and ASH. Ablation of *Hes-1* leads to a marked increase in enteroendocrine cells,[31] and SCLC cells are characteristically deficient in Hes-1.[35]

Collectively, these data delineate a pathway of origin of neuroendocrine tumor cells and identify transcription factors that may be directly involved in up-regulating expression in neuroendocrine cells. However, examples of direct regulation of hormonal expression by such genes have not yet been adduced.

Criteria for Diagnosis of Ectopic Hormone Secretion

Criteria for the diagnosis of ectopic hormone secretion, arranged in increasing order of stringency, are summarized in Table 43–3. The association of a clinical syndrome of hormone excess with a neoplasm provokes a search for inappropriate plasma or urinary hormone levels. In many cases, the clinician performs suppression tests, because glandular hypersecretion of hormones is often suppressible, whereas the secretion of hormones by neoplasms is typically autonomous and nonsuppressible. In the usual clinical circumstance, the last step is to exclude other possible causal mechanisms for hormone excess.

TABLE 43–3 CRITERIA FOR DIAGNOSIS OF ECTOPIC HORMONE SECRETION

CLINICAL CRITERIA
A clinical syndrome of hormone excess is associated with a neoplasm.
Serum or urine levels of the hormone are inappropriately elevated.
The hormone level is not suppressible.
Other possible causal mechanisms are excluded.
The syndrome is reversed by resection of the tumor (rare).
RESEARCH CRITERIA
The hormone can be detected in tumor tissue.
Messenger RNA for the hormone is present in tumor tissue.
The hormone is secreted from tumor cells in culture.
There is an arteriovenous gradient for the hormone across the tumor.

The coincidental occurrence of an endocrine tumor and a cancer is not uncommon; for example, primary hyperparathyroidism can be present in a patient who also has cancer and can be detected with ease using modern assays for PTH. Occasionally, the presence of an ectopic hormone syndrome can be confirmed by showing that resection of the tumor reverses the clinical syndrome. Because such syndromes are typically late manifestations of widespread neoplasms, these opportunities are sadly rare.

The remaining criteria for ectopic hormone secretion are useful mainly for research purposes. The detection of a hormone in tumor tissue by immunoassay methods provides evidence that the tumor is a site of its production, although caution must be exercised because of the possibility of false-positive reactions in immunohistochemistry and radioimmunoassay. An additional theoretical concern is that the tumor might accumulate hormone from the circulation; no examples of this phenomenon have been reported, however. Detection of mRNA for the hormone confirms that the tumor is indeed a site of synthesis of the peptide. For this evidence to be compelling, hormone mRNA should be detectable in solution hybridization or RNA blotting assays. The technique of reverse transcription and PCR is so sensitive that a signal can be obtained from samples containing only a few molecules of hormone mRNA, a level that may be insignificant. In addition, identification of hormone mRNA without hormone protein leaves open the possibility that the mRNA is not translated; for example, many normal tissues express a form of POMC mRNA that cannot be translated into protein.

Demonstration of the presence of both hormone mRNA and protein provides strong evidence for synthesis in the tumor but does not directly establish that the hormone is secreted. The most rigorous criterion for ectopic hormone secretion is the demonstration of an arteriovenous gradient of the hormone across the tumor or of production and secretion of the hormone by tumor cells cultured in vitro. Unfortunately, selective catheterization to obtain a true arteriovenous gradient is often impossible, because many of the tumors are present in the pulmonary or splanchnic bed or are widely metastatic. Establishing tumor cells in culture provides an important research tool but requires an element of good fortune; many tumor cells, exuberant as their growth may be in the host, are difficult to propagate in cell culture.

Malignancy-Associated Hypercalcemia

Clinical Features

Hypercalcemia is probably the most common endocrine complication of malignant tumors, occurring in as many as 5% of all cancers. The incidence of hypercalcemia in malignancy is 15 cases per 100,000 person-years, about one half the incidence of primary hyperparathyroidism, and malignant tumors are the most common cause of hypercalcemia in hospitalized patients (see Chapter 27).[36,37]

Hypercalcemia in malignancy usually has a rapid onset and can cause confusion, stupor, nausea, vomiting, and dehydration. The offending neoplasm is almost always evident clinically, even when hypercalcemia is the initial manifestation. Thus, physical examination and a chest radiograph disclose the underlying tumor in about 98% of patients. Because hypercalcemia usually occurs in advanced malignancy, the prognosis is poor, with a median survival of only 4 to 8 weeks after the discovery of hypercalcemia. Exceptions are breast carcinoma and multiple myeloma, in which successful treatment of the underlying malignancy can allow long survival of the hypercalcemic patient.

The incidence of individual tumors in patients with hypercalcemia is shown in Table 43–4. Lung carcinoma, breast carcinoma, and multiple myeloma account for more than 50% of all cases of malignancy-associated hypercalcemia. Lung carcinomas that produce hypercalcemia have squamous or large cell histology, whereas small cell carcinoma almost never causes hypercalcemia. About two thirds of lung cancer patients have bone metastasis at the time hypercalcemia develops. Among other solid tumors, the most common are squamous and renal carcinomas. Gastrointestinal tumors and prostate carcinoma are less common causes of hypercalcemia.

Hypercalcemia is uncommon in lymphomas and leukemia but occurs in two thirds of patients with adult T-cell leukemia syndrome, which is caused by the retrovirus HTLV-1 (human T-lymphotropic virus type 1).[38] Another rare variety of leukemia in which hypercalcemia is common is the M7 variant of acute myelogenous leukemia, megakaryocytic leukemia.[39] Hypercalcemia is a common complication of multiple myeloma. Hypercalcemia in myeloma has been ascribed to a local osteolytic cause, but a substantial fraction of cases have increased PTHrP levels, as discussed later. Pheochromocytomas can produce hypercalcemia by secretion of PTHrP.[40]

TABLE 43–4 MALIGNANCY-ASSOCIATED HYPERCALCEMIA

Primary Site	No. (%) of Cases	Known Metastatic Disease (%)
Lung	111 (25.0)	62
Breast	87 (19.6)	92
Multiple myeloma	43 (9.7)	100
Head and neck	36 (8.1)	73
Renal and urinary tract	35 (7.9)	36
Esophagus	25 (5.6)	53
Female genitalia	24 (5.2)	81
Unknown primary	23 (5.2)	—
Lymphoma	14 (3.2)	91
Colon	8 (1.8)	—
Liver, biliary	7 (1.6)	—
Skin	6 (1.4)	—
Other	25 (5.6)	—
Total	444 (100)	

Data from Fisken RA, Heath DA, Bold AM. Hypercalcaemia: a hospital survey. Q J Med 1980;49:405-418; Fisken RA, Heath DA, Somers S. Hypercalcemia in hospital patients: clinical and diagnostic aspects. Lancet 1981;1:202-207; and Singer FR, Sharp CF Jr, Rude RK. Pathogenesis of hypercalcemia of malignancy. Miner Electrolyte Metab 1979;2:161-168.

Data on metastatic disease from Fisken RA, Heath DA, Somers S. Hypercalcemia in hospital patients: clinical and diagnostic aspects. Lancet 1981;1:202-207; and Singer FR, Sharp CF Jr, Rude RK. Pathogenesis of hypercalcemia of malignancy. Miner Electrolyte Metab 1979;2:161-168.

From Strewler GJ. Nonparathyroid hypercalcemia. Adv Intern Med 1987;32:235-258.

Laboratory Features

Overall, about 80% of patients, including most patients with solid tumors, have increased serum levels of PTHrP, which can be measured in two-site, amino-terminal or midregion assays (Fig. 43–1).[41,42] Hypophosphatemia is common because of the phosphaturic effect of PTHrP. Although the combination of hypercalcemia and hypophosphatemia is consistent with the presence of primary hyperparathyroidism, the level of intact PTH is suppressed to less than 2 pM/L (20 pg/mL) in patients with malignancy-associated hypercalcemia.[41,42] The serum level of $1,25(OH)_2D_3$ is also suppressed in hypercalcemic patients, except in lymphoma, in which $1,25(OH)_2D_3$ levels are often high. Renal function may be impaired by hypercalcemia; the decreased glomerular filtration rate can lead to normalization of blood phosphate in patients with PTHrP-mediated hypercalcemia.

Pathogenesis

Hypercalcemia in malignancy is caused by excessive bone resorption. Multiple myeloma and some breast cancers induce hypercalcemia by local osteolytic mechanisms, but in most patients bone resorption is induced by humoral factors. The most common humoral factor is PTHrP, but $1,25(OH)_2D_3$ is a hypercalcemic factor in lymphomas, and in rare instances PTH is secreted ectopically by nonparathyroid tumors.

Parathyroid Hormone–Related Protein

PTHrP is related to PTH structurally (see Fig. 24-13) and shares a common receptor with PTH (see Chapter 27 for a discussion of the chemistry of PTHrP).[44] Because PTH and PTHrP share a receptor, their biologic actions are similar. PTHrP produces hypercalcemia by increasing resorption of bone throughout the skeleton and by increasing the renal resorption of calcium and causes hypophosphatemia through a phosphaturic effect at the kidney. The hypocalciuric effect of PTHrP probably plays a significant role in the pathogenesis of hypercalcemia, albeit secondary to the role of bone resorption. In some but not all studies of bisphosphonate treatment of hypercalcemia, the effect of treatment was negatively correlated with the serum level of PTHrP, suggesting that increased renal calcium reabsorption might limit the response of some patients to treatment with inhibitors of bone resorption.

PTHrP functions in normal physiology as a tissue factor that regulates cellular proliferation and differentiation in fetal development and in tissues such as the breast, skin, and hair follicle in the adult (see Chapter 27).[44] PTHrP locally regulates development, remarkably acting via the same receptor that PTH uses systemically to regulate its target tissues, bone and kidney. However, when PTHrP is produced by a tumor of sufficient mass, it enters the systemic circulation, where it activates PTH-

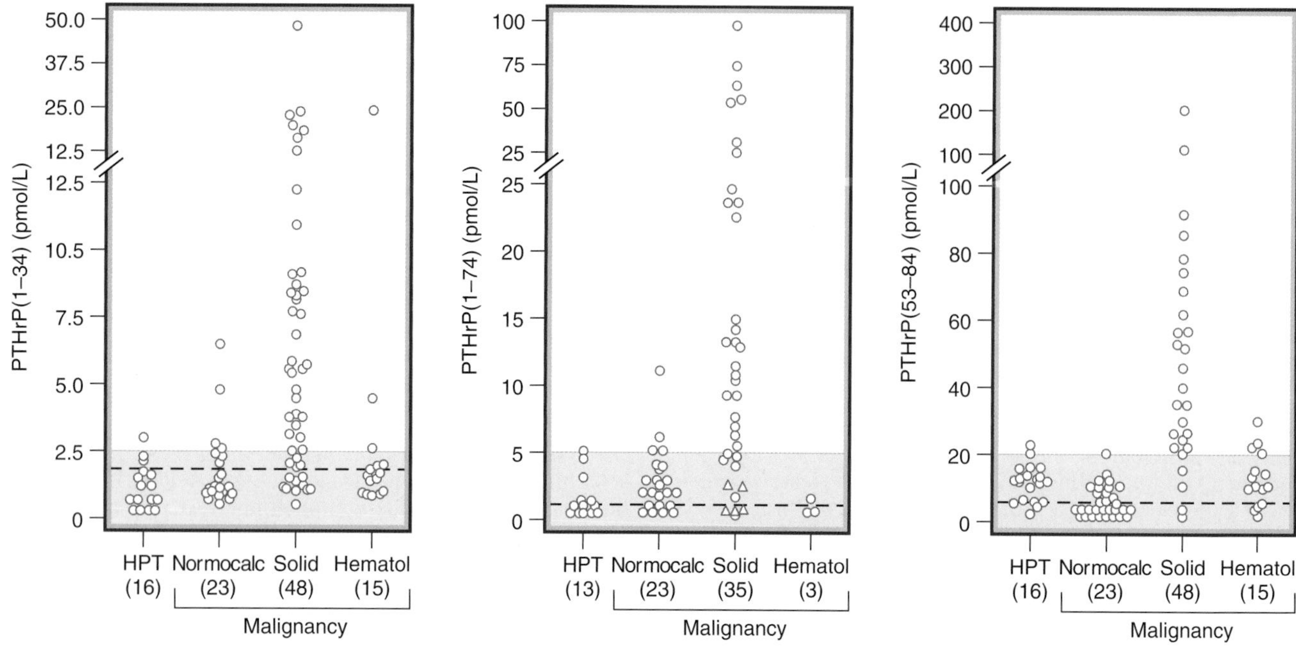

Figure 43–1 ▪ Plasma concentration of parathyroid hormone–related protein (PTHrP) in patients with hyperparathyroidism (HPT), normocalcemic patients with malignancy (Normocalc), and patients with hypercalcemia of malignancy caused by a solid tumor (Solid) or a hematologic malignancy (Hematol). Radioimmunoassay for amino-terminal PTHrP(1-34) *(left panel),* an immunoradiometric assay for PTHrP(1-74) *(center panel),* and a radioimmunoassay for midregion PTHrP(53-84) *(right panel).* The *hatched* area represents the normal ranges; the *dashed line* denotes the limits of detection; the numbers attached to each group indicate the number of patients. In the PTHrP(1-74) assay, the group Solid includes five patients classified as having local osteolytic type of hypercalcemia (Δ). Note the different scales of the *y*-axes. (Data from Budayr AA, Nissenson RA, Klein RF, et al. Increased serum levels of a parathyroid hormone–like protein in malignancy-associated hypercalcemia. Ann Intern Med 1989;111:807-812; Burtis WJ, Brady TG, Orloff JJ, et al. Immunochemical characterization of circulating parathyroid hormone–related protein in patients with humoral hypercalcemia of cancer. N Engl J Med 1990;322:1106-1112; Blind E, Raue F, Gotzmann J, et al. Circulating levels of midregional parathyroid hormone–related protein in hypercalcaemia of malignancy. Clin Endocrinol [Oxf] 1992;37:290-297. Reprinted from Blind E, Nissenson RA, Strewler GJ. Parathyroid hormone–related protein. In Becker KL, Bremner WJ, Hung W, et al [eds]. Principles and Practice of Endocrinology and Metabolism, 2nd ed. Philadelphia, JB Lippincott, 1985.)

PTHrP receptors in bone and kidney and produces hypercalcemia.

PTHrP can either produce humoral hypercalcemia or cause local osteolytic hypercalcemia by direct activation of osteoclasts in the vicinity of bone metastases. In lung and renal carcinoma, PTHrP often acts as a humoral factor because hypercalcemia can occur without evidence of bone metastasis (see Table 43–1). Even when bone metastases are present, hypercalcemia is predominantly humoral because the serum calcium level correlates better with the level of PTHrP than with the number or size of bone metastases.

There is experimental evidence that PTHrP, when expressed in bone metastasis, can also be a local osteolytic factor. In an experimental model, transfection of PTHrP complementary DNA into breast carcinoma cells increased their propensity for bone metastasis, and bone metastasis induced local osteolysis without an increase in the circulating level of PTHrP.[45] This result is in agreement with the biology of human breast carcinoma, in which about 50% of hypercalcemic patients have extensive bone metastases without increased serum levels of PTHrP and are presumed to have local osteolytic hypercalcemia (see Table 43–4). Metastases of breast cancer to bone are immunohistochemically positive for PTHrP in 92% of cases, compared with 17% for nonosseous metastases. Tumor cells that secrete PTHrP have a selective advantage in bone, probably because they induce local resorption.[45] Moreover, transforming growth factor β (TGF-β) released from bone matrix as a result of bone resorption induces the expression of PTHrP, setting up a positive feedback loop to perpetuate the process.[46]

At least two aspects of the hypercalcemia syndrome associated with PTHrP are paradoxical. First, plasma levels of $1,25(OH)_2D_3$ tend to be low in malignancy, despite the acute effect of PTHrP to stimulate renal synthesis of $1,25(OH)_2D_3$. This finding contrasts with normal to high levels of $1,25(OH)_2D_3$ in primary hyperparathyroidism. The difference may be due to the capacity of hypercalcemia itself to suppress production of $1,25(OH)_2D_3$, tending to counteract the acute stimulatory effect of PTH or PTHrP. Thus, a continuous chronic infusion of PTH, in contrast to the effects of primary hyperparathyroidism, suppresses $1,25(OH)_2D_3$ levels, but clamping the serum calcium in the normal range prevents this suppression. Acute infusion of PTHrP(1-36) produces a smaller increase in the serum $1,25(OH)_2D_3$ level than infusion of an equimolar concentration of PTH(1-34), despite attainment of similar plasma levels.[47] Thus, another possible explanation of the lack of elevation of $1,25(OH)_2D_3$ in PTHrP-mediated hypercalcemia may be actions unique to PTHrP.

A second paradox concerns bone turnover in the setting of high PTHrP levels. Despite avid bone resorption, bone formation is reduced in postmortem bone biopsy specimens from patients with malignancy and hypercalcemia.[48] This uncoupled state contrasts with primary hyperparathyroidism and most other resorptive states, which are characterized by coupled increases in bone formation. The precise mechanism whereby hyperparathyroidism leads to increased bone formation is not well understood. In fact, acute infusion of PTH or of PTHrP can cause suppression of bone formation.[47] Thus, this aspect of PTH/PTHrP action might be important in malignant states. It is also possible that immobilization, inanition, illness, or other cytokines secreted by neoplasms depress osteoblastic activity.

Mechanisms involved in the activation of PTHrP gene expression in malignant tumors might include *trans*-activation by tumor-specific factors and differential methylation. The best example of *trans*-activation is adult T-cell leukemia, which is commonly characterized by PTHrP-dependent hypercalcemia.[38] A specific *trans*-activating protein, called tax, in the genome of HTLV-1 is capable of direct activation of PTHrP transcription, acting primarily at an Ets-1 site near the most downstream promoter, though tax-independent activation of PTHrP gene transcription can apparently also occur.[49] The keratinocyte is a prominent site of normal PTHrP expression, and secretion of PTHrP by squamous carcinomas can hence be regarded as eutopic. However, only a fraction of patients with squamous carcinomas have hypercalcemia. When PTHrP promoter constructs were fused to a reporter gene and transfected into squamous carcinoma cell lines, the relative level of expression of the reporter gene correlated with the intensity of endogenous PTHrP gene expression in the same cell lines,[50] suggesting that in this circumstance also, the expression of PTHrP is regulated in *trans* by a factor or factors that are differentially expressed in different squamous carcinomas. PTHrP expression in human squamous carcinoma cells is also repressed by mutant forms of the tumor suppressor gene p53.[51] Renal carcinomas are sharply divided between PTHrP expressors and nonexpressors. The PTHrP gene is undermethylated in renal carcinomas that express PTHrP compared with those that do not.[40] This finding suggests that hypomethylation may be a mechanism by which the gene is expressed in some renal carcinomas.

1,25-Dihydroxyvitamin D_3

About 50% of lymphoma patients who become hypercalcemic have inappropriately high serum $1,25(OH)_2D_3$ levels.[52] In a few cases, lymph node tissue from such patients has been shown to produce $1,25(OH)_2D_3$ in vitro from 25(OH)D.[53] Challenge of normocalcemic lymphoma patients with the precursor sterol 25(OH)D resulted in increased serum $1,25(OH)_2D_3$ levels, increased serum calcium levels, and suppression of PTH.[53] This response is in marked contrast to that of normal persons, who regulate the conversion of substrate to $1,25(OH)_2D_3$ tightly.

The enhanced responsiveness of normocalcemic lymphoma patients to vitamin D indicates that the fundamental abnormality in lymphoma, unregulated extrarenal production of $1,25(OH)_2D_3$, is more common than hypercalcemia. As would be expected from this interpretation, hypercalciuria is also more common than hypercalcemia in lymphoma patients[52] and presumably compensates at least in part for the inappropriate synthesis of $1,25(OH)_2D_3$. This syndrome resembles the hypercalcemia of sarcoidosis, which is also due to enhanced extrarenal production of $1,25(OH)_2D_3$. As in sarcoidosis, hypercalcemia in lymphoma is often responsive to administration of glucocorticoids, but it might not respond well to treatment with hydroxychloroquine.

Parathyroid Hormone

Secretion of PTH from extraparathyroid tumors is extremely rare,[54-56] although one case fulfilled the most rigorous criterion: demonstration of an arteriovenous gradient for PTH across the tumor.[54] Most nonparathyroid tumors that secrete PTH are neuroendocrine tumors, although one was an ovarian adenocarcinoma and one a hepatocellular carcinoma. The diagnosis should be considered in patients with malignant tumors (particularly small cell tumors), hypercalcemia, and elevated PTH levels. However, most patients with these findings have a malignant tumor with coincident primary hyperparathyroidism, because this coincidence is more likely than the truly rare syndrome of ectopic PTH secretion. Consequently, exploration of the parathyroid glands may be indicated in patients who require treatment for hypercalcemia.

Local Osteolytic Hypercalcemia

Osteolytic lesions cause hypercalcemia by secretion of bone-resorbing cytokines that activate osteoclasts. Cytokines with osteoclast-activating activity include interleukin-1, tumor necrosis factor α (TNF-α), interleukin-6, TGF-α, macrophage inflammatory protein-1, receptor activator of nuclear factor κB (NFκB) ligand (RANKL), and PTHrP. As discussed earlier, PTHrP appears to be an important local osteolytic factor in breast carcinoma.[57] The other classic example of local osteolytic hypercalcemia is multiple myeloma. Although at least one third of myeloma patients have hypercalcemia at some time during their disease, the offending cytokine has not been identified with certainty. Leading candidates are the chemokine macrophage inflammatory protein-1 and the osteoclastogenic cytokine RANKL.[58] Moreover, a fraction of hypercalcemic patients with multiple myeloma have high serum PTHrP levels and thus humoral rather than local osteolytic hypercalcemia.[59] PTHrP is expressed commonly in myeloma cells and could also function locally as an osteolytic factor in multiple myeloma and lymphoma.

Diagnosis

The diagnosis of malignancy-associated hypercalcemia is usually not difficult because the offending neoplasm is clinically evident. A low serum phosphorus level in conjunction with suppressed PTH levels suggests that the causative factor is PTHrP. It is important to exclude intercurrent primary hyperparathyroidism by showing that the level of intact PTH is suppressed below 2 pM/L (20 pg/mL). Demonstration of elevated levels of PTHrP confirms the diagnosis in patients with solid tumors, but this is often unnecessary clinically. PTHrP is processed to amino-terminal, midregion, and carboxyl-terminal peptides, and similar assay performance has been achieved with assays of the amino terminus[41] and midregion[43] and two-site immunoradiometric assays (see Fig. 43–1). Two-site assays for PTHrP have become the standard.[42]

Treatment

The treatment of hypercalcemia is discussed in Chapter 27. The mainstays of therapy for tumor patients, in whom hypercalcemia is often acute and severe, are rehydration, institution of a saline diuresis, and institution of chronic treatment. In general, the treatment of choice is the second-generation bisphosphonate pamidronate, 60 to 90 mg by intravenous infusion, or intravenous zoledronic acid. Patients with multiple myeloma or lymphoma often respond to glucocorticoid treatment.

■ Syndrome of Inappropriate Vasopressin Secretion

This syndrome is discussed fully in Chapter 9.

Clinical Features

The syndrome of inappropriate vasopressin secretion (commonly termed the *syndrome of inappropriate antidiuretic hormone* [SIADH]) is probably the second most common endocrine complication in cancer patients.[5,60,61] The secretion of vasopressin impairs the ability to dilute the urine, leading to a state of water intoxication, with hypotonicity and hyponatremia. Patients with hyponatremia may be asymptomatic if the condition has developed gradually. Patients may experience weight gain because of water retention, but because the retained water is distributed among both extracellular and intracellular spaces, there is no edema. However, when the serum sodium level falls rapidly to less than 120 mM/L, somnolence, coma, and seizures can occur. Symptomatic hyponatremia carries a mortality rate of 10% to 15%, but this rate is higher when the serum sodium level is below 110 mM/L.

By far, the most common tumor that causes SIADH is SCLC. SIADH occurs in 5% to 15% of patients with SCLC and in less than 1% of patients with non–small cell lung cancer (non-SCLC).[62] Other neuroendocrine tumors, including carcinoids and small cell carcinomas of the prostate and cervix, can also cause SIADH. SIADH also occurs occasionally in a wide range of carcinomas, including as many as 2% of squamous carcinomas of the head and neck, adenocarcinoma of the colon, Hodgkin's disease, non-Hodgkin's lymphomas, and several varieties of brain tumors.[62] The finding of hyponatremia in cancer is nonspecific, and central secretion of vasopressin from various nonosmotic stimuli may be at fault in some of these patients, for example, patients with thoracic or intracranial tumors. However, vasopressin and associated neurophysins have been found in non-neuroendocrine tumor cells, and some epithelial tumors can secrete vasopressin.

Laboratory Features

The cardinal features of SIADH are hypotonicity with hyponatremia and an inappropriately concentrated urine. It is often unnecessary to measure serum osmolality directly in a hyponatremic patient because the effective serum osmolality closely approximates direct measurements. Serum osmolality can be calculated as:

$$\text{Serum osmolality} = (\text{serum Na}^+ \times 2) + (\text{glucose}/18)$$

where serum sodium and serum glucose are in millimoles per liter. A urine osmolality greater than 100 mOsm/L water is inappropriate in the setting of serum hypotonicity, which should inhibit the release of vasopressin and permit the excretion of a maximally dilute urine. The urine osmolality in SIADH is often higher than the serum osmolality, but that is not a necessary feature of the syndrome. If measured directly, vasopressin levels are inappropriately elevated, as are the levels of the associated neurophysins. However, it is rarely necessary to measure vasopressin. As discussed later, other causes of hypotonicity can generally be excluded with reasonable certainty by reliance on clinical and biochemical criteria.

Several other laboratory features of SIADH are helpful in diagnosis. The urinary sodium concentration is typically high, reflecting the natriuresis induced by expansion of extracellular fluid volume. However, the ability to conserve sodium in SIADH is usually unimpaired,[5] and the urinary sodium excretion can fall to low levels in the setting of reduced dietary sodium intakes. The blood urea nitrogen and serum uric acid levels are low, again reflecting expanded extracellular fluid volumes and decreased tubular resorption of these solutes. Other electrolytes are diluted in proportion to the serum sodium, except for serum bicarbonate, which is normal.

Pathogenesis

Vasopressin is synthesized as a prohormone of 166 amino acids that is processed to produce three peptides: the mature octapeptide hormone, a midregion peptide of molecular weight 10,000 with vasopressin-binding activity called neurophysin II, and a C-terminal glycopeptide (see Chapter 9). Vasopressin and its neurophysin are packaged together in neurosecretory granules, stored in nerve termini in the posterior pituitary, and released in response to hypotonicity or nonosmotic stimuli (baroreceptor stimulation, pain, nausea). Vasopressin is similarly processed in neuroendocrine tumor cells, but these cells commonly secrete not only vasopressin and neurophysin II but also vasopressin's sister peptide oxytocin together with its binding protein, neurophysin I.

The molecular basis for inappropriate secretion of vasopressin from tumor cells is poorly understood. Immunoreactive vasopressin is identifiable in a portion of bronchial neuroendocrine cells, the presumed precursors of SCLC. Thus, like other hormonal products of neuroendocrine neoplasms, vasopressin may be regarded as secreted eutopically from neuroendocrine tumors. The usual coordinate expression of vasopressin and oxytocin precursors in tumor cells may be related to the physical linkage of the two genes, which are found within 12 kb of each other in the human genome with an inverted arrangement of the coding strands. Either DNA rearrangements or *trans*-acting factors expressed in malignant tumors could simultaneously activate both promoters.

An E-box in the vasopressin promoter, a binding motif for bHLH transcription factors, is necessary for increased vasopressin gene expression in high-expressing SCLC cell lines.[63] This motif appears to bind the transcription factor USF (upstream transcription factor); a nearby sequence appears to interact and is a candidate for binding other bHLH factors. A neuron-specific silencer element has also been identified in the arginine vasopressin promoter.

It is not known whether the secretion of neurohypophyseal peptides from tumor cells is under regulatory control. Four patterns of vasopressin release have been identified in SIADH.[61] Most commonly (37%), vasopressin levels fluctuate widely and independently of the serum osmolality. In a second group (33%), vasopressin is released in response to changes in osmolality, but the osmotic threshold for vasopressin release is decreased (reset osmostat). Other patients with SIADH manifest a constant leak of vasopressin or have no demonstrable abnormality in vasopressin secretion and could conceivably produce a different antidiuretic substance.

Patients with cancer and SIADH fall into all four categories. It is conceivable that those with a reset osmostat express both the vasopressin gene and an osmoreceptor in their tumors; more likely, however, vasopressin is released centrally in these patients because of stimulation of baroreceptors in the pulmonary bed or periphery, invasion of the vagus nerve, or metastasis to regulatory centers, for example, the hypothalamus.

Expression and secretion of vasopressin are more common than hyponatremia in SCLC.[64] More than 50% of SCLC patients have elevated plasma vasopressin levels, and plasma levels of the neurophysins are increased in 44% to 65% of untreated patients with SCLC. Some tumors also express the gene for oxytocin, but no clinical syndrome of inappropriate oxytocin release has been reported in tumor patients.

In patients with elevated vasopressin levels who do not have hyponatremia, abnormalities in water metabolism can be elicited by water loading, which discloses an impaired diuretic response in 47% of patients with limited SCLC and 86% of patients with extensive disease.[65] Patients with milder degrees of vasopressin excess probably compensate for reduced free water excretion by reducing fluid intake; only if free water intake exceeds the maximum excretion of free water does hyponatremia result. Thus, the development of hyponatremia is a function not only of the level of vasopressin but also of fluid intake.

Although some tumors secrete abnormally processed forms of vasopressin with reduced biologic activity, it is likely that compensatory mechanisms of this type account for the disparity in the frequency of biochemical and clinical abnormalities in SIADH.

When water is retained, extracellular and intracellular volumes are expanded. The expansion of extracellular fluid volume, probably by causing suppression of aldosterone and an increase in atrial natriuretic peptide (ANP), induces the natriuresis that is characteristic of patients with SIADH who have an adequate intake of sodium. Plasma levels of ANP are normal or high in SIADH.[66] It is not clear whether high ANP levels are a compensatory response to extracellular fluid volume expansion or a consequence of release of ANP from the tumor. Many tumors that express the vasopressin gene also express the gene for ANP. Restriction of sodium intake in patients with SIADH causes weight loss, however, and as the extracellular fluid volume returns to normal, natriuresis is reversed and sodium is conserved appropriately.[5] This suggests that the secretion of ANP is compensatory in most patients and that an ANP-induced natriuresis does not contribute significantly to the genesis of hyponatremia.

Acute water retention causes neurologic symptoms by rapidly increasing the intracellular volumes of brain cells and thus inducing cerebral edema. Chronic hyponatremia is probably less symptomatic because there is time for activation of compensatory volume-regulatory mechanisms in the central nervous system. Brain cells compensate for volume gain by activating ion transport processes that pump out intracellular potassium chloride (KCl) and sodium chloride (NaCl) and later by secreting organic osmolytes. This compensation has therapeutic importance because rapid correction of hyponatremia by infusion of hypertonic saline produces a transient hypertonic encephalopathy as water is drawn out of the already contracted intracellular space.[60] This can cause permanent neurologic damage (e.g., central pontine myelinolysis) and death.

Diagnosis

The diagnosis of SIADH is usually made on clinical grounds. The first step is to establish that the urine is inappropriately concentrated in the presence of hypotonicity. In a hyponatremic patient, a urine osmolality higher than 100 mOsm/L water is inappropriate, and many patients with SIADH have urine osmolalities higher than the plasma osmolality. Next, other causes of hypotonicity must be excluded. The differential diagnosis of hyponatremia includes states of true volume contraction; edematous states such as congestive heart failure and hepatic failure, in which the effective central plasma volume is diminished; adrenal insufficiency; hypothyroidism; drug effects; and SIADH (see Chapter 9).

Measurements of vasopressin are of little value in the differential diagnosis because vasopressin levels are increased in most hyponatremic states. True volume contraction and edematous states can usually be excluded on clinical grounds. It is appropriate to exclude adrenal insufficiency with a corticotropin stimulation test in patients with malignant tumors and SIADH, particularly because patients with bilateral adrenal metastases are at risk for adrenal insufficiency. Thyrotropin should be measured to exclude hypothyroidism. Among the drugs that stimulate the nonosmotic release of vasopressin are the cancer chemotherapeutic agents vincristine and cyclophosphamide and the SSRIs. Euvolemic patients without hormonal disorders or drug causes are presumed to have SIADH.

SIADH is a common cause of hyponatremia in hospitalized patients, but only a small minority of these patients develop the syndrome as the result of inappropriate secretion of vasopressin by a tumor. Furthermore, not all patients with cancer who meet the criteria for SIADH have ectopic secretion of vasopressin from a tumor. Not only are benign forms of SIADH more common, but also the response of vasopressin to osmotic stimuli in some patients with malignant tumors is consistent with eutopic secretion of the hormone from the pituitary.

The uncertainty regarding the etiology in an individual patient may be intellectually unsatisfying but is not of great practical importance. Patients with severe and symptomatic hyponatremia are more likely to have a true ectopic source of vasopressin. The treatment of hyponatremia in SIADH is similar regardless of the cause of the syndrome.

Treatment

Symptomatic hyponatremia in patients with a serum sodium level less than 120 mM/L requires immediate treatment (see Chapter 9). The therapeutic options include infusion or administration of hypertonic saline (3% or 5% saline) or of saline and furosemide.[60] The latter regimen has the advantage of not rapidly expanding extracellular fluid volume in an already volume-expanded patient. The goal of acute treatment is to reverse symptoms and raise the serum sodium level above 125 mM/L. Such an increase takes the patient out of immediate danger, and further correction can be accomplished in a more leisurely fashion.

How rapidly the initial phase of correction should be carried out is controversial; too rapid correction of hyponatremia can predispose to central pontine myelinolysis and other neurologic sequelae (see Chapter 9). As discussed earlier, the risk of rapid correction probably has to do with brain shrinking in the presence of high concentrations of extracellular sodium and intracellular dehydration, which is exacerbated by prior loss of cell solute, the adaptive response of the central nervous system to hyponatremia. Patients with chronic hyponatremia have had more opportunity to adapt and are at greater risk of neurologic damage when the serum osmolality is raised too rapidly. Under most circumstances, it seems best to correct hyponatremia at a rate of 0.5 mM/L per hour until the serum sodium concentration reaches 120 to 125 mM/L.

In asymptomatic patients or after acute correction of hyponatremia in symptomatic patients, the mainstay of chronic therapy is water restriction. Moderate fluid restriction may be reasonably well tolerated. The goal is to establish a fluid intake at which the intake of free water does not exceed the maximum free water clearance, which is determined by the circulating vasopressin level. If necessary, most patients can be maintained with severe restrictions to 800 to 1000 mL of fluid intake daily. At this level, the free water intake is actually negative because the patient is ingesting osmoles from food in excess of water. Therefore, even a patient who is obliged to excrete a concentrated urine and thus has negative free water excretion may be maintained in zero net water balance. However, severe fluid restrictions are onerous and difficult to maintain.

As an adjunct to water restriction, it can be beneficial to interfere with vasopressin action. The drug of choice for this purpose is demeclocycline, an antibiotic that blocks the action of vasopressin and produces nephrogenic diabetes insipidus. At a dose of 150 to 300 mg four times a day, demeclocycline has a reproducible effect on the urine-concentrating mechanism,[67] but up to 2 weeks may be necessary for the full effect. Side effects include azotemia, photosensitive rashes, and liver toxicity. Lithium also produces nephrogenic diabetes insipidus, but its effects are less predictable than those of demeclocycline and the drug should be given only in refractory cases. SCLC is now treated with aggressive combination chemotherapy, and SIADH often remits in responders to chemotherapy.

Ectopic Corticotropin Syndrome and Ectopic Secretion of Corticotropin-Releasing Hormone

Clinical Features

The ectopic corticotropin syndrome accounts for 10% to 20% of cases of Cushing's syndrome.[68-70] Unlike Cushing's disease, with an 8:1 female preponderance, this syndrome is more common in men than in women. The typical presentation also differs; the onset is sudden, and progression is rapid. Patients complain of proximal myopathy and peripheral edema. Hypertension, hypokalemia, and severe glucose intolerance are often present. Hyperpigmentation can occur, but hirsutism is unusual. Other manifestations of cancer, such as anorexia, weight loss, and anemia, are common.

The somatic features of Cushing's syndrome are notably absent in the typical patient, perhaps because of the rapid evolution of the clinical picture. Patients with slowly growing carcinoid tumors of the bronchus or thymus have a more indolent disease and often present with the classic habitus of Cushing's syndrome: moon facies, centripetal obesity, proximal myopathy, polydipsia, and polyuria. Hyperpigmentation is common in these patients, as is hirsutism in women.

The tumors that produce the ectopic corticotropin syndrome are primarily of neuroendocrine cell origin. In published series, approximately 45% are SCLC, 15% are thymic carcinoids, 10% are bronchial carcinoids, 10% are islet cell tumors, 5% are other carcinoid tumors, 2% are pheochromocytomas, and 1% are ovarian adenocarcinomas. However, adenocarcinoma and squamous carcinoma are also occasionally associated with the syndrome. It appears that SCLC is greatly underrepresented in these referral series; it probably accounts for well over 50% of unselected cases.

Laboratory Features

Both the level of cortisol secretion and the level of corticotropin tend to be higher in ectopic than in pituitary Cushing's syndrome, although there is some overlap. In most ectopic cases, both cortisol and corticotropin levels are elevated to two to four times the normal morning values, and the normal diurnal variation in their levels is lost. Urinary excretion of adrenal steroid metabolites is increased correspondingly. Two-site immunoradiometric assays, which are in common use for detection of corticotropin, give lower values for corticotropin in ectopic cases than older radioimmunoassays, probably because they do not detect partially processed forms that are common in the ectopic syndrome.

Despite the abnormal processing of corticotropin by nonpituitary tumors, there is no other POMC peptide in serum whose presence is decisive in the diagnosis of the ectopic syndrome. More than one half of nonpituitary tumors that secrete corticotropin also secrete other peptides, including carcinoembryonic antigen, GRP, calcitonin, somatostatin, and corticotropin-releasing hormone (CRH), and the presence of these peptides is suggestive of the ectopic corticotropin syndrome.

Hypokalemia occurs in 80% to 100% of cases in various series, and potassium wasting is more severe than in pituitary Cushing's disease. The hypokalemia is probably explained by the mineralocorticoid effects of cortisol, which are more evident both because cortisol levels tend to be higher in ectopic than in pituitary Cushing's syndrome and because 11β-hydroxysteroid dehydrogenase activity appears for unknown reasons to be decreased in patients with ectopic corticotropin secretion.[71] A deficiency of 11β-hydroxysteroid dehydrogenase activity impairs the inactivation of cortisol in the renal tubule, leading to increased exposure of mineralocorticoid receptors to cortisol. In disorders such as congenital deficiency of 11β-hydroxysteroid dehydrogenase and licorice intoxication, in which the activity of the enzyme is inhibited, normal levels of cortisol produce a state of pseudohyperaldosteronism.

Pathogenesis

Although many nonpituitary tissues contain POMC mRNA, most are short transcripts (800 nucleotides) that are initiated by a downstream promoter at the third exon of the *POMC* gene and do not include coding sequences for the signal peptide that is necessary for direction of POMC into the secretory pathway.[72] Thus, nonpituitary POMC transcripts probably do not generate bioactive POMC products that can be secreted. In contrast, nonpituitary tumors that secrete corticotropin contain a 1150-nucleotide mRNA similar to the predominant pituitary species, and many nonpituitary tumors also contain 1350-nucleotide transcripts initiated from an upstream promoter that is largely quiescent in pituitary cells.[72,73]

Two regions of the POMC promoter contribute to activity in SCLC; the region that confers high POMC promoter activity on pituitary cells is not active. One region binds the transcription factor E2F[74] in a methylation-sensitive fashion.[22] E2F is inactivated by the tumor suppressor gene Rb, which is inactive in 90% of cases of SCLC. Thus, both loss of Rb and differential methylation of the POMC promoter are potential mechanisms of POMC expression in SCLC.

Consistent with the nonsuppressibility of most nonpituitary tumors by glucocorticoids, the sensitivity of *POMC* gene expression to inhibition by glucocorticoids is reduced in SCLC cell lines. In some cell lines, glucocorticoid receptors are absent; in others, glucocorticoid receptor action appears to be defective.[73] Negative glucocorticoid regulatory elements are typically composite elements that require binding of regulatory factors in addition to the glucocorticoid receptor, leading to the possibility that such accessory factors may be abnormal in transformed cell lines. However, glucocorticoids also fail to stimulate transcription from classic glucocorticoid regulatory elements in SCLC cell lines, and this defect is overcome by overexpression of the wild-type glucocorticoid receptor.

POMC processing in nonpituitary tumors is often incomplete, with the release into blood of POMC fragments with reduced biologic activity.[75] These incompletely processed forms are larger than corticotropin by gel filtration and were first described in the serum of cancer patients with the ectopic corticotropin (ACTH) syndrome as *big ACTH*.[76] Some incompletely processed POMC peptides can be detected by radioimmunoassay techniques for corticotropin but not by two-site immunoradiometric assays. In one study, the ratio of corticotropin precursors to corticotropin in plasma was 58:1 in the ectopic ACTH syndrome and 5:1 in pituitary Cushing's disease.[77]

Unusual small peptides are also produced from POMC in nonpituitary tumors (Fig. 43–2).[72] In anterior pituitary corticotrope cells, four of the six dibasic sites in POMC are cleaved by the prohormone convertase PC1/PC3, and the predominant products are six peptides: an NH_2-terminal peptide, a joining peptide, corticotropin, β-lipotropin (β-LPH), smaller amounts of γ-LPH, and β-endorphin.

Additional products that are detected routinely in extracts of nonpituitary tumors include the corticotropin-like intermediate lobe polypeptide (CLIP) and β-melanocyte-stimulating hormone (β-MSH) (5-22).[78] Both peptides are present in the intermediate lobe in the rodent pituitary gland, and their presence in nonpituitary tumors indicates that nonpituitary tumors contain the PC2 convertase, which is normally present in intermediate but not anterior pituitary cells. These peptides are not secreted in large amounts and are not useful as tumor markers in blood,

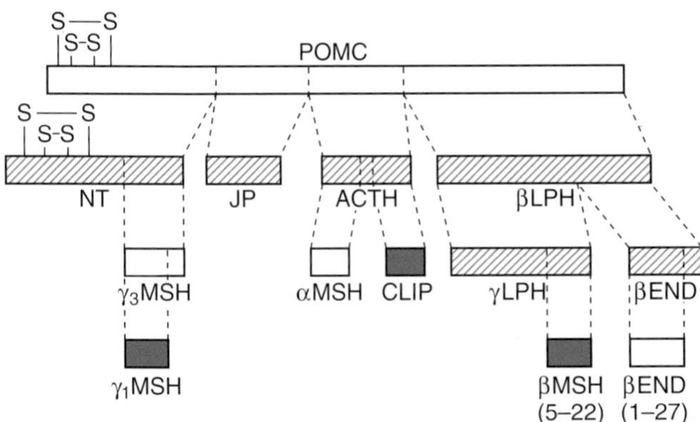

Figure 43–2 ▪ Processing of pro-opiomelanocortin (POMC) in normal pituitary *(hatched bars)*, intermediate lobe *(open bars)*, and nonpituitary neoplasms *(solid bars)*. ACTH, adrenocorticotropic hormone (corticotropin); CLIP, corticotropin-like intermediate lobe peptide; END, endorphin; LPH, lipotropin; MSH, melanocyte-stimulating hormone. (Adapted from Schteingart DE. Ectopic secretion of peptides of the proopiomelanocortin family. Endocrinol Metab Clin North Am 1991;20:453-471.)

but the serum LPH-to-corticotropin ratio in the ectopic corticotropin syndrome is higher than in pituitary tumors, possibly reflecting the increased PC2 activity in nonpituitary tumors.[78]

Corticotropin-like activity can be identified in extracts of many non-SCLCs and in virtually all SCLCs, and at least one third of all SCLCs show POMC mRNA by in situ hybridization.[79] Yet only 1% to 3% of patients with SCLC have clinical evidence of corticotropin excess. Thus, the ectopic corticotropin syndrome is a good example of the principle that ectopic production of hormones is more common than clinical syndromes of hormone excess. Differences between tumors in *trans*-acting nuclear factors or epigenetic regulation of the POMC promoter by DNA methylation may account for differential expression of the POMC gene.[22,74]

Patients with corticotropin-producing neoplasms are protected from the consequences of hormone excess by several mechanisms. Malignant tumors contain much smaller quantities of POMC mRNA and peptides than the pituitary and are thus inefficient in producing corticotropin. Tumor cells are much poorer in neurosecretory granules than pituitary corticotropes and are relatively deficient in the ability to process POMC efficiently and secrete the peptide products. Inefficient cleavage of POMC leads to incompletely processed forms of corticotropin with little biologic activity. Processing of POMC by tumors can also lead to production of biologically inactive products. For example, some tumors produce significant amounts of corticotropin but cleave it to the CLIP.

Laboratory Diagnosis

The diagnosis of the ectopic corticotropin syndrome is described in Chapters 8 and 14.

The first step consists of determining whether cortisol excess is present and whether it is corticotropin-dependent. Increased basal cortisol secretion can often be shown by measurement of serum cortisol or urinary free cortisol, both of which are increased in the ectopic corticotropin syndrome. When the basal levels are not markedly increased, the presence of cortisol excess can be established with a low-dose dexamethasone suppression test, for example, the 1-mg overnight dexamethasone suppression test. The corticotropin dependence of cortisol excess can be established by measurement of corticotropin in the same sample in which cortisol is measured.

Corticotropin-dependent Cushing's syndrome results from either pituitary or ectopic secretion of corticotropin. In the classic form of the syndrome (e.g., corticotropin-secreting SCLC), secretion is nonsuppressible and there is little or no response of serum or urinary cortisol to the administration of high-dose dexamethasone, whereas the secretion of corticotropin by pituitary adenomas is dexamethasone-responsive. In a patient with a recognized malignancy and clinical features suggesting the ectopic syndrome, the finding of nonsuppressible hypercortisolism with elevated corticotropin levels usually suffices to make the diagnosis.

In occasional lung cancers and in about 50% of bronchial or thymic carcinoid tumors, the secretion of corticotropin can be suppressed with high-dose dexamethasone. This circumstance has been called the *occult ectopic corticotropin syndrome* and presents a major diagnostic challenge because the clinical presentation and secretory dynamics may be identical to those of pituitary Cushing's syndrome and because neither these small tumors nor pituitary corticotroph adenomas may be evident on routine radiologic studies. Hence, patients with pituitary and ectopic Cushing's syndrome might have identical biochemical profiles and no evident tumor when imaged.

Although a number of noninvasive methods are used in this circumstance, none is definitive.[80,81] Because nonpituitary tumors are not as well suppressed by glucocorticoids as corticotrope adenomas of the pituitary gland, it is useful to apply stringent criteria for glucocorticoid suppressibility, namely suppression of urinary free cortisol by more than 80% after administration of high-dose dexamethasone.[80] Stimulation with the ovine CRH test is valuable because nonpituitary tumors do not respond well to CRH. An increase in plasma cortisol of 14% after administration of hCRH was reported to have a sensitivity of 80% and a specificity of 100% for the diagnosis of pituitary Cushing's syndrome.[82]

The definitive study for distinguishing pituitary from nonpituitary forms of hypercortisolism is *inferior petrosal sinus sampling* with administration of ovine CRH.[80,81,83] The ratio of corticotropin in the inferior petrosal sinus to that in peripheral blood after administration of CRH is greater than 3 in patients with pituitary tumors and less than 2 in patients with corticotropin-secreting nonpituitary tumors. *Cavernous sinus sampling* has also been successful. Localization of bronchial and thymic carcinoids may be difficult. Thin-section computed tomography of the chest and scanning with labeled octreotide have sometimes been useful but have a high failure rate.

Treatment

The management of Cushing's syndrome is discussed in Chapters 8 and 14.

When possible, the treatment of the ectopic corticotropin syndrome is surgical. With slow-growing carcinoid tumors of the bronchus, thymomas, or pheochromocytomas, surgical resection can be curative. If the tumor cannot be identified, it is necessary to block cortisol secretion with adrenolytic agents. Some patients ultimately require surgical adrenalectomy to control hypercortisolism.

Malignant nonpituitary neoplasms that secrete corticotropin are rarely amenable to resection because the tumor is usually advanced and inoperable by the time the clinical syndrome appears. With malignant neoplasms, the aim is to palliate hypercortisolism by *medical adrenalectomy* using adrenolytic drugs, such as aminoglutethimide (250 mg tid) or metyrapone (250-500 mg tid). Ketoconazole (200-400 mg bid) has also been useful for treating ectopic corticotropin syndrome. A replacement dose of hydrocortisone should be administered with these drugs to avoid adrenal insufficiency. Mitotane inhibits mineralocorticoid as well as glucocorticoid synthesis, and replacement of both is required. Some patients respond to the long-acting somatostatin agonist octreotide, and the glucocorticoid antagonist mifepristone has also been used.

Ectopic Secretion of Corticotropin-Releasing Hormone

Nonendocrine tumors rarely cause Cushing's syndrome by secretion of CRH.[68,84] Patients have increased CRH levels in tumor tissue or in plasma and high plasma corticotropin levels. It is important to document that the site of corticotropin secretion is the pituitary gland because many nonendocrine tumors that secrete CRH also secrete corticotropin itself. Presumptive evidence of a pituitary source of corticotropin can come from demonstration that the gradient of corticotropin between the inferior petrosal sinus and peripheral blood is more than 3:1, from finding pituitary corticotropic hyperplasia in patients who underwent pituitary surgery for a presumed corticotropic adenoma, or from the failure to detect corticotropin in the nonendocrine tumor. When the nonendocrine tumor secretes both CRH and corticotropin, the true role of CRH in the clinical syndrome may be indeterminate.

Cushing's syndrome resulting from ectopic secretion of CRH does not have a distinctive presentation. In most cases, the hypercortisolism is unresponsive to dexamethasone suppression, but a normal response to high-dose dexamethasone has also been reported. The response to metyrapone is also variable. Tumors that secrete CRH include small cell carcinomas of the prostate and lung, medullary thyroid carcinoma, carcinoids, and a hypothalamic gangliocytoma. These neuroendocrine tumors are similar to the tumors that cause Cushing's syndrome by direct secretion of corticotropin.

The diagnosis of ectopic CRH secretion as the cause of Cushing's syndrome is usually made retrospectively. In view of the rarity of the disorder, it is probably inappropriate to measure CRH routinely in Cushing's syndrome. However, it may be worthwhile to determine the plasma CRH level when pituitary surgery has disclosed diffuse corticotropic hyperplasia in a patient with Cushing's syndrome.

Hypoglycemia with Nonislet Cell Tumors

Clinical Features

Fasting hypoglycemia produced by non–islet cell tumors typically causes neuroglycopenic symptoms of obtundation, confusion, or behavioral aberrations, which may have been present for some time before the diagnosis is made.[8,85,86] Non-islet cell tumors rarely secrete insulin, but cases of small cell carcinoma with high levels of insulin, proinsulin, and C peptide have been reported. One tumor was found to contain insulin mRNA by in situ hybridization and immunoreactive insulin by immunohistochemical methods; the other had a demonstrable gradient in venous effluent after selective arterial calcium stimulation.[10,11]

Most extrapancreatic tumors that cause hypoglycemia do so by secreting IGF-II. The offending neoplasms are usually bulky, slow-growing mesenchymal tumors. Fibrosarcomas, rhabdomyosarcomas, leiomyosarcomas, mesotheliomas, and hemangiopericytomas account for more than 50% of cases. Hepatocellular carcinomas (hepatomas), carcinoid tumors, and adrenocortical carcinomas account for about 25% of cases, and the remainder are made up of various carcinomas, leukemias, and lymphomas. More than one third of the tumors are retroperitoneal, about one third are intra-abdominal, and the remainder are intrathoracic.

Pathogenesis

Fasting hypoglycemia produced by non–islet cell tumors results from increased peripheral utilization of glucose, primarily in skeletal muscle, coupled with decreased hepatic glucose output.[87] Lipolysis is inhibited and free fatty acid levels are low. Although it had been suspected that bulky tumors themselves, sometimes weighing many kilograms, might metabolize enough glucose to exceed the capacity for hepatic glucose production, this phenomenon has not been documented. Despite insulin-like effects on glucose utilization, hepatic glucose production, and lipolysis, fasting insulin levels during hypoglycemia are appropriately suppressed. For this reason, it has seemed that an insulin-like factor is probably responsible for hypoglycemia.

It appears that IGF-II is the causative agent of hypoglycemia. Hypoglycemia is caused by increased secretion of IGF-II, altered IGF-II processing and increased bioavailability. Sera from patients with non–islet cell tumors contain elevated levels of an insulin-like activity by radioreceptor assay. IGF-II levels are sometimes elevated during hypoglycemia but may be normal,[88,89] and the levels of IGF-I are typically suppressed.[88,89] The level of IGF-II mRNA in non–islet cell tumors is often increased, even in patients with normal IGF-II levels.[90,91]

Altered binding of IGF-II in the tumor-hypoglycemia syndrome increases its bioavailability to peripheral receptors.[8,86] In normal serum, IGFs are bound largely in one of two complexes. Most IGF is normally bound to a heterotrimeric 150-kd complex consisting of the IGF, the binding protein IGFBP3, and an acid-labile glycoprotein. Because this large complex is retained in the circulation, the half-life of the IGF-II complex is relatively long—12 to 15 hours. A minority of IGF circulates in a smaller 50-kd complex that contains mainly IGF and a different binding protein, IGFBP2. The small complex can cross capillaries and deliver IGF to tissue receptors, and IGF-II bound to this complex has a half-life of only about 30 minutes. In sera from patients with non–islet cell tumors and hypoglycemia, the fraction of IGF-II bound to the small, bioavailable complex is increased, on average by threefold,[92] presumably increasing the access of IGF-II to the receptor, even in the setting of normal total IGF-II levels.

A substantial fraction of IGF-II in both tumors and sera is present in a high-molecular-weight form, *big IGF-II*,[88,89,91,93] a partially processed form that contains a 21-amino-acid carboxyl-terminal extension from the E domain.[88] Big IGF-II was reported to lack *O*-linked glycosylation, which might give it increased bioactivity, but *O*-linked glycosylation was reported to be normal in another study. Whether a decreased ability of big IGF-II to form a normal ternary complex contributes directly to its increased bioavailability remains to be determined.

Current concepts of the alteration in IGF-II binding are summarized in Figure 43–3.[8,94] Oversecretion of big IGF-II suppresses the secretion of insulin, growth hormone (GH), and IGF-I. In turn, suppression of GH and IGF-I down-regulates the synthesis of IGFBP3 and the acid-labile subunit, both of which are GH-dependent, and up-regulates the synthesis of IGFBP2. Consistent with this proposal regarding the role of GH is the response of a patient to GH therapy.[95] Thus, IGF-II oversecretion leads to altered binding and increased bioactivity of IGF-II and can cause hypoglycemia even when total IGF-II levels are normal. The level of free IGF-II in serum is also increased.

Laboratory Diagnosis

The fasting levels of insulin and C peptide are appropriately suppressed in samples obtained during hypoglycemia (insulin <36 pM/L [6 μU/mL], C peptide <0.2 nM/L [0.6 ng/mL]). The IGF-II level may be normal or increased. In patients with normal

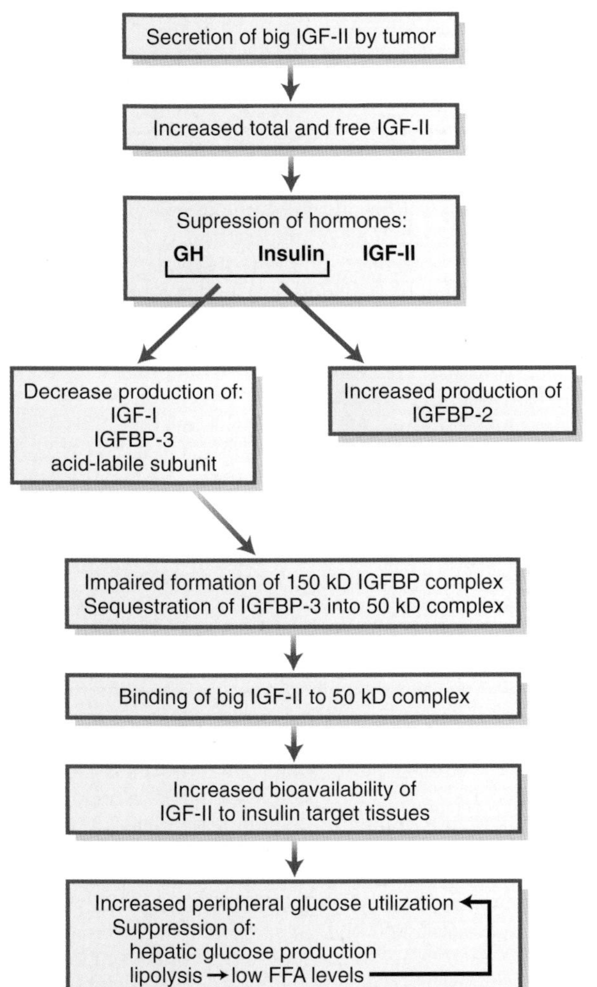

Figure 43–3 ▪ Proposed explanation for the pathogenesis of hypoglycemia with non–islet cell tumors. FFA, free fatty acid; GH, growth hormone; IGF, insulin-like growth factor; IGFBP, IGF-binding protein. (Adapted from Zapf J. IGFs: function and clinical importance. 3. Role of insulin-like growth factor (IGF) II and IGF binding proteins in extrapancreatic tumour hypoglycaemia. J Intern Med 1993;234:543-552.)

levels of IGF-II, the diagnosis is supported by finding low levels of IGF-I, GH, and IGFBP3.

Treatment

The mainstay of treatment is resection of the tumor. Even partial debulking can ameliorate hypoglycemia. In patients with unresectable tumors, several maneuvers based on the pathogenetic scheme have been attempted. Therapy with GH, glucagon, glucocorticoids, or somatostatin has been effective in individual patients with unresectable tumors. These measures are temporary, however, until the unresectable tumor can be treated with chemotherapy.

Syndromes Caused By Growth Hormone-Releasing Hormone, Growth Hormone, and Human Placental Lactogen

Since 1980, more than 40 cases of acromegaly have been associated with nonpituitary tumors.[96,97] There are only two well-documented cases of acromegaly resulting from secretion of GH by a nonpituitary tumor.[98,99] The other tumors caused acromegaly by secreting growth hormone-releasing hormone (GHRH), which was first isolated from extracts of pancreatic tumors.

Overall, secretion of GHRH accounts for less than 1% of cases of acromegaly.[100] The clinical findings, aside from the presence of a nonpituitary tumor, do not differ from those in acromegaly caused by somatotropic adenomas. The mean duration of acromegalic features before diagnosis is 7.9 years, about the same as in pituitary acromegaly. Diabetes mellitus, amenorrhea, and galactorrhea are common. In about 50% of cases, the extrapituitary neoplasm is symptomatic. Other syndromes of hormone excess, including Cushing's syndrome, primary hyperparathyroidism, and the Zollinger-Ellison syndrome, can occur in conjunction with acromegaly.

Carcinoids are the most common extrapituitary tumors that produce acromegaly (69% of cases), followed by islet cell tumors (23%), pheochromocytoma, and paraganglioma.[96] GHRH immunoreactivity can often be demonstrated in neuroendocrine tumors from patients without acromegaly, usually in smaller amounts than in tumors associated with acromegaly. However, high plasma levels of GHRH have been reported in SCLC patients without acromegaly.[101] Some of these patients have abnormal GH secretory dynamics, such as a paradoxical GH increase after administration of thyrotropin-releasing hormone (TRH), suggesting that subclinical or incomplete forms of acromegaly may be present. All three isoforms of GHRH have been identified in nonpituitary tumors, but the predominant species in most tumors is GHRH(1-40), whereas the dominant hypothalamic form is GHRH(1-44).

Serum levels of GHRH in acromegaly caused by extrapituitary tumors are markedly elevated, from 0.3 to 5 μg/L (0.3 to 50 ng/mL).[100] Normal fasting GHRH levels are less than 60 ng/L (0.06 ng/mL), and the peripheral level is less than 200 ng/L (0.2 ng/mL) in typical acromegaly.

The dynamics of GH secretion in acromegaly induced by nonpituitary secretion of GHRH are not distinctive. GH and IGF-I levels are high, and the normal circadian rhythm of GH secretion is lost. Prolactin levels are elevated in 80% of patients. Virtually all patients display a paradoxical increase of GH after administration of TRH, compared with approximately 40% of patients with classic acromegaly. Many patients with GHRH-induced acromegaly do not respond to exogenous GHRH, but this is not a uniform finding and cannot be used diagnostically. GHRH-induced acromegaly should be considered in patients with a small sella turcica, but oftentimes the sella is enlarged in these patients and pituitary imaging is nondiagnostic. In most cases, the nonpituitary tumor can be identified by imaging studies of the chest and abdomen. About 90% of carcinoid tumors that cause acromegaly are located in the chest (see Chapter 8).

The primary therapy is surgical. About half of patients have resectable tumors. For patients with nonresectable disease, the therapy of choice is octreotide, the somatostatin agonist. In about half of patients, GH levels return to normal with octreotide or lanreotide treatment, and most of the remainder have a partial response.[102] The level of GHRH is often reduced less than that of GH, which suggests that the drug affects primarily the pituitary response to GHRH.

One case of extrapituitary acromegaly caused by nonpituitary secretion of GH itself involved a pancreatic islet cell tumor that contained both GH and GH mRNA. At surgery, an arteriovenous GH gradient was demonstrated across the tumor, and tumor cells in culture secreted immunoreactive GH.[99,103] GHRH was not detectable in plasma. The other well-documented case was a patient with follicular non-Hodgkin's lymphoma in which the cells expressed the GH gene, but not the GHRH gene, and secreted large amounts of GH in culture. Hypersecretion of GH was abolished by successful chemotherapy of the lymphoma.[98]

The propensity of other members of the GH family for secretion by nonendocrine tumors is variable. Prolactin has not been conclusively shown to be secreted into the blood by nonpituitary tumors. However, prolactin and its receptor are expressed in human breast carcinoma cells,[104] and an autocrine pathway has been described in which prolactin induces constitutive phosphorylation of erbB2 (Her/Neu).[20] Prolactin receptor antagonists have been developed to target this pathway.[105] Neoplastic production of human placental lactogen (hPL) (or chorionic somatomammotropin) appears to be relatively common.[106] In large series, hPL was detectable in plasma in 9% of patients with malignant disease, most commonly lung carcinoma but also carcinoma of the thyroid, breast, stomach, pheochromocytoma, carcinoids, and leukemia.[106] Fourteen percent of patients with breast carcinoma had increased blood hPL levels. hPL has weak GH activity but substantial lactotropic activity. Patients with elevated hPL levels in blood do not have galactorrhea, however, because the circulating hPL levels in such patients are lower than the equivalent levels of prolactin that produce galactorrhea. It is also possible that neoplasms secrete hPL in biologically inactive forms.

Syndromes Caused By Human Chorionic Gonadotropin and Other Glycoprotein Hormones

hCG is produced eutopically by trophoblastic and germ cell tumors, including testicular embryonal carcinoma and extragonadal germinomas. For these tumors, hCG is a very useful marker. Clinical syndromes of gonadotropin excess are rare in nontrophoblastic cancer. Gynecomastia has been reported in a few adult patients, and incomplete sexual precocity has occurred in children, mostly with hepatoblastomas.[13,258]

hCG can be detected in serum or urine of about 20% of cancer patients, but secretion of intact, biologically active hCG is rare. Most cancers secrete hCGβ, and immunoreactive hCGβ is also present in urine as a core fragment. Serum hCGβ is increased in 60% of biliary, 46% of pancreatic, and 40% of gastric carcinomas, 10% to 75% of bladder cancers, about 25% of renal carcinomas, and about 12% of small cell lung carcinomas.[9] hCG can sometimes be a useful tumor marker; in one study, the receiver operating characteristics of hCGβ were equivalent to CEA and CA 19-9 in gastrointestinal carcinomas.[107] In contrast, malignant neuroendocrine tumors characteristically secrete hCGα, and secretion of hCGα has been used to distinguish benign and malignant insulinomas.[9,108]

Adrenal and pancreatic tumors can cause anovulation or sexual precocity by secreting luteinizing hormone (LH) ectopically. Three cases have been well documented. Two were young boys with adrenal tumors that contained LH and presented with precocious puberty[109,110]; the other was a woman with infertility and high LH levels in serum, in whom the syndrome was cured by resection of a neuroendocrine tumor from the pancreatic tail.[111]

Oncogenic Osteomalacia

More than 50 cases of hypophosphatemic osteomalacia or rickets have been reported in patients with tumors of mesenchymal origin, usually small, benign skeletal tumors of the extremities or head.[112,113] The disorder has been termed *oncogenic osteomalacia, oncogenous osteomalacia,* or *tumor-induced osteomalacia.* Histologically, the causative tumors have been called *hemangiopericytomas, ossifying and nonossifying fibromas,* or *giant cell tumors,* but a recent review suggests that most have a similar histology and has grouped them as *phosphaturic mesenchymal tumors* (mixed connective tissue variant).[114] Hypophosphatemic osteomalacia has also been reported in patients with disseminated prostatic carcinoma,[115] a situation in which the disorder may be due to renal phosphate wasting or phosphate uptake by osteoblastic metastases.

Most patients with oncogenic osteomalacia are middle-aged and present with bone pain and proximal myopathy, which may have been present for years before diagnosis. However, the disorder has been described in children. The serum phosphorus level is markedly reduced because of renal phosphate wasting. The serum alkaline phosphatase is increased, but the serum calcium and PTH levels are normal. The level of $1,25(OH)_2D_3$ is typically low and the level of 25-hydroxyvitamin D is normal. Osteomalacia is present in bone biopsies. The fact that the syndrome is reversed by resection of the tumor indicates that it has a humoral basis.

Although rare, oncogenic osteomalacia is probably the most common cause of acquired hypophosphatemic osteomalacia. The manifestations are similar to those of hereditary phosphate-wasting disorders such as X-linked hypophosphatemic rickets, but the primary event is the induction of severe phosphaturia by a humoral factor, phosphatonin, secreted by the tumor. The dominant phosphatonin in tumors associated with oncogenic osteomalacia has been identified as fibroblast growth factor 23 (FGF-23).[116,117] Most patients have markedly increased serum levels of FGF-23.[118] FGF-23 causes phosphate wasting in the disorders autosomal dominant hypophosphatemic rickets and fibrous dysplasia, and it has been implicated in the most common form of inherited phosphate wasting, X-linked hypophosphatemia.[117] Removal of the FGF-23 gene causes severe hyperphosphatemia and high $1,25(OH)_2D_3$ levels, which eventuate in hypercalcemia and subsequently death from nephrocalcinosis.[119] Although FGF-23 is apparently necessary for phosphate and vitamin D homeostasis, its precise physiological role is not yet clear (Chapter 27).

Syndromes Caused By Other Hormones

Erythropoietin and Erythrocytosis

Erythrocytosis occurs in 1% to 4% of renal carcinomas, 2% to 10% of hepatocellular carcinomas, and 10% to 20% of cerebellar hemangioblastomas. It has been observed in patients with uterine fibromyomas, adrenocortical carcinomas, or ovarian tumors. Renal and hepatocellular carcinomas account for 71% of cases; thus, erythrocytosis is most common in tumors arising from the tissues that normally secrete erythropoietin, the fetal liver and the adult kidney.

In cerebellar hemangioblastomas and renal carcinomas, there is increased expression not only of the erythropoietin gene but also other genes upregulated by hypoxia, including vascular endothelial growth factor.[16] In the von Hippel-Lindau syndrome, expression of the hypoxia-associated genes is directly linked to the inherited oncogenic mutation, loss of the *VHL* tumor suppressor gene. VHL-negative renal carcinomas and hemangioblastomas have constitutively high levels of hypoxia-inducible factor-1 (HIF-1), a heterodimeric member of the bHLH PAS (*Period [per]* gene, *Aryl hydrocarbon receptor,* and *Single-minded [sim]* gene) family of transcription factors that is composed of α and β subunits.[25] In ordinary circumstances, HIF-1α is stable under hypoxic conditions and consequently able to activate transcription of hypoxia-sensitive genes like erythropoietin. Normoxia destabilizes HIF-1α by hydroxylation of critical prolyl residues; this causes the VHL protein to bind HIF-1, thereby targeting the protein for ubiquitination and proteosomal degradation. Because loss of VHL stabilizes HIF-1, and thereby activates erythropoietin gene expression, renal carcinomas and hemangioblastomas represent rare examples of direct activation of inappropriate hormone secretion by an oncogenic mutation.

The majority of sporadic renal carcinomas and hemangioblastomas are VHL-negative, providing a ready explanation for the occurrence of erythropoietin-dependent polycythemia.[120] The *VHL* gene also displays loss of heterozygosity in some hepatocellular carcinomas,[121] and tissue-specific inactivation of the *VHL* gene in hepatocytes gives rise to cavernous hemangioma of the liver and up-regulation of the erythropoietin gene.[122] It is thus likely that inactivation of *VHL* plays a central role in the induction of erythropoietin synthesis in each of the tumors classically associated with erythropoietin-dependent polycythemia, by either transcriptional or post-transcriptional mechanisms. Genetic data on *VHL* in hepatocellular carcinoma are scarce, however.

Early studies reported that erythropoietic bioactivity was often present in tumor extracts from polycythemic patients; erythropoietin mRNA has been demonstrated in extracts of renal carcinomas,[123] hepatocellular carcinoma, and cerebellar hemangioblastoma. Erythrocytosis has been produced in nude mice by transplantation of erythropoietin-positive renal carcinoma cells and hepatocarcinoma cells.[124] Some patients with tumors and erythrocytosis have increased serum erythropoietin levels.[123] However, in the best-studied group, patients with hepatocellular carcinoma, it has been difficult to demonstrate a consistent relationship between the red blood cell mass and serum levels of erythropoietin. Increased serum levels of erythropoietin are common in patients with hepatocellular carcinoma, but few of the patients with high erythropoietin levels have erythrocytosis, and some patients with erythrocytosis have normal levels of erythropoietin. Absence of erythrocytosis in the presence of high erythropoietin levels could reflect secretion of biologically inactive (e.g., precursor) forms of erythropoietin. Low-level expression of erythropoietin and its receptor are commonplace in other cancers, raising the possibility of paracrine effects of erythropoietin to increase proliferation of tumor cells, and several recent studies have suggested negative outcomes for erythropoietin treatment of anemia associated with cancer.[125]

Calcitonin

Calcitonin is present in neuroendocrine cells of the normal bronchial epithelium and is often secreted by neuroendocrine tumors, including 18% to 60% of SCLCs. Calcitonin is also secreted by other lung carcinomas, breast cancers, leukemias, and a broad spectrum of other neoplasms. Estimates of the frequency of calcitonin secretion are lower in studies that rigorously control for assay artifacts,[126] but it is clear that some tumors express the gene for calcitonin and calcitonin gene-related peptide (CGRP) and secrete calcitonin in vitro.[127]

Tumors often secrete large forms of calcitonin[126] and are less sensitive to stimulation than in patients with hypercalcitoninemia resulting from medullary thyroid carcinoma.[128] CGRP, which is derived from alternative splicing of the calcitonin gene, is expressed in normal bronchial epithelium and has been detected in tumor extracts and serum.[129] The levels of calcitonin in the sera of patients with lung carcinoma are lower than those in medullary thyroid carcinoma, and no clinical syndrome is associated with the secretion of calcitonin or CGRP.

Endothelin

The potent vasoconstrictor peptide endothelin is expressed in hepatocellular carcinoma,[19,130] breast carcinoma, ovarian carcinoma,[131] and prostate carcinoma.[19] Endothelin receptors are often coexpressed on tumor cells, and endothelin-1 was reported to have paracrine effects on tumor cell growth.[19,131] Increased serum levels of endothelin-1 and a partially processed form of the peptide big endothelin-1 have been found in hepatocellular carcinoma.[130] Arteriovenous differences, albeit small, have been found across the liver of patients with hepatocellular carcinoma. No clinical manifestations of systemic secretion of endothelin have been reported, but endothelin-1 has been implicated as the factor causing the osteoblastic response to bone metastasis in breast carcinoma,[132] and a similar role was suggested in prostate carcinoma, where an endothelin A receptor antagonist has been used therapeutically.[133]

Vasoactive Intestinal Peptide

Inappropriate secretion of VIP produces pancreatic cholera, also known as the *WDHA syndrome* (watery diarrhea, hypokalemia, and achlorhydria) or *Verner-Morrison syndrome* (see Chapter 38). In addition to pancreatic islet cell tumors, other neuroendocrine tumors including ganglioneuroma, ganglioneuroblastoma, neuroblastoma, pheochromocytoma, and medullary thyroid carcinoma can produce the syndrome.[134,135] These tumors stain for VIP, and removal of the tumor causes return of peripheral VIP levels to normal and reverses the clinical syndrome. Increased VIP levels have also been reported in lung carcinoma and in a neuroendocrine tumor of the kidney. VIP is present in the central and peripheral nervous systems; thus, its production by neuroendocrine tumors may be regarded as eutopic rather than ectopic.

Other Gut Hormones

Somatostatin is frequently detectable in extracts of lung tumor and is secreted by cultured SCLC cells,[136] but elevated serum somatostatin concentrations are uncommon in lung cancer.[137] Only one case of the *somatostatinoma syndrome* has been attributed to SCLC. The *glucagonoma syndrome* occurred in a patient with a renal neuroendocrine tumor and in a patient with a large cell lung carcinoma.[138]

GRP is often found in lung carcinomas, cultured SCLC cells, and prostate, breast, and other tumors, but elevated serum levels are uncommon.[18] Pro-GRP may be a better tumor marker.[18,139] GRP receptors are widely distributed in lung, prostate, and breast carcinomas, and the peptide is a mitogen for SCLC cells.[17,18] Neutralizing studies with antibodies and antagonists suggest that GRP is an autocrine growth factor; GRP antagonists, antibodies, and a small molecule have been used to block tumor growth in experimental models and early clinical trials, primarily in SCLC. GRP is also reported to affect the motility of tumor cells and to have angiogenic effects.[18,140] GRP is expressed in neuroendocrine cells of bronchial mucosa, particularly at branch points, and appears to have a developmental role in the regulation of branching morphogenesis of airways and possibly in the innate immune system.[28] Pancreatic polypeptide is occasionally detectable in the sera of patients with carcinoid tumors.

REFERENCES

1. Brown WH. A case of pluriglandular syndrome: "Diabetes of bearded woman." Lancet 1928;2:1022.
2. Case Records of the Massachusetts General Hospital. Case 27461. N Engl J Med 1941;225:789-791.

3. Plimpton CH, Gellhorn A. Hypercalcemia in malignant disease without evidence of bone destruction. Am J Med 1956;21: 750-759.
4. Connor TB, Thomas WC Jr. Etiology of hypercalcemia associated with lung carcinoma. J Clin Invest 195635:697-701.
5. Schwartz WB, Bennett W, Curelop S, Bartter FC. A syndrome of renal sodium loss and hyponatremia probably resulting from inappropriate secretion of antidiuretic hormone. Am J Med 9157; 23:529-542.
6. Meador CK, Liddle GW, Island DP, et al. Cause of Cushing's syndrome in patients with tumors arising from nonendocrine tissue. J Clin Endocrinol Metab 196222:693-700.
7. Liddle GW, Nicholson WE, Island DP, et al. Clinical and laboratory studies of ectopic humoral syndromes. Recent Prog Horm Res 1969;25:283-314.
8. Zapf J. Insulinlike growth factor binding proteins and tumor hypoglycemia. Trends Endocrinol Metab 1995;6:37-42.
9. Stenman UH, Alfthan H, Hotakainen K. Human chorionic gonadotropin in cancer. Clin Biochem 2004;37:549-61.
10. Seckl MJ, Mulholland PJ, Bishop AE, et al. Hypoglycemia due to an insulin-secreting small-cell carcinoma of the cervix [see comments]. N Engl J Med 1999;341:733-736.
11. Furrer J, Hattenschwiler A, Komminoth P, et al. Carcinoid syndrome, acromegaly, and hypoglycemia due to an insulin-secreting neuroendocrine tumor of the liver. J Clin Endocrinol Metab 2001;86:2227-2230.
12. Baylin SB, Mendelsohn G. Ectopic (inappropriate) hormone production by tumors: mechanisms involved and the biological and clinical implications. Endocr Rev 1980;1:45-77.
13. Feinberg AP, Ohlsson R, Henikoff S. The epigenetic progenitor origin of human cancer. Nat Rev Genet 2006;7:21-33.
14. Reya T, Morrison SJ, Clarke MF, Weissman IL. Stem cells, cancer, and cancer stem cells. Nature 2001;414:105-111.
15. Krieg M, Marti HH, Plate KH. Coexpression of erythropoietin and vascular endothelial growth factor in nervous system tumors associated with von Hippel-Lindau tumor suppressor gene loss of function. Blood 1998;92:3388-3393.
16. Kim WY, Kaelin WG. Role of VHL gene mutation in human cancer. J Clin Oncol 2004;22:4991-5004.
17. Cuttitta F, Desmond NC, Mulshine J, et al. Bombesin-like peptides can function as autocrine growth factors in human small-cell lung cancer. Nature 1985;316:823-826.
18. Patel O, Shulkes A, Baldwin GS: Gastrin-releasing peptide and cancer. Biochim Biophys Acta 2006;1766:23-41.
19. Nelson J, Bagnato A, Battistini B, Nisen P. The endothelin axis: emerging role in cancer. Nat Rev Cancer 2003;3:110-116.
20. Yamauchi T, Yamauchi N, Ueki K, et al. Constitutive tyrosine phosphorylation of ErbB-2 via Jak2 by autocrine secretion of prolactin in human breast cancer. J Biol Chem 2000;275: 33937-33944.
21. Newell-Price J, King P, Clark AJ. The CpG island promoter of the human proopiomelanocortin gene is methylated in nonexpressing normal tissue and tumors and represses expression. Mol Endocrinol 2001;15:338-348.
22. Ye L, Li X, Kong X, et al. Hypomethylation in the promoter region of POMC gene correlates with ectopic overexpression in thymic carcinoids. J Endocrinol 2005;185:337-343.
23. Holt EH, Vasavada RC, Bander NH, et al. Region-specific methylation of the parathyroid hormone–related peptide gene determines its expression in human renal carcinoma cell lines. J Biol Chem 1993;268:20639-20645.
24. Dannies PS. Protein hormone storage in secretory granules: mechanisms for concentration and sorting. Endocr Rev 1999;20:3-21.
25. Hannah MJ, Schmidt AA, Huttner WB. Synaptic vesicle biogenesis. Annu Rev Cell Dev Biol 1999;15:733-798.
26. Taupenot L, Harper KL, O'Connor DT. The chromogranin-secretogranin family. N Engl J Med 2003;348:1134-1149.
27. Taylor NA, Van De Ven WJM, Creemers JWM. Curbing activation: proprotein convertases in homeostasis and pathology. FASEB J 2003;17:1215-1227.
28. Linnoila RI. Functional facets of the pulmonary neuroendocrine system. Lab Invest 2006;86:425-444.
29. Meuwissen R, Linn SC, Linnoila RI, et al. Induction of small cell lung cancer by somatic inactivation of both Trp53 and Rb1 in a conditional mouse model. Cancer Cell 2003;4:181-189.
30. Wikenheiser-Brokamp KA. Rb family proteins differentially regulate distinct cell lineages during epithelial development. Development 2004;131:4299-4310.
31. Ball DW. Achaete-scute homolog-1 and Notch in lung neuroendocrine development and cancer. Cancer Lett 2004;204:159-169.
32. Linnoila RI, Zhao B, DeMayo JL, et al. Constitutive achaete-scute homologue-1 promotes airway dysplasia and lung neuroendocrine tumors in transgenic mice. Cancer Res 2000;60:4005-4009.
33. Ball DW, Azzoli CG, Baylin SB, et al. Identification of a human achaete-scute homolog highly expressed in neuroendocrine tumors. Proc Natl Acad Sci U S A 1993;90:5648-5652.
34. Artavanis-Tsakonas S, Rand MD, Lake RJ. Notch signaling: cell fate control and signal integration in development. Science 1999; 284:770-776.
35. Chen H, Thiagalingam A, Chopra H, et al. Conservation of the *Drosophila* lateral inhibition pathway in human lung cancer: a hairy-related protein (HES-1) directly represses achaete- scute homolog-1 expression. Proc Natl Acad Sci U S A 1997;94: 5355-5360.
36. Stewart AF. Hypercalcemia associated with cancer. N Engl J Med 2005;352:373-379.
37. Body JJ. Hypercalcemia of malignancy. Semin Nephrol 2004;24: 48-54.
38. Matsuoka M. Human T-cell leukemia virus type I and adult T-cell leukemia. Oncogene 2003;22:5131-5140.
39. Kumar S, Mow BM, Kaufmann SH. Hypercalcemia complicating leukemic transformation of agnogenic myeloid metaplasia-myelofibrosis. Mayo Clin Proc 1999;74:1233-1237.
40. Kimura S, Nishimura Y, Yamaguchi K, et al. A case of pheochromocytoma producing parathyroid hormone–related protein and presenting with hypercalcemia. J Clin Endocrinol Metab 1990;70:1559-1563.
41. Budayr AA, Nissenson RA, Klein RF, et al. Increased serum levels of a parathyroid hormone–like protein in malignancy-associated hypercalcemia. Ann Intern Med 1989;111:807-812.
42. Burtis WJ, Brady TG, Orloff JJ, et al. Immunochemical characterization of circulating parathyroid hormone–related protein in patients with humoral hypercalcemia of cancer. N Engl J Med 1990;322:1106-1112.
43. Blind E, Raue F, Gotzmann J, et al. Circulating levels of midregional parathyroid hormone–related protein in hypercalcaemia of malignancy. Clin Endocrinol (Oxf) 1992;37:290-297.
44. Wysolmerski JJ, Stewart AF. The physiology of parathyroid hormone–related protein—an emerging role as a developmental factor. Annu Rev Physiol 1998;60:431-460.
45. Guise TA, Yin JJ, Taylor SD, et al. Evidence for a causal role of parathyroid hormone–related protein in the pathogenesis of human breast cancer–mediated osteolysis. J Clin Invest 1996; 98:1544-1549.
46. Yin JJ, Selander K, Chirgwin JM, et al. TGF-β signaling blockade inhibits PTHrP secretion by breast cancer cells and bone metastases development. J Clin Invest 1999;103:197-206.
47. Horwitz MJ, Tedesco MB, Sereika SM, et al. Continuous PTH and PTHrP infusion causes suppression of bone formation and discordant effects on 1,25$(OH)_2$ vitamin D. J Bone Miner Res 2005; 20:1792-1803.
48. Stewart AF, Vignery A, Silverglate A, et al. Quantitative bone histomorphometry in humoral hypercalcemia of malignancy. J Clin Endocrinol Metab 55:219-227, 1982.
49. Richard V, Rosol TJ, Foley J. PTHrP gene expression in cancer: do all paths lead to Ets? Crit Rev Eukaryot Gene Expr 2005;15: 115-132.
50. Wysolmerski JJ, Vasavada RC, Foley J, et al. Transactivation of the *PTHrP* gene in squamous carcinoma predicts the occurrence of hypercalcemia in athymic mice. Cancer Res 1996;56:1043-1049.
51. Foley J, Wysolmerski JJ, Broadus AE, Philbrick WM. Parathyroid hormone–related protein gene expression in human squamous carcinoma cells is repressed by mutant isoforms of p53. Cancer Res 1996;56:4056-4062.
52. Seymour JF, Gagel RF, Hagemeister FB, et al. Calcitriol production in hypercalcemic and normocalcemic patients with non-Hodgkin lymphoma. Ann Intern Med 1994;121:633-640.
53. Davies M, Hayes ME, Yin JA, et al. Abnormal synthesis of 1,25-dihydroxyvitamin D in patients with malignant lymphoma. J Clin Endocrinol Metab 1994;78:1202-1207.

54. Nussbaum SR, Gaz RD, Arnold A. Hypercalcemia and ectopic secretion of parathyroid hormone by an ovarian carcinoma. N Engl J Med 1990;323:1324-1238.
55. Strewler GJ, Budayr AA, Clark OH, Nissenson RA. Production of parathyroid hormone by a malignant nonparathyroid tumor in a hypercalcemic patient. J Clin Endocrinol Metab 1993;76: 1373-1375.
56. VanHouten JN, Yu N, Rimm D, et al. Hypercalcemia of malignancy due to ectopic transactivation of the parathyroid hormone gene. J Clin Endocrinol Metab 2006;91:580-583.
57. Clines GA, Guise TA. Hypercalcaemia of malignancy and basic research on mechanisms responsible for osteolytic and osteoblastic metastasis to bone. Endocr Relat Cancer 2005;12:549-583.
58. Barille-Nion S, Bataille R. New insights in myeloma-induced ostelysis. Leuk Lymphoma 2003;44:1463-467.
59. Horiuchi T, Miyachi T, Arai T, et al. Raised plasma concentrations of parathyroid hormone related peptide in hypercalcemic multiple myeloma. Horm Metab Res 1997;29:469-471.
60. Adrogue HJ, Madias NE. Hyponatremia. N Engl J Med 2000;342: 1581-1589.
61. Robertson GL. Antidiuretic hormone. Normal and disordered function. Endocrinol Metab Clin North Am 2001;30:671-694, vii.
62. Sorensen JB, Andersen MK, Hansen HH. Syndrome of inappropriate secretion of antidiuretic hormone (SIADH) in malignant disease. J Intern Med 1995;238:97-110.
63. Coulson JM, Edgson JL, Marshall-Jones ZV, et al. Upstream stimulatory factor activates the vasopressin promoter via multiple motifs, including a non-canonical E-box. Biochem J 2003;369:549-561.
64. North WG. Neuropeptide production by small cell carcinoma: vasopressin and oxytocin as plasma markers of disease. J Clin Endocrinol Metab 1991;73:1316-1320.
65. Comis RL, Miller M, Ginsberg SJ. Abnormalities in water homeostasis in small cell anaplastic lung cancer. Cancer 1980;45: 2414-2421.
66. Chute JP, Taylor E, Williams J, et al. A metabolic study of patients with lung cancer and hyponatremia of malignancy. Clin Cancer Res 2006;12:888-896.
67. Forrest JN Jr, Cox M, Hong C, et al. Superiority of demeclocycline over lithium in the treatment of chronic syndrome of inappropriate secretion of antidiuretic hormone. N Engl J Med 1978;298: 173-177.
68. Wajchenberg BL, Mendonca BB, Liberman B, et al. Ectopic adrenocorticotropic hormone syndrome. Endocr Rev 1994;15:752-787.
69. Magiakou MA, Mastorakos G, Oldfield EH, et al. Cushing's syndrome in children and adolescents. Presentation, diagnosis, and therapy. N Engl J Med 1994;331:629-636.
70. Beuschlein F, Hammer GD. Ectopic pro-opiomelanocortin syndrome. Endocrinol Metab Clin North Am 2002;31:191-234.
71. Stewart PM, Walker BR, Holder G, et al. 11β-Hydroxysteroid dehydrogenase activity in Cushing's syndrome: explaining the mineralocorticoid excess state of the ectopic adrenocorticotropin syndrome. J Clin Endocrinol Metab 1995;80:3617-3620.
72. Raffin-Sanson ML, de Keyzer Y, Bertagna X. Proopiomelanocortin, a polypeptide precursor with multiple functions: from physiology to pathological conditions. Eur J Endocrinol 2003;149:79-90.
73. Ray DW, Littlewood AC, Clark AJ, et al. Human small cell lung cancer cell lines expressing the proopiomelanocortin gene have aberrant glucocorticoid receptor function. J Clin Invest 1994;93:1625-1630.
74. Picon A, Bertagna X, de Keyzer Y. Analysis of the human proopiomelanocortin gene promoter in a small cell lung carcinoma cell line reveals an unusual role for E2F transcription factors. Oncogene 1999;18:2627-2633.
75. Raffin-Sanson ML, Massias JF, Dumont C, et al. High plasma proopiomelanocortin in aggressive adrenocorticotropin-secreting tumors. J Clin Endocrinol Metab 1996;81:4272-4277.
76. Yalow RS, Berson SA. Size heterogeneity of immunoreactive human ACTH in plasma and in extracts of pituitary glands and ACTH-producing thymoma. Biochem Biophys Res Commun 1971;44:439-45.
77. White A, Clark AJ. The cellular and molecular basis of the ectopic ACTH syndrome. Clin Endocrinol (Oxf) 1993;39:131-141.
78. Vieau D, Seidah NG, Mbikay M, et al. Expression of the prohormone convertase PC2 correlates with the presence of corticotropin-like intermediate lobe peptide in human adrenocorticotropin-secreting tumors. J Clin Endocrinol Metab 1994;79: 1503-1506.
79. Black M, Carey FA, Farquharson MA, et al. Expression of the proopiomelanocortin gene in lung neuroendocrine tumours: in situ hybridization and immunohistochemical studies. J Pathol 1993; 169:329-334.
80. Arnaldi G, Angeli A, Atkinson AB, et al. Diagnosis and complications of Cushing's syndrome: A consensus statement. J Clin Endocrinol Metab 2003;88:5593-602.
81. Ilias I, Torpy DJ, Pacak K, et al. Cushing's syndrome due to ectopic corticotropin secretion: twenty years' experience at the National Institutes of Health. J Clin Endocrinol Metab 2005;90:4955-4962.
82. Newell-Price J, Morris DG, Drake WM, et al. Optimal response criteria for the human CRH test in the differential diagnosis of ACTH-dependent Cushing's syndrome. J Clin Endocrinol Metab 2002;87:1640-1645.
83. Oldfield EH, Doppman JL, Nieman LK, et al. Petrosal sinus sampling with and without corticotropin-releasing hormone for the differential diagnosis of Cushing's syndrome. N Engl J Med 1991;325:897-905.
84. Carey RM, Varma SK, Drake CR Jr, et al. Ectopic secretion of corticotropin-releasing factor as a cause of Cushing's syndrome. N Engl J Med 1984;311:13-20.
85. Service FJ. Diagnostic approach to adults with hypoglycemic disorders. Endocrinol Metab Clin North Am 1999;28:519-532, vi.
86. Daughaday WH. Hypoglycemia in patients with non–islet cell tumors. Endocrinol Metab Clin North Am 1989;18:91-101.
87. Eastman RC, Carson RE, Orloff DG, et al. Glucose utilization in a patient with hepatoma and hypoglycemia: assessment by a positron emission tomography. J Clin Invest 1992;89:1958-1963.
88. Daughaday WH, Trivedi B. Measurement of derivatives of proinsulin-like growth factor-II in serum by a radioimmunoassay directed against the E-domain in normal subjects and patients with nonislet cell tumor hypoglycemia. J Clin Endocrinol Metab 1992;75: 110-115.
89. Hizuka N, Fukuda I, Takano K, et al. Serum insulin-like growth factor II in 44 patients with non–islet cell tumor hypoglycemia. Endocr J 1998;45(suppl):S61-S65.
90. Lowe WL Jr, Roberts CT Jr, LeRoith D, et al. Insulin-like growth factor-II in nonislet cell tumors associated with hypoglycemia: increased levels of messenger ribonucleic acid. J Clin Endocrinol Metab 1989;69:1153-1159.
91. Shapiro ET, Bell GI, Polonsky KS, et al. Tumor hypoglycemia: relationship to high molecular weight insulin-like growth factor-II. J Clin Invest 1990;85:1672-1679.
92. Baxter RC, Daughaday WH. Impaired formation of the ternary insulin-like growth factor—binding protein complex in patients with hypoglycemia due to nonislet cell tumors. J Clin Endocrinol Metab 1991;73:696-702.
93. Miraki-Moud F, Grossman AB, Besser M, et al. A rapid method for analyzing serum pro-insulin-like growth factor-II in patients with non–islet cell tumor hypoglycemia. J Clin Endocrinol Metab 2005;90:3819-3823.
94. Zapf J. Role of insulin-like growth factor (IGF) II and IGF binding proteins in extrapancreatic tumour hypoglycaemia. J Intern Med 1993;234:543-552.
95. Katz LE, Liu F, Baker B, et al. The effect of growth hormone treatment on the insulin-like growth factor axis in a child with nonislet cell tumor hypoglycemia. J Clin Endocrinol Metab 1996;81: 1141-116.
96. Faglia G, Arosio M, Bazzoni N. Ectopic acromegaly. Endocrinol Metab Clin North Am 1992;21:575-595.
97. Melmed S. Extrapituitary acromegaly. Endocrinol Metab Clin North Am 1991;20:507-518.
98. Beuschlein F, Strasburger CJ, Siegerstetter V, et al. Acromegaly caused by secretion of growth hormone by a non-Hodgkin's lymphoma. N Engl J Med 2000;342:1871-1876.
99. Melmed S, Ezrin C, Kovacs K, et al. Acromegaly due to secretion of growth hormone by an ectopic pancreatic islet-cell tumor. N Engl J Med 1985;312:9-17.
100. Thorner MO, Frohman LA, Leong DA, et al. Extrahypothalamic growth-hormone–releasing factor (GRF) secretion is a rare cause of acromegaly: plasma GRF levels in 177 acromegalic patients. J Clin Endocrinol Metab 1984;59:846-849.

101. Schopohl J, Losa M, Frey C, et al. Plasma growth hormone (GH)–releasing hormone levels in patients with lung carcinoma. Clin Endocrinol (Oxf)1991; 34:463-467.
102. Drange MR, Melmed S. Long-acting lanreotide induces clinical and biochemical remission of acromegaly caused by disseminated growth hormone–releasing hormone–secreting carcinoid. J Clin Endocrinol Metab 1998;83:3104-3109.
103. Ezzat S, Ezrin C, Yamashita S, Melmed S. Recurrent acromegaly resulting from ectopic growth hormone gene expression by a metastatic pancreatic tumor. Cancer 1993;71:66-70.
104. Clevenger CV, Furth PA, Hankinson SE, Schuler LA. The role of prolactin in mammary carcinoma. Endocr Rev 2003;24:1-27.
105. Goffin V, Bernichtein S, Touraine P, Kelly PA. Development and potential clinical uses of human prolactin receptor antagonists. Endocr Rev 2005;26:400-422.
106. Weintraub BD, Rosen SW. Ectopic production of human chorionic somatomammotropin by nontrophoblastic cancers. J Clin Endocrinol Metab 1971;32:94-101.
107. Louhimo J, Finne P, Alfthan H, et al. Combination of hCGβ, CA 19-9 and CEA with logistic regression improves accuracy in gastrointestinal malignancies. Anticancer Res 2002;22:1759-1764.
108. Kahn CR, Rosen SW, Weintraub BD, et al. Ectopic production of chorionic gonadotropin and its subunits by islet-cell tumors. A specific marker for malignancy. N Engl J Med 1977;297:565-569.
109. Gadner H, Weber B, Riehm H. Adrenocortical carcinoma with ectopic LH production. Z Kinderheilkd 1974;118:63-70.
110. Romer TE, Sachnowska K, Savage MO, et al. Luteinizing hormone secreting adrenal tumour as a cause of precocious puberty. Clin Endocrinol (Oxf) 1998;48:367-372.
111. Hirshberg B, Conn PM, Uwaifo GI, et al. Ectopic Luteinizing hormone secretion and anovulation. N Engl J Med 2003;348: 312-317.
112. Schapira D, Ben Izhak O, Nachtigal A, et al. Tumor-induced osteomalacia. Semin Arthritis Rheum 1995;25:35-46.
113. Drezner MK. Tumor-induced osteomalacia. Rev Endocr Metab Disord 2001;2:175-186.
114. Folpe AL, Fanburg-Smith JC, Billings SD, et al. Most osteomalacia-associated mesenchymal tumors are a single histopathologic entity: an analysis of 32 cases and a comprehensive review of the literature. Am J Surg Pathol 2004;28:1-30.
115. Lyles KW, Berry WR, Haussler M, et al. Hypophosphatemic osteomalacia: association with prostatic carcinoma. Ann Intern Med 1980;93:275-278.
116. Shimada T, Mizutani S, Muto T, et al. Cloning and characterization of FGF23 as a causative factor of tumor-induced osteomalacia. Proc Natl Acad Sci U S A 2001;98:6500-6505.
117. White KE, Larsson TE, Econs MJ. The roles of specific genes implicated as circulating factors involved in normal and disordered phosphate homeostasis: frizzled related protein-4, matrix extracellular phosphoglycoprotein, and fibroblast growth factor 23. Endocr Rev 2006;27:221-241.
118. Jonsson KB, Zahradnik R, Larsson T, et al. Fibroblast growth factor 23 in oncogenic osteomalacia and X-linked hypophosphatemia. N Engl J Med 2003;348:1656-1663.
119. Shimada T, Kakitani M, Yamazaki Y, et al. Targeted ablation of FGF23 demonstrates an essential physiological role of FGF23 in phosphate and vitamin D metabolism. J Clin Invest 2004;113: 561-568.
120. Cohen HT, McGovern FJ. Renal-cell carcinoma. N Engl J Med 2005;353:2477-2490.
121. Piao Z, Kim H, Jeon BK, et al. Relationship between loss of heterozygosity of tumor suppressor genes and histologic differentiation in hepatocellular carcinoma. Cancer 1997;80:865-872.
122. Haase VH, Glickman JN, Socolovsky M, Jaenisch R. Vascular tumors in livers with targeted inactivation of the von Hippel-Lindau tumor suppressor. Proc Natl Acad Sci U S A 2001;98:1583-1588.
123. Da Silva JL, Lacombe C, Bruneval P, et al. Tumor cells are the site of erythropoietin synthesis in human renal cancers associated with polycythemia. Blood 75:577-582, 1990.
124. Horinouchi A, Miyamoto S, Sekiguchi M, et al. Erythropoietin mRNA in hepatocellular carcinomas and kidney in male B6C3F1 mice with secondary polycythemia. Toxicol Pathol 1998;26: 682-686.
125. Hardee ME, Arcasoy MO, Blackwell KL, et al. Erythropoietin biology in cancer. Clin Cancer Res 2006;12:332-339.
126. Roos BA, Lindall AW, Baylin SB, et al. Plasma immunoreactive calcitonin in lung cancer. J Clin Endocrinol Metab 1980;50: 659-666.
127. Symes AJ, Craig RK, Brickell PM. Loss of transcriptional repression contributes to the ectopic expression of the calcitonin/a-CGRP gene in a human lung carcinoma cell line. FEBS Lett 1992;306: 229-233.
128. Machens A, Haedecke J, Holzhausen HJ, et al. Differential diagnosis of calcitonin-secreting neuroendocrine carcinoma of the foregut by pentagastrin stimulation. Langenbecks Arch Surg 2000;385:398-401.
129. Ghatei MA, Stratton MR, Allen JM, et al. Co-secretion of calcitonin gene-related peptide, gastrin-releasing peptide and ACTH by a carcinoid tumor metastasizing to the cerebellum. Postgrad Med J 63:123-130, 1987.
130. Ishibashi M, Fujita M, Nagai K, et al. Production and secretion of endothelin by hepatocellular carcinoma. J Clin Endocrinol Metab 1993;76:378-383.
131. Bagnato A, Salani D, Di Castro V, et al. Expression of endothelin 1 and endothelin A receptor in ovarian carcinoma: evidence for an autocrine role in tumor growth. Cancer Res 1999;59:720-727.
132. Yin JJ, Mohammad KS, Kakonen SM, et al. A causal role for endothelin-1 in the pathogenesis of osteoblastic bone metastases. Proc Natl Acad Sci U S A 2003;100:10954-10959.
133. Carducci MA, Padley RJ, Breul J, et al. Effect of endothelin-A receptor blockade with atrasentan on tumor progression in men with hormone-refractory prostate cancer: a randomized, phase II, placebo-controlled trial. J Clin Oncol 2003;21:679-689.
134. Said SI, Faloona GR. Elevated plasma and tissue levels of vasoactive intestinal polypeptide in the watery-diarrhea syndrome due to pancreatic, bronchogenic and other tumors. N Engl J Med 1975;293:155-160.
135. Pratz KW, Ma C, Aubry MC, et al. Large cell carcinoma with calcitonin and vasoactive intestinal polypeptide–associated Verner-Morrison syndrome. Mayo Clin Proc 2005;80:116-120.
136. Szabo M, Berelowitz M, Pettengill OS, et al. Ectopic production of somatostatin-like immuno- and bioactivity by cultured human pulmonary small cell carcinoma. J Clin Endocrinol Metab 1980; 51:978-987.
137. Penman E, Wass JA, Besser GM, Rees LH. Somatostatin secretion by lung and thymic tumours. Clin Endocrinol (Oxf) 1980;13: 613-620.
138. Hunstein W, Trumper LH, Dummer R, Schwechheimer K. Glucagonoma syndrome and bronchial carcinoma. Ann Intern Med 1988;109:920-921.
139. Stieber P, Dienemann H, Schalhorn A, et al. Pro–gastrin-releasing peptide (ProGRP)—a useful marker in small cell lung carcinomas. Anticancer Res 1999;19:2673-2678.
140. Martinez A, Zudaire E, Julian M, et al. Gastrin-releasing peptide (GRP) induces angiogenesis and the specific GRP blocker 77427 inhibits tumor growth in vitro and in vivo. Oncogene 2005;24: 4106-4113.

CHAPTER 44

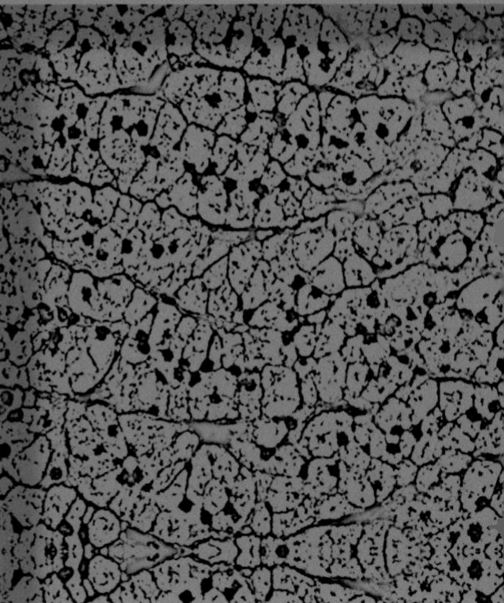

CARCINOID TUMORS, THE CARCINOID SYNDROME, AND RELATED DISORDERS

Kjell Öberg

The first clinical and histopathologic description of carcinoid tumor was made by Otto Lubarsch in 1888.[1] He was impressed by the multicentric origin of carcinoid tumors of the gastrointestinal (GI) tract, their lack of gland formation, and their lack of similarity with the usual adenocarcinoma of the alimentary system.

The term *Karzinoide* was introduced in 1907 by the pathologist Oberndorffer[2] as a descriptive name for what he considered to be a benign type of neoplasm of the ileum, which could nevertheless behave like a carcinoma. It was subsequently generally accepted that the carcinoid tumor was a very slow growing and benign neoplasm with no potential for invasiveness and no tendency to give rise to metastases. This myth of benignity has survived to the present, even though in 1949 Pearson and Fitzgerald[3] described a large series of metastasizing carcinoid tumors.

Carcinoid tumors have subsequently been reported in a wide range of organs, but they most commonly involve the lungs and GI tract. Carcinoid tumors of the thymus, ovaries, testes, heart, and middle ear have also been described. The clinically well known *carcinoid syndrome* was described by Thorson and associates[4] in 1954; 1 year earlier, Lembeck[5] had extracted serotonin from a carcinoid tumor.

Phylogenesis and Embryology

Carcinoid tumors are derived from neuroendocrine cells, and Gosset and Masson[6] in 1914 were the first to point out the neuroendocrine properties of carcinoid tumors. Masson[7] later described the remarkable affinity for silver salts displayed by intracytoplasmic granules in tumor cells and noted that carcinoid tumors originate from enterochromaffin cells, the Kulchitsky cells in the crypts of Lieberkühn in the intestinal epithelium. Furthermore, he suggested that the tumors were of endocrine origin (Fig. 44–1).

The mammalian GI tract and pancreas contain a large number of endocrine cell types, which initially were believed to originate from the neuroectoderm. This observation gave rise to the *APUD concept* (*a*mine *p*recursor *u*ptake and *d*ecarboxylation) because of the ability of these cells to take up and decarboxylate amino acid precursors of biogenic amines such as serotonin and catecholamines.[8] The APUD concept was later revised by others, who postulated that these endocrine cells might also be derived from mesoderm and endoderm.[9] The neuronal phenotype is clearly seen when culturing carcinoid tumor cells in vitro. The enterochromaffin cells, from which many carcinoid tumors derive, have the property of producing

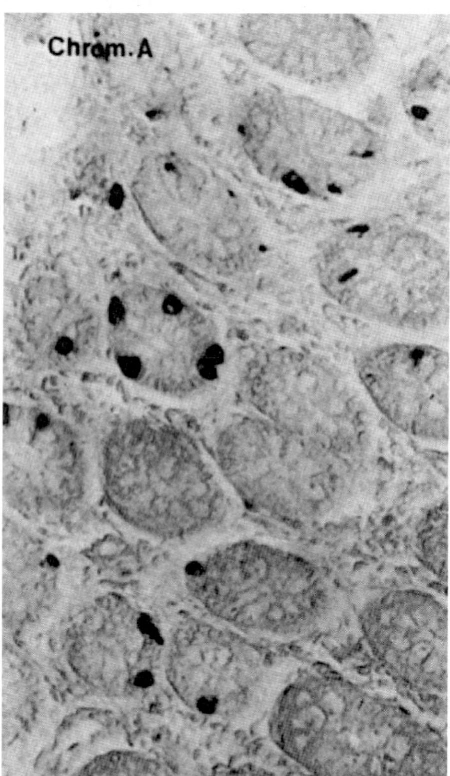

Figure 44–1 ▪ Normal human intestine stained with chromogranin A (Chrom. A) to delineate neuroendocrine cells. The cells are scattered in the intestinal mucosa.

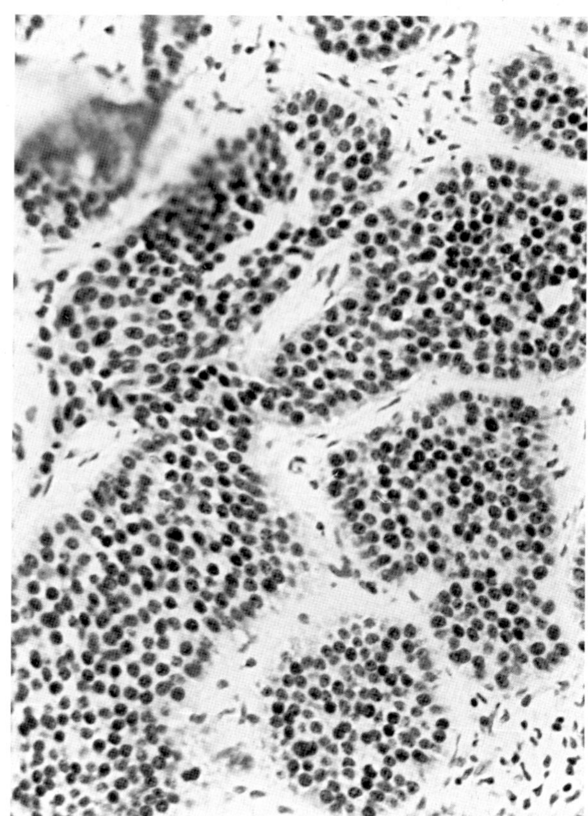

Figure 44–2 ▪ Histopathology of classic well-differentiated midgut carcinoid tumor.

and secreting amines (such as serotonin) and polypeptides (such as neurokinin-A and substance P).

Carcinoid tumors might also originate from other neuroendocrine cells, such as the enterochromaffin-like (ECL) cells of the gut and endocrine cells in the bronchi. The tumors derived from these cells can produce a wide range of hormones, such as gastrin, gastrin-releasing peptide (GRP), ghrelin, calcitonin, pancreatic polypeptide, adrenocorticotropic hormone (ACTH), corticotropin-releasing hormone (CRH), and growth hormone–releasing hormone (GHRH), as well as somatostatin, glucagon, and calcitonin gene–related peptide (CGRP).[10] A common secretory product from all types of carcinoid tumors is the glycoprotein chromogranin-A (CgA)—the most important general tumor marker in these patients (see later).

Molecular Genetics

Despite advances in the diagnosis, localization, and treatment of carcinoid tumors, no etiologic factor associated with the development of these tumors has been identified. Little is known about molecular genetic changes underlying tumorigenesis. Sporadic foregut carcinoids as well as the familial-type multiple endocrine neoplasia type 1 (MEN-1) often display allelic losses at chromosome 11q13, and somatic *MEN-1* gene mutations have been reported in one third of sporadic foregut tumors.[11] In contrast with foregut carcinoids, molecular and cytogenetic data for midgut carcinoids are quite limited, and these tumors are not included in MEN-1 syndrome. Deletions of chromosomes 18q and 18p have been reported in 38% and 33%, respectively, of GI carcinoids.[12]

In one publication, deletions on chromosome 18 were found in 88% of midgut carcinoid tumors, but the Smad 4/DPC4 locus was not deleted.[13] In addition to the consistent finding of deletions on chromosome 18, multiple deletions on other chromosomes (4, 5, 7, 9, 14, 20) were noticed in single tumors. The region telomeric to Smad 4/DPC 4/DCC loci must be further explored for possible losses of a tumor suppressor gene in this area. Gene expression arrays in carcinoid tumors have demonstrated up-regulation of the *RET* proto-oncogene, but no mutations have been detected so far. Recent data indicate that the Notch signaling pathway is a significant regulator of neuroendocrine differentiation and serotonin production in GI carcinoid tumors.[14,15]

Classification

In 1963, Williams and Sandler reported a relationship between the embryonic origin of carcinoid tumors and the histologic, biochemical, and, to some extent, clinical features of the tumors.[16] Three distinct groups were formed (Table 44–1): foregut carcinoids (i.e., intrathoracic, gastric, and duodenal carcinoids), midgut carcinoids (carcinoids of the small intestine, appendix, and proximal colon), and hindgut carcinoids (carcinoid tumors of the distal colon and rectum).

Although this original classification has been useful in the clinical assessment of patients with carcinoid tumors, it has demonstrated significant shortcomings. As a result, a new classification system has emerged that takes into account not only the site of origin but also variations in the histopathologic characteristics of carcinoid tumors (World Health Organization [WHO] classification).[17] In this revised system, typical tumors are classified as *well-differentiated* neuroendocrine tumors, with their characteristic growth pattern (Fig. 44–2). These tumors are usually slow growing, with low proliferation capacity (proliferation index <2%). They are usually confined to the mucosa and

TABLE 44–1 CLASSIFICATION OF CARCINOID TUMORS

Foregut	Midgut	Hindgut
	HISTOPATHOLOGY	
Argyrophilic CgA positive NSE positive	Argentaffin positive CgA positive NSE positive	Argyrophilic SVP-2 positive CgA positive, NSE positive
	MOLECULAR GENETICS	
Chromosome 11q13 deletion	Chromosome 18q, 18p deletion	Unknown
	SECRETORY PRODUCTS	
CgA, 5-HT, 5-HTP, histamine, ACTH, GHRH, CGRP, somatostatin, AVP, glucagon, gastrin, NKA, substance P, neurotensin, GRP	CgA, 5-HT, NKA, substance P, prostaglandin E_1 and F_2, bradykinin	PP, YY, somatostatin
	CARCINOID SYNDROME	
Present (30%)	Present (70%)	Absent

ACTH, adrenocorticotropic hormone; AVP, arginine vasopressin; CgA, chromogranin A; CGRP, calcitonin gene–releasing hormone; GRP, gastrin-releasing peptide; 5-HT, 5-hydroxytryptamine; 5-HTP, 5-hydroxytryptophan; NKA, neurokinin; NSE, neuron-specific enolase; PP, pancreatic peptide; YY, peptide YY; SVP-2, synaptic vesicle protein 2.

submucosa and are less than 1 to 2 cm in diameter (classical midgut carcinoid). Well-differentiated endocrine carcinomas are larger than 2 cm and show widely invasive growth and a high proliferation index (PI 2% to 15%). Poorly differentiated carcinomas are large tumors with metastases and a proliferation index of greater than 15% (Table 44–2).

The incidence of carcinoid tumors is similar in Western countries and is estimated to be 2.8 to 4.5 per 100000 people.[18,19] Because many carcinoid tumors are indolent, the true incidence may be higher. In particular, appendiceal carcinoids have not been included in many studies, but a higher incidence of 8.2 per 100000 was found in an autopsy study when appendiceal carcinoids were included.[20] The incidence of patients with a carcinoid syndrome is about 0.5 per 100,000.[21] Data from the United States, based on results from the End Results Group and the Third National Cancer Survey, 1950 to 1969 and 1969 to 1971, respectively, found that the appendix was the most common site of carcinoid tumors, followed by the rectum, ileum, lungs, and bronchi.[22]

An analysis done in the Surveillance, Epidemiology, and End Results (SEER) program of the National Cancer Institute between 1973 and 1999 reported an increase in the percentage of pulmonary and gastric carcinoids and a decrease in the percentage of appendiceal carcinoids.[19] Age-specific incidence rates showed a peak between 65 and 75 years (7.5-9.5/100,000), with a male predominance. In persons younger than 50 years, a female predominance has been observed both for appendiceal and lung carcinoids.[23]

TABLE 44–2 WORLD HEALTH ORGANIZATION CLINICOPATHOLOGIC CLASSIFICATION OF INTESTINAL NEUROENDOCRINE TUMORS

WELL-DIFFERENTIATED ENDOCRINE TUMOR
Functioning or nonfunctioning Confined to mucosa-submucosa Nonangioinvasive <1 or 2 cm in diameter PI<2% (Ki-67) Serotonin-producing tumor (midgut carcinoid)
WELL-DIFFERENTIATED ENDOCRINE CARCINOMA
Functioning or nonfunctioning >2 cm in size Invasive growth Metastases PI>2%<15% Examples: Serotonin-producing carcinoma with or without carcinoid syndrome; bronchial carcinoid
POORLY DIFFERENTIATED ENDOCRINE CARCINOMA
Large and invasive tumors PI>15% (small cell tumors)
MIXED ENDOCRINE–EXOCRINE TUMORS
TUMOR-LIKE LESIONS

Biochemistry

The production of hormones appears to be a highly organized function of carcinoid cells. In 1953, Lembeck isolated serotonin from a carcinoid tumor; since then, the carcinoid syndrome has been related to serotonin overproduction.[5] The biosynthesis of serotonin and its metabolic degradation are outlined in Figure 44–3.

Carcinoid tumors of the midgut and foregut region with metastatic disease secrete serotonin and show elevated urinary excretion of 5-hydroxyindoleacetic acid (5-HIAA) in 76% and 30%, respectively.[24] Carcinoid tumors arising from the foregut, however, commonly have low levels of L-amino-acid decarbox-

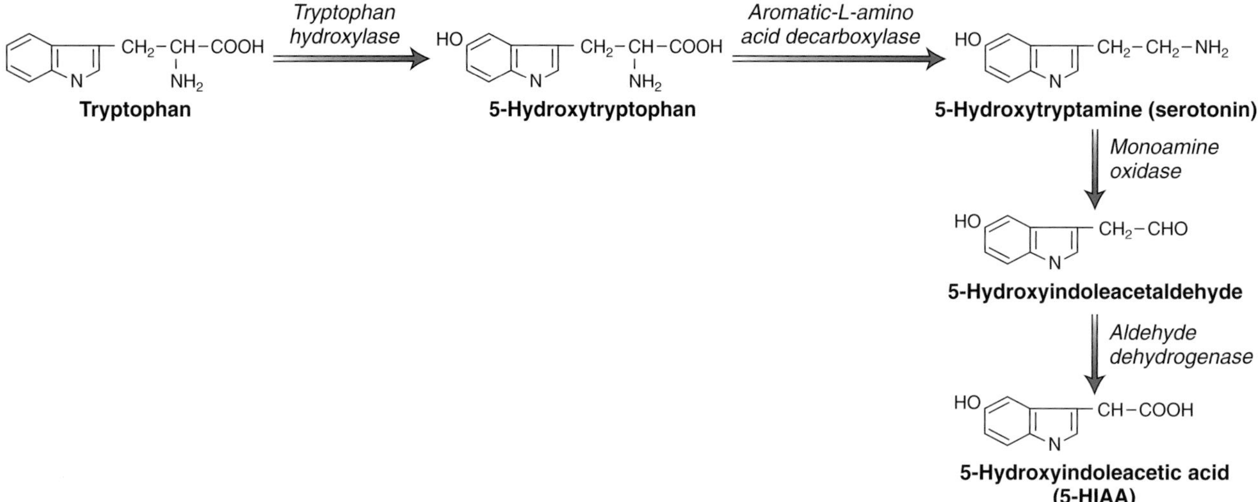

Figure 44–3 ▪ Biosynthesis and metabolism of 5-hydroxytryptamine (5-HT) (serotonin).

ylase, which converts 5-hydroxytryptophan (5-HTP) to serotonin. Thus, these tumors secrete primarily 5-HTP.[25,26]

For many years, it was believed that the entire carcinoid syndrome could be explained by the secretion of these biologically active amines. However, further studies have indicated that serotonin is mainly involved in the pathogenesis of diarrhea and that other biologically active substances play a more important part in the carcinoid flush and bronchoconstriction.

Oates and associates[27] proposed that *kallikrein*, an enzyme found in carcinoid tumors, is released in association with flush and stimulates plasma kininogen to liberate lysyl-bradykinin and bradykinin. These are biologically active substances that cause vasodilation, hypotension, tachycardia, and edema.[27-29] Furthermore, prostaglandins (E_1, E_2, F_1, F_2) might also play a role in the carcinoid syndrome.[30] Gastric carcinoids and lung carcinoids have been found to contain and secrete histamine, which might be responsible for the characteristic bright red flush seen in these patients.[31-33] Metabolites of histamine are often present in high concentration in the urine from these patients. Dopamine and norepinephrine have also been found in carcinoid tumors.[34]

The occurrence of *substance P* in carcinoid tumors was first demonstrated by Håkansson and coworkers in 1977.[35] Substance P belongs to a family of polypeptides that share the same carboxyl terminus and are called *tachykinins* (Fig. 44–4). A number of tachykinin-related peptides have been isolated from carcinoid tumors, such as neurokinin A, neuropeptide K, and eledoisin. During stimulation of flush in patients with midgut carcinoids, multiple forms of tachykinins are released to the circulation (Fig. 44–5).[36-38]

Many different polypeptides (e.g., insulin, gastrin, somatostatin, S-100 protein, polypeptide YY, pancreatic polypeptide, human chorionic gonadotropin α subunit [hCG-α], motilin, calcitonin, vasoactive intestinal polypeptide [VIP], and endorphins) have been demonstrated in carcinoid tumors by immunohistochemical staining and sometimes in tumor extracts.[10] Ectopic ACTH or CRH production may be found in foregut carcinoids; in particular, patients with bronchial carcinoids seem susceptible to Cushing's syndrome.[39] Patients with carcinoid tumors of the foregut type might also present with acromegaly due to ectopic secretion of GHRH from the tumor.[40] Duodenal carcinoids as part of von Recklinghausen's disease can secrete somatostatin.[41]

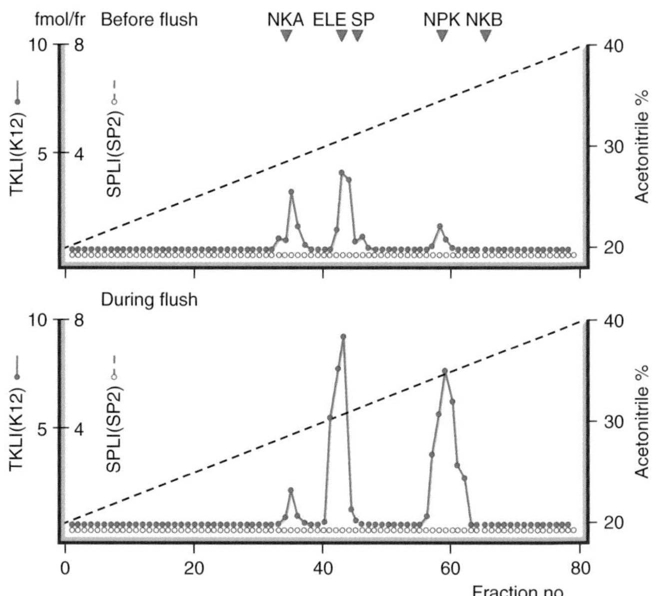

Figure 44–5 ▪ Chromatography samples of plasma from a patient with carcinoid before flush *(upper panel)* and during flush *(lower panel)*. Note the significant increase in eledoisin-like peptide as well as in neuropeptide K. ELE, eledoisin; NKA, neurokinin A; NKB, neurokinin B; NPK, neuropeptide K; SP, substance P.

The *chromogranin/secretogranin* family consists of CgA, CgB (sometimes called *secretogranin I*), secretogranin II (sometimes

```
Substance P          Arg-Pro-Lys-Pro-Gln-Gln-Phe-Phe-Gly-Leu-Met-NH2
Neurokinin A                 His-Lys-Thr-Asp-Ser-Phe-Val-Gly-Leu-Met-NH2
Neurokinin B                     Asp-Met-His-Asp-Phe-Val-Gly-Leu-Met-NH2
Eledoisin            Pyr-Pro-Ser-Lys-Asp-Ala-Phe-Ile-Gly-Leu-Met-NH2
Kassinin         Asp-Val-Pro-Lys-Ser-Asp-Glu-Phe-Val-Gly-Leu-Met-NH2
Physalemin           Pyr-Ala-Asp-Pro-Asn-Lys-Phe-Tyr-Gly-Leu-Met-NH2
Neuropeptide K       Arg-His-Lys-Thr-Asp-Ser-Phe-Val-Gly-Leu-Met-NH2
                    1-Lys-His-Ser-Ile-Gln-Gly-His-Gly-Tyr-Leu-Ala-Lys
                 Asp-Ala-Asp-Ser-Ser-Ile-Glu-Lys-Gln-Val-Ala-Leu-Leu1
```

Figure 44–4 ▪ The tachykinin family of peptides shares the same carboxyl terminus. Neuropeptide K is a prohormone containing neurokinin A, which can be spliced off.

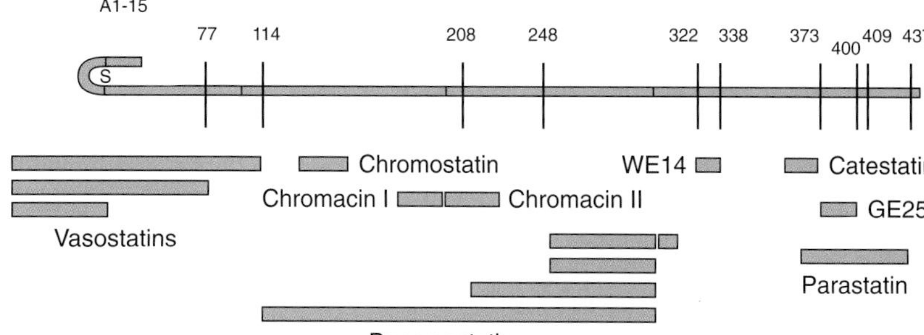

Figure 44–6 ▪ The glycoprotein chromogranin A and related peptides. GE25, WE14.

called *CgC*), and some other members. CgA was first isolated in 1965 as a water-soluble protein present in chromaffin cells from bovine adrenal medulla.[42] Its immunoreactivity has been found in all parts of the GI tract and pancreas and has also been isolated from all endocrine glands.[43]

CgA is an acidic glycoprotein of 439 amino acids with a molecular weight of 48 kd. It can be spliced into smaller fragments at dibasic cleavage sites, generating multiple bioactive fragments such as vasostatins, chromostatin, and pancreastatin (Fig. 44–6).[43-47]

Amines and hormones are stored intracellularly in two types of vesicles: large dense-core vesicles and small synaptic-like vesicles. These vesicles release amines and hormones on stimulation. Large dense-core vesicles contain the hormones and one or more members of the chromogranin/secretogranin family of proteins.[44,48] Both amines and peptides are coreleased (Fig. 44–7).

The physiologic function of CgA is not fully elucidated. Its ubiquitous presence in neuroendocrine tissues and its cosecretion with peptide hormones and amines indicate a storage role of the peptide within the secretory granule.[43,44,48] It also acts as a prohormone that can generate bioactive smaller fragments. CgA is an important tissue and serum marker for different types of carcinoid tumors, including those of the foregut, midgut, and hindgut (see Table 44–1 and later discussion).

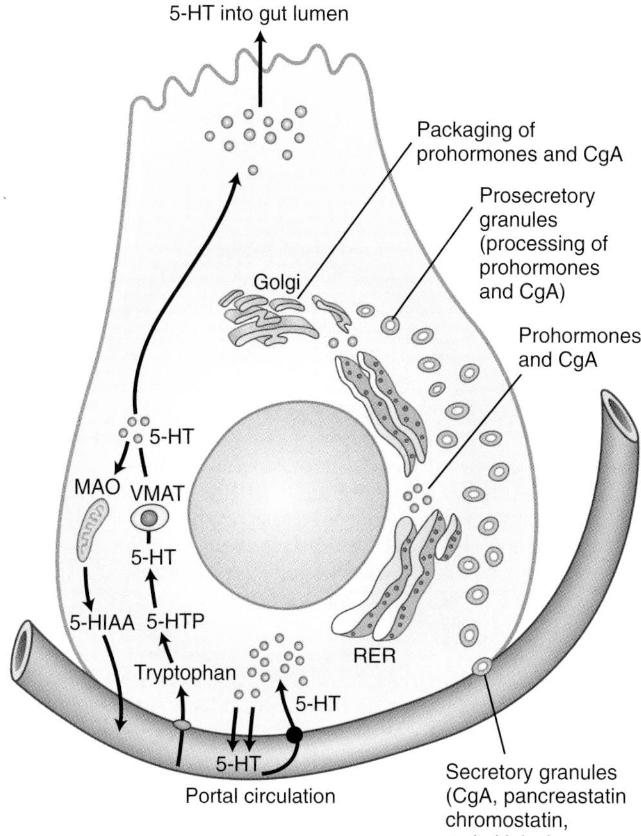

Figure 44–7 ▪ Schematic drawing of an enterochromaffin cell. The initial step in 5-hydroxytryptamine (5-HT) synthesis is carrier transport of the amino acid tryptophan from blood into the cell across the cell membrane. Intracellular tryptophan is first converted to 5-hydroxytryptophan (5-HTP), in turn converted to 5-HT and stored in secretory granules. The transport of 5-HT into granules requires vesicular monoamine transporters (VMATs). Via the basal lateral membrane, 5-HT can be released into the circulation. There is also a membrane pump mechanism in the cell membrane responsible for amine reuptake. A minor part of 5-HT can also be released into the gut lumen. Monoamine oxidase (MAO) degrades 5-HT to 5-hydroxyindoleacetic acid (5-HIAA). Peptide prohormones are synthesized in the rough endoplasmic reticulum (RER) together with chromogranin A (CgA) and other granule proteins. The products are transported to the Golgi apparatus (GA) for packaging into prosecretory granules. On stimulation, the secretory products are released from the granules by exocytosis.

Clinical Presentation

The clinical presentation of carcinoid tumors depends on localization, hormone production, and extent of the disease. Usually, a lung carcinoid is diagnosed incidentally on routine pulmonary radiography, whereas a midgut carcinoid may be identified as a bowel obstruction or as a cause of abdominal discomfort or pain. Rectal carcinoids might cause bleeding or obstruction. However, lung carcinoids can also manifest clinically with Cushing's syndrome, due to secretion of CRH or ACTH, or with the carcinoid syndrome, due to production of serotonin, 5-HTP, or histamine.[49] A midgut carcinoid often manifests with the carcinoid syndrome, due to production of serotonin and tachykinins.

The clinical manifestations at referral depend on the type of referral center. At my institution, which cares for patients with malignant tumors, 74% of the patients present with the carcinoid syndrome, 13% with abdominal pain, 12% with carcinoid heart disease, and 2% with bronchial constriction.[24] When unbiased material is analyzed, bowel obstruction is the most common problem leading to the diagnosis of ileal carcinoid tumor. The second most common symptom is abdominal pain. Flushing and diarrhea, which are components of the carcinoid syndrome, make up only the third most common presentations.[18,50-52] Because many patients have vague symptoms, however, diagnosis of the tumor may be delayed by approximately 2 to 3 years.[21]

The Carcinoid Syndrome

In 1954, Thorson and coworkers for the first time described the carcinoid syndrome as having the following features: malignant carcinoid of the small intestine with metastasis to the liver; valvular disease of the right heart (pulmonary stenosis and tricuspid insufficiency without septal defect); peripheral vasomotor symptoms; bronchial constriction; and an unusual type of cyanosis.[4] One year later, Dr. William Bean[53] gave this colorful description of the carcinoid syndrome: "This witch's brew of unlikely signs and symptoms, intriguing to the most fastidious connoisseur of clinical esoterica—the skin underwent rapid and extreme changes—resembling in clinical miniature the fecal phantasmagoria of the aurora borealis."

The syndrome is thus well characterized and includes flushing, diarrhea, right-sided heart failure, and sometimes bronchial constriction and increased urinary levels of 5-HIAA.[54,55] This is the classic carcinoid syndrome, but some patients display only one or two of the features. Other symptoms related to the syndrome are weight loss, sweating, and pellagra-like skin lesions.

Development of the carcinoid syndrome is a function of tumor mass, extent and localization of metastases, and localization of the primary tumor. The syndrome is most common in tumors originating in the small intestine and proximal colon; 40% to 60% of patients with these tumors experience the syndrome.[24,51,54,55] The disorders are less common in patients with bronchial carcinoids and do not occur in patients with rectal carcinoids.[49,56,57] The syndrome rarely occurs in patients with midgut carcinoids and a small tumor burden, such as only regional lymph node metastases.[52] Patients with the full syndrome usually have multiple liver metastases. The association with hepatic metastases is due to efficient inactivation by the liver of amines and peptides released into the portal circulation. The venous drainage of liver metastases is directly into the systemic circulation and bypasses hepatic inactivation.[58]

Other carcinoid tumors likely to be associated with the carcinoid syndrome in the absence of liver metastases are ovarian carcinoids and bronchial carcinoids, which release mediators directly into the systemic rather than the portal circulation. Retroperitoneal metastases from classic midgut carcinoids also release mediators directly into the circulation and might cause the carcinoid syndrome without any liver metastases.[54,55]

Flushing

Four types of flushing have been described in the literature.[54,55] They are erythematous, violaceous, prolonged, and bright red.

The first and most well-known type is the sudden, diffuse, erythematous flush, usually affecting the face, neck, and upper chest (i.e., the normal flushing area) (Fig. 44–8). This type of flush is commonly of short duration, lasting from 1 to 5 minutes, and is related to early-stage midgut carcinoids. Patients usually experience a sensation of warmth during flushing and sometimes heart palpitations. This type of flushing is reported in 20% to 70% of patients with midgut carcinoid at manifestation of the disease.[21,54,55,56]

The second type is the violaceous flush, which affects the same area of the body. It has roughly the same time course or sometimes lasts a little longer. Patients may also have facial telangiectasia. This flush is related to the later stages of midgut carcinoid (Fig. 44–9) and is normally not felt by patients because they have become accustomed to the flushing reaction.

The third type is prolonged flushing that usually lasts a couple of hours but can last up to several days. This flush sometimes involves the whole body and is associated with profuse lacrimation, swelling of the salivary gland, hypotension, and facial edema (Fig. 44–10). These symptoms are usually associated with malignant bronchial carcinoids.

The fourth type of flushing is a bright red, patchy flush, seen in patients with chronic atrophic gastritis and ECL-cell hyperplasia, or ECLoma (derived from ECL [enterochromaffin-like] cells). This type of flushing is related to an increased release of histamine and histamine metabolites.

Flushes may be spontaneous or may be precipitated by stress (physical and mental); infection; alcohol; certain foods (spicy); or drugs, such as by injections of catecholamines, calcium, or pentagastrin (see later). The pathophysiology of flushing in the carcinoid syndrome is not yet elucidated.[59-61] It was previously believed to be totally related to excess production of serotonin or serotonin metabolites.[60] However, several patients with high levels of plasma serotonin did not have any flushing, nor did a serotonin antagonist (e.g., methysergide, cyproheptadine, or ketanserin) have any effect on the flushing.[59,62]

In a study from my own group in which we measured the release of tachykinins, neuropeptide K, and substance P during flushing provoked by pentagastrin or alcohol, a clear correlation was found between the onset and intensity of the flushing reaction and the release of tachykinins (see Fig. 44–5). Furthermore,

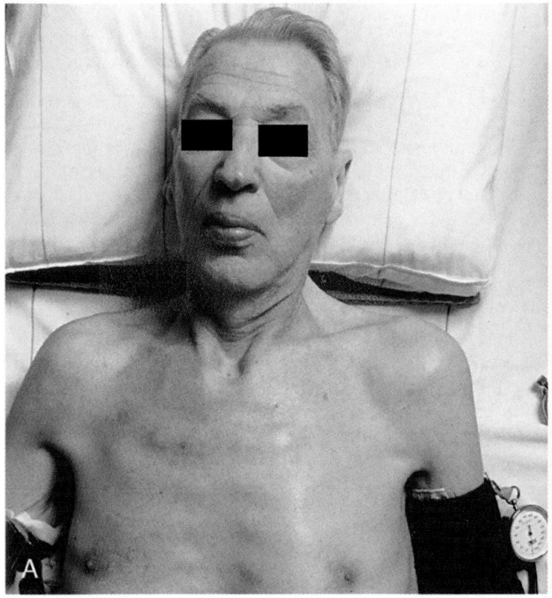

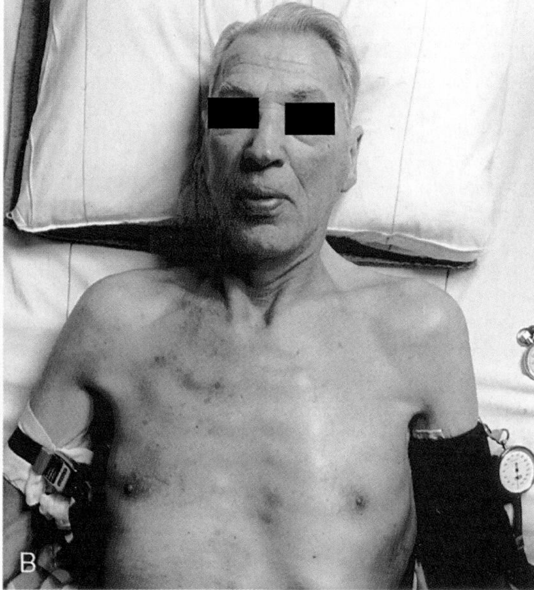

Figure 44–8 ▪ Carcinoid syndrome before and after provocation. **A,** Before flush provocation. **B,** The same patient after pentagastrin-stimulated flush.

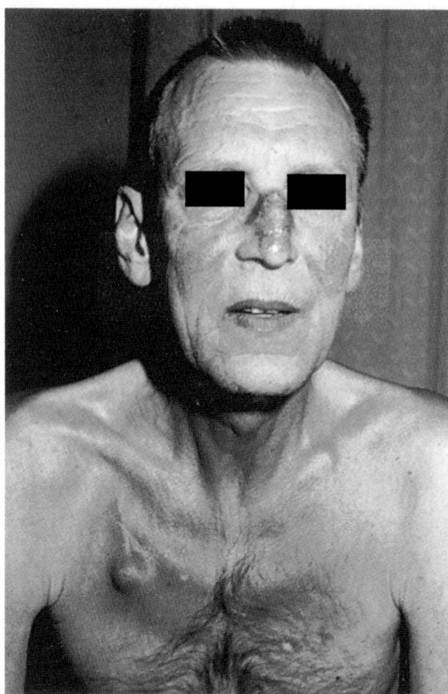

Figure 44–9 ▪ Long-lasting chronic flushing in a patient with long-standing carcinoid disease. Note the telangiectases.

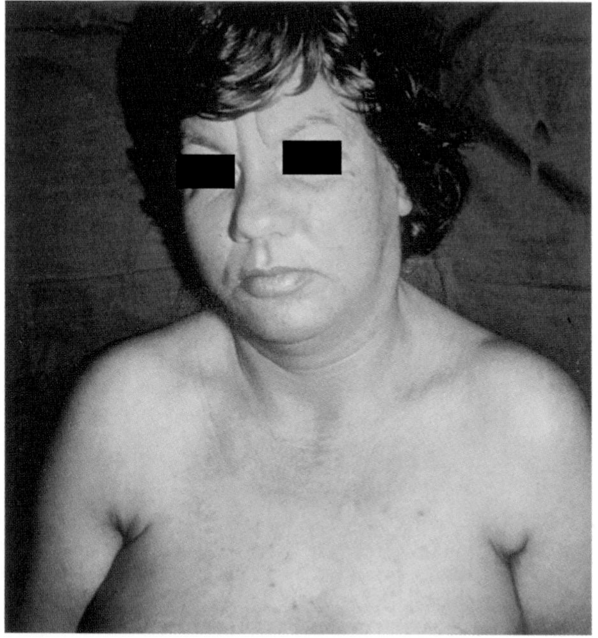

Figure 44–10 ▪ The patient has lung carcinoid and carcinoid syndrome with severe, long-standing flushing, lacrimation, and a swollen face.

when the release of tachykinins was blocked by prestimulatory administration of octreotide, little or no flushing was observed in the same patient (Fig. 44–11).[36-38] Other mediators of the flushing reaction may be kallikrein and bradykinins, which are released during provoked flushing.[27-29]

Histamine may be a mediator of the flushes seen in lung carcinoids and in gastric carcinoids (ECLomas).[31-33] Tachykinins, bradykinins, and histamines are well-known vasodilators, and somatostatin analogues might alleviate flushing by reducing circulating levels of these agents (see later).[36-38,61-66] Furschgott and Zawadski have suggested that flushing is caused by an indirect vasodilation mediated by endothelium-derived relaxing factor (EDRF) or by nitric oxide released by 5-HTP during platelet activation.[67]

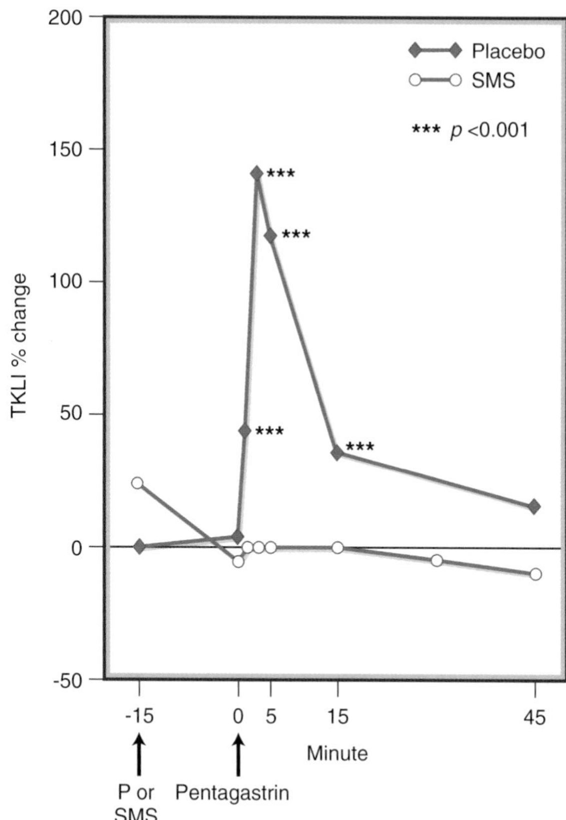

Figure 44–11 ▪ Tachykinin levels (TKLI) after stimulation with pentagastrin in patients with classic midgut carcinoids. Pretreatment for 15 minutes with somatostatin (SMS) causes inhibition of tachykinin release and inhibition of the flush reaction (0-0). P, placebo.

The facial flushing associated with carcinoid tumors should be distinguished from idiopathic flushing and menopausal hot flushes. Patients with idiopathic flushes usually have a long history of flushing starting early in life and sometimes with a family history without occurrence of a tumor. Menopausal hot flushes usually involve the whole body and are accompanied by intense sweating. Postmenopausal women in whom a true carcinoid syndrome is developing can tell the difference between the two types of flushes.

Diarrhea

Diarrhea occurs in 30% to 80% of patients with the carcinoid syndrome.[21,24,54,55] Its pathophysiology is poorly understood but is probably multifactorial. The diarrhea is often accompanied by abdominal cramping, and endocrine, paracrine, and mechanical factors contribute to this condition. A variety of tumor products, including serotonin, tachykinins, histamines, kallikrein, and prostaglandins, can stimulate peristalsis, electromechanical activity, and tone in the intestine.[61,68-70] Secretory diarrhea can occur with fluid and electrolyte imbalance. Malabsorption can result from intestinal resections, from lymphangiectasia, secondary to mesenteric fibrosis, from bacterial overgrowth, and secondary to a tumor partially obstructing the small bowel or rapid intestinal transit. Increased secretion by the small bowel, malabsorption, or accelerated transit can overwhelm the normal storage and absorptive capacity of proximal colon and result in diarrhea, which may be aggravated if the reabsorptive function of the colon is impaired.

In a study of patients with elevated serotonin levels and the carcinoid syndrome, transit time in the small bowel and colon was significantly decreased in comparison with that of normal subjects.[71] The volume of the ascending colon was significantly smaller than in normal subjects, and the postprandial colonic tone was markedly increased. This indicates that in patients in whom the carcinoid syndrome is associated with diarrhea, major alterations in gut motor function occur that affect both the small intestine and the colon. Many patients with carcinoid tumors have undergone wide resection of the small intestine, and they may be affected by the symptoms of short-bowel syndrome.

Serotonin is believed to be responsible for the diarrhea in the carcinoid syndrome by its effects on gut motility and intestinal electrolyte and fluid secretion.[55,68-70] Serotonin receptor antagonists, such as ondansetron and ketanserin, relieve the diarrhea to a certain degree.[68,72-74]

Carcinoid Heart Disease

A unique endocrine effect of carcinoid tumors is the development of plaquelike thickenings of the endocardium, valve leaflets, atria, and ventricles in 10% to 20% of the patients.[75,76] This fibrotic involvement causes stenosis and regurgitation of the blood flow. Findings of new collagen beneath the endothelium of the endocardium is almost pathognomonic for carcinoid heart disease.[75-77] The incidence of these lesions depends on the diagnostic methodology. Echocardiography can demonstrate early lesions in about 70% of patients with the carcinoid syndrome, whereas routine clinical examinations detect them in only 30% to 40%.[75,76,78] These figures have significantly dropped to 10% to 15%, probably because of earlier diagnosis and the use of biologic antitumor treatments such as somatostatin analogues and α-interferons. Both of these agents control the hormonal release and excess that might be involved in the fibrotic process.

In a study performed 15 years ago,[21] 40% of patients with carcinoid tumors died of cardiac complications related to the carcinoid disease. More recent data reveal that this complication is a rare event, and patients usually die of the effects of a progressive tumor.[24]

The precise mechanism behind the fibrosis in the right heart has not been solved yet, but it occurs mainly in patients with liver metastases who usually also have the carcinoid syndrome.[75,76] Substances inducing fibrosis are believed to be released directly into the right heart and are then neutralized or degraded through the lung circulation, because few patients present with similar lesions of the left heart.[75,76] However, patients with lung carcinoids occasionally display the same fibrotic changes in the left heart. Histologically, the plaquelike thickenings in the endocardium consist of myofibroblasts and fibroblasts embedded in a stroma that is rich in mucopolysaccharides and collagen.[75]

We have previously shown that the transforming growth factor β (TGF-β) family of growth factors is up-regulated in carcinoid fibrous plaques on the right heart.[79] The TGF-β family of growth factors is known to stimulate matrix formation and collagen deposition. The substances that induce TGF-β locally in the heart are not known, but serotonin, tachykinins, and insulin-like growth factor I (IGF-I) may be mediators.[75,80]

A correlation has been found between circulating levels of serotonin and tachykinins and the degree and frequency of carcinoid heart lesions. The weight-reducing drugs fenfluramine and dexfenfluramine appear to interfere with normal serotonin metabolism and have been associated with valvular lesions identical to those seen in carcinoid heart disease.[81,82] However, treatment resulting in decreased urinary 5-HIAA excretion does not result in regression of cardiac lesions.[83] Two animal studies indicate that serotonin might play a significant role in the development of carcinoid heart disease. Serotonin is also known to induce TGF-β_1 in in-vitro experiments.[84-86]

Bronchial Constriction

A true asthma episode is rare in patients with the carcinoid syndrome.[21,54,55] The causative agents of bronchial constriction are not known, but tachykinins and bradykinins have been suggested as mediators.[87,88] These agents can constrict smooth muscle in the respiratory tract and can also cause local edema in the airways.

Other Manifestations of the Carcinoid Syndrome

Fibrotic complications other than heart lesions may be found in patients with carcinoid tumors. These include intra-abdominal and retroperitoneal fibroses, occlusion of the mesenteric arteries and veins, Peyronie's disease, and carcinoid arthropathy.[54,55]

Intraabdominal fibrosis can lead to intestinal adhesions and bowel obstruction and is a more common cause of bowel obstruction than is the primary carcinoid tumor itself.[52,89,90] Retroperitoneal fibrosis can result in urethral obstruction that impairs kidney function, which sometimes requires treatment with urethral stents.

Narrowing and occlusion of arteries and veins by fibrosis are potentially life-threatening. Ischemic loops of the bowel might have to be removed, and this procedure ultimately causes short-bowel syndrome.[52,90]

Other rare features of the syndrome are pellagra-like skin lesions with hyperkeratosis and pigmentation, myopathy, and sexual dysfunction.[55]

Carcinoid Crisis

Carcinoid crisis has become rare since the introduction of treatment with somatostatin analogues.[91] It might occur spontaneously or during induction of anesthesia, embolization procedures, chemotherapy, or infection. Carcinoid crisis is a clinical condition characterized by severe flushing, diarrhea, hypotension, hyperthermia, and tachycardia. Without treatment, patients might die during the crisis.[91-93]

Intravenous (IV) or subcutaneous somatostatin analogues (or both) are given before, during, and after surgery to prevent the development of carcinoid crisis.[91,93-95] Patients with metastatic lung carcinoids are particularly difficult to treat during crisis. IV infusions of octreotide at doses of 50 to 100 μg/hour, supplemented with histamine H_1-receptor and H_2-receptor blockers and IV sodium chloride, are recommended.[96]

Other Clinical Manifestations of Carcinoid Tumors

Ectopic secretion of CRH and ACTH from pulmonary carcinoid tumors and thymic carcinoids accounts for 1% of all cases of Cushing's syndrome.[39,97] Acromegaly due to ectopic secretion of GHRH has also been reported in foregut carcinoids.[40,98] Gastric carcinoid tumors make up less than 1% of gastric neoplasms.[19] They can be separated into three distinct groups or types on the basis of clinical and histologic characteristics and originate from gastric ECL cells.[99] Type I is associated with chronic atrophic gastritis type A (80%). Type II is associated with Zollinger-Ellison syndrome as part of MEN-1 syndrome

(6%). Type III represents sporadic gastric carcinoids occurring without hypergastrinemia and pursue a more malignant course, with 50% to 60% developing metastases.[99,100]

About 80% of gastric carcinoids are associated with chronic atrophic gastritis type A, and more than 50% of patients with these carcinoids also have pernicious anemia. These tumors are more common in women than in men and are usually identified endoscopically during diagnostic evaluation for anemia or abdominal pain.[99,101] They are often multifocal and localized in the gastric fundus area, and they are derived from ECL cells. Patients have hypochlorhydria and hypergastrinemia. Gastrin hypersecretion has been postulated to result in hyperplasia of the ECL cells, which might later develop into carcinoid tumors.[102,103] Hyperplasia of ECL cells has been noticed in patients on long-standing proton-pump inhibitor therapy.[104,105]

Diagnosis

The diagnosis of a suspected carcinoid tumor must take into consideration molecular genetics, tumor biology, histopathology, biochemistry, and localization. The diagnosis of a carcinoid tumor may be suspected from clinical symptoms suggesting the carcinoid syndrome or from the presence of other clinical symptoms, or it can be made in relatively asymptomatic patients from the histopathology at surgery or after liver biopsy for unknown hepatic lesions.

In one study involving 154 consecutive patients with GI carcinoids found at surgery, 60% were asymptomatic.[106] In patients with symptomatic tumors, the time from onset of symptoms until diagnosis is often delayed 1 to 2 years.[18,21] The current tumor biology program includes growth factors (platelet-derived growth factor, epidermal growth factor, IGF-I, TGF-β)[107,109] and proliferation factors (measurements of the nuclear antigen Ki-67) as a proliferation index. Such an index correlates with tumor aggressiveness and survival.[107,108] Adhesion molecules such as CD-44, particularly exon-V6 and exon-V9, have been related to improved survival.[110] Determination of the expression of angiogenic factors basic fibroblast growth factor (b-FGF) and vascular endothelial growth factor (VEGF) should also be included in a tumor biology program. Somatostatin analogues are cornerstones in the treatment of the carcinoid syndrome; therefore, determination of the different subtypes of somatostatin receptors (sst-1 to sst-5) with specific antibodies is warranted.[111,112] Rare cases with familial carcinoids should be analyzed with respect to loss of heterozygosity on chromosome 11q13 and chromosome 18.

The histopathologic diagnosis of carcinoids is based on immunohistochemistry using antibodies against CgA, synaptophysin, and neuron-specific enolase. These immunohistochemical stains have replaced the old silver stains, the argyrophil stains by Grimelius and Sevier-Munger. The argentaffin stain by Masson to demonstrate content of serotonin has also been replaced by immunocytochemistry with serotonin antibodies.[10] These neuroendocrine markers can be supplemented by specific immunocytochemistry to different hormones such as substance P, gastrin, and ACTH.

Biochemical Diagnosis

In patients with flushing and other manifestations of the carcinoid syndrome, the diagnosis can be established by measuring the urinary excretion of 5-HIAA because levels are invariably elevated under these circumstances.[113] Patients with carcinoid tumors usually have urinary 5-HIAA levels of 100 to 3000 μM/24 hours (15 to 60 mg/24 hours) (reference range <50 μM/24 hours [10 mg/24 hours]). Assays for urinary 5-HIAA include high-pressure liquid chromatography (HPLC) with electrochemical detection and colorimetric and fluorescence methods.[114] Various foods and drugs can interfere with the measurement of urinary 5-HIAA, and patients should avoid these agents during the 24-hour sampling (Table 44–3).[115] Normally, two 24-hour urine collections are recommended. In a study of patients with malignant midgut carcinoid tumors, 60% to 73% presented with increased urinary 5-HIAA levels,[24,54,55] with a specificity of almost 100%.

Today, measurement of urinary 5-HIAA for diagnosis of carcinoid tumor is the predominant biochemical analytic procedure. However, urinary and platelet measurements of serotonin itself can give additional information. In some studies, platelet serotonin levels were more sensitive than urinary 5-HIAA and urinary serotonin levels and were not affected by the patient's diet, as are 5-HIAA levels.

In a comparative study of 44 consecutive patients with carcinoid tumor, the platelet serotonin, urinary 5-HIAA, and urinary serotonin levels were measured. In foregut carcinoids the sensitivities were 50%, 29%, and 55%, respectively. For midgut carcinoids, the sensitivities were 100%, 92%, and 82%, respectively, and for hindgut carcinoids they were 20%, 0%, and 60%, respectively.[116]

Elevations of 5-HIAA can occur in malabsorption states and a number of other conditions. Foregut carcinoids tend to produce an atypical carcinoid syndrome with increased plasma 5-HTP, but not serotonin, because they lack the appropriate decarboxylase.[25,34] That results in normal urinary 5-HIAA. However, some of the 5-HTP is decarboxylated in the intestine and other tissues, and many of these patients have slightly elevated urinary 5-HT or 5-HIAA levels.

Attempts have been made to identify more specific and sensitive serum markers for carcinoid tumors that might allow earlier

TABLE 44–3 FACTORS THAT INTERFERE WITH DETERMINATION OF URINARY 5-HIAA

Foods	Drugs
FACTORS THAT PRODUCE FALSE-POSITIVE RESULTS	
Avocado	Acetaminophen
Banana	Acetanilid
Chocolate	Caffeine
Coffee	Fluorouracil
Eggplant	Guaifenesin
Pecan	L-Dopa
Pineapple	Melphalan
Plum	Mephenesin
Tea	Methamphetamine
Walnuts	Methocarbamol
	Methysergide maleate
	Phenmetrazine
	Reserpine
	Salicylates
FACTORS THAT CAUSE FALSE-NEGATIVE RESULTS	
Corticotropin	None
p-Chlorophenylalanine	
Chlorpromazine	
Heparin	
Imipramine	
Isoniazid	
Methenamine mandelate	
Methyldopa	
Monoamine oxidase inhibitors	
Phenothiazine	
Promethazine	

5-HIAA, 5-hydroxyindoleacetic acid.

diagnosis. One such marker is CgA. It has been shown that CgA and CgB are more abundant than CgC in human neuroendocrine tissues.[43,44,117] In 44 patients with carcinoid tumors, CgA was increased in 99%, CgB in 88%, and CgC in only 6% (Fig. 44–12).[117] It has been proposed that CgA levels in plasma might reflect tumor size. In a study of 75 patients with midgut carcinoids and the carcinoid syndrome, CgA was elevated in 87% of carcinoid patients. Furthermore, a correlation between levels of plasma chromogranin and extent of disease was found ($P<.0001$).[24] In the same study, urinary 5-HIAA was elevated in 76% of midgut carcinoids, and there were no correlations with tumor size or extent of disease.

CgA is a more sensitive marker than urinary 5-HIAA in detecting carcinoid tumors, but because CgA is released and secreted from various types of neuroendocrine tumors, the specificity is lower.[117-120] Therefore, in a work-up of patients with the carcinoid syndrome, one should combine the determination of plasma CgA with urinary 5-HIAA or serotonin. Plasma neuron-specific enolase shows a lower sensitivity and specificity than does plasma CgA.[119] Serum hCG-α has been reported to be increased in 60% of patients with foregut carcinoid tumors and 50% of hindgut carcinoids but in only 11% of those patients with midgut carcinoids and the carcinoid syndrome. Plasma neuropeptide K levels have been reported to be elevated in 46% of patients with midgut carcinoids, whereas only 9% of patients with foregut carcinoids displayed elevated levels.[118,121] Plasma substance P has a sensitivity of 32% and a specificity of 85%.[24,36-38] Pancreatic polypeptide levels are also elevated in about one third of patients with midgut carcinoids and in as many with foregut carcinoids.[122,123]

During therapy with somatostatin analogues, neither plasma CgA nor urinary 5-HIAA is a reliable marker of tumor size because somatostatin inhibits the synthesis and release of the hormones without changes in tumor size.

Localization Procedures

Numerous imaging techniques, including endoscopy, barium enema, chest radiography, ultrasonography, computed tomography (CT), magnetic resonance imaging (MRI), and angiography, have been used to determine the location of the primary tumor as well as the metastases in patients with carcinoid tumors. In more recent years, somatostatin-receptor scintigraphy (SRS) and iodinated meta-iodobenzylguanidine (^{131}I-MIBG) scanning have been used to localize and stage the disease.[124-127] Bronchial carcinoids are usually detected by chest radiography, CT, or, occasionally, by bronchoscopy.[128] The primary midgut tumor is usually small and difficult to localize with traditional diagnostic methods such as barium enema, CT scan, or MRI. Some of these tumors can be localized by angiography, capsule endoscopy, or SRS. Liver metastases are usually detected by CT or MRI. At present, CT or MRI and SRS are the primary diagnostic modalities for tumor staging (Fig. 44–13).

A more sensitive method is positron emission tomography (PET) using ^{11}C-5-HTP, the precursor of serotonin synthesis (Fig. 44–14).[129,130] This isotope accumulates in carcinoid tumors, and with the recent development of PET cameras, tumors as small as 0.5 cm in diameter can be detected.[129] During treatment, a close relation has been found among changes in the PET scan, transport rate constant, and urinary 5-HIAA, suggesting that PET scanning may be useful in monitoring the results of therapy. PET scanning using fluorodeoxyglucose 18 (^{18}FDG) is not useful in detecting low-proliferating neuroendocrine tumors, but it can be beneficial in identifying poorly differentiated anaplastic tumors.

Carcinoid tumors contain high-affinity receptors for somatostatin in 80% to 100% of cases.[111,112,131] The receptors are present in both the primary tumor and metastases. Five subtypes of somatostatin receptors have been cloned (sst-1 to sst-5), and somatostatin receptor type 2 is the predominant subtype expressed in carcinoid tumors.

The most commonly available somatostatin analogue, *octreotide,* binds with high affinity to sst-2 and with lower affinity to sst-3 and sst-5.[132-134] SRS with ^{111}In-DTPA-Phe-octreotide has been reported to detect carcinoids with a sensitivity of 80% to 90% in patients.[134,135] Many studies have demonstrated that SRS has greater sensitivity for localizing carcinoids compared with conventional imaging studies.[135,137-140] False-positive scans can be encountered in patients with granulomas (e.g., sarcoidosis, tuberculosis), activated lymphocytes (lymphomas, chronic infection), thyroid diseases (goiter, thyroiditis), endocrine pancreatic tumors, and other endocrine tumors. Because of its high sensitivity and ability to image, whole-body SRS should be the initial imaging procedure to localize and establish the stage of

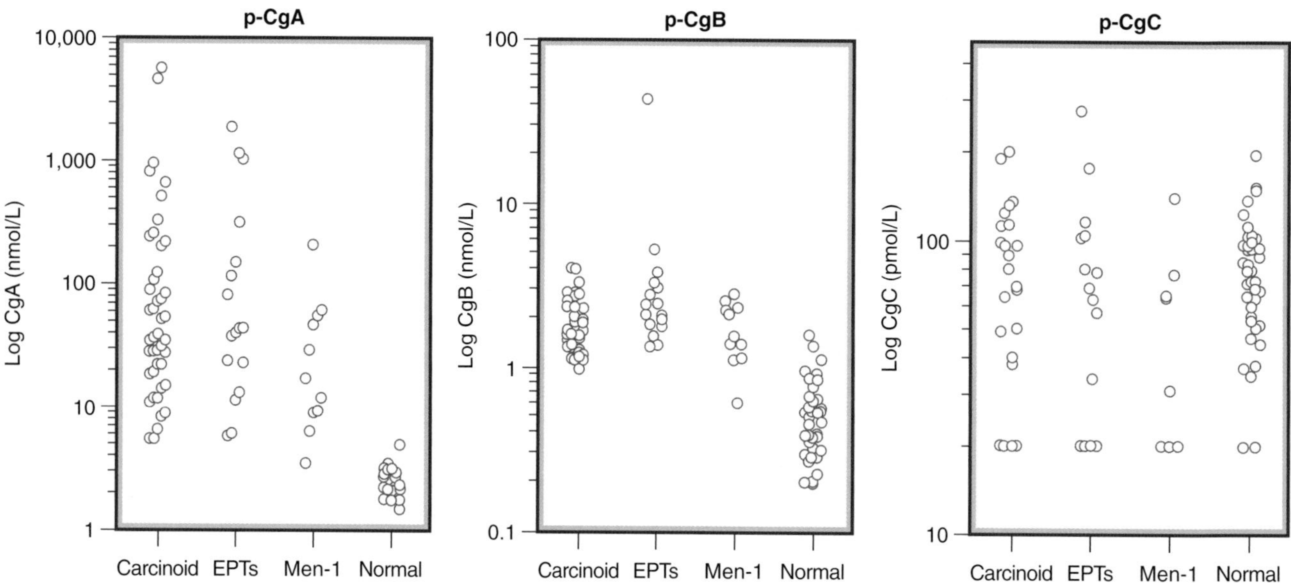

Figure 44–12 ■ Plasma (p) levels of chromogranin A (CgA), CgB, and CgC in patients with various neuroendocrine tumors. EPTs, endocrine pancreatic tumors; MEN-1, multiple endocrine neoplasia type 1.

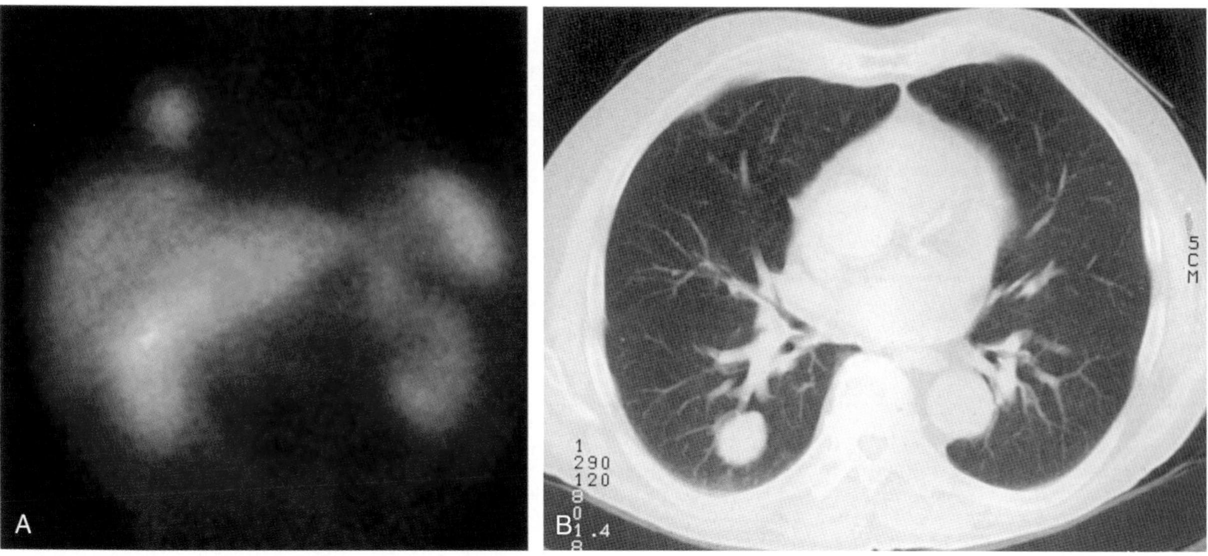

Figure 44–13 ▪ Bronchial carcinoid. **A,** Somatostatin-receptor scintigraphy in a patient with a bronchial carcinoid. **B,** CT scan in the same patient.

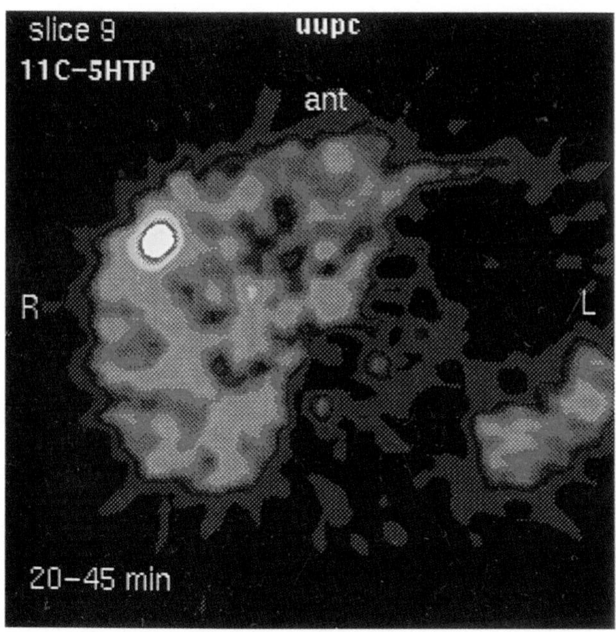

Figure 44–14 ▪ Positron emission tomography (PET) scan with ^{11}C-5-hydroxytryptophan. Note the metastasis in the liver.

the disease. Bone metastases, which are common with carcinoid tumors, are efficiently detected by SRS, which is as sensitive as traditional bone scanning with technetium.[136,138]

Scintigraphy with ^{123}I-MIBG has been applied in patients with midgut carcinoids with a sensitivity of about 50%, which is lower than that for SRS (80% to 90%). However, it can pick up carcinoids in patients that are sensitive to therapy with ^{123}I-MIBG.[141]

A diagnostic algorithm is outlined in Figure 44–15.

Treatment

Treatment of carcinoid tumors with the carcinoid syndrome requires a multimodal approach, including symptomatic control as well as tumor reduction. Most patients with the carcinoid syndrome have metastatic disease. The therapeutic goals are to ameliorate and improve clinical symptoms, abrogate the tumor growth, improve quality of life, and if possible, prolong overall survival.

Symptomatic control of the carcinoid syndrome includes lifestyle changes, diet supplementation, and specific medical treatment that reduces the clinical symptoms related to the different components of the carcinoid syndrome. Avoiding stress, both psychological and physical, as well as substances such as alcohol, spicy foods, and medications that precipitate a flushing reaction might be sufficient in early cases.[55]

Production of serotonin by the tumor consumes tryptophan. Normally, about 1% of body tryptophan is used for production of serotonin; in carcinoid tumors, however, as much as 60% of the available tryptophan may be consumed for the synthesis of serotonin, and this can result in tryptophan and niacin deficiencies. Therefore, supplemental niacin to prevent the development of pellagra has been recommended over the years. Many patients have undergone resection of the terminal ileum, which can result in vitamin B_{12} and folic acid deficiencies. Supplementation is needed in these patients.

Heart failure due to carcinoid heart disease can require diuretics or angiotensin-converting enzyme (ACE) inhibitors. A few patients need bronchodilators such as salbutamol, which interacts with β-adrenergic receptors and does not induce flushing. The diarrhea seen in the carcinoid syndrome might be controlled by loperamide or diphenoxylate.[142] If patients still have the carcinoid syndrome, they receive somatostatin analogue treatment, which has replaced most of the earlier types of serotonin and serotonin receptor inhibitors. Serotonin inhibitors (e.g., parachlorophenylalanine and α-methyldopa), which inhibit serotonin synthesis, and serotonin receptor antagonists (e.g., cyproheptadine, methysergide, and ketanserin) are not used routinely clinically.

These earlier treatments had limited efficacy in terms of inhibiting flushing and diarrhea and were accompanied by significant side effects. A combination of histamine H_1 and H_2 receptor antagonists is effective in the carcinoid syndrome that is caused by foregut carcinoids due to concomitant secretion of histamine and serotonin. Prednisolone in doses of 15 to 30 mg/day gives occasional relief in some cases with severe flushing and diarrhea.[142]

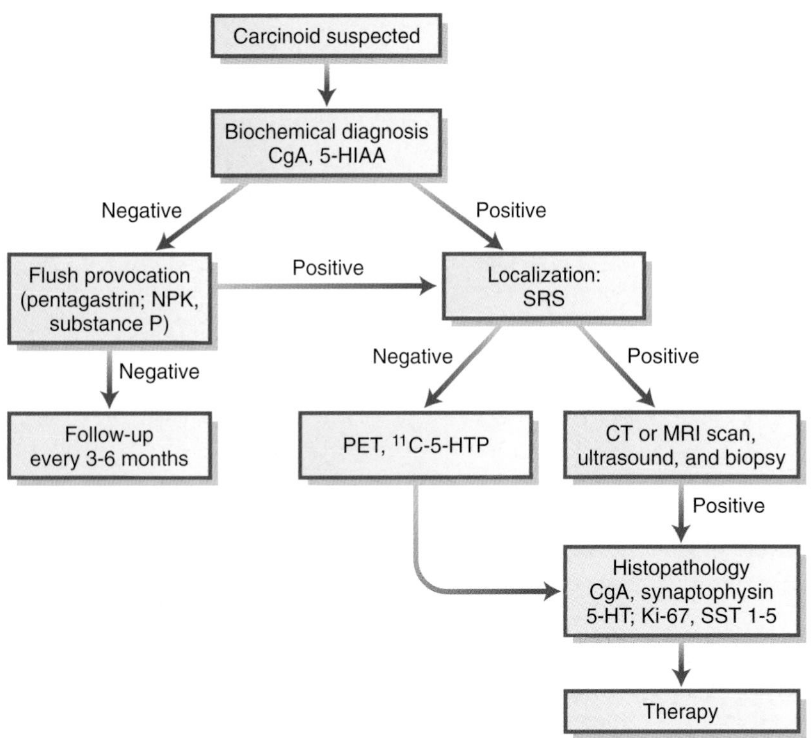

Figure 44–15 ▪ Diagnostic algorithm for patients with carcinoid tumors. CgA, chromogranin A; ^{11}C-5-HTP, ^{11}C-5-hydroxytryptophan; 5-HIAA, 5-hydroxyindoleacetic acid; 5-HT, 5-hydroxytryptamine; NPK, neuropeptide-K; PET, positron emission tomography; SRS, somatostatin-receptor scintigraphy; sst 1-5, somatostatin-receptor subtypes 1-5.

Somatostatin Analogues

Although natural somatostatin-14 reduces symptoms in patients with the carcinoid syndrome,[143] its use is limited by its short half-life (~2.5 minutes). During the last two decades, synthetic somatostatin analogues (octapeptides) have been developed for clinical use. Octreotide is the most commonly available drug; other analogues are lanreotide and vapreotide.[144-146]

The somatostatin analogues used in clinical practice (octreotide, lanreotide) (Fig. 44–16) bind to receptors sst-1 and sst-5 and, with lower affinity, to sst-3. They exert their cellular action through interaction with specific cell and transmembrane receptors belonging to the superfamily of G protein–coupled membrane receptors. They inhibit adenylate cyclase activity, activate phosphotyrosine phosphatases (PTPs), and modulate mitogen-activated protein kinases (MAPKs).[132,147-149] Receptor subtypes 2 and 5 modulate K^+ and Ca^{2+} fluxes in the cell.[147] Activation of all these pathways results in inhibition of known growth factor production and release and has antiproliferative effects.[149-152]

Somatostatin receptor subtype 3 is known to mediate PTP-dependent apoptosis accompanied by activation of p53 and Bax.[153] Four of the five somatostatin receptor subtypes (sst-2 to sst-5) undergo rapid internalization after ligand binding, which has been explored by tumor-targeted radioactive somatostatin analogue therapy.[147,149,154]

An antiproliferative effect has been reported, probably through a combination of receptor subtypes 2 and 5 activities, which inhibits MAPK and K^+ and Ca^{2+} fluxes leading to cell cycle arrest[150-152]; the precise antitumor mechanism, however, is not known.

It is now known that different subtypes of somatostatin receptors form heterodimers (sst-1 and sst-5) and heterodimers with dopamine receptor D2R. This cross-talk modulates the intracellular signal and gives a "fine tuning" of the mediated effects.[155]

All five subtypes of somatostatin receptors are expressed in carcinoid tumors; they are expressed in various combinations, although some tumors express all five subtypes.[147,156-158] The

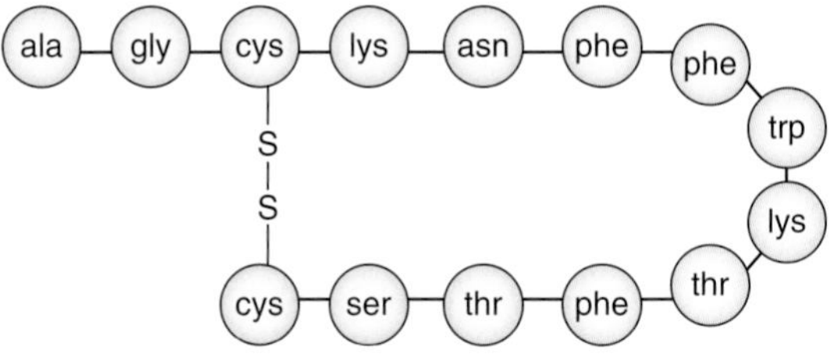

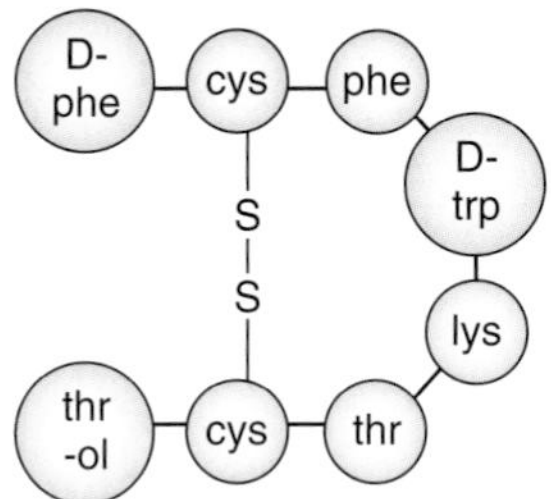

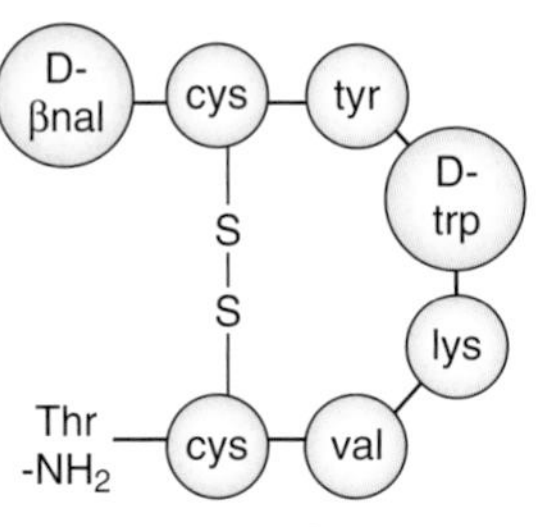

Figure 44–16 ▪ Molecular structure of human somatostatin-14, octreotide acetate, and lanreotide.

receptors are expressed not only on tumor cells but also in peritumoral veins.[159] Antiangiogenesis might be another antitumor mechanism of somatostatin analogues.[160]

Subcutaneous administration of octreotide and lanreotide every 8 to 12 hours can control the clinical symptoms in about 60% to 70% of patients with the carcinoid syndrome; these agents are considered the drugs of choice.[161-166] Octreotide and lanreotide decrease serotonin and urinary 5-HIAA levels as well as plasma tachykinin and CgA levels. The recommended dose for octreotide is 100 to 150 µg two or three times a day, a standard treatment for controlling clinical symptoms.[165] However, some patients require higher doses, up to a total of 3000 µg/day, to control the clinical symptoms and tumor growth, particularly during long-term therapy.

Tachyphylaxis (reduced sensitivity) to somatostatin analogues can develop during long-term therapy.[149] Long-acting, slow-release formulations of octreotide and lanreotide have been developed, and doses of octreotide of 20 to 30 mg given once a month or lanreotide Autogel 90 to 120 mg once a month, control clinical symptoms and hormone levels in 50% to 60% of patients with the carcinoid syndrome.[167-169] The long-acting formulations of somatostatin analogues have clearly improved the quality of life of patients by reducing the number of injections and provide more stable control of clinical symptoms.[168] A new somatostatin analogue (SOM230) binding to sst-1, -2, -3 and -5 has recently come into clinical trials in carcinoid tumors.

High-dose therapy with lanreotide (12 mg/day) and octreotide (3 mg/day) has increased the percentage of patients demonstrating a significant reduction in tumor size (12% versus 5% for the standard dose).[170-173] Induction of apoptosis has been reported during high-dose therapy,[174] possibly mediated through activation of receptor subtype 3. Ultra-high dose octreotide has generated significant antitumor responses in patients resistant to standard dose therapy.[175]

For patients at risk for carcinoid crisis, somatostatin analogue therapy is the treatment of choice. Carcinoid crisis is a life-threatening complication of the carcinoid syndrome and can occur spontaneously or may be associated with stress and anesthesia, chemotherapy, and infections (see earlier). Patients usually experience severe flushing, diarrhea, abdominal pain, and hypotension. Continuous infusion with somatostatin analogues, 50 to 100 µg/hour, is recommended and usually alters the life-threatening condition. It is also recommended that patients be given subcutaneous somatostatin analogues before surgery or other stressful situations.

Side effects of somatostatin analogue therapy have generally not been serious and occur in 20% to 40% of patients. They include pain at the injection site, gas formation, diarrhea, and abdominal cramping. Significant long-term side effects include gallstone formation, sludge in the gallbladder, steatorrhea, deterioration of glucose tolerance, and hypocalcemia.[165,167,168] The incidence of gallstones in patients treated over the long term has varied from 5% to 70%, and the incidence of symptomatic gallstones requiring surgical treatment is less than 10%.[176]

Interferons

Interferon α—alone or in combination with somatostatin analogue—is effective in the treatment of the carcinoid syndrome. Symptomatic and biochemical control may be obtained in 40% to 50% of patients with the recommended doses of 3 to 5 million units of recombinant IFN-α-2a or IFN-α-2b three to five times per week subcutaneously.[177-183] Significant tumor reduction is reported in 10% to 20% of the patients.[177,183]

IFN-α exerts a direct effect on the tumor cells by blocking cell division in the G_1/S-phase, by inhibiting protein and hormone synthesis, and by reducing angiogenesis through inhibition of angiogenic factors β-FGF and VEGF. It has also an indirect effect through stimulation of the immune system, particularly T cells and natural killer cells.[184-187] Response to IFN-α can be predicted by analyzing induction of 2′,5′-oligoadenylate synthetase or P68 (PKR) protein kinase, enzymes involved in cell cycle regulation and protein synthesis.[188,189] Long-acting formulations of IFN-α are now available (pegylated interferons) that can be applied at doses of 80 to 150 µg/week subcutaneously.

Treatment with IFN-α induces an intratumoral fibrosis that is not picked up by regular CT scanning or ultrasonography; therefore, tumor size may remain unchanged.[190] The side effects of α-interferons are more pronounced than with somatostatin analogues and include chronic fatigue syndrome, anemia, leukopenia, and thrombocytopenia as well as the development of autoimmune reactions in 10% to 15% of the patients.[178,191] Most of the side effects are dose-dependent and can be managed by individualizing the dose.

Patients with the carcinoid syndrome who have not responded to octreotide or IFN-α alone may be given a combination of both agents. Such combinations have generated symptomatic control in 70% of patients and stabilization of tumor growth in 40% to 50% of patients.[192,193] The combination also offers better tolerance of α-interferons when somatostatin analogues are added. Moreover, somatostatin analogue treatment is hampered by development of tachyphylaxis with time, which means less sensitivity to the somatostatin analogue, necessitating escalating doses and, finally, withdrawal of the compound for several months, when IFN-α therapy can continue. Conversely, IFN-α can be withdrawn and the somatostatin analogue can be continued if severe side effects to IFN-α (mainly chronic fatigue syndrome or mental depression) develop.[194]

Chemotherapy

Most agree that patients with classic midgut carcinoids and the carcinoid syndrome, in which tumors show low proliferation capacity, should not receive chemotherapy. The results in various studies have been disappointing; response rates are not more than 5% to 10%, are short lived, and are accompanied by considerable side effects.[195,196] The combination of streptozotocin and 5-fluorouracil, which has demonstrated antitumor effect in endocrine pancreatic tumors, has not shown similar effects in classic midgut carcinoids.[197] In foregut carcinoids, which usually manifest a more malignant behavior, however, cytotoxic treatment may be attempted. Such combinations include streptozotocin plus 5-fluorouracil, doxorubicin, cisplatin plus etoposide, and dacarbazine plus 5-fluorouracil.[198-200] Temozolamide has significant efficacy in thymic carcinoids clinical cancer research all for published. All of these cytotoxic treatments can be combined with a somatostatin analogue.

Other Agents

Tyrosine kinase receptors (PDGFR α/β, EGFR, VEGFR) are expressed in carcinoid tumor cells. Therefore, tyrosine kinase receptor inhibitors might be attempted in the future.[201,202]

Surgery

Because most tumors in patients with the carcinoid syndrome are malignant at the time of clinical presentation, surgical cure is seldom obtained. Resection of local disease or regional nodular metastatic disease can cure some patients; however, even if radical surgery cannot be performed, debulking procedures and bypass should always be considered and can be performed at any time during the course of treatment.[203-205]

In recent years, a more proactive attitude among surgeons has emerged, and wider resections and debulking procedures are being performed today than in the 1990s.[204,206] In contrast to other metastatic tumors to the liver, in which liver transplantation has generally given poor results, an interest in liver transplantation is increasing for patients with metastatic carcinoids.[207,208] In a review of 103 patients with malignant neuroendocrine tumors, including both carcinoids and pancreatic endocrine tumors, 5- and 2-year survival rates were 16% and 47%, respectively; however, recurrence-free survival was less than 24%.[207] Liver transplantation might be considered in younger patients (<50 years of age) with a life-threatening uncontrolled carcinoid syndrome during medical therapy or tumor-targeted radioactive treatment without known metastatic spread outside the liver.

Another means of tumor reduction is hepatic artery embolization, which not only improves the carcinoid syndrome in about 50% of the patients but also reduces the tumor size in as many. The therapeutic effect may last for 9 to 12 months, and the procedure can be repeated.[209,210] Chemoembolization, simultaneous embolization with surgical gel (Gelfoam), and chemotherapy (doxorubicin, mitomycin C, cisplatin, 5-fluorouracil), or IFN-α has resulted in symptomatic improvement in a significant number of patients with the carcinoid syndrome.[211,212] However, hepatic artery occlusion or embolization can result in serious side effects (nausea, vomiting, liver pain, fever) and major complications (hepatorenal syndrome, sepsis, gallbladder perforation, and intestinal necrosis). Complications are seen in 5% to 7% of patients.[210-212]

Other cytoreductive treatments include cryotherapy and radiofrequency ablation.[213] However, these procedures are limited to patients with smaller tumor burden, tumors less than 4 cm in diameter, and a limited number of metastases.

Irradiation

External irradiation has demonstrated limited efficacy and is used mainly to palliate symptoms related to bone and brain metastases.[214,215] MIBG is taken up by carcinoids and is concentrated. The possibility of radiolabeled MIBG therapy has been evaluated in a limited number of patients. The response rate has been reported to be about 30% with ^{125}I-MIBG or ^{131}I-MIBG.[216,217]

Somatostatin analogue–based tumor-targeted radioactive treatment has been applied over the last few years using ^{111}In-DTPA-octreotide. Symptomatic improvement is reported in about 40% of the patients and tumor stabilization in about 30%.[218] Indium 111 (^{111}In) is a weak irradiator (Auger electrons) and seems to be replaced by yttrium 90 (^{90}Y) (γ and β emitters).

Studies with ^{90}Y-DOTA-octreotide have been reported with promising results.[219,220] Most recently a new isotope, Lu^{177}-DOTA-octreotate (β-emitted), has come into clinical use with further improved results. Significant tumor reduction occurs in 30% to 40% of patients with advanced disease. However, it is more effective for small tumors. It is an attractive mode of treatment because the radioactive ligand, after binding to the receptor, is internalized and transported to the cell nucleus, causing DNA damage.[221] Because tumor cells usually have higher-density somatostatin receptors (sst-2 and sst-5) than do surrounding normal tissues, the treatment might be better tolerated.

Prognosis

Clinically, the carcinoid syndrome is generally a manifestation of advanced disease. Carcinoids from various sites differ not only in the percentage developing the carcinoid syndrome but also in their aggressiveness. Survival rates for patients with various carcinoids depend on the site and the extent of the tumor. In patients with only localized disease, the 5-year survival rate for midgut carcinoids is about 65%, not essentially higher than that for patients with regional metastases. In patients with distant metastases, the 5-year survival rate is reduced to 39%.[10,18,19,22,24] The relative 5 to 10, and 15-year survival rates for midgut carcinoids were 67%, 54%, and 44%, respectively.[221]

One of the main determinants of survival in carcinoid patients is the presence of metastases. Female gender and a younger age are associated with a better prognosis. Other factors that correlate with impaired survival are high CgA level at diagnosis and high proliferation index (Ki-67).[32,223] During the 1990s, there was a reduced incidence of death from carcinoid heart disease, possibly a result of earlier diagnosis, active surgery, and the introduction of somatostatin analogues and α-interferons. In an earlier study performed by our group, 30% of the patients died of carcinoid heart complications.[21] In a more recent study, this rate was reduced to less than 10%.[24] Clinically significant carcinoid heart disease is now rare. Five percent to 10% of patients with carcinoids are at an increased risk for developing simultaneous adenocarcinoma of the large intestine. The occurrence of a second malignancy is associated with a worse prognosis.[19,22]

Other Flushing Disorders

Medullary Thyroid Carcinoma and VIPoma

Other neuroendocrine tumors, such as medullary thyroid carcinoma (MTC) and VIP-producing tumors (ganglioneuroma, endocrine pancreatic tumors), can manifest with flushing syndromes (Figure 44–17).[224,225] Patients might also have diarrhea, particularly those with VIP-producing tumors, which are accompanied by a severe secretory diarrhea. In patients with MTC, flushing and diarrhea are infrequent symptoms and are seen mainly in patients with high circulating levels of calcitonin and CGRP.

The mechanism behind the flushing and diarrhea is unknown, but it has been postulated to be mediated through prostaglandins stimulated by calcitonin. The frequency of flushing and diarrhea is usually less than 5% in patients with advanced metastatic MTC.[224,226] Treatment is directed against tumor growth and can consist of surgical resection, embolization of liver metastases, and cytotoxic treatment (doxorubicin-based combination therapies). Somatostatin analogue therapy can alleviate the diarrhea.

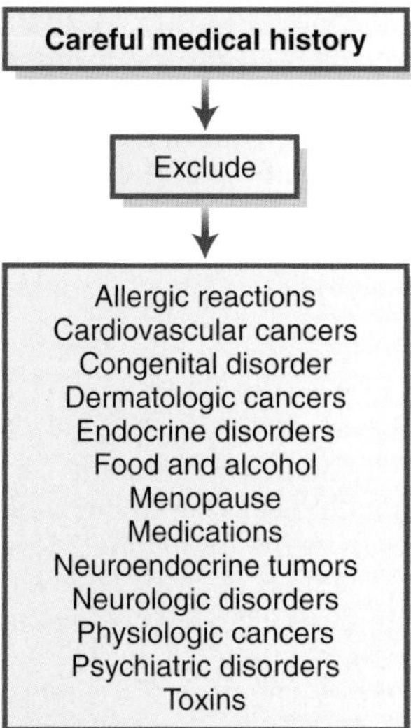

Figure 44–17 ■ Flushing disorders. (From Yale SH, Vasudeva S, Mazza JJ, et al. Disorders of flushing. Compr Ther 2005;31(1):59-71.)

VIPoma or WDHA (*w*atery *d*iarrhea, *h*ypokalemia, and *a*chlorhydria) syndrome (Verner-Morrison syndrome) is associated with severe secretory diarrhea (up to 15 L/day), and some patients also display a continuous whole-body violaceous flushing and hypotension.[225,227] The syndrome also includes achlorhydria, hypokalemia, and metabolic acidosis and is related to overproduction of VIP and a related peptide-peptide histidine methionine. These patients have tumors in the pancreas, lung, or sympathetic ganglia.[225,226]

The diagnosis is confirmed by measuring plasma VIP, usually exceeding 70 pmol/L.[228]

Treatment is directed against the tumor and hormone excess. Administration of somatostatin analogues by either subcutaneous or intravenous infusion in the worst cases can control clinical symptoms.[229] Cytotoxic treatment with streptozotocin-based combinations, 5-fluorouracil, or doxorubicin is recommended for malignant cases.[195]

Mastocytosis and Related Disorders

Mastocytosis as well as other systemic mast cell activation is clinically related to flushing disorders. Most patients with mastocytosis have an indolent course, but some forms of mastocytosis are aggressive. Symptoms are attributed primarily to paroxysmal mast cell activation.[230,231]

Most patients with mastocytosis have evidence of cutaneous involvement, the most common being multiple, small pigmented lesions that produce urticaria on stroking with a blunt object (Darier's sign); this condition is called *urticaria pigmentosa.*[232] Another form of cutaneous mastocytosis is a more telangiectatic form called *telangiectasia macularis eruptiva persistans.* Hepatomegaly and splenomegaly can be due to infiltration of mast cells, and hepatic fibrosis is also common.[233,234]

Bone involvement can be manifested by either osteoporosis or osteosclerosis.[235] Systemic mastocytosis can also involve the GI tract with mucosal nodules in the ileum, stomach, and large bowel.[236]

Hematologic abnormalities are nonspecific, with marked mast cell infiltration of the bone, anemia, leukocytosis, sometimes lymphadenopathy, and eosinophilia.[237] In a subgroup of patients, the mastocytosis is secondary to primary hematologic disorders, usually myeloproliferative or myelodysplastic disease.[238,239] Mast cell leukemia has been reported in rare cases.[240] Some cases with Fip 1–like-1 platelet derived growth factor α (FIP 1L1-PDGFRA)$^+$ overlap to chronic eosinophilic leukemia. They also manifest elevated serum tryptase levels.[241]

Clinical signs of systemic mastocytosis include flushing, tachycardia, hypotension, and sometimes nausea, vomiting, and diarrhea. This syndrome resembles the carcinoid syndrome. Histamine is a potent vasodilator and is released from mast cells. Other mediators of the syndrome are the release of prostaglandin D_2, tryptase, and heparin.[242] Prostaglandin D_2 is a more potent mediator than is histamine.

The diagnosis is made by measurement of histamine and histamine metabolites in the urine.[242,243] Quantification of histamine metabolites (*N*-methylhistamine and methylimidazoleacetic acid) appears to be more sensitive for overproduction of histamine in patients with mastocytosis.[243] Measurement of endogenous production of prostaglandin D_2 can be assessed by quantifying the major urinary metabolite (9α-hydroxy-11,15-dioxo-2,3,18,19-tetranorprost-5-ene-1,20-dioic acid).[244] However, these measurements can be done only in specialized laboratories. Measurement of the tryptase release is easier to perform, and increased quantities of this granule-associated enzyme tryptase can be detected by immunoassay.[245] Bone marrow analysis of CD25$^+$cells might support the diagnosis of mast cell disease.[241]

Treatment depends on the severity of the disease. As in the treatment of allergic anaphylaxis, epinephrine is effective in reversing the hypotension associated with mast cell mediator release[246]; thus, these patients should have constant access to epinephrine in the form of subcutaneous injection or inhalation. Chronic therapy to prevent acute attacks includes antihistamine therapy combined with inhibition of prostaglandin biosynthesis. Blockade of both histamine H_1 and H_2 receptors is required to prevent the vasodilator effect of histamine.[241,247]

Nonsteroidal antiinflammatory drugs (NSAIDs) inhibit the cyclooxygenase enzyme that catalyzes the formation of prostaglandins. Aspirin has been used, but some patients cannot tolerate it because of side effects in the gut and allergic reactions.[248] In patients resistant to both antihistamines and NSAIDs, IFN-α has been attempted with a reduction in mast cell numbers as well as excretion of mast cell mediators. Treatment with IFN-α is still considered experimental.[241,249] A subset of patients who carry the FIP1L1-PDGFRA oncogene will achieve complete clinical, histologic, and molecular remission with imatinib mesylate therapy, in contrast to those with C-kit D816V-mutation.[241]

REFERENCES

1. Lubarsch O. Über den primären Krebs des Ileum, nebst Bemerkungen über das gleichzeitige Vorkommen von Krebs und Tuberculose. Virchows Arch Path Anat Ill 1888;280-317.
2. Oberndorfer S. Karcinoide Tumoren des Dunndarms. Frankfurt II Pathol 1907;1:1426-1429.
3. Pearson CM, Fitzgerald PJ. Carcinoid tumors, a re-emphasis of their malignant nature: review of 140 cases. Cancer 1949;2: 1005-1026.
4. Thorson A, Bjork G, Bjorkman G, et al. Malignant carcinoid of the small intestine with metastases to the liver, valvular disease of the right side of the heart (pulmonary stenosis and tricuspid regurgitation with septal defects), peripheral vasomotor symptoms, bronchoconstriction, and an unusual type of cyanosis: a clinical and pathologic syndrome. Am Heart J 1954;47:795-817.
5. Lembeck F. 5-Hydroxytryptamine in carcinoid tumor. Nature 1953;172:910-911.
6. Gosset A, Masson P. Tumeurs endocrines de l'appendice. Presse Med 1914;22:237-240.
7. Masson P. Carcinoid (argentaffin-cell tumors) and nerve hyperplasia of appendicular mucosa. Am J Pathol 1928;4:181-212.
8. Pearse AGE. The cytochemistry and ultrastructure of polypeptide hormone–producing cells of the APUD series, and the embryonic physiologic and pathologic implications of this concept. J Histochem Cytochem 1969;17:303-313.
9. Andrew A. The APUD concept: where has it led us? Br Med Bull 1982;38:221-225.
10. Wilander E, Lundqvist M, Öberg K. Gastrointestinal carcinoid tumours. Prog Histochem Cytochem 1989;19:1-85.
11. Debelenko LV, Brambilla E, Agarwal SK, et al. Identification of *MEN-1* gene mutations in sporadic carcinoid tumors of the lung. Hum Mol Genet 1997;6:2285-2290.
12. Zhao J, Krijger RR, Meier D, et al. Genomic alterations in well-differentiated gastrointestinal and bronchial neuroendocrine tumors (carcinoids). Am J Pathol 2000;157:1431-1438.
13. Lollgen RM, Hessman O, Szabo E, et al. Chromosome 18 deletions are common events in classical midgut carcinoid tumors. Int J Cancer 2001;92(6):812-815.
14. Gartner W, Mineva I, Daneva T, et al. A newly identified RET proto-oncogene polymorphism is found in a high number of endocrine tumor patients. Hum Genet 2005;117(2-3):143-153.
15. Nakakura EK, Sriuranpong VR, Kunnimalaiyaan M, et al. Regulation of neuroendocrine differentiation in gastrointestinal carcinoid tumor cells by notch signaling. J Clin Endocrinol Metab 2005;90(7):4350-4356.
16. Williams ED, Sandler M. The classification of carcinoid tumours. Lancet 1963;1:238-239.
17. Solcia E, Kloppel G, Sobin L. Histological typing of endocrine tumours. In: Verlag S, editor. World Health Organization Histological Classification of Tumours, 2nd ed. Berlin: Springer, 2000: 38-74.

18. Moertel CG. Karnofsky memorial lecture: an odyssey in the land of small tumors. J Clin Oncol 1987;5:1502.
19. Modlin IM, Lye KD, Kidd M. A 5-decade analysis of 13,715 carcinoid tumors. Cancer 2003;97(4):934-959.
20. Berge T, Linell F. Carcinoid tumours: frequency in a defined population during a 12-year period. Acta Pathol Microbiol Scand 1976; 84:322.
21. Norheim I, Oberg K, Theodorsson-Norheim E, et al. Malignant carcinoid tumors: an analysis of 103 patients with regard to tumor localization, hormone production, and survival. Ann Surg 1987; 206:215.
22. Godwin J. Carcinoid tumors: an analysis of 2837 cases of carcinoid tumors. Cancer 1975;36:560-569.
23. Quaedvlieg PF, Visser O, Lamers CB, et al. Epidemiology and survival in patients with carcinoid disease in the Netherlands: an epidemiological study with 2391 patients. Ann Oncol 2001;12(9): 1295-300.
24. Tiensuu Janson E, Holmberg L, Stridsberg M, et al. Carcinoid tumors: an analysis of prognostic factors and survival in 301 patients from a referral center. Ann Oncol 1997;8:685-690.
25. Sandler M, Scheuer PJ, Watt PJ. 5-Hydroxytryptophan–secreting bronchial carcinoid tumour. Lancet 1961;2:1067-1069.
26. Oates JA, Sjoerdsma A. A unique syndrome associated with secretion of 5-hydroxytryptophan by metastatic gastric carcinoids. Am J Med 1962;32:333-344.
27. Oates JA, Melmon KL, Sjoerdsma A. Release of a kinin peptide in the carcinoid syndrome. Lancet 1964;1:514-517.
28. Lucas KJ, Feldman JM. Flushing in the carcinoid syndrome and plasma kallikrein. Cancer 1986;58:2290-2293.
29. Gustafsen J, Boesby S, Nielsen F, et al. Bradykinin in carcinoid syndrome. Gut 1987;28:1417-1419.
30. Metz SA, McRae JR, Robertson RP. Prostaglandins as mediators of paraneoplastic syndromes: review and update. Metabolism 1981; 30:299.
31. Roberts LJ II, Bloomgarden ZT, Marney SR Jr, et al. Histamine release from a gastric carcinoid: provocation by pentagastrin and inhibition by somatostatin. Gastroenterology 1983;84:272-275.
32. Gilligan CJ, Lawton GP, Tang LH, et al. Gastric carcinoid tumors: the biology and therapy of an enigmatic and controversial lesion. Am J Gastroenterol 1995;90:338-352.
33. Todd TR, Cooper JD, Weissberg D, et al. Bronchial carcinoid tumors: twenty years' experience. J Thorac Cardiovasc Surg 1980; 79:532-536.
34. Kema IP, deVries GE, Sloof MJH, et al. Serotonin, catecholamines, histamine, and their metabolites in urine, platelets, and tumor tissue of patients with carcinoid tumors. Clin Chem 1994;40: 86-95.
35. Håkansson R, Bergmark S, Brodin E, et al. Substance-P–like immunoreactivity in intestinal carcinoid tumors. In von Euler US, Pernow B, eds. Substance-P. New York: Raven, 1977:55-58.
36. Norheim I, Theodorsson-Norheim E, Brodin E, et al. Tachykinins in carcinoid tumors: use as a tumor marker and possible role in carcinoid flush. J Clin Endocrinol Metab 1986;63:605-612.
37. Theodorsson-Norheim E, Norheim I, Öberg K, et al. Neuropeptide-K: a major tachykinin in plasma and tumor tissues from carcinoid patients. Biochem Biophys Res Comm 1985;131:77-83.
38. Conlon JM, Deacon CF, Richter G, et al. Measurement and partial characterization of the multiple forms of neurokinin A–like immunoreactivity in carcinoid tumors. Regul Pept 1986;13:183-196.
39. Becker M, Aron DC. Ectopic ACTH syndrome and CRH-mediated Cushing's syndrome. Endocrinol Metab Clin North Am 1994;23: 585.
40. Jensen RT, Norton JA. Endocrine neoplasms of the pancreas. In Yamada T, Alpers DH, Owyang C, et al, eds. Textbook of Gastroenterology. Philadelphia: JB Lippincott, 1998:2193.
41. Mao C, Shah A, Hanson DJ, et al. Von Recklinghausen's disease associated with duodenal somatostatinoma: contrast of duodenal versus pancreatic somatostatinoma. J Surg Oncol 1995;59:67-73.
42. Banks P, Helle KB. The release of protein from stimulated adrenal medulla. Biochem J 1965;97:40C-41C.
43. Fisher-Colbrie R. Chromogranins A, B, and C: widespread constituents of secretory vesicles. Ann NY Acad Sci 1987;493:120-134.
44. Iacangelo AL, Eiden LE. Chromogranin A: current status as a precursor for bioactive peptides, a granulogenic/sorting factor in the regulated secretory pathway. Regul Pept 1995;58:65-88.
45. Tatemoto K, Efendic S, Mutt V, et al. Pancreastatin, a novel pancreatic peptide that inhibits insulin secretion. Nature 1986;324: 476-478.
46. Angeletti RH, Mints L, Aber C, et al. Determination of residues in chromogranin A (16-40) required for inhibition of parathyroid secretion. Endocrinol 1996;137:2918-2922.
47. Aardal S, Helle KB, Elsayed S, et al. Vasostatins comprising the *N*-terminal domain of chromogranin A, suppress tension in isolated human blood vessel segments. J Neuroendocrinol 1993;5:105-112.
48. Wiedenmann B, Huttner WB. Synaptophysin and chromogranins/secretogranins: widespread constituents of distinct types of neuroendocrine vesicles and new tools in tumor diagnosis. Virchows Archiv B Cell Pathol 1989;58:95-121.
49. Harpole DH Jr, Feldman JM, Buchanan S, et al. Bronchial carcinoid tumors: a retrospective analysis of 126 patients. Ann Thorac Surg 1992;54:50-55.
50. Barcklay TH, Shapira DV. Malignant tumors of the small intestine. Cancer 1983;51:878-881.
51. Moertel CG, Sauer WG, Dockerty MB, et al. Life history of the carcinoid tumor of the small intestine. Cancer 1961;14:901-912.
52. Makridis C, Öberg K, Juhlin C, et al. Surgical treatment of midgut carcinoid tumors. World J Surg 1990;14:377-385.
53. Bean WB, Olch D, Weinberg HB. The syndrome of carcinoid and acquired valve lesions of the right side of the heart. Circulation 1955;12:1-6.
54. Grahame-Smith DG. The carcinoid syndrome. Am J Cardiol 1968; 21:376.
55. Feldman JM. Carcinoid tumors and syndrome. Semin Oncol 1987;14:237-246.
56. Smith RA. Bronchial carcinoid tumours. Thorax 1969;24:43-50.
57. Caldarola VT, Jackman RJ, Moertel CG, et al. Carcinoid tumors of the rectum. Am J Surg 1964;107:844-849.
58. Levin RJ, Elsas LJ, Duvall CP, et al. Malignant carcinoid tumors with and without flushing. JAMA 1963;186:905-907.
59. Matuchansky C, Luanay JM. Serotonin, catecholamines, and spontaneous midgut carcinoid flush: plasma studies from flushing and nonflushing sites. Gastroenterology 1995;108:743.
60. Robertson JIS, Peast WS, Andrews TM. The mechanism of facial flushes in the carcinoid syndrome. Q J Med 1962;31: 103-123.
61. Makridis C, Theodorsson E, Akerström G, et al. Increased intestinal non–substance P tachykinin concentrations in malignant midgut carcinoid disease. J Gastroenterol Hepatol 1999;14: 500.
62. Creutzfeldt W, Stockmann F. Carcinoids and carcinoid syndrome. Am J Med 1987;82:4.
63. Emson PC, Gilbert RF, Martensson H, et al. Elevated concentrations of substance P and 5-HT in plasma in patients with carcinoid tumors. Cancer 1984;54:715-718.
64. Schaffalizky de Muckadell OB, Aggestrup P, Stentoft P. Flushing and plasma substance P concentration during infusion of synthetic substance P in normal man. Scand J Gastroenterol 1986;21:498.
65. Frolich JC, Bloomgarden ZT, Oates JA, et al. The carcinoid flush: provocation by pentagastrin and inhibition by somatostatin. N Engl J Med 1978;299:1055-1057.
66. Nawa H, Doteucki M, Iganok, et al. Substance-K: a novel mammalian tachykinin that differs from substance-P in its pharmacological profile. Life Sci 1984;34:1153-1160.
67. Furschgott RF, Zawadski JU. The obligatory role of endothelial cells in the relaxation of arterial smooth muscle by acetylcholine. Nature 1980;288:373-376.
68. Jensen RT. Overview of chronic diarrhea caused by functional neuroendocrine neoplasms. Semin Gastrointest Dis 1999;10:156.
69. Donowitz M, Binder HJ. Jejunal fluid and electrolyte secretion in carcinoid syndrome. Am J Dig Dis 1975;20:1115-1122.
70. Debonguie JC, Philips SF. Capacity of the human colon to absorb fluid. Gastroenterology 1978;74:698-703.
71. Von der Otte MR, Camilieri M, Kvols LK, et al. Motor dysfunction of the small bowel and colon in patients with the carcinoid syndrome and diarrhea. N Engl J Med 1993;329:1073-1078.
72. Wymenga AN, de Vries EG, Leijsma MK, et al. Effects of ondansetron on gastrointestinal symptoms in carcinoid syndrome. Eur J Cancer 1998;34:1293.

73. Wilde MI, Markham A. Ondansetron: a review of its pharmacology and preliminary clinical findings in novel applications. Drugs 1996;52:773.
74. Gustafsen J, Lindorf A, Raskev H, Boesby S. Ketanserin versus placebo in carcinoid syndrome: a clinical controlled trial. Scand J Gastroenterol 1986;21:816.
75. Lundin L, Norheim I, Landelius J, et al. Carcinoid heart disease: relationship of circulating vasoactive substances to ultrasound-detectable cardiac abnormalities. Circulation 1988;77:264-269.
76. Roberts WC, Sjoerdsma A. The cardiac disease associated with the carcinoid syndrome (carcinoid heart disease). Am J Med 1964;36:5-34.
77. Ferrans VJ, Roberts WC. The carcinoid endocardial plaque: an ultrastructural study. Hum Pathol 1976;7:387-409.
78. Lundin L, Landelius J, Andren B, et al. Transoesophageal echocardiography improves the diagnostic value of cardiac ultrasound in patients with carcinoid heart disease. Br Heart J 1990;64:190-194.
79. Waltenberger J, Lundin L, Öberg K, et al. Involvement of transforming growth factor-β in the formation of fibrotic lesions in carcinoid heart disease. Am J Pathol 1993;142:71-78.
80. Robiolo PA, Rigolin VH, Wilson JS, et al. Carcinoid heart disease: correlation of high serotonin levels with valvular abnormalities deleted by cardiac catheterization and echocardiography. Circulation 1995;92:790-795.
81. Connoly HM, Crary JL, McGoon MD, et al. Valvular heart disease associated with fenfluramine-phentermine. N Engl J Med 1997; 337:581-588. (Erratum, N Engl J Med 1997;337:1783.)
82. Khan MA, Herzog CA, St. Peter JV, et al. The prevalence of cardiac valvular insufficiency assessed by transthoracic echocardiography in obese patients treated with appetite-suppressant drugs. N Engl J Med 1998;339:713-718.
83. Pellikka PA, Tajik AJ, Khandheria BK, et al. Carcinoid heart disease: clinical and echocardiographic spectrum in 74 patients. Circulation 1993;87:1188-1196.
84. Musunuru S, Carpenter JE, Sippel RS, et al. A mouse model of carcinoid syndrome and heart disease. J Surg Res 2005;126(1): 102-105.
85. Gustafsson BI, Tommeras K, Nordrum I, et al. Long-term serotonin administration induces heart valve disease in rats. Circulation 2005;111(12):1517-1522.
86. Jian B, Xu J, Connolly J, et al. Serotonin mechanisms in heart valve disease I: serotonin-induced up-regulation of transforming growth factor-β_1 via G-protein signal transduction in aortic valve interstitial cells. Am J Pathol 2002;161(6):2111-2121.
87. Hua XI, Lundberg JM, Theodorsson-Norheim E, et al. Comparison of cardiovascular and bronchoconstrictor effects of substance P, substance K, and other tachykinins. Naunyn Schmiedebergs Arch Pharmacol 1984;328:196-201.
88. Gardner B, Dollinger M, Silen W, et al. Studies of the carcinoid syndrome: its relationship to serotonin, bradykinin, and histamine. Surgery 1967;61:846-852.
89. Vinik AK, McLeod MK, Fig LM, et al. Clinical features, diagnosis, and localization of carcinoid tumors and their management. Gastroenterol Clin North Am 1989;18:865-896.
90. Andaker L, Lamke LO, Smeds S. Follow-up of 102 patients operated on for gastrointestinal carcinoid. Acta Chir Scand 1985;151:469.
91. Kvols LK, Martin JK, Mash HM, et al. Rapid reversal of carcinoid crisis with a somatostatin analogue (letter). N Engl J Med 1985;313:1229-1230.
92. Vaughan DJ, Brunner MD. Anaesthesia for patients with carcinoid syndrome. Int Anesthesiol Clin 1997;35:129.
93. Veall GRQ, Peacock JE, Bax NDS, et al. Review of the anaesthetic management of 21 patients undergoing laparotomy for carcinoid syndrome. Br J Anaesth 1994;72:335.
94. Harris AG, Redfern JS. Octreotide treatment of carcinoid syndrome: analysis of published dose-titration data. Aliment Pharmacol Ther 1995;9:387.
95. Kvols LK. Therapy of the malignant carcinoid syndrome. Endocrinol Metab Clin North Am 1989;18:557.
96. Roberts LJ, Marney SR Jr, Oates JA. Blockade of the flush associated with metastatic gastric carcinoid by combined histamine H_1 and H_2 receptor antagonists: evidence for an important role of H_2 receptors in human vasculature. N Engl J Med 1979;300: 236-238.
97. Limper AH, Carpenter PC, Scheithauer B, et al. The Cushing syndrome induced by bronchial carcinoid tumors. Ann Intern Med 1992;117:209-214.
98. Carroll DG, Delahunt JW, Teague CA, et al. Resolution of acromegaly after removal of a bronchial carcinoid shown to secrete growth hormone–releasing factor. Aust N Z J Med 1987;17:63-67.
99. Rindi G, Bordi C, Rappel S, et al. Gastric carcinoids and neuroendocrine carcinoma pathogenesis, pathology, and behaviour. World J Surg 1996;20:168.
100. Granberg D, Wilander E, Stridsberg M, et al. Clinical symptoms, hormone profiles, treatment, and prognosis in patients with gastric carcinoids. Gut 1998;43:223.
101. Thomas RM, Baybick JH, Elsayed AM, et al. Gastric carcinoids: an immunohistochemical and clinicopathologic study of 104 patients. Cancer 1994;73:2053-2058.
102. Sjoblom SM, Sipponen P, Karonen SL, et al. Mucosal argyrophil endocrine cells in pernicious anaemia and upper gastrointestinal carcinoid tumors. J Clin Pathol 1989;42:371-377.
103. Solcia E, Fiocca R, Villani L, et al. Morphology and pathogenesis of endocrine hyperplasia, precarcinoid lesions, and carcinoids arising in chronic atrophic gastritis. Scand J Gastroenterol Suppl 1991;180:146-159.
104. Havu N. Enterochromaffin-like cell carcinoids of gastric mucosa in rats after life-long inhibition of gastric secretion. Digestion 1986;35(Suppl 1):42-55.
105. Rindi G, Luinetti O, Cornaggia M, et al. Three subtypes of gastric argyrophil carcinoid and the gastric neuroendocrine carcinoma: a clinicopathologic study. Gastroenterology 1993;104: 994-1006.
106. Thompson GB, Van Heerden JA, Martin JK Jr, et al. Carcinoid tumors of the gastrointestinal tract: presentation, management, and prognosis. Surgery 1985;98:1054.
107. Chaudhry A, Oberg K, Wilander E, et al. A study of biological behaviour based on the expression of a proliferating antigen in neuroendocrine tumors of the digestive system. Tumour Biol 1992;13:27.
108. von Herbay A, Sieg B, Shurmann G, et al. Proliferative activity of neuroendocrine tumours of the gastroenteropancreatic endocrine system: DNA flow cytometric and immunohistological investigations. Gut 1991;32:949.
109. Chaudry A, Öberg K, Gobl A, et al. Expression of transforming growth factors β_1, β_2, β_3, in neuroendocrine of the digestive tract. Anticancer Res 1994;14:2085-2092.
110. Granberg D, Wilander E, Öberg K, Skogseid B. Prognostic markers in patients with typical bronchial carcinoid tumors. J Clin Endocrinol Metab 2000;85:3425-3430.
111. Patel YC, Srikant CB. Somatostatin receptors. Trends Endocrinol Metab 1997;8:398-405.
112. Schaer JC, Waser B, Mengod G, Reubi JC. Somatostatin receptor subtypes, sst_1, sst_2, sst_1, sst_5 expression in human pituitary, gastro-entero-pancreatic, and mammary tumors: comparison of mRNA analysis with receptor autoradiography. Int J Cancer 1997;50: 530-537.
113. Feldman JM. Urinary serotonin in the diagnosis of carcinoid tumors. Clin Chem 1986;32:840.
114. Mailman RB, Kilts CD. Analytical considerations for quantitative determination of serotonin and its metabolically related products in biological matrices. Clin Chem 1985;31:1849-1854.
115. Nuttall KL, Pingree SS. The incidence of elevations in urine 5-hydroxyindoleacetic acid. Am J Clin Nutr 1985;42:639.
116. De Vries EGE, Kema IP, Slooff MJH, et al. Recent developments in diagnosis and treatment of metastatic carcinoid tumors. J Gastroenterol 1993;28:87.
117. Stridsberg M, Öberg K, Li Q, et al. Measurements of chromogranin A, chromogranin B (secretogranin I), chromogranin C (secretogranin II), and pancreastatin in plasma and urine from patients with carcinoid tumors and endocrine pancreatic tumors. J Endocrinol 1995;144:49-59.
118. Nobels FR, Kwekkeboom DJ, Coopmans W, et al. Chromogranin A as serum marker for neuroendocrine neoplasia: comparison with neuron-specific enolase and the alpha-subunit of glycoprotein hormones. J Clin Endocrinol Metab 1997;82:2622.
119. Baudin E, Gigliotti A, Ducreux M, et al. Neuron-specific enolase and chromogranin A as markers of neuroendocrine tumours. Br J Cancer 1998;78:1102.

120. Öberg K, Stridsberg M. Chromogranins as diagnostic and prognostic markers in neuroendocrine tumours. Adv Exp Med Biol 2000;482:329-337.
121. Grossman M, Trautmann ME, Poertl S, et al. Alpha-subunit and human chorionic gonadotropin-β immunoreactivity in patients with malignant endocrine gastroentero-pancreatic tumours. Eur J Clin Invest 1994;24:131.
122. Feldman JM, O'Dorisio TM. Role of neuropeptides and serotonin in the diagnosis of carcinoid tumors. Am J Med 1986;81:41.
123. Öberg K, Grimelius L, Lundquist G, et al. Update on pancreatic polypeptide as a specific marker for endocrine tumours of the pancreas and gut. Acta Medica Scand 1981;210:145-152.
124. Mani S, Modlin IM, Ballantyne G, et al. Carcinoids of the rectum. J Am Coll Surg 1994;179:231-248.
125. Krenning EP, Kwekkeboom DJ, Oei HY, et al. Somatostatin-receptor scintigraphy in gastroenteropancreatic tumors. Ann N Y Acad Sci 1994;733:416.
126. Westlin JE, Janson ET, Arnberg H, et al. Somatostatin receptor scintigraphy of carcinoid tumours using the [^{111}In-DTPA-D-Phe^{1}]-octreotide. Acta Oncol 1993;32:783.
127. Taal BG, Hoefnagel CA, Valdés Olmos RA, et al. Combined diagnostic imaging with ^{121}I-metaiodobenzyl guanidine and ^{111}In-pentectreotide in carcinoid tumours. Eur J Cancer 1996;32A: 1924-1932.
128. Nessi R, Basso Ricci P, Basso Ricci S, et al. Bronchial carcinoid tumors: radiologic observations in 49 cases. J Thorac Imaging 1991; 6:47.
129. Orlefors H, Sundin A, Garske U, et al. Whole-body ^{11}C-5-hydroxytryptophan positron emission tomography as a universal imaging technique for neuroendocrine tumors: comparison with somatostatin receptor scintigraphy and computed tomography. J Clin Endocrinol Metab 2005;90(6):3392-400.
130. Eriksson B, Bergström M, Örlefors H, et al. Use of PET in neuroendocrine tumors: in vivo applications and in vitro studies. Q J Nucl Med 2000;44:68-76.
131. Reubi JC, Kvols LK, Waser B, et al. Detection of somatostatin receptors in surgical and percutaneous needle biopsy samples of carcinoids and islet cell carcinomas. Cancer Res 1990;50: 5969-5977.
132. Reisine T, Bell G. Molecular biology of somatostatin receptors. Endocr Rev 1995;16:427-442.
133. Patel YC, Srikant CB. Subtype selectivity of peptide analogs for all five cloned human somatostatin receptors (sst 1-5) Endocrinology 1994;135:2814-2817.
134. Kubota A, Yamada Y, Kagimoto S, et al. Identification of somatostatin receptor subtypes and an implication for the efficacy of somatostatin analogue SMS 201-995 in treatment of human endocrine tumors. J Clin Invest 1994;93:1321-1325.
135. Janson ET, Westlin JE, Eriksson B, et al. [^{111}In-DTPA-D-Phe] octreotide scintigraphy in patients with carcinoid tumours: the predictive value for somatostatin analogue treatment. Eur J Endocrinol 1994;131:577-581.
136. Gibril F, Doppman JL, Reynolds JC, et al. Bone metastases in patients with gastrinomas: a prospective study of bone scanning, somatostatin receptor scanning, and MRI in their detection, their frequency, location, and effect of their detection on management. J Clin Oncol 1998;16:1040.
137. Kisker O, Weinel RJ, Geks J, et al. Value of somatostatin receptor scintigraphy for preoperative localization of carcinoids. World J Surg 1996;20:162.
138. Lebtahi R, Cadiot G, Delahaye N, et al. Detection of bone metastases in patients with endocrine gastroenteropancreatic tumors: bone scintigraphy compared with somatostatin receptor scintigraphy. J Nucl Med 1999;40:1602.
139. Nilsson O, Kolby L, Wangberg B, et al. Comparative studies on the expression of somatostatin receptor subtypes, outcome of octreotide scintigraphy, and response to octreotide treatment in patients with carcinoid tumors. Br J Cancer 1998;77:1632-1637.
140. Janson ET, Gobl A, Kälkner KM, Öberg K. A comparison between the efficacy of somatostatin receptor scintigraphy and that of in situ hybridization for somatostatin receptor subtype 2 messenger RNA to predict therapeutic outcome in carcinoid patients. Cancer Res 1996;56:2561-2565.
141. Kaltsas G, Korbonits M, Heintz E, et al. Comparison of somatostatin analog and meta-iodobenzylguanidine radionuclides in the diagnosis and localization of advanced neuroendocrine tumors. J Clin Endocrinol Metab 2001;86(2):895-902.
142. Gregor M. Therapeutic principles in the management of metastasizing carcinoid tumors: drugs for symptomatic treatment. Digestion 1994;55(Suppl 3):60.
143. Frolich JC, Bloomgarden ZT, Oates JA, et al. The carcinoid flush: provocation by pentagastrin and inhibition by somatostatin. N Engl J Med 1978;299:1055.
144. Bauer WG, Briner U, Doepfner W, et al. SMS 201-995: a very potent and selective octapeptide analogue of somatostatin with prolonged action. Life Sci 1982;31:1133-1140.
145. Murphy WA, Heiman ML, Lance V, et al. Octapeptide analogs of somatostatin exhibiting greatly enhance in vivo and in vitro inhibition of growth hormone secretion in the rat. Biochem Biophys Res Commun 1985;132:922-928.
146. Cai RZ, Szoke B, Liu R, et al. Synthesis and biological activity of highly potent octapeptide analogs of somatostatin. Proc Natl Acad Sci U S A 1986;83:1896-1900.
147. Patel YC. Somatostatin and its receptor family. Front Neuroendocrinol 1999;20:157-198.
148. Coy DH, Taylor JE. Receptor-specific somatostatin analogs: correlation with biological activity. Metabolism 1996;45(Suppl 1): 21-23.
149. Scarpignato C, Pelosini I. Somatostatin analogues for cancer treatment and diagnosis-an overview. Chemotherapy 2001;47: 1-29.
150. Buscail L, Esteve JP, Saint-Laurent N, et al. Inhibition of cell proliferation by somatostatin analogue RC-160 is mediated by somatostatin receptor subtypes SSTR2 and SSTR5 through different mechanisms. Proc Natl Acad Sci U S A 1995;92:1580-1584.
151. Cordelier P, Esteve JP, Bousguel C. Characterization of the antiproliferative signal mediated by somatostatin receptor subtype sst5. Proc Natl Acad Sci U S A 1997;94:9343.
152. Cattaneo MG, Amoroso D, Gussoni G, et al. A somatostatin analogue inhibits MAP kinase activation and cell proliferation in human neuroblastoma and in human small cell carcinoma cell lines. FEBS Lett 1996;397:164-168.
153. Sharma K, Patel YC, Srikant CB. Subtype selective induction of p53-dependent apoptosis but not cell cycle arrest by human somatostatin receptor 3. Mol Endocrinol 1996;10:1688-1696.
154. Hofland LJ, Van Koetsveld PM, Waaijers M, et al. Internalization of radioiodinated somatostatin analogue [^{125}I-Tyr^{3}] octreotide by mouse and human pituitary tumor cells: increase by unlabelled octreotide. Endocrinology 1995;136:3698-3700.
155. Rockeville M, Lange DC, Kumar U, et al. Receptors for dopamine and somatostatin: formation of hetero-oligomers with enhanced functional activity. Science 2000;288:154-157.
156. Schaer JC, Waser B, Mengod G, et al. Somatostatin receptor subtypes, SSTR-1, SSTR-2, SSTR-3 and SSTR-5 expression in human pituitary, gastroenteropancreatic and mammary tumors: comparison of mRNA analysis with receptor autoradiography. Int J Cancer 1997;70:530-537.
157. Janson ET, Stridsberg M, Gobl M, et al. Determination of somatostatin receptor subtype 2 in carcinoid tumors by immunohistochemical investigation with somatostatin receptor subtype 2 antibodies. Cancer Res 1998;58:2375-2378.
158. Reubi JC, Koppeler A, Waser B, et al. Immunohistochemical localization of somatostatin receptors SSTR-2A in human tumors. Am J Pathol 1998;153:233-245.
159. Denzler B, Reubi JC. Expression of somatostatin receptors in peritumoral veins of human tumors. Cancer 1999;85:188-198.
160. Fassler JE, Hughes JH, Cataland S, et al. Somatostatin analogue: an inhibitor of angiogenesis? Biomed Res 1988; II (Suppl): 181-185.
161. Lamberts SW, van der Lely AJ, De Herder WW, et al. Octreotide. N Engl J Med 1996;334:246-254.
162. Kvols LK, Moertel CG, O'Connel MJ, et al. Treatment of the malignant carcinoid syndrome: evaluation of a long-acting somatostatin analogue. N Engl J Med 1986;315:663-666.
163. Öberg K, Norheim I, Lundqvist G, et al. Treatment of the carcinoid syndrome with SMS 201-995, a somatostatin analogue. Scand J Gastroenterol 1986;119:191-192.
164. Scarpignato C. Somatostatin analogues in the management of endocrine tumors of the pancreas. In Mignon M, Jensen RT (eds): Endocrine Tumors of the Pancreas. Basel: Karger, 1995:385-414.

165. Harris A, Redfern JS. Octreotide treatment of arcinoid syndrome: analysis of published dose-titration data. Aliment Pharmacol Ther 1995;9:387-394.
166. Lamberts SWJ, Krenning EP, Reubi JC. The role of somatostatin and its analogs in the diagnosis and treatment of tumors. Endocrinol Rev 1991;12:450-482.
167. Ruszniewski P, Ducreux M, Chayvialle JA, et al. Treatment of the carcinoid syndrome with the long-acting somatostatin analogue lanreotide: a prospective study in 39 patients. Gut 1996;39: 279-283.
168. Wymenga ANM, Eriksson B, Salmela PI, et al. Efficacy and safety of lanreotide: prolonged release in patients with gastrointestinal neuroendocrine tumors with hormone-related symptoms. J Clin Oncol 1999;17(4):1111.
169. Rubin J, Ajani J, Schimer W, et al. Octreotide acetic long-acting formulation versus open-label subcutaneous octreotide acelate in malignant carcinoid syndrome. J Clin Oncol 1999;17:600-606.
170. Eriksson B, Renstrup J, Imam H, et al. High-dose treatment with lanreotide of patients with advanced neuroendocrine gastrointestinal tumors: clinical and biological effects. Ann Oncol 1997; 8:1-4.
171. Anthony L, Johnson D, Hande K, et al. Somatostatin analogue phase 1 trials in neuroendocrine neoplasms. Acta Oncol 1993;32: 217-223.
172. Faiss S, Wiedenmann B. Dose-dependent and antiproliferative effects of somatostatin. J Endocrinol Invest 1997;20:68-70.
173. Eriksson B, Janson ET, Bax NDS, et al. The use of new somatostatin analogues, lanreotide and octastatin, in neuroendocrine gastrointestinal tumors. Digestion 1996;57:77-80.
174. Imam H, Eriksson B, Lukinius A, et al. Induction of apoptosis in neuroendocrine tumors of the digestive system during treatment with somatostatin analogs. Acta Oncol 1997;16:607-614.
175. Welin SV, Janson ET, Sundin A, et al. High-dose treatment with a long-acting somatostatin analogue in patients with advanced midgut carcinoid tumours. Eur J Endocrinol 2004;151(1):107-112.
176. Trendle MC, Moertel CG, Kvols LK. Incidence and morbidity of cholelithiasis in patients receiving chronic octreotide for metastatic carcinoid and malignant islet cell tumors. Cancer 1997;79: 830-834.
177. Öberg K, Norheim I, Lind E, et al. Treatment of malignant carcinoid tumors human leukocyte interferon: long-term results. Cancer Treat Rep 1986;70:1297.
178. Öberg K, Eriksson B. The role of interferons in the management of carcinoid tumors. Acta Oncol 1991;30:519.
179. Nobin A, Lindblom A, Mansson B, et al. Interferon treatment in patients with malignant carcinoids. Acta Oncol 1989;28:445.
180. Hanssen LE, Schrumpf E, Jacobsen MB, et al. Extended experience with recombinant α2b interferon with or without hepatic artery embolization in the treatment of midgut carcinoid tumors. Acta Oncol 1991;30:523.
181. Öberg K, Eriksson B, Janson ET. The clinical use of interferons in the management of neuroendocrine gastroenteropancreatic tumors. Ann N Y Acad Sci 1994;733:471-478.
182. Hanssen LE, Schrumpf E, Kolbenstvedt AN, et al. Treatment of malignant metastatic midgut carcinoid tumors with recombinant human α2b interferon with or without prior hepatic artery embolization. Scand J Gastroenterol 1989;24:787.
183. Moertel CS, Rubin J, Kvols LK. Therapy of metastatic carcinoid tumor and the malignant carcinoid syndrome with recombinant leukocyte A interferon. J Clin Oncol 1989;7:865.
184. Fleischmann WR Jr, Fleischmann CM. Mechanism of interferon's antitumor actions. In Baron S, Coppenhaver DH, Dianzani F, et al, eds. Interferon: Principles and Medical Application. Galveston: UTMB, 1992:299-310.
185. Öberg K. The action of interferon-α on human carcinoid tumors. Semin Cancer Biol 1992;3:35-41.
186. Grander D, Sangfelt O, Erickson S. How does interferon exert its cell growth inhibitory effect? Eur J Haematol 1997;59:129-135.
187. Hobeika AC, Subramaniam PS, Johnson HM. IFNα induces the expression of the cyclin-dependent kinase inhibitor p21 in human prostate cancer cells. Oncogene 1997;14:1165-1170.
188. Grandér D, Öberg K, Lundqvist ML. Interferon-induced enhancement of 2′,5′-oligoadenylate synthetase in midgut carcinoid tumors. Lancet 1990;336:337-340.
189. Zhou Y, Gobl A, Wang S, et al. Expression of p68 protein kinase and its prognostic significance during IFN-α therapy in patients with carcinoid tumors. Cancer 1998;34:2046-2052.
190. Andersson T, Wilander E, Eriksson B, et al. Effects of interferon on tumor tissue content in liver metastases of carcinoid tumors. Cancer Res 1990;50:3413-3415.
191. Rönnblom L, Alm GV, Öberg K. Autoimmunity after α-interferon therapy for malignant carcinoid tumors. Ann Intern Med 1991;115:178-183.
192. Tiensuu Janson E, Ahlström H, Andersson T, et al. Octreotide and interferon alfa: a new combination for the treatment of malignant carcinoid tumors. Eur J Cancer 1992;28A:1647-1650.
193. Frank M, Klose KJ, Wied M, et al. Combination therapy with octreotide and α-inteferon: effect on tumor growth in metastatic endocrine gastroenteropancreatic tumors. Am J Gastroenterol 1999;94:1382-1387.
194. Öberg K. Interferon in the management of neuroendocrine GEP-tumors: a review. Digestion 2000;62(Suppl 1):92-97.
195. Öberg K. The use of chemotherapy in the management of neuroendocrine tumors. Endocrinol Metab Clin North Am 1993;22: 941.
196. Rougier P, Ducreux M. Systemic chemotherapy of advanced digestive neuroendocrine tumours. Ital J Gastroenterol Hepatol 1999;31: S202.
197. Engstrom PF, Lavin PT, Moertel CG, et al. Streptozocin plus fluorouracil versus doxorubicin therapy for metastatic carcinoid tumor. J Clin Oncol 1984;2:1255.
198. Moertel CG, Kvols LK, O'Connell MJ, et al. Treatment of neuroendocrine carcinomas with combined etoposide and cisplatin: evidence of major therapeutic activity in the anaplastic variants of these neoplasms. Cancer 1991;68:227.
199. Di Bartolomeo M, Bajetta E, Bochicchio AM, et al. A phase II trial of dacarbazine, fluorouracil, and epirubicin in patients with neuroendocrine tumours: a study by the Italian Trials in Medical Oncology (ITMO) Group. Ann Oncol 1995;6:77.
200. Bajetta E, Rimassa L, Carnaghi C, et al. 5-Fluorouracil, dacarbazine, and epirubicin in the treatment of patients with neuroendocrine tumors. Cancer 1998;83:372.
201. Carr K, Yao JC, Rashid A, et al. A phase II trial with imatinib in patients with advanced carcinoid tumour. American Society for Clinical Oncology Annual Meeting, New Orleans, June 2-8, 2004.
202. Yao JC, Ng C, Hoff PM, et al. Improved progression free survival (PFS) and rapid, sustained decrease in tumour perfusion among patients with advanced carcinoid treated with Bevacizumab. J Clin Oncol 2005;23(116S):309s
203. Norton JA. Surgical management of carcinoid tumors: role of debulking and surgery for patients with advanced disease. Digestion 1994;55(Suppl 3):98.
204. Makridis C, Öberg K, Juhlin C, et al. Surgical treatment of midgut carcinoid tumors. World J Surg 1990;14:377.
205. Andaker L, Lamke LO, Smeds S. Follow-up of 102 patients operated on for gastrointestinal carcinoid. Acta Chir Scand 1985;151:469.
206. Wangberg B, Westberg G, Tylen U, et al. Survival of patients with disseminated midgut carcinoid tumors after aggressive tumor reduction. World J Surg 1996;20:892.
207. Lehnert T. Liver transplantation for metastatic neuroendocrine carcinoma. Transplantation 1998;66:1307.
208. Anthuber M, Jauch KW, Briegel J, et al. Results of liver transplantation for gastroenteropancreatic tumor metastases. World J Surg 1996;20:73.
209. Drougas JG, Anthony LB, Blair TK, et al. Hepatic artery chemoembolization for management of patients with advanced metastatic carcinoid tumors. Am J Surg 1998;175:408.
210. Eriksson BK, Larsson EG, Skogseid BM, et al. Liver embolizations of patients with malignant neuroendocrine gastrointestinal tumors. Cancer 1998;83:2293.
211. Kim YH, Ajani JA, Carrasco CH, et al. Selective hepatic arterial chemoembolization for liver metastases in patients with carcinoid tumor or islet cell carcinoma. Cancer Invest 1999;17:474.
212. Diamandidou E, Ajani JA, Yang DJ, et al. Two-phase study of hepatic artery vascular occlusion with microencapsulated cisplatin in patients with liver metastases from neuroendocrine tumors. AJR Am J Roentgenol 1998;170:339.
213. Seifert JK, Cozzi PJ, Morris DL. Cryotherapy for neuroendocrine liver metastases. Semin Surg Oncol 1998;14:175.

214. Schupak KD, Wallner KE. The role of radiation therapy in the treatment of locally unresectable or metastatic carcinoid tumors. Int J Radiat Oncol Biol Phys 1991;20:489.
215. Kimmig BN. Radiotherapy for gastroenteropancreatic neuroendocrine tumors. Ann N Y Acad Sci 1994;733:488.
216. Hoefnagel CA, den Hartog Jager FC, Taal BG, et al. The role of ^{131}I-MIBG in the diagnosis and therapy of carcinoids. Eur J Nucl Med 1987;13:187.
217. Taal BG, Hoefnagel CA, Valdes Olmes RA. Palliative effect of metaiodobenzyl guanidine in metastatic carcinoid tumors. J Clin Oncol 1996;14:1829-1835.
218. Krenning EP, Valkema R, Kooij PPM, et al. Scintigraphy and radionuclide therapy with [Indium-111-labelled-diethyl triamine pentaacetic acid-*D*-Phe^1]-octreotide. Ital J Gastroenterol Hepatol 1999; 31(Suppl 2):S219-S223.
219. Otte A, Müller-Brand J, Dellas S, et al. Ytrium-90–labelled somatostatin analogue for cancer treatment. Lancet 1998;351:417-418.
220. Leimer M, Kurtaran A, Smith-Jones P, et al. Response to treatment with yttrium-90-DOTA-lanreotide of a patient with metastatic gastrinoma. J Nucl Med 1998;39:2090-2094.
221. Zar N, Garmo H, Holmberg L, et al. Long-term survival of patients with small intestinal carcinoid tumors. World J Surg 2004;28(11): 1163-8.
222. Kwekkeboom DJ, Teunissen JJ, Bakker WH, et al. Radiolabeled somatostatin analog [^{177}Lu-DOTA0,Tyr3]octreotate in patients with endocrine gastroenteropancreatic tumors. J Clin Oncol 2005; 23(12):2754-62.
223. Chaudhry A, Öberg K, Wilander E. A study of biological behaviour based on the expression of a proliferating antigen in neuroendocrine tumors of the digestive system. Tumour Biol 1992;13:27.
224. Williams ED. Medullary caricinoma of the thyroid. J Clin Pathol 1996;20:395-398.
225. Verner JV, Morrison AB. Islet cell tumor and a syndrome of refractory watery diarrhea and a syndrome of refractory watery diarrhea and hypokalemia. Am J Med 1958;28:529.
226. Gray TK, Bieberdorf FA, Fordhan JS. Thyrocalcitonin and the jejunal absorption of calcium, water, and electrolytes in normal subjects. J Clin Invest 1973;52:3084-3088.
227. Long RG, Bryant MG, Mitchbell SJ, et al. Clinicopathological study of pancreatic and ganglioneuroblastoma tumors secreting vasoactive intestinal polypeptide (VIP-omas). Br Med J 1981;282:1767.
228. Krejs GJ, Fordtran JS. Effect of VIP infusion on water and ion transport in the human jejunum. Gastroenterology 1980;78: 722-727.
229. Maton PN, Gardner JD, Jensen RT. Use of long-acting somatostatin analogue SMS 201-995 in patients with pancreatic islet cell tumors. Dis Sci 1989;34:285-291.
230. Friedman BS, Metcalfe DD. Mastocytosis. Prog Clin Biol Res 1989;297:163-173.
231. Metcalfe DD. Classification and diagnosis of mastocytosis: current status. J Invest Dermatol 1991;96:2S-4S.
232. Soter NA. The skin in mastocytosis. J Invest Dermatol 1991;96: 32S-39S.
233. Mican JM, Di Bisceglie AD, Fong TL, et al. Hepatic involvement in mastocytosis: clinicopathologic correlations in 41 cases. Hepatology 1995;22:1163-1170.
234. Metcalfe DD. The liver, spleen, and lymph nodes in mastocytosis. J Invest Dermatol 1991;96:45S-46S.
235. Sostre MS, Handler HL. Bony lesions in systemic mastocytosis. Arch Dermatol 1977;113:1245-1247.
236. Ammann RW, Vetter D, Deyhle P, et al. Gastrointestinal involvement in systemic mastocytosis. Gut 1976;17:107-112.
237. Czarnetski BM, Kolde G, Schoemann A, et al. Bone marrow findings in adult patients with urticaria pigmentosa. J Am Acad Dermatol 1988;18:45-51.
238. Travis WD, Li CY, Yam LT, et al. Significance of systemic mast cell disease with associated hematologic disorders. Cancer 1988;62: 965-972.
239. Hutchinson RM. Mastocytosis and co-existent non-Hodgkin's lymphoma and myeloproliferative disorders. Leuk Lymphoma 1992;7:29-36.
240. Travis WD, Li CY, Hoagland HC, et al. Mast cell leukemia: report of a case and review of the literature. Mayo Clin Proc 1986;61: 957-966.
241. Pardanani A. Systemic mastocytosis: bone marrow pathology, classification, and current therapies. Acta Haematol 2005;114(1): 41-51.
242. Roberts LJ II, Oates JA. Biochemical diagnosis of systemic mast cell disorder. J Invest Dermatol 1991;96:19S-25S.
243. Keyzer JJ, deMonchy JGR, van Doormaal JJ, et al. Improved diagnosis of mastocytosis by measurement of urinary histamine metabolites. N Engl J Med 1983;309:1603-1605.
244. Awad JA, Morrow JD, Roberts LJ II. Detection of the major urinary metabolite of prostaglandin D_2 in the circulation: demonstration of elevated levels in patients with disorders of systemic mast cell activation. J Allergy Clin Immunol 1994;93:817-824.
245. Schwartz LB, Metcalf DD, Miler JJ, et al. Tryptase levels as an indicator of mast cell activation in systemic anaphylaxis and mastocytosis. N Engl J Med 1987;316:1622-1626.
246. Turk J, Oates JA, Roberts LJ II. Intervention with epinephrine in hypotension associated with mastocytosis. J Allergy Clin Immunol 1983;71:189-192.
247. Roberts LJ II, Marney SR Jr, Oates JA. Blockade of the flush associated with a metastatic gastric carcinoid by combined histamine H_1 and H_2 receptor antagoninsts: evidence for an important role of H_2 receptors in human vasculature. N Engl J Med 1979;300: 236-238.
248. Butterfield JH, Kao PC, Klee GC, et al. Aspirin idiosyncrasy in systemic mast cell disease: a new look at mediator release during aspirin desensitization. Mayo Clin Proc 1995;70:481-487.
249. Czarnetski BM, Algermissen B, Jeep S, et al. Interferon treatment of patients with chronic urticaria and mastocytosis. J Am Acad Dermatol 1994;30:500-501.
250. Yale SH, Vasudeva S, Mazza JJ, et al. Disorders of flushing. Compr Ther 2005;31(1):59-71.

DISCLOSURE INDEX

The following contributors have indicated that they have a relationship that, in the context of their participation in the writing of a chapter for the eleventh edition Williams Textbook of Endocrinology, could be perceived by some people as a real or apparent conflict of interest. Codes for the disclosure information (institution[s] and nature of relationship[s]) are provided below.

RELATIONSHIP CODES

A Stock, stock options, or bond holdings
B Research grants
C Employment (full- or part-time)
D Ownership or partnership
E Consulting fees or other remuneration received by the contributor or immediate family
F Nonremunerative positions, such as board member, trustee, or public spokesperson
G Receipt of royalties
H Participation in a "speakers' bureau"

INSTITUTION AND COMPANY CODES

001 Abbott Diagnostics
002 Abbott Laboratories
003 Acceleron Pharma
004 Alliance for Better Bone Health
005 Altus
006 Amgen Inc.
007 Amylin Pharmaceuticals
008 Arisaph Pharmaceuticals Inc.
009 Astellas Pharma USA
010 AstraZeneca
011 Bayer Schering
012 Bayhill Therapeutics
013 BD Research Laboratories
014 Beckman-Coulter
015 Biogen
016 Biopartners
017 Bristol Meyers Squibb
018 Canadian Institute of Health Research
019 Chugai Pharmaceuticals, Inc
020 Conjuchem Inc
021 Consults for Alliance for Better Bone Health
022 Dexcom
023 Eli Lilly Inc
024 Emisphere Technologies Inc.
025 Esoterix
026 Ferring Research Institute
027 Genentech
028 Genzyme
029 GlaxoSmithKline
030 Glenmark Pharmaceuticals
031 GSK/Roche
032 Hoffman LaRoche
033 Insulet Corporation
034 Ipsen Biomeasures
035 Isis Pharmaceuticals Inc.
036 Johnson & Johnson
037 Juvenile Diabetes Research Foundation
038 Kronus Corp
039 LG Life Sciences
040 LipoScience
041 MannKind
042 Macrogenics
043 MannKind Corp.
044 Marcadia Biotech
045 Merck and Co.
046 Merck Fr.
047 Merck Research Laboratories
048 Metabolex
049 Novartis
050 Novartis Pharma AG
051 Novo Nordisk Inc.
052 NPS Pharmaceuticals Inc.
053 Orexigen Therapeutics, Inc.
054 Organon Inc.
055 Otsuka
056 Pfizer
057 Phenomix Inc
058 ProteoGenix
059 Quest Diagnostics
060 Sanofi
061 Sanofi-Aventis
062 Serono
063 Speaker Bureau Alliance for Better Bone Health
064 Takeda Pharmaceuticals
065 Takeda North America
066 Tercica
067 Theratechnologies, Inc.
068 Thiakis, Ltd.
069 TolerRx Inc.
070 Transition Pharmaceuticals Inc
071 Transition Therapeutics
072 Wyeth Pharmaceuticals
073 World Anti Doping Agency
074 Yamanouchi Pharma America
075 Zydus Pharmaceuticals

CONTRIBUTORS

Barker, Jennifer M., B-037
Basson, Rosemary, B-018
Braunstein, Glenn D., E-001, E-025
Bulun, Serdar, E-029, E-049, E-062
Burant, Charles, E-007, E-017, E-064, E-075
Buse, John B., A-033; B-007, B-013, B-017, B-022, B-023, B-032, B-049, B-051, B-056, B-071; E-033, E-036, E-045, E-061; F-002, F-007, F-013, F-017, F-023, F-032, F-040, F-043, F-072; H-045
Canalis, Ernesto, E-003, E-004, E-049; H-004, H-031, H-045
Cryer, Philip E., E-006, E-043, E-044, E-045, E-051, E-065, E-069
Darney, Philip D., B-054; E-011, E-054; H-011, H-054
Davies, Terry F., E-002, E-038; H-002
Drucker, Daniel J., B-023, B-036, B-047, B-051; E-006, E-007, E-008, E-019, E-023, E-024, E-029, E-30, E-035, E-036, E-046, E-047, E-049, E-051, E-052, E-057, E-064, E-070; G-008
Eisenbarth, George S., A-012; E-012, E-042; G-059
Fisher, Delbert A., A-059; C-059
Grinspoon, Steven, B-017, B-029, B-067; E-062, E-067
Grumbach, Melvin M., E-050
Kleinberg, David L., B-049; E-023, E-027, E-034, E-039, E-049, E-066
Kronenberg, Henry M., B-019; E-015, E-019, E-049
Lamberts, S. W. J., E-034, E-023, E-049
Lazar, Mitchell A., B-029, E-002, E-072
Low, Malcolm J., A-053, A-068; G-053, G-068
Mahley, Robert W., B-045
Melmed, Shlomo, B-023, B-034, B-049; E-023, E-049, E-066
Nesto, Richard, H-029, H-056, H-060, H-061
Öberg, Kjell, E-049, H-049
Polonsky, Kenneth S., A-007, A-048; E-007, E-029, E-048
Reiter, Edward O., E-005, E-010, E-056; H-027
Rosenfeld, Ron, A-058; B-066; E-014, E-023, E-027, E-051, E-066; H-027, H-066
Schlumberger, Martin-Jean, H-028
Strasburger, Christian J., B-023, B-056, B-073; E-016; F-023, F-056
Verbalis, Joseph G., B-009, B-074; E-009, E-026, E-029, E-055, E-061, E-074; H-009
Weisgraber, Karl H., A-029; B-045, B-056; E-056; G-045

INDEX

Note: Page numbers followed by f indicate figures; those followed by t indicate tables.

B

D

E

G

I

J

K

N

O

P

Q

R

S

T

U

Z